Contents in Brief

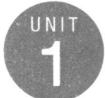
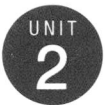

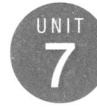

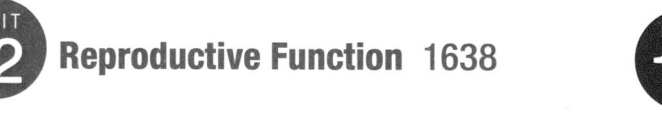

BRUNNER & SUDDARTH'S

TEXTBOOK OF
Medical-Surgical
Nursing

15TH EDITION

BRUNNER & SUDDARTH'S

TEXTBOOK OF
Medical-Surgical Nursing

15TH EDITION

Janice L. Hinkle, PhD, RN, CNRN
Fellow
Villanova University M. Louise Fitzpatrick
  College of Nursing
Villanova, Pennsylvania

Kerry H. Cheever, PhD, RN
Professor *Emerita*
Helen S. Breidegam School of Nursing
Moravian University
Bethlehem, Pennsylvania

Kristen J. Overbaugh, PhD, RN, ACNS-BC, CHPN
Assistant Professor
School of Nursing and Health Sciences
La Salle University
Philadelphia, Pennsylvania

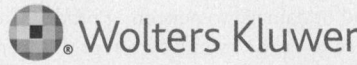

. Wolters Kluwer

Philadelphia • Baltimore • New York • London
Buenos Aires • Hong Kong • Sydney • Tokyo

Vice President, Nursing Segment: Julie K. Stegman
Director, Nursing Education and Practice Content: Jamie Blum
Senior Acquisitions Editor: Jonathan Joyce
Senior Development Editor: Meredith L. Brittain
Freelance Development Editor: Rose G. Foltz
Senior Editorial Coordinator: Julie Kostelnik
Marketing Manager: Brittany Clements
Editorial Assistant: Molly Kennedy
Senior Production Project Manager: David Saltzberg
Manager, Graphic Arts and Design: Steve Druding
Art Director: Jennifer Clements
Manufacturing Coordinator: Margie Orzech
Prepress Vendor: Aptara, Inc.

15th Edition

Copyright © 2022 Wolters Kluwer

11 10 9 8 7 6 5 4 3

Printed in Mexico

978-1-9751-6103-3
Library of Congress Cataloging-in-Publication Data
available upon request

Library of Congress Control Number: 2021911700

shop.lww.com

To our fellow nurses who provide comfort and care, and who instill hope for a healthier world . . .

To our nursing faculty colleagues who nurture, guide, and steer the future of our profession . . .

To nursing students who challenge themselves with courage and conviction . . .

You inspire us!

Contributors

Contributors to the 15th Edition

Marianne T. Adam, PhD, RN, FNP, CNE
Associate Teaching Professor of Nursing
Campus Coordinator, Nursing
Pennsylvania State University Schuylkill
Schuylkill Haven, Pennsylvania

Chapter 38: Assessment of Digestive and Gastrointestinal Function

Rachel Barish, RN, MSN, ANP-BC, AACC
Nurse Practitioner, Division of Cardiology
MedStar Georgetown University Hospital Physicians Group
Washington, District of Columbia

Chapter 24: Management of Patients with Structural, Infectious, and Inflammatory Cardiac Disorders

Jennifer L. Bartlett, PhD, RN-BC, CNE, CHSE
Associate Professor
Georgia Baptist College of Nursing of Mercer University
Atlanta, Georgia

Chapter 39: Management of Patients with Oral and Esophageal Disorders

Susan Bartos, PhD, RN, CCRN
Adjunct Professor
Egan School of Nursing & Health Sciences
Fairfield University
Fairfield, Connecticut

Chapter 25: Management of Patients with Complications from Heart Disease

Cynthia Bautista, PhD, APRN, FNCS, FCNS
Associate Professor
Egan School of Nursing and Health Studies
Fairfield University
Fairfield, Connecticut

Chapter 63: Management of Patients with Neurologic Trauma

Tricia Bernecker, PhD, RN
Associate Professor
DeSales University
Center Valley, Pennsylvania

Chapter 22: Management of Patients with Arrhythmias and Conduction Problems

Lisa Bowman, RN, MSN, CRNP, CNRN
Nurse Practitioner
Jefferson Hospital for Neuroscience
Thomas Jefferson University Hospital
Philadelphia, Pennsylvania

Chapter 62: Management of Patients with Cerebrovascular Disorders

Carolyn Bradley, MSN, RN, CCRN
Heart & Vascular Center Nursing Professional Development Specialist
Yale New Haven Hospital
New Haven, Connecticut

Chapter 21: Assessment of Cardiovascular Function

Sherry Burrell, PhD, RN, CNE
Assistant Professor
Villanova University M. Louise Fitzpatrick College of Nursing
Villanova, Pennsylvania

Chapter 12: Oncologic Management

Theresa Capriotti, DO, CRNP, MSN, RN
Clinical Professor
Villanova University M. Louise Fitzpatrick College of Nursing
Villanova, Pennsylvania

Chapter 10: Fluid and Electrolytes
Chapter 33: Assessment and Management of Patients with Allergic Disorders

Jean Colaneri, ACNP-BC, CNN
Acute Care Nurse Practitioner
Albany Medical Center Hospital
Albany, New York

Chapter 48: Management of Patients with Kidney Disorders

Linda Carman Copel, PhD, RN, PMHCNS, BC, CNE, ANEF, NCC, FAPA
Professor
Villanova University M. Louise Fitzpatrick College of Nursing
Villanova, Pennsylvania

Chapter 3: Health Education and Health Promotion
Chapter 5: Stress and Inflammatory Responses
Chapter 53: Assessment and Management of Patients with Male Reproductive Disorders

Patricia Dillon, PhD, RN
Chair of Graduate, RN to BSN, and RN to MSN Programs, & Professor
School of Nursing and Health Sciences
La Salle University
Philadelphia, Pennsylvania

Chapter 56: Management of Patients with Dermatologic Disorders

Nancy Donegan, MPH, RN
Independent Consultant
Washington, District of Columbia

Chapter 66: Management of Patients with Infectious Diseases

Paulette Dorney, PhD, RN, CCRN-K
Associate Professor & Director, Accelerated BSN Program
Helen S. Breidegam School of Nursing
Moravian University
Bethlehem, Pennsylvania

*Chapter 19: Management of Patients with Chest and Lower
Respiratory Tract Disorders*

Phyllis Dubendorf, MSN, RN, CCNS, CNRN, ACNP-BC
Clinical Nurse Specialist
Hospital of the University of Pennsylvania
Philadelphia, Pennsylvania

*Chapter 61: Management of Patients with Neurologic
Dysfunction*

Kimberly Silver Dunker, DNP, MSN, RN, CNE, CNEcl
Dean of Nursing
Fortis Institute
Nashville, Tennessee

Unit-opening case studies

Elizabeth C. Evans, CNP, DNP
Nephrology Nurse Practitioner
Renal Medicine Associates
Albuquerque, New Mexico

*Chapter 27: Assessment and Management of Patients with
Hypertension*

Janice Farber, PhD, RN, CNOR
Associate Professor
Helen S. Breidegam School of Nursing
Moravian University
Bethlehem, Pennsylvania

*Chapter 4: Adult Health and Physical, Nutritional, and Cultural
Assessment*

**Eleanor Fitzpatrick, DNP, RN, CCRN, AGCNS-BC,
ACNP-BC**
Clinical Nurse Specialist
Thomas Jefferson University Hospital
Philadelphia, Pennsylvania

*Chapter 43: Assessment and Management of Patients with Hepatic
Disorders*

Chapter 44: Management of Patients with Biliary Disorders

Anessa M. Foxwell, MSN, CRNP, ACHPN
Predoctoral Fellow, NewCourtland Center for Transitions &
Health
University of Pennsylvania School of Nursing
Nurse Practitioner, Clinical Practices of the University of
Pennsylvania
Philadelphia, Pennsylvania

Chapter 13: Palliative and End-of-Life Care

Stacy M. Fusner, DNP, APRN, CNP
Assistant Professor of Clinical Practice
The Ohio State University College of Nursing
Columbus, Ohio

*Chapter 58: Assessment and Management of Patients with Eye and
Vision Disorders*

Trudy Gaillard, PhD, RN, CDCES, FAHA
Associate Professor
Nicole Wertheim College of Nursing and Health Sciences
Florida International University
Miami, Florida

Chapter 46: Management of Patients with Diabetes

Dawn M. Goodolf, PhD, RN
Associate Professor and Chairperson
Helen S. Breidegam School of Nursing
Moravian University
Bethlehem, Pennsylvania

Chapter 35: Assessment of Musculoskeletal Function
Chapter 67: Emergency Nursing
Chapter 68: Disaster Nursing

Beth Gotwals, PhD, RN
Associate Professor
Helen S. Breidegam School of Nursing
Moravian University
Bethlehem, Pennsylvania

Chapter 2: Medical-Surgical Nursing

Karen D. Groller, PhD, RN, CV-BC, CMSRN
Assistant Professor
Helen S. Breidegam School of Nursing
Moravian University
Bethlehem, Pennsylvania

Chapter 42: Assessment and Management of Patients with Obesity

Debbie A. Gunter, APRN, FNP-BC, ACHPN
Family & Palliative Care Nurse Practitioner
Emory Healthcare Cognitive Neurology Clinic
Nursing Instructor
Emory University School of Nursing
Atlanta, Georgia

*Chapter 18: Management of Patients with Upper Respiratory Tract
Disorders*

Jamie Heffernan, MSN, RN, CCRN-K, NE-BC
Burn Program Manager
New York-Presbyterian Weill Cornell Medicine
New York, New York

Chapter 57: Management of Patients with Burn Injury

Kristina Hidalgo, ACNP-BC
Nurse Practitioner, Division of Cardiology/Electrophysiology
MedStar Washington Hospital Center
Washington, District of Columbia

*Chapter 24: Management of Patients with Structural, Infectious, and
Inflammatory Cardiac Disorders*

Janice L. Hinkle, PhD, RN, CNRN
Fellow
Villanova University M. Louise Fitzpatrick College of Nursing
Villanova, Pennsylvania

*Chapter 34: Assessment and Management of Patients with
    Inflammatory Rheumatic Disorders*

Michael Johnson, PhD, RN, PMH-BC, CNE
Assistant Professor
Director of Clinical Partnerships
School of Nursing
Nevada State College
Henderson, Nevada

*Chapter 54: Assessment and Management of Patients Who Are
    LGBTQ*

Debra P. Kantor, PhD, RN, CNE
Associate Professor of Nursing
Molloy College
The Barbara H. Hagan School of Nursing and Health
    Sciences
Rockville Centre, New York

*Chapter 45: Assessment and Management of Patients with Endocrine
    Disorders*

Sarah Kweeder, MSN, RN-BC, CNOR
Lead Clinical Nurse Educator, Surgical Services
Main Line Health
Bryn Mawr, Pennsylvania

Chapter 14: Preoperative Nursing Management
Chapter 15: Intraoperative Nursing Management
Chapter 16: Postoperative Nursing Management

Audra Lewis, PhD, RN, CHSE
Director, Highland Campus Regional Simulation Center
Austin Community College
Austin, Texas

*Chapter 59: Assessment and Management of Patients with Hearing
    and Balance Disorders*

**Mary Beth Flynn Makic, PhD, CCNS, CCRN-K, FAAN,
    FNAP, FCNS**
Professor
University of Colorado College of Nursing
Aurora, Colorado

Chapter 11: Shock, Sepsis, and Multiple Organ Dysfunction Syndrome

Jane F. Marek, DNP, MSN, RN
Assistant Professor
Frances Payne Bolton School of Nursing
Case Western Reserve University
Cleveland, Ohio

*Chapter 41: Management of Patients with Intestinal and Rectal
    Disorders*

Katrina Nice Masterson, DNP, RN, FNP-BC, DCNP
Educational Coordinator
Randall Dermatology
West Lafayette, Indiana

Chapter 55: Assessment of Integumentary Function

Jennifer McCaughey, MSN, BS, RNC-MNN, CCE
Clinical Educator
Women and Children's Services
Inova Fair Oaks Hospital
Fairfax, Virginia

*Chapter 50: Assessment and Management of Patients with Female
    Physiologic Processes*
Chapter 51: Management of Patients with Female Reproductive Disorders

Salimah H. Meghani, PhD, MBE, RN, FAAN
Professor & Term Chair of Palliative Care
University of Pennsylvania School of Nursing
Philadelphia, Pennsylvania

Chapter 13: Palliative and End-of-Life Care

Carin Molfetta, MSN, CRNP, BC
Nurse Practitioner
Penn Medicine Lancaster General Health
Lancaster, Pennsylvania

*Chapter 52: Assessment and Management of Patients with Breast
    Disorders*

Sue Monaro, PhD, MN, RN
Vascular Clinical Nurse Consultant
Concord Repatriation General Hospital
Concord
Senior Clinical Lecturer
Susan Wakil School of Nursing and Midwifery
University of Sydney
New South Wales, Australia

*Chapter 26: Assessment and Management of Patients with Vascular
    Disorders and Problems of Peripheral Circulation*

**Melissa V. Moreda, MSN, APRN, ACCNS-AG, CCRN,
    CNRN, SCRN**
Diabetes Educator Clinical Nurse Specialist
Duke Raleigh Hospital
Raleigh, North Carolina

*Chapter 65: Management of Patients with Oncologic or Degenerative
    Neurologic Disorders*

Kathleen Nokes, PhD, RN, FAAN
Professor *Emerita*
Hunter College and Graduate Center, CUNY
New York, New York

Chapter 32: Management of Patients with Immune Deficiency Disorders

Geraldine M. O'Leary, MSN, RN, FNP-BC
Clinical Instructor
School of Nursing and Health Sciences
La Salle University
Philadelphia, Pennsylvania

Chapter 23: Management of Patients with Coronary Vascular Disorders

Mae Ann Pasquale, PhD, RN
Associate Professor
School of Nursing
Cedar Crest College
Allentown, Pennsylvania

Chapter 37: Management of Patients with Musculoskeletal Trauma

Sue Pugh, MSN, RN, CNRN, CRRN, CNS-BC, FAHA
Neuro Clinical Nurse Specialist/Stroke Coordinator
Sinai Hospital of Baltimore
Baltimore, Maryland

*Chapter 64: Management of Patients with Neurologic Infections,
    Autoimmune Disorders, and Neuropathies*

Katrina A. Pyo, PhD, RN, CCRN
Associate Professor
Robert Morris University
Moon Township, Pennsylvania

Chapter 17: Assessment of Respiratory Function

Ann Quinlan-Colwell, PhD, RN-BC, AHN-BC
Pain Management Clinical Nurse Specialist
Educator and Consultant
Wilmington, North Carolina

Chapter 9: Pain Management

Rebecca Wildman Repetti, RN, ANP-BC
Nurse Practitioner, Thoracic Oncology Service
Memorial Sloan Kettering Cancer Center
New York, New York

Chapter 31: Assessment of Immune Function

Denise Rhew, PhD, RN, CNS, CEN
Clinical Nurse Specialist – Emergency Services
Director, Neuro-Progressive Care
Cone Health
Greensboro, North Carolina

Chapter 8: Management of the Older Adult Patient

Marylou V. Robinson, PhD, FNP-C
Olympia, Washington

Chapter 36: Management of Patients with Musculoskeletal Disorders

Tami J. Rogers, PhD, DVM, RN, CNE
Professor of Nursing, Curriculum QA/Course Development
Rasmussen University
Bloomington, Minnesota

Chapter 28: Assessment of Hematologic Function and Treatment Modalities

Sally Russel, MN, CMSRN, CNE
Director, Education Services
American Nephrology Nurses Association
Pitman, New Jersey

Chapter 49: Management of Patients with Urinary Disorders

Catherine Sargent, PhD, RN, BC, AOCNS
Assistant Professor
Gwynedd Mercy University
Gwynedd Valley, Pennsylvania

Chapter 30: Management of Patients with Hematologic Neoplasms

Susan Parnell Scholtz, PhD, RN
Associate Professor
Helen S. Breidegam School of Nursing
Moravian University
Bethlehem, Pennsylvania

Chapter 1: Professional Nursing Practice

Lindsey R. Siewert, RN, MSN, APRN, CCNS, SCRN
Clinical Nurse Specialist Neuroscience/Stroke Coordinator
Norton Healthcare
Louisville, Kentucky

Chapter 60: Assessment of Neurologic Function

Suzanne C. Smeltzer, RN, EdD, ANEF, FAAN
Richard and Marianne Kreider Endowed Professor in
    Nursing for Vulnerable Populations
Villanova University M. Louise Fitzpatrick College of
    Nursing
Villanova, Pennsylvania

Chapter 7: Disability and Chronic Illness

Nancy Colobong Smith, MN, ARNP, CNN
Clinical Nurse Specialist – Renal, Dialysis, Transplant
University of Washington Medical Center
Seattle, Washington

Chapter 47: Assessment of Kidney and Urinary Function

Kimberly A. Subasic, PhD, MS, RN, CNE
Professor & Chairperson
Swain Department of Nursing
The Citadel
Charleston, South Carolina

Chapter 6: Genetics and Genomics in Nursing

Mindy L. Tait, PhD, MBA, CRNP, FNP-BC
Associate Professor
School of Nursing and Health Sciences
La Salle University
Philadelphia, Pennsylvania

*Chapter 40: Management of Patients with Gastric and Duodenal
    Disorders*

M. Eileen Walsh, PhD, APRN, CVN, FAHA
Associate Dean, Research and Scholarship
Director, College of Nursing Honors Program
Professor, College of Nursing
University of Toledo
Toledo, Ohio

*Chapter 26: Assessment and Management of Patients with Vascular
    Disorders and Problems of Peripheral Circulation*

Camille Wendekier, PhD, CNE, RN
Program Director, MSN Leadership/Education
Department of Nursing
St. Francis University
Loretto, Pennsylvania

*Chapter 20: Management of Patients with Chronic Pulmonary
    Disease*

Mary Lynn Wilby, PhD, MPH, MSN, CRNP, ANP-BC, RN
Associate Professor
School of Nursing and Health Sciences
La Salle University
Philadelphia, Pennsylvania

*Chapter 29: Management of Patients with Nonmalignant Hematologic
    Disorders*

Contributors to the 14th Edition

Marianne Adam, PhD, RN, CRNP
Schuylkill Haven, Pennsylvania

Chapter 43: Assessment of Digestive and Gastrointestinal Function

Julie Adkins, DNP, APN, FNP-BC, FAANP
West Frankfort, Illinois

Chapter 63: Assessment and Management of Patients with Eye and Vision Disorders

Jennifer L. Bartlett, PhD, RN-BC, CNE, CHSE
Atlanta, Georgia

Chapter 45: Management of Patients with Oral and Esophageal Disorders

Tara Bilofsky, ACNP-BC, MS
Allentown, Pennsylvania

Chapter 21: Respiratory Care Modalities

Susan Bonini, MSN, RN
Aurora, Colorado

Chapter 31: Assessment and Management of Patients with Hypertension

Lisa Bowman, RN, MSN, CRNP, CNRN
Philadelphia, Pennsylvania

Chapter 67: Management of Patients with Cerebrovascular Disorders

Jo Ann Brooks, PhD, RN, FAAN, FCCP
Indianapolis, Indiana

Chapter 23: Management of Patients with Chest and Lower Respiratory Tract Disorders
Chapter 24: Management of Patients with Chronic Pulmonary Disease

Sherry Burrell, PhD, RN, CNE
Villanova, Pennsylvania

Chapter 46: Management of Patients with Gastric and Duodenal Disorders

Wendy Cantrell, DNP, CRNP
Birmingham, Alabama

Chapter 61: Management of Patients with Dermatologic Disorders

Lauren Cantwell, RN, MS, ACNP-BC, ACNPC, CNS, CCNS, CCRN, CHFN
Falls Church, Virginia

Chapter 28: Management of Patients with Structural, Infectious, and Inflammatory Cardiac Disorders

Kim Cantwell-Gab, MN, ACNP-BC, ANP-BC, CVN, RVT, RDMS
Medford, Oregon

Chapter 30: Assessment and Management of Patients with Vascular Disorders and Problems of Peripheral Circulation

Patricia E. Casey, MSN, RN, CPHQ, AACC
Washington, District of Columbia

Chapter 26: Management of Patients with Dysrhythmias and Conduction Problems

Jill Cash, RN, MSN, APRN-BC
Franklin, Tennessee

Chapter 38: Assessment and Management of Patients with Rheumatic Disorders
Chapter 64: Assessment and Management of Patients with Hearing and Balance Disorders

Kerry H. Cheever, PhD, RN
Bethlehem, Pennsylvania

Chapter 1: Health Care Delivery and Evidence-Based Nursing Practice
Chapter 47: Management of Patients with Intestinal and Rectal Disorders
Chapter 48: Assessment and Management of Patients with Obesity

Elise Colancecco, MSN, RN
Bethlehem, Pennsylvania

Chapter 42: Management of Patients with Musculoskeletal Trauma

Moya Cook RN, MSN, APN
Marion, Illinois

Chapter 13: Fluid and Electrolytes: Balance and Disturbance

Linda Carman Copel, PhD, RN, PMHCNS, BC, CNE, ANEF, NCC, FAPA
Villanova, Pennsylvania

Chapter 4: Health Education and Health Promotion
Chapter 6: Individual and Family Homeostasis, Stress, and Adaptation
Chapter 59: Assessment and Management of Problems Related to Male Reproductive Processes

Elizabeth Petit deMange, PhD, RN
Villanova, Pennsylvania

Chapter 52: Assessment and Management of Patients with Endocrine Disorders

Nancy Donegan, MPH, RN
Washington, District of Columbia

Chapter 71: Management of Patients with Infectious Diseases

Paulette Dorney, PhD, RN, CCRN
Bethlehem, Pennsylvania

Chapter 21: Respiratory Care Modalities

Diane Dressler, MSN, RN, CCRN-R
Milwaukee, Wisconsin

Chapter 27: Management of Patients with Coronary Vascular Disorders
Chapter 29: Management of Patients with Complications from Heart Disease

Debra Drew, MS, RN-BC (retired), ACNS-BC (retired), AP-PMN
Minneapolis, Minnesota

Chapter 12: Pain Management

Phyllis Dubendorf, MSN, RN, CCNS, CNRN, CRNP-BC
Philadelphia, Pennsylvania

Chapter 66: Management of Patients with Neurologic Dysfunction

Susan M. Fallone, MS, RN, CNN
Albany, New York

Chapter 53: Assessment of Kidney and Urinary Function

Janice Farber, PhD, RN, CNOR
Bethlehem Pennsylvania

Chapter 7: Overview of Transcultural Nursing

Eleanor Fitzpatrick, RN, MSN, CCRN, AGCNS-BC, ACNP-BC
Philadelphia, Pennsylvania

Chapter 49: Assessment and Management of Patients with Hepatic Disorders
Chapter 50: Assessment and Management of Patients with Biliary Disorders

Trudy Gaillard, PhD, RN, CDE
Cincinnati, Ohio

Chapter 51: Assessment and Management of Patients with Diabetes

Dawn Goodolf, PhD, RN
Bethlehem, Pennsylvania

Chapter 39: Assessment of Musculoskeletal Function

Beth Gotwals, PhD, RN
Bethlehem Pennsylvania

Chapter 2: Community-Based Nursing Practice
Home Care Checklists

Theresa Lynn Green, PhD, MScHRM, BScN, RN
Queensland, Australia

Chapter 10: Principles and Practices of Rehabilitation

Debbie Gunter, MSN, APRN, ACHPN
Atlanta, Georgia

Chapter 22: Management of Patients with Upper Respiratory Tract Disorders

Jamie Heffernan, MSN, RN, CCRN-K, NE-BC
New York, New York

Chapter 62: Management of Patients with Burn Injury

Janice L. Hinkle, PhD, RN, CNRN
Villanova, Pennsylvania
Chapter 55: Management of Patients with Urinary Disorders

Lisa J. Jesaitis, RN, MS, CHFN, ACNP
Washington, District of Columbia
Chapter 28: Management of Patients with Structural, Infectious, and Inflammatory Cardiac Disorders

Tamara Kear, PhD, RN, CNS, CNN
Villanova, Pennsylvania
Chapter 54: Management of Patients with Kidney Disorders

Elizabeth Keech, RN, PhD
Villanova, Pennsylvania
Chapter 11: Health Care of the Older Adult

Kathleen Kelleher, DMH, WHNP-BC, CBCN, DVS
Pompton Plains, New Jersey
Chapter 58: Assessment and Management of Patients with Breast Disorders

Lynne Kennedy, PhD, MSN, RN, RNFA, CHPN, CNOR, CLNC, CHTP, Alumnus CCRN
Fairfax, Virginia
Chapter 17: Preoperative Nursing Management
Chapter 18: Intraoperative Nursing
Chapter 19: Postoperative Nursing Management

Mary Beth Flynn Makic, PhD, CNS, CCNS, CCRN-K, FAAN, FNAP
Professor
Denver, Colorado
Chapter 14: Shock and Multiple Organ Dysfunction Syndrome

Katrina Nice Masterson, RN, DNP, FNP-BC, DCNP
West Lafayette, Indiana
Chapter 60: Assessment of Integumentary Function

Jennifer McCaughey, MSN, BS, RNC-MNN, CCE
Fairfax, Virginia
Chapter 57: Management of Patients with Female Reproductive Disorders

Melissa V. Moreda, BSN, RN, CCRN, CNRN, SCRN
Raleigh, North Carolina
Chapter 70: Management of Patients with Oncologic or Degenerative Neurologic Disorders

Donna Nayduch, MSN, RN, ACNP, TCRN
Ocala, Florida
Chapter 72: Emergency Nursing
Chapter 73: Terrorism, Mass Casualty, and Disaster Nursing

Kathleen Nokes, PhD, RN, FAAN
New York, New York
Chapter 36: Management of Patients with Immunodeficiency Disorders

Kristen J. Overbaugh, PhD, RN, ACNS-BC, CHPN
San Antonio, Texas
Chapter 20: Assessment of Respiratory Function

Janet Parkosewich, DNSc, RN, FAHA
New Haven, Connecticut
Chapter 25: Assessment of Cardiovascular Function

Mae Ann Pasquale, PhD, RN
Allentown, Pennsylvania
Chapter 40: Musculoskeletal Care Modalities

Beth A. Bednarz Pruski, RN, MSN, CCRN
Washington, District of Columbia
Chapter 26: Management of Patients with Dysrhythmias and Conduction Problems

Sue Pugh, MSN, RN, CNRN, CRRN, CNS-BC, FAHA
Baltimore, Maryland
Chapter 69: Management of Patients with Neurologic Infections, Autoimmune Disorders, and Neuropathies

JoAnne Reifsnyder, PhD, RN, FAAN
Kennett Square, Pennsylvania
Chapter 16: End-of-Life Care

Rebecca Wildman Repetti, RN, ANP-BC
New York, New York
Chapter 35: Assessment of Immune Function

Marylou V. Robinson, PhD, FNP
Tacoma, Washington
Chapter 41: Management of Patients with Musculoskeletal Disorders

Erin Sarsfield, MSN, RN, CCRN-K
Hershey, Pennsylvania
Chapter 44: Digestive and Gastrointestinal Treatment Modalities

Susan Scholtz, PhD, RN
Bethlehem, Pennsylvania
Chapter 3: Critical Thinking, Ethical Decision Making, and the Nursing Process
Ethical Dilemma charts

Lindsey R. Siewert, RN, MSN, APRN, CCNS, CCRN-K
Louisville, Kentucky
Chapter 65: Assessment of Neurologic Function

Suzanne C. Smeltzer, RN, EdD, ANEF, FAAN
Villanova, Pennsylvania
Chapter 9: Chronic Illness and Disability

Jennifer Specht, PhD, RN
Chester, Pennsylvania
Chapter 5: Adult Health and Nutritional Assessment
Chapter 48: Assessment and Management of Patients with Obesity

Cindy Stern, RN, MSN, CCRP
Philadelphia, Pennsylvania
Chapter 15: Management of Patients with Oncologic Disorders

Julie G. Stover, RN, MSN, CRNP
Lancaster, Pennsylvania
Chapter 56: Assessment and Management of Female Physiologic Processes

Kimberly A. Subasic, PhD, MS, RN
Scranton, Pennsylvania
Chapter 8: Overview of Genetics and Genomics in Nursing
Genetics in Nursing Practice charts

Carole Sullivan, DNP, RN
Eldorado, Illinois
Chapter 37: Assessment and Management of Patients with Allergic Disorders
Unit-opening case studies, Units 1–9

Mary Laudon Thomas, MS, CNS, AOCN
Palo Alto, California
Chapter 32: Assessment of Hematologic Function and Treatment Modalities
Chapter 33: Management of Patients with Nonmalignant Hematologic Disorders
Chapter 34: Management of Patients with Hematologic Neoplasms

Kristin Weitmann, RN, MSN, ACNP
Wauwatosa, Wisconsin
Chapter 27: Management of Patients with Coronary Vascular Disorders
Chapter 29: Management of Patients with Complications from Heart Disease

Marie Wilson, RN, MSN, CCRN, CNRN, CRNP
Philadelphia, Pennsylvania
Chapter 68: Management of Patients with Neurologic Trauma

Reviewers

Julie Baldwin, DNP
Associate Professor
Missouri Western State University
St. Joseph, Missouri

Tamara Baxter, MSN, RN, CNE
Assistant Professor
Northwestern State University
Natchitoches, Louisiana

Rachel Coats, MS, RN, CEN, CNE
Lecturer
Lander University
Greenwood, South Carolina

Debra Connell-Dent, MSN, RN
Assistant Teaching Professor
University of Missouri St. Louis
St. Louis, Missouri

Sarah Darrell, MSN, RN, CNOR
Faculty
Ivy Tech Community College Valparaiso
Valparaiso, Indiana

Amanda Finley, MSN, RN
Assistant Teaching Professor
University of Missouri St. Louis
St. Louis, Missouri

Cassie Flock, MSN, RN
Assistant Professor
Vincennes University
Jasper, Indiana

Belinda Fuller, RN, MSN
Nurse Educator
Gadsden State Community College
Gadsden, Alabama

Melissa Gorton, MS, RN
Assistant Professor of Nursing
Castleton University
Castleton, Vermont

Lori Hailey, RN, MSN, CHSE
Assistant Professor
Arkansas State University
Jonesboro, Arkansas

Carol Heim, MA, RN
Associate Professor
Mount Mercy University
Cedar Rapids, Iowa

Melissa Humfleet, DNP, RN
Assistant Professor of Nursing
Lincoln Memorial University
Harrogate, Tennessee

Elizabeth D. Katrancha, DNP, CCNS, RN, CNE
Assistant Professor
University of Pittsburgh at Johnstown
Johnstown, Pennsylvania

Llynne C. Kiernan, DNP, MSN, RN-BC
Assistant Professor
Norwich University
Northfield, Vermont

Tammy Killen, MSN, RN
Instructor
Jacksonville State University
Jacksonville, Alabama

Tina Marie Kline, MSN, RN, CMSRN, CNE
Associate Professor
Pennsylvania College of Technology
Williamsport, Pennsylvania

Angie Koller, DNP, MSN, RN
Dean and Professor
Ivy Tech Community College
Indianapolis, Indiana

Trudy Kuehn, RN, BSN, MSN
Associate Professor of Nursing
Paul D. Camp Community College
Franklin, Virginia

Dana Law-Ham, PhD, RN, FNP-BC, CNE
Assistant Clinical Professor
University of New England
Portland, Maine

Phyllis Magaletto, MS, RN, BC
Nursing Instructor
Cochran School of Nursing
Yonkers, New York

Julie Page, EdD, MSN, RN
Assistant Professor
University of North Carolina at Chapel Hill
Chapel Hill, North Carolina

Judith Pahlck, MSN-Ed, RN
Dean of Nursing
Jersey College
Teterboro, New Jersey

Annette M. Peacock-Johnson, DNP, RN
Associate Professor of Nursing
Saint Mary's College
Notre Dame, Indiana

Amanda Pribble, MSN, FNP-C
Assistant Professor of Nursing
University of Lynchburg
Lynchburg, Virginia

Karen Robertson, MSN, MBA, PhD/ABD
Associate Professor
Rock Valley College
Rockford, Illinois

Nancy Ross, PhD, RN
Assistant Clinical Professor
University of New England
Portland, Maine

Susan Self, DNP, RN
Assistant Professor in Nursing
Arkansas Tech University
Russellville, Arkansas

Leah Shreves, MSN, RN
Associate Professor of Nursing
Edison State Community College
Piqua, Ohio

Janice A. Sinoski, MSN/Ed, BSN, CCRN, CEN
Assistant Professor of Nursing
University of Lynchburg
Lynchburg, Virginia

Mendy Stanford, DNP, MSN/Ed, CNE
Executive Director of Nursing and Allied Health
Treasure Valley Community College
Ontario, Oregon

Charles Tucker, DNP, RN, CNE
Associate Professor
Mars Hill University
Mars Hill, North Carolina

Heather Vitko, PhD, RN, CCRN, TCRN, CNL
Assistant Professor of Nursing
Saint Francis University
Windber, Pennsylvania

Mina Wayman, APRN, MSN
Associate Professor
Utah Valley University
Orem, Utah

Heather Wierzbinski-Cross, MSN, RN, CNE
Dean for the School of Nursing
Ivy Tech Community College Richmond
Richmond, Indiana

Kennetta Wiggins, MSN, RN
Nursing Instructor and Registered Nurse
Northwest Arkansas Community College
Bentonville, Arkansas

Renee Wright, EdD, RN
Associate Professor
York College, City University of New York
Jamaica, New York

Preface

Since 1964, when Lillian Sholtis Brunner and Doris Smith Suddarth introduced the first edition of the *Textbook of Medical-Surgical Nursing*, the practice of nursing has flexed, changed, evolved, and advanced to meet changing health needs and expectations for health care. With each subsequent edition of this textbook, Lillian and Doris, and their successors, Suzanne Smeltzer and Brenda Bare (and eventually we, the current authors), admirably updated and revised content to reflect changes and challenges that shaped the practice of nursing, considering complex and interconnected influences and maintaining a focus upon salient social, cultural, economic, and environmental factors. Never have we, nor our distinguished and capable predecessors, had to revise and update seminal medical-surgical nursing concepts, principles, and practices during a global pandemic—until now. Most assuredly, this has been a daunting task. Yet, compared to what many of our phenomenally creative, determined, and resilient professional colleagues have had to confront and contend with as a result of this pandemic, our work was much less onerous. We would also like to recognize the long overdue and growing awareness of structural racism within healthcare and the impact of systemic racism on perpetuating stereotypes and health disparities. We encourage nurse educators and students to thoughtfully consider and discuss these issues when exploring epidemiological factors of specific disorders and nursing care throughout the textbook. Now that we have sent this edition to print and have time to reflect upon our work, we find ourselves humbled to call ourselves your peers and so proud of the important and sacred work that you do today and every day. We have decided to break with a long tradition in this textbook that tends to not provide dedications. To YOU our fellow nurses, nursing faculty, and nursing students, we dedicate this book.

Organization

Brunner & Suddarth's Textbook of Medical-Surgical Nursing, 15th Edition, is organized into 16 units. These units mirror those found in previous editions with the incorporation of some changes. Content was updated throughout all units, with cross-references to specific chapters included as appropriate. Units 1 through 3 cover foundational principles and core concepts related to medical-surgical nursing practice. Units 4 through 15 discuss adult health conditions that are treated medically or surgically. Unit 16 describes community-based challenges that affect medical-surgical nursing practice.

Units 4 through 15 are structured in the following way to better facilitate comprehension:

- The first chapter in the unit covers assessment and includes a review of normal anatomy and physiology of the body system being discussed.
- Subsequent chapters in the unit cover management of specific disorders. Pathophysiology, clinical manifestations, assessment and diagnostic findings, medical management, and nursing management are presented. Nursing Process sections, provided for select conditions, clarify and expand on the nurse's role in caring for patients with these conditions.

There are fewer chapters in this edition than in the past several editions; however, the seminal content within the deleted chapters remains, and is updated and revised. Notably, core content in previous-edition chapters that focused exclusively on *therapeutic modalities* has now been incorporated into chapters focused on health conditions and disorders, where its application dovetails seamlessly into nursing management and the nursing process. Thus, the application of these modalities to medical-surgical nursing practice is readily apparent.

Special Features

When caring for patients, nurses assume many different roles, including practitioner, educator, advocate, and researcher. Many of the features in this textbook have been developed to help nurses fulfill these varied responsibilities. Key updates to practice-oriented features in the 15th edition include new unit-opening Case Studies with QSEN Competency Focus—a feature that highlights a competency from the Quality and Safety Education for Nurses (QSEN) Institute that is applicable to the case study and poses questions for students to consider about relevant knowledge, skills, and attitudes (KSAs). Quality and Safety Nursing Alerts, Genetics in Nursing Practice charts, Ethical Dilemma charts, and Home Care Checklist charts offer updated information.

Plans of Nursing Care, provided for select disorders, illustrate how the nursing process is applied to meet the patient's health care and nursing needs. New to the 15th edition, nursing diagnoses used in the Plans of Nursing Care and throughout the textbook are those devised and validated by the International Council of Nurses in the *International Classification for Nursing Practice (ICNP) Catalogue*. (Please note that because of the global foci of these nursing diagnoses, select terms in these diagnoses are spelled in the British manner.)

A new addition to the textbook this cycle is a chapter focused exclusively on the unique health care needs of persons who identify as lesbian, gay, bisexual, transgender, and/or queer (LGBTQ). As is the case with other chapters of this textbook, the roles of the professional nurse as a practitioner, educator, advocate, and researcher when providing care for persons who are LGBTQ provide the framework for this new chapter.

In addition, two new features in this edition highlight content related to COVID-19 and care of veterans. *COVID-19 Considerations* sections identify evidence-based information at the time this material was written related to the severe acute respiratory syndrome coronavirus 2 (SARS-CoV-2) or the nursing care of patients with coronavirus disease 2019 (COVID-19). *Veterans Considerations* sections include information applicable to the special care needs of military veterans. Veterans—who may include persons from all age groups, genders, races, and socioeconomic strata—may have unique health risks based upon dates of service and assignment locale.

The textbook also provides pedagogical features developed to help readers engage and learn critical content. Concept Mastery Alerts continue to clarify fundamental nursing concepts to improve the reader's understanding of potentially confusing topics, as identified by Misconception Alerts in Lippincott's Adaptive Learning Powered by PrepU. An enhanced suite of online, interactive multimedia resources is also highlighted with icons placed in text near relevant topics. Unfolding Patient Stories (case study vignettes) based on vSim for Nursing patients are part of this suite of resources.

Read the User's Guide that follows the Preface for a full explanation and visual representation of all special features. See also the "Special Charts in This Book" and "Case Studies in This Book" sections of this front matter for the location of these items in the text.

A Comprehensive Package for Teaching and Learning

To further facilitate teaching and learning, a carefully designed ancillary package has been developed to assist faculty and students.

Instructor Resources

Tools to assist you with teaching your course are available upon adoption of this text on the Point at http://thepoint. lww.com/Brunner15e.

- An **e-Book** on the Point gives you access to the book's full text and images online.
- A thoroughly revised and augmented **Test Generator** contains more than 2900 NCLEX-style questions mapped to chapter learning outcomes.
- An extensive collection of materials is provided for each book chapter:
  - **Lesson Plans** outline learning outcomes and identify relevant resources from the robust instructor and student resource packages to help you prepare for your class.
  - **Pre-Lecture Quizzes** (and answers) allow you to check students' reading.
  - **PowerPoint Presentations** provide an easy way to integrate the textbook with your students' classroom experience; multiple-choice and true/false questions are included to promote class participation.
  - **Guided Lecture Notes** are organized by outcome and provide corresponding PowerPoint slide numbers to simplify preparation for lecture.
  - **Discussion Topics** (and suggested answers) can be used in the classroom or in online discussion boards to facilitate interaction with your students.
  - **Assignments** (and suggested answers) include group, written, clinical, and Web assignments to engage students in varied activities and assess their learning.
  - **Case Studies** with related questions (and suggested answers) give students an opportunity to apply their knowledge to a client case similar to one they might encounter in practice.
- Sample **Syllabi** are provided for one- and two-semester courses.

- A **QSEN Competency Map** identifies content and special features in the book related to competencies identified by the QSEN Institute.
- An **Image Bank** lets you use the photographs and illustrations from this textbook in your course materials.
- Access to all **Student Resources** is provided so that you can understand the student experience and use these resources in your course as well.

Student Resources

An exciting set of free learning resources is available on the Point to help students review and apply vital concepts in medical-surgical nursing. Multimedia engines have been optimized so that students can access many of these resources on mobile devices. Students can access all these resources at http://thepoint.lww.com/Brunner15e using the codes printed in the front of their textbooks.

- **NCLEX-Style Review Questions** for each chapter, totaling more than 1800 questions, help students review important concepts and practice for NCLEX.
- Interactive learning resources appeal to a variety of learning styles. Icons in the text direct readers to relevant resources:
  - **Concepts in Action Animations** bring physiologic and pathophysiologic concepts to life.
  - **Practice & Learn Case Studies** present case scenarios and offer interactive exercises and questions to help students apply what they have learned.
  - **Watch & Learn Video Clips** reinforce skills from the textbook and appeal to visual and auditory learners.
- **Procedural Guidelines** charts review key nursing interventions and rationales for specific patient care situations.
- **Appendix A, Diagnostic Studies and Interpretation**, provides reference ranges and lab values for common laboratory tests.
- **Journal Articles** offer access to current articles relevant to each chapter and available in Wolters Kluwer journals to familiarize students with nursing literature.

Study Guide

A comprehensive study aid for reviewing key concepts, *Study Guide for Brunner & Suddarth's Textbook of Medical-Surgical Nursing*, 15th Edition, has been thoroughly revised and presents a variety of exercises, including case studies and practice NCLEX-style questions, to reinforce textbook content and enhance learning.

vSim for Nursing

Available for separate purchase, vSim for Nursing, jointly developed by Laerdal Medical and Wolters Kluwer, offers innovative scenario-based learning modules consisting of Web-based virtual simulations, course learning materials, and curriculum tools designed to develop critical thinking skills and promote clinical confidence and competence. vSim for Nursing | Medical-Surgical includes 10 virtual simulations based on the National League for Nursing Volume I Complex patient scenarios. Students can progress through suggested readings, pre- and postsimulation assessments, documentation assignments, and guided reflection questions, and will receive an individualized feedback log immediately upon completion of the simulation. Throughout the student learning experience, the product offers remediation back to trusted Lippincott resources, including *Brunner & Suddarth's Textbook of Medical-Surgical Nursing*, as well as Lippincott Nursing Advisor and Lippincott Nursing Procedures—two online, evidence-based, clinical information solutions used in health care facilities throughout the United States. This innovative product provides a comprehensive patient-focused solution for learning and integrating simulation into the classroom.

Contact your Wolters Kluwer sales representative or visit http://thepoint.lww.com/vsim for options to enhance your medical-surgical nursing course with vSim for Nursing.

Lippincott DocuCare

Available for separate purchase, Lippincott DocuCare combines Web-based academic EHR simulation software with clinical case scenarios, allowing students to learn how to use an EHR in a safe, true-to-life setting, while enabling instructors to measure their progress. Lippincott DocuCare's nonlinear solution works well in the classroom, simulation lab, and clinical practice.

Contact your Wolters Kluwer sales representative or visit http://thepoint.lww.com/DocuCare for options to enhance your medical-surgical nursing course with DocuCare.

A Comprehensive, Digital, Integrated Course Solution

Lippincott® CoursePoint+ is an integrated, digital curriculum solution for nursing education that provides a completely interactive experience geared to help students understand, retain, and apply their course knowledge and be prepared for practice. The time-tested, easy-to-use, and trusted solution includes engaging learning tools, evidence-based practice, case studies, and in-depth reporting to meet students where they are in their learning, combined with the most trusted nursing education content on the market to help prepare students for practice. This easy-to-use digital learning solution of *Lippincott® CoursePoint+*, combined with unmatched support, gives instructors and students everything they need for course and curriculum success!

Lippincott® CoursePoint+ includes:

- Leading content provides a variety of learning tools to engage students of all learning styles.
- A personalized learning approach gives students the content and tools they need at the moment they need it, giving them data for more focused remediation and helping to boost their confidence and competence.
- Powerful tools, including varying levels of case studies, interactive learning activities, and adaptive learning powered by PrepU, help students learn the critical thinking and clinical judgment skills to help them become practice-ready nurses.
- Preparation for Practice tools improve student competence, confidence, and success in transitioning to practice.
  - vSim for Nursing: Co-developed by Laerdal Medical and Wolters Kluwer, vSim for Nursing simulates real nursing scenarios and allows students to interact with virtual patients in a safe, online environment.
  - Lippincott Advisor for Education: With over 8500 entries covering the latest evidence-based content and drug information, Lippincott Advisor for Education provides students with the most up-to-date information possible, while giving them valuable experience with the same point-of-care content they will encounter in practice.
- Unparalleled reporting provides in-depth dashboards with several data points to track student progress and help identify strengths and weaknesses.
- Unmatched support includes training coaches, product trainers, and nursing education consultants to help educators and students implement CoursePoint+ with ease.

Janice L. Hinkle, PhD, RN, CNRN
Kerry H. Cheever, PhD, RN
Kristen J. Overbaugh, PhD, RN, ACNS-BC, CHPN

User's Guide

Brunner & Suddarth's Textbook of Medical-Surgical Nursing, 15th Edition, has been revised and updated to reflect the complex nature of nursing practice today. This textbook includes many features to help you gain and apply the knowledge that you need to pass NCLEX and successfully meet the challenges and opportunities of clinical practice. In addition, features have been developed specifically to help you fulfill the varied roles that nurses assume in practice.

Opening Features That Start with the End in Mind

Unit-opening features put the patient first and highlight competent nursing as well as application of the nursing process.

- **All new! A Case Study with QSEN Competency Focus** opens each unit and provides discussion points focusing on one competency from the QSEN Institute: patient-centered care, interdisciplinary teamwork and collaboration, evidence-based practice, quality improvement, safety, or informatics. This feature helps you consider the KSAs required for the delivery of safe, quality patient care. For your convenience, a list of these case studies, along with their location in the book, appears in the "Case Studies in This Book" section later in this front matter.

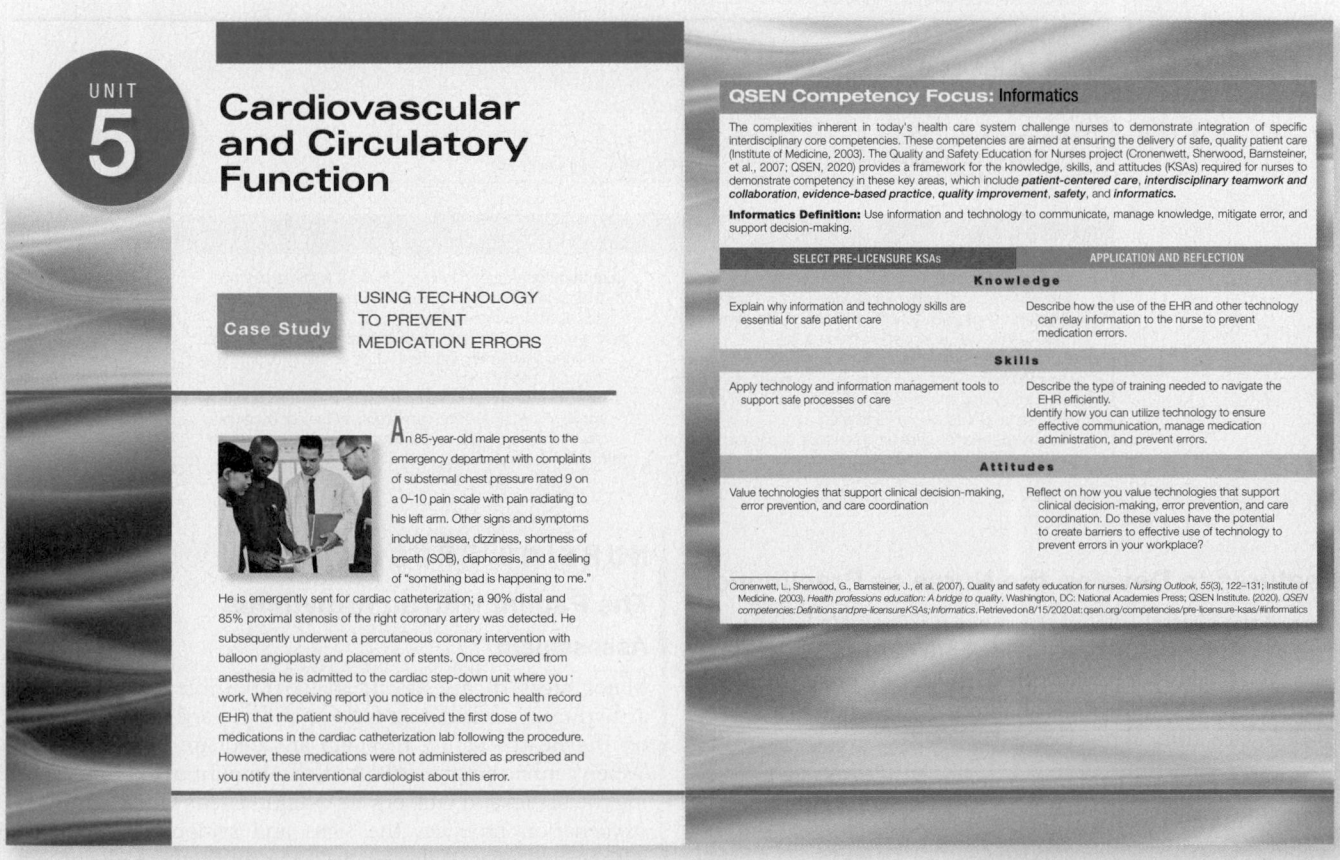

- **Learning Outcomes**, succinctly focused and condensed in this edition, provide an overview of each chapter and identify what you will be able to do after completing the material, to help focus reading and studying.
- **NEW! Nursing Concepts** listed at the beginning of each chapter make clear how content applies to Concepts-based curricula.

- A **Glossary** provides a list of key terms and definitions at the beginning of each chapter, providing a review of vocabulary words before reading the material and a useful reference and study tool.

54   Assessment and Management of Patients Who Are LGBTQ

LEARNING OUTCOMES

On completion of this chapter, the learner will be able to:

1. Describe the importance of providing inclusive health-care environments for people who are lesbian, gay, bisexual, transgender, and queer.
2. Use inclusive terminology when communicating and conducting an assessment with a person who is lesbian, gay, bisexual, transgender, and queer.
3. Explain and demonstrate the proper techniques to perform a health history and physical assessment and discriminate between normal and abnormal findings

identified in the patient who is lesbian, gay, bisexual, transgender, and queer.
4. Describe the various medical procedures and hormone treatments available for the person who is undergoing gender reassignment.
5. Compare and contrast surgical procedures available to people seeking gender reassignment in terms of indications and preoperative and postoperative complications.
6. Use the nursing process as a framework for care of the patient who undergoes gender reassignment surgery.

NURSING CONCEPTS

Assessment	Family	Sexuality
Communication	Identity	
Development/Human Development	Professionalism/Professional Behaviors	

GLOSSARY

bisexual: people who are romantically, emotionally, or sexually attracted to both male and female genders
cisgender: people who identify with the gender that matches the sex assigned to them at birth
gay: people who are romantically, emotionally, or sexually attracted to the same gender, such as men attracted to men
gender: set of socially constructed norms and behaviors that are taught to women and men
gender dysphoria: distress a person feels due to a mismatch between their gender identity and sex assigned at birth

questioning: a person who is unsure or is still exploring their sexual orientation or is concerned about applying a social label to themselves
sex: refers to the physical or biological characteristics that distinguish women and men, such as chromosomes, genitals, and hormones
sexual orientation: umbrella term that refers to romantic, emotional, or sexual attraction to persons of the opposite gender, the same gender, or to both or more than one gender
third-person pronouns: a way of referencing a person

Features to Develop the Nurse as Practitioner

One of the central roles of the nurse is to provide holistic care to patients and their families, both independently and through collaboration with other health care professionals. Special features throughout chapters are designed to assist readers with clinical practice.

- **Nursing Process sections** are organized according to the nursing process framework—the basis for all nursing practice—and help clarify the nurse's responsibilities in caring for patients with select disorders.

NURSING PROCESS

The Patient with an Arrhythmia

Assessment

Major areas of assessment include possible causes of the arrhythmia, contributing factors, and the arrhythmia's effect on the heart's ability to pump an adequate blood volume. When cardiac output is reduced, the amount of oxygen reaching the tissues and vital organs is diminished. This diminished oxygenation produces the signs and symptoms associated with arrhythmias. If these signs and symptoms are severe or if they occur frequently, the patient may experience significant distress and disruption of daily life.

- **Plans of Nursing Care**, provided for select disorders, illustrate how the nursing process is applied to meet the patient's health care and nursing needs.

Chart 45-4	PLAN OF NURSING CARE
	Care of the Patient with Hypothyroidism

NURSING DIAGNOSIS: Impaired breathing associated with depressed ventilation
GOAL: Improved respiratory status and maintenance of normal breathing pattern

Nursing Interventions	Rationale	Expected Outcomes
1. Assess respiratory rate, depth, pattern, pulse oximetry, and arterial blood gases.	1. Identifies patient's baseline to monitor further changes and evaluate effectiveness of interventions.	• Shows improved respiratory status and normal respiratory rate, depth, and pattern
2. Encourage deep breathing, coughing, and the use of incentive spirometry.	2. Prevents atelectasis and promotes adequate ventilation.	• Takes deep breaths, coughs and uses incentive spirometry
3. Verify with the provider orders to administer any hypnotic and sedative until euthyroid state achieved. If these medications are needed, monitor for adverse side effects.	3. Patients with hypothyroidism are susceptible to respiratory depression with the use of hypnotics and sedatives.	• Explains rationale for cautious use of medications
4. Maintain patient airway through suction and ventilator support if needed (see Chapter 19 for care of patients requiring mechanical ventilation).	4. The use of artificial airway and ventilator support may be necessary.	• Maintains adequate oxygenation

- **Assessment charts** focus on data that should be collected as part of the assessment step of the nursing process.

- **Risk Factors charts** outline factors that can impair health and should be considered in the context of social determinants of health and systemic racism.

Chart 35-3	ASSESSMENT
	Assessing for Peripheral Nerve Function

Assessment of peripheral nerve function has two key elements: evaluation of sensation and evaluation of motion. The nurse may perform one or all of the following during a musculoskeletal assessment.

Nerve	Test of Sensation	Test of Movement
Peroneal	Prick the skin midway between the great and second toe.	Ask the patient to dorsiflex the foot and extend the toes.

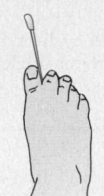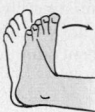

Chart 49-1	RISK FACTORS
	Urinary Tract Infection

- Contributing conditions such as:
  - Female gender
  - Diabetes
  - Pregnancy
  - Neurologic disorders
  - Gout
  - Altered states caused by incomplete emptying of the bladder and urinary stasis
- Decreased natural host defenses or immunosuppression
- Inability or failure to empty the bladder completely
- Inflammation or abrasion of the urethral mucosa
- Instrumentation of the urinary tract (e.g., catheterization, cystoscopic procedures)
- Obstructed urinary flow caused by:
  - Congenital abnormalities
  - Urethral strictures
  - Contracture of the bladder neck
  - Bladder tumors
  - Calculi (stones) in the ureters or kidneys
  - Compression of the ureters

- **Genetics in Nursing Practice charts** summarize and highlight nursing assessments and management issues related to the role of genetics in select disorders.

Chart 8-1   **GENETICS IN NURSING PRACTICE**

Genetics Concepts and the Older Adult

Genetic conditions in the older adult may occur from a specific gene mutation or arise as a result of a genetic predisposition combined with other factors (multifactorial). The following are examples of some adult-onset genetic conditions:

- Colon cancer
- Hemochromatosis
- Huntington disease
- Polycystic kidney disease
- Alzheimer's disease

The following are some examples of diseases with multifactorial components, which may include a genetic predisposition, in the older adult:

- Diabetes
- Emphysema
- Heart disease

Nursing Assessments

Refer to Chapter 4, Chart 4-2: Genetics in Nursing Practice: Genetic Aspects of Health Assessment

Family History Assessment Specific to the Older Adult

- Collect and assess family history on both maternal and paternal sides of the family for three generations.
- Determine whether genetic testing has occurred with other family members.
- Assess for individual and family perceptions and beliefs around topics related to genetics.

Patient Assessment Specific to the Older Adult and Genetic Illness

- Assess older adult patient's knowledge and understanding of genetics, genetic testing, and gene-based therapies.

- Assess the patient's understanding of genetic information and decipher health literacy needs.
- Perform cultural, social, and spiritual assessment.
- Assess patient's communication capacities so that communication strategies about genetics are tailored to their needs and abilities.
- Identify patient's support system.

Management Issues Specific to Genetics and the Older Adult

- Refer for further genetic counseling and evaluation as warranted so that family members can discuss inheritance, risk to other family members, and availability of genetic testing and gene-based interventions.
- Offer appropriate genetic information and resources that take into consideration older patient's literacy needs.
- Evaluate older patient's understanding before, during, and after the introduction of genetic information and services.
- Take the time to clearly explain the concepts of genetic testing to older patients and provide written information that reinforces the topic of discussion.
- Participate in the management and coordination of care of older patients with genetic conditions and individuals predisposed to develop or pass on a genetic condition.

Genetics Resources

See Chapter 6, Chart 6-7: Components of Genetic Counseling for additional resources.

- **Pharmacology charts and tables** display important considerations related to administering medications and monitoring drug therapy.

TABLE 42-2 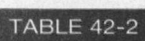 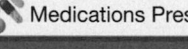 Medications Prescribed to Treat Obesity

Medication	Adverse Effects	Nursing Considerations[a]
Gastrointestinal Lipase Inhibitor		
Mechanism of Action: Diminishes intestinal absorption and metabolism of fats, particularly triglycerides		
Orlistat *Note: Also available in lower dosages over-the-counter*	Diarrhea Flatus Oily stools Fecal incontinence	Patients may have associated problems with malabsorption of nutrients; advise them to take a concomitant daily multivitamin. Caution in patients with known history of renal insufficiency, liver disease, or gallbladder disease as concomitant use is associated with renal calculi, liver failure, and cholelithiasis. Do not administer with cyclosporine.
Selective Serotonin Receptor Agonist		
Mechanism of Action: Stimulates serotonin 5-HT2C receptors, causing excretion of the alpha-melanocortin–stimulating hormone (alpha-MSH) and elicits appetite suppression		
Lorcaserin	Fatigue Dizziness Nausea Headaches Cough Dry mouth Constipation	Encourage patient to stay well hydrated. Can be associated with deficits in attention or memory; administer with caution in patients who drive or work with hazardous equipment when first prescribed until effects are realized. Can cause hypoglycemia in patients with diabetes. Contraindicated for patients taking antidepressants or migraine medications due to synergistic effects. Discontinue in patients who express suicidal ideation. Rarely, serotonin syndrome may develop—be alert for high fevers, brisk reflexes, agitation, and diarrhea; notify primary provider immediately and hold medication if these occur.

- **Updated! Quality and Safety Nursing Alerts** offer tips for best clinical practice and red-flag safety warnings to help avoid common mistakes.

> ⚑ *Quality and Safety Nursing Alert*
>
> *Any signed form required for surgery is placed in a prominent place on the patient's medical record and accompanies the patient to the OR.*

- **NEW! Veterans Considerations sections** highlight information applicable to the special care needs of veterans of the military. Veterans—who may include persons from all age groups, genders, races, and socioeconomic strata—may have unique health risks, based upon dates of service and assignment locale.

 ## Veterans Considerations

Many American veterans who served in Iraq and Afghanistan are experiencing respiratory disorders as a result of exposure to pollutants in situations such as sand storms and car bombings. Their illnesses can range from a new onset of asthma to constrictive bronchiolitis (Harrington, Schmidt, Szema, et al., 2017). These veterans could also have been exposed to organic contamination within the sand that could further irritate airways. When providing care to a veteran, it is important to assess exposure to airway irritants, particularly when the patient is complaining of chronic respiratory symptoms.

- **Obesity Considerations icons** identify content related to obesity or to the nursing care of patients with obesity.

 Obesity contributes to back strain by overtaxing the relatively weak back muscles in the absence of abdominal muscle support. Exercises are less effective and more difficult to perform when the patient is overweight. Weight reduction through diet modification is important to minimize recurrence of back pain. A sound nutritional plan that includes a change in eating habits and low-impact activities is vital. Noting achievement of weight reduction and providing positive reinforcement facilitate adherence. Back

- **NEW! COVID-19 Considerations sections** identify evidence-based information at the time this material was written related to the severe acute respiratory syndrome coronavirus 2 (SARS-CoV-2) or the nursing care of patients with coronavirus disease 2019 (COVID-19).

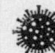 COVID-19 Considerations

The coronavirus disease 2019 (COVID-19) pandemic began in Wuhan, China, in late 2019. Since that time, several risks for both severe acute respiratory syndrome coronavirus 2 (SARS-CoV-2) infection and pathogenesis to coronavirus disease (COVID-19) have been posed. Epidemiologic findings from early data in China suggest that having a history of hypertension could be an important risk factor for becoming infected with SARS-CoV-2 as well as for being hospitalized to manage COVID-19 (Guo, Huang, Lin, et al., 2020;

- **Critical Care icons** identify nursing considerations for the patient who is critically ill.

 Pulmonary Edema

Pulmonary edema is an acute event, reflecting a breakdown of physiologic compensatory mechanisms; hence, it is sometimes referred to as acute decompensated heart failure. It can occur following acute MI or as an exacerbation of chronic HF. When the left ventricle begins to fail, blood backs up into the pulmonary circulation, causing pulmonary interstitial edema. This may occur quickly in some patients, a condition sometimes called *flash pulmonary edema*. Pulmonary edema can also develop slowly, especially when it is caused by noncardiac disorders such as kidney injury and other conditions that cause fluid overload. The left ventricle cannot handle the volume overload, and blood volume and pressure build up in the left atrium. The rapid increase in atrial pressure results in an acute increase in pulmonary venous pressure, which produces an increase in hydrostatic pressure that forces fluid out of the pulmonary capillaries and into the interstitial spaces and alveoli (Norris, 2019).

- **Gerontologic Considerations icons** highlight information that pertains specifically to the care of the older adult patient. In the United States, older adults comprise the fastest-growing segment of the population.

 Gerontologic Considerations

During the normal aging process, the nervous system undergoes many changes and is more vulnerable to illness. Age-related changes in the nervous system vary in degree and must be distinguished from those due to disease. It is important for clinicians not to attribute abnormality or dysfunction to aging without appropriate investigation. For example, although diminished strength and agility are a normal part of aging, localized weakness can only be attributed to disease.

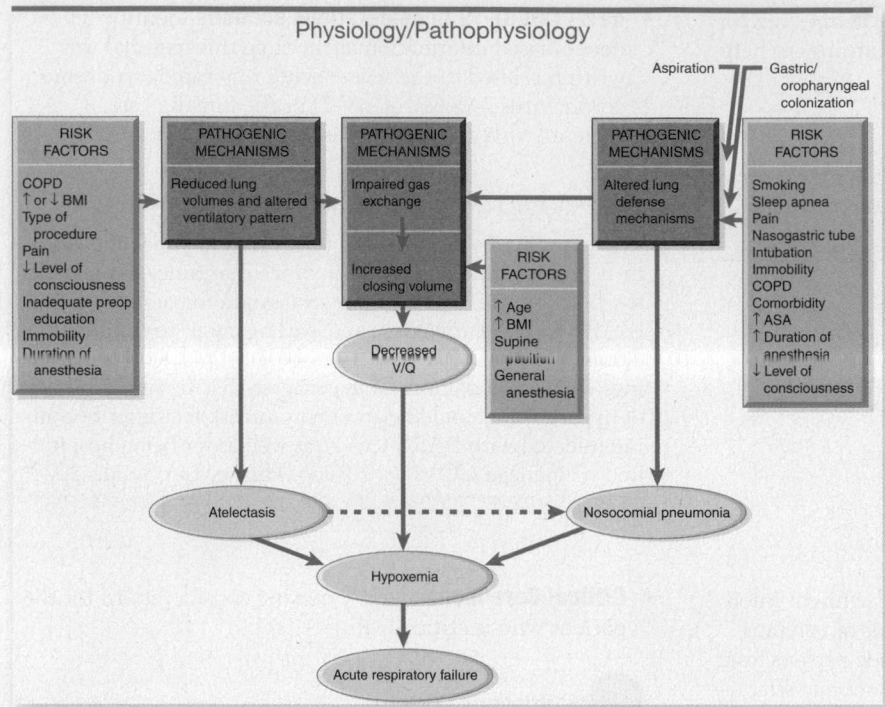

Physiology/Pathophysiology

- **Physiology/Pathophysiology figures** include illustrations and algorithms describing normal physiologic and pathophysiologic processes.

Features to Develop the Nurse as Educator

Health education is a primary responsibility of the nursing profession. Nursing care is directed toward promoting, maintaining, and restoring health; preventing illness; and helping patients and families adapt to the residual effects of illness. Patient education and health promotion are central to all of these nursing activities.

- **Patient Education charts and sections** help the nurse prepare the patient and family for procedures, assist them in understanding the patient's condition, and explain to them how to provide self-care.

Chart 20-5   **PATIENT EDUCATION**
Breathing Exercises

General Instructions

The nurse instructs the patient to:

- Breathe slowly and rhythmically to exhale completely and empty the lungs completely.
- Inhale through the nose to filter, humidify, and warm the air before it enters the lungs.
- Breathe more slowly by prolonging the exhalation time when feeling out of breath.
- Keep the air moist with a humidifier.

Diaphragmatic Breathing

Goal: To use and strengthen the diaphragm during breathing
The nurse instructs the patient to:

- Place one hand on the abdomen (just below the ribs) and the other hand on the middle of the chest to increase the awareness of the position of the diaphragm and its function in breathing.
- Breathe in slowly and deeply through the nose, letting the abdomen protrude as far as possible.
- Breathe out through pursed lips while tightening (contracting) the abdominal muscles.
- Press firmly inward and upward on the abdomen while breathing out.
- Repeat for 1 min; follow with a rest period of 2 min.

- Gradually increase duration up to 5 min, several times a day (before meals and at bedtime).

Pursed-Lip Breathing

Goal: To prolong exhalation and increase airway pressure during expiration, thus reducing the amount of trapped air and the amount of airway resistance
The nurse instructs the patient to:

- Inhale through the nose while slowly counting to 3—the amount of time needed to say "Smell a rose."
- Exhale slowly and evenly against pursed lips while tightening the abdominal muscles. (Pursing the lips increases intratracheal pressure; exhaling through the mouth offers less resistance to expired air.)
- Count to 7 slowly while prolonging expiration through pursed lips—the length of time to say "Blow out the candle."
- While sitting in a chair:
  Fold arms over the abdomen.
  Inhale through the nose while counting to 3 slowly.
  Bend forward and exhale slowly through pursed lips while counting to 7 slowly.
- While walking:
  Inhale while walking two steps.
  Exhale through pursed lips while walking four or five steps.

- **Health Promotion charts** review important points that the nurse should discuss with the patient to prevent common health problems from developing.

Chart 12-2 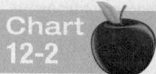 **HEALTH PROMOTION**

American Cancer Society Guidelines on Nutrition and Physical Activity for Cancer Prevention

Individual Choices

Achieve and Maintain a Healthy Weight Throughout Life

- Be as lean as possible throughout life without being underweight.
- Avoid excessive weight gain at all ages. For those who are currently overweight or have obesity, losing even a small amount of weight has health benefits and is a good place to start.
- Engage in regular physical activity and limit consumption of high-calorie foods and beverages as key strategies for maintaining a healthy weight.

Adopt a Physically Active Lifestyle

- Adults should engage in at least 150 minutes of moderate-intensity or 75 minutes of vigorous-intensity physical activity each week, or an equivalent combination, preferably spread throughout the week.
- Children and adolescents should engage in at least 1 hour of moderate- or vigorous-intensity physical activity each day, with vigorous-intensity activity at least 3 days each week.
- Limit sedentary behavior such as sitting, lying down and watching television, and other forms of screen-based entertainment.
- Doing any intentional physical activity above usual activities, no matter what one's level of activity, can have many health benefits.

Consume a Healthy Diet, with an Emphasis on Plant Sources

- Choose foods and beverages in amounts that help achieve and maintain a healthy weight.
- Limit consumption of processed meat and red meats.
- Eat at least 2½ cups of vegetables and fruits each day.
- Choose whole grains in preference to processed (refined) grains.

If You Drink Alcoholic Beverages, Limit Consumption

- Drink no more than one drink per day for women or two per day for men.

Community Action

Public, private, and community organizations should work collaboratively at national, state, and local levels to implement policy environmental changes that:

- Increase access to affordable, healthy foods in communities, worksites, and schools, and decrease access to and marketing of foods and beverages of low nutritional value, particularly to youth.
- Provide safe, enjoyable, and accessible environments for physical activity in schools and worksites, and for transportation and recreation in communities.

Adapted from American Cancer Society. (2019i). ACS guidelines on nutrition and physical activity for cancer. Retrieved on 9/28/2018 at: Prevention www.cancer.org/healthy/eat-healthy-get-active/acs-guidelines-nutrition-physical-activity-cancer-prevention.html.

- **Home Care Checklists** review points that should be covered as part of home care education prior to discharge from the health care facility.

Chart 41-9 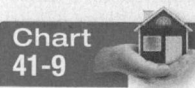 **HOME CARE CHECKLIST**

Managing Ostomy Care

At the completion of education, the patient and/or caregiver will be able to:

- Name the procedure that was performed and identify changes in anatomic structure or function as well as changes in ADLs, IADLs, roles, relationships, and spirituality.
  - Describe the frequency and character of effluent.
- Identify sources for obtaining ostomy care/appliance supplies.
- State the name, dose, side effects, frequency, and schedule for all medications.
- Demonstrate ostomy care, including wound cleansing, irrigation, and appliance changing.
- Describe the importance of assessing and maintaining peristomal skin integrity.
- Identify dietary restrictions (foods that can cause diarrhea and constipation), process for reintroduction of foods, as well as foods that may be encouraged.

- Identify measures to be used to promote fluid and electrolyte balance.
- Describe potential complications and necessary actions to be taken if complications occur.
- Relate how to reach primary provider with questions or complications.
  - Identify how to contact wound-ostomy-continence or home health nurse.
- State time and date of follow-up medical appointments, therapy, and testing.
- Identify sources of support (e.g., friends, relatives, faith community, ostomy support, caregiver support).
- Identify the need for health promotion, disease prevention, and screening activities.

ADLs, activities of daily living; IADLs, instrumental activities of daily living.

Features to Develop the Nurse as Patient Advocate

Nurses advocate for patients by protecting their rights (including the right to health care) and assisting patients and their families in making informed decisions about health care.

- **All new! Ethical Dilemma charts** provide a clinical scenario, discussion points, and questions to help analyze fundamental ethical principles related to the dilemma.

Chart 48-9 · **ETHICAL DILEMMA**
How Can Patient Rights Be Discerned during a Pandemic?

Case Scenario

B.J. is a 74-year-old widow with chronic kidney disease (CKD) managed with HD three times weekly in an outpatient dialysis center. She is admitted to the medical unit where you work as a staff nurse with fluid retention and dyspnea. It is reported that B.J. had been a "no show" at the dialysis center for at least the past week. As part of her therapeutic plan, she is supposed to be dialyzed while in the hospital. As you enter her room to prepare her for transport to the hospital's dialysis center, you find B.J. humming to herself, clapping her hands, and smiling. When you explain to her that she is going to be transported to the dialysis center, she says "Honey, I am not going anywhere. I want to see Jesus. It is my time and I am ready to see the Lord." You have heard from the medical social worker that this is not B.J.'s first admission to the hospital for poor adherence to her outpatient dialysis treatment. During past hospitalizations, her three adult daughters would visit her together and effectively cajole her into receiving dialysis treatments. Reportedly, the daughters have a loving and supportive relationship with each other and their mother. However, there is an outbreak of coronavirus disease 2019 (COVID-19) within your community and the hospital has responded with a no-visitor policy throughout the facility, so B.J.'s daughters may not visit her.

Discussion

The principle of autonomy is considered sacrosanct. Patients have the right to refuse treatments, even if those treatments are life-saving. However, in this particular instance, B.J. could be delirious as a manifestation of her poorly managed CKD. If she is delirious, it may be determined that she lacks the capacity to

make her own decisions. Her daughters might be her surrogates and legally responsible to make health care decisions for her. However, her daughters' prohibition to visit her while she is hospitalized hampers their ability to discuss her options with her and gain her assent for treatment.

Analysis

- Describe the ethical principles that are in conflict in this case (see Chapter 1, Chart 1-7). Can the principle of beneficence and wishing to "do good" for B.J. trump her autonomous right to refuse treatment? Can she be forced to undergo dialysis?
- What if it is determined that B.J. lacks the capacity to make informed decisions? On the contrary, what if it is determined that B.J. is not delirious and has the capacity to refuse to be dialyzed? Describe methods that you might employ to engage B.J.'s daughters so that they might be able to communicate with her and with each other as a family unit.
- What resources might be mobilized to be of assistance to B.J., her daughters, and the health care team so that a treatment plan that preserves B.J.'s dignity during this pandemic might be devised?

References

Hulkower, A. (2020). Learning from COVID. *Hastings Center Report, 50*(3), 16–17.

Resources

See Chapter 1, Chart 1-10 for Steps of an Ethical Analysis and Ethics Resources.

Chart 30-2 · **NURSING RESEARCH PROFILE**
Fatigue and Sleep Disturbances in Adults with Acute Leukemia

Bryant, A., Gosselin, T., Coffman, E., et al. (2018). Symptoms, mobility, and function, and quality of life in adults with acute leukemia during initial hospitalization. *Oncology Nursing Forum, 45*(5), 653–664.

Purpose

Patients newly diagnosed with acute leukemia require hospitalization, typically for 4 to 6 weeks, for managing aggressive induction therapy and its toxicities. These symptoms can greatly impact the patient's quality of life and ability to perform activities of daily living. The purpose of this study was to evaluate global, physical, and mental health symptoms in adults with newly diagnosed acute leukemia.

Design

This was a prospective, longitudinal study with a total of 49 adult participants, including 36 males and 13 females. Data were collected at time of hospitalization (baseline), then weekly until discharge from hospital. Evaluation tools for data included: the Patient-Reported Outcomes Measurement Information System (PROMIS) to determine several self-reported quality-of-life measures such as fatigue, anxiety, depression, pain, sleep disturbances, and global physical and mental health; the Functional Assessment of Cancer Therapy-Leukemia (FACT-Leu) to measure symptom concerns that are leukemic specific; Karnofsky Performance Status Scale (KPS) to measure function; and the Timed UP and Go Test (TUG) to measure physical mobility.

Findings

This study was the largest, to date, to evaluate the symptoms and quality of life of patients newly diagnosed with acute leukemia during hospitalization. All participants had one or more comorbidities, as well as a group mean body mass index of 30.8 (SD = 6.7), indicative of being overweight or having obesity, at time of hospitalization. No significant differences were seen in global mental health, pain, or KPS during hospitalization. There were significant decreases in fatigue ($p < 0.001$), anxiety ($p < 0.001$), depression ($p = 0.004$), and sleep disturbance ($p = 0.005$) from baseline to hospital discharge. Also significant were a decrease in leukemic symptoms ($p < 0.001$), indicating improved leukemic outcomes, which is the goal of therapy.

Nursing Implications

Nurses need to be aware of factors that can impact sleep in patients with cancer, both during and following treatment. As fatigue plays a major role in sleep disturbances, the nurse needs to assess for and develop strategies to address both concerns, especially while the patient is in the hospital. Poor sleep, fatigue, and pain can all contribute to the increased risk for falls, so safety issues should also be addressed with the patient and the patient's family. The nurse should encourage the patient to exercise and have some physical activity as part of the daily routine, to decrease fatigue while enhancing sleep. Additionally, the nurse should have a good understanding of the symptoms common to patients with leukemia and interventions to manage them as they occur.

Features to Develop the Nurse as Researcher

Nurses identify potential research problems and questions to increase nursing knowledge and improve patient care. The use and evaluation of research findings in nursing practice are essential to further the science of nursing.

- **All new and in every chapter! Nursing Research Profiles** identify the implications and applications of nursing research findings for evidence-based nursing practice.

Features to Facilitate Learning

In addition to practice-oriented features, special features have been developed to help readers learn key information.

- **Concept Mastery Alerts** highlight and clarify fundamental nursing concepts to improve understanding of difficult topics, as identified by Misconception Alerts in Lippincott's Adaptive Learning Powered by PrepU, an adaptive quizzing platform.

 Concept Mastery Alert

It is important to remember the different types of cholesterol and the role of each as a risk factor for heart disease. HDL is the "good cholesterol," and higher levels are better; LDL is the "bad cholesterol," and lower levels are better.

- **Unfolding Patient Stories**, written by the National League for Nursing, are an engaging way to begin meaningful conversations in the classroom. These vignettes, which appear throughout the text near related content, feature patients from Wolters Kluwer's vSim for Nursing | Medical-Surgical (co-developed by Laerdal Medical) and DocuCare products; however, each Unfolding Patient Story in the book stands alone, not requiring purchase of these products. For your convenience, a list of these case studies, along with their location in the book, appears in the "Case Studies in This Book" section later in this front matter.

- Interactive learning tools available online enrich learning and are identified with icons in the text:

   Concepts in Action Animations bring physiologic and pathophysiologic concepts to life.

   Practice & Learn Case Studies present case scenarios and offer interactive exercises and questions to help you apply what you have learned.

   Watch & Learn Video Clips reinforce skills from the textbook and appeal to visual and auditory learners.

- **All new! Critical Thinking Exercises** foster critical thinking and challenge you to apply textbook knowledge to clinical scenarios. Evidence-based practice (EBP) questions encourage you to apply best evidence from research findings to nursing interventions. Prioritization (PQ) questions ask you to consider the priorities for nursing care for specific patients and conditions. Interprofessional collaboration (IPC) exercises challenge you to identify the roles and responsibilities of the professional nurse and of interprofessional colleagues in collaboratively delivering quality patient-centered care.

- **References** cited are listed at the end of each chapter and include updated, current sources.

- **Resources** lists at the end of each chapter include sources of additional information, Web sites, agencies, and patient education materials.

Unfolding Patient Stories: Doris Bowman • Part 2

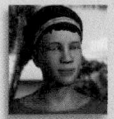

Recall from Chapter 12 **Doris Bowman**, who is undergoing a total abdominal hysterectomy with bilateral salpingo-oophorectomy. What are potential postoperative complications that the nurse should consider? What assessments and interventions are done by the nurse to monitor for early detection or to prevent these complications? Describe the discharge education provided by the nurse on self-care monitoring required of the patient at home and what should be reported to the health care provider.

Care for Doris and other patients in a realistic virtual environment: ***vSim** for Nursing* (**thepoint.lww.com/vSimMedicalSurgical**). Practice documenting these patients' care in DocuCare (**thepoint.lww.com/DocuCareEHR**).

CRITICAL THINKING EXERCISES

1 IPC You are caring for a 53-year-old woman in the outpatient clinic where you work; she is newly diagnosed with urinary incontinence. What type of referrals might be appropriate for this patient? What members of the interprofessional health care team do you anticipate as being integral to the care of this patient?

2 ebp You notice an increase in the number of CAUTIs among patients on the medical-surgical unit where you work. What are the evidence-based management techniques used in CAUTI prevention? Identify the criteria used to evaluate the strength of the evidence for these practices. How will you individualize these techniques for your unit?

3 pq A 65-year-old man is admitted to the medical-surgical nursing unit where you work with bladder cancer. He is scheduled for a radical cystectomy with an orthotopic neobladder reconstruction. Identify the priorities, approach, and techniques you would use to provide care for this patient in the preoperative phase of care. How will your priorities, approach, and techniques differ in the postoperative phase of care?

REFERENCES

*Asterisk indicates nursing research.

Books

American College of Surgeons. (2018). *Advanced trauma life support* (10th ed.). Chicago, IL: Author.

Atanelov, Z., & Rebstock, S. E. (2020) Nasopharyngeal airway. *StatPearls [Internet]*. Treasure Island, FL: StatPearls Publishing. Retrieved on 4/6/2020 at: www.ncbi.nlm.nih.gov/books/NBK513220/

Emergency Nurses Association (ENA). (2017). *Emergency nursing scope and standards of practice* (2nd ed.). Des Plaines, IL: Author.

Emergency Nurses Association (ENA). (2020a). *Sheehy's manual of emergency care* (7th ed.). St. Louis, MO: Mosby.

Holleran, R., Wolfe, A., & Frakes, M. (2018). *Patient transport: Principles & practice* (5th ed.). St Louis, MO: Elsevier.

Resources

American Association of Poison Control Centers (AAPCC), www.aapcc.org

American College of Emergency Physicians (ACEP), www.acep.org

American College of Surgeons (ACS), Injury Prevention and Control, www.facs.org/quality-programs/trauma/ipc

American Heart Association, www.heart.org

American Trauma Society (ATS), www.amtrauma.org/default.aspx

American Red Cross, Prepare for Emergencies, www.redcross.org/get-help/prepare-for-emergencies/types-of-emergencies

Divers Alert Network (DAN), www.diversalertnetwork.org

Emergency Nurses Association (ENA), www.ena.org

National Capital Poison, Poison Control Center, poison.org

National Center on Elder Abuse (NCEA), ncea.acl.gov

National Center for Health Statistics (NCHS), cdc.gov/nchs/

National Human Trafficking Hotline, www.humantraffickinghotline.org

Contents

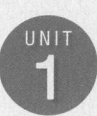

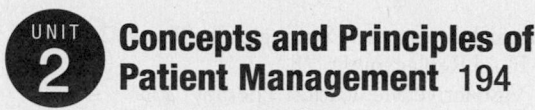

Concepts and Principles of Patient Management 194

UNIT 3 Perioperative Concepts and Nursing Management 394

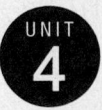

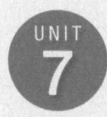

UNIT 7 Immunologic Function 984

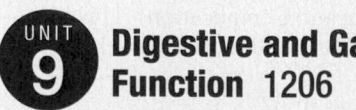

UNIT 9 Digestive and Gastrointestinal Function 1206

UNIT 10 Metabolic and Endocrine Function 1340

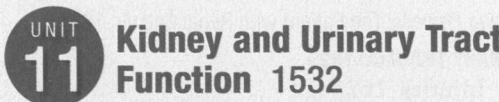

UNIT 11 Kidney and Urinary Tract Function 1532

47 Assessment of Kidney and Urinary Function 1534

48 Management of Patients with Kidney Disorders 1554

UNIT 12 Reproductive Function 1638

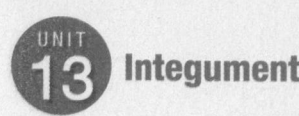

UNIT 13 Integumentary Function 1796

UNIT 14 Sensory Function 1894

UNIT 15 Neurologic Function 1964

Case Studies in This Book

Special Charts in This Book

Health Promotion

Home Care Checklist

Nursing Research Profile

Patient Education

Pharmacology

BRUNNER & SUDDARTH'S

TEXTBOOK OF

Medical-Surgical Nursing

15TH EDITION

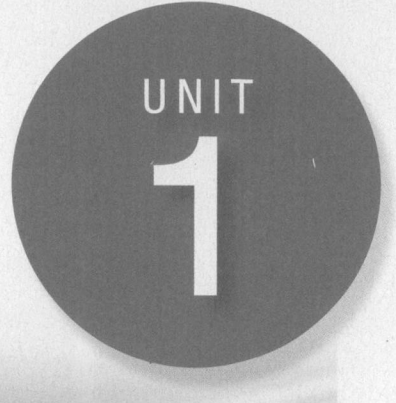

UNIT

1

Principles of Nursing Practice

Case Study

EDUCATING OLDER ADULTS TO NAVIGATE THEIR ELECTRONIC HEALTH RECORDS

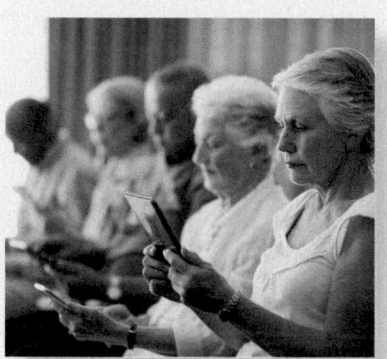

Y ou are a nurse working in a community health center that provides services for older adults. A recent needs assessment indicates that patrons of the health center are underutilizing electronic resources available to them. Furthermore, these individuals need education about resources such as their electronic health records (EHRs) including how to access, maintain, and utilize this tool. EHRs enable patients to be more aware and have better control over their health management. You implement a plan for educating older adults in the community on this technology. The main goal of this project is to empower older adults to easily access their own EHRs and manage their appointments, medications, and follow-up visits. An additional goal is that use of this technology will enable patients, families, and communities to have up-to-date information and increased access to health-related resources.

QSEN Competency Focus: Patient-Centered Care

The complexities inherent in today's health care system challenge nurses to demonstrate integration of specific interdisciplinary core competencies. These competencies are aimed at ensuring the delivery of safe, quality patient care (Institute of Medicine, 2003). The Quality and Safety Education for Nurses project (Cronenwett, Sherwood, Barnsteiner, et al., 2007; QSEN, 2020) provides a framework for the knowledge, skills, and attitudes (KSAs) required for nurses to demonstrate competency in these key areas, which include **patient-centered care**, **interdisciplinary teamwork and collaboration**, **evidence-based practice**, **quality improvement**, **safety,** and **informatics.**

Patient-Centered Care Definition: Recognize the patient or designee as the source of control and full partner in providing compassionate and coordinated care based on respect for patient's preferences, values, and needs.

SELECT PRE-LICENSURE KSAs	APPLICATION AND REFLECTION
Knowledge	
Describe strategies to empower patients or families in all aspects of the health care process	How does providing access to patient information empower patients, families, and communities to manage their health? What are the advantages to having immediate access to patient information?
Skills	
Engage patients or designated surrogates in active partnerships that promote health, safety and well-being, and self-care management	What is the responsibility of the nurse in helping patients navigate their EHR? Discuss how you would advocate for patients so they have the resources to access, understand, and utilize their EHR.
Attitudes	
Seek learning opportunities with patients who represent all aspects of human diversity	Think about your own experience and training with patients, families, and communities that have technology barriers. Why is it important for nurses to provide opportunities to patients, families, and communities of diverse backgrounds about the use of technology to access information?

Cronenwett, L., Sherwood, G., Barnsteiner, J., et al. (2007). Quality and safety education for nurses. *Nursing Outlook*, *55*(3), 122–131; Institute of Medicine. (2003). *Health professions education: A bridge to quality*. Washington, DC: National Academies Press; QSEN Institute. (2020). *QSEN competencies: Definitions and pre-licensure KSAs; Patient-centered care*. Retrieved on 8/15/2020 at: qsen.org/competencies/pre-licensure-ksas/#patient-centered_care

1 Professional Nursing Practice

LEARNING OUTCOMES

On completion of this chapter, the learner will be able to:

1. Define nursing, patient, health, wellness, health promotion, and health care.
2. Describe salient influences on the delivery of health care.
3. Discuss practices that improve quality and safety and ensure the use of evidence-based practices within the health care system.
4. Discuss behavioral competencies and characteristics of professional nursing practice and the nurse's role as a collaborative member of the interprofessional health care team.
5. Define the characteristics of critical thinking, the critical thinking process, and clinical decision making.
6. Describe the components of the nursing process.
7. Identify strategies that can be implemented in ethical decision making.

NURSING CONCEPTS

Accountability
Advocacy
Assessment
Caring
Clinical Decision Making
Collaboration

Critical Thinking
Ethics
Evidence-Based Practice
Health Care Systems
Health Policy
Health Promotion

Informatics
Legal Issues
Nursing Process
Quality Improvement
Safety

GLOSSARY

assessment: the systematic collection of data, through interview, observation, and examination, to determine the patient's health status and any actual or potential problems

bundle: a set of three to five evidence-based practices that, when implemented appropriately, can measurably improve patient outcomes

critical thinking: a cognitive process that utilizes thinking that is purposeful, insightful, reflective, and goal directed to develop conclusions, solutions, and alternatives that are appropriate to the given solution

ethics: the formal, systematic process used to understand, analyze, and evaluate decisions regarding matters of right and wrong as they apply to well-being

evaluation: determination of the patient's response to nursing interventions and the extent to which the outcomes have been achieved

evidence-based practice (EBP): a best practice derived from valid and reliable research studies that also considers the health care setting, patient preferences and values, and clinical judgment

health: according to the World Health Organization (2006), a "state of complete physical, mental, and social well-being and not merely the absence of disease and infirmity" (p. 1)

health informatics: the use of health information technology to improve the quality, efficiency, or delivery of health care

health promotion: focuses on the potential for wellness and targets appropriate alterations in personal habits, lifestyle, and environment in ways that reduce risks and enhance health and well-being

implementation: actualization or carrying out of the nursing plan of care through nursing interventions

interprofessional collaborative practice: employing multiple health professionals to work together with patients, families, and communities to deliver best practices, thus ensuring best patient outcomes

morality: specific beliefs or actions whose outcomes are often examined utilizing the principles of autonomy, beneficence, nonmaleficence, double effect, and distributive justice

moral dilemma: situation in which two or more ethically plausible principles are in opposition to each other and only one may be chosen

moral distress: internal response that occurs when a health care provider believes they inherently know the correct ethical action that is needed but cannot act on that knowledge

moral integrity: virtue composed of veracity, fidelity, benevolence, wisdom, and moral courage

moral problem: competing moral claim or principle; one principle is clearly dominant

moral uncertainty: internal conflict that arises when the person cannot define what the moral situation is or what moral principles apply but has a strong feeling that something is not right

nursing: according to the American Nurses Association (2015b), "the protection, promotion, and optimization of health and abilities, prevention of illness and injury, facilitation of healing, alleviation of suffering through the diagnosis and treatment of human response, and advocacy in the care of individuals, families, groups, communities, and populations" (p. 1)

nursing diagnosis: a clinical judgment concerning a person's, family's, or community's actual or potential health problems, state of health promotion, or potential risk that can be managed by independent nursing interventions

nursing process: a systematic, problem-solving approach for meeting people's health care and nursing needs; components involve assessment, diagnosis, planning, implementation, and evaluation

patient: a traditional term used to identify someone who is a recipient of health care

planning: development of measurable goals and outcomes as well as a plan of care designed to assist the patient in resolving the diagnosed problems and achieving the identified goals and outcomes

precision medicine: using advances in research, technology, and policies to develop individualized plans of care to prevent and treat disease

Quality and Safety Education for Nurses (QSEN): a project whose aim is to develop curricula that prepare future nurses with the knowledge, skills, and attitudes (KSA) required to continuously improve the quality and safety of the health care system through demonstrating competency in patient-centered care, teamwork and collaboration, evidence-based practice, quality improvement, safety, and informatics

telehealth: the use of technology to deliver health care, health information, or health education at a distance

The Joint Commission: a nonprofit organization that accredits hospitals and health care organizations

wellness: the ability to perform well, adjust and adapt to varying situations, and report feeling well and harmonious

As American society has undergone changes, so has the nation's health care system. Nursing, as the health care profession with the greatest number of employees and a major contributor to the health care delivery system, has been significantly affected by these changes. Nursing has played an important role in the health care system and will continue to do so. This chapter provides an overview of the practice of nursing in the United States today, as well important factors and issues that will continue to affect its practice into the future.

Nursing

Since the time of Florence Nightingale, who wrote in 1858 that the goal of nursing was "to put the patient in the best condition for nature to act upon him," nursing scholars and leaders have described nursing as both an art and a science. However, the definition of nursing has evolved over time. In the American Nurses Association (ANA) Scope and Standards of Practice (ANA, 2015b, p. 1), **nursing** is defined as "the protection, promotion, and optimization of health and abilities, prevention of illness and injury, facilitation of healing, alleviation of suffering through the diagnosis and treatment of human response, and advocacy in the care of individuals, families, groups, communities, and populations." Nurses have a responsibility to carry out their role as described in Nursing's Social Policy Statement (ANA, 2010; Fowler, 2015), to comply with the nurse practice act of the state in which they practice, and to comply with the Code of Ethics for Nurses as spelled out by the ANA (2015a) and the International Council of Nurses (ICN, 2012). Advocacy, promotion of a safe environment, research, education, and participation in patient and health systems management as well as shaping health policy are also key nursing roles (ICN, 2012).

The Patient: Consumer of Nursing and Health Care

The term **patient**, derived from a Latin verb meaning "to suffer," has traditionally been used to describe a person who is a recipient of care. The connotation commonly attached to the word is one of dependence. For this reason, many nurses prefer to use the term *client*, which is derived from a Latin verb meaning "to lean," connoting alliance and interdependence. The term *patient* is used purposely throughout this book; it is most commonly used by clinicians, as evidenced by its usage by the Interprofessional Education Collaborative (IPEC, 2016a), whose members include 15 national associations of schools of the health professions, including nursing, allopathic medicine, osteopathic medicine, pharmacy, dentistry, and public health, to name a few (see later discussion of IPEC).

The patient who seeks care for a health problem or problems (increasing numbers of people have multiple health problems or comorbidities) is also an individual person, a member of a family, a member of various social groups, and a citizen of the community. Patients' needs vary depending on problems, associated circumstances, and past experiences. Many patients, who as consumers of health care have become more knowledgeable about health care options, expect a collaborative approach with the nurse in the quest for optimal health (Majid & Gagliardi, 2019). Among the nurse's important functions in health care delivery are identifying the patient's immediate, ongoing, and long-term needs and working together with the patient to address them.

The Patient's Basic Needs: Maslow Hierarchy of Needs

Certain needs are basic to all people. Some of these needs are more important than others. Once an essential need is met, people often experience a need on a higher level of priority. Addressing needs by priority reflects Maslow's Hierarchy of Needs (Fig. 1-1).

Maslow ranked human needs to include physiologic needs, safety and security, sense of belonging and affection, esteem and self-respect, and self-actualization. Self-actualization includes self-fulfillment, desire to know and understand, and aesthetic needs. Lower-level needs always remain; however, a person's ability to pursue higher-level needs indicates movement toward psychological health and well-being (Maslow, 1954). Such a hierarchy of needs is a useful framework that can be applied to many nursing models for assessment of a patient's strengths, limitations, and need for nursing interventions.

Health

How health is perceived depends on how health is defined. The World Health Organization (WHO, 2006) defines **health** in the preamble to its constitution as a "state of complete physical, mental, and social well-being and not merely the absence of disease and infirmity" (p. 1). This definition implies that health and illness are not polar opposites. Theoretically, therefore, it is possible for a patient to have a physical illness and yet strive for and perhaps attain health in another domain (e.g., mental, social). Although commonly

cited worldwide, this definition has been criticized for being too utopian—after all, it is not possible for anyone to achieve *complete* physical, mental, and social well-being (Murdaugh, Parsons, & Pender, 2019).

Wellness

Wellness has been defined as being equivalent to health. Wellness involves being proactive and being involved in self-care activities aimed toward a state of physical, psychological, social, and spiritual well-being. Wellness is conceptualized as having four components: (1) the capacity to perform to the best of one's ability, (2) the ability to adjust and adapt to varying situations, (3) a reported feeling of well-being, and (4) a feeling that "everything is together" and harmonious (Hood, 2018). With this in mind, nurses must aim to promote positive changes that are directed toward health and well-being. The sense of wellness has a subjective aspect that addresses the importance of recognizing and responding to patient individuality and diversity in health care and nursing.

Health Promotion

Today, increasing emphasis is placed on health, wellness, health promotion, and self-care. Health is seen as resulting from a lifestyle oriented toward wellness. **Health promotion** focuses on the potential for wellness and targets appropriate alterations in personal habits, lifestyle, and environment in ways that reduce risks and enhance health and well-being (see Chapter 3).

People are increasingly knowledgeable about health and take more interest in and responsibility for health and well-being. Organized self-care wellness education programs emphasize health promotion, disease prevention, management of illness, self-care, and collaborative use of the professional health care system. Web sites, chat groups, open forums, and social media support groups promote sharing of experiences and information about self-care with others who have similar conditions, chronic diseases, or disabling conditions. The advent of mobile wireless computer technologies (e.g., Fitbit™) and novel informatics tools (e.g., Carb Manager) have had the effect of tailoring health promotion activities to meet individual preferences (Murdaugh et al., 2019). Researchers have begun to take advantage of these popular technologic advancements by developing population-based registries. The use of mobile health apps has demonstrated a positive impact on health-related behaviors, specifically, physical activity, dietary management, adherence to medication or therapy, and knowledge related to medications and diagnostic testing. Moreover, most mobile health apps seem to promote better clinical health outcomes (Han & Lee, 2018). According to the WHO (2019), "primary health care ensures people receive comprehensive care—ranging from promotion and prevention to treatment, rehabilitation and palliative care—as close as feasible to people's everyday environment" (p. 1). Primary health care includes a lifelong commitment to meeting individuals' health needs across the lifespan; empowerment of individuals to assume accountability for their own health care; and attention to societal needs for health care through social policy and action.

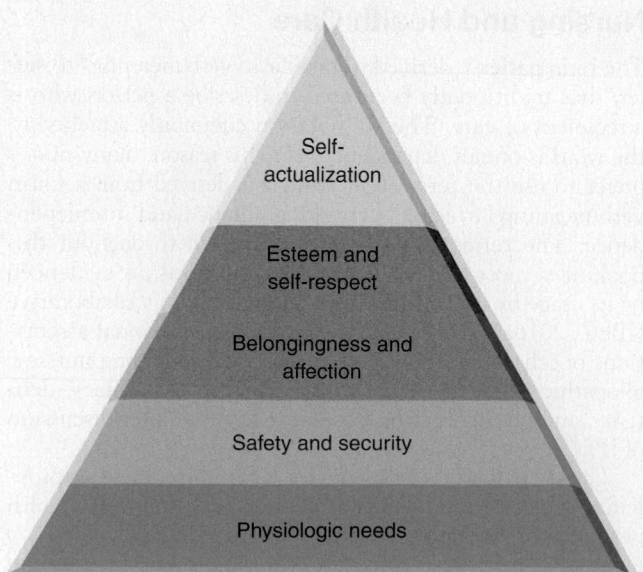

Figure 1-1 • This scheme of Maslow's hierarchy of needs shows how a person moves from fulfillment of basic needs to higher levels of needs, with the ultimate goal being integrated human functioning and health.

Health Care

Health care describes services that are offered to individuals, families, and communities to help them maintain health and wellness, prevent and manage illness and complications, and provide support through rehabilitation, recovery, and transitions to palliative care. Health care can be provided in inpatient, outpatient, and community settings by a variety of health professionals, including but not limited to nurses, primary providers, pharmacists, dieticians, social workers, psychologists, and physical, occupational, speech and respiratory therapists.

Influences on Health Care Delivery

The health care delivery system is constantly adapting to changes in health care needs and expectations. Shifting population demographics; changing patterns of disease and wellness; advances in technology and genetics; and greater emphasis on health care quality, costs, reform efforts, and interprofessional collaborative practices have impacted health care delivery and the practice of nursing.

Population Demographics

Changes in the population in general are affecting the need for and the delivery of health care. According to the United States (U.S.) Census Bureau (2020), over 329 million people reside in the country. Not only is the population increasing, but its composition is also changing. The decline in birth rate and the increase in lifespan have resulted in proportionately fewer school-age children and more senior citizens, many of whom are women. Much of the population resides in highly congested urban areas, with a steady migration of members of ethnic minorities to urban settings. Poverty is a growing concern. According to the U.S. Department of Housing and Urban Development's (HUD's) 2019 Annual Homeless Assessment Report, on a given night, approximately 568,000 individuals were documented as homeless in the United States. Homelessness increased by 3% from 2018 to 2019, with almost 40% of this population staying on the streets or other unsheltered locations; in addition, a higher percentage of minority populations compared to the total U.S. population are impacted by homelessness today (U.S. Department of Housing and Urban Development, 2020).

 Gerontologic Considerations

Both the number and proportion of Americans 65 years of age and older have grown substantially in the past century. In 2017, an estimated 47.8 million older adults resided in the United States; this number continues to climb, with the greatest growth in the Hispanic population (U.S. Census Bureau, 2017).

The health care needs of older adults are complex and demand significant investments, both professional and financial (see Chapter 8 for further discussion). Many older adults suffer from multiple chronic conditions that are exacerbated by acute episodes. In particular, older women are frequently underdiagnosed and undertreated. According to the United Nations' (2017) report on world population aging, globally, the number of people 80 years of age or older is projected to increase more than threefold between 2017 and 2050, rising from 137 to 425 million.

 Veterans Considerations

Veterans of the U.S. armed services comprise a unique population with health care needs that vary dependent upon branch of military service, whether service occurred during wartime eras, time and place of service, and individual experiences (Olenick, Flowers, & Diaz, 2015). According to the U.S. Census Bureau (2019), there are currently 18 million veterans, 1.8 million of whom are female. Substance use disorders (SUDs), posttraumatic stress disorder (PTSD), traumatic brain injury (TBI), suicide, depression, hazardous substance exposure, and amputations are common health care problems found among veterans (Olenick et al., 2015) (see Chapter 4). According to a Pew Research Center (2017) report, the proportion of Americans who served in the U.S. military has been steadily declining since 1980, when 18% of American adults were veterans. In 2016, 7% of Americans were veterans. That proportion is projected to continue to decline, and by 2045 the U.S. Department of Veteran Affairs estimates that there will be approximately 12 million veterans, roughly a 40% decrease from 2016 (Pew Research Center, 2017).

Cultural Diversity

An appreciation for the diverse characteristics and needs of people from varied ethnic and cultural backgrounds is important in health care and nursing. Some projections indicate that by 2030, racial and ethnic minority populations in the United States will triple. The latest U.S. census classified five distinct races as White, Black or African American, Asian, Native American or Alaska Native, and Native Hawaiian/Pacific Islander. The Asian race had the largest growth rate among these five racial groups. The Hispanic population, classified primarily under the White race, was noted to account for more than half of the increased population growth. The non-Hispanic Caucasian population will proportionally decrease so that they will no longer comprise the majority population, and other ethnic and racial minority populations will collectively comprise the majority of all Americans by approximately 2044 (Colby & Ortman, 2015). As the cultural composition of the population changes, it is increasingly important to address cultural considerations in the delivery of health care. Patients from diverse sociocultural groups not only bring various health care beliefs, values, and practices to the health care setting but also have unique risk factors for some disease conditions and unique reactions to treatment. These factors significantly affect a person's responses to health care problems or illnesses, to caregivers, and to the care itself. Unless these factors are assessed, understood, and respected by nurses, the care delivered may be ineffective, and health care outcomes may be negatively affected (see Chapter 4 for additional information on cultural assessment).

Changing Patterns of Disease and Wellness

During the past several decades, the health problems of Americans have changed significantly. Chronic diseases, including cardiovascular disease, cancers, diabetes, and chronic lung diseases account for 7 out of the 10 leading causes of death (Centers for Disease Control and Prevention [CDC], 2019).

Nearly half of all adults live with one diagnosed chronic condition; 60 million live with two or more (CDC, 2019). Tobacco use, SUD (e.g., alcohol, illicit drugs), poor physical activity and nutrition habits, and obesity have become major health concerns (CDC, 2019).

As the prevalence of chronic conditions increases, health care broadens from a focus on cure and eradication of disease to include health promotion and the prevention or rapid treatment of exacerbations of chronic conditions. Nursing, which has always encouraged patients to take control of health and wellness, has a prominent role in the current focus on management of chronic illness and disability (see Chapter 7).

Healthy People 2030

The *Healthy People* initiatives identify important periodic goals that, if reached, could have major impacts on the health and overall well-being of people in the United States (U.S. Department of Health and Human Services [HHS], 2020a). Since their inception over four decades ago, these initiatives have contributed to substantial decreases in cancer and cardiovascular deaths, infant and maternal mortality, and improvements in vaccinations (HHS, 2020a). Leading health indicators (LHIs) or goals outlined in the *Healthy People 2020* initiative aimed to improve access to health services, environmental quality, use of preventive services, nutrition and physical activity, and to address social determinants of health, while decreasing rates of injury and violence, obesity, tobacco use, and substance abuse, among others (HHS, 2020b). This initiative considered social influences that shape health, such as poverty and social injustices, rather than simply focusing on disease states. To date, significant progress has been made in decreasing the number of adults who are smoking and in improving physical activity of adults (HHS, 2020b). The *Healthy People 2030* framework, guided the development of the *Healthy People 2030* initiative and identified the need to collaborate more effectively with a variety of stakeholders across diverse agencies to accomplish its vision of helping all people in the United States optimize their health and well-being across developmental life stages, with a continued emphasis on reducing health disparities and improving health equity and health literacy (HHS, 2020a). The development of *Healthy People 2030* is in progress, data-driven national objectives have been established, and updates can be found by visiting its website. Enacting the goals set by the LHIs and other health care reforms have contributed to continuous change in health care organizations and delivery in the United States.

Advances in Technology and Genetics

Advances in technology and genetics have occurred rapidly during the past several decades. Sophisticated techniques and devices, such as robot assisted technology, have revolutionized treatments making it possible to perform many procedures and tests on an outpatient basis. Increased knowledge and understanding of genetics and genomics have resulted in expanded screening, diagnostic testing, and treatments for a variety of conditions (see Chapter 6 for information on genetics and genomics and nursing practice implications; in addition, note that there are charts that focus upon *Genetics in Nursing Practice* throughout the book, which highlight various relevant genetic disorders).

In January 2015, President Obama announced the launching of the *Precision Medicine Initiative (PMI)*, which aimed to leverage advances in research, technology, and policies to develop individualized plans of care to prevent and treat disease (Genetics Home Reference, 2020). **Precision medicine** is possible because of the recent development of biologic databases (e.g., human genome sequencing), technologic advances that can identify unique characteristics of individual people (e.g., genomics, cellular assay tests), and computer-driven systems that can mine and analyze data sets. The immediate goal of the PMI is to focus on preventing and curing cancers; however, there are long-term implications that hold promise for preventing and treating many other conditions and diseases (Ciupka, 2018).

Health Informatics

The sophisticated communication systems that connect most parts of the world, with the capability of rapid storage, retrieval, and dissemination of information, have stimulated advances in health information technology (HIT). Using HIT to improve the quality, efficiency, or delivery of health care is an interdisciplinary field of study called **health informatics**. Key examples of recent advances in HIT include artificial intelligence, blockchain, cloud technology, disease management technology, and improved operability of electronic health records (EHRs). The *Technology Informatics Guiding Education Reform (TIGER)* initiative, now a subsidiary of the Healthcare Information Management Systems Society (HIMSS), provides expert panel reports and guidelines for incorporating HIT into nursing practice (HIMSS, 2020).

The *International Classification of Diseases (ICD)* (WHO) launched its 10th iteration for use in the United States in 2015. The ICD-10 classifies diseases and conditions into nearly 70,000 codes. In June 2018, WHO released a version of ICD-11, which was presented to the World Health Assembly in 2019 for adoption by countries (WHO, 2018). Currently, the Centers for Medicare & Medicaid Services (CMS, 2015) and most other major health insurance programs require utilization of ICD-10 codes when treatment is rendered for providers to claim reimbursement. This system provides for common nomenclature and tracking of the incidence and prevalence of various diseases and conditions globally. CMS (2020) also requires that clinicians and health care systems use EHRs; its final rule for stage 3 of the *EHR Incentive Program*, now known as the *Promoting Interoperability Program*, required that by 2018 providers use EHRs or face reductions in reimbursement.

In addition to these HIT advancements, **telehealth**, which uses technology to deliver health care, health information, or health education at a distance, is being utilized by both individual clinicians and health care systems more and more frequently. In particular, home health services use telehealth to develop more individualized care plans for patients. One type of telehealth application uses *real-time communication*, characterized by an exchange of information between people at one point in time. For instance, a nurse practitioner in a rural clinic may consult with a specialist on a webcam about a patient's condition. Another type of telehealth application uses *store-and-forward*, characterized by transmission of digital images that may be retrieved and reviewed at later points in time (HealthIT.gov, 2018).

Quality, Safety, and Evidence-Based Practice

At the turn of the millennium, the Institute of Medicine (IOM, 2000) reported an alarming breakdown in quality control in the American health care system. The IOM report *To Err Is Human: Building a Safer Health System* (2000) noted that nearly 100,000 Americans died annually from preventable errors in hospitals, and many more suffered nonfatal injuries from errors. A subsequent IOM report, *Crossing the Quality Chasm: A New Health System for the 21st Century* (2001), described an inefficient, fragmented, health care system fraught with inequities and inaccessibility. It envisioned a reformed health care system that is evidence-based and systems oriented. Its proposed six aims for improvement included ensuring that patient care is safe, effective, patient centered, timely, efficient, and equitable (IOM, 2001). The following sections describe a series of key practices that are aimed at improving quality and safety and ensuring use of evidence-based practices (EBPs) within the U.S. health care system.

Principles of Evidence-Based Nursing Practice

An **evidence-based practice (EBP)** is a best practice derived from valid and reliable research studies that also considers the health care setting, patient preferences and values, and clinical judgment. The facilitation of EBP involves identifying and evaluating current literature and research findings, and then incorporating these findings into patient care as a means of ensuring quality care (Melnyk & Fineout-Overholt, 2018).

Evidence-Based Practice Bundles

The Institute for Healthcare Improvement (IHI) has developed numerous sets of readily implemented EBP sets for use by hospitals (IHI, 2020). These **bundles** include a set of three to five EBPs that, when implemented appropriately, can measurably improve patients' outcomes. Many of these practices are within the scope of independent nursing practice. For instance, the IHI Ventilator Bundle advocates that the head of the bed should be elevated, and that oral care should be provided using chlorhexidine for all patients on ventilators (IHI, 2012; see Chapter 19).

EBP tools used for planning patient care may include not only bundles but also clinical guidelines, algorithms, care mapping, multidisciplinary action plans (MAPs), and clinical pathways. These tools are used to move patients toward predetermined, measurable outcomes. Algorithms are used more often in acute situations to determine a particular treatment based on patient information or response. Care maps, clinical guidelines, and MAPs (the most detailed of these tools) help to facilitate coordination of care and education throughout hospitalization and after discharge. Nurses who provide direct care have an important role in the development and use of these tools through participation in researching the literature and then developing, piloting, implementing, and revising the tools as needed.

Quality and Safety Education for Nurses

The **Quality and Safety Education for Nurses (QSEN)** project was initially funded by the nonprofit Robert Wood Johnson Foundation (RWJF) to develop curricula that prepare future nurses with the knowledge, skills, and attitudes (KSA) required to continuously improve the quality and safety of the health care system. In particular, nurses educated under QSEN concepts demonstrate the KSA consonant with competency in patient-centered care, teamwork and collaboration, EBP, quality improvement, safety, and informatics (QSEN, 2020). Each of the Unit Openers in this book highlights a case study that demonstrates the application of QSEN competencies germane to prelicensure nursing practice. Table 1-1 highlights the QSEN definition of teamwork and collaboration and its associated KSA.

Interprofessional Collaborative Practice

The IOM report, *Health Professions Education: A Bridge to Quality* (IOM, 2003), challenged health professions education programs to integrate interdisciplinary core competencies into respective curricula to include patient-centered care, interdisciplinary teamwork and collaboration, EBP, quality improvement, safety, and informatics. In response to this report, the Interprofessional Education Collaborative Expert Panel (IPEC) published *Core Competencies for Interprofessional Collaborative Practice* (IPEC, 2011) with the goal to "prepare all health professions students for deliberately working together with the common goal of building a safer and better patient-centered and community/population-oriented US health care system" (p. 3). **Interprofessional collaborative practice** involves employing multiple health professionals to work together with patients, families, and communities to deliver best practices, thus assuring best patient outcomes. In 2016, the IPEC updated this document by organizing the four original competencies under the essential domain of interprofessional collaboration; topics within this central domain, as displayed in Figure 1-2, include values/ethics for

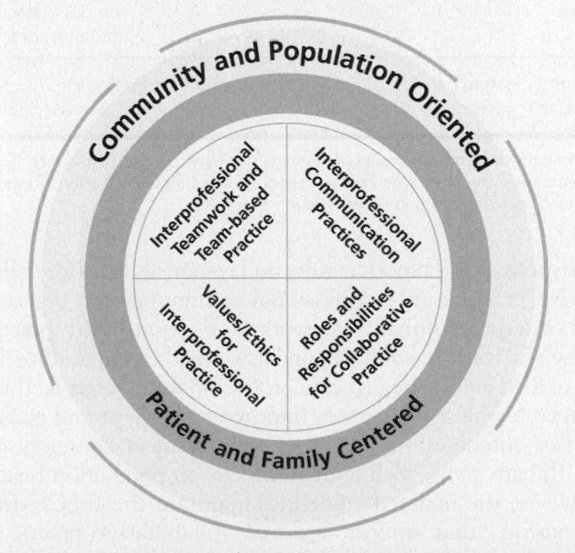

The Learning Continuum pre-licensure through practice trajectory

Figure 1-2 • Interprofessional Collaboration Competency Domain. Interprofessional Education Collaborative. (2016b). *Core competencies for interprofessional collaborative practice: 2016 update.* Washington, DC: Author. All rights reserved. Reproduced with permission.

TABLE 1-1	Quality and Safety Education for Nurses (QSEN) Definition of Safety and Knowledge, Skills, and Attitudes (KSA) for Pre-Licensure Nursing Students

Teamwork and Collaboration

Definition: Function effectively within nursing and inter-professional teams, fostering open communication, mutual respect, and shared decision making to achieve quality patient care.

Knowledge	Skills	Attitudes
Describe own strengths, limitations, and values in functioning as a member of a team	Demonstrate awareness of own strengths and limitations as a team member Initiate plan for self-development as a team member Act with integrity, consistency and respect for differing views	Acknowledge own potential to contribute to effective team functioning Appreciate importance of intra- and inter-professional collaboration
Describe scopes of practice and roles of health care team members Describe strategies for identifying and managing overlaps in team member roles and accountabilities Recognize contributions of other individuals and groups in helping patient/family achieve health goals	Function competently within own scope of practice as a member of the health care team Assume role of team member or leader based on the situation Initiate requests for help when appropriate to situation Clarify roles and accountabilities under conditions of potential overlap in team member functioning Integrate the contributions of others who play a role in helping patient/family achieve health goals	Value the perspectives and expertise of all health team members Respect the centrality of the patient/family as core members of any health care team Respect the unique attributes that members bring to a team, including variations in professional orientations and accountabilities
Analyze differences in communication style preferences among patients and families, nurses and other members of the health team Describe impact of own communication style on others Discuss effective strategies for communicating and resolving conflict	Communicate with team members, adapting own style of communicating to needs of the team and situation Demonstrate commitment to team goals Solicit input from other team members to improve individual, as well as team, performance Initiate actions to resolve conflict	Value teamwork and the relationships upon which it is based Value different styles of communication used by patients, families and health care providers Contribute to resolution of conflict and disagreement
Describe examples of the impact of team functioning on safety and quality of care Explain how authority gradients influence teamwork and patient safety	Follow communication practices that minimize risks associated with handoffs among providers and across transitions in care Assert own position/perspective in discussions about patient care Choose communication styles that diminish the risks associated with authority gradients among team members	Appreciate the risks associated with handoffs among providers and across transitions in care
Identify system barriers and facilitators of effective team functioning	Participate in designing systems that support effective teamwork	Value the influence of system solutions in achieving effective team functioning

Reprinted with permission from Cronenwett, L., Sherwood, G., Barnsteiner, J., et al. (2007). Quality and safety education for nurses. *Nursing Outlook, 55*(3), 122–131; QSEN Institute & Frances Payne Bolton School of Nursing, Case Western Reserve University (2020). Competencies: Prelicensure KSAs. Retrieved on 2/26/20 at: qsen.org/competencies/pre-licensure-ksas/#safety

interprofessional practice, roles and responsibilities for collaborative practice, interprofessional communication practices, and interprofessional teamwork and team-based practice (IPEC, 2016b). In addition, updates aimed to standardize language used among health care professionals to better facilitate interprofessional education, improve assessment and evaluation of outcomes, and more effectively meet contemporary health care goals, with a greater focus on population health. However, the updated guidelines maintain the IPEC's original vision "that interprofessional collaborative practice is key to the safe, high-quality, patient-centered care desired by all" (IPEC, 2016b, p. 4). Many of the end-of-chapter Critical Thinking Exercises that are presented throughout this book highlight the role of the nurse as a member of the interprofessional collaborative team.

The Practice of Nursing

As scientific advances in health care technology continue to evolve, nurses face increasingly complex issues and situations. Greater acuity of patients in both hospital and community settings, an aging population, complex disease processes, and end-of-life concerns, as well as ethical issues and cultural factors must be considered. The decision making component of nurses' problem-solving activities has become increasingly multifaceted and requires critical thinking based upon sound ethical principles.

Critical Thinking

Critical thinking is a cognitive process that utilizes thinking that is purposeful, insightful, reflective, and goal directed in order to develop conclusions, solutions, and alternatives that are appropriate for the given situation. Critical thinking, which includes reasoning and judgment, is based upon a body of knowledge and includes analysis of all information and ideas. Critical thinking leads to the formulation of conclusions and alternatives that are the most appropriate for the situation and is used to plan patient-centered care. Critical thinking has been identified as an essential core competency for nurses by the National League for Nursing (NLN) and the American Association of Colleges of Nursing (AACN, 2008; NLN, 2012). This cognitive process is critical to effective use of the nursing process and clinical reasoning (Flanders, Gunn, Wheeler, et al., 2017).

Critical thinking includes metacognition—the examination of one's own reasoning or thought processes—to help refine thinking skills. Independent nursing judgments and decisions evolve from a sound knowledge base and the ability to synthesize information within the context in which it is presented. Nursing practice in today's society requires the use of high-level critical thinking skills. Critical thinking enhances clinical decision making, helping to identify patient needs and the best nursing actions that will assist patients in meeting those needs. Because critical thinking is a deliberate, outcome-oriented activity, it is logical, organized, and iterative. "In nursing, critical thinking is the ability to think systematically and reflect on the reasoning process used to ensure safe nursing practice" (Zarifsanaiey, Amini, & Saadat, 2016, p. 2). The process of critical thinking gives nurses the tools to make sound decisions and implement quality nursing care.

Critical thinkers are inquisitive truth seekers who are open to the alternative solutions that might surface. Critical thinking is influenced by "habits of the mind including: confidence, perseverance, inquisitiveness, intuition, flexibility, creativity, intellectual integrity, contextual perspective, open-mindedness and reflection" (Griffits, Hines, Maloney, et al., 2017, p. 2832). Clinical reasoning is a thought process that is a specific method of critical thinking. The process of clinical reasoning results in clinical judgment, which is nursing actions. Clinical reasoning is the core of the nursing process (see later discussion) (Alfaro-LeFevre, 2017).

The following factors are identified as critical components of clinical reasoning: communication and relationships, educational level, knowledge and ability to use critical thinking, familiarity with the environment and the context of care, experience and exposure to a variety of situations, as well as professionalism (Griffits et al., 2017). The skills involved in critical thinking are developed over time through effort, practice, and experience.

Rationality and Insight

Skills needed in critical thinking include interpretation, analysis, inference, explanation, evaluation, self-reflection, and self-regulation. Critical thinking requires strong background knowledge and knowledge of key concepts as well as logical thinking. Nurses use this disciplined process to validate the accuracy of data and the reliability of any assumptions they have made, and they then carefully evaluate the effectiveness of what they have identified as the necessary

actions to take. Nurses also evaluate the reliability of sources, being mindful of and questioning inconsistencies. Nurses use interpretation to determine the significance of data that are gathered, analysis to identify patient problems suggested by the data, and inference to draw conclusions. Explanation is the justification of actions or interventions used to address patient problems and to help patients move toward desired outcomes. Evaluation is the process of determining whether outcomes have been or are being met. Self-regulation is the process of examining the care provided and adjusting the interventions as needed. All processes are iterative.

Critical thinking is also reflective, involving metacognition, active evaluation, and refinement of the thinking process. Metacognition involves reflective thinking as well as awareness of the nursing skills needed for patient-centered care (Alfaro-LeFevre, 2017). Nurses engaged in critical thinking consider the possibility of cultural differences and personal bias when interpreting data and determining appropriate actions (see Chapter 4 for further discussion). Critical thinkers must be insightful and have a sense of fairness and integrity; the courage to question personal ethics; and the perseverance to strive continuously to minimize the effects of egocentricity, ethnocentricity, and other biases on the decision making process (Alfaro-LeFevre, 2017).

Components of Critical Thinking

Certain cognitive or mental activities are key components of critical thinking as it relates to nurses. Critical thinkers (Alfaro-LeFevre, 2017):

- Identify the priorities that will determine the nurse's plan of patient-centered care.
- Gather pertinent data from the patient's chart and assessments to determine why certain developments have occurred and to determine if additional data are needed to address the situation accurately.
- Validate the information presented to make sure that it is accurate and compare it with any preexisting data. Information should be evidence based.
- Analyze the information to determine its significance and to identify the formation of clusters or patterns that point to certain conclusions.
- Utilize logical thinking, past clinical experiences, theoretical knowledge, and intuitive thinking to assess the status of the patient's condition. Anticipate the patient's needs and outcomes while acknowledging personal bias and cultural influences.
- Maintain a flexible attitude that facilitates thinking and inquiry and consider all possibilities.
- Utilize inductive and deductive reasoning to identify available options and analyze each in terms of its advantages and disadvantages.
- Formulate decisions that reflect creativity and independent decision making.
- Demonstrate personal humility in terms of one's knowledge deficits and willingly seek additional information to assist with decision making.
- Exhibit the courage to seek new, innovative approaches to patient-centered care. Detach their personal viewpoints

from situations and look at things objectively, a process called *bracketing*.

Critical thinking requires going beyond basic problem solving into a realm of inquisitive exploration, looking for all relevant factors that affect the issue, and being an "out-of-the-box" thinker. Nurses' ongoing quest for "best practice" clearly demonstrates intellectual integrity, a component of critical thinking.

Critical Thinking and Clinical Reasoning in Nursing Practice

Critical thinking and decision making are thought to be associated with improved clinical expertise. Critical thinking is the foundation of the process of clinical reasoning and clinical judgment (Alfaro-LeFevre, 2017). Using critical thinking to develop a plan of nursing care requires considering the human factors that might influence the plan. Nurses interact with patients, families, and other health care providers in the process of providing appropriate, individualized nursing care.

Nurses must use critical thinking skills in all practice settings—acute care, ambulatory care, extended care, and the home and community—and must view each patient situation as unique and dynamic. The unique factors that patients and nurses bring to the health care situation are considered, studied, analyzed, interpreted, and evaluated. Interpretation of the information then allows nurses to focus on those factors that are most relevant and most significant to the clinical situation. Decisions about a nursing plan, priority of actions, and measurable outcomes are developed into an action plan.

In decision making related to the nursing process, nurses use cognitive and metacognitive skills as well as logical reasoning to set priorities. These skills include systematic and comprehensive assessment, recognition of assumptions, inconsistencies and biases, verification of reliability and accuracy, identification of missing information, distinguishing relevant from irrelevant information, support of the evidence with facts and conclusions, priority setting with timely decision making, determination of patient-specific outcomes, and reassessment of responses and outcomes (Alfaro-LeFevre, 2017). All of these data are examined within the context of a solid knowledge base. For example, Goodrich, Wagner-Johnston, and Delibovi (2017) describe how oncology nurses use critical thinking, clinical reasoning, and decision making skills in identifying and managing complications of novel and complex therapies for cancer treatment when they:

- Develop greater knowledge of potential adverse events by examining evidence-based guidelines.
- Partner with the patient and family to better understand how treatments impact activities of daily living, quality of life, and overall symptom burden.
- Distinguish potential complications from expected manifestations associated with the underlying cancer diagnosis.
- Collaborate with interprofessional team members to modify treatment plans based on assessment data.

Because developing the skill of critical thinking involves experiential learning and practice, critical thinking exercises are offered at the end of each chapter as a means of honing the reader's ability to think critically. Some exercises include questions that stimulate the reader to seek information about EBP relative to the clinical situation described, others challenge the reader to identify priority assessments and interventions, while others challenge the reader to describe the role of the nurse as a member of the interprofessional collaborative team, as noted previously. Additional exercises may be found in the study guide that accompanies the text. The questions listed in Chart 1-1 can serve as a guide in working through the exercises. It is important to remember that each clinical situation is unique and calls for an individualized approach that fits its unique set of circumstances. As critical thinking may require consideration of ethical principles and cultural contexts, these concepts are discussed in this chapter and in Chapter 4.

The Nursing Process

The **nursing process** is a deliberate problem-solving approach for meeting people's health care and nursing needs. Although the steps of the nursing process have been stated in various ways by different writers, the common components cited are assessment, diagnosis, planning, implementation, and evaluation (Carpenito, 2017). The ANA's *Scope and Standards of Practice* (ANA, 2015b) includes an additional component entitled outcome identification, defined as identification of expected outcomes for a plan that is tailored to the patient's needs. The sequence of steps in this process is assessment, diagnosis, outcome identification, planning, implementation, and evaluation. For the purposes of this text, the nursing process is based on the traditional five steps and delineates two components in the diagnosis step: nursing diagnoses and collaborative problems. After the diagnoses or problems have been determined, the desired outcomes are often evident. The traditional steps are defined as follows:

1. *Assessment:* The systematic collection of data through interview, observation, and examination to determine the patient's health status as well as any actual or potential health problems. (Analysis of data is included as part of the assessment. Analysis may also be identified as a separate step of the nursing process.)
2. *Diagnosis:* Identification of the following two types of patient problems:
   - *Nursing diagnoses:* According to Carpenito (2017), "Are clinical judgments about individual, family, or community responses to actual or potential health problems/life processes" that can be managed by independent nursing interventions (p. 9).
   - *Collaborative problems:* According to Carpenito (2017), "Certain physiologic complications that nurses monitor to detect onset or changes in status. Nurses manage collaborative problems using physician- and nurse-prescribed interventions to minimize the complications of the events" (p. 9).
3. *Planning:* Development of measurable goals and outcomes as well as a plan of care designed to assist

Chart 1-1 The Inquiring Mind: Critical Thinking in Action

Throughout the critical thinking process, a continuous flow of questions evolves in the thinker's mind. It is not sufficient to rely solely on the acquisition of knowledge or a set of problem-solving skills; rather, it is the combination of one's application of knowledge, analysis of the situation, synthesis, and evaluation that promotes effective critical thinking inquiry. Although posing questions will vary according to the particular clinical situation, certain general inquiries can serve as a basis for reaching conclusions and determining a course of action.

When faced with a patient situation, seeking answers to some or all of the following questions may help to determine those actions that are most appropriate:

- What relevant assessment information do I need, and how do I interpret this information? What is the most effective way to gather this information? What does this information tell me? What contextual factors must be considered when gathering this information? What are the priority assessments?
- Have I identified the most important assessments and findings? Does the information I have gathered point to any other problems that I should consider?
- Have I gathered all of the necessary information (signs and symptoms, laboratory values, medication history, emotional factors, mental status)? Is anything missing?
- Is there anything that needs to be reported immediately? Do I need to seek additional assistance?

- What risks factors are specific to this patient? Which risk factors are of the highest priority? What must I do to minimize these risks?
- What possible complications must I anticipate?
- What are the most important problems in this situation? Do the patient and the patient's family recognize the same problems?
- What are the desired outcomes for this patient? Which have the highest priority? Do the patient and I agree on these points?
- What is going to be my first action in this situation? Why is this action a priority?
- How can I construct a plan of care to achieve the goals?
- Are there any age-related factors involved, and will they require some special approach? Will I need to make some change in the plan of care to take these factors into account?
- How do the family dynamics affect this situation, and will they affect my actions or the plan of care?
- Are there cultural factors that I must address and consider?
- Am I dealing with an ethical issue here? If so, how am I going to resolve it?
- Has any nursing research been conducted on this subject? What are the nursing implications of this research for care of this patient? What is the strength of the evidence found from research?

Adapted from Alfaro-LeFevre, R. (2017). *Critical thinking and clinical judgment: A practical approach* (6th ed.). Philadelphia, PA: Elsevier; Alfaro-LeFevre, R. (2019). Promoting critical thinking in frontline nurses. Retrieved on 2/29/2020 at: www.alfaroteachsmart.com

---

the patient in resolving the diagnosed problems and achieving the identified goals and desired outcomes.

4. *Implementation:* Actualization or carrying out of the plan of care through nursing interventions.
5. *Evaluation:* Determination of the patient's responses to the nursing interventions and the extent to which the outcomes have been achieved.

Dividing the nursing process into distinct steps serves to emphasize the essential nursing actions that must be taken to address the patient's nursing diagnoses and manage any collaborative problems or complications. However, dividing the process into separate steps is artificial: The process functions as an integrated whole, with the steps being interrelated, interdependent, and recurrent (Fig. 1-3). Chart 1-2 presents an overview of the nursing activities involved in applying the nursing process. Note that the use of the nursing process requires critical thinking and consideration of common ethical principles to ensure that a truly comprehensive plan of care is developed.

Assessment

According to Carpenito (2017), the initial or baseline assessment is a systematic process of collecting predetermined data during the first contact with the patient. Data are gathered through the health history and the physical assessment. In addition, ongoing assessment and monitoring are crucial to remain aware of changing patient needs and the effectiveness of nursing care.

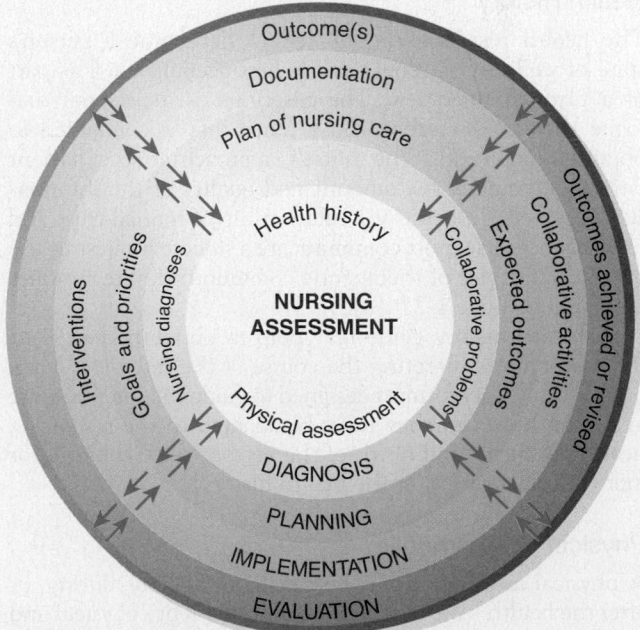

Figure 1-3 • The nursing process is depicted schematically in this circle. Starting from the innermost circle, nursing assessment, the process moves outward through the formulation of nursing diagnoses and collaborative problems; planning, with setting of goals and priorities in the nursing plan of care; implementation and documentation; and, finally, the ongoing process of evaluation and outcomes.

Chart 1-2 Steps of the Nursing Process

Assessment

1. Conduct the health history.
2. Perform the physical assessment.
3. Interview the patient's family or significant others.
4. Study the health record.
5. Organize, analyze, synthesize, and summarize the collected data.

Diagnosis

Nursing Diagnoses

1. Identify the patient's nursing problems or potential problems.
2. Identify the defining characteristics of the nursing problems.
3. Identify the etiology of the nursing problems.
4. State nursing diagnoses concisely and precisely.

Collaborative Problems

1. Identify potential problems or complications that require collaborative interventions.
2. Identify health care members with whom collaboration is essential.

Planning

1. Assign priority to the nursing diagnoses.
2. Specify the goals.
   a. Develop immediate, intermediate, and long-term goals.
   b. State the goals in realistic and measurable terms.
3. Identify nursing interventions appropriate for goal attainment.
4. Establish expected outcomes.
   a. Make sure that the outcomes are realistic and measurable.
   b. Identify critical times for the attainment of outcomes.

5. Develop the written plan of nursing care.
   a. Include nursing diagnoses, goals, nursing interventions, expected outcomes, and critical times.
   b. Write all entries precisely, concisely, and systematically.
   c. Keep the plan current and flexible to meet the patient's changing problems and needs.
6. Involve the patient, family or significant others, nursing team members, and other health care team members in all aspects of planning.

Implementation

Put the plan of nursing care into action.

1. Coordinate the activities of the patient, family or significant others, nursing team members, and other health care team members.
2. Record the patient's responses to the nursing actions.

Evaluation

1. Collect data.
2. Compare the patient's actual outcomes with the expected outcomes. Determine the extent to which the expected outcomes were achieved.
3. Include the patient, family or significant others, nursing team members, and other health care team members in the evaluation.
4. Identify alterations that need to be made in the nursing diagnoses, collaborative problems, goals, nursing interventions, and expected outcomes.
5. Continue all steps of the nursing process: assessment, diagnosis, planning, implementation, and evaluation.

Health History

The health history is conducted to determine a person's state of wellness or illness and is best accomplished as part of a planned interview. The interview is a personal dialogue between a patient and a nurse that is conducted to obtain information. The nurse's approach to the patient largely determines the amount and quality of the information received. To achieve a relationship of mutual trust and respect, the nurse must communicate a sincere interest in the patient. Examples of therapeutic communication techniques are found in Table 1-2.

A health history guide may help in obtaining pertinent information and directing the course of the interview. Various health history formats designed to guide the interview are available; however, they must be adapted to the responses, health problems, and needs of the person (see Chapter 4 for more information about the health history).

Physical Assessment

A physical assessment may be carried out before, during, or after the health history, depending on a patient's physical and emotional status and the immediate priorities of the situation. The purpose of the physical assessment is to identify those aspects of a patient's physical, psychological, and emotional state that indicate a need for nursing care. It requires the use of sight, hearing, touch, and smell as well as appropriate interview skills and techniques. Physical examination techniques, as well as techniques and strategies for assessing behaviors

and role changes, are presented in Chapter 4 and in the first chapter of each unit of this book, beginning with Unit 4 and continuing through Unit 15.

Other Components of the Assessment

Additional relevant information should be obtained from the patient's family or significant others, from other members of the health care team, and from the patient's EHR. Depending on the patient's immediate needs, this information may have been completed before the health history and the physical assessment were obtained. A review of a past medical history or records from previous admissions may provide important information for consideration. Whatever the sequence of events, the nurse should use all available sources of pertinent data to complete the nursing assessment.

Recording the Data

After the health history and physical assessment are completed, the information obtained is recorded in the patient's permanent record. These records are more commonly becoming electronic (i.e., EHRs). The ANA (2009) advocates that when EHRs are used, "patients should receive written, easily understood notification of how their health records are used and when their individually identifiable health information is disclosed to third parties" (p. 1). It is imperative that the patient's right to privacy and confidentiality are not violated through the use of EHRs. Regardless of whether the record is in a traditional paper format or an EHR, it must provide a

TABLE 1-2	Select Therapeutic Communication Techniques	
Technique	**Definition**	**Therapeutic Value**
Listening	Active process of receiving information and examining one's reactions to the messages received	Nonverbally communicates nurse's interest in the patient
Silence	Periods of no verbal communication among participants for therapeutic reasons	Gives patient time to think and gain insights, slows the pace of the interaction, and encourages the patient to initiate conversation while conveying the nurse's support, understanding, and acceptance
Restating	Repeating to the patient what the nurse believes is the main thought or idea expressed	Demonstrates that the nurse is listening and validates, reinforces, or calls attention to something important that has been said
Reflection	Directing back to the patient their feelings, ideas, questions, or content	Validates the nurse's understanding of what the patient is saying and signifies empathy, interest, and respect for the patient
Clarification	Asking the patient to explain what they mean or attempting to verbalize vague ideas or unclear thoughts of the patient to enhance the nurse's understanding	Helps to clarify the patient's feelings, ideas, and perceptions and to provide an explicit correlation between them and the patient's actions
Focusing	Questions or statements to help the patient develop, explore, or expand an idea or verbalize feelings	Allows the patient to discuss central issues and keeps communication goal directed
Broad openings	Encouraging the patient to select topics for discussion	Indicates acceptance by the nurse and the value of the patient's initiative
Humor	Discharge of energy through the comic enjoyment of the imperfect	Promotes insight by bringing repressed material to consciousness, resolving paradoxes, tempering aggression, and revealing new options; a socially acceptable form of sublimation
Informing	Providing information	Helpful in health teaching or patient education about relevant aspects of the patient's well-being and self-care
Sharing perceptions	Asking the patient to verify the nurse's understanding of what the patient is thinking or feeling	Conveys the nurse's understanding to the patient and has the potential to clarify confusing communication; may promote additional reflection
Theme identification	Underlying issues or problems experienced by the patient that emerge repeatedly during the course of the nurse–patient relationship	Allows the nurse to best promote the patient's exploration and understanding of important problems
Suggesting	Presentation of alternative ideas for the patient's consideration relative to problem solving	Increases the patient's perceived options or choices

Adapted from Stuart, G. W. (2012). *Principles and practice of psychiatric nursing* (10th ed.). St. Louis, MO: CV Mosby.

means of communication among members of the health care team and facilitate coordinated planning and continuity of care (Räsänen & Günther, 2019). The record fulfills other functions as well:

- Serves as the legal and business record for a health care agency and for the professional staff members who are responsible for the patient's care. Various systems are used for documenting patient care, and each health care agency selects the system that best meets its needs.
- Serves as a basis for evaluating the quality and appropriateness of care and for reviewing the effective use of patient care services.
- Provides data that are useful in research, education, and short- and long-range planning.

Diagnosis

The assessment component of the nursing process serves as the basis for identifying nursing diagnoses and collaborative problems. Soon after the completion of the health history and the physical assessment, nurses organize, analyze, synthesize, and summarize the data collected and determine the patient's need for nursing care.

Nursing Diagnoses

Nursing diagnoses, the first taxonomy created in nursing, have fostered autonomy and accountability in nursing and have helped to delineate the scope of practice. Many state nurse practice acts include nursing diagnosis as a nursing function, and nursing diagnosis is included in the ANA's *Scope and Standards of Practice* (2015b) and the standards of nursing specialty organizations. Nursing diagnoses are routinely validated, refined, and updated to reflect current clinical practice and research.

NANDA International (NANDA-I; formerly known as the North American Nursing Diagnosis Association) was the first official organization responsible for developing the taxonomy of nursing diagnoses. In 2000, the International Classification for Nursing Practice (ICNP®) was established as an alternative system to support nursing care and standardization in documentation for practicing nurses at the point of care and across specialties (Coenen, 2003; International Council of Nurses [ICN], 2019). ICNP offers nursing diagnoses, intervention statements, and outcome statements designed to assist nurses within each step of the nursing process and all phases of care and was most recently updated in 2019. The nursing diagnoses used throughout this book are ICNP diagnoses. Because ICNP is proprietary to ICN, which has a global health focus, ICNP terms are spelled using the British method.

Choosing a Nursing Diagnosis

When identifying a nursing diagnosis for a particular patient, nurses must first identify the commonalities among the assessment data collected. These common features lead to the categorization of related data that reveal the existence of a problem and the need for nursing intervention. The identified problems are then defined as specific nursing diagnoses. Nursing diagnoses represent actual or potential health problems, state of health promotion, or potential risks that can be managed by independent nursing actions.

It is important to remember that nursing diagnoses are not medical diagnoses; they are not medical treatments prescribed by the primary provider, and they are not diagnostic studies. Rather, they are succinct statements of specific patient problems that guide nurses in the development of the plan of nursing care.

To give additional meaning to the nursing diagnosis, the characteristics and etiology of the problem are identified and included as part of the diagnosis. For example, the nursing diagnoses and their defining characteristics and etiology for a patient who has anemia may include the following:

- Activity intolerance associated with imbalance between supply and demand of oxygen
- Impaired peripheral tissue perfusion associated with decreased hemoglobin
- Impaired nutritional status associated with fatigue and inadequate intake of essential nutrients

Collaborative Problems

In addition to nursing diagnoses and their related nursing interventions, nursing practice involves certain situations and interventions that do not fall within the definition of nursing diagnoses. These activities pertain to potential problems or complications that are medical in origin and require collaborative interventions with the primary provider and other members of the health care team. The term *collaborative problem* is used to identify these situations.

Collaborative problems are certain physiologic complications that nurses monitor to detect changes in the status or onset of complications. Nurses manage collaborative problems using primary provider- and nurse-prescribed interventions to minimize complications (Carpenito, 2017). When treating collaborative problems, the primary nursing focus is monitoring patients for the onset of complications or changes in the status of existing complications. The complications are usually related to the disease process, treatments, medications, or diagnostic studies. The nurse recommends nursing interventions that are appropriate for managing the complications and implements the treatments prescribed by the

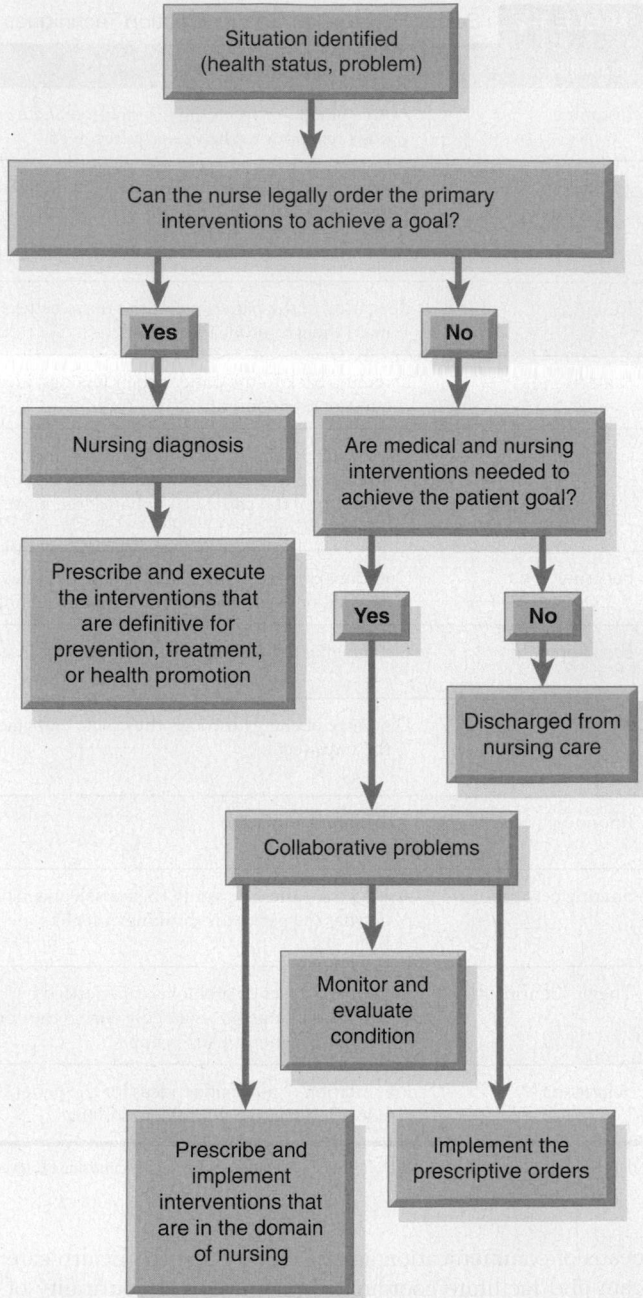

Figure 1-4 • Differentiating nursing diagnoses and collaborative problems. Redrawn with permission from Carpenito, L. J. (2017). *Nursing diagnosis: Application to clinical practice* (15th ed., p. 25). Philadelphia, PA: Lippincott Williams & Wilkins.

patient's primary provider. According to Carpenito (2017), collaborative problems do not have patient goals; therefore, the approach to evaluation is different from a nursing diagnosis. The algorithm in Figure 1-4 depicts the differences between nursing diagnoses and collaborative problems. After the nursing diagnoses and collaborative problems have been identified, they are recorded on the plan of nursing care.

Planning

Once the nursing diagnoses have been identified, the planning component of the nursing process begins. This phase involves the following steps:

1. Assigning priorities to the nursing diagnoses and collaborative problems
2. Specifying realistic and measurable expected outcomes
3. Specifying the immediate, intermediate, and long-term goals of nursing action
4. Identifying specific nursing interventions appropriate for attaining the outcomes
5. Identifying interdependent interventions
6. Documenting the nursing diagnoses, collaborative problems, expected outcomes, nursing goals, and nursing interventions on the plan of nursing care
7. Communicating to appropriate personnel any assessment data that point to health care needs that can best be met by other members of the health care team

Setting Priorities

Assigning priorities to the nursing diagnoses and collaborative problems is a joint effort by the nurse and the patient or family members. Any disagreement about priorities is resolved in a way that is mutually acceptable. Consideration must be given to the urgency of the problems, with the most critical problems receiving the highest priority. Maslow Hierarchy of Needs provides one framework to prioritize problems (see previous discussion).

Establishing Expected Outcomes

Expected outcomes of the nursing interventions, identified either as long term or short term, are written in terms of the patient's behaviors and the time period in which the outcomes are to be met. The outcomes must be attainable and quantifiable (Carpenito, 2017). Resources for identifying appropriate expected outcomes include the ICNP and the standard outcome criteria developed by the Nursing Outcomes Classification (NOC) (Moorhead, Swanson, Johnson, et al., 2018) (Chart 1-3) and by health care agencies for people with specific health problems. These outcomes can be associated with nursing diagnoses and interventions and can be used when appropriate. However, the NOC may need to be adapted to establish realistic criteria for the specific patient involved.

The expected outcomes that define the patient's desired behavior are used to measure the progress made toward resolving the problem. The expected outcomes also serve as the basis for evaluating the effectiveness of the nursing interventions and for deciding whether additional nursing care is needed or whether the plan of care needs to be revised.

Establishing Goals

After the priorities of the nursing diagnoses and expected outcomes have been established, goals (immediate, intermediate, and long term) and the nursing actions appropriate for attaining the goals are identified. The patient and family are included in establishing goals for the nursing actions. Immediate goals are those that can be attained within a short time frame. Intermediate and long-term goals require a longer time frame to be achieved and usually involve preventing complications and other health problems and promoting self-care and rehabilitation. For example, goals for a patient with a nursing diagnosis of impaired mobility associated with pain and edema following total knee replacement may be stated as follows:

- Immediate goal: Stands at bedside for 5 minutes 6 to 12 hours after surgery
- Intermediate goal: Ambulates 15 to 20 minutes with walker or crutches in hospital and home
- Long-term goal: Ambulates independently 1 to 2 miles each day

Determining Nursing Actions

In planning appropriate nursing actions to achieve the desired goals and outcomes, the nurse, with input from the patient and significant others, identifies individualized interventions based on the patient's circumstances and preferences that address each outcome. Interventions should identify the activities needed, who will implement them, as well as the frequency. Determination of interdisciplinary activities is made in collaboration with other health care providers as needed. The patient's medications and other prescribed treatments should be integrated into the plan of care to assist the nurse in determining how all interventions contribute to resolution of the identified problems.

The nurse identifies and plans patient education as needed to assist the patient in learning certain self-care activities. Planned interventions should be ethical and appropriate to the patient's culture, age, developmental level, and gender. Standardized interventions, such as those found on standardized care plans, the ICNP, or in the Nursing Interventions Classification (NIC) (Butcher, Bulechek, Dochterman, et al., 2018) can be used. Chart 1-4 describes the NIC system and provides an example of an NIC system intervention. It is important to individualize prewritten interventions to promote optimal effectiveness for each patient. Actions of nurses should be based on established standards.

Implementation

The implementation phase of the nursing process involves carrying out the proposed plan of nursing care. The nurse assumes responsibility for implementation and coordinates the activities of all those involved in implementation, including the patient and family, and other members of the health care team so that the schedule of activities facilitates the patient's recovery. The plan of nursing care serves as the basis for implementation as such:

- The immediate, intermediate, and long-term goals are used as a focus for the implementation of the designated nursing interventions.
- While implementing nursing care, the nurse continually assesses the patient and the patient's individual response to the nursing care.
- Revisions are made in the plan of care as the patient's condition, problems, and responses change and when reordering of priorities is required.

Implementation includes direct or indirect execution of the planned interventions. It is focused on resolving the patient's nursing diagnoses and collaborative problems and achieving expected outcomes, thus meeting the patient's health needs. The following are examples of nursing interventions:

- Supervise the patient performing active range-of-motion exercises three times a day.

Chart 1-3 Nursing Outcomes Classification

The Nursing Outcomes Classification (NOC) is a classification of patient outcomes that are sensitive to nursing interventions. Each outcome is a neutral statement about a variable patient condition, behavior, or perception, coupled with a rating scale. The outcome statement and scale can be used to identify baseline functioning, expected outcomes, and actual outcomes for individual patients. The following table is an example of a nursing-sensitive outcome.

Cardiac Pump Effectiveness (0400)

Definition: Adequacy of blood volume ejected from the left ventricle to support systemic perfusion pressure.

Outcome Target Rating   *Maintain at* _____   *Increase to* _____

Cardiac Pump Effectiveness Overall Rating		Severe Deviation From Normal Range 1	Substantial Deviation From Normal Range 2	Moderate Deviation From Normal Range 3	Mild Deviation From Normal Range 4	No Deviation From Normal Range 5	
Indicators							
040001	Systolic blood pressure	1	2	3	4	5	NA
040019	Diastolic blood pressure	1	2	3	4	5	NA
040002	Apical heart rate	1	2	3	4	5	NA
040003	Cardiac index	1	2	3	4	5	NA
040004	Ejection fraction	1	2	3	4	5	NA
040006	Peripheral pulses	1	2	3	4	5	NA
040007	Heart size	1	2	3	4	5	NA
040020	Urine output	1	2	3	4	5	NA
040022	24-hour intake and output balance	1	2	3	4	5	NA
040025	Central venous pressure	1	2	3	4	5	NA
		Severe	**Substantial**	**Moderate**	**Mild**	**None**	
040009	Neck vein distention	1	2	3	4	5	NA
040010	Dysrhythmia	1	2	3	4	5	NA
040011	Abnormal heart sounds	1	2	3	4	5	NA
040012	Angina	1	2	3	4	5	NA
040013	Peripheral edema	1	2	3	4	5	NA
040014	Pulmonary edema	1	2	3	4	5	NA
040015	Diaphoresis	1	2	3	4	5	NA
040016	Nausea	1	2	3	4	5	NA
040017	Fatigue	1	2	3	4	5	NA
040023	Dyspnea at rest	1	2	3	4	5	NA
040026	Dyspnea with mild exertion	1	2	3	4	5	NA
040024	Weight gain	1	2	3	4	5	NA
040027	Ascites	1	2	3	4	5	NA
040028	Hepatomegaly	1	2	3	4	5	NA
040029	Impaired cognition	1	2	3	4	5	NA
040030	Activity intolerance	1	2	3	4	5	NA
040031	Pallor	1	2	3	4	5	NA
040032	Cyanosis	1	2	3	4	5	NA
040033	Flushed	1	2	3	4	5	NA

Used with permission from Moorhead, S., Swanson, E., Johnson, M., et al. (Eds.). (2018). *Nursing outcomes classification (NOC)* (6th ed.). St. Louis, MO: Mosby-Elsevier.

- Teach the patient who is postoperative to use an incentive spirometer 10 times every hour while awake.
- Monitor the patient for adverse effects of opioid analgesic medications, including sedation and respiratory depression.
- Assist the patient in developing a plan to reduce dietary sodium and increase daily activity.
- Administer sublingual nitroglycerin as prescribed to the patient who complains of angina.
- Assess electrolyte levels prior to administering scheduled intravenous diuretics.

<table>
<tr><td colspan="2">

Chart 1-4   Nursing Interventions Classification

</td></tr>
</table>

The Nursing Interventions Classification (NIC) is an in-depth, evidence-based taxonomy of interventions that includes independent and collaborative interventions. These interventions are performed in a variety of health care settings. Intervention labels are terms such as *bleeding precautions, medication administration,* or *pain management: acute.* Listed under each intervention are multiple discrete nursing actions that together constitute a comprehensive approach to the treatment of a particular condition. Not all actions are applicable to every patient; nursing judgment and critical thinking will determine which actions to implement. The following is an example of a nursing intervention:

Fluid Resuscitation

Definition

Administering prescribed intravenous (IV) fluids rapidly

Activities

Obtain and maintain a large-bore IV.
Collaborate with primary providers to ensure administration of both crystalloids (e.g., normal saline and lactated Ringer's) and colloids (e.g., Hesban, and Plasmanate), as appropriate.
Administer IV fluids, as prescribed.
Obtain blood specimens for crossmatching, as appropriate.
Administer blood products, as prescribed.
Monitor hemodynamic response.
Monitor oxygen status.
Monitor for fluid overload.
Monitor output of various body fluids (e.g., urine, nasogastric drainage, and chest tube).
Monitor BUN, creatinine, total protein, and albumin levels.
Monitor for pulmonary edema and third spacing.

Used with permission from Butcher, H. K., Bulecheck, G. M., Dochterman, J. M., et al. (Eds.). (2018). *Nursing interventions classification (NIC)* (7th ed.). St. Louis, MO: Elsevier.

- Check gastric residuals in the patient receiving tube feedings before each feeding.

Clinical judgment, critical thinking, and good decision-making skills are essential in the selection of appropriate evidence-based and ethical nursing interventions. All nursing interventions are patient centered and outcome directed and are implemented with compassion, skill, confidence, and a willingness to accept and understand the patient's responses.

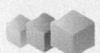 *Concept Mastery Alert*

Implementation is nursing action. Therefore, statements involving implementation always start with a verb.

Although many nursing actions are independent, others are interdependent, such as carrying out prescribed treatments, administering medications and therapies, and collaborating with other health care team members to accomplish specific expected outcomes and to monitor and manage potential complications. Such interdependent functioning is just that—interdependent. Requests or prescriptions from other health care team members should

not be followed blindly but must be assessed critically and questioned when necessary. The implementation phase of the nursing process ends when the nursing interventions have been completed.

Evaluation

Evaluation, the final step of the nursing process, allows the nurse to determine the patient's response to the nursing interventions and the extent to which the objectives have been achieved. The plan of nursing care is the basis for evaluation. The nursing diagnoses, collaborative problems, priorities, nursing interventions, and expected outcomes provide the specific guidelines that dictate the focus of the evaluation. Through evaluation, the nurse can answer the following questions:

- Were the nursing diagnoses and collaborative problems accurate?
- Did the patient achieve the expected outcomes within the critical time periods?
- Have the patient's nursing diagnoses been resolved?
- Have the collaborative problems been resolved?
- Do priorities need to be reordered?
- Have the patient's nursing needs been met?
- Should the nursing interventions be continued, revised, or discontinued?
- Have new problems evolved for which nursing interventions have not been planned or implemented?
- What factors influenced the achievement or lack of achievement of the objectives?
- Should changes be made to the expected outcomes and outcome criteria?

Objective data that provide answers to these questions are collected from all available sources (e.g., patients, families, significant others, health care team members). These data are included in patients' records and must be substantiated by direct patient observation before the outcomes are documented.

Documentation of Outcomes and Revision of the Plan

Outcomes are documented concisely and objectively. Documentation should relate outcomes to the nursing diagnoses and collaborative problems, describe the patient's responses to the interventions, indicate whether the outcomes were met, and include any additional pertinent data. As noted previously, the nurse individualizes a plan of care for each patient's particular circumstances. Chart 1-5 gives an example of a plan of nursing care that has been developed for a 22-year-old woman admitted to a postoperative surgical unit after having an emergent laparoscopic appendectomy.

The plan of care is subject to change as a patient's needs change, as the priorities of needs shift, as needs are resolved, and as additional information about a patient's state of health is collected. As the nursing interventions are implemented, the patient's responses are evaluated and documented, and the plan of care is revised accordingly. A well-developed, continuously updated plan of care is the greatest assurance that the patient's nursing diagnoses, and collaborative problems are addressed, and their basic needs are met.

(text continued on page 23)

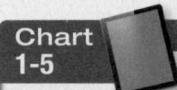

Chart 1-5 | PLAN OF NURSING CARE

Example of a Plan of Nursing Care for a Patient Post Laparoscopic Appendectomy

NURSING DIAGNOSIS: Acute pain
GOAL: Relief of pain and discomfort

Nursing Interventions	Rationale	Expected Outcomes
1. When taking vital signs, use pain scale to assess pain and discomfort characteristics: location, quality, frequency, durations, etc., at baseline and on an ongoing basis.	1. Provides baseline data.	• Reports decreased level of pain and discomfort on pain scale. • Reports less disruption in activity and quality of life from pain and discomfort. • Reports decrease in other symptoms and psychosocial distress.
2. Assure the patient that you know that pain is real and will assist in reducing it.	2. Fear that pain will not be considered real increases anxiety and reduces pain tolerance.	• Adheres to analgesic regimen as prescribed. • Barriers to adequately addressing pain do not interfere with strategies for managing pain.
3. Assess other factors contributing to patient's pain: fear; fatigue; other symptoms; psychosocial and/or spiritual distress, etc.	3. Provides data about factors that decrease patient's ability to tolerate pain and increase pain level.	• Takes an active role in administration of analgesia. • Identifies additional effective pain relief strategies.
4. Administer prescribed analgesic regimen, and provide education to patient and family regarding regimen.	4. Analgesics tend to be more effective when given early in pain cycle, around the clock at regular intervals, or when given in long-acting forms; breaks the pain cycle; premedication with analgesics is used for activities that cause increased pain or breakthrough pain.	• Uses previously employed successful pain relief strategies appropriately. • Reports effective use of nonpharmacologic pain relief strategies and a decrease in pain. • Reports that decreased level of pain permits early ambulation postoperatively.
5. Address myths or misconceptions and lack of knowledge about use of opioid analgesics.	5. Barriers to adequate pain management involve patients' fear of side effects, fatalism about the possibility of achieving pain control, fear of distracting providers from treating the postoperative pain, belief that pain is indicative of progressive disease, and fears about addiction. Professional health providers also have demonstrated limited knowledge about pain management, potential analgesic side effects, and management and risk of addiction.	
6. Collaborate with patient, primary provider/surgeon, and other health care team members when changes in pain management are necessary.	6. New methods of administering analgesia must be acceptable to the patient, primary provider/surgeon, and health care team to be effective; patient's participation decreases sense of powerlessness.	
7. Encourage strategies of pain relief that patient has used successfully in previous pain experience.	7. Encourages success of pain relief strategies accepted by patient and family.	
8. Offer nonpharmacologic strategies to relieve pain and discomfort: distraction, guided imagery, relaxation, cutaneous stimulation, therapeutic touch, Reiki, etc.	8. Increases options and strategies available to patient that serve as adjuncts to pharmacologic interventions.	

NURSING DIAGNOSIS: Risk for infection (i.e., wound infection, pneumonia, urinary tract infection [UTI])
GOAL: No evidence of infection

Nursing Interventions	Rationale	Expected Outcomes
1. Assess wound site for signs of infection or increased inflammation:	1. Some manifestations of inflammation are to be expected (e.g., wound tenderness, slight erythema, and edema); however, this should decrease over time and there should be no evidence of an infection at the wound site.	• No drainage, increased erythema, or edema at the laparoscopic wound site. • Temperature within normal limits (i.e., between 36.1°C [97°F] and 38.0°C [100.4°F]). • Lung sounds clear to auscultation; no cough. • Voids clear yellow urine without complaints of burning on micturition or feelings of bladder fullness. • Laboratory results, if assessed, are within normal limits.
a. If there is a dressing or bandage present, verify whether and when it will be changed by the primary provider/surgeon.	a. The primary provider/surgeon may wish to remove the first dressing or bandage, to assess the status of the wound and presence of drainage firsthand.	

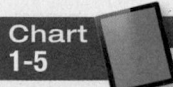

Chart 1-5   **PLAN OF NURSING CARE** (continued)

Example of a Plan of Nursing Care for a Patient Post Laparoscopic Appendectomy

Nursing Interventions	Rationale	Expected Outcomes
b. Note the color, consistency, and amount of drainage, if present; if so, also note if any odor is present; notify the primary provider/surgeon as indicated.	**b.** Drainage may indicate an infectious process, particularly if it is malodorous.	
c. Note any changes in appearance of wound over time, particularly if it becomes increasingly edematous or erythematous.	**c.** Increased wound edema or erythema may indicate an infection.	
2. Monitor vital signs, temperature, and laboratory results (if available) for signs of infection.	**2.** Changes in vital signs, particularly temperature, may suggest an infection; if these changes are marked, they may suggest sepsis (see Chapter 11 for further discussion of the clinical manifestations of sepsis); laboratory results, particularly the presence of leukocytosis with a shift to the left on the differential of the white blood cell count (WBC) on the complete blood count (CBC), may suggest an infection is present. Postoperatively, most patients will have a slightly elevated temperature (up to 38.0°C [100.4°F]), which is consistent with the inflammatory process. A temperature higher than this in a previously healthy adult suggests some type of underlying infectious process.	
3. Monitor for manifestations of atelectasis or pneumonia.	**3.** Atelectasis and pneumonia are prevalent postoperative pulmonary complications (see Chapter 16, Table 16-4).	
a. Assess for adventitious lung sounds (e.g., rales, wheezes) or for decreased air movement.	**a.** Lung sounds should be clear to auscultation bilaterally; the presence of adventitious sounds may suggest the development of atelectasis or pneumonia; diminished lung sounds may suggest poor air movement from splinting respirations, which can lead to respiratory compromise.	
b. Encourage early movement (e.g., demonstrate and encourage use of incentive spirometer, encourage early ambulation).	**b.** Movement mobilizes respiratory secretions and respiratory effort.	
c. Preemptively treat postoperative pain, as described above.	**c.** Pain interferes with the ability to move; pain results in splinting of respiratory effort.	
4. Monitor micturition status; note when patient first voids, the amount, and if there are any complaints of burning or bladder fullness; notify the primary provider/surgeon as indicated; monitor laboratory results, including the CBC and urinalysis as indicated.	**4.** Urinary retention and urinary tract infections are prevalent postoperative complications (see Chapter 16, Table 16-4); CBC results may reveal leukocytosis with a shift to the left on the WBC differential; urinalysis results may reveal the presence of blood cells (e.g., red blood cells [RBCs], WBCs) that may suggest a urinary tract infection.	

(continued on page 22)

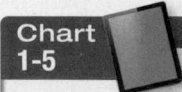

Chart 1-5

PLAN OF NURSING CARE (continued)
Example of a Plan of Nursing Care for a Patient Post Laparoscopic Appendectomy

NURSING DIAGNOSIS: Impaired nutritional status associated with perioperative *nil per os* (NPO) status
GOAL: Will consume typical diet by discharge

Nursing Interventions	Rationale	Expected Outcomes

1. Assess for return of gastrointestinal function postoperatively.
  a. Auscultate for the presence of bowel sounds.
  b. Ask the patient if they have passed flatus.
  c. Encourage early ambulation as this will assist with return of gastrointestinal function.
2. Advance diet as tolerated and prescribed by primary provider/surgeon.
 	
  a. Assess for complaints of nausea. If present, may give antiemetic medications as prescribed (e.g., ondansetron) and delay advancement of diet.
	1. Gastrointestinal motility is diminished post surgery; peristalsis should return within hours and is evidenced by return of bowel sounds and passing of flatus.
	
	2. Patient will need to demonstrate ability to tolerate fluids and food prior to discharge.
	  a. Complaints of nausea are prevalent post laparoscopic surgery; if patient vomits, that may delay recovery (e.g., disrupt wound, delay intake of nutrients); administering antiemetic medications may preempt complications.
		• Will advance diet, as tolerated.
		• No complaints of nausea.

NURSING DIAGNOSIS: Activity intolerance associated with fatigue post surgery
GOAL: Participation in activities of daily living within tolerance

Nursing Interventions	Rationale	Expected Outcomes

1. Assess factors contributing to activity intolerance and fatigue.
2. Promote atmosphere conducive to physical and mental rest:
  a. Encourage alternation of rest and activity.
  b. Encourage limitation of visitors and stress-producing interactions.
	1. Indicates factors contributing to severity of fatigue
	2. Promotes rest, activity tolerance, and decreased overall stress
		• Identifies factors contributing to fatigue
		• Alternates periods of rest and activity
		• Limits visitors to ensure adequate rest periods

NURSING DIAGNOSIS: Lack of knowledge regarding methods to ensure postoperative recovery
GOAL: Increased knowledge about expected postoperative recovery and transition back to preoperative baseline functional status

Nursing Interventions	Rationale	Expected Outcomes

1. Educate patient on expectations for recovery, discharge, and transition to home.
  a. Demonstrate wound care to patient, as prescribed by primary provider/surgeon; ask patient to return demonstrate wound care.
  b. Educate patient on use of prescribed analgesic medications (e.g., oxycodone), including actions, indications, side effects, and when to take them (e.g., prior to ambulation).
  c. Educate patient on activity restrictions (e.g., bathing, lifting, return to work or school) as prescribed by primary provider/surgeon.
  d. Educate patient on when to follow up with primary provider/surgeon postoperatively, for scheduled postoperative appointment and as needed.
	1. Inpatient recovery time after a laparoscopic appendectomy is short (e.g., 1 day, assuming there are no complications [see Chapter 16, Table 16-4]); therefore, preparing patient for discharge must commence expeditiously.	• Demonstrates appropriate care of wound.
		• Verbalizes understanding of continued analgesic regimen, including when to take prescriptive analgesic medications (e.g., oxycodone), and whether there are any activity restrictions associated with their use (e.g., no driving).
		• Verbalizes understanding of activity restrictions, including bathing, lifting, return to work/school, as prescribed by primary provider/surgeon.
		• Verbalizes adherence to scheduled postoperative appointment.

Frameworks for a Common Approach to Nursing

Various frameworks or taxonomies can be used for determining nursing diagnoses, establishing outcomes, designing interventions, and guiding clinical decision making. Ultimately, a framework that uses a language common to all aspects of nursing, regardless of the classification system, is desirable. In 2001, a taxonomy of nursing practice was developed for the harmonization of NANDA-I, NIC, and NOC. This three-part combination links nursing diagnoses, accompanying interventions, and outcomes, organizing them in the same way. Similarly, the ICNP has developed catalogues that align nursing diagnoses, outcome statements, and intervention statements. Such organization of concepts in a common language or taxonomy may facilitate the process of clinical judgment and critical thinking, because interventions and outcomes are more accurately matched with appropriately developed nursing diagnoses (Carpenito, 2017). More recently, the National Council of State Boards of Nursing (NCSBN®) developed the NCSBN Clinical Judgment Measurement Model, which offers a framework to measure clinical decision making and clinical judgment in the context of the National Council Licensure Examination (NCLEX-RN® examination; see Chart 1-6). Figure 1-5 illustrates the application of this model to the nursing process.

Ethical Nursing Care

In the complex health care world, nurses are faced with numerous ethical issues. Consequently, there has been a heightened interest in the field of ethics in an attempt to gain

---

Chart 1-6 The NCSBN Clinical Judgment Measurement Model

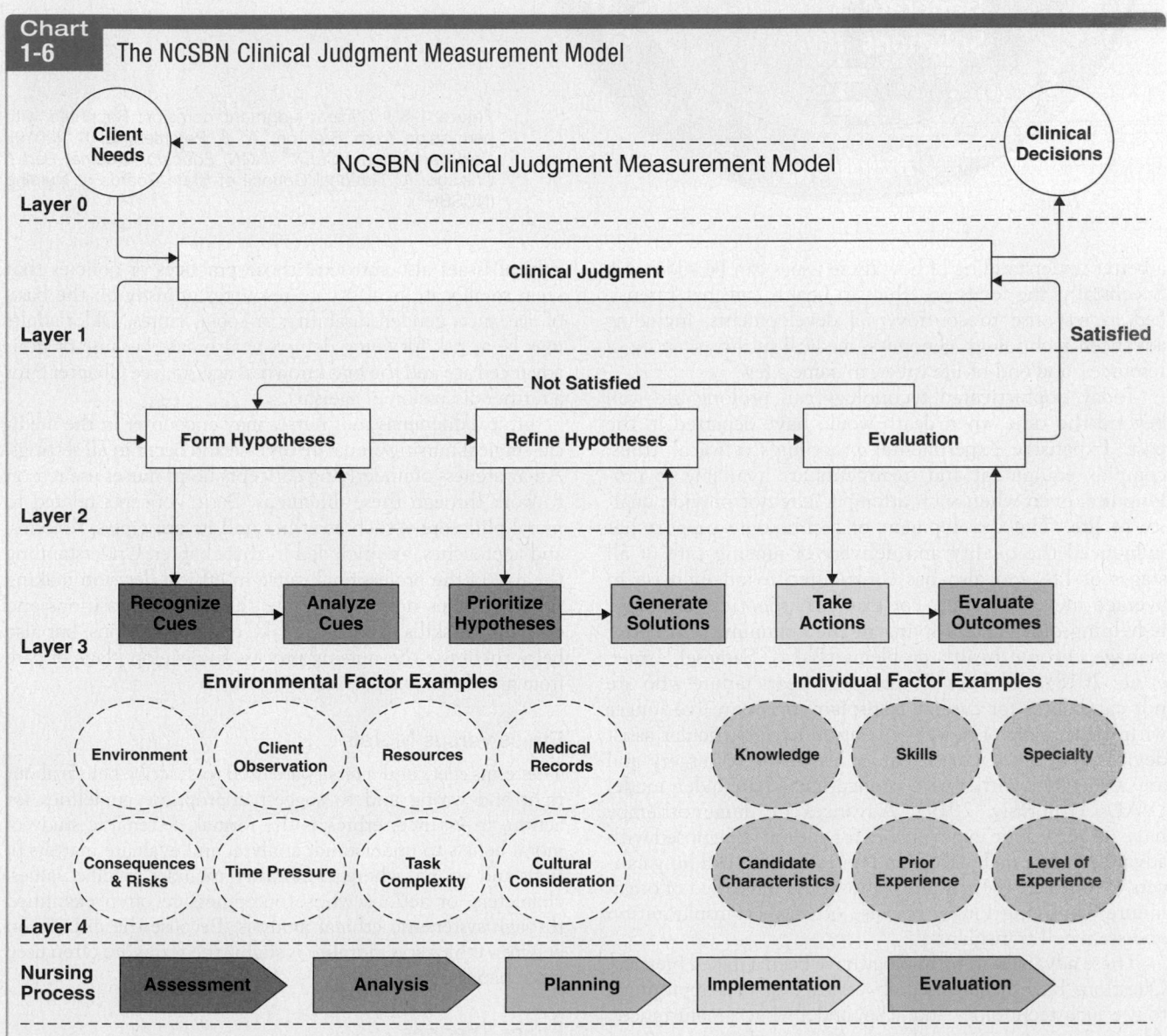

Reprinted with permission from the National Council of State Boards of Nursing (NCSBN®). (2021). NCSBN clinical judgment measurement model. Retrieved on 3/22/2021 at: www.ncsbn.org/14798.htm

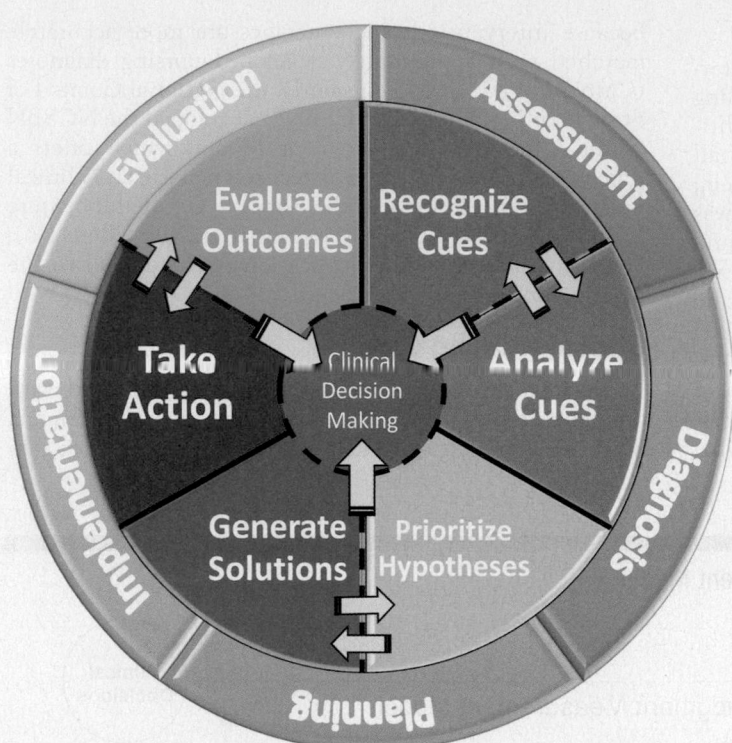

Figure 1-5 • Clinical judgment domains. Reprinted with permission from Brenton, A. & Petersen, E. K. (2019). *Next generation NCLEX® (NGN) Educator Webinar Part I.* Chicago, IL: National Council of State Boards of Nursing (NCSBN®).

a better understanding of how these issues can be addressed. Specifically, the focus on ethics in health care has intensified in response to controversial developments, including advanced technology, genomics, medical futility, scarcity of resources, and end-of-life issues, to name a few.

Today, sophisticated technology can prolong life well beyond the time when death would have occurred in the past. Expensive experimental procedures, clinical trials, complex equipment and treatments are available to prolong life, even when such attempts may not provide quality of life. The development of technologic support has influenced the quality and delivery of nursing care at all stages of life and also has contributed to an increase in average life expectancy. For example, robotic technology is helping older adults living in the community to better manage chronic health problems (Bakas, Sampsel, Israel, et al., 2018). Adults with end-stage heart failure who are not candidates for cardiac transplantation can live longer with the support of newer generation left ventricular assist devices (LVADs), which require less invasive surgery and are associated with less complications than older model LVADs (Kubrusly, 2019). Advances in immunotherapy have increased life expectancies for patients diagnosed with advanced stage melanomas and nonsquamous cell lung cancers (Munro, 2019). Patients who would have died of organ failure are living longer because of organ transplantation and stem cell transplant.

These advances in technology have been a mixed blessing. Questions have been raised about whether it is appropriate to use such technology and, if so, under what circumstances. Although many patients do achieve a good quality of life, others face extended suffering as a result of efforts to prolong life, usually at great expense both emotionally and financially.

Ethical issues also surround those practices or policies that seem to allocate health care resources unjustly on the basis of age, race, gender, disability, or social mores. Older adults may be at risk for being denied health care because of their advanced age and the bias known as ageism (see Chapter 8 for a further discussion of ageism).

Ethical dilemmas that nurses may encounter in the medical-surgical nursing arena are diverse and occur in all settings. An awareness of underlying concepts helps nurses use reason to work through these dilemmas. Basic concepts related to moral philosophy, such as ethics and its principles, theories, and approaches, are included in this chapter. Understanding the role of the professional nurse in ethical decision making not only helps nurses articulate their ethical positions and develop the skills needed to make ethical decisions, but also helps them use the nursing process to develop plans of care from an ethical perspective.

Ethics versus Morals

The terms *ethics* and *morality* are used to describe beliefs about right and wrong and to suggest appropriate guidelines for action. In essence, **ethics** is the formal, systematic study of moral beliefs to understand, analyze, and evaluate matters of right and wrong; whereas, **morality** includes specific values, characters, or actions whose outcomes are often examined through systematic ethical analysis. Because the distinction between ethics and morality is slight, the terms are often used interchangeably.

Ethics Theories

One classic theory in ethics is teleologic theory or consequentialism, which focuses on the ends or consequences of

---

Chart 1-7	**ETHICAL DILEMMA**

Common Ethical Principles

The following common ethical principles may be used to validate moral claims.

Autonomy

This word *autonomy* is derived from the Greek words *autos* ("self") and *nomos* ("rule" or "law") and therefore refers to self-determination. The principle of autonomy entails the right of patients to receive adequate and accurate information so that they have the ability to make a choice free from external constraints. It is synonymous with self-determination.

Beneficence and Nonmaleficence

Beneficence is the duty to perform acts that can be of benefit others. It also entails taking positive action to prevent patients from harming themselves or others, including society as a whole. There is also an implied commitment to help people with disability.

Nonmaleficence is the duty to not inflict harm. The only time when it is considered morally permissible to exercise power over a competent person against their will is when by doing so, harm to others is prevented.

Double Effect

The double effect is a principle that may morally justify some actions that produce both good and evil effects.

All four of the following criteria must be fulfilled:

1. The action itself is good or morally neutral.
2. The agent sincerely intends the good and not the evil effect (the evil effect may be foreseen but is not intended).
3. The good effect is not achieved by means of the evil effect.
4. There is proportionate or favorable balance of good over evil.

Distributive Justice

From a broad perspective, justice states that like cases should be treated alike. More specifically, distributive justice is an ethical principle commonly applicable to clinical situations. This principle is upheld when benefits and burdens are distributed equitably and fairly without consideration of age, gender, socioeconomic status, religion, ethnicity, or sexual orientation. Simply stated, there is an ethical obligation to distribute or allocate resources fairly.

Adapted from Beauchamp, T. L., & Childress, J. F. (2019). *Principles of biomedical ethics* (8th ed.). New York: Oxford University Press.

---

actions. The best-known form of this theory, utilitarianism, is based on the concept of "the greatest good for the greatest number." The choice of action is clear under this theory, because the action that maximizes good over bad is the correct one. The theory poses difficulty when one must judge intrinsic values and determine whose good is the greatest. In addition, it is important to ask whether good consequences can justify any amoral actions that might be used to achieve them.

Another theory in ethics is the deontologic or formalist theory, which argues that ethical standards or principles exist independently of the ends or consequences. In a given situation, nurses have a "sense of duty" to act based on the one relevant principle, or the most relevant of several ethical principles. Their actions must be independent of the ends or consequences. Problems arise with this theory when personal and cultural biases influence the choice of the most primary ethical principle.

Approaches to Ethics

Two approaches to ethics are meta-ethics and applied ethics. An example of meta-ethics (understanding the concepts and linguistic terminology used in ethics) in the health care environment is analysis of the concept of informed consent. Nurses are aware that patients must give consent before surgery; however, sometimes a question arises as to whether a patient is truly informed and mentally competent. Delving more deeply into the concept of informed consent would be a meta-ethical inquiry (see Chapter 14 for more information about informed consent before surgery).

Applied ethics refers to identification of ethical problems relevant to a specific discipline and that discipline's practice. It addresses the implications of actions or practices in terms of their moral permissibility. Various disciplines use the frameworks of general ethical theories and principles and apply them to specific problems within their domain. Nursing ethics may be considered a form of applied ethics because it addresses moral situations that are specific to the nursing profession and patient care. Common ethical principles that can be used to validate moral claims in clinical practice include autonomy, beneficence and nonmaleficence, double effect, and distributive justice. Brief definitions of these important principles can be found in Chart 1-7.

Moral Situations

Many situations exist in which ethical analysis is needed. Some are **moral dilemmas,** or situations in which a clear conflict exists between two or more moral principles or competing moral claims, and nurses must choose the lesser of two evils. Other situations represent **moral problems,** in which there may be competing moral claims or principles, although one claim or principle is clearly dominant. Some situations result in **moral uncertainty,** when one cannot accurately define what the moral situation is or what moral principles apply but has a strong feeling that something is not right. Still other situations may result in **moral distress,** in which one is aware of the correct course of action, but institutional constraints stand in the way of pursuing the correct action. Altaker, Howie-Esquivel, and Cataldo (2018) found that moral distress in critical-care nurses was related to perceptions of a poor ethical climate and poor personal empowerment (see Nursing Research Profile in Chart 1-8).

Many scenarios may occur in clinical practice that require an ethical analysis. For example, an older adult patient with a history of advanced dementia and heart failure is admitted to the hospital with shortness of breath and diagnosed with

---

Chart 1-8 NURSING RESEARCH PROFILE
Moral Distress in Critical-Care Nurses

Altaker, K. W., Howie-Esquivel, J., & Cataldo, J. K. (2018). Relationships among palliative care, ethical climate, empowerment, and moral distress in intensive care unit nurses. *American Journal of Critical Care*, 27(4), 295–302.

Purpose

Between 10% and 29% of patients admitted to intensive care units (ICUs) die. Difficulty delivering adequate end-of-life comfort care can cause moral distress among nurses who work in ICUs. Delivering quality comfort care can be predicated upon the ability of the critical-care nurses to appropriately access palliative care services. Moral distress may also be affected by the overall ethical climate in the ICU, as well as by the personal sense of empowerment by the individual critical-care nurse. Therefore, the purpose of this study was to evaluate relationships between critical-care nurses' moral distress, palliative care service access, ICU ethical climate, and personal empowerment.

Design

A Web-based survey was sent to a nationally representative sample of critical-care nurses who belonged to the American Association of Critical-Care Nurses. In order to be eligible for the study, participants had to be currently working as a direct provider of nursing care in an adult ICU and had to have provided care to at least one dying patient within the past 6 months. Of those who agreed to participate, 235 completed all survey items. Items included in the survey were derived from psychometrically validated instruments including the Moral Distress Scale-Revised, the Hospital Ethical Climate Survey, and the Psychological Empowerment Instrument. In addition, survey items that assessed participants' perceptions of access to, use of, and barriers to palliative care in the ICU were developed and included in the survey.

Findings

Moral distress was negatively associated with feelings of empowerment ($r = -0.145$; $p = 0.02$) and with the ICU ethical climate ($r = -0.354$; $p < 0.001$). Multiple regression analysis found that the factors that contributed to variance in moral distress included the ICU ethical climate, access to palliative care services, size of the ICU, and personal characteristics of the nurse, such as ethnicity and educational level. The factor that contributed the most to moral distress was the ICU ethical climate, with a positive ICU ethical climate correlating with lower levels of moral distress.

Nursing Implications

Findings from this study suggest that critical-care nurses who feel less empowered also feel greater moral distress; however, this relationship was not clear when the variable of ICU ethical climate was analyzed. It seems that personal characteristics of the critical-care nurse, including feelings of empowerment, as well as the ethical climate within the ICU, have roles in determining whether the critical-care nurse experiences moral distress. An unexpected finding was that critical-care nurses who reported access to palliative care services reported greater moral distress. The quality of the interprofessional relationships between critical-care nurses and interdisciplinary members of palliative care teams must be explored. Further studies must be conducted to better discern the causes of moral distress among critical-care nurses so that appropriate interventions may be targeted to mitigate moral distress, which can cause nurse burnout and patient care avoidance.

---

aspiration pneumonia. This is the patient's third hospitalization in the last year for aspiration pneumonia. The patient fails a swallow evaluation and the speech-language pathologist recommends that the patient remain NPO (nothing by mouth). The primary provider coordinates a family meeting to discuss options for nutrition which include inserting a percutaneous feeding tube or carefully hand feeding the patient to promote comfort. The team learns that the patient never completed a living will or assigned a health care representative. The patient's son recalls his mother telling him once on a trip to Italy that "eating was one of her greatest pleasures." However, the patient's daughter is adamant that her mother receives a feeding tube, despite learning that feeding tubes do not increase survival and are associated with complications in patients with significant cognitive deficits. Both the son and daughter have a close relationship with their mother, but neither have had a formal discussion with her about her end-of-life wishes. They do not have any other siblings and their father died several years ago suddenly from a cerebral aneurysm. The son is reluctant to go against his sister's wishes. The nurse has worked with other patients and families in similar situations and knows that his role is to advocate for his patient. He is familiar with current literature which suggests enteral feedings do not improve nutritional or functional status in this population and feels strongly that a feeding tube will not enhance the patient's quality of life. The primary provider is concerned that the daughter will create "problems" for the hospital if a feeding tube is not inserted and states that "he does not have time to deal with her" so schedules the patient for the procedure. The nurse feels strongly that this is the wrong decision and that the daughter would benefit from more education and time to process this complex decision. However, the nurse does not feel empowered to voice his concerns to the primary provider and is left feeling a sense of moral distress; he knows the right course of action, but institutional factors, including existing power hierarchies among nurses and primary providers and lack of time and additional supportive services, prevent him from acting. The nurse wishes that he had had more time to discuss this case with his charge nurse or nurse manager, or to consult the palliative care team which is not in the hospital on the weekends, and today is a Saturday.

It is essential that nurses freely engage in dialogue concerning moral situations, even though such dialogue is difficult for everyone involved. Improved interdisciplinary collaboration is supported when all members of the health care team can voice their concerns and come to an understanding of the moral situation. Consultation with an ethics committee could be helpful to assist the health care team, patient, and family to identify the moral dilemma and possible approaches to the dilemma (see the Ethics Committees section). Nurses should be familiar with agency policy supporting patient self-determination and resolution of ethical issues.

Types of Ethical Problems in Nursing

As a profession, nursing is accountable to society. Nursing has identified its standards of accountability through formal codes of ethics that explicitly state the profession's values and goals. The ICN has endorsed a globally applicable *Code of Ethics for Nurses* (ICN, 2012). Likewise, the ANA established a *Code of Ethics for Nurses* that includes ethical standards, each with its own interpretive statements (ANA, 2015a). The interpretive statements provide guidance to address and resolve ethical dilemmas by incorporating universal moral principles. In addition, the ANA sponsors a Center for Ethics and Human Rights that contains a repository of position statements that can be used to guide nursing practice (Chart 1-9).

Ethical issues have always affected the role of professional nurses. The accepted definition of professional nursing not only supports the advocacy role for nurses, but also the claim that nurses must be actively involved in the decision making process regarding ethical concerns surrounding health care and human responses. Nurses are morally obligated to present ethical conflicts within a logical, systematic framework. Health care settings in which nurses are valued members of the team promote interdisciplinary communication and may enhance patient care. The nurse presented in the case study in the previous section is morally obligated to address his concerns constructively. He should carve out the time to discuss his concerns within his chain of command, through notifying his charge nurse of his concerns for the patient. To practice effectively in these settings, nurses must be aware of ethical issues and serve as patient advocates to assist patients in asserting their autonomy in decision making.

Nursing theories that incorporate the biopsychosocial–spiritual dimensions emphasize a holistic viewpoint, with humanism or caring at the core. Caring and compassion are often cited as virtues inherent within the moral foundation for professional nursing practice. For nurses to embrace this professional ethos, they must be aware not only of major ethical dilemmas but also of those daily interactions with health care consumers that frequently give rise to less easily identifiable ethical challenges. Although technologic advances and diminished resources have been instrumental in raising numerous ethical questions and controversies, including life-and-death issues, nurses should not ignore the many routine situations that involve ethical considerations. Some of the most common issues faced by nurses today include confidentiality, the use of restraints, truth-telling, refusing to provide care, and end-of-life decisions and palliative care.

Confidentiality

All nurses should be aware of the confidential nature of information obtained in daily practice. Confidentiality acknowledges and respects each person's privacy. If information is not pertinent, nurses should question whether it is prudent to document it in a patient's record. In the practice setting, discussion of patients with other members of the health care team is often necessary. However, these discussions should occur in a private area where it is unlikely that the conversation will be overheard. Nurses should also be aware that the use of family members or hospital ancillary personnel as interpreters for patients who are not fluent in English language or who are deaf violates patients' rights of confidentiality. Translation services should be provided for non–English-speaking patients, and interpreters should be provided for those who use sign language by the hospital or institution.

Another threat to confidentiality is the widespread use of computer-based technologies, particularly EHRs, and people's easy access to them. The growing demand for telehealth innovations and the increasing use of this method can result in unchecked access to health information. In addition, personal and health information is often made available to numerous individuals and corporate stakeholders, which may increase the potential for misuse of health care information. Because of these possibilities of maleficence, sensitivity to the principle of confidentiality is

Chart 1-9	Position Statements from the American Nurses Association Center for Ethics and Human Rights	

Position Statement	Latest Approval/ Revision Date
Addressing Nurse Fatigue to Promote Safety and Health	Revised 9/10/14
Capital Punishment and Nurses' Participation in Capital Punishment	Revised 2016
Euthanasia, Assisted Suicide, and Aid in Dying	Revised 4/24/19
Nurse's Role in Providing Ethically and Developmentally Appropriate Care to People with Intellectual and Developmental Disabilities	Approved 10/10/19
Nursing Advocacy for LGBTQ+ Populations	Approved 4/19/18
Nursing Care and Do Not Resuscitate (DNR) and Allow Natural Death (AND)	Approved 3/12/12
Nutrition and Hydration at the End of Life	Revised 6/7/17
Privacy and Confidentiality	Revised 6/2015
Reduction of Patient Restraint and Seclusion in Health Care Settings	Approved 3/12/12
Registered Nurses' Role and Responsibilities in Providing Expert Care and Counseling at End of Life	Revised 2016
Risk and Responsibility in Providing Nursing Care	Approved 6/2015
Stem Cell Research	Approved 1/10/07
The Nurses' Role in Ethics and Human Rights: Protecting and Promoting Individual Worth, Dignity, and Human Rights in Practice Setting	Approved 2/2016
Therapeutic Use of Marijuana and Related Cannabinoids	Revised 2016

essential. The ANA (2015) published a position statement that addresses patients' rights to privacy and confidentiality of their health information.

Federal legislation has been developed to protect the right of confidentiality. According to the Health Insurance Portability and Accountability Act (HIPAA) (HHS, 2003), efforts must be made to protect each patient's private health information (PHI), whether it is transmitted by verbal, written, or electronic means of communication. Communication should be confined to the appropriate settings and with appropriate individuals and should occur for the appropriate purposes of facilitating patient care. Violations of protection of any patient's privacy could result in criminal or civil litigation (HHS, 2003).

Restraints

The use of restraints (including physical and pharmacologic measures) and patient seclusion are additional issues with ethical overtones because of the limits on a person's autonomy and human dignity when these measures are used. Nurses must weigh carefully the risks of limiting autonomy and increasing the risks of injury by using restraints against the risks of injury if not using restraints, which have been documented as resulting in physical harm and death. The ANA (2012) advocates that in situations where restraints and seclusion must be used, all staff must be educated on safety measures. In addition, there must be adequate staff that are vigilant in monitoring their use. These interventions may be utilized only when there is no other viable option available. **The Joint Commission**, a nonprofit organization that accredits hospitals and health care organizations, and CMS have designated standards for the use of restraints (see The Joint Commission and CMS Web sites listed in the Resources section).

Trust Issues

Truth-telling or veracity is one of the basic principles in the nurse–patient relationship. Truth-telling is based upon the principle of autonomy; it requires that the nurse understands and supports patient self-determination (Beauchamp & Childress, 2019). For example, failure to disclose a diagnosis to a patient deprives the person of the right to make informed decisions. Three ethical dilemmas in clinical practice that can directly conflict with this principle are the use of placebos (nonactive substances used for treatment), not revealing a diagnosis to a patient, and revealing a diagnosis to people other than the patient with the diagnosis. All involve the issue of trust, which is an essential element in the nurse–patient relationship.

Placebos may be used in experimental research, in which a patient is involved in the decision making process and is aware that placebos are being used in the treatment regimen. However, the use of a placebo as a substitute for an active drug to show that a patient does not have actual symptoms of a disease is deceptive, has both ethical and legal implications, and severely undermines the nurse–patient relationship.

Informing a patient of his or her diagnosis when the family and primary provider have chosen to delay full disclosure of pertinent information is an ethical dilemma that can occur in nursing practice. The nurse may experience moral distress when asked by the patient for a truthful diagnosis. The nurse may use evasive comments with the patient in these situations. This area is indeed complex, because it challenges a nurse's **moral integrity**. Nurses could consider the following strategies:

- Avoid lying to the patient.
- Provide all information related to nursing procedures and diagnoses.
- Act as a patient advocate and communicate the patient's requests for information to the family and primary provider. The family is often unaware of the patient's repeated questions to the nurse. With a better understanding of the situation, the family members may change their perspective.
- Make a referral to the institution's ethics committee.

Although providing the information may be the morally appropriate behavior, the manner in which the patient is told is important. Nurses must be compassionate and caring when informing patients; disclosure of information merely for the sake of patient autonomy does not convey respect for others and in some circumstances may result in emotional distress. Family support or the support of a spiritual advisor (e.g., chaplain) may be needed to reduce the impact of distressing information or a poor prognosis.

Disclosing the patient's diagnosis to others without the patient's consent is a HIPAA violation and therefore is not only unethical but also illegal. Failure to protect the patient's right to privacy and a breach of confidentiality is unethical.

Refusing to Provide Care

Any nurse who feels morally obliged to refuse to provide care for a particular type of patient faces an ethical dilemma. Reasons for refusal range from a conflict of personal values to a fear that the nurse would place either the patient or self in jeopardy. Feelings related to care of people of different ethnicities or sexual orientation also surface as societal changes emerge. The ethical obligation to care for all patients is clearly identified in the *Code of Ethics for Nurses* (ANA, 2015a). Accordingly, the nurse must give patient-centered care to all patients, regardless of their socioeconomic status, sexual orientation, gender expression, ethnicity, or proximity to death. In particular, patients facing end-of-life decisions must receive supportive care, which must be extended to their family and surrogate decision makers (ANA, 2015a).

End-of-Life Issues

Dilemmas that center on death and dying are prevalent in medical-surgical nursing practice. With the availability of increasingly sophisticated and advanced technology, it may be difficult to accept that nothing more can be done to prolong life or that technology may prolong life but at the expense of the patient's comfort and quality of life. When providing end-of-life care, nurses serve as the patient's advocate and manage pain and suffering. Nurses have the moral obligation to facilitate a patient's right to self-determination.

Furthermore, nurses should facilitate end-of-life discussions between the patient and the family in order to prevent suffering and preserve the patient's dignity (ANA, 2015a).

Many people who are terminally ill seek legal options for a peaceful and dignified death. Nurses who deliver palliative care must understand that their actions are targeted at relieving pain and suffering and not hastening death. According to Provision 1.4 of the *Code of Ethics for Nurses*, "The nurse should provide interventions to relieve pain and other symptoms in the dying patient consistent with palliative care practice standards and may not act with the sole intent to end life (2015a, p. 3)," even if the intent to end life is motivated by compassion or respect for patient autonomy.

End-of-life issues shift the focus from curative care to palliative and end-of-life care. Focusing on the caring as well as the curing role may help nurses deal with these difficult moral situations. Needs of patients and families require holistic and interdisciplinary approaches. End-of-life issues that often involve ethical dilemmas include pain control, "do not resuscitate" (DNR) orders, life support measures, and administration of food and fluids. These issues are discussed in detail in Chapter 13.

Preventive Ethics

When a nurse is faced with two conflicting alternatives, it is the nurse's moral responsibility to choose the lesser of the two evils. These situations often result in feelings of moral distress in the nurse who is obliged to make a choice.

Patient Self-Determination

Frequently, dilemmas occur when health care practitioners are unsure of the patient's wishes because the patient is unconscious or mentally incompetent and cannot communicate. The Patient Self-Determination Act, enacted in December 1991, encourages people to prepare advance directives in which they indicate their wishes concerning the degree of supportive care they wish if they become incapacitated. This legislation requires that patients be informed about advance directives by the staff of the health care facility.

Advance directives are legal documents that specify a person's wishes before hospitalization and provide valuable information that may assist health care providers in decision making. A living will is one type of advance directive. Typically, living wills are limited to situations in which the patient's medical condition is deemed terminal. Because it is difficult to define *terminal* accurately, living wills are not always honored. Another potential drawback is that living wills are frequently written while people are in good health. It is not unusual for people to change their minds as an illness progresses; therefore, patients retain the option to nullify these documents.

Identifying a health care representative, in which one person identifies another person to make health care decisions on his or her behalf, is another type of advance directive. It is the responsibility of the health care representative to act as the patient stated in the advance directive. For example, patients may have clarified their wishes concerning various medical situations. If there is no advance directive, the health care representative must act in good faith and make decisions that they believe the patient would make if mentally competent. Laws concerning advance directives vary among state jurisdictions. However, even in states where these documents are not legally binding, they provide helpful information to determine the patient's prior expressed wishes in situations in which this information can no longer be obtained.

Advance directives are limited in scope to hospital and long-term care facility environments. Emergency medical system (EMS) personnel (e.g., paramedics) therefore cannot legally follow advance directives. Yet, there are many patients with debilitating long-term chronic and eventually fatal illnesses who reside at home. Some of these patients may not wish to have invasive, life-sustaining emergency interventions should their status rapidly deteriorate. To protect the wishes of these patients to forego life-sustaining treatments, a document titled Physician Orders for Life-Sustaining Treatment (POLST) has been legally endorsed by many states. POLST gives EMS personnel the ability to rapidly determine whether a patient wishes to have cardiopulmonary resuscitation (CPR) or receive any type of emergency interventions that may sustain life in the event when the patient suddenly becomes incapacitated (National POLST Paradigm, 2019).

Ethics Committees

Institutional ethics committees exist in many hospitals to assist clinicians with ethical dilemmas. The purpose of these multidisciplinary committees varies among institutions. In some hospitals, the committees exist solely for the purpose of developing policies; whereas in others, they may have a strong educational or consultation focus. Consultations can be conducted on the nursing unit, at the patient's bedside, or in a designated conference room. These committees usually are composed of people with some advanced training in ethics and are important resources for the health care team, patient, and family. Nurses with a particular interest or expertise in the area of ethics can serve as members of these committees, which are valuable resources for staff nurses. In addition, primary providers, social workers, and hospital chaplains are often members of the team.

Ethical Decision Making

Ethical dilemmas are common and diverse in nursing practice. Situations vary, and experience indicates that there are no clear solutions to these dilemmas (Beauchamp & Childress, 2019). However, the fundamental philosophical principles are the same, and the process of moral reflection helps nurses justify their actions. The systematic approach to ethical decision making can follow the steps of the nursing process. Ethics charts contained in all units within this text present case scenarios that challenge the reader to identify the ethical principles involved that may or may not be in conflict (Chart 1-10). Chart 1-10 outlines the steps of an ethical analysis that may be used to resolve the moral dilemmas presented in these charts.

Chart 1-10 ETHICAL DILEMMA
Steps of an Ethical Analysis

The following guidelines reflect an active process in decision making, similar to the nursing process detailed in this chapter. Nurses can use these guidelines to engage in ethical decision making. Key resources that may assist in ethical decision making are also included.

Assessment

1. Once the ethical issue has been identified, assess the ethical/moral situations of the problem. This step entails recognition of the ethical, legal, and professional dimensions involved.
   a. Does the situation entail substantive moral problems (conflicts among ethical principles or professional obligations)? Examine the ethical issue using the principles of autonomy, beneficence, justice, and nonmaleficence.
   b. Are there procedural conflicts? (e.g., Who should make the decisions? Any conflicts among the patient, health care providers, family, and guardians?)
   c. Identify the significant people involved and those affected by the decision.
   d. Identify agency or hospital policy or protocol to use when a conflict exists. Is there an ethics committee or council? How is an ethics consult made, and who may request this consultation? What other resources are available to help resolve this conflict?

Planning

2. Collect information.
   a. Include the following information: the medical facts, treatment options, nursing diagnoses, legal data, and the values, beliefs, cultures, and religious components.
   b. Make a distinction between the factual information and the values/beliefs.
   c. Validate the patient's capacity, or lack of capacity, to make decisions.
   d. Identify any other relevant information that should be elicited.
   e. Identify the ethical/moral issues and the competing claims.

f. If it is an end-of-life issue, determine whether an advance directive exists and whether a medical power of attorney or a health care representative has been identified.

Implementation

3. List the alternatives. Compare alternatives with applicable ethical principles and the 2015 ANA *Code of Ethics for Nurses*. Choose either of the frameworks that follow, or other frameworks, and compare outcomes.
   a. *Utilitarian approach:* Predict the consequences of the alternatives; assign a positive or negative value to each consequence; choose the consequence that predicts the highest positive value or "the greatest good for the greatest number."
   b. *Deontologic approach:* Identify the relevant moral principles; compare alternatives with moral principles; appeal to the "higher-level" moral principle if there is a conflict.

Evaluation

4. Decide and evaluate the decision.
   a. What is the best or morally correct action?
   b. Give the ethical reasons for your decision.
   c. What are the ethical reasons against your decision or your biases?
   d. How do you respond to the reasons against your decision?

Resources

American Nurses Association, Center for Ethics and Human Rights: An online resource that contains a repository of positions papers, codes, and other materials aimed at improving the ethical competence of nurses, www.nursingworld.org/ethics
The Hastings Center: A nonprofit, nonpartisan research institute dedicated to interdisciplinary bioethics, www.thehastingscenter.org
National Center for Ethics in Health Care: Provides key analysis of topics in health care ethics, publishes ethics-related news, and posts seminal national reports in ethics, www.ethics.va.gov

Adapted from Beauchamp, T. L., & Childress, J. F. (2019). *Principles of biomedical ethics* (8th ed.). New York: Oxford University Press.

CRITICAL THINKING EXERCISES

1 **ebp** Recently a team of staff nurses working on a pulmonary step-down unit was asked to examine the incidence of tracheotomy-related skin breakdown and found a 30% increase over the last year. The team reported these findings to the evidence-based practice council who determined the need to examine nursing interventions to improve skin integrity. As part of this team, what steps will you take to identify best practices? Based on this review, how will you determine which nursing practices would be most effective in helping to reduce the incidence of tracheotomy-related skin breakdown on your unit?

2 **ipc** You are part of an interprofessional team discussing the plan of care for a patient who experienced an ischemic stroke. After the meeting, the physical therapist asks you to explain how you formulate a nursing diagnosis and prioritize goals and interventions for your patients. How do you respond? The physical therapist also asks you for suggestions on ways the team could improve communication and teamwork to better address collaborative problems. Using professional practice guidelines, what recommendations do you share with the physical therapist?

REFERENCES

*Asterisk indicates nursing research article.
**Double asterisk indicates classic reference.

Books

Alfaro-LeFevre, R. (2017). *Critical thinking and clinical judgment: A practical approach* (6th ed.). Philadelphia, PA: Elsevier.
American Nurses Association (ANA). (2010). *Nursing's social policy statement* (3rd ed.). Silver Springs, MD: Nursesbooks.org
American Nurses Association (ANA). (2015a). *Code of ethics for nurses with interpretive statements*. Washington, DC: Nursesbooks.org
American Nurses Association (ANA). (2015b). *Nursing: Scope and standards of practice* (3rd ed.). Silver Springs, MD: Nursesbooks.org
Beauchamp, T. L., & Childress, J. F. (2019). *Principles of biomedical ethics* (8th ed.). New York: Oxford University Press.

Butcher, H. K., Bulechek, G. M., Dochterman, J. M., et al. (Eds.). (2018). *Nursing interventions classification (NIC)* (7th ed.). St. Louis, MO: Elsevier.

Carpenito, L. J. (2017). *Nursing diagnosis: Application to clinical practice* (15th ed.). Philadelphia, PA: Lippincott Williams & Wilkins.

Fowler, M. D. (2015). *Guide to nursing's social policy statement: Understanding the profession from social contract to social covenant.* Silver Springs, MD: Author.

Hood, L. (2018). *Leddy & Pepper's conceptual bases of professional nursing* (9th ed.). Philadelphia, PA: Lippincott Williams & Wilkins.

**Institute of Medicine (IOM). (2000). *To err is human: Building a safer health system.* Washington, DC: National Academies Press.

**Institute of Medicine (IOM). (2001). *Crossing the quality chasm: A new health system for the 21st century.* Washington, DC: National Academies Press.

**Institute of Medicine (IOM). (2003). *Health professions education: A bridge to quality.* Washington, DC: National Academies Press.

**International Council of Nurses (ICN). (2012). *Code of ethics for nurses.* Geneva: Author.

International Council of Nurses (ICN). (2019). Nursing diagnosis and outcome statements. Retrieved on 3/11/2021 at: www.icn.ch/sites/default/files/inline-files/ICNP2019-DC.pdf

**Interprofessional Education Collaborative Expert Panel (IPEC). (2011). *Core competencies for interprofessional collaborative practice: Report of an expert panel.* Washington, DC: Author.

Interprofessional Education Collaborative (IPEC). (2016b). *Core competencies for interprofessional collaborative practice: 2016 update.* Washington, DC: Author.

**Maslow, A. (1954). *Motivation and personality.* New York: Harper.

Melnyk, B. M., & Fineout-Overholt, E. (2018). *Evidence-based practice in nursing and healthcare: A guide to best practice* (4th ed.). Philadelphia, PA: Wolters Kluwer.

Moorhead, S., Swanson, E., Johnson, M., et al. (Eds.). (2018). *Nursing outcomes classification (NOC)* (6th ed.). St. Louis, MO: Mosby-Elsevier.

Murdaugh, C. L., Parsons, M. A., & Pender, N. L. (2019). *Health promotion in nursing practice* (8th ed.). Upper Saddle River, NJ: Pearson Education.

National Academy of Medicine. (2020). *The future of nursing 2020–2030.* Retrieved on 2/29/20 at: https://nam.edu/publications/the-future-of-nursing-2020-2030/Pender

Stuart, G. W. (2012). *Principles and practice of psychiatric nursing* (10th ed.). St. Louis, MO: CV Mosby.

**World Health Organization (WHO). (2006). *Constitution of the World Health Organization* (45th ed.). New York: Author.

Journals and Electronic Documents

Alfaro-LeFevre, R. (2019). Promoting critical thinking in frontline nurses. Retrieved on 2/29/2020 at: www.alfaroteachsmart.com

*Altaker, K. W., Howie-Esquivel, J., & Cataldo, J. K. (2018). Relationships among palliative care, ethical climate, empowerment, and moral distress in intensive care unit nurses. *American Journal of Critical Care, 27*(4), 295–302.

**American Association of College of Nurses (AACN). (2008). The essentials of baccalaureate education for professional nursing practice. Retrieved on 2/16/2020 at: www.aacnnursing.org/Portals/42/Publications/BaccEssentials08.pdf

**American Nurses Association (ANA). (2009). Position statement on electronic health record. Retrieved on 8/18/2019 at: www.nursingworld.org/practice-policy/nursing-excellence/official-position-statements/id/electronic-health-record

**American Nurses Association (ANA). (2012). Position statement on reduction of patient restraint and seclusion in health care settings. Retrieved on 8/18/2019 at: www.nursingworld.org/practice-policy/nursing-excellence/official-position-statements/id/reduction-of-patient-restraint-and-seclusion-in-health-care-settings

American Nurses Association (ANA). (2015). Position statement on privacy and confidentiality. Retrieved on 8/18/2019 at: www.nursingworld.org/~4ad4a8/globalassets/docs/ana/position-statement-privacy-and-confidentiality.pdf

*Bakas, T., Sampsel, D., Israel, J., et al. (2018). Satisfaction and technology evaluation of a telehealth robotic program to optimize healthy independent living for older adults. *Journal of Nursing Scholarship, 50*(6), 666–675.

Brenton, A. & Petersen, E. K. (2019). *Next generation NCLEX® (NGN) Educator Webinar Part I.* Chicago, IL: National Council of State Boards of Nursing (NCSBN®).

Centers for Disease Control and Prevention (CDC). (2019). National Center for Chronic Disease Prevention and Health Promotion. At a glance. Prevalence of chronic illnesses. Retrieved on 3/9/2020 at: www.cdc.gov/chronicdisease/resources/infographic/chronic-diseases.htm

Centers for Medicare & Medicaid Services (CMS). (2015). ICD-10 next steps for providers: Assessment and maintenance toolkit. Retrieved on 8/18/2019 at: www.cms.gov/Medicare/Coding/ICD10/Downloads/ICD-10NextStepsToolkit20170324.pdf

Centers for Medicare & Medicaid Services (CMS). (2020). Promoting interoperability programs. Retrieved on 4/15/2020 at: www.cms.gov/Regulations-and-Guidance/Legislation/EHRIncentivePrograms

Ciupka, B. (2018). Precision Medicine 101. Retrieved on 2/2/2020 at: www.nfcr.org/blog/precision-medicine-101

**Coenen, A. (2003). The International Classification for Nursing Practice (ICNP®) Programme: Advancing a unifying framework for nursing. *Online Journal of Issues in Nursing.* Retrieved on 3/11/2021 at: ojin.nursingworld.org/MainMenuCategories/ANAMarketplace/ANAPeriodicals/OJIN/TableofContents/Volume82003/No2May2003/ArticlesPreviousTopics/TheInternationalClassificationforNursingPractice.html

Colby, S. L., & Ortman, J. M. (2015). *Projections of the Size and Composition of the U.S. Population: 2014 to 2060.* Current Population Reports P25-114 (March). Washington, DC: U.S. Census Bureau.

**Cronenwett, L., Sherwood, G., Barnsteiner, J., et al. (2007). Quality and safety education for nurses. *Nursing Outlook, 55*(3), 122–131.

Flanders, S. A., Gunn, S., Wheeler, M., et al. (2017). Accelerating the development of higher-level clinical thinking in novice nurses. *Journal for Nurses in Professional Development, 33*(5), 240–246.

Genetics Home Reference. (2020). Help me understand genetics. Precision medicine. Retrieved on 2/23/2020 at: ghr.nlm.nih.gov/primer/precisionmedicine/initiative

Goodrich, A., Wagner-Johnston, N., & Delibovi, D. (2017). Lymphoma therapy and adverse events: Nursing strategies for thinking critically and acting decisively. *Clinical Journal of Oncology Nursing, 21*(1), 2–12.

Griffits, S., Hines, S., Mahoney, C., et al. (2017). Characteristics and processes of clinical reasoning in nursing and factors related to its use: A scoping review protocol. *JBI Database of Systematic Reviews and Implementation Reports, 15*(12), 2832–2836.

Han, M. S., & Lee, E. (2018). Effectiveness of mobile health application use to improve health behavior changes: A systematic review of randomized controlled trials. *Healthcare Informatics Research, 24*(3), 207–226. Retrieved on 2/16/20 at: www.researchgate.net/publication/326915461_Effectiveness_of_Mobile_Health_Application_Use_to_Improve_Health_Behavior_Changes_A_Systematic_Review_of_Randomized_Controlled_Trials/link/5b735392299bf14c6da24a32/download

Haskins, J. (2017). Healthy People 2030 to create objectives for health of nation: Process underway for next 10-year plan. *The Nation's Health, 47*(6), 1–14.

Healthcare Information Management Systems Society (HIMSS). (2020). TIGER initiative for technology and health informatics education. Retrieved on 2/16/2020 at: www.himss.org/what-we-do-Initiatives/tiger

HealthIT.gov. (2018). Telemedicine and telehealth. Retrieved on 2/16/2020 at: www.healthit.gov/topic/health-it-initiatives/telemedicine-and-telehealth

**Institute for Healthcare Improvement (IHI). (2012). How-to guide: Prevent ventilator-associated pneumonia. Retrieved on 2/16/2020 at: www.ihi.org/Topics/Bundles/Pages/default.aspx

Institute for Healthcare Improvement (IHI). (2020). Evidence-based care bundles. Retrieved on 2/16/2020 at: www.ihi.org/Topics/Bundles/Pages/default.aspx

**International Council of Nurses (ICN). (2012). The ICN code of ethics for nurses: Revised 2012. Retrieved on 8/18/2019 at: www.icn.ch/sites/default/files/inline-files/2012_ICN_Codeofethicsfornurses_%20eng.pdf

Interprofessional Education Collaborative (IPEC). (2016a). Interprofessional Education Collaborative announces expansion: Nine new members join organization dedicated to improving patient care. Press release: February 22, 2016, Washington, DC. Retrieved on 8/18/2019 at: nebula.wsimg.com/526457f846fbb60c0baed44008b0d890?AccessKeyId=DC06780E69ED19E2B3A5&disposition=0&alloworigin=1

Kubrusly, L. F. (2019). Ventricular assist devices: An evolving field. *Brazilian Journal of Cardiovascular Surgery, 34*(1), 3–5.

Majid, U., & Gagliardi, A. (2019). Conceptual frameworks and degrees of patient engagement in the planning and designing of health services: A scoping review of qualitative studies. *Patient Experience Journal, 6*(3), 82–90.

Munro, N. (2019). Immunology and immunotherapy in critical care: An overview. AACN *Advanced Critical Care, 30*(2), 113–125.

National Alliance to END HOMELESSNESS. (2019). State of homelessness. Retrieved on 8/18/2019 at: www.endhomelessness.org/homelessness-in-america/homelessness-statistics/state-of-homelessness-report

National Council of State Boards of Nursing (NCSBN®). (2021). NCSBN clinical judgment measurement model. Retrieved on 3/22/2021 at: www.ncsbn.org/14798.htm

**National League for Nurses. (2012). Outcomes and competencies for graduates of practical/vocational, diploma, baccalaureate, master's practice doctorate, and research doctorate programs in nursing. Retrieved on 2/16/2020 at: nln.lww.com/Outcomes-and-Competencies-for-Graduates-of-Practical-Vocational–Diploma–Baccalaureate–Master-s-Practice-Doc/p/9781934758120

National POLST Paradigm. (2019). About POLST. Retrieved on 8/18/2019 at: www.polst.org

Olenick, M., Flowers, M., & Diaz, V. J. (2015). US veterans and their unique issues: Enhancing health care professional awareness. *Advances in Medical Education and Practice, 6*, 635–639. Retrieved on 2/16/2020 at: www.dovepress.com/us-veterans-and-their-unique-issues-enhancing-health-care-professional-peer-reviewed-fulltext-article-AMEP

Pew Research Center. (2017). The changing face of America's veteran population. Retrieved on 2/16/2020 at: www.pewresearch.org/fact-tank/2017/11/10/the-changing-face-of-americas-veteran-population

QSEN Institute & Frances Payne Bolton School of Nursing, Case Western Reserve University. (2020). Competencies: Prelicensure KSAs. Retrieved on 2/16/2020 at: qsen.org/competencies/pre-licensure-ksas

Räsänen, J. M., & Günther, K. (2019). Inter-organisational use of electronic health record in mental health. *Communication & Medicine, 15*(1), 65–76.

United Nations, Department of Economic and Social Affairs, Population Division. (2017). World Population Ageing 2017—Highlights (ST/ESA/SER.A/397). Retrieved on 2/16/2020 at: www.un.org/en/development/desa/population/publications/pdf/ageing/WPA2017_Highlights.pdf

U.S. Census Bureau. (2017). 2017 National Population Projections Tables: Main series. Retrieved on 3/20/20 at: www.census.gov/data/tables/2017/demo/popproj/2017-summary-tables.html

U.S. Census Bureau. (2019). Quick facts United States. Retrieved on 2/16/2020 at: https://www.census.gov/quickfacts/fact/table/US/VET605218

U.S. Census Bureau. (2020). United States® Census 2020. Retrieved on 2/16/2020 at: www.census.gov

**U.S. Department of Health and Human Services (HHS). (2003). Summary of the HIPAA privacy rule. Retrieved on 8/18/2019 at: www.hhs.gov/sites/default/files/privacysummary.pdf

U.S. Department of Health and Human Services (HHS), Office of Disease Prevention and Health Promotion. (2020a). Healthy People 2030 framework. Retrieved on 2/16/2020 at: www.healthypeople.gov/2020/About-Healthy-People/Development-Healthy-People-2030/Framework

U.S. Department of Health and Human Services (HHS), Office of Disease Prevention and Health Promotion. (2020b). Leading health indicators. Retrieved on 3/9/2020 at: www.healthypeople.gov/2020/Leading-Health-Indicators

U.S. Department of Housing and Urban Development (HUD), Office of Community Planning and Development. (2020). The 2019 annual homeless assessment report (AHAR) to congress. Retrieved on 3/20/20 at: https://www.huduser.gov/portal/sites/default/files/pdf/2019-AHAR-Part-1.pdf

World Health Organization (WHO). (2018). International classification of diseases. Retrieved on 8/18/2019 at: www.who.int/classifications/icd/en

World Health Organization (WHO). (2019). Primary health care key facts. Retrieved on 2/16/2020 at: www.who.int/news-room/fact-sheets/detail/primary-health-care

Zarifsanaiey, N., Amini, M., & Saadat, F. (2016). A comparison of educational strategies for the acquisition of nursing student's performance and critical thinking: Simulation-based training vs. integrated training (simulation and critical thinking strategies). *BMC Medical Education, 16*(294), 1–7.

Resources

American Association of Colleges of Nursing (AACN), www.aacn.nche.edu

American Nurses Association (ANA), www.nursingworld.org

American Nurses Association Center for Ethics and Human Rights, www.nursingworld.org/ethics

Campaign for Action: Future of Nursing, campaignforaction.org

Centers for Medicare & Medicaid Services (CMS), www.cms.hhs.gov

Development of Healthy People 2030, https://www.healthypeople.gov/2020/About-Healthy-People/Development-Healthy-People-2030/Framework

Healthy People 2030, www.healthypeople.gov

Institute for Healthcare Improvement (IHI), www.ihi.org

International Council of Nurses (ICN), www.icn.ch

Interprofessional Education Collaborative (IPEC), ipecollaborative.org

NANDA International, www.nanda.org

National Academy of Sciences, Engineering, Medicine (formerly the Institute of Medicine [IOM]), iom.nationalacademies.org

National Center for Ethics in Health Care (NCEHC), www.ethics.va.gov

National League for Nursing, nln.org

QSEN Institute: Quality and Safety Education for Nurses, qsen.org

The Hastings Center, www.thehastingscenter.org

The Joint Commission, www.jointcommission.org

The TIGER Initiative, www.himss.org/professional-development/tiger-initiative

World Health Organization (WHO), who.int

2 Medical-Surgical Nursing

On completion of this chapter, the learner will be able to:

1. Discuss principles of medical-surgical nursing practice as well as characteristics and settings of select nursing practice specialties in today's health care delivery system.
2. Describe the significance of the nurse as coordinator of care transitions.
3. Specify the components of a comprehensive assessment of functional capacity.
4. Use the nursing process as a framework for care of the patient with self-care deficits or with impaired physical mobility.
5. Describe the role and practice settings of home health nursing and the significance of continuity of care in transition into community or home settings.

NURSING CONCEPTS

Accountability
Collaboration

Evidence-Based Practice
Functional Ability

Mobility
Safety

GLOSSARY

activities of daily living (ADLs): personal care activities, such as bathing, dressing, grooming, eating, toileting, and transferring

adaptive device: a type of assistive technology that is used to change the environment or help the person modify the environment

assistive device: a type of assistive technology that helps people with disability perform a given task

assistive technology: any item, piece of equipment, or product system that is used to improve the functional capabilities of individuals with disability; this term encompasses both assistive devices and adaptive devices

critical-care nursing: a specialty area of practice that provides nursing services to critically ill patients across the lifespan in acute care settings such as the hospital intensive unit; current practice settings have expanded to include virtual care and community settings

home health nursing: a specialty area of practice that provides nursing services to patients across the lifespan in a home setting; practice roles include holistic care planning which incorporates resource and service coordination as part of an interdisciplinary team

impairment: loss or abnormality of psychological, physiologic, or anatomic structure or function at the organ level (e.g., dysphagia, hemiparesis); an abnormality of body structure, appearance, an organ, or system function resulting from any cause

instrumental activities of daily living (IADLs): complex skills needed for independent living, such as shopping, cooking, housework, using the telephone, managing medications and finances, and being able to travel by car or public transportation

medical-surgical nursing: a specialty area of practice that provides nursing services to patients from adolescence through the end of life in hospital-based and community-based settings

orthosis: an external appliance that provides support, prevents or corrects joint deformities, and improves function

prosthesis: a device used to replace a body part

rehabilitation: making able again; learning or relearning skills or abilities or adjusting existing functions to meet maximum potential

rehabilitation nursing: a specialty area of evidence-based practice that provides holistically-focused nursing services to patients who have been incapacitated by illness or injury or are facing potentially life-altering health conditions throughout their lifespan

rehospitalization: admission to the hospital within 30 days of a prior discharge from a hospitalization

telehealth: the use of technology to provide health care services

third-party payer: an organization or insurance company that provides reimbursement for services covered by a health plan

transfer: movement of a patient from one place to another, such as a bed to chair, chair to commode, or wheelchair to tub

transitional care: a process of ensuring consistency and coordination of care as patients move within and between health care settings

The profession of nursing is ever expanding to meet the health needs of patients, families, and communities. The practice of medical-surgical nursing continues to evolve, too, and is no longer restricted to the traditional environment of the inpatient hospital-based medical-surgical unit. The shift in delivery of medical-surgical nursing from only inpatient settings to also include outpatient settings is a result of multiple factors, including population trends (the growing number of older adults), changes in federal legislation, tighter insurance regulations, and decreasing hospital revenues. Transitions in the health care industry, the nursing profession, and changing patterns of disease and wellness have also affected the shift in care delivery settings. On an increasing basis, hospitals, health care organizations, and providers are held accountable for providing health care using best practices, as evidenced by meeting performance benchmarks for quality and efficiency; this system is known as pay for performance or value-based purchasing. Under this system, hospitals, health care organizations, and providers can reduce costs and earn additional income by carefully monitoring the types of services they provide, discharging patients as soon as possible, and keeping patients who are discharged from the hospital from being readmitted. Consequently, patients who transition from the hospital to the home or to residential or long-term care facilities are in the early stages of recovery. With these changes in health care delivery and accountability, specialty practices under the scope of medical-surgical nursing practice have arisen to further identify evidence-based nursing care and interventions. This chapter provides an overview of medical-surgical nursing and other associated nursing specialty practices.

The Practice of Nursing in Today's Health Care Delivery System

Novice, entry-level registered nurses, as well as those with advanced degrees who work in highly specialized settings, all engage in the practice of nursing. The American Nurses Association (ANA, 2015b) notes that the profession of nursing's scope of practice encompasses the full range of nursing practice, pertinent to general and specialty practice. "The depth and breadth in which individual registered nurses and advanced practice registered nurses engage in the total scope of nursing practice is dependent on education, experience, role, and the population served" (p. 2). The ANA (2015b, pp. 7–9) also identifies the following tenets characteristic of all nursing practice:

- Caring and health are central to the practice of the registered nurse.
- Nursing practice is individualized.
- Registered nurses use the nursing process to plan and provide individualized care for health care consumers (see Chapter 1).

- Nurses coordinate care by establishing partnerships.
- A strong link exists between the professional work environment and the registered nurse's ability to provide quality health care and achieve optimal outcomes.

The profession of nursing has a distinct disciplinary body of knowledge, education, and specialty standards of practice (ANA, 2015b); social contract (ANA, 2010; Fowler, 2015); and code of ethics (ANA, 2015a). Nursing's Standards of Practice describe basic competencies in delivering nursing care using the nursing process, whereas the Standards of Professional Performance describe expectations for behavioral competencies (ANA, 2015b, pp. 5–6), which include that the registered nurse:

- Practices ethically
- Practices in a manner that is congruent with cultural diversity and inclusion principles
- Communicates effectively in all areas of practice
- Collaborates with the health care consumer and other key stakeholders in the conduct of nursing practice
- Leads within the professional practice setting and the profession
- Seeks knowledge and competence that reflect current nursing practice and promote futuristic thinking
- Integrates evidence and research findings into practice
- Contributes to quality nursing practice
- Evaluates one's own and others' nursing practice
- Utilizes appropriate resources to plan, provide, and sustain evidence-based nursing services that are safe, effective, and fiscally responsible
- Practices in an environmentally safe and healthy manner

Medical-Surgical Nursing

Medical-surgical nursing is a specialty area of practice that provides nursing services to patients from adolescence through the end of life in a variety of inpatient and outpatient clinical settings. These settings may include traditional hospital medical-surgical units as well as intensive care units (ICUs), acute and subacute care rehabilitation units, clinics, ambulatory care units, urgent care centers, home health care agencies, and long-term care facilities (Academy of Medical-Surgical Nurses [AMSN], 2018; AMSN 2019). The *Scope and Standards of Medical-Surgical Nursing Practice* (AMSN, 2018) mirror the scope of practice and standards for practice set by the ANA (2015b) for professional nursing practice; the AMSN (2018) further delineates specific role expectations for the medical-surgical nurse. Medical-surgical nurses can demonstrate proficiency in their role by completing certification requirements. They may also enhance practice by completing graduate degree programs in nursing (AMSN, 2018).

The Nurse as Coordinator of Care Transitions

Nearly one third of the $3.5 trillion spent on health care in the United States is spent on hospitalizations, including hospital readmissions within 30 days of a prior hospital discharge, called **rehospitalizations** (Centers for Medicare & Medicaid Services [CMS], 2018a). Rehospitalizations raise concerns not only about costs, but also about health care quality (Bailey, Weiss, Barrett, et al., 2019). Approximately 20% of patients insured by Medicare experience rehospitalization. Rehospitalizations in those over 65 years of age are not only costly; these patients may experience weakness and stress which can make them vulnerable to falls and other adverse events (Agency for Healthcare Research and Quality [AHRQ], 2019). Medicare is one example of a health insurance plan holding hospitals accountable for readmissions within 30 days of hospital discharge through a reduction in reimbursement for costs associated with these readmissions (Bailey et al., 2019). Rehospitalizations can result from breakdowns in care transitions including during the discharge planning processes, as evidenced by patients' inability to manage their own care; and, as a result of poor communication between the hospital and the next level of care (e.g., home health agency, primary care office) regarding patients' needs and resources (AHRQ, 2019). Altogether, these factors have led to an increasing focus on **transitional care**, a process of ensuring consistency and coordination of care as patients move within and between care settings (Carr, 2019). For example, transitional care takes place as a patient is transferred from intensive care to a medical-surgical unit within an acute care setting. Another important time of transitional care occurs with patient discharge from the acute care setting

to continued care out in the community. See Chart 2-1 for a Nursing Research Profile on transitional care and the important components needed to assure positive outcomes during this transition process. A number of models and programs of transitional care describe the process as an interdisciplinary team approach in which team members include both the patient and the caregivers. Nurses in a variety of settings are important transitional care team members, managing many aspects of the transition process (Carr, 2019).

Patient care must be coordinated seamlessly from the inpatient hospital environment through transitions into the community setting. Various nursing roles have evolved to provide improved care coordination and care transitions, including the nurse navigator, case manager, and the clinical nurse leader (CNL). Nurse navigators are registered nurses employed by hospitals and health networks who work with a given population of patients with a common diagnosis or disease (e.g., cancer). Their role involves helping the patient and the patient's family transition through different levels of care (e.g., from hospital to a skilled nursing facility, from home care to assisted care). One example of an essential role function for the oncology nurse navigator (ONN) is education. In this role, the ONN assesses patients, families, and caregivers for their educational needs and recognizes barriers to education, which can impact health in areas such as diagnosis, treatment, and management of treatment associated side effects (Baileys, McMullen, Lubejko, et al., 2018).

Case management is a system of coordinating health care services to ensure cost-effectiveness, accountability, and quality care. Case managers may be nurses or may have backgrounds in other health professions, such as social work. The case manager coordinates the care of a caseload of patients through facilitating communication between nurses, other health care personnel who provide care, and insurance companies. In some settings, particularly the community setting,

---

Chart 2-1 · NURSING RESEARCH PROFILE
Important Components of Transitional Care

Naylor, M. D., Shaid, E. C., Carpenter, D., et al. (2017). Components of comprehensive and effective transitional care. *Journal of the American Geriatrics Society, 65*(6), 1119–1125.

Purpose

Transitional care is recognized as important in assuring improved health care outcomes and health care quality while decreasing costs associated with unnecessary hospital readmissions. A national study called Project ACHIEVE that focused on Medicare beneficiaries was conducted to identify key aspects of transitional care that lead to positive patient and caregiver outcomes.

Design

Project ACHIEVE included experts, patients, and caregivers in a multimethod approach that included interviews, focus groups, and review of literature, which led to the identification and definition of critical components of transitional care. The working group collected case studies to evaluate how these components connect to the real experience of transitional care, selecting one case study for concept mapping of the components, all leading to further refinement of the critical components.

Findings

Eight core components were identified and visualized on a transitional care model: patient engagement, caregiver engagement, complexity management, patient education, caregiver education, patient and caregiver well-being, care continuity, and accountability. Each of the eight components was defined with examples of the issues as they related to patients and caregivers. Additional information provided suggestions for interdisciplinary interventions from the reviewed evidence.

Nursing Implications

Transitional care is a team approach that includes the patient and caregiver, and so research into transitional care should include these important stakeholders. The model and definitions for transitional care yielded from Project ACHIEVE provide a common framework for interdisciplinary health care team members who can then focus on providing optimal patient outcomes. Nurses who work in transitional care can utilize these core components in assessment of individual patients, and then tailor interventions to needed components. The model also provides a framework for program development, evaluation, and future refinement through additional investigation of transitional care.

the case manager focuses on coordinating the treatment plan of the patient with complex conditions. The case manager may follow the patient throughout hospitalization and at home after discharge in an effort to coordinate health care services that will avert or delay rehospitalization. The caseload is usually limited in scope to patients with similar diagnoses, needs, and therapies (Case Management Society of America [CMSA], 2019).

A CNL is a certified nurse generalist with a master's degree in nursing educated to help patients navigate the complex health care system (American Association of Colleges of Nursing [AACN], 2019a). The CNL coordinates care for a distinct group of patients, may provide direct care as the situation warrants, and assumes a leadership role among members of the health care team. The CNL integrates evidence-based practices with advocacy, care coordination, outcomes measurement, risk assessment, quality improvement, and interprofessional communication skills (AACN, 2019a). Currently, CNLs are being utilized in hospital-based environments as well as in community settings.

Critical-Care Nursing

Critical-care nursing is a specialty area of practice that provides nursing services to critically ill patients across the lifespan, traditionally delivered in acute care settings such as the hospital ICU. Current practice settings for critical-care nursing have now expanded to include virtual care and a variety of community settings, including the home (American Association of Critical-Care Nurses [AACN], 2019b). When patients face actual or potential life-threatening illness, critical-care nurses provide holistic nursing interventions individualized to each patient.

The *Scope and Standards for Progressive and Critical-Care Nursing* (AACN, 2019b) mirror the scope and standards set by the ANA (2015b) for professional nursing practice; these are revised as needed based on health care trends and technologic advances in the care of patients facing critical illness. The AACN (2019b) further delineates specific role expectations with the nursing process as the foundation and guide. For example, the standard of assessment includes competencies in holistic data collection based on current evidence and the recognition of assessment priorities for each individual patient. The current *Scope and Standards* (AACN, 2019b) recognize two types of nursing care provided by the progressive care nurse and the critical-care nurse. The progressive care nurse provides care for the acutely ill patient who is moving toward physiologic stability yet still at risk for life-threatening illness. The critical-care nurse provides care for those acute care patients with an actual or at high risk of life-threatening illness. The AACN also sets the standards for proficiency in progressive and critical-care nursing that may lead to specialty certification. In addition to specialty certification, there are opportunities for nurses to enhance critical-care nursing practice by completing graduate nursing programs leading to advanced practice as a critical-care clinical nurse specialist or acute care nurse practitioner.

The AACN recognizes the role of the critical-care nurse in care transitions and the need to begin discharge planning early, even during the critical or acute phase of hospitalization (Alspach, 2018). With caregiver tasks ranging from activities of daily living (ADLs) and instrumental activities of daily living (IADLs) (see later discussion) to advocacy and coordination, the critical-care nurse can involve family members or significant others of the patient who is critically ill in rounds and patient care planning, begin to assess their capabilities, and start the education needed so that family members or significant others can manage the role of caregiver.

Rehabilitation Nursing

Rehabilitation means to make able again; it involves learning or relearning skills or abilities or adjusting existing functions to meet maximum potential. Thus, rehabilitation is a goal-oriented process of caring for people with disability or chronic disorders. This philosophy of practice works to restore or optimize abilities rather than focus on disability (Association of Rehabilitation Nursing [ARN], 2013). Rehabilitation is an integral part of nursing because every major illness or injury carries the threat of disability or **impairment**, which involves a loss of function or an abnormality in body structure or function. **Rehabilitation nursing** is a specialty area of practice that focuses on returning patients to optimal functionality through a holistic approach to care that is based on scientific evidence (ARN, 2019a). The ARN has developed an *ARN Competency Model for Professional Rehabilitation Nurses* with resources. The domains in the model (nurse-led interventions, promotion of successful living, leadership and interprofessional care) encompass all competencies needed to promote rehabilitation nursing of people with disability and/or chronic illness (ARN, 2019b). The ARN further describes the roles of the rehabilitation nurse as teacher, caregiver, collaborator, and patient advocate working in a variety of inpatient and outpatient settings (ARN, 2019a).

Rehabilitation services are required by more people than ever before because of advances in technology that save or prolong the lives of seriously ill and injured patients and patients with disability. Increasing numbers of patients who are recovering from serious illnesses or injuries are returning to their homes and communities with ongoing needs. Significant disability caused by war and terrorism also increases the demand for rehabilitation services. All patients, regardless of age, gender, ethnic group, socioeconomic status, or diagnosis, have a right to rehabilitation services.

A person is considered to have a disability, such as a restriction in performance or function in everyday activities, if they have difficulty talking, hearing, seeing, walking, climbing stairs, lifting or carrying objects, performing ADLs, doing schoolwork, or working at a job. The disability is considered severe if the person cannot perform one or more activities, receives federal benefits because of an inability to work, uses an assistive device for mobility, or needs help from another person to accomplish basic activities. The purpose of **assistive technology** is to incorporate devices to improve the functional capabilities of people with disability; these may include any item, piece of equipment, or product system that may be acquired commercially, off the shelf, modified, or customized. Types of assistive technology may include **adaptive devices**, which help a person with a disability to either modify or change the environment (e.g., an access ramp used in place of steps for a person who uses a wheelchair), and assistive devices, which help a person with a disability perform a given task (e.g., a lap board with pictures used to assist a person who cannot talk to communicate) (see Chapter 7 for further discussion on disability).

Assessment of Functional Ability

Comprehensive assessment of functional capacity is the basis for developing a rehabilitation program. Functional capacity is a person's ability to perform ADLs and IADLs. **Activities of daily living (ADLs)** are those self-care activities that the patient must accomplish each day to meet personal needs; they include personal hygiene/bathing, dressing/grooming, feeding, toileting, and transferring. Many patients cannot perform such activities easily. **Instrumental activities of daily living (IADLs)** include those complex skills needed for independent living, such as meal preparation, grocery shopping, household and financial management, medication management, telephone usage, and transportation.

The nurse observes the patient performing specific activities (e.g., eating, dressing) and notes the degree of independence; the time taken; the patient's mobility, coordination, and endurance; and the amount of assistance required. The nurse also carefully assesses joint motion, muscle strength, cardiovascular reserve, and neurologic function, because functional ability depends on these factors as well. Observations are recorded on a functional assessment tool. These tools provide a way to standardize assessment parameters and include a scale or score against which improvements may be measured. They also clearly communicate the patient's level of functioning to all members of the rehabilitation team. Rehabilitation staff members use these tools to provide an initial assessment of the patient's abilities and to monitor the patient's progress in achieving independence.

One of the most frequently used tools to assess the patient's level of independence is the Functional Independence Measure (FIM™) (Keith, Granger, Hamilton, et al., 1987). The FIM is a minimum data set, measuring 18 self-care items including eating, bathing, grooming, dressing upper body, dressing lower body, toileting, bladder management, and bowel management. The FIM addresses transfers and the ability to ambulate and climb stairs and also includes communication and social cognition items. Scoring is based on a seven-point scale, with items used to assess the patient's level of independence. The Alpha FIM, a short version of the FIM, is used frequently within 72 hours of admission in acute care settings to measure functional independence and the amount of assistance the patient needs to perform ADLs.

Although there are many disease-specific tools used to assess the patient's functional ability, some frequently used generic measures include the following (Fidecki, Wysokiński, Wrońska, et al., 2017):

- The Katz Index of Independence in Activities of Daily Living (Katz Index) (Katz, Downs, Cash, et al., 1970) is used to assess six areas of ADLs (i.e., bathing, dressing, toileting, transferring, continence, feeding) and rate them as done independently or done with assistance.
- The Barthel Index (Mahoney & Barthel, 1965) is used to measure the patient's level of independence in ADLs, continence, toileting, transfers, and ambulation (or wheelchair mobility). This scale does not address communicative or cognitive abilities.

A detailed functional evaluation of secondary conditions related to the patient's disability, such as muscle atrophy and deconditioning, skin integrity, bowel and bladder control, and sexual function, together with residual strengths unaffected by disease or disability, is necessary. In addition, the nurse assesses the patient's physical, mental, emotional, spiritual, social, and economic status, as well as cultural and familial environment. These elements may provide a context to the functional findings and influence the rehabilitation plan. For example, the patient's perception of what it means to have a disability and the implications that this might have on familial and social roles can influence the rehabilitation process.

NURSING PROCESS

The Patient with Self-Care Deficits in Activities of Daily Living

An ADL program is started as soon as the rehabilitation process begins, because the ability to perform ADLs is frequently the key to independence, return to the home, and transition into the community.

Assessment

The nurse must observe and assess the patient's ability to perform ADLs to determine the level of independence in self-care and the need for nursing intervention. Chart 2-2 depicts behaviors that may indicate struggles with function or movement and thus should be assessed. For example, bathing requires obtaining bath water and items used for bathing (e.g., soap, washcloth), washing, and drying the body after bathing. Dressing requires getting clothes from the closet, putting on and taking off clothing, and fastening the clothing. Self-feeding requires using utensils to bring food to the mouth and chewing and swallowing the food. Toileting includes removing clothing to use the toilet, cleansing oneself, and readjusting clothing. Grooming activities include combing hair, brushing one's teeth, shaving or applying makeup, and handwashing. Patients who can sit up and raise their hands to their head can begin self-care activities. Assistive devices are often essential in achieving some level of independence in ADLs.

Additional assessment should include gaining an understanding of the patient's and family members' perspectives on the patient's condition and how it affects functional ability. The nurse should also be aware of the patient's medical conditions or other health problems, the effect that they have on the ability to perform ADLs, and the family's involvement in the patient's ADLs. This information is valuable in setting goals and developing the plan of care to maximize self-care.

Nursing Diagnoses

Based on the assessment data, major nursing diagnoses may include the following:

- Impaired ability to perform hygiene
- Impaired ability to dress
- Impaired self feeding
- Impaired self toileting
- Impaired health maintenance

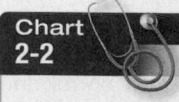

> ### Chart 2-2 · ASSESSMENT
> ### Assessing Potential Struggles in Function or Movement
>
> Be alert for the following behaviors:
>
> - Holding onto a hand rail to pull the body while going up stairs
> - Holding onto a bedside rail or bedcovers to pull to a sitting position in bed
> - Leaning to one side and using both hands on the hand rail while going down the stairs or a ramp
> - Holding onto furniture or doorways and watching the feet while walking in the house
> - Lifting a leg (or arm) by using the other leg (or arm) as support or by lifting with the pants leg (or sleeve)
> - Tilting the head to reach the back or side of the hair while grooming
> - Pushing up, rocking forward and back, and/or leaning the body over for momentum ("nose over toes") when rising to stand from a chair
> - Leaning over from the waist without bending the knees and then placing one hand on the thigh, as if it were a prop, and pushing against the thigh to assist in moving to the upright position
> - Turning to reach for an object and then using the other arm or an object to support the reaching arm at the elbow or wrist
> - Positioning a chair before sitting down by using the front or back of the knees and then using the back of the knees to guide sitting down; using the torso and hips to lean against a table or chair
> - Reaching and leaning with the body rather than with an arm
> - Walking with a lean to one side, a limp, a waddle, or other variation of a gait
> - Scanning (i.e., observing or being aware of surroundings) ineffectively while eating or grooming
> - Rolling or scooting the body, sliding forward in a seat, or other maneuvers to move off a bed or out of a chair
>
> Adapted from Weber, J. R., & Kelley, J. H. (2018). *Health assessment in nursing* (6th ed.). Philadelphia, PA: Lippincott Williams & Wilkins.

Planning and Goals

Major goals for the patient include performing the following activities independently or with assistance, using adaptive or assistive devices as appropriate: bathing/hygiene, dressing/grooming, feeding, and toileting. A related goal is patient expression of satisfaction with the extent of independence achieved in self-care activities. Another major goal is that the patient acknowledges adjustments in new lifestyle and ADLs and can identify resources to facilitate optimal functioning (Carpenito, 2017).

Nursing Interventions

Repetition, practice, and demonstrations help patients achieve maximum independence in personal care activities. The nurse's role is to provide an optimal learning environment that minimizes distractions. The nurse can identify the patient's optimal time to work on activities, encourage concentration, identify endurance issues that may affect safety, and provide cues and reminders to patients with specific disability, such as alteration in or loss of sensation that may occur with stroke (Gregory & Galloway, 2017). Patients with impaired mobility, sensation, strength, or dexterity may need to use assistive devices to accomplish self-care.

FOSTERING SELF-CARE ABILITIES

A patient's approach to self-care may be affected by altered or impaired mobility and influenced by family or cultural expectations. The inability to perform self-care as carried out previously may lead to ineffective coping behaviors, such as social isolation, dependency on caregivers, or depression. The nurse must motivate the patient to learn and accept responsibility for self-care. It helps to encourage an "I'd rather do it myself" attitude. The nurse must also help the patient identify the safe limits of independent activity; knowing when to ask for assistance is particularly important.

The nurse educates, guides, and supports the patient who is learning or relearning how to perform self-care activities while maintaining a focus on patient strengths and optimal level of function. Consistency in instructions and assistance given by health care providers, including rehabilitation therapists (e.g., physiotherapists, occupational therapists, recreation therapists, speech-language pathologists, primary providers) facilitates the learning process. Recording the patient's performance provides data for evaluating progress and may be used as a source for motivation and morale building. Guidelines for educating patients and families about ADLs are presented in Chart 2-3.

Often, performing a simple maneuver requires the patient with a disability to concentrate intensely and exert considerable effort; therefore, self-care techniques need to be adapted to accommodate the individual patient's lifestyle. Because a self-care activity usually can be accomplished in several ways, common sense and a little ingenuity may promote increased independence. For example, a person who cannot quite reach his or her head may be able to do so by leaning forward. Encouraging the patient to participate in a support group may also help the patient discover creative solutions to self-care problems.

> ### Chart 2-3 · PATIENT EDUCATION
> ### Educating Patients About Activities of Daily Living
>
> The nurse instructs the patient to:
>
> 1. Be realistic about the goal of the activity and set short-term goals that can be accomplished in the near future.
> 2. Identify several approaches to accomplish the task (e.g., there are several ways to put on a given garment).
> 3. Select the approach most likely to succeed.
> 4. Identify the motions necessary to accomplish the activity (e.g., to pick up a glass, extend arm with hand open; place open hand next to glass; flex fingers around glass; move arm and hand holding glass vertically; flex arm toward body).
> 5. Focus on gross functional movements initially, and gradually include activities that use finer motions (e.g., buttoning clothes, eating with a fork).
>
> The nurse should also be sure to:
>
> 1. Specify the approach selected to accomplish the task on the patient's plan of care and the patient's level of accomplishment on the progress notes.
> 2. Encourage the patient to perform the activity up to maximal capacity within the limitations of the disability.
> 3. Monitor the patient's tolerance.
> 4. Minimize frustration and fatigue.
> 5. Support the patient by giving appropriate praise for effort put forth and for acts accomplished.
> 6. Assist the patient to perform and practice the activity in real-life situations and in a safe environment.

Preexisting cultural norms may influence the degree of self-care the patient is willing to consider. Cultural and ethnic beliefs about hygiene can vary among individuals and families. The nurse must recognize these beliefs, work through any issues with the patient and family, and communicate pertinent findings to the rehabilitation team.

RECOMMENDING ADAPTIVE AND ASSISTIVE DEVICES

If the patient has difficulty performing an ADL, an adaptive or assistive device (self-help device) may be useful. Such devices may be obtained commercially or can be constructed by the nurse, occupational therapist, patient, or family. The devices may include built-up handles on toothbrushes or razors; long, curved handles on mirrors or shoe horns; suction cups to hold items in place; shower chairs; raised toilet seats; and universal cuffs to grip self-care items. Some of these are shown in Figure 2-1. To assist premenopausal women with managing menstruation, clothing adaptations (e.g., Velcro crotch flaps for ease of access), mirrors, self-sticking sanitary pads, packaged wipes, and loose underwear may be used.

> ### ◤ Quality and Safety Nursing Alert
>
> *To avoid injury or bleeding, people who take anticoagulant medication should be encouraged to use an electric razor. Women may wish to consider depilatory creams or electrolysis.*

A wide selection of computerized devices is available, or devices can be designed to help individual patients with severe disability to function more independently. The Able-Data project (see Resources list at the end of this chapter) offers a computerized listing of commercially available aids and equipment for patients with disability.

The nurse should be alert to "gadgets" coming on the market and evaluate their potential usefulness. The nurse must exercise professional judgment and caution in recommending devices, because in the past, unscrupulous vendors have marketed unnecessary, overly expensive, or useless items to patients.

HELPING PATIENTS ACCEPT LIMITATIONS

If the patient has a severe disability, independent self-care may be an unrealistic goal. In this situation, the nurse educates the patient how to take charge by directing their care. The patient may require a personal caregiver to perform ADLs. Family members may not be appropriate for providing bathing/hygiene, dressing/grooming, feeding, and toileting assistance, and spouses may have difficulty providing bowel and bladder care for patients and maintaining the role of sexual partners. If a personal caregiver is necessary, the patient and family members must learn how to manage an employee effectively. The nurse helps the patient accept self-care dependency. Independence in other areas, such as social interaction, should be emphasized to promote a positive self-concept.

ENSURING EFFECTIVE HEALTH MANAGEMENT

The nurse ensures effective health management by educating the patient and caregiver in appropriate language so that they understand the nature of the health condition or disorder and the resulting changes in ADLs. This understanding facilitates transition to a new way of life upon discharge. Barriers that may impede successful health maintenance are identified and strategies employed to mitigate them. The transition team, under the guidance of the nurse, collaborates on identifying and securing resources that are needed to make the transition successful and prevent complications (Carpenito, 2017).

Evaluation

Expected patient outcomes may include:
1. Demonstrates independent self-care in bathing/hygiene or with assistance, using adaptive devices as appropriate
   a. Bathes self at maximal level of independence
   b. Uses adaptive and assistive devices effectively
   c. Reports satisfaction with level of independence in bathing/hygiene

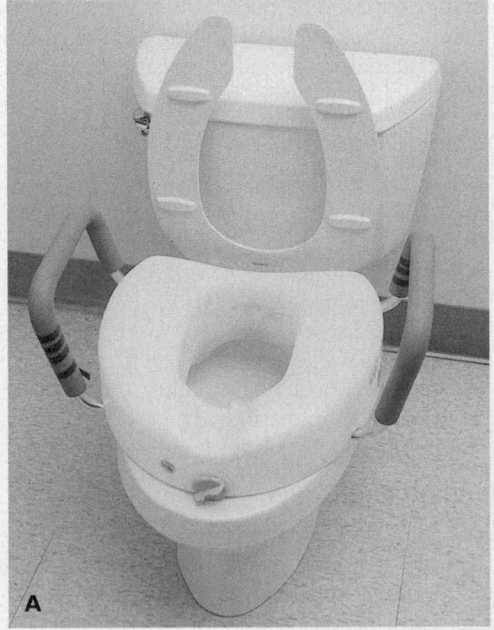
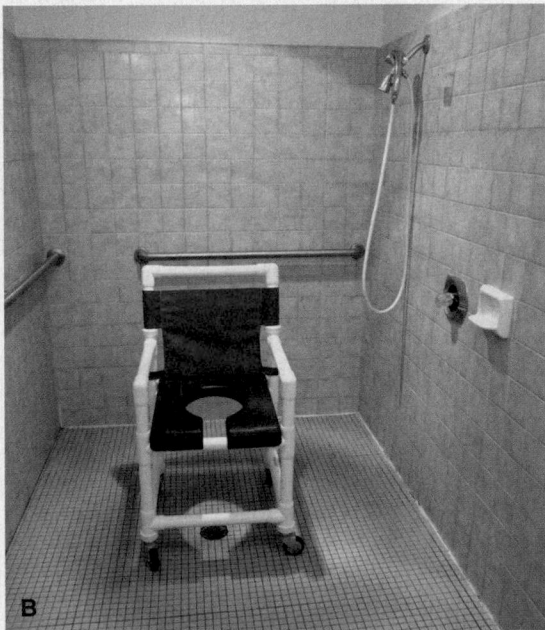

Figure 2-1 • Adaptive and assistive devices. **A.** Raised toilet seat. **B.** Shower chair.

2. Demonstrates independent self-care in dressing/grooming or with assistance, using adaptive devices as appropriate
   a. Dresses/grooms self at maximal level of independence
   b. Uses adaptive devices effectively
   c. Reports satisfaction with level of independence in dressing/grooming
   d. Demonstrates increased interest in appearance
3. Demonstrates independent self-care in feeding or with assistance, using adaptive and assistive devices as appropriate
   a. Feeds self at maximal level of independence
   b. Uses adaptive and assistive devices effectively
   c. Demonstrates increased interest in eating
   d. Maintains adequate nutritional intake
4. Demonstrates independent self-care in toileting or with assistance, using adaptive and assistive devices as appropriate
   a. Toilets self at maximal level of independence
   b. Uses adaptive and assistive devices effectively
   c. Indicates positive feelings regarding level of toileting independence
   d. Experiences adequate frequency of bowel and bladder elimination
   e. Does not experience incontinence, constipation, urinary tract infection, or other complications
5. Demonstrates knowledge about effective health maintenance
   a. Verbalizes knowledge of health problem/disorder and resulting changes in functional abilities and lifestyle
   b. Identifies and secures resources needed to maintain health upon discharge

NURSING PROCESS

The Patient with Impaired Physical Mobility

Problems commonly associated with immobility include weakened muscles, joint contracture, and deformity. Each joint of the body has a normal range of motion; if the range is limited, the functions of the joint and the muscles that move the joint are impaired, and painful deformities may develop. The nurse must identify patients at risk for such complications. The nurse needs to assess, plan, and intervene to prevent complications of immobility.

Another problem frequently seen in rehabilitation nursing is an altered ambulatory/mobility pattern. Patients with disability may be either temporarily or permanently unable to walk independently and unaided. The nurse assesses the mobility of the patient and designs care that promotes independent mobility within the prescribed therapeutic limits. If a patient cannot exercise and move his or her joints through their full range of motion, contractures may develop. A contracture is a shortening of the muscle and tendon that leads to deformity and limits joint mobility. When the contracted joint is moved, the patient experiences pain; in addition, more energy is required to move when joints are contracted.

Disability brings change to the patient and family unit as well as adjustments in lifestyle, mobility, and interactions as members of a community. Whether temporary or permanent, patients can grieve the loss of health and will need to process the loss as part of the adaptation process and plan of care (Carpenito, 2017).

Assessment

Mobility may be restricted owing to pain, paralysis, loss of muscle strength, systemic disease, an immobilizing device (e.g., cast, brace), or prescribed limits to promote healing. Assessment of mobility includes positioning, ability to move, muscle strength and tone, joint function, and the prescribed mobility limits. The nurse must collaborate with physical therapists or other team members to assess mobility.

During position change, transfer, and ambulation activities, the nurse assesses the patient's abilities, the extent of disability, and residual capacity for physiologic adaptation. The nurse observes for orthostatic hypotension, pallor, diaphoresis, nausea, tachycardia, and fatigue.

In addition, the nurse assesses the patient's ability to use various assistive devices that promote mobility. If the patient cannot ambulate without assistance, the nurse assesses the patient's ability to balance, transfer, and use assistive devices (e.g., crutches, walker). Crutch walking requires high energy expenditure and produces considerable cardiovascular stress; therefore, people with reduced exercise capacity, decreased arm strength, and problems with balance because of aging or multiple diseases may be unable to use crutches. A walker is more stable and may be a better choice for such patients. If the patient uses an orthosis, the nurse monitors the patient for effective use and potential problems associated with its use.

The assessment process includes gaining an understanding of the meaning of illness or disability for the patient and family, whether it be a temporary or permanent loss of normal functioning or lifestyle. Signs and symptoms evidenced by the patient or family members such as disbelief, crying, expressions of emotions such as sorrow and anger can be part of the grieving process. The nurse collaborates with the interdisciplinary team to develop a holistic plan of care that addresses relevant actual or potential nursing diagnoses (Carpenito, 2017).

Nursing Diagnosis

Based on the assessment data, major nursing diagnoses may include the following:
- Impaired mobility
- Activity intolerance or risk for activity intolerance
- Risk for injury
- Risk for disuse
- Impaired walking
- Impaired wheelchair mobility
- Impaired mobility in bed
- Grief

Planning and Goals

Major goals for the patient may include absence of contracture and deformity, maintenance of muscle strength and joint mobility, independent mobility, increased activity tolerance, and prevention of further disability. A major goal for the patient and family may include that they express an understanding of the meaning of the illness or disability and its associated losses.

Nursing Interventions

POSITIONING TO PREVENT MUSCULOSKELETAL COMPLICATIONS

Deformities and contractures can often be prevented by proper positioning. Maintaining correct body alignment when the patient is in bed is essential regardless of the position selected. During each patient contact, the nurse evaluates the patient's position and assists the patient to achieve and maintain proper positioning and alignment. The most common positions that patients assume in bed are supine (dorsal), side-lying (lateral), and prone. The nurse helps the patient assume these positions and uses pillows to support the body in correct alignment. At times, a splint (e.g., wrist or hand splint) may be made by the occupational therapist to support a joint and prevent deformity. The nurse must ensure proper use of the splint and provide skin care.

Preventing External Rotation of the Hip. The patient who is in bed for an extended period of time may develop external rotation deformity of the hip because the ball-and-socket joint of the hip tends to rotate outward when the patient lies on their back. A trochanter roll (i.e., a flannel sheet or bath towel folded in thirds lengthwise and rolled toward the patient or a commercially manufactured roll) extending from the crest of the ilium to the midthigh prevents this deformity; with correct placement, it serves as a mechanical wedge under the projection of the greater trochanter.

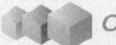 **Concept Mastery Alert**

Abduction moves the body part away from the body; adduction moves the body part toward the body. External rotation occurs as the leg moves outward. To prevent external rotation deformity, the patient's hip should *not* be abducted or moved away from the body.

Preventing Footdrop. Footdrop is a deformity in which the foot is plantar flexed (the ankle bends in the direction of the sole of the foot). If the condition continues without correction, the patient will not be able to hold the foot in a normal position and will be able to walk only on their toes, without touching the ground with the heel of the foot. The deformity is caused by contracture of both the gastrocnemius and soleus muscles. Damage to the peroneal nerve or loss of flexibility of the Achilles tendon may also result in footdrop. To prevent this disabling deformity, the patient is positioned to sit at a 90-degree angle in a wheelchair with the feet on the footrests or flat on the floor.

When the patient is supine in bed, padded splints or protective boots are used to keep the patient's feet at right angles to the legs. Frequent skin inspection of the feet must also be performed to determine whether positioning devices have created any unwanted pressure areas.

The patient is encouraged to perform the following ankle exercises several times each hour: dorsiflexion and plantar flexion of the feet, flexion and extension (curl and stretch) of the toes, and eversion and inversion of the feet at the ankles. The nurse provides frequent passive range-of-motion exercises if the patient cannot perform active exercises.

> ▶ *Quality and Safety Nursing Alert*
>
> *Prolonged bed rest, lack of exercise, incorrect positioning in bed, and the weight of bedding that forces the toes into plantar flexion must be avoided to prevent footdrop. Patients should be encouraged to wear shoes for support and protection to prevent footdrop.*

MAINTAINING MUSCLE STRENGTH AND JOINT MOBILITY

Optimal function depends on the strength of the muscles and joint motion, and active participation in ADLs promotes maintenance of muscle strength and joint mobility. Range-of-motion exercises and specific therapeutic exercises may be included in the nursing plan of care.

Performing Range-of-Motion Exercises. Range of motion involves moving a joint through its full range in all appropriate planes (Chart 2-4). To maintain or increase the motion of a joint, range-of-motion exercises are initiated as soon as the patient's condition permits. The exercises are planned for individual patients to accommodate the wide variation in the degrees of motion that people of varying body builds and age groups can attain.

Range-of-motion exercises may be active (performed by the patient under the supervision of the nurse), assisted (with the nurse helping if the patient cannot do the exercise independently), or passive (performed by the nurse). Unless otherwise prescribed, a joint should be moved through its range of motion three times, at least two times a day. The joint to be exercised is supported, the bones above the joint are stabilized, and the body part distal to the joint is moved through the range of motion of the joint. For example, the humerus must be stabilized while the radius and ulna are moved through their range of motion at the elbow joint.

A joint should not be moved beyond its free range of motion; the joint is moved to the point of resistance and stopped at the point of pain. If muscle spasms are present,

Chart 2-4	Range-of-Motion Terminology

Abduction: movement away from the midline of the body
Adduction: movement toward the midline of the body
Flexion: bending of a joint so that the angle of the joint diminishes
Extension: the return movement from flexion; the joint angle is increased
Rotation: turning or movement of a part around its axis
Internal: turning inward, toward the center
External: turning outward, away from the center
Dorsiflexion: movement that flexes or bends the hand back toward the body or the foot toward the leg
Palmar flexion: movement that flexes or bends the hand in the direction of the palm
Plantar flexion: movement that flexes or bends the foot in the direction of the sole
Pronation: rotation of the forearm so that the palm of the hand is down
Supination: rotation of the forearm so that the palm of the hand is up
Opposition: touching the thumb to each fingertip on same hand
Inversion: movement that turns the sole of the foot inward
Eversion: movement that turns the sole of the foot outward

the joint is moved slowly to the point of resistance. Gentle, steady pressure is then applied until the muscle relaxes, and the motion is continued to the joint's final point of resistance.

To perform assisted or passive range-of-motion exercises, the patient must be in a comfortable supine position with the arms at the sides and the knees extended. Good body posture is maintained during the exercises. The nurse also uses good body mechanics during the exercise session.

Performing Therapeutic Exercises. Therapeutic exercises are prescribed by the primary provider and performed with the assistance and guidance of the physical therapist or nurse. The patient should have a clear understanding of the goal of the prescribed exercise. Written instructions about the frequency, duration, and number of repetitions, as well as simple line drawings of the exercise, help to ensure adherence to the exercise program. Return demonstration of the exercises also helps the patient and family to follow the instructions correctly.

When performed correctly, exercise assists in maintaining and building muscle strength, maintaining joint function, preventing deformity, stimulating circulation, developing endurance, and promoting relaxation. Exercise is also valuable in helping to restore motivation and the well-being of the patient. Weight-bearing exercises may slow the bone loss that occurs with disability. There are five types of exercise: passive, active-assistive, active, resistive, and isometric. The description, purpose, and action of each of these exercises are summarized in Table 2-1.

PROMOTING INDEPENDENT MOBILITY

When the patient's condition stabilizes, their physical condition permits, and the patient is able to stand, the patient is assisted to sit up on the side of the bed and then to stand.

Tolerance of this activity is assessed. Orthostatic (postural) hypotension may develop when the patient assumes a vertical position. Because of inadequate vasomotor reflexes, blood pools in the splanchnic (visceral or intestinal) area and in the legs, resulting in inadequate cerebral circulation. If indicators of orthostatic hypotension (e.g., drop in blood pressure, pallor, diaphoresis, nausea, tachycardia, dizziness) are present, the activity is stopped, and the patient is assisted to a supine position in bed.

Some disabling conditions, such as spinal cord injury (SCI), acute brain injury, and other conditions that require extended periods in the recumbent position, prevent the patient from assuming an upright position at the bedside. Several strategies can be used to help the patient assume a 90-degree sitting position. A reclining wheelchair with elevating leg rests allows a slow and controlled progression from a supine position to a 90-degree sitting position. A tilt table (a board that can be tilted in 10-degree increments from a horizontal to a vertical position) may also be used. The tilt table promotes vasomotor adjustment to positional changes and helps patients with limited standing balance and limited weight-bearing activities avoid the decalcification of bones and low bone mass associated with disuse syndrome and lack of weight-bearing exercise. Physical therapists may use a tilt table for patients who have not been upright owing to illness or disability. Gradual elevation of the head of the bed may help. When getting patients with SCI out of bed, it is important to gradually raise the head of the bed to a 90-degree angle; this may take approximately 10 to 15 minutes.

Graduated compression stockings are used to prevent venous stasis. For some patients, a compression garment (leotard) or snug-fitting abdominal binder and elastic compression bandaging of the legs are needed to prevent venous stasis

TABLE 2-1	Therapeutic Exercises		
	Description	**Purposes**	**Action**
Passive	An exercise carried out by the therapist or the nurse without assistance from the patient	To retain as much joint range of motion as possible; to maintain circulation	Stabilize the proximal joint and support the distal part; move the joint smoothly, slowly, and gently through its full range of motion; avoid producing pain.
Active-assistive	An exercise carried out by the patient with the assistance of the therapist or the nurse	To encourage normal muscle function	Support the distal part, and encourage the patient to take the joint actively through its range of motion; give no more assistance than is necessary to accomplish the action; short periods of activity should be followed by adequate rest periods.
Active	An exercise accomplished by the patient without assistance; activities include turning from side to side and from back to abdomen and moving up and down in bed	To increase muscle strength	When possible, active exercise should be performed against gravity; the joint is moved through full range of motion without assistance; make sure that the patient does not substitute another joint movement for the one intended.
Resistive	An active exercise carried out by the patient working against resistance produced by either manual or mechanical means	To provide resistance to increase muscle power	The patient moves the joint through its range of motion, while the therapist resists slightly at first and then with progressively increasing resistance; sandbags and weights can be used and are applied at the distal point of the involved joint; the movements should be performed smoothly.
Isometric or muscle setting	Alternately contracting and relaxing a muscle while keeping the part in a fixed position; this exercise is performed by the patient	To maintain strength when a joint is immobilized	Contract or tighten the muscle as much as possible without moving the joint, hold for several seconds, then let go and relax; breathe deeply.

and orthostatic hypotension. When the patient is standing, the feet are protected with a pair of properly fitted shoes. Extended periods of standing are avoided because of venous pooling and pressure on the soles of the feet. The nurse monitors the patient's blood pressure and pulse and observes for signs and symptoms of orthostatic hypotension and cerebral insufficiency (e.g., the patient reports feeling faint and weak), which suggest intolerance of the upright position. If the patient does not tolerate the upright position, the nurse should return the patient to the reclining position and elevate their legs.

Assisting Patients with Transfer. A **transfer** is movement of the patient from one place to another (e.g., bed to chair, chair to commode, wheelchair to tub). As soon as the patient is permitted out of bed, transfer activities are started. The nurse assesses the patient's ability to participate actively in the transfer and determines, in conjunction with occupational therapists or physical therapists, the adaptive equipment required to promote independence and safety. A lightweight wheelchair with brake extensions, removable and detachable armrests, and leg rests minimize structural obstacles during the transfer. Tub seats or benches make transfers in and out of the tub easier and safer. Raised, padded commode seats may also be warranted for patients who must avoid flexing the hips greater than 90 degrees when transferring to a toilet. It is important that the nurse educate the patient about hip precautions (e.g., no adduction past the midline, no flexion greater than 90 degrees, and no internal rotation); abduction pillows can be used to keep the hip in correct alignment if precautions are warranted.

It is important that the patient maintains muscle strength and, if possible, performs push-up exercises to strengthen the arm and shoulder extensor muscles. The push-up exercises require the patient to sit upright in bed; a book is placed under each of the patient's hands to provide a hard surface, and the patient is instructed to push down on the book, raising the body. The nurse should encourage the patient to raise and move the body in different directions by means of these push-up exercises.

The nurse or physical therapist instructs the patient how to transfer. There are several methods of transferring from the bed to the wheelchair when the patient cannot stand, and the technique chosen should consider the patient's abilities and disability. It is helpful to demonstrate the technique to the patient. If the physical therapist is involved in teaching the patient to transfer, the nurse and physical therapist must collaborate so that consistent instructions are given to the patient. During transfer, the nurse assists and coaches the patient. Figure 2-2 shows weight-bearing and non–weight-bearing transfers. For example, with a weight-bearing transfer from bed to chair, the patient stands up, pivots until his back is opposite the new seat, and sits down. If the patient's muscles are not strong enough to overcome the resistance of body weight, a polished lightweight board (transfer board, sliding board) may be used to bridge the gap between the bed and the chair. The patient slides across on the board with or without assistance from a caregiver. This board may also be used to transfer the patient from the chair to the toilet or bathtub bench. It is important to avoid the effects of shear on the patient's skin while sliding across the board. The nurse should make sure that the patient's fingers do not curl around the edge of the board during the transfer, because the patient's body weight can crush the fingers as they move across the board.

Safety is a primary concern during a transfer, and the following guidelines are recommended:

- Wheelchairs and beds must be locked before transfer begins.
- Detachable arm- and footrests are removed to make getting in and out of the chair easier.
- One end of the transfer board is placed under the buttocks and the other end on the surface to which the transfer is being made (e.g., the chair).
- The patient is instructed to lean forward, push up with his or her hands, and then slide across the board to the other surface.

Nurses frequently assist patients who are weak and incapacitated out of bed. The nurse supports and gently assists the patient during position changes, protecting the patient from injury. The nurse avoids pulling on a weak or paralyzed upper extremity to prevent dislocation of the shoulder. The patient is assisted to move toward the stronger side.

In the home setting, getting in and out of bed and performing chair, toilet, and tub transfers are difficult for patients with weak muscles and loss of hip, knee, and ankle motion. A rope attached to the headboard of the bed enables a patient to move toward the center of the bed, and the use of a rope attached to the footboard facilitates getting in and out of bed. The height of a chair can be raised with cushions on the seat or with hollowed-out blocks placed under the chair legs. Grab bars can be attached to the wall near the toilet and tub to provide leverage and stability.

Preparing for Ambulation. Regaining the ability to walk is a prime morale builder. However, to be prepared for ambulation—whether with a brace, walker, cane, or crutches—the patient must strengthen the muscles required. Therefore, exercise is the foundation of preparation. The nurse and physical therapist instruct and supervise the patient in these exercises.

For ambulation, the quadriceps muscles, which stabilize the knee joint, and the gluteal muscles are strengthened. To perform quadriceps-setting exercises, the patient contracts the quadriceps muscle by attempting to push the popliteal area against the mattress and at the same time raising the heel. The patient maintains the muscle contraction for a count of five and relaxes for a count of five. The exercise is repeated 10 to 15 times hourly. Exercising the quadriceps muscles prevents flexion contractures of the knee. In gluteal setting, the patient contracts or "pinches" the buttocks together for a count of five, relaxes for a count of five; the exercise is repeated 10 to 15 times hourly.

If assistive devices (i.e., walker, cane, crutches) will be used, the muscles of the upper extremities are exercised and strengthened. Push-up exercises are especially useful. While in a sitting position, the patient raises the body by pushing the hands against the chair seat or mattress. The patient should be encouraged to do push-up exercises while in a prone position as well. Pull-up exercises done on a trapeze while lifting the body are also effective for conditioning. The patient is taught to raise the arms above the head and then lower them in a slow, rhythmic manner while holding weights. Gradually, the weight is increased. The hands are strengthened by squeezing a rubber ball.

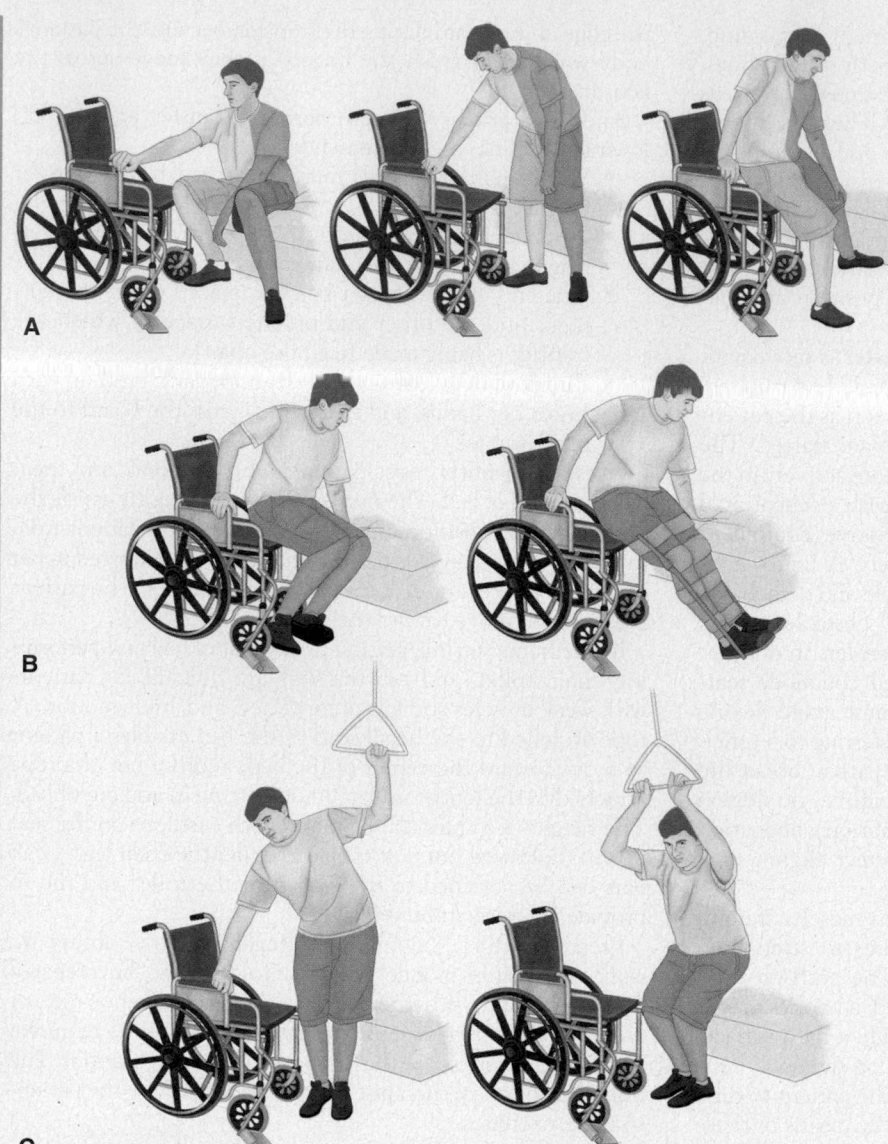

Figure 2-2 • Methods of patient transfer from the bed to a wheelchair. The wheelchair is in a locked position. Colored areas indicate non–weight-bearing body parts. **A.** Weight-bearing transfer from bed to chair. The patient stands up, pivots until his back is opposite the new seat, and sits down. **B. (Left)** Non–weight-bearing transfer from chair to bed. **(Right)** With legs braced. **C. (Left)** Non–weight-bearing transfer, combined method. **(Right)** Non–weight-bearing transfer, pull-up method. One of the wheelchair arms is removed to make getting in and out of the chair easier.

Typically, the physical therapist designs exercises to help the patient develop sitting and standing balance, stability, and coordination needed for ambulation. After sitting and standing balance is achieved, the patient is able to use parallel bars. Under the supervision of the physical therapist, the patient practices shifting weight from side to side, lifting one leg while supporting weight on the other, and then walking between the parallel bars.

A patient who is ready to begin ambulation must be fitted with the appropriate assistive device, instructed about the prescribed weight-bearing limits (e.g., non–weight-bearing, partial weight-bearing ambulation), and taught how to use the device safely. Figure 2-3 illustrates some of the more common assistive devices used in rehabilitation settings. The nurse continually assesses the patient for stability and adherence to weight-bearing precautions and protects the patient from falling. The nurse provides contact guarding by holding on to a gait belt that the patient wears around the waist. The patient should wear sturdy, well-fitting shoes and be advised of the dangers of wet or highly polished floors and throw rugs.

The patient should also learn how to ambulate on inclines, uneven surfaces, and stairs.

AMBULATING WITH AN ASSISTIVE DEVICE: CRUTCHES, A WALKER, OR A CANE

Crutches are for partial weight-bearing or non–weight-bearing ambulation. Good balance, adequate cardiovascular reserve, strong upper extremities, and erect posture are essential for crutch walking. Ambulating a functional distance (at least the length of a room or house) or maneuvering stairs on crutches requires significant arm strength, because the arms must bear the patient's weight (Fig. 2-4). The nurse or physical therapist determines which gait is best (Chart 2-5).

A walker provides more support and stability than a cane or crutches. A pick-up walker is best for patients with poor balance and poor cardiovascular reserve, and a rolling walker, which allows automatic walking, is best for patients who cannot lift. A cane helps the patient walk with balance and support and relieves the pressure on weight-bearing joints by redistributing weight.

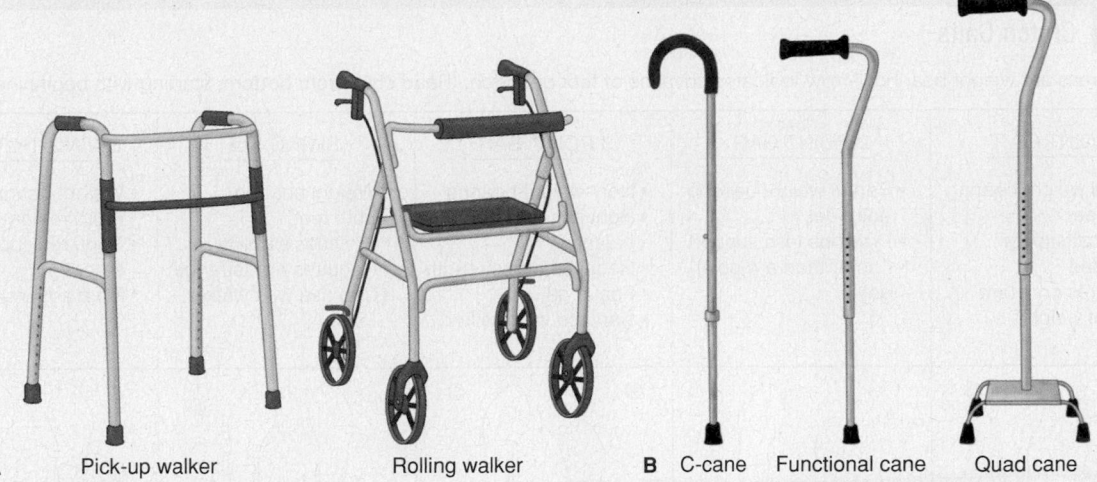

A   Pick-up walker   Rolling walker   **B** C-cane   Functional cane   Quad cane

Figure 2-3 • Mechanical aids to walking. **A.** Two types of walkers: pick-up and rolling. **B.** Three types of canes: C-cane, functional cane, and quad cane.

Before patients can be considered to be independent in walking with crutches, a walker, or a cane, they should learn to sit, stand from sitting, and go up and down stairs using the device. Table 2-2 describes how patients can ambulate and maneuver using each of the three devices and nursing actions to support using assistive devices.

ASSISTING PATIENTS WITH AN ORTHOSIS OR PROSTHESIS

Orthoses and prostheses are designed to facilitate mobilization and to maximize the patient's quality of life. An **orthosis** is an external appliance that provides support, prevents or corrects deformities, and improves function. Orthoses include braces, splints, collars, corsets, and supports that are designed and fitted by orthotists or prosthetists. Static orthoses (no moving parts) are used to stabilize joints and prevent contractures.

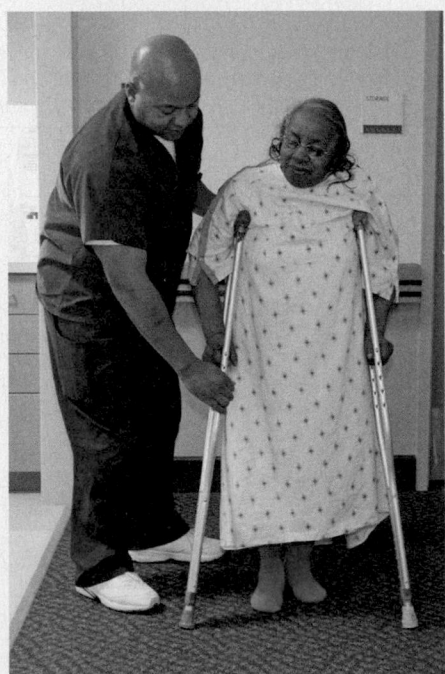

Figure 2-4 • For a person walking with crutches, the tripod stance, with crutches out to the sides and in front of the toes, increases stability.

Dynamic orthoses are flexible and are used to improve function by assisting weak muscles. A **prosthesis** is an artificial body part that may be internal, such as an artificial knee or hip joint, or external, such as an artificial leg or arm.

In addition to learning how to apply and remove the orthosis and maneuver the affected body part correctly, patients must learn how to properly care for the skin that comes in contact with the appliance. Skin problems or pressure injuries may develop if the device is applied too tightly or too loosely, or if it is adjusted improperly. The nurse instructs the patient to clean and inspect the skin daily, to make sure the brace fits snugly without being too tight, to check that the padding distributes pressure evenly, and to wear a cotton garment without seams between the orthosis and the skin.

If the patient has had an amputation, the nurse promotes tissue healing, uses compression dressings to promote residual limb shaping, and minimizes contracture formation. A permanent prosthetic limb cannot be fitted until the tissue has healed completely and the residual limb shape is stable and free from edema. The nurse also helps the patient cope with the emotional issues surrounding loss of a limb and encourages acceptance of the prosthesis. The prosthetist, nurse, and primary provider collaborate to provide instructions related to skin care and care of the prosthesis.

SUPPORTING THE GRIEVING PROCESS

Developing a trusting nurse–patient relationship provides an opportunity to support patients and families as they grieve and process the meaning of the illness or disability, whether it be a temporary or permanent loss of normal functioning and lifestyle. The nurse helps the grieving process by providing clear, simple communications that do not minimize the loss. The nurse also educates the patient and family about the grieving process, normal grief reactions, and signs and symptoms of complicated grieving. Time should be planned to share feelings in a safe setting which provides needed privacy. In many cases, just being present and listening supports the grieving process. Patients and families may benefit from community resources such as support groups as well as connection to their local faith community for spiritual support through the changes associated with disability (Carpenito, 2017).

(*text continued on page 48*)

Chart 2-5 Crutch Gaits

Shaded areas are weight bearing. Arrow indicates advance of foot or crutch. (Read chart from bottom, starting with beginning stance.)

4-POINT GAIT	2-POINT GAIT	3-POINT GAIT	SWING-TO	SWING-THROUGH
• Partial weight bearing both feet • Maximal support provided • Requires constant shift of weight	• Partial weight bearing both feet • Provides less support • Faster than a 4-point gait	• Non–weight bearing • Requires good balance • Requires arm strength • Faster gait • Can use with walker	• Weight bearing both feet • Provides stability • Requires arm strength • Can use with walker	• Weight bearing • Requires arm strength • Requires coordination/balance • Most advanced gait
4. Advance right foot	4. Advance right foot and left crutch	4. Advance right foot	4. Lift both feet/swing forward/land feet next to crutches	4. Lift both feet/swing forward/land feet in front of crutches
3. Advance left crutch	3. Advance left foot and right crutch	3. Advance left foot and both crutches	3. Advance both crutches	3. Advance both crutches
2. Advance left foot	2. Advance right foot and left crutch	2. Advance right foot	2. Lift both feet/swing forward/land feet next to crutches	2. Lift both feet/swing forward/land feet in front of crutches
1. Advance right crutch	1. Advance left foot and right crutch	1. Advance left foot and both crutches	1. Advance both crutches	1. Advance both crutches
Beginning stance	Beginning stance	Beginning stance	Beginning stance	Beginning stance

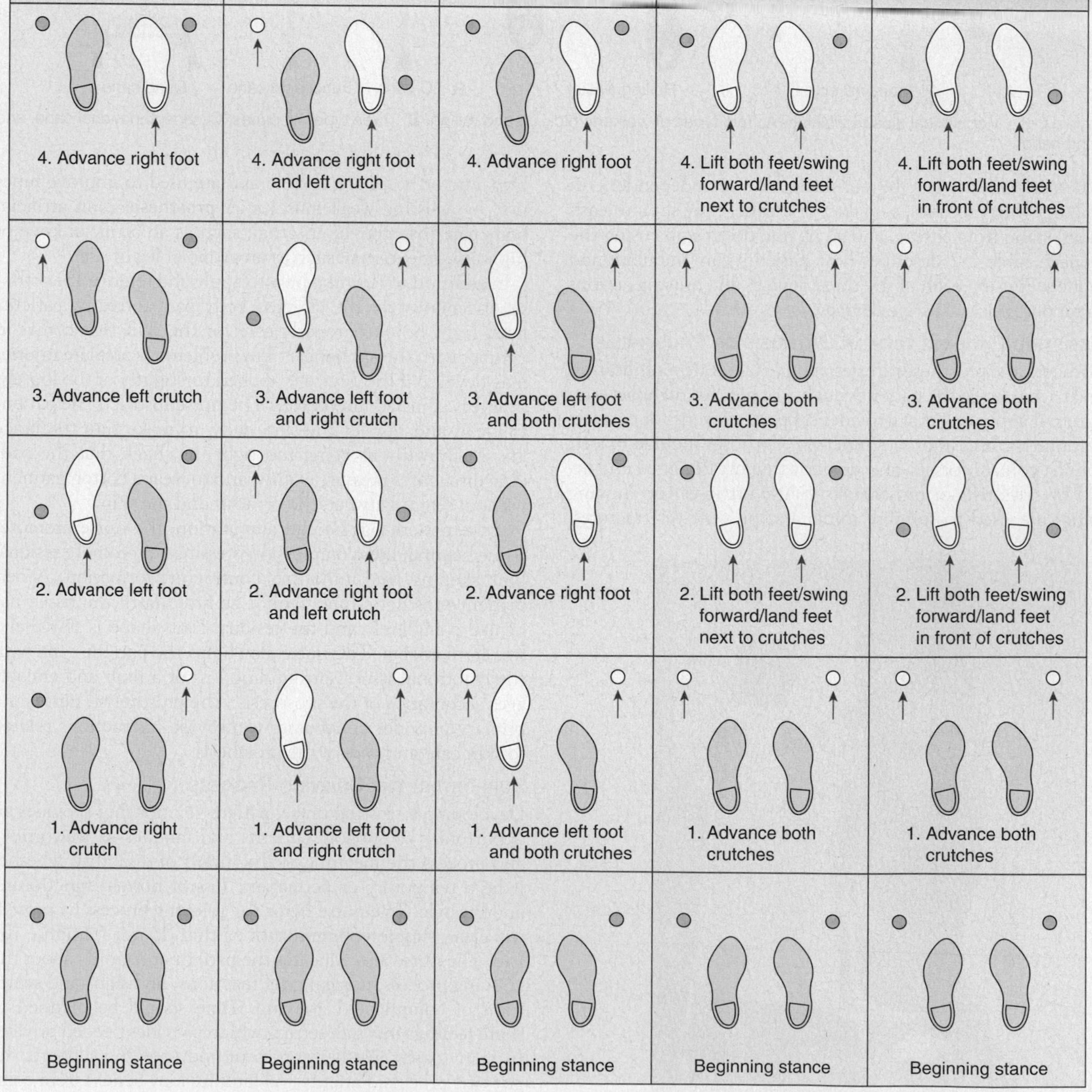

TABLE 2-2	Nursing Actions Involved in Using Assistive Devices		
	Crutches	**Walker**	**Cane**
Patient Preparation Adjusting device to fit patient	Measure patient standing or lying down: If standing, set crutch length approximately 5 cm (2 inches) below axilla. If lying down, measure from anterior fold of axilla to sole of the foot and add 5 cm. If using patient's height, subtract 40 cm (16 inches) to obtain crutch height. Adjust hand grip to allow 20 to 30 degrees of flexion at elbow. Use foam rubber pad on underarm piece to relieve pressure of crutch.	Adjust height to individual patient. Patient's arms should be in 20 to 30 degrees of flexion at elbows when hands are resting on hand grips.	With patient flexing elbow at 30-degree angle, hold handle of cane level with greater trochanter and place tip of cane 15 cm (6 inches) lateral to base of 5th toe. Fit cane with gently flaring tip that has flexible, concentric rings to provide stability, absorb shock, and enable greater speed and less fatigue with walking.
Assessment	Assess safety. Crutches should have large rubber tips, and patients should wear firm-soled, well-fitting shoes. Assess balance by asking patient to stand on unaffected leg by a chair. Assess stability and stamina (tolerance). Sweating and shortness of breath indicate that rest is necessary.	Assess safety. Patients should wear firm-soled, well-fitting shoes. Assess stability and stamina (tolerance). Sweating and shortness of breath indicate that rest is necessary.	Assess safety. Patients should wear firm-soled, well-fitting shoes. Assess stability and stamina (tolerance). Sweating and shortness of breath indicate that rest is necessary.
Interventions and patient education	Assist with balance by using a transfer belt or holding patient near waist. Have patient practice shifting weight and maintaining balance. Protect patient from falls. To maximize stability, encourage patient to use tripod stance, with crutches to the front and sides of toes. Have patient perform prescribed preparatory exercises to strengthen shoulder girdle and upper extremity muscles.[a]	Walk with patient, holding at waist if needed for balance. Instruct patient to never pull self up using walker and to look up when walking. Discuss full, partial, or non–weight bearing as prescribed. Protect patient from falls.	Walk with patient, holding at waist if needed for balance. Have patient hold cane in hand opposite to affected extremity, if possible, to widen the base of support and reduce stress on involved extremity. Instruct patient to move opposite arm and leg together. Protect patient from falls.
Ambulation Gait/action used	Determine which gait is best (see Chart 2-5, Tripod Gait)[b] Four-point Three-point Two-point Swing-to Swing-through	Instruct patient to: Pick-up walker: lift device and move it forward with each step. Rolling walker: roll device forward and walk automatically.	Instruct patient to: Advance cane at same time that affected leg is moved forward. Keep cane fairly close to body to prevent leaning. Bear down on cane when unaffected extremity begins swing phase.
Sitting	Instruct patient to: Grasp hand-piece for control. Bend forward slightly while assuming sitting position. Place affected leg forward to prevent weight bearing and flexion while sitting.	Instruct patient to hold walker on hand grips for stability.	
Standing	Instruct patient to: Move forward to edge of chair, and keep unaffected leg slightly under seat. Place both crutches on side of affected extremity. Push down on hand-piece while rising to standing position.	Instruct patient to: Push off chair or bed to come to a standing position. Rolling walker: if walker has a brake, apply it before standing. Lift walker, placing it in front of self while leaning slightly forward. Walk into walker, supporting weight on hands when advancing. Balance on feet. Lift walker and place it in front of self again.	Instruct patient to: Push off chair or bed to come to a standing position. Hold cane for stability. Step forward on unaffected extremity. Swing cane and affected extremity forward in a normal walking gait.
Going down stairs	Instruct patient to: Walk forward as far as possible. Advance crutches to lower step; advance affected leg, then unaffected leg.	Continue pattern.	Instruct patient to: Step down on affected extremity. Place the cane and then unaffected extremity on down step.
Going up stairs	Instruct patient to: Advance unaffected leg first up next step. Advance crutches and affected extremity. Unaffected leg goes up first.	n/a	Instruct patient to: Step up on unaffected extremity. Place cane and affected extremity up on step.

[a]For patients who cannot support their weight through the wrist and hand because of arthritis or fracture, platform crutches that support the forearm and allow the weight to be borne through the elbow are available. If weight is borne on the axilla, the pressure of the crutch can damage the brachial plexus nerves, producing "crutch paralysis."
[b]Teach patients two gaits so that they can change from one to another to avoid fatigue. In addition, a faster gait can be used when walking an uninterrupted distance, and a slower gait can be used for shorter distances or in crowded places.
n/a, not applicable.

Evaluation

Expected patient outcomes may include:

1. Demonstrates improved physical mobility
   a. Maintains muscle strength and joint mobility
   b. Does not develop contractures
   c. Participates in exercise program
2. Transfers safely
   a. Demonstrates assisted transfers
   b. Performs independent transfers
3. Ambulates with maximum independence
   a. Uses ambulatory aid safely
   b. Adheres to weight-bearing prescription
   c. Requests assistance as needed
4. Demonstrates increased activity tolerance
   a. Does not experience episodes of orthostatic hypotension
   b. Reports absence of fatigue with ambulatory efforts
   c. Gradually increases distance and speed of ambulation
5. Patient and family members verbalize loss and express feelings of grief
   a. Describe the meaning of the loss as it relates to function or lifestyle
   b. Share grief with each other and those who are important to well-being
   c. Acquire knowledge of resources for support after discharge

Promoting Home, Community-Based, and Transitional Care

An important goal of rehabilitation is to assist the patient to return to the home environment after learning to manage the disability. A referral system maintains continuity of care when the patient is transferred to the home or to a long-term care facility. The plan for discharge is formulated when the patient is first admitted to the hospital, and discharge plans are made with the patient's functional potential in mind.

 ### Educating Patients About Self-Care

Significant expenditures of time and resources are necessary to ensure that patients gain the skills and confidence to self-manage their health effectively after discharge from the hospital (Naylor, Shaid, Carpenter, et al., 2017). Formal programs provide patients with effective strategies for interpreting and managing disease-specific issues and skills needed for problem solving, as well as building and maintaining self-awareness and self-efficacy. Self-care programs often use multifaceted approaches, including didactic teaching, group sessions, individual learning plans, and Web-based resources. When planning the approach to self-care, the nurse must consider the individual patient's knowledge, experience, social and cultural background, level of formal education, and psychological status. The preparation for self-care must also be spread out over the course of the recovery period, and it must be monitored and updated regularly as the patient masters aspects of self-care. Preparation for self-care is also highly relevant for informal caregivers of patients in rehabilitation.

When a patient is discharged from acute care or a rehabilitation facility, informal caregivers, typically family members, often assume the care and support of the patient. Although the most obvious care tasks involve physical care (e.g., personal hygiene, dressing, meal preparation), other elements of the caregiving role include psychosocial support and a commitment to this supportive role. Thus, the nurse must assess the patient's support system (family, friends) well in advance of discharge. The positive attitudes of family and friends toward the patient, the patient's disability, and the return home are important in making a successful transition to home. Not all families can carry out the arduous programs of exercise, physical therapy, and personal care that the patient may need. They may not have the resources or stability to care for family members with a severe disability. The physical, emotional, economic, and energy strains of a disabling condition may overwhelm even a stable family. Members of the rehabilitation team must not judge the family but rather should provide supportive interventions that help the family to attain its highest level of function.

The family members need to know as much as possible about the patient's condition and care so that they do not fear the patient's return home. The nurse develops methods to help the patient and family cope with problems that may arise. For example, the nurse may develop an ADLs checklist individualized for the patient and family to ensure that the family is proficient in assisting the patient with certain tasks (Chart 2-6).

Continuing and Transitional Care

A home health or transitional care nurse may visit the patient prior to discharge, interview the patient and the family, and review the ADLs sheet to learn which activities the patient can perform. This helps to ensure that continuity of care is provided and that the patient does not regress yet maintains the independence gained while in the hospital or rehabilitation setting. The family may need to purchase, borrow, or improvise needed equipment, such as safety rails, a raised toilet seat or commode, or a tub bench. Ramps may need to be built or doorways widened to allow full access.

Family members are taught how to use equipment and are given a copy of the equipment manufacturer's instruction booklet, the names of resource people, lists of equipment-related supplies, and locations where they may be obtained. A written summary of the care plan is included in family education. The patient and family members are reminded about the importance of routine health screening and other health promotion strategies.

A network of support services and communication systems may be required to enhance opportunities for independent living. The nurse uses collaborative, administrative skills to coordinate these activities and pull together the network of care. The nurse also provides skilled care, initiates additional referrals when indicated, and serves as a patient advocate and counselor when obstacles are encountered. The nurse continues to reinforce prior patient education and helps the patient to set and achieve attainable goals. The degree to which the patient adapts to the home and community environment depends on the confidence and self-esteem developed during the rehabilitation process and on the acceptance, support,

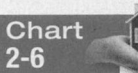

Chart 2-6 HOME CARE CHECKLIST
Managing the Therapeutic Regimen at Home

At the completion of education, the patient and/or caregiver will be able to:

- State the impact of disability on physiologic functioning, ADLs, IADLs, roles, relationships, and spirituality.
- State changes in lifestyle (e.g., diet, activity) necessary to maintain health.
- State the name, dose, side effects, frequency, and schedule for all medications.
- State how to obtain medical supplies after discharge.
- Identify durable medical equipment needs, proper usage, and maintenance necessary for safe utilization:
  - Wheelchair—manual/power
  - Cushion
  - Grab bars
  - Sliding board
  - Mechanical lift
  - Raised padded commode seat
  - Padded commode wheelchair
  - Bedside commode
  - Crutches
  - Walker
  - Cane
  - Prosthesis
  - Orthosis
  - Shower chair
  - Specialty bed
- Demonstrate usage of adaptive equipment for activities of daily living:
  - Long-handled sponge
  - Reacher
  - Universal cuff
  - Plate mat and guard
  - Rocker knife, spork, weighted utensils
  - Special closures for clothing
  - Other
- Demonstrate mobility skills:
  - Transfers: bed to chair; in and out of toilet and tub; in and out of car
  - Negotiate ramps, curbs, stairs
  - Assume sitting from supine position
  - Turn side to side in bed
  - Maneuver wheelchair; manage armrests and leg rests; lock brakes
  - Ambulate safely using assistive devices

- Perform range-of-motion exercises
- Perform muscle-strengthening exercises
- Identify community resources for peer and caregiver/family support:
  - Identify sources of support (e.g., friends, relatives, faith community)
  - Identify phone numbers of support groups for people with disability and their caregivers/families
  - State meeting locations and times
- Demonstrate how to access transportation:
  - Identify locations of wheelchair accessibility for public buses or trains
  - Identify phone numbers for private wheelchair van
  - Contact Division of Motor Vehicles for handicapped parking permit
  - Contact Division of Motor Vehicles for driving test when appropriate
  - Identify resources for adapting private vehicle with hand controls or wheelchair lift
- Identify vocational rehabilitation resources:
  - State name and phone number of vocational rehabilitation counselor
  - Identify educational opportunities that may lead to future employment
- Identify community resources for recreation:
  - State local recreation centers that offer programs for people with disability
  - Identify leisure activities that can be pursued in the community
  - State how to reach primary provider with questions or if complications arise
  - State time and date of follow-up appointments
  - Identify the need for health promotion, disease prevention, and screening activities

ADLs, activities of daily living; IADLs, instrumental activities of daily living.

---

and reactions of family members, employers, and community members.

There is a growing trend toward independent living by people with severe disability, either alone or in groups that share resources. Preparation for independent living should include training in managing a household and working with personal caregivers as well as training in mobility. The goal is integration into the community—living and working in the community with accessible housing, employment, public buildings, transportation, and recreation.

State rehabilitation administration agencies provide services to assist people with disability in obtaining the help they need to engage in gainful employment. These services include diagnostic, medical, and mental health services. Counseling, training, placement, and follow-up services are available to help people with disability select and obtain jobs.

If the patient is transferred to a long-term care facility, the transition is planned to promote continued progress. Independence gained continues to be supported, and progress is fostered. Adjustment to the facility is promoted through communication. Family members are encouraged to visit, to

be involved, and to take the patient home on weekends and holidays if possible.

Home Health Nursing

Home health care is a unique component of posthospital care for patients who return home to complete recuperation following an acute illness episode or exacerbation of chronic illness. Home health agencies can also provide advanced technologies in the home setting. All together, these services provided in the home setting work to maximize the patient's ability to function at his highest level of wellness (Rector, 2018).

The ANA defines **home health nursing** as a specialty area of practice that provides nursing services to patients across the lifespan in a home setting (Wilson, 2019). Home health nursing practice roles include holistic care planning, which incorporates resource and service coordination as part of a collaborative interdisciplinary team. This team includes home health aides; social workers; physical, speech, and occupational therapists; and primary providers. The approach provides health and social services with oversight of the total health care plan by a case manager, clinical nurse specialist, or nurse practitioner. Interdisciplinary collaboration is required if a home health agency is to receive Medicare certification (Rector, 2018).

Most home health agencies are reimbursed by various sources, including Medicare and Medicaid programs, private insurance, and direct patient payment. Older adults are the most frequent users of home care expenditures financed by Medicare, which allows nurses to manage and evaluate care of seriously ill patients who have complex, labile conditions and are at high risk for rehospitalization. Each funding source has its own requirements for services rendered, number of visits allowed, and amount of reimbursement the agency receives. The Omaha System's care documentation, referred to as the Outcome and Assessment Information Set (OASIS), has been a requirement for some time to ensure that outcome-based care is provided for all care reimbursed by Medicare. This system uses sociodemographic, environment, support system, health status, and functional status domains to assess and plan care for adult patients. OASIS is also used to collect data and improve performance or quality outcomes (CMS, 2018b).

Services Provided

Many home care patients are acutely ill or have chronic health problems or disability requiring that nurses provide more education and monitoring to patients and families. Home health nurses make home visits to provide skilled nursing care, follow-up care, and education to promote health and prevent complications. Home health care visits may be intermittent or periodic, and case management via telephone or Internet may be used to promote communication with home care consumers. The nurse instructs the patient and family about skills, self-care strategies, and health maintenance and promotion activities (e.g., nutritional counseling, exercise programs, stress management). Nursing care includes skilled assessment of the patient's physical, psychological, social, and environmental status (Fig. 2-5). Nursing interventions may include intravenous (IV) therapy and injections, parenteral nutrition, venipuncture, catheter insertion, pressure injury treatment, wound care, ostomy care, and patient and family

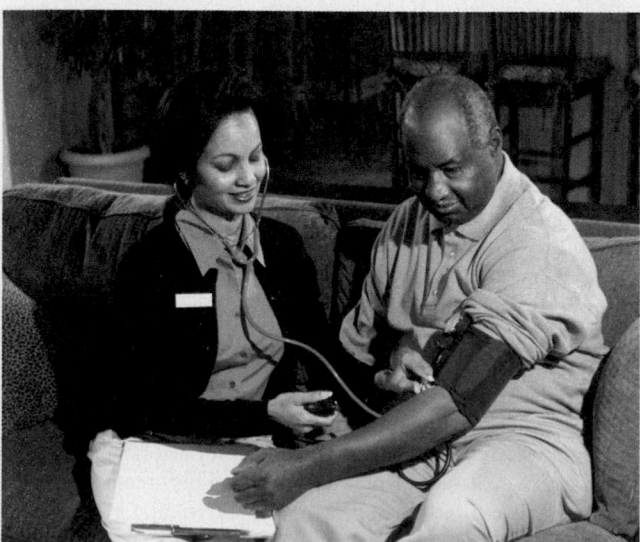

Figure 2-5 • Assessment is an important part of any home health visit.

education. Complex technical equipment such as mechanical ventilation and procedures such as peritoneal dialysis may be involved in home health care. Nurses have a role in evaluating the safety and effectiveness of technology in the home setting. In addition, **telehealth** is useful in home health care in facilitating exchange of information via telephone or computers between patients and nurses regarding health information such as blood glucose readings, vital signs, and cardiac parameters. The use of a broad spectrum of computer and Internet resources, such as webcams, also facilitates exchange of information (Rector, 2018).

The Home Setting

The home health nurse is a guest in the patient's home and must have permission to visit and give care. The nurse has minimal control over the lifestyle, living situation, and health practices of the visited patients. This lack of full decision making authority can create a conflict for the nurse and lead to problems in the nurse–patient relationship. To work successfully with patients in any setting, the nurse must be nonjudgmental and convey respect for patients' beliefs, even if they differ sharply from those of the nurse. This can be difficult when a patient's lifestyle involves activities that a nurse considers harmful or unacceptable, such as smoking, excessive use of alcohol, use of illicit drugs or misuse of prescription drugs, or overeating (Rector, 2018).

The cleanliness of a patient's home may not meet the standards of a hospital. Although the nurse can provide education points about maintaining clean surroundings, the patient and family decide if they will implement the nurse's suggestions. The nurse must accept their decisions and deliver the care required regardless of the conditions of the setting. The kind of equipment and the supplies or resources that usually are available in acute care settings are often unavailable in the patient's home. The nurse has to learn to improvise when providing care, such as when changing a dressing or catheterizing a patient in a regular bed that is not adjustable and lacks a bedside table (Rector, 2018).

Infection control is as important in the home as it is in the hospital; however, it can be more challenging in the home and requires creative approaches. As in any situation, it is important to perform hand hygiene before and after giving direct patient care, even in a home that does not have running water. If aseptic technique is required, the nurse must have a plan for implementing this technique before going to the home. This applies to universal precautions, transmission-based precautions, and disposal of bodily secretions and excretions. If injections are given, the nurse must use a closed container to dispose of syringes. Injectable and other medications must be kept out of the reach of children during visits and stored in a safe place if the medications remain in the home.

> ▶ **Quality and Safety Nursing Alert**
>
> *Friends, neighbors, or family members may ask the nurse about the patient's condition. The patient has a right to confidentiality, and information should be shared only with the patient's permission. The nurse should be mindful of any sensitive information (e.g., electronic health records [EHRs]) taken into the home and prevent it from being misplaced or picked up by others.*

Home Health Visits

Most agencies have a policy manual that identifies the agency's philosophy and procedures and defines the services provided. The eligibility of a patient and provision of services may be prescribed by the type of insurance the patient carries. For example, Medicare beneficiaries must meet certain eligibility requirements such as homebound criteria and may be permitted only intermittent skilled services of a registered nurse or licensed therapist (CMS, 2019). Becoming familiar with these policies is essential before initiating a home visit. It is also important to know the state laws regarding what actions to take if the nurse finds a patient dead, suspects abuse, determines that a patient cannot safely remain at home, or observes a situation that possibly indicates harm to the community at large.

Preparing for a Home Visit

Before making a home visit, the nurse should review pertinent data about the patient that is typically provided on a referral form. It may be necessary to contact the referring agency if the purpose for the referral is unclear or important information is missing. The nurse calls the patient to obtain permission to visit, schedules a time for the visit, and verifies the address. This initial phone conversation provides an opportunity to introduce oneself, identify the agency, and explain the reason for the visit. If the patient does not have a telephone, the nurse should see if the person who made the referral is able to contact the patient regarding the visit. If an unannounced visit to a patient's home must be made, the nurse should ask permission to come in before entering the house. Explaining the purpose of the referral at the outset and setting up the times for future visits before leaving are also recommended.

Conducting a Home Visit

Personal Safety Precautions

Home health nurses must pay attention to personal safety, because they often practice in unknown environments. Based on the principle of due diligence, agencies should investigate at-risk working environments prior to making the assignment and must inform employees accordingly. Agencies have policies and procedures concerning the promotion of safety for clinical staff, and training is provided to facilitate personal safety. The individual nurse and agency must proactively assess environments for safety. Suggested precautions to take when making a home visit are presented in Chart 2-7.

Initial Home Visit

The first visit sets the tone for subsequent visits and is crucial in establishing the nurse–patient relationship. The situations encountered depend on numerous factors. Patients may be in pain and have additional factors that make them unable to care for themselves. Family members may be overwhelmed and doubt their ability to care for loved ones. They may not understand why the patient was sent home from the hospital before being totally rehabilitated. They may not comprehend what home care is or why they cannot have 24-hour nursing services. It is critical that the nurse conveys an understanding of what patients and families are experiencing and how the illness is affecting their lives.

Chart 2-7 Safety Precautions in Home Health Care

- Learn, or preprogram a phone with, the telephone numbers of the agency, police, and emergency services. Most agencies provide phones for nurses so that the agency can contact the nurse and the nurse can easily contact the agency.
- Carry agency identification and a charged phone to make telephone calls if you become lost or have problems; a mobile phone charger provides additional backup.
- Let the agency know your daily schedule and the telephone numbers of your patients (if available) so that you can be located if you do not return when expected.
- Know where the patient lives before leaving to make the visit, and either carry a map or use the navigation system in your car or the GPS software on your smartphone for quick referral.
- Keep your car in good working order, and have sufficient gas in the tank.
- Park the car near the patient's home, and lock the car during the visit.
- Do not drive an expensive car or wear expensive jewelry when making visits.
- Know the regular bus schedule, and know the routes when using public transportation or walking to the patient's house.
- When making visits in high-crime areas, visit with another person rather than alone (if possible).
- Try to schedule visits during daylight hours (when possible).
- Never walk into a patient's home uninvited; be vigilant for unrestrained pets.
- If you do not feel safe entering a patient's home, leave the area.
- Become familiar with the layout of the house, including exits from the house.
- If a patient or family member is visibly intoxicated, under the influence, or hostile, leave and reschedule the visit.
- If a family is having a serious argument or abusing the patient or anyone else in the household, leave, reschedule the visit, contact your supervisor, and report the abuse to the appropriate authorities.

GPS, Global Positioning System.

During the initial home visit, which may take 1 hour or more, the patient is evaluated and a plan of care is established that may be modified on subsequent visits. The nurse informs the patient of the agency's practices, policies, and hours of operation. If the agency is to be reimbursed for the visit, the nurse asks for insurance information, such as a Medicare or Medicaid card. The initial assessment includes evaluating the patient, the home environment (Chart 2-8), the patient's self-care abilities or the family's ability to provide care, and the patient's need for additional resources. After the assessment, necessary skilled interventions are accomplished. Most agencies provide nurses with bags that contain standard supplies and equipment needed during home visits. It is important to keep the bag properly supplied and to bring any additional items that might be needed for the visit. Depending on insurance coverage, supplies may be delivered to the home or may need to be purchased by the patient. Home health nurses need to be prepared for the inevitability that a patient may not have the medical supplies needed for treatment, and work to procure all needed items.

One important aspect of the transition from hospital to home is self-management of the medication regimen. Older

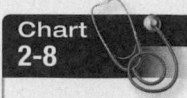

Chart 2-8 ASSESSMENT
Assessing the Home Environment

Physical Facilities (check all that apply)

Exterior
- Steps
- Unsafe steps
- Porch
- Litter
- Noise
- Adequate lighting
- Other

Interior
- Accessible bathroom
- Level, safe floor surface
- Number of rooms
- Privacy
- Sleeping arrangements
- Refrigeration
- Trash management
- Animals
- Adequate lighting
- Steps/stairs
- Other

Safety Hazards (check all that apply)

- None
- Inadequate floor, roof, or windows
- Inadequate lighting
- Unsafe gas/electric appliances
- Inadequate heating
- Inadequate cooling
- Lack of fire safety devices
- Unsafe floor coverings
- Inadequate stair rails
- Lead-based paint (particularly for homes built prior to 1978) or lead in drinking water (particularly in homes built prior to 1986)
- Improperly stored hazardous material
- Improper wiring/electrical cords
- Other

Safety Factors (check all that apply)

- Fire/smoke detectors
- Working telephone
- Placement of electrical cords
- Emergency plan
- Emergency phone numbers displayed
- Safe portable heaters
- Oxygen in use
- Obstacle-free paths
- Other

medication reconciliation at each skilled nursing visit. As patients and families observe medication reconciliation, they begin to understand the importance of medication management. Managing the medication regimen is an important part of a successful transition home; without it, there is risk for readmission to the hospital.

Determining the Need for Future Visits

While assessing a patient's situation, the home health nurse evaluates and clearly documents the need for future visits and the optimal frequency for those visits. To make these judgments, the nurse should consider the questions listed in Chart 2-9. With each subsequent visit, these same factors are evaluated to determine the continuing health needs of the patient. As progress is made and the patient—with or without the help of significant others—becomes more capable of self-care and more independent, the need for home visits may decline.

Ending the Visit

As the visit comes to a close, the nurse summarizes the main points of the visit for the patient and family and identifies expectations for future visits or patient achievements. The following points should be considered at the end of each visit:
- What are the main points the patient or family should remember from the visit?
- What positive attributes have been noted about the patient and the family that will give a sense of accomplishment?
- What were the main points of the education plan or the treatments needed to ensure that the patient and family understand what they must do? A written set of instructions should be left with the patient or family, provided they can read and see (alternative formats include video or audio recordings). Printed material must be in the patient's primary language and in large print when indicated.
- Whom should the patient or family call if someone needs to be contacted immediately? Are current emergency telephone numbers readily available? Is telephone service available, or can an emergency phone service be provided?
- What signs of complications should be reported immediately?
- How frequently will visits be made? How long will they last (approximately)?
- What is the day and time of the next visit? Will a different nurse make the visit?

Documenting the Visit

Documentation considerations for home visits follow fairly specific regulations. The patient's needs and the nursing care provided must be documented to ensure that the agency qualifies for payment for the visit. Medicare, Medicaid, and other **third-party payers** (i.e., organizations that provide reimbursement for services covered under a health care insurance plan) require documentation of the patient's homebound status and the need for skilled professional nursing care. The medical diagnosis and specific detailed information on the functional limitations of the patient are usually part of the documentation. The goals and the actions appropriate for attaining those goals must be identified. Expected outcomes

adults may have multiple prescribers, or may use alternative therapies such as herbal remedies as well as vitamins and other over-the-counter medications. While the patient is under the care of the home health agency, the home health nurse promotes medication management through the process of medication reconciliation. The nurse reviews current medication orders and assists with solving problems or medication discrepancies such as wrong dosages, duplicate medications, omissions, or use of a medication for something other than the prescribed reason (Kollerup, Curtis, & Schantz Laursen, 2018). Home health agencies may mandate

Chart 2-9 ASSESSMENT
Assessing the Need for Home Visits

Current Health Status

- How well is the patient progressing?
- How serious are the present signs and symptoms?
- Has the patient shown signs of progressing as expected, or does it seem that recovery will be delayed?

Home Environment

- Are safety concerns apparent?
- Are family or friends available to provide care, or is the patient alone?

Level of Self-Care Ability

- Is the patient capable of self-care?
- What is the patient's level of independence?
- Is the patient ambulatory or bedridden?
- Does the patient have sufficient energy, or are they frail and easily fatigued?
- Does the patient need and use assistive devices?

Level of Nursing Care Needed

- What level of nursing care does the patient require?
- Does the care require basic skills or more complex interventions?

Prognosis

- What is the expectation for recovery in this particular instance?
- What are the chances that complications may develop if nursing care is not provided?

Educational Needs

- How well has the patient or family grasped the education points made?
- Is there a need for further follow-up and retraining?
- What level of proficiency does the patient or family show in carrying out the necessary care?

Mental Status

- How alert is the patient?
- Are there signs of confusion or thinking difficulties?
- Does the patient tend to be forgetful or have a limited attention span?

Level of Adherence

- Is the patient following the instructions provided?
- Does the patient seem capable of following the instructions?
- Are the family members helpful, or are they unwilling or unable to assist in caring for the patient as expected?

of the nursing interventions must be stated in terms of patient behaviors and must be realistic and measurable. In addition, the goals must reflect the nursing diagnosis or the patient's problems and must specify those actions that address the patient's problems. Inadequate documentation may result in nonpayment for the visit and care services.

Discharge Planning for Transition to the Community or Home Care Setting

Discharge planning is an essential component of facilitating the transition of the patient from the acute care to the community or home care setting, or for facilitating the transfer of the patient from one health care setting to another. A documented discharge plan is mandatory for patients who receive Medicare or Medicaid health insurance benefits. Discharge planning begins with the patient's admission to the hospital or health care setting and must consider the potential for necessary follow-up care in the home or another community setting. Several different personnel (e.g., social workers, home health nurses, case managers) or agencies may be involved in the planning process.

The development of a comprehensive discharge plan requires collaboration between professionals at the referring agency and the home care agency, as well as other community agencies that provide specific resources upon discharge. The process involves identifying the patient's needs and developing a thorough plan to meet them. It is essential to have open lines of communication with family members to ensure understanding and cooperation.

Continuing the Transition through Community Resources and Referrals

Case managers and discharge planners often make referrals to other team members, such as home health aides and social workers. These nurses work collaboratively with the health care team and the referring agency or person. Continuous coordinated care among all health care providers involved in a patient's care is essential to avoid duplication of effort by the various personnel caring for the patient. These nurses must also be knowledgeable about community resources available to patients, as well as services provided by local agencies, eligibility requirements for those services, and any charges for the services (i.e., co-pays). Most communities have directories, which may include online directories or resource booklets, that list local health and social service agencies and their offerings. The Internet is useful in helping patients identify the location and accessibility of grocery and drug stores, banks, health care facilities, ambulances, primary providers, dentists, pharmacists, social service agencies, and senior citizens' programs. In addition, a patient's place of worship or faith community may be an important resource for services. The process includes informing the patient and family about the community resources available to meet their needs. When appropriate, nurses may make the initial contact.

CRITICAL THINKING EXERCISES

1 **PG** An 80-year-old community-dwelling woman with a new diagnosis of heart failure was transferred to your medical-surgical unit from the intensive care unit (ICU). The transfer report from the ICU nurse included the notation that prior to this admission and diagnosis, the patient lived alone at home. The patient has one son who lives locally. Both the patient and son agree with a plan to transition the patient from living alone to living with her son at his home. She has been prescribed new medications to take at home and will need to see her primary provider in 2 weeks. What are your priorities as you work on discharge planning for this patient? What referrals will you consider to achieve a successful transition from hospital to home?

2 `ebp` An 82-year-old man newly diagnosed with diabetes is being referred for home care after discharge from the hospital. He needs regular monitoring and diabetes education. He has several family members at home who have assisted with IADLs in the past; however, they all work. You are concerned about his ability to manage his diabetes as his family reports he will be home alone during the day and has decreased activity tolerance related to ADLs since his hospitalization and new diagnosis of diabetes. Identify a specific evidence-based question related to this patient in order to conduct a relevant and focused literature search. What key words would you use in this search, and what sources would be appropriate to search? What resources could you use to assist him to remain in his home for as long as possible? How would you go about obtaining this information? What is the strength of the evidence?

3 `ipc` You are a home health nurse caring for a 75-year-old man who has transitioned home from inpatient rehabilitation following a fall in which his hip was fractured. He had surgery to reduce the fracture and stabilize the hip. He lives with his wife who is also 75 and who has memory impairment. Both need assistance with IADLs. He needs assistance with ADLs as he continues the rehabilitation process at home. As the home health nurse and case manager, develop a list of resources and interdisciplinary services that will enhance this transition to the home setting.

REFERENCES

*Asterisk indicates nursing research.
**Double asterisk indicates classic reference.

Books

Academy of Medical-Surgical Nurses (AMSN). (2018). *Scope and standards of medical-surgical nursing practice* (6th ed.). Pitman, NJ: Author.
American Association of Critical-Care Nurses (AACN). (2019b). *AACN scope and standards for acute and critical care nursing practice* (3rd ed.). Aliso Viejo, CA: Author.
American Nurses Association (ANA). (2010). *Nursing's social policy statement* (3rd ed.). Silver Springs, MD: Nursesbooks.org
American Nurses Association (ANA). (2015a). *Code of ethics for nurses with interpretive statements*. Washington, DC: Nursesbooks.org
American Nurses Association (ANA). (2015b). *Nursing: Scope and standards of practice* (3rd ed.). Silver Springs, MD: Nursesbooks.org
Carpenito, J. L. (2017). *Handbook of nursing diagnosis* (15th ed.). Philadelphia, PA: Wolters Kluwer.
Fowler, M. D. (2015). *Guide to nursing's social policy statement: Understanding the profession from social contract to social covenant*. Silver Springs, MD: Author.
Rector, C. (2018). *Community and public health nursing: Promoting the public's health* (9th ed.). Philadelphia, PA: Wolters Kluwer.
Weber, J. R., & Kelley, J. H. (2018). *Health assessment in nursing* (6th ed.). Philadelphia, PA: Lippincott Williams & Wilkins.

Journals and Electronic Documents

Academy of Medical-Surgical Nurses (AMSN). (2019). What is medical-surgical nursing? Retrieved on 6/12/2019 at: www.amsn.org/practice-resources/what-medical-surgical-nursing
Agency for Healthcare Research and Quality (AHRQ). (2019). *Readmissions and adverse events after discharge*. Rockville, MD: AHRQ. Retrieved on 6/25/19 at: psnet.ahrq.gov/primers/primer/11/Readmissions-and-Adverse-Events-After-Discharge

Alspach, J. G. (2018). Overlooking an integral lynchpin of patient care: The caregiver at home. *Critical Care Nurse, 38*(1), 10–15.
American Association of Colleges of Nursing (AACN). (2019a). Clinical nurse leader (CNL). Retrieved on 6/25/2019 at: www.aacnnursing.org/CNL
Association of Rehabilitation Nurses (ARN). (2013). *The essential role of the rehabilitation nurse in facilitating care transitions: A white paper by the association of rehabilitation nurses*. Chicago, IL: ARN. Retrieved on 7/1/19 at: rehabnurse.org/uploads/membership/ARN_Care_Transitions_White_Paper_Journal_Copy_FINAL.pdf
Association of Rehabilitation Nurses (ARN). (2019a). What does a rehabilitation staff nurse do? Retrieved on 6/28/19 at: rehabnurse.org/about/roles/rehabilitation-staff-nurse
Association of Rehabilitation Nurses (ARN). (2019b). Professional rehabilitation nursing competency model. Retrieved on 6/28/19 at: rehabnurse.org/advance-your-practice/practice-tools/competency-model
Bailey, M. K., Weiss, A. J., Barrett, M. L., et al. (2019, February). *Characteristics of 30-day all-cause hospital readmissions, 2010–2016.* (Statistical Brief No. 248). Rockville, MD: AHRQ. Retrieved on 6/25/19 at: hcup-us.ahrq.gov/reports/statbriefs/sb248-Hospital-Readmissions-2010-2016.jsp
Baileys, K., McMullen, L., Lubejko, B., et al. (2018). Nurse navigators core competencies. *Clinical Journal of Oncology Nursing, 22*(3), 272–281.
Carr, D. D. (2019). High-quality care transitions promote continuity of care and safer discharges. *Journal of the New York State Nurses Association, 46*(2), 4–11.
Case Management Society of America. (2019). What is a case manager? Retrieved on 7/29/2019 at: www.cmsa.org/who-we-are/what-is-a-case-manager
Centers for Medicare & Medicaid Services. (2018a). *National health care expenditures highlights*. Woodlawn, MD: CMS. Retrieved on 6/25/19 at: www.cms.gov/Research-Statistics-Data-and-Systems/Statistics-Trends-and-Reports/NationalHealthExpendData/Downloads/highlights.pdf
Centers for Medicare & Medicaid Services. (2018b). Outcome and assessment information set (OASIS-D) guidance manual. Retrieved on 7/17/2019 at: www.cms.gov/Medicare/Quality-Initiatives-Patient-Assessment-Instruments/HomeHealthQualityInits/Downloads/draft-OASIS-D-Guidance-Manual-7-2-2018.pdf
Centers for Medicare & Medicaid Services. (2019). Medicare benefit policy manual chapter 7—home health services. Retrieved on 7/17/2019 at: www.cms.gov/Regulations-and-Guidance/Guidance/Manuals/downloads/bp102c07.pdf
*Fidecki, W., Wysokiński, M., Wrońska, I., et al. (2017). Functional efficiency of elderly patients hospitalized in neurological departments. *The Journal of Neurological and Neurosurgical Nursing, 6*(3), 102–106.
Gregory, M., & Galloway, T. (2017). Stroke survivors: The long road to recovery. *Practice Nurse, 47*(7), 29–32.
**Katz, S., Downs, T. D., Cash, H. R., et al. (1970). Progress in the development of the index of ADL. *Gerontologist, 10*(1), 20–30.
**Keith, R. A., Granger, C. V., Hamilton, B. B., et al. (1987). The functional independence measure: A new tool for rehabilitation. *Advances in Clinical Rehabilitation, 1*, 6–18.
*Kollerup, M. G., Curtis, T., & Schantz Laursen, B. (2018). Visiting nurses' posthospital medication management in home health care: An ethnographic study. *Scandinavian Journal of Caring Sciences, 32*(1), 222–232.
**Mahoney, F., & Barthel, D. (1965). Functional evaluation: The Barthel Index. *Maryland State Medical Journal, 14*, 61–65.
*Naylor, M. D., Shaid, E. C., Carpenter, D., et al. (2017). Components of comprehensive and effective transitional care. *Journal of the American Geriatrics Society, 65*(6), 1119–1125.
Wilson, D. R. (2019). Home health nursing: Scope and standards of practice. *Activities, Adaptation & Aging, 43*(1), 78–79.

Resources

AbleData, abledata.acl.gov
Academy of Medical-Surgical Nurses (AMSN), www.amsn.org
Agency for Healthcare Research and Quality (AHRQ), www.ahrq.gov
American Association of Colleges of Nursing (AACN), www.aacnnursing.org
American Association of Critical-Care Nurses (AACN), www.aacn.org

American Association of People with Disabilities (AAPD),
   www.aapd.com
American Nurses Association (ANA), www.nursingworld.org
Assistive Technology Industry Association (ATIA), www.atia.org
Association of Rehabilitation Nurses (ARN), www.rehabnurse.org
Case Management Society of America (CMSA), www.cmsa.org
Center on Knowledge Translation for Disability and Rehabilitation
   Research (KTDRR), www.ncddr.org
Centers for Medicare & Medicaid Services (CMS), www.cms.gov

Inpatient Rehabilitation Facilities (IRF) Quality Reporting Program (QRF),
   www.cms.gov/Medicare/Quality-Initiatives-Patient-Assessment-
   Instruments/IRF-Quality-Reporting
National Association for Home Care and Hospice (NAHC),
   www.nahc.org
National Council on Disability (NCD), www.ncd.gov
National Rehabilitation Information Center (NARIC), www.naric.com
World Health Organization, health topics: rehabilitation, www.who.int/
   topics/rehabilitation/en

Health Education and Health Promotion

On completion of this chapter, the learner will be able to:

1. Describe the purposes and significance of health education.
2. Distinguish between the concepts of adherence to a therapeutic regimen and health literacy.
3. Explain the variables that affect learning and apply them to the teaching—learning process.
4. Describe the components of health promotion and discuss major health promotion models.
5. Specify the variables that affect health promotion activities across the life cycle, and describe the role of the nurse in health promotion.

NURSING CONCEPTS

Community-Based Practice
Family
Health Promotion

Health, Wellness, and Illness
Managing Care

Stress and Coping
Teaching and Learning

GLOSSARY

adherence: the process of faithfully following guidelines or directions
community: an interacting population of individuals living together within a larger society
feedback: the return of information given to a person
health education: various learning experiences designed to promote behaviors that facilitate health
health literacy: the capability of a person to obtain, communicate, process, and understand essential health information for the purpose of securing health care services and for making health care decisions
health promotion: activities that assist people in developing resources to maintain or enhance well-being and improve quality of life
learning: the act of acquiring knowledge, attitudes, or skills

learning readiness: the optimum time for learning to occur; usually corresponds to the learner's perceived need and desire to obtain specific knowledge
nutrition: the science that deals with food and nourishment in humans
physical fitness: the condition of being physically healthy as a result of proper exercise and nutrition
self-responsibility: personal accountability for one's actions or behavior
stress management: behaviors and techniques used to strengthen a person's resources against stress
teaching: helping another person learn
therapeutic regimen: a routine that promotes health and healing

Effective health education lays a solid foundation for individual and **community** (population of individuals living together within a larger society) wellness. All nurses use teaching as a tool to assist patients and families in developing effective health behaviors and altering lifestyle patterns that predispose people to health risks. Health education is an influential factor directly related to positive health outcomes.

Purpose of Health Education

Today's health care environment mandates the use of an organized approach to **health education** (learning experiences designed to promote behaviors that facilitate health) so that patients can meet their specific health care needs. There are many reasons for providing health education.

Meeting Nursing Standards

Teaching, as a function of nursing, is included in all state nurse practice acts and in the American Nurses Association's (ANA's) *Scope and Standards of Practice* (ANA, 2015). Health teaching and health promotion are independent functions of nursing practice and essential nursing responsibilities. All nursing care is directed toward promoting, maintaining, and restoring health; preventing illness; and helping people adapt to the residual effects of illness. Many of these nursing activities are accomplished through patient education. Nurses are challenged to focus on the health education needs of communities and to provide specific patient and family education. Health education is important to nursing care because it affects the abilities of people and families to perform important self-care activities.

Every contact a nurse has with a health care consumer, whether or not that person is ill, should be considered an opportunity for health education. Although people have a right to decide whether to learn, nurses have the responsibility to present information that motivates people to recognize the need to learn. Therefore, nurses must use opportunities in all health care settings to promote wellness. There are many educational environments. Some examples include homes, hospitals, community health centers, schools, places of business, service agencies, shelters, and consumer action or support groups (deChesnay & Anderson, 2020).

Supporting Informed Decision Making and Self-Care

The emphasis on health education stems in part from the public's right to comprehensive health care, which includes up-to-date health information. It also reflects the emergence of an informed public that is asking more questions about health and health care. Because of the importance that American society places on health and the responsibility that all people must maintain and promote their own health, members of the health care team, specifically nurses, are obligated to make health education available. Significant factors to consider when planning patient education include the availability of health care, the use of diverse health care providers to accomplish care management goals, and the increased use of complementary and alternative strategies rather than traditional approaches to care. Without adequate knowledge and training in self-care skills, consumers cannot make informed decisions about their health. Guidance from nurses may assist consumers to obtain health information from trustworthy, credible, and timely Internet resources, as well as from appropriate health promotion practitioners and researchers (Cohn, Lyman, Broshek, et al., 2018). People with chronic illnesses and disability are among those most in need of health education. As the lifespan of the population increases, the number of people with such illnesses also increases. Health information targeted at identifying and managing the exacerbations or issues commonly associated with having a chronic illness or disability is a major focus of health education. People with chronic illness need health care information to participate actively in and assume responsibility for self-care. Health education can help those with chronic illness adapt to their illness, prevent complications, carry out prescribed therapy, and solve problems when confronted with new situations. It can also help to prevent crisis situations and reduce the potential for rehospitalization resulting from inadequate information about self-care. The goal of health education is to teach people to live a healthy life and strive toward achieving their maximum health potential.

In addition to the public's right to and desire for health education, patient education is also a strategy for promoting self-care at home and in the community, reducing health care costs by preventing illness, effectively managing necessary therapies, avoiding expensive medical interventions, decreasing lengths of hospital stay, and facilitating earlier discharge. For health care agencies, offering community wellness programs is a public relations tool for increasing patient satisfaction and for developing a positive image of the institution. Patient education is also a cost-avoidance strategy in that positive staff–patient relationships may avert malpractice suits. Some insurance companies support health education through reimbursement for programs, such as diabetes management classes and fitness and weight management programs.

Promoting Adherence to the Therapeutic Regimen

One of the goals of patient education is to encourage people to adhere to their **therapeutic regimen** (a routine that promotes health and healing). **Adherence** (the process of faithfully following guidelines or directions) to treatment usually requires that a person make one or more lifestyle changes to carry out specific activities that promote and maintain health. Common examples of behaviors facilitating health include taking prescribed medications, maintaining a healthy diet, increasing daily activities and exercise, self-monitoring for signs and symptoms of illness and changes in baseline health status, practicing specific hygiene measures, seeking recommended health evaluations and screening, and performing other therapeutic and preventive measures.

Factors Affecting Adherence

Many people do not adhere to their prescribed regimens; rates of adherence are generally low, especially when the regimens are complex or of long duration (e.g., therapy for chronic inflammatory rheumatic diseases, hypertension, breast cancer, human immune deficiency virus [HIV] infection, hemodialysis). Nonadherence to prescribed therapy has been the subject of many studies (Al-Noumani, Wu, Barksdale, et al., 2019; Hine, Smith, Eshun-Wilson, et al., 2018; Lambert, Balneaves, Howard, et al., 2018; Lavielle, Puyraimond-Zenmour, Romand, et al., 2018). For the most part, findings have been inconclusive, and no one predominant causative factor has been identified. Instead, a wide range of variables influences the degree of adherence, including the following:

- Demographic variables, such as age, gender, race, socioeconomic status, and level of education
- Illness variables, such as the severity of the illness and the relief of symptoms afforded by the therapy
- Therapeutic regimen variables, such as the complexity of the regimen, treatment fatigue, and uncomfortable side effects
- Psychosocial variables, such as intelligence, motivation, availability of significant and supportive people (especially family members and significant others),

competing or conflicting demands, attitudes toward health professionals, acceptance or denial of illness, substance abuse, and religious or cultural beliefs

- Financial variables, especially the direct and indirect costs associated with a prescribed regimen

Another factor to consider when the nurse is developing strategies to promote patient adherence is the concept of **health literacy** or the capability of a person to obtain, communicate, process, and understand essential health information for the purpose of securing health care services and for making health care decisions. A challenge for all health care providers is to improve the health literacy of patients. In establishing suitable health education materials, technologic innovations and services, providers must communicate health information in plain language and work with patients to promote accurate processing and understanding of the health information. Nurses must consider their knowledge of the myriad factors that affect health literacy in any given population. The primary factors influencing health literacy are the effective use of communication and cultural skills, along with the presentation of health care information, and a basic background of mathematical skills. Without such skills, patients are at risk for being unable to share personal health information, perform self-care management for both acute and chronic health conditions, navigate through health systems and complete health forms, and calculate information such as nutritional information on food labels (Carrara & Schulz, 2018; Osborne, 2018).

Health literacy skills are basic to understanding the body and how it functions, assessing lifestyle choices along with the variables that cause and perpetuate disease, as well as making health care decisions. If people have low health literacy, the consequence is poor overall health. Deconstructing this cycle of low health literacy leading to poor health status and higher risk of health problems is essential. To increase health literacy, providers must design and distribute accurate health information and must ensure that these health materials are culturally appropriate for various populations. It is imperative to build community partnerships to support education and public health activities. Nurses can be instrumental in performing evaluation research on the educational undertakings that support individuals, groups, or communities. Furthermore, nurses must be directly involved in facilitating change through the development of health care policies that address the promotion of a health literate society (Patton, Zalon, & Ludwick, 2019).

Nurses' success with health education is determined by both the development of strong health literacy and the ongoing assessment of the variables that affect patients' ability to adopt specific behaviors to obtain resources, and maintain a healthy social environment (Edelman & Kudzma, 2018). Programs are more likely to succeed if patients have improved health literacy and providers pay careful attention to the variables affecting patient adherence. Both health literacy and the concept of adherence must be considered in the patient's teaching plan. Teaching strategies are discussed later in the chapter.

Motivation

The problem of nonadherence to therapeutic regimens is substantial and must be addressed before patients can achieve their maximum health potential. Patients' need for knowledge has not been found to be a sufficient stimulus for acquiring knowledge and thereby enabling complete adherence to a health regimen. Teaching directed toward stimulating patient motivation results in varying degrees of adherence. Research suggests that factors such as personal relevance of strategies for self-care, perceived control, and type of health problem must also be considered (Seibre, Toumpakari, Turner, et al., 2018; Whiteley, Brown, Lally, et al., 2018). The variables of choice, establishment of mutual goals, and quality of the patient–provider relationship also influence the behavioral changes that can result from patient education. Many factors are linked to motivation for learning.

Using a learning contract or agreement can also be a motivator for learning. Such a contract is based on assessment of patient needs; health care data; and specific, measurable goals (Miller & Stoeckel, 2019). The learning contract is recorded in writing and contains methods for ongoing evaluation. A well-designed learning contract is realistic and positive. In a typical learning contract, a series of measurable goals is established, beginning with small, easily attainable objectives and progressing to more advanced goals. Frequent, positive reinforcement is provided as the person moves from one goal to the next. For example, incremental goals such as weight loss of 1 to 2 pounds per week are more appropriate in a weight reduction program than a general goal such as a 30-pound weight loss.

 Gerontologic Considerations

Nonadherence to therapeutic regimens is a significant problem for older adults, leading to increased morbidity, mortality, and cost of treatment (Abada, Clark, Sinha, et al., 2019; Taylor, Coogle, Cotter, et al., 2019). Many admissions to nursing homes and hospitals are associated with nonadherence.

Older adults frequently have one or more chronic illnesses that are managed with numerous medications, and their disease course may be complicated by periodic acute episodes (Miller, 2019). Older adults may have additional issues that affect adherence to therapeutic regimens, such as increased sensitivity to medications and their side effects, difficulty in adjusting to change and stress, financial constraints, forgetfulness, inadequate support systems, lifetime habits of self-treatment with over-the-counter medications, visual and hearing impairments, and mobility limitations. To promote adherence among older adults, all variables that may affect health behavior should be assessed (Fig. 3-1). Nurses must also consider that cognitive impairment may result in the older adult's inability to draw inferences, apply information, or understand the major points (Mauk, 2017; Touhy & Jett, 2018). The person's strengths and limitations must be assessed to encourage the use of existing strengths to compensate for limitations. Above all, health care professionals must work together to provide continuous, coordinated care; otherwise, the efforts of one health care professional may be negated by those of another.

The Nature of Teaching and Learning

Learning can be defined as acquiring knowledge, attitudes, or skills. **Teaching** is defined as helping another person learn. These definitions indicate that the teaching–learning

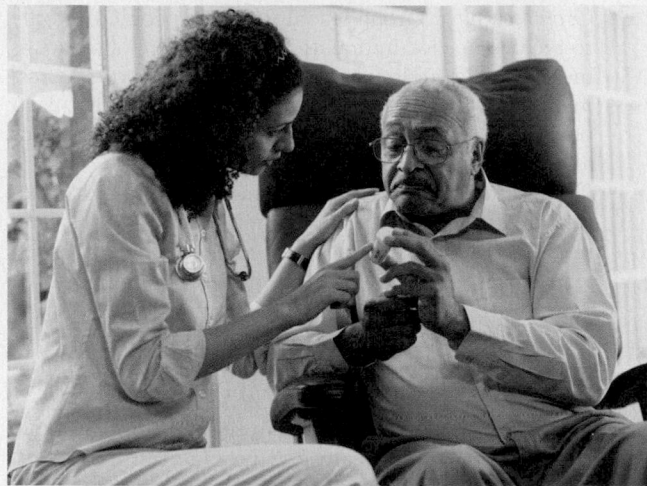

Figure 3-1 • Taking time to teach patients about their medication and treatment program promotes interest and cooperation. Older adults who are actively involved in learning about their medication and treatment program and the expected effects may be more likely to adhere to the therapeutic regimen.

process is an active one, requiring the involvement of both the teacher and the learner in the effort to reach the desired outcome—a change in behavior. The teacher does not simply give knowledge to the learner but instead serves as a facilitator of learning. Although learning can take place without teachers, most people who are attempting to learn new or altered health behaviors benefit from contact with a nurse. The interpersonal interaction between the person and the nurse who is attempting to meet the person's learning needs may be formal or informal, depending on the method and techniques of teaching.

There is no definitive theory about how learning occurs and how it is affected by teaching. However, learning can be affected by factors, such as readiness to learn, the learning environment, and the teaching techniques used (Miller & Stoeckel, 2019).

Learning Readiness

One of the most significant factors influencing learning is a person's **learning readiness** or the optimum time for learning to occur, which usually corresponds to the learner's perceived need and desire to obtain specific knowledge. For adults, readiness is based on culture, personal values, physical and emotional status, and past experiences in learning. The "teachable moment" occurs when the content and skills being taught are congruent with the task to be accomplished (Miller & Stoeckel, 2019).

Culture encompasses values, ideals, and behaviors, and the traditions within each culture provide the framework for solving the issues and concerns of daily living. Because people with different cultural backgrounds have different values and lifestyles, choices about health care vary. Culture is a major variable influencing readiness to learn because it affects how people learn and what information can be learned. Sometimes people do not accept health teaching because it conflicts with culturally mediated values. Before beginning health teaching, nurses must conduct an individual cultural assessment instead of relying only on generalized assumptions about a particular culture. A patient's social and cultural patterns must be appropriately incorporated into the teaching–learning interaction. See Chapter 4, Chart 4-7, which describes cultural assessment components to consider when formulating a teaching plan.

A person's values include beliefs about behaviors that are desirable and undesirable. The nurse must know what value the patient places on health and health care. In clinical situations, patients express their values through their actions and the level of knowledge pursued (deChesnay & Anderson, 2020). When the nurse is unaware of the patient's values (cultural and personal), misunderstanding, lack of cooperation, and negative health outcomes may occur (McFarland & Wehbe-Alamah, 2018). A person's values and behaviors can be either an asset or a deterrent to readiness to learn. Therefore, patients are unlikely to accept health education unless their values and beliefs about health and illness are respected (Kersey-Matusiak, 2018).

Physical readiness is of vital importance, because until the person is physically capable of learning, attempts at teaching and learning may be both futile and frustrating. For example, a person in acute pain is unable to focus attention away from the pain long enough to concentrate on learning. Likewise, a person who is short of breath concentrates on breathing rather than on learning.

Emotional readiness also affects the motivation to learn. A person who has not accepted an existing illness or the threat of illness is not motivated to learn. A person who does not accept a therapeutic regimen, or who views it as conflicting with their present lifestyle, may consciously avoid learning about it. Until the person recognizes the need to learn and demonstrates an ability to learn, teaching efforts may be thwarted. However, it is not always wise to wait for the person to become emotionally ready to learn, because that time may never come unless the nurse makes an effort to stimulate the person's motivation. For example, a person with colon cancer who has a fasting blood sugar twice the expected normal value may focus only on the cancer diagnosis and exclude or deny the health consequences of an abnormal blood sugar.

Illness and the threat of illness are usually accompanied by anxiety and stress. Nurses who recognize such reactions can use simple explanations and instructions to alleviate these anxieties and provide further motivation to learn. Because learning involves behavior change, it often produces mild anxiety, which can be a useful motivating factor.

Emotional readiness can be promoted by creating a warm, accepting, positive atmosphere and by establishing realistic learning goals. When learners achieve success and a feeling of accomplishment, they are often motivated to participate in additional learning opportunities. One example of a strategy that facilitates learner success is the teach-back technique. This technique is used to evaluate the recall and understanding of the learner after health teaching has occurred. It is a useful, in-the-moment feedback and evaluation method because it allows the educator to discover if the learner can effectively verbalize information or demonstrate a particular health behavior (Miller & Stoeckel, 2019). In addition, the teach-back strategy can be used with family members and caregivers to ascertain if they have retained and understood the health content. Having a strategy to actively involve the adult learner in making health care decisions and performing self-management skills promotes learner receptivity and motivation to integrate health principles into one's daily life. Furthermore, **feedback** (the return of information given to a person) about progress also motivates learning. Such feedback should be presented in the form of positive reinforcement when the learner is successful, and in the form of constructive suggestions for improvement when the learner is unsuccessful.

Experiential readiness refers to past experiences that influence a person's ability to learn. Previous educational experiences and life experiences in general are significant determinants of a person's approach to learning. People with little or no formal education may not be able to understand the instructional materials presented. People who have had difficulty learning in the past may be hesitant to try again. Many behaviors required for reaching maximum health potential require knowledge, physical skills, and positive attitudes. In their absence, learning may be very difficult and very slow. For example, a person who does not understand the basics of normal **nutrition** (the science that deals with food and nourishment in humans) may not be able to understand the restrictions of a specific diet. A person who does not view the desired learning as personally meaningful may reject teaching efforts. A person who is not future oriented may be unable to appreciate many aspects of preventive health teaching. Experiential readiness is closely related to emotional readiness, because motivation tends to be stimulated by an appreciation for the need to learn and by those learning tasks that are familiar, interesting, and meaningful.

The Learning Environment

Learning may be optimized by minimizing factors that interfere with the learning process. For example, the room temperature, lighting, noise levels, use of functional assistive devices such as glasses and hearing aids, and other environmental conditions should be appropriate to the learning situation. In addition, the time selected for teaching should be suited to the needs of the individual person. Scheduling a teaching session at a time of day when a patient is fatigued, uncomfortable, or anxious about a pending diagnostic or therapeutic procedure, or when visitors are present, is not conducive to learning. However, if the family is to participate in providing care, the sessions should be scheduled when family members are present so that they can learn any necessary skills or techniques.

Teaching Techniques and Resources

Teaching techniques and methods enhance learning if they are appropriate to the patient's needs. Nurses use a variety of teaching techniques to educate patients in many different settings. Techniques that are available include the following:

- *Lectures:* Lectures are explanation methods of teaching and should be accompanied by discussion, because discussion affords learners opportunities to express their feelings and concerns, ask questions, and receive clarification.

- *Group teaching:* Group teaching allows people not only to receive needed information but also to feel secure as members of a group (promoting moral support). Assessment and follow-up are imperative to ensure that each person has gained sufficient knowledge and skills. Not all patients relate or learn well in groups.

- *Demonstration and practice:* Demonstration and practice are especially important when teaching skills. The nurse should demonstrate the skill and then give the learner ample opportunity for practice. When special equipment is involved, such as syringes or colostomy bags, it is important to teach with the same equipment that will be used in the home setting to avoid confusion, frustration, and mistakes.

- *Reinforcement and follow-up:* Nurses must allow ample time for patients to learn and provide reinforcement. Follow-up sessions are imperative to promote the learner's confidence in their abilities and to plan for additional teaching sessions.

- *Motivational interviewing:* Pilot research suggests that using motivational interviewing as an enhanced educational method in an acute inpatient setting can increase both patient and caregiver knowledge as well as patient self-care (McKillop, Grace, de Melo Ghisi, 2018).

- *Electronic, online, or Internet information:* Electronic technologies are used to provide health information. Examples are interactive or noninteractive Internet learning, an online self-paced program, or a structured online course. There are also DVD, CD-ROM, podcasts, and recorded programs available over a television channel.

- *Teaching aids:* Teaching aids include books, pamphlets, pictures, films, slides, audiotapes, models, programmed instruction, other visual aids (e.g., charts), mobile device applications, and computer-assisted learning modules. They are invaluable when used appropriately and can save a significant amount of personnel time and related cost. However, all such aids should be reviewed before use to ensure that they meet the patient's learning needs and are free of advertisements that may confuse the patient. (See Resources section at the end of the chapter for additional information.)

The likelihood of success for educating patients is maximized when nurses, families, and other health care professionals work collaboratively to facilitate learning. Successful learning should result in improved self-care management skills, enhanced self-esteem, confidence, and a willingness to learn in the future. There are specific considerations for educating special populations. Table 3-1 outlines some of the strategies to use when educating people with disability. (See Chapters 7 and 8 for additional teaching strategies for people with disability and older adults.)

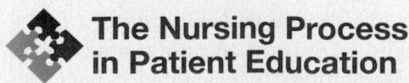

The Nursing Process in Patient Education

The nurse relies on the steps of the nursing process when constructing an individualized teaching plan to meet the patient's teaching and learning needs (Chart 3-1).

TABLE 3-1	Educating People with Disability
Type of Disability	**Educational Strategy**
Physical, Emotional, or Cognitive Disability	Adapt information to accommodate the person's cognitive, perceptual, and behavioral disabilities. Give clear written and oral information. Highlight significant information for easy reference. Avoid medical terminology or "jargon."
Hearing Impairment	Use slow, directed, deliberate speech. Use sign language or interpreter services if appropriate. Position yourself so that the person can see your mouth if speech reading. Use telecommunication devices (TTY or TDD) for the person with hearing impairment. Use written materials and visual aids, such as models and diagrams. Use captioned videos, films, and computer-generated materials. Speak on the side of the "good ear" if unilateral deafness is present.
Sensory Disability	Use optical devices such as a magnifying lens. Use proper lighting and proper contrast of colors on materials and equipment. Use or convert information to auditory and tactile formats if appropriate (e.g., Braille or large-print materials). Obtain audiotapes, CDs, digital audio available on smartphones or tablets, and talking books. Explain noises associated with procedures, equipment, and treatments. Arrange materials in clockwise pattern.
Learning Disabilities Input disability	If visual perceptual disorder: Explain information verbally; repeat and reinforce frequently. Use audiotapes, CDs, and digital audio. Encourage learner to verbalize information received. If auditory perceptual disorder: Speak slowly with as few words as possible; repeat and reinforce frequently. Use direct eye contact (as appropriate for the person's culture) to help focus on the task. Use demonstration and return demonstration, such as modeling, role-playing, and hands-on experiences. Use visual tools; written materials; and computers, tablets, and smartphones.
Output disability	Use all senses as appropriate. Use written, audiotape, and computerized or other electronic information. Review information and give time verbally to interact and ask questions. Use hand gestures and motions.
Developmental disability	Base information and teaching on developmental stage, not chronologic age. Use nonverbal cues, gestures, signing, and symbols as needed. Use simple explanations and concrete examples with repetition. Encourage active participation. Demonstrate information, and have person perform return demonstrations.

Assessment

Assessment in the teaching–learning process is directed toward the systematic collection of data about the patient's and family's learning needs and readiness to learn. The nurse identifies all internal and external variables that affect the patient's readiness to learn. Many learning assessment guides are available. Some guides are directed toward the collection of general health information (e.g., healthy eating), whereas others are specific to medication regimens or disease processes (e.g., stroke risk assessments). Such guides facilitate assessment but must be adapted to the responses, problems, and needs of each person. The nurse organizes, analyzes, synthesizes, and summarizes the assessment data collected and determines the patient's need for teaching.

Nursing Diagnosis

The process of formulating nursing diagnoses makes educational goals and evaluations of progress more specific and meaningful. Teaching is an integral intervention implied by all nursing diagnoses, and for some diagnoses, education is the primary intervention. Examples of nursing diagnoses that help in planning for educational needs are impaired health maintenance and decisional conflict. A nursing diagnosis that relates specifically to a patient's and family's learning needs serves as a guide in the development of the teaching plan.

Planning

Once the nursing diagnoses have been identified, the planning component of the teaching–learning process is established in accordance with the steps of the nursing process:

1. Assigning priorities to the diagnoses
2. Specifying the immediate, intermediate, and long-term goals of learning
3. Identifying specific teaching strategies appropriate for attaining goals
4. Specifying the expected outcomes
5. Documenting the diagnoses, goals, teaching strategies, and expected outcomes of the teaching plan

The assignment of priorities to the diagnoses should be a collaborative effort by the nurse and the patient or family members. Consideration must be given to the urgency of

---

Chart 3-1

Summary of the Nursing Process for Individualized Patient Education

Assessment

1. Assess the person's readiness for health education.
   a. What are the person's health beliefs and behaviors?
   b. What physical and psychosocial adaptations does the person need to make?
   c. Is the learner ready to learn?
   d. Is the person able to learn these behaviors?
   e. What additional information about the person is needed?
   f. Are there any variables (e.g., hearing or visual impairment, cognitive issues, literacy issues) that will affect the choice of teaching strategy or approach?
   g. What are the person's expectations?
   h. What does the person want to learn?
2. Organize, analyze, synthesize, and summarize the collected data.

Nursing Diagnosis

1. Formulate the nursing diagnoses that relate to the person's learning needs.
2. Identify the learning needs, their characteristics, and their etiology.

Planning

1. Assign priority to the nursing diagnoses that relate to the person's learning needs.
2. Specify the immediate, intermediate, and long-term learning goals established by teacher and learner together.
3. Identify teaching strategies appropriate for goal attainment.
4. Establish expected outcomes.
5. Develop the written teaching plan.
   a. Include diagnoses, goals, teaching strategies, and expected outcomes.
   b. Put the information to be taught in logical sequence.
   c. Write down the key points.
   d. Select appropriate teaching aids.

   e. Keep the plan current and flexible to meet the person's changing learning needs.
6. Involve the learner, family or significant others, nursing team members, and other health care team members in all aspects of planning.

Implementation

1. Put the teaching plan into action.
2. Use language that the person can understand.
3. Use appropriate teaching aids and provide Internet resources if appropriate.
4. Use the same equipment that the person will use after discharge.
5. Encourage the person to participate actively in learning.
6. Record the learner's responses to the teaching actions.
7. Provide feedback.

Evaluation

1. Collect objective data.
   a. Observe the person.
   b. Ask questions to determine whether the person understands.
   c. Use rating scales, checklists, anecdotal notes, and written tests when appropriate.
2. Compare the person's behavioral responses with the expected outcomes. Determine the extent to which the goals were achieved.
3. Include the person, family or significant others, nursing team members, and other health care team members in the evaluation.
4. Identify alterations that need to be made in the teaching plan.
5. Make referrals to appropriate sources or agencies for reinforcement of learning after discharge.
6. Continue all steps of the teaching process: assessment, diagnosis, planning, implementation, and evaluation.

---

the patient's learning needs; the most critical needs should receive the highest priority.

 Concept Mastery Alert

> The nurse needs to keep in mind that before the teaching strategy can be determined, the goals of learning must be developed.

After the diagnostic priorities have been mutually established, it is important to identify the immediate and long-term goals and the teaching strategies appropriate for attaining the goals. Teaching is most effective when the objectives of both the patient and the nurse are in agreement (Bastable, 2017). Learning begins with the establishment of goals that are appropriate to the situation and realistic in terms of the patient's ability and desire to achieve them. Involving the patient and family in establishing goals and in planning teaching strategies promotes their cooperation in the implementation of the teaching plan.

Outcomes of teaching strategies can be stated in terms of expected behaviors of patients, families, or both. Outcomes should be realistic and measurable, and the critical time periods for attaining them should be identified. The desired outcomes and the critical time periods serve

as a basis for evaluating the effectiveness of the teaching strategies.

During the planning phase, the nurse must consider the sequence in which the subject matter is presented. Critical information (e.g., survival skills for a patient with diabetes) and material that the person or family identifies to be of particular importance must receive high priority. An outline is often helpful for arranging the subject matter and for ensuring that all necessary information is included. In addition, appropriate teaching aids to be used in implementing teaching strategies are prepared or selected at this time. Patient Education charts throughout this textbook guide teaching about self-care.

The entire planning phase concludes with the formulation of the teaching plan. This teaching plan communicates the following information to all members of the nursing team:

- The nursing diagnoses that specifically relate to the patient's learning needs and the priorities of these diagnoses
- The goals of the teaching strategies
- The teaching strategies that are appropriate for goal attainment
- The expected outcomes, which identify the desired behavioral responses of the learner
- The critical time period within which each outcome is expected to be met

- The patient's behavioral responses (which are documented on the teaching plan)

The same rules that apply to writing and revising the plan of nursing care apply to the teaching plan.

Implementation

In the implementation phase of the teaching–learning process, the patient, family, and other members of the nursing and health care team carry out the activities outlined in the teaching plan. The nurse coordinates these activities.

Flexibility during the implementation phase of the teaching–learning process and ongoing assessment of patient responses to the teaching strategies support modification of the teaching plan as necessary. Creativity in promoting and sustaining the patient's motivation to learn is essential. New learning needs that may arise after discharge from the hospital or after home care visits have ended should also be taken into account.

The implementation phase ends when the teaching strategies have been completed and when the patient's responses to the actions have been recorded. This serves as the basis for evaluating how well the defined goals and expected outcomes have been achieved.

Evaluation

Evaluation of the teaching–learning process determines how effectively the patient has responded to teaching and to what extent the goals have been achieved. An evaluation must be made to determine what was effective and what needs to be changed or reinforced. It cannot be assumed that patients have learned just because teaching has occurred; learning does not automatically follow teaching. An important part of the evaluation phase addresses the question, "What could be done to improve teaching and enhance learning?" Answers to this question direct the changes to be made in the teaching plan.

Various measurement techniques can be used to identify changes in patient behavior as evidence that learning has taken place. These techniques include directly observing the behavior; using rating scales, checklists, or anecdotal notes to document the behavior; and indirectly measuring results using oral questioning and written tests. All direct measurements should be supplemented with indirect measurements whenever possible. Using more than one measuring technique enhances the reliability of the resulting data and decreases the potential for error from a measurement strategy.

In many situations, measurement of actual behavior is the most accurate and appropriate evaluation technique. Nurses often perform comparative analyses using patient admission data as the baseline: Selected data points observed when nursing care is given and self-care is initiated are compared with the patient's baseline data. In other cases, indirect measurement may be used. Some examples of indirect measurement are patient satisfaction surveys, attitude surveys, and instruments that evaluate specific health status variables.

Measurement is only the beginning of evaluation, which must be followed by data interpretation and judgments about learning and teaching. These aspects of evaluation should be conducted periodically throughout the teaching–learning program, at its conclusion, and at varying periods after the teaching has ended.

Evaluation of learning after teaching that occurs in any setting (e.g., clinics, offices, nursing centers, hospitals) is essential, because the analysis of teaching outcomes must extend into aftercare. With shortened lengths of hospital stay and with short-stay and same-day surgical procedures, follow-up evaluation is especially important. Coordination of efforts and sharing of information between hospital- and community-based nursing personnel facilitate postdischarge teaching and home care evaluation.

Evaluation is not the final step in the teaching–learning process but is the beginning of a new patient assessment. The information gathered during evaluation should be used to redirect teaching actions, with the goal of improving the patient's responses and outcomes.

Health Promotion

Health teaching and health promotion are linked by a common goal—to encourage people to achieve as high a level of wellness as possible so that they can live maximally healthy lives and avoid preventable illnesses. The call for health promotion has become a cornerstone in health policy because of the need to control costs and reduce unnecessary sickness and death.

Health goals for the nation are established in the publication *Healthy People 2030*. The priorities from this initiative were identified as health promotion, health protection, and the use of preventive services. *Healthy People 2030* defines the current national health promotion and disease prevention initiative for the nation. Measurable goals for key health topics for the nation are shown in Chart 3-2. The overall goals are to (1) increase the quality and years of healthy life for people and (2) eliminate health disparities among various segments of the population (Haskins, 2017; U.S. Department of Health and Human Services, 2017).

Definition

Health promotion may be defined as those activities that assist people in developing resources that maintain or enhance well-being and improve their quality of life. These activities involve people's efforts to remain healthy in the absence of

---

Chart 3-2

Select Topics from the Proposed Objectives for *Healthy People 2030*

Access to Health Services
Adolescent Health
Arthritis, Osteoporosis, and Chronic Back Conditions
Blood Disorders and Blood Safety
Cancer
Chronic Kidney Disease
Dementias, Including Alzheimer's Disease
Diabetes
Disability and Health
Educational and Community-Based Programs

Adapted from Haskins, J. (2017). Healthy People 2030 to create objectives for health of nation: Process underway for next 10-year plan. *The Nation's Health, 47*(6), 1–14; U.S. Department of Health and Human Services. (2017). *Healthy People 2030*. Retrieved on 7/15/2019 at: www.healthypeople.gov/2020/About-Healthy-People/Development-Healthy-People-2030/framework

symptoms, may not require the assistance of a health care team member, and occur within or outside of the health system (Haber, 2019; O'Donnell, 2017).

The purpose of health promotion is to focus on the person's potential for wellness and to encourage appropriate alterations in personal habits, lifestyle, and environment in ways that reduce risks and enhance health and well-being. As discussed in Chapter 1, health is viewed as a dynamic, ever-changing condition that enables people to function at an optimal potential at any given time, whereas wellness, a reflection of health, involves a conscious and deliberate attempt to maximize one's health. Health promotion is an active process—that is, it is not something that can be prescribed or dictated. It is up to each person to decide whether to make changes to promote a higher level of wellness. Only the individual can make these choices.

Health Promotion Models

Several health promotion models identify health-protecting behaviors and seek to explain what makes people engage in preventive behaviors. A health-protecting behavior is defined as any behavior performed by people, regardless of their actual or perceived health condition, for the purpose of promoting or maintaining their health, whether or not the behavior produces the desired outcome (Murdaugh, Parsons, & Pender, 2019).

The Health Belief Model was designed to foster understanding of why some healthy people choose actions to prevent illness while others do not. Developed by Becker (1974), the model is based on the premise that four variables influence the selection and use of health promotion behaviors. Demographic and disease factors, the first variable, include patient characteristics, such as age, gender, education, employment, severity of illness or disability, and length of illness. Barriers, the second variable, are defined as factors leading to unavailability or difficulty in gaining access to a specific health promotion alternative. Resources, the third variable, encompass such factors as financial and social support. Perceptual factors, the fourth variable, consist of how the person views his or her health status, self-efficacy, and the perceived demands of the illness. Further research has demonstrated that these four variables have a positive correlation with a person's quality of life (Becker, Stuifbergen, Oh, et al., 1993).

Another model, the Resource Model of Preventive Health Behavior, addresses the ways in which people use resources to promote health (Murdaugh et al., 2019). It is based on Social Learning Theory and emphasizes the importance of motivational factors in acquiring and sustaining health promotion behaviors. This model explores how cognitive-perceptual factors affect the person's view of the importance of health. It also examines perceived control of health, self-efficacy, health status, and the benefits and barriers to health-promoting behaviors. Nurse educators can use this model to assess how demographic variables, health behaviors, and social and health resources influence health promotion.

The Canadian health promotion initiative, Achieving Health for All, builds on the work of Lalonde (1977), in which four determinants of health—human biology, environment, lifestyle, and the health care delivery system—were identified. Determinants of health were defined as factors and conditions that have an influence on the health of individuals and communities. Since the 1970s, a total of 12 health determinants have been identified, and this number will continue to increase as population health research progresses. Determinants of health provide a framework for assessing and evaluating the population's health.

A model crafted to address organizational and individual health behavior change is the Awareness, Motivation, Skills, and Opportunity (AMSO) Model. The four components of this model focus on empowering people, understanding their individual priorities, and assisting them to change in personal ways that promote and maintain their optimal level of health. The dimensions of optimal health are physical, emotional, social, intellectual, and spiritual. This model promotes the process of creating and maintaining a balance among these five dimensions (O'Donnell, 2017). Optimal health is a dynamic condition kept in balance by a combination of efforts to sustain awareness, maintain motivation, build skills, and have opportunities to practice positive health behaviors.

The Transtheoretical Model of Change, also known as the Stages of Change Model, is a framework that focuses on the motivation of a person to make decisions that promote healthy behavior change (DiClemente, 2007). Table 3-2 shows the six stages in the model. Research indicates that people working with health professionals progress through these stages of change (Blake, Stanulewicz, & McGill, 2017; Chen, Palmer, & Lin, 2018; Das, Rouseff, Guzman, et al., 2019; Wen, Li, Wang, et al., 2018). Any of the models can serve as an organizing framework for clinical work and research that support the enhancement of health. Research suggests that the application of health promotion models, concepts, and frameworks increases the nurse's understanding of the health promotion behaviors of families and communities (Støle, Nilsen, & Joranger, 2019).

TABLE 3-2	Stages in the Transtheoretical Model of Change
Stage	**Description**
1. Precontemplative	The person is not thinking about making a change.
2. Contemplative	The person is only thinking about change in the near future.
3. Decision making	The person constructs a plan to change behavior.
4. Action	The person takes steps to operationalize the plan of action.
5. Maintenance	The person works to prevent relapse and to sustain the gains made from the actions taken.
6. Termination	The person has the ability to resist relapse back to unhealthy behavior(s).

Adapted from DiClemente, C. (2007). The transtheoretical model of intentional behavior change. *Drugs & Alcohol Today, 7*(1), 29–33; Miller, C. A. (2019). *Nursing for wellness in older adults* (8th ed.). Philadelphia, PA: Wolters Kluwer.

Components of Health Promotion

Health promotion as an active process includes the following components: self-responsibility, nutritional awareness, stress reduction and management, and physical fitness.

Self-Responsibility

Taking responsibility for oneself is the key to successful health promotion. The concept of **self-responsibility**, personal accountability for one's actions or behavior, is based on the understanding that individuals control their lives. Each person alone must make the choices that determine the health of his or her lifestyle. As more people recognize that lifestyle and behavior significantly affect health, they may assume responsibility for avoiding high-risk behaviors, such as smoking or use of any electronic nicotine delivery systems (ENDS) (including e-cigarettes, e-pens, e-pipes, e-hookah, and e-cigars), misuse of alcohol as well as prescription drugs and illegal drugs, overeating, driving under the influence, risky sexual practices, and other unhealthy habits. They may also assume responsibility for adopting routines that have been found to have a positive influence on health, such as engaging in regular exercise, wearing seat belts, and eating a healthy diet.

Various techniques have been used to encourage people to accept responsibility for their health, including public service announcements, educational programs, and reward systems. No one technique has been found to be superior to any other. Instead, self-responsibility for health promotion is individualized and depends on a person's desires and inner motivations. Health promotion programs are important tools for encouraging people to assume responsibility for their health and to develop behaviors that improve health.

Nutritional Awareness

Nutrition, as a component of health promotion, has become the focus of considerable attention and publicity with the growing epidemic of obesity in the United States. A vast array of books and magazine articles address the topics of special diets; natural foods; and the hazards associated with certain substances, such as sugar, salt, cholesterol, trans fats, carbohydrates, artificial colors, and food additives. Research suggests that good nutrition is the single most significant factor in determining health status, longevity, and weight control (U.S. Department of Agriculture and U.S. Department of Health and Human Services, 2015).

Nutritional awareness involves an understanding of the importance of a healthy diet that supplies all essential nutrients. Understanding the relationship between diet and disease is an important facet of a person's self-care. Some clinicians believe that a healthy diet is one that substitutes "natural" foods for processed and refined ones and reduces the intake of sugar, salt, fat, cholesterol, caffeine, alcohol, food additives, and preservatives.

Chapter 4 contains further information about the assessment of a person's nutritional status. It describes the physical signs indicating nutritional status, assessment of food intake (food record, 24-hour recall), the dietary guidelines presented in the MyPlate plan (see Fig. 4-5), and calculation of body mass index (see Table 4-1).

Stress Reduction and Management

Stress management (behaviors and techniques used to strengthen a person's resources against stress), and stress reduction are important aspects of health promotion. Studies suggest the negative effects of stress on health and a cause-and-effect relationship between stress and infectious diseases, traumatic injuries (e.g., motor vehicle crashes), and some chronic illnesses. Stress has become inevitable in contemporary societies in which demands for productivity have become excessive. More and more emphasis is placed on encouraging people to manage stress appropriately and to reduce the pressures that are counterproductive. Research suggests that including techniques such as relaxation training, exercise, yoga, and modification of stressful situations in health promotion programs assist patients in dealing with stress (Davidson, Graham, Montross-Thomas, et al., 2017; Hoogland, Lechner, Gonzalez, et al., 2018; Kim, Lee, Lee, et al., 2019; Morgan, Hourani, & Tueller, 2017; Moscoso, Goese, Van Hyfte, et al., 2019; Yadav, Yadav, Sarvottam, et al., 2017). Further information on stress management, including health risk appraisal and stress reduction methods such as the Benson Relaxation Response, can be found in Chapter 5.

Physical Fitness

Physical fitness (the condition of being physically healthy as a result of proper exercise and nutrition) is an important component of health promotion. Clinicians and researchers (Katsura, Takeda, Hara, et al., 2019; Loprinzi & Wade, 2019; Wisnieski, Dalimente-Merckling, & Robbins, 2019) who have examined the relationship between health and physical fitness have found that a regular exercise program can promote health in the following ways:

- Improve the function of the circulatory system and the lungs
- Decrease cholesterol and low-density lipoprotein levels
- Decrease body weight by increasing calorie expenditure
- Delay degenerative changes such as osteoporosis
- Improve flexibility and overall muscle strength and endurance

An appropriate exercise program can have a positive effect on a person's performance capacity, appearance, and level of stress and fatigue, as well as their general state of physical, mental, and emotional health (Gilbertson, Mandelson, Hilovsky, et al., 2019; Ma, West, Martin Ginis, et al., 2019; Pettigrew, Burton, Farrier, et al., 2019). An exercise program should be designed specifically for a given person, with consideration to age, physical condition, and any known cardiovascular or other risk factors. Exercise can be harmful if it is not started gradually and increased slowly in accordance with a person's response.

A significant amount of research suggests that people, by virtue of what they do or fail to do, influence their own health. Many diseases and disorders (e.g., diabetes, coronary artery disease, lung and colon cancer, chronic obstructive pulmonary diseases, hypertension, cirrhosis, traumatic injury, HIV infection) have been closely related to lifestyle behaviors. To a large extent, a person's health status may be reflective of their lifestyle. For example, there is research examining how emerging adult patients with inflammatory bowel disease self-manage their chronic condition through the use of social support (Kamp, Luo, Holmstrom, et al., 2019). (See the Nursing Research Profile in Chart 3-3.)

Chart 3-3 NURSING RESEARCH PROFILE
Adherence to a Medication Regimen and Informational Support

Kamp, K. J., Luo, Z., Holmstrom, A., et al. (2019). Self-management through social support among emerging adults with inflammatory bowel disease. *Nursing Research, 68*(4), 285–295.

Purpose

The purpose of this study was to examine the relationship between two conceptualizations of social support, (the first type was received social support and the second type was perceived availability of social support) and the self-management behaviors by emerging adults ages 18 to 29 years with inflammatory bowel disease (IBD).

Design

In this quantitative, cross-sectional study the researchers administered an online survey to 61 emerging adults with IBD who lived in the United States. This convenience sample was recruited from ResearchMatch, Facebook, and through word of mouth. The participants completed a composite survey consisting of a demographic data form, the Inventory of Dimensions of Emerging Adulthood, the Inventory of Socially Supportive Behaviors, the Medical Outcomes: Social Support Survey, the Medication Adherence Report Scale, and the Dietary Screener Questionnaire.

Findings

Of the 61 study participants, 90% were female and 10% were male. The sample was noted to be primarily single and educated. The major findings of the study indicated that emerging adults who had received high informational support reported greater adherence to the prescribed medication regimen as compared to participants who had received low informational support. Within this study the researchers controlled for medications, time since diagnosis, symptom frequency, and feeling in-between adolescence and adulthood. Neither one of the two types of social support were related to modification of participants' diet.

Nursing Implications

Nurses should be aware of the needs of emerging adults living with IBD. Often emerging adults allow others to make decisions about their health management. By providing informational support, the nurse may significantly influence their patients' ability to more actively learn about themselves and how to manage their IBD through the use of group interventions and peer-to-peer mentoring. From this study it was noted that only the received social support was useful in the participants' self-management behaviors for medication adherence. More research must be directed toward the benefits of received social support for effective self-management of chronic conditions faced by emerging adults.

Unfolding Patient Stories: Vincent Brody • Part 1

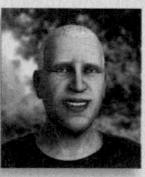

Vincent Brody, a 67-year-old male with chronic obstructive pulmonary disease (COPD), is experiencing increased fatigue. He spends most of the day in a recliner chair watching television and smoking 1 to 2 packs/d. His nutritional intake is poor due to shortness of breath. What patient education can the nurse provide to promote self-care behaviors for symptom improvement and a healthier lifestyle? (Vincent Brody's story continues in Chapter 55.)

Care for Vincent and other patients in a realistic virtual environment: **vSim for Nursing (thepoint.lww.com/vSimMedicalSurgical)**. Practice documenting these patients' care in DocuCare (**thepoint.lww.com/DocuCareEHR**).

Health Promotion Strategies Throughout the Lifespan

Health promotion is a concept and a process that extends throughout the lifespan. The health of a child can be affected either positively or negatively by the health practices of the mother during the prenatal period. Therefore, health promotion starts before birth and extends through childhood, adolescence, adulthood, and old age (Haber, 2019).

Health promotion includes health screening, counseling, immunizations, and preventive medications. The U.S. Preventive Services Task Force (2019) evaluates clinical research to assess the merits of preventive measures. Table 3-3 presents general population guidelines, including adult immunization recommendations (Centers for Disease Control and Prevention [CDC], 2021; U.S. Preventive Services Task Force, 2019).

Adolescents

Health screening has traditionally been an important aspect of adolescent health care. The goal has been to detect health problems at an early age so that they can be treated at that time. Today, health promotion goes beyond the mere screening for illnesses and disability and includes extensive efforts to promote positive health practices at an early age. Because health habits and practices are formed early in life, adolescents should be encouraged to develop positive health attitudes. For this reason, more programs are being offered to adolescents to help them develop good health habits. Although the negative results of practices such as smoking, risky sex, misuse of drugs and alcohol, and poor nutrition are explained in these educational programs, emphasis is also placed on values training, self-esteem, and healthy lifestyle practices. The projects are designed to appeal to a particular age group, with emphasis on learning experiences that are fun, interesting, and relevant.

Young and Middle-Aged Adults

Young and middle-aged adults represent an age group that not only expresses an interest in health and health promotion but also responds enthusiastically to suggestions that show how lifestyle practices can improve health. Adults are frequently motivated to change their lifestyles in ways that are believed to enhance their health and wellness. Many adults who wish to improve their health turn to health promotion programs to help them make the desired changes in their lifestyles. Many have responded to programs that focus on topics such as general wellness, smoking cessation, exercise, physical conditioning, weight control, conflict resolution, and stress

TABLE 3-3 Select Health Promotion Screening for Adults

Type of Screening	Suggested Time Frame
Routine health examination	Yearly
Blood chemistry profile	Baseline at age 20 y, then as mutually determined by patient and clinician
Complete blood count	Baseline at age 20 y, then as mutually determined by patient and clinician
Lipid profile	Baseline at age 20 y, then as mutually determined by patient and clinician
Hemoccult screening	Yearly after age 50 y
Electrocardiogram	Baseline at age 40 y, then as mutually determined by patient and clinician
Blood pressure	Yearly at age 45, then as mutually determined by patient and clinician
Tuberculosis skin test	Every 2 y, or as mutually determined by patient and clinician
Chest x-ray or film	For positive PPD results
Mammogram	Every year for women beginning at age 45, or earlier or more often as indicated; women age 55 and older may continue yearly screening or transition to every 2 y
Clinical breast examination	Yearly
Gynecologic examination	Yearly
Papanicolaou (Pap) test	Every 3 y
Bone density screening	Based on identification of primary and secondary risk factors (prior to onset of menopause, if indicated)
Nutritional screening	As mutually determined by patient and clinician
Digital rectal examination	Yearly
Colonoscopy	Every 5–10 y after age 50 y or as mutually determined by patient and clinician
Prostate examination	Yearly
Testicular examination	Monthly
Skin examination	Yearly or as mutually determined by patient and clinician
Vision screening: Glaucoma	Every 2–3 y
Hearing screening	As needed
Health risk appraisal	As needed

Select Adult Immunizations

Hepatitis B (if not received as a child)	Series of 2 doses one month apart
Human papillomavirus (HPV)	3 doses for males up to the age of 21 y, females up to the age of 26 y; men who have sex with men between 22 and 26 y; if lacking documentation of prior immunization
Influenza vaccine	Yearly
Meningococcal	1 or more doses after age 19 y
Td or Tdap vaccine (Tetanus, diphtheria, and pertussis)	Every 10 y
Zoster	After age 50 y
Pneumococcal conjugate vaccine (PCV13)	Given once to adults 65 y and older regardless of health status Given to those ages 19 to 64 y if immunocompromised, with cerebrospinal fluid (CSF) leakage or cochlear implants
Pneumococcal polysaccharide vaccine (PPSV23)	Given once to adults 65 years and older if they have previously received the PCV13, regardless of health status. For those adults 65 years and older who have not received either PCV13 or PPSV23, the PCV13 should be given first and the PPSV23 should be given at least 1 y later. Given to adults younger than 65 years who have chronic heart, lung or liver disease; diabetes; alcoholism, and smoking.
COVID-19	Administer within the scope of the Emergency Use Authorization or Biologics License Application for the particular vaccine.

Note: Any of these screenings may be performed more frequently if deemed necessary by the patient or recommended by the health care provider.

Adapted from Adult Immunization Schedule approved by CDC Advisory Committee on Immunization Practices. (2021). Recommendations. Retrieved on 4/19/2021 at: www.cdc.gov/vaccines/schedules/hcp/imz/adult.html; American Cancer Society (ACS). (2019). Breast Cancer Facts & Figures 2019-2020. Retrieved on 9/9/2019 at: www.cancer.org/content/dam/cancer-org/research/cancer-facts-and-statistics/breast-cancer-facts-and-figures/breast-cancer-facts-and-figures-2019-2020.pdf; Centers for Disease Control and Prevention (CDC). (2017). Pneumococcal disease: Pneumococcal vaccination. Retrieved on 9/23/2019 at: www.cdc.gov/pneumococcal/vaccination.html; Ezeanolue, E., Harriman, K., Hunter, P., et al. (2019). General best practice guidelines for Immunization Advisory Committee on Immunization Practices (ACIP). Retrieved on 05/19/2019 at: www.cdc.gov/vaccines/hcp/acip-recs/general-recs/downloads/general-recs.pdf; U.S. Preventive Services Task Force. (2019). Recommendations. Retrieved on 7/10/2019 at: www.uspreventiveservicestaskforce.org/BrowseRec/Index/browse-recommendations

management. Because of the nationwide emphasis on health during the reproductive years, young adults actively seek programs that address prenatal health, parenting, family planning, and women's or men's health issues.

Programs that provide health screening, such as those that screen for cancer, high cholesterol, hypertension, diabetes, abdominal aneurysm, and visual and hearing impairments, are quite popular with young and middle-aged adults. Programs that involve health promotion for people with specific chronic illnesses such as cancer, diabetes, heart disease, and pulmonary disease are also popular. Chronic disease and disability do not preclude health and wellness; rather, positive health attitudes and practices can promote optimal health for people who must live with the limitations imposed by their chronic illnesses and disability.

Health promotion programs can be offered almost anywhere in the community, or in online venues. Common physical sites include local clinics, schools, colleges, recreation centers, places of worship, and even private homes. Health fairs are frequently held in civic centers and shopping malls. The outreach idea for health promotion programs has served to meet the needs of many adults who otherwise would not avail themselves of opportunities to strive toward a healthier lifestyle.

The workplace has become a center for health promotion activity for several reasons. Employers have become increasingly concerned about the rising costs of health care insurance to treat illnesses related to lifestyle behaviors, and they are also concerned about increased absenteeism and lost productivity. Some employers use health promotion specialists to develop and implement these programs, some contract with employee assistance programs, and others purchase packaged programs that have already been developed by health care agencies or private health promotion corporations.

Programs offered at the workplace usually include employee health screening and counseling, physical fitness, nutritional awareness, work safety, and stress management and stress reduction. In addition, efforts are made to promote a safe and healthy work environment. Many large businesses provide exercise facilities for their employees and offer their health promotion programs to retirees.

 Gerontologic Considerations

Health promotion is as important for older adults as it is for others. Although 80% of people older than 65 years have one or more chronic illnesses and many are limited in their activity, the older adult population experiences significant gains from health promotion. Older adults are very health conscious, and most view their health positively and are willing to adopt practices that will improve their health and well-being (Touhy & Jett, 2018). Although their chronic illness and disability cannot be eliminated, these adults can benefit from activities and education that help them maintain independence and achieve an optimal level of health (Harbottle, Bartholomaeus, Van Agteren, et al., 2019).

Various health promotion programs have been developed to meet the needs of older Americans. Both public and private organizations continue to be responsive to health promotion, and more programs that serve this population are emerging. Many of these programs are offered by health care agencies, places of worship, community centers, senior citizen residences, and various other organizations. The activities directed toward health promotion for older adults are the same as those for other age groups: physical fitness and exercise, nutrition, safety, and stress management (Fig. 3-2).

Nursing Implications of Health Promotion

By virtue of their expertise in health and health care and their long-established credibility with consumers, nurses play a vital role in health promotion. In many instances, they initiate health promotion and health screening programs or participate with other health care personnel in developing and providing wellness services in various settings.

As health care professionals, nurses have a responsibility to promote activities that foster well-being, self-actualization, and personal fulfillment. Every interaction with consumers of health care must be viewed as an opportunity to promote positive health attitudes and behaviors. Health Promotion charts and tables throughout this textbook identify opportunities for promoting health.

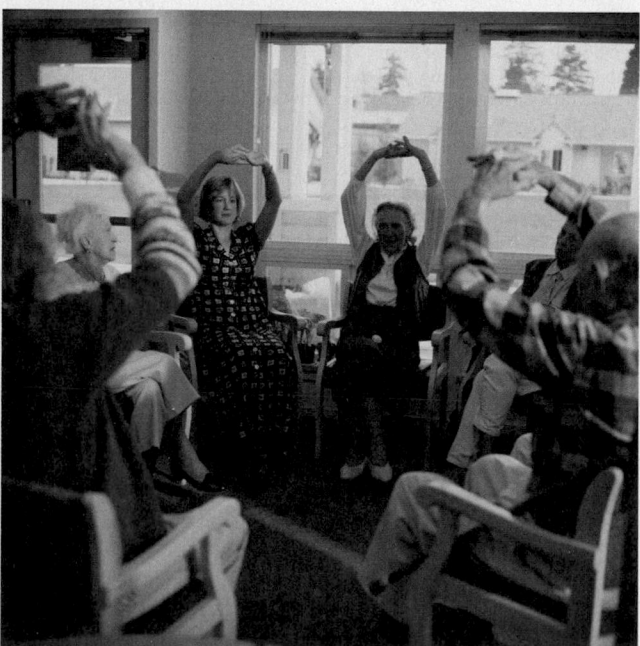

Figure 3-2 • Health promotion for older adults includes physical fitness. Here, a nurse teaches simple exercises at a senior center.

CRITICAL THINKING EXERCISES

1 **ebp** A male college student has been to the student health center three times in 2 months for sore throats, mild headaches, coughing and other cold symptoms. He tells you that he does not smoke cigarettes anymore, but he has started vaping on an almost daily basis. However, he does not think that vaping is contributing to his respiratory problems, and he thinks that his symptoms are due to stress. What health promotion factors can guide you in educating the student about his health situation? What is the evidence base to use for providing health promotion information to help this student make appropriate health decisions and engage in positive health behaviors? Identify the criteria used to evaluate the strength of the evidence for this practice.

2 **ipc** At the cardiology clinic where you work as a nurse navigator, a 45-year-old woman presents with a history of cardiac disease, depression, and recent addiction to alcohol due to her anxiety and self-medicating her depression. You think it prudent to consult other health team members to provide services for her health care needs. What interdisciplinary health team members are the essential providers to facilitate interdisciplinary care? How will the team best address the patient's health care needs? What care modalities must be established to treat the patient's cardiac needs, addiction, rehabilitation process, and psychological health treatment?

REFERENCES

*Asterisk indicates nursing research.
**Double asterisk indicates classic reference.

Books

American Nurses Association (ANA). (2015). *Nursing: Scope and standards of practice* (3rd ed.). Silver Spring, MD: ANA.

Bastable, S. B. (2017). *Nurse as educator: Principles of teaching and learning for nursing practice* (5th ed.). Sudbury, MA: Jones & Bartlett.

**Becker, M. H. (Ed.). (1974). *The health belief model and personal health behavior.* Thorofare, NJ: Charles B. Slack.

deChesnay, M., & Anderson, B. A. (2020). *Caring for the vulnerable: Perspectives in nursing theory, practice, and research* (5th ed.). Sudbury, MA: Jones & Bartlett.

Edelman, C. L., & Kudzma, E. C. (2018). *Health promotion throughout the life span* (9th ed.). Philadelphia, PA: Elsevier Health Sciences.

Haber, D. (2019). *Health promotion and aging: Practical application for health professionals* (8th ed.). New York: Springer.

Kersey-Matusiak, G. (2018). *Delivering culturally competent nursing care: Working with diverse and vulnerable populations* (2nd ed.). New York: Springer.

**Lalonde, M. (1977). *New perspectives on the health of Canadians: A working document.* Ottawa, Canada: Minister of Supply and Services.

Mauk, K. L. (2017). *Gerontological nursing: Competencies for care* (4th ed.). Sudbury, MA: Jones & Bartlett.

McFarland, M. R., & Wehbe-Alamah, H. B. (2018). *Leininger's transcultural nursing: Concepts, theories, research and practice* (4th ed.). New York: McGraw-Hill.

Miller, C. A. (2019). *Nursing for wellness in older adults* (8th ed.). Philadelphia, PA: Wolters Kluwer.

Miller, M. A., & Stoeckel, P. R. (2019). *Client education: Theory and practice* (3rd ed.). Sudbury, MA: Jones & Bartlett.

Murdaugh, C. L., Parsons, M. A., & Pender, N. J. (Eds.). (2019). *Health promotion in nursing practice* (8th ed.). Upper Saddle River, NJ: Prentice-Hall Health.

O'Donnell, M. P. (Ed.). (2017). *Health promotion in the workplace* (5th ed.). Troy, MI: American Journal of Health Promotion.

Osborne, H. (2018). *Health literacy from A to Z: Practical ways to communicate your health message.* Lake Placid, NY: Aviva Publishing.

Patton, R. M., Zalon, M. L., & Ludwick, R. (2019). *Nurses making policy: From bedside to boardroom* (2nd ed.). New York: Springer.

Touhy, T. A., & Jett, K. F. (2018). *Ebersole and Hess' gerontological nursing and healthy aging* (5th ed.). St. Louis, MO: Mosby.

U.S. Department of Agriculture and U.S. Department of Health and Human Services. (2015). *Dietary guidelines for Americans 2015–2020* (8th ed.). Washington, DC: U.S. Government Printing Office.

Journals and Electronic Documents

*Abada, S., Clark, L. E., Sinha, S. K., et al. (2019). Medication regimen complexity and low adherence in older community-dwelling adults with substantiated self-neglect. *Journal of Applied Gerontology, 38*(6), 866–883.

Adult Immunization Schedule approved by CDC Advisory Committee on Immunization Practices. (2021). Recommendations. Retrieved on 4/19/2021 at: www.cdc.gov/vaccines/schedules/hcp/imz/adult.html

Al-Noumani, H., Wu, J. W., Barksdale, D., et al. (2019). Health beliefs and medication adherence in patients with hypertension: A systematic review of quantitative studies. *Patient Education and Counseling, 102*(6), 1045–1056.

American Cancer Society (ACS). (2019). Breast Cancer Facts & Figures 2019–2020. Retrieved on 9/9/2019 at: www.cancer.org/content/dam/cancer-org/research/cancer-facts-and-statistics/breast-cancer-facts-and-figures/breast-cancer-facts-and-figures-2019-2020.pdf

**Becker, H. A., Stuifbergen, A. K., Oh, H., et al. (1993). The self-rated abilities for health practices scale: A health self-efficacy measure. *Health Values, 17*, 42–50.

*Blake, H., Stanulewicz, N., & McGill, F. (2017). Predictors of physical activity and barriers to exercise in nursing and medical students. *Journal of Advanced Nursing, 73*(4), 917–929.

Carrara, A., & Schulz, P. J. (2018). The role of health literacy in predicting adherence to nutritional recommendations: A systematic review. *Patient Education and Counseling, 101*(1), 16–24.

Centers for Disease Control and Prevention (CDC). (2021). Recommended adult immunization schedule—United States, 2021. Retrieved on 7/12/2019 at: www.cdc.gov/vaccines/schedules/hcp/limz/adult.html

Centers for Disease Control and Prevention (CDC). (2017). Pneumococcal disease: Pneumococcal vaccination. Retrieved on 9/23/2019 at: www.cdc.gov/pneumococcal/vaccination.html

Chen, M., Palmer, M. H., & Lin, S. (2018). Creating a conceptual model for family caregivers of older adults. *Geriatric Nursing, 39*(5), 521–527.

*Cohn, W. F., Lyman, J., Broshek, D. K., et al. (2018). Tailored educational approaches for consumer health: A model to address health promotion in an era of personalized medicine. *American Journal of Health Promotion, 32*(1), 188–197.

*Das, S., Rouseff, M., Guzman, H. E., et al. (2019). The impact of lifestyle modification on cardiometabolic risk factors in health-care employees with type 2 diabetes. *American Journal of Health Promotion, 33*(5), 745–748.

*Davidson, J. E., Graham, P., Montross-Thomas, L., et al. (2017). Code lavender: Cultivating intentional acts. *Explore, 13*(3), 181–185.

**DiClemente, C. (2007). The transtheoretical model of intentional behavior change. *Drugs & Alcohol Today, 7*(1), 29–33.

Ezeanolue, E., Harriman, K., Hunter, P., et al. (2019). General best practice guidelines for Immunization Advisory Committee on Immunization Practices (ACIP). Retrieved on 05/19/2019 at: www.cdc.gov/vaccines/hcp/acip-recs/general-recs/downloads/general-recs.pdf

*Gilbertson, N. M., Mandelson, J. A., Hilovsky, K., et al. (2019). Combining supervised run interval training or moderate intensity continuous training with the diabetes prevention program on clinical outcomes. *European Journal of Applied Physiology, 119*(7), 1503–1512.

Harbottle, L., Bartholomaeus, J. D., Van Agteren, J. E. M., et al. (2019). Positive aging: The impact of a community wellbeing and resilience program. *Clinical Gerontologist, 42*(4), 377–386.

Haskins, J. (2017). Healthy People 2030 to create objectives for health of nation: Process underway for next 10-year plan. *The Nation's Health, 47*(6), 1–14.

*Hine, P., Smith, R., Eshun-Wilson, I., et al. (2018). Measures of antiretroviral adherence for detecting viral non-suppression in people living with HIV. *Cochrane Database of Systematic Reviews, 7,* CD013080.

*Hoogland, A. I., Lechner, S. C., Gonzalez, B. D., et al. (2018). Efficacy of a Spanish-language self-administered stress management training intervention for Latinas undergoing chemotherapy. *Psycho-Oncology, 27*(4), 1305–1311.

Kamp, K. J., Luo, Z., Holmstrom, A., et al. (2019). Self-management through social support among emerging adults with inflammatory bowel disease. *Nursing Research, 68*(4), 285–295.

*Katsura, Y., Takeda, N., Hara, T., et al. (2019). Comparison between eccentric and concentric resistance exercise training without equipment for changes in muscle strength and functional fitness of older adults. *European Journal of Applied Physiology, 119*(7), 1581–1590.

*Kim, J. Y., Lee, M. K., Lee, D. H., et al. (2019). Effects of a 12-week home-based exercise program on quality of life psychological health, and the level of physical activity in colorectal cancer survivors: A randomized controlled trial. *Supportive Care in Cancer, 27*(8), 2933–2940.

Lambert, L. K., Balneaves, L. G., Howard, A. F., et al. (2018). Patient-reported factors associated with adherence to adjuvant endocrine therapy after breast cancer: An integrative review. *Breast Cancer Research and Treatment, 167*(3), 615–633.

Lavielle, M., Puyraimond-Zenmour, D., Romand, X., et al. (2018). Methods to improve medication adherence in patients with chronic inflammatory rheumatic diseases: A systematic literature review. *Rheumatic & Musculoskeletal Diseases, 4*, 1–8.

*Loprinzi, P. D., & Wade, B. (2019). Exercise and cardiorespiratory fitness on subjective memory complaints. *Psychology, Health & Medicine, 24*(6), 749–756.

*Ma, J. K., West, C. R., Martin Ginis, K. A., et al. (2019). The effects of a patient and provider co-developed, behavioral physical activity intervention on physical activity, psychosocial predictors, and fitness in individuals with spinal cord injury: A randomized controlled trial. *Sports Medicine, 49*(7), 1117–1131.

McKillop, A., Grace, S. L., de Melo Ghisi, G. L. (2018). Adapted motivational interviewing to promote exercise in adolescents with congenital heart disease: A pilot trial. *Pediatric Physical Therapy, 30*(4), 326–334.

*Morgan, J. K., Hourani, L., & Tueller, S. (2017). Health-related coping behaviors and mental health in military personnel. *Military Medicine*, 182(3–4), e1620–e1627.

Moscoso, D. I., Goese, D., Van Hyfte, G. J., et al. (2019). The impact of yoga in medically underserved populations: A mixed-methods study. *Complementary Therapies in Medicine*, 43, 201–207.

*Pettigrew, S., Burton, E., Farrier, K., et al. (2019). Encouraging older people to engage in resistance training: A multi-stakeholder perspective. *Aging and Society*, 39(8), 1806–1825.

*Seibre, S. J., Toumpakari, Z., Turner, K. M., et al. (2018). "I've made this my lifestyle now": A prospective qualitative study of motivation for lifestyle change among people with newly diagnosed type two diabetes mellitus. *BMC Public Health*, 18(204), 1–10.

*Støle, H. S., Nilsen, L. T. N., & Joranger, P. (2019). Beliefs, attitudes and perceptions to sun-tanning behavior in the Norwegian population: A cross-sectional study using the health belief model. *BMC Public Health*, 19(206), 1–12.

Taylor, S. F., Coogle, C. L., Cotter, J. J., et al. (2019). Community-dwelling older adults' adherence to environmental fall prevention. *Journal of Applied Gerontology*, 38(6), 755–774.

U.S. Department of Health and Human Services. (2017). Healthy People 2030 Framework. What is the Healthy People 2030 framework? Healthy People 2030. Retrieved on 11/03/2020 at: www.healthypeople.gov/2020/About-Healthy-People/Development-Healthy-People-2030/Framework

U.S. Preventive Services Task Force. (2019). Recommendations. Retrieved on 7/12/2019 at: www.uspreventiveservicestaskforce.org/BrowseRec/Index/browse-recommendations

*Wen, S., Li, J., Wang, A., et al. (2018). Effects of transtheoretical model-based intervention on the self-management of patients with an ostomy: A randomised controlled trial. *Journal of Clinical Nursing*, 28(9–10), 1936–1951.

Whiteley, L., Brown, L., Lally, M., et al. (2018). A mobile gaming intervention to increase adherence to antiretroviral treatment for youth living with HIV: Development guided by the information, motivation, and behavioral skills model. *JMIR Mhealth Uhealth*, 6(4), E96.

*Wisnieski, L., Dalimente-Merckling, D., & Robbins, L. B. (2019). Cardiorespiratory fitness as a mediator of the association between physical activity and overweight and obesity in adolescent girls. *Childhood Obesity*, 15(5), 338–345.

*Yadav, R., Yadav, R. K., Sarvottam, K., et al. (2017). Framingham risk score and estimated 10-year cardiovascular disease risk reduction by a short-term yoga-based lifestyle intervention. *Journal of Alternative and Complementary Medicine*, 23(9), 730–737.

Resources

Centers for Disease Control and Prevention (CDC), www.cdc.gov/chronicdideaser/index.htm

Health Education Resource Exchange, Washington State Department of Health, www.doh.wa.gov/Publications/HERE

Healthy People 2030, www.healthypeople.gov/2020/About-Healthy-People/Development-Healthy-People-2030/framework

Take Charge of Your Life by Making Healthy Choices, www.helpguide.org

U.S. Army Public Health Command (USAPHC), phc.amedd.army.mil/topics/healthyliving/Pages/default.aspx

U.S. Department of Agriculture (USDA), www.choosemyplate.gov

U.S. Department of Health and Human Services, National Institutes of Health, www.nih.gov/icd

U.S. Department of Health and Human Services, Office of Disease Prevention and Health Promotion, www.health.gov

World Health Organization, www.who.int

4 Adult Health and Physical, Nutritional, and Cultural Assessment

LEARNING OUTCOMES

On completion of this chapter, the learner will be able to:

1. Describe the components of a holistic and comprehensive health history and assessment.
2. Describe the techniques of inspection, palpation, percussion, and auscultation to perform a basic physical assessment.
3. Discuss the techniques of measurement of body mass index, biochemical assessment, clinical examination, and assessment of food intake to assess a person's nutritional status.
4. Describe the techniques of conducting a cultural assessment.

NURSING CONCEPTS

Culture
Diversity

Health, Wellness, and Illness
Nutrition

GLOSSARY

auscultation: listening to sounds produced within different body structures created by the movement of air or fluid

body mass index (BMI): a calculation done to estimate the amount of body fat of a person

culture: the knowledge, belief, art, morals, laws, customs, and any other capabilities and habits acquired by humans as members of society

cultural assessment: a systematic appraisal or examination of individuals, families, groups, and communities in terms of their cultural beliefs, values, and practices

culturally competent care: effective, individualized care that demonstrates respect for the dignity, personal rights, preferences, beliefs, and practices of the person receiving care while acknowledging the biases of the caregiver and preventing these biases from interfering with the care provided

electronic health record (EHR): computerization of health records; also referred to as electronic medical record (EMR)

ethnicity: affiliation relating to large groups of people classed according to common racial, national, tribal, religious, linguistic, or cultural background

faith: trust in God, belief in a higher power or something that a person cannot see

health history: the collection of subjective data, most often a series of questions that provides an overview of the patient's current health status

inspection: visual assessment of different aspects of the patient (e.g., visual assessment of the patient's body systems and body movements)

palpation: examination of different organs of the body using the sense of touch

percussion: the use of sound to examine different organs of the body

physical examination: collection of objective data about the patient's health status

self-concept: a person's view of themself/themselves

spirituality: connectedness with self, others, a life force, or God that allows people to find meaning in life

substance use disorder: a maladaptive pattern of substance use that causes physical and emotional harm with the potential for disruption of daily life

---

The ability to assess patients in a holistic manner is a skill integral to nursing, regardless of the practice setting. Eliciting a complete health history, using appropriate physical assessment skills, while respecting spiritual and cultural considerations, is critical to identifying physical and psychological problems and concerns experienced by the patient. As the first step in the nursing process, a holistic patient assessment is necessary to obtain data that enable the nurse to make accurate nursing diagnoses, identify and implement appropriate interventions, and assess their effectiveness. This chapter covers health assessment, including the complete health history and basic physical assessment techniques. Because a patient's nutritional status and culture are important factors in overall health and well-being, specific components of nutritional and cultural assessments are addressed.

The Role of the Nurse Conducting a Health Assessment

The role of the nurse in today's health care system is rooted in a health care model that emphasizes wellness, health promotion, and disease prevention. The professional nurse uses foundational knowledge of scientific evidence and best clinical judgment when assessing patients (Weber & Kelley, 2018). Various formats for obtaining the **health history** (the collection of subjective data about the patient's health status) and performing the **physical examination** (the collection of objective data about the patient's health status) have been developed. Regardless of the format, the information obtained by the nurse complements the data obtained by other members of the health care team and focuses on nursing's unique concerns for the patient. The nurse completes a health assessment by obtaining the patient's health history and performing a physical assessment, which can be carried out in a variety of settings. These settings may include an acute care facility, a clinic or outpatient office, a long-term care facility, a school, or the patient's home. The nursing process is a systematic process used by the nurse for assessing, planning, implementing, and evaluating care for the patient (see Chapter 1). Data are collected and documented in the patient's health record. This record may be on paper or in the **electronic health record (EHR)**, also called the electronic medical record (EMR), enabling clear communication among care team members and the collection of data for continuous improvement in patient care (Ackley, Ladwig, Flynn Makic, et al., 2019).

Effective Communication

People who seek health care for a specific problem are often anxious. Their anxiety may be increased by fear about potential diagnoses, possible disruption of lifestyle, and other concerns. With this in mind, the nurse attempts to establish rapport, put the patient at ease, encourage honest communication, make eye contact, and listen carefully to the patient's responses to questions about health issues (Fig. 4-1).

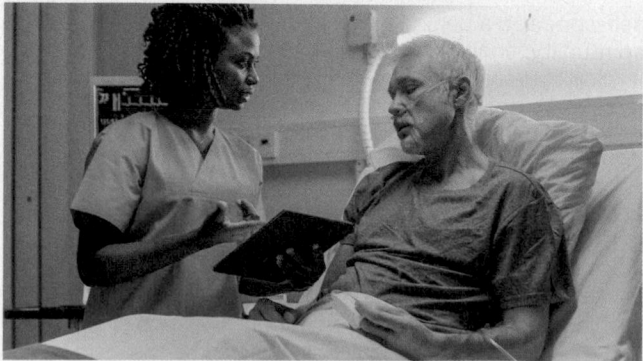

Figure 4-1 • A comfortable, relaxed atmosphere and an attentive interviewer are essential for a successful clinical interview.

When obtaining a health history or performing a physical examination, nurses must be aware of their own nonverbal communication, as well as that of the patient. The nurse should take into consideration the patient's educational background, language proficiency, and cultural background (see following discussion on Cultural Concepts and Cultural Competence). Questions and instructions to the patient should be phrased so that they are easily understandable. Technical terms and medical jargon should be avoided. In addition, the nurse must consider any disability or impairments (hearing, vision, cognitive, and physical limitations). At the end of the assessment, the nurse summarizes and clarifies the information obtained and asks the patient whether they have any questions; this gives the nurse the opportunity to correct misinformation and add facts that may have been omitted.

Cultural Concepts

The concept of culture and its relationship to the health care beliefs and practices of patients and their family or significant others provide the foundation for transcultural nursing. This awareness of culture in the delivery of nursing care has been described in different terms and phrases, including respect for cultural diversity or cultural humility; cultural awareness or sensitivity; comprehensive care; cultural consciousness or culturally congruent nursing care (Alexander-Ruff & Kinion, 2019; Henderson, Horne, Hills, et al., 2018).

Culture is commonly defined as the knowledge, belief, art, morals, laws, customs, and any other capabilities and habits acquired by humans as members of society. Such groups may distinguish themselves by socioeconomic class, race, ethnicity, religion, gender, sexual orientation, nationality, physical disability, or some other specific characteristic (Fioravanti, Puskar, Knapp, et al., 2018). During the past century, many other definitions of culture have been offered that integrate these themes as well as the themes of ethnic variations of a population. Culture also implies that something is learned or developed, a process that occurs over time. Leininger (2002), founder of the specialty known as transcultural nursing, noted that culture involves learned and transmitted knowledge about values, beliefs, rules of behavior, and lifestyle practices that guide designated groups in their thinking and actions in patterned ways. Culture guides each person's thinking, doing, and being, and becomes patterned expressions of who that person is and becomes.

Ethnicity is defined as an affiliation relating to large groups of people classed according to common racial, national, tribal, religious, linguistic, or cultural background.

Ethnic culture has four basic characteristics:

- Learned from birth through language and socialization
- Shared by members of the same cultural group, and it includes an internal sense and external perception of distinctiveness
- Influenced by specific conditions related to environmental and technical factors and to the availability of resources
- Dynamic and ever changing

With the exception of the first characteristic, culture related to age, physical appearance, and lifestyle, as well as other less frequently acknowledged aspects, also shares these characteristics.

Cultural Competence

By the middle of the 21st century, the non–Hispanic Caucasian population is projected to proportionally decrease so that it will no longer comprise the *majority* population, and other ethnic and racial populations (i.e., *minority* populations as compared to non–Hispanic Caucasians) will collectively comprise the majority of all Americans. This projected phenomenon is called the *majority–minority* crossover (Colby & Ortman, 2015).

According to the 2017 National Nursing Workforce Survey, more than 80% of all nurses are Caucasian (Smiley, Lauer, Bienemy, et al., 2018). Progress toward increasing the percentage of culturally diverse nurses has been significantly slower than the increasing percentage of ethnic minorities in the United States. Educational institutions must prepare nurses to deliver culturally competent care and must work to increase the number of ethnic minority providers in the nursing workforce. **Culturally competent care** is defined as effective, individualized care that demonstrates respect for the dignity, personal rights, preferences, beliefs, and practices of the person receiving care while acknowledging the biases of the caregiver and preventing these biases from interfering with the care provided. Nurse educators are exploring creative ways to promote cultural competence and humanistic care in nursing students, including offering multicultural health studies in their curricula. Simulation methods and role-playing could be effective methods to practice person-centered culturally competent care (Fioravanti et al., 2018).

Cultural diversity remains an important issue in health care today. Nurses are expected to provide culturally competent care for patients. To do so, nurses must work effectively with the increasing number of patients, nurses, and health care team members whose ancestry reflects the multicultural complexion of contemporary society.

Ethical Use of Health Assessment Data

Whenever information is elicited from a person through a health history or physical examination, the person has the right to know why the information is sought and how it will be used. Information is only shared with appropriate health care team members (Weber & Kelly, 2018). It is also important that the person knows that the decision to participate is voluntary. A private setting for the history interview and physical examination should promote trust and encourage open, honest communication. After the history and examination are completed, the nurse selectively records the data pertinent to the patient's health status. This record of the patient's history and physical examination findings is then securely maintained and made available only to those health professionals directly involved in the care of the patient. The Health Insurance Portability and Accountability Act (HIPAA), passed in 1996, established national standards to protect individuals' medical records and other personal health information and applies to health plans, health care clearinghouses, and those health care providers that conduct certain health care transactions electronically. The act requires appropriate safeguards to protect the privacy of personal health information and sets limits and conditions on the uses and disclosures that may be made of such information without patient authorization. HIPAA outlines patients' rights over their health information, including rights to examine and obtain a copy of their health records and to request corrections (U.S. Department of Health & Human Services [HHS], 2019a).

The Role of Technology

The use of technology to augment the information-gathering process, particularly through the use of EHRs, has become an increasingly important aspect of obtaining a health history and physical examination. An EHR offers convenient access to health data for the patient and for providers who can use the information more effectively to improve the quality and efficiency of patient care. The information in EHRs also can be shared with other organizations involved in care of the patients if the systems interface (HHS, 2019b). Nurses must be sensitive to the needs of older adults and others who may not be comfortable with newer technology. Nurses may need to allow extra time, provide detailed instructions, explanations, or assistance. It is important to establish and maintain eye contact with the patient during the health history and to not focus solely on the computer screen for data entry.

Assessment in the Home or Community

Assessment of patients in community settings, including the home, consists of collecting information specific to existing health problems, including data on the patient's physiologic and emotional status, the community and home environment, the adequacy of support systems or care given by family and other care providers, and the availability of needed resources. In addition, it is important to evaluate the ability of the person and the family to cope with and address their respective needs. The physical assessment in the community and the home consists of similar techniques to those used in the hospital, outpatient clinic, or office setting. Privacy is provided, and the patient is made as comfortable as possible. See Chapter 2 for more information on community-based nursing practice.

Health History

The health history is a series of questions used to provide an overview of the patient's current health status. Many nurses are responsible for obtaining a detailed history of the patient's current health problems, past health history and family history, and a review of the patient's functional status. This results in a total health profile that focuses on lifestyle and health, as well as on illness.

While obtaining the health history, attention is focused on the impact of psychosocial and cultural background and ethnicity on a patient's health, illnesses, and health promotion behaviors. The interpersonal and physical environments, as well as the patient's lifestyle and activities of daily living, are explored in depth.

The format of the health history traditionally combines the medical history and the nursing assessment. Both the review of systems and the patient profile are expanded to include individual and family relationships, lifestyle patterns, health practices and nutritional assessment, and coping strategies. These components of the health history are the basis of nursing assessment and can be easily adapted to address the needs of any patient population in any setting, institution, or agency (Hogan-Quigley, Palm, & Bickley, 2017; Weber & Kelley, 2018).

The health history format discussed in this chapter is only one approach that is useful in obtaining and organizing information about a patient's health status. Some experts consider this traditional format to be inappropriate for nurses, because it does not focus exclusively on the assessment of human responses to actual or potential health problems. Several attempts have been made to develop an assessment format and database with this focus in mind. One example is a nursing database developed by NANDA International and its 13 domains: health promotion, nutrition, elimination and exchange, activity/rest, perception/cognition, self-perception, role relationships, sexuality, coping/stress tolerance, life principles, safety/protection, comfort, and growth/development (Ackley et al., 2019) (see Chapter 1, Chart 1-6 for further details). Although there is support in nursing for using this approach, no consensus for its use has been reached.

The National Information Center on Health Services Research and Health Care Technology (NICHSR) and other groups from the public and private sectors have focused on assessing not only biologic health but also other dimensions of health. These dimensions include physical, functional, emotional, mental, and social health. Efforts to assess health status have focused on the manner in which disease or disability affects a patient's functional status—that is, the ability of patients to function normally and perform their usual physical, mental, and social activities. An emphasis on functional assessment is viewed as more holistic than the traditional medical history. Instruments to assess health status in these ways may be used by nurses along with their own clinical assessment skills to determine the impact of illness, disease, disability, and health problems on functional status (U.S. National Library of Medicine, 2019).

Regardless of the assessment format used, the focus of nurses during data collection is different from that of primary providers and other health care team members. Combining the information obtained by the primary provider and the nurse into one health history prevents duplication of information and minimizes efforts on the part of the patient to provide this information repeatedly. This also encourages collaboration among members of the health care team who share in the collection and interpretation of the data.

The Informant

The informant, or the person providing the health history, may not always be the patient, as in the case of a patient with a developmental or cognitive disability or those who are disoriented, confused, unconscious, or comatose. The interviewer should assess the reliability of the informant and the usefulness of the information provided. For example, a patient who is disoriented is often unable to provide reliable information; people who use alcohol and illicit drugs often deny using these substances. The interviewer must make a clinical judgment about the reliability of the information (based on the context of the entire interview) and include this assessment in the record. Chart 4-1 provides special considerations for obtaining a health history from an older adult.

Chart 4-1 **Health Assessment in the Older Adult**

- Obtain the health history from older adult patients in a calm, unrushed manner.
- Consider possible vision or hearing impairments. Ensure that lighting is adequate but not glaring, and keep distracting noises to a minimum.
- Assume a position that enables the older adult patient to read lips and facial expressions. Sometimes sitting at a 90-degree angle to the patient is helpful because some visual impairments, such as macular degeneration, can limit the patient's vision to only peripheral vision. It is best to ask the patient where the interviewer should sit in relation to the patient to optimize the patient's view of the interviewer.
- Determine if the patient uses a hearing aid and ask the patient to use it during the interview. Check if the patient usually wears glasses and ensure that they are worn as well.
- Be aware that older adults often assume that new physical problems are a result of age rather than a treatable illness. Some of these problems may limit their activities of daily living and lifestyle patterns.
- Ask questions related to changes in the level of functioning. The signs and symptoms of illness in older adults are often more subtle than those in younger adults and may go unreported. A question such as "What interferes most in your daily activities?" may be useful in focusing the clinical evaluation.
- Obtain a complete history of medications used, because many older adult patients take many different kinds of prescription and over-the-counter (OTC) medications.
- Consider including a member of the family in the interview process. Although older adults may experience a decline in mental function, it should not be assumed that they are unable to provide an adequate history. Including a spouse, adult child, sibling, or caretaker may validate information and provide missing details. However, this should be done after obtaining the patient's permission (further details about assessment of the older adult are provided in Chapter 8).

Adapted from Weber, J. R., & Kelley, J. H. (2018). *Health assessment in nursing* (6th ed.). Philadelphia, PA: Lippincott Williams & Wilkins.

Components of the Health History

When a patient is seen for the first time by a member of the health care team, the first requirement is that baseline information be obtained (except in emergency situations). The sequence and format of obtaining data about a patient may vary; however, the content, regardless of format, usually addresses the same general topics. A traditional health history includes the following: biographical data, chief complaint, present health concern (or history of present illness), past health history, family history, review of systems, and patient profile.

Biographical Data

Biographical information puts the patient's health history into context. This information includes the person's name, address, age, gender, marital status, occupation, and ethnic origins. Some interviewers prefer to ask more personal questions at this part of the interview, whereas others wait until more trust and confidence have been established or until a patient's immediate or urgent needs are first addressed.

A patient who is in severe pain or has another urgent problem is unlikely to have a great deal of patience for an interviewer who is more concerned about marital or occupational status than with quickly addressing the problem at hand.

Chief Complaint

The chief complaint is the issue that caused the patient to seek the care of the health care provider. Questions such as "Why have you come to the health center today?" or "Why were you admitted to the hospital?" usually elicit the chief complaint. However, a statement such as "My doctor sent me" should be followed up with questions that identify and clarify the chief complaint (Weber & Kelley, 2018). In the home setting, the initial question might be, "What is bothering you most today?" When a problem is identified, the person's exact words are usually recorded in quotation marks. Sometimes patients have no specific complaints. The nurse should report their goals instead. For example, patients might report that "I have come for my regular checkup" or "I've been admitted for a thorough evaluation of my heart" (Hogan-Quigley et al., 2017).

Present Health Concern or Illness

The history of the present health concern or illness is the single most important factor in helping the health care team arrive at a diagnosis or determine the patient's current needs. The physical examination is also helpful and often validates the information obtained from the history. A careful history and physical examination assist in the correct selection of appropriate diagnostic tests. Although diagnostic test results can be helpful, they often support rather than establish the diagnosis.

If the present illness is only one episode in a series of episodes, the nurse records the entire sequence of events. For example, a history from a patient whose chief complaint is an episode of chest pain should describe the entire course of their disease to put the current episode into context. The history of the present illness or problem includes information such as the date and type of onset (sudden or gradual) in which the problem occurred, the setting in which the problem occurred (at home, at work, after an argument, after exercise), manifestations of the problem, and the course of the illness or problem. This should include self-treatment (including complementary and alternative therapies), medical interventions, progress and effects of treatment, and the patient's perceptions of the cause or meaning of the problem.

Specific symptoms such as headaches, fever, or changes in bowel habits are described in detail. The interviewer should also ask whether the symptom is persistent or intermittent, what factors aggravate or alleviate it, and whether any associated manifestations exist. If the patient complains of pain, the location, quality, severity, and duration of the pain are determined (see Chapter 9 for a more detailed discussion of pain).

Associated manifestations are symptoms that occur simultaneously with the chief complaint. The presence or absence of such symptoms may help determine the origin or extent of the problem, as well as the diagnosis. These symptoms are referred to as significant positive or negative findings and are obtained from a review of systems directly related to the chief complaint. For example, if a patient reports a vague symptom such as fatigue or weight loss, all body systems are reviewed.

On the contrary, if a patient's chief complaint is something specific, such as chest pain, then the cardiopulmonary and gastrointestinal systems will be the focus of the history of the present illness. In either situation, both positive and negative findings are recorded to further define the issue.

Past Health History

A detailed summary of a patient's past health is an important part of the health history. After determining the patient's general health status, the interviewer should inquire about immunization status and compare it with the General Best Practice Guidelines for Immunization Advisory Committee on Immunization Practices (ACIP) (Ezeanolue, Harriman, Hunter, et al., 2019) (see Chapter 3, Table 3-3 for an adult immunization schedule) and then record the dates of immunization (if known). The interviewer should also inquire about any known allergies to medications or other substances, along with the nature of the allergy and associated adverse reactions. Other relevant material includes information, if known, about the patient's last physical examination, chest x-ray, electrocardiogram, eye examination, hearing test, dental checkup, Papanicolaou (Pap) smear and mammogram (if female), digital rectal examination of the prostate gland (if male), bone density testing, colon cancer screening, and any other pertinent tests.

The interviewer discusses previous illnesses and records negative as well as positive responses to a list of specific diseases. The dates of illnesses, or the age of the patient at the time, as well as the names of the primary providers and hospitals, the diagnoses, and the treatments, are noted. The interviewer elicits a history of the following areas:

- Childhood illnesses—rubeola, rubella, polio, whooping cough, mumps, measles, chickenpox, scarlet fever, rheumatic fever, strep throat
- Adult illnesses
- Psychiatric illnesses
- Injuries—burns, fractures, head injuries, traumatic injuries
- Hospitalizations
- Surgical and diagnostic procedures

If a particular hospitalization or major medical intervention is related to the present illness, the account of it is not repeated here; rather, the report refers to the appropriate part of the record, such as (see present health concern or illness) on the patient's health record.

Family History

To identify diseases that may be genetic, communicable, or possibly environmental in origin, the interviewer asks about the age and health status, or the age and cause of death, of first-order relatives (parents, siblings, spouse, children) and second-order relatives (grandparents, cousins). The nurse records the age and health, or age and cause of death, of each relative. In addition, each of the following conditions should be reviewed with the patient to determine whether they are present or absent among family members: hypertension, coronary artery disease, elevated cholesterol levels, stroke, diabetes, thyroid or renal disease, arthritis, tuberculosis, asthma or lung disease, headache, seizure disorder, mental illness, substance use disorder, cancer and the site or type, genetic diseases, and allergies; the nurse should also determine if there is

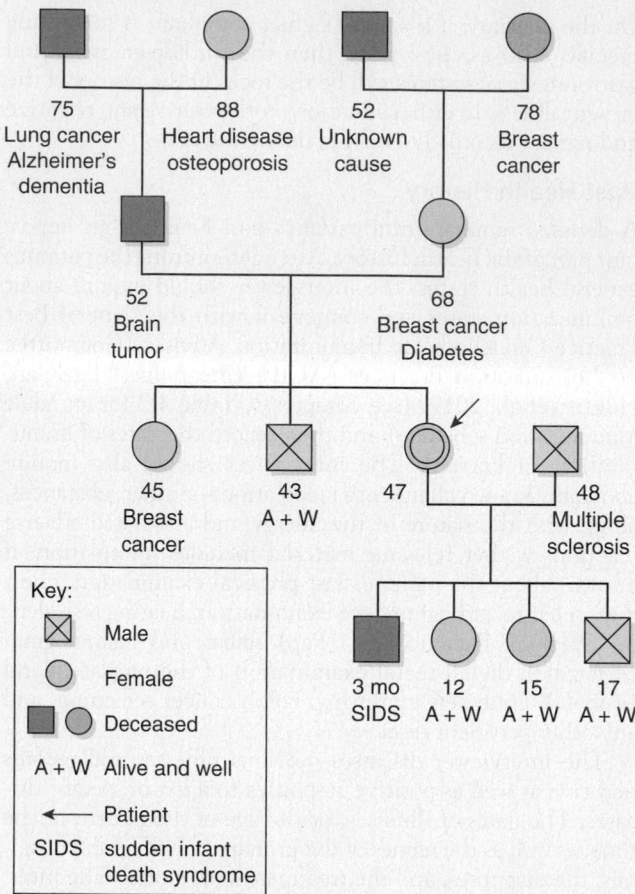

Key:

⊠	Male
○	Female
■ ●	Deceased
A + W	Alive and well
←	Patient
SIDS	sudden infant death syndrome

Figure 4-2 • Diagram (called a *genogram*) used to record history of family members, including their age and cause of death or, if living, their current health status.

a family history of suicide (Hogan-Quigley et al., 2017). One of the easiest methods of recording such data is by using the family tree, genogram, or pedigree (Fig. 4-2). The results of genetic testing or screening, if known, are recorded. Chart 4-2 provides genetic considerations related to health assessment (see Chapter 6 for a detailed discussion of genetics).

Review of Systems

The review of systems includes an overview of general health as well as symptoms related to each body system. Questions are asked about each of the major body systems for information about past and present symptoms. Negative and positive answers should be recorded. If a patient responds positively to questions about a particular system, the information is analyzed carefully. If any illnesses were previously mentioned or recorded, it is not necessary to repeat them in this part of the history.

A review of systems can be organized in a formal checklist, which becomes part of the health history. One advantage of a checklist is that it can be easily audited and is less subject to error than a system that relies heavily on the interviewer's memory.

Patient Profile

In the patient profile, more biographical information is gathered. A complete composite, or profile, of the patient is critical to the analysis of the chief complaint and of the patient's ability to deal with the problem. A complete patient profile is summarized in Chart 4-3.

At this point in the interview, the information elicited is highly personal and subjective. People are encouraged to express feelings honestly and to discuss significant health events. It is best to begin with general, open-ended questions and to move to direct questioning when specific facts are needed. Interviews that progress from information that is less personal (birthplace, occupation, education) to information that is more personal (sexuality, body image, coping abilities) often reduce anxiety.

A general patient profile consists of the following content areas: past life events related to health; current medications; complementary, alternative and integrative health therapies; education and occupation; financial resources; environment (physical, spiritual, interpersonal); lifestyle patterns; presence of a physical or mental disability; self-concept; sexuality, risk for abuse or intimate partner violence (IPV); and stress and coping response.

Past Life Events Related to Health

The patient profile begins with a brief life history. Questions about place of birth and past places of residence help focus attention on the earlier years of life. Personal experiences during childhood or adolescence that have special significance may be elicited by asking a question such as, "Were there any events that occurred when you were a child or adolescent that would be helpful for me to know about?" The interviewer's intent is to encourage the patient to make a quick review of their earlier life, highlighting information of particular significance. Although many patients may not recall anything significant, others may share information such as a personal achievement, a failure, a developmental crisis, or an instance of physical, emotional, or sexual abuse. The life history should include a brief medication history as appropriate for the patient.

Current Medications

A review of the patient's current medications is necessary to complete a comprehensive health history. Particular attention is given to allergies or adverse reactions to medications. The interviewer should inquire about the use of over-the-counter (OTC) medications and herbal supplements and complementary therapies (see next section); patients often include only prescription medications when they list their current medications.

When gathering information on use of current medications, the nurse must also consider the physiologic impact of ethnicity and culture on patients' response to medications. Data have been collected for many years regarding differences in the effect that some medications have on people of diverse ethnic or cultural origins. Genetic predispositions to different rates of metabolism cause some patients to be prone to adverse reactions to the standard dose of a medication, whereas other patients are likely to experience a greatly reduced benefit from the standard dose of the medication (Giger, 2016). For example, an antihypertensive agent may work well at reducing blood pressure to acceptable levels for a Caucasian man within a 4-week time span, but may take much longer to work or not work at all for an African American man with hypertension. In the future, genomic research may capitalize on the work of transdisciplinary teams that are building the skills needed to design and assess multilevel interventions aimed at improving the health of minorities and reducing health disparities (Agurs-Collins, Persky, Paskett, et al., 2019). Nurses

Chart 4-2 GENETICS IN NURSING PRACTICE
Genetic Aspects of Health Assessment

Nursing Assessments

Family History Assessment

- Obtain information about maternal and paternal sides of family for three generations.
- Obtain history of known diseases or disorders for three generations for:
  - Clustering of diseases or disorders.
  - Early onset of disease or illness (e.g., blood clots in an active, otherwise apparently healthy 30 year old, or colon cancer in a 40 year old).
  - Similar disorder or disease in two or more close relatives.
  - History of multiple miscarriages, birth defects, or developmental delays.
  - Close biologic relationship between parents.
- Assess for individual and family perceptions and beliefs around genetics topics through a cultural, social, and spiritual assessment.
- Acknowledge ethnic risk for particular genetic disorders.
- Determine whether the patient or a direct family member has had an unexpected response to medications or anesthesia.
- Recognize and evaluate for patterns of inheritance.
- Ascertain family relationships (family structure, roles, communication patterns, support system).

Patient Assessment

- Assess physical findings that may suggest a genetic condition (e.g., unusually tall stature—Marfan syndrome, low set ears, and epicanthal folds—Down syndrome).
- Is there a presence of two or more dysmorphic features?
- Is there a presence of disability (physical or intellectual) or a history of developmental delay?

- Assess for conditions that occur in a less-often affected gender (e.g., stuttering in females, breast cancer in males, inguinal hernia in females).
- Presence of disease without known risk factors (e.g., hyperlipidemia).
- Acknowledge genetic-related risk related to ethnic background.
- Identify religious health, spiritual health, beliefs, and practices.

Management Issues Specific to Genetics

- Assess patient's understanding of genetic information and factors related to their health risks.
- Refer for risk assessment when a hereditary disease or disorder is suspected.
- Determine if genetic testing has been performed and if other family members are affected.
- Educate patient and family about the *Genetic Information Nondiscrimination Act (GINA),* passed in 2008.
- Offer appropriate genetic information and resources.
- Refer to a genetic counselor.
- Ensure that consent obtained for genetic testing is voluntary and informed.
- Provide support to patients and families with known genetic test results for hereditary disease or disorders, and refer to support groups as indicated.
- Participate in the management and coordination of risk-reduction measures for those with known gene mutations.

Genetics Resources

Genetic Information Nondiscrimination Act. Retrieved on 6/17/2019 at: www.ginahelp.org
For additional genetic resources, see Chapter 6, Chart 6-7: Components of Genetics Counseling.

---

must be aware that ethnicity and related factors such as values and beliefs regarding the use of herbal supplements, dietary intake, and genetic factors can affect the effectiveness of treatment and adherence to the prescribed medication regimen (Giger, 2016).

Complementary, Alternative, and Integrative Health Therapies

Interventions for alterations in health and wellness vary among cultures. Interventions most commonly used in the United States have been labeled as *conventional medicine,* which is also variously referred to as allopathy, Western medicine, regular medicine, mainstream medicine, and biomedicine (National Center for Complementary and Integrative Health [NCCIH], 2019). Therapy used to supplement conventional medicine is referred to as *complementary therapy,* whereas therapy used to replace conventional medicine is referred to as *alternative therapy* (NCCIH, 2019). Interest in interventions that are not an integral part of conventional medicine prompted the National Institutes of Health to create the Office of Alternative Medicine and then to establish the National Center for Complementary and Alternative Medicine, which is now called the National Center for Complementary and Integrative Health (NCCIH, 2019). Integrative health care is viewed as a comprehensive, interdisciplinary approach to preventing and treating illness and promoting health that brings together complementary, alternative, and conventional therapies. The use of an integrative approach to health and wellness has grown within mainstream health care settings in the United States (NCCIH, 2019). More than 30% of adults use health care approaches that are not typically part of conventional medical care or that may have origins outside of usual Western practice. Most people who use nonmainstream approaches also use conventional health care (NCCIH, 2019).

Integrative health therapies are classified by product or practice type into two subgroups—natural products or mind and body practices (NCCIH, 2019):

- *Natural products* include herbs (also known as botanicals), vitamins and minerals, and probiotics. These are widely marketed to consumers and often sold and used as dietary supplements.
- *Mind and body practices* include large and diverse procedures and techniques given or taught by trained practitioners or teachers and include practices such as yoga, meditation, chiropractic and osteopathic manipulation, massage therapy, acupuncture, relaxation techniques, and T'ai chi.

Patients may choose to seek a complementary or alternative approach to conventional medical or surgical therapies. Nurses must assess all patients for the use of complementary therapies, be alert to the danger of natural product–drug interactions or conflicting treatments, and be prepared to provide information to patients about treatments that may be harmful

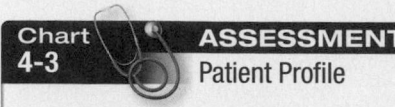

Chart 4-3

ASSESSMENT
Patient Profile

Past Life Events Related to Health

Place of birth
Places lived
Significant childhood/adolescent events

Current Medications

Prescription, over-the-counter, home remedies, complementary and alternative therapies

Education and Occupation

Jobs held in past
Current position/job
Length of time at position
Educational preparation
Work satisfaction and career goals

Financial Resources

Income
Insurance coverage
Concerns

Environment

Physical—living arrangements (type of housing, neighborhood, presence of hazards)
Spiritual—extent to which religion or spirituality is a part of a person's life; religious or spiritual beliefs related to perception of health and illness; religious or spiritual practices
Interpersonal—ethnicity (language spoken, customs and values held, folk practices used to maintain health or cure illness); support systems (family relationships and friendships)

Lifestyle Patterns

Sleep (time person retires, hours per night, comfort measures, awakens rested)
Nutrition (24-h diet recall, idiosyncrasies, restrictions)
Health promotion (exercise and recreation: type, duration, frequency; health screenings)

Caffeine (type: coffee, tea, cola, chocolate), amount
Alcohol (type, amount, pattern over past year)
Smoking (type: cigarette, pipe, cigar, marijuana, or electronic nicotine delivery systems (ENDS) including e-cigarettes, e-pens, e-pipes, e-hookah, and e-cigars; amount per day; number of years; desire to quit)
Drugs (type, amount, route of administration)

Physical or Mental Disability

Presence of a disability (physical or mental)
Effect of disability on function and health access
Accommodations needed to support functioning

Self-Concept

View of self in present
View of self in future
Body image (level of satisfaction, concerns)

Sexuality

Perception of self as a heterosexual, lesbian, gay, bisexual or transgender
Quality of sexual relationships
Concerns related to sexuality or sexual functioning

Risk for Intimate Partner Violence (IPV)

Physical injury in past
Afraid of partner, caregiver, or family member
Refusal of caregiver to provide necessary equipment or assistance

Stress and Coping Response

Major concerns or problems at present
Daily "hassles"
Past experiences with similar problems
Past coping patterns and outcomes
Present coping strategies and anticipated outcomes
Person's expectations of family/friends and health care team in problem resolution

---

or helpful, based upon best evidence from research findings. However, nurses must be accepting of patients' beliefs and right to autonomy—that is, to control their own care. As patient advocates, nurses facilitate the integration of conventional medical, complementary, and alternative therapies.

Education and Occupation

Inquiring about a patient's current occupation can reveal much about their economic status and educational preparation. A statement such as "Tell me about your job" often elicits information about role, job tasks, and satisfaction with the position. Direct questions about past employment and career goals may be asked if the person does not provide this information.

It is important to learn about a patient's educational background. Asking what kind of educational requirements were necessary for a patient to attain their present job is a more sensitive approach than asking whether they graduated from high school.

Financial Resources

Information about the patient's general financial status may be obtained by asking questions such as "Do you have any

financial concerns at this time?" Inquiries about the person's insurance coverage and plans for health care payment are also appropriate.

Environment

The concept of environment includes a person's physical environment and its potential hazards. It also includes a person's spiritual awareness, ethnicity, and support systems.

Physical Environment

Information is elicited about the type of housing (e.g., apartment, duplex, single family) in which the person lives, its location, the level of safety and comfort within the home and neighborhood, and the presence of environmental hazards (e.g., social isolation, potential fire risks, inadequate sanitation). If the patient is homeless, details about available resources are important to ascertain.

Spiritual Environment

Spirituality is defined as connectedness with self, others, a life force, or God that allows people to experience self-transcendence and find meaning in life. Spirituality helps many people discover a purpose in life, understand the ever-changing qualities of life, and develop their relationship with God or a higher power. Spirituality in nursing practice includes concerns with the personal spiritual and religious needs of the patient and nurse, as well as the spiritual dimension of the nurse–patient interaction (O'Brien, 2017).

Spiritual behavior can be expressed through devotion, sacrifice, self-discipline, and spending time in activities that focus on the inner self or the soul. Although religion and nature are two vehicles that people use to connect themselves with God or a higher power, bonds to religious institutions, beliefs, or dogma are not required to experience the spiritual sense of self. **Faith,** considered the foundation of spirituality, is trust in God and belief in a higher power or something that a person cannot see. The spiritual part of a person views life as a mystery that unfolds over one's lifetime, encompassing questions about meaning, hope, relatedness to a higher power, acceptance or forgiveness, and transcendence.

A person's spiritual environment refers to the degree to which they think about or contemplate existence, accept challenges in life, and seek and find answers to personal questions. Spirituality may be expressed through identification with a particular religion. Spiritual values and beliefs often direct a person's behavior and approach to health problems and can influence responses to sickness. A strong sense of spirituality or religious faith can have a positive impact on health. Spirituality is also a component of hope, and, especially during chronic, serious, or terminal illness, patients and their families often find comfort and emotional strength in their religious traditions or spiritual beliefs. At other times, illness and loss can cause a loss of faith or meaning in life and a spiritual crisis, which can place considerable stress on a person's internal resources and beliefs. It is important that the spiritual beliefs of people and families be acknowledged, valued, and respected for the comfort and guidance they provide. Inquiring about spirituality can identify possible support systems as well as beliefs and customs that need to be considered in planning care. Information is gathered about the extent to which religion is a part of the person's life as well as religious beliefs and practices related to health and illness.

A spiritual assessment may involve asking the following questions:

- Is religion or spirituality important to you?
- If no, what is the most important thing in your life?
- If yes, in what way? For instance:
- Are there any religious or spiritual practices that are important to you?
- Do you belong to a faith community or have a place of worship?
- Do you have any religious or spiritual concerns because of your present health problem?

The nurse should assess spiritual strength further by inquiring about the patient's sense of spiritual well-being, hope, and peacefulness. It is also necessary to assess whether spiritual beliefs and values have changed in response to illness or loss. The nurse assesses current and past participation in religious or spiritual practices and notes the patient's responses to questions regarding spiritual needs to help determine the patient's need for spiritual care. Another simple assessment technique is to inquire about the patient's and family's desire for spiritual support (O'Brien, 2017).

Interpersonal Environment

A patient's ethnicity and support system are considered when obtaining a health history. Attitudes and beliefs about health, illness, health care, hospitalization, the use of medications, and the use of complementary and alternative therapies, which are derived from personal experiences, vary according to ethnicity. A person from another culture may have different views of personal health practices from those of the health care practitioner (Hogan-Quigley et al., 2017; Weber & Kelley, 2018) (see later discussion on Cultural Assessment).

The beliefs, customs, and practices that have been shared from generation to generation are known as ethnic patterns. The influence of these patterns on health-related behaviors and patient's perceptions of health and illness, as well as on how a patient reacts to health problems and interacts with health care providers, cannot be underestimated. Ethnic patterns can be expressed through language, dress, dietary choices, and role behaviors. The following questions may assist in obtaining relevant information:

- Where did your parents or ancestors come from? When?
- What language do you speak at home?
- Are there certain customs or values that are important to you?
- Do you have any specific practices to keep in good health or for treating illness?

Support systems are another important aspect of a patient's interpersonal environment. The evaluation of a patient's family structure (members, ages, and roles), patterns of communication, and the quality of the patient's relationships is an integral part of assessing support systems. Although the traditional family is recognized as a mother, a father, and children, many different types of living arrangements exist within our society. "Family" may mean two or more people bound by emotional ties or commitments. Live-in companions, roommates, and close friends can also play a significant role in a person's support system. Keeping this in mind, nurses should use neutral terms and be sensitive when evaluating family structure. For example, the interview can begin with an open-ended question, such as "Tell me about your family and social support system." Neutral terms should also be used when asking follow-up questions about partners/significant others and parents/guardians (for further discussion, see Chapter 54, Table 54-1).

Lifestyle Patterns

The lifestyle section of the patient profile provides information about health-related behaviors. These behaviors include patterns of sleep, nutrition, and health promotion, as well as personal habits such as smoking and the use of illicit drugs, alcohol, and caffeine. Adequate sleep and nutrition are important to maintain optimal health; therefore, it is important to inquire about usual sleep habits and bedtime routines, as well as perform a nutritional assessment. Although most people readily describe their exercise patterns or recreational activities, many are unwilling to report their smoking, alcohol use, and illicit drug use, and many deny or understate the degree to which they use such substances. The Centers for Disease Control and Prevention (CDC) reports that abuse of prescription drugs has replaced abuse of illicit drugs as a leading cause of drug-induced deaths (CDC, 2019c). Questions such as "What kind of alcohol do you enjoy drinking?"

may elicit more accurate information than "Do you drink?" Determining the specific type of alcohol (e.g., wine, liquor, beer) the patient drinks and the last time they had a drink is an important aspect of the assessment. Every patient should be asked about alcohol use, substance use disorder, and misuse of prescription drugs (Hogan-Quigley et al., 2017).

The lifestyle of some people includes the use of mood-altering substances. People with **substance use disorder** (SUD) use illegally obtained drugs, prescribed or OTC medications, and alcohol alone or in combination with other drugs in ineffective attempts to cope with the pressures, strains, and burdens of life. Over time, physiologic, emotional, cognitive, and behavioral problems develop as a result of SUD.

If alcohol abuse is suspected, additional information may be obtained by using common alcohol screening questionnaires such as the CAGE (Cutting down, Annoyance by criticism, Guilty feeling, and Eye-openers) (Ewing, 1984), AUDIT (Alcohol Use Disorders Identification Test), or the shorter AUDIT-C questionnaire (Drug and Alcohol Clinical Advisory Service [DACAS], 2019).

Similar questions can be used to elicit information about smoking and caffeine consumption. Questions about illicit drug use follow naturally after questions about smoking, caffeine consumption, and alcohol use. A nonjudgmental approach makes it easier for a person to respond truthfully and factually. If street names or unfamiliar terms are used to describe drugs, the person is asked to define the terms used.

Investigation of the patient's lifestyle patterns should also include questions about complementary, alternative, and integrative health therapies, which may include energy and breath work, botanical and manual healing, and mind–body therapies (Fontaine, 2018).

Marijuana is used for the management of symptoms, especially pain and anorexia, in several chronic conditions. Since the marijuana plant contains chemicals, called cannabinoids, that may help treat a range of illnesses or symptoms, many people have argued that it should be legal for medical purposes. This has led to the legalization of marijuana for medical use in many states. The U.S. Food and Drug Administration (FDA) has not recognized or approved the marijuana plant as medicine; however, the FDA has approved medications that contain cannabinoids in pill form. Currently, the two main cannabinoids from the marijuana plant that are of medical interest are delta-9-tetrahydrocannabinol (THC) and cannabidiol (CBD). The FDA-approved drugs dronabinol and nabilone both contain THC. They are indicated specifically to treat nausea caused by chemotherapy and to increase appetite in patients with extreme weight loss caused by acquired immune deficiency syndrome (AIDS). THC also may decrease pain, inflammation, and muscle control problems. Unlike THC, drugs that contain CBD are not intoxicating and do not make people "high." CBD is useful in reducing pain, inflammation, controlling epileptic seizures, and possibly even treating mental illness and addiction (National Institute on Drug Abuse, 2019).

The assessment of a patient's lifestyle patterns also includes questions about continuing health promotion and health-screening practices. The health history assessment should include the type, frequency, and duration of exercise and recreational activities. Inquiry should also include the types of health screenings the patient has completed. If the person has not been involved in these practices in the past, they should be educated about their importance and referred to the appropriate health care providers. Nurses should recognize the importance of encouraging culturally competent care and health promotion activities (Giger, 2016).

Disability

The general patient profile needs to contain information about any hearing, vision, or other type of physical disability. In addition, developmental, intellectual, sensory, or cognitive disabilities need to be addressed. The presence of an obvious physical limitation (e.g., using crutches to walk or using a wheelchair to get around) necessitates further investigation. The initial cause or onset of the disability, as well as the impact on functional ability, should be established. Chart 4-4 presents specific issues that the nurse should consider when obtaining health histories and conducting physical assessments of patients with disability.

 ## Veterans Considerations

When conducting a health assessment, a key part of the nurse's role is to ask all adult patients if they have served in the U.S. military, and, if so, their branch of service, length of service, and assigned duty stations (i.e., geographic locations and type of assignments). Patients who are veterans should be specifically asked about their experiences with violence and war, regardless of their ages, genders, lengths of service, and assignments. Asking about violent experiences works best when it is viewed as a normal and natural part of the nursing assessment. The nurse's approach to gathering this information should be similar to that used when asking patients about sleep or activity difficulties or dietary or sexual concerns. It is important to try to establish a connection with the patient first. Taking time to listen in a nonjudgmental, nondirective way and noting that confidentiality of responses will be ensured helps create a safe, supportive atmosphere. Traumatic experiences from witnessing violence are common for combat veterans and veterans who have experienced other forms of violence, placing them at risk for posttraumatic stress disorder (PTSD), alcohol abuse (Possemato, Maisto, Wade, et al., 2015), pain (Flynn, Cook, Kallen, et al., 2017), and increased suicide risk compared with nonveterans (Kang, Bullman, Smolenski, et al., 2015). Pain is a leading cause of disability among active duty service members and veterans (Flynn et al., 2017) (see Chapter 9 for further discussion).

Veterans may be eligible for Veterans Administration (VA) benefits, including access to VA financial aid services and health care through the Veterans Health Administration (VHA), the largest integrated health care system in the United States. The VHA provides care to veterans at more than 1200 health care facilities, including 170 medical centers and 1000 outpatient sites that provide health care services of varying complexity. In addition, benefits-eligible veterans who reside in rural areas may opt to receive some VHA services through mobile vans and telehealth services. Less than half of the 20 million benefits-eligible U.S. veterans are enrolled in VA benefits services (Chokshi & Sommers, 2015).

Self-Concept

Self-concept, a person's view of themself/themselves, is an image that develops over many years. To assess self-concept,

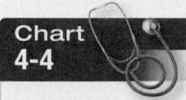

Chart 4-4 ASSESSMENT
Assessing the Health of People with Disability

Overview

People with disability are entitled to the same level of health assessment and physical examination as people without disability. Physical and mental disability should be explained in the health history. Patients with mental disability are often marginalized from mainstream health care services because of the complexities of their disability. It is appropriate to ask the patient, or caregiver when necessary, what assistance they need rather than assuming that help is needed for all activities or that, if assistance is needed, the patient will ask for it.

Health History

Communication between the nurse and the patient is essential. To ensure that the patient is able to respond to assessment questions and provide needed information, interpreters, assistive listening devices, or other alternative formats (e.g., Braille, large-print forms) may be required.

When interpreters are needed, interpretation services should be arranged. Health care facilities have a responsibility to provide these services without charge to the patient. Family members (especially children) should *not* be used as interpreters, because doing so violates the patient's right to privacy and confidentiality.

The nurse should speak directly to the patient and not to family members or others who have accompanied the patient. If patients have impaired hearing, they should be encouraged to use their hearing aids or hearing assistance technology during the assessment. The patient should be able to see the nurse's face clearly during the health history so that speech reading and nonverbal clues can be used to aid communication.

The health history should address general health issues that are important to all patients, including sexual history and risk for abuse, including intimate partner violence. It should also address the impact of the patient's disability on health issues and access to care, as well as the effect of the patient's current health problem on their disability. An assessment of whether the patient's quality of life meets their expectations should be included in the health history.

The nurse should verify what the patient has said; if the patient has difficulty communicating verbally, the nurse should ask for clarification rather than assume that it is too difficult for the patient to do so. Most people would rather be asked to explain again than run the risk of being misunderstood.

Physical Examination

Inaccessible facilities remain a major barrier to health care for people with disability. Barriers include lack of ramps and grab bars, inaccessible restrooms, small examination rooms, and examination tables that cannot be lowered to allow the patient to move himself or herself onto, or be transferred easily and safely to, the examination table. The patient may need help getting undressed for the physical examination (and dressed again), moving on and off the examination table, and maintaining positions usually required during physical examination maneuvers. It is important to ask the patient what assistance is needed.

If the patient has impaired sensory function (e.g., lack of sensation, hearing or vision loss), it is important to inform the patient that you will be touching them. Furthermore, it is important to explain all procedures and maneuvers.

Gynecologic examinations should *not* be deferred because a patient has a disability or is assumed to be sexually inactive. Explanations of the examination are important for all women, and even more so for women with disability, because they may have had previous negative experiences. Slow, gentle moving and positioning of the patient for the gynecologic examination and warming the speculum before attempting insertion often minimize spasticity in women with neurologically related disability.

Health Screenings and Testing

Many people with disability report that they have not been weighed for years or even decades because they are unable to stand for this measurement. Alternative methods (e.g., use of wheelchair scales) are needed to monitor weight and body mass index. This is particularly important because of the increased incidence of obesity and its effects on health status and transfer of people with disabilities.

Patients with disability may require special assistance if urine specimens are to be obtained as part of the visit. They are often able to suggest strategies to obtain urine specimens based on previous experience.

If it is necessary for the nurse to wear a mask during a procedure or if the patient is unable to see the face of the nurse during a procedure, it is important to explain the procedure and the expected role of the patient ahead of time. If the patient is unable to hear or communicate with the nurse or other health care provider verbally during an examination or diagnostic test, a method of communication (e.g., signaling the patient by tapping the arm, signaling the nurse by using a bell) should be established beforehand.

People with disability experience difficulties related to obtaining care, challenges accessing health care facilities, perceptions that health professionals are insensitive to their needs, and concerns about the quality of care they receive. Therefore, it is important to ask about health screening and recommendations for screening. In addition, people with disability should be asked about their participation in health promotion activities, because inaccessible environments and other barriers may limit their participation in exercise, health programs, and other health promotion efforts such as health screenings.

Adapted from Amieva, H., Ouvrard, C., Meillon, C., et al. (2018). Death, depression, disability, and dementia associated with self-reported hearing problems: A 25-year study. *Journals of Gerontology Series A: Biological Sciences & Medical Sciences, 73*(10), 1383–1389; Axmon, A., Björkman, M., & Ahlström, G. (2019). Hospital readmissions among older people with intellectual disability in comparison with the general population. *Journal of Intellectual Disability Research, 63*(6), 593–602; Mitra, M., Akobirshoev, I., Moring, N. S., et al. (2017). Access to and satisfaction with prenatal care among pregnant women with physical disabilities: Findings from a national survey. *Journal of Women's Health, 26*(12), 1356–1363; Zetterlund, C., Lundqvist, L., Richter, H. O., et al. (2019). Visual, musculoskeletal and balance symptoms in individuals with visual impairment. *Clinical & Experimental Optometry, 102*(1), 63–69.

the interviewer might ask how a person views life, using a question such as "How do you feel about your life in general?" A person's self-concept can be threatened very easily by changes in physical function, appearance, or other threats to health. The impact of certain medical conditions or surgical interventions, such as a colostomy or a mastectomy, can threaten body image. In addition, patients with implantable devices may have body image concerns, particularly those with implantable cardioverter defibrillators (ICDs) and ventricular assist devices (VADs) (Alonso,

Mollard, Zimmerman, et al., 2019; Frydensberg, Skovbakke, Pedersen, et al., 2018). The question, "Do you have any particular concerns about your body?" may elicit useful information about self-image.

Sexuality

The sexual history is an extremely personal area of assessment. Interviewers are frequently uncomfortable with such questions and ignore this area of the patient profile or conduct a very cursory interview about this subject. It is the nurse's professional and clinical responsibility to discuss issues of sexuality with patients.

Sexual function may be affected negatively by disease (or treatment), surgery, or aging. In order for the patient to maintain sexual function and optimize quality of life, sexual issues must be addressed. In addition, the interviewer should project a positive attitude related to sexual orientation or toward those who may be lesbian, gay, bisexual, transgender, or queer (LGBTQ). In addition, if a patient's sexual orientation and gender identity is not yet known, use of neutral language will help put the patient at ease and enhance the therapeutic relationship (see Chapter 54, Table 54-1, for examples of gender neutral language and assessment questions).

Sexual assessment can be approached at the end of the interview or at the time interpersonal or lifestyle factors are assessed; otherwise, it may be easier to discuss sexuality as a part of the genitourinary history within the review of systems. In cisgender female patients, a discussion of sexuality could follow questions about menstruation. In cisgender male patients, a similar discussion could follow questions about the urinary system.

Obtaining the sexual history provides an opportunity to discuss sexual matters openly and gives the person permission to express sexual concerns to an informed professional. The assessment begins with an orienting sentence such as "Next, I would like to ask about your sexual health and practices." This type of opening may lead to a discussion of concerns related to sexual expression or the quality of a relationship, or to questions about contraception, risky sexual behaviors, and safer sex practices. Examples of other questions include "Do you have one or more sexual partners?" and "Are you satisfied with your sexual relationships?"

Determining whether a person is sexually active should precede any attempts to explore issues related to sexuality and sexual function. Care should be taken to initiate conversations about sexuality with older adult patients and patients with disability and not to treat them as asexual people. Questions should be worded in such a way that the person feels free to discuss sexuality regardless of marital status or sexual orientation. Direct questions are usually less threatening when prefaced with such statements as "Some people feel that…" or "Many people worry about…." This suggests the normalcy of such feelings or behavior and encourages the person to share information that might otherwise be omitted because of fear of seeming "different."

If a person answers abruptly or does not wish to carry the discussion any further, then the interviewer should move to the next topic. However, introducing the subject of sexuality indicates to the person that a discussion of sexual concerns is acceptable and can be approached again in the future if so desired (further discussion of the sexual history is presented in Chapters 50, 53, and 54).

 Gerontologic Considerations

Effective health care for older adults requires assessment of sexual health (Weber & Kelley, 2018). Older adults may be stereotyped by misconceptions that they are sick and disabled, have dementia, have lower intelligence and are resistant to change, are not able to have sexual intercourse, or are not interested in sex (Eliopoulos, 2018); however, sexual activity continues in later life, and sexual satisfaction depends on age-related changes (Skałacka & Gerymski, 2019). Literature supports that people not only remain sexually active for a long time into their old age, but also that various forms of sexual activity is associated with their global life satisfaction (Lee, Vanhoutte, Nazroo, et al., 2016; Skałacka & Gerymski, 2019). Many older adults prefer to engage in more subtle forms of sexual activity (e.g., kissing, cuddling) rather than having intercourse. The frequency of intercourse may diminish because of body changes and health issues that may result from the aging process and/or sexual dysfunction in one or both partners (Skałacka & Gerymski, 2019).

Risk for Intimate Partner Violence

Physical, sexual, and psychological violence affects people of both genders and those who identify as gender fluid or nonbinary, as well as people of all ages and from all socioeconomic and ethnic groups. IPV, also called domestic violence, is common in the United States. One in four women in the United States experiences IPV (Smith, Chen, Basile, et al., 2017). IPV includes physical, sexual, or emotional abuse, as well as sexual coercion and stalking by a current or former intimate partner (HHS, 2019c). Patients rarely discuss this topic unless specifically asked about it. Therefore, it is important to ask direct questions, such as:

- Is anyone physically hurting you or forcing you to engage in sexual activities?
- Has anyone ever hurt you physically or threatened to do so?
- Are you ever afraid of anyone close to you (your partner, caregiver, or other family members)?

Patients who are older or have disability are at increased risk for IPV and should be asked about it as a routine part of assessment (Truong, Burnes, Alaggia, et al., 2019). However, when older patients are questioned directly, they rarely admit to abuse. Health care professionals should assess for risk factors, such as high levels of stress or alcoholism in caregivers, or evidence of violence, emotional outbursts, or financial, emotional, or physical dependency in patients.

Two additional questions have been found to be effective in uncovering specific types of IPV that may occur only in people with disability:

- Does anyone prevent you from using a wheelchair, cane, respirator, or other assistive device?
- Does anyone you depend on refuse to help you with an important personal need, such as taking your medicine, getting to the bathroom, getting in or out of bed, bathing, dressing, or getting food or drink?

If a person's response indicates that IPV is a risk, further assessment is warranted, and efforts are made to ensure the patient's safety and provide access to appropriate community and professional resources and support systems (further discussion of IPV is presented in Chapters 50 and 67).

Stress and Coping Responses

Each person handles stress differently. How well people adapt to stress depends on their ability to cope. During a health history, past coping patterns and perceptions of current stresses and anticipated outcomes are explored to identify the person's overall ability to handle stress. It is especially important to identify the expectations that a person may have related to family, friends, and caregivers in terms of providing financial, emotional, or physical support (further discussion of stress and coping is presented in Chapter 5).

Physical Assessment

Physical assessment, or the physical examination (collection of objective data about the patient's health status), is an integral part of nursing assessment. The basic techniques and tools used in performing a physical examination are described in general in this chapter. The examinations of specific systems, including special maneuvers, are described in the respective system assessment chapters throughout the book.

Examination Considerations

The physical examination is usually performed after the health history is obtained. It is carried out in a well-lighted, warm area. The patient is asked to (or helped to) undress and is draped appropriately so that only the area to be examined is exposed. The patient's physical and psychological comfort are considered at all times. It is necessary to describe procedures to the patient and explain what sensations to expect before each part of the examination. The examiner washes his or her hands before and immediately after the examination. Fingernails are kept short to avoid injuring the patient. If there is a possibility of coming into contact with blood or other body secretions during the physical examination, gloves should be worn.

An organized and systematic examination is the key to obtaining appropriate data in the shortest time. Such an approach encourages cooperation and trust on the part of the patient. The patient's health history provides the examiner with a health profile that guides all aspects of the physical examination.

A "complete" physical examination is not routine. Many of the body systems are selectively assessed on the basis of the presenting problem. For example, if a healthy 20-year-old college student requires an examination to study abroad and reports no history of neurologic abnormality, the neurologic assessment is brief. Conversely, a history of transient numbness and diplopia (double vision) usually necessitates a complete neurologic investigation. Similarly, a patient with chest pain receives a much more intensive examination of the chest and the heart than one with an earache. In general, the health history guides the examiner in obtaining additional data for a complete picture of the patient's health.

The process of learning to perform a physical examination requires repetition and reinforcement in a simulated or clinical setting. Only after basic physical assessment techniques are mastered can the examiner tailor the routine examination to include thorough assessments of particular systems, including special maneuvers (Hogan-Quigley et al., 2017; Weber & Kelley, 2018).

Components of the Physical Examination

The components of a physical examination include general observations and then a more focused assessment of the pertinent body systems. The tools of the physical examination are the human senses of vision, hearing, touch, and smell. These may be augmented by special tools (e.g., stethoscope, ophthalmoscope, reflex hammer) that are extensions of the human senses; they are simple tools that anyone can learn to use well. Expertise comes with practice, and sophistication comes with the interpretation of what is seen and heard.

Initial Observations

General inspection begins with the first contact with the patient. Introducing oneself and shaking hands provide opportunities for making initial observations: Is the person old or young? How old? How young? Does the person appear to be their stated age? Is the person thin or obese? Does the person appear anxious or depressed? Is the person's body structure normal or abnormal—in what way and how different from normal? It is essential to pay attention to the details in observation. Vague, general statements are not a substitute for specific descriptions based on careful observation. Consider the following examples:

- "The patient appears sick." In what way do they appear sick? Is the skin clammy, pale, jaundiced, or cyanotic? Is the patient grimacing in pain or having difficulty breathing? Do they have edema? What specific physical features or behavioral manifestations indicate that the patient is "sick?"
- "The patient appears chronically ill." In what way do they appear chronically ill? Does the patient appear to have lost weight? Patients who lose weight secondary to muscle-wasting diseases (e.g., AIDS, malignancy) have a different appearance than those who are merely thin, and weight loss may be accompanied by loss of muscle mass or atrophy. Does the skin have the appearance of chronic illness (i.e., is it pale, or does it give the appearance of dehydration or loss of subcutaneous tissue)?

These important specific observations are documented in the patient's chart or health record. Among general observations that should be noted in the initial examination of the patient are posture, body movements, nutritional status, speech pattern, and vital signs.

Posture

The posture that a patient assumes often provides valuable information. Patients who have dyspnea (breathing difficulties) secondary to cardiac disease prefer to sit and may report feeling short of breath when lying flat for even a brief time. Patients with abdominal pain owing to peritonitis prefer to lie perfectly still; even slight jarring of the bed or examination table causes agonizing pain. In contrast, patients with abdominal pain owing to renal or biliary colic are often restless and may pace the room.

Body Movements

There are two kinds of abnormalities of body movement: generalized disruption of voluntary or involuntary movement and asymmetry of movement. The first category includes various tremors; some tremors may occur at rest (Parkinson's disease), whereas others occur only on voluntary movement (cerebellar ataxia). Other tremors may exist during both rest and activity (alcohol withdrawal syndrome, thyrotoxicosis). Some voluntary or involuntary movements are fine and others are quite coarse. Extreme examples include the convulsive movements of generalized seizures and the choreiform (involuntary and irregular) movements of patients with rheumatic fever or Huntington disease.

Asymmetry of movement, in which only one side of the body is affected, may occur with disorders of the central nervous system (CNS), primarily in those patients who have had a stroke. Patients may have drooping of one side of the face, weakness or paralysis of the extremities on one side of the body, or a foot-dragging gait.

Nutritional Status

Nutritional status is important to note. Obesity may be generalized as a result of excessive intake of calories, or it may be specifically localized to the trunk in patients who have an endocrine disorder (Cushing's disease) or who have been taking corticosteroids for long periods. Loss of weight may be generalized as a result of inadequate caloric intake, or it may be seen in loss of muscle mass with disorders that affect protein synthesis. Nutritional assessment is discussed in more detail later in this chapter.

Speech Pattern

Speech may be slurred because of CNS disease or because of damage to cranial nerves. Recurrent damage to the laryngeal nerve results in hoarseness, as do disorders that produce edema or swelling of the vocal cords. Speech may be halting, slurred, or interrupted in flow in patients with some CNS disorders (e.g., multiple sclerosis, stroke).

Vital Signs and Pain Assessment

The recording of vital signs is a part of every physical examination (Hogan-Quigley et al., 2017). Blood pressure, pulse rate, respiratory rate, and body temperature measurements are obtained and recorded. Acute changes and trends over time are documented, and unexpected changes and values that deviate significantly from a patient's normal values are brought to the attention of the patient's primary provider. Pain is also assessed and documented, if indicated (see Chapter 9 for further discussion).

Focused Assessment

Following the general inspection, a more focused assessment is conducted. Although the sequence of physical examination depends on the circumstances and the patient's reason for seeking health care, the complete examination usually proceeds as follows:

- Skin
- Head and neck
- Thorax and lungs
- Breasts
- Cardiovascular system
- Abdomen
- Rectum
- Genitalia
- Neurologic system
- Musculoskeletal system

In clinical practice, all relevant body systems are tested throughout the physical examination, not necessarily in the sequence described (Weber & Kelley, 2018). For example, when the face is examined, it is appropriate to check for facial asymmetry and, thus, for the integrity of the fifth and seventh cranial nerves; the examiner does not need to repeat this as part of a neurologic examination. When systems are combined in this manner, the patient does not need to change positions repeatedly, which can be exhausting and time-consuming.

The traditional sequence in the focused portion of the examination is inspection, palpation, percussion, and then auscultation, except in the case of an abdominal examination (in which auscultation precedes palpation and percussion).

Inspection

The first fundamental technique is **inspection**, or observation of each relevant body system in more detail as indicated from the health history or the general inspection. Characteristics such as skin color, presence and size of lesions, edema, erythema, symmetry, and pulsations are noted. Specific body movements that are noted on inspection include spasticity, muscle spasms, and an abnormal gait (Norris, 2019).

Palpation

Palpation, which utilizes the sense of touch, is a vital part of the physical examination. Many structures of the body, although not visible, may be assessed through the techniques of light and deep palpation (Fig. 4-3). Examples include the

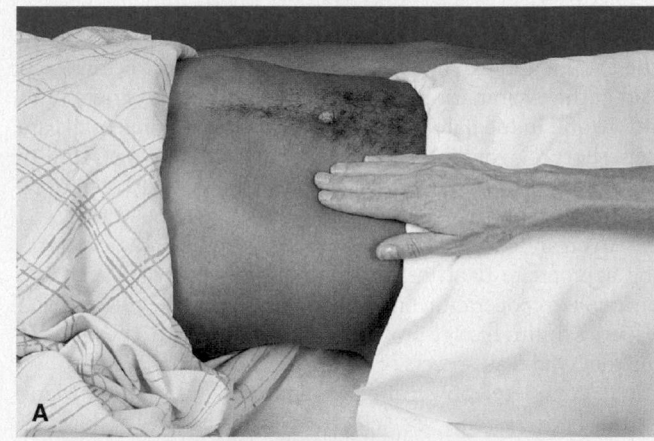

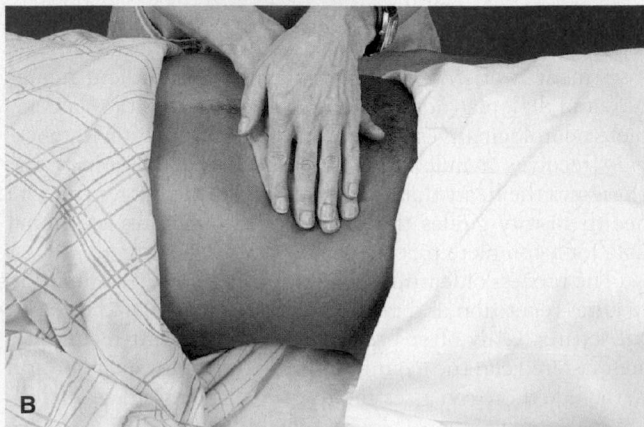

Figure 4-3 • **A.** Light palpation. **B.** Deep palpation.

superficial blood vessels, lymph nodes, thyroid gland, organs of the abdomen and the pelvis, and rectum. When the abdomen is examined, auscultation is performed before palpation and percussion to avoid altering bowel sounds (Hogan-Quigley et al., 2017; Weber & Kelley, 2018).

Some sounds generated within the body, if within specified frequency ranges, may also be detected through touch. For example, turbulent flow in the heart or within blood vessels (thrills) may be detected. Thrills cause a sensation to the hand much like the purring of a cat. Voice sounds are transmitted along the bronchi to the periphery of the lung. These may be perceived by touch and may be altered by disorders affecting the lungs. The phenomenon is called *tactile fremitus* and is useful in assessing diseases of the chest. The significance of these findings is discussed in Chapters 17 and 21.

Percussion

The technique of **percussion** translates the application of physical force into sound. It is a skill requiring practice that yields much information about disease processes in the chest and the abdomen (Hogan-Quigley et al., 2017; Weber & Kelley, 2018). The principle is to set the chest wall or abdominal wall into vibration by striking it with a firm object. The sound produced reflects the density of the underlying structure. Certain densities produce sounds as percussion notes. These sounds, listed in a sequence that proceeds from the least to the densest, are tympany, hyperresonance, resonance, dullness, and flatness. Tympany is the drumlike sound produced by percussing the air-filled stomach. Hyperresonance is audible when one percusses over inflated lung tissue in a person with emphysema. Resonance is the sound elicited over air-filled lungs. Percussion of the liver produces a dull sound, whereas percussion of the thigh produces a flat sound.

Percussion allows the examiner to assess such normal anatomic details as the borders of the heart and the movement of the diaphragm during inspiration. It is also possible to determine the level of a pleural effusion (fluid in the pleural cavity) and the location of a consolidated area caused by pneumonia or atelectasis (collapse of alveoli). The use of percussion is described further with disorders of the thorax and the abdomen (see Chapters 17 and 38).

 Concept Mastery Alert

> Whereas auscultation involves listening to sounds produced within the body by the movement of air, percussion involves applying physical force to the body in order to discern what sounds are made, thereby assessing internal organs. Hyperresonance is audible when one percusses over inflated lung tissue in a person with emphysema.

Auscultation

Auscultation is the skill of listening to sounds produced within the body created by the movement of air or fluid (Fig. 4-4). A stethoscope is typically used to enhance this technique. Examples include breath sounds, the spoken voice, bowel sounds, heart sounds, and cardiac murmurs. Physiologic sounds may be normal (e.g., first and second heart sounds) or pathologic (e.g., heart murmurs in diastole, crackles in the

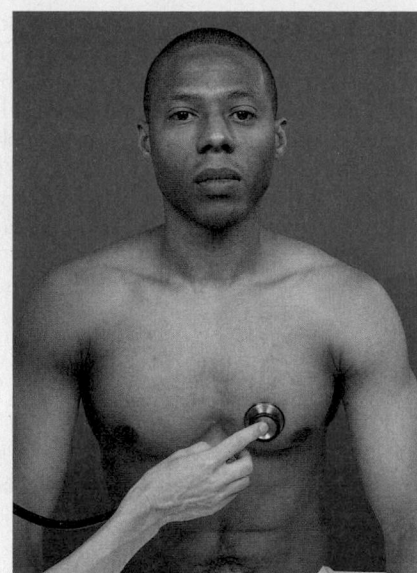

Figure 4-4 • Auscultation of the heart in forward sitting position.

lung). Some normal sounds may be distorted by abnormalities of structures through which the sound must travel (e.g., changes in the character of breath sounds as they travel through the consolidated lung of a patient with lobar pneumonia).

Sound produced within the body, if of sufficient amplitude, may be detected with the stethoscope, which functions as an extension of the human ear and channels sound. The nurse must avoid touching the tubing or rubbing other surfaces (hair, clothing) during auscultation to minimize extraneous noises. Sounds detected by auscultation are classified according to their intensity (loud or soft), pitch (high or low), duration (length), and quality (musical, raspy, crackling) (Hogan-Quigley et al., 2017; Weber & Kelley, 2018).

Nutritional Assessment

Nutrition is important to maintain health and to prevent disease and premature death. When illness or injury occurs, optimal nutrition is essential for recovery, healing, and for resisting infection and other complications. An in-depth nutritional assessment is often integrated into the health history and physical examination. Assessment of a patient's nutritional status provides information about obesity, undernutrition, and malnutrition.

Certain signs that suggest possible nutritional deficiency, such as muscle wasting, poor skin integrity, loss of subcutaneous tissue, and obesity, are easy to note because they are evident and objective. Other physical signs may be subtle, or the patient may report subjective symptoms, which must be carefully assessed. It is important to note that some signs and symptoms that appear to indicate nutritional deficiency may actually reflect other systemic conditions (e.g., endocrine disorders, infectious disease). Others may result from impaired digestion, absorption, excretion, or storage of nutrients in the body (Norris, 2019; Weber & Kelley, 2018). Disorders caused by nutritional deficiency, overeating, or eating unhealthy foods are among the leading causes of illness and death in the United States today. Examples of health problems associated with poor nutrition include obesity, osteoporosis, cirrhosis, diverticulitis, and eating disorders.

Obesity is a major concern for children, adolescents, and adults in the United States and globally. The World Health Organization (WHO) defines obesity as abnormal or excessive fat accumulation that may impair health. Obesity and being overweight are leading risk factors for global deaths; most of the world's population lives in countries where overweight and obesity kill more people than underweight. In addition, coronary artery disease, diabetes, musculoskeletal disorders, and certain cancers can be attributable to obesity (WHO, 2019) (see Chapter 42 for a detailed discussion of obesity).

Lifespan Considerations

When the nurse conducts a nutritional assessment, two age groups merit special consideration: adolescents and older adults. Key considerations for each group are highlighted below.

Adolescents

Adolescence is a time of critical growth and when lifelong eating and exercise habits are established. Nutritional assessment is particularly important during this time period. In general, adolescents gain 40% of their adult weight and 15% of their adult height during this developmental stage of life (Lassi, Moin, & Bhutta, 2017). It is vital to assess for obesity in adolescents to prevent complications from obesity as they grow and develop, as well as when they enter adulthood.

Adolescent girls should consume approximately 1400 to 2400 calories daily; whereas, adolescent boys require between 1600 to 3200 calories each day to support their greater growth needs in terms of both overall size and muscle mass. Athletes of either gender may need to consume up to 5000 calories daily to support their metabolic demands. In adolescents of both genders, sufficient micronutrients such as calcium, B-complex vitamins, iron, and folate are necessary to support increased metabolic activity during this time of growth. Adolescent girls are at particular nutritional risk, because they are thought to be exposed to expectations to diet and maintain a thin body. As a consequence, many adolescent girls are purposely deficient in their intake of dairy products, because they are caloric-rich. However, dairy products provide an important source of calcium that is necessary in order to build bone mass. Adolescents of both genders are at risk for behavioral eating disorders, such as anorexia, bulimia, and binge-eating disorders, although girls are at greater risk (Lassi et al., 2017).

Older Adults

Older adults are also at risk for altered nutrition. Nutritional assessment in the older adult should include inquiry about the patient's current dietary practices as well as a nutritional screening to assess for adequate nutrition. The Mini Nutritional Assessment is a commonly used, well-validated tool developed specifically for this purpose (Chart 4-5). Many older adults adhere to specific diets, such as those low in saturated fat or sodium, for improving or maintaining health. Proper nutrition for an older adult meets daily requirements, maintains ideal body weight, and addresses specific health concerns such as cardiovascular or renal disease (Eliopoulos, 2018).

Older adults are particularly at high risk for poor nutrition due to factors that may include social isolation, frailty, cognitive impairment, polypharmacy (i.e., use of multiple prescription and OTC medications), reduced functional status, and financial instability (Astrup & O'Connor, 2018). Disorders affecting any part of the gastrointestinal tract can alter nutritional requirements and health status in people of any age; however, such disorders are likely to occur more quickly and more frequently in older adults. Acute and chronic diseases may affect the metabolism and utilization of nutrients, which already are altered by the aging process. Even well older adults may be nutritionally at risk because of decreased odor perception, poor dental health, limited ability to shop and cook, financial hardship, and the fact that they often eat alone (Eliopoulos, 2018).

Polypharmacy also may place older adults at risk nutritionally. The number of adverse reactions increases proportionately with the number of medications taken. Age-related physiologic and pathophysiologic changes may alter the metabolism and elimination of many medications (Eliopoulos, 2018). Medications can influence food intake by producing side effects such as nausea, vomiting, decreased appetite, and changes in cognition. They may also interfere with the distribution, utilization, and storage of nutrients.

Components of Nutritional Assessment

The sequence of the assessment may vary; however, evaluation of a patient's nutritional status includes the use of one or more of the following methods: measurement of body mass index (BMI) and waist circumference, biochemical assessment, clinical examination findings, and dietary data. Measurement of BMI and waist circumference is recommended to determine whether a patient has obesity (CDC, 2019a).

Body Mass Index, Ideal Weight, and Waist Circumference

Body mass index (BMI) is a ratio based on body weight and height (Table 4-1). The obtained value is compared to established standards; however, trends or changes in values

TABLE 4-1	How Is BMI Calculated?[a]
Measurement Units	**Formula and Calculation**
Kilograms and meters (or centimeters)	Formula: weight (kg)/[height (m)]^2 With the metric system, the formula for BMI is weight in kilograms divided by height in meters squared. Because height is commonly measured in centimeters, divide height in centimeters by 100 to obtain height in meters. Example: Weight = 68 kg, Height = 165 cm (1.65 m) Calculation: $68/(1.65)^2 = 24.98$
Pounds and inches	Formula: weight (lb)/[height (in)]$^2 \times 703$ Calculate BMI by dividing weight in pounds (lb) by height in inches (in) squared and multiplying by a conversion factor of 703. Example: Weight = 150 lb, Height = 65 in Calculation: $[150/(65)^2] \times 703 = 24.96$

[a]BMI is calculated the same way for both adults and children. The calculation is based on formulas within this table.

BMI, body mass index.

Adapted from the Centers for Disease Control and Prevention (CDC). (2019b). About body mass index (BMI). Retrieved on 6/9/2019 at: www.cdc.gov/healthyweight/assessing/bmi/adult_bmi/index.html

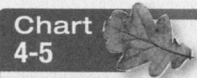

Chart 4-5   Mini Nutritional Assessment

The Mini Nutritional Assessment (MNA) is a six-item tool designed to identify adults aged 65 y and older who are either malnourished or at risk for becoming malnourished. It is available in several languages and there are several methods of delivery, including self-assessment as well as an electronic health record (EHR) version. It provides a more sensitive measure than body mass index (BMI) in identifying older adults in long-term care facilities at risk for malnutrition (Nestlé Nutrition Institute, 2011).

Mini Nutritional Assessment MNA®

Nestlé Nutrition Institute

Last name: _____   First name: _____

Sex: _____ Age: _____ Weight, kg: _____ Height, cm: _____ Date: _____

Complete the screen by filling in the boxes with the appropriate numbers. Total the numbers for the final screening score.

Screening

A Has food intake declined over the past 3 months due to loss of appetitie, digestive problems, chewing or swallowing difficulties?
0 = severe decrease in food intake
1 = moderate decrease in food intake
2 = no decrease in food intake ☐

B Weight loss during the last 3 months
0 = weight loss greater than 3 kg (6.6 lbs)
1 = does not know
2 = weight loss between 1 and 3 kg (2.2 and 6.6 lbs)
3 = no weight loss ☐

C Mobility
0 = bed or chair bound
1 = able to get out of bed / chair but does not go out
2 = goes out ☐

D Has suffered psychological stress or acute disease in the past 3 months?
0 = yes   2 = no ☐

E Neuropsychological problems
0 = severe dementia or depression
1 = mild dementia
2 = no psychological problems ☐

F1 Body Mass Index (BMI) (weight in kg) / (height in m²)
0 = BMI less than 19
1 = BMI 19 to less than 21
2 = BMI 21 to less than 23
3 = BMI 23 or greater ☐

IF BMI IS NO AVAILABLE, REPLACE QUESTION F1 WITH QUESTION F2.
DO NOT ANSWER QUESTION F2 IF QUESTION F1 IS ALREADY COMPLETED.

F2 Calf circumference (CC) in cm
0 = CC less than 31
3 = CC 31 or greater ☐

Screening score (max. 14 points)

12 - 14 points: Normal nutritional status
8 - 11 points: At risk of malnutrition
0 - 7 points: Malnourished ☐☐

References
1. Vellas B, Villars H, Abellan G, *et al.* Overview of MNA® - Its History and Challenges. *J Nutr Health Aging.* 2006;**10**:456-465.
2. Rubenstein LZ, Harker JO, Salva A, Guigoz Y, Vellas B. Screening for Undernutrition in Geriatric Practice: Developing the Short-Form Mini Nutritional Assessment (MNA-SF). *J Geront.* 2001;**56A**:M366-377.
3. Guigoz Y. The Mini-Nutritional Assessment (MNA®) Review of the Literature - What does it tell us? *J Nutr Health Aging.* 2006;**10**:466-487.
4. Kaiser MJ, Bauer JM, Ramsch C, et al. Validation of the Mini Nutritional Assessment Short-Form (MNA®-SF): A practical tool for identification of nutritional status. *J Nutr Health Aging.* 2009;**13**:782-788.
® Société des Produits Nestlé, S.A., Vevey, Switzerland, Trademark Owners © Nestlé, 1994, Revision 2009. N67200 12/99 10M
For more information: www.mna-elderly.com

over time are considered more useful than isolated or one-time measurements. BMI is highly correlated with body fat, although increased lean body mass or a large body frame can also increase the BMI. People who have a BMI lower than 18.5 (or who are 80% or less of their desirable body weight for height) are at increased risk for problems associated with poor nutritional status. In addition, a low BMI is associated with a higher mortality rate among hospitalized patients and community-dwelling older adults. Those who have a BMI between 25 and 29.9 are considered overweight. Obesity is defined as a BMI of greater than 30 (WHO, 2019). Although there are no current standard recommendations for BMI based on race or ethnicity, there is literature to support that BMI and body fat percentages can vary between genders and among people of different ages and from different ethnic groups (McConnell-Nzunga, Naylor, Macdonald, et al., 2018). In analyzing BMI, the nurse must be aware that there may be weight variance that could be dependent upon age, gender, and ethnicity.

It is important to assess for usual body weight and height and to compare these values with ideal weight (see Chapter 42, Fig. 42-3). Current weight does not provide information about recent changes in weight; therefore, patients are asked about their usual body weight and any recent weight loss or gain. Loss of height may be attributable to osteoporosis—an important problem related to nutrition, especially in postmenopausal women (Hogan-Quigley et al., 2017; Weber & Kelley, 2018).

In addition to the calculation of BMI, waist circumference measurement is a useful assessment tool. To measure waist circumference, a tape measure is placed in a horizontal plane around the abdomen at the level of the iliac crest. A waist circumference greater than 40 inches for men or 35 inches for women indicates excess abdominal fat. Those with a high waist circumference are at an increased risk for diabetes, dyslipidemias, hypertension, heart attack, and stroke (Hogan-Quigley et al., 2017; Weber & Kelley, 2018).

Biochemical Assessment

Biochemical measurements are applicable to a patient's nutritional assessment as they can test the level of a given nutrient and reflect abnormalities of metabolism in relation to the utilization of nutrients. Tests of serum and urine are done to determine whether the values are within an acceptable range. Some of these tests, while reflecting recent intake of the elements detected, can also identify a long-term deficiency (below-normal levels) even when there are no clinical symptoms of deficiency.

Low serum albumin and prealbumin levels are most often used as measures of protein deficit in adults. Albumin synthesis depends on normal liver function and an adequate supply of amino acids. Because the body stores a large amount of albumin, the serum albumin level may not decrease until malnutrition is severe; therefore, its usefulness in detecting recent protein depletion is limited. Decreased albumin levels may be caused by overhydration, liver or renal disease, or excessive protein loss due to burns, major surgery, infection, or cancer. Serial measurements of prealbumin levels are used to assess the effectiveness of nutritional therapy.

Additional laboratory data, such as levels of transferrin and retinol-binding protein, and complete blood and electrolyte counts, are used in many institutions. Transferrin is a protein that binds and carries iron from the intestine through the serum. Because of its short half-life, transferrin levels decrease more quickly than albumin levels in response to protein depletion. Low levels of transferrin can also lead to a deficiency in iron; low availability of iron in the body limits the synthesis of functioning hemoglobin causing anemia. Although measurement of retinol-binding protein is not available from many laboratories, it may be a useful means of monitoring acute, short-term changes in protein status. The total lymphocyte count may be reduced in people who are acutely malnourished as a result of stress and low-calorie feeding, as well as in those with impaired cellular immunity. Anergy, or the absence of an immune response to injection of small concentrations of recall antigen under the skin, may also indicate malnutrition because of delayed antibody synthesis and response. Serum electrolyte levels provide information about fluid and electrolyte balance and kidney function.

A 24-hour urine collection can be utilized to calculate the creatinine/height index that assesses metabolically active tissue and indicates the degree of protein depletion. The amount of creatinine is measured and the index is calculated on the basis of the patient's height and gender. The patient's creatinine/height index is then compared to normal ranges based on the expected body weight by height. Values lower than normal may indicate loss of lean body mass and protein malnutrition (Fischbach & Fischbach, 2018).

Clinical Examination

The state of nutrition is often reflected in a person's appearance. Although the most obvious physical sign of good nutrition is a normal body weight with respect to height, body frame, and age, other tissues can serve as indicators of general nutritional status and adequate intake of specific nutrients; these include the hair, skin, teeth, gums, mucous membranes, mouth and tongue, skeletal muscles, abdomen, lower extremities, and thyroid gland (Table 4-2).

Dietary Data

Commonly used methods of determining individual eating patterns include the food record, the 24-hour food recall, and a dietary interview. Each of these methods helps estimate whether food intake is adequate and appropriate. If these methods are used to obtain the dietary history, instructions must be given to the patient about measuring and recording food intake.

Methods of Collecting Data

The nurse may employ multiple methods to collect a patient's dietary data. Two common methods described here include the food record and the 24-hour recall.

Food Record

The food record, also called the food diary, is used most often in nutritional status studies. A person is instructed to keep a record of food consumed over a period of time, varying from 3 to 7 days, and to accurately estimate and describe the specific foods consumed. Food records are fairly accurate if the person is willing to provide factual information and is able to estimate food quantities.

TABLE 4-2	Physical Indicators of Nutritional Status	
Indicator	**Signs of Good Nutrition**	**Signs of Poor Nutrition**
General appearance	Alert, responsive	Listless, appears acutely or chronically ill
Hair	Shiny, lustrous; firm, healthy scalp	Dull and dry, brittle, dyspigmentation, alopecia (hair loss)
Face	Skin color uniform; healthy appearance	Skin dark over cheeks and under eyes, skin flaky, face swollen or hollow/sunken cheeks, moon face, pallor
Eyes	Bright, clear, moist	Xerophthalmia (pale conjunctiva, dry mucosa), increased vascularity, xanthelasma (yellow subdermal fat deposits around the lids)
Lips	Good color (pink), smooth	Swollen and puffy, angular stomatitis (cracks at corners), cheilosis (angular lesion at corners of mouth)
Tongue	Deep red in appearance; surface papillae present	Glossitis (smooth appearance, swollen, beefy-red or magenta), sores, atrophic papillae
Teeth	Straight, no crowding, no dental caries, bright	Delayed eruption, dental caries, fluorosis (mottled appearance), malpositioned
Gums	Firm, good color (pink)	Spongy, scorbutic (bleeding), marginal redness, recession
Thyroid	No enlargement of the thyroid	Simple goiter (thyroid enlargement)
Skin	Smooth, good color, moist	Rough, dry, flaky, swollen, pale, pigmented; lack of fat under skin
Nails	Firm, pink	Spoon shaped, ridged, brittle
Skeleton	Good posture, no malformation	Stunted growth, poor posture, rachitic rosary (beading of ribs), bowed legs (rickets), narrow chest (pigeon breast), loss of fat, muscle wasting
Muscles	Well developed, firm	Flaccid, poor tone, wasted, underdeveloped
Extremities	No tenderness	Weak and tender, loss of fat, muscle wasting, edematous
Abdomen	Flat	Swollen
Nervous system	Normal reflexes	Decreased or absent ankle and knee reflexes, confusion, neuropathy, tetany
Weight	Normal for height, age, and body build	Overweight or underweight

Adapted from Fenske, C., Watkins, K., Saunders, T., et al. (2020). *Health & physical assessment in nursing* (4th ed.). Hoboken, NJ: Pearson Education, Inc.

24-Hour Recall

As the name implies, the 24-hour recall method is a recall of food intake over a 24-hour period. A person is asked to recall all foods eaten during the previous day and to estimate the quantities of each food consumed. Because information does not always represent usual intake, at the end of the interview the patient is asked whether the previous day's food intake was typical. To obtain supplementary information about the typical diet, it is also necessary to ask how frequently the person eats foods from the major food groups.

Dietary Interview

The success of the interviewer in obtaining information for dietary assessment depends on effective communication, which requires that good rapport be established to promote respect and trust. The interview is conducted in a nondirective and exploratory way, allowing the respondent to express feelings and thoughts while encouraging them to answer specific questions. The manner in which questions are asked influences the respondent's cooperation. The interviewer must be nonjudgmental and avoid expressing disapproval by verbal comments or facial expression.

Several questions may be necessary to elicit the information needed. When attempting to elicit information about the type and quantity of food eaten at a particular time, open-ended questions should be utilized. In addition, assumptions should not be made about the size of servings; instead, questions are phrased to clearly determine the quantities. For example, to help determine the size of one hamburger, the patient may be asked, "How many servings were prepared with the pound of meat you bought?" Another approach to determining quantities is to use food models of known sizes in estimating portions of meat, cake, or pie, or to record quantities in common measurements, such as cups or spoonfuls (or the size of containers when discussing intake of bottled beverages).

In recording a particular combination dish, such as a casserole, it is useful to ask about the ingredients, recording the largest quantities first. When recording quantities of ingredients, the interviewer notes whether the food item was raw or cooked and the number of servings provided by the recipe. When a patient lists the foods for the recall questionnaire, it may help read back the list of foods and ask whether anything was forgotten, such as condiments, fruit, cake, candy, between-meal snacks, or alcoholic beverages.

Cultural, Ethnic, and Religious Considerations

Individuals' culture, ethnicity, or personal beliefs determine to a large extent which foods are eaten and how they are prepared and served. Cultural and religious practices can determine whether certain foods are prohibited (Chart 4-6) and whether certain foods and spices are eaten on holidays or at specific family gatherings. Because of the value of food pattern choices to many individuals, the nurse must be sensitive to these choices when obtaining a dietary history. Equally important, the nurse must not stereotype individuals and assume that because they are from a certain culture or religious group, they adhere to specific dietary customs. Specific eating patterns, such as vegan or vegetarian, should be explored so that appropriate dietary recommendations can be offered (U.S. Department of Agriculture [USDA] & HHS,

---

Chart 4-6 **Prohibited Foods and Beverages of Select Religious Groups**

Hinduism

All meats
Animal shortenings/fats

Islam

Pork
Alcoholic products and beverages (including extracts, such as vanilla and lemon)
Animal shortenings
Gelatin made from pork, marshmallow, and other confections made with gelatin
Note: Halal is lawful food that may be consumed according to tenets of the Koran, whereas *Haram* is food that is unlawful to consume.

Judaism

Pork
Predatory fowl
Shellfish and scavenger fish (e.g., shrimp, crab, lobster, escargot, catfish). Fish with fins and scales are permissible.
Mixing milk and meat dishes at same meal
Blood by ingestion (e.g., blood sausage, raw meat).
Note: Packaged foods will contain labels identifying kosher ("properly preserved" or "fitting") and pareve (made without meat or milk) items.

Church of Jesus Christ of Latter-Day Saints (formerly known as Mormonism)

Alcohol
Beverages containing caffeine stimulants (coffee, tea, colas, and selected carbonated soft drinks)

Seventh-Day Adventism

Alcohol
Beverages containing caffeine stimulants (coffee, tea, colas, and selected carbonated soft drinks)
Pork
Certain seafood, including shellfish
Fermented beverages
Note: Optional vegetarianism is encouraged.

Adapted from Giger, J. (2016). *Transcultural nursing: Assessment and intervention* (7th ed.). St. Louis, MO: Elsevier; Holland, K. (2018). *Cultural awareness in nursing and healthcare: An introductory text* (3rd ed.). New York: Taylor & Francis.

2019). Deficiencies in certain diets may cause disorders such as anemia (see Chapter 29 for further discussion).

The cultural context of food varies widely but usually includes one or more of the following: relief of hunger; promotion of health and healing; prevention of disease or illness; expression of caring for another; promotion of interpersonal closeness among individual people, families, groups, communities, or nations; and promotion of kinship and family alliances. Food is also associated with strengthening of social ties; observance of life events (e.g., birthdays, marriages, funerals); expression of gratitude or appreciation; recognition of achievement or accomplishment; validation of social, cultural, or religious ceremonial functions; facilitation of business negotiations; and expression of affluence, wealth, or social status.

Culture influences which foods are served and when they are served, the number and frequency of meals, who eats with whom, and who receives the choicest portions. Culture also may influence how foods are prepared and served, how they are eaten (with chopsticks, hands, or fork, knife, and spoon), and where people shop (e.g., ethnic grocery stores, specialty food markets). Culture also determines the impact of excess weight and obesity on self-esteem and social standing. In some cultures, physical bulk is viewed as a sign of affluence and health (e.g., a chubby baby is a healthy baby).

Religious practices may include fasting (e.g., Catholics, Buddhists, Jews, Muslims) and abstaining from selected foods at particular times (e.g., Catholics abstain from meat on Ash Wednesday and on Fridays during Lent). Practices may also include the ritualistic use of food and beverages (e.g., Passover dinner, consumption of bread and wine during religious ceremonies; see Chart 4-6).

Most groups feast, often in the company of family and friends, on selected holidays. For example, many Christians eat large dinners on Christmas and Easter and consume other traditional high-calorie, high-fat foods, such as seasonal cookies, pastries, and candies. These culturally based dietary practices are especially significant in the care of patients with diabetes, hypertension, gastrointestinal disorders, obesity, and other conditions in which diet plays a key role in the treatment and health maintenance regimen.

Evaluating Dietary Information

After obtaining basic dietary information, the nurse evaluates the patient's dietary intake and communicates the information to the dietitian and the rest of the health care team for more detailed assessment and clinical nutrition intervention. If the goal is to determine whether the patient generally eats a healthful diet, their food intake may be compared with the dietary guidelines outlined in the USDA's Center for Nutrition Policy & Promotion's MyPlate (Fig. 4-5). Foods are divided into five major groups (fruits, vegetables, grains, protein foods, and dairy), plus oils. Recommendations are provided related to variety in the diet, proportion of food from each food group, and moderation in eating fats, oils, and sweets. A patient's food intake is compared with recommendations based on various food groups for different age groups and activity levels (Weber & Kelley, 2018).

If nurses or dietitians are interested in knowing about the intake of specific nutrients, such as vitamin A, iron, or calcium, the patient's food intake is analyzed by consulting a list

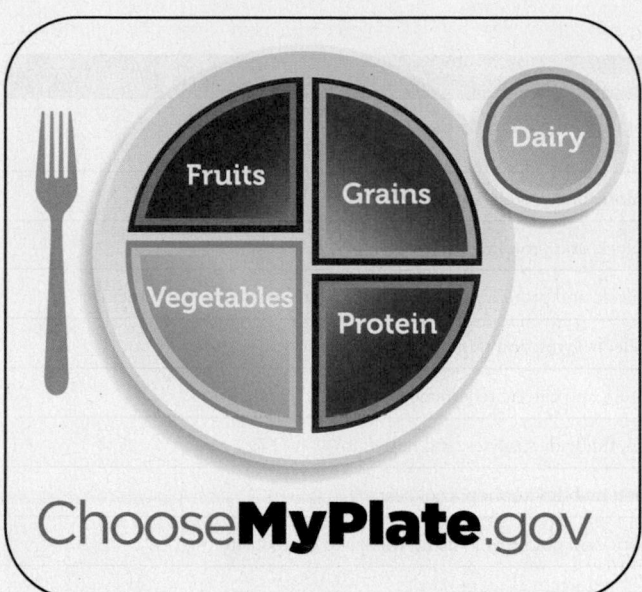

Figure 4-5 • MyPlate, a simple reminder for healthy eating. From the U.S. Department of Agriculture's Center for Nutrition Policy & Promotion. Retrieved on 7/24/2019 at: www.choosemyplate.gov

of foods and their composition and nutrient content. The diet is analyzed in terms of grams and milligrams of specific nutrients. The total nutritive value is then compared with the recommended dietary allowances specific for the patient's age category, gender, and special circumstances such as pregnancy or lactation.

Fat intake and cholesterol levels are additional aspects of the nutritional assessment. Trans fats are produced when hydrogen atoms are added to monounsaturated or polyunsaturated fats to produce a semisolid product, such as margarine. Partially hydrogenated oils (PHOs), the primary source of industrially produced trans fats, are found in many popular processed foods, such as baked goods and frozen foods. This is a concern because increased amounts of trans fats have been associated with increased risk for heart disease and stroke. In 2015, the FDA released its final determination that PHOs were not *Generally Recognized as Safe (GRAS)*.

At that time, the FDA announced that manufacturers must stop adding PHOs to processed food, providing a 3-year compliance period so that food manufacturers could gradually phase out the use of PHOs. However, to allow for an orderly transition in the marketplace, FDA extended the compliance date for these foods (FDA, 2019).

Factors Influencing Nutritional Status in Various Situations

Patients who are hospitalized may have an inadequate dietary intake because of the illness or disorder that necessitated the hospital stay. Patients who are at home may feel too sick or fatigued to shop and prepare food, or they may be unable to eat because of other physical problems or limitations. Limited or fixed incomes or the high costs of medications may result in insufficient money to buy nutritious foods. Culturally influenced food patterns can also affect nutritional status. Because complex treatments (e.g., mechanical ventilation, intravenous infusions, chemotherapy) once used only in the hospital setting are now being provided in the home and outpatient settings, nutritional assessment of patients in these settings is an important aspect of home and community-based care. Many of the factors that contribute to poor nutritional status are identified in Table 4-3.

Analysis of Nutritional Status

Physical measurements (BMI, waist circumference) and biochemical and dietary data are used in combination to determine a patient's nutritional status. Often, these data provide more information about the patient's nutritional status than the clinical examination, which may not detect subclinical deficiencies unless they become so advanced that overt signs develop. A low intake of nutrients over a long period may lead to low biochemical levels and, without nutritional intervention, may result in characteristic and observable signs and symptoms. A plan of action for nutritional intervention is based on the results of the dietary assessment and the patient's clinical examination. To be effective, the plan should include a healthy diet, maintenance (or control) of weight, and compensation for increased nutritional needs.

Cultural Assessment

Cultural assessment refers to a systematic appraisal or examination of individuals, families, groups, and communities in terms of their cultural beliefs, values, and practices. Nurses need to ensure that patients of all cultures understand what the nurse is trying to accomplish by gathering cultural data during the assessment process in order to avoid misunderstanding (Holland, 2018). In an effort to establish a database for determining a patient's cultural background, nurses have developed cultural assessment tools or modified existing assessment tools (Leininger, 2002) to ensure that transcultural considerations are included in the plan of care. Giger and Davidhizar's Transcultural Assessment Model can be used to help nurses perform cultural assessments. Questions derived from this model may be used to direct nursing assessment of a person's ethnic, cultural, or religious beliefs and its relationship to their personal and health care traditions (Chart 4-7) (Giger, 2016). In addition, nurses should gather data on patients' cultural perceptions and family ancestry throughout the assessment process. Nurses should recognize that advancing knowledge about culturally congruent care is important for promoting care that is consistent with the cultural needs of each patient's heritage (Jakub, Turk, Fapohunda, et al., 2018) (see Chart 4-8 for a Nursing Research Profile).

Culturally Mediated Considerations

Nurses should be aware that patients act and behave in various ways, in part because of the influence of culture on behaviors and attitudes. However, although certain attributes and attitudes are frequently associated with particular cultural groups, it is important to remember that not all people from the same cultural background share the same behaviors and views. Although nurses who fail to consider patients' cultural preferences and beliefs are considered insensitive and possibly indifferent, nurses who assume that all members of any one culture act and behave in the same way run the risk of stereotyping people. As stated previously, the best way to avoid

TABLE 4-3	Factors Associated with Potential Nutritional Deficits
Factor	Possible Consequences
Dental and oral problems (missing teeth, ill-fitting dentures, impaired swallowing or chewing)	Inadequate intake of high-fiber foods
Nothing by mouth (NPO) for diagnostic testing	Inadequate caloric and protein intake; dehydration
Prolonged use of glucose and saline intravenous fluids	Inadequate caloric and protein intake
Nausea and vomiting	Inadequate caloric and protein intake; loss of fluid, electrolytes, and minerals
Diarrhea	Loss of fluid, electrolytes, and minerals; malabsorption of nutrients
Stress of illness, surgery, and/or hospitalization	Increased protein and caloric requirement; increased catabolism
Wound drainage	Loss of protein, fluid, electrolytes, and minerals
Pain	Loss of appetite; inability to shop, cook, eat
Fever	Increased caloric and fluid requirement; increased catabolism
Gastrointestinal intubation	Loss of protein, fluid, and minerals
Tube feedings	Inadequate amounts; variation of nutrients in each formula
Gastrointestinal disease	Inadequate intake and malabsorption of nutrients
Alcoholism	Inadequate intake of nutrients; increased consumption of calories without other nutrients; vitamin deficiencies
Depression	Loss of appetite; inability to shop, cook, eat
Eating disorders (anorexia, bulimia)	Inadequate caloric and protein intake; loss of fluid, electrolytes, and minerals
Medications	Inadequate intake due to medication side effects, such as dry mouth, loss of appetite, decreased taste perception, difficulty swallowing, nausea and vomiting, malabsorption of nutrients
Restricted ambulation or disability	Limited ability to shop, cook, or help self to food, liquids, other nutrients

Chart 4-7 ASSESSMENT
Assessing for Patients' Cultural Beliefs

Communication
- Do you like communicating with friends, family, and acquaintances?
- When asked a question, do you usually respond?
- If you have something important to discuss with your family, how would you approach them?

Space
- When you talk with family members, how close do you stand?
- When you talk with acquaintances, how close do you stand?
- If a stranger touches you, how do you react or feel?
- If a loved one touches you, how do you react or feel?
- Are you comfortable with the distance between us now?

Social Organization
- What are some activities that you enjoy?
- What are your hobbies, or what do you do when you have free time?
- Do you believe in a Supreme Being?
- How do you worship that Supreme Being?
- What is your role in your family/unit system?

Time
- Do you wear a timepiece daily?
- If a nurse tells you that you will receive a medication "in about a half hour," how much time will you allow before calling the nurse?

Environmental Control
- Is it acceptable for you to have visitors drop in unexpectedly?
- Do you use home remedies? Which home remedies worked? Will you use them in the future?
- What is your definition of "good health"?
- What is your definition of illness or "poor health"?

Biologic Variations
- What diseases or illnesses are common in your family?
- Who usually helps you to cope during a difficult time?
- What foods do you and your family like to eat? What foods are family favorites or are considered traditional?

Nursing Process Utilization
- Note whether the patient has become culturally assimilated or observes own cultural practices.
- Incorporate data into the plan of nursing care.

Adapted from Giger, J. (2016). *Transcultural nursing: Assessment and intervention* (6th ed.). St. Louis, MO: Elsevier.

Chart 4-8	NURSING RESEARCH PROFILE
	Cultural Beliefs, Perceptions, and Practices of Adult Children of African Immigrants

Jakub, K. E., Turk, M. T., Fapohunda, A., et al. (2018). Cultural beliefs, perceptions, and practices of young adult offspring of African immigrants regarding healthy eating and activity. *Journal of Transcultural Nursing, 29*(6), 548–554.

Purpose

The purpose of this study was to understand and explore the beliefs, perceptions, and practices of young adult offspring of African immigrants regarding healthy eating and activities in the context of their environment and culture. The researchers also examined what influences the beliefs, perceptions, and practices of the study population.

Design

Using a focused ethnography design, five small group interviews consisting of two to six participants were conducted yielding a total of 20 college-age students who were offspring of African immigrants. Focused group semistructured interviews were digitally recorded during the data collection. Data collection was completed upon determination of data saturation. Leininger's four phases of qualitative data analysis were used to analyze the data.

Findings

The 20 participants, between the ages of 18 and 23, reported parental ancestry from eight different countries of the African continent: 11 from Nigeria, 3 from Ghana, and 1 participant each from Ethiopia, Cameroon, Egypt, Sudan, Liberia, and Eritrea. Seventeen categories, six patterns, and four themes emerged from the data. The four themes included (1) family, community, and religious ties to traditional African foods; (2) traditional African cuisine as healthy and American foods as nonhealthy; (3) eating patterns vary according to availability and resources; and (4) exercise patterns have familial, peer-driven, and generational influences significant to this college-age group. Participants also reported balancing acculturation into a university setting. Food choices were influenced by living arrangements, availability, financial resources, and time constraints.

Nursing Implications

Nurses should assess cultural perceptions and family ancestry that may affect a patient's perceptions of health and activity levels. Advancing knowledge about culturally congruent care is important and may promote healthy behaviors that include better eating habits and activity for college-age offspring of immigrants. Efforts should be made to identify the country of origin of patients and develop educational or health promoting programs to manage wellness specific to each patient's heritage.

---

stereotyping is to view each patient as a person and to assess the patient's cultural preferences. A thorough cultural assessment using a culture assessment tool or questionnaire can be beneficial.

Information Disclosure

Many aspects of care may be influenced by the diverse cultural perspectives held by health care providers, patients, families, or significant others. One example is the issue of communication and full disclosure. In general, nurses may argue that patients have the right to full disclosure concerning their disease and prognosis and may believe that advocacy means working to provide that disclosure. However, family members in some cultural backgrounds may believe that it is their responsibility to protect and spare the patient (their loved one) knowledge about a terminal illness. In some cultures, the head of the family group, older adult, or husband is expected to receive all information and make decisions. Patients may in fact not want to know about their condition and may expect their family members to "take the burden" of that knowledge and related decision making. Nurses should not decide that a family or patient is simply wrong or that a patient must know all of the details of their illness regardless of the patient's preference. Similar concerns may be noted when patients refuse pain medication or treatment because of cultural beliefs regarding pain or beliefs in divine intervention or faith healing.

Determining the most appropriate and ethical approach to patient care requires an exploration of the cultural aspects of these situations. Self-examination and recognition of one's own cultural bias and worldview play a major part in helping the nurse resolve cultural and ethical conflicts. Nurses must promote open dialogue and work with patients, families, primary providers, and other health care providers to reach the culturally appropriate solution for the individual patient.

Space and Distance

Personal space is the area that surrounds a person's body and includes the space and the objects within the space (Giger, 2016). People tend to regard the space in their immediate vicinity as an extension of themselves. The amount of space that they need between themselves and others to feel comfortable is a culturally determined phenomenon.

Because nurses and patients usually are not consciously aware of their personal space requirements, they frequently have difficulty understanding different behaviors. For example, one patient may perceive the nurse sitting close to them as an expression of warmth and care; another patient may perceive the nurse's act as a threatening invasion of personal space. Research reveals that people from the United States, Canada, and Great Britain require the most personal space between themselves and others, whereas those from Latin America, Japan, and the Middle East need the least amount of space and feel comfortable standing close to others (Giger, 2016).

If the patient appears to position himself or herself too close or too far away, the nurse should consider cultural preferences for space and distance. Ideally, the patient should be permitted to assume a position that is comfortable to them in terms of personal space and distance. The nurse should be aware that the wheelchair of a person with a disability is considered an extension of the person; therefore, the nurse should ask the person's permission before moving or touching the wheelchair. Because a significant amount of communication during nursing care requires close physical contact, the nurse should be aware that having personal space promotes self-identity by allowing opportunities for patient self-expression (Giger, 2016).

Eye Contact

Eye contact is also a culturally determined behavior. Although most nurses have been taught to maintain eye contact when speaking with patients, some people from certain cultural backgrounds may interpret this behavior differently. For example, some Asians, Native Americans, Indo-Chinese, Arabs, and Appalachians may consider direct eye contact impolite or aggressive, and they may avert their own eyes when talking with nurses and others whom they perceive to be in positions of authority. Some Native Americans stare at the floor during conversations—a cultural behavior conveying respect and indicating that the listener is paying close attention to the speaker. Some Hispanic patients maintain downcast eyes as a sign of culturally appropriate deferential behavior toward others on the basis of age, gender, social position, economic status, and position of authority (Giger, 2016). Eye contact is an important tool in a transcultural assessment and is used for both observation and to initiate interaction (Giger, 2016). The nurse who is aware that eye contact may be culturally determined can better understand the patient's behavior and provide an atmosphere in which the patient can feel comfortable.

Time

Attitudes about time vary widely among cultures and can be a barrier to effective communication between nurses and patients. Views about punctuality and the use of time are culturally determined, as is the concept of waiting. Symbols of time, such as watches, sunrises, and sunsets, represent methods for measuring the duration and passage of time (Giger, 2016).

For most health care providers, time and promptness are extremely important. For example, nurses frequently expect patients to arrive at an exact time for an appointment, although patients may be kept waiting by health care providers who are running late. Health care providers are likely to function according to an appointment system in which there are short intervals. However, for patients from some cultures, time is a relative phenomenon, with little attention paid to the exact hour or minute. Time may also be determined according to traditional times for meals, sleep, and other activities or events. For people from some cultures, the present is of the greatest importance, and time is viewed in broad ranges rather than in terms of a fixed hour. Being flexible in regard to schedules is the best way to accommodate these differences.

Value differences also may influence a person's sense of priority when it comes to time. For example, responding to a family matter may be more important to a patient than meeting a scheduled health care appointment. Allowing for these different views is essential in maintaining an effective nurse–patient relationship. Scolding or acting annoyed at patients for being late undermines their confidence and may result in further missed appointments or indifference to health care suggestions.

Touch

Touch is the most personal of all sensations, is central to the human communication process, and is often used as a method of communication (Giger, 2016). The meaning that people associate with touching is culturally determined to a great degree. In some cultures (e.g., Hispanic, Arab), male health care providers may be prohibited from touching or examining certain parts of the female body. Similarly, it may be inappropriate for females to care for males. Among many Asians, it is impolite to touch a person's head because the spirit is believed to reside there. Therefore, assessment of the head or evaluation of a head injury requires permission of the patient or a family member, if the patient is not able to give permission.

The patient's culturally defined sense of modesty must also be considered when providing nursing care. For example, some Jewish and Muslim women believe that modesty requires covering their head, arms, and legs with clothing. It is important for the nurse to recognize cultural variances and to understand that touch can be perceived as intrusive to some patients.

Observance of Holidays

People from all cultures observe certain civil and religious holidays. Nurses should familiarize themselves with major observances for members of the cultural groups they serve. Information about these observances is available from various sources, including religious organizations, hospital chaplains, and patients themselves. Routine health appointments, diagnostic tests, surgery, and other major procedures should be scheduled to avoid observances that patients identify as significant. If not contraindicated, efforts should also be made to accommodate patients and families or significant others who wish to perform cultural and religious rituals in the health care setting.

CRITICAL THINKING EXERCISES

1 **pq** You are conducting an admission assessment on a 66-year-old Vietnamese woman who was recently discharged from the hospital with a diagnosis of congestive heart failure. The patient's blood pressure is elevated, and the patient has a productive cough. The patient speaks very little English, but the patient's son is able to interpret. What types of assessments are necessary to complete a comprehensive admission assessment? What are the priorities in this patient's care? What interventions should you incorporate into the plan of care for this patient?

2 **ebp** A 28-year-old woman is admitted to the hospital with diverticulitis. She is visibly undernourished with poor skin turgor and loss of subcutaneous tissue. After calculating her ideal body weight, you note that her weight is well below average for her height. What standardized assessment tools would you use to determine her health risk? Identify her health risks, given her decreased weight, based on the most recent evidence. Evaluate the strength of the evidence for these risks.

REFERENCES

*Asterisk indicates nursing research.
**Double asterisk indicates classic reference.

Books

Ackley, B., Ladwig, G., Flynn Makic, M., et al. (2019). *Nursing diagnosis handbook: An evidence-based guide to planning care* (12th ed.). St. Louis, MO: Elsevier, Inc.

Eliopoulos, C. (2018). *Gerontological nursing* (9th ed.). Philadelphia, PA: Lippincott Williams & Wilkins.

Fenske, C., Watkins, K., Saunders, T., et al. (2020). *Health & physical assessment in nursing* (4th ed.). Hoboken, NJ: Pearson Education, Inc.

Fischbach, F., & Fischbach, M. (2018). *A manual of laboratory and diagnostic tests* (10th ed.). Philadelphia, PA: Lippincott Williams & Wilkins.

Fontaine, K. L. (2018). *Complementary and alternative therapies for nursing practice* (5th ed.). Upper Saddle River, NJ: Prentice Hall.

Giger, J. (2016). *Transcultural nursing: Assessment and intervention* (7th ed.). St. Louis, MO: Elsevier.

Hogan-Quigley, B., Palm, M. L., & Bickley, L. (2017). *Bates' nursing guide to physical examination and history taking* (2nd ed.). Philadelphia, PA: Lippincott Williams & Wilkins.

Holland, K. (2018). *Cultural awareness in nursing and healthcare: An introductory text* (3rd ed.). New York: Taylor & Francis.

Lassi, Z., Moin, A., & Bhutta, Z. (2017). Nutrition in middle childhood and adolescence. In A. D. Bundy, N. de Silva, S. Horton, et al. (Eds.). *Disease control priorities: Child and adolescent health and development* (3rd ed., *Vol.* 8). Washington, DC: The World Bank Group.

Norris, T. (2019). *Porth's pathophysiology concepts of altered health states* (10th ed.). Philadelphia, PA: Lippincott Williams & Wilkins.

O'Brien, M. E. (2017). *Spirituality in nursing* (6th ed.). Sudbury, MA: Jones & Bartlett.

Weber, J. R., & Kelley, J. H. (2018). *Health assessment in nursing* (6th ed.). Philadelphia, PA: Lippincott Williams & Wilkins.

Journals and Electronic Documents

Agurs-Collins, T., Persky, S., Paskett, E. D., et al. (2019). Designing and assessing multilevel interventions to improve minority health and reduce health disparities. *American Journal of Public Health, 109*(S1), S86–S93.

Alexander-Ruff, J. H., & Kinion, E. S. (2019). Developing a cultural immersion service-learning experience for undergraduate nursing students. *Journal of Nursing Education, 58*(2), 117–120.

Alonso, W., Mollard, E., Zimmerman, L., et al. (2019). Self-care management after ventricular assist device implantation: Recipient needs and experiences after hospital discharge. *Journal of Heart & Lung Transplantation, 38*(4), S303–S304.

*Amieva, H., Ouvrard, C., Meillon, C., et al. (2018). Death, depression, disability, and dementia associated with self-reported hearing problems: A 25-Year Study. *Journals of Gerontology Series A: Biological Sciences & Medical Sciences, 73*(10), 1383–1389.

*Astrup, C., & O'Connor, M. (2018). Fuel for life: A literature review of nutrition education and assessment among older adults living at home. *Home Health Care Management & Practice, 30*(2), 61–69.

*Axmon, A., Björkman, M., & Ahlström, G. (2019). Hospital readmissions among older people with intellectual disability in comparison with the general population. *Journal of Intellectual Disability Research, 63*(6), 593–602.

Centers for Disease Control and Prevention (CDC). (2019a). Assessing your weight. Retrieved on 6/9/2019 at: www.cdc.gov/healthyweight/assessing/index.html

Centers for Disease Control and Prevention (CDC). (2019b). About body mass index (BMI). Retrieved on 6/9/2019 at: www.cdc.gov/healthyweight/assessing/bmi/adult_bmi/index.html

Centers for Disease Control (CDC). (2019c). Prescription painkiller use in the US. Retrieved on 5/28/2019 at: www.cdc.gov/vitalsigns/PainkillerOverdoses/index.html

Chokshi, D. A., & Sommers, B. D. (2015). Universal health coverage for US veterans: A goal within reach. *Lancet, 385*(9984), 2320–2321.

Colby, S., & Ortman, J. (2015). Projections of the size and composition of the U.S. population: 2014–2020. U.S. Census Bureau. Retrieved on 9/16/2019 at: www.census.gov/programs-surveys/popproj.html

Drug and Alcohol Clinical Advisory Service (DACAS). (2019). Screening and assessment. Retrieved on 5/28/2019 at: www.dacas.org.au/clinical-resources/screening-assessment

**Ewing, J. A. (1984). Detecting alcoholism: The CAGE questionnaire. *JAMA, 252*(14), 1905–1907.

Ezeanolue, E., Harriman, K., Hunter, P., et al. (2019). General best practice guidelines for Immunization Advisory Committee on Immunization Practices (ACIP). Retrieved on 5/19/2019 at: www.cdc.gov/vaccines/hcp/acip-recs/general-recs/downloads/general-recs.pdf

*Fioravanti, M. A., Puskar, K., Knapp, E., et al. (2018). Creative learning through the use of simulation to teach nursing students screening, brief intervention, and referral to treatment for alcohol and other drug use in a culturally competent manner. *Journal of Transcultural Nursing, 29*(4), 387–394.

Flynn, D. M., Cook, K., Kallen, M., et al. (2017). Use of the pain assessment screening tool and outcomes registry in an army interdisciplinary pain management center, lessons learned and future implications of a 10-month beta test. *Military Medicine, 182*(Suppl 1), 167–174.

Frydensberg, V. S., Skovbakke, S. J., Pedersen, S. S., et al. (2018). Body image concerns in patients with an implantable cardioverter defibrillator: A scoping review. *Pacing & Clinical Electrophysiology, 41*(9), 1235–1260.

Henderson, S., Horne, M., Hills, R., et al. (2018). Cultural competence in healthcare in the community: A concept analysis. *Health & Social Care in the Community, 26*(4), 590–603.

*Jakub, K. E., Turk, M. T., Fapohunda, A., et al. (2018). Cultural beliefs, perceptions, and practices of young adult offspring of African immigrants regarding healthy eating and activity. *Journal of Transcultural Nursing, 29*(6), 548–554.

Kang, H. K., Bullman, T. A., Smolenski, D. J., et al. (2015). Suicide risk among 1.3 million veterans who were on active duty during the Iraq and Afghanistan wars. *Annals of Epidemiology, 25*(2), 96–100.

Lee, D. M., Vanhoutte, B., Nazroo, J., et al. (2016). Sexual health and positive subjective well-being in partnered older men and women. *Journals of Gerontology Series B: Psychological Sciences & Social Sciences, 71*(4), 698–710.

**Leininger, M. (2002). Culture care theory: A major contribution to advance transcultural nursing knowledge and practices. *Journal of Transcultural Nursing, 13*(3), 189–192.

McConnell-Nzunga, J., Naylor, P. J., Macdonald, H., et al. (2018). Classification of obesity varies between body mass index and direct measures of body fat in boys and girls of Asian and European ancestry. *Measurement in Physical Education and Exercise Science, 22*(2), 154–166.

Mitra, M., Akobirshoev, I., Moring, N. S., et al. (2017). Access to and satisfaction with prenatal care among pregnant women with physical disabilities: Findings from a national survey. *Journal of Women's Health, 26*(12), 1356–1363.

National Center for Complementary and Integrative Health (NCCIH). (2019). Complementary, alternative, or integrative health: What's in a name? Retrieved on 6/16/2019 at: nccih.nih.gov/health/integrative-health

National Institute on Drug Abuse. (2019). DrugFacts: Marijuana as medicine. Retrieved on 5/28/2019 at: www.drugabuse.gov/publications/drugfacts/marijuana-medicine

Nestlé Nutrition Institute. (2011). MNA® mini nutritional assessment: Overview. Retrieved on 6/16/2019 at: www.mna-elderly.com

Possemato, K., Maisto, S. A., Wade, M., et al. (2015). Ecological momentary assessment of PTSD symptoms and alcohol use in combat veterans. *Psychology of Addictive Behaviors, 29*(4), 894–905.

*Skałacka, K., & Gerymski, R. (2019). Sexual activity and life satisfaction in older adults. *Psychogeriatrics, 19*(3), 195–201.

Smiley, R. A., Lauer, P., Bienemy, C., et al. (2018). The 2017 National Nursing Workforce Survey. *Journal of Nursing Regulation, 9*(3), S1–S88.

Smith, S. G., Chen, J., Basile, K. C., et al. (2017). *The National Intimate Partner and Sexual Violence Survey (NISVS): 2010–2012 State Report.* Atlanta, GA: National Center for Injury Prevention and Control, Centers for Disease Control and Prevention. Retrieved on 9/16/2019 at: www.cdc.gov/violenceprevention/datasources/nisvs/index.html

Truong, C., Burnes, D., Alaggia, R., et al. (2019). Disclosure among victims of elder abuse in healthcare settings: A missing piece in the overall effort toward detection. *Journal of Elder Abuse & Neglect, 31*(2), 181–190.

U.S. Department of Agriculture (USDA). (2019). Dietary guidelines for Americans 2015–2020: Dietary guidelines and MyPlate. Retrieved on 6/13/2019 at: www.choosemyplate.gov/dietary-guidelines

U.S. Department of Agriculture (USDA) & U.S. Department of Health & Human Services (HHS). (2019). *2015–2020 Dietary Guidelines for Americans* (8th ed.). Retrieved on 6/13/2019 at: health.gov/dietaryguidelines/2015

U.S. Department of Health & Human Services (HHS). (2019a). Your health information privacy rights. Retrieved on 5/15/2019 at: www.healthit.gov/patients-families/your-health-information-privacy

U.S. Department of Health & Human Services (HHS). (2019b). Privacy and security of electronic health records. Retrieved on 5/15/2019 at: www.hhs.gov/sites/default/files/ocr/privacy/hipaa/understanding/consumers/privacy-security-electronic-records.pdf

U.S. Department of Health & Human Services (HHS). (2019c). Domestic and intimate partner violence. Retrieved on 6/3/2019 at: www.womenshealth.gov/violence-against-women/types-of-violence/ domestic-intimate-partner-violence.html

U.S. Food and Drug Administration (FDA). (2019). Final determination regarding partially hydrogenated oils (removing trans fats). Retrieved on 6/13/2019 at: www.fda.gov/food/food-additives-petitions/final-determination-regarding-partially-hydrogenated-oils-removing-trans-fat

U.S. National Library of Medicine. (2019). National Information Center on Health Services Research and Health Care Technology (NICHSR). Retrieved on 5/15/2019 at: www.nlm.nih.gov/nichsr

World Health Organization (WHO). (2019). Obesity and overweight. Retrieved on 6/4/2019 at: www.who.int/news-room/fact-sheets/detail/ obesity-and-overweight

Zetterlund, C., Lundqvist, L., Richter, H. O., et al. (2019). Visual, musculoskeletal and balance symptoms in individuals with visual impairment. *Clinical & Experimental Optometry, 102*(1), 63–69.

Resources

Academy of Nutrition and Dietetics, www.eatright.org

Advisory Committee on Immunization Practices (ACIP), Centers for Disease Control and Prevention, National Immunization Program, Division of Epidemiology and Surveillance, www.cdc.gov/vaccines/acip/ index.html

Alcoholics Anonymous, www.aa.org

Al-Anon Family Groups, www.al-anon.org

American Heart Association, heart.org

Center on Addiction and the Family, www.phoenixhouse.org

Co-Anon Family Groups, www.co-anon.org

Cocaine Anonymous, www.ca.org

Council on Nursing and Anthropology (CONAA), www.conaa.org

Dual Recovery Anonymous World Network Central Office, www.draonline.org

Genetic Alliance, www.geneticalliance.org

Healthcare Information and Management Systems Society, Inc. (HIMSS), www.himss.org

LanguageLine Solutions, www.languageline.com

Narcotics Anonymous World Services, www.na.org

National Cancer Institute, Cancer Information Service, www.cancer.gov

National Center for Complementary and Integrative Heath, nccih.nih.gov

National Center for Cultural Competence (NCCC), Georgetown University Center for Child and Human Development, nccc.georgetown.edu

National Institute on Drug Abuse, www.drugabuse.gov

Office of Minority Health (OMH), minorityhealth.hhs.gov

Substance Abuse and Mental Health Services Administration (SAMHSA), www.samhsa.gov

Transcultural Nursing Society, www.tcns.org

5 Stress and Inflammatory Responses

LEARNING OUTCOMES

On completion of this chapter, the learner will be able to:

1. Describe the significance of the principles of internal constancy, homeostasis, stress, and adaptation in promoting and maintaining steady state in the body.
2. Describe the General Adaptation Syndrome and the sympathetic–adrenal–medullary and hypothalamic-pituitary responses to stress.
3. Identify ways in which maladaptive responses to stress can increase the risk of illness and cause disease.
4. Compare the adaptive processes of atrophy, hypertrophy, hyperplasia, metaplasia, and dysplasia within the body's inflammatory and reparative processes.
5. Assess the health patterns of individuals and families, identifying strategies that are useful in reducing stress.

NURSING CONCEPTS

Anxiety

Cellular Regulation

Communication

Family

Immunity

Inflammation

Stress and Coping

GLOSSARY

adaptation: a change or alteration designed to assist in adjusting to a new situation or environment

adrenocorticotropic hormone (ACTH): a hormone produced by the anterior lobe of the pituitary gland that stimulates the secretion of cortisol and other hormones by the adrenal cortex

antidiuretic hormone (ADH): a hormone secreted by the posterior lobe of the pituitary gland that constricts blood vessels, elevates blood pressure, and reduces the excretion of urine

catecholamines: any of the group of amines (such as epinephrine, norepinephrine, or dopamine) that serve as neurotransmitters

coping: the cognitive and behavioral strategies used to manage the stressors that tax a person's resources

corticosteroids: the group of steroid hormones, such as cortisol, that are produced by the adrenal cortex; they are involved in carbohydrate, protein, and fat metabolism and have anti-inflammatory properties

disease: an abnormal variation in the structure or function of any part of the body

dysplasia: bizarre cell growth resulting in cells that differ in size, shape, or arrangement from other cells of the same tissue type

family: a group whose members are related by reciprocal caring, mutual responsibilities, and loyalties

fight-or-flight response: the alarm stage in the General Adaptation Syndrome described by Selye

gluconeogenesis: the formation of glucose by the liver from noncarbohydrate sources, such as amino acids and the glycerol portion of fats

guided imagery: the mindful use of a word, phrase, or visual image to achieve relaxation or direct attention away from uncomfortable sensations or situations

homeostasis: a steady state within the body; the stability of the internal environment

hyperplasia: an increase in the number of new cells in an organ or tissue

hypoxia: inadequate supply of oxygen to the cell

inflammation: a localized reaction of tissue to injury, irritation, or infection that is manifested by five cardinal signs of redness, warmth, swelling, pain, and loss of function

metaplasia: a cell transformation in which one type of mature cell is converted into another type of cell

negative feedback: mechanisms that monitor the internal environment and restore homeostasis when conditions shift out of the normal range

positive feedback: mechanisms that perpetuate a chain of events

steady state: a stable condition that does not change over time, or when change in one direction is balanced by change in an opposite direction

---

stress: a disruptive condition that occurs in response to adverse influences from the internal or external environments

stressor: an internal or external event or situation that creates the potential for physiologic, emotional, cognitive, or behavioral changes

---

When the body is threatened or suffers an injury, its response may involve functional and structural changes; these changes may be adaptive (having a positive effect) or maladaptive (having a negative effect). The defense mechanisms that the body uses determine the difference between adaptation and maladaptation—health and disease. This chapter addresses individual homeostasis, stress, adaptation, health problems associated with maladaptation, and ways that nurses intervene with patients and families to reduce stress and its health-related effects.

Fundamental Concepts

Each body system performs specific functions to sustain optimal life for an organism. Compensatory mechanisms for adjusting internal conditions promote the steady state of the organism, ensure its survival, and restore balance in the body. Pathophysiologic processes result when cellular injury occurs at such a rapid rate that the body's compensatory mechanisms cannot make the adaptive changes necessary to remain healthy.

Physiologic mechanisms must be understood in the context of the body as a whole. Each person has both an internal and external environment, between which information and matter are continuously exchanged. Within the internal environment, each organ, tissue, and cell is also a system or subsystem of the whole, each with its own internal and external environment, each exchanging information and matter (Fig. 5-1). The goal of the interaction of the body's

subsystems is to produce a dynamic balance or **steady state** (even in the presence of change) so that all subsystems are in harmony with each other. Four concepts—constancy, homeostasis, stress, and adaptation—are key to the understanding of steady state.

Constancy and Homeostasis

Claude Bernard, a 19th-century French physiologist, first developed the biologic principle that for life there must be a constancy or "fixity of the internal milieu" despite changes in the external environment. The internal milieu is the fluid that bathed the cells, and the constancy the balanced internal state maintained by physiologic and biochemical processes. His principle implies a static process.

Bernard's principle of "constancy" underpins the concept of **homeostasis**, which refers to a steady state within the body. When a change or stress occurs that causes a body function to deviate from its stable range, processes are initiated to restore and maintain dynamic balance. An example of this restorative effort is the development of hyperpnea (rapid breathing) after intense exercise in an attempt to compensate for an oxygen deficit and excess lactic acid accumulated in the muscle tissue. When these adjustment processes or compensatory mechanisms are not adequate, steady state is threatened, function becomes disordered, and dysfunctional responses occur. For example, in heart failure, the body reacts by retaining sodium and water and increasing venous pressure, which worsens the condition. Dysfunctional responses can lead to **disease** (an abnormal variation in the structure or function of any part of the body), which is a threat to steady state.

Stress and Adaptation

Stress is a disruptive condition produced by a change in the environment that is perceived as challenging, threatening, or damaging to a person's dynamic balance or equilibrium. The person may feel unable to meet the demands of the new situation. The change or stimulus that evokes this state is the stressor. A person appraises and copes with changing situations. The desired goal is **adaptation** or adjustment to the change so that the person is again in equilibrium and has the energy and ability to meet new demands. This is the process of coping with the stress, a compensatory process that uses cognitive and behavioral strategies.

Because both stress and adaptation may exist at different levels of a system, it is possible to study these reactions at the cellular, tissue, and organ levels. Biologists are concerned mainly with subcellular components or with subsystems of the total body. Behavioral scientists, including many nurse researchers, study stress and adaptation in individuals, families, groups, and societies; they focus on how a group's organizational features are modified to meet the requirements of the social and physical environment in which the group exists. In any system, the desired goals of adaptation are survival, growth, and reproduction.

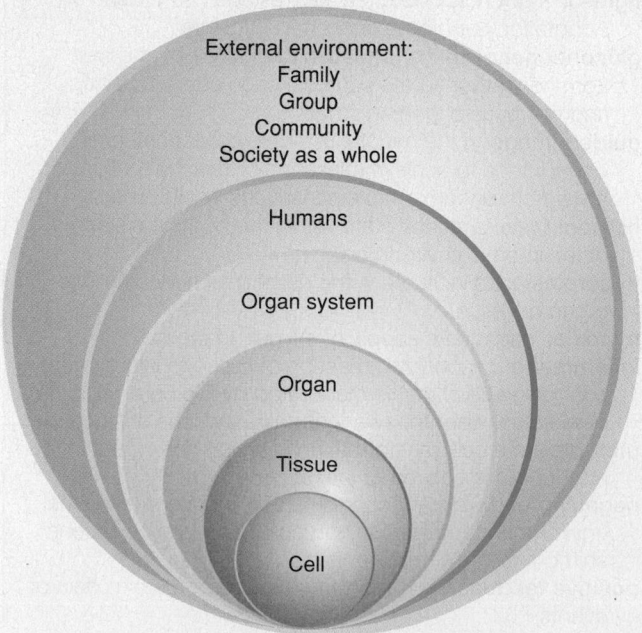

Figure 5-1 • Constellation of systems. Each system is a subsystem of the larger system (suprasystem) of which it is a part. The cells represent the smallest system and are a subsystem of all other systems.

Overview of Stress

Each person operates at a certain level of adaptation and regularly encounters a certain amount of change. Such change is expected; it contributes to growth and enhances life. A stressor can upset this equilibrium. A **stressor** may be defined as an internal or external event or situation that creates the potential for physiologic, emotional, cognitive, or behavioral changes.

Types of Stressors

Stressors exist in many forms and categories. They may be described as physical, physiologic, or psychosocial. Physical stressors include cold, heat, and chemical agents; physiologic stressors include pain and fatigue. An example of a psychosocial stressor is fear (e.g., fear of failing an examination, losing a job, waiting for a diagnostic test result). Stressors can also occur as normal life transitions that require some adjustment, such as going from childhood into puberty, getting married, or giving birth.

Stressors have also been classified as day-to-day frustrations or hassles, major complex occurrences involving large groups, and stressors that occur less frequently and involve fewer people. Day-to-day stressors include common occurrences as getting caught in a traffic jam, experiencing computer downtime, and having an argument with a spouse or roommate. These experiences vary in effect. For example, encountering a rainstorm while you are vacationing at the beach will most likely evoke a more negative response than it might at another time. These daily hassles have been shown to have a greater health impact than major life events because of the cumulative effect they have over time. They can lead to high blood pressure, palpitations, or other physiologic problems (Sarid, Slonim-Nevo, Sergienko, et al., 2018; Terrill & Molton, 2019).

Major stressors influence larger groups of individuals, families, and sometimes even entire nations. These include events of history, such as terrorism and war, experienced either directly in the war zone or indirectly through live news coverage. The demographic, economic, and technologic changes occurring in society also serve as stressors. The tension produced by any stressor is sometimes a result not only of the change itself, but also of the speed with which the change occurs.

Stressors concerning relatively infrequent situations that directly affect people have been studied extensively. This category includes the influence of life events such as death, birth, military service, marriage, divorce, and retirement. It also includes the psychosocial crises that occur in the life cycle stages of the human experience. More enduring chronic stressors may include having a permanent disability or coping with the need to provide long-term care for a child who has a developmental disability or for an older parent who is frail.

Duration may also be used to categorize stressors, as in the following:

- An acute, time-limited stressor, such as studying for final examinations
- A stressor sequence—a series of stressful events that result from an initial event such as job loss or divorce
- A chronic intermittent stressor, such as daily hassles
- A chronic enduring stressor that persists over time, such as chronic illness, a disability, or poverty

Stress as a Stimulus for Disease

Relating life events to illness (the theoretical approach that defines stress as a stimulus) has been a major focus of psychosocial studies. Research suggests that people under constant stress have a high incidence of disease (Kalinowski, Taylor, & Spruill, 2019; Kibler, Ma, Tursich, et al., 2018).

Holmes and Rahe (1967) developed life events scales that assign numerical values, called *life-change units*, to typical life events. Because the items in the scales reflect events that require a change in a person's life pattern, and stress is viewed as an accumulation of changes in one's life that require psychological adaptation, one can theoretically predict the likelihood of illness by checking off the number of recent events and deriving a total score. The Recent Life Changes Questionnaire (RLCQ) (Tausig, 1982) contains 118 items such as death, birth, marriage, divorce, promotions, serious arguments, and vacations. The items include both desirable and undesirable events. Both the life events scale and the RLCQ have formed the basis for the development of two additional scales: the Positive–Negative Relationship Quality Scale (PNRQS) (Fincham & Rogge, 2010), which measures stress related to relationship quality, and the Stress Overload Scale (SOS) (Amirkhan, 2012; Amirkhan, Urizar, & Clark, 2015), which measures excessive stress. A tool developed by Vohra and colleagues (2019) called the Stressometer® (SOM) was designed to measure stress and mental health. This instrument is composed of subscales related to a person's individual nature, personal circumstances, clinical symptoms, home life and work life. The underlying premise of the PNRQS, SOS, and SOM instruments is that sources of stress, such as stressful life events and a person's personal vulnerabilities, can influence and even undermine engaging in adaptive processes.

Sources of stress for people have been well researched (Anniko, Boersma, & Tillfors, 2019; Pitt, Oprescu, Tapia, et al., 2018). People typically experience distress related to alterations in their physical and emotional health status, changes in their level of daily functioning, and decreased social support or the loss of significant others (Albdour, Hong, Lewin, et al., 2019; Benham & Charak, 2019; Reblin, Stanley, Galligan, et al., 2019; Sikes & Hall, 2017). Fears of immobilization, isolation, loneliness, sensory changes, financial problems, and death or disability increase a person's anxiety level. Loss of one's role or perceived purpose in life can cause intense discomfort. Any of these identified variables, plus a myriad of other conditions or demands, are likely to cause ineffective coping, and a lack of effective coping skills is often a source of additional distress for the person. When a person endures prolonged or unrelenting suffering, the outcome is frequently the development of a stress-related illness. Nurses have the skills to assist people to alter their distressing circumstances and manage their responses to stress, as discussed later in the chapter.

Psychological Responses to Stress

After recognizing a stressor, a person consciously or unconsciously reacts to manage the situation. This is termed the *mediating process*. A theory developed by Lazarus (1991) emphasizes cognitive appraisal and coping as important mediators of stress. Appraisal and coping are influenced by antecedent variables, including the internal and external resources of the individual person.

Appraisal of the Stressful Event

Cognitive appraisal (Lazarus, 1991; Lazarus & Folkman, 1984) is a process by which an event is evaluated with respect to what is at stake (primary appraisal) and what might and can be done (secondary appraisal). What a person sees as being at stake is influenced by their personal goals, commitments, or motivations. Important factors include how important or relevant the event is to the person, whether the event conflicts with what the person wants or desires, and whether the situation threatens the person's own sense of strength and ego identity.

Primary appraisal results in the situation being identified as either nonstressful or stressful. Secondary appraisal is an evaluation of what might and can be done about the situation. Reappraisal—a change of opinion based on new information—may occur. The appraisal process is not necessarily sequential; primary and secondary appraisal and reappraisal may occur simultaneously.

The appraisal process contributes to the development of an emotion. Negative emotions such as fear and anger accompany harm/loss appraisals, and positive emotions accompany challenge. In addition to the subjective component or feeling that accompanies a particular emotion, each emotion also includes a tendency to act in a certain way. For example, unprepared students may view an unexpected quiz as threatening. They might feel fear, anger, and resentment and might express these emotions through hostile behavior or comments.

Lazarus (1991) expanded his initial ideas about stress, appraisal, and coping into a more complex model relating emotion to adaptation. He called this model a "cognitive–motivational–relational theory," with the term *relational* "standing for a focus on negotiation with a physical and social world" (p. 13). A theory of emotion was proposed as the bridge to connect psychology, physiology, and sociology: "More than any other arena of psychological thought, emotion is an integrative, organismic concept that subsumes psychological stress and coping within itself and unites motivation, cognition, and adaptation in a complex configuration" (p. 40).

Coping with the Stressful Event

Coping consists of the cognitive and behavioral efforts made to manage the specific external or internal demands that tax a person's resources and may be emotion focused or problem focused. Emotion-focused coping seeks to make the person feel better by lessening the emotional distress. Problem-focused coping aims to make direct changes in the environment so that the situation can be managed more effectively. Both types of coping usually occur in a stressful situation. Even if the situation is viewed as challenging or beneficial, coping efforts may be required to develop and sustain the challenge—that is, to maintain the positive benefits of the challenge and to ward off any threats. In harmful or threatening situations, successful coping reduces or eliminates the source of stress and relieves the emotion generated.

Appraisal and coping are affected by internal characteristics such as health, energy, personal belief systems, commitments, or life goals, self-esteem, control, mastery, knowledge, problem-solving skills, and social skills. The characteristics that have been studied in nursing research are health-promoting lifestyles and resilience (Callaghan, Fellin, & Alexander, 2019; Marques, Perolta, Santos, et al., 2019; Shen, 2019; Sima, Yu, Marwitz, et al., 2019). Resilience is considered both a personal trait and a process. Researchers have defined resilience as the ability of a person to function well in stressful situations such as traumatic events and other types of adverse situations (Kim, Lin, Kim, et al., 2019). A resilient person maintains flexibility even in difficult circumstances and controls strong emotional reactions using appropriate communication and problem-solving skills. Factors that play a role in building a person's resilience are having strong, supportive relationships with family members and other individuals and being exposed to positive role models. A resilient person knows when to act, when to step back and rely on others, and when to stop to re-energize and nurture the self. Researchers have found positive support for resilience as a significant variable that positively influences rehabilitation and overall improvement after a challenging or traumatic experience (Kok, Reed, Wickham, et al., 2019; Liu, Zhou, Zhang, et al., 2019; McNeil, Bartram, Cregan, et al., 2019; Vaughan, Koczwara, Kemp, et al., 2019).

A health-promoting lifestyle buffers the effect of stressors. From a nursing practice standpoint, this outcome—buffering the effect of stressors—supports nursing's goal of promoting health. In many circumstances, promoting a healthy lifestyle is more achievable than altering the stressors.

Physiologic Response to Stress

The physiologic response to a stressor, whether it is physical, psychological, or psychosocial, is a protective and adaptive mechanism to maintain the body's homeostatic balance. When a stress response occurs, it activates a series of neurologic and hormonal processes within the brain and body systems. The duration and intensity of the stress can cause both short- and long-term effects.

Selye's Theory of Adaptation

Selye (1976) developed a theory of adaptation to biologic stress that profoundly influenced the scientific study of stress.

General Adaptation Syndrome

Selye's theory, called the *General Adaptation Syndrome* (GAS), has three phases: alarm, resistance, and exhaustion. During the alarm phase, the sympathetic **fight-or-flight response** is activated with release of **catecholamines** (i.e., epinephrine, norepinephrine, and dopamine), that serve as neurotransmitters and the onset of the **adrenocorticotropic hormone (ACTH)**–adrenal cortical response. ACTH is produced by the anterior lobe of the pituitary gland and stimulates the secretion of cortisol as well as other hormones by the adrenal cortex. The alarm reaction is defensive and anti-inflammatory but self-limited. Because living in a continuous state of alarm would result in death, people move into the second stage—resistance. During the resistance stage, adaptation to the noxious stressor occurs, and cortisol activity is still increased. If exposure to the stressor is prolonged, the third stage—exhaustion—occurs. During the exhaustion stage, endocrine activity increases, and this has negative effects on the body systems (i.e., the circulatory, digestive, and immune systems) that can lead to death. The first two stages of this syndrome are repeated, in different degrees, throughout life as the person encounters stressors.

Selye compared the GAS with the life process. During childhood, too few encounters with stress occur to promote the development of adaptive functioning, and children are vulnerable. During adulthood, numerous stressful events occur, and people develop resistance or adaptation. During the later years, the accumulation of life's stressors and wear and tear on the organism again decrease people's ability to adapt, resistance falls, and eventually death occurs.

Local Adaptation Syndrome

According to Selye, a *Local Adaptation Syndrome* also occurs. This syndrome includes the inflammatory response and repair processes that occur at the local site of tissue injury. This syndrome occurs in small, topical injuries, such as contact dermatitis. If the local injury is severe enough, the GAS is activated as well.

Selye emphasized that stress is the nonspecific response common to all stressors, regardless of whether they are physiologic, psychological, or psychosocial. The many conditioning factors in each person's environment account for why different demands are experienced by different people as stressors. Conditioning factors also account for differences in the tolerance of different people for stress: Some people may develop diseases of adaptation, such as hypertension and migraine headaches, whereas others are unaffected.

Interpretation of Stressful Stimuli by the Brain

Physiologic responses to stress are mediated by the brain through a complex network of chemical and electrical messages. The neural and hormonal actions that maintain homeostatic balance are integrated by the hypothalamus, which is located in the center of the brain, surrounded by the limbic system and the cerebral hemispheres. The hypothalamus is made up of a number of nuclei and integrates autonomic nervous system mechanisms that maintain the chemical constancy of the internal environment of the body. Together with the limbic system, which contains the amygdala, hippocampus, and septal nuclei, along with other structures, the hypothalamus regulates emotions and many visceral behaviors necessary for survival (e.g., eating, drinking, temperature control, reproduction, defense, aggression).

Each of the brain structures responds differently to stimuli. The cerebral hemispheres are concerned with the cognitive functions of thought processes, learning, and memory. The limbic system has connections with both the cerebral hemispheres and the brain stem. In addition, the reticular activating system, a network of cells that forms a two-way communication system, extends from the brain stem into the midbrain and limbic system. This network controls the alert or waking state of the body.

In the stress response, afferent impulses are carried from sensory organs (eye, ear, nose, skin) and internal sensors (baroreceptors, chemoreceptors) to nerve centers in the brain. The response to the perception of stress is integrated in the hypothalamus, which coordinates the adjustments necessary to return to homeostatic balance. The degree and duration of the response vary; initially, there is a sympathetic nervous system discharge, followed by a sympathetic–adrenal–medullary discharge. If the stress persists, the hypothalamic-pituitary system is activated (Fig. 5-2).

Sympathetic Nervous System Response

The sympathetic nervous system response is rapid and short-lived. Norepinephrine is released at nerve endings that are in direct contact with their respective end organs to cause an increase in function of the vital organs and a state of general body arousal (Norris, 2019). Heart rate increases and peripheral vasoconstriction occurs, raising the blood pressure. Blood is also shunted away from abdominal organs. The purpose of these responses is to provide better perfusion of vital organs (brain, heart, skeletal muscles). Blood glucose is increased, supplying more readily available energy. The pupils dilate, and mental activity increases; a greater sense of awareness exists. Constriction of the blood vessels of the skin limits bleeding in the event of trauma. The person is likely to experience cold feet, clammy skin and hands, chills, palpitations, and "knots" in the stomach. Typically, the person appears tense, with the muscles of the neck, upper back, and shoulders tightened; respirations may be rapid and shallow, with the diaphragm tense.

Sympathetic–Adrenal–Medullary Response

In addition to directly affecting major end organs, the sympathetic nervous system stimulates the adrenal medulla to release the hormones epinephrine and norepinephrine into the bloodstream. These hormones act similarly to the sympathetic nervous system, sustaining and prolonging its actions. Because these hormones are catecholamines, they stimulate the nervous system and produce metabolic effects that increase the blood glucose level and metabolic rate. The effect of the sympathetic–adrenal–medullary responses is summarized in Table 5-1. This effect is called the *fight-or-flight response* (Norris, 2019).

Hypothalamic-Pituitary Response

The longest-acting phase of the physiologic response, which is more likely to occur in persistent stress, involves the hypothalamic-pituitary pathway. The hypothalamus secretes corticotropin-releasing factor, which stimulates the anterior pituitary to produce ACTH, which in turn stimulates the adrenal cortex to produce **corticosteroids**, primarily cortisol (Norris, 2019). Cortisol stimulates protein catabolism, releasing amino acids; stimulates liver uptake of amino acids and their conversion to glucose (**gluconeogenesis**); and inhibits glucose uptake (anti-insulin action) by many body cells but not those of the brain and the heart (Norris, 2019). These cortisol-induced metabolic effects provide the body with a ready source of energy during a stressful situation. This effect has some important implications. For example, a person with diabetes who is under stress, such as that caused by an infection, needs more insulin than usual. Any patient who is under stress (e.g., illness, surgery, trauma, prolonged psychological stress) catabolizes body protein and needs supplements.

The actions of the catecholamines (epinephrine and norepinephrine) and cortisol are the most important in the general response to stress. Other hormones that play a role are **antidiuretic hormone (ADH)** released from the posterior pituitary and aldosterone released from the adrenal cortex. ADH and aldosterone promote sodium and water retention, which is an adaptive mechanism in the event of hemorrhage or loss of fluids through excessive perspiration. ADH constricts blood vessels, elevates blood pressure, and reduces the excretion of urine. ADH has also been shown to influence

Physiology/Pathophysiology

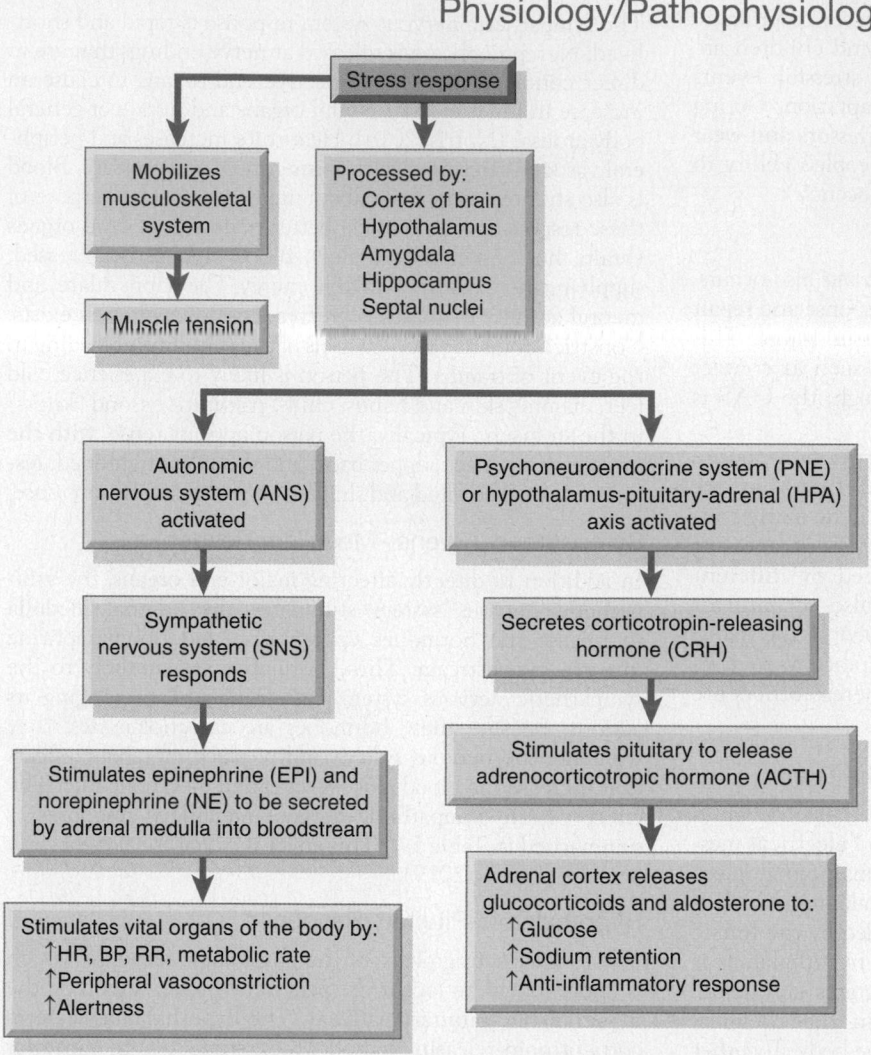

Figure 5-2 • The physiologic response to stress. The body is prepared through brain activation of the autonomic nervous system and psychoneuroendocrine system commonly referred to as the hypothalamus–pituitary–adrenal axis to cope with stress.

TABLE 5-1	Sympathetic–Adrenal–Medullary Reaction to Stress or Fight-or-Flight Response	
Effect	**Purpose**	**Mechanism**
Increased heart rate and blood pressure	More perfusion to vital organs	Increased cardiac output owing to increased myocardial contractility and heart rate; increased venous return (peripheral vasoconstriction)
Increased blood glucose level	Increased available energy	Increased liver and muscle glycogen breakdown; increased breakdown of adipose tissue triglycerides
Mental acuity	Alert state	Increase in amount of blood shunted to the brain from the abdominal viscera and skin
Dilated pupils	Increased awareness	Contraction of radial muscle of iris
Increased tension of skeletal muscles	Preparedness for activity, decreased fatigue	Excitation of muscles; increase in amount of blood shunted to the muscles from the abdominal viscera and skin
Increased ventilation (may be rapid and shallow)	Provision of oxygen for energy	Stimulation of respiratory center in medulla; bronchodilation
Increased coagulability of blood	Prevention of hemorrhage in event of trauma	Vasoconstriction of surface vessels

Adapted from Norris, T. L. (2019). *Porth's pathophysiology: Concepts of altered health status* (10th ed.). Philadelphia, PA: Wolters Kluwer.

learning and may thus facilitate coping in new and threatening situations. Secretion of growth hormone and glucagon stimulates the uptake of amino acids by cells, helping to mobilize energy resources. Endorphins, which are endogenous opioids, increase during stress and enhance the threshold for tolerance of painful stimuli. They may also affect mood and have been implicated in the so-called high that long-distance runners experience. The secretion of other hormones is also affected; however, their adaptive function is less clear.

Immunologic Response

The immune system is connected to the neuroendocrine and autonomic systems. Lymphoid tissue is richly supplied by autonomic nerves capable of releasing a number of different neuropeptides that can have a direct effect on leukocyte regulation and the inflammatory response. Neuroendocrine hormones released by the central nervous system and endocrine tissues can inhibit or stimulate leukocyte function. The various stressors a person experiences may result in different alterations in autonomic activity and subtle variations in neurohormone and neuropeptide synthesis. All of these possible autonomic and neuroendocrine responses can interact to initiate, weaken, enhance, or terminate an immune response.

The study of the relationships among the neuroendocrine system, the central and autonomic nervous systems, and the immune system and the effects of these relationships on overall health outcomes are called *psychoneuroimmunology*. Because one's perception of events and one's coping styles determine whether, and to what extent, an event activates the stress response system, and because the stress response affects immune activity, one's perceptions, ideas, and thoughts can have profound neurochemical and immunologic consequences. Some studies have demonstrated altered immune function in people who are under stress (Atkinson, Rodman, Thuras, et al., 2019; Christensen, Flensborg-Madsen, Garde, et al., 2019; Frishman, 2019; Ubel & Rosenthal, 2019). Other studies have identified certain personality traits, such as decisiveness, assertiveness, compassion, helpfulness, and conscientiousness, as having positive effects on health (Antoni & Dhabhar, 2019; Champagne, 2019; Wilson, Woody, Padin, et al., 2019). As research continues, this field of study will likely uncover to what extent and by what mechanisms people can consciously influence their immunity.

Maladaptive Responses to Stress

The stress response, as indicated earlier, facilitates adaptation to threatening situations and is retained from humans' evolutionary past. The fight-or-flight response, for example, is an anticipatory response that mobilized the bodily resources of our ancestors to deal with predators and other harsh factors in their environment. This same mobilization comes into play in response to emotional stimuli unrelated to danger. For example, a person may get an "adrenaline rush" when competing over a decisive point in a ball game or when excited about attending a party.

When responses to stress are ineffective, they are referred to as *maladaptive*. Maladaptive responses are chronic, recurrent responses or patterns of response that do not promote the goals of adaptation. The goals of adaptation are somatic or physical health (optimal wellness); psychological health or having a sense of well-being (happiness, satisfaction with life, morale); and enhanced social functioning, which includes work, social life, and family (positive relationships). Maladaptive responses that threaten these goals include faulty appraisals and inappropriate coping (Lazarus, 1991).

The frequency, intensity, and duration of stressful situations contribute to the development of emotions and subsequent patterns of neurochemical discharge. By appraising situations adequately and coping appropriately, it is possible to anticipate and defuse some of these situations. For example, frequent stressful encounters (e.g., marital discord) might be avoided with better communication and problem solving, or a pattern of procrastination (e.g., delaying work on tasks) could be corrected to reduce stress when deadlines approach.

Coping processes that include the use of alcohol or drugs to reduce stress increase the risk of illness. Other inappropriate coping patterns may increase the risk of illness less directly. For example, people who demonstrate "type A" behaviors, including impatience, competitiveness, and achievement orientation, have an underlying aggressive approach to life. Type A behaviors increase the output of catecholamines, the adrenal–medullary hormones, with their attendant effects on the body. Additional forms of inappropriate coping include denial, avoidance, and distancing.

Models of illness frequently include stress and maladaptation as precursors to disease. A general model of illness, based on Selye's theory, suggests that any stressor elicits a state of disturbed physiologic equilibrium. If this state is prolonged or the response is excessive, it increases the susceptibility of the person to illness. This susceptibility, coupled with a predisposition in the person (from genetic traits, health, or age), leads to illness. If the sympathetic–adrenal–medullary response is prolonged or excessive, a state of chronic arousal develops that may lead to high blood pressure, arteriosclerotic changes, and cardiovascular disease. If the production of ACTH is prolonged or excessive, behavior patterns of withdrawal and depression are seen. In addition, the immune response is decreased, and infections and tumors may develop.

Selye (1976) proposed a list of disorders known as diseases of maladaptation: high blood pressure (including hypertension of pregnancy), diseases of the heart and blood vessels, diseases of the kidney, rheumatic diseases and inflammatory diseases of the skin and eyes, infections, allergic and hypersensitivity diseases, nervous and mental diseases, sexual dysfunction, digestive diseases, metabolic diseases, and cancer. Research continues on the complex interconnections between stress, coping (adaptive and maladaptive), and disease (Torkzadeh, Danesh, Mirbagher, et al., 2019; Tormohlen, Tobin, & Latkin, 2019).

Indicators of Stress

Indicators of stress and the stress response include both subjective and objective measures. Chart 5-1 lists signs and symptoms that may be observed directly or reported by a person. They are psychological, physiologic, or behavioral and reflect social behaviors and thought processes. Some of these reactions may be coping behaviors. Over time, each person tends to develop a characteristic pattern of behavior during stress to warn that the system is out of balance.

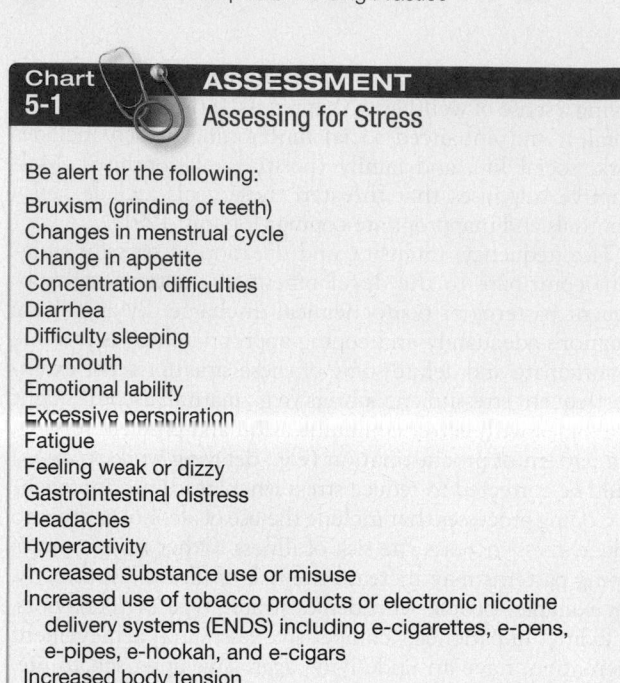

Adapted from Rice, V. H. (Ed.). (2012). *Handbook of stress, coping, and health: Implications for theory, research, and practice* (2nd ed.). Thousand Oaks, CA: Sage; Selye, H. (1976). *The stress of life, Rev. ed.* New York: McGraw-Hill.

Chart 5-1 ASSESSMENT — Assessing for Stress

Be alert for the following:

Bruxism (grinding of teeth)
Changes in menstrual cycle
Change in appetite
Concentration difficulties
Diarrhea
Difficulty sleeping
Dry mouth
Emotional lability
Excessive perspiration
Fatigue
Feeling weak or dizzy
Gastrointestinal distress
Headaches
Hyperactivity
Increased substance use or misuse
Increased use of tobacco products or electronic nicotine delivery systems (ENDS) including e-cigarettes, e-pens, e-pipes, e-hookah, and e-cigars
Increased body tension
Intense or increased anxiety
Impulsive behaviors
Loss of interest in life activities
Nausea or vomiting
Nervous habits
Nervous laughter
Overpowering urge to act out
Pain in back, neck, or other parts of the body
Palpitations
Prone to injury
Restlessness
Strong startle response
Tremors
Unintentional weight loss or gain
Urinary frequency

Laboratory measurements of indicators of stress have helped in understanding this complex process. Blood and urine analyses can be used to demonstrate changes in hormonal levels and hormonal breakdown products. Blood levels of catecholamines, corticosteroids, ACTH, and eosinophils are reliable measures of stress. Serum cholesterol and free fatty acid levels can be used to measure stress. Distress can cause an increase in adrenal hormones, including cortisol and aldosterone, which can lead to high serum cholesterol levels. Both physical and psychological distress can trigger an elevated cholesterol level. In addition, the results of immunoglobulin assays are increased when a person is exposed to various stressors, especially infections and immune deficiency conditions.

In addition to using laboratory tests, researchers have developed questionnaires to identify and assess stressors, stress, and coping strategies. The work of Rice (2012) includes a compilation of information gained from research on stress, coping, and health, and includes some of these questionnaires.

Physiology/Pathophysiology

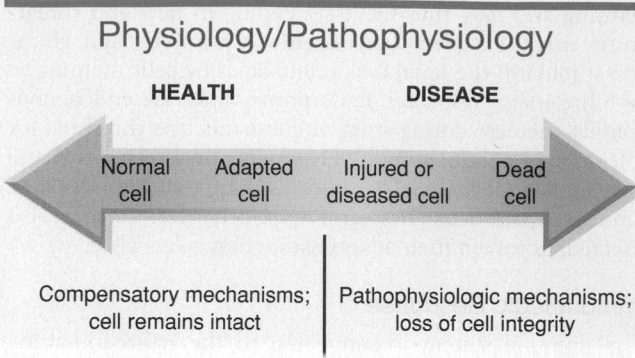

Figure 5-3 • The cell on a continuum of function and structure. Changes in the cell are not as easily discerned as the diagram depicts, and the point at which compensation subsides and pathophysiology begins is not clearly defined.

Stress at the Cellular Level

The cell exists on a continuum of function and structure, ranging from the normal cell, to the adapted cell, to the injured or diseased cell, to the dead cell (Fig. 5-3). Changes from one state to another may occur rapidly and may not be readily detectable, because each state does not have discrete boundaries, and disease represents disruption of normal processes. The earliest changes occur at the molecular or subcellular level and are not perceptible until steady-state functions or structures are altered. With cell injury, some changes may be reversible; in other instances, the injuries are lethal. For example, tanning of the skin is an adaptive, morphologic response to exposure to the rays of the sun. However, if the exposure is continued, sunburn and injury occur, and some cells may die, as evidenced by desquamation ("peeling").

Different cells and tissues respond to stimuli with different patterns and rates of response, and some cells are more vulnerable to one type of stimulus or stressor than others. The cell involved, its ability to adapt, and its physiologic state are determinants of the response. For example, cardiac muscle cells respond to **hypoxia** (inadequate cellular oxygenation) more quickly than do smooth muscle cells.

Other determinants of cellular response are the type or nature of the stimulus, its duration, and its severity. For example, neurons that control respiration can develop a tolerance to regular, small amounts of a barbiturate; however, one large dose may result in respiratory depression and death.

Control of the Steady State

The concept of the cell as existing on a continuum of function and structure includes the relationship of the cell to compensatory mechanisms, which occur continuously in the body to maintain the steady state. Compensatory processes are regulated primarily by the autonomic nervous system and the endocrine system, with control achieved through negative feedback.

Negative Feedback

Negative feedback mechanisms throughout the body monitor the internal environment and restore homeostasis when conditions shift out of the normal range. These mechanisms sense deviations from a predetermined set point or range of adaptability and trigger a response to offset the deviation. Functions regulated through such compensatory mechanisms include blood pressure, acid–base balance, blood glucose level, body temperature, and fluid and electrolyte balance.

Most of the human body's control systems are integrated by the brain with feedback from the nervous and endocrine systems. Control activities involve detecting deviations from the predetermined reference point and stimulating compensatory responses in the muscles and glands of the body. The major organs affected are the heart, lungs, kidneys, liver, gastrointestinal tract, and skin. When stimulated, these organs alter their rate of activity or the amount of secretions they produce. Because of this, these major organs are considered the *"organs of homeostasis or adjustment"* (Norris, 2019).

In addition to the responses influenced by the nervous and endocrine systems, local responses consisting of small feedback loops in a group of cells or tissues occur. The cells detect a change in their immediate environment and initiate an action to counteract its effect. For example, the accumulation of lactic acid in an exercised muscle stimulates dilation of blood vessels in the area to increase blood flow and improve the delivery of oxygen and removal of waste products.

The net result of negative feedback loops is homeostasis. A steady state is achieved by the continuous, variable action of the organs involved in making the adjustments and by the continuous exchange of chemical substances among cells, interstitial fluid, and blood. For example, an increase in the carbon dioxide (CO_2) concentration of the extracellular fluid leads to increased pulmonary ventilation, which decreases the CO_2 level. On a cellular level, increased CO_2 raises the hydrogen ion concentration of the blood. This is detected by chemosensitive receptors in the brain's medullary respiratory control center. The chemoreceptors then stimulate an increase in the rate of discharge of the neurons that innervate the diaphragm and intercostal muscles, which increases the respiratory rate. Excess CO_2 is exhaled, the hydrogen ion concentration returns to normal, and the chemically sensitive neurons are no longer stimulated (Norris, 2019).

Positive Feedback

Another type of feedback, **positive feedback**, perpetuates the chain of events set in motion by the original disturbance instead of compensating for it. As the system becomes more unbalanced, disorder and disintegration occur. There are some exceptions to this; blood clotting in humans, for example, is an important positive feedback mechanism.

Cellular Adaptation

Cells are complex units that dynamically respond to the changing demands and stresses of daily life. They possess a maintenance function and a specialized function. The maintenance function refers to the activities that the cell performs with respect to itself; specialized functions are those that the cell performs in relation to the tissues and organs of which it is a part. Individual cells may cease to function without posing a threat to the organism. However, as the number of dead cells increases, the specialized functions of the tissues are altered and health is threatened.

Cells can adapt to environmental stress through structural and functional changes. Some of these adaptations include

cellular atrophy, hypertrophy, hyperplasia, metaplasia, and dysplasia. Such adaptations reflect changes in the normal cell in response to stress (Fig. 5-4A). If the stress is unrelenting, cellular injury and death may occur.

Atrophy can be the consequence of disease, decreased use, decreased blood supply, loss of nerve supply, or inadequate nutrition. Disuse of a body part is often associated with the aging process and immobilization. Cell size and organ size decrease (Fig. 5-4B), and the structures principally affected are the skeletal muscles, the secondary sex organs, the heart, and the brain.

Atrophy and **hypertrophy** lead to changes in the size of cells (Fig. 5-4C) and hence the size of the organs they form.

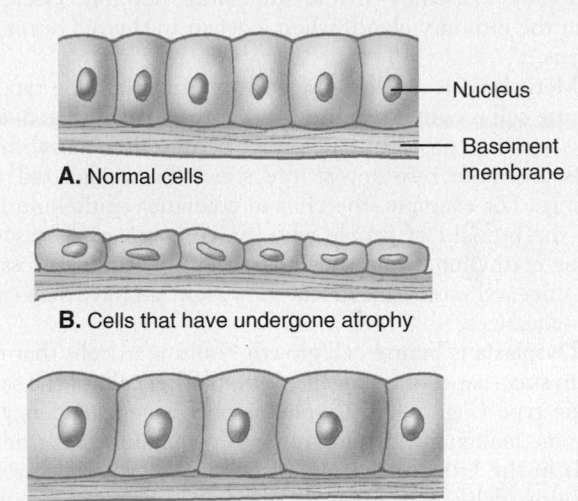

A. Normal cells — Nucleus, Basement membrane

B. Cells that have undergone atrophy

C. Cells that have undergone hypertrophy

D. Hyperplasia at the cellular level

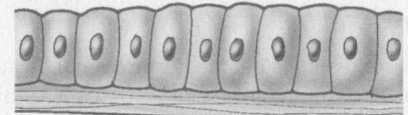

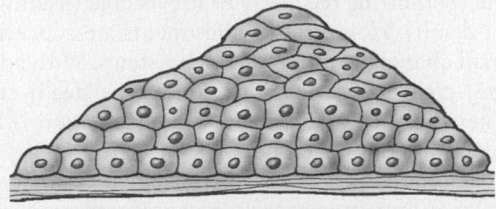

E. Metaplasia at the cellular level

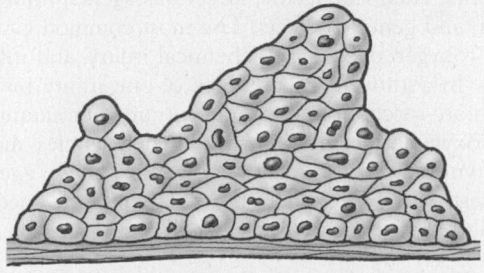

F. Dysplasia at the cellular level.

Figure 5-4 • Adaptation at the cellular level. Adapted with permission from Stewart J, Anatomical Chart Company. *Atlas of pathophysiology* (4th ed., p. 5). Wolters Kluwer Health, Inc., 2017.

Compensatory hypertrophy is the result of an enlarged muscle mass and commonly occurs in skeletal and cardiac muscle that experiences a prolonged, increased workload. One example is the bulging muscles of an athlete.

Hyperplasia is an increase in the number of new cells in an organ or tissue (Fig. 5-4D). As cells multiply and are subjected to increased stimulation, the tissue mass enlarges. This mitotic response (a change occurring with mitosis) is reversible when the stimulus is removed. This distinguishes hyperplasia from neoplasia or malignant growth, which continues after the stimulus is removed. Hyperplasia may be hormonally induced. An example is the increased size of the thyroid gland caused by thyroid-stimulating hormone (secreted from the pituitary gland) when a deficit in thyroid hormone occurs.

Metaplasia is a cell transformation in which one type of mature cell is converted into another type of cell (Fig. 5-4E). This serves a protective function, because less-transformed cells are more resistant to the stress that stimulated the change. For example, the ciliated columnar epithelium lining the bronchi of people who smoke is replaced by squamous epithelium. The squamous cells can survive; loss of the cilia and protective mucus, however, can have damaging consequences.

Dysplasia is bizarre cell growth resulting in cells that differ in size, shape, or arrangement from other cells of the same tissue type (Fig. 5-4F). Dysplastic cells have a tendency to become malignant; dysplasia is seen commonly in epithelial cells in the bronchi of people who smoke or use electronic nicotine delivery systems (ENDS) including e-cigarettes, e-pens, e-pipes, e-hookah, and e-cigars.

Cellular Injury

Injury is defined as a disorder in steady-state regulation. Any stressor that alters the ability of the cell or system to maintain optimal balance of its adjustment processes leads to injury. Structural and functional damage then occurs, which may be reversible (permitting recovery) or irreversible (leading to disability or death). Homeostatic adjustments are concerned with the small changes within the body's systems. With adaptive changes, compensation occurs, and a new steady state may be achieved. With injury, steady-state regulation is lost and changes in functioning ensue.

Causes of disorder and injury in the system (cell, tissue, organ, body) may arise from the external or internal environment (Fig. 5-5) and include hypoxia, nutritional imbalance, physical agents, chemical agents, infectious agents, immune mechanisms, and genetic defects. The most common causes are hypoxia (oxygen deficiency), chemical injury, and infectious agents. In addition, the presence of one injury makes the system more susceptible to another injury. For example, inadequate oxygenation and nutritional deficiencies make the system vulnerable to infectious agents. These agents damage or destroy the integrity of the cell membrane (necessary for ionic balance) as well as the cell's ability to do the following:
- Transform energy (aerobic respiration, production of adenosine triphosphate)
- Synthesize enzymes and other necessary proteins
- Grow and reproduce (genetic integrity)

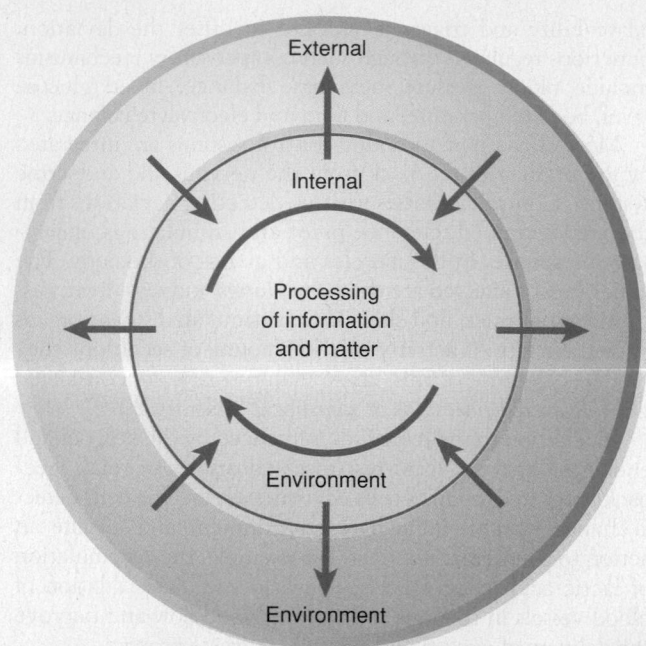

Figure 5-5 • Influences leading to disorder may arise from the internal and external environments of the system. Excesses or deficits of information and matter may occur, or there may be faulty regulation of processing.

Hypoxia

Hypoxia interferes with the cell's ability to transform energy. Hypoxia may be caused by a decrease in blood supply to an area, a decrease in the oxygen-carrying capacity of the blood (decreased hemoglobin), a ventilation–perfusion or respiratory problem that reduces the amount of arterial oxygen available, or a problem in the cell's enzyme system that makes it unable to use oxygen.

The usual cause of hypoxia is ischemia or deficient blood supply. Ischemia is commonly seen in myocardial cell injury in which arterial blood flow is decreased because of atherosclerotic narrowing of blood vessels. Ischemia also results from intravascular clots (thrombi or emboli) that may form and interfere with blood supply. Thromboemboli are common causes of cerebrovascular disease (strokes). The length of time in which different tissues can survive without oxygen varies. For example, brain cells most often succumb in 3 to 6 minutes. If the condition leading to hypoxia is slow and progressive, collateral circulation may develop, whereby blood is supplied by other blood vessels in the area. However, this mechanism is not highly reliable.

Nutritional Imbalance

Nutritional imbalance refers to a relative or absolute deficiency or excess of one or more essential nutrients. This may be manifested as undernutrition (inadequate consumption of food or calories) or overnutrition (caloric excess). Caloric excess to the point of obesity overloads cells in the body with lipids. By requiring more energy to maintain the extra tissue, obesity places a strain on the body and has been associated with the development of disease, especially pulmonary and cardiovascular disease as well as several types of cancer. (See Chapter 42 for further discussion of obesity.)

Specific deficiencies arise when an essential nutrient is deficient or when a nutrient imbalance exists. Protein deficiencies and avitaminosis (deficiency of vitamins) are typical examples. An energy deficit leading to cell injury can occur if there is insufficient glucose or insufficient oxygen to transform the glucose into energy. A lack of insulin, or the inability to use insulin, may also prevent glucose from entering the cell from the blood. This occurs in diabetes, a metabolic disorder that can lead to nutritional deficiency, as well as a host of short- and long-term life-threatening complications. (See Chapter 46 for further discussion of diabetes.)

Physical Agents

Physical agents, including temperature extremes, radiation, electrical shock, and mechanical trauma, can cause injury to the cells or to the entire body. The duration of exposure and the intensity of the stressor determine the severity of damage.

Temperature

When a person's temperature is elevated, hypermetabolism occurs and the respiratory rate, heart rate, and basal metabolic rate increase. With fever induced by infections, the hypothalamic thermostat may be reset at a higher temperature and then return to normal when the fever abates. The increase in body temperature is achieved through physiologic mechanisms. Body temperatures greater than 41°C (106°F) indicate hyperthermia, because the physiologic function of the thermoregulatory center breaks down and the temperature soars (Norris, 2019). This physiologic condition occurs in people who have heatstroke. Eventually, the high temperature causes coagulation of cell proteins, and cells die.

The local response to burn injury is similar. Increased metabolic activity occurs, and, as heat increases, proteins coagulate and enzyme systems are destroyed. In extreme situations, charring or carbonization occurs. See Chapter 57 for more information about burn injuries.

Extreme low environmental temperature (cold) causes vasoconstriction. Blood flow becomes sluggish and clots form, leading to ischemic damage in the involved tissues. With still lower temperatures, ice crystals may form and cells may burst.

Radiation and Electrical Shock

Radiation is used for diagnosis and treatment of diseases. Ionizing forms of radiation may cause injury by their destructive action. Radiation decreases the protective inflammatory response of the cell, creating a favorable environment for opportunistic infections. Electrical shock produces burns as a result of the heat generated when electrical current travels through the body. It may also abnormally stimulate nerves, leading, for example, to fibrillation of the heart.

Mechanical Trauma

Mechanical trauma can result in wounds that disrupt the cells and tissues of the body. The severity of the wound, amount of blood loss, and extent of nerve damage are significant factors in determining the extent of injury.

Chemical Agents

Chemical injuries are caused by poisons, such as lye, that have a corrosive action on epithelial tissue, or by heavy metals, such as mercury, arsenic, and lead, each of which has its own specific destructive action. Many other chemicals are toxic in certain amounts, in certain people, and in specific tissues. For example, excessive secretion of hydrochloric acid can damage the stomach lining; large amounts of glucose can cause osmotic shifts, affecting the fluid and electrolyte balance; and too much insulin can cause subnormal levels of glucose in the blood (hypoglycemia) and can lead to coma.

Drugs, including prescribed medications, can also cause chemical poisoning. Some people are less tolerant of medications than others and manifest toxic reactions at the usual or customary dosages. Aging tends to decrease tolerance to medications. Polypharmacy (taking many medications at one time) occurs frequently in older adults, and the unpredictable effects of the resulting medication interactions can cause injury.

Alcohol (ethanol) is also a chemical irritant. In the body, alcohol is broken down into acetaldehyde, which has a direct toxic effect on liver cells that leads to various liver abnormalities, including cirrhosis in susceptible people. Disordered liver cell function leads to complications in other organs of the body.

Infectious Agents

Biologic agents known to cause disease in humans are viruses, bacteria, rickettsiae, mycoplasmas, fungi, protozoa, and nematodes. The severity of the infectious disease depends on the number of microorganisms entering the body, their virulence, and the host's defenses (e.g., health, age, immune responses; see Chapter 66 for further discussion of infectious diseases).

An infection exists when the infectious agent is living, growing, and multiplying in the tissues and is able to overcome the body's normal defenses. Some bacteria, such as those that cause tetanus and diphtheria, produce exotoxins that circulate and create cell damage. Others, such as gram-negative bacteria, produce endotoxins when they die. Tubercle bacilli induce an immune reaction.

Viruses are among the smallest living organisms known and survive as parasites of the living cells they invade. Viruses infect specific cells. Through a complex mechanism, viruses replicate within cells and then invade other cells, where they continue to replicate. As the body mounts an immune response to eliminate the viruses, cells harboring the viruses can be injured in the process. Typically, an inflammatory response and immune reaction are the body's physiologic responses to viral infection.

Disordered Immune Responses

The immune system is an exceedingly complex system, the purpose of which is to defend the body from invasion by any foreign object or foreign cell type, such as cancerous cells. This is a steady-state mechanism; however, like other adjustment processes, it can become disordered and cellular injury results. The immune response detects foreign bodies by distinguishing non-self substances from self substances and destroying the non-self entities. The entrance of an antigen (foreign substance) into the body evokes the production of antibodies that attack and destroy the antigen (antigen–antibody reaction).

The immune system may function normally, or it may be hypoactive or hyperactive. When it is hypoactive, immune deficiency diseases occur; when it is hyperactive, hypersensitivity disorders occur. A disorder of the immune system can result in damage to the body's own tissues. Such disorders are labeled autoimmune diseases (see Unit 7).

Genetic Disorders

There is intense interest in genetic defects as causes of disease and modifiers of genetic structure. Many of these defects produce mutations that have no recognizable effect, such as lack of a single enzyme; others contribute to more obvious congenital abnormalities, such as Down syndrome. (For further information on genetics, see Chapter 6.)

Cellular Response to Injury: Inflammation

Cells or tissues of the body may be injured or killed by any of the agents (physical, chemical, infectious) described earlier. When this happens, an inflammatory response (or inflammation) naturally occurs in the healthy tissues adjacent to the site of injury. **Inflammation** is a localized reaction intended to neutralize, control, or eliminate the offending agent to prepare the site for repair. It is a nonspecific response (not dependent on a particular cause) that is meant to serve a protective function. For example, inflammation may be observed at the site of a bee sting, in a sore throat, in a surgical incision, and at the site of a burn. Inflammation also occurs in cell injury events, such as stroke, deep vein thrombosis, and myocardial infarction.

Inflammation is not the same as infection. An infectious agent is only one of several agents that may trigger an inflammatory response. Regardless of the cause, a general sequence of events occurs in the local inflammatory response. This sequence involves changes in the microcirculation, including vasodilation, increased vascular permeability, and leukocytic cellular infiltration (Fig. 5-6). As these changes take place, five cardinal signs of inflammation are produced: redness, warmth, swelling, pain, and loss of function (Norris, 2019).

The transient vasoconstriction that occurs immediately after injury is followed by vasodilation and an increased rate of blood flow through the microcirculation to the area of tissue damage. Local warmth and redness result. Next, the structure of the microvascular system changes to accommodate the movement of plasma protein from the blood into the tissues. Following this increase in vascular permeability, plasma fluids (including proteins and solutes) leak into the inflamed tissues, producing swelling. Leukocytes migrate through the endothelium and accumulate in the tissue at the site of the injury. The pain that occurs is attributed to the pressure of fluids or swelling on nerve endings and to the irritation of nerve endings by chemical mediators released at the site. Bradykinin is one of the chemical mediators suspected of causing pain. Loss of function is most likely related to the pain and swelling; however, the exact mechanism is not completely known.

As blood flow increases and fluid leaks into the surrounding tissues, the formed elements (red blood cells, white blood cells, and platelets) remain in the blood, causing it to become more viscous. Leukocytes (white blood cells) collect in the vessels, exit, and migrate to the site of injury to engulf offending organisms and to remove cellular debris in a process called *phagocytosis*. Fibrinogen in the leaked plasma fluid coagulates, forming fibrin for clot formation, which serves to wall off the injured area and prevent the spread of infection.

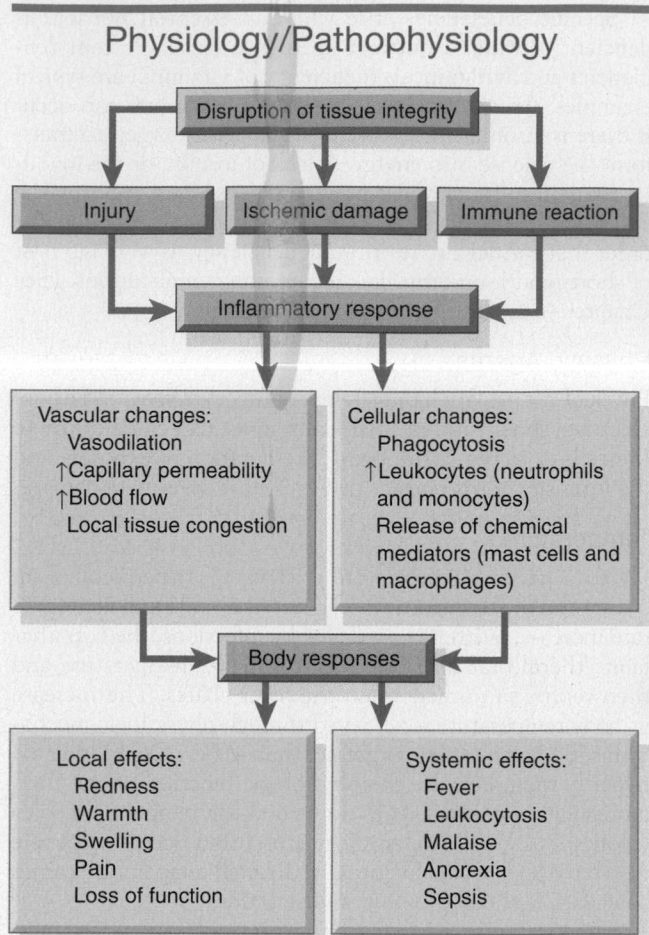

Physiology/Pathophysiology

Figure 5-6 • Inflammatory response. Source: Norris, T. L. (2019). *Porth's pathophysiology: Concepts of altered health status* (10th ed.). Philadelphia, PA: Wolters Kluwer.

Chemical Mediators of Inflammation

Injury initiates the inflammatory response; however, chemical substances released at the site induce vascular changes. Foremost among these chemicals are histamine and kinins. Histamine is present in many tissues of the body but is concentrated in the mast cells. It is released when injury occurs and is responsible for the early changes in vasodilation and vascular permeability. Kinins cause vasodilation and increased vascular permeability, and they attract neutrophils to the area. Prostaglandins—another group of chemical substances—are also suspected of causing increased vascular permeability (Norris, 2019).

Systemic Response to Inflammation

The inflammatory response is often confined to the site, causing only local signs and symptoms. However, systemic responses can also occur. Fever is the most common sign of a systemic response to injury, and it is most likely caused by endogenous pyrogens (internal substances that cause fever) released from neutrophils and macrophages (specialized forms of leukocytes). These substances reset the hypothalamic thermostat, which controls body temperature, and produce fever. Leukocytosis, an increase in the synthesis and release of neutrophils from bone marrow, may occur, enhancing the body's ability to fight infection. During this process, general, non-specific symptoms develop, including malaise, loss of appetite, aching, and weakness.

Types of Inflammation

Inflammation is categorized primarily by its duration and the type of exudate produced. It is most often acute or chronic. Acute inflammation is characterized by the local vascular and exudative changes described previously and usually lasts less than 2 weeks. An acute inflammatory response is immediate and serves a protective function. After the causative agent is removed, the inflammation subsides and healing takes place with the return of normal or near-normal structure and function.

Chronic inflammation develops if the injurious agent persists and the acute response is perpetuated. Symptoms are present for many months or years. Chronic inflammation may also begin insidiously and never have an acute phase. The chronic response does not serve a beneficial and protective function; on the contrary, it is debilitating and can produce long-lasting effects. As the inflammation becomes chronic, changes occur at the site of injury, and the nature of the exudate becomes proliferative. A cycle of cellular infiltration, necrosis, and fibrosis begins, with repair and breakdown occurring simultaneously. Considerable scarring may occur, resulting in permanent tissue damage.

Cellular Healing

The reparative process begins at approximately the same time as the injury. Healing proceeds after the inflammatory debris has been removed. Healing may occur by regeneration, in which the defect is gradually repaired by proliferation of the same type of cells as those destroyed, or by replacement, in which cells of another type, usually connective tissue, fill in the tissue defect and result in scar formation.

Regeneration

The ability of cells to regenerate depends on whether they are labile, permanent, or stable. Labile cells multiply constantly to replace cells worn out by normal physiologic processes; these include epithelial cells of the skin and those lining the gastrointestinal tract. Permanent cells include neurons—the nerve cell bodies, not their axons. Destruction of neurons is permanent; however, axons may regenerate. If normal activity is to return, tissue regeneration must occur in a functional pattern, especially in the growth of several axons. Stable cells in some organ systems have a latent ability to regenerate. Under normal physiologic processes, they are not shed and do not need replacement; if they are damaged or destroyed, they are able to regenerate. Examples include functional cells of the kidney, liver, and pancreas. Cells in other organs, such as the brain, do not regenerate.

Replacement

The condition of the host, the environment, and the nature and severity of the injury affect the processes of inflammation, repair, and replacement. Depending on the extent of damage, repair and replacement may occur by primary or secondary intention. In primary intention healing, the wound edges are approximated, as in a surgical wound (see Chapter 16). Little scar formation occurs, and the wound healing occurs without granulation. In secondary intention healing, there is tissue loss so the edges are not approximated and the wound fills with granulation tissue (Norris, 2019). The process of repair takes longer and may result in scar formation, with loss of specialized function. For example, people who have recovered from myocardial infarction have abnormal electrocardiographic tracings because the electrical signal cannot be conducted through the connective tissue that has replaced the infarcted area.

Nursing Management

Stress or the potential for stress is ubiquitous—that is, it is both everywhere and anywhere. It is essential for all people, particularly student nurses, to engage in strategies for stress relief. Nursing students experience stressors that can negatively affect their academic and clinical performance (Kinchen & Loerzel, 2019). See the Nursing Research Profile in Chart 5-2. Anxiety, frustration, anger, and feelings of inadequacy, helplessness, or powerlessness are emotions often associated with stress. In the presence of these emotions, the customary activities of daily living may be disrupted—for example, a sleep disturbance may occur, eating and activity patterns may be altered, and family processes or role performance may be disrupted.

The optimal point of intervention to promote health is during the stage when a person's own compensatory processes are still functioning effectively. A major role of nurses is the early identification of both physiologic and psychological stressors. Nurses should be able to relate the presenting signs and symptoms of distress to the physiology they represent and identify a person's position on the continuum of function, from health and compensation to pathophysiology and disease.

In the assessment of people who seek health care, both objective signs and subjective symptoms are the primary indicators of existing physiologic processes. The following questions are addressed:

- Are the heart rate, respiratory rate, and temperature normal?
- What emotional distress may be contributing to the patient's health problems?
- Are there other indicators of steady-state deviation?
- What are the patient's blood pressure, height, and weight?
- Are there any problems in movement or sensation?
- Are there any problems with affect, behavior, speech, cognitive ability, orientation, or memory?
- Are there obvious impairments, lesions, or deformities?

Objective evidence can be obtained from laboratory data, such as electrolytes, blood urea nitrogen, blood glucose, and urinalysis results. Further signs of injury are seen in diagnostic studies such as computed tomography (CT) scanning, magnetic resonance imaging (MRI), and positron emission tomography (PET). Further information on diagnostic evaluation can be found in assessment chapters of each unit of this book. Many nursing diagnoses are possible for patients suffering from stress. One nursing diagnosis associated with stress is anxiety, which is defined as a vague, uneasy feeling,

Chart 5-2   NURSING RESEARCH PROFILE

Nursing Students' Attitudes and Use of Holistic Therapies for Stress Relief

Kinchen, E. V., & Loerzel, V. (2019). Nursing students' attitudes and use of holistic therapies for stress relief. *Journal of Holistic Nursing, 37*(1), 6–17.

Purpose

The purpose of this mixed methods research study was to determine nursing students' openness to using or making recommendations to use holistic strategies to manage school or work stress, along with their perceptions of engaging in the use of holistic therapies for their own personal health.

Design

In this quasi-experimental, mixed methods study, a convenience sample of nursing students was recruited from a senior undergraduate class and provided an email to obtain information about the study, the consent form, and the survey link. Participants completed the quantitative electronic survey and answered the accompanying three open-ended questions. The questions asked the participants about their personal use or recommendation to use holistic therapies for stress relief, the strategies they utilized for managing their stress, and their perceptions of the influence that holistic therapies have on personal health. Students who participated in the study were given two extra credit points; nonparticipants who desired to obtain the extra credit points were permitted to write a one-page essay as an alternative assignment on the holistic therapy of their choice.

Findings

The reported findings were only from the qualitative portion of the study. Of the 116 participants, 81 (70%) were very open or open to using or recommending holistic therapies, while 32 (28%) were somewhat open, and 3 (2%) were not open to using

or recommending holistic modalities. From the data, eight categories of stress management activities were obtained: physical activity, prayer and meditation, time management, distraction, socialization, artistic/creative pursuits, interactions with animals, and other behaviors such as napping, taking a day off, stress eating, and crying. It was noted that 62% of the identified stress management actions are designated as holistic therapies. Overall, 85 of the participants (73%) held the view that holistic therapies had a positive influence on personal health, while 25 participants (22%) believed that holistic therapies had a potential influence on their health, and the remaining 6 (5%) perceived that holistic therapies had no effect on personal health. Four recurring themes were extracted from the data: wholeness, self-empowerment, relaxation/restoration, and alternative/complement to traditional medicine. The student participants were open to recommending these strategies to others. There also were barriers identified, such as a lack of knowledge and a lack of time, which interfered with using holistic methods for managing stress.

Nursing Implications

Information from this study supports that, in addition to the traditional behavioral health and pharmacologic interventions used for managing stress, many nursing students found holistic strategies useful for managing stress in their daily lives. This study lends support to the recommendations from many nursing organizations, such as the American Holistic Nurses Association (AHNA) and the American Nurses Association (ANA), to promote self-care and stress-relief strategies while providing students with the knowledge necessary to educate their patients about the use of holistic therapies. It is important for nursing education programs to establish and implement curriculum content and practical experiences related to holistic therapies.

---

the source of which may be nonspecific or not known to the person. Stress may also be manifested as difficulty coping patterns, decisional conflict, or relationship problem. These human responses are reflected in the nursing diagnoses of anxiety, difficulty coping, and denial, all of which indicate poor adaptive responses. Other possible nursing diagnoses include social isolation, risk for spiritual distress, readiness for positive family processes, decisional conflict, lack of resilience, and risk for powerlessness, among others. Because human responses to stress are varied, as are the sources of stress, arriving at an accurate diagnosis allows interventions and goals to be more specific and leads to improved outcomes.

Stress management is directed toward reducing and controlling stress and improving coping. The need to prevent illness, improve the quality of life, and decrease the cost of health care makes efforts to promote health essential, and stress control a significant health promotion goal. Stress reduction methods and coping enhancements can derive from either internal or external sources. For example, healthy eating habits and relaxation techniques are internal resources that help reduce stress, and a broad social network is an external resource that helps reduce stress. Goods and services that can be purchased are also external resources for stress management. It may be easier for people with adequate financial resources to cope with constraints in the environment, because their sense of vulnerability to threat

is decreased compared to those without adequate financial resources.

Promoting a Healthy Lifestyle

A health-promoting lifestyle provides internal resources that aid in coping, and it buffers or cushions the impact of stressors. Lifestyles or habits that contribute to the risk of illness can be identified through a health risk appraisal, which is an assessment method designed to promote health by examining a person's habits and recommending changes when a health risk is identified.

Health risk appraisals involve the use of health risk questionnaires to estimate the likelihood that people with a given set of characteristics will become ill. People who receive this information may be influenced to adopt healthy behaviors (e.g., stop smoking, have periodic screening examinations) to improve their health. Questionnaires typically address the information presented in Chart 5-3.

The personal information is compared with average population risk data, and the risk factors are identified and weighted. From this analysis, a person's risks and major health hazards are identified. Further comparisons with population data can estimate how many years will be added to a person's lifespan if the suggested changes are made. However, research has not yet demonstrated that providing people with such information ensures that they will change their behaviors. The single most important factor for determining health

<table>
<tr><td>

Chart 5-3

Information Addressed in Health Risk Questionnaires

Demographic data such as age, gender, race/ethnic background
Personal and family history of diseases and health problems
Lifestyle choices:

- Eating, sleeping, exercise, smoking, drinking, use of illicit drugs, sexual activity, recreation activity, and driving habits
- Stressors at home and on the job
- Roles, role relationships, and associated stressors
- Living and family situation
- Family and social supports

Physical measurements:

- Blood pressure
- Height, weight, body mass index
- Laboratory analyses of blood and urine

Participation in high-risk behaviors (e.g., engaging in unprotected sexual activity, not using seat belts while riding in a motor vehicle, using illicit drugs)

</td></tr>
</table>

status is social class, and within a social class, research suggests that the major factor influencing health is level of education (Bastable, Gramet, Jacobs, et al., 2019).

Enhancing Coping Strategies

Bulechek, Butcher, Dochterman, and colleagues (2018) identified coping enhancement as a nursing intervention and defined it as handling perceived and actual stressors, changes, or threats that affect how one meets daily life demands and roles (Chart 5-4). The nurse can build on

Chart 5-4

Coping Enhancement: Nursing Interventions

Definition

Facilitation of cognitive and behavioral efforts to manage perceived stressors, changes, or threats that interfere with meeting life's demands and roles.

Select Activities

Assist the patient in identifying appropriate short- and long-term goals.
Assist the patient to solve problems in a constructive manner.
Provide information concerning diagnosis, treatment, and prognosis.
Encourage an attitude of realistic hope as a way of dealing with feelings of helplessness.
Acknowledge the patient's spiritual/cultural background and encourage the use of spiritual resources if desired.
Foster constructive outlets for anger and hostility.
Assist the patient in examining available resources to meet goals.
Appraise the needs and desires for social support, and assist the patient to identify available support systems.
Assist the patient to identify positive strategies to deal with limitations, manage needed lifestyle or role changes, and work through the losses of chronic illness and/or disability if appropriate.

Adapted from Bulechek, G. M., Butcher, H. K., Dochterman, J. M., et al. (Eds.). (2018). *Nursing interventions classification (NIC)* (7th ed.). St. Louis, MO: Mosby-Elsevier.

the patient's existing coping strategies, as identified in the health appraisal, or provide education about new strategies for coping if necessary.

The five predominant ways of coping with illness identified in a review of 57 nursing research studies were as follows (Jalowiec, 1993):

- Trying to be optimistic about the outcome
- Using social support
- Using spiritual resources
- Trying to maintain control either over the situation or over feelings
- Trying to accept the situation

Other ways of coping included seeking information, reprioritizing needs and roles, lowering expectations, making compromises, comparing oneself to others, planning activities to conserve energy, taking things one step at a time, listening to one's body, and using self-talk for encouragement.

Unfolding Patient Stories: Skyler Hansen • Part 1

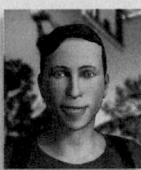

Skyler Hansen is an 18-year-old male recently diagnosed with type 1 diabetes. He lives with his parents and two younger siblings and is active in high school sports. He now requires insulin injections, glucose monitoring, and a diabetic diet. Examine how the psychological, physical, and educational needs for managing a new diagnosis can be a great source of stress to the patient and the family. How can the nurse enhance his ability to cope with and adapt to diabetes management? (Skyler Hansen's story continues in Chapter 46.)

Care for Skyler and other patients in a realistic virtual environment: *vSim for Nursing* (**thepoint.lww.com/vSimMedicalSurgical**). Practice documenting these patients' care in DocuCare (**thepoint.lww.com/DocuCareEHR**).

Educating About Relaxation Techniques

Relaxation techniques are a major method used to relieve stress. The goal of using relaxation techniques is to produce a response that counters the stress response. When this goal is achieved, the action of the hypothalamus adjusts, decreasing sympathetic and parasympathetic nervous system activity. The sequence of physiologic effects and their signs and symptoms are then interrupted, thus reducing psychological stress. This is a learned response and requires practice to achieve. Commonly used techniques include progressive muscle relaxation, the Benson relaxation response, and relaxation with guided imagery (all discussed later). Other relaxation techniques include meditation, breathing techniques, massage, Reiki, music therapy, biofeedback, and the use of humor.

The different relaxation techniques share four similar elements: (1) a quiet environment, (2) a comfortable position, (3) a passive attitude, and (4) a mental device (something on which to focus one's attention, such as a word, phrase, or sound).

> ### Chart 5-5 The Benson Relaxation Response
>
> 1. Pick a brief phrase or word that reflects your basic belief system.
> 2. Choose a comfortable position.
> 3. Close your eyes.
> 4. Relax your muscles.
> 5. Become aware of your breathing and start using your selected focus word.
> 6. Maintain a passive demeanor.
> 7. Continue for a set period of time.
> 8. Practice the technique twice daily.
>
> Adapted from Benson, H. (1993). The relaxation response. In D. Goleman, & J. Gurin. (Eds.). *Mind-body medicine: How to use your mind for better health.* Yonkers, NY: Consumer Reports Books.

Progressive Muscle Relaxation

Progressive muscle relaxation involves tensing and releasing the muscles of the body in sequence and sensing the difference in feeling. It is best if the person lies on a soft cushion in a quiet room, breathing easily. Someone usually reads the instructions in a low tone in a slow and relaxed manner, or a recording of the instructions may be played. The person tenses the muscles in the entire body (one muscle group at a time), holds, senses the tension, and then relaxes. As each muscle group is tensed, the person keeps the rest of the body relaxed. Each time the focus is on feeling the tension and relaxation. When the exercise is completed, the entire body should be relaxed (Benson, 1993; Benson & Stark, 1996).

The Benson Relaxation Response

The Benson relaxation response (Chart 5-5) combines meditation with relaxation. Along with the repeated word or phrase, a passive demeanor is essential. If other thoughts or distractions (noises, pain) occur, Benson recommends not fighting the distraction but simply continuing to repeat the focus phrase. Time of day is not important; however, the exercise works best on an empty stomach (Benson, 1993; Benson & Proctor, 1984; Benson & Stark, 1996).

Guided Imagery

Simple **guided imagery** is the mindful use of a word, phrase, or visual image for the purpose of distracting oneself from distressing situations or consciously taking time to relax or re-energize. A nurse can help a person select a pleasant scene or experience, such as watching the ocean or dabbling the feet in a cool stream. The image serves as the mental device in this technique. As the person sits comfortably and quietly, the nurse guides the person to review the scene, trying to feel and relive the imagery with all of the senses. A recording may be made of the description of the image, or commercial recordings for guided imagery and relaxation can be used.

Educating About Stress Management

Two commonly prescribed nursing educational interventions—providing sensory information and providing procedural information (e.g., preoperative education)—aim to reduce stress and improve the patient's coping ability. This preparatory education includes giving structured content, such as a lesson in childbirth preparation to expectant parents, a review of how an implantable cardioverter defibrillator works to a patient with heart disease, or a description of sensations a patient will experience during cardiac catheterization. These techniques may alter the person–environment relationship such that something that might have been viewed as harmful or a threat will now be perceived more positively. Giving patients information also reduces the emotional response so that they can concentrate and solve problems more effectively (Kittleson, 2019; Miller & Stoeckel, 2017; Rhee, Marottoli, Van Ness, et al., 2018).

 Veterans Considerations

Veterans have similar educational needs to nonveterans. Yet one study revealed that, in a postsecondary education setting, women service members and veterans received less health information compared to women who were not service members or veterans (Albright, Thomas, McDaniel, et al., 2019). In this cross-sectional study, women service members and veterans received less education about alcohol and illicit drug use, depression and anxiety, sexual assault and relational violence prevention, and stress reduction. Nurses who work on college campuses should be attuned to the educational needs of women veterans.

Promoting Family Health

In addition to individual concepts of homeostasis, stress, adaptation, and health problems associated with maladaptation, the concept of family is also important. Nurses can intervene with both individuals and families to reduce stress and its health-related effects. The **family** (group whose members are related by reciprocal caring, mutual responsibilities, and loyalties) plays a central role in the life of the patient and is a major part of the context of the patient's life. It is within families that people grow, are nurtured, acquire a sense of self, develop beliefs and values about life, and progress through life's developmental stages (Fig. 5-7). Families are also the first source for socialization and education about health and illness.

Ideally, the health care team conducts a careful and comprehensive family assessment (including coping style), develops interventions tailored to handle the stressors, implements

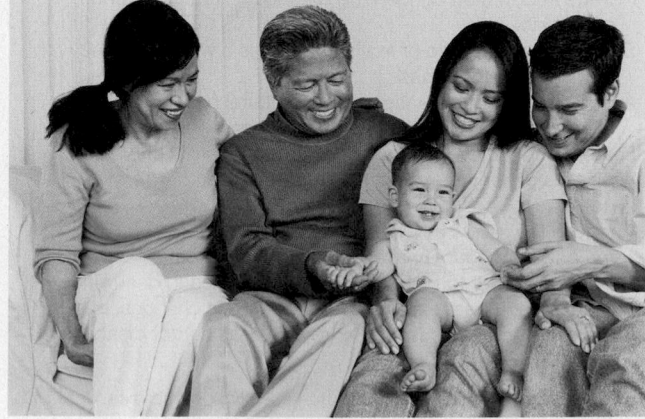

Figure 5-7 • Within families, individuals progress through life's developmental stages.

the specified treatment protocols, and facilitates the construction of social support systems. The use of existing family strengths, resources, and education is augmented by therapeutic family interventions. The nurse's primary goals are to maintain and improve the patient's present level of health and to prevent physical and emotional deterioration. Next, the nurse intervenes in the cycle that the illness creates: patient illness, stress for other family members, new illness in other family members, and additional patient stress.

Helping the family members manage the myriad stressors that bombard them daily involves working with family members to develop coping skills. Seven traits that enhance coping of family members under stress have been identified (Burr, Klein, Burr, et al., 1994). Communication skills and spirituality were frequently useful traits. Cognitive abilities, emotional strengths, relationship capabilities, willingness to use community resources, and individual strengths and talents were also associated with effective coping. As nurses work with families, they must not underestimate the impact of their therapeutic interactions, educational information, positive role modeling, provision of direct care, and education on promoting health. Maladaptive coping may result if health care team members are not perceived as actively supporting family members. Often, denial and blaming of others occur. Sometimes, physiologic illness, emotional withdrawal, and physical distancing are the results of severe family conflict, violent behavior, or addiction to drugs and alcohol. Substance abuse may develop in family members who feel unable to cope or solve problems. People may engage in these dysfunctional behaviors when faced with difficult or problematic situations.

Enhancing Social Support

The nature of social support and its influence on coping have been studied extensively. Social support has been demonstrated to be an effective moderator of life stress. Such support has been found to provide people with several different types of emotional information (Nicks, Wray, Peavler, et al., 2019; Warner, Roberts, Jeanblanc, et al., 2017). The first type of information leads people to believe that they are cared for and loved. This emotional support appears most often in a relationship between two people in which mutual trust and attachment are expressed by helping each other to meet their emotional needs. The second type of information leads people to believe that they are esteemed and valued. This is most effective when others in a group recognize a person's favorable position within that group, demonstrating the person's value. Known as esteem support, this elevates the person's sense of self-worth. The third type of information leads people to feel that they belong to a network of communication and mutual obligation. Members of this network share information and make goods and services available to the members as needed.

Social support also facilitates a person's coping behaviors; however, this depends on the nature of the social support. People can have extensive relationships and interact frequently; however, the necessary support comes only when people feel a deep level of involvement and concern, not when they merely touch the surface of each other's lives.

The critical qualities within a social network are the exchange of intimate communications and the presence of solidarity and trust.

Emotional support from family and significant others provides love and a sense of sharing the burden. The emotions that accompany stress are unpleasant and often increase in a spiraling fashion if relief is not provided. Being able to talk with someone and express feelings openly may help a person gain mastery of the situation. Nurses can provide this support but also must identify the person's social support system and encourage its use. People who are "loners," who are isolated, or who withdraw in times of stress have a high risk of coping failure.

Because anxiety can also distort a person's ability to process information, it helps to seek information and advice from others who can assist with analyzing the threat and developing a strategy to manage it. Again, this use of others helps people maintain mastery of a situation and self-esteem.

Thus, social networks assist with management of stress by providing people with:
- A positive social identity
- Emotional support
- Material aid and tangible services
- Access to information
- Access to new social contacts and new social roles

Recommending Support and Therapy Groups

Support groups exist especially for people in similar stressful situations. Groups have been formed by people with ostomies; women who have had mastectomies; and people with cancer or other serious diseases, chronic illness and disability. There are groups for single parents, substance abusers and their family members, homicide bereavement, and victims of child abuse. Professional, civic, and religious support groups are active in many communities (Mavandadi, Wray, & Toseland, 2019; Supiano & Overfelt, 2018). Encounter groups, assertiveness training programs, and consciousness-raising groups help people modify their usual behaviors in their transactions with their environment. Many find that being a member of a group with similar problems or goals has a releasing effect that promotes freedom of expression and exchange of ideas.

 Veterans Considerations

Due to the loss of their military community and associated support systems, veterans are at higher risk compared to civilians of experiencing psychiatric symptoms (such as posttraumatic stress disorder [PTSD]) and interpersonal distress. One group of researchers reported that in a study of 117 veterans, group psychotherapy helped to reduce the symptoms of PTSD and interpersonal distress, mainly by increasing social support among the veterans (Cox, Owen, & Ogrodniczuk, 2017).

The Role of Stress in Health Patterns

As noted previously, a person's psychological and biologic health, internal and external sources of stress management, and relationships with the environment are predictors of health outcomes. These factors are directly related to the person's health patterns. The nurse has a significant role and responsibility in identifying the health patterns of patients receiving care as well as those of their families. If those patterns are not achieving physiologic, psychological, and social balance, the nurse is obligated, with the assistance and agreement of the patient, to seek ways to promote individual and family balance.

This chapter has presented some physiologic mechanisms and perspectives on health and disease, the way that one copes with stress. Nurses should keep in mind that the way that one relates to others and the values and goals held are also interwoven into those physiologic patterns. To evaluate a patient's health patterns and to intervene if a disorder exists requires a total assessment of the person. Specific disorders and their nursing management are addressed in greater depth in other chapters.

CRITICAL THINKING EXERCISES

1 **ebp** You are the nurse in a student health center, and a female veteran comes in after experiencing 1 week of persistent discomfort in her shoulder after spiking a ball during a volleyball game. During the appointment, the student tells you, "I play hard as this is the only form of exercise that I get during the week. I have been putting ice on it at night, but that has stopped helping. I'm very stressed-out about this injury, and I am afraid that I may have torn my rotator cuff. How serious do you think this is?" What is the evidence base for offering guidelines for managing this student's health situation and her high level of stress? What educational information can you share to assist her to make appropriate health decisions and establish positive health behaviors? Identify the criteria used to evaluate the strength of the evidence for this practice.

2 **pq** An 82-year-old man recently moved out of his daughter's home into an assisted living program where you are working. His reason for coming to see you is "because I haven't been feeling well and sometimes my chest is sore." During his interview, he states, "I am a stomach cancer survivor and I have heart disease. I chose to move into assisted living rather than being with my daughter and her crazy family. Those people make me upset and anxious. They raise my blood pressure and make me sick." Identify this older man's health priorities and state the next steps you will take to meet his identified needs and other health promotion needs.

3 **ipc** You are the nurse working in an outpatient clinic. You tell a 30-year-old woman that during her routine physical examination a thyroid nodule was found. How will you educate this patient about this finding? What referrals do you anticipate will be made? What steps will the interdisciplinary team take to address the patient's health care needs?

REFERENCES

*Asterisk indicates nursing research.
**Double asterisk indicates classic reference.

Books

Bastable, S., Gramet, P., Jacobs, K., et al. (2019). *Health professional as educator: Principles of teaching and learning* (5th ed.). Sudbury, MA: Jones & Bartlett.

**Benson, H. (1993). The relaxation response. In D. Goleman, & J. Gurin. (Eds.). *Mind-body medicine: How to use your mind for better health.* Yonkers, NY: Consumer Reports Books.
**Benson, H., & Proctor, W. (1984). *Beyond the relaxation response.* New York: Berkley Books.
**Benson, H., & Stark, M. (1996). *Timeless healing.* New York: Scribner.
Bulechek, G. M., Butcher, H. K. K., Dochterman, J. M., & Wagner, C. M. (Eds.). (2018). *Nursing interventions classification (NIC)* (7th ed.). St. Louis, MO: Elsevier.
**Burr, W., Klein, S., Burr, R., et al. (1994). *Reexamining family stress: New theory and research.* Thousand Oaks, CA: Sage.
**Jalowiec, A. (1993). Coping with illness: Synthesis and critique of the nursing literature from 1980–1990. In J. D. Barnfather, & B. L. Lyon. (Eds.). *Stress and coping: State of the science and implications for nursing theory, research, and practice.* Indianapolis, IN: Sigma Theta Tau International.
**Lazarus, R. S. (1991). *Emotion and adaptation.* New York: Oxford University Press.
**Lazarus, R. S., & Folkman, S. (1984). *Stress, appraisal, and coping.* New York: Springer.
Miller, M. A., & Stoeckel, P. R. (2017). *Client education: Theory and practice* (3rd ed.). Sudbury, MA: Jones & Bartlett.
Norris, T. L. (2019). *Porth's pathophysiology: Concepts of altered health status* (10th ed.). Philadelphia, PA: Wolters Kluwer.
Rice, V. H. (Ed.). (2012). *Handbook of stress, coping, and health: Implications for theory, research, and practice* (2nd ed.). Thousand Oaks, CA: Sage.
**Selye, H. (1976). *The stress of life,* Rev. ed. New York: McGraw-Hill.

Journals and Electronic Documents

*Albdour, M., Hong, S. J., Lewin, L., et al. (2019). The impact of cyberbullying on physical and psychological health of Arab American Adolescents. *Journal of Immigrant and Minority Health, 21*(4), 706–715.
Albright, D. L., Thomas, K. H., McDaniel, J., et al. (2019). When women veterans return: The role of postsecondary education in transition in their civilian lives. *Journal of American College Health, 67*(5), 479–485.
Amirkhan, J. H. (2012). Stress overload: A new approach to the assessment of stress. *American Journal of Community Psychology, 49*(1–2), 55–71.
*Amirkhan, J. H., Urizar, G. G., & Clark, S. (2015). Criterion validation of a stress measure: The Stress Overload Scale. *Psychological Assessment, 27*(3), 985–996.
*Anniko, M. K., Boersma, K., & Tillfors, M. (2019). Sources of stress and worry in the development of stress-related mental health problems: A longitudinal investigation from early to mid-adolescence. *Anxiety, Stress & Coping, 32*(2), 155–167.
Antoni, M. H., & Dhabhar, F. S. (2019). The impact of psychosocial stress and stress management on immune responses in patients with cancer. *Cancer, 125*(9), 1417–1431.
*Atkinson, D. M., Rodman, J. L., Thuras, P. D., et al. (2019). Examining burnout, depression, and self-compassion in Veterans Affairs mental health staff. *Journal of Alternative and Complementary Medicine, 23*(7), 551–557.
*Benham, G., & Charak, R. (2019). Stress and sleep remain significant predictors of health after controlling for negative affect. *Stress & Health: Journal of the International Society for the Investigation of Stress, 35*(1), 59–68.
Callaghan, J. E. M., Fellin, L. C., & Alexander, J. H. (2019). Promoting resilience and agency in children and young people who have experienced domestic violence and abuse. *Journal of Family Violence, 34*(6), 521–537.
Champagne, D. (2019). Stress and perceived social isolation (loneliness). *Archives of Gerontology and Geriatrics, 82,* 192–199.
Christensen, D. S., Flensborg-Madsen, T., Garde, E., et al. (2019). Big five personality traits and allostatic load in midlife. *Psychological Health, 34*(8), 1011–1028.
Cox, D. W., Owen, J. J., & Ogrodniczuk, J. S. (2017). Group psychotherapeutic factors and perceived social support among veterans with PTSD symptoms. *The Journal of Nervous and Mental Disease, 205*(2), 127–132.
**Fincham, F. D., & Rogge, R. (2010). Understanding relationship quality: Theoretical challenges and new tools for assessment. *Journal of Family Theory and Review, 2,* 227–242.

Frishman, W. H. (2019). Ten secrets to a long life. *The American Journal of Medicine, 132*(5), 564–566.

**Holmes, T. H., & Rahe, R. H. (1967). The social readjustment rating scale. *Journal of Psychosomatic Research, 11*, 213–218.

Kalinowski, J., Taylor, J. Y., & Spruill, T. M. (2019). Why are young black women at high risk for cardiovascular disease? *Circulation, 139*(8), 1003–1004.

*Kibler, J. L., Ma, M., Tursich, M., et al. (2018). Cardiovascular risks in relation to posttraumatic stress severity among young trauma-exposed women. *Journal of Affective Disorders, 241*, 147–153.

Kim, G. M., Lim, J. Y., Kim, E. J., et al. (2019). Resilience of patients with chronic diseases: A systematic review. *Health & Social Care in the Community, 27*(4), 797–807.

*Kinchen, E. V., & Loerzel, V. (2019). Nursing students' attitudes and use of holistic therapies for stress relief. *Journal of Holistic Nursing, 37*(1), 6–17.

Kittleson, M. J. (2019). Mental health v. mental illness: A health education perspective. *American Journal of Health Education, 50*(4), 210–212.

Kok, B. C., Reed, D. E., Wickham, R. E., et al. (2019). Adult ADHD symptomatology in active duty army personnel: Results from the army study to assess risk and resilience in service members. *Journal of Attention Disorders, 23*(9), 968–975.

*Liu, Z., Zhou, X., Zhang, W., et al. (2019). Factors associated with quality of life early after ischemic stroke: The role of resilience. *Topics in Stroke Rehabilitation, 26*(5), 335–341.

Marques, A., Perolta, M., Santos, T., et al. (2019). Self-rated health and health-related quality of life are related with adolescents' healthy lifestyle. *Public Health, 170*, 89–94.

*Mavandadi, S., Wray, L. O., & Toseland, R. W. (2019). Measuring self-appraised changes following participation in an intervention for caregivers of individuals with dementia. *Journal of Gerontological Social Work, 62*(3), 324–337.

*McNeil, N., Bartram, T., Cregan, C., et al. (2019). Caring for aged people: The influence of personal resilience and workplace climate on 'doing good' and 'feeling good.' *Journal of Advanced Nursing, 75*(7), 1450–1461.

*Nicks, S. E., Wray, R. J., Peavler, O., et al. (2019). Examining peer support and survivorship for African American women with breast cancer. *Psycho-Oncology, 28*(2), 358–364.

*Pitt, A., Oprescu, F., Tapia, G., et al. (2018). An exploratory study of students' weekly stress levels and sources of stress during the semester. *Active Learning in Higher Education, 19*(1), 61–75.

*Reblin, M., Stanley, N. B., Galligan, A., et al. (2019). Family dynamics in young adult cancer caregiving: "It should be teamwork." *Journal of Psychosocial Oncology, 37*(4), 526–540.

Rhee, T. G., Marottoli, R. A., Van Ness, P. H., et al. (2018). Patterns and perceived benefits of utilizing seven major complementary health approaches in U.S. older adults. *Gerontological Journal of Medical Sciences, 73*(8), 1119–1124.

*Sarid, O., Slonim-Nevo, V., Sergienko, R., et al., (2018). Daily hassles score associates with the somatic and psychological health of patients with Crohn's disease. *Journal of Clinical Psychology, 74*(6), 969–988.

*Shen, A. (2019). Religious attendance, healthy lifestyles, and perceived health: A comparison of baby boomers with the silent generation. *Journal of Religion and Health, 58*(4), 1235–1245.

*Sikes, P., & Hall, M. (2017). 'Every time I see him he's the worst he's ever been and the best he'll ever be': Grief and sadness in children and young people who have a parent with dementia. *Mortality, 22*(4), 324–338.

*Sima, A. P., Yu, G., Marwitz, J. H., et al. (2019). Outcome prediction from post-injury resilience in patients with TBI. *Rehabilitation Psychology, 64*(3), 320–328.

Supiano, K. P., & Overfelt, V. K. (2018). Honoring grief, honoring ourselves: Mindfulness-based stress reduction education for grief group clinician-facilitators. *Social Work in Mental Health, 16*(1), 62–73.

**Tausig, M. (1982). Measuring life events. *Journal of Health and Social Behavior, 23*(1), 52–64.

Terrill, A. L., & Molton, I. R. (2019). Frequency and impact of midlife stressors among men and women with physical disability. *Disability and Rehabilitation, 41*(5), 1760–1767.

*Torkzadeh, F., Danesh, M., Mirbagher, L., et al. (2019). Relations between coping skills, symptom severity, psychological symptoms, and quality of life in patients with irritable bowel syndrome. *International Journal of Preventive Medicine, 17*(10), 72–83.

*Tormohlen, K. N., Tobin, K. E., & Latkin, C. (2019). Sources of stress among adults with co-occurring drug use and depressive symptoms. *Journal of Urban Health, 96*(3), 379–389.

Ubel, P. A., & Rosenthal, M. B. (2019). Beyond nudges—When improving health calls for greater assertiveness. *New England Journal of Medicine, 380*(4), 309–311.

Vaughan, E., Koczwara, B., Kemp, E., et al. (2019). Exploring emotion regulation as a mediator of the relationship between resilience and distress in cancer. *Psycho-Oncology, 28*(7), 1506–1512.

Vohra, S., Kelling, A. W., Varma, M. M., et al. (2019). Measuring reliability and validity of "Stressometer®": A computer-based mass screening and assessment tool for stress levels and sources of stress. *Indian Journal of Psychiatry, 61*(3), 295–299.

Warner, C. B., Roberts, A. R., Jeanblanc, A. B., et al. (2017). Coping resources, loneliness, and depressive symptoms of older women with chronic illness. *Journal of Applied Gerontology, 38*(3), 295–322.

*Wilson, S. J., Woody, A., Padin, A. C., et al. (2019). Loneliness and telomere length: Immune and parasympathetic function in associations with accelerated aging. *Annals of Behavioral Medicine, 53*(6), 541–550.

Resources

American Holistic Nurses Association (AHNA), www.ahna.org

Anxiety and Depression Association of America (ADAA), www.adaa.org

Grief Recovery Institute, www.griefrecoverymethod.com

Help Guide: A Nonprofit Guide to Mental Health and Well Being, www.helpguide.org

Institute of HeartMath: Connecting Hearts and Minds, www.heartmath.org

National Hospice and Palliative Care Organization (NHPCO), www.nhpco.org

Physiological Stress Response: Its Effects on the Body, www.stressfocus.com/stress_focus_article/stress-removal.htm

Psych Central: Tips to Decrease Stress, www.psychcentral.com/lib/20-tips-to-tame-your-stress

Stress: The Silent Killer, www.holisticonline.com/Stress/stress_home.htm

The Compassionate Friends, www.compassionatefriends.org

The Psychology of "Stress," www.guidetopsychology.com/stress.htm

Widowed Persons Service, 3950 Ferrara Dr., Silver Spring, MD; 1-301-949-7398; www.wpsgr.org

Women's Health Network, www.womentowomen.com/inflammation/default.aspx

6 Genetics and Genomics in Nursing

GLOSSARY

carrier: a person who is heterozygous; possessing two different alleles of a gene pair, with one allele typically altered/mutated; therefore, the expression of the altered gene may not be expressed

chromosome: microscopic structures in the cell nucleus that contain genetic information; humans have 46 chromosomes in all somatic cells

deoxyribonucleic acid (DNA): the primary genetic material in humans consisting of nitrogenous bases, a sugar group, and phosphate combined into a double helix

dominant: a genetic trait that is normally expressed when a person has a gene mutation on one of a pair of chromosomes and the "normal" form of the gene is on the other chromosome

epigenetics: the study of changes in gene expression that are not directly related to changes in the DNA genetic code

genetics: the scientific study of heredity; how specific traits or predispositions are transmitted from parents to offspring

genome: the total genetic complement of an individual genotype

genomics: the study of the human genome, including gene sequencing, mapping, and function

genotype: the genetic structure and the variations therein that a person inherits from their parents

mutation: a heritable alteration in a DNA sequence

nondisjunction: the failure of a chromosome pair to separate appropriately during cell division, resulting in abnormal chromosome numbers in daughter cells

pedigree: a diagrammatic representation of a family history

pharmacogenetics: the study of the safety and efficacy of medication administration based on a person's genotype

phenotype: a person's entire physical, biochemical, and physiologic genetic makeup that generates the physical presentation of the person

preimplantation genetic testing: a testing procedure used to identify genetic alterations in embryos

prenatal screening: testing that is used to identify whether a fetus is at risk for a birth defect (e.g., Down syndrome or spina bifida)

presymptomatic testing: genetic testing that is used to determine whether a person with a family history of a disorder, but no current symptoms, has the gene mutation (e.g., testing for Huntington disease)

recessive: a genetic trait that is expressed only when a person has two copies of a mutant autosomal gene or a single copy of a mutant X-linked gene in the absence of another X chromosome

variable expression: variation in the degree to which a trait is manifested; clinical severity

X-linked: located on the X chromosome

The completion of the Human Genome Project, which was an international research project focused on identifying and characterizing the DNA of the human genome, generated rapid advances in the application of genetics and genomics in health care, and stimulated the growth of translational genetic research (Khoury, Bowen, Clyne, et al., 2018). This genetic revolution gave rise to understanding how genetics and genomics influence health and to the development of tests and screening tools to diagnose genetic alterations and mutations. **Pharmacogenetics**, the study of the safety and efficacy of medication administration based on a person's genotype, preimplantation genetic testing, a testing procedure used to identify genetic alterations in embryos, and the use of biobanking, the storage of genetic material for research or personal use, are just a few examples of the advances in genetic and genomic technologies since the discovery of the human genome.

The anticipated rapid growth of genetics and genomics led to the creation of the Genetic Information Nondiscrimination Act (GINA), a law created to protect the privacy and confidentiality of a person's genetic information (Rothstein, 2018). The Precision Medicine Initiative is a national effort intended to advance personalized medicine through the understanding of genetic makeup, lifestyle, and the environment (National Institutes of Health [NIH], U.S. National Library of Medicine [NLM], 2019a).

Identification of genetic and genomic factors associated with disease, including gene–gene function and gene–environment interactions, contributes to the development of more effective therapies customized to that person's genetic makeup and the genomic profile of his or her disease. The term **genetics** (i.e., the study of heredity) generally applies to single genes and their impact on relatively rare single gene disorders, whereas **genomics** is the study of the interaction of all genes in the human **genome** (i.e., the total genetic complement of a person), environmental factors, and their interactions with each other (NIH, National Human Genome Research Institute [NHGRI], 2019a). **Epigenetics** refers to changes in the expression of a given gene due to environmental exposures or personal health activity rather than the alteration of a specific gene (NIH, NLM, 2019b). Over time, epigenetic influences can cause alterations to DNA. Genetic and genomic profiles allow health care providers to prescribe individualized and effective treatment for each patient, to identify and follow individuals at high risk for disease, and to avoid adverse drug reactions (NIH, NLM, 2019a). New genomic-based strategies for disease detection, management, and treatment are being utilized, making personalized medicine a reality (Table 6-1).

To meet the challenges of personalized medicine, nurses must understand how genetics and genomics can influence the health of the patient and the family. Nurses must stay abreast of new genetic and genomic technologies and understand how these influence treatments that support personalized medicine. Nurses are a vital link between the patient and health care services; patients often turn to nurses first with questions about a family history of risk factors, information regarding genetics, and genetic tests and interpretations. The incorporation of genetics and genomics is relevant to all aspects of the nursing process. For instance, genetics and genomics should be included in conducting health assessments, in devising nursing diagnoses (as appropriate) in planning nursing interventions that are specific to the patient and based on the patient's diagnosis and genetic makeup, in implementing interventions that support the identification of and in response to genetic-related health needs, and in evaluating responses to medications based on pharmacogenetics (Consensus Panel on Genetic/Genomic Nursing Competencies [Consensus Panel], 2009). This chapter offers a foundation for the clinical application of genetic and genomic principles in medical-surgical nursing; outlines the nurse's role in genetic counseling and evaluation; addresses important legal, ethical, and social issues; and provides related information and resources for nurses and patients.

Genomic Framework for Nursing Practice

Nurses' contribution to genomic focused health care offers a holistic perspective that takes into account each person's intellectual, physical, spiritual, social, cultural, biopsychological, ethical, and aesthetic experiences. Because genomics addresses all of the genes of a given person's human genome working together as a whole, genomics expands nursing's holistic view. Genetics and genomics are the basis of normal and pathophysiologic development, human health and disease, and health outcomes. Knowledge and interpretation of genetic and genomic information, gene-based testing, diagnosis, and treatment broaden the holistic view of nursing. It is a professional expectation that nurses understand genetics and genomics, and can apply this information in the clinical setting (American Nurses Association [ANA], 2017; Rogers, Lizer, Doughty, et al., 2017).

The *Essentials of Genetic and Genomic Nursing* (Consensus Panel, 2009) provides a framework for integrating genetics and genomics into nursing practice (Chart 6-1). This document includes a philosophy of care that recognizes when genetic and genomic factors play a role or could play a role

TABLE 6-1	Transition from the Medical Era to the Genomic Era of Personalized Medicine	
	Medical Era	**Genomic Era of Personalized Medicine**
Defining characteristics	• Considers single genes • Waits for disease symptoms to appear • Treats symptoms of presenting disease • Uses trial-and-error approach to treatment • Tailors medication administration according to clinical trials	• Considers interaction of genes with each other and the environment • Identifies genetic predisposition and optimizes risk reduction to prevent disease • Treats underlying genetic cause of disease • Uses personalized approach tailored to the genetic/genomic profile of the person and the disease • Adapts medication administration per clinical trials *and* personalized genetic response to medication

---

Chart 6-1
Essential Nursing Competencies for Genetics and Genomics

Professional Responsibilities

- Recognition of attitudes and beliefs related to genetic and genomic science
- Advocacy for genetic and genomic services
- Incorporation of genetic and genomic technologies and information into practice
- Demonstration of personalizing genetic and genomic information and services
- Providing autonomous, informed genetics- and genomics-related decision making

Professional Practice

- Integrate and apply genetic and genomic knowledge to nursing assessment.
- Identify patients who may benefit from specific genetic and genomic resources, services, or technologies.
- Facilitate referrals for genetic and genomic services.
- Provide education, care, and support related to the interpretation of genetic or genomic tests, services, interventions, or treatments.

Adapted from Consensus Panel on Genetic/Genomic Nursing Competencies (Consensus Panel). (2009). *Essentials of genetic and genomic nursing: Competencies, curricular guidelines, and outcome indicators* (2nd ed.). Silver Spring, MD: American Nurses Association.

---

in a person's health. This means assessing predictive genetic and genomic factors using family history and the results of genetic tests effectively, informing patients about genetic and genomic concepts, understanding the personal and societal impact of genetics and genomic information, and valuing the privacy and confidentiality of genetics and genomic information. There is also formal consensus regarding higher-level competencies in the application of genetics and genomics for nurses with graduate degrees. In addition, nurses need to be aware of genetic and genomic standards of practice as it relates to their specific area of clinical practice (Kerber & Ledbetter, 2017).

A person's response to genetic and genomic information, genetic testing, or genetic-related conditions may be either empowering or disabling. Genetic and genomic information may stigmatize people if it affects how they view themselves or how others view them. Nurses help individuals and families learn how genetic traits and conditions are passed on within families as well as how genetic and environmental factors influence health and disease (Consensus Panel, 2009). Nurses facilitate communication among family members, the health care system, and community resources, and they offer valuable support to patients and families. All nurses should be able to apply genetic and genomic knowledge by (ANA, 2017):

- providing basic genetic or genomic information to a patient or family member,
- obtaining family health histories that are inclusive of genetic information for at least three generations,
- conducting physical and developmental assessments and then correlating relevant assessment findings to genetic alterations,
- formulating nursing diagnoses based on actual or potential genetic risk,

- implementing nursing care that is reflective of genetic and genomic competencies,
- facilitating genetic and genomic referrals, and
- collaborating with other health professionals.

For example, when nurses assess patients' cardiovascular risk, they can expand their assessment to include information about family history of hypertension, hypercholesterolemia, clotting disorders, or premature sudden cardiac death. Knowledge that genes are involved in the control of lipid metabolism, insulin resistance, blood pressure regulation, clotting factors, cardiac structure, and vascular lining function helps individualize care based on the patient's genetic and genomic risk profile.

Essential to a genetic and genomic framework in nursing is the awareness of one's attitudes, experience, and assumptions about genetics and genomic concepts and how these are manifested in one's own practice (Consensus Panel, 2009). To develop awareness of these attitudes, experiences, and assumptions, nurses must examine their own:

- Beliefs or values about health as well as family, religious, or cultural beliefs about the cause of illness and how one's values or biases affect understanding of genetic conditions
- Philosophical, theologic, cultural, and ethical perspectives related to health and how these perspectives influence one's use of genetic information or services
- Level of expertise about genetics and genomics
- Experiences with birth defects, chronic illnesses, and genetic conditions, along with one's view of such conditions as disabling or empowering
- Attitudes about the right to access and other rights of individuals with genetic disorders
- View and assumptions about deoxyribonucleic acid (DNA) and beliefs about the value of information about one's risk for genetic disorders
- Beliefs about reproductive options
- View of genetic testing and engineering
- Approach to patients with disability

Integrating Genetic and Genomic Knowledge

Scientific developments and advances in technology have increased our understanding of genetics, promoted prompt genetic screening and genetic testing for common and rare genetic disorders, and improved patient health outcomes (Khoury et al., 2018). Scientists are able to characterize inherited metabolic variations that interact over time and lead to common diseases such as cancer, heart disease, and dementia. The transition from genetics to genomics has increased understanding of how multiple genes act and control biologic processes. Many diseases are the result of a combination of genetic and environmental influences (Khoury, 2019).

Genes and Their Role in Human Variation

Genes are central components of human health and disease. The Human Genome Project has linked basic human genetics to human development, health, and disease (NIH, NHGRI, 2018). Knowledge that specific genes are associated with specific genetic conditions makes diagnosis possible, even in the unborn. Many common conditions have genetic causes, and many more associations between genetics, health, and disease continue to be identified.

Genes and Chromosomes

A person's unique genetic composition, called a **genotype,** is made up of approximately 25,000 genes (NIH, NLM, 2019c). A person's **phenotype**—the observable characteristics or expression of their genotype—includes physical appearance and other biologic, physiologic, and molecular traits. Environmental influences modify every person's phenotype, even phenotypes with a major genetic component. This concept of genotype and phenotype applies to a person's total genome and the respective traits of their genetic makeup.

The concepts of genotype and phenotype also apply to specific diseases. For example, in hypercholesterolemia, the genotype refers to specific apolipoprotein genes (*LDLR, APOB, LDLRAP1,* or *PCSK9*) that involve mutations in low-density lipoprotein (LDL) receptors which control lipid metabolism (NIH, NLM, 2019d). Whereas, phenotype is characterized by early onset of cardiovascular disease, high levels of LDL, skin xanthomas, and a family history of heart disease. A person's genotype, consisting of normal functioning genes as well as some mutations, is characterized by physical and biologic traits that may predispose to disease.

Human growth and development and disease occur as a result of both genetic and environmental influences and interactions. The contribution of genetic factors may be large or small. For example, in a person with cystic fibrosis or phenylketonuria (PKU), the genetic contribution is significant. In contrast, the genetic contribution underlying a person's response to infection may be less applicable.

A single gene is conceptualized as a unit of heredity. A gene is composed of a segment of **deoxyribonucleic acid (DNA)** that contains a specific set of instructions for making the protein or proteins needed by body cells for proper functioning. Genes regulate both the types of proteins made and the rate at which proteins are produced. The structure of the DNA molecule is referred to as a double helix. The essential components of the DNA molecule are sugar–phosphate molecules and pairs of nitrogenous bases. Each nucleotide contains a sugar (deoxyribose), a phosphate group, and one of four nitrogenous bases: adenine (A), cytosine (C), guanine (G), and thymine (T). DNA is composed of two paired strands, each made up of a number of nucleotides. The strands are held together by hydrogen bonds between pairs of bases (Fig. 6-1).

Genes are arranged in a linear order within **chromosomes,** which are microscopic structures located in the cell nucleus. In humans, 46 chromosomes occur in pairs in all body cells except oocytes (eggs) and sperm, which each contains only 23 unpaired chromosomes. Twenty-two pairs of chromosomes, called *autosomes,* are the same in females and males. The 23rd pair is referred to as the sex chromosomes. A female has two X chromosomes, whereas a male has one X chromosome and one Y chromosome. At conception, each parent normally gives one chromosome of each pair to their child. As a result, children receive half of their chromosomes from fathers and half from mothers (Fig. 6-2).

Careful examination of DNA sequences from many people shows that these sequences have multiple versions in a

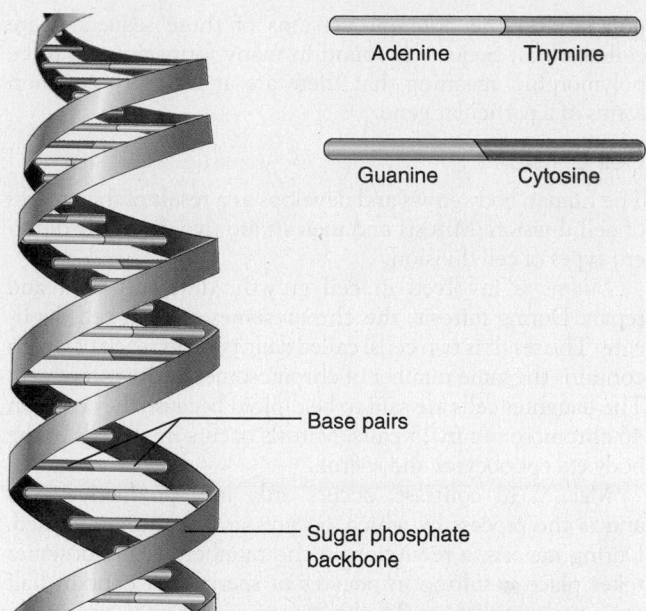

Figure 6-1 • DNA is a double helix formed by base pairs attached to a sugar-phosphate backbone. DNA carries the instructions that allow cells to make proteins. DNA is made up of four chemical bases. Redrawn from Genetics Home Reference, retrieved on 7/29/2020 at www.ghr.nlm.nih.gov/primer/basics/dna

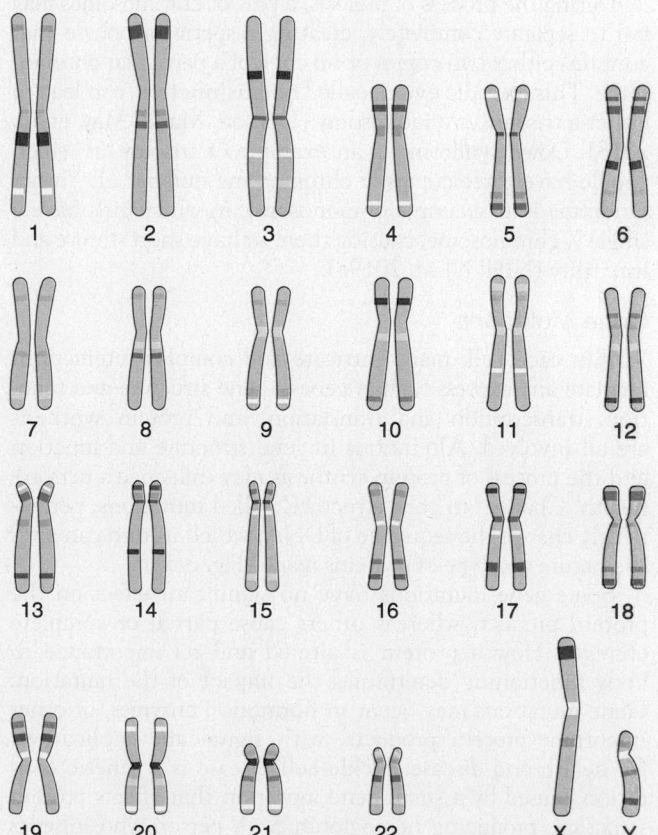

Figure 6-2 • Each human cell contains 23 pairs of chromosomes, which can be distinguished by their size and unique banding patterns. This set is from a male, because it contains a Y chromosome. Females have two X chromosomes.

population. The different versions of these sequences are called *alleles*. Sequences found in many forms are said to be polymorphic, meaning that there are at least two common forms of a particular gene.

Cell Division

The human body grows and develops as a result of the process of cell division. Mitosis and meiosis are two distinctly different types of cell division.

Mitosis is involved in cell growth, differentiation, and repair. During mitosis, the chromosomes of each cell duplicate. The result is two cells, called *daughter cells*, each of which contains the same number of chromosomes as the parent cell. The daughter cells are said to be diploid because they contain 46 chromosomes in 23 pairs. Mitosis occurs in all cells of the body except oocytes and sperm.

Meiosis, in contrast, occurs only in reproductive cells and is the process by which oocytes and sperm are formed. During meiosis, a reduction in the number of chromosomes takes place, resulting in oocytes or sperm that contain half the usual number, or 23 chromosomes. Oocytes and sperm are referred to as haploid because they contain a single copy of each chromosome, compared to the usual two copies in all other body cells. During meiosis, as the paired chromosomes come together in preparation for cell division, portions cross over, and an exchange of genetic material occurs before the chromosomes separate. This event, called *recombination*, creates greater diversity in the makeup of oocytes and sperm.

During the process of meiosis, a pair of chromosomes may fail to separate completely, creating a sperm or oocyte that contains either two copies or no copy of a particular chromosome. This sporadic event, called **nondisjunction**, can lead to either a trisomy or a monosomy (Jackson, Marks, May, et al., 2018). Down syndrome is an example of trisomy, in which people have three copies of chromosome number 21. Turner syndrome is an example of monosomy, in which girls have a single X chromosome, causing them to have short stature and infertility (NIH, NLM, 2019e).

Gene Mutations

Within each cell, many intricate and complex interactions regulate and express human genes. Gene structure and function, transcription and translation, and protein synthesis are all involved. Alterations in gene structure and function and the process of protein synthesis may influence a person's health. Changes in gene structure, called **mutations**, permanently change the sequence of DNA, which in turn can alter the nature and type of proteins made (Fig. 6-3).

Some gene mutations have no significant effect on the protein product, whereas others cause partial or complete changes. How a protein is altered and its importance to body functioning determines the impact of the mutation. Gene mutations may occur in hormones, enzymes, or other important protein products, with significant implications for health and disease. Sickle cell disease is a genetic condition caused by a small gene mutation that affects protein structure, producing hemoglobin S. A person who inherits two copies of the hemoglobin S gene mutation has sickle cell disease and experiences the symptoms of severe anemia and thrombotic organ damage resulting from hypoxia (NIH, NLM, 2019f).

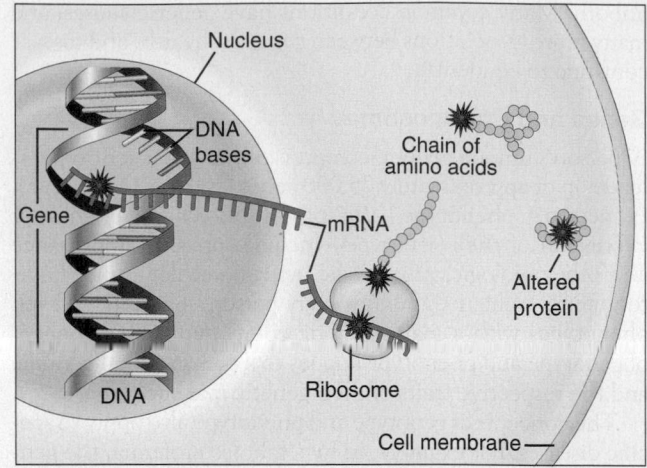

Figure 6-3 • When a gene contains a mutation, the protein encoded by that gene is likely to be abnormal. Sometimes the protein is able to function, although it does so imperfectly. In other cases, it is totally disabled. The outcome depends not only on how the mutation alters the protein's function but also on how vital that particular protein is to survival.

Other gene mutations include deletion (loss), insertion (addition), duplication (multiplication), or translocation (rearrangement) of a longer DNA segment (Jackson et al., 2018). Duchenne muscular dystrophy, myotonic dystrophy, Huntington disease, and fragile X syndrome are examples of conditions caused by gene mutations.

Gene mutations may be inherited or acquired. Inherited or germline gene mutations are present in the DNA of all body cells and are passed on in reproductive cells from parent to child. Germline or hereditary mutations are passed on to all daughter cells when body cells replicate (Fig. 6-4). The gene that causes Huntington disease is one example of a germline mutation.

Spontaneous mutations take place in individual oocytes or sperm at the time of conception. A person who carries the new "spontaneous" mutation may pass on the mutation to his

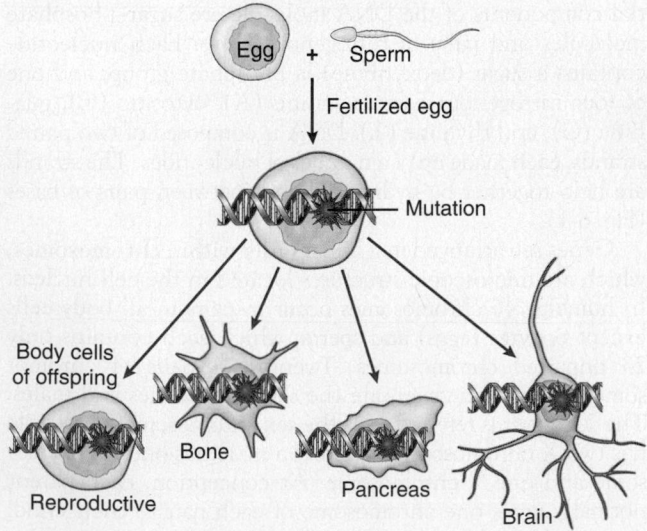

Figure 6-4 • Hereditary mutations are carried in the DNA of the reproductive cells. When reproductive cells containing mutations combine to produce offspring, the mutation is present in all of the offspring's body cells.

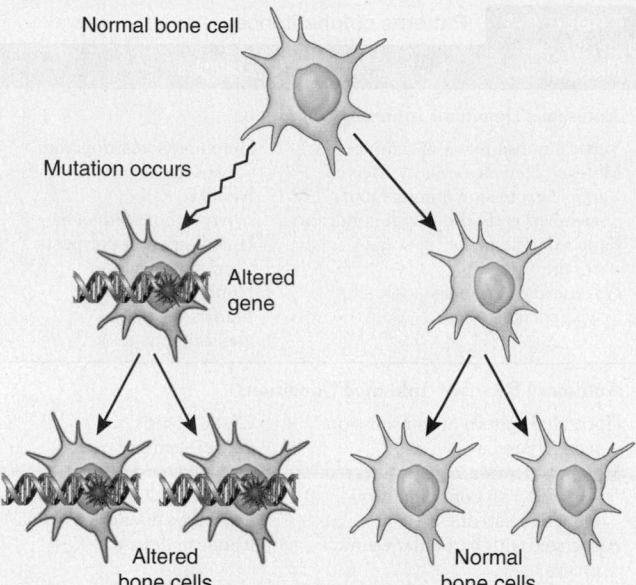

Figure 6-5 • Acquired mutations develop in DNA during a person's lifetime. If the mutation arises in a body cell, copies of the mutation will exist only in the descendants of that particular cell.

or her children. Achondroplasia, Marfan syndrome, and neurofibromatosis type 1 are examples of genetic conditions that may occur in a single family member as a result of spontaneous mutation.

Acquired mutations take place in somatic cells and involve changes in DNA that occur after conception, during a person's lifetime. Acquired mutations develop as a result of cumulative changes in body cells other than reproductive cells (Fig. 6-5). Somatic gene mutations are passed on to the daughter cells derived from that particular cell line.

Gene mutations occur in the human body all the time. Cells have built-in mechanisms by which they can recognize mutations in DNA, and in most situations, they correct the changes before they are passed on by cell division. However, over time, body cells may lose their ability to repair damage from gene mutations, causing an accumulation of genetic changes that result in diseases such as cancer, Alzheimer's disease, and disorders associated with aging (Khoury, 2019).

Genetic Variation

Genetic variations occur among all people. Single nucleotide polymorphisms (SNPs, referred to as "snips") is the term used to identify common genetic variations that occur most frequently throughout the human genome (Jackson et al., 2018). SNPs are changes in a single nucleotide (an A, T, C, or G) of the DNA sequence. For example, a normal DNA sequence of AAGG could change to ATGG; in this case, there is one single nucleotide change from A to T. Most SNPs do not alter normal cell function. Some SNPs do alter gene function and may influence disease development. Knowledge about SNPs that affect biologic function will help pinpoint individuals who may be more prone to common diseases such as cancer, diabetes, and heart disease. Information on SNPs has helped to clarify why some individuals metabolize drugs differently (Centers for Disease Control and Prevention [CDC], 2018a). For example, a polymorphism or SNP can alter protein or enzyme activity of medications. If the SNP causes a variation in drug transport or drug metabolism, the drug's action, half-life, or excretion could lead to lack of drug response or drug toxicity.

Epigenetics

Epigenetics refers to generational changes within the genetic instruction (NIH, NLM, 2019b). Over time, epigenetic influences can cause cellular change throughout the lifetime of the affected person and be passed on to subsequent generations. Epigenomics, which is the study of epigenetics, is an expanding area of research that correlates epigenetics to cancer, psychiatric disorders, obesity, diabetes, and autoimmune disease (Jackson et al., 2018).

Inheritance Patterns

Nursing assessment of the patient's health includes obtaining and recording family history information in the form of a **pedigree** (i.e., a diagrammatic representation of a family history). This is a first step in establishing the pattern of inheritance. Nurses must be familiar with mendelian patterns of inheritance and pedigree construction and analysis to help identify patients and families who may benefit from further genetic counseling, testing, and treatment (Consensus Panel, 2009).

Mendelian conditions are genetic conditions that are inherited in fixed proportions among generations. They result from gene mutations that are present on one or both chromosomes of a pair. A single gene inherited from one or both parents can cause a mendelian condition. Mendelian conditions are classified according to their pattern of inheritance: autosomal dominant, autosomal recessive, and X-linked. The terms dominant and recessive refer to the trait, genetic condition, or phenotype but not to the genes or alleles that cause the observable characteristics (Jackson et al., 2018).

Autosomal Dominant Inheritance

The term **dominant** refers to the trait of the gene that is expressed when two genes do not mirror each other on matched chromosomes. Autosomal dominant inherited conditions affect female and male family members equally and follow a vertical pattern of inheritance in families (Fig. 6-6).

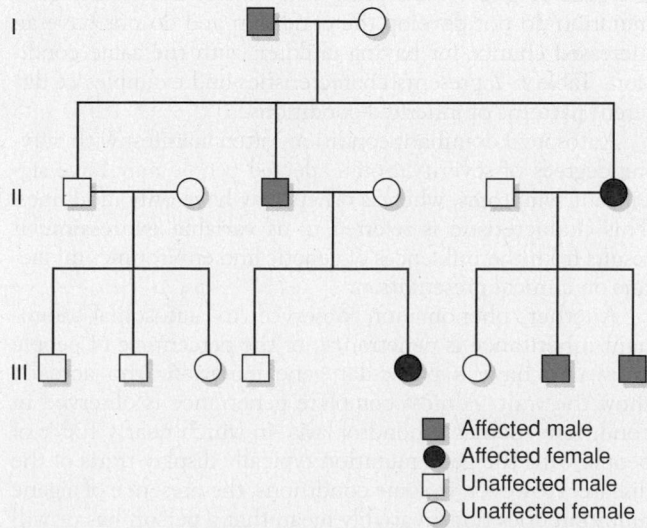

■ Affected male
● Affected female
□ Unaffected male
○ Unaffected female

Figure 6-6 • Three-generation pedigree illustrating autosomal dominant inheritance.

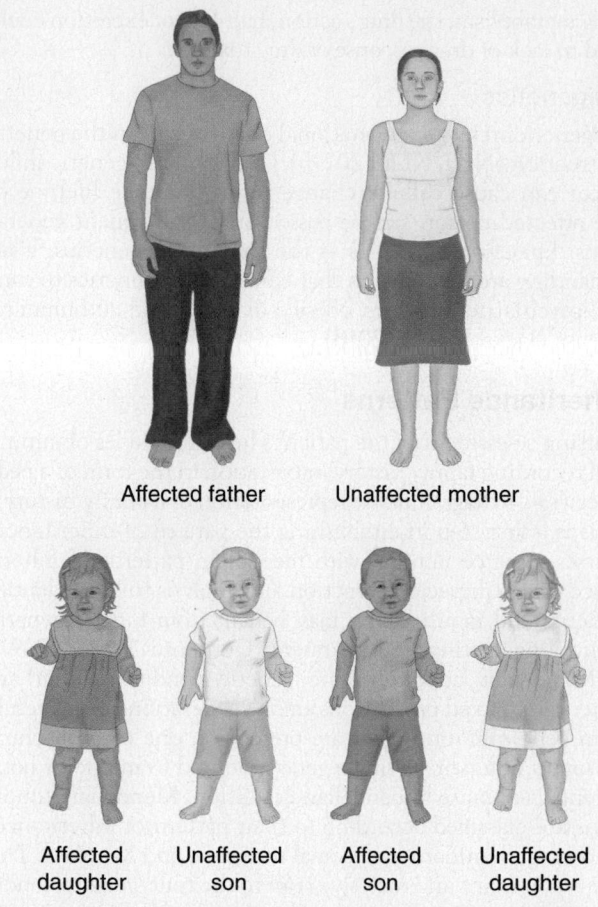

Affected father   Unaffected mother

Affected daughter   Unaffected son   Affected son   Unaffected daughter

Figure 6-7 • In dominant genetic disorders, if one affected parent has a disease-causing allele that dominates its normal counterpart, each child in the family has a 50% chance of inheriting the disease allele and the disorder.

The presence of an autosomal dominant inherited condition only requires a genetic mutation on one of the chromosomes associated with that pair. Each of that person's offspring has a 50% chance of inheriting the gene mutation for the condition and a 50% chance of inheriting the normal version of the gene (Fig. 6-7). Offspring who do not inherit the gene mutation do not develop the condition and do not have an increased chance for having children with the same condition. Table 6-2 presents characteristics and examples of different patterns of inherited conditions.

Autosomal dominant conditions often manifest with varying degrees of severity. Some affected people may have significant symptoms, whereas others may have only mild ones. This characteristic is referred to as **variable expression**; it results from the influences of genetic and environmental factors on clinical presentation.

Another phenomenon observed in autosomal dominant inheritance is penetrance, or the percentage of people known to have a particular gene mutation who actually show the trait. Almost complete penetrance is observed in conditions such as achondroplasia, in which nearly 100% of people with the gene mutation typically display traits of the disease. However, in some conditions, the presence of a gene mutation does not invariably mean that a person has or will develop an autosomal inherited condition. For example, a woman who has the *BRCA1* hereditary breast cancer gene

TABLE 6-2	Patterns of Inheritance
Characteristics	**Examples**
Autosomal Dominant Inherited Conditions	
Vertical transmission in families	Hereditary breast/ovarian
Males and females equally affected	cancer syndrome
Variable expression among family	Familial
members and others with condition	hypercholesterolemia
Reduced penetrance (in some	Hereditary non-polyposis
conditions)	colorectal cancer
Advanced paternal age associated	Huntington disease
with sporadic cases	Marfan syndrome
	Neurofibromatosis
Autosomal Recessive Inherited Conditions	
Horizontal pattern of transmission	Cystic fibrosis
seen in families	Galactosemia
Males and females equally affected	Phenylketonuria
Associated with consanguinity	Sickle cell disease
(genetic relatedness)	Tay-Sachs disease
Associated with particular ethnic	Canavan disease
groups	
X-Linked Inherited Conditions	
Vertical transmission in families	Duchenne muscular
Males predominantly affected	dystrophy
	Hemophilia A
	Wiskott–Aldrich syndrome
	Color blindness
	Fragile X
Mitochondrial Inherited Conditions	
Transmission occurs through the	Leber's hereditary optic
mother	neuropathy
All children have the condition	Leigh syndrome
	Kearns–Sayre syndrome
Multifactorial Inherited Conditions	
Occur as a result of combination of	Congenital heart defects
genetic and environmental factors	Cleft lip and/or palate
May recur in families	Neural tube defects (anen-
Inheritance pattern does not dem-	cephaly and spina bifida)
onstrate characteristic pattern of	Diabetes
inheritance seen with other mende-	Osteoarthritis
lian conditions	High blood pressure
	Alzheimer's disease
	Hypothyroidism

Adapted from Learn.Genetics, Genetic Science Learning Center. (2019). Genetic disorders. Retrieved on 8/30/2019 at: www.learn.genetics.utah.edu/content/disorders; National Institutes of Health (NIH), U.S. National Library of Medicine (NLM); Genetics Home Reference. (2015). What are the different ways in which a genetic condition can be inherited? Retrieved on 8/30/2019 at: www.ghr.nlm.nih.gov/primer/inheritance/inheritancepatterns

mutation has a lifetime risk of breast cancer that can be as high as 80%, not 100%. This quality, known as reduced or incomplete penetrance, indicates the probability that a given gene will produce disease. In other words, a person may inherit the gene mutation that causes an autosomal dominant condition but may not have any of the observable physical or developmental features of that condition. However, this person carries the gene mutation and still has a 50% chance of passing the gene for the condition to each of their children (NIH, NLM, 2019g). One of the effects of incomplete penetrance is that the gene appears to "skip" a generation, thus leading to errors in interpreting family history and in genetic counseling.

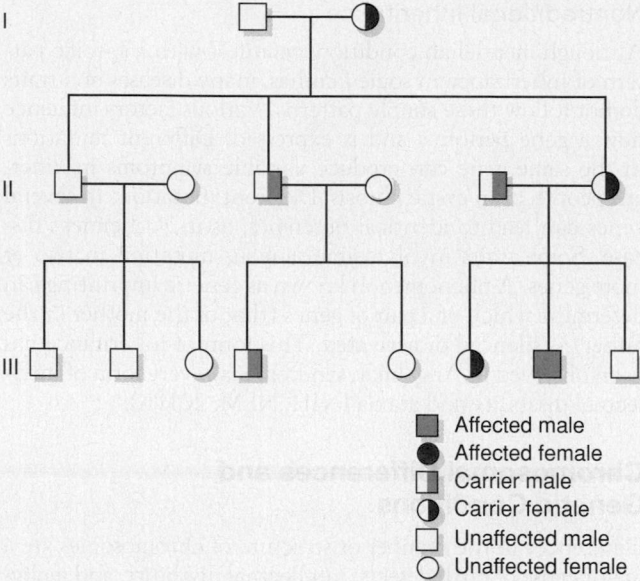

Affected male
Affected female
Carrier male
Carrier female
Unaffected male
Unaffected female

Figure 6-8 • Three-generation pedigree illustrating autosomal recessive inheritance.

Autosomal Recessive Inheritance

The term **recessive** refers to a genetic trait that is expressed only when a person has two copies of a mutant autosomal gene or a single copy of a mutant X-linked gene in the absence of another X chromosome. In contrast to autosomal dominant conditions, autosomal recessive conditions have a pattern that is more horizontal than vertical; relatives of a single generation tend to have the condition (Fig. 6-8). Autosomal recessive conditions are frequently seen among particular ethnic groups and usually occur more often in children of parents who are related by blood, such as first cousins (see Table 6-2).

In autosomal recessive inheritance, each parent carries a gene mutation on one chromosome of the pair and a normal gene on the other chromosome. The parents are said to be **carriers** of the gene mutation. Unlike people with an autosomal dominant condition, carriers of a gene mutation for a recessive condition do not have symptoms of the genetic condition. When carriers have children together, there is a 25% chance that each child may inherit the gene mutation from both parents and have the condition (Fig. 6-9). Cystic fibrosis, sickle cell disease, and PKU are examples of autosomal recessive conditions (Jackson et al., 2018).

X-Linked Inheritance

X-linked conditions may be inherited in recessive or dominant patterns (see Table 6-2). In both, the gene mutation is located on the X chromosome. All males inherit an X chromosome from mothers and a Y chromosome from fathers for a normal sex constitution of 46, XY. Because males have only one X chromosome, they do not have a counterpart for its genes, as do females. This means that a gene mutation on the X chromosome of a male is expressed even though it is present in only one copy. Females, on the contrary, inherit one X chromosome from each parent for a normal sex constitution of 46, XX. A female may be an unaffected carrier of a gene mutation, or she may be affected if the condition results from a gene mutation causing an X-linked dominant

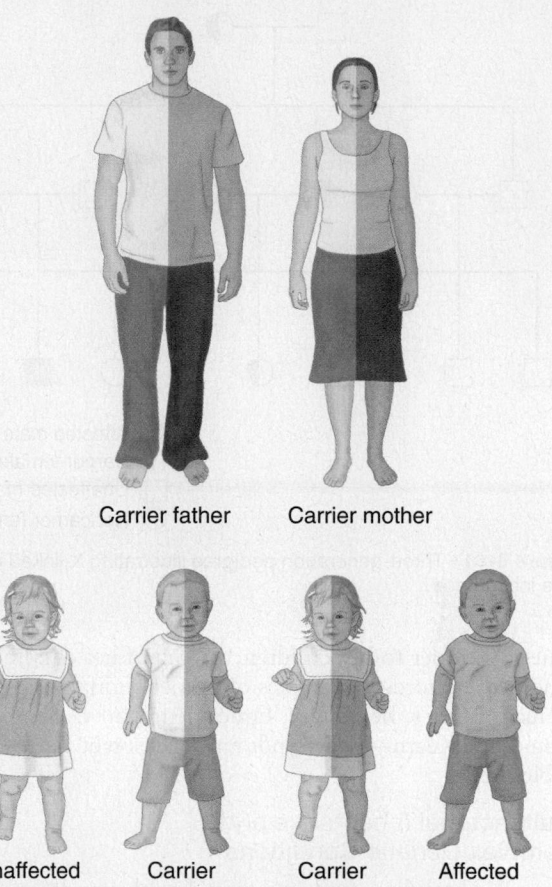

Carrier father   Carrier mother

Unaffected   Carrier   Carrier   Affected
daughter   son   daughter   son

Figure 6-9 • In diseases associated with altered recessive genes, both parents—although disease free themselves—carry one normal allele and one altered allele. Each child has one chance in four of inheriting two abnormal alleles and developing the disorder; one chance in four of inheriting two normal alleles; and two chances in four of inheriting one normal and one altered allele—therefore, being a carrier like both parents.

condition. Either the X chromosome that she received from her mother or the X chromosome she received from her father may be passed on to each of her offspring, and this is a random occurrence.

The most common pattern of X-linked inheritance is that in which a female is a carrier for a gene mutation on one of her X chromosomes. This is referred to as X-linked recessive inheritance, in which a female carrier has a 50% chance of passing on the gene mutation to a son, who would be affected, or to a daughter, who would be a carrier like her mother (Fig. 6-10). Examples of X-linked recessive conditions include factor VIII and factor IX hemophilia, severe combined immunodeficiency, and Duchenne muscular dystrophy (Jackson et al., 2018).

Mitochondrial Inheritance

The mitochondrium is an organelle, a cellular component associated with generating cellular energy. Although it is not a part of the nucleus, genetic alterations can occur in the mitochondria and be passed to offspring. These disorders are typically associated with muscle or nerve tissue. Unique to mitochondrial inheritance is that only the mother will pass the mitochondrial DNA to her offspring, and thus the

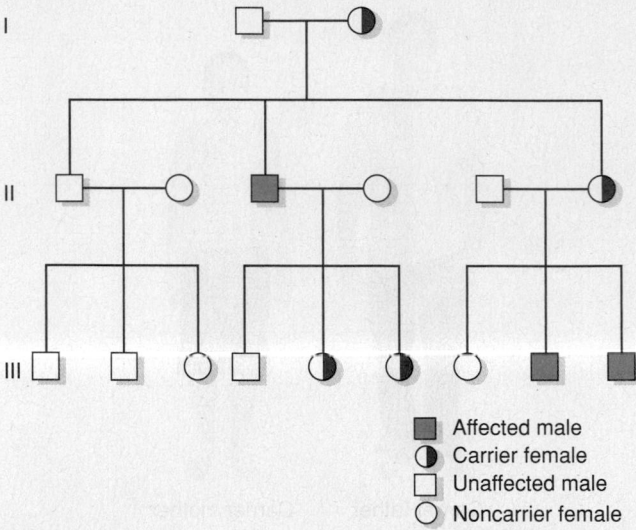

Affected male
Carrier female
Unaffected male
Noncarrier female

Figure 6-10 • Three-generation pedigree illustrating X-linked recessive inheritance.

genetic disorder to her children, and all of her children will inherit the disorder. Examples of mitochondrial inheritance include Leber's hereditary optic neuropathy, Leigh syndrome, and Kearns–Sayre syndrome (Jackson et al., 2018; see Table 6-2).

Multifactorial Inheritance and Complex Genetic Conditions

Many birth defects and common health conditions such as heart disease, high blood pressure, cancer, osteoarthritis, and diabetes occur as a result of interactions of multiple gene mutations and environmental influences. Thus, they are called *multifactorial* or *complex conditions* (see Table 6-2). Other examples of multifactorial genetic conditions include neural tube defects such as spina bifida and anencephaly. Multifactorial conditions may cluster in families; however, they do not always result in the characteristic pattern of inheritance seen in families who have mendelian inherited conditions (Fig. 6-11).

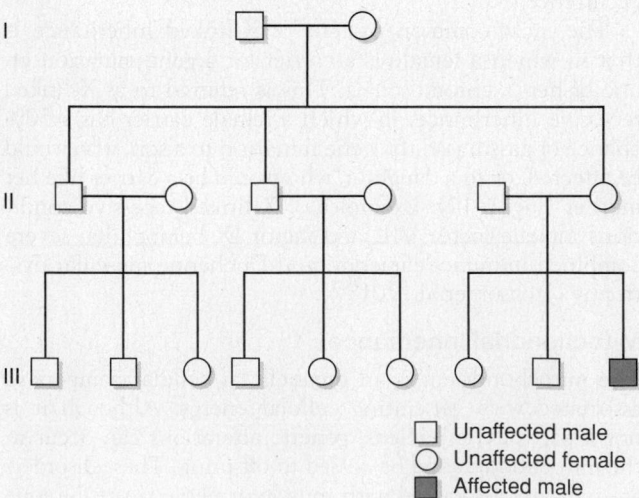

Unaffected male
Unaffected female
Affected male

Figure 6-11 • Three-generation pedigree illustrating multifactorial conditions.

Nontraditional Inheritance

Although mendelian conditions manifest with a specific pattern of inheritance in some families, many diseases and traits do not follow these simple patterns. Various factors influence how a gene performs and is expressed. Different mutations in the same gene can produce variable symptoms in different people, as in cystic fibrosis. Different mutations in several genes can lead to identical outcomes, as in Alzheimer's disease. Some traits involve simultaneous mutation in two or more genes. A phenomenon known as genetic imprinting can determine which of a pair of genes (that of the mother or the father) is silenced or activated. This form of inheritance has been observed in Angelman syndrome, a severe form of intellectual disability and ataxia (NIH, NLM, 2019h).

Chromosomal Differences and Genetic Conditions

Differences in the number or structure of chromosomes are a major cause of birth defects, intellectual disability, and malignancies. Chromosomal differences most commonly involve an extra or missing chromosome; this is called *aneuploidy*. These genetic alterations are neither inherited nor passed down through generations. Whenever there is an extra or missing chromosome, there is always associated intellectual or physical disability to some degree (NIH, National Center for Advancing Translational Sciences [NCATS], 2017).

Down syndrome, or trisomy 21, is a common chromosomal condition that occurs with greater frequency in pregnancies of women who are 35 years of age or older. A person with trisomy 21 has a complete extra chromosome 21, which causes a particular facial appearance and increased risk of congenital heart defects, thyroid and vision problems, and intellectual disability. Other examples of chromosomal differences include trisomy 13 and trisomy 18, both more severe than Down syndrome, and conditions involving extra or missing sex chromosomes, such as Turner syndrome (Jackson et al., 2018).

Chromosomal differences may also involve a structural rearrangement within or between chromosomes. These are less common than chromosomal conditions in which there is an extra or missing chromosome (NIH, NCATS, 2017). People who carry "balanced" chromosome rearrangements have all of their chromosomal material; however, it is rearranged. Women with a "balanced" chromosomal rearrangement have an increased risk of spontaneous pregnancy loss and of having children with an unbalanced chromosomal arrangement that may result in physical or intellectual disability. Known carriers of these chromosomal differences are offered prenatal counseling and testing.

Chromosome studies may be needed at any age, depending on the indication. Two common indications for these studies include a suspected diagnosis of Down syndrome or a history of two or more unexplained pregnancy losses. Chromosome studies are accomplished by obtaining a tissue sample (e.g., blood, skin, and amniotic fluid), preparing and staining the chromosomes, and analyzing them under a microscope. The microscopic study of chromosomes, called *cytogenetics*, is used with molecular techniques such as fluorescent in situ hybridization (FISH), which permits more detailed examination of chromosomes (Jackson et al., 2018). FISH is useful to detect small abnormalities and to characterize chromosomal rearrangements.

Genetic and Genomic Technologies in Practice

Genetic tests are used to detect a trait, to diagnose a genetic condition, or to identify people who have a genetic predisposition to a particular disease or condition. A plethora of genetic tests are available; some may be purchased directly by the consumer. The Genetic Testing Registry recognizes genetic tests for almost 12,000 genetic conditions (National Center for Biotechnology Information [NCBI], NLM, 2019a). Advances in the application of genetic testing are noted in pharmacogenetics, preimplantation genetic diagnosis, newborn screening, direct-to-consumer testing, and prenatal screening. Forms of genetic testing or genetic screening are available across the lifespan, extending from preimplantation genetic screening during pregnancy to posthumous testing (Bilkey, Burns, Coles, et al., 2019). Future applications may include the use of gene chips to map a person's individual genome for genetic variations that may lead to disease. Nurses are involved in caring for patients who are undergoing genetic testing and gene-based treatments. Knowledge of the clinical applications of modern genetic and genomic technologies enables nurses to inform and to support patients and their family members, and to provide high-quality genetic-related health care.

Genetic Testing

Genetic testing is the primary tool used to identify individuals who are predisposed to specific genetic diseases. Genetic tests provide information leading to the diagnosis of inherited conditions or other conditions with a known genetic contribution.

Approaches to genetic testing may focus on genotype or phenotype. Genotypic methods involve analysis of the chromosomes and genes directly, using specific laboratory techniques to learn whether a genetic alteration related to a specific disease or condition is present. This testing may be DNA based, chromosomal, or biochemical. Awareness of molecular biomarkers that can enhance the sensitivity and specificity of genetic-related tests allows for early detection of genetic illness, and for researchers to understand genetic pathways that may be useful in the treatment of specific disorders (van Lanschot, Bosch, de Wit, et al., 2017). Phenotypic methods examine the familial or biologic presentation of disease and include assessment of the patient's personal or family history and medical factors influencing their disease as well as testing for gene products such as protein markers in body fluids or diseased tissues. The family history, which is considered the first genetic test, is discussed later in this chapter (see the Family History Assessment section). It is expected that all nurses are able to create and interpret a three-generation family pedigree (Consensus Panel, 2009).

Another phenotypic approach involves searching for gene products, such as proteins and enzymes that can clinically indicate a genetic abnormality. For example, germline mutations in the repair genes *MLH1, MSH2, MSH6,* and *PMS2* are responsible for hereditary early-onset colorectal cancer or Lynch syndrome. Colorectal tumors are now tested to measure the presence or absence of these proteins using immunohistochemistry, which is a routine type of pathology test. Specific colon cancer gene mutations are used to identify other genetic forms of colon cancer which increases the

likelihood of cancer in other areas of the body. These include not only Lynch syndrome, but also familial adenomatous polyposis (FAP), Peutz–Jeghers, Cowden syndrome, and juvenile polyposis syndrome (Edwards & Maradiegue, 2018).

Genetic testing can be used for various purposes in prenatal, pediatric, and adult populations. Prenatal testing is widely used for **prenatal screening** and diagnosis of conditions such as Down syndrome. **Preimplantation genetic testing**, a form of prenatal genetic testing, detects the presence of genetic abnormalities in embryos (Parikh, Athalye, Naik, et al., 2018). Carrier testing is used to determine if a person carries a recessive allele for an inherited condition (e.g., cystic fibrosis, sickle cell disease, Tay-Sachs disease) and, therefore, risks passing it on to his or her children. Genetic testing is also used widely in newborn screening. Newborn testing is performed on infants to identify conditions, such as PKU, in which interventions can be implemented to prevent severe outcomes.

Diagnostic testing is used to detect the presence or absence of a particular genetic alteration or allele to identify or confirm a diagnosis of a disease or condition (e.g., myotonic dystrophy, fragile X syndrome) (Chart 6-2). Increasingly, genetic tests are being used to predict drug response and to design specific and individualized treatment plans or personalized medicine. For example, genetic testing is used to identify specific gene variants that can predict the effectiveness of treatments of human immunodeficiency virus infection, atherothrombosis, thrombophilia, hyperlipidemia, breast cancer, pain management, hepatitis C, rheumatoid arthritis, leukemia, depression, and bipolar disorder (NCBI, NLM, 2019b). Select examples of current uses of genetic tests are shown in Table 6-3.

TABLE 6-3	Select Genetic Tests: Examples of Current Uses
Purpose of Genetic Test	**Type of Genetic Test**
Carrier Testing	
Cystic fibrosis	DNA analysis
Tay-Sachs disease	Hexosaminidase A activity testing and DNA analysis
Canavan disease	DNA analysis
Sickle cell disease	Hemoglobin electrophoresis
Thalassemia	Complete blood count and hemoglobin electrophoresis
Diagnosis	
Down syndrome	Chromosomal analysis
Fragile X syndrome	DNA analysis
Myotonic dystrophy	DNA analysis
Presymptomatic Testing	
Huntington disease	DNA analysis
Myotonic dystrophy	DNA analysis
Susceptibility Testing	
Hereditary breast/ovarian cancer	DNA analysis
Hereditary non-polyposis colorectal cancer	DNA analysis

DNA, deoxyribonucleic acid.
Adapted from National Institutes of Health (NIH), U.S. National Library of Medicine (NLM); Genetics Home Reference. (2019j). Help me understand genetics. Retrieved on 8/30/2019 at: www.ghr.nlm.nih.gov/primer#testing; National Institutes of Health (NIH), U.S. National Library of Medicine (NLM). (2019k). Genetic testing. *MedlinePlus.* Retrieved on 8/30/2019 at: www.medlineplus.gov/genetictsting.html

Chart 6-2   ETHICAL DILEMMA
Can Predictive Genetic Testing Threaten Patient Autonomy?

Case Scenario

M.T., a high school biology teacher, brings her 11-year-old daughter to the family practice clinic where you are employed as the nurse manager. M.T. insists that she wants her daughter to have predictive genetic testing (PGT) for familial adenomatous polyposis (FAP), an autosomal dominant disorder associated with aggressive colorectal cancer that typically evidences pathology during young adulthood. M.T. tells you that her husband's sister, who is 36 years old, was recently diagnosed with FAP and advanced colorectal cancer. She also tells you that she recently discovered that her husband's father and his father's only sibling both died of colorectal cancer before they were 50. Her husband is 34 years old; according to M.T., he has not been seen by a health care provider since he was a teenager and refuses to do so or to be tested for FAP.

Discussion

There are many legal and ethical concerns raised by health care providers regarding PGT in children. Some genetic disorders are not amenable to treatment during childhood (e.g., carrying a *BRCA* genetic mutation, which is associated with various cancers in adulthood). In these instances, it is generally advisable to forego offering PGT to a child until such time that the child reaches adulthood and is able to make the autonomous decision to either be tested or not be tested. The American College of Medical Genetics contends that ultimately, the best interest of the person tested must be the focus of PGT.

In this particular case, it is presumed that the father has not consented to be tested for the FAP genetic mutation. However, should he consent to testing and find out that he does not have the genetic mutation associated with FAP, then the daughter could not have that mutated gene, since it is conferred through autosomal dominant inheritance. By contrast, if the father does carry the gene for FAP, then the daughter would have a 50% chance of having the gene; moreover, if she has the gene, she and her parents should be advised that she should begin screening colonoscopies. Precancerous colonic polyps can be found and excised before they become malignant in children with FAP, which can be a lifesaving treatment.

Analysis

- Describe the ethical principles that are in conflict in this case (see Chapter 1, Chart 1-7). Which principle do you believe should have preeminence in deciding whether or not parents have the right to have PGT done for a child?
- In this case, do the benefits outweigh the risks of PGT for a child? Would your viewpoint on PGT be different if the child assented to be tested? What if she tells you that she would rather not be tested and wants to follow her father's example?
- Identify the stakeholders in this case. Does the father have the right to forego being tested for the genetic mutation? What if the daughter has PGT performed despite the father's refusal to be tested, and it is found that she has the genetic mutation? In that case, the father must also have the genetic mutation. Does he have the right to be told or to not be told these results and their implications?
- Are there any professional guidelines that you can turn to for help in determining the ethical issues that revolve around PGT? If so, what are they, and how can they help?

References

Beamer, L. C. (2017). Ethics and genetics: Examining a crossroads in nursing through a case study. *Clinical Journal of Oncology Nursing, 21*(6), 730–737.

Keogh, L. A., Niven, H., Rutstein, A., et al. (2017). Choosing not to undergo predictive genetic testing for hereditary colorectal cancer syndromes: Expanding our understanding of decliners and declining. *Journal of Behavioral Medicine, 40*(4), 583–594.

Resources

See Chapter 1, Chart 1-10 for Steps of an Ethical Analysis and Ethics Resources.

Nurses are increasingly involved in taking family histories and educating the patient about aspects of genetic testing. They contribute by ensuring informed health choices and consent, advocating for privacy and confidentiality with regard to genetic test results, assessing genetic risk, and helping patients understand the complex issues involved (Edwards & Maradiegue, 2018). The rapid uptake of direct-to-consumer genetic testing mandates that nurses educate patients about the pros and cons of the selected type of genetic testing, navigate the psychosocial needs of patients and their families, and make referrals to genetic specialists as indicated (Mahon, 2018).

Genetic Screening

Genetic screening, in contrast to genetic testing, is performed independent of having a positive family history or symptom manifestation based on a personal risk or based on the person having a risk associated with a specific population or group of people that they belong to. There are multiple forms of genetic screening which are useful at different points across the lifespan. Most commonly, genetic screening occurs in prenatal and newborn programs. For example, shortly after birth, newborns are screened for a variety of conditions, including PKU, congenital hypothyroidism, and galactosemia as a means to identify treatable genetic conditions that could prove dangerous to their health if left untreated. Prenatal genetic screening is provided as a reproductive option to people with a high probability of having children with severe, untreatable diseases and for whom genetic counseling, prenatal diagnosis, and other reproductive options could be helpful. Genetic screening of pregnant women is used to detect birth defects such as neural tube defects and Down syndrome. Cascade screening is a cost-effective strategy to identify those at risk for genetic illness based on the identification of another family member with the disorder (Silva, Jannes, Oliveira, et al., 2018). This form of genetic screening is most useful for autosomal dominant disorders such as familial hypercholesterolemia or Lynch syndrome. The results of genetic screening may also be used for public health purposes to determine the incidence and prevalence of a birth defect or to investigate the feasibility and value of new genetic testing methods. Table 6-4 gives examples of types of genetic screening.

 Concept Mastery Alert

Genetic testing and *genetic screening* are terms that are often confused. Nurses need to remember that testing is individual; screening is population based.

TABLE 6-4	Applications for Genetic Screening	
Timing of Screening	**Purpose**	**Examples**
Preconception/preimplantation screening	Preconception screening may be done to test for autosomal recessive inherited genetic conditions that occur with greater frequency among individuals of certain ethnic groups; furthermore, through the use of in vitro fertilization, embryos may be tested for specific genetic or chromosomal abnormalities	Cystic fibrosis—all couples, but especially northern European Caucasian and Ashkenazi Jewish Tay-Sachs disease—Ashkenazi Jewish Sickle cell disease—African American, Puerto Rican, Mediterranean, Middle Eastern Alpha-thalassemia—Southeast Asian, African American
Prenatal screening	For genetic conditions that are common and for which prenatal diagnosis is available when a pregnancy is identified at increased risk	Neural tube defects—spina bifida, anencephaly Down syndrome Other chromosomal abnormalities—trisomy 18
Newborn screening	For genetic conditions for which there is specific treatment	Phenylketonuria (PKU) Galactosemia Homocystinuria Biotinidase deficiency
Diagnostic screening	To determine whether a specific genetic mutation exists or to confirm diagnosis when phenotypic presentation exists	Hypertrophic cardiomyopathy
Carrier testing	To determine if a person carries a mutated gene; this type of testing is useful for couples to ascertain genetic risk of having a child with a genetic disorder; particularly useful with autosomal recessive disorders	Cystic fibrosis—all couples, but especially northern European Caucasian and Ashkenazi Jewish Tay-Sachs disease—Ashkenazi Jewish Sickle cell disease—African American, Puerto Rican, Mediterranean, Middle Eastern
Predictive testing	For genetic conditions that appear later in life or for genetic disorders that have minimal phenotypic presentation	Colorectal cancer Huntington disease Hemochromatosis

Adapted from National Institutes of Health (NIH), U.S. National Library of Medicine (NLM); Genetics Home Reference. (2019l). What are the types of genetic tests? Retrieved on 8/30/2019 at: www.ghr.nlm.nih.gov/handbook/testing/uses

Population Screening

Population screening—the use of genetic testing for large groups or entire populations—to identify late-onset conditions is under development. For a test to be considered for population screening, there must be (1) sufficient information about gene distribution within populations, (2) accurate prediction about the development and progression of disease, and (3) appropriate medical management for asymptomatic people with a mutation. Currently, population screening is considered in some ethnic groups to identify cancer-predisposing genes. For example, individuals of Ashkenazi Jewish ancestry have a greater chance of inheriting breast and ovarian cancer than other ethnic groups (Manchanda & Gaba, 2019). The identification of one of these mutations gives patients options that may include cancer screening, chemoprevention, or prophylactic mastectomy or oophorectomy. In addition, population screening for this group could also include screening for conditions such as Tay-Sachs disease and Canavan disease. Population screening is being explored for other adult-onset conditions such as type 2 diabetes, heart disease, and hereditary hemochromatosis (i.e., iron overload disorder). In some countries, there is a push to conduct population screening as a form of precision medicine focused on prevention (Silva et al., 2018; Turnball, Sud, & Houlston, 2019).

Testing and Screening for Adult-Onset Conditions

Adult-onset conditions with a genetic or genomic basis are manifested during adulthood and the disease is clearly observed to run in families. Some conditions typically associated with advanced age that manifest earlier in life may also have a genetic correlation and require further examination. For example, hypercholesterolemia is often considered an adult-onset disorder associated with a diet high in fat. A form of hypercholesterolemia with excessively high cholesterol levels and lack of lifestyle risk factors correlates with a genetic alteration referred to as familial hypercholesterolemia (Knowles, Rader, & Khoury, 2017). This is an autosomal dominant disorder, suggesting that there is a 50% likelihood that each child of a parent with the disorder will inherit this disorder. Cascade screening of children of parents with familial hypercholesterolemia would be indicated to identify whether or not they have the disorder so that they may be promptly identified and treated (Setia, Saxena, Sawhney, et al., 2018). Adult-onset genetic conditions can be attributed to specific genetic mutations and follow either an autosomal dominant or an autosomal recessive inheritance pattern; however, most adult-onset conditions are considered to be genomic or multifactorial—that is, they result from a combination of genes or gene–environment interactions. Examples of multifactorial conditions include heart disease, diabetes, and arthritis. Genomic or multifactorial influences involve interactions among several genes (gene–gene interactions) and between genes and the environment (gene–environment interactions), the person's lifestyle. Furthermore, some adult-onset conditions occur due to sporadic changes to a gene (Gael & Veltman, 2019).

Nursing assessment for adult-onset conditions is based on family history, personal and medical risk factors, and identification of associated diseases or clinical manifestations (the phenotype). Knowledge of adult-onset conditions and their genetic bases (i.e., mendelian vs. multifactorial conditions) influences the nursing considerations for genetic testing and health promotion. Table 6-5 describes select adult-onset conditions, their age of onset, patterns of inheritance, molecular genetics, and test availability.

Single Gene Conditions

If a single gene accounts for an adult-onset condition in a symptomatic person, testing is used to confirm a diagnosis to assist in the plan of care and management. Diagnostic testing for adult-onset conditions is most frequently used with autosomal dominant conditions, such as Huntington disease or Factor V Leiden thrombophilia, and with autosomal recessive conditions such as hemochromatosis. Other single gene conditions are associated with a confirmed genetic mutation in an affected family member or with a family history suggestive of an inherited pattern of adult-onset disease, such as a particular type of cancer. **Presymptomatic testing** provides information to people without symptoms about the presence of a genetic mutation and about the likelihood of developing the disease. Presymptomatic testing is considered for people in families with a known adult-onset condition in which either a positive or a negative test result indicates an increased or reduced risk of developing the disease, affects medical management, or allows earlier treatment of a condition.

Huntington disease has long served as the model for presymptomatic testing because the presence of the genetic mutation predicts disease onset and progression. Although preventive measures are not yet available for Huntington disease, the genetic information enables health care providers to develop a clinical, supportive, and psychological plan of care. Indeed, the presence of a single gene mutation has implications for the risk of developing many types of cancer; therefore, presymptomatic testing has become more common as a means to start early planning and implementation of select medical measures that may reduce that risk (Edwards & Maradiegue, 2018).

Genomic Conditions

The foremost factor that may influence the development and severity of disease is a person's genomic makeup. In the absence of a single disease-causing gene, it is thought that multiple genes and other environmental factors are related to the onset of most adult diseases. For some diseases, the interactions among several genes and other environmental or metabolic events affect disease onset and progression. Specific gene–gene interactions or SNPs can confer susceptibility to disease. Genomic testing helps distinguish variations within the same disease or response to treatment. For example, no single gene is associated with osteoporosis. Several polymorphisms on candidate genes related to the vitamin D receptor, estrogen and androgen receptors, and regulation of

TABLE 6-5	Select Adult-Onset Disorders				
Clinical Description		**Age of Onset**	**Genetic Inheritance**	**Associated Gene**	**Test Availability**
Neurologic Conditions					
Alzheimer's Disease Progressive dementia, memory failure, personality disturbance, loss of intellectual functioning associated with cerebral cortical atrophy, beta-amyloid plaque formation, and intraneuronal neurofibrillary tangles		<60–65 y; often <55 y	A.D.	APOE PSEN1 APP PSEN2	Presymptomatic and diagnostic
Parkinson's Disease Dementia and/or parkinsonism: Slowly progressive behavioral changes, language disturbances and/or extrapyramidal signs, rigidity, bradykinesia, and saccadic eye movements		40–60 y	A.D.	MAPT PARK	Diagnostic and presymptomatic
Huntington Disease Widespread degenerative brain change with progressive motor loss; both voluntary disability and involuntary disability, cognitive decline, chorea (involuntary movements) at later stage, psychiatric disturbances		Mean age, 35–44 y	A.D.	HTT	Diagnostic and presymptomatic
Neuromuscular Disorders					
Spinocerebellar Ataxia Type 6 Progressive cerebellar ataxia, dysarthria, nystagmus, bulbar dysfunction, peripheral neuropathy, decreased deep tendon reflexes, dementia		Mean age, 30–52 y	A.D.	CACNA1A ATXN	Diagnostic and presymptomatic
Myotonic Muscular Dystrophy Type 1 Cataracts and myotonia or muscle wasting and weakness, frontal balding and electrocardiographic changes (heart block or arrhythmia), diabetes in 5% of all cases		20–70 y	A.D. with variable penetrance	DMPK CNBP	Diagnostic
Familial Amyotrophic Lateral Sclerosis Progressive loss of motor function with predominantly lower motor neuron manifestations		45–60 y	Both A.D. and A.R.	ALS1 ALS2 SOD1 SETX	Diagnostic

TABLE 6-5	Select Adult-Onset Disorders (continued)				
Clinical Description	**Age of Onset**	**Genetic Inheritance**	**Associated Gene**	**Test Availability**	

Hematologic Conditions

Hereditary Hemochromatosis

Clinical Description	Age of Onset	Genetic Inheritance	Associated Gene	Test Availability
High absorption of iron by gastrointestinal mucosa resulting in excessive iron storage in liver, skin, pancreas, heart, joints, and testes. Abdominal pain, weakness, lethargy, and weight loss are early symptoms. Untreated individuals can present with skin pigmentation, diabetes, hepatic fibrosis or cirrhosis, congestive heart failure, arrhythmias, or arthritis.	40–60 y in males; after menopause in females	A.R.	*HFE*	Diagnostic and presymptomatic

Factor V Leiden Thrombophilia

Clinical Description	Age of Onset	Genetic Inheritance	Associated Gene	Test Availability
Poor anticoagulant response to activated protein C with increased risk for venous thromboembolism and increased risk for fetal loss during pregnancy	30s; during pregnancy in females	A.D.	*F5*	Diagnostic and presymptomatic

Polycystic Kidney Disease Dominant

Clinical Description	Age of Onset	Genetic Inheritance	Associated Gene	Test Availability
Most common genetic disease in humans. Manifests with renal cysts, liver cysts, and occasionally intracranial/aortic aneurysm and hypertension. Loss of glomerular filtration can lead to kidney failure.	Variable onset; all carriers have detectable disease by ultrasonography at age 30 y	A.D.	*PKD1* *PKD2*	Diagnostic and presymptomatic

Cardiovascular Disease

Familial Hypercholesterolemia

Clinical Description	Age of Onset	Genetic Inheritance	Associated Gene	Test Availability
Elevated low-density lipoprotein levels leading to coronary artery disease, xanthoma, and corneal arcus	40–50 y	A.D.	*LDLR* *PCSK* *APOB*	Diagnostic

Hyperlipidemia

Clinical Description	Age of Onset	Genetic Inheritance	Associated Gene	Test Availability
Elevated cholesterol and triglycerides associated with premature coronary disease and peripheral vascular disease	30–40 y	A.R.	*APOE* *APOA*	Clinical testing related to Alzheimer's/ research

Alpha₁-Antitrypsin Deficiency

Clinical Description	Age of Onset	Genetic Inheritance	Associated Gene	Test Availability
Small airway and alveolar wall destruction; emphysema, especially at base; chronic obstructive pulmonary disease	35-year-old smoker; 45-year-old nonsmoker	M.F. in A.R. fashion	*SERPINA-1*	Diagnostic and presymptomatic

Oncology Conditions

Multiple Endocrine Neoplasia

Clinical Description	Age of Onset	Genetic Inheritance	Associated Gene	Test Availability
Familial medullary thyroid cancer: Medullary thyroid cancer, pheochromocytoma, and parathyroid abnormalities	Early adulthood 40–50 y	A.D.	*MEN1* *MEN2*	Presymptomatic

Breast Cancer

Clinical Description	Age of Onset	Genetic Inheritance	Associated Gene	Test Availability
BRCA1/2 hereditary breast/ovarian cancer: Breast, ovarian, prostate, and colon (*BRCA1*); breast, ovarian, and other cancers (*BRCA2*)	30–70 y; often <50 y	A.D.	*BRCA1* *BRCA2*	Presymptomatic Presymptomatic

Lynch Syndrome

Clinical Description	Age of Onset	Genetic Inheritance	Associated Gene	Test Availability
Colorectal, endometrial, bladder, gastric, biliary, and renal cell cancers as well as atypical endometrial hyperplasia and uterine leiomyosarcoma	<50 y	A.D.	*MLH1* *MSH2* *MSH6* *PMS2*	Presymptomatic and diagnostic

Li–Fraumeni Syndrome

Clinical Description	Age of Onset	Genetic Inheritance	Associated Gene	Test Availability
Soft tissue sarcoma, breast cancer, leukemia, osteosarcoma, melanoma, and other cancers often including colon, pancreas, adrenal cortex, and brain	Often <40 y	A.D.	*TP53* *CHEK2*	Presymptomatic and diagnostic

Cowden Syndrome

Clinical Description	Age of Onset	Genetic Inheritance	Associated Gene	Test Availability
Breast, nonmedullary (papillary or follicular) thyroid cancer; breast fibroadenomas and noncancerous thyroid modules or goiter; multiple buccal mucosa papillomas (cobblestone-line papules), facial trichilemmomas, gastrointestinal polyps; high-arched palate, thickened furrowed tongue, megalencephaly, and pectus excavatum	40–50 y for cancer; teens—20 y for mucocutaneous lesions	A.D.	*PTEN*	Presymptomatic and research

AD, autosomal dominant; AR, autosomal recessive; MF, multifactorial.
Adapted from National Center for Biotechnology Information (NCBI), U.S. National Library of Medicine (NLM). (2019a). Genetic Testing Registry. Retrieved on 8/30/2019 at: www.ncbi.nlm.gov/gtr

bone mineral density (BMD) have been shown to contribute to osteoporosis and fracture risk. Moreover, diet and exercise have a strong interaction with the polymorphisms regulating BMD (Cho, Lee, & Kang, 2017).

Some genomic tests may predict treatment response. For example, people may present with similar clinical signs and symptoms of asthma but have different responses to corticosteroid treatment. Mutations in genes that regulate corticosteroid receptors can help classify people with asthma as sensitive or resistant to treatment with corticosteroids (NCBI, NLM, 2019b).

The Nursing Role in Testing and Screening for Adult-Onset Conditions

Nurses participate in explaining risk and genetic predisposition, supporting informed health decisions and opportunities for prevention and early intervention, clarifying legal protections and risks related to genetic testing or health concerns, and protecting patients' privacy. Nurses assess family histories, which may indicate that multiple generations (autosomal dominant inheritance) or multiple siblings (autosomal recessive inheritance) are affected with the same condition or that onset of disease is earlier than expected (e.g., multiple generations with early-onset hyperlipidemia). Possible adult-onset conditions are discussed with other members of the health care team for appropriate resources and referral. When a family history of disease is identified, a patient is made aware that this is a risk factor for disease; resources and referral are then provided. It is the patient's decision whether or not to pursue a genetic testing workup. For example, if a 45-year-old woman presents for her annual gynecology visit and reports a family history of colon cancer in multiple paternal relatives, including her father, the nurse should discuss the family history with the gynecologist. In addition, the woman should be alerted to the risk of colon cancer on the basis of the family history and given information about possible genetic testing and referral for a colonoscopy.

If the existence of a mutation for an adult-onset condition in a family is identified, at-risk family members can be referred for cascade screening for a specific genetic disorder based on genetic susceptibility or genetic predisposition. If the patient is found to carry the mutation, the nurse provides them with information and referral for risk-reduction measures and educates the person about the risk to other family members. In that discussion, the nurse assures the patient that the test results are private and confidential and will not be shared with others, including family members, without the patient's permission. If the patient is an unaffected family member, the nurse discusses inheritance and the risk of developing the disease, provides support for the decision making process, and offers referral for genetics services.

 Concept Mastery Alert

Cascade screening is used for at-risk family members if the existence of a mutation for an adult-onset condition in a family is identified. Presymptomatic testing provides information to people without symptoms about the presence of a genetic mutation and about the likelihood of developing the disease.

Personalized Genomic Treatments

Information about genes and their variations helps researchers identify genetic differences that predispose certain people to more aggressive diseases and affect their responses to treatment. Genetics and genomics have revolutionized the field of oncology because genetic mutations are the basis for the development and progression of all cancers. In the medical era, individuals with cancer faced treatment based on the stage of the cancer, lymph node involvement, and spread to distant organs. Treatments of a particular type of cancer, stage for stage, were similar. Now, in the genomic era of personalized medicine, cancer is treated on the basis of genetic makeup. For example, women with early stage breast cancer (i.e., tumor diameter less than 2 cm, estrogen receptor–positive tumors, no lymph node involvement) have often received chemotherapy. In the past, deciding which of these women would benefit the most from chemotherapy was unclear. Currently, a gene tumor profile of these women's tumors can be used to predict which women are more likely to have an aggressive cancer. Genetic testing helps clinicians to provide personalized care and the most effective treatment based on the genetic signature of the tumor treatment, called *targeted therapy*, which tries to match the treatment to the specific malfunctioning genes expressed in the tumor, or to selectively inhibit genetic factors that promote cancer growth (Dodson, 2017; National Cancer Institute, 2019). Progressive personalized genomic treatment has expanded into genome editing, known as CRISPR (clustered regularly interspaced short palindromic repeats), which shows promise for single gene disorders and cancer by repairing, replacing, or deleting genes that are altered or damaged (Foss, Hochstrasser, & Wilson, 2019).

Pharmacogenomics

The difference between genetics and genomics, described earlier in this chapter, corresponds to the terms *pharmacogenetics* and *pharmacogenomics*, which combine pharmacology and genetics or genomics. Pharmacogenetics refers to the study of the effect of variations in a single gene on drug response and toxicity. The field of pharmacogenetics has evolved so that it has become a broader genomic-based approach that recognizes the interaction of multiple genes and the environment on drug response. Pharmacogenomics refers to the study of the combined effect of variations in many genes on drug response and toxicity and involves methods that rapidly identify which genetic variations influence a drug's effect. The aim of pharmacogenomics is to deliver safe, effective medication and dosages that are specifically tailored to a person's genetic makeup (Dodson, 2017). The clinical application of pharmacogenetics has provided a better understanding of drug pathways, leading to the development of new drugs that do not have toxic side effects and that have the potential to change current standards of treatment (Conyers, Devaraja, & Elliott, 2018; Mannino, Andreozzi, & Sesti, 2019; Pickard, 2017). Drug pathways target specific gene biomarkers to elicit a specific and therapeutic response (U.S. Food and Drug Administration [FDA], 2019).

It has long been known that patients differ in their response to medications. The genetic and genomic variations in drug metabolism account largely for the differences in drug response and drug-related toxicities. Drug metabolism involves genetically controlled protein/enzyme activity for absorption, distribution, drug–cell interaction, inactivation, and excretion—metabolic processes that are known as pharmacokinetics. The cytochrome P450 (CYP) genes play a key role in the pharmacokinetic process of drug metabolism (Clinical Pharmacogenetics Implementation Consortium [CPIC], 2019). Once a drug reaches its target cell, other genes such as those regulating cell receptors and cell signaling control the drug's effect. This process is known as pharmacodynamics. Single genes may affect drug response. More commonly, drug response involves the interaction of multiple genes, the host, and the effects of other drugs. Figure 6-12 is a schematic display of the genetic and genomic influences on drug metabolism and treatment effect.

SNPs, described earlier, are common genetic variations that occur most frequently throughout the human genome and often contribute to variations in enzymatic activity that affect drug metabolism. The CYPs, a family of enzymes, play a key role in the pharmacokinetic process of drug metabolism. Numerous variations (SNPs) of genes that control CYP activation and deactivation have been identified. Researchers have created a catalog of CYP variations because of their role in drug metabolism (CPIC, 2019).

Four classes of CYP metabolic activity levels have been identified based on a person's CYP genotype and the corresponding drug response: (1) poor metabolizers, (2) intermediate metabolizers, (3) extensive metabolizers, and (4) ultrarapid

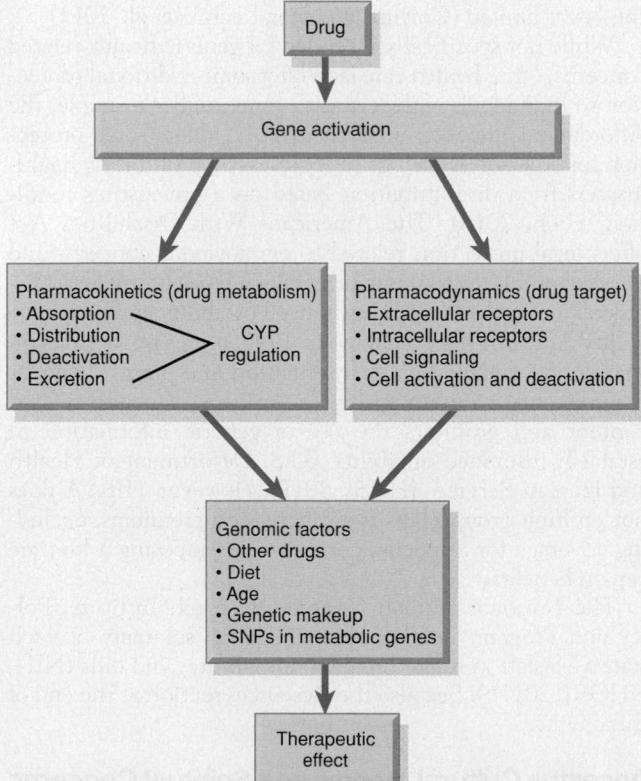

Figure 6-12 • Simplified schematic representation of the multiple, complex, genetic-regulated mechanisms involved in pharmacokinetics (cytochrome [CYP] dependent) and pharmacodynamics, along with other genomic and environmental factors affecting drug metabolism and treatment effect. SNPs, single nucleotide polymorphisms.

metabolizers. Poor metabolizers have a specific SNP variation in a CYP gene that causes little or no function, resulting in very little or no drug metabolism and higher blood levels of active drug because the drug cannot be absorbed or excreted. Conversely, ultrarapid metabolizers have SNP variations that cause increased enzyme activity, resulting in rapid absorption, distribution, and excretion of a drug. Ultrarapid metabolizers have lower drug blood levels, usually with inadequate therapeutic response or longer treatment time to achieve therapeutic results. Both poor metabolizers and ultrarapid metabolizers are predisposed to adverse drug reactions. Poor metabolizers may have adverse effects or toxicities from high blood levels of drugs and need a lower dose, whereas ultrarapid metabolizers have inadequate treatment response because of lower drug blood levels and may need a higher dose or more frequent dosing. Intermediate metabolizers have reduced enzyme activity levels and metabolize drugs at a slower than normal rate. Because intermediate metabolizers have some enzyme activity, they may have differences in treatment response. Extensive metabolizers have normal enzyme activity levels and normal drug metabolism. Differences in metabolism of other medications occur with other genetic variations.

Nurses have traditionally monitored and reported drug response and drug adverse effects. Pharmacogenomic (drug–gene) testing is currently available for more than 16 drugs (Mayo Clinic, 2019). This type of testing offers patients and health care providers more information about a specific drug and whether the medication is the best option for the patient based on genetic interactions that may influence the absorption, metabolism, or excretion of the drug, and the likelihood of an adverse effect from the medication. Nurses are in a position not only to provide education about a particular patient's genomic profile for drug metabolism, but also to explain the rationale for the recommended dosage and discuss associated symptoms related to potential adverse effects. Nurses will continue to incorporate information about gender differences, food interactions, and drug adherence into patient education (Consensus Panel, 2009).

Ethical, Legal, and Social Issues Surrounding Genetics

The rapid application of genetics and genomics across all sectors of health care has had implications for gathering, recording, and sharing personal health information. An ethical foundation provides nurses with a holistic framework for handling these issues with integrity and provides a basis for communicating genetic and genomic information to a patient, a family, other care providers, community agencies and organizations, and for society. Nurses must consider their responsibilities in handling genetic and genomic information and strive to ensure that informed decision making occurs, that patient and family health information is kept private and confidential, and that access to and justice in health care is available to everyone (ANA, 2017).

Ethical Concerns

Ethical principles of beneficence (i.e., to do good) and nonmaleficence (i.e., to do no harm), as well as autonomy, justice, fidelity, and veracity, are used to resolve ethical dilemmas that may arise in clinical care. Respect for persons is the ethical principle underlying all nursing care. Using these principles and the values of caring, nurses can promote thoughtful discussions that are useful when patients and families are facing genetics- and genomics-related health and reproductive decisions and consequences (ANA, 2017; Consensus Panel, 2009). The ethical principles of autonomy, fidelity, and veracity are also important (ANA, 2015). (Further information about ethics is included in Chapter 1.)

Ethical questions relating to genetics and genomics occur in all settings and at all levels of nursing practice. At the level of direct patient care, nurses participate in providing genetic information, testing, and gene-based therapeutics. They offer patient care based on the values of self-determination and personal autonomy. To be as fully informed as possible, patients need appropriate, accurate, and complete information given at a level and in a form so that they and their families can make well-informed personal, medical, and reproductive health decisions. Nurses can help patients clarify values and goals, assess understanding of information, protect their rights, and support their decisions. Nurses can advocate for patient autonomy in health decisions. Several resources and position statements have been developed to guide genetic-related nursing practice (International Society of Nurses in Genetics [ISONG], 2019).

Respecting the patient's right to self-determination—that is, supporting decisions that reflect the patient's personal beliefs, values, and interests—is a central principle in directing how nurses provide genetic and genomic information and counseling. Nurses and others participating in genetic counseling make every attempt to respect the patient's ability to make autonomous decisions. Recognizing one's own attitudes and beliefs and how communication of genetic and genomic information may be influenced by those attitudes and beliefs is a first step toward assuring patients' autonomous decision making.

Confidentiality of genetic and genomic information and respect for privacy are other essential principles underlying genetic counseling. Patients have the right to not have test results divulged to anyone, including insurers, primary providers, employers, or family members. Some patients pay for testing themselves so that insurers will not learn of the test, and others use a different name for testing to protect their privacy.

Ethical challenges may occur for family members and health care providers when the findings of one person's test may inadvertently disclose another family member's risk or carrier status. A nurse may want to disclose genetic information to family members who could experience significant harm if they do not know such information. However, the patient may have other views and may wish to keep this information from the family, resulting in an ethical dilemma for both patient and nurse. The nurse must honor the patient's wishes, while explaining to the patient the potential benefit this information may have for other family members (ANA, 2017; ISONG, 2019).

Ethical considerations must be reviewed as part of genetic and genomic research. For example, before a person participates in genetic and genomic clinical research, the research team must discuss how incidental findings will be addressed. Incidental findings are genetic-related illnesses which are found secondary to the intended goals of the research project or purpose of the test (Boardman & Hale, 2018). The American College of Medical Genetics and Genomics (American College of Medical Genetics and Genomics Policy Statement [ACMG], 2017) issued a policy statement that lists conditions known to be treatable and should be reported to the patient if found incidentally during clinical research.

Legal Aspects of Personalized Health Care

The Genetic Information Nondiscrimination Act (GINA), a law passed in 2008, protects individuals from genetic discrimination (Rothstein, 2018). Its purpose is to protect Americans against improper use of genetic and genomic information in insurance and employment decisions. GINA is particularly helpful for people who carry a gene mutation but are asymptomatic for the illness. The act prohibits health insurers from denying coverage to a healthy person or charging higher insurance rates based on a person's genetic predisposition to a disease. GINA offers legal protection with regard to health insurance and employment; however, gaps in protection exist with regard to disability, life, and long-term care insurance. The act also prevents employers from using a person's genetic and genomic information to make decisions about hiring, job placement, promotion, or firing. Protection provided by GINA does not apply to employers with less than 15 employees, to people in the military, Veterans Health Administration, Indian Health Services, and Federal Employees Health Benefits Programs (Rothstein, 2018). As a result of GINA, most Americans are free to use genetic and genomic information in health care without the fear of misuse; however, public awareness of this law is limited (Cragun, Weidner, Kechik, et al., 2019).

While not specifically intended for genetic health-related concerns, other health care laws offer some additional protection to individuals with regard to genetics. For example, the Affordable Care Act, enacted in 2010, offers some protection for a person with a genetic illness by prohibiting health insurers from discrimination based on a preexisting condition (Rich, 2018). The Americans With Disabilities Act offers legal protection related to employment concerns and physical or intellectual impairment as a result of a genetic disorder. Finally, the Health Insurance Portability and Accountability Act (HIPAA), enacted in 1996, places restrictions on sharing identifiable health information and places stringent requirements on maintaining the privacy of health-related content and prohibits the use of genetic information to establish insurance eligibility (U.S. Department of Health and Human Services [HHS], 2017). However, HIPAA does not prohibit group plans from increasing premiums, excluding coverage for a specific condition, or imposing a lifetime cap on benefits.

The National Human Genome Research Institute, Policy and Program Analysis branch, has a summary of each state's legislation related to genomic statutes and bills (NIH, NHGRI, 2019b). See also the Resources section at the end of this chapter.

Ancestry, Cultural, Social, and Spiritual Concerns Related to Genetic and Genomic Practice

Genetic assessment addresses the ancestry of patients and families, as well as their ethnicity. This information helps identify individual patients and groups who could benefit from genetic testing for carrier identification, prenatal diagnosis, and susceptibility testing. For example, carrier testing for sickle cell disease is routinely offered to people of African American descent, and carrier testing for Tay-Sachs disease and Canavan disease is offered to people of Ashkenazi Jewish descent. The American College of Obstetricians and Gynecologists ([ACOG], 2019) recognizes the benefit of a thorough family history in correlation with the identification of personalized risks and the option of genetic testing prior to conception. Health care providers must be aware of at-risk status based on racial and ethnic population. Ideally, carrier testing is offered before conception to allow people who are carriers to make decisions about reproduction. Prenatal diagnosis is offered and discussed when both partners of a couple are found to be carriers.

It is important to inquire about the patient's ethnic backgrounds when assessing for susceptibilities to adult-onset conditions such as hereditary breast or ovarian cancer. For example, a *BRCA1* cancer–predisposing gene mutation seems to occur more frequently in women of Ashkenazi Jewish descent. Therefore, asking about ethnicity can help identify people with an increased risk of cancer gene mutations.

Nurses should consider patients' views about the significance of a genetic condition and its effect on self-concept, as well as patients' perception of the role of genetics in health and illness, reproduction, and disability. For instance, among women without a history of breast cancer but with a strong family history of breast cancer, negative results for the *BRCA1* and *BRCA2* genetic mutations may not be a relief, since those women's risks for having breast cancer is estimated to be four times as high as women who do not have a family history. Among these women, negative findings for known genetic mutations may simply seem uninformative and cause frustration (Schroeder, Duggleby, & Cameron, 2017; see Chart 6-3: Nursing Research Profile: Living with Breast Cancer Risk). Patients' social and cultural backgrounds determine their interpretations and values about information obtained from genetic testing and evaluation and thus influence their perceptions of health, illness, and risk. Family structure, decision making, and educational background contribute in the same way (Consensus Panel, 2009).

Assessment of the patients' beliefs, values, and expectations regarding genetic testing and genetic and genomic

Chart 6-3 — NURSING RESEARCH PROFILE
Living with Breast Cancer Risk

Schroeder, D., Duggleby, W., & Cameron, B. L. (2017). Moving in and out of the what-ifs: The experiences of unaffected women living in families where a breast cancer 1 or 2 genetic mutation was not found. *Cancer Nursing, 40*(5), 386–393.

Purpose

The genetic mutations of *BRCA1* and *BRCA2* account for approximately 15% of cases of familial breast cancer in women. For women without these mutations and without breast cancer but with a strong family history, the risk of eventually having breast cancer remains high. These risks may be related to another currently unidentified *BRCA* mutation or to a mutation in another gene not yet identified. Little is known about the effects that living with a high breast cancer risk has on these women. Therefore, the aims of this study were to discover the day-to-day lived experience of having breast cancer risk on women with a strong family history of breast cancer but who are *BRCA1* and *BRCA2* negative, and to elucidate how they cope with the knowledge of their breast cancer risk.

Design

This was a hermeneutic phenomenologic study that used van Manen's methods to explore the lived experiences among *BRCA1* and *BRCA2* negative women without breast cancer but with a strong family history of breast cancer and to uncover the meanings this knowledge had on their everyday lives. Purposive sampling was used to recruit participants eligible to be included in the study. The researchers hoped to recruit between five and eight participants. Ten patients who received care in a hereditary breast and ovarian cancer clinic (HBOC) in Western Canada consented to participate in this study, although one dropped out prior to data collection, resulting in a total of nine participants.

Findings

Participants ($N = 9$) engaged in a total of 20 interviews with the researchers. Each participant engaged in at least two conversations. After each session, participants were given copies of the summaries of the conversations and proposed emerging themes that researchers posited for corroboration, in order to ensure trustworthiness of findings. Researchers identified one main overarching theme of *Moving In and Out of the What-Ifs,* which identified the tensions between "normal" living, as expressed in the subtheme *Just Moving Along: Living a Normal Life,* that was juxtaposed with the "what-ifs" subthemes, which included *Moving Into Those Dark Spaces, Is There Something Wrong with Me?* and *Markings in Time.* For instance, all participants identified that most of the time they had an awareness of their familial breast cancer risk, but kept it in the background, expressing the need to "live a normal life." The "dark spaces" were described as triggers that provoked anxiety about their risks, such as anticipating an appointment at the HBOC, or hearing news of a close relative newly diagnosed with cancer. Although all participants identified themselves as "healthy," they found that many times, others who knew of their risks tended to label them as not healthy, causing conflict within them "Is there something wrong with me?" Lastly, there were key milestones in participants' lives that caused tension, or "time marks," such as approaching or surpassing an age when a family member was diagnosed with cancer, or when a family member died of cancer. Coping through the "dark spaces" the "wrongness" and the "marks in time" was facilitated through the methods employed in the subthemes *Living in the Moment,* or slowing down to enjoy the "here and now"; *Being Cared For,* or feeling cared for by significant others as well as the staff at the HBOC; and, *Keeping Me Grounded,* expressed by having family and significant others find ways to keep them out of the "dark spaces," supporting their view of themselves as healthy, and celebrating significant "time marks" with them.

Nursing Implications

Findings from this study suggest that being *BRCA1* and *BRCA2* negative can be seen as both a blessing and a curse for women who are nonetheless at risk for familial breast cancer. These women must deal with conflicting emotions and anxieties that surround the uncertainty of living with this risk. Nurses who care for women at risk for familial breast cancer who are *BRCA1* and *BRCA2* negative should aim to foster their coping mechanisms by encouraging them to focus on the positives in the "here and now" of their lives, by keeping them grounded, and by demonstrating a caring relationship with them.

information helps nurses provide appropriate information about the specific genetics or genomics topic. For example, in some cultures, people believe that health means the absence of symptoms and that the cause of illness is supernatural. Patients with these beliefs may initially reject suggestions for presymptomatic or carrier testing. However, by including resources such as family and cultural and religious community leaders when providing genetics- or genomics-related health care, nurses can help ensure that patients receive information in a way that transcends social, cultural, and economic barriers (Tluczek, Twal, Beamer, et al., 2019).

Applications of Genetics and Genomics in Nursing Practice

Nurses who provide genetics- and genomics-related health care blend the principles of human genetics with nursing care in collaboration with other professionals, including genetic specialists, to foster improvement, maintenance, and restoration of patients' health (Tluczek et al., 2019). Genetic-related nursing practice involves the care of people who have genetic conditions, those who may be predisposed to develop or pass on genetic conditions, and those who are seeking genetic information and referral for additional genetics services. The application of genomic information has been integrated into clinical practice areas of preconception, preimplantation, and prenatal testing, newborn screening, disease susceptibility, screening and diagnosis, prognosis and therapeutic decisions, and in monitoring disease recurrence (see Table 6-4). In the near future, nurses will need to engage in public health efforts to improve genetic literacy within the public domain so that patients can make informed genetic-genomic related decisions (Boerwinkel, Yarden, & Waarlo, 2017).

Nurses are positioned to support patients and families with genetics- and genomics-related health concerns by ensuring not only that their health choices are informed ones but by also advocating for the privacy and confidentiality of genetic and genomic information and for equal access to genetic testing and treatments. Nurses are expected to attend to the genetic and genomic health care needs of the patient (ANA, 2017).

Genetics and Genomics in Health Assessment

Assessment of a person's genetic and genomic health status is an ongoing process. Nurses collect information that can help identify individuals and families who have actual or potential genetics- or genomics-related health concerns or who may benefit from further genetic information, counseling, testing, and treatment. This process can begin before conception and continue throughout the lifespan. Nurses evaluate family and past medical histories, including prenatal history, childhood illnesses, developmental history, adult-onset conditions, past surgeries, treatments, and medications; this information may relate to the genetic or genomic condition at hand or to a condition being considered (see Chapter 4 for more information on assessing past medical history). Nurses also identify the patient's ethnic background and conduct a physical assessment to gather pertinent genetic information. The assessment also includes information about culture, spiritual beliefs, and ancestry. Health assessment includes determining a patient's or family's understanding of actual or potential genetics- or

genomics-related health concerns and awareness of how these issues are communicated within a family (ANA, 2017).

Family History Assessment

Nurses in any practice setting can assess families' genetics histories to identify a genetic trait, inherited condition, or predisposition. Obtaining a thorough family health history is the first, most important tool when determining the potential risk for a genetic illness. Targeted questions are used to identify genetic and genomic conditions for which further information, education, testing, or treatment can be offered (Chart 6-4). A three-generation family history should be collected that includes ages of each family member, medical illnesses, age and cause of death, history of miscarriages or stillbirths, and ethnicity (ACOG, 2018). After consultation and collaboration with other health care providers and specialists, further genetic testing and evaluation is offered for the trait or condition in question. A genetic family history is used to make a diagnosis, identify testing strategies, and establish a pattern of inheritance. Nurses can also inquire about medical conditions that are known to have a heritable component and for which genetic testing may be available. Information is obtained about the presence of birth defects, intellectual disability, familial traits, or similarly affected family members (Consensus Panel, 2009).

Nurses need to consider the closeness of the relationship (genetic relatedness or consanguinity) among family members when assessing the risk of genetic conditions in couples or families. For example, when obtaining a preconception or prenatal family history, it is important for the nurse to ask if the prospective parents have common ancestors (i.e., are they cousins?). This is key because, as noted previously, people who are related have more genes in common than those who are unrelated, thus increasing their chance of having children with an autosomal recessive inherited condition such as cystic fibrosis. Ascertaining genetic relatedness provides direction for genetic counseling and evaluation. It may also serve as an explanation for parents who have a child with a rare autosomal recessive inherited condition or for an adult who is similarly affected.

When the assessment of family history reveals that a patient has been adopted, genetic- and genomic-based health assessment becomes more challenging. Every effort is made to help the patient obtain as much information as possible about their biologic parents, including their ethnic backgrounds.

Questions about previous miscarriage or stillbirth are included in genetics health assessments to identify possible chromosomal conditions. Nurses can also inquire about any history of family members with inherited conditions or birth defects; maternal health conditions such as type 1 diabetes, seizure disorders, or PKU, which may increase the risk for birth defects in children; and about exposure to alcohol or other drugs during pregnancy. Maternal age is also noted; women who are 35 years of age or older who are considering pregnancy and childbearing or who are already pregnant should be offered prenatal diagnosis (e.g., testing through amniocentesis) because of the association between advanced maternal age and chromosomal abnormalities such as Down syndrome. Advanced paternal age, which includes men over 40 years of age, is associated with a slightly higher risk for a child to have autism, schizophrenia, or leukemia (Mayo Clinic, 2018).

Chart 6-4 GENETICS FAMILY HISTORY
An Essential Tool for All Nurses

A Well-Documented Family History Can Be Used to:

- Assess risk of certain diseases
- Decide on testing strategies, such as what genetic and other diagnostic tests to order
- Establish a pattern of inheritance
- Identify other family members who are at increased risk
- Identify shared environmental risk factors
- Calculate risks
- Assess risk of passing on conditions to children
- Determine and recommend treatments that modify disease risk
- Make decisions about management or surveillance
- Develop patient rapport
- Educate patients

Key Questions to Ask About Each Family Member Include:

- What is the current age, or what was the age at death?
- What is the ethnic background (some genetic conditions are more common in certain ethnic groups)?

- Is there a history of:
  - Multiple pregnancy losses/stillbirths?
  - Unexplained infertility?
  - Birth defects?
  - Intellectual disability or developmental delay?
  - Learning disability?
  - Medical problems in children whose parents are closely related (second cousins or closer)?
  - Congenital or juvenile blindness, cataracts, hearing loss, or deafness?
  - Very short or very tall stature?
  - Several close relatives with the same or related conditions (e.g., breast or colon cancer, diabetes, heart disease, asthma, stroke, high blood pressure, kidney disease)?
  - Occurrence of a common condition with earlier age of onset than is usual (e.g., breast or colon cancer, hearing loss, dementia, heart disease)?

Adapted from Ginsburg, G. S., Wu, R. R., & Orlando, L. A. (2019). Family health history: Underused for actionable risk assessment. *Lancet, 394*(10198), 596–603.

Physical Assessment

Physical assessment may provide clues that a particular genetic or genomic condition is present in a person and family. Family history assessment may serve as a guide to focus the physical assessment. For example, a history of familial hypercholesterolemia would alert the nurse to assess for symptoms of hyperlipidemias (xanthomas, corneal arcus, and abdominal pain of unexplained origin). A family history of neurofibromatosis type 1, an inherited condition involving tumors of the central nervous system, would prompt the nurse to carry out a detailed assessment of closely related family members.

Skin findings such as *café-au-lait* spots, axillary freckling, or tumors of the skin (neurofibromas) would warrant referral for further evaluation, including genetic evaluation and counseling (NIH, NLM, 2019i).

If a genetic or genomic condition is suspected as a result of a family history or physical assessment, the nurse, as a part of their role, and in collaboration with the health care team, may initiate further discussion of genetics and genomic information, offering and discussing genetic tests, and suggesting a referral for further genetic evaluation (Chart 6-5).

Chart 6-5 Indications for Making a Genetics Referral

Prepregnancy and Prenatal

- Maternal age of 35 y or older at expected time of delivery
- Previous child with a chromosome problem
- Positive alpha-fetoprotein profile screening test
- Previous child with a birth defect or family history of birth defects
- Pregnancy history of two or more unexplained miscarriages
- Maternal conditions such as diabetes, epilepsy, or alcoholism
- Exposures to certain medications or drugs during pregnancy
- Family history of intellectual disability
- Either member of the couple has a birth defect such as cleft lip or palate, spina bifida, or congenital heart defect
- Either member of the couple has a chromosome abnormality

Pediatric

- Positive newborn screening test
- One or more major birth defects
- Unusual (dysmorphic) facial features
- Developmental delay/intellectual disability
- Suspicion of a metabolic disorder
- Unusually tall or short stature, or growth delays
- Known chromosomal abnormality

Adult

- Intellectual disability without a known cause
- Unexplained infertility or multiple pregnancy losses
- A personal or family history of thrombotic events
- Adult-onset conditions such as hemochromatosis, hearing loss, and visual impairment
- Family history of an adult-onset neurodegenerative disorder (e.g., Huntington disease)
- Features of a genetic condition such as neurofibromatosis (*café-au-lait* spots, neurofibromas on the skin), Marfan syndrome (unusually tall stature, dilation of the aortic root), others
- Personal or family history of cardiovascular disorders known to be associated with genetic factors such as cardiomyopathy or long QT syndrome
- Family history of cancers known to be associated with specific genes such as hereditary breast/ovarian cancer or Lynch syndrome
- Family history of early-onset cancers and familial clustering of related tumors

Adapted from Centers for Disease Control and Prevention (CDC). (2017). Family health history. Retrieved on 8/30/2019 at: www.cdc.gov/genomics/famhistory; McClatchey, T., Lay, E., Strassberg, M., et al. (2018). Missed opportunities: Unidentified genetic risk factors in prenatal care. *Prenatal Care, 38*, 75–79.

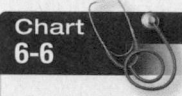

Chart 6-6

ASSESSMENT
Assessing Psychosocial Genetic Health

The nurse's assessment of psychosocial factors impacting a patient's genetic health is based on the nurse's professional responsibility to "demonstrate in practice the importance of tailoring genetic and genomic information and services to patients based on their culture, religion, knowledge level, literacy and preferred language." (Consensus Panel, 2009; p. 11).

The nurse assesses:

- Educational level and understanding of the genetic condition or concern in the family.
- Desired goals and health outcomes in relation to the genetic condition or concern.
- Family rules regarding disclosure of medical information (e.g., some families may not reveal a history of a disease such as cancer or mental illness during the family history assessment).
- Family rules, boundaries, and cultural practices as well as personal preference about knowing genetic information.
- Past coping mechanisms and social support.
- Ability to make an informed decision (e.g., is the patient under stress from family situations, acute or chronic illness, or medications that may impair the patient's ability to make an informed decision?).

Adapted from Consensus Panel on Genetic/Genomic Nursing Competencies (Consensus Panel). (2009). *Essentials of genetic and genomic nursing: Competencies, curricular guidelines, and outcome indicators* (2nd ed.). Silver Spring, MD: Author.

Psychosocial Assessment

Psychosocial assessment is an essential nursing component of the genetics health assessment. The assessment findings can help identify the potential impact of new genetic and genomic information on the patient and the family and how they may cope with this information (Chart 6-6).

Genetic Counseling and Evaluation Services

People seek genetic counseling for various reasons and at different stages of life. Some are seeking preconception or prenatal information, others are referred after the birth of a child with a birth defect or suspected genetic condition, and still others are seeking information for themselves or their families because of the presence of, or a family history of, a genetic condition. Regardless of the timing or setting, genetic counseling is offered to all people who have questions about genetics or genomics and their health.

As the contribution of genetics and genomics to the health–illness continuum is recognized, genetic counseling will become a responsibility of all health care professionals in clinical practice. Nurses are in an ideal position to assess the patient's health and genetics family history and to make referrals for specialized diagnosis and treatment. They offer anticipatory guidance by explaining the purpose and goals of a referral. They collaborate with other health care providers in giving support and follow-up counseling; additionally, they coordinate follow-up and case management.

Genetic Services

Genetic services provide genetic information, education, and support to patients and families. Medical geneticists, genetic counselors, and advanced practice nurses in genetics provide specific genetics services to patients and families who are referred by their primary or specialty health care providers. A team approach is often used to obtain and interpret complex family history information, evaluate and diagnose genetic conditions, interpret and discuss complicated genetic test results, support patients throughout the evaluation process, and offer professional and family support. Patients participate as team members and decision makers throughout the process. Genetics services enable patients and their families to learn and understand relevant aspects of genetics and genomics, to make informed health decisions, and to receive support as they integrate personal and family genetic and genomic information into daily living.

Genetic counseling may take place over an extended period and may entail more than one counseling session, which may include other family members. The components of genetic counseling are outlined in Chart 6-7. Although genetic counseling may be offered at any point during the lifespan, counseling issues are often relevant to the life stage in which counseling is sought (CDC, 2018b). Examples are presented in Chart 6-8.

Providing Precounseling Information

All genetic specialists, including nurses who participate in the genetic counseling process and those with access to a person's genetic information, must honor a patient's desire for confidentiality. Genetic information should not be revealed to family members, insurance companies, employers, and schools if the patient so desires, even if keeping the information confidential is difficult.

Preparing the patient and the family, promoting informed decision making, and obtaining informed consent are essential in genetic counseling. Nurses assess the patient's capacity and ability to give voluntary consent. This includes assessment of factors that may interfere with informed consent, such as hearing loss, language differences, cognitive impairment, and the effects of medication. Nurses make sure that a person's decision to undergo testing is not affected by coercion, persuasion, or manipulation. Because information may need to be repeated over time, nurses offer follow-up discussion as needed (ANA 2017; Consensus Panel, 2009).

The genetic service to which a patient or a family is referred for genetic counseling will ask the nurse for background information for evaluation. Genetic specialists need to know the reason for referral, the patient's or family's reason for seeking genetic counseling, and potential genetic-related health concerns. For example, a nurse may refer a family with a new diagnosis of hereditary breast or ovarian cancer for counseling or to discuss the likelihood of developing the disease and the implications for other family members. The family may have concerns about confidentiality and privacy. The nurse and the genetic specialist tailor the genetic counseling to respond to these concerns.

With the patient's permission, genetic specialists will request the relevant test results and medical evaluations. Nurses obtain permission from the patient and, if applicable, from other family members to provide medical records that document the genetic condition of concern. In some situations, evaluation of more than one family member may be necessary to establish a diagnosis of a genetic disorder. Nurses

Chart 6-7 Components of Genetic Counseling

Information and Assessment Sources

- Reason for referral
- Family history
- Medical history/records
- Relevant test results and other medical evaluations
- Social and emotional concerns
- Relevant cultural, educational, and financial factors

Analysis of Data

- Family history
- Physical examination as needed
- Additional laboratory testing and procedures (e.g., echocardiogram, ophthalmology, or neurologic examination)

Communication of Genetic Finding

- Natural history of disorder
- Pattern of inheritance
- Reproductive and family health issues and options
- Testing options
- Management and treatment issues

Counseling and Support

- Identify individual and family questions and concerns
- Identify existing support systems
- Provide emotional and social support
- Refer for additional support and counseling as indicated

Follow-Up

- Written summary to referring primary providers and family
- Coordination of care with primary providers and specialists
- Additional discussions of test results or diagnosis

Genetics Resources

Genetic and Rare Diseases Information Center: provides links with experienced information specialists who can answer questions in English and Spanish to patients, families, and health care providers regarding specific genetic diseases, rarediseases.info.nih.gov

Genetics Home Reference: provides a layman's online encyclopedic guide to understanding genetic conditions, ghr.nlm.nih.gov

National Human Genome Research Institute, Genome Statute and Legislative Database: summarizes each state's legislation on employment and insurance discrimination, www.genome.gov/about-genomics/policy-issues/Genome-Statute-Legislation-Database

National Organization for Rare Disorders (NORD): a directory of support groups and information for patients and families with rare genetic disorders, rarediseases.org

Online Mendelian Inheritance in Man (OMIM): a complete listing of inherited genetic conditions, omim.org

Chart 6-8 Genetic Counseling across the Lifespan

Prenatal Issues

- Understanding prenatal screening and diagnosis testing
- Implications of reproductive choices
- Potential for anxiety and emotional distress
- Effects on partnership, family, and parental–fetal bonding

Newborn Issues

- Understanding newborn screening results
- Potential for disrupted parent–newborn relationship on diagnosis of a genetic condition
- Parental guilt
- Implications for siblings and other family members
- Coordination and continuity of care

Pediatric Issues

- Caring for children with complex medical needs
- Coordination of care
- Potential for impaired parent–child relationship
- Potential for social stigmatization

Adolescent Issues

- Potential for impaired self-image and decreased self-esteem
- Potential for altered perception of family
- Implications for lifestyle and family planning

Adult Issues

- Potential for ambiguous test results
- Identification of a genetic susceptibility or diagnosis without an existing cure
- Effect on marriage, reproduction, parenting, and lifestyle
- Potential impact on insurability and employability

Adapted from Dwyer, T. M., Glaser, R. L., & Mason, T. M. (2016). Inheritance patterns in human phenotypes and types of genetic disorders. In C. E. Kasper, T. A. Schneidereith, & F. R. Lashley. (Eds.). (2015). *Lashley's essentials of clinical genetics in nursing practice* (pp. 65–114). New York: Springer Publishing Company.

for patients with hearing loss, a sign interpreter's services may have to be arranged. For those with vision loss, alternative forms of communication may be necessary. Genetics professionals prepare for the genetic counseling and evaluation with these relevant issues in mind (CDC, 2018b).

Preparing Patients for Genetics Evaluation

Before a genetic counseling appointment, the nurse discusses with the patient and the family the type of family history information that will be collected during the consultation. Family history collection and analysis are comprehensive and focus on information that may be relevant to the genetics- or genomics-related concern in question. The genetic analysis always includes assessment for any other potentially inherited conditions for which testing, prevention, and treatment may be possible.

A physical examination may be performed by the medical geneticist to identify specific clinical features commonly associated with a genetic condition. The examination also helps determine if further testing is needed to diagnose a genetic disorder. This examination generally involves assessment of all body systems, with a focus on specific physical characteristics. Nurses describe the diagnostic evaluations that are part of a genetics consultation and explain their purposes.

explain that the medical information is needed to ensure that appropriate information and counseling (including risk interpretation) are provided.

The genetic service asks nurses about the emotional and social status of the patient and the family. Genetic specialists want to know the coping skills of patients and families who have recently learned of the diagnosis of a genetic disorder as well as what type of genetic information is being sought. Nurses help identify cultural and other issues that may influence how information is provided and by whom. For example,

Communicating Genetic and Genomic Information to Patients

After the family history and the physical examination are completed, the genetics team reviews the information gathered before beginning genetic counseling with the patient and the family. The genetic specialists meet with the patient and the family to discuss their findings. If information gathered confirms a genetic condition in a family, genetic specialists discuss with the patient the natural history of the condition, the pattern of inheritance, and the implications of the condition for reproductive and general health. When appropriate, specialists also discuss relevant testing and management options.

Providing Support

The genetics team provides support throughout the counseling session and identifies personal and family concerns. Genetic specialists use active listening to interpret patient concerns and emotions, seek and provide feedback, and demonstrate understanding of those concerns. They suggest referral for additional social and emotional support. In addition, genetic specialists discuss pertinent patient and family concerns and needs with nurses and primary health care teams so that they can provide additional support and guidance (CDC, 2018b). Nurses assess the patient's understanding of the information given during the counseling session, clarify information, answer questions, assess patient reactions, and identify support systems.

Follow-Up After Genetic Evaluation

As a follow-up to genetic evaluation and counseling, genetic specialists prepare a written summary of the evaluation and counseling session for the patient and, with the patient's consent, send this summary to the primary provider as well as other providers identified by the patient as participants in care. The consultation summary outlines the results of the family history and physical and laboratory assessments, provides a discussion of any specific diagnosis made, reviews the inheritance and associated risk of recurrence for the patient and the family, presents reproductive and general health options, and makes recommendations for further testing and management. The nurse reviews the summary with the patient and identifies information, education, and counseling for which follow-up genetic counseling may be useful (ANA, 2017).

Follow-up genetic counseling is always offered because some patients and families need more time to understand and discuss the specifics of a genetic test or diagnosis, or they may wish to review reproductive options again later, when pregnancy is being considered. Follow-up counseling is also offered to patients when further evaluation and counseling of extended family members is recommended (ANA, 2017).

During follow-up sessions, nurses can educate patients about sources of information related to genetic and genomic issues. Some resources that provide the most up-to-date and reliable genetic and genomic information are available on the Internet (see the Resources section at the end of this chapter).

Genetics and Genomics Tomorrow

The pace of genetic and genomic research is transforming our understanding of the role of genetics and genomics in health and disease. In addition, it is increasing clinical opportunities for presymptomatic prediction of illness based on a patient's genetic makeup. Genetic research is now focused on identifying the genetic and environmental causes of common diseases such as diabetes, heart disease, and asthma. The studies are opening the doors for many advances in the prevention and treatment of both rare and common diseases (NIH, NHGRI, 2019c). Genetic testing as a part of palliative care is being discussed as having the potential to inform future generations of genetic health risk (Morrow, Jacobs, Best, et al., 2018). For example, a person dying of a rare cancer may biobank a DNA sample that could be helpful to future generations as research and technology advances to treat that specific illness. Additionally, advances are ongoing in the microbiome, the genetic structure of the gut, which is now known to play a key role in many absorption and malabsorption disorders (Greathouse, Faucher, & Hastings-Tolsma, 2017; Sun, 2018). In addition, alterations to the telomere, the end unit or cap on each chromosome, referred to as telomeropathies, is providing insight to understanding the molecular mechanism of rare genetic disorders (Armando, Gomez, Maggio, et al., 2019).

As applications of genetics and genomics to health and disease develop, genetic testing may be used to scan all of a patient's genetic material so that disease risk variants can be identified and early interventions and treatments can be determined. It is estimated that the cost of testing a patient's entire genome is less than $1000. Personalized medicine will continue to expand, and many treatments and interventions for medical conditions will be chosen on the basis of what genetic testing indicates about a patient's genetic makeup. Nurses will be on the front line in communicating genetic and genomic information to patients, families, and communities. Patients, families, and communities will also expect that health care providers, including nurses, will use new genetic and genomic information and technologies in the provision of care. It is, therefore, imperative that all nurses become fluent in the language of genetics and genomics so that they can provide effective nursing care (ANA 2017; Consensus Panel, 2009).

CRITICAL THINKING EXERCISES

1 **ipc** A 34-year-old male reports urinary difficulty. Following a medical examination and subsequent laboratory work, he is diagnosed with early stages of kidney failure. After a further, more extensive workup, he is diagnosed with polycystic kidney disease, an autosomal dominant disorder. You work as a nurse in the nephrology clinic where he is now being treated. How should this inheritance pattern be explained to the patient? Utilizing knowledge of the inheritance pattern, whom should you include as part of the family assessment of this patient as it relates to this genetic condition? What comorbidities should you be alert to and include in future assessments? Understanding the progressive nature of this illness, what additional members of the health care team should be included in the care of this patient?

2 **pq** You work as a nurse in a family practice office setting. Linda, the mother of three children, tells you during a well-child physical that her 2-year-old son tends to have bleeding gums. She relates this to aggressive brushing because he is still learning how to brush his teeth. Through further questioning, you begin to suspect that the child may have hemophilia A, an X-linked recessive disorder. Based on the inheritance pattern of X-linked recessive disorders, what would be critical to know in this family history? Linda states that she has a brother who has two daughters, ages 9 and 12, and she has a sister with an infant son. Her father died when she was young and sadly, she doesn't recall much about his family history. Her mother is 77 years of age and has rheumatoid arthritis. How could you use knowledge of the inheritance pattern to guide the care of Linda and her family? Create a three-generation pedigree to determine if anyone else in the family should be screened for hemophilia.

3 ebp A 50-year-old female is being screened in the neurology clinic where you work for progressive neurologic impairment and physical decline. Through DNA analysis and chromosomal testing, a diagnosis of Huntington chorea is made. This illness has an autosomal dominant inheritance pattern. What is the best evidence you find to guide the care of this patient and her family? What ethical concerns must be taken into consideration when caring for a patient with this genetic disorder? This patient has two daughters who are 17 and 20 years of age. Should the age of her daughters have an impact as to whether or not they should have genetic testing?

REFERENCES

*Asterisk indicates nursing research.
**Double asterisk indicates classic reference.

Books

American Nurses Association (ANA). (2015). *Code of ethics for nurses with interpretive statements*. Washington, DC: American Nurses Publishing.

American Nurses Association (ANA). (2017). *Genetics and genomics nursing scope and standards of practice* (2nd ed.). Silver Spring, MD: American Nurses Publishing.

**Consensus Panel on Genetic/Genomic Nursing Competencies (Consensus Panel). (2009). *Essentials of genetic and genomic nursing: Competencies, curricular guidelines, and outcome indicators* (2nd ed.). Silver Spring, MD: American Nurses Association.

Edwards, Q. T., & Maradiegue, A. H. (2018). *Genetics and genomics in nursing*. New York: Springer Publishing Company.

Journals and Electronic Documents

American College of Medical Genetics and Genomics Policy Statement (ACMG). (2017). Recommendations for reporting of secondary findings in clinical exome and genome sequencing, 2016 update (ACMG SF v2.0): A policy statement of the American College of Medical Genetics and Genomics. *Genetics in Medicine, 19*(2), 249–255.

American College of Obstetricians and Gynecologists Committee on Genetics (ACOG). (2018). Committee opinion. Committee on Genetics. Number 478. Family history as a risk assessment tool. Retrieved on 8/28/2019 at: www.acog.org/Clinical-Guidance-and-Publications/Committee-Opinions/Committee-on-Genetics/Family-History-as-a-Risk-Assessment-Tool

American College of Obstetricians and Gynecologists Committee on Genetics (ACOG). (2019). Committee opinion. Committee on Genetics. Number 691 (replaces 486). Carrier screening for genetic conditions. Retrieved on 8/28/2019 at: www.cancer.gov/types/breast/hp/breast-ovarian-genetics-pdq#link/_113_toc

Armando, R. G., Gomez, D. L., Maggio, J., et al. (2019). Telomeropathies: Etiology, diagnosis, treatment and follow-up. Ethical and legal considerations. *Clinical Genetics, 96*(1), 3–16.

Beamer, L. C. (2017). Ethics and genetics: Examining a crossroads in nursing through a case study. *Clinical Journal of Oncology Nursing, 21*(6), 730–737.

Bilkey, G. A., Burns, B. L., Coles, E. P., et al. (2019). Genomic testing for human health and disease across the life cycle: Applications and ethical, legal, and social challenges. *Frontiers in Public Health, 7*, 40.

Boardman, F., & Hale, R. (2018). Responsibility, identity, and genomic sequencing: A comparison of published recommendations and patient perspectives on accepting or declining incidental findings. *Molecular Genetics and Genomic Medicine, 6*, 1079–1096.

Boerwinkel, D. J., Yarden, A., & Waarlo, A. J. (2017). Reaching a consensus on the definition of genetic literacy that is required from a twenty-first-century citizen. *Science and Education, 26*(10), 1087–1114.

Centers for Disease Control and Prevention (CDC). (2017). Family health history. Retrieved on 8/30/2019 at: www.cdc.gov/genomics/famhistory

Centers for Disease Control and Prevention (CDC). (2018a). Public health genomics. Pharmacogenomics: What does it mean for your health? Retrieved on 8/24/2019 at: www.cdc.gov/genomics/disease/pharma.htm

Centers for Disease Control and Prevention (CDC). (2018b). Public health genomics. Genetic counseling. Retrieved on 8/27/2019 at: www.cdc.gov/genomics/gtesting/genetic_counseling.htm

Cho, J., Lee, I., & Kang, H. (2017). ACTN3 gene and susceptibility to sarcopenia and osteoporotic status in older Korean adults. *BioMed Research International*, Article ID 4239648, 8 pages. doi: 10.1155/2017/4239648

Clinical Pharmacogenetics Implementation Consortium (CPIC). (2019). Guidelines. Retrieved on 8/25/2019 at: www.cpicpgx.org/guidelines

Conyers, R., Devaraja, S., & Elliott, D. (2018). Systematic review of pharmacogenomics and adverse drug reactions in paediatric oncology patients. *Pediatric Blood Cancer, 65*(4), 1–12.

Cragun, D., Weidner, A., Kechik, J., et al. (2019). Genetic testing across young Hispanic and non-Hispanic white breast cancer survivors: Facilitators, barriers, and awareness of the Genetic Information Nondiscrimination Act. *Genetic Testing and Molecular Biomarkers, 23*(2), 75–83.

Dodson, C. H. (2017). Pharmacogenomics: Principles and relevance to oncology nursing. *Clinical Journal of Oncology Nursing, 21*(6), 739–745.

Foss, D. V., Hochstrasser, M. L., & Wilson, R. C. (2019). Clinical applications of CRISPR-based genome editing and diagnostics. *Transfusion, 59*(4), 1389–1399.

Gael, N., & Veltman, J. A. (2019). The role of de novo mutations in adult-onset neurodegenerative disorders. *Acta Neuropathologica, 137*(2), 183–207.

Ginsburg, G. S., Wu, R. R., & Orlando, L. A. (2019). Family health history: Underused for actionable risk assessment. *Lancet, 394*(10198), 596–603.

Greathouse, K. L., Faucher, M. A., & Hastings-Tolsma, M. (2017). The gut microbiome, obesity, and weight control in women's reproductive health. *Western Journal of Nursing Research, 39*(8), 1094–1119.

International Society of Nurses in Genetics (ISONG). (2019). Position statements. Retrieved on 8/27/2019 at: www.isong.org/page-135072

Jackson, M., Marks, L., May, G. H. W., et al. (2018). The genetic basis of disease. *Essays in Biochemistry, 62*(5), 643–723.

Keogh, L. A., Niven, H., Rutstein, A., et al. (2017). Choosing not to undergo predictive genetic testing for hereditary colorectal cancer syndromes: Expanding our understanding of decliners and declining. *Journal of Behavioral Medicine, 40*(4), 583–594.

Kerber, A. S., & Ledbetter, N. J. (2017). Standards of practice: Applying genetics and genomics resources to oncology. *Clinical Journal of Oncology Nursing, 2*(2), 169–173.

Khoury, M. J. (2019). Precision medicine versus preventive medicine. *Journal of the American Medical Association, 321*(4), 406.

Khoury, M. J., Bowen, M. S., Clyne, M., et al. (2018). From public health genomics to precision public health: A 20-year journey. *Genetics in Medicine, 20*(6), 574–582.

Knowles, J. W., Rader, D. J., & Khoury, M. J. (2017). Cascade screening for familial hypercholesterolemia and the use of genetic testing. *Journal of the American Medical Association, 318*(4), 381–382.

Learn.Genetics, Genetic Science Learning Center. (2019). Genetic disorders. Retrieved on 8/30/2019 at: www.learn.genetics.utah.edu/content/disorders

Mahon, S. M. (2018). Direct-to-consumer genetic testing. *Clinical Journal of Oncology Nursing, 22*(1), 33–36.

Manchanda, R., & Gaba, F. (2019). A commentary on population genetic testing for primary prevention: Changing landscape and the need to change paradigm. *British Journal of Obstetrics and Gynaecology, 126*(6), 686–689.

Mannino, G. C., Andreozzi, F., & Sesti, G. (2019). Pharmacogenetics of type 2 diabetes mellitus, the route toward tailored medicine. *Diabetes Metabolic Research Review, 35*(3), e3109.

Mayo Clinic. (2018). Getting pregnant. Retrieved on 8/27/19 at: www.mayoclinic.org/healthy-lifestyle/getting-pregnant/expert-answers/paternal-age/faq-20057873

Mayo Clinic. (2019). Pharmacogenomics: Drug-gene testing. Retrieved on 8/27/19 at: www.mayo.edu/research/cent3ers-programs/center-individualized-medicine/patinet-care/pharmacogenomidcs/drug-gene-testing

McClatchey, T., Lay, E., Strassberg, M., et al. (2018). Missed opportunities: Unidentified genetic risk factors in prenatal care. *Prenatal Care, 38*(1), 75–79.

Morrow, A., Jacobs, C., Best, M., et al. (2018). Genetics in palliative oncology: A missing agenda? A review of the literature and future directions. *Supportive Care in Cancer, 26*, 721–730.

National Cancer Institute. (2019). Targeted cancer therapies. Retrieved on 8/26/2019 at: www.cancer.gov/about-cancer/treatment/types/targeted-therapies/targeted-therapies-fact-sheet

National Center for Biotechnology Information (NCBI), U.S. National Library of Medicine (NLM). (2019a). Genetic Testing Registry. Retrieved on 8/25/2019 at: www.ncbi.nlm.nih.gov/gtr

National Center for Biotechnology Information (NCBI), U.S. National Library of Medicine (NLM). (2019b). Online Mendelian Inheritance in Man. Retrieved on 8/25/2019 at: www.ncbi.nlm.nih.gov/omim

National Institutes of Health (NIH), National Center for Advancing Translational Sciences (NCATS); Genetic and Rare Diseases Information Center. (2017). FAQs about chromosome disorders. Retrieved on 8/25/2019 at: www.rarediseases.info.nih.gov/guides/pages/73/faqs-about-chromosome-disorders

National Institutes of Health (NIH), National Human Genome Research Institute (NHGRI). (2018). What is the human genome project? Retrieved on 8/24/2019 at: www.genome.gov/human-genome-project/What

National Institutes of Health (NIH), National Human Genome Research Institute (NHGRI). (2019a). Introduction to genomics. Retrieved on 8/24/2019 at: www.genome.gov/About-Genomics/Introduction-to-Genomics#one

National Institutes of Health (NIH), National Human Genome Research Institute (NHGRI). (2019b). Genome statute and legislation database. Retrieved on 8/26/2019 at: www.genome.gov/about-genomics/policy-issues/Genome-Statute-Legislation-Database

National Institutes of Health (NIH), National Human Genome Research Institute (NHGRI). (2019c). Research at NHGRI. Retrieved on 8/29/2019 at: www.genome.gov/research-at-nhgri

National Institutes of Health (NIH), U.S. National Library of Medicine (NLM); Genetics Home Reference. (2015). What are the different ways in which a genetic condition can be inherited? Retrieved on 8/30/2019 at: www.ghr.nlm.nih.gov/primer/inheritance/inheritancepatterns

National Institutes of Health (NIH), U.S. National Library of Medicine (NLM); Genetics Home Reference. (2019a). What is the precision medicine initiative? Retrieved on 8/24/2019 at: www.ghr.nlm.nih.gov/primer/precisionmedicine/initiative

National Institutes of Health (NIH), U.S. National Library of Medicine (NLM); Genetics Home Reference. (2019b). What is epigenetics? Retrieved on 8/24/2019 at: www.ghr.nlm.nih.gov/primer/howgeneswork/epigenome

National Institutes of Health (NIH), U.S. National Library of Medicine (NLM); Genetics Home Reference. (2019c). What is a gene? Retrieved on 8/24/2019 at: www.ghr.nlm.nih.gov/primer/basics/gene

National Institutes of Health (NIH), U.S. National Library of Medicine (NLM); Genetics Home Reference. (2019d). Hypercholesterolemia. Retrieved on 8/24/2019 at: www.ghr.nlm.nih.gov/condition/hypercholesterolemia#inheritance

National Institutes of Health (NIH), U.S. National Library of Medicine (NLM); Genetics Home Reference. (2019e). Turner syndrome. Retrieved on 8/24/2019 at: www.ghr.nlm.nih.gov/condition/turner-syndrome

National Institutes of Health (NIH), U.S. National Library of Medicine (NLM); Genetics Home Reference. (2019f). Sickle cell disease. Retrieved on 8/24/2019 at: www.ghr.nlm.nih.gov/condition/sickle-cell-disease

National Institutes of Health (NIH), U.S. National Library of Medicine (NLM); Genetics Home Reference. (2019g). What are reduced penetrance and variable expressivity? Retrieved on 8/24/2019 at: www.ghr.nlm.nih.gov/primer/inheritance/penetranceexpressivity

National Institutes of Health (NIH), U.S. National Library of Medicine (NLM); Genetics Home Reference. (2019h). Angelman syndrome. Retrieved on 8/24/2019 at: www.ghr.nlm.nih.gov/condition/angelman-syndrome

National Institutes of Health (NIH), U.S. National Library of Medicine (NLM); Genetics Home Reference. (2019i). Neurofibromatosis type 1. Retrieved on 8/29/2019 at: www.ghr.nlm.nih.gov/condition/neurofibromatosis-type-1

National Institutes of Health (NIH), U.S. National Library of Medicine (NLM); Genetics Home Reference. (2019j). Help me understand genetics. Retrieved on 8/30/2019 at: www.ghr.nlm.nih.gov/primer#testing

National Institutes of Health (NIH), U.S. National Library of Medicine (NLM). (2019k). Genetic testing. *MedlinePlus.* Retrieved on 8/30/2019 at: www.medlineplus.gov/genetictsting.html

National Institutes of Health (NIH), U.S. National Library of Medicine (NLM); Genetics Home Reference. (2019l). What are the types of genetic tests? Retrieved on 8/30/2019 at: www.ghr.nlm.nih.gov/handbook/testing/uses

Parikh, F. R., Athalye, A. S., Naik, N. J., et al. (2018). Preimplantation genetic testing: Its evolution, where are we today? *Journal of Human Reproductive Sciences, 11*(4), 306–314.

Pickard, B. S. (2017). Genomics of lithium action and response. *Neurotherapeutics, 14*(3), 582–587.

Rich, K. (2018). Genetic Nondiscrimination Act and the Affordable Care Act: When two is better than one. *Genetic Testing and Molecular Biomarkers, 22*(6), 331–332.

*Rogers, M. A., Lizer, S., Doughty, A., et al. (2017). Expanding RN scope of knowledge—genetics and genomics: The new frontier. *Journal for Nurses in Professional Development, 33*(2), 56–63.

Rothstein, M. (2018). GINA at ten and the future of Genetic Nondiscrimination Law. *Hastings Center Report, 48*(3), 5–7.

*Schroeder, D., Duggleby, W., & Cameron, B. L. (2017). Moving in and out of the what-ifs: The experiences of unaffected women living in families where a breast cancer 1 or 2 genetic mutation was not found. *Cancer Nursing, 40*(5), 386–393.

Setia, N., Saxena, R., Sawhney, J. P. S., et al. (2018). Familial hypercholesterolemia: Cascade screening in children and relatives of the affected. *The Indian Journal of Pediatrics, 85*(5), 339–343.

Silva, P. R., Jannes, C. E., Oliveira, T. G. M., et al. (2018). Predictors of family enrollment in a genetic cascade screening program for familial hypercholesterolemia. *Arquivos Brasileiros De Cardiologia, 111*(4), 578–584.

Sun, J. (2018). Dietary vitamin D, vitamin D receptor, and microbiome. *Current Opinion Clinical Nutrition and Metabolic Care, 21*(6), 471–474.

Tluczek, A., Twal, M. E., Beamer, L. C., et al. (2019). How American Nurses Association Code of Ethics informs genetic/genomic nursing. *Nursing Ethics, 26*(5), 1505–1517.

Turnball, C., Sud, A., & Houlston, R. S. (2019). Cancer genetic, precision prevention and a call to action. *Nature Genetics, 50*(9), 1212–1218.

U.S. Department of Health and Human Services (HHS). (2017). HIPAA for professionals. Retrieved on 8/27/2019 at: www.hhs.gov/hipaa/for-professionals/index.html

U.S. Food and Drug Administration (FDA). (2019). Table of pharmacogenomic biomarkers in drug labeling. Retrieved on 8/26/2019 at: www.fda.gov/drugs/science-research-drugs/table-pharmacogenomic-biomarkers-drug-labeling

van Lanschot, M. C. J., Bosch, L. J. W., de Wit, M., et al. (2017). Early detection: The impact of genomics. *Virchows Archiv: An International Journal of Pathology, 471*(2), 165–173.

Resources

Association of Women's Health, Obstetric and Neonatal Nurses (AWHONN), awhonn.org

Centers for Disease Control and Prevention, Public Health Genomics, www.cdc.gov/genomics

Genetic and Rare Diseases Information Center, www.rarediseases.info.nih.gov

International Society of Nurses in Genetics (ISONG), www.isong.org

Learn.Genetics, Genetic Learning Science Center, learn.genetics.utah.edu

National Cancer Institute (NCI), www.cancer.gov

National Center for Biotechnology Information, www.ncbi.nlm.nih.gov

National Human Genome Research Institute, Genome Statute and Legislative Database, www.genome.gov/about-genomics/policy-issues/Genome-Statute-Legislation-Database

National Organization for Rare Disorders (NORD), www.rarediseases.org

Oncology Nursing Society (ONS), www.ons.org

Online Mendelian Inheritance in Man, www.omim.org

The Human Genome Project, www.genome.gov/human-genome-project

Disability and Chronic Illness

Disability and chronic illness affect people of all ages—the very young, the middle aged, older adults, and the very old. Disability and chronic illness are found in all ethnic, cultural, racial, and socioeconomic groups, although some disorders occur more frequently in some groups than in others. Nurses in all settings will encounter patients with disability and chronic illness. This chapter presents concepts about disability and chronic illness and ways that nurses can address the health issues of these patients and their families.

Disability

Definitions of Disability

A person is considered to have a **disability** (limitation in performance or function in everyday activities) if they have difficulty talking, hearing, seeing, walking, climbing stairs, lifting or carrying objects, performing activities of daily living (ADLs), such as feeding oneself, bathing, dressing, grooming, toileting, doing school work, or working at a job. A severe disability is present if a person is unable to perform one or more activities, uses an assistive device for mobility, or needs help from another person to accomplish basic activities. People are also considered severely disabled if they receive federal benefits because of an inability to work.

According to the World Health Organization (WHO, 2018a), *disability* is the interaction between individuals with a health condition (e.g., cerebral palsy, spinal cord injury, Down syndrome) personal and environmental factors (e.g., negative attitudes on the part of society, inaccessible transportation and public buildings, and limited social supports). In 2001, WHO developed the International Classification of Functioning, Disability and Health (ICF), which defined disability as an umbrella term for impairments, activity limitations, participation restrictions, and environmental factors.

The term *impairment* describes a loss or abnormality in body structure or physiologic function, including mental function. The term *societal participation* is used in the WHO classification system in place of *handicap* to acknowledge the fact that the environment is always interacting with people to either assist or hinder participation in life activities. The environment may have a greater impact on a person's ability to participate in life activities than do physical, mental, or emotional factors or conditions (WHO, 2018a).

In the United States, federal legislation uses multiple definitions of disability, which makes common understanding of disability difficult. The Americans With Disabilities Act of 1990 (ADA; discussed later in this chapter) defines a person with a disability as one who (1) has a physical or mental impairment that substantially limits one or more major life activities, (2) has a record of such an impairment, or (3) is regarded as having such an impairment. Other phrases used to describe people with disabilities that are not universally accepted, understood or recommended are "people who are physically challenged" and "people with special needs."

Prevalence of Disability

According to the WHO (2018a), over one billion people, or about 15% of the global population, have some type of disability. Between 110 and 190 million adults worldwide have significant difficulties in function due to disability. The number of people with disabilities is increasing and is expected to continue to climb as people with early-onset disability, chronic disorders, and severe trauma survive. People with disability comprise the world's largest minority (United Nations, n.d.).

The Centers for Disease Control and Prevention (CDC, 2017) reported that in 2016, one in four noninstitutionalized adults, or 61 million adults in the United States, had a disability that negatively affected major life activities. This reflects an increase from 2013 in which one in five noninstitutionalized adults in the United States had a disability (Okoro, Hollis, Cyrus, et al., 2018). The estimate is likely low as these figures do not include people who are living in institutions or are active duty military personnel.

The last U.S. Census indicated that more than 46% of people with one disability have other disabilities. Although the prevalence of disability is higher in men than in women for people younger than 65 years, the prevalence is higher in women than in men for people older than 65 years (U.S.

Census Bureau, 2018a). In the United States, the prevalence of disability is higher among American Indians as well as Alaska Natives, adults with incomes below the federal poverty level, and people living in the southwestern U.S. census region (Okoro et al., 2018). In addition, the prevalence of disability in the United States is higher for African Americans and Whites than for Hispanics and Asians (U.S. Department of Labor, Bureau of Labor Statistics, 2019). Globally, more than 80% of the one billion people worldwide with disability live in low- and middle-income countries, in which all people have limited access to basic health care and social services. However, limited access to basic health care and support services has a more profound effect on those with disability.

The proportion of individuals with disability employed in 2018 was 19.1%. In contrast, 65.9% of those without disability were employed. About 8 in 10 people with a disability were not in the labor force in 2018, compared to about 3 in 10 of those with no disability. Individuals with disability are more likely to be employed part time than those with no disability. These discrepancies exist across all educational attainment groups (U.S. Department of Labor, Bureau of Labor Statistics, 2019). A consequence of lack of employment or only part-time employment is that those with a disability earn less money than people without disabilities. Low income along with limited access to basic health care and support services has a profound effect on those with disability. In 2017, the poverty rate of those individuals of working age, generally considered 18 to 64 years, with disability was 29.6%. In contrast, the poverty rate in 2017 of those without disability was 13.2% (Houtenville & Boege, 2019). See Chart 7-1 for a summary of additional facts about people with disabilities.

Characteristics of Disability

The characteristics of disability include an understanding of the categories, types, and models of disability. Additional characteristics include understanding the broad concept of disability.

Categories and Types of Disability

There are many categories and types of disabilities that include cognitive, developmental, intellectual, sensory, acquired, psychiatric, and physical. A **cognitive disability** is defined as limitations in mental functioning and difficulties with communication, self-care, and difficulty with social skills.

Developmental disabilities are those that occur any time from birth to 22 years of age and result in impairment of physical or mental health, cognition, speech, language, or self-care. This is an umbrella term that includes intellectual disabilities but can be a physical disability only. Examples of developmental disabilities include spina bifida, cerebral palsy, Down syndrome, muscular dystrophy, dwarfism, and osteogenesis imperfecta. Some developmental disabilities occur as a result of birth trauma or severe illness or injury at a very young age, whereas many developmental disabilities are genetic in origin (see Chapter 6). Some developmental disabilities overlap with cognitive and/or intellectual disabilities that affect intellectual functioning and adaptive behavior. An **intellectual disability** occurs before 18 years of age and is characterized by significant limitations in both intellectual functioning as well as in adaptive behavior, including

Chart 7-1 Summary of Facts About People with Disability

- Approximately 61 million people in the United States have a disability, or one in every four people.
- The prevalence of disabilities in adults is approximately 10% of people 18–64 years of age and 38% of adults 65 years of age and older.
- The prevalence of disabilities varies by state and by gender, with higher prevalence in the South and among females.
- More than 11 million people with disabilities require personal assistance with everyday activities (e.g., getting around inside the home, bathing or showering, preparing meals, and performing light housework).
- Approximately 3.3 million people use a wheelchair; another 10 million use a walking aid such as cane, crutches, or walker.
- More than 1.8 million people report being unable to see printed words because of vision impairment, 1 million are unable to hear conversations because of hearing impairment, and 2.5 million have difficulty with their speech being understood.
- More than 16 million people have limitations in cognitive function or have a mental or emotional illness that interferes with daily activities, including those with Alzheimer's disease and intellectual disabilities.
- Self-reported health status among adults with disabilities differs from that of people without disabilities, with fewer people with disabilities describing their health as excellent or good.
- The percentage of people with disabilities who are employed ranges from 17.8% to 23.4%; of those without disabilities, the percent ranges from 63.5% to 66.2%.
- Among all age groups, people with a disability are much less likely to be employed than those without a disability. People with a disability who work are more likely than those without disability to work part time. People with a disability who were not in the labor force (neither employed nor unemployed) are about 8 in 10, compared with about 3 in 10 of those without a disability.
- Many people with disabilities would like to work but are hampered in doing so by limited access, lack of accommodations in the workplace, lack of transportation, and reluctance of employers to hire them.
- The percentage of people with disabilities below the poverty level is more than twice that of people without disabilities.

Adapted from Centers for Disease Control and Prevention (CDC), National Center for Health Statistics. (2017). Disability and functioning (non-institutionalized adults aged 18 and over). Retrieved on 7/15/2019 at: www.cdc.gov/nchs/fastats/disability.htm; Centers for Disease Control and Prevention (CDC). (2018). Disability and health. Common barriers to participation experienced by people with disabilities. Retrieved on 7/16/2019 at: www.cdc.gov/ncbddd/disabilityandhealth/disability-barriers.html; Lauer, E. A., & Houtenville, A. J. (2018). Estimates of prevalence, demographic characteristics and social factors among people with disabilities in the USA: A cross-survey comparison. *BMJ Open, 8,* e017828; Na, L., Hennessy, S., Boner, H. R., et al. (2017). Disability stage and receipt of recommended care among elderly Medicare beneficiaries. *Disability & Health Journal, 10*(1), 48–57; U.S. Department of Labor, Bureau of Labor Statistics. (2019). Persons with a disability: Labor force characteristics—2018. Retrieved on 7/5/2019 at: www.bls.gov/news.release/pdf/disabl.pdf; United Nations. (n.d.). Factsheet on persons with disabilities. Retrieved on 7/20/2019 at: www.un.org /development/desa/disabilities/resources/factsheet-on-persons-with-disabilities.html

many everyday social and practical skills. Because individuals with developmental and intellectual disabilities are living well into adulthood and aging with a disability, all nurses and other health care providers will encounter them in practice and must be knowledgeable and prepared to provide high quality health care.

A sensory disability is characterized by impairment of the sense of sight, hearing, smell, touch, and/or taste. Sensory disabilities most commonly affect hearing or vision; however, they also include learning disabilities that affect the ability to learn, remember, or concentrate; disabilities that affect the ability to speak or communicate; and disabilities that affect the ability to work, shop, and care for oneself, or access health care. Risks associated with sensory disabilities include isolation, reduced cognitive function, poor physical and psychological health, and increased risk of falls and hospitalization (McKee, 2019).

Psychiatric disability is defined as a mental illness or impairment that substantially limits one's ability to complete major life activities, such as learning, working, and communicating (WHO, 2018b). Although psychiatric disability and mental health disorders are not the focus of this chapter, it is important to note that a person may have more than one type of disability at the same time, requiring health care providers to be prepared to care for patients with several types of disabilities.

Whether a disability is cognitive, developmental, intellectual, physical, or sensory it may also be characterized as acquired. Acquired disabilities may occur as a result of an acute and sudden injury (e.g., traumatic brain injury [TBI]; spinal cord injury; and traumatic amputation due to traffic crashes, falls, burns, or acts of violence such as intimate partner violence and war and military conflicts), acute nontraumatic disorders (e.g., stroke, myocardial infarction), or progression of a chronic disorder (e.g., arthritis, multiple sclerosis, Parkinson's disease, chronic obstructive pulmonary disease, heart disease, blindness due to diabetic retinopathy).

Many disabilities are visible; however, invisible disabilities are often as disabling as those that can be seen. Some disabilities affect only instrumental activities of living (IADLs), such as shopping for food, doing laundry, housekeeping, and handling financial matters. Other disabilities affect ADLs only. People can be temporarily disabled because of an injury or acute exacerbation of a chronic disorder but later return to full functioning.

A common challenge for people with disability is the need to hire and oversee caregivers who come into their homes to assist with ADLs and IADLs. For many, it is difficult to be in a position of hiring, supervising, and sometimes firing people who may provide them with intimate physical care. The need to balance the roles of receiving care and overseeing the person providing that care may lead to blurring of role boundaries.

Many people with disabilities are at risk for **secondary health conditions** (e.g., pressure injuries, urinary tract infections, low bone density, depression) because of a narrow margin of health. Many of these conditions are predictable and with treatment are preventable with appropriate assessment for risk, prevention and treatment strategies (WHO, 2018a). Some conditions can be both primary and secondary conditions depending on circumstances. For example, a mobility disability could lead to social isolation and absence of participation in activities. This in turn could lead to depression as a secondary condition (Krahn, 2019). Comorbidities (e.g., cardiac disease, cancer, hearing loss) are not due to disability and thus can occur in those with or without disability.

Although different impairments may result from different types of disabilities, there are some similarities across disabilities. People with disabilities are often considered by society to be dependent and needing to be cared for by others; however, many people with disabilities are highly functioning, independent, productive people who are capable of caring for themselves and others, having children and raising families, holding full-time jobs, and making significant and major contributions to society. Like other people, most individuals with disabilities prefer to live in their own homes with family members. Most of them are able to live at home independently. Some individuals with disabilities live alone in their own homes and use home care services. However, alternative living arrangements may be necessary; these include assisted living facilities, long-term care facilities, and group homes.

Models of Disability

Several models of disability have been used to address or explain the issues encountered by people with disabilities. Chart 7-2 describes several models of disability. The Interface Model (Goodall, 1995), developed by a nurse, promotes care designed to be empowering rather than care that promotes dependency. It takes into account the disabling condition and its disabling effects. Furthermore, it promotes the view that people with disabilities are capable, responsible people who are able to function effectively despite having a disability. The Interface Model can serve as a basis for the role of nurses as advocates for the removal of barriers to health care and for the examination of how society and health care professionals contribute to discrimination by viewing disability as an abnormal state. Several other models of disability exist and serve as a guide for reflection on what disability means as well as its antecedents and outcomes (Retief & Letšosa, 2018).

Disability versus Disabling Disorders

Regardless of which definition or model of disability is adopted, it is important to realize that one can understand

---

Chart 7-2   Models of Disability

Medical Model

The Medical Model equates people who are disabled with their disabilities and views disability as a problem of the person, directly caused by disease, trauma, or other health condition, that requires medical care provided in the form of individual treatment by professionals. Health care providers, rather than people with disabilities, are viewed as the experts or authorities. Management of the disability is aimed at cure or the person's adjustment and behavior change. The model is viewed as promoting passivity and dependency. People with disabilities are viewed as tragic.

Rehabilitation Model

The Rehabilitation Model emerged from the medical model. It regards disability as a deficiency that requires a rehabilitation specialist or other helping professional to fix the problem. People with disabilities are often perceived as having failed if they do not overcome the disability.

Social Model

The Social Model, which is also referred to as the barriers or disability model, views disability as socially constructed and as a political issue that is a result of social and physical barriers in the environment. Its perspective is that disability can be overcome by removal of these barriers.

Biopsychosocial Model

The Biopsychosocial Model integrates the medical and social models to address perspectives of health from a biologic, individual, and social perspective. Critiques of this model have suggested that the disabling condition, rather than the person and the experience of the person with a disability, remains the defining construct of the Biopsychosocial Model.

Functional Model

The Functional Model is driven by the World Health Organization's *International Classification of Functioning, Disability and Health* (*ICF*). Disability is considered an umbrella term for impairments, activity limitations, participation restrictions, and their interaction with environmental factors. The ICF addresses components of health rather than consequence of disease.

Interface Model

The Interface Model is based on the life experience of the person with a disability and views disability at the intersection (i.e., interface) of the medical diagnosis of a disability and environmental barriers. It considers rather than ignores the diagnosis. The person with a disability, rather than others, defines the problems and seeks or directs solutions.

Other Models of Disability

Other models include the Identity Model (views disability as a positive rather than negative identity), the Human Rights Model (emphasizes the human dignity of individuals with disability and policy change), the Cultural Model (focuses on different views of disability within the context of a specific culture), the Charity Model (encourages humane treatment of people with disabilities, but views people with disabilities as victims of their impairment), and the Economic Model (approaches disability from the perspective of the ability of people with disabilities to work and contribute to society). Each of these models introduces elements that affect how individuals with disability are perceived and, as a result, how they are treated. Therefore, the underlying views and implications suggested by each model need to be examined and critiqued. Importantly, an analysis of these models helps promote introspection and discussion of the concept of disability.

Adapted from Drum, C. F. (2014). The dynamics of disability and chronic conditions. *Disability and Health Journal, 7*(1), 2–5; Goodall, C. J. (1995). Is disability any business of nurse education? *Nurse Education Today, 15*(5), 323–327; Retief, M., & Letšosa, R. (2018). Models of disability: A brief overview. *HTS Teologiese Studies/Theological Studies, 74*(1), a4738; Smeltzer, S. C. (2007). Improving the health and wellness of persons with disabilities: A call to action too important for nursing to ignore. *Nursing Outlook, 55*(4), 189–193; Smeltzer, S. C. (2021). *Delivering quality healthcare for people with disability*. Indianapolis, IN: Sigma Theta Tau International. World Health Organization. (2001). *International Classification of Functioning, Disability and Health—ICF*. Geneva, Switzerland: Author.

the pathophysiology and physical changes related to a disabling condition or injury without understanding the concept of disability. The nurse caring for patients with pre-existing disabilities or new disabilities must recognize the impact of a disability on patients' well-being and their current and future health, their ability to participate in self-care or self-management, and their ability to obtain required health care and recommended health screening. Nursing management—from assessment through evaluation of the effectiveness of nursing interventions—must be monitored frequently to ensure that appropriate modifications

have been made so that people with disabilities can receive health care equal to that of people without disabilities. Furthermore, nurses as well as other health care providers need to examine their facilities and procedures to ensure that the needs of people with various disabilities can be adequately addressed. Although the health care needs of people with disabilities generally do not differ from those of the general population, some disabilities create special needs and necessitate the use of special accommodations. Chart 7-3 reviews questions to ask to ensure quality health care for people with disabilities.

Chart 7-3 Questions to Ask to Ensure Quality Health Care for People with Disability

Communication Strategies

- Does the patient with a disability require or prefer accommodations (e.g., a sign language interpreter) to ensure full participation in conversations about their health care?
- Are appropriate accommodations made to communicate with the patient?
- Are efforts made to direct all conversations to the patient rather than to others who have accompanied the patient to the health care facility?
- Is appropriate language (people-first language) used in referring to the patient?

Accessibility of the Health Care Facility

- Are clinics, hospital rooms, offices, restrooms, laboratories, and imaging facilities accessible to people with disabilities, as legally required by the Americans With Disabilities Act and Rehabilitation Act?
- Has accessibility been verified by a person with a disability?
- Is a sign language interpreter other than a family member available to assist in obtaining a patient's health history and in conducting a physical assessment?
- Does the facility include appropriate equipment to permit people with disabilities to obtain health care (including mammography, gynecologic examination and care, dental care) in a dignified and safe manner?

Assessment

Usual Health Considerations

- Does the health history address the same issues that would be included when obtaining a history from a person without disabilities, including recent preventive health screening, sexuality, sexual function, and reproductive health issues?

Disability-Related Considerations

- Does the health history address the patient's specific disability and the effect of disability on the patient's ability to obtain health care, manage self-care activities, and obtain preventive health screening and follow-up care?
- What physical modifications and positioning are needed to ensure a thorough physical examination, including pelvic or testicular and rectal examination?

Abuse

- Is the increased risk for abuse (physical, emotional, financial, and sexual) by various people (family, paid care providers, strangers) addressed in the assessment?
- If abuse is detected, are men and women with disability who are survivors of abuse directed to appropriate resources, including accessible shelters and hotlines?

Depression

- Is the patient experiencing depression? If so, is treatment offered just as it would be to a patient without a disability, without assuming that depression is normal and a result of having a disability?

Aging

- What concerns does the patient have about aging with a preexisting disability?
- What effect has aging had on the patient's disability, and what effect has the disability had on the patient's aging?

Secondary Health Conditions

- Does the patient have secondary health conditions related to their disability or its treatment?
- Is the patient at risk for secondary health conditions because of environmental barriers or lack of access to health care or health promotion activities?
- Are strategies in place to reduce the risk for secondary health conditions or to treat existing secondary health conditions?

Accommodations in the Home

- What accommodations does the patient have at home to encourage or permit self-care?
- What additional accommodations does the patient need at home to encourage or permit self-care?

Cognitive Status

- Is it assumed that the patient is able to participate in discussion and conversation rather than assuming that they are unable to do so because of a disability?
- Are appropriate modifications made in written and verbal communication strategies?

Modifications in Nursing Care

- Are modifications made during hospital stays, acute illness or injury, and other health care encounters to enable a patient with disability to be as independent as they prefer?
- Is "people-first language" used in referring to a patient with disability, and do nurses and other staff talk directly to the patient rather than to those who accompanied the patient?
- Are all staff informed about the activities of daily living for which the patient will require assistance?
- Are accommodations made to enable the patient to use his or her assistive devices (hearing/visual aids, prostheses, limb support devices, ventilators, service animals)?
- If a patient with disability is immobilized because of surgery, illness, injury, or treatments, are risks of immobility addressed and strategies implemented to minimize those risks?

(continued on page 146)

Chart 7-3	Questions to Ask to Ensure Quality Health Care for People with Disabilities (continued)

- Is the patient with a disability assessed for other illnesses and health issues (e.g., other acute or chronic illness, depression, psychiatric-mental health, cognitive disorders) not related to the primary disability?

Patient Education

- Are accommodations and alternative formats of instructional materials (large print, Braille, visual materials, audiotapes) provided for patients with disabilities?
- Does patient instruction address the modifications (e.g., use of assistive devices) needed by patients with disabilities to enable them to adhere to recommendations?
- Are modifications made in educational strategies to address learning needs, cognitive changes, and communication impairment?

Health Promotion and Disease Prevention

- Are health promotion strategies discussed with people with disabilities along with their potential benefits: improving quality of life and preventing secondary health conditions (health problems that result because of preexisting disability)?

- Are patients aware of accessible community-based facilities (e.g., health care facilities, imaging centers, public exercise settings, transportation) to enable them to participate in health promotion?

Independence versus Dependence

- Is independence, rather than dependence, of the patient with a disability the focus of nursing care and interaction?
- Are care and interaction with the patient focused on empowerment rather than promoting dependence of the patient?
- Is the patient aware of available resources and supports and do they know how to access them?

Insurance Coverage

- Does the patient have access to the health insurance coverage and other services for which they qualify?
- Is the patient aware of various insurance and other available programs?
- Would the patient benefit from talking to a social worker about eligibility for Medicaid, Medicare, disability insurance, and other services?

Federal Legislation

Because of widespread discrimination against people with disabilities, the U.S. Congress has enacted legislation to address health care disparities in this population. This legislation includes the Rehabilitation Act of 1973 and the ADA. The Rehabilitation Act of 1973 protects people from discrimination based on their disability. This act applies to employers and organizations that receive financial assistance from any federal department or agency, including many hospitals, long-term care facilities, mental health centers, and human service programs. It forbids organizations from excluding or denying people with disabilities equal access to program benefits and services. It also prohibits discrimination related to availability, accessibility, and delivery of services, including health care services.

The ADA, implemented in 1990, mandates that people with disabilities have access to job opportunities and to the community without discrimination based on having a disability. The ADA also requires that "reasonable accommodations" be provided for transportation and to facilitate employment of a person with a disability. Examples of reasonable accommodations in health care settings include accessible facilities and equipment (e.g., accessible restrooms, adjustable examination tables, access ramps, grab bars, elevated toilet seats) and alternative communication methods (e.g., telecommunication devices and sign language interpreters for use by people who are deaf). Failure to make reasonable accommodations can result in poor care for patients with disabilities. For example, lack of accommodation for people who have hearing loss or are deaf can lead to failed communication and inadequate sharing of important information between them and their health care providers (McKee, 2019).

Although the ADA took effect in 1992, compliance has been slow, and some facilities continue to be inaccessible although all new construction and modifications of public facilities must address access for people with disabilities. Because some courts previously interpreted the definition

of disability in the ADA so narrowly that few people could meet it, the ADA Amendments Act was signed into law in 2008 and enacted in January 2009 (U.S. Department of Justice, 2009). The act broadly defines *disability* to encompass impairments that substantially limit a major life activity. This wording states that effective use of assistive devices, auxiliary aids, accommodations, medical therapies, and supplies (other than eyeglasses and contact lenses) does not alter the determination of whether a disability qualifies under the law. The purpose of these amendments was to cover more people and to shift the attention from focusing on who has a disability to making accommodations and avoiding discrimination.

Right of Access to Health Care

People with disabilities have the right of access to health care that is equal in quality to that of other people. The United Nations Convention on the Rights of Persons with Disabilities (CRPD, 2006) identifies the rights of people with disabilities to receive the highest standard of health care, without discrimination. More than 30 years after the passage of the ADA, the United States has not ratified the CRPD. Despite the rights identified by the CRPD and the ADA in the United States, people with disabilities continue to experience health disparities (Kaye, 2019; McClintock, Kurichi, Barg, et al., 2018).

For years, people with disabilities around the world have been discriminated against in employment, public accommodations, and public and private services, including health care (WHO, 2018a). Unmet needs of people with disabilities include but are not limited to medical, dental, and prescription medication needs. The needs of people with disabilities in health care settings present challenges to health care providers: how to communicate effectively if there are communication deficits, how to address the additional physical requirements for mobility, and how to ensure sufficient time to provide assistance with self-care routines during

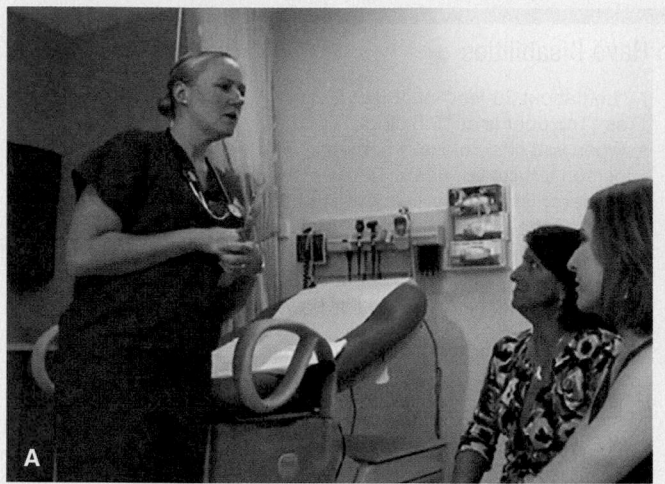
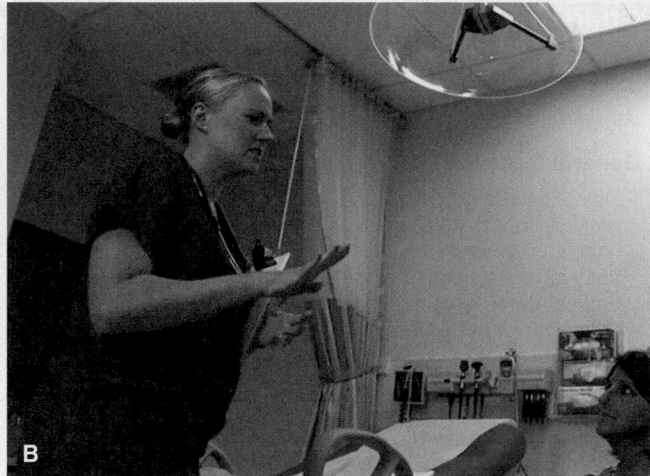

Figure 7-1 • Examples of inappropriate communication by nurse with young woman with a disability in a wheelchair. The nurse stands instead of sitting at the patient's eye level (**A**) and talks to the patient's mother rather than directly to the patient (**B**).

hospitalization. Nurses and other clinicians need to be aware of the specific needs of people with disabilities and to provide appropriate care and services for them. People with disabilities have a legally mandated right to accessible health care facilities for all medical care and screening procedures. Furthermore, they have the right to health care provided by knowledgeable clinicians who are sensitive to the effects of disability on access to health care, including care that addresses their reproductive issues and sexuality. As multiple recent studies have demonstrated, however, improvements are needed to provide women with disabilities with quality care targeting their sexuality and reproductive health care needs (Hayward, Chen, Forbes, et al., 2017; LaPierre, Zimmerman, & Hall, 2017; Mitra, Smith, Smeltzer, et al., 2017; Morris, Maragh-Bass, Griffin, et al., 2017; Tarasoff, 2017).

Reasonable accommodations are mandated by law and are the financial responsibility of the health care provider or facility. People with disabilities should not be expected to provide their own accommodations (e.g., sign language interpreters, assistants). Family members should not be

expected to serve as interpreters because of concern for the patient's privacy and confidentiality and the risk of errors in interpreting information by either the patient or the health care provider. Chart 7-4 identifies strategies to communicate effectively with people with disabilities. Figures 7-1A,B and 7-2A,B illustrate inappropriate and appropriate communication, respectively, with a person with a disability who uses a wheelchair or is seated.

In response to continued accessibility issues, the U.S. Surgeon General issued *Call to Action to Improve the Health and Wellness of Persons with Disabilities* (Smeltzer, 2007; U.S. Department of Health and Human Services [HHS], 2005). This report recognized that all people with disabilities need to have access to comprehensive health care so that they are able to have full, engaged, and productive lives in their own communities. Among strategies to accomplish this, the call to action stipulated that health care professionals need to become knowledgeable about disability. It further recommended that schools educating health care professionals educate about disability and address the need for increased

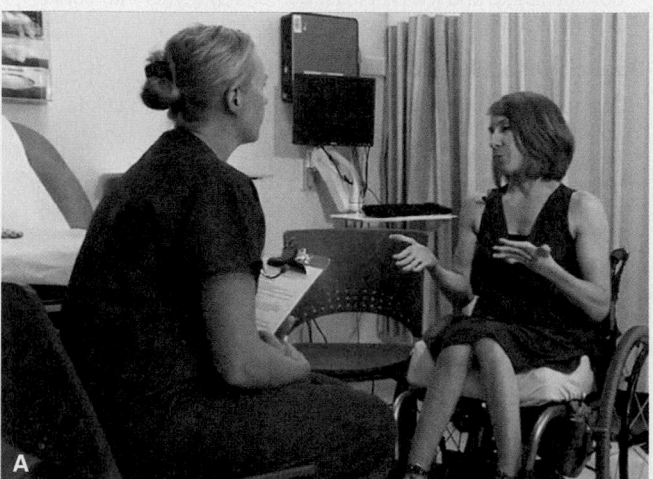
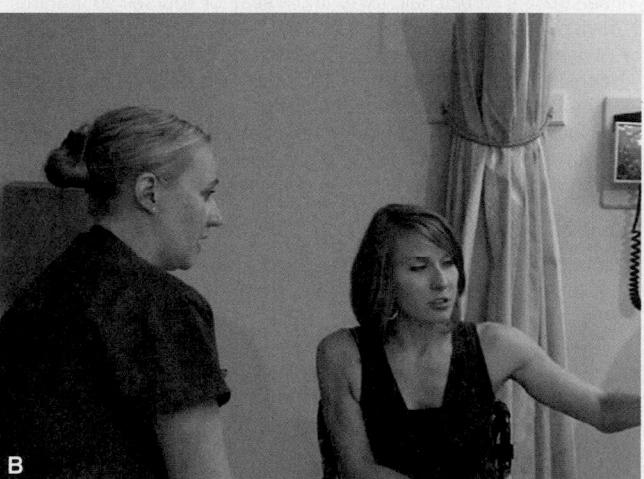

Figure 7-2 • Examples of appropriate communication by nurse with young woman with a disability in a wheelchair. **A.** The nurse is sitting at patient's eye level and talks directly to the patient after asking her mother to step out of the room during the history. **B.** The nurse explains to the patient how the examination table moves up and down, which allows the patient to be as independent as possible in moving the table.

**Chart
7-4**   ## Interacting and Communicating with People Who Have Disabilities

Patients will feel most comfortable receiving health care if you consider the following suggestions.

General Considerations

- Do not be afraid to make a mistake when interacting and communicating with someone with a disability or chronic medical condition. Keep in mind that a person with a disability is a person first and is entitled to the dignity, consideration, respect, and rights you expect for yourself.
- Treat adults as adults. Address people with disabilities by their first names only if extending the same familiarity to all others present. Never patronize people by patting them on the head or the shoulder.
- Relax. If you do not know what to do, allow the person who has a disability to identify how you may be of assistance and to put you at ease.
- If you offer assistance and the person declines, do not insist. If your offer is accepted, ask how you can best help, and follow directions. Do not take over.
- If someone with a disability is accompanied by another person, address the person with a disability directly rather than speaking through the accompanying companion.
- Be considerate of the extra time it might take for a person with a disability to get things done or said. Let the person set the pace.
- Do not be embarrassed to use common expressions, such as "See you later" or "Got to be running," that seem to relate to the person's disability.
- Use people-first language: Refer to "a person with a disability" rather than "a disabled person" and avoid referring to people by the disability or disorder they have (e.g., "the diabetic").

Mobility Limitations

- Do not make assumptions about what a person can and cannot do.
- Do not push a person's wheelchair or grab the arm of someone walking with difficulty without first asking whether you can be of assistance and how you can assist. Personal space includes a person's wheelchair, scooter, crutches, walker, cane, or other mobility aid.
- Never move someone's wheelchair, scooter, crutches, walker, cane, or other mobility aid without permission.
- When speaking for more than a few minutes to a person who is seated in a wheelchair, try to find a seat for yourself so that the two of you are at eye level (see Fig. 7-2A,B).
- When giving directions to people with mobility limitations, consider distance, weather conditions, and physical obstacles such as stairs, curbs, and steep hills.
- Shake hands when introduced to a person with a disability. People who have limited hand use or who wear an artificial limb do shake hands.

Vision Loss (Low Vision and Blindness)

- Identify yourself when you approach a person who has low vision or blindness. If a new person approaches, introduce them.
- Touch the person's arm lightly when you speak so that they know to whom you are speaking before you begin.
- Face the person and speak directly to them. Use a normal tone of voice.
- Do not leave without saying that you are leaving.
- If you are offering directions, be as specific as possible and point out obstacles in the path of travel. Use specifics such as "Left about 20 feet" or "Right 2 yards." Use clock cues, such as "The door is at 10 o'clock."
- When you offer to assist someone with vision loss, allow the person to take your arm. This will help you guide rather than propel or lead the person. When offering seating, place the person's hand on the back or the arm of the seat.
- Alert people with low vision or blindness to posted information.
- Never pet or otherwise distract a canine companion or service animal unless the owner has given you permission.

Hearing Loss (Hard of Hearing, Deaf, Deaf–Blind)

- Ask the person how they prefer to communicate.
- If you are speaking through a sign language interpreter, remember that the interpreter may lag a few words behind—especially if there are names or technical terms to be finger spelled—so pause occasionally to allow the interpreter time to translate completely and accurately.
- Talk directly to the person who has hearing loss, not to the interpreter. However, although it may seem awkward to you, the person who has hearing loss will look at the interpreter and may not make eye contact with you during the conversation.
- Before you start to speak, make sure that you have the attention of the person you are addressing. A wave, a light touch on the arm or the shoulder, or other visual or tactile signals are appropriate ways of getting the person's attention.
- Speak in a clear, expressive manner. Do not over enunciate or exaggerate words. Unless you are specifically requested to do so, do not raise your voice. Speak in a normal tone; do not shout.
- To facilitate lip reading, face the person and keep your hands and other objects away from your mouth. Maintain eye contact. Do not turn your back or walk around while talking. If you look away, the person might assume that the conversation is over.
- Avoid talking while you are writing a message for someone with hearing loss, because the person cannot read your note and your lips at the same time.
- Try to eliminate background noise.
- Encourage feedback to assess clear understanding.
- If you do not understand something that is said, ask the person to repeat it or to write it down. The goal is communication; do not pretend to understand if you do not.
- If you know any sign language, try using it. It may help you communicate, and it will at least demonstrate your interest in communicating and your willingness to try.

Speech Disabilities or Speech Difficulties

- Talk to people with speech disabilities as you would talk to anyone else.
- Be friendly; start up a conversation.
- Be patient; it may take the person a while to answer. Allow extra time for communication. Do not speak for the person.
- Give the person your undivided attention.
- Ask the person for help in communicating with them. If the person uses a communication device such as a manual or electronic communication board, ask the person the best way to use it.
- Speak in your regular tone of voice.
- Tell the person if you do not understand what they are trying to say. Ask the person to repeat the message, spell it, tell you in a different way, or write it down. Use hand gestures and notes.
- Repeat what you understand. The person's reactions will clue you in and guide you to understanding.

Chart 7-4   Interacting and Communicating with People Who Have Disabilities (continued)

- To obtain information quickly, ask short questions that require brief answers or a head nod. Avoid insulting the person's intelligence with oversimplification.
- Keep your manner encouraging rather than correcting.

Intellectual/Cognitive Disabilities

- Treat adults with intellectual/cognitive disabilities as adults.
- Be alert to the person's responses so that you can adjust your method of communication as necessary. For example, some people may benefit from simple, direct sentences or from supplementary visual forms of communication, such as gestures, diagrams, or demonstrations.
- Use concrete rather than abstract language. Be specific, without being too simplistic. When possible, use words that relate to things you both can see. Avoid using directional terms such as right, left, east, or west.
- Be prepared to give the person the same information more than once in different ways.
- When asking questions, phrase them to elicit accurate information. People with intellectual/cognitive disabilities may be eager to please and may tell you what they think you want to hear. Verify responses by repeating the question in a different way.
- Give exact instructions. For example, "Be back for lab work at 4:30," not "Be back in 15 min."
- Avoid giving too many directions at one time, which may be confusing.
- Keep in mind that the person may prefer information provided in written or verbal form. Ask the person how you can best relay the information.
- Using humor is fine, but do not interpret a lack of response as rudeness. Some people may not grasp subtleties of language.
- Know that people with brain injuries may have short-term memory deficits and may repeat themselves or require information to be repeated.
- Recognize that people with auditory perceptual problems may need to have directions repeated and may take notes to help them remember directions or the sequence of tasks. They may benefit from watching a task demonstrated.
- Understand that people with perceptual or "sensory overload" problems may become disoriented or confused if there is too much to absorb at once. Provide information gradually and clearly. Reduce background noise if possible.
- Repeat information using different wording or a different communication approach if necessary. Allow time for the information to be fully understood.

- Do not pretend to understand if you do not. Ask the person to repeat what was said. Be patient, flexible, and supportive.
- Be aware that some people who have an intellectual disability are easily distracted. Try not to interpret distraction as rudeness.
- Do not expect all people to be able to read well. Some people may not read at all.

Psychiatric-Mental Health Disabilities

- Speak directly to the person. Use clear, simple communication.
- Offer to shake hands when introduced. Use the same good manners in interacting with a person who has a psychiatric-mental health disability that you would with anyone else.
- Make eye contact and be aware of your own body language. Like others, people with psychiatric-mental health disabilities will sense your discomfort.
- Listen attentively, and wait for the person to finish speaking. If needed, clarify what the person has said. Never pretend to understand.
- Treat adults as adults. Do not patronize, condescend, or threaten. Do not make decisions for the person or assume that you know the person's preferences.
- Do not give unsolicited advice or assistance. Do not panic or summon an ambulance or the police if a person appears to be experiencing a mental health crisis. Calmly ask the person how you can help.
- Do not blame the person. A person with a psychiatric disability has a complex, biomedical condition that is sometimes difficult to control. The person cannot just "shape up." It is rude, insensitive, and ineffective to tell or expect a person to do so.
- Question the accuracy of media stereotypes of psychiatric-mental health disabilities: Movies and media often sensationalize psychiatric-mental health disabilities. Most people never experience symptoms that include violent behavior.
- Relax. Be yourself. Do not be embarrassed if you happen to use common expressions that seem to relate to a psychiatric-mental health disability.
- Recognize that beneath the symptoms and behaviors of psychiatric disabilities is a person who has many of the same wants, needs, dreams, and desires as anyone else. If you are afraid, learn more about psychiatric-mental health disabilities.

This material is adapted and based in part on U.S. Department of Labor, Office of Disability Employment Policy. *Effective Interaction: Communicating With and About People with Disabilities in the Workplace.* Retrieved on 11/26/20 at: www.dol.gov/general/aboutdol/majorlaws

---

availability of methods to screen, diagnose, and treat the whole person with a disability with dignity.

Health care in people with disabilities received further national attention through specific national objectives in *Healthy People 2020* (HHS, 2010). The midcourse review of those objectives indicated some improvement in health and health-related outcomes for people with disabilities (Sinclair, Fox, Jonas, et al., 2018). For example, the midcourse review revealed that national goals for health were improved or exceeded for 44.6% of objectives for people without disabilities compared to only 30.6% for people with disabilities (National Center for Health Statistics, 2016). These results indicate that work toward achieving equity in health care for individuals with disability is still needed.

Thirty years after the passage of the ADA in 1990, significant health status and health care disparities persist for people with disabilities. Furthermore, progress has been slow in ensuring that health care professionals receive adequate education about providing quality health care to them.

Barriers to Health Care

People with disabilities often encounter barriers in their daily lives and in their efforts to obtain health care, health promotion, and preventive health screening. For example, structural barriers such as stairs, lack of ramps, and narrow doorways may prevent people who are wheelchair users from entering facilities. Other structural barriers include restroom facilities that lack grab bars or sufficiently large restroom stalls, elevated toilet seats, and accessible sinks (CDC, 2018; WHO, 2018a).

Structural barriers to accessibility are most easily identified and eliminated. Other less visible barriers include negative and stereotypic attitudes (e.g., believing that all people with disabilities have a poor quality of life and are dependent and nonproductive) on the part of the public. Health care providers with similar negative attitudes make it difficult for people with disabilities to obtain health care equal in quality to that of people without disabilities. The Rehabilitation Act and the ADA were passed more than 46 and 30 years ago, respectively, to ensure equal access to people with disabilities; however, people with disabilities continue to encounter and report multiple barriers to health care facilities and providers. This legislation, the U.S. Surgeon General's call to action (HHS, 2005) and the ADA Amendments Act of 2008 are examples of efforts to eliminate barriers encountered by people with disabilities.

People with disabilities have also reported lack of access to information, transportation difficulties, inability to pay because of limited income, difficulty finding a health care provider knowledgeable about their particular disability, previous negative health care encounters, reliance on caregivers, and the demands of coping with the disability itself (HHS, 2005). These issues affect both men and women with severe disabilities; however, women are at higher risk for receiving a lower level of health care than men. Women with disabilities are significantly less likely to receive pelvic examinations than women without disabilities; the more severe the disability, the less frequent the examination. In particular, minority women and older women with disabilities are less likely to have regular pelvic examinations and Papanicolaou (Pap) tests. Reasons given by women for not having regular pelvic examinations are difficulty transferring on to the examination table, belief that they do not need pelvic examinations because of their disability, difficulty in accessing the office or the clinic, and difficulty finding transportation (HHS, 2005). Health care providers often underestimate the effect of disabilities on women's ability to access health care, including health screening and health promotion, and they focus on women's disabilities while ignoring women's general health issues and concerns. Furthermore, women with disabilities have reported lack of knowledge about disability and insensitivity on the part of health care providers.

Individuals with disabilities living in rural settings also face barriers associated with having fewer resources and less access to care than those living in larger communities or urban settings. Therefore, establishing and maintaining involvement in their community can help ensure that they remain active and connected to others living around them, as described by Thurman, Harrison, and Walker (2019) (see the Nursing Research Profile in Chart 7-5). Additionally, those living in rural areas are less likely to have many types of recommended screenings (Goyat, Vyas, & Sambamoorthi, 2016; Magaña, Parish, Morales, et al., 2016; WHO, 2018a, 2018b).

Costs of care continue to be a factor in delaying or forgoing health care despite changes brought about by legislation, including the ADA and the Patient Protection and Affordable Care Act (ACA) (see later discussion in this chapter). Working individuals with disability are two to four times

more likely to delay necessary health care than those without disabilities. Lack of transportation and being refused care are also associated with failure to obtain needed health care among those with disabilities. Further, individuals with multiple limitations and more severe disabilities are less likely to obtain or receive health care than those without disabilities and those without multiple limitations or less severe disability (Na, Hennessy, Boner, et al., 2017; Reichard, Stransky, Phillips, et al., 2017).

Race, gender, and type of disability also affect prevalence, health status and receipt of health care and screening. For example, African American women with intellectual disabilities are less likely to receive mammography than Caucasian women with intellectual disabilities.

Because of the persistence of these and other barriers, it is essential that nurses and other health care providers take steps to ensure that clinics, offices, hospitals, and other health care facilities are accessible to people with disabilities. This includes removal of structural barriers by the addition of ramps, designation of accessible parking spaces, and modification of restrooms to make them usable by people with disabilities. Alternative communication methods (e.g., sign language interpreters, teletypewriter devices, assistive listening devices) and types of patient education (e.g., audiotapes, large print, Braille) are essential to provision of appropriate health-related information to people with disabilities. Such accommodations are mandated by the ADA, which requires their provision without cost to the patient.

People with intellectual and developmental disabilities often need assistance in obtaining health care, including preventive health screening. They often lack knowledge about cancer screening, including breast cancer screening. Educational materials and interventions modified to accommodate patients with intellectual and developmental disabilities are needed to enable them to make informed decisions about screening. Major barriers to breast cancer screening by this population of women include fear, anxiety, and embarrassment, primarily due to lack of understanding about cancer and the importance of its early detection.

Federal Assistance Programs

Lack of financial resources, including health insurance, is an important barrier to health care for people with chronic illness and disabilities. However, several federal assistance programs provide financial assistance for health-related expenses for people with some chronic illnesses, acquired disabling acute and chronic diseases, and childhood disabilities.

Medicare is a federal health insurance program that is available to most people 65 years of age and older, people with permanent kidney injury, and qualified people with disabilities. Title II of the Social Security Disability Insurance program pays benefits to those people who meet medical criteria for disability, who have worked long enough (40 quarters of covered employment) to qualify, and who have paid Social Security taxes. Title II also provides benefits to people disabled since childhood (younger than 22 years), who are dependents of a deceased insured parent or a parent entitled to disability or retirement benefits, and disabled widows or widowers, 50 to 60 years of age, if their deceased spouse was insured under Social Security. Title XVI of the Social Security

Chart 7-5	NURSING RESEARCH PROFILE
	Well-Being among Adults with Disabilities in Rural Settings

Thurman, W. A., Harrison, T. C., Walker, V. G., et al. (2019). Pursuing well-being among rural-dwelling adults with disabilities. *Qualitative Health Research, 29*(12), 1699–1710.

Purpose

The rate of disabilities is higher in rural areas globally than in more urban settings across gender, race, and type of disability or impairment. Individuals with disability who reside in rural communities are at a greater disadvantage for receiving services than those who live in urban settings. Although sociocultural and environmental factors affect the well-being of individuals with disabilities, little is known about the experience of adults with disabilities who live in rural areas. This qualitative study was conducted to explore the experience of living with a disability in rural America with the goal of greater understanding of how disability affects social roles, adaptation to impairments, and use of resources to improve well-being in individuals. The researchers' goal was to examine how working-age adults (35–70 years of age) with mobility and sensory disabilities living in rural areas of the United States define and pursue well-being.

Design

The researchers used a constructivist grounded theory approach with constant comparison analysis to study the well-being of community-residing adults with disabilities living in rural settings, defined as communities with fewer than 10,000 residents. The study participants were recruited through community organizations, newspaper announcements, word of mouth, and professional networks of the researchers. Twelve individuals who met inclusion criteria, including the ability to understand spoken or written English, participated in up to three one-to-one interviews. The interview questions addressed participants' perceptions of how their disability affected their lives over time, activities they enjoyed, qualities of their rural communities, and people who interacted with them regularly. Demographic data (e.g., age, race/ethnicity, length of time they lived in their rural setting, level of education, income, housing, employment status, occupation, age

at onset of their disability, and the structure of their family) were collected to describe the sample. The study participants had a variety of mobility and sensory impairments, including osteoarthritis, paraplegia, multiple sclerosis, hearing loss, diabetes, and heart disease. Ten of the participants used some type of assistive device.

Findings

Six concepts related to well-being were identified: values, rural attitude, demands, set expectations, strategic participation, and membership. Membership in the rural community, identified as the core category, refers to a feeling of belonging and being part of something greater than one's self. This was sustained by ongoing contributions to the rural community. Establishing and maintaining membership in the community described participants' sense of belonging to a group, and they felt that they were regarded as contributing participants in their communities. Membership also provided access to support from other community members when needed. These findings support previous research on rural settings indicating the importance of a sense of belonging to well-being. In the rural setting, social processes are used to mobilize resources needed to overcome functional limitations secondary to disability to establish group membership and create a sense of well-being. Meaningful social relationships contributed to participants' well-being, self-confidence, and self-valuing.

Nursing Implications

The findings indicate the importance of having social support, being a member of a group, and belonging to a network in which there is a reciprocal exchange of support and services for individuals with disabilities from rural communities. Thus, nurses and other health professionals working in rural settings could encourage individuals with disabilities to maintain social relationships, memberships, and participation in meaningful activities. Such participation could promote confidence and a sense of well-being and facilitate access to material and psychological support.

Disability Insurance program provides supplemental security income payments to people who are disabled and have limited income and resources.

Medicaid provides home and community-based services to people with disabilities and long-term illnesses to enable them to lead meaningful lives in their families and communities (Krahn, Walker, & Correa-De-Araujo, 2015). The ACA has expanded insurance options for people with disabilities and made these options more affordable. Furthermore, although the ACA stipulates that people with preexisting chronic conditions and disabilities can no longer be dropped by insurance companies and no longer have a lifetime cap on benefits, comparison of pre-ACA and post-ACA access to health care indicates that health disparities based on disability status persist (Kaye, 2019). Because of differences in states' implementation of the ACA, differences in access to health care among people with disability also differ (Lindner, Rowland, Spurlock, et al., 2018). See later discussion of the ACA in this chapter, and the Resources section at the end of this chapter.

Despite the availability of these federal programs, people with disabilities often have health-related costs and other expenses related to disability that result in low-income status.

Furthermore, people must undergo a disability determination process to establish eligibility for benefits, and the process can be prolonged and cumbersome for those who may need assistance in establishing their eligibility.

Nursing Care of Patients with Disability

As active members of society, people with disabilities are no longer an invisible minority. An increased awareness of their needs will bring about changes to improve access and accommodations. Modification of the physical environment permits access to public and private facilities and services, including health care, and nurses can serve as advocates for people with disabilities to eliminate discriminatory practices.

Nursing Considerations during Hospitalization

During hospitalization, as well as during periods of acute illness or injury or while recovering from surgery, patients with preexisting disabilities may require assistance with carrying out ADLs that they could otherwise manage at home independently and easily. Patients should be asked preferences about approaches to carrying out their ADLs, and assistive devices they require should be readily available. Careful planning with patients to ensure that the hospital room is arranged with their input enables them to manage as independently as possible. For example, patients who have paraplegia may be able to transfer independently from bed to their wheelchair; however, if the bed is left in an elevated position, they may be unable to do so. If patients usually use service animals to assist them with ADLs, it is necessary to make arrangements for the accommodation of these animals.

If patients with hearing loss or vision impairment are hospitalized, it is essential to establish effective communication strategies. Alternative methods for these patients to communicate with the health care team must be put in place and used, and all staff members must be aware that some patients are not able to respond to the intercom or telephone. If patients have vision impairment, it is necessary to orient them to the environment and talk to them in a normal tone of voice. When a patient has a disability that affects speech, referral with a speech-language therapist or communication specialist may assist in identifying alternative communication methods (use of sounds, gestures, eye movements) between the nurse and the patient. When a person with intellectual, cognitive, or psychiatric-mental health disability is hospitalized, the health care team must determine what strategies are effective in ensuring that the patient understands what is happening and can communicate his or her needs, promoting a safe and nonstressful environment, adhering as closely as possible to the patient's daily patterns, and consulting with the patient's family caregiver.

Health Promotion and Prevention

Health care providers often neglect health promotion concerns of people with disabilities, who may be unaware of these concerns. For example, people who have had hearing loss since childhood may lack exposure to information about new immunizations through television and podcasts. People with lifelong disabilities may not have received information about general health issues as children, and people with new onset as well as lifelong disabilities may not receive encouragement to participate in health promotion activities. Because individuals with disabilities, including those with intellectual and developmental disabilities, are living longer and aging with their disability, the need for health promotion takes on increasing importance. Therefore, nurses should take every opportunity to emphasize the importance of participation in health promotion activities (e.g., healthy diet, exercise, social interactions) and preventive health screening.

The management of some disabilities increases the risk of illness, and in some people, health screening (e.g., bone density testing, gynecologic examinations, mammography) may be required earlier in life or more frequently (HHS, 2005). Referrals by nurses to accessible sites for screening may be needed, because many imaging centers are inaccessible or staff are unprepared to make modifications for women who need assistance for screening (McClintock et al., 2018). In addition, nursing consultation with physical therapists may be needed to identify creative ways of enabling people with disabilities to exercise safely, because exercise facilities are also often inaccessible for people with disabilities.

General health promotion strategies and health-screening recommendations for all men and women also apply to those with disabilities. Although physical limitations, cognitive impairments, and structural and attitudinal barriers existing in clinical facilities may make it difficult for some men and women to obtain health care and preventive health screening, the presence of a disability should not be used as a reason or excuse to defer recommended screening. Rather, the presence of a disability may *increase* the risk of secondary health conditions or disorders that require screening and follow-up. Just as people without disabilities should have regular screening tests, such as mammography or testicular and prostate examinations, so should people with disabilities. Nurses are often in a position to influence decisions about how equipment and procedures can be adapted to meet the special needs of their patients, whether these needs are cognitive, motor, or communicative.

The effect of the disabling condition on health risks should be considered. For example, the risk of osteoporosis may be increased in women and men whose disabilities limit their ability to participate in weight-bearing exercise or who use medications that contribute to bone loss (Smeltzer & Qi, 2014). Individuals with intellectual disabilities have several additional risk factors, such as taking medications to treat seizures that contribute to bone loss. Although people with certain disabilities have an increased risk of osteoporosis at a younger age than people without disabilities, little attention is given to prevention, detection, and treatment of osteoporosis, despite the increased risk for falls associated with many disabling disorders.

Nurses can provide expert health promotion education classes that are targeted to people with disabilities and refer them to accessible online resources. Classes on nutrition and weight management are extremely important to people who are wheelchair users and need assistance with transfers. Safer sex classes are needed by adolescents and young adults who have spinal cord injury, TBI, or developmental disabilities, because the threats of sexually transmitted infections and unplanned pregnancy exist for these populations just as they do for the population in general.

The need for health promotion in the areas of establishing relationships, sex, pregnancy, and childbearing is as great in people with disabilities, including those with intellectual and cognitive disabilities, as in people without disabilities. However, societal attitudes and biases against sexual relationships and childbearing in people with disabilities often result in health care providers either excluding such individuals from discussions about these issues, or failing to take their interest and questions seriously. Approaching these topics at the point of interest and knowledge level of a patient with a disability is important for sexual health. Furthermore, addressing sexual issues is important to prepare people with disabilities, who are at risk for sexual and other forms of abuse, to distinguish between healthy and abusive or exploitative sexual interactions and relationships. The increased risk for abuse and violence affects both men and women with disabilities; such abuse and violence has potential physical and psychological consequences that must be assessed and addressed (Dembo, Mitra, & McKee, 2018).

Other healthy behaviors about which people with neurologic disabilities need education include avoiding alcohol and nonprescription medications while taking antispasmodic and anticonvulsant medications, which are commonly prescribed for those with disabilities.

 Veterans Considerations

Growing attention has addressed health issues of veterans, those individuals who have served in the military, including service-connected disability and chronic illness. There are currently 18.5 million U.S. veterans. Over 41% of those who served in the military after September 11, 2001 ("911") in Afghanistan, Iraq, and other war zones have disabilities, which is significantly higher than the rate of 25% of veterans from earlier eras (U.S. Census Bureau, 2018b). Many have more severe disabilities than previous veterans, because of survival of those who previously would have died from their injuries. In addition, the increased use of explosive devices in warfare has increased the number of veterans with limb loss and TBI. The impact of disability on the lives of veterans and their families is considerable and multifaceted and must be considered when providing care to them. Asking patients, "Have you ever served in the military?" is the first step to identifying health-related issues that veterans face when seeking health care; asking this question also acknowledges the importance of military service to veterans.

Significance of "People-First" Language

It is important to all people, both those with and those without disabilities, that they not be equated with their illness or physical condition. Therefore, nurses should refer to all people using "people-first" language. That means referring to the person first: "the patient with diabetes" rather than "the diabetic" or "the diabetic patient," "the person with a disability" rather than the "disabled person," "women with disabilities" rather than "disabled women," and "people who are wheelchair users" rather than "the wheelchair bound." This simple use of language conveys the message that the person, rather than the illness or disability, is of greater importance to the nurse.

 Gerontologic Considerations

The demographic profile in the United States reflects an increased number of older adults with disabilities, with two thirds of Americans 85 years of age and older experiencing functional limitations. Age-related disabilities are those that occur in the older adult population and are thought to be attributable to the aging process. Examples of age-related disabilities include osteoarthritis, osteoporosis, and hearing loss.

Although disability is often perceived as being associated with old age, it occurs across the lifespan; in fact, the majority of people with disabilities are younger than 65 years, with one third between 44 and 65 years of age (Krahn et al., 2015). While many people with intellectual and developmental disabilities (cerebral palsy, Down syndrome, autism spectrum disorder) have a slightly shorter lifespan than other people from their age cohort, others live well into adulthood and old age. The number of adults with intellectual and developmental disabilities aged 60 years and older is expected to nearly double from 850,600 in 2010 to 1.4 million by 2030 (Heller, 2017).

Aging is an important issue that affects people with preexisting disabilities, as they often develop changes associated with aging at a younger age than do those without disabilities. Therefore, people with preexisting disability should be evaluated for early onset of changes related to aging. The nurse must also consider the effects of aging on a preexisting disability and in turn the effects of disability on aging. The following are examples of changes that occur with aging in people with preexisting disabilities:

- People who use crutches for ambulation because of spina bifida, polio, and lower extremity amputation may experience muscle or joint problems as they age because of long-time overuse of the upper extremities; symptoms may not occur for many years but may cause discomfort and interfere with the person's ability to perform ADLs.
- People who experienced respiratory compromise with the onset of polio decades earlier may experience increasing respiratory symptoms with aging (National Institute of Neurological Disorders and Stroke, 2019). Others experience increased muscle weakness and fatigue, making it necessary to begin to use more extensive assistive devices for mobility (Duncan & Batliwalla, 2018).
- Women with long-standing mobility limitations, lack of weight-bearing exercise, and issues associated with intellectual disabilities may experience bone loss and osteoporosis prior to menopause, yet their rate of screening is low (Dreyfus, Lauer, & Wilkinson, 2014; Heller, 2017; Smeltzer & Qi, 2014).

Concern about what the future holds is common in people aging with preexisting disabilities, who may have questions about what physical, financial, and emotional supports they will have as they age (Nosek, 2000). For example, if their disability becomes more severe, they may be concerned about entering an assisted living or a long-term care facility. The nurse should recognize the concerns of people with disabilities about their future and encourage them to make suitable plans, which may relieve some of their fears about what will happen to them as they age.

Aging parents of adult children with intellectual or developmental disabilities often fear what will happen when they are no longer available and able to care for their children. Limited long-term care resources, increased life expectancy for people with developmental disabilities, changing family patterns, and competition with the older adult population for similar resources increase the fears of these parents. Thus, nurses must identify needed community resources and services. Identifying these issues and concerns and assessing arrangements made by aging parents of adult children with disabilities can help reduce some of parents' fears about their children's futures.

Disability in Medical-Surgical Nursing Practice

Disability is often considered an issue that is specific or confined to rehabilitation, pediatrics, or gerontologic nursing. However, as noted previously, disability can occur across the lifespan and is encountered in all settings. Patients with preexisting disabilities due to conditions that have been present from birth or to illnesses or injuries experienced as an adolescent or young adult or during middle age often require health care and nursing care in medical-surgical settings. It is important to note that even if a disability has been present for patients' entire lives and they have adapted to it, the disability may still have implications for nursing care and needs to be considered in planning and providing care.

Although in the past many people with lifelong disabilities or adult onset of severe disabilities may have had shortened lifespans, today most can expect to have normal or near-normal lifespans and to live productive and meaningful lives. They are also at risk for the same acute illnesses that can affect all people and are at increased risk for aging-related chronic diseases due to smoking, obesity, and lack of physical activity. In addition, they are at increased risk for unintentional injuries, with fall-related injuries the most common type of injury.

Because of unfavorable interactions with health care providers, including negative attitudes, insensitivity, and lack of knowledge, people with disabilities may avoid seeking medical intervention or health care services. For this reason, and because the number of people with disabilities is increasing, nurses must acquire knowledge and skills and be available to assist them in maintaining a high level of wellness. Nurses are in key positions to influence the architectural design of health care settings and the selection of equipment that promotes ease of access and health. Padded examination tables that can be raised or lowered make transfers easier for people with disabilities. Birthing chairs benefit women with disability during yearly pelvic examinations and Pap smears and during urologic evaluations. Ramps, grab bars, and raised and padded toilet seats benefit many people who have neurologic or musculoskeletal disabilities and need routine physical examination and monitoring. When a patient with a disability is admitted to the hospital for any reason, the patient's needs for these modifications should be assessed and addressed.

Men and women with disabilities may be encountered in hospitals, clinics, offices, and nursing centers when they seek health care to address a problem related to their disability. However, they may also be encountered in these settings when they seek care for a health problem that is not related in any way to their disability. For example, a woman with spina bifida, spinal cord injury, or post-polio syndrome might seek health care related to a gynecologic issue, such as vaginal bleeding. Although her disability should be considered in the course of assessment and delivery of health and nursing care, it should not be the exclusive focus of the assessment or care that she receives. Furthermore, neither a severe physical disability that affects a woman's ability to transfer to an examination table for a gynecologic examination nor a cognitive disability should be a reason to defer a complete health assessment and physical examination, including a pelvic examination. Reproductive care for women with disabilities is notoriously lacking due to absence of appropriate accessible equipment and facilities, health care providers' unfamiliarity with health issues of women with disabilities, and negative attitudes toward women with disabilities who are sexually active or who are pregnant or considering pregnancy (Hasson-Ohayon, Hason-Shaked, Silberg, et al., 2018; Hayward et al., 2017; LaPierre et al., 2017; Mitra et al., 2017; Nosek, 2000; Tarasoff, 2017). Nurses who are knowledgeable about these issues and other barriers can make a significant impact on the quality of health care these women receive.

Health care, including preventive health screening and health promotion, is essential to enable people with disabilities to live the highest quality of life within the limitations imposed by their disabling conditions. Men and women with disabilities have the same needs and same rights for health care and preventive health screening as others, although in some cases, the consequences of their disability increase rather than decrease their need for health screening and participation in health-promoting activities. Therefore, it is essential that medical-surgical nurses be knowledgeable about disability and how it affects people across the lifespan as well as how to provide sensitive and quality nursing care for patients with preexisting and new-onset disability. In an effort to address these issues, specific information on health care of people with disabilities has been included throughout this book.

Home, Community-Based, and Transitional Care

 Educating Patients About Self-Care

Chart 7-6 contains points the nurse should consider when educating patients about managing disability at home. A major and often overlooked issue in educating patients about a health problem, a treatment regimen, or health promotion strategies is the need for alternative formats to accommodate people with various disabilities. Patients with disabilities are in need of the same information as other patients; however, they often require large print, Braille, audiotapes, or the assistance of a sign language interpreter. Materials may be obtained from a variety of sources for patients who need these educational strategies and for patients with cognitive impairments attributable to developmental disabilities or newly acquired disabilities.

Nurses should ensure that all people—whether or not they have disabilities—recognize the warning signs and symptoms of stroke, heart attack, and cancer, as well as how to access help. In addition, nurses should educate all patients who are stroke survivors and those with diabetes how to monitor their own blood pressure or glucose levels.

Continuing and Transitional Care

When caring for patients with disabilities and helping them plan for discharge and continuing care in the home, it is important to consider how a particular disability affects a patient's ability to adhere to recommended treatment regimens and keep follow-up appointments. Furthermore, it is important to consider how the health issue or treatment regimen affects the disability. Although many people with disabilities are independent and able to make decisions, arrangements for transportation, and appointments to accessible facilities, others may have difficulty doing so, particularly if they are experiencing a health problem. The nurse should recognize the effect that the disability has on the patient's ability to follow-up. The nurse should ask the patient whether they anticipate having any difficulties arranging for follow-up care. It is important for the nurse to assist the patient with disabilities to identify unmet needs and to find and use resources (community and social resources, and transportation services) that enable the patient to obtain needed services while remaining in his or her home, if preferred. The nurse should have a list of accessible sites and services available and share

Chart 7-6	HOME CARE CHECKLIST

Managing Disability and Chronic Illness at Home

At the completion of education, the patient and/or caregiver will be able to:

- State the impact of disability or chronic illness on physiologic functioning, ADLs, IADLs, roles, relationships, and spirituality.
- State changes in lifestyle (e.g., diet, activity) necessary to maintain health.
- State the name, dose, side effects, frequency, and schedule for all medications.
- State how to carry out prescribed regimens (e.g., skin care, bladder/bowel care, daily weights).
- State how to obtain medical supplies after discharge.
- Identify durable medical equipment needs, proper usage, and maintenance necessary for safe utilization.
- Demonstrate safe usage of adaptive equipment for ADLs.
- Identify community resources for peer and caregiver/family support:
  - Identify sources of support (e.g., friends, relatives, faith community)

- Identify phone numbers of support groups for people with chronic illness/disabilities and their caregivers/families
- State meeting locations and times
- Demonstrate safe mobility skills and/or how to access transportation.
- Identify community resources for recreation:
  - State local recreation centers that offer programs for people with disabilities
  - Identify leisure activities that can be pursued in the community
- State how to reach health care provider with questions or complications.
- State time and date of follow-up appointments.
- Identify the need for health promotion, disease prevention, and preventive screening activities.

those resources with the patient and the family. In collaboration with other health care providers (occupational and physical therapists, speech therapists), the nurse can identify needed home modifications, including those that are simple and inexpensive, that will enable the patient to participate in self-care at home.

Transitional care, if available, is ideal for patients with severe disabilities being discharged home. Patients hospitalized for an acute or secondary health condition may be more vulnerable to deterioration in health status or developing other health conditions because of their narrow margin of health or deconditioning that occurs with hospitalization. Important roles of the transitional care nurse are to ensure that required services are available in the home at the time of the patient's discharge, to assess and monitor the patient through home visits, and to provide support and assistance to the patient and the family in the aftermath of hospitalization and discharge (Naylor, Shaid, Carpenter, et al., 2017).

Chronic Disease and Chronic Illness

Chronic disease refers to **noncommunicable diseases** (conditions not caused by an acute infection or injury), chronic conditions, or chronic disorders. In contrast, **chronic illness** refers to the human experience of living with a chronic disease or condition. Chronic illness includes the person's perception of the experience of having a chronic disease or condition and the person's and others' responses to it, including health care professionals (Larsen, 2019). Persons' and their families' values and previous experiences determine their perceptions and beliefs about the condition, which in turn affect their illness and wellness behaviors. Their values are influenced by a number of demographic, socioeconomic, technologic, cultural, and environmental variables. Only the person and the family really know what it is like to live with chronic illness (Larsen, 2019).

The following section of this chapter discusses chronic illness and its implications for nursing practice. Because some degree of disability is often present in severe or advanced chronic illness, the previous discussion about disability is relevant to chronic disease as well.

Chronic diseases are long-term health conditions that affect one's well-being and function in an episodic, continuous, or progressive way over many years of life. Although each chronic disease or condition has its own specific physiologic characteristics, many chronic conditions share common features. For example, common symptoms typically include pain, fatigue, sleep disturbances, and difficulty adjusting to the onset and uncertainty of a chronic condition (Larsen, 2019). Many people with chronic health conditions and disability function independently with little or no inconvenience to their everyday lives; others, however, require frequent and close monitoring or placement in long-term care facilities. Certain conditions require advanced technology for survival, as in the late stages of chronic obstructive lung disease or end-stage renal disease, or intensive care or mechanical ventilation for periods of weeks, months, or years. People with disorders such as these have been described as being chronically critically ill, although there is no consensus on a definition of chronic critical illness. An overview of chronic disease in the United States is presented in Chart 7-7.

Multiple Chronic Conditions

Having **multiple chronic conditions (MCC)** increases the complexity of care and often necessitates care by multiple health care specialists, a variety of treatment regimens, and prescription medications that may not interact. Thus, patients with MCC are at risk for conflicting medical advice, adverse effects of medications, unnecessary and duplicative tests, and preventable hospitalizations, all of which can negatively affect their health (CDC, 2019b). Patients with MCC and their families may have to keep track of different medications with different schedules and multiple appointments with various health care professionals. Costs of health care increase with the number of chronic conditions a person has; those with five or more chronic conditions account for 41% of total health expenditures in the United States (Buttorff, Ruder, & Bauman, 2017). Approximately 80% of health care costs in the

Chart 7-7

Overview of Chronic Illness in the United States

- Chronic diseases are the leading causes of death and disability in the United States.
- Chronic disease and conditions (e.g., heart disease, stroke, cancer, diabetes, obesity, arthritis) are among the most common, costly, and preventable of all health problems.
- Heart disease, cancer, stroke, chronic lower respiratory diseases, Alzheimer's disease, and diabetes pose greater risks as people age.
- Chronic disease, specifically diabetes, is the leading cause of kidney failure, amputation of lower extremities, and new causes of blindness among adults.
- Obesity is a serious health concern with one third of adults and one of five youths having obesity.
- Lack of exercise or physical activity, poor nutrition, use of tobacco, and excessive alcohol use contribute to the growing prevalence of chronic diseases and resulting disability. Tobacco remains the leading cause of six million preventable deaths per year globally. Although cigarette smoking among U.S. youths has declined steadily over the past two decades, the recent introduction of electronic nicotine delivery systems (ENDS) has resulted in increased exposure of youth to nicotine, considered an epidemic by the U.S. Surgeon General's office.
- Americans living in rural communities are more likely to have chronic disease, such as high blood pressure, heart disease, and diabetes, than those living in nonrural areas.
- Eighty-six percent of all health care spending is related in general to chronic disease.
- People with chronic disease may have other health problems that may or may not be related to the primary chronic disease; these include alcohol abuse and substance use or addiction disorders, mental illness, dementia or other cognitive impairments, and developmental disabilities.

Adapted from AARP. (2017). Chronic conditions among older adults. Retrieved on 11/25/20 at: www.assets.aarp.org/rgcenter/health/beyond_50_hcr_conditions.pdf; Agency for Healthcare Research and Quality. (2018). *2017 National healthcare quality and disparities report*. Rockville, MD: Agency for Healthcare Research and Quality; American Heart Association. (2019). Cardiovascular diseases affect nearly half of American adults, statistics show. Retrieved on 7/19/2019 at: www.heart.org/en/news/2019/01/31/cardiovascular-diseases-affect-nearly-half-of-american-adults-statistics-show; Buttorff, C., Ruder, T., Bauman, M. (2017). Multiple chronic conditions in the United States. Retrieved on 01/01/2018 at: www.rand.org/pubs/tools/TL221.html; Centers for Disease Control and Prevention (CDC), National Center for Chronic Disease Prevention and Health Promotion (NCCDPHP). (2019a). At a glance. Prevalence of chronic illnesses. Retrieved on 7/19/2019 at: www.cdc.gov/chronicdisease/resources/infographic/chronic-diseases.htm; Centers for Disease Control and Prevention (CDC), National Center for Chronic Disease Prevention and Health Promotion (NCCDPHP). (2019b). Multiple chronic conditions. Retrieved on 7/19/2019 at: www.cdc.gov/chronicdisease/about/multiple-chronic.htm; Raghupathi, W., & Raghupathi, V. (2018). An empirical study of chronic diseases in the United States: A visual analytics approach to public health. *International Journal of Environmental Research and Public Health, 15*(3), 431–455.

Chart 7-8

Facts About Multiple Chronic Conditions (MCC)

- About half of all adults—117 million people—have one or more chronic health conditions. One of every four adults has two or more chronic health conditions.
- The occurrence of MCC increases with age. Three in every four Americans 65 years of age and older have MCC.
- The number of people with MCC is predicted to increase substantially over the next decade, adding to the pressures on the health care system to deliver high quality of care, at optimal cost, while improving the health of this complex population.
- Women are more likely than men to have MCC.
- Non-Hispanic White adults, non-Hispanic Black adults, and non-Hispanic adults of other races have a high prevalence of MCC.
- As the number of chronic conditions a person has increases, the greater the risk of dying prematurely, being hospitalized, and having poor day-to-day functioning.
- Many patients with MCC have mobility limitations and require assistance with dressing, bathing, or preparing meals.
- People with MCC account for the majority of health care visits, prescriptions, home health visits, and hospital stays in the United States.

Adapted from Buttorff, C., Ruder, T., & Bauman, M. (2017). Multiple chronic conditions in the United States. Retrieved on 11/25/20 at: www.rand.org/pubs/tools/TL221.html; Centers for Disease Control and Prevention (CDC), National Center for Chronic Disease Prevention and Health Promotion (NCCDPHP). (2019b). Multiple chronic conditions. Retrieved on 11/25/20 at: www.cdc.gov/chronicdisease/about/multiple-chronic.htm

Health Disparities and Chronic Disease

Although chronic disease occurs in all socioeconomic groups, people from low-income and disadvantaged backgrounds are more likely to report poor health. Factors such as poverty and inadequate health insurance decrease the likelihood that people with chronic illness or disability receive health care and preventive health-screening measures such as mammography, cholesterol testing, and routine checkups (National Academies of Sciences, Engineering, and Medicine [NASEM], 2017; Raghupathi & Raghupathi, 2018). In addition, chronic conditions can lead to poverty for the patient and the family. There also are implications for society or the nation as a whole, because chronic conditions or subsequent premature deaths occur most commonly during the most productive years for people with chronic conditions.

Disparities in health and health outcomes are associated with social, economic, and environmental disadvantages. Although the gap between health outcomes in African Americans and Caucasians has decreased in some areas, in others (e.g., mortality due to breast cancer) the gaps have increased. Disparities in health and health outcomes are associated with higher incidence and prevalence, earlier onset, faster progression, and poorer outcomes of disease and conditions (NASEM, 2017; Raghupathi & Raghupathi, 2018).

Some chronic conditions have little effect on quality of life, whereas others have a major effect because they result in disability. However, not all disabilities are a result of chronic illness, and not all chronic illnesses cause disability. Unlike

United States are associated with having MCC. Approximately 93% of the total health care expenditures for those who are covered by Medicare are associated with MCC. In addition, out-of-pocket health-related expenses increase with the number of MCC. Facts about MCC are summarized in Chart 7-8.

the term *acute*, which implies a curable and relatively short disease course, the term *chronic* describes a long disease course that may be incurable. This often makes managing chronic conditions difficult for those who live with them. Yet nurses can and do make a difference in the experience of chronic illness by providing quality nursing care in the absence of a cure (Larsen, 2019).

Psychological and emotional reactions of patients to acute and chronic conditions and changes in their health status are described in Chapter 5. People who develop chronic conditions or disabilities may react with shock, disbelief, anger, resentment, or other emotions. How people react to and cope with chronic illness is usually similar to how they react to other events in their lives, depending, in part, on their understanding of the condition and their perceptions of its potential impact on their own and their family's lives. Adjustment to chronic illness (and disability) is affected by various factors:

- Suddenness, extent, and duration of lifestyle changes necessitated by the illness
- Uncertainty related to the course and outcome of chronic illnesses
- Family and individual resources for dealing with stress
- Availability of support from family, friends, and the community
- Stages of individual/family life cycle
- Previous experience with illness and crises
- Underlying personality characteristics
- Unresolved anger or grief from the past

Psychological, emotional, and cognitive reactions to chronic conditions are likely to occur at their onset and to recur if symptoms worsen or return after a period of remission. Symptoms associated with chronic health conditions are often unpredictable and may be perceived as crisis events by patients and their families, who must contend with both the uncertainty of chronic illness and the changes it brings to their lives. The possible effects of chronic conditions can guide nursing assessment and interventions for the patient who has a chronic illness.

Definitions of Chronic Diseases or Conditions

Chronic diseases or conditions are often defined as medical conditions or health problems with associated symptoms or disabilities that require long-term management. Chronic diseases are those that persist for months or years rather than days or weeks (Larson, 2019). The National Center for Health Statistics defines chronic disease as a condition lasting 3 or more months; the CDC's National Center for Chronic Disease Prevention and Health Promotion (NCCDPHP) (CDC, 2019a) defines it as a condition that lasts for a year or more and that can usually be controlled but not cured. Definitions of chronic disease or chronic illness share the characteristics of being irreversible, having a prolonged course, and remaining unlikely to resolve spontaneously (Larsen, 2019). The specific chronic condition may be a result of illness, genetic factors, or injury; it may be a consequence of conditions or unhealthy behaviors that began during childhood and young adulthood.

The social determinants of health (SDOH) provide a useful framework to identify factors that affect a person's or a population's health, including the prevalence of chronic disease, its management, the quality of health care that is available, and the outcomes of chronic disease. The main SDOH that have been identified include income and social status, employment and working conditions, education and literacy, childhood experiences, physical environment, social supports and coping skills, healthy behaviors, access to health services, biology and genetic makeup, gender, culture, race and ethnicity (Office of Disease Prevention and Health Promotion, 2019).

The effect of SDOH is illustrated by large discrepancies in life expectancy, up to a 48-year difference among countries and 20 years or more within countries. Deaths due to chronic disease are expected to increase globally, from 41 million deaths reported in 2016 (many of which were premature) to 52 million per year by 2030 (Raghupathi & Raghupathi, 2018; WHO, 2018c, 2019).

Management of chronic conditions includes learning to live with symptoms or resulting disabilities and coming to terms with identity changes resulting from having a chronic condition. Management also consists of carrying out the lifestyle changes and regimens designed to control symptoms and prevent complications. Although some people assume what might be called a "sick role" identity, most people with chronic conditions do not consider themselves to be sick or ill and try to live as normal a life as possible. Only when complications develop or symptoms interfere with ADLs do most people with chronic health conditions think of themselves as being sick or having a disability.

Prevalence and Causes of Chronic Conditions

Chronic conditions occur in people of every age group, socioeconomic level, race, and culture. Six in 10 adults in the United States have a chronic disease. Chronic diseases are the most common causes of death in the United States; the most frequently occurring chronic diseases account for 7 of the 10 leading causes of death, with cancer and heart disease together accounting for nearly half of all deaths. Globally, chronic diseases are responsible for more than two thirds of deaths. Chronic diseases include cancers, cardiovascular disease, diabetes, and chronic lung diseases (CDC, 2019a).

Chronic diseases or disorders are one of the major health and development challenges of this century because of their global impact on human, social, and financial well-being and status. Although chronic diseases affect all countries, their impact is more severe in low- and middle-income countries, with devastating consequences in poor and vulnerable populations. Chronic diseases cause more deaths than all other causes combined, and lifespan is shortened by chronic illnesses in those countries.

It is predicted that by the year 2030, about half the population will have a chronic disease or disorder. One fifth of those with chronic disease also have an activity limitation. As the incidence of chronic diseases increases, the costs associated with these chronic conditions (e.g., hospital costs, equipment, medications, supportive services) also increase. These costs represent four of every five health care dollars expended. In the United States, chronic diseases are also leading drivers of the nation's $3.5 trillion in annual health care costs (NCCDPHP, 2020; Raghupathi & Raghupathi, 2018).

Although some chronic diseases are associated with non-modifiable factors, including genetic and physiologic factors, many are the result of unhealthy lifestyles. Most chronic diseases are caused by four major behaviors: use of tobacco, electronic nicotine delivery systems (ENDS), and exposure to secondhand smoke; poor nutrition (diets high in sodium and saturated fats and low in fruits and vegetables); lack of physical activity; and excessive consumption of alcohol (CDC, 2019a; WHO, 2018c). Because these behaviors are modifiable, nurses have a major role in the prevention of chronic disorders associated with these behaviors (for more detailed information, see later discussion in section on Prevention of Chronic Disease).

Some chronic health conditions cause little or no inconvenience; others are severe enough to cause major activity limitations that may prevent people from meeting their needs for health care and personal services. For example, they may be unable to carry out their therapeutic regimens or have their prescriptions filled on time, may miss appointments and office visits with their health care providers, and may be unable to manage ADLs.

Chronic diseases are a global issue that affects both rich and poor nations. The total number of people dying from chronic disease is twice that of patients dying from infectious (including human immunodeficiency virus infection), maternal, and perinatal conditions, and nutritional deficiencies combined (WHO, 2019). Most of these chronic diseases and complications of chronic illness are preventable, emphasizing the importance of health promotion across the globe. Although chronic diseases or illnesses are common, people have many myths or misunderstandings about them (Table 7-1).

Causes of the increasing number of people with chronic conditions include the following:

- A decrease in mortality from infectious diseases (e.g., smallpox, diphtheria, acquired immune deficiency syndrome [AIDS]–related infections) because of immunizations and new drug development and from acute conditions (e.g., myocardial infarction, trauma) because of prompt and aggressive management.
- Lifestyle factors such as smoking, chronic stress, poor nutrition, and sedentary lifestyle that increase the risk of chronic health problems such as respiratory disease, hypertension, cardiovascular disease, and obesity. Although signs and symptoms of chronic illness often first appear during older age, risks typically begin earlier in life, even during fetal development.
- Obesity, often due to lifestyle issues, has become a major health issue across the lifespan and across the globe with about 2.1 billion people overweight and one third of them having obesity. Obesity is no longer limited to high-income countries but increasingly occurs in low- and middle-income countries. The proportion of adults with a body mass index (BMI) of 25 or greater increased between 1980 and 2013 from about 29% to 37% in men and about 30% to 38% in women (Kushner & Kahan, 2018). It is estimated that unless this trend is reversed, almost half of the world's population will be overweight or have obesity by 2030. Approximately 5% of deaths worldwide are due to obesity (Tremmel, Gerdtham, Nilsson, et al., 2017). The increasing prevalence of obesity has increased the incidence of heart

---

TABLE 7-1 Myths and Truths About Chronic Disease

Common Misconceptions About Chronic Disease	The Reality About Chronic Disease
1. Everyone dies of something.	Chronic illnesses typically do not result in sudden death but often result in progressive illness and disability. People with chronic disease often die slowly, painfully, and prematurely.
2. People can live to old age even if they lead unhealthy lives (smoke, have obesity).	While there are exceptions (some people who live unhealthy lives live to old age, and some people who live healthy lives develop chronic illnesses), most chronic illnesses can be traced to modifiable risk factors and can be prevented by eliminating these risks.
3. Solutions for chronic disease prevention and control are expensive and not feasible for low- and middle-income countries.	A full range of chronic disease interventions are very cost-effective for all regions of the world, including the poorest. Many of these interventions are inexpensive to implement.
4. Nothing can be done to prevent chronic diseases.	The major causes of chronic diseases are known, and if these risk factors were eliminated, at least more than 80% of heart disease, stroke, and type 2 diabetes and more than 40% of cancers would be prevented.
5. If individuals develop chronic disease as a result of unhealthy "lifestyles," they have only themselves to blame.	Individual responsibility can have its full effect only if individuals have equal access to a healthy life and are supported to make healthy choices. People who are poor often have limited choices about the food they eat, their living conditions, and access to education and health care.
6. Certain chronic diseases primarily affect men.	Chronic diseases, including heart disease, affect women and men almost equally. Almost half of all deaths attributed to chronic illness occur in women.
7. Chronic diseases primarily affect people who are old.	Almost half of chronic disease deaths occur prematurely in people younger than 70 years of age.
8. Chronic diseases mainly affect people who are rich (affluent).	People who are poor are much more likely than those who are wealthy to develop chronic diseases and as a result are more likely to die prematurely. Chronic diseases cause substantial financial burden and result in extreme poverty.
9. The priority of low- and middle-income countries should be on control of infectious diseases.	Although infectious diseases are an issue, low- and middle-income countries are experiencing a dramatic increase in chronic disease risk factors and deaths, especially in urban settings.
10. Chronic diseases affect mostly high-income countries.	Eighty percent of deaths attributed to chronic disease are in low- and middle-income countries. The prevalence of chronic diseases in low- and middle-income countries is rapidly growing.

Adapted from World Health Organization (WHO). (2005). Face the facts #2: Widespread misunderstandings about chronic disease—and the reality. Retrieved on 7/15/2019 at: www.who.int/chp/chronic_disease_report/media/Factsheet2.pdf

disease, strokes, diabetes, and hypertension. Obesity also affects one's self-esteem, achievement, and emotional state. In 2015, high BMI contributed to four million deaths globally, which was over 7% of deaths from any cause (Kushner & Kahan, 2018).

- Longer lifespans because of advances in technology and pharmacology, improved nutrition, safer working conditions, and greater access (for some people) to health care.
- Improved screening and diagnostic procedures enabled early detection and treatment of diseases, resulting in improved outcomes of management of cancer and other disorders.

Physiologic changes in the body often occur before the appearance of symptoms of chronic disease. Therefore, the goal of emphasizing healthy lifestyles early in life is to improve overall health status and slow the development of such disorders. In addition, serious psychiatric or mental illness disorders puts people at greater risk for chronic illness than the general population and leads to higher morbidity and mortality rates of chronic diseases (National Prevention Council, 2016).

Prevention of Chronic Disease

The CDC (2019a) has identified risk factors for common chronic diseases and pointed out that most American adults have more than one of the following risk factors:

- Hypertension (high blood pressure)
- Tobacco and ENDS use or exposure to secondhand smoke
- Overweight or obesity (high BMI)
- Lack of physical activity
- Excessive alcohol use
- Consumption of diets low in fruits and vegetables
- Consumption of food high in sodium and saturated fats

The WHO (2005, 2013) has identified high-impact, cost-effective interventions to prevent premature death due to chronic disease or chronic conditions that can be implemented even in settings with limited resources. These interventions, summarized in Chart 7-9, are consistent with the risk factors for chronic disease identified by the CDC.

Patient education to prevent chronic disease or reduce its severity or effects is another important component of the nurse's role in working with patients to identify risks for chronic disease and to identify strategies to reduce those risks. Health promotion and patient education are discussed in detail in Chapter 3 in this book.

Characteristics of Chronic Conditions

Sometimes it is difficult for people who are disease free to understand the profound effect that chronic illness often has on the lives of patients and their families. It is easy for health professionals to focus on the illness or disability itself while overlooking the person who has the disorder. In all illnesses, but even more so with chronic conditions, the illness cannot be separated from the person. People with chronic illness must contend with it daily (Larsen, 2019). To properly manage their chronic condition, individuals often have to find the time, as well as the social and financial resources, to participate in physically and psychologically beneficial activities, work with health care professionals to follow treatment guidelines, monitor their health and

---

Chart 7-9 **Interventions According to Risk Factors**

Tobacco

- Reduce affordability of tobacco and electronic nicotine delivery systems (ENDS) including e-cigarettes, e-pens, e-pipes, e-hookah, and e-cigars by increasing their costs.
- Legally mandate smoke-free environments in all indoor workplaces, public places, and public transport.
- Disseminate warnings about dangers of tobacco, tobacco smoke, and ENDS through mass media campaigns and ban all forms of tobacco advertising, promotion, and sponsorship.

Harmful Use of Alcohol

- Reduce affordability of alcohol by increasing its costs.
- Limit availability of alcohol.
- Ban all forms of alcohol advertising and promotions.

Diet and Physical Activity

- Promote reduction of dietary salt intake and replacement of trans fats with unsaturated fats.
- Implement public awareness programs on diet and physical activity.
- Promote and protect breast-feeding (reduces risk of obesity later in life).

Cardiovascular Disease and Diabetes

- Promote glycemic control for diabetes and control of hypertension using medication therapy.
- Counsel individuals who have had a heart attack or stroke and those people at high risk of a fatal and nonfatal cardiovascular event in the next 10 years.
- Initiate acetylsalicylic acid (aspirin) use for acute myocardial infarction.

Cancer

- Promote hepatitis B immunization to prevent liver cancer.
- Promote screening, immunization with the HPV vaccine, and early treatment of precancerous lesions to prevent cervical cancer.

Adapted from World Health Organization (WHO). (2013). Global action plan for the prevention and control of noncommunicable diseases, 2013–2020. Geneva, Switzerland: Author.

---

make decisions about their health and lifestyle and those of their family, and manage the effects of the illness on their physical, psychological, and social well-being. To relate to what people must cope with or to plan effective interventions, nurses must understand the multiple characteristics of a chronic illness.

- Psychological and social issues: Managing chronic illness involves more than treating medical problems. Associated psychological and social issues must also be addressed, because living for long periods with illness symptoms and disability can threaten identity, bring about role changes, alter body image, and disrupt lifestyles, work, and family life. These changes require continuous adaptation and accommodation, depending on the patient's age and situation in life. Each change or decline in functional ability requires physical, emotional, and social adaptation for patients and their families (Corbin, 2003; Larsen, 2019).

- Course of chronic disease: Chronic health conditions usually involve many different phases over the course of a person's lifetime. There can be acute periods, stable and unstable periods, flare-ups, and remissions. Each phase brings its own set of physical, psychological, and social problems, and each requires its own regimens and types of management. Individuals with chronic illnesses may experience high levels of stress or anxiety with each change in the course of their illness.
- Progression of chronic disease: The rate of progression of chronic diseases can vary from a rapid downhill course leading quickly to disability and death within a few months of onset to those with a slow downhill progression over years. Others may be characterized by disappearance of signs and symptoms with a return to "normal" with later return of symptoms, or relapses.
- Therapeutic regimens: Keeping chronic conditions under control requires persistent adherence to therapeutic regimens that may be complex and may interfere with usual activities or even life goals. Failing to adhere to a treatment plan or to do so consistently increases the risks of developing complications and accelerating the disease process. However, the realities of daily life, including the impact of culture, values, and socioeconomic factors, affect the degree to which people adhere to a treatment regimen. Managing a chronic illness takes time, requires knowledge and often planning, and can be uncomfortable and inconvenient. It is not unusual for patients to stop taking medications or alter dosages because of side effects that are more disturbing or disruptive than symptoms of the illness, or to cut back on regimens they consider overly time-consuming, fatiguing, or costly (Corbin, 2003; Larsen, 2019).
- Development of other chronic conditions: One chronic disease can lead to the development of other chronic conditions. Diabetes, for example, can lead to neurologic and vascular changes that may result in visual, cardiac, and kidney diseases and erectile dysfunction. The presence of a chronic illness also contributes to a higher risk of morbidity and mortality in patients admitted to the intensive care unit with acute health conditions as well as greater utilization of clinical services during hospitalization.
- Family life: Chronic illness affects the entire family. Family life can be dramatically altered as a result of role reversals, unfilled roles, loss of income, time required to manage the illness, decreases in family socialization activities, and the costs of treatment. Family members often become caregivers for the person with chronic illness while trying to continue to work and keep the family intact. Over 16.6% of the U.S. adult population are considered caregivers for a family member with a chronic illness, or with a disability, or who is an older adult. Although many caregivers derive positive effects from providing care, many are employed and attempting to maintain as normal a life as possible for their families. Stress, depression, fatigue, and loss of sleep as well as missed days of work are not uncommon. Thus, the wellbeing of caregivers merits attention by nurses and other health care providers (Hopps, Iadeluca, & McDonald, 2017).
- Home life: The day-to-day management of illness is largely the responsibility of people with chronic disorders and their families. As a result, the home, rather than the hospital, is the center of care in chronic conditions. Hospitals, clinics, primary care providers' offices, nursing homes, nursing centers, and community agencies (home care services, social services, and disease-specific associations and societies) are considered adjuncts or backup services to daily home management.
- Self-management: The management of chronic conditions is a continual process. People can be taught how to manage their conditions. However, each patient must discover how his or her own body reacts under varying circumstances—for example, what it is like to be hypoglycemic, what activities are likely to bring on angina, and how these or other conditions can best be prevented and managed.
- Collaborative process: Managing chronic conditions must be a collaborative process that involves many different health care professionals working together with patients and their families to provide the services and supports that are often needed for management at home. The medical, social, and psychological aspects of chronic health problems are often complex, especially in severe conditions.
- Health care costs: The management of chronic conditions is expensive. Many expenses incurred by an individual patient (e.g., costs for hospital stays, diagnostic tests, equipment, medications, and supportive services) may be covered by health insurance and by federal and state agencies. The Patient Protection and Affordable Care Act (ACA), passed in 2010, the most significant change to health care policy in the United States since the establishment of Medicare and Medicaid, has made available health insurance for many previously uninsured individuals who were unable to obtain health insurance. The ACA has ended lifetime and most annual limits on health care, provided patients with access to recommended preventive services, and banned the practice of denying coverage because of the presence of a preexisting health condition (Krahn et al., 2015).
- Lost income: Direct out-of-pocket expenses can represent a significant percent of income, especially in low- and middle-income families. These expenses include high copays and deductibles that must be paid out of pocket. Those with serious chronic disorders may have difficulty paying for care, resulting in bankruptcy or having to rely on family or friends to pay for health insurance or health care. People from low-income groups who do not receive adequate health care get sicker and die sooner from chronic diseases than those from groups with higher levels of education, greater financial resources, and access to care (WHO, 2017a). If a family's primary income earner becomes ill, chronic diseases can result in drastic loss in income with inadequate funds for food, education, and health care. Furthermore, affected families may become unstable and impoverished.
- Ethical issues: Chronic conditions raise difficult ethical issues for patients, families, health care professionals, and society. Issues include how to control costs, how to allocate scarce resources (e.g., organs for transplantation), what constitutes quality of life, and if and when life support should be withdrawn.

- Living with uncertainty: Having a chronic illness means living with uncertainty. Although health care providers may be aware of the usual progression of a chronic disease such as Parkinson's disease or multiple sclerosis, no one can predict with certainty the course of a person's illness. Even when a patient is in remission or symptom free, the person often fears that symptoms will reappear.

Implications of Managing Chronic Conditions

Chronic conditions have implications for everyday living and management for people and their families as well as for society at large (Larsen, 2019). Most importantly, individual efforts should be directed at preventing chronic conditions, because many—but not all—chronic illnesses or disorders are linked to unhealthy lifestyles or behaviors such as smoking and overeating. Therefore, changes in lifestyle can prevent some chronic disorders or at least delay onset until a later age. Because most people resist change, bringing about alterations in people's lifestyles is a major challenge for nurses.

Once a chronic condition has occurred, the focus shifts to managing symptoms, avoiding complications (e.g., eye complications in a person with diabetes), and preventing other acute illnesses (e.g., pneumonia in a person with chronic obstructive lung disease). Quality of life—often overlooked by health care professionals in their approach to people with chronic conditions—is also important. Health-promoting behaviors, such as exercise, are essential to quality of life even in people who have chronic illnesses or disabilities, because it helps maintain functional status (Larsen, 2019).

Although coworkers, extended family, and health care professionals are affected by chronic illnesses, the problems of living with chronic conditions are most acutely experienced by individuals and their immediate families. They experience the greatest impact, with lifestyle changes that directly affect quality of life. Nurses provide not only direct care, especially during acute episodes, but also education and they help secure the resources and other supports that enable people to integrate their illness into their lives and to have an acceptable quality of life despite their chronic condition. To understand essential nursing care, it is important to recognize and appreciate the issues that people with chronic illness and their families contend with and manage, often on a daily basis (Larsen, 2019). Ultimately the course of the chronic illness and its outcomes, including end-of-life decisions, are determined in large part by the patient and family.

Many people with chronic disease or chronic illness must face an additional challenge: the need to deal with more than one chronic condition at a time (CDC, 2019b; Raghupathi & Raghupathi, 2018). The symptoms or treatment of a second chronic condition may aggravate the first chronic condition. Patients need to be able to deal with their various chronic conditions separately as well as in combination and to coordinate the health care and directions they receive, often from more than one health care professional.

Often challenging for many people with chronic illness is the need to hire and oversee caregivers who come into their homes to assist with ADLs and IADLs, such as shopping for food, doing laundry, housekeeping, and handling financial matters. It is difficult for many people to be in a position of hiring, supervising, and sometimes firing people who may provide them with intimate physical care. The need to balance the role of recipient of care and oversight of the person providing care may lead to blurring of role boundaries.

The challenges of living with and managing a chronic illness are well known, and people with chronic illnesses often report receiving inadequate care, information, services, and counseling. This provides an opportunity for nurses to assume a more active role in addressing many of the issues experienced, coordinating care, and serving as advocates for patients who need additional assistance to manage their illness while maintaining a quality of life that is acceptable to them.

 ## Veterans Considerations

Gulf War Illness (GWI) is a chronic illness or syndrome that has been reported in veterans who served in the U.S. military in the Gulf War following the September 11, 2001 ("911") terrorist attacks (Baldwin, Rudquist, Lava-Parmele, et al., 2019). Similar to GWI, the term chronic multisymptom illness (CMI) defines a set of nonspecific symptoms experienced by veterans who served in the Gulf War in 1990–1991 and report one or more symptom lasting more than 6 months in at least two of three categories: fatigue, depressed mood and altered cognition, and musculoskeletal pain. The term, CMI, may be employed when the symptoms are moderate to severe and have no other explanation. There is speculation that GWI and CMI may be a consequence of exposure of veterans to biologic and chemical toxins during their military service. Veterans with symptoms of both GWI and CMI want and need to be taken seriously by health care professionals.

 ## Gerontologic Considerations

The U.S. demographic profile reflects an increased number of older adults with chronic illnesses and those with MCC. By 2060, the number of older adults is expected to more than double to 98.2 million; the number of people 85 years of age and older is expected to triple to 19.7 million. The ratio of women and men who are 65 years of age and older is 127 women for every 100 men. In 2014, there were 75.4 million baby boomers (people born between 1946 and 1964) accounting for almost one quarter of the population. Baby boomers began turning 65 years old in 2011, contributing to the increase in numbers of older adults. Most older adults have at least one chronic condition and three in every four older Americans have MCC (AARP, 2017; Raghupathi & Raghupathi, 2018). Some of the most frequently occurring conditions among older Americans are arthritis, cancer, cardiac disease, type 2 diabetes, and hypertension.

Treatment for older adults with chronic illness accounts for 66% of total U.S. health care expenditures (CDC, 2018). The cost of providing health care for a person 65 years of age or older is estimated to be three to five times higher than costs for someone younger than 65 years. Chronic conditions increase the risk for death due to influenza and pneumonia among older adults, although effective vaccines for them exist. The WHO (2017b) has issued guidelines for community-level interventions aimed at preventing declines in older people as they age.

In 2014, about 28% (12.6 million) of all older adults in the United States lived alone (8.8 million women, 3.8 million men). They represented 35% of older women and 19% of older men. Almost half of women aged 75 and older live alone; many of them live below the poverty level (Administration for Community Living, 2018). The living arrangements of older adults with chronic illness have important nursing implications for preparing those who are hospitalized for discharge and for ensuring coordination of services.

Nursing Care of Patients with Chronic Conditions

Nursing care of patients with chronic conditions is varied and occurs in a variety of settings. Care may be direct or supportive. Direct care may be provided in the clinic or primary care provider's office, a nurse-managed center or clinic, a hospital, long-term care facility, or the patient's home. Direct care includes assessing the patient's physical status, providing wound care, managing and overseeing medication regimens, providing education to the patient and family, and performing technical tasks. The availability of this type of nursing care may allow the patient to remain at home and return to a more normal life after an acute episode of illness.

Because much of the day-to-day responsibility for managing chronic conditions rests with the patient and the family, nurses often provide supportive care at home. Supportive care may include ongoing monitoring, education, counseling, serving as an advocate for the patient, making referrals, and case management. Giving supportive care is just as important as giving direct physical care. For example, through ongoing monitoring either in the home or in a clinic, a nurse might detect early signs of impending complications and make a referral (e.g., contact the primary health care clinician or consult the medical protocol in a clinic) for medical evaluation, thereby preventing a lengthy and costly hospitalization.

Keeping in mind the many facets and implications of chronic health conditions and their potential impact on patients and families will enable the nurse to provide direct physical care to the patient when warranted, to address the emotional and psychological needs of the patient and family, and to prepare and assist patients and family caregivers to assume management of the condition. By doing so, the nurse can help patients and families maintain as normal a life as possible and as they desire.

Working with people with chronic illness requires not only dealing with the medical aspects of their disorder but also working with the whole person—physically, emotionally, and socially. This holistic approach to care requires nurses to draw on their knowledge and skills, including knowledge from the social sciences and psychology, in particular. People often respond to illness, health education, and regimens in ways that differ from the expectations of health care providers. Although quality of life is usually affected by chronic illness, especially if the illness is severe, patients' perceptions of what constitutes quality of life often drive their management behaviors or affect how they view advice about health care. Nurses and other health care professionals need to recognize this, even though it may be difficult to see patients make unwise choices and decisions about lifestyles and disease management. People have the right to receive care without fearing ridicule or refusal of treatment, even if their behaviors (e.g., smoking, substance abuse, overeating, failure to follow health care providers' recommendations) may have contributed to their chronic disorder.

Home, Community-Based, and Transitional Care

 Educating Patients About Self-Care

Because chronic conditions are so costly to people, families, and society, two of the major goals of nursing are the prevention of chronic conditions and the care of people with them. This requires promoting healthy lifestyles and encouraging the use of safety and disease prevention measures, such as wearing seat belts and obtaining immunizations. Prevention should also begin early in life and continue throughout life. Education on self-care may need to address interactions among the patient's chronic conditions as well as skills necessary to manage the individual diseases and their interactive effects.

Patient and family education is an important nursing role that may make the difference in the ability of the patient and the family to adapt to chronic conditions. Well-informed, educated patients are more likely than uninformed patients to be concerned about their health and do what is necessary to maintain it. They are also more likely to manage symptoms, recognize the onset of complications, and seek health care early. Knowledge is the key to making informed choices and decisions during all phases of the chronic illness trajectory.

Despite the importance of educating the patient and the family, the nurse must recognize that patients recently diagnosed with serious chronic conditions and their families may need time to understand the significance of their condition and its effect on their lives. Education must be planned carefully so that it is not acute. Furthermore, it is important to assess the impact of a new diagnosis of chronic illness on a patient's life and the meaning of self-management to the patient.

The nurse who cares for patients with chronic conditions in the hospital, clinic, home, or any other setting should assess patient's knowledge about their illness and its management; the nurse cannot assume that patients with a long-standing chronic condition have the knowledge necessary to manage the condition. Patients' learning needs change as the chronic condition changes and their personal situations change. The nurse must also recognize that patients may know how their body responds under certain conditions and how best to manage their symptoms. Contact with patients in any setting offers nurses the ideal opportunity to reassess patients' learning needs and provide additional education about a chronic condition and its management.

Educational strategies and materials should be adapted to the individual patient so that the patient and the family can understand and follow recommendations from health care providers. For instance, educational materials should be tailored for people with low literacy levels and available in several languages and in various alternative formats (e.g., Braille, large print, audiotapes). It may be necessary to provide sign language interpreters.

Continuing and Transitional Care

Chronic illness management is a collaborative process between the patient, family, nurse, and other health care providers. Collaboration extends to all settings and throughout the illness trajectory. Keeping an illness stable over time requires careful monitoring of symptoms and attention to management regimens. Detecting problems early and helping patients develop appropriate management strategies can make a significant difference in outcomes.

Most chronic conditions are managed in the home. Therefore, care and education during hospitalization should focus on essential information about the condition so that management can continue once the patient is discharged home. Nurses in all settings should be aware of the resources and services available in a community and should make the arrangements (before hospital discharge, if the patient is hospitalized) to secure those resources and services. When appropriate, home care services are contacted directly. The home health nurse reassesses how the patient and the family are adapting to the chronic condition and its treatment and continues or revises the plan of care accordingly.

Because chronic conditions occur worldwide and the world is increasingly interconnected, nurses should think beyond the personal level to the community and global levels. In terms of illness prevention and health promotion, this entails wide-ranging efforts to assess people for risks of chronic illness (e.g., blood pressure and diabetes screening, stroke risk assessments) and group education related to illness prevention and management. In addition, nurses should remind patients with chronic illnesses or disabilities and their families about the need for ongoing health promotion and preventive health screening recommended for all people, because chronic illness and disability are often considered the main concern while other health-related issues are ignored (see Chart 7-6).

Telehealth or telehomecare (use of electronic data and telecommunications technologies to support long-distance clinical health care, patient and professional health-related education, public health, and health administration) has been used effectively to provide care for patients with chronic illness. It is particularly useful in monitoring patients with chronic conditions living in rural areas (Health Resources & Services Administration, 2013). It has also been used to deliver select medical and nursing interventions (e.g., counseling) and provide ongoing education and support.

Transitional care, if available, should be considered and implemented when the patient has MCC, has impaired cognitive status as well as physical limitations, has complex therapies, or is frail or unstable prior to discharge from the hospital to home. Transitional care nurses serve as the primary coordinator of care. These nurses conduct assessments of the patient as well as the family caregivers' ability to assist in management of the patient in the home. Nurses in this role help the patient and the family set goals during hospitalization, identify the reasons for the patient's current health status, design a plan of care that addresses them, make home visits, provide telephone support, and coordinate various care providers and services (Naylor et al., 2017) (see Chapter 2).

Nursing Care for Special Populations with Chronic Illness

When providing care and education, the nurse must consider multiple factors (e.g., age; gender; culture and ethnicity; cognitive status; the presence of physical, sensory, and cognitive limitations; health literacy) that influence susceptibility to chronic illness and the ways patients respond to chronic disorders. Certain populations, for example, tend to be more susceptible to certain chronic conditions. Populations at high risk for specific conditions can be targeted for special education and monitoring programs; this includes those at risk because of their genetic profile (see Chapter 6 for further discussion of genomics and genetics). People of different cultures and genders may respond to illness differently, and being aware of these differences is essential. For cultures in which patients rely heavily on the support of their families, the families must be involved and made part of the nursing plan of care. As the United States becomes more multicultural and ethnically diverse, and as the general population ages, nurses need to be aware of how a person's culture and age affect chronic illness management and be prepared to adapt their care accordingly.

It is important to consider the effect of a preexisting disability, or a disability associated with recurrence of a chronic condition, on the patient's ability to manage ADLs, self-care, and the therapeutic regimen. These issues were discussed earlier in this chapter.

CRITICAL THINKING EXERCISES

1 **ebp** A 70-year-old man is hospitalized for congestive heart failure. He has an above-the-knee amputation because of an injury that occurred 40 years ago as well as significant hearing loss due to exposure to loud noise in his work and lack of ear protection. In providing discharge planning for him, what evidence-based education is warranted to ensure that he is able to monitor his cardiac status? What evidence-based safety precautions are warranted? How would you modify education because of his hearing loss?

2 **ipc** A 28-year-old woman with paraplegia experienced since she was 14 years of age is hospitalized with a large sacral pressure injury due to her failure to relieve pressure points when in her wheelchair. She is scheduled for surgery to débride the pressure injury followed by placement of a graft to the area. She acknowledges that she has difficulty following medical advice and is eager to be discharged from the hospital as soon as possible to return home because she becomes depressed when she is away from her home and her boyfriend. What nursing and interprofessional assessments are indicated during your initial interactions with her? What interventions, including education, will you implement during her postoperative recovery? What other interprofessional services might you try to engage so she can make the best transition back to her home setting?

3 **qsen** A 48-year-old woman with multiple sclerosis has experienced frequent relapses, increasing mobility limitations with each relapse, and mild cognitive impairment. She is now hospitalized with a diagnosis of possible pneumonia and a urinary tract infection. Her daughter has asked you, her mother's primary nurse, for assistance in making alternative living arrangements for her mother; the daughter tells you she is exhausted and frustrated by providing care for her mother and her own two children while trying to maintain her full-time job as an administrative assistant. How would you approach this situation? What is your priority in assessing the situation and taking action to assist this family?

REFERENCES

*Asterisk indicates nursing research.
**Double asterisk indicates classic reference.

Books

Agency for Healthcare Research and Quality. (2018). *2017 National healthcare quality and disparities report*. Rockville, MD: Agency for Healthcare Research and Quality.

Larsen, P. D. (2019). *Lubkin's chronic illness—Impact and intervention* (10th ed.). Burlington, MA: Jones & Bartlett Learning.

National Academies of Sciences, Engineering, and Medicine (NASEM). (2017). *Communities in action: Pathways to health equity*. Washington, DC: The National Academies Press.

National Center for Health Statistics. (2016). Chapter III: Overview of midcourse progress and health disparities. *Healthy People 2020 Midcourse Review*. Hyattsville, MD: U.S. Department of Health and Human Services.

Smeltzer, S. C. (2021). *Delivering quality healthcare for people with disability*. Indianapolis, IN: Sigma Theta Tau International.

The Patient Protection and Affordable Care Act. (2010). Public Law 111-148—March 23, 2010. 111–148—11th Congress. U.S. Government Publishing Office

United Nations Convention on the Rights of Persons with Disabilities (CRPD). (2006). *Final report of the Ad Hoc Committee on a comprehensive and integral international convention on the protection and promotion of the rights and dignity of persons with disabilities*. New York: United Nations.

**U.S. Department of Health & Human Services (HHS). (2005). *Surgeon general's call to action to improve the health and wellness of people with disabilities*. Rockville, MD: Author.

**U.S. Department of Health & Human Services (HHS), Office of Disease Prevention and Health Promotion. (2010). *Healthy People 2020*. Washington, DC: Author.

**U.S. Department of Justice, Civil Rights Division, Disability Rights Section. (2009). *A guide to disability rights law*. Washington, DC: Author.

World Health Organization (WHO). (2013). *Global action plan for the prevention and control of noncommunicable diseases 2013–2020*. Geneva, Switzerland: Author.

Journals and Electronic Documents

AARP. (2017). Chronic conditions among older adults. Retrieved on 7/18/2019 at: www.assets.aarp.org/rgcenter/health/beyond_50_hcr_conditions.pdf

AARP Public Policy Institute. (2018). Chronic care: A call to action for health reform. Chronic Conditions among Older Americans. Retrieved on 11/26/20 at: https://assets.aarp.org/rgcenter/health/beyond_50_hcr.pdf

Administration for Community Living, U.S. Department of Health and Human Services. (2018). 2018 Profile of older Americans. Retrieved on 7/16/2019 at: www.acl.gov/sites/default/files/Aging%20and%20Disability%20in%20America/2018OlderAmericansProfile.pdf

American Heart Association. (2019). Cardiovascular diseases affect nearly half of American adults, statistics show. Retrieved on 7/19/2019 at: www.heart.org/en/news/2019/01/31/cardiovascular-diseases-affect-nearly-half-of-american-adults-statistics-show

Americans with Disabilities Act of 1990 (ADA). (1990). Retrieved on 11/25/20 at: www.ada.gov/pubs/ada.htm

Americans with Disabilities Act of 1990 (ADA), As Amended. (2009). Retrieved on 11/26/20 at: www.ada.gov/pubs/ada.htm

Baldwin, N., Rudquist, R., Lava-Parmele, S., et al. (2019). Improving health care for Veterans with Gulf War Illness. *Federal Practitioner*, 36(5), 212–219.

Buttorff, C., Ruder, T., & Bauman, M. (2017). Multiple chronic conditions in the United States. Retrieved on 01/01/2018 at: www.rand.org/pubs/tools/TL221.html

Centers for Disease Control and Prevention (CDC). (2018). Disability and health. Common barriers to participation experienced by people with disabilities. Retrieved on 7/16/2019 at: www.cdc.gov/ncbddd/disabilityandhealth/disability-barriers.html

Centers for Disease Control and Prevention (CDC), National Center for Chronic Disease Prevention and Health Promotion (NCCDPHP). (2019a). At a glance. Prevalence of chronic illnesses. Retrieved on 7/19/2019 at: www.cdc.gov/chronicdisease/resources/infographic/chronic-diseases.htm

Centers for Disease Control and Prevention (CDC), National Center for Chronic Disease Prevention and Health Promotion (NCCDPHP). (2019b). Multiple chronic conditions. Retrieved on 7/19/2019 at: www.cdc.gov/chronicdisease/about/multiple-chronic.htm

Centers for Disease Control and Prevention (CDC), National Center for Health Statistics. (2017). Disability and functioning. Retrieved on 11/26/20 at: www.cdc.gov/nchs/fastats/disability.htm

**Corbin, J. M. (2003). The body in health and illness. *Qualitative Health Research*, 13(2), 256–267.

Dembo, R. S., Mitra, M., & McKee, M. M. (2018). The psychological consequences of violence against people with disabilities. *Disability & Health Journal*, 11(3), 390–397.

Dreyfus, D., Lauer, E., & Wilkinson, J. (2014). Characteristics associated with bone mineral density screening in adults with intellectual disabilities. *Journal of the American Board of Family Medicine*, 27(1), 104–114.

Drum, C. F. (2014). The dynamics of disability and chronic conditions. *Disability and Health Journal*, 7(1), 2–5.

Duncan, A., & Batliwalla, Z. (2018). Growing older with post-polio syndrome: Social and quality-of-life implications. *SAGE Open Medicine*, 6, 2050312118793563. eCollection 2018.

**Goodall, C. J. (1995). Is disability any business of nurse education? *Nurse Education Today*, 15(5), 323–327.

Goyat, R., Vyas, A., & Sambamoorthi, U. (2016). Racial/ethnic disparities in disability prevalence. *Journal of Racial and Ethnic Disparities*, 3(4), 635–645.

Hasson-Ohayon, I., Hason-Shaked, M., Silberg, T., et al. (2018). Attitudes toward motherhood of women with physical versus psychiatric disabilities. *Disability & Health Journal*, 11(4), 612–617.

Hayward, K., Chen, A.Y., Forbes, E., et al. (2017). Reproductive healthcare experiences of women with cerebral palsy. *Disability & Health Journal*, 10(3), 413–418.

Health Resources & Services Administration. (2013). *The Telehealth Network Grant Program (TNGP). A report summarizing performance of the TNGP*. Office of the Advancement of Telehealth. Office of Rural Health. HRSA. Washington, DC. http://www.pbtrc.org/wp-content/uploads/2014/06/The-Telehealth-Network-Grant-Program-Performance-Report-2013.pdf. Accessed on 11/25/20.

Heller, T. (2017). Service and support needs of adults aging with intellectual/developmental disabilities. Testimony to the U.S. Senate Committee on Aging. Working and Aging with Disabilities: From school to retirement. Retrieved on 11/25/20 at: https://www.aging.senate.gov/imo/media/doc/SCA_Heller_10_25_17.pdf

Hopps, M., Iadeluca, L., McDonald, M. (2017). The burden of family caregiving in the United States: Work productivity, health care resource utilization, and mental health among employed adults. *Journal of Multidisciplinary Health Care*, 10, 437–444.

Houtenville, A., & Boege, S. (2019). *Annual report on people with disabilities in America: 2018*. Durham, NH: University of New Hampshire, Institute on Disability. Retrieved on 7/19/2019 at: www.iod.unh.edu/facts-and-figures

Kaye, H. S. (2019). Disability-related disparities in access to health care before (2008–2010) and after (2015–2017) the Affordable Care Act. *American Journal of Public Health*, 109(7), 1015–1021.

Krahn, G. L. (2019). Digging deeper on the impact of the Affordable Care Act on disability-related health care access disabilities. *American Journal of Public Health*, 109(7), 956–958.

Krahn, G. L., Walker, D. K., & Correa-De-Araujo, R. (2015). Persons with disabilities as an unrecognized health disparity population. *American Journal of Public Health*, 105(S2), S198–S206.

Kushner, R. F., & Kahan, S. (2018). Introduction: The state of obesity in 2017. *Medical Clinics of North America*, 102(1), 1–11.

LaPierre, T. A., Zimmerman, M. K., & Hall, J. P. (2017). "Paying the price to get there": Motherhood and the dynamics of pregnancy deliberations among women with disabilities. *Disability & Health Journal*, 10(3), 419–425.

Lauer, E. A., & Houtenville, A. J. (2018). Estimates of prevalence, demographic characteristics and social factors among people with disabilities in the USA: A cross-survey comparison. *BMJ Open*, 8, e017828. Retrieved on 7/19/2019 at: www.ncbi.nlm.nih.gov/pmc/articles/PMC5829676/pdf/bmjopen-2017-017828.pdf

Lindner, S., Rowland, R., Spurlock, M., et al. (2018). "Canaries in the mine…" the impact of Affordable Care Act implementation on people with disabilities: Evidence from interviews with disability advocates. *Disability & Health Journal*, 11(1), 86–92.

Magaña, S., Parish, S., Morales, M. A., et al. (2016). Racial and ethnic health disparities among people with intellectual and developmental disabilities. *Intellectual and Developmental Disabilities*, 54(3), 161–172.

McClintock, H. F., Kurichi, J. R., Barg, F. K., et al. (2018). Health care access and quality for persons with disability: Patient and provider recommendations. *Disability & Health Journal, 11*(3), 382–389.

McKee, M. M. (2019). The invisible costs of hearing loss. *JAMA Otolaryngology–Head & Neck Surgery, 145*(1), 35.

McKee, M. M., Lin, F. K., & Zazive, P. (2018). State of research and program development for adults with hearing loss. *Disability & Health Journal, 11*(4), 519–524.

Mitra, M., Smith, L. D., Smeltzer, S. C., et al. (2017). Barriers to providing care to women with physical disabilities: Perceptions from health care practitioners. *Disability & Health Journal, 10*(3), 445–450.

Morris, M. A., Maragh-Bass, A. C., Griffin, J. M., et al. (2017). Use of accessible examination tables in the primary care setting: A survey of physical evaluations and patient attitudes. *Journal General Internal Medicine, 32*(12), 1342–1348.

Na, L., Hennessy, S., Boner, H. R., et al. (2017). Disability stage and receipt of recommended care among elderly Medicare beneficiaries. *Disability & Health Journal, 10*(1), 48–57.

National Center for Chronic Disease Prevention and Health Promotion (NCCDPHP). (2020). Health and economic costs of chronic diseases. Retrieved on 11/26/20 at: www.cdc.gov/chronicdisease/about/costs/index.htm.

National Institute of Neurological Disorders and Stroke. (2019). Post-polio syndrome fact sheet. Retrieved on 7/19/2019 at: www.ninds.nih.gov/Disorders/Patient-Caregiver-Education/Fact-Sheets/Post-Polio-Syndrome-Fact-Sheet

National Prevention Council, U.S. Department of Health and Human Services. Office of the Surgeon General. (2016). Healthy aging in action. Retrieved on 11/26/20 at: https://www.cdc.gov/aging/pdf/healthy-aging-in-action508.pdf

*Naylor, M. D., Shaid, E. C., Carpenter, D., et al. (2017). Components of comprehensive and effective transitional care. *Journal of the American Geriatrics Society, 65*(6), 1119–1125.

**Nosek, M. A. (2000). Overcoming the odds: The health of women with physical disabilities in the United States. *Archives of Physical Medicine and Rehabilitation, 81*(2), 135–138.

Office of Disease Prevention and Health Promotion. (2019). Development of the National Health Promotion and Disease Prevention Objectives for 2030. Retrieved on 7/16/2019 at: www.healthypeople.gov/2020/about/foundation-health-measures/Determinants-of-Health

Okoro, C. A., Hollis, N. D., Cyrus, A. C., et al. (2018). Prevalence of disabilities and health care access by disability status and type among adults—United States, 2016. *MMWR Morbidity Mortality Weekly Report, 67*, 882–887.

Raghupathi, W., & Raghupathi, V. (2018). An empirical study of chronic diseases in the United States: A visual analytics approach to public health. *International Journal of Environmental Research and Public Health, 15*(3), 431–455.

Reichard, A., Stransky, M., Phillips, K., et al. (2017). Prevalence and reasons for delaying or forgoing necessary care in the presence and type of disability among working-age adults. *Disability & Health Journal, 10*(1), 39–47.

Retief, R., & Letšosa, R. (2018). Models of disability: A brief overview. *Theological Studies, 74*(1), 2–8.

Sinclair, L. B., Fox, M. H., Jonas, B. S., et al. (2018). Considering disability and health: Reflections on the Healthy People 2020 Midcourse review. *Disability & Health Journal, 11*(3), 333–338.

**Smeltzer, S. C. (2007). Improving the health and wellness of persons with disabilities: A call to action too important for nursing to ignore. *Nursing Outlook, 55*(4), 189–193.

Smeltzer, S. C., & Qi, B. B. (2014). The practical implications for nurses caring for patients being treated for osteoporosis. *Nursing: Research and Reviews, 4*(4), 19–33.

Tarasoff, L. A. (2017). "We don't know. We've never had anybody like you before": Barriers to perinatal care for women with physical disabilities. *Disability & Health Journal, 10*(3), 426–433.

*Thurman, W. A., Harrison, T. C., Walker, V. G., et al. (2019). Pursuing well-being among rural-dwelling adults with disabilities. *Qualitative Health Research, 29*(12), 1699–1710.

Tremmel, M., Gerdtham, U-G., Nilsson, P. M., et al. (2017). Economic burden of obesity: A systematic literature review. *International Journal of Environmental Research and Public Health, 14*(4), 435.

United Nations. (n.d.). Factsheet on persons with disabilities. Retrieved on 7/20/2019 at: www.un.org/development/desa/disabilities/resources/factsheet-on-persons-with-disabilities.html

U.S. Census Bureau. (2018a). Americans with disabilities: 2014. Retrieved on 7/20/2019 at: www.census.gov/library/publications/2018/demo/p70-152.html

U.S. Census Bureau. (2018b). Facts for features: Veterans Day 2018: Nov. 11. Retrieved on 7/20/2019 at: www.census.gov/newsroom/facts-for-features/2018/veterans-day.html

U.S. Department of Health and Human Services (HHS), National Prevention Council. (2015). Healthy aging in action: Advancing the national prevention strategy. Office of the Surgeon General. Healthy Aging in Action. Retrieved on 7/20/2019 at: www.hhs.gov/sites/default/files/healthy-aging-in-action-final.pdf

U.S. Department of Labor, Bureau of Labor Statistics. (2020). Persons with a disability: Labor force characteristics—2019. Retrieved on 11/26/20 at: www.bls.gov/news.release/pdf/disabl.pdf

**World Health Organization (WHO). (2001). *International Classification of Functioning, Disability and Health—ICF*. Geneva, Switzerland: Author.

**World Health Organization (WHO). (2005). Preventing chronic diseases: A vital investment: WHO global report. Retrieved on 7/20/2019 at: www.who.int/chp/chronic_disease_report/full_report.pdf?ua=1

World Health Organization (WHO). (2017a). Tackling NCDs. Retrieved on 11/26/20 at: www.who.int/nmh/publications/ncd-progress-monitor-2017/en

World Health Organization (WHO). (2017b). Integrated care for older people—Guidelines on community-level interventions to manage declines in intrinsic capacity. Retrieved on 11/26/20 at: https://www.who.int/nutrition/publications/guidelines/integrated-care-older-people/en/

World Health Organization (WHO). (2018a). Fact sheets: Disability and health. Retrieved on 11/26/20 at: https://www.who.int/news-room/fact-sheets/detail/disability-and-health

World Health Organization (WHO). (2018b). Fact sheets: Mental disorders. Retrieved on 11/26/20 at: https://www.who.int/topics/mental_health/factsheets/en/

World Health Organization (WHO). (2018c). Noncommunicable diseases country profiles 2018. Retrieved on 7/20/2019 at: www.who.int/nmh/publications/ncd-profiles-2018/en

World Health Organization (WHO). (2019). Face the facts #2: Widespread misunderstandings about chronic disease—and the reality. Retrieved on 7/19/2019 at: www.who.int/chp/chronic_disease_report/media/Factsheet2.pdf

Resources

AbleData, www.abledata.com or www.healthfinder.gov/FindServices/Organizations/Organization.aspx?code=HR2423

Advancing Care Excellence for Persons with Disabilities (ACE.D) (National League for Nursing), www.nln.org/professional-development-programs/teaching-resources/ace-d

Alliance for Disability in Health Care Education, Inc., www.ADHCE.org

American Academy of Developmental Medicine & Dentistry (AADMD), www.aadmd.org

American Association of the DeafBlind, www.aadb.org

American Association on Intellectual and Developmental Disabilities, www.aaidd.org

American Foundation® for the Blind, www.afb.org

American Speech-Language-Hearing Association, www.asha.org

Americans With Disabilities Act | National Network, www.adata.org

Arc of the United States, www.thearc.org

Association of Late-Deafened Adults, ALDA, Inc., www.alda.org

Center for Research on Women with Disabilities (CROWD), www.bcm.edu/crowd

Centers for Medicare & Medicaid Services (CMS), www.cms.gov

Developmental Disabilities Nurses Association (DDNA), www.ddna.org

Fact Sheet: The Affordable Care Act and The Disability Community, www.advocacymonitor.com/fact-sheet-the-affordable-care-act-and-the-disability-community

National Aphasia Association (NAA), www.aphasia.org

National Center for Learning Disabilities, www.ncld.org

National Organization for Rare Disorders (NORD), Through the Looking Glass, www.rarediseases.org/organizations/through-the-looking-glass

The Lurie Institute for Disability Policy | The Heller School for Social Policy and Management. Brandeis University, www.lurie.brandeis.edu

United Cerebral Palsy (UCP), www.ucp.org

United Spinal Association, www.unitedspinal.org

U.S. Department of Labor, Office of Disability Employment Policy, www.dol.gov/odep/topics/disability.htm

LEARNING OUTCOMES

On completion of this chapter, the learner will be able to:

1. Specify the demographic trends and the physiologic aspects of aging in the United States.
2. Describe the significance of preventive health care and health promotion for the older adult.
3. Compare and contrast the common physical and mental health problems of aging and their effects on the functioning of older adults and their families.
4. Identify the role of the nurse in meeting the health care needs of the older patient.
5. Examine common health issues of older adults and their families in the home and the community, in the acute care setting, and in the long-term care facility.

NURSING CONCEPTS

Development
Ethics and Legal Issues

Family
Health, Wellness, and Illness

GLOSSARY

activities of daily living (ADLs): personal care activities such as bathing, dressing, grooming, eating, toileting, and transferring

ageism: a bias that discriminates, stigmatizes, and disadvantages older adults based solely on their chronologic age

comorbidity: having more than one illness at the same time (e.g., diabetes, congestive heart failure)

depression: the most common affective (mood) disorder of old age; results from changes in reuptake of the neurochemical serotonin in response to chronic illness and emotional stresses

durable power of attorney: a formal, legally endorsed document that identifies a proxy decision maker who can make decisions if the signer becomes incapacitated

elder abuse: the physical, emotional, or financial harm to an older person by one or more of the person's children, caregivers, or others; includes neglect

geriatric syndromes: common conditions found in older adults that tend to be multifactorial and do not fall under discrete disease categories; these conditions include falls, delirium, frailty, dizziness, and urinary incontinence

geriatrics: a field of practice that focuses on the physiology, pathology, diagnosis, and management of the disorders and diseases of older adults

gerontologic/geriatric nursing: the field of nursing that relates to the assessment, planning, implementation, and evaluation of older adults in all environments, including acute, intermediate, and skilled care, as well as within the community

gerontology: the combined biologic, psychologic, and sociologic study of older adults within their environment

instrumental activities of daily living (IADLs): complex skills needed for independent living, such as shopping, cooking, housework, using the telephone, managing medications and finances, and being able to travel by car or public transportation

orientation: a person's ability to recognize who and where they are in a time continuum; used to evaluate one's basic cognitive status

polypharmacy: the use of multiple prescription and over-the-counter (OTC) medications

presbycusis: decreased ability to hear high-pitched tones that naturally begins in midlife as a result of irreversible inner ear changes

presbyopia: decrease in visual accommodation that occurs with advancing age

urinary incontinence: unplanned, involuntary, or uncontrolled loss of urine

Aging, the normal process of time-related change, begins with birth and continues throughout life. Americans are living longer than any previous generation. With the baby boomers turning 65 years of age beginning in 2010, older Americans are the most rapidly expanding portion of the population. In 2016, 3.5 million people celebrated their 65th birthdays. It is projected that 10,000 older adults will celebrate their 65th birthday each year until the year 2030 (Administration on Aging [AoA], 2020). Whenever nurses work with adults, they are likely to encounter older adult patients. This chapter presents demographics of aging, normal age-related changes, health problems associated with aging, and ways that nurses can influence the quality of life and address the health issues of older adults.

Overview of Aging

Demographics of Aging

The proportion of Americans 65 years of age and older has increased from 37 million in 2006 to 49.2 million in 2016 (a 33% increase). It is projected that by 2060, the older adult population will double to 98 million. Currently one in every seven persons is an older adult, or 15.2% of the population. As the older adult population increases, the number of people who live to a very old age is also dramatically increasing. The greatest growth in the older adult population is for those aged 85 years and older; this population is projected to more than double from 6.4 million in 2016 to 14.6 million in 2040, a 129% increase (AoA, 2020). Life expectancy—the average number of years that a person can expect to live—varies by gender and race, with women living longer than men and White women having the longest life expectancy. The difference in life expectancy between the genders is a full 5 years. Life expectancy has risen dramatically in the past 100 years. In 1900, average life expectancy was 47 years and by 2009, that figure had increased to 78.8 years. In 2016, life expectancy decreased by 0.2% to 78.6% (Xu, Murphy, Kochanek, et el., 2018).

The older adult population is becoming more diverse, reflecting changing demographics in the United States. Although this population will increase in number for all minority groups, the rate of growth is projected to be fastest in the Hispanic population, which is expected to increase by 112% between 2016 and 2030. Proportionally, there will be a significant decline in the percentage of the White non-Hispanic population, which is anticipated to increase only by 39% by 2030 (AoA, 2020).

Health Status of the Older Adult

Although many older adults enjoy good health, most have at least one chronic illness, and many have multiple health conditions. Chronic conditions, many of which are preventable or treatable, are the major cause of disability and pain among older adults (see Fig. 8-1).

Most deaths in the United States occur in people 65 years of age and older. However, improvements in the prevention, early detection, and treatment of diseases have impacted the health of people in this age group. In the past 60 years, there has been a significant decline in overall deaths—specifically, deaths from heart disease and cancer, the two leading causes of deaths. In addition, deaths from chronic lower respiratory diseases, stroke, influenza, pneumonia, and sepsis, have declined (Xu et al., 2018). Deaths from unintentional injuries and chronic lower pulmonary diseases exchanged places, making unintentional injuries the third leading cause of death. Deaths from Alzheimer's disease (AD) have risen and are projected to quadruple by the year 2050, affecting 14 million U.S. adults aged 65 years and older (Centers for Disease Control and Prevention [CDC], 2017).

Between the years 2012 and 2014, 78% of noninstitutionalized Americans aged 65 years and older rated their health as good, very good, or excellent (AoA, 2020). Men and women reported comparable levels of health; however, positive health reports declined with advancing age. Even at the age of 85 years and more, the majority of Americans reported good or better health. Blacks, Hispanics, and Latinos appeared less likely to report good health than their White counterparts. Most Americans 75 years of age and older remained functionally independent regardless of how they perceived their health. The proportion of older Americans reporting a

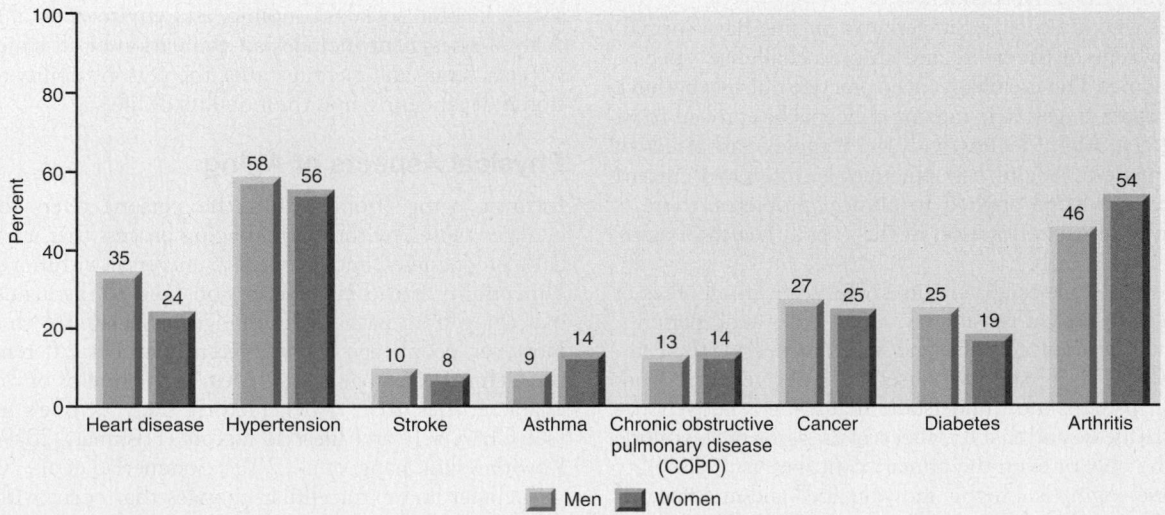

Figure 8-1 • Percentage of people 65 years of age and older who reported having selected chronic health conditions, by sex, 2018. From National Center for Health Statistics. (2020). Older Americans 2020: Key indicators of well-being. Washington, DC: U.S. Government Printing Office. Retrieved 11/30/2020 at: https://www.agingstats.gov/data.html

limitation in activities declined from 49% in 1992 to 44% in 2013 (AoA, 2020). These declines in limitations may reflect trends in health promotion and disease prevention activities, such as improved nutrition, decreased smoking, increased exercise, and early detection and treatment of risk factors such as hypertension and elevated serum cholesterol levels.

Many chronic conditions commonly found among older people can be managed, limited, and even prevented. Older people are more likely to maintain good health and functional independence if encouraged to do so and if appropriate community-based support services are available (Miller, 2019). Nurses need to promote positive lifelong health behaviors, because the impact of unhealthy behaviors and choices can result in chronic disease.

Nursing Care of the Older Adult

Gerontology, the study of the aging process, is a multidisciplinary field that draws from the biologic, psychologic, and sociologic sciences. **Geriatrics** is the practice (medical or nursing) that focuses on the physiology, pathology, diagnosis, and management of the disorders and diseases of older adults. Care for older adults should not be limited to one discipline but is best provided through a cooperative effort. An interdisciplinary approach to providing care combines expertise and resources to provide comprehensive geriatric assessment and intervention. Nurses collaborate with the team to obtain appropriate services for patients and provide a holistic approach to care.

Gerontologic/geriatric nursing is the field of nursing that specializes in the care of older adults. The Scope and Standards of Gerontological Nursing Practice was originally developed in 1969 by the American Nurses Association (ANA) and revised in 2010 (ANA, 2010). The nurse gerontologist can be either a specialist or a generalist providing comprehensive nursing care to older adults by combining the basic nursing process with a specialized knowledge of aging. Gerontologic nursing is provided in acute care, skilled and assisted living, the community, and home settings. The goals of care include promoting and maintaining functional status as well as helping older adults identify and use their strengths to achieve optimal independence.

Nurses who are certified in geriatric nursing have specialized knowledge of the acute and chronic challenges specific to older adults. The use of advanced practice nurses who have been educated in geriatric nursing concepts has proved to be very effective when dealing with the complex care needs of an older patient. When best practices are used and current scientific knowledge applied to clinical problems, there is significantly less deterioration in the overall health of aging patients (ANA, 2010).

In addition to specialists, nurses who work in all areas of adult medical-surgical nursing encounter older adult patients. Nurses must be knowledgeable and skilled in meeting the complex needs of these patients. Nurses and caregivers who work with older patients must understand that aging is not synonymous with disease and that the effects of the aging process alone are not the only or even the primary contributors to disability and disease. Aging is a highly individualized and multifaceted process (Sommerlad, Sabia, Singh-Manoux, et al., 2019).

Functional assessment is a common framework for assessing older adults. Age-related changes, as well as additional risk factors such as disease and the effects of medications, can reduce function. Assessing the functional consequences of aging and proposing practical interventions helps to maintain and improve the health of older adults (Miller, 2019). The goal is to help older adults sustain maximum functional level and dignity despite physical, social, and psychological losses. Early intervention can prevent complications of many health problems and help maximize the quality of life.

Theories of Aging

Aging has been defined chronologically by the passing of time—subjectively, as in how a person feels, and functionally, as in changes in physical or mental capabilities. Many theories attempt to provide a framework in which to understand aging from different perspectives. Clinicians can use each theory to gain insight into different aspects of aging.

In addition to the biologic, developmental, and sociologic theories of aging, Miller (2019) developed the Functional Consequences Theory, which encourages nurses to consider the effects of normal age-related changes as well as the damage incurred through disease or environmental and behavioral risk factors when planning care. This theory suggests that nurses can alter the outcome for patients through nursing interventions that address the consequences of these changes. Age-related changes and risk factors may negatively interfere with patient outcomes and impair patient activity and quality of life. For example, normal age-related changes in vision may increase sensitivity to glare. Alterations in the environment that reduce glare may enhance patient comfort and safety. In contrast, the development of cataracts, which is not a normal age-related change, also may increase sensitivity to glare. The nurse must differentiate between normal, irreversible age-related changes and modifiable risk factors. Doing so helps the nurse design appropriate nursing interventions that have a positive impact on outcomes for older patients—most importantly, for their quality of life.

Age-Related Changes

The well-being of older adults depends on physical, psychosocial, mental, social, economic, and environmental factors. A total assessment includes an evaluation of all major body systems, social and mental status, the person's ability to function independently, and their quality of life.

Physical Aspects of Aging

Intrinsic aging (from within the person) refers to those changes caused by the normal aging process that are genetically programmed and essentially universal within a species. Universality is the major criterion used to distinguish normal aging from pathologic changes associated with illness. However, people age quite differently and at different rates; thus, chronologic age is often less predictive of obvious age characteristics than other factors, such as one's genetics (see Chart 8-1) and lifestyle factors (Frishman, 2019; Seah, Kowitlawakul, Jiang, et al., 2019; Sommerlad et al., 2019).

Cellular and extracellular changes that occur with aging cause functional decline and measurable changes in physical appearance, including changes in shape and body makeup. Cellular aging and tissue deficits also diminish the body's

Chart 8-1 GENETICS IN NURSING PRACTICE
Genetics Concepts and the Older Adult

Genetic conditions in the older adult may occur from a specific gene mutation or arise as a result of a genetic predisposition combined with other factors (multifactorial). The following are examples of some adult-onset genetic conditions:

- Colon cancer
- Hemochromatosis
- Huntington disease
- Polycystic kidney disease
- Alzheimer's disease

The following are some examples of diseases with multifactorial components, which may include a genetic predisposition, in the older adult:

- Diabetes
- Emphysema
- Heart disease

Nursing Assessments

Refer to Chapter 4, Chart 4-2: Genetics in Nursing Practice: Genetic Aspects of Health Assessment

Family History Assessment Specific to the Older Adult

- Collect and assess family history on both maternal and paternal sides of the family for three generations.
- Determine whether genetic testing has occurred with other family members.
- Assess for individual and family perceptions and beliefs around topics related to genetics.

Patient Assessment Specific to the Older Adult and Genetic Illness

- Assess older adult patient's knowledge and understanding of genetics, genetic testing, and gene-based therapies.

- Assess the patient's understanding of genetic information and decipher health literacy needs.
- Perform cultural, social, and spiritual assessment.
- Assess patient's communication capacities so that communication strategies about genetics are tailored to their needs and abilities.
- Identify patient's support system.

Management Issues Specific to Genetics and the Older Adult

- Refer for further genetic counseling and evaluation as warranted so that family members can discuss inheritance, risk to other family members, and availability of genetic testing and gene-based interventions.
- Offer appropriate genetic information and resources that take into consideration older patient's literacy needs.
- Evaluate older patient's understanding before, during, and after the introduction of genetic information and services.
- Take the time to clearly explain the concepts of genetic testing to older patients and provide written information that reinforces the topic of discussion.
- Participate in the management and coordination of care of older patients with genetic conditions and individuals predisposed to develop or pass on a genetic condition.

Genetics Resources

See Chapter 6, Chart 6-7: Components of Genetic Counseling for additional resources.

---

ability to maintain homeostasis and prevent organ systems from functioning at full efficiency. As cells become less able to replace themselves, they accumulate a pigment known as lipofuscin. A degradation of elastin and collagen causes connective tissue to become stiffer and less elastic. These changes result in diminished capacity for organ function and increased vulnerability to disease and stress. Age-related changes in the hematopoietic system influence red blood cell production, leading to increased rates of anemia (Norris, 2019).

Table 8-1 summarizes subjective and objective findings related to age-related changes in the body systems. More in-depth information about age-related changes can be found in the chapters pertaining to each organ system.

When assessing the physical aspects of aging, nurses should know that tactile sensation is reduced and changes in the ability to sense pressure, pain, and temperature all lead to a decreased ability to identify and attend to physical symptoms (Kennedy-Malone, Martin-Plank, & Duffy, 2019)

Cardiovascular System

Heart disease is the leading cause of death in older adults. Age-related changes reduce the efficiency of the heart and contribute to decreased compliance of the heart muscle. These changes include myocardial hypertrophy, which changes left ventricular strength and function; increased fibrosis and calcified tissues that infiltrate muscles and conductive tissues causing stenosis of the valves; and decreased pacemaker cells. As a result, the heart valves become thicker and stiffer, and the heart muscle and arteries lose their elasticity, resulting in a reduced stroke volume. Calcium and fat deposits accumulate within arterial walls, and veins become increasingly stiff and tortuous, increasing arterial resistance; this leads to hypertension and increases the workload of the heart (Capriotti & Frizzell, 2016).

It is difficult to differentiate between age- and disease-related changes in cardiovascular function because of the significant influence of behavioral factors on cardiovascular health. When cross-cultural studies are conducted, cardiovascular changes that in the past were thought to be age related do not consistently appear. For example, the higher blood pressure found in older adults in Western societies does not occur in less-developed societies and may be a result of different lifestyle behaviors rather than normal age-related changes (Miller, 2019). The cardiovascular system can adapt to many normal age-related changes and often an older person is unaware of any significant decline in cardiovascular performance. However, when challenged, for instance, during exercise or stress, the cardiovascular system of an older person is less efficient and may be unable to respond sufficiently when life-sustaining activities are needed.

Careful assessment of older adults is necessary because they often present with different symptoms than those seen in younger patients. Older adults are more likely to have dyspnea or neurologic symptoms associated with heart disease,

TABLE 8-1	Age-Related Changes in Body Systems and Health Promotion Strategies	
Changes	**Subjective and Objective Findings**	**Health Promotion Strategies**
Cardiovascular System Decreased cardiac output; diminished ability to respond to stress; heart rate and stroke volume do not increase with maximum demand; slower heart recovery rate; increased blood pressure	Complaints of fatigue with increased activity Increased heart rate recovery time *Optimal blood pressure:* <130/80 mm Hg	Exercise regularly; pace activities; avoid smoking; eat a low-fat, low-salt diet; participate in stress-reduction activities; check blood pressure regularly; adherence to medications; weight control (body mass index <25 kg/m^2)
Respiratory System Increase in residual lung volume; decrease in muscle strength, endurance, and vital capacity; decreased gas exchange and diffusing capacity; decreased cough efficiency	Fatigue and breathlessness with sustained activity; decreased respiratory excursion and chest/lung expansion with less effective exhalation; difficulty coughing up secretions	Exercise regularly; avoid smoking; take adequate fluids to liquefy secretions; receive yearly influenza immunization and pneumonia vaccine at 65 years of age; avoid exposure to upper respiratory tract infections
Integumentary System Decreased subcutaneous fat, interstitial fluid, muscle tone, glandular activity, and sensory receptors, resulting in atrophy and decreased protection against trauma, sun exposure, and temperature extremes; diminished secretion of natural oils and perspiration; capillary fragility	Thin, wrinkled, and dry skin; increased fragility, more easily bruised, and sunburned; complaints of intolerance to heat; prominent bone structure	Limit sun exposure to 10–15 min daily for vitamin D (use protective clothing and sunscreen); dress appropriately for temperature; stay hydrated; maintain a safe indoor temperature; take shower rather than hot tub bath if possible; lubricate skin with lotions that contain petroleum or mineral oil
Reproductive System *Female:* Vaginal narrowing and decreased elasticity; decreased vaginal secretions *Male:* Gradual decline in fertility, less firm testes, and decreased sperm production *Male and female:* Slower sexual response	*Female:* Painful penile-vaginal intercourse; vaginal bleeding following intercourse; vaginal itching and irritation; delayed orgasm *Male:* Less firm erection and delayed erection and achievement of orgasm	*Female:* May require vaginal estrogen replacement; gynecology/urology follow-up; use a lubricant with sexual intercourse
Musculoskeletal System Loss of bone density; loss of muscle strength and size; degenerated joint cartilage	Height loss; prone to fractures; kyphosis; back pain; loss of strength, flexibility, and endurance; joint pain	Weight-bearing exercise regularly (3 times a week); recommend bone density screening; take calcium and vitamin D supplements as prescribed
Genitourinary System Decrease in detrusor muscle contractility, bladder capacity, flow rate, ability to withhold voiding; increase in residual urine *Male:* Benign prostatic hyperplasia *Female:* Relaxed perineal muscles; detrusor instability leads to urge incontinence; urethral dysfunction (stress urinary incontinence)	Urinary retention; irritative voiding symptoms including frequency, feeling of incomplete bladder emptying, multiple nighttime voiding Urgency/frequency syndrome; decreased "warning time"; drops of urine lost with cough, laugh, position change	Drink adequate fluids but limit drinking in evening; avoid bladder irritants (e.g., caffeinated beverages, alcohol, artificial sweeteners); do not wait long periods between voiding; empty bladder completely when voiding; wear easily manipulated clothing; consider urologic workup. Women: perform pelvic floor muscle exercises, preferably learned via biofeedback
Gastrointestinal System Decreased sense of thirst, smell, and taste; decreased salivation; difficulty swallowing food; delayed esophageal and gastric emptying; reduced gastrointestinal motility	Risk of dehydration, electrolyte imbalances, and poor nutritional intake; complaints of dry mouth; complaints of fullness, heartburn, and indigestion; constipation, flatulence, and abdominal discomfort; risk for aspiration	Use ice chips, mouthwash; brush, floss, and massage gums daily; receive regular dental care; eat small, frequent meals; sit up while and after eating and avoid heavy activity after eating; limit antacids; eat a high-fiber, low-fat diet; limit laxatives; toilet regularly; drink adequate fluids
Nervous System Decrease in brain volume and cerebral blood flow. Reduced speed in nerve conduction	Slower to respond and react; learning may take longer; increased vulnerability to delirium with illness, anesthesia, even changes in environmental cues such as a room change; increased risk of fainting and falls	Pace education; with hospitalization, encourage visitors; enhance sensory stimulation; with sudden confusion, look for cause; encourage slow rising from a resting position and practice fall prevention measures

TABLE 8-1 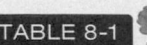 Age-Related Changes in Body Systems and Health Promotion Strategies (continued)		
Changes	**Subjective and Objective Findings**	**Health Promotion Strategies**
Special Senses		
Vision: Presbyopia; diminished ability to focus on close objects; decreased ability to tolerate glare; pupils become more rigid and lenses more opaque; decreased contrast sensitivity; decrease in aqueous humor	Holds objects far away from face; complains of glare; poor night vision and "dry" eye; difficulty adjusting to changes in light intensity; decreased ability to distinguish colors	Wear eyeglasses and use sunglasses outdoors; avoid abrupt changes from dark to light; use adequate indoor lighting with area lights and nightlights; use large-print books; use magnifier for reading; avoid night driving; use contrasting colors for color coding; avoid glare of shiny surfaces and direct sunlight
Hearing: Presbycusis; decreased ability to hear high-frequency sounds; tympanic membrane thinning and loss of resiliency; difficulty with sound discrimination especially in noisy environment	Gives inappropriate responses; asks people to repeat words; strains forward to hear; can result in social isolation and increases vulnerability for delirium during hospitalization	Recommend a hearing examination; reduce background noise; face person; enunciate clearly; speak with a low-pitched voice; use nonverbal cues; rephrase questions
Taste and smell: Decreased ability to taste and smell	Decreased recognition of familiar smells including recognizing spoiled food or a gas stove left on; decreased enjoyment of food; uses excessive sugar and salt	Encourage use of lemon, spices, herbs; recommend smoking cessation

Adapted from Weber, J. R., & Kelley, J. H. (2019). *Health assessment in nursing* (6th ed.). Philadelphia, PA: Wolters Kluwer.

and they may experience mental status changes or report vague symptoms such as fatigue, nausea, and syncope. Rather than the typical substernal chest pain associated with myocardial ischemia, older patients may report burning or sharp pain or discomfort in an area of the upper body. Complicating the assessment is the fact that many older patients have more than one underlying disease. When a patient complains of symptoms related to digestion and breathing and upper extremity pain, cardiac disease must be considered. The absence of chest pain in an older patient is not a reliable indicator of the absence of heart disease.

Orthostatic and postprandial hypotension may be a concern as well because of decreased baroreflex sensitivity and risk factors such as medications (Miller, 2019). Therefore, it is important to assess blood pressure in two positions. A patient experiencing hypotension should be counseled to rise slowly (from a lying, to a sitting, to a standing position), avoid straining when having a bowel movement, and consider having five or six small meals each day, rather than three, to minimize the hypotension that can occur after a large meal. Extremes in temperature, including hot showers and whirlpool baths, should be avoided.

Respiratory System

The respiratory system compensates well for the functional changes of aging. In general, healthy, nonsmoking older adults show very little decline in respiratory function; however, there are substantial individual variations and aerobic capacity declines with each decade by about 10% from peak performance in the early to mid-20s (Capriotti & Frizzell, 2016). The age-related changes that do occur are subtle and gradual, and healthy older adults are able to compensate for these changes. Diminished respiratory efficiency and reduced maximal inspiratory and expiratory force may occur as a result of calcification and weakening of the muscles of the chest wall. Lung mass decreases and residual volume increases (Norris, 2019).

Conditions of stress, such as illness, may increase the demand for oxygen and affect the overall function of other systems. Like cardiovascular diseases, respiratory diseases manifest more subtly in older adults than in younger adults and do not necessarily follow the typical pattern of cough, chills, and fever. Older adults may exhibit fatigue, lethargy, anorexia, dehydration, and mental status changes (Miller, 2019).

Smoking is the most significant risk factor for respiratory diseases and older adults have a higher rate of smoking, about 20%, compared to the national average of 18% (Bowler, Hansel, Jacobson, et al., 2017). Therefore, a major focus of health promotion activities should be on smoking cessation and avoidance of environmental smoke. Despite marketing by manufacturers, e-cigarettes are not an effective smoking cessation aid nor do they promote health (Bowler et al., 2017).

Additional activities that help older adults maintain adequate respiratory function include regular exercise, appropriate fluid intake, pneumococcal vaccination, yearly influenza immunizations, and avoidance of people who are ill. Hospitalized older adults should be frequently reminded to cough and take deep breaths, particularly postoperatively, because their decreased lung capacity and decreased cough efficiency predispose them to atelectasis and respiratory infections.

Integumentary System

The functions of the skin include protection, temperature regulation, sensation, and excretion. Aging can interrupt all functions of the skin and affect appearance (Norris, 2019). Epidermal proliferation decreases, and the dermis becomes thinner. Elastic fibers are reduced in number and collagen becomes stiffer. Subcutaneous fat diminishes, particularly in the extremities, and less vasodilation renders the body less able to produce or conserve body heat. These changes lead to lack of fever in circumstances in which fever would normally be present in younger individuals and reduced tolerance to temperature extremes, which increases the likelihood of hypothermia and hyperthermia (Capriotti & Frizzell, 2016). There is also a loss of resiliency with wrinkling and sagging of the skin. The skin becomes drier and more susceptible to burns, injury, and infection. Hair pigmentation may change and balding may occur; genetic factors strongly influence these changes. These changes in the integument reduce tolerance to temperature extremes and sun exposure.

Lifestyle practices have a large impact on skin changes. Strategies to promote healthy skin function include not smoking, limiting alcohol consumption, avoiding exposure to the sun, using a sun protection factor of 15 or higher, wearing protective clothing, using emollient skin cream containing petrolatum or mineral oil, avoiding hot soaks in the bathtub, and maintaining optimal nutrition and hydration (Farage, Miller, & Maibach, 2017). Older adults should be encouraged to have any changes in the skin examined, because early detection and treatment of precancerous or cancerous lesions are essential for the best outcome.

Reproductive System

An outdated perception is that older adults are asexual, but older adults report that a fairly stable and active sex life is an important quality of life issue. Sexual activity declines with the loss of a partner, primarily for women as a result of widowhood and for men as a result of poor heath, poor sleep, erectile dysfunction, medications, and emotional factors. However, although good health is a predictor of sexual activity, older adults with chronic illnesses may be able to have a sexually active life as well. Because of the many factors that influence the ability to be sexually active, nurses and the older person need to understand the physiologic, psychologic, and social factors that affect reproductive and sexual functioning as aging progresses (Bozorgmehri, Fink, Parimi, et al., 2017; Kennedy-Malone et al., 2019; Miller, 2019).

Ovarian production of estrogen and progesterone declines with menopause. Changes that occur in the female reproductive system include thinning of the vaginal wall, along with a shortening of the vagina and a loss of elasticity; decreased vaginal secretions, resulting in vaginal dryness, itching, and decreased acidity; involution (atrophy) of the uterus and ovaries; and decreased pubococcygeal muscle tone, resulting in a relaxed vagina and perineum. Without the use of water-soluble lubricants, these changes may contribute to vaginal bleeding and painful penile-vaginal intercourse.

In older men, the testes become less firm but may continue to produce viable sperm up to 90 years of age. At about 50 years of age, production of testosterone begins to diminish (Mark, 2017). Decreased libido and erectile dysfunction may develop but are more likely to be associated with factors other than age-related changes. These risk factors include obesity, smoking, cardiovascular disease, neurologic disorders, diabetes, respiratory disease, chronic pain, and many medications (i.e., vasodilators, antihypertensive agents, and tricyclic antidepressants) (Bozorgmehri et al., 2017; Miller, 2019).

In both older men and women, it may take longer to become sexually aroused, longer to complete sexual intercourse, and longer before sexual arousal can occur again. Although a less intense response to sexual stimulation and a decline in sexual activity occurs with increasing age, sexual desire does not disappear. Many couples are unaware of the causes of decreased libido or erectile dysfunction and are often reluctant to discuss decreased sexual function. Many nonpharmacologic, pharmacologic, and surgical methods are available to improve sexual relationships. Assessment and communication require sensitivity and expert knowledge in the field of sexual dysfunction. If sexual dysfunction is present, referral to a gynecologist, urologist, or sex therapist may be warranted.

Genitourinary System

The genitourinary system continues to function adequately in older adults, although kidney mass is decreased, primarily because of a loss of nephrons. However, the loss of nephrons does not typically become significant until about 90 years of age, and changes in kidney function vary widely; approximately one third of older adults show no decrease in renal function (Mark, 2017). Changes in renal function may be attributable to a combination of aging and pathologic conditions such as hypertension. The changes most commonly seen include a decreased filtration rate, diminished tubular function with less efficiency in reabsorbing and concentrating the urine, and a slower restoration of acid base balance in response to stress. In addition, older adults who take medications may experience serious consequences owing to decline in renal function because of impaired absorption, decreased ability to maintain fluid and electrolyte balance, and decreased ability to concentrate urine.

Certain genitourinary disorders are more common in older adults than in the general population. In the United States, **urinary incontinence** (i.e., unplanned, involuntary, or uncontrolled loss of urine) affects women more than men at a ratio of 2:1 until after age 80, when both are equally affected. This condition should not be mistaken as a normal consequence of aging (Resnick, 2019). Costly and often embarrassing, it should be evaluated, because in many cases it is reversible or can be treated. When treatable, this condition needs to be addressed as the risk of mortality associated with urinary incontinence can be as high as 44% in patients living in long-term care facilities (Damián, Pator-Barriuso, Garcia López, et al., 2017). See Chapter 49 for further discussion of urinary incontinence. Benign prostatic hyperplasia (enlarged prostate gland), a common finding in older men, causes a gradual increase in urine retention and overflow incontinence. Changes in the urinary tract increase the susceptibility to urinary tract infections (UTIs). Adequate consumption of fluids is an important nursing intervention that reduces the risk of bladder infections and also helps decrease urinary incontinence.

Gastrointestinal System

Digestion of food is less influenced by changes associated with aging than by the risk of poor nutrition. Older adults can adjust to changes in the gastrointestinal (GI) system but may have difficulty purchasing, preparing, and enjoying their meals. The sense of smell diminishes as a result of neurologic changes and environmental factors such as smoking, medications, and vitamin B_{12} deficiencies. The ability to recognize sweet, sour, bitter, or salty foods diminishes over time, altering satisfaction with food. Salivary flow does not decrease in healthy adults; however, approximately one third of older adults may experience a dry mouth as a result of medications and diseases (Miller, 2019). Difficulties with chewing and swallowing are generally associated with lack of teeth and diseases.

Experts disagree on the extent of gastric changes that occur as a result of normal aging. However, gastric motility appears to slow modestly, which results in delayed emptying of stomach contents and early satiety (feeling of fullness). Diminished secretion of gastric acid and pepsin, seemingly the result of pathologic conditions rather than normal aging, reduces the absorption of iron, calcium, and vitamin B_{12}. Absorption of nutrients in the small intestine, particularly calcium and vitamin D, appears to diminish with age. Functions of the liver, gallbladder, and pancreas are generally maintained, although absorption and tolerance to fat may decrease. The incidence of gallstones and common bile duct stones increases progressively with advancing years.

Dysphagia, or difficulty swallowing, increases with age and is a major health care problem in older patients. Normal aging alters some aspects of the swallowing function. In addition, dysphagia is a frequent complication of stroke and a significant risk factor for the development of aspiration pneumonia that can be life-threatening. Dysphagia is caused by interruption or dysfunction of neural pathways. It may also result from dysfunction of the striated and smooth muscles of the GI tract in patients with Parkinson's disease. Aspiration of food or fluid is the most serious complication and can occur in the absence of coughing or choking.

Constipation is a common condition affecting many older adults; it is influenced by multiple risk factors rather than age-related changes alone. Symptoms of mild constipation are abdominal discomfort and flatulence; more serious constipation leads to fecal impaction that contributes to diarrhea around the impaction, fecal incontinence, and obstruction. Predisposing factors for constipation include lack of dietary bulk, prolonged use of laxatives, some medications, inactivity, insufficient fluid intake, and excessive dietary fat. Ignoring the urge to defecate may also be a contributing factor (Miller, 2019).

Practices that promote GI health include regular tooth brushing and flossing; receiving regular dental care; drinking sufficient fluids; eating small, frequent meals that are high in fiber and low in fat; avoiding heavy activity or lying flat after eating; and avoiding the use of laxatives and antacids. Understanding that there is a direct correlation between loss of smell and taste perception and food intake helps caregivers intervene to maintain the nutritional health of older patients.

Nutritional Health

The social, psychologic, and physiologic functions of eating influence the dietary habits of older adults. Increasing age alters nutrient requirements; older adults require fewer calories and a more nutrient-rich, healthy diet in response to alterations in body mass and a more sedentary lifestyle. Recommendations include reducing fat intake while consuming sufficient protein, vitamins, minerals, and dietary fiber for health and prevention of disease. Decreased physical activity and a slower metabolic rate reduce the number of calories needed by older adults to maintain an ideal weight. As stated previously, age-related changes that alter pleasure in eating include a decrease in taste and smell. Older adults are likely to require more sugar to achieve a sweet flavor due to blunted taste. They also may lose the ability to differentiate sour, salty, and bitter tastes. Apathy, immobility, depression, loneliness, poverty, inadequate knowledge, and poor oral health also contribute to suboptimal nutrient intake. Budgetary constraints and physical limitations may interfere with food shopping and meal preparation.

Health promotion for older adults is based on the person's physical, emotional, social, spiritual, and intellectual health. The main focus of health promotion is engaging the older adult in improving their health (Meiner & Yeager, 2019). The goals of nutrition therapy are to maintain or restore maximal independent functioning and health and to maintain the sense of dignity and quality of life by imposing as few restrictions as possible. Dietary changes should be incorporated into the older adult's existing food pattern as much as possible. Figure 8-2 lists modified dietary guidelines for older adults.

Women older than 50 years and men older than 70 years should have a daily calcium intake of 1200 mg. To foster the absorption of calcium, adults should have 600 IU of vitamin D until 70 years of age and 800 IU after 70 years of age to maintain bone health (National Institutes of Health [NIH], 2018a).

Undernutrition, which can lead to malnutrition, may be a problem for older adults. Hospitalized older adults are at particular risk of malnutrition, especially those with cognitive impairment or dementia (Tatum, Talebreza, & Ross, 2018). A recent unintentional weight loss may be a result of an illness or other factors, such as depression, that may have serious consequences and affect a person's ability to maintain health and fight illness (Norris, 2019). Many people are unaware of dietary deficits. Nurses are in an ideal position to identify nutritional problems among their patients and to work within the patient's own framework of knowledge of their health status to improve health behaviors. (See Chapter 4 for more information on nutritional assessment.)

Sleep

Older adults have increased complaints about their sleep as they age, and as many as 50% of those living at home and 65% of those living in nursing homes complain of sleep disturbances (Devlin, Skrobik, Gelinas, et al., 2018; Štefan, Vrgoč, Rupčić, et al., 2018). Many factors affect sleep quality in older adults including respiratory problems during sleep, restless leg syndrome, nocturia, pain, osteoarthritis, heart failure, incontinence, prostatic hyperplasia, menopause-related problems, pruritus, allergies, AD, depression, dementia, social isolation, loneliness, being bedridden, experiences of loss, drug use, and living in nursing homes (e.g., inadequate lighting, keeping light on during the night, noises). Some of the consequences of poor sleep quality in older adults include cognitive decline, increased risk of falls, daytime fatigue, reduced physical and mental health and health-related quality-of-life status, and poor ICU outcomes (Devlin et al., 2018; Štefan et al., 2018).

The incidence of sleep apnea (a sleep disorder characterized by brief periods in which respirations are absent) increases with age. Having insomnia symptoms and a sleep-related disorder (snoring, choking, or pauses in breathing) is associated with significantly impaired daytime functioning and longer psychomotor reaction times compared with having either condition. Sleep apnea is discussed in more detail in Chapter 18.

The nurse often observes patients while they are sleeping and can identify problems. Health education can be provided on sleep hygiene behaviors such as avoiding use of the bed for activities other than sleeping (or sex), maintaining a consistent bedtime routine, avoiding or limiting daytime napping, and limiting alcohol intake to one drink a day. Additional suggestions include avoiding stimulants such as caffeine and nicotine after noon; curbing the amount of liquids in the

MyPlate for Older Adults

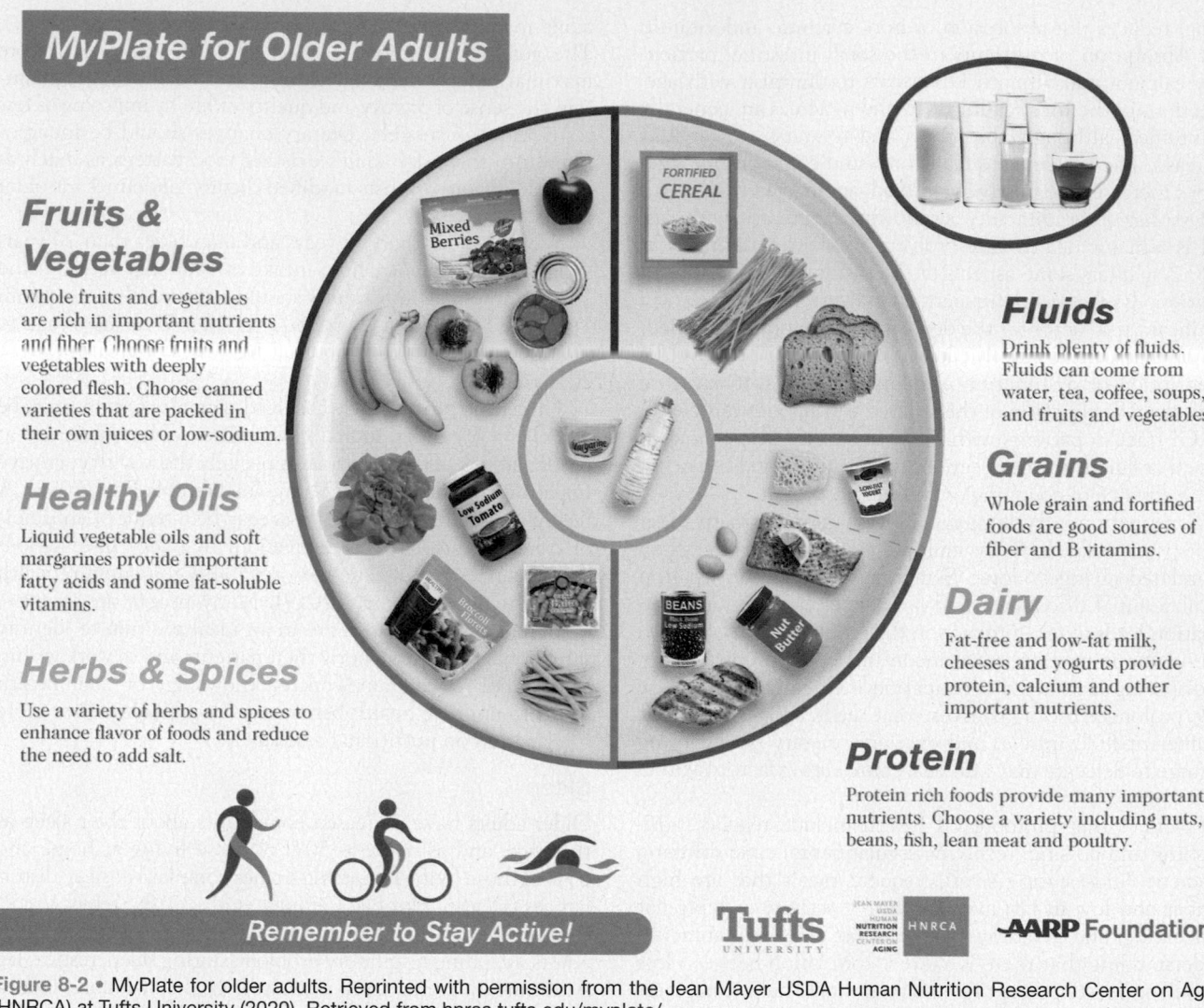

Fruits & Vegetables

Whole fruits and vegetables are rich in important nutrients and fiber. Choose fruits and vegetables with deeply colored flesh. Choose canned varieties that are packed in their own juices or low-sodium.

Healthy Oils

Liquid vegetable oils and soft margarines provide important fatty acids and some fat-soluble vitamins.

Herbs & Spices

Use a variety of herbs and spices to enhance flavor of foods and reduce the need to add salt.

Fluids

Drink plenty of fluids. Fluids can come from water, tea, coffee, soups, and fruits and vegetables.

Grains

Whole grain and fortified foods are good sources of fiber and B vitamins.

Dairy

Fat-free and low-fat milk, cheeses and yogurts provide protein, calcium and other important nutrients.

Protein

Protein rich foods provide many important nutrients. Choose a variety including nuts, beans, fish, lean meat and poultry.

Remember to Stay Active!

Tufts UNIVERSITY   JEAN MAYER USDA HUMAN NUTRITION RESEARCH CENTER ON AGING HNRCA   AARP Foundation

Figure 8-2 • MyPlate for older adults. Reprinted with permission from the Jean Mayer USDA Human Nutrition Research Center on Aging (HNRCA) at Tufts University (2020). Retrieved from hnrca.tufts.edu/myplate/

evening to avoid nocturia; and engaging in regular physical activity, preferably in bright outside light. Aromatherapy trials have reported that the use of lavender essential oil can improve the quality of sleep (Karadag, Samancioglu, Ozden, et al., 2017).

Musculoskeletal System

Intact musculoskeletal and neurologic systems are essential for the maintenance of safe mobility, performance of **activities of daily living (ADLs)** (basic personal care activities), and **instrumental activities of daily living (IADLs)** (complex skills such as shopping, cooking, housework, using the telephone, managing medications and finances, and being able to travel by car or public transportation), thus allowing older adults to remain safe and live independently in the community. Age-related changes that affect mobility include alterations in bone remodeling, leading to decreased bone density, loss of muscle mass, deterioration of muscle fibers and cell membranes, and degeneration in the function and efficiency of joints. These factors are discussed in detail in Unit 8.

Without exercise, a gradual, progressive decrease in bone mass begins before 40 years of age. The cartilage of joints also progressively deteriorates in middle age. Degenerative joint disease is found in most adults older than 70 years, and weight-bearing joint and back pain is a common complaint. Excessive loss of bone density results in osteoporosis, which leads to potentially life-altering hip and vertebral fractures. Osteoporosis is preventable.

The axiom "use it or lose it" is very relevant to the physical capacity of older adults. Nurses play an important role by encouraging older adults to participate in a regular exercise program. The benefits of regular exercise cannot be overstated. Aerobic exercises are the foundation of programs of cardiovascular conditioning; however, resistance and strength training and flexibility exercises are essential components of an exercise program. Even late in life, in adults who may be frail, it is believed that exercise has benefits of increasing strength, aerobic capacity, flexibility, and balance. In addition, older adults who are hospitalized benefit from getting out of bed as soon as possible and in-hospital physical activity.

Nervous System

Homeostasis is difficult to maintain with aging, but older people have a tremendous ability to adapt and function adequately, retaining their cognitive and intellectual abilities in the absence of pathologic changes. However, normal aging changes in the nervous system can affect all parts of the body. The structure, chemistry, and function of the nervous system change with advanced age. Nerve cells in the brain decrease but the decrease is compensated for by other neurons; there is high variability among individuals and the quantity of neuronal loss varies in different parts of the brain. Overall, the decreases contribute to a small loss of brain mass (Capriotti & Frizzell, 2016). Chemical changes include a decrease in the synthesis and metabolism of the major neurotransmitters. Because nerve impulses are conducted more slowly, older people take longer to respond and react (Miller, 2019). The autonomic nervous system performs less efficiently, and orthostatic hypotension, discussed earlier, may occur. Neurologic changes can affect gait and balance, which may interfere with mobility and safety. Nurses must advise older adults to allow a longer time to respond to a stimulus and to move more deliberately. Adequate nutrition and absorption of vitamin B_{12} is important for neurologic health. Nurses should advise older adults about proper nutrition and intake of vitamin B_{12}, especially for older adults who follow a vegetarian diet.

Slowed reaction time puts older adults at risk for falls and injuries, as well as driving errors. Although older adults spend less time driving than younger people, older adults are just as likely to be involved in motor vehicle crashes that result in serious injury or death. Older adults who are suspected of driving unsafely should receive a driving fitness evaluation (Miller, 2019). The evaluation is often performed by an occupational therapist in conjunction with a neuropsychologist, who conducts more detailed cognitive testing.

Mental function may be threatened by physical or emotional stresses. A sudden onset of confusion may be the first symptom of an infection or change in physical condition (e.g., pneumonia, UTI, medication interactions, dehydration).

Sensory System

People interact with the world through their senses. Losses associated with old age affect all sensory organs, and it can be devastating not to be able to see to read or watch television, hear conversation well enough to communicate, or discriminate taste well enough to enjoy food. Nearly half of older men and one third of older women report difficulty hearing without a hearing aid. Most older adults have a decrease in visual acuity, a narrowing of the visual field, and may have trouble seeing at night. An uncompensated sensory loss negatively affects the functional ability and quality of life of the older adult. However, assistive devices such as visual and hearing aids can compensate for a sensory loss (Miller, 2019).

Sensory Loss Versus Sensory Deprivation

In contrast to sensory loss, sensory deprivation is the absence of stimuli in the environment or the inability to interpret existing stimuli (perhaps as a result of a sensory loss). Sensory deprivation can lead to boredom, confusion, irritability, disorientation, and anxiety. A decline in sensory input can mimic a decline in cognition that is in fact not present. Meaningful sensory stimulation provided to the older person is often helpful in correcting this problem. In some situations, one sense can substitute for another in observing and interpreting stimuli. Nurses can enhance sensory stimulation in the environment with colors, pictures, textures, tastes, smells, and sounds. The stimuli are most meaningful if they are appropriate for older adults and the stimuli are changed often. Cognitively impaired people tend to respond well to touch and to familiar music.

Vision

As new cells form on the outside surface of the lens of the eye, the older central cells accumulate and become yellow, rigid, dense, and cloudy, leaving only the outer portion of the lens elastic enough to change shape (accommodate) and focus at near and far distances. As the lens becomes less flexible, the near point of focus gets farther away. This common condition—**presbyopia**—usually begins in the fifth decade of life and requires the person to wear reading glasses to magnify objects (Miller, 2019). In addition, the yellowing, cloudy lens causes light to scatter and is sensitive to glare. The ability to distinguish colors decreases, particularly blue from green. The pupil dilates slowly and less completely because of increased stiffness of the muscles of the iris, thus the older person takes more time to adjust when going to and from light and dark settings and needs brighter light for close vision. Pathologic visual conditions are not a part of normal aging; however, the incidence of eye disease (most commonly cataracts, glaucoma, diabetic retinopathy, and age-related macular degeneration) increases in older adults.

Age-related macular degeneration (AMD) is the leading cause of vision loss and blindness in older adults 65 and older. It is predicted that cases of AMD will double from 48 million to 88 million people by 2050 (CDC, 2017). Macular degeneration does not affect peripheral vision, which means that it does not cause blindness. However, it affects central vision, color perception, and fine detail, greatly affecting common visual skills such as reading, driving, and seeing faces. Risk factors include sunlight exposure, cigarette smoking, and heredity. People with fair skin and blue eyes may be at increased risk. Sunglasses and hats with visors provide some protection, and stopping smoking is paramount in preventing the disease. Although there is no definitive treatment and no cure that restores vision, several treatment options are available, depending on factors such as the location of the abnormal blood vessels. Laser photocoagulation and photodynamic therapy are commonly used (CDC, 2017). The earlier this condition is diagnosed, the greater the chances of preserving sight. See Chapter 58 for more information on altered vision.

Hearing

Auditory changes begin to be noticed at about 40 years of age. Environmental factors, such as exposure to noise, medications, and infections, as well as genetics, may contribute to hearing loss as much as age-related changes. **Presbycusis** is a gradual sensorineural loss that progresses from the loss of the ability to hear high-frequency tones to a generalized loss of hearing. It is attributed to irreversible inner ear changes. Older adults often cannot follow conversation because tones of high-frequency consonants (the sounds *f, s, th, ch, sh, b, t, p*) all sound alike. Hearing loss may cause older adults to respond inappropriately, misunderstand conversation, and avoid social interaction. This behavior may be erroneously interpreted as confusion. Wax buildup or other correctable problems may also be responsible for hearing difficulties. A systematic review reported the prevalence of under detection of hearing loss and the under use of hearing aids in long-term care facilities (Punch & Horstmanshof, 2019). A properly prescribed and fitted hearing aid may be useful in reducing some types of hearing deficits and increasing quality of life (Punch & Horstmanshof, 2019). See Chapter 59 for discussion of alterations in hearing.

Taste and Smell

The senses of taste and smell are reduced in older adults. Of the four basic tastes (sweet, sour, salty, and bitter), sweet tastes are particularly dulled in older adults. Blunted taste may contribute to the preference for salty, highly seasoned foods, but herbs, onions, garlic, and lemon can be used as substitutes for salt to flavor food.

Changes in the sense of smell, generally greater than the loss of taste, are related to cell loss in the nasal passages and in the olfactory bulb in the brain (Norris, 2019). Environmental factors such as long-term exposure to toxins (e.g., dust, pollen, smoke) contribute to the cellular damage.

Psychosocial Aspects of Aging

Successful psychological aging is reflected in the ability of older adults to adapt to physical, social, and emotional losses and to achieve life satisfaction. Because changes in life patterns are inevitable over a lifetime, older adults need resiliency and coping skills when confronting stresses and change. A positive self-image enhances risk taking and participation in new, untested roles.

Although attitudes toward older adults differ in ethnic subcultures, a subtle theme of **ageism**—prejudice or discrimination against older adults—predominates in society, and many myths surround aging. Ageism is based on stereotypes—simplified and often untrue beliefs that reinforce society's negative image of older adults. Although older adults make up an extremely heterogeneous and increasingly a racially and ethnically diverse group, these negative stereotypes are sometimes attributed to all older adults.

Fear of aging and the inability of many to confront their own aging process may trigger ageist beliefs. Retirement and perceived nonproductivity are also responsible for negative feelings, because a younger working person may falsely see older people as not contributing to society, as draining economic resources, and may actually feel that they are in competition with children for resources. Concern about the large numbers of older people leaving the workforce (baby boomers began to turn 65 years of age in 2010) is fueling this debate.

Negative images are so common in society that older adults themselves often believe and perpetuate them. An understanding of the aging process and respect for each person as an individual can dispel the myths of aging. Nurses can facilitate successful aging by recommending health promotion strategies such as anticipatory planning for retirement, including ensuring adequate income, developing routines not associated with work, replacing work-related friends with new acquaintances, and relying on other people and groups in addition to spouse to fill leisure time (Meiner & Yeager, 2019).

Stress and Coping in the Older Adult

Coping patterns and the ability to adapt to stress develop over the course of a lifetime and remain consistent later in life. Experiencing success in younger adulthood helps a person develop a positive self-image that remains solid through old age. A person's abilities to adapt to change, make decisions, and respond predictably are also determined by past experiences. A flexible, well-functioning person will probably continue as such. However, losses may accumulate within a short period of time and become acute. The older person often has fewer choices and diminished resources to deal with stressful events. Common stressors of old age include normal aging changes that impair physical function, activities, and appearance; disability from injury or chronic illness; social and environmental losses related to loss of income and decreased ability to perform previous roles and activities; and the deaths of significant others. Many older adults rely strongly on their families and spiritual beliefs for comfort during stressful times.

An additional aspect of coping that nurse researchers have examined is self-efficacy, which is the confidence to perform well at a particular task or life domain (Hladek, Gill, Bandeen-Roche, et al., 2019). Chart 8-2 is a Nursing Research Profile about the associations between coping self-efficacy and frailty in a group of community-dwelling older adults.

Living Arrangements

Many older adults have more than adequate financial resources and good health even until very late in life; therefore, they have many housing options. In 2017, 93% of older adults lived in the community, with a relatively small percentage (2.3%) residing in nursing homes and a comparable percentage living in some type of senior housing. Seventy-six percent of those older than 65 years own their homes. In 2018, 28% of noninstitutionalized older people lived alone, and widowed women predominated. In 2018, 70% of men older than 65 years were married compared with 40% of women in the same age group. This difference in marital status increases with age and is a result of several factors: Women have a longer life expectancy than men; women tend to marry older men; and women tend to remain widowed, whereas men often remarry (AoA, 2020).

Many older adults relocate in response to changes in their lives such as retirement or widowhood, a significant deterioration in health, or disability. The type of housing they choose depends on their reason for moving. With increasing disability and illness, older adults may move to retirement facilities or assisted living communities that provide some support such as meals, transportation, and housekeeping but otherwise allow them to live somewhat independently. If they develop a serious illness or disability and can no longer live independently or semi-independently, they may need to move to a setting where additional support is available, such as a relative's home or a long-term care or assisted living facility. Often they will seek a location near an adult child's home.

Living at Home or With Family

Most older adults want to remain in their own homes; in fact, they function best in their own environment. The family home and familiar community may have strong emotional significance for them, and this should not be ignored. However, with advanced age and increasing disability, adjustments to the environment may be required to allow older adults to remain in their own homes or apartments. Additional family support or more formal support may be necessary to compensate for declining function and mobility. Many services and

---

Chart 8-2

NURSING RESEARCH PROFILE

The Association Between Coping Self-efficacy and Frailty in Community-Dwelling Older Adults

Hladek, M.D., Gill, J., Bandeen-Roche, K., et al. (2019). High coping self-efficacy associated with lower odds of pre-frailty/ frailty in older adults with chronic disease. *Aging & Mental Health*. doi.org/10.108 0/13607863.2019.1639136

Purpose

Self-efficacy is the confidence to perform well at a particular task or life domain while frailty is a state of decreased physiologic reserve and vulnerability to negative health outcomes. The purpose of this study was to evaluate associations between self-efficacy and frailty in a group of community-dwelling older adults.

Design

This quantitative study used a cross-sectional design to study 146 older adults who lived in retirement communities. Instruments included the five-item Fatigue, Resistance, Ambulation, Illness, and Loss of weight (FRAIL) scale as well as two self-efficacy instruments that measured confidence in one's ability to problem solve, emotionally regulate, and ask for support when problems in life occur. Additional variables measured included illness intrusiveness, depressive symptoms, financial strain, life events, social support, heart rate, tobacco use, and

body mass index (BMI). Logistic regression was used for model development.

Findings

Approximately half of the participants were in the frail or pre-frail range on the FRAIL scale. High coping self-efficacy was associated with a 92% reduction in the odds of participants being in the frail or pre-frail range on the FRAIL scale after adjusting for age, race, comorbidities, heart rate, life events count, and BMI. This relationship remained a significant finding even after the inclusion of illness intrusiveness and depressive symptoms (OR: 0.10, p-value = 0.014). Higher age, number of comorbidities, heart rate, and BMI were also significantly associated with participants being in the frail or pre-frail range on the FRAIL scale.

Nursing Implications

When working with older adults, nurses should keep in mind the association of high self-efficacy with healthy aging. Nurses can be instrumental in developing interventions to help older adults increase self-efficacy, as measured by their confidence in their ability to problem solve, emotionally regulate, and ask for support when problems in life occur.

---

organizations can assist older adults to successfully "age in place" in their own homes or in assisted living facilities (see Resources at the end of this chapter).

Sometimes older adults or couples move in with adult children. This can be a rewarding experience as the children, their parents, and the grandchildren interact and share household responsibilities (see Fig. 8-3). It can also be stressful, depending on family dynamics. Adult children and their older parents may choose to pool their financial resources by moving into a house that has an attached "in-law suite." This arrangement provides security for the older adult and privacy for both families. Many older adults and their adult children make housing decisions in times of crisis, such as during a serious illness or after the death of a spouse. Caring for an older adult may also be stressful; older adults and

their families often are unaware of the emotional and physical demands of shared housing and assuming care for an increasingly dependent person, especially given the uncertain and extended length of time that may be associated with caring for a person with a chronic illness. Families can be helped by anticipatory guidance and long-term planning before a crisis occurs. Older adults should participate in decisions that affect them as much as possible.

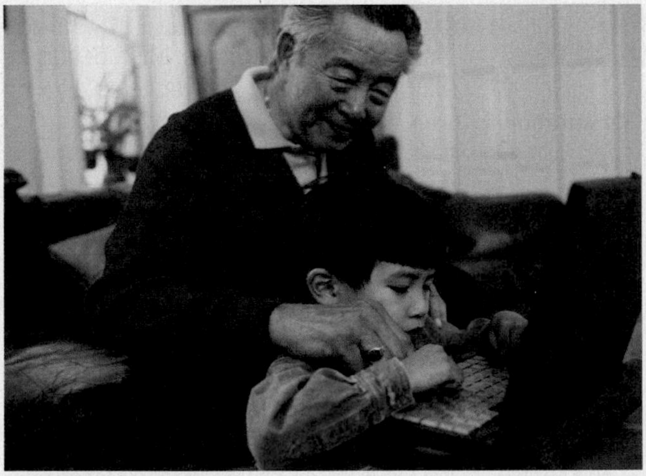

Continuing Care Retirement Communities

Continuing care retirement communities (CCRCs) offer three levels of living arrangements and care that provide for aging in place (Miller, 2019). CCRCs consist of independent single-dwelling houses or apartments for people who can manage their day-to-day needs, assisted living apartments for those who need limited assistance with their daily living needs, and skilled nursing services when continuous nursing assistance is required. CCRCs usually contract for a large down payment before the resident moves into the community. This payment gives a person or couple the option of residing in the same community from the time of total independence through the need for assisted or skilled nursing care. Decisions about living arrangements and health care can be made before any decline in health status occurs. CCRCs also provide continuity at a time in an older adult's life when many other factors, such as health status, income, and availability of friends and family members, may be changing.

Assisted Living Facilities

Assisted living facilities are an option when an older person's physical or cognitive changes necessitate at least minimal supervision or assistance. Assisted living allows for a degree of independence while providing minimal nursing assistance with administration of medication, assistance with ADLs, or other chronic health care needs. Other services, such as laundry, cleaning, and meals, may also be included.

Figure 8-3 • Families are an important source of psychosocial and physical support for all people. Caring interaction among grandchildren, grandparents, and other family members typically contributes to the health of all.

Both assisted living and CCRCs are costly and primarily paid out-of-pocket.

Long-Term Care Facilities

Many types of nursing homes, nursing facilities, or long-term care facilities offer continuous nursing care. Contrary to the myth of family abandonment and the fear of "ending up in a nursing home," the actual percentage of older adults residing in long-term care facilities has declined, from 5.4% in 1985 to 2.3% in 2018 (AoA, 2020). However, the actual number of older people who reside in long-term care facilities has risen owing to the large increase in the population of older adults and the use of nursing homes for short-term rehabilitation.

Short-term nursing facility care is often reimbursed by Medicare if the patient is recovering from an acute illness such as a stroke, myocardial infarction (MI), or cancer and requires skilled nursing care or therapy for recuperation. Usually, if an older adult suffers a major health event and is hospitalized and then goes to a nursing facility, Medicare covers the cost of the first 30 to 90 days in a skilled nursing facility as long as ongoing therapy is needed. The requirement for continued Medicare coverage during this time is documentation of persistent improvement in the condition that requires therapy, most often physical therapy, occupational therapy, respiratory therapy, or cognitive therapy. Some adults choose to have long-term care insurance as a means of paying, at least in part, for the cost of these services should they become necessary. Costs of long-term care for older adults who are living in nursing homes and are medically stable, despite having multiple chronic and debilitating health issues, are primarily paid out-of-pocket by the patient. When a person's financial resources become exhausted as a result of prolonged nursing home care, the patient, the institution, or both may apply for Medicare and Medicaid reimbursement depending on the situation. Family members are not responsible for nursing home costs.

An increasing number of skilled nursing facilities offer subacute care. This area of the facility offers a high level of nursing care that may either avoid the need for a resident to be transferred to a hospital from the nursing home or allow a hospitalized patient to be transferred back to the nursing facility sooner.

The Role of the Family

Planning for care and understanding the psychosocial issues confronting older adults must be accomplished within the context of the family. If dependency needs occur, the spouse often assumes the role of primary caregiver. In the absence of a surviving spouse, an adult child may assume caregiver responsibilities and need help in providing or arranging for care and support.

Two common myths in American society are that adult children and their aged parents are socially alienated, and that adult children abandon their parents when health and other dependency problems arise. In reality, the family has been and continues to be an important source of support for older adults; similarly, older family members provide a great deal of support to younger family members.

Although adult children are not financially responsible for their older parents, social attitudes and cultural values often dictate that adult children should provide services and

assume the burden of care if their aged parents cannot care for themselves. It is estimated that in 2018, informal caregivers provided 18.5 billion hours of unpaid care (Alzheimer's Association, 2019). Caregiving, which may continue for many years, can become a source of family stress and is a well-known risk for psychiatric and physical morbidity. Evidence-based interventions to reduce distress and enhance well-being in caregivers have been identified. Three broad types of effective programs include psychoeducational skill building, cognitive behavioral therapy, and using a combination of at least two approaches such as education, family meetings, and skill building sessions (Bakas, McCarthy, & Miller, 2018). Researchers have reported that web-based interventions are effective, efficient, and a better fit for the hectic lives of families and caregivers (Wasilewski, Stinson, & Cameron, 2017).

Cognitive Aspects of Aging

Cognition can be affected by many variables, including sensory impairment, physiologic health, environment, sleep, and psychosocial influences. Older adults may experience temporary changes in cognitive function (i.e., delirium) when hospitalized or admitted to skilled nursing facilities, rehabilitation centers, or long-term care facilities. These changes are related to differences in the environment or in medical therapy or to alteration in role performance. A commonly used assessment tool is the Mini-Mental State Examination (MMSE) (see Chart 8-3).

Good sleep hygiene can improve cognition, as can treatment of depression and anxiety. Several researchers are evaluating memory enhancement programs for older adults. In addition, researchers have found that eating a healthy balanced diet, being physically active for at least 30 minutes each day, and getting plenty of sleep can assist in preventing chronic illnesses as well as improving cognitive function (McDougall, 2017).

When intelligence test scores from people of all ages are compared, test scores for older adults show a progressive decline beginning in midlife. However, research has shown

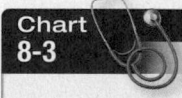

Chart 8-3   **ASSESSMENT**
Assessing Mental Status: Mini-Mental State Examination Sample Items

Orientation to Time

"What is the date?"

Naming

"What is this?" (Point to a pencil or pen.)

Reading

"Please read this and do what it says." (Show examinee the words on the stimulus form.) CLOSE YOUR EYES.

that environment and health have a considerable influence on scores, and that certain types of intelligence (e.g., spatial perceptions and retention of nonintellectual information) decline, whereas others (e.g., problem-solving ability based on past experiences, verbal comprehension, mathematical ability) do not. Cardiovascular health, a stimulating environment, and high levels of education, occupational status, and income all appear to have a positive effect on intelligence scores in later life.

Significant age-related declines in intelligence, learning, and memory are not inevitable. Many factors affect the ability of older adults to learn and remember and to perform well in testing situations. Older adults who have higher levels of education, good sensory function, good nutrition, and jobs that require complex problem-solving skills continue to demonstrate intelligence, memory, and the capacity for learning. Part of the challenge in testing older adults is determining what is actually being tested (e.g., speed of response) and whether the test results are indicative of a normal age-related change, a sensory deficit, or poor health. However, age differences continue to emerge even with untimed tests and when the tests are controlled for variations in motor and sensory function. In general, fluid intelligence—the biologically determined intelligence used for flexibility in thinking and problem solving—declines. Preventing or managing circulatory and nervous system disorders may positively affect the decline in fluid intelligence. Crystallized intelligence—gained through education and lifelong experiences (e.g., verbal skills)—remains intact. These differences exemplify the classic aging pattern of intelligence. Despite these slight declines, many older adults continue to learn and participate in varied educational experiences. Good health and motivation are important influences on learning (see Chart 8-4).

Pharmacologic Aspects of Aging

Because an increasing number of chronic conditions affect older adults, they use more medications than any other age group. Although medications improve health and well-being by relieving pain and discomfort, treating chronic illnesses, and curing infectious processes, adverse drug reactions are common because of medication interactions, multiple medication effects, incorrect dosages, and the use of multiple medications.

Drug Interactions and Adverse Effects

Polypharmacy is the use of multiple prescription or over-the-counter (OTC) medications. Over or incorrect prescribing occurs commonly in older adults (Miller, 2019). The potential for drug–drug interactions increases with increased medication use and with multiple coexisting diseases (**comorbidity**) that affect the absorption, distribution, metabolism, and elimination of the medications. Such interactions are responsible for numerous emergency department and primary provider visits, which cost billions of dollars annually.

Any medication is capable of altering nutritional status, and the nutritional health of an older adult may already be compromised by a marginal diet or by chronic disease and its treatment. Medications can affect the appetite, cause nausea and vomiting, irritate the stomach, cause constipation or diarrhea, and decrease absorption of nutrients. In addition, these medications may alter electrolyte balance as well as carbohydrate and fat metabolism. For example, antacids may cause thiamine deficiency; laxatives diminish absorption; antibiotics and phenytoin reduce utilization of folic acid; and phenothiazines, estrogens, and corticosteroids increase appetite and cause weight gain.

Combining multiple medications with alcohol, as well as with OTC and herbal medications, further complicates GI problems. For example, St. John's wort, a common herbal supplement effective for mild depression, decreases the anticoagulant effect of warfarin and interacts with many other medications metabolized in the liver (Miller, 2019).

Tools such as the American Geriatrics Society (AGS) Beers Criteria® are available to evaluate the patterns of drug use in older adults (Fick, Selma, Steinman, et al., 2019). The criteria rate the evidence for potentially harmful medications according to body systems. They are updated every 4 years in an attempt to improve the care of older adults by limiting their exposure to potentially inappropriate medications.

Altered Pharmacokinetics

Alterations in absorption, metabolism, distribution, and excretion occur as a result of normal aging and may also result from drug and food interactions (Comerford & Durkin, 2020). Absorption may be affected by changes in gastric pH and a decrease in GI motility. Drug distribution may be altered as a result of decrease in body water and increase in body fat. Normal age-related changes and diseases that alter blood flow, liver and renal function, or cardiac output (CO) may affect distribution and metabolism (see Table 8-2).

Nursing Implications

Principles that have been identified as appropriate for older patients include starting with a low dose, going slowly, keeping the medication regimen as simple as possible, and reconciling new and previous medication regimens at the time of discharge from an acute hospital stay (Comerford & Durkin, 2020; Fick et al., 2019). A comprehensive assessment that begins with a thorough medication history, including use

---

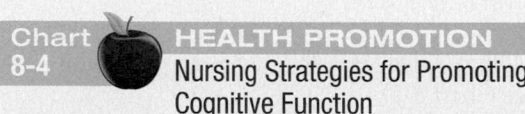

Chart 8-4 **HEALTH PROMOTION**

Nursing Strategies for Promoting Cognitive Function

Nurses can support the processes by which older adults learn by using the following strategies:

- Supply mnemonics to enhance recall of related data.
- Encourage ongoing learning.
- Link new information with familiar information.
- Use visual, auditory, and other sensory cues.
- Encourage learners to wear prescription glasses and hearing aids.
- Provide glare-free lighting.
- Provide a quiet, nondistracting environment.
- Set short-term goals with input from the learner.
- Prioritize the most important information and focus on the priority information.
- Keep education periods short.
- Pace learning tasks according to the endurance of the learner.
- Encourage verbal participation by learners.
- Reinforce successful learning in a positive manner.

TABLE 8-2   Altered Drug Responses in Older Adults

Age-Related Changes	Effect of Age-Related Changes	Applicable Medications
Absorption		
Reduced gastric acid; increased pH (less acid)	Rate of drug absorption—possibly delayed	Vitamins
Reduced gastrointestinal motility; prolonged gastric emptying	Extent of drug absorption—not affected	Calcium
Distribution		
Decreased circulating plasma proteins and total body water	Serious alterations in drug binding to plasma proteins (the unbound drug gives the pharmacologic response); highly protein-bound medications have fewer binding sites, leading to increased effects and accelerated metabolism and excretion	*Select highly protein-binding medications:* Oral anticoagulants (warfarin) Oral hypoglycemic agents (sulfonylureas) Barbiturates Calcium channel blockers Furosemide Nonsteroidal anti-inflammatory drugs (NSAIDs) Sulfonamides Quinidine Phenytoin
Reduced cardiac output Impaired peripheral blood flow Increased or decreased percentage of body fat	Decreased perfusion of many bodily organs Decreased perfusion Proportion of body fat increases with age, resulting in increased ability to store fat-soluble medications; this causes drug accumulation, prolonged storage, and delayed excretion	*Select fat-soluble medications:* Barbiturates Diazepam Lidocaine Phenothiazines (antipsychotics) Ethanol Morphine
Decreased lean body mass	Decreased body volume allows higher peak levels of medications	
Metabolism		
Decreased cardiac output; decreased size of the liver; diminished intestinal and portal vein blood flow	Decreased metabolism and delay of breakdown of medications, resulting in prolonged duration of action, accumulation, and drug toxicity	All medications metabolized by the liver
Excretion		
Decreased renal blood flow; loss of functioning nephrons; decreased renal efficiency	Decreased rates of elimination and increased duration of action; danger of accumulation and drug toxicity	*Select medications with prolonged action:* Aminoglycoside antibiotics Cimetidine Chlorpropamide Digoxin Lithium Procainamide

Adapted from Comerford, K. C., & Durkin, M. T. (2020). *Nursing 2020 drug handbook*. Philadelphia, PA: Wolters Kluwer.

of alcohol, recreational drugs, and OTC and herbal medications, is essential. It is best to ask the patient or reliable informants to provide all medications for review. Assessing the patient's understanding of when and how to take each prescription and OTC medication, as well as the purpose of each medication, allows the nurse to assess the patient's health literacy and adherence to the medication regimen. The patient's beliefs and concerns about the medications should be identified, including beliefs on whether a given medication is helpful.

Nonadherence with medication regimens can lead to significant morbidity and mortality among older adults. The many contributing factors include the number of medications prescribed, the complexity of the regimen, difficulty opening containers, inadequate patient education, financial cost, and the disease or medication interfering with the patient's life. Visual and hearing problems may make it difficult to read or to hear directions. Multifaceted interventions tailored to the individual patient are the most effective strategies in improving adherence. Allowing enough time for the older adult to

learn new skills, particularly when technology is involved, is essential (see Chart 8-5).

Mental Health Problems in the Older Adult

Severe mood swings, uncontrolled laughing or crying, changes in cognitive ability, and excessive forgetfulness are not a part of normal aging. These symptoms should not be dismissed as age-related changes; a thorough assessment may reveal a treatable, reversible condition. Changes in mental status can be related to many factors, such as alterations in diet and fluid and electrolyte balance, fever, or low oxygen levels associated with many cardiovascular and pulmonary diseases. Older adults are less likely than younger people to acknowledge or seek treatment for mental health symptoms. Changes may be reversible when the underlying condition is identified and treated. Nurses must recognize, assess, refer, collaborate, treat, and support older adults who exhibit signs and symptoms of depression, substance abuse, delirium, or dementia.

Chart 8-5 Nursing Strategies for Improving Medication Management and Adherence

The following strategies can help patients manage their medications and improve adherence:

- Assess self-management abilities, psychomotor skills, and current medication knowledge.
- Destroy or remove old, unused medications.
- Encourage the use of standard containers without safety lids (if there are no children in the household).
- Encourage the patient to inform the primary provider about the use of OTC medications and herbal agents, alcohol, and recreational drugs.
- Encourage the patient to keep a current list of all medications, including OTC and herbal medications, in their purse or wallet to share with the primary provider at each visit and in case of an emergency.
- Explain the purpose, adverse effects, and dosage of each medication, particularly those that are newly prescribed.
- If the patient's competence is doubtful, identify a reliable family member or friend who might assist the patient with adherence.
- Provide the medication schedule in writing.
- Reconcile medication schedule upon discharge from hospital or rehabilitation facility.
- Recommend using one supplier for prescriptions; pharmacies frequently track patients and are likely to notice a prescription problem such as duplication or contraindications in the medication regimen.
- Suggest the use of a multiple-day, multiple-dose medication dispenser to help the patient adhere to the medication schedule.

OTC, over-the-counter.
Adapted from Eliopoulos, C. (2018). *Gerontological nursing* (9th ed). Philadelphia, PA: Wolters Kluwer.

Depression

Depression is the most common affective or mood disorder of old age (Eliopoulos, 2018). The percentage of older adults with depressive symptoms varies widely depending upon the measures used and the population studied. Estimates range from 15% to 25% in community-dwelling older adults, and up to 25% of those living in long-term care facilities (Eliopoulos, 2018). Depression among older adults can follow a major precipitating event or loss and is often related to chronic illness or pain. It may also be secondary to a medication interaction or an undiagnosed physical condition. Rather than obvious sadness, an older person may exhibit more subtle signs of depression such as fatigue, diminished memory and concentration, feelings of worthlessness, sleep disturbances, appetite disturbances with excessive weight loss or gain, restlessness, impaired attention span, and suicidal ideation. Mild depression with symptoms that do not meet the criteria for a major depression is often underrecognized and undertreated, which results in reduced quality of life and function (Eliopoulos, 2018).

The risk of suicide is increased in older adults. There is a need for routine assessment of patients for depression and risk for suicide. Geriatric depression may be confused with dementia. However, the cognitive impairment resulting from depression is related to apathy rather than decline in brain function. When depression and medical illnesses coexist, as they often do, neglect of the depression can impede physical recovery. Assessing the patient's mental status, including depression, is vital and must not be overlooked. A commonly used assessment tool is the Geriatric Depression Scale (GDS) (Yesavage, Brink, Rose, et al., 1983). (See Chart 8-6.)

Older adults with depression can respond appropriately to treatment. Initial management involves evaluation of the patient's medication regimen and eliminating or changing any medications that contribute to depression. Furthermore, treatment of underlying medical conditions that may produce depressive symptoms may alleviate the depression. For mild depression, nonpharmacologic measures such as exercise, bright lighting, increasing interpersonal interactions, cognitive therapy, and reminiscence therapy are effective. However, for major depression, antidepressants and short-term psychotherapy, particularly in combination, are effective in older adults. Antidepressants, such as bupropion hydrobromide, venlafaxine hydrochloride, and mirtazapine, as well as selective serotonin reuptake inhibitors, such as paroxetine hydrochloride, can be effective (Comerford & Durkin, 2020). Tricyclic antidepressants can be useful for treating major depression in some patients. Electroconvulsive therapy is highly effective when antidepressant medications are not tolerated, not effective, or pose a significant medical risk (Miller, 2019).

Most antidepressant medications have anticholinergic, cardiac, and orthostatic adverse effects (Comerford & Durkin, 2020). They also interact with other medications and, therefore, should be used with care to avoid medication toxicity, hypotensive events, and falls. Older patients prescribed antidepressants should be carefully monitored for side effects. Good patient education is needed to make sure older adults understand that it may take even longer than the typical 4 to 6 weeks for symptoms to diminish. During this period, nurses should offer support, encouragement, and strategies to maintain safety, such as changing positions slowly and maintaining adequate hydration (Miller, 2019).

Substance Use Disorder

Substance use disorders caused by misuse of alcohol and drugs may be related to depression. A national survey indicated that between 7% and 14% of adults age 65 and older reported alcohol abuse, dependence, binge drinking, or were at least at risk for alcohol dependence (Miller, 2019). Approximately 50% of adults age 65 and older drink alcohol on a regular basis (Kennedy-Malone et al., 2019). Moderate alcohol consumption has shown to have positive health benefits, such as lowering the risks for cardiovascular disease. Alcohol abuse is especially dangerous in older adults because of age-related changes in renal and liver function as well as the high risk of interactions with prescription medications and the resultant adverse effects. Alcohol and drug misuse in older adults often remains hidden because many older adults deny their habit when questioned. Using screening tools may help provide a rapid, sensitive, and inexpensive method for screening alcohol misuse. Alcohol use should be addressed during routine physical examinations (Resnick, 2019). See Chapter 4 for more information and specific assessment tools.

Chart 8-6 Geriatric Depression Scale

Choose the best answer for how you felt this past week.

[a]1.	Are you basically satisfied with your life?	YES	NO
2.	Have you dropped many of your activities and interests?	YES	NO
3.	Do you feel that your life is empty?	YES	NO
4.	Do you often get bored?	YES	NO
[a]5.	Are you hopeful about the future?	YES	NO
6.	Are you bothered by thoughts you can't get out of your head?	YES	NO
[a]7.	Are you in good spirits most of the time?	YES	NO
8.	Are you afraid that something bad is going to happen to you?	YES	NO
[a]9.	Do you feel happy most of the time?	YES	NO
10.	Do you often feel helpless?	YES	NO
11.	Do you often get restless and fidgety?	YES	NO
12.	Do you prefer to stay at home, rather than going out and doing new things?	YES	NO
13.	Do you frequently worry about the future?	YES	NO
14.	Do you feel you have more problems with memory than most?	YES	NO
[a]15.	Do you think it is wonderful to be alive now?	YES	NO
16.	Do you often feel downhearted and blue?	YES	NO
17.	Do you feel pretty worthless the way you are now?	YES	NO
18.	Do you worry a lot about the past?	YES	NO
[a]19.	Do you find life very exciting?	YES	NO
20.	Is it hard for you to get started on new projects?	YES	NO
[a]21.	Do you feel full of energy?	YES	NO
22.	Do you feel that your situation is hopeless?	YES	NO
23.	Do you think that most people are better off than you are?	YES	NO
24.	Do you frequently get upset over little things?	YES	NO
25.	Do you frequently feel like crying?	YES	NO
26.	Do you have trouble concentrating?	YES	NO
[a]27.	Do you enjoy getting up in the morning?	YES	NO
28.	Do you prefer to avoid social gatherings?	YES	NO
[a]29.	Is it easy for you to make decisions?	YES	NO
[a]30.	Is your mind as clear as it used to be?	YES	NO

Score: _____ (Number of "depressed" answers)

Norms
Normal: 5 ± 4
Mildly depressed: 15 ± 6
Very depressed: 23 ± 5

[a]Appropriate (nondepressed) answers = yes; all others = no.
From Yesavage, J., Brink, T. L., Rose, T. L., et al. (1983). Development and validation of a geriatric screening scale: A preliminary report. *Journal of Psychiatric Research, 17*(1), 37–49.

Delirium

Delirium occurs secondary to numerous causes, including physical illness, surgery, medication or alcohol toxicity, dehydration, fecal impaction, malnutrition, infection, head trauma, lack of environmental cues, and sensory deprivation or overload. Older adults are particularly vulnerable to acute confusion because of their decreased biologic reserve and the large number of medications they may take. Nurses must recognize the symptoms of delirium and report them immediately. The Confusion Assessment Method (CAM) is a commonly used screening tool (Inouye, van Dyck, Alessi, et al., 1990). (See Chart 8-7.) Because of the acute and unexpected onset of symptoms and the unknown underlying cause, delirium is a medical emergency. If the delirium goes unrecognized and the underlying cause is not treated, permanent, irreversible brain damage or death can follow.

Alzheimer's Disease

AD is the sixth leading cause of death in the United States. For adults 65 years of age and older it is the fifth leading cause

of death. AD is a progressive, irreversible, degenerative neurologic disease that begins insidiously and is characterized by gradual losses of cognitive function and disturbances in behavior and affect. AD can occur in people as young as 40 years of age but is less common before 65 years of age. Although the prevalence of AD increases dramatically with increasing age, affecting as many as half of those 85 years and older, AD is not a normal part of aging. Without a cure or any preventive measures, it is estimated that 13.8 million Americans will have this disease by 2050 (Alzheimer's Association, 2019).

There are numerous theories about the cause of age-related cognitive decline. Although the greatest risk factor for AD is increasing age, many environmental, dietary, and inflammatory factors also may determine whether a person suffers from this cognitive disease. AD is a complex brain disorder caused by a combination of various factors that may include genetics, neurotransmitter changes, vascular abnormalities, stress hormones, circadian changes, head trauma, and the presence of seizure disorders.

AD can be classified into two types: familial or early-onset AD and sporadic or late-onset AD (see Chapter 6, Table 6-5). Familial AD is rare, accounting for less than 2% of all cases,

Chart 8-7 ASSESSMENT
Confusion Assessment Method (CAM)

Acute Onset

1. Is there evidence of an acute change in mental status from the patient's baseline?

Inattention[a]

2. **A.** Did the patient have difficulty focusing attention, for example, being easily distractible, or having difficulty keeping track of:
   What was being said?
   Not present at any time during interview.
   Present at some time during interview but in mild form.
   Present at some time during interview, in marked form.
   Uncertain.

   B. (If present or abnormal) Did this behavior fluctuate during the interview, that is, tend to come and go or increase and decrease in severity?
   Yes.
   No.
   Uncertain.
   Not applicable.

   C. (If present or abnormal) Please describe this behavior:

Disorganized Thinking

3. Was the patient's thinking disorganized or incoherent, such as rambling or irrelevant conversation, unclear or illogical flow of ideas, or unpredictable switching from subject to subject?

Altered Level of Consciousness

4. Overall, how would you rate this patient's level of consciousness?
   Alert (normal).
   Vigilant (hyperalert, overly sensitive to environmental stimuli, startled very easily).
   Lethargic (drowsy, easily aroused).
   Stupor (difficult to arouse).
   Coma (unarousable).
   Uncertain.

Disorientation

5. Was the patient disoriented at any time during the interview, such as thinking that they were somewhere other than the hospital, using the wrong bed, or misjudging the time of day?

Memory Impairment

6. Did the patient demonstrate any memory problems during the interview, such as inability to remember events in the hospital or difficulty remembering instructions?

Perceptual Disturbances

7. Did the patient have any evidence of perceptual disturbances, for example, hallucinations, illusions, or misinterpretations (such as thinking something was moving when it was not)?

Psychomotor Agitation

8. Part 1.
   At any time during the interview, did the patient have an unusually increased level of motor activity, such as restlessness, picking at bedclothes, tapping fingers, or making frequent sudden changes of position?

Psychomotor Retardation

8. Part 2.
   At any time during the interview, did the patient have an unusually decreased level of motor activity, such as sluggishness, staring into space, staying in one position for a long time, or moving very slowly?

Altered Sleep–Wake Cycle

9. Did the patient have evidence of disturbance of the sleep–wake cycle, such as excessive daytime sleepiness with insomnia at night?

[a]The questions listed under this topic were repeated for each topic where applicable.
From Inouye, S. K., van Dyck, C. H., Alessi, C. A., et al. (1990). Clarifying confusion: The confusion assessment method. *Annals of Internal Medicine,* 113(12), 941–948. Used with permission.

---

and is frequently associated with genetic mutations. It can occur in middle-aged adults. If family members have at least two other relatives with AD, then there is a familial component, which may include both environmental triggers and genetic determinants (NIH, 2017).

Pathophysiology

The pathogenesis of AD is uncertain but the disease includes specific neuropathologic and biochemical changes that interfere with neurotransmission. These changes consist of neurofibrillary tangles (tangled masses of nonfunctioning neurons) and senile or neuritic plaques (deposits of amyloid protein, part of a larger protein called *amyloid precursor protein* in the brain). The neuronal damage occurs primarily in the cerebral cortex and results in decreased brain size. Similar changes are found in the normal brain tissue of nonsymptomatic older adults, although to a lesser extent. Cells that use the neurotransmitter acetylcholine are principally affected by AD. At the biochemical level, the enzyme active in producing acetylcholine, which is specifically involved in memory processing, is decreased.

Scientists have been studying complex neurodegenerative diseases such as AD and have focused on two key issues: whether a gene might influence a person's overall risk of developing the disease, and whether a gene might influence some particular aspect of a person's risk, such as the age at which the disease begins (age at onset). There are genetic differences in early- and late-onset forms of AD (NIH, 2017). Researchers are investigating what predisposes people to develop the plaques and neurofibrillary tangles that can be seen at autopsy in the brains of patients with AD. Understanding the complex ways in which aging as well as genetic and nongenetic factors affect brain cells over time, eventually leading to AD, continues to increase.

Clinical Manifestations

In the early stages of AD, forgetfulness and subtle memory loss occur. Patients may experience small difficulties in work or social activities but have adequate cognitive function to compensate for the loss and continue to function independently. With further progression of AD, the deficits can no longer be concealed. Forgetfulness is manifested in many daily actions; patients may lose their ability to recognize familiar faces, places, and objects and they may become lost in a familiar environment. They may repeat the same stories or ask the same question repeatedly. Trying to reason with people with AD and using reality **orientation** (a person's ability to recognize who and where they are in a time continuum) only increase their anxiety without increasing function. Conversation becomes difficult, and word-finding difficulties occur. The ability to formulate concepts and think abstractly disappears—for example, a patient can interpret a proverb only in concrete terms. Patients are often unable to recognize the consequences of their actions and, therefore, exhibit impulsive behavior—for example, on a hot day a patient may decide to wade in the city fountain fully clothed. Patients have difficulty with everyday activities, such as operating simple appliances and handling money.

Personality changes are also usually evident. Patients may become depressed, suspicious, paranoid, hostile, and even combative. Progression of the disease intensifies the symptoms: Speaking skills deteriorate to nonsense syllables, agitation and physical activity increase, and patients may wander at night. Eventually, assistance is needed for most ADLs, including eating and toileting, because dysphagia and incontinence develop. The terminal stage, in which patients are usually immobile and require total care, may last months or years. Occasionally, patients may recognize family members or caregivers. Death occurs as a result of complications such as pneumonia, malnutrition, or dehydration.

Assessment and Diagnostic Findings

A definitive diagnosis of AD can be made only at autopsy; however, an accurate clinical diagnosis can be made in the majority of cases. The most important goal is to rule out other causes of dementia that are reversible, such as depression, delirium, alcohol or drug abuse, or inappropriate drug dosage or drug toxicity. AD is a diagnosis of exclusion; a diagnosis of probable AD is made when the medical history, physical examination, and laboratory tests have excluded all known causes of other dementias.

The health history—including medical history, family history, social and cultural history, and medication history—and the physical examination, including functional and mental health status, are essential to the diagnosis of probable AD. Diagnostic tests, including complete blood count, chemistry profile, and vitamin B_{12} and thyroid hormone levels, as well as screening with electroencephalography, computed tomography (CT), magnetic resonance imaging (MRI), and examination of the cerebrospinal fluid (CSF), may all refute or support a diagnosis of probable AD.

Depression can closely mimic early-stage AD and coexists in many patients. Therefore, assessing the patient for underlying depression is important. The GDS is a useful tool to assess for depression (see Chart 8-6). Tools such as the MMSE (see Chart 8-3) are useful for assessing cognitive status and screening for AD. Both CT and MRI of the brain are useful for excluding hematoma, brain tumor, stroke, normal-pressure hydrocephalus, and atrophy but are not reliable in making a definitive diagnosis of AD. Infections and physiologic disturbances, such as hypothyroidism, Parkinson's disease, and

vitamin B_{12} deficiency, can cause cognitive impairment that may be misdiagnosed as AD. Biochemical abnormalities can be excluded through examination of the blood and CSF.

Medical Management

In AD, the primary goal is to help maintain mental function as well as manage the cognitive and behavioral symptoms, and slow down the symptoms of the disease. Although there is no cure, several medications slow the progression of the disease. Cholinesterase inhibitors such as donepezil hydrochloride and rivastigmine tartrate, for example, enhance acetylcholine uptake in the brain, thus maintaining memory skills for a period of time. Cognitive ability may improve within 6 to 12 months of therapy. Rivastigmine is indicated for severe AD and it is recommended that treatment continue as long as possible (NIH, 2018b).

Behavioral problems such as agitation and psychosis can be managed by behavioral and other interventions such as music therapy (Weise, Jakob, Töpfer, et al., 2018). Associated depression and behavioral problems can also be treated pharmacologically if other interventions fail. Because symptoms change over time, all patients with AD should be reevaluated routinely, and the nurse should document and report both positive and negative responses to medications.

Nursing Management

Nurses play an important role in the recognition of AD, particularly in hospitalized older adults, by assessing for signs (e.g., repeating or asking the same thing over and over). Nursing interventions for AD are aimed at promoting patient function and independence for as long as possible. Other important goals include promoting the patient's physical safety, promoting independence in self-care activities, reducing anxiety and agitation, improving communication, providing for socialization and intimacy, promoting adequate nutrition, promoting balanced activity and rest, and supporting and educating family caregivers. These nursing interventions apply to all patients with AD, regardless of cause.

Supporting Cognitive Function

Because dementia of any type is degenerative and progressive, patients display a decline in cognitive function over time. In the early phase of dementia, minimal cuing and guidance may be all that are needed for the patient to function fairly independently for a number of years. However, as the patient's cognitive ability declines, family members must provide more and more assistance and supervision. A calm, predictable environment helps people with dementia interpret their surroundings and activities. Environmental stimuli are limited, and a regular routine is established. A quiet, pleasant manner of speaking, clear and simple explanations, and the use of memory aids and cues help minimize confusion and disorientation and give patients a sense of security. Prominently displayed clocks and calendars may enhance orientation to time. Color-coding the doorway may help patients who have difficulty locating their room. Active participation may help patients maintain cognitive, functional, and social interaction abilities for a longer period. Physical activity and communication have also been demonstrated to slow some of the cognitive decline of AD.

Promoting Physical Safety

A safe home and hospital environment allow the patient to move about as freely as possible and relieves the family of constant worry about safety. For the patient residing at home, in order to prevent falls and other injuries, all obvious hazards are removed and hand rails are installed. A hazard-free environment allows the patient maximum independence and a sense of autonomy. Adequate lighting, especially in halls, stairs, and bathrooms, is necessary. Nightlights are helpful, particularly if the patient has increased confusion at night, sometimes referred to as sundowning. Driving is prohibited, and smoking is allowed only with supervision. The patient may have a short attention span and be forgetful; therefore, the nurse and the family must be patient, repeat instructions as needed, and use reminders (i.e., post-it notes, electronic reminders) for daily activities. Doors leading from the house must be secured. Outside the home, all activities must be supervised to protect the patient, and the patient should wear some type of identification in case of separation from the caregiver.

If the patient is hospitalized, additional precautionary measures should be taken. Wandering behavior, which may be worse in the hospital due to unfamiliar surroundings, can often be reduced by gentle persuasion, distraction, or by placing the patient close to the nursing station. Restraints should be avoided because they can increase agitation and lead to injury.

Promoting Independence in Self-Care Activities

Pathophysiologic changes in the brain make it difficult for people with AD to maintain physical independence. Patients should be assisted to remain functionally independent for as long as possible. One way to do this is to simplify daily activities by organizing them into short, achievable steps so that the patient experiences a sense of accomplishment. Frequently, occupational therapists can suggest ways to simplify tasks or recommend adaptive equipment. Direct patient supervision is sometimes necessary; however, maintaining personal dignity and autonomy is important for people with AD, who should be encouraged to make choices when appropriate and to participate in self-care activities as much as possible.

Reducing Anxiety and Agitation

Despite profound cognitive losses, patients are sometimes aware of their diminishing abilities. Patients need constant emotional support that reinforces a positive self-image. When loss of skills occurs, goals are adjusted to fit the patient's declining ability.

The environment should be kept familiar and noise free. Excitement and confusion can be upsetting and may precipitate a combative, agitated state known as a catastrophic reaction (overreaction to excessive stimulation). The patient may respond by screaming, crying, or becoming abusive (physically or verbally); this may be the patient's only way of expressing an inability to cope with the environment. When this occurs, it is important to remain calm and unhurried. Forcing the patient to proceed with the activity only increases the agitation. It is better to postpone the activity until later, even to another day. Frequently, the patient quickly forgets what triggered the reaction. Measures such as moving to a familiar environment, listening to music, stroking, rocking, or distraction may quiet the patient. Research suggests that the use of activities and music therapy, both individualized and in groups, help decrease agitation (Zhang, Cai, An, et al., 2017). Becoming familiar with a particular patient's usual responses to certain stressors helps caregivers avoid stressful situations.

Improving Communication

To promote the patient's interpretation of messages, the nurse should remain unhurried and reduce noises and distractions. Use of clear, easy-to-understand sentences to convey messages is essential because patients frequently forget the meaning of words or have difficulty organizing and expressing thoughts. In the earlier stages of dementia, lists and simple written instructions that serve as reminders may be helpful. In later stages, the patient may be able to point to an object or use nonverbal language to communicate. Tactile stimuli, such as hugs or hand pats, are usually interpreted as signs of affection, concern, and security.

Providing for Socialization and Intimacy Needs

Because socialization with friends can be comforting, visits, letters, and phone calls are encouraged. Recreation is important, and people with dementia are encouraged to participate in simple activities. Realistic goals for activities that provide satisfaction are appropriate. Hobbies and activities such as walking, exercising, and socializing can improve quality of life. The nonjudgmental friendliness of a pet may provide stimulation, comfort, and contentment. Care of plants or a pet can also be satisfying and an outlet for energy.

AD does not eliminate the need for intimacy. Patients and their spouses may continue to enjoy sexual activity. Spouses should be encouraged to talk about any sexual concerns, and sexual counseling may be necessary. Simple expressions of love, such as touching and holding, are often meaningful.

Promoting Adequate Nutrition

Mealtime can be a pleasant social occasion or a time of upset and distress, and it should be kept simple and calm, without confrontations. Patients prefer familiar foods that look appetizing and taste good. Cueing may be necessary to encourage adequate nutrition and hydration. Food is cut into small pieces to prevent choking. Liquids may be easier to swallow if they are thickened. Hot food and beverages are served warm, and the temperature of the foods should be checked to prevent burns.

When lack of coordination interferes with self-feeding, adaptive equipment is helpful (see Fig. 8-4). Some patients may do well eating with a spoon or with their fingers. If this is the case, an apron or a smock, rather than a bib, is used to protect clothing. As deficits progress, it may become necessary to feed the patient. Forgetfulness, disinterest, dental problems, lack of coordination, overstimulation, and choking all serve as barriers to good nutrition and hydration.

Promoting Balanced Activity and Rest

Many patients with dementia exhibit sleep disturbances, wandering, and behaviors that may be considered inappropriate. These behaviors are most likely to occur when there are unmet underlying physical or psychological needs. Caregivers must identify the needs of patients who are exhibiting these behaviors because further health decline may occur if the

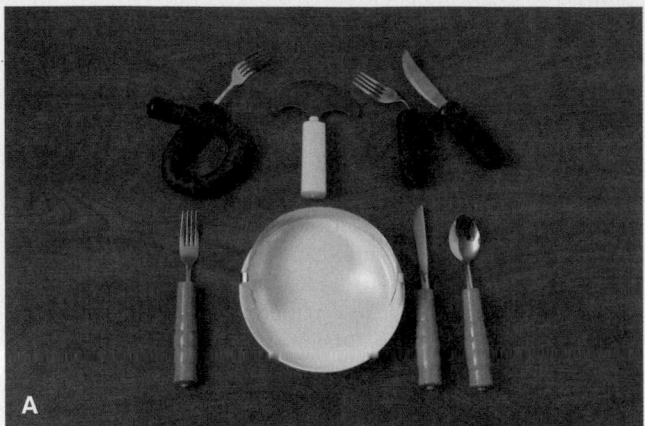

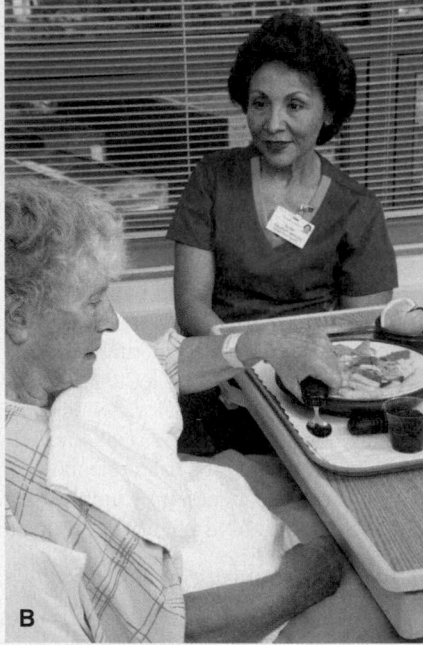

Figure 8-4 • **A.** Assistive feeding devices make it easy for patients to grasp and get food on utensils. **B.** Assistive feeding devices may be required for patients who are weak, fatigued, or paralyzed or have neuromuscular impairment.

source of the problem is not corrected. Adequate sleep and physical exercise are essential. If sleep is interrupted or the patient cannot fall asleep, music, warm milk, or a back rub may help the patient relax. During the day, patients should be encouraged to participate in exercise because a regular pattern of activity and rest enhances nighttime sleep. Long periods of daytime sleeping are discouraged.

Promoting Home, Community-Based, and Transitional Care

The emotional burden on the families of patients with all types of dementia is enormous. The physical health of the patient is often very stable and the decline gradual. Family members may cling to the hope that the diagnosis is incorrect and that their relative will improve with greater effort. Family members provide at least 83% of the home care that is required by patients with AD (Alzheimer's Association, 2019). They are faced with numerous difficult decisions (e.g.,

when the patient should stop driving, when to assume responsibility for the patient's financial affairs). Aggression and hostility exhibited by the patient are often misunderstood by caregivers, who may feel unappreciated, frustrated, and angry. Feelings of guilt, nervousness, and worry contribute to caregiver fatigue, depression, and family dysfunction. Researchers have identified that a Web-based intervention can be effective in helping with anxiety and stress, reducing depressive symptoms, and identifying care needs and planning interventions that promote balance and congruence in the lives of caregivers (Ploeg, Markle-Reid, Valaitis, et al., 2017).

Neglect or abuse of the patient can occur, and this has been documented in home situations as well as in institutions. If neglect or abuse of any kind—including physical, emotional, sexual, neglect, or financial abuse—is suspected, the local adult protective services agency must be notified. The responsibility of the nurse is to report the suspected abuse, not to prove it.

The Alzheimer's Association is a coalition of family members and professionals who share the goals of family support and service, education, research, and advocacy. Family support groups, respite (relief) care, and adult day care may be available through different community resources, such as the Area Agency on Aging, in which concerned volunteers are trained to provide structure to caregiver support groups (see Resources section at the end of chapter). Respite care is a commonly provided service in which caregivers can get away from the home for short periods while someone else tends to the needs of the patient.

Vascular Dementia

Vascular dementia is the second most common cause of dementia and is characterized by an uneven, stepwise downward decline in mental function (Norris, 2019). Multi-infarct dementia, the most common form of vascular dementia, has an unpredictable course and is characterized by variable impairment depending on the affected sites in the brain. The patient may present with a deficit in only one domain such as word retrieval whereas other cognitive abilities may be intact. Diagnosis may be even more difficult if a patient has both vascular dementia and AD.

Because vascular dementia is associated with hypertension and cardiovascular disease, risk factors (e.g., hypercholesterolemia, smoking, heart disease, diabetes) are similar. Prevention and management are also similar (see Chapter 27). Measures to decrease blood pressure, control diabetes, and lower cholesterol levels may slow cognitive decline.

Additional Aspects of Health Care of the Older Adult

The nurse needs to consider other health issues of older adults. These include geriatric syndromes, elder neglect and abuse, as well as ethical and legal issues.

Geriatric Syndromes

Older adults tend to acquire multiple problems and illnesses as they age. The decline of physical function leads to a loss of independence and increasing frailty as well as to susceptibility to both acute and chronic health problems, which generally result from several factors rather than from a single cause. When combined with a decrease in host resistance, these factors can lead to illness or injury. Some problems commonly experienced by older adults are becoming recognized as **geriatric syndromes**. These conditions do not fit into discrete disease categories and require a multidisciplinary and comprehensive assessment to identify the underlying cause or causes. Examples include skin impairment (e.g., pressure injuries), poor nutrition, falls or functional decline, urinary incontinence, defecation incontinence, cognitive impairment (e.g., delirium), and sleep disturbances (Tang, Tang, Hu, et al., 2017). Although these conditions may develop slowly, the onset of symptoms is often acute. Furthermore, the presenting symptoms may appear in other body systems before becoming apparent in the affected system. For example, an older patient may present with confusion, and the underlying disease may be a UTI, dehydration, or a heart attack (van Seben, Reichardt, Aarden, et al., 2019).

The term *geriatric triad* includes changes in cognitive status, falls, and incontinence. This term is used to focus awareness on these three conditions, which need particular attention, and the implementation of prevention measures during the hospitalization of older patients.

Impaired Mobility

The causes of decreased mobility are many and varied. Common causes include strokes, Parkinson's disease, diabetic neuropathy, cardiovascular compromise, osteoarthritis, osteoporosis, and sensory deficits. To avoid immobility, older people should be encouraged to stay as active as possible. During illness, bed rest should be kept to a minimum, even with hospitalized patients, because brief periods of bed rest quickly lead to deconditioning and, consequently, to a wide range of complications. When bed rest cannot be avoided, patients should perform active range-of-motion and strengthening exercises with the unaffected extremities, and nurses or family caregivers should perform passive range-of-motion exercises on the affected extremities. Frequent position changes help offset the hazards of immobility. Both the health care staff and the patient's family can assist in maintaining the current level of mobility.

Dizziness

Older adults frequently seek help for dizziness, which presents a particular challenge because there are numerous possible causes. For many, the problem is complicated by an inability to differentiate between true dizziness (a sensation of disorientation in relation to position) and vertigo (a spinning sensation). Other similar sensations include near-syncope and disequilibrium. The causes for these sensations range in severity from minor (e.g., buildup of ear wax) to severe (e.g., dysfunction of the cerebral cortex, cerebellum, brain stem, proprioceptive receptors, or vestibular system). Even a minor reversible cause, such as ear wax impaction, can result in a loss of balance and a subsequent fall and injury. Because dizziness has many predisposing factors, nurses should seek to identify any potentially treatable factors related to the condition.

Falls and Falling

Inadvertent injuries rank third as a cause of death for older people, and falls are the most common cause of nonfatal injuries and hospital admissions. The incidence of falls rises with increasing age.

Many older adults who fall do not sustain an injury; however, between 20% and 30% of older adults who fall sustain moderate to serious injury such as bruises, hip fractures, or head trauma. One out of five falls in older adults results in serious injury such as broken bones or a head injury (Heron, 2019). Overall, older women who fall sustain a greater degree of injury than do older men; however, men are more likely to die of a fall injury (World Health Organization [WHO], 2019). Hip fracture is a common type of fracture that can occur as a result of a fall. Fifty percent of adults who fall but cannot get up on their own and sustain a hip fracture are then unable to return to the same functional level after this type of injury. Causes of falls are multifactorial. Both extrinsic factors such as changes in the environment or poor lighting and intrinsic factors such as physical illness, neurologic changes, or sensory impairment play a role. Mobility difficulties, medication effects, foot problems or unsafe footwear, orthostatic hypotension, visual problems, and tripping hazards are common and treatable causes. Polypharmacy, medication interactions, and the use of alcohol precipitate falls by causing drowsiness, decreased coordination, and orthostatic hypotension. Falls have physical dangers as well as serious psychological and social consequences. It is not uncommon for an older person who has experienced a fall to become fearful and lose self-confidence (Miller, 2019).

Nurses can encourage older adults and their families to make lifestyle and environmental changes to prevent falls. Adequate lighting with minimal glare and shadow can be achieved through the use of small area lamps, indirect lighting, sheer curtains to diffuse direct sunlight, dull rather than shiny surfaces, and nightlights. Sharply contrasting colors can be used to mark the edges of stairs. Grab bars by the bathtub, shower, and toilet are useful. Loose clothing, improperly fitting shoes, scatter rugs, small objects, and pets create hazards and increase the risk of falls. Older adults function best in familiar settings when the arrangement of furniture and objects remains unchanged.

> ► *Quality and Safety Nursing Alert*
>
> *In hospitalized and institutionalized older adults, physical restraints (lap belts; geriatric chairs; side rails, vest, waist, and jacket restraints) and chemical restraints (medications) precipitate many of the injuries they were meant to prevent. Because of the acute negative consequences of restraint use, accrediting agencies of nursing homes and acute care facilities now maintain stringent guidelines for correct application and use.*

Urinary Incontinence

Urinary incontinence may be acute, occurring during an illness, or may develop chronically over a period of years. Older patients often do not report this very common problem unless specifically asked. Transient causes may be attributed to *d*elirium and *d*ehydration; *r*estricted mobility; *i*nflammation, *i*nfection, and *i*mpaction; and *p*harmaceuticals and *p*olyuria (the acronym *drip* may be used to remember them). Once identified, the causative factor can be eliminated.

Older patients with incontinence should be urged to seek help from appropriate health care providers because incontinence can be both emotionally devastating and physically debilitating. Nurses who specialize in behavioral approaches to urinary incontinence management can help patients regain full continence or significantly improve the level of continence. Although medications such as anticholinergics may decrease some of the symptoms of urge incontinence (detrusor instability), the adverse effects of these medications (dry mouth, slowed GI motility, and confusion) may make them inappropriate choices for older adults (Fick et al., 2019). Various surgical procedures are also used to manage urinary incontinence, particularly stress urinary incontinence.

Detrusor hyperactivity with impaired contractility is a type of urge incontinence that is seen predominantly in the older adult population. In this variation of urge incontinence, patients have no warning that they are about to urinate. They often void only a small volume of urine or none at all and then experience a large volume of incontinence after leaving the bathroom. Nurses should be familiar with this form of incontinence and not show disapproval when it occurs. Many patients with dementia suffer from this type of incontinence, because both incontinence and dementia are a result of dysfunction in similar areas of the brain. Prompted, timed voiding can be of assistance in these patients, although clean intermittent catheterization may be necessary because of postvoid residual urine. See Chapter 49 for information on management of urinary disorders.

Increased Susceptibility to Infection

Infectious diseases present a significant threat of morbidity and mortality to older adults, in part because of the blunted response of host defenses caused by a reduction in both cell-mediated and humoral immunity (see Chapters 31 and 32). Age-related loss of physiologic reserve and chronic illnesses also contribute to increased susceptibility. Pneumonia, UTIs, GI infections, and skin infections are some of the common infections in older adults.

Because of a weakened immune response, the effects of influenza and pneumococcal infections on older adults are significant. Vaccination can help prevent both infections. There is a national goal to increase vaccination rates among people 65 years of age and older. More than 71% of those 65 years of age and older reported receiving an influenza vaccination between January and June 2018 and 69% reported that they had received a pneumococcal vaccination (AoA, 2020).

Influenza and pneumococcal vaccinations lower the risks of hospitalization and death in older adults. The influenza vaccine, which is prepared yearly to adjust for the specific immunologic characteristics of the influenza viruses at that time, should be given annually in autumn. A systematic review and meta-analysis on the effectiveness of high-dose versus standard-dose influenza vaccine suggests that better protection is provided with the high-dose, trivalent, inactivated influenza vaccine versus the standard vaccine in older adults (Lee, Lam, Shin, et al., 2018). The pneumococcal vaccine should be administered as recommended (see Chapter 3, Table 3-3). Both of these injections can be received at the same time in separate injection sites. Nurses should urge older adults to be vaccinated. All health care providers working with older adults or high-risk chronically ill people should also be immunized.

AIDS occurs across the age spectrum. It is increasingly recognized that AIDS does not spare the older segment of society, and many who are living with HIV/AIDS are aging.

Atypical Responses

Many altered physical, emotional, and systemic reactions to disease are attributed to age-related changes in older adults. Physical indicators of illness that are useful and reliable in young and middle-aged people cannot be relied on for the diagnosis of potential life-threatening problems in older adults. The response to pain in older adults may be lessened because of reduced acuity of touch, alterations in neural pathways, and diminished processing of sensory data.

Older adults who are experiencing an MI may not have chest pain but present with confusion. Hiatal hernia or upper GI distress is often the cause of chest pain. Therefore, acute abdominal conditions may go unrecognized in older adults because of atypical signs and absence of pain.

The baseline body temperature for older adults is about 1°F lower than it is for younger people (Weber & Kelley, 2019). In the event of illness, the body temperature of an older person may not be high enough to qualify as a traditionally defined fever. A temperature of 37.8°C (100°F) in combination with systemic symptoms may signal infection. A temperature of 38.3°C (101°F) almost certainly indicates a serious infection that needs prompt attention. A blunted fever in the face of an infection often indicates a poor prognosis. Temperatures rarely exceed 39.5°C (103°F). Nurses must be alert to other subtle signs of infection, such as mental confusion, increased respirations, tachycardia, and a change in skin color.

Altered Emotional Impact

The emotional component of illness in older adults may differ from that in younger people. Many older adults equate good health with the ability to perform their daily activities and believe that "you are as old as you feel." An illness that requires hospitalization or a change in lifestyle is an imminent threat to well-being. Older adults admitted to the hospital are at high risk for disorientation, confusion, change in level of consciousness, and other symptoms of delirium, as well as anxiety and fear. In addition, economic concerns and fear of becoming a burden to families often lead to high anxiety in older adults. Nurses must recognize the implications of fear, anxiety, and dependency in older patients. They should encourage autonomy, independent decision making, and early mobilization. A positive and confident demeanor in nurses and family members promotes a positive mental outlook in older patients.

Altered Systemic Response

In an older person, illness has far-reaching repercussions. The decline in organ function that occurs in every system of the aging body eventually depletes the body's ability to respond at full capacity. Illness places new demands on body systems that have little or no reserve to meet the crisis. Homeostasis is jeopardized. Older adults may be unable to respond effectively to an acute illness or, if a chronic health condition is present, they may be unable to sustain appropriate responses over a long period. Furthermore, their ability to respond to definitive treatment is impaired. The altered responses of older adults reinforce the need for nurses to monitor all body system functions closely, being alert to signs of impending systemic complication.

Elder Neglect and Abuse

Older adults are at risk for abuse and neglect both in the community setting and in nursing homes (Burnes, Pillemer, & Lachs, 2017). Because of different definitions and terminology and the pattern of underreporting, a clear picture of the incidence and prevalence of abuse among older adults is lacking. Furthermore, one of the major barriers to fully understanding elder abuse is that most professionals in all professions, including law enforcement, are not equipped to recognize and report this type of abuse. Often victims are reluctant to report the abuse and clinicians are unaware of the frequency of the problems.

Neglect is the most common type of abuse. Other forms of abuse include physical, psychological or emotional, sexual, abandonment, and financial exploitation or abuse. Burnes and colleagues (2017) reported factors associated with physical and emotional abuse included being separated or divorced, living in a low-income household, functional impairment, and younger age for community-dwelling older adults. Neglect was associated with poor health, living below the poverty level, being separated or divorced, and younger age. Neglect was lowest in Hispanic households (Burnes et al., 2017).

Physical abuse associated with staff misconduct in long-term care facilities has received much attention in the past decade. Braaten and Malmedal (2017) did a qualitative study to understand the perspective of staff regarding prevention of physical abuse of nursing home residents. Staff were asked what measures they considered useful to implement in their daily work to prevent abusive behaviors. Staff shared that there was a need for increased competence among staff about the concept of abuse, known risk factors, good communication skills, and trusting relationships, as well as a work environment/culture that promotes openness where ethical dilemmas can be discussed (Braaten & Malmedal, 2017). Factors associated with resident on resident abuse in a nursing home setting were reported as previous staff physical or emotional abuse; younger age; limitations in ADLs and IADLs; and the emotional closeness of the resident to their family (Braaten & Malmedal, 2017). Older adults with disability of all types are at increased risk for abuse from family members, paid caregivers, and staff, whether they live in the community or a long-term care facility.

Nurses should be alert to possible **elder abuse** and neglect. During the health history, the older adult should be asked about abuse during a private portion of the interview. Most states require that care providers, including nurses, report suspected abuse. Preventive action should be taken when caregiver strain is evident—before elder abuse occurs. Early detection and intervention may provide sufficient resources to the family or the person at risk to ensure patient safety. Interdisciplinary team members, including the psychologist, social worker, or chaplain, can be enlisted to help the caregiver develop self-awareness, increased insight, and an understanding of the disease or aging process. Community resources such as caregiver support groups, respite services, and local offices of Area Agencies on Aging (AAAs) are useful for both the older adult and the caregiver.

Social Services

Many social programs exist for older Americans, including Medicare, Medicaid, the Older Americans Act, Supplemental Security Income, Social Security amendments, Section 202 housing, and Title XX social services legislation. These federal programs have increased health care options and financial support for older Americans. The Older Americans Act mandated creation of a federal aging network, resulting in the establishment of the AAAs, a national system of social services and networks providing many community services for older adults. Each state has an advisory network that is charged with overseeing statewide planning and advocacy for older adults throughout the state. Among the services provided by the AAAs are assessment of need, information and referral, case management, transportation, outreach, homemaker services, day care, nutritional education and congregate meals, legal services, respite care, senior centers, and part-time community work. The agencies target low-income, ethnic minority, rural living, and frail older adults who are at risk for institutionalization; however, the assessment and information services are available to all older adults. Similar services such as homemaker, home health aide, and chore services can be obtained at an hourly rate through these agencies or through local community nursing services if the family does not meet the low-income criteria. Informal sources of help, such as family, friends, mail carriers, church members, and neighbors, all keep an informal watch on community-dwelling senior citizens. (See Resources section at the end of the chapter.)

Other community support services are available to help older adults outside the home. Senior centers have social and health promotion activities, and some provide a nutritious noontime meal. Adult day care facilities offer daily supervision and social opportunities for older adults who cannot be left alone. Adult day care services, although expensive, provide respite and enable family members to carry on daily activities while the older person is at the day care center.

Health Care Costs of Aging

Health care is a major expenditure for older adults, especially for those with chronic illness and limited financial resources. Older adults, who make up about 15% of the population, accounted for 38% of health care costs, particularly in the last year of life (Centers for Medicaid & Medicare Services [CMS], 2018).

The two major programs that finance health care in the United States are Medicare and Medicaid, both of which are overseen by the CMS. Both programs cover acute care needs such as inpatient hospitalization, primary provider care, outpatient care, home health services, and skilled nursing care in a nursing facility. Medicare is federally funded, whereas

Medicaid is given by states; therefore, eligibility and reimbursements for Medicaid services vary from state to state. For older adults with limited incomes, even with the support of Medicare or Medicaid, paying out-of-pocket expenses can be a hardship. Out-of-pocket health care expenses represent 28% of the income of poor and near-poor older adults. Despite changes to the Medicare prescription benefit plan, out-of-pocket expenditures and prescription costs can be burdensome (AoA, 2020).

Home Health Care

The use of home care services and skilled nursing home care increases with age. Because of the rapidly growing older adult population and the availability of Medicare funding for acute care, home health care in the United States has rapidly expanded. (See Chapter 2 for more information on home health care.)

Hospice Services

Hospice and palliative care have much in common. Both are for people with serious illnesses. Both follow treatment goals that aim to relieve pain, increase comfort, and improve quality of life for the patient and family. The goal of hospice is to improve the quality of life by focusing on symptom management, pain control, and emotional support. In most hospice cases, patients are not expected to live longer than 6 months. Hospice care focuses on quality of life, and by necessity, it usually includes realistic emotional, social, spiritual, and financial preparation for death. Palliative care is for people at any stage of a serious illness, and their condition does not have to be incurable. Palliative care aims to relieve pain and other symptoms to maintain the highest quality of life for the longest period of time (Casey, 2019). Under Medicare and Medicaid, medical and nursing services are provided to keep patients as pain free and comfortable as possible. (For an in-depth discussion of palliative and end-of-life care, see Chapter 13.)

Aging With a Disability

As the life expectancy of people with all types of physical, cognitive, and mental disability has increased, individuals must deal with the normal changes associated with aging in addition to their preexisting disability. There are still large gaps in our understanding of the interaction between disability and aging, including how this interaction varies depending on the type and degree of disability and other factors such as socioeconomics and gender. For adults without disability, the changes associated with aging may be minor inconveniences. For adults with disorders such as spinal cord injuries, aging is associated with higher rates of secondary health conditions compared to those aging without a disability (Jorgensen, Iwarsson, & Lexell, 2019). Many people with disability are greatly concerned about what will happen to them as they age and whether assistance will be available when they need care.

It has been proposed that nurses view people with disability as capable, responsible individuals who are able to function effectively despite having a disability. Both the Interface and the Biopsychosocial models of disability can serve as a basis for the role of nurses as advocates for removal of barriers to health care. The use of such models would also encourage public policies that support full participation of all citizens through greater availability of personal assistants and affordable and accessible transportation. See Chapter 7, Chart 7-2 for discussion of other disability models.

Today, children born with intellectual and physical disability and those who acquire them early in life are also living into middle and older age. Often, their care has been provided by the family, primarily by the parents. As parents age and can no longer provide the needed care, they seek additional help with the care or long-term care alternatives for their children. However, few services are available at present to support a smooth transition between caregiving by parents and then by others. Research and public policy must focus on supports and interventions that allow people with disability who are aging to increase or maintain function within their personal environment as well as in the outside community. Important questions include who will provide the care and how will it be financed. The National Institute on Aging has identified aging with a disability as a focus and is striving to provide streamlined information and access to those with a disability and their family caregivers.

Ethical and Legal Issues Affecting the Older Adult

Nurses play an important role in supporting and informing patients and families when making treatment decisions. This nursing role becomes even more important in the care of aging patients who are facing life-altering and possibly end-of-life decisions. Loss of rights, victimization, and other serious problems might occur if a patient has not made plans for personal and property management in the event of disability or death. As advocates, nurses should encourage end-of-life discussions and educate older adults to prepare advance directives before incapacitation (Miller, 2019).

An advance directive is a formal, legally endorsed document that provides instructions for care (living will) or names a proxy decision maker (**durable power of attorney**). It is to be implemented if the signer becomes incapacitated. This written document must be signed by the person and by two witnesses, and a copy should be given to the primary provider and placed in the medical record. The advance directive is not meant to be used only when certain (or all) types of medical treatment are withheld; rather, it allows for a description of health care preferences, including requesting full use of all available medical interventions. The health care proxy may have the authority to interpret the patient's wishes on the basis of medical circumstances and should be guided by the decisions or situations stated in the living will (see Chart 8-8).

When such serious decisions are made, possibilities exist for significant conflict of values among patients, family members, health care providers, and the legal representative. Autonomy and self-determination are Western concepts, and people from different cultures may view advance directives as a method for denial of care. Older adults from some cultures

Chart 8-8 ETHICAL DILEMMA
Does Stopping of Eating and Drinking Violate the Principle of Nonmaleficence?

Case Scenario

You work as a staff nurse in a skilled nursing facility in the Alzheimer care unit. C.R. is an 82-year-old woman with advanced Alzheimer's disease who has been a resident in the facility for over a year. Her status has deteriorated significantly over the past 2 months. C.R.'s daughter has been visiting her mother at dinnertime most evenings, bringing her favorite foods and drinks to feed her by hand. One evening, C.R.'s son visits during dinnertime and finds his sister feeding their mother. This was the first time C.R.'s son has visited her in over 2 months. He reacts angrily, noting that C.R. had noted in her advance directive that she did not wish to receive nutrition and fluids if she became incapacitated. He admonishes his sister "Mom does not even recognize either one of us—she would not want to keep going on this way!" C.R.'s daughter notes that although their mother does not recognize anyone or understand what is happening, she opens her mouth and seems to enjoy the food and fluids that she is receiving. C.R.'s son is his mother's sole designated proxy; he was authorized by her with her power-of-attorney to make health care decisions during a time when she had the mental capacity to make that decision. He reminds you and C.R.'s daughter of this, and tells you that he wants his sister to stop giving food and fluids to his mother.

Discussion

Whether or not a patient may autonomously decide to forego artificial nutrition and hydration therapy (ANH) is not subject to much debate at present. Most bioethicists tend to agree that a patient with mental capacity may decide to forego ANH, even if doing so may hasten the patient's death. Advance directives for health care that specify no ANH written by patients before such time as they lose capacity is considered binding. Proxy decision makers for patients who lose capacity may also make the decision to withhold ANH.

However, decisions to voluntarily stop eating and drinking (VSED), or taking nutrition and fluids by the "natural" oral route, can be more complicated. While ANH may only be delivered using medical interventions (e.g., intravenous fluids, feeding tubes), taking food and fluids orally might not be considered "medical care." In these instances, whether or not a designated proxy or person

vested with power-of-attorney for health care agrees that this type of feeding can continue may be inconsequential. The ANA (2017) declares that "VSED, with the intention of hastening death can only be made by those patients with decision making capacity, not by surrogates." (p.1). In that same position statement, however, the ANA (2017) also states that "the patient's decision regarding VSED remains binding, even if the patient subsequently loses capacity." (p.1). It is important for a person who wishes to VSED to specify that in an advance directive.

Analysis

- Describe the ethical principles that are in conflict in this case (see Chapter 1, Chart 1-7). Which principle do you believe should have preeminence as you proceed to work with C.R. and her adult children? Does VSED in a patient who now lacks capacity violate the principle of nonmaleficence?
- Is C.R.'s son authorized to specify that his sister may not hand feed their mother? What if C.R.'s advance directive specifically states that, should she lose capacity, she would not wish to receive *oral* food and fluids? C.R. opens her mouth and willingly accepts the foods and fluids given to her by her daughter; does this imply that she now consents to be hand fed?
- What resources might be available to you and the health care team to help C.R.'s adult children determine what is in her best interests?

References

American Nurses Association (ANA). (2017). Position statement: Nutrition and hydration at end of life. Retrieved on 7/31/2020 at: www.nursingworld.org/~4af0ed/globalassets/docs/ana/ethics/ps_nutrition-and-hydration-at-the-end-of-life_2017 june7.pdf

Christensen, J. (2019). An ethical discussion on voluntarily stopping eating and drinking by proxy decision maker or by advance directive. *Journal of Hospice and Palliative Nursing, 21*(3), 188–192.

Resources

See Chapter 1, Chart 1-10 for Steps of an Ethical Analysis and Ethics Resources.

---

may be unwilling to consider the future, or they may wish to protect relatives and not want them to be informed about a serious illness. Nurses can facilitate the decision making process by being sensitive to the complexity of patients' values and respecting their decisions. Directives must be focused on the wishes of the patient, not those of the family or the designated proxy.

If no advance arrangement has been made and the older person appears unable to make decisions, the court may be petitioned for a competency hearing. If the court rules that an older adult is incompetent, the judge appoints a guardian—a third party who is given powers by the court to assume responsibility for making financial or personal decisions for that person.

People with communication difficulties or mild dementia tend to be viewed as incapable of self-determination. However, people with mild dementia may have sufficient cognitive capability to make some, but perhaps not all, decisions.

For example, a patient may be able to identify a proxy decision maker and yet be unable to select specific treatment options. People with mild dementia may be competent to understand the nature and significance of different options for care.

In 1990, the Patient Self-Determination Act (PSDA), a federal law, was enacted to require patient education about advance directives at the time of hospital admission, as well as documentation of this education. Nursing homes are also mandated to enhance residents' autonomy by increasing their involvement in health care decision making. In both nursing homes and hospitals, the documentation and placement of advance directives in the medical record and the education of patients about advance directives vary considerably. Periodically, it is important to ensure that the directives reflect the current wishes of the patient and that all providers have a copy so that they are aware of the patient's wishes.

CRITICAL THINKING EXERCISES

1 **ebp** You notice an increase in the number of older patients who are confused on the medical-surgical unit where you work. What do you suspect may be the cause of this increase in patients who are confused? What screening tool(s) would you recommend for these patients? Would you recommend that these tools be used for every older patient? Why? What is the strength of the evidence base guiding your assessment, actions, and recommendations?

2 **inc** A 90-year-old man has been admitted to your medical unit with urinary retention. What nursing and interprofessional assessments are indicated during your initial interactions with him? What other interprofessional services might you try to engage?

3 **pq** During a home visit, an 81-year-old woman with diabetes and a lower limb amputation admits to you that she has fallen three times in the past 6 months. Identify priorities and strategies that may help to prevent further falls for this patient.

REFERENCES

*Asterisk indicates nursing research.
**Double asterisk indicates classic reference.

Books

American Nurse Association (ANA). (2010). *Gerontological nursing: Scope and standards of practice.* Silver Spring, MD: Author.

Capriotti, T., & Frizzell, J. P. (2016). *Pathophysiology: Introductory concepts and clinical perspectives.* Philadelphia, PA: FA Davis.

Comerford, K. C., & Durkin, M. T. (2020). *Nursing 2020 drug handbook.* Philadelphia, PA: Wolters Kluwer.

Eliopoulos, C. (2018). *Gerontological nursing* (9th ed.). Philadelphia, PA: Wolters Kluwer.

Farage, M., Miller, K. W., & Maibach, H. (2017). *Textbook of aging skin* (2nd ed.). Berlin: Springer.

Kennedy-Malone, L., Martin-Plank, L., & Duffy, E. (2019). *Advanced practice nursing in the care of older adults* (2nd ed.). Philadelphia, PA: F.A. Davis.

Mark, K. (2017). *Gerontological nursing: Competencies for care* (4th ed.). Boston, MA: Jones and Bartlett Learning, LCC.

Meiner, S. E., & Yeager, J. J. (2019). *Gerontologic nursing* (6th ed.). St. Louis, MO: Elsevier Mosby.

Miller, C. A. (2019). *Nursing for wellness in older adults* (8th ed.). Philadelphia, PA: Wolters Kluwer.

Norris, T. T. (2019). *Porth's pathophysiology: Concepts of altered health states* (10th ed.). Philadelphia, PA: Wolters Kluwer.

Resnick, B. (2019). *Geriatric nursing review syllabus: A core curriculum in advanced practice geriatric nursing* (6th ed.). New York: American Geriatric Society.

Weber, J. R., & Kelley, J. H. (2019). *Health assessment in nursing* (6th ed.). Philadelphia, PA: Wolters Kluwer.

Journal and Electronic Documents

Administration on Aging (AoA). (2020). A profile of older Americans: 2019. Retrieved on 11/30/2020 at: www.acl.gov/sites/default/files/Aging%20and%20Disability%20in%20America/2019ProfileOlderAmericans508.pdf

Alzheimer's Association. (2019). Alzheimer's and dementia facts and figures. Retrieved on 11/30/2020 at: www.alz.org/alzheimers-dementia/facts-figures

American Nurses Association (ANA). (2017). Position statement: Nutrition and hydration at end of life. Retrieved on 7/31/2020 at: www.nursingworld.org/~4af0ed/globalassets/docs/ana/ethics/ps_nutrition-and-hydration-at-the-end-of-life_2017june7.pdf

Bakas, T., McCarthy, M., & Miller, E. T. (2018). An update on the state of the evidence for stroke family caregiver and dyad interventions. *Stroke, 48*(5), e122–e125.

Bowler, R. P., Hansel, N. N., Jacobson, S., et al. (2017). Electronic cigarette use in US adults at risk for COPD: Analysis from two observational cohorts. *Journal of General Internal Medicine, 32*(12), 1315–1322.

Bozorgmehri, S., Fink, H. A., Parimi, N. C., et al. (2017). Association of sleep disordered breathing with erectile dysfunction in community dwelling older men. *The Journal of Urology, 197*(3 Pt 1), 776–782.

Braaten, K. L., & Malmedal, W. (2017). Preventing physical abuse of nursing home residents- as seen from the nursing staff's perspective. *Nursing Open, 4*(4), 274–281.

Burnes, D., Pillemer, K., & Lachs, M. S. (2017). Elder abuse severity: A critical but understudied dimension of victimization for clinicians and researchers. *The Gerontologist, 57*(4), 745–756.

Casey, D. (2019). Hospice and palliative care: What's the difference? *MedSurg Nursing, 28*(3), 196–197.

Centers for Disease Control and Prevention (CDC). (2017). Alzheimer's disease. Retrieved 11/30/2020 at: www.cdc.gov/aging/aginginfo/alzheimers.htm

Centers for Medicare & Medicaid Services (CMS). (2018). National health expenditure data. Retrieved 11/30/2020 at: www.cms.gov/newsroom/press-releases/cms-office-actuary-releases-2018-national-health-expenditures

Christensen, J. (2019). An ethical discussion on voluntarily stopping eating and drinking by proxy decision maker or by advance directive. *Journal of Hospice and Palliative Nursing, 21*(3), 188–192.

Damián, J., Pator-Barriuso, R., Garcia López, F. J., et al. (2017). Urinary incontinence and mortality among older adults residing in care homes. *Journal of Advanced Nursing, 73*(3), 688–699.

Devlin, J. W., Skrobik, Y., Gelinas, C., et al. (2018). Clinical practice guidelines for the prevention and management of pain, agitation/sedation, delirium, immobility, and sleep disruption in adult patients in the ICU. *Critical Care Medicine, 46*(9), e825–e873.

Fick, D. M., Semla, T. P., Steinman, M., et al. (2019). American Geriatrics Society 2019 Updated AGS Beers Criteria® for potentially inappropriate medication use in older adults. *Journal of the American Geriatrics Society, 67*(4), 674–694.

Frishman, W. H. (2019). Ten secrets to a long life. *The American Journal of Medicine, 132*(5), 564–566.

Heron, M. (2019). Death: Leading causes for 2017. National Vital Statistics Reports (NVSS). Retrieved on 7/2/2019 at: www.cdc.gov/nchs/data/nvsr/nvsr68/nvsr68_06-508.pdf

*Hladek, M. D., Gill, J., Bandeen-Roche, K., et al. (2019). High coping self-efficacy associated with lower odds of pre-frailty/frailty in older adults with chronic disease. *Aging & Mental Health.* doi.org/10.1080/13607863.2019.1639136

**Inouye, S. K., van Dyck, C. H., Alessi, C. A., et al. (1990). Clarifying confusion: The confusion assessment method. *Annals of Internal Medicine, 113*(12), 941–948.

Jorgensen, S., Iwarsson, S., & Lexell, J. (2019). Secondary health conditions, activity limitations, and life satisfaction in older adults with long-term spinal cord injury. *Journal of Injury, Function, & Rehabilitation, 9*(4), 356–366.

Karadag, E., Samancioglu, S., Ozden, D., et al. (2017). Effects of aromatherapy on sleep quality and anxiety of patients. *Nursing in Critical Care, 22*(2), 105–112.

Lee, J. K. H., Lam, G. K. L., Shin, T., et al. (2018). Efficacy and effectiveness of high-dose versus standard-dose influenza vaccination for older adults: A systematic review and meta-analysis. *Expert Review of Vaccines, 17*(5), 435–443.

McDougall, G. J. (2017). Assessing and addressing cognitive impairment in the elderly. A look at the research into cognitive impairment. *American Nurse Today, 12*(11), 12–17.

National Institutes of Health (NIH). (2017). Late-onset familial Alzheimer disease. Retrieved on 7/2/2019 at: rarediseases.info.nih.gov/diseases/12799/late-onset-familial-alzheimer-disease

National Institutes of Health (NIH). (2018a). Dietary supplement fact sheet: Vitamin D. Retrieved on 7/2/2019 at: www.grc.com/health/pdf/NIH_GOV_Dietary_Supplement_Fact_Sheet.pdf

National Institutes of Health (NIH). (2018b). How is Alzheimer's disease treated? Retrieved on 7/2/2019 at: www.nia.nih.gov/health/how-alzheimers-disease-treated

Ploeg, J., Markle-Reid, M., Valaitis, R. et al. (2017). Web-based interventions to improve mental health, general caregiving outcomes, and general health for informal caregivers of adults with chronic conditions living in the community: Rapid evidence review. *Journal of Medical Internet Research, 19*(7), e263.

Punch, R., & Horstmanshof, L. (2019). Hearing loss and its impact on residents in long term care facilities: A systematic review of literature. *Geriatric Nursing, 40*(2), 138–147.

Seah, B., Kowitlawakul, Y., & Jiang, Y., et al. (2019). A review on healthy ageing interventions addressing physical, mental and social health of independent community-dwelling older adults. *Geriatric Nursing, 40*(1), 37–50.

Sommerlad, A., Sabia, S., Singh-Manoux, A., et al. (2019). Association of social contact with dementia and cognition: 28 year follow-up of the Whitehall II cohort study. *PLoS Medicine, 16*(8), 1–12.

Štefan, L., Vrgoč, G., Rupčić, T., et al. (2018). Sleep duration and sleep quality are associated with physical activity in elderly people living in nursing homes. *International Journal of Environmental Research and Public Health, 15*(11), 2512.

Tang, H. J., Tang, H-Y. J, Hu, F. W., et al. (2017). Changes of geriatric syndromes in older adults survived from intensive care unit. *Geriatric Nursing, 38*(3), 219–224.

Tatum, P. E., Talebreza, S., & Ross, J. S. (2018). Geriatric assessment: An office-based approach. *American Family Physician, 97*(12), 776–784.

van Seben, R., Reichardt, L. A., Aarden, J. J., et al. (2019). The course of geriatric syndromes in acutely hospitalized older adults: The hospital-ADL Study. *Journal of the American Medical Directors Association, 20*(2), 152–158.

Wasilewski, M. B., Stinson, J. N., & Cameron, J. L. (2017). Web-based health interventions for family caregivers of elderly individuals: A scoping review. *International Journal of Medical Informatics, 103*(7), 109–138.

Weise, L., Jakob, E., Töpfer, N. F., et al. (2018). Study protocol: individualized music for people with dementia – improvement of quality of life and social participation for people with dementia in institutional care. *BMC Geriatrics, 18*(1), 313.

World Health Organization (WHO). (2019). Falls. Retrieved on 10/21/2019 at: www.who.int/news-room/fact-sheets/detail/falls

Xu, J., Murphy, B. S., Kochanek, M. A., et al. (2018). Deaths: Final data for 2016. *National Vital Statistics Reports, 67*(5), 1–20.

**Yesavage, J., Brink, T. L., Rose, T. L., et al. (1983). Development and validation of a geriatric screening scale: A preliminary report. *Journal of Psychiatric Research, 17*(1), 37–49.

Zhang, Y., Cai, J., An, L., et al. (2017). Does music therapy enhance behavioral and cognitive function in elderly dementia patients? A systematic review and meta-analysis. *Ageing Research Reviews, 35*, 1–11.

Resources

Administration on Aging (AoA), www.aoa.gov

Alzheimer's Association, www.alz.org

American Association for Geriatric Psychiatry (AAGP), www.aagponline.org

American Association of Retired Persons (AARP), www.aarp.org

American Federation for Aging Research (AFAR), www.afar.org

American Geriatrics Society (AGS), www.americangeriatrics.org

Association for Gerontology in Higher Education (AGHE), www.aghe.org

Children of Aging Parents (CAPS), www.caps4caregivers.org

Family Caregiver Alliance (FCA), www.caregiver.org

Gerontological Society of America (GSA), www.geron.org

Hartford Institute for Geriatric Nursing, www.hign.org

Hospital Elder Life Program (HELP), www.hospitalelderlifeprogram.org

LeadingAge (formerly American Association of Homes and Services for the Aging), www.leadingage.org

MedicAlert + Alzheimer's Association Safe Return (program for locating lost patients), www.alz.org/care/dementia-medic-alert-safe-return.asp

National Caucus and Center on Black Aging (NCBA), www.ncba-aged.org

National Council on Aging (NCOA), www.ncoa.org

National Gerontological Nursing Association (NGNA), www.ngna.org

National Institute on Aging (NIA), Alzheimer's Disease Education and Referral (ADEAR) Center, www.nia.nih.gov/Alzheimers

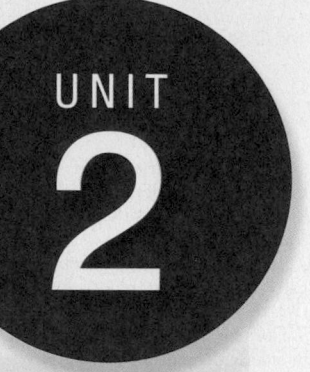

Concepts and Principles of Patient Management

PROMOTING TEAMWORK AND COLLABORATION IN PALLIATIVE CARE

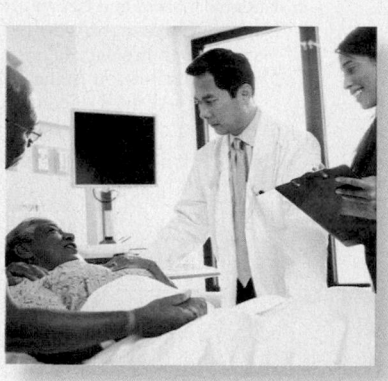

A 56-year-old woman diagnosed with advanced adenocarcinoma of the lung arrives at her outpatient palliative care appointment with delirium, lethargy, and confusion. Her blood work is drawn, and she is transferred to the inpatient oncology unit where you work for further evaluation. The admission profile reports that she is prescribed gabapentin 300 mg three times daily and fentanyl 50 mcg transdermal patch to be replaced every 72 hours. Upon assessment you find the patient confused and unable to rate her pain. The family is concerned about the confusion and worried that she is unable to tolerate the medications ordered for pain. Because this patient has many underlying components to her care, you request a case conference with the family, palliative care team, pharmacist, and the oncologist to determine the best plan of care at this time.

QSEN Competency Focus: Teamwork and Collaboration

The complexities inherent in today's health care system challenge nurses to demonstrate integration of specific interdisciplinary core competencies. These competencies are aimed at ensuring the delivery of safe, quality patient care (Institute of Medicine, 2003). The Quality and Safety Education for Nurses project (Cronenwett, Sherwood, Barnsteiner, et al., 2007; QSEN, 2020) provides a framework for the knowledge, skills, and attitudes (KSAs) required for nurses to demonstrate competency in these key areas, which include *patient-centered care, interdisciplinary teamwork and collaboration, evidence-based practice, quality improvement, safety,* and *informatics.*

Teamwork and Collaboration Definition: Function effectively within nursing and interprofessional teams, fostering open communication, mutual respect, and shared decision-making to achieve quality patient care.

SELECT PRE-LICENSURE KSAs	APPLICATION AND REFLECTION
Knowledge	
Recognize contributions of other individuals and groups in helping patient/family achieve health goals	Describe the nursing role in participating in a case conference. How do the various health care team members work with the patient and family and as a team to develop the best plan to manage care for this patient's pain while managing and minimizing the deleterious effects of delirium?
Skills	
Function competently within own scope of practice as a member of the health care team	Even though the patient is unable to rate her pain, what other methods of assessment can you use and rely on to assess pain in this patient? What interventions for pain can a nurse implement as part of a nursing care plan?
Attitudes	
Contribute to resolution of conflict and disagreement	After the case conference, the palliative care team recommends that the pain medication be administered to the patient as prescribed. The family is in conflict with the decision because the patient is confused and is not rating her pain. How can you best resolve the conflict? Are there other members of the team that may be instrumental in communicating with the family?

Cronenwett, L., Sherwood, G., Barnsteiner, J., et al. (2007). Quality and safety education for nurses. *Nursing Outlook*, *55*(3), 122–131; Institute of Medicine. (2003). *Health professions education: A bridge to quality*. Washington, DC: National Academies Press; QSEN Institute. (2020). *QSEN competencies: Definitions and pre-licensure KSAs; Teamwork and collaboration*. Retrieved on 8/15/2020 at: qsen.org/competencies/pre-licensure-ksas/#teamwork_collaboration

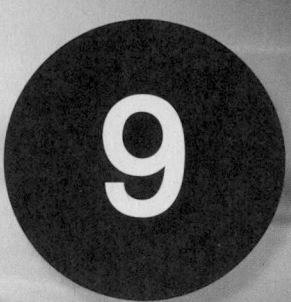

9 Pain Management

LEARNING OUTCOMES

On completion of this chapter, the learner will be able to:

1. Describe the fundamental concepts of pain including the types of pain, the four processes of nociception, and neuropathic pain.
2. Explain and demonstrate methods to perform a pain assessment.
3. List the first-line agents from the three groups of analgesic agents.
4. Identify the unique effects of select analgesic agents on older adults.
5. Describe practical nonpharmacologic methods that can be used in the clinical setting in patients with pain.
6. Use the nursing process as a framework for care of the patient with pain.

NURSING CONCEPTS

Addiction
Comfort

GLOSSARY

acute pain: pain that results from tissue damage that generally abates as healing occurs; serves as a warning signal that something is wrong or needs attention

adjuvant analgesic agent: a substance or medication added to an analgesic medication regimen to improve analgesia (*synonym:* co-analgesic agent)

agonist: a medication that binds to an opioid receptor mimicking the way endogenous substances provide analgesia

agonist–antagonist: a type of opioid (e.g., nalbuphine and butorphanol) that binds to the kappa opioid receptor site acting as an agonist (capable of producing analgesia) and simultaneously to the mu opioid receptor site acting as an antagonist (reversing mu agonist effects)

allodynia: pain due to a stimulus that does not normally provoke pain, such as touch; typically experienced in the skin around areas affected by nerve injury and commonly seen with many neuropathic pain syndromes

antagonist: a medication that competes with agonists for opioid receptor binding sites; can displace agonists, thereby inhibiting their action

breakthrough pain: a transitory increase in pain that occurs in the context of otherwise controlled persistent pain

ceiling effect: an analgesic dose above which further dose increments produce no change in effect

central sensitization: a key central mechanism of neuropathic pain; the abnormal hyperexcitability of central neurons in the spinal cord, which results from complex changes induced by the incoming afferent barrages of nociceptors and results in an increased nociceptive neuron response

chronic or persistent pain: pain that may or may not be time limited but that persists beyond the usual course/time of tissue healing

co-analgesic agent: one of many medications that can either improve the effectiveness of another analgesic agent or independently have analgesic action (*synonym:* adjuvant analgesic agent)

comfort–function goal: the pain rating identified by the individual patient above which the patient experiences interference with function and quality of life (e.g., activities the patient needs or wishes to perform)

efficacy: the extent to which a medication or another treatment "works" and can produce the intended effect—analgesia in this context

half-life: the time it takes for the plasma concentration (amount of medication in the body) to be reduced by 50% (after starting a medication, or increasing its dose; four to five half-lives are required to approach a steady-state level in the blood, irrespective of the dose, dosing interval, or route of administration; after four to five half-lives, a medication that has been discontinued generally is considered to be mostly eliminated from the body)

hydrophilic: a substance or medication that is readily absorbed in aqueous solution

hyperalgesia: an increasingly intense experience of pain resulting from a noxious stimulus

intraspinal: "within the spine"; refers to the spaces or potential spaces surrounding the spinal cord into which medications can be given

lipophilic: a substance or medication that is readily absorbed in fatty tissues

metabolite: the product of biochemical reactions during medication metabolism

mu agonist: any opioid that binds to the mu opioid receptor subtype and produces analgesic effects (e.g., morphine); used interchangeably with the terms *full agonist, pure agonist,* and *morphinelike medication*

multimodal analgesia or multimodal pain management: the intentional, concurrent use of more than one pharmacologic or nonpharmacologic intervention with different methods of action with the goal to achieve better analgesia while using lower doses of medications with fewer adverse effects

neuraxial: of the central nervous system

neuropathic (pathophysiologic) pain: pain caused by injury or dysfunction (lesion or disease) of one or more nerves of the peripheral or central nervous systems with resultant impaired processing of sensory input

neuroplasticity: the ability of the peripheral and central nervous systems to change both structure and function as a result of noxious stimuli

nociceptive (physiologic) pain: pain that is sustained by ongoing activation of the sensory system that conducts the perception of noxious stimuli; implies the existence of damage to somatic or visceral tissues sufficient to activate the nociceptive system

nociceptor: a type of primary afferent neuron that has the ability to respond to a noxious stimulus or to a stimulus that would be noxious if prolonged

nonopioid: refers to analgesic medications that include acetaminophen and nonsteroidal anti-inflammatory drugs (NSAIDs)

NSAID: an acronym for nonsteroidal anti-inflammatory drug (pronounced "en said")

opioid: refers to morphine and other natural, semisynthetic, and synthetic medications that relieve pain by binding to multiple types of opioid receptors; term is preferred to "narcotic"

opioid dose–sparing effect: occurs when a nonopioid or co-analgesic medication is prescribed in addition to an opioid, enabling the opioid dose to be lower without diminishing analgesic effects

opioid-induced hyperalgesia: a phenomenon in which exposure to an opioid induces increased sensitivity, or a lowered threshold, to the neural activity conducting pain perception; it is the "flip side" of tolerance

opioid naïve: denotes a person who has not recently taken enough opioid on a regular enough basis to become tolerant to the opioid's effects

opioid tolerant: denotes a person who has taken opioids long enough at doses high enough to develop tolerance to many of the opioid's effects, including analgesia and sedation

pain: an unpleasant experience that is either emotional or sensory resulting from actual or possible damage to tissues and is uniquely experienced and described by each person

peripheral sensitization: a key peripheral mechanism of neuropathic pain that occurs when there are changes in the number and location of ion channels; in particular, sodium channels abnormally accumulate in injured nociceptors, producing a lower nerve depolarization threshold, ectopic discharges, and an increase in the response to stimuli

physical dependence: the body's normal response to administration of an opioid for 2 or more weeks; withdrawal symptoms may occur if an opioid is abruptly stopped or an antagonist is given

placebo: any medication or procedure, including surgery, that produces an effect in a patient because of its implicit or explicit intent and not because of its specific physical or chemical properties

preemptive analgesic agents: pre-injury pain treatments (e.g., preoperative epidural analgesia and preincision local anesthetic infiltration) to prevent the development of peripheral and central sensitization of pain

refractory: nonresponsive or resistant to therapeutic interventions such as analgesic agents

substance use disorder (SUD): problematic use of substances such as opioids, benzodiazepines, or alcohol based on identification of at least two of the diagnostic criteria listed by the American Psychiatric Association. It is characterized by craving the substance; continuing use despite harm; inability to stop using; and experiencing withdrawal symptoms when abruptly not using the substance; formerly known as addiction

titration: upward or downward adjustment of the amount (dose) of an analgesic agent

tolerance: a normal physiologic process characterized by decreasing effects of a medication at its previous dose, or the need for a higher dose of medication to maintain an effect

withdrawal: result of abrupt cessation or rapid decrease in dose of a substance upon which one is physically dependent. It is not necessarily indicative of substance use disorder

Pain serves as a survival tactic that guides individuals not only to avoid damage in the moment, but also to learn to avoid danger in the future (Martin, Power, Boyle, et al., 2017). Nurses in all settings play a key role in the management of pain as experts in assessment, medication administration, and patient education. They are uniquely positioned to assume this role as members of the health care team most consistently at the patient's bedside. These characteristics have led to nurses' distinction as the primary managers of patients who are experiencing pain (Curtis & Wrona, 2018).

Fundamental Concepts

Understanding the definition, effects, and types of pain lays the foundation for proper pain assessment and management.

Definition of Pain

The American Pain Society (APS, 2016) defines **pain** as "an unpleasant sensory and emotional experience associated with actual or potential tissue damage or described in terms of such damage" (p. 2). This definition describes pain as a complex phenomenon that can impact a person's psychosocial, emotional, and physical functioning. The clinical definition of pain reinforces that pain is a highly personal and subjective experience: "Pain is whatever the experiencing person says it is, existing whenever he says it does" (McCaffery, 1968, p. 8). The self-report by the patient is the standard; it is considered to be the most reliable indicator of pain and the most essential component of pain assessment (DiMaggio, Clark, Czarenecki, et al., 2018).

Effects of Pain

Pain affects individuals of every age, gender, race, and socioeconomic class (APS, 2016). It is the primary reason people seek health care and one of the most common conditions that nurses treat (U.S. Department of Health & Human Services [HHS], 2019). Unrelieved pain has the potential to affect every system in the body and cause numerous harmful effects, some of which may last a lifetime (Table 9-1). Despite many advances in the understanding of the underlying mechanisms of pain and the availability of improved analgesic agents and technology, as well as nonpharmacologic pain management methods, all types of pain continue to be undertreated (Jungquist, Vallerand, Sicoutris, et al., 2017).

Types and Categories of Pain

Pain can be categorized in many ways, and clear distinctions are not always possible. Pain often is described from the perspective of duration, as being acute or chronic (persistent) (APS, 2016). **Acute pain** involves tissue damage as a result of surgery, trauma, burn, or venipuncture, and is expected to have a relatively short duration and resolve with normal healing. **Chronic or persistent pain** is subcategorized as being of cancer or noncancer origin and can persist throughout the course of a person's life. Examples of noncancer chronic pain include peripheral neuropathy from diabetes, back or neck pain after injury, and osteoarthritis pain from joint degeneration. Chronic pain may be intermittent, occurring with flares, or it may be continuous. Some conditions can produce both acute and chronic pain. For example, some patients with cancer have continuous chronic pain and also experience more intense acute exacerbations of pain periodically, which is called **breakthrough pain** (BTP). Patients may also endure acute pain from repetitive painful procedures during cancer treatment (APS, 2016).

Pain is also classified by its inferred pathology as being either nociceptive pain or neuropathic pain (Table 9-2). **Nociceptive (physiologic) pain** refers to the normal functioning of physiologic systems that leads to the perception of noxious stimuli (tissue injury) as being painful (International Association for the Study of Pain [IASP], 2017). This is the reason why nociception is described as "normal" pain transmission. **Neuropathic (pathophysiologic) pain** is pathologic and results from abnormal processing of sensory input by the nervous system as a result of damage to the

peripheral or central nervous system (CNS) or both (IASP, 2017).

Patients may have a combination of nociceptive and neuropathic pain. For example, a patient may have nociceptive pain as a result of tumor growth, and also report radiating sharp and shooting neuropathic pain if the tumor is pressing against a nerve plexus. Sickle cell disease pain is usually a combination of nociceptive pain from the various hematologic changes of sickled cells as well as neuropathic pain from nerve ischemia (Belvis, Henderson, & Benzon, 2018).

Nociceptive Pain

Nociception includes four specific processes: transduction, transmission, perception, and modulation (Ellison, 2017).

TABLE 9-1	Harmful Effects of Unrelieved Pain
Domains Affected	**Specific Responses to Pain**
Endocrine	↑ Adrenocorticotrophic hormone (ACTH), ↑ cortisol, ↑ antidiuretic hormone (ADH), ↑ epinephrine, ↑ norepinephrine, ↑ growth hormone (GH), ↑ catecholamines, ↑ renin, ↑ angiotensin II, ↑ aldosterone, ↑ glucagon, ↑ interleukin-1; ↓ insulin, ↓ testosterone
Metabolic	Gluconeogenesis, hepatic glycogenolysis, hyperglycemia, glucose intolerance, insulin resistance, muscle protein catabolism, ↑ lipolysis
Cardiovascular	↑ Heart rate, ↑ cardiac workload, ↑ peripheral vascular resistance, ↑ systemic vascular resistance, hypertension, ↑ coronary vascular resistance, ↑ myocardial oxygen consumption, hypercoagulation, deep vein thrombosis
Respiratory	↓ Flows and volumes, atelectasis, shunting, hypoxemia, ↓ cough, sputum retention, infection
Genitourinary	↓ Urinary output, urinary retention, fluid overload, hypokalemia
Gastrointestinal	↓ Gastric and bowel motility
Musculoskeletal	Muscle spasm, impaired muscle function, fatigue, immobility
Cognitive	Reduction in cognitive function, mental confusion
Immune	Depression of immune response
Developmental	↑ Behavioral and physiologic responses to pain, altered temperaments, higher somatization; possible altered development of the pain system, ↑ vulnerability to stress disorders, addictive behavior, and anxiety states
Future pain	Debilitating chronic pain syndromes: postmastectomy pain, post thoracotomy pain, phantom pain, postherpetic neuralgia
Quality of life	Sleeplessness, anxiety, fear, hopelessness, ↑ thoughts of suicide

Copyright 1999, Pasero, C., & McCaffery, M. Used with permission from Pasero, C., & McCaffery, M. (2011). *Pain assessment and pharmacologic management.* St. Louis, MO: Mosby-Elsevier.

TABLE 9-2	Classification of Pain by Inferred Pathology		
	Nociceptive Pain	**Neuropathic Pain**	**Mixed Pain**
Physiologic Processes	Normal processing of stimuli that damages tissues or has the potential to do so if prolonged; can be somatic or visceral	Abnormal processing of sensory input by the peripheral or central nervous system or both	Components of both nociceptive and neuropathic pain; poorly defined
Categories and Examples	*Somatic Pain:* Arises from bone joint, muscle, skin, or connective tissue. It is usually described as aching or throbbing in quality and is well localized *Examples:* Surgical, trauma; wound and burn pain; cancer pain (tumor growth) and pain associated with bony metastases; labor pain (cervical changes and uterine contractions); osteoarthritis and rheumatoid arthritis pain; osteoporosis pain; pain of Ehlers–Danlos syndrome; ankylosing spondylitis *Visceral Pain:* Arises from visceral organs, such as the GI tract and pancreas. This may be subdivided: • Tumor involvement of the organ capsule that causes aching and fairly well-localized pain • Obstruction of hollow viscus, which causes intermittent cramping and poorly localized pain *Examples:* Organ-involved cancer pain; ulcerative colitis; irritable bowel syndrome; Crohn's disease; pancreatitis	*Centrally Generated Pain* *Deafferentation pain:* Injury to either the peripheral or central nervous system; burning pain below the level of a spinal cord lesion reflects injury to the central nervous system *Examples:* Phantom pain as a result of peripheral nerve damage; poststroke pain; pain following spinal cord injury *Sympathetically maintained pain:* Associated with dysregulation of the autonomic nervous system *Example:* Complex regional pain syndrome *Peripherally Generated Pain* *Painful polyneuropathies:* Pain is felt along the distribution of many peripheral nerves. *Examples:* Diabetic neuropathy; postherpetic neuralgia; alcohol–nutritional neuropathy; some types of neck, shoulder, and back pain; pain of Guillain–Barré syndrome *Painful mononeuropathies:* Usually associated with a known peripheral nerve injury; pain is felt at least partly along the distribution of the damaged nerve *Examples:* Nerve root compression, nerve entrapment; trigeminal neuralgia; some types of neck, shoulder, and back pain	No identified categories *Examples:* Fibromyalgia; some types of neck, shoulder, and back pain; some headaches; pain associated with HIV; some myofascial pain; pain associated with Lyme disease
Pharmacologic Treatment	Most responsive to nonopioids, opioids, and local anesthetics	Co-analgesic agents, such as antidepressants, anticonvulsants, and local anesthetics, but there is wide variability in terms of efficacy and adverse-effect profiles	Co-analgesic agents, such as antidepressants, anticonvulsants, and local anesthetics, but there is wide variability in terms of efficacy and adverse-effect profiles

GI, gastrointestinal; HIV, human immune deficiency virus.
Copyright 1999, Pasero, C., & McCaffery, M. Used with permission from Pasero, C., & McCaffery, M. (2011). *Pain assessment and pharmacologic management.* St. Louis, MO: Mosby-Elsevier.

Figure 9-1 illustrates these processes and following is an overview of each.

Transduction

Transduction refers to the processes by which noxious stimuli, such as a surgical incision or burn, activate primary afferent neurons called **nociceptors**, located throughout the body in the skin, subcutaneous tissue, and visceral (organ), and somatic (musculoskeletal) structures (Montgomery, Mallick-Searle, Peltier, et al., 2018). These neurons have the ability to respond selectively to noxious stimuli generated as a result of tissue damage from mechanical (e.g., incision, tumor growth), thermal (e.g., burn, frostbite), chemical (e.g., toxins, chemotherapy), and infectious sources. Noxious stimuli cause the release of a number of excitatory compounds (e.g., serotonin, bradykinin, histamine, substance P, and prostaglandins), which move pain along the pain pathway (Ringkamp, Dougherty, & Raja, 2018) (see Fig. 9-1A). In addition, sodium, calcium, and potassium ion channels are stimulated to open, resulting in electrical impulses that are transmitted through the large, rapid conducting A-delta and smaller, peripheral C-fiber nociceptors (Ellison, 2017).

Prostaglandins are lipid compounds that initiate inflammatory responses that increase tissue swelling and pain at the site of injury (Baral, Udit, & Chiu, 2019). They form when the enzyme phospholipase breaks down phospholipids into arachidonic acid. In turn, the enzyme cyclo-oxygenase (COX) acts on arachidonic acid to produce prostaglandins (Fig. 9-2). COX-1 and COX-2 are isoenzymes of COX and play an important role in producing the effects of the **nonopioid** analgesic agents, which include the nonsteroidal anti-inflammatory drugs (**NSAIDs**) and acetaminophen. NSAIDs produce pain relief by mediating inflammation at the site of trauma, primarily by blocking the formation of prostaglandins (Leppert, Malec-Milewska, Zajaczkowska, et al., 2018). The nonselective NSAIDs, such as ibuprofen, naproxen,

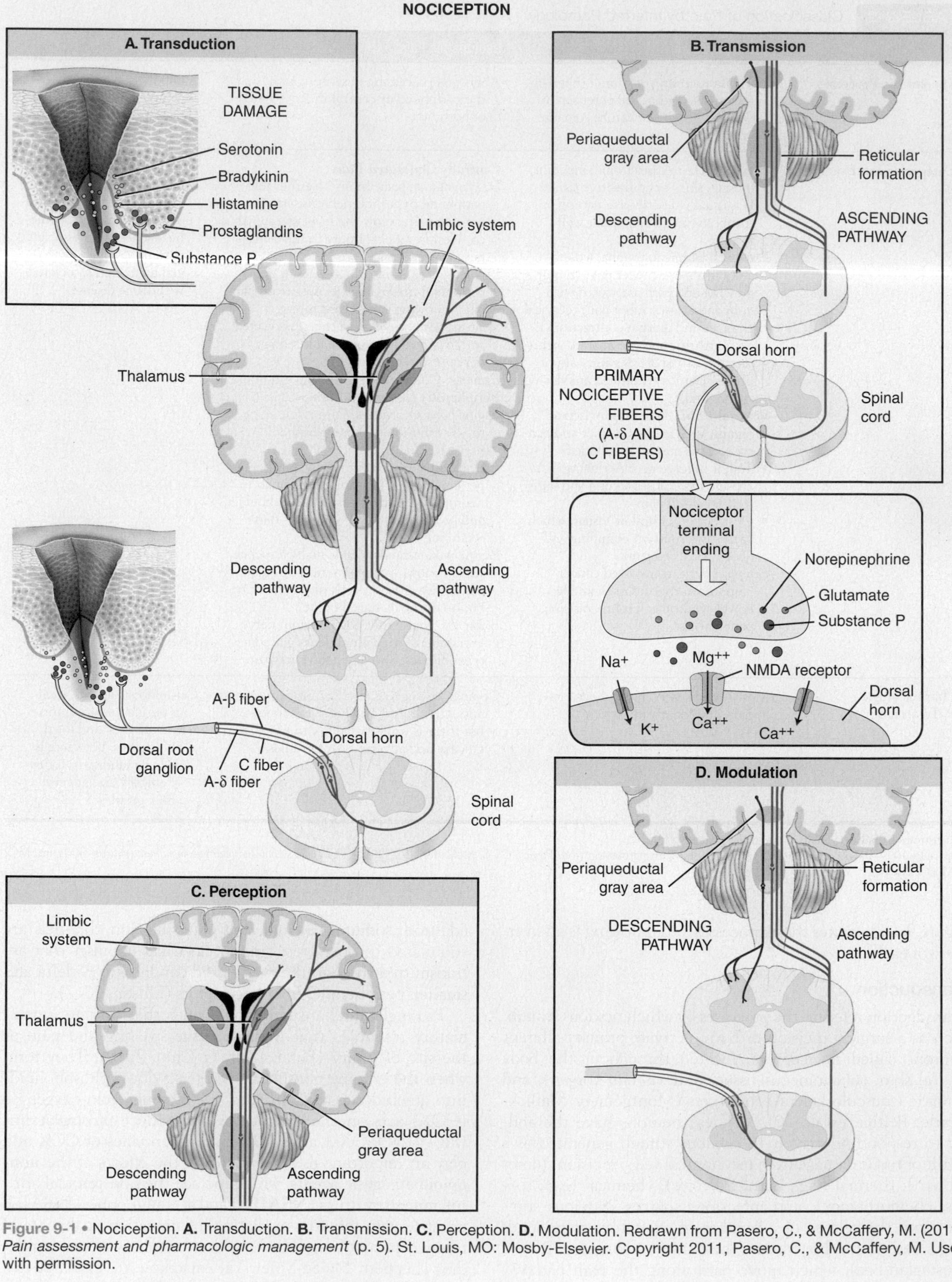

NOCICEPTION

Figure 9-1 • Nociception. **A.** Transduction. **B.** Transmission. **C.** Perception. **D.** Modulation. Redrawn from Pasero, C., & McCaffery, M. (2011). *Pain assessment and pharmacologic management* (p. 5). St. Louis, MO: Mosby-Elsevier. Copyright 2011, Pasero, C., & McCaffery, M. Used with permission.

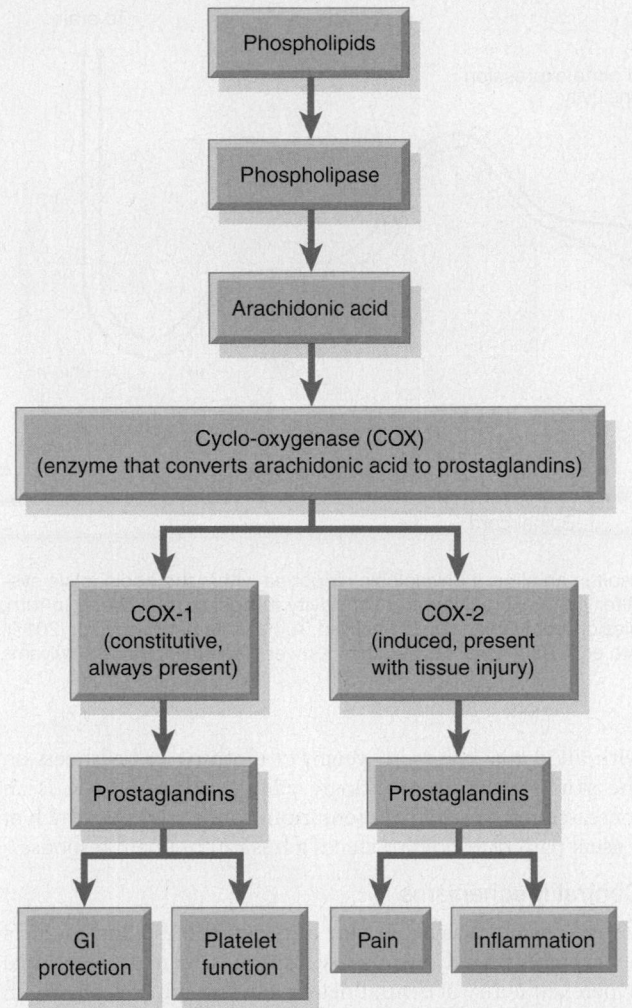

Figure 9-2 • Enzyme pathway: COX-1 and COX-2. Redrawn from Pasero, C., & McCaffery, M. (2011). *Pain assessment and pharmacologic management* (p. 6). St. Louis, MO: Mosby-Elsevier. Copyright 2004, Pasero, C., & McCaffery, M. Used with permission.

diclofenac, and ketorolac, inhibit both COX-1 and COX-2, and the COX-2 selective NSAIDs, such as celecoxib, inhibit only COX-2. As Figure 9-2 illustrates, both types of NSAIDs produce anti-inflammation and pain relief through the inhibition of COX-2. Acetaminophen is known to be a COX inhibitor that has minimal peripheral effect, is not anti-inflammatory, and can both relieve pain and reduce fever by preventing the formation of prostaglandins in the CNS (Slattery & Klegeris, 2018).

Other analgesic agents work at the site of transduction by affecting the flux of ions. For example, sodium channels are closed and inactive at rest but undergo changes in response to nerve membrane depolarization. Transient channel opening leads to an influx of sodium that results in nerve conduction (Nouri, Osuagwu, Boyette-Davis, et al., 2018). Local anesthetics reduce nerve conduction by blocking sodium channels. The calcium channel blocking anticonvulsants that are used to treat neuropathic pain facilitate analgesia by reducing the flux of calcium ions and limiting glutamate, norepinephrine, and substance P release (Peterson, Benson, & Hurley, 2018).

Transmission

Transmission is another process involved in nociception. Effective transduction generates an action potential that is transmitted along the lightly myelinated rapid conducting A-delta fibers and the unmyelinated slower impulse conducting C fibers (Ellison, 2017) (see Fig. 9-1B). The endings of A-delta fibers detect thermal and mechanical injury, allow relatively quick localization of pain, and are responsible for a rapid reflex withdrawal from the painful stimulus. Unmyelinated C fibers respond to mechanical, thermal, and chemical stimuli. They produce poorly localized and often aching or burning pain. A-beta (β) fibers are the largest of the fibers and respond to touch, movement, and vibration but do not normally transmit pain (Ellison, 2017; Vardeh & Naranjo, 2017).

The action potential impulse with the noxious information passes through the dorsal root ganglia, then synapses in the dorsal horn of the spinal cord, and then ascends up to the spinal cord and transmits the information to the brain, where pain is perceived (Ellison, 2017; Ringkamp et al., 2018) (see Fig. 9-1B). Extensive modulation occurs in the dorsal horn via complex neurochemical mechanisms (see Fig. 9-1B inset). The primary A-delta fibers release glutamate and C fibers release substance P and other neuropeptides (Schliessbach & Maurer, 2017). Glutamate is a key neurotransmitter because it binds to the *N*-methyl-*D*-aspartate (NMDA) receptor and promotes pain transmission (Zhou, 2017).

Perception

An additional process involved in nociception is perception, which is the result of the neural activity associated with transmission of noxious stimuli (Ringkamp et al., 2018). It requires activation of higher brain structures for the occurrence of awareness, emotions, and impulses associated with pain (see Fig. 9-1C). Although the physiology of pain perception continues to be studied, it can be targeted by nonpharmacologic therapies, such as distraction, which are based on the belief that innate brain processes can strongly influence pain perception (Chayadi & McConnell, 2019).

Modulation

Modulation is another process involved in nociception. Modulation of the information generated in response to noxious stimuli occurs at every level from the periphery to the cortex and involves many different neurochemicals (Damien, Colloca, Bellei-Rodriguez, et al., 2018) (see Fig. 9-1D). For example, serotonin and norepinephrine are inhibitory neurotransmitters that are released in the spinal cord and the brain stem by the descending (efferent) fibers of the modulatory system (Nouri et al., 2018). Some antidepressants provide pain relief by blocking the body's reuptake (resorption) of serotonin and norepinephrine, extending their availability to fight pain (Martin et al., 2017). Endogenous opioids are located throughout the peripheral and central nervous systems, and like exogenous opioids, they bind to opioid receptors in the descending system and inhibit pain transmission (Nouri et al., 2018).

Neuropathic Pain

Neuropathic pain is caused by either a lesion or a disease involving the somatosensory nervous system (Bouhassira, 2019).

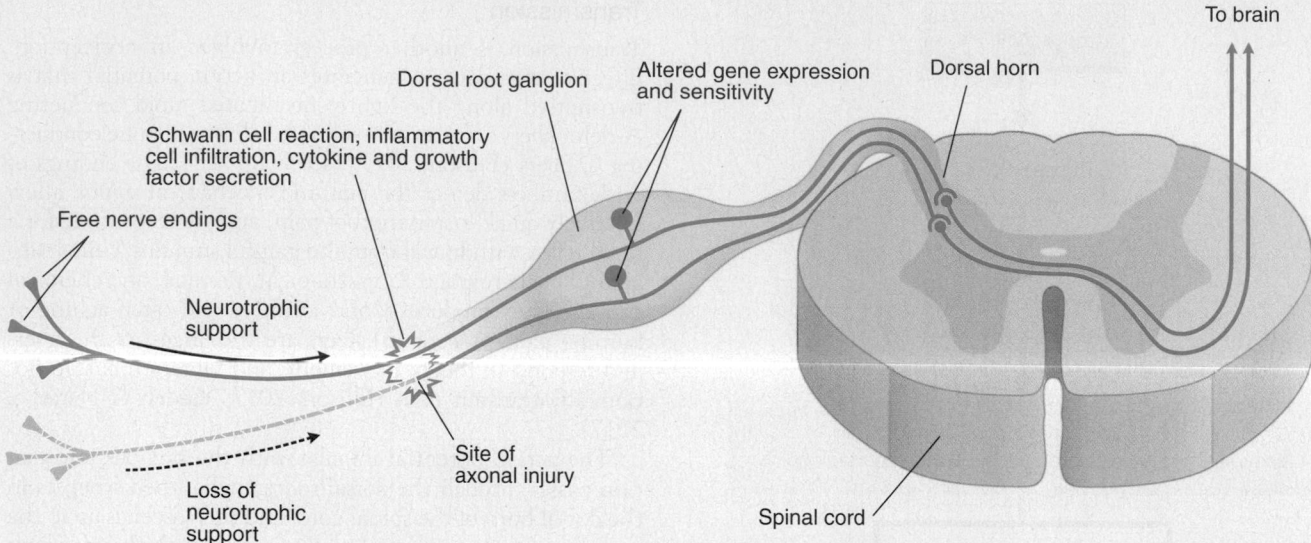

Figure 9-3 • Neuropathic pain. Nociceptive injury or inflammation may result in an altered physiologic response within the nociceptive system. These changes cause release of inflammatory cytokines that may alter gene expression and sensitivity in nociceptive fibers. In turn, these alter nociceptive activity, causing neuropathic pain. Used with permission from Golan, D. E., Tashjian, A. H., & Armstrong, E. J. (2017). *Principles of pharmacology: The pathophysiologic basis of drug therapy* (4th ed.). Baltimore, MD: Wolters Kluwer Health | Lippincott Williams & Wilkins.

Injuries to peripheral nerves can either be traumatic or non-traumatic, such as diabetic or compression neuropathies (Osborne, Anastakis, & Davis, 2018). Although specific causes may vary based on the underlying pathology, it is theorized that there are changes in the ion channels; imbalance of the stimuli processing between excitatory and inhibitory somatosensory signals; activity of glial cells; or potential differences in modulation of pain that occur with neuropathic pain (Colloca, Ludman, Bouhassira, et al., 2017; Liu, Zhu, Ju, et al., 2019) (Fig. 9-3). Recent research findings suggest that dysfunction in autophagy (i.e., cellular degradation of unnecessary materials) is involved with neuropathic pain (Liu et al., 2019). Research is ongoing to better define the peripheral and central mechanisms that initiate and maintain neuropathic pain (García, Gutiérrez-Lara, Centurión, et al., 2019; Kwiatkowski & Mika, 2018; Liu et al., 2019; Nishimura, Kawasaki, Suzuki, et al., 2019).

Peripheral Mechanisms

At any point from the periphery to the CNS, the potential exists for the development of neuropathic pain. Nerve endings in the periphery can become damaged, leading to abnormal reorganization in the nervous system called maladaptive **neuroplasticity**, an underlying mechanism of some neuropathic pain states (Osborne et al., 2018). Changes in ion channels can occur, such as increased sodium channel activity in sensory nerves resulting in heightened excitability, increased transduction, and release of neurotransmitters (Colloca et al., 2017). These and many other processes lead to a phenomenon called **peripheral sensitization**, which is thought to contribute to the maintenance of neuropathic pain and is thought to be reflected in allodynia and hyperalgesia (Osborne et al., 2018). **Allodynia**, or pain from a normally non-noxious stimulus (e.g., touch), is one such type of abnormal sensation and a common feature of neuropathic pain (Chekka & Benzon, 2018; Osborne et al., 2018). In patients

with allodynia, the mere weight of clothing or bedsheets on the skin can be excruciatingly painful. **Hyperalgesia** is an increased response of pain sensation from a stimulus which at a usual pain threshold produces a less intense pain response.

Central Mechanisms

Central mechanisms also play a role in the establishment of neuropathic pain. **Central sensitization** is defined as abnormal hyperexcitability of central neurons in the spinal cord, which results from complex changes induced by incoming afferent barrages of nociceptors, which also can result in allodynia and hyperalgesia (Osborne et al., 2018). Extensive release and binding of excitatory neurotransmitters, such as glutamate, activate the NMDA receptor and cause an increase in intracellular calcium levels into the neuron, resulting in pain (Yan, Li, Zhou, et al., 2017). Similar to what happens in the peripheral nervous system, an increase in the influx of sodium is thought to lower the threshold for nerve activation, increase response to stimuli, and enlarge the receptive field served by the affected neuron (Osborne et al., 2018; Yan et al., 2017).

As in the peripheral nervous system, anatomic changes can occur in the CNS. For example, when the NMDA receptor cells are continuously activated, reorganization in the dorsal horn of the spinal cord can occur (Nouri et al., 2018). Nerve fibers can invade other locations and create abnormal sensations, such as allodynia, in the area of the body served by the injured nerve.

Pain Assessment

The highly subjective nature of pain causes challenges in assessment and management; however, the patient's self-report is the undisputed standard for assessing the existence and intensity of pain (APS, 2016; Herr, Coyne, McCaffery, et al., 2011; McCaffery, Herr, & Pasero, 2011). Self-report

Chart 9-1 — Strategies to Use When the Patient's Report of Pain Is Not Accepted

- Acknowledge that everyone is entitled to a personal opinion, but personal opinion does not form the basis for professional practice.
- Clarify that the sensation of pain is subjective and cannot be proved or disproved.
- Quote recommendations from clinical practice guidelines, especially those published by the American Pain Society.
- Ask, "Why is it so difficult to believe that this person hurts?"

Copyright 2011, Pasero, C., & McCaffery, M. Used with permission from Pasero, C., & McCaffery, M. (2011). *Pain assessment and pharmacologic management.* St. Louis, MO: Mosby-Elsevier.

is considered the most reliable measure of the existence and intensity of the patient's pain and is recommended by The Joint Commission (Baker, 2017). Accepting and acting on the patient's report of pain are sometimes difficult. Because pain cannot be proven, clinicians may feel vulnerable to inaccurate or untruthful reports of pain. Although clinicians are entitled to their personal opinions, those thoughts cannot interfere with appropriate patient care. Chart 9-1 provides strategies to use when the patient's report of pain is not accepted.

◣ *Quality and Safety Nursing Alert*

Although accepting and responding to the report of pain may result in administering analgesic agents to an occasional patient who does not have pain, doing so helps to ensure that everyone who does have pain receives appropriate care. Health care professionals do not have the right to deprive any patient of appropriate assessment and treatment simply because they believe a patient is not being truthful. Pain is an extremely personal experience manifested uniquely by each person. It is important to carefully assess and reassess pain when administering analgesic medications.

Performing the Comprehensive Pain Assessment: Patient Interview

A comprehensive pain assessment should be conducted during the admission assessment or initial interview with the patient, with each new report of pain, and whenever indicated by changes in the patient's condition or treatment plan. It serves as the foundation for developing and evaluating the effectiveness of the pain treatment plan. The following are components of a comprehensive pain assessment and tips on how to elicit the information from the patient:

- *Location(s) of pain:* Ask the patient to state or point to the area(s) of pain on the body. Sometimes allowing patients to make marks on a body diagram is helpful in gaining this information.
- *Intensity:* Ask the patient to rate the severity of the pain using a reliable and valid pain assessment tool. Chart 9-2 provides guidance for educating patients and their families on how to use a pain rating scale. Various scales translated in several languages have been evaluated

Chart 9-2 — PATIENT EDUCATION: Educating Patients and Their Families How to Use a Pain Rating Scale[a]

Step 1. Show the pain rating scale to the patient and the family and explain its primary purpose.
Example: "This is a pain rating scale that many of our patients use to help us understand their pain and to set goals for pain relief. We will ask you regularly about pain, but any time you have pain you must let us know. We do not always know when you hurt."

Step 2. Explain the parts of the pain rating scale. If the patient does not like it or understand it, switch to another scale (e.g., vertical presentation, VDS, or faces).
Example: "On this pain rating scale, 0 means no pain and 10 means the worst possible pain. The middle of the scale, around 5, means moderate pain. A 2 or 3 would be mild pain, but 7 or higher means severe pain."

Step 3. Discuss pain as a broad concept that is not restricted to a severe and intolerable sensation.
Example: "Pain refers to any kind of discomfort anywhere in your body. Pain also means aching and hurting. Pain can include pulling, tightness, burning, knifelike feelings, and other unpleasant sensations."

Step 4. Verify that the patient understands the broad concept of pain. Ask the patient to mention two examples of pain they have experienced. If the patient is already in pain that requires treatment, use the present situation as the example.
Example: "I want to be sure that I have explained this clearly, so would you give me two examples of pain you have had recently?" If the patient's examples include various parts of the body and various pain characteristics, that indicates that they understand pain as a fairly broad concept. An example of what a patient might say is "I have a mild, sort of throbbing headache now, and yesterday my back was aching."

Step 5. Ask the patient to practice using the pain rating scale with the present pain or select one of the examples mentioned.
Example: "Using the scale, what is your pain right now? What is it at its worst?" OR "Using the pain rating scale and one of your examples of pain, what is that pain usually? What is it at its worst?"

Step 6. Set goals for comfort and function/recovery/quality of life. Ask patients what pain rating would be acceptable or satisfactory, considering the activities required for recovery or for maintaining a satisfactory quality of life.
Example for a surgical patient: "I have explained the importance of coughing and deep breathing to prevent pneumonia and other complications. Now we need to determine the pain rating that will not interfere with this so that you may recover quickly."
Example for patient with chronic pain or terminal illness: "What do you want to do that pain keeps you from doing? What pain rating would allow you to do this?"

[a]When a patient is obviously in pain or not focused enough to learn to use a pain rating scale, pain treatment should proceed without pain ratings. Education can be undertaken when pain is reduced to a level that facilitates understanding how to use a pain scale.
VDS, verbal descriptor scale.
Copyright 2011, Pasero, C., & McCaffery, M. Used with permission from Pasero, C., & McCaffery, M. (2011). *Pain assessment and pharmacologic management.* St. Louis, MO: Mosby-Elsevier.

and made available for use in clinical practice and for educational practice. The most common include the following:

- *Numeric Rating Scale (NRS):* The NRS is most often presented as a horizontal 0- to 10-point scale, with word anchors of "no pain" at one end of the scale, "moderate pain" in the middle of the scale, and "worst possible pain" at the end of the scale. It may also be put on a vertical axis, which may be helpful for patients who read from right to left.
- *Wong–Baker FACES Pain Rating Scale:* The FACES scale consists of six cartoon faces with word descriptors, ranging from a smiling face on the left for "no pain (or hurt)" to a frowning, tearful face on the right for "worst pain (or hurt)." Patients are asked to choose the face that best reflects their pain. The faces are most commonly numbered using a 0, 2, 4, 6, 8, 10 metric, although 0 to 5 can also be used. Patients are asked to choose the face that best describes their pain. The FACES scale is used in adults and children as young as 3 years (McCaffery et al., 2011). It is important to appreciate that FACES scales are self-report tools; clinicians should not attempt to match a face shown on a scale to the patient's facial expression to determine pain intensity. Patients may be able to understand the tool better if it is displayed vertically with no pain as the anchor at the bottom.
- *Faces Pain Scale—Revised (FPS-R):* The FPS-R has six faces to make it consistent with other scales using the 0 to 10 metric. The faces range from a neutral facial expression to one of intense pain and are numbered 0, 2, 4, 6, 8, and 10. As with the Wong–Baker FACES scale, patients are asked to choose the face that best reflects their pain. Faces scales have been shown to be reliable and valid measures in children as young as 3 years of age; however, the ability to optimally quantify pain (identify a number) is not acquired until approximately 8 years of age (Spagrud, Piira, & Von Baeyer, 2003). Ongoing research suggests that the FPS-R is preferred by both patients who are cognitively intact and older adults who are cognitively impaired, and by minority populations (Kang & Demiris, 2018).
- *Verbal descriptor scale (VDS):* A VDS uses different words or phrases to describe the intensity of pain, such as "no pain, mild pain, moderate pain, severe pain, very severe pain, and worst possible pain." The patient is asked to select the phrase that best describes pain intensity.
- *Visual Analogue Scale (VAS):* The VAS is a horizontal (sometimes vertical) 10-cm line with word anchors at the extremes, such as "no pain" on one end and "pain as bad as it could be" or "worst possible pain" on the other end. Patients are asked to make a mark on the line to indicate intensity of pain, and the length of the mark from "no pain" is measured and recorded in centimeters or millimeters. Although often used in research, the VAS is impractical for use in daily clinical practice and rarely used in that setting.
- *Quality:* Ask the patient to describe how the pain feels. Descriptors such as "sharp," "shooting," or "burning" may help identify the presence of neuropathic pain.

- *Onset and duration:* Ask the patient when the pain started and whether it is constant or intermittent.
- *Aggravating and relieving factors:* Ask the patient what makes the pain worse and what makes it better.
- *Effect of pain on function and quality of life:* The effect of pain on the ability to perform recovery activities should be regularly evaluated in the patient with acute pain. It is particularly important to ask patients with persistent pain about how pain has affected their lives, what they could do before the pain began that they can no longer do, or what they would like to do but cannot do because of the pain.
- *Comfort–function goal* (pain intensity): For patients with acute pain, identify short-term functional goals and reinforce to the patient that good pain control will more likely lead to successful achievement of the goals. For example, surgical patients are told that they will be expected to ambulate or participate in physical therapy postoperatively. Patients with chronic pain can be asked to identify their unique functional or quality-of-life goals, such as being able to work or walk the dog. Success is measured by progress toward meeting those functional goals (Topham & Drew, 2017).
- *Other information:* The patient's culture, past pain experiences, and pertinent medical history such as comorbidities, laboratory tests, and diagnostic studies are considered when establishing a treatment plan.

Patients who are unable to report their pain are at higher risk for undertreated pain than those who can report (Horgas, 2017; McCaffery et al., 2011). In the adult population, this includes patients who are cognitively impaired, critically ill (intubated, unresponsive), comatose, or imminently dying. Patients who are receiving neuromuscular blocking agents or are sedated from anesthesia and other medications given during surgery are also among this at-risk population.

The Hierarchy of Pain Measures is recommended as a framework for assessing pain in patients who are nonverbal (Herr et al., 2011; McCaffery et al., 2011). The key components of the hierarchy require the nurse to (1) attempt to obtain self-report, (2) consider underlying pathology or conditions and procedures that might be painful (e.g., surgery), (3) observe behaviors, (4) evaluate physiologic indicators, and (5) conduct an analgesic trial. Chart 9-3 provides detailed information on each component of the Hierarchy of Pain Measures.

When patients cannot self-report their pain, some observational tools may be used to help with clinical decision making. Some of these assign a score by observing behaviors that tend to be associated with pain. These observational scores are not considered equivalent to a patient's self-reported pain intensity score, however.

It is imperative to remember that behaviors can indicate the presence of pain, but the absence of behavior does not indicate the absence of pain. Patients who are not moving or making any sounds may still be experiencing intense pain. For instance, older adults with moderate and severe dementia frequently have comorbid disorders that may cause pain (Mueller, Schumacher, Holzer, et al., 2017). Accurately assessing and treating their pain can be difficult to achieve (see Chart 9-4 Nursing Research Profile: Evaluation of a Tool to Assess Pain in Older Adults with Dementia). The following tools are examples of validated measures that are appropriate for different populations of patients unable to self-report their

Chart 9-3   Hierarchy of Pain Measures

1. Attempt to obtain the patient's self-report, the single most reliable indicator of pain. Do not assume that a patient cannot provide a report of pain; many patients who are cognitively impaired are able to use a self-report tool if simple actions are taken.
   - Try using standard pain assessment tools (see text).
   - Increase the size of the font and other features of the scale.
   - Present the tool in vertical format (rather than the frequently used horizontal).
   - Try using alternative words, such as "ache," "hurt," and "sore," when discussing pain.
   - Ensure eyeglasses and hearing aids are functioning.
   - Ask about pain in the present.
   - Repeat instructions and questions more than once.
   - Allow ample time to respond.
   - Remember that head nodding and eye blinking or squeezing the eyes tightly can also be used to signal presence of pain and sometimes used to rate intensity.
   - Ask patients who are intubated and who are awake and oriented to point to a number on the numerical scale if they are able.
   - Repeat instructions and show the scale each time pain is assessed.
2. Consider the patient's condition or exposure to a procedure that is thought to be painful. If appropriate, assume pain is present and document as such when approved by institution policy and procedure. As an example, pain should be assumed to be present in a patient who is unresponsive, mechanically ventilated, and critically ill due to trauma.
3. Observe behavioral signs, for example, facial expressions, crying, restlessness, and changes in activity. A pain behavior in one patient may not be in another. Try to identify pain behaviors that are unique to the patient ("pain signature"). Many behavioral pain assessment tools are available that will yield a pain behavior score and may help determine whether pain is present. However, it is important to remember that a behavioral score is not the same as a pain intensity score. Behavioral tools are used to help identify the presence of pain, but the pain intensity is unknown if the patient is unable to provide it.
   - A surrogate who knows the patient well (e.g., parent, spouse, or caregiver) may be able to provide information about underlying painful pathology or behaviors that may indicate pain.
4. Evaluate physiologic indicators with the understanding that they are the *least* sensitive indicators of pain and may signal the existence of conditions other than pain or a lack of it (e.g., hypovolemia, blood loss). Patients quickly adapt physiologically despite pain and may have normal or below normal vital signs in the presence of severe pain. The overriding principle is that the absence of an elevated blood pressure or heart rate does not mean the absence of pain.
5. Conduct an analgesic trial to confirm the presence of pain and to establish a basis for developing a treatment plan if pain is thought to be present. An analgesic trial involves the administration of a low dose of nonopioid or opioid and observing patient response. The initial low dose may not be enough to elicit a change in behavior and should be increased if the previous dose was tolerated, or another analgesic agent may be added. If behaviors continue despite optimal analgesic doses, other possible causes should be investigated. In patients who are completely unresponsive, no change in behavior will be evident and the optimized dose of the analgesic agent should be continued.

Adapted from Pasero, C. (2009). Challenges in pain assessment. *Journal of PeriAnesthesia Nursing, 24*(1), 50–54; Pasero, C., & McCaffery, M. (2011). *Pain assessment and pharmacologic management*. St. Louis, MO: Mosby-Elsevier.

Chart 9-4   NURSING RESEARCH PROFILE
Evaluation of a Tool to Assess Pain in Older Adults with Dementia

Mueller, G., Schumacher, P., Holzer, E., et al. (2017). The inter-rater reliability of the observation instrument for assessing pain in elderly with dementia: An investigation in the long-term care setting. *Journal of Nursing Measurement, 25*(3), E173–E184.

Purpose

The aim of this study was to examine the interrater reliability of the German version of the observation instrument for assessing pain in older adults with dementia called the BISAD for the German (Beobachtungsinstrument für das Schmerzassessment bei alten Menschen mit Demenz). This is a tool that is commonly used to assess pain among older adults with moderate and severe dementia who reside in long-term care facilities in both Germany and Austria; however, interrater reliability was not previously done to ensure its validity.

Design

This study used a quantitative multicenter-descriptive cross-sectional design with a convenience sample of 71 participants who resided in one of three nursing homes in Austria. The nursing participants consisted of 46 registered nurses who had been working at one of the same three nursing homes for at least 2 y. Nurse participants were paired to independently evaluate a resident participant within the same hour using the eight-item BISAD observational pain assessment tool.

Findings

Although modest agreement between raters was noted, the absolute concordance of the total was only 25.32%. The analysis of interrater reliability was low and did not support reliability of the items in the BISAD. There was agreement that pain was greater with movement than when the participant residents were at rest.

Nursing Implications

Findings of this study are important since they indicate the items used in the BISAD tool are not reliable for assessing pain in older adult residents with moderate and severe dementia in nursing homes in Austria, although it is commonly used. This is an important finding since use of this tool with that population could yield inaccurate data upon which nurses could base pain management care. One interesting aspect of this study was that behaviors did demonstrate greater pain with activity than when at rest. Finally, the authors note that there may be cultural and language issues that affected the results and encourage a translated version of the tool be assessed in long-term care facilities where English is the primary language.

pain (Fry & Elliott, 2018; Kochman, Howell, Sheridan, et al., 2017; Rijkenberg, Stilma, Bosman, et al., 2017; Schofield & Abdulla, 2018).

- FLACC: indicated for use in young children. Scores are assigned after assessing Facial expression, Leg movement, Activity, Crying, and Consolability, with each of these five categories assigned scores from 0 to 2, yielding a total composite score of 0 to 10. Scores of "0" are interpreted as reflecting that the patient is relaxed and comfortable, scores of "1" to "3" are interpreted as consistent with mild discomfort, scores from "4" to "6" are considered consistent with moderate pain, and scores from "7" to "10" are considered consistent with severe discomfort or pain.
- PAINAD (Pain Assessment IN Advanced Dementia): indicated for use in adults with advanced dementia who are not able to verbalize their needs. Patterned after the FLACC, this tool was developed by the U.S. Department of Veterans Affairs for patients who have dementia.
- CPOT (Critical Care Pain Observation Tool): indicated for use in patients in critical-care units who cannot self-report pain, whether or not they may be intubated. It is also patterned after the FLACC.

Reassessing Pain

Following initiation of the pain management plan, pain is reassessed and documented on a regular basis to evaluate the effectiveness of treatment. At a minimum, pain should be reassessed with each new report of pain and before and after the administration of analgesic agents (McCaffery et al., 2011). The frequency of reassessment depends on the stability of the patient and the timing of peak effect of the medication administered, which is generally between 15 and 30 minutes following parenteral administration and between 1 and 2 hours following oral administration (Chou, Gordon, de Leon-Casasola, et al., 2016). For example, in the postanesthesia care unit (PACU), reassessment may be necessary as often as every 10 minutes when pain is unstable during intravenous (IV) opioid **titration** but may be done an hour following administration of oral medication in patients with satisfactory and stable pain control the day following surgery.

 Veterans Considerations

Nurses should be aware that research has demonstrated a high prevalence of pain associated disorders, including arthritis, fibromyalgia, headaches and generalized abdominal, back, and joint pain in veteran populations (Nahin, 2017). In addition, reports of severe pain are more common in military veterans compared to nonveterans, especially in those who served, more recently, in conflicts in Iraq and Afghanistan (Nahin, 2017). In particular, younger veterans (18 to 39 years of age) and male veterans report significantly higher levels of pain compared to matched age groups and men in the general public (Nahin, 2017). As a result, it is important for the nurse to determine during assessment if a patient has served in the U.S. military, to recognize that this group may have unique needs related to their service, and to advocate for multimodal and multidisciplinary approaches to help veterans better cope with pain. For example, Groessi, Liu, Change, and colleagues (2017) found that yoga was a safe and beneficial intervention in helping veterans to reduce pain and disability, while taking fewer opioid medications.

Pain Management

Achieving optimal pain relief is best viewed on a continuum, with the primary objective being to provide both effective and safe analgesia (Pozek, De Ruyter, & Khan, 2018). The quality of pain control should be addressed whenever patient care is passed on from one clinician to another, such as at change of shift and transfer from one clinical area to another. Optimal pain relief is the responsibility of *every* member of the health care team and begins with titration of the analgesic agent, followed by continued prompt assessment, analgesic agent administration, and nonpharmacologic interventions during the course of care to safely achieve pain intensities that allow patients to meet their functional goals with relative ease.

Although it may not always be possible to achieve a patient's pain intensity goal within the short time the patient is in an area like the PACU or emergency department, this goal provides direction for ongoing analgesic care. Important information to provide during transfer report is the patient's comfort–function goal, how close the patient is to achieving it, what has been done thus far to achieve it (analgesic agents and doses and/or nonpharmacologic interventions), and how well the patient has tolerated administration of the analgesic agent (adverse effects). There is growing interest among both clinicians and researchers in linking pain management to functional goals. One effort in this work is the Clinically Aligned Pain Assessment (CAPA) Tool, which is used to assess various degrees of comfort, pain control, function, and sleep (Topham & Drew, 2017). Pain management interventions should improve and not inhibit progress toward healing and rehabilitation.

Pharmacologic Management of Pain: Multimodal Analgesia

Pain is a complex phenomenon involving multiple underlying mechanisms that requires more than one analgesic agent to manage it safely and effectively. The recommended approach for the treatment of all types of pain in all age groups is called **multimodal analgesia or multimodal pain management**. A multimodal regimen intentionally and simultaneously combines medications with different underlying mechanisms, along with nonpharmacologic interventions, which allows for lower doses of each of the medications in the treatment plan, reducing the potential for adverse effects. Furthermore, multimodal analgesia can result in comparable or greater pain relief with fewer adverse effects than can be achieved with any single analgesic agent (Beverly, Kaye, Ljungqvist, et al., 2017; Blackburn, 2018).

Routes of Administration

Oral is the preferred route of analgesic administration and should be used whenever feasible (Chou et al., 2016). Medications administered via the oral route are generally best tolerated, easiest to administer, and most cost-effective. When the oral route is not possible, such as when patients cannot swallow, are NPO (nothing by mouth), or nauseated, other routes of administration are used. For example, patients with cancer pain who are unable to swallow may take analgesic agents by the transdermal, rectal, or subcutaneous route of administration (Burchum & Rosenthal, 2019).

In the immediate postoperative period, the IV route is most often the first-line route of administration for analgesic delivery, and patients are transitioned to the oral route as tolerated (see Chapter 16 for the management of postoperative pain).

The rectal route of analgesic administration is an alternative route when oral or IV analgesic agents are not an option (e.g., for palliative purposes during end-of-life care). The rectum allows passive diffusion of medications and absorption into the systemic circulation. This route can be less expensive and does not involve the skill and expertise required of the parenteral route of administration. Limitations are that medication absorption can be unreliable and depends on many factors including rectal tissue health and administrator technique. Some patients may be resistant to or fearful of rectal administration. The rectal route is contraindicated in patients who are neutropenic or thrombocytopenic because of potential rectal bleeding. Diarrhea, perianal abscess or fistula, and abdominoperineal resection are also relative contraindications (Burchum & Rosenthal, 2019).

The topical route of administration is used for both acute and chronic pain. For example, the nonopioid diclofenac is available in patch and gel formulations for application directly over painful areas. Local anesthetic creams, such as eutectic mixture or emulsion of local anesthetics and lidocaine cream 4%, can be applied directly over the injection site prior to painful needle stick procedures; the lidocaine patch 5% is often used for well-localized types of neuropathic pain, such as postherpetic neuralgia. It is important to distinguish between topical and transdermal medication delivery. Although both routes require the medication to cross the stratum corneum to produce analgesia, transdermal delivery requires absorption into the systemic circulation to achieve effects, whereas topical agents produce effects in the tissues immediately under the site of application (referred to as targeted peripheral analgesia). Compounding pharmacies may be consulted to custom blend antispasmodic agents, such as topical morphine or gabapentin, for topical application at the painful site.

A more invasive method used to manage pain is accomplished using **neuraxial** analgesia, which involves administering medication in the epidural or subarachnoid space (American Society of Regional Anesthesia and Pain Medicine, 2016). Delivery of analgesic agents by the neuraxial route is accomplished by inserting a needle into the subarachnoid space (for intrathecal [spinal] analgesia) or the epidural space, and either injecting the analgesic medication directly, or threading a catheter through the needle to enable bolus dosing or continuous administration (Conlin, Grant, & Wu, 2018; Hernandez, Grant, & Wu, 2018). Intrathecal catheters for acute pain management are used most often for providing anesthesia or a single bolus dose of an analgesic agent. Implanted intrathecal pumps deliver very small amounts of medication in a constant infusion for treatment of end-of-life pain or persistent pain (Jamison, Cohen, & Rosenow, 2018). Temporary epidural catheters for acute pain management are removed after 2 to 4 days. Epidural analgesia is administered by clinician-given bolus, continuous infusion (basal rate), and patient-controlled epidural analgesia (PCEA). The most common opioids given intraspinally are morphine, fentanyl, and hydromorphone. These are often combined with a local anesthetic, most often ropivacaine or bupivacaine (Jamison et al., 2018). The multimodal use of local anesthetics with opioids improves analgesia and produces an **opioid dose-sparing effect**.

A pain management technique that involves the use of an indwelling catheter is the continuous peripheral nerve block (also called *perineural anesthesia*), whereby an initial local anesthetic block is established and followed by the placement of a catheter or catheters through which an infusion of local anesthetic, usually ropivacaine or bupivacaine, is infused continuously to the targeted site of innervation. The effect of local anesthetic is dose dependent: at lower doses, the smaller sensory nerve fibers are affected before the larger motor fibers. Patients thus medicated are able to walk but have well controlled pain (Burchum & Rosenthal, 2019; Ilfeld & Mariano, 2018).

Dosing Regimen

Achieving, then maintaining, optimal pain management that is safe, effective, and progresses toward realistic functional goals requires patient education with continuing reassessment of analgesic effect and development of any untoward effects (Chou et al., 2016). Accomplishing these goals may require the mainstay analgesic agent to be given on a scheduled around-the-clock (ATC) basis, rather than PRN (as needed) to maintain stable analgesic blood levels when pain is continuous (Eksterowicz & DiMaggio, 2018). ATC dosing regimens are designed to control pain for patients who report pain being present 12 hours or more during a 24-hour period. PRN dosing of analgesic agents is appropriate for intermittent pain, such as prior to painful procedures and for BTP (pain that "breaks through" the pain being managed by the mainstay analgesic agent), for which supplemental doses of analgesia are provided (Palat, 2018).

Patient-Controlled Analgesia

Patient-controlled analgesia (PCA) is an interactive method of pain management that allows patients to treat their pain by self-administering doses of analgesic agents (Burchum & Rosenthal, 2019). It is used to manage all types of pain by multiple routes of administration, including oral, IV, subcutaneous, epidural, and perineural (Fernandes, Hernandes, de Almeida, et al., 2017). Current guidelines from the APS, the American Society of Regional Anesthesia and Pain Medicine, and the American Society of Anesthesiologists strongly recommended IV PCA for postoperative pain management when it is necessary to use the parenteral route to deliver analgesic medications (Chou et al., 2016). A PCA infusion device is programmed so that the patient can press a button (pendant) to self-administer a dose of an analgesic agent (PCA dose) at a set time interval (demand or lockout) as needed. Patients who use PCAs must be able to understand the relationships among pain, pushing the PCA button or taking the analgesic agent, and pain relief, and must be cognitively and physically able to use any equipment that is necessary to administer the therapy (ECRI Institute Patient Safety Organization, 2017).

A basal rate (continuous infusion) may be used for patients who are opioid tolerant, and when PCEA is used. It is discouraged for patients who are opioid naïve and receiving IV

PCA due to the risk of oversedation with subsequent respiratory depression (Chou et al., 2016; ECRI Institute Patient Safety Organization, 2017). Essential to the safe use of a basal rate with PCA is close monitoring by nurses of sedation and respiratory status and prompt decreases in opioid dose (e.g., discontinue basal rate) if increased sedation is detected (Pasero, Quinn, Portenoy, et al., 2011).

The primary benefit of PCA is that it recognizes that only the patient can feel the pain and only the patient knows how much analgesic will relieve it. This reinforces that PCA is for patient use only and that unauthorized activation of the PCA device by anyone other than the patient (PCA by proxy) should be discouraged (Burchum & Rosenthal, 2019).

> ### ◢ Quality and Safety Nursing Alert
>
> *Staff, family, and other visitors should be instructed to contact the nurse if they have concerns about pain control rather than activating the PCA device for the patient.*

However, for some patients who are candidates for PCA but unable to use the PCA equipment, the nurse or a capable family member may be authorized to manage the patient's pain using PCA equipment. This is referred to as Authorized Agent Controlled Analgesia; guidelines are available for the safe administration of this therapy (Cooney, Czarnecki, Dunwoody, et al., 2013).

Analgesic Medications

Analgesic medications are categorized into three main groups: (1) nonopioid antispasmodic agents, which include acetaminophen and NSAIDs; (2) opioid antispasmodic agents, which include, among others, morphine, hydromorphone, fentanyl, and oxycodone; and (3) co-analgesic agents (also referred to as **adjuvant analgesic agents**). The co-analgesic agents comprise the largest group and include various agents with unique and widely differing mechanisms of action. Examples are local anesthetics, some anticonvulsants, and some antidepressants (APS, 2016).

Nonopioid Analgesic Agents

Acetaminophen and NSAIDs comprise the group of nonopioid analgesic agents (refer to earlier discussion of the two categories of NSAIDs; see Fig. 9-2).

Indications and Administration

Nonopioid medications are analgesic agents used for a wide variety of painful conditions. They are appropriate alone for mild to some moderate nociceptive pain (e.g., from surgery, trauma, or osteoarthritis) and are added to opioids, local anesthetics, and/or anticonvulsants as part of a multimodal analgesic regimen for more severe nociceptive pain (APS, 2016; Chou et al., 2016; Comerford & Durkin, 2020). Since acetaminophen and NSAIDs have different mechanisms of action, they may be administered concomitantly (Chou et al., 2016). Although there is no research supporting staggering the two medications, it may be helpful for some patients. Unless contraindicated, surgical patients should routinely be given acetaminophen and an NSAID in scheduled doses throughout the postoperative course, which can be initiated preoperatively (Chou et al., 2016).

Nonopioids are often combined in a single tablet with opioids, such as oxycodone or hydrocodone, and are very popular for the treatment of mild to moderate acute pain. They are traditionally a common choice after invasive pain management therapies are discontinued and for pain treatment after hospital discharge and dental surgery when an opioid is prescribed. Many people with persistent pain also take a combination nonopioid–opioid analgesic agent; however, it is important to remember that these combination medications are not appropriate for severe pain of any type because the maximum daily dose of the nonopioid limits the escalation of the opioid dose (Burchum & Rosenthal, 2019; Comerford & Durkin, 2020).

Acetaminophen is versatile in that it can be given by multiple routes of administration, including oral, rectal, and IV. Oral acetaminophen has a long history of safety in recommended doses in all age groups. It is a useful addition to multimodal treatment plans for postoperative pain (Wick, Grant, & Wu, 2017). Findings from one research study suggest that patients who receive scheduled acetaminophen with PRN opioids will use less opioids than if they receive PRN acetaminophen plus opioids (Valentine, Carvalho, Lazo, et al., 2015). These results were supported in a more recent study evaluating opioid use among women who underwent Cesarean deliveries (Holland, Bateman, Cole, et al., 2019).

IV acetaminophen is approved for the treatment of pain and fever and is given by a 15-minute infusion in single or repeated doses. It may be given alone for mild to moderate pain or in combination with opioid analgesic agents for more severe pain. The results of several research studies have been inconsistent regarding the opioid sparing effects of IV acetaminophen (Nelson & Wu, 2018). Recommended dosing is 1000 mg every 6 hours for a maximum of 4000 mg in adult patients (Comerford & Durkin, 2020).

A benefit of the NSAID group is the availability of a wide variety of agents for administration via noninvasive routes. Ibuprofen, naproxen, and celecoxib are the most widely used oral NSAIDs in the United States. When rectal formulations are unavailable, an intact oral tablet or a crushed tablet in a gelatin capsule may be inserted into the rectum. The rectal route may require higher doses than the oral route to achieve similar analgesic effects (Pasero et al., 2011). Diclofenac can be prescribed in patch and gel form for topical administration, and an intranasal patient-controlled formulation of ketorolac has been approved for the treatment of postoperative pain.

IV formulations of ketorolac and ibuprofen are available for acute pain treatment. Both have been shown to produce excellent analgesia alone for moderate nociceptive pain, and significant opioid dose–sparing effects when given as part of a multimodal analgesia plan for more severe nociceptive pain (Comerford & Durkin, 2020; Williams, 2018).

Adverse Effects of Nonopioid Analgesic Agents

Acetaminophen is widely considered one of the safest, best tolerated, and most cost effective of the analgesic agents (APS, 2016; Williams, 2018). Its most serious complication is hepatotoxicity (liver damage) as a result of overdose. In the healthy adult, a maximum daily dose below 4000 mg is rarely associated with liver toxicity. Nevertheless, one manufacturer of oral acetaminophen voluntarily changed its dosing recommendations in 2011, calling for a maximum daily dose of

3000 mg (Shiffman, Battista, Kelly, et al., 2018). In 2014, the U.S. Food and Drug Administration (FDA) recommended that health care professionals stop prescribing and pharmacists stop dispensing prescription combination medication products that contain more than 325 mg of acetaminophen per tablet, capsule, or other dosage unit in order to reduce the risk of hepatotoxicity (FDA, 2014). Acetaminophen does not increase bleeding time and has a low incidence of gastrointestinal (GI) adverse effects, making it the analgesic agent of choice in many individuals with comorbidities. There are two potential interactions with acetaminophen that warrant caution. Acetaminophen should be avoided when consuming alcohol because the combination can result in serious liver damage; acetaminophen also should be avoided when warfarin is prescribed because it can inhibit metabolism of warfarin resulting in toxicity with bleeding risk (Burchum & Rosenthal, 2019).

NSAIDs have considerably more adverse effects than acetaminophen, with gastric toxicity and ulceration being the most common (Comerford & Durkin, 2020). The primary underlying mechanism of NSAID-induced gastric ulceration is the inhibition of COX-1, which leads to a reduction in GI-protective prostaglandins (see Fig. 9-2). This is a systemic (rather than local) effect and can occur regardless of the route of administration of the NSAID. Risk factors include advanced age (older than 60 years), presence of prior ulcer disease, and cardiovascular (CV) disease and other comorbidities (Williams, 2018). In patients with elevated risks, the use of a COX-2 selective NSAID (e.g., celecoxib) or the least ulcerogenic nonselective NSAID (e.g., ibuprofen) plus a proton pump inhibitor is recommended; however, there are risks with proton pump inhibitors as well (Gwee, Goh, Lima, et al., 2018). Proton pump inhibitors may decrease the absorption of some other medications such as itraconazole and rilpivirine (Burchum & Rosenthal, 2019). As with all medications, it is important to frequently reassess the need for continued use and to discontinue when appropriate. GI adverse effects are also related to the dose and duration of NSAID therapy; the higher the NSAID dose and the longer the duration of NSAID use, the higher the risk of GI toxicity (Williams, 2018). A principle of nonopioid analgesic use is to administer the lowest dose for the shortest time necessary (Pasero, Portenoy, & McCaffery, 2011).

All NSAIDs carry a risk of CV adverse effects through prostaglandin inhibition, and the risk is increased with COX-2 inhibition, whether it is produced by a COX-2 selective NSAID (e.g., celecoxib) or by NSAIDs that are nonselective inhibitors of both COX-1 and COX-2 (e.g., ibuprofen, naproxen, and ketorolac). Findings from a recent meta-analysis suggest that the risk of acute myocardial infarction is greatest during the first month of treatment with NSAIDs, with this risk developing during the first week of treatment (Bally, Dendukuri, Rich, et al., 2017). All patients prescribed NSAIDs should receive the lowest effective dose for the shortest time period to decrease risks.

NSAIDs can negatively impact renal function, and are associated with diminished renal prostaglandin formation, interstitial nephritis, reduced secretion of renin, and greater reabsorption of water and sodium (APS, 2016). NSAID-induced renal toxicity can occur, but is relatively rare in otherwise healthy adults who are given NSAIDs for short-term

pain management (e.g., in the perioperative period); however, individuals with acute or chronic volume depletion or hypotension rely on prostaglandin synthesis to maintain adequate renal blood flow, and NSAID inhibition of prostaglandin synthesis in such patients can cause acute kidney injury (Burchum & Rosenthal, 2019). Attention to adequate hydration is essential when administering NSAIDs to prevent this complication (Pasero et al., 2011).

Most nonselective NSAIDs increase bleeding time through inhibition of COX-1. This is both medication and dose related, so the lowest dose of nonopioids with minimal or no effect on bleeding time should be used in patients having procedures with high risk for bleeding. Options include acetaminophen, celecoxib, choline magnesium trisalicylate, salsalate, and nabumetone (APS, 2016; Burchum & Rosenthal, 2019).

Opioid Analgesic Agents

Although it is often used, the term *narcotic* is inaccurate and considered obsolete when discussing the use of **opioids** for pain management, in part because it is a term used loosely by law enforcement and the media to refer to various substances of potential abuse, which include opioids as well as cocaine and other illicit substances. Legally, controlled substances classified as narcotics include opioids, cocaine, and others. The accurate term, when discussing these agents in the context of pain management, is *opioid analgesics* (Burchum & Rosenthal, 2019).

Opioid analgesic agents are divided into two major groups: (1) **mu agonist** opioids (also called *morphinelike medications*) and (2) **agonist–antagonist** opioids. The mu agonist opioids comprise the larger of the two groups and include morphine, hydromorphone, hydrocodone, fentanyl, oxycodone, and methadone, among others. The agonist–antagonist opioids include buprenorphine, nalbuphine, and butorphanol (APS, 2016).

Opioid analgesic agents exert their effects by interacting with opioid receptor sites located throughout the body, including in the peripheral tissues, GI system, and CNS; they are abundant in the dorsal horn of the spinal cord. There are three major classes of opioid receptor sites involved in analgesia: the mu, delta, and kappa. The pharmacologic differences in the various opioids are the result of their interaction with these opioid receptor types (Burchum & Rosenthal, 2019; Sheth, Holtsman, & Mahajan, 2018). When an opioid binds to the opioid receptor sites, it produces analgesia as well as unwanted effects, such as constipation, nausea, sedation, and respiratory depression (Arthur & Hui, 2018).

The opioid analgesic agents that are designated as first line (e.g., morphine, hydromorphone, fentanyl, and oxycodone) belong to the mu opioid agonist class because they bind primarily to the mu-type opioid receptors. The agonist–antagonist opioids are designated as "mixed" because they bind to more than one opioid receptor site. They bind as **agonists**, producing analgesia, at the kappa opioid receptor sites, and as weak antagonists at the mu opioid receptor sites. Their propensity to antagonize the effects of mu opioid analgesic agents limits their usefulness in pain management (Burchum & Rosenthal, 2019). They should be avoided in patients receiving long-term mu opioid therapy because their use may trigger severe pain and opioid **withdrawal** syndrome characterized by rhinitis, abdominal cramping, nausea, agitation, and restlessness.

Antagonists (e.g., naloxone, naltrexone, naloxegol) are medications that also bind to opioid receptors but produce no analgesia. If an antagonist is present, it competes with opioid molecules for binding sites on the opioid receptors and has the potential to block analgesia and other effects. Antagonists are used most often to reverse adverse effects, such as respiratory depression (Burchum & Rosenthal, 2019). Antagonists have been incorporated in the manufacture of some opioids in an effort to deter abuse of the opioid (Li, 2019)

Administration

Safe and effective use of opioid analgesic agents requires the development of an individualized treatment plan based on a comprehensive pain assessment, which includes clarifying the goals of treatment and discussing options with the patient and the family when appropriate (Chou et al., 2016; Sheth et al., 2018). Goals are periodically reevaluated, and changes made depending on patient response and in some cases disease progression.

Many factors are considered when determining the appropriate opioid analgesic agent for the patient with pain. These include the unique characteristics of the various opioids and patient factors, such as pain intensity, age, coexisting disease, current medication regimen and potential medication interactions, prior treatment outcomes, and patient preference (APS, 2016; Sheth et al., 2018). In all cases, a multimodal approach that may rely on the selection of appropriate analgesic agents from the nonopioid, opioid, and co-analgesic agent groups is recommended to manage all types of pain (APS, 2016; Li, 2019). Chart 9-5 lists the key considerations when developing an opioid pain treatment plan.

Titration of the opioid dose is usually required at the start and throughout the course of treatment when opioids are given. Whereas patients with cancer pain most often

---

Chart 9-5 Use of Opioids

- Perform a comprehensive assessment that addresses pain, comorbidities, and functional status.
- Develop an individualized treatment plan that includes specific goals related to pain intensity, activities (function/quality of life), and adverse effects (e.g., pain intensity rating of 3 on a 0–10 numerical rating scale to ambulate accompanied by minimal or no sedation).
- Use multimodal analgesia (e.g., add acetaminophen and NSAID; anticonvulsant in patients at risk for persistent postsurgical pain).
- Assess for presence preoperatively of underlying persistent pain in surgical patients and optimize its treatment.
- Consider **preemptive analgesic agents** before surgery, particularly for those at risk for severe postoperative pain or a persistent postsurgical pain syndrome.
- Provide analgesic agents prior to all painful procedures.
- Medication selection
  - Consider diagnosis, condition, or surgical procedure, current or expected pain intensity, age, presence of major organ dysfunction or failure, and presence of coexisting disease.
  - Consider pharmacologic issues (e.g., accumulation of metabolites and effects of concurrent medications).
  - Consider prior treatment outcomes and patient preference.
  - Be aware of available routes of administration (oral, transdermal, rectal, intranasal, IV subcutaneous, perineural, intraspinal) and formulations (e.g., short acting, modified release).
  - Be aware of cost differences.
- Route of administration selection
  - Use least invasive route possible.
  - Consider convenience and patient's ability to adhere to the regimen.
  - Consider staff's (or patient's or caregiver's) ability to monitor and provide care required.
- Dosing and titration
  - Consider previous dosing requirement and relative analgesic potencies when initiating therapy.
  - Use equianalgesic dose chart (Table 9-3) to determine starting dose with consideration of patient's current status (e.g., sedation and respiratory status) and comorbidities

(e.g., medical frailty), and then titrate until adequate analgesia is achieved or dose-limiting adverse effects are encountered.
  - Use appropriate dosing schedule (e.g., around-the-clock for continuous pain; PRN for intermittent pain).
  - When dose is safe but additional analgesia is desired, titrate upward as prescribed by 25% for slight increase, 50% for moderate increase, and 100% for considerable increase in analgesia.
  - Provide supplemental doses for breakthrough pain; consider PCA if appropriate.
- Treatment of adverse effects
  - Be aware of the prevalence and impact of opioid adverse effects.
  - Remember that most opioid adverse effects are dose dependent; always consider decreasing the opioid dose as a method of treating or eliminating an adverse effect; adding nonopioid analgesic agents for additive analgesia facilitates this approach.
  - Use a preventive approach in the management of constipation, including for patients receiving short-term opioid treatment.
  - Prevent respiratory depression by monitoring sedation levels and respiratory status frequently and decreasing the opioid dose as soon as increased sedation is detected.
- Monitoring
  - Continually and consistently evaluate the plan on the basis of the specific goals identified at the outset and assess pain intensity, adverse effects, and activity levels.
  - Make necessary modifications to treatment plan to maintain efficacy and safety.
- Tapering and cessation of treatment
  - If a decrease in dose or cessation of treatment is appropriate, do so in accordance with decreased pain intensity and after evaluation of functional outcomes.
  - Be aware of the potential for withdrawal syndrome (rhinitis, abdominal cramping, diarrhea, restlessness, agitation) and need for tapering schedule in patients who have been receiving opioid therapy for more than a few days.

IV, intravenous; NSAID, nonsteroidal anti-inflammatory drug; PCA, patient-controlled analgesia; PRN, as needed.

are titrated upward over time for progressive pain, patients with acute pain, particularly postoperative pain, are eventually titrated downward and discontinued as pain resolves (Chou et al., 2016; FDA, 2017; Sheth et al., 2018). The dose and analgesic effect of mu agonist opioids have no **ceiling effect,** although the dose may be limited by adverse effects. The absolute dose given is based on a balance between pain relief and tolerability of adverse effects. The goal of titration is to use the smallest dose that provides satisfactory pain relief with the fewest adverse effects (Sheth et al., 2018). The time at which the dose can be increased is determined by the onset and peak effects of the opioid and its formulation.

Equianalgesia. The term *equianalgesia* means approximately "equal analgesia." An equianalgesic chart provides a list of doses of analgesic agents, both oral and parenteral (IV, subcutaneous, and intramuscular), that are approximately equal to each other in ability to provide pain relief. Equianalgesic conversion of doses is developed from the ratio representing the difference in the potency of the two medications (Treillet, Laurent, & Hadjiat, 2018). The information is used to help ensure that patients are not overdosed or underdosed when they are switched from one opioid or route of administration to another. It requires a series of calculations based on the daily dose of the current opioid to determine the equianalgesic dose of the opioid to which the patient is to be switched. Several excellent guidelines are available to assist in calculating equianalgesic doses (Burchum & Rosenthal, 2019) (see Table 9-3). Equianalgesic tools available in electronic health records enable all clinicians at any facility to easily convert analgesic dosages (APS, 2016).

Formulation terminology. The terms *short acting, immediate release,* and *normal release* have been used interchangeably to describe oral opioids that have an onset of action of approximately 30 minutes and a relatively short duration of 3 to 4 hours. The term *immediate release* is misleading because none of the oral analgesic agents have an immediate onset of analgesia; *short acting* is preferred. The terms *modified release, extended release, sustained release, controlled release,* and *long acting* are used to describe opioids that are formulated to release over a prolonged period of time. For the purposes of this chapter, the term *modified release* will be used when discussing these opioid formulations.

Substance Use Disorder, Physical Dependence, and Tolerance

In 2013 the American Psychological Association (APA) renamed *addiction* as *substance use disorder* (SUD) (Lo Coco, Melchiori, Oiendi, et al., 2019). SUD includes a number of subcategories, including *opioid use disorder*. The terms *physical dependence* and *tolerance* often are confused with *substance use disorder*, previously understood as *addiction*; thus, clarification of definitions is important (Burchum & Rosenthal, 2019).

- **Physical dependence** is a normal response that occurs with repeated administration of the opioid, with intensity and duration dependent upon the half-life of the medication and how long it has been used. It is manifested by the occurrence of withdrawal symptoms when

---

TABLE 9-3   Equianalgesic Dose Chart for Common mu Opioid Analgesic Agents

- *Equianalgesic* means approximately the same pain relief.
- The equianalgesic chart is a guideline for selecting doses for patients who are opioid-naïve. Doses and intervals between doses are titrated according to individuals' responses.
- The equianalgesic chart is helpful when switching from one medication or route of administration to another.

Opioid	Oral	Parenteral	Comments
Morphine	30 mg	10 mg	Standard for comparison; first-line opioid via multiple routes of administration; once- and twice-daily oral formulations; clinically significant metabolites
Fentanyl	No formulation	100 mcg IV 100 mcg/h of transdermal fentanyl is approximately equal to 4 mg/h of IV morphine; 1 mcg/h of transdermal fentanyl is approximately equal to 2 mg/24 h of oral morphine	First-line opioid via IV, transdermal, and intraspinal routes; available in oral transmucosal and buccal formulations for breakthrough pain in patients who are opioid-tolerant; no clinically relevant metabolites
Hydrocodone	30 mg (not recommended)	No formulation	Available only in combination with acetaminophen and as such is appropriate only for mild to some moderate pain
Hydromorphone	7.5 mg	1.5 mg	First-line opioid via multiple routes of administration; once-daily oral formulation; clinically significant metabolites noted with long-term and high-dose infusion
Oxycodone	20 mg	No formulation in the United States	Short-acting and twice-daily oral formulations
Oxymorphone	10 mg	1 mg	Parenteral and short-acting and twice-daily oral formulations

IV, intravenous.

Adapted from Comerford, K. C., & Durkin, M. T. (2020). *Nursing 2020 drug handbook.* Philadelphia, PA: Wolters Kluwer; Pasero, C., & McCaffery, M. (2011). *Pain assessment and pharmacologic management.* St. Louis, MO: Mosby-Elsevier.

the opioid is suddenly stopped or rapidly reduced, or an antagonist such as naloxone is given. Withdrawal symptoms may be suppressed by the natural, gradual reduction of the opioid as pain decreases or by gradual, systematic reduction, referred to as tapering (Burchum & Rosenthal, 2019). Withdrawal occurs with prolonged use of opioids, regardless of whether the use of opioids is prescribed for pain management or because of SUD (Sheth et al., 2018).

- **Tolerance** is also a normal physiologic response that can occur with regular administration of an opioid and consists of a decrease in one or more effects of the opioid (e.g., decreased analgesia, sedation, or respiratory depression). Although it may occur in conjunction with SUD, it cannot be equated with SUD. It may be treated with increases in dose to attain the previous effect. With the exception of constipation, tolerance to the opioid adverse effects develops with regular daily dosing of opioids over several days (Burchum & Rosenthal, 2019; Sheth et al., 2018).

- **Substance Use Disorder (SUD)** was historically known as addiction or addictive disease, and defined as a chronic, relapsing, treatable neurologic disease. The APA has since described SUD as the impaired use of a substance, such as opioids, even while experiencing major problems, characterized by impaired control over use, compulsive use, continued use despite harm, and craving for the substance. With SUD, use of the opioid is for nontherapeutic reasons and is thus independent of pain relief. The development and characteristics of SUD are influenced by genetic, psychosocial, and environmental factors (Auriacombe, Serre, Denis, et al., 2019; Lo Coco et al., 2019; Sheth et al., 2018).

- **Withdrawal** occurs when a medication or substance to which the body has become dependent is abruptly reduced or discontinued. This is true of prescribed medications as well as illicitly obtained substances. Withdrawal is exhibited by a cascade of unpleasant symptoms including anxiety, nausea, vomiting, rhinitis, sneezing, chills, hot flashes, abdominal cramping, tremors, diaphoresis, hyperreflexia, diarrhea, piloerection, and/or insomnia (APS, 2016; Burchum & Rosenthal, 2019; Sheth et al., 2018).

- *Pseudoaddiction* is a mistaken diagnosis of substance use disorder that occurs when a patient's pain is not well controlled; the patient may begin to manifest symptoms suggestive of SUD. In an effort to obtain adequate pain relief, the patient may respond with demanding behavior, escalating demands for more or different medications, and repeated requests for opioids on time or before the prescribed interval between doses has elapsed. Pain relief typically eliminates these behaviors and is often accomplished by increasing opioid doses or decreasing intervals between doses (Sheth et al., 2018; Weissman & Haddox, 1989).

Pain management specialists have increasingly come to realize that the progression from prescribed opioid use to the disease of opioid SUD is poorly understood and complex. The National Institute on Drug Abuse (2014) estimated that the rates of SUD among patients with chronic pain vary widely, from 3% to 40%. A government effort to address the issue

of SUD is the *Comprehensive Addiction and Recovery Act of 2016* which provides prevention, treatment, and rehabilitative support (Burchum & Rosenthal, 2019). There is real concern for adequately treating the 2 million Americans who are living with opioid SUD and the 50 million people who are living with chronic pain (National Institutes of Health [NIH], 2019). The patients in both groups need and deserve to receive informed, evidence-based, compassionate nursing care.

Opioid naïve versus opioid tolerant. Patients are often characterized as being either *opioid naïve* or *opioid tolerant.* Whereas an **opioid naïve** person has not recently taken enough opioid on a regular basis to become tolerant to the effects of an opioid, an **opioid tolerant** person has taken an opioid long enough at doses high enough to develop tolerance to many of the effects, including analgesia and sedation. There is no set time for the development of tolerance, and there is great individual variation, with some not developing tolerance at all. By convention, most clinicians consider a patient who has taken opioids regularly for approximately 7 or more days to be opioid tolerant (Pasero et al., 2011).

Opioid-Induced Hyperalgesia

Opioid-induced hyperalgesia (OIH) is a paradoxical situation in which increasing doses of an opioid result in increasing sensitivity to pain. The incidence of clinically significant OIH has not been determined; however, it is a serious consequence of opioid administration. At this time, it is not possible to predict who will develop OIH as a result of opioid exposure, and the mechanisms underlying OIH are largely unknown. In general, OIH is thought to be the result of changes in the central and peripheral nervous systems that produce increased transmission of nociceptive signals (APS, 2016; Higgins, Smith, & Matthews, 2018; Ringkamp et al., 2018; Spofford & Hurley, 2018).

Some experts characterize OIH and analgesic tolerance as "opposite sides of the coin" (Pasero et al., 2011). In tolerance, increasing doses of opioid are needed to provide the same level of pain relief because opioid exposure induces neurophysiologic changes that reverse analgesia; in OIH, opioid exposure induces neurophysiologic changes that produce pain or increase sensitivity to noxious input (APS, 2016). In other words, tolerance may be inferred clinically when opioid treatment leads to decreased sensitivity to opioid analgesia over time (in the absence of another process that would explain this), whereas OIH may be inferred clinically when opioid treatment leads to increased pain or sensitivity to pain. Patients with OIH may report an increase in pain that increases with increased dosing of opioids (APS, 2016). Recent research findings have reported the onset of postoperative OIH following intraoperative administration of opioids (Spofford & Hurley, 2018). OIH is an area in which additional research is much needed.

Select Opioid Analgesic Agents

Morphine is the standard against which all other opioid medications are compared. It is used worldwide, particularly for cancer pain, and its use is established by extensive research and clinical experience. It is available in a wide variety of short-acting and modified-release oral formulations and is given by multiple routes of administration. It was the first

TABLE 9-4	Characteristics of Select First-Line Opioid Analgesic Agents[a]		
Opioid	**Onset (Minutes)**	**Peak (Minutes)**	**Duration (Hours)**
Morphine	30 (PO) 5 (IV)	60–120 (PO) 20 (IV)	4–12 (PO) 4–5 (IV)
Fentanyl	5–15 (OT) 1–2 (IV)	20–30 (OT) 3–5 (IV)	2–5 (OT) 1/2–1 (IV)
Hydromorphone	15–30 (PO) 10–15 (IV)	30–60 (PO) 15–30 (IV)	4–5 (PO) 2–3 (IV)

[a]Characteristics do not apply to modified-release formulations.
IV, intravenous; OT, oral transmucosal; PO, oral.
Adapted from Comerford, K. C., & Durkin, M. T. (2020). *Nursing 2020 drug hand-book*. Philadelphia, PA: Wolters Kluwer; Pasero, C., & McCaffery, M. (2011). *Pain assessment and pharmacologic management*. St. Louis, MO: Mosby-Elsevier.

medication to be given intraspinally and remains a first-line choice for long-term **intraspinal** analgesia. It is the only opioid uniquely formulated to produce analgesia for up to 48 hours following epidural administration for acute pain management (extended-release epidural morphine). Morphine is a **hydrophilic** medication (readily absorbed in aqueous solution), which accounts for its slow onset and long duration of action when compared with other opioid analgesic agents (Tables 9-3 and 9-4). It has two principal, clinically significant **metabolites:** morphine-3-glucuronide (M3G) and morphine-6-glucuronide (M6G). M6G may be responsible for some of the analgesic effect of morphine; accumulation of M3G can produce neurotoxicity, which necessitates switching the patient to a different opioid (Burchum & Rosenthal, 2019; Conlin et al., 2018; Howard & Brant, 2019; Sheth et al., 2018).

Fentanyl, in contrast to morphine, is a **lipophilic** (readily absorbed in fatty tissues) opioid and as such has a fast onset and short duration of action (see Tables 9-3 and 9-4). These characteristics make it the most commonly used IV opioid when rapid analgesia is desired, such as for the treatment of severe, escalating acute pain, and for procedural pain when a short duration of action is desirable. This medication is a good choice for patients with end-organ failure because it has no clinically relevant metabolites. It also produces minimal hemodynamic adverse effects; thus, fentanyl is often preferred in patients who are hemodynamically unstable, such as the critically ill (Chou et al., 2016; Conlin et al., 2018; Howard & Brant, 2019).

Its lipophilicity makes fentanyl ideal for medication delivery by transdermal patch for long-term opioid administration and by the oral transmucosal and buccal routes for BTP treatment in patients who are opioid tolerant. Following application of the transdermal patch, a subcutaneous depot of fentanyl is established in the skin near the patch. After absorption from the depot into the systemic circulation, the medication distributes to fat and muscle. When the first patch is applied, 12 to 18 hours are required for clinically significant analgesia to be obtained; attention must be paid to providing adequate supplemental analgesia during that time. Conversely, when the patch is removed, the serum levels of fentanyl remain for a minimum of 16 hours, so it is important to not administer additional long-acting opioids during that time. Another important caution is that heat (e.g., heating pads, hot water

blankets, hot tubs, fever) may increase the rate of absorption leading to serious adverse events. The patch is changed every 48 to 72 hours depending on patient response. It is important to note that the patch is not appropriate for treating acute pain or rapidly changing pain (Burchum & Rosenthal, 2019; Howard & Brant, 2019; Sheth et al., 2018).

Hydromorphone is less hydrophilic than morphine but less lipophilic than fentanyl, which contributes to an onset and duration of action that is intermediate between morphine and fentanyl (see Tables 9-3 and 9-4). This medication is often used as an alternative to morphine, especially for acute pain because the two medications produce similar analgesia and have comparable adverse effect profiles. It is a first- or second-choice opioid (after morphine) for postoperative pain management via IV PCA and is available in a once-daily modified-release oral formulation for chronic pain management. Accumulation of its neuroexcitatory metabolite hydromorphone-3-glucuronide (H3G) may occur with high-dose, long-term infusion therapy, which would necessitate a switch to another opioid (Burchum & Rosenthal, 2019; Sheth et al., 2018).

Oxycodone is available in the United States for administration by the oral route only and is used to treat all types of pain. Single-entity short-acting and modified-release oxycodone formulations are used most often for moderate to severe cancer pain and in some patients with moderate to severe noncancer pain (see Table 9-3). When it is combined with acetaminophen, the dose of oxycodone is limited by the acetaminophen dose to avoid exceeding the maximum daily dose of that agent. Oxycodone has been used successfully as part of a multimodal treatment plan for postoperative pain as well (Burchum & Rosenthal, 2019; Sheth et al., 2018).

Oxymorphone has been available for many years in parenteral formulation and more recently in short-acting and modified-release oral tablets for the treatment of moderate to severe chronic pain (see Table 9-3). It must be taken on an empty stomach (1 hour before or 2 hours after a meal), and coingestion of alcohol at the time of dosing must be avoided because food and alcohol can increase the serum concentration of the medication up to 300% (Burchum & Rosenthal, 2019; Comerford & Durkin, 2020; Sheth et al., 2018).

Hydrocodone is commercially available only in combination with nonopioids (e.g., with acetaminophen or ibuprofen), which limits its use to the treatment of mild to some moderate pain (see Table 9-3). It is one of the more commonly prescribed analgesic agents in the United States; however, its prescription for the treatment of persistent pain (except for breakthrough dosing) should be carefully evaluated because of its ceiling on **efficacy** and safety concerns inherent in the nonopioid constituent. In the rare situation when a patient can only tolerate hydrocodone and needs a dose higher than is possible with the acetaminophen or ibuprofen combination, hydrocodone alone can be obtained from a compounding pharmacy with a prescription. In 2014, the U.S. Drug Enforcement Agency changed hydrocodone from a schedule III to the more restrictive schedule II classification to reduce abuse of this pain medication (Federal Register, 2014). It is now also available as two extended-release products (Burchum & Rosenthal, 2019; Comerford & Durkin, 2020).

Methadone is a unique synthetic opioid analgesic medication that may have advantages over other opioids in carefully selected patients. In addition to being a mu opioid, it is an antagonist at the NMDA receptor site and thus has the potential to produce analgesic effects as a second- or third-line option for some neuropathic pain states. It may be used as an alternative when it is necessary to switch a patient to a new opioid because of inadequate analgesia or unacceptable adverse effects. The use of conventional equianalgesic dose conversion is not recommended when switching patients to and from methadone. Extensive guidelines on how to safely accomplish this are available elsewhere. In 2014, the APS, in conjunction with the Heart Rhythm Society and the College on Problems of Drug Dependence, issued clinical practice guidelines to encourage safe use of methadone (APS, 2016).

Methadone is usually given orally but has also been given by virtually every other route of administration. Although it has no active metabolites, methadone has a very long and highly variable **half-life** (5 to 100-plus hours; average is 20 hours), which makes it a good choice for the treatment of SUD; patients must be watched closely for excessive sedation, a sign of medication accumulation during this time period. (The medication is described as "long acting" because of its exceptionally long half-life.) When methadone is used to treat opioid use disorder, it is dosed once daily and is not intended to manage pain; acute pain management with other analgesic medications is needed in addition to daily methadone dosing. Other limitations are its propensity to interact with a large number of medications and prolong the QTc interval on the electrocardiogram (ECG). Some medications (e.g., clarithromycin and some antifungal medications) that inhibit CYP3A4, the enzyme that metabolizes methadone, should be avoided as they can inadvertently increase methadone levels in the blood. Despite these characteristics, methadone can be an effective and safe medication when prescribed by providers who have an appreciation of the unique characteristics of the medication and who are experienced in prescribing it (APS, 2016; Burchum & Rosenthal, 2019; Comerford & Durkin, 2020; Sheth et al., 2018).

Dual-Mechanism Analgesic Agents

The dual-mechanism analgesic agents tramadol and tapentadol bind weakly to the mu opioid receptor site and block the reuptake (resorption) of the inhibitory neurotransmitters serotonin and norepinephrine at central synapses in the spinal cord and brain stem of the modulatory descending pain pathway (APS, 2016; Holtsman & Hale, 2018). This makes these neurotransmitters more available to counteract pain. Dual-mechanism analgesic agents have been described as providing automatic "built-in" multimodal analgesia because a single tablet produces an effect on more than one analgesic action site (Varrassi, Hanna, Macheras, et al., 2017). The underlying mechanisms of tapentadol and tramadol differ in that tramadol blocks the reuptake of both serotonin and norepinephrine, but tapentadol blocks the reuptake of only norepinephrine. This is pertinent because norepinephrine may play a more significant role than serotonin in the endogenous analgesia pathways. Serotonin may be the more powerful mediator of depression; low serotonin levels are associated with depression. This helps explain why selective serotonin reuptake inhibitors (SSRIs), such as fluoxetine and paroxetine, which block only serotonin, are effective for the treatment of depression but not pain (APS, 2016; Burchum & Rosenthal, 2019; Comerford & Durkin, 2020; Holtsman & Hale, 2018).

Tramadol is used for both acute and chronic pain and is available in oral short-acting and modified-release formulations, including a short-acting tablet in combination with acetaminophen. It has demonstrated good efficacy for the treatment of neuropathic pain (Comerford & Durkin, 2020). The medication can lower seizure threshold and interact with other medications that block the reuptake of serotonin, such as the SSRIs, putting the patient at risk for serotonin syndrome, characterized by agitation, diarrhea, heart and blood pressure changes, and loss of coordination (Holtsman & Hale, 2018).

Tapentadol is available in short-acting and modified-release oral formulations. This medication has been shown to produce dose-dependent analgesia comparable to oxycodone. Major benefits are that it has no active metabolites and a significantly more favorable adverse effect profile (particularly GI) compared with opioid analgesic agents. These characteristics make tapentadol an attractive alternative to traditional oral opioid analgesic agents for many patients with pain (Comerford & Durkin, 2020; Holtsman & Hale, 2018).

Opioids to Avoid

Codeine is a prodrug, which means it is pharmacologically inactive when given. It must be metabolized to morphine for the patient to experience pain relief. It is estimated that 5% to 10% of patients lack the enzymatic ability to convert codeine to morphine via the CYP2D6 metabolic pathway, meaning that in this population of patients, codeine is an ineffective analgesic agent. In contrast, codeine has been associated with overdoses in some children due to rapid metabolism of the medication to morphine.

Meperidine has either been removed from or severely restricted on hospital formularies for the treatment of pain in an effort to improve patient safety. However, it is an accepted practice to use it in low doses (12.5 to 25 mg IV) to treat *rigors* (shivering) associated with general anesthesia. A major limitation to the use of meperidine is its active metabolite, normeperidine, which is a CNS stimulant and can cause delirium, irritability, tremors, myoclonus, and generalized seizures. Concern for meperidine's neurotoxicity risks has dramatically reduced its use (APS, 2016; Burchum & Rosenthal, 2019; Comerford & Durkin, 2020; Sheth et al., 2018).

Adverse Effects of Opioid Analgesic Agents

The most common adverse effects of opioids are constipation, nausea, vomiting, pruritus, hypotension, and sedation. Respiratory depression, while less common, is the most serious and feared of the opioid adverse effects (Pasero, 2009). The risk of respiratory depression is increased when other medications that have depressive effects on the CNS, such as benzodiazepines (e.g., diazepam), alcohol, and barbiturates, are used concurrently with opioids. In surgical patients, postoperative ileus can become a major complication as well (Burchum & Rosenthal, 2019; Comerford & Durkin, 2020; Sheth et al., 2018). Morphine lowers blood pressure by dilating peripheral arterioles and veins. In the presence of dehydration or with concomitant use of hypotensive medications, orthostatic hypotension may result (Burchum & Rosenthal, 2019). Long-term use of opioids may result in opioid-induced androgen deficiency and sleep disordered breathing (Chowdhuri & Javaheri, 2017; Hsieh, DiGiorgio, Fakunle, et al., 2018; Nagappa, Weingarten, Montandon, et al., 2017).

Opioids can result in delayed gastric emptying, slowed bowel motility, and decreased peristalsis, all of which result in slow-moving, hard stool that is difficult to pass. Risk is elevated with advanced age, and immobility; however, it is an almost universal opioid adverse effect (i.e., tolerance rarely develops). Constipation is a primary reason people stop taking their pain medication, which underscores the importance of taking a preventive approach and aggressive management if symptoms are detected. Prevention includes reminding patients to take a daily stool softener plus mild peristaltic stimulant for as long as they are taking opioids (APS, 2016; Burchum & Rosenthal, 2019).

Postoperative nausea and vomiting (PONV) occur following opioid administration due to medulla chemoreceptor trigger zone stimulation. PONV are among the most unpleasant of the adverse effects associated with surgery, and can have a negative impact on patient outcomes, and increase the need for nursing intervention. Guidelines from the American Society of PeriAnesthesia Nurses (ASPAN) recommend that all patients be evaluated for PONV risk, risk factors be reduced if possible, multimodal analgesia be provided (so that no opioid or the lowest effective opioid dose can be given), and prophylactic treatment (e.g., dexamethasone and a serotonin receptor antagonist, such as ondansetron, at the end of surgery) be given to patients with moderate risk (APS, 2016; ASPAN, 2006; Gan, Diemunsch, Habib, et al., 2014). More aggressive interventions should be utilized in patients with high risk (Pasero et al., 2011). (See Chapter 16 for further discussion of PONV.)

Pruritus is an adverse effect of opioids, not an allergic reaction to them. Although antihistamines such as diphenhydramine are commonly used, and patients may report being less bothered by itching after taking an antihistamine, this may be the result of sedating effects. Any additional coadministered sedating medication can be problematic in people already at risk for excessive sedation, such as postoperative patients, because this can lead to life-threatening respiratory depression (APS, 2016). Loratadine and cetirizine are considered nonsedating histamines and might be selected. Often the most effective, safest, and least expensive treatment of pruritus is opioid dose reduction. In fact, simply decreasing the opioid dose is sufficient to eliminate or make most of the adverse effects tolerable for many patients. Opioid rotation is another possible treatment. Nonsedating analgesic agents can be added to facilitate this approach. Parenteral low dose nalbuphine, an agonist–antagonist opioid, has been reported to be superior to placebo, control, antihistamines, and naloxone in the treatment of pruritus caused by neuraxial opioids (APS, 2016).

In addition to dose reduction strategies, most opioid pain treatment plans include prescriptions for medications that can be used to treat adverse effects should they occur. Recent research with animals demonstrated successful prevention of opioid induced pruritis through administration of capsaicin (Melo, Basso, Iftinca, et al., 2018). Nonpharmacologic interventions may also be effective, such as the application of a cool damp cloth over affected areas to help relieve the discomfort of pruritus.

With the exception of constipation, as patients become opioid tolerant, an accompanying tolerance to the opioid adverse effects develops. It is reassuring for patients receiving long-term opioid therapy to know that most of the adverse effects will subside with regular daily doses of opioids over several days.

Sedation and respiratory depression. Most patients experience sedation at the beginning of opioid therapy and whenever the opioid dose is increased significantly. If left untreated, excessive sedation can progress to clinically significant respiratory depression. Like other opioid adverse effects, sedation and respiratory depression are dose related. In most cases (exceptions may apply at the end of life), nurses should promptly reduce opioid doses or stop titration whenever advancing sedation is detected to prevent respiratory depression (Pasero, 2009; Pasero et al., 2011). In some patients (e.g., those with obstructive sleep apnea, pulmonary dysfunction), monitoring with capnography is warranted (Jarzyna, Junquist, Pasero, et al., 2011). When supplemental oxygen is needed to maintain the patient's oxygen saturation, pulse oximetry may not detect hypoventilation. Patients receiving opioid therapy and supplemental oxygen can benefit from capnography, which reflects the adequacy of ventilation and airflow, in conjunction with monitoring of sedation and respiratory function (Gupta & Edwards, 2018).

> ### ▶ Quality and Safety Nursing Alert
>
> *Opioid-induced respiratory depression is dose related and preceded by increasing sedation. Prevention of clinically significant opioid-induced respiratory depression begins with the administration of the lowest effective opioid dose, careful titration, close monitoring of sedation and respiratory function and status (i.e., rate, depth, regularity, excursion) throughout therapy, and prompt dose reduction when advancing sedation is detected (Nagappa et al., 2017).*

The knowledge that excessive sedation precedes opioid-induced respiratory depression reinforces that systematic sedation assessment is an essential aspect of the care of patients receiving opioid therapy (Gupta & Edwards, 2018; Pasero, 2009). Nursing assessment of sedation is convenient, inexpensive, and takes minimal time to perform. A simple, easy-to-understand sedation scale, developed for the assessment of *unintended* sedation, which includes what should be done at each level of sedation, is recommended to enhance accuracy and consistency of assessment, better monitor trends, and improve communication among members of the health care team (Garcia & McMullan, 2019; Jarzyna et al., 2011; Pasero, 2009; Pasero et al., 2011; Quinlan-Colwell, Thear, Miller-Baldwin, et al., 2017). Chart 9-6 presents a widely used sedation scale.

Chart 9-6

Pasero Opioid-Induced Sedation Scale with Interventions

Each level of sedation is followed by the appropriate action in italics.

S = Sleep, easy to arouse
Acceptable; no action necessary; may increase opioid dose if needed

1 = Awake and alert
Acceptable; no action necessary; may increase opioid dose if needed

2 = Slightly drowsy, easily aroused
Acceptable, no action necessary; may increase opioid dose if needed

3 = Frequently drowsy, arousable, drifts off to sleep during conversation
Unacceptable; monitor respiratory status and sedation level closely until sedation level is stable at less than 3 and respiratory status is satisfactory; decrease opioid dose 25–50%[1] or notify primary[2] or anesthesia provider for orders; consider administering a nonsedating, opioid-sparing nonopioid, such as acetaminophen or an NSAID, if not contraindicated; ask patient to take deep breaths every 15–30 min.

4 = Somnolent, minimal, or no response to verbal and physical stimulation
Unacceptable; stop opioid; consider administering naloxone[3,4]; call Rapid Response Team (Code Blue); stay with patient, stimulate, and support respiration as indicated by patient status; notify primary[2] or anesthesia provider; monitor respiratory status and sedation level closely until sedation level is stable at less than 3 and respiratory status is satisfactory.

[1]Opioid analgesic agent prescriptions or a hospital protocol should include the expectation that a nurse will decrease the opioid dose if a patient is excessively sedated.

[2]For example, the primary provider, nurse practitioner, advanced practice nurse, or physician assistant responsible for the pain management prescription.

[3]For adults experiencing respiratory depression, mix 0.4 mg of naloxone and 10 mL of normal saline in syringe and administer this dilute solution very slowly (0.5 mL over 2 min) while observing the patient's response (titrate to effect).

[4]Hospital protocols should include the expectation that a nurse will administer naloxone to any patient suspected of having life-threatening opioid-induced sedation and respiratory depression.

Copyright 1994, Pasero, C. Used with permission from Pasero, C., & McCaffery, M. (2011). *Pain assessment and pharmacologic management.* St. Louis, MO: Mosby-Elsevier.

Respiratory depression is assessed on the basis of what is normal for a particular person and is usually described as clinically significant when there is a decrease in the rate, depth, and regularity of respirations from baseline, rather than just by a specific number of respirations per minute (Pasero et al., 2011). There are many risk factors for opioid-induced respiratory depression, including older age (65 years of age or older), obesity, obstructive sleep apnea, and preexisting pulmonary dysfunction, or other comorbidities (APS, 2016; Jarzyna et al., 2011). Risk is elevated during the first 24 hours following surgery and in patients who require a high dose of opioid in a short period of time (e.g., more than 10 mg of IV morphine or equivalent in the PACU). Patients who receive regularly scheduled opioids often develop tolerance to this

effect in approximately 1 week (APS, 2016; Nagappa et al., 2017).

A comprehensive respiratory assessment constitutes more than counting a patient's respiratory rate (Pasero, 2009). A proper assessment requires watching the rise and fall of the patient's chest to determine rate, depth, and regularity of respirations. Listening to the sound of the patient's respirations is critical as well—snoring indicates airway obstruction and must be attended to promptly with repositioning and, depending on severity, a request for respiratory therapy consultation and further evaluation (Pasero, 2009; Pasero et al., 2011).

In most cases (exceptions may apply at the end of life), the opioid antagonist naloxone is promptly given IV to reverse clinically significant opioid-induced respiratory depression (Burchum & Rosenthal, 2019). The goal is to reverse only the sedation and respiratory depressant effects of the opioid. To this end, it should be diluted and titrated very slowly to prevent severe pain and other adverse effects, which can include hypertension, tachycardia, ventricular arrhythmias, pulmonary edema, and cardiac arrest (APS, 2016) (see Chart 9-6, footnote 3, for correct technique). Sometimes more than one dose of naloxone is necessary, because naloxone has a shorter duration of action (1 hour in most patients) than most opioids. In particular, this is true with transdermal fentanyl for which reversal requires repeated doses or an infusion of naloxone to insure appropriate reversal (Burchum & Rosenthal, 2019).

Co-Analgesic Medications

The **co-analgesic agents** comprise the largest group of analgesic agents, which offers many options. Medication selection and dosing is based on both experience and evidence-based guideline recommendations. There is considerable variability among individuals in their response to co-analgesic agents, including to agents within the same class; often a "trial and error" strategy is used in the outpatient setting. Treatment in the outpatient setting often is primarily for patients who have a neuropathic component of pain and involves the use of low initial doses and gradual dose escalation to allow tolerance to the adverse effects. Patients must be forewarned in this setting that the onset of analgesia is likely to require time to achieve analgesic benefit (Pasero, Polomano, Portenoy, et al., 2011). Following is a brief overview of the most commonly used co-analgesic agents.

Local Anesthetics

Local anesthetics have a long history of safe and effective use for all types of pain management. Local anesthetics are sodium channel blockers that affect the formation and propagation of action potentials. They are given by various routes of administration and are generally well tolerated by most individuals (Pasero et al., 2011). Injectable and topical local anesthetics are commonly used for procedural pain treatment. Local anesthetics are added to opioid analgesic agents and other agents to be given intraspinally for the treatment of both acute and chronic pain. They are also infused for continuous peripheral nerve blocks, primarily after surgery (Chou et al., 2016).

The lidocaine patch 5% is placed directly over or adjacent to the painful area for absorption into the tissues directly below. This medication produces minimal systemic absorption and adverse effects. The patch is left in place for 12 hours and then removed for as long as 12 hours (12 hours on, 12 hours off regimen). This application process is repeated as needed for continuous analgesia (Burchum & Rosenthal, 2019). The medication is FDA approved for the neuropathic pain syndrome and postherpetic neuralgia; however, research suggests that it is effective and safe for a variety of other painful neuropathic conditions (APS, 2016). Lidocaine is also available in topical preparations as cream, gel, solution, ointment, and aerosol (APS, 2016; Burchum & Rosenthal, 2019). More recent liposomal formulations of local anesthetics such as bupivacaine, which can be instilled in a surgical wound, are reported to have longer duration of action, supporting improved analgesia (Shah, Votta-Velis, & Borgeat, 2018).

Allergy to local anesthetics is rare. Cardiac and CNS adverse effects are dose related (Burchum & Rosenthal, 2019). CNS signs of systemic toxicity include ringing in the ears, metallic taste, irritability, and seizures. Signs of cardiotoxicity include circumoral tingling and numbness, bradycardia, cardiac arrhythmias, and CV collapse (Pasero et al., 2011).

Membrane Stabilizer Anticonvulsant Medications

The anticonvulsant calcium channel blockers gabapentin and pregabalin are first-line analgesic agents for neuropathic pain (Peterson et al., 2018). They are increasingly being added to postoperative pain treatment plans to address the neuropathic component of surgical pain and can be considered as part of a multimodal approach for postoperative analgesia (Chou et al., 2016). Although further research is needed, their addition has been shown to improve analgesia, allow lower doses of other analgesic agents, and help prevent persistent neuropathic postsurgical pain syndromes, such as phantom limb, post thoracotomy, posthernia, and postmastectomy pain. They may be effective in improving the acute pain associated with burn injuries and as treatment for the neuropathic pain and pruritis following major burn injuries (Griggs, Goverman, Bittner, et al., 2017; Kaul, Amin, Rosenberg, et al., 2018; Wang, Beekman, Hew, et al., 2018). Analgesic anticonvulsant therapy is initiated with low doses and titrated according to patient response. Initial doses of gabapentin may not provide analgesia; titration to effective dosing may take up to 2 months. Pregabalin has a more rapid onset of action with expected maximum effect typically reached in 2 weeks. Primary adverse effects of anticonvulsants are sedation and dizziness, which are usually transient and most notable during the titration phase of treatment (Peterson et al., 2018).

Antidepressant Medications

From an analgesic perspective, antidepressant co-analgesic medications are divided into two major groups: the tricyclic antidepressants (TCAs) and the serotonin and norepinephrine reuptake inhibitors (SNRIs). Evidence-based guidelines recommend the TCAs desipramine and nortriptyline and the SNRIs duloxetine and venlafaxine as first-line options for neuropathic pain treatment (Cruccu & Truini, 2017). Their delayed onset of action makes them inappropriate for acute pain treatment. Analgesic antidepressant therapy

is initiated with low doses and titrated according to patient response (Comerford & Durkin, 2020; Issa, Marshall, & Wasan, 2018).

Primary adverse effects of TCAs are dry mouth, sedation, dizziness, mental clouding, weight gain, and constipation. Orthostatic hypotension is a potentially serious TCA adverse effect. The most serious adverse effect is cardiotoxicity, and patients with significant heart disease are at high risk. SNRIs are thought to have a more favorable adverse effect profile and to be better tolerated than the TCAs. Due to the side effects, including delirium and confusion, amitriptyline is not indicated for use in older adults (Aguiar, Costa, da Costa, et al., 2019; Burchum & Rosenthal, 2019). The 2015 Beers Criteria® identified amitriptyline as potentially inappropriate for prescription among older adults (Fick, Semla, Steinman, et al., 2019) (see Chapter 8 for further information on the Beers Criteria). The most common SNRI adverse effects are nausea, headache, sedation, insomnia, weight gain, impaired memory, sweating, and tremors (Comerford & Durkin, 2020).

Ketamine

Ketamine is a dissociative anesthetic with dose-dependent analgesic, sedative, and amnestic properties (Burchum & Rosenthal, 2019). As an NMDA antagonist, it blocks the binding of glutamate at the NMDA receptors and thus prevents the transmission of pain to the brain via the ascending pathway (see Fig. 9-1B, inset). At high doses, this medication can produce psychomimetic effects (e.g., hallucinations, dreamlike feelings); however, these are minimized when low doses are given. A benefit of the medication is that it does not produce respiratory depression. Ketamine is given most often by the IV route but can also be given by the oral, rectal, intranasal, and subcutaneous routes. In addition to intraoperative and procedural use, ketamine has been used for the treatment of persistent neuropathic pain, but its adverse effect profile makes it less favorable than other analgesic agents for long-term therapy. It is, however, increasingly used as a third-line analgesic agent for **refractory** acute pain among patients who are very opioid-tolerant or for patients who are not able to be treated with opioids. It does have a potential for abuse (APS, 2016; Burchum & Rosenthal, 2019).

Gerontologic Considerations

Older adults often live with chronic pain, yet physiologic changes and comorbidities make management more complicated among them (HHS, 2019). Older adults are often sensitive to the effects of co-analgesic agents that produce sedation and other CNS effects, such as antidepressants and anticonvulsants. Since they are also at risk for undertreatment of pain, therapy should be initiated with low doses, and titration should proceed slowly with systematic assessment of patient response (Burchum & Rosenthal, 2019).

Older adults are also at increased risk for NSAID-induced GI toxicity. Acetaminophen should be used for mild pain and is recommended as first line for musculoskeletal pain (e.g., osteoarthritis). If an NSAID is needed for inflammatory pain, it is recommended that a COX-2 selective NSAID (if not contraindicated by an increased CV risk) or the nonselective NSAID least likely to cause a peptic ulcer should be used. The addition of a proton pump inhibitor to NSAID therapy, or opioid analgesic agents rather than an NSAID, is recommended for high-risk patients. The American Geriatric Society (AGS) recommends using extreme caution when prescribing NSAIDs among older adults (Jones, Ehrhardt, Ripoll, et al., 2016). NSAIDs are safest when used for short-term pain flares that may occur during transient worsening in severity of chronic diseases or conditions (e.g., osteoarthritis, fibromyalgia, low back pain). A number of NSAIDs are available in topical formulations which may be preferred for older adults (Burchum & Rosenthal, 2019; Horgas, 2017; HSS, 2019; Sowa, Weiner, & Camacho-Soto, 2018).

Age is considered an important factor to consider when selecting an opioid dose. The starting opioid dose should be reduced by 25% to 50% in adults older than 70 years because they are more sensitive to opioid adverse effects than younger adults; the number of subsequent doses is based on patient response (American Geriatrics Society [AGS], 2009; Burchum & Rosenthal, 2019).

Use of Placebos

A **placebo** is "any sham medication or procedure designed to be void of any known therapeutic value" (Lang, Christopher, Emmott, et al., 2018, p. 55). A saline injection is one example of a placebo. Administration of a medication at a known subtherapeutic dose (e.g., 0.10 mg of morphine in an adult) is also considered a placebo.

Placebos only are appropriately used as controls in research evaluating the effects of a new medication. The new substance or treatment is compared with the effects of a placebo and must show more favorable effects than placebos to warrant further investigation or marketing of the substance or treatment (Enck, Klosterhalfen, & Weimer, 2017). When a person responds to a placebo in accordance with its intent, it is called a *positive placebo response*

(Arnstein, Broglio, Wuhrman, et al., 2011). Individuals who participate in placebo-controlled research must be able to give informed consent or have a guardian who can provide informed consent.

Placebos should never be used clinically in a deceitful manner and without informed consent. It is disrespectful and harmful to use them. Pain relief resulting from a placebo is mistakenly believed to invalidate a patient's report of pain. This typically results in the patient being deprived of pain-relief measures, despite research showing that many patients who have obvious physical stimuli for pain (e.g., abdominal surgery) report pain relief after placebo administration. The reason for this is a mystery, but it is one of the many reasons that pain guidelines, position papers, nurse practice acts, and hospital policies nationwide agree that there are no individuals for whom and no condition for which placebos are the recommended treatment. The deceptive use of placebos has both ethical and legal implications, violates the nurse–patient relationship, and inevitably deprives patients of appropriate assessment and treatment (Arnstein et al., 2011; Enck et al., 2017; Lang et al., 2018).

Nonpharmacologic Methods of Pain Management

Most individuals use self-management strategies to deal with their health issues and promote well-being. According to national health information, it is estimated that American adults spent $30.2 billion on complementary health practices to treat painful conditions (O'Conner-Von, Heck, & Peltier, 2018). Nonpharmacologic complementary and alternative interventions include using natural products (e.g., herbs or botanicals, vitamins, probiotics) or using mind and body practices (e.g., acupuncture, behavior-based therapies, chiropractic manipulation, massage therapy, spirituality, yoga, T'ai chi) (HHS, 2019). Table 9-5

TABLE 9-5	Nonpharmacologic Methods of Pain Management	
Type	**Examples**	**Nursing Considerations**
Physical modalities	Proper body alignment; application of heat and/or cold; massage; transcutaneous electrical nerve stimulation (TENS); acupuncture; physical therapy; and aqua therapy	Be aware that some of these methods require a prescription in the inpatient setting, as inappropriate use can cause harm (e.g., burns or frostbite from extreme temperatures and prolonged thermal application).
Cognitive and behavioral methods	Relaxation breathing; distraction; listening, singing, or rhythmic tapping to music; imagery; humor; pet therapy; prayer; meditation; hypnosis	Prior to use, evaluate patient's cognitive ability to learn and perform necessary activities.
Movement therapy	Yoga, T'ai chi	Prior to use, evaluate patient's physical ability to perform necessary activities.
Biologically based therapies	Taking herbs, vitamins, and proteins; aromatherapy; diet modifications	Evaluate use to identify potential adverse effects.
Energy therapies	Therapeutic touch, Reiki, and healing touch	Obtain patient's permission before using intervention.

Adapted from National Center for Complementary and Integrative Health (NCCIH). (2015). *Complementary, alternative, or integrative health: What's in a name?* Retrieved on 11/9/2019 at: www.nccih.nih.gov/health/integrative-health#types; O'Conner-Von, S., Heck, C. R., & Peltier, C. H. (2018). *Complementary and integrative therapies for pain management.* In M. L. Czarnecki, & H. N. Turner (Eds.). *Core curriculum for pain management nursing* (3rd ed.). St. Louis, MO: Elsevier.

<table>
<tr><td colspan="2">

Chart 9-7   **Considerations in Selecting and Using Nonpharmacologic Methods**

</td></tr>
<tr><td>

- Do the patient, family, and health care team understand the relationship between nonpharmacologic pain management and antispasmodic agents? Patients who have been taking analgesic agents may mistakenly assume that when clinicians suggest a nonpharmacologic method, the purpose is to reduce the use or dose of analgesic agents. All involved must understand that nonpharmacologic methods are used to complement—not replace—pharmacologic methods.
- Does the patient understand the limitations of nonpharmacologic methods? Nonpharmacologic methods are valuable as comfort measures; however, not all such measures relieve pain and should not be promoted as such.
- Is the patient interested in using a nonmedication method, and have any been tried previously? If so, what happened? Is the patient using nonmedication methods because of unfounded fears about analgesic agents? Willingness and interest are important for successful use of nonpharmacologic methods; however, patients may fear taking analgesic agents that clearly are indicated for their pain, such as nonsteroidal anti-inflammatory drugs (NSAIDs) for an inflammatory painful condition. Such fears should be explored, and accurate information and appropriate treatment provided. Alternately, the reasons a patient refuses to use a nonpharmacologic method also should be explored, but the patient's right to refuse must be respected.

</td><td>

- What are the patient's preferences and coping styles? Encouraging patients to choose from a variety of techniques allows them to match the technique to their individual and cultural preferences. If none of the choices appeal to the patient, the patient's right to refuse use should be respected.
- Does the patient have the physical and cognitive abilities necessary for using the nonpharmacologic method? Does the patient have sufficient energy to learn and perform any tasks involved? For example, physical and mental fatigue can interfere with the use of distraction and relaxation imagery techniques. Does the patient want to dedicate the necessary time required for the nonpharmacologic method? For example, those who do not find a 20-min self-sustained relaxation technique appealing may be more suited for passive application of cold or heat.
- Do others (e.g., family, friends) want to be involved in helping the patient? Is the method a potential vehicle for improving relationships between the patient and others? For example, a method that patients cannot do for themselves, such as massage, may be a burden to some caregivers in the home, whereas others may welcome that opportunity to be physically close to a loved one.
- Are support materials and patient education resources available? Whenever possible, verbal, written, and in some cases, online or video education should be provided.

</td></tr>
<tr><td colspan="2">

Adapted from McCaffery, M. (2002). What is the role of nondrug methods in the nursing care of patients with acute pain? *Pain Management Nursing, 3*(3), 77–80; McCaffery, M., & Pasero, C. (1999). *Pain: Clinical manual*. St. Louis, MO: Mosby.

</td></tr>
</table>

lists examples of select complementary and alternative therapies.

Nonpharmacologic therapies are usually effective alone for mild to some moderate-intensity pain. They should not be a replacement or alternative but complement pharmacologic therapies as part of a multimodal approach for more severe pain. The effectiveness of nonpharmacologic methods can be unpredictable, and although not all will relieve pain, they offer many benefits to patients with pain. For example, research suggests that nonpharmacologic methods can facilitate relaxation and reduce anxiety and stress. Many patients find that the use of nonpharmacologic methods helps them cope better with their pain and feel greater control over the pain experience (HHS, 2019; O'Conner-Von et al., 2018).

Several nonpharmacologic methods can be used in the clinical setting to provide comfort and pain relief for all types of pain; however, time is often limited in this setting for implementation of these methods. Nurses play an important role in providing them and educating patients about their use. Many of the methods are relatively easy for nurses to incorporate into daily clinical practice and may be used individually or in combination with other nonpharmacologic therapies to facilitate patient-centered care utilizing a multimodal approach (HHS, 2019; O'Conner-Von et al., 2018). Chart 9-7 provides points for nurses to consider before using nonpharmacologic methods.

Unfolding Patient Stories: Stan Checketts • Part 1

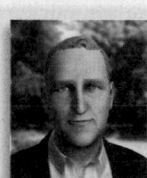

Stan Checketts, a 52-year-old man, is in the emergency department with severe abdominal pain. The provider has prescribed buprenorphine 0.3-mg IV push for pain. Explain the assessments performed by the nurse prior to, during, and following the administration of the medication. Also consider nonpharmacologic interventions the nurse can incorporate to assist with his pain relief. (Stan Checketts' story continues in Chapter 41.)

Care for Stan and other patients in a realistic virtual environment: *vSim for Nursing* (**thepoint.lww.com/vSimMedicalSurgical**). Practice documenting these patients' care in DocuCare (**thepoint.lww.com/DocuCareEHR**).

Nursing Implications of Pain Management

The provision of optimal pain management requires a collaborative approach between patients with pain, their families, and members of the health care team. Everyone involved must share common goals, a common knowledge base, and a common language with regard to the antispasmodic agents and nonpharmacologic methods used to manage pain.

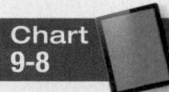

Chart 9-8

PLAN OF NURSING CARE
Care of the Patient with Acute Pain

NURSING DIAGNOSIS: Acute Pain
GOAL: Achievement and maintenance of patient's comfort–function goal

Nursing Intervention	Rationale	Expected Outcomes

1. Perform and document a comprehensive pain assessment.
 	
  a. Use a reliable and valid tool to determine pain intensity.
  b. Accept the patient's report of pain.
  c. Assist the patient in establishing a comfort–function goal.
 	
  d. Apply the Hierarchy of Pain Measures in patients who are unable to report their pain.
2. Administer analgesic agents as prescribed.
3. Offer and educate patient how to use appropriate nonpharmacologic interventions.
4. Reassess for degree of pain relief and presence of adverse effects at peak effect time of intervention.
5. Obtain additional prescriptions as needed.
 	
6. Prevent and treat adverse effects.
 	
7. Educate patient and family about the effects of analgesic agents and the goals of care; explain how adverse effects will be prevented and treated; address fears of substance use disorder.
	1. The comprehensive pain assessment is the foundation of the pain treatment plan; documentation ensures communication between team members.
	  a. The use of valid and reliable tools helps ensure accuracy and consistency in assessment.
	  b. Accepting the patient's report of pain is the undisputed standard of pain assessment.
	  c. The comfort–function goal links function to pain control and provides direction for necessary adjustments in the treatment plan to maximize function.
	  d. The use of the Hierarchy of Pain Measures provides a process to ensure pain treatment in the patient who cannot report pain.
	2. Pharmacologic interventions are the cornerstone of pain management.
	3. Nonpharmacologic methods are used to supplement pharmacologic interventions.
	4. Reassessment permits evaluation of both the effectiveness and safety of interventions.
	5. Prescriptions for additional analgesic agents or adjustment in dose are often needed to maximize pain control.
	6. Adverse effects are prevented whenever possible and promptly treated to reduce patient discomfort and prevent harm.
	7. An understanding of the treatment plan and goals of care educates patients and their families how to partner with the health care team to optimize pain control.
		• If able, provides information about the pain
		• Expresses understanding of the link between function and pain control and establishes a realistic comfort–function goal
		• Reports a pain intensity that allows participation in important functional activities
		• If not able to report pain, demonstrates behaviors that indicate pain relief and participation in important functional activities
		• Expresses satisfaction with the use of nonpharmacologic methods
		• Tolerates pharmacologic and nonpharmacologic interventions without adverse effects
		• Demonstrates an understanding of the treatment plan and goals of care

Whether nurses provide care in the home, hospital, or any other setting, they are in a unique position to coordinate a comprehensive, evidence-based approach to meet the needs of people with pain. Chart 9-8 provides a plan of nursing care for the patient with pain.

CRITICAL THINKING EXERCISES

1 **ebp** An 88-year-old woman arrives in the emergency department following a motor vehicle crash in which she was the restrained front seat passenger. She repeatedly says "owie" and her daughter reports that this is her mom's way of expressing pain. Her daughter also reports that her mother was recently diagnosed with dementia after family members began noticing increasing forgetfulness and confusion at home. When asked to rate the intensity of her pain, the patient replies "owie, yes" but she is not able to easily assign a number to her pain. What pain assessment tool would be most helpful in assessing this patient's pain and in evaluating the effectiveness of interventions? What

is the strength of the evidence supporting the assessment tool you selected?

2 **pq** A 62-year-old woman who has chronic abdominal pain following multiple surgeries resulting from an abusive domestic situation is admitted to the medical floor for reports of worsening pain at home. She reports pain and nausea but denies diarrhea or vomiting. In addition to the 50-mcg fentanyl transdermal patch she has used to control pain at home for the last 2 years, the primary provider has prescribed: 1 mg intravenous hydromorphone every 2 hours PRN pain; promethazine 25 mg IV every 4 hours PRN nausea; lorazepam 0.5 mg IV every 6 hours PRN anxiety; and zolpidem 1.75 mg sublingual nightly prior to sleep. The patient asks you to give her all her medications at the same time so that she can sleep. She asserts that "the nurses always give me the medication that way when I am in the hospital." You are concerned that all these medications are central nervous system depressants and that given together, they could lead to oversedation and possibly result in respiratory depression. How would you prioritize administering the medications that she is requesting and your ongoing assessments to ensure adequate symptom relief while maintaining patient safety and minimizing the risks of adverse outcomes?

3 **ipc** A 28-year-old man is hospitalized with a diagnosis of an epidural abscess. He reports a 5-year history of daily intravenous self-administration of heroin. He tells you that the oxycodone his primary provider prescribed is "not doing anything" and his pain "is 100/10." How will you collaborate with other members of the interprofessional health care team to manage his pain? Using a multimodal approach for analgesia, what other interventions, both pharmacologic and nonpharmacologic, can the team incorporate into his plan of care to better manage his severe pain?

REFERENCES

*Asterisk indicates nursing research.
**Double asterisk indicates classic reference.

Books

American Pain Society (APS). (2016). *Principles of analgesic use* (7th ed.) Chicago, IL: American Pain Society.

Auriacombe, M., Serre, F., Denis, C., et al. (2019). Diagnosis of addictions. In H. Pickard, & S. H. Ahmed (Eds.). *The Routledge handbook of the philosophy and science of addiction.* New York: Routledge.

Belvis, D., Henderson, K. J., & Benzon, H. A. (2018). Sickle cell disease. In H. T. Benzon, S. N. Raja, S. M. Fishman, et al. (Eds.). *Essentials of pain medicine* (4th ed.). Philadelphia, PA: Elsevier.

Burchum, J. R., & Rosenthal, L. D. (2019). *Lehne's pharmacology for nursing care* (10th ed.). St. Louis, MO: Elsevier Saunders.

Chekka, K., & Benzon, H. T. (2018). Taxonomy: Definition of pain terms and chronic pain syndromes. In H. T. Benzon, S. N. Raja, S. M. Fishman, et al. (Eds.). *Essentials of pain medicine* (4th ed.). Philadelphia, PA: Elsevier.

Comerford, K. C., & Durkin, M. T. (2020). *Nursing 2020 drug handbook.* Philadelphia, PA: Wolters Kluwer.

Conlin, N., Grant, M. C., & Wu, C. L. (2018). Intrathecal opioids for postoperative pain. In H. T. Benzon, S. N. Raja, S. M. Fishman, et al. (Eds.). *Essentials of pain medicine* (4th ed.). Philadelphia, PA: Elsevier.

Curtis, C. P., & Wrona, S. (2018). Pain management education. In M. L. Czarnecki, & H. N. Turner (Eds.). *Core curriculum for pain management nursing* (3rd ed.). St. Louis, MO: Elsevier.

DiMaggio, T. J., Clark, L. M., Czarenecki, M. L., et al. (2018). Acute pain management. In M. L. Czarnecki, & H. N. Turner (Eds.). *Core curriculum for pain management nursing* (3rd ed.). St. Louis, MO: Elsevier.

Eksterowicz, N., & DiMaggio, T. J. (2018). Acute pain management. In M. L. Czarnecki, & H. N. Turner (Eds.). *Core curriculum for pain management nursing* (3rd ed.). St. Louis, MO: Elsevier.

Fernandes, M. T. P., Hernandes, F. B., de Almeida, T. N., et al. (2017). Patient-controlled analgesia (PCA) in acute pain: Pharmacological and clinical aspects. In C. Maldonado (Ed.). *Pain relief: From analgesics to alternative therapies.* INTECH. Retrieved on 11/9/19 at: www.dx.doi.org/10.5772/67299

Golan, D. E., Tashjian, A. H., & Armstrong, E. J. (2017). *Principles of pharmacology: The pathophysiologic basis of drug therapy* (4th ed.). Baltimore, MD: Wolters Kluwer.

Hernandez, G. A., Grant, M. C., & Wu, C. L. (2018). Epidural opioids for postoperative pain. In H. T. Benzon, S. N. Raja, S. M. Fishman, et al. (Eds.). *Essentials of pain medicine* (4th ed.). Philadelphia, PA: Elsevier.

Holtsman, M., & Hale, C. (2018). Major opioids in pain management. In H. T. Benzon, S. N. Raja, S. M. Fishman, et al. (Eds.). *Essentials of pain medicine* (4th ed.). Philadelphia, PA: Elsevier.

Ilfeld, B. M., & Mariano, E. R. (2018). Continuous peripheral nerve blocks. In H. T. Benzon, S. N. Raja, S. M. Fishman, et al. (Eds.). *Essentials of pain medicine* (4th ed.). Philadelphia, PA: Elsevier.

Issa, M. A., Marshall, Z., & Wasan, A. D. (2018). Psychopharmacology for pain medicine. In H. T. Benzon, S. N. Raja, S. M. Fishman, et al. (Eds.). *Essentials of pain medicine* (4th ed.). Philadelphia, PA: Elsevier.

Jamison, D. E., Cohen, S. P., & Rosenow, J. (2018). Implanted medication delivery systems for control of chronic pain. In H. T. Benzon, S. N. Raja, S. M. Fishman, et al. (Eds.). *Essentials of pain medicine* (4th ed.). Philadelphia, PA: Elsevier.

Lang, K. R., Christopher, M. J., Emmott, H. C., et al. (2018). Acute pain management. In M. L. Czarnecki, & H. N. Turner (Eds.). *Core curriculum for pain management nursing* (3rd ed.). St. Louis, MO: Elsevier.

**McCaffery, M. (1968). *Nursing practice theories related to cognition, bodily pain, and man-environment interactions.* Los Angeles, CA: University of California, Los Angeles.

**McCaffery, M., Herr, K., & Pasero, C. (2011). Assessment. In C. Pasero, & M. McCaffery (Eds.). *Pain assessment and pharmacologic management.* St. Louis, MO: Mosby-Elsevier.

**McCaffery, M., & Pasero, C. (1999). *Pain: Clinical manual.* St. Louis, MO: Mosby.

Montgomery, R., Mallick-Searle, T., Peltier, C. H., et al. (2018). Physiology of pain. In M. L. Czarnecki, & H. N. Turner (Eds.). *Core curriculum for pain management nursing* (3rd ed.). St. Louis, MO: Elsevier.

National Institute on Drug Abuse. (2014). *Prescription drug abuse.* Washington, DC: NIH publication.

Nouri, K. H., Osuagwu, U., Boyette-Davis, J., et al. (2018). Neurochemistry of somatosensory and pain processing. In H. T. Benzon, S. N. Raja, S. M. Fishman, et al. (Eds.). *Essentials of pain medicine* (4th ed.). Philadelphia, PA: Elsevier.

O'Conner-Von, S., Heck, C. R., & Peltier, C. H. (2018). Complementary and integrative therapies for pain management. In M. L. Czarnecki, & H. N. Turner (Eds.). *Core curriculum for pain management nursing* (3rd ed.). St. Louis, MO: Elsevier.

Palat, G. (2018). Addressing breakthrough pain leads to successful outcome. In S. Bhatnagar (Ed.). *Cancer pain management in developing countries.* Philadelphia, PA: Wolters Kluwer.

**Pasero, C., & McCaffery, M. (2011). *Pain assessment and pharmacologic management.* St. Louis, MO: Mosby-Elsevier.

**Pasero, C., Polomano, R. C., Portenoy, R. K., et al. (2011). Adjuvant analgesics. In C. Pasero, & M. McCaffery (Eds.). *Pain assessment and pharmacologic management.* St. Louis, MO: Mosby-Elsevier.

**Pasero, C., & Portenoy, R. K. (2011). Neurophysiology of pain and analgesia and the pathophysiology of neuropathic pain. In C. Pasero, & M. McCaffery (Eds.). *Pain assessment and pharmacologic management.* St. Louis, MO: Mosby-Elsevier.

**Pasero, C., Portenoy, R. K., & McCaffery, M. (2011). Nonopioid analgesics. In C. Pasero, & M. McCaffery (Eds.). *Pain assessment and pharmacologic management.* St. Louis, MO: Mosby-Elsevier.

**Pasero, C., Quinn, T. E., Portenoy, R. K., et al. (2011). Opioid analgesics. In C. Pasero, & M. McCaffery (Eds.). *Pain assessment and pharmacologic management.* St. Louis, MO: Mosby-Elsevier.

Peterson, S., Benson, H. T., & Hurley, R. W. (2018). Membrane stabilizers. In H. T. Benzon, S. N. Raja, S. M. Fishman, et al. (Eds.). *Essentials of pain medicine* (4th ed.). Philadelphia, PA: Elsevier.

Ringkamp, M., Dougherty, P. M., & Raja, S. N. H. A. (2018). Anatomy and physiology of the pain signaling process. In H. T. Benzon, S. N. Raja, S. M. Fishman, et al. (Eds.). *Essentials of pain medicine* (4th ed.). Philadelphia, PA: Elsevier.

Schliessbach, J., & Maurer, K. (2017). Pharmacology of pain transmission and modulation. In R. J. Young, M. Nguyen, E. Nelson, et al. (Eds.). *Pain medicine: An essential review* (1st ed.). Cham, Switzerland: Springer International Publishing.

Sheth, S., Holtsman, M., & Mahajan, G. (2018). Major opioids in pain management. In H. T. Benzon, S. N. Raja, S. M. Fishman, et al. (Eds.). *Essentials of pain medicine* (4th ed.). Philadelphia, PA: Elsevier.

Sowa, G. A., Weiner, D. K., & Camacho-Soto, A. (2018). Geriatric pain management. In H. T. Benzon, S. N. Raja, S. M. Fishman, et al. (Eds.). *Essentials of pain medicine* (4th ed.). Philadelphia, PA: Elsevier.

Spofford, C. M., & Hurley, R. W. (2018). Preventive analgesia. In H. T. Benzon, S. N. Raja, S. M. Fishman, et al. (Eds.). *Essentials of pain medicine* (4th ed.). Philadelphia, PA: Elsevier.

Vardeh, D., & Naranjo, J. F. (2017). Pharmacology of pain transmission and modulation. In R. J. Young, M. Nguyen, E. Nelson, & R. D. Uman

(Eds.). *Pain medicine: An essential review* (1st ed.). Cham, Switzerland: Springer International Publishing.

Williams, B. S. (2018). Nonopioid analgesics: Nonsteroidal antiinflammatory drugs, cyclooxygenase-2 inhibitors, and acetaminophen. In H. T. Benzon, S. N. Raja, S. M. Fishman, et al. (Eds.). *Essentials of Pain Medicine* (4th ed.). Philadelphia, PA: Elsevier.

Journals and Electronic Documents

Aguiar, J. P., Costa, L. H., da Costa, F. A., et al. (2019). Identification of potentially inappropriate medications with risk of major adverse cardiac and cerebrovascular events among elderly patients in ambulatory setting and long-term care facilities. *Clinical Interventions in Aging, 14*, 535–547.

**American Geriatrics Society (AGS). (2009). Pharmacological management of persistent pain in older persons. *Journal of the American Geriatrics Society, 57*(6), 1331–1346.

**American Society of PeriAnesthesia Nurses. (2006). ASPAN's evidence-based clinical practice guideline for the prevention and/or management of PONV/PDNV. *Journal of PeriAnesthesia Nursing, 21*(4), 230–250.

American Society of Regional Anesthesia and Pain Medicine. (2016). Practice guidelines for the prevention, detection, and management of respiratory depression associated with neuraxial opioid administration: An updated report by the American Society of Anesthesiologists Task Force on Neuraxial Opioids and the American Society of Regional Anesthesia and Pain Medicine. *Anesthesiology, 124*(3), 535–552.

*Arnstein, P., Broglio, K., Wuhrman, E., et al. (2011). Use of placebos in pain management. *Pain Management Nursing, 12*(4), 225–229.

Arthur, J., & Hui, D. (2018). Safe opioid use: Management of opioid-related adverse effects and aberrant behaviors. *Hematology/Oncology Clinics, 32*(3), 387–403.

Baker, D. W. (2017). History of The Joint Commission's pain standards: Lessons for today's prescription opioid epidemic. *Journal of the American Medical Association, 317*(11), 1117–1118.

Bally, M., Dendukuri, N., Rich, B., et al. (2017). Risk of acute myocardial infarction with NSAIDs in real world use: Bayesian meta-analysis of individual patient data. *British Medical Journal, 357*, 1–13.

Baral, P., Udit, S., & Chiu, I. M. (2019). Pain and immunity: Implications for host defence. *Nature Reviews Immunology, 19*, 433–447.

Beverly, A., Kaye, A. D., Ljungqvist, O., et al. (2017). Essential elements of multimodal analgesia in enhanced recovery after surgery (ERAS) guidelines. *Anesthesiology Clinics, 35*(2), e115–e143.

Blackburn, J. P. (2018). The diagnosis and management of chronic pain. *Medicine, 46*(12), 786–791.

Bouhassira, D. (2019). Neuropathic pain: Definition, assessment and epidemiology. *Revue Neurologique, 175*(1), 16–25.

Chayadi, E., & McConnell, B. L. (2019). Gaining insights on the influence of attention, anxiety, and anticipation on pain perception. *Journal of Pain Research, 12*, 851–854.

Chou, R., Gordon, D. B., de Leon-Casasola, et al. (2016). Management of postoperative pain: A clinical practice guideline from the American Pain Society, the American Society of Regional Anesthesia and Pain Medicine, and the American Society of Anesthesiologists' committee on regional anesthesia, executive committee, and administrative council. *The Journal of Pain, 17*(2), 131–157.

Chowdhuri, S., & Javaheri, S. (2017). Sleep disordered breathing caused by chronic opioid use: Diverse manifestations and their management. *Sleep Medicine Clinics, 12*(4), 573–586.

Colloca, L., Ludman, T., Bouhassira, D., et al. (2017). Neuropathic pain. *Nature Reviews Disease Primers, 3*, 17002.

Cooney, M. F., Czarnecki, M., Dunwoody, C., et al. (2013). American Society for Pain Management Nursing position statement with clinical practice guidelines: Authorized agent controlled analgesia. *Pain Management Nursing, 14*(3), 176–181.

Cruccu, G., & Truini, A. (2017). A review of neuropathic pain: from guidelines to clinical practice. *Pain and Therapy, 6*(1), 35–42.

Damien, J., Colloca, L., Bellei-Rodriguez, C. E., et al. (2018). Pain modulation: From conditioned pain modulation to placebo and nocebo effects in experimental and clinical pain. *International Review of Neurobiology, 139*, 255–296.

ECRI Institute Patient Safety Organization. (2017). *ECRI PSO deep dive: Opioid use in acute care.* Plymouth Meeting, PA: ECRI Institute. Retrieved on 11/14/19 at: www.ecri.org/opioids-deep-dive

Ellison, D. L. (2017). Physiology of pain. *Critical Care Nursing Clinics, 29*(4), 397–406.

Enck, P., Klosterhalfen, S., & Weimer, K. (2017). Unsolved, forgotten, and ignored features of the placebo response in medicine. *Clinical Therapeutics, 39*(3), 458–468.

Federal Register. (2014). *Schedules of controlled substances: Rescheduling of hydrocodone combination products from Schedule III to Schedule II. Final Rule.* 2014. Retrieved on 7/22/2019 at: www.gpo.gov/fdsys/pkg/FR-2014-08-22/pdf/2014-19922.pdf

Fick, D. M., Semla, T. P., Steinman, M., et al. (2019). American Geriatrics Society 2019 Updated AGS Beers Criteria® for potentially inappropriate medication use in older adults. *Journal of the American Geriatrics Society, 67*(4), 674–694.

Fry, M., & Elliott, R. (2018). Pragmatic evaluation of an observational pain assessment scale in the emergency department: The Pain Assessment in Advanced Dementia (PAINAD) scale. *Australasian Emergency Care, 21*(4), 131–136.

Gan, T. J., Diemunsch, P., Habib, A. S., et al. (2014). Consensus guidelines for the management of postoperative nausea and vomiting. *Anesthesia & Analgesia, 118*(1), 85–113.

García, G., Gutiérrez-Lara, E. J., Centurión, D., et al. (2019). Fructose-induced insulin resistance as a model of neuropathic pain in rats. *Neuroscience, 404*, 233–245.

Garcia, M. G., & McMullan, T. W. (2019). Pasero Opioid-Induced Sedation Scale in a pediatric surgical ward: A quality improvement project. *Journal of Pediatric Surgical Nursing, 8*(2), 29–39.

Griggs, C., Goverman, J., Bittner, E. A., et al. (2017). Sedation and pain management in burn patients. *Clinics in Plastic Surgery, 44*(3), 535–540.

Groessi, E. J., Liu, L., Change, D. G., et al. (2017). Yoga for military veterans with chronic low back pain: A randomized clinical trial. *American Journal of Preventative Medicine, 53*(5), 599–608.

Gupta, R. K., & Edwards, D. A. (2018). Monitoring for opioid-induced respiratory depression. *APSF Newsletter, 32*(3), 70–73.

Gwee, K. A., Goh, V., Lima, G., et al. (2018). Coprescribing proton-pump inhibitors with nonsteroidal anti-inflammatory medications: Risks versus benefits. *Journal of Pain Research, 11*, 361.

**Herr, K., Coyne, P. J., McCaffery, M., et al. (2011). Pain assessment in the patient unable to self-report: Position statement with clinical practice recommendations. *Pain Management Nursing, 12*(4), 230–250.

Higgins, C., Smith, B. H., & Matthews, K. (2018). Evidence of opioid-induced hyperalgesia in clinical populations after chronic opioid exposure: A systematic review and meta-analysis. *British Journal of Anaesthesia, 122*(6), e114–e126.

Holland, E., Bateman, B. T., Cole, N., et al. (2019). Evaluation of a quality improvement intervention that eliminated routine use of opioids after cesarean delivery. *Obstetrics & Gynecology, 133*(1), 91–97.

Horgas, A. L. (2017). Pain management in older adults. *Nursing Clinics, 52*(4), e1–e7.

Howard, A., & Brant, J. M. (2019). Pharmacologic management of cancer pain. *Seminars in Oncology Nursing, 35*(3), 235–240.

Hsieh, A., DiGiorgio, L., Fakunle, M., et al. (2018). Management strategies in opioid abuse and sexual dysfunction: A review of opioid-induced androgen deficiency. *Sexual Medicine Reviews, 6*(4), 618–623.

International Association for the Study of Pain (IASP). (2017). IASP terminology. Retrieved on 5/20/2019 at: www.iasp-pain.org/Education/Content.aspx?ItemNumber=1698&navItemNumber=576#Peripheralsensitization

**Jarzyna, D., Junquist, C., Pasero, C., et al. (2011). American Society for Pain Management evidence-based guideline on monitoring for opioid-induced sedation and respiratory depression. *Pain Management Nursing, 12*(3), 118–145.

Jones, M. R., Ehrhardt, K. P., Ripoll, J. G., et al. (2016). Pain in the elderly. *Current Pain and Headache Reports, 20*(4), 23.

Jungquist, C. R., Vallerand, A. H., Sicoutris, C., et al. (2017). Assessing and managing acute pain: A call to action. *The American Journal of Nursing, 117*(3), S4–S11.

Kang, Y., & Demiris, G. (2018). Self-report pain assessment tools for cognitively intact older adults: Integrative review. *International Journal of Older People Nursing, 13*(2), 1–29.

Kaul, I., Amin, A., Rosenberg, M., et al. (2018). Use of gabapentin and pregabalin for pruritus and neuropathic pain associated with major burn injury: A retrospective chart review. *Burns, 44*(2), 414–422.

Kochman, A., Howell, J., Sheridan, M., et al. (2017). Reliability of the Faces, Legs, Activity, Cry, and Consolability scale in assessing acute pain in the pediatric emergency department. *Pediatric Emergency Care*, 33(1), 14–17.

Kwiatkowski, K., & Mika, J. (2018). The importance of chemokines in neuropathic pain development and opioid analgesic potency. *Pharmacological Reports*, 70(4), 821–830.

Leppert, W., Malec-Milewska, M., Zajaczkowska, R., et al. (2018). Transdermal and topical medication administration in the treatment of pain. *Molecules*, 23(3), 681.

Li, J. X. (2019). Combining opioids and non-opioids for pain management: Current status. *Neuropharmacology*, 158, 107619.

Liu, X., Zhu, M., Ju, Y., et al. (2019). Autophagy dysfunction in neuropathic pain. *Neuropeptides*, 75(1), 41–48.

Lo Coco, G., Melchiori, F., Oiendi, V., et al. (2019). Group treatment for substance use disorder in adults: A systematic review and meta-analysis of randomized-controlled trials. *Journal of Substance Abuse Treatment*, 99(1), 104–116.

Martin, S. L., Power, A., Boyle, Y., et al. (2017). 5-HT modulation of pain perception in humans. *Psychopharmacology*, 234(19), 2929–2939.

**McCaffery, M. (2002). What is the role of nondrug methods in the nursing care of patients with acute pain? *Pain Management Nursing*, 3(3), 77–80.

Melo, H., Basso, L., Iftinca, M., et al. (2018). Itch induced by peripheral mu opioid receptors is dependent on TRPV1-expressing neurons and alleviated by channel activation. *Scientific Reports*, 8(1), 15551.

*Mueller, G., Schumacher, P., Holzer, E., et al. (2017). The inter-rater reliability of the observation instrument for assessing pain in elderly with dementia: An investigation in the long-term care setting. *Journal of Nursing Measurement*, 25(3), E173–E184.

Nagappa, M., Weingarten, T. N., Montandon, G., et al. (2017). Opioids, respiratory depression, and sleep-disordered breathing. *Best Practice & Research Clinical Anaesthesiology*, 31(4), 469–485.

Nahin, R. L. (2017). Severe pain in Veterans: The impact of age and sex, and comparisons to the general population. *Journal of Pain*, 18(3), 247–254.

National Center for Complementary and Integrative Health (NCCIH). (2015). Complementary, alternative, or integrative health: What's in a name? Retrieved on 6/8/2019 at: www.nccih.nih.gov/health/integrative-health#types

National Institutes of Health (NIH). (2019). *HEAL Initiative Research Plan*. Washington, DC: NIH publication. Retrieved on 6/6/2019 at: www.nih.gov/research-training/medical-research-initiatives/heal-initiative/heal-initiative-research-plan

Nelson, A. M., & Wu, C. L. (2018). "Randomization at the Expense of Relevance." L. J. Cronbach and intravenous acetaminophen as an opioid-sparing adjuvant. *Anesthesia & Analgesia*, 127(5), 1099–1100.

Nishimura, H., Kawasaki, M., Suzuki, H., et al. (2019). Neuropathic pain upregulates hypothalamo-neurohypophysial and hypothalamo-spinal oxytocinergic pathways in oxytocin-monomeric red fluorescent protein 1 transgenic rat. *Neuroscience*, 406(1), 50–61.

Osborne, N. R., Anastakis, D. J., & Davis, K. D. (2018). Peripheral nerve injuries, pain, and neuroplasticity. *Journal of Hand Therapy*, 31(2), 184–194.

***Pasero, C. (2009). Assessment of sedation during opioid administration for pain management. *Journal of PeriAnesthesia Nursing*, 24(3), 186–190.

Pozek, J. P. J., De Ruyter, M., & Khan, T. W. (2018). Comprehensive acute pain management in the perioperative surgical home. *Anesthesiology Clinics*, 36(2), 295–307.

Quinlan-Colwell, A., Thear, G., Miller-Baldwin, E., et al. (2017). Use of the Pasero Opioid-induced Sedation Scale (POSS) in pediatric patients. *Journal of Pediatric Nursing*, 33, 83–87.

Rijkenberg, S., Stilma, W., Bosman, R. J., et al. (2017). Pain measurement in mechanically ventilated patients after cardiac surgery: Comparison of the Behavioral Pain Scale (BPS) and the Critical-Care Pain Observation Tool (CPOT). *Journal of Cardiothoracic and Vascular Anesthesia*, 31(4), 1227–1234.

Schofield, P., & Abdulla, A. (2018). Pain assessment in the older population: What the literature says. *Age and Ageing*, 47(3), 324–327.

Shah, J., Votta-Velis, E. G., & Borgeat, A. (2018). New local anesthetics. *Best Practice & Research Clinical Anaesthesiology*, 32(2), 179–185.

Shiffman, S., Battista, D. R., Kelly, J. P., et al. (2018). Exceeding the maximum daily dose of acetaminophen with use of different single-ingredient OTC formulations. *Journal of the American Pharmacists Association*, 58(5), 499–504.

Slattery, W. T., & Klegeris, A. (2018). Acetaminophen metabolites p-aminophenol and AM404 inhibit microglial activation. *Neuroimmunology and Neuroinflammation*, 5(4), 11.

**Spagrud, L. J., Piira, T., & Von Baeyer, C. L. (2003). Children's self-report of pain intensity. The faces pain scale—revised. *American Journal of Nursing*, 103(12), 62–64.

Topham, D., & Drew, D. (2017). Quality improvement project: Replacing the numeric rating scale with a clinically aligned pain assessment (CAPA) tool. *Pain Management Nursing*, 18(6), 363–371.

Treillet, E., Laurent, S., & Hadjiat, Y. (2018). Practical management of opioid rotation and equianalgesia. *Journal of Pain Research*, 11, 2587–2601.

U.S. Department of Health & Human Services (HSS). (2019, May). Pain Management Best Practices Inter-agency Task Force Report: Updates, gaps, inconsistencies and recommendations. Retrieved on 7/22/2019 at: www.hhs.gov/ash/advisory-committees/pain/reports/index.html

U.S. Food and Drug Administration (FDA). (2014). *Drug Information Update: FDA reminds health care professionals to stop dispensing prescription combination drug products with more than 325 mg of acetaminophen*. Retrieved on 11/26/2020 at: aapmr.org

U.S. Food and Drug Administration (FDA). (2017). Blueprint for prescriber education for extended-release and long-acting opioid analgesics. Retrieved on 7/22/2019 at: www.fmda.org/2017/Blueprint%20Opioid%20LA.ER%20REMS%20as%20of%201.20.2017.pdf

Valentine, A. R., Carvalho, B., Lazo T. A., et al. (2015). Scheduled acetaminophen with as-needed opioids compared to as-needed acetaminophen plus opioids for post-cesarean pain management. *International Journal of Obstetric Anesthesia*, 24(3), 210–216.

Varrassi, G., Hanna, M., Macheras, G., et al. (2017). Multimodal analgesia in moderate-to-severe pain: A role for a new fixed combination of dexketoprofen and tramadol. *Current Medical Research and Opinion*, 33(6), 1165–1173.

Wang, Y., Beekman, J., Hew, J., et al. (2018). Burn injury: Challenges and advances in burn wound healing, infection, pain and scarring. *Advanced Drug Delivery Reviews*, 123, 3–17.

**Weissman, D. E., & Haddox, J. D. (1989). Opioid pseudoaddiction—an iatrogenic syndrome. *Pain*, 36(3), 363–366.

Wick, E. C., Grant, M. C., & Wu, C. L. (2017). Postoperative multimodal analgesia pain management with nonopioid analgesics and techniques: A review. *JAMA Surgery*, 152(7), 691–697.

Yan, Y. Y., Li, C. Y., Zhou, L., et al. (2017). Research progress of mechanisms and medication therapy for neuropathic pain. *Life Sciences*, 190, 68–77.

Zhuo, M. (2017). Ionotropic glutamate receptors contribute to pain transmission and chronic pain. *Neuropharmacology*, 112, 228–234.

Resources

American Academy of Pain Medicine (AAPM), www.painmed.org

American Chronic Pain Association, www.theacpa.org

American Pain Foundation (APF), www.painfoundation.org

American Society for Pain Management Nursing (ASPMN), www.aspmn.org

City of Hope Pain & Palliative Care Resource Center, www.cityofhope.org/

National Center for Complementary and Integrative Health (NCCIH), www.nccih.nih.gov

Pain Treatment Topics, www.pain-topics.org

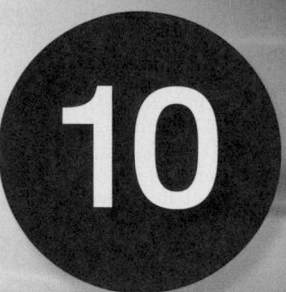

10 Fluid and Electrolytes

LEARNING OUTCOMES

On completion of this chapter, the learner will be able to:

1. Differentiate between osmosis, diffusion, filtration, and active transport.
2. Describe the role of the kidneys, lungs, and endocrine glands in regulating the body's fluid composition and volume.
3. Plan effective care of patients with the following imbalances: fluid volume deficit and fluid volume excess, sodium deficit (hyponatremia) and sodium excess (hypernatremia), and potassium deficit (hypokalemia) and potassium excess (hyperkalemia).
4. Describe the cause, clinical manifestations, management, and nursing interventions for the following imbalances: calcium deficit (hypocalcemia) and calcium excess (hypercalcemia), magnesium deficit (hypomagnesemia) and magnesium excess (hypermagnesemia), phosphorus deficit (hypophosphatemia) and phosphorus excess (hyperphosphatemia), and chloride deficit (hypochloremia) and chloride excess (hyperchloremia).
5. Explain the roles of the lungs, kidneys, and chemical buffers in maintaining acid–base balance; and compare metabolic as well as respiratory acidosis and alkalosis with regard to causes, clinical manifestations, diagnosis, and management.
6. Interpret arterial blood gas measurements.

NURSING CONCEPTS

Acid–Base
Cellullar Regulation

Fluids and Electrolytes
Metabolism

GLOSSARY

acidosis: an acid–base imbalance characterized by an increase in H⁺ concentration (decreased blood pH) (A low arterial pH due to increased H⁺ concentration or reduced bicarbonate concentration is called *metabolic acidosis;* a low arterial pH due to increased PCO₂ is called *respiratory acidosis.*)

active transport: physiologic pump that uses energy to move fluid or electrolytes from one region to another

alkalosis: an acid–base imbalance characterized by a reduction in H⁺ concentration or increase in bicarbonate concentration (increased blood pH) (A high arterial pH with either decreased H⁺ ion concentration or increased bicarbonate concentration is called *metabolic alkalosis;* a high arterial pH due to reduced PCO₂ is called *respiratory alkalosis.*)

colloid: a fluid containing particles that are nonsoluble and evenly distributed throughout the solution

colloid oncotic pressure: osmotic pressure created by the protein (mainly albumin) in the bloodstream (*synonym:* colloidal osmotic pressure)

crystalloid: a fluid containing soluble mineral ions and water in solution

diffusion: the process by which solutes move from an area of higher concentration to one of lower concentration; does not require expenditure of energy

homeostasis: maintenance of a constant internal equilibrium in a biologic system

hydrostatic pressure: the pressure created by the weight of fluid against the wall that contains it. In the body, hydrostatic pressure in blood vessels results from the weight of fluid itself and the force resulting from cardiac contraction (*synonym:* hydraulic pressure)

hypertonic solution: a solution with an osmolality higher than that of serum

hypotonic solution: a solution with an osmolality lower than that of serum

isotonic solution: a solution with the same osmolality as blood

osmolality: the number of milliosmoles (the standard unit of osmotic pressure) per kilogram of solvent; expressed as milliosmoles per kilogram (mOsm/kg).

(The term *osmolality* is used more often than *osmolarity* to evaluate serum and urine.)

osmolarity: the number of milliosmoles (the standard unit of osmotic pressure) per liter of solution; expressed as milliosmoles per liter (mOsm/L); describes the concentration of solutes or dissolved particles

osmosis: the process by which fluid moves across a semipermeable membrane from an area of low solute concentration to an area of high solute concentration; the process continues until the solute concentrations are equal on both sides of the membrane

tonicity: fluid tension or the effect that osmotic pressure of a solution with impermeable solutes exerts on cell size because of water movement across the cell membrane

Fluid and electrolyte balance are dependent on dynamic processes that are crucial for life and **homeostasis** (the maintenance of a constant internal equilibrium in a biologic system). Potential and actual disorders of fluid and electrolyte balance occur in every setting, with every disorder, and with a variety of changes that affect healthy people as well as those who are ill.

Nurses need to understand the physiology of fluid and electrolyte balance and acid–base balance to anticipate, identify, and respond to imbalances. Maintaining the balance of fluid and electrolytes is crucial to the care of patients of every age and in every clinical setting.

Fundamental Concepts

Basic concepts of chemistry are involved in fluid and electrolyte balance and imbalance. A solution is a mixture of solvent, which is a fluid medium, and solutes, which are particles. Blood is composed of blood cells that are suspended in plasma. The blood cells include erythrocytes, leukocytes, and platelets. Plasma is composed of 92% water, which is a solvent that contains solutes including proteins (mainly albumin), glucose, lipoproteins, and mineral ions, termed electrolytes.

Amount and Composition of Body Fluids

Approximately 60% of a typical adult's weight consists of fluid (water and electrolytes) (Fig. 10-1). Factors that influence the amount of body fluid are age, gender, and body fat. In general, younger people have a higher percentage of body fluid than older adults, and men have proportionately more body fluid than women. The skeleton has low water content. Muscle, skin, and blood contain the highest amounts of water (Norris, 2019).

Body fluid is located in two fluid compartments: the intracellular space (fluid in the cells) and the extracellular space (fluid outside the cells). Approximately two thirds of body fluid is in the intracellular fluid (ICF) compartment. Approximately one third is in the extracellular fluid (ECF) compartment (Norris, 2019).

The ECF compartment is further divided into the intravascular (blood), interstitial, and transcellular fluid spaces:

- The intravascular space (the fluid within the blood vessels) contains plasma, the effective circulating volume. Approximately 3 L of the average 6 L of blood volume in adults is made up of plasma. The remaining 3 L is made up of the blood cells: erythrocytes, leukocytes, and thrombocytes (platelets).
- The interstitial space contains the fluid that surrounds the cell and totals about 11 to 12 L in an adult. Lymph is an interstitial fluid.

- The transcellular space is the smallest division of the ECF compartment and contains approximately 1 L. Examples of transcellular fluids include cerebrospinal, pericardial, synovial, intraocular, and pleural fluids, sweat, and digestive secretions.

As the next section describes, the ECF transports electrolytes; it also carries other substances, such as enzymes and hormones.

Body fluid normally moves between the two major compartments (i.e., ICF and ECF) in an effort to maintain equilibrium between the spaces. A semipermeable membrane surrounding each of the cells allows certain fluids and electrolytes to move between the ICF and ECF. Loss of fluid from the ICF or ECF can disrupt equilibrium. The body constantly works to keep fluid and electrolytes in a homeostatic balance. If too much fluid moves from ICF to ECF, cellular dehydration can occur. If too much fluid moves from ECF to ICF, cell swelling can occur (Papadakis, McPhee, & Rabow, 2019).

Sometimes fluid is not lost from the body but is unavailable for use by either the ICF or ECF. Loss of ECF into a space that does not contribute to equilibrium between the ICF and the ECF is referred to as a third-space fluid shift, or third spacing. Third-space fluid accumulates within membrane-bound spaces in the body such as the peritoneal cavity and pleural space. Examples of third-spaced fluid include ascites, pleural effusion, pericardial effusion, and angioedema (Papadakis et al., 2019).

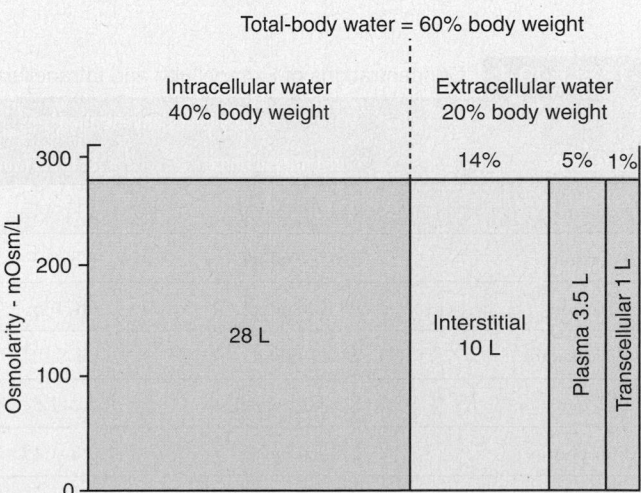

Figure 10-1 • Approximate sizes of body compartments in a 70-kg adult. Reprinted with permission from Norris, T. L. (2019). *Porth's pathophysiology: Concepts of altered health states* (10th ed., Fig. 8-4, p. 162). Philadelphia, PA: Wolters Kluwer.

Early evidence of a third-space fluid shift is a decrease in urine output despite adequate fluid intake. Urine output decreases because fluid shifts out of the intravascular space; the kidneys then receive less blood and attempt to compensate by decreasing urine output. Other signs and symptoms of third spacing that indicate an intravascular fluid volume deficit (FVD) include increased heart rate, decreased blood pressure, decreased central venous pressure, edema, increased body weight, and imbalances in fluid intake and output (I&O). Third-space fluid is reabsorbed back into the bloodstream over a period of a few days to a few weeks. However, the acute volume depletion must be restored to prevent further complications (Sterns, 2017a).

Electrolytes

Electrolytes in body fluids are active chemicals (cations that carry positive charges and anions that carry negative charges). The major cations in body fluid are sodium, potassium, calcium, magnesium, and hydrogen ions. The major anions are chloride, bicarbonate, phosphate, sulfate, and negatively charged protein ions.

These chemicals unite in varying combinations. Therefore, electrolyte concentration in the body is expressed in terms of milliequivalents (mEq) per liter, a measure of chemical activity, rather than in terms of milligrams (mg), and a unit of weight. More specifically, a milliequivalent is defined as being equivalent to the electrochemical activity of 1 mg of hydrogen. In a solution, cations and anions are equal in milliequivalents per liter.

Electrolyte concentrations in the ICF differ from those in the ECF, as reflected in Table 10-1. Because special techniques are required to measure electrolyte concentrations in the ICF, it is customary to measure the electrolytes in the most accessible portion of the ECF—namely, the plasma (Norris, 2019).

Sodium ions, which are positively charged, far outnumber the other cations in the ECF. Because sodium concentration affects the overall concentration of the ECF, sodium is important in regulating the volume of body fluid. Water follows movement of sodium in the body fluids. Retention of sodium

is associated with fluid retention, and excessive loss of sodium is usually associated with decreased volume of body fluid.

As shown in Table 10-1, one of the major electrolytes in the ICF is potassium. The ECF has a low concentration of potassium, and patients can tolerate only small changes in potassium concentration. Changes in potassium within the ECF can cause cardiac rhythm disturbances and hyperkalemia can cause cardiac arrest. Therefore, the release of large stores of intracellular potassium, typically caused by trauma to the cells and tissues, can be extremely dangerous.

The body expends a great deal of energy maintaining the high extracellular concentration of sodium and the high intracellular concentration of potassium. It does so by means of a cell membrane pump that exchanges sodium and potassium ions, termed the sodium–potassium pump (see discussion later in this chapter).

Osmosis, Osmolality, and Osmolarity

When two different solutions are separated by a membrane that is semi-permeable; fluid shifts from the region of less concentrated solution to a more concentrated solution, until the solutions are of equal concentration. This diffusion of water caused by fluid and solute concentration gradients is known as **osmosis** (Fig. 10-2). Osmolality and osmolarity are terms that describe the concentration of solutes or dissolved particles in a solution. **Osmolality** is the number of milliosmoles of solute (the standard unit of osmotic pressure) per kilogram of solvent; it is expressed as milliosmoles per kilogram (mOsm/kg). **Osmolarity** is the number of milliosmoles (the standard unit of osmotic pressure) per liter of solution; it is expressed as milliosmoles per liter (mOsm/L). The term *osmolality* is used more often than *osmolarity* to evaluate the solutes in the blood or urine (Emmett & Palmer, 2018a).

Regulation of Fluid within the Body Compartments

Normal movement of fluids through the capillary wall into the tissues depends on Starling's Laws of Capillary Forces. Capillary forces are the two forces at every capillary

TABLE 10-1	Concentrations of Extracellular and Intracellular Electrolytes in Adults			
	Extracellular Concentration[a]		**Intracellular Concentration**[a]	
Electrolyte	**Conventional Units**	**SI Units (mmol/L)**	**Conventional Units**	**SI Units (mmol/L)**
Sodium	135–145 mEq/L	135–145	10–14 mEq/L	10–14
Potassium	3.5–5.0 mEq/L	3.5–5.0	140–150 mEq/L	140–150
Chloride	98–106 mEq/L	98–106	3–4 mEq/L	3–4
Bicarbonate	24–31 mEq/L	24–31	7–10 mEq/L	7–10
Calcium	8.8–10.5 mg/dL	2.2–2.6	<1 mEq/L	<0.25
Phosphorus	2.5–4.5 mg/dL	0.8–1.45	Variable	Variable
Magnesium	1.8–3.6 mg/dL	0.75–1.07	40 mEq/kg[b]	20

[a]Values may vary among laboratories, depending on the method of analysis used.
[b]Values vary among various tissues and with nutritional status.
Reprinted with permission from Norris, T. L. (2019). *Porth's pathophysiology: Concepts of altered health states* (10th ed.). Philadelphia, PA: Wolters Kluwer.

OSMOSIS

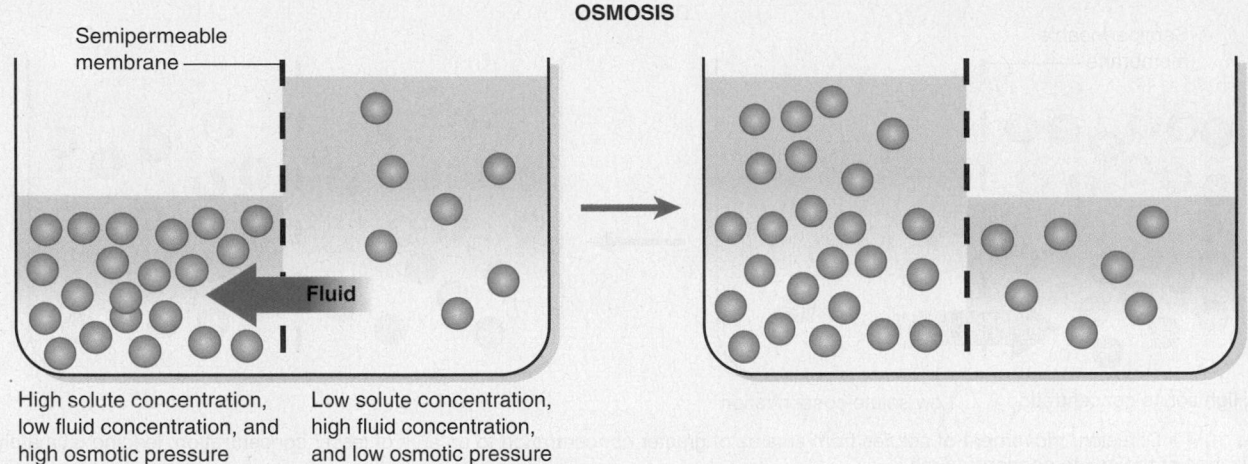

High solute concentration, low fluid concentration, and high osmotic pressure

Low solute concentration, high fluid concentration, and low osmotic pressure

Figure 10-2 • Osmosis: when two different solutions are separated by a semi-permeable fluid shifts from the region of less concentrated solution to a more concentrated solution, until the solutions are of equal concentration.

membrane: hydrostatic pressure (also called hydraulic pressure) and osmotic pressure. **Hydrostatic pressure** is the pressure exerted by fluid on the walls of the blood vessel, and osmotic pressure is the pressure exerted by the solutes within the plasma. Hydrostatic pressure pushes fluid out of the capillary toward the ICF. Osmotic pressure pulls fluid into the capillary from the ICF. These forces oppose each other at every capillary membrane and balance each other out in healthy (homeostatic) conditions. The direction of fluid movement depends on the differences in the two opposing forces of hydrostatic and osmotic pressure (Fig. 10-3). If hydrostatic pressure is greater than osmotic pressure, then the movement of fluid is from ECF toward the ICF.

Oncotic Pressure

Osmotic pressure specifically exerted by the albumin within the bloodstream is termed **colloid oncotic pressure** or **colloid osmotic pressure**. A **colloid** is fluid consisting of nonsoluble substances that are evenly distributed within a solvent. Blood is an example of a colloid solution. It is a mixture of blood cells and plasma which contains water, proteins, enzymes, and other solutes.

Crystalloid versus Colloid Solutions

Fluid replacement in the body depends on what type of fluid is lost. If a large amount of blood is lost, for example,

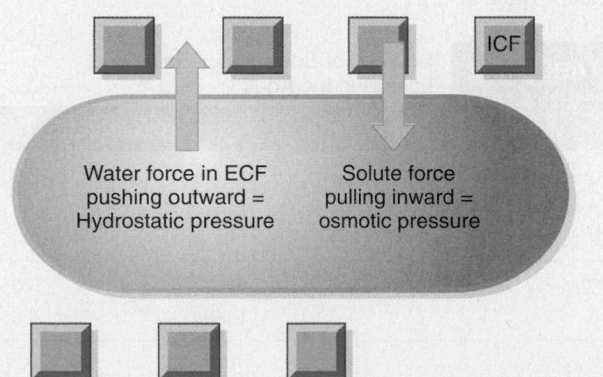

Water force in ECF pushing outward = Hydrostatic pressure

Solute force pulling inward = osmotic pressure

ICF

Figure 10-3 • The forces of osmotic and hydrostatic pressure constantly oppose each other. ECF, extracellular fluid; ICF, intracellular fluid.

the preferred treatment is replacement with matching blood (commonly packed red blood cells). However, crystalloid or colloid solutions can be used to temporarily replace blood or replenish fluid losses from the body. **Crystalloid** solutions are mineral ions dissolved in water. Examples include normal saline (0.9% NaCl), half normal saline (0.45% NaCl), and lactated Ringer's solution (Plasma-Lyte). Crystalloid solutions are commonly used to replace fluid in hypovolemia. Examples of colloid solutions include albumin solutions, hyperoncotic starch, and dextran. Colloid solutions are commonly used as temporary blood replacement until the correct type of blood is available for infusion (Mandel & Palevsky, 2019).

Tonicity

Tonicity is the ability of solutes to cause an osmotic driving force that promotes water movement from one compartment to another. Movement of water is either from ICF to ECF or ECF to ICF. The tonicity of a solution can be used to drive water movement between compartments to change the state of cellular hydration and cell size. Tonicity most commonly refers to the NaCl content of the solution. The tonicity of a solution is determined by how it compares to physiologic fluid which is 0.9% NaCl (Sterns, 2017b). Fluids can be isotonic, hypotonic, or hypertonic compared to physiologic fluid of 0.9% NaCl.

Tonicity commonly pertains to intravenous (IV) solutions. IV solutions of different tonicities can be infused into the bloodstream to produce movement of water from one compartment to the other.

Isotonic solutions are composed of 0.9% NaCl; the same sodium and chloride concentration as the bloodstream and the same water concentration as the bloodstream. Isotonic solutions do not provoke water movement between ICF or ECF compartments. Isotonic solutions expand the plasma volume of the blood (Sterns, 2017b).

Hypotonic solutions are composed of less sodium chloride concentration compared to the blood; for example, 0.45% NaCl or 0.225% NaCl. Hypotonic solutions contain less solute but more water than the bloodstream. IV hypotonic solution infusions can be used to move water from the ECF into the ICF. IV hypotonic solutions can be used to hydrate a patient as they contain high water concentration (Sterns, 2017b).

DIFFUSION

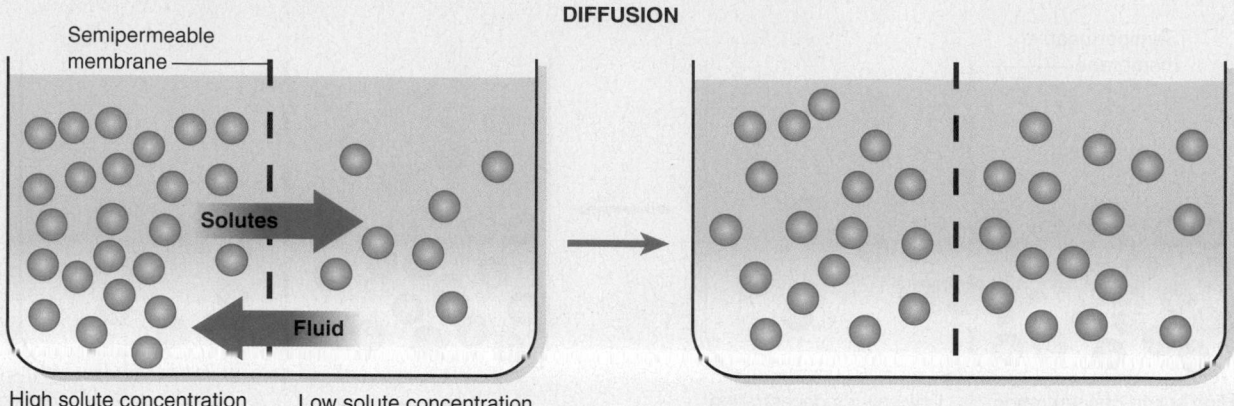

Figure 10-4 • Diffusion: movement of solutes from an area of greater concentration to an area of lesser concentration, leading ultimately to equalization of the solute concentrations.

Hypertonic solutions are composed of greater concentration of NaCl compared to blood (e.g., 3% NaCl). Hypertonic solutions contain more solute concentration and less water than the bloodstream. IV hypertonic solution can be infused into the bloodstream to pull water from the ICF into the ECF. The movement of water from ICF to ECF will cause dehydration of the cells. This is useful in disorders of severe edema; particularly cerebral edema, which requires immediate treatment. Sodium, glucose, and mannitol are examples of solutes capable of affecting water movement from ICF to ECF. Mannitol, a nonresorbable sugar alcohol, in water is an IV solution that can be used to move water from ICF to ECF rapidly. IV mannitol can induce a condition termed osmotic diuresis; it is most commonly used to decrease cerebral edema (Brater & Ellison, 2019). (See discussion of parenteral therapy later in this chapter.)

Osmotic diuresis is the increase in urine output caused by the excretion of solutes, such as glucose or mannitol. In high concentrations, glucose or mannitol can act as solutes within the bloodstream. These solutes exert a force that pulls water out of the ICF and brings it into the ECF (bloodstream). The water then is filtered out of the bloodstream at the kidneys and excreted into the urine. The urine contains extra water that is derived from the ICF; this increased urine volume is called diuresis (Brater & Ellison, 2019).

Diffusion

Diffusion is the natural tendency of a substance to move from an area of higher concentration to one of lower concentration (Fig. 10-4). It occurs through the random movement of ions and molecules. Examples of diffusion are the exchange of oxygen (O_2) and carbon dioxide (CO_2) between the pulmonary capillaries and alveoli and the tendency of sodium to move from the ECF compartment, where the sodium concentration is high, to the ICF, where its concentration is low (Hall, 2016).

Filtration

Hydrostatic pressure in the capillaries tends to filter fluid out of the intravascular compartment into the interstitial fluid. Movement of water and solutes occurs from an area of high hydrostatic pressure to an area of low hydrostatic pressure. The kidneys filter approximately 180 L of plasma per day. Another example of filtration is the passage of water and electrolytes from the capillary bed to the interstitial fluid; in this instance, the hydrostatic pressure results from the pumping action of the heart (Hall, 2016).

Sodium–Potassium Pump

The sodium concentration is greater in the ECF than in the ICF; because of this, sodium tends to enter the cell by diffusion. To maintain cellular function, more potassium needs to be inside the cell and more sodium needs to be outside the cell. The sodium–potassium pump maintains the electrolyte gradient of high extracellular Na^+ compared to low intracellular Na^+, and high intracellular K^+ compared to low extracellular K^+. The pump maintains the different concentrations of cations Na^+ and K^+ in and out of the cell. For every 3 Na^+ pumped out of the cell, 2 K^+ ions are pumped into the cell (Pirahanchi & Aeddula, 2019).

The sodium–potassium pump uses energy to maintain this electrolyte gradient and is powered by the enzyme termed Na^+K^+-ATPase. The sodium–potassium pump performs **active transport** which actively moves sodium from the ICF into the ECF and actively moves potassium from the ECF to the ICF. Active transport is the use of energy to create movement against a concentration gradient (Hall, 2016; Norris, 2019).

Systemic Routes of Gains and Losses

Water and electrolytes are gained in various ways. Healthy people gain fluids by drinking and eating, and their daily average intake and output (I & O) of water are approximately equal (Table 10-2).

TABLE 10-2	Sources of Body Water Gains and Losses in the Adult		
Intake (mL)		**Output (mL)**	
Oral intake		Urine	1500
As water	1000	Insensible losses	
In food	1300	Lungs	300
Water of oxidation	200	Skin	500
		Feces	200
Total gain[a]	2500	Total loss[a]	2500

[a]Approximate volumes.
Adapted from Norris, T. L. (2019). *Porth's pathophysiology: Concepts of altered health state* (10th ed.). Philadelphia, PA: Wolters Kluwer.

Kidneys

The daily urine volume excreted by the adult varies according to hydration status. A well-hydrated person excretes 1 to 2 L urine per day. A general rule is that the output is approximately 1 mL of urine per kilogram of body weight per hour (1 mL/kg/h) in all age groups (Sterns, 2017a). For example, a 70-kg adult will excrete 70 mL/h; over 24 hours this equals approximately 1680 mL of urine.

Skin

Perspiration is visible water and electrolyte loss through the skin (sweating). The chief solutes in sweat are sodium, chloride, and potassium. Actual sweat losses can vary from 0 to 1000 mL or more every hour, depending on factors such as the environmental and body temperature. Continuous water loss by evaporation through the skin (approximately 500 mL/day) occurs through perspiration, referred to as insensible water loss (Norris, 2019). Fever, high environmental temperature, and exercise greatly increase insensible water loss through the skin. Burn injury, which causes the loss of the natural skin barrier, also causes a large water loss (Sterns, 2017b).

Lungs

The lungs normally eliminate water vapor, also referred to as insensible water loss, at a rate of approximately 300 mL daily (Norris, 2019). The loss is much greater with increased respiratory rate or depth, or in a dry climate. Similar to water loss through the skin, fever, high environmental temperature, and exercise all increase insensible water loss through the lungs.

Gastrointestinal Tract

Loss of fluid from the gastrointestinal (GI) tract is about 100 to 200 mL daily. Approximately 8 L of fluid circulates through the GI system every 24 hours. However, most of the fluid is reabsorbed into the bloodstream from the small intestine.

Diarrhea and fistulas of the intestine can cause large losses of fluids (Sterns, 2018a).

 Quality and Safety Nursing Alert

When fluid balance is critical, all routes of systemic gain and loss must be recorded and all volumes compared. Organs of fluid loss include the kidneys, skin, lungs, and GI tract.

Laboratory Tests for Evaluating Fluid Status

Serum osmolality primarily reflects the concentration of sodium, although blood urea nitrogen (BUN) and glucose also play a major role in determining serum osmolality. Urine osmolality is determined by urea, creatinine, and uric acid. When measured with serum osmolality, urine osmolality is the most reliable indicator of urine concentration. In healthy adults, normal serum osmolality is 275 to 290 mOsm/kg (Emmett & Palmer, 2018a). The value of osmolarity is usually within 10 mOsm of the value of osmolality (Emmett & Palmer, 2018a). Factors that increase and decrease serum and urine osmolality are identified in Table 10-3. Serum osmolality may be measured directly through laboratory tests or estimated at the bedside by doubling the serum sodium level or by using the following formula:

$$Na^+ \times 2 = \frac{Glucose}{18} + \frac{BUN}{3} = \text{Approximate value of serum osmolality}$$

Urine specific gravity measures the density of urine compared to water. It is a measure of the concentration of solutes in the urine. It is one way to assess the kidneys' ability to excrete or conserve water. The specific gravity of urine is compared to that of distilled water, which has a specific gravity of 1.000. The normal range of urine specific gravity is 1.005 to 1.030 (Van Leeuwen & Bladh, 2017). Urine with a specific gravity of 1.005 is very dilute or high in water

TABLE 10-3	Factors Affecting Serum and Urine Osmolality	
Fluid	**Factors Increasing Osmolality**	**Factors Decreasing Osmolality**
Serum (275–290 mOsm/kg water)	Severe dehydration Free water loss Diabetes insipidus Hypernatremia Hyperglycemia Stroke or head injury Acute tubular necrosis Consumption of methanol or ethylene glycol (antifreeze) High ion gap metabolic acidosis Mannitol therapy Advanced liver disease Alcoholism Burns	Fluid volume excess Syndrome of inappropriate antidiuretic hormone (SIADH) Acute kidney injury Diuretic use Adrenal insufficiency Hyponatremia Overhydration Paraneoplastic syndrome associated with lung cancer
Urine (200–800 mOsm/kg water)	Fluid volume deficit SIADH Congestive heart failure Acidosis Prerenal kidney injury	Fluid volume excess Diabetes insipidus Hyponatremia Aldosteronism Pyelonephritis Acute tubular necrosis

Adapted from Norris, T. L. (2019). *Porth's pathophysiology: Concepts of altered health states* (10th ed.). Philadelphia, PA: Wolters Kluwer.

content, whereas urine with a specific gravity of 1.030 is very concentrated or low in water content. Under normal conditions, a well-hydrated person excretes urine with a low specific gravity, whereas a dehydrated person excretes urine with high specific gravity. Urine specific gravity can be measured by sending approximately 20 mL of urine to the laboratory for urinalysis testing or assessed using a urine dipstick test. Specific gravity is a less reliable indicator of urine concentration than urine osmolality; increased glucose or protein in urine can cause a falsely elevated specific gravity. Factors that increase or decrease urine osmolality are the same as those for urine specific gravity (Sterns, 2017a).

BUN is a laboratory value that measures the amount of urea in the bloodstream. The normal range of BUN is 10 to 20 mg/dL (3.6 to 7.2 mmol/L). BUN level can vary with renal function, amount of cellular breakdown, protein intake, and hydration status. If urine output decreases, as occurs in renal dysfunction, then urea is not excreted and accumulates in the bloodstream causing an increase. Increased BUN can also occur if water content in the bloodstream decreases due to dehydration. If a person is consuming a high protein diet, there is an increased amino acid content in the bloodstream, which in turn increases nitrogen content of the blood, thereby increasing BUN (Inker & Perrone, 2018).

Additional factors that increase BUN include GI bleeding, fever, and sepsis. Factors that decrease BUN include end-stage liver disease, a low protein diet, starvation (due to low protein), and any condition that results in expanded fluid volume which dilutes urea in the blood (e.g., pregnancy). Because of all these variables, BUN is not an optimal gauge of kidney function (Inker & Perrone, 2018).

Creatinine is a breakdown product of muscle metabolism that is almost totally cleared from the bloodstream and excreted by the kidney. It is a better indicator of renal function than BUN because it does not vary with protein intake or hydration status. The normal serum creatinine is approximately 0.7 to 1.4 mg/dL (62 to 124 mmol/L); however, its concentration depends on lean body mass and varies from person to person. Serum creatinine levels increase when renal function decreases in most people and is an accurate gauge of kidney function (Norris, 2019).

Hematocrit measures the percentage of red blood cells (RBCs) (erythrocytes) in a volume of whole blood and normally ranges from 42% to 52% in men and 35% to 47% in women. Conditions that increase the hematocrit value are dehydration and polycythemia. Dehydration causes decreased water content of the blood which concentrates the RBCs in the bloodstream. Polycythemia is a disorder in which there is an abnormally high number of RBCs made by the bone marrow, which in turn increases the number of RBCs in the bloodstream. Conversely, over hydration (which increases the volume of water within the bloodstream) will decrease the hematocrit. Anemia (which is a lack of sufficient production of RBCs by the bone marrow) causes decreased hematocrit (Schrier, 2018).

Urine sodium values change with sodium intake and the status of fluid volume: As sodium intake increases, excretion increases; as the circulating fluid volume decreases, sodium is conserved. Normal urine sodium levels range from 75 to 200 mEq/24 h (75 to 200 mmol/24 h). A random specimen usually contains more than 40 mEq/L of sodium. Urine sodium levels are used to assess volume status and are useful in the diagnosis of hyponatremia and acute kidney injury (Sterns, 2017a).

Homeostatic Mechanisms

The body is equipped with remarkable homeostatic mechanisms to keep the composition and volume of body fluid within narrow limits of normal. Organs involved in homeostasis include the kidneys, heart, lungs, pituitary gland, adrenal glands, and parathyroid glands (Norris, 2019).

Kidney Functions

Vital to the regulation of fluid and electrolyte balance, the kidneys normally filter 180 L of plasma every day in the adult and excrete 1 to 2 L of urine (Inker & Perrone, 2018). They act both autonomously and in response to hormones, such as aldosterone and antidiuretic hormone (ADH) (Norris, 2019). Major functions of the kidneys in maintaining normal fluid balance include the following:

- Regulation of ECF volume and osmolality by selective retention and excretion of body fluids
- Regulation of normal electrolyte levels in the ECF by selective electrolyte retention and excretion of hydrogen ions
- Regulation of pH of the ECF by retention and excretion of hydrogen ions
- Excretion of metabolic wastes and toxic substances (Inker & Perrone, 2018)

Given these functions, failure of the kidneys results in multiple fluid and electrolyte abnormalities.

Heart and Blood Vessel Functions

The pumping action of the heart circulates blood through the kidneys under sufficient pressure to allow for urine formation. Failure of this pumping action interferes with renal perfusion and thus with water and electrolyte regulation.

Lung Functions

The lungs are also vital in maintaining homeostasis. Through exhalation, the lungs remove approximately 300 mL of water daily in the normal adult as insensible water loss (Sterns, 2017a). Abnormal conditions, such as hyperventilation (abnormally deep respiration) or continuous coughing, increase this water loss. The lungs also play a major role in acid–base balance. Because the lungs regulate carbon dioxide (CO_2), which directly influences acid content of the bloodstream, they influence acid–base balance. When the lungs have a decrease in breathing rate, CO_2 is retained in the alveoli and bloodstream, which increases acid content of the blood. When the lungs have an increase in breathing rate, CO_2 is blown off, lost from the bloodstream, which decreases acid content of the blood (Norris, 2019).

Pituitary Functions

The hypothalamus manufactures ADH, which is stored in the posterior pituitary gland and released as needed to conserve water. ADH is secreted by the pituitary gland in reaction to dehydration or blood loss and acts at the nephrons. At the collecting duct of the nephron, ADH causes increased reabsorption of water from the tubules into the bloodstream (Norris, 2019). This increases the water content of the bloodstream (Fig. 10-5).

Physiology/Pathophysiology

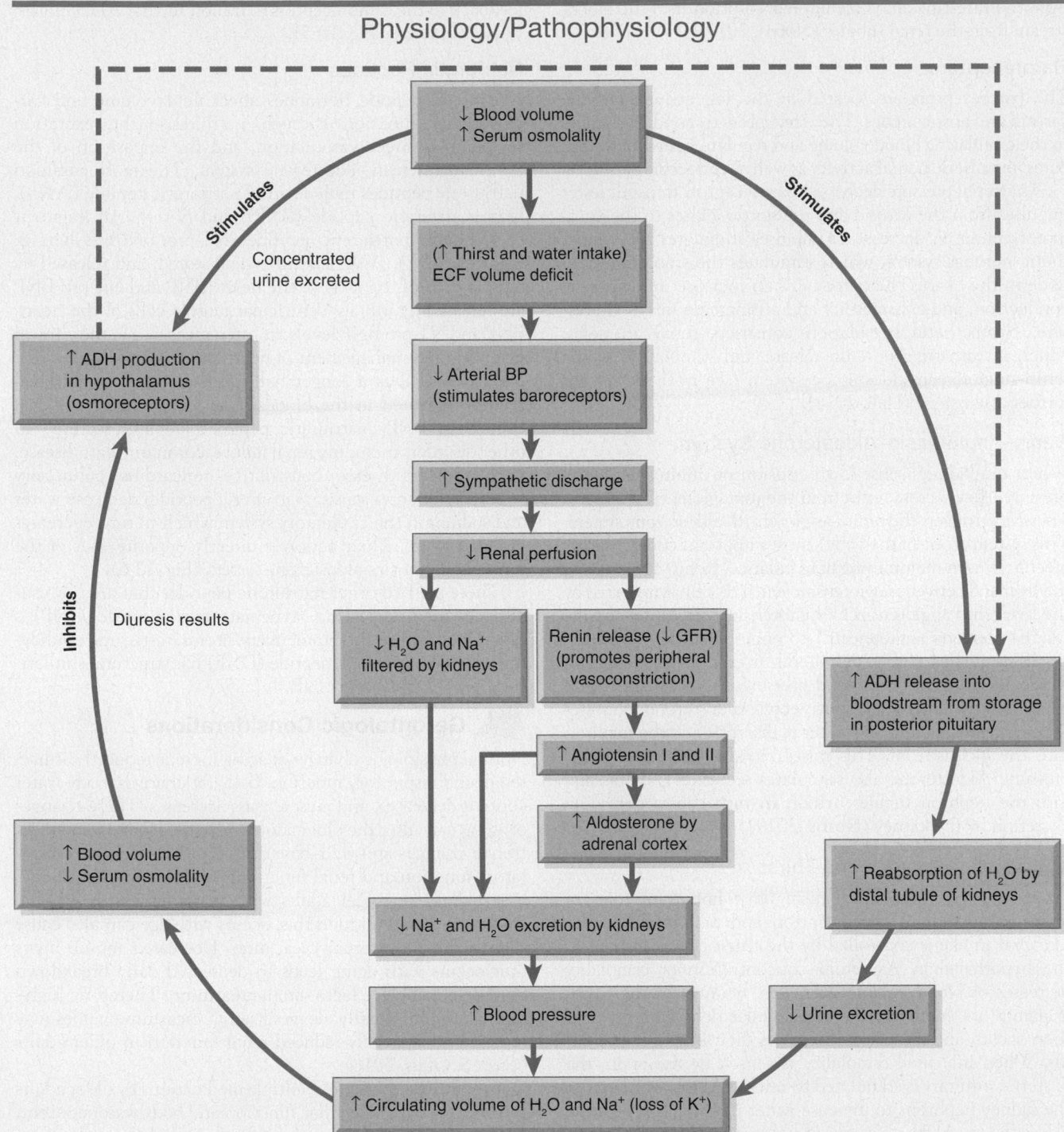

Figure 10-5 • Fluid regulation cycle. ADH, antidiuretic hormone; BP, blood pressure; ECF, extracellular fluid; GFR, glomerular filtration rate.

Adrenal Functions

Aldosterone, a mineralocorticoid secreted by the zona glomerulosa (outer zone) of the adrenal cortex, has a profound effect on fluid balance. Increased secretion of aldosterone causes sodium retention (and thus water retention) and potassium loss. Conversely, decreased secretion of aldosterone causes sodium and water loss and potassium retention.

Cortisol, another adrenocortical hormone, has less mineralocorticoid action. However, when secreted in large quantities (or administered as corticosteroid therapy), it can also produce sodium and fluid retention (Norris, 2019).

Parathyroid Functions

The parathyroid glands, embedded in the thyroid gland, regulate calcium and phosphate balance by means of parathyroid hormone (PTH). PTH influences reabsorption of calcium from the bones into the bloodstream, calcium absorption from the intestine, and calcium reabsorption into the bloodstream from the renal tubules (Norris, 2019).

Baroreceptors

The baroreceptors are located in the left atrium and the carotid and aortic arches. These receptors respond to changes in the circulating blood volume and regulate sympathetic and parasympathetic neural activity as well as endocrine activities.

As arterial pressure decreases, baroreceptors transmit fewer impulses from the carotid and the aortic arches to the vasomotor center. A decrease in impulses stimulates the sympathetic nervous system, which stimulates the sinoatrial (SA) node in the heart. The outcome is an increase in heart rate, conduction, and contractility and an increase in blood pressure. Sympathetic stimulation constricts renal arterioles, which in turn triggers renin release and stimulation of the renin–angiotensin–aldosterone system (see next section for further discussion) (Hall, 2016).

Renin–Angiotensin–Aldosterone System

When the kidneys sense low perfusion or diminished blood pressure, they secrete renin from the juxtaglomerular apparatus, which triggers the renin–angiotensin–aldosterone system. This system is one of the body's most important compensatory mechanisms in maintaining fluid balance. Renin circulates to the liver and converts angiotensinogen, a protein synthesized by the liver, into angiotensin I. Angiotensin-converting enzyme (ACE) converts angiotensin I to angiotensin II. Angiotensin II stimulates potent peripheral arterial vasoconstriction which increases arterial blood pressure. Angiotensin II also stimulates the adrenal gland to secrete aldosterone. Aldosterone increases sodium and water reabsorption at the nephron into the bloodstream. This raises blood volume and blood pressure. Aldosterone also stimulates secretion of potassium into the nephron tubules, which in turn causes potassium excretion by the kidney (Norris, 2019).

Antidiuretic Hormone and Thirst

ADH and the thirst mechanism have important roles in maintaining sodium concentration and oral intake of fluids. Oral intake is controlled by the thirst center located in the hypothalamus. As serum concentration or osmolality increases or blood volume decreases, neurons in the hypothalamus are stimulated by intracellular dehydration; thirst then occurs, and the person increases their intake of oral fluids. When increased osmolality is sensed by the brain, the posterior pituitary is stimulated to release ADH. ADH acts at the kidney nephrons to increase water reabsorption into the bloodstream. ADH raises blood volume and decreases urine output (Hall, 2016; Norris, 2019).

Osmoreceptors

Located on the surface of the hypothalamus, osmoreceptors sense changes in sodium concentration. As osmotic pressure increases, the neurons become dehydrated and quickly release impulses to the posterior pituitary, which increases the release of ADH, which then travels in the blood to the kidneys, where it alters permeability to water, causing increased reabsorption of water and decreased urine output. The retained water dilutes the ECF and returns its concentration to normal. Restoration of normal osmotic pressure provides

feedback to the osmoreceptors to inhibit further ADH release (Hall, 2016) (see Fig. 10-5).

Natriuretic Peptides

Natriuretic peptide hormones affect fluid volume and cardiovascular function through natriuresis (the excretion of sodium), direct vasodilation, and the opposition of the renin–angiotensin–aldosterone system. The most common natriuretic peptides include atrial natriuretic peptide (ANP), brain natriuretic peptide (BNP), and N-terminal fragment of pro-brain natriuretic peptide (NT-pro BNP) (Chen & Colucci, 2017). ANP is synthesized, stored, and released by muscle cells of the atria of the heart. BNP and NT-pro BNP are released mainly by ventricular muscle cells of the heart. BNP and NT-pro BNP levels are often measured in the clinical diagnosis and management of heart failure (see Chapter 25). NT-pro BNP has a longer half-life than BNP, so its level remains elevated in the bloodstream for a longer period of time than BNP. Natriuretic peptides are also secreted in other disorders including renal failure, coronary heart disease, valvular heart disease, constrictive pericarditis, pulmonary hypertension, and sepsis. Natriuretic peptides decrease water and sodium in the circulatory system which in turn decreases blood pressure. Their action is directly opposite that of the renin–angiotensin–aldosterone system (Fig. 10-6).

There are two other natriuretic peptides that are not usually measured clinically. C-type natriuretic peptide (CNP) is distributed within the brain, ovary, uterus, testis, and epididymis. D-type natriuretic peptide (DNP) has structural similarities to ANP, BNP, and CNP.

Gerontologic Considerations

Normal physiologic changes of aging include reduced cardiac, renal, and respiratory function. Body fat changes, body water content decreases, and muscle mass decreases. These changes of aging may alter the older adult's responses to fluid and electrolyte changes and acid–base disturbances. Decreased respiratory function and renal function can cause impaired acid–base balance in older adults with major illness or trauma. Decreased renal function that occurs with age can also cause slightly elevated serum creatinine. Decreased muscle mass that occurs with aging leads to decreased daily breakdown of muscle, which reduces serum creatinine. Therefore, high-normal and minimally elevated serum creatinine values may indicate substantially reduced renal function in older adults (Cash & Glass, 2018).

In addition, the use of multiple medications by older adults can affect renal and cardiac function and body water content, thereby increasing susceptibility to fluid and electrolyte disturbances. Routine procedures, such as the vigorous administration of laxatives or enemas before colon x-ray studies, may produce a serious FVD, necessitating the use of IV fluids to prevent hypotension and other effects of hypovolemia.

Alterations in fluid and electrolyte balance that may produce minor changes in young and middle-aged adults may produce profound changes in older adults. In many older patients, the clinical manifestations of fluid and electrolyte disturbances may be subtle or atypical. For example, fluid deficit may not trigger thirst sensation and can lead to delirium in the older adult (see Chapter 8). Rapid infusion of an excessive volume of IV fluids can cause fluid overload and cardiac

Physiology/Pathophysiology

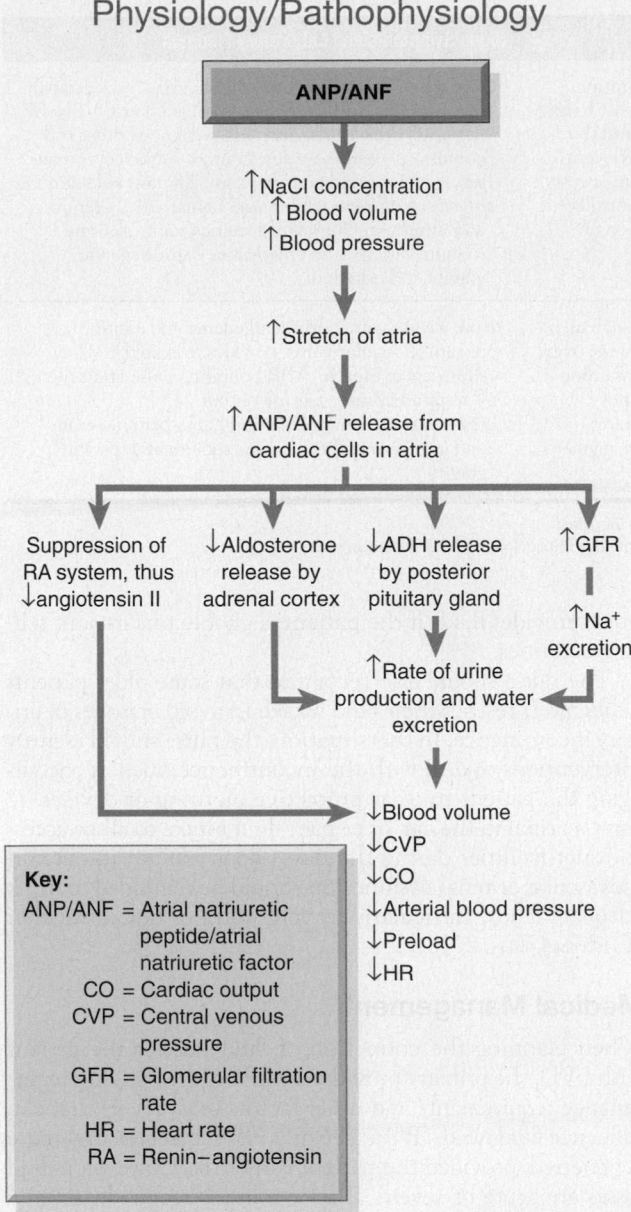

Figure 10-6 • Role of atrial natriuretic peptide in maintenance of fluid balance.

failure in older patients. These reactions are likely to occur more quickly and with the administration of smaller volumes of fluid than in healthy young and middle-aged adults because of the decreased cardiac reserve and reduced renal function that accompany aging (Cash & Glass, 2018).

Dehydration is the rapid loss of body weight due to the loss of either water or sodium. This results in an elevated sodium concentration (Sterns, 2017c). Dehydration in older adults is common because of decreased kidney mass, decreased glomerular filtration rate, decreased renal blood flow, decreased ability to concentrate urine, inability to conserve sodium, decreased excretion of potassium, and a decrease of total-body water. Loss of subcutaneous tissue and resultant thinning of the skin occurs with aging; the dermis is dehydrated and loses strength and elasticity.

FLUID VOLUME DISTURBANCES

Hypovolemia

FVD, or hypovolemia, occurs when loss of ECF volume exceeds the intake of fluid. It occurs when water and electrolytes are lost in the same proportion as they exist in normal body fluids; thus, the ratio of serum electrolytes to water remains the same. FVD should not be confused with dehydration, which refers to loss of water alone, with increased serum sodium levels. FVD may occur alone or in combination with other imbalances. Serum electrolyte concentrations can remain normal, increase, or increase in FVD (Sterns, 2017a).

Pathophysiology

FVD results from loss of body fluids and occurs more rapidly when coupled with decreased fluid intake. FVD can also develop with a prolonged period of inadequate intake. Causes of FVD include abnormal fluid losses, such as those resulting from vomiting, diarrhea, GI suctioning, and sweating; decreased intake, as in nausea or lack of access to fluids; and third-space fluid shifts, or the movement of fluid from the vascular system to other body spaces (e.g., with edema formation in burns, ascites with liver dysfunction). Additional causes include diabetes insipidus (a decreased ability to concentrate urine due to either a deficit of ADH or nephron resistance to ADH), adrenal insufficiency, osmotic diuresis, hemorrhage, and coma (Sterns, 2017a).

Clinical Manifestations

FVD can develop rapidly, and its severity depends on the degree of fluid loss. Clinical signs and symptoms and laboratory findings are presented in Table 10-4.

Assessment and Diagnostic Findings

Laboratory data used to evaluate fluid volume status include BUN and its relation to serum creatinine concentration. Normal BUN to serum creatinine concentration ratio is 10:1. A volume-depleted patient has a BUN elevated out of proportion to the serum creatinine (ratio greater than 20:1) because urea becomes concentrated in FVD (Sterns, 2017a).

The presence and cause of hypovolemia may be determined through the health history and physical examination. In addition, the hematocrit level is greater than normal because there is a decreased plasma volume, which concentrates the volume of RBCs.

Serum electrolyte changes may also exist. Potassium and sodium levels can be reduced (hypokalemia, hyponatremia) or elevated (hyperkalemia, hypernatremia).

- Hypokalemia can occur with GI and renal losses as these organs are major regulators of potassium.
- Hyperkalemia can occur with adrenal insufficiency due to aldosterone deficiency which causes lack of potassium excretion.
- Hyponatremia can occur with increased thirst and ADH release, which increases water content of the bloodstream.
- Hypernatremia can result from increased insensible water losses and diabetes insipidus.

TABLE 10-4 Fluid Volume Disturbances

Imbalance	Contributing Factors	Signs/Symptoms and Laboratory Findings
Fluid volume deficit (hypovolemia)	Loss of water and electrolytes, as in vomiting, diarrhea, fistulas, fever, excess sweating, burns, blood loss, gastrointestinal suction, and third-space fluid shifts; and decreased intake, as in anorexia, nausea, and inability to gain access to fluid. Diabetes insipidus and uncontrolled diabetes both contribute to a depletion of extracellular fluid volume.	Acute weight loss, ↓ skin turgor, oliguria, concentrated urine, capillary filling time prolonged, low CVP, ↓ BP, flattened neck veins, dizziness, weakness, thirst and confusion, ↑ pulse, muscle cramps, sunken eyes, nausea, increased temperature; cool, clammy, pale skin *Labs indicate:* ↑ hemoglobin and hematocrit, ↑ serum and urine osmolality and specific gravity, ↓ urine sodium, ↑ BUN and creatinine, ↑ urine specific gravity and osmolality
Fluid volume excess (hypervolemia)	Compromised regulatory mechanisms, such as kidney injury, heart failure, and cirrhosis; over-zealous administration of sodium-containing fluids; and fluid shifts (i.e., treatment of burns). Prolonged corticosteroid therapy, severe stress, and hyperaldosteronism augment fluid volume excess.	Acute weight gain, peripheral edema and ascites, distended jugular veins, crackles, elevated CVP, shortness of breath, ↑ BP, bounding pulse and cough ↑ respiratory rate, ↑ urine output *Labs indicate:* ↓ hemoglobin and hematocrit, ↓ serum and urine osmolality, ↓ urine sodium and specific gravity

BP, blood pressure; BUN, blood urea nitrogen; CVP, central venous pressure; ↓, decreased; ↑, increased.
Adapted from Norris, T. L. (2019). *Porth's pathophysiology: Concepts of altered health states* (10th ed.). Philadelphia, PA: Wolters Kluwer.

Oliguria, the excretion of less than 400 mL urine per day in the adult, may or may not be present in hypovolemia. Urine specific gravity will change in relation to the kidneys' attempt to conserve water. If the kidney does not reabsorb water, urine contains more water, and urine specific gravity is low. If the kidney does reabsorb water, urine will be concentrated and specific gravity increases. Due to lack of ADH in diabetes insipidus, urine water content increases, which decreases urine specific gravity. Aldosterone is secreted when fluid volume is low, causing reabsorption of sodium and chloride and resulting in decreased urinary sodium and chloride. When the kidneys conserve water, urine osmolality can increase to greater than 450 mOsm/kg and urine specific gravity increases (Sterns, 2017a). Normal values for laboratory data are listed in Appendix A on thePoint.

 Gerontologic Considerations

Increased sensitivity to fluid and electrolyte changes in older patients requires careful physical assessment, measurement of I&O of fluids from all sources, assessment of daily weight, careful monitoring of side effects and interactions of medications, and prompt reporting and management of disturbances. In most adult patients, it is useful to monitor skin turgor to detect subtle changes. However, assessment of skin turgor is not as valid in older adults because the skin has lost elasticity; therefore, other assessment measures (e.g., slowness in filling of veins of the hands and feet) become more useful in detecting FVD (Cash & Glass, 2018; Weber & Kelley, 2018).

The nurse also performs a functional assessment of the older patient's ability to determine fluid and food needs and to obtain adequate intake in addition to assessments discussed earlier in this chapter. For example, the nurse assesses whether or not the patient is cognitively intact, able to ambulate and to use both arms and hands to reach fluids and foods, and able to swallow with an intact gag reflex. Results of this functional assessment have a direct bearing on how the patient will be able to meet their own need for fluids and foods (Weber & Kelley, 2018). During an older patient's hospital stay, the nurse provides fluids if the patient is unable to carry out self-care activities.

The nurse should also recognize that some older patients deliberately restrict their fluid intake to avoid episodes of urinary incontinence. In this situation, the nurse should identify interventions to deal with the incontinence, such as encouraging the patient to wear protective clothing or devices, to carry a urinal in the car, or to pace fluid intake to allow access to toilet facilities during the day. Older adults without cardiovascular or renal dysfunction should be reminded to drink adequate fluids, particularly in very warm or humid weather (Cash & Glass, 2018).

Medical Management

When planning the correction of fluid loss for the patient with FVD, the primary provider considers the patient's maintenance requirements and other factors (e.g., fever) that can influence fluid needs. If the deficit is not severe, the oral route is preferred, provided the patient can drink. However, if fluid losses are acute or severe, the IV route is required. Isotonic electrolyte crystalloid solutions (e.g., lactated Ringer's solution or 0.9% sodium chloride) are frequently the first-line choice to treat the hypotensive patient with FVD because they expand plasma volume. As soon as the patient becomes normotensive, a hypotonic electrolyte solution (e.g., 0.45% sodium chloride) is often used to provide both electrolytes and water for renal excretion of metabolic wastes (Sterns, 2017a; Sterns, 2017b). These and additional fluids are listed in Table 10-5.

Accurate and frequent assessments of I&O, weight, vital signs, central venous pressure, level of consciousness, breath sounds, and skin color are monitored to determine when therapy should be slowed to avoid volume overload. The rate of fluid administration is based on the severity of loss and the patient's hemodynamic response to volume replacement (Sterns, 2017a; Sterns, 2017b).

If the patient with severe FVD is not excreting enough urine and is therefore oliguric, the primary provider needs to determine whether the depressed renal function is caused by

TABLE 10-5	Select Water and Electrolyte Solutions
Solution	**Considerations**
Isotonic Solutions 0.9% NaCl (isotonic, also called *normal saline* [NS]) Na^+ 154 mEq/L Cl^- 154 mEq/L (308 mOsm/L) Also available with varying concentrations of dextrose (a 5% dextrose concentration is commonly used)	• An isotonic solution that expands the extracellular fluid (ECF) volume; used in hypovolemic states, resuscitative efforts, shock, diabetic ketoacidosis, metabolic alkalosis, hypercalcemia, mild Na^+ deficit • Supplies an excess of Na^+ and Cl^-; can cause fluid volume excess and hyperchloremic acidosis if used in excessive volumes, particularly in patients with compromised renal function, heart failure, or edema • When mixed with 5% dextrose, the resulting solution becomes temporarily hypertonic in relation to plasma and, in addition to the previously described electrolytes, provides 170 cal/L. After dextrose is metabolized it leaves an isotonic solution. • Only solution that may be given with blood products • Tonicity similar to plasma
Lactated Ringer's solution Na^+ 130 mEq/L K^+ 4 mEq/L Ca^{++} 3 mEq/L Cl^- 109 mEq/L Lactate (metabolized to bicarbonate) 28 mEq/L (274 mOsm/L) Also available with varying concentrations of dextrose (the most common is 5% dextrose)	• An isotonic solution that contains multiple electrolytes in roughly the same concentration as found in plasma (note that solution is lacking in Mg^{++}); provides 9 cal/L • Used in the treatment of hypovolemia, burns, fluid lost as bile or diarrhea, and for acute blood loss replacement • Lactate is rapidly metabolized into HCO_3^- in the body. Lactated Ringer's solution should not be used in lactic acidosis because the ability to convert lactate into HCO_3^- is impaired in this disorder • Not to be given with a pH >7.5 because bicarbonate is formed as lactate breaks down, causing alkalosis • Should not be used in kidney injury because it contains potassium and can cause hyperkalemia • Tonicity similar to plasma
5% dextrose in water (D_5W) No electrolytes 50 g of dextrose	• An isotonic solution that supplies 170 cal/L and free water to aid in renal excretion of solutes • Used in treatment of hypernatremia, fluid loss, and dehydration • Should not be used in excessive volumes in the early postoperative period (when antidiuretic hormone secretion is increased due to stress reaction) • Should not be used solely in treatment of fluid volume deficit because it dilutes plasma electrolyte concentrations • Contraindicated in head injury because it may cause increased intracranial pressure • Should not be used for fluid resuscitation because it can cause hyperglycemia • Should be used with caution in patients with renal or cardiac disease because of risk of fluid overload • Electrolyte-free solutions may cause peripheral circulatory collapse, anuria in patients with sodium deficiency, and increased body fluid loss • Converts to hypotonic solution as dextrose is metabolized by body. Over time, D_5W without NaCl can cause water intoxication (intracellular fluid volume excess [FVE]) because the solution is hypotonic • Fluid therapy for an extended period of time without electrolytes may result in hypokalemia
Hypotonic Solutions 0.45% NaCl (half-strength saline) Na^+ 77 mEq/L Cl^- 77 mEq/L (154 mOsm/L) Also available with varying concentrations of dextrose (the most common is a 5% concentration)	• Provides Na^+, Cl^-, and free water • Free water is desirable to aid the kidneys in elimination of solute • Lacking in electrolytes other than Na^+ and Cl^- • When mixed with 5% dextrose, the solution becomes slightly hypertonic to plasma temporarily until dextrose is metabolized. It leaves a hypotonic solution after dextrose metabolism. Provides 170 cal/L • Used to treat hypertonic dehydration, Na^+ and Cl^- depletion, and gastric fluid loss • Not indicated for third-space fluid shifts or increased intracranial pressure • Administer cautiously, because hypotonic solution can cause fluid shifts from vascular system into cells, resulting in cardiovascular collapse and increased intracranial pressure
Hypertonic Solutions 3% NaCl (hypertonic saline) Na^+ 513 mEq/L Cl^- 513 mEq/L (1026 mOsm/L) 5% NaCL (hypertonic solution) Na^+ 855 mEq/L Cl^- 855 mEq/L (1710 mOsm/L) IV Mannitol 5–25% (hypertonic solution) (1372 mOsm/L contained in 25% solution)	• Used to increase ECF volume, decrease cellular swelling • Highly hypertonic solution used only in critical situations to treat hyponatremia • Must be given slowly and cautiously, because it can cause intravascular volume overload and pulmonary edema • Assists in removing intracellular fluid excess • Highly hypertonic solution used to treat symptomatic hyponatremia • Administer slowly and cautiously because it can cause intravascular volume overload and pulmonary edema • Supplies no calories
Colloid Solutions Dextran in NS or D_5W Available in low-molecular-weight (Dextran 40) and high-molecular-weight (Dextran 70) forms	• Colloid solution used as volume/plasma expander for intravascular part of ECF • Affects clotting by coating platelets and decreasing ability to clot • Remains in circulatory system up to 24 h • Used to treat hypovolemia in early shock to increase pulse pressure, cardiac output, and arterial blood pressure • Improves microcirculation by decreasing red blood cell aggregation • Contraindicated in hemorrhage, thrombocytopenia, renal disease, and severe dehydration • Not a substitute for blood or blood products

reduced renal blood flow secondary to FVD (prerenal azotemia) or, more seriously, by acute tubular necrosis (intrarenal azotemia) from prolonged FVD (Norris, 2019). The test used in this situation is referred to as a fluid challenge test. During a fluid challenge test, volumes of fluid are given at specific rates and intervals while the patient's hemodynamic response to this treatment is monitored (i.e., vital signs, breath sounds, orientation status, central venous pressure, urine output) (Sterns, 2017b).

An example of a typical fluid challenge test involves administering 100 to 200 mL of normal saline solution over 15 minutes. The goal is to provide fluids rapidly enough to attain adequate tissue perfusion without compromising the cardiovascular system. The response by a patient with FVD but normal renal function is increased urine output and an increase in blood pressure and central venous pressure.

Shock can occur when the volume of fluid lost exceeds 25% of the intravascular volume or when fluid loss is rapid (Mandel & Palevsky, 2019). (Shock and its causes and treatment are discussed in detail in Chapter 11.)

Nursing Management

To assess for FVD, the nurse monitors and measures fluid I&O at least every 8 hours, and sometimes hourly. Maintaining an accurate I&O is a particular challenge with patients in critical-care settings. As FVD develops, body fluid losses exceed fluid intake through excessive urination (polyuria), diarrhea, vomiting, or other mechanisms. Once FVD has developed, the kidneys attempt to conserve body fluids, leading to a urine output of less than 1 mL/kg/h in an adult. Urine in this instance is concentrated and represents a healthy renal response.

Vital signs should be closely monitored in FVD.

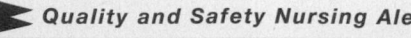

Quality and Safety Nursing Alert

The nurse observes for a weak, rapid pulse and orthostatic hypotension (i.e., a decrease in systolic pressure exceeding 20 mm Hg when the patient moves from a lying to a sitting position).

A decrease in body temperature often accompanies FVD, unless there is a concurrent infection.

Skin and tongue turgor are monitored on a regular basis. In a healthy person, pinched skin immediately returns to its normal position when released (Weber & Kelley, 2018). This elastic property, referred to as turgor, is partially dependent on interstitial fluid volume. In a person with FVD, the skin flattens more slowly after the pinch is released. In a person with severe FVD, the skin may remain elevated for many seconds. Tissue turgor is best measured by pinching the skin over the sternum, dorsal surface of the hand, inner aspects of the thighs, or forehead. It is important to recognize skin turgor is normally diminished in old age. Tongue turgor is not affected by age, and evaluating this may be more valid than evaluating skin turgor (Sterns, 2017a). In a normal person, the tongue has one longitudinal furrow. In the person with FVD, there are additional longitudinal furrows and the tongue is smaller because of fluid loss. The degree of oral mucous membrane moisture is also assessed; a dry mouth may indicate either FVD or mouth breathing.

Quality and Safety Nursing Alert

It is useful to monitor daily body weight when monitoring fluid volume; an acute loss of 0.5 kg (1.1 lb) represents a fluid loss of approximately 500 mL. One liter (1000 mL) of fluid weighs approximately 1 kg, or 2.2 lb. A weight loss or gain of 1–2 lb/day is mainly due to water loss or gain.

Urine concentration is monitored by measuring the urine specific gravity. In a volume-depleted patient, the urine specific gravity should be greater than 1.020, indicating healthy renal conservation of fluid. Dark amber-colored urine is highly concentrated; whereas, clear yellow urine indicates a dilute urine.

Mental function is eventually affected, resulting in confusion, lack of cognition, and delirium in severe FVD as a result of decreasing cerebral perfusion. Behavioral changes are particularly evident in older adults with FVD. Decreased peripheral perfusion can result in cold extremities. In patients with relatively normal cardiopulmonary function, a low central venous pressure is indicative of hypovolemia (Sterns, 2017a). Patients with acute cardiopulmonary decompensation require more extensive hemodynamic monitoring of pressures in both sides of the heart to determine whether hypovolemia exists. Hemodynamic monitoring is particularly important in critically ill patients (Mandel & Palevsky, 2019) (see Chapters 11 and 21).

Preventing Hypovolemia

To prevent FVD, the nurse identifies patients at risk and takes measures to minimize fluid losses. For example, if the patient has diarrhea, measures should be implemented to control diarrhea and replacement fluids given. This includes administering antidiarrheal medications and small volumes of oral fluids at frequent intervals.

Correcting Hypovolemia

When possible, oral fluids are given to help correct FVD, with consideration given to the patient's likes and dislikes. The type of fluid the patient has lost is also considered, and fluids most likely to replace the lost electrolytes are appropriate. If the patient is reluctant to drink because of oral discomfort, the nurse assists with frequent mouth care and provides nonirritating fluids. The patient may be offered small volumes of oral rehydration solutions (e.g., Rehydralyte, Elete, and Cytomax). These solutions provide fluid, glucose, and electrolytes in concentrations that are easily absorbed. If nausea is present, an antiemetic may be needed before oral fluid replacement can be tolerated (Sterns, 2017a; Sterns, 2017b).

If the deficit cannot be corrected by oral fluids, therapy may need to be initiated by an alternative route (enteral or parenteral) until adequate circulating blood volume and renal perfusion are achieved. Isotonic fluids are prescribed to increase ECF volume (Sterns, 2017b).

Hypervolemia

Fluid volume excess (FVE), or hypervolemia, refers to an expansion of the ECF caused by the abnormal retention of water and sodium in approximately the same proportions in which they normally exist in the ECF. It is most often secondary to an increase in the total-body sodium content, which, in turn, leads to an increase in total-body water. This can be referred to as an isotonic accumulation of fluids. Because there is isotonic retention of body substances, the serum sodium concentration remains essentially normal.

Pathophysiology

FVE may be related to simple fluid overload or diminished function of the homeostatic mechanisms responsible for regulating fluid balance. Contributing factors can include heart failure, kidney dysfunction, and cirrhosis of the liver. Another contributing factor is consumption of excessive amounts of table or other sodium salts. Excessive administration of sodium-containing fluids in a patient with impaired regulatory mechanisms may predispose them to a serious FVE as well (Sterns, 2018a).

Clinical Manifestations

Clinical manifestations of FVE result from expansion of the ECF and may include edema, distended jugular veins, and crackles (abnormal lung sounds due to interstitial pulmonary fluid). In patients who are ambulatory, edema is most evident in the ankles; in patients who are supine, edema occurs over the sacrum (Weber & Kelley, 2018). Further discussion of clinical signs and symptoms and laboratory findings can be found in Table 10-4.

Assessment and Diagnostic Findings

Laboratory data useful in diagnosing FVE include BUN and hematocrit levels. In FVE, both of these values may be decreased because of plasma dilution. In chronic kidney disease, both serum osmolality and the sodium level are decreased due to excessive retention of water. The urine sodium level is increased if the kidneys are attempting to excrete excess volume. A chest x-ray may reveal pulmonary congestion in FVE. Hypervolemia occurs when aldosterone is chronically stimulated—for example, in conditions such as cirrhosis, heart failure, and nephrotic syndrome. Aldosterone increases both sodium and water reabsorption into the bloodstream from the nephron; therefore, the urine sodium level is normal in these conditions (Emmett & Palmer, 2019; Sterns, 2018a).

Medical Management

Management of FVE is directed at the causes, and if related to excessive administration of sodium-containing fluids, discontinuing the infusion may be all that is needed. Symptomatic treatment consists of administering diuretics and restricting fluids and sodium. Diuretics are medications that reduce sodium and water reabsorption at the nephron and thereby enhance water loss via the kidneys (Brater & Ellison, 2019).

Pharmacologic Therapy

Diuretics are prescribed when dietary restriction of sodium alone is insufficient to reduce edema. The choice of diuretic is based on the severity of the hypervolemic state, the degree of impairment of renal function, and the potency of the diuretic. Thiazide diuretics block sodium and water reabsorption into

the bloodstream at the distal tubule of the nephron, where 5% to 10% of sodium is normally reabsorbed. This leads to a small amount of sodium and water loss via the urine. Loop diuretics, such as furosemide, bumetanide, or torsemide, can cause a greater loss of both sodium and water because they block sodium reabsorption in the ascending limb of the loop of Henle, where 20% to 30% of filtered sodium is normally reabsorbed. Generally, thiazide diuretics, such as hydrochlorothiazide, are prescribed for mild to moderate hypervolemia and loop diuretics for severe hypervolemia (Brater & Ellison, 2019).

Electrolyte imbalances may result from side effects of diuretics. Hypokalemia can occur with all diuretics except those that inhibit aldosterone. Potassium supplements can be prescribed with diuretics to avoid this complication. Hyperkalemia can occur with diuretics that inhibit aldosterone (e.g., spironolactone, a potassium-sparing diuretic), especially in patients with decreased renal function. Hyponatremia occurs with diuresis due to increased release of ADH secondary to reduction in circulating volume. Decreased magnesium levels occur with administration of loop and thiazide diuretics due to decreased reabsorption and increased excretion of magnesium by the kidney (Brater & Ellison, 2019; Vallerand & Sanoski, 2019).

Azotemia (increased nitrogen levels in the blood) can occur with FVE when urea and creatinine are not excreted due to decreased perfusion by the kidneys and decreased excretion of waste, as occurs in renal failure. High uric acid levels (hyperuricemia) can also occur from increased reabsorption and decreased excretion of uric acid by the kidneys.

Dialysis

If renal function is so severely impaired that pharmacologic agents cannot act efficiently, other modalities are considered to remove sodium and fluid from the body. Hemodialysis or peritoneal dialysis may be used to remove nitrogenous wastes and control potassium and acid–base balance, and to remove sodium and fluid. Continuous renal replacement therapy may also be required (see Chapter 48 for a discussion of these treatment modalities).

Nutritional Therapy

Treatment of FVE usually involves dietary restriction of sodium. An average daily diet not restricted in sodium contains 6 to 15 g of salt, whereas low sodium diets can range from a mild restriction (less than 2000 mg/day) to as little as 250 mg of sodium per day, depending on the patient's needs. A mild sodium-restricted diet allows only light salting of food (about half the usual amount) in cooking and at the table, and no addition of salt to commercially prepared foods that are already seasoned. Foods high in sodium must be avoided. It is the sodium salt (sodium chloride) rather than sodium itself that contributes to edema. Therefore, patients are instructed to read food labels carefully to determine salt content (Olendzki, 2017).

Because about half of ingested sodium is in the form of seasoning, seasoning substitutes can play a major role in decreasing sodium intake. Lemon juice, onions, and garlic are excellent substitute flavorings, although some patients prefer salt substitutes. Most salt substitutes contain potassium and must therefore be used cautiously by patients taking potassium-sparing diuretics (e.g., spironolactone, triamterene, amiloride). These substitutes should not be used in conditions associated with potassium retention, such as advanced kidney disease. Salt substitutes containing ammonium chloride can be harmful to patients with liver damage (Olendzki, 2017; Vallerand & Sanoski, 2019).

In some communities, drinking water may contain too much sodium for a sodium-restricted diet. Depending on its source, water may contain as little as 1 mg or more than 1500 mg of sodium per quart. Patients may need to use distilled water if the local water supply is very high in sodium. Bottled water can have a sodium content that ranges from 0 to 1200 mg/L; therefore, if sodium is restricted, the label must be carefully examined for sodium content before purchasing and drinking bottled water. Also, patients on sodium-restricted diets should be cautioned to avoid water softeners that add sodium to water in exchange for other ions, such as calcium. Protein intake may be increased in patients who are malnourished or who have low serum protein levels in an effort to increase capillary oncotic pressure. Increasing oncotic pressure in the bloodstream will pull fluid out of the tissues into vessels for excretion by the kidneys (Sterns, 2018a).

Nursing Management

To assess for FVE, the nurse measures I&O at regular intervals to identify excessive fluid retention. The patient is weighed daily, and rapid weight gain is noted. Breath sounds are assessed at regular intervals in at-risk patients, particularly if parenteral fluids are being given. The nurse monitors the degree of edema in the most dependent parts of the body, such as the feet and ankles in ambulatory patients and the sacral region in patients confined to bed. Pitting edema is assessed by pressing a finger into the affected part, creating a pit or indentation that is evaluated on a scale of 1+ (minimal) to 4+ (severe) (see Chapter 25, Fig. 25-2). Peripheral edema is monitored by measuring the circumference of the extremity with a tape measure marked in millimeters (Weber & Kelley, 2018).

> **Quality and Safety Nursing Alert**
>
> An acute weight gain of 1 kg (2.2 lb) is equivalent to a gain of approximately 1 L of fluid.

Preventing Hypervolemia

Specific interventions vary with the underlying condition and the degree of FVE. However, most patients require sodium-restricted diets in some form, and adherence to the prescribed diet is encouraged. Patients are instructed to avoid over-the-counter (OTC) medications without first checking with a health care provider, because they may contain sodium (e.g., Alka-Seltzer). If fluid retention persists despite adherence to a prescribed diet, hidden sources of sodium, such as the water supply or use of water softeners, should be considered.

Detecting and Controlling Hypervolemia

It is important to detect FVE before the condition becomes severe. Interventions include promoting rest, restricting sodium intake, monitoring parenteral fluid therapy, and administering appropriate medications.

Regular rest periods may be beneficial, because bed rest favors diuresis of fluid. The mechanism is related to diminished venous pooling and the subsequent increase in effective circulating blood volume and renal perfusion. Sodium and fluid restriction should be instituted as indicated. Because most patients with FVE require diuretics, the patient's response to these agents is monitored. The rate of parenteral fluids and the patient's response to these fluids are also closely monitored (Frandsen & Pennington, 2018). If dyspnea or orthopnea is present, the patient is placed in a semi-Fowler position to promote lung expansion. The patient is turned and repositioned at regular intervals because edematous tissue is more prone to skin breakdown than normal tissue. Because conditions predisposing to FVE are likely to be chronic, patients are taught to monitor their response to therapy by documenting fluid I&O and body weight changes. The importance of adhering to the treatment regimen is emphasized.

 Educating Patients About Edema

Because edema is a common manifestation of FVE, patients need to recognize its symptoms and understand its importance. The nurse gives special attention to edema when instructing the patient with FVE. Edema can occur as a result of increased capillary fluid pressure, decreased capillary oncotic pressure, or increased interstitial oncotic pressure, causing expansion of the interstitial fluid compartment (Hall, 2016). Edema can be localized (e.g., in the ankle, as in rheumatoid arthritis) or generalized (as in cardiac failure and kidney injury) (Sterns, 2018b). Severe generalized edema is called *anasarca*.

Edema occurs when there is a change in the capillary membrane, increasing the formation of interstitial fluid or decreasing the removal of interstitial fluid. Sodium retention is a frequent cause of the increased ECF volume. Burns and infection are examples of conditions associated with increased interstitial fluid volume. Obstruction to lymphatic outflow, a plasma albumin level less than 1.5 to 2 g/dL, or a decrease in plasma oncotic pressure contributes to increased interstitial fluid volume. If there is decreased cardiac output as in heart failure, the kidneys sense low perfusion and secrete renin which triggers the renin–angiotensin–aldosterone system that increases sodium and water retention (Sterns, 2018b). A thorough medication history is necessary to identify any medications that could cause edema, such as nonsteroidal anti-inflammatory drugs (NSAIDs), estrogens, corticosteroids, and antihypertensive agents (Vallerand & Sanoski, 2019).

Ascites is a type of edema in which fluid accumulates in the peritoneal cavity; it results from heart failure, nephrotic syndrome, cirrhosis, and some malignant tumors. The patient commonly reports shortness of breath and a sense of pressure because of pressure on the diaphragm.

The goal of treatment is to preserve or restore the circulating intravascular fluid volume. Thus, in addition to treating the cause of the edema, other treatments may include diuretic therapy, restriction of fluids and sodium, elevation of the extremities, application of anti-embolic stockings, paracentesis (pulling fluid out of the peritoneal cavity using a needle and syringe), dialysis, and continuous renal replacement therapy in cases of kidney injury or life-threatening fluid volume overload (Sterns, 2018b).

ELECTROLYTE IMBALANCES

Disturbances in electrolyte balances are common in clinical practice and may need to be corrected based on history, physical examination findings, and laboratory values (with comparison to previous values).

Sodium Imbalances

Sodium (Na$^+$) is the most abundant electrolyte in the ECF; its concentration ranges from 135 to 145 mEq/L (135 to 145 mmol/L), and it is the primary determinant of ECF volume and osmolality. Sodium has a major role in controlling water distribution throughout the body, because it does not easily cross the plasma membrane and because of its abundance and high concentration in the body. Sodium is regulated by ADH, thirst, and the renin–angiotensin–aldosterone system. A loss or gain of sodium is usually accompanied by a loss or gain of water. Sodium also functions in establishing the electrochemical state necessary for muscle contraction and the transmission of nerve impulses (Hall, 2016).

The syndrome of inappropriate secretion of antidiuretic hormone (SIADH) may be associated with sodium imbalance. When there is a decrease in the circulating plasma osmolality, blood volume, or blood pressure, ADH (also called arginine vasopressin [AVP]) is released from the posterior pituitary. Oversecretion of ADH can cause SIADH. Patients at risk for SIADH include older adults; those who have had brain surgery or have a brain tumor, pulmonary malignancy, or acquired immune deficiency syndrome (AIDS); those on mechanical ventilation; and those taking selective serotonin reuptake inhibitors (SSRIs) (Sterns, 2017d). (SIADH is discussed in more detail in Chapter 45.)

Sodium imbalance can develop under simple or complex circumstances. The two most common sodium imbalances are sodium deficit and sodium excess (Table 10-6).

Sodium Deficit (Hyponatremia)

Hyponatremia refers to a serum sodium level that is less than 135 mEq/L (135 mmol/L) (Sterns, 2017e). Hyponatremia can present as an acute or chronic form. Acute hyponatremia is commonly the result of a fluid overload in a surgical patient. This is a dilutional hyponatremia because the excess water dilutes the sodium in the bloodstream. Chronic hyponatremia is seen more frequently in patients outside the hospital setting, has a longer duration, and has less serious neurologic sequelae. Another type of hyponatremia is exercised-associated hyponatremia, which is more frequently found in women and those of smaller stature. It can occur during extreme temperatures, because of excessive fluid intake before exercise, or prolonged exercise that results in excess loss of sodium through perspiration (Apostu, 2014; McDermott, Anderson, Armstrong, et al., 2017).

Pathophysiology

Hyponatremia primarily occurs due to an imbalance of water rather than sodium. Checking the urine sodium value can assist in differentiating renal from nonrenal causes of hyponatremia. Low sodium in the urine occurs as the nephrons of the kidney retain sodium to compensate for nonrenal fluid loss (i.e., vomiting, diarrhea, sweating). High sodium concentration in the urine is associated with renal salt wasting that occurs in renal dysfunction or diuretic use. In dilutional hyponatremia, the ECF volume has excess water but there is no edema, and the excess water dilutes the sodium (Sterns, 2017e).

A deficiency of aldosterone, as occurs in adrenal insufficiency, also predisposes to sodium deficiency. Lack of aldosterone causes lack of sodium and water reabsorption into the bloodstream at the nephrons. In addition, the use of certain medications, such as anticonvulsants (e.g., carbamazepine, oxcarbazepine, levetiracetam), SSRIs (e.g., fluoxetine, sertraline, paroxetine), or desmopressin acetate, have side effects

TABLE 10-6	Sodium Imbalances		
Imbalance	**Contributing Factors**		**Signs/Symptoms and Laboratory Findings**
Sodium deficit (hyponatremia) Serum sodium <135 mEq/L	Loss of sodium, as in use of diuretics, loss of GI fluids, renal disease, and adrenal insufficiency. Gain of water, as in excessive administration of D$_5$W and water supplements for patients receiving hypotonic tube feedings; disease states associated with SIADH, such as head trauma and oat-cell lung tumor; medications associated with water retention (oxytocin and certain tranquilizers); and psychogenic polydipsia. Hyperglycemia and heart failure cause a loss of sodium.		Anorexia, nausea and vomiting, headache, lethargy, dizziness, confusion, muscle cramps and weakness, muscular twitching, seizures, papilledema, dry skin, ↑ pulse, ↓ BP, weight gain, edema *Labs indicate:* ↓ serum and urine sodium, ↓ urine specific gravity and osmolality
Sodium excess (hypernatremia) Serum sodium >145 mEq/L	Fluid deprivation in patients who cannot respond to thirst, hypertonic tube feedings without adequate water supplements, diabetes insipidus, heatstroke, hyperventilation, watery diarrhea, burns, and diaphoresis. Excess corticosteroid, sodium bicarbonate, and sodium chloride administration, and saltwater nonfatal drowning victims.		Thirst, elevated body temperature, swollen dry tongue and sticky mucous membranes, hallucinations, lethargy, restlessness, irritability, simple partial or tonic–clonic seizures, pulmonary edema, hyperreflexia, twitching, nausea, vomiting, anorexia, ↑ pulse, and ↑ BP *Labs indicate:* ↑ serum sodium, ↓ urine sodium, ↑ urine specific gravity and osmolality, ↓ CVP

BP, blood pressure; CVP, central venous pressure; ↓, decreased; D$_5$W, dextrose 5% in water; GI, gastrointestinal; ↑, increased; SIADH, syndrome of inappropriate secretion of antidiuretic hormone.
Adapted from Norris, T. L. (2019). *Porth's pathophysiology: Concepts of altered health state* (10th ed.). Philadelphia, PA: Wolters Kluwer.

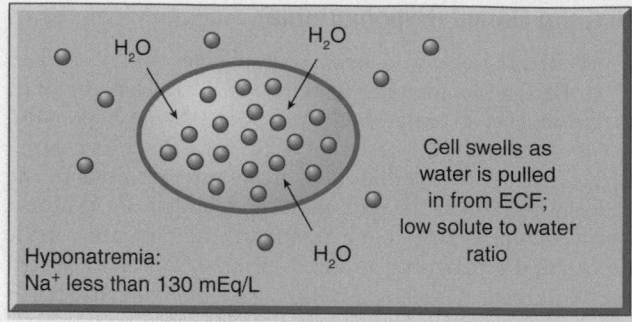

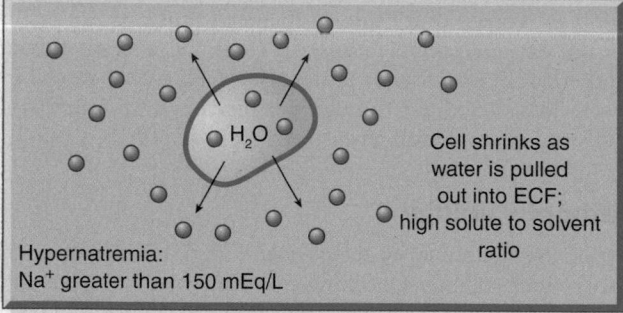

Figure 10-7 • Effect of extracellular sodium level on cell size.

that increase the risk of hyponatremia (Liamis, Megapanou, Elisaf, et al., 2019).

Clinical Manifestations

Clinical manifestations of hyponatremia depend on the cause, magnitude, and speed with which the deficit occurs. Poor skin turgor, dry mucosa, headache, decreased saliva production, orthostatic fall in blood pressure, nausea, vomiting, and abdominal cramping can occur. Neurologic changes, including altered mental status, status epilepticus, and coma, are related to the cellular swelling and cerebral edema associated with hyponatremia. As the extracellular sodium level decreases, the cellular fluid becomes relatively more concentrated and pulls water into the cells (Fig. 10-7). In general, patients with an acute decrease in serum sodium levels have more cerebral edema and higher mortality rates than do those with more slowly developing hyponatremia. Acute decreases in sodium, developing in less than 48 hours, may be associated with cerebral edema. Cerebral edema can lead to compression of brain stem structures and brain herniation. Chronic decreases in sodium, developing over 48 hours or more, can occur in status epilepticus and other neurologic conditions (Sterns, 2017e).

Clinical features of hyponatremia associated with sodium loss and water gain include anorexia, muscle cramps, and a feeling of exhaustion. The severity of symptoms increases with the degree of hyponatremia and the speed with which it develops. When the serum sodium level decreases to less than 115 mEq/L (115 mmol/L), signs of increasing intracranial pressure, such as lethargy, confusion, muscle twitching, focal weakness, hemiparesis, papilledema, seizures, and death, may occur (Sterns, 2017e).

Assessment and Diagnostic Findings

Targeted assessment includes the history and physical examination with a focused neurologic examination; evaluation of signs and symptoms as well as laboratory test results; identification of current IV fluids, if applicable; and a review of all medications the patient is taking. Regardless of the cause of hyponatremia, the serum sodium level is less than 135 mEq/L; in SIADH, it may be lower than 100 mEq/L (100 mmol/L). Serum osmolality is usually decreased. When hyponatremia is due to lack of sodium ingestion, the urinary sodium content is less than 20 mEq/L (20 mmol/L) and the specific gravity is low (1.002 to 1.004). However, when hyponatremia is due to SIADH, the urinary sodium content is greater than 20 mEq/L, and the urine specific gravity is usually greater than 1.012. Although the patient with SIADH retains water abnormally there is no peripheral edema; instead, fluid accumulates inside the cells. This phenomenon sometimes manifests as pitting edema (Sterns, 2017d).

Medical Management

The key to treating hyponatremia is an assessment that focuses on the clinical symptoms of the patient and signs of hyponatremia (including laboratory values). As a general rule, treating the underlying condition will bring the sodium level back to normal.

Sodium Replacement

The most common treatment for hyponatremia is careful administration of sodium by mouth, nasogastric tube, or a parenteral route. For patients who can eat and drink, sodium is easily replaced, because sodium is consumed abundantly in a normal diet. For those who cannot consume sodium, lactated Ringer's solution or isotonic saline (0.9% sodium chloride) solution may be prescribed. Serum sodium must not be increased by more than 12 mEq/L in 24 hours to avoid neurologic damage due to demyelination (Jain, Phadke, Chauhan, et al., 2018). This condition may occur when the serum sodium concentration is overcorrected (exceeding 140 mEq/L) too rapidly or in the presence of hypoxia or anoxia. It may produce lesions that show symmetric myelin destruction affecting all fiber tracts that can present with altered cognition and decreased alertness, ataxia, paraparesis, dysarthria, horizontal gaze paralysis, pseudobulbar palsy, and coma. The usual daily sodium requirement in adults is approximately 100 mEq, provided there are not excessive losses (Sterns, 2020). Select water and electrolyte solutions are described in Table 10-5.

In SIADH, the administration of hypertonic saline solution alone cannot change the plasma sodium concentration. Excess sodium would be excreted rapidly in highly concentrated urine. With the addition of the diuretic furosemide, urine is not concentrated and isotonic urine is excreted to effect a change in water balance. In patients with SIADH, in whom water restriction is difficult, lithium can antagonize the osmotic effect of ADH on the nephrons' collecting ducts (Sterns, 2017d).

Water Restriction

In patients with normal or excess fluid volume, hyponatremia is usually treated effectively by restricting fluid. However, if neurologic symptoms are severe (e.g., seizures, delirium, coma), or in patients with traumatic brain injury, it may be necessary to administer small volumes of a hypertonic sodium solution with the goal of alleviating cerebral edema. Incorrect use of these fluids is extremely dangerous, because 1 L of 3%

sodium chloride solution contains 513 mEq of sodium and 1 L of 5% sodium chloride solution contains 855 mEq of sodium. The recommendation for hypertonic saline administration in patients with craniocerebral trauma is 3% saline between 0.10 and 1.0 mL/kg of body weight per hour (Sterns, 2017d).

 Quality and Safety Nursing Alert

In patients with hyponatremia, highly hypertonic sodium solutions (2–23% sodium chloride) should be administered slowly. The patient needs close monitoring, because only small volumes are needed to elevate the serum sodium concentration.

Pharmacologic Therapy

AVP receptor antagonists (also called ADH receptor antagonists) are pharmacologic agents that treat hyponatremia by blocking the effect of ADH at the nephron, which in turn allows diuresis to occur and leads to water excretion. Use of IV conivaptan HCl, an AVP receptor antagonist, is limited to the treatment of hospitalized patients. It may be a useful therapy for those patients with moderate to severe symptomatic hyponatremia but is contraindicated in patients with seizures, delirium, or coma, which warrants the use of hypertonic saline. Tolvaptan is an oral medication indicated for clinically significant hypervolemic and euvolemic hyponatremia that must be initiated and monitored in the hospital setting (Frandsen & Pennington, 2018; Vallerand & Sanoski, 2019).

Nursing Management

The nurse needs to identify and monitor patients at risk for hyponatremia. The nurse monitors I&O as well as daily body weight. I&O can be used to identify excess water input or lack of sufficient water output.

The nurse needs to get a thorough history to identify if the patient is a performance athlete. Performance athletes (i.e., marathon runners) may use salt tablets to compensate for loss of sodium with sweating, hoping to decrease sodium loss during prolonged exercise; however, there is no evidence that this practice works and it is not recommended (Hew-Butler, Loi, Pani, et al., 2017).

Hyponatremia is a frequently overlooked cause of confusion in older patients, who are at increased risk because of decreased renal function and subsequent inability to excrete excess fluids. Administration of prescribed and OTC medications that cause sodium loss or water retention is often the predisposing factor. A diminished sense of thirst or decreased ability to access food or fluids may also contribute to the problem (Cash & Glass, 2018).

Detecting and Controlling Hyponatremia

Early detection and treatment of hyponatremia are necessary to prevent serious consequences. For patients at risk, the nurse closely monitors fluid I&O as well as daily body weight. It is also necessary to monitor laboratory values (i.e., sodium) and be alert for GI manifestations such as anorexia, nausea, vomiting, and abdominal cramping. The nurse must be alert for central nervous system changes, such as lethargy, confusion, muscle twitching, and seizures. Neurologic signs are associated with very low sodium levels that have fallen rapidly because of fluid overloading. Serum sodium is monitored very closely in patients who are at risk for hyponatremia; when indicated, urine sodium and specific gravity are also monitored.

For a patient with abnormal losses of sodium who can consume a general diet, the nurse encourages foods and fluids with high sodium content to control hyponatremia. For example, broth made with one beef cube contains approximately 900 mg of sodium; 8 oz of tomato juice contains approximately 700 mg of sodium. The nurse also needs to be familiar with the sodium content of parenteral fluids (see Table 10-5).

If the primary cause of hyponatremia is water retention, it is safer to restrict fluid intake than to administer sodium. In normovolemia or hypervolemia, administration of sodium predisposes a patient to fluid volume overload. In severe hyponatremia, the aim of therapy is to elevate the serum sodium level only enough to alleviate neurologic signs and symptoms. It is generally recommended that the serum sodium concentration be increased to no greater than 125 mEq/L (125 mmol/L) with a hypertonic saline solution (Sterns, 2020).

 Quality and Safety Nursing Alert

When administering fluids to patients with cardiovascular disease, the nurse assesses for hemodynamic signs of circulatory overload (e.g., cough, dyspnea, jugular venous distention, dependent edema, 1–2 lb weight gain in 24 h). The lungs should be auscultated for crackles as this can indicate pulmonary edema.

For the patient taking lithium, the nurse observes for lithium toxicity, particularly when sodium is lost. In such instances, supplemental salt and fluid are given. Because diuretics promote sodium loss, the patient taking lithium is instructed not to use diuretics without close medical supervision. For all patients on lithium therapy, normal salt and oral fluid intake (approximately 6- to 15-g sodium and 2.5- to 3.0-L fluid/day) should be encouraged and a sodium restricted diet should be avoided (Frandsen & Pennington, 2018; Vallerand & Sanoski, 2019).

Excess water supplements are avoided in patients receiving isotonic or hypotonic enteral feedings, particularly if abnormal sodium loss occurs or water is being abnormally retained (as in SIADH). Actual fluid needs are determined by evaluating fluid I&O, urine specific gravity, and serum sodium levels.

Sodium Excess (Hypernatremia)

Hypernatremia is a serum sodium level higher than 145 mEq/L (145 mmol/L). It can be caused by a gain of sodium in excess of water or by a loss of water in excess of sodium. It can occur in patients with normal fluid volume or in those with FVD or FVE. With water loss, the patient loses more water than sodium; as a result, the serum sodium concentration increases and the increased concentration pulls fluid out of the cell. This is both an extracellular and an intracellular FVD. In sodium excess, the patient ingests or retains more sodium than water (Mushin & Mount, 2018; Sterns, 2017e).

Chart 10-1 Dysnatremia

Dysnatremia is lack of normal sodium level in the bloodstream; either hypernatremia or hyponatremia. In performance athletes who lose excessive water via perspiration, sodium can become concentrated in the bloodstream causing hypernatremia. This can lead to the following life-threatening conditions:

- Encephalopathy
- Confusion
- Disorientation
- Stupor

In performance athletes who lose excess sodium via perspiration during exercise, this can lead to excess sodium depletion from the bloodstream causing hyponatremia. This can also manifest as the following:

- Confusion
- Disorientation
- Stupor

Testing of the blood and urine can differentiate hyponatremia from hypernatremia, determine the severity of the dysnatremia, and guide appropriate therapy.

Adapted from Apostu, M. (2014). A strategy for maintaining fluid and electrolyte balance in aerobic effort. *Procedia—Social and Behavioral Sciences, 117*(2014), 323–328; Hew-Butler, T., Loi, V., Pani, A., et al. (2017). Exercise-induced hyponatremia: 2017 update. *Frontiers in Medicine (Lausanne), 4*, 21.

Pathophysiology

A common cause of hypernatremia is fluid deprivation in patients who do not respond to thirst. Most often affected are patients who are very old, very young, or cognitively impaired. Administration of hypertonic enteral feedings without adequate water supplements leads to hypernatremia, as does watery diarrhea and greatly increased insensible water loss through the lungs or skin (e.g., hyperventilation, burns). In addition, diabetes insipidus, which is a lack of ADH due to posterior pituitary dysfunction, can lead to lack of adequate reabsorption of water into the bloodstream at the level of the nephron. This leads to inadequate water volume in the bloodstream which leads to hypernatremia if the patient does not respond to thirst, or if fluids are excessively restricted (Sterns, 2017c).

Less common causes of hypernatremia are heatstroke, nonfatal drowning in seawater (which contains a sodium concentration of approximately 500 mEq/L), and malfunction of hemodialysis or peritoneal dialysis systems. IV administration of hypertonic saline or excessive use of sodium bicarbonate also causes hypernatremia. Exertional dysnatremia can occur in performance athletes (Apostu, 2014) (Chart 10-1).

Clinical Manifestations

The clinical manifestations of hypernatremia are due to increased plasma osmolality caused by an increase in plasma sodium concentration. Water moves out of the cell into the ECF, resulting in cellular dehydration (Norris, 2019) (see Fig. 10-7). Clinical signs and symptoms as well as laboratory findings can be found in Table 10-6. Dehydration (resulting in hypernatremia) is often overlooked as the cause of mental status and behavioral changes in older patients (Cash & Glass, 2018). Body temperature may increase mildly, but it returns to normal after the hypernatremia is corrected.

A primary characteristic of hypernatremia is thirst. Thirst is a strong defender of normal serum sodium levels in healthy people. Because of thirst, hypernatremia does not occur unless the person is unconscious or cannot access water. However, those who are ill and older adults may have an impaired thirst mechanism (Cash & Glass, 2018).

Assessment and Diagnostic Findings

In hypernatremia, the serum sodium level exceeds 145 mEq/L (145 mmol/L) and the serum osmolality exceeds 300 mOsm/kg (300 mmol/L). The urine specific gravity and urine osmolality are increased as the kidneys attempt to conserve water (provided the water loss is from a route other than the kidneys). Patients with diabetes insipidus do not reabsorb water into the bloodstream at the nephron. These patients consequently develop excess urine output, dehydration, and hypernatremia. Without ADH, these patients excrete very dilute urine with a urine osmolality less than 250 mOsm/kg (Emmett & Palmer, 2018a).

Medical Management

Treatment of hypernatremia consists of a gradual lowering of the serum sodium level by the infusion of a hypotonic solution (e.g., 0.45% sodium chloride) or an isotonic nonsaline solution (e.g., dextrose 5% in water [D_5W]). D_5W can be used when water needs to be replaced without sodium. However, hypotonic sodium chloride solution (0.45% NaCl) is thought to be safer than D_5W because it allows a gradual reduction in the serum sodium level. Gradual reduction in serum sodium decreases the risk of cerebral edema. Hypotonic sodium chloride solution (0.45% NaCl) is the IV solution of choice in severe hyperglycemia with hypernatremia. A rapid reduction in the serum sodium level that occurs with D_5W temporarily decreases the plasma osmolality below that of the fluid in the brain tissue, causing dangerous cerebral edema. Alternatively in hypernatremia, diuretics can be prescribed to treat the excess sodium (Sterns & Hoorn, 2019).

There is no consensus about the exact rate at which serum sodium levels should be reduced. As a general rule, the serum sodium level is reduced at a rate no faster than 0.5 to 1 mEq/L/h to allow sufficient time for readjustment through diffusion across fluid compartments. Desmopressin acetate, a synthetic ADH, may be prescribed to treat diabetes insipidus if it is the cause of hypernatremia (Bichet, 2017; Mushin & Mount, 2018).

Nursing Management

Fluid losses and gains are carefully monitored in patients who are at risk for hypernatremia. The nurse should assess for abnormal losses of water or low water intake and for large gains of sodium, as might occur with ingestion of OTC medications that have a high sodium content (e.g., Alka-Seltzer). In addition, the nurse obtains a medication history, because some prescription medications have a high sodium content. The nurse also notes the patient's thirst or elevated body temperature and evaluates it in relation to other clinical signs and symptoms. The patient is monitored closely for changes in behavior, such as restlessness, disorientation, and lethargy (Sterns, 2017c; Sterns & Hoorn, 2019).

Preventing Hypernatremia

The nurse attempts to prevent hypernatremia by providing oral fluids at regular intervals, particularly in patients who are unable to perceive or respond to thirst. If fluid intake remains inadequate or the patient is unconscious, the nurse consults with the primary provider to plan an alternative route for intake, either by enteral feedings or by the parenteral route. If enteral feedings are used, sufficient water should be given to keep the serum sodium and BUN within normal limits. As a rule, the higher the osmolality of the enteral feeding, the greater is the need for water supplementation (Emmett & Palmer, 2018a; Sterns & Hoorn, 2019). Some herbal medications can also increase serum sodium levels.

For patients with diabetes insipidus, adequate water intake must be ensured. If the patient is alert and has an intact thirst mechanism, merely providing access to water may be sufficient. If the patient has a decreased level of consciousness or other disability interfering with adequate fluid intake, parenteral fluid replacement may be prescribed. This therapy can be anticipated in patients with neurologic disorders, particularly in the early postoperative period (Bichet, 2017).

Correcting Hypernatremia

When parenteral fluids are necessary for managing hypernatremia, the nurse monitors the patient's response to the infusion of fluids by reviewing serial serum sodium levels and by observing for changes in neurologic status, such as confusion, disorientation, and possible decreased level of consciousness (Mushin & Mount, 2018). With a gradual decrease in the serum sodium level, neurologic status should improve. However, too rapid reduction in the serum sodium level renders the plasma temporarily hypoosmotic compared to the intracellular fluid within the brain cells. This can cause fluid in the plasma to shift into the brain cells which can produce the dangerous state of cerebral edema (Hutto & French, 2017).

Potassium Imbalances

Potassium (K^+) is the major intracellular electrolyte; in fact, 98% of the body's potassium is inside the cells. The remaining 2% is in the ECF and is important to neuromuscular and cardiac function. Potassium influences both skeletal and cardiac

muscle activity. For example, alterations in K^+ concentration can change myocardial irritability and rhythm. Under the influence of the sodium–potassium pump, potassium is constantly being pumped into the cells. The normal serum potassium concentration ranges from 3.5 to 5 mEq/L (3.5 to 5 mmol/L), and even minor variations are significant (Norris, 2019). Potassium imbalances are commonly associated with various diseases, injuries, medications (e.g., NSAIDs and ACE inhibitors), and acid–base imbalances (Mount, 2017a). The two types of potassium imbalances are potassium deficit and potassium excess (Table 10-7).

To maintain potassium balance, the renal system must function, because 80% of the potassium excreted daily leaves the body by way of the kidneys; the other 20% is lost through the bowel and in sweat. The kidneys regulate potassium balance by adjusting the amount of potassium that is excreted in the urine. As serum potassium levels increase, so does the potassium level in the renal tubular cell. A concentration gradient occurs, favoring the movement of potassium into the renal tubule and excretion of potassium in the urine. Aldosterone also increases the excretion of potassium by the kidney. Because the kidneys do not conserve potassium as well as they conserve sodium, potassium may still be lost in urine in the presence of a potassium deficit (Norris, 2019).

Potassium Deficit (Hypokalemia)

Hypokalemia (serum potassium level below 3.5 mEq/L [3.5 mmol/L]) usually indicates a deficit in total potassium stores. However, it may occur in patients with normal potassium stores: When **alkalosis** (high blood pH) is present, a temporary shift of serum potassium into the cells occurs (see later discussion).

Pathophysiology

Potassium-losing diuretics, such as the thiazides and loop diuretics, can induce hypokalemia. Other medications that can lead to hypokalemia include corticosteroids, sodium penicillin, and amphotericin B (Vallerand & Sanoski, 2019). GI loss of potassium is another common cause of potassium depletion. Vomiting and gastric suction frequently lead to

TABLE 10-7	Potassium Imbalances	
Imbalance	**Contributing Factors**	**Signs/Symptoms**
Potassium deficit (hypokalemia) Serum potassium <3.5 mEq/L	Diarrhea, vomiting, gastric suction, corticosteroid administration, hyperaldosteronism, carbenicillin, amphotericin B, bulimia, osmotic diuresis, alkalosis, starvation, diuretics, and digoxin toxicity	Fatigue, anorexia, nausea and vomiting, muscle weakness, polyuria, decreased bowel motility, ventricular asystole or fibrillation, paresthesias, leg cramps, ↓ BP, ileus, abdominal distention, hypoactive reflexes. ECG: flattened T waves, prominent U waves, ST depression, prolonged PR interval
Potassium excess (hyperkalemia) Serum potassium >5.0 mEq/L	Pseudohyperkalemia, oliguric kidney injury, use of potassium-conserving diuretics in patients with renal insufficiency, metabolic acidosis, Addison disease, crush injury, burns, stored bank blood transfusions, rapid IV administration of potassium, and certain medications such as ACE inhibitors, NSAIDs, cyclosporine	Muscle weakness, tachycardia → bradycardia, arrhythmias, flaccid paralysis, paresthesias, intestinal colic, cramps, abdominal distention, irritability, anxiety. ECG: tall tented T waves, prolonged PR interval and QRS duration, absent P waves, ST depression

ACE, angiotensin-converting enzyme; BP, blood pressure; ↓, decreased; ECG, electrocardiogram; →, followed by; IV, intravenous; NSAIDs, nonsteroidal anti-inflammatory drugs.
Adapted from Norris, T. L. (2019). *Porth's pathophysiology: Concepts of altered health state* (10th ed.). Philadelphia, PA: Wolters Kluwer.

hypokalemia, because potassium is lost when gastric fluid is lost and because potassium is lost through the kidneys in response to metabolic alkalosis. Because relatively large amounts of potassium are contained in intestinal fluids, potassium deficit occurs frequently with diarrhea, which may contain as much potassium as 30 mEq/L. Potassium deficit also occurs from prolonged intestinal suctioning, recent ileostomy, and villous adenoma (a tumor of the intestinal tract characterized by excretion of potassium-rich mucus) (Mount, 2017b).

Alterations in acid–base balance have a significant effect on potassium distribution due to shifts of hydrogen and potassium ions between the cells and the ECF. Respiratory or metabolic alkalosis promotes the transcellular shift of potassium and can have a variable and unpredictable effect on serum potassium. For example, hydrogen ions move out of the cells into the bloodstream in alkalotic states to help correct the high pH, and potassium ions move into the cells to maintain an electrically neutral state (Mount, 2017c) (see later discussion of acid–base balance).

Aldosterone from the adrenal gland acts on the nephron to increase sodium and water reabsorption into the bloodstream. It simultaneously secretes potassium into the renal tubules which in turn is excreted in the urine. In hyperaldosteronism, potassium is constantly secreted into the nephron tubule fluid which leads to loss of potassium into the urine. Hyperaldosteronism causes renal potassium wasting and can lead to severe potassium depletion. Primary hyperaldosteronism is seen in patients with adrenal adenomas (tumors). Secondary hyperaldosteronism occurs in patients with cirrhosis, nephrotic syndrome, heart failure, or malignant hypertension (Dick, Queiroz, Bernardi, et al., 2018).

Insulin promotes the entry of potassium into cells from the bloodstream; therefore, patients with persistent insulin hypersecretion may experience hypokalemia. Patients receiving high carbohydrate parenteral nutrition will have increased secretion of insulin. This will cause the shift of potassium into the cells from the bloodstream, causing hypokalemia. In diabetic ketoacidosis (DKA), potassium moves out of the cell since H^+ ions are high; during this acute phase it seems as though the patient has hyperkalemia. With insulin treatment of DKA, potassium moves back into the cells, causing hypokalemia (Palmer & Clegg, 2016a).

Patients who are not able to eat a normal diet for a prolonged period are at risk for hypokalemia. This may occur in debilitated older adults and in patients with alcoholism or anorexia nervosa. In addition to poor intake, people with bulimia frequently experience increased potassium loss through self-induced vomiting and overuse of laxatives, diuretics, and enemas. These patients may also be deficient in magnesium. Magnesium depletion also causes renal potassium loss and must be corrected first; otherwise, urine loss of potassium will continue (Mount, 2017d).

Clinical Manifestations

Potassium deficiency can result in widespread derangements in physiologic function. Severe hypokalemia can cause death through cardiac or respiratory arrest. Clinical signs develop when the potassium level decreases to less than 3 mEq/L (3 mmol/L) (Mount, 2017b). Clinical signs and symptoms can be found in Table 10-7. If prolonged, hypokalemia can lead to an inability of the kidneys to concentrate urine, causing

dilute urine (resulting in polyuria, nocturia) and excessive thirst. Potassium depletion suppresses the release of insulin and results in glucose intolerance (Palmer & Clegg, 2016a).

Assessment and Diagnostic Findings

In hypokalemia, the serum potassium concentration is less than the lower limit of normal, which is 3.5 mEq/L. Electrocardiographic (ECG) changes can include flat T waves or inverted T waves or both, suggesting ischemia, and depressed ST segments (Fig. 10-8). An elevated U wave is specific to hypokalemia.

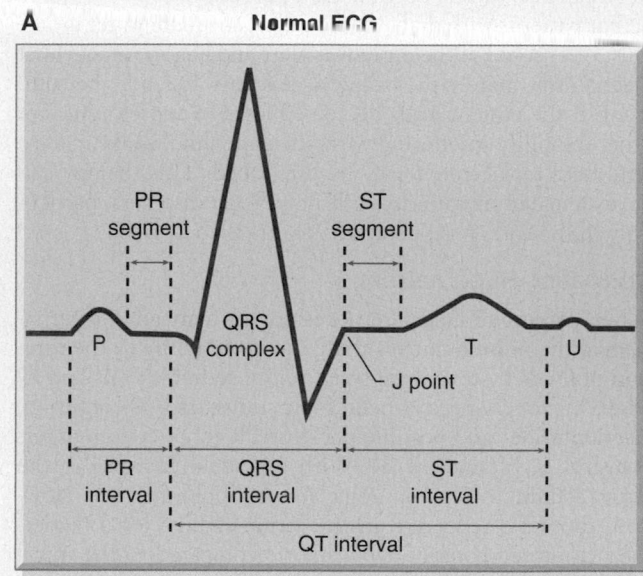

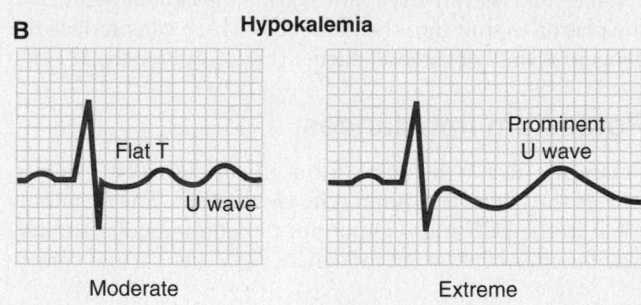

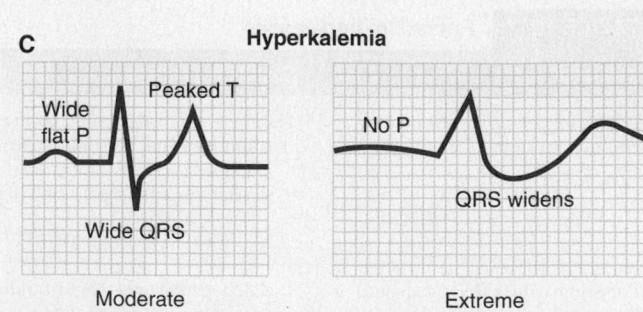

Figure 10-8 • Effect of potassium on the electrocardiogram (ECG). **A.** Normal tracing. **B.** Hypokalemia: serum potassium level below normal. **Left:** Flattening of the T wave and the appearance of a U wave. **Right:** Further flattening with prominent U wave. **C.** Hyperkalemia: serum potassium level above normal. **Left:** Moderate elevation with wide, flat P wave; wide QRS complex; and peaked T wave. **Right:** ECG changes seen with extreme potassium elevation: widening of QRS complex and absence of P wave.

Quality and Safety Nursing Alert

Hypokalemia increases sensitivity to digitalis, predisposing the patient to digitalis toxicity at lower digitalis levels.

Metabolic alkalosis is commonly associated with hypokalemia. This is discussed further in the section on acid–base disturbances in this chapter.

The source of the potassium loss is usually evident from a careful history. However, if the cause of the loss is unclear, a 24-hour urinary potassium excretion test can be performed to distinguish between renal and extrarenal loss. Urinary potassium excretion exceeding 20 mEq/day with hypokalemia suggests that renal potassium loss is the cause.

Medical Management

If hypokalemia cannot be prevented by conventional measures such as increased intake in the daily diet or by oral potassium supplements for deficiencies, then it is treated cautiously with IV replacement therapy (Mount, 2017b). Potassium loss must be corrected daily; administration of 40 to 60 mEq/day of potassium is adequate in the adult if there are no abnormal losses of potassium.

For patients who are at risk for hypokalemia, a diet containing sufficient potassium should be provided. Dietary intake of potassium in the average adult is 50 to 100 mEq/day. Foods high in potassium include most fruits and vegetables, legumes, whole grains, milk, and meat (Palmer & Clegg, 2016b).

When dietary intake is inadequate for any reason, oral or IV potassium supplements may be prescribed. Many salt substitutes contain 50 to 60 mEq of potassium per teaspoon and may be sufficient to prevent hypokalemia. If oral administration of potassium is not feasible, the IV route is indicated. The IV route is mandatory for patients with severe hypokalemia (e.g., serum level of 2 mEq/L). Although potassium chloride (KCl) is usually used to correct potassium deficits, potassium acetate or potassium phosphate may be prescribed (Mount, 2017e; Vallerand & Sanoski, 2019).

Nursing Management

Because hypokalemia can be life-threatening, the nurse needs to monitor for its early presence in patients at risk. Fatigue, anorexia, muscle weakness, decreased bowel motility, paresthesias, and arrhythmias are signals that warrant assessing the serum potassium concentration. When available, the ECG may provide useful information (Mount, 2017b). For example, patients receiving digitalis who are at risk for potassium deficiency should be monitored closely for signs of digitalis toxicity, because hypokalemia potentiates the action of digitalis.

Preventing Hypokalemia

The nurse helps prevent hypokalemia by encouraging patients at risk to eat foods rich in potassium (when the diet allows). Consumption of foods high in potassium should be encouraged; examples include bananas, melon, citrus fruits, fresh and frozen vegetables (avoid canned vegetables), lean meats, milk, and whole grains. If the hypokalemia is caused by abuse of laxatives or diuretics, patient education may help alleviate

the problem. Part of the health history and assessment should be directed at identifying problems that are amenable to prevention through education. Careful monitoring of fluid I&O is necessary, because 40 mEq of potassium is lost for every liter of urine output. The ECG is monitored for changes, and arterial blood gas (ABG) values are checked for elevated bicarbonate and pH levels.

Correcting Hypokalemia

The oral route is ideal to treat mild to moderate hypokalemia because oral potassium supplements are well absorbed. Care should be exercised when administering potassium, particularly in older adults, who have lower lean body mass and total-body potassium levels and therefore lower potassium requirements. In addition, because of the physiologic loss of renal function with advancing years, potassium may be retained more readily in older than in younger people (Cash & Glass, 2018).

Quality and Safety Nursing Alert

Oral potassium supplements can produce small bowel lesions; therefore, the patient must be assessed for and cautioned about abdominal distention, pain, or GI bleeding.

Administering Intravenous Potassium

Potassium should be given only after adequate urine output has been established. A decrease in urine volume to less than 20 mL/h for 2 consecutive hours is an indication to stop the potassium infusion and notify the primary provider. Potassium is primarily excreted by the kidneys; when oliguria occurs, potassium administration can cause the serum potassium concentration to rise to dangerous levels (Mount, 2017e).

Quality and Safety Nursing Alert

Potassium is never given by IV push or intramuscularly to avoid replacing potassium too quickly. Potassium is extremely irritating to tissues. IV potassium must be given using an infusion pump.

Each health care facility has its own policy for the administration of potassium, which must be consulted. Administration of IV potassium is done with extreme caution using an infusion pump with the patient monitored by continuous ECG. Caution must be used when selecting a premixed solution of IV fluid containing KCl, as the concentrations range from 10 to 40 mEq/100 mL. Renal function should be monitored through BUN and serum creatinine levels and urine output if the patient is receiving potassium replacement. During replacement therapy, the patient should be monitored for signs of worsening hypokalemia as well as hyperkalemia.

Potassium Excess (Hyperkalemia)

Hyperkalemia (serum potassium level greater than 5 mEq/L [5 mmol/L]) seldom occurs in patients with normal renal function. In older adults, there is an increased risk of hyperkalemia due to decreases in renin and aldosterone as well as an increased number of comorbid cardiac conditions. Like hypokalemia, hyperkalemia is often caused by iatrogenic (treatment-induced) causes. Although hyperkalemia is less common than hypokalemia, it is usually more dangerous because cardiac arrest is more frequently associated with high serum potassium levels (Mount, 2017a).

Pathophysiology

Major causes of hyperkalemia are decreased renal excretion of potassium, rapid administration of potassium, and movement of potassium from the ICF compartment to the ECF compartment. Hyperkalemia is commonly seen in patients with untreated kidney injury, particularly those in whom potassium levels increase as a result of infection or excessive intake of potassium in food or medications (Mount, 2017a). Patients with hypoaldosteronism or Addison disease are at risk for hyperkalemia because of a lack of aldosterone. Lack of aldosterone activity at the nephron causes inadequate sodium and water reabsorption into the bloodstream and inadequate excretion of potassium in the urine. Therefore, deficient adrenal hormones lead to sodium loss and potassium retention (Norris, 2019).

Medications have been identified as a probable contributing factor in more than 60% of hyperkalemic episodes. Medications commonly implicated are KCl, heparin, ACE inhibitors, NSAIDs, beta-blockers, cyclosporine, tacrolimus, and potassium-sparing diuretics (Comerford & Durkin, 2020). Potassium regulation is compromised in acute and chronic kidney disease, with a glomerular filtration rate less than 10% to 20% of normal (Mount, 2017c).

Improper use of potassium supplements predisposes all patients to hyperkalemia, especially if salt substitutes are used. Not all patients receiving potassium-losing diuretics require potassium supplements, and patients receiving potassium-conserving diuretics should not receive supplements.

> ▶ *Quality and Safety Nursing Alert*
>
> *Potassium supplements are extremely dangerous for patients who have impaired renal function and thus decreased ability to excrete potassium. Even more dangerous is the IV administration of potassium to such patients, because serum levels can rise very quickly. It is possible to exceed the renal tolerance of any patient with rapid IV potassium administration, as well as when large amounts of oral potassium supplements are ingested.*

In **acidosis** (low blood pH), potassium moves out of the cells and into the ECF. This occurs as hydrogen ions enter the cells to buffer the pH of the ECF (see later discussion).

An elevated ECF potassium level should be anticipated when extensive tissue trauma has occurred, as in burns, crushing injuries, or severe infections. Similarly, it can occur with lysis of malignant cells after chemotherapy (i.e., tumor lysis syndrome). Any disorder that causes high amounts of cellular lysis or deterioration can cause hyperkalemia (Mount, 2017a).

Pseudohyperkalemia (a false hyperkalemia) has several causes, including the improper collection or transport of a blood sample, a traumatic venipuncture, and use of a tight tourniquet around an exercising extremity while drawing a blood sample, producing hemolysis of the sample before analysis. Other causes include marked leukocytosis (white

blood cell count exceeding 200,000/mm³) and thrombocytosis (platelet count exceeding 1 million/mm³); drawing blood above a site where potassium is infusing; and familial pseudohyperkalemia, in which potassium leaks out of the RBCs while the blood is awaiting analysis. Lack of awareness of these causes of pseudohyperkalemia can lead to aggressive treatment of a nonexistent hyperkalemia, resulting in serious lowering of serum potassium levels. Therefore, measurements of grossly elevated levels of potassium in the absence of clinical manifestations (e.g., normal ECG) should be verified by retesting (Mount, 2017a).

Clinical Manifestations

Clinical signs and symptoms can be found in Table 10-7. The most important consequence of hyperkalemia is its effect on the myocardium. Cardiac effects of elevated serum potassium are usually not significant when the level is less than 7 mEq/L (7 mmol/L); however, they are almost always present when the level is 8 mEq/L (8 mmol/L) or greater. As the plasma potassium level rises, disturbances in cardiac conduction occur. The earliest changes, often occurring at a serum potassium level greater than 6 mEq/L (6 mmol/L), are peaked, narrow T waves; ST-segment depression; and a shortened QT interval. If the serum potassium level continues to increase, the PR interval becomes prolonged and is followed by disappearance of the P waves. Finally, there is decomposition and widening of the QRS complex (see Fig. 10-7). Ventricular arrhythmias and cardiac arrest may occur (Mount, 2017a).

Assessment and Diagnostic Findings

Serum potassium levels and ECG changes are crucial to the diagnosis of hyperkalemia, as discussed previously. ABG analysis may reveal either a metabolic or a respiratory acidosis. These are discussed further in the section on acid–base disturbances in this chapter. Correcting the acidosis helps correct the hyperkalemia.

Medical Management

In disorders involving potassium level changes, an ECG should be obtained immediately. Shortened repolarization and peaked T waves are seen initially in hyperkalemia. To verify results, a repeat serum potassium level should be obtained from a vein that is not concomitantly infusing an IV solution containing potassium (Mount, 2017e).

In nonacute situations, restriction of dietary potassium and potassium-containing medications may correct the imbalance. For example, eliminating the use of potassium-containing salt substitutes in a patient who is taking a potassium-conserving diuretic may be all that is needed to deal with mild hyperkalemia.

Administration, either orally or by retention enema, of cation exchange resins (e.g., sodium polystyrene sulfonate) may be necessary. The use of cation exchange resins requires normal bowel function. For instance, cation exchange resins cannot be used if the patient has a paralytic ileus (i.e., absence of peristalsis in the intestine), because intestinal perforation can occur. Sodium polystyrene sulfonate binds with potassium and then is eliminated in the feces. Other cations in the GI tract can also be depleted which can cause hypomagnesemia and hypocalcemia. Sodium polystyrene sulfonate may also cause sodium retention and fluid overload and should be used with caution in patients with heart failure (Frandsen & Pennington, 2018; Mount, 2017e).

Patiromer sorbitex calcium is another oral agent that is a potassium-removing resin used to treat hyperkalemia. It exchanges calcium for potassium in the lower intestine, thereby increasing fecal excretion of potassium. Side effects include GI intolerance, hypomagnesemia, and edema (Depret, Peacock, Liu, et al., 2019).

Emergency Pharmacologic Therapy

If serum potassium levels are dangerously elevated, it may be necessary to administer IV calcium gluconate. Within minutes after administration, calcium antagonizes the action of hyperkalemia on the heart but does not reduce the serum potassium concentration. Calcium chloride and calcium gluconate are not interchangeable; calcium gluconate contains 4.5 mEq of calcium, and calcium chloride contains 13.6 mEq of calcium. Therefore, caution is required when using calcium preparations to reduce potassium levels (Ashurst, Sergent, & Sergent, 2016).

Monitoring the blood pressure is essential to detect hypotension, which may result from the rapid IV administration of calcium gluconate. The ECG should be continuously monitored during administration; the appearance of bradycardia is an indication to stop the infusion. The myocardial protective effects of calcium last about 30 minutes. Extra caution is required if the patient has received an accelerated dose of a digitalis-based cardiac glycoside to reach a desired serum digitalis level rapidly as parenteral administration of calcium sensitizes the heart to digitalis and may precipitate digitalis toxicity (Ashurst et al., 2016).

IV administration of sodium bicarbonate may be necessary in severe metabolic acidosis to alkalinize the plasma, shift potassium into the cells, and furnish sodium to antagonize the cardiac effects of potassium. Effects of this therapy begin within 30 to 60 minutes and may persist for hours; however, they are temporary. Circulatory overload and hypernatremia can occur when large amounts of hypertonic sodium bicarbonate are given. Bicarbonate therapy should be guided by the bicarbonate concentration or calculated base deficit obtained from blood gas analysis or laboratory measurement (Mount, 2017c).

IV administration of regular insulin and a hypertonic dextrose solution causes a temporary shift of potassium into the cells. Glucose and insulin therapy have an onset of action within 30 minutes and lasts for several hours. Loop diuretics, such as furosemide, increase excretion of water by inhibiting sodium, potassium, and chloride reabsorption in the ascending loop of Henle and distal renal tubule (Ashurst et al., 2016).

Beta-2 agonists, such as albuterol, are highly effective in decreasing potassium; however, their use is not without risk as they can cause tachycardia and chest discomfort (Depret et al., 2019; Long, Warix, & Koyfman, 2018). Beta-2 agonists, administered intravenously or via nebulizer, move potassium into the cells and may be used in the absence of ischemic cardiac disease. Their use is a stopgap measure that only temporarily protects the patient from hyperkalemia.

If the hyperkalemic condition is not transient, removal of potassium from the body can also be done through peritoneal dialysis, hemodialysis, or other forms of renal replacement therapy.

Nursing Management

Patients at risk for potassium excess (e.g., those with kidney disease) need to be identified and closely monitored for signs of hyperkalemia. The nurse monitors I&O and observes for signs of muscle weakness and arrhythmias. When measuring vital signs, an apical pulse should be taken. The presence of paresthesias and GI symptoms such as nausea and intestinal cramping should be noted. Serum potassium levels, as well as BUN, serum creatinine, serum glucose, and ABG values, should be monitored for patients at risk for developing hyperkalemia.

Preventing Hyperkalemia

Measures should be taken to prevent hyperkalemia in patients at risk, when possible, by encouraging the patient to adhere to the prescribed potassium restriction. Potassium-rich foods to be avoided include many fruits and vegetables, legumes, whole-grain breads, lean meat, milk, eggs, coffee, tea, and cocoa. Conversely, foods with minimal potassium content include butter, margarine, cranberry juice or sauce, ginger ale, gumdrops or jelly beans, hard candy, root beer, sugar, and honey. Labels of cola beverages must be checked carefully because some are high in potassium and some are not (McDonough & Youn, 2017).

Correcting Hyperkalemia

It is possible to exceed the tolerance for potassium if given rapidly by the IV route. Therefore, careful monitoring is necessary when administering potassium solutions. Particular attention is paid to the solution's concentration and rate of administration. IV administration should only be via an infusion pump (Mount, 2017e).

The nurse must caution patients to use salt substitutes sparingly if they are taking other supplementary forms of potassium or potassium-conserving diuretics. In addition, potassium-conserving diuretics, potassium supplements, and salt substitutes should not be given to patients with kidney injury (Mount, 2017e).

Calcium Imbalances

More than 99% of the body's calcium (Ca^{++}) is located in the skeletal system; it is a major component of bones and teeth. About 1% of skeletal calcium is rapidly exchangeable with blood calcium, and the rest is more stable and only slowly exchanged. The small amount of calcium located outside the bone circulates in the serum, partly bound to protein and partly ionized. Calcium plays a major role in transmitting nerve impulses and helps regulate muscle contraction and relaxation, including cardiac muscle. Calcium is instrumental in activating enzymes that stimulate many essential chemical reactions in the body, and it also plays a role in blood coagulation. Because many factors affect calcium regulation, both hypocalcemia and hypercalcemia are relatively common disturbances (Norris, 2019) (Table 10-8).

The normal adult total serum calcium level is 8.8 to 10.4 mg/dL (2.2 to 2.6 mmol/L) (Fischbach & Fischbach, 2018). Calcium exists in plasma in three forms: ionized,

TABLE 10-8 Calcium Imbalances

Imbalance	Contributing Factors	Signs/Symptoms and Laboratory Findings
Calcium deficit (hypocalcemia) Serum calcium <8.8 mg/dL	Hypoparathyroidism (may follow thyroid surgery or radical neck dissection), malabsorption, pancreatitis, alkalosis, vitamin D deficiency, massive subcutaneous infection, generalized peritonitis, massive transfusion of citrated blood, chronic diarrhea, decreased parathyroid hormone, diuretic phase of acute kidney injury, $\uparrow PO_4$, fistulas, burns, alcoholism	Numbness, tingling of fingers, toes, and circumoral region; positive Trousseau sign and Chvostek sign; seizures, carpopedal spasms, hyperactive deep tendon reflexes, irritability, bronchospasm, anxiety, impaired clotting time, $\downarrow$ prothrombin, diarrhea, $\downarrow$ BP. ECG: prolonged QT interval and lengthened ST *Labs indicate:* $\downarrow Mg^{++}$
Calcium excess (hypercalcemia) Serum calcium > 10.1 mg/dL	Hyperparathyroidism, malignant neoplastic disease, prolonged immobilization, overuse of calcium supplements, vitamin D excess, oliguric phase of acute kidney injury acidosis, corticosteroid therapy, thiazide diuretic use, increased parathyroid hormone, and digoxin toxicity	Muscular weakness, constipation, anorexia, nausea and vomiting, polyuria and polydipsia, dehydration, hypoactive deep tendon reflexes, lethargy, deep bone pain, pathologic fractures, flank pain, calcium stones, hypertension. ECG: shortened ST segment and QT interval, bradycardia, heart blocks

BP, blood pressure; $\downarrow$, decreased; ECG, electrocardiogram; $\uparrow$, increased.
Adapted from Norris, T. L. (2019). *Porth's pathophysiology: Concepts of altered health state* (10th ed.). Philadelphia, PA: Wolters Kluwer.

bound, and complex. Approximately 50% of the serum calcium exists in a physiologically active ionized form that is important for neuromuscular activity and blood coagulation; this is the only physiologically and clinically significant form. The normal ionized serum calcium level is 4.5 to 5.1 mg/dL (1.1 to 1.3 mmol/L). Less than half of the plasma calcium is bound to serum proteins, primarily albumin. The remainder is combined with nonprotein anions: phosphate, citrate, and carbonate (Hogan & Goldfarb, 2018).

Calcium is absorbed from foods in the presence of normal gastric acidity and vitamin D. It is excreted primarily in the feces, with the remainder excreted in the urine. The serum calcium level is controlled by PTH and calcitonin. As ionized serum calcium decreases in the bloodstream, the parathyroid glands secrete PTH. This, in turn, increases calcium absorption from the GI tract, increases calcium reabsorption from the renal tubule, and releases calcium from the bone. The resultant increase in calcium ion concentration in the bloodstream then suppresses PTH secretion. When calcium increases excessively, the thyroid gland secretes calcitonin, which inhibits calcium reabsorption from bone and decreases the serum calcium concentration (Norris, 2019).

Calcium Deficit (Hypocalcemia)

Hypocalcemia (serum calcium value lower than 8.8 mg/dL [2.20 mmol/L]) occurs in a variety of clinical situations. A patient may have a total-body calcium deficit (as in osteoporosis) but a normal serum calcium level. Older adults and those with disability have an increased risk of hypocalcemia because immobility, particularly lack of weight-bearing activity, increases bone resorption (Cash & Glass, 2018; Goltzman, 2017).

Pathophysiology

The parathyroid glands are instrumental in regulating blood and body calcium levels. Several factors can cause hypocalcemia, including primary hypoparathyroidism and surgical hypoparathyroidism. Surgical hypoparathyroidism is more common as a result of unintentional trauma or devascularization of the parathyroid glands (Kazaure & Sosa, 2018). Not only is hypocalcemia associated with thyroid and parathyroid surgery, but it can also occur after radical neck dissection and is most likely in the first 24 to 48 hours after surgery. Transient hypocalcemia can occur with massive administration of citrated blood (i.e., massive hemorrhage and shock), because citrate can combine with ionized calcium and temporarily remove it from the circulation (Goltzman, 2017).

Inflammation of the pancreas causes the breakdown of proteins and lipids. It is thought that calcium ions combine with the fatty acids released by lipolysis, forming soaplike compounds. As a result of this process, hypocalcemia occurs and is common in pancreatitis. Hypocalcemia may also be related to excessive secretion of glucagon from the inflamed pancreas, which results in increased secretion of calcitonin from the thyroid gland.

Hypocalcemia is common in patients with acute kidney injury, because these patients frequently have elevated serum phosphate levels. Hyperphosphatemia usually causes a reciprocal drop in the serum calcium level. Other causes of hypocalcemia include inadequate vitamin D consumption, magnesium deficiency, medullary thyroid carcinoma, low serum albumin levels, alkalosis, and alcohol abuse. Medications predisposing to hypocalcemia include aluminum-containing antacids, aminoglycosides, caffeine, cisplatin, corticosteroids, mithramycin, phosphates, isoniazid, loop diuretics, and proton pump inhibitors (Goltzman, 2017).

Clinical Manifestations

Tetany, the most characteristic manifestation of hypocalcemia and hypomagnesemia, refers to the entire symptom complex induced by increased neural excitability. Clinical signs and symptoms are caused by spontaneous discharges of both sensory and motor fibers in peripheral nerves and are outlined in Table 10-8.

Chvostek sign (Fig. 10-9A) consists of twitching of muscles innervated by the facial nerve in response to tapping of the muscle just below the zygomatic arch. Trousseau sign (Fig. 10-9B) can be elicited by inflating a blood pressure cuff on the upper arm to about 20 mm Hg above systolic pressure; within 2 to 5 minutes, carpal spasm will occur as ischemia of the ulnar nerve develops (Goltzman, 2019a).

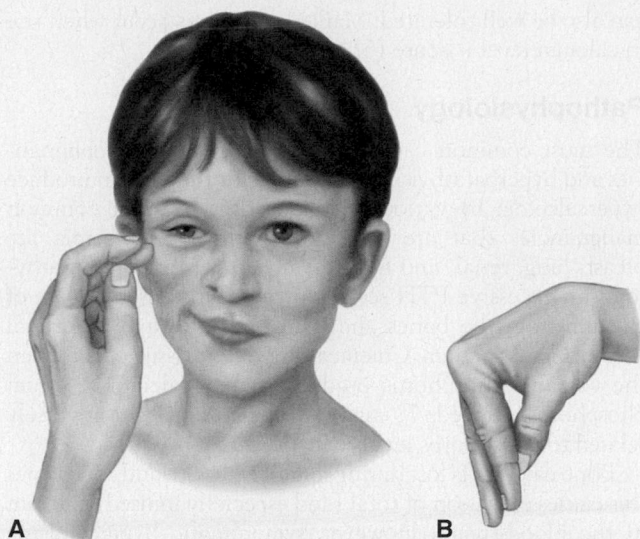

Figure 10-9 • A. Chvostek sign: a contraction of the facial muscles elicited in response to light tap over the facial nerve in front of the ear. **B.** Trousseau sign: a carpopedal spasm induced by inflating a blood pressure cuff above systolic blood pressure. Adapted from Bullock, B. A., & Henze, R. J. (2000). *Focus on pathophysiology* (p. 173). Philadelphia, PA: Lippincott Williams & Wilkins.

Chart 10-2 **Calculating Corrected Serum Calcium Level**

Abnormalities in serum albumin levels may affect interpretation of the serum calcium level. Below is a method for calculating the corrected serum calcium level if the serum albumin level is abnormal.

Quick Calculation Method

Measured total serum Ca^{++} level (mg/dL) + 0.8
× (4.0 − Measured albumin level [g/dL])
= Corrected total calcium concentration (mg/dL)

Example Calculation

A patient's reported serum albumin level is 2.5 g/dL; the reported serum calcium level is 10.5 mg/dL. First, the decrease in serum albumin level from normal (i.e., the difference from the normal albumin concentration of 4 g/dL) is calculated: 4 g/dL − 2.5 g/dL = 1.5 g/dL. Next, the following ratio is calculated:

0.8 mg/dL:1 g/dL = X mg/dL:1.5 mg/dL
X = 0.8 × 1.5 mg/dL
X = 1.2 mg/dL calcium

Finally, 1.2 mg/dL is added to 10.5 mg/dL (the reported serum calcium level) to obtain the corrected total serum calcium level: 1.2 mg/dL + 10.5 mg/dL = 11.7 mg/dL.

Hypocalcemia can cause seizures because low calcium levels increase irritability of the central and peripheral nervous systems. Other changes associated with hypocalcemia include mental changes such as depression, impaired memory, confusion, delirium, and hallucinations. A prolonged QT interval is seen on the ECG due to prolongation of the ST segment, and torsades de pointes, a type of ventricular tachycardia, may occur. Respiratory effects with decreasing calcium include dyspnea and laryngospasm. Signs and symptoms of chronic hypocalcemia include hyperactive bowel sounds, dry and brittle hair and nails, and abnormal clotting (Goltzman, 2019a).

Osteoporosis is associated with prolonged low intake of calcium and represents a total-body calcium deficit, even though serum calcium levels are usually normal. This disorder occurs in millions of Americans and is most common in postmenopausal women. It is characterized by loss of bone mass, which causes bones to become porous and brittle and therefore susceptible to fracture (Black & Rosen, 2016) (see Chapter 36 for further discussion of osteoporosis).

Assessment and Diagnostic Findings

When evaluating serum calcium levels, the serum albumin level and the arterial pH must also be considered. Because abnormalities in serum albumin levels may affect interpretation of the serum calcium level, it may be necessary to calculate the corrected serum calcium if the serum albumin level is abnormal. For every decrease in serum albumin of 1 g/dL below 4 g/dL, the total serum calcium level is underestimated by approximately 0.8 mg/dL (Hogan & Goldfarb, 2018). Chart 10-2 displays a quick method that nurses can use to calculate the corrected serum calcium level.

Clinicians often discount a low serum calcium level in the presence of a similarly low serum albumin level. The ionized calcium level is usually normal in patients with reduced total serum calcium levels and concomitant hypoalbuminemia.

When the arterial pH increases (alkalosis), more calcium becomes bound to protein. As a result, the ionized portion decreases. Symptoms of hypocalcemia may occur with alkalosis. Acidosis has the opposite effect—that is, less calcium is bound to protein and therefore more exists in the ionized form. However, relatively small changes in serum calcium levels occur in these acid–base abnormalities (Yu & Stubbs, 2019).

Ideally, the ionized level of calcium should be measured in the laboratory. However, in many laboratories, only the total calcium level is reported; therefore, the concentration of the ionized fraction must be estimated by simultaneous measurement of the serum albumin level. Magnesium and phosphorus levels need to be assessed to identify possible causes of decreased calcium (Yu & Stubbs, 2019).

Medical Management

Emergency Pharmacologic Therapy

Acute symptomatic hypocalcemia is life-threatening and requires prompt treatment with IV administration of a calcium salt. Parenteral calcium salts include calcium gluconate and calcium chloride (Duval, Bach, Masson, et al., 2018; Goltzman, 2019b). Although calcium chloride produces a significantly higher ionized calcium level than calcium gluconate does, it is not used as often because it is more irritating and can cause sloughing of tissue if it infiltrates.

IV administration of calcium is particularly dangerous in patients receiving digitalis-derived medications, because calcium ions exert an effect similar to that of digitalis and can cause digitalis toxicity, with adverse cardiac effects. The IV site that delivers calcium must be observed often for any evidence of infiltration because of the risk of extravasation and resultant cellulitis or necrosis. A 0.9% sodium chloride solution should not be used with calcium because it increases renal calcium loss. Solutions containing phosphates or bicarbonate should not be used with calcium because they cause precipitation when calcium is added. The nurse must clarify with the primary provider and pharmacist which calcium salt to administer, because calcium gluconate yields 4.5 mEq of calcium and calcium chloride provides 13.6 mEq of calcium. Calcium replacement can cause orthostatic hypotension; therefore, the patient should remain in bed during IV infusion, and blood pressure is monitored (Duval et al., 2018).

> ### ▶ Quality and Safety Nursing Alert
>
> *Too rapid IV administration of calcium can cause cardiac arrest, preceded by bradycardia. Therefore, calcium should be diluted in D$_5$W and given as a slow IV bolus or a slow IV infusion using an infusion pump. A 0.9% sodium chloride solution should not be used when administering calcium.*

Nutritional Therapy

Vitamin D therapy may be instituted to increase calcium absorption from the GI tract; otherwise, the amount of calcium absorbed may not satisfy the body's calcium requirement. In addition, aluminum hydroxide, calcium acetate, or calcium carbonate antacids may be prescribed to decrease elevated phosphorus levels before treating hypocalcemia in the patient with chronic kidney disease. Increasing the dietary intake of calcium to at least 1000 to 1500 mg/day in the adult is recommended. Calcium supplements must be given in divided doses of no higher than 500 mg to promote calcium absorption. Calcium-containing foods include milk products; green, leafy vegetables; canned salmon; canned sardines; and fresh oysters. Hypomagnesemia can also cause tetany; if the tetany responds to IV calcium, then a low magnesium level is considered as a possible cause in chronic kidney dysfunction (Goltzman, 2019b; Rosen & Drezner, 2019).

Nursing Management

It is important to assess for hypocalcemia in at-risk patients. Seizure precautions are initiated if hypocalcemia is severe. The status of the airway is closely monitored because laryngospasm can occur. Safety precautions are taken, as indicated, if confusion is present (Duval et al., 2018).

The nurse must educate the patient with hypocalcemia about foods that are rich in calcium. The nurse must also advise the patient to consider calcium supplements if sufficient calcium is not consumed in the diet. Such supplements should be taken in divided doses with meals. Alcohol and caffeine in high doses inhibit calcium absorption, and moderate cigarette smoking increases urinary calcium excretion. The patient is also cautioned to avoid the overuse of laxatives and antacids that contain phosphorus, because their use decreases calcium absorption (Rosen & Drezner, 2019).

Calcium Excess (Hypercalcemia)

Hypercalcemia (serum calcium value greater than 10.4 mg/dL [2.6 mmol/L]) can affect many organ systems. Symptoms depend on the degree of hypercalcemia and the rate of rise of calcium in the bloodstream. Mild hypercalcemia usually causes no apparent symptoms if the rise in calcium level is chronic over a long period of time. Moderate hypercalcemia can also be well tolerated. Marked symptoms occur when rise in calcium level is acute (Shane, 2019b).

Pathophysiology

The most common causes of hypercalcemia are malignancies and hyperparathyroidism. Malignant tumors can produce hypercalcemia by various mechanisms. The most common malignancies that are associated with hypercalcemia are breast, lung, renal, and multiple myeloma. In hyperparathyroidism, excessive PTH secretion causes increased release of calcium from the bones and increased intestinal and renal absorption of calcium. Calcifications of soft tissue occur when the calcium–phosphorus product (serum calcium × serum phosphorus) exceeds 70 mg/dL. Calcium levels are inversely related to phosphorus levels (Shane, 2019a).

Bone calcium is lost during immobilization, and sometimes this causes elevation of total (and especially ionized) calcium in the bloodstream. However, symptomatic hypercalcemia from immobilization is rare; when it does occur, it is limited to people with high calcium turnover rates (e.g., adolescents during a growth spurt). Most cases of hypercalcemia secondary to immobility occur after severe or multiple fractures or spinal cord injury (Shane, 2019a).

Thiazide diuretics can cause a slight elevation in serum calcium levels because they potentiate the action of PTH on the kidneys, reducing urinary calcium excretion. Vitamin A and D intoxication, as well as chronic lithium use and theophylline toxicity, can cause calcium excess.

Hypercalcemia reduces neuromuscular excitability because it suppresses activity at the myoneural junction. Decreased tone in smooth and striated muscle may cause symptoms such as muscle weakness, incoordination, anorexia, and constipation. Lethal arrhythmias (e.g., ventricular fibrillation) can occur when the serum calcium level is about 18 mg/dL (4.5 mmol/L). Calcium enhances the inotropic effect of digitalis; therefore, hypercalcemia aggravates digitalis toxicity (Shane, 2019a).

Clinical Manifestations

Clinical signs and symptoms can be found in Table 10-8. The symptoms of hypercalcemia are proportional to the degree of elevation of the serum calcium level. The more severe symptoms tend to appear when the serum calcium level climbs rapidly and may be as high as 16 mg/dL (4 mmol/L) or higher. However, some patients become profoundly disturbed with serum calcium levels of only 12 mg/dL (3 mmol/L). These symptoms resolve as serum calcium levels return to normal after treatment (Shane, 2019b).

Hypercalcemic crisis refers to an acute rise in the serum calcium level. Severe thirst and polyuria are often present. Other findings may include muscle weakness, intractable nausea, abdominal cramps, severe constipation, diarrhea, peptic ulcer symptoms, and bone pain. Lethargy, confusion, and coma may also occur. This condition is dangerous and may result in cardiac arrest. Emergency treatment with calcitonin is indicated (Shane & Berenson, 2019) (see later discussion under Pharmacologic Therapy).

Assessment and Diagnostic Findings

In hypercalcemia, the serum calcium level is greater than 10.4 mg/dL (2.6 mmol/L). Cardiovascular changes may include a variety of arrhythmias (e.g., heart blocks) and shortening of the QT interval and ST segment. The PR interval is sometimes prolonged. The double-antibody PTH test may be used to differentiate between primary hyperparathyroidism and malignancy as a cause of hypercalcemia: PTH levels are increased in primary or secondary hyperparathyroidism and suppressed in malignancy. X-rays may reveal bone changes if the patient has hypercalcemia secondary to a malignancy, bone cavitations, or urinary calculi. Urine calcium can be normal or elevated in hyperparathyroidism and hypercalcemia caused by malignancy (Shane, 2019b).

Medical Management

Therapeutic aims include decreasing the serum calcium level and reversing the process causing the hypercalcemia. Treating the underlying cause (e.g., chemotherapy for a malignancy, partial parathyroidectomy for hyperparathyroidism) is essential.

Pharmacologic Therapy

To treat hypercalcemia, measures include administering fluids to dilute serum calcium and promote its excretion by the kidneys, mobilizing the patient, and restricting dietary calcium intake. IV administration of 0.9% sodium chloride solution temporarily dilutes the serum calcium level and increases urinary calcium excretion by inhibiting tubular reabsorption of calcium. Administering IV phosphate can cause a reciprocal drop in serum calcium. Furosemide is often used in conjunction with administration of a saline solution; in addition to causing diuresis, furosemide increases calcium excretion. Although often overlooked, fluids and medications that contain calcium and dietary sources of calcium should be halted (Shane & Berenson, 2019).

Calcitonin can be used to lower the serum calcium level and is particularly useful for patients with heart disease or acute kidney injury who cannot tolerate large sodium loads. Calcitonin reduces bone resorption, increases the deposition of calcium and phosphorus in the bones, and increases urinary excretion of calcium and phosphorus. Although several forms are available, calcitonin derived from salmon is commonly used. Skin testing for allergy to salmon calcitonin may be necessary before the hormone is given. Systemic allergic reactions are possible because this hormone is a protein; resistance to the medication may develop later because of antibody formation. Calcitonin is administered by intramuscular injection or intranasal spray rather than subcutaneously, because patients with hypercalcemia have poor perfusion of subcutaneous tissue (Shane & Berenson, 2019).

For patients with cancer, treatment is directed at controlling the condition by surgery, chemotherapy, or radiation therapy. Corticosteroids may be used to decrease bone turnover and tubular reabsorption for patients with sarcoidosis, myelomas, lymphomas, and leukemias; patients with solid tumors are less responsive. Some bisphosphonates (e.g., pamidronate disodium, ibandronate sodium) inhibit osteoclast activity. IV forms of bisphosphonates can cause fever, transient leukopenia, eye inflammation, nephrotic syndrome, and jaw osteonecrosis (Shane & Berenson, 2019).

Mithramycin, a cytotoxic antibiotic, inhibits bone resorption and thus lowers the serum calcium level. This agent must be used cautiously because it has significant side effects, including thrombocytopenia, nephrotoxicity, rebound hypercalcemia when discontinued, and hepatotoxicity. Inorganic phosphate salts can be given orally or by nasogastric tube (in the form of Phospho-Soda or Neutra-Phos), rectally (as retention enemas), or IV. IV phosphate therapy is used with extreme caution in the treatment of hypercalcemia, because it can cause severe calcification in various tissues, hypotension, tetany, and acute kidney injury (Frandsen & Pennington, 2018; Vallerand & Sanoski, 2019).

Nursing Management

The nurse must monitor for hypercalcemia in at-risk patients. Interventions such as increasing patient mobility and encouraging fluids can help prevent hypercalcemia, or at least minimize its severity. Hospitalized patients at risk should be encouraged to ambulate as soon as possible. Those who are outpatients and receive home care are educated about the importance of frequent ambulation (Daly, 2017).

When encouraging oral fluids, the nurse considers the patient's likes and dislikes. Fluids containing sodium should be given unless contraindicated, because sodium assists with calcium excretion. Patients are encouraged to drink 2.8 to 3.8 L (3 to 4 quarts) of fluid daily (Sterns, 2017b). Adequate fiber in the diet is encouraged to offset the tendency for constipation. Safety precautions are implemented, as necessary, when altered mental status is present. The patient and family are informed that these mental changes are reversible with treatment. Increased calcium increases the effects of digitalis; therefore, the patient on digitalis should be frequently assessed for signs and symptoms of digitalis toxicity. Because ECG changes (premature ventricular contractions, paroxysmal atrial tachycardia, and heart block) can occur, the cardiac rate and rhythm are monitored for any abnormalities (Shane & Berenson, 2019; Vallerand & Sanoski, 2019).

Magnesium Imbalances

Magnesium (Mg^{++}) is an abundant intracellular cation. It acts as an activator for many intracellular enzyme systems and plays a role in both carbohydrate and protein metabolism. The normal serum magnesium level is 1.8 to 2.6 mg/dL (0.74 to 1.07 mmol/L) (Fischbach & Fischbach, 2018). Approximately one third of serum magnesium is bound to protein; the remaining two thirds exist as free cations—the active component (Mg^{++}). Magnesium balance is important in neuromuscular function. Because magnesium acts directly on the myoneural junction, variations in the serum level affect neuromuscular irritability and contractility. For example, an excess of magnesium diminishes the excitability of the muscle cells, whereas a deficit increases neuromuscular irritability and contractility. Magnesium produces its sedative effect at the neuromuscular junction, probably by inhibiting the release of the neurotransmitter acetylcholine. It also increases the stimulus threshold in nerve fibers. Magnesium imbalances are magnesium deficit and magnesium excess (Norris, 2019) (Table 10-9).

Magnesium also affects the cardiovascular system, acting peripherally to produce vasodilation and decreased peripheral resistance. Most magnesium in the body is stored within bone, whereas magnesium ions in the blood are bound to protein, such as albumin, or free as Mg^{++} ions (Yu, 2019a).

TABLE 10-9 Magnesium Imbalances

Imbalance	Contributing Factors	Signs/Symptoms
Magnesium deficit (hypomagnesemia) Serum magnesium <1.8 mg/dL	Chronic alcoholism, hyperparathyroidism, hyperaldosteronism, diuretic phase of acute kidney injury, malabsorptive disorders, diabetic ketoacidosis, refeeding after starvation, parenteral nutrition, chronic laxative use, diarrhea, acute myocardial infarction, heart failure, decreased serum K^+ and Ca^{++} and certain pharmacologic agents (e.g., gentamicin, cisplatin, cyclosporine)	Neuromuscular irritability, positive Trousseau sign and Chvostek sign, insomnia, mood changes, anorexia, vomiting, increased tendon reflexes, and ↑ BP. ECG: PVCs, flat or inverted T waves, depressed ST segment, prolonged PR interval, and widened QRS
Magnesium excess (hypermagnesemia) Serum magnesium >2.6 mg/dL	Oliguric phase of acute kidney injury (particularly when magnesium-containing medications are given), adrenal insufficiency, excessive IV magnesium administration, diabetic ketoacidosis, and hypothyroidism	Flushing, hypotension, muscle weakness, drowsiness, hypoactive reflexes, depressed respirations, cardiac arrest and coma, diaphoresis. ECG: tachycardia → bradycardia, prolonged PR interval and QRS, peaked T waves

BP, blood pressure; ECG, electrocardiogram; →, followed by; ↑, increased; IV, intravenous; PVCs, premature ventricular contractions.
Adapted from Norris, T. L. (2019). *Porth's pathophysiology: Concepts of altered health state* (10th ed.). Philadelphia, PA: Wolters Kluwer.

Magnesium Deficit (Hypomagnesemia)

Hypomagnesemia refers to a below-normal serum magnesium concentration and is frequently associated with hypokalemia and hypocalcemia. Magnesium is similar to calcium in two aspects: (1) it is the ionized fraction of magnesium that is primarily involved in neuromuscular activity and other physiologic processes, and (2) magnesium levels should be evaluated in combination with albumin levels. Because about 30% of magnesium is protein bound, principally to albumin, a decreased serum albumin level can reduce the measured total magnesium concentration; however, it does not reduce the ionized plasma magnesium concentration. Magnesium is essential for the function of the Na^+/K^+ pump, and low Mg^{++} levels have effects on intracellular influxes of K^+ and myocardial ion fluxes (Norris, 2019; Yu, 2019a).

Pathophysiology

An important route of magnesium loss is the GI tract; such loss can occur with nasogastric suction, diarrhea, or fistulas. Because fluid from the lower GI tract has a higher concentration of magnesium (10 to 14 mEq/L) than fluid from the upper tract (1 to 2 mEq/L), losses from diarrhea and intestinal fistulas are more likely to induce magnesium deficit than are those from gastric suction. Although magnesium losses are relatively small in nasogastric suction, hypomagnesemia occurs if losses are prolonged and magnesium is not replaced through IV infusion. Because the distal small bowel is the major site of magnesium absorption, any disruption in small bowel function (e.g., intestinal resection or inflammatory bowel disease) can lead to hypomagnesemia. Hypomagnesemia is a common yet often overlooked imbalance in acutely and critically ill patients. Studies suggest that up to 65% of patients in intensive care are magnesium deficient (Upala, Jaruvongvanich, Wijarnpreecha, et al., 2016). Hypomagnesemia may occur with withdrawal from alcohol and administration of tube feedings or parenteral nutrition (Yu, 2019a).

Chronic alcohol abuse is a major cause of symptomatic hypomagnesemia in the United States. The serum magnesium level should be measured at least every 2 or 3 days in patients undergoing withdrawal from alcohol. The level may be normal on admission but may decrease as a result of metabolic changes, such as the intracellular shift of magnesium associated with IV glucose administration (Yu, 2019a).

During nutritional replacement, the major cellular electrolytes move from the serum to intracellular compartments of newly synthesized cells. Therefore, if the enteral or parenteral feeding formula is deficient in magnesium content, serious hypomagnesemia can occur. Because of this, serum magnesium levels should be measured at regular intervals in patients who are receiving parenteral or enteral feedings, especially those who have undergone a period of starvation (Yu, 2019a).

Other causes of hypomagnesemia include the administration of aminoglycosides, cyclosporine, cisplatin, diuretics, digitalis, proton pump inhibitors, and amphotericin, as well as the rapid administration of citrated blood, especially to patients with renal or hepatic disease. Magnesium deficiency often occurs in DKA, secondary to increased renal excretion during osmotic diuresis and shifting of magnesium into the cells with insulin therapy (Yu, 2019a). A magnesium IV solution can be used to counteract seizures due to preeclampsia or eclampsia, the cardiac arrhythmia torsades de pointes, asthma, and hypertension (Vallerand & Sanoski, 2019).

Clinical Manifestations

Clinical signs and symptoms can be found in Table 10-9. Some clinical manifestations of hypomagnesemia are due directly to the low serum magnesium level; others are due to secondary changes in potassium and calcium metabolism. Symptoms do not usually occur until the serum magnesium level has dropped to less than 1.8 mEq/L (0.75 mmol/L). Chvostek and Trousseau signs (see earlier discussion) occur, in part, because of accompanying hypocalcemia (Norris, 2019).

Hypomagnesemia may be accompanied by marked alterations in psychological status. Apathy, depressed mood, apprehension, and extreme agitation have been noted, as well as ataxia, dizziness, insomnia, and confusion. At times, delirium, auditory or visual hallucinations, and frank psychoses may occur (Yu & Yarlagadda, 2019).

Magnesium deficiency can disturb the ECG by prolonging the QRS, depressing the ST segment, and predisposing to cardiac arrhythmias, such as premature ventricular contractions, supraventricular tachycardia, torsades de pointes, and ventricular fibrillation. Increased susceptibility to digitalis toxicity is associated with low serum magnesium levels. Patients receiving digoxin are also likely to be receiving diuretic therapy, predisposing them to renal loss of magnesium. Concurrent hypokalemia and hypocalcemia must be addressed in addition to hypomagnesemia. These electrolyte disturbances are difficult to correct until magnesium has been replenished. Additionally, hypocalcemia can be worsened by isolated treatment of hypomagnesemia with IV magnesium sulfate because sulfate binds ionized calcium (Yu & Yarlagadda, 2019).

Assessment and Diagnostic Findings

On laboratory analysis, the serum magnesium level is less than 1.8 mg/dL (0.74 mmol/L). Urine magnesium may help identify the cause of magnesium depletion, and levels are measured after a loading dose of magnesium sulfate is given. Additional diagnostic techniques (nuclear magnetic resonance spectroscopy and the ion-selective electrode) are sensitive and direct means of measuring ionized serum magnesium levels (Yu, 2019b).

Medical Management

Mild magnesium deficiency can be corrected by diet alone. Principal dietary sources of magnesium include green leafy vegetables, beans, lentils, white potatoes, wheat bran, dry roasted almonds, and peanut butter (National Institutes of Health [NIH], 2019).

If necessary, magnesium salts can be given orally in an oxide or gluconate form to replace continuous losses but can produce diarrhea. Patients receiving parenteral nutrition require magnesium in the IV solution to prevent hypomagnesemia

Vital signs must be assessed frequently during magnesium administration to detect changes in cardiac rate or rhythm, hypotension, and respiratory distress. Monitoring urine output is essential before, during, and after magnesium administration as this is how Mg^{++} is excreted; the primary provider is notified if urine volume decreases to less than 100 mL over 4 hours. Calcium gluconate must be readily available to treat hypocalcemic tetany or hypermagnesemia.

> ### ◤ Quality and Safety Nursing Alert
>
> Inadvertent overdosage of IV magnesium can result in serious patient harm and death. Whenever a patient is prescribed IV magnesium, a second nurse should independently double check the IV magnesium prescription, including dose calculations, and check infusion pump settings. Milligrams (mg) and grams (g) are not equivalent to milliequivalent (mEq) dosages.

Nursing Management

The nurse should be aware of patients at risk for hypomagnesemia and observe them for its signs and symptoms. Patients receiving digitalis are monitored closely, because a deficit of magnesium can predispose them to digitalis toxicity. If hypomagnesemia is severe, seizure precautions are implemented. Other safety precautions are instituted, as indicated, if confusion is observed. Patients should be screened for dysphagia (difficulty in swallowing), as this may occur in those with magnesium depletion.

Patient education plays a major role in treating magnesium deficit. The patient is educated about sources of magnesium-rich foods, including green vegetables, nuts, legumes, bananas, and oranges.

Magnesium Excess (Hypermagnesemia)

Hypermagnesemia (serum magnesium level higher than 2.6 mg/dL [1.07 mmol/L]) is a rare electrolyte abnormality, because the kidneys efficiently excrete magnesium (Norris, 2019). A serum magnesium level can appear falsely elevated if blood specimens are allowed to hemolyze or are drawn from an extremity with a tourniquet that was applied too tightly.

Pathophysiology

The most common cause of hypermagnesemia is kidney injury (Yu & Gupta, 2019). In fact, most patients with advanced kidney injury have at least a slight elevation in serum magnesium levels. This condition is aggravated when such patients receive magnesium to control seizures.

Hypermagnesemia can occur in patients with untreated DKA when catabolism causes the release of cellular magnesium that cannot be excreted because of profound fluid volume depletion and resulting oliguria. A surplus of magnesium can also result from excessive magnesium given to treat hypertension of pregnancy or to treat hypomagnesemia. Increased serum magnesium levels can also occur in adrenocortical insufficiency, Addison disease, or hypothermia.

Excessive use of magnesium-based antacids or laxatives and medications that decrease GI motility, including opioids and anticholinergics, can also increase serum magnesium levels. Decreased elimination of magnesium or its increased absorption due to intestinal hypomotility from any cause can contribute to hypermagnesemia. Lithium intoxication can also cause an increase in serum magnesium levels. Extensive soft tissue injury or necrosis as with trauma, shock, sepsis, cardiac arrest, or severe burns can also result in hypermagnesemia (Yu & Gupta, 2019).

Clinical Manifestations

Acute elevation of the serum magnesium level depresses the central nervous system as well as the peripheral neuromuscular junction. Clinical signs and symptoms can be found in Table 10-9. The respiratory center is depressed when serum magnesium levels exceed 10 mEq/L (5 mmol/L). Coma, atrioventricular heart block, and cardiac arrest can occur when the serum magnesium level is greatly elevated and not treated. High levels of magnesium also result in platelet clumping and delayed thrombin formation (Yu & Gupta, 2019).

Assessment and Diagnostic Findings

In hypermagnesemia, the serum magnesium level is greater than 2.6 mg/dL (1.07 mmol/L). Increased potassium and calcium are present concurrently. As creatinine clearance decreases to less than 3.0 mL/min, the serum magnesium levels increase. ECG findings may include a prolonged PR interval, tall T waves, a widened QRS, and a prolonged QT interval, as well as an atrioventricular block (Norris, 2019).

Medical Management

Hypermagnesemia can be prevented by avoiding the administration of magnesium to patients with kidney injury and by carefully monitoring seriously ill patients who are receiving magnesium salts. In patients with severe hypermagnesemia, all parenteral and oral magnesium salts are discontinued. In emergencies, such as respiratory depression or defective cardiac conduction, ventilatory support and IV elemental calcium as a magnesium antagonist are indicated. In addition, hemodialysis with a magnesium-free dialysate can reduce the serum magnesium to a safe level within hours. Administration of loop diuretics (e.g., furosemide) and sodium chloride or lactated Ringer's IV solution enhances magnesium excretion in patients with adequate renal function. IV calcium antagonizes the cardiovascular and neuromuscular effects of magnesium (Yu & Gupta, 2019).

Nursing Management

Patients at risk for hypermagnesemia should be monitored closely. If hypermagnesemia is suspected, the nurse should monitor the vital signs, noting hypotension and shallow respirations. The nurse should be aware that arrhythmias, bradycardia, and heart block can occur. The nurse also observes for decreased deep tendon reflexes (DTRs), muscle weakness, and changes in the level of consciousness. Medications that contain magnesium are not given to patients with compromised renal function, and patients with kidney injury are cautioned to check with their primary providers before taking OTC supplements. Administration of fluids and diuretics are often used in treatment, and monitoring of I&O is important. Hemodialysis may be necessary in severe hypermagnesemia, particularly if cardiovascular or neurologic manifestations are present. Hemodialysis is also necessary in patients with severe hypermagnesemia and kidney injury (Yu & Gupta, 2019).

Phosphorus Imbalances

Phosphorus (HPO_4^-) is a critical constituent of all body tissues and is plentiful in the average diet of people living in developed countries. Intake of phosphorus usually exceeds body requirements and the kidney excretes the excess. Phosphorus is essential to the function of muscle and RBCs; the formation of adenosine triphosphate (ATP) and of 2,3-diphosphoglycerate, which facilitates the release of oxygen from hemoglobin; and the maintenance of acid–base balance, as well as the nervous system and the intermediary metabolism of carbohydrate, protein, and fat. It is a major component of the cell structure, phospholipids, nucleotides, and nucleic acids (DNA and RNA). It provides structural support to bones and teeth. Phosphorus is the primary anion of the ICF and requires active transport mechanisms to maintain its presence inside the cells. Most intracellular phosphorus is bound to proteins and lipids. About 85% of phosphorus is located in bones and teeth, 14% in soft tissue, and less than 1% in the ECF (Norris, 2019).

The normal serum phosphorus level is 2.7 to 4.5 mg/dL (0.87 to 1.45 mmol/L) in adults (Fischbach & Fischbach, 2018). Phosphorus homeostasis is maintained through absorption and secretion in the GI tract, filtration and absorption in the kidneys, and shifts into and out of bone. PTH and vitamin D assist in phosphate homeostasis by varying phosphate reabsorption in the proximal tubule of the kidney. PTH allows the shift of phosphate from bone to plasma. Phosphorus deficit and phosphorus excess are less common electrolyte imbalances (Table 10-10).

Phosphorus Deficit (Hypophosphatemia)

Hypophosphatemia is indicated by a value below 2.7 mg/dL (0.87 mmol/L). Although it often indicates phosphorus deficiency, hypophosphatemia may occur under a variety of circumstances in which total-body phosphorus stores are normal. Phosphorus deficiency can also occur as an abnormally low content of phosphorus in lean tissues without evidence of low phosphate in the bloodstream. Hypophosphatemia can be due to lack of sufficient intake, excess excretion (renal phosphate wasting), shift of phosphorus from extracellular to intracellular spaces, or by decreased intestinal absorption of phosphorus (Yu & Stubbs, 2019).

Pathophysiology

Hypophosphatemia rarely occurs due to inadequate intake, as there are many dietary sources of phosphate (e.g., meats, dairy products, beans). However, phosphate can become depleted in GI malabsorption disorders such as chronic diarrhea, Crohn's

TABLE 10-10	Phosphorus Imbalances	
Imbalance	**Contributing Factors**	**Signs/Symptoms**
Phosphorus deficit (hypophosphatemia) Serum phosphorus <2.7 mg/dL	Refeeding after starvation, alcohol withdrawal, diabetic ketoacidosis, respiratory and metabolic alkalosis, ↓ magnesium, ↓ potassium, hyperparathyroidism, vomiting, diarrhea, hyperventilation, vitamin D deficiency associated with malabsorptive disorders, burns, acid–base disorders, parenteral nutrition, and diuretic and antacid use	Paresthesias, muscle weakness, bone pain and tenderness, chest pain, confusion, cardiomyopathy, respiratory failure, seizures, tissue hypoxia, and increased susceptibility to infection, nystagmus
Phosphorus excess (hyperphosphatemia) Serum phosphorus >4.5 mg/dL	Acute kidney injury and chronic kidney disease, excessive intake of phosphorus, vitamin D excess, respiratory and metabolic acidosis, hypoparathyroidism, volume depletion, leukemia/lymphoma treated with cytotoxic agents, increased tissue breakdown, rhabdomyolysis	Tetany, tachycardia, anorexia, nausea and vomiting, muscle weakness, signs and symptoms of hypocalcemia; hyperactive reflexes; soft tissue calcifications in lungs, heart, kidneys, and cornea

↓, decreased.
Adapted from Norris, T. L. (2019). *Porth's pathophysiology: Concepts of altered health state* (10th ed.). Philadelphia, PA: Wolters Kluwer.

disease, or celiac disease. Hypophosphatemia can also occur in anorexia, bulimia, and alcoholism. Vitamin D deficit can cause low phosphate levels in the bloodstream. Vitamin D regulates intestinal absorption of calcium and phosphate ion; therefore, a deficiency of vitamin D can cause both decreased calcium and phosphorus levels. These deficiencies can lead to osteomalacia (softened and brittle bones) in the adult (Norris, 2019).

Hypophosphatemia can occur if there is high intake of antacids—particularly those containing calcium, magnesium, or aluminum. Excess phosphorus binding by antacids may decrease the phosphorus available from the diet to an amount lower than required to maintain serum phosphorus balance. The degree of hypophosphatemia depends on the amount of phosphorus in the diet compared to the dose of antacid (Yu & Stubbs, 2019).

Hypophosphatemia can also occur during the administration of calories to patients who have had severe protein–calorie malnutrition. This syndrome can be induced in any person with severe malnutrition (e.g., patients with anorexia nervosa or alcoholism, older patients who are debilitated and unable to eat). Feeding a patient who is nutritionally deprived stimulates a large insulin release that can cause shift of phosphate from the extracellular to the intracellular compartment. Also, marked hypophosphatemia can develop in patients who are malnourished who receive parenteral nutrition that does not contain sufficient phosphorus (Aubry, Friedli, Schetz, et al., 2018).

Other causes of hypophosphatemia include heatstroke, prolonged intense hyperventilation, alcohol withdrawal, DKA, respiratory alkalosis, hepatic encephalopathy, and major thermal burns. Hyperparathyroidism can also cause increased urinary losses of phosphorus leading to hypophosphatemia. Loss of phosphorus through the kidneys also occurs with acute volume expansion, osmotic diuresis, the use of carbonic anhydrase inhibitors (acetazolamide), and some malignancies.

Respiratory alkalosis can cause a decrease in phosphorus in the bloodstream because of an intracellular shift of phosphorus. Respiratory alkalosis, commonly caused by extreme hyperventilation, can reduce serum phosphate concentrations to very low levels and is a common cause of marked hypophosphatemia in patients who are hospitalized.

Some genetic disorders, such as Fanconi syndrome and X-linked hypophosphatemic rickets, cause renal phosphate wasting. Acquired oncogenic osteomalacia, a paraneoplastic syndrome that occurs with some types of cancer, can also cause low phosphate levels. Hypophosphatemia is also a frequent complication of renal transplantation (Yu & Stubbs, 2019).

Clinical Manifestations

Most of the signs and symptoms of phosphorus deficiency result from a deficiency of ATP, 2,3-diphosphoglycerate, or both (Yu & Stubbs, 2019). ATP deficiency impairs cellular energy resources; diphosphoglycerate deficiency impairs oxygen delivery to tissues, resulting in generalized weakness and neurologic manifestations. Clinical signs and symptoms can be found in Table 10-10.

Muscle damage may develop as the ATP level in the muscle tissue declines. Clinical manifestations are muscle weakness, which may be subtle or profound and may affect any muscle group; muscle pain; and at times acute rhabdomyolysis (breakdown of skeletal muscle). Weakness of the diaphragm and intercostal muscles may greatly impair ventilation. Bone pain, altered mental status, seizures, focal neurologic signs, and heart failure can occur with severe hypophosphatemia (Yu & Stubbs, 2019).

Assessment and Diagnostic Findings

On laboratory analysis, the serum phosphorus level is less than 2.7 mg/dL (0.87 mmol/L). When reviewing laboratory results, the nurse should keep in mind that glucose or insulin administration causes a decrease in the serum phosphorus level. Acute hypophosphatemia can occur during the treatment of DKA due to high doses of insulin. Elevated PTH levels that occur as a result of hyperparathyroidism can lower blood levels of phosphate. A 24-hour urine collection for phosphorus can be done if renal-phosphate wasting is suspected. Fanconi syndrome causes loss of glucose, amino acids, uric acid, and phosphate in the urine. X-rays and bone density studies may show skeletal changes of reduced bone mineralization caused by osteomalacia or rickets. A technetium (Tc99m) sestamibi scan of the neck can be done to check for hyperparathyroidism. CT scan, MRI, or indium-111 octreotide scan may show oncogenic osteomalacia (decreased bone density due to cancer) (Sharma & Castro, 2019).

Medical Management

Prevention of hypophosphatemia is the goal. In patients at risk for hypophosphatemia, serum phosphate levels should be closely monitored and correction initiated before deficits become severe. Adequate amounts of phosphorus should be added to parenteral solutions, and attention should be paid to the phosphorus levels in enteral feeding solutions.

Medical management of hypophosphatemia depends on the etiology, and treatment of the cause is essential. Severe hypophosphatemia is dangerous and requires prompt attention. Oral phosphate supplements are usually adequate for mild hypophosphatemia. Sources of phosphorus include dairy foods, meats, and beans. Oral supplements may be sufficient to treat renal-wasting disorders, malabsorption, or oncogenic osteomalacia until an exact etiology is found. Vitamin D may also be necessary to enhance absorption of phosphorus and calcium.

Aggressive IV phosphorus correction is usually limited to the patient whose serum phosphorus levels decrease to less than 1 mg/dL (0.3 mmol/L). Possible effects of IV administration of phosphorus include tetany from hypocalcemia and calcifications in tissues (blood vessels, heart, lung, kidney, eyes) from hyperphosphatemia.

Recently a monoclonal antibody-type drug, burosumab, has been approved for patients with renal phosphate wasting disorders and hypophosphatemic rickets. This drug has been found to normalize phosphate levels, improve bone mineralization, and heal fractures in rickets (Perwad & Portale, 2019).

If hyperparathyroidism is caused by parathyroid tumor, surgery may be necessary. A parathyroid tumor, termed an adenoma, can cause hyperparathyroidism with resulting demineralization of bone (osteomalacia). Patients with hyperparathyroidism can also be given calcimimetic medications, such as cinacalcet, which activate the calcium receptor in the gland and decrease PTH secretion (Wang & Yuan, 2019).

Patients with oncogenic osteomalacia should be treated for the cancer causing this syndrome. If malabsorption is the cause of hypophosphatemia, treatment of the GI disorder is necessary. Because patients with osteomalacia are at high risk for fracture, fall precautions should be observed. If hypophosphatemia is caused by an eating disorder, the patient should obtain behavioral counseling and nutritional therapy.

Nursing Management

The nurse should identify patients at risk for hypophosphatemia and monitor them. Because patients who are malnourished and receiving parenteral nutrition are at risk when calories are introduced too aggressively, preventive measures involve gradually introducing the solution to avoid rapid shifts of phosphorus into the cells. Vitamin D and calcium levels should also be monitored as phosphate levels are influenced by these levels. Vitamin D supplementation may be needed to enhance calcium and phosphate absorption (Aubry et al., 2018).

In patients requiring correction of phosphorus losses, the nurse frequently monitors serum phosphorus levels and documents and reports early signs of hypophosphatemia (apprehension, confusion, change in level of consciousness). If the patient experiences mild hypophosphatemia, foods such as milk and milk products, organ meats, beans, nuts, fish, poultry, and whole grains should be encouraged. With moderate hypophosphatemia, supplements such as Neutra-Phos capsules, K-Phos, and Fleet Phospho-Soda may be prescribed (Vallerand & Sanoski, 2019; Yu & Stubbs, 2019).

For patients with severe hypophosphatemia, IV preparations of phosphorus are available as sodium or potassium phosphate. The rate of phosphorus administration should not exceed 3 mmol/h, and the site should be carefully monitored because tissue sloughing and necrosis can occur with infiltration. Serum calcium and phosphate blood levels should be monitored every 6 hours with IV therapy.

Phosphorus Excess (Hyperphosphatemia)

Hyperphosphatemia is a serum phosphorus level that exceeds 4.5 mg/dL (1.45 mmol/L). Abnormally high levels of phosphate in the bloodstream can arise from excessive intake of phosphorus, decreased excretion of phosphorus, or a disorder that shifts intracellular phosphate into the extracellular space.

Pathophysiology

Various conditions can lead to hyperphosphatemia; however, the most common is kidney injury, which diminishes urinary phosphate excretion (Stubbs & Yu, 2019). When renal insufficiency progresses to 40% to 50% of renal function, hyperphosphatemia can occur. Other causes include increased intake or a shift of phosphate from the intracellular to extracellular space. Conditions such as excessive vitamin D intake, administration of total parenteral nutrition, chemotherapy for neoplastic disease, hypoparathyroidism, pseudohypoparathyroidism, metabolic or respiratory acidosis, DKA, acute hemolysis, high phosphate intake, profound muscle necrosis,

and increased phosphorus absorption may also lead to this phosphorus imbalance. Hypoparathyroidism causes hyperphosphatemia by failure of the kidneys to inhibit renal reabsorption of phosphate. The kidneys reabsorb excessive phosphate into the bloodstream. Pseudohypoparathyroidism is a disorder caused by end-organ resistance to PTH. Excessive use of phosphate-containing laxatives or enemas can also lead to hyperphosphatemia. False elevation of phosphate in the bloodstream can occur with elevated protein or bilirubin levels, dyslipidemia, or hemolysis. The primary complication of increased phosphorus is metastatic calcification in the organs, soft tissues, joints, and arteries. Arterial calcification is a risk factor for myocardial infarction, stroke, and peripheral arterial disease (Norris, 2019; Stubbs & Yu, 2019).

Clinical Manifestations

Clinical signs and symptoms can be found in Table 10-10. Most symptoms result from decreased calcium levels and soft tissue calcifications. The most important short-term consequence is tetany (severe muscle cramping). Because of the reciprocal relationship between phosphorus and calcium, a high serum phosphorus level tends to cause a low serum calcium concentration. Hypocalcemia causes neuromuscular irritability and muscle spasms (Bove-Fenderson & Mannstadt, 2018).

The major long-term consequence is soft tissue calcification, which occurs mainly in patients with a reduced glomerular filtration rate. High serum levels of inorganic phosphorus promote precipitation of calcium phosphate in nonosseous sites, which can decrease urine output, impair vision, and produce palpitations. Skin and soft tissue deposits of calcium can cause pruritus (Marcucci, Cianferotti, & Brandi, 2018).

Assessment and Diagnostic Findings

On laboratory analysis, the serum phosphorus level exceeds 4.5 mg/dL (1.5 mmol/L). The serum calcium level is useful also for diagnosing the primary disorder and assessing the effects of treatments. X-rays may show skeletal changes with abnormal bone development. PTH levels are decreased in hypoparathyroidism. BUN and creatinine levels are used to assess renal function (Marcucci et al., 2018).

Medical Management

Phosphate intake should be reduced and phosphate binders can be given with meals to reduce hyperphosphatemia. When possible, treatment is directed at the underlying disorder. For example, hyperphosphatemia may be related to volume depletion or respiratory or metabolic acidosis. Correction of these disorders may normalize the blood level of phosphate.

Calcium carbonate or calcium citrate are phosphate binders that can be used to lower blood phosphate levels. However, careful monitoring of calcium is essential as hypercalcemia can result. Phosphate binding resins that do not contain calcium include sevelamer and lanthanum. Sucroferric oxyhydroxide can also be used particularly in patients who require iron supplementation. Forced diuresis with a loop diuretic or saline diuresis can be used in patients with normal renal function. Hemodialysis can also lower phosphorus (Carfagna, Del Vecchio, Pontoriero, et al., 2018).

Nursing Management

The nurse monitors patients at risk for hyperphosphatemia. If a low phosphorus diet is prescribed, the patient is instructed to avoid phosphorus-rich foods, such as hard cheeses, cream, nuts, meats, whole-grain cereals, dried fruits, dried vegetables, kidneys, sardines, and dairy foods (Shimada, Shutto-Uchita, & Yamabe, 2019). When appropriate, the nurse instructs the patient to avoid phosphate-containing laxatives and enemas. When administering phosphate binders, calcium levels should be monitored as well. During diuresis the nurse monitors urine output. The nurse also educates the patient about recognizing the signs of hypocalcemia, such as muscle cramping (Goltzman, 2019a).

Chloride Imbalances

Chloride (Cl⁻) is the major anion of the ECF compartment. It maintains cellular integrity by providing water balance and maintains acid–base balance. Sodium and chloride make up the electrolytes that exert osmotic pressure. Chloride is also contained in gastric and pancreatic juices, sweat, bile, and saliva. Chloride is produced in the stomach, where it combines with hydrogen to form hydrochloric acid. Chloride control depends on the intake of chloride and the excretion and reabsorption of its ions in the kidneys. A small amount of chloride is lost in the feces (Norris, 2019).

The normal serum chloride level is 97 to 107 mEq/L (97 to 107 mmol/L). Inside the cell, the chloride level is 4 mEq/L. The serum level of chloride reflects a change in dilution or concentration of the ECF and does so in direct proportion to the sodium concentration. Serum osmolality parallels chloride levels as well. Aldosterone secretion increases sodium reabsorption, thereby increasing chloride reabsorption (Hall, 2016).

The choroid plexus, which secretes cerebrospinal fluid in the brain, depends on sodium and chloride to attract water to form the fluid portion of the cerebrospinal fluid.

Bicarbonate has an inverse relationship with chloride. As chloride moves from plasma into the RBCs (called the *chloride shift*), bicarbonate moves back into the plasma. Hydrogen ions are formed, which then help release oxygen from hemoglobin (Emmett & Szerlip, 2017a). When the level of one of these three electrolytes (sodium, bicarbonate, or chloride) is disturbed, the other two are also affected. Chloride assists in maintaining acid–base balance and works as a buffer in the exchange of oxygen and CO_2 in RBCs (Fischbach & Fischbach, 2018). Chloride is primarily obtained from the diet as table salt. The chloride imbalances are chloride deficit and chloride excess (Table 10-11).

Chloride Deficit (Hypochloremia)

Hypochloremia is a serum chloride level below 97 mEq/L (97 mmol/L).

Pathophysiology

Hypochloremia can occur with GI tube drainage, gastric suctioning, gastric surgery, and severe vomiting and diarrhea. Administration of chloride-deficient IV solutions, low sodium intake, decreased serum sodium levels, DKA, chronic respiratory acidosis, massive blood transfusions, diuretic therapy, excessive sweating, burns, SIADH, and fever may cause hypochloremia. Administration of aldosterone, ACTH, corticosteroids, bicarbonate, excess diuretics, or laxatives decreases serum chloride levels as well. As chloride decreases (usually because of volume depletion), sodium and bicarbonate ions are retained by the kidney to balance the loss. Bicarbonate accumulates in the ECF, which raises the pH and can lead to hypochloremic metabolic alkalosis (Emmett & Szerlip, 2017a).

Clinical Manifestations

The signs and symptoms of hypochloremia are outlined in Table 10-11. The signs and symptoms of hyponatremia, hypokalemia, and metabolic alkalosis may also be present. Metabolic alkalosis is a disorder that results in a high pH and a high serum bicarbonate level as a result of excess alkali intake

TABLE 10-11   Chloride Imbalances

Imbalance	Contributing Factors	Signs/Symptoms and Laboratory Findings
Chloride deficit (hypochloremia) Serum chloride <96 mEq/L	Addison disease, reduced chloride intake or absorption, untreated diabetic ketoacidosis, chronic respiratory acidosis, excessive sweating, vomiting, gastric suction, diarrhea, sodium and potassium deficiency, metabolic alkalosis; loop, osmotic, or thiazide diuretic use; overuse of bicarbonate, rapid removal of ascitic fluid with a high sodium content, IV fluids that lack chloride (dextrose and water), draining fistulas and ileostomies, heart failure, cystic fibrosis	Agitation, irritability, tremors, muscle cramps, hyperactive deep tendon reflexes, hypertonicity, tetany, slow shallow respirations, seizures, arrhythmias, coma *Labs indicate:* ↓ serum chloride, ↓ serum sodium, ↑ pH, ↑ serum bicarbonate, ↑ total carbon dioxide content, ↓ urine chloride level, ↓ serum potassium
Chloride excess (hyperchloremia) Serum chloride >108 mEq/L	Excessive sodium chloride infusions with water loss, head injury (sodium retention), hypernatremia, kidney injury, corticosteroid use, dehydration, severe diarrhea (loss of bicarbonate), respiratory alkalosis, administration of diuretics, overdose of salicylates, sodium polystyrene sulfonate, acetazolamide, phenylbutazone and ammonium chloride use, hyperparathyroidism, metabolic acidosis	Tachypnea, lethargy, weakness, deep rapid respirations, decline in cognitive status, ↓ cardiac output, dyspnea, tachycardia, pitting edema, arrhythmias, coma *Labs indicate:* ↑ serum chloride, ↑ serum potassium and sodium, ↓ serum pH, ↓ serum bicarbonate, normal anion gap, ↑ urinary chloride level

↓, decreased; ↑, increased; IV, intravenous.
Adapted from Norris, T. L. (2019). *Porth's pathophysiology: Concepts of altered health state* (10th ed.). Philadelphia, PA: Wolters Kluwer.

or loss of hydrogen ions. With compensation, the partial pressure of CO_2 in arterial blood ($PaCO_2$) increases to 50 mm Hg. Hyperexcitability of muscles, tetany, hyperactive DTRs, weakness, twitching, and muscle cramps may result. Hypokalemia can cause hypochloremia, resulting in cardiac arrhythmias. In addition, because low chloride levels parallel low sodium levels, a water excess may occur. Hyponatremia can cause seizures and coma (Squiers, 2017).

Assessment and Diagnostic Findings

In addition to the chloride level, sodium and potassium levels are also evaluated, because these electrolytes are lost along with chloride. ABG analysis identifies the acid–base imbalance, which is usually metabolic alkalosis. The urine chloride level, which is also measured, decreases in hypochloremia.

Medical Management

Treatment involves correcting the cause of hypochloremia and the contributing electrolyte and acid–base imbalances. Normal saline (0.9% sodium chloride) or half-strength saline (0.45% sodium chloride) solution is given by IV to replace the chloride. If the patient is receiving a diuretic (loop, osmotic, or thiazide), it may be discontinued or another diuretic prescribed (Squiers, 2017).

Ammonium chloride, an acidifying IV agent, may be prescribed to treat metabolic alkalosis; the dosage depends on the patient's weight and serum chloride level. This agent is metabolized by the liver, and its effects last for about 3 days. Its use should be avoided in patients with impaired liver or renal function (Emmett & Szerlip, 2017b).

Nursing Management

The nurse monitors the patient's I&O, ABG values, and serum electrolyte levels. Changes in the patient's level of consciousness and muscle strength and movement are reported to the primary provider promptly. Vital signs are monitored, and respiratory assessment is carried out frequently. The nurse provides and educates the patient about foods with high chloride content, which include tomato juice, bananas, dates, eggs, cheese, milk, salty broth, canned vegetables, and processed meats. A person who drinks free water (water without electrolytes) or bottled water and excretes large amounts of chloride needs instruction to avoid drinking this kind of water (Squiers, 2017).

Chloride Excess (Hyperchloremia)

Hyperchloremia exists when the serum level of chloride exceeds 107 mEq/L (107 mmol/L). Hypernatremia, bicarbonate loss, and metabolic acidosis can occur with high chloride levels.

Pathophysiology

High serum chloride levels are almost exclusively a result of iatrogenically induced hyperchloremic metabolic acidosis, stemming from excessive administration of chloride relative to sodium, most commonly as 0.9% normal saline solution, 0.45% normal saline solution, or lactated Ringer's solution. This condition can also be caused by the loss of bicarbonate

ions via the kidney or the GI tract with a corresponding increase in chloride ions. Chloride ions in the form of acidifying salts accumulate, and acidosis occurs with a decrease in bicarbonate ions. Head trauma, increased perspiration, excess adrenocortical hormone production, and decreased glomerular filtration can lead to a high serum chloride level (Squiers, 2017).

Clinical Manifestations

The signs and symptoms of hyperchloremia are the same as those of metabolic acidosis: hypervolemia and hypernatremia. Tachypnea, weakness, lethargy, deep and rapid respirations, diminished cognitive ability, and hypertension occur. If untreated, hyperchloremia can lead to a decrease in cardiac output, arrhythmias, and coma. A high chloride level is accompanied by a high sodium level and fluid retention (Squiers, 2017).

Assessment and Diagnostic Findings

The serum chloride level is 108 mEq/L (108 mmol/L) or greater, the serum sodium level is greater than 145 mEq/L (145 mmol/L), the serum pH is less than 7.35, and the serum bicarbonate level is less than 22 mEq/L (22 mmol/L). Urine chloride levels are elevated.

Medical Management

Correcting the underlying cause of hyperchloremia and restoring electrolyte, fluid, and acid–base balance are essential. Hypotonic IV solutions may be given to restore balance. Lactated Ringer's solution may be prescribed to convert lactate to bicarbonate in the liver, which increases the bicarbonate level and corrects the acidosis. IV sodium bicarbonate may be given to increase bicarbonate levels, which leads to the renal excretion of chloride ions because bicarbonate and chloride compete for combination with sodium. Diuretics may be given to eliminate chloride as well. Sodium, chloride, and fluids are restricted (Squiers, 2017).

Nursing Management

Monitoring vital signs, ABG values, and I&O is important to assess the patient's status and the effectiveness of treatment. Assessment findings related to respiratory, neurologic, and cardiac systems are documented, and changes are discussed with the primary provider. The nurse educates the patient about the diet that should be followed to manage hyperchloremia and maintain adequate hydration.

 ACID–BASE DISTURBANCES

Acid–base disturbances are commonly encountered in clinical practice, especially in critical-care units. Identification of the specific acid–base imbalance is important in ascertaining the underlying cause of the disorder and determining appropriate treatment.

Plasma pH is an indicator of hydrogen ion (H^+) concentration and measures the acidity or alkalinity of the blood. Homeostatic mechanisms keep pH within a normal range (7.35 to 7.45). These mechanisms consist of buffer systems, the kidneys, and the lungs. The H^+ concentration is extremely important: The greater the concentration, the more acidic the solution and the lower the pH. The lower the H^+ concentration, the more alkaline the solution and the higher the pH (Larkin & Zimmanck, 2015; Norris, 2019).

Buffer systems prevent major changes in the pH of body fluids by removing or releasing H^+; they can act quickly to prevent excessive changes in H^+ concentration. Hydrogen ions are buffered by both intracellular and extracellular buffers. The body's major extracellular buffer system is the bicarbonate–carbonic acid buffer system, which is assessed when ABGs are measured. Normally, there are 20 parts of bicarbonate (HCO_3^-) to 1 part of carbonic acid (H_2CO_3). If this ratio is altered, the pH will change. It is the ratio of HCO_3^- to H_2CO_3 that is important in maintaining pH, not absolute values (Larkin & Zimmanck, 2015; Norris, 2019).

CO_2 is a potential acid; when dissolved in water, it becomes carbonic acid ($CO_2 + H_2O = H_2CO_3$). Therefore, when CO_2 is increased, the carbonic acid content is also increased. When the CO_2 level decreases, carbonic acid decreases. If either bicarbonate or carbonic acid is increased or decreased so that the 20:1 ratio is no longer maintained, acid–base imbalance results (Larkin & Zimmanck, 2015; Theodore, 2019).

Less important buffer systems in the ECF include the inorganic phosphates and the plasma proteins. Intracellular buffers include proteins, organic and inorganic phosphates, and, in RBCs, hemoglobin (Norris, 2019).

The kidneys regulate the bicarbonate level in the ECF; they can regenerate bicarbonate ions as well as reabsorb them from the renal tubular cells. In respiratory acidosis and most cases of metabolic acidosis, the kidneys excrete hydrogen ions and conserve bicarbonate ions to help restore balance. In respiratory and metabolic alkalosis, the kidneys retain hydrogen ions and excrete bicarbonate ions to help restore balance. The kidneys cannot compensate for the metabolic acidosis created by kidney injury. Renal compensation for imbalances is relatively slow (a matter of hours or days) (Larkin & Zimmanck, 2015; Norris, 2019).

The lungs, under the control of the medulla, control the CO_2 and thus the carbonic acid content of the ECF. They do so by adjusting ventilation in response to the amount of CO_2 in the arterial blood. A rise in the partial pressure of CO_2 in arterial blood (designated $PaCO_2$) is a powerful stimulant to respiration. Of course, the partial pressure of oxygen in arterial blood (designated PaO_2) also influences respiration. However, its effect is not as marked as that produced by the $PaCO_2$ (Theodore, 2019).

In metabolic acidosis, the lungs compensate by raising respiratory rate, causing greater elimination of CO_2 (to reduce the acid load). In metabolic alkalosis, the lungs compensate by decreasing respiratory rate, causing CO_2 to be retained (to increase the acid load).

In order to understand acid–base imbalances, it is important to comprehend the chemical reaction that occurs in the bloodstream to maintain homeostasis. The bicarbonate buffer system is demonstrated by the following chemical equation:

$$CO_2 + H_2O \longleftrightarrow H_2CO_3 \longleftrightarrow H^+ \text{ and } HCO_3^-$$

In this chemical equation, carbon dioxide (CO_2) and water form carbonic acid (H_2CO_3) which dissociates into H^+ and

TABLE 10-12	Normal Values for Arterial and Mixed Venous Bloods	
Parameter	Arterial Blood	Mixed Venous Blood
pH	7.35–7.45	7.32–7.42
PCO_2	35–45 mm Hg	38–52 mm Hg
PO_2^a	>80 mm Hg	24–48 mm Hg
HCO_3^-	22–26 mEq/L	19–25 mEq/L
Base excess/deficit	±2 mEq/L	±5 mEq/L
Oxygen saturation (SaO_2%)	>94%	65–75%

[a]At altitudes of 3000 feet and higher; age dependent.
Adapted from Fischbach, F., & Fischbach, M. (2018). *A manual of laboratory and diagnostic tests* (10th ed.). Philadelphia, PA: Lippincott Williams & Wilkins.

HCO_3^-. It is also important to recognize that the major organs that control acid–base balance are the lungs, in control of CO_2, and the kidneys, which can excrete or reabsorb the ions needed to balance the pH. ABGs are laboratory tests that can provide values of blood pH, $PaCO_2$, PaO_2, and HCO_3^-. ABGs are used to diagnose acid–base imbalances of the bloodstream. The saturation of Hgb with oxygen can also be measured by pulse oximetry and designated as SaO_2. Normal range of SaO_2 is 95% to 100% (Theodore, 2019) (Table 10-12).

If the lungs slow down breathing rate, a condition termed hypoventilation, CO_2 will increase. Hypoventilation increases CO_2 retention. Normal $PaCO_2$ range is 35 to 45 mm Hg. Hypoventilation can increase the $PaCO_2$ greater than 45 mm Hg. Increased CO_2 will move the chemical equation to the right, which produces more H^+ ions and an acidotic bloodstream. The normal pH of the bloodstream is 7.35 to 7.45. An acidotic bloodstream has a pH less than 7.35 (Larkin & Zimmanck, 2015; Norris, 2019).

If the lungs increase breathing rate, a condition called hyperventilation, CO_2 is lost via the lungs. If CO_2 decreases it moves the equation to the left, pulling H^+ out of the bloodstream and creating an alkalotic bloodstream. An alkalotic bloodstream has a pH greater than 7.45 (Larkin & Zimmanck, 2015; Norris, 2019).

If H^+ ions increase in the bloodstream due to lactic acid accumulation, DKA, toxicity, or other source, it will push the equation to the left and increase CO_2 to be eliminated by the lungs. The lungs will increase breathing rate to rid the body of CO_2 in attempt to compensate for the high acid (Larkin & Zimmanck, 2015; Theodore, 2019).

If H^+ ions decrease in the bloodstream, it will pull the equation to the right using up some CO_2 to create more H^+. The lungs will slow breathing rate in an attempt to compensate by accumulating CO_2, which will produce H^+ (Larkin & Zimmanck, 2015; Theodore, 2019).

Acute and Chronic Metabolic Acidosis (Base Bicarbonate Deficit)

Metabolic acidosis is a common clinical disturbance characterized by a low pH due to an increased H^+ concentration and a low plasma bicarbonate concentration. Metabolic acidosis can occur by a gain of hydrogen ions or a loss of bicarbonate ions in the bloodstream. It can be divided clinically into two forms, according to the values of the serum anion gap: high anion gap metabolic acidosis and normal anion gap metabolic acidosis. The anion gap refers to the difference between the sum of all measured positively charged electrolytes (cations) and the sum of all negatively charged electrolytes (anions) in blood. Because the sum of measured cations is typically greater than the sum of measured anions in the bloodstream, there normally exists a disparity with predominance of cations; this is referred to as the anion gap. The anion gap reflects unmeasured anions (phosphates, sulfates, and proteins) in plasma that replace bicarbonate in metabolic acidosis. Measuring the anion gap is necessary when analyzing conditions of metabolic acidosis as it can help determine the cause of the acidosis (Emmett & Szerlip, 2018).

The anion gap can be calculated by either of the following equations:

$$\text{Anion gap} = Na^+ + K^+ - (Cl^- + HCO_3^-)$$
$$\text{Anion gap} = Na^+ - (Cl^- + HCO_3^-)$$

Potassium is often omitted from the equation because of its low level in the plasma; therefore, the second equation is used more often than the first (Theodore, 2019).

The normal value for an anion gap is 8 to 12 mEq/L (8 to 12 mmol/L) without potassium in the equation. If potassium is included in the equation, the normal value for the anion gap is 12 to 16 mEq/L (12 to 16 mmol/L). The unmeasured anions in the serum normally account for less than 16 mEq/L of the anion production. Metabolic acidotic conditions can be differentiated according to the anion gap; there is either a normal anion gap or high anion gap. A person diagnosed with metabolic acidosis is determined to have normal anion gap metabolic acidosis if the anion gap is within this normal range (8 to 12 mEq/L). An anion gap greater than 16 mEq (16 mmol/L) suggests excessive accumulation of unmeasured anions and would indicate high anion gap metabolic acidosis. An anion gap occurs because not all electrolytes are measured. More anions are left unmeasured than cations (Emmett & Szerlip, 2018).

Pathophysiology

Normal anion gap metabolic acidosis results from the direct loss of bicarbonate, as in diarrhea, lower intestinal fistulas, ureterostomies, use of diuretics, early renal insufficiency, excessive administration of chloride, and the administration of parenteral nutrition without bicarbonate or bicarbonate-producing solutes (e.g., lactate) (Emmett & Szerlip, 2018).

High anion gap metabolic acidosis occurs when there is an excessive accumulation of acids. High anion gap occurs in lactic acidosis, salicylate poisoning (acetylsalicylic acid), renal failure, methanol, ethylene or propylene glycol toxicity, DKA, and ketoacidosis that occurs with starvation. The high amount of hydrogen ions due to the acids present are neutralized and buffered by HCO_3^- causing the bicarbonate concentration to fall and become exhausted. Other anions in the bloodstream are called upon to neutralize the high acid in the blood. In all of these instances, abnormally high levels of anions are used to neutralize the H^+, which increases the anion gap above normal limits (high anion gap) (Emmett & Szerlip, 2019).

 **Concept Mastery Alert**

Metabolic acidosis is characterized by a low pH and low plasma bicarbonate concentration. Nurses need to remember that an anion gap is calculated primarily to identify the cause (pathology) of metabolic acidosis.

	Reduced or Negative Anion Gap	Normal Anion Gap	High Anion Gap
Anion gap without potassium	<8	8–12 mEq/L	>12
Anion gap with potassium	<12	12–16 mEq/L	>16
Clinical significance	Hypoproteinemia	Normal anion gap metabolic acidosis	High anion gap metabolic acidosis

Clinical Manifestations

Signs and symptoms of metabolic acidosis vary with the severity of the acidosis but include headache, confusion, drowsiness, increased respiratory rate and depth, nausea, and vomiting. Peripheral vasodilation and decreased cardiac output occur when the pH drops to less than 7. Additional physical assessment findings include decreased blood pressure, cold and clammy skin, arrhythmias, and shock. Chronic metabolic acidosis is primarily caused by chronic kidney disease because dysfunctional kidneys do not excrete acid (Emmett & Szerlip, 2018; Kovesdy, 2018).

Assessment and Diagnostic Findings

ABG measurements are used in the diagnosis of acid–base imbalances such as metabolic acidosis. Expected ABG changes include a low bicarbonate level (less than 22 mEq/L) and a low blood pH (less than 7.35). The cardinal feature of metabolic acidosis is a decrease in the serum bicarbonate level. In conditions of acidosis there is elevated H^+ and the sodium–potassium cellular pump brings H^+ into the cells in place of K^+. Therefore, high K^+ accumulates in the bloodstream in metabolic acidosis as a result of the shift of potassium out of the cells (Theodore, 2019). Later, when the acidosis is corrected and pH normalized, the cellular pump causes potassium to move back into the cells and hypokalemia may occur. Blood levels of potassium need to be closely monitored. ECG monitoring is recommended as changes of potassium in the bloodstream can cause arrhythmias (Palmer & Clegg, 2016a).

In metabolic acidosis, the lungs compensate for the high H^+ through hyperventilation to decrease the CO_2 level, which in turn reduces H^+ (see carbonic acid equation). Calculation of the anion gap is helpful in determining the cause of metabolic acidosis. There are certain conditions that cause high anion gap metabolic acidosis and others that cause normal anion gap metabolic acidosis (Table 10-13).

TABLE 10-13	Summary of Single Acid–Base Disturbances and Their Compensatory Responses		
Acid–Base Imbalance	Primary Disturbance	Respiratory Compensation and Predicted Response[a]	Renal Compensation and Predicted Response[a,b]
Metabolic acidosis	↓ pH and HCO_3^- HCO_3^- <22 mEq/L	↑ ventilation and ↓ PCO_2 *1 mEq/L ↓ HCO_3^- → 1–1.2 mm Hg ↓ PCO_2*	↑ H^+ excretion and ↑ HCO_3^- reabsorption if no renal disease
Metabolic alkalosis	↑ pH and HCO_3^- HCO_3^- >26 mEq/L	↓ ventilation and ↑ PCO_2 *1 mEq/L ↑ HCO_3^- → 0.7 mm Hg ↑ PCO_2*	↓ H^+ excretion and ↓ HCO_3^- reabsorption if no renal disease
Respiratory acidosis	↓ pH and ↑ PCO_2 PCO_2 >45 mm Hg	None	↑ H^+ excretion and ↑ HCO_3^- reabsorption *Acute: 1 mm Hg ↑ PCO_2 → 0.1 mEq/L ↑ HCO_3^-* *Chronic: 1 mm Hg ↑ PCO_2 → 0.3 mEq/L ↑ HCO_3^-*
Respiratory alkalosis	↑ pH and ↓ PCO_2 PCO_2 <35 mm Hg	None	↓ H^+ excretion and ↓ HCO_3^- reabsorption *Acute: 1 mm Hg ↓ PCO_2 → 0.2 mEq/L ↓ HCO_3^-* *Chronic: 1 mm Hg ↓ PCO_2 → 0.4 mEq/L ↓ HCO_3^-*

Note: Predicted compensatory responses are in *italics*.
[a]If blood values are the same as predicted compensatory values, a single acid–base disorder is present; if values are different, a mixed acid–base disorder is present.
[b]Acute renal compensation refers to duration of minutes to several hours; chronic renal compensation refers to a duration of several days.
Reprinted with permission from Norris, T. L. (2019). *Porth's pathophysiology: Concepts of altered health state* (10th ed.). Philadelphia, PA: Wolters Kluwer.

Medical Management

Treatment is directed at correcting the metabolic imbalance. If the problem results from excessive intake of chloride, treatment is aimed at eliminating the source of the chloride. When necessary, bicarbonate is given; however, the administration of sodium bicarbonate during cardiac arrest can result in paradoxical intracellular acidosis. Hyperkalemia may occur with acidosis and hypokalemia with reversal of the acidosis and subsequent movement of potassium back into the cells. Therefore, the serum potassium level is monitored closely, and hypokalemia is corrected as acidosis is reversed (Mount, 2017c).

In chronic metabolic acidosis, low serum calcium levels are treated before the chronic metabolic acidosis is treated to avoid tetany resulting from an increase in pH and a decrease in ionized calcium. Alkalizing agents may be given. Treatment modalities may also include hemodialysis or peritoneal dialysis (Goltzman, 2019b).

Acute and Chronic Metabolic Alkalosis (Base Bicarbonate Excess)

Metabolic alkalosis is a clinical disturbance characterized by a high pH (decreased H^+ concentration) and a high plasma bicarbonate concentration. It is caused by a gain of bicarbonate or a loss of H^+ (Emmett & Szerlip, 2017a; Norris, 2019).

Pathophysiology

A common cause of metabolic alkalosis is severe vomiting or gastric suction that causes loss of stomach HCl (hydrogen and chloride ions). The disorder also occurs in pyloric stenosis, in which only gastric fluid is lost. Gastric fluid has an acid pH (usually 1 to 3), and loss of this highly acidic fluid pulls H^+ ions from the bloodstream to replenish the gastric acid. As a result, the bloodstream loses H^+ ions and becomes alkalotic. Other situations predisposing to metabolic alkalosis include those associated with loss of potassium, such as diuretic therapy that promotes excretion of potassium (e.g., thiazides, furosemide), and ACTH secretion (as in hyperaldosteronism and Cushing's syndrome) (Emmett & Szerlip, 2017a; Norris, 2019).

Hypokalemia produces alkalosis in two ways: (1) when the bloodstream is low in K^+, the nephrons reabsorb K^+ into the bloodstream and secrete H^+ into the tubule fluid which is excreted in the urine and (2) when the bloodstream is low in K^+, intracellular potassium moves out of the cells into the ECF, and as potassium ions leave the cells, hydrogen ions must enter to maintain electroneutrality (Mount, 2017c). Excessive alkali ingestion from antacids containing bicarbonate or from the use of sodium bicarbonate during cardiopulmonary resuscitation can also cause metabolic alkalosis (Emmett & Szerlip, 2017b).

Chronic metabolic alkalosis can occur with long-term diuretic therapy (thiazides or furosemide), villous adenoma in the GI tract, external drainage of gastric fluids, significant potassium depletion, cystic fibrosis, and the chronic ingestion of milk and calcium carbonate (Emmett & Szerlip, 2017b).

Clinical Manifestations

In alkalosis, H^+ ions are decreased in the bloodstream, leaving negatively charged proteins attracting other positive ions. Calcium (Ca^{++}) ions bind to these proteins. As calcium ions bind to proteins in the bloodstream, free Ca^{++} ions decrease in the bloodstream and hypocalcemia develops. Alkalosis is primarily manifested by symptoms related to hypocalcemia, such as tingling of the fingers and toes, dizziness, and tetany (cramping muscles). Because it is the ionized fraction of calcium that is diminished in metabolic alkalosis, neuromuscular symptoms due to hypocalcemia are often the predominant symptoms (Emmett & Szerlip, 2017c).

In metabolic alkalosis, the lungs attempt to compensate by slowing respiratory rate, which increases CO_2 retention, and in turn increases H^+ content of the blood (see carbonic acid equation). If the kidneys are functional, there is increased renal excretion of HCO_3^- and conservation of H^+ in an attempt to reduce the alkalinity of the bloodstream. As the pH of blood increases in metabolic alkalosis, H^+ ions are reabsorbed into the bloodstream to neutralize the blood. As the nephrons increase H^+ ion reabsorption, they excrete K^+, and hypokalemia develops (Larkin & Zimmanck, 2015). In hypokalemia a prominent U wave often develops on the ECG and ventricular rhythm disturbances, such as PVCs, may occur. Hypokalemia also can lead to decreased GI motility and paralytic ileus (Emmett & Szerlip, 2017c).

Assessment and Diagnostic Findings

In metabolic alkalosis, evaluation of ABGs reveals a pH greater than 7.45 and a serum bicarbonate concentration greater than 26 mEq/L (see Table 10-12 for normal values of ABGs). The $PaCO_2$ increases as the lungs attempt to compensate for the excess bicarbonate by retaining CO_2. This hypoventilation is more pronounced in patients who are semiconscious, unconscious, or debilitated than in patients who are alert. Because of hypoventilation the patient may develop hypoxemia (Emmett & Szerlip, 2017c).

Urine chloride levels may help identify the cause of metabolic alkalosis if the patient's history provides inadequate information. Metabolic alkalosis is the setting in which urine chloride concentration may be a more accurate estimate of fluid volume than the urine sodium concentration. Urine chloride concentrations can help to determine the source of the metabolic alkalosis. Urine chloride concentrations can be used to differentiate between vomiting, diuretic therapy, and excessive adrenocorticosteroid secretion as the cause of the metabolic alkalosis. In patients with vomiting or cystic fibrosis, those receiving nutritional repletion, and those receiving diuretic therapy, hypovolemia and hypochloremia produce urine chloride concentrations lower than 25 mEq/L. Signs of hypovolemia are not present, and the urine chloride concentration exceeds 40 mEq/L in patients with mineralocorticoid excess or alkali loading; these patients usually have expanded fluid volume (Emmett & Palmer, 2019).

Medical Management

Treatment of both acute and chronic metabolic alkalosis is aimed at correcting the underlying acid–base disorder. Because volume depletion is commonly present with GI losses of H^+, the patient's I&O must be monitored carefully.

Treatment includes restoring normal fluid volume by administering normal saline because continued volume depletion perpetuates the alkalosis. In patients with hypokalemia, potassium is given as KCl to replace both K^+ and Cl^- losses. Proton pump inhibitors (e.g., omeprazole) are recommended to reduce the production of gastric hydrogen chloride (HCl). This decreased HCl will in turn decrease the loss of HCl with gastric suction in metabolic alkalosis. Carbonic anhydrase inhibitors (e.g., acetazolamide) are useful in treating metabolic alkalosis in patients who cannot tolerate rapid volume expansion (e.g., patients with heart failure). Carbonic anhydrase inhibitors act at the nephron to enhance bicarbonate excretion (Mehta & Emmett, 2018).

Acute and Chronic Respiratory Acidosis (Carbonic Acid Excess)

Respiratory acidosis is a clinical disorder in which the pH is less than 7.35 and the $PaCO_2$ is greater than 45 mm Hg. It may be either acute or chronic.

Pathophysiology

Respiratory acidosis is due to inadequate excretion of CO_2 with inadequate ventilation, resulting in elevated plasma CO_2 concentrations and, consequently, increased levels of carbonic acid. In addition to an elevated $PaCO_2$, inadequate ventilation usually causes a decrease in PaO_2. Acute respiratory acidosis occurs in emergency situations, such as acute pulmonary edema, aspiration of a foreign object, atelectasis, pneumothorax, and overdose of sedatives, as well as in nonemergent situations, such as sleep apnea associated with severe obesity, severe pneumonia, and acute respiratory distress syndrome. Respiratory acidosis commonly occurs in patients with severe chronic obstructive pulmonary disease (COPD) when patients acutely decompensate due to respiratory infection or heart failure. Respiratory acidosis can also occur in diseases that impair respiratory muscle function and cause hypoventilation. These disorders include severe scoliosis, muscular dystrophy, multiple sclerosis, myasthenia gravis, and Guillain-Barré syndrome (Feller-Kopman & Schwartzstein, 2017).

Clinical Manifestations

Clinical signs in acute and chronic respiratory acidosis vary. Acute respiratory acidosis can occur due to sudden hypercapnia (elevated $PaCO_2$) that will increase pulse, blood pressure, and respiratory rate. The patient may complain of confusion, disorientation, or may exhibit diminished level of consciousness. An elevated $PaCO_2$, greater than 60 mm Hg causes reflexive cerebrovascular vasodilation and increased cerebral blood flow. Ventricular fibrillation may be the first sign of respiratory acidosis in anesthetized patients (Feller-Kopman & Schwartzstein, 2017).

If respiratory acidosis is severe, intracranial pressure may increase, resulting in papilledema and dilated conjunctival blood vessels. Acidosis can cause hyperkalemia as the hydrogen ion concentration overwhelms the compensatory mechanisms. Acidosis causes H^+ ion to move into the cells, causing a shift of potassium out of the cell. The bloodstream then gains increased potassium ions (i.e., hyperkalemia) (Mount, 2017c).

Chronic respiratory acidosis occurs with pulmonary diseases such as COPD, including emphysema and chronic bronchitis; obstructive sleep apnea; and obesity. As long as the $PaCO_2$ does not exceed the body's ability to compensate, the patient will be asymptomatic. However, if the $PaCO_2$ increases rapidly, reflexive cerebral vasodilation will increase intracranial pressure, and cyanosis and tachypnea will develop. Patients with slowly progressive COPD gradually accumulate CO_2 over a prolonged period of time (months to years) and the body becomes used to high CO_2 levels. Patients with long-term COPD may not develop symptoms of hypercapnia because compensatory renal changes have had time to occur (Feller-Kopman & Schwartzstein, 2017).

> ⚑ *Quality and Safety Nursing Alert*
>
> If the $PaCO_2$ is chronically greater than 50 mm Hg, the respiratory center becomes relatively insensitive to CO_2 as a respiratory stimulant, leaving hypoxemia as the major drive for respiration. Patients with long-term COPD breathe independently based on a hypoxic drive. High oxygen concentration administration can remove the stimulus of hypoxemia. The patient can lose the independent stimulus to breathe and incur respiratory failure. Therefore, oxygen is given with extreme caution in patients with long-term COPD.

Assessment and Diagnostic Findings

In respiratory acidosis, ABG analysis reveals a pH less than 7.35, a $PaCO_2$ greater than 45 mm Hg, and variation in the bicarbonate level, depending on the duration of the acute respiratory acidosis. When compensation occurs over a prolonged period and renal retention of bicarbonate has fully occurred, the bicarbonate neutralizes the acidosis. Arterial pH is within the lower limits of normal (e.g., pH 7.35). Depending on the cause of respiratory acidosis, other diagnostic measures include monitoring of serum electrolyte levels, chest x-ray for determining respiratory infection or other disease, and a drug screen if an overdose is suspected. ECG monitoring is recommended to identify any cardiac involvement as a result of COPD (Feller-Kopman & Schwartzstein, 2017).

Medical Management

Treatment is directed at improving ventilation in acute and chronic respiratory acidosis. Exact measures vary according to the cause of inadequate ventilation. Pharmacologic agents are commonly used. For example, bronchodilators help reduce bronchial spasm and increase ventilation, antibiotics are used for respiratory infections, and thrombolytics or anticoagulants are used for pulmonary emboli (Stoller, 2019).

Pulmonary physiotherapy and nebulizer treatment can be used to clear the respiratory tract of mucus and purulent drainage. Adequate hydration (2 to 3 L/day) is indicated to keep the mucous membranes moist and decrease viscosity of mucous, thereby facilitating removal of secretions. Low concentration of supplemental oxygen is given as necessary (Aboussouan, 2018).

Mechanical ventilation, used appropriately, may be necessary to improve pulmonary ventilation. $PaCO_2$ should be reduced slowly and gradually using a mechanical ventilator. Mechanical ventilation can cause too rapid ventilatory loss of CO_2, which pulls H^+ out of the bloodstream too rapidly. If there is a rapid loss of H^+ the bloodstream becomes too alkalotic. The kidneys are unable to eliminate bicarbonate quickly enough to prevent alkalosis and seizures (Feller-Kopman & Schwartzstein, 2017).

Acute and Chronic Respiratory Alkalosis (Carbonic Acid Deficit)

Respiratory alkalosis is a clinical condition in which the arterial pH is greater than 7.45 and the $PaCO_2$ is less than 35 mm Hg. As with respiratory acidosis, acute and chronic conditions can cause this acid–base disturbance.

Pathophysiology

Respiratory alkalosis is caused by hyperventilation, which causes excessive loss or "blowing off" of CO_2 and, hence, there is a decrease in the plasma carbonic acid concentration (see carbonic acid equation). Causes include extreme anxiety such as panic disorder, hypoxemia, salicylate intoxication, gram-negative sepsis, and inappropriate ventilator settings.

Chronic respiratory alkalosis results from chronic hypocapnia which leads to decreased serum H^+ ion, resulting in alkalosis. Chronic hepatic insufficiency and cerebral tumors can cause chronic hyperventilation that leads to chronic respiratory alkalosis (Schwartzstein, Richards, Edlow, et al., 2018).

Clinical Manifestations

Clinical signs of respiratory alkalosis consist of lightheadedness and inability to concentrate due to cerebral artery vasoconstriction and decreased cerebral blood flow, numbness and tingling from decreased calcium ionization in the bloodstream, tinnitus, and sometimes loss of consciousness. Cardiac effects of respiratory alkalosis include tachycardia and ventricular and atrial arrhythmias (Schwartzstein et al., 2018).

Assessment and Diagnostic Findings

Analysis of ABGs assists in the diagnosis of both acute and chronic respiratory alkalosis. In the acute state, the pH is elevated above normal (greater than 7.45) as a result of a low $PaCO_2$ and a normal bicarbonate level. The kidneys take days to compensate for acid–base imbalances. Therefore, the kidneys cannot alter the bicarbonate level in the bloodstream quickly enough and medical intervention is necessary (Norris, 2019).

In the compensated state of chronic respiratory alkalosis, the kidneys have had sufficient time to lower the bicarbonate level to a near-normal level. Evaluation of serum electrolytes is indicated to identify any decrease in potassium, as hydrogen is pulled out of the cells in exchange for potassium. A decreased calcium level may occur as severe alkalosis inhibits calcium ionization, resulting in carpopedal spasms and tetany. A decreased phosphate level can occur due to alkalosis because there is increased uptake of phosphate by the cells. A toxicology screen should be performed to rule out salicylate intoxication due to aspirin poisoning (Schwartzstein et al., 2018).

Medical Management

Treatment depends on the exact underlying cause of respiratory alkalosis. If the cause is anxiety, the patient is instructed to breathe more slowly to allow CO_2 to accumulate or to breathe into a closed system (such as a paper bag or CO_2 rebreather mask). An antianxiety agent may be required to relieve hyperventilation in very anxious patients. Treatment of other causes of respiratory alkalosis is directed at correcting the underlying problem.

Mixed Acid–Base Disorders

Patients can simultaneously experience two or more independent acid–base disorders. A normal pH in the presence of changes in the $PaCO_2$ and plasma HCO_3^- concentration immediately suggests a mixed disorder. An example of a mixed disorder is the simultaneous occurrence of metabolic acidosis due to lactic acid accumulation and respiratory acidosis due to hypoventilation. Both of these disorders result in excessive acid accumulation in the bloodstream due to respiratory failure and cardiac arrest (Emmett & Palmer, 2018b).

Compensation

Generally, the pulmonary and renal systems compensate for each other to return the pH to normal. In a single acid–base disorder, the system not causing the problem tries to compensate by returning the ratio of bicarbonate to carbonic acid to the normal 20:1. The lungs compensate for metabolic disturbances by changing CO_2 excretion; hypoventilation accumulates CO_2, hyperventilation causes loss of CO_2. The kidneys compensate for respiratory disturbances by altering bicarbonate reabsorption and H^+ secretion (Norris, 2019; Theodore, 2019).

In respiratory acidosis, excess hydrogen in the blood is excreted in the urine in exchange for bicarbonate ions which are conserved. In respiratory alkalosis, the renal excretion of bicarbonate increases, and hydrogen ions are retained. In metabolic acidosis, the lungs compensate by increasing the ventilation rate and the kidneys retain bicarbonate. In metabolic alkalosis, the respiratory system compensates by decreasing ventilation to conserve CO_2 and increase the $PaCO_2$, which in turn increases carbonic acid. Because the lungs respond to acid–base disorders within minutes, compensation for metabolic imbalances occurs faster than renal compensation for respiratory imbalances (Norris, 2019; Theodore, 2019).

Table 10-13 summarizes compensation effects.

Blood Gas Analysis

Blood gas analysis is often used to identify the specific acid–base disturbance and the degree of compensation that has occurred. The analysis is usually based on an arterial blood sample; however, if an arterial sample cannot be obtained, a mixed venous sample may be used (Theodore, 2019). Results of ABG analysis provide information about alveolar ventilation, oxygenation, and acid–base balance. It is necessary to evaluate the concentrations of serum electrolytes (e.g., sodium, potassium, chloride) along with ABG data because electrolytes are commonly affected by acid–base imbalances. The health history, physical examination, previous blood gas results, and serum electrolytes should always be part of the assessment used to determine the cause of the acid–base disorder (Larkin & Zimmanck, 2015). Responding to isolated sets of blood gas results without these data can lead to serious errors in interpretation. Treatment of the underlying condition usually corrects acid–base disorders (Chart 10-3).

PARENTERAL FLUID THERAPY

When patients cannot take oral fluid or oral feedings, their status is termed NPO (*nil per os*), meaning nothing by mouth.

In patients who are NPO, **parenteral fluid therapy,** also termed IV fluid therapy, is used to administer fluids. IV fluid therapy can be initiated to replace fluids in various clinical settings such as hospitals, outpatient diagnostic and surgical settings, clinics, and home health care. IV fluids can also be used to administer medications and provide nutrients.

Purpose

The choice of an IV solution depends on the purpose of its administration. Generally, IV fluids are given to achieve one or more of the following goals:
- To provide water, electrolytes, and nutrients to meet daily requirements
- To replace water and correct electrolyte deficits
- To administer medications and blood products

IV solutions contain dextrose and/or electrolytes mixed in various proportions with water. Pure, electrolyte-free water can never be given by IV because it rapidly enters RBCs and causes them to rupture (Sterns, 2017b).

Types of Intravenous Solutions

IV solutions are categorized as isotonic, hypotonic, or hypertonic, according to whether their total osmolality is the same as, less than, or greater than that of blood, respectively (see earlier discussion of osmolality and tonicity). Electrolyte solutions are considered isotonic if the total electrolyte content (anions + cations) is between 250 and 375 mEq/L, hypotonic if the total electrolyte content is less than 250 mEq/L, and hypertonic if the total electrolyte content is greater than 375 mEq/L. The nurse must also consider a solution's osmolality, keeping in mind that the osmolality of plasma is approximately 300 mOsm/L (300 mmol/L). For example, a 10% dextrose solution has an osmolality of approximately 505 mOsm/L, which is greater than the osmolality of the bloodstream (Emmett & Palmer, 2018a).

Isotonic Fluids

Fluids that are classified as isotonic have a total osmolality close to that of the ECF and do not cause cells to shrink or swell. When isotonic fluids are administered they expand the ECF volume. One liter of isotonic fluid expands the ECF by 1 L; however, isotonic solution expands the plasma component of ECF by only 0.25 L. An isotonic solution is a crystalloid solution (water containing soluble mineral salts). Plasma is a colloidal solution. A colloidal solution is a mixture of fluid containing insoluble large particles, such as proteins. Colloidal solutions exert oncotic pressure; crystalloids do not exert oncotic pressure (Siparsky, 2019; Sterns, 2018a).

 Quality and Safety Nursing Alert

It is important for the nurse to recognize that in blood loss, 3 L of isotonic fluid (crystalloid solution) is needed to replace 1 L of blood (colloidal solution).

Because isotonic fluids expand the water volume in the intravascular space, patients with heart failure or hypertension

---

Chart 10-3

ASSESSMENT

Assessing Arterial Blood Gases

The following steps are recommended to evaluate arterial blood gas values. They are based on the assumption that the average values are:

pH = 7.35–7.45
$PaCO_2$ = 35–45 mm Hg
HCO_3^- = 24 to 27 mEq/L

1. *First, note the pH.* It can be high, low, or normal, as follows:

   A normal pH may indicate perfectly normal blood gases, *or* it may indicate a *compensated* imbalance. A compensated imbalance is one in which the body has been able to correct the pH by either respiratory or metabolic changes (depending on the primary problem). For example, a patient with primary metabolic acidosis starts out with a low bicarbonate level but a normal CO_2 level. Soon afterward, the lungs try to compensate for the imbalance by exhaling large amounts of CO_2 (hyperventilation). As another example, a patient with primary respiratory acidosis starts out with a high CO_2 level; soon afterward, the kidneys attempt to compensate by retaining bicarbonate. If the compensatory mechanism is able to restore the bicarbonate to carbonic acid ratio back to 20:1, full compensation (and thus normal pH) will be achieved.
   pH > 7.45 (alkalosis)
   pH < 7.35 (acidosis)
   pH = 7.4 (normal)

2. The next step is to determine the primary cause of the disturbance. This is done by evaluating the $PaCO_2$ and HCO_3^- in relation to the pH.

   Example: pH > 7.45 (alkalosis)
   a. If the $PaCO_2$ is less than 35 mm Hg, the primary disturbance is respiratory alkalosis. (This situation occurs when a patient hyperventilates and "blows off" too much CO_2. Recall that CO_2 dissolved in water becomes carbonic acid, the acid side of the "carbonic acid–bicarbonate buffer system.")
   b. If the HCO_3^- is greater than 27 mEq/L, the primary disturbance is metabolic alkalosis. (This situation occurs when the body gains too much bicarbonate, an alkaline substance. Bicarbonate is the basic or alkaline side of the "carbonic acid–bicarbonate buffer system.")

   Example: pH < 7.35 (acidosis)
   c. If the $PaCO_2$ is greater than 40 mm Hg, the primary disturbance is respiratory acidosis. (This situation occurs when a

patient hypoventilates and thus retains too much CO_2, an acidic substance.)
   d. If the HCO_3^- is less than 24 mEq/L, the primary disturbance is metabolic acidosis. (This situation occurs when the body's bicarbonate level drops, either because of direct bicarbonate loss or because of gains of acids such as lactic acid or ketones.)

3. The next step involves determining if compensation has begun. This is done by looking at the value other than the primary disorder. If it is moving in the same direction as the primary value, compensation is under way. Consider the following gases:

   The first set (1) indicates acute respiratory acidosis without compensation (the $PaCO_2$ is high, the HCO_3^- is normal). The second set (2) indicates chronic respiratory acidosis. Note that compensation has taken place—that is, the HCO_3^- has elevated to an appropriate level to balance the high $PaCO_2$ and produce a normal pH.

	pH	$PaCO_2$	HCO_3^-
(1)	7.2	60 mm Hg	24 mEq/L
(2)	7.4	60 mm Hg	37 mEq/L

4. Two distinct acid–base disturbances may occur simultaneously. These can be identified when the pH does not explain one of the changes. When the $PaCO_2$ is ↑ and the HCO_3 is ↓, respiratory acidosis and metabolic acidosis coexist. When the $PaCO_2$ is ↓ and the HCO_3 is ↑, respiratory alkalosis and metabolic alkalosis coexist.

   Example: Metabolic and respiratory acidosis

a.	pH	7.2	decreased pH (indicates acidosis)
b.	$PaCO_2$	52	increased pH (indicates respiratory acidosis)
c.	HCO_3	13	decreased HCO_3 (indicates metabolic acidosis)

5. If metabolic acidosis exists, then calculate the anion gap (AG) to determine the cause of the metabolic acidosis (AG vs. non-AG):

   $$AG = Na - (Cl^- + HCO_3^-)$$
   Normal AG = 10–14 mmol/L

6. Evaluate the patient to determine if the clinical signs and symptoms are compatible with the acid–base analysis.

Adapted from Fischbach, F., & Fischbach, M. (2018). *A manual of laboratory and diagnostic tests* (10th ed.). Philadelphia, PA: Lippincott Williams & Wilkins.

---

who receive isotonic solutions should be carefully monitored for signs of fluid overload (Siparsky, 2019).

D_5W

A solution of D_5W is unique in that it may be both isotonic and hypotonic (Hoorn, 2017). Once given, the glucose is rapidly metabolized, and this initially isotonic solution (same osmolality as serum) then disperses as a hypotonic fluid—one third extracellular and two thirds intracellular. It is essential to consider this action of D_5W, especially if the patient is at risk for increased intracranial pressure. During fluid resuscitation, this solution should not be used because hyperglycemia can result. Therefore, D_5W is used mainly to supply water and to correct an increased serum osmolality. About 1 L of D_5W

provides less than 170 kcal and is a minor source of the body's daily caloric requirements (Hoorn, 2017).

Normal Saline Solution

Normal saline (0.9% sodium chloride) solution contains water, sodium, and chloride. Because the osmolality is entirely contributed by electrolytes, the solution remains within the ECF and expands the intravascular volume. For this reason, normal saline solution is often used to correct an extracellular volume deficit but is not identical to ECF. It is used with administration of blood transfusions and to replace large sodium losses, such as in burn injuries. It should not be used in heart failure, pulmonary edema, renal impairment, or sodium retention. Normal saline does not supply calories (Hoorn, 2017).

Other Isotonic Solutions

Several other solutions contain ions in addition to sodium and chloride and are somewhat similar to the ECF in composition. Lactated Ringer's solution contains potassium and calcium in addition to sodium chloride. It is used to correct dehydration, blood loss, and sodium depletion and to replace GI losses.

Hypotonic Fluids

One purpose of hypotonic solution is to replace fluid, because it is hypotonic compared with plasma. Another purpose of hypotonic solution is to provide free water. At times, hypotonic sodium solutions are used to treat hypernatremia and other hyperosmolar conditions. Half-strength saline (0.45% sodium chloride) solution is frequently used.

Hypertonic Fluids

Hypertonic fluids include 3% NaCl and IV mannitol. If a patient is sodium depleted, a hypertonic sodium IV solution might be used. If a patient is experiencing acute cerebral edema, IV mannitol is often used. Hypertonic solutions pull water from the interstitial and intracellular compartments into the bloodstream. These solutions draw water out of intracellular compartments causing cellular dehydration (Hoorn, 2017). Normal saline and lactated Ringer's solution are considered isotonic solutions. When 5% dextrose (D_5W) is added to normal saline solution or lactated Ringer's solution, the total osmolality exceeds that of the ECF. With the added dextrose, these are then considered hypertonic solutions. However, the dextrose is quickly metabolized, and after the dextrose is depleted, only the isotonic solution remains. Therefore, any effect on the intracellular compartment is temporary. Similarly, with hypotonic electrolyte solutions containing 5% dextrose, once the dextrose is metabolized, these solutions disperse as hypotonic fluids. However, higher concentrations of dextrose, such as 50% dextrose ($D_{50}W$) in water, are strongly hypertonic. Hypertonic solutions should be administered into central veins so that they can be diluted by large amounts of rapid blood flow (Hoorn, 2017).

Saline solutions are also available in osmolar concentrations greater than that of the ECF. These solutions draw water from the ICF to the ECF and cause cells to shrink. If given rapidly or in large quantity, they may cause an extracellular volume excess and precipitate circulatory overload and dehydration. As a result, these solutions must be given cautiously and usually only when the serum osmolality has decreased to dangerously low levels. Hypertonic solutions exert an osmotic pressure greater than that of the ECF (Hoorn, 2017).

Other Intravenous Therapies

When the patient is unable to tolerate food, nutritional requirements are often met using the IV route. Solutions may include high concentrations of glucose (such as 50% dextrose in water), protein, or fat to meet nutritional requirements (see Chapter 41). The IV route may also be used to administer colloids, plasma expanders, and blood products (Hoorn, 2017). Examples of blood products include whole blood, packed RBCs, fresh-frozen plasma, albumin,

and cryoprecipitate (these are discussed in more detail in Chapter 28).

Many medications are also delivered by the IV route, either by continuous infusion or by intermittent bolus directly into the vein. Because IV medications enter the circulation rapidly, administration by this route is potentially hazardous. All medications can produce adverse reactions; however, medications given by the IV route can cause these reactions quickly after administration, because the medications are delivered directly into the bloodstream. Administration rates and recommended dilutions for individual medications are available in specialized texts pertaining to IV medications and in manufacturers' package inserts; these should be consulted to ensure safe IV administration of medications (Institute for Safe Medication Practices [ISMP], 2019).

> ▶ **Quality and Safety Nursing Alert**
>
> *The nurse must assess the patient for a history of allergic reactions to medications. Although obtaining drug allergy information is important when administering any medication, it is especially critical with IV administration, because the medication is delivered directly into the bloodstream. This can trigger an immediate hypersensitivity reaction.*

Nursing Management of the Patient Receiving Intravenous Therapy

In many settings, the ability to perform venipuncture to gain access to the venous system for administering fluids and medication is an expected nursing skill. This responsibility includes selecting the appropriate venipuncture site and type of cannula and being proficient in the technique of vein entry. The nurse should demonstrate competency in and knowledge of IV catheter placement according to the Nurse Practice Act applicable in their state and should follow the rules and regulations, organizational policies and procedures, and practice guidelines of that state's board of nursing (Gorski, Hadaway, Hagle, et al., 2016).

Managing Systemic Complications

Fluid Overload

Overloading the circulatory system with excessive IV fluids causes increased blood pressure and central venous pressure. Signs and symptoms of fluid overload include moist crackles on auscultation of the lungs, cough, restlessness, distended neck veins, edema, weight gain, dyspnea, and rapid, shallow respirations. Possible causes include rapid infusion of an IV solution or hepatic, cardiac, or renal disease. The risk of fluid overload and subsequent pulmonary edema is especially increased in older patients with cardiac disease; this is referred to as circulatory overload. Its treatment includes decreasing the IV rate, monitoring vital signs frequently, assessing breath sounds, and placing the patient in a high Fowler position. The primary provider is contacted immediately. This complication can be avoided by using an infusion pump and by carefully monitoring all infusions. Complications of circulatory overload include heart failure and pulmonary edema (Connelly, 2018).

Air Embolism

The risk of air embolism is rare but ever-present. It is most often associated with cannulation of central veins and directly related to the size of the embolus and the rate of entry. Air entering into central veins gets to the right ventricle, where it lodges against the pulmonary valve and blocks the flow of blood from the ventricle into the pulmonary arteries. Manifestations of air embolism include palpitations, dyspnea, continued coughing, jugular venous distention, wheezing, and cyanosis; hypotension; weak, rapid pulse; altered mental status; and chest, shoulder, and low back pain. Treatment calls for immediately clamping the cannula and replacing a leaking or open infusion system, placing the patient on the left side in the Trendelenburg position, assessing vital signs and breath sounds, and administering oxygen. Air embolism can be prevented by using locking adapters on all lines, filling all tubing completely with solution, and using an air detection alarm on an IV infusion pump. Complications of air embolism include shock and death. The amount of air necessary to induce death in humans is not known; however, the rate of entry is probably as important as the actual volume of air (Malik, Claus, Illman, et al., 2017).

Infection

Pyogenic substances in either the infusion solution or the IV administration set can cause bloodstream infections. Signs and symptoms include an abrupt temperature elevation shortly after the infusion is started, backache, headache, increased pulse and respiratory rate, nausea and vomiting, diarrhea, chills and shaking, and general malaise. Additional symptoms include erythema, edema, and induration or drainage at the insertion site. In sepsis, vascular collapse and septic shock may occur (Connelly, 2018). (See Chapter 11 for a discussion of septic shock.)

Infection ranges in severity from local involvement of the insertion site to systemic dissemination of organisms through the bloodstream, as in sepsis. Measures to prevent infection are essential at the time the IV line is inserted and throughout the entire infusion (Hugill, 2017).

Managing Local Complications

Local complications of IV therapy include phlebitis, infiltration and extravasation, thrombophlebitis, hematoma, and clotting of the needle (Simin, Milutinović, Turkulov, et al., 2019). Chart 10-4 provides a Nursing Research Profile about complications of peripheral IVs.

Phlebitis

Phlebitis, or inflammation of a vein, can be categorized as chemical, mechanical, or bacterial; however, two or more of these types of irritation often occur simultaneously. Chemical phlebitis can be caused by an irritating medication or solution (increased pH or high osmolality of a solution), rapid infusion rates, and medication incompatibilities. Mechanical phlebitis results from long periods of cannulation, catheters in flexed areas, catheter gauges larger than the vein lumen, and poorly secured catheters. Bacterial phlebitis can develop from poor hand hygiene, lack of aseptic technique, failure to check all equipment before use, and failure to recognize early signs and symptoms of phlebitis. Other factors include poor venipuncture technique, catheter in place for a prolonged period, and failure to adequately secure the catheter (Hugill, 2017). Phlebitis is characterized by a reddened, warm area around the insertion site or along the path of the vein, pain or tenderness at the site or along the vein, and swelling. The incidence of phlebitis increases with the length of time the IV line is in place, the composition of the fluid or medication infused (especially its pH and tonicity), catheter material, emergency insertions, the size and site of the cannula inserted, ineffective filtration, inadequate anchoring of the line, and the introduction of microorganisms at the time of insertion (Mihala, Ray-Barruel, Chopra, et al., 2018).

Chart 10-4 — NURSING RESEARCH PROFILE
Complication Rates of Peripheral IVs

Simin, D., Milutinović, D., Turkulov, V., et al. (2019). Incidence, severity and risk factors of peripheral intravenous cannula-induced complications: An observational prospective study. *Journal of Clinical Nursing, 28*(9–10), 1585–1599.

Purpose

The incidence and severity of complications of peripheral IV insertion is not known. The purpose of this study was to determine the incidence, severity, and risk factors of peripheral IV cannula-induced complications in hospitalized adult patients.

Design

This was an observational prospective study. Observations were made of 1428 IV insertions among 368 adult patients hospitalized in a tertiary medical center.

Findings

Phlebitis was the most common complication, with a rate of 44%, followed by infiltration with a rate of 16%, while the incidence of occlusion and catheter dislodgement were 7.6% and 5.6%, respectively. The risk factors for phlebitis were identified as the presence of a comorbidity (i.e., diabetes), a current infection, and an indwelling urinary catheter. The frequency of infiltration increased with the age of the patient, the number of attempts at the IV insertion in the same anatomic site, and the number of medications and IV solutions administered per day.

Nursing Implications

Medical-surgical nurses assess for all complications following IV insertion but should be particularly alert for phlebitis, which is the most common. This study provides evidence that older patients are at higher risk of infiltration and that attempting multiple IV sticks in the same anatomic site may lead to higher complication rates. The nurse should also be aware that patients who have comorbidities (such as diabetes) and those who are receiving multiple medications and IV solutions are at higher risk for IV complications.

Chart 10-5

ASSESSMENT

Assessing for Phlebitis

Grade	Clinical Criteria
0	No clinical symptoms
1	Erythema at access site with or without pain
2	Pain at access site Erythema, edema, or both
3	Pain at access site Erythema, edema, or both Streak formation Palpable venous cord
4	Pain at access site with erythema Streak formation Palpable venous cord (longer than 1 inch) Purulent drainage

Adapted from Gorski, L. A., Hadaway, L., Hagle, M., et al. (2016). Infusion therapy standards of practice. *Journal of Infusion Nursing, 39*(1 Suppl), S1–S159.

The Infusion Nurses Society (INS) has identified specific standards for assessing phlebitis (Gorski et al., 2016); these appear in Chart 10-5. Phlebitis is graded according to the most severe presenting indication.

Treatment consists of discontinuing the IV line and restarting it in another site, and applying a warm, moist compress to the affected site (INS, 2016). Phlebitis can be prevented by using aseptic technique during insertion, using the appropriate-size cannula or needle for the vein, considering the composition of fluids and medications when selecting a site, observing the site hourly for any complications, anchoring the cannula or needle well, and changing the IV site according to agency policy and procedures (Mihala et al., 2018).

Infiltration and Extravasation

Infiltration is the unintentional administration of a nonvesicant solution or medication into surrounding tissue. This can occur when the IV cannula dislodges or perforates the wall of the vein. Infiltration is characterized by edema around the insertion site, leakage of IV fluid from the insertion site, discomfort and coolness in the area of infiltration, and a significant decrease in the flow rate. When the solution is particularly irritating, sloughing of tissue may result. Close monitoring of the insertion site is necessary to detect infiltration before it becomes severe (Nickel, 2019; Simin et al., 2019).

Infiltration is usually easily recognized if the insertion area is larger than the same site of the opposite extremity but is not always so obvious. A common misconception is that a backflow of blood into the tubing proves that the catheter is properly placed within the vein. However, if the catheter tip has pierced the wall of the vessel, IV fluid will seep into tissues and flow into the vein. Although blood return occurs, infiltration may have occurred as well. A more reliable means of confirming infiltration is to apply a tourniquet above (or proximal to) the infusion site and tighten it enough to restrict venous flow. If the infusion continues to drip despite the venous obstruction, infiltration is present.

As soon as the nurse detects infiltration, the infusion should be stopped, the IV catheter removed, and a sterile dressing applied to the site after careful inspection to determine the extent of infiltration. The infiltration of any amount of blood product, irritant, or vesicant is considered the most severe (Brooks, 2018; Odom, Lowe, & Yates, 2018).

The IV infusion should be started in a new site or proximal to the infiltration site if the same extremity must be used again. A warm compress may be applied to the site if small volumes of noncaustic solutions have infiltrated over a long period, or if the solution was isotonic with a normal pH; the affected extremity should be elevated to promote the absorption of fluid. If the infiltration is recent and the solution was hypertonic or had an increased pH, a cold compress may be applied to the area (Gorski et al., 2016; Odom et al., 2018).

Infiltration can be detected and treated early by inspecting the site every hour for redness, pain, edema, blood return, coolness at the site, and IV fluid leaking from the IV site. Using the appropriate size and type of cannula for the vein prevents this complication. The use of electronic infusion devices (EIDs) does not cause an infiltration or extravasation; however, these devices will exacerbate the problem until the infusion is turned off. The Infusion Nursing Standards of Practice state that a standardized infiltration scale should be used to document the infiltration (Brooks, 2018; Gorski et al., 2016) (Chart 10-6).

Extravasation is similar to infiltration, with an inadvertent administration of vesicant or irritant solution or medication into the surrounding tissue. Medications such as vasopressors, potassium and calcium preparations, and chemotherapeutic agents can cause pain, burning, and redness at the site. Blistering, inflammation, and necrosis of tissues can occur. Older patients, comatose or anesthetized patients, patients with diabetes, and patients with peripheral vascular or cardiovascular disease are at greater risk for extravasation; other risk factors include high pressure infusion pumps, palpable cording of

Chart 10-6

ASSESSMENT

Assessing for Infiltration

Grade	Clinical Criteria
0	No clinical symptoms
1	Skin blanched, edema less than 1 inch in any direction, cool to touch, with or without pain
2	Skin blanched, edema 1 to 6 inches in any direction, cool to touch, with or without pain
3	Skin blanched, translucent, gross edema greater than 6 inches in any direction, cool to touch, mild to moderate pain, possible numbness
4	Skin blanched, translucent, skin tight, leaking, skin discolored, bruised, swollen, gross edema greater than 6 inches in any direction, deep pitting tissue edema, circulatory impairment, moderate to severe pain, infiltration of any amount of blood products, irritant, or vesicant

Adapted from Gorski, L. A., Hadaway, L., Hagle, M., et al. (2016). Infusion therapy standards of practice. *Journal of Infusion Nursing, 39*(1 Suppl), S1–S159.

vein, and fluid leakage from the insertion site. The extent of tissue damage is determined by the concentration of the medication, the quantity that extravasated, the location of the infusion site, the tissue response, and the duration of the process of extravasation (Gorski et al., 2016; Odom et al., 2018).

When extravasation occurs, the infusion must be stopped and the provider notified promptly. The agency's protocol to treat extravasation is initiated; the protocol may specify specific treatments, including antidotes specific to the medication that extravasated, and may indicate whether the IV line should remain in place or be removed before treatment. The protocol often specifies infiltration of the infusion site with an antidote prescribed after assessment by the provider, removal of the cannula, and application of warm compresses to sites of extravasation from alkaloids or cold compresses to sites of extravasation from alkylating and antibiotic vesicants. The affected extremity should not be used for further cannula placement. Thorough neurovascular assessments of the affected extremity must be performed frequently (Gorski et al., 2016).

Reviewing the institution's IV policy and procedures and incompatibility charts and checking with the pharmacist before administering any IV medication, whether peripherally or centrally, are recommended to determine incompatibilities and vesicant potential to prevent extravasation. Careful, frequent monitoring of the IV site, avoiding insertion of IV devices in areas of flexion, securing the IV line, and using the smallest catheter possible that accommodates the vein help minimize the incidence and severity of this complication. In addition, when vesicant medication is given by IV push, it should be given through a side port of an infusing IV solution to dilute the medication and decrease the severity of tissue damage if extravasation occurs. Extravasation is rated as grade 4 on the infiltration scale. Complications of an extravasation may include blister formation, skin sloughing and tissue necrosis, functional or sensory loss in the injured area, and disfigurement or loss of limb (Gorski et al., 2016; Nickel, 2019).

Thrombophlebitis

Thrombophlebitis refers to the presence of a clot plus inflammation in the vein. It is evidenced by localized pain, redness, warmth, and swelling around the insertion site or along the path of the vein, immobility of the extremity because of discomfort and swelling, sluggish flow rate, fever, malaise, and leukocytosis (Brooks, 2018).

Treatment includes discontinuing the IV infusion; applying a cold compress first to decrease the flow of blood, followed by a warm compress; elevating the extremity; and restarting the line in the opposite extremity. If the patient has signs and symptoms of thrombophlebitis, the IV line should not be flushed (although flushing may be indicated in the absence of phlebitis to ensure cannula patency and to prevent mixing of incompatible medications and solutions). The catheter should be cultured after the skin around the catheter is cleaned with alcohol. If purulent drainage exists, the site is cultured before the skin is cleaned (Brooks, 2018; Hugill, 2017).

Thrombophlebitis can be prevented by avoiding trauma to the vein at the time the IV line is inserted, observing the site every hour, and checking medication additives for compatibility (Gorski et al., 2016).

Hematoma

Hematoma results when blood leaks into tissues surrounding the IV insertion site. Leakage can result if the vein wall is perforated during venipuncture, the needle slips out of the vein, a cannula is too large for the vessel, or insufficient pressure is applied to the site after removal of the needle or cannula. The signs of a hematoma include ecchymosis, immediate swelling at the site, and leakage of blood at the insertion site.

Treatment includes removing the needle or cannula and applying light pressure with a sterile, dry dressing; applying ice for 24 hours to the site to avoid extension of the hematoma; elevating the extremity to maximize venous return, if tolerated; assessing the extremity for any circulatory, neurologic, or motor dysfunction; and restarting the line in the other extremity if indicated. A hematoma can be prevented by carefully inserting the needle and by frequently monitoring patients who have a bleeding disorder, are taking anticoagulant medication, or have advanced liver disease (Nickel, 2019).

Clotting and Obstruction

Blood clots may form in the IV line as a result of kinked IV tubing, a very slow infusion rate, an empty IV bag, or failure to flush the IV line after intermittent medication or solution administrations. The signs are decreased flow rate and blood backflow into the IV tubing (Brooks, 2018).

If blood clots in the IV line, the infusion must be discontinued and restarted in another site with a new cannula and administration set. The tubing should not be irrigated or milked. Neither the infusion rate nor the solution container should be raised, and the clot should not be aspirated from the tubing. Clotting of the needle or cannula may be prevented by not allowing the IV solution bag to run dry, taping the tubing to prevent kinking and maintain patency, maintaining an adequate flow rate, and flushing the line after intermittent medication or other solution administration. In some cases, a specially trained nurse or primary provider may inject a thrombolytic agent into the catheter to clear an occlusion resulting from fibrin or clotted blood (Brooks, 2018; Gorski et al., 2016).

Promoting Home, Community-Based, and Transitional Care

 Educating Patients About Self-Care

At times, IV therapy must be given in the home setting, in which case much of the daily management rests with the patient and family. Education becomes essential to ensure that the patient and family can manage the IV fluid and infusion correctly and avoid complications. Written instructions as well as demonstration and return demonstration help reinforce the key points for all of these functions (Payne, 2019).

Continuing and Transitional Care

Home infusion therapies cover a wide range of treatments, including antibiotic, analgesic, and antineoplastic medications; blood or blood component therapy; and parenteral nutrition. When direct nursing care is necessary, arrangements are made to have an infusion nurse visit the home and administer the IV therapy as prescribed. In addition to implementing and monitoring the IV therapy, the nurse carries out a comprehensive assessment of the patient's condition and continues to educate the patient and family about the skills involved in overseeing the IV therapy setup. Any dietary changes that may be necessary because of fluid or electrolyte imbalances are explained or reinforced during such sessions (Payne, 2019).

Periodic laboratory testing may be necessary to assess the effects of IV therapy and the patient's progress. Blood specimens may be obtained by a laboratory near the patient's home, or a home visit may be arranged to obtain blood specimens for analysis (Payne, 2019).

The nurse collaborates with the case manager in assessing the patient, family, and home environment; developing a plan of care in accordance with the patient's treatment plan and level of ability; and arranging for appropriate referral and follow-up if necessary. Any necessary equipment may be provided by the agency or purchased by the patient, depending on the terms of the home care arrangements. Appropriate documentation is necessary to assist in obtaining third-party payment for the service provided.

CRITICAL THINKING EXERCISES

1 **ebp** A 34-year-old woman comes to the walk-in clinic where you work. She is going to run her first marathon and asks about using salt tablets to compensate for loss of sodium through sweat. What is the best evidence for the use of salt tablets in performance athletes? What is the strength of the evidence base guiding your recommendation?

2 **ipc** An 82-year-old man with hypovolemia has been admitted to the medical unit where you work. What nursing and interprofessional assessments are indicated during your initial interactions with him? What other interprofessional services might you try to engage?

3 **pg** A 55-year-old woman is sent to the emergency department by her primary provider. The patient has a history of congestive heart failure. The primary provider has requested laboratory tests. Blood gas results are as follows: pH 7.46; HCO_3^- 26; $PaCO_2$ 40 mm Hg. Blood chemistry results are as follows: potassium 4.5 mEq/L; sodium 140 mEq/L; glucose 110 mg/dL. Vital signs: BP 140/92, HR 90 bpm, RR 18 bpm. What is your priority for this patient? Give your rationale. What further diagnostic testing is indicated?

REFERENCES

*Asterisk indicates nursing research.

Books

Cash, J., & Glass, C. (2018). *Adult gerontology practice guidelines* (2nd ed.). New York: Springer.

Comerford, K. C., & Durkin, M. T. (2020). *Nursing 2020 drug handbook*. Philadelphia, PA: Wolters Kluwer.

Fischbach, F., & Fischbach, M. (2018). *A manual of laboratory and diagnostic tests* (10th ed.). Philadelphia, PA: Lippincott Williams & Wilkins.

Frandsen, G., & Pennington, S. S. (2018). *Abram's clinical drug therapy: Rationales for nursing practice* (11th ed.). Philadelphia, PA: Wolters Kluwer.

Hall, J. E. (2016). *Guyton and Hall textbook of medical physiology* (13th ed.). Philadelphia, PA: Saunders Elsevier.

Norris, T. L. (2019). *Porth's pathophysiology: Concepts of altered health states* (10th ed.). Philadelphia, PA: Wolters Kluwer.

Papadakis, M. A., McPhee, S. J., & Rabow, M. W. (2019). *Current medical diagnosis and treatment* (58th ed.). New York: McGraw-Hill.

Pirahanchi, Y., & Aeddula, N. R. (2019). *Physiology, sodium potassium pump. StatPearls [Internet]*. Treasure Island, FL: StatPearls Publishing.

Sharma, S., & Castro, D. (2019). *Hypophosphatemia. StatPearls [Internet]*. Treasure Island, FL: StatPearls Publishing.

Vallerand, A. H., & Sanoski, C. A. (2019). *Davis drug guide for nurses* (16th ed.). Philadelphia, PA: FA Davis.

Van Leeuwen, A. M., & Bladh, M. L. (2017). *Davis's comprehensive handbook of laboratory and diagnostic tests*. Philadelphia, PA: FA Davis.

Weber, J., & Kelley, J. (2018). *Health assessment in nursing* (6th ed.). Philadelphia, PA: Wolters Kluwer.

Journals and Electronic Documents

Aboussouan, L. S. (2018). Role of mucoactive agents and secretion clearance techniques in chronic obstructive pulmonary disease. *UpToDate*. Retrieved on 6/18/2019 at: www.uptodate.com/contents/role-of-mucoactive-agents-and-secretion-clearance-techniques-in-copd

Apostu, M. (2014). A strategy for maintaining fluid and electrolyte balance in aerobic effort. *Procedia—Social and Behavioral Sciences, 117*(2014), 323–328.

Ashurst, J., Sergent, S. R., & Sergent, B. R. (2016). Evidence-based management of potassium disorders in the emergency department. *Emergency Medical Practice, 18*(11), 1–24.

Aubry, E., Friedli, N., Schetz, P., et al. (2018). Refeeding syndrome in the frail elderly population: Prevention, diagnosis and management. *Clinical and Experimental Gastroenterology, 11*, 255–264.

Bichet, D. G. (2017). Treatment of central diabetes insipidus. *UpToDate*. Retrieved on 6/15/2019 at: www.uptodate.com/contents/treatment-of-central-diabetes-insipidus

Black, D. M., & Rosen, C. J. (2016). Clinical practice. Postmenopausal osteoporosis. *New England Journal of Medicine, 374*(3), 254–262.

Bove-Fenderson, E., & Mannstadt, M. (2018). Hypocalcemic disorders. Best practice and research. *Clinical Endocrinology & Metabolism, 32*(5), 639–656.

Brater, D. C., & Ellison, D. H. (2019). Mechanism of action of diuretics. *UpToDate*. Retrieved on 6/14/2019 at: www.uptodate.com/contents/mechanism-of-action-of-diuretics

Brooks, N. (2018). Remember the risks of intravenous therapy and how to reduce them. *British Journal of Nursing, 27*(8), S20–S21.

Carfagna, F., Del Vecchio, L., Pontoriero, G., et al. (2018). Current and potential treatment options for hyperphosphatemia. *Expert Opinion on Drug Safety, 17*(6), 597–607.

Chen, H. H., & Colucci, W. S. (2017). Natriuretic peptide measurement in heart failure. *UpToDate*. Retrieved on 6/15/2019 at: www.uptodate.com/contents/natriuretic-peptide-measurement-in-heart-failure

Connelly, K. (2018). Intravenous fluid administration: Improving patient outcomes with evidence-based care. *Journal for Nurse Practitioners, 14*(8), 598–604.

Daly, R. M. (2017). Exercise and nutritional approaches to prevent frail bones, falls and fractures: An update. *Climacteric, 20*(2), 119–124.

Depret, F., Peacock, W. F., Liu, K. D., et al. (2019). Management of hyperkalemia in the acutely ill patient. *Annals of Intensive Care, 9*(1), 32.

Dick, S. M, Queiroz, M., Bernardi, B. L., et al. (2018). Update in diagnosis and management of primary aldosteronism. *Clinical Chemistry and Laboratory Medicine, 56*(3), 360–372.

Duval, M., Bach, K., Masson, D., et al. (2018). Is severe hypocalcemia immediately life threatening? *Endocrine Connections, 7*(10), 1067–1074.

Emmett, M., & Palmer, B. F. (2018a). Serum osmol gap. *UpToDate*. Retrieved on 6/14/2019 at: www.uptodate.com/contents/serum-osmol-gap

Emmett, M., & Palmer, B. F. (2018b). Simple and mixed acid-base disorders. *UpToDate*. Retrieved on 6/18/2019 at: www.uptodate.com/contents/simple-and-mixed-acid-base-disorders

Emmett, M., & Palmer, B. F. (2019). Urine anion and osmolal gaps in metabolic acidosis. *UpToDate*. Retrieved on 6/14/2019 at: www.uptodate.com/contents/urine-anion-and-osmolal-gaps-in-metabolic-acidosis

Emmett, M., & Szerlip, H. (2017a). Approach to the adult with metabolic alkalosis. *UpToDate*. Retrieved on 6/17/2019 at: www.uptodate.com/contents/approach-to-the-patient-with-metabolic-alkalosis

Emmett, M., & Szerlip, H. (2017b). Causes of metabolic alkalosis. *UpToDate*. Retrieved on 6/17/2019 at: www.uptodate.com/contents/causes-of-metabolic-alkalosis

Emmett, M., & Szerlip, H. (2017c). Clinical manifestations and evaluation of metabolic alkalosis. *UpToDate*. Retrieved on 6/17/2019 at: www.uptodate.com/contents/clinical-maniferstations-and-evaluation-of-metabolic-alkalosis

Emmett, M., & Szerlip, H. (2018). Approach to the patient with metabolic acidosis. *UpToDate*. Retrieved on 6/17/2019 at: www.uptodate.com/contents/approach-to-the-patient-with-metabolic-acidosis

Feller-Kopman, D. J., & Schwartzstein, R. M. (2017). Mechanisms, causes, and effects of hypercapnia. *UpToDate*. Retrieved on 6/18/2019 at: www.uptodate.com/contents/mechanisms-causes-and-effects-of-hypercapnia

Ferguson, G. T., & Make, B. (2019). Management of stable chronic obstructive pulmonary disease. *UpToDate*. Retrieved on 6/18/2019 at: www.uptodate.com/contents/management-of-stable-chronic-obstructive-pulmonary-disease

Goltzman, D. (2017). Etiology of hypocalcemia in adults. *UpToDate*. Retrieved on 6/16/2019 at: www.uptodate.com/contents/etiology-of-hypocalcemia-in-adults

Goltzman, D. (2019a). Clinical manifestations of hypocalcemia. *UpToDate*. Retrieved on 6/16/2019 at: www.uptodate.com/contents/clinical-manifestations-of-hypocalcemia

Goltzman, D. (2019b). Treatment of hypocalcemia. *UpToDate*. Retrieved on 6/16/2019 at: www.uptodate.com/contents/treatment-of-hypocalcemia

Gorski, L. A., Hadaway, L., Hagle, M., et al. (2016). Infusion therapy standards of practice. *Journal of Infusion Nursing, 39*(1 Suppl), S1–S159.

Hew-Butler, T., Loi, V., Pani, A., et al. (2017). Exercise-induced hyponatremia: 2017 update. *Frontiers in Medicine (Lausanne), 4*, 21.

Hogan, J., & Goldfarb, S. (2018). Regulation of calcium and phosphate balance. *UpToDate*. Retrieved on 9/01/2019 at: www.uptodate.com/contents/regulation-of-calcium-and-phosphate-balance

Hoorn, E. J. (2017). Intravenous fluids: Balancing solutions. *Journal of Nephrology, 30*(4), 485–492.

Hugill, K. (2017). Preventing bloodstream infection in intravenous therapy. *British Journal of Nursing, 26*(4), S4–S10.

Hutto, C., & French, M. (2017). Neurologic intensive care unit electrolyte management. *Nursing Clinics of North America, 52*(3), 321–329.

Infusion Nurses Society (INS). (2016). Infusion therapy: Standards of practice. *Journal of Infusion Nursing, 39*(1S), S1–S92.

Inker, L., & Perrone, R. (2018). Assessment of kidney function. *UpToDate*. Retrieved on 6/14/2019 at: www.uptodate.com/contents/assessment-of-kidney-function

Institute for Safe Medication Practices (ISMP). (2019). 2018–2019 Targeted medication safety best practices for hospitals. Retrieved on 8/02/2019 at: www.ismp.org

Jain, N., Phadke, R. V., Chauhan, G., et al. (2018). Osmotic demyelination syndrome in the setting of hypernatremia. *Neurology India, 66*(2), 559–560.

Kazaure, H. S., & Sosa, J. A. (2018). Surgical hypoparathyroidism. *Endocrinologic and Metabolic Clinics of North America, 4*(4), 783–796.

Kovesdy, C. (2018). Pathogenesis, consequences, and treatment of metabolic acidosis in chronic kidney disease. *UpToDate*. Retrieved on 6/17/2019 at: www.uptodate.com/contents/pathogenesis-consequences-and-treatment-of-metabolic-acidosis-in-chronic-kidney-disease

Langer, T., Santini, A., Scotti, E., et al. (2015). Intravenous balanced solutions: From physiology to clinical evidence. *Anaesthesiol Intensive Therapy, 47*, s78–s88.

Larkin, B. G., & Zimmanck, R. J. (2015). Interpreting arterial blood gases successfully. *AORN Journal, 102*(4), 343–357.

Liamis, G., Megapanou, E., Elisaf, M., et al. (2019). Hyponatremia-inducing drugs. In A. Peri, C. J. Thompson, & J. G. Verbalis (Eds.). *Disorders of fluid and electrolyte metabolism. Focus on hyponatremia. Frontiers of Hormone Research, 52*, 167–177.

Long, B., Warix, J. R., & Koyfman, A. (2018). Controversies in management of hyperkalemia. *Journal of Emergency Medicine, 55*(2), 192–205.

Malik, N., Claus, P. L., Illman, J. E., et al. (2017). Air embolism: Diagnosis and management. *Future Cardiology, 13*(4), 365–378.

Mandel, J., & Palevsky, P. M. (2019). Treatment of severe hypovolemia or hypovolemic shock. *UpToDate*. Retrieved on 6/15/19 at: www.uptodate.com/contents/treatment-of-severe-hypovolemia-or-hypovolemic-shock

Marcucci, G., Cianferotti, L., & Brandi, M. L. (2018). Clinical presentation and management of hypoparathyroidism. *Best Practice & Research. Clinical Endocrinology & Metabolism, 32*(6), 927–939.

McDermott, B. P., Anderson, S. A., Armstrong, L. E., et al. (2017). National Athletic Trainers' Association Position Statement: Fluid replacement for the physically active. *Journal of Athletic Training, 52*(9), 877–895.

McDonough, A. A., & Youn, J. H. (2017). Potassium homeostasis: The knowns, the unknowns, and the health benefits. *Physiology (Bethesda), 32*(2), 100–111.

Mehta, A., & Emmett, M. (2018). Treatment of metabolic alkalosis. *UpToDate*. Retrieved on 6/14/2019 at: www.uptodate.com/contents/treatment-of-metabolic-alkalosis

*Mihala, G., Ray-Barruel, G., Chopra, V., et al. (2018). Phlebitis signs and symptoms with peripheral intravenous catheters: Incidence and correlation study. *Journal of Infusion Nursing, 41*(4), 260–263.

Mount, D. B. (2017a). Causes and evaluation of hyperkalemia in adults. *UpToDate*. Retrieved on 6/14/2019 at: www.uptodate.com/contents/causes-and-evaluation-of-hyperkalemia-in-adults

Mount, D. B. (2017b). Clinical manifestations and treatment of hypokalemia in adults. *UpToDate*. Retrieved on 6/15/2019 at: www.uptodate.com/contents/clinical-manifestations-and-treatment-of-hypokalemia-in-adults

Mount, D. B. (2017c). Potassium balance in acid-base disorders. *UpToDate*. Retrieved on 6/15/2019 at: www.uptodate.com/contents/potassium-balance-in-acid-base-disorders

Mount, D. B. (2017d). Causes of hypokalemia in adults. *UpToDate*. Retrieved on 6/15/2019 at: www.uptodate.com/contents/causes-of-hypokalemia-in-adults

Mount, D. B. (2017e). Treatment and prevention of hyperkalemia in adults. *UpToDate*. Retrieved on 6/15/2019 at: www.uptodate.com/contents/treatment-and-prevention-of-hyperkalemia-in-adults

Mushin, S. A., & Mount, D. B. (2018). Diagnosis and treatment of hypernatremia. *Best Practice & Research. Clinical Endocrinology & Metabolism, 30*(2), 189–203.

National Institutes of Health (NIH), Office of Dietary Supplements. (2019). Magnesium. Retrieved on 8/1/2019 at: www.ods.od.nih.gov/factsheets/Magnesium-HealthProfessional

Nickel, B. (2019). Peripheral intravenous access: Applying infusion therapy standards of practice to improve patient safety. *Critical Care Nurse, 39*(1), 61–71.

*Odom, B., Lowe, L., & Yates, C. (2018). Peripheral infiltration and extravasation injury methodology: A retrospective study. *Journal of Infusion Nursing, 41*(4), 247–252.

Olendzki, B. (2017). Patient education: Low sodium diet (beyond the basics). *UpToDate*. Retrieved on 6/15/2019 at: www.uptodate.com/contents/patient-education-low-sodium-diet

Palmer, B. F., & Clegg, D. J. (2016a). Physiology and pathophysiology of potassium homeostasis. *Advances in Physiology Education, 40*(4), 480–490.

Palmer, B. F., & Clegg, D. J. (2016b). Achieving the benefits of a high-potassium, Paleolithic diet, without the toxicity. *Mayo Clinic Proceedings, 91*(4), 496–508.

Payne, D. (2019). Administering intravenous therapy in the patient's home. *British Journal of Community Nursing, 24*(2), 67–71.

Perwad, F., & Portale, A. (2019). Burosumab therapy for X-linked hypophosphatemia and therapeutic implications for CKD. *Clinical Journal of American Society of Nephrology, 14* (7), 1–3.

Rosen, H., & Drezner, M. K. (2019). Overview of the management of osteoporosis in postmenopausal women. *UpToDate*. Retrieved on 6/16/2019 at: www.uptodate.com/contents/overview-of-the-management-of-osteoporosis-in-postmenopausal-women

Schrier, S. L. (2018). Approach to the adult with anemia. *UpToDate*. Retrieved on 6/15/2019 at: www.uptodate.com/contents/approach-to-the-adult-with-anemia

Schwartzstein, R. M., Richards, J., Edlow, J. A., et al. (2018). Hyperventilation syndrome. *UpToDate*. Retrieved on 6/18/2019 at: www.uptodate.com/contents/hyperventilation-syndrome

Shane, E. (2019a). Etiology of hypercalcemia. *UpToDate*. Retrieved on 6/16/2019 at: www.uptodate.com/contents/etiology-of-hypercalcemia

Shane, E. (2019b). Clinical manifestations of hypercalcemia. *UpToDate*. Retrieved on 6/16/2019 at: www.uptodate.com/contents/clinicla-manifestations-of-hypercalcemia

Shane, E., & Berenson, J. R. (2019). Treatment of hypercalcemia. *UpToDate*. Retrieved on 9/01/2019 at: www.uptodate.com/contents/treatment-of-hypercalcemia

Shimada, M., Shutto-Uchita, Y., & Yamabe, H. (2019). Lack of awareness of dietary sources of phosphorus is a clinical concern. *In Vivo (Athens, Greece)*, 33(1), 11–16.

*Simin, D., Milutinović, D., Turkulov, V., et al. (2019). Incidence, severity and risk factors of peripheral intravenous cannula-induced complications: An observational prospective study. *Journal of Clinical Nursing*, 28(9–10), 1585–1599.

Siparsky, N. (2019). Overview of postoperative fluid therapy in adults. *UpToDate*. Retrieved on 6/18/2019 at: www.uptodate.com/contents/overview-of-postoperative-fluid-therapy-in-adults

Squiers, J. (Ed.). (2017). Fluids and electrolytes. *Nursing Clinics of North America*, 52(2), 237–348.

Sterns, R. H. (2017a). Etiology, clinical manifestations, and diagnosis of volume depletion in adults. *UpToDate*. Retrieved on 6/14/2019 at: www.uptodate.com/contents/etiology-clinical-manifestations-and-diagnosis-of-volume-depletion-in-adults

Sterns, R. H. (2017b). Maintenance and replacement fluid therapy in adults. *UpToDate*. Retrieved on 6/14/2019 at: www.uptodate.com/contents/maintenance-and-replacement-fluid-therapy-in-adults

Sterns, R. H. (2017c). Etiology and evaluation of hypernatremia in adults. *UpToDate*. Retrieved on 6/15/2019 at: www.uptodate.com/contents/etiology-and-evaluation-of-hypernatremia-in-adults

Sterns, R. H. (2017d). Pathophysiology and etiology of syndrome of inappropriate antidiuretic hormone. *UpToDate*. Retrieved on 6/15/2019 at: www.uptodate.com/contents/pathophysiology-and-etiology-of-syndrome-of-inappropriate-antidiuretic-hormone

Sterns, R. H. (2017e). Manifestations of hyponatremia and hypernatremia. *UpToDate*. Retrieved on 6/15/2019 at: www.uptodate.com/contents/manifestations-of-hyponatremia-and-hypernatremia

Sterns, R. H. (2018a). General principles of disorders of water balance (hyponatremia and hypernatremia) and sodium balance (hypovolemia and edema). *UpToDate*. Retrieved on 6/14/2019 at: www.uptodate.com/contents/general-principles-of-disorders-of-water-balance

Sterns, R. H. (2018b). Pathophysiology and etiology of edema in adults. *UpToDate*. Retrieved on 6/14/2019 at: www.uptodate.com/contents/pathophysiology-and-etiology-of-edema-in-adults

Sterns, R. H. (2018c). Diagnostic evaluation of adults with hyponatremia. *UpToDate*. Retrieved on 6/14/2019 at: www.uptodate.com/contents/evaluation-of-adults-with-hyponatremia

Sterns, R. H. (2020). Overview of treatment of hyponatremia. *UpToDate*. Retrieved on 12/9/2020 at: www.uptodate.com/overview-of-treatment-of-hyponatremia

Sterns, R. H., & Hoorn, E. J. (2019). Treatment of hypernatremia in adults. *UpToDate*. Retrieved on 6/15/2019 at: www.uptodate.com/contents/treatment-of-hypernatremia-in-adults

Stoller, J. K. (2019). Management of exacerbations of chronic obstructive pulmonary disease. *UpToDate*. Retrieved on 6/18/2019 at: www.uptodate.com/contents/management-of-exacerbations-of-chronic-obstructive-pulmonary-disease

Stubbs, J., & Yu, A. (2019). Overview of the causes and treatment of hyperphosphatemia. *UpToDate*. Retrieved on 6/18/2019 at: www.uptodate.com/contents/overview-of-the-causes-and-treatment-of-hyperphosphatemia

Theodore, A. C. (2019). Arterial blood gases. *UpToDate*. Retrieved on 6/17/19 at: www.uptodate.com/contents/arterial-blood-gases

Upala, S., Jaruvongvanich, V., Wijarnpreecha, K., et al. (2016). Hypomagnesemia and mortality in patients admitted to intensive care unit: A systematic review and meta-analysis. *Quarterly Journal of Medicine*, 109(7), 453–459.

Wang, A., & Yuan, L. (2019). Primary hyperthyroidism. *Clinical Case Reports*, 7(4), 849–850.

Yu, A. (2019a). Hypomagnesemia: Causes of hypomagnesemia. *UpToDate*. Retrieved on 8/1/19 at: www.uptodate.com/contents/causes-of-hypomagnesemia

Yu, A. (2019b). Hypomagnesemia: Evaluation and treatment. *UpToDate*. Retrieved on 6/16/19 at: www.uptodate.com/contents/evaluation-and-treatment-of-hypomagnesemia

Yu, A., & Gupta, A. (2019). Hypermagnesemia: Causes, symptoms, and treatment. *UpToDate*. Retrieved on 6/17/2019 at: www.uptodate.com/contents/causes-and-treatment-of-hypermagnesemia

Yu, A., & Stubbs, J. (2019). Relation between total and ionized serum calcium concentrations. *UpToDate*. Retrieved on 6/16/19 at: www.uptodate.com/contents/relation-between-total-and-ionized-serum-calcium-concentrations

Yu, A., & Yarlagadda, S. G. (2019). Clinical manifestations of magnesium depletion. *UpToDate*. Retrieved on 8/1/19 at: www.uptodate.com/contents/clinical-manifestations-of-magnesium-depletion

Resources

Infusion Nurses Society (INS), www.ins1.org

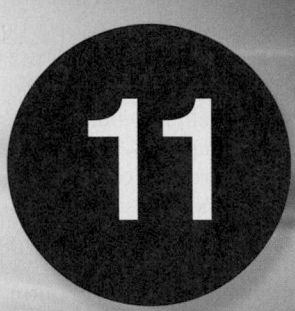

11 Shock, Sepsis, and Multiple Organ Dysfunction Syndrome

LEARNING OUTCOMES

On completion of this chapter, the learner will be able to:

1. Describe the pathophysiology, clinical manifestations, and collaborative management of progressive stages of various types of shock, of sepsis, and of multiple organ dysfunction syndrome.
2. Compare and contrast the pathophysiology, clinical manifestations, and collaborative management of shock states in hypovolemic, cardiogenic, and distributive shock.
3. Identify medical and nursing management priorities in treating patients across the continuum of shock.
4. Describe medical and nursing management priorities in the treatment and prevention of sepsis and septic shock.
5. Discuss the role of nurses in providing psychosocial support to patients experiencing shock, sepsis, and multiple organ dysfunction syndrome, and their families.
6. Discuss the role of nurses in providing transitional care to patients and their families after having been managed in a critical-care unit for shock, sepsis, or multiple organ dysfunction syndrome.

NURSING CONCEPTS

Cellular Regulation

Fluids and Electrolytes

Infection

Medical Emergencies

Perfusion

GLOSSARY

anaphylactic shock: distributive shock state resulting from a severe allergic reaction producing an acute systemic vasodilation and relative hypovolemia

cardiogenic shock: shock state resulting from impairment or failure of the myocardium

colloids: intravenous solutions that contain molecules that are too large to pass through capillary membranes

crystalloids: intravenous electrolyte solutions that move freely between the intravascular compartment and interstitial spaces

cytokines: messenger substances that may be released by a cell to create an action at that site or may be carried by the bloodstream to a distant site before being activated; (*synonyms:* biochemical mediators, inflammatory mediators)

distributive shock: shock state resulting from displacement of intravascular volume creating a relative hypovolemia and inadequate delivery of oxygen to the cells

hypovolemic shock: shock state resulting from decreased intravascular volume due to fluid loss

multiple organ dysfunction syndrome: presence of altered function of two or more organs in an acutely ill patient such that interventions are necessary to support continued organ function

neurogenic shock: shock state resulting from loss of sympathetic tone causing relative hypovolemia

sepsis: life-threatening organ dysfunction caused by a dysregulated host response to infection

septic shock: a subset of sepsis in which underlying circulatory and cellular metabolic abnormalities are profound enough to substantially increase mortality

shock: life-threatening physiologic condition in which there is inadequate blood flow to tissues and cells of the body

systemic inflammatory response syndrome: a syndrome resulting from a clinical insult that initiates an inflammatory response that is systemic, rather than localized to the site of the insult; a type of cytokine release syndrome also referred to as cytokine storm

Shock is a life-threatening condition that results from inadequate tissue perfusion. Many conditions may cause shock; irrespective of the cause, tissue hypoperfusion prevents adequate oxygen delivery to cells, leading to cell dysfunction and death. The progression of shock is neither linear nor predictable, and shock states, especially septic shock (the most life-threatening form of sepsis), comprise an area of ongoing clinical research. Nurses caring for patients with shock and those at risk for shock must understand the underlying mechanisms of the various shock states (i.e., hypovolemic, cardiogenic, obstructive [see Chapter 25], and distributive shock [i.e., septic, neurogenic, anaphylactic]) and recognize the subtle as well as more obvious signs of each of these states. If shock is not effectively treated, **multiple organ dysfunction syndrome (MODS)** which is the presence of altered function of two or more organs in an acutely ill patient such that interventions are necessary to support continued organ function may ensue, often resulting in patient death. MODS may be a complication of any form of shock but is most commonly seen in patients with sepsis. Rapid assessment with early recognition and response to shock states and sepsis is essential to the patient's recovery.

Overview of Shock

Shock can best be defined as a clinical syndrome that results from inadequate tissue perfusion, creating an imbalance between the delivery of oxygen and nutrients needed to support cellular function (Kislitsina, Rich, Wilcox, et al., 2019; Massaro, 2018). Adequate blood flow to the tissues and cells requires an effective cardiac pump, adequate vasculature or circulatory system, and sufficient blood volume. If one of these components is impaired, perfusion to the tissues is threatened or compromised. Without treatment, inadequate blood flow to the cells results in poor delivery of oxygen and nutrients, cellular hypoxia, and cell death that progresses to organ dysfunction and eventually death.

Shock affects all body systems. It may develop rapidly or slowly, depending on the underlying cause. During shock, the body struggles to survive, calling on all its homeostatic mechanisms to restore blood flow. Any insult to the body can create a cascade of events resulting in poor tissue perfusion. Therefore, any patient with any disease state may be at risk for developing shock. The primary underlying pathophysiologic process and underlying disorder are used to classify the shock state (e.g., hypovolemic shock, cardiogenic shock, obstructive shock [see Chapter 25], distributive shock [i.e., septic, neurogenic, anaphylactic]; all discussed later in the chapter).

Regardless of the initial cause of shock, certain physiologic responses are common to all types of shock. These physiologic responses include hypoperfusion of tissues, hypermetabolism, and activation of the inflammatory response. The body responds to shock states by activating the sympathetic nervous system and mounting a hypermetabolic and inflammatory response. Failure of compensatory mechanisms to effectively restore physiologic balance is the final pathway of all shock states and results in end-organ dysfunction and death (Massaro, 2018; Seymour & Angus, 2018).

Nursing care of patients with shock requires ongoing systematic assessment. Many of the interventions required in caring for patients with shock call for close collaboration with other members of the health care team and rapid implementation of prescribed therapies. Nurses are in key positions to identify early signs of shock and anticipate rapid therapy.

Normal Cellular Function

Energy metabolism occurs within the cell, where nutrients are chemically broken down and stored in the form of adenosine triphosphate (ATP). Cells use this stored energy to perform necessary functions, such as active transport, muscle contraction, and biochemical synthesis, as well as specialized cellular functions, such as the conduction of electrical impulses. ATP can be synthesized aerobically (in the presence of oxygen) or anaerobically (in the absence of oxygen). Aerobic metabolism yields far greater amounts of ATP per mole of glucose than does anaerobic metabolism; therefore, it is a more efficient and effective means of producing energy. In addition, anaerobic metabolism results in the accumulation of the toxic end product lactic acid, which must be removed from the cell and transported to the liver for conversion into glucose and glycogen.

Pathophysiology

The pathophysiology of shock involves cellular changes, vascular responses, and changes in blood pressure.

Cellular Changes

In shock, the cells lack an adequate blood supply and are deprived of oxygen and nutrients; therefore, they must produce energy through anaerobic metabolism. This results in low-energy yields from nutrients and an acidotic intracellular environment. Because of these changes, normal cell function ceases (Fig. 11-1). The cell swells and the cell membrane becomes more permeable, allowing electrolytes and fluids to seep out of and into the cell. The sodium–potassium pump becomes impaired; cell structures, primarily the mitochondria, are damaged, and death of the cell results.

Glucose is the primary substrate required for the production of cellular energy in the form of ATP. In stress states, catecholamines, cortisol, glucagon, and inflammatory **cytokines** (i.e., biochemical or inflammatory mediators) are released, causing hyperglycemia and insulin resistance to mobilize glucose for cellular metabolism. Activation of these substances promotes gluconeogenesis, which is the formation of glucose from noncarbohydrate sources such as proteins and fats. Glycogen that has been stored in the liver is converted to glucose through glycogenolysis to meet metabolic needs, increasing the blood glucose concentration (i.e., hyperglycemia).

Continued activation of the stress response by shock states causes a depletion of glycogen stores, resulting in increased proteolysis and eventual organ failure (Massaro, 2018). The deficit of nutrients and oxygen for normal cellular metabolism causes a buildup of metabolic end products in the cells and interstitial spaces. The clotting cascade, also associated with the inflammatory process, becomes activated, which compounds this pathologic cycle. With significant cell injury or death caused by shock, the clotting cascade is overproductive, resulting in small clots lodging in microcirculation, further hampering cellular perfusion (Seymour & Angus, 2018). This upregulation of the clotting cascade further compromises microcirculation of tissues, exacerbating cellular hypoperfusion (Seymour & Angus, 2018). Cellular metabolism is impaired, and a self-perpetuating negative situation (i.e., a positive feedback loop) is initiated.

Vascular Responses

Local regulatory mechanisms, referred to as autoregulation, stimulate vasodilation or vasoconstriction in response to biochemical mediators released by the cell, communicating the need for oxygen and nutrients (Kislitsina et al., 2019). A cytokine is a substance released by a cell or immune cells such as macrophages; the substance triggers an action at a cell site

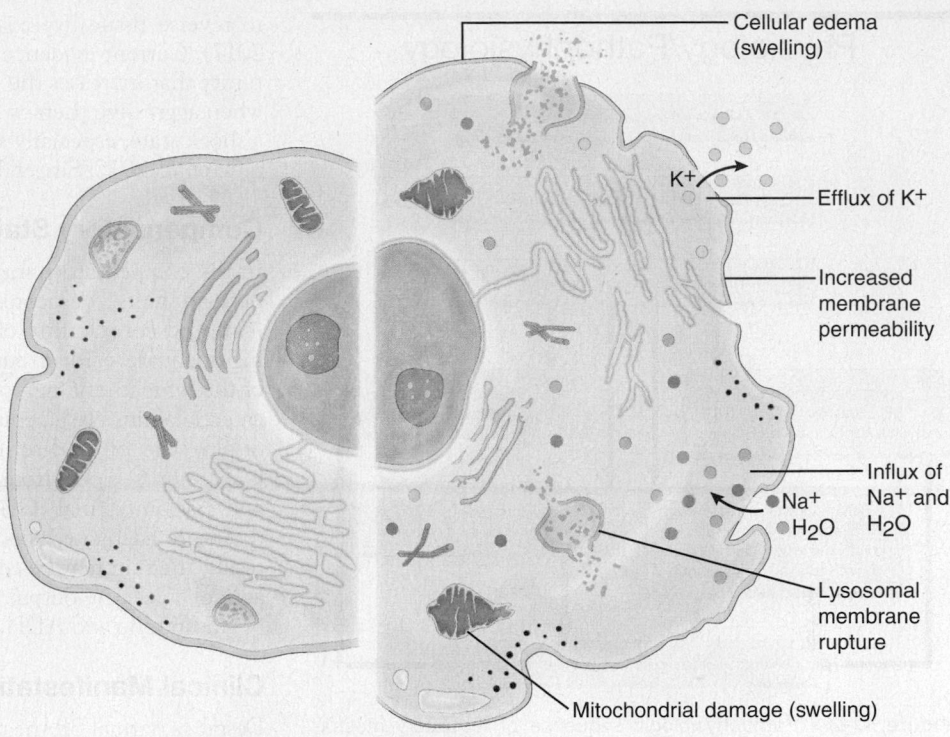

Figure 11-1 • Cellular effects of shock. The cell swells and the cell membrane becomes more permeable; fluids and electrolytes seep from and into the cell. Mitochondria and lysosomes are damaged and the cell dies.

or travels in the bloodstream to a distant site, where it triggers action. Researchers are learning more every day about the physiologic actions of numerous proinflammatory and anti-inflammatory biochemical mediators that are responsible for the complex clinical presentation of shock states (Honore, Hoste, Molnár, et al., 2019).

Blood Pressure Regulation

Three major components of the circulatory system—blood volume, the cardiac pump, and the vasculature—must respond effectively to complex neural, chemical, and hormonal feedback systems to maintain an adequate blood pressure (BP) and perfuse body tissues. BP is regulated through a complex interaction of neural, chemical, and hormonal feedback systems affecting both cardiac output and peripheral resistance. This relationship is expressed in the following equation:

Mean arterial BP = Cardiac output × Peripheral resistance

Cardiac output is a product of the stroke volume (the amount of blood ejected from the left ventricle during systole) and heart rate. Peripheral resistance is primarily determined by the diameter of the arterioles.

Tissue perfusion and organ perfusion depend on mean arterial pressure (MAP), or the average pressure at which blood moves through the vasculature. MAP must exceed 65 mm Hg for cells to receive the oxygen and nutrients needed to metabolize energy in amounts sufficient to sustain life (Hallisey & Greenwood, 2019). True MAP can be calculated only by complex methods; however, most digital BP machines provide a MAP reading to guide clinical decisions.

BP is regulated by baroreceptors (pressure receptors) located in the carotid sinus and aortic arch. These pressure receptors are responsible for monitoring the circulatory

volume and regulating neural and endocrine activities (see Chapter 27 for further description). When BP drops, catecholamines (e.g., epinephrine, norepinephrine) are released from the adrenal medulla. These increase heart rate and cause vasoconstriction, restoring BP. Chemoreceptors, also located in the aortic arch and carotid arteries, regulate BP and respiratory rate using much the same mechanism in response to changes in oxygen and carbon dioxide (CO_2) concentrations in the blood. These primary regulatory mechanisms can respond to changes in BP on a moment-to-moment basis.

The kidneys regulate BP by releasing renin, an enzyme needed for the eventual conversion of angiotensin I to angiotensin II, a potent vasoconstrictor. This stimulation of the renin–angiotensin mechanism and the resulting vasoconstriction indirectly lead to the release of aldosterone from the adrenal cortex, which promotes the retention of sodium and water (i.e., hypernatremia). Hypernatremia then stimulates the release of antidiuretic hormone (ADH) by the pituitary gland. ADH causes the kidneys to retain water further in an effort to raise blood volume and BP. These secondary regulatory mechanisms may take hours or days to respond to changes in BP. The relationship between the initiation of shock and the responsiveness of primary and secondary regulatory mechanisms that compensate for deficits in blood volume, the pumping effectiveness of the heart, or vascular tone, which may result because of the shock state, is noted in Figure 11-2.

Stages of Shock

Shock progresses along a continuum and can be identified as early or late, depending on the signs and symptoms and the overall severity of organ dysfunction. A convenient way to

Physiology/Pathophysiology

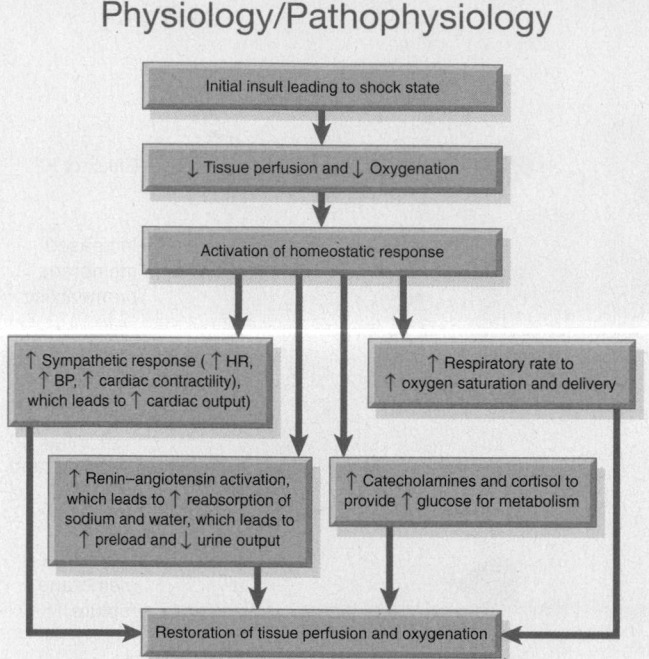

Figure 11-2 • Pathophysiologic sequence of regulatory mechanisms in shock.

understand the physiologic responses and subsequent clinical signs and symptoms of shock is to divide the continuum into separate stages: compensatory (stage 1), progressive (stage 2), and irreversible (stage 3). The earlier that interventions are initiated along this continuum, the greater the patient's chance of survival. Current research and evidence-based practice focuses on assessing patients at greatest risk for shock and implementing early and aggressive interventions

to reverse tissue hypoxia (Zhang, Hong, Smischney, et al., 2017). Current evidence suggests that the window of opportunity that increases the likelihood of patient survival occurs when aggressive therapy begins within 3 hours of identifying a shock state, especially septic shock (Rhodes, Evans, Alhazzani, et al., 2017; Singer, Deutschman, Seymour, et al., 2016).

Compensatory Stage

In the compensatory stage of shock, the BP remains within normal limits. Vasoconstriction, increased heart rate, and increased contractility of the heart contribute to maintaining adequate cardiac output. This results from stimulation of the sympathetic nervous system and subsequent release of catecholamines (e.g., epinephrine, norepinephrine). Patients display the often-described "fight-or-flight" response. The body shunts blood from organs such as the skin, kidneys, and gastrointestinal (GI) tract to the brain, heart, and lungs to ensure adequate blood supply to these vital organs. As a result, the skin may be cool and pale, bowel sounds are hypoactive, and urine output decreases in response to the release of aldosterone and ADH.

Clinical Manifestations

Despite a normal BP, the patient shows numerous clinical signs indicating inadequate organ perfusion (Table 11-1). The result of inadequate perfusion is anaerobic metabolism and a buildup of lactic acid, producing metabolic acidosis. The respiratory rate increases in response to the need to increase oxygen to the cells and in compensation for metabolic acidosis. This rapid respiratory rate facilitates removal of excess CO_2 but raises the blood pH and often causes a compensatory respiratory alkalosis. The patient may experience a change in effect, feel anxious, or be confused. If treatment begins in this stage of shock, the prognosis for the patient is better than in later stages.

TABLE 11-1 Clinical Findings in Stages of Shock

Finding	Stage		
	Compensatory	Progressive	Irreversible
Blood pressure	Normal	Systolic ≤100 mm Hg; MAP ≤65 mm Hg Requires fluids resuscitation to support blood pressure	Requires mechanical or pharmacologic support
Heart rate	>100 bpm	>150 bpm	Erratic
Respiratory status	≥22 breaths/min PaCO₂ <32 mm Hg	Rapid, shallow respirations; crackles PaO₂ <80 mm Hg PaCO₂ >45 mm Hg	Requires intubation and mechanical ventilation and oxygenation
Skin	Cold, clammy Capillary refill ≤3.5 s	Mottling, petechiae Capillary refill ≥3.5 s	Jaundice
Urinary output	Decreased	<0.5 mL/kg/h	Anuric; requires dialysis
Mentation	Confusion and/or agitation	Lethargy	Unconscious
Acid–base balance	Respiratory alkalosis	Metabolic acidosis	Profound acidosis

MAP, mean arterial pressure; PaCO₂, partial pressure of arterial carbon dioxide; PaO₂, partial pressure of arterial oxygen.
Adapted from Bridges, E. (2017). Assessing patients during septic shock resuscitation. *American Journal of Nursing, 117*(10), 34–40; Makic, M. B. F., & Bridges, E. (2018). Managing sepsis and septic shock: Current guidelines and definitions. *American Journal of Nursing, 118*(2), 34–39; Rhodes, A., Evans, L., Alhazzani, W., et al. (2017). Surviving Sepsis Campaign. (2017). Retrieved on 11/27/20 at: www.sccm.org/getattachment/SurvivingSepsisCampaign/Guidelines/Adult-Patients/SSC-Guidelines-FAQ.pdf?lang=en-US; Simmons, J., & Ventetuolo, C. E. (2017). Cardiopulmonary monitoring of shock. *Current Opinion, 23*(3), 223–231.

Medical Management

Medical treatment is directed toward identifying the cause of the shock, correcting the underlying disorder so that shock does not progress, and supporting those physiologic processes that thus far have responded successfully to the threat. Because compensation cannot be maintained indefinitely, measures such as fluid replacement, supplemental oxygen, and medication therapy must be initiated to maintain an adequate BP and reestablish and maintain adequate tissue perfusion (Makic & Bridges, 2018; Rhodes et al., 2017).

Nursing Management

Early intervention along the continuum of shock is the key to improving the patient's prognosis (Makic & Bridges, 2018; Rhodes et al., 2017). The nurse must systematically assess the patient at risk for shock, recognizing subtle clinical signs of the compensatory stage before the patient's BP drops. Early interventions include identifying the cause of shock, administering intravenous (IV) fluids and oxygen, and obtaining necessary laboratory tests to rule out and treat metabolic imbalances or infection. Special considerations related to recognizing early signs of shock in the older adult patient are discussed in Chart 11-1.

Monitoring Tissue Perfusion

In assessing tissue perfusion, the nurse observes for subtle changes in level of consciousness, vital signs (including pulse pressure), urinary output, skin (including assessment of capillary refill and signs of mottling), respiratory rate, and laboratory values (e.g., base deficit, lactic acid levels). In the compensatory stage of shock, serum sodium and blood glucose levels are elevated in response to the release of aldosterone and catecholamines. If infection is suspected, blood cultures should be obtained prior to administration of prescribed antibiotics; both of these interventions should be given priority in the care of the patient (Bridges, 2017; Levy, Evans, & Rhodes, 2018).

The nurse should monitor the patient's hemodynamic status and promptly report deviations to the primary provider, assist in identifying and treating the underlying disorder by continuous in-depth assessment of the patient, administer prescribed fluids and medications, and promote patient safety. Vital signs are key indicators of hemodynamic status, and BP is an indirect measure of tissue hypoxia. The nurse should report a systolic BP of 100 mm Hg or lower, or a drop in systolic BP of 40 mm Hg from baseline, or a MAP of 65 mm Hg or less (Hallisey & Greenwood, 2019; Rhodes et al., 2017). If the patient is concurrently diagnosed with an infection or if an infection is suspected, the nurse should promptly notify the primary provider if the patient exhibits any two of the three following signs (Singer et al., 2016) (see later discussion of Septic Shock):

- Respiratory rate greater than or equal to 22 breaths/min
- Altered mentation
- Systolic BP less than or equal to 100 mm Hg

Pulse pressure correlates well with stroke volume. Pulse pressure is calculated by subtracting the diastolic measurement from the systolic measurement; the difference is the pulse pressure. Normally, the pulse pressure is 30 to 40 mm Hg. Narrowing or decreased pulse pressure is an earlier indicator

Chart 11-1 — Recognizing Shock in Older Adults

The physiologic changes associated with aging, coupled with pathologic and chronic disease states, place older adults at increased risk for developing a state of shock and possibly multiple organ dysfunction syndrome. Older adults can recover from shock if it is detected and treated early with aggressive and supportive therapies. Nurses play an essential role in assessing and interpreting subtle changes in older adults' responses to illness.

- Medications such as beta-blocking agents (e.g., metoprolol) used to treat hypertension may mask tachycardia, a primary compensatory mechanism to increase cardiac output, during hypovolemic states.
- The aging immune system may not mount a truly febrile response (temperature greater than 38.3°C [101°F]); however, a lack of a febrile response (temperature less than 37°C [98.6°F]) or an increasing trend in body temperature should be addressed. The patient may also report increased fatigue and malaise in the absence of a febrile response.
- The heart does not function well in hypoxemic states, and the aging heart may respond to decreased myocardial oxygenation with arrhythmias that may be misinterpreted as a normal part of the aging process.
- There is a progressive decline in respiratory muscle strength, maximal ventilation, and response to hypoxia. Older adults have a decreased respiratory reserve and decompensate more quickly.
- Changes in mentation may be inappropriately misinterpreted as dementia. Older adults with a sudden change in mentation should be aggressively assessed for acute delirium (hypo- and hyperdelirium states) and treated for the presence of infection and organ hypoperfusion.

Adapted from Rhodes, A., Evans, L., Alhazzani, W., et al. (2017). Surviving Sepsis Campaign: International guidelines for management of sepsis and septic shock: 2016. *Critical Care Medicine, 45*(3), 486–552; Rowe, T. A., & McKoy, J. M. (2017). Sepsis in older adults. *Infectious Disease Clinics of North America, 31*(4), 731–742.

of shock than a drop in systolic BP (Simmons & Ventetuolo, 2017). Decreased or narrowing pulse pressure, an early indication of decreased stroke volume, is illustrated in the following example:

$$\text{Systolic BP} - \text{Diastolic BP} = \text{Pulse pressure}$$

Normal pulse pressure:

$$120 \text{ mm Hg} - 80 \text{ mm Hg} = 40 \text{ mm Hg}$$

Narrowing of pulse pressure:

$$90 \text{ mm Hg} - 70 \text{ mm Hg} = 20 \text{ mm Hg}$$

Elevation of the diastolic BP with release of catecholamines and attempts to increase venous return through vasoconstriction is an early compensatory mechanism in response to decreased stroke volume, BP, and overall cardiac output.

Quality and Safety Nursing Alert

By the time BP drops, damage has already been occurring at the cellular and tissue levels. Therefore, the patient at risk for shock must be assessed and monitored closely before the BP falls.

Continuous central venous oximetry (ScⅴO₂) monitoring may be used to evaluate mixed venous blood oxygen saturation and severity of tissue hypoperfusion states. A central catheter is introduced into the superior vena cava (SVC), and a sensor on the catheter measures the oxygen saturation of the blood in the SVC as blood returns to the heart and pulmonary system for reoxygenation. A normal $Sc\overline{v}O_2$ value is 70% (Zhang et al., 2017). Body tissues use approximately 25% of the oxygen delivered to them during normal metabolism. During stressful events, such as shock, more oxygen is consumed and the $Sc\overline{v}O_2$ saturation is lower, indicating that the tissues are consuming more oxygen.

Interventions focus on decreasing tissue oxygen requirements and increasing perfusion to deliver more oxygen to the tissues. For instance, sedating agents may be given to lower metabolic demands, or the patient's pain may be treated with opioid, nonopioid, or sedating agents (e.g., propofol, dexmedetomidine, acetaminophen) to decrease metabolic demands for oxygen. Supplemental oxygen and mechanical ventilation may be required to increase the delivery of oxygen in the blood. Administration of IV fluids and medications supports BP and cardiac output, and the transfusion of packed red blood cells enhances oxygen transport. Monitoring tissue oxygen consumption with $Sc\overline{v}O_2$ is an invasive measure to more accurately assess tissue oxygenation in the compensatory stage of shock before changes in vital signs detect altered tissue perfusion (Rhodes et al., 2017; Zhang et al., 2017).

In the patient who has an arterial line present, arterial pulse waveform analysis or pulse contour may be used to determine the patient's stroke volume and responsiveness to IV fluid replacement to meet tissue perfusion needs (Simmons & Ventetuolo, 2017). More commonly, passive leg raising (PLR) is used to determine which patients will or will not respond to IV fluid bolus challenges. PLR involves raising the patient's legs to a 30- to 45-degree angle to increase venous return and thus cardiac output (Fig. 11-3). If the blood pressure improves with PLR, the patient will respond to additional fluids. If the blood pressure does not improve, giving more IV fluids will not improve the patient's condition and can precipitate fluid overload (Laher, Watermeyer, Buchanan, et al., 2017; Pickett, Bridges, Kritek, et al., 2018). If the patient is mechanically ventilated, functional hemodynamic monitoring will be used to assess fluid volume needs and the patient's response to IV fluid administration (i.e., preload, cardiac output, and blood pressure). An improvement in preload, cardiac output, and blood pressure indicates a favorable response. Functional hemodynamic monitoring has replaced static measures obtained from central venous pressure (CVP) or pulmonary artery (PA) monitoring. Functional hemodynamic monitoring assesses real-time dynamic changes between the patient's

breathing patterns and circulating blood volume. Assessing functional hemodynamic parameters requires the patient to be mechanically ventilated and have an invasive arterial catheter placed and connected to monitoring devices that measure fluid volume (Bridges, 2013; Hallisey & Greenwood, 2019; Simmons & Ventetuolo, 2017).

Although treatments are prescribed and initiated by the primary provider, the nurse usually implements them, operates and troubleshoots equipment used in treatment, monitors the patient's status during treatment, and evaluates the immediate effects of treatment. In addition, the nurse assesses the response of the family to the crisis and its treatment.

Reducing Anxiety

Patients and their families often become anxious and apprehensive when they face a major threat to health and well-being and are the focus of attention of many health care providers. Providing brief explanations about the diagnostic and treatment procedures, supporting the patient during these procedures, and providing information about their outcomes are usually effective in reducing stress and anxiety and thus promoting the patient's physical and mental well-being. Speaking in a calm, reassuring voice and using gentle touch also help ease the patient's concerns. These actions may provide comfort for patients who are critically ill and frightened (Reaza-Alarcón & Rodríguez-Martín, 2019). Evidence suggests that family members have certain needs during a health-related crisis, which include that health care professionals provide honest, consistent, and thorough communication; are present with the patient to facilitate physical and emotional support; demonstrate caring behaviors, see the patient frequently, and know the daily, short-term, and long-term plan of care for the patient (Reaza-Alarcón & Rodríguez-Martín, 2019; Wong, Redley, Digby, et al., 2019).

The nurse should advocate for family members to be present during procedures and routine patient care activities. The presence of family provides an important connection and support for the patient during a time of crisis. Clinical practice guidelines suggest that sharing decision making with the patient and the family enhances communication with the health care team, reduces patient anxiety, and improves overall satisfaction with care (Davidson, Aslakson, Long, et al., 2017).

Clarifying Advance Directives

Because shock can progress rapidly and its course may be unpredictable, it is important for the nurse to ask patients on admission if they have advance directives, including durable power of attorney for health care or living wills, or if they have had conversations with anyone about their health care wishes. When appropriate, the patient and family (with patient permission) should be approached regarding preferences for resuscitation and Physician Orders for Life-Sustaining Treatment (POLST) (see Chapter 13). The POLST helps ensure that the patient's wishes are honored if their condition deteriorates rapidly and they lose the ability to speak for themselves (Turner & Hylton, 2019).

Promoting Safety

The nurse must be vigilant for potential threats to the patient's safety, because a high anxiety level and changes in

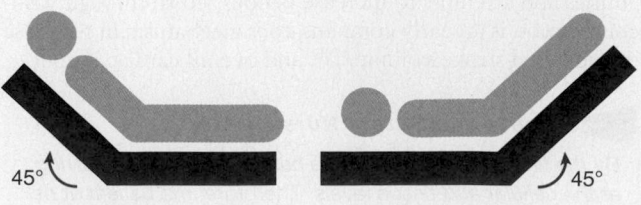

| Semirecumbent position | Passive leg raising |

Figure 11-3 • Passive leg raise.

mental status may impair judgment. Patients who were previously cooperative and followed instructions may now disrupt IV lines and catheters, increasing the risk for potential complications. Close monitoring, frequent reorientation, hourly rounding, and implementing interventions to prevent falls (e.g., bed alarms) are essential.

Progressive Stage

In the second stage of shock, the mechanisms that regulate BP can no longer compensate, and the MAP falls below normal limits. Patients are clinically hypotensive; this is defined as a systolic BP of 100 mm Hg or lower, or a decrease in systolic BP of 40 mm Hg from baseline. The patient shows signs of declining mental status (Rhodes et al., 2017; Singer et al., 2016).

Pathophysiology

Although all organ systems suffer from hypoperfusion at this stage, several events perpetuate the shock syndrome. First, the overworked heart becomes dysfunctional, the body's inability to meet increased oxygen requirements produces ischemia, and biochemical mediators cause myocardial depression (Massaro, 2018). This leads to failure of the heart, even if the underlying cause of the shock is not of cardiac origin. Second, the autoregulatory function of the microcirculation fails in response to the numerous biochemical mediators released by the cells, resulting in increased capillary permeability, with areas of arteriolar and venous constriction further compromising cellular perfusion (Massaro, 2018). At this stage, the prognosis worsens. The relaxation of precapillary sphincters causes fluid to leak from the capillaries, creating interstitial edema and decreased return to the heart. In addition, the inflammatory response is activated, and proinflammatory and anti-inflammatory mediators are released, which activate the coagulation system in an effort to reestablish homeostasis (Seymour & Angus, 2018). The body mobilizes energy stores and increases oxygen consumption to meet the increased metabolic needs of the underperfused tissues and cells. Anaerobic metabolism ensues, resulting in a buildup of lactic acid and disruption of normal cell function.

Even if the underlying cause of the shock is reversed, the sequence of compensatory responses to the decrease in tissue perfusion perpetuates the shock state, and a vicious cycle ensues. The cellular reactions that occur during the progressive stage of shock are an active area of clinical research. It is believed that the body's response to shock or lack of response in this stage of shock may be the primary factor determining the patient's survival. Early recognition of shock signs and symptoms is essential to improving morbidity and mortality.

Clinical Manifestations

Chances of survival depend on the patient's general health before the shock state as well as the amount of time it takes to restore tissue perfusion. As shock progresses, organ systems decompensate (see Table 11-1).

Respiratory Effects

The lungs, which become compromised early in shock, are affected at this stage. Subsequent decompensation of the lungs increases the likelihood that mechanical ventilation will be needed. Respirations are rapid and shallow. Crackles are heard over the lung fields. Decreased pulmonary blood flow causes arterial oxygen levels to decrease and CO_2 levels to increase. Hypoxemia and biochemical mediators cause an intense inflammatory response and pulmonary vasoconstriction, perpetuating pulmonary capillary hypoperfusion and hypoxemia. The hypoperfused alveoli stop producing surfactant and subsequently collapse. Pulmonary capillaries begin to leak, causing pulmonary edema, diffusion abnormalities (shunting), and additional alveolar collapse. This condition is called *acute lung injury* (ALI); as ALI continues, interstitial inflammation and fibrosis are common consequences, leading to acute respiratory distress syndrome (ARDS) (Mitchell & Seckel, 2018). Further explanation of ALI and ARDS, as well as their nursing management, can be found in Chapter 19.

Cardiovascular Effects

A lack of adequate blood supply leads to arrhythmias and ischemia. The heart rate is rapid, sometimes exceeding 150 bpm. The patient may complain of chest pain and even suffer a myocardial infarction (MI). Levels of cardiac biomarkers (e.g., cardiac troponin I [cTn-I]) increase. In addition, myocardial depression and ventricular dilation may further impair the heart's ability to pump enough blood to the tissues to meet increasing oxygen requirements.

Neurologic Effects

As blood flow to the brain becomes impaired, mental status deteriorates. Changes in mental status occur with decreased cerebral perfusion and hypoxia. Initially, the patient may exhibit subtle changes in behavior, become agitated, confused, or demonstrate signs of delirium. (See Chapter 61 for more information about delirium.) Subsequently, lethargy increases, and the patient begins to lose consciousness.

Renal Effects

When the MAP falls below 65 mm Hg (Hallisey & Greenwood, 2019), the glomerular filtration rate of the kidneys cannot be maintained, and significant changes in renal function occur. Acute kidney injury (AKI) is characterized by an increase in blood urea nitrogen (BUN) and serum creatinine levels, fluid and electrolyte shifts, acid–base imbalances, and a loss of the renal–hormonal regulation of BP. Urinary output usually decreases to less than 0.5 mL/kg/h (or less than 30 mL/h) but may vary depending on the phase of AKI. (See Chapter 48 for further information about AKI.)

Hepatic Effects

Decreased blood flow to the liver impairs the ability of liver cells to perform metabolic and phagocytic functions. Consequently, the patient is less able to metabolize medications and metabolic waste products, such as ammonia and lactic acid. Metabolic activities of the liver, including gluconeogenesis and glycogenolysis, are impaired. The patient becomes more susceptible to infection as the liver fails to filter bacteria from the blood. Liver enzymes (aspartate aminotransferase, alanine aminotransferase, lactate dehydrogenase) and bilirubin levels are elevated, and the patient develops jaundice.

Gastrointestinal Effects

GI ischemia can cause stress ulcers in the stomach, putting the patient at risk for GI bleeding. In the small intestine, the mucosa can become necrotic and slough off, causing bloody diarrhea. Beyond the local effects of impaired perfusion, GI ischemia leads to bacterial translocation and organ dysfunction, in which bacterial toxins enter the bloodstream through the lymphatic system. In addition to causing infection, bacterial toxins can cause cardiac depression, vasodilation, increased capillary permeability, and an intense inflammatory response with activation of additional biochemical mediators. The net result is interference with healthy cellular functioning and the ability to metabolize nutrients (Rhodes et al., 2017).

Hematologic Effects

The combination of hypotension, sluggish blood flow, metabolic acidosis, coagulation system imbalance, and generalized hypoxemia can interfere with normal hemostatic mechanisms. In shock states, the inflammatory cytokines activate the clotting cascade, causing deposition of microthrombi in multiple areas of the body and consumption of clotting factors. The alterations of the hematologic system, including imbalance of the clotting cascade, are linked to the overactivation of the inflammatory response (Massaro, 2018; Seymour & Angus, 2018). Disseminated intravascular coagulation (DIC) may occur either as a cause or as a complication of shock. In this condition, widespread clotting and bleeding occur simultaneously. Ecchymoses (bruises) and petechiae (bleeding) may appear in the skin. Coagulation times (e.g., prothrombin time, activated partial thromboplastin time) are prolonged. Clotting factors and platelets are consumed and require replacement therapy to achieve hemostasis. (Further discussion of DIC appears in Chapter 29.)

 Medical Management

Specific medical management in the progressive stage of shock depends on the type of shock, its underlying cause, and the degree of decompensation in the organ systems. Medical management specific to each type of shock is discussed later in this chapter. Although medical management in the progressive stage differs by type of shock, some medical interventions are common to all types. These include the use of appropriate IV fluids and medications to restore tissue perfusion by the following methods:

- Supporting the respiratory system
- Optimizing intravascular volume
- Supporting the pumping action of the heart
- Improving the competence of the vascular system

Other aspects of management may include early enteral nutritional support, targeted hyperglycemic control with IV insulin and use of antacids, histamine-2 (H_2) blockers, or antipeptic medications to reduce the risk of GI ulceration and bleeding.

Tight glycemic control (i.e., maintaining serum glucose close to the normal parameters of 80 to 100 mg/dL) is not recommended in patients who are critically ill because this therapy has been found to result in adverse patient outcomes (Griesdale, DeSouza, VanDam, et al., 2009). Current evidence suggests that maintaining serum glucose less than 180 mg/dL with insulin therapy and close monitoring is indicated in the management of the patient who is critically ill (American Diabetes Association, 2019; Rhodes et al., 2017).

 Quality and Safety Nursing Alert

Glycemic control is linked to outcomes in the patient in shock. Although tight glycemic control is not indicated, evidence shows that maintaining serum glucose less than 180 mg/dL is linked to best outcomes.

 Nursing Management

Nursing care of patients in the progressive stage of shock requires expertise in assessing and understanding shock and the significance of changes in assessment data. Early interventions are essential to the survival of patients; therefore, suspecting that a patient may be in shock and reporting subtle changes in assessment are imperative. Patients in the progressive stage of shock are cared for in the intensive care setting to facilitate close monitoring (hemodynamic monitoring, electrocardiographic [ECG] monitoring, arterial blood gases, serum electrolyte levels, physical and mental status changes); rapid and frequent administration of various prescribed medications and fluids; and possibly interventions with supportive technologies, such as mechanical ventilation, dialysis (e.g., continuous renal replacement therapy), and intra-aortic balloon pump (IABP).

Working closely with other members of the health care team, the nurse carefully documents treatments, medications, and fluids that are given; the time, dosage or volume, and patient responses are recorded. In addition, the nurse coordinates care, including the scheduling of diagnostic procedures that may occur at the bedside, and communication among health care personnel, family members, and the patient.

Preventing Complications

The nurse monitors the patient for early signs of complications to help reduce potential risks to the patient. Monitoring includes evaluating blood levels of medications, observing invasive vascular lines and catheters for signs of infection, and checking neurovascular status if arterial lines are inserted, especially in the lower extremities. Simultaneously, the nurse promotes the patient's safety and comfort by ensuring that all procedures, including invasive procedures and arterial and venous punctures, are carried out using correct aseptic techniques and that venous and arterial puncture and infusion sites are maintained with the goal of preventing infection. Nursing interventions that reduce the incidence of ventilator-associated pneumonia (VAP) must also be implemented. These include frequent oral care with a toothbrush, aseptic suction technique, turning, elevating the head of the bed at least 30 degrees to prevent aspiration, and implementing daily interruption of sedation as prescribed to evaluate patient readiness for extubation (Mitchell, Russo, Cheng, et al., 2019). See Chart 19-6 for an overview of the evidence-based ("bundled") interventions aimed at preventing VAP. Positioning and repositioning of the patient to promote comfort and maintain skin integrity are essential.

The nurse must also be vigilant in assessing for acute delirium, characterized by an acute change in mental status, inattention, disorganized thinking, and altered level of consciousness. Delirium is potentially preventable (Devlin, Skrobik, Gelians, et al., 2018; Makic, 2018). Patients who are critically ill and have delirium have longer mechanical ventilation support needs, experience higher functional decline, and have higher rates of morbidity and mortality than those without delirium. Furthermore, they are at a higher risk of developing postintensive care syndrome (PICS), which manifests as new or worsening impairments in the patient's physical, cognitive, or mental status after a critical illness has resolved and that persists beyond the acute hospitalization (Devlin et al., 2018). Delirium should be assessed at a minimum each shift using a standardized delirium assessment tool, such as the Confusion Assessment Method (CAM)-ICU (Critical Illness, Brain Dysfunction, and Survivorship (CIBS) Center, 2020). The CAM-ICU is a modified version of the CAM, specifically designed for use in patients who are critically ill (see Chapter 8, Chart 8-7 for discussion of the CAM). Nursing interventions that can prevent delirium include engaging the patient in frequent reorientation activities (e.g., to date, time, place), assessing and treating pain, promoting sleep, providing early mobilization activities, and limiting sedation, especially sedation with benzodiazepines (e.g., lorazepam) (Devlin et al., 2018; Makic, 2018).

Promoting Rest and Comfort

Efforts are made to minimize the cardiac workload by reducing the patient's physical activity and treating pain and anxiety. Because promoting patient rest and comfort is a priority, the nurse performs essential nursing activities in blocks of time, allowing the patient to have periods of uninterrupted sleep, which may prevent acute delirium, as noted previously (Devlin et al., 2018). To conserve the patient's energy, the nurse should protect the patient from temperature extremes (e.g., excessive warmth or cold, shivering), which can increase the metabolic rate and oxygen consumption and thus the cardiac workload.

Supporting Family Members

Because patients in shock receive intense attention by the health care team, families may be overwhelmed and frightened. Family members may be reluctant to ask questions or seek information for fear that they will be in the way or will interfere with the attention given to the patient. The nurse should make sure that the family is comfortably situated and kept informed about the patient's status. Often, families need encouragement from the health care team to get some rest; family members are more likely to take this advice if they feel that the patient is being well cared for and that they will be notified of any significant changes in the patient's status. A visit from the hospital chaplain may be comforting and provides some attention to the family while the nurse concentrates on the patient. Ensuring patient- and family-centered care is central to the delivery of high-quality care. This helps meet the emotional well-being as well as the physiologic needs of the patient and the family (Wong et al., 2019).

Irreversible Stage

The irreversible (or refractory) stage of shock represents the point along the shock continuum at which organ damage is so severe that the patient does not respond to treatment and cannot survive. Despite treatment, BP remains low. Renal and liver dysfunction, compounded by the release of biochemical mediators, creates an acute metabolic acidosis. Anaerobic metabolism contributes to a worsening lactic acidosis. Reserves of ATP are almost totally depleted, and mechanisms

for storing new supplies of energy have been destroyed. Respiratory system dysfunction prevents adequate oxygenation and ventilation despite mechanical ventilatory support, and the cardiovascular system is ineffective in maintaining an adequate MAP for tissue perfusion. Multiple organ dysfunction progressing to complete organ failure has occurred, and death is imminent. Multiple organ dysfunction can occur as a progression along the shock continuum or as a syndrome unto itself and is described in more detail later in this chapter.

 ## Medical Management

Medical management during the irreversible stage of shock is similar to interventions and treatments used in the progressive stage. Although the patient may have progressed to the irreversible stage, the judgment that the shock is irreversible can only be made after the patient has failed to respond to treatment. Strategies that may be experimental (e.g., investigational medications, such as immunomodulation therapy) may be tried to reduce or reverse the severity of shock.

 ## Nursing Management

As in the progressive stage of shock, the nurse focuses on carrying out prescribed treatments, monitoring the patient, preventing complications, protecting the patient from injury, and providing comfort. Offering brief explanations to the patient about what is happening is essential even if there is no certainty that the patient hears or understands what is being said. Simple comfort measures, including reassuring touches, should continue to be provided despite the patient's nonresponsiveness to verbal stimuli (Wong et al., 2019).

As it becomes obvious that the patient is unlikely to survive, the family needs to be informed about the prognosis and likely outcome. Opportunities should be provided throughout the patient's care for the family to see, touch, and talk to the patient. Close friends or spiritual or religious advisors may be of comfort to the family members in dealing with the inevitable death of their loved one.

During this stage of shock, the family may misinterpret the actions of the health care team. They have been told that nothing has been effective in reversing the shock and that the patient's survival is very unlikely, yet they find primary providers and nurses continuing to work feverishly on the patient. Distraught, grieving families may interpret this as a chance for recovery when none exists, and family members may become angry when the patient dies. Conferences with all members of the health care team and the family promote better understanding by the family of the patient's prognosis and the purpose for management interventions. Engaging palliative care specialists can be beneficial in developing a plan of care that maximizes comfort and effective symptom management as well as assisting the family with difficult decisions (Ivany & Aitken, 2019). During these conferences, it is essential to explain that the equipment and treatments being provided are intended for patient comfort and do not suggest that the patient will recover. Family members should be encouraged to express their views of life-support measures. In some cases, ethics committees may be consulted to assist families and health care teams make complex end-of-life decisions (Ivany & Aitken, 2019; Turner & Hylton, 2019).

General Management Strategies in Shock

As described previously and in the discussion of types of shock to follow, management in all types and all phases of shock includes the following:

- Support of the respiratory system with supplemental oxygen and/or mechanical ventilation to provide optimal oxygenation (see Chapter 19)
- Fluid replacement to restore intravascular volume
- Vasoactive medications to restore vasomotor tone and improve cardiac function
- Nutritional support to address the metabolic requirements that are often dramatically increased in shock

Therapies described in this section require collaboration among all members of the health care team.

Fluid Replacement

Fluid replacement, also referred to as fluid resuscitation, is given in all types of shock. The type of fluids administered, and the speed of delivery vary; however, fluids are given to improve cardiac and tissue oxygenation, which in part depends on flow. The fluids given may include **crystalloids** (electrolyte solutions that move freely between intravascular compartment and interstitial spaces), **colloids** (large-molecule IV solutions), and blood components (packed red blood cells, fresh-frozen plasma, and platelets).

Crystalloid and Colloid Solutions

In emergencies, the "best" fluid is often the fluid that is readily available. Fluid resuscitation should be initiated early in shock to maximize intravascular volume. Isotonic crystalloid solutions are often selected because they contain the same concentration of electrolytes as the extracellular fluid and, therefore, can be given without altering the concentrations of electrolytes in the plasma. IV crystalloids commonly used for resuscitation in hypovolemic shock include 0.9% sodium chloride solution (normal saline) and lactated Ringer's solution. Lactated Ringer's is an electrolyte solution containing the lactate ion, which should not be confused with lactic acid. The lactate ion is converted to bicarbonate, which helps buffer the overall acidosis that occurs in shock. Lactated Ringer's solution more closely resembles plasma and is considered a more appropriate first choice solution over 0.9% normal saline (de-Madaria, Herrera-Marante, Gonzalez-Camacho, et al., 2018). While normal saline is an isotonic solution, large infusions may cause hypernatremia, hypokalemia, and hyperchloremic metabolic acidosis (de-Madaria et al., 2018; Sethi, Owyang, Meyers, et al., 2018). Hypertonic crystalloid solution, often 3% sodium chloride, does not improve patient outcomes and may result in unintended complications and is not recommended as a fluid for resuscitation (Bauer, MacLaren, & Erstad, 2019). A disadvantage of using isotonic crystalloid solutions is that some of the volume given is lost to the interstitial compartment and some remains in the intravascular compartment. This occurs as a consequence of cellular permeability that occurs during shock. Diffusion of crystalloids into the interstitial space means that more fluid may need to be given than the amount lost to support tissue perfusion (Lewis, Pritchard, Evans, et al., 2018).

Care must be taken when rapidly administering isotonic crystalloids to avoid both underresuscitating and overresuscitating the patient in shock. Insufficient fluid replacement is associated with a higher incidence of morbidity and mortality from lack of tissue perfusion, whereas excessive fluid administration can cause systemic and pulmonary edema that progresses to ALI (see Chapter 19), intra-abdominal hypertension (IAH) and abdominal compartment syndrome (ACS), and MODS (see later discussion).

ACS is a serious complication that may occur when large volumes of fluid are given. It may also occur after trauma, abdominal surgery, pancreatitis, or sepsis (Harrell & Miller, 2017). In ACS, fluid leaks into the intra-abdominal cavity, increasing pressure that is displaced onto surrounding vessels and organs. Venous return, preload, and cardiac output are compromised. The pressure also elevates the diaphragm, making it difficult to breathe effectively. The renal and GI systems also begin to show signs of dysfunction (e.g., decreased urine output, absent bowel sounds, intolerance of tube feeding). Abdominal compartment pressure can be measured. Normally, it is 0 to 5 mm Hg, and a pressure of 12 mm Hg is considered to be indicative of IAH (Harrell & Miller, 2017). If ACS is present, interventions that usually include surgical decompression are necessary to relieve the pressure.

Generally, IV colloidal solutions are similar to plasma proteins, in that they contain molecules that are too large to pass through capillary membranes. Colloids expand intravascular volume by exerting oncotic pressure, thereby pulling fluid into the intravascular space, increasing intravascular volume. In addition, colloids have a longer duration of action than crystalloids, because the molecules remain within the intravascular compartment longer. Typically, if colloids are used to treat tissue hypoperfusion, albumin is the agent prescribed. Albumin is a plasma protein; an albumin solution is prepared from human plasma and is heated during production to reduce its potential to transmit disease. The disadvantage of albumin is its high cost compared to crystalloid solutions. Resuscitation with colloid solutions has not reduced the risk of morbidity or death compared to resuscitation with crystalloid solutions; moreover, colloids can be considerably more expensive than crystalloid solutions (Annane, Siami, Jaber, et al., 2013; Lewis et al., 2018).

 Quality and Safety Nursing Alert

With all colloidal solutions, side effects include the rare occurrence of anaphylactic reactions. Nurses must monitor patients closely.

Complications of Fluid Administration

Close monitoring of the patient during fluid replacement is necessary to identify side effects and complications. The most common and serious side effects of fluid replacement are cardiovascular overload, pulmonary edema, and ACS. The patient receiving fluid replacement must be monitored frequently for adequate urinary output, changes in mental status, skin perfusion, and changes in vital signs. Lung sounds are auscultated frequently to detect signs of fluid accumulation. Adventitious lung sounds, such as crackles, may indicate pulmonary edema and ALI and ARDS.

> ⚑ *Quality and Safety Nursing Alert*
>
> *When administering large volumes of crystalloid solutions, the nurse must monitor the lungs for adventitious sounds, signs and symptoms of interstitial edema, work of breathing (i.e., increasing effort required for the patient to breathe, depth of breathing, respiratory rate), and changes in oxygen saturation.*

Often, a CVP line is inserted (typically into the subclavian or jugular vein) and is advanced until the tip of the catheter rests near the junction of the SVC and the right atrium. CVP measurements have traditionally been used to assess preload in the right side of the heart and fluid responsiveness during shock states. However, research confirms there is no direct relationship between CVP, circulating blood volume, and fluid responsiveness; thus, CVP is no longer used as a reliable measure to guide fluid replacement therapy (Laher et al., 2017; Marik, Baram, & Vahid, 2008; Marik & Cavallazzi, 2013; Simmons & Ventetuolo, 2017). CVP devices provide access for large volumes of fluid replacement, and administration of blood products and vasoactive agents. If CVP measurements are still used to evaluate fluid needs of the patient, assessment variables such as BP, urine output, heart rate, and PLR should be considered when interpreting the CVP for clinical decisions (Laher et al., 2017; Simmons & Ventetuolo, 2017). Some CVP catheters allow the monitoring of intravascular measures and venous oxygen levels. Assessment of venous oxygenation (venous oxygen saturation $S\bar{v}O_2$, or $Sc\bar{v}O_2$ with a CVP line) may be helpful in evaluating the adequacy of intravascular volume (Rhodes et al., 2017; Rivers, McIntyre, Morro, et al., 2005). Hemodynamic monitoring with arterial lines may be implemented to allow close monitoring of the patient's BP and tissue perfusion. A pulmonary artery catheter may be inserted to assist with closer monitoring of a patient's cardiac status as well as response to therapy. Advances in noninvasive or minimally invasive technology (e.g., esophageal Doppler, arterial pulse contour analysis, cardiac output devices, intrathoracic impedance monitoring) provide additional hemodynamic monitoring options (Hallisey & Greenwood, 2019; Laher et al., 2017; Zhang et al., 2017). (For additional information about hemodynamic monitoring, see Chapter 21.)

Placement of central lines for fluid administration and monitoring requires collaborative practice between the provider and the nurse to ensure that all measures to prevent central line–associated bloodstream infection (CLABSI) are implemented. Several interventions aimed at preventing CLABSI should be implemented collaboratively while the central line is being placed as well as during ongoing nursing management of the central line itself. Chart 11-2 describes the evidence-based ("bundled") interventions that have been found to reduce CLABSI.

Vasoactive Medication Therapy

Vasoactive medications are given in all forms of shock to improve the patient's hemodynamic stability when fluid therapy alone cannot maintain adequate MAP. Specific medications are selected to correct the particular hemodynamic alteration that is impeding cardiac output. These medications help increase the strength of myocardial contractility, regulate the heart rate, reduce myocardial resistance, and initiate vasoconstriction.

Vasoactive medications are selected for their action on receptors of the sympathetic nervous system. These receptors are known as alpha-adrenergic and beta-adrenergic receptors. Beta-adrenergic receptors are further classified as beta-1 and beta-2 adrenergic receptors. When alpha-adrenergic receptors are stimulated, blood vessels constrict in the cardiorespiratory and GI systems, skin, and kidneys. When beta-1 adrenergic receptors are stimulated, heart rate and myocardial contraction increase. When beta-2 adrenergic receptors are stimulated, vasodilation occurs in the heart and skeletal muscles, and the bronchioles relax. The medications used in treating shock consist of various combinations of vasoactive medications to maximize tissue perfusion by stimulating or blocking the alpha- and beta-adrenergic receptors.

When vasoactive medications are given, vital signs must be monitored frequently (at least every 15 minutes until stable, or more often if indicated). Vasoactive medications should be given through a central venous line, because infiltration and extravasation of some vasoactive medications can cause tissue necrosis and sloughing (Maclaren, Mueller, & Dasta, 2019). Individual medication dosages are usually titrated by the nurse, who adjusts drip rates on the basis of the prescribed dose and target outcome parameter (e.g., BP, heart rate) and the patient's response. Dosages are changed to maintain the MAP at a physiologic level that ensures adequate tissue perfusion (usually greater than 65 mm Hg).

> ⚑ *Quality and Safety Nursing Alert*
>
> *Vasoactive medications should never be stopped abruptly, because this could cause severe hemodynamic instability, perpetuating the shock state.*

Dosages of vasoactive medications must be tapered. When vasoactive medications are no longer needed or are necessary to a lesser extent, the infusion should be weaned with frequent monitoring of BP (e.g., every 15 minutes). Table 11-2 presents some of the commonly prescribed vasoactive medications used in the treatment of shock.

Nutritional Support

Nutritional support is an important aspect of care for critically ill patients. Increased metabolic rates during shock increase energy requirements and therefore caloric requirements. Patients in shock may require more than 3000 calories daily. The release of catecholamines early in the shock continuum causes rapid depletion of glycogen stores. Nutritional energy requirements are then met by breaking down lean body mass. In this catabolic process, skeletal muscle mass is broken down even when the patient has large stores of fat or adipose tissue. Loss of skeletal muscle greatly prolongs the patient's recovery time.

Parenteral or enteral nutritional support should be initiated as soon as possible. Enteral nutrition is preferred, promoting GI function through direct exposure to nutrients and limiting infectious complications associated with parenteral feeding (Reintam, Blaser, Starkopf, et al., 2017). Implementation of an evidence-based enteral feeding protocol that

Chart 11-2 Collaborative Practice Interventions to Prevent Central Line–Associated Bloodstream Infections (CLABSIs)

Current best practices can include the implementation of specific evidence-based bundle interventions that when used together (i.e., as a "bundle") improve patient outcomes. This chart outlines specific parameters for the central line bundled collaborative interventions that have been found to reduce central line–associated bloodstream infections (CLABSI).

What are the five key elements of the central line bundle?

- Hand hygiene
- Maximal sterile barrier precautions during line insertion (see later discussion)
- Chlorhexidine skin antisepsis
- Optimal catheter site selection with avoidance of using the femoral vein for central venous access in adult patients
- Daily review of line necessity, with prompt removal of unnecessary lines

When should hand hygiene be performed in the care of a patient with a central line?

- All clinicians who provide care to the patient should adhere to good hand hygiene practices, particularly:
  - Before and after palpating the catheter insertion site
  - With all dressing changes to the intravascular catheter access site
  - When hands are visibly soiled or contamination of hands is suspected
  - Before donning and after removing gloves

What changes can be made to improve hand hygiene?

- Implement a central line procedure checklist that requires that clinicians perform hand hygiene as an essential step in care.
- Post signage stating the importance of hand hygiene.
- Have soap and alcohol-based hand sanitizers prominently placed to facilitate hand hygiene practices.
- Model hand hygiene practices.
- Provide patient and family education and engage family in hand hygiene practices during visitation.

What are maximal sterile barrier precautions?

- These are implemented during central line insertion:
  - For the primary provider, this means strict adherence with wearing a cap, mask, sterile gown, and sterile gloves. The cap should cover all hair, and the mask should cover the nose and the mouth tightly. The nurse should also wear a cap and a mask.
  - For the patient, this means covering the patient from head to toe with a sterile drape, with a small opening for the site of insertion. If a full-size drape is not available, two drapes may be applied to cover the patient, or the operating room may be consulted to determine how to procure full-size sterile drapes, because these are routinely used in surgical settings.

- Nurses should be empowered to enforce use of a central line checklist to be sure that all processes related to central line placement are properly executed for every line placed.

Which antiseptic should be used to prepare the patient's skin for central line insertion?

- Chlorhexidine skin antisepsis has been proven to provide better skin antisepsis than other antiseptic agents, such as povidone–iodine solution.
- An alcohol chlorhexidine antiseptic should be applied using a back and forth friction scrub for at least 30 s; this should not be wiped or blotted dry.
- The antiseptic solution should be allowed time to dry completely before the insertion site is punctured/accessed (approximately 2 min).

What nursing interventions are essential to reduce the risk of infection?

- Maintaining sterile technique when changing the central line dressing
- Always performing hand hygiene before manipulating or accessing the line ports
- Wearing clean gloves before accessing the line port
- Performing a 15- to 30-s "hub scrub" using chlorhexidine or alcohol and friction in a twisting motion on the access hub (reduces biofilm on the hub that may contain pathogens)
- Using chlorhexidine-containing dressings in patients older than 2 mo
- Consider using antiseptic-containing port protectors to cover connectors

When should central lines be discontinued?

- Assessment for removal of central lines should be included as part of the nurse's daily goal sheets.
- The time and date of central line placement should be recorded and evaluated by staff to aid in decision making.
- The need for the central line access should be reviewed as part of multidisciplinary rounds.
- During these rounds, the "line day" should be stated to remind everyone how long the central line has been in place (e.g., "Today is line day 6").
- An appropriate time frame for regular review of the necessity for a central line should be identified, such as weekly, when central lines are placed for long-term use (e.g., chemotherapy, extended antibiotic administration).

Quality improvement processes that trend CLABSI rates and the adherence with CLABSI bundle prevention strategies have been found to effectively engage the multidisciplinary team in achieving goals to reduce infections related to central lines.

Adapted from Institute for Healthcare Improvement (IHI). (2012). How-to guide: Prevent central line-associated bloodstream infection. Retrieved on 9/10/2019 at: www.ihi.org/resources/Pages/Tools/HowtoGuidePreventCentralLineAssociatedBloodstreamInfection.aspx; Marschall, J., Mermel, L. A., Fakih, M., et al. (2014). Strategies to prevent central-line associated bloodstream infections in acute care hospitals: 2014 update. *Infection Control and Hospital Epidemiology, 35*(7), 753–771.

is tolerant of increased gastric residual volumes ensures the delivery of adequate nutrition to patients who are critically ill (Wang, Ding, Fang, et al., 2019). Gastric residual volume does not predict a patient's risk of aspiration (Wang et al., 2019). Implementing early enteral nutrition has been found to promote gut-mediated immunity, reduce metabolic response to stress, and improve overall patient morbidity and mortality (Reintam et al., 2017). (See Chapter 39 for further discussion of monitoring gastric residual volumes.)

Stress ulcers occur frequently in acutely ill patients because of the compromised blood supply to the GI tract. Therefore, antacids, H_2 blockers (e.g., famotidine), and proton pump

TABLE 11-2 Select Vasoactive Agents Used in Treating Shock		
Medication	**Desired Action in Shock**	**Disadvantages**
Inotropic Agents Dobutamine Dopamine Epinephrine Milrinone	Improve contractility, increase stroke volume, increase cardiac output	Increase oxygen demand of the heart
Vasodilators Nitroglycerin Nitroprusside	Reduce preload and afterload, reduce oxygen demand of heart	Cause hypotension
Vasopressor Agents Norepinephrine Dopamine Phenylephrine Vasopressin Epinephrine Angiotensin II	Increase blood pressure by vasoconstriction	Increase afterload, thereby increasing cardiac workload; compromise perfusion to skin, kidneys, lungs, gastrointestinal tract

Adapted from Annane, D., Ouanes-Besbes, L., DeBacker, D., et al. (2018). A global perspective on vasoactive agents in shock. *Intensive Care Medicine, 44*(6), 833–346; Maclaren, R., Mueller, S. W., & Dasta, J. F. (2019). Use of vasopressors and inotropes in the pharmacotherapy of shock. In J. T. DiPiro, R. L. Talbert, G. C. Yee, et al. (Eds.). *Pharmacotherapy: A pathophysiologic approach* (11th ed.). New York: McGraw-Hill Medical.

inhibitors (e.g., lansoprazole, esomeprazole magnesium) are prescribed to prevent ulcer formation by inhibiting gastric acid secretion or increasing gastric pH.

Hypovolemic Shock

Hypovolemic shock, the most common type of shock, is characterized by decreased intravascular volume. Body fluid is contained in the intracellular and extracellular compartments. Intracellular fluid accounts for about two thirds of the total body water. The extracellular body fluid is found in one of two compartments: intravascular (inside blood vessels) or interstitial (surrounding tissues). The volume of interstitial fluid is about three to four times that of intravascular fluid. Hypovolemic shock occurs when there is a reduction in intravascular volume by 15% to 30%, which represents an approximate loss of 750 to 1500 mL of blood in a 70-kg (154-lb) person (American College of Surgeons, 2018).

Pathophysiology

Hypovolemic shock can be caused by external fluid losses, as in traumatic blood loss, or by internal fluid shifts, as in severe dehydration, severe edema, or ascites (Chart 11-3). Intravascular volume can be reduced by both fluid loss and fluid shifting between the intravascular and interstitial compartments.

Chart 11-3 ⚠️ **RISK FACTORS** Hypovolemic Shock	
External: Fluid Losses	**Internal: Fluid Shifts**
Trauma	Hemorrhage
Surgery	Burns
Vomiting	Ascites
Diarrhea	Peritonitis
Diuresis	Dehydration
Diabetic ketoacidosis	Necrotizing pancreatitis
Diabetes insipidus	

The sequence of events in hypovolemic shock begins with a decrease in the intravascular volume. This results in decreased venous return of blood to the heart and subsequent decreased ventricular filling. Decreased ventricular filling results in decreased stroke volume (amount of blood ejected from the heart) and decreased cardiac output. When cardiac output drops, BP drops and tissues cannot be adequately perfused (Fig. 11-4).

Medical Management

Major goals in the treatment of hypovolemic shock are to restore intravascular volume to reverse the sequence of events leading to inadequate tissue perfusion, to redistribute

Physiology/Pathophysiology

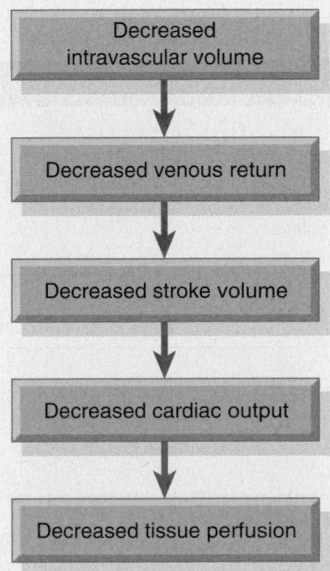

Figure 11-4 • Pathophysiologic sequence of events in hypovolemic shock.

fluid volume, and to correct the underlying cause of the fluid loss as quickly as possible. Depending on the severity of shock and the patient's condition, often all three goals are addressed simultaneously.

Treatment of the Underlying Cause

If the patient is hemorrhaging, efforts are made to stop the bleeding. This may involve applying pressure to the bleeding site or surgical interventions to stop internal bleeding. If the cause of the hypovolemia is diarrhea or vomiting, medications to treat diarrhea and vomiting are given while efforts are made to identify and treat the cause. In older adult patients, dehydration may be the cause of hypovolemic shock.

Fluid and Blood Replacement

Beyond reversing the primary cause of the decreased intravascular volume, fluid replacement is of primary concern. At least two large-gauge IV lines are inserted to establish access for fluid administration. If an IV catheter cannot be quickly inserted, an intraosseous catheter may be used for access in the sternum, legs (tibia), or arms (humerus) to facilitate rapid fluid replacement (Clemency, Tanaka, May, et al., 2017). Multiple IV lines allow simultaneous administration of fluid, medications, and blood component therapy if required. Because the goal of the fluid replacement is to restore intravascular volume, it is necessary to administer fluids that will remain in the intravascular compartment to avoid fluid shifts from the intravascular compartment into the intracellular compartment. Table 11-3 summarizes the fluids commonly used in the treatment of shock.

As discussed earlier, crystalloid solutions such as lactated Ringer's solution or 0.9% sodium chloride solution are commonly used to treat hypovolemic shock, as large amounts of fluid must be given to restore intravascular volume. If hypovolemia is primarily due to blood loss, the American College of Surgeons (2018) recommends administration of 3 mL of crystalloid solution for each milliliter of estimated blood loss. This is referred to as the 3:1 rule. Colloid solutions (e.g., albumin) may also be used. Hetastarch and dextran solutions are not indicated for fluid administration because these agents interfere with platelet aggregation.

Blood products, which are also colloids, may need to be given, particularly if the cause of the hypovolemic shock is hemorrhage. The decision to give blood is based on the patient's lack of response to crystalloid resuscitation, the volume of blood lost, the need for hemoglobin to assist with oxygen transport, and the necessity to correct the patient's coagulopathy. Patients requiring massive transfusion respond better when blood products are given in a 1:1:1 ratio, meaning units of plasma, platelets, and packed red blood cells (Holcomb, Tiley, Baraniuk, et al., 2015).

Packed red blood cells are given to replenish the patient's oxygen-carrying capacity in conjunction with other fluids that will expand volume. Plasma and platelets are transfused to assist with coagulation and hemostasis. The need for transfusions is based on the patient's oxygenation needs and coagulation status, which are determined by vital signs, blood gas, chemistry, coagulation laboratory values, and clinical appearance.

Redistribution of Fluid

In addition to administering fluids to restore intravascular volume, positioning the patient properly assists fluid redistribution. PLR may be used to evaluate the patient's responsiveness to fluids and continued resuscitation efforts (Simmons & Ventetuolo, 2017). The nurse assesses for an improvement in the patient's vital signs, specifically a rise in the BP. Trendelenburg is not indicated as this position makes breathing difficult and does not increase BP or cardiac output (Bridges & Jarquin-Valdivia, 2005).

Pharmacologic Therapy

If fluid administration fails to reverse hypovolemic shock, then vasoactive medications that prevent cardiac failure are given. Medications are also given to reverse the cause of the dehydration. For example, insulin is given if dehydration is secondary to hyperglycemia, desmopressin is given for diabetes insipidus, antidiarrheal agents for diarrhea, and antiemetic medications for vomiting.

TABLE 11-3 Fluid Replacement in Shock[a]

Fluids	Advantages	Disadvantages
Crystalloids		
Lactated Ringer's	Widely available; Lactate ion that helps buffer metabolic acidosis	Requires large volume of infusion; overresuscitation can result in pulmonary edema, abdominal compartment syndrome
0.9% Sodium chloride (normal saline solution)	Widely available	Requires large volume of infusion; can cause hypernatremia, hypokalemia, hyperchloremic metabolic acidosis; overresuscitation can result in pulmonary edema, abdominal compartment syndrome
Colloids		
Albumin (5%, 25%)	Rapidly expands plasma volume	Expensive; requires human donors; limited supply; can cause heart failure
Blood Products		
Plasma, packed red blood cells, and platelets	Rapidly replaces volume lost due to hemorrhage	Crossmatch type-specific blood is desired for optimal massive transfusion protocols to reduce transfusion-related complications (e.g., transfusion-related acute lung injury, hemolytic reactions, transfusion-associated circulatory overload)

[a]Deliver a minimum of 30 mL/kg of crystalloid.

Adapted from Holcomb, J. B., Tiley, B. C., Baraniuk, S., et al. (2015). Transfusion of plasma, platelets, and red blood cells in a 1:1:1 vs a 1:1:2 ratio and mortality in patients with severe trauma. *JAMA, 313*(5), 471–482; Lewis, S. R., Pritchard, M. W., Evans, D. J. W., et al. (2018). Colloids versus crystalloids for fluid resuscitation in critically ill people. The *Cochrane Database of Systematic Reviews*, 8(8), CD000567;

Rhodes, A., Evans, L., Alhazzani, W., et al. (2017). Surviving Sepsis Campaign: International guidelines for management of sepsis and septic shock: 2016. *Critical Care Medicine,* 45(3), 486–552.

Nursing Management

Primary prevention of shock is an essential focus of nursing care. Hypovolemic shock can be prevented in some instances by closely monitoring patients who are at risk for fluid deficits and assisting with fluid replacement before intravascular volume is depleted. In other circumstances, nursing care focuses on assisting with treatment targeted at the cause of the shock and restoring intravascular volume.

General nursing measures include ensuring safe administration of prescribed fluids and medications and documenting their administration and effects. Volumetric IV pumps should be used to administer prescribed vasopressor medications. Another important nursing role is monitoring for complications and side effects of treatment and reporting them promptly.

Administering Blood and Fluids Safely

Administering blood transfusions safely is a vital nursing role. In emergency situations, it is important to acquire blood specimens quickly, to obtain a baseline complete blood count, and to type and crossmatch the blood in anticipation of blood transfusions. A patient who receives a transfusion of blood products must be monitored closely for adverse effects (see Chapter 28).

Fluid replacement complications can occur, especially when large volumes are given rapidly. Therefore, the nurse monitors the patient closely for cardiovascular overload and signs of difficulty breathing, a condition known as transfusion-associated circulatory overload. Transfusion-related ALI may occur and is characterized by pulmonary edema, hypoxemia, respiratory distress, and pulmonary infiltrates, usually within hours after massive transfusion (Vlaar & Kleinman, 2019). The risk of these complications is increased in older adults, in patients with preexisting cardiac disease, and with increasing number of blood products given. ACS is also a possible complication of excessive fluid resuscitation and may initially present with respiratory symptoms (difficulty breathing) and decreased urine output. Hemodynamic pressure, vital signs, arterial blood gases, serum lactate levels, hemoglobin and hematocrit levels, bladder pressure monitoring, and fluid intake and output (I&O) are among the parameters monitored. Temperature should also be monitored closely to ensure that rapid fluid resuscitation does not cause hypothermia. IV fluids may need to be warmed when large volumes are given. Physical assessment focuses on observing the jugular veins for distention and monitoring jugular venous pressure. Jugular venous pressure is low in hypovolemic shock; it increases with effective treatment and is significantly increased with fluid overload and heart failure. The nurse must monitor cardiac and respiratory status closely and report changes in BP, pulse pressure, CVP, heart rate and rhythm, and lung sounds to the primary provider.

Implementing Other Measures

Oxygen is given to increase the amount of oxygen carried by available hemoglobin in the blood. A patient who is confused may feel apprehensive with an oxygen mask or cannula in place, and frequent explanations about the need for the mask may reduce some of the patient's fear and anxiety. Simultaneously, the nurse must direct efforts to the safety and comfort of the patient.

Cardiogenic Shock

Cardiogenic shock occurs when the heart's ability to contract and to pump blood is impaired and the supply of oxygen is inadequate for the heart and the tissues. The causes of cardiogenic shock are known as either coronary or noncoronary. Coronary cardiogenic shock is more common than noncoronary cardiogenic shock and is seen most often in patients with acute MI resulting in damage to a significant portion of the left ventricular myocardium (Wilcox, 2019). Patients who experience an anterior wall MI are at greatest risk for cardiogenic shock because of the potentially extensive damage to the left ventricle caused by occlusion of the left anterior descending coronary artery. Noncoronary causes of cardiogenic shock are related to conditions that stress the myocardium (e.g., severe hypoxemia, acidosis, hypoglycemia, hypocalcemia, tension pneumothorax) as well as conditions that result in ineffective myocardial function (e.g., cardiomyopathies, valvular damage, cardiac tamponade, arrhythmias).

Pathophysiology

In cardiogenic shock, cardiac output, which is a function of both stroke volume and heart rate, is compromised. When stroke volume and heart rate decrease or become erratic, BP falls and tissue perfusion is reduced. Blood supply for tissues and organs and for the heart muscle itself is inadequate, resulting in impaired tissue perfusion. Because impaired tissue perfusion weakens the heart and impairs its ability to pump, the ventricle does not fully eject its volume of blood during systole. As a result, fluid accumulates in the lungs. This sequence of events can occur rapidly or over a period of days (Fig. 11-5).

Clinical Manifestations

Patients in cardiogenic shock may experience the pain of angina, develop arrhythmias, complain of fatigue, express feelings of doom, and show signs of hemodynamic instability.

Physiology/Pathophysiology

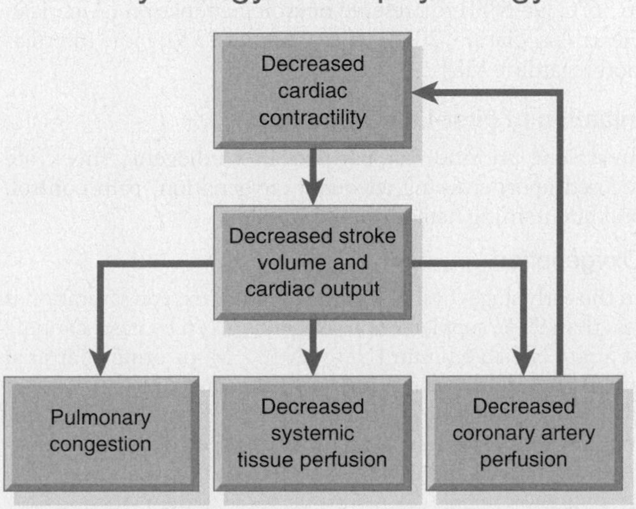

Figure 11-5 • Pathophysiologic sequence of events in cardiogenic shock.

Assessment and Diagnostic Findings

To assess the degree of myocardial damage, laboratory biomarkers for ventricular dysfunction (e.g., B-type natriuretic peptide), cardiac enzyme levels and biomarkers (cTn-I), and serum lactate are measured. In addition, a transthoracic echocardiography may be performed at the bedside, and serial 12-lead electrocardiograms are obtained (Bellumkonda, Gul, & Masri, 2018; Wilcox, 2019). Continuous ECG and ST segment monitoring is also done to closely monitor the patient for ischemic changes.

 Medical Management

The goals of medical management in cardiogenic shock are to limit further myocardial damage and preserve the healthy myocardium and to improve cardiac function by increasing cardiac contractility, decreasing ventricular afterload, or both (Wilcox, 2019). In general, these goals are achieved by increasing oxygen supply to the heart muscle while reducing oxygen demands.

Correction of Underlying Causes

As with all forms of shock, the underlying cause of cardiogenic shock must be corrected. It is necessary first to treat the oxygenation needs of the heart muscle to ensure its continued ability to pump blood to other organs. In the case of coronary cardiogenic shock (e.g., acute coronary syndromes, ischemic cardiomyopathy, nonischemic cardiomyopathies, and myocarditis), the patient may require thrombolytic (fibrinolytic) therapy, a percutaneous coronary intervention, coronary artery bypass graft surgery, IABP therapy, ventricular assist device, or some combination of these treatments (Bellumkonda et al., 2018; Wilcox, 2019). In the case of noncoronary cardiogenic shock, interventions focus on correcting the underlying cause, such as replacement of an impaired cardiac valve, correction of an arrhythmia, correction of acidosis and electrolyte disturbances, or treatment of a tension pneumothorax. If the cause of the cardiogenic shock was related to a cardiac arrest, once the patient is successfully resuscitated, targeted temperature management, also called *therapeutic hypothermia,* may be initiated to actively lower the body temperature to a targeted core temperature (e.g., 32°C [89.6°F] to 36°C [96.8°F]) to preserve neurologic function (American Heart Association, 2018). (See Chapter 23 for more information regarding MI.)

Initiation of First-Line Treatment

Treatment priorities for patients in cardiogenic shock are focused upon ensuring adequate oxygenation, pain control, and maintaining hemodynamic stability.

Oxygenation

In the early stages of shock, if the patient's oxygen saturation is less than 90%, supplemental oxygen is given by nasal cannula at a rate of 2 to 6 L/min (Neto, 2018). Monitoring of arterial blood gas values, pulse oximetry values, and ventilatory effort (i.e., work of breathing) helps determine whether the patient requires a more aggressive method of oxygen delivery (including noninvasive and invasive mechanical ventilation).

Pain Control

If a patient experiences chest pain, IV morphine may be given for pain relief. In addition to relieving pain, morphine may dilate the blood vessels, reducing the workload of the heart by both decreasing the cardiac filling pressure (preload) and reducing the pressure against which the heart muscle has to eject blood (afterload). However, recent evidence suggests morphine may adversely affect antiplatelet agents used to treat the ischemic event; thus, the benefits of morphine may not outweigh its risks (McCarthy, Bhambhani, Pomerantsev, et al., 2018; Neto, 2018).

Hemodynamic Monitoring

Hemodynamic monitoring is initiated to assess the patient's response to treatment. In many institutions, this is performed in the intensive care unit (ICU), where an arterial line can be inserted. The arterial line enables accurate and continuous monitoring of BP and provides a port from which to obtain frequent arterial blood samples without having to perform repeated arterial punctures. A multilumen CVP and PA catheter may be inserted to allow measurement of myocardial filling pressures, pulmonary artery pressures, cardiac output, and pulmonary and systemic resistance. (For more information, see Chapter 21.)

Fluid Therapy

Appropriate fluid administration is also necessary in the treatment of cardiogenic shock. Administration of fluids must be monitored closely to detect signs of fluid overload. Incremental IV fluid boluses are cautiously given to determine optimal filling pressures for improving cardiac output.

 Quality and Safety Nursing Alert

A fluid bolus should never be given rapidly, because rapid fluid administration in patients with cardiac failure may result in acute pulmonary edema.

Pharmacologic Therapy

Vasoactive medication therapy consists of multiple pharmacologic strategies to restore and maintain adequate cardiac output. In coronary cardiogenic shock, the aims of vasoactive medication therapy are improved cardiac contractility, decreased preload and afterload, and stabilized heart rate and rhythm.

Because improving contractility and decreasing cardiac workload are opposing pharmacologic actions, two types of medications may be given in combination: inotropic agents and vasodilators. Inotropic medications increase cardiac output by mimicking the action of the sympathetic nervous system, activating myocardial receptors to increase myocardial contractility (inotropic action), or increasing the heart rate (chronotropic action). These agents may also enhance vascular tone, increasing preload. Vasodilators are used primarily to decrease afterload, reducing the workload of the heart and oxygen demand. Vasodilators also decrease preload. Medications commonly combined to treat cardiogenic shock include dobutamine, nitroglycerin, and dopamine (see Table 11-2).

Dobutamine

Dobutamine produces inotropic effects by stimulating myocardial beta-receptors, increasing the strength of myocardial activity and improving cardiac output. Myocardial alpha-adrenergic receptors are also stimulated, resulting in decreased pulmonary and systemic vascular resistance (decreased afterload) (Maclaren et al., 2019).

Nitroglycerin

IV nitroglycerin in low doses acts as a venous vasodilator and therefore reduces preload. At higher doses, nitroglycerin causes arterial vasodilation and therefore reduces afterload as well. These actions, in combination with dobutamine, increase cardiac output while minimizing cardiac workload. In addition, vasodilation enhances blood flow to the myocardium, improving oxygen delivery to the weakened heart muscle (Maclaren et al., 2019; Wilcox, 2019).

Dopamine

Dopamine is a sympathomimetic agent that has varying vasoactive effects depending on the dosage. It may be used with dobutamine and nitroglycerin to improve tissue perfusion. Doses of 2 to 8 μg/kg/min improve contractility (inotropic action), slightly increase the heart rate (chronotropic action), and may increase cardiac output. Doses that are higher than 8 μg/kg/min predominantly cause vasoconstriction, which increases afterload and thus increases cardiac workload. Because this effect is undesirable in patients with cardiogenic shock, dopamine doses must be carefully titrated.

In severe metabolic acidosis, which occurs in the later stages of shock, metabolic acidosis must first be corrected to ensure maximum effectiveness of vasoactive medications (Maclaren et al., 2019).

Other Vasoactive Medications

Additional vasoactive agents that may be used in managing cardiogenic shock include norepinephrine, epinephrine, milrinone, vasopressin, phenylephrine, and angiotensin II. Each of these medications stimulates different receptors of the sympathetic nervous system. A combination of these medications may be prescribed, depending on the patient's response to treatment. All vasoactive medications have adverse effects, making specific medications more useful than others at different stages of shock (see Table 11-2). Diuretics such as furosemide may be given to reduce the workload of the heart by reducing fluid accumulation.

Antiarrhythmic Medications

Multiple factors, such as hypoxemia, electrolyte imbalances, and acid–base imbalances, contribute to serious cardiac arrhythmias in all patients with shock. In addition, as a compensatory response to decreased cardiac output and BP, the heart rate increases beyond normal limits. This impedes cardiac output further by shortening diastole and thereby decreasing the time for ventricular filling. Consequently, antiarrhythmic medications are required to stabilize the heart rate. General principles regarding the administration of vasoactive medications are discussed later in this chapter. (For a full discussion of cardiac arrhythmias as well as commonly prescribed medications, see Chapter 22.)

Mechanical Assistive Devices

If cardiac output does not improve despite supplemental oxygen, vasoactive medications, and fluid boluses, mechanical assistive devices are used temporarily to improve the heart's ability to pump. Intra-aortic balloon counterpulsation with an IABP is one means of providing temporary circulatory assistance (Hochman & Reyentovich, 2019). The IABP is a catheter with an inflatable balloon at the end. The catheter is usually inserted through the femoral artery and threaded toward

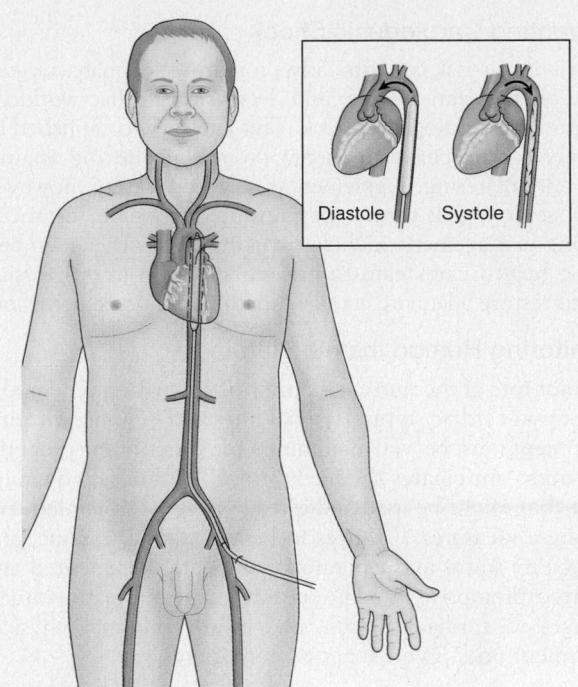

Figure 11-6 • The intra-aortic balloon pump inflates at the beginning of diastole, which results in increased perfusion of the coronary and peripheral arteries. It deflates just before systole, which results in a decrease in afterload (resistance to ejection) and in the left ventricular workload.

the heart, and the balloon is positioned in the descending thoracic aorta (Fig. 11-6). The IABP uses internal counterpulsation through the regular inflation and deflation of the balloon to augment the pumping action of the heart. It inflates during diastole, increasing the pressure in the aorta during diastole and therefore increasing blood flow through the coronary and peripheral arteries. It deflates just before systole, lessening the pressure within the aorta before left ventricular contraction, decreasing the amount of resistance the heart has to overcome to eject blood and therefore decreasing left ventricular workload. The device is connected to a console that synchronizes the inflation and deflation of the balloon with the ECG or the arterial pressure (as indicators for systole and diastole). Hemodynamic monitoring is often used to determine the patient's response to the IABP. The IABP provides short-term (days) support for the failing myocardium.

Other means of mechanical assistance include left and right ventricular assist devices and total temporary artificial hearts (see Chapters 24 and 25). Another short-term means of providing cardiac or pulmonary support to the patient in cardiogenic shock is through an extracorporeal device similar to the cardiopulmonary bypass (CPB) system used in open-heart surgery (see Chapter 23). CPB is used only in emergency situations until definitive treatment, such as heart transplantation, can be initiated.

Nursing Management

The role of the nurse managing the care of a patient with cardiogenic shock revolves around preventing its serious complications, monitoring hemodynamics, administering medications and fluids, maintaining intra-aortic counterpulsation as indicated, and promoting safety and comfort.

Preventing Cardiogenic Shock

Identifying at-risk patients early, promoting adequate oxygenation of the heart muscle, and decreasing cardiac workload can prevent cardiogenic shock. This can be accomplished by conserving the patient's energy, promptly relieving angina, and administering supplemental oxygen. Often, however, cardiogenic shock cannot be prevented. In such instances, nursing management includes working with other members of the health care team to prevent shock from progressing and to restore adequate cardiac function and tissue perfusion.

Monitoring Hemodynamic Status

A major role of the nurse is monitoring the patient's hemodynamic and cardiac status. Arterial lines and ECG monitoring equipment must be well maintained and functioning properly. The nurse anticipates the medications, IV fluids, and equipment that might be used and is ready to assist in implementing these measures. Changes in hemodynamic, cardiac, and pulmonary status and laboratory values are documented and reported promptly. In addition, adventitious breath sounds, changes in cardiac rhythm, and other abnormal physical assessment findings are reported immediately.

Administering Medications and Intravenous Fluids

The nurse plays a critical role in the safe and accurate administration of IV fluids and medications. Fluid overload and pulmonary edema are risks because of ineffective cardiac function and accumulation of blood and fluid in the pulmonary tissues. The nurse documents medications and treatments that are given as well as the patient's response to treatment.

The nurse must be knowledgeable about the desired effects as well as the side effects of medications. For example, the nurse monitors the patient for decreased BP after administering morphine or nitroglycerin. Arterial and venous puncture sites must be observed for bleeding, and pressure must be applied at the sites if bleeding occurs. IV infusions must be observed closely because tissue necrosis and sloughing may occur if vasopressor medications infiltrate the tissues. When possible, vasoactive medications should be given using central IV lines (Bauer et al., 2019). Furthermore, the need for the central IV access devices should be reviewed daily to reduce the risk of CLABSIs (Marschall, Mermel, Fakih, et al., 2014). The nurse must also monitor urine output, serum electrolytes, BUN, and serum creatinine levels to detect decreased renal function secondary to the effects of cardiogenic shock or its treatment.

Maintaining Intra-Aortic Balloon Counterpulsation

The nurse plays a critical role in caring for the patient receiving intra-aortic balloon counterpulsation. The nurse makes ongoing timing adjustments of the balloon pump to maximize its effectiveness by synchronizing it with the cardiac cycle. The patient is at risk for circulatory compromise to the leg on the side where the catheter for the balloon has been inserted; therefore, the nurse must check the neurovascular status of the lower extremities frequently.

Enhancing Safety and Comfort

The nurse must take an active role in safeguarding the patient, enhancing comfort, and reducing anxiety. This includes administering medication to relieve chest pain, preventing infection at the multiple arterial and venous line insertion sites, protecting the skin, and monitoring respiratory and renal function. Proper positioning of the patient promotes effective breathing without decreasing BP and may also increase patient comfort while reducing anxiety.

Brief explanations about procedures that are being performed and the use of comforting touch often provide reassurance to the patient and the family. The family is usually anxious and benefits from opportunities to see and talk to the patient. Explanations of treatments and the patient's responses are often comforting to family members.

Family presence during a patient's critical illness has been a concern for family members, patients, nurses and other health care providers. Evidence-based clinical practice guidelines have outlined several elements that may enhance and support the patient and family experience during critical illness. Davidson and colleagues (2017) identified the importance of frequent, clear communication, an environment which encourages comfortable visitation, flexible visitation policies, including the option for family to stay overnight, and patient and family engagement in clinical decisions as mechanisms to enhance family support. A qualitative research study conducted by Wong and colleagues (2020) explored family perspectives of participation in patient care in the adult ICU. The nurse researchers interviewed and observed 30 family members. Findings demonstrated that families' perceptions of their contribution to the patient's psychosocial and emotional well-being were influenced by their engagement in care. See the Nursing Research Profile in Chart 11-4.

Distributive Shock

Distributive shock occurs when intravascular volume pools in peripheral blood vessels. This abnormal displacement of intravascular volume causes a relative hypovolemia because not enough blood returns to the heart, which leads to inadequate tissue perfusion. The ability of the blood vessels to constrict helps return the blood to the heart. Vascular tone is determined both by central regulatory mechanisms, as in BP regulation, and by local regulatory mechanisms, such as tissue demands for oxygen and nutrients. Therefore, distributive shock can be caused by either a loss of sympathetic tone or a release of biochemical mediators from cells that causes vasodilation.

The varied mechanisms leading to the initial vasodilation in distributive shock provide the basis for the further subclassification of shock into three types: septic shock, neurogenic shock, and anaphylactic shock. These subtypes of distributive shock cause variations in the pathophysiologic chain of events and are explained below separately. In all types of distributive shock, massive arterial and venous dilation promotes peripheral pooling of blood. Arterial dilation reduces systemic vascular resistance. Initially, cardiac output can be high, both from the reduction in afterload (systemic vascular resistance) and from the heart muscle's increased effort to maintain perfusion despite the incompetent vasculature. Pooling of blood in the periphery results in decreased venous return. Decreased venous return results in decreased stroke volume and decreased cardiac output. Decreased cardiac output, in turn, causes decreased BP and ultimately decreased tissue perfusion. Figure 11-7 presents the pathophysiologic sequence of events in distributive shock.

Chart 11-4 · NURSING RESEARCH PROFILE

Family Participation in the Intensive Care Unit

Wong, P., Redley, B., Digby, R., et al. (2020). Families' perspectives of participation in patient care in an adult intensive care unit: A qualitative study. *Australian Critical Care, 33*(4), 317–325.

Purpose

The aim of this study was to describe family participation in patient care in the adult intensive care unit (ICU).

Design

This was a qualitative, descriptive observational study that enrolled a convenience sample of 30 family members who had an adult family member admitted to the ICU for more than 72 h. Researchers observed the family members' engagement in patient care activities and conducted semi-structured interviews focused on their experiences and perceptions of providing care.

Findings

Most of the family participants (77%) were female. Ages of the patient and family member were similar ranging from 28 to 73, with a median age for family members of 53. Researchers observed 193 activities in which 25% involved physical care for the patient, while the remaining 75% of activities were intangible care interventions such as communication and psychosocial/emotional care. Themes that emerged from the interviews revealed that the families felt part of the health care team and thus wanted to support the care and recovery of the loved one. Family members reported being motivated to provide care because they wanted the best care for the patient, desired to know the prognosis, treatment, and condition of the patient, and desired to help the patient recover. Lastly, family members wanted to advocate for their relatives, provide psychosocial and emotional care, and be supportive during medical treatments. The researchers observed that the physical environment was either a contributor or barrier to the family member's ability to engage in care. Equipment sometimes created physical barriers that made it hard for family to get close to the patient. Staff support and communication either encouraged or discouraged family participation in care. When nurses communicated openly, keeping families informed, family members felt more welcomed and better able to support the patient's treatment plans.

Nursing Implications

Most families wish to be engaged and to advocate for their loved ones in the treatment decision making process. The ability for family to feel part of the health care team and develop trust in the plan of care is influenced by positive relationships with the nursing and medical staff as well as the welcoming nature of the environment. Patient- and family-centered care is facilitated when families are considered collaborative partners in the care of adult patients who are critically ill.

Physiology/Pathophysiology

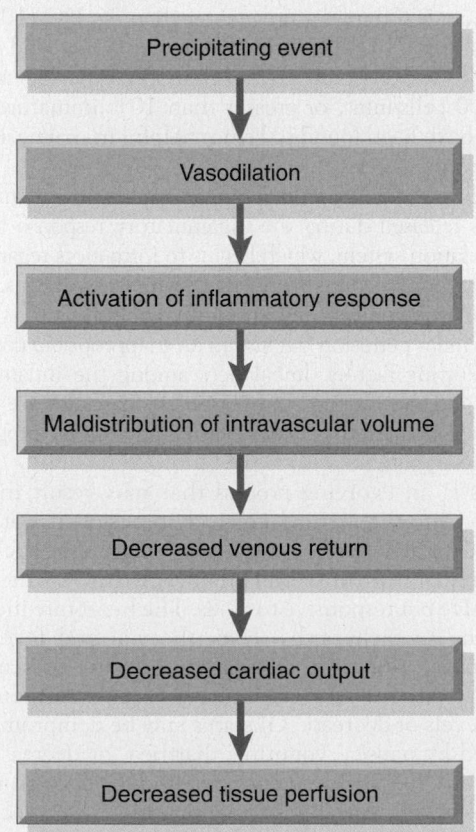

Figure 11-7 • Pathophysiologic sequence of events in distributive shock.

Sepsis and Septic Shock

Septic shock, the most common type of distributive shock, is caused by widespread infection or sepsis. According to the Third International Consensus Definitions for Sepsis and Septic Shock (*Sepsis-3*) Task Force, **sepsis** is "life-threatening organ dysfunction caused by a dysregulated host response to infection (Singer et al., 2016, p. 804)," and **septic shock** is "a subset of sepsis in which underlying circulatory and cellular metabolism abnormalities are profound enough to substantially increase mortality (Singer et al., 2016, p. 806)."

Despite the increased sophistication of antibiotic therapy, the incidence of both sepsis and septic shock has continued to rise; today sepsis and septic shock are the leading causes of death in noncoronary ICU patients. Worldwide, sepsis impacts more than 31 million people, and more than 6 million people die from it annually (Global Sepsis Alliance, 2017). The number of hospital admissions related to sepsis has increased threefold over the last decade (Surviving Sepsis Campaign, 2019). Identifying and aggressively treating the source of infection and quickly restoring tissue perfusion are important interventions that may positively influence clinical outcomes.

Hospital-acquired conditions, which may include hospital-associated infections (i.e., infections not present at the time of admission to the health care setting) in critically ill patients that may progress to septic shock, most frequently originate in the bloodstream (bacteremia), lungs (pneumonia), and urinary tract (urosepsis). Other infections include intra-abdominal infections and wound infections. Of increasing concern are bacteremias associated with intravascular catheters and indwelling urinary catheters (Centers for Disease Control and Prevention [CDC], 2019).

Additional risk factors that contribute to the growing incidence of sepsis are the increased use of invasive procedures and indwelling medical devices, the increased number of antibiotic-resistant microorganisms, and the aging population (CDC, 2019). Older adult patients are at particular risk for sepsis because of decreased physiologic reserves, an aging immune system, comorbid conditions and often nonspecific presentation of infection (Rowe & McKoy, 2017) (see Chapter 8). Other patients at risk are those undergoing surgical and other invasive procedures, especially patients who have undergone emergency surgery or multiple surgeries (Rhodes et al., 2017); those with malnutrition or immunosuppression; and those with chronic illness such as diabetes, hepatitis, chronic kidney disease, and immunodeficiency disorders (Keeley, Hine, & Nsutebu, 2017) (Chart 11-5).

The incidence of sepsis can be reduced by using strict infection control practices, beginning with thorough hand hygiene techniques (Dunne, Kingston, Slevin, et al., 2018). Other interventions include implementing programs to prevent central line infections and ventilator-associated events (e.g., aspiration) and pneumonia; ensuring early removal of invasive devices that are no longer necessary (e.g., indwelling urinary catheters); promoting early ambulation and timely débridement of wounds; and adhering to standard precautions and infection prevention/control practices, including the use of meticulous aseptic technique and proper cleaning of equipment and the patient environment.

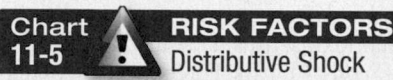

Chart 11-5 · RISK FACTORS
Distributive Shock

Septic Shock

- Immunosuppression
- Extremes of age (<1 y and >65 y)
- Malnourishment
- Chronic illness
- Invasive procedures
- Emergent and/or multiple surgeries

Neurogenic Shock

- Spinal cord injury
- Spinal anesthesia
- Depressant action of medications

Anaphylactic Shock

- History of medication sensitivity
- Transfusion reaction
- History of reaction to insect bites/stings
- Food allergies
- Latex sensitivity

Adapted from Keeley, A., Hine, P., & Nsutebu, E. (2017). The recognition and management of sepsis and septic shock: A guide for non-intensivists. *Postgraduate Medicine Journal, 93*(1104), 626–634; Pajno, G. B., Fernandez-Rivas, M., Arasi, S., et al. (2018). EAACI guidelines on allergen immunotherapy: IgE-mediated food allergy. *Allergy, 73*(4), 799–815; Rhodes, A., Evans, L., Alhazzani, W., et al. (2017). Surviving Sepsis Campaign: International guidelines for management of sepsis and septic shock: 2016. *Critical Care Medicine, 45*(3), 486–552; Singer, M., Deutschman, C. S., Seymour, C. W., et al. (2016). The Third International Consensus Definitions for Sepsis and Septic Shock (Sepsis-3). *JAMA, 315*(8), 801–810.

Pathophysiology

Gram-negative bacteria traditionally were the most commonly implicated microorganisms in sepsis. However, there is an increased incidence of gram-positive bacterial infections, viral infections, and fungal infections that can also cause sepsis (Keeley et al., 2017). Although a site of infection is identified in most cases, in up to 30% of patients with sepsis an identifiable source of infection is not determined (Surviving Sepsis Campaign, 2019).

When microorganisms invade body tissues, patients exhibit an immune response. This immune response provokes the activation of biochemical cytokines and mediators associated with an inflammatory response and produces a complex cascade of physiologic events that leads to poor tissue perfusion. Increased capillary permeability results in fluid seeping from the capillaries. Capillary instability and vasodilation interrupt the body's ability to provide adequate perfusion, oxygen, and nutrients to the tissues and cells. The widespread inflammatory response that occurs is called the **systemic inflammatory response syndrome** (SIRS). SIRS, which is a type of cytokine release syndrome and is often referred to as cytokine storm, results from a clinical insult that initiates an inflammatory response that is systemic, rather than localized to the site of the insult (see Chapter 12 for further discussion of cytokine release syndrome). The insult may be a significant injury (e.g., multitrauma) or an infection (e.g., sepsis). A patient presenting with manifestations of SIRS may be exhibiting a protective inflammatory response to the initiating insult or may be exhibiting a response to infection, which may lead to sepsis. The clinical criteria used to identify SIRS, which include a temperature greater than 38.3°C (101°F) or less than 36°C (96.8°F), tachycardia, tachypnea, and a white blood cell (WBC) count greater than 12,000 cells/mm^3, less than 4000 cells/mm^3, or greater than 10% immature WBC (bands), have been found to be not helpful in diagnosing sepsis, however (Singer et al., 2016).

In addition to SIRS, proinflammatory and anti-inflammatory cytokines released during the inflammatory response activate the coagulation system, which begins to form clots regardless of whether or not bleeding is present (Seymour & Angus, 2018). This results not only in microvascular occlusions that further disrupt cellular perfusion but also in an inappropriate consumption of clotting factors. Imbalances among the inflammatory response and the clotting and fibrinolysis cascades are considered critical elements of the devastating physiologic progression that occurs in patients with sepsis.

Sepsis is an evolving process that may result in septic shock and life-threatening organ dysfunction if not recognized and treated early. In the early stage of septic shock, BP may remain within normal limits, or the patient may be hypotensive but responsive to fluids. The heart rate increases, progressing to tachycardia. Hyperthermia and fever, with warm, flushed skin and bounding pulses, are present. The respiratory rate is elevated. Urinary output may remain at normal levels or decrease. GI status may be compromised, as evidenced by nausea, vomiting, diarrhea, or decreased gastric motility. Hepatic dysfunction is evidenced by rising bilirubin levels and worsening coagulopathies (e.g., decreasing platelet counts). Signs of hypermetabolism include increased serum glucose and insulin resistance. Subtle changes in mental status, such as confusion or agitation, may be present.

The lactate level is elevated because of the maldistribution of blood. Inflammatory markers such as WBC counts, plasma C-reactive protein (CRP), and procalcitonin levels are also elevated (Rhodes et al., 2017; Seymour & Angus, 2018; Singer et al., 2016).

As sepsis progresses, tissues become less perfused and acidotic, compensation begins to fail, and the patient begins to show signs of organ dysfunction. The cardiovascular system also begins to fail, the BP does not respond to fluid resuscitation and vasoactive agents, and signs of end-organ damage are evident (e.g., AKI, pulmonary dysfunction, hepatic dysfunction, confusion progressing to nonresponsiveness). As sepsis progresses to septic shock, the BP drops and the skin becomes cool, pale, and mottled. Temperature may be normal or below normal. Heart and respiratory rates remain rapid. Urine production ceases, and multiple organ dysfunction progressing to death occurs.

 Medical Management

A significant body of research has been conducted in the past few decades that is aimed at reducing the morbidity and mortality caused by sepsis and septic shock. In 1991, 2003, 2008, 2012, and again in 2016 (i.e., *Sepsis-3*), critical-care experts systematically reevaluated the body of research and provided evidence-based recommendations for the acute management of patients with sepsis and septic shock (Rhodes et al., 2017; Singer et al., 2016; Surviving Sepsis Campaign, 2019). Developing and implementing protocols, sepsis bundles, that focus on prevention and early detection and management of patients with sepsis have reduced the mortality of hospitalized patients (Kahn, Davis, Yabes, et al., 2019). *Sepsis-3* provides an overview of key concepts and principles germane to sepsis that must be understood in order for primary providers and nurses to be able to identify and manage patients with sepsis, including the following (Levy & Townsend, 2019; Singer et al., 2016):

- As the leading cause of death from infection, sepsis must be recognized and treated promptly.
- Sepsis is different from infection in that in sepsis there is a dysregulated host response with organ dysfunction. An infection may cause specific organ dysfunction without a dysregulated host response.
- Sepsis is caused by an interplay between infectious pathogens and a myriad of patient-specific risks, including genetics, age, and the presence of other diseases/disorders.
- The organ dysfunction that occurs with sepsis may not be readily apparent; on the contrary, a new onset of organ dysfunction may be caused by an unrecognized infectious process.

Research efforts are focusing on better identification and early aggressive treatment of patients with sepsis, rapid and effective restoration of tissue perfusion, evaluation and treatment of the patient's immune response, and treatment of dysregulation of the coagulation system that occurs with sepsis (Keeley et al., 2017; Makic & Bridges, 2018).

Correction of Underlying Causes

Current treatment of sepsis and septic shock involves rapid identification and elimination of the cause of infection. Current goals are to identify and initiate treatment for patients in early sepsis within 1 hour to optimize patient outcomes (Levy et al., 2018; Levy & Townsend, 2019). Several evidence-based screening tools can be used to help identify patients for sepsis (see later discussion of assessment tools under the section Nursing Management).

In an effort to continue to reduce deaths from sepsis, Centers for Medicare and Medicaid Services (CMS) has identified sepsis and sepsis bundle adherence as a *Core Measure*. The focus on adherence with these evidence-based bundled interventions is to foster early recognition and interventions in patients with sepsis so that patient outcomes improve. These assessments and interventions are collectively referred to as the *Sepsis Bundles* (Chart 11-6).

Rapid identification of the infectious source is a critical element in managing sepsis. Specimens of blood, sputum, urine, wound drainage, and tips of invasive catheters are collected for culture using aseptic technique. IV lines are removed and reinserted at alternate sites. If possible, urinary catheters are removed or changed. Any abscesses are drained, and necrotic areas are débrided. All cultures should be obtained prior to antibiotic administration. Current guidelines suggest that antibiotics should be initiated within the first hour of treatment of a patient with sepsis (Surviving Sepsis Campaign, 2019).

Fluid Replacement Therapy

Fluid replacement must be instituted to correct tissue hypoperfusion that results from the incompetent vasculature and the inflammatory response. Reestablishing tissue perfusion through aggressive fluid resuscitation is key to the management of sepsis and septic shock (Rhodes et al., 2017; Singer et al., 2016). An initial fluid challenge, which includes an IV infusion of at least 30 mL/kg of crystalloids over 30 minutes, may be required to aggressively treat sepsis-induced tissue hypoperfusion. In addition to monitoring BP, patient mentation, respiratory rate, fluid responsiveness after PLR, urine output, and serum lactate levels are monitored to assess effectiveness of fluid resuscitation.

Pharmacologic Therapy

If the infecting organism is unknown, broad-spectrum antibiotic agents are started until culture and sensitivity reports are received (Levy & Townsend, 2019; Rhodes et al., 2017), at which time the antibiotic agents may be changed to agents that are more specific to the infecting organism and less toxic to the patient.

If fluid therapy alone does not effectively improve tissue perfusion, vasopressor agents, specifically norepinephrine or dopamine, may be initiated to achieve a MAP of 65 mm Hg or higher. Inotropic agents may also be given to provide pharmacologic support to the myocardium. Packed red blood cells may be prescribed to support oxygen delivery and transport to the tissues. Neuromuscular blockade agents and sedation agents may be required to reduce metabolic demands and provide comfort to the patient. Deep vein thrombosis (DVT) prophylaxis with low-dose unfractionated heparin or low-molecular-weight heparin, in combination with mechanical prophylaxis (e.g., sequential compression devices) should be initiated, as well as medications for stress ulcer prophylaxis (e.g., H_2-blocking agents, proton pump inhibitors).

Chart 11-6 Surviving Sepsis Campaign Bundle and CMS Core Measure Monitoring Metrics

Complete within 1 h of patient presentation/symptoms
- Measure lactate level. Remeasure if initial lactate is >2 mmol/L
- Obtain blood cultures prior to administration of antibiotics
- Administer broad-spectrum antibiotics
- Begin rapid administration of 30 mL/kg crystalloid for hypotension or lactate ≥4 mmol/L (within 30 min)
- Administer vasopressors if patients is hypotensive during or after fluid resuscitation to maintain MAP ≥65 mm Hg

Reprinted with permission from Levy, M., Evans, L., & Rhodes, A. (2018). The Surviving Sepsis Campaign bundle: 2018 update. *Critical Care Medicine, 46*(6), 997–1000.

CMS Core Measure Metrics and Surviving Sepsis Bundles 2016:

Complete within 3 h of patient presentation/symptoms
- Obtain serum lactate level
- Obtain blood culture prior to administration of antibiotics
- Administer prescribed broad-spectrum antibiotics
- Initiate aggressive fluid resuscitation in patients with hypotension or elevated serum lactate (>4 mmol/L):
  - Minimum initial fluid bolus of 30 mL/kg using crystalloid solutions

Complete as soon as possible or within the first 6 h of patient presentation/symptoms
- Begin vasopressor agents if hypotension is not improved (MAP <65 mm Hg) after initial fluid resuscitation
- If hypotension persists after initial fluid administration (MAP <65 mm Hg) or initial lactate was ≥4 mmol/L, reassess intravascular volume status and tissue perfusion using two of the following assessment parameters, including vital signs, capillary refill, pulse, and skin findings, or two of the following:
  - Measurement of CVP and/or ScvO$_2$ (goal >70%)
  - Bedside cardiovascular ultrasound
  - Dynamic assessment of fluid responsiveness with passive leg raise or fluid challenge

Additional interventions and targets for therapy in the early management of sepsis
- Support blood pressure to achieve a urine output of >0.5 mL/kg/h over a 6-h period
- Administer vasopressor agents if fluid resuscitation does not restore an effective BP and cardiac output:
  - Norepinephrine centrally given is the initial vasopressor of choice.
  - Epinephrine, phenylephrine, or vasopressin should not be given as the initial vasopressor in septic shock.
- Obtain blood, sputum, urine, and wound cultures and administer broad-spectrum antibiotics:
  - Cultures should be obtained prior to antibiotic administration.
  - Antibiotic administration should occur within 3 h of admission to the emergency department or within 1 h of inpatient admission.
- Support the respiratory system with supplemental oxygen and mechanical ventilation.
- Transfuse with packed red blood cells when hemoglobin is <7 g/dL to achieve a target hemoglobin of 7–9 g/dL in adults.
- Provide adequate IV sedation and analgesia; avoid the use of neuromuscular blockade agents when possible.
- Control serum glucose <180 mg/dL with IV insulin therapy.
- Implement interventions and medications to prevent deep vein thrombosis and stress ulcer prophylaxis.
- Discuss advance care planning with patients and families.

BP, blood pressure; CVP, central venous pressure; IV, intravenous; MAP, mean arterial pressure.
Adapted from Centers for Medicare & Medicaid Services (CMS). (2019). Hospital Toolkit for Adult Sepsis Surveillance. Retrieved on 9/10/19 at: www.cdc.gov/sepsis/clinicaltools/index.html; Levy, M., Evans, L., & Rhodes, A. (2018). The Surviving Sepsis Campaign bundle: 2018 update. *Critical Care Medicine, 46*(6), 997–1000; Levy, M. M., & Townsend, S. R. (2019). Early identification of sepsis on the hospital floors: Insights for implementation of the hour-1 bundle. *Society of Critical Care Medicine.* Retrieved on 9/10/19 at: www.survivingsepsis.org/SiteCollectionDocuments/Surviving-Sepsis-Early-Identify-Sepsis-Hospital-Floor.pdf

---

Nutritional Therapy

Aggressive nutritional supplementation should be initiated within 24 to 48 hours of ICU admission to address the hypermetabolic state present with septic shock (Reintam et al., 2017; Wang et al., 2019). Malnutrition further impairs the patient's resistance to infection. Enteral feedings are preferred to the parenteral route because of the increased risk of iatrogenic infection associated with IV catheters; however, enteral feedings may not be possible if decreased perfusion to the GI tract reduces peristalsis and impairs absorption.

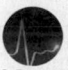 ### Nursing Management

Nurses caring for patients in any setting must keep in mind the risks of sepsis and the high mortality rate associated with sepsis and septic shock. All invasive procedures must be carried out with aseptic technique after careful hand hygiene. In addition, IV lines, arterial and venous puncture sites, surgical incisions, traumatic wounds, and urinary catheters must be monitored for signs of infection. Nursing interventions to prevent infection need to be implemented in the care of all patients. Nurses should identify patients who are at particular risk for sepsis and septic shock (i.e., older adults and immunosuppressed patients

and those with extensive trauma, burns, or diabetes), keeping in mind that these high-risk patients may not develop typical or classic signs of infection and sepsis. However, confusion with or without agitation along with an increased respiratory rate may be the first sign of infection and sepsis in any adult patient (Ferguson, Coates, Osborn, et al., 2019).

Sepsis-3 recommends that patients in the ICU setting with infection be monitored for the development of sepsis by using the *Sepsis-Related Organ Failure Assessment Score* (also known as the *Sequential Organ Failure Assessment [SOFA] score*) (Singer et al., 2016; Vincent, Moreno, Takala, et al., 1996) (Table 11-4). The parameters that are monitored on the SOFA which include assessment of respiratory rate, platelets, bilirubin, MAP (and use of any vasopressors), serum creatinine, urine output, and Glasgow Coma Scale (GCS) score (see Chapter 63), may all be gathered and assessed by the nurse in the ICU setting. A drop of 2 points or more in a patient's SOFA score from baseline is suggestive of organ dysfunction. In a patient with infection, the presence of organ dysfunction suggests the development of sepsis (Singer et al., 2016).

For a patient not in the ICU setting who has an infection, *Sepsis-3* recommends that the Quick SOFA (qSOFA) scale be used to screen for the development of sepsis. The qSOFA is an easy measurement tool that nurses may readily use; the presence of any two of the three parameters on this

TABLE 11-4 The Sepsis-Related Organ Failure Assessment Score (Sequential Organ Failure Assessment [SOFA] Score)

SOFA Score	1	2	3	4
Respiration PaO$_2$/FiO$_2$, mm Hg	<400	<300	<200	<100 ——with respiratory support——
Coagulation Platelets × 10^3/mm^3	<150	<100	<50	<20
Liver Bilirubin, mg/dL (μmol/L)	1.2–1.9 (20–32)	2.0–5.9 (33–101)	6.0–11.9 (102–204)	>12.0 (<204)
Cardiovascular Hypotension	MAP <70 mm Hg	Dopamine ≤5 or dobutamine (any dose)^a	Dopamine >5 or epinephrine ≤0.1 or norepinephrine ≤0.1	Dopamine >15 or epinephrine >0.1 or norepinephrine >0.1
Central Nervous System Glasgow Coma Scale	13–14	10–12	6–9	<6
Renal Creatinine, mg/dL (μmol/L) or urine output	1.2–1.9 (110–170)	2.0–3.4 (171–299)	3.5–4.9 (300–440) or <500 mL/day	>5.0 (>440) or <200 mL/day

MAP, mean arterial pressure.

^{a}Adrenergic agents given for at least 1 h (doses given are in μg/kg/min).

Reprinted with permission from Vincent, J. L., Moreno, R., Takala, J., et al. (1996). The SOFA (Sepsis-related Organ Failure Assessment) score to describe organ dysfunction/failure. On behalf of the Working Group on Sepsis-Related Problems of the European Society of Intensive Care Medicine. *Intensive Care Medicine, 22*(7), 707–710.

scale suggests the development of sepsis. These parameters include a respiratory rate of 22 breaths/min or higher, a GCS score of less than 15 (any change in the patient's mentation), and a systolic BP of 100 mm Hg or less. In order to facilitate ease of use, therefore, *Sepsis-3* recommends that any change in the patient's mentation status be used when computing the qSOFA scale score (Singer et al., 2016). Another assessment tool that is frequently used in hospital-based settings that can identify patients with sepsis is the *Modified Early Warning System* (MEWS) (Institute for Healthcare Improvement [IHI], 2017). The nurse assesses the patient for changes in respiratory rate, heart rate, BP, consciousness, temperature, and urine output. Scores ranging from 0 to 3 are assigned to each variable, and a MEWS score greater than 4 is suggestive of the development of sepsis (IHI, 2017) (Table 11-5).

When caring for a patient with sepsis or septic shock, the nurse collaborates with other members of the health care team to identify the site and source of sepsis and the specific organisms involved. The nurse often obtains appropriate specimens for culture and sensitivity. Prescribed antibiotics are not given until these specimens are obtained. Hyperthermia (elevated body temperature) is common with sepsis and raises the patient's metabolic rate and oxygen consumption. Efforts may be made to reduce the temperature by administering acetaminophen or applying a hypothermia blanket. During these therapies, the nurse monitors the patient closely for shivering, which increases oxygen consumption. Efforts to increase comfort are important if the patient experiences fever, chills, or shivering.

The nurse administers prescribed IV fluids and medications, including antibiotic agents and vasoactive medications, to restore vascular volume. Because of decreased perfusion, serum concentrations of antibiotic agents that are normally cleared by the kidneys and liver may increase and produce toxic effects. Therefore, the nurse monitors blood levels

TABLE 11-5 The MEWS (Modified Early Warning System)

	MEWS (Modified Early Warning System)						
	3	2	1	0	1	2	3
Respiratory rate per minute		<8		9–14	15–20	21–29	>30
Heart rate per minute		<40	40–50	51–100	101–110	111–129	>129
Systolic blood pressure	<70	71–80	81–100	101–199		>200	
Conscious level (AVPU)	Unresponsive	Responds to **Pain**	Responds to **Voice**	**Alert**	New agitation; Confusion		
Temperature (°C)		<35.0	35.1–36	36.10–38	38.1–38.5	>38.6	
Hourly urine for 2 h	<10 mL/h	<30 mL/h	<45 mL/h				

Developed by Ysbyty Glan Clwyd, Conwy & Denbighshire National Health Service Trust, North Wales. Reprinted with permission from Institute for Healthcare Improvement (IHI). (2017). *Improvement stories: Early warning systems: Scorecards that save lives.* Retrieved on 11/6/19 at: http://www.ihi.org/resources/Pages/ImprovementStories/EarlyWarningSystemsScorecardsThatSaveLives.aspx

(serum levels of antibiotic agents, procalcitonin, CRP, BUN, creatinine, WBC count, hemoglobin, hematocrit, platelet levels, coagulation studies) and reports changes to the primary provider. As with other types of shock, the nurse monitors the patient's hemodynamic status, fluid I&O, daily weight, and nutritional status. Close monitoring of serum albumin and prealbumin levels helps determine the patient's protein requirements.

Neurogenic Shock

In **neurogenic shock,** vasodilation occurs as a result of a loss of balance between parasympathetic and sympathetic stimulation. Sympathetic stimulation causes vascular smooth muscle to constrict, and parasympathetic stimulation causes vascular smooth muscle to relax or dilate. The patient experiences a predominant parasympathetic stimulation that causes vasodilation lasting for an extended period, leading to a relative hypovolemic state. However, blood volume is adequate, because the vasculature is dilated; the blood volume is displaced, producing a hypotensive (low BP) state. The overriding parasympathetic stimulation that occurs with neurogenic shock causes a drastic decrease in the patient's systemic vascular resistance and bradycardia. Inadequate BP results in the insufficient perfusion of tissues and cells that is common to all shock states.

Neurogenic shock can be caused by spinal cord injury, spinal anesthesia, or other nervous system damage. It may also result from the depressant action of medications or from lack of glucose (e.g., insulin reaction) (see Chart 11-5). Neurogenic shock may have a prolonged course (spinal cord injury) or a short one (syncope or fainting). Normally, during states of stress, the sympathetic stimulation causes the BP and heart rate to increase. In neurogenic shock, the sympathetic system is not able to respond to body stressors. Therefore, the clinical characteristics of neurogenic shock are signs of parasympathetic stimulation. It is characterized by dry, warm skin rather than the cool, moist skin seen in hypovolemic shock. Another characteristic is hypotension with bradycardia, rather than the tachycardia that characterizes other forms of shock.

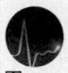 **Medical Management**

Treatment of neurogenic shock involves restoring sympathetic tone, either through the stabilization of a spinal cord injury or, in the instance of spinal anesthesia, by positioning the patient properly. Specific treatment depends on the cause of the shock. (Further discussion of management of patients with a spinal cord injury is presented in Chapter 63.)

 Nursing Management

It is important to elevate and maintain the head of the bed at least 30 degrees to prevent neurogenic shock when a patient receives spinal or epidural anesthesia. Elevation of the head helps prevent the spread of the anesthetic agent up the spinal cord. In suspected spinal cord injury, neurogenic shock may be prevented by carefully immobilizing the patient to prevent further damage to the spinal cord (Kessler, Traini, Welk, et al., 2018). Nursing interventions are directed toward supporting cardiovascular and neurologic function until the usually transient episode of neurogenic shock resolves.

Patients with neurogenic shock have a higher risk for venous thromboembolism (VTE) formation because of increased pooling of blood from vascular dilation; this risk is greater in patients with neurogenic shock related to spinal cord injury. The nurse must assess the patient daily for any lower extremity pain, redness, tenderness, and warmth. If the patient complains of pain and objective assessment of the calf is suspicious, the patient should be evaluated for DVT. Passive range of motion of the immobile extremities helps promote circulation. Early interventions to prevent VTE include the application of pneumatic compression devices often combined with antithrombotic agents (e.g., low-molecular-weight heparin).

A patient who has experienced a spinal cord injury may not report pain caused by internal injuries. Therefore, in the immediate post-injury period, the nurse must monitor the patient closely for signs of internal bleeding that could lead to hypovolemic shock.

Anaphylactic Shock

Anaphylactic shock is caused by a severe allergic reaction when patients who have already produced antibodies to an antigen (foreign substance) develop a systemic antigen–antibody reaction; specifically, an immunoglobulin E (IgE)-mediated response. This antigen–antibody reaction provokes mast cells to release potent vasoactive substances, such as histamine or bradykinin, and activates inflammatory cytokines, causing widespread vasodilation and capillary permeability. The most common triggers are foods (especially peanuts), medications, and insect stings and bites (Pajno, Fernandez-Rivas, Arasi, et al., 2018) (see Chart 11-5). Anaphylaxis has three defining characteristics:
- Acute onset of symptoms
- Presence of two or more symptoms that include respiratory compromise, reduced BP, GI distress, and skin or mucosal tissue irritation
- Cardiovascular compromise from minutes to hours after exposure to the antigen

Signs and symptoms of anaphylaxis may present within 2 to 30 minutes of exposure to the antigen; however, occasionally some reactions may not develop for several hours (Chan & John, 2020). The patient may report headache, lightheadedness, nausea, vomiting, acute abdominal pain or discomfort, pruritus, and feeling of impending doom. Assessment may reveal diffuse erythema and generalized flushing, dyspnea (laryngeal edema), bronchospasm, cardiac arrhythmias, and hypotension. Characteristics of severe anaphylaxis usually include rapid onset of hypotension, neurologic compromise, respiratory distress, and cardiac arrest (Chan & John, 2020). Anaphylactoid reactions present similarly to anaphylaxis but are not mediated by IgE responses. Anaphylaxis and anaphylactoid reactions are often clinically indistinguishable (Pajno et al., 2018).

 Medical Management

Treatment of anaphylactic shock requires removing the causative antigen (e.g., discontinuing an antibiotic agent), administering medications that restore vascular tone, and providing emergency support of basic life functions. Fluid management is critical, as massive fluid shifts can occur within minutes due to increased vascular permeability (Pajno et al., 2018).

Intramuscular epinephrine is given for its vasoconstrictive action. Diphenhydramine is given intravenously to reverse the effects of histamine, thereby reducing capillary permeability. Nebulized medications, such as albuterol, may be given to reverse histamine-induced bronchospasm.

If cardiac arrest and respiratory arrest are imminent or have occurred, cardiopulmonary resuscitation (CPR) is performed. Endotracheal intubation may be necessary to establish an airway. IV lines are inserted to provide access for administering fluids and medications. See Chapter 33 for further discussion of anaphylaxis and specific chemical mediators.

Nursing Management

The nurse has an important role in prevention and early recognition of anaphylactic shock. The nurse must assess all patients for allergies or previous reactions to antigens (e.g., medications, blood products, foods, contrast agents, latex) and communicate the existence of these allergies or reactions to others. In addition, the nurse assesses the patient's understanding of previous reactions and steps taken by the patient and the family to prevent further exposure to antigens. When new allergies are identified, the nurse advises the patient to wear or carry identification that names the specific allergen or antigen.

When administering any new medication, the nurse observes all patients for allergic reactions. This is especially important with antibiotics, beta-blockers, angiotensin-converting enzyme inhibitors, angiotensin receptor blockers, aspirin, and nonsteroidal anti-inflammatory drugs (Chan & John, 2020). Previous adverse drug reactions increase the risk that the patient will develop a reaction to a new medication. If the patient reports an allergy to a medication, the nurse must be aware of the risks involved in the administration of similar medications.

At any diagnostic testing site, the nurse must identify patients who are at risk for anaphylactic reactions to contrast agents (radiopaque, dyelike substances that may contain iodine) used for diagnostic tests. The nurse must be knowledgeable about the clinical signs of anaphylaxis, must take immediate action if signs and symptoms occur, and must be prepared to begin CPR if cardiorespiratory arrest occurs.

Quality and Safety Nursing Alert

Patients with a known allergy to iodine or fish and those who have had previous allergic reactions to contrast agents are at high risk for anaphylactic reactions. The nurse should ask the patient about the allergy, signs and symptoms and severity, and if the patient has been tested for the allergy or carries an autoinjectable epinephrine device. This information must be communicated to the staff at the diagnostic testing site, including x-ray personnel.

Community health and home health nurses who administer medications, including antibiotic agents, in the patient's home or other settings, must be prepared to administer epinephrine intramuscularly in the event of an anaphylactic reaction.

After recovery from anaphylaxis, the patient and the family require an explanation of the event. Furthermore, the nurse provides education about avoiding future exposure to antigens and administering emergency medications to treat anaphylaxis (see Chapter 33).

Multiple Organ Dysfunction Syndrome

MODS is altered organ function in acutely ill patients that requires medical intervention to support continued organ function. It is another phase in the progression of shock states. The actual incidence of MODS is difficult to determine, because it develops with acute illnesses that compromise tissue perfusion. Dysfunction of one organ system is associated with 20% mortality, and if more than four organs fail, the mortality is at least 60% (Sauaia, Moore, & Moore, 2017).

Pathophysiology

The precise mechanism by which MODS occurs remains unknown, but it is most commonly seen in patients with sepsis as a result of inadequate tissue perfusion. MODS frequently occurs toward the end of the continuum of septic shock when tissue perfusion cannot be effectively restored. It is not possible to predict which patients who experience shock will develop MODS, partly because much of the organ damage occurs at the cellular level and, therefore, cannot be directly observed or measured.

The clinical presentation of MODS is insidious; tissues become hypoperfused at both a microcellular and macrocellular level, eventually causing organ dysfunction that requires mechanical and pharmacologic intervention to support organ function. Organ failure usually begins in the lungs, and cardiovascular instability, as well as failure of the hepatic, GI, renal, immunologic, and central nervous systems, follows (Sauaia et al., 2017).

Clinical Manifestations

While it is not possible to predict MODS, clinical severity assessment tools may be used to anticipate patient risk of organ dysfunction and mortality. These clinical assessment tools include APACHE (Acute Physiology and Chronic Health Evaluation); SAPS (Simplified Acute Physiology Score); PIRO (Predisposing factors, the Infection, the host Response, and Organ dysfunction); and SOFA score (see Table 11-4) (Gustot, 2011; Kress & Hall, 2018).

In MODS, the sequence of organ dysfunction varies depending on the patient's primary illness and comorbidities before experiencing shock. Advanced age, malnutrition, and coexisting disease appear to increase the risk of MODS in acutely ill patients. For simplicity of presentation, the classic pattern is described. Typically, the lungs are the first organs to show signs of dysfunction. The patient experiences progressive dyspnea and respiratory failure that are manifested as ALI or ARDS, requiring intubation and mechanical ventilation (see Chapters 19). The patient usually remains hemodynamically stable but may require increasing amounts of IV fluids and vasoactive agents to support BP and cardiac output. Signs of a hypermetabolic state, characterized by hyperglycemia (elevated blood glucose level), hyperlactic acidemia (excess lactic acid in the blood), and increased BUN, are present. The metabolic rate may be 1.5 to 2 times the basal metabolic rate. At this time, there is a severe loss of skeletal muscle mass (autocatabolism) to meet the high energy demands of the body.

After approximately 7 to 10 days, signs of hepatic dysfunction (e.g., elevated bilirubin and liver function tests) and renal dysfunction (e.g., elevated creatinine and anuria) are evident. As the lack of tissue perfusion continues, the hematologic system becomes dysfunctional, with worsening immunocompromise, increasing the risk of bleeding. The cardiovascular system becomes unstable and unresponsive to vasoactive agents, and the patient's neurologic response progresses to a state of unresponsiveness or coma.

The goal of all shock states is to reverse the tissue hypoperfusion and hypoxia. If effective tissue perfusion is restored before organs become dysfunctional, the patient's condition stabilizes. Along the septic shock continuum, the onset of organ dysfunction is an ominous prognostic sign; the more organs that fail, the worse the outcome.

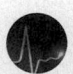 ## Medical Management

Prevention remains the top priority in managing MODS. Older adult patients are at increased risk for MODS because of the lack of physiologic reserve and the natural degenerative process, especially immune compromise (Kress & Hall, 2018). Early detection and documentation of initial signs of infection are essential in managing MODS in older adult patients. Subtle changes in mentation and a gradual rise in temperature are early warning signs. Other patients at greater risk for MODS are those with chronic illness, malnutrition, immunosuppression, or surgical or traumatic wounds.

If preventive measures fail, treatment measures to reverse MODS are aimed at (1) controlling the initiating event, (2) promoting adequate organ perfusion, (3) providing nutritional support, and (4) maximizing patient comfort.

 ## Nursing Management

The general plan of nursing care for patients with MODS is the same as that for patients with shock. Primary nursing interventions are aimed at supporting the patient and monitoring organ perfusion until primary organ insults are halted. Providing information and support to family members is a critical role of the nurse. The health care team must address end-of-life decisions to ensure that supportive therapies are congruent with the patient's wishes (see Chapter 13).

Promoting Communication

Nurses should encourage frequent and open communication about treatment modalities and options to ensure that the patient's wishes regarding medical management are met. Patients who survive MODS must be informed about the goals of rehabilitation and expectations for progress toward these goals, because massive loss of skeletal muscle mass makes rehabilitation a long, slow process. A strong nurse–patient relationship built on effective communication provides needed encouragement during this phase of recovery.

Promoting Home, Community-Based, and Transitional Care

 ### Educating Patients About Self-Care

Patients who experience and survive any type of shock or sepsis may have been unable to get out of bed for an extended period of time and are likely to have a slow, prolonged recovery. The patient and the family are educated about strategies

to prevent further episodes of shock or sepsis by identifying the factors implicated in the initial episode (Ferguson et al., 2019). In addition, the patient and the family require education about assessments needed to identify the complications that may occur after the patient is discharged from the hospital. Depending on the type of shock and its management, the patient or the family may require education about treatment modalities such as emergency administration of medications, IV therapy, parenteral or enteral nutrition, skin care, exercise, and ambulation. The patient and the family are also educated about the need for gradual increases in ambulation and other activity. The need for adequate nutrition is another crucial aspect of education.

Continuing and Transitional Care

Because of the physical toll associated with recovery from shock and sepsis, patients may be cared for in a long-term care facility or rehabilitation setting after hospital discharge. Alternatively, a referral may be made for home, community-based, or transitional care. Patients may also experience PICS, a condition that is gaining increased recognition. PICS occurs after critically ill patients are discharged from the hospital. PICS involves physical, cognitive, and mental impairments that may adversely impact the patient's long-term recovery (Inoue, Hatakeyama, Kondo, et al., 2019). Nursing interventions to prevent PICS occur during the patient's critical illness and include early mobilization, assessment and management of delirium, promoting adequate sleep, and assisting with mechanical ventilation liberation (e.g., weaning) as soon as possible. The nurse assesses the patient's physical status and monitors recovery. The adequacy of treatments continued at home and the ability of the patient and the family to cope with these treatments are also assessed. The patient is likely to require close medical supervision until complete recovery occurs. The nurse reinforces the importance of continuing medical care and helps the patient and the family identify and mobilize community resources.

CRITICAL THINKING EXERCISES

1 `pq` A 32-year-old patient is admitted after falling from a second-story balcony. The patient has a fractured femur, several fractured ribs, and possible head injury. The primary provider has prescribed lactated Ringer's solution to be infused at 250 mL/h to maintain a blood pressure >120 mm Hg and urine output >50 mL/h. Two large-bore IVs are started in each arm and IV fluids are initiated. The patient is alert to name only. The patient is typed and crossed for blood products, and a series of metabolic labs and a lactate level are drawn for analysis. The patient becomes unresponsive to name and begins moaning and grimacing. Vital signs are as follows: BP 92/72, HR 132 bpm, RR 32 bpm, SpO_2 92% on 40% FiO_2 via a facemask with a urine output of 15 mL over the last hour. Identify 3–5 priority interventions that you should implement, the order in which they should be implemented, and explain how you made these decisions.

2 `ebp` A 76-year-old patient is scheduled for surgery for benign prostatic enlargement that is causing significant obstruction to his urinary function. The patient's past medical history includes chronic obstructive pulmonary disease, hypertension, and type 2 diabetes. Due to his medical history and surgical risks, he is not a candidate for general anesthesia and instead receives spinal anesthesia. Midway through the surgery his vital signs decrease abruptly to BP 88/32 mm Hg and HR 62 bpm, while his RR remains stable controlled by anesthesia with ventilatory support. Surgery is aborted for suspected neurogenic shock. The patient is transferred to the postanesthesia care unit (PACU) for monitoring. The surgeon explains the complication that has occurred to the patient's wife and tells her that a nurse will continue to provide updates to her by phone. The wife asks to see her husband, but the waiting room clerk says that family is not allowed in the PACU. An hour passes and the nurse does not call to update the wife. The clerk observes the wife quietly crying in a corner and calls the nurse caring for the patient to inform her of the wife's distress. As the nurse, what actions would you implement to facilitate patient- and family-centered care? What evidence supports these actions?

3 **ipc** An 88-year-old woman is admitted from an assisted living facility with acute decline in mental status. On admission vital signs are as follows: BP 100/76 mm Hg, HR 126 bpm, and RR 26 bpm. The patient is also incontinent of urine. As the nurse, you suspect a possible urinary tract infection and immediately assess the patient for sepsis. What other members of the interprofessional team will you need to collaborate with to facilitate early interventions to minimize the risk of complications? To implement a sepsis protocol, what additional information should you obtain prior to calling the provider? What should you anticipate from the provider? How will you effectively communicate your assessment and recommendations to the provider and other members of the interprofessional team?

REFERENCES

*Asterisk indicates nursing research.
**Double asterisk indicates classic reference.

Books

American College of Surgeons, Committee on Trauma. (2018). *Advanced trauma life support: Student course manual* (10th ed.). Chicago, IL: American College of Surgeons.

Bauer, S. R., MacLaren, R., & Erstad, B. L. (2019). Shock syndromes. In J. T. DiPiro, R. L. Talbert, G. C. Yee, et al. (Eds.). *Pharmacotherapy: A pathophysiologic approach* (11th ed.). New York: McGraw-Hill Medical.

Kress, J. P., & Hall, J. B. (2018). Approach to the patient with critical illness. In L. J. Jameson, A. S. Fauci, K. L. Kasper, et al. (Eds.). *Harrison's principles of internal medicine* (20th ed.). New York: McGraw-Hill Medical.

Maclaren, R., Mueller, S. W., & Dasta, J. F. (2019). Use of vasopressors and inotropes in the pharmacotherapy of shock. In J. T. DiPiro, R. L. Talbert, G. C. Yee, et al. (Eds.). *Pharmacotherapy: A pathophysiologic approach* (11th ed.). New York: McGraw-Hill Medical.

Massaro, A. F. (2018). Approach to the patient with shock. In L. J. Jameson, A. S. Fauci, K. L. Kasper, et al. (Eds.). *Harrison's principles of internal medicine* (20th ed.). New York: McGraw-Hill Medical.

Seymour, C. W., & Angus, D. C. (2018). Sepsis and septic shock. In L. J. Jameson, A. S. Fauci, K. L. Kasper, et al. (Eds.). *Harrison's principles of internal medicine* (20th ed.). New York: McGraw-Hill Medical.

Journals and Electronic Documents

American Diabetes Association. (2019). Diabetes care in the hospital: Standards of medical care. *Diabetes Care*, 42(Suppl 1), S173–S181.

American Heart Association. (2018). Highlights of the 2018 American Heart Association Guidelines update for CPR and ECC. Retrieved on 9/10/2019 at: www.eccguidelines.heart.org/circulation/cpr-ecc-guidelines

Annane, D., Ouanes-Besbes, L., DeBacker, D., et al. (2018). A global perspective on vasoactive agents in shock. *Intensive Care Medicine*, 44(6), 833–846.

**Annane, D., Siami, S., Jaber, S., et al. (2013). Effects of fluid resuscitation with colloids vs crystalloids on mortality in critically ill patients presenting with hypovolemic shock: The CRISTAL randomized trial. *JAMA*, 310(17), 1809–1817.

Bellumkonda, L., Gul, B., & Masri, S. C. (2018). Evolving concepts in diagnosis and management of cardiogenic shock. *American Journal of Cardiology*, 122(6), 1104–1110.

Bridges, E. (2013). Using functional hemodynamic indicators to guide fluid therapy. *American Journal of Nursing*, 113(5), 42–50.

Bridges, E. (2017). Assessing patients during septic shock resuscitation. *American Journal of Nursing*, 117(10), 34–40.

**Bridges, N., & Jarquin-Valdivia, A. A. (2005). Use of the Trendelenburg position as the resuscitation position: To T or not to T. *American Journal of Critical Care*, 14(3), 364–367.

Centers for Disease Control and Prevention (CDC). (2019). Sepsis. Retrieved on 9/10/19 at: www.cdc.gov/sepsis/index.html

Centers for Medicare & Medicaid Services (CMS). (2019). Hospital Toolkit for Adult Sepsis Surveillance. Retrieved on 9/10/19 at: www.cdc.gov/sepsis/clinicaltools/index.html

Chan, S., & John, R. M. (2020). Idiopathic anaphylaxis: What you do not know may hurt you. *Journal of the American Association of Nurse Practitioners*, 32(1), 81–88.

Clemency, B., Tanaka, K., May, P., et al. (2017). Intravenous vs. intraosseous access and return of spontaneous circulation during out of hospital cardiac arrest. *American Journal of Emergency Medicine*, 35(2), 222–226.

Davidson, J. E., Aslakson, R. A., Long, A. C., et al. (2017). Guidelines for family-centered care in the neonatal, pediatric, and adult ICU. *Critical Care Medicine*, 45(1), 103–128.

de-Madaria, E., Herrera-Marante, I., Gonzalez-Camacho, V., et al. (2018). Fluid resuscitation with lactated Ringer's solution vs normal saline in acute pancreatitis: A triple-blind, randomized controlled trial. *United European Gastroenterology Journal*, 6(1), 63–72.

Devlin, J. W., Skrobik, Y., Gelians, C., et al. (2018). Clinical practice guidelines for the prevention and management of pain, agitation/sedation, delirium, immobility, and sleep disruption in adult patients in the ICU. *Critical Care Medicine*, 46(9), e825–e873.

Dunne, C. P., Kingston, L., Slevin, B., et al. (2018). Hand hygiene and compliance behaviours are the under-appreciated human factors pivotal to reducing hospital-acquired infections. *Journal of Hospital Infection*, 98(4), 328–330.

Ferguson, A., Coates, D. E., Osborn, S., et al. (2019). Early, nurse-directed sepsis care. *American Journal of Nursing*, 119(1), 52–58.

Global Sepsis Alliance. (2017). WHA adopts resolution on sepsis. Retrieved on 9/16/19 at: www.global-sepsis-alliance.org/news/2017/5/26/wha-adopts-resolution-on-sepsis

**Griesdale, D. E., DeSouza, R. J., VanDam, R. M., et al. (2009). Intensive insulin therapy and mortality among critically ill patients: A meta-analysis including NICE-Sugar study data. *Canadian Medical Association Journal*, 180(8), 821–827.

**Gustot, T. (2011). Multiple organ failure in sepsis: Prognosis and role of systemic inflammatory response. *Current Opinion in Critical Care*, 17(2), 153–159.

Hallisey, S. D., & Greenwood, J. C. (2019). Beyond mean arterial pressure and lactate: Perfusion end points for managing the shocked patient. *Emergency Medicine Clinics of North America*, 37(3), 394–408.

Harrell, B. R., & Miller, S. (2017). Abdominal compartment syndrome as a complication of fluid resuscitation. *Nursing Clinics of North America*, 52(2), 331–338.

Hochman, J. S., & Reyentovich, A. (2019). Prognosis and treatment of cardiogenic shock complicating myocardial infarction. *UpToDate*. Retrieved on 9/11/19 at: www.uptodate.com/contents/prognosis-and-treatment-of-cardiogenicshock-complicating-acute myocardial infarction

**Holcomb, J. B., Tiley, B. C., Baraniuk, S., et al. (2015). Transfusion of plasma, platelets, and red blood cells in a 1:1:1 vs a 1:1:2 ratio and mortality in patients with severe trauma. *JAMA*, 313(5), 471–482.

Honore, P. M., Hoste, E., Molnár, Z., et al. (2019). Cytokine removal in human septic shock: Where are we and where are we going? *Annals of Intensive Care, 9*(56), 1–13.

Inoue, S., Hatakeyama, J., Kondo, Y., et al. (2019). Post-intensive care syndrome: Its pathophysiology, prevention, and future directions. *Acute Medicine & Surgery, 6*(3), 233–246.

Institute for Healthcare Improvement (IHI). (2012). How-to guide: Prevent central line–associated bloodstream infection. Retrieved on 9/10/2019 at: www.ihi.org/knowledge/Pages/Tools/HowtoGuidePrevent CentralLineAssociatedBloodstreamInfection.aspx

Institute for Healthcare Improvement (IHI). (2017). Improving stories: Early warning systems: Scorecards that save lives. Retrieved on 11/7/19 at: www.ihi.org/resources/Pages/ImprovementStories/EarlyWarningSyst emsScorecardsThatSaveLives.aspx

Ivany, E., & Aitken, L. (2019). Challenges and facilitators in providing effective end of life care in intensive care units. *Nursing Standard, 34*(6), 44–50.

Kahn, J. M., Davis, B. S., Yabes, J. G., et al. (2019). Association between state-mandated protocolized sepsis care and in-hospital mortality among adults with sepsis. *JAMA, 322*(3), 240–250.

Keeley, A., Hine, P., & Nsutebu, E. (2017). The recognition and management of sepsis and septic shock: A guide for non-intensivists. *Postgraduate Medical Journal, 93*(1104), 626–634.

Kessler, T. M., Traini, L. R., Welk, B., et al. (2018). Early neurological care of patients with spinal cord injury. *World Journal of Urology, 36*(10), 1529–1536.

Kislitsina, O. N., Rich, J. D., Wilcox, J. E., et al. (2019). Shock—Classification and pathophysiological principles of therapeutics. *Current Cardiology Reviews, 15*(2), 102–113.

Laher, A. E., Watermeyer, M. J., Buchanan, S. K., et al. (2017). A review of hemodynamic monitoring techniques, methods and devices for the emergency physician. *American Journal of Emergency Medicine, 35*(9), 1135–1347.

Levy, M., Evans, L., & Rhodes, A. (2018). The surviving sepsis campaign bundle: 2018 update. *Critical Care Medicine, 46*(6), 997–1000.

Levy, M. M., & Townsend, S. R. (2019). Early identification of sepsis on the hospital floors: Insights for implementation of the hour-1 bundle. *Society of Critical Care Medicine.* Retrieved on 9/10/19 at: www. survivingsepsis.org/SiteCollectionDocuments/Surviving-Sepsis-Early-Identify-Sepsis-Hospital-Floor.pdf

Lewis, S. R., Pritchard, M. W., Evans, D. J. W., et al. (2018). Colloids versus crystalloids for fluid resuscitation in critically ill people. The *Cochrane Database of Systematic Reviews, 8*(8), CD000567.

Makic, M. B. F. (2018). Delirium: Are we doing enough? *Journal of Perianesthesia Nursing, 33*(6), 990–992.

Makic, M. B. F., & Bridges, E. (2018). Managing sepsis and septic shock: Current guidelines and definitions. *American Journal of Nursing, 118*(2), 34–39.

**Marik, P. E., Baram, M., & Vahid, B. (2008). Does central venous pressure predict fluid responsiveness? A systematic review of the literature and the tale of seven mares. *Chest, 134*(1), 172–178.

**Marik, P. E., & Cavallazzi, R. (2013). Does the central venous pressure predict fluid responsiveness? An updated meta-analysis and a plea for some common sense. *Critical Care Medicine, 41*(7), 1774–1782.

Marschall, J., Mermel, L. A., Fakih, M., et al. (2014). Strategies to prevent central-line associated blood stream infections in acute care hospitals: 2014 update. *Infection Control and Hospital Epidemiology, 35*(7), 753–771. Retrieved on 9/10/2019 at: www.cambridge.org/ core/journals/infection-control-and-hospital-epidemiology/article/ strategies-to-prevent-central-lineassociated-bloodstream-infections-in-acute-care-hospitals-2014-update/CB398EB001FEADE0D9B4FF1A09 6ECA52

McCarthy, C. P., Bhambhani, V., Pomerantsev, E., et al. (2018). In-hospital outcomes in invasively managed acute myocardial infarction patients who receive morphine. *Journal of Interventional Cardiology, 31*(2), 150–158.

Mitchell, B. G., Russo, P. L., Cheng, A. C., et al. (2019). Strategies to reduce non-ventilator-associated hospital-acquired pneumonia: A systematic review. *Infection, Disease, & Health, 24*(4), 229–239.

Mitchell, D. A., & Seckel, M. A. (2018). Acute respiratory distress syndrome and prone positioning. *AACN Advanced Critical Care, 29*(4), 415–425.

Neto, J. N. A. (2018). Morphine, oxygen, nitrates, and mortality reducing pharmacological treatment for acute coronary syndrome: An evidence-based review. *Cureus. 10*(1), e2114. Retrieved on 9/10/19 at: www.ncbi.

nlm.nih.gov/pmc/articles/PMC5866121/pdf/cureus-0010-00000002114. pdf

Pajno, G. B., Fernandez-Rivas, M., Arasi, S., et al. (2018). EAACI guidelines on allergen immunotherapy: IgE-mediated food allergy. *Allergy, 73*(4), 799–815.

*Pickett, J. D., Bridges, E., Kritek, P. A., et al. (2018). Noninvasive blood pressure monitoring and prediction of fluid responsiveness to passive leg raising. *American Journal of Critical Care, 27*(3), 228–237.

*Reaza-Alarcón, A., & Rodríguez-Martín, B. (2019). Effectiveness of nursing educational interventions in managing post-surgical pain. Systematic review. *Universidad de Antioquia, 37*(2), e10. Retrieved on 10/5/19 at: www.aprendeenlinea.udea.edu.co/revistas/index.php/iee/ article/view/338899/20793899

Reintam, B. A., Blaser, A., Starkopf, J., et al. (2017). Early enteral nutrition in critically ill patients: ESICM clinical practice guidelines. *Intensive Care Medicine, 43*(3), 380 398.

Rhodes, A., Evans, L., Alhazzani, W., et al. (2017). Surviving Sepsis Campaign: International guidelines for management of sepsis and septic shock: 2016. *Critical Care Medicine, 45*(3), 486–552.

**Rivers, E. P., McIntyre, L., Morro, D. C., et al. (2005). Early and innovative interventions for severe sepsis and septic shock: Taking advantage of a window of opportunity. *Canadian Medical Association Journal, 173*(9), 1054–1065.

Rowe, T. A., & McKoy, J. M. (2017). Sepsis in older adults. *Infectious Disease Clinics of North America, 31*(4), 731–742.

Sauaia, A., Moore, F. A., & Moore, E. E. (2017). Postinjury inflammation and organ dysfunction. *Critical Care Clinics, 33*(1), 167–191.

Sethi, M., Owyang, C. G., Meyers, C., et al. (2018). Choice of resuscitative fluids and mortality in emergency department patients with sepsis. *American Journal of Emergency Medicine, 36*(4), 625–629.

Simmons, J., & Ventetuolo, C. E. (2017). Cardiopulmonary monitoring of shock. *Current Opinion, 23*(3), 223–231.

**Singer, M., Deutschman, C. S., Seymour, C. W., et al. (2016). The Third International Consensus Definitions for Sepsis and Septic Shock (Sepsis-3). *JAMA, 315*(8), 801–810.

Surviving Sepsis Campaign. (2017). Retrieved on 11/27/20 at: www. sccm.org/getattachment/SurvivingSepsisCampaign/Guidelines/Adult-Patients/SSC-Guidelines-FAQ.pdf?lang=en-US

Surviving Sepsis Campaign. (2019). Retrieved on 9/20/2019 at: www. survivingsepsis.org

Turner, K., & Hylton, C. (2019). "Why are we doing this?" Creating new narratives to meet futility with integrity. *AACN Advanced Critical Care, 30*(2), 198–203.

Vanderbilt University Medical Center. (2019). ICU delirium and cognitive impairment study group. Retrieved on 8/15/2019 at: www.icude-lirium.org/delirium/monitoring.html

**Vincent, J. L., Moreno, R., Takala, J., et al. (1996). The SOFA (Sepsis-related Organ Failure Assessment) score to describe organ dysfunction/ failure. On behalf of the Working Group on Sepsis-Related Programs of the European Society of Intensive Care Medicine. *Intensive Care Medicine, 22*(7), 707–710.

Vlaar, A. P. J., & Kleinman, S. (2019). An update of the transfusion-related acute lung injury (TRALI) definition. *Transfusion and Apheresis Science, 58*(5), 632–633.

*Wang, Z., Ding, W., Fang, Q., et al. (2019). Effects of not monitoring gastric residual volume in intensive care patients: A meta-analysis. *International Journal of Nursing Studies, 91*(3), 86–93.

Wilcox, S. R. (2019). Nonischemic causes of cardiogenic shock. *Emergency Medical Clinics of North America, 37*(3), 493–509.

*Wong, P., Redley, B., Digby, R., et al. (2020). Families' perspectives of participation in patient care in an adult intensive care unit: A qualitative study. *Australian Critical Care, 33*(4), 317–325.

Zhang, Z., Hong, Y., Smischney, N. J., et al. (2017). Early management of sepsis with emphasis on early goal directed therapy: AME evidence series 002. *Journal of Thoracic Disease, 9*(2), 392–405.

Resources

American Association of Critical-Care Nurses Resources for Sepsis, www.aacn.org/clinical-resources/sepsis

Institute for Healthcare Improvement, www.ihi.org

Sepsis Alliance, www.sepsis.org

Surviving Sepsis Campaign, www.survivingsepsis.org

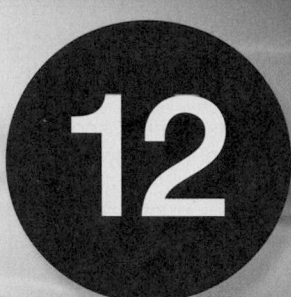

12 Management of Patients with Oncologic Disorders

nadir is most often used to describe the lowest absolute neutrophil count following chemotherapy

neoplasia: uncontrolled cell growth that follows no physiologic demand; cancer

neutropenia: abnormally low absolute neutrophil count

oncology: field or study of cancer

palliation: relief of symptoms and promotion of comfort and quality of life regardless of the disease stage

precision medicine: using advances in research, technology, and policies to develop individualized plans of care to prevent and treat disease

radiation therapy: the use of ionizing radiation to kill malignant cells

staging: process of determining the extent of disease, including tumor size and spread or metastasis to distant sites

stomatitis: inflammation of the oral tissues, often associated with some chemotherapeutic agents and radiation therapy to the head and neck region

targeted therapies: the use of medications or other agents to kill or prevent the spread of cancer cells by targeting specific part of the cell, with less negative effects on healthy cells

thrombocytopenia: decrease in the number of circulating platelets; associated with the potential for bleeding

toxicity: an unfavorable and unintended sign, symptom, or condition associated with cancer treatment

vesicant: substance that can cause inflammation, damage, and necrosis with extravasation from blood vessels and contact with tissues

Cancer is a large group of disorders with different causes, manifestations, treatments, and prognoses. Because cancer can involve any organ system and treatment approaches have the potential for multisystem effects, cancer nursing practice overlaps with numerous nursing specialties. Cancer nursing practice covers all age groups and is carried out in various settings, including acute care institutions, outpatient centers, physician offices, rehabilitation facilities, the home, and long-term care facilities. The scope, responsibilities, and goals of cancer nursing, also called **oncology** nursing, are as diverse and complex as those of any nursing specialty. Nursing management of the patient with oncologic disorders includes care of patients throughout the cancer trajectory from prevention through end-of-life care (see Fig. 12-1).

Precision medicine is possible because of the recent development of biologic databases (e.g., human genome sequencing), technologic advances that can identify unique characteristics of individual persons (e.g., genomics, cellular assay tests), and computer-driven systems that can mine and analyze datasets (see Chapter 1). This is an exciting time for oncology as the overall goal of the precision medicine initiative is to focus on preventing and curing cancers (Ginsburg & Phillips, 2018).

Epidemiology

Cancer is a common health problem worldwide. In the United States, it was estimated in 2019 that more than 1,700,000 new cancer cases would be diagnosed, and that

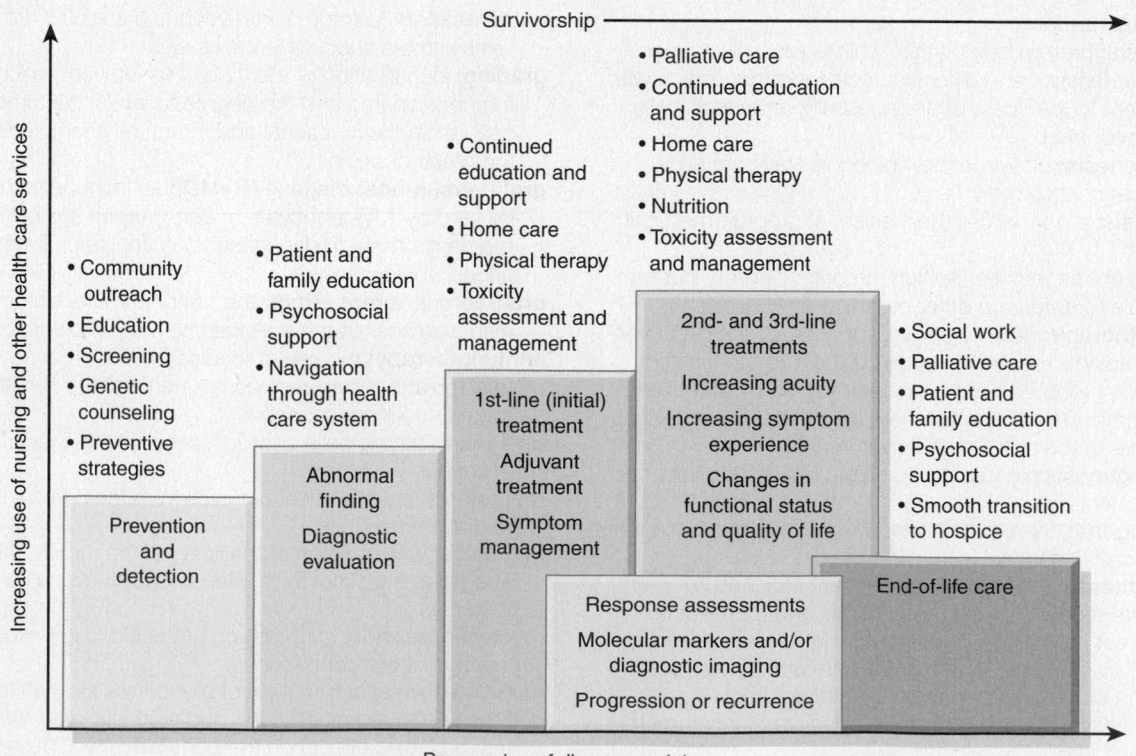

Figure 12-1 • Cancer care trajectory. The cancer care trajectory reflects the phases and care required during the continuum of the cancer experience from prevention and early detection through end-of-life care. Specialized nursing care is provided throughout the entire trajectory.

more than 600,000 Americans would die as a result of cancer (Siegel, Miller, & Jemal, 2019). Despite significant advances in science and technology, cancer is the second leading cause of death in the United States. The leading causes of cancer-related death in the United States in order of frequency and location are lung, prostate, and colorectal cancer in men and lung, breast, and colorectal cancer in women. Most cancer occurs in older adults; according to the American Cancer Society (ACS), 80% of all cancer diagnoses are in people 55 years of age or older (2019a). Overall, the incidence of cancer is slightly higher in women than in men (ACS, 2019a).

Cancer affects all groups of people; however, some groups are more adversely affected by cancer than others (National Cancer Institute [NCI], 2019a). Differences in cancer measures (e.g., incidence, screening rates, stage of diagnosis, morbidity, mortality) or cancer-related health conditions are termed *cancer health disparities*. These disparities often result from multiple, complex interrelated factors, including indicators of socioeconomic status (e.g., income, educational level, health care access), culture, diet, stress, the environment, and biology.

Cancer health disparities are most often observed among people of low-socioeconomic status, certain races/ethnicities, and those who reside in particular geographical locations (NCI, 2019a). For example, even though the overall rate of cancer deaths has declined, cancer death rates in non-Hispanic Black men and women remain substantially higher compared to all other racial and ethnic groups for most cancer types (DeSantis, Miller, Goding Sauer, et al., 2019). Hispanic/Latino Americans have a lower overall cancer incidence when compared to non-Hispanic White Americans; however, the incidence of infection-related cancers (e.g., liver cancer) is two times higher in those of Hispanic/Latino origin compared to non-Hispanic White Americans (Miller, Goding Sauer, Ortiz, et al., 2018).

Cancer incidence and death rates also vary by geography. In states where the prevalence of tobacco use is high (e.g., Kentucky), the incidence of lung cancer tends to be greater than in states where smoking is not as common (e.g., Utah) (Siegel et al., 2019). In locations where there is greater socio-economic disparity, the incidence of cancer and overall cancer death rates are higher than in regions where there is not such a disparity (Siegel et al., 2019). For example, the incidence of cancers of the lung, colon and rectum, and cervix are substantially higher in Appalachian Ohio (southwestern region of the state) than in more affluent and more populated regions of the state (NCI, 2019a).

Pathophysiology of the Malignant Process

Cancer is a disease process that begins when a cell is transformed by genetic mutations of the cellular deoxyribonucleic acid (DNA). Genetic mutations may be inherited or acquired, leading to abnormal cell behavior (Norris, 2019). The initial genetically altered cell forms a clone and begins to proliferate abnormally, evading normal intracellular and extracellular growth-regulating processes or signals as well as the immune system defense mechanisms of the body. Genetic mutations may lead to abnormalities in cell signaling transduction processes (signals from outside and within cells that turn cell activities either on or off) that can in turn lead to cancer development. Ultimately cells acquire a variety of capabilities that allow them to invade surrounding tissues or gain access to lymph and blood vessels, which carry the cells to other areas of the body resulting in **metastasis** or spread of the cancer (Pachmayr, Treese, & Stein, 2017).

Benign (noncancerous) and **malignant** (cancerous) cells differ in many cellular growth characteristics, including the method and rate of growth, ability to metastasize or spread, destruction of tissue, and ability to cause death. These differences are summarized in Table 12-1. The degree of **anaplasia**

TABLE 12-1	Characteristics of Benign and Malignant Cells	
Characteristics	**Benign**	**Malignant**
Cell	Well-differentiated cells resemble normal cells of the tissue from which the tumor originated.	Cells are undifferentiated and may bear little resemblance to the normal cells of the tissue from which they arose.
Mode of growth	Tumor grows by expansion and does not infiltrate the surrounding tissues; usually encapsulated.	Grows at the periphery and overcomes contact inhibition to invade and infiltrate surrounding tissues
Rate of growth	Rate of growth is usually slow.	Rate of growth is variable and depends on level of differentiation; the more anaplastic the tumor, the faster its growth.
Metastasis	Does not spread by metastasis.	Gains access to the blood and lymphatic channels and metastasizes to other areas of the body or grows across body cavities such as the peritoneum.
General effects	Usually a localized phenomenon that does not cause generalized effects unless its location interferes with vital functions.	Often causes generalized effects, such as anemia, weakness, systemic inflammation, weight loss, and CACS.
Tissue destruction	Does not usually cause tissue damage unless its location interferes with blood flow.	Often causes extensive tissue damage as the tumor outgrows its blood supply or encroaches on blood flow to the area; may also produce substances that cause cell damage.
Ability to cause death	Does not usually cause death unless its location interferes with vital functions.	Eventually causes death unless growth can be controlled.

CACS, cancer-related anorexia-cachexia syndrome.
Adapted from Norris, T. L. (2019). *Porth's pathophysiology: Concepts of altered health states* (10th ed.). Philadelphia, PA: Lippincott Williams & Wilkins.

(a pattern of growth in which cells lack normal characteristics and differ in shape and organization with respect to their cells of origin) is associated with increased malignant potential.

Carcinogenesis

Understanding the pathophysiology of cancer involves knowledge of the molecular process and proliferation patterns of cancers as well as the numerous etiologic factors that induce the malignant transformation of cells.

Molecular Process

Malignant transformation, or **carcinogenesis**, is thought to be at least a three-step cellular process, involving initiation, promotion, and progression (Norris, 2019). Agents that initiate or promote malignant transformation are referred to as **carcinogens**. A complete carcinogen is an agent that both initiates and promotes the development of cancer (e.g., cigarette smoking, asbestos).

During *initiation*, carcinogens (substances that can cause cancer), such as chemicals, physical factors, or biologic agents, cause mutations in the cellular DNA. Normally, these alterations are reversed by DNA repair mechanisms or the changes initiate **apoptosis** (programmed cellular death) or cell senescence. Cells can escape these protective mechanisms with permanent cellular mutations occurring, but these mutations usually are not significant to cells until the second step of carcinogenesis.

During *promotion*, repeated exposure to promoting agents (co-carcinogens) causes proliferation and expansion of initiated cells with increased expression or manifestations of abnormal genetic information, even after long latency periods. Promoting agents are not mutagenic and do not need to interact with the DNA. Promotion is reversible if the promoting substance is removed (a key focus in the prevention of cancer). Latency periods for the promotion of cellular mutations vary with the type of agent, the dosage of the promoter, and the innate characteristics and genetic stability of the target cell.

During *progression*, the altered cells exhibit increasingly malignant behavior. These cells acquire the ability to stimulate **angiogenesis** (growth of new blood vessels that allow cancer cells to grow), to invade adjacent tissues, and to metastasize. Cellular oncogenes are responsible for vital cell functions, including proliferation and differentiation. Cellular proto-oncogenes, such as those for the epidermal growth factor receptor (EGFR), transcription factors such as *c-Myc*, or cell signaling proteins such as *Kirsten ras* (*KRAS*), act as "on switches" for cellular growth. Amplification of proto-oncogenes or overexpression of growth factors, such as epidermal growth factor (EGF), can lead to uncontrolled cell proliferation. Mutations that increase the activity of oncogenes also deregulate cell proliferation. Genetic alterations in the gene for *KRAS* have been associated with pancreatic, lung, and colorectal cancers (Mainardi, Mulero-Sánchez, Prahallad, et al., 2018). Just as proto-oncogenes "turn on" cellular growth, cancer suppressor genes "turn off," or regulate, unneeded cellular proliferation. When suppressor genes are mutated, resulting in loss of function or expression, the cells begin to produce mutant cell populations that are different from their original cellular ancestors. See Chart 12-1 for further discussion of genetics concepts and cancer.

Proliferative Patterns

During the lifespan, various body tissues normally undergo periods of rapid or proliferative growth that must be distinguished from malignant growth activity. Several patterns of cellular adaptation include atrophy, hypertrophy, hyperplasia, metaplasia, and dysplasia (see Chapter 5, Fig. 5-4). Cancerous cells, described as malignant, demonstrate **neoplasia**, or uncontrolled cell growth that follows no physiologic demand. Although both benign and malignant growths are classified and named by tissue of origin, the *International Classification of Diseases for Oncology* (Fritz, Percy, Jack et al., 2013) is used by scientists and clinicians around the world as the nomenclature for malignant disease (see Table 12-2).

Etiology

Factors implicated or known to induce carcinogenesis include viruses and bacteria, physical agents, chemicals, genetic or familial factors, lifestyle factors, and hormones. Additional research is needed for a better understanding of the relationships among etiologic factors and cancer.

Viruses and Bacteria

It is estimated that 10% to 12% of all cancers worldwide are linked to viral infections (Lunn, Jahnke, & Rabkin, 2017). After infecting individuals, DNA viruses insert a part of their own DNA near the infected cell genes causing cell division. The newly formed cells that now carry viral DNA lack normal controls on growth. Examples of these viruses that are known to cause cancer include human papillomavirus (HPV) (cervical and head and neck cancers), hepatitis B virus (HBV) (liver cancer), and Epstein–Barr virus (EBV) (Burkitt lymphoma and nasopharyngeal cancer).

While there is little evidence to support a direct link between most bacteria and cancer, secondary responses to certain bacterial infections, such as the production of carcinogenic metabolites and inflammatory reactions, are suspected mechanisms of cancer development (van Elsland & Neefjes, 2018). Examples of bacteria that are associated with an increased risk of cancer include: *Helicobacter pylori* (stomach cancer), *Salmonella enteritidis* (colon cancer), and *Chlamydia trachomatis* (ovarian and cervical cancers).

Physical Agents

Physical factors associated with carcinogenesis include exposure to sunlight, radiation, chronic irritation or inflammation, tobacco carcinogens, industrial chemicals, and asbestos (ACS, 2019b).

Excessive exposure to the ultraviolet rays of the sun is associated with skin cancers in all individuals, although those with fair-skin are at highest risk. Factors such as clothing styles (sleeveless shirts or shorts), the use of sunscreens, occupation, recreational habits, and environmental variables, including humidity, altitude, and latitude, all play a role in the amount of exposure to ultraviolet light (ACS, 2019c).

Chart 12-1 GENETICS IN NURSING PRACTICE
Genetics Concepts and Oncologic Disorders

Cancer is a genetic disease. Every phase of carcinogenesis is affected by multiple gene mutations. Some of these mutations are inherited (present in germ-line cells) and present a greater risk for a person to develop oncologic disorders; however, most (90%) are somatic mutations that are acquired mutations in specific cells. Examples of cancers influenced by genetics include:

Autosomal dominant:

- Breast and ovarian cancer
- Colorectal cancer
- Familial adenomatous polyposis
- Cowden syndrome
- Li–Fraumeni syndrome
- Lynch syndrome (hereditary nonpolyposis colon cancer)
- Multiple endocrine neoplasia types 1 and 2
- Neurofibromatosis types 1 and 2
- Prostate cancer
- Retinoblastoma
- Von Hippel–Lindau syndrome
- Wilms tumor

Autosomal recessive:

- Ataxia telangiectasis
- Endometrial cancer
- Gastrointestinal stromal tumor
- Familial melanoma syndrome
- Xeroderma pigmentosum

Nursing Assessments

Refer to Chapter 4, Chart 4-2: Genetics in Nursing Practice: Genetic Aspects of Health Assessment

Family History Assessment Specific to Oncologic Disorders

- Obtain information about both maternal and paternal sides of family for three generations.
- Obtain cancer history for at least three generations.
- Look for clustering of cancers that occur at young ages, multiple primary cancers in one individual, cancer in paired organs, and two or more close relatives with the same type of cancer suggestive of hereditary cancer syndromes.

Patient Assessment

- Assess for the following:
  - Physical findings that may predispose the patient to cancer, such as multiple colon polyps or the presence of more than one tumor. If a tumor was previously diagnosed, inquire about the age of the patient when the first tumor was noted.
  - Skin findings, such as atypical moles, that may be related to familial melanoma syndrome.
  - Multiple *café-au-lait* spots, axillary freckling, and two or more neurofibromas associated with neurofibromatosis type 1.
  - Facial trichilemmomas, mucosal papillomatosis, multinodular thyroid goiter or thyroid adenomas, macrocephaly, fibrocystic breasts, and other fibromas or lipomas related to Cowden syndrome.
- Assess for lifestyle risks (e.g., smoking, obesity, alcohol use).
- Determine potential occupational or environmental hazards that may generate exposure to inhaled chemicals, gases, or other irritants (e.g., toxic metals, asbestos, radon).

Management Issues Specific to Oncologic Disorders

- Assess patient's understanding of genetics factors related to their cancer.
- Offer appropriate genetics information and resources.
- Refer for cancer risk assessment when a hereditary cancer syndrome is suspected so that patient and family can discuss inheritance risk with other family members and availability of genetic testing.
- Provide support to patients and families with known genetic test results for hereditary cancer syndromes. Refer to support groups as appropriate.
- Participate in the management and coordination of risk reduction measures for those with known gene mutations.

Genetics Resources Specific to Oncologic Disorders

American Cancer Society: www.cancer.org
National Cancer Institute: www.cancer.gov
See also Chapter 6, Chart 6-7 for additional components of genetic counseling.

Exposure to ionizing radiation from repeated diagnostic x-ray procedures or with radiation therapy used to treat disease can cause cancer (ACS, 2019c). Improved x-ray equipment minimizes the risk of extensive radiation exposure. Radiation therapy used in cancer treatment and exposure to radioactive materials at nuclear weapon manufacturing sites or nuclear power plants in the past have been associated with a higher incidence of leukemia, multiple myeloma, and cancers of the breast, thyroid, and other tissues. Background radiation from the natural decay processes that produce radon has also been associated with lung cancer. Ventilation is advised in homes with high levels of trapped radon to allow the gas to disperse into the atmosphere.

Chemical Agents

Most cancers are thought to be related to environmental factors (ACS, 2019b). Most hazardous chemicals produce their toxic effects by altering DNA structure. This can occur in body sites distant from that of initial chemical exposure.

Tobacco use is thought to be the single most lethal chemical carcinogen; it accounts for about 30% of all cancer-related deaths (ACS, 2019a). Cigarette smoking is strongly associated with 12 different cancer types including: cancers of the oral cavity and pharynx, larynx, lung, esophagus, pancreas, uterine cervix, kidney, bladder, stomach, colorectal, liver, and myeloid leukemia.

Environmental tobacco smoke (ETS), otherwise known as secondhand smoke, has been linked to lung cancer—even in people who never smoked (ACS, 2019d). Nonsmokers who were exposed to ETS in the home or workplace have about a 20% to 30% greater risk of developing lung cancer (Centers for Disease Control and Prevention [CDC], 2019). There is also some evidence that ETS may be linked with cancers of the larynx, pharynx, nasal sinuses, brain, bladder, rectum, stomach, and breast (ACS, 2019d).

Other combustible forms of tobacco, such as cigars, pipes, roll-your-own products, and water pipes (or hookah), are also associated with increased cancer risk (ACS, 2019d).

TABLE 12-2	Classification of Cancer by Tissue of Origin			
Classification	**Tissue of Origin**	**Characteristics**	**Term**	**Examples**
Carcinoma	Epithelial	Account for 80–90% of all cancers		
	• Glandular epithelium	Organs or glands capable of secretion	Adenocarcinoma	Adenocarcinoma of the breast, lung, prostate
	• Squamous epithelium	Covers or lines all external and internal body surfaces	Squamous cell carcinoma	Squamous cell cancer of the skin, lung, esophagus
Sarcoma	Connective or Supportive			
	• Bone	Most common form of cancer of the bone	Osteosarcoma	Osteosarcoma of the femur, humerus
	• Cartilage	Rare, arises from within bones	Chondrosarcoma	Chondrosarcoma of the femur, pelvis
	• Adipose	Arises from deep soft tissue	Liposarcoma	Liposarcoma of the retroperitoneum, thigh
	• Smooth muscle	Very rare	Leiomyosarcoma	Leiomyosarcoma of the uterus, intestines, stomach
	• Skeletal muscle	Most common in young children	Rhabdosarcoma	Rhabdosarcoma of the head and neck, limbs
	• Fibrous tissue	Often involves long or flat bones	Fibrosarcoma	Fibrosarcoma of the femur, tibia, mandible
	• Membranes lining body cavities	Most often related to asbestos exposure	Mesothelial sarcoma or mesothelioma	Mesothelioma of the pleura or peritoneum
	• Blood vessels	With liver involvement may be related to occupational exposure to vinyl chloride monomer	Angiosarcoma	Angiosarcoma of the liver, heart
Myeloma	Plasma cells	Produced by B-cell lymphocytes; plasma cells produce antibodies	Not applicable (N/A)	N/A
Lymphoma	Lymphocytes	Two main classifications; may involve lymph nodes or body organs	Non-Hodgkin lymphoma	B-cell lymphoma, T–cell lymphoma
			Hodgkin lymphoma	N/A
Leukemia	Hematopoietic cells in the bone marrow	May involve various cell lines produced in the bone marrow		
	• White blood cells (WBCs)	N/A	Myelogenous	Acute myelogenous leukemia
	• Lymphocytes	N/A	Lymphocytic	Acute lymphocytic leukemia
	• Red blood cells (RBCs)	Involves overproduction of RBCs and is associated with increased levels of WBCs and platelets; also risk of additional bone marrow disease	Erythremia	Polycythemia vera

Adapted from Fritz, A., Percy, C., Jack, A., et al.; World Health Organization. (2013). International classification of diseases for oncology (ICD-O)–3rd edition, 1st revision. Retrieved on 7/22/2019 at: codes.iarc.fr/home

Electronic nicotine delivery systems (ENDS) including e-cigarettes, e-pens, e-pipes, e-hookah and e-cigars have gained increased popularity as an alternative to tobacco. While ENDS do not contain tobacco, most contain nicotine, which is highly addictive, and other potentially harmful substances, such as volatile organic compounds, formaldehyde, and flavoring chemicals (ACS, 2019d). Given that ENDS are relatively new to the market, the long-term health effects of these products remain unknown.

Smokeless tobacco products, such as chewing tobacco, snuff and snus, used most often by young adults aged 18 to 25 years, are associated with an increased risk of oral, pancreatic, and esophageal cancer (ACS, 2019d; Lipari & Van Horn, 2017).

Many chemical substances found in the workplace are carcinogens or co-carcinogens (ACS, 2019e). In the United States, carcinogens are classified by two federal agencies: the National Toxicology Program of the Department of Health and Human Services (HHS) and the Environmental Protection Agency's (EPA) Integrated Risk Information System (IRIS) (CDC, 2017). The CDC established the National Institute for Occupational Safety and Health (NIOSH) to provide occupational exposure limits and guidelines for protection of the workforce as regulated by the Occupational Safety and Health Act of 1970 (U.S. EPA, 2017). The extensive list of suspected chemical substances continues to grow and includes aromatic amines and aniline dyes; pesticides and formaldehydes; arsenic, soot, and tars; asbestos; benzene; cadmium; chromium compounds; nickel and zinc ores; wood dust; beryllium compounds; and polyvinyl chloride (ACS, 2019e). Betel quid, which are chewed as stimulants in some cultures, are also included (ACS, 2019e; Chen, Mahmood, Mariottini, et al., 2017).

Genetics and Familial Factors

Almost every cancer type has been shown to run in families. This may be due to a combination of genetic, environmental, and lifestyle factors. Genetic factors play a fundamental role in cancer cell development. Cancer has been associated with extra chromosomes, too few chromosomes, or translocated chromosomes (NCI, 2019b).

Approximately 5% to 10% of cancers in adults display a pattern of cancers suggestive of a familial predisposition (NCI, 2019b). Hereditary cancer syndromes represent a cluster of cancers identified by a specific genetic alteration that is inherited across generations. In these families, the associated genetic mutation is found in all cells in the body (germline mutation) and represents an inherited susceptibility to cancer for all family members who carry the mutation.

There are more than 50 hereditary syndromes identified by scientists that may predispose individuals to develop certain cancers (NCI, 2019b). The hallmarks of families with a hereditary cancer syndrome include cancer in two or more first-degree relatives (the parent, sibling, or child of an individual), onset of cancer in family members younger than 50 years, the same type of cancer in several family members, individual family members with more than one type of cancer, and a rare cancer in one or more family members. There is also evidence of an autosomal dominant inheritance pattern of cancers affecting several generations of a family (NCI, 2019b).

There have been considerable advances in the recognition of inherited cancer susceptibility syndromes and in the ability to isolate and identify the inherited genetic mutations responsible. These advances have enabled the appropriate identification of families at risk for certain syndromes. Examples include hereditary breast and ovarian cancer syndrome (*BRCA1* and *BRCA2*) and multiple endocrine neoplasia syndrome (*MEN1* and *MEN2*) (see Chart 12-1). Other cancers associated with familial inheritance syndromes include nephroblastomas, pheochromocytomas, and colorectal, stomach, thyroid, renal, prostate, and lung cancers (NCI, 2019b).

Lifestyle Factors

Lifestyle factors (e.g., obesity, alcohol intake, poor diet, physical inactivity) were estimated to account for 16% of all cancer cases and 18% of all cancer deaths in 2017 (Islami, Goding Sauer, Miller, et al., 2018). These lifestyle factors were second only to cigarette smoking as a major modifiable risk factor associated with both cancer development and cancer mortality.

The risk of cancer increases with long-term ingestion of carcinogens or co-carcinogens or the absence of protective substances in the diet. Dietary substances that appear to increase the risk of cancer include fats, alcohol, salt-cured or smoked meats, nitrate- and nitrite-containing foods, and red and processed meats (World Cancer Research Fund [WCRF], 2018). Heavy alcohol use increases the risk of cancers of the mouth, pharynx, larynx, esophagus, liver, colon, rectum, and breast (WCRF, 2018).

Obesity has been linked to the development of cancers of the breast (in postmenopausal women), colon and rectum, endometrium, esophagus, kidney, and pancreas (WCRF, 2018). Obesity may be also associated with an increased risk for cancers of the gallbladder, liver, ovary, and cervix, and for multiple myeloma, Hodgkin lymphoma, and aggressive forms of prostate cancer. While there is a clear relationship between obesity and cancer, the etiology of cancer in the context of obesity remains poorly understood (NCI, 2017). Several possible mechanisms have been suggested,

however, including that excess fat may cause chronic inflammation resulting in DNA damage, increased levels of certain hormones (e.g., estrogen, insulin, adipokines), and disruptions in levels of cell growth regulators (e.g., mammalian target of rapamycin and AMP-activated protein kinase)—all of which may increase the development of certain types of cancer. Multiple studies have long linked a sedentary lifestyle and lack of regular exercise to cancer development (Cannioto, Etter, Guterman, et al., 2017; Cannioto, Etter, LaMonte, et al., 2018).

Hormonal Agents

Tumor growth may be promoted by disturbances in hormonal balance, either by the body's own (endogenous) hormone production or by administration of exogenous hormones (Norris, 2019). Cancers of the breast, prostate, ovaries, and endometrium are thought to depend on endogenous hormonal levels for growth. Prenatal exposure to diethylstilbestrol (a synthetic form of the female hormone estrogen) has long been recognized as a risk factor for clear cell adenocarcinoma of the lower genital tract (Huo, Anderson, Palmer, et al., 2017).

Hormonal changes related to the female reproductive cycle are also associated with cancer incidence. Early onset of menses before age 12 and delayed onset of menopause after age 55, null parity (never giving birth), and delayed childbirth after age 30 are all associated with an increased risk of breast cancer (Chen, 2019). Increased numbers of pregnancies are associated with a decreased incidence of breast, endometrial, and ovarian cancers.

Women who take estrogen after menopause appear to have a decreased risk of breast cancer, but an increased risk of developing endometrial cancers (NCI, 2018). Thus, estrogen replacement alone is not used in women who have not had a hysterectomy. Combination estrogen and progesterone therapy is linked to a higher risk of breast cancer. The longer the combined therapy is used, the higher the risk of developing breast cancer. However, the risk substantially decreases when therapy is discontinued (NCI, 2018).

Role of the Immune System

In humans, transformed cells arise on a regular basis, but are recognized by surveillance cells of the immune system that destroy them before cell growth becomes uncontrolled (immune surveillance) (Norris, 2019). When the immune system fails to identify and stop the growth of transformed cells, a tumor can develop and progress.

Patients who are immunocompromised have an increased incidence of cancer. Transplant recipients who receive immunosuppressive therapy to prevent rejection of the transplanted organ have an increased incidence of cancer (Norris, 2019). Patients with acquired immune deficiency syndrome (AIDS) have an increased incidence of Kaposi sarcoma and other cancers. Patients who were previously treated for one cancer are at increased risk for secondary cancers (Norris, 2019).

Normal Immune Responses

Through the process of immune surveillance, an intact immune system usually has the ability to recognize and combat cancer cells through multiple, interacting cells and actions of the innate, humoral, and cellular components of the immune system (Jameson, Fauci, Kasper, et al., 2018; Norris, 2019). Tumor-associated antigens (TAAs; also called *tumor cell antigens*) are found on the membranes of many cancer cells. TAAs are processed by antigen-presenting cells (APCs) (e.g., macrophages and dendritic cells [very specialized cells of the immune system] that present antigens to both T and B lymphocytes) and are presented to T lymphocytes that recognize the antigen-bearing cells as foreign. Multiple TAAs have been identified—some are found in many types of cancer, some exist in the normal tissues of origin as well as the cancer cells, some exist in both normal and cancer cells but are overexpressed (exist in higher concentrations) in cancer cells, and others are very specific to certain cancer types (Norris, 2019).

In response to recognizing TAAs as foreign, T lymphocytes release several cytokines that elicit various immune system actions, including (1) proliferation of cytotoxic (cell-killing) T lymphocytes capable of direct destruction of cancer cells, (2) induction of cancer cell apoptosis, and (3) recruitment of additional immune system cells (B-cell lymphocytes that produce antibodies, natural killer cells, and macrophages) that contribute to the destruction and degradation of cancer cells (Jameson et al., 2018; Norris, 2019).

Immune System Evasion

Several theories postulate how malignant cells survive and proliferate, evading the elaborate immune system defense mechanisms (Jameson et al., 2018; Norris, 2019). If the body fails to recognize the TAAs on cancer cells or the function of the APCs is impaired, the immune response is not stimulated. Some cancer cells have been found to have altered cell membranes that interfere with APC binding and presentation to T lymphocytes. Tumors can also express molecules that induce T-lymphocyte anergy or tolerance such as PD-1 ligand. These molecules bind to PD-1 proteins on T lymphocytes and either block the killing of the tumor or induce cell death in the lymphocyte. In addition, cancer cells have been found to release cytokines that inhibit APCs as well as other cells of the immune system. When tumors do not possess TAAs that label them as foreign, the immune response is not alerted. This allows the tumor to grow too large to be managed by normal immune mechanisms.

The immunogenicity (immunologic appearance) of cancer cells can be altered through genetic mutations, allowing the cells to evade immune cell recognition (Norris, 2019). Conversely, mutations are the source for some TAAs. Tumor antigens may combine with the antibodies produced by the immune system and hide or disguise themselves from normal immune defense mechanisms. The tumor antigen–antibody complexes that evade recognition lead to a false message to decrease further production of antibodies as well as other immune system components.

Overexpression (abnormally high concentrations) of host suppressor T lymphocytes induced through the release of cytokines by malignant cells is thought to downregulate the immune response, thus permitting uncontrolled cell growth (Jameson et al., 2018). Suppressor T lymphocytes normally assist in regulating lymphocyte production and diminishing immune responses (e.g., antibody production) when they are no longer required. Low levels of antibodies and high levels of suppressor cells have been found in patients with multiple myeloma, which is a cancer associated with hypogammaglobulinemia (low amounts of serum antibodies). Conversely, there is evidence that proliferation of helper T lymphocytes, which promote the immune response, is impaired by cytokines produced by cancer cells (Jameson et al., 2018). Without helper T lymphocytes, the immune system response is limited, and the cancer cells continue to proliferate. Understanding the role of the immune system and identification of the ways in which cancer evades the body's natural defenses provide the foundation for therapeutic approaches that seek to support and enhance the immune system's role in combating cancer (see Chapter 31).

Detection and Prevention of Cancer

Nurses in all settings play a key role in cancer detection and prevention. Primary, secondary, and tertiary prevention of cancer are all important.

Primary Prevention

Primary prevention is about reducing the risks of disease through health promotion and risk reduction strategies. Guidelines on nutrition and physical activity for cancer prevention can be found in Chart 12-2.

An example of primary prevention is the use of immunization to reduce the risk of cancer through prevention of infections associated with cancer. The HPV vaccine is recommended to prevent cervical and head and neck cancers (Hashim, Genden, Posner, et al., 2019). The vaccine to prevent HBV infection is recommended by the CDC (2018) to reduce the risk of hepatitis and subsequent development of liver cancer.

Secondary Prevention

Secondary prevention involves screening and early detection activities that seek to identify precancerous lesions and early-stage cancer in individuals who lack signs and symptoms of cancer. ACS screening is advocated for many types of cancer (see Table 12-3) (ACS, 2018). Detection of cancer at an early stage may reduce costs, use of resources, and the morbidity associated with advanced stages of cancer and their associated complex treatment approaches. Many screening and detection programs target people who do not regularly practice health-promoting behaviors or lack access to health care. Nurses continue to develop community-based screening and detection programs that address barriers to health care or reflect the socioeconomic and cultural beliefs of the target population (Rees, Jones, Jones, et al., 2018; So, Kwong, Chen, et al., 2019).

The evolving understanding of the role of genetics in cancer cell development has contributed to prevention and screening efforts. Many centers offer cancer risk evaluation programs that provide interdisciplinary in-depth assessment, screening, education, and counseling as well as follow-up monitoring for people at high risk for cancer (National Comprehensive Cancer Network [NCCN] 2019a,b). The NCI provides guidance for cancer risk assessment, counseling, education, and genetic testing (NCI, 2019b).

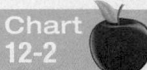

Chart 12-2 · HEALTH PROMOTION
American Cancer Society Guidelines on Nutrition and Physical Activity for Cancer Prevention

Individual Choices

Achieve and Maintain a Healthy Weight Throughout Life

- Be as lean as possible throughout life without being underweight.
- Avoid excessive weight gain at all ages. For those who are currently overweight or have obesity, losing even a small amount of weight has health benefits and is a good place to start.
- Engage in regular physical activity and limit consumption of high-calorie foods and beverages as key strategies for maintaining a healthy weight.

Adopt a Physically Active Lifestyle

- Adults should engage in at least 150 minutes of moderate-intensity or 75 minutes of vigorous-intensity physical activity each week, or an equivalent combination, preferably spread throughout the week.
- Children and adolescents should engage in at least 1 hour of moderate- or vigorous-intensity physical activity each day, with vigorous-intensity activity at least 3 days each week.
- Limit sedentary behavior such as sitting, lying down and watching television, and other forms of screen-based entertainment.
- Doing any intentional physical activity above usual activities, no matter what one's level of activity, can have many health benefits.

Consume a Healthy Diet, with an Emphasis on Plant Sources

- Choose foods and beverages in amounts that help achieve and maintain a healthy weight.
- Limit consumption of processed meat and red meats.
- Eat at least $2\frac{1}{2}$ cups of vegetables and fruits each day.
- Choose whole grains in preference to processed (refined) grains.

If You Drink Alcoholic Beverages, Limit Consumption

- Drink no more than one drink per day for women or two per day for men.

Community Action

Public, private, and community organizations should work collaboratively at national, state, and local levels to implement policy environmental changes that:

- Increase access to affordable, healthy foods in communities, worksites, and schools, and decrease access to and marketing of foods and beverages of low nutritional value, particularly to youth.
- Provide safe, enjoyable, and accessible environments for physical activity in schools and worksites, and for transportation and recreation in communities.

Adapted from American Cancer Society. (2019i). ACS guidelines on nutrition and physical activity for cancer. Retrieved on 9/28/2018 at: Prevention www.cancer.org/healthy/eat-healthy-get-active/acs-guidelines-nutrition-physical-activity-cancer-prevention.html.

Unfolding Patient Stories: Doris Bowman • Part 1

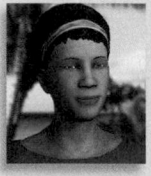

Doris Bowman, a 39-year-old diagnosed with uterine fibroids, dysmenorrhea, and menorrhagia, is scheduled for a total abdominal hysterectomy with bilateral salpingoopherectomy. She has a family history of uterine and ovarian cancer. She asks the nurse what she can do to further reduce her risk for cancer and is also concerned for her family members. What patient and family education should the nurse present on risk reduction strategies, health promotion, and cancer screening? (Doris Bowman's story continues in Chapter 51.)

Care for Doris and other patients in a realistic virtual environment: ***vSim** for Nursing* (**thepoint.lww.com/vSimMedicalSurgical**). Practice documenting these patients' care in DocuCare (**thepoint.lww.com/DocuCareEHR**).

Tertiary Prevention

Improved screening, diagnosis, and treatment approaches have led to an estimated 16.9 million cancer survivors in the United States (ACS, 2019f). Tertiary prevention efforts focus on monitoring for and preventing recurrence of the primary cancer as well as screening for the development of second malignancies in cancer survivors. Survivors are assessed for the development of second malignancies such as lymphoma and leukemia, which have been associated with certain chemotherapy agents and the use of radiation therapy (ACS, 2019f). Survivors may also develop second malignancies not related to treatment,

but rather genetic mutations related to inherited cancer syndromes, environmental exposures, and lifestyle factors.

Diagnosis of Cancer

A cancer diagnosis is based on assessment of physiologic and functional changes and results of the diagnostic evaluation. Patients with suspected cancer undergo extensive testing to (1) determine the presence and extent of cancer, (2) identify possible disease metastasis, (3) evaluate the function of involved and uninvolved body systems and organs, and (4) obtain tissue and cells for analysis, including evaluation of tumor stage and grade. The diagnostic evaluation includes a review of systems; physical examination; imaging studies; laboratory tests of blood, urine, and other body fluids; procedures; and pathologic analysis. A selection of diagnostic tests is found in Table 12-4.

Patients undergoing extensive testing may be fearful of the procedures and anxious about possible test results. Nurses help address the patient's fear and anxiety by explaining the tests to be performed, the sensations likely to be experienced, and the patient's role in the test procedures. The nurse encourages the patient and family to voice their fears about the test results, supports the patient and family throughout the diagnostic evaluation, and reinforces and clarifies information conveyed by the primary provider. The nurse also encourages the patient and family to communicate, share their concerns, and discuss their questions and concerns with one another.

Tumor Staging and Grading

A complete diagnostic evaluation includes identifying the stage and grade of the tumor. This is accomplished prior to

TABLE 12-3	American Cancer Society Screening Guidelines for the Early Detection of Cancer[a]		
Cancer Site	**Population**	**Test or Procedure**	**Recommendation**
Breast	Women, ages 40–54	Mammography	Women should undergo regular screening mammography starting at age 45 yrs. Women ages 45–54 should be screened annually. Women should have the opportunity to begin annual screening between the ages of 40 and 44.
	Women age 55 and over	Mammography	Transition to biennial screening or can continue annual screening. Continue screening if overall health is good and life expectancy is 10+ yrs.
Cervix	Women, ages 21–29	Papanicolaou (Pap) test	Screening should be done every 3 yrs with conventional or liquid based Pap tests. HPV DNA testing only for abnormal Pap test.
	Women ages 30–65 Women ages 66+	Pap test and HPV DNA test	Screening should be done every 5 yrs with both the HPV test and the Pap test (preferred), or every 3 yrs with the Pap test alone (acceptable). Women ages 66+ who have regular cervical cancer screening with negative results should stop cervical cancer screening. Women who have had a total hysterectomy should stop cervical cancer screening.
Colorectal[b]	Men and women, ages 45–75. People aged 76–84, should discuss continued screening with their provider. People 85+ should no longer participate in colorectal cancer screenings.	Highly sensitive guaiac-based fecal occult blood test (gFOBT) or highly sensitive fecal immuno-chemical test (FIT)	Annual highly sensitive gFOBT or FIT testing.
		Multi-targeted stool DNA test (MT-sDNA) test	MT-sDNA testing every 3 yrs.
		Flexible sigmoidoscopy (FSIG), or Colonoscopy, or CT colonography (virtual colonoscopy)	Every 5 yrs. Every 10 yrs. Every 5 yrs.
Endometrial	Women, at menopause	At the time of menopause, women at average risk should be informed about risks and symptoms of endometrial cancer and encouraged to report any unexpected bleeding or spotting to their providers.	Not applicable (N/A)
Lung	Current or former smokers (quit within past 15 yrs) ages 55–74 in fairly good health with at least a 30 pack-year history.	Low-dose CT (LDCT)	LDCT annually. Providers with access to high-volume, high-quality lung cancer screening and treatment centers should initiate a discussion about lung cancer screening with apparently healthy patients aged 55–74 who have at least a 30 pack-year smoking history, and who currently smoke or have quit within the past 15 yrs. Patient has been involved in the process of informed and shared decision making with a provider related to the potential benefits, limitations, and harms associated with screening for lung cancer with LDCT should occur before any decision is made to initiate lung cancer screening. Smoking cessation counseling remains a high priority for clinical attention in discussions with current smokers, who should be informed of their continuing risk of lung cancer. Screening should not be viewed as an alternative to smoking cessation.
Prostate	Men, age 50+, African American Men, age 45+	Digital rectal examination (DRE) and prostate-specific antigen (PSA) test	Men who have at least a 10-yr life expectancy should have an opportunity to make an informed decision with their providers about whether to be screened for prostate cancer, after receiving information about the potential benefits, risks, and uncertainties associated with prostate cancer screening. Prostate cancer screening should not occur without an informed decision making process.

TABLE 12-3	American Cancer Society Screening Guidelines for the Early Detection of Cancer[a] (continued)		
Cancer Site	**Population**	**Test or Procedure**	**Recommendation**
Cancer-related checkup	Men and women, age 20+	On the occasion of a periodic health examination, the cancer-related checkup should include examination for cancers of the thyroid, testicles, ovaries, lymph nodes, oral cavity, and skin, as well as health counseling about tobacco, sun exposure, diet and nutrition, risk factors, sexual practices, and environmental and occupational exposures.	N/A

CT, computed tomography; DNA, deoxyribonucleic acid; HPV, human papillomavirus.
[a]All individuals should become familiar with the potential benefits, limitations, and harms associated with cancer screening.
[b]All positive tests (other than colonoscopy) should be followed up with colonoscopy.
Adapted from American Cancer Society (ACS). (2018). American Cancer Society guidelines for the early detection of cancer. Retrieved on 7/5/2019 at: www.cancer.org/healthy/find-cancer-early/cancer-screening-guidelines/american-cancer-society-guidelines-for-the-early-detection-of-cancer.html

TABLE 12-4	Select Diagnostic Tests Used to Detect Cancer	
Test	**Description**	**Examples of Diagnostic Uses**
Tumor marker identification	Analysis of biochemical mediators found in tumor tissue, blood, or other body fluids that are indicative of cancer cells or specific characteristics of cancer cells. These biochemical mediators may also be found in some normal body tissues.	Breast, colon, lung, ovarian, testicular, prostate cancers
Genetic tumor markers (also called prognostic indicators)	Analysis for the presence of mutations (alterations) in genes found in tumors or body tissues. Assists in diagnosis, selection of treatment, prediction of response to therapy, and risk of progression or recurrence.	Breast, lung, kidney, ovarian, brain cancers; leukemia; and lymphoma. Many uses of genetic profiling are considered investigational.
Mammography	Use of x-ray images of the breast.	Breast cancer
Magnetic resonance imaging (MRI)	Use of magnetic fields and radiofrequency signals to create sectioned images of various body structures.	Neurologic, pelvic, abdominal, thoracic, breast cancers
Computed tomography (CT) scan	Use of narrow-beam x-ray to scan successive layers of tissue for a cross-sectional view.	Neurologic, pelvic, skeletal, abdominal, thoracic cancers
Fluoroscopy	Use of x-rays that identify contrasts in body tissue densities; may involve the use of contrast agents.	Skeletal, lung, gastrointestinal cancers
Ultrasonography (ultrasound)	High-frequency sound waves echoing off body tissues are converted electronically into images; used to assess tissues deep within the body.	Abdominal and pelvic cancers
Endoscopy	Direct visualization of a body cavity or passageway by insertion of an endoscope into a body cavity or opening; allows tissue biopsy, fluid aspiration, and excision of small tumors. Used for diagnostic and therapeutic purposes.	Bronchial, gastrointestinal cancers
Nuclear medicine imaging	Uses IV injection or ingestion of radioisotopes followed by imaging of tissues that have concentrated the radioisotopes.	Bone, liver, kidney, spleen, brain, and thyroid cancers
Positron emission tomography (PET)	Through the use of a tracer, provides black-and-white or color-coded images of the biologic activity of a particular area, rather than its structure. Used in detection of cancer or its response to treatment.	Lung, colon, liver, pancreatic, head and neck cancers; Hodgkin and non-Hodgkin lymphoma and melanoma
PET fusion	Use of a PET scanner and a CT scanner in one machine to provide an image combining anatomic detail, spatial resolution, and functional metabolic abnormalities.	See PET
Radioimmunoconjugates	Monoclonal antibodies are labeled with a radioisotope and injected IV into the patient; the antibodies that aggregate at the tumor site are visualized with scanners.	Colorectal, breast, ovarian, head and neck cancers; lymphoma and melanoma
Vascular imaging	Use of contrast agents that are injected into veins or arteries and monitored by fluoroscopy, CT, or MRI imaging in order to assess tumor vasculature. Used to assess tumor vascularity prior to surgical procedures.	Liver and brain cancers

Adapted from Fischbach, F. T., & Fischbach, M. A. (2018). *Fischbach's manual of laboratory and diagnostic tests* (10th ed.). Philadelphia, PA: Wolters Kluwer Health.

treatment to provide baseline data for evaluating outcomes of therapy and to maintain a systematic and consistent approach to ongoing diagnosis and treatment. Cancer treatment options and prognosis are based on the cancer type; stage and grade of cancer; as well as the individual's health status and response to treatment (NCI, 2019c).

Staging describes the size of the tumor, the existence of local invasion, lymph node involvement, and distant metastasis. Several systems exist for classifying the anatomic extent of disease. The tumor, nodes, and metastasis (TNM) system (see Chart 12-3) is the most common system used to describe the stage of many solid tumors (Amin, Greene, Edge, et al., 2017; NCCN, 2019c).

Staging provides a common language used by health care providers and scientists to accurately communicate about cancer across clinical settings and in research. These systems also provide a convenient shorthand notation that condenses lengthy descriptions into manageable terms for comparisons of treatments and prognoses.

Grading is the pathologic classification of tumor cells (NCI, 2019c). Grading systems seek to define the type of tissue from which the tumor originated and the degree to which the tumor cells retain the functional and histologic characteristics of the tissue of origin (differentiation). Samples of cells used to establish the tumor grade may be obtained from tissue scrapings, body fluids, secretions, washings, biopsy, or surgical excision. This information helps providers predict the behavior and prognosis of various tumors. The grade corresponds with a numeric value ranging from I to IV. Grade I tumors, also known as well-differentiated tumors, closely resemble the tissue of origin in structure and function. Tumors that do not clearly resemble the tissue of origin in structure or function

are described as poorly differentiated or undifferentiated and are assigned grade IV. These tumors tend to be more aggressive, less responsive to treatment, and associated with a poorer prognosis as compared to well-differentiated, grade I tumors. Various staging and grading systems are used to characterize cancers.

Anatomic Stage Group

Once the diagnosis, clinical stage, and histologic grade have been determined, the anatomic stage group, designated by I through IV (representing increasing severity of disease), is assigned to facilitate communication, treatment decisions, and estimation of prognosis. The anatomic stage group is also useful for comparing clinical outcomes.

Management of Cancer

Treatment options offered to patients with cancer are based on treatment goals for each specific type, stage, and grade of cancer. The range of possible treatment goals includes cure, a complete eradication of malignant disease; control, which includes prolonged survival and containment of cancer cell growth; or **palliation**, which involves relief of symptoms associated with the disease and improvement of quality of life. Treatment approaches are not initiated until the diagnosis of cancer has been confirmed and staging and grading have been completed.

The health care team and the patient and family must have a clear understanding of the treatment options and goals. Open communication and support are vital as those involved periodically reassess treatment plans and goals when complications of therapy develop or disease progresses.

Multiple modalities are commonly used in cancer treatment. Various approaches, including surgery, radiation therapy, chemotherapy, hematopoietic stem cell transplantation (HSCT), immunotherapy, and targeted therapy may be used together or at different times throughout treatment. Understanding the principles of each and how they interrelate is important in understanding the rationale and goals of treatment.

Surgery

Surgical removal of the entire cancer remains the ideal and most frequently used treatment method. However, the specific surgical approach may vary for several reasons. Diagnostic surgery is the definitive method for obtaining tissue to identify the cellular characteristics that influence all treatment decisions. Surgery may be the primary method of treatment, or it may be prophylactic, palliative, or reconstructive.

Diagnostic Surgery

Diagnostic surgery, or biopsy, is performed to obtain a tissue sample for histologic analysis of cells suspected to be malignant. In most instances, the biopsy is taken from the actual tumor; however, in some situations, it is necessary to take a sample of lymph nodes near a suspicious tumor. Many cancers can metastasize from the primary site to other areas of the body through the lymphatic circulation. Knowing whether adjacent lymph nodes contain tumor cells helps the health care team plan the best therapeutic approach to combat cancer that has spread beyond the primary tumor site. The use of injectable dyes and nuclear medicine imaging can help identify the sentinel lymph node or the initial lymph node to which the primary tumor and surrounding tissue drain. Sentinel lymph node biopsy (SLNB), also known as sentinel lymph node mapping, is a minimally invasive surgical approach that in many instances has replaced lymphadenectomy (more invasive lymph node dissections) and the associated complications such as lymphedema and delayed healing. SLNB has been widely adopted for regional lymph node staging in selected cases of melanoma and breast cancer (NCCN, 2019d, 2019e).

Biopsy Types

Biopsy methods include excisional, incisional, and needle biopsy. The biopsy type is determined by the size and location of the tumor, the type of treatment anticipated if the cancer diagnosis is confirmed, and the need for surgery and general anesthesia. The biopsy method that allows for the least invasive approach while permitting the most representative tissue sample is chosen. Diagnostic imaging techniques can be used to assist in locating the suspicious lesion and to facilitate accurate tissue sampling. The patient and family are provided the opportunity and time to discuss the options before definitive plans are made.

Excisional biopsy is used for small, easily accessible tumors. In many cases, the surgeon can remove the entire tumor as well as the surrounding marginal tissues. The removal of normal tissue beyond the tumor area decreases the possibility that residual microscopic malignant cells may lead to a recurrence of the tumor. This approach not only provides the pathologist with the entire tissue specimen for the determination of stage and grade but also decreases the chance of seeding tumor cells (disseminating cancer cells throughout surrounding tissues).

Incisional biopsy is performed if the tumor mass is too large to be removed. In this case, a wedge of tissue from the tumor is removed for analysis. The cells of the tissue wedge must be representative of the tumor mass so that the pathologist can provide an accurate diagnosis. If the specimen does not contain representative tissue and cells, negative biopsy results do not guarantee the absence of cancer.

Excisional and incisional approaches are often performed through endoscopy. However, a surgical procedure may be required to determine the anatomic extent or stage of the tumor. For example, a diagnostic or staging laparotomy (the surgical opening of the abdomen to assess malignant abdominal disease) may be necessary to assess malignancies such as gastric or colon cancer.

Needle biopsy is performed to sample suspicious masses that are easily and safely accessible, such as some masses in the breasts, thyroid, lung, liver, and kidney. Needle biopsies are most often performed on an outpatient basis. They are fast, relatively inexpensive, easy to perform, and may require only local anesthesia. In general, the patient experiences slight and temporary physical discomfort. In addition, the surrounding tissues are minimally disturbed, thus decreasing the likelihood of seeding cancer cells. Fine-needle aspiration (FNA) biopsy involves aspirating cells rather than intact tissue through a needle that is guided into a suspected diseased area. This type of specimen can only be analyzed by cytologic

examination (viewing only cells, not tissue). Often, x-ray, computed tomography (CT) scanning, ultrasonography, or magnetic resonance imaging (MRI) is used to help locate the suspicious area and guide placement of the needle. FNA does not always yield enough material to permit accurate diagnosis, necessitating additional biopsy procedures. A core needle biopsy uses a specially designed needle to obtain a small core of tissue that permits histologic analysis. Most often, this specimen is sufficient to permit accurate diagnosis.

Surgery as Primary Treatment

When surgery is the primary approach in treating cancer, the goal is to remove the entire tumor or as much as is feasible (a procedure sometimes called *debulking*) as well as any involved surrounding tissue, including regional lymph nodes.

Two common surgical approaches used for treating primary tumors are local and wide excisions. Local excision, often performed on an outpatient basis, is warranted when the mass is small. It includes removal of the mass and a small margin of normal tissue that is easily accessible. Wide or radical excisions (en bloc dissections) include removal of the primary tumor, lymph nodes, adjacent involved structures, and surrounding tissues that may be at high risk for tumor spread. This surgical method may result in disfigurement and altered functioning, necessitating rehabilitation, reconstructive procedures, or both. However, wide excisions are considered if the tumor can be removed completely and the chances of cure or control are good.

Minimally invasive surgical techniques are increasingly replacing traditional surgery associated with large incisions for a variety of cancers (Yarbro, Wujcik, & Gobel, 2018). Advantages of minimally invasive approaches include less surgical trauma, decreased blood loss, decreased incidence of wound infection and other complications associated with surgery, decreased surgical time and requirement for anesthesia, decreased postoperative pain and limited mobility, and shorter periods of recovery (Pache, Hübner, Jurt, et al., 2017).

Endoscopic surgery, an example of minimally invasive surgery, uses an endoscope with intense lighting and an attached multichip mini camera that is inserted into the body through a small incision. The surgical instruments are inserted into the surgical field through one or two additional small incisions, each about 1 to 2 cm in length. The camera transmits the image of the involved area to a monitor so that the surgeon can manipulate the instruments to perform the necessary procedure. Endoscopic surgery is used to treat many cancer-related conditions of the thorax (thoracoscopy) and abdomen (laparoscopy).

The use of robotics is another advancement in the surgical treatment of cancer (Yarbro, et al., 2018). The use of robotics during laparoscopic procedures permits the removal of tumors with more precision and dexterity than could be accomplished by laparoscopic surgery alone. Laparoscopic robotic-assisted surgery has been used to treat cancers of the colon, prostate and uterus; however, it remains unclear if long-term cancer-related outcomes are improved with robotic surgery when compared to more conventional surgical approaches (U.S. Food and Drug Administration [FDA], 2019).

Salvage surgery is an additional treatment option that uses an extensive surgical approach to treat the local recurrence of cancer after the use of a less extensive primary approach. Mastectomy to treat recurrent breast cancer after primary lumpectomy and radiation is an example of salvage surgery.

Surgery may completely excise limited areas of metastatic disease (referred to as oligometastatic disease) as well. An example would be colon cancer with one to three small areas of liver metastasis and no evidence of cancer elsewhere. In the past, patients with recurrent or metastatic disease were treated with palliation only as their disease was considered incurable. However, evidence now suggests that there is a possibility of a cure or prolonged survival for select subgroups of patients with certain cancer types (Jang, Kim, Jeong, et al., 2018; Ruiz, Sebagh, Wicherts, et al., 2018).

In addition to surgery that uses surgical blades or scalpels to excise the mass and surrounding tissues, several other types of techniques are available. Table 12-5 provides examples of select techniques.

A multidisciplinary approach to patient care is essential for the patient undergoing cancer-related surgery. The effects of surgery on the patient's body image, self-esteem, and functional abilities are addressed. If necessary, a plan for postoperative rehabilitation is made before the surgery is performed. The growth and dissemination of cancer cells may have produced distant micrometastases by the time the patient seeks treatment. Therefore, attempting to remove wide margins of tissue in the hope of "getting all the cancer" may not be feasible. This reality substantiates the need for a coordinated multidisciplinary approach to cancer therapy.

Once the surgery has been completed, one or more additional (or adjuvant) modalities may be chosen to increase the likelihood of eradicating the remaining microscopic cancer cells that are undetectable by available diagnostic procedures. However, some cancers that are treated surgically in the very early stages (e.g., skin and testicular cancers) are curable without additional therapy.

Prophylactic Surgery

Prophylactic or risk reduction surgery involves removing nonvital tissues or organs that are at increased risk of developing cancer. The following factors are considered when discussing possible prophylactic surgery:

- Family history and genetic predisposition
- Presence or absence of signs and symptoms
- Potential risks and benefits
- Ability to detect cancer at an early stage
- Alternative options for managing increased risk
- The patient's acceptance of the postoperative outcome

Colectomy, mastectomy, and oophorectomy are examples of prophylactic surgeries. Identification of genetic markers indicative of inherited cancer syndromes or a predisposition to develop some types of cancer plays a role in decisions concerning prophylactic surgeries. However, what is adequate justification for prophylactic surgery remains controversial. For example, several factors are considered when deciding to proceed with a prophylactic mastectomy, including a family history of breast cancer; positive *BRCA1* or *BRCA2* findings; severity of overall breast cancer risk; a personal history of breast cancer; and individual factors (e.g., younger age, psychological well-being that may influence the patient's decision making process) (Chagpar, 2018; Schott, Vetter, Keller, et al., 2017). Prophylactic surgery is discussed with patients and families along with other approaches for managing increased risk of cancer development. Preoperative education and counseling, as well as long-term follow-up, are provided.

Palliative Surgery

The overall goal of palliative surgery in cancer care is to relieve symptoms and to improve the patient's quality of life (Fahy, 2019; Hanna, Blazer, & Mosca, 2012). Palliative surgery is often performed in an attempt to relieve symptoms such as ulceration, obstruction, hemorrhage, pain, and malignant effusions (see Table 12-6). When surgical cure is not possible, honest and informative communication with

---

TABLE 12-5 Select Techniques Used for Localized Destruction of Tumor Tissue

Type of Procedure	Description	Examples of Use
Chemosurgery	Use of chemicals or chemotherapy applied directly to tissue to cause destruction.	Intraperitoneal chemotherapy for ovarian cancer involving the abdomen and peritoneum.
Cryoablation	Use of liquid nitrogen or a very cold probe to freeze tissue and cause cell destruction.	Cervical, prostate, and rectal cancers.
Electrosurgery	Use of an electric current to destroy tumor cells.	Basal and squamous cell skin cancers.
Laser surgery	Use of light and energy aimed at an exact tissue location and depth to vaporize cancer cells (also referred to as photocoagulation or photoablation).	Dyspnea associated with endobronchial obstructions.
Photodynamic therapy	Intravenous (IV) administration of a light-sensitizing agent (hematoporphyrin derivative) that is taken up by cancer cells, followed by exposure to laser light within 24–48 h; causes cancer cell death.	Palliative treatment of dysphagia associated with esophageal and dyspnea associated with endobronchial obstructions.
Radiofrequency ablation (RFA)	Uses localized application of thermal energy that destroys cancer cells through heat: temperatures exceed 50°C (122°F).	Nonresectable liver tumors, pain control with bone metastasis.

Adapted from DeVita, V. T., Rosenberg S. A., & Lawrence, T. S., (Eds.). (2018). *Cancer: Principles & practice of oncology* (11th ed.). Philadelphia, PA: Lippincott Williams & Wilkins.

TABLE 12-6	Types of Palliative Surgery and Interventions
Procedure	**Indications**
Abdominal shunt placement	Ascites
Biliary stent placement	Biliary obstruction
Bone stabilization	Displaced bone fracture related to metastatic disease
Colostomy or ileostomy	Bowel obstruction
Cordotomy	Pain
Epidural catheter placement (for administering epidural analgesics)	Pain
Excision of solitary metastatic lesion	Metastatic lung, liver, or brain lesion
Gastrostomy, jejunostomy tube placement	Upper gastrointestinal tract obstruction
Hormone manipulation (removal of ovaries, testes, adrenals, pituitary)	Tumors that depend on hormones for growth
Nerve block	Pain
Percutaneous enteral gastrostomy (PEG) tube placement	Enteral nutrition
Pericardial drainage tube placement	Pericardial effusion
Peritoneal drainage tube placement	Ascites
Pleural drainage tube placement	Pleural effusion
Ureteral stent placement	Ureteral obstruction
Venous access device placement (for administering parenteral analgesics)	Pain

the patient and family about the goal of palliative surgery is essential to avoid false hope and disappointment. In certain cases, however, surgical intervention with palliative intent may also be performed as a supportive treatment to relieve symptoms along with other potentially curative cancer treatments (Fahy, 2019; Hanna et al., 2012). Thus, the role of palliative surgery today is no longer limited to end-of-life care.

Reconstructive Surgery

Reconstructive surgery may follow curative or extensive surgery in an attempt to improve function or obtain a more desirable cosmetic effect. It may be performed in one operation or in stages. The surgeon who will perform the surgery discusses possible reconstructive surgical options with the patient before the primary surgery is performed. Reconstructive surgery may be indicated for breast, head and neck, and skin cancers.

The nurse assesses the patient's needs and the impact that altered functioning and body image may have on quality of life. Nurses provide patients and families with opportunities to discuss these issues. The individual needs of the patient

undergoing reconstructive surgery and their families must be accurately recognized and addressed.

Nursing Management

Patients undergoing surgery for cancer require general perioperative nursing care (see Chapters 14, 15, and 16). Surgical care is individualized according to age, organ impairment, specific deficits, comorbidities, cultural implications, and altered immunity. Combining other treatment methods, such as radiation and chemotherapy, with surgery also contributes to postoperative complications, such as infection, impaired wound healing, altered pulmonary or renal function, and the development of venous thromboembolism (VTE). The nurse completes a thorough preoperative assessment for factors that may affect the patient undergoing the surgical procedure.

Preoperatively, the nurse provides the patient and family with verbal and written information about the surgical procedure as well as other interventions that may take place intraoperatively (e.g., radiation implants). Instructions concerning prophylactic antibiotic requirements, diet, and bowel preparation are also provided.

Patients who are undergoing surgery for the diagnosis or treatment of cancer may be anxious about the surgical procedure, possible findings, postoperative limitations, changes in normal body functions, and prognosis. The patient and family require time and assistance to process this information, possible changes, and expected outcomes resulting from the surgery.

The nurse serves as the patient advocate and liaison and encourages the patient and family to take an active role in decision making when possible. If the patient or family asks about the results of diagnostic testing and surgical procedures, the nurse's response is guided by the information that was conveyed previously. The nurse may be asked to explain and clarify information for patients and families that was provided initially but was not grasped because of intense anxiety. It is important that the nurse, as well as other members of the health care team, provide information that is consistent.

Postoperatively, the nurse assesses patient responses to surgery and monitors the patient for possible complications, such as infection, bleeding, thrombophlebitis, wound dehiscence, fluid and electrolyte imbalance, and organ dysfunction. The nurse also provides for the patient's comfort. Postoperative education addresses wound care, pain management, activity, nutrition, and medication information.

Plans for discharge, follow-up, home care, and subsequent treatment and rehabilitation are initiated as early as possible to ensure continuity of care from hospital to home or from a cancer referral center to the patient's local hospital and health care provider. Patients and families are encouraged to use community resources such as the ACS for support and information (see the Resources section at the end of this chapter).

Radiation Therapy

Approximately 60% of patients with cancer receive **radiation therapy** at some point during treatment (Halperin, Wazer, Perez, et al., 2019). Radiation may be used to cure cancer, as in thyroid carcinomas, localized cancers of the head and neck, and cancers of the cervix. Radiation therapy may also be used to control cancer when a tumor cannot be removed surgically or when local nodal metastasis is present. Neoadjuvant (prior to local definitive treatment) radiation therapy, with or without chemotherapy, is used to reduce tumor size in order to facilitate surgical resection. Radiation therapy may be given prophylactically to prevent local recurrence or spread of microscopic cells from the primary tumor to a distant area (e.g., irradiating the breast and axilla following lumpectomy or mastectomy for breast cancer). Palliative radiation therapy is used to relieve the symptoms of locally advanced or metastatic disease, especially when the cancer has spread to the brain, bone, or soft tissue, or to treat oncologic emergencies, such as superior vena cava syndrome, bronchial airway obstruction, or spinal cord compression.

Two types of ionizing radiation—electromagnetic radiation (x-rays and gamma rays) and particulate radiation (electrons, beta particles, protons, neutrons, and alpha particles)—can be used to kill cells. The most lethal damage is the direct alteration of the DNA molecule within the cells of both malignant and normal tissues. Ionizing radiation can directly break the strands of the DNA helix, leading to cell death. It can also indirectly damage DNA through the formation of free radicals. If the DNA cannot be repaired, the cell may die immediately or may initiate apoptosis (Yarbro et al., 2018).

Replicating cells are most vulnerable to the disruptive effects of radiation (during DNA synthesis and mitosis, e.g., early S, G_2, and M phases of the cell cycle; see Fig. 12-2). Therefore, those body tissues that undergo frequent cell division are most sensitive to radiation therapy. These tissues include bone marrow, lymphatic tissue, epithelium of the gastrointestinal tract, hair follicles, and gonads. Slower-growing tissues and tissues at rest (e.g., muscle, cartilage, nervous system, connective tissues) are relatively radioresistant (less sensitive to the effects of radiation). However, it is important to remember that radiation therapy is localized treatment, and only the tissues that are within the treatment field are affected.

A radiosensitive tumor is one that can be destroyed by a dose of radiation that still allows for cell repair and regeneration in the surrounding normal tissue. If the radiation is delivered when most tumor cells are cycling through the cell cycle, the number of cancer cells destroyed (cell kill) is maximal. Radiation sensitivity is enhanced in tumors that are smaller in size and that contain cells that are rapidly dividing (highly proliferative) and poorly differentiated (no longer resembling the tissue of origin).

Radiation Dosage

The radiation dosage depends on the sensitivity of the target tissues to radiation, the size of the tumor, radiation tolerance of the surrounding normal tissues, and critical structures adjacent to the tumor target. The lethal tumor dose is defined as the dose that will eradicate 95% of the tumor yet preserve normal tissue. In external-beam radiation therapy (EBRT), the total radiation dose is delivered over several weeks in daily doses called *fractions*. This allows healthy tissue to repair and achieves greater cell kill by exposing more cells to the radiation as they begin active cell division. Repeated radiation treatments over time (fractionated doses) also allow for the periphery of the tumor to be reoxygenated repeatedly, because tumors shrink from the outside inward. This increases

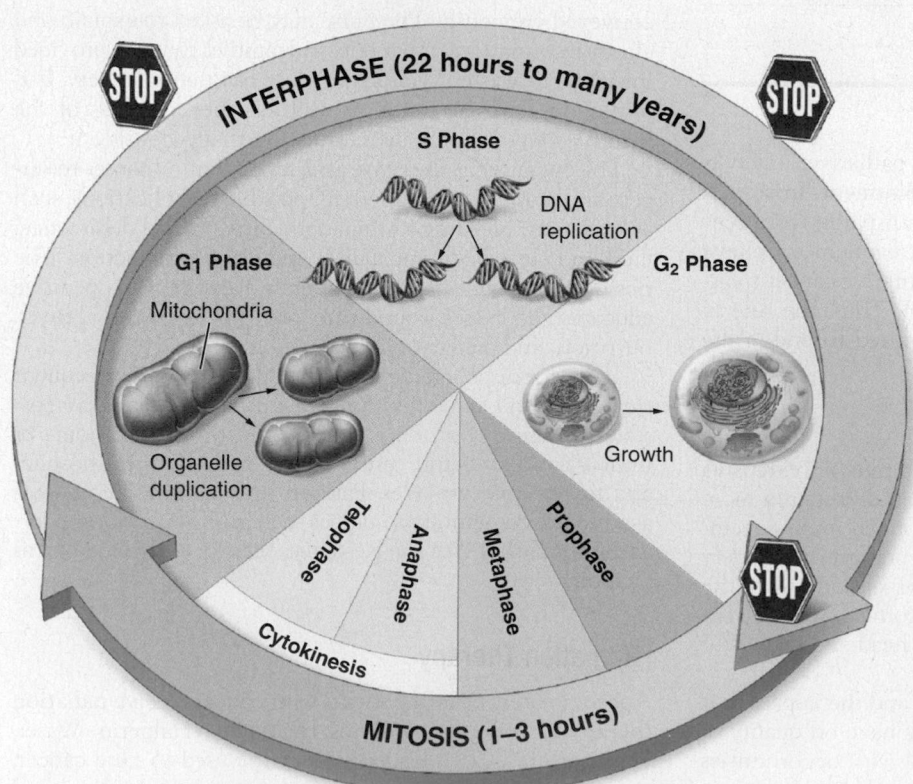

Figure 12-2 • Cell cycle. The cell cycle's four steps are illustrated beginning with G_1 and proceeding to M. The first growth phase (G_1), DNA synthesis phase (S), second growth phase (G_2), and mitosis (M) are illustrated. Reprinted with permission from Grossman, S. G., & Porth, C. M. (2014). *Porth's pathophysiology: Concepts of altered health states* (9th ed.). Philadelphia, PA: Lippincott Williams & Wilkins.

the radiosensitivity of the tumor, thereby increasing tumor cell death (Morgan, Ten Haken, & Lawrence, 2018). Newer approaches take advantage of increased radiation beam conformality (better tumor targeting) to administer radiation in fewer doses with larger fractions sizes (hypo-fractionation and stereotactic body radiotherapy [SBRT]).

Administration of Radiation

Radiation therapy can be given in various ways depending on the source of radiation used, the location of the tumor, and the type of cancer. The primary radiotherapy modalities include EBRT, **brachytherapy** (a form of internal radiation), systemic (radioisotopes), and contact or surface molds.

External Radiation

EBRT is the most commonly used form of radiation therapy. The energy utilized in EBRT is generated either from a linear accelerator or from a unit that generates energy directly from a core source of radioactive material such as a GammaKnife™ unit. Through computerized software programs, both approaches can shape an invisible beam of highly charged photons or gamma rays to penetrate the body and target the tumor with pinpoint accuracy.

Advances in computer technology allow multiple imaging modalities (CT, MRI, and PET scans) to be used to provide three-dimensional images of the tumor, neighboring tissues at risk for microscopic spread, and surrounding normal tissues or organs at risk for radiation-induced injury. These images, referred to as volumetric images, allow the radiation oncologist to plan for multiple radiation beams directed from different angles and different planes so that the beams conform precisely around the tumor (referred to as conformal radiation). The dose of radiation that reaches the surrounding normal tissues is reduced, leading to much less tissue injury than in older forms of radiation therapy (Halperin et al., 2019). Treatment enhancements in EBRT include the ability to control different intensity or energy levels of radiation beams at different angles directed at the tumor, a process known as intensity-modulated radiation therapy (IMRT), which enables higher doses to be delivered to the tumor while sparing the important healthy structures surrounding the tumor (Halperin et al., 2019). IMRT can be given as standard daily fractions or as "hyperfractionated" twice-daily fractions, which shortens the duration of the patient's treatment schedule. Image-guided radiation therapy (IGRT) uses continuous monitoring of the tumor with ultrasound, x-ray, or CT scans during the treatment to allow for automatic adjustment of the beams as the tumor changes shape or position in an effort to spare the healthy surrounding tissue and reduce side effects. Additional treatment enhancements include respiratory gating, where the treatment delivery is synchronized with the patient's respiratory cycle, enabling the beam to be adjusted as the tumor or organ moves. These treatment advancements improve tumor destruction while reducing acute and long-term toxicities (Halperin et al., 2019).

Gamma rays generated from the spontaneous decay of naturally occurring solid source of radioactivity, such as cobalt-60, are one of the oldest forms of EBRT. With the advent of modern linear accelerators, the use of solid radioactive elements is confined primarily to the GammaKnife™

stereotactic radiosurgery unit, which is used as a one-time, high-dose delivery of EBRT for treatment of both benign and malignant intracranial lesions.

SBRT is another form of EBRT that uses higher doses of radiation to penetrate very deeply into the body to control deep-seated tumors that cannot be treated by other approaches such as surgery. SBRT is delivered with considerably higher treatment fraction doses over a short span of time, usually 1 to 5 treatment days, in contrast to daily treatments for 5 days per week for 6 to 8 weeks for conventional EBRT. Specialized linear accelerators with the capability of robotically moving around the patient are used to deliver SBRT, such as the CyberKnife™, Trilogy™, and TomoTherapy™ delivery systems, which are now more commonly available.

Proton therapy is another approach to EBRT. Proton therapy utilizes high linear energy transfer (LET) in the form of charged protons generated by a large magnetic unit called a *cyclotron*. The advantage of proton therapy is that it is capable of delivering its high-energy dose to a deep-seated tumor, with decreased doses of radiation to the tissues in front of the tumor while virtually no energy exits through the patient's healthy tissue behind the tumor (Halperin et al., 2019). Proton therapy permits treatment of deep tumors near critical structures, such as the heart or major blood vessels.

Internal Radiation

Internal radiation includes localized implantation or systemic radionuclide administration. Brachytherapy delivers the dose of radiation to a localized area while systemic radiotherapy relies on strategies for getting the radionuclides closer to the tumor. The specific radioisotope used is selected based on its half-life, which is the time it takes for half of its radioactivity to decay, and the depth of penetration of the radiation.

Brachytherapy

Brachytherapy is the placement of radioactive sources within or immediately next to the cancer site in order to provide a highly targeted, intense dose of radiation beyond a dose that is usually provided by EBRT. In addition, this form of radiation delivery helps to spare exposure to normal surrounding tissue. The radiation source can be implanted by means of needles or rods, seeds, beads, ribbons, or catheters placed into body cavities (vagina, abdomen, pleura), lumens within organs, or interstitial tissue compartments (breast, prostate). Multiple imaging techniques such as ultrasound, CT, or MRI are used to guide placement of radiation sources. Patients may have many fears or concerns about internal radiation, and the nurse explains the various approaches and safety precautions that will be used to protect the patient, family, and health care staff.

Brachytherapy may be delivered as a temporary or a permanent implant. Temporary applications are delivered as high-dose radiation (HDR) for short periods of time, while low-dose radiation (LDR) is delivered over a more extended period. The primary advantage of HDR brachytherapy is that treatment time is shorter, there is reduced exposure to personnel, and the procedure can be performed on an outpatient basis over several days. HDR brachytherapy can be used for intraluminal, surface, interstitial, and intracavitary lesions. Intraluminal HDR brachytherapy involves the insertion of catheters or hollow tubes into the lumens of organs so that the radioisotope can be delivered as close to the tumor bed as possible. Lesions in the bronchus, esophagus, rectum, or bile duct can be treated with this approach. Contact or surface application is used for treatment of tumors of the eye, such as retinoblastoma in children or ocular melanoma in adults.

Interstitial HDR implants, used in treating such malignancies as prostate, pancreatic, or breast cancer, may be temporary or permanent, depending on the site and radioisotope used. Based on the dose to be delivered (LDR or HDR), the implants may consist of seeds, needles, wires, strands, or small catheters positioned to provide a local radiation source. Prostate HDR therapy is one form of interstitial brachytherapy, in which radioactive strands or wires are placed, while the patient is under anesthesia, into hollow catheters that have been inserted in the perineum close to the prostate gland (Halperin et al., 2019).

Intracavitary radioisotopes are used to treat gynecologic cancers. In these malignancies, the radioisotopes are inserted into specially positioned applicators within the vagina. The applicator placement is verified by x-ray. Treatment can be achieved with either HDR or LDR brachytherapy sources, depending on the extent of disease. LDR therapy requires hospitalization because the patient is treated over several days. HDR intraoperative radiotherapy (IORT) has been used as a treatment approach for advanced gynecologic cancer that has spread to the paraaortic area or pelvic wall (Krengli, Pisani, Deantonio, et al., 2017).

Systemic radiotherapy (radiopharmaceutical therapy) involves oral or intravenous (IV) administration of a therapeutic radioactive isotope targeted to a specific tumor. Radioactive iodine (I-131) is a widely used form of systemic brachytherapy that is the primary treatment for thyroid cancer (Divgi, 2018). Radium-223 dichloride selectively targets prostate cancer bone metastases with high-energy, short-range alpha particles and is approved for the treatment of patients with symptomatic bone metastases and no known visceral metastatic disease (NCCN, 2019f). Radioisotopes are also used as a form of radioimmunotherapy for the treatment of refractory non-Hodgkin lymphoma (see Chapter 30 for more information on lymphoma).

Toxicity

A **toxicity** is an unfavorable and unintended sign, symptom, or condition associated with cancer treatment. Toxicities associated with radiation therapy are most often localized in the region being irradiated and may be increased if concomitant chemotherapy is given (Yarbro et al., 2018). Acute or early toxicities most often begin within 2 weeks of the initiation of treatment and occur when normal cells within the treatment area are damaged and cellular death exceeds regeneration. Body tissues most affected are those that normally proliferate rapidly, such as the skin, the epithelial lining of the gastrointestinal tract, and the bone marrow.

Altered skin integrity is common and can include **alopecia** (hair loss) associated with whole brain radiation. Other skin reactions, referred to as radiodermatitis, occur along a continuum ranging from erythema and dry desquamation (flaking of skin) to moist or wet desquamation (dermis exposed, skin oozing serous fluid) to, potentially, ulceration. Factors that contribute to the severity of radiodermatitis include the

dose and form of radiation; use of concurrent chemotherapy, immunotherapy, or targeted therapy; inclusion of skin folds in the irradiated area; increased age, poor nutritional status, chronic sun exposure, current smoking status, and the presence of medical comorbidities, such as diabetes or kidney failure (Yarbro et al., 2018). Symptoms of radiodermatitis may necessitate treatment interruption, delays, or cessation of therapy. Re-epithelialization occurs after treatments have been completed. Hyperpigmentation, a less severe radiation-associated skin reaction, may develop about 2 to 4 weeks after the initiation of treatment.

Alterations in oral mucosa secondary to radiation therapy in the head and neck region include stomatitis (inflammation of the oral tissues), decreased salivation and xerostomia (dryness of the mouth), and change in or loss of taste. Depending on the targeted region, any portion of the gastrointestinal mucosa may be involved, causing **mucositis** (inflammation of the lining of the mouth, throat, and gastrointestinal tract). For example, patients receiving thoracic irradiation for lung cancer may experience acute esophageal irritation—associated chest pain and dysphagia. Anorexia, nausea, vomiting, and diarrhea may occur if the stomach or colon is in the radiation field. Symptoms subside and gastrointestinal re-epithelialization occurs after treatments have been completed. Bone marrow cells proliferate rapidly, and if sites containing bone marrow (e.g., the iliac crest or sternum) are included in the radiation field, anemia, leukopenia (decreased white blood cells [WBCs]), and thrombocytopenia (a decrease in platelets) may result. The patient is then at increased risk for infection and bleeding until blood cell counts return to normal.

Systemic side effects are commonly experienced by patients receiving radiation therapy. These include fatigue, malaise, and anorexia that may be secondary to biochemical mediators released when tumor cells are destroyed. Fatigue is commonly reported as one of the most distressing cancer-related symptoms. According to Kessels, Husson, and Van Der Feltz-Cornelis (2018), up to 99% of patients with cancer undergoing radiation therapy will experience fatigue. Additionally, patients often report increased severity of fatigue when radiation therapy is used along with other cancer treatments. These early effects tend to be temporary and most often subside within 6 months of the cessation of treatment.

Late effects (approximately 6 months to years after treatment) of radiation therapy may occur in body tissues that were in the field of radiation. These effects are chronic, usually a result of permanent damage to tissues, loss of elasticity, and changes secondary to a decreased vascular supply. Severe late effects include fibrosis, atrophy, ulceration, and necrosis and may affect the lungs, heart, central nervous system, and bladder. With advances in treatment planning and the accuracy of treatment delivery, the occurrence of late toxicities has diminished. However, late or chronic symptoms, such as dysphagia, incontinence, cognitive impairment, and sexual dysfunction, may persist for several years with implications for survivors' overall health and quality of life (Kessels et al., 2018).

Nursing Management

Nurses anticipate, prevent, and work collaboratively with other providers to manage symptoms associated with radiation therapy in order to promote healing, patient comfort, and quality of life. Symptoms that are not appropriately managed may lead to poor outcomes as a result of interruptions, decreased doses, or early cessation of treatment (Lazarev, Gupta, Ghiassi-Nejad, et al., 2018; Wagner, Zhao, Goss, et al., 2018).

Ideally, nurses consider factors that may be predictive of radiation toxicities or radiosensitivity of tissues. In particular, advanced age, elevated radiation dose, and BMI have been associated with greater toxicity and symptoms (O'Gorman, Sasiadek, Denieffe, et al., 2015). The nature of the relationship between body mass index (BMI) and radiation toxicities is less clear. For example, a decreased BMI was found to be associated with an increased incidence of toxicities in women with cervical cancer (Rubinsak, Kang, Fields, et al., 2018); whereas, an increased BMI (obesity) was associated with increased incidence of late toxicities in men being treated for prostate cancer (Akthar, Liao, Eggener, et al., 2019). Consequently, the area of the body being irradiated must be used as the focus of nursing assessments of radiation toxicities.

In patients receiving EBRT, the nurse assesses the patient's skin, nutritional status, and general feelings of well-being throughout the course of treatment. Evidence-based protocols for nursing management of the toxicities associated with radiation therapy are used. If systemic symptoms such as fatigue occur the nurse explains that these symptoms are a result of the treatment and do not represent deterioration or progression of the disease. The nurse should recommend evidence-based interventions for the management of fatigue, which should include aerobic exercise, which is most effective when adherence is high (Kessels et al., 2018).

Protecting Caregivers

When the patient has a radioactive implant in place, the nurse and other health care providers need to protect themselves, as well as the patient, from the effects of radiation. Patients receiving internal radiation emit radiation while the implant is in place; therefore, contact with the health care team is guided by principles of time, distance, and shielding to minimize exposure of personnel to radiation. Specific instructions are provided by the radiation safety officer from the radiology department and specify the maximum time that can be spent safely in the patient's room, the shielding equipment to be used, and special precautions and actions to be taken if the implant is dislodged (Halperin et al., 2019). Safety precautions used in caring for a patient receiving brachytherapy include assigning the patient to a private room, posting appropriate notices about radiation safety precautions, having staff members wear dosimeter badges, making sure that pregnant staff members are not assigned to the patient's care, prohibiting visits by children or pregnant visitors, limiting visits from others to 30 minutes daily, and seeing that visitors maintain a 6-foot distance from the radiation source.

Patients with seed implants typically return home; radiation exposure to others is minimal. Information about any precautions, if needed, is provided to the patient and family members to ensure safety. Depending on the dose and energy emitted by a systemic radionuclide, patients may or may not require special precautions or hospitalization (Halperin et al., 2019). The nurse should explain the rationale for these precautions to keep the patient from feeling unduly isolated.

Chemotherapy

Chemotherapy involves the use of antineoplastic drugs in an attempt to destroy cancer cells by interfering with cellular functions, including replication and DNA repair (Norris, 2019). Chemotherapy is used primarily to treat systemic disease rather than localized lesions that are amenable to surgery or radiation. Chemotherapy may be combined with surgery, radiation therapy, or both to reduce tumor size preoperatively (neoadjuvant), to destroy any remaining tumor cells postoperatively (adjuvant), or to treat some forms of leukemia or lymphoma (primary). The goals of chemotherapy (cure, control, or palliation) must be realistic because they will determine the medications that are used and the aggressiveness of the treatment plan.

Cell Kill and the Cell Cycle

Each time a tumor is exposed to chemotherapy, a percentage of the tumor cells (20% to 99%, depending on dosage and agent) are destroyed. Repeated doses of chemotherapy are necessary over a prolonged period to achieve regression of the tumor. Eradication of 100% of the tumor is almost impossible; the goal of treatment is eradication of enough of the tumor so that the remaining malignant cells can be destroyed by the body's immune system (Norris, 2019).

Actively proliferating cells within a tumor are the most sensitive to chemotherapy (the ratio of dividing cells to resting cells is referred to as the growth fraction). Nondividing cells capable of future proliferation are the least sensitive to antineoplastic medications and consequently are potentially dangerous. However, the nondividing cells must be destroyed to eradicate the disease. Repeated cycles of chemotherapy or sequencing of multiple chemotherapeutic agents is used to achieve more tumor cell destruction by destroying the nondividing tumor cells as they begin active cell division.

Reproduction of both healthy and malignant cells follows the cell cycle pattern (see Fig. 12-2). All cells in the body (healthy and malignant) are affected by chemotherapy. The effect of chemotherapy on the body's cells is best described in relation to the cell cycle. The cell cycle time is the time required for one cell to divide and reproduce two identical daughter cells. The cell cycle of any cell has four distinct phases, each with a vital underlying function (Norris, 2019):

- G_1 phase—RNA and protein synthesis occurs
- S phase—DNA synthesis occurs
- G_2 phase—premitotic phase; DNA synthesis is complete, mitotic spindle forms
- Mitosis—duplicated chromosomes separate, and cell division occurs

Classification of Chemotherapeutic Agents

Chemotherapeutic agents may be classified by their mechanism of action in relation to the cell cycle. Agents that exert their maximal effect during specific phases of the cell cycle are termed *cell cycle–specific agents* (e.g., docetaxal, vinblastine, etoposide). These agents destroy cells that are actively reproducing by means of the cell cycle; most affect cells in the S phase by interfering with DNA and RNA synthesis. Other agents, such as plant alkaloids, are specific to the M phase, where they halt mitotic spindle formation. Chemotherapeutic agents that act independently of the cell cycle phases are termed *cell cycle–nonspecific agents* (e.g., busulfan, cisplatin, bleomycin). These agents usually have a prolonged effect on cells, leading to cellular damage or death. Many treatment plans combine agents that target different phases of the cell cycle to increase the number of vulnerable tumor cells killed during a treatment period (Dickens & Ahmed, 2018).

Chemotherapeutic agents are also classified by chemical group, each with a different mechanism of action. These include the alkylating agents, nitrosoureas, antimetabolites, antitumor antibiotics, topoisomerase inhibitors, plant alkaloids (also referred to as mitotic inhibitors), hormonal agents, and miscellaneous agents. The classification, mechanism of action, cell cycle specificity, and common side effects of select antineoplastic agents are listed in Table 12-7.

Chemotherapeutic agents from multiple categories may be used together to maximize cell destruction. Combination chemotherapy relies on agents with varying mechanisms, potential synergistic actions, and differing toxicities. The use of combination therapy also helps prevent the development of drug-resistant cells (Dickens & Ahmed, 2018).

Adjunct Chemotherapeutic Agents

In certain regimens, additional medications are given with chemotherapy agents to enhance activity or protect normal cells from injury. For example, leucovorin is often given with fluorouracil to treat colorectal cancer. Leucovorin, a compound similar to folic acid, helps fluorouracil bind with an enzyme inside of cancer cells and enhances the ability of fluorouracil to remain in the intracellular environment. Leucovorin also rescues normal cells from the toxic effects of high doses of methotrexate. When given at certain doses for the treatment of some forms of leukemia or lymphoma, methotrexate causes a folic acid deficiency in cells, resulting in cell death. Significant toxicity, including severe bone marrow suppression, mucositis, diarrhea and liver, and lung and kidney damage, can occur. Leucovorin helps to prevent or lessen these toxicities.

Administration of Chemotherapeutic Agents

Chemotherapy may be given in the hospital, outpatient center, or home setting by multiple routes. The route of administration depends on the type of agent; the required dose; and the type, location, and extent of malignant disease being treated. Standards for the safe administration of chemotherapy have been developed by the Oncology Nursing Society (ONS) and the American Society of Clinical Oncology (ASCO) (Neuss, Gilmore, Belderson, et al., 2017). Patient education is essential to maximize safety when chemotherapy is given in the home.

Dosage

The dosage of chemotherapeutic agents is based primarily on the patient's total body surface area, weight, previous exposure and response to chemotherapy or radiation therapy, and function of major organ systems. Dosages are determined to maximize cell kill while minimizing impact on healthy tissues and subsequent toxicities. The therapeutic effect may be compromised if modified and inadequate dosing is required due to

toxicities. Modification of dosage is often required if critical laboratory values or the patient's symptoms indicate unacceptable or dangerous toxicities. Chemotherapy treatment regimens include standard-dose therapy, dose-dense regimens (giving chemotherapy more frequently than standard treatment regimens), and myeloablative therapy for HSCT. For certain chemotherapeutic agents, there is a maximum lifetime dose limit that must be adhered to because of the danger of long-term irreversible organ complications (e.g., because of the risk of cardiomyopathy, doxorubicin has a cumulative lifetime dose limit of 550 mg/m^2).

Extravasation

Intravenously administered chemotherapy agents are additionally classified by their potential to damage tissue if they inadvertently leak from a vein into surrounding tissue; this leakage is called **extravasation**. The consequences of extravasation range from mild discomfort to severe tissue destruction, depending on whether the agent is classified as an irritant or vesicant. Irritant agents induce a localized inflammatory reaction at the infusion or injection site, but usually do not cause permanent tissue damage (Olsen, LeFebvre, & Brassil, 2019).

Unlike irritants, **vesicants** are agents that cause inflammation, tissue damage, and possibly necrosis of tendons, muscles, nerves, and blood vessels if extravasation occurs (Olsen et al., 2019). Although the mechanism of vesicant actions varies with each drug, some agents bind to cell DNA and cause cell death that progresses to involve neighboring cells, whereas other agents are metabolized into cells and cause a localized, painful reaction that usually improves over time. Sloughing and ulceration of the tissue may progress to tissue necrosis that is so severe that skin grafting becomes necessary. The full extent of tissue damage may take several weeks to become apparent. Examples of commonly used agents classified as vesicants include dactinomycin, daunorubicin, doxorubicin, nitrogen mustard, mitomycin, vinblastine, and vincristine. Chemotherapy administration safety standards require the availability of defined extravasation management procedures, including antidote order sets and accessibility of antidotes in all settings where vesicant chemotherapy is given (Neuss et al., 2017; Olsen et al., 2019).

Chemotherapy is given only by those who have the knowledge and established competencies for vesicant and extravasation management (Neuss et al., 2017; Olsen et al., 2019). Prevention and management of extravasation are essential. Vesicant chemotherapy should never be given in peripheral veins involving the hand or wrist. Peripheral administration is permitted for short-duration infusions only, and placement of the venipuncture site should be on the forearm area using a soft, plastic catheter. For any frequent or prolonged administration of antineoplastic vesicants, right atrial silastic catheters, implanted venous access devices, or peripherally inserted central catheters (PICCs) should be inserted to promote safety during medication administration and reduce problems with access to the circulatory system (Figs. 12-3 and 12-4).

Hypersensitivity Reactions

Although hypersensitivity reactions (HSRs) can occur with any medication, many chemotherapy agents pose a high risk and have been associated with life-threatening outcomes (Olsen et al., 2019). HSRs are a subgroup of adverse drug

TABLE 12-7 Select Antineoplastic Agents

Drug Class and Examples	Mechanism of Action	Cell Cycle Specificity	Common Side Effects
Alkylating Agents Busulfan, carboplatin, chlorambucil, cisplatin, cyclophosphamide, dacarbazine, altretamine ifosfamide, melphalan, nitrogen mustard, oxaliplatin, thiotepa	Bond with DNA, RNA, and protein molecules leading to impaired DNA replication, RNA transcription, and cell functioning; all resulting in cell death	Cell cycle— nonspecific	Bone marrow suppression, nausea, vomiting, cystitis (cyclophosphamide, ifosfamide), stomatitis, alopecia, gonadal suppression, renal toxicity (cisplatin), and development of secondary malignancies
Nitrosoureas Carmustine, lomustine or CCNU, semustine, streptozocin	Similar to alkylating agents; cross the blood–brain barrier	Cell cycle—nonspecific	Delayed and cumulative myelosuppression, especially thrombocytopenia; nausea, vomiting, pulmonary, hepatic, and renal damage
Topoisomerase I Inhibitors Irinotecan Topotecan **Topoisomerase II Inhibitors** Etoposide Teniposide	Induce breaks in the DNA strand by binding to enzyme topoisomerase, preventing cells from dividing	Cell cycle—specific (S phase)	Bone marrow suppression, diarrhea, nausea, vomiting, flulike symptoms (topotecan), rash (etoposide), hepatotoxicity (teniposide)
Antimetabolites 5-Azacytidine, capecitabine, cytarabine, edatrexate fludarabine, 5-fluorouracil (5-FU), gemcitabine, hydroxyurea, cladribine, 6-mercaptopurine, methotrexatepentostatin, 6-thioguanine	Interferes with the biosynthesis of metabolites or nucleic acids necessary for RNA and DNA synthesis; inhibits DNA replication and repair	Cell cycle—specific (S phase)	Nausea, vomiting, diarrhea, bone marrow suppression, stomatitis, renal toxicity (methotrexatepentostatin), hepatotoxicity (6-thioguanine), hand-foot syndrome (capecitibine)
Antitumor Antibiotics Bleomycin, dactinomycin, daunorubicin, doxorubicin, epirubicin, idarubicin, mitomycin, mitoxantrone, plicamycin	Interfere with DNA synthesis by binding DNA; prevent RNA synthesis	Cell cycle—nonspecific	Bone marrow suppression, nausea, vomiting, alopecia, anorexia, cardiac toxicity (daunorubicin, doxorubicin), red urine (doxorubicin, idarubicin, epirubicin), pulmonary fibrosis (bleomycin)
Mitotic Spindle Inhibitors *Plant alkaloids:* vinblastine, vincristine, vinorelbine	Arrest metaphase by inhibiting mitotic tubular formation (spindle); inhibit DNA and protein synthesis	Cell cycle—specific (M phase)	Bone marrow suppression (mild with vincristine), peripheral neuropathies, nausea and vomiting
Taxanes: paclitaxel, docetaxel	Arrest metaphase by inhibiting tubulin depolymerization	Cell cycle—specific (M phase)	Hypersensitivity reactions, bone marrow suppression, alopecia, peripheral neuropathies, mucositis
Epothilones: ixabepilone	Alters microtubules and inhibits mitosis	Cell cycle—specific (M phase)	Peripheral neuropathies, bone marrow suppression, hypersensitivity reactions, hepatic impairment
Hormonal Agents Androgens and antiandrogens, estrogens and antiestrogens, progestins and antiprogestins, aromatase inhibitors, luteinizing hormone-releasing hormone analogues, steroids	Bind to hormone receptor sites that alter cellular growth; block binding of estrogens to receptor sites (antiestrogens); inhibit RNA synthesis; suppress cytochrome P450 system	Cell cycle—nonspecific	Hypercalcemia, jaundice, increased appetite, masculinization, feminization, sodium and fluid retention, nausea, vomiting, hot flashes, vaginal estrogen dryness
Miscellaneous Agents Asparaginase, procarbazine	Inhibits protein, DNA, and RNA synthesis	Varies	Anorexia, nausea, vomiting, bone marrow suppression, hepatotoxicity, hypersensitivity reaction, pancreatitis
Arsenic trioxide	Causes fragmentation of DNA resulting in cell death; in acute promyelocytic leukemia, it corrects protein changes and changes malignant T-cells into normal white blood cells.		Nausea, vomiting, electrolyte imbalances, fever, headache, cough, dyspnea, electrocardiogram abnormalities

DNA, deoxyribonucleic acid; RNA, ribonucleic acid.

Adapted from Comerford, K. C., & Durkin, M. T. (2020). *Nursing 2020 drug handbook.* Philadelphia, PA: Wolters Kluwer; Neuss, M. N., Gilmore, T. R., Belderson, K., et al. (2017). 2016 updated American Society of Clinical Oncology/Oncology Nursing Society chemotherapy administration safety standards, including standards for pediatric oncology. *Oncology Nursing Forum, 44*(1), 31–43.

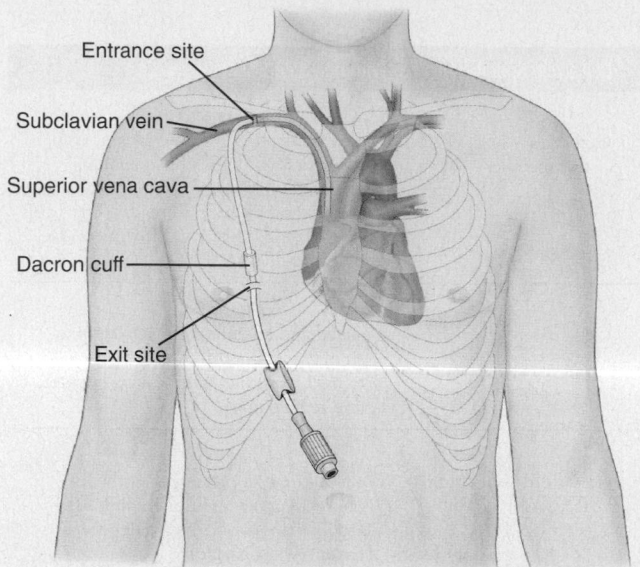

Figure 12-3 • Right atrial catheter. The right atrial catheter is inserted into the subclavian vein and advanced until its tip lies in the superior vena cava just above the right atrium. The proximal end is then tunneled from the entry site through the subcutaneous tissue of the chest wall and brought out through an exit site on the chest. The Dacron cuff anchors the catheter in place and serves as a barrier to infection.

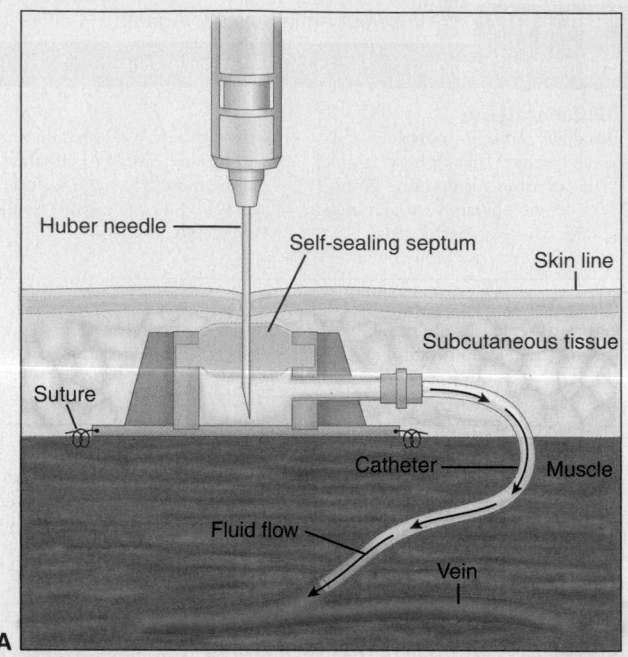

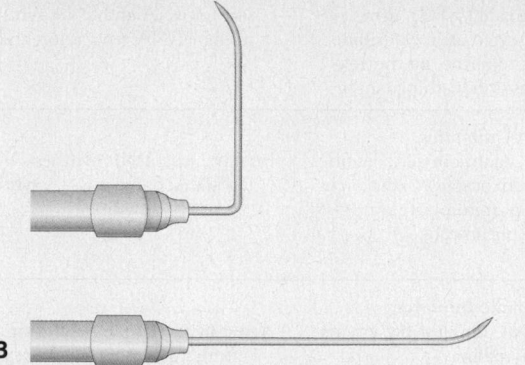

Figure 12-4 • Implanted vascular access device. **A.** A schematic diagram of an implanted vascular access device used for administration of medications, fluids, blood products, and nutrition. The self-sealing septum permits repeated puncture by Huber needles without damage or leakage. **B.** Huber needles used to enter the implanted vascular port. The 90-degree needle is used for top-entry ports for continuous infusions.

reactions that are unexpected and associated with mild or progressively worsening signs and symptoms, such as rash, urticaria, fever, hypotension, cardiac instability, dyspnea, wheezing, throat tightness, and syncope. Immediate HSRs may appear within 5 minutes and up to 6 hours of an infusion. Delayed HSRs may occur after the completion of the infusion. Although patients may or may not react to the first infusion of a chemotherapy agent, repeated exposure increases the likelihood of a reaction.

Most immediate HSRs are immunoglobulin E (IgE)-mediated reactions—an allergic reaction (Olsen et al., 2019). Examples of agents that may cause an allergic, IgE-mediated response include carboplatin, oxaliplatin, and L-asparaginase. However, some HSRs, such as anaphylactoid reactions, are non–IgE-mediated (nonallergic) and a result of cytokine release syndrome (CRS). Rituximab and cetuximab are examples of agents associated with non–IgE-mediated (nonallergic) HSRs. When signs and symptoms of HSR occur, the medication should be discontinued immediately, and emergency procedures initiated. Many institutions have developed specific protocols for responding to HSRs, including standing orders for administration of emergency medications (Roselló, Blasco, García Fabregat, et al., 2017). (See Chapter 33 for further discussion of allergic reactions.)

For some chemotherapeutic agents, especially if they are essential in the treatment plan, desensitization procedures may be possible, and the patient is retreated with the agent at reduced dosages or slower infusion rates. Premedication regimens are used for certain chemotherapy agents to prevent or minimize reactions.

Toxicity

Toxicity associated with chemotherapy can be acute or chronic. Cells with rapid growth rates (e.g., epithelium, bone marrow, hair follicles, sperm) are very susceptible to damage, and the effects may manifest in virtually any body system.

Gastrointestinal System

The most common side effects of chemotherapy are nausea and vomiting, which may persist for 24 to 48 hours; delayed nausea and vomiting may occur up to 1 week after administration. The experience of chemotherapy-induced nausea and vomiting (CINV) may affect quality of life, psychological status, nutrition, fluid and electrolyte status, functional ability, compliance with treatment, and utilization of health care resources (Natale, 2018). Comorbidities, the underlying malignancy, other treatment modalities, and medications, as well as symptoms (e.g., pain), may contribute to CINV. Acute CINV is experienced in the first 24 hours after chemotherapy with a maximal intensity after 5 to 6 hours; delayed CINV occurs 24 hours posttreatment and may last as many as 7 days with a maximal intensity 48 to 72 hours after drug administration (anticipatory nausea and vomiting, occurring prior to administration of chemotherapy, may be a conditioned response triggered by a stimulus such as the smell of the infusion setting, the sight of the nurse, or the outpatient center waiting room) (Olsen et al., 2019).

Several mechanisms are responsible for the occurrence of nausea and vomiting, including activation of multiple receptors found in the vomiting center of the medulla, the chemoreceptor trigger zone, the gastrointestinal tract, the pharynx, and the cerebral cortex. Activation of neurotransmitter receptors in these areas is thought to induce CINV. Stimulation may originate through peripheral, autonomic, vestibular, or cognitive pathways. The primary neuroreceptors known to be implicated in CINV are 5-hydroxytryptamine (5-HT or serotonin) and dopamine receptors (Olsen et al., 2019).

The approach for managing CINV is based on the knowledge of the probability of emesis of the chemotherapy agents used. Algorithms are used to prevent and treat CINV based on national guidelines that consider this classification of chemotherapy agents (NCCN, 2019g).

Corticosteroids, phenothiazines, sedatives, and histamines are helpful, especially when used in combination with serotonin blockers to provide antiemetic protection (NCCN, 2019g). In order to manage delayed nausea and vomiting, antiemetic medications may be combined and are given for the first week at home after chemotherapy. Nonpharmacologic approaches such as relaxation techniques, imagery, acupressure, or acupuncture can help decrease stimuli contributing to symptoms and may be most helpful for patients with anticipatory nausea and vomiting. Small, frequent meals, bland foods, and comfort foods may reduce the frequency or severity of symptoms.

Stomatitis is commonly associated with some chemotherapy agents because of the rapid turnover of epithelium that lines the oral cavity. The entire gastrointestinal tract is susceptible to mucositis. Antimetabolites and antitumor antibiotics are the major culprits in mucositis and other gastrointestinal symptoms, which can be severe in some patients.

Hematopoietic System

Many chemotherapy agents cause some degree of **myelosuppression** (depression of bone marrow function), resulting in leukopenia (decreased WBCs), **neutropenia** (decreased granulocytes), anemia (decreased red blood cells [RBCs]), thrombocytopenia (decreased platelets), and increased risk of infection and bleeding (Olsen et al., 2019). Depression of these cells is the usual reason for limiting the dose of the chemotherapy. Myelosuppression is predictable; for most agents, patients usually reach the point at which blood counts are lowest 7 to 14 days after chemotherapy has been given. During these 2 weeks, nurses anticipate associated toxicities, especially a fever associated with neutrophil count less than 1,500 cells/mm^3. Frequent monitoring of blood cell counts is essential, and patients are educated about strategies to protect against infection, injury, and blood loss, particularly while counts are low.

Other agents—colony-stimulating factors (granulocyte colony-stimulating factor [G-CSF] and granulocyte-macrophage colony-stimulating factor [GM-CSF])—can be given after chemotherapy to stimulate the bone marrow to produce WBCs, especially neutrophils, at an accelerated rate, thus decreasing the duration of neutropenia. G-CSF and GM-CSF decrease the episodes of infection and the need for antibiotics and allow for more timely treatment cycles of chemotherapy with less need to reduce the dosage. Erythropoietin (EPO) stimulates RBC production, thus decreasing the symptoms of treatment-induced chronic anemia and reducing the need for blood transfusions. Interleukin 11 (IL-11) (oprelvekin) stimulates the production of megakaryocytes (precursors to platelets) and can be used to prevent and treat severe thrombocytopenia but has had limited use because of toxicities, such as HSR; capillary leak syndrome; pulmonary edema; atrial arrhythmias; and nausea, vomiting, and diarrhea (Olsen et al., 2019).

Renal System

Some chemotherapy agents can cause renal dysfunction by damaging the blood vessels or filtering structures of the kidneys (Olsen et al., 2019). Clinical manifestations of renal dysfunction from conventional chemotherapy can range from the asymptomatic elevation of serum electrolytes and creatinine levels to acute kidney injury (Merchan, Jhaveri, Berns, et al., 2017). Cisplatin, methotrexate, and mitomycin are particularly toxic to the kidneys (Olsen et al., 2019). Damage to the kidneys may also result in impaired water secretion, leading to syndrome of inappropriate secretion of antidiuretic hormone (SIADH). Rapid tumor cell lysis after chemotherapy results in increased urinary excretion of uric acid, which can cause renal damage. In addition, intracellular contents are released into circulation, resulting in hyperkalemia, hyperphosphatemia, and hypocalcemia and obstructive nephropathy. (See later discussion of tumor lysis syndrome.)

The monitoring of laboratory values, including blood urea nitrogen (BUN), serum creatinine, creatinine clearance, and serum electrolytes is essential (Olsen et al., 2019). Adequate hydration and diuresis to prevent formation of uric acid crystals and administration of allopurinol may be used to prevent renal toxicity. Amifostine has demonstrated an ability to minimize renal toxicities associated with cisplatin, cyclophosphamide, and ifosfamide therapy.

Hemorrhagic cystitis is a bladder toxicity that can result from cyclophosphamide and ifosfamide, and alkylating agent (e.g., busulfan and thiotepa) therapy (Olsen et al., 2019). Hematuria can range from microscopic to frank bleeding with symptoms ranging from transient irritation during urination, dysuria, and suprapubic pain to life-threatening hemorrhage. Protection of the bladder focuses on aggressive IV hydration, frequent voiding, and diuresis.

Cardiopulmonary System

Several chemotherapy agents are associated with cardiac toxicity. Anthracyclines (e.g., daunorubicin, doxorubicin) are known to cause irreversible cumulative cardiac toxicities when total dosage reaches 400 mg/m^2 (Henriksen, 2018). If these agents are given in the presence of thoracic radiation therapy or other agents with cardiotoxicity potential, the cumulative dose limit is lower. Patients at increased risk for the development of cardiac toxicities include: extreme ages >65 years or <18 years, female gender, African American race, chest radiation, kidney failure, and preexisting cardiac disease (including hypertension) (Henriksen, 2018).

Dexrazoxane has been used on a limited basis as a cardio-protectant when doxorubicin is needed in individuals who have already received a cumulative dose limit and continuation of therapy is deemed beneficial. Patients with known cardiac disease (e.g., heart failure) are treated with lower doses or agents not known to be associated with cardiac toxicity. Cardiac ejection fraction (volume of blood ejected from the heart with each beat) and other signs of heart failure must be monitored closely.

Bleomycin, carmustine, busulfan, mitomycin C, and paclitaxel/docetaxel, among other agents, have toxic effects on lung function, such as alveolar damage, bronchospasm, pneumonitis, and pulmonary fibrosis (Olsen et al., 2019). Therefore, patients are monitored closely for changes in pulmonary function, including pulmonary function test results. Patients with known lung disease are treated with alternative agents not known to cause pulmonary toxicity. When pulmonary toxicity occurs, the agent is discontinued and patients are treated with steroids and other supportive therapies.

Capillary leak syndrome with resultant pulmonary edema is an effect of cytarabine, mitomycin C, cyclophosphamide, and carmustine (Olsen et al., 2019). Subtle onset of dyspnea and cough may progress rapidly to acute respiratory distress and subsequent respiratory failure. Patients who are at significant risk for capillary leak syndrome are monitored closely.

Reproductive System

Testicular and ovarian function can be affected by chemotherapeutic agents, resulting in possible infertility (Olsen et al., 2019). Women may develop problems with ovulation or early menopause, whereas men may develop temporary or permanent azoospermia (absence of spermatozoa). Because treatment may damage reproductive cells, banking of sperm is often recommended for men before treatment is initiated (Oktay, Harvey, Partridge, et al., 2018). Options available for women prior to initiation of chemotherapy include cryopreservation (freezing) of oocytes, embryos, or ovarian tissue. Patients and their partners are informed about potential changes in reproductive function resulting from chemotherapy. In addition, many chemotherapy agents are known or thought to be teratogenic. Therefore, patients are advised to use reliable methods of birth control while receiving chemotherapy and not to assume that infertility has resulted (Olsen et al., 2019).

Neurologic System

Chemotherapy-induced neurotoxicity, a potentially dose-limiting toxicity, can affect the central, peripheral, and autonomic nervous systems (Olsen et al., 2019). Neurotoxicity characterized by metabolic encephalopathy can occur with ifosfamide, high-dose methotrexate, and cytarabine. With repeated doses, the taxanes and plant alkaloids, especially vincristine, can cause cumulative peripheral nervous system damage with sensory alterations in the feet and hands. These sensations can be described as tingling, pricking, or numbness of the extremities; burning or freezing pain; sharp, stabbing, or electric shock–like pain; and extreme sensitivity to touch. If unreported by patients or undetected, progressive motor axon damage can lead to loss of deep tendon reflexes, with muscle weakness, loss of balance and coordination, and paralytic ileus.

Some chemotherapy agents (e.g., paclitaxel and gemcitabine) can cause severe peripheral neuropathies that may lead to diminished quality of life and functional abilities and result in dose reductions, a change in chemotherapy regimen, or early cessation of treatment (Haryani, Fetzer, Wu, et al., 2017). Although often reversible, these side effects may take many months to resolve or persist indefinitely. Along with the usual paresthesias of the hands and feet, oxaliplatin has a unique and frightening neurotoxicity presentation that is often precipitated by exposure to cold and is characterized by pharyngolaryngeal dysesthesia consisting of lip paresthesia, discomfort or tightness in the back of the throat, inability to breathe, and jaw pain (Olsen et al., 2019).

> ▶ *Quality and Safety Nursing Alert*
>
> *Patients receiving oxaliplatin must be instructed to avoid drinking cold fluids or going outside with hands and feet exposed to cold temperatures to avoid exacerbation of these symptoms for 3 to 4 days after therapy (Olsen et al., 2019). Cisplatin may cause peripheral neuropathies and hearing loss due to damage to the acoustic nerve.*

Cognitive Impairment

Many patients with cancer have trouble with remembering dates, multitasking, managing numbers and finances, organization, face or object recognition, inability to follow directions, feeling easily distracted, and motor and behavioral changes. Although not completely understood, these are viewed as symptoms of cognitive impairment. Cognitive impairment is a multidimensional concept involving a decline in information-handling processes in several domains, including attention and concentration, executive function, information processing speed, language, motor function, visuospatial skill, learning, and memory (Jansen, 2017). Commonly referred to by patients as "chemo brain" or "chemo fog," cognitive impairment has been associated with both cancer and cancer treatments, including surgery, radiation, chemotherapy, and targeted agents. The symptoms may be subtle or profound with potential negative effects on functional abilities, employment, independence, quality of life, and psychosocial status. Comorbidities, age, medications, pain, impaired nutrition, anemia, fatigue, fluid and electrolyte disturbances, organ dysfunction, infection, and hormonal imbalances are factors that may contribute to the experience of cognitive impairment and make it difficult to fully understand. Underlying mechanisms of cognitive impairment in patients with cancer being explored include neurotoxic effects, oxidative stress, hormonal changes, immune dysregulation, cytokine release, clotting, genetic predisposition, and accelerated aging processes (Jansen, 2017).

Fatigue

Cancer-related fatigue has been defined as an unusual, persistent, and subjective sense of tiredness that is not proportional to recent activity and interferes with usual functioning (NCCN, 2019f). Fatigue is a distressing side effect for most patients that greatly affects quality of life, during treatment and for months after treatment. The health care team works together to identify effective pharmacologic and nonpharmacologic approaches for fatigue management.

Nursing Management

Nurses play an important role in assessing and managing many of the problems experienced by patients receiving chemotherapy. Chemotherapy agents affect both normal and malignant cells; therefore, their effects are often widespread, affecting many body systems.

Laboratory and physical assessments of metabolic indices and the dermatologic, hematologic, hepatic, renal, cardiovascular, neurologic, and pulmonary systems are critical in evaluating the body's response to chemotherapy. These assessments are performed prior to, during, and after a course of chemotherapy to determine optimal treatment options, evaluate the patient's response, and monitor toxicity. Patients are monitored for long-term effects of chemotherapy after active treatment has been completed during the period of survivorship (see Chart 12-4).

Assessing Fluid and Electrolyte Status

Anorexia, nausea, vomiting, altered taste, mucositis, and diarrhea put patients at risk for nutritional and fluid and electrolyte disturbances. Therefore, it is important for the nurse to assess the patient's nutritional and fluid and electrolyte status on an ongoing basis and to identify creative ways to encourage an adequate fluid and dietary intake.

Assessing Cognitive Status

Nurses should assess patients routinely for indications of cognitive impairment. Prior to the initiation of treatment, patients and families should be informed about the possibility of cognitive impairment. Nursing assessment plays an important role in determining the need for referral for neurocognitive evaluation and intervention (Jansen, 2017).

Modifying Risks for Infection and Bleeding

Suppression of the bone marrow and immune system is expected and frequently serves as a guide in determining appropriate chemotherapy dosage but increases the risk of anemia, infection, and bleeding disorders. Nursing assessment and care address factors that would further increase the patient's risk. The nurse's role in decreasing the risk of infection and bleeding is discussed further in the Nursing Care of the Patient with Cancer section.

Administering Chemotherapy

Nurses must be aware of chemotherapy and other agents most associated with HSRs, strategies for prevention, signs and symptoms characteristic of HSRs, and the appropriate early and time-sensitive interventions for preventing progression to anaphylaxis. Nurses provide patient and family education that emphasizes two key points: the importance of adhering to prescribed self-administered premedication before presenting to the infusion center and recognizing and reporting the signs and symptoms to the nurse once the infusion has started. Patients and families are also educated about signs and symptoms that may occur at home following discharge from the infusion area that may warrant medication administration or immediate transport to the emergency department for further assessment and treatment.

The local effects of the chemotherapeutic agent are also of concern. The patient is observed closely during administration of the agent because of the risk and consequences of extravasation. Prevention of extravasation is essential and relies on vigilant nursing care (Neuss et al., 2017). Selection of peripheral veins, skilled venipuncture, and careful administration of medications are essential. Peripheral administration is limited to short duration (less than 1 hour; IV push or bolus) infusions using only a soft, plastic catheter placed in the forearm area (Olsen et al., 2019). Continuous infusion of vesicants that takes longer than 1 hour or are given frequently are given only via a central line, such as a right atrial silastic catheter, implanted venous access device, or PICC. These long-term venous access devices promote safety during medication administration and reduce problems with repeated access to the circulatory system (see Figs. 12-3 and 12-4). Indwelling or subcutaneous venous access devices require consistent nursing care. Complications include infection and thrombosis (Voog, Campion, Du Rusquec, et al., 2018).

Indications of extravasation during administration of vesicant agents include the following:

- Absence of blood return from the IV catheter
- Resistance to flow of IV fluid
- Burning or pain, swelling, or redness at the site

> ⚑ **Quality and Safety Nursing Alert**
>
> *If extravasation is suspected, the medication administration is stopped immediately.*

> **Chart 12-4**
>
> ## Potential Long-Term Complications of Cancer Chemotherapy
>
> Abnormalities in senses of taste, smell, and touch
> Abnormal balance, tremors, or weakness
> Avascular necrosis
> Cardiovascular toxicity (coronary artery disease, myocardial infarction, congestive heart failure, valvular heart disease, peripheral arterial disease)
> Decreased libido
> Dental caries
> Dry mouth
> Dysphagia
> Dyspnea on exertion
> Growth retardation in children
> Herpes infections (zoster and varicella)
> Hypothyroidism
> Immune dysfunction
> Infertility
> Osteoporosis
> Pericarditis (acute or chronic)
> Pneumococcal sepsis
> Pneumonitis (acute or chronic)
> Secondary cancers:
>   Acute myeloid leukemia
>   Myelodysplastic syndromes
>   Non-Hodgkin lymphomas
>   Solid tumors (especially bone and soft tissue, lung, breast)
>   Thyroid cancer
>   Thymic hyperplasia
>
> Adapted from Yarbro, C. H., Wujcik, D., & Gobel, B. H. (2018). *Cancer nursing: Principles and practice.* Burlington, MA: Jones & Bartlett Publishers.

An extravasation kit should be readily available with emergency equipment and antidote medications, as well as a quick reference for how to properly manage an extravasation of the specific vesicant agent used (although evidence-based data regarding effective antidotes are limited) (Neuss et al., 2017; Olsen et al., 2019). Nurses should refer to their organization's policy and procedures for reporting, managing, and documenting extravasation. Safety standards require the availability of defined extravasation management procedures, including antidote order sets and accessibility of antidotes in all settings where vesicant chemotherapy is given (Neuss et al., 2017). Recommendations and guidelines for managing vesicant extravasation, which vary with each agent, have been issued by individual medication manufacturers, pharmacies, and the ONS (Neuss et al., 2017; Olsen et al., 2019).

Difficulties or problems with administration of chemotherapeutic agents are brought to the attention of the primary provider promptly so that corrective measures can be taken to minimize local tissue damage.

The nurse evaluates the patient receiving neurotoxic chemotherapy, communicates findings with the medical oncologist, provides education to patients and families, and makes appropriate referrals for complete neurologic evaluation and occupational or rehabilitative therapies.

Preventing Nausea and Vomiting

Nurses are integral to the prevention and management of CINV. They collaborate with other members of the oncology care team to identify factors contributing to the experience of CINV and select effective antiemetic regimens that maximize currently available therapies. Nurses provide education for patients and families regarding antiemetic regimens and care for delayed CINV that may continue at home after the chemotherapy infusion has completed (NCCN, 2019g).

Managing Cognitive Changes

Although several approaches have been explored, no evidence-based guidelines for the prevention, treatment, or management of cognitive impairment have been established. Examples of nonpharmacologic approaches that nurses recommend to patients include exercise, natural restorative environmental intervention (walking in nature or gardening), and cognitive training programs (Jansen, 2017). Nurses should assist patients to address factors, such as fluid and electrolyte imbalances, nutrition deficits, fatigue, pain, and infection to minimize their contribution to cognitive impairment.

Managing Fatigue

Fatigue is a common side effect of chemotherapy. Nurses assist patients to explore the role that the underlying disease processes, combined treatments, other symptoms, and psychosocial distress play in the patient's experience of fatigue. In addition, nurses work with the patient and other team members to identify effective approaches for fatigue management (NCCN, 2019h).

Protecting Caregivers

Nurses involved in handling chemotherapeutic agents may be exposed to low doses of the agents by direct contact, inhalation, or ingestion (Menonna-Quinn, Polovich, & Marshall, 2019). Skin and eye irritation, nausea, vomiting, nasal mucosal ulcerations, infertility, low-birth-weight babies, congenital anomalies, spontaneous abortions, and mutagenic substances in urine have been reported in nurses preparing and handling chemotherapy agents. The Occupational and Safety Health Administration (OSHA), the ONS, hospitals, and other health care agencies have developed specific precautions for health care providers involved in the preparation and administration of chemotherapy and for handling materials exposed to body fluids of those who have received these hazardous agents (see Chart 12-5) (Neuss et al., 2017; Olsen et al., 2019). Nurses must be familiar with their institutional policies and procedures regarding personal protective equipment, handling and disposal of chemotherapy agents and supplies, and management of accidental spills or exposures. Emergency spill kits should be readily available in any treatment area where chemotherapy is prepared or given. Precautions must also be taken when handling any bodily fluids or excreta from the patient, as many agents are excreted unaltered in urine and feces. Nurses in all treatment settings have a responsibility to educate patients, families, caregivers, assistive personnel, and housekeepers concerning precautions.

Hematopoietic Stem Cell Transplantation

HSCT has been used to treat several malignant and nonmalignant diseases for many years (Yarbro et al., 2018). In adults, HSCT is most commonly used to treat certain hematologic malignancies (e.g., malignant myeloma, acute leukemia, non-Hodgkin lymphoma), and less commonly some solid tumors (e.g., germ cell tumors, breast cancer, neuroblastomas).

The process of obtaining hematopoietic stem cells (HSCs) has evolved over the years (Yarbro et al., 2018). Historically, HSCs were obtained in the operating room by harvesting large amounts of bone marrow tissue from a donor under general anesthesia. However, peripheral blood stem cell collection using the process of apheresis now accounts for the vast majority of HSCT procedures (Yarbro et al., 2018). The cells collected are specially processed and reinfused into the patient. This method of collecting HSCs is a safe and a more cost-effective means of collection than the process of harvesting of marrow. Stem cells can also be collected from umbilical cord blood harvested from the placenta of newborns at birth that is cryopreserved and stored for later use (Yarbro et al., 2018).

Types of Hematopoietic Stem Cell Transplantation

Types of HSCT are based on the source of donor cells and the treatment (conditioning) regimen used to prepare the patient for stem cell infusion and eradicate malignant cells (Yarbro et al., 2018). These include:

- *Allogeneic HSCT* (AlloHSCT): From a donor other than the patient (may be a related donor such as a family member or a matched unrelated donor from the National Bone Marrow Registry or Cord Blood Registry)
- *Autologous:* From the patient
- *Syngeneic:* From an identical twin
- *Myeloablative:* Consists of giving patients high-dose chemotherapy and, occasionally, total-body irradiation
- *Nonmyeloablative:* Also called *mini-transplants;* does not completely destroy bone marrow cells

Chart 12-5 Safety in Handling Chemotherapy for Health Care Providers

- When preparing (compounding, reconstituting) chemotherapy for administration, use the following safety equipment to prevent exposure through inhalation, direct contact, and ingestion:
  - Class II or III biologic safety cabinet (BSC)
  - Closed-system transfer devices
  - Puncture and leak-proof containers, IV bags
  - Needleless systems (e.g., IV tubing and syringes)
- If BSC is not available when preparing chemotherapy for administration, use the following safety equipment to minimize exposure:
  - Surgical N-95 respirator to provide respiratory and splash protection
  - Eye and face protection (both face shield and goggles) working at or above eye level or cleaning a spill
- When preparing or administering chemotherapy or handling linens and other materials contaminated with chemotherapy or blood and body fluids of patients receiving chemotherapy, wear the following for personal protection:
  - Double layer of powder-free gloves specifically designated for chemotherapy handling (the inner glove is worn under the gown cuff and the outer glove is worn over the cuff)
  - Long sleeve, disposable gowns (without seams or closures that can allow drugs to pass through) made of polyethylene-coated polypropylene or other laminate materials
- Linens contaminated with chemotherapy or blood and body fluids of patients receiving chemotherapy should be placed in the following:
  - Closed-system, puncture- and leak-proof containers labeled "hazardous: chemotherapy contaminated linens"

- Above referenced container maintained in the infusion center soiled utility room for outpatient settings
- Above referenced container maintained in the patient room or soiled utility room for inpatient settings
- Chemotherapy preparation equipment (e.g., syringes, tubing, empty vials, etc.), gowns, and gloves should be disposed of in:
  - Closed-system, puncture- and leak-proof containers labeled "hazardous: chemotherapy contaminated waste"
- Wash hands with soap and water after removing gloves used to prepare or administer chemotherapy or clean contaminated linens and other materials
- "Spill kits" with the appropriate gowns, gloves, disposable absorbent materials for cleansing large areas, and hazard sign should be kept in all areas where chemotherapy is prepared and given
- Implement a quality improvement program addressing safe chemotherapy handling that includes the following:
  - Standard operating policies and procedures for:
    - Chemotherapy handling, preparation, and disposal
    - Handling and disposal of chemotherapy spills
    - Handling and disposal of blood and body fluids and contaminated materials of patients receiving chemotherapy
- Conduct competency-based education, training, and performance evaluations regarding chemotherapy safety procedures at orientation and at subsequent regular intervals
- Medical monitoring program to identify indicators of exposure
- Root cause analysis for all chemotherapy spills and exposure incidents

Adapted from National Institute for Occupational Safety and Health. (2008). Personal protective equipment for health care workers who work with hazardous drugs. Retrieved on 7/11/2019 at: www.cdc.gov/niosh/docs/wp-solutions/2009-106/pdfs/2009-106.pdf?id=10.26616/NIOSHPUB2009106; Olsen, M. M., LeFebvre, K. B., & Brassil, K. (Eds.) (2019). *Chemotherapy and immunotherapy guidelines and recommendations for practice*. Pittsburgh, PA: Oncology Nursing Society.

AlloHSCTs are used primarily for diseases of the bone marrow and are dependent on the availability of a human leukocyte antigen–matched donor, which greatly limits the number of possible transplants. An advantage of AlloHSCT is that the transplanted cells should not be immunologically tolerant of a patient's malignancy and should cause a lethal **graft-versus-tumor effect** in which the donor cells recognize the malignant cells and act to eliminate them.

AlloHSCT may involve either myeloablative (high-dose) or nonmyeloablative (mini-transplant) chemotherapy (Yarbro et al., 2018). In ablative AlloHSCT, the recipient receives high doses of chemotherapy and possibly total-body irradiation to completely eradicate (ablate) the bone marrow and any malignant cells and help prevent rejection of the donor stem cells. The collected HSCs that are infused IV into the recipients travel to sites in the body where they produce bone marrow and establish themselves through the process of engraftment. Once engraftment is complete (8 to 10 days, sometimes longer), the new bone marrow becomes functional and begins producing RBCs, WBCs, and platelets. In nonablative AlloHSCT, the chemotherapy doses are lower and aimed at destroying malignant cells (without completely eradicating the bone marrow), thus suppressing the recipient's immune system to allow engraftment of donor stem cells. The lower doses of chemotherapy, associated with less organ toxicity and infection, can be used for older patients or those with underlying organ dysfunction for whom high-dose chemotherapy would be prohibitive (Yarbro et al., 2018). After engraftment, it is hoped that the donor cells will create a graft-versus-tumor effect. Before engraftment, patients are at high risk for infection, sepsis, and bleeding. Side effects of the high-dose chemotherapy and total-body irradiation can be acute and chronic (Negrin, 2018; Yarbro et al., 2018). Acute side effects include headache, alopecia, nausea, vomiting, mucositis, diarrhea, fluid and electrolyte imbalances, and acute kidney injury. Chronic side effects include infertility; pulmonary, cardiac, liver, and kidney dysfunction; osteoporosis and avascular bone necrosis; diabetes; and secondary malignancies.

During the first 30 days after the conditioning regimen, AlloHSCT patients are at risk for developing hepatic sinusoidal obstructive syndrome (HSOS) (previously referred to as veno-oclusive disease) related to chemotherapy-induced inflammation of the sinusoidal epithelium (Negrin & Bonis, 2019). Inflammation causes embolization of RBCs, resulting in destruction, fibrosis, and occlusion of the sinusoids. Clinical manifestations of HSOS may include weight gain, hepatomegaly, increased bilirubin, and ascites. Although various approaches have been used to treat HSOS, evidence-based strategies have not emerged. The use of peripheral stem cells, specific chemotherapy dosing, and nonmyeloablative regimens have been associated with a decreased incidence (Negrin, 2018; Yarbro et al., 2018).

Graft-versus-host disease (GVHD), a major cause of morbidity and mortality in 30% to 50% of the allogeneic transplant population, occurs when the donor lymphocytes initiate an immune response against the recipient's tissues (e.g., skin, gastrointestinal tract, liver) during the beginning of engraftment (Yarbro et al., 2018). The donor cells view the recipient's tissues as foreign or immunologically different from what they recognize as "self" in the donor. To prevent GVHD, patients receive immunosuppressant drugs, such as cyclosporine, methotrexate, tacrolimus, or mycophenolate mofetil.

GVHD may be acute, occurring within the first 100 days, or chronic, occurring after 100 days (Yarbro et al., 2018). Clinical manifestations of acute GVHD include diffuse rash progressing to blistering and desquamation similar to second-degree burns; mucosal inflammation of the eyes and the entire gastrointestinal tract with subsequent diarrhea that may exceed 2 L per day; and biliary stasis with abdominal pain, hepatomegaly, and elevated liver enzymes progressing to obstructive jaundice. The first 100 days or so after AlloHSCT is crucial for patients; the immune system and blood-making capacity (hematopoiesis) must recover sufficiently to prevent infection and hemorrhage.

Autologous HSCT (AuHSCT) is considered for patients with disease of the bone marrow who do not have a suitable donor for AlloHSCT or for patients who have healthy bone marrow but require bone marrow–ablative doses of chemotherapy to cure an aggressive malignancy (Yarbro et al., 2018). The most common malignancies treated with AuHSCT include lymphoma and multiple myeloma. However, the use of AuHSCT has gained increasing acceptance in treating neuroblastoma, Ewing sarcoma, and germ cell tumors. Stem cells are collected from the patient and preserved for reinfusion; if necessary, they are treated to kill any malignant cells within the marrow, called *purging*. The patient is then treated with ablative chemotherapy and, possibly, total-body irradiation to eradicate any remaining tumor. Stem cells are then reinfused. Until engraftment occurs in the bone marrow sites of the body, there is a high risk of infection, sepsis, and bleeding. Acute and chronic toxicities from chemotherapy and radiation therapy may be severe. The risk of HSOS is also present after autologous transplantation. No immunosuppressant medications are necessary after AuHSCT, because the patient does not receive foreign tissue. A disadvantage of AuHSCT is the risk that tumor cells may remain in the bone marrow despite high-dose chemotherapy (conditioning regimens).

Syngeneic transplants result in less incidence of GVHD and graft rejection; however, there is also less graft-versus-tumor effect to fight the malignancy. For this reason, even when an identical twin is available for marrow donation, another matched sibling or even an unrelated donor may be the most suitable donor to combat an aggressive malignancy (Yarbro et al., 2018).

Nursing Management

Nursing care of the patient undergoing HSCT is complex and demands a high level of skill. The success of HSCT is greatly influenced by nursing care throughout the transplantation process.

Implementing Care Before Treatment

All patients must undergo extensive evaluations before HSCT to assess the current clinical status of the disease. Nutritional assessments, extensive physical examinations, organ function tests, and psychological evaluations are conducted. Blood work includes assessing past infectious antigen exposure (e.g., hepatitis virus, cytomegalovirus, herpes simplex virus, human immunodeficiency virus, syphilis). The patient's social support systems and financial and insurance resources are also evaluated. Informed consent and patient education about the procedure and care before and after HSCT are vital.

Providing Care During Treatment

Skilled nursing care is required during the treatment phase of HSCT when high-dose chemotherapy (conditioning regimen) and total-body irradiation are given. The acute toxicities of nausea, diarrhea, mucositis, and hemorrhagic cystitis require close monitoring and symptom management by the nurse.

Nursing management during stem cell infusion consists of monitoring the patient's vital signs and blood oxygen saturation; assessing for adverse effects, such as fever, chills, shortness of breath, chest pain, cutaneous reactions, nausea, vomiting, hypotension or hypertension, tachycardia, anxiety, and taste changes; and providing strategies for symptom control, ongoing support, and patient education. During stem cell infusion, patients may experience adverse reactions to the cryoprotectant dimethylsulfoxide (DMSO) used to preserve the harvested stem cells. Less common toxicities include neurologic and renal impairment (Yarbro et al., 2018).

> ► **Quality and Safety Nursing Alert**
>
> *Until engraftment of the new marrow occurs, the patient undergoing HSCT is at high risk for death from sepsis and bleeding.*

A cluster of symptoms referred to as engraftment syndrome may occur during the neutrophil recovery phase in both allogeneic and autologous transplants. Clinical features of this syndrome vary widely but may include noninfectious fever associated with skin rash, weight gain, diarrhea, and pulmonary infiltrates, with improvement noted after the initiation of corticosteroid therapy rather than antibiotic therapy (Mutahar & Al-Anazi, 2017). Until engraftment is well established, the patient requires support with blood products and hematopoietic growth factors.

Potential infections may be bacterial, viral, fungal, or protozoan in origin. During the first 30 days following transplant, the patient is most at risk for developing reactivations of viral infections, including herpes simplex, EBV, cytomegalovirus, and varicella zoster. Mucosal denudement poses a risk for *Candida* (yeast) infection locally and systemically. Pulmonary toxicities offer the opportunity for fungal infections such as *Aspergillus*. Renal complications arise from the nephrotoxic chemotherapy agents used in the conditioning regimen or those used to treat infection (amphotericin B, aminoglycosides). A neutropenic diet is usually prescribed for patients to decrease the risk of exposure to foodborne infections from bacteria, yeast, molds, viruses, and parasites (Yarbro et al., 2018).

Tumor lysis syndrome and acute tubular necrosis are also potential complications after HSCT. Nursing assessment for signs of these complications is essential for early identification and treatment. GVHD requires skillful nursing assessment to detect early effects on the skin, liver, and gastrointestinal tract. HSOS resulting from the conditioning regimens used can result in fluid retention, jaundice, abdominal pain, ascites, tender and enlarged liver, and encephalopathy. Pulmonary complications, such as pulmonary edema, interstitial pneumonia, and other pneumonias, often complicate recovery.

Providing Care After Treatment

Nursing care following HSCT includes care of recipients and donors. These are discussed in the following sections.

Caring for Recipients

Ongoing nursing assessment during follow-up visits is essential to detect late effects of therapy after HSCT, which may occur 100 days or more after the procedure (Yarbro et al., 2018). Late effects include infections (e.g., varicella-zoster infection), restrictive pulmonary abnormalities, and recurrent pneumonias. Infertility often results due to total-body irradiation, chemotherapy, or both as components of the ablative regimen. Chronic GVHD can involve the skin, liver, intestine, esophagus, eyes, lungs, joints, and vaginal mucosa. Cataracts may also develop after total-body irradiation.

There is a high potential of psychological distress following an HSCT, which has been associated with delayed recovery, mortality, and increased rates of complications, such as GVHD (Hermioni, Christina, Melanie, et al., 2019). Thus, psychosocial assessments by nursing staff must be ongoing and a priority. In addition to the multiple physical and psychological stressors affecting patients at each phase of the transplantation experience, the nature of the treatment and patient experience can place extreme emotional, social, financial, and physical demands on family, friends, and donors. Nurses assess the family and other caregivers' needs and provide education, support, and information about resources.

Caring for Donors

Like HSCT recipients, donors also require nursing care. They may experience mood alterations, decreased self-esteem, and guilt from feelings of failure if the transplantation fails. Family members must be educated and supported to reduce anxiety and promote coping during this difficult time. In addition, they must also be assisted to maintain realistic expectations of themselves as well as of the patient.

Immunotherapy and Targeted Therapy

Immunotherapy

Immunotherapy involves the use of medications or biochemical mediators to stimulate or suppress components of the immune system to kill cancer cells (ACS, 2019g). Over the past decade, advances in the understanding of the immune system and about its interaction with cancer have led to significant advances in immunotherapy. This has dramatically changed how patients with cancer are treated and has resulted in improvements in overall survival for many forms of cancer. There are several types of immunotherapy currently being used to treat cancer, including nonspecific immunotherapies, monoclonal antibodies, checkpoint inhibitors, cancer vaccines, and chimeric antigen receptor (CAR) T–cell therapy. Many immunotherapies are targeted therapies. Targeted therapies are discussed later in this chapter.

Nonspecific Immunotherapy

Nonspecific immunotherapy does not target the cancer cell directly, but rather boosts the immune system to enhance cancer cell destruction alone or along with other cancer treatments, such as chemotherapy or radiation therapy (ACS, 2019f). Common nonspecific immunotherapy agents include bacille Calmette-Guérin (BCG) and cytokines (interferon, interleukins, and colony-stimulating factors).

BCG is one of the earliest immunotherapy agents used to treat cancer. BCG is a live attenuated strain of *Mycobacterium bovis*, which is closely related to the bacterium that causes tuberculosis in people. BCG is most commonly used to treat localized bladder cancer (ACS, 2019h). When instilled into the bladder, BCG serves as an antigen to stimulate an immune response. The intention is that the stimulated immune system will then eradicate malignant cells. Common toxicities associated with BCG therapy include mild flulike symptoms (e.g., fever, chills, malaise), bladder burning/discomfort, urinary frequency, and blood tinged urine, which typically last 2 to 3 days after treatment (ACS, 2019h).

The most commonly used nonspecific immunotherapy agents are cytokines. **Cytokines** are messenger substances that may be released by a cell to create an action at that site or may be carried by the bloodstream to a distant site before being activated; they are also called *biochemical* or *inflammatory mediators*. These substances are produced primarily by cells of the immune system to enhance or suppress the production and functioning of other components of the immune system and thus can be used to treat cancer or the adverse effects of some cancer treatments. Cytokines are grouped into families, such as interferons (IFNs), interleukins (ILs), and colony-stimulating factors. Colony-stimulating factors were described earlier in this chapter for their supportive role in myelosuppressive treatment modalities. (Refer to Chapter 31 for more detailed discussion of the immune system.)

IFNs are cytokines with antiviral, antitumor, and immunomodulatory (inhibition or stimulation of the immune system) properties. Multiple antitumor effects of IFNs include antiangiogenesis, direct destruction of tumor cells, inhibition of growth factors, and disruption of the cell cycle (Yarbro et al., 2018). IFNs are used on a limited basis for the treatment of some solid and hematologic cancers. Similar to IFNs, ILs have immunomodulatory effects on other components of the immune response. IL-2, an interleukin made in a laboratory, has been approved as a treatment option for advanced kidney cancer and metastatic melanoma in adults.

Adverse effects such as fever, myalgia, nausea, and vomiting, as seen with IFN and IL-2 therapy, may not be life-threatening. However, other adverse effects with these therapies (e.g., capillary leak syndrome, pulmonary edema, hypotension) may become life-threatening. These severe toxicities have restricted the use of IFN and IL-2 clinically and have prompted clinicians to seek alternative anticancer therapies (Waldmann, 2018).

Monoclonal Antibodies (MoAbs)

MoAbs, another type of immunotherapy, have become available through technologic advances, enabling investigators to grow and produce targeted antibodies for specific malignant cells. Theoretically, this type of specificity allows MoAbs to destroy the cancer cells and spare normal cells. The specificity of MoAbs is dependent on identifying key antigen proteins on the surface (outside) of tumors that are not present on normal tissues. When the MoAb attaches to the cell surface antigen, an important signal transduction pathway for communication between the malignant cells and the extracellular environment is blocked. The results may include an inability to initiate apoptosis, reproduce, or invade surrounding tissues.

The production of MoAbs involves injecting tumor cells that act as antigens into mice. B-cell lymphocytes in the spleen of the mouse produce immunoglobulin (antibodies) made in response to the injected antigens. Antibody-producing B-cells are combined with a cancer cell that can grow indefinitely in culture medium and continue producing more antibodies.

The combination of spleen cells and the cancer cells is referred to as a hybridoma. From hybridomas that continue to grow in the culture medium, the desired antibodies are harvested, purified, and prepared for diagnostic or therapeutic use (see Fig. 12-5). Advances in genetic engineering have led to the production of MoAbs with combinations of mouse and human components (*chimeric MoAbs*) or all-human components (*human MoAbs*). MoAbs made with human genes have greater immunologic properties and are less likely to cause allergic and infusion reactions (Norris, 2019).

MoAbs (with names usually ending in -mab) are large particles that work on extracellular molecules, which are usually administered intravenously. Several MoAbs are used for the treatment in cancer using various extracellular (on the cell membrane) and intracellular targets. Trastuzumab targets the HER2 protein, an error of gene overexpression found in breast and other cancers (ACS, 2019g). Rituximab is a MoAb that binds specifically with the CD20 antigen expressed by non-Hodgkin lymphoma and B-cell chronic lymphocytic leukemia.

Some MoAbs are used alone (termed naked MoAbs), whereas others are used in combination with agents that facilitate their antitumor actions (termed conjugated MoAbs). Ibritumomab tiuxetan, a MoAb conjugated with a radioactive isotope, is used in the treatment of certain types of lymphoma (ACS, 2019g). MoAbs are also used as aids in

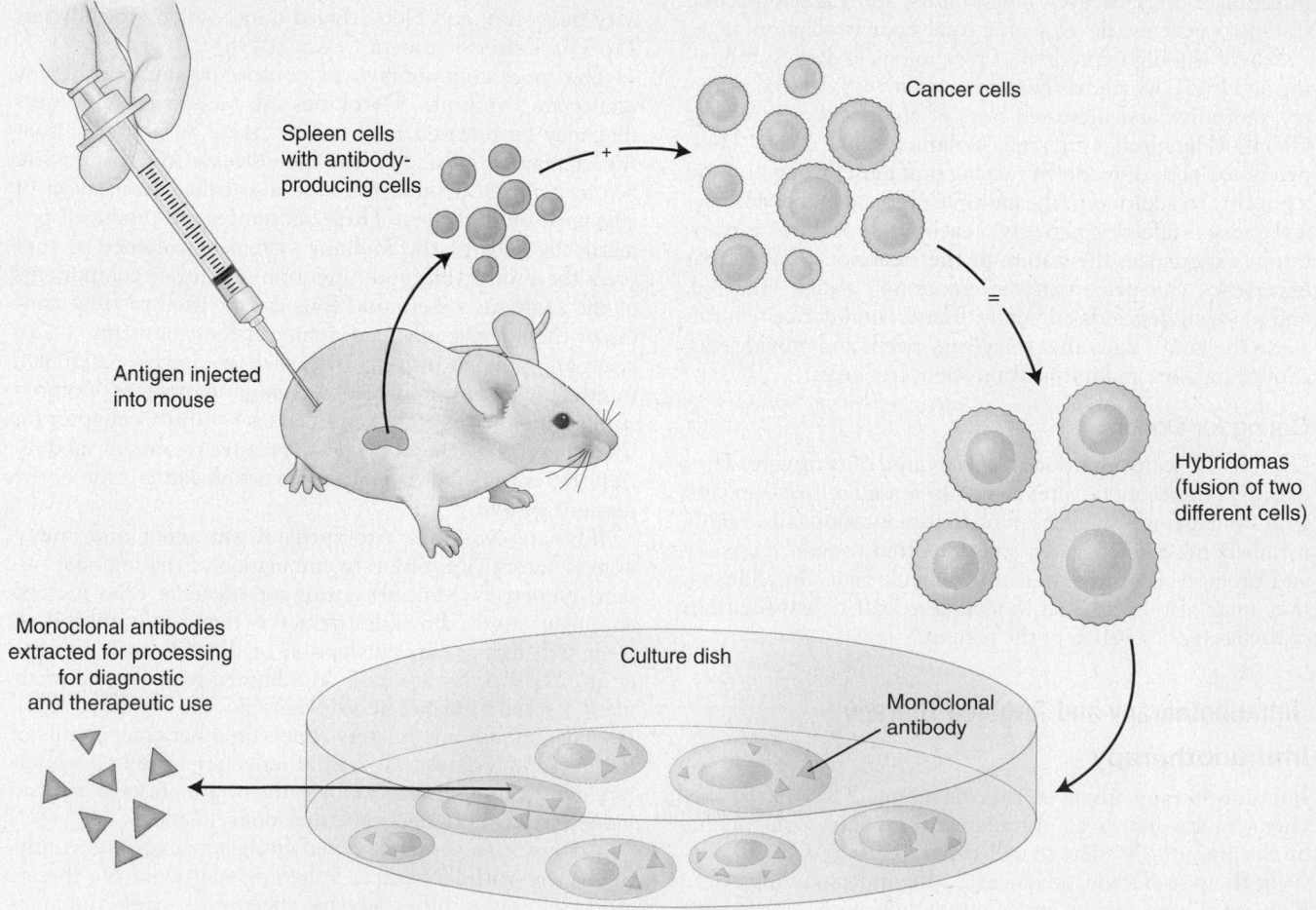

Figure 12-5 • Antibody-producing spleen cells are fused with cancer cells. This process produces cells called *hybridomas*. These cells, which can grow indefinitely in a culture medium, produce antibodies that are harvested, purified, and prepared for diagnostic or treatment purposes.

diagnostic evaluation of both primary and metastatic tumors through radiologic imaging and laboratory techniques (Olsen et al., 2019). For example, the process of immunohistochemistry uses a MoAb tagged with a stain that binds with the protein of interest, providing a visual stain for the presence or absence of the protein (Bishop, Cole, Zhang, et al., 2018). This type of test is used to identify the presence of estrogen and progesterone receptors on breast cancer cells to see if the cells will be responsive to hormonal agents. Immunohistochemistry testing is also used to detect several proteins associated with hereditary nonpolyposis colon cancers. MoAbs are used to assist in the diagnosis of ovarian, colorectal, breast, and prostate cancers and some types of leukemia and lymphoma. MoAbs are also used in purging residual tumor cells from peripheral stem cell collections for patients who are undergoing HSCT after high-dose cytotoxic therapy. Researchers continue to explore the development and use of MoAbs, either alone or in combination with other substances such as radioactive materials, chemotherapy agents, toxins, and hormones.

MoAbs are associated with both common and unique toxicities (ACS, 2019g). Common toxicities associated with MoAbs include flulike symptoms (e.g., chills, weakness, malaise) headache, nausea and vomiting, diarrhea, rash, proteinuria, hypothyroidism, hypertension, and hepatoxicity. Although mild to moderate allergic and infusion reactions are more commonly associated with chimeric MoAbs, severe HSRs have been seen with MoAb infusions. Other toxicities are specific to the substance attached to the MoAbs.

Checkpoint Inhibitors

The immune system uses inhibitory and acceleratory pathways and immune checkpoints to regulate the antitumor response (ACS, 2019g; Bayer, Amaya, Baniewicz, et al., 2017). Checkpoints are specific proteins on T–cells that need to be blocked (or inactivated) to initiate an immune response against cancer cells. Cancer cells use different mechanisms to avoid recognition by the immune system, thus allowing them to grow unchecked. Immune checkpoint inhibitors block proteins that diminish immune system function and prevent T lymphocytes from identifying and destroying cancer cells. When these mechanisms are blocked, the "brakes are off" and T–cells are released, allowing the immune system to identify and mount an immune response against cancer cells (this is termed an antitumor response).

Recently, special type of MoAbs were developed that block specific checkpoints on T–cells to enhance cancer cell surveillance and destruction by the immune system. These MoAbs are called check point inhibitors. Three classes of checkpoint inhibitors have been approved by the FDA for the treatment of cancer, including cytotoxic T-lymphocyte antigen-4 (CTLA-4), anti-programmed cell death protein 1 (PD-1) receptor, and anti-programmed cell death ligand 1(PD-L1) (Olsen et al., 2019). The CTLA-4 is an intracellular protein within resting T lymphocytes. CTLA receptors on certain T–cells prevent the overactivation of the immune response; thus, blocking this receptor allows for a persistent T–cell antitumor response (Bayer et al., 2017). An example of an immune check point inhibitor that blocks CTLA-4 is ipilimumab. Ipilimumab is currently approved for some forms of melanoma, colorectal cancer, and kidney cancer.

PD-1 is a checkpoint protein on activated T–cells that when bound to another protein called PD-L1 prevents the immune system from mounting a response against normal cells (Olsen et al., 2019). PD-L1 is also located on some cancer cells, which disrupts immune surveillance and the antitumor response, thus allowing cancer cells to grow unchecked. Immune checkpoint inhibitors that block PD-1 (e.g., nivolumab and pembrolizumab) and PD-L1 (e.g., atezolizumab, avelumab, durvvalumab) are used to treat a wide range of cancers, including: melanoma of the skin, non–small cell lung cancer, kidney cancer, bladder cancer, head and neck cancers, and Hodgkin lymphoma.

Immune checkpoint inhibitors exhibit a different toxicity profile from other anticancer therapies. Thus, the unique toxicities associated with immune checkpoint inhibitors are termed "immune-related adverse events" (irAes). These irAes are thought to be related to an inflammatory response to immune-related activity that can affect any organ or organ system; however, the exact etiology is not fully known (Olsen et al., 2019). IrAes often present with a delayed onset and the severity of toxicities can range from mild to potentially life-threatening. The most common irAes include dermatologic (e.g., rash and pruritus); gastrointestinal (e.g., diarrhea and colitis); pulmonary (e.g., pneumonitis); renal (e.g., nephritis); endocrine (e.g., hypophysitis [inflammation of the pituitary gland], thyroiditis, hyper- and hypothyroidism) toxicities. Prompt recognition of immune-related toxicities is essential to prevent treatment delays and to ensure prompt initiation of effective management strategies, which often include the use of anti-inflammatory medications, such as corticosteroids (Olsen et al., 2019).

Cancer Vaccines

Cancer vaccines mobilize the body's immune response to prevent or treat cancer. These vaccines contain either portions of cancer cells alone or portions of cells in combination with other substances (adjuvants) that can augment or boost immune responses. *Autologous* vaccines are made from the patient's own cancer cells, which are taken from tumor tissue obtained during biopsy or surgical intervention. The cancer cells are killed and prepared for injection back into the patient. *Allogeneic* vaccines are made from cancer cell lines that are immortalized cells that were originally obtained from other people who had a specific type of cancer. These cancer cells are grown in a laboratory and eventually killed and prepared for injection.

Prophylactic vaccines prevent disease. Three vaccines have been approved by the FDA for the prevention of HPV. HPV2 (Cervarix), recommended for use in females only, protects against HPV types 16 and 18 that are responsible for about 70% of all cervical cancers (ACS, 2019g). HPV4 (Gardasil) provides protection against four HPV types (6, 11, 16, and 18) and is recommended for use in both genders. HPV9 (Gardasil-9), recommended for both males and females, protects against nine HPV types associated with cervical, anal, vaginal, and vulvar cancers. HPV9 also protects against genital warts. All of the HPV vaccines are given as a series of three doses over 6 months. Although the role of HPV vaccines in prevention of oropharyngeal cancers related to HPV16 has not been fully established, there are preliminary data to suggest effectiveness (Wang, Dickie, Sutavani, et al., 2018).

Vaccines are also used to treat existing disease. Therapeutic vaccines kill existing cancer cells and inhibit further cancer development. Sipuleucel-T (ACS, 2019g) is indicated for men with metastatic prostate cancer that is no longer responding to hormone therapy. It is the only therapeutic vaccine currently FDA approved. Therapeutic vaccines do not cure cancer but are associated with improved patient survival.

Chimeric Antigen Receptor (CAR) T–Cell Immunotherapy

A new addition to the treatment of cancer with immunotherapy is chimeric antigen receptor (CAR) T–cell therapy. CAR T–cell is a type of targeted immunotherapy that uses tumor-specific antigen recognition to target specific malignancies. CAR T–cell therapy involves the use of genetically modified T–cells to kill cancer cells (Lamprecht & Dansereau, 2019; Olsen et al., 2019). For example, in CART-19 therapy, cluster of differentiation (CD)–19 is the target antigen. This antigen is commonly overexpressed in acute lymphoblastic leukemia and certain types of non-Hodgkin lymphoma (Bayer et al., 2017). The only two CAR T–cell immunotherapy agents currently FDA-approved both target CD19 (tisagenlecleucel and axicabtagene ciloleucel). Tisagenlecleucel is approved to treat adults with relapsed or refractory non-Hodgkin lymphoma and young adults (up to 25 years old) with relapsed or refractory acute lymphoblastic leukemia. Axicabtagene and ciloleucel are approved to treat certain types of relapsed or refractory B-cell lymphoma (Olsen et al., 2019).

The process of making CAR genetically modified T–cells begins with collecting T–cells. T–cells may be collected from the patient (autologous) or collected from a healthy donor (allogeneic) using leukapheresis. The T–cells are sent to the laboratory where they are genetically altered by adding a specific chimeric antigen receptor. This process takes several weeks to make enough CAR T–cells needed for therapy. When there are enough CAR T–cells (based on the patient's body weight), the cells are infused to the patient in a procedure similar to a blood transfusion (Lamprecht & Dansereau, 2019). A few days before a CAR T–cell infusion, the patient may be given chemotherapy to reduce the number of other immune cells to make room for the new CAR T–cells to expand and proliferate. Once infused, the CAR T–cells will continue to grow (up to a year or more postinfusion) while binding with tumor-specific antigen to kill cancer cells.

The two most common toxicities related to CAR T–cell therapy are CRS and neurologic toxicities (Anderson & Latchford, 2019). CRS, also referred to as cytokine storm, is the most common toxicity of CAR T–cell therapy and is experienced to some degree by most patients. During therapy, the infused CAR T–cells and other immune cells stimulate the release of inflammatory cytokines resulting in a systemic inflammatory response, which usually occurs within a few days of treatment. Clinical manifestations of CRS most commonly include fever (hallmark sign), tachycardia, chills, myalgias, arthralgias, and fatigue. Although, if the CRS is severe, hypotension, dyspnea, hypoxia, respiratory distress, coagulopathies, and end-organ toxicities may occur (Anderson & Latchford, 2019). Neurologic toxicities can range from a headache and mild confusion to cerebral edema or intracranial hemorrhage. Although the exact etiology of neurologic toxicities related to CAR T–cell therapy is not yet known, it has been postulated that increased vascular permeability, increased cytokine levels, and the ability of the cells to cross the blood–brain barriers may be factors (Anderson & Latchford, 2019). Other toxicities seen with CAR T–cell therapy include tumor lysis syndrome, myelosuppression (neutropenia, anemia, and thrombocytopenia), and hypogammaglobulinemia.

Targeted Therapies

Normal cell growth is regulated by well-defined communication pathways between the environment surrounding the cell and the internal cell environment, the nucleus, and the intracellular cytoplasm. The cell membrane contains important protein receptors that respond to signals transmitted from the external cell environment and transmit that signal to the internal cell environment using enzymatic pathways called *signal transduction pathways*. Although normal cells have transduction pathways, scientific advances have led to the recognition that cancer, at the cellular level, is characterized by deregulated cell signaling transduction pathways (both intra- and extracellular pathways), as well as altered cell membrane receptors and proteins that play an important role in tumor initiation, growth, and spread (Norris, 2019). This improved understanding of cancer cell behavior has allowed scientists to develop molecular-based therapies, called targeted therapies.

Targeted therapies involve the use of agents to kill or prevent the spread of cancer cells by targeting a specific part of the cell, with less negative effects on healthy cells than conventional chemotherapy. These agents specifically target (like a lock and key mechanism) receptors, proteins, signal transduction pathways, and other processes to prevent the continued growth of cancer cells (NCI, 2019d). Targeted therapies allow for cancer treatment to be "personalized" to the unique molecular basis of the patient's cancer. To determine if a patient would benefit from a targeted therapy, the patient's cancer cells must be evaluated in the laboratory to determine if they have enough of the target molecule for the therapy to be effective. Thus, not all patients with the same type of cancer may benefit from the same targeted treatment. New unique molecular targets are regularly being identified, resulting in the discovery of many new targeted agents over the past decade (Olsen et al., 2019).

There are two main types of targeted therapies: monoclonal antibodies (previously discussed in the immunotherapy section) and small molecule drugs. Small molecule drugs (with names usually ending in -nib) target specific molecules on the inside of the cancer cells and are usually administered orally. Targeted therapies are further classified in accordance with their mechanism of action (or the unique molecule targeted) (Olsen et al., 2019). There is a good amount of overlap in the mechanism of action of these agents because many targeted therapies work via complex pathways and have more than one target molecule. An overview of common categories of targeted therapies including tyrosine kinase inhibitors, EGFR inhibitors, vascular endothelial growth factor/receptor inhibitors, multikinase inhibitors, and proteasome inhibitors are discussed below using small molecule drugs as exemplars.

Tyrosine kinase inhibitors block a group of enzymes called tyrosine kinases, which regulate many cellular functions including signaling cellular growth and division (Olsen et al., 2019). Overexpression (too much) of tyrosine kinase is found in some cancer cells. Blocking these enzymes may prevent cancer cell growth. An example of a tyrosine kinase inhibitor is imatinib mesylate, which is used to treat cancers with an overexpression of BCR-ABL, such as chronic myeloid leukemias, acute lymphoblastic leukemias, and gastrointestinal stromal tumors (Comerford & Durkin, 2020).

Epidermal growth factor receptor (EGFR) inhibitors block a specific surface protein called epidermal growth factor (EGF), which is present on both normal and cancer cells. The overexpression of EGF in cancer cells promotes division and growth; thus, blocking EGFR can result in decreased cancer cell proliferation (Olsen et al., 2019). For example, erlotinib blocks the tyrosine kinase domain of the EGF protein to reduce cancer cell growth. Elotinib is approved to treat advanced non–small cell lung cancer and advanced pancreatic cancer in combination with chemotherapy (Comerford & Durkin, 2020).

Vascular endothelial growth factor/receptor inhibitors (VEGFRIs) are agents that block vascular endothelial growth factor, which is produced by cells to stimulate **angiogenesis** (the growth of new blood vessels). As such, VEGFRIs inhibit angiogenesis, which prevents cancer cells from receiving adequate amounts of oxygen and nutrients needed for growth. VEGFRIs are used to treat various types of cancer, including soft tissue sarcomas, and thyroid, lung, kidney, and colorectal cancers. For example, axitinib is a VEGFRI approved to treat advanced renal cell carcinoma (kidney cancer) after failure of one prior systemic therapy (Comerford & Durkin, 2020; Olsen et al., 2019).

Multikinase inhibitors (MKIs) inhibit several intracellular and extracellular (surface) kinases that play a role in cellular growth and metastatic processes to reduce cancer cell growth and replication (Comerford & Durkin, 2020; Olsen et al., 2019). Sorafenib is an example of an MKI that inhibits several kinase receptor pathways (e.g., c-KIT, PDGFR, RAF, RET, VEGFR-1, VEGFR-2, VEGFR-3). Sorafenib is used to treat several different cancer types including liver, kidney, and thyroid cancers.

Proteasome inhibitors inhibit proteasome cellular complexes, that prevent certain enzymes from making proteins (Comerford & Durkin, 2020; Olsen et al., 2019). Proteasome helps maintain intracellular homeostasis by regulating proteins that facilitate cell division and prevent cell death. Thus, blocking proteasome interferes with cell division and enhances cancer cell death. An example of a proteasome inhibitor is bortezomib, which is approved to treat multiple myeloma and certain types of lymphoma (e.g., mantle cell lymphoma).

Common toxicities that occur with targeted therapies include mucositis, nausea, vomiting, diarrhea, abdominal pain, electrolyte and fluid imbalances, skin rash, impaired wound healing, hypertension, and myelosuppression (decreased red blood cells, WBCs, and platelets) (Comerford & Durkin, 2020; Olsen et al., 2019). Peripheral neuropathy can also occur with some proteasome inhibitors. More serious complications of targeted therapy include cardiotoxicity (e.g., brotezomib) and hepatoxicity (e.g., sorafenib).

Nursing Management

Patients receiving immunotherapy and targeted therapy have many of the same needs as patients undergoing other conventional cancer treatments. However, manipulation and stimulation of the immune system also creates unique challenges (Bayer et al., 2017; Olsen et al., 2019). Nurses must be aware of the adverse effects of these therapies and recognize the signs and symptoms of serious reactions to emergently institute appropriate interventions and supportive care. Nurses monitor patients for the impact of adverse effects on performance status and quality of life so that appropriate measures can be implemented to improve patient outcomes. The nurse must also assist in planning and evaluating patient care, and assess the need for education, support, and additional resources for both the patient and the family.

Patient education is important, as many of the toxicities are not only a source of physical discomfort, but they may also affect quality of life and patient adherence to treatment (Olsen et al., 2019; Yarbro et al., 2018). Key points of education related to immunotherapy and targeted therapy include providing information about (Bayer et al., 2017; Olsen et al., 2019; Yarbro et al., 2018):

- prescribed treatment(s) and associated toxicities to allow for prompt recognition of potentially treatment-limiting (e.g., peripheral neuropathy) and life-threatening (i.e., heart and liver failure) toxicities;
- the importance of reporting new symptoms or the exacerbation of existing symptoms promptly to the health care provider;
- how and when to contact the primary provider and seek the assistance of emergency medical services; and
- how to provide self-care during and after treatment.

Patient and family education should also include attention to general standards of care relevant to all anticancer treatment (such as principles of infection control, hand hygiene, nutrition and hydration, safe sexual practices, good skin care) and instructions to notify the health care provider about any newly prescribed or over-the-counter medications, including herbs, vitamins, and dietary supplements (Bayer et al., 2017).

Promoting Home, Community-Based, and Transitional Care

The nurse educates patients about self-care and assists in providing for continuing care. Some cancer immunotherapy and targeted therapies can be given subcutaneously (e.g., trastuzumab and denosumab) by the patient or family members at home. As needed, the home health nurse educates the patient and family how to administer these agents and monitors the use of appropriate technique as well as safe disposal of sharps and contaminated materials. The nurse also provides education about toxicities and helps the patient and family identify strategies to manage common side effects of immunotherapy and targeted therapy.

The use of oral medications to treat cancer has risen greatly in the past several years, especially with advances in targeted therapies, many of which are given by mouth. Since 2015, more than 50 oral anticancer medications were approved by FDA and it is estimated between 25% and 35% of all anticancer therapies being developed are orally administered (Dusetzina, Huskamp, Winn, et al., 2018; Kays, 2018). The rising use of oral therapies shifts the responsibility for delivery of treatment to patients and families in the home setting. Treatment approaches with newer mechanisms of action and associated toxicities, as well as the transition of responsibility to patients and families, increase the need for nurses to identify factors affecting adherence and to develop strategies to address adherence barriers (see Table 12-8).

TABLE 12-8	Strategies for Promoting Adherence to Oral Antineoplastic Agents

Assess for factors that may interfere with adherence to oral antineoplastic agents; develop plan of care that identifies and addresses specific assessment findings.

Barriers to Adherence	Strategies for Promoting Adherence
Sociodemographic Factors • Limited financial resources • Competing priorities for financial resources • Joblessness • Limited or no insurance • Racial or ethnic disparities • Lower level of education • Poor health literacy • Illiteracy • Non–English speaking • Lack of transportation • Lack of or limited social support • Rural residence	• Refer to financial counseling through health care facility, local nonprofit health/oncology support/advocacy, or other nonprofit community advocacy organizations. • Refer to social worker for referrals as described above and/or for disability applications through employer or Social Security Administration, Medicaid, or Medicare applications. • Explore patient assistance programs for costs of health care, copays, medications, household costs, transportation services (costs or availability), and home care available through nonprofit organizations, oncology support/advocacy or other nonprofit community advocacy organizations, religious institutions, philanthropic organizations, pharmaceutical industry–sponsored programs, health care institution–specific programs; assist with financial documentation and application procedures as needed. • Explore assistance programs for other priorities competing for financial resources (e.g., for utility costs, gas, child care, food). • Assist patient to identify family, friends, or other available supports to assist with activities of daily living, household responsibilities, errands, shopping, meals, transportation or other responsibilities; assist with delegation of needs and schedules of availability if needed. • Assess preferred method of learning (e.g., verbal, visual, written materials); tailor instructional materials to patient needs, including language. • Include family, significant other, and friends in education whenever feasible. • Use return demonstration of behaviors and devices used to support adherence. • Provide contact information that spans 24 h for questions or problems. • Contact patient by phone or other means (e-mail, texting, video conference, telehealth) to assess for concerns in between follow-up visits to provider. • Encourage patient to use adherence reminders, such as pill boxes, medication calendars, checklists, medication diaries, alarms on cell phone or other devices/timers; explore availability of programmed telephone reminder services, text messages from family member, friend, or other caregiver; review diary at each visit. • Instruct patient to bring pill bottles to each follow-up visit; perform pill counts to monitor adherence. • Send postcard reminder to patient weekly (or less often) or 1 wk prior to due date for medication refill. • Refer to home care for continued education and follow-up on adherence. • Identify local pharmacies that supply oral medications for cancer therapies. Instruct patients to contact nurse if the pharmacy cannot fill the prescription within 24 h. • Remind patients to anticipate need for adequate supply of medications prior to travel or vacation.
Age • Older adults; especially those >75 yrs	• Ensure that printed education materials and instructions are printed in black using at least 14-point sans serif font such as Arial or Calibri. • Use illustrated education materials. • Review and revise adherence strategies if patient status declines or changes. • Explore availability of alarmed medication box.
Beliefs • Oral medications less effective or important than IV treatments • Fatalism about disease outcomes	• Provide education regarding oral versus IV medications. • Discuss goals of care and ongoing assessment of response to treatment.
Comorbidities • Preexisting chronic disease • Vision or hearing impairments	• Communicate with primary care and other providers involved in care of patient regarding current cancer disease status and treatment; collaborate with other providers for ongoing management of nononcology issues or exacerbation of issues that may impact cancer treatment adherence. • Collaborate with appropriate resources to assist with special needs and assistive devices for vision or hearing impairments.
Polypharmacy • Multiple medications for comorbidities or cancer treatment and symptom management	• Review all medications prescribed by oncology physicians and other providers involved in care of patient for preexisting chronic disease. • Assess patient use of over-the-counter medications and other agents. • Consult with pharmacist to identify medications and other agents that may be contraindicated or that may interfere with antineoplastic regimen. • Collaborate with all providers prescribing medications in order to simplify or reduce number of required medications if possible. • Provide patient, family, or other caregiver education regarding specific instructions when multiple medications are required. • Provide written checklist for patient to utilize daily to check off each medication when taken. • Check if patient prescriptions allow for refills; prescriptions should be for a finite period of time that concludes with next scheduled visit.

TABLE 12-8	Strategies for Promoting Adherence to Oral Antineoplastic Agents (continued)
Barriers to Adherence	**Strategies for Promoting Adherence**
Psychiatric, Psychological, or Cognitive Concerns • Psychiatric disease • Depression • Cognitive impairments • Anxiety	• Avoid initial education regarding oral medications at the same time of first provider visit; have patient and other learners return for another appointment to see nurse for education and follow-up with subsequent visit if deemed to be at high risk for adherence challenges. • Discuss with provider the necessity for referral to psychiatrist to evaluate need for psychotropic medications. • Refer patient for professional mental health counseling as needed. • Identify additional supports for care and education as discussed earlier.
Disease Factors • Symptoms such as pain, nausea, fatigue, skin rashes, etc. • Impaired mobility	• Proactively assess and manage symptoms related to underlying disease or treatments. • Provide patient, family, or other caregivers education about expected side effects and management strategies. • Instruct patient to premedicate with antiemetic as prescribed 30 min prior to taking oral antineoplastic agent if needed for nausea or vomiting. • Identify additional supports for care as discussed earlier. • Assess need for referral to home physical or occupational therapy to address impaired mobility and need for assistive devices.
Communication Issues • Patient–Clinician • Clinician–Clinician	• Establish rapport and allow patients, families, and other caregivers time and opportunity to ask questions. • Do not assume adherence to oral antineoplastic agents; emphasize the value and importance of adherence and assess potential barriers consistently throughout course of treatment at each follow-up visit. • Communicate with primary provider regarding current cancer disease status, treatment and information regarding antineoplastic agents, such as drug–drug interactions, expected toxicities, and toxicities requiring prompt intervention.

IV, intravenous.

Adapted from Olsen, M. M., LeFebvre, K. B., & Brassil, K. (Eds.). (2019). *Chemotherapy and immunotherapy guidelines and recommendations for practice.* Pittsburgh, PA: Oncology Nursing Society.

The nurse collaborates with physicians, social workers, third-party payers, and pharmaceutical companies to help the patient obtain reimbursement or support for the cost of oral cancer therapies and other required medications (Dusetzina et al., 2018). The nurse also reminds the patient about the importance of keeping follow-up appointments with the primary provider and assesses the patient's need for symptom management related to the underlying diseases or adverse effects of treatment. Home health nurses maintain communication with the primary provider regarding patient adherence and tolerance of treatment so that changes in care can be implemented in a timely fashion.

Complementary, Alternative, and Integrative Health Therapies

Integrative health care is viewed as a comprehensive, interdisciplinary approach to preventing and treating illness and promoting health that brings together complementary, alternative, and conventional therapies. The use of an integrative approach to health and wellness has grown within mainstream health care settings in the United States, particularly within oncology care (National Center for Complementary and Integrative Health [NCCIH], 2018).

Individuals use complementary approaches to prevent and treat cancer, although there are no data to support efficacy. Patients also use complementary approaches to manage symptoms related to cancer and associated treatments; some approaches are supported by clinical research while others

are not. It is estimated that as many as 67% of people diagnosed with cancer use some form of complementary medicine (Wanchai, Armer, Smith, et al., 2017). However, many patients do not routinely communicate complementary practices to their health care providers because they usually are not asked about its use; they withhold the information, fearing that their provider would not approve, or they feel that the use of these approaches will not affect the conventional treatment they are receiving.

Although many complementary modalities can be a source of comfort and emotional support for patients, assessment of complementary therapy use is important for patient safety. Patients often perceive vitamins and dietary supplements as harmless, natural products that have no side effects or potential toxicities. In patients receiving any conventional therapies, the use of herbs or botanicals may interfere with drug metabolism, decrease or increase desired effects, or contain elements of uncertain pharmacologic capacities (NCCIH, 2018). Deep tissue massage and other manipulative therapies are contraindicated in patients with open wounds, radiodermatitis, thrombocytopenia, VTE, and coagulation disorders, and in those taking anticoagulants. See Chapter 4 for more information on complementary, alternative, and integrative health therapies.

COVID-19 Considerations

The novel coronavirus disease 2019 (COVID-19) pandemic began in Wuhan, China, in late 2019. Since that time, several risks for both severe acute respiratory syndrome coronavirus 2 (SARS-CoV-2) infection and pathogenesis to COVID-19 have been posed (see Chapter 66). Epidemiologic findings from early data in China suggest that having cancer could be an important risk factor for becoming infected with SARS-CoV-2 as well as increasing the risk of mortality from COVID-19 (Deng, Yin, Chen, et al., 2020). Many cancer clinicians and researchers worldwide recognized during the early days of the pandemic that there was an urgent need to identify idiosyncratic risks and treatment issues that revolve around managing adults with both COVID-19 and cancer. As a result, the COVID-19 and Cancer Consortium (CCC19) was established (see Resources section for link to CCC19). An early cohort study sponsored by CCC19 of 928 patients from the United States, Canada, and Spain with either a history of cancer or active malignancy identified prognostic factors for mortality and severe COVID-19 (Kuderer, Choueiri, Shah, et al., 2020). Overall 13% of the patients died (Kuderer et al., 2020), a higher mortality rate than the 5.6% case fatality rate for all adult patients in the United States with COVID-19 (Johns Hopkins University & Medicine Coronavirus Resource Center, 2020). The researchers identified the following factors as associated with an increase in 30-day mortality: older age, male sex, a history of smoking, having two or more comorbidities, having an active cancer, and having received azithromycin plus hydroxychloroquine during treatment for COVID-19 (Kuderer et al., 2020). The four most common presenting symptoms of COVID-19 in these patients included fever, cough, fatigue or malaise, and dyspnea; the same as for all patients with COVID-19 (Kuderer et al., 2020). There was no association between having recently had surgery and either having severe COVID-19 or dying, suggesting that surgery indicated for patients with cancer should not be postponed due to pandemic concerns (Kuderer et al., 2020). CCC19 will continue to analyze registry data of patients with COVID-19 and cancer and publicize noteworthy findings as they become available, to facilitate optimal management of patients with COVID-19 and cancer (Kuderer et al., 2020).

Nursing Care of the Patient with Cancer

The outlook for patients with cancer has greatly improved because of scientific and technologic advances. However, as a result of the underlying disease or various treatment modalities, patients with cancer may experience a variety of secondary problems such as reduced WBC counts, infection, bleeding, skin and nutritional problems, pain, fatigue, and psychological stress. Chart 12-6 provides a nursing care plan for the patient with cancer.

Maintaining Tissue Integrity

Some of the most frequently encountered disturbances of tissue integrity include stomatitis, skin and tissue reactions to radiation therapy, cutaneous toxicities associated with targeted therapy, alopecia, and metastatic skin lesions.

Stomatitis

Mucositis, a common side effect of radiation and some types of chemotherapy, refers to an inflammatory process involving the mucous membranes of the oral cavity and the gastrointestinal tract. **Stomatitis**, a form of mucositis, is an inflammatory process of the mouth, including the mucosa and tissues surrounding the teeth. Stomatitis is characterized by changes in sensation, erythema (mild redness), and edema or, if severe, by painful ulcerations, bleeding, and secondary infection. Stomatitis commonly develops within 3 to 14 days after patients receive certain chemotherapeutic agents (e.g., 5-fluorouracil and doxorubicin), immunotherapies (e.g., IL-2 and nivolumab); and targeted therapies (e.g., temsirolimus and everolimus). Stomatitis affects up to 100% of patients undergoing high-dose chemotherapy with HSCT, 90% of patients with malignancies of the head and neck receiving radiotherapy, and up to 40% of patients receiving standard-dose chemotherapy (Eilers, Asakura, Blecher, et al., 2017; Olsen et al., 2019). Stomatitis may be worse in patients with head and neck cancers who receive combined modality therapy of both radiation and chemotherapy. When severe, stomatitis can lead to interruptions, delays, and modifications in the course of treatment, all of which may contribute to less desirable patient outcomes. Severe oral pain can significantly affect swallowing, nutritional intake, speech, quality of life, coping abilities, and willingness to adhere to treatment regimens. In addition, stomatitis may lead to more frequent health care visits, hospitalizations, and increased health care costs (Berger, Schopohl, Bollig, et al., 2018). Stomatitis and mucositis are attributed to a cascade of molecular processes and submucosal endothelial cell destruction that begin almost immediately after the initiation of radiation and certain types of chemotherapy, prior to the development of signs and symptoms. Mucositis develops because of a sequence of related and interacting biologic events, culminating in injury and apoptosis of basal epithelial cells, leading to the loss of epithelial renewal, atrophy, and ulceration. Gram-positive and gram-negative organisms can invade the ulcerated tissue and result in infection.

Nursing assessment begins with an understanding of the patient's usual practices for oral hygiene and identification of individuals at risk for stomatitis. Oral cavity assessment is performed daily or at each patient visit (Olsen et al., 2019). Risk factors and comorbidities associated with stomatitis include poor oral hygiene, general debilitation, existing dental disease, prior irradiation to the head and neck region, impaired salivary gland function, the use of other medications that dry mucous membranes, myelosuppression, tobacco use, previous cancer treatment with a stomatotoxic agent or radiation therapy, diminished renal function, impaired nutritional status, and both older (>65 years) and younger (<20 years) ages (Olsen et al., 2019). The patient is also assessed for dehydration, infection, pain, and nutritional impairment resulting from mucositis.

Optimal evidence-based prevention and treatment approaches for stomatitis remain limited but continue to be studied across disciplines (Bowen, Gibson, Coller, et al., 2019; Eilers et al., 2017). Most clinicians agree that maintenance of good oral hygiene, including brushing, flossing, rinsing, and dental care, is necessary to minimize the risk of oral complications associated with cancer therapies.

Palifermin, an IV-administered synthetic form of human keratinocyte growth factor, is beneficial in the prevention and management of stomatitis in patients with hematologic malignancies who are preparing for HSCT and in those

(text continued on page 349)

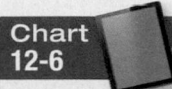

Chart 12-6   PLAN OF NURSING CARE
The Patient with Cancer

NURSING DIAGNOSIS: Risk for infection associated with inadequate defenses related to myelosuppression secondary to radiation or antineoplastic agents

GOAL: Prevention of infection

Nursing Interventions	Rationale	Expected Outcomes

1. Assess patient for evidence of infection.
  a. Check vital signs every 4 hours.
  b. Monitor white blood cell (WBC) count and differential each day.
  c. Inspect all sites that may serve as entry ports for pathogens (IV sites, wounds, skin folds, bony prominences, perineum, and oral cavity).
2. Report fever (≥38.3°C [101°F] or ≥38°C [100.4°F] for >1 hour) (see Table 12-10), chills, diaphoresis, swelling, heat, pain, erythema, exudate on any body surfaces. Also report change in respiratory or mental status, urinary frequency or burning, malaise, myalgias, arthralgias, rash, or diarrhea.
3. Obtain cultures and sensitivities as indicated before initiation of antimicrobial treatment (wound exudate, sputum, urine, stool, blood).
 	
4. Initiate measures to minimize infection.
  a. Discuss with patient and family:
    1. Placing patient in private room if absolute WBC count <1000/mm³.
    2. Importance of patient avoiding contact with people who have known or recent infection or recent vaccination.
  b. Instruct all personnel in careful hand hygiene before and after entering room.
  c. Avoid rectal or vaginal procedures (rectal temperatures, examinations, suppositories; vaginal tampons).
 	
  d. Use stool softeners to prevent constipation and straining.
  e. Assist patient in practice of meticulous personal hygiene.
  f. Instruct patient to use electric razor.
  g. Encourage patient to ambulate in room unless contraindicated.
  h. Provide patient and family education on food hygiene and safe food handling.
 	
  i. Each day change water pitcher, denture cleaning fluids, and respiratory equipment containing water.
	1. Signs and symptoms of infection may be diminished in the immunocompromised host. Prompt recognition of infection and subsequent initiation of therapy will reduce morbidity and mortality associated with infection.
	
	2. Early detection of infection facilitates early intervention.
	
	3. Tests identify the organism and indicate the most appropriate antimicrobial therapy. The use of inappropriate antibiotics enhances proliferation of additional flora and encourages growth of antibiotic-resistant organisms.
	
	4. Exposure to infection is reduced.
	  a. Preventing contact with pathogens helps prevent infection.
	
	  b. Hands are significant source of contamination.
	
	  c. Incidence of rectal and perianal abscesses and subsequent systemic infection is high. Manipulation may cause disruption of membrane integrity and enhance progression of infection.
	  d. Minimizes trauma to tissues
	
	  e. Prevents skin irritation
	
	  f. Minimizes skin trauma
	  g. Minimizes chance of skin breakdown and stasis of pulmonary secretions
	  h. No evidence supports dietary restrictions of avoiding raw or fresh fruit and vegetables for patients who are neutropenic. General precautions regarding food handling and storage are recommended.
	  i. Stagnant water is a source of infection.
		• Demonstrates normal temperature and vital signs
		• Exhibits absence of signs of inflammation: local edema, erythema, pain, and warmth
		• Exhibits normal breath sounds on auscultation
		• Takes deep breaths and coughs every 2 hours to prevent respiratory dysfunction and infection.
		• Exhibits absence of pathogens on cultures
		• Avoids contact with others with infections
		• Avoids crowds
		• All personnel carry out hand hygiene after each voiding and bowel movement.
		• Excoriation and trauma of skin are avoided.
		• Trauma to mucous membranes is avoided (avoidance of rectal thermometers, suppositories, vaginal tampons, perianal trauma).
		• Uses evidence-based procedures and techniques if participating in management of invasive lines or catheters
		• Uses electric razor
		• Is free of skin breakdown and stasis of secretions
		• Adheres to dietary and environmental precautions
		• Exhibits no signs of sepsis or septic shock
		• Exhibits normal vital signs, cardiac output, and arterial pressures when monitored
		• Demonstrates ability to administer colony-stimulating factor
		• Has bowel movements at regular intervals without constipation or straining
		• Patient hygiene is maintained.
		• Absence of IV catheter–related infection
		• Absence of skin abscesses
		• Absence of urinary catheter–related infection

(continued on page 338)

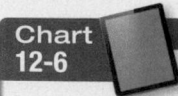

Chart 12-6

PLAN OF NURSING CARE (continued)
The Patient with Cancer

Nursing Interventions	Rationale	Expected Outcomes

5. Assess IV sites every day for evidence of infection.
  a. Change peripheral short-term IV sites every other day.
  b. Cleanse skin with chlorhexidine before arterial puncture or venipuncture.
  c. Change central venous catheter dressings every 48 hours.
  d. Change all solutions and infusion sets every 72–96 hours.
 	
  e. Follow Infusion Nursing Society guidelines for care of peripheral and central venous access devices.
6. Avoid intramuscular injections.
7. Avoid insertion of urinary catheters; if catheters are necessary, use aseptic technique.
8. Educate patient or family member to administer granulocyte (or granulocyte-macrophage) colony-stimulating factor when prescribed.
9. Advise patient to avoid exposure to animal excreta, discuss dental procedures with primary provider, avoid vaginal douche, and avoid vaginal or rectal manipulation during sexual contact during the period of neutropenia.
	5. Hospital-acquired sepsis is closely associated with IV catheters.
	  a. Incidence of infection is increased when catheter is in place >72 hours.
	  b. Chlorhexidine is effective against many gram-positive and gram-negative pathogens.
	  c. Allows observation of site and removes source of contamination.
	  d. Once introduced into the system, microorganisms can grow in infusion sets despite replacement of container and high flow rates.
	  e. Infusion Nursing Society collaborates with other nursing subspecialties in determining guidelines for IV access care.
	6. Reduces risk for skin abscesses.
	7. Rates of infection greatly increase after urinary catheterization.
	
	8. Granulocyte colony-stimulating factor decreases the duration of neutropenia and the potential for infection.
	
	9. Minimizes exposure to potential sources of infection and disruption of skin integrity	

NURSING DIAGNOSIS: Risk for impaired skin integrity: erythematous and wet desquamation reactions to radiation therapy
GOAL: Maintenance of skin integrity

Nursing Intervention	Rationale	Expected Outcomes

1. In erythematous areas:
 	
  a. Avoid the use of soaps, cosmetics, perfumes, powders, lotions, and ointments; non–aluminum-based deodorant may be used on intact skin.
  b. Use only lukewarm water to bathe the area.
  c. Avoid rubbing or scratching the area.
 	
  d. Avoid shaving the area with a straight-edged razor.
 	
  e. Avoid applying hot-water bottles, heating pads, ice, and adhesive tape to the area.
  f. Avoid exposing the area to sunlight or cold weather.
  g. Avoid tight clothing in the area. Use cotton clothing.
  h. Topical agents such as Aquaphor, radiacare gel, aloe vera, or biafine may be used, and low- or medium-potency corticosteroid cream may be given if pruritus is present.
	1. Care to the affected areas must focus on preventing further skin irritation, drying, and damage.
	  a. These substances may cause pain and additional skin irritation and damage.
	
	  b. Avoiding water of extreme temperatures and soap minimizes additional skin damage, irritation, and pain.
	  c. Rubbing, scratching, or both will lead to additional skin irritation, damage, and increased risk of infection.
	  d. The use of razors may lead to additional irritation and disruption of skin integrity and increased risk of infection.
	  e. Avoiding extreme temperatures minimizes additional skin damage, irritation, burns, and pain.
	  f. Sun exposure or extreme cold weather may lead to additional skin damage and pain.
	  g. Allows air circulation to affected area
	  h. May aid healing; however, evidence supporting the benefits of topical agents is lacking.
		• Avoids use of soaps, powders, and other cosmetics on site of radiation therapy
		• States rationale for special care of skin
		• Exhibits minimal change in skin
		• Avoids trauma to affected skin region (avoids shaving, constricting and irritating clothing, extremes of temperature, and the use of adhesive tape)
		• Reports change in skin promptly
		• Demonstrates proper care of blistered or open areas
		• Exhibits absence of infection of blistered and opened areas.
		• Wound is free of development of eschar

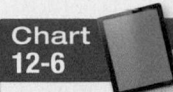

Chart 12-6 PLAN OF NURSING CARE (continued)
The Patient with Cancer

Nursing Intervention	Rationale	Expected Outcomes
2. If wet desquamation occurs:	2. Open weeping areas are susceptible to bacterial infection. Care must be taken to prevent introduction of pathogens.	
a. Do not disrupt any blisters that have formed.	a. Disruption of skin blisters disrupts skin integrity and may lead to increased risk of infection.	
b. Avoid frequent washing of the area.	b. Frequent washing may lead to increased irritation and skin damage, with increased risk of infection.	
c. Report any blistering.	c. Blistering of skin represents progression of skin damage.	
d. Use prescribed creams or ointments; topical antibacterial creams may help to dry a wet wound (e.g., Silvadene cream).	d. Anecdotally believed to decrease irritation and inflammation of the area and promote healing; although a variety of products are used in many settings, there are few randomized controlled trials with evidence to support one product or intervention over another.	
e. If area weeps, apply a nonadhesive absorbent dressing.	e. Easier to remove and associated with less pain and trauma when drainage dries and adheres to dressing.	
f. If the area is without drainage, moisture and vapor-permeable dressings, such as hydrocolloids and hydrogels on noninfected areas, have been used in many settings.	f. May promote healing; however, randomized controlled clinical trial support is lacking in the setting of moist desquamation. Hydrocolloid dressings may enhance comfort.	
g. Consult with wound-ostomy-continence nurse (WOCN) and primary provider if eschar forms.	g. Eschar must be removed to promote healing and prevent infection. WOCNs have expertise in the care of wounds.	

NURSING DIAGNOSIS: Impaired oral mucous membrane integrity: stomatitis
GOAL: Maintenance of intact oral mucous membranes

Nursing Intervention	Rationale	Expected Outcomes
1. Assess oral cavity daily using the same assessment criteria or rating scale.	1. Provides baseline for later evaluation; maintains consistency in assessment findings	• States rationale for frequent oral assessment and hygiene
2. Identify individuals at increased risk for stomatitis and related complications.	2. Patient and treatment variables are associated with the incidence and severity of stomatitis as well as related complications such as delayed healing and infection.	• Factors associated with the incidence, severity, and complications are identified prior to initiation of cancer treatment • Oral mucosal assessment is conducted at baseline and on an ongoing basis
3. Instruct patient to report oral burning, pain, areas of redness, open lesions on oropharyngeal mucosa and lips, pain associated with swallowing, or decreased tolerance to temperature extremes of food.	3. Identification of initial stages of stomatitis will facilitate prompt interventions, including modification of treatment as prescribed by primary provider.	• Oral hygiene practices are initiated prior to development of stomatitis. • Identifies signs and symptoms of stomatitis to report to nurse or primary provider
4. Encourage and assist as needed in oral hygiene.	4. Patients who are having discomfort or pain, or other symptoms related to the disease and treatment, may require encouragement and assistance in performing oral hygiene. Oral hygiene is maintained to prevent complications of stomatitis, such as infection.	• Participates in recommended oral hygiene regimen • Avoids mouthwashes with alcohol • Brushes teeth and mouth with soft toothbrush • Uses lubricant to keep lips soft and nonirritated • Avoids hard-to-chew, spicy, hot foods or other irritating foods • Maintains adequate hydration

(continued on page 340)

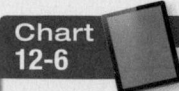

PLAN OF NURSING CARE (continued)

Chart 12-6

The Patient with Cancer

Nursing Intervention	Rationale	Expected Outcomes
Preventive		• Exhibits clean, intact oral mucosa
1. Advise patient to avoid irritants such as commercial mouthwashes, alcoholic beverages, and tobacco.	1. Alcohol content of mouthwashes and tobacco smoke will dry oral tissues and potentiate breakdown.	• Exhibits no ulcerations or infections of oral cavity
2. Brush with soft toothbrush using non-abrasive toothpaste for 90 seconds after meals and at bedtime; allow toothbrush to air dry before storing; floss at least once daily or as advised by the clinician; patients who have not previously flossed regularly should not initiate flossing during stomatoxic treatment; rinse mouth four times a day with a bland rinse (normal saline, sodium bicarbonate, or saline and sodium bicarbonate); avoid irritating foods (acidic, hot, rough, and spicy); use water-based moisturizers to protect lips.	2. Limits trauma and removes debris. Patients who have not previously flossed regularly should not initiate flossing during stomatoxic treatment due to potential for injury to the oral mucosa and increased susceptibility to infection.	• Exhibits no evidence of bleeding • Reports absent or decreased oral pain • Reports no difficulty swallowing • Exhibits healing (reepithelialization) of oral mucosa within 5–7 days (mild stomatitis)
3. Consider use of oral ice chips during stomatoxic chemotherapy infusions.	3. Oral cryotherapy has demonstrated reduced oral mucositis incidence, severity, and pain; improved quality of life; and minimizes chances of complications of oral mucositis	
4. Consider use of low-level laser therapy.	4. Low-energy level laser therapy has demonstrated decreased severity, duration, and pain associated with stomatitis.	
5. Consider administration of palifermin as prescribed for patients receiving high-dose chemotherapy.	5. Palifermin, a recombinant keratinocyte growth factor (KGF) that stimulates the growth of cells lining the mouth and intestinal tract, has been shown to decrease the severity and duration of stomatitis.	
6. Maintain adequate hydration.	6. Maintenance of hydration prevents mucosal drying and breakdown.	
7. Provide written instruction and education to patients on the above items.	7. Written information reinforces patient education and provides the patient and family with a source.	
Mild stomatitis (generalized erythema, limited ulcerations, small white patches: *Candida*)		• Exhibits healing of oral tissues within 10–14 days (severe stomatitis)
1. Use normal saline mouth rinses every 1–4 hours.	1. Assists in removing debris, thick secretions, and bacteria	• Exhibits no bleeding or oral ulceration
2. Use soft toothbrush or toothette.	2. Minimizes trauma	• Consumes adequate fluid and food
3. Remove dentures except for meals; be certain that dentures fit well.	3. Minimizes friction and discomfort	• Exhibits absence of dehydration and weight loss
4. Apply water-soluble lip lubricant.	4. Promotes comfort	• Exhibits no evidence of infection
5. Avoid foods that are spicy or hard to chew and those with extremes of temperature.	5. Prevents local trauma	
Severe stomatitis (confluent ulcerations with bleeding and white patches covering >25% of oral mucosa)		a. Adheres to oral care regimen
1. Obtain tissue samples for culture and sensitivity tests of areas of infection.	1. Assists in identifying need for antimicrobial therapy	b. Exhibits healing of oral tissues within 10–14 days (severe stomatitis)
2. Assess ability to chew and swallow; assess gag reflex.	2. Patient may be in danger of aspiration	• Consumes adequate fluid and food
3. Use oral rinses (may combine in solution saline, anti-*Candida* agent, such as mycostatin, and topical anesthetic agent [described later]) as prescribed, or place patient on side and irrigate mouth; have suction available.	3. Facilitates cleansing and provides for safety and comfort	• Exhibits absence of dehydration and weight loss • Exhibits no evidence of infection • Reports absent or decreased discomfort or pain

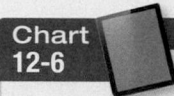

Chart 12-6

PLAN OF NURSING CARE (continued)

The Patient with Cancer

Nursing Intervention	Rationale	Expected Outcomes
4. Remove dentures.	4. Prevents trauma from ill-fitting dentures	
5. Use toothette or gauze soaked with solution for cleansing.	5. Limits trauma and promotes comfort	
6. Use water-soluble lip lubricant.	6. Promotes comfort and minimizes loss of skin integrity	
7. Provide liquid or pureed diet.	7. Ensures intake of easily digestible foods without chewing	
8. Monitor for dehydration.	8. Decreased oral intake and ulcerations potentiate fluid deficits	
9. Minimize discomfort.	9. Promotes healing	
a. Consult primary provider for use of topical anesthetic, such as dyclonine and diphenhydramine, or viscous lidocaine.	a. Alleviates pain and increases sense of well-being; promotes participation in oral hygiene and nutritional intake	
b. Administer systemic analgesics as prescribed.	b. Adequate management of pain related to severe stomatitis can facilitate improved quality of life, participation in other aspects of activities of daily living, oral intake, and verbal communication.	
c. Perform mouth care as described.	c. Promotes removal of debris, healing, and comfort	

NURSING DIAGNOSIS: Impaired skin integrity associated with rash
GOALS: Maintenance of skin integrity

Nursing Intervention	Rationale	Expected Outcomes
Prevention		
1. Instruct patients to avoid sunlight through use of protective clothing, use of sun screen with SPF of 30 with physical blockers (zinc oxide, titanium dioxide), or avoidance of direct sun exposure.	1. Many agents are associated with photosensitivity; sunburn would intensify inflammation associated with rash and potentiate loss of skin integrity	• Sun exposure will be limited; no development of sun burn • Absence of dehydration • Participates in skin care regimen as instructed • Absence of dryness, flaking
2. Maintain adequate oral hydration.	2. Prevents skin dryness related to dehydration	
3. Avoid long hot showers or baths, harsh soaps and laundry detergents, perfumes, and nonhypoallergenic cosmetics.	3. Prevents skin irritation, dryness, flaking, and inflammation	
4. Apply emollients; apply hydrocortisone 1% cream with moisturizer at least twice daily; administer doxycycline 100 mg twice per day or minocycline, as prescribed	4. Minimizes dryness, flaking, and disruption of skin integrity	
Treatment		
1. Apply topical treatment as prescribed: clindamycin 1%, fluocinonide 0.05% cream twice a day, or alclometasone 0.05% cream twice a day	1. Recommended as treatment to minimize skin disruption and prevent infection by Multinational Association of Supportive Care in Cancer (MASCC)	• Rash severity does not interfere with level of comfort and adherence to targeted therapy as prescribed; absence of local or systemic infection • Rash severity does not interfere with level of comfort and adherence to targeted therapy as prescribed; absence of local or systemic infection • Local infection is controlled; absence of sepsis
2. For severe papulopustular rash: Administer systemic treatment as prescribed: doxycycline 100 mg twice per day; minocycline 100 mg daily; or isotretinion at low doses of 20–30 mg per day	2. Recommended as treatment to minimize skin disruption and prevent infection by Multinational Association of Supportive Care in Cancer (MASCC)	
3. Assess for development of infection: obtain cultures of pustules and administer appropriate antibiotics as prescribed by the physician	3. Prompt recognition and treatment of infection are necessary to prevent bacteremia, sepsis, and further patient compromise	

(continued on page 342)

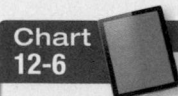

Chart 12-6

PLAN OF NURSING CARE (continued)

The Patient with Cancer

NURSING DIAGNOSIS: Impaired tissue integrity: alopecia
GOAL: Maintenance of tissue integrity; coping with hair loss

Nursing Intervention	Rationale	Expected Outcomes
1. Discuss potential hair loss and regrowth with patient and family; advise that hair loss may occur on body parts other than the head.	1. Provides information so that patient and family can begin to prepare cognitively and emotionally for loss	• Identifies alopecia as potential side effect of treatment
2. Explore potential impact of hair loss on self-image, interpersonal relationships, and sexuality.	2. Facilitates coping and maintenance of interpersonal relationships	• Identifies positive and negative feelings and threats to self-image
3. Prevent or minimize hair loss through the following:	3. Retains hair as long as possible.	• Verbalizes meaning that hair and possible hair loss have for them
a. Use scalp cooling (hypothermia), if appropriate.	a. Decreases hair follicle uptake of chemotherapy (not used for patients with leukemia or lymphoma because tumor cells may be present in blood vessels or scalp tissue)	• States rationale for modifications in hair care and treatment
b. Cut long hair before treatment.	b. Minimizes hair loss due to the weight and manipulation of hair	• Uses mild shampoo and conditioner, and shampoos hair only when necessary
c. Use mild shampoo and conditioner, gently pat dry, and avoid excessive shampooing.		• Avoids hair dryer, curlers, sprays, and other stresses on hair and scalp
d. Avoid electric curlers, curling irons, dryers, clips, barrettes, hair sprays, hair dyes, hair extensions, weaves, braids, dreadlocks, hair straightening products, and permanent waves.		• Wears hat or scarf over hair when exposed to sun
e. Avoid excessive combing or brushing; use wide-toothed comb.		• Takes steps to deal with possible hair loss before it occurs; purchases wig or hairpiece if desired
4. Prevent trauma to scalp.	4. Preserves tissue integrity	• Maintains hygiene and grooming
a. Use sunscreen or wear hat when in the sun.	a. Assists in maintaining skin integrity	• Interacts and socializes with others
	b. Prevents ultraviolet light exposure	
5. Suggest ways to assist in coping with hair loss.	5. Minimizes change in appearance	
a. Purchase wig or hairpiece before hair loss.	a. Wig that closely resembles hair color and style is more easily selected if hair loss has not begun.	
b. If hair loss has occurred, take photograph to wig shop to assist in selection.	b. Facilitates adjustment	
c. Begin to wear wig before hair loss.	c. Enables patient to be prepared for loss and facilitates adjustment	
d. Contact the American Cancer Society for donated wigs or a store that specializes in this product.	d. Provides options to patient and assists with financial burden if necessary	
e. Wear hat, scarf, or turban.	e. Conceals loss and protects scalp	
6. Encourage patient to wear own clothes and retain social contacts.	6. Assists in maintaining personal identity	
7. Explain that hair growth usually begins again once therapy is completed.	7. Reassures patient that hair loss is usually temporary	

NURSING DIAGNOSIS: Impaired nutritional status associated with nausea and vomiting
GOAL: Patient experiences less nausea and vomiting associated with therapies; weight loss is minimized

Nursing Intervention	Rationale	Expected Outcomes
1. Assess the patient's previous experiences and expectations of nausea and vomiting, including causes and interventions used.	1. Identifies patient concerns, misinformation, and potential strategies for intervention; also gives patient sense of empowerment and control.	• Identifies previous triggers of nausea and vomiting
2. Adjust diet before and after drug administration according to patient preference and tolerance.	2. Each patient responds differently to food after chemotherapy. A diet containing foods that relieve or prevent nausea or vomiting is most helpful.	• Exhibits decreased apprehension and anxiety
3. Prevent unpleasant sights, odors, and sounds in the environment.	3. Unpleasant sensations can stimulate the nausea and vomiting center.	• Identifies previously used successful interventions for nausea and vomiting
		• Reports decrease in nausea
		• Reports decrease in incidence of vomiting

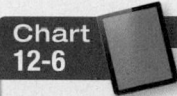

**Chart
12-6**

PLAN OF NURSING CARE (continued)

The Patient with Cancer

Nursing Intervention	Rationale	Expected Outcomes
4. Use distraction, music therapy, biofeedback, self-hypnosis, relaxation techniques, and guided imagery before, during, and after chemotherapy.	4. Decreases anxiety, which can contribute to nausea and vomiting. Psychological conditioning may also be decreased.	• Consumes adequate fluid and food when nausea subsides
5. Administer prescribed antiemetics, sedatives, and corticosteroids before chemotherapy and afterward as needed.	5. Administration of antiemetic regimen before onset of nausea and vomiting limits the adverse experience and facilitates control. Combination drug therapy reduces nausea and vomiting through various triggering mechanisms.	• Demonstrates use of distraction, relaxation, and imagery when indicated • Exhibits normal skin turgor and moist mucous membranes • No additional weight loss
6. Ensure adequate fluid hydration before, during, and after drug administration; assess intake and output.	6. Adequate fluid volume dilutes drug levels, decreasing stimulation of vomiting receptors.	
7. Encourage frequent oral hygiene.	7. Reduces unpleasant taste sensations	
8. Provide pain-relief measures, if necessary.	8. Increased comfort increases physical tolerance of symptoms.	
9. Consult with dietician as needed.	9. Interdisciplinary collaboration is essential in addressing complex patient needs.	
10. Assess and address other contributing factors to nausea and vomiting, such as other symptoms, constipation, gastrointestinal irritation, electrolyte imbalance, radiation therapy, medications, and central nervous system metastasis.	10. Multiple factors may contribute to nausea and vomiting.	

NURSING DIAGNOSIS: Impaired nutritional status associated with anorexia, cachexia, or malabsorption
GOAL: Maintenance of nutritional status and of weight within 10% of pretreatment weight

Nursing Intervention	Rationale	Expected Outcomes
1. Assess and address factors that interfere with oral intake or are associated with increased risk of decreased nutritional status.	1. Multiple patient or treatment-related factors are associated with increased risk of impaired nutritional intake, such as radiation to the head, neck, and thorax; stomatoxic or emetogenic chemotherapy; prior oral, head, and neck surgery; mucositis; impaired swallowing or dysphagia; poor dentition; cough or dyspnea.	• Factors associated with increased risk for impaired nutritional intake are identified • Factors associated with increased risk of impaired nutritional intake are identified and addressed, whenever possible, through interdisciplinary collaboration
2. Initiate appropriate referrals for interdisciplinary collaboration to manage factors that interfere with oral intake.	2. Other disciplines may be more appropriate for assessment and management of issues such as swallowing impairments (speech therapy), fatigue and decreased physical ability (physical and occupational therapy), nutritional assessment and determination of patient needs (nutritionist), cough and dyspnea (respiratory therapy), poor dentition (dental medicine), depression/anxiety (social worker, psychologist, or psychiatrist).	• Patient and family identify minimal nutritional requirements • Maintains or increases weight and body cell mass as per goals identified by nutritionist • Reports decreasing anorexia and increased interest in eating • Demonstrates normal skin turgor • Identifies rationale for dietary modifications; patient and family verbalize strategies to minimize nutritional deficits • Participates in calorie counts and diet histories • Uses relaxation techniques and guided imagery before meals
3. Educate patient to avoid unpleasant sights, odors, and sounds in the environment during mealtime.	3. Anorexia can be stimulated or increased with noxious stimuli.	• Exhibits laboratory and clinical findings indicative of adequate nutritional intake:
4. Suggest foods that are preferred and well tolerated by the patient, preferably high-calorie and high-protein foods. Respect ethnic and cultural food preferences.	4. Foods preferred, well tolerated, and high in calories and protein maintain nutritional status during periods of increased metabolic demand.	normal serum levels of protein, albumin, transferrin, iron, blood urea nitrogen (BUN), creatinine, vitamin D, electrolytes, hemoglobin, hematocrit, and lymphocytes; normal urinary creatinine levels

(continued on page 344)

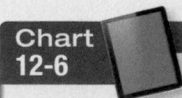

Chart 12-6

PLAN OF NURSING CARE (continued)

The Patient with Cancer

Nursing Intervention	Rationale	Expected Outcomes
5. Encourage adequate fluid intake, but limit fluids at mealtime.	5. Fluids are necessary to eliminate wastes and prevent dehydration. Increased fluids with meals can lead to early satiety.	• Consumes diet containing required nutrients • Carries out oral hygiene before meals • Reports decreased pain or other symptoms; symptoms do not interfere with oral intake • Reports decreasing episodes of nausea and vomiting • Participates in increasing levels of activity as measured by assessment of performance status • Family and friends do not focus efforts on encouraging food intake • States rationale for use of tube feedings or parenteral nutrition • Demonstrates ability to manage enteral feedings or parenteral nutrition, if prescribed • Maintains body position and alignment needed to facilitate chewing and swallowing
6. Suggest smaller, more frequent meals.	6. Smaller, more frequent meals are better tolerated because early satiety is less likely to occur.	
7. Promote relaxed, quiet environment during mealtime with increased social interaction as desired.	7. A quiet environment promotes relaxation. Social interaction at mealtime may foster appetite, divert focus on food, and promote enjoyment of eating.	
8. If patient desires, serve alcoholic beverages at mealtime with foods.	8. Alcoholic beverages may stimulate appetite and add calories.	
9. Consider cold foods, if desired.	9. Cold, high-protein foods are often more tolerable and less odorous than hot foods.	
10. Encourage nutritional supplements and high-protein foods between meals.	10. Supplements and snacks add protein and calories to meet nutritional requirements.	
11. Encourage frequent oral hygiene, particularly prior to meals.	11. Oral hygiene may stimulate appetite and increase saliva production.	
12. Address pain and other symptom management needs.	12. Pain and other symptoms impair appetite and nutritional intake.	
13. Increase activity level as tolerated.	13. Increased activity promotes appetite.	
14. Decrease anxiety by encouraging verbalization of fears and concerns; use relaxation techniques and guided imagery at mealtime.	14. Relief of anxiety may increase appetite.	
15. Instruct patient and family about body alignment and proper positioning at mealtime.	15. Proper body position and alignment are necessary to aid chewing and swallowing.	
16. Collaborate with dietician to provide nutritional counseling; instruct patient and family regarding enteral tube feedings of commercial liquid diets, elemental diets, or other foods as prescribed.	16. Nutritional counseling may improve outcomes. Tube feedings may be necessary in the severely debilitated patient who has a functioning gastrointestinal system but is unable to maintain adequate oral intake.	
17. Collaborate with dietician or nutrition support team to instruct patient and family regarding home parenteral nutrition with lipid supplements as prescribed.	17. Parenteral nutrition with supplemental fats supplies needed calories and proteins to meet nutritional demands, especially in the nonfunctional gastrointestinal system.	
18. Administer appetite stimulants as prescribed by primary provider.	18. Although the mechanism is unclear, medications such as megestrol acetate have been noted to improve appetite in patients with cancer and human immunodeficiency virus infection.	
19. Encourage family and friends not to nag or cajole patient about eating.	19. Pressuring patient to eat may cause conflict and unnecessary stress.	
20. Assess and address other contributing factors to nausea, vomiting, and anorexia such as electrolyte imbalance, radiation therapy, medications, and central nervous system metastasis.	20. Multiple factors contribute to anorexia and nausea.	

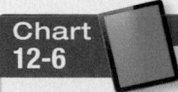

Chart 12-6

PLAN OF NURSING CARE (continued)
The Patient with Cancer

NURSING DIAGNOSIS: Fatigue
GOAL: Decreased fatigue level

Nursing Intervention	Rationale	Expected Outcomes
1. Assess patient and treatment factors that are associated with or increase fatigue (e.g., anemia, fluid and electrolyte imbalances, pain, anxiety, etc.)	1. Multiple factors are associated with or contribute to cancer-related fatigue. Although fatigue is common in patients receiving chemotherapy or radiation therapy, there are several factors that can be modified or addressed, such as dehydration, electrolyte abnormalities, organ impairment, anemia, impaired nutrition, pain and other symptoms, depression, anxiety, impaired mobility, and dyspnea	• Factors contributing to fatigue are assessed and managed whenever possible • Exhibits acceptable serum value levels for nutritional indices (see Imbalanced Nutrition) • Reports decreased pain or other symptoms • Consumes diet with recommended nutritional intake • Achieves or maintains appropriate weight and body mass • Maintains adequate hydration • Reports decreasing levels of fatigue • Adopts healthy lifestyle practices • Rests when fatigued • Reports adequate sleep • Requests assistance with activities appropriately • Uses relaxation exercises and imagery to decrease anxiety and promote rest • Reports no breathlessness during activities • Reports improved ability to relax and rest • Exhibits improved mobility and decreased fatigue Fatigue does not interfere with ability to participate in activities of daily living or pleasure
2. Institute interventions to address factors contributing to fatigue (e.g., correct electrolyte imbalance, manage pain, collaborative management of anemia, administer prescribed antidepressants, anxiolytics, hypnotics, or psychostimulants, as indicated)	2. Addressing factors contributing to fatigue assists in managing fatigue (e.g., lowered hemoglobin and hematocrit predispose patient to fatigue due to decreased oxygen availability especially in a setting of impaired mobility that requires increased energy expenditure).	
3. Encourage balance of rest and exercise; avoiding extended periods of inactivity. At minimum, promote patient's normal sleep habits.	3. Sleep helps to restore energy levels. Prolonged napping during the day may interfere with sleep habits.	
4. During active treatment, rearrange daily schedule and organize activities to conserve energy expenditure; encourage patient to ask for others' assistance with necessary chores, such as housework, child care, shopping, and cooking. During periods of profound fatigue, consider reduced job workload, if necessary and possible, by reducing number of hours worked per week.	4. Reorganization of activities can reduce energy losses and stressors.	
5. Encourage protein, fat, and calorie intake at least equal to that recommended for the general public.	5. Protein and calorie depletion decreases activity tolerance; preventing malnutrition, achieving and maintaining recommended weight and body mass assist in management of fatigue.	
6. Encourage the use of relaxation techniques and guided imagery.	6. Promotion of relaxation and psychological rest limits contribution to physical fatigue.	
7. Encourage participation in planned exercise programs involving aerobic, resistance, and flexibility training based on individual limitations and safety measures. a. Minimum exercise for survivors depending on individual capabilities ranges from 10 minutes of light exercise, yoga, or stretching daily to 30 minutes of moderate to vigorous of activity	7. Various approaches to exercise programs have demonstrated increases in endurance and stamina and lower fatigue.	
8. Collaborate with other cancer providers to encourage them to give patients a prescription to exercise and explain role of exercise in cancer treatment.	8. Many providers fail to discuss the role of exercise and healthy lifestyle practices for patients during and after cancer treatment. Patients may be more likely to utilize the benefits of exercise in addressing fatigue if they receive a formal prescription.	

(continued on page 346)

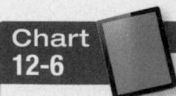

Chart 12-6

PLAN OF NURSING CARE (continued)

The Patient with Cancer

Nursing Intervention	Rationale	Expected Outcomes
9. Partner with community organizations (e.g., YMCA) to develop and offer cancer survivor specific rehab/exercise programs.	9. Creates community partnerships, a nonclinical environment of support, fosters increased awareness of survivorship needs, and provides referral sources that can reach more survivors.	
10. Collaborate with physical and occupational therapy or refer to American College of Sports Medicine (ACSM) Certified Cancer Exercise Trainer (CET) to identify safe and appropriate activities.	10. A CET designs and administers fitness assessments and exercise programs specific to an individual's cancer diagnosis, treatment, current recovery status; possesses basic understanding of cancer diagnoses, treatments, and potential adverse effects.	

NURSING DIAGNOSIS: Chronic pain
GOAL: Relief of pain and discomfort

Nursing Intervention	Rationale	Expected Outcomes
1. Use pain scale to assess pain and discomfort characteristics: location, quality, frequency, duration, etc., at baseline and on an ongoing basis.	1. Provides baseline for assessing changes in pain level and evaluation of interventions	• Reports decreased level of pain and discomfort on pain scale • Reports less disruption in activity and quality of life from pain and discomfort • Reports decrease in other symptoms and psychosocial distress
2. Assure patient that you know the pain is real and will assist them in reducing it.	2. Fear that pain will not be considered real increases anxiety and reduces pain tolerance.	• Adheres to analgesic regimen as prescribed
3. Assess prior pain experiences and previous management strategies the patient found successful.	3. Helps to individualize pain management approaches and identify potential challenges or approaches that should not be utilized because of safety or other issues	• Barriers to adequately addressing pain do not interfere with strategies for managing pain.
4. Assess other factors contributing to patient's pain: fear, fatigue, other symptoms, psychosocial distress, etc.	4. Provides data about factors that decrease the patient's ability to tolerate pain and increase pain level	• Takes an active role in administration of analgesia
5. Provide education to patient and family about prescribed analgesic regimen.	5. Analgesics tend to be more effective when given early in pain cycle, around the clock at regular intervals, or when given in long-acting forms; breaks the pain cycle; premedication with analgesics is used for activities that cause increased pain or breakthrough pain.	• Identifies additional effective pain-relief strategies • Uses previously employed successful pain-relief strategies appropriately • Identifies or utilizes nonpharmacologic pain-relief strategies and reports successful decrease in pain • Reports that decreased level of pain permits participation in other activities and events and quality of life
6. Address myths or misconceptions and lack of knowledge about the use of opioid analgesics.	6. Barriers to adequate pain management involve patients' fear of side effects, fatalism about the possibility of achieving pain control, fear of distracting providers from treating the cancer, belief that pain is indicative of progressive disease, and fears about addiction. Professional health providers also have demonstrated limited knowledge about evidence-based approaches to pain.	
7. Collaborate with patient, primary provider, and other health care team members when changes in pain management are necessary.	7. New methods of administering analgesia must be acceptable to patient, primary provider, and health care team to be effective; patient's participation decreases the sense of powerlessness.	
8. Consult with palliative care providers or team throughout the cancer continuum.	8. Palliative care specialists provide expertise and contribute to symptom management regardless of stage of disease or treatment within the cancer continuum, not only during end-stage disease. Palliative care can improve quality of life, length of survival, symptom burden, mood, and efficient utilization of health services.	
9. Explore nonpharmacologic and complementary strategies to relieve pain and discomfort: distraction, imagery, relaxation, cutaneous stimulation, acupuncture, etc.	9. Increases the number of options and strategies available to patient that serve as adjuncts to pharmacologic interventions.	

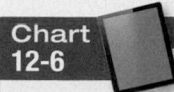

Chart 12-6

PLAN OF NURSING CARE (continued)
The Patient with Cancer

NURSING DIAGNOSIS: Grief associated with loss; altered role functioning
GOAL: Appropriate progression through grieving process

Nursing Intervention	Rationale	Expected Outcomes
1. Encourage verbalization of fears, concerns, and questions regarding disease, treatment, and future implications.	1. An increased and accurate knowledge base decreases anxiety and dispels misconceptions.	The patient and family:
2. Explore previous successful coping strategies.	2. Provides frame of reference and examples of coping.	• Progress through the phases of grief as evidenced by increased verbalization and expression of grief.
3. Encourage active participation of patient or family in care and treatment decisions.	3. Active participation maintains patient independence and control.	• Identify resources available to aid coping strategies during grieving.
4. Visit family and friends to establish and maintain relationships and physical closeness.	4. Frequent contacts promote trust and security and reduce feelings of fear and isolation.	• Use resources and supports appropriately.
5. Encourage ventilation of negative feelings, including projected anger and hostility, within acceptable limits.	5. This allows for emotional expression without loss of self-esteem.	• Discuss the future openly with each other.
6. Allow for periods of crying and expression of sadness.	6. These feelings are necessary for separation and detachment to occur.	• Discuss concerns and feelings openly with each other.
7. Involve spiritual advisor as desired by the patient and family.	7. This facilitates the grief process and spiritual care.	• Use nonverbal expressions of concern for each other.
8. Refer patient and family to professional counseling as indicated to alleviate pathologic or nonadaptive grieving.	8. Goal is to facilitate the grief process or adaptive methods of coping.	• Develop positive or adaptive coping mechanisms for processing of grief.
9. Allow for progression through the grieving process at the individual pace of the patient and family.	9. Grief work is variable. Not every person uses every phase of the grief process, and the time spent in dealing with each phase varies with every person. To complete grief work, this variability must be allowed.	

NURSING DIAGNOSIS: Disturbed body image and situational low self-esteem associated with changes in appearance, function, and roles
GOAL: Improved body image and self-esteem

Nursing Intervention	Rationale	Expected Outcomes
1. Assess patient's feelings about body image and level of self-esteem.	1. Provides baseline assessment for evaluating changes and assessing effectiveness of interventions.	• Identifies concerns of importance
		• Takes active role in activities
2. Identify potential threats to patient's self-esteem (e.g., altered appearance, decreased sexual function, hair loss, decreased energy, role changes). Validate concerns with patient.	2. Anticipates changes and permits patient to identify importance of these areas to them.	• Maintains participation in decision making
		• Verbalizes feelings and reactions to losses or threatened losses
3. Encourage continued participation in activities and decision making.	3. Encourages and permits continued control of events and self.	• Participates in self-care activities
4. Encourage patient to verbalize concerns.	4. Identifying concerns is an important step in coping with them.	• Permits others to assist in care when they are unable to be independent
5. Individualize care for the patient.	5. Prevents or reduces depersonalization and emphasizes patient's self-worth.	• Exhibits interest in appearance, maintains grooming, and uses aids (cosmetics, scarves, etc.) appropriately if desired
6. Assist patient in self-care when fatigue, lethargy, nausea, vomiting, and other symptoms prevent independence.	6. Physical well-being improves self-esteem.	• Participates with others in conversations and social events and activities
7. Assist patient in selecting and using cosmetics, scarves, hair pieces, hats, and clothing that increase their sense of attractiveness.	7. Promotes positive body image.	• Verbalizes concern about sexual partner or significant others
8. Encourage patient and partner to share concerns about altered sexuality and sexual function and to explore alternatives to their usual sexual expression.	8. Provides opportunity for expressing concern, intimacy, affection, and acceptance.	• Explores alternative ways of expressing concern and affection
9. Refer to collaborating specialists as needed.	9. Interdisciplinary collaboration is essential in meeting patient needs.	• The patient and significant other can maintain level of intimacy and express affection and acceptance

(continued on page 348)

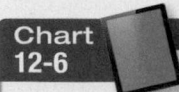

Chart 12-6

PLAN OF NURSING CARE (continued)

The Patient with Cancer

COLLABORATIVE PROBLEM: Potential complication: risk for bleeding problems
GOAL: Prevention of bleeding

Nursing Intervention	Rationale	Expected Outcomes
1. Monitor for factors increasing risk of bleeding (thrombocytopenia, elevated INR/PT/PTT, decreased fibrinogen or other clotting factors, use of medications affecting platelets or other clotting indices)	1. The underlying cancer, antineoplastic agents or other medications may interfere with normal mechanisms of clotting.	• Signs and symptoms of bleeding are identified • Exhibits no blood in feces, urine, or emesis • Exhibits no bleeding of gums or injection/venipuncture sites
2. Assess for and educate patient/family about signs and symptoms of bleeding: a. Petechiae or ecchymosis (bruising) b. Decrease in hemoglobin or hematocrit c. Prolonged bleeding from invasive procedures, venipunctures, minor cuts or scratches d. Frank or occult blood in any body fluids e. Bleeding from any body orifice f. Altered mental status g. Hypotension; tachycardia	2. Early detection promotes early intervention. a. Petechiae and ecchymosis indicate injury to microcirculation and larger vessels. b. Decreased hemoglobin or hematocrit may indicate blood loss. c. Prolonged bleeding may indicate abnormal clotting indices. d. Occult blood in body fluids indicates bleeding. e. Indicates blood loss f. Altered mental status may indicate decreased cerebral tissue oxygenation or bleeding. g. Hypotension or tachycardia may indicate blood loss.	• Exhibits no ecchymosis (bruising) or petechiae • Patient and family identify ways to prevent bleeding • Uses recommended measures to reduce risk of bleeding (uses soft toothbrush, shaves with electric razor only) • Exhibits normal vital signs • Reports that environmental hazards have been reduced or removed • Maintains hydration • Reports absence of constipation • Avoids substances interfering with clotting • Absence of tissue destruction • Exhibits normal mental status and absence of signs of intracranial bleeding • Avoids medications that interfere with clotting (e.g., aspirin) • Absence of epistaxis and cerebral bleeding
3. Instruct patient and family about ways to minimize risk of bleeding. a. Use soft toothbrush for mouth care. b. Avoid commercial mouthwashes. c. Use electric razor for shaving. d. Use emery board for nail care. e. Avoid foods that are difficult to chew. f. Keep lips moisturized with water-based lubricant g. Maintain fluid intake of at least 3 L per 24 hours unless contraindicated h. Use stool softeners or increase bulk in diet. i. Recommend use of water-based lubricant before sexual intercourse.	3. Patient can participate in self-protection. a. Prevents trauma to oral tissues b. Contain high alcohol content that will dry oral tissues c. Prevents trauma to skin d. Reduces risk of trauma to nail beds e. Prevents oral tissue trauma f. Prevents skin from drying g. Prevents skin and oral tissue membranes from drying h. Prevents trauma to rectal mucosa from straining i. Prevents friction and tissue trauma	
4. Initiate measures to minimize bleeding. Draw all blood for lab work with one daily venipuncture for hospitalized patients. a. Avoid taking temperature rectally or administering suppositories and enemas. b. Avoid intramuscular injections; use smallest needle possible. c. Apply direct pressure to injection and venipuncture sites for at least 5 minutes. d. Avoid bladder catheterizations; use smallest catheter if catheterization is necessary. e. Avoid medications that will interfere with clotting (e.g., aspirin). f. Recommend use of water-based lubricant before sexual intercourse.	4. Measures are taken to minimize bleeding a. Minimizes blood loss b. Bleeding may occur from intramuscular injection sites, particularly if large bore needles are used c. Bleeding may occur if direct pressure is not applied for a long enough time period d. Prevents trauma to urethra e. Minimizes risk of bleeding f. Helps prevent bleeding from small skin tears	

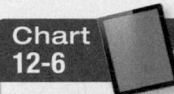

Chart 12-6 PLAN OF NURSING CARE (continued)
The Patient with Cancer

Nursing Intervention	Rationale	Expected Outcomes
g. Platelet transfusions as prescribed; administer prescribed diphenhydramine hydrochloride or hydrocortisone sodium succinate to prevent reaction to platelet transfusion.	**g.** Platelet count <20,000/mm^3 (0.02 × 1012/L) is associated with increased risk of spontaneous bleeding. Allergic reactions to blood products are associated with antigen–antibody reaction that causes platelet destruction	
h. Supervise activity when out of bed.	**h.** Reduces risk of falls	
i. Caution against forceful nose blowing.	**i.** Prevents trauma to nasal mucosa and increased intracranial pressure	

Adapted from Corbitt, N., Harrington, J., Kendall, T. (2017). Putting evidence into practice: Prevention of bleeding. Retrieved on 7/23/2019 at: www.ons.org/pep/bleeding; Eilers, J. G., Asakura, Y., Blecher, C. S., et al. (2017). Putting evidence into practice: Mucositis. Retrieved on 7/7/2019 at: www.ons.org/pep/mucositis; Gosselin, T., Beamer, L., Ciccolini, K., et al. (2017). Putting evidence into practice: Radiodermatitis. Retrieved on 7/29/2019 at: www.ons.org/pep/radiodermatitis; Miaskowski, C. A., Brant, J. M., Caldwell, P., et al. (2017). Putting evidence into practice: Chronic pain. Retrieved on 7/19/2019 at: www.ons.org/pep/chronic-pain; Mitchell, S. A., Albrecht, T. A., Omar Alkaiyat, M., et al. (2017). Putting evidence into practice: Fatigue. Retrieved on 7/2/2019 at: www.ons.org/pep/fatigue; Thorpe, D. M., Conley, S. B., Drapek, L., et al. (2017). Putting evidence into practice: Anorexia. Retrieved on 7/28/2019 at: www.ons.org/pep/anorexia; Williams, L., Ciccolini, K., Johnson, L. A., et al. (2017). Putting evidence into practice: Skin reactions. Retrieved on 7/23/2019 at: www.ons.org/pep/skin-reactions; and Wilson, B. J., Ahmed, F., Crannell, C. E., et al. (2017). Putting evidence into practice: Preventing infection – general. Retrieved on 7/5/2019 at: www.ons.org/pep/prevention-infection-general

undergoing chemotherapy for head and neck cancer (Bowen et al., 2019; Eilers et al., 2017). Palifermin promotes epithelial cell repair and accelerated replacement of cells in the mouth and gastrointestinal tract. Careful timing of administration and monitoring are essential for effectiveness and to detect adverse effects. Other approaches recommended for practice include cryotherapy (topical application of oral ice during infusions), consistent oral hygiene, low-level laser therapy, and sodium bicarbonate mouth rinses (Bowen et al., 2019; Eilers et al., 2017; Olsen et al., 2019). Additional aspects of care are discussed in Chart 12-6: nursing care plan for patients with cancer.

Radiation-Associated Impairment of Skin Integrity

Although advances in radiation therapy have resulted in decreased incidence and severity of skin impairments, patients may still develop radiodermatitis, formerly called radiation dermatitis, associated with pain, irritation, pruritus, burning, skin sloughing without drainage (dry desquamation) or with drainage (wet desquamation), and diminished quality of life (Gosselin, Beamer, Ciccolini, et al., 2017; Olsen et al., 2019). Nursing care for patients with radiodermatitis includes maintenance of skin integrity, cleansing, promotion of comfort, pain reduction, prevention of additional trauma, prevention and management of infection, and promotion of a moist wound-healing environment (Olsen et al., 2019). In order to prevent impaired skin integrity, patients are advised to use moisturizer on the skin, avoid sun exposure to the area of treatment, and avoid tape or bandages and other sources of irritation or trauma. Although a variety of methods and products are used in clinical practice for patients with radiation-induced skin impairment, there is limited evidence to support their value (Gosselin et al., 2017). Patients with skin and tissue reactions to radiation therapy require careful skin care to prevent further skin irritation, drying, and damage, as discussed in the nursing care plan (see Chart 12-6, Risk for impaired skin integrity: erythematous and wet desquamation reactions to radiation therapy).

Alopecia

The temporary or permanent thinning or complete loss of hair is a potential adverse effect of whole brain radiation therapy, various chemotherapies and targeted agents. Alopecia usually begins 1 to 3 weeks after the initiation of chemotherapy and radiation therapy; regrowth most often begins within 8 weeks after the last treatment (Olsen et al., 2019). Some patients who undergo radiation to the head may sustain permanent hair loss. The onset of gradually progressing alopecia and body hair loss associated with targeted therapies generally occurs 1 to 3 months after the start of treatment and may be patchy appearing as temporal or frontal hair loss (Barton-Burke, Ciccolini, Mekas, et al., 2017). This type of hair loss is usually reversible after the end of therapy and in some cases beginning sooner. Several targeted agents are associated with changes in hair growth rate, curliness, texture, and pigmentation. Although health care providers may view hair loss as a minor issue, for many patients it is a major assault on body image, challenging to self-esteem, and resulting in psychosocial distress and depression. Despite the significant psychosocial impact of alopecia, few studies have addressed methods to prevent or minimize the impact of alopecia. The use of cryotherapy to the head (scalp cooling) has been shown to be effective in reducing alopecia during chemotherapy administration (Ross & Fischer-Cartlidge, 2017; Rugo, Melin, & Voigt, 2017). However, due to reports of scalp metastasis and a lack of safety data, cryotherapy is not recommended for use in patients with hematologic malignancies (Rugo et al., 2017). Nurses provide information about hair loss and support the patient and family in coping with changes in body image. Patients are assisted to identify proactive choices that may empower them to improve responses to cancer and perceived lack of control as discussed in the nursing care plan (see Chart 12-6, Impaired tissue integrity: alopecia).

Malignant Skin Lesions

Skin lesions may occur with local extension or metastasis of the tumor into the epithelium and its surrounding lymph and blood vessels. Either locally invasive or metastatic cancer to the skin may result in erythema, discolored nodules, or progression to wounds involving edema, exudates, and tissue necrosis. The most extensive lesions involve ulceration (referred to as fungating lesions) with an overgrowth of malodorous microorganisms. These lesions are a source of considerable pain, discomfort, and embarrassment. Although skin lesions occur in various malignancies, they are most commonly associated with breast cancer.

Ulcerating skin lesions usually indicate advanced or disseminated disease that is unlikely to be eradicated but may be controlled or palliated through systemic treatment (chemotherapy and targeted therapy) or radiation therapy. Local care of these lesions is a nursing priority. Nurses carefully assess malignant skin lesions for the size, appearance, condition of surrounding tissue, odor, bleeding, drainage, and associated pain or other symptoms, including evidence of infection. The potential for serious complications such as hemorrhage, vessel compression/obstruction, or airway obstruction, especially in head and neck cancer, should be noted so that the caregiver can be instructed in palliative measures to maintain patient comfort.

Nursing care (see Chart 12-6) also includes wound cleansing, reduction of superficial bacteria, control of bleeding, odor reduction, protection from further skin trauma, and pain management. The patient and family require emotional support, assistance, and guidance in providing wound care and addressing comfort measures at home.

Promoting Nutrition

Most patients with cancer experience some weight loss during their illness. Thus nurses need to promote good nutrition throughout treatment.

Nutritional Impairment

Anorexia, malabsorption, and cancer-related anorexia-cachexia syndrome (CACS) are some common nutritional problems. Impaired nutritional status may contribute to both physical and psychosocial consequences (see Chart 12-7). Nutritional concerns include decreased protein and caloric intake, metabolic or mechanical effects of the cancer, systemic disease, side effects of the treatment, or the patient's emotional status.

Chart 12-7

Potential Consequences of Impaired Nutrition in Patients with Cancer

- Anemia
- Decreased survival
- Immune incompetence and increased incidence of infection
- Delayed tissue and wound healing
- Fatigue
- Diminished functional ability
- Decreased capacity to continue antineoplastic therapy
- Increased hospital admissions
- Increased length of hospital stay
- Impaired psychosocial functioning

Anorexia

Among the many causes of anorexia in patients with cancer are alterations in taste, manifested by increased salty, sour, and metallic taste sensations, and altered responses to sweet and bitter flavors. Taste changes contribute to decreased appetite and nutritional intake and subsequently protein–calorie malnutrition. Taste alterations may result from mineral (e.g., zinc) deficiencies, increases in circulating amino acids and cellular metabolites, or the administration of chemotherapeutic agents. Patients undergoing radiation therapy to the head and neck may experience "mouth blindness," which is a severe impairment of taste.

Anorexia may occur because patients develop early satiety after eating only a small amount of food. This sense of fullness occurs secondary to a decrease in digestive enzymes, abnormalities in the metabolism of glucose and triglycerides, and prolonged stimulation of gastric volume receptors, which convey the feeling of being full. Psychological distress (e.g., fear, pain, depression, isolation) throughout illness may also have a negative impact on appetite. Patients may develop an aversion to food because of nausea and vomiting associated with treatment.

Malabsorption

Some patients with cancer are unable to absorb nutrients from the gastrointestinal system as a result of tumor activity, cancer treatments, or both. Malignancy can affect gastrointestinal activity in several ways (e.g., impaired enzyme production, interference with both protein and fat digestion) that can lead to increased gastrointestinal irritation, peptic ulcer disease, and fistula formation.

Chemotherapy and radiation associated with mucositis cause damage to mucosal cells of the bowel, resulting in impaired nutrient absorption. Abdominal irradiation has been associated with sclerosis of intestinal blood vessels and fibrotic changes in the gastrointestinal tissue, both impacting nutrient absorption. Surgical intervention may change peristaltic patterns, alter gastrointestinal secretions, and reduce the absorptive surfaces of gastrointestinal mucosa, all of which contribute to malabsorption.

Cancer-Related Anorexia-Cachexia Syndrome

CACS is a complex biologic process that results from a combination of increased energy expenditure and decreased intake (Mattox, 2017; Olsen et al., 2019). This syndrome can occur in both the curative and palliative stages of treatment and care. Combined immunologic, neuroendocrine, and metabolic processes give rise to anorexia, unintentional weight loss, and increased metabolic demand with impaired metabolism of glucose and lipids. As this syndrome continues, altered metabolic processes and tumor responses lead to cytokine release, causing generalized systemic inflammation. The patient experiences continued weight loss and malnutrition characterized by loss of adipose tissue, visceral protein, and skeletal muscle mass. Patients with CACS complain of loss of appetite, early satiety, and fatigue. It is estimated that 50% of patients with cancer experience anorexia and cachexia; this percentage increases to as high as 86% in patients with advanced cancer at the end of life (Olsen et al., 2019). Protein losses are associated with the development of anemia, peripheral edema, and progressive debilitation. The signs and symptoms of cancer cachexia and progressive debilitation result in decreased quality of life, psychological distress, and anxiety for both patient and family as they respond to actual and perceived impending losses, fear, lack of control, and helplessness.

Nursing care is integral to an interdisciplinary approach that addresses the multiple factors contributing to impaired nutritional status in patients with cancer (see Chart 12-6).

General Nutrition Considerations

Assessment of the patient's nutritional status is conducted at diagnosis and monitored throughout the course of treatment and follow-up. Early identification of patients at risk for problems with intake, absorption, and cachexia, particularly during the early stages of disease, can facilitate timely implementation of specifically targeted interventions that attempt to improve quality of life, treatment outcomes, and survival (Krishnasamy, Yoong, Chan, et al., 2017). Current weight, weight loss, diet and medication history, patterns of anorexia, nausea and vomiting, diarrhea, and situations and foods that aggravate or relieve symptoms are assessed and addressed.

The type of cancer, stage, and treatment approaches are considered so that proactive measures to support nutrition can be identified. For example, patients with head and neck cancers who are treated with radiation therapy, or some combination of surgery, radiation, chemotherapy or targeted agents, are at high risk for inadequate oral intake and nutritional deficits. In many centers, these patients have a percutaneous endoscopic gastrostomy (PEG) tube placed for enteral nutrition prior to initiation of treatment and the onset of mucositis, weight loss, and other consequences of impaired oral intake. A speech therapy consult may be helpful for patients with oropharyngeal or laryngeal tumors or surgical interventions that are anticipated to effect swallowing, secretion management, speech, or respiratory function.

Whenever possible, every effort is made to maintain adequate nutrition through the oral route. Prokinetic agents such as metoclopramide are used to increase gastric emptying in patients with early satiety and delayed gastric emptying. Other pharmacologic interventions such as megestrol acetate or corticosteroids (on a short-term basis) may be used to improve appetite. Oral nutritional supplements are encouraged to meet nutritional needs and to maintain or improve weight gain and physical functioning. Approaches incorporate nutritional counseling, exercise, pharmacologic interventions to combat anorexia, and symptom management when feasible (NCCN, 2019g). If adequate nutrition cannot be maintained by oral intake, nutritional support via the enteral route may be necessary as discussed previously. When needed, the patient and family are taught to administer enteral nutrition in the home. Home health nurses assist with patient education and monitor the patient's symptoms and response to enteral nutrition.

When malabsorption is a problem, enzyme and vitamin replacement may be instituted. Additional strategies include changing the feeding schedule, using simple diets, and relieving diarrhea. If malabsorption is severe, or the cancer involves the upper gastrointestinal tract, parenteral nutrition may be necessary. However, patients receiving parenteral nutrition are at increased risk for complications, including catheter-related and systemic infection. The use of parenteral nutrition in patients with advanced or end-stage cancer is seldom

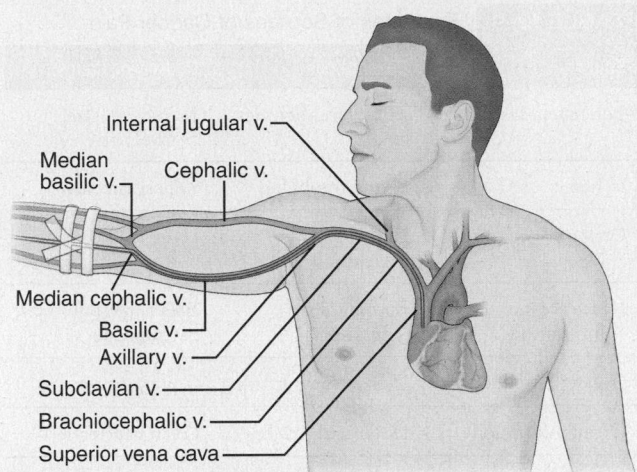

Figure 12-6 • A peripherally inserted central catheter is advanced through the cephalic or basilic vein to the axillary, subclavian, or brachiocephalic vein or the superior vena cava.

used and controversial (Jatoi & Kelly, 2019). Parenteral nutrition can be given in several ways: by a long-term venous access device such as a right atrial catheter (see Fig. 12-3), implanted venous port (see Fig. 12-4), or PICC (see Fig. 12-6). The nurse educates the patient and family to care for the venous access device and to administer parenteral nutrition. Home health nurses provide education and assist with or supervise parenteral nutrition administration in the home.

Relieving Pain

More than half of patients with cancer experience pain throughout the cancer trajectory. Moderate to severe pain is reported by approximately 28% of patients with cancer during treatment and as many as 52% of those with advanced disease (van den Beuken-van Everdingen, Hochstenbach, Joosten, et al., 2016). Although cancer pain may be acute, it is more frequently characterized as chronic. (See Chapter 9 for more information on pain.) As in other situations involving pain, the experience of cancer pain is influenced by physical, psychosocial, cultural, and spiritual factors.

Cancer can cause pain in various ways (see Table 12-9). Initially, pain is most often related to the underlying cancer process. Pain is also associated with various cancer treatments. Acute pain is linked with trauma from surgery. Occasionally, chronic pain syndromes, such as postsurgical neuropathies (pain related to nerve tissue injury), occur. Some chemotherapeutic agents cause tissue necrosis, peripheral neuropathies, and stomatitis—all potential sources of pain—whereas radiation therapy can cause pain secondary to skin, nervous tissue, or organ inflammation. Patients with cancer may have other sources of pain, such as arthritis or migraine headaches, that are unrelated to the underlying cancer or its treatment.

The nurse assesses the patient for the source and site of pain as well as those factors that influence the patient's perception and experience of pain, such as fear and apprehension, fatigue, anger, and social isolation. Pain assessment scales are useful for assessing the patient's pain before and after pain-relieving interventions are instituted to assess the effectiveness of interventions. Other symptoms that contribute to the

TABLE 12-9 Examples of Sources of Cancer Pain

Source	Descriptions	Underlying Cancer
Bone metastasis	Throbbing, aching	Breast, prostate, myeloma
Ischemia	Sharp, throbbing	Kaposi sarcoma
Lymphatic or venous obstruction	Dull, aching, tightness	Lymphoma, breast, Kaposi sarcoma
Nerve compression, infiltration	Burning, sharp, tingling	Breast, prostate, lymphoma
Organ obstruction	Dull, crampy, gnawing	Colon, gastric
Organ infiltration	Distention, crampy	Liver, pancreatic
Skin inflammation, ulceration, infection, necrosis	Burning, sharp	Breast, head and neck, Kaposi sarcoma

Adapted from van den Beuken-van Everdingen, M. H., Hochstenbach, L. M., Joosten, E. A., et al. (2016). Update on prevalence of pain in patients with cancer: Systematic review and meta-analysis. *Journal of Pain and Symptom Management, 51*(6), 1070–1090; Yarbro, C. H., Wujcik, D., & Gobel, B. H. (2018). *Cancer nursing: Principles and practice.* Burlington, MA: Jones & Bartlett Publishers.

pain experience, such as nausea and fatigue, are assessed and addressed as well.

Today, most people expect pain to disappear or resolve quickly. Although it is often controllable, advanced cancer pain is commonly irreversible and not quickly resolved. For many patients, pain is often seen as a signal that cancer is advancing, and that death is approaching. As patients anticipate pain and anxiety increases, pain perception heightens, producing fear and further pain. Thus, chronic cancer pain can lead to a cycle progressing from pain to anxiety to fear and back to pain, especially when the pain is not adequately managed. Inadequate pain management is most often the result of misconceptions and insufficient knowledge about pain assessment and management on the part of patients, families, and health care providers (Scarborough & Smith, 2018). Chapter 9 provides information regarding factors contributing to the pain experience, pain perception, and tolerance as well as pharmacologic and nonpharmacologic nursing interventions addressing pain. The nursing care plan (see Chart 12-6) also provides strategies for nursing assessment and management of chronic pain. Analgesics are administered based on the patient's reported level of pain. A cancer pain algorithm, developed as a set of analgesic guiding principles, is given in Figure 12-7.

Pharmacologic and nonpharmacologic approaches, even those that may be invasive, are considered in managing cancer-related pain regardless of the patient's status along the cancer trajectory. The nurse assists the patient and family to take an active role in managing pain. The nurse provides education and support to correct fears and misconceptions about opioid use. Inadequate pain management leads to a diminished quality of life characterized by distress, suffering, anxiety, fear, immobility, isolation, and depression.

Decreasing Fatigue

Fatigue is one of the most frequent and distressing symptoms experienced by patients receiving cancer therapy. Patients report that fatigue persists and interferes with activities of daily living for months to years after the completion of treatment (Wang, Yang, Miao, et al., 2018). Fatigue rarely exists in isolation; patients typically experience other symptoms concurrently, such as pain, dyspnea, anemia, sleep disturbances, or depression. The relationship between sleep disturbances, fatigue, and depression (as well as other clinical factors) in older adults with cancer is an active area of research.

In assessing fatigue, the nurse distinguishes between *acute fatigue*, which occurs after an energy-demanding experience, and *cancer-related fatigue*, which is defined as "a distressing persistent, subjective sense of physical, emotional or cognitive tiredness or exhaustion related to cancer or cancer treatment that is not proportional to recent activity and interferes with usual functioning" (NCCN, 2019h). Acute fatigue serves a protective function, whereas cancer-related fatigue does not. The exact mechanisms of fatigue are not well understood and are multifactorial in nature.

Despite the commonly occurring experience of fatigue in patients with cancer, a reliable assessment tool has not been identified. The experience of fatigue is highly subjective, with patient descriptors varying greatly (NCCN, 2019h). The nurse assesses physiologic and psychological factors that can contribute to fatigue (see Chart 12-8).

Exercise is an effective approach to the management of cancer-related fatigue (Mitchell, Albrecht, Omar Alkaiyat, et al., 2017). Psychoeducational approaches, cognitive-behavioral therapy to address sleep, progressive muscle relaxation, yoga, and mindfulness meditation may be effective measures to facilitate fatigue management (Mitchell et al., 2017). Nurses assist patients with strategies to minimize fatigue or help the patient cope with fatigue as described in the nursing care plan (see Chart 12-6, Fatigue). Occasionally, pharmacologic interventions are utilized, including antidepressants for patients with depression, anxiolytics for those with anxiety, hypnotics for patients with sleep disturbances, and psychostimulants for some patients with advanced cancer or fatigue that does not respond to other interventions

---

Chart 12-8 **Sources of Fatigue in Patients with Cancer**

- Anxiety associated with fear, diagnosis, role changes, uncertainty of future
- Disturbed sleep pattern related to cancer therapies, anxiety, and pain
- Electrolyte imbalances due to vomiting, diarrhea
- Risk for impaired nutritional intake due to nausea, vomiting, cancer-related anorexia-cachexia syndrome
- Impaired physical mobility due to neurologic impairments, surgery, bone metastasis, pain, and analgesic use
- Impaired tissue integrity due to stomatitis, mucositis
- Ineffective breathing associated with cough and dyspnea
- Ineffective protection secondary to neutropenia, thrombocytopenia, anemia
- Pain, pruritus
- Uncertainty and education needs related to disease process, treatment

Adapted from the National Comprehensive Cancer Network (NCCN). (2019h). NCCN guidelines for supportive care: Cancer related fatigue – version 1.2019. Retrieved on 7/20/2019 at: www.nccn.org/professionals/physician_gls/pdf/fatigue.pdf

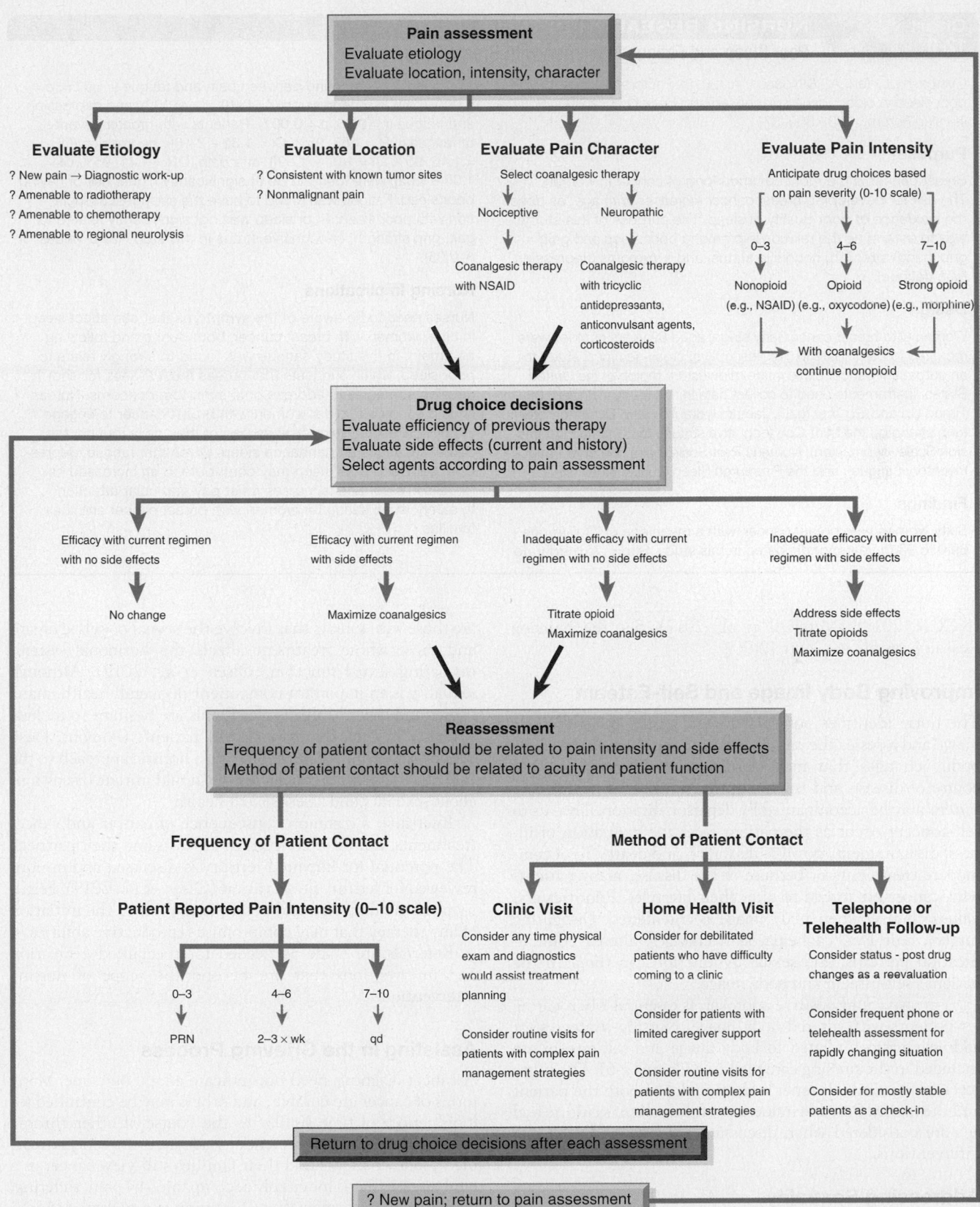

Figure 12-7 • The cancer pain algorithm (highest-level view) is a decision-tree model for pain treatment. NSAID; nonsteroidal anti-inflammatory drug; PRN, as needed; qd, once a day; wk, week. Adapted from DuPen, A. R., DuPen, S., Hansberry, J., et al. (2000). An educational implementation of a cancer pain algorithm for ambulatory care. *Pain Management Nursing, 1*(4), 118.

Chart 12-9 NURSING RESEARCH PROFILE
Poor Sleep and Fatigue in Women with Breast Cancer

Overcash, J., Tan, A., & Noonan, A. (2018). Factors associated with poor sleep in older women diagnosed with breast cancer. *Oncology Nursing Forum, 45*(3), 359–371.

Purpose

Breast cancer is the most common form of cancer in women. The risk for developing breast cancer increases with age, as does the incidence of poor quality of sleep. The purpose of this study was to determine the relationship among poor sleep and gait, grip (hand) strength, cognitive status, and symptoms (depression, pain, fatigue).

Design

Women with breast cancer (any stage) aged 69 years or older were recruited to participate in this descriptive, cross-sectional study for an outpatient cancer clinic in the midwestern region of the United States. Instruments used to collect data in this study included: the Timed Up and Go Test (gait), Jamar Hydraulic Hand Dynamometer (grip strength), the Mini-Cog (cognitive status), the Geriatric Depression Scale (depression), Numeric Pain Scale (pain), the Brief Fatigue Inventory (fatigue), and the Pittsburgh Sleep Quality Index (sleep).

Findings

Sixty women with breast cancer, with a mean age of 77.6 (range 69.0 to 93.0) years, participated in this study. Strong to moderate relationships were found between pain and fatigue ($r = 0.58$, $p = 0.001$); pain and depression ($r = 0.40$, $p = 0.002$); and depression and fatigue ($r = 0.66$, $p = 0.001$). Patients with greater severity of fatigue (OR = 1.57, 95% CI = 1.32 – 2.16]), depression (OR = 1.46, 95% CI = 1.07 – 1.99]), and pain (OR = 1.41, 95% CI = 1.04 – 1.92]) were found to be at significantly higher risk of having poor sleep. Fatigue was found to have the strongest association with poor sleep. Poor sleep was not significantly related to gait, grip strength, or cognitive status in this study (all p-values > 0.05).

Nursing Implications

Nurses need to be aware of the symptoms that can affect sleep in older women with breast cancer, both during and following treatment. In this study, fatigue was found to strongly relate to poor sleep, which suggests that nurses must assess for and develop strategies to address both symptom concerns. Nurses should encourage older women with breast cancer to engage in physical activity (exercise) as part of their daily routine, to decrease fatigue and enhance sleep. Given that fatigue, depression, pain, and poor sleep may contribute to an increased risk for falls in older adults, nurses must pay particular attention to safety when caring for women with breast cancer and their families.

(NCCN, 2019h; Mitchell et al., 2017). See the Nursing Research profile in Chart 12-9.

Improving Body Image and Self-Esteem

The nurse identifies potential threats to the patient's body image and assesses the patient's ability to cope with the many bodily changes that may be experienced throughout the course of disease and treatment. Entry into the health care system may be accompanied by depersonalization. Threats to self-concept occur as the patient faces the realization of illness, disfigurement, possible disability, and death. To accommodate treatments or because of the disease, many patients with cancer are forced to alter their lifestyles. Priorities and values change when body image is threatened. Disfiguring surgery, hair loss, cachexia, skin changes, altered communication patterns, and sexual dysfunction can threaten the patient's self-esteem and body image.

A creative and positive approach is essential when caring for patients with altered body image. Nursing strategies for addressing issues related to body image and self-esteem are included in the nursing care plan (see Chart 12-6). The nurse serves as an active listener and counselor to both the patient and the family. Possible influences of the patient's culture and age are considered when discussing concerns and potential interventions.

Addressing Sexuality

The physiologic processes associated with cancer; potential short- and long-term effects of cancer treatments; and psychosocial, emotional, and spiritual responses to the entire experience may lead patients to confront a variety of sexuality-based issues. Patients at the greatest risk of sexual dysfunction are those with tumors that involve the sexual or pelvic organs and those whose treatment affects the hormonal systems mediating sexual function (Olsen et al., 2019). Although sexuality is an important component of overall health, many nurses and other health professionals are hesitant to include sexuality in their discussions with patients (Almont, Farsi, Krakowski, et al., 2019). In offering a holistic approach to the care of patients with cancer, nurses should initiate discussions about sexuality and assess sexual health.

Infertility, a common consequence of cancer and cancer treatments, can be of concern to patients and their partners. The potential for impaired fertility is discussed and options reviewed for fertility preservation (Olsen et al., 2019). Fertility plans are discussed and determined prior to the initiation of any therapy that may compromise reproductive abilities.

Referrals are made as needed for specialized evaluation and interventions that are beyond the scope of nursing intervention.

Assisting in the Grieving Process

A cancer diagnosis need not indicate a fatal outcome. Many forms of cancer are curable, and others may be controlled for long periods of time similar to the course of other chronic diseases. Despite the tremendous advances in cancer treatment, many patients and their families still view cancer as a fatal disease that is inevitably accompanied by pain, suffering, debilitation, and emaciation. Grieving is a normal response to these fears and to actual or potential losses: loss of health, normal sensations, body image, social interaction, intimacy, independence, and usual social roles. Patients, families, and friends may grieve for the loss of quality time to spend with others, the loss of future and unfulfilled plans, and the loss of control over the patient's body and emotional reactions. Nurses continue to assess the patient and family for positive or maladaptive coping behaviors, interpersonal communication, and evidence of the need for additional psychosocial support or interventions such as referral for professional counseling.

If the patient enters the terminal phase of disease, the nurse may assess that the patient and family members are at different stages of grief. In such cases, the nurse assists the patient and family to acknowledge and cope with their reactions and feelings. The nurse also empowers the patient and family to explore preferences for issues related to end-of-life care, such as withdrawal of active disease treatment, desire for the use of life-support measures, and symptom management approaches. Oncology nurses respectfully support the patient's spiritual or religious views and facilitate contact with their preferred clergy member, if desired. In addition, nurses consider the patient's cultural beliefs and practices when addressing issues related to grief. After the death of a patient with cancer, home health or hospice nurses follow up with surviving family members for bereavement counseling to facilitate expression and coping with feelings of loss and grief. (See Chapter 13 for further discussion of end-of-life issues.)

Management of Psychosocial Distress

Despite advances in cancer care, patients experience varying levels of psychosocial distress related to actual or potential losses, fear of the unknown, symptoms due to cancer or cancer treatments, changes in usual family and social roles, financial concerns, and a sense of loss of control. Psychosocial distress is defined as a multifactorial unpleasant emotional experience of a psychological (cognitive, behavioral, emotional), social, or spiritual nature that may interfere with the ability to cope effectively with cancer, its physical symptoms and its treatment (NCCN, 2019i). Distress occurs along a continuum, ranging from common normal feelings of vulnerability, sadness, and fears to problems that can become disabling, such as depression, anxiety, panic, social isolation, and existential and spiritual crisis. Distress that is not addressed can have a significant impact on the overall well-being, interpersonal relationships, cognitive abilities, and adherence to treatment regimens, leading to poor outcomes.

Nurses need to screen patients for psychosocial distress during the cancer experience. Patients are supported in managing various sources and levels of distress. Referral to mental health providers may be helpful to address specific concerns (NCCN, 2019i).

Monitoring and Managing Potential Complications

Nurses need to pay particular attention to monitoring for and helping manage complications such as infection, septic shock, bleeding, and thrombocytopenia.

Infection

For patients in all stages of cancer, the nurse assesses factors associated with the development of infection. Although infection-associated morbidity and mortality have greatly decreased, prevention and prompt treatment of infection are essential in patients with cancer (Olsen et al., 2019). Often, more than one predisposing factor is present in patients with cancer. The nurse monitors laboratory studies to detect early changes in WBC counts. Common sites of infection, such as the pharynx, skin, perianal area, urinary, and respiratory tracts, are assessed on a regular basis. However, the typical signs of infection (swelling, redness, drainage, and pain) may not occur in myelosuppressed patients because of decreased circulating WBCs and a diminished local inflammatory response. Fever may be the only sign of infection (NCCN, 2019j). The nurse monitors the patient for sepsis, particularly if invasive catheters or long-term IV catheters are in place.

WBC function is often impaired in patients with cancer. Among the five types of WBCs (neutrophils [granulocytes], lymphocytes, monocytes, basophils, and eosinophils), neutrophils serve as the body's primary initial defense against invading organisms. Comprising 60% to 70% of the body's WBCs, neutrophils act by engulfing and destroying infective organisms through phagocytosis. Both the total WBC count and the concentration of neutrophils are important in determining the patient's ability to fight infection. A decrease in circulating WBCs is referred to as leukopenia. The terms granulocytopenia and neutropenia refer to a decrease in neutrophils.

A differential WBC count identifies the relative numbers of WBCs and permits tabulation of polymorphonuclear neutrophils (PMNs) or segmented neutrophils (mature neutrophils, reported as "polys," PMNs, or "segs") and immature forms of neutrophils (reported as bands, metamyelocytes, and "stabs"). The absolute neutrophil count (ANC) is calculated by the following formula:

$$\text{ANC} = (\text{segmented neutrophils [\%]} + \text{band [\%]}) \times \text{WBC count (cell/mm}^3)$$

$$\text{Example: } (25\% \text{ seg} + 25\% \text{ bands}) \times 6000 \text{ WBC cell/mm}^3 = 3000 \text{ ANC}$$

Neutropenia, an abnormally low ANC, is associated with an increased risk of infection. The risk of infection rises as the ANC decreases. As the ANC declines below 1500 cells/mm^3, the risk of infection rises. An ANC less than 500 cells/mm^3 reflects a severe risk of infection (NCCN, 2019j). The *nadir* is the lowest ANC following chemotherapy, targeted therapy, or radiation therapy that suppresses bone marrow function. Severe neutropenia may necessitate delays in administration of myelosuppressive therapies or treatment dose adjustments, although the use of the hematopoietic growth factors (e.g., colony-stimulating factors; see previous discussion) has reduced the severity and duration of treatment-associated neutropenia as well as infection-related morbidity and early death (NCCN, 2019j). The administration of these growth factors assists in maintaining treatment schedules, drug dosages, treatment effectiveness, and quality of life.

Patients with febrile neutropenia are assessed for factors that increase the risk of infection and for sources of infection through cultures of blood, sputum, urine, stool, IV and urinary or other catheters, and wounds, if appropriate (see Table 12-10). In addition, a chest x-ray is usually obtained to assess for pulmonary infection.

Defense against infection is compromised in many ways. The integrity of the skin and mucous membranes is challenged by multiple invasive diagnostic procedures, by the adverse effects of all cancer treatment modalities, and by the detrimental effects of immobility. Impaired nutrition as a result of

TABLE 12-10	Assessment of Neutropenic Fever in Patients with Cancer

Fever Criteria	Neutropenia Criteria
• Any one-time temperature of 38.3°C (101°F) or • Any temperature of ≥38°C (100.4°F) or ≥1 h	• <500 neutrophils/mcL or • <1000 neutrophils/mcL and predicted to decline to ≤500 neutrophils/mcL over the next 48 h

Assessment Targets for Neutropenic Fever Evaluation

Infection Risk Factors	Physical Assessment	Diagnostic Procedures	Microbiologic Cultures
• Chronic comorbid illnesses • Underlying hematologic malignancies • Immunosuppression related to factors other than neutropenia (e.g., immunosuppressive therapy following allogeneic HSCT or hypogammaglobulinemia [decreased gammaglobulin production]) • Solid tumors causing obstructions of the bronchial tree, ureters, colon, or biliary ducts • Advanced or refractory underlying malignancy • Prolonged duration of neutropenia • Age ≥65 yrs • Limited mobility or debilitation • Medications (e.g., corticosteroids such as prednisone) • Antibiotic therapy or prophylaxis • Recent surgery for diagnosis or treatment • Chemotherapy or targeted therapy received within the last 7–10 days • Prior treatment with multiple types of chemotherapy regimens • Recent radiation therapy; especially to areas associated with bone marrow reserves • Prior documented infections • Impaired skin integrity • Invasive drainage or urinary catheters • Peripheral or central venous access devices • Exposures (travel, others with infection, blood administration, pets) • Diarrhea • Poor nutritional status • Recent lumbar puncture or indwelling Ommaya reservoir™ (long-term intraventricular catheter for administration of chemotherapy into CSF and ventricles)	• Skin, pressure points, wounds • Surgical or biopsy incision sites • IV access or reservoir sites • Drainage catheter sites • Tracheostomy site • Lungs and sinuses • Perivaginal and perirectal area • Alimentary canal, abdomen • Neurologic assessment • Vital signs	• Diagnostic imaging as appropriate to identify abscesses, fistulas, pneumonia, obstruction, etc. • Complete blood count/differential • Serum chemistries, liver function tests • Renal function tests • Pulse oximetry or arterial blood gases • Lumbar puncture for CSF analysis	• Blood (peripheral and central venous access if applicable) • Urine (especially with indwelling catheter) • Skin wounds, lesions, incision sites, catheter exit sites • Catheter tips when feasible • Drainage from catheters • Stool, diarrhea • Sputum • CSF

CSF, cerebrospinal fluid; HSCT, hematopoietic stem cell transplantation; IV, intravenous.
Adapted from National Comprehensive Cancer Network (NCCN). (2019j). NCCN clinical practice guidelines in oncology: Prevention and treatment of cancer-related infection—version 1.2019. Retrieved on 7/14/2019 at: www.nccn.org/professionals/physician_gls/pdf/infections.pdf; Palmore, T. N., Parta, M., Cuellar-Rodriguez, J., et al. (2018). Infections in the cancer patient. In DeVita, V. T., Lawrence, T. S., Rosenberg, S. A. (Eds.). *Cancer: Principles & practice of oncology* (11th ed.). Philadelphia, PA: Lippincott Williams & Wilkins.

CACS, nausea, vomiting, diarrhea, and the underlying disease alters the body's ability to combat invading organisms. Medications such as antibiotics disturb the balance of normal flora, allowing the overgrowth of normal flora and pathogenic organisms. Other medications can also alter the immune response (see Chapter 31). Cancer itself may lead to defects in cellular and humoral immunity. Advanced cancer may cause obstruction of hollow viscera (e.g., intestines), blood, and lymphatic vessels, creating a favorable environment for proliferation of pathogenic organisms. In some patients, tumor cells infiltrate bone marrow and prevent normal production of WBCs.

Nurses are in a key position to assist in preventing and identifying symptoms of infection, as discussed in the nursing care plan (see Chart 12-6). Clinical practice guidelines developed by the ONS, the Infusion Nurses Society (INS), the NCCN, and the ASCO are used to guide prevention and management of infection. Interventions to prevent infection and alternative patient education formats for infection-related instruction are high nursing research priorities.

Gram-positive bacteria (*Streptococcus*, enterococci, and *Staphylococcus* species) and gram-negative organisms (*Escherichia coli*, *Klebsiella pneumoniae*, *Enterobacter*, and *Pseudomonas aeruginosa*) are the most frequently isolated causes of infection. Fungal organisms, such as *Candida albicans*, also contribute to the incidence of serious infection. Viral infections in immunocompromised patients are caused most often by herpes simplex, respiratory syncytial, parainfluenza, and influenza A and B viruses.

Fever is reported promptly as it is an important sign of infection in patients when associated with neutropenia (Olsen et al., 2019). Patients with neutropenic fever (see Table 12-10) are assessed for infection and reported promptly (NCCN, 2019j). Antibiotics may be prescribed after cultures of wound drainage, exudates, sputum, urine, stool, or blood are obtained. Careful consideration is given to the underlying malignancy, prior antineoplastic treatment, ANC, comorbidities, and other patient-related factors prior to the identification of the most appropriate antibiotic therapy. Evidence-based guidelines are available for prevention and treatment of cancer-related infections (NCCN, 2019j). Patients with neutropenia are treated with broad-spectrum antibiotics before the infecting organism is identified because of the increased risk of mortality associated with untreated infection. Broad-spectrum antibiotic therapy targets the most likely major pathogenic organisms. It is important for these medications to be given and taken promptly as scheduled to achieve adequate blood levels. Once the offending organism is identified, more specific antimicrobial therapy is prescribed as appropriate. Nurses provide education for patients and families regarding prevention of infection, signs and symptoms to report, and the importance of adherence to prescribed antimicrobial therapy.

 Septic Shock

The nurse assesses the patient frequently for signs and symptoms of infection and inflammation throughout the trajectory of cancer care. Sepsis and septic shock are life-threatening complications that must be prevented or detected and treated promptly. Although all patients with cancer are at risk, patients who are neutropenic or who have hematologic malignancies are at the greatest risk. Patients with signs and symptoms of impending sepsis and septic shock require immediate hospitalization and aggressive treatment in the intensive care setting. See Chapter 11 for discussion of sepsis and septic shock.

Bleeding and Thrombocytopenia

Platelets are essential for normal blood clotting and coagulation (hemostasis). **Thrombocytopenia**, a decrease in the circulating platelet count, is the most common cause of bleeding in patients with cancer and is usually defined as a platelet count less than $100,000/mm^3$ ($0.1 \times 10^{12}/L$). The risk of bleeding increases when the platelet count decreases below $50,000/mm^3$ ($0.05 \times 10^{12}/L$). At platelet counts lower than $10,000/mm^3$ ($0.02 \times 10^{12}/L$), the risk for spontaneous bleeding is increased (Olsen et al., 2019).

Thrombocytopenia often results from bone marrow depression after certain types of chemotherapy and radiation therapy and with tumor infiltration of the bone marrow. In some cases, platelet destruction is associated with hypersplenism (enlarged spleen) and abnormal antibody function, which occur with leukemia and lymphoma. Bacterial and viral infections may lead to early platelet destruction or impaired bone marrow production of platelets and subsequent thrombocytopenia. Some medications (e.g., heparin, vancomycin) may cause bone marrow toxicity leading to decreases in circulating platelets. Less commonly, posttransfusion complications may lead to antibody destruction of platelets causing profound thrombocytopenia (Mones & Soff, 2019). The nursing care plan addresses nursing assessment parameters and interventions for patients at risk for bleeding (see Chart 12-6).

 Quality and Safety Nursing Alert

Although laboratory test results confirm the diagnosis of thrombocytopenia, the patient who is developing thrombocytopenia may display early signs and symptoms. Thus, nurses need to observe keenly for petechiae and ecchymoses, which are early indicators of decreasing platelet levels. Early detection promotes early intervention.

Additional medications may be prescribed to address bleeding or thrombocytopenia based on the underlying etiology. See Chapter 29 for further discussion of assessment and treatment of thrombocytopenia and coagulopathies.

VTE, a common problem for patients with cancer, includes deep venous thrombosis (DVT), pulmonary embolism (PE), superficial venous thrombosis (SVT), and thrombosis in other abdominal or thoracic venous tributaries such as the mesenteric veins or the superior vena cava. The incidence of VTE has been linked to an increased likelihood of death in patients with cancer (NCCN, 2019k). Factors associated with risk for VTEs in cancer patients include preexisting underlying or cancer-related coagulopathies, medications including chemotherapy, hospitalizations, surgical procedures, increased age, debilitation, immobility, infection, and peripheral and central venous catheters (NCCN, 2019k). Patients with cancer are monitored for associated risk factors and are assessed on an ongoing basis for VTE. Nurses provide patient and family education regarding symptoms of VTE to report to the provider. Recommendations for prophylaxis are based on national guidelines and patient risk factors. Nursing assessment findings associated with VTE are reported promptly so that VTE evaluation and treatment can be initiated expeditiously.

Promoting Home, Community-Based, and Transitional Care

 Educating Patients About Self-Care

Most commonly, patients with cancer are diagnosed and treated in the outpatient setting. Nurses in outpatient settings often have the responsibility for patient education and helping coordinate care in the home (see Chart 12-10). The shift of care from acute care facilities to the home or outpatient settings as well as the increasing use of oral antineoplastic agents places significant responsibility for care on the patient and family. In order to maintain optimal patient outcomes and quality of life, patients and families require support and information that will prepare them to engage in self-care. Education initially focuses on the most immediate care needs likely to be encountered at home.

Approaches to preparing patients for self-care responsibilities are chosen with consideration of the patient's preferred learning strategies, level of education, and health literacy (Howell, Harth, Brown, et al., 2017). Nurses are in a prime role to promote self-care by ensuring that the educational needs of patients and families are met across time points of the cancer continuum (Eller, Lev, Yuan, et al., 2018; White, Cohen, Berger, et al., 2017). Easily understood, concrete, objective information that assists patients to understand what to expect and includes sensory and temporal components is important. Symptoms, side effects of treatment, and changes in the patient's status that should be reported are discussed and reinforced with printed materials that can be referred to in the home. Nurses help to empower patients by sharing strategies to manage side effects or other symptoms. Additional learning needs are based on the priorities conveyed by the patient and family as well as on the complexity of care required (Howell et al., 2017).

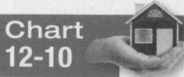

Chart 12-10

HOME CARE CHECKLIST

The Patient Receiving Care for an Oncologic Disorder

At the completion of education, the patient or caregiver will be able to:

- State the impact of cancer treatment on physiologic functioning, ADLs, IADLs, roles, relationships, and spirituality.
- State changes in lifestyle (e.g., diet, activity) necessary to maintain health.
- State the name, dose, side effects, frequency, and schedule for all medications.
- Demonstrate how to administer the chemotherapy agent in the home:
  - Describe safe storage and handling of oral chemotherapy/immunotherapy/targeted therapy agents in the home.
  - Demonstrate safe disposal of needles, syringes, IV supplies, or unused chemotherapy medications.
  - List possible side effects of chemotherapy/immunotherapy/targeted therapy agents and suggested management approaches.
- List possible side effects of radiation therapy and suggested management approaches.
- List complications of medications/therapeutic regimen necessitating a call to the nurse or primary provider.
- List complications of medications/therapeutic regimen necessitating a visit to the emergency department.

- Locate list of names and contact details of resource personnel involved in care (e.g., home health nurse, infusion services, IV vendor, equipment company, radiation therapy department).
- Explain treatment plan and importance of upcoming visits to the primary provider.
- State how to obtain medical supplies after discharge.
- Identify durable medical equipment needs, proper usage, and maintenance necessary for safe utilization.
- Demonstrate usage of adaptive equipment for ADLs.
- Identify community resources for peer and caregiver/family support:
  - Identify sources of support (e.g., friends, relatives, faith community)
  - Identify phone numbers of support groups for people with cancer and their caregivers/families
  - State meeting locations and times
- Identify the need for health promotion, disease prevention, and screening activities

ADL, activities of daily living; IADL, independent activities of daily living.

Technologic advances allow home administration of IV chemotherapy, blood products, and antibiotics; enteral or parenteral nutrition; and parenteral analgesics. Patients and families are taught to care for vascular access devices, infusion pumps, various types of drainage catheters, and on occasion complex wounds. The importance of patient safety and infection control is included in patient and family education. Although nurses are often available to provide some assistance with cancer care in the home, patients and families need to acquire the requisite knowledge and skills that will enable them to develop a strong sense of self-efficacy to not only foster self-care, but also to promote a more positive health status and better quality of life (Eller et al., 2018; White et al., 2017).

Continuing and Transitional Care

Referral for home or transitional care is often indicated for patients with cancer. The responsibilities of the nurse include assessing the home environment and suggesting modifications in the home or in care to help address the patient's physical and safety needs. Home health nurses also assess the psychosocial impact of cancer on the patient and family so that appropriate interventions can be identified or referrals for support services are instituted.

Ongoing nursing visits or phone contact from the home or transitional care nurse assist in prevention, early identification, prompt reporting, and management of patient problems. Timely modifications in therapy to manage symptoms and adverse effects of treatment may decrease patient suffering and decrease emergency department visits or hospital admissions. Continued contact facilitates evaluation of the patient's progress, responses to treatment, and assessment of the ongoing needs of the patient and family. It is necessary to assess the patient's and family's understanding of the treatment plan and management strategies and to reinforce previous education. The nurse facilitates coordination of patient care by maintaining close communication with all involved health care providers. The nurse may make referrals and coordinate available community resources (e.g., local office of the ACS, home aides, church groups, faith community nurses, support groups) to assist patients and caregivers.

Gerontologic Considerations

Approximately 55% of cancer incidence and 70% of cancer deaths occur in persons aged 65 years or older (ACS, 2019a). The rising number of individuals over age 65 with cancer has led to the emergence of geriatric oncology, a multidimensional and multidisciplinary approach to treating growing numbers of older adults with cancer.

Nurses working with older adults must understand the normal physiologic changes that occur with aging and the implications for the patient with cancer (see Table 12-11). These changes that affect all body systems may ultimately influence older patients' responses to cancer treatment. In addition, many older patients have other chronic diseases requiring multiple medications. The existence of comorbidities and multiple medications may contribute to drug interactions and toxicities in older patients.

The understanding of the effects and tolerance of chemotherapy, immunotherapy, targeted therapies, and radiation in the older adult is limited, as older adults have been underrepresented in oncology clinical trials. Potential chemotherapy-related toxicities, such as renal impairment, myelosuppression, fatigue, and cardiomyopathy, may increase as a result of declining organ function and diminished physiologic reserves. The recovery of normal tissues after radiation therapy may be delayed, and older adult patients may experience more severe adverse effects, such as mucositis, nausea and vomiting, and

TABLE 12-11 Age-Related Changes and Their Effects on Patients with Cancer

Age-Related Changes	Implications
Impaired immune system	Use special precautions to avoid infection; monitor for atypical signs and symptoms of infection.
Altered drug absorption, distribution, metabolism, and elimination	Mandates careful calculation of chemotherapy and frequent assessment for drug response and side effects; dose adjustments may be necessary.
Increased prevalence of other chronic diseases	Monitor for effect of cancer or its treatment on patient's other chronic diseases; monitor patient's tolerance for cancer treatment; monitor for interactions with medications used to treat chronic diseases.
Diminished renal, respiratory, and cardiac reserve	Be proactive in prevention of decreased renal function, atelectasis, pneumonia, and cardiovascular compromise; monitor for side effects of cancer treatment.
Decreased skin and tissue integrity; reduction in body mass; delayed healing	Prevent pressure ulcers secondary to immobility; monitor skin and mucous membranes for changes related to radiation or chemotherapy; monitor nutritional status.
Decreased musculoskeletal strength	Prevent falls; assess support for performing activities of daily living in home setting; encourage safe use of assistive mobility devices.
Decreased neurosensory functioning: loss of vision, hearing, and distal extremity tactile senses	Provide instruction modified for patient's hearing and vision changes; provide instruction concerning safety and skin care for distal extremities; assess home for safety.
Altered social and economic resources	Assess for financial concerns, living conditions, and resources for support.
Potential changes in cognitive and emotional capacity	Provide education and support modified for patient's level of functioning and safety.

Adapted from Eliopoulos, C. (2018). *Gerontological nursing* (10th ed.). Philadelphia, PA: Wolters Kluwer.

myelosuppression. Because of impaired healing and declining pulmonary and cardiovascular functioning, older patients are slower to recover from surgery. Older patients are also at increased risk for complications, such as atelectasis, pneumonia, and wound infections.

Cancer Survivorship

In the United States, there are currently an estimated 16.9 million adult cancer survivors; by 2030, that number is estimated to be 22.1 million (ACS, 2019f). Advances in cancer screening, treatment, and management of complications have contributed to a lengthened survival period for many, with long-term survival becoming possible for many patients. *Cancer survivorship* has been defined as the period from cancer diagnosis through the remaining years of life and focuses on the health and life of a person beyond diagnostic and treatment phases. Although individuals vary and many types of cancers and treatments exist, the acute, long-term, and late effects of cancer and its treatment may have multiple long-term physical, cognitive, psychological, social, and financial consequences that can impact activities of daily living, ultimately affecting quality of life (ACS, 2019f).

Survivorship care is often based on expert opinion and experience rather than on evidence-based practices. Knowledge regarding survivorship concerns continues to evolve. The Institute of Medicine has identified four components of survivorship care, the period that follows primary treatment for cancer and lasts until end of life. In addition to a summary of prior diagnosis and treatment, survivorship care includes monitoring and treatment for late effects related to disease and prior treatments, physical and vocational rehabilitation, psychosocial support and counseling as necessary, surveillance

and screening for new and recurrent cancer, and coordination between specialists and primary care providers to ensure that all of the survivor's needs are met (Hewitt, Greenfield, & Stovall, 2006) (see Table 12-12). Advocacy organizations across the country have recommended that a survivorship

TABLE 12-12 Components of Survivorship Care

Component	Examples of Care
Prevention and detection of new and recurrent cancer	Mammography (per ACS guidelines) Papanicolaou (Pap) smears (per ACS guidelines) Smoking cessation programs Nutrition counseling
Surveillance for cancer spread, recurrence, or second cancers	Colonoscopy post colon cancer Mammography post breast cancer Liver function tests post colon cancer Prostate-specific antigen post prostate cancer
Intervention for consequences of cancer and its treatments	Lymphedema therapy Pain management Enterostomal therapy Fertility care Psychosocial support or counseling Reconstructive surgery
Coordination between specialists and primary providers to meet health needs	Care for comorbidities (e.g., diabetes) Influenza vaccination Bone densitometry Monitoring for chemotherapy induced cardiotoxicity

ACS, American Cancer Society.
Adapted from Hewitt, M., Greenfield, S., & Stovall, E. (Eds.). (2006). *From cancer patient to cancer survivor: Lost in translation.* Washington, DC: Institute of Medicine and National Research Council, National Academies Press. Components of survivorship care provided by the Institute of Medicine report on cancer survivorship.

care plan be provided to all patients with cancer and their primary provider at the completion of treatment. The survivorship care plan includes a summary of cancer diagnosis, treatment, recommendations for follow-up care, including approaches to treat symptoms, rehabilitative needs, monitoring for late effects, and surveillance and screening for new and recurrent cancer. Referrals for specific services such as lymphedema therapy, chronic pain management, and genetic counseling are also provided. Nurses assist in the development of the survivorship care plan and provide education and care for cancer survivors. Nurses, other health care providers, public health professionals, and patient advocates design and conduct research to identify needs of cancer survivors and evidence-based approaches to care.

Providing Care to the Patient with Advanced Cancer

The patient with advanced cancer needs to be monitored for oncologic emergencies and have appropriate treatment should emergencies occur. These patients may have end-of-life and palliative care needs that must be addressed.

Providing Care in Oncologic Emergencies

Table 12-13 discusses select nursing and medical care of oncologic emergencies.

As a result of advances in all aspects of cancer care, it is more common that individuals are living with cancer that has advanced beyond the original site of development to regional or distant sites. Patients with advanced cancer are likely to experience many of the problems described previously, although more often and to a greater degree. Symptoms of pain, anorexia, weight loss, CACS, fatigue, and impaired functional status and mobility make patients more susceptible to depressive symptoms, skin breakdown, fluid and electrolyte imbalances, and infection.

Treatment for the patient with advanced cancer is likely to be palliative rather than curative, with an emphasis on prevention and appropriate management of pain. The use of long-acting analgesic agents at set intervals, rather than on an "as needed" basis, is recommended in addressing pain

TABLE 12-13	Oncologic Emergencies: Manifestations and Management	
Oncologic Emergency	**Clinical Manifestations and Diagnostic Findings**	**Medical and Nursing Management**
Superior Vena Cava Syndrome (SVCS) Compression or invasion of the superior vena cava by tumor; enlarged lymph nodes; intraluminal thrombus that obstructs venous circulation; or drainage of the head, neck, arms, and thorax. Most often associated with lung cancer, SVCS is also associated with lymphoma, thymoma, and testicular cancers and mediastinal metastases from breast cancer. If untreated, SVCS may lead to cerebral anoxia (because not enough oxygen reaches the brain), laryngeal edema, bronchial obstruction, and death.	**Clinical Manifestations:** Gradually or suddenly impaired venous drainage giving rise to: progressive dyspnea (shortness of breath), cough, hoarseness, chest pain, and facial swelling Edema of the neck, arms, hands, and thorax and reported sensation of skin tightness, difficulty swallowing, and stridor. Possibly engorged and distended jugular, temporal, and arm veins. Dilated thoracic vessels causing prominent venous patterns on the chest wall. Increased intracranial pressure, associated visual disturbances, headache, and altered mental status **Diagnostic Findings:** Diagnosis confirmed by: Clinical findings Chest x-ray Thoracic CT scan Thoracic MRI Venogram if intraluminal thrombosis is suspected	**Medical Management:** Radiation therapy to shrink tumor or enlarged lymph nodes and relieve symptoms. Chemotherapy for sensitive cancers (e.g., lymphoma, small cell lung cancer) or when the mediastinum has been irradiated to maximum tolerance. Anticoagulant or thrombolytic therapy for central venous catheter–related intraluminal thrombosis. Percutaneously placed intravascular stents may be priority consideration rather than surgery unless symptoms are rapidly progressing. Supportive measures such as oxygen therapy, corticosteroids, and diuretics (in cases of fluid overload). **Nursing Management:** Identify patients at risk for SVCS. Provide patient and family education regarding signs and symptoms to report. Monitor and report clinical manifestations of SVCS. Monitor cardiopulmonary and neurologic status. Avoid upper extremity venipuncture and blood pressure measurement; instruct patient to avoid tight or restrictive clothing and jewelry on fingers, wrist, and neck. Facilitate breathing and drainage from upper portion of body by instructing patient to maintain some elevation of head and upper body with semi-Fowler position; avoid completely supine or prone position (this helps to promote comfort and reduce anxiety associated with dependent and progressive edema). Promote energy conservation to minimize dyspnea. Monitor the patient's fluid volume status; administer fluids cautiously to minimize edema. Assess for thoracic radiation-related problems such as mucositis with resultant dysphagia (difficulty swallowing) and esophagitis. Monitor for chemotherapy-related problems, such as myelosuppression. Provide postoperative care as appropriate.

TABLE 12-13	Oncologic Emergencies: Manifestations and Management (continued)	
Oncologic Emergency	**Clinical Manifestations and Diagnostic Findings**	**Medical and Nursing Management**
Spinal Cord Compression Most commonly caused by compression of the cord and its nerve roots by a metastatic paravertebral tumor that extends into the epidural space; vertebral bone metastasis leading to bone collapse and displacement impinging on the spinal cord or nerve roots; and less commonly, primary malignancy of the cord. May potentially lead to significant and permanent neurologic impairment associated with multiple physical, psychosocial consequences. Most often associated with cancers that metastasize to the bone such as breast, lung, and prostate cancers and lymphoma. Also seen in nasopharyngeal cancer and multiple myeloma. About 60% of spinal cord compressions occur at the thoracic level, 30% in the lumbosacral level, and 10% in the cervical and sacral regions. The prognosis depends on the severity and rapidity of onset.	**Clinical Manifestations:** Local inflammation, edema, venous stasis, and impaired blood supply to nerve tissues. Local or radicular back or neck pain along the dermatomal areas innervated by the affected nerve root (e.g., thoracic radicular pain extends in a band around the chest or abdomen). Pain exacerbated by movement, supine recumbent position, coughing, sneezing, or the Valsalva maneuver. Neurologic dysfunction and related motor and sensory deficits (numbness, tingling, feelings of coldness in the affected area, inability to detect vibration, loss of positional sense). Motor loss ranging from subtle weakness to flaccid paralysis. Bladder or bowel dysfunction depending on level of compression (above S2, overflow incontinence; from S3 to S5, flaccid sphincter tone and bowel incontinence). **Diagnostic Findings:** Percussion tenderness at the level of compression; abnormal reflexes; and sensory and motor abnormalities. MRI is a preferred diagnostic tool; may also utilize x-rays, bone scans, and CT scan.	**Medical Management:** Radiation therapy to reduce tumor size and halt progression; corticosteroid therapy to decrease inflammation and swelling at the compression site. Surgery to debulk tumor and stabilize the spine if symptoms progress despite radiation therapy or if vertebral fracture or bone fragments lead to additional nerve damage; surgery is also an option when the tumor is not radiosensitive or is located in an area that was previously irradiated. Minimally invasive surgical procedures, referred to as vertebral augmentation, may be used for patients with vertebral fractures to attain stability of the bone, prevent nerve compression, and decrease pain. Procedures include: Vertebroplasty: involves percutaneous injection of polymethyl methacrylate (PMMA), a bone cement filler, into the vertebral body. Kyphoplasty: a balloon is inserted into the damaged vertebral body and then inflated to create a cavity within the bone that can be filled with bone cement. The balloon helps to compress the fracture fragments together as the cavity is created. Radiofrequency vertebral augmentation: similar to kyphoplasty; instead of the balloon, a small navigational cannula is inserted into the vertebra to create small pathways for cement. The cement is heated with radiofrequency to create an ultra-high viscosity that is thought to promote bone stability. Chemotherapy as adjuvant to other local therapies for patients with chemosensitive cancers, such as lymphoma or small cell lung cancer. *Note:* Despite treatment, patients with poor neurologic function before treatment are less likely to regain complete motor and sensory function; patients who develop complete paralysis usually do not regain all neurologic function. **Nursing Management:** Perform ongoing assessment of neurologic function to identify existing and progressing dysfunction. Control pain with pharmacologic and nonpharmacologic measures. Prevent complications of immobility resulting from pain and decreased function (e.g., skin breakdown, urinary stasis, thrombophlebitis, decreased clearance of pulmonary secretions). Maintain muscle tone by assisting with range-of-motion exercises in collaboration with physical and occupational therapists; patients with unstable vertebral fractures do not initiate physical therapy until spine stabilization procedures have been completed. Institute intermittent urinary catheterization and bowel training programs for patients with bladder or bowel dysfunction. Provide encouragement and support to the patient and family coping with pain and altered functioning, lifestyle, roles, and independence. Institute appropriate referrals for home care and physical and occupational therapy. Provide patient and family education about pharmacologic and nonpharmacologic interventions

(continued on page 362)

TABLE 12-13 Oncologic Emergencies: Manifestations and Management (continued)

Oncologic Emergency	Clinical Manifestations and Diagnostic Findings	Medical and Nursing Management
Hypercalcemia Hypercalcemia is a potentially life-threatening metabolic abnormality resulting when the calcium released from the bones is more than the kidneys can excrete or the bones can reabsorb. It may result from production of cytokines, hormonal substances, and growth factors by cancer cells, or by the body in response to biochemical mediators produced by cancer cells, which lead to bone breakdown and calcium release. Occurs in about 20% of patients with cancer; most commonly seen in patients with multiple myeloma and cancers of the lung and breast.	**Clinical Manifestations:** Fatigue, weakness, confusion, decreased level of responsiveness, hyporeflexia, nausea, vomiting, constipation, ileus, polyuria (excessive urination), polydipsia (excessive thirst), dehydration, and arrhythmias. **Diagnostic Findings:** Total serum calcium level >10.4 mg/dL (2.6 mmol/L) Ionized serum calcium >1.29 mmol/L	**Medical Management:** Identify patients at risk for hypercalcemia and assess for signs and symptoms of hypercalcemia. Treatment of the underlying malignancy (e.g., chemotherapy, radiation therapy, hormone therapy, immunotherapy or targeted therapy). Reduce serum calcium levels: Oral hydration (3–4 L of fluid daily unless contraindicated by existing renal or cardiac disease) or IV hydration followed by diuretics (forced diuresis). Avoid dietary supplements and medications that can increase serum calcium levels (e.g., thiazide diuretics, nonsteroidal anti-inflammatory drugs; and vitamins A and D, and calcium supplements). Bisphosphonate therapy may be indicated for the long-term management. Maintenance of nutritional intake without restricting normal calcium intake. Dietary and pharmacologic interventions such as stool softeners and laxatives for constipation. Antiemetic therapy for nausea and vomiting. **Nursing Management:** Monitor closely for changes in mental status; fluid and electrolyte imbalances; and renal, gastrointestinal, cardiac dysfunction. Monitor treatment effectiveness and for the presence of side effects. Ensure proper hydration and monitor fluid and electrolyte balance closely. Educate patients who are at-risk and their families to recognize and report signs and symptoms of hypercalcemia. Encourage mobilization / weight-bearing activities, as tolerated, to limit bone resorption. Maintain patient safety and ensure comfort. Educate patient and families about prescribed management strategies.
Tumor Lysis Syndrome (TLS) Potentially fatal complication that occurs spontaneously or more commonly following radiation, immunotherapy, targeted therapy, or chemotherapy-induced cell destruction of large or rapidly growing cancers such as leukemia, lymphoma, and small cell lung cancer. The release of tumor intracellular contents (nuclei acids, electrolytes, and debris) leads to rapidly induced electrolyte imbalances—hyperkalemia, hyperphosphatemia (leading to hypocalcemia), and hyperuricemia—that can have life-threatening end-organ effects on the myocardium, kidneys, and central nervous system.	**Clinical Manifestations:** Clinical manifestations depend on the extent of metabolic abnormalities. *Neurologic:* Fatigue, weakness, memory loss, altered mental status, muscle cramps, tetany, paresthesias (numbness and tingling), and seizures. *Cardiac:* Elevated blood pressure, shortened QT complexes, widened QRS waves, altered T waves, arrhythmias, and cardiac arrest. *Gastrointestinal:* Anorexia, nausea, vomiting, abdominal cramps, diarrhea, and increased bowel sounds *Renal:* Flank pain, oliguria, anuria, kidney injury, and acidic urine pH. *Other:* Gout, malaise, and pruritis. **Diagnostic Findings:** Electrolyte imbalances identified by serum electrolyte measurement and urinalysis (see Chapter 10); electrocardiogram to detect cardiac arrhythmias. Clinical TLS is diagnosed when ≥1 of 3 conditions arise either 3 days prior to or 7 days after cytotoxic cancer therapy: acute kidney injury (defined as a rise in creatinine to ≥1.5 times the upper limit of normal that is not attributable to medications, arrhythmias, and seizures).	**Medical Management:** To prevent kidney injury and restore electrolyte balance. Aggressive fluid hydration is initiated 24–48 h before and after the initiation of cytotoxic therapy to increase urine volume and eliminate uric acid and electrolytes. Diuresis with a loop diuretic or osmotic diuretic, if urine output is inadequate. Allopurinol therapy to inhibit the conversion of nucleic acids to uric acid (oral or IV). Rasburicase may be used to convert already formed uric acid to allantoin, which is highly water soluble and eliminated in urine. Administration of a cation-exchange resin, such as sodium polystyrene sulfonate to treat hyperkalemia by binding and eliminating potassium through the bowel. Administration of IV sodium bicarbonate, hypertonic dextrose, and regular insulin temporarily shifts potassium into cells and lowers serum potassium levels if a rapid decrease in potassium is necessary. Administration of phosphate-binding gels, such as aluminum hydroxide, to treat hyperphosphatemia by promoting phosphate excretion in the feces. Hemodialysis when patients are unresponsive to the standard approaches for managing uric acid and electrolyte abnormalities. Identify at-risk patients. Institute essential preventive measures (e.g., fluid hydration, medications) as prescribed. Assess patient for signs and symptoms of electrolyte imbalances. **Nursing Management:** Monitor for signs and symptoms of TLS in patients who are at-risk (e.g., those with hematologic malignancies). Monitor vital signs, laboratory values (i.e., electrolyte), fluid balance closely (i.e., daily weights, intakes and outputs), and cardiac status closely. Educate patients and families about risk factors for TLS; teach about current treatments (e.g., hydration, dietary restrictions [e.g., potassium and phosphorous], and pharmacologic therapy); signs and symptoms of complications; and when to report symptoms indicating electrolyte disturbances to the provider.

CT, computed tomography; IV, intravenous; MRI, magnetic resonance imaging.

Adapted from Kaplan, M. (Ed.). (2018). *Understanding and managing oncologic emergencies: A resource for nurses.* Pittsburgh, PA: Oncology Nursing Society; Rimmer, A., & Yahalom, J. (2018). Superior vena cava syndrome. In DeVita, V. T., Lawrence, T. S., Rosenberg, S. A. (Eds.). *Cancer: Principles & practice of oncology* (11th ed.). Philadelphia, PA: Lippincott Williams & Wilkins; Stein, S., & Deshpande, H. A. (2018). Metabolic emergencies. In DeVita, V. T., Lawrence, T. S., Rosenberg, S. A. (Eds.). *Cancer: Principles & practice of oncology* (11th ed.). Philadelphia, PA: Lippincott Williams & Wilkins; and Szerlip, N., Beeler, W. H., & Spratt, D. E. (2018). Spinal cord compression. In DeVita, V.T., Lawrence, T. S., Rosenberg, S. A. (Eds.). *Cancer: Principles & practice of oncology* (11th ed.). Philadelphia, PA: Lippincott Williams & Wilkins.

management. Working with the patient and family, as well as with other health care providers, to manage pain is essential to increase the patient's comfort and offer some sense of control. Other medications (e.g., sedatives, tranquilizers, muscle relaxants, antiemetics) are added to assist in palliating additional symptoms and promoting quality of life.

If the patient is a candidate for radiation therapy or surgical interventions to relieve pain or other symptoms, the potential benefits and risks of these procedures (e.g., percutaneous nerve block, cordotomy) are explained to the patient and family. Measures are taken to prevent complications that result from altered sensation, immobility, and changes in bowel and bladder function.

Weakness, altered mobility, fatigue, and inactivity typically increase with advanced cancer as a result of the disease, treatment, inadequate nutritional intake, or dyspnea. The nurse works with the patient and family to identify realistic goals and promote comfort. Measures include use of energy conservation methods to accomplish tasks and activities that the patient values most.

Efforts are made to provide the patient with as much control and independence as desired but with assurance that support and assistance are available when needed. In addition, health care teams work with the patient and family to ascertain and comply with the patient's wishes about treatment methods and care as the terminal phase of illness and death approach.

Hospice

The needs of patients with end-stage illness are best met by a comprehensive interdisciplinary specialty program that focuses on quality of life; palliation of symptoms; and provision of physical, psychosocial, and spiritual support for patients and families when cure and control of the disease are no longer possible. The concept of hospice best addresses these needs.

Hospice care is often delivered through coordination of specialty services provided by hospitals, home care programs, and the community. Patients need to be referred to hospice services in a timely fashion so that complex patient and family needs can be addressed. See Chapter 13 for detailed discussion of end-of-life care.

CRITICAL THINKING EXERCISES

1 ebp A 38-year-old man with early-onset colorectal cancer completed his first cycle of chemotherapy 2 days ago. He is now being admitted to the inpatient oncology unit with febrile neutropenia. What interventions and education should be considered for febrile neutropenia? What is the evidence for these interventions and education that you identified for febrile neutropenia? How strong is that evidence, and what criteria will you use to assess the strength of that evidence?

2 pq A 76-year-old woman, with a past medical history that is significant for cataracts, arthritis, and hypertension, was recently diagnosed with stage II breast cancer. She is being discharged today from the hospital following a bilateral mastectomy with several surgical drains in place. What are the priorities for the assessment of this patient to ensure her readiness for discharge to home? What will be your priorities when educating this patient for self-care?

3 ipc You are caring for a 53-year-old man with diffuse large B-cell lymphoma who received CAR T–cell therapy 2 days ago. How does CAR T–cell therapy differ from conventional chemotherapy? What type of referrals might be appropriate for this patient? What members of the interprofessional health care team do you anticipate as being integral to the care of this patient?

REFERENCES

*Asterisk indicates nursing research.
**Double asterisk indicates classic reference.

Books

Comerford, K. C., & Durkin, M. T. (2020). *Nursing 2020 drug handbook.* Philadelphia, PA: Wolters Kluwer.

DeVita, V. T., Rosenberg S. A., & Lawrence, T. S. (Eds.). (2018). *Cancer: Principles & practice of oncology* (11th ed.). Philadelphia, PA: Lippincott Williams & Wilkins.

Eliopoulos, C. (2021). *Gerontological nursing* (10th ed.). Philadelphia, PA: Wolters Kluwer.

Fischbach, F. T., & Fischbach, M. A. (2018). *Fischbach's manual of laboratory and diagnostic tests* (10th ed.). Philadelphia, PA: Wolters Kluwer.

Halperin, E. C., Wazer, D. E., Perez, C. A., et al. (Eds.). (2019). *Perez and Brady's principles and practice of radiation oncology* (6th ed.). Philadelphia, PA: Lippincott Williams & Wilkins.

**Hewitt, M., Greenfield, S., & Stovall, E. (Eds.). (2006). *From cancer patient to cancer survivor: Lost in translation.* Washington, DC: Institute of Medicine and National Research Council, National Academies Press.

Jameson, J. L., Fauci, A. S., Kasper, D. L., et al. (Eds.). (2018). *Harrison's principles of internal medicine* (20th ed.). New York: McGraw Hill Education.

Jansen, C. (2017). Cognitive changes. In J. Eggert (Ed.). *Cancer basics* (2nd ed.). Pittsburg, PA: Oncology Nursing Society.

Kaplan, M. (Ed.) (2018). *Understanding and managing oncologic emergencies: A resource for nurses.* Pittsburgh, PA: Oncology Nursing Society.

Mones, J. V., & Soff, G. (2019). Management of thrombocytopenia in cancer patients. In *Thrombosis and hemostasis in cancer* (pp. 139–150). Basel, Switzerland: Springer Publishing International.

Morgan, M. A., Ten Haken, R. K., & Lawrence, T. S. (2018). Essentials of radiation therapy. In V. T. DeVita, S. A. Rosenberg, & T. S. Lawrence (Eds.). *Cancer: Principles & practice of oncology* (11th ed.). Philadelphia, PA: Lippincott Williams & Wilkins.

Norris, T. L. (2019). *Porth's pathophysiology: Concepts of altered health states* (10th ed.). Philadelphia, PA: Lippincott Williams & Wilkins.

Olsen, M. M., LeFebvre, K. B., & Brassil, K. (Eds.). (2019). *Chemotherapy and immunotherapy guidelines and recommendations for practice.* Pittsburgh, PA: Oncology Nursing Society.

Palmore, T. N., Parta, M., Cuellar-Rodriguez, J., et al. (2018). Infections in the cancer patient. In V. T. DeVita, S. A. Rosenberg, & T. S. Lawrence (Eds.). *Cancer: Principles & practice of oncology* (11th ed.). Philadelphia, PA: Lippincott Williams & Wilkins.

Rimmer, A., & Yahalom, J. (2018). Superior vena cava syndrome. In V. T. DeVita, S. A. Rosenberg, & T. S. Lawrence (Eds.). *Cancer: Principles & practice of oncology* (11th ed.). Philadelphia, PA: Lippincott Williams & Wilkins.

Stein, S., & Deshpande, H. A. (2018). Metabolic emergencies. In V. T. DeVita, S. A. Rosenberg, & T. S. Lawrence (Eds.). *Cancer: Principles & practice of oncology* (11th ed.). Philadelphia, PA: Lippincott Williams & Wilkins.

Szerlip, N., Beeler, W. H., & Spratt, D. E. (2018). Spinal cord compression. In V. T. DeVita, S. A. Rosenberg, & T. S. Lawrence (Eds.). *Cancer: Principles & practice of oncology* (11th ed.). Philadelphia, PA: Lippincott Williams & Wilkins.

Yarbro, C. H., Wujcik, D., & Gobel, B. H. (2018). *Cancer nursing: Principles and practice.* Burlington, MA: Jones & Bartlett Publishers.

Journals and Electronic Documents

Akthar, A. S., Liao, C., Eggener, S. E., et al. (2019). Patient-reported outcomes and late toxicity after postprostatectomy intensity-modulated radiation therapy. *European Urology, 8404*, E1–E7.

Almont, T., Farsi, F., Krakowski, I., et al. (2019). Sexual health in cancer: The results of a survey exploring practices, attitudes, knowledge, communication, and professional interactions in oncology healthcare providers. *Supportive Care in Cancer, 27*(3), 887–894.

American Cancer Society (ACS). (2018). American Cancer Society Guidelines for the early detection of cancer. Retrieved on 7/14/2019 at: www.cancer.org/healthy/find-cancer-early/cancer-screening-guidelines/american-cancer-society-guidelines-for-the-early-detection-of-cancer.html

American Cancer Society (ACS). (2019a). Cancer facts and figures 2019. Retrieved on 7/5/2019 at: www.cancer.org/research/cancer-facts-statistics/all-cancer-facts-figures/cancer-facts-figures-2019.html

American Cancer Society (ACS). (2019b). What causes cancer? Retrieved on 7/6/2019 at: www.cancer.org/cancer/cancer-causes.html

American Cancer Society (ACS). (2019c). Ultraviolet (UV) radiation sun and other types of radiation. Retrieved on 7/7/2019 at: www.cancer.org/cancer/cancer-causes/radiation-exposure/uv-radiation.html

American Cancer Society (ACS). (2019d). Tobacco and cancer. Retrieved on 7/8/2019 at: www.cancer.org/cancer/cancer-causes/tobacco-and-cancer.html

American Cancer Society (ACS). (2019e). Known and probable human carcinogens. Retrieved on 7/22/2019 at: www.cancer.org/cancer/cancer-causes/general-info/known-and-probable-human-carcinogens.html

American Cancer Society (ACS). (2019f). Cancer treatment and survivorship: Facts and figures 2019–2021. Retrieved on 7/10/2019 at: www.cancer.org/research/cancer-facts-statistics/survivor-facts-figures.html

American Cancer Society (ACS). (2019g). Cancer immunotherapy. Retrieved on 7/15/2019 at: www.cancer.org/treatment/treatments-and-side-effects/treatment-types/immunotherapy.html

American Cancer Society (ACS). (2019h). Intravesical therapy for bladder cancer. Retrieved on 7/20/2019 at: www.cancer.org/cancer/bladder-cancer/treating/intravesical-therapy.html

American Cancer Society (ACS). (2019i). ACS guidelines on nutrition and physical activity for cancer. Retrieved on 9/28/2018 at: https://www.cancer.org/healthy/eat-healthy-get-active/acs-guidelines-nutrition-physical-activity-cancer-prevention.html

Amin, M. B., Greene, F. L., Edge, S. B., et al. (2017). The eighth edition AJCC cancer staging manual: Continuing to build a bridge from a population-based to a more "personalized" approach to cancer staging. *CA: A Cancer Journal for Clinicians, 67*(2), 93–99.

Anderson, K., & Latchford, T. (2019). Associated toxicities: Assessment and management related to CAR T cell therapy. *Clinical Journal of Oncology Nursing, 23*(2-suppl.), 13–19.

Armenian, S., & Bhatia, S. (2018). Predicting and preventing anthracycline-related cardiotoxicity. *American Society of Clinical Oncology Educational Book, 38*, 3–12.

Barton-Burke, M., Ciccolini, K., Mekas, M., et al. (2017). Dermatologic reactions to targeted therapy: A focus on epidermal growth factor receptor inhibitors and nursing care. *Nursing Clinics, 52*(1), 83–113.

Bayer, V., Amaya, B., Baniewicz, D., et al. (2017). Cancer immunotherapy: An evidence-based overview and implications for practice. *Clinical Journal of Oncology Nursing, 21*(2 Suppl), 13–21.

Berger, K., Schopohl, D., Bollig, A., et al. (2018). Burden of oral mucositis: A systematic review and implications for future research. *Oncology Research and Treatment, 41*(6), 399–405.

Bishop, D. P., Cole, N., Zhang, T., et al. (2018). A guide to integrating immunohistochemistry and chemical imaging. *Chemical Society Reviews, 47*(11), 3770–3787.

Bowen, J. M., Gibson, R. J., Coller, J. K., et al. (2019). Systematic review of agents for the management of cancer treatment-related gastrointestinal mucositis and clinical practice guidelines. *Supportive Care in Cancer, 27*(10), 4011–4012.

Cannioto, R., Etter, J. L., Guterman, L. B., et al. (2017). The association of lifetime physical inactivity with bladder and renal cancer risk: A hospital-based case-control analysis. *Cancer Epidemiology, 49*, 24–29.

Cannioto, R., Etter, J. L., LaMonte, M. J., et al. (2018). Lifetime physical inactivity is associated with lung cancer risk and mortality. *Cancer Treatment and Research Communications, 14*, 37–45.

Centers for Disease Control and Prevention (CDC). (2017). NIOSH chemical carcinogen policy: DHHS (NIOSH) publication number 2017-100. Retrieved on 7/13/2019 at: www.cdc.gov/niosh/docs/2017-100/default.html

Centers for Disease Control and Prevention (CDC). (2018). Hepatitis B vaccine saves lives. Retrieved on 7/28/2019 at: www.cdc.gov/features/hepatitisb/index.html

Centers for Disease Control and Prevention (CDC). (2019). Smoking and tobacco use. Retrieved on 7/5/2019 at: www.cdc.gov/tobacco/data_statistics/fact_sheets/secondhand_smoke/health_effects/index.html

Chagpar, A. B. (2018). Contralateral prophylactic mastectomy. UpToDate. Waltham, MA. Retrieved on 7/17/2019 at: www.uptodate.com/contents/contralateral-prophylactic-mastectomy

Chen, P. H., Mahmood, Q., Mariottini, G. L., et al. (2017). Adverse health effects of betel quid and the risk of oral and pharyngeal cancers. *BioMed Research International, 2017*, 1–25.

Chen, W. Y. (2019). Factors that modify breast cancer risk in women. UpToDate, Waltham, MA. Retrieved on 7/27/2019 at: www.uptodate.com/contents/factors-that-modify-breast-cancer-risk-in-women

*Corbitt, N., Harrington, J., & Kendall, T. (2017). Putting evidence into practice: Prevention of bleeding. Retrieved on 7/23/2019 at: www.ons.org/pep/bleeding

Deng, G., Yin, M., Chen, X., et al. (2020). Clinical determinants for fatality of 44,672 patients with COVID-19. *Critical Care, 24*, 179–181.

DeSantis, C. E., Miller, K. D., Goding Sauer, A., et al. (2019). Cancer statistics for African Americans, 2019. *CA: A Cancer Journal for Clinicians, 69*(3), 211–233.

Dickens, E., & Ahmed, S. (2018). Principles of cancer treatment by chemotherapy. *Surgery (Oxford), 36*(3), 134–138.

Divgi, C. (2018). The current state of radiopharmaceutical therapy. *Journal of Nuclear Medicine, 59*(11), 1706–1707.

**DuPen, A. R., DuPen, S., Hansberry, J., et al. (2000). An educational implementation of a cancer pain algorithm for ambulatory care. *Pain Management Nursing, 1*(4), 116–128.

Dusetzina, S. B., Huskamp, H. A., Winn, A. N., et al. (2018). Out-of-pocket and health care spending changes for patients using orally administered anticancer therapy after adoption of state parity laws. *JAMA Oncology, 4*(6), e173598.

Eilers, J. G., Asakura, Y., Blecher, C. S., et al. (2017). Putting evidence into practice: Mucositis. Retrieved on 7/7/2019 at: www.ons.org/pep/mucositis

Eller, L. S., Lev, E. L., Yuan, C., et al. (2018). Describing self-care self-efficacy: Definition, measurement, outcomes, and implications. *International Journal of Nursing Knowledge, 29*(1), 38–48.

Fahy, B. N. (2019). Introduction: Role of palliative care for the surgical patient. *Journal of Surgical Oncology, 120*(1), 5–9.

Fritz, A., Percy, C., & Jack, A. (2013). International classification of diseases for oncology (ICD-O)–3rd edition, 1st revision. Retrieved at: https://apps.who.int/iris/bitstream/handle/10665/96612/9789241548496_eng.pdf;jsessionid=60D66DA21C5A4BA7486F40A4DC258752?sequence=1

Ginsburg, G. S., & Phillips, K. A. (2018). Precision medicine: From science to value. *Health Affairs, 37*(5), 694–701.

Gosselin, T., Beamer, L., Ciccolini, K., et al. (2017). Putting evidence into practice: Radiodermatitis. Retrieved on 6/28/2019 at: www.ons.org/pep/radiodermatitis

Hanna, J., Blazer, D. G., & Mosca, P. J. (2012). Overview of palliative surgery: principles and priorities. *J Palliative Care Med, 2*(7), 1–6.

Haryani, H., Fetzer, S. J., Wu, C. L., et al. (2017). Chemotherapy-induced peripheral neuropathy assessment tools: A systematic review. *Oncology Nursing Forum, 44*(3), E111–E123.

Hashim, D., Genden, E., Posner, M., et al. (2019). Head and neck cancer prevention: From primary prevention to impact of clinicians on reducing burden. *Annals of Oncology, 30*(5), 744–756.

Henriksen, P. A. (2018). Anthracycline cardiotoxicity: An update on mechanisms, monitoring and prevention. *Heart, 104*(12), 971–977.

Hermioni, A., Christina, M., Melanie, F., et al. (2019). Psychological considerations in hematopoietic stem cell transplantation. *Psychosomatics, 60*(4), 331–342.

Howell, D., Harth, T., Brown, J., et al. (2017). Self-management education interventions for patients with cancer: A systematic review. *Supportive Care in Cancer, 25*(4), 1323–1355.

Huo, D., Anderson, D., Palmer, J. R., et al. (2017). Incidence rates and risks of diethylstilbestrol-related clear-cell adenocarcinoma of the vagina and cervix: Update after 40-year follow-up. *Gynecologic Oncology, 146*(3), 566–571.

Islami, F., Goding Sauer, A., Miller, K. D., et al. (2018). Proportion and number of cancer cases and deaths attributable to potentially modifiable risk factors in the United States. *CA: A Cancer Journal for Clinicians, 68*(1), 31–54.

Jang, W. S., Kim, M. S., Jeong, W. S., et al. (2018). Does robot-assisted radical prostatectomy benefit patients with prostate cancer and bone oligometastases? *BJU International, 121*(2), 225–231.

Jatoi, A., & Kelly, D. (2019). The role of parenteral and enteral/oral nutritional support in patients with cancer. UpToDate. Waltham, MA. Retrieved on 7/19/2019 at: www.uptodate.com/contents/the-role-of-parenteral-and-enteral-oral-nutritional-support-`tients-with-cancer

Johns Hopkins University & Medicine Coronavirus Resource Center. (2020). Maps and trends: Mortality analysis. Retrieved on 6/12/2020 at: coronavirus.jhu.edu/data/mortality

Kays, L. B. (2018). Advancements come with a cost: Oral chemotherapy parity laws. Retrieved on 6/28/2019 at: www.pharmacytimes.com/publications/issue/2018/february2018/advancements-come-with-a-cost-oral-chemotherapy-parity-laws

Kessels, E., Husson, O., & Van der Feltz-Cornelis, C. M. (2018). The effect of exercise on cancer-related fatigue in cancer survivors: A systematic review and meta-analysis. *Neuropsychiatric Disease and Treatment, 14*, 479–494.

Krengli, M., Pisani, C., Deantonio, L., et al. (2017). Intraoperative radiotherapy in gynaecological and genitourinary malignancies: Focus on endometrial, cervical, renal, bladder and prostate cancers. *Radiation Oncology, 12*(1), 2–10.

Krishnasamy, K., Yoong, T. L., Chan, C. M., et al. (2017). Identifying malnutrition. *Clinical Journal of Oncology Nursing, 21*(1), E23–E29.

Kuderer, N. M., Choueiri, T. K., Shah, D. P., et al. (2020). Clinical impact of COVID-19 on patients with cancer (CC-19): A cohort study. *Lancet, 6736*(20), 31187-9.

Lamprecht, M., & Dansereau, C. (2019). CAR T cell therapy. *Clinical Journal of Oncology Nursing, 23*(2), 6–10.

Lazarev, S., Gupta, V., Ghiassi-Nejad, Z., et al. (2018). Premature discontinuation of curative radiation therapy: Insights from head and neck irradiation. *Advances in Radiation Oncology, 3*(1), 62–69.

Lipari, R. N., & Van Horn, S. L. (2017). Trends in smokeless tobacco use and initiation: 2002 to 2012. *The Center for Behavioral Health Statistics and Quality Report.* Retrieved on 6/18/2019 at: www.samhsa.gov/data/sites/default/files/report_2740/ShortReport-2740.html

Lunn, R. M., Jahnke, G. D., & Rabkin, C. S. (2017). Tumour virus epidemiology. *Philosophical Transactions of the Royal Society B: Biological Sciences, 372*(1732), 1–11.

Mainardi, S., Mulero-Sánchez, A., Prahallad, A., et al. (2018). SHP2 is required for growth of KRAS-mutant non-small-cell lung cancer in vivo. *Nature Medicine, 24*(7), 961–967.

Mattox, T. W. (2017). Cancer cachexia: Cause, diagnosis, and treatment. *Nutrition in Clinical Practice, 32*(5), 599–606.

*Menonna-Quinn, D., Polovich, M., & Marshall, B. (2019). Personal protective equipment: Evaluating usage among inpatient and outpatient oncology nurses. *Clinical Journal of Oncology Nursing, 23*(3), 260–265.

Merchan, J. R., Jhaveri, K. D., Berns, J. S., et al. (2017). Chemotherapy nephrotoxicity and dose modification in patients with renal insufficiency: Molecularly targeted agents. UpToDate. Waltham, MA. Retrieved on 6/29/2019 at: www.uptodate.com/contents/chemotherapy-nephrotoxicity-and-dose-modification-in-patients-with-renal-insufficiency-molecularly-targeted-agents

*Miaskowski, C. A., Brant, J. M., Caldwell, P., et al. (2017). Putting evidence into practice: Chronic pain. Retrieved on 7/19/2019 at: www.ons.org/pep/chronic-pain

Miller, K. D., Goding Sauer, A., Ortiz, A. P., et al. (2018). Cancer statistics for Hispanics/Latinos, 2018. *CA: A Cancer Journal for Clinicians, 68*(6), 425–445.

*Mitchell, S. A., Albrecht, T. A., Omar Alkaiyat, M., et al. (2017). Putting evidence into practice: Fatigue. Retrieved on 7/2/2019 at: www.ons.org/pep/fatigue

Mutahar, E., & Al-Anazi, K. A. (2017). Engraftment syndrome: An updated review. *Journal of Stem Cell Biology and Transplantation, 1*(3), E1–E5.

Natale, J. J. (2018). Overview of the prevention and management of CINV. *The American Journal of Managed Care, 24*(18 Suppl), S391–S397.

National Cancer Institute (NCI). (2017). Obesity and cancer. Retrieved on 7/13/2019 at: www.cancer.gov/about-cancer/causes-prevention/risk/obesity/obesity-fact-sheet

National Cancer Institute (NCI). (2018). Menopausal hormone therapy and cancer. Retrieved on 7/7/2019 at: www.cancer.gov/about-cancer/causes-prevention/risk/hormones/mht-fact-sheet

National Cancer Institute (NCI). (2019a). Cancer disparities. Retrieved on 7/4/2019 at: www.cancer.gov/about-cancer/understanding/disparities

National Cancer Institute (NCI). (2019b). Cancer genetics overview for health professionals. Retrieved on 7/3/2019 at: www.cancer.gov/about-cancer/causes-prevention/genetics/overview-pdq

National Cancer Institute (NCI). (2019c). Understanding cancer prognosis. Retrieved on 7/2/2019 at: www.cancer.gov/about-cancer/diagnosis-staging/prognosis

National Cancer Institute (NCI). (2019d). Targeted cancer therapies. Retrieved 7/17/2019 at: www.cancer.gov/about-cancer/treatment/types/targeted-therapies/targeted-therapies-fact-sheet

National Comprehensive Cancer Network (NCCN). (2019a). Clinical practice guidelines in oncology: Genetic/familial high-risk assessment: Breast and ovarian—version 1.2019. Retrieved on 7/12/2019 at: www.nccn.org/professionals/physician_gls/pdf/genetics_screening.pdf

National Comprehensive Cancer Network (NCCN). (2019b). Clinical practice guidelines in oncology: Genetic/familial high-risk assessment: Colorectal—version 1.2019. Retrieved on 7/22/2019 at: www.nccn.org/professionals/physician_gls/pdf/genetics_colon.pdf

National Comprehensive Cancer Network (NCCN). (2019c). Cancer staging guide. Retrieved on 7/20/2019 at: www.nccn.org/patients/resources/diagnosis/staging.aspx

National Comprehensive Cancer Network (NCCN). (2019d). Clinical practice guidelines in oncology: Breast cancer – version 1.2019. Retrieved on 7/17/2019 at: www.nccn.org/professionals/physician_gls/pdf/breast_blocks.pdf

National Comprehensive Cancer Network (NCCN). (2019e). NCCN clinical practice guidelines in oncology: Cutaneous melanoma – version 1.2019. Retrieved on 7/2/2019 at: www.nccn.org/professionals/physician_gls/pdf/cutaneous_melanoma_blocks.pdf

National Comprehensive Cancer Network (NCCN). (2019f). NCCN clinical practice guidelines in oncology: Prostate cancer – version 1.2019. Retrieved7/23/2019 at: www.nccn.org/professionals/physician_gls/pdf/prostate_blocks.pdf

National Comprehensive Cancer Network (NCCN). (2019g). NCCN clinical practice guidelines in oncology: Antiemesis – version 1.2019. Retrieved on 7/19/2019 at: www.nccn.org/professionals/physician_gls/pdf/antiemesis.pdf

National Comprehensive Cancer Network (NCCN). (2019h). NCCN guidelines for supportive care: Cancer related fatigue – version 1.2019. Retrieved on 7/20/2019 at: www.nccn.org/professionals/physician_gls/pdf/fatigue.pdf

National Comprehensive Cancer Network (NCCN). (2019i). NCCN clinical practice guidelines in oncology: Distress – version 1.2019. Retrieved on 7/11/2019 at: www.nccn.org/professionals/physician_gls/pdf/distress.pdf

National Comprehensive Cancer Network (NCCN). (2019j). NCCN clinical practice guidelines in oncology: Prevention and treatment of cancer-related infection—version 1.2019. Retrieved on 7/14/2019 at: www.nccn.org/professionals/physician_gls/pdf/infections.pdf

National Comprehensive Cancer Network (NCCN). (2019k). NCCN clinical practice guidelines in oncology: Cancer-associated thromboembolic disease – version 1.2019. Retrieved on 7/10/2019 at: www.nccn.org/professionals/physician_gls/pdf/vte.pdf

National Institutes of Health, National Center for Complementary and Integrative Health (NCCIH). (2018). Complementary, alternative, or integrative health: What's in a name? Retrieved on 7/12/2019 at: www.nccih.nih.gov/health/complementary-alternative-or-integrative-health-whats-in-a-name

Negrin, R. S. (2018). Early and late complications of hematopoietic cell transplantation. UpToDate. Waltham, MA. Retrieved on 7/27/2019 at: www.uptodate.com/contents/early-and-late-complications-of-hematopoietic-cell-transplantation

Negrin, R. S., & Bonis, P. A. L. (2019). Diagnosis of hepatic sinusoidal obstruction syndrome (veno-occlusive disease) following hematopoietic cell transplant. UpToDate. Waltham, MA. Retrieved on7/19/2019 at: www.uptodate.com/contents/diagnosis-of-hepatic-sinusoidal-obstruction-syndrome-veno-occlusive-disease-following-hematopoietic-cell-transplantation

Neuss, M. N., Gilmore, T. R., Belderson, K. M., et al. (2017). 2016 updated American Society of Clinical Oncology/Oncology Nursing Society chemotherapy administration safety standards, including standards for pediatric oncology. *Oncology Nursing Forum, 44*(1), 31–43

O'Gorman, C., Sasiadek, W., Denieffe, S., et al. (2015). Predicting radiotherapy-related clinical toxicities in cancer: A literature review. *Clinical Journal of Oncology Nursing, 18*(3), 37–44.

Oktay, K., Harvey, B. E., Partridge, A. H., et al. (2018). Fertility preservation in patients with cancer: ASCO clinical practice guideline update. *Journal of Clinical Oncology, 36*(19), 1994–2001.

*Overcash, J., Tan, A., & Noonan, A. (2018). Factors associated with poor sleep in older women diagnosed with breast cancer. *Oncology Nursing Forum, 45*(3), 359–371.

Pache, B., Hübner, M., Jurt, J., et al. (2017). Minimally invasive surgery and enhanced recovery after surgery: The ideal combination? *Journal of Surgical Oncology, 116*(5), 613–616.

Pachmayr, E., Treese, C., & Stein, U. (2017). Underlying mechanisms for distant metastasis-molecular biology. *Visceral Medicine, 33*(1), 11–20.

Rees, I., Jones, D., Chen, H., et al. (2018). Interventions to improve the uptake of cervical cancer screening among lower socioeconomic groups: A systematic review. *Preventive Medicine, 111*, 323–335.

Roselló, S., Blasco, I., García Fabregat, L., et al. (2017). Management of infusion reactions to systemic anticancer therapy: ESMO Clinical Practice Guidelines. *Annals of Oncology, 28*(suppl_4), iv100–iv118.

Ross, M., & Fischer-Cartlidge, E. (2017). Scalp cooling. *Clinical Journal of Oncology Nursing, 21*(2), 226–233.

Rubinsak, L. A., Kang, L., Fields, E. C., et al. (2018). Treatment-related radiation toxicity among cervical cancer patients. *International Journal of Gynecologic Cancer, 28*(7), 1387–1393.

Rugo, H. S., Melin, S. A., & Voigt, J. (2017). Scalp cooling with adjuvant/neoadjuvant chemotherapy for breast cancer and the risk of scalp metastases: Systematic review and meta-analysis. *Breast Cancer Research and Treatment, 163*(2), 199–205.

Ruiz, A., Sebagh, M., Wicherts, D. A., et al. (2018). Long-term survival and cure model following liver resection for breast cancer metastases. *Breast Cancer Research and Treatment, 170*(1), 89–100.

Scarborough, B. M., & Smith, C. B. (2018). Optimal pain management for patients with cancer in the modern era. *CA: A Cancer Journal for Clinicians, 68*(3), 182–196.

Schott, S., Vetter, L., Keller, M., et al. (2017). Women at familial risk of breast cancer electing for prophylactic mastectomy: Frequencies, procedures, and decision-making characteristics. *Archives of Gynecology and Obstetrics, 295*(6), 1451–1458.

Siegel, R. L., Miller, K. D., & Jemal, A. (2019). Cancer statistics, 2019. *CA: A Cancer Journal for Clinicians, 69*(1), 7–34.

*So, W. K., Kwong, A. N., Chen, J. M., et al. (2019). A theory-based and culturally aligned training program on breast and cervical cancer prevention for South Asian community health workers: A feasibility study. *Cancer Nursing, 42*(2), E20–E30.

*Thorpe, D. M., Conley, S. B., Drapek, L., et al. (2017). Putting evidence into practice: Anorexia. Retrieved on 7/28/2019 at: www.ons.org/pep/anorexia

United States Environmental Protection Agency (EPA). (2017). Summary of the Occupational Safety and Health Act: 29 U.S.C. §651 et seq. (1970). Retrieved on 7/11/2019 at: www.epa.gov/laws-regulations/summary-occupational-safety-and-health-act

U.S. Food and Drug Administration (FDA). (2019). Caution when using robotically-assisted surgical devices in women's health including mastectomy and other cancer-related surgeries: FDA safety communication. Retrieved on 7/26/2019 at: www.fda.gov/medical-devices/safety-communications/caution-when-using-robotically-assisted-surgical-devices-womens-health-including-mastectomy-and-other-cancer-related-surgeries

van den Beuken-van Everdingen, M. H., Hochstenbach, L. M., Joosten, E. A., et al. (2016). Update on prevalence of pain in patients with cancer: Systematic review and meta-analysis. *Journal of Pain and Symptom Management, 51*(6), 1070–1090.

van Elsland, D., & Neefjes, J. (2018). Bacterial infections and cancer. *European Molecular Biology Organization Reports, 19*(11), e46632.

Voog, E., Campion, L., Du Rusquec, P., et al. (2018). Totally implantable venous access ports: A prospective long-term study of early and late complications in adult patients with cancer. *Supportive Care in Cancer, 26*(1), 81–89.

Wagner, L. I., Zhao, F., Goss, P. E., et al. (2018). Patient-reported predictors of early treatment discontinuation: Treatment-related symptoms and health-related quality of life among postmenopausal women with primary breast cancer randomized to anastrozole or exemestane on NCIC Clinical Trials Group (CCTG) MA. 27 (E1Z03). *Breast Cancer Research and Treatment, 169*(3), 537–548.

Waldmann, T. A. (2018). Cytokines in cancer immunotherapy. *Cold Spring Harbor Perspectives in Biology, 10*(12), a028472.

Wanchai, A., Armer, J. M., Smith, K. M., et al. (2017). Complementary health approaches: Overcoming barriers to open communication during cancer therapy. *Clinical Journal of Oncology Nursing, 21*(6), E287–E298.

Wang, C., Dickie, J., Sutavani, R. V., et al. (2018). Targeting head and neck cancer by vaccination. *Frontiers in Immunology, 9*, 830, 1–12.

*Wang, N., Yang, Z., Miao, J., et al. (2018). Clinical management of cancer-related fatigue in hospitalized adult patients: A best practice implementation project. *JBI Database of Systematic Reviews and Implementation Reports, 16*(10), 2038–2049.

White, L. L., Cohen, M. Z., Berger, A., et al. (2017). Perceived self-efficacy: A concept analysis for symptom management in patients with cancer. *Clinical Journal of Oncology Nursing, 21*(6), E272–E279.

*Williams, L., Ciccolini, K., Johnson, L. A., et al. (2017). Putting evidence into practice: Skin reactions. Retrieved on 7/23/2019 at: www.ons.org/pep/skin-reactions

*Wilson, B. J., Ahmed, F., Crannell, C. E., et al. (2017). Putting evidence into practice: Preventing infection – general. Retrieved on 7/5/2019 at: www.ons.org/pep/prevention-infection-general

World Cancer Research Fund (WCRF)/American Institute for Cancer Research. (2018). Diet, nutrition, physical activity and cancer: A global perspective. Retrieved on 7/19/2019 at: www.wcrf.org/dietandcancer

Resources

American Association of Cancer Research (AACR), www.aacr.org
American Cancer Society (ACS), www.cancer.org
American College of Surgeons Commission on Cancer (CoC), www.facs.org/quality-programs/cancer/coc
American Pain Society (APS), www.ampainsoc.org
American Society of Clinical Oncology (ASCO), www.asco.org
American Society for Radiation Oncology (ASTRO), www.astro.org
Association of Oncology Social Work (AOSW), www.aosw.org
Cancer Care, www.cancercare.org/
Centers for Disease Control and Prevention (CDC): Cancer Control and Prevention, www.cdc.gov/cancer/
Hospice and Palliative Nurses Association (HPNA), www.hpna.org
LIVESTRONG Survivorship Centers of Excellence, www.livestrong.org
National Cancer Institute (NCI), www.cancer.gov
National Coalition for Cancer Survivorship, www.canceradvocacy.org
National Comprehensive Cancer Network (NCCN), www.nccn.org
National Hospice and Palliative Care Organization, www.nhpco.org
National Institutes of Health, National Center for Complementary and Integrative Health (NCCIH), nccih.nih.gov
OncoLink (cancer resources), www.oncolink.org
Oncology Nursing Society (ONS), www.ons.org
Quackwatch, www.quackwatch.org
The Bone Marrow Foundation, bonemarrow.org/
The Cancer Support Community, www.cancersupportcommunity.org
The COVID-19 and Cancer Consortium, ccc19.org
The Leukemia and Lymphoma Society, www.lls.org

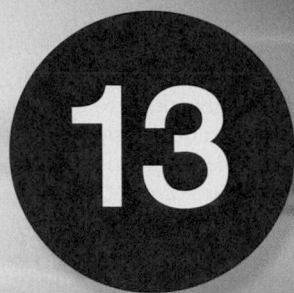

13 Palliative and End-of-Life Care

Nurses have a significant and lasting effect on the way patients live until they die, the manner in which death occurs, and the enduring memories of that death for patients' families. The contemporary definition of nursing includes "...the diagnosis and treatment of human responses, and advocacy in the care of individuals, families, groups, communities, and populations" (American Nurses Association [ANA], 2015, p. 1). There may be no group more important than seriously ill and dying patients.

Knowledge about palliative and end-of-life principles of care and the ability to recognize the unique response of each patient and family to a given illness are essential components

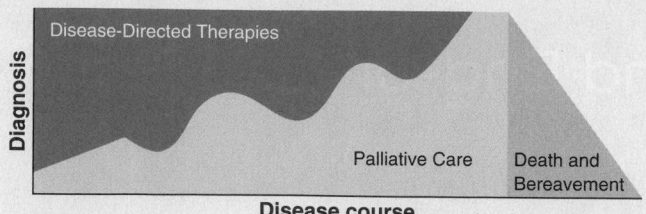

Figure 13-1 • This model shows the intersection of disease-directed therapies and palliative care beginning at diagnosis and continuing to death and bereavement. Adapted from Ferrell, B. R., Twaddle, M. L., Melnick., A., et al. (2018). National consensus project clinical practice guidelines for quality palliative care guidelines, 4th edition. *Journal of Palliative Medicine, 21*(12), 1684–1689.

required to support the unique values, preferences, and goals of a person's care. Nurses have an opportunity to bring research, education, and practice together to impact the culture of dying, allowing for much-needed improvement to care that is relevant across practice settings, age groups, cultural backgrounds, and illnesses. Nurses in all settings are likely to encounter patients who are seriously ill and families who can benefit from palliative care during advanced illness and at end-of-life. This chapter presents concepts about death and dying in the United States, settings for end-of-life care of the dying, and ways that nurses can address the health issues of patients who are terminally ill.

Palliative Care and End-of-Life Care

Palliative care uses an interdisciplinary model of care, focusing on symptom management and psychosocial/spiritual support for those with serious, life-limiting illnesses. Palliative care aims to improve quality of life for people and families through early integration into the plan of care strategies for managing pain and symptoms and for reducing burdensome care

transitions through interdisciplinary teamwork, care coordination, clinician–patient communication, and decisional support. It is appropriate for patients at any age and at any stage in a serious illness, even while pursuing disease-directed or curative therapies, and extending into bereavement for families (Fig. 13-1). Palliative care can be viewed as both an approach to care and as a structured system for care delivery that aims to optimize quality of life by anticipating, preventing, and treating suffering (National Consensus Project for Quality Palliative Care [NCP], 2018). **Interdisciplinary collaboration** is an essential component which is rooted in communication and cooperation among the various disciplines, with each member of the team contributing to a single integrated care plan that addresses the needs of the patient and the family. In contrast, multidisciplinary care refers to participation of clinicians with varied backgrounds and skill sets but without coordination and integration of care into a unified plan.

Hospice is a type of palliative care, focusing on comfort at the end-of-life. When patients enroll in hospice, they have made the decision to forego disease-directed therapies and focus solely on the relief of symptoms associated with their illness and the dying process. Both palliative care and hospice clinicians are skilled in the delivery of end-of-life care (which may include the months or weeks prior to death), expert pain and symptom management, life review and bereavement support. Focus on care of the dying is motivated by the aging of the population, the prevalence of and publicity surrounding life-threatening illnesses, and the increasing likelihood of a prolonged period of chronic illness prior to death. Figure 13-2 depicts four illness trajectories: sudden death, terminal illness, organ failure, and frailty. Sudden death is unexpected and accounts for the minority of deaths in this day and age. The other trajectories depict a common course in three types of chronic life-limiting illness: (1) terminal illness (e.g., cancer)

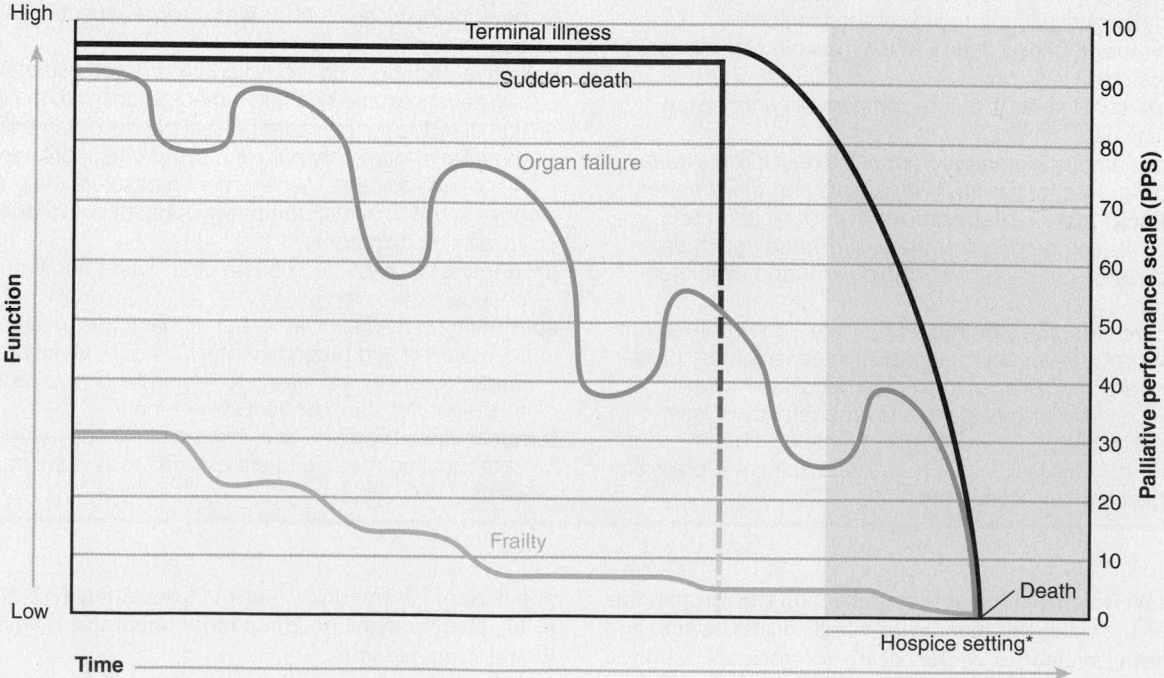

*May be eligible for hospice at this stage

Figure 13-2 • The four trajectories of illness.

is generally diagnosed when one is highly functioning, with a short steady decline before death; (2) organ failure (e.g., heart failure, end-stage kidney disease, or chronic lung disease) usually follows a slow decline after diagnosis, with episodic illnesses, perhaps exacerbation or hospitalization, where one has difficulty returning back to functional baseline; and (3) frailty (e.g., dementia) is typically diagnosed when one is already frail, with a slow decline over years. With the exception of sudden death, functional status can be a good prognostic indication; one such scale, the Palliative Performance Scale, is based on ambulation, activity, outward evidence of disease, self-care, intake, and level of consciousness (10-point increments, with 100% being fully functional and independent) (Hui, Park, Liu, et al., 2016).

The Evolution of End-of-Life Care

In the 20th century, chronic, degenerative diseases replaced communicable diseases as the major causes of death. In the earlier part of the 20th century, most deaths occurred at home and most families had direct experience with death, through providing care to family members at the end-of-life and then mourning their losses together as a family unit. As the place of death shifted from home to hospitals, families became increasingly distanced from the death experience, placing the care of the patient into the health care provider's hands.

In the latter half of the 20th century, a technologic imperative practice pattern among health care professionals emerged, along with an expectation among patients and families that every available means to extend life must be tried. In the 21st century, technologic intervention at the end-of-life continues to have profound implications, affecting how clinicians care for the dying, how family and friends participate in care, how patients and families understand and choose among end-of-life care options, how families prepare for **terminal illness** (a progressive, irreversible illness that despite medical treatment will result in the patient's death) and death, and how they heal after the death of a loved one. Palliative and end-of-life care continues to evolve with the technology and medical interventions that are used to care for the seriously ill.

Between 2000 and 2050, the number of people older than 85 years is expected to quadruple (West, Cole, Goodkind, et al., 2014). More than half of the aged population has one or more chronic, serious illness (West et al., 2014). The incidence of life-limiting illness is expected to continue to rise. Numerous initiatives aimed at improving end-of-life care have been launched in recent years, spurred by a widespread call for substantive change in the way Americans deal with death. In 2014, the Institute of Medicine (IOM) released a consensus report titled *Dying in America: Improving Quality and Honoring Individual Preferences Near the End of Life.* The report presented a summary of findings from a review of the evidence and provided recommendations for improving palliative and end-of-life care. The authors noted that patients experienced many transitions in settings, frequent and potentially avoidable hospital readmission, and inconsistent referral to palliative care. Recommendations include widespread and timely access to, and comprehensive coverage for palliative care services, improved clinician–patient communication, greater emphasis on advance care planning, professional education and development, and stronger public education and engagement (IOM, 2014).

The NCP identified eight key domains that underline a more comprehensive and humane approach to the care of the seriously ill patient at any stage, age, setting or prognosis, with the most recent update released in 2018 and outlined in Chart 13-1 (NCP, 2018). These practice guidelines have been endorsed by more than 80 national organizations, such as the Institute for Healthcare Improvement (IHI), American Cancer Society (ACS), Hospice and Palliative Nurses Association (HPNA), and the National Hospice and Palliative Care Organization (NHPCO), to structure and evaluate quality palliative and end-of-life programs for all those with serious illness at any stage, age, setting or prognosis.

In 2017, the ANA in collaboration with HPNA developed a *Call for Action—Nurses Lead and Transform Palliative Care,* which outlined the five areas of palliative nursing care: clinical practice, education, policy, research, and administration. In the document, the ANA and HPNA outline ways that nurses can transform palliative care, both as primary and specialty palliative care clinicians (ANA, 2017a). Primary palliative care is defined as the fundamental palliative care skills that all health care providers should have, including basic symptom assessment and management and the ability to explore goals of care through therapeutic communication. In contrast, the palliative care specialist addresses complex symptoms and navigates difficult goals of care conversations and family conflict. As a measure to better incorporate primary palliative care into nursing education, the American Association of Colleges of Nursing (AACN) recommended a new curriculum for palliative education for undergraduate nurses, including developing an online version of the End-of-Life Nursing Education Consortium (ELNEC) (Ferrell, Malloy, Mazanec, et al., 2016). See Resources section at end of chapter.

Settings for Palliative Care and End-of-Life Care

As the landscape of care at the end-of-life moved from the home to a more institutionalized death, the models of palliative care delivery changed as well. At hospice's inception, end-of-life care was home based or at a free-standing hospice. Palliative care was largely hospital based; it was born out of academic medical centers, where some health care providers felt that everyone deserves to receive treatment based on the tenets of hospice care throughout the progression of serious illness (Morrison, 2013). Current models for palliative and end-of-life care delivery will be described in greater detail in the following sections and include (NCP, 2018):

- Institution-based palliative care programs (e.g., programs within hospitals or long-term care facilities)
- Outpatient-based palliative care programs (e.g., outpatient clinics, ambulatory settings)
- Community-based palliative care program (consultative teams collaborate with hospice or home health agencies, to support patients not yet receiving hospice care in their place of residence)
- Hospice care (under Medicare Part A)

As our population ages and is expected to develop multiple comorbidities, the need for a palliative care workforce also grows. Yet, experts project a workforce shortage of all

Chart 13-1   Overview of National Consensus Project Guidelines, Fourth Edition

Domain 1: Structure and Processes of Care

- *Overview:* Palliative care is based on a comprehensive interdisciplinary assessment of the patient and the family, by all clinicians with assistance from palliative care specialists as needed.
- *Clinical Implications:* Palliative care may improve quality of life for patients and families when well-trained interdisciplinary clinicians create care plans based on patient-stated values and preferences.

Domain 2: Physical Aspects of Care

- *Overview:* Pain, other symptoms, and side effects are managed based on the best available evidence, with attention to disease-specific pain and symptoms, which is skillfully and systematically applied.
- *Clinical Implications:* Interdisciplinary teams treat physical symptoms through recognition that physical symptoms impact a patient's emotional and spiritual well-being. Clinicians also consider goals, cultural, and developmental needs when choosing pharmacologic and nonpharmacologic treatments.

Domain 3: Psychological and Psychiatric Aspects of Care

- *Overview:* Psychological status, including need for assistance with distress, coping, family conflict, grief support and resources is assessed and managed based on the best available evidence, which is skillfully and systematically applied. When necessary, psychiatric issues are addressed and treated.
- *Clinical Implications:* Initial assessment is usually performed by social workers with assistance from psychologists and psychiatrists as needed.

Domain 4: Social Aspects of Care

- *Overview:* Comprehensive interdisciplinary assessment identifies the environmental and social factors that may impact the patient's and family members' quality of life, and a plan of care is developed to respond to these needs as effectively as possible.
- *Clinical Implications:* Coordination of care to address social and environmental vulnerabilities.

Domain 5: Spiritual, Religious, and Existential Aspects of Care

- *Overview:* Spiritual and existential dimensions are assessed and responded to based on the best available evidence, which is skillfully and systematically applied.
- *Clinical Implications:* The interdisciplinary team assesses each patient's sources of meaning and purpose, while respecting patient-specific beliefs, values, and traditions.

Domain 6: Cultural Aspects of Care

- *Overview:* Palliative care team members assess and attempt to meet the needs of the patient, family, and community in a culturally sensitive manner.
- *Clinical Implications:* Health care providers must examine their own biases to work to avoid judgment and provide culturally sensitive care.

Domain 7: Care of the Patient Nearing the End-of-Life

- *Overview:* Care is provided by interdisciplinary team members skilled in end-of-life care domains including expert symptom management, skilled communication, and grief/bereavement support.
- *Clinical Implications:* Signs and symptoms of impending death are recognized and communicated in developmentally appropriate language for the patient, family, and children, if applicable, with respect to information preferences.

Domain 8: Ethical and Legal Aspects of Care

- *Overview:* The patient's goals, preferences, and choices are respected within the limits of applicable state and federal law, within current accepted standards of medical care, and form the basis for the plan of care.
- *Clinical Implications:* Knowledge of ethical principles (beneficence, nonmaleficence, justice, self-determination) as well as pertinent health care laws is required. Clinicians must determine moral agency and understand when to engage surrogate decision makers to employ substituted judgment.

Adapted from Ferrell, B. R., Twaddle, M. L., Melnick., A., et al. (2018). National consensus project clinical practice guidelines for quality palliative care guidelines, 4th edition. *Journal of Palliative Medicine, 21*(12), 1684–1689.

---

palliative clinicians that may not recover for nearly three decades. Proposed policy changes include (Kamal, Wolf, Troy, et al., 2019):

- The adoption of the Palliative Care and Hospice Education and Training Act (PCHETA), which if passed would increase the field by over 9000 practitioners.
- Policy to financially support palliative fellowship training across disciplines.
- Further research defining nonphysician palliative care specialist clinicians (nurses, social workers, chaplaincy).
- Creative reimbursement models that support the full interdisciplinary team.
- Policy to promote resiliency and, in turn, prevent burnout. (For more on burnout see later section entitled "Professional Caregiver Issues.")

Institution-Based Palliative Care

The landmark Study to Understand Prognoses and Preferences for Outcomes and Risks of Treatments (SUPPORT)

documented troubling deficiencies in the care of the dying in hospital settings (SUPPORT Principal Investigators, 1995). Subsequently, the IOM's *Dying in America* (2014), the NCP *Clinical Practice Guidelines* (2018), and the ANA-HPNA *Call for Action* (2017a) have been shaping palliative and end-of-life care through developing and encouraging adherence to standards of care for patients with advanced illness and at end-of-life that will apply regardless of where the patients are receiving care (ANA, 2017a; IOM, 2014; NCP, 2018). There has been a steady increase in American hospital-based palliative care, with reportedly 90% of hospitals with 300 beds or more offering palliative care, compared to 56% of hospitals with fewer than 300 beds (Dumanovsky, Augustin, Rogers, et al., 2016).

In the hospital, the delivery of palliative care is typically through an interdisciplinary consultation service where primary teams consult specialists for one or more of the following reasons:

- Pain management
- Symptom management

- Goals of care discussions
- End-of-life issues
- Psychosocial distress
- Spiritual or existential distress

The core interdisciplinary team usually consists of physicians, nurses, advanced practice nurses, social workers, and chaplains (National Palliative Care Registry, 2017). Additional team members may include pharmacists, nutritionists, music or art therapists, ethicists, and psychologists. Occasionally, institutions have palliative care units where palliative care clinicians oversee a patient's care when palliative care needs supersede other hospital conditions. The most common reason for palliative care consultation in the hospital setting is goals of care discussion; those referred for care planning are most often older with a serious illness other than cancer and typically have a full code status (Bischoff, O'Riordan, Marks, et al., 2017).

In 2011, The Joint Commission launched an advanced certification program for palliative care to recognize hospitals that provide exceptional patient and family-centered care (The Joint Commission, 2018). The Center to Advance Palliative Care (CAPC) has a plethora of institutional resources for developing hospital–hospice partnerships to provide high-quality palliative care for hospitalized patients and for addressing the palliative care needs of other specialized populations. See Resources section at the end of the chapter.

According to the National Palliative Care Registry in 2017, the most common primary diagnoses seen by palliative care specialists included cancer (26%), cardiac diseases (15%), pulmonary conditions (9%), neurologic diagnoses (9%), and infectious causes (7%). For patients with diagnoses for which palliative care specialists have rarely been consulted, the efficacy of palliative care has been demonstrated. In one study, for example, patients undergoing stem cell transplant at an academic medical center reported better quality of life during transplant hospitalization after palliative care intervention (El-Jawahri, LeBlanc, VanDusen, et al., 2016).

Researchers have reported that seriously ill hospitalized patients who receive palliative care consultations for goals of care have lower future health care utilization and cost (O'Connor, Junker, Appel, et al., 2018). Despite the growth of palliative care, many believe that palliative care resources are still lacking; in a survey of administrators and clinicians, respondents felt that 60% of patients who may benefit from palliative or end-of-life care do not receive this type of support (Compton-Phillips & Mohta, 2019). Additionally, there is ample room for improvement in end-of-life care delivery. Hospital end-of-life care has been found to be of higher quality in hospitals with better rated nurse practice environments (as measured by the Practice Environment Scale of the Nursing Work Index survey, where nurse workload, autonomy, and interdisciplinary collaboration are favored); however, the majority of nurses rated overall end-of-life care in hospitals unfavorably (Lasater, Sloane, McHugh, et al., 2019).

Experts estimate that the number of people who will need some form of short- or long-term skilled nursing care in their lifetimes, whether in the community or in a residential care facility, is likely to increase exponentially (West et al., 2014). As a result, the likely place of death for a growing number of Americans after the age of 65 years will be a skilled nursing facility. A 2018 study by Teno and colleagues found that,

among Medicare fee-for-service beneficiaries, the proportion of death in acute care hospitals has decreased, yet one in five beneficiaries continues to die in acute care settings. More than one in four (29%) fee-for-service beneficiaries are admitted to intensive care units in the last 30 days of their life. Based on recent trends, about two in five (40%) of fee-for-service beneficiaries die at home and community settings, including assisted living facilities. Nursing homes remain the site of death for 25% of Medicare beneficiaries. Thus, while dying at home has increased for those older than age 65 in recent years, deaths in other locations still exceed the number of deaths occurring at home (Teno, Gozalo, Trivedi, et al., 2018).

Residents of skilled nursing facilities typically have poor access to palliative care. Regulations that govern how care in these facilities is organized and reimbursed tend to emphasize restorative measures and serve as a disincentive to palliative care. Since 1989, home hospice programs have been permitted to enroll long-term care facility residents in hospice programs and to provide interdisciplinary services to residents who qualify for hospice care. Of over one million Medicare beneficiaries who received hospice services in 2016, close to a third resided in long-term care facilities, an increase from 14.5% in 2013 to 32.8% (NHPCO, 2018). Because hospices provide some services that may overlap with services provided by the skilled nursing provider, payment models have been developed to define and reconcile duplication of services. In 1997, the Office of Inspector General (OIG), an oversight arm of the federal government, questioned whether hospice services in nursing homes were an unnecessary duplication of services already provided by long-term care facility staff. Hospice/skilled nursing facility contracts continue to be scrutinized by federal regulators. More recently, facilities are under increasing public pressure to improve care of the dying and are beginning to develop palliative care units or services; continuing to contract with home hospice programs to provide palliative care consultations and hospice care in the facilities; and to educate staff, residents, and their families about pain and symptom management and end-of-life care. Many skilled nursing providers have implemented culture change innovations such as resident-centered care plans and consistent staff assignments to change the experience of long-term skilled nursing care. In nursing homes, "comfort measures" are used to identify residents who do not wish to receive life-sustaining interventions. Nevertheless, hospitalizations continue to occur and research reports that 77% of events (i.e., fall, change in mental status, or development of a new symptom) are unavoidable, yet opportunities exist for improvement in communication and monitoring (Unroe, O'Kelly Phillips, Effler, et al., 2019). Palliative care education and training for nursing home staff may improve the quality of care residents receive at the end-of-life.

Outpatient-Based Palliative Care

As palliative care has become more prevalent in hospitals, skilled nursing settings, and in home hospice programs, outpatient palliative care has emerged as an approach to providing services and support to patients and families who opt not to, or are not eligible for, home hospice but could benefit from comprehensive palliative care in the community. Outpatient palliative care benefits both patients and their families and other providers by providing expert consultation and management of symptoms and other needs. A growing body of evidence supports the role of palliative care that is delivered *concurrently* with standard medical treatment. For example, in a landmark study of outpatient referral to palliative care for patients newly diagnosed with metastatic non–small cell lung carcinoma (a disease with very poor prognosis), researchers found that those patients randomized to the palliative care plus standard oncology care arm of the trial not only showed improved quality of life and mood, but also had longer median survival than those who received standard oncology care alone (Temel, Greer, Muzikansky, et al., 2010). Such studies underscore the value of palliative care.

Models for palliative care in ambulatory clinics vary and include independent clinics, colocated clinics and embedded practices (Finlay, Newport, Sivendran, et al., 2019). Each model differs in the referral process, financial makeup, staffing and population served (Finlay et al., 2019). In addition, clinics may follow a consultative only, comanagement with one or shared opioid prescribing (Finlay et al., 2019). Although many outpatient palliative care clinics start with oncology patients, as palliative care has gained traction in many disease states in the hospital, other medical specialties (cardiologists, pulmonologist, nephrologists, etc.) are lacking proper palliative care follow-up and requesting nononcology palliative care clinics.

Community-Based Palliative Care

Home-based primary care has become more common due to the aging of society and a desire for people to remain at home rather than live in an institution (Schuchman, Fain, & Cornwell, 2018). Home-based primary care incorporates palliative care skills, and specialty palliative care home programs have developed with the goal of managing symptoms and providing support in the home. The Affordable Care Act, passed in 2010, also included new payment models for home-based palliative care in an effort to reduce hospital readmissions and mortality (Morrison, 2013).

Hospice Care

The broadening of the application of palliative care in the United States actually *followed* the development of hospice programs. All hospice care is palliative care; however, not all palliative care is hospice care. The difference is that hospice care is an application of palliative care delivered at the end-of-life. Hospice care focuses on quality of life, and by necessity, it usually includes realistic emotional, social, spiritual, and financial preparation for death. Hospice in the United States is not a *place* but a philosophy of care in which the end-of-life is viewed as a developmental stage.

Originally, the concept of hospice care as an alternative to depersonalized death in institutions began in the early 1970s as a volunteer-based, grassroots, and spiritually centered movement (Meghani, 2004). In 2016, there were 4382 hospice programs in operation across all 50 states (as well as Washington, DC and Puerto Rico), serving an estimated 1.43 million patients (NHPCO, 2018). Currently the most common diagnosis for hospice patients in the United States is cancer (Table 13-1). While median length of hospice

TABLE 13-1	Hospice Admission Diagnosis Prevalence
Diagnosis	**Percent of Hospice Patients (%)**
Cancer	27.2
Cardiac/circulatory	18.7
Dementia	18.0
Respiratory	11.0
Stroke	9.5
Other	15.6

Adapted from National Hospice and Palliative Care Organization (NHPCO). (2018). *NHPCO facts and figures: Hospice care in America.* Alexandria, VA: Author.

stay in 2016 was approximately 24 days across diagnoses, for patients with dementia, the average length of stay was 104 days (NHPCO, 2018).

After hospice care was recognized as a distinct program of services under Medicare in early 1983, organizations providing hospice care were able to receive Medicare reimbursement if they could demonstrate that the hospice program met the Medicare conditions of participation, or regulations for hospice providers as enforced by the Centers for Medicare & Medicaid Services (CMS, 2019). In many aspects, Medicare standards have come to largely define hospice philosophy and services. State Medical Assistance (Medicaid) also provides coverage for hospice care, as do most commercial insurers.

Hospice is a coordinated program of interdisciplinary services provided by professional caregivers and trained volunteers to patients with serious, progressive illnesses that are not responsive to cure. The root of the word *hospice* is *hospes*, meaning "host." According to Cicely Saunders, who founded the world-renowned St. Christopher's Hospice in London, the principles underlying hospice are as follows:

- Death must be accepted.
- The patient's total care is best managed by an interdisciplinary team whose members communicate regularly with one another.
- Pain and other symptoms of terminal illness must be managed.
- The patient and the family should be viewed as a single unit of care.
- Home care of the dying is necessary.
- Bereavement care must be provided to family members.
- Research and education should be ongoing.

The goal of hospice is to enable the patient to remain at home, surrounded by the people and objects that have been important to them throughout life. The patient and the family comprise the unit of care. Hospice care does not seek to hasten death or encourage the prolongation of life through artificial means.

Despite more than 45 years of existence in the United States and the early calls for its concurrent integration with disease-modifying treatments (Meghani, 2004), hospice remains an option for end-of-life care that has not been fully integrated into mainstream health care. Reasons include the difficulties in making a terminal prognosis (especially for those patients with noncancer diagnoses), the strong association of hospice with death, advances in "curative" treatment options in late-stage illness, and financial pressures on health care providers that may cause them to retain rather than refer patients who are eligible for hospice. Moreover, there are significant racial differences in the utilization of hospice care; for example, Asian Americans tend to have shorter lengths of hospice stay, and non-White patients have a higher incidence of revoking hospice when compared to White patients (Wang, Hsu, Aldridge, et al., 2019).

The Medicare-certified hospice is paid a predetermined dollar amount for each day of hospice care that each patient receives. Four levels of hospice care are covered under Medicare and Medicaid hospice benefits: (1) routine care, (2) continuous care, (3) respite care, and (4) general inpatient hospice care. Most hospice care is provided at the "routine home care" level; routine and continuous care are outlined in greater detail in Chart 13-2. According to federal guidelines, hospices may provide no more than 20% of the aggregate annual patient-days at the inpatient level. Respite care allows primary caregivers a break through admission of the patient to an inpatient unit or nursing facility.

Federal rules for hospices require that eligibility be reviewed periodically. Patients who live longer than 6 months under hospice care are *not* discharged, provided that their primary provider and the hospice medical director continue to certify that they are terminally ill with a life expectancy of 6 months or less (assuming that the disease continues its expected course). Thus, the patient is re-certified and continues to receive hospice benefits. Once a patient meets eligibility criteria and elects to use the benefit, the Medicare-certified hospice program assumes responsibility for providing and paying for the care and treatment to palliate the terminal illness for which hospice care was elected. Patients may revoke their hospice benefits at any time, resuming traditional coverage under Medicare or Medicaid for the terminal illness. Those who revoke their benefits may also reelect to use them at a later time.

The **Medicare Hospice Benefit** requirement that beneficiaries make a choice between palliative care (to enroll in hospice) and cure-focused treatment has long been a barrier to earlier hospice enrollment. A Medicare beneficiary could not receive BOTH palliative care and cure-focused care under their hospice benefit. The Affordable Care Act authorized a study of concurrent palliative and curative care services. Under this federally funded study, titled Medicare Care Choices, CMS is evaluating whether beneficiaries would choose palliative care under hospice guidelines while they *continue to receive* cure-focused care (CMS, 2018). The model is being tested with 104 hospices currently participating and 1092 Medicare patients receiving this concurrent care, with a hope to reach 150,000 in the coming years (CMS, 2018).

 Veterans Considerations

The Veterans Administration (VA) offers concurrent care, whereby a veteran has the option to receive disease-directed therapy, such as radiation or chemotherapy, while receiving hospice care. The VA reported that veterans with cancer at the end-of-life received radiation and chemotherapy at the same rate as before concurrent care was offered, but the utilization of hospice increased, thus allowing patients to receive

---

Chart 13-2 — Eligibility Criteria for Hospice Care

Who? A Patient with a Serious, Progressive Life-Limiting Illness Must Meet Two Criteria:
- Two primary providers certify that prognosis is less than 6 mo if the disease runs usual course
- Patient and family agree with comfort as the goal of care

When? The patient wishes to pursue comfort-focused care and prognosis is believed to be months. If a patient survives >6 mo they may be re-enrolled in hospice care.

What? Medicare and Medicaid Hospice Benefits
- Medicare Part A; Medical Assistance eligibility
- Waiver of traditional Medicare/Medicaid benefits for the terminal illness (e.g., surgery, skilled nursing care, hospital stay)
- Care must be provided by a Medicare-certified hospice program

Where? Hospice settings vary depending on a person's care needs and may include:
- Home (*Routine Hospice Care,* delivered in a private residence, nursing home)
  - The majority of patients receive hospice at home
  - Care is primarily delivered by family and friends
  - Hospice staff (nurses, aides, social workers and chaplains) provide additional support as needed
  - All services (staff visits, medications, durable medical equipment) provided are included in the daily rate to the hospice
  - Phone hotline available for caregivers to reach a hospice nurse 24 hours a day
  - *Continuous care:* This is a temporary level of care provided in the patient's home where continuous nursing care is provided in the home for the management of a medical crisis (e.g., the hospice patient seizes and a hospice nurse comes to the home to monitor the patient and administer medications; nursing need is reevaluated every shift). Care reverts to the routine home care level after the crisis is resolved
- Long-term care facility
  - Hospice staff is added as additional layer of support for established residents
  - Facility staff continue to provide 24-h care
  - Facility room and board paid separately from hospice care
- Residential hospice
  - Residences for long-term stay
  - Payment is typically prorated based on income
  - Not many exist and travel may be prohibitive for family or friends
- General inpatient hospice
  - Indicated for acute pain or symptom management requiring 24-h care
  - Usually in a free-standing inpatient hospice unit or in a Medicare certified hospital

---

significant support in the last weeks of life (Mor, Joyce, Cote, et al., 2016).

Communication in Palliative Care

Expert communication is a tenet of palliative and end-of-life care. Historically, communication was thought of as an innate art. Experts now view communication as a set of skills that can be taught, practiced, and built upon. Nurses need to develop skill and comfort in assessing patients' and families' responses to serious illness and planning interventions that support their values and choices throughout the continuum of care (Wittenberg-Lyles, Goldsmith, Ferrell, et al., 2013). To develop a level of comfort and expertise in communicating with seriously and terminally ill patients and their families, nurses must first consider their own experiences with and values concerning illness and death through reflection, discussion with colleagues, reading, and self-discovery.

Skills for Communicating with the Seriously Ill

Throughout the course of a serious illness, patients and their families encounter complicated treatment options and bad news about disease progression. They may have to make difficult decisions at the time of diagnosis, when disease-focused treatment fails, when the effectiveness of a particular intervention is being discussed, and when decisions about hospice care are presented. These critical points on the treatment continuum demand patience, empathy, and honesty from nurses. Over the years, many communication training models have been developed to improve goals of care and end-of-life conversations (Table 13-2). One such program, the Serious Illness Conversation Project (SICP) communication guide, has helped clinicians have earlier, more thorough, and more accessible conversations around patients' values,

worries, and preferences (Paladino, Bernacki, Neville, et al., 2019).

Therapeutic communication can be learned and, like other skills, must be practiced to gain expertise. Like other skills, communication should be practiced in a safe setting, such as a classroom or clinical skills laboratory with other students and clinicians. One skill that nurses have the opportunity to master is responding to emotion. Nurses often meet patients in vulnerable states experiencing strong emotions such as anxiety, anger, fear, and sadness. The NURSE framework (Table 13-3) should be considered when a patient expresses an emotion. Typically, the nurse would choose one response listed at a time.

Patients often direct questions or concerns to nurses before they have been able to fully discuss the details of their diagnosis and prognosis with their primary providers or the entire health care team. Using open-ended questions allows the nurse to elicit the patient's and family's concerns, explore misconceptions and needs for information, and form the basis for collaboration with primary providers and other team members. Chart 13-3 provides sample language for exploring a patient's values and preferences. In practice, communication with each patient and family should be tailored to their particular level of understanding and values concerning disclosure.

TABLE 13-2	Interdisciplinary Communication Training Models			
Model Name	**Target Clinicians**	**Format**	**Curriculum**	**Considerations**
Center to Advance Palliative Care Continuing Medical Education modules[a]	All disciplines	Online, case-based, open-ended answers	Five modules on foundational communication skills. Additional PC modules available	Included in institutional CAPC membership
Education on Palliative and End-of-Life Care[b]	All disciplines	Classroom didactic	Overview of communication skills embedded in PC curriculum	A separate 2-d facilitator training is available
End-of-Life Nursing Education Consortium (ELNEC)[c]	RN, NP	Classroom didactic	Communication is focus during 1 h of a 2-d course. Various tracks including: ELNEC-Core, ELNEC-APRN, ELNEC Critical Care, ELNEC-Geriatrics	"Train-the-trainer" model. ELNEC added a communication-only course called COMFORT
Respecting Choices	RN, SW, APP, MD	Classroom didactic	First steps (RN/SW focused), next steps (RN/SW focused), last steps (MD focused). From advanced care planning to decision making	Usually paired with system implementation
Serious Illness Care Program at Ariadne Labs[d]	All disciplines	3-h workshop with didactic and roleplay	Training on the Serious Illness Conversation Guide (see Chart 13-3) with scripted exploratory questions	Usually paired with system implementation. Faculty members have 2+ d training
VitalTalk[e]	MD, APP, and ICU RN	Online video, Smartphone application, small-group workshop (0.5–2 d) with simulated patient actors	Content across disease continuum customized to learner needs organized by clinical task. Includes five-step talking map	Core workshop with actors, constructive feedback, and opportunity to replay

[a]Available at: www.capc.org/providers/courses/communication-skills-34
[b]Available at: www.bioethics.northwestern.edu/programs/epec/index.html
[c]Available at: www.aacnnursing.org/ELNEC
[d]Available at: www.ariadnelabs.org/areas-of-work/serious-illness-care
[e]Available at: www.vitaltalk.org
APP, advanced practice provider; ICU, intensive care unit; MD, medical doctor; NP, nurse practitioner; RN, registered nurse; SW, social worker.
Adapted from Back, A. L., Fromme, E. K., & Meier, D. E. (2019). Training clinicians with communication skills needed to match medical treatments to patient values. *Journal of American Geriatric Society, 67*(S2), S435–S441.

Chart 13-3 ASSESSMENT
Preferred Language for Assessing Goals of Care

Assess understanding of diagnosis and prognosis: Seek patient's knowledge of illness.

- What is your understanding of your condition?
- What did your provider say about your illness?
- How have things been going with your treatment?
- What is the plan moving forward?

Exploratory questions: Ask for clarifications and allow patient the space to tell narrative.

- Tell me more.
- Can you say more about that?
- I heard you say [x], can we go back to that?
- Will you tell me more about how you are feeling about [x]?

Ask about patient's values, preferences, and concerns: These questions allow health care providers to match patient values to treatment options, often called goals of care.

- What is most important to you?
- What are you hoping for, in terms of your illness?
- What you hoping from this treatment?
- What concerns you when you think about the future?
- What is most important to you?

Assess coping and support system: In learning more about how a person has coped in the past, you can incorporate appropriate supports (e.g., social work, chaplain)

- How have you coped with challenges in the past?
- What gives you strength?
- What gives you meaning and purpose?
- Is there anything we should consider or anyone we should include when making decisions about your care?
- If you cannot participate in health care decisions, with whom should we speak?

Important questions for family members when patient is unable to participate in conversation.

- Tell me about your loved one.
- What did they value?
- Did they ever talk about what they would or would not want if they were in a situation like this?
- Did they ever discuss states of living that would not be acceptable (e.g., being bedbound, unable to toilet, inability to speak)?

Adapted from Peereboom, K., & Coyle, N. (2012). Facilitating goals-of-care discussions for patients with life-limiting disease—Communication strategies for nurses. *Journal of Hospice and Palliative Nursing, 14*(4), 251–258.

The Role of the Nurse in Family Meetings

Family meetings, prompted by either the patient and family or the care team, are often held to clarify goals, address concerns, and formulate a plan. The objectives of a family meeting are to both gather information and share information. Family meetings may be held at any time during a serious illness and should especially be arranged when new diagnostic information is available. More often than not, difficult news is shared at a family meeting. As such, patient and family members may become emotional and the nurse has the unique opportunity to offer support (see Table 13-3).

Before a family meeting, the nurse in collaboration with the primary team can perform a stakeholder analysis to ensure that important people are present. The nurse can ask the patient who helps them make decisions and help arrange for their presence. Engaging integral medical team members and consults is important to ensure that experts can answer all patient and family questions. The nurse can assure the patient that they will be present at the meeting to support the patient. The nurse can also ensure the setting is right—free from disturbances, private, ample seating. Additional roles for the nurse in a family meeting are listed in Chart 13-4.

Advanced Care Planning

The process of thinking through, and possibly documenting, the medical interventions that one would or would not want

TABLE 13-3 Responding to Emotions

Patient Statement: "I just can't handle any more setbacks."

	Empathic Response	Sample Language
N	NAME the emotion	It sounds like you are worried about the future.
U	UNDERSTAND the emotion	You have been through so much already.
R	RESPECT (or praise) the patient	I am so impressed with how you have dealt with so many ups and downs.
S	SUPPORT the patient	I hope you don't have any more setbacks and I'm here for you no matter what the future holds.
E	EXPLORE the emotion	You seem more worried than usual; can you tell me more about what's different about today than yesterday?

Adapted from Back, A., Arnold, R., Tulsky, J. (2009). *Mastering communication with seriously ill patients: Balancing empathy and hope.* New York: Cambridge University Press.

Chart 13-4 The Role of the Nurse in a Family Meeting

- Advocate for patient based on values shared by patient and family.
- Act as interpreter when medical jargon is not clearly understood by patient and family.
- Respond to emotion expressed in meeting.
- Prior to meeting, encourage and assist patient and family with developing questions to ask of interdisciplinary teams during meeting.
- Express concerns.
- Share clinical nursing updates.

Adapted from Nelson, J. E., Cortez, T. B., Curtis, J. R., et al. (2011). Integrating palliative nursing in the ICU: The nurse in a leading role. *Journal of Hospice and Palliative Nursing, 13*(2), 89–94; Wittenberg-Lyles, E., Goldsmith, J., Ferrell, B. R., et al. (2013). *Communication in palliative nursing.* New York: Oxford.

Advance directives: written documents that allow the person of sound mind to document preferences regarding end-of-life care that should be followed when the signer is terminally ill and unable to verbally communicate their wishes. The documents are generally completed in advance of serious illness but may be completed after a diagnosis of serious illness if the signer is still of sound mind. The most common types are the durable power of attorney for health care and the living will.

Do not resuscitate: a medical order to withhold cardiopulmonary resuscitation (CPR) in the event of cardiac arrest. In some settings, the term "allow natural death" (AND) is used in place of "do not resuscitate" (DNR).

Durable power of attorney for health care: a legal document through which the signer appoints and authorizes another person to make medical decisions on their behalf when they are no longer able to speak for themselves. This is also known as a health care power of attorney, medical power of attorney, or a proxy directive.

Living will: a type of advance directive in which the individual documents treatment preferences. It provides instructions for care in the event that the signer is terminally ill and not able to communicate their wishes directly and often is accompanied by a durable power of attorney for health care. This is also known as a medical directive or treatment directive.

Physician orders for life-sustaining treatment (POLST): a form that translates patient preferences expressed in advance directives to medical "orders" that are transferable across settings and readily available to all health care providers, including emergency medical personnel. The POLST form is a brightly colored form that specifies preferences related to CPR, intubation, artificial nutrition and hydration, antibiotics, and other medical interventions. The form is signed by the patient or surrogate and the primary provider, advanced practice nurse, or physician assistant. The use of the POLST is subject to state laws and regulations. Numerous states have endorsed the POLST or a similar form and some states have implemented electronic registries and electronic versions of POLST forms (e.g., New York's e-MOLST program).

Information about the advance care planning and state-specific advance directive documents and instructions is available at www.caringinfo.org. Information about the POLST is available at www.polst.org

in the case one is no longer able to voice one's own decisions is called advanced care planning (ACP). Nurses play an integral role in ACP. With the proper training and understanding of ACP, nurses should feel empowered to engage with patients about their goals of care and, when applicable, assist patients with completion of ACP documentation (Izumi, 2017). Two components of ACP are designating a health care surrogate and documenting end-of-life preferences (Chart 13-5).

Now legally sanctioned in every state and federally sanctioned through the Patient Self-Determination Act of 1991, advance directives are written documents that allow competent people to document their preferences regarding the use or abatement of medical treatment at the end-of-life, specify their preferred setting for care, and communicate other valuable insights into their values and beliefs. These documents are widely available from health care providers, community organizations, bookstores, and from trusted Web

sites. Unfortunately, ACP documents remain underutilized, as a systematic review found that only one in three Americans have completed any advanced directive (Yadav, Gabler, Cooney, et al., 2017). Data was similar for those with chronic illnesses and healthy adults in this study. The underuse of advanced directives may reflect society's continued discomfort with openly confronting the subject of death. Furthermore, the existence of a properly executed advance directive does not reduce the complexity of end-of-life decisions.

The Patient Self-Determination Act requires that health care entities receiving Medicare or Medicaid reimbursement must ask whether patients have advance directives, provide information about advance directives, and incorporate advance directives into the medical record. However, advance directives should not be considered a substitute for ongoing communication among the health care provider, patient, and family as the end-of-life approaches.

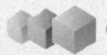 *Concept Mastery Alert*

An advance directive states a patient's wishes for treatment. A proxy directive appoints another person to make medical decisions on behalf of the patient and is added to the advance directive.

Symptom Assessment and Management

Expected Physiologic Changes

Patients approaching the end-of-life experience many of the same symptoms, regardless of their underlying disease processes. Symptoms in terminal illness may be caused by the disease, either directly (e.g., dyspnea owing to chronic obstructive lung disease) or indirectly (e.g., nausea and vomiting related to pressure in the gastric area), by the treatment for the disease, or by a coexisting disorder that is unrelated to the disease. Symptoms should be carefully and systematically assessed and managed. Pharmacologic and nonpharmacologic methods of symptom management may be used in combination with medical interventions to modify the physiologic causes of symptoms. The principles of pharmacologic symptom management are the use of the smallest dose of the medication to achieve the desired effect, avoidance of polypharmacy, anticipation and management of adverse effects, and creation of a therapeutic regimen that is acceptable to the patient based on the patient's goals for maximizing quality of life.

The patient's goals should guide symptom management. The clinician should help the patient and the family weigh the benefits and risks of continued diagnostic testing and disease-focused medical treatment in the context of their goals for care. The patient and the family may be extremely reluctant to forego monitoring that has become routine throughout the illness (e.g., blood testing, x-rays) but that may contribute little to a primary focus on comfort. Medical interventions may be aimed at treating the underlying causes of the symptoms or reducing the impact of symptoms. For example, a medical intervention such as thoracentesis (an invasive procedure in which fluid is drained from the pleural space) may be performed to temporarily relieve dyspnea in a patient with pleural effusion secondary to lung cancer.

For the procedural guidelines for assisting the patient undergoing thoracentesis, go to **thepoint.lww.com/Brunner15e**.

Anticipating and planning interventions for symptoms is a cornerstone of both palliative and end-of-life care. Patients and family members cope more effectively with new symptoms and exacerbations of existing symptoms when they know what to expect and how to manage them. At the end-of-life, hospice programs typically provide a *comfort kit* which contains ready-to-administer doses of various medications that are useful to treat symptoms in advanced illness. For example, a kit might contain small doses of oral morphine liquid for pain or shortness of breath, a benzodiazepine for anxiety, and an acetaminophen suppository for fever. Family members can be instructed to administer a prescribed dose from the emergency kit, often avoiding prolonged suffering for the patient.

Although clinicians may believe that symptoms must be completely relieved whenever possible, the patient might choose instead to decrease symptoms to a tolerable level rather than to relieve them completely if the side effects of medications are unacceptable to them. This often allows the patient to have greater independence, mobility, and alertness and to devote attention to issues that they consider of higher priority and greater importance. For instance, a mother may choose to wait to take pain medication until bedtime so that she can be awake and engaged when her children return home from school.

As death approaches and organ systems begin to fail, observable, expected changes in the body take place (Table 13-4). The nurse should prepare the family for the normal, expected changes that accompany the period immediately preceding death. Although the exact time of death cannot be predicted, it is often possible to identify when the patient is very close to death. When death is imminent, patients may become increasingly somnolent and unable to clear sputum or oral secretions, which may lead to further impairment of breathing from pooled secretions. The sound and appearance of the secretions are often more distressing to family members than is the presence of the secretions to the patient. Family distress over the changes in the patient's condition may be eased by supportive nursing care. Continuation of comfort-focused interventions and reassurance that the patient is not in any distress can do much to ease family concerns. Hospice programs frequently provide written information for families so that they know what to expect and what to do as death nears.

Pain

In the final stages of illnesses such as cancer, heart disease, chronic obstructive pulmonary disease (COPD), and renal

TABLE 13-4	Stages of the Dying Process	
Time Frame	**Symptoms:** *How the patient is feeling*	**Nursing Interventions:** *What you can do*
Months before death	• Gradual generalized weakness • Fatigue • Social isolation • Decreased appetite	• Provide education to patient and family that symptoms are expected. • Allow patient choice in activity level and sleep schedule. • Assist with life review. Provide support to family who are distressed by patient's withdrawal. • Educate patient/family on eating for comfort.
Weeks before death	• Neurologic: ↑ sleepiness, possible delirium, dulled senses (except hearing) • Cardiopulmonary: ↑ pulse and ↑ RR, ↓ BP, Periodic apnea or agonal breathing, inability to clear secretions • Renal: ↓ urinary output + incontinence or retention • Skin: feverish or cold, possible perspiration, pallor	• Provide education on terminal delirium. Engage family in periods of lucidity. Talk to patient even when appears to be sleepy (to avoid leaving anything unsaid). • Assess and treat dyspnea as appropriate. Cluster care. Assess if ANH is contributing to pulmonary congestion. Position patient in side-lying position with HOB elevated. • Insert urinary catheter for comfort if indicated. Use absorbent pads and change as needed. Consider retention if patient is restless. • Bath and change linens as needed. Engage family in scheduling.
Days before death	• Neurologic: somnolence, restlessness, further dulled senses (except hearing), possible "rally" in energy • Cardiopulmonary: ↑ pulse and ↑ or ↓ RR, ↓ BP, more frequent periods of apnea or agonal breathing, inability to clear secretions • Renal: ↓ urinary output + incontinence or retention • Skin: feverish or cold, mottling of extremities, pallor	• Normalize the dying process for family. If patient has a "rally" in energy, guide family to take patient's lead in preference for this time (e.g., a favorite meal). • Assess and treat dyspnea as appropriate. Cluster care. Position patient in side-lying position with HOB elevated. Avoid suctioning; administer anticholinergics for impaired secretions as prescribed. • Provide education to family. Use absorbent pads and change as needed. Consider retention if patient is restless. • Change linens as needed. Bed bath for comfort.
Hours before death (or *actively dying* phase)	• Neurologic: obtunded, nonresponsive, hearing may remain • Cardiopulmonary: ↑ pulse (may be irregular or difficult to palpate) and ↑ or ↓ RR, ↓ BP, periods of apnea (>40 s) or agonal breathing • Renal: oliguria/anuria • Skin: worsening mottling of extremities	Interventions as above. Continue to provide education that these signs and symptoms are a normal part of the dying process. If certain family wishes to be present at the time of death, alert them of prognosis. Encourage family self-care during vigil. Additionally, the nurse may engage in conversation with family around funeral/burial preferences and cultural rituals at the end-of-life. Offer chaplaincy support if helpful to family.

ANH, artificial nutrition and hydration; BP, blood pressure; ↓, decreased; HOB, head of bed; ↑, increased; +, plus; RR, respiratory rate.
Adapted from Berry, P., & Griffie, J. (2019). Planning for the actual death. In B. R. Ferrell, N. Coyle, & J. Paice (Eds.). *Oxford textbook of palliative nursing* (5th ed.). New York: Oxford.

disease, pain is a common symptom. Pain results from the disease state as well as the modalities used to treat them. The Worldwide Palliative Care Alliance, World Health Organization (2014) called attention to the continuing, worldwide high prevalence of pain at the end-of-life and the inadequate supply of opioids, particularly in developing nations. A primary role for nurses in end-of-life care is to ensure that pain is assessed, prevented where possible, and managed. Chapter 9 presents the importance of pain assessment, assessment principles for pain that include identifying the effect of the pain on the patient's life, and the importance of believing the patient's report of the pain and its effect. Poorly managed pain affects the psychological, emotional, social, and financial well-being of patients. Every clinician should be able to assess and oversee the basic management of pain (IOM, 2014).

Management of moderate to severe pain in the United States is complicated by public policy and legal challenges due to an opioid crisis (Foxwell, Uritsky, & Meghani, 2019) and federal prescribing guidelines aimed at reducing opioid use (Centers for Disease Control and Prevention [CDC], 2016). While patients receiving palliative care are exempt from the opioid guidelines, there are reports of the misapplication of the guidelines for patients with serious illnesses (Dowell, Haegerich, & Chou, 2019). The current context of pain management is also feared to worsen the widely documented disparities in pain treatment in the United States (Meghani & Vapiwala, 2018). Simultaneously, there are concerns about opioid misuse in the palliative care setting (Hui, Arthur, & Bruera, 2019). Thus, palliative care clinicians are also challenged with the imperative to provide effective pain relief while balancing societal risks.

All patients on opioid therapy and their family caregivers should receive comprehensive education and support to ensure safe use of opioids while addressing fears and concerns about opioid use. Personalized treatment plans should include longitudinal assessment and documentation of pain management goals and needs, management of treatment side effects, use of integrative therapies and interventional techniques when appropriate, monitoring risk of opioid misuse, and longitudinal counseling.

In their recent position statement, the American Society for Pain Management Nursing (ASPMN) and HPNA maintain that nurses and other health care professionals "must advocate for effective, efficient, and safe pain and symptom management to alleviate suffering for every patient receiving end-of-life care regardless of their age, diseases, history of substance misuse, or site of care" (Coyne, Mulvenon, & Paice, 2018). The statement underscores the indispensable role of comprehensive and continuous pain and symptom management in all patients and, specifically, in the patient who is nonverbal during the dying phase (Coyne et al., 2018).

The nurse educates the family caregivers about continuation of comfort measures as the patient approaches the end-of-life, how to administer antispasmodic agents via alternative routes, and how to assess for pain when the patient cannot verbally report pain intensity. Short-acting antispasmodic agents are most effective for uncontrolled pain. At the end-of-life, patients may receive frequent dosing. There is always a strong possibility that a patient approaching the end-of-life will die in close proximity to the time of analgesic administration. If the patient is at home, family members administering antispasmodic agents should be prepared for this possibility. They need reassurance that they did not cause the death of the patient by administering a dose of analgesic medication. In the hospital, nurses need to understand that there is always a last dose of medication in a patient who is dying, but the last dose does not cause death.

Dyspnea

Dyspnea, an uncomfortable awareness of breathing, is one of the most prevalent symptoms at the end-of-life and can be challenging to manage. A highly subjective symptom, dyspnea often is not associated with visible signs of distress, such as tachypnea, diaphoresis, or cyanosis. Although the underlying cause of the dyspnea can be identified and treated in some cases, the burdens of additional diagnostic evaluation and treatment aimed at the physiologic problem may outweigh the benefits. The treatment of dyspnea varies depending on the underlying cause, the patient's general physical condition, and imminence of death. For example, a blood transfusion may provide temporary symptom relief for a patient with anemia earlier in the disease process; however, as the patient approaches the end-of-life, the benefits are typically short-lived or absent.

Similar to the assessment of pain, reports of dyspnea are typically a subjective report. Also, as is true for physical pain, the meaning of dyspnea to an individual patient may increase their suffering. For example, the patient may interpret increasing dyspnea as a sign that death is approaching. For some patients, sensations of breathlessness may invoke frightening images of drowning or suffocation, and the resulting cycle of fear and anxiety may increase the sensation of breathlessness. Therefore, the nurse should conduct a careful assessment of the psychosocial and spiritual components of the dyspnea. Physical assessment parameters include symptom intensity, distress, and interference with activities; auscultation of lung sounds; assessment of fluid balance, including measurement of dependent edema (circumference of lower extremities) and abdominal girth; temperature; skin color; sputum quantity and character; and cough.

To determine the intensity of dyspnea and its interference with daily activities, the patient can be asked to report the severity of the dyspnea using a scale of 0 to 10 (similar to the pain scale), where 0 is no dyspnea and 10 is the worst imaginable dyspnea. There is new evidence that the use of the Respiratory Distress Observation Scale may be effective as well (Birkholz & Haney, 2018) (see the Nursing Research Profile in Chart 13-6). The nurse should assess the patient's baseline rating before treatment and should elicit subsequent measurements taken during exacerbation of the symptom, periodically during treatment, and whenever the treatment plan changes; these parameters provide ongoing objective evidence for the efficacy of the treatment plan. In addition, physical assessment findings may assist in locating the source of the dyspnea and selecting nursing interventions to relieve the symptom. The components of the assessment change as the patient's condition changes. Like other symptoms at the end-of-life, dyspnea can be managed effectively in the absence of assessment and diagnostic data (e.g., arterial blood gases) that are standard when a patient's illness or symptom is acute and considered reversible.

Nursing management of dyspnea at the end-of-life is directed toward administering medical treatment for the

Chart 13-6
NURSING RESEARCH PROFILE
Comparison of Dyspnea Assessment Tools

Birkholz, L., & Haney, T. (2018). Using a dyspnea assessment tool to improve care at the end of life. *Journal of Hospice and Palliative Nursing, 20*(3), 219–227.

Purpose

There is no standard for the assessment of dyspnea, the subjective sensation of breathlessness. Generally, patients experiencing shortness of breath tell providers. However, when a person is no longer able to report symptoms at the end-of-life, nurses rely on experiential practice to guide dyspnea management. The purpose of this study was to compare end-of-life dyspnea assessment and management before and after educational implementation of Respiratory Distress Observation Scale (RDOS).

Design

This was a pre-experimental study which used a pretest/posttest format to examine the use of the RDOS. Nurses ($n = 39$) who provide end-of-life care where there is no standardized dyspnea assessment tool were recruited from centers: (1) a hospice agency in the Northeastern region of United States with both home hospice and an inpatient hospice unit, and (2) a medical-surgical unit in a community hospital in the Rural Western United States. RDOS was taught by video where standardized patients simulated mild, moderate, and severe levels of dyspnea in six scenarios. Nurses watched the simulated scenarios and recorded a dyspnea assessment based on experiential knowledge, in a pretest. Then, RDOS education was provided by a palliative nurse educator. Finally, the nurses rewatched the video of simulated scenarios and documented a dyspnea assessment using the RDOS in a posttest.

Findings

Researchers found a statistically significant difference in both the nurse's ability to accurately assess level of dyspnea ($p < 0.001$) and the nurse's ability to choose the most appropriate treatment ($p = 0.021$), after RDOS education. There was no statistically significant difference after education in the nurses' determination of overall comfort. The final research question addressed the nurse's evaluation of the RDOS education, where almost all agreed that the RDOS was easy to use with strong recommendation to use in end-of-life dyspnea assessment.

Nursing Implications

Nurses working in end-of-life care treat dyspnea frequently and tend to rely on previous experiences for assessment and management of dyspnea. The RDOS is a validated dyspnea assessment tool which helps nurses to systematically assess dyspnea. When nurses used the RDOS, there was a significant improvement in both the ability to assess degree of dyspnea and select the appropriate treatment.

---

underlying pathology, monitoring the patient's response to treatment, helping the patient and the family manage anxiety (which exacerbates dyspnea), altering the perception of the symptom, and conserving energy (Chart 13-7). Pharmacologic intervention is aimed at modifying lung physiology and improving performance as well as altering the perception of the symptom. Bronchodilators and corticosteroids are used to treat underlying obstructive pathology, thereby improving overall lung function. Low doses of opioids effectively relieve dyspnea, although the mechanism of relief is not entirely clear. Although dyspnea in terminal illness is typically not associated with diminished blood oxygen saturation, low-flow oxygen often provides psychological comfort to both patients and families, particularly in the home setting.

As mentioned previously, dyspnea may be exacerbated by anxiety, and anxiety may trigger episodes of dyspnea, setting off a respiratory crisis in which the patient and the family may panic. For patients receiving care at home, patient and family education should include anticipation and management of crisis situations and a clearly communicated emergency plan. The patient and the family should be educated about medication administration, condition changes that should be reported to the primary provider and the nurse, and strategies for coping with diminished reserves and increasing symptomatology as the disease progresses. The patient on hospice and their family require reassurance that the symptom can be effectively managed at home without the need for activation of the emergency medical services or hospitalization and that a nurse will be available at all times via telephone and to make a visit.

Impaired Secretions at the End-of-Life

In the last stage of dying, patients typically experience impaired secretions. This may be manifested by noisy, gurgling breathing or moaning. In most cases, the sounds of breathing at the end-of-life are related to oropharyngeal relaxation with inability to clear secretions through cough or swallowing due to somnolence. Treatment of impaired secretions in the actively dying is usually achieved with the use of anticholinergic medications to dry secretions (Table 13-5). Sounds caused by impaired secretions are generally most distressing

Chart 13-7
Palliative Nursing Interventions for Dyspnea

Treat Underlying Cause

- Administer prescribed bronchodilators and corticosteroids (obstructive pathology).
- Administer blood products as prescribed for anemia.
- Administer prescribed diuretics and monitor fluid balance.

Interdisciplinary Resources

- Respiratory Therapists: pulmonary rehabilitation, noninvasive ventilation, chest wall vibration
- Physical and Occupational Therapists: energy conservation techniques, walking aids (rolling walker, cane), exercise
- Social Work or Psychologists: cognitive-behavioral therapy, meditation/mindfulness training
- Integrative Medicine Treatments: Biofeedback, Reiki, Chiropractic, Acupuncture, Yoga, T'ai Chi, and Qi gong

Self-Management (Nursing Role: Provide Education and Foster Practices)

- Forward-leaning posture
- Pursed lips or abdominal accessory muscle breathing
- Cool air movement: portable fan, air-conditioning unit, opening window in fall/winter
- Lifestyle changes: adapting socialization practices and/or accepting limitations

TABLE 13-5	Medications to Control Secretions and Terminal Respiratory Congestion
Medication	**Suggested Initial Dosing**
Atropine 1% ophthalmic	1–2 drops PO/SL every 4 h, scheduled or PRN
Atropine injection	0.4 mg IV/SC/IM every 4 h, scheduled or PRN
Glycopyrrolate	1 mg PO TID, scheduled or PRN, up to 6 mg/day or 0.1 mg SC/IM/IV TID or PRN
Hyoscyamine	0.125 mg PO/SL every 4 h PRN, up to 1.5 mg/day
Hyoscyamine extended-release	0.375 mg PO every 12 h, up to 1.5 mg/day
Scopolamine transdermal	Apply 1 patch topically behind the ear every 72 h, up to 3 patches/72 h

IM, intramuscularly; IV, intravenously; PO, by mouth; PRN, as needed; SC, subcutaneously; SL, sublingually; TID, twice a day.
Reprinted with permission from Enclara Pharmacia, Inc. (2015). *Enclara Pharmacia medication use guidelines* (1st ed.). Philadelphia, PA: Author.

to family members. Nurses need to educate family members about impaired secretions, provide assurance on the normalcy of the symptom, and distinguish it from dyspnea.

Anorexia and Cachexia at the End-of-Life

Anorexia and cachexia are common in the seriously ill. The profound changes in the patient's appearance and a lack of interest in the socially important rituals of mealtime are particularly disturbing to families. The approach to the problem varies depending on the patient's stage of illness, level of disability associated with the illness, and desires. The anorexia–cachexia syndrome (Table 13-6) is characterized by disturbances in carbohydrate, protein, and fat metabolism; endocrine dysfunction; and anemia. The syndrome results in severe asthenia (loss of energy).

Anorexia and cachexia differ from starvation (simple food deprivation) in several important ways. Anorexia is defined as inadequate nutritional intake, while cachexia refers to severe lean muscle loss. In chronic illness, appetite is lost early in the process, the body becomes catabolic in a dysfunctional way, and supplementation by enteral feeding or parenteral nutrition in advanced disease does not replenish lean body mass that has been lost. Similarly, appetite stimulants are ineffective at this stage. Cachexia is associated with anabolic and catabolic changes in metabolism that relate to activity of neurohormones and proinflammatory cytokines, resulting in profound protein loss.

Near the end-of-life, the body's nutritional needs change, and the desire for food and fluid may diminish. People may no longer be able to use, eliminate, or store nutrients and fluids adequately. Eating and sharing meals are important social activities in families and communities, and food preparation and enjoyment are linked to happy memories, strong emotions, and hope for survival. For patients with serious illness, food preparation and mealtimes often become a constant struggle in which well-meaning family members argue, plead,

TABLE 13-6	Anorexia/Cachexia Syndrome
Mechanism	**Effect**
Loss of appetite	• Generalized tissue wasting • Queasiness • Decreased pleasure at meals yielding decreased socialization
Reduced voluntary motor activity	• Sarcopenia (muscle wasting) • Skeletal muscle fatigue
Reduced rate of muscle protein synthesis	• Sarcopenia • Skeletal muscle weakness
Decreased immune response	• Increased risk of infection
Decreased response or intolerability to treatments	• Increased morbidity • Increased mortality

Nursing Interventions for Anorexia/Cachexia Syndrome:
Assess the impact of current medications (e.g., chemotherapy, antiretroviral).
Consider impact of additional therapies on appetite (e.g., radiation, dialysis).
Assess for concomitant symptoms including nausea, anxiety, depression, constipation, and diarrhea.
Perform oral assessment (e.g., presence of ulcers or thrush); administer and monitor effects of topical and systemic treatment for oropharyngeal pain.
Ensure that dentures fit properly, if applicable.
Administer antiemetics or laxatives when appropriate.
Explore barriers to eating with patient and develop plan.
Remove unpleasant odors including soiled tissues, bedpans, and emesis basin.
Position to enhance gastric emptying.
Provide frequent mouth care, especially after eating.

Adapted from Schack, E. E., & Wholihan, D. (2019). Anorexia and cachexia. In B. R. Ferrell, N. Coyle, & J. Paice (Eds.). *Oxford textbook of palliative nursing* (5th ed.). New York: Oxford.

and cajole to encourage ill people to eat. Patients who are seriously ill often lose their appetites entirely, develop strong aversions to foods that they have enjoyed in the past, or crave a particular food to the exclusion of all other foods.

As the patient approaches the end-of-life, the family and the health care providers should offer the patient what they prefer and can most easily tolerate. The nurse should educate the family about ways to separate feeding from caring and how to demonstrate love, sharing, and caring by being with the loved one in other ways. Preoccupation with appetite, feeding, and weight loss diverts energy and time that the patient and the family could use in other meaningful activities. Encourage patients to eat what brings them joy. For family members who are struggling with seeing their loved one eat less, the nurse ensures they understand that patients are allowed to refuse foods and fluids. The nurse may also instruct family members how to make ice cubes from frozen fruit juices or smoothies and to offer these to the patient.

Anxiety and Depression

Almost half of patients in hospice experience significant anxiety and/or depression at the end-of-life as reported by proxy (Kozlov, Phongtankuel, Prigerson, et al., 2019). Anxiety may be exacerbated by other symptoms such as pain or dyspnea, as well as anticipating symptoms at the end-of-life. A systematic approach to anxiety involves treating the underlying cause, providing psychosocial support, referral to counseling as needed, and administering medications as prescribed.

Clinical depression should neither be accepted as an inevitable consequence of dying nor confused with sadness and anticipatory grieving, which are normal reactions to the losses associated with impending death. Emotional and spiritual support and control of disturbing physical symptoms are appropriate interventions for situational depression associated with terminal illness. Patients and their families must be given space and time to experience sadness and to grieve; however, patients should not have to endure untreated depression at the end of their lives. An effective approach to clinical depression includes relief of physical symptoms, attention to emotional and spiritual distress, psychotherapy, and pharmacologic intervention with antidepressants.

Delirium

Many patients remain alert, arousable, and able to communicate until very close to death. Others sleep for long intervals and awaken only intermittently, with eventual somnolence until death. Delirium refers to concurrent disturbances in the level of consciousness, attention, awareness, and cognitive capability that develop over a relatively short period of time (Bush, Tierney, & Lawlor, 2017). Confusion may be related to underlying, treatable conditions such as medication side effects or interactions, pain or discomfort, hypoxia or dyspnea, or a full bladder or impacted stool. In patients with cancer, confusion may be secondary to brain metastases. Delirium may also be related to metabolic changes, infection, and organ failure. In some patients, a period of agitated delirium precedes death, sometimes causing families to be hopeful that suddenly active patients may be getting better.

Nursing interventions are aimed at identifying the underlying causes of delirium; acknowledging the family's distress over its occurrence; reassuring family members about what is normal; educating family members how to interact with and ensure safety for the patient with delirium; and monitoring the effects of medications used to treat severe agitation, paranoia, and fear. Confusion may mask the patient's unmet spiritual needs and fears about dying. Spiritual intervention, music therapy, gentle massage, and therapeutic touch may provide some relief. Reduction of environmental stimuli, avoidance of harsh lighting or very dim lighting (which may produce disturbing shadows), presence of familiar faces, and gentle reorientation and reassurance are also helpful.

Patients with delirium may become hypoactive and/or hyperactive, restless, irritable, and fearful. Sleep deprivation and hallucinations may occur. When treating delirium, it is important to attempt to treat underlying factors contributing to symptoms first. Much controversy remains on the pharmacologic treatment of delirium at the end-of-life. One study compared the use of haloperidol plus lorazepam to haloperidol alone and found improved relief of symptoms with the medication combination (Hui, Frisbee-Hume, Wilson, et al., 2017). Unfortunately, delirium is a common symptom at the end-of-life; providing education on this may be the most reassuring intervention for family members.

Additional Common Symptoms

Patients may experience other common symptoms. Progressive fatigue occurs in most chronic, progressive illnesses, worsening in the last weeks and months of life. At the end-of-life, many patients suffer from constipation as a side effect of medications, such as opioids, as well as the sedentary nature of advanced chronic illness. Nurses should be performing a physical assessment including abdominal examination and last bowel movement. The nurse can administer laxatives (either by mouth or per rectum) as prescribed if patients show signs of constipation.

Nausea and vomiting may be common at the end-of-life, especially in patients who experienced nausea during disease progression. Patients with malignant bowel obstructions may experience refractory nausea at the end-of-life requiring antiemetics to target multiple hormone receptors or decompression via a gastric tube. Further, skin breakdown occurs as the organs, including skin begin to fail. Diligent nursing care of wounds includes assessment, treatment of pain, dressing changes for comfort, and consultation with wound care specialists.

Time of Death

For patients who have received adequate management of symptoms and for families who have received adequate preparation and support, the actual time of death is commonly peaceful and occurs without struggle. Nurses may or may not be present at the time of a patient's death. In many states, nurses are authorized to make the pronouncement of death and sign the death certificate when death is expected. The determination of death is made through a physical examination that includes auscultation for the absence of breathing and heart sounds. Home care or hospice programs in which nurses make the time-of-death visit and pronounce death have policies and procedures to guide the nurse's actions during this visit. Immediately on cessation of vital functions, the body begins to change. It becomes dusky or bluish, waxen appearing, and cool; blood darkens and pools in dependent areas of the body (e.g., the back and the sacrum if the body is in a supine position); and urine and stool may be evacuated.

Immediately after death, family members should be allowed and encouraged to spend time with the deceased. Normal responses of family members at the time of death vary widely and range from quiet expressions of grief to overt expressions that include wailing and prostration. The family members' desire for privacy during their time with the deceased should be honored. Family members may wish to independently manage or assist with care of the body after death. In the home, after-death care of the body frequently includes culturally specific rituals such as bathing the body. Home care agencies and hospices vary in the policies surrounding removal of tubes. In the absence of specific guidance from the organization, the nurse should shut off infusions of any kind (intravenous or tube feeding) and leave intravenous access devices, feeding tubes, catheters, and wound dressings in place. When an expected death occurs in the home setting, the family generally will have received assistance with funeral arrangements in advance of the death. The funeral home should be called and the funeral director will transport the body directly to the funeral home. In the hospital or long-term care facility, nurses follow the respective facility's procedure for preparation of the body and transportation to the facility's morgue. However, the needs of families to remain with the deceased, to wait until other family members arrive before the body is moved, and to perform after-death rituals should be honored.

Some patients may have elected to donate tissue such as corneas, bone, veins, or heart valves for transplant. Typically, this information would be known to the care team before the patient dies. In some cases, such as late referral or an unexpectedly rapid progression, the patient's wishes with respect to donation might be unknown. If the patient died at home or in a nursing home and the deceased's wishes are known, a team member should contact the organ procurement organization through which the deceased had arranged to donate tissue. That organization will ordinarily transport the body for tissue procurement and to the funeral home.

Providing Psychosocial and Spiritual Support

Many patients suffer unnecessarily when they do not receive adequate attention for the symptoms accompanying serious illness. Careful evaluation of the patient should include not only the physical problems but also the psychosocial and spiritual dimensions of the patient's and family's experience of serious illness. This approach contributes to a more comprehensive understanding of how the patient's and family's life has been affected by illness and leads to nursing care that addresses their needs in every dimension.

Hope and Meaning in Illness

Clinicians and researchers have observed that although specific hopes may change over time, hope generally persists in some form across every stage of illness. In terminal illness, hope represents the patient's imagined future, forming the basis of a positive, accepting attitude and providing the patient's life with meaning, direction, and optimism. When hope is viewed in this way, it is not limited to cure of the disease; instead, it focuses on what is achievable in the time remaining. Many patients find hope in working on important relationships and creating legacies. Patients who are terminally ill can be extremely resilient, reconceptualizing hope repeatedly as they approach the end-of-life.

Numerous nurse researchers have studied the concept of hope, and they have related its presence to spirituality, quality of life, and transcendence (Tarbi & Meghani, 2019). Hope is a multidimensional construct that provides comfort as a person endures life threats and personal challenges. The following are hope-fostering and hope-hindering activities among patients who are terminally ill and in hospice with various diagnoses:

- *Hope-fostering categories:* Love of family and friends, spirituality/faith, setting goals and maintaining independence, positive relationships with clinicians, humor, personal characteristics, and uplifting memories
- *Hope-hindering categories:* Abandonment and isolation, uncontrollable pain/discomfort, and devaluation of personhood

Nurses can support hope for the patient and the family by using effective listening and communication skills, thus encouraging realistic hope that is specific to their needs for information, expectations for the future, and values and preferences concerning the end-of-life. Nurses must engage in self-reflection and identify their own biases and fears concerning illness, life, and death. As nurses become more skilled in working with patients who are seriously ill, they can become less determined to *fix* and more willing to listen; more comfortable with silence, grief, anger, and sadness; and more fully present with patients and their families.

Nursing interventions for enabling and supporting hope include the following:

- Answering questions about illness in terms the patient understands
- Listening attentively
- Encouraging sharing of feelings
- Providing accurate information
- Encouraging and supporting patients' control over their circumstances, choices, and environment whenever possible
- Assisting patients to explore ways for finding meaning in their lives
- Facilitating effective communication within families
- Making referrals for psychosocial and spiritual counseling
- Assisting with the development of supports in the home or community when none exist

Providing Culturally Sensitive Care at the End-of-Life

Nurses are responsible for educating patients and their caregivers and for supporting them as they adapt to life with the illness. Nurses can assist patients and families with life review, values clarification, treatment decision making, and end-of-life goals. The only way to do this effectively is to try to appreciate and understand the illness from the patient's perspective.

The nurse's role is to assess the values, preferences, and practices of every patient, regardless of ethnicity, gender identity, socioeconomic status, or background. The nurse can share knowledge about a patient's and family's cultural beliefs and practices with the health care team and facilitate the adaptation of the care plan to accommodate these practices.

Although death, grief, and mourning are universally accepted aspects of living, the values, expectations, and practices during serious illness as death approaches and after death are culturally bound and expressed. Health care providers may share similar values concerning end-of-life care and may find that they are inadequately prepared to assess for and implement care plans that support culturally diverse perspectives. Historical mistrust of the health care system and unequal access to even basic medical care may underlie the beliefs and attitudes among ethnically diverse populations. In addition, lack of education or knowledge about end-of-life care treatment options and language barriers may influence decisions among many socioeconomically disadvantaged groups.

Nurses should be both culturally aware and sensitive in their approaches to communication with patients and families about death. To provide effective patient- and family-centered care at the end-of-life, nurses must be willing to set aside their own assumptions and attitudes so that they can discover what type and amount of disclosure is most meaningful to each patient and family within their unique belief systems. For example, a nurse may find that a female patient prefers to have her eldest son make all of her care decisions. Institutional practices and laws governing informed consent are also rooted in the Western notion of autonomous decision making and informed consent. If a patient wishes to defer decisions to her son, the nurse can work with the team to negotiate informed consent, respecting the patient's right not to participate in decision making and honoring her family's cultural practice.

Every person has unique needs at the end-of-life and deserves to be respected as a person. Those who identify as lesbian, gay, bisexual, transgender, and queer may need special attention to psychological stressors of serious illness and ACP to designate a preferred surrogate, as this may be outside of the biologic family. An additional concern for some transgender patients is loss of identity after death; for instance, not being buried in clothes of their preferred gender or honored with the name they chose (Higgins & Hynes, 2019).

The nurse should assess and document the patient's and family's specific beliefs, preferences, and practices regarding end-of-life care, preparation for death, and after-death rituals. Chart 13-8 identifies suggested language for cultural and spiritual assessment. The discomfort of novice nurses with asking questions and discussing this type of sensitive content can be reduced by prior practice in a classroom or clinical skills laboratory, observation of interviews conducted by experienced nurses, and partnering with experienced nurses during the first few assessments.

Spiritual Care

Attention to the spiritual component of the illness experienced by the patient and the family is not new within the context of nursing care, yet many nurses lack the comfort or skills to assess and intervene in this dimension. Spirituality contains features of religiosity; however, the two concepts are not interchangeable. **Spirituality** includes domains such as how a person derives meaning and purpose from life, one's beliefs and faith, sources of hope, and attitudes toward death (Puchalski, 2015).

The spiritual assessment is a key component of comprehensive nursing assessment for patients who are terminally ill and their families. While the nursing assessment should include religious affiliation, the nurse keeps in mind that spirituality is a broader concept than just religion (see Chart 13-8). In addition to the assessment of the role of religious faith and practices, important religious rituals, and connection to a religious community, the nurse should further explore:

- The harmony or discord between the patient's and the family's beliefs
- Other sources of meaning, hope, and comfort
- The presence or absence of a sense of peace of mind and purpose in life
- Spiritual or religious beliefs about illness, medical treatment, and care of the sick

A four-step spiritual assessment process using the acronym FICA involves asking the following questions (Puchalski & Romer, 2000):

- Faith and belief: Do you consider yourself to be a spiritual or religious person? What is your *faith* or belief? What gives your life meaning?

Chart 13-8

ASSESSMENT

Cultural and Spiritual Issues at the End-of-Life

Cultural Assessment

- Tell me more about yourself and your family.
- How are decisions made in your family?
- In order to provide you with the best care, are there any customs or practices important to you that should be included in your care plan?

Spiritual Assessment

- How is your spirit?
- Are you at peace?
- What gives you meaning and purpose?
- What are you most hoping for?
- Is anything worrying you?
- Is there anything you have not done that you wish/need to do?

Assessing Cultural and Spiritual Practices Surrounding Death

- What do you believe happens after death?
- Would you like your family to be involved in the care of your body?
- Are there certain people you would like to care for your body after death (e.g., women only or spiritual care provider)?
- Immediately after death are there any rituals, practices, or ceremonies that should be performed? Are there ways that we can help facilitate these?

Culturally Competent Communication Skills

- Respect uniqueness of each patient.
- Listen attentively to patient's narratives.
- Assess values and preferences for care.
- Address concerns.
- Anticipate when communication may be difficult and engage interdisciplinary team to provide support.

Adapted from Cormack, C., Mazanec, P., & Panke, J. T. (2019). Cultural considerations in palliative care. In B. R. Ferrell, N. Coyle, & J. Paice (Eds.). *Oxford textbook of palliative nursing* (5th ed.). New York: Oxford; Taylor, E. J. (2019). Spiritual screening, history, and assessment. In B. R. Ferrell, N. Coyle, & J. Paice (Eds.). *Oxford textbook of palliative nursing* (5th ed.). New York: Oxford.

- Importance and Influence: What *importance* does faith have in your life? Have your beliefs *influenced* the way you take care of yourself and your illness? What role do your beliefs play in regaining your health?
- Community: Are you a part of a spiritual or religious *community*? Is this of support to you and how? Is there a group of people you really love or who are important to you?
- Address in care: How would you like me to *address* these issues in your health care?

For most people, contemplating one's own death raises many issues, such as the meaning of existence, the purpose of suffering, and the existence of an afterlife. When faced with a grave prognosis, many patients experience spiritual or existential distress where a sense of meaning or purpose is lost. Other manifestations of spiritual distress include questioning or blaming their god. Nurses may identify distress when patients ask questions like, "Why me?" or "Why is God punishing me?" When hearing such questions, nurses should engage a spiritual care provider. Near the end-of-life, many draw strength from religion and spirituality and may turn to spiritual care providers for support; however, one study showed that 75% of clergy want more education surrounding end-of-life issues (Sanders, Chow, Enzinger, et al., 2017). Nurses may be perfectly poised to deliver point-of-care education to spiritual care providers. Further, the interdisciplinary team can organize a debriefing session to enrich education for all disciplines.

Another phenomenon associated with spirituality at the end-of-life is spiritual pain, defined as a pain deep in one's soul not manifested as physical symptoms, which may be experienced in the seriously ill. Although prevalence is not known in all illnesses, in those with advanced cancer as many as 67% of patients may experience spiritual pain, which is correlated with lower quality of life (Perez-Cruz, Langer, Carrasco, et al., 2019).

Grief, Mourning, and Bereavement

A wide range of feelings and behaviors are normal, adaptive, and healthy reactions to the loss of a loved one. **Grief** refers to the personal feelings that accompany an anticipated or actual loss; see Table 13-7 for types of grief. **Mourning** refers to individual, family, group, and cultural expressions of grief and associated behaviors. **Bereavement** refers to the period of time during which mourning for a loss takes place. Both grief

TABLE 13-7	Characteristics of Types of Grief and Nursing Interventions
Type of Grief	**Characteristics**
Anticipatory	Unconsciously preparing for what might happen *Examples:* Grief at diagnosis at loss of "normal" life; preparing for the loss of a limb for amputation
Uncomplicated	Range of emotions experienced after a loss moving toward adjustment; brief periods of relapse common *Examples:* Missing a deceased grandparent during holidays
Complicated or Prolonged	Intense response after loss where profound emotions persist usually >1 y *Example:* Widow who stops caring for herself after the death of her husband and sobs at any mention of his name a year later
Disenfranchised	Grieving person feels that society does not acknowledge or support person's right to grieve *Examples:* Mistress, homosexual partner, colleagues
Unresolved	Traumatic or unexpected losses *Examples:* Death of a child; suicide; disaster-related death

Nursing Interventions: Assessment of self-care and social supports. Employ assessment tools, such as the Inventory of Complicated Grief. Referral to professional counseling services.

Adapted from Corless, I. B., & Meisenh, J. B. (2019). Bereavement. In B. R. Ferrell, N. Coyle, & J. Paice (Eds.). *Oxford textbook of palliative nursing* (5th ed.). New York: Oxford; Limbo, R., Kobler, K., & Davies, B. (2019). Grief and bereavement in perinatal and pediatric palliative care. In B. R. Ferrell, N. Coyle, & J. Paice (Eds.). *Oxford textbook of palliative nursing* (5th ed.). New York: Oxford.

reactions and mourning behaviors change over time as people learn to live with the loss. Although the pain of the loss may be tempered by the passage of time, loss is an ongoing developmental process, and time does not heal the bereaved person completely. That is, the bereaved do not get over a loss entirely, nor do they return to who they were before the loss. Rather, they develop a new sense of who they are and where they fit in a world that has changed dramatically and permanently.

Anticipatory Grief and Mourning

People experience grief in different ways. Kübler-Ross (1969) originally described five stages of grief including (1) denial, (2) anger, (3) bargaining, (4) depression, and (5) acceptance. Newer models of grief acknowledge that grieving is not a linear process and many more emotions may be present than originally identified by Kübler-Ross. Additionally, people many feel conflicting emotions, such as hope and guilt when thinking about the future, at the same time. The Dual Process Model (Fig. 13-3) of coping with bereavement allows oscillation between the loss-oriented process and the restoration-oriented process (Stroebe & Schut, 1999). The Dual Process Model assumes fluidity in bereavement and normalizes the individual experience by offering that people will experience competing and complicated emotions after the death of a loved one.

Individual and family coping with the anticipation of death is complicated by the varied and conflicting trajectories that grief and mourning may assume in families. For example, the patient may be experiencing sadness while contemplating role changes that have been brought about by the illness, and the patient's spouse or partner may be expressing or suppressing feelings of anger about the current changes in role and impending loss of the relationship. Others in the family may cope with fear using withdrawal. Each person copes in their own way as there is no *right* way to cope.

The nurse should assess the characteristics of the family system and intervene in a manner that supports and enhances the cohesion of the family unit. The nurse can suggest that family members talk about their feelings and understand them in the broader context of anticipatory grief and mourning. Acknowledging and expressing feelings, continuing to interact with the patient in meaningful ways, and planning for the time of death and bereavement are adaptive family behaviors. Professional support provided by grief counselors, whether in the community, at a local hospital, in the long-term care facility, or associated with a hospice program, can help both the patient and the family sort out and acknowledge feelings and make the end-of-life as meaningful as possible.

Grief and Mourning After Death

When a loved one dies, family members enter a new phase of grief and mourning as they begin to accept the loss, feel the pain of permanent separation, and prepare to live a life without the deceased. Even if the loved one dies after a long illness, preparatory grief experienced during the terminal illness does not preclude the grief and mourning that follow the death. With a death after a long or difficult illness, family members may experience conflicting feelings of relief that the loved one's suffering has ended, compounded by guilt and grief

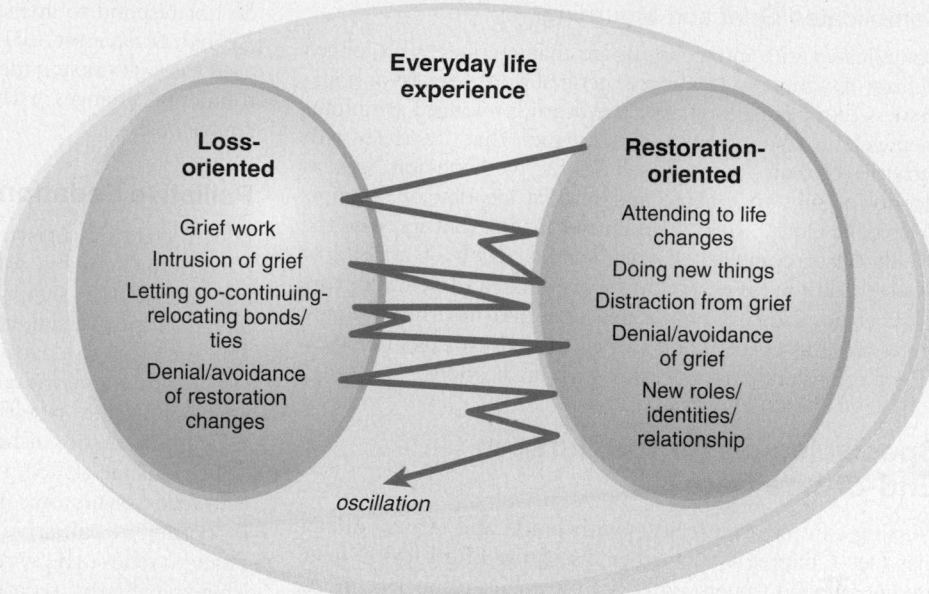

Figure 13-3 • The Dual Process Model of coping with bereavement. Adapted with permission from Stroebe, M. S., & Schut, H. (1999). The Dual Process Model of coping with bereavement: Rationale and description. *Death Studies*, 23, 197–224, by permission of Taylor & Francis Ltd (http://www.tandfonline.com) and Stroebe MS & Schut H. doi: 10.1080/074811899201046.

related to unresolved issues or the circumstances of death. Grief work may be especially difficult if a patient's death was painful, prolonged, accompanied by unwanted interventions, or unattended. Families that had no preparation or support during the period of imminent death may have a more difficult time finding a place for the painful memories.

Feelings of grief are often profound; however, bereaved people eventually reconcile the loss and find a way to reengage with their lives. Grief and mourning are affected by several factors, including individual characteristics, coping skills, and experiences with illness and death; the nature of the relationship to the deceased; factors surrounding the illness and the death; family dynamics; social support; and cultural expectations and norms.

After-death rituals, including preparation of the body, funeral practices, and burial rituals, are socially and culturally significant ways in which family members begin to accept the reality and finality of death. Preplanning of funerals is common, and hospice professionals, in particular, help the family make plans for death, often involving the patient, who may wish to play an active role. Preplanning of the funeral relieves the family of the burden of making decisions in the intensely emotional period after a death.

In general, the period of mourning is an adaptive response to loss during which mourners come to accept the loss as real and permanent, acknowledge and experience the painful emotions that accompany the loss, experience life without the deceased, overcome impediments to adjustment, and find a new way of living in a world without the loved one. Particularly immediately after the death, mourners begin to recognize the reality and permanence of the loss by talking about the deceased in past terms and telling and retelling the story of the illness and death. Societal norms in the United States are frequently at odds with the normal grieving processes of people; time excused from work obligations is typically measured in days, and mourners are often expected to get over the loss quickly and get on with life.

In reality, the work of grief and mourning takes time, and avoiding grief work after the death often leads to long-term

adjustment difficulties. According to Rando (2000), mourning for a loss involves the "undoing" of psychosocial ties that bind mourners to the deceased, personal adaptation to the loss, and learning to live in the world without the deceased. Six key processes of mourning allow people to accommodate to the loss in a healthy way (Rando, 2000):

• Recognition of the loss
• Reaction to the separation and experiencing and expressing the pain of the loss
• Recollection and reexperiencing the deceased, the relationship, and the associated feelings
• Relinquishing old attachments to the deceased
• Readjustment to adapt to the new world without forgetting the old
• Reinvestment

Although many people complete the work of mourning with the informal support of families and friends, many find that talking with others who have had a similar experience, such as in formal support groups, normalizes the feelings and experiences and provides a framework for learning new skills to cope with the loss and create a new life. Hospitals, hospices, religious organizations, and other community organizations often sponsor bereavement support groups. When a person dies while enrolled in hospice, families receive proactive bereavement from the hospice agency for an average of 13 months after the death. Hospice bereavement programs vary, yet bereavement support usually starts with scheduled calls to deceased primary contact. Bereavement may then be set up as individual counseling or group sessions, such as widow or parents support groups. Hospices may offer specialized child bereavement support services. Bereavement staff may consist of specially trained nurses, child psychologists, counselors, child life specialists, and/or music or art therapists. If a person dies and is not enrolled in hospice, some palliative care teams offer bereavement or help to connect families with a hospice for bereavement resources. When one cancer center implemented a bereavement program, surveyed bereaved family members felt that acknowledgment of their loved one through a formal condolence letter had a positive impact (Morris & Block, 2015).

Complicated Grief and Mourning

Complicated grief and mourning are characterized by prolonged feelings of sadness and feelings of general worthlessness or hopelessness that persist long after the death, prolonged symptoms (depression, anxiety, insomnia, fatigue) that interfere with activities of daily living, or self-destructive behaviors such as alcohol or substance abuse and suicidal ideation or attempts (Mason & Duffy, 2019). Certain risk factors that increase the likelihood of complicated grief include death of a child or spouse, multiple losses, and history of trauma (Tofthagen, Kip, Witt, et al., 2017). Complicated grief and mourning require professional assessment and can be treated with psychological interventions and, in some cases, with medications.

Special Issues for the Nurse in End-of-Life Care

Nursing care often intersects with moral and ethical dilemmas (see Chapter 1 for further discussion of ethics). Nurses are encouraged to personally examine their respective moral compasses in order to provide the best, unbiased care for patients and families. In caring for patients at the end-of-life, questions of *right* and *wrong* may arise in relation to treatment options. The ANA's *Code of Ethics for Nurses* provides a framework for the nurse to support patients, with guiding principles being the patient's right to self-determination and the nurse's adherence to professional nursing standards (ANA, 2015). When approaching an ethical dilemma, the nurse should take the following steps: define the problem, clarify facts and assumptions, compile a list of all options, evaluate options with interdisciplinary team input, and choose the most appropriate option and implement the plan (Prince-Paul & Daly, 2019). The most common ethical dilemmas a nurse will encounter are determining decisional capacity, withholding or withdrawing life-prolonging measures—including, but not limited to, ventilator support, dialysis, artificial nutrition and hydration—requests for hastening death, and concerns related to proxy decision making. Select ethical issues are discussed in greater detail in the following sections.

Medically Administered Nutrition and Hydration

Although nutritional supplementation may be an important part of the treatment plan in early or chronic illness, unintended weight loss and dehydration are expected characteristics of progressive illness. As illness progresses, patients, families, and clinicians may believe that without artificial nutrition and hydration, patients who are terminally ill will *starve*, causing profound suffering and hastened death. The use of artificial nutrition and hydration (tube and intravenous fluids and feeding) carries considerable risks and generally does not contribute to comfort at the end-of-life (Casarett, Kapo, & Kaplan, 2005; Marcolini, Putnam, & Aydin, 2018). Similarly, survival is not increased when patients who are terminally ill with advanced dementia receive enteral feeding, and no data support an association between tube feeding and improved quality of life in these patients (De & Thomas, 2019). Furthermore, in patients who are close to death, symptoms associated with dehydration such as dry mouth, confusion, and diminished alertness are common and typically do not respond to artificial nutrition and hydration (Danis, Arnold, & Savarese, 2018). Dry mouth can generally be managed through nursing measures such as mouth care, and environmental changes with medications can help to diminish confusion.

Palliative Sedation at the End-of-Life

Effective control of symptoms can be achieved under most conditions; however, some patients may experience distressing, intractable symptoms. Although **palliative sedation** remains controversial, it is offered in some settings to patients who are close to death or who have symptoms that do not respond to conventional pharmacologic and nonpharmacologic approaches, resulting in unrelieved suffering. Palliative sedation is distinguished from euthanasia and physician-assisted suicide (PAS) in that the intent of palliative sedation is to relieve symptoms, not to hasten death (see Chart 13-9). Proportionate palliative sedation uses the minimum drug necessary to relieve the symptom while preserving consciousness, whereas palliative sedation induces unconsciousness, which is more controversial (Quill, Lo, Brock, et al., 2009). Palliative sedation is most commonly used when the patient exhibits intractable pain, dyspnea, seizures, or delirium, and it is generally considered appropriate in only the most difficult situations. Palliative sedation is accomplished through an infusion of one or more pharmacologic agents in doses adequate to eliminate signs of discomfort. Before implementing palliative sedation, the health care team should assess for the presence of underlying and treatable causes of suffering, such as depression or spiritual distress. Finally, the patient and the family should be fully informed about the use of this treatment and alternatives. A retrospective study of Italian hospice patients reported that palliative sedation was documented as discussed in only half of the cases where it was implemented (Ingravallo, de Nooijer, Pucci, et al., 2018).

Published guidelines for pharmacologic management of palliative sedation vary widely internationally (Abarshi, Rietjens, Robijn, et al., 2017) but most mention the use of midazolam, a short-acting benzodiazepine (Lux, Protus, Kimbrel, et al., 2017). Nurses act as collaborating members of the interdisciplinary health care team, providing emotional support to patients and families, facilitating clarification of values and preferences, and providing comfort-focused physical care. Once sedation has been induced, the nurse should continue to comfort the patient, monitor the physiologic effects of the sedation, support the family during the final hours or days of their loved one's life, and ensure communication within the health care team and between the team and the family.

Requests for Assistance in Dying

A major debate in palliative and end-of-life care is the acceptability of a patient's requests to hasten death. Health care recognizes the right to choose for or against medical treatments when a patient is of sound mind and can relay a rationale for or against treatments. Further, patients may choose to withdraw or withhold life-sustaining treatments and allow natural death if such therapies are not aligned with their wishes. When faced with a progressive life-limiting illness, some cannot fathom suffering at the end-of-life and explore options to hasten death. Language around assistance in dying has

Chart 13-9 ETHICAL DILEMMA
Does Intent Matter When Palliative Care Leads to Death?

Case Scenario

You are a staff nurse working for an outpatient home hospice service. G.R. is a 68-year-old man admitted to home hospice service two months ago with advanced multiple myeloma. As a consequence of his disease he also has extensive destruction of bony matrix resulting in widespread pain, numerous vertebral fractures, and spinal cord compression. For the first six weeks that G.R. was managed in hospice, you and the hospice staff have successfully kept his pain and other symptoms under reasonable control. However, over the past two weeks his pain has been more difficult to control, despite escalating dosages of opioids. He has not been able to sleep, and is restless, dyspneic, and anxious. The hospice physician was consulted, and G.R. and his husband agreed to intravenous opioids, sedatives, and anxiolytics to relieve G.R.'s suffering, knowing that he would also lose consciousness as a consequence of this treatment. However, they stated that though they were not pleased that G.R. would never regain consciousness, that result was offset by their hope was the G.R. might die peacefully. You administer the prescribed intravenous medications, and slowly administer the minimum dosages of these medications to relieve symptoms. G.R. loses consciousness and dies peacefully 48 hours later with his husband holding his hand at his bedside.

Discussion

There is a great deal of apprehension among both clinicians and laypersons around what constitutes comfort care (i.e., palliative care) at end-of-life and what may constitute either assisted suicide or euthanasia. The premise is that palliative care should ameliorate pain and suffering in the patient who is terminally ill, but it should not significantly shorten the patient's life.

The principle of double-effect highlights that some actions have two effects - one good, the other evil. The good and evil consequences are not considered in terms of proportions; if they were, and the evil outcome is death, then the good outcome could never be considered sufficient to justify the action. Rather, the intention behind the action is given paramount consideration. If the intention is to cause death, then the act is not morally justifiable. However, if the intention is to relieve suffering, then the act might be sanctioned.

Analysis

- Describe how the ethical principles of autonomy, beneficence, and nonmaleficence may intersect or be at odds with each other in this case. Discuss how palliative sedation meets the moral justification of the four criteria for the principle of double effect (see Chapter 1, Chart 1-7).
- Would you describe your role in this case as complicit in assisted suicide, euthanasia, or providing palliation? What distinction, if any, might there be among these three acts?
- Note that the ANA (2015) *Code of Ethics* clearly states that nurses should not *intentionally* cause a patient's death. What were your "intentions" in this case? How might intentionality be instrumental in making this act of titrating medications that provided palliation morally defensible? Are there resources you could identify that might be of assistance to you if you were to feel moral distress about your actions?

References

American Nurses Association (ANA). (2015). *Code of ethics for nurses with interpretive statements*. Silver Spring, MD: Author.

Rodrigues, P., Crokaert, J., & Gastmans, C. (2018). Palliative sedation for existential suffering: A systematic review of argument-based ethics literature. *Journal of Pain and Symptom Management, 55*(6), 1577–1590.

Wholihan, D. & Olson, E. (2017). The doctrine of double effect: A review for the bedside nurse providing end-of-life care. *Journal of Hospice and Palliative Nursing, 19*(3), 205–211.

Resources

See Chapter 1, Chart 1-10 for Steps of an Ethical Analysis and Ethics Resources.

---

evolved over the years and it is important to recognize the following terms:

- *Physician aid in dying (PAD), medical aid in dying (MAD), and physician-assisted dying:* A physician prescribes a lethal dose of oral medication that the patient self-administers, for the purpose of ending someone's life.
- *PAS:* A physician prescribes medications, that the patient self-administers, to end their life at the person's voluntary and competent request.
- *Euthanasia:* Greek for "good death"; has evolved to mean the intentional killing by act or omission of a dependent human being for their alleged benefit.

Although assisted suicide is expressly prohibited under statutory or common law in the majority of states, calls for legalized aid in dying have highlighted inadequacies in end-of-life care. In 1994, Oregon voters approved the Oregon Death with Dignity Act, the first and—until 2009 only such legislative initiative to pass. This law provides for access to PAS by terminally ill patients under very controlled circumstances. After numerous challenges, the law was enacted in 1997. Of 2127 Oregonians who have received written prescriptions under the terms of the law since it was passed in 1997, 1459 have self-administered physician-prescribed lethal medication and have died (Oregon Public Health Division, 2018).

In recent years, additional states have adopted MAD laws, and Montana's Supreme Court has ruled that PAD is not a crime. International MAD is legal in Canada, the Netherlands, Belgium, Luxembourg, Switzerland, Columbia, and Victoria in Australia. Proponents of PAS argue that people who are terminally ill should have a legally sanctioned right to make independent decisions about the value of their lives and the timing and circumstances of their deaths, and its opponents argue for greater access to symptom management and psychosocial support for people approaching the end-of-life.

In its 2013 position statement on *Euthanasia, Assisted Suicide, and Aid in Dying*, the ANA acknowledged the complexity of the assisted suicide debate but clearly stated that nursing participation in assisted suicide is a violation of the Code for Nurses. The ANA position statement further stressed the important role of the nurse in supporting effective symptom management, contributing to the creation of environments for care that honor the patient's and family's wishes, as well as identifying their concerns and fears (ANA, 2013). Per the ANA, "Nurses have an obligation to provide humane, comprehensive, and compassionate care that respects the rights of patients but upholds the standards of the profession in the presence of chronic, debilitating illness and at end-of-life" (ANA, 2013, p. 1).

Similarly, the HPNA favors the value of comprehensive end-of-life care, as opposed to physician-assisted death (HPNA, 2017). The HPNA acknowledges that nurses may care for patients exploring or choosing physician-assisted death and thus concludes that nurses must be able to provide unbiased education yet not take an active role in this end-of-life option. American Academy of Hospice and Palliative Medicine (AAHPM, 2016) has taken a position of "studied neutrality" on assisted death, recommending that clinicians carefully assess the fear and suffering that have led patients to request assisted suicide and to address these without hastening death.

The International Association for Hospice and Palliative Care (IAHPC) released a position statement on euthanasia and PAS, in which they recommend access to palliative care and medication, such as opioids, prior to the legalization of both euthanasia and/or PAS. Further, they recommend that these acts should not be carried out on palliative care units (De Lima, Woodruff, Pettus, et al., 2017).

Voluntary Stopping of Eating and Drinking

Another potential, however quite controversial, option of last resort is voluntary stopping of eating and drinking (VSED) when a person cannot imagine prolonged dying and suffering for a life-limiting illness. Patient inquiry about VSED should be met with thorough assessment of both decisional capacity and presence of mental illness (Quill, Ganzini, Troug, et al., 2018; Wax, An, Koiser, et al., 2018). Aggressive palliative treatments for all types of suffering—physical, psychological, social, spiritual, and existential—should be explored and offered before pursing VSED. Typically, a person will die 10 to 14 days after starting VSED during which the most distressing symptoms include thirst and delirium (Quill et al., 2018; Wax et al., 2018). Given this expected prognosis, patients may have the opportunity to complete legacy work prior to initiating VSED.

The ANA included VSED in a 2017 position statement on *Nutrition and Hydration at the End of Life* in which the organization upholds respect for autonomy, relief of suffering, and expert care at the end of life. Nurses involved in the care of a patient who self-initiates VSED should support the family while providing expert symptom assessment and management. One example of a patient who may choose to pursue VSED is a patient who has been diagnosed with a progressive disease, such as ALS, and who finds a slow decline intolerable.

COVID-19 Considerations

The coronavirus disease 2019 (COVID-19) pandemic has altered the delivery of palliative and end-of-life care. Patients with severe COVID-19 pneumonia are managed with endotracheal intubation and mechanical ventilation and have a high case fatality rate (see Chapter 19) (Bajwah, Wilcock, Towers, et al., 2020; Richardson, Hirsch, Narasimhan, et al., 2020). Common end-of-life symptoms for those with severe COVID-19 include dyspnea, cough, anxiety, and delirium (Bajwah et al., 2020). During the pandemic, symptom management at the end-of-life has required revisions due to logistical challenges such as medication shortages and preservation of personal protective equipment (Chidiac, Feuer, Naismith, et al., 2020). Due to high risk of infectious transmission, family members may not be permitted to see loved ones at the end-of-life (Richardson et al., 2020; Wakam, Montgomery, Biesterveld, et al., 2020). Furthermore, family meetings are primarily virtual, where proxies must make difficult decisions such as resuscitation and intubation, and even removal of life support (Richardson et al., 2020). Communication guides for proactive goals of care discussions related to possible COVID-19 infection (Back, Tulsky, & Arnold, 2020), recommendations for "webside" manner (Chua, Jackson, & Kamdar, 2020), innovative use of virtual reality to stimulate previously unachieved dreams or allow families to virtually share one last moment together (Wang, Teo, Teo, et al., 2020). Meanwhile, health care providers are struggling from high physical workload demands while simultaneously experiencing moral and psychological distress (Adams & Walls, 2020). Clinicians working with patients with COVID-19 voice concerns about the risk of infecting self and family and stress due to constant change as health care systems evolve to meet patient needs during a pandemic situation (Foxwell, 2020). Health systems have developed innovative processes to support staff at the front lines of working with patients with COVID-19 and at end-of-life, such as a 24-hour hotlines and pet therapy.

Clinicians' Attitudes toward Death

Clinicians' attitudes toward the terminally ill and dying remain the greatest barrier to improving care at the end-of-life. Kübler-Ross illuminated the concerns of the seriously ill and dying in her seminal work, *On Death and Dying,* first published in 1969. At that time, it was common for patients to be kept uninformed about life-threatening diagnoses, particularly cancer, and for primary providers and nurses to avoid open discussion of death and dying with their patients. Kübler-Ross's work revealed that, given open discussion, adequate time, and some help in working through the process, patients could reach a stage of acceptance in which they were neither angry nor depressed about their fate.

The growth of palliative and hospice care programs has led to greater numbers of health care providers becoming comfortable with and skilled in assessing patients' and families' information needs and disclosing honest information about the seriousness of illness (Brighton & Bristowe, 2016). However, in many settings, clinicians still avoid the topic of death in the hope that patients will ask or find out on their own. Despite progress on many health care fronts, many who work with patients who are seriously ill and dying recognize a persistent conspiracy of silence about dying.

How to communicate truthfully with patients and encourage patient **autonomy** (the right of the person to make choices) in a way that acknowledges where they are on the continuum of acceptance is a challenge. Despite continued reluctance of health care providers to engage in open discussion about end-of-life issues, patients want information about their illness and end-of-life choices and are not harmed by open discussion about death (Hamel, Wu, & Brodie, 2017; The Conversation Project National Survey, 2018). Timing of sensitive discussion takes experience, but speaking the truth can be a relief to patients and families, enhancing their autonomy by making way for truly informed consent as the basis for decision making.

Patient and Family Concerns

Terminal illness is experienced uniquely by each person and their loved ones. Family members are key stakeholders in honoring patients' wishes, caring for patients, and engaging in care planning. Family members are impacted by a loved one's illness and require support throughout the course of caregiving. Recognizing maladaptive coping in family members and providing resources for the family whether through social work staff or palliative care specialists is key to preventing worsening distress at the time of death. Palliative care interventions have been reported to improve communication, improve person-centeredness and decrease length of ICU stay without significantly impacting caregiver psychological distress (White, Angus, Shields, et al., 2018).

Patient and family awareness of **prognosis** is a key factor in acceptance of and planning for death. For patients who have been informed about terminal illness, their understanding of treatment goals and prognosis is dynamic and may sometimes require reinforcement. Even when patients have been told that the intent of a therapy is palliative, they may think *I'll be the one to beat the odds*. As many as 37% of patients with metastatic cancer receiving palliative therapies misperceive their cancer as potentially curable (Yennurajalingam, Lu, Prado, et al., 2018). Just as patients and families may have differing perspectives on prognosis, they may also have different perceptions of severity of symptoms. Family caregivers tend to report distress and quality of life as worse than patient reports at the end-of-life (Hack, McClement, Chochinov, et al., 2018). This may be due to the family member's distress or anticipatory grief.

Historically, the approach in the United States to serious illness has been described as *death denying*—that is, the health care system has been built on management of acute illness and the use of technology to cure (when possible) and to extend life. As a result, life-threatening illness, life-sustaining treatment decisions, dying, and death occur in a social environment in which illness is largely considered an enemy. Many common expressions reflect this dominant sociocultural view. For example, people talk about the *war* against cancer or *fighting* illness, and when patients choose not to pursue the most aggressive course of medical treatment available, many health care providers and indeed patients and families perceive this as *giving up*. A care/cure dichotomy has persisted in which health care providers may view cure as the ultimate good and care as second best, a good only when cure is no longer possible. In such a model, alleviating suffering is not as valued as curing disease. Patients who cannot be cured feel distanced from the health care team, and when curative treatments have failed, they may feel that they too have failed. Patients and families may fear that any shift from curative goals to comfort-focused care will result in no care or lower-quality care, and that the clinicians on whom they have come to rely will abandon them if they withdraw from a focus on cure.

The statement in late-stage illness that exemplifies this care versus cure dichotomy is *nothing more can be done*. This all-too-frequently used statement communicates the belief of many clinicians that there is nothing of value to offer patients beyond cure; however, in a care-focused perspective, there is always more that can be done. This expanded notion of healing implies that healing can take place throughout life. There are many opportunities for physical, spiritual, emotional, and social healing, even as body systems begin to fail at the end-of-life.

TABLE 13-8	Select Resiliency Skills
Individual Skills	**System Level Opportunities**
• Assessing personal strengths • Recognizing clinical emotional triggers • Applying mindfulness skills at work • Establishing health boundaries and reasonable expectations • Finding meaning in daily work • Continuing to adapt and cultivate resiliency skills	• Supporting autonomy • Structuring rewards • Promoting collaboration among peers and other disciplines • Establishing fairness in the workplace • Acknowledging that patient-centered care takes time to explore patient's individual values • Allowing flexibility

Adapted from Back, A. L., Stienhauser, K. E., Kamal, A. H., et al. (2017). Why burnout is so hard to fix. *Journal of Oncology Practice, 13*(6), 348–351.

Professional Caregiver Issues

Issues of importance to professional caregivers include burnout, promoting resiliency, and nurses supporting themselves.

Burnout and Promoting Resiliency

Burnout is defined as the triad of emotional exhaustion, cynicism, and ineffectiveness at work. By the time one notices burnout it is usually too late. In order to prevent burnout, there is a body of work to promote resilience, thereby providing clinicians with the skills needed to have work–life balance and the opportunity to remain productive and satisfied with their career (Back, Steinhauser, Kamal, et al., 2017). See Table 13-8 for select resiliency skills and workplace factors to prevent burnout.

While the prevalence of burnout among nurses working in palliative care and hospice is unknown, researchers have attempted to assess the prevalence of burnout among all clinicians working in palliative care. One study found that physicians were more likely to exhibit signs of burnout; however, factors for both physicians and clinicians from other disciplines (advanced practice provider, nurse, chaplain, social worker) that contributed to burnout are younger age, working weekends or overtime, and feeling isolated (Kamal, Bull, Wolf, et al., 2020). Overall, hospice and palliative clinicians were found to have a burnout rate of approximately 39% (Kamal et al., 2020).

The ANA (2017a) published *A Call to Action: Exploring Moral Resilience toward a Culture of Ethical Practice*, which highlights potential for burnout among nurses and makes recommendations for both individuals and institutions to foster resilience, as well as recommendations for research. This document also contains a toolkit for resources for the nurse and proposed actions.

Supporting Ourselves

In addition to healthy work environments that promote resiliency, nurses are often encouraged to develop self-care practices. Self-care can be any number of activities or practices that a person maintains while not at work; examples include practicing yoga or meditation, engaging in hobbies, or simply not checking email when away from work. A recent qualitative study found palliative care clinicians (primary providers and nurses) seek practices that promote well-being and allow restoration of self so as to better care for patients (Mills,

Wand, & Fraser, 2018). The palliative care clinicians sought meaning through work–life balance and building relationships; they sought self-care during work (such as establishing boundaries, negotiating workload, and reflecting on practice) and outside of work (such as meditation, rest, separating self from work, and positive social relationships) (Mills et al., 2018).

Whether practicing in a trauma center, ICU, or other acute care setting, home care, hospice, long-term care, or the many locations where patients and their families receive ambulatory services, nurses are closely involved with complex and emotionally laden issues surrounding loss of life. To be most effective and satisfied with the care they provide, nurses should attend to their own emotional responses to the losses witnessed every day. In hospice settings, where death, grief, and loss are expected outcomes of patient care, interdisciplinary colleagues rely on one another for support by learning coping skills from one another and speaking about how they were affected by the lives of those patients who have died. In many settings, staff members organize periodic memorial services to support bereaved families and other caregivers, who find comfort in joining one another to remember and celebrate the lives of patients.

CRITICAL THINKING EXERCISES

1 **ipc** Your patient is a 60-year-old woman with lung cancer who is hospitalized with increasing shortness of breath. She is currently receiving second-line chemotherapy treatment and recently completed palliative radiation to rib metastases. She lives with her husband and has two adult children who live out of state. As you are administering her morning medications, she asks, "Why did God do this to me? What did I do to deserve this?" How will you facilitate an interprofessional discussion to address the patient's spiritual concerns? What members of the interdisciplinary team are essential to include?

2 **ebp** Your patient is a 52-year-old man with idiopathic pulmonary fibrosis who is being evaluated for a lung transplant. He arrives at the lung transplant clinic with his friend from work. He is a security guard, but has been calling out frequently as he can't make hourly rounds. He lives alone in a two-story home with one bathroom on the second floor. Due to dyspnea on exertion, he has not been able to go upstairs and now sleeps on a recliner and hasn't showered in weeks. He has an estranged daughter whom he has not spoken to in over 10 years. Dyspnea also interferes with his appetite and he has been drinking sports drinks and eats fast food when his friends bring it over. How would you complete an evidence-based symptom assessment? What interventions would you consider to treat his dyspnea based on the evidence?

3 **pq** You are a new hospice nurse in your third month making home hospice visits. Your patient is a 73-year-old woman who has had multiple strokes. She previously expressed to her family that she would not want to live on prolonged life support. She has four devoted children who have set up a schedule so that someone will be with her 24 hours a day. When you enter the room, the patient is somnolent with periods of apnea. Her daughter at the bedside tells you that her mother was screaming out last night, calling for her parents and trying to get out of bed. The daughter feels that her mother is more comfortable now. She is intermittently tearful as she talks with you. At one point she asks, "Do you think she's angry with us? That must be why she was agitated last night. . . . I knew I shouldn't have listened to my siblings—My mom wants to live!" What stage of dying is this patient experiencing? How would you educate the daughter about stages of dying? How would you assess for bereavement needs?

REFERENCES

*Asterisk indicates nursing research.
**Double asterisk indicates classic reference.

Books

American Nurses Association (ANA). (2015). *Nursing scope and standards of practice* (3rd ed.). Silver Spring, MD: Author.

American Nurses Association (ANA). (2015). *Code of ethics for nurses with interpretive statements.* Silver Spring, MD: Author.

Back, A., Arnold, R., & Tulsky, J. (2009). *Mastering communication with seriously ill patients: Balancing empathy and hope.* New York: Cambridge University Press.

Berry, P., & Griffie, J. (2019). Planning for the actual death. In B. R. Ferrell, N. Coyle, & J. Paice (Eds.). *Oxford textbook of palliative nursing* (5th ed.). New York: Oxford.

Cormack, C., Mazanec, P., & Panke, J. T. (2019). Cultural considerations in palliative care. In B. R. Ferrell, N. Coyle, & J. Paice (Eds.). *Oxford textbook of palliative nursing* (5th ed.). New York: Oxford.

**Glaser, B. G., & Strauss, A. (1965). *Awareness of dying.* Chicago, IL: Aldine.

**Kübler-Ross, E. (1969). *On death and dying.* New York: Macmillan.

National Hospice and Palliative Care Organization (NHPCO). (2018). *NHPCO facts and figures: Hospice care in America.* Alexandria, VA: Author.

Prince-Paul, M., & Daly, B. J. (2019). Ethical consideration in palliative care. In B. R. Ferrell, N. Coyle, & J. Paice (Eds.). *Oxford textbook of palliative nursing* (5th ed.). New York: Oxford.

**Rando, T. A. (2000). Promoting healthy anticipatory mourning in intimates of the life-threatened or dying person. In T. A. Rando (Ed.). *Clinical dimensions of anticipatory mourning.* Champaign, IL: Research Press.

Schack, E. E., & Wholihan, D. (2019). Anorexia and cachexia. In B. R. Ferrell, N. Coyle, & J. Paice (Eds.). *Oxford textbook of palliative nursing* (5th ed.). New York: Oxford.

Taylor, E. J. (2019). Spiritual screening, history, and assessment. In B. R. Ferrell, N. Coyle, & J. Paice (Eds.). *Oxford textbook of palliative nursing* (5th ed.). New York: Oxford.

Wittenberg-Lyles, E., Goldsmith, J., Ferrell, B. R., et al. (2013). *Communication in palliative nursing.* New York: Oxford.

Journals and Electronic Documents

Abarshi, E., Rietjens, J., Robijn, L., et al. (2017). International variations in clinical practice guidelines for palliative sedation: A systematic review. *BMJ Supportive & Palliative Care, 7*(3), 223–229.

Adams, J. G., & Walls, R. M. (2020). Supporting the health care workforce during the COVID-19 global epidemic. *JAMA, 323,* 1439–1440.

American Academy of Hospice and Palliative Medicine (AAHPM). (2016). Position statements: Physician-assisted dying. Retrieved on 6/25/2019 at: www.aahpm.org/positions/default/suicide.html

**American Nurses Association (ANA). (2010). Position statement: Registered nurses' roles and responsibilities in providing expert care and counseling at the end of life. Retrieved on 6/21/2019 at: www.nursingworld.org/~4af078/globalassets/docs/ana/ethics/endoflife-positionstatement.pdf

American Nurses Association (ANA). (2013). Position statement: Euthanasia, assisted suicide, and aid in dying. Retrieved on 6/27/2019 at: www.nursingworld.org/~4af287/globalassets/docs/ana/ethics/euthanasia-assisted-suicideaid-in-dying_ps042513.pdf

American Nurses Association (ANA). (2017a). Call for action: Nurses lead and transform palliative care. Retrieved on 6/20/19 at: www.nursingworld.org/~497158/globalassets/practiceandpolicy/health-policy/palliativecareprofessionalissuespanelcallforaction.pdf

American Nurses Association (ANA). (2017b). A call to action: Exploring moral resilience toward a culture of ethical practice. Retrieved on 6/26/2019 at: www.nursingworld.org/~4907b6/globalassets/docs/ana/ana-call-to-action–exploring-moral-resilience-final.pdf

Back, A. L., Fromme, E. K., & Meier, D. E. (2019). Training clinicians with communication skills needed to match medical treatments to patient values. *Journal of the American Geriatrics Society, 67*(S2), S441.

Back, A. L., Steinhauser, K. E., Kamal, A. H., et al. (2017). Why burnout is so hard to fix. *Journal of Oncology Practice, 13*(6), 348–351.

Back, A., Tulsky, J. A., & Arnold, R. M. (2020). Communication skills in the age of COVID-19. *Annals of Internal Medicine, 172*(11), 759–760.

Bajwah, S., Wilcock, A., Towers, R., et al. (2020). Managing the supportive care needs of those affected by COVID-19. *European Respiratory Journal, 55*(4), 2000815.

Balboni, T. A., Fitchett, G., Handzo, G. F., et al. (2017). State of the Science of Spirituality and Palliative Care Research Part II: Screening, assessment, and interventions. *Journal of Pain & Symptom Management, 54*(3), 441–453.

*Birkholz, L., & Haney, T. (2018). Using a dyspnea assessment tool to improve care at the end of life. *Journal of Hospice and Palliative Nursing, 20*(3), 219–227.

Bischoff, K., O'Riordan, D. L., Marks, A. K., et al. (2017). Care planning for inpatients referred for palliative care consultation. *JAMA Internal Medicine, 178*(1), 48–54.

Brighton, L. J., & Bristowe, K. (2016). Communication in palliative care: Talking about the end of life, before the end of life. *Postgraduate Medicine Journal, 92*(1090), 466–470.

Bush, S. H., Tierney, S., & Lawlor, P. G. (2017). Clinical assessment and management of delirium in the palliative care setting. *Drugs, 77*(15), 1623–1643.

**Casarett, D. J., Kapo, J., & Kaplan, A. (2005). Appropriate use of artificial nutrition and hydration—fundamental principles and recommendations. *New England Journal of Medicine, 353*(24), 2607–2612.

Centers for Disease Control and Prevention (CDC). (2016). CDC Guideline for prescribing opioids for chronic pain—United States, 2016. Centers for Disease Control and Prevention Morbidity and Mortality Weekly Report. Retrieved on 3/28/2019 at: www.cdc.gov/mmwr/volumes/65/rr/rr6501e1.htm

Centers for Medicare & Medicaid Services (CMS). (2018). Evaluation of the Medicare care choices model: Annual report #1. Retrieved on 6/30/2019 at: www.innovation.cms.gov/Files/reports/mccm-firstannrpt.pdf

Centers for Medicare & Medicaid Services (CMS). (2019). Hospice. Retrieved on 6/24/2019 at: www.cms.gov/Medicare/Medicare-Fee-for-Service-Payment/Hospice/index.html

Chidiac, C., Feuer, D., Naismith, J., et al. (2020). Emergency palliative care planning and support in a COVID-19 pandemic. *Journal of Palliative Medicine, 23*, 752–753.

Chua, I. S., Jackson, V., & Kamdar, M. (2020). Webside manner during the COVID-19 pandemic: Maintaining human connection during virtual visits. *Journal of Palliative Medicine.* doi: 10.1089/jpm.2020.0298

Compton-Phillips, A., & Mohta, N. S. (2019). Care redesign survey: The power of palliative care. *NEJM Catalyst.* Retrieved on 6/27/2019 at: www.catalyst.nejm.org/power-palliative-end-of-life-care-program

Coyne, P., Mulvenon, C., & Paice, J. A. (2018). American Society for Pain Management Nursing and Hospice and Palliative Nurses Association position statement: Pain management at the end of life. *Pain Management Nursing, 19*(1), 3–7.

Danis, R., Arnold, R. M., & Savarese, D. M. F. (2018). Stopping artificial nutrition and hydration at the end of life.

Retrieved on 6/27/2019 at: www.uptodate.com/contents/stopping-nutrition-and-hydration-at-the-end-of-life#topicContent

De, D., & Thomas, C. (2019). Enhancing the decision-making process when considering artificial nutrition in advanced dementia care. *International Journal of Palliative Nursing, 25*(5), 216–223.

De Lima, L. D., Woodruff, R., Pettus, K., et al. (2017). International Association for Hospice and Palliative Care position statement: Euthanasia and physician-assisted suicide. *Journal of Palliative Medicine, 20*(1), 8–14.

Dowell, D., Haegerich, T., & Chou, R. (2019). No shortcuts to safer opioid prescribing. *New England Journal of Medicine, 380*(24), 2285–2287.

Dumanovsky, T., Augustin, R., Rogers, M., et al. (2016). The growth of palliative care in U.S. hospitals: A status report. *Journal of Palliative Medicine, 19*(1), 8–15.

El-Jawahri, A., LeBlanc, T., VanDusen, H., et al. (2016). Effect of inpatient palliative care on quality of life 2 weeks after hematopoietic stem cell transplantation: A randomized clinical trial. *JAMA, 316*(20), 2094–2103.

Enclara Pharmacia, Inc. (2015). *Enclara Pharmacia medication use guidelines* (1st ed.). Philadelphia, PA: Author.

Ferrell, B., Malloy, P., Mazanec, P., et al. (2016). CARES: AACN's new competencies and recommendations for educating undergraduate nursing students to improve palliative care. *Journal of Professional Nursing, 32*(5), 327–333.

Ferrell, B. R., Twaddle, M. L., Melnick, A., et al. (2018). National consensus project clinical practice guidelines for quality palliative care guidelines, 4th edition. *Journal of Palliative Medicine, 21*(12), 1684–1689.

Finlay, E., Newport, K., Sivendran, S., et al. (2018). Models of outpatient palliative care clinics for patients with cancer. *Journal of Oncology Practice, 15*(4), 187–193.

Foxwell, A. M. (2020). On the coronavirus front lines: Part-time nurse, full-time worry | Expert Opinion. *The Philadelphia Inquirer.* Retrieved on 7/15/2020 at: www.inquirer.com/health/coronavirus/coronavirus-covid19-frontline-nurse-practitioner-20200417.html

Foxwell, A. M., Uritsky, T., & Meghani, S. H. (2019). Opioids and cancer pain management in the United States: Public policy and legal challenges. *Seminars in Oncology Nursing, 35*(3), 322–326.

Hack, T. F., McClement, S. E., Chochinov, H. M., et al. (2018). Assessing symptoms, concerns, and quality of life in noncancer patients at end of life: How concordant are patients and family proxy members? *Journal of Pain and Symptom Management, 56*(5), 760–766.

Hamel, L., Wu, B., & Brodie, M. (2017). Views and experiences with end-of-life medical care in Japan, Italy, the United States, and Brazil: A cross-country survey. *The Henry J. Kaiser Family Foundation Report.* Retrieved on 9/12/2019 at: www.kff.org

*Higgins, A., & Hynes, G. (2019). Meeting the needs of people who identify as lesbian, gay, bisexual, transgender, and queer in palliative care. *Journal of Hospice and Palliative Nursing, 21*(4), 286–290.

Hospice and Palliative Nurses Association (HPNA). (2017). HPNA position statement: Physician-assisted death/physician assisted suicide. Retrieved on 6/22/2019 at: www.file:///Users/anessa/Downloads/Physician%20Assisted%20Death%20Physician%20Assisted%20Suicide.pdf

Hui, D., Arthur, J., & Bruera, E. (2019). Palliative care for patients with opioid misuse. *JAMA, 321*(5), 511.

Hui, D., Frisbee-Hume, S., Wilson, A., et al. (2017). Effect of lorazepam with haloperidol vs haloperidol alone on agitated delirium in patients with advanced cancer receiving palliative care: A randomized clinical trial. *JAMA, 318*(11), 1047–1056.

Hui, D., Park, M., Liu, D., et al. (2016). Clinician prediction of survival versus the palliative prognostic score: Which approach is more accurate? *European Journal of Cancer, 64*, 89–95.

Ingravallo, F., de Nooijer, K., Pucci, V., et al. (2018). Discussions about palliative sedation in hospice: Frequency, timing and factors associated with patient involvement. *European Journal of Cancer Care, 28*(3), e13019.

**Institute of Medicine (IOM). (2014). Dying in America: Improving quality and honoring individual preferences near the end of life. Retrieved on 6/13/2019 at: www.nationalacademies.org/hmd/Reports/2014/Dying-In-America-Improving-Quality-and-Honoring-Individual-Preferences-Near-the-End-of-Life.aspx

Izumi, S. (2017). Advance care planning: The nurse's role. *The American Journal of Nursing, 117*(6), 56–61.

Kamal, A. H., Bull, J. H., Wolf, S. P., et al. (2020). Prevalence and predictors of burnout among hospice and Palliative Care clinicians in the U.S. *Journal of Pain and Symptom Management, 59*(5), e6–e13.

Kamal, A. H., Wolf, S. P., Troy, J., et al. (2019). Policy changes key to promoting sustainability and growth of the specialty palliative care workforce. *Health Affairs, 38*(6), 910–918.

Kozlov, E., Phongtankuel, V., Prigerson, H., et al. (2019). Prevalence, severity, and correlates of symptoms of anxiety and depression at the very end of life. *Journal of Pain and Symptom Management, 58*(1), 80–85.

*Lasater, K. B., Sloane, D. M., McHugh, M. D., et al. (2019). Quality of end-of-life care and its association with nurse practice environments in U.S. hospitals. *Journal of the American Geriatrics Society, 67*(2), 302–308.

Lux, M. R., Protus, B. M., Kimbrel, J., et al. (2017). A survey of hospice and palliative care physicians regarding palliative sedation practices. *American Journal of Hospice and Palliative Medicine, 34*(3), 217–222.

Marcolini, E. G., Putnam, A. T., & Aydin, A. (2019). History and perspectives on nutrition and hydration at the end of life. *Journal of Biology and Medicine, 91*(2), 173–176.

Mason, T. M., & Duffy, A. R. (2019). Complicated grief and cortisol response: An integrative review of the literature. *Journal of the American Psychiatric Nurses Association, 25*(3), 181–188.

**Meghani, S. H. (2004). A concept analysis of palliative care in the United States. *Journal of Advanced Nursing, 46*(2), 152–161.

*Meghani, S. H., & Vapiwala, N. (2018). Building the critical divide in pain management guidelines from the CDC, NCCN, and ASCO for cancer survivors. *JAMA Oncology, 4*(10), 1323–1324.

Mills, J., Wand, T., & Fraser, J. A. (2018). Exploring the meaning and practice of self-care among palliative care nurses and doctors: A qualitative study. *BMC Palliative Care, 17*(63), 1–12.

Mor, V., Joyce, N. R., Cote, D. L., et al. (2016). The rise of concurrent care for veterans with advanced cancer at the end of life. *Cancer, 122*(5), 782–790.

Morris, S. E., & Block, S. D. (2015). Adding value to palliative care services: The development of an institutional bereavement program. *Journal of Palliative Medicine, 18*(11), 655–662.

Morrison, S. R. (2013). Models of palliative care delivery in the United States. *Current Opinion Supportive and Palliative Care, 7*(2), 201–206.

National Consensus Project for Quality Palliative Care (NCP). (2018). *Clinical practice guidelines for quality palliative care* (4th ed.). Retrieved on 6/22/2019 at: www.nationalcoalitionhpc.org

National Palliative Care Registry. (2017). National Hospice and Palliative Care Organization. Retrieved on 6/29/2019 at: www.registry.capc.

Nelson, J. E., Cortez, T. B., Curtis, J. R., et al. (2011). Integrating palliative nursing in the ICU: The nurse in a leading role. *Journal of Hospice and Palliative Nursing, 13*(2), 89–94.

O'Connor, N. R., Junker, P., Appel, S. M., et al. (2018). Palliative care consultation for goals of care and future acute care costs: A propensity-matched study. *American Journal of Hospice and Palliative Medicine, 35*(7), 966–971.

Oregon Public Health Division. (2018). Oregon's Death with Dignity Act—2018 Data Summary. Retrieved on 6/30/2019 at: www.oregon.gov/oha/PH/PROVIDERPARTNERRESOURCES/EVALUATIONRESEARCH/DEATHWITHDIGNITYACT/Documents/year21.pdf

Paladino, J., Bernacki, R., Neville, B. A., et al. (2019). Evaluating an intervention to improve communication between oncology clinicians and patients with life-limiting cancer: A cluster randomized clinical trial of the serious illness care program. *JAMA Oncology, 5*(6), 801–809.

Peereboom, K., & Coyle, N. (2012). Facilitating goals-of-care discussions for patients with life-limiting disease—Communication strategies for nurses. *Journal of Hospice and Palliative Nursing, 14*(4), 251–258.

Perez-Cruz, P. E., Langer, P., Carrasco, C., et al. (2019). Spiritual pain is associated with decreased quality of life in advanced cancer patients in palliative care: An exploratory study. *Journal of Palliative Medicine, 22*(6), 663–669.

Puchalski, C. M. (2015). Spirituality in geriatric palliative care. *Clinical Geriatric Medicine, 31*(2), 245–252.

**Puchalski, C., & Romer, A. L. (2000). Taking a spiritual history allows clinicians to understand patients more fully. *Journal of Palliative Medicine, 3*(1), 129–137.

Quill, T. E., Ganzini, L., Troug, R. D., et al. (2018). Voluntarily stopping eating and drinking among patients with serious advanced illness—Clinical, ethical, and legal aspects. *JAMA Internal Medicine, 178*(1), 123–127.

Quill, T. E., Lo, B., Brock, D. W., et al. (2009). Last-resort options for palliative sedation. *Annals of Internal Medicine, 151*, 421–424.

Richardson, S., Hirsch, J. S., Narasimhan, M., et al. (2020). Presenting characteristics, comorbidities, and outcomes among 5700 patients hospitalized with COVID-19 in the New York City area. *JAMA, 323*, 2052.

Rodrigues, P., Crokaert, J., & Gastmans, C. (2018). Palliative sedation for existential suffering: A systematic review of argument-based ethics literature. *Journal of Pain and Symptom Management, 55*(6), 1577–1590.

Sanders, J. J., Chow, V., Enzinger, A. C., et al. (2017). Seeking and accepting: U.S. clergy theological and moral perspectives informing decision making at the end of life. *Journal of Palliative Medicine, 20*(10), 1059–1067.

Schuchman, M., Fain, M., & Cornwell, T. (2018). The resurgence of home-based primary care models in the United States. *Geriatrics (Basel, Switzerland), 3*(3), 41.

Steinhauser, K. E., Fitchett, G., Handzo, G. F., et al. (2017). State of the Science of Spirituality and Palliative Care Research Part I: Definitions, measurement, and outcomes. *Journal of Pain & Symptom Management, 54*(3), 428–440.

**Stroebe, M., & Schut, H. (1999). The dual process of coping with bereavement: Rationale and description. *Death Studies, 23*(3), 197–224.

**SUPPORT Principal Investigators. (1995). A controlled trial to improve care for seriously ill hospitalized patients. *JAMA, 274*(20), 1591–1598.

Tarbi, E. C., & Meghani, S. H. (2019). Existential experience in adults with advanced cancer: A concept analysis. *Nursing Outlook, 67*(5), 540–557.

**Temel, J. S., Greer, J. A., Muzikansky, A., et al. (2010). Early palliative care for patients with metastatic non-small-cell lung cancer. *New England Journal of Medicine, 363*(8), 733–742.

Teno, J. M., Gozalo, P., Trivedi, A. N., et al. (2018). Site of death, place of care, and health care transitions among US Medicare beneficiaries, 2000-2015. *JAMA, 320*(3), 264–271.

The Conversation Project National Survey. (2018). *Institute for Healthcare Improvement.* The conversation project. Retrieved on 9/13/19 at: www.theconversationproject.org

The Joint Commission. (2018). Facts about the advanced certification program for palliative care. Retrieved on 6/28/2019 at: www.jointcommission.org/assets/1/18/Palliative_Care.pdf

Tofthagen, C. S., Kip, K., Witt, A., et al. (2017). Complicated grief: Risk factors, interventions and resources for oncology nurses. *Clinical Journal of Oncology Nursing, 21*(3), 331–337.

Unroe, K. T., O'Kelly Phillips, E., Effler, S., et al. (2019). Comfort measures orders and hospital transfers: Insights from the OPTIMISTIC demonstration project. *Journal of Pain and Symptom Management, 58*(4), 559–566.

Wakam, G. K., Montgomery, J. R., Biesterveld, B. E., et al. (2020). Not dying alone—Modern compassionate care in the Covid-19 pandemic. *New England Journal of Medicine, 382*, e88.

Wang, S., Hsu, S., Aldridge, M. D., et al. (2019). Racial differences in health care transitions and hospice use at the end of life. *Journal of Palliative Medicine, 22*(6), 619–627.

Wang, S. S. Y., Teo, W. Z. W., Teo, W. Z. Y., et al. (2020). Virtual reality as a bridge in palliative care during COVID-19. *Journal of Palliative Medicine, 23*(6), 756.

Wax, J. W., An, A. W., Koiser, N., et al. (2018). Voluntary stopping eating and drinking. *Journal of the American Geriatric Society, 66*(3), 441–445.

West, L. A., Cole, S., & Goodkind, D., et al. (2014). 65+ in the United States: 2010. Retrieved on 6/29/2019 at: www.commongroundhealth.org/Media/Default/documents/Senior%20Health/2010%20Census%20Report_%2065-lowest_Part1.pdf

White, D. B., Angus, D. C., Shields, A. M., et al. (2018). A randomized trial of a family-support intervention in intensive care units. *The New England Journal of Medicine, 378*(25), 2365–2375.

Wholihan, D. & Olson, E. (2017). The doctrine of double effect: A review for the bedside nurse providing end-of-life care. *Journal of Hospice and Palliative Nursing, 19*(3), 205–211.

Worldwide Palliative Care Alliance, World Health Organization. (2014). Global atlas of palliative care at the end of life. Retrieved on 6/25/2019 at: www.who.int/nmh/Global_Atlas_of_Palliative_Care.pdf

Yadav, K. N., Gabler, N. B., Cooney, E., et al. (2017). Approximately one in three US adults completes any type of advanced directive for end-of-life care. *Health Affairs*, 36(7), 1244–1251.

Yennurajalingam, S., Lu, Z., Prado, B., et al. (2018). Association between advanced cancer patients' perceptions of curability and patients' characteristics, decisional control preferences, symptoms, and end-of-life quality care. *Journal of Palliative Medicine*, 21(11), 1609–1616.

Resources

American Academy of Hospice and Palliative Medicine (AAHPM), www.aahpm.org

American Hospice Foundation, www.americanhospice.org

Americans for Better Care of the Dying (ABCD), www.abcd-caring.org

Association for Death Education and Counseling (ADEC), www.adec.org/default.aspx

Caring Connections: A program of the National Hospice and Palliative Care Organization, www.caregiver.org/caring-connections-0

Center to Advance Palliative Care (CAPC), www.capc.org

Children's Hospice International (CHI), www.chionline.org

Compassion & Choices, www.compassionandchoices.org

End-of-Life Nursing Education Consortium (ELNEC), www.aacnnursing.org/ELNEC

Family Caregiver Alliance (FCA), www.caregiver.org

Get Palliative Care (Blog and resources for palliative care), www.getpalliativecare.org

Harvard Medical School Center for Palliative Care, Dana Farber Cancer Institute, /pallcare.hms.harvard.edu

Hospice and Palliative Credentialing Center (HPCC), www.advancingexpertcare.org/HPNA/HPNA/About_Us/About.aspx

Hospice and Palliative Nurses Association (HPNA), www.advancingexpertcare.org

Hospice Association of America, http://hospice.nahc.org/

Hospice Compare (Medicare ratings), www.medicare.gov/hospicecompare

Hospice Education Institute, www.guidestar.org/profile/22-2701794

Hospice Foundation of America (HFA), www.hospicefoundation.org

International Association for Hospice & Palliative Care (IAHPC), www.hospicecare.com/home

National Association for Home Care & Hospice, www.nahc.org

National Consensus Project for Quality Palliative Care, www.nationalcoalitionhpc.org/ncp

National Hospice and Palliative Care Organization (NHPCO), www.nhpco.org

National Prison Hospice Association, www.npha.org

Office of End-of-Life and Palliative Care Research (OEPCR), www.ninr.nih.gov/researchandfunding/desp/oepcr

Palliative Care NOW Fast Facts and Concepts, www.mypcnow.org/fast-facts

POLST (Physician Orders for Life-Sustaining Treatment Paradigm), www.polst.org

Promoting Excellence in End-of-Life Care, www.promotingexcellence.org

Supportive Care Coalition, www.supportivecarecoalition.org

TIME: Toolkit of Instruments to Measure End of Life Care (Brown University), www.chcr.brown.edu/pcoc/resourceguide/resourceguide.pdf

We Honor Veterans (Partnership between Veterans Administration and NHPCO), www.wehonorveterans.org

World Health Organization (WHO) Palliative Care, www.who.int/news-room/fact-sheets/detail/palliative-care

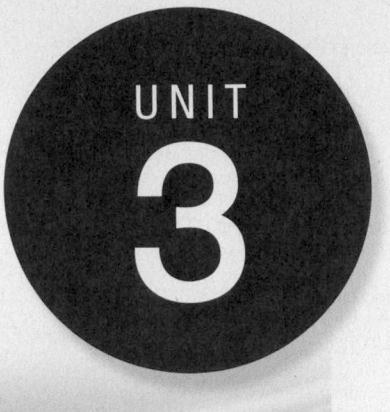

UNIT
3

Perioperative Concepts and Nursing Management

Case Study

MAINTAINING A CULTURE OF SAFETY USING THE SURGICAL SAFETY CHECKLIST

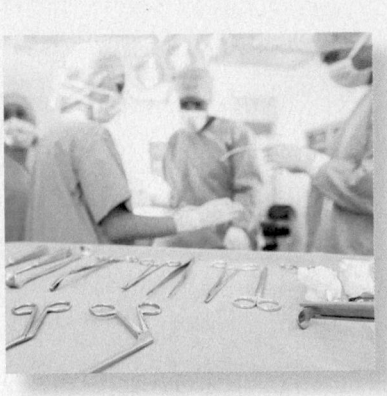

A 32-year-old woman is admitted to the hospital with nausea, vomiting, and right upper quadrant pain. She is diagnosed with acute cholecystitis and is scheduled for a laparoscopic procedure to remove her gallbladder. After completing the preoperative procedures and preprocedure verification, the patient is brought to the operating room (OR) where you work. The surgical safety checklist involves members of the team including the surgeon, anesthesia provider, circulating nurse, and OR technician. Prior to induction of anesthesia the team confirms the patient's identity, procedure, and consent. In addition, the incision site is marked, the anesthesia machine and medication check is completed, and the pulse oximeter is placed on the patient and is confirmed to be working. The team also checks if the patient has a known allergy, if there are any airway or aspiration risks, and whether there is risk of a >500 mL blood loss.

QSEN Competency Focus: Safety

The complexities inherent in today's health care system challenge nurses to demonstrate integration of specific interdisciplinary core competencies. These competencies are aimed at ensuring the delivery of safe, quality patient care (Institute of Medicine, 2003). The Quality and Safety Education for Nurses project (Cronenwett, Sherwood, Barnsteiner, et al., 2007; QSEN, 2020) provides a framework for the knowledge, skills, and attitudes (KSAs) required for nurses to demonstrate competency in these key areas, which include *patient-centered care*, *interdisciplinary teamwork and collaboration*, *evidence-based practice*, *quality improvement*, *safety*, and *informatics.*

Safety Definition: Minimizes risk of harm to patients and providers through both system effectiveness and individual performance.

SELECT PRE-LICENSURE KSAs	APPLICATION AND REFLECTION
Knowledge	
Describe factors that create a culture of safety (such as, open communication strategies and organizational error reporting systems)	Describe your role in participating in a surgical safety checklist. Identify the additional checks that need to be conducted before the surgical skin incision is made and further safety measures that must be addressed before the patient leaves the OR to help facilitate a culture of safety.
Skills	
Communicate observations or concerns related to hazards and errors to patients, families, and the health care team	Identify your role in communicating to the members of the OR team important assessments, potential hazards, and errors that may occur because of surgery.
Attitudes	
Value relationship between national safety campaigns and implementation in local practices and practice settings	A goal of the Joint Commission is to ensure the safety of patients by eliminating potential errors. The surgical safety checklist is supported by accrediting bodies such as the Joint Commission and the World Health Organization. What other practices can you implement to ensure safety in the OR setting?

Cronenwett, L., Sherwood, G., Barnsteiner, J., et al. (2007). Quality and safety education for nurses. *Nursing Outlook, 55*(3), 122–131; Institute of Medicine. (2003). *Health professions education: A bridge to quality.* Washington, DC: National Academies Press; QSEN Institute. (2020). *QSEN competencies: Definitions and pre-licensure KSAs; Safety.* Retrieved on 8/15/2020 at: qsen.org/competencies/pre-licensure-ksas/#safety

14 Preoperative Nursing Management

LEARNING OUTCOMES

On completion of this chapter, the learner will be able to:

1. Define the phases of perioperative patient care.
2. Perform a comprehensive preoperative assessment to identify pertinent health and surgical risk factors.
3. Describe considerations related to preoperative nursing care of older adult patients, patients with obesity, and patients with disability.
4. Identify the regulatory documents that are required prior to a patient entering surgery.
5. Initiate the immediate preoperative preparation and education of the patient.

NURSING CONCEPTS

Communication   Managing Care   Mobility

GLOSSARY

ambulatory surgery: includes outpatient, same-day, or short-stay surgery that does not require an overnight hospital stay

bariatrics: having to do with patients with obesity

history and physical: mandatory form completed by the surgeon that gives a comprehensive overview of the patient's history, current physical status, and plan of care

informed consent: the patient's autonomous decision about whether to undergo a surgical procedure, based on the nature of the condition, the treatment options, and the risks and benefits involved

intraoperative phase: period of time that begins with transfer of the patient to the operating room area and continues until the patient is admitted to the postanesthesia care unit

minimally invasive surgery: surgical procedures that use specialized instruments inserted into the body either through natural orifices or through small incisions

perioperative phase: period of time that constitutes the surgical experience; includes the preoperative, intraoperative, and postoperative phases of nursing care

postoperative phase: period of time that begins with the admission of the patient to the postanesthesia care unit and ends after follow-up evaluation in the clinical setting or home

preadmission testing: diagnostic testing performed before admission to the hospital

preoperative phase: period of time from when the decision for surgical intervention is made to when the patient is transferred to the operating room table

As techniques to perform surgery have evolved with improved technology and expertise, surgery has become less invasive and less debilitating. The increased use of **minimally invasive surgery** (procedures that use specialized instruments inserted into the body either through natural orifices or through small incisions) enables many procedures to be performed on an outpatient basis. Surgery remains a complex, stressful experience, whether minimally invasive, elective, or emergent. Even healthy patients having elective outpatient surgery may experience unanticipated complications during otherwise benign procedures. Many patients enter the hospital 90 minutes prior to surgery and have necessary medical assessments and analyses preceding the surgical intervention. The surgery is followed by a recovery period in the postanesthesia care unit (PACU). Later that day the patient goes home. When comorbidities exist or procedures are more complex, the patient may have laboratory studies completed prior to admission, and may be admitted to the hospital for postoperative recovery.

Traumatic and emergency surgery most often results in prolonged hospital stays. Patients who are acutely ill or undergoing major surgery and patients with concurrent medical disorders may require supportive supplementary care from other medical disciplines, which can be coordinated more easily within the hospital setting. The high acuity level of surgical inpatients and the greater complexity of procedures have placed greater demands on the practice of nursing in this setting.

Although each setting (ambulatory, outpatient, or inpatient) offers its own unique advantages for the delivery of patient care, all patients require a comprehensive preoperative nursing assessment, patient education, and nursing interventions to prepare for surgery.

Perioperative Nursing

Communication, teamwork, and patient assessment are crucial to ensure good patient outcomes in the perioperative setting. Professional perioperative and perianesthesia nursing standards encompass the domains of behavioral response, physiologic response, and patient safety and are used as guides toward development of nursing diagnoses, interventions, and plans. Perioperative nursing, which spans the entire surgical experience, consists of three phases that begin and end at particular points in the sequence of surgical experience events. The **preoperative phase** begins when the decision to proceed with surgical intervention is made and ends with the transfer of the patient onto the operating room (OR) bed. The **intraoperative phase** begins when the patient is transferred onto the OR bed and ends with admission to the PACU. Intraoperative nursing responsibilities involve acting as scrub nurse, circulating nurse, or registered nurse first assistant (see Chapter 15 for the description of these roles). The **postoperative phase** begins with the admission of the patient to the PACU and ends with a follow-up evaluation in the clinical setting or home (see Chapter 16).

Each **perioperative phase** includes the many diverse activities a nurse performs, using the nursing process, and is based on the recommended practice standards of the Association of periOperative Registered Nurses (AORN), formerly known as the Association of Operating Room Nurses (AORN, 2019) and the American Society of PeriAnesthesia Nurses (ASPAN, 2019). Chart 14-1 presents examples of nursing activities characteristic of the three perioperative phases of care. The phases of the surgical experience are reviewed in more detail in this chapter and in the other chapters in this unit.

A conceptual model of patient care, published by AORN, helps delineate the relationships between various components of nursing practice and patient outcomes into four domains: safety, physiologic responses, behavioral responses, and health care systems. The first three domains reflect phenomena of concern to perioperative nurses and are composed of nursing diagnoses, interventions, and outcomes. The fourth domain—the health care system—consists of structural data elements and focuses on clinical processes and outcomes. The model is used to depict the relationship of nursing process components to the achievement of optimal patient outcomes (Rothrock, 2019).

Advances in Surgical and Anesthesia Approaches

Technologic advancements continue to lead health care industry providers toward performing more complex procedures that are less invasive, and therefore cause less morbidity

during the recovery phase of surgery (Rothrock, 2019). Minimally invasive and robotic surgeries are continuing to replace traditional surgical procedures. Advancements in surgical technology allow for shorter hospital stays and promote patient comfort (Sadler, 2017).

The fastest growing trend in recent years is the use of robotic surgery (see Fig. 14-1). Robotic surgery offers many advantages over laparoscopic surgery including more precise accuracy for dissecting and suturing, better range of motion of the instruments, enhanced ability to access deep structures, and attain three-dimensional visual feedback (Rothrock, 2019). Robotic surgery is used in a wide variety of surgical specialties such as cardiac; gastrointestinal; urologic; gynecologic; ear, nose, and throat (ENT); thoracic; and orthopedic.

Enhanced anesthesia methodology complements advances in surgical technology. Modern methods of achieving airway patency, sophisticated monitoring devices, and new pharmacologic agents, such as short-acting anesthetics, have created a safer atmosphere in which to operate. Effective antiemetics have reduced postoperative nausea and vomiting (PONV). Improved postoperative pain management and shortened procedure and recovery times have improved the operative experience for surgical patients.

Surgical Classifications

The decision to perform surgery may be based on facilitating a diagnosis (a diagnostic procedure such as biopsy, exploratory laparotomy, or laparoscopy), a cure (e.g., excision of a tumor or an inflamed appendix), or repair (e.g., multiple wound repair). It may be reconstructive or cosmetic (such as mammoplasty or a facelift) or palliative (to relieve pain or correct a problem—such as debulking a tumor to achieve comfort, or removal of a dysfunctional gallbladder). In addition, surgery might be rehabilitative (e.g., total joint replacement surgery to correct crippling pain or progression of degenerative osteoarthritis). Surgery can also be classified based upon the degree of urgency involved: emergent, urgent, required, elective, and optional (see Table 14-1).

Preadmission Testing

Concurrent with the increase in **ambulatory surgeries** (surgery that does not require an overnight hospital stay) have been changes in the delivery of and payment for health care. Incentives to reduce hospital stays and contain costs have resulted in diagnostic **preadmission testing** (PAT) and preoperative preparation prior to admission. Many facilities have a presurgical services department to facilitate PAT and to initiate the nursing assessment process, which focuses on admission data such as patient demographics, health history, and other information pertinent to the surgical procedure (i.e., appropriate consent forms, diagnostic and laboratory tests) (Rothrock, 2019). During the PAT visit, patients learn what to expect on the day of surgery and receive answers to questions they may have. Nurses in the PAT department are responsible for communicating information related to the surgical procedure and the effect that the surgical procedure and anesthetic may have on the patient's health status, functional status, and family dynamics (Malley, Kenner, Kim, et al., 2015).

Chart 14-1 — Examples of Nursing Activities in the Perioperative Phases of Care

Preoperative Phase

Preadmission Testing

1. Performs initial preoperative assessment
2. Initiates education appropriate to patient's needs
3. Involves family in interview
4. Verifies completion of preoperative diagnostic testing according to patient's needs
5. Confirms understanding of surgeon-specific preoperative prescribed therapies (e.g., bowel preparation, preoperative shower)
0. Discusses and reviews advance directive document
7. Begins discharge planning by assessing patient's need for postoperative transportation and care

Admission to Surgical Center

1. Completes preoperative assessment
2. Assesses for risks for postoperative complications
3. Reports unexpected findings or any deviations from normal
4. Verifies that operative consent has been signed
5. Coordinates patient education and plan of care with nursing staff and other health team members
6. Reinforces previous education
7. Explains phases in perioperative period and expectations
8. Answers patient's and family's questions

In the Preoperative Area

1. Identifies patient
2. Assesses patient's physical and emotional status, baseline pain, and nutritional status
3. Reviews medical record
4. Verifies surgical site and that it has been marked per institutional policy
5. Establishes IV line
6. Administers medications if prescribed
7. Takes measures to ensure patient's comfort
8. Provides psychological support
9. Communicates patient and family's needs to other appropriate members of the health care team

Intraoperative Phase

Maintenance of Safety

1. Maintains aseptic, controlled environment
2. Effectively manages human resources, equipment, and supplies for individualized patient care
3. Transfers patient to operating room bed or table
4. Positions patient based on functional alignment and exposure of surgical site
5. Applies grounding device to patient
6. Ensures that the sponge, needle, and instrument counts are correct
7. Completes intraoperative documentation

Physiologic Monitoring

1. Communicates amount of fluid instillation and blood loss
2. Distinguishes normal from abnormal cardiovascular data
3. Reports changes in patient's vital signs
4. Institutes measures to promote normothermia

Psychological Support (Before Induction and When Patient is Conscious)

1. Provides emotional support to patient
2. Stands near or touches patient during procedures and induction

3. Continues to assess patient's emotional status
4. Notifies the patient's family or significant others of updates throughout the procedure

Postoperative Phase

Transfer of Patient to Postanesthesia Care Unit

1. Communicates intraoperative information:
   a. Identifies patient by name
   b. States type of surgery performed
   c. Identifies type and amounts of anesthetic and analgesic agents used
   d. Reports patient's vital signs and response to surgical procedure and anesthesia
   e. Describes intraoperative factors (e.g., insertion of drains or catheters, administration of blood, medications during surgery, or occurrence of unexpected events)
   f. Describes physical limitations
   g. Reports patient's preoperative level of consciousness
   h. Communicates necessary equipment needs
   i. Communicates presence of family or significant others

Postoperative Assessment Recovery Area

1. Determines patient's immediate response to surgical intervention
2. Monitors patient's vital signs and physiologic status
3. Assesses patient's pain level and administers appropriate pain-relief measures
4. Maintains patient's safety (airway, circulation, prevention of injury)
5. Administers medications, fluid, and blood component therapy, if prescribed
6. Provides oral fluids if prescribed for ambulatory surgery patient
7. Assesses patient's readiness for transfer to inhospital unit or for discharge home based on institutional policy (e.g., Aldrete score, see Chapter 16)

Surgical Nursing Unit

1. Continues close monitoring of patient's physical and psychological response to surgical intervention
2. Assesses patient's pain level and administers appropriate pain-relief measures
3. Provides education to patient during immediate recovery period
4. Assists patient in recovery and preparation for discharge home
5. Determines patient's psychological status
6. Assists with discharge planning

Home or Clinic

1. Provides follow-up care during office or clinic visit or by telephone contact
2. Reinforces previous education and answers patient's and family's questions about surgery and follow-up care
3. Assesses patient's response to surgery and anesthesia and their effects on body image and function
4. Determines family's perception of surgery and its outcome

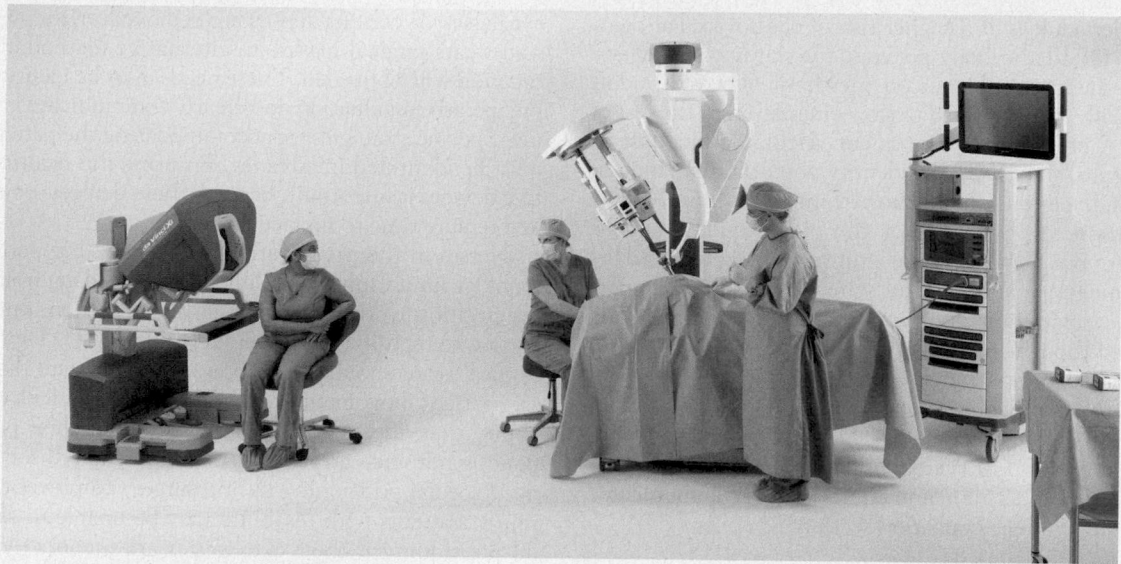

Figure 14-1 • The daVinci surgical system. Reprinted with permission from ©2022 Intuitive Surgical, Inc.

Special Considerations during the Perioperative Period

In an effort to reduce surgical complications, The Joint Commission and the Centers for Medicare and Medicaid Services (CMS) developed National Patient Safety Goals. The goals are updated yearly and identify performance measures aimed at preventing surgical complications, including venous thromboembolism (VTE), surgical site infections (SSIs), and wrong-site surgery related to positive patient identification (Joint Commission, 2019). On the day of surgery, the preoperative nurse should verify the list of home medications with the patient and, if applicable, confirm which medications the patient discontinued and when they were last taken. This information assists providers in understanding the patient's

medical conditions and helps to avoid medication interactions between what patients take at home and what is administered to them during surgery (Ubaldi, 2019). For example, particular beta-blockers taken within 24 hours of surgery are associated with improved perioperative cardiovascular outcomes. If the patient has not taken the usual dosage of this medication, the anesthesiologist or certified registered nurse anesthetist (CRNA) must evaluate whether or not it should be administered prior to surgery or during the perioperative period. The nurse in the perioperative area needs to be alert for appropriate preoperative prescriptions aimed at preventing VTE and SSIs. If these prescriptions are not present, they should be requested so that appropriate treatment begins before the start of surgery.

Gerontologic Considerations

The hazards of surgery for older adults are proportional to the number and severity of comorbidities and the nature and duration of the operative procedure. Anesthesia associated with these surgeries can precipitate the dysregulation of older adult physiology. Identification of at-risk older adult patients is important in determining the appropriate operative risk and management (Vernon, Rice, Titch, et al., 2019). Cardiac reserves are lower, renal and hepatic functions are depressed, and gastrointestinal activity is likely to be reduced. Therefore, a comprehensive assessment that focuses on the cardiovascular, respiratory, and renal systems may help improve immediate perioperative outcomes (Odom-Forren, 2018). See Chapter 8, Table 8-1 for additional age-related changes.

In the preoperative period, the nurse pays careful attention to the integumentary system of the patient as it can reveal pertinent data about the patient's health status. Assessment includes the overall condition of the skin, and determination of any bruises, abrasions, and discolorations (Phillips, 2017). Precautions are taken when moving an older adult. Decreased subcutaneous fat makes older adults more susceptible to temperature changes. A lightweight cotton blanket is an appropriate cover when an older patient is moved to and from the OR but never replaces asking patients if they feel sufficiently warm and attending to their needs.

	Indications for Surgery	Examples
TABLE 14-1		Categories of Surgery Based on Urgency
Classification		
I. Emergent—Patient requires immediate attention; disorder may be life-threatening	Without delay	Severe bleeding Bladder or intestinal obstruction Fractured skull Gunshot or stab wounds Extensive burns
II. Urgent—Patient requires prompt attention	Within 24–30 h	Closed fractures Infected wound exploration/irrigation
III. Required—Patient needs to have surgery	Plan within a few weeks or months	Prostatic hyperplasia Thyroid disorders Cataracts
IV. Elective—Patient should have surgery	Failure to have surgery not catastrophic	Repair of scars Simple hernia Vaginal repair
V. Optional—Decision rests with patient	Personal preference	Cosmetic surgery

The older adult is at a higher risk of cardiovascular complications. Of all the body systems, the cardiovascular system exerts the most influence on anesthesia. The older adult patient usually has decreased or slow circulation to the rest of the body. A preoperative assessment, including blood tests, blood pressure, and EKG, can identify potential risks including anemia, hypertension, and arrhythmias (Phillips, 2017).

In addition to physical risks, the older adult should be assessed for poor memory and cognition. When older adults are in a vulnerable and stressful state, such as preparing for surgery, they may show poor concentration, confusion, and disorganized thought patterns (Odom-Forren, 2018). Nurses must educate patients and caregivers about appropriate pain management and encourage good communication to obtain greater postoperative pain relief. Older adults may need multiple education formats (verbal and print) along with extra time in order to understand and retain what is communicated (see Providing Patient Education section).

 ### Bariatric Patients

Bariatrics is a specialty that revolves around diagnosing, treating, and managing patients with obesity. The prevalence of obesity is approximately 39.8% and affects about 93.3 million adults in the United States (Centers for Disease Control and Prevention [CDC], 2018). Obesity increases the risk and severity of complications associated with surgery. Preoperative assessment of the patient with obesity should pay careful attention to pulmonary, cardiovascular, psychological, and integumentary systems.

Patients with obesity have more subcutaneous fat. The increase in adipose tissue can result in difficult intravenous (IV) access and delayed wound healing at the incision site (Odom-Forren, 2018). Obesity is also associated with increased SSIs and joint replacement failure. Patients with a body mass index (BMI) of greater than 45 are at a significantly increased risk for total joint replacement failure and postoperative infection (Boudreaux & Simmons, 2019).

The patient with obesity tends to have shallow respirations when supine, increasing the risk of hypoventilation and postoperative pulmonary complications. Additionally, diagnosed and undiagnosed obstructive sleep apnea (OSA) is common among patients with obesity. Since these apnea and hypopnea events occur during sleep, most patients with OSA may not be aware that they have the condition. It has been estimated that up to 80% of individuals with moderate to severe OSA may remain undiagnosed and untreated (Chung, Abdullah, & Liao, 2016). Positive identification of OSA and OSA risks can dramatically reduce intubation and postoperative complications (see Chapter 18).

Patients with Disability

Special considerations for patients with mental or physical disability include the need for appropriate assistive devices, modifications in preoperative education, and additional assistance with and attention to positioning or transferring. Assistive devices include hearing aids, eyeglasses, braces, prostheses, and other devices. People who are hearing impaired may need and are entitled by law to a sign interpreter or some alternative communication system perioperatively. If the patient relies on signing or speech (lip) reading and their

eyeglasses or contact lenses are removed or the health care staff wears surgical masks, an alternative method of communication will be needed. These needs must be identified in the preoperative evaluation and clearly communicated to personnel. Specific strategies for accommodating the patient's needs must be identified in advance. Ensuring the security of assistive devices is important, because these devices are expensive and require time to replace if lost.

Nurses in the preoperative area report that patients with mobility limitations have difficulty transferring from a standing position to the transport gurney and then, once on the gurney, to reposition themselves (Link, 2018). Therefore, the surgical team should incorporate a plan of care that ensures safe patient movement and handling. The patient with a disability that affects body position (e.g., cerebral palsy, postpolio syndrome, and other neuromuscular disorders) may need special positioning during surgery to prevent pain and injury. Patients with disability may be unable to sense painful positioning if their extremities are incorrectly adjusted, or they may be unable to communicate their discomfort. A comprehensive care plan should be developed preoperatively addressing the type of disability and patient specific needs.

Patients with respiratory problems related to a disability (e.g., multiple sclerosis, muscular dystrophy) may experience difficulties unless the problems are made known to the anesthesiologist or CRNA and adjustments are made (Barash, Cullen, Stoelting, et al., 2017). These factors need to be clearly identified in the preoperative period and communicated to the appropriate personnel.

Patients Undergoing Ambulatory Surgery

Ambulatory surgery includes outpatient, same-day, or short-stay surgery not requiring admission for an overnight hospital stay but may entail observation in a hospital setting for 23 hours or less. During the brief time the patient and family spend in the ambulatory setting, the nurse must quickly and comprehensively assess and anticipate the needs of the patient and at the same time begin planning for discharge and follow-up home care.

The nurse needs to be sure that the patient and family understand that the patient will first go to the preoperative area before going to the OR for the surgical procedure and then will spend some time in the PACU before being discharged home with the family member later that day. Other preoperative education content should also be verified and reinforced as needed (see later discussion). The nurse should ensure that any plans for follow-up home care or new assistive devices are in place if needed.

Patients Undergoing Emergency Surgery

Emergency surgeries are unplanned and occur with little time for preparation of the patient or the perioperative team. The unpredictable nature of trauma and emergency surgery poses unique challenges throughout the perioperative period. It is important for the nurse to communicate with the patient and team members as calmly and effectively as possible in these situations. (See Chapter 15 for the duties of the members of the perioperative team.)

Factors that affect patients preparing to undergo surgery also apply to patients undergoing emergency surgery, although usually in a very condensed time frame. The only opportunity for preoperative assessment may take place at the same time as resuscitation in the emergency department. A quick visual survey of the patient is essential to identify all sites of injury if the emergency surgery is due to trauma (see Chapter 67 for more information). The patient, who may have undergone a traumatic experience, may need extra support and explanation of the surgery. For the patient who is unconscious, essential information, such as pertinent past medical history and allergies, need to be obtained from a family member, if one is available.

Required Preoperative Documents

Informed consent is the patient's autonomous decision about whether to undergo a surgical procedure. Voluntary and written informed consent from the patient is necessary before nonemergent surgery can be performed to protect the patient from unsanctioned surgery and protect the surgeon from claims of an unauthorized operation or battery. Consent is a legal mandate, but it also helps the patient to prepare psychologically, because it helps to ensure that the patient understands the surgery to be performed (Rothrock, 2019).

It is the surgeon's and the anesthesiologist's responsibility to provide a clear and simple explanation of what the surgery will entail prior to the patient giving consent. The surgeon must also inform the patient of the benefits, alternatives, possible risks, complications, disfigurement, disability, and removal of body parts as well as what to expect in the early and late postoperative periods. The nurse clarifies the information provided, verifies the presence of the patient's or designee's signature, and may be asked to sign as a witness. If at any point the patient requests additional information, or if the nurse feels that the patient may not understand, the nurse notifies the physician. The nurse ascertains that the consent form has been signed before administering psychoactive premedication, because consent is not valid if it is obtained while the patient is under the influence of medications that can affect judgment and decision making capacity.

> ▶ **Quality and Safety Nursing Alert**
>
> *Any signed form required for surgery is placed in a prominent place on the patient's medical record and accompanies the patient to the OR.*

Many ethical principles are integral to informed consent. Informed consent is necessary in the following circumstances:

- Invasive procedures, such as a surgical incision, a biopsy, a cystoscopy, or paracentesis
- Procedures requiring sedation or anesthesia (see Chapter 15 for a discussion of anesthesia)
- A nonsurgical procedure, such as an arteriography, that carries more than a slight risk to the patient
- Procedures involving radiation
- Blood product administration

The patient personally signs the consent if of legal age and mentally capable. Permission is otherwise obtained from a surrogate, who most often is a responsible family member (preferably next of kin) or legal guardian (see Chart 14-2 for criteria for valid informed consent). State regulations and agency policy must be followed. In an emergency, it may be

---

Chart 14-2

Valid Informed Consent

Voluntary Consent

Valid consent must be freely given, without coercion. Patient must be at least 18 years of age (unless an emancipated minor), a physician must obtain consent, and a professional staff member must witness patient's signature.

Patient Who Is Incompetent

Legal definition: individual who is *not* autonomous and cannot give or withhold consent (e.g., individuals who are cognitively impaired, mentally ill, or neurologically incapacitated).

Informed Subject

Informed consent should be in writing. It should contain the following:

- Explanation of procedure and its risks
- Description of benefits and alternatives
- An offer to answer questions about procedure
- Instructions that the patient may withdraw consent
- A statement informing the patient if the protocol differs from customary procedure

Patient Able to Comprehend

If the patient is non-English speaking, it is necessary to provide consent (written and verbal) in a language that is understandable to the patient. A trained medical interpreter may be consulted. Alternative formats of communication (e.g., Braille, large print, sign interpreter) may be needed if the patient has a disability that affects vision or hearing. Questions must be answered to facilitate comprehension if material is confusing.

---

necessary for the surgeon to operate as a lifesaving measure without the patient's informed consent. However, every effort must be made to contact the patient's family. In such a situation, contact can be made by telephone, fax, or other electronic means and consent obtained.

If the patient has doubts and has not had the opportunity to investigate alternative treatments, a second opinion may be requested. No patient should be urged or coerced to give informed consent. Refusing to undergo a surgical procedure is a person's legal right and privilege. Such information must be documented and relayed to the surgeon so that other arrangements can be made. Additional explanations may be provided to the patient and family, or the surgery may be rescheduled. Consents for specific procedures such as sterilization, therapeutic abortion, disposal of severed body parts, organ donation, and blood product administration provide additional protection for the patient (Rothrock, 2019). States and regions may vary in their mandates.

Discussion with patients and their family members may be supplemented with audiovisual materials. Consent forms should be written in easily understandable words and concepts to facilitate the consent process and should use other strategies and resources as needed to help the patient understand the content (see Chart 14-2). Asking patients to describe in their own words the surgery they are about to have promotes nurses' understanding of patients' comprehension.

A completed, updated and signed **History and Physical** must be present prior to the patient entering the OR. Not more than 30 days before the date of the scheduled surgery, each patient must have a comprehensive medical history and physical assessment. The primary provider is required to update the form within 24 hours of scheduled surgery on all non-inpatient clients (Joint Commission, 2019). The History and Physical consists of the history of present illness; surgical, medical, social, and family histories; allergies; current medications; and plan of care. It is the surgical team's responsibility to make sure the presence of these forms and all other supporting documentation (medication reconciliation, Power of Attorney form, etc.) are current and accurate in the preoperative area.

Preoperative Assessment

The goal in the preoperative period is for the patient to be as healthy as possible. Every attempt is made to assess for and address risk factors that may contribute to postoperative complications and delay recovery (see Chart 14-3). The preoperative assessment provides information regarding underlying conditions that may affect the patient's response to surgery techniques and anesthesia (AORN, 2019). During the physical examination, many factors that have the potential to affect the patient undergoing surgery are considered, such

as joint mobility. Genetic considerations are also taken into account during assessment to prevent complications with anesthesia (see Chart 14-4).

Asking the patient about use of prescription and over-the-counter (OTC) medications, including herbal and other supplements, provides useful information. Activity and functional levels should be determined, including that involving regular aerobic exercise. Known allergies and sensitivities to drugs, foods, adhesives, and latex could avert an anaphylactic response (Barash et al., 2017). Patients may have early manifestations of a latex allergy and be unaware of this. If a patient states that he or she is allergic to kiwi, avocado, or banana, or cannot blow up balloons, there may be an association with an allergy to latex.

The patient should be assessed for latex allergy and sensitivities. Latex is found in some food (such as bananas and kiwi) as well as in some hospital materials and equipment. Most hospital products today are latex-free, especially in ORs; however, special precautions are still taken to eliminate the risk of exposure to the patient. These precautions include thorough cleaning of the surgical areas between cases, awareness of allergy among surgical team members, ensuring the materials used are latex-free, and eliminating the use of latex powdered gloves during the case (Mendez, Martinez, Lopez, et al., 2018).

> ### Quality and Safety Nursing Alert
>
> A latex allergy can manifest as a rash, asthma, or anaphylactic shock.

The preoperative assessment should pay attention to the possible presence of undiagnosed OSA. The STOP-Bang is one assessment that may be performed (Snoring, Tired, Observed, Pressure, BMI, Age, Neck, Gender) to assess for the presence of OSA (Chung et al., 2016).

Health care providers also should be alert for signs of interpersonal violence, including intimate partner violence, which can occur at any age, in either sex, and in any socioeconomic, ethnic, and cultural group. Findings need to be reported accordingly (see Chapter 4 for further discussion of signs of interpersonal violence). Laboratory tests and other diagnostic tests are prescribed when indicated by information obtained from the history and physical examination. Autologous blood donation or patient self-donation is discussed as needed for the type of surgical procedure planned. See Chapter 28 for further discussion of autologous blood donation.

Nutritional and Fluid Status

Optimal nutrition is an essential factor in promoting healing and resisting infection and other surgical complications. Assessment of a patient's nutritional status identifies factors that can affect the patient's surgical course, such as obesity, weight loss, malnutrition, deficiencies in specific nutrients, metabolic abnormalities, and the effects of medications on nutrition. Nutritional needs may be determined by measurement of BMI and waist circumference. (See Chapter 4 for further discussion of nutritional assessment.)

Any nutritional deficiency should be corrected before surgery to provide adequate protein for tissue repair. The nutrients needed for wound healing are summarized in Table 14-2.

Assessment of a patient's hydration status is also essential. The patient's NPO (Nothing by Mouth or *nil per os*)

Chart 14-3 ⚠ **SELECT RISK FACTORS**
Surgical Complications

- Arthritis
- Cardiovascular disease:
  - Coronary artery disease or previous myocardial infarction
  - Cardiac failure
  - Cerebrovascular disease
  - Arrhythmias
  - Hemorrhagic disorders
  - Hypertension
  - Prosthetic heart valve
  - Venous thromboembolism (VTE)
- Dehydration or electrolyte imbalance
- Endocrine dysfunction:
  - Adrenal disorders
  - Diabetes
  - Thyroid malfunction
- Extremes of age (very young, very old)
- Extremes of weight (underweight, obese)
- Hepatic disease:
  - Cirrhosis
  - Hepatitis
- Hypovolemia
- Immunologic abnormalities
- Infection and sepsis
- Low socioeconomic status
- Medications
- Nicotine use
- Nutritional deficits
- Pregnancy:
  - Diminished maternal physiologic reserve
- Preexisting cognitive, developmental, intellectual, physical, or sensory disability
- Pulmonary disease:
  - Obstructive disease
  - Restrictive disorder
  - Respiratory infection
- Renal or urinary tract disease:
  - Decreased kidney function
  - Urinary tract infection
  - Obstruction
  - Toxic conditions

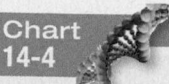

Chart 14-4 GENETICS IN NURSING PRACTICE
Genetics Concepts and Perioperative Nursing

Nurses who are caring for patients undergoing surgery need to take various genetic considerations into account when assessing patients throughout the operative experience. Genetic disorders can impact pre-, intra-, and postoperative surgical outcomes. In particular, consideration must be given to genetic disorders associated with the delivery of anesthesia as well as other genetic disorders that may increase the risk of postoperative complications. Examples of genetic conditions that may cause complications with anesthesia include the following:

Autosomal Dominant

- Central core disease
- Hyperkalemic periodic paralysis
- Malignant hyperthermia

Examples of other genetic conditions that must be evaluated and are associated with perioperative risks include the following:

- Cystic fibrosis (autosomal recessive)
- Duchenne muscular dystrophy (X-linked recessive)
- Ehlers–Danlos syndrome
- Factor V Leiden (autosomal dominant)
- Hemophilia (X-linked)
- Scleroderma

Nursing Assessments

Refer to Chapter 4, Chart 4-2: Genetics in Nursing Practice: Genetic Aspects of Health Assessment

Family History Assessment Specific to Genetics and Perioperative Nursing

- Obtain a thorough assessment of personal and family history for three generations, inquiring about prior problems with surgery or anesthesia with specific attention to complications, such as fever, rigidity, dark urine, and unexpected reactions.
- Inquire about any history of musculoskeletal complaints, history of heat intolerance, fevers of unknown origin, or unusual drug reactions.

- Assess for family history of any sudden or unexplained death, especially during participation in athletic events.
- Assess whether any family members have been diagnosed with King–Denborough syndrome, as this is a form of congenital myopathy that places the patient at risk for malignant hyperthermia.

Patient Assessment Specific to Genetics and Perioperative Nursing

- Identify the presence of other inherited genetic disorders that may impact surgical outcomes (e.g., inherited connective tissue, metabolic, bleeding, or neurologic disorders).
- Assess for subclinical muscle weakness.
- Assess for other physical features suggestive of an underlying genetic condition, such as contractures, kyphoscoliosis, and pterygium with progressive weakness.

Management Issues Specific to Genetics and Perioperative Nursing

- Inquire as to whether DNA mutation or other genetic testing has been performed on an affected family member.
- If indicated, refer for further genetic counseling and evaluation so that family members can discuss inheritance, risk to other family members, and availability of diagnostic/genetic testing.
- Provide support to families of patients with newly diagnosed malignant hyperthermia.
- Participate in management and coordination of care of patients with genetic conditions and individuals predisposed to develop or pass on a genetic condition.

Genetics Resources

Malignant Hyperthermia Association, www.mhaus.org
See Chapter 6, Chart 6-7: Components of Genetic Counseling for genetics resources.

---

status should be confirmed preoperatively. Preoperative fasting helps prevent the risk of aspiration but it also induces stress on the body, including the loss of glycogen stores, and the body sacrifices lean muscle to meet the energy needs of the surgery. This may lead to dehydration, which may be exhibited day of surgery by low blood pressure or blood tests revealing fluid and electrolyte imbalances. The depletion of fluids and electrolytes following bowel preparation, especially when combined with prolonged fasting, can result in dehydration and chemical imbalances, even among healthy surgical patients.

Dentition

The condition of the mouth is an important health factor to assess. Dental caries, dentures, and partial plates are particularly significant to the anesthesiologist or CRNA, because decayed teeth or dental prostheses may become dislodged during intubation and occlude the airway. This is especially important for older patients as well as those who may not have regular dental care. The condition of the mouth is also important because any bodily infection, even in the mouth, can be a source of postoperative infection.

Drug or Alcohol Use

Excessive alcohol consumption can cause arrhythmias, infections, and withdrawal. These factors can lead to extended hospital stays and increased complications. Identifying patients who have excessive alcohol use presurgically and implementing interventions can reduce the incidence of complications by about 50% (Cuomo, Abate, Springer, et al., 2018). In addition, the use of illicit drugs and alcohol may impede the effectiveness of some medications. Because acutely intoxicated people are susceptible to injury, surgery is postponed if possible. If surgery is required, local, spinal, or regional block anesthesia is used for minor surgery (Norris, 2019). In an emergency, to prevent vomiting and potential aspiration, a nasogastric tube is inserted before general anesthesia is given.

The person with a history of alcohol abuse often suffers from malnutrition and other systemic problems or metabolic imbalances that increase surgical risk. People who have a substance abuse problem may deny or attempt to hide it. In such situations, the nurse who is obtaining the patient's health history needs to ask frank questions with patience, care, and a nonjudgmental attitude. Such questions should include asking whether the patient has had two drinks per day or more

TABLE 14-2	Nutrients Important for Wound Healing	
Nutrient	**Rationale for Increased Need**	**Possible Deficiency Outcome**
Protein	Allows collagen deposition and wound healing to occur	Collagen deposition leading to impaired/delayed wound healing Decreased skin and wound strength Increased wound infection rates
Arginine (amino acid)	Provides necessary substrate for collagen synthesis and nitric oxide (crucial for wound healing) at wound site Increases wound strength and collagen deposition Stimulates T-cell response Associated with various essential reactions of intermediary metabolism	Impaired wound healing
Carbohydrates and fats	Primary source of energy in the body and consequently in the wound-healing process Meets demand for increased essential fatty acids needed for cellular function after an injury Spares protein Restores normal weight	Signs and symptoms of protein deficiency due to the use of protein to meet energy requirements Extensive weight loss
Water	Replaces fluid lost through vomiting, hemorrhage, exudates, fever, drainage, diuresis Helps maintain homeostasis	Signs, symptoms, and complications of dehydration, such as poor skin turgor, dry mucous membranes, oliguria, anuria, weight loss, increased pulse rate, decreased central venous pressure
Vitamin C	Important for capillary formation, tissue synthesis, and wound healing through collagen formation Needed for antibody formation	Impaired/delayed wound healing related to impaired collagen formation and increased capillary fragility and permeability Increased risk for infection related to decreased antibodies
Vitamin B complex	Indirect role in wound healing through their influence on host resistance	Decreased enzymes available for energy metabolism
Vitamin A	Increases inflammatory response in wounds, reduces anti-inflammatory effects of corticosteroids on wound healing	Impaired/delayed wound healing related to decreased collagen synthesis; impaired immune function Increased risk for infection
Vitamin K	Important for normal blood clotting Impaired intestinal synthesis associated with the use of antibiotics	Prolonged prothrombin time Hematomas contributing to impaired healing and predisposition to wound infections
Magnesium	Essential cofactor for many enzymes that are involved in the process of protein synthesis and wound repair	Impaired/delayed wound healing (impaired collagen production)
Copper	Required cofactor in the development of connective tissue	Impaired wound healing
Zinc	Involved in DNA synthesis, protein synthesis, cellular proliferation needed for wound healing Essential to immune function	Impaired immune response

DNA, deoxyribonucleic acid.
Adapted from Norris, T. L. (2019). *Porth's pathophysiology: Concepts of altered health states* (10th ed.). Philadelphia, PA: Wolters Kluwer.

on a regular basis in the 2 weeks prior to surgery (see Chapter 4 for an assessment of alcohol and drug use).

Respiratory Status

The patient is educated about breathing exercises and the use of an incentive spirometer, if indicated, to achieve optimal respiratory function prior to surgery. The potential compromise of ventilation during all phases of surgical treatment necessitates a proactive response to respiratory infections. Surgery is usually postponed for elective cases if the patient has a respiratory infection. Patients with underlying respiratory disease (e.g., asthma, chronic obstructive pulmonary disease) are assessed carefully for current threats to their pulmonary status.

Preoperative smoking cessation interventions can be effective in changing smoking behavior and reducing the incidence of postoperative complications. Patients who smoke are more likely to experience poor wound healing, a higher incidence of SSI, and complications that include VTE

and pneumonia. During the preoperative assessment, patients should be asked about current and previous tobacco use. The PAT visit is an optimal time to advocate for smoking cessation (Cuomo et al., 2018). Patients undergoing elective cases may have their surgery delayed or cancelled due to the potential complications associated with smoking. Those at highest risk of complications are patients scheduled to receive artificial implants such as grafts, total joint replacements, or breast enhancements (Devlin & Smeltzer, 2017).

Cardiovascular Status

Patient preparation for surgical intervention includes ensuring that the cardiovascular system can support the oxygen, fluid, and nutritional needs of the perioperative period. Patients are assessed for cardiac comorbidities including congestive heart failure, shortness of breath upon movement, and arrhythmias (Clifford, 2018). Preoperatively, patients may receive a chest x-ray and electrocardiogram (ECG) to rule out any undiagnosed cardiac condition. Before surgery, the patient's baseline vital signs and blood pressure are taken. In elective situations, surgery may be postponed if there is evidence of cardiac decomposition or unexplained elevated blood pressure (Phillips, 2017).

Hepatic and Renal Function

The presurgical goal is optimal function of the liver and urinary systems so that medications, anesthetic agents, body wastes, and toxins are adequately metabolized and removed from the body. The liver, lungs, and kidneys are the routes for elimination of drugs and toxins.

The liver is important in the biotransformation of anesthetic compounds. Disorders of the liver may substantially affect how anesthetic agents are metabolized. Acute liver disease is associated with high surgical mortality; preoperative improvement in liver function is a goal. Careful assessment may include various liver function tests (see Chapter 43).

The kidneys are involved in excreting anesthetic medications and their metabolites; therefore, surgery is contraindicated if a patient has acute nephritis, acute renal insufficiency with oliguria or anuria, or other acute renal problems (see Chapter 48). Exceptions include surgeries performed as lifesaving measures, surgery to enable easier access for dialysis, or those necessary to improve urinary function (e.g., obstructive uropathy or hydronephrosis).

Endocrine Function

Dysfunction of the endocrine system is associated with overproduction or underproduction of a hormone or hormones. This dysfunction may be the primary reason for surgery or it may coexist in patients who need surgery on other organ systems (Odom-Forren, 2018). Patients who have received corticosteroids are at risk for adrenal insufficiency. The use of corticosteroids for any purpose during the preceding year must be reported to the anesthesiologist or CRNA and surgeon. The patient is monitored for signs of adrenal insufficiency (see Chapter 45).

Patients with uncontrolled thyroid disorders are at risk for thyrotoxicosis (with hyperthyroid disorders) or respiratory failure (with hypothyroid disorders). The patient with an associated history of a thyroid disorder is assessed preoperatively (see Chapter 45).

The patient with diabetes who is undergoing surgery is at risk for both hypoglycemia and hyperglycemia. Hypoglycemia may develop during anesthesia or postoperatively from inadequate carbohydrates or excessive administration of insulin. Hyperglycemia, which can increase the risk of SSI, may result from the stress of surgery, which can trigger increased levels of catecholamine. Other risks are acidosis and glucosuria. Although the surgical risk in the patient with controlled diabetes is no greater than in the patient without diabetes, strict glycemic control leads to better outcomes (ASPAN, 2019). Frequent monitoring of blood glucose levels is important before, during, and after surgery. (See Chapter 46 for a discussion of the patient with diabetes.)

Immune Function

An important function of the preoperative assessment is to determine the presence of infection or allergies. Routine laboratory tests used to detect infection include the white blood cell (WBC) and the urinalysis. Surgery may be postponed in the presence of infection or elevated temperature.

It is important to identify and document any sensitivity to medications, solutions, adhesives, and past adverse reactions (ASPAN, 2019). The patient is asked to identify any substances that precipitated previous allergic reactions, including medications, blood transfusions, contrast agents, latex, and food products, and to describe the signs and symptoms produced by these substances. A sample latex allergy screening questionnaire is shown in Figure 14-2.

Latex Allergy Assessment

Ask the patient the following questions. Check "Yes" or "No" in the box.	YES	NO
1. Has a doctor ever told you that you are allergic to latex?		
2. Do you have on-the-job exposure to latex?		
3. Were you born with problems involving your spinal cord?		
4. Have you ever had allergies, asthma, hay fever, eczema, or problems with rashes?		
5. Have you ever had respiratory distress, rapid heart rate, or swelling?		
6. Have you ever had swelling, itching, hives, or other symptoms after contact with a balloon?		
7. Have you ever had swelling, itching, hives, or other symptoms after a dental examination or procedure?		
8. Have you ever had swelling, itching, hives, or other symptoms following a vaginal or rectal examination or after contact with a diaphragm or condom?		
9. Have you ever had swelling, itching, hives, or other symptoms during or within 1 hour after wearing rubber gloves?		
10. Have you ever had a rash on your hands that lasted longer than 1 week?		
11. Have you ever had swelling, itching, hives, runny nose, eye irritation, wheezing, or asthma after contact with any latex or rubber product?		
12. Have you ever had swelling, itching, hives, or other symptoms after being examined by someone wearing rubber or latex gloves?		
13. Are you allergic to bananas, avocados, kiwi, or chestnuts?		
14. Have you ever had an unexplained anaphylactic episode?		

Preop RN Signature: _____

Patient Name: _____

Procedure: _____

Scheduled Date / Time: _____

Surgeon: _____

Figure 14-2 • Example of a latex allergy assessment form. Courtesy of Inova Fair Oaks Hospital, Fairfax, VA.

TABLE 14-3	Examples of Medications with the Potential to Affect the Surgical Experience
Agent	**Effect of Interaction with Anesthetics**
Corticosteroids Dexamethasone	Cardiovascular collapse can occur if discontinued suddenly. Therefore, a bolus of corticosteroids may be administered IV immediately before and after surgery.
Diuretics Hydrochlorothiazide	During anesthesia, may cause excessive respiratory depression resulting from an associated electrolyte imbalance.
Phenothiazines Chlorpromazine hydrochloride	May increase the hypotensive action of anesthetics.
Tranquilizers Diazepam	May cause anxiety, tension, and even seizures if withdrawn suddenly.
Insulins Insulin	Interaction between anesthetics and insulin must be considered when a patient with diabetes is undergoing surgery. IV insulin may need to be given to keep the blood glucose within the normal range.
Anticoagulants Warfarin	Can increase the risk of bleeding during the intraoperative and postoperative periods; should be discontinued in anticipation of elective surgery. The surgeon will determine how long before the elective surgery the patient should stop taking an anticoagulant, depending on the type of planned procedure and the medical condition of the patient.
Anticonvulsant Medications Carbamazepine	IV administration of medication may be needed to keep the patient seizure-free in the intraoperative and postoperative periods.
Thyroid Hormone Levothyroxine sodium	IV administration may be needed during the postoperative period to maintain thyroid levels.
Opioids Morphine sulfate	Long-term use of opioids for chronic pain (≥6 mo) in the preoperative period may alter the patient's response to analgesic agents.

IV, intravenous.
Adapted from Comerford, K. C., & Durkin, M. T. (2020). *Nursing 2020 drug handbook*. Philadelphia, PA: Wolters Kluwer.

Immunosuppression is common with corticosteroid therapy, organ transplantation, radiation therapy, chemotherapy, and disorders affecting the immune system, such as acquired immunodeficiency syndrome and leukemia. The mildest symptoms or slightest temperature elevation must be investigated.

Previous Medication Use

A medication history is obtained because of the possible interactions with medications that might be given during surgery and the effects of any of these medications on the patient's perioperative course. Any medications the patient is using or has used in the past are documented, including OTC preparations and herbal agents, as well as the frequency with which they are used. Many medications have an effect on physiologic functions; interactions of such medications with anesthetic agents can cause serious problems, such as hypotension and circulatory collapse. Medications that cause particular concern are listed in Table 14-3.

Aspirin, clopidogrel, and other medications that inhibit platelet aggregation should be prudently discontinued 7 to 10 days before surgery; otherwise, the patient may be at increased risk for bleeding (Rothrock, 2019). Any use of aspirin or other OTC medications is noted in the patient's

medical record and conveyed to the intraoperative team. The anesthesia provider evaluates the potential effects of prior medication therapy, considering the length of time the patient has used the medication, the physical condition of the patient, and the nature of the proposed surgery.

> ### ◄ Quality and Safety Nursing Alert
>
> *The possible adverse interactions of some medications require the nurse to assess and document the patient's use of prescription medications, OTC medications (especially aspirin), herbal agents, and the frequency with which medications are used. The nurse must clearly communicate this information to the intraoperative team.*

Preprocedure evaluation needs to include dietary and herbal supplements that may increase surgical risks (Odom-Forren, 2018). Commonly used herbal medications and supplements along with their indications for use and possible surgical risks can be found in Table 14-4. Additional herbal medications may include echinacea and licorice extract (*Glycyrrhizic acid*). Many patients fail to report the use of herbal medicines to health care service providers; therefore, the nurse must ask surgical patients specifically about the use of these agents.

TABLE 14-4	Herbs or Supplements and Possible Surgical Risks	
Herb or Supplement	**Indication for Use**	**Possible Surgical Risk**
Ephedra (Ma-Huang)	Appetite suppressant	May interact with medications to cause increased BP and HR
Garlic (*Allium sativum*)	Reported to lower BP and cholesterol levels	Can increase bleeding
Ginkgo biloba	Used to improve memory	Can increase bleeding
Ginseng	Used to increase concentration	Can increase HR and risk of bleeding
Kava kava (*Piper methysticum*)	Used to decrease anxiety	Can increase the effect of anesthesia
St. John's wort (*Hypericum perforatum*)	Used to decrease anxiety, help with depression and sleep problems	May prolong the effects of anesthesia
Valerian (*Valeriana officinalis*)	Used as a sleep aid	May prolong the effects of some types of anesthesia
Vitamin E	Thought to slow the aging process	Can increase bleeding and may cause BP problems

BP, blood pressure; HR, heart rate.
Adapted from American Society of Anesthesiologists. (2017). Herbal and dietary supplements and anesthesia. Retrieved on 6/3/2019 at: www.asahq.org/when secondscount/wp-content/uploads/2017/10/asa_supplements-anesthesia_final.pdf.

The American Society of Anesthesiologists (ASA) issued a statement cautioning patients who take herbal products to refrain from taking them for at least 2 weeks before surgery (American Society of Anesthesiologists [ASA], 2017).

Psychosocial Factors

The nurse anticipates that most patients have emotional reactions prior to surgery—obvious or veiled, normal or abnormal. Fear may be related to the unknown, lack of control, or of death and may be influenced by anesthesia, pain, complications, cancer, or prior surgical experience. Preoperative anxiety can be a preemptive response to a threat to the patient's role in life, a permanent incapacity or body integrity, increased responsibilities or burden on family members, or life itself. Less obvious concerns may occur because of previous experiences with the health care system and people the patient has known with the same condition. Psychological distress directly influences body functioning. Identification of anxiety by the health care team using supportive guidance at every juncture of the perioperative process helps to ease anxiety. Research suggests that negative postoperative outcomes can result from fear and anxiety preoperatively. Anxiety triggers a physical response, stimulating the release of epinephrine and norepinephrine, which in turn raises blood pressure and increases heart rate, cardiac output, and blood glucose

levels. Therefore, overall healing may be impaired while pain and risk of infection may increase postoperatively (Bagheri, Ebrahimi, Abbasi, et al., 2019).

People express fear in different ways. Some patients may ask repeated questions, regardless of information already shared with them. Others may withdraw, deliberately avoiding communication by reading, watching television, or talking about trivialities. Consequently, the nurse must be empathetic, listen well, and provide information that helps alleviate concerns.

An important outcome of the psychosocial assessment is the determination of the extent and role of the patient's support network. The value and reliability of available support systems are assessed. Other information, such as knowledge of the usual level of functioning and typical daily activities, may assist in the patient's care and recovery. Assessing the patient's readiness to learn and determining the best approach to maximize comprehension provide the basis for preoperative patient education. This is of particular importance in patients who are developmentally delayed and those who are cognitively impaired, where the approach to patient education and consent will include the legal guardian.

Spiritual and Cultural Beliefs

Showing respect for a patient's cultural values and beliefs facilitates rapport and trust. Assessment includes identifying the ethnic group to which the patient relates and the customs and beliefs the patient holds about illness and health care providers. Knowledge of the patient's physiologic, psychosocial, cultural, spiritual, and educational needs allows the perioperative nurse to provide a holistic approach to care. A holistic picture of the patient allows the perioperative nurse the opportunity to identify patient care issues that extend beyond the medical diagnosis and planned surgical procedure and choose a nursing diagnosis based on key elements of the patient's needs and goals. The nurse advocates for the patient and develops a holistic care plan that is communicated to members of the intraoperative and postoperative team. Perioperative patient advocacy entails paying respect to other human beings, preserving the patient's expressed values, and treating all patients equally (Sundqvist, Holmefur, Nilsson, et al., 2016).

Certain ethnic groups are unaccustomed to expressing feelings openly with strangers, and nurses need to consider this pattern of communication when assessing pain. In some cultural groups, it is seen as impolite to make direct eye contact with others and doing so is seen as disrespectful. The nurse should know that this lack of eye contact is not avoidance nor does it reflect a lack of interest. Other ethnicities view the top of the head as sacred; therefore, a nurse would not put the surgical cap on the patient but would ask the patient to don the cap.

Perhaps the most valuable skill at the nurse's disposal is listening carefully to the patient and observing body language, especially when obtaining the history. Invaluable information and insights may be gained through effective communication and interviewing skills. An unhurried, understanding, and caring nurse promotes confidence on the part of the patient.

Preoperative Nursing Interventions

A wide range of interventions are used to prepare the patient physically and psychologically and to maintain safety. Beginning with the nursing history and physical examination, listing of medications taken routinely, history of allergies, and surgical and anesthetic histories, the patient's overall health status and level of experience and understanding may be established.

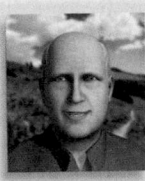 **Providing Patient Education**

Nurses have long recognized the value of preoperative education (Rothrock, 2019). Each patient's education is individualized, with consideration for any unique concerns or learning needs. Multiple education strategies should be used (e.g., verbal, written, return demonstration), depending on the patient's needs and abilities.

Preoperative education is initiated as soon as possible, beginning in the physician's office, in the clinic, or at the time of PAT when diagnostic tests are performed. During PAT, the nurse or health care provider makes resources available related to patient education, such as written instructions (designed to be copied and given to patients), audiovisual and online resources, and telephone numbers, to ensure that education continues until the patient arrives for the surgical intervention. When possible, education is spaced over a period of time to allow the patient to assimilate information and ask questions as they arise.

Frequently, education sessions are combined with various preparation procedures to allow for an easy and timely flow of information. The nurse should guide the patient through the experience and allow ample time for questions. Education should go beyond descriptions of the procedure and should include explanations of the sensations the patient will experience. Telling the patient that a preoperative medication will cause relaxation before the operation is not as effective as also noting that a medication will act quickly and may result in light-headedness, dizziness, and drowsiness. Knowing what to expect will help the patient anticipate these reactions and attain a superior degree of relaxation. Overly detailed descriptions may increase anxiety in some patients; therefore, the nurse should be sensitive to this, by watching and listening, and provide less detail based on the individual patient's needs.

Unfolding Patient Stories: Vernon Watkins • Part 1

Vernon Watkins, a 69-year-old male, came to the emergency department with severe abdominal pain, and a bowel perforation was diagnosed. He is being prepared for surgery. Significant medical history includes controlled hypertension and smoking for 50 years. What preoperative education should the nurse discuss with Mr. Watkins prior to his emergent surgery? (Vernon Watkins' story continues in Chapter 58.)

Care for Vernon and other patients in a realistic virtual environment: **vSim** *for Nursing* (**thepoint.lww. com/vSimMedicalSurgical**). Practice documenting these patients' care in DocuCare (**thepoint.lww.com/ DocuCareEHR**).

Deep Breathing, Coughing, and Incentive Spirometry

One goal of preoperative nursing care is to educate the patient how to promote optimal lung expansion and resulting blood oxygenation after anesthesia. The patient assumes a sitting position to enhance lung expansion. The nurse then demonstrates how to take a deep, slow breath and how to exhale slowly. After practicing deep breathing several times, the patient is instructed to breathe deeply, exhale through the mouth, take a short breath, and cough deeply in the lungs (see Chart 14-5). The nurse or respiratory therapist also demonstrates how to use an incentive spirometer, a device that provides measurement and feedback related to breathing effectiveness (see Chapter 19). In addition to enhancing respiration, these exercises may help the patient relax.

If a thoracic or abdominal incision is anticipated, the nurse demonstrates how to splint the incision to minimize pressure and control pain. The patient should put the palms of both hands together, interlacing the fingers snugly. Splinting or placing the hands across the incision site acts as an effective support when coughing. The patient is informed that medications are available to relieve pain and should be taken regularly for pain relief so that effective deep-breathing and coughing exercises can be performed comfortably. The goal in promoting coughing is to mobilize secretions so that they can be removed. Deep breathing before coughing stimulates the cough reflex. If the patient does not cough effectively, atelectasis (collapse of the alveoli), pneumonia, or other lung complications may occur.

Mobility and Active Body Movement

The goals of promoting mobility postoperatively are to improve circulation, prevent venous stasis, and promote optimal respiratory function. The patient should be taught that early and frequent ambulation postoperatively, as tolerated, will help prevent complications.

The nurse explains the rationale for frequent position changes after surgery and then shows the patient how to turn from side to side and how to assume the lateral position without causing pain or disrupting IV lines, drainage tubes, or other equipment. Any special position the patient needs to maintain after surgery (e.g., adduction or elevation of an extremity) is discussed, as is the importance of maintaining as much mobility as possible despite restrictions. Reviewing the process before surgery is helpful, because the patient may be too uncomfortable or drowsy after surgery to absorb new information.

Exercise of the extremities includes extension and flexion of the knee and hip joints (similar to bicycle riding while lying on the side) unless contraindicated by type of surgical procedure (e.g., hip replacement). The great toe is pointed and rotated as though tracing a large circle (see Chart 14-5). The elbow and shoulder are also put through their range of motion. At first, the patient is assisted and reminded to perform these exercises. Later, the patient is encouraged to do them independently. Muscle tone is maintained so that ambulation will be easier. The nurse should remember to use proper body mechanics and to instruct the patient to do the same. Whenever the patient is positioned, their body needs to be properly aligned.

Chart 14-5

PATIENT EDUCATION

Preoperative Instructions to Prevent Postoperative Complications

Diaphragmatic Breathing

Diaphragmatic breathing refers to a flattening of the dome of the diaphragm during inspiration, with resultant enlargement of the upper abdomen as air rushes in. During expiration, the abdominal muscles contract.

1. Practice in the same position you would assume in bed after surgery: a semi-Fowler position, propped in bed with the back and shoulders well supported with pillows.
2. Feel the movement with your hands resting lightly on the front of the lower ribs and fingertips against the lower chest.

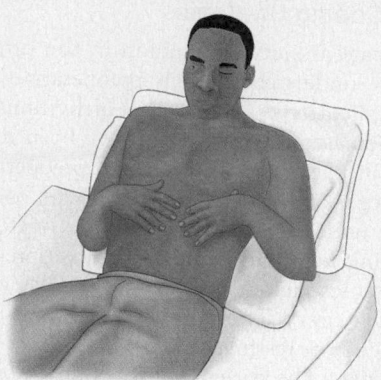

Diaphragmatic breathing

3. Breathe out gently and fully as the ribs sink down and inward toward midline.
4. Then take a deep breath through your nose and mouth, letting the abdomen rise as the lungs fill with air.
5. Hold this breath for a count of five.
6. Exhale and let out *all* the air through your nose and mouth.
7. Repeat this exercise 15 times with a short rest after each group of five.
8. Practice this twice a day preoperatively.

Coughing

1. Lean forward slightly from a sitting position in bed, interlace your fingers together, and place your hands across the incision site to act as a splint for support when coughing.

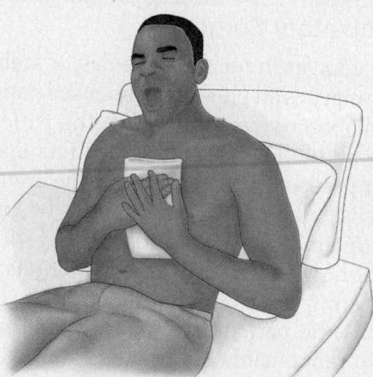

Splinting of chest when coughing

2. Breathe with the diaphragm as described under "Diaphragmatic Breathing."

3. With your mouth slightly open, breathe in fully.
4. "Hack" out sharply for three short breaths.
5. Then, keeping your mouth open, take in a quick deep breath and immediately give a strong cough once or twice. This helps clear secretions from your chest. It may cause some discomfort but will not harm your incision.

Leg Exercises

1. Lie in a semi-Fowler position and perform the following simple exercises to improve circulation.
2. Bend your knee and raise your foot—hold it a few seconds, then extend the leg and lower it to the bed.

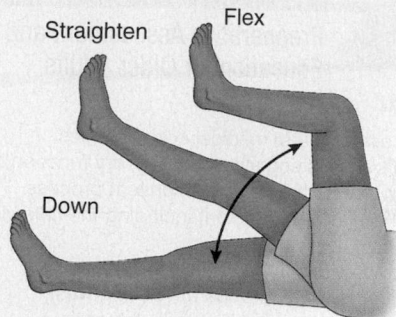

Straighten   Flex

Down

Leg exercises

3. Do this five times with one leg and then repeat with the other leg.
4. Then trace circles with the feet by bending them down, in toward each other, up, and then out.
5. Repeat these movements five times.

Turning to the Side

1. Turn on your side with the uppermost leg flexed most and supported on a pillow.
2. Grasp the side rail as an aid to maneuver to the side.
3. Practice diaphragmatic breathing and coughing while on your side.

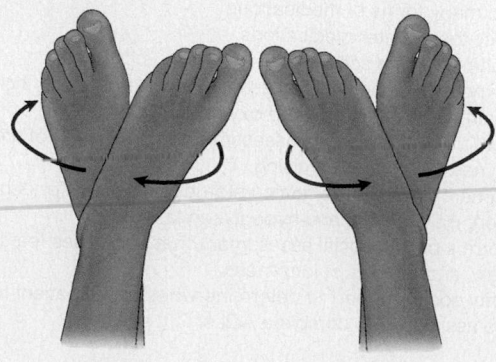

Foot exercises

Getting Out of Bed

1. Turn on your side.
2. Push yourself up with one hand as you swing your legs out of bed.

Pain Management

A pain assessment should include differentiation between acute and chronic pain. A pain intensity scale should be introduced and explained to the patient to promote more effective postoperative pain management. (See Chapter 9 for examples of pain scales.) Preoperative patient education also needs to include the difference between acute and chronic pain so that the patient is prepared to differentiate acute postoperative pain from a chronic condition such as back pain. Preoperative pain assessment and education for the older patient may require additional attention (see Chart 14-6).

Chart 14-6 · Preoperative Assessment and Education for Older Adults

Assessment

- Assess for allergies and medical comorbidities.
- Assess the patient's cognitive and sensory function before the surgeon begins the informed consent process.
- Perform a Fall Risk Assessment including the following factors:
  - History of previous falls
  - Medication use (e.g., preoperative sedatives)
  - Level of consciousness (e.g., alert, lethargic)
  - Ability to follow directions (e.g., cognitive impairment, language barrier)
  - Sensory impairments (e.g., vision, hearing)
  - Level of coordination or balance
  - Toileting needs (e.g., incontinence, frequency, need for assistance)
  - Presence of external devices (e.g., catheters, drains)
- Determine the need for a designated support person or power of attorney to complete the informed consent process.
- Review medications to identify potential polypharmaceutical risks to include the following:
  - Multiple medications
  - Multiple prescribers
  - Several filling pharmacies
  - Too many forms of medications
  - Over-the-counter medications
  - Multiple dosing schedules
- Document baseline physical assessment parameters, including pain, cardiac rhythm, and oxygen saturation level.
- Document a detailed skin assessment with notation of areas of dryness, lesions, or bruising.
- Document preoperative fasting status and assess for dehydration, malnutrition, and hypoglycemia.
- Perform a psychosocial assessment that addresses fears, anxiety, and feelings of loneliness.
- Identify social support to determine whether the patient has home assistance to complete ADLs.

Education

- Discuss advanced directives and code status to identify the patient's wishes.
- Educate the patient about the benefits of controlling pain.
- Be prepared to spend additional time, increase the amount of therapeutic touch utilized, and encourage family members to be present to decrease anxiety.

ADLs, activities of daily living.
Adapted from Ogg, M. (2018). Clinical issues. *AORN Journal,* *108*(2), 195–203; Phillips, N. (2017). *Berry and Kohn's operating room technique.* St. Louis, MO: Elsevier.

Postoperatively, medications are given to relieve pain and maintain comfort without suppressing respiratory function. The patient is instructed to take the medication as frequently as prescribed during the initial postoperative period for pain relief. Anticipated methods of administration of analgesic agents for inpatients include patient-controlled analgesia (PCA), epidural catheter bolus or infusion, or patient-controlled epidural analgesia (PCEA; see Chapter 9 for discussion of PCA and PCEA). A patient who is expected to go home will likely receive oral analgesic agents. These methods are discussed with the patient before surgery, and the patient's interest and willingness to use them are assessed.

Cognitive Coping Strategies

Although some anxiety is common in the surgical setting, untreated or undertreated high preoperative anxiety can lead to complications. Tachycardia, arrhythmias, hypertension, and increased levels of pain have been reported postoperatively in patients with increased preoperative anxiety (Jaruzel, Gregoski, Mueller, et al., 2019). Cognitive strategies may be useful for relieving tension, overcoming anxiety, decreasing fear, and achieving relaxation. Examples of general strategies include:

- *Guided Imagery:* The patient concentrates on a pleasant experience or restful scene.
- *Distraction:* The patient thinks of an enjoyable story or recites a favorite poem or song.
- *Optimistic Self-Recitation:* The patient recites optimistic thoughts ("I know all will go well").
- *Music Therapy:* The patient listens to soothing music (an easy-to-administer, inexpensive, noninvasive intervention).
- *Aromatherapy:* The patient inhales aromatic oils to trigger emotional and physical relaxation responses through the olfactory system and brain.
- *Reiki:* The practitioner places hands over the patient to (theoretically) transfer energy to promote healing and relaxation.

Alternative interventions may include acupuncture, yoga therapy, muscle relaxation, and therapeutic touch.

Education for Patients Undergoing Ambulatory Surgery

Preoperative education for the same-day or ambulatory surgical patient comprises all previously discussed patient education as well as collaborative planning with the patient and family for discharge and follow-up home care. The major difference in outpatient preoperative education is the environment.

Preoperative education content may be presented in a group class, in a media presentation, at PAT, or by telephone in conjunction with the preoperative interview. In addition to answering questions and describing what to expect, the nurse tells the patient when and where to report, what to bring (insurance card, list of medications and allergies), what to leave at home (jewelry, watch, medications, contact lenses), and what to wear (loose-fitting, comfortable clothes; flat shoes). The nurse in the surgeon's office may initiate education before the perioperative telephone contact.

During the final preoperative telephone call, education is completed or reinforced as needed and last-minute instructions are given. The patient is reminded not to eat or drink for a specified period of time and about skin cleansing techniques prior to surgery (see later section on preparing the skin).

Providing Psychosocial Interventions

The nurse assesses for and provides interventions to enhance coping mechanisms to deal effectively with anxiety and fears, and thus provide emotional comfort (Phillips, 2017). Preoperatively, the nurse assesses any patient specific needs that may affect the emotional, psychosocial, or physical surgical experience.

Reducing Anxiety and Decreasing Fear

Perioperative nurses in the preoperative department have a limited amount of time to acquire information and establish trust. Nurses must introduce themselves, giving their title and a brief synopsis of their professional role and background. Each preoperative patient should be acknowledged as an individual, and each patient's needs and desires must be assessed. The patient should be thanked for choosing that particular hospital or surgical center. These methods facilitate establishing a positive nurse–patient relationship. Discussion of the surgical experience, its length, and explanation of what will happen may diminish the patient's anxiety.

During the preoperative assessment of psychological factors and spiritual and cultural beliefs, the nurse assists the patient to identify coping strategies that he or she has previously used to decrease fear. Discussions with the patient to help determine the source of fears can help with expression of concerns. The patient benefits from knowing when family and friends will be able to visit after surgery and that a spiritual advisor will be available if desired. Knowing ahead of time about the possible need for a ventilator, drainage tubes, or other types of equipment helps decrease anxiety related to the postoperative period. Careful attention should be placed on patients who experience a delay in surgery as prolonged wait times in the preoperative area can lead to increased fear and anxiety.

Respecting Cultural, Spiritual, and Religious Beliefs

The nurse assesses for any patient specific needs that may affect the spiritual, emotional, or physical surgical experience. In some cultures, for example, people are stoic in regard to pain, whereas in others they are more expressive. These responses should be recognized as normal for those patients and families and should be respected by perioperative personnel. If patients decline blood transfusions for religious reasons (Jehovah's Witnesses), this information needs to be clearly identified in the preoperative period, documented, and communicated to the appropriate personnel. Although minimally invasive surgery has significantly lowered blood loss, any surgical procedure has the potential for hemorrhage.

Maintaining Patient Safety

Protecting patients from injury is one of the major roles of the perioperative nurse. Adherence to AORN-recommended practices and The Joint Commission's National Patient Safety Goals (see Chart 14-7) are crucial (Rothrock, 2019). These apply to hospitals as well as to ambulatory surgery centers and office-based surgery facilities (Joint Commission, 2019).

Chart 14-7

Summary of the 2019 National Patient Safety Goals

- Identify patients correctly
- Improve staff communication
- Use medicines safely
- Use alarms safely
- Prevent infection
- Identify patient safety risks
- Prevent mistakes in surgery

Adapted from Joint Commission (2019). 2019 National Patient Safety Goals. Retrieved on 5/22/19 at: www.jointcommission.org/assets/1/6/2019_HAP_NPSGs_final2.pdf

---

Managing Nutrition and Fluids

The purpose of withholding food and fluid before surgery is to prevent aspiration. Specific recommendations for restrictions depend on the age of the patient and the type of food eaten. For example, adults may be advised to fast for 8 hours after eating fatty food and 6 hours after ingesting milk products. Healthy patients are allowed clear liquids up to 2 hours before an elective procedure. New methods of "carbohydrate loading" have been implemented preoperatively in surgeries that do not involve the gastrointestinal system (i.e., thoracic, urologic, obstetric, orthopedic). A carbohydrate-rich drink has been used as a safe fasting process before surgery. It has been reported that these solutions do not pose a risk for aspiration and decrease insulin resistance when the duration of gastric emptying and the amount of liquid intake are controlled (Cakar, Yilmaz, Cakar, et al., 2017). Preoperative carbohydrate loading in patients undergoing surgery as part of an enhanced recovery after surgery protocol has demonstrated positive outcomes including decreased LOS, decreased incidence of PONV, and decreased pain (Pachella, Mehran, Curtin, et al., 2019).

Preparing the Bowel

Enemas are not commonly prescribed preoperatively unless the patient is undergoing abdominal or pelvic surgery. In this case, a cleansing enema or laxative may be prescribed the evening before surgery and may be repeated the morning of surgery. The goals of this preparation are to allow satisfactory visualization of the surgical site and to prevent trauma to the intestine or contamination of the peritoneum by fecal material. Unless the condition of the patient presents some contraindication, the toilet or bedside commode, rather than the bedpan, is used for evacuating the enema if the patient is hospitalized during this time. In addition, antibiotics may be prescribed to reduce intestinal flora.

Preparing the Skin

The goal of preoperative skin preparation is to decrease bacteria without injuring the skin. If the surgery is not performed as an emergency, most health care facilities and ambulatory surgical centers have implemented preoperative antiseptic skin cleansing protocols. At a minimum, preoperative bathing should consist of a full-body wash using antimicrobial soap the night before the planned surgery (Berríos-Torres,

Umscheid, Bratzler, et al., 2018). Additional body cleansing with chlorhexidine wipes may occur in the preoperative area via the nurse or by the patient under the direction of the nurse. Surgical site hair removal should occur in the preoperative area. Electric clippers, not skin razors, are the preferred method for hair removal. Special consideration is given to those undergoing gynecologic, urologic, and cranial surgeries. To ensure the correct site, the surgical site is typically marked by the patient and the surgeon prior to the procedure.

Immediate Preoperative Nursing Interventions

The nurse confirms the patient identity upon entry and dons "alert" bracelets on the patient when applicable: medication allergies, fall risk, extremity precautions (for needle sticks and blood pressures), and code status. The patient changes into a hospital gown, covers the head with a disposable bouffant, and nail polish is removed (if present) as it may interfere with hemodynamic monitoring. The mouth is inspected, and dentures or plates are removed. If left in the mouth, these items could easily fall to the back of the throat during induction of anesthesia and cause respiratory obstruction.

Jewelry is not worn to the OR; wedding rings and jewelry or body piercings should be removed to prevent injury. If a patient objects to removing jewelry, the patient must be notified of the risks associated with it. All articles of value, including assistive devices, dentures, glasses, and prosthetic devices, are given to family members or are labeled clearly with the patient's name and stored in a safe and secure place according to the institution's policy.

Preoperative Checklist

1. Patient's name: _____ Date: _____ Height: _____ Weight: _____
   Identification band present: _____
2. Informed consent signed: _____ Special permits signed: _____
3. Surgical site: _____ (Ex: Sterilization)
4. History & physical examination report present: _____ Date: _____
5. Laboratory records present:_____
   CBC: _____ Hgb: _____ Urinalysis: _____ Hct: _____
6. Traveled Outside of the United States in the last 14 days: Yes/No
7. NPO Status: Date/Time last liquid: _____ Date/Time last solid: _____

8. Item	Present	Removed
a. Natural teeth		
Dentures; upper, lower, partial		
Bridge, fixed; crown		
b. Contact lenses		
c. Other prostheses—type: _____		
d. Jewelry:		
Wedding band (taped/tied)		
Rings		
Earrings: pierced, clip-on		
Neck chains		
Any other body piercings		
e. Make-up		
Nail polish		
9. Clothing		
a. Clean patient gown		
b. Cap		
c. Sanitary pad, etc.		

10. Family instructed where to wait? _____
11. Valuables secured? _____
12. Blood available? _____ Ordered? _____ Where? _____
13. Preanesthetic medication given: _____
    Type: _____ Time: _____
14. Voided: _____ Amount: _____ Time: _____ Catheter: _____
    Mouth care given: _____
15. Vital signs: Temperature: _____ Pulse: _____ Resp: _____ Blood Pressure: _____
16. Special problems/precautions: (Allergies, deafness, etc.): _____
17. Area of skin preparation: _____
18. _____ Date: _____ Time:_____
    Signature: Nurse releasing patient

Figure 14-3 • Example of a preoperative checklist.

All patients (except those with urologic disorders) should void immediately before going to the OR. This is particularly important in promoting visibility of anatomy and continence during low abdominal surgery. Urinary catheterization is performed in the OR only as necessary.

Administering Medication

The use of preanesthetic medication is minimal with ambulatory or outpatient surgery but may be used to help some patients remain calm and comfortable (Phillips, 2017). If a preanesthetic medication is given, the patient is kept in bed with the side rails raised, because the medication can cause lightheadedness or drowsiness. During this time, the nurse observes the patient for any untoward reaction to the medications.

Antibiotics are given preoperatively, as needed, to help reduce the risk of SSIs. The antibiotic is typically prescribed prior to the patient arriving and is prepared by the pharmacy so that it can be administered in a timely fashion prior to surgery. Administration of the appropriate antibiotic should occur so that the peak efficacy of the medication is in the patient's tissues and bloodstream immediately before incision (Bashaw & Keister, 2018).

Maintaining the Preoperative Record

Preoperative checklists contain critical elements that must be checked and verified before the procedure (Rothrock, 2019). The nurse completes a preoperative checklist (see Fig. 14-3). The completed medical record (with the preoperative checklist and verification form) accompanies the patient to the OR with the surgical consent form attached, along with all laboratory reports and nurses' records. These documents may also be found in the patient's electronic health record; however, they must be easily accessed and verified by the surgical team. Any patient alerts (allergies, safety precautions) and individual needs are "flagged" on either the paper or electronic record.

Preoperative Patient Warming

Preoperative patient warming for a period of at least 30 minutes can be beneficial to prevent hypothermia development after anesthesia induction. Various techniques include warm blankets, forced air warming, and warmed IV fluid administration. Unintended hypothermia is associated with increased adverse patient outcomes, including bleeding, delayed surgical wound healing, increased length of stay (LOS) in the PACU, cardiac dysfunction, and longer inpatient hospital stay (Williams, 2018). Patients should be educated about the purpose of the warming intervention and should be assessed for abnormal temperatures, profuse sweating, and discomfort (Williams, 2018). Research suggests that nurses play a crucial part in the reduction of unintended hypothermia, below 36°C (96.8°F), by applying prewarming techniques in the preoperative area (Rosenkilde, Vamosi, Lauridsen, et al., 2017). See the Nursing Research Profile in Chart 14-8.

The patient is taken to the preoperative area, greeted by name, and positioned comfortably on the stretcher or bed. The surrounding area should be kept quiet if the preoperative medication is to have maximal effect. Unpleasant sounds or conversation should be avoided, because a patient who is sedated may misinterpret them.

Attending to Family Needs

Most hospitals and ambulatory surgery centers have a waiting room where family members and significant others can wait while the patient is undergoing surgery. This room may be equipped with comfortable chairs, televisions, telephones, and light refreshments. Volunteers may remain with the family, offer them coffee, and keep them informed of the patient's progress. After surgery, the surgeon may meet the family in the waiting room and discuss the outcome.

The family and significant others should never judge the seriousness of an operation by the length of time the patient

---

Chart 14-8 **NURSING RESEARCH PROFILE**

The Efficacy of Prewarming in the Preoperative Setting

Rosenkilde, C., Vamosi, M., Lauridsen, J. T., et al. (2017). Efficacy of prewarming with a self-warming blanket for the prevention of unintended perioperative hypothermia in patients undergoing hip or knee arthroplasty. *Journal of PeriAnesthesia Nursing, 32*(5), 419–428.

Purpose

Unintended perioperative hypothermia (UPH) is defined as a core temperature of less than 36°C (96.8°F) in patients in the surgical setting when cooling is not associated with the procedure. Many risks are associated with UPH including increased wound infections, pain, coagulation disorders, and cardiac complications. The purpose of this study was to evaluate UPH rates when a self-warming blanket was utilized by patients undergoing hip or knee joint replacement surgeries.

Design

This was a secondary analysis of two cross-sectional studies. A control group of patients did not receive any warming methods, and another group of patients received a prewarming

intervention. Core temperatures of both groups were taken preoperatively, every 30 minutes throughout the procedure, and postoperatively.

Findings

Sixty patients were included in the study, 30 in each group. The incidence of UPH was identified in 13% of the patients in the prewarmed group and 43% of the patients in the control group. Mean core temperature in the prewarmed group was significantly higher and remained above 36°C in the perioperative period.

Nursing Implications

Careful attention needs to be paid to maintaining normothermia in the patient throughout the entire perioperative phase of care. The findings of this study showed a reduction in UPH rates when patients were prewarmed with a self-warming blanket. Nurses at both outpatient and inpatient surgical settings could use this study to help develop interdisciplinary prewarming techniques and protocols.

is in the OR. A patient may be in the OR much longer than the actual operating time for several reasons:

- Patients are routinely transported well in advance of the actual operating time.
- The anesthesiologist or CRNA often makes additional preparations that may take 30 to 60 minutes.
- The preceding case may take longer than expected, which delays the start of the next surgical procedure.

After surgery, the patient is taken to the PACU to ensure safe emergence from anesthesia. Family members and significant others waiting to see the patient after surgery should be informed that the patient may have certain equipment or devices (e.g., IV lines, indwelling urinary catheter, nasogastric tube, oxygen lines, monitoring equipment, blood transfusion lines) in place when he or she returns from surgery. When the patient returns to the room, the nurse provides explanations regarding the frequent postoperative observations that will be made. However, it is the responsibility of the surgeon, not the nurse, to relay the surgical findings and the prognosis, even when the findings are favorable.

Expected Patient Outcomes

Expected patient activities to decrease anxiety and fear, as well as increase knowledge in the preoperative phase of care are summarized in Chart 14-9. Nurse-sensitive outcomes often include central line–associated bloodstream

infections (CLABSI), catheter-associated urinary tract infections (CAUTI), hospital-acquired pressure ulcers and unit-acquired pressure ulcers.

CRITICAL THINKING EXERCISES

1 **pq** A 55-year-old man who is a patient on the surgical unit where you work is scheduled for a prostatectomy; he is showing signs of increased anxiety, fear, and insomnia. What are the priorities of the perioperative nurse? What further assessments are priorities? What are your priorities for nursing intervention?

2 **ebp** A 60-year-old woman with obesity has been admitted for a minimally invasive hysterectomy. She was diagnosed during her PAT visit with severe OSA. What resources would you use to identify evidence-based practices for prevention of complications during the perioperative period? Identify the evidence, as well as the criteria used to evaluate the strength of the evidence, for the practices identified.

3 **ipc** A 38-year-old man is admitted for knee surgery following a horse riding accident. He is in good physical condition but reports a family history of "problems with anesthesia." What are your immediate preoperative assessments? What should you include in the interprofessional handoff to the surgical team?

Chart 14-9 Expected Patient Activities in the Preoperative Phase of Care

Relief of anxiety, evidenced when the patient:

- Discusses with the anesthesiologist or CRNA concerns related to types of anesthesia and induction
- Verbalizes an understanding of the preanesthetic medication and general anesthesia
- Discusses last-minute concerns with the nurse or physician
- Discusses financial concerns with the social worker, when appropriate
- Requests visit with spiritual advisor, when appropriate
- Appears relaxed when visited by health care team members

Decreased fear, evidenced when the patient:

- Discusses fears with health care professionals or a spiritual advisor, or both
- Verbalizes an understanding of any expected bodily changes, including expected duration of bodily changes

Understanding of the surgical intervention, evidenced when the patient:

- Participates in preoperative preparation as appropriate (e.g., bowel preparation, shower)
- Demonstrates and describes exercises that he or she is expected to perform postoperatively
- Reviews information about postoperative care
- Accepts preanesthetic medication, if prescribed
- Remains in bed once premedicated
- Relaxes during transportation to the operating room or unit
- States rationale for use of side rails
- Discusses postoperative expectations

CRNA, certified registered nurse anesthetist.

REFERENCES

*Asterisk indicates nursing research.

Books

American Society of PeriAnesthesia Nurses (ASPAN). (2019). *2015–2019 Perianesthesia nursing standards, practice recommendations and interpretive statements.* Cherry Hill, NJ: Author.

Association of periOperative Registered Nurses (AORN). (2019). *Association of PeriOperative Registered Nurses (AORN) standards, recommended practice, and guidelines.* Denver, CO: Author.

Barash, P. G., Cullen, B. F., Stoelting, R. K., et al. (2017). *Clinical anesthesia* (8th ed.). Philadelphia, PA: Lippincott Williams & Wilkins.

Comerford, K. C., & Durkin, M. T. (2020). *Nursing 2020 drug handbook.* Philadelphia, PA: Wolters Kluwer.

Norris, T. L. (2019). *Porth's pathophysiology: Concepts of altered health states* (10th ed.). Philadelphia, PA: Wolters Kluwer.

Odom-Forren, J. (2018). *Drain's perianesthesia nursing: A critical care approach.* St Louis, MO: Elsevier.

Phillips, N. (2017). *Berry and Kohn's operating room technique.* St. Louis, MO: Elsevier.

Rothrock, J. (2019). *Alexander's care of the patient in surgery* (16th ed.). St. Louis, MO: Elsevier.

Journals and Electronic Documents

American Society of Anesthesiologists (ASA). (2017). Herbal and dietary supplements and anesthesia. Retrieved on 6/3/2019 at: www.asahq.org/whensecondscount/wp-content/uploads/2017/10/asa_supplements-anesthesia_final.pdf.

Bagheri, H., Ebrahimi, H., Abbasi, A., et al. (2019). Effect of preoperative visitation by operating room staff on preoperative anxiety in patients receiving elective hernia surgery. *Journal of PeriAnesthesia Nursing,* 34(2), 272–280.

Bashaw, M., & Keister, K. (2018). Perioperative strategies to reduce surgical site infections. *AORN Journal,* 109(1), 68–78.

Berríos-Torres, S. I., Umscheid, C. A., Bratzler, D. W., et al. (2017). Centers for Disease Control and Prevention guideline for the prevention of surgical site infection, 2017. *JAMA Surgery, 152*(8), 784–791.

Boudreaux, A. M., & Simmons, J. W. (2019). Prehabilitation and optimization of modifiable patient risk factors: The importance of effective preoperative evaluation to improve patient outcomes. *AORN Journal, 109*(4), 500–507.

Cakar, E., Yilmaz, E., Cakar, E., et al. (2017). The effect of preoperative oral carbohydrate solution intake on patient comfort: A randomized controlled study. *Journal of Perianesthesia Nursing, 32*(6), 589–599.

Centers for Disease Control and Prevention (CDC). (2018). Adult obesity facts. Retrieved on 6/1/19 at: https://www.cdc.gov/obesity/data/adult.html

Chung, F., Abdullah, H., & Liao, P. (2016). STOP-Bang questionnaire: A practical approach to screen for obstructive sleep apnea. *Chest, 149*(3), 631–638.

Clifford, T. (2018). Preoperative optimization. *Journal of PeriAnesthesia Nursing, 33*(6), 1006–1007.

Cuomo, S., Abate, M., Springer, C., et al. (2018). Nurse practitioner–driven optimization of presurgical testing. *Journal of PeriAnesthesia Nursing, 33*(6), 887–894.

Devlin, C. A., & Smeltzer, S. C. (2017). Temporary perioperative tobacco cessation: A literature review. *AORN Journal, 106*(5), 415–423.e5.

Huang, L., Kim, R., & Berry, W. (2013). Creating a culture of safety by using checklists. *AORN Journal, 97*(3), 365–368.

Jaruzel, C., Gregoski, M., Mueller, M., et al. (2019). Aromatherapy for preoperative anxiety: A pilot study. *Journal of PeriAnesthesia Nursing, 34*(2), 259–264.

Joint Commission. (2019). 2019 national patient safety goals. Retrieved on 5/22/19 at: www.jointcommission.org/assets/1/6/2019_HAP_NPSGs_final2.pdf

Link, T. (2018). Guideline implementation: Safe patient handling and movement. *AORN Journal, 108*(6), 663–674.

Malley, A., Kenner, C., Kim, T., et al. (2015). The role of the nurse and the preoperative assessment in patient transitions. *AORN Journal, 102*(2), 181.

Mendez, C., Martinez, E., Lopez, E., et al. (2018). Analysis of environmental conditions in the operating room for latex-allergic patients' safety. *Journal of PeriAnesthesia Nursing, 33*(4), 490–498.

Ogg, M. (2018). Clinical issues. *AORN Journal, 108*(2), 195–203.

Pachella, L., Mehran, R., Curtin, K., et al. (2019). Preoperative carbohydrate loading in patients undergoing thoracic surgery: A quality-improvement project. *Journal of PeriAnesthesia Nursing.* Retrieved on 8/22/19 at: www.sciencedirect.com/science/article/pii/S1089947219301364?via%3DihubxLaura

*Rosenkilde, C., Vamosi, M., Lauridsen, J. T., et al. (2017). Efficacy of prewarming with a self-warming blanket for the prevention of unintended perioperative hypothermia in patients undergoing hip or knee arthroplasty. *Journal of PeriAnesthesia Nursing, 32*(5), 419–428.

Sadler, D. (2017). Advanced surgical technology. *OR Today.* Retrieved on 6/8/19 at: ortoday.com/advanced-surgical-technology/

Sundqvist, A., Holmefur, M., Nilsson, U., et al. (2016). Perioperative patient advocacy: An integrative a review. *Journal of PeriAnesthesia Nursing, 31*(5), 422–433.

Ubaldi, K. (2019). Safe medication management at ambulatory surgery centers. *AORN Journal, 109*(4), 435–442.

Vernon, T., Rice, A., Titch, J., et al. (2019). Implementation of Vulnerable Elders Survey-13 frailty tool to identify at-risk geriatric surgical patients. *Journal of PeriAnesthesia Nursing, 34*(5), 911–918.

Williams, A. (2018). Benefits of passive warming on surgical patients undergoing regional anesthetic procedures. *Journal of PeriAnesthesia Nursing, 33*(6), 928–934.

Resources

American Academy of Ambulatory Care Nursing (AACN), www.aaacn.org
American Association of Gynecologic Laparoscopy (AAGL), www.aagl.org
American Society for Metabolic and Bariatric Surgery (ASMBS), asmbs.org
American Society of Anesthesiologists (ASA), www.asahq.org
American Society of PeriAnesthesia Nurses (ASPAN), www.aspan.org
Association of periOperative Registered Nurses (AORN), www.aorn.org
Joint Commission, www.jointcommission.org

15 Intraoperative Nursing Management

LEARNING OUTCOMES

On completion of this chapter, the learner will be able to:

1. Describe the roles of the surgical team members during the intraoperative phase of care.
2. Identify adverse effects of surgery and anesthesia.
3. Describe ways to decrease the risk of surgical site infections.
4. Compare types of anesthesia with regard to uses, advantages, disadvantages, and nursing responsibilities.
5. Use the nursing process to optimize patient outcomes during the intraoperative period.

NURSING CONCEPTS

Assessment
Comfort

Managing Care
Safety

GLOSSARY

anesthesia: a state of narcosis or severe central nervous system depression produced by pharmacologic agents

anesthesiologist: physician trained to deliver anesthesia and to monitor the patient's condition during surgery

anesthetic agent: the substance, such as a chemical or gas, used to induce anesthesia

certified registered nurse anesthetist (CRNA): advanced practice registered nurse who delivers anesthesia care under the direction of an anesthesiologist

circulating nurse : registered nurse who coordinates and documents patient care in the operating room (*synonym*: circulator)

laparoscope: a thin endoscope inserted through a small incision into a cavity or joint using fiber-optic technology to project live images of structures onto a video monitor; other small incisions allow additional instruments to be inserted to facilitate laparoscopic surgery

malignant hyperthermia: a rare life-threatening condition triggered by exposure to most anesthetic agents inducing a drastic and uncontrolled increase in skeletal muscle oxidative metabolism that can overwhelm the body's capacity to supply oxygen, remove carbon dioxide, and regulate body temperature, eventually leading to circulatory collapse and death if untreated; often inherited as an autosomal dominant disorder

moderate sedation: previously referred to as conscious sedation, involves the use of sedation to depress the level of consciousness without altering the patient's ability to maintain a patent airway and to respond to physical stimuli and verbal commands

monitored anesthesia care: moderate sedation given by an anesthesiologist or CRNA

multimodal anesthesia: the intentional practice of using a combination of nonopioid pharmaceuticals and regional anesthesia techniques

registered nurse first assistant: a member of the operating room team whose responsibilities may include handling tissue, providing exposure at the operative field, suturing, and maintaining hemostasis

restricted zone: area in the operating room where scrub attire and surgical masks are required; includes operating room and sterile core areas

scrub role: registered nurse, licensed practical nurse, or surgical technologist who scrubs and dons sterile surgical attire, prepares instruments and supplies, and hands instruments to the surgeon during the procedure

semirestricted zone: area in the operating room where scrub attire is required; may include areas where surgical instruments are processed

sterile technique: measures taken to maintain an area free from living microorganisms, including all spores

surgical asepsis: absence of microorganisms in the surgical environment to reduce the risk of infection

unrestricted zone: area in the operating room that interfaces with other departments; includes patient reception area and holding area

The intraoperative experience has undergone many changes and advances that make it safer and less disturbing to patients. Even with these advances, anesthesia and surgery still place the patient at risk for several complications or adverse events. Consciousness or full awareness, mobility, protective biologic functions, and personal control are totally or partially relinquished by the patient when entering the operating room (OR). Staff from the departments of anesthesia, nursing, and surgery work collaboratively to implement professional standards of care, to control iatrogenic and individual risks, to prevent complications, and to promote high-quality patient outcomes.

The Surgical Team

The surgical team consists of the patient, the anesthesiologist (physician) or certified registered nurse anesthetist (CRNA), the surgeon, nurses, surgical technicians, and registered nurse first assistants (RNFAs) or certified surgical technologists (assistants). The anesthesiologist or CRNA administers the **anesthetic agent** (substance used to induce anesthesia) and monitors the patient's physical status throughout the surgery. The surgeon, nurses, technicians, and assistants scrub and perform the surgery. The person in the scrub role, either a nurse or a surgical technician, provides sterile instruments and supplies to the surgeon during the procedure by anticipating the surgical needs as the surgical case progresses. The circulating nurse coordinates the care of the patient in the OR. Care provided by the circulating nurse includes planning for and assisting with patient positioning, preparing the site for surgery, managing surgical specimens, anticipating the needs of the surgical team, documenting intraoperative events, and updating the plan of care. Collaboration of the core surgical team using evidence-based practices tailored to the specific case results in optimum patient care and improved outcomes (see Chart 15-1).

The Patient

As the patient enters the OR, they may feel either relaxed and prepared or fearful and highly stressed. These feelings depend to a large extent on the amount and timing of preoperative sedation, preoperative education, and the individual patient. Fears about loss of control, the unknown, pain, death, changes in body structure, appearance, or function, and disruption of lifestyle all contribute to anxiety. These fears can increase the amount of anesthetic medication needed, the level of postoperative pain, and overall recovery time (see Chapter 5 for more information on stress).

The patient is subject to several risks. Infection, failure of the surgery to relieve symptoms or correct a deformity, temporary or permanent complications related to the procedure or the anesthetic agent, and death are uncommon but potential outcomes of the surgical experience (see Chart 15-2). In

---

Chart 15-1   ETHICAL DILEMMA

Can Lack of Civility in the OR Threaten Patient Safety?

Case Scenario

You are a registered nurse who has worked in the operating room (OR) for the past five years. You have enjoyed an ancillary role precepting students for the past two years. Recently, you volunteered to serve as a preceptor for a nurse who is transferring to the OR after working as a registered nurse on a general medical-surgical unit for the past two years since graduating from nursing school. The new nurse was accepted into the hospital's onsite perioperative nursing internship program three months ago and has completed most of the classroom portion of the program, reportedly receiving excellent test scores. Today, she is assigned to the role of scrub nurse. A staff nurse with 20 years of experience in the OR is the circulating nurse assigned to the OR suite where the new nurse is assigned. As you are preparing to enter the OR suite to check on the new nurse and to verify that she has setup the instruments properly, the circulating nurse storms angrily out of the room, rolls her eyes and tells you "that newbie badly bungled" and did not set up instruments correctly for the case. You immediately walk into the OR suite to investigate and find the surgeon and the CRNA are there, as well as the new nurse, who is blinking back tears. The new nurse tells you that the circulating nurse "chewed me out in front of everyone." The surgeon requests to have a different nurse assigned to be the scrub nurse.

Discussion

In the *Code of Ethics for Nurses*, the American Nurses Association (ANA; 2015) stresses that it is the responsibility of the nurse to treat colleagues with civility, dignity, and respect and that doing so creates an ethical work environment. By contrast, incivility, which can be evidenced by harassment, intimidation, and bullying, is considered morally unacceptable behaviors for the nurse to exhibit. Clark and Kenski (2017) take these tenets further, and note that incivility, which can consist of both overt behaviors (e.g., yelling, making disparaging remarks) as well as covert behaviors (e.g., eye rolling, withholding communication) can disrupt important professional transactions and communication, which may then threaten patient safety. They assert that "nurses have an ethical responsibility to foster healthy work environments in which conflict is managed in a respectful way and communication is clear, direct, and concise." (p. 62).

Analysis

- Identify the ethical principles that are in conflict in this case (see Chapter 1, Chart 1-7). Who are the stakeholders who might have been adversely affected by this event? Do nurses have a moral obligation to foster beneficent relationships? Can incivility threaten nonmaleficence?
- Describe how you would proceed and what you would say to the nurse you are precepting. Would your communication with her be different if you were to find that she had set up the instruments correctly or incorrectly? Would you honor the surgeon's request and ask the charge nurse to change the new nurse's assignment?
- What resources might be of help to you so that a civil work environment may be cultivated? Should the nurse manager or other administrators be consulted to help resolve this conflict?

References

American Nurses Association (ANA). (2015). *Code of ethics for nurses with interpretive statements*. Silver Spring, MD: Author.

Clark, C. M. & Kenski, D. (2017). Promoting civility in the OR: An ethical imperative. *AORN Journal, 105*(1), 60–66.

Resources

See Chapter 1, Chart 1-10 for Steps of an Ethical Analysis and Ethics Resources.

Chart 15-2

Potential Adverse Effects of Surgery and Anesthesia

Anesthesia and surgery disrupt all major body systems. Although most patients can compensate for surgical trauma and the effects of anesthesia, all patients are at risk during the operative procedure. These risks include the following:

- Agitation or disorientation, especially in older adult patients
- Allergic reactions
- Anesthesia awareness
- Bleeding
- Cardiac arrhythmia from electrolyte imbalance or adverse effect of anesthetic agents
- Central nervous system agitation, seizures, and respiratory arrest
- Drug toxicity, faulty equipment, and other types of human error
- Electrical shock or burns
- Hypotension from blood loss or adverse effect of anesthesia
- Hypothermia from cool operating room temperatures, exposure of body cavities, and impaired thermoregulation secondary to anesthetic agents
- Hypoxemia or hypercarbia from hypoventilation and inadequate respiratory support during anesthesia
- Infection
- Laryngeal trauma, oral trauma, and broken teeth from difficult intubation
- Laser burns
- Malignant hyperthermia secondary to adverse effect of anesthesia
- Myocardial depression, bradycardia, and circulatory collapse
- Nerve damage and skin breakdown from prolonged or inappropriate positioning
- Oversedation or undersedation
- Retained foreign body or object
- Thrombosis from compression of blood vessels or stasis

Adapted from Association of PeriOperative Registered Nurses (AORN). (2019a). *Association of PeriOperative Registered Nurses (AORN) standards, recommended practice, and guidelines.* Denver, CO: Author.

addition to fears and risks, the patient undergoing sedation and anesthesia temporarily loses both cognitive function and biologic self-protective mechanisms. Loss of the sense of pain, reflexes, and the ability to communicate subjects the intraoperative patient to possible injury. The OR nurse is the patient's advocate while surgery proceeds.

Gerontologic Considerations

One in 10 patients undergoing surgery is age 65 or older (American Society of Anesthesiologists [ASA], 2019). Older adult patients are at higher risk for complications from anesthesia and surgery compared with younger adult patients due to several factors (Rothrock, 2019). One factor is age-related decline in physiologic reserve that weakens the normal response to stressors, acute illness, anesthesia, and surgery (Vernon, Rice, Titch, et al., 2019). Risks include delirium, hypothermia, positioning injury, deep vein thrombosis (DVT) formation, electrolyte imbalance, and circulatory compromise. Further discussion of age-related physiologic changes can be found in Chapter 8.

Biologic variations of particular importance include age-related cardiovascular and pulmonary changes. The aging heart and blood vessels have decreased ability to respond to stress. Cardiac output and pulmonary capacity diminish with age, with a decline in maximal oxygen uptake. Slow circulation and hypotension predispose the patient to thrombus formation and emboli (Phillips, 2017). Excessive or rapid administration of intravenous (IV) solutions can cause pulmonary edema. A sudden or prolonged decline in blood pressure may lead to cerebral ischemia, thrombosis, embolism, infarction, and anoxia. Reduced gas exchange can result in cerebral hypoxia.

Lower doses of anesthetic agents are required in older adults due to decreased tissue elasticity (lung and cardiovascular systems) and reduced lean tissue mass. Older patients often experience an increase in the duration of clinical effects of medications. With decreased plasma proteins, more of the anesthetic agent remains free or unbound, and the result is more potent action (Barash, Cullen, Stoelting, et al., 2017).

In addition, body tissues of the older adult are made up predominantly of water, and those tissues with a rich blood supply, such as skeletal muscle, liver, and kidneys, shrink as the body ages. Reduced liver size decreases the rate at which the liver can inactivate many anesthetic agents, and decreased kidney function slows the elimination of waste products and anesthetic agents. Nursing management for the older surgical patient in the intraoperative period includes the following (Phillips, 2017):

- Application of intraoperative warming techniques to reduce unintentional hypothermia
- Careful transfer and positioning on the OR bed. Protect pressure points and bony prominences with extra padding. Support the back and neck to prevent stiffness while maintaining respiratory and circulatory support
- Use of antiembolic stockings or a sequential compression device to prevent VTE formation
- Careful fluid and electrolyte monitoring via accurate blood loss measurement, urinary output, and blood gases

Nursing Care

Throughout surgery, nursing responsibilities include providing for the safety and well-being of the patient, coordinating the OR personnel, and performing scrub and circulating activities. Because the patient's emotional state remains a concern, the intraoperative nursing staff provides the patient with information and reassurance, continuing the care initiated by preoperative nurses. The nurse supports coping strategies and reinforces the patient's ability to influence outcomes by encouraging active participation in the plan of care, incorporating cultural, ethnic, and religious considerations as appropriate. The establishment of an environment of trust and relaxation through visualization techniques is another method of patient reassurance that can be used as the patient is anesthetically induced.

As patient advocates, intraoperative nurses monitor factors that have the potential to cause injury, such as patient position, equipment malfunction, and environmental hazards. Nurses also protect the patient's dignity and interests while the patient is under anesthesia. Additional nursing responsibilities include maintaining surgical standards of care, identifying risks, and minimizing complications.

Cultural Diversity

Cultural, ethnic, and religious diversities are important considerations for all health care professionals. Nurses in the perioperative area should be aware of medications that may

Surgical Safety Checklist

World Health Organization | **Patient Safety**
A World Alliance for Safer Health Care

Before induction of anaesthesia

(with at least nurse and anaesthetist)

Has the patient confirmed his/her identity, site, procedure, and consent?
☐ Yes

Is the site marked?
☐ Yes
☐ Not applicable

Is the anaesthesia machine and medication check complete?
☐ Yes

Is the pulse oximeter on the patient and functioning?
☐ Yes

Does the patient have a:

Known allergy?
☐ No
☐ Yes

Difficult airway or aspiration risk?
☐ No
☐ Yes, and equipment/assistance available

Risk of >500ml blood loss (7ml/kg in children)?
☐ No
☐ Yes, and two IVs/central access and fluids planned

Before skin incision

(with nurse, anaesthetist and surgeon)

☐ **Confirm all team members have introduced themselves by name and role.**

☐ **Confirm the patient's name, procedure, and where the incision will be made.**

Has antibiotic prophylaxis been given within the last 60 minutes?
☐ Yes
☐ Not applicable

Anticipated Critical Events

To Surgeon:
☐ What are the critical or non-routine steps?
☐ How long will the case take?
☐ What is the anticipated blood loss?

To Anaesthetist:
☐ Are there any patient-specific concerns?

To Nursing Team:
☐ Has sterility (including indicator results) been confirmed?
☐ Are there equipment issues or any concerns?

Is essential imaging displayed?
☐ Yes
☐ Not applicable

Before patient leaves operating room

(with nurse, anaesthetist and surgeon)

Nurse Verbally Confirms:
☐ The name of the procedure
☐ Completion of instrument, sponge and needle counts
☐ Specimen labelling (read specimen labels aloud, including patient name)
☐ Whether there are any equipment problems to be addressed

To Surgeon, Anaesthetist and Nurse:
☐ What are the key concerns for recovery and management of this patient?

This checklist is not intended to be comprehensive. Additions and modifications to fit local practice are encouraged.   Revised 1 / 2009   © WHO, 2009

Figure 15-1 • Surgical safety checklist. Reproduced with permission from the World Health Organization. WHO Bulletin, 86[7]. New checklist to help make surgery safer, 496–576. © 2015. Retrieved on 5/22/19 at: whqlibdoc.who.int/publications/2009/9789241598590_eng_Checklist.pdf

be prohibited by certain groups (e.g., Muslims and those of the Jewish faith may not wish to use porcine-based products [heparin (porcine or bovine)]; Buddhists may choose not to use bovine products). In certain cultures, the head is a sacred area, and staff should allow patients to apply their own surgical cap in this case. When English is the second language of the patient having surgery under local anesthesia, certified medical translators can be provided to maintain understanding and comprehension by the patient. Translator devices are also available at most hospitals. Family members may have the ability to translate but should not be used as medical translators, as they may wish to save the patient anxiety and not provide an accurate translation, resulting in the patient not receiving complete information.

The Circulating Nurse

The **circulating nurse (or circulator)**, a qualified registered nurse, works in collaboration with surgeons, anesthesia providers, and other health care providers to plan the best course of action for each patient (Rothrock, 2019). In this leadership role, the circulating nurse manages the OR and protects the patient's safety and health by monitoring the activities of the surgical team, checking the OR conditions, and continually assessing the patient for signs of injury and implementing appropriate interventions. A foremost responsibility includes

verifying consent; if not obtained, surgery may not commence. The team is coordinated by the circulating nurse, who ensures cleanliness, proper temperature, humidity, appropriate lighting, safe function of equipment, and the availability of supplies and materials.

The circulating nurse monitors aseptic practices to avoid breaks in technique while coordinating the movement of related personnel (medical, x-ray, and laboratory), as well as implementing fire safety precautions. The circulating nurse also monitors the patient and documents specific activities throughout the operation to ensure the patient's safety and well-being.

In addition, the circulating nurse is responsible for ensuring that the second verification of the surgical procedure and site takes place and is documented (see Fig. 15-1). In some institutions, this is referred to as a time-out, surgical pause, or universal protocol that takes place among the surgical team prior to induction of anesthesia with a briefing about anticipated problems, potential complications, allergies, and comorbidities. Every member of the surgical team verifies the patient's name, procedure, and surgical site using objective documentation and data before beginning the surgery. Identifying patients correctly is a 2019 National Patient Safety Goal (see Chapter 14, Chart 14-7). The Surgical Safety Checklist (SSC) (see Fig. 15-1) has been adopted in ORs worldwide to reduce medical errors, increase patient safety, and improve interprofessional communication (Ziman, Espin,

Grant, et al., 2018). A team debriefing session, led by the circulating nurse, often follows the completion of surgery to identify potential problems with the postsurgical care of the patient and potential areas for improvement (American Society of PeriAnesthesia Nurses [ASPAN], 2019).

> ◤ *Quality and Safety Nursing Alert*
>
> *It is imperative that the correct patient identity, surgical procedure, and surgical site be verified prior to surgery. The surgical site should be marked by the physician and confirmed by the patient prior to coming to the OR suite during the consent process. The marking should be visible after the sterile drapes are applied and verified by the surgical team members during the time-out.*

The Scrub Role

The registered nurse, licensed practical nurse, or surgical technologist (or assistant) performs the activities of the **scrub role**, including performing hand hygiene; setting up the sterile equipment, tables, and sterile field; preparing sutures, ligatures, and special equipment (e.g., a **laparoscope**, which is a thin endoscope inserted through a small incision into a cavity or joint using fiber-optic technology to project live images of structures onto a video monitor); and assisting the surgeon and the surgical assistants during the procedure by anticipating the instruments and supplies that will be required, such as sponges, drains, and other equipment. As the surgical incision is closed, the scrub person and the circulating nurse count all needles, sponges, and instruments to be sure that they are accounted for and not retained as a foreign body in the patient (Association of PeriOperative Registered Nurses [AORN], 2019a; Rothrock, 2019). Standards call for all sponges used in surgery to be visible on x-ray and for sponge counts to take place at the beginning of surgery and twice at the end (when wound closure begins and again as the skin is being closed). Tissue specimens obtained during surgery are labeled by the person in the scrub role and sent to the laboratory by the circulating nurse. Medications and solutions are transferred to the sterile table by the circulating nurse and the name, strength, dosage, and expiration date are labeled by the person in the scrub role. Implants are handled in a similar fashion whereby the name, type, size, expiration date, and sterility are verified prior to handoff to the person in the scrub role.

The Surgeon

The surgeon performs the surgical procedure, heads the surgical team, and is a licensed physician (MD or DO), oral surgeon (DDS or DMD), or podiatrist (DPM) who is specially trained and qualified. Qualifications and training must adhere to The Joint Commission standards, hospital standards, and local and state admitting practices and procedures (Rothrock, 2019).

The Registered Nurse First Assistant

The **registered nurse first assistant (RNFA)** is another member of the OR team. Although the scope of practice of the RNFA depends on each state's nurse practice act, the RNFA practices under the direct supervision of the surgeon. RNFA responsibilities may include handling tissue, providing exposure at the operative field, suturing, and maintaining hemostasis (Rothrock, 2019). The role requires a thorough understanding of anatomy and physiology, tissue handling, and the principles of surgical asepsis. The RNFA must be aware of the objectives of the surgery, must have the knowledge and ability to anticipate needs and to work as a skilled member of a team, and must be able to handle any emergency situation in the OR.

The Anesthesiologist and CRNA

An **anesthesiologist** is a physician specifically trained in the art and science of anesthesiology. A **certified registered nurse anesthetist (CRNA)** is a qualified and specifically trained health care professional who administers anesthetic agents, has graduated from an accredited nurse anesthesia program, and has passed examinations sponsored by the American Association of Nurse Anesthetists. The anesthesiologist or CRNA assesses the patient before surgery, selects the anesthesia, administers it, intubates the patient if necessary, manages any technical problems related to the administration of the anesthetic agent, and supervises the patient's condition throughout the surgical procedure. Before the patient enters the OR, often at preadmission testing, the anesthesiologist or CRNA visits the patient to perform an assessment, supply information, and answer questions. The type of anesthetic agent to be given, previous reactions to anesthetic medications, and known anatomic abnormalities that would make airway management difficult are among topics addressed.

The anesthesiologist or CRNA uses the American Society of Anesthesiologists (ASA) Physical Classification System to determine the patient's status. A patient who is classified as P2, P3, or P4 has a systemic disease that may or may not be related to the cause of surgery. If a patient with a classification of P1, P2, P3, P4, or P5 requires emergency surgery, an E is added to the physical status designation (e.g., P1E, P2E). P6 refers to a patient who is brain dead and is undergoing surgery as an organ donor. The abbreviations ASA1 through ASA6 are often used interchangeably with P1 to P6 to designate physical status (Rothrock, 2019).

When the patient arrives in the OR, the anesthesiologist or CRNA reassesses the patient's physical condition immediately prior to initiating anesthesia. The anesthetic agent is given, and the patient's airway is maintained through an intranasal intubation (if the surgeon is using an oral approach to surgery), intubation with an endotracheal tube (ET), or a laryngeal mask airway (LMA). During surgery, the anesthesiologist or CRNA monitors the patient's blood pressure, pulse, and respirations, as well as the electrocardiogram (ECG), blood oxygen saturation level, tidal volume, blood gas levels, blood pH, alveolar gas concentrations, and body temperature. End tidal CO_2 monitoring by electroencephalography (EEG) is sometimes required. Levels of anesthetic medications in the body can also be determined; a mass spectrometer can provide instant readouts of critical concentration levels on display terminals. This information is used to assess the patient's ability to breathe unassisted or the need for mechanical assistance if ventilation is poor and the patient is not breathing well independently.

Safety and Infection Prevention

Within the OR, many factors prevent the spread of microorganisms that may cause surgical site infections (SSIs). These factors involve a combination of facility structure and personnel practices, which are regulated by professional guidelines and overseen by facility members.

The Surgical Environment

The surgical suite is behind double doors, and access is limited to authorized, appropriately clad personnel. The OR is considered a restricted area where careful attention to infection prevention is at the highest standard. In the OR environment, microbial contamination can occur through an airborne or contact route; as a result, the OR has special air filtration devices to screen out contaminating particles, dust, and pollutants. ORs are designed with laminar flow ventilation to circulate particles away from the patient and surgical field. Personnel also follow strict aseptic practices, including hand scrubbing, machine and room cleaning, sterile supply and instrumentation use, and limited movement. Reducing traffic and door openings has been linked to maintaining optimal airflow with minimal circulating particles and contaminants (Armellino, 2017). Policies governing this environment address such issues as the health of the staff; the cleanliness of the rooms; the sterility of equipment and surfaces; processes for scrubbing, gowning, and gloving; and OR attire (AORN, 2019a).

The surgical environment is known for its stark appearance and cool temperature. Therefore, it is important to maintain patient normothermia. Research supports warming the patient starting in the preoperative area, and throughout all perioperative phases of care. Examples of intraoperative warming techniques are raising room temperature, using forced-air warming blankets, and administering warmed irrigation and IV solutions (Phillips, 2017; Williams, 2018).

To provide the best possible conditions for surgery, the OR is situated in a location that is central to all supporting services (e.g., pathology, x-ray, and laboratory).

Many National Patient Safety Goals pertain to the perioperative areas (see Chapter 14, Chart 14-7); however, the one with the most direct relevance to the OR is to identify patient safety risks. A unique risk is the risk of fire in the OR due to three factors: a source of fuel, an oxygen source, and a mechanism to ignite a fire (AORN, 2019b; ASPAN, 2019).

Prevention of OR Fires

AORN recommends the use of the Fire Risk Assessment Tool to assess the dangers of fires for each surgical case (see Fig. 15-2). The fire risk is discussed during the surgical time-out, and an indication of whether or not the patient has a fire risk is placed on the team communication board in the OR. A regulatory requirement endorsed by The Joint Commission is that every OR perform an annual fire drill to ensure staff familiarity with evacuation plans and to test facility safeguards in the event of a fire (Joint Commission, 2019). To further improve safety, electrical hazards, emergency exit clearances, and storage of equipment and anesthetic gases are monitored periodically by official agencies, such as the respective state Department of Health and The Joint Commission.

Surgical Attire

To help decrease microbes, the surgical area is divided into three zones: the **unrestricted zone**, where street clothes are allowed; the **semirestricted zone**, where attire consists of

---

Fire Prevention Assessment Tool

Is an alcohol-based skin antiseptic or other flammable solution being used preoperatively?
☐ Yes
☐ No

Is the operative or other invasive procedure being performed above the xiphoid process or in the oropharynx?
☐ Yes
☐ No

Is open oxygen or nitrous oxide being administered?
☐ Yes
☐ No

Is an electrosurgical unit, laser, or fiber-optic light being used?
☐ Yes
☐ No

Are there other possible contributors (e.g., defibrillators, drills, saws, burrs)?
☐ Yes
☐ No

Figure 15-2 • AORN fire risk assessment tool. Reprinted with permission from Association of PeriOperative Registered Nurses (AORN). (2019b). Fire safety tool kit: Fire prevention assessment tool. Retrieved on 5/29/19 at: www.aorn.org/guidelines/clinical-resources/tool-kits/fire-safety-tool-kit

---

scrub clothes and caps; and the **restricted zone**, where scrub clothes, shoe covers, caps, and masks are worn. The surgeons and other surgical team members wear additional sterile clothing and protective devices during surgery.

The AORN recommends specific practices for personnel wearing surgical attire to promote a high level of cleanliness in a particular practice setting (AORN, 2019a). OR attire includes close-fitting cotton scrub shirts and pants, gowns, and jackets. Knitted cuffs on sleeves prevent organisms from shedding and being released into the immediate surroundings. Shirts and waist drawstrings should be tucked inside the pants to prevent accidental contact with sterile areas and to contain skin shedding. Wet or soiled garments should be changed.

Masks are worn at all times in the restricted zone of the OR. High-filtration masks decrease the risk of postoperative wound infection by containing and filtering microorganisms from the oropharynx and nasopharynx. Masks should fit tightly; should cover the nose and mouth completely; and should not interfere with breathing, speech, or vision. Masks must be adjusted to prevent venting from the sides. Disposable masks have a filtration efficiency exceeding 95%. Masks are changed between patients and should not be worn outside the surgical department. The mask must be either on or off; it must not be allowed to hang around the neck.

Headgear should completely cover the hair (head and neckline, including beard) so that hair, bobby pins, clips, and particles of dandruff or dust do not fall on the sterile field.

Shoes designated for use inside the OR (not worn home) should be comfortable and supportive. Shoe covers are used when spills or splashes are anticipated. If worn, the covers should be changed whenever they become wet, torn, or soiled (AORN 2019a; Rothrock, 2019).

Barriers such as scrub attire and masks do not entirely protect the patient from microorganisms. Upper respiratory tract infections, sore throats, and skin infections in staff and patients are sources of pathogens and must be reported.

Because artificial fingernails harbor microorganisms and can cause nosocomial infections, a ban on artificial nails by OR personnel is supported by the Centers for Disease Control and Prevention (CDC), AORN, and the Association for Professionals in Infection Control and Epidemiology (APIC). Research provides support for policies prohibiting artificial nails for health care workers (AORN, 2019a). Short, natural fingernails are encouraged.

Principles of Surgical Asepsis and Sterile Technique

Surgical asepsis prevents the contamination of surgical wounds. **Sterile technique** implies that the area is free of living microorganisms. The patient's natural skin flora or a previously existing infection may cause postoperative SSI. Rigorous adherence to the principles of sterility by OR personnel is basic to preventing SSIs.

All surgical supplies, instruments, needles, sutures, dressings, gloves, covers, and solutions that may come in contact with the surgical wound or exposed tissues must be sterilized before use (Rothrock, 2019). The surgeon, surgical assistants, scrub personnel, and nurses prepare themselves by scrubbing their hands and arms with antiseptic soap and water or alcohol-based (waterless) product. OR personnel must follow the product manufacturer's recommendations in order to achieve hand antisepsis (AORN, 2019a).

The skin of patients, OR team members, and visitors constitutes a microbiologic hazard. In an average individual, an estimated 4000 to 10,000 viable contaminated particles are shed by the skin each minute. *Staphylococcus aureus*, a bacterium, is the most common type of particle on dispersed skin cells (Phillips, 2017). Surgical team members wear long-sleeved, sterile gowns and gloves. Head and hair are covered with a cap, and a mask is worn over the nose and mouth to minimize the possibility that bacteria from the upper respiratory tract will enter the wound. During surgery, only personnel who have scrubbed, gloved, and gowned touch sterilized objects. Nonscrubbed personnel refrain from touching or contaminating anything sterile.

An area of the patient's skin larger than that requiring exposure during the surgery is meticulously cleansed, and an antiseptic solution is applied (Rothrock, 2019). Close attention is paid to the application dry time of the agent, in particular chlorhexidine and other alcohol-based products. If hair removal needs to take place and this was unable to be performed before the patient arrived in the OR suite, this is done immediately before the procedure with electric clippers (not shaved) to minimize the risk of infection (AORN, 2019a). The remainder of the patient's body is covered with sterile drapes.

Environmental Controls

In addition to the protocols described previously, surgical asepsis requires meticulous cleaning and maintenance of the OR environment. Floors and horizontal surfaces are cleaned between cases with detergent, soap, and water or a detergent germicide. Sterilized equipment is inspected regularly to ensure optimal operation and performance.

All equipment that comes into direct contact with the patient must be sterile. Sterilized linens, drapes, and solutions are used. Instruments are cleaned and sterilized in a unit near the OR. Individually wrapped sterile items are used when additional individual items are needed.

Airborne bacteria are a concern. To decrease the amount of bacteria in the air, standard OR ventilation provides 15 air exchanges per hour, at least three of which are fresh air (AORN, 2019a; Rothrock, 2019). A room temperature of 20° to 24°C (68° to 73°F), humidity between 30% and 60%, and positive pressure relative to adjacent areas are maintained. With the standard air exchanges, air counts of bacteria are reduced to 50 to 150 colony-forming units (CFUs) per cubic foot per minute. Systems with high-efficiency particulate air (HEPA) filters are needed to remove particles larger than 0.3 μm (Rothrock, 2019). Unnecessary personnel and physical movement may be restricted to minimize bacteria in the air and achieve an OR infection rate no greater than 3% to 5% in clean, infection-prone surgery.

Some ORs have laminar airflow units. These units provide 400 to 500 air exchanges per hour (Rothrock, 2019). When used appropriately, laminar airflow units result in fewer than 10 CFUs per cubic foot per minute during surgery. The goal for a laminar airflow–equipped OR is an infection rate of less than 1%. An OR equipped with a laminar airflow unit is frequently used for total joint replacement or organ transplant surgery.

Even using all precautions, wound contamination may inadvertently occur. Constant surveillance and conscientious technique in carrying out aseptic practices are necessary to reduce the risk of contamination and infection.

Basic Guidelines for Maintaining Surgical Asepsis

All practitioners involved in the intraoperative phase have a responsibility to provide and maintain a safe environment. Adherence to aseptic practice is part of this responsibility. The basic principles of aseptic technique follow (AORN, 2019a):

- All materials in contact with the surgical wound or used within the sterile field must be sterile. Sterile surfaces or articles may touch other sterile surfaces or articles and remain sterile; contact with unsterile objects at any point renders a sterile area contaminated.
- Gowns of the surgical team are considered sterile in front from the chest to the level of the sterile field. The sleeves are also considered sterile from 2 inches above the elbow to the stockinette cuff.
- Sterile drapes are used to create a sterile field (see Fig. 15-3). Only the top surface of a draped table is considered sterile. During draping of a table or patient, the sterile drape is held well above the surface to be covered and is positioned from front to back.
- Items are dispensed to a sterile field by methods that preserve the sterility of the items and the integrity of the sterile field. After a sterile package is opened, the edges are considered unsterile. Sterile supplies, including solutions, are delivered to a sterile field or handed to a scrubbed person in such a way that the sterility of the object or fluid remains intact.

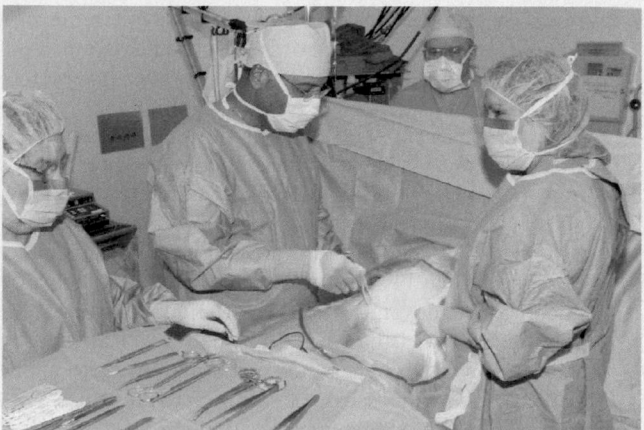

Figure 15-3 • Proper draping exposes only the surgical site, which decreases the risk of infection.

- The movements of the surgical team are from sterile to sterile areas and from unsterile to unsterile areas. Scrubbed people and sterile items contact only sterile areas; circulating nurses and unsterile items contact only unsterile areas.
- Movement around a sterile field must not cause contamination of the field. Sterile areas must be kept in view during movement around the area. At least a 1-ft distance from the sterile field must be maintained to prevent inadvertent contamination.
- Whenever a sterile barrier is breached, the area must be considered contaminated. A tear or puncture of the drape permitting access to an unsterile surface underneath renders the area unsterile. Such a drape must be replaced.
- Every sterile field is constantly monitored and maintained. Items of doubtful sterility are considered unsterile. Sterile fields are prepared as close as possible to the time of use.
- The routine administration of hyperoxia (high levels of oxygen) is *not* recommended to reduce SSIs.

Health Hazards Associated with the Surgical Environment

Faulty equipment, improper use of equipment, exposure to toxic substances, surgical plume (smoke generated by electrosurgical cautery), as well as infectious waste, cuts, needlestick injuries, and lasers are some of the associated hazards in the surgical environment (Rothrock, 2019). Internal monitoring of the OR includes the analysis of surface swipe samples and air samples for infectious and toxic agents. In addition, policies and procedures for minimizing exposure to body fluids and reducing the dangers associated with lasers and radiation are identified in AORN standards (AORN, 2019a).

Regardless of the size or location of an incision, unintentional retention of an object (e.g., sponge, instrument) can occur. A retained object can cause wound infection or disruption, an abscess can form, and fistulas may develop between organs (Rothrock, 2019). Safety measures should be in place to reduce the risk of a retained object. Best practices include minimized distractions during the counting process, radiofrequency (RF) technology, and clear communication that includes the willingness to raise concerns among the surgical team members.

RF technology acts as a "back-up method" for sponge counting using low-frequency RF chips inside sponges that can be detected via a wand or other scanning detection device. The technology is used in many institutions and can increase patient safety by detecting retained sponges before the surgeon closes the incision (Steelman, Schaapveld, Storm, et al., 2019).

Laser Risks

The AORN has recommended practices for laser safety (AORN, 2019a). When lasers are in use, warning signs must be posted on the doors and safety goggles must be available for staff to don prior to room entry. Personnel must also wear a protective mask to prevent inhalation of the plume emitted from the laser. The type of laser in use and the safety precautions in place are verified by all team members during the time-out (Burlingame, 2017). Several types of lasers are available for clinical use; perioperative personnel should be familiar with the unique features, specific operation, and safety measures for each type of laser used in the practice setting and wear appropriate laser goggles for the type of laser beam in use. Registered nurses trained and certified in laser safety maintain the established standards in the OR (AORN, 2019a).

Surgical Smoke

Approximately 500,000 health care workers are exposed to surgical smoke each year. This smoke is created from thermal destruction of tissue. Smoke plumes may contain toxic gases and vapors such as benzene, hydrogen cyanide, formaldehyde, bioaerosols, dead and live cellular material, and viruses. It is estimated that in an average day, the effect of breathing surgical smoke could be comparable to smoking 30 unfiltered cigarettes. Perioperative nurses are twice as likely as the general population to report experiencing respiratory problems (Davis, 2018; US Department of Labor, Occupational Safety and Health Administration, 2018).

Smoke evacuators are used in some procedures to remove the plume from the operative field. If a smoke evacuator is not available, surgical team members should don an N95 respirator mask rather than a surgical mask, which does not prevent smoke from entering the airway orifices. In recent years, this technology has been extended to all surgical cases to protect the surgical team from the potential hazards associated with the generalized smoke plume generated by standard electric cautery units. Evacuating surgical smoke not only protects the perioperative team, but also patients (Spruce, 2018).

Exposure to Blood and Body Fluids

Basic scrub attire worn by sterile "scrubbed-in" OR personnel include double sterile gloves, eye protection, surgical mask, a sterile gown, and shoe covers. These help to protect against splashing, drilling, and blood loss exposure. In hospitals where numerous total joint procedures are performed, a complete bubble mask may be used. This mask provides full-barrier protection from bone fragments and splashes. Ventilation is accomplished through an accompanying hood with a separate air filtration system.

An estimated 380,000 sharps injuries occur in health care per year, and roughly one third of these occur in the OR setting. Interventions such as using sharps with safety engineered devices, passing sharps using a "neutral zone" or "safe zone," and placing used sharps in puncture-resistant containers can help to reduce these incidents (Davis, 2018). The "neutral zone" or "safe zone" techniques are designated spaces established for sharps to be put down and picked up (AORN, 2019).

Robotics

Several types of surgical robots are used to facilitate the performance of minimally invasive procedures. These techniques were first introduced in the 1980s in an effort to overcome the disadvantages of traditional laparoscopic surgery, such as limited arm movement and view (Carlos & Saulan, 2018). Many surgical specialties have the ability to use robotic technology for surgical cases, particularly those in the cardiac, urologic, thoracic, and gynecologic specialties. Several types of robotic-driven tools assist in making surgery more precise and less invasive for patients. Technologic advancements of the robot include 3D high-definition imaging and better motion control of instrumentation. The articulated arms offer a 360-degree wristlike movement for precision grasping, manipulation, dissection, and suturing of tissue (Phillips, 2017).

The Surgical Experience

During the surgical procedure, the patient will need sedation, anesthesia, or some combination of these. There are many low-risk anesthesia agents to choose from.

Types of Anesthesia and Sedation

Research estimates anesthesia-related death rates in the United States to be less than 1 per 10,000 surgeries (Barash et al., 2017). For the patient, the anesthesia experience consists of having an IV line inserted, if it was not inserted earlier; receiving a sedating agent prior to induction with an anesthetic agent; losing consciousness; being intubated, if indicated; and then receiving a combination of anesthetic agents. Typically, the experience is a smooth one, and the patient has no recall of the events. The main types of anesthesia are general anesthesia (inhalation, IV), regional anesthesia (epidural, spinal, and local conduction blocks), moderate sedation (monitored anesthesia care [MAC]), and local anesthesia.

General Anesthesia

Anesthesia is a state of narcosis (severe central nervous system depression produced by pharmacologic agents), analgesia, relaxation, and reflex loss. Patients under general anesthesia are not arousable, not even to painful stimuli. They lose the ability to maintain ventilatory function and require assistance in maintaining a patent airway. Cardiovascular function may be impaired as well.

General anesthesia consists of four stages, each associated with specific clinical manifestations (Rothrock, 2019). Understanding of these stages is necessary for nurses because of the emotional support that the patient might need as anesthesia progresses. These stages occur in reverse as the patient wakes up at the end of surgery, so the nurse must be aware of the need for appropriate patient support.

- *Stage I: beginning anesthesia.* Dizziness and a feeling of detachment may be experienced during induction. The patient may have a ringing, roaring, or buzzing in the ears and, although still conscious, may sense an inability to move the extremities easily. These sensations can

result in agitation. During this stage, noises are exaggerated; even low voices or minor sounds seem loud and unreal. For these reasons, unnecessary noises and motions are avoided when anesthesia begins.

- *Stage II: excitement.* The excitement stage, characterized variously by struggling, shouting, talking, singing, laughing, or crying, is often avoided if IV anesthetic agents are given smoothly and quickly. The pupils dilate, but they constrict if exposed to light; the pulse rate is rapid; and respirations may be irregular. Because of the possibility of uncontrolled movements of the patient during this stage, the anesthesiologist or CRNA must always be assisted by someone ready to help restrain the patient or to apply cricoid pressure in the case of vomiting to prevent aspiration. Manipulation increases circulation to the operative site and thereby increases the potential for bleeding.

- *Stage III: surgical anesthesia.* Surgical anesthesia is reached by administration of anesthetic vapor or gas and supported by IV agents as necessary. The patient is unconscious and lies quietly on the table. The pupils are small but constrict when exposed to light. Respirations are regular, the pulse rate and volume are normal, and the skin is pink or slightly flushed. With proper administration of the anesthetic agent, this stage may be maintained for hours in one of several planes, ranging from light (1) to deep (4), depending on the depth of anesthesia needed.

- *Stage IV: medullary depression.* This stage is reached if too much anesthesia has been given. Respirations become shallow, the pulse is weak and thready, and the pupils become widely dilated and no longer constrict when exposed to light. Cyanosis develops and, without prompt intervention, death rapidly follows. If this stage develops, the anesthetic agent is discontinued immediately and respiratory and circulatory support is initiated to prevent death. Stimulants, although rarely used, may be given; narcotic antagonists can be used if the overdose is due to opioids. It is not a planned stage of surgical anesthesia.

When opioid agents (narcotics) and neuromuscular blockers (relaxants) are given, several of the stages are absent. During smooth administration of an anesthetic agent, there is no sharp division between stages. The patient passes gradually from one stage to another, and it is through close observation of the signs exhibited by the patient that an anesthesiologist or CRNA controls the situation. The responses of the pupils, the blood pressure, and the respiratory and cardiac rates are among the most reliable guides to the patient's condition.

Anesthetic medications produce anesthesia because they are delivered to the brain at a high partial pressure that enables them to cross the blood–brain barrier. Relatively large amounts of anesthetic medication must be given during induction and the early maintenance phases because the anesthetic agent is recirculated and deposited in body tissues. As these sites become saturated, smaller amounts of the anesthetic agent are required to maintain anesthesia because equilibrium or near-equilibrium has been achieved between brain, blood, and other tissues. When possible, the anesthesia induction (initiation) begins with IV anesthesia and is then maintained at the desired stage by inhalation methods, achieving a smooth transition and eliminating the obvious stages of anesthesia (see Table 15-1). All are given in combination with oxygen and usually nitrous oxide as well.

TABLE 15-1		Inhalation Anesthetic Agents		
Agent	Administration	Advantages	Disadvantages	Implications/Considerations
Volatile Liquids				
Halothane	Inhalation; special vaporizer	Not explosive or flammable Induction rapid and smooth Useful in almost every type of surgery Low incidence of postoperative nausea and vomiting	Requires skillful administration to prevent overdose May cause liver damage May produce hypotension Requires special vaporizer for administration	In addition to observation of pulse and respiration postoperatively, blood pressure must be monitored frequently
Enflurane	Inhalation	Rapid induction and recovery Potent analgesic agent Not explosive or flammable	Respiratory depression may develop rapidly, along with electrocardiogram abnormalities Not compatible with epinephrine	Observe for possible respiratory depression. Administration with epinephrine may cause ventricular fibrillation
Isoflurane	Inhalation	Rapid induction and recovery Muscle relaxants are markedly potentiated	A profound respiratory depressant	Monitor respirations closely, support when necessary, and monitor for malignant hyperthermia
Sevoflurane[a]	Inhalation	Rapid induction and excretion; minimal side effects	Coughing and laryngospasm; trigger for malignant hyperthermia	Monitor for malignant hyperthermia
Desflurane	Inhalation	Rapid induction and emergence; rare organ toxicity	Respiratory irritation; trigger for malignant hyperthermia	Monitor for malignant hyperthermia and arrhythmias
Gases				
Nitrous oxide (N_2O)	Inhalation (semiclosed method)	Induction and recovery rapid Nonflammable Useful with oxygen for short procedures Useful with other agents for all types of surgery	Poor relaxant Weak anesthetic May produce hypoxia	Most useful in conjunction with other agents with longer action Monitor for chest pain, nausea and vomiting, hypertension, and stroke
Oxygen (O_2)	Inhalation	Can increase O_2 available to tissues	High concentrations are hazardous	Increased fire risk when used with lasers

[a]Currently most popular choice.
Adapted from Association of PeriOperative Registered Nurses (AORN). (2019a). *Association of PeriOperative Registered Nurses (AORN) standards, recommended practice, and guidelines.* Denver, CO: Author.

Any condition that diminishes peripheral blood flow, such as vasoconstriction or shock, may reduce the amount of anesthetic medication required. Conversely, when peripheral blood flow is unusually high, as in a muscularly active or apprehensive patient, induction is slower, and greater quantities of anesthetic agents are required because the brain receives a smaller quantity of anesthetic agent.

Inhalation

Inhaled anesthetic agents include volatile liquid agents and gases. Volatile liquid anesthetic agents produce anesthesia when their vapors are inhaled. Some commonly used inhalation agents are included in Table 15-1. All are given in combination with oxygen and usually nitrous oxide as well.

Gas anesthetic agents are given by inhalation and are always combined with oxygen. Nitrous oxide, sevoflurane, and desflurane are the most commonly used gas anesthetic agents. When inhaled, the anesthetic agents enter the blood through the pulmonary capillaries and act on cerebral centers to produce loss of consciousness and sensation. When anesthetic administration is discontinued, the vapor or gas is eliminated through the lungs.

The vapor from inhalation anesthetic agents can be given to the patient by several methods. The inhalation anesthetic agent may be given through an LMA—a flexible tube with an inflatable silicone ring and cuff that can be inserted into the larynx (see Fig. 15-4A). The endotracheal technique for administering anesthetic medications consists of introducing

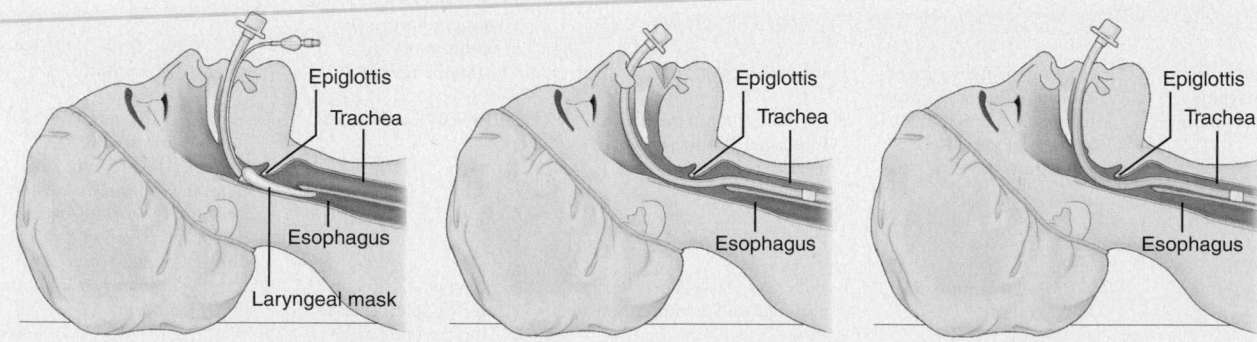

A. Laryngeal Mask Airway (LMA)   **B.** Intranasal intubation   **C.** Oral intubation

Figure 15-4 • Anesthetic delivery methods. **A.** Laryngeal mask airway (LMA). **B.** Nasal endotracheal catheter used when oral access will be required by the surgeon (in position with cuff inflated). **C.** Oral endotracheal intubation (tube is in position with cuff inflated).

a soft rubber or plastic ET into the trachea, usually by means of a laryngoscope. The ET may be inserted through either the nose (see Fig. 15-4B) or mouth (see Fig. 15-4C). When in place, the tube seals off the lungs from the esophagus so that if the patient vomits, stomach contents do not enter the lungs.

Intravenous Administration

General anesthesia can also be produced by the IV administration of various anesthetic and analgesic agents, such as barbiturates, benzodiazepines, nonbarbiturate hypnotics, dissociative agents, and opioid agents. Table 15-2 lists

TABLE 15-2 Commonly Used Intravenous Medications

Medication	Common Usage	Advantages	Disadvantages	Comments
Opioid Analgesic Agents				
Alfentanil	Surgical analgesia in ambulatory patients	Ultra–short-acting (5–10 min) analgesic agent, duration of action 0.5 h; bolus or infusion	—	Potency: 750 µg; half-life 1.6 h
Fentanyl	Surgical analgesia: epidural infusion for postoperative analgesia; add to SAB	Good cardiovascular stability; duration of action 0.5 h	May cause muscle or chest wall rigidity	Most commonly used opioid; potency: 100 µg = 10 mg morphine sulfate; elimination half-life 3.6 h
Morphine sulfate	Preoperative pain; pre-medication; postoperative pain	Inexpensive; duration of action 4–5 h; euphoria; good cardiovascular stability	Nausea and vomiting; histamine release; postural $\downarrow$ BP and $\downarrow$ SVR	Epidural and intrathecal administration for postoperative pain; elimination half-life 3 h
Remifentanil	IV infusion for surgical analgesia; small boluses for brief, intense pain	Easily titrated; very short duration; good cardiovascular stability. Ultiva is rapidly metabolized by hydrolysis of the propanoic acid–methyl ester linkage by nonspecific blood and tissue esterases	Expensive; requires mixing; may cause muscle rigidity	Potency: 25 µg = 10 mg morphine sulfate; 20–30 times potency of alfentanil; elimination half-life 3–10 min
Sufentanil	Surgical analgesia	Duration of action 0.5 h; prolonged analgesia exceptionally potent (5–10 times more than fentanyl); provides good stability in cardiovascular surgery	Prolonged respiratory depression	Potency: 15 µg = 10 mg morphine sulfate; elimination half-life 2.7 h
Depolarizing Muscle Relaxants				
Succinylcholine	Relax skeletal muscles for surgery and orthopedic manipulations; short procedures; intubation	Short duration; rapid onset	No known effect on consciousness, pain threshold, or cerebration; fasciculations, postoperative myalgias, arrhythmias; raises serum K$^+$ in tissue trauma, muscular disease, paralysis, burns; histamine release is slight; requires refrigeration	Prolonged muscle relaxation with serum cholinesterase deficiency and some antibiotics; may trigger malignant hyperthermia
Nondepolarizing Muscle Relaxants—Intermediate Onset and Duration				
Atracurium besylate	Intubation; maintenance of skeletal muscle relaxation	No significant cardiovascular or cumulative effects; good with kidney injury	Requires refrigeration; slight histamine release; pregnancy risk category C; do not mix with lactated Ringer's solution or alkaline solutions such as barbiturates	Rapid IV bolus; use cautiously with older adult patients and those who are debilitated
Cisatracurium besylate	Intubation; maintenance of skeletal muscle relaxation	Similar to atracurium	No histamine release	Similar to atracurium
Mivacurium	Intubation; maintenance of skeletal muscle relaxation	Short acting; rapid metabolism by plasma cholinesterase; used as bolus or infusion	Expensive in longer cases	Competes with acetylcholine for receptor sites at the motor end plate, blocking neuromuscular transmission; new; rarely need to reverse; prolonged effect with plasma cholinesterase deficiency
Rocuronium	Intubation; maintenance of relaxation	Rapid onset (dose dependent); elimination via kidney and liver	No known effect on consciousness, pain threshold, or cerebration; vagolytic; may $\uparrow$ HR	Duration similar to atracurium and vecuronium
Vecuronium	Intubation; maintenance of relaxation	No significant cardiovascular or cumulative effects; no histamine release	Requires mixing	Mostly eliminated in bile, some in urine

TABLE 15-2	Commonly Used Intravenous Medications (continued)			
Medication	**Common Usage**	**Advantages**	**Disadvantages**	**Comments**
Nondepolarizing Muscle Relaxants—Longer Onset and Duration				
d-Tubocurarine	Adjunct to anesthesia; maintenance of relaxation	—	No known effect on consciousness, pain threshold, or cerebration; might cause histamine release and transient ganglionic blockade	Mostly used for pretreatment with succinylcholine
Metocurine	Maintenance of relaxation	Good cardiovascular stability	Slight histamine release	Most commonly used opioid; potency: 100 μg = 10 mg morphine sulfate; elimination half-life 3.6 h
Pancuronium	Maintenance of relaxation	—	May cause ↑ HR and ↑ BP	Used intrathecally and epidurally for postoperative pain; elimination half-life 3 h
Intravenous Anesthetic Agents				
Diazepam	Amnesia; hypnotic; relieves anxiety; preoperative	Good sedation	Long acting	Residual effects for 20–90 h; increased effect with alcohol
Etomidate	Induction of general anesthesia; indicated to supplement low-potency anesthetic agents	Short-acting hypnotic; good cardiovascular stability; fast, smooth induction and recovery	May cause brief period of apnea; pain with injection and myotonic movements	—
Ketamine	Induction; occasional maintenance (IV or IM)	Short acting; profound analgesia; patient maintains airway; good in small children and burn patients	Large doses may cause hallucinations and respiratory depression; chest wall rigidity; laryngeal spasm	Need darkened, quiet room for recovery; often used in trauma cases
Midazolam	Hypnotic; anxiolytic; sedation; often used as adjunct to induction	Excellent amnesia; water soluble (no pain with IV injection); short acting	Slower induction than thiopental	Often used for amnesia with insertion of invasive monitors or regional anesthesia; depresses all levels of CNS, including limbic and reticular formation, probably through increased action of GABA, which is major inhibitory neurotransmitter in brain
Propofol	Induction and maintenance; sedation with regional anesthesia or MAC	Rapid onset; awakening in 4–8 min; produces sedation/hypnosis rapidly (within 40 s) and smoothly with minimal excitation; decreases intraocular pressure and systemic vascular resistance; rarely is associated with malignant hyperthermia and histamine release	May cause pain when injected; suppresses cardiac output and respiratory drive	Short elimination half-life (34–64 min)
Methohexital sodium	Induction; methohexital slows the activity of brain and nervous system	Ultra–short-acting barbiturate	May cause hiccups	Can be given rectally
Thiopental sodium	Induction; stops seizures	—	May cause laryngospasm	Large doses may cause apnea and cardiovascular depression; can be given rectally

BP, blood pressure; CNS, central nervous system; GABA, gamma-aminobutyric acid; HR, heart rate; IM, intramuscular; IV, intravenous; K+, potassium; MAC, monitored anesthesia care; SAB, subarachnoid block; SVR, stroke volume ratio.
Adapted from Association of PeriOperative Registered Nurses (AORN). (2019a). *Association of PeriOperative Registered Nurses (AORN) standards, recommended practice, and guidelines.* Denver, CO: Author.

commonly used IV anesthetic and analgesic agents, including IV medications used as muscle relaxants in the intraoperative period. These medications may be given to induce or maintain anesthesia. Although they are often used in combination with inhalation anesthetic agents, they may be used alone. They may also be used to produce moderate sedation, as discussed later in this chapter.

An advantage of IV anesthesia is that the onset of anesthesia is pleasant; there is none of the buzzing, roaring, or dizziness known to follow administration of an inhalation anesthetic agent. The duration of action is brief, and the patient awakens with little nausea or vomiting.

The IV anesthetic agents are nonexplosive, require little equipment, and are easy to administer. The low incidence of postoperative nausea and vomiting (PONV) makes the method useful in eye surgery, because in this setting vomiting would increase intraocular pressure and endanger vision in the operated eye. IV anesthesia is useful for short procedures but is used less often for the longer procedures of abdominal surgery. It is not indicated for those who require intubation because of their susceptibility to respiratory obstruction. The combination of IV and inhaled anesthetic agents produces an effective and smooth experience for the patient, with a controlled emergence following surgery.

IV neuromuscular blockers (muscle relaxants) block the transmission of nerve impulses at the neuromuscular junction of skeletal muscles. Muscle relaxants are used to relax muscles in abdominal and thoracic surgery, relax eye muscles in certain types of eye surgery, facilitate endotracheal intubation, treat laryngospasm, and assist in mechanical ventilation.

Multimodal Anesthesia

Multimodal analgesia regimens in surgical patients often use a combination of scheduled, nonopioid analgesic agents and regional anesthesia techniques (Wolfe, 2018). Multimodal analgesia aims to reduce opioid requirements and associated risks such as sedation, respiratory depression, nausea, vomiting, and potential of overuse of opioids. Multimodal anesthesia is a growing trend in the enhanced recovery after surgery (ERAS) pathways, as it decreases the risks of general anesthesia and aids in opioid reduction strategies. Analysis of opioid-naive surgical patients and opioid-naive nonsurgical patients found that those undergoing surgery had an increased risk of chronic opioid use during the first year after surgery (Sun, Darnall, Baker, et al., 2016). ERAS pathways are evidence based and facility specific; the patient follows these pathways from pre-, intra-, postoperative, and home phases of care. ERAS pathways are developed by multidisciplinary teams to optimize the recovery from surgery by reducing the patient's stress response. Instead of general anesthesia, regional/local anesthesia (LA) (discussed below) is administered. Nonopioid medications such as acetaminophen and nonsteroidal anti-inflammatory drugs (NSAIDs), ketamine, and gabapentinoids are preferred pain control methods in ERAS pathways (American Association of Nurse Anesthetists [AANA], 2019b).

Regional Anesthesia

In regional anesthesia, an anesthetic agent is injected around nerves so that the region supplied by these nerves is anesthetized. The effect depends on the type of nerve involved. Motor fibers are the largest fibers and have the thickest myelin sheath. Sympathetic fibers are the smallest and have a minimal covering. Sensory fibers are intermediate. A local anesthetic agent blocks motor nerves least readily and sympathetic nerves most readily. An anesthetic agent is not considered metabolized until all three systems (motor, sensory, and autonomic) are no longer affected.

The patient receiving regional anesthesia is awake and aware of their surroundings unless medications are given to produce mild sedation or to relieve anxiety. The health care team must avoid careless conversation, unnecessary noise, and unpleasant odors; these may be noticed by the patient in the OR and may contribute to a negative response to the surgical experience. A quiet environment is therapeutic. The diagnosis must not be stated aloud if the patient is not to know it at this time.

Epidural Anesthesia

Epidural anesthesia is achieved by injecting a local anesthetic agent into the epidural space that surrounds the dura mater of the spinal cord (see Fig. 15-5). The given medication diffuses across the layers of the spinal cord to provide anesthesia and pain relief (AORN, 2019; ASPAN, 2019). In contrast, spinal anesthesia involves injection through the dura mater into the subarachnoid space surrounding the spinal cord. Epidural anesthesia blocks sensory, motor, and autonomic functions; it differs from spinal anesthesia by the site of the injection and the amount of anesthetic agent used. Epidural doses are much higher because the epidural anesthetic agent does not make direct contact with the spinal cord or nerve roots (AORN, 2019a; ASPAN, 2019).

An advantage of epidural anesthesia is the absence of headache that can result from spinal anesthesia. A disadvantage is the greater technical challenge of introducing the

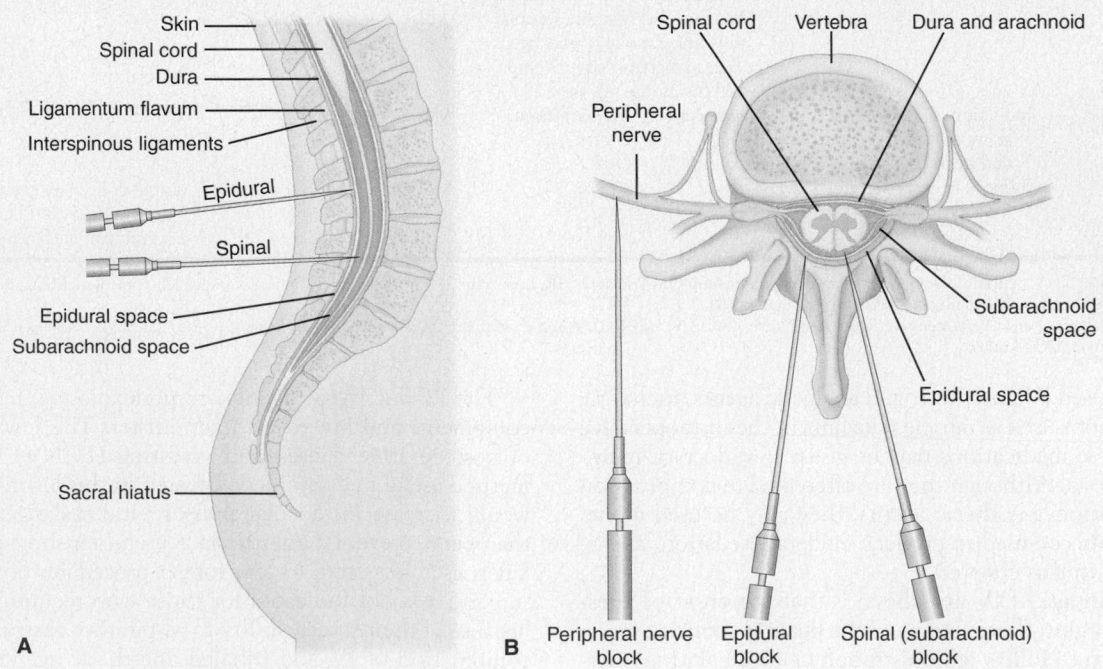

A Skin / Spinal cord / Dura / Ligamentum flavum / Interspinous ligaments / Epidural / Spinal / Epidural space / Subarachnoid space / Sacral hiatus

B Spinal cord / Vertebra / Dura and arachnoid / Peripheral nerve / Subarachnoid space / Epidural space / Peripheral nerve block / Epidural block / Spinal (subarachnoid) block

Figure 15-5 • A. Injection sites for spinal and epidural anesthesia. **B.** Cross-section of injection sites for peripheral nerve, epidural, and spinal blocks.

TABLE 15-3 Select Regional and Local Anesthetic Agents

Age	Administration	Advantages	Disadvantages	Implications/Considerations
Lidocaine	Epidural, spinal, peripheral IV anesthesia, and local infiltration	Rapid Longer duration of action (compared with procaine) Free of local irritative effect	Occasional allergic reaction	Useful topically for cystoscopy Observe for untoward reactions—drowsiness, depressed respiration, seizures
Bupivacaine	Epidural, spinal, peripheral IV anesthesia, and local infiltration	Duration is 2–3 times longer than lidocaine	Use cautiously in patients with known drug allergies or sensitivities	A period of analgesia persists after return of sensation; therefore, the need for strong analgesic agents is reduced Greater potency and longer action than lidocaine
Tetracaine	Topical, infiltration, and nerve block	Long acting, produces good relaxation	Occasional allergic reaction	>10 times as potent as procaine
Procaine	Local infiltration	—	Occasional allergic reaction	Commonly used in oral or dental surgery

IV, intravenous.

anesthetic agent into the epidural space rather than the subarachnoid space. If inadvertent puncture of the dura occurs during epidural anesthesia and the anesthetic agent travels toward the head, high spinal anesthesia can result; this can produce severe hypotension and respiratory depression and arrest. Treatment of these complications includes airway support, IV fluids, and the use of vasopressors.

Spinal Anesthesia

Spinal anesthesia is an extensive conduction nerve block that is produced when a local anesthetic agent is introduced into the subarachnoid space at the lumbar level, usually between L4 and L5 (see Fig. 15-5). It produces anesthesia of the lower extremities, perineum, and lower abdomen. For the lumbar puncture procedure, the patient usually lies on the side in a knee–chest position. Sterile technique is used as a spinal puncture is made and the medication is injected through the needle. As soon as the injection has been made, the patient is positioned on their back. If a relatively high level of block is sought, the head and shoulders are lowered.

The spread of the anesthetic agent and the level of anesthesia depend on the amount of agent injected, the speed with which it is injected, the positioning of the patient after the injection, and the specific gravity of the agent. If the specific gravity is greater than that of cerebrospinal fluid (CSF), the agent moves to the dependent position of the subarachnoid space. If the specific gravity is less than that of CSF, the anesthetic agent moves away from the dependent position. The anesthesiologist or CRNA controls the administration of the agent. Table 15-3 presents select regional anesthesia agents.

A few minutes after induction of a spinal anesthetic agent, anesthesia and paralysis affect the toes and perineum and then gradually the legs and abdomen.

Headache may be an aftereffect of spinal anesthesia. Several factors are related to the incidence of headache: the size of the spinal needle used, the leakage of fluid from the subarachnoid space through the puncture site, and the patient's hydration status. Measures that increase cerebrospinal pressure are helpful in relieving headache. These include maintaining a quiet environment, keeping the patient lying flat, and keeping the patient well hydrated.

In continuous spinal anesthesia, the tip of a plastic catheter remains in the subarachnoid space during the surgical procedure so that more anesthetic medication may be injected as needed. This technique allows greater control of the dosage; however, there is greater potential for postanesthetic headache because of the large-gauge needle used.

Peripheral Nerve Blocks

Peripheral nerve blocks (PNBs) are used in conjunction with general or MAC anesthesia, or as a stand-alone method. Instead of a single nerve being targeted, a bundle of nerves is located via ultrasound and injected with an anesthetic, opioid, or steroid. Traditionally, anesthesia would place the block in the OR setting. However, current research and best practices indicate that placing regional blocks in the preoperative department has greater efficacy. Patients emerge from anesthesia with less pain, decreasing the need for opioids. Research also suggests that patients spend less time in the postanesthesia care unit (PACU) and inpatients are discharged earlier (Gutierrez, Biehn, Eluna, et al., 2018).

Examples of common local conduction blocks include:
- Brachial plexus block, which produces anesthesia of the arm
- Paravertebral anesthesia, which produces anesthesia of the nerves supplying the chest, abdominal wall, and extremities
- Transsacral (caudal) block, which produces anesthesia of the perineum and, occasionally, the lower abdomen

Moderate Sedation

Moderate sedation, previously referred to as conscious sedation, is a form of anesthesia that involves the IV administration of sedatives or analgesic medications to reduce patient anxiety and control pain during diagnostic or therapeutic procedures. It is commonly used for many short-term surgical procedures in hospitals and ambulatory care centers (Rothrock, 2019). The goal is to depress a patient's level of consciousness to a moderate level to enable surgical, diagnostic, or therapeutic procedures to be performed while ensuring the patient's comfort during and cooperation with the procedures. With moderate sedation, the patient is able to maintain a patent airway, retain protective airway reflexes, and respond to verbal and physical stimuli.

Moderate sedation can be given by an anesthesiologist, CRNA, or other specially trained and credentialed physician or nurse. The practitioner who administers the sedation must be trained in resuscitative efforts as these patients are at risk for slipping into a deeper level of sedation (AORN, 2017). The continual assessment of the patient's vital signs, level of consciousness, and cardiac and respiratory function is an essential component of moderate sedation. Pulse oximetry, a continuous ECG monitor, and frequent measurement of vital signs are used to monitor the patient. Regulations for the use and administration of moderate sedation differ from state to state, and its administration is governed by standards issued by The Joint Commission and by institutional policies and nursing specialty organizations (AORN, 2017; ASPAN, 2018).

Monitored Anesthesia Care

Monitored anesthesia care (MAC), also referred to as monitored sedation, is moderate sedation given by an anesthesiologist or CRNA who must be prepared and qualified to convert to general anesthesia if necessary. The skills of an anesthesiologist or CRNA may be necessary to manage the effects of a level of deeper sedation to return the patient to the appropriate level of sedation (Barash et al., 2017). MAC may be used for healthy patients undergoing relatively minor surgical procedures and for some critically ill patients who may be unable to tolerate anesthesia without extensive invasive monitoring and pharmacologic support (Rothrock, 2019).

Local Anesthesia

LA is the injection of a solution containing the anesthetic agent into the tissues at the planned incision site. Often it is combined with a local regional block by injecting around the nerves immediately supplying the area. A monitoring nurse (in addition to a circulating nurse) must be present during these cases. The monitoring nurse is responsible for documenting the patient's condition, pain level, level of consciousness, and vital signs throughout the procedure (AORN, 2019a). Advantages of LA are as follows:

- It is simple, economical, and nonexplosive.
- Equipment needed is minimal.
- Postoperative recovery is brief.
- Undesirable effects of general anesthesia are avoided.
- It is ideal for short and minor surgical procedures.

LA is often given in combination with epinephrine. Epinephrine constricts blood vessels, which prevents rapid absorption of the anesthetic agent and thus prolongs its local action and prevents seizures. Select local anesthetic agents are listed in Table 15-3; some of the same agents used in regional anesthesia are used as local anesthetic agents.

The skin is prepared as for any surgical procedure, and a small-gauge needle is used to inject a modest amount of the anesthetic medication into the skin layers. This produces blanching or a wheal. Additional anesthetic medication is then injected into the skin until an area surrounding the proposed incision is anesthetized. A larger, longer needle then is used to infiltrate deeper tissues with the anesthetic agent. The action of the agent is almost immediate, so surgery may begin shortly after the injection is complete. The anesthetic may be mixed with a fast-acting analgesic of short duration to circumvent the burning felt when the longer-acting anesthetics are injected.

Local Anesthetic Systemic Toxicity

Local Anesthetic Systemic Toxicity (LAST) is a potentially life-threatening event. LAST occurs when a bolus of LA is inadvertently injected into peripheral tissue or venous or arterial circulation during a PNB or spinal nerve block procedure and is rapidly absorbed into systemic circulation, resulting in cardiovascular or neurologic collapse (Ferguson, Coogle, Leppert, et al., 2019).

Signs and symptoms of LAST are:
- Metallic taste
- Oral numbness
- Auditory changes
- Slurred speech
- Arrhythmias
- Seizure
- Respiratory arrest

LAST is a rare event that occurs in approximately 1 of every 1000 patients (Wadlund, 2017). Early detection and treatment may prevent symptom progression and can lead to a better outcome for the patient. Initial treatment of LAST should focus on airway management. Hypoxemia and acidosis intensify the effects of LAST. The nurse calls for help and maintains the patient's airway while administering 100% oxygen and confirming IV access. Additional resources include members of the anesthesia team and critical-care nurses in the event that CPR or airway interventions take place. An IV infusion of lipid emulsions (an emulsion of soybean oil, egg phospholipids, and glycerin) can reverse the effects of LAST on the heart and central nervous system (AORN, 2019a; Wadlund, 2017).

Potential Intraoperative Complications

The surgical patient is subject to several risks. The major potential intraoperative complications include anesthesia awareness, nausea and vomiting, anaphylaxis, hypoxia, hypothermia, and malignant hyperthermia (MH). Targeted areas include SSIs as well as cardiac, respiratory, and venous thromboembolic complications (Joint Commission, 2019).

Anesthesia Awareness

It is important to discuss concerns about intraoperative awareness with patients preoperatively so that they realize that only general anesthesia is meant to create a state of oblivion. All other forms of anesthesia will eliminate pain, but sensation of pushing and pulling tissues may still be recognized and they may hear conversations among the operative team. In many cases, patients may be able to respond to questions and involve themselves in the discussion. This is normal and is not what is referred to as anesthesia awareness.

Unintended intraoperative awareness refers to a patient becoming cognizant of surgical interventions while under general anesthesia and then recalling the incident. Neuromuscular blocks, sometimes required for surgical muscle relaxation, intensify the fear of the patient experiencing awareness because they are then unable to communicate during the episode. Patients may or may not feel pain, and some patients experience a feeling of pressure. It has been estimated that roughly 1 patient per 1000 receiving general anesthesia experiences some level of awareness that is most commonly fleeting (AANA, 2019a).

Indications of the occurrence of anesthesia awareness include an increase in the blood pressure, rapid heart rate, and patient movement. However, hemodynamic changes can be masked by paralytic medication, beta-blockers, and calcium channel blockers, thus the awareness may remain undetected. Premedication with amnesic agents and avoidance of muscle paralytics except when essential help to preclude its occurrence.

Nausea and Vomiting

Nausea and vomiting, or regurgitation, may affect patients during the intraoperative period. The patient should be assessed preoperatively for risk factors of PONV so that the surgical team can formulate a plan for intraoperative prevention. Risk factors include female gender, age less than 50 years, history of PONV, and opioid administration (Finch, Parkosewich, Perrone, et al., 2019).

If gagging occurs, the patient is turned to the side, the head of the table is lowered, and a basin is provided to collect the vomitus. Suction is used to remove saliva and vomited gastric contents. In some cases, the anesthesiologist or CRNA administers antiemetics preoperatively or intraoperatively to counteract possible aspiration. If the patient aspirates vomitus, an attack with severe bronchial spasms and wheezing is triggered. Pneumonitis and pulmonary edema can subsequently develop, leading to extreme hypoxia. Increasing medical attention is being paid to silent regurgitation of gastric contents (not related to preoperative fasting times), which occurs more frequently than previously realized. The volume and acidity of the aspirate determine the extent of damage to the lungs. Patients may be given citric acid and sodium citrate, a clear, nonparticulate antacid to increase gastric fluid pH or a histamine-2 (H_2) receptor antagonist such as cimetidine, or famotidine to decrease gastric acid production (Rothrock, 2019).

Anaphylaxis

Any time the patient comes into contact with a foreign substance, there is potential for an anaphylactic reaction. An anaphylactic reaction can occur in response to many medications, latex, or other substances. The reaction may be immediate or delayed. Anaphylaxis can be a life-threatening reaction.

Latex allergy—the sensitivity to natural rubber latex products—has become more prevalent, creating the need for alert responsiveness among health care professionals. If patients state that they have allergies to latex, even if they are wearing latex in their clothing, treatment must be latex free. In the OR, many products are latex free with the notable exception of softer latex catheters. Surgical cases should use latex-free gloves in anticipation of a possible allergy, and if no allergy is present, then personnel can switch to other gloves after the case starts if desired.

Fibrin sealants are used in various surgical procedures, and cyanoacrylate tissue adhesives are used to close wounds without the use of sutures. These sealants have been implicated in allergic reactions and anaphylaxis (Rothrock, 2019). Although these reactions are rare, the nurse must be alert to the possibility and observe the patient for changes in vital

signs and symptoms of anaphylaxis when these products are used. In the OR, the team should remove potential causative agents promptly—within 3 minutes or less—of becoming aware of an anaphylactic reaction. The surgical team should be aware of the importance of prompt intervention to prevent cardiovascular and respiratory collapse (Seifert, 2017). (Chapters 11 and 33 provide more details about the signs, symptoms, and treatment of anaphylaxis and anaphylactic shock.)

Hypoxia and Other Respiratory Complications

Inadequate ventilation, occlusion of the airway, inadvertent intubation of the esophagus, and hypoxia are significant potential complications associated with general anesthesia. Many factors can contribute to inadequate ventilation. Respiratory depression caused by anesthetic agents, aspiration of respiratory tract secretions or vomitus, and the patient's position on the operating table can compromise the exchange of gases. Anatomic variation can make the trachea difficult to visualize and result in insertion of the artificial airway into the esophagus rather than into the trachea. In addition to these dangers, asphyxia caused by foreign bodies in the mouth; spasm of the vocal cords; relaxation of the tongue; or aspiration of vomitus, saliva, or blood can occur. Brain damage from hypoxia occurs within minutes; therefore, vigilant monitoring of the patient's oxygenation status is a primary function of the anesthesiologist or CRNA and the circulating nurse. Peripheral perfusion is checked frequently, and capnography readings are monitored continuously. Capnography provides instantaneous information about carbon dioxide production, pulmonary perfusion, and respiratory patterns that detect hypoventilation and apnea (Odom-Forren, 2018).

Hypothermia

During anesthesia, the patient's temperature may fall. Glucose metabolism is reduced, and as a result, metabolic acidosis may develop. This condition is called *hypothermia* and is indicated by a core body temperature that is lower than normal (36.6°C [98°F] or less). Risks of intraoperative hypothermia include cardiovascular events, SSIs, bleeding, and delayed arousal from anesthesia (Williams, 2018). Unintended hypothermia may occur as a result of a low temperature in the OR, infusion of cold fluids, inhalation of cold gases, open body wounds or cavities, decreased muscle activity, advanced age, or the pharmaceutical agents used (e.g., vasodilators, phenothiazines, general anesthetic medications). Hypothermia can depress neuronal activity and decrease cellular oxygen requirements below the minimum levels normally required for continued cell viability. As a result, it is used to protect function during some surgical procedures (e.g., carotid endarterectomy, cardiopulmonary bypass) (Barash et al., 2017).

Unintended hypothermia needs to be avoided. If it occurs, it must be minimized or reversed. If hypothermia is intentional, the goal is safe return to normal body temperature. Environmental temperature in the OR can temporarily be set at 25° to 26.6°C (78° to 80°F). IV and irrigating fluids are warmed to 37°C (98.6°F). Wet gowns and drapes are removed promptly and replaced with dry materials, because wet materials promote heat loss. Warm air blankets and thermal blankets can also be used on the areas not exposed for surgery, and minimizing the area of the patient that is exposed will help maintain core temperature. Whatever methods are used to rewarm the patient, warming must be accomplished gradually, not rapidly. Conscientious monitoring of core temperature, urinary output, ECG, blood pressure, arterial blood gas levels, and serum electrolyte levels is required.

Malignant Hyperthermia

Malignant hyperthermia is a rare inherited muscle disorder that is chemically induced by anesthetic agents (Rothrock, 2019). This disorder can be triggered by myopathies, emotional stress, heatstroke, neuroleptic malignant syndrome, strenuous exercise exertion, and trauma. The incidence rate is 1 in every 170,698 general anesthetic cases (Phi, Carvalho, Sun, et al., 2018). MH occurs because of a genetic autosomal dominant disorder involving a mutation on the ryanodine receptor that causes an atypical increase in release of calcium in muscle cells (Mullins, 2018). Susceptible people include those with strong and bulky muscles, a history of muscle cramps or muscle weakness and unexplained temperature elevation, and an unexplained death of a family member during surgery that was accompanied by a febrile response (Ho, Carvalho, Sun, et al., 2018).

Pathophysiology

During anesthesia, potent agents such as inhalation anesthetic agents (i.e., halothane, enflurane, isoflurane) and muscle relaxants (succinylcholine) may trigger the symptoms of malignant hyperthermia (Rothrock, 2019). Stress and some medications, such as sympathomimetics (epinephrine), theophylline, aminophylline, anticholinergics (atropine), and cardiac glycosides (digitalis), can induce or intensify a reaction.

The pathophysiology of MH is related to a hypermetabolic condition that involves altered mechanisms of calcium function in skeletal muscle cells. This disruption of calcium causes clinical symptoms of hypermetabolism, which in turn increases muscle contraction (rigidity) and causes hyperthermia and subsequent damage to the central nervous system.

Clinical Manifestations

The initial symptoms of MH are often cardiovascular, respiratory, and abnormal musculoskeletal activity. Tachycardia (heart rate greater than 150 bpm) may be an early sign. Sympathetic nervous stimulation also leads to ventricular arrhythmia, hypotension, decreased cardiac output, oliguria, and, later, cardiac arrest. Hypercapnia, an increase in carbon dioxide (CO_2), may be an early respiratory sign. With the abnormal transport of calcium, rigidity or tetanuslike movements occur, often in the jaw. Generalized muscle rigidity is one of the earliest signs. The rise in temperature is actually a late sign that develops rapidly; body temperature can increase 1° to 2°C (2° to 4°F) every 5 minutes, and core body temperature can exceed 42°C (107°F) (Rothrock, 2019).

Medical Management

Goals of treatment are to decrease metabolism, reverse metabolic and respiratory acidosis, correct arrhythmias, decrease body temperature, provide oxygen and nutrition to tissues, and correct electrolyte imbalance. The treatment for MH is well known. Use of dantrolene has lowered mortality rates to 10% in current practice (Ho et al., 2018). The Malignant Hyperthermia Association of the United States (MHAUS) publishes a treatment protocol that should be posted in the OR and be readily available on a MH cart (see Resources section).

Anesthesia and surgery should be postponed. However, if end-tidal CO_2 monitoring and dantrolene sodium are available and the anesthesiologist is experienced in managing MH, the surgery may continue using a different anesthetic agent (Barash et al., 2017). Although MH usually manifests about 10 to 20 minutes after induction of anesthesia, it can also occur during the first 24 hours after surgery.

Nursing Management

Although MH is uncommon, the nurse must identify patients at risk, recognize the signs and symptoms, have the appropriate medication and equipment available, and be knowledgeable about the protocol to follow. Preparation and early intervention may be lifesaving for the patient.

NURSING PROCESS

The Patient during Surgery

Intraoperative nurses focus on nursing diagnoses, interventions, and outcomes that surgical patients and their families experience. Additional priorities include collaborative problems and expected goals.

Assessment

Nursing assessment of the intraoperative patient involves obtaining data from the patient and the patient's medical record to identify factors that can affect care. These serve as guidelines for an individualized plan of patient care. The intraoperative nurse uses the focused preoperative nursing assessment documented on the patient record. This includes assessment of physiologic status (e.g., health–illness level, level of consciousness), psychosocial status (e.g., anxiety level, verbal communication problems, coping mechanisms), physical status (e.g., surgical site, skin condition, and effectiveness of preparation; mobility of joints), and ethical concerns.

Diagnosis

NURSING DIAGNOSES

Based on the assessment data, major nursing diagnoses may include the following:

- Anxiety associated with surgical or environmental concerns
- Risk for latex allergy
- Risk for perioperative positioning injury associated with positioning in the OR
- Risk for injury associated with anesthesia and surgical procedure
- Risk for compromised dignity associated with general anesthesia or sedation

COLLABORATIVE PROBLEMS/POTENTIAL COMPLICATIONS

Based on the assessment data, potential complications may include the following:

- Anesthesia awareness
- Nausea and vomiting

- Anaphylaxis
- Hypoxia
- Unintentional hypothermia
- Malignant hyperthermia
- Infection

Planning and Goals

The major goals for care of the patient during surgery include reduced anxiety, absence of latex exposure, absence of positioning injuries, freedom from injury, maintenance of the patient's dignity, and absence of complications.

Nursing Interventions

REDUCING ANXIETY

Preoperatively, the intraoperative nurse visiting the patient can help decrease anxiety and promote a relationship of communication and trust. The effect of familiarizing patients revealed significant decreased preoperative and postoperative anxiety (Bagheri, Ebrahimi, Abbasi, et al., 2019). The patient should be notified of what to expect when entering the operating room, and the nurse should inquire about any patient-specific relaxation preferences. The OR environment can seem cold, stark, and frightening to the patient, who may be feeling isolated and apprehensive. Introducing yourself, addressing the patient by name warmly and frequently, verifying details, providing explanations, and encouraging and answering questions provide a sense of professionalism and friendliness that can help the patient feel safe and secure. When discussing what the patient can expect in surgery, the nurse uses basic communication skills, such as touch and eye contact, to reduce anxiety. Attention to physical comfort (warm blankets, padding, position changes) helps the patient feel more comfortable. Telling the patient who else will be present in the OR, how long the procedure is expected to take, and other details helps the patient prepare for the experience and gain a sense of control.

The circulating nurse may assist to decrease anxiety during induction by using techniques such as guided imagery, decreasing room stimuli by dimming the lights, having the patient's favorite music playing, or by talking in a soft voice and using eye contact, if culturally appropriate.

REDUCING LATEX EXPOSURE

Patients with latex allergies require early identification and communication to all personnel about the presence of the allergy according to standards of care for patients with latex allergy (AORN, 2019a). In most ORs, there are few latex items currently in use, but because there still remain some instances of latex use, maintenance of latex allergy precautions throughout the perioperative period must be observed. For safety, manufacturers and hospital materials managers need to take responsibility for identifying the latex content in items used by patients and health care personnel. (See Chapters 14 and 33 for assessment for latex allergy.)

Quality and Safety Nursing Alert

It is the responsibility of all nurses, and particularly perianesthesia and perioperative nurses, to be aware of latex allergies, necessary precautions, and products that are latex free. Hospital staff are also at risk for development of a latex allergy secondary to repeated exposure to latex products.

PREVENTING PERIOPERATIVE POSITIONING INJURY

The patient's position on the operating table depends on the surgical procedure to be performed as well as the patient's physical condition (see Fig. 15-6). One type of injury, peripheral nerve injury, is defined as the interruption of electrical activity that affects either the sensory, motor, or both nerve functions resulting in a deficit. Studies suggest a correlation between total OR time and tissue breakdown (Grap, Schubert, Munro, et al., 2019). See Chart 15-3 for a Nursing Research Profile that investigated these occurrences. The potential for transient discomfort or permanent injury is present because many surgical procedures require awkward

---

Chart 15-3 · NURSING RESEARCH PROFILE

Sacral Tissue Pressure Injury Prevalence in Surgical Patients

Grap, M. J., Schubert, C., Munro, C. L., et al. (2019). OR time and sacral pressure injuries in critically ill surgical patients. *AORN Journal, 109*(2), 229–239.

Purpose

The ability to identify early changes associated with pressure injury and OR time may enhance pressure injury prevention strategies. The purpose of this study was to explore the relationship between OR time and sacral pressure injuries in critically ill patients using high-frequency ultrasound (HFU) to identify early tissue changes.

Design

A secondary analysis was used to evaluate the effect of backrest elevation on 150 ventilated patients in the ICU post surgery. All of the patients had recorded OR time and the Braden Score was collected to identify patients at risk for surgical pressure injury.

Findings

One hundred and fifty participants were enrolled and 132 had skin evaluations. The majority of participants were middle-aged White males (58%), overweight, and had a Braden Scale score showing moderate risk for pressure injury. Total OR time ranged from just under 1 hour to more than 13 hours, with an average time of more than 4 hours. For those participants who developed pressure injuries, time between the OR and injury observed was approximately 2 to 3 days on average. Approximately 63% of participants did not have sacral pressure injuries at any point during the observation period. Using multivariable models, the model containing OR bed time, BMI, and Braden Scale score produced the best prediction of pressure injury. A higher BMI, shorter OR bed time, and lower Braden Scale score were associated with a greater chance of pressure injury.

Nursing Implications

Preventing pressure injuries are a priority for nurses in all setting and is particularly challenging for critical-care patients. These preliminary results demonstrate that the use of HFU may help nurses identify the development of tissue changes before observable skin changes, leading to earlier pressure injury prevention strategies.

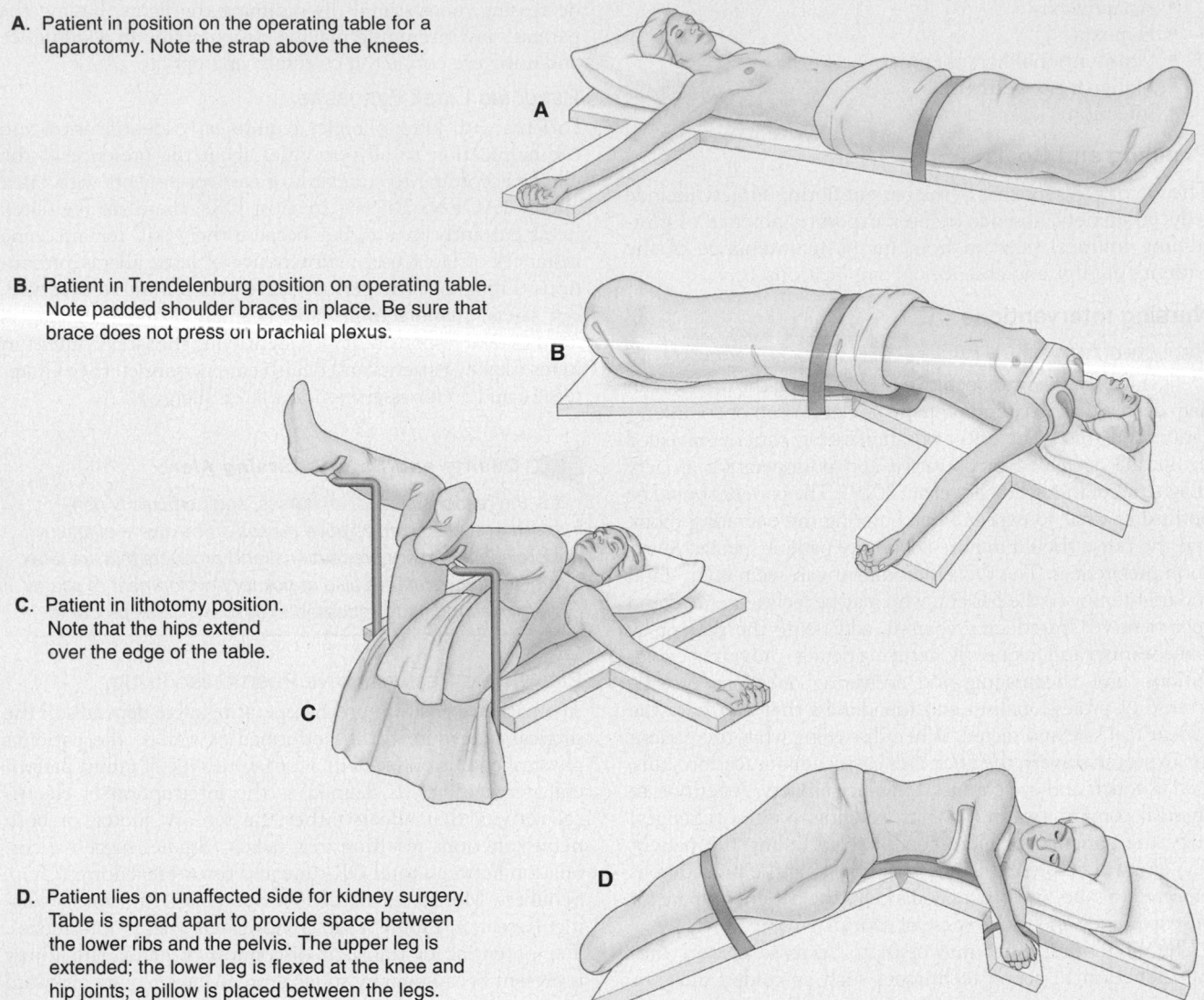

A. Patient in position on the operating table for a laparotomy. Note the strap above the knees.

B. Patient in Trendelenburg position on operating table. Note padded shoulder braces in place. Be sure that brace does not press on brachial plexus.

C. Patient in lithotomy position. Note that the hips extend over the edge of the table.

D. Patient lies on unaffected side for kidney surgery. Table is spread apart to provide space between the lower ribs and the pelvis. The upper leg is extended; the lower leg is flexed at the knee and hip joints; a pillow is placed between the legs.

Figure 15-6 • Patient positions on the operating table. Captions call attention to safety and comfort features. All surgical patients wear caps to cover the hair completely.

anatomical positions. Hyperextending joints, compressing arteries, or pressing on nerves and bony prominences usually results in discomfort simply because the position must be sustained for a long period of time (Rothrock, 2019). Factors to consider include the following:

- The patient should be in as comfortable a position as possible, whether conscious or unconscious.
- The operative field must be adequately exposed.
- An awkward anatomical position, undue pressure on a body part, or the use of stirrups or traction should not obstruct the vascular supply.
- Respiration should not be impeded by pressure of arms on the chest or by a gown that constricts the neck or chest.
- Nerves must be protected from undue pressure. Improper positioning of the arms, hands, legs, or feet can cause serious injury or paralysis. Shoulder braces must be well padded to prevent irreparable nerve injury, especially when the Trendelenburg position is necessary.

- Precautions for patient safety must be observed, particularly with older adults, patients who are thin or obese, and those with a physical deformity.
- The patient may need light restraint before induction in case of excitement.

The usual position for surgery, called the *dorsal recumbent position*, is flat on the back. Both arms are positioned at the side of the table: one with the hand placed palm down and the other carefully positioned on an armboard to facilitate IV infusion of fluids, blood, or medications. This position is used for most abdominal surgeries, except for surgery of the gallbladder or pelvis (see Fig. 15-6A).

The Trendelenburg position usually is used for surgery on the lower abdomen and pelvis to obtain good exposure by displacing the intestines into the upper abdomen. In this position, the head and body are lowered. The patient is supported in position by padded shoulder braces (see Fig. 15-6B), bean bags, and foam padding. Reverse Trendelenburg position provides the space to operate on the upper abdomen by shifting the intestines into the pelvis. A padded footboard and other supportive cushioning preserve a safe environment for the patient.

The lithotomy position is used for nearly all perineal, rectal, and vaginal surgical procedures (see Fig. 15-6C). The patient is positioned on the back with the legs and thighs flexed. The position is maintained by placing the feet in stirrups.

The Sims or lateral position is used for renal surgery. The patient is placed on the nonoperative side with an air pillow 12.5 to 15 cm (5 to 6 inches) thick under the loin, or on a table with a kidney or back lift (see Fig. 15-6D).

PROTECTING THE PATIENT FROM INJURY

Various activities are used to address the diverse patient safety issues that arise in the OR. The nurse protects the patient from injury by providing a safe environment. Verifying information, checking the medical record for completeness, and maintaining surgical asepsis and an optimal environment are critical nursing responsibilities. Verification that all the required documentation is completed is an important function of the intraoperative nurse. A surgical checklist is used prior to induction of anesthesia, before the skin incision is made, and before the patient leaves the OR (see Fig. 15-1). It is important to review the patient's record for the following:

- Allergies (including latex)
- Correct informed surgical consent, with patient's signature
- Completed records for health history and physical examination
- Results of diagnostic studies

In addition to checking that all necessary patient data are complete, the perioperative nurse obtains the necessary equipment specific to the procedure. The need for nonroutine medications, blood components, instruments, and other equipment and supplies is assessed, and the readiness of the room, completeness of physical setup, and completeness of instrument, suture, and dressing setups are determined. Any aspects of the OR environment that may negatively affect the patient are identified. These include physical features, such as room temperature and humidity; electrical hazards; potential contaminants (dust, blood, and discharge on floor or surfaces; uncovered hair; nonsterile attire of personnel; jewelry worn by personnel; chipped or artificial fingernails); and unnecessary traffic. The circulating nurse also sets up and maintains suction equipment in working order, initiates appropriate physical comfort measures for the patient, and prepares any potential implantable devices and medications used at the surgical field.

Preventing physical injury includes using safety straps and side rails and not leaving the sedated patient unattended. Transferring the patient from the stretcher to the OR table requires safe transferring practices. Other safety measures include properly positioning a grounding pad under the patient to prevent electrical burns and shock, removing excess antiseptic solution from the patient's skin, and promptly and completely draping exposed areas after the sterile field has been created to decrease the risk of hypothermia.

Nursing measures to prevent injury from excessive blood loss include blood conservation using equipment such as a cell saver (a device for recirculating the patient's own blood cells) and administration of blood products (Rothrock, 2019). Fewer patients undergoing an elective procedure require blood transfusion, but those undergoing high-risk procedures (such as orthopedic or cardiac surgeries) may require an intraoperative transfusion. The circulating nurse anticipates this need, checks that blood has been cross-matched and held in reserve, and is prepared to administer blood.

SERVING AS PATIENT ADVOCATE

The patient undergoing general anesthesia or moderate sedation experiences temporary sensory or perceptual alteration or loss, and has an increased need for protection and advocacy. Patient advocacy in the OR entails maintaining the patient's physical and emotional comfort, privacy, rights, and dignity. Patients, whether conscious or unconscious, should not be subjected to excess noise, inappropriate conversation, or, most of all, derogatory comments. Other advocacy activities include minimizing the clinical, dehumanizing aspects of being a surgical patient by making sure that the patient is treated as a person, respecting cultural and spiritual values, providing physical privacy, maintaining confidentiality, and contacting approved family or support personnel about updates throughout the procedure.

PREVENTING RETAINED SURGICAL ITEMS

It is the entire surgical team's responsibility to provide vigilance and communication regarding items entering and leaving the surgical site. As part of their responsibilities, the circulating nurse and scrub personnel must account for items introduced to the sterile field. This includes sponges, needles, instruments, and access devices. Some of these items are radiopaque (visible under x-ray), others are not. All items must be accounted for at the beginning of surgery, prior to wound closure, and again at skin closure. The nurse serves as a patient advocate to alert the team of any missing items. Technology can assist in surgical item identification; however, it should not be used as the primary source for counting.

MONITORING AND MANAGING POTENTIAL COMPLICATIONS

It is the responsibility of the surgeon and the anesthesiologist or CRNA to monitor and manage complications. However, intraoperative nurses also play an important role. Being alert to and reporting changes in vital signs, cardiac arrhythmias, symptoms of nausea and vomiting, anaphylaxis, hypoxia, hypothermia, and MH and assisting with their management are important nursing functions. Each of these complications was discussed earlier. Maintaining asepsis and preventing infection are responsibilities of all members of the surgical team (Rothrock, 2019). Evidence-based interventions to decrease SSIs include appropriate skin preparation and antibiotic administration. These interventions are discussed by the surgical team and documented by the nurse in the intraoperative record.

Evaluation

Expected patient outcomes may include:

1. Exhibits low level of anxiety while awake during the intraoperative phase of care
2. Has no symptoms of latex allergy
3. Remains free of perioperative positioning injury
4. Experiences no unexpected threats to safety
5. Has dignity preserved throughout OR experience
6. Is free of complications (e.g., cardiac arrhythmias, nausea and vomiting, anaphylaxis, hypoxia, hypothermia, or MH or experiences successful management of adverse effects of surgery and anesthesia should they occur)

CRITICAL THINKING EXERCISES

1 `ebp` A 48-year-old man is scheduled to have robotic-assisted abdominal surgery. What is the best evidence for how his vital signs should be monitored? As the OR nurse, what best practices should you implement to support the patient and OR team during this minimally invasive surgery?

2 `ipc` A 66-year-old woman with chronic obstructive pulmonary disease (COPD) is scheduled for an elective procedure to remove a lipoma on her chest. She is having problems breathing, is agitated, and cannot lie flat on the surgical bed. How will you, as the circulating nurse, facilitate an interprofessional discussion to improve the patient's breathing and relieve her agitation? Which members of the surgical team are essential to include?

3 `pq` Identify the priorities, assessments, and nursing interventions you would implement for a 76-year-old female patient who is hard of hearing and is having spinal anesthesia for total knee replacement surgery. How would your priorities, approach, and techniques differ if the patient is having general anesthesia? What other risks should be considered based on this patient's age?

REFERENCES

*Asterisk indicates nursing research.

Books

American Society of PeriAnesthesia Nurses (ASPAN). (2019). *2015–2019 Perianesthesia nursing standards, practice recommendations and interpretive statements.* Cherry Hill, NJ: Author.

Association of PeriOperative Registered Nurses (AORN). (2019a). *Association of PeriOperative Registered Nurses (AORN) standards, recommended practice, and guidelines.* Denver, CO: Author.

Barash, P. G., Cullen, B. F., Stoelting, R. K., et al. (2017). *Clinical anesthesia* (8th ed.). Philadelphia, PA: Lippincott Williams & Wilkins.

Odom-Forren, J. (2018). *Drain's perianesthesia nursing: A critical care approach.* St Louis, MO: Elsevier.

Phillips, N. M. (2017). *Operating room technique* (13th ed.). St. Louis, MO: Elsevier.

Rothrock, J. (2019). *Alexander's care of the patient in surgery* (16th ed.). St. Louis, MO: Elsevier.

Journals and Electronic Documents

American Association of Nurse Anesthetists (AANA). (2019a). Anesthetic awareness fact sheet. Retrieved on 8/21/19 at: www.aana.com/patients/all-about-anesthesia/anesthetic-awareness/anesthetic-awareness-fact-sheet

American Association of Nurse Anesthetists (AANA). (2019b). Enhanced recovery after surgery. Retrieved on 8/15/19 at: www.aana.com/practice/clinical-practice-resources/enhanced-recovery-after-surgery

American Society of Anesthesiologists (ASA). (2019). Preparing for surgery: Risks: Age. Retrieved on 8/26/19 at: www.asahq.org/whensecondscount/preparing-for-surgery/risks/age/

Armellino, D. (2017). Minimizing sources of airborne, aerosolized, and contact contaminants in the OR environment. *AORN Journal, 106*(6), 494–501.

Association of PeriOperative Registered Nurses (AORN). (2017). Guideline at a glance: Moderate sedation/analgesia. *AORN Journal, 105*(6), 638–642.

Association of PeriOperative Registered Nurses (AORN). (2019b). Fire safety tool kit: Fire prevention assessment tool. Retrieved on 5/29/19 at: www.aorn.org/guidelines/clinical-resources/tool-kits/fire-safety-tool-kit

*Bagheri, H., Ebrahimi, H., Abbasi, A., et al. (2019). Effect of preoperative visitation by operating room staff on preoperative anxiety in patients receiving elective hernia surgery. *Journal of PeriAnesthesia Nursing, 34*(2), 272–280.

Burlingame, B. L. (2017). Guideline implementation: Energy-generating devices, Part 2-lasers. *AORN Journal, 105*(4), 392–401.

Carlos, G., & Saulan, M. (2018). Robotic emergencies: Are you prepared for disaster? *AORN Journal, 108*(5), 493–501.

Clark, C. M. & Kenski, D. (2017). Promoting civility in the OR: An ethical imperative. *AORN Journal, 105*(1), 60–66.

Davis, S. (2018). The key to safety: A healthy workforce. *AORN Journal, 108*(2), 120–122.

Ferguson, W., Coogle C., Leppert J., et al. (2019). Local anesthetic systemic toxicity (LAST): Designing an educational effort for nurses that will last. *Journal of PeriAnesthesia Nursing, 34*(1), 180–187.

Finch, C., Parkosewich, J. A., Perrone, D., et al. (2019). Incidence, timing, and factors associated with postoperative nausea and vomiting in the ambulatory surgery setting. *Journal of PeriAnesthesia Nursing, 34*(6), 1146–1155.

*Grap M. J., Schubert, C., Munro, C. L., et al. (2019). OR time and sacral pressure injuries in critically ill surgical patients. *AORN Journal, 109*(2), 229–239.

Gutierrez, M., Biehn, S., Eluna, A., et al. (2018). Placing regional anesthesia blocks in the preoperative unit. *Journal of PeriAnesthesia Nursing, 33*(4), e14–e15.

Ho, P. T., Carvalho, B., Sun, E. C., et al. (2018). Cost-benefit analysis of maintaining a fully stocked malignant hyperthermia cart versus an initial dantrolene treatment dose for maternity units. *Anesthesiology, 129*(2), 249–259.

Joint Commission. (2019). 2019 National Patient Safety Goals. Retrieved on 5/22/19 at: www.jointcommission.org/assets/1/6/2019_HAP_NPSGs_final2.pdf

Mullins, M. F. (2018). Malignant hyperthermia: A review. *Journal of PeriAnesthesia Nursing, 33*(5), 582–589.

Seifert, P. (2017). Crisis management of anaphylaxis in the operating room. *AORN Journal, 105*(2), 219–227.

Spruce, L. (2018). Back to basics: Protection from surgical smoke. *AORN Journal, 108*(1), 24–32.

*Steelman, V., Schaapveld, A., Storm, H. E., et al. (2019). The effect of radiofrequency technology on time spent searching for surgical sponges and associated costs. *AORN Journal, 109*(6), 718–727.

Sun, E. C., Darnall, B. D., Baker, L. C., et al. (2016). Incidence of and risk factors for chronic opioid use among opioid-naïve patients in the postoperative period. *JAMA Internal Medicine, 176*(9), 1286–1293.

US Department of Labor, Occupational Safety and Health Administration. (2018). Laser/Electrosurgery plume. Retrieved on 5/29/2019 at: www.osha.gov/SLTC/laserelectrosurgeryplume/index.html

Vernon, T. L., Rice, A. N., Titch, J. F., et al. (2019). Implementation of vulnerable elders survey-13 frailty tool to identify at-risk geriatric surgical patients. *Journal of PeriAnesthesia Nursing, 34*(5), 911–918.

Wadlund, D. (2017). Local anesthetic systemic toxicity. *AORN Journal, 106*(5), 367–377.

*Williams, A. (2018). Benefits of passive warming on surgical patients undergoing regional anesthetic procedures. *Journal of PeriAnesthesia Nursing, 33*(6), 928–934.

Wolfe, R. (2018). Multimodal anesthesia in the perioperative setting. *Journal of PeriAnesthesia Nursing, 33*(4), 563–569.

World Health Organization (WHO). (2019). Surgical safety checklist. Retrieved on 5/22/19 at: www.who.int/patientsafety/topics/safe-surgery/checklist/en/

Ziman, R., Espin, S., Grant, R., et al. (2018). Looking beyond the checklist: An ethnography of interprofessional operating room safety cultures. *Journal of Interprofessional Care, 32*(5), 575–583.

Resources

American Association of Nurse Anesthetists (AANA), www.aana.com
American Society of Anesthesiologists (ASA), www.asahq.org
American Society of PeriAnesthesia Nurses (ASPAN), www.aspan.org
Association of PeriOperative Registered Nurses, www.aorn.org
Centers for Disease Control and Prevention, Injury and Violence Prevention and Control, www.cdc.gov/injury
Joint Commission, www.jointcommission.org
Malignant Hyperthermia Association of the United States (MHAUS), www.mhaus.org
World Health Organization (WHO), www.who.int/en/

16 Postoperative Nursing Management

The postoperative period extends from the time the patient leaves the operating room (OR) until the last follow-up visit with the surgeon. This may be as short as a day or two or as long as several months. During the postoperative period, nursing care focuses on reestablishing the patient's physiologic equilibrium, alleviating pain, preventing complications, and educating the patient about self-care. Careful assessment and immediate intervention assist the patient in returning to optimal function quickly, safely, and as comfortable as possible. Ongoing care in the community through home care, clinic visits, office visits, or telephone follow-up facilitates an uncomplicated recovery.

Care of the Patient in the Postanesthesia Care Unit

The **postanesthesia care unit** (PACU) is located adjacent to the OR suite. Patients still under anesthesia or recovering from anesthesia are placed in this unit for easy access to experienced, highly skilled nurses, anesthesia providers, surgeons, advanced hemodynamic and pulmonary monitoring and support, special equipment, and medications.

Phases of Postanesthesia Care

In some hospitals and ambulatory surgical centers, postanesthesia care is divided into two phases (Rothrock, 2019). In the **phase I PACU**, used during the immediate recovery phase, intensive nursing care is provided. After this phase, the patient transitions to the next phase of care as either an inpatient to a nursing unit or phase II PACU. In the **phase II PACU**, the patient is prepared for transfer to an inpatient nursing unit, an extended care setting, or discharge. Recliners rather than stretchers or beds are standard in many phase II units, which may also be referred to as step-down, sit-up, or progressive care units. Patients remain in PACU until they have met predetermined discharge criteria, depending on the type of surgery and any preexisting conditions or comorbidities. In facilities without separate phase I and II units, the patient remains in the PACU and may be discharged home directly from this unit.

Admitting the Patient to the Postanesthesia Care Unit

Transferring the postoperative patient from the OR to the PACU is the responsibility of the anesthesiologist or certified registered nurse anesthetist (CRNA) and other licensed members of the OR team. During transport from the OR to the PACU, the anesthesia provider remains at the head of the stretcher (to maintain the airway), and a surgical team member remains at the opposite end. Transporting the patient involves special consideration of the incision site, potential vascular changes, and exposure. The surgical incision is considered every time the postoperative patient is moved; many wounds are closed under considerable tension, and every effort is made to prevent further strain on the incision. The patient is positioned so that they are not lying on and obstructing drains or drainage tubes. Orthostatic hypotension may occur when a patient is moved too quickly from one position to another (e.g., from a lithotomy position to a horizontal position or from a lateral to a supine position), so the patient must be moved slowly and carefully. As soon as the patient is placed on the stretcher or bed, the soiled gown is removed and replaced with a dry gown. The patient is covered with lightweight blanket or a forced air warming blanket.

The nurse who admits the patient to the PACU reviews essential information with the anesthesiologist or CRNA (see Chart 16-1) and the circulating nurse. Oxygen is applied, monitoring equipment is attached, and an immediate physiologic assessment is conducted.

Chart 16-1

Anesthesia Provider-to-Nurse Report and Nurse-to-Nurse Report: Information to Convey

Patient name, gender, age
Allergies
Surgical procedure
Position during the procedure
Length of time in the operating room
Anesthetic agents and reversal agents used
Estimated blood loss/fluid loss
Fluid/blood replacement
Last set of vital signs and any problems during the procedure (e.g., nausea and/or vomiting)
Any complications encountered (anesthetic or surgical)
Medical comorbidities (e.g., diabetes, hypertension)
List of allergies and medications taken at home (including pain medications, antihypertensives, and anticoagulants)
Considerations for immediate postoperative period (pain management, reversals, ventilator settings)
Language barrier
Location of patient's family

Ideally, the anesthesia provider should not leave the patient until the nurse is satisfied with the patient's airway and immediate condition.

Nursing Management in the Postanesthesia Care Unit

The nursing management objectives for the patient in the PACU are to provide care until the patient has recovered from the effects of anesthesia. PACU nurses have unique competencies as they care for patients who have undergone a wide range of surgical procedures. Recovery criteria include a return to baseline cognitive function, the airway is clear, nausea and vomiting is controlled, and vital signs are stabilized. The nurse in the PACU uses critical care skills and training to detect early subtle changes that could lead to complications (i.e., hemorrhage or respiratory distress) without intervention (American Society of PeriAnesthesia Nurses [ASPAN], 2019; Odom-Forren, 2018).

Some patients, particularly those who have had extensive or lengthy surgical procedures, may be transferred from the OR directly to the intensive care unit (ICU) or from the PACU to the ICU while still intubated and receiving mechanical ventilation. In most facilities, the patient is awakened and extubated in the OR (except in cases of trauma or critical illness) and arrives in the PACU breathing without ventilatory support.

Assessing the Patient

The nurse performs frequent, basic assessments of every postoperative patient. These assessments include airway, level of consciousness, cardiac, respiratory, wound, and pain. The patient's comorbidities and type of procedure will dictate additional assessments such as peripheral pulses, hemodynamics, and surgical drain placements (Odom-Forren, 2018). A baseline of any postanesthesia assessment scoring tool, such as the Aldrete score, is performed at this time as well (Aldrete & Wright, 1992). See discussion of this score later in this chapter.

The nurse performs and documents a baseline assessment, checks all drainage tubes, and verifies that monitoring lines are connected and functioning. IV fluids and medications currently infusing are checked, and the nurse verifies that they are infusing at the correct dosage and rate. Vital signs are assessed at time of arrival to PACU and repeated at intervals (i.e., every 5 or 15 minutes) per institutional protocol. The nurse must be aware of any pertinent information from the patient's history that may be significant (e.g., patient is deaf or hard of hearing, has a history of seizures, has diabetes, or is allergic to certain medications or to latex).

 Concept Mastery Alert

> Following surgery, patients who had ketamine as anesthesia must be placed in a quiet, darkened area of the PACU. See Chapter 15, Table 15-2 for more information about anesthetic agents.

Maintaining a Patent Airway

The primary objective in the immediate postoperative period is to maintain ventilation and thus prevent hypoxemia (reduced oxygen in the blood) and hypercapnia (excess carbon dioxide in the blood). Both can occur if the airway is obstructed and ventilation is reduced (hypoventilation). Besides administering supplemental oxygen as prescribed, the

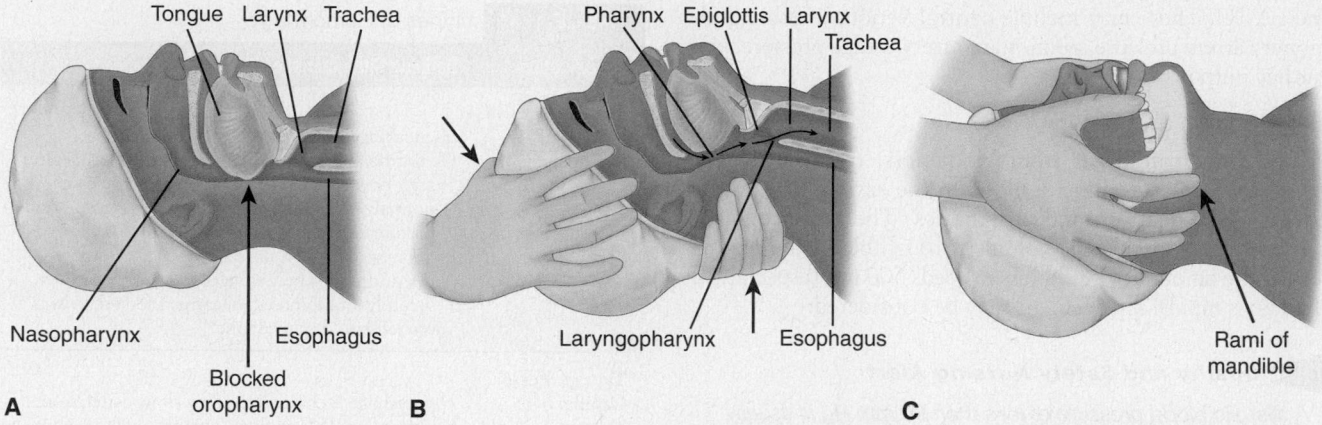

Tongue Larynx Trachea

Nasopharynx   Esophagus

Blocked
oropharynx

A

Pharynx Epiglottis Larynx
Trachea

Laryngopharynx   Esophagus

B

Rami of
mandible

C

Figure 16-1 • **A.** A hypopharyngeal obstruction occurs when neck flexion permits the chin to drop toward the chest; obstruction almost always occurs when the head is in the midposition. **B.** Tilting the head back to stretch the anterior neck structure lifts the base of the tongue off the posterior pharyngeal wall. The direction of the *arrows* indicates the pressure of the hands. **C.** Opening the mouth is necessary to correct a valvelike obstruction of the nasal passage during expiration, which occurs in about 30% of unconscious patients. Open the patient's mouth (separate lips and teeth) and move the lower jaw forward so that the lower teeth are in front of the upper teeth. To regain backward tilt of the neck, lift with both hands at the ascending rami of the mandible.

nurse assesses respiratory rate and depth, ease of respirations, oxygen saturation, and breath sounds.

Patients who have experienced prolonged anesthesia usually are unconscious, with all muscles relaxed. This relaxation extends to the muscles of the pharynx. When the patient lies on the back, the lower jaw and the tongue fall backward and the air passages become obstructed (Fig. 16-1A). This is called *hypopharyngeal obstruction*. Signs of occlusion include choking; noisy and irregular respirations; decreased oxygen saturation scores; and, within minutes, a blue, dusky color (cyanosis) of the skin. Because movement of the thorax and the diaphragm does not necessarily indicate that the patient is breathing, the nurse needs to place the palm of the hand at the patient's nose and mouth to feel the exhaled breath.

> ◣ *Quality and Safety Nursing Alert*
>
> *The treatment of hypopharyngeal obstruction involves tilting the head back and pushing forward on the angle of the lower jaw, as if to push the lower teeth in front of the upper teeth (see Fig. 16-1B,C). This maneuver pulls the tongue forward and opens the air passages.*

The anesthesiologist or CRNA may place a temporary, hard rubber or plastic airway in the patient's mouth to maintain a patent airway (see Fig. 16-2). Such a device should not be removed until signs such as gagging indicate that reflex action is returning. Alternatively, the patient may enter the PACU with an endotracheal tube still in place and may require continued mechanical ventilation. The nurse assists in initiating the use of the ventilator as well as the weaning and extubation processes.

If the teeth are clenched, the mouth may be opened manually but cautiously with a padded tongue depressor. The head of the bed is elevated 15 to 30 degrees unless contraindicated, and the patient is closely monitored to maintain the airway as well as to minimize the risk of aspiration. If vomiting occurs, the patient is turned to the side to prevent aspiration and the vomitus is collected in the emesis basin. Mucus or vomitus obstructing the pharynx or the trachea is suctioned with

a pharyngeal suction tip or a nasal catheter introduced into the nasopharynx or oropharynx to a distance of 15 to 20 cm (6 to 8 inch). Caution is necessary in suctioning the throat of a patient who has had a tonsillectomy or other oral or laryngeal surgery because of the risk of bleeding and discomfort.

Maintaining Cardiovascular Stability

To monitor cardiovascular stability, the nurse assesses the patient's level of consciousness; vital signs; cardiac rhythm; skin temperature, color, and moisture; and urine output. The nurse also assesses the patency of all IV lines. The primary cardiovascular complications seen in the PACU include hypotension and shock, hemorrhage, hypertension, and arrhythmias.

In patients who are critically ill, have significant comorbidity, or have undergone riskier procedures, additional monitoring may have been done in the OR and will continue in

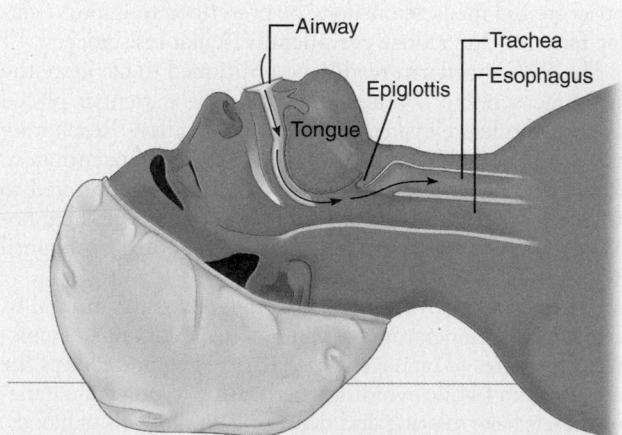

Airway   Trachea
Epiglottis   Esophagus
Tongue

Figure 16-2 • The use of an airway to maintain a patent airway after anesthesia. The airway passes over the base of the tongue and permits air to pass into the pharynx in the region of the epiglottis. Patients often leave the operating room with an airway in place. The airway should remain in place until the patient recovers sufficiently to breathe normally. As the patient regains consciousness, the airway usually causes irritation and should be removed.

the PACU. These may include central venous pressure, pulmonary artery pressure, pulmonary artery wedge pressure, and cardiac output.

Hypotension and Shock

Hypotension can result from blood loss, hypoventilation, position changes, pooling of blood in the extremities, or side effects of medications and anesthetics. The most common cause is loss of circulating volume through blood and plasma loss. If the amount of blood loss exceeds 500 mL (especially if the loss is rapid), replacement may be considered.

> ▶ **Quality and Safety Nursing Alert**
>
> *A systolic blood pressure of less than 90 mm Hg is usually considered immediately reportable. However, the patient's preoperative or baseline blood pressure is used to make informed postoperative comparisons. A previously stable blood pressure that shows a downward trend of 5 mm Hg at each 15-minute reading should also be reported.*

Types of shock are classified as hypovolemic, cardiogenic, neurogenic, anaphylactic, and septic. The most common type of shock in the postoperative setting is hypovolemic and is associated with hemorrhage from the surgical site (Odom-Forren, 2018). The classic signs of hypovolemic shock are pallor; cool, moist skin; rapid breathing; cyanosis of the lips, gums, and tongue; rapid, weak, thready pulse; narrowing pulse pressure; low blood pressure; and concentrated urine (see Chapter 11 for a detailed discussion of shock).

Hypovolemic shock can be avoided largely by the timely administration of IV fluids, blood, blood products, and medications that elevate blood pressure. The primary intervention for hypovolemic shock is volume replacement, with an infusion of lactated Ringer solution, 0.9% sodium chloride solution, colloids, or blood component therapy (see Chapter 11, Table 11-3). Oxygen is given by nasal cannula, facemask, or mechanical ventilation. If fluid administration fails to reverse hypovolemic shock, then various cardiac, vasodilator, and corticosteroid medications may be prescribed to improve cardiac function and reduce peripheral vascular resistance.

The PACU bed can readily be positioned to facilitate the use of measures to counteract shock. The patient is placed flat with the legs elevated, usually with a pillow. Respiratory rate, pulse rate, blood pressure, blood oxygen concentration, urinary output, and level of consciousness are monitored to provide information on the patient's respiratory and cardiovascular status. Vital signs are monitored continuously until the patient's condition has stabilized.

Other factors can contribute to hemodynamic instability, such as body temperature and pain. The PACU nurse implements measures to manage these factors. The nurse keeps the patient warm (while avoiding overheating to prevent cutaneous vessels from dilating and depriving vital organs of blood), avoids exposure, and maintains normothermia (to prevent vasodilation). Pain control measures are implemented, as discussed later in this chapter.

Hemorrhage

Hemorrhage is an uncommon yet serious complication of surgery that can result in hypovolemic shock and death. It can

TABLE 16-1	Types of Hemorrhage
Classification	**Defining Characteristic**
Time Frame	
Primary	Hemorrhage occurs at the time of surgery.
Intermediary	Hemorrhage occurs during the first few hours after surgery when the rise of blood pressure to its normal level dislodges insecure clots from nonanastomosed vessels.
Secondary	Hemorrhage may occur sometime after surgery if a suture slips because a blood vessel was not securely anastomosed, became infected, or was eroded by a drainage tube.
Type of Vessel	
Capillary	Hemorrhage is characterized by slow, general ooze.
Venous	Darkly colored blood flows quickly.
Arterial	Blood is bright red and appears in spurts with each heartbeat.
Visibility	
Evident	Hemorrhage is on the surface and can be seen.
Concealed	Hemorrhage is in a body cavity and cannot be seen.

present insidiously or emergently at any time in the immediate postoperative period or up to several days after surgery (see Table 16-1). The patient presents with hypotension; rapid, thready pulse; disorientation; restlessness; oliguria; and cold, pale skin. The early phase of shock will manifest in feelings of apprehension, decreased cardiac output, and vascular resistance. Breathing becomes labored, and "air hunger" will be exhibited; the patient will feel cold (hypothermia) and may experience tinnitus. Laboratory values may show a sharp drop in hemoglobin and hematocrit levels. If shock symptoms are left untreated, the patient will continually grow weaker but can remain conscious until near death (Rothrock, 2019).

Determining the cause of hemorrhage includes assessing the surgical site and incision for bleeding. If bleeding is evident, a sterile gauze pad and a pressure dressing are applied, and the site of the bleeding is elevated to heart level if possible. The patient is placed in the shock position (flat on back; legs elevated at a 20-degree angle; knees kept straight). Severe bleeding requires immediate action by the nurse. The surgeon is called and preparations are made to return the patient to the OR for ligation of bleeding veins and arteries, hematoma evacuation, or other necessary surgical interventions to stop the bleeding (Odom-Forren, 2018).

If hemorrhage is suspected, the nurse should be aware of any special considerations related to blood loss replacement. The treatment of hemorrhage is infusion of crystalloid and possibly blood product. Patients with blood loss of over 1500 mL should be considered for blood administration (Henry, 2018). Nurses in the PACU should be aware that patients may decline blood transfusions for religious or cultural reasons and may identify this request on their advance directives or living will.

Hypertension and Arrhythmias

Hypertension is common in the immediate postoperative period secondary to sympathetic nervous system stimulation from pain, hypoxia, or bladder distention. Arrhythmias are associated with electrolyte imbalance, altered respiratory function, pain, hypothermia, stress, and anesthetic agents. Both hypertension and arrhythmias are managed by treating the underlying causes.

Relieving Pain and Anxiety

The nurse in the PACU monitors the patient's physiologic status, manages pain, and provides psychological support in an effort to relieve the patient's fears and concerns. The nurse checks the electronic health record (EHR) for special needs and concerns of the patient. Opioid analgesic medications are given mostly by IV in the PACU (Rothrock, 2019). IV opioids provide immediate pain relief and are short acting, thus minimizing the potential for drug interactions or prolonged respiratory depression while anesthetics are still active in the patient's system (Barash, Cullen, Stoelting, et al., 2017). (See Chapter 9 for more information about pain management.) When the patient's condition permits, a close member of the family may visit in the PACU to decrease the family's anxiety and make the patient feel more secure. The nurse should consider providing nonpharmacologic, emotional, and psychological support to the patient. These include massage, acupuncture, heat or cold packs, relaxation and breathing techniques, guided imagery, and soothing music (Odom-Forren, 2018).

Controlling Nausea and Vomiting

Postoperative nausea and vomiting (PONV) occurs in about 30% to 50% of surgical patients (Thomas, Maple, Williams, et al., 2019). The nurse should intervene at the patient's first report of nausea to control the problem rather than wait for it to progress to vomiting.

> ### Quality and Safety Nursing Alert
>
> *At the slightest indication of nausea, the patient is turned completely to one side to promote mouth drainage and prevent aspiration of vomitus, which can cause pneumonia, asphyxiation, and death.*

PONV is controlled via medication administered intraoperatively and postoperatively. Table 16-2 contains select medications prescribed to control PONV. Studies suggest that nonpharmacologic measures, such as aromatherapy, may be effective for PONV prevention and treatment (Asay, Olson, Donnelly, et al., 2019). Aromatherapy inhalers with ginger, lavender, spearmint, and peppermint are a complementary, homeopathic, and a nonpharmacologic option (de la Vega, Gilliand, Martinez, et al., 2019).

Risk factors for PONV are female gender, age less than 50 years, history of nausea or vomiting after previous anesthesia, and opioid administration (Finch, Parkosewich, Perrone, et al., 2019). Surgical risks are increased with PONV due to an increase in intra-abdominal pressure, elevated central venous pressure, the potential for aspiration, increased heart rate, and systemic blood pressure, which increase the risk of myocardial ischemia and arrhythmias. Aside from PONV as an unpleasant and uncomfortable experience, it may lead to dehydration, electrolyte imbalances, airway compromise, stress on suture lines or incision dehiscence, esophageal tears, hypotension, and increased length of stay in the recovery room (Asay et al., 2019). Chart 16-2 contains a Nursing Research Profile about PONV.

Gerontologic Considerations

The older patient, like all patients, is transferred from the OR table to the bed or stretcher slowly and gently. The effects of this action on blood pressure and ventilation are monitored. Special attention is given to keeping the patient warm, because older adults are more susceptible to hypothermia. The patient's position is changed frequently to stimulate respirations as well as promote circulation and comfort.

Immediate postoperative care for the older adult is the same as for any surgical patient; however, additional support is given if cardiovascular, pulmonary, or renal function is impaired. With careful monitoring, it is possible to

---

TABLE 16-2 Select Medications Used to Control Postoperative Nausea and Vomiting

Drug Classes	Name	Nursing Implications
GI stimulant	Metoclopramide	Acts by stimulating gastric emptying and increasing GI transit time. Administration recommended at the end of procedure. Available in oral, IM, and IV forms.
Phenothiazine antiemetic	Prochlorperazine	Indicated for control of severe nausea and vomiting. Available in oral, SR, rectal, IM, and IV forms.
Phenothiazine antiemetic antimotion sickness	Promethazine	Recommended every 4–6 h for nausea and vomiting associated with anesthesia and surgery. Available in oral, IM, and IV forms.
Antimotion sickness	Dimenhydrinate	Indicated for prevention of nausea, vomiting, or vertigo of motion sickness. Available in oral, IM, and IV forms.
Antiemetic	Hydroxyzine	Control of nausea and vomiting and as adjunct to analgesia preoperatively and postoperatively to allow decreased opioid dosage. Available in oral and IM forms.
Antiemetic antimotion sickness	Scopolamine	Used to prevent and control of nausea and vomiting associated with motion sickness and recovery from surgery. Available in oral, transdermal SC, and IM forms.
Antiemetic	Ondansetron	Prevention of postoperative nausea and vomiting. Available in oral, IM, and IV forms. With few side effects, frequently the drug of choice.

GI, gastrointestinal; IM, intramuscular; IV, intravenous; SR, sustained release; SC, subcutaneous.
Adapted from Comerford, K. C., & Durkin, M. T. (2020). *Nursing 2020 drug handbook.* Philadelphia, PA: Wolters Kluwer.

Chart 16-2

NURSING RESEARCH PROFILE
An Investigation of PONV in Ambulatory Surgery

Finch, C., Parkosewich, J. A., Perrone, D., et al. (2019). Incidence, timing, and factors associated with postoperative nausea and vomiting in the ambulatory surgery setting. *Journal of PeriAnesthesia Nursing, 34*(6), 1146–1155.

Purpose

Postoperative nausea and vomiting (PONV) is a major concern for patients having surgery under general anesthesia. The purpose of this study was to investigate the incidence, timing, and factors associated with PONV in an ambulatory surgery PACU.

Design

The study used a prospective descriptive correlational, cross-sectional design. A random sample of 139 patients admitted to a 10-bed ambulatory PACU participated.

Findings

The mean age of participants was 50 years and 70% were female. Only 3 participants had nausea upon arrival to the PACU, but this number increased to 10 by 90 minutes in the PACU, and then went back down to 3 at 150 minutes in the PACU. A total of 4 participants vomited after reporting nausea. Participants with nausea had more hydration and longer PACU stays. Younger age and the presence of gastroesophageal reflux disease (GERD) were significantly associated with nausea.

Nursing Implications

Nurses working with postoperative patients should be aware that PONV can and does occur in both ambulatory and inpatient surgery settings. Nurses should take the age of patients into consideration with anticipating PONV. This study provides evidence that a history of GERD may be a risk factor and thus should be included in preoperative assessment.

---

detect cardiopulmonary deficits before signs and symptoms are apparent. Changes associated with the aging process, the prevalence of chronic diseases, alteration in fluid and nutrition status, and the increased use of medications result in the need for postoperative vigilance. Nurses should keep in mind that older adults may have slower recovery from anesthesia due to the prolonged time it takes to eliminate sedatives and anesthetic agents. Thermoregulation is important to maintain immune function, adequate pain relief, and tissue oxygenation. Special care to maintain normothermia can minimize the risk of postoperative ischemia and angina in older patients (Odom-Forren, 2018).

Postoperative confusion and delirium may occur in up to half of all older adult patients. Signs and symptoms include cognitive deficits, hallucinations, and fluctuating state of consciousness. It is important for the nurse to verify the preoperative psychological assessment as it can help differentiate between postoperative cognitive dysfunction (POCD) and postoperative delirium. With both conditions, patients exhibit signs of cognitive impairment; however, POCD is of sudden onset in the postsurgical period and is associated with the use of several anesthetic agents (Alalawi & Yasmeen, 2018). Providing adequate hydration, reorienting to the environment, and reassessing the doses of sedative, anesthetic, and analgesic agents may reduce the risk of confusion. Hypoxia can present as confusion and restlessness, as can blood loss and electrolyte imbalances. Exclusion of all other causes of confusion must precede the assumption that confusion is related to age, circumstances, and medications.

Maintaining a safe environment for older adults requires alertness and planning. Arthritis is a common condition among older patients, and it affects mobility, creating difficulty turning from one side to the other or ambulating without discomfort. The nurse provides mobility support and is vigilant for patients with an increased risk for falls. Fall prevention methods include using a fall risk identification method, providing assistance with ambulation, and allowing legs to dangle off of the stretcher prior to standing (DeSilva, Seabra, Thomas, et al., 2019).

 Bariatric Considerations

Patients with obesity are seen in the PACU for a wide variety of conditions, including bariatric and nonbariatric procedures (Tjeertes, Hoeks, Beks, et al., 2015). Properly sized blood pressure cuffs, gowns, transfer devices, and wheelchairs may be needed for the recovery and transitioning care of these patients. Patients with obesity have unique postoperative risks including an increased risk of venous thromboembolism (VTE), deep vein thrombosis (DVT), and pulmonary embolus (PE).

Patients with obesity are at particular risk for obstructive sleep apnea (OSA) in the postoperative period. A direct correlation exists between the incidence of pulmonary complications and the degree of obesity. The mortality rate after upper abdominal operations in patients with severe obesity is 2.5 times that of their normal weight counterparts (Odom-Forren, 2018). As discussed in Chapter 14, careful preoperative assessment for OSA should occur in patients with obesity in order to detect and manage the manifestations that may occur during the surgical stay. A combination of pulse oximetry and capnography should be utilized when patients are on supplemental oxygen therapy as respiratory depression may be masked when measured only by pulse oximetry (Jungquist, Card, Charchaflieh, et al., 2018). Research suggests that the combination of continuous monitoring tools alerts PACU nurses to respiratory changes allowing for timely interventions (Wortham, Rice, Gupta, et al., 2019). Patients with OSA, many of whom also have obesity, are prone to hypoventilation and airway obstruction (ASPAN, 2019).

Determining Readiness for Postanesthesia Care Unit Discharge

A patient remains in the PACU until fully recovered from the anesthetic agent. Indicators of recovery include stable blood pressure, adequate respiratory function, and adequate oxygen saturation level compared with baseline.

The Aldrete score is used to determine the patient's general condition and readiness for transfer from the PACU (Aldrete & Wright, 1992). Throughout the recovery period, the patient's physical signs are observed and evaluated by

Post Anesthesia Care Unit
MODIFIED ALDRETE SCORE

Patient: _____   Final score: _____

Room: _____   Surgeon: _____

Date: _____   PACU nurse: _____

Area of Assessment	Point Score	Upon Admission	After			
			15 min	30 min	45 min	60 min
Activity						
(Able to move spontaneously or on command)						
• Ability to move all extremities	2					
• Ability to move 2 extremities	1					
• Unable to control any extremity	0					
Respiration						
• Ability to breathe deeply and cough	2					
• Limited respiratory effort (dyspnea or splinting)	1					
• No spontaneous effort	0					
Circulation						
• BP 20% of preanesthetic level	2					
• BP 20% –49% of preanesthetic level	1					
• BP 50% of preanesthetic level	0					
Consciousness						
• Fully awake	2					
• Arousable on calling	1					
• Not responding	0					
O_2 Saturation						
• Able to maintain O_2 sat >92% on room air	2					
• Needs O_2 inhalation to maintain O_2 sat >90%	1					
• O_2 sat <90% even with O_2 supplement	0					
Totals:						

Required for discharge from Post Anesthesia Care Unit: 7–8 points

_____   _____
Time of release   Signature of nurse

Figure 16-3 • Postanesthesia care unit record; modified Aldrete score. O_2 sat, oxygen saturation; BP, blood pressure. Adapted from Aldrete, A., & Wright, A. (1992). Revised Aldrete score for discharge. *Anesthesiology News, 18*(1), 17.

means of a scoring system based on a set of objective criteria. This evaluation guide allows an objective assessment of the patient's condition in the PACU (see Fig. 16-3). The patient is assessed at regular intervals, and a total score is calculated and recorded on the assessment record. The Aldrete score is usually between 7 and 10 before discharge from the PACU. The unit policy and the established PACU discharge criteria determine appropriate postanesthesia recovery score parameters. Scores or conditions lower than the preestablished level necessitate evaluation by the anesthesia provider or surgeon and can result in an extension of the PACU stay or possible disposition to a special care or critical care unit (Odom-Forren, 2018).

The patient is discharged from the phase I PACU by the anesthesiologist or CRNA to the critical care unit, the medical-surgical unit, or the phase II PACU.

Preparing the Postoperative Patient for Direct Discharge

Ambulatory surgical centers frequently have a step-down PACU similar to a phase II PACU. Patients seen in this type of unit are usually healthy, and the plan is to discharge them directly to home. Prior to discharge, the patient will require verbal and written instructions and information about follow-up care.

Promoting Home, Community-Based, and Transitional Care

To ensure patient safety and recovery, expert patient education and discharge planning are necessary when a patient undergoes same-day or ambulatory surgery (Association of PeriOperative Registered Nurses [AORN], 2019; ASPAN, 2019). Because anesthetics cloud memory for concurrent events, verbal and written instructions should be given to both the patient and the adult who will be accompanying the patient home. Alternative formats (e.g., large print, Braille) of instructions or the use of a sign language interpreter may be required to ensure patient and family understanding. A translator may be required if the patient and family members do not understand English.

Discharge Preparation

The patient and caregiver (e.g., family member, friend) are informed about expected outcomes and immediate postoperative changes anticipated (AORN, 2019; ASPAN, 2019). Chart 16-3 identifies important educational points; before discharging the patient, the nurse provides written instructions covering each of those points. Prescriptions are given to the patient. Contact information for the hospital and surgeon's office are provided, and the patient and caregiver are encouraged to call with questions and to schedule follow-up appointments. A list of possible complications and how to manage them (e.g., call the surgeon's office, report to the emergency department [ED]), including elevated temperature, bleeding, and wound care instructions, are key focal points during discharge education.

Although recovery time varies depending on the type and extent of surgery and the patient's overall condition, instructions usually advise limited activity for 24 to 48 hours. During this time, the patient should not drive a vehicle, drink alcoholic beverages, or perform tasks that require high levels of energy or skill. Fluids may be consumed as desired and smaller than normal amounts may be eaten at mealtime. Patients are cautioned not to make important decisions at this time because the medications, anesthesia, and surgery may affect their decision-making ability. Follow-up phone calls from the nurse are also used to assess the patient's progress and to answer any questions.

Continuing and Transitional Care

Although most patients who undergo ambulatory surgery recover quickly and without complications, some patients require referral for some type of continuing or transitional care. These may be older or frail patients, those who live alone, and patients with other health care problems or disabilities that might interfere with self-care or resumption of usual activities. The home, community, or transitional care nurse assesses the patient's physical status (e.g., respiratory and cardiovascular status, adequacy of pain management, the surgical incision, surgical complications) and the patient's and family's ability to adhere to the recommendations given at the time of discharge. Previous education is reinforced as needed. Nursing interventions may include changing surgical dressings, monitoring the patency of a drainage system, or administering medications. The patient and family are reminded about the importance of keeping follow-up appointments with the surgeon.

Care of the Hospitalized Postoperative Patient

The majority of surgical patients who require hospital stays are trauma patients, acutely ill patients, patients undergoing major surgery, patients who require emergency surgery, and patients with a concurrent medical disorder. Seriously ill patients and those who have undergone major cardiovascular, pulmonary, or neurologic surgery may be admitted to specialized ICUs for close monitoring and advanced interventions and support. The care required by these patients in the immediate postoperative period is discussed in specific chapters of this book.

Chart 16-3 **HOME CARE CHECKLIST**
Discharge After Surgery

At the completion of education, the patient and/or caregiver will be able to:

- Name the procedure that was performed and identify any permanent changes in anatomic structure or function as well as changes in ADLs, IADLs, roles, relationships, and spirituality.
- Identify interventions and strategies (e.g., durable medical equipment, adaptive equipment) used in adapting to any permanent change in structure or function.
- Describe ongoing postoperative therapeutic regimen, including diet and activities to perform (e.g., walking and breathing exercises) and to limit or avoid (e.g., lifting weights, driving a car, contact sports).

- State the name, dose, side effects, frequency, and schedule for all medications.
- State how to obtain medical supplies and carry out dressing changes, wound care, and other prescribed regimens.
- Describe signs and symptoms of complications.
- State time and date of follow-up appointments.
- Relate how to reach health care provider with questions or complications.
- State understanding of community resources and referrals (if any).

Identify the need for health promotion (e.g., weight reduction, smoking cessation, stress management), disease prevention, and screening activities. ADLs, activities of daily living; IADLs, instrumental activities of daily living.

Patients admitted to the clinical unit for postoperative care have multiple needs and require frequent assessment and care interventions by nursing staff. Postoperative care for those surgical patients returning to the general medical-surgical unit is discussed later in this chapter.

Receiving the Patient in the Clinical Unit

The patient's room is readied by assembling the necessary equipment and supplies: IV pumps, drainage receptacle holder, suction equipment, oxygen, emesis basin, tissues, disposable pads, blankets, and postoperative documentation forms. When the call comes to the unit about the patient's transfer from the PACU, the need for any additional items is communicated. The PACU nurse reports relevant data about the patient to the receiving nurse (see Chart 16-1).

Usually, the surgeon speaks to the family after surgery and relates the general condition of the patient. The receiving nurse gets a report about the patient's condition, reviews the postoperative orders, admits the patient to the unit, performs an initial assessment, and attends to the patient's immediate needs (see Chart 16-4).

Nursing Management After Surgery

During the first 24 hours after surgery, nursing care of the hospitalized patient on the medical-surgical unit involves continuing to help the patient recover from the effects of anesthesia (Barash et al., 2017), frequently assessing the patient's physiologic status, monitoring for complications, managing pain, and implementing measures designed to achieve the long-range goals of independence with self-care, successful management of the therapeutic regimen, discharge to home, and full recovery. In the initial hours after admission to the clinical unit, adequate ventilation, hemodynamic stability, incisional pain, surgical site integrity, nausea and vomiting, neurologic status, and spontaneous voiding are primary concerns. The pulse rate, blood pressure, and respiration rate are assessed at intervals determined by the institution.

Patients usually begin to return to their usual state of health several hours after surgery or after awaking the next morning. Although pain may still be intense, many patients feel more alert, less nauseous, and less anxious. They have begun their breathing and leg exercises as appropriate for the type of surgery, and most will have dangled their legs over the edge of the bed, stood, and ambulated a few feet or been assisted out of bed to the chair at least once. Many will have tolerated a light meal and had IV fluids discontinued. The focus of care shifts from intense physiologic management and symptomatic relief of the adverse effects of anesthesia to regaining independence with self-care and preparing for discharge.

Chart 16-4 Immediate Postoperative Nursing Interventions

Nursing Interventions	Rationale
1. Assess breathing and administer supplemental oxygen, if prescribed.	1. Assessment provides a baseline and helps identify signs and symptoms of respiratory distress early.
2. Monitor vital signs and note skin warmth, moisture, and color.	2. A careful baseline assessment helps identify signs and symptoms of shock early.
3. Assess the surgical site and wound drainage systems. Connect all drainage tubes to gravity or suction as indicated and monitor closed drainage systems.	3. Assessment provides a baseline and helps identify signs and symptoms of hemorrhage early.
4. Assess level of consciousness, orientation, and ability to move extremities.	4. These parameters provide a baseline and help identify signs and symptoms of neurologic complications.
5. Assess pain level; pain characteristics (location, quality); and timing, type, and route of administration of the last dose of analgesic.	5. Assessment provides a baseline of current pain level and assesses effectiveness of pain management strategies.
6. Administer analgesic medications as prescribed and assess their effectiveness in relieving pain.	6. Administration of analgesic agents helps decrease pain.
7. Place the call light, emesis basin, ice chips (if allowed), and bedpan or urinal within reach.	7. Attending to these needs provides for comfort and safety.
8. Position the patient to enhance comfort, safety, and lung expansion.	8. This promotes safety and reduces risk of postoperative complications.
9. Assess IV sites for patency and infusions for correct rate and solution.	9. Assessing IV sites and infusions helps detect phlebitis and prevents errors in rate and solution type.
10. Assess urine output in closed drainage system or use bladder scanner to detect distention.	10. Assessment provides a baseline and helps identify signs of urinary retention.
11. Reinforce the need to begin deep breathing and leg exercises.	11. These activities help prevent complications related to immobility (e.g., atelectasis, VTE).
12. Provide information to the patient and family.	12. Patient education helps decrease the patient's and family's anxiety.

VTE, venous thromboembolism.
Adapted from Association of PeriOperative Registered Nurses (AORN). (2019). *Association of PeriOperative Registered Nurses (AORN) standards, recommended practice, and guidelines*. Denver, CO: Author.

NURSING PROCESS

The Hospitalized Patient Recovering from Surgery

Nursing care of the hospitalized patient recovering from surgery takes place in a compressed time frame, with much of the healing and recovery occurring after the patient is discharged to home or to a rehabilitation center.

Assessment

Assessment of the hospitalized postoperative patient includes monitoring vital signs and completing a review of systems upon the patient's arrival to the clinical unit (see Chart 16-4) and at regular intervals thereafter.

Respiratory status is important because pulmonary complications are among the most frequent and serious problems encountered by the surgical patient. The nurse monitors for airway patency and any signs of laryngeal edema. The quality of respirations, including depth, rate, and sound, is assessed regularly. Chest auscultation verifies that breath sounds are normal (or abnormal) bilaterally, and the findings are documented as a baseline for later comparisons. Often, because of the effects of analgesic and anesthetic medications, respirations are slow. Shallow and rapid respirations may be caused by pain, constricting dressings, gastric dilation, abdominal distention, or obesity. Noisy breathing may be due to obstruction by secretions or the tongue. Another possible complication is flash pulmonary edema that occurs when protein and fluid accumulate in the alveoli unrelated to elevated pulmonary artery occlusive pressure. Signs and symptoms include agitation; tachypnea; tachycardia; decreased pulse oximetry readings; frothy, pink sputum; and crackles on auscultation.

The nurse assesses the patient's pain level using a verbal or visual analog scale and assesses the characteristics of the pain. The patient's appearance, pulse, respirations, blood pressure, skin color (adequate or cyanotic), and skin temperature (cold and clammy, warm and moist, or warm and dry) are clues to cardiovascular function. When the patient arrives in the clinical unit, the surgical site is assessed for bleeding, type and integrity of dressings, and drains.

The nurse also assesses the patient's mental status and level of consciousness, speech, and orientation and compares them with the preoperative baseline. Although a change in mental status or postoperative restlessness may be related to anxiety, pain, or medications, it may also be a symptom of oxygen deficit or hemorrhage. These serious causes must be investigated and excluded before other causes are pursued.

General discomfort that results from lying in one position on the operating table, the handling of tissues by the surgical team, the body's reaction to anesthesia, and anxiety are also common causes of restlessness. These discomforts may be relieved by administering the prescribed analgesic medication, changing the patient's position frequently, and assessing and alleviating the cause of anxiety. If tight, drainage-soaked bandages are causing discomfort, reinforcing or changing the dressing completely as prescribed by the provider may make the patient more comfortable. The bladder is assessed for distention (usually with a bladder scanner) because urinary retention can also cause restlessness and change in mental status (AORN, 2019).

Diagnosis

NURSING DIAGNOSES

Based on the assessment data, major nursing diagnoses may include the following:

- Impaired airway clearance associated with to depressed respiratory function, pain, and bed rest
- Acute pain associated with surgical incision
- Impaired cardiac output associated with shock or hemorrhage
- Risk for activity intolerance associated with generalized weakness secondary to surgery
- Impaired skin integrity associated with surgical incision and drains
- Impaired thermoregulation associated with surgical environment and anesthetic agents
- Risk for impaired nutritional status associated with decreased intake and increased need for nutrients secondary to surgery
- Risk for constipation associated with effects of medications, surgery, dietary change, and immobility
- Impaired urinary system function associated with anesthetic agents
- Risk for injury associated with surgical procedure/positioning or anesthetic agents
- Anxiety associated with surgical procedure
- Lack of knowledge associated with wound care, dietary restrictions, activity recommendations, medications, follow-up care, or signs and symptoms of complications in preparation for discharge

COLLABORATIVE PROBLEMS OR POTENTIAL COMPLICATIONS

Based on the assessment data, potential complications may include the following:

- Pulmonary infection/hypoxia
- Venous thromboembolism (VTE) (e.g., deep vein thrombosis [DVT], pulmonary embolism [PE])
- Hematoma or hemorrhage
- Infection
- Wound dehiscence or evisceration

Planning and Goals

The major goals for the patient include optimal respiratory function, relief of pain, optimal cardiovascular function, increased activity tolerance, unimpaired wound healing, maintenance of body temperature, and maintenance of nutritional balance (Dudek, 2017). Further goals include resumption of usual pattern of bowel and bladder elimination, identification of any perioperative positioning injury, acquisition of sufficient knowledge to manage self-care after discharge, and absence of complications.

Nursing Interventions

PREVENTING RESPIRATORY COMPLICATIONS

Respiratory depressive effects of opioid medications, decreased lung expansion secondary to opioid pain medication, and decreased mobility combine to put the patient at risk for respiratory complications, particularly atelectasis (alveolar collapse; incomplete expansion of the lung), pneumonia, and hypoxemia (Rothrock, 2019). Atelectasis remains a risk for the patient who is not moving well or ambulating or who is not performing deep-breathing and coughing exercises or using an incentive spirometer. Signs and symptoms include decreased breath sounds over the affected area, crackles, and cough. Pneumonia is characterized by chills and fever, tachycardia, and tachypnea. Cough may or may not be present and may or may not be productive. Pulmonary congestion may occur if secretions are not cleared from the airway. The symptoms are often vague, with perhaps a slight elevation of temperature, pulse, and respiratory rate as well as a cough. Physical examination reveals dullness and crackles at the base of the lungs. If the condition progresses, the outcome may be fatal.

The types of hypoxemia that can affect postoperative patients are subacute and episodic. Subacute hypoxemia is a constant low level of oxygen saturation when breathing appears normal. Episodic hypoxemia develops suddenly, and the patient may be at risk for cerebral dysfunction, myocardial ischemia, and cardiac arrest. Risk for hypoxemia is increased in patients who have undergone major surgery (particularly abdominal), have obesity, or have preexisting pulmonary problems. Unidentified hypoxemia in the postanesthesia patient is not common since the advent of noninvasive oxygen saturation monitoring with pulse oximetry (Odom-Forren, 2018). Factors that may affect the accuracy of pulse oximetry readings include cold extremities, tremors, atrial fibrillation, acrylic nails, and nail polish.

Preventive measures and timely recognition of signs and symptoms help avert pulmonary complications. Crackles indicate static pulmonary secretions that need to be mobilized by coughing and deep-breathing exercises. When a mucus plug obstructs one of the bronchi entirely, the pulmonary tissue beyond the plug collapses, resulting in atelectasis.

To clear secretions and prevent pneumonia, the nurse encourages the patient to turn frequently, take deep breaths, cough, and use the incentive spirometer at least every 2 hours. These pulmonary exercises should begin as soon as the patient arrives on the clinical unit and continue until the patient is discharged. Even if they are not fully awake from anesthesia, the patient can be asked to take several deep breaths. This helps expel residual anesthetic agents, mobilize secretions, and prevent atelectasis. Careful splinting of abdominal or thoracic incision sites helps the patient overcome the fear that the exertion of coughing might open the incision (see Chapter 14, Chart 14-5). Analgesic agents are given to permit more effective coughing, and oxygen is given as prescribed to prevent or relieve hypoxia. To encourage lung expansion, the patient is encouraged to yawn or take sustained maximal inspirations to create a negative intrathoracic pressure of −40 mm Hg and expand lung volume to total capacity. Chest physical therapy may be prescribed if indicated (see Chapter 19).

Coughing is contraindicated in patients who have head injuries or have undergone intracranial surgery (because of the risk for increasing intracranial pressure), as well as in patients who have undergone eye surgery (because of the risk for increasing intraocular pressure) or plastic surgery (because of the risk for increasing tension on delicate tissues).

Early ambulation increases metabolism and pulmonary aeration and, in general, improves all body functions. Assessment for readiness to ambulate as soon as the patient arrives in the PACU provides consistency and increased patient safety (Persico, Miller, Way, et al., 2019). Ambulation occurs as soon as the patient returns to a safe physical state and level of consciousness.

RELIEVING PAIN

Most patients experience some pain after a surgical procedure. Complete absence of pain in the area of the surgical incision

may not occur for a few weeks, depending on the site and nature of the surgery, but the intensity of postoperative pain gradually subsides on subsequent days. A comprehensive pain assessment provides the foundation of good pain control and includes obtaining information regarding the location, intensity, and quality (e.g., sharp, shooting) (Odom-Forren, 2018). Many patients are unable to accurately report their level of pain in the postoperative setting due to sedatives and other medications given during surgery. Nurses must be able to accurately assess other indicators such as behavior, vital signs, level of consciousness, and preoperative baseline pain report (see Chapter 9).

The degree and severity of postoperative pain and the patient's tolerance for pain depend on the incision site, the nature of the surgical procedure, the extent of surgical trauma, the type of anesthesia, and the route of administration.

Intense pain stimulates the stress response, which adversely affects the cardiac and immune systems. When pain impulses are transmitted, both muscle tension and local vasoconstriction increase, further stimulating pain receptors. This increases myocardial demand and oxygen consumption. The hypothalamic stress response also results in an increase in blood viscosity and platelet aggregation, increasing the risk of thrombosis and PE.

In some states, providers may prescribe different medications or dosages to cover various levels of pain. After the medication is delivered, the nurse should periodically assess the patient's level of pain using a validated pain scale.

Opioid Analgesic Medications. Opioid analgesic agents are commonly prescribed for pain and immediate postoperative restlessness. A realistic goal for postoperative pain management is toleration rather than the elimination of pain. A preventive approach, rather than an "as needed" (PRN) approach, is more effective in relieving pain. With a preventive approach, the medication is given at prescribed intervals rather than when the pain becomes severe or unbearable. In the postoperative setting, intravenous (IV) route is the first-line route of administration for analgesia delivery (Odom-Forren, 2018).

Prior to opioid delivery, the nurse should assess the patient's level of sedation. Sedation assessment tools, such as the POSS (Pasero Opioid-Induced Sedation Scale), are used by the nurse to assess sedation level at frequent intervals to safely care for patients in the PACU. The POSS is a tool developed to identify advancing sedation before it is compounded by continued opioid administration and results in clinically significant respiratory depression or apnea. The POSS indicates the nurse may administer opioids to a patient at sedation level S (*sleep, easy to arouse*) if it has been determined that the patient's respiratory status (rate, depth, regularity, and airway patency) is optimal. Patients assigned a sedation level of 1 or 2 may receive opioid administration; however, beginning at sedation level 3, the recommendation is that the nurse should provide nonopioid therapies to treat pain because the patient is becoming too sedated. Other sedation scales commonly used in the PACU are the RASS (Richmond Agitation–Sedation Scale), Aldrete Scale (see Fig. 16-3), and Glasgow Coma Scale (Hall & Stanley, 2019).

Patient-Controlled Analgesia. The goal is pain prevention rather than sporadic pain control. Patients recover more quickly when adequate pain relief measures are used, and patient-controlled analgesia (PCA) permits patients to administer their own pain medication when needed. Most patients are candidates for PCA. The two requirements for PCA are an understanding of the need to self-dose and the physical ability to self-dose. The amount of medication delivered by the IV or epidural route and the time span during which the opioid medication is released are controlled by the PCA device. PCA promotes patient participation in care; eliminates delayed administration of analgesic medications; maintains a therapeutic drug level; and enables the patient to move, turn, cough, and take deep breaths with less pain, thus reducing postoperative pulmonary complications (Rothrock, 2019).

Multimodal Analgesia. The use of more than one method of analgesia, referred to as multimodal analgesia, is a growing trend to manage postoperative pain. Some of these methods are started in the preoperative area; however, the effects are seen in the postoperative area. The most common analgesics used for postoperative pain are a mixture of opioid and nonopioid analgesics (i.e., acetaminophen and NSAIDs) and local anesthetics. A multimodal approach may combine agents in any of the analgesic groups to provide effective pain relief and minimize adverse effects (Odom-Forren, 2018). A balanced, multimodal approach to pain management within the larger framework of an Enhanced Recovery After Surgery (ERAS) pathway has become standard at many institutions for perioperative care, to control postsurgical pain, reduce opioid-related adverse events, hasten postsurgical recovery, and shorten length of hospital stay (Montgomery & McNamara, 2016). ERAS is an evidence-based, multimodal care model resulting in substantial improvements in clinical outcomes and cost savings (Ljungqvist, Scott, & Fearon, 2017).

Epidural Infusions and Intrapleural Anesthesia. Epidural analgesia involves a continuous infusion of local anesthetics through a catheter and is the most widely used neuraxial technique for acute postoperative pain (Wolfe, 2018). A local opioid or a combination anesthetic (opioid plus local anesthetic agent) is used in the epidural infusion. Epidural infusions are used with caution in chest procedures because the analgesic may ascend along the spinal cord and affect respiration. Intrapleural anesthesia involves the administration of a local anesthetic by a catheter between the parietal and visceral pleura. It provides sensory anesthesia without affecting motor function to the intercostal muscles. This anesthesia allows more effective coughing and deep breathing in conditions such as cholecystectomy, renal surgery, and rib fractures, in which pain in the thoracic region would interfere with these exercises.

Postoperative nurses may also care for patients who received a preoperative local anesthetic block. The intended effects of pain relief may last for hours or up to days, depending on the method used. Nurses should include the location of the block, when it was administered, current pain level, and insertion site assessment when providing report to the inpatient nursing unit. Patient discharge instructions include information about when to expect the return of sensation, mobility precautions with decreased sensation, and care of the dressing at the insertion site.

Other Pain Relief Measures. For pain that is difficult to control, a subcutaneous pain management system may be used. In this system, a nylon catheter is inserted at the site of the affected area. The catheter is attached to a pump that delivers a continuous amount of local anesthetic at a specific amount determined and prescribed by the primary provider (see Fig. 16-4).

Nonpharmacologic pain management approaches may be used as components of multimodal pain management plans of care. Effective methods include music therapy, guided

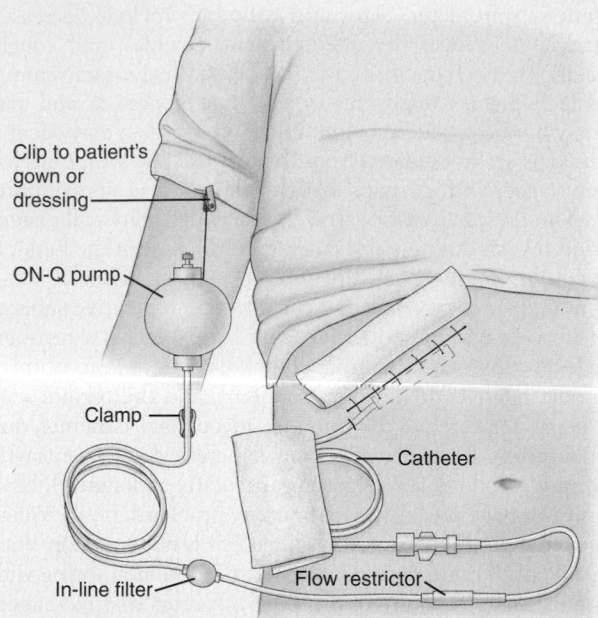

Figure 16-4 • Subcutaneous pain management system consists of a pump, filter, and catheter that delivers a specific amount of prescribed local anesthetic at the rate determined by the physician. Redrawn with permission from Kimberly-Clark Corporation, Neenah, WI.

imagery, Reiki, and therapeutic massage (Poulson, Coto, & Cooney, 2019). Changing the patient's position, using distraction, applying cool washcloths to the face, and providing back massage may be useful in relieving general discomfort temporarily, promoting relaxation, and rendering medication more effective when it is given.

PROMOTING CARDIAC OUTPUT

If signs and symptoms of shock or hemorrhage occur, treatment and nursing care are implemented as described in the discussion of care in the PACU and in Chapter 11.

Although most patients do not hemorrhage or go into shock, changes in circulating volume, the stress of surgery, and the effects of medications and preoperative preparations all affect cardiovascular function. Volume status assessment in the PACU can be difficult because vasoconstriction from surgical stress and hypothermia can compensate for hypovolemia (Odom-Forren, 2018). Close monitoring is indicated to detect and correct conditions such as fluid volume deficit, altered tissue perfusion, and decreased cardiac output, all of which can increase the patient's discomfort, place him or her at risk of complications, and prolong the hospital stay. Consequently, fluid replacement must be carefully managed, and intake and output records must be accurate. IV fluid replacement may be prescribed for up to 24 hours after surgery or until the patient is stable and tolerating oral fluids.

Nursing management includes assessing the patency of the IV lines and ensuring that the correct fluids are given at the prescribed rate. Intake and output, including emesis and output from wound drainage systems, are recorded separately and totaled to determine fluid balance. If the patient has an indwelling urinary catheter, hourly outputs are monitored and should not be less than 0.5 mL/kg/h or 25 mL/h; oliguria is reported immediately (Odom-Forren, 2018). Electrolyte levels and hemoglobin and hematocrit levels are monitored. Decreased hemoglobin and hematocrit levels can indicate blood loss or dilution of circulating volume by IV fluids. If dilution is contributing to the decreased levels, the hemoglobin and hematocrit will rise as the stress response abates and fluids are mobilized and excreted.

Venous stasis from dehydration, immobility, and pressure on leg veins during surgery put the patient at risk for VTE. Leg exercises and frequent position changes are initiated early in the postoperative period to stimulate circulation. Patients should avoid positions that compromise venous return, such as raising the bed's knee gatch, placing a pillow under the knees, sitting for long periods, and dangling the legs with pressure at the back of the knees. Venous return is promoted by antiembolism stockings and early ambulation.

ENCOURAGING ACTIVITY

Early ambulation has a significant effect on recovery and the prevention of complications (e.g., atelectasis, hypostatic pneumonia, gastrointestinal [GI] discomfort, circulatory problems) (Rothrock, 2019). Postoperative activity orders are checked before the patient is assisted to get out of bed, in many instances, on the evening following surgery. Sitting up at the edge of the bed for a few minutes may be all that the patient who has undergone a major surgical procedure can tolerate at first.

Ambulation reduces postoperative abdominal distention by increasing GI tract and abdominal wall tone and stimulating peristalsis. Early ambulation prevents stasis of blood, and thromboembolic events occur less frequently. Pain is often decreased when early ambulation is possible, and the hospital stay is shorter and less costly.

Despite the advantages of early ambulation, patients may be reluctant to get out of bed on the evening of surgery. Reminding them of the importance of early mobility in preventing complications may help patients overcome their fears. When a patient gets out of bed for the first time, orthostatic hypotension, also called *postural hypotension*, is a concern. Orthostatic hypotension is an abnormal drop in blood pressure that occurs as the patient changes from a supine to a standing position. It is common after surgery because of changes in circulating blood volume and bed rest. Signs and symptoms include a decrease of 20 mm Hg in systolic blood pressure or 10 mm Hg in diastolic blood pressure, weakness, dizziness, and fainting (Weber & Kelley, 2018). Patients may report a sense of dizziness or fainting, along with a marked drop in blood pressure. Older adults are at increased risk for orthostatic hypotension secondary to age-related changes in vascular tone. To detect orthostatic hypotension, the nurse assesses the patient's blood pressure first in the supine position, after the patient sits up, again after the patient stands, and 2 to 3 minutes later. Gradual position change gives the circulatory system time to adjust. If the patient becomes dizzy, they are returned to the supine position, and ambulation is delayed for several hours.

To assist the postoperative patient in getting out of bed for the first time after surgery, the nurse:

- Helps the patient move gradually from the lying position to the sitting position by raising the head of the bed and encourages the patient to splint the incision when applicable.
- Positions the patient completely upright (sitting) and turned so that both legs are hanging over the edge of the bed.
- Helps the patient stand beside the bed.

After becoming accustomed to the upright position, the patient may start to walk. The nurse should be at the patient's side to give physical support and encouragement. Care must be taken not to tire the patient; the extent of the first few periods of ambulation varies with the type of surgical procedure and the patient's physical condition and age.

Whether or not the patient can ambulate early in the postoperative period, bed exercises are encouraged to improve circulation. Bed exercises consist of the following:

- Arm exercises (full range of motion, with specific attention to abduction and external rotation of the shoulder)
- Hand and finger exercises
- Foot exercises to prevent VTE, footdrop, and toe deformities and to aid in maintaining good circulation
- Leg flexion and leg-lifting exercises to prepare the patient for ambulation
- Abdominal and gluteal contraction exercises

Hampered by pain, dressings, IV lines, or drains, many patients cannot engage in activity without assistance. Helping the patient increase the activity level on the first postoperative day is important to prevent complications related to prolonged inactivity. One way to increase the patient's activity is to have the patient perform as much routine hygiene care as possible. Setting up the patient to bathe with a bedside wash basin or, if possible, assisting the patient to the bathroom to sit in a chair at the sink not only gets the patient moving but helps restore a sense of self-control and prepares the patient for discharge.

For a safe discharge to home, patients need to be able to ambulate a functional distance (e.g., length of the house or apartment), get in and out of bed unassisted, and be independent with toileting. Patients can be asked to perform as much as they can and then to call for assistance. The patient and the nurse can collaborate on a schedule for progressive activity that includes ambulating in the room and hallway and sitting out of bed in a chair. Assessing the patient's vital signs before, during, and after a scheduled activity helps the nurse and patient determine the rate of progression. By providing physical support, the nurse maintains the patient's safety; by communicating a positive attitude about the patient's ability to perform the activity, the nurse promotes the patient's confidence. The nurse encourages the patient to continue to perform bed exercises, wear pneumatic compression or prescribed antiembolism stockings when in bed, and rest as needed. If the patient has had orthopedic surgery of the lower extremities or will require a mobility aid (i.e., walker, crutches) at home, a physical therapist may be involved the first time the patient gets out of bed to educate him or her to ambulate safely or to use the mobility aid correctly.

CARING FOR WOUNDS

Wound Healing. Wounds heal by different mechanisms, depending on the condition of the wound.

The healing of skin wounds follows three general phases, the inflammatory phase, the proliferative phase, and then wound contraction and remodeling phase. Each of these phases is mediated through cytokines and growth factors (Norris, 2019). See Chart 16-5 for explanations and illustrations of these three phases.

Surgical wound healing occurs in two ways, by **first-intention or second-intention wound healing** (Norris, 2019). A sutured

Chart 16-5   Three Phases of Wound Healing

Inflammatory Phase

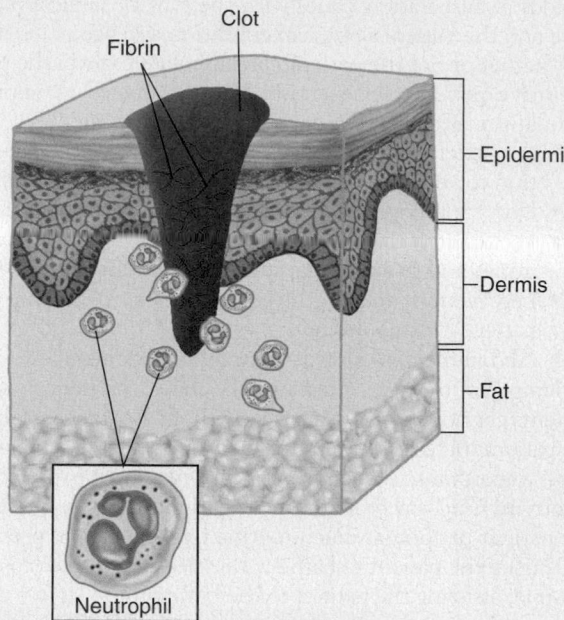

The inflammatory phase begins at the time of injury with the formation of a blood clot and the migration of phagocytic white blood cells into the wound site. The first cells to arrive, the neutrophils, ingest and remove bacteria and cellular debris. After 24 hours, the neutrophils are joined by macrophages, which continue to ingest cellular debris and play an essential role in the production of growth factors for the proliferative phase.

Proliferative Phase

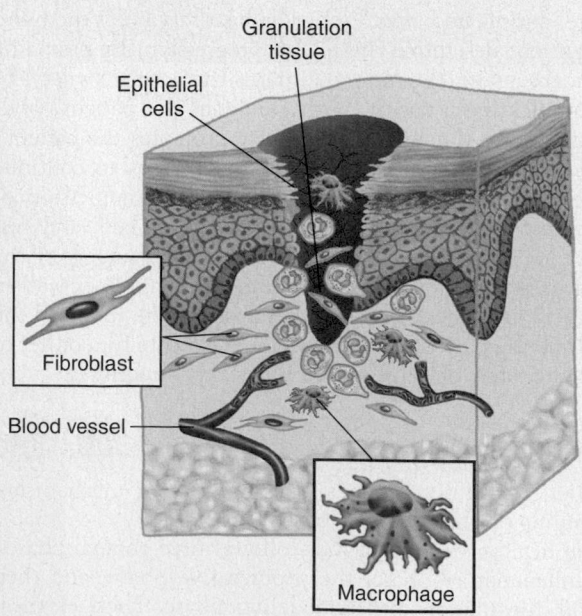

The primary processes during this phase focus on the building of new tissue to fill the wound space. The key cell during

this phase is the *fibroblast*, a connective tissue cell that synthesizes and secretes the collagen, proteoglycans, and glycoproteins needed for wound healing. Fibroblasts also produce a family of growth factors that induce angiogenesis (growth of new blood vessels) and endothelial cell proliferation and migration. The final component of the proliferative phase is epithelialization, during which epithelial cells at the wound edges proliferate to form a new surface layer that is similar to that which was destroyed by the injury.

Wound Contraction and Remodeling Phase

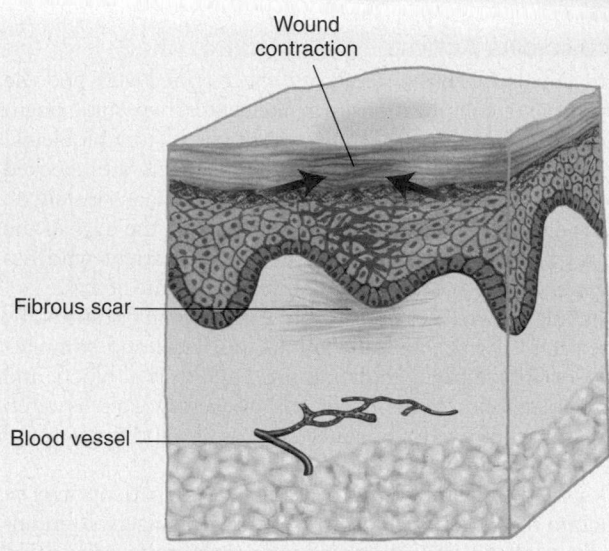

This phase begins approximately 3 weeks after injury with the development of the fibrous scar and can continue for 6 months or longer, depending on the extent of the wound. During this phase, there is a decrease in vascularity and continued remodeling of scar tissue by simultaneous synthesis of collagen by fibroblasts and lysis by collagenase enzymes. As a result of these two processes, the architecture of the scar is capable of increasing its tensile strength, and the scar shrinks so it is less visible.

surgical incision is an example of first-intention healing. A larger wound, such as a burn heals by secondary intention.

With shorter hospital stays, much of the healing takes place at home, and both the hospital and the transitional or home health nurse needs to be well versed in the principles of wound healing.

Ongoing assessment of the surgical site involves inspection for approximation of wound edges, integrity of sutures or staples, redness, discoloration, warmth, swelling, unusual tenderness, or drainage. The area around the wound should also be inspected for a reaction to tape or trauma from tight bandages. Risk factors for altered wound healing include poor nutrition, smoking, diabetes, and poor hygiene (Nasser, Kosty, Shah, et al., 2018; Norris, 2019). Specific nursing assessments and interventions that address these factors and help promote wound healing are presented in Table 16-3.

TABLE 16-3 Factors Affecting Wound Healing

Factors	Rationale	Nursing Interventions
Age of patient	The older the patient, the less resilient the tissues.	Handle all tissues gently.
Bathing protocol	Use of chlorhexidine gluconate shower and preoperative wipes as a means for antimicrobial skin antisepsis.	Educate patient regarding use and importance. Confirm use with patient in preoperative area.
Hemorrhage	Accumulation of blood creates dead spaces as well as dead cells that must be removed. The area becomes a growth medium for organisms.	Monitor vital signs. Observe incision site for evidence of bleeding and infection.
Hypovolemia	Insufficient blood volume leads to vasoconstriction and reduced oxygen and nutrients available for wound healing.	Monitor for volume deficit (circulatory impairment). Correct by fluid replacement as prescribed.
Temperature Management	Hypothermia causes poor tissue oxygenation and thus poor perfusion needed for wound healing.	Assess the patient's temperature pre-, intra-, and postoperatively. Implement warm blanket or forced air warming measures.
Local Factors		
Edema	Reduces blood supply by exerting increased interstitial pressure on vessels.	Elevate part; apply cool compresses.
Inadequate dressing technique:		
Too small	Permits bacterial invasion and contamination.	Follow guidelines for proper dressing technique.
Too tight	Reduces blood supply carrying nutrients and oxygen.	
Nutritional deficits	Protein–calorie depletion may occur. Insulin secretion may be inhibited, causing blood glucose to rise.	Correct deficits; this may require parenteral nutritional therapy. Monitor blood glucose levels. Administer vitamin supplements as prescribed.
Foreign bodies	Foreign bodies retard healing.	Keep wounds free of dressing threads, ensure sterility of implanted items.
Oxygen deficit (tissue oxygenation insufficient)	Insufficient oxygen may be due to inadequate lung and cardiovascular function as well as localized vasoconstriction.	Encourage deep breathing, turning, and controlled coughing.
Drainage accumulation	Accumulated secretions hamper healing process.	Monitor closed drainage systems for proper functioning. Institute measures to remove accumulated secretions.
Medications		
Corticosteroids	May mask presence of infection by impairing normal inflammatory response.	Be aware of action and effect of medications patient is receiving.
Anticoagulants	May cause hemorrhage.	
Broad-spectrum and specific antibiotics	Effective if given immediately before surgery for specific pathology or bacterial contamination. Ineffective if given after wound is closed due to intravascular coagulation at the periphery of the surgical site.	
Patient overactivity	Prevents approximation of wound edges. Resting favors healing.	Use measures to keep wound edges approximated: taping, bandaging, splints. Encourage rest.
Systemic Disorders		
Hemorrhagic shock	These depress cell functions that directly affect wound healing.	Be familiar with the nature of the specific disorder. Administer prescribed treatment. Cultures may be indicated to determine appropriate antibiotic.
Acidosis		
Hypoxia		
Kidney injury		
Hepatic disease		
Sepsis		
Immunosuppressed state	Patient is more vulnerable to bacterial and viral invasion; defense mechanisms are impaired.	Provide maximum protection to prevent infection. Restrict visitors with colds; institute mandatory hand hygiene by all staff.
Wound Stressors		
Vomiting	Produce tension on wounds, particularly of the torso.	Encourage frequent turning and ambulation, and administer antiemetic medications as prescribed. Assist patient in splinting incision.
Valsalva maneuver		
Heavy coughing		
Straining		

Adapted from Padgette, P., & Wood, B. (2018). Conducting a surgical site infection prevention tracer. *AORN Journal, 107*(5), 580–590.

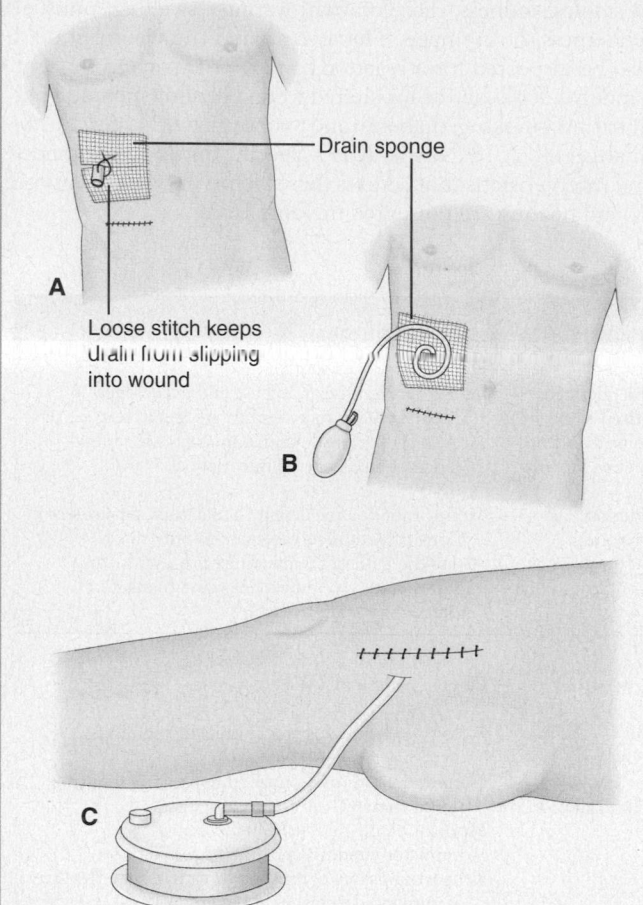

Drain sponge

A

Loose stitch keeps drain from slipping into wound

B

C

Figure 16-5 • Types of surgical drains: **A.** Penrose. **B.** Jackson–Pratt. **C.** Hemovac.

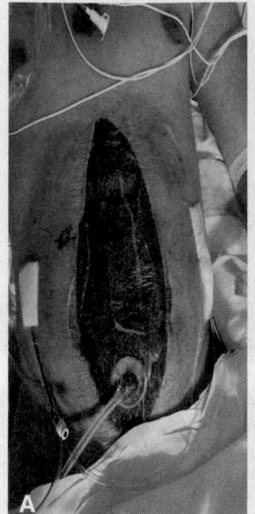
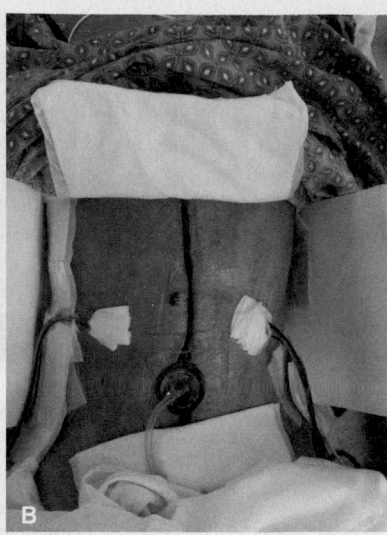

Figure 16-6 • Example of an abdominal wound with a vacuum-assisted closure (VAC). **A.** Abdominal gunshot wound showing VAC following initial laparotomy that allows for swelling. **B.** Abdominal gunshot wound showing VAC following partial closure 3 days later. Photos courtesy of Blaine Thomas.

Caring for Surgical Drains. Nursing interventions to promote wound healing also include management of surgical drains. Drains are tubes that exit the peri-incisional area, either into a portable wound suction device (closed) or into the dressings (open). The principle involved is to allow the escape of fluids that could otherwise serve as a culture medium for bacteria. In portable wound suction, the use of gentle, constant suction enhances drainage of these fluids and collapses the skin flaps against the underlying tissue, thus removing "dead space." Types of wound drains include the Penrose, Jackson-Pratt, and Hemovac drains (see Fig. 16-5). Output (drainage) from wound systems is recorded.

Wound vacuum-assisted closure (VAC) devices are used on open wounds allowed to heal on their own. The wound VAC is a foam dressing that uses negative pressure suction at the wound surface. The vacuum removes debris while promoting granulation tissue growth and blood flow. Wound VACs are placed intraoperatively and the foam dressing is changed periodically as the wound shrinks in size (see Fig. 16-6). The amount, pressure, and color of drainage should be assessed and recorded. Patients should be assessed for pain as nerve endings may grow into the sponge as tissue regrows.

The amount of bloody drainage on the surgical dressing is assessed frequently. Spots of drainage on the dressings are outlined with a pen, and the date and time of the outline are recorded on the dressing so that increased drainage can be easily seen. A certain amount of bloody drainage in a wound drainage system or on the dressing is expected, but excessive amounts should be reported to the surgeon. Increasing amounts of fresh blood on the dressing should be reported immediately. Some wounds are irrigated heavily before closure in the OR, and open drains exiting the wound may be embedded in the dressings. These wounds may drain large amounts of blood-tinged fluid that saturate the dressing. The dressing can be reinforced with sterile gauze bandages; the time at which they were reinforced should be documented. If drainage continues, the surgeon should be notified so that the dressing can be changed. Multiple similar drains are numbered or otherwise labeled (e.g., left lower quadrant, left upper quadrant) so that output measurements can be reliably and consistently recorded.

CHANGING THE DRESSING

The surgical dressing is placed in the operating suite by a member of the surgical team. Dressing changes (if needed) in the immediate postoperative period are performed by the nurse. A dressing is applied to a wound for one or more of the following reasons: (1) to provide a proper environment for wound healing; (2) to absorb drainage; (3) to splint or immobilize the wound; (4) to protect the wound and new epithelial tissue from mechanical injury; (5) to protect the wound from bacterial contamination and from soiling by feces, vomitus, and urine; (6) to promote hemostasis, as in a pressure dressing; and (7) to provide mental and physical comfort for the patient.

The patient is told that the dressing is to be changed and that changing the dressing is a simple procedure associated with little discomfort. The dressing change is performed at a suitable time (e.g., not at mealtimes or when visitors are present). Privacy is provided, and the patient is not unduly exposed. Assurance is given that the incision will shrink as it heals and that the redness will fade.

The nurse performs hand hygiene before and after the dressing change and wears disposable gloves (sterile or clean as needed) for the dressing change itself. Most dressing changes following surgery are sterile. In accordance with standard precautions, dressings are never touched by ungloved hands because of the danger of transmitting pathogenic organisms. The tape or adhesive portion of the dressing is removed by pulling it parallel with the skin surface and in the direction of hair growth rather than at right angles. Alcohol wipes or nonirritating solvents aid in removing adhesive painlessly and quickly. The soiled dressing is removed and deposited in a container designated for disposal of biomedical waste.

Gloves are changed, and a new dressing is applied. If the patient is sensitive to adhesive tape, the dressing may be held in place with hypoallergenic tape. Many tapes are porous to prevent skin maceration. Some wounds become edematous after having been dressed, causing considerable tension on the tape. If the tape is not flexible, the stretching bandage will also cause a shear injury to the skin. This can result in denuded areas or large blisters and should be avoided. An elastic adhesive bandage (Elastoplast, 3M Microfoam) may be used to hold dressings in place over mobile areas, such as the neck or the extremities, or where pressure is required.

While changing the dressing, the nurse has an opportunity to educate the patient on how to care for the incision and change the dressings at home. The nurse observes for indicators of the patient's readiness to learn, such as looking at the incision, expressing interest, or assisting in the dressing change. Information on self-care activities and possible signs of infection is summarized in Chart 16-6.

MAINTAINING NORMAL BODY TEMPERATURE

The patient is still at risk for malignant hyperthermia and hypothermia in the postoperative period. Efforts are made to identify malignant hyperthermia and to treat it early and promptly (Rothrock, 2019).

Patients who have received anesthesia are susceptible to chills and drafts. Interventions to avoid hypothermia, temperatures below 36°C (98.6°F), begin in the preoperative area (see Chapter 14) and continue throughout the intraoperative period (see Chapter 15). Low body temperature is reported to the primary provider. The room is maintained at a comfortable temperature, and blankets are provided to prevent chilling. Treatment includes oxygen administration, adequate hydration, and proper nutrition including glycemic control. The patient is also monitored for cardiac arrhythmias. The risk of hypothermia is greater in older adults and in patients who were in the cool OR environment for a prolonged period.

MANAGING GASTROINTESTINAL FUNCTION AND RESUMING NUTRITION

Discomfort of the GI tract (nausea, vomiting, and hiccups) and resumption of oral intake are issues for the patient and affect their outcome following surgery. (See the earlier discussion of PONV in the PACU.)

If the risk of vomiting is high due to the nature of surgery, a nasogastric tube is inserted preoperatively and remains in place throughout the surgery and the immediate postoperative period. A nasogastric tube also may be inserted before surgery if postoperative distention is anticipated. In addition, a nasogastric tube may be inserted if a patient who has food in the stomach requires emergency surgery.

Hiccups, produced by intermittent spasms of the diaphragm secondary to irritation of the phrenic nerve, can occur after surgery. The irritation may be direct, such as from stimulation

---

Chart 16-6

PATIENT EDUCATION
Wound Care Instructions

Until Sutures Are Removed

1. Keep the wound dry and clean.
   - If there is no dressing, ask your nurse or physician if you can bathe or shower.
   - If a dressing or splint is in place, do not remove it unless it is wet or soiled.
   - If wet or soiled, change dressing yourself if you have been taught to do so; otherwise, call your nurse or physician for guidance.
   - If you have been taught, instruction might be as follows:
     - Cleanse area *gently* with sterile normal saline once or twice daily.
     - Cover with a sterile Telfa pad™ or gauze square large enough to cover wound.
     - Apply hypoallergenic tape (Dermicel™ or paper). Adhesive is not recommended because it is difficult to remove without possible injury to the incisional site.
2. Immediately report any of these signs of infection:
   - Redness, marked swelling exceeding 0.5 inch (2.5 cm) from incision site; tenderness; or increased warmth around wound
   - Red streaks in skin near wound
   - Pus or discharge, foul odor
   - Chills or temperature higher than 37.7°C (100°F)
3. If soreness or pain causes discomfort, apply a dry cool pack (containing ice or cold water) or take prescribed acetaminophen tablets every 4 to 6 hours. Avoid using aspirin without direction or instruction because bleeding can occur with its use.
4. Swelling after surgery is common. To help reduce swelling, elevate the affected part to the level of the heart.
   - Hand or arm:
     - Sleep—elevate arm on pillow at side
     - Sitting—place arm on pillow on adjacent table
     - Standing—rest affected hand on opposite shoulder; support elbow with unaffected hand
   - Leg or foot:
     - Sitting—place a pillow on a facing chair; provide support underneath the knee
     - Lying—place a pillow under affected leg

After Sutures Are Removed

Although the wound appears to be healed when sutures are removed, it is still tender and will continue to heal and strengthen for several weeks.

- Follow recommendations of physician or nurse regarding extent of activity.
- Keep suture line clean; do not rub vigorously; pat dry. Wound edges may look red and may be slightly raised. This is normal.
- If the site continues to be red, thick, and painful to pressure after 8 weeks, consult the health care provider. (This may be due to excessive collagen formation and should be checked.)

Adapted from American Society of PeriAnesthesia Nurses (ASPAN). (2019). *Perianesthesia nursing standards, practice recommendations and interpretive statements*. Cherry Hill, NJ: Author.
Association of PeriOperative Registered Nurses (AORN). (2019). *Association of PeriOperative Registered Nurses (AORN) standards, recommended practice, and guidelines*. Denver, CO: Author.

---

of the nerve by a distended stomach, subdiaphragmatic abscess, or abdominal distention; indirect, such as from toxemia or uremia that stimulates the nerve; or reflexive, such as from irritation from a drainage tube or obstruction of the intestines. These occurrences usually are mild, transitory attacks that cease spontaneously. If hiccups persist, they may produce considerable distress and serious effects, such as vomiting, exhaustion, and wound dehiscence. Chlorpromazine (a phenothiazine) is the only drug approved to treat intractable hiccups (Aroke & Hicks, 2019).

> ### ▶ Quality and Safety Nursing Alert
>
> *Any condition that is persistent or considered intractable, such as hiccups, should be reported to the primary provider so that appropriate measures can be implemented.*

Once PONV has subsided and the patient is fully awake and alert, the sooner they can tolerate a usual diet, the more quickly normal GI function will resume. Taking food by mouth stimulates digestive juices and promotes gastric function and intestinal peristalsis. The return to normal dietary intake should proceed at a pace set by the patient. The nature of the surgery and the type of anesthesia directly affect the rate at which normal gastric activity resumes. Enhanced recovery programs encourage early nutrition as a way to maintain fluid balance, prevent postoperative ileus, and decrease overall length of stay (Persico et al., 2019).

Clear liquids are typically the first substances desired and tolerated by the patient after surgery. Water, juice, and tea may be given in increasing amounts. Cool fluids are tolerated more easily than those that are ice cold or hot. Soft foods (gelatin, custard, milk, and creamed soups) are added gradually after clear fluids have been tolerated. As soon as the patient tolerates soft foods well, solid food may be given.

Assessment and management of GI function are important after surgery because the GI tract is subject to uncomfortable or potentially life-threatening complications. Any postoperative patient may suffer from distention. Postoperative distention of the abdomen results from the accumulation of gas in the intestinal tract. Manipulation of the abdominal organs during surgery may produce a loss of normal peristalsis for 24 to 48 hours, depending on the type and extent of surgery. Even though nothing is given by mouth, swallowed air and GI tract secretions enter the stomach and intestines; if not propelled by peristalsis, they collect in the intestines, producing distention and causing the patient to complain of fullness or pain in the abdomen. Most often, the gas collects in the colon. Abdominal distention is further increased by immobility, anesthetic agents, and the use of opioid medications.

After major abdominal surgery, distention may be avoided by having the patient turn frequently, exercise, and ambulate as early as possible. This also alleviates distention produced by swallowing air, which is common in anxious patients. A nasogastric tube inserted before surgery may remain in place until full peristaltic activity (indicated by the passage of flatus) has resumed. The nurse detects bowel sounds by listening to the abdomen with a stethoscope. Bowel sounds are documented so that diet progression can occur.

Paralytic ileus and intestinal obstruction are potential postoperative complications that occur more frequently in patients undergoing intestinal or abdominal surgery (see Chapter 41).

PROMOTING BOWEL FUNCTION

Constipation can occur after surgery as a minor or a serious complication. Decreased mobility, decreased oral intake, and opioid analgesic medications can contribute to difficulty having a bowel movement. In addition, irritation and trauma to the bowel during surgery may inhibit intestinal movement for several days. The combined effect of early ambulation, improved dietary intake, and a stool softener (if prescribed) promotes bowel elimination. Multimodal analgesia regimens in surgical patients minimize opioid-related adverse effects such as nausea, vomiting, and reduced gastric motility (Wolfe, 2018). The nurse should assess the abdomen for distention and the presence and frequency of bowel sounds. If the patient does not have a bowel movement by the second or third postoperative day, the primary provider should be notified and a laxative or other test or intervention may be needed.

MANAGING VOIDING

The type of procedure, length of case, and patient position may have warranted a catheter being placed in the patient's urinary tract in the OR. In the postoperative period, any urine that was collected using a catheter (indwelling or straight) during the operative procedure should be noted. This information will assist the nurse to anticipate the patient's voiding needs.

Urinary retention after surgery can occur for various reasons. Anesthetics, anticholinergic agents, and opioids interfere with the perception of bladder fullness and the urge to void and inhibit the ability to initiate voiding and completely empty the bladder. Abdominal, pelvic, and hip surgery may increase the likelihood of retention secondary to pain. In addition, some patients find it difficult to use the bedpan or urinal in the recumbent position.

Bladder distention and the urge to void should be assessed at the time of the patient's arrival at the unit and frequently thereafter. The patient is expected to void within 8 hours after surgery (this includes time spent in the PACU). If the patient has an urge to void and cannot, or if the bladder is distended and no urge is felt or the patient cannot void, catheterization is not delayed solely on the basis of the 8-hour time frame. All methods to encourage the patient to void should be tried (e.g., letting water run, applying heat to the perineum). The bedpan should be warm; a cold bedpan causes discomfort and automatic tightening of muscles (including the urethral sphincter). If the patient cannot void on a bedpan, it may be possible to use a commode or a toilet (if there is one in the PACU). Male patients are often permitted to sit up or stand beside the bed to use the urinal; however, safeguards should be taken to prevent the patient from falling or fainting due to loss of coordination from medications or orthostatic hypotension. If the patient has not voided within the specified time frame, a portable bladder ultrasound is performed to check for urinary retention (see Chapter 47, Fig. 47-8). The patient is catheterized, and the catheter is removed after the bladder has emptied. Straight intermittent catheterization is preferred over indwelling catheterization because the risk of infection is increased with an indwelling catheter.

Even if the patient voids, the bladder may not empty. The nurse notes the amount of urine voided and palpates the suprapubic area for distention or tenderness. Postvoid residual urine may be assessed by using either straight catheterization or a portable bladder ultrasound scanner and is considered diagnostic of urinary retention. Bladder scanning is an effective way to detect urinary retention in patients who have had general and regional anesthesia. Research suggests that frequent bladder scanning decreases incontinence as retention is detected early and treated before an incontinent episode (Wishart, 2019).

MAINTAINING A SAFE ENVIRONMENT

During the immediate postoperative period, the patient recovering from anesthesia should have two side rails up, and the bed should be in the low position. The nurse assesses the patient's level of consciousness and orientation and determines whether the patient can resume wearing assistive devices as needed (e.g., eyeglasses, hearing aid). Impaired vision, inability to hear postoperative instructions, or inability to communicate verbally places the patient at risk for injury. All objects the patient may need should be within reach, especially the call light. Any immediate postoperative prescribed therapies concerning special positioning, equipment, or interventions should be implemented as soon as possible. The patient is instructed to ask for assistance with any activity. Although restraints are occasionally necessary for a patient who is disoriented, they should be avoided if at all possible (see Chapter 1 for further discussion on use of restraints). Agency policy on the use of restraints must be consulted and followed.

Any surgical procedure has the potential for injury due to disrupted neurovascular integrity resulting from prolonged awkward positioning in the OR, manipulation of tissues, inadvertent severing of nerves or blood vessels, or tight bandages. Any orthopedic or neurologic surgery or surgery involving the extremities carries a risk of peripheral nerve damage. Vascular surgeries, such as replacement of sections of diseased peripheral arteries or insertion of an arteriovenous graft, put the patient at risk for thrombus formation at the surgical site and subsequent ischemia of tissues distal to the thrombus. Assessment includes having the patient move the hand or foot distal to the surgical site through a full range of motion, assessing all surfaces for intact sensation, and assessing peripheral pulses (Rothrock, 2019).

PROVIDING EMOTIONAL SUPPORT TO THE PATIENT AND FAMILY

Although patients and families are undoubtedly relieved that surgery is over, stress and anxiety levels may remain high in the immediate postoperative period. Many factors contribute to this stress and anxiety, including pain, being in an unfamiliar environment, inability to control one's circumstances or care for oneself, fear of the long-term effects of surgery, fear of complications, fatigue, spiritual distress, altered role responsibilities, ineffective coping, and altered body image, and all are potential reactions to the surgical experience. The nurse helps the patient and family work through their stress and anxieties by providing reassurance and information and by spending time listening to and addressing their concerns. The nurse describes hospital routines and what to expect in the time until discharge and explains the purpose of nursing assessments and interventions. Informing patients when they will be able to drink fluids or eat, when they will be getting out of bed, and when tubes and drains will be removed helps them gain a sense of control and participation in recovery and engages them in the plan of care. Acknowledging family members' concerns and accepting and encouraging their

TABLE 16-4	Select Postoperative Complications
Body System/Type	**Complications**
Respiratory	Atelectasis, pneumonia, pulmonary embolism, aspiration
Cardiovascular	Shock, thrombophlebitis, DVT, pulmonary embolism
Neurologic	Delirium, stroke
Skin/Wound	Breakdown, infection, dehiscence, evisceration, delayed healing, hemorrhage, hematoma
Gastrointestinal	Constipation, paralytic ileus, bowel obstruction
Urinary	Acute urine retention, urinary tract infection
Functional	Weakness, fatigue, functional decline

DVT, deep vein thrombosis.

participation in the patient's care assist them in feeling that they are helping their loved one. The nurse can modify the environment to enhance rest and relaxation by providing privacy, reducing noise, adjusting lighting, providing enough seating for family members, and encouraging a supportive atmosphere.

MANAGING POTENTIAL COMPLICATIONS

The postoperative patient is at risk for complications as outlined next and summarized in Table 16-4.

Venous Thromboembolism. Serious potential VTE complications of surgery include DVT and PE (Rothrock, 2019).

Prevention of DVT and PE development includes pharmacologic prophylaxis (e.g., subcutaneous heparin) (Odom-Forren, 2018). External pneumatic compression and antiembolism stockings can be used alone or in combination with low-dose heparin. The stress response that is initiated by surgery inhibits the thrombolytic (fibrinolytic) system, resulting in blood hypercoagulability. Dehydration, low cardiac output, blood pooling in the extremities, and bed rest add to the risk of thrombosis formation. Although all postoperative patients are at some risk, factors such as a history of thrombosis, malignancy, trauma, obesity, indwelling venous catheters, and hormone use (e.g., estrogen) increase the risk. The first symptom of DVT may be a pain or cramp in the calf, although many patients are asymptomatic. Other signs and symptoms include tachypnea, chest pain, hemoptysis, shortness of breath, and a sense of impending doom (Odom-Forren, 2018).

The benefits of early ambulation and leg exercises in preventing DVT cannot be overemphasized, and these activities are recommended for all patients, regardless of their risk. It is important to avoid the use of blanket rolls, pillow rolls, or any form of elevation that can constrict vessels under the knees. Even prolonged "dangling" (having the patient sit on the edge of the bed with legs hanging over the side) can be dangerous and is not recommended in susceptible patients because pressure under the knees can impede circulation. Adequate hydration is also encouraged; the patient can be offered juices and water throughout the day to avoid dehydration. (Refer to Chapter 26 for discussion of DVT and PE.)

Hematoma. At times, concealed bleeding occurs beneath the skin at the surgical site. This hemorrhage usually stops spontaneously but results in clot (hematoma) formation within the wound. If the clot is small, it will be absorbed and need not be treated. If the clot is large, the wound usually bulges somewhat, and healing will be delayed unless the clot is removed. Evacuation of the clot requires surgery where several sutures are removed by the surgeon, the clot is evacuated, and the wound is packed lightly with gauze. Healing occurs usually by granulation, or a secondary closure may be performed.

Infection (Wound Sepsis). The creation of a surgical wound disrupts the integrity of the skin, bypassing the body's primary defense and protection against infection. Exposure of deep body tissues to pathogens in the environment places the patient at risk for infection of the surgical site, and a potentially life-threatening complication such as infection can increase the length of hospital stay, costs of care, and risk of further complications.

Joint Commission–approved hospitals measure surgical site infections (SSIs) for the first 30 or 90 days following surgical procedures based on national standards. Reduction of SSIs remains an important National Patient Safety Goal (see Chapter 14, Chart 14-7) (Joint Commission, 2019).

Multiple factors, including the type of wound, place the patient at potential risk for infection. Surgical wounds are classified according to the degree of contamination. Table 16-5 defines the classification of surgical wounds and SSI rates per category. Patient-related factors include age, nutritional status, diabetes, smoking, obesity, remote infections, endogenous mucosal microorganisms, altered immune response, length of preoperative stay, and severity of illness (Rothrock, 2019). Factors related to the surgical procedure are proper ventilation in the surgical space, aseptic technique of personnel, sterile instrument use, and overall room cleanliness (Armellino, 2017). The focus of infection prevention has transitioned from controlling infections to preventing their occurrence. Prevention efforts include skin antisepsis, preoperative bathing, hair removal, antimicrobial prophylaxis, and patient temperature management (Padgette & Wood, 2018). (Preoperative and intraoperative risks and interventions are discussed in Chapters 14 and 15.) Postoperative care of the wound centers on assessing the wound, preventing contamination and infection before wound edges have sealed, and enhancing healing.

Signs and symptoms of wound infection include increased pulse rate and temperature; an elevated white blood cell count; wound swelling, warmth, tenderness, or discharge; and increased incisional pain. Local signs may be absent if the infection is deep. *Staphylococcus aureus* accounts for many postoperative wound infections. Other infections may result from *Escherichia coli*, *Proteus vulgaris*, *Aerobacter aerogenes*, *Pseudomonas aeruginosa*, and other organisms. Although they are rare, beta-hemolytic streptococcal or clostridial infections can be rapid and deadly and need strict infection control practices to prevent the spread of infection to others. Intensive medical and nursing care is essential if the patient is to survive (Ackley & Ladwig, 2017).

When a wound infection is diagnosed in a surgical incision, the surgeon may remove one or more sutures or staples and, using aseptic precautions, separate the wound edges with a pair of blunt scissors or a hemostat. Once the incision is opened, a drain may be inserted. If the infection is deep, an incision and drainage procedure may be necessary. Antimicrobial therapy and a wound care regimen are also initiated.

Wound Dehiscence and Evisceration. Wound **dehiscence** (disruption of surgical incision or wound) and **evisceration** (protrusion of wound contents) are serious surgical complications (see Fig. 16-7). Dehiscence and evisceration are especially serious when they involve abdominal incisions or wounds. These complications result from sutures giving way, from infection, or, more frequently, from marked distention or strenuous cough. They may also occur because of increasing age, anemia, poor nutritional status, obesity, malignancy, diabetes, the use of steroids, and other factors in patients undergoing abdominal surgery.

TABLE 16-5	Wound Classification and Associated Surgical Site Infection Risk	
Surgical Category	**Determinants of Category**	**Expected Risk of Postsurgical Infection (%)**
Clean	Nontraumatic site Uninfected site No inflammation No break in aseptic technique No entry into respiratory, alimentary, genitourinary, or oropharyngeal tracts	1–3
Clean contaminated	Entry into respiratory, alimentary, genitourinary, or oropharyngeal tracts without unusual contamination Appendectomy Minor break in aseptic technique Mechanical drainage	3–7
Contaminated	Open, newly experienced traumatic wounds Gross spillage from gastrointestinal tract Major break in aseptic technique Entry into genitourinary or biliary tract when urine or bile is infected	7–16
Dirty	Traumatic wound with delayed repair, devitalized tissue, foreign bodies, or fecal contamination Acute inflammation and purulent drainage encountered during procedure	16–29

Adapted from Edmiston, C. E., Jr., & Spencer, M. (2014). Patient care interventions to help reduce the risk of surgical site infections. *AORN Journal, 100*(6), 590–602.

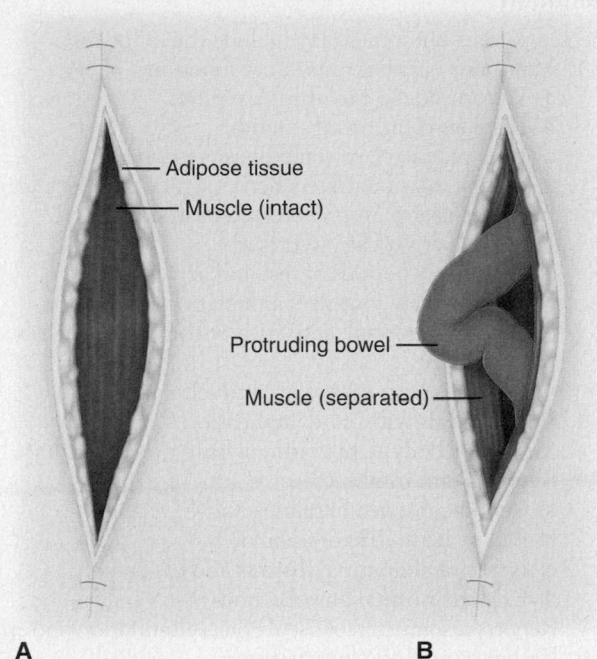

Figure 16-7 • A. Wound dehiscence. **B.** Wound evisceration.

When the wound edges separate slowly, the intestines may protrude gradually or not at all, and the earliest sign may be a gush of bloody (serosanguineous) peritoneal fluid from the wound. When a wound ruptures suddenly, coils of intestine may push out of the abdomen. The patient may report that "something gave way." The evisceration causes pain and may be associated with vomiting.

> ▶ **Quality and Safety Nursing Alert**
>
> *If disruption of a wound occurs, the patient is placed in the low Fowler position and instructed to lie as still as possible. These actions minimize protrusion of body tissues. The protruding coils of intestine are covered with sterile dressings moistened with sterile saline solution, and the surgeon is notified at once.*

An abdominal binder can provide support and guard against dehiscence and may be used along with the primary dressing, especially in patients with weak or pendulous abdominal walls or when rupture of a wound has occurred.

Gerontologic Considerations. Older patients recover more slowly, have longer hospital stays, and are at greater risk for development of postoperative complications. Cardiovascular, respiratory, renal, hepatic, thermoregulatory, sensory, and cognition problems unique to the older adult can cause complications throughout the recovery phase (Odom-Forren, 2018). Expert nursing care can help the older adult avoid these complications or minimize their effects (Rothrock, 2019).

Potential causes of postoperative delirium are multifactorial (see Chart 16-7). Skilled and frequent assessment of mental status and of all physiologic factors helps the nurse plan care because delirium may be the initial or only indicator of infection, fluid and electrolyte imbalance, or deterioration of respiratory or hemodynamic status in the older adult patient. Factors

---

Chart 16-7   Potential Causes of Postoperative Delirium

- Acid–base disturbances
- Acute myocardial infarction
- Age >80 years
- Alcohol withdrawal
- Blood loss
- Cerebral hypoxia
- Decreased cardiac output
- Dehydration
- Emergent surgery
- Fecal impaction
- Fluid and electrolyte imbalance
- Heart failure
- High stress or anxiety levels
- History of dementia like symptoms
- Hypercarbia
- Hypothermia or hyperthermia
- Hypoxia
- Infection (urinary tract, wound, respiratory)
- Medications (anticholinergics, benzodiazepines, central nervous system depressants)
- Polypharmacy
- Presence of multiple diseases
- Sensory impairments
- Unfamiliar surroundings and sensory deprivation
- Unrelieved pain
- Urinary retention

---

that determine whether a patient is at risk for delirium include age, history of alcohol abuse, preoperative cognitive function, physical function, serum chemistries, and type of surgery.

Recognizing postoperative delirium and identifying and treating its underlying cause are the goals of care. Postoperative delirium is sometimes mistaken for preexisting dementia or is attributed to age. In addition to monitoring and managing identifiable causes, the nurse implements supportive interventions. Keeping the patient in a well-lit room and in close proximity to staff can reduce sensory deprivation. At the same time, distracting and unfamiliar noises should be minimized. Because pain can contribute to postoperative delirium, adequate pain control without oversedation is essential (Rothrock, 2019).

The patient is reoriented as often as necessary, and staff should introduce themselves each time they come in contact with the patient. Engaging the patient in conversation and care activities and placing a clock and calendar nearby may improve cognitive function. Physical activity should not be neglected while the patient is confused because physical deterioration can worsen delirium and place the patient at increased risk for other complications. Restraints should be avoided because they can worsen confusion. A staff member is asked to stay with the patient instead. Medications may be given during episodes of acute confusion but should be discontinued as soon as possible to avoid side effects.

Other problems confronting the older postoperative patient, such as pneumonia, altered bowel function, DVT, weakness, and functional decline, often can be prevented by early and progressive ambulation. Prolonged sitting positions are avoided as they promote venous stasis in the lower extremities. A physical therapy referral may be indicated to promote safe, regular exercise for the older adult.

Urinary incontinence can be prevented by providing easy access to the call bell and the commode and by prompting voiding. Early ambulation and familiarity with the room help the patient become self-sufficient sooner.

Optimal nutrition can help promote wound healing and anesthesia recovery. The nurse and patient can consult with the dietitian to plan appealing, high-protein meals that provide sufficient fiber, calories, and vitamins. Nutritional supplements, such as Ensure™ or Sustacal™, may be recommended. Multivitamins, iron, and vitamin C supplements may be prescribed to aid in tissue healing, formation of new red blood cells, and overall nutritional status.

In addition to monitoring and managing physiologic recovery of the older adult, the nurse identifies and addresses psychosocial needs. The older adult may require much encouragement and support to resume activities, and the pace may be slow. Sensory deficits may require frequent repetition of instructions, and decreased physiologic reserve may necessitate frequent rest periods. The older adult may require extensive discharge planning to coordinate both professional and family care providers, and the nurse, social worker, or case management resource may institute the plan for continuing and transitional care.

PROMOTING HOME, COMMUNITY-BASED, AND TRANSITIONAL CARE

Educating Patients About Self-Care. Patient education is critical during postoperative care and includes what can be expected at every stage of the surgical process, including after discharge. It is important for nurses to assess patients preoperatively, especially outpatients, to determine their ability to manage at home and begin educating them about managing any postoperative wound care, drains, or other daily care needs (Lahr & Elliot, 2018). Although needs are specific to individual patients and the procedures they have undergone, general patient education needs prior to discharge have been identified (see Chart 16-3).

Continuing and Transitional Care. Community-based and transitional care services are frequently necessary after surgery. Older patients, patients who live alone, patients without family support, and patients with preexisting chronic illness or disabilities are often in greatest need. Planning for discharge involves arranging for necessary services early in the acute care hospitalization for wound care, drain management, catheter care, infusion therapy, and physical or occupational therapy. The home, community-based, or transitional care nurse coordinates these activities and services.

During home visits, the nurse assesses the patient for postoperative complications by assessment of the surgical incision, respiratory and cardiovascular status, adequacy of pain management, fluid and nutritional status, and the patient's progress in returning to preoperative status. The nurse evaluates the patient's ability to administer prescribed medications, manage dressing changes, drainage systems and other devices. The nurse may change dressings or catheters if needed. The nurse identifies any additional services that are needed and assists the patient and family to arrange for them. Previous education is reinforced, and the patient is reminded to keep follow-up appointments. The patient and family are educated about signs and symptoms to be reported to the surgeon. In addition, the nurse provides information about how to obtain needed supplies and suggests resources or support groups.

Evaluation

Expected patient outcomes may include the following:

1. Maintains optimal respiratory function
   a. Performs deep-breathing exercises
   b. Displays clear breath sounds
   c. Uses incentive spirometer as prescribed
   d. Splints incisional site when coughing to reduce pain
2. Indicates that pain is decreased in intensity
3. Increases activity as prescribed
   a. Alternates periods of rest and activity
   b. Progressively increases ambulation
   c. Resumes normal activities within the prescribed time frame
   d. Performs activities related to self-care
4. Wound heals without complication
5. Maintains body temperature within normal limits
6. Resumes oral intake
   a. Reports absence of nausea and vomiting
   b. Eats at least 75% of usual diet
   c. Is free of abdominal distress and gas pains
   d. Exhibits normal bowel sounds
7. Reports resumption of usual bowel elimination pattern
8. Resumes usual voiding pattern
9. Is free of injury
10. Exhibits decreased anxiety
11. Acquires knowledge and skills necessary to manage regimen after discharge
12. Experiences no complications

CRITICAL THINKING EXERCISES

1 **ipc** A 38-year-old woman is admitted to the PACU following open abdominal surgery for excision of a benign tumor and lysis of adhesions. The patient has been a smoker for many years and begins coughing as soon as she is transferred from the OR stretcher to the bed in PACU. How will you, as the nurse receiving this patient, facilitate an interprofessional discussion to improve her care and increase her chance of a good surgical outcome? What information is essential to obtain from the OR team during handoff report?

2 **pq** A 60-year-old man with obesity and a history of diabetes is admitted to the PACU following a right shoulder repair. He received multimodal analgesia, including a peripheral nerve block, and is scheduled to be discharged home. Identify the essential information you would need reported from the OR team. What are your immediate priorities in delivering care to this patient? He is transferred to Phase II PACU. What are your priorities for discharge instructions and education for this patient?

3 **ebp** An 80-year-old man has had a right total knee replacement. The anesthesia given was a spinal anesthetic. What signs and symptoms might he exhibit as he awakens from the surgery? As the PACU nurse, what complications should you observe for as he recovers? Describe an evidence-based nursing care plan for the patient during his hospital stay.

REFERENCES

*Asterisk indicates nursing research.
**Double asterisk indicates classic reference.

Books

Ackley, B. J., & Ladwig, G. B. (2017). *Nursing diagnosis handbook: An evidence-based guide to planning care* (11th ed.). St. Louis, MO: Mosby.

American Society of PeriAnesthesia Nurses (ASPAN). (2019). *Perianesthesia nursing standards, practice recommendations and interpretive statements.* Cherry Hill, NJ.

Association of PeriOperative Registered Nurses (AORN). (2019). *Association of perioperative registered nurses (AORN) standards, recommended practice, and guidelines.* Denver, CO.

Barash, P. G., Cullen, B. F., Stoelting, R. K., et al. (2017). *Clinical anesthesia* (8th ed.). Philadelphia, PA: Lippincott Williams & Wilkins.

Comerford, K. C., & Durkin, M. T. (2020). *Nursing 2020 drug handbook.* Philadelphia, PA: Wolters Kluwer.

Dudek, S. G. (2017). *Nutrition essentials for nursing practice* (8th ed.). Philadelphia, PA: Lippincott Williams & Wilkins.

Norris, T. L. (2018). *Porth's pathophysiology: Concepts of altered health states* (10th ed.). Philadelphia, PA: Wolters Kluwer.

Odom-Forren, J. (2017). *Drain's perianesthesia nursing: A critical care approach.* St Louis, MO: Elsevier.

Rothrock, J. (2019). *Alexander's care of the patient in surgery* (16th ed.). St. Louis, MO: Elsevier.

Weber, J. R., & Kelley, J. H. (2018). *Health assessment in nursing* (6th ed.). Philadelphia, PA: Wolters Kluwer.

Journals and Electronic Documents

Alalawi, R., & Yasmeen, N. (2018). Postoperative cognitive dysfunction in the elderly: A review comparing the effects of desflurane and sevoflurane. *Journal of Perianesthesia Nursing, 33*(5), 732–740.

**Aldrete, A., & Wright, A. (1992). Revised Aldrete score for discharge. *Anesthesiology News, 18*(1), 17.

Armellino, D. (2017). Minimizing sources of airborne, aerosolized, and contact contaminants in the OR environment. *AORN Journal, 106*(6), 494–501.

Aroke, E., & Hicks, T. (2019). Pharmacogenetics of postoperative nausea and vomiting. *Journal of PeriAnesthesia Nursing, 34*(6), 1088–1105.

Asay, K., Olson, C., Donnelly, J., et al. (2019). The use of aromatherapy in postoperative nausea and vomiting: A systematic review. *Journal of PeriAnesthesia Nursing, 34*(3), 502–516.

De la Vega, J., Gilliand, C., Martinez, L., et al. (2019). Aromatherapy in the PACU (Abstract). *Journal of PeriAnesthesia Nursing, 34*(4), e51.

DeSilva, R., Seabra, T., Thomas, L., et al. (2019). "I feel fine": Fall preventative measures in the post anesthesia care unit (PACU). *Journal of PeriAnesthesia Nursing, 34*(4), e10.

Edmiston, C. E., Jr., & Spencer, M. (2014). Patient care interventions to help reduce the risk of surgical site infections. *AORN Journal, 100*(6), 590–602.

*Finch, C., Parkosewich, J. A., Perrone, D., et al. (2019). Incidence, timing, and factors associated with postoperative nausea and vomiting in the ambulatory surgery setting. *Journal of PeriAnesthesia Nursing, 34*(6), 1146–1155.

Hall, K. R., & Stanley, A. Y. (2019). Literature review: Assessment of opioid-related sedation and the Pasero Opioid Sedation Scale. *Journal of PeriAnesthesia Nursing, 34*(1), 132–142.

Henry, S. (2018). *ATLS 10th edition offers new insights into managing trauma patients. Bulletin of the American College of Surgeons:* Retrieved on 8/16/19 at: bulletin.facs.org/2018/06/atls-10th-edition-offers-new-insights-into-managing-trauma-patients/

Joint Commission. (2019). 2019 national patient safety goals. Retrieved on 5/22/2019 at: www.jointcommission.org/assets/1/6/2019_HAP_NPSGs_final2.pdf

Jungquist, C. R., Card, E., Charchaflieh, J., et al. (2018). Preventing opioid-induced respiratory depression in the hospitalized patient with obstructive sleep apnea. *Journal of PeriAnesthesia Nursing, 33*(5), 601–607.

Lahr, J., & Elliott, B. (2018). Perspectives from home care for guiding patients and families to a successful transition home after same-day surgery. *Journal of PeriAnesthesia Surgery, 33*(3), 348–352.

Ljungqvist, O., Scott, M., & Fearon, K. C. (2017). Enhanced recovery after surgery: A review. *JAMA Surgery, 152*(3), 292–298.

Montgomery, R., & McNamara, S. (2016). Multimodal pain management for enhanced recovery: Reinforcing the shift from traditional pathways through nurse-led interventions. *AORN Journal, 104*(6S), S9–S16.

Nasser, R., Kosty, J. A., Shah, S., et al. (2018). Risk factors and prevention of surgical site infections following spinal procedures. *Global Spine Journal, 8*(4), 44S–48S.

Padgette, P., & Wood, B. (2018). Conducting a surgical site infection prevention tracer. *AORN Journal, 107*(5), 580–590.

Persico, M., Miller, D., Way, C., et al. (2019). Implementation of enhanced recovery after surgery in a community hospital: An evidence-based approach. *Journal of PeriAnesthesia Nursing, 34*(1), 188–197.

Poulson, M., Coto, J., & Cooney, M. (2019). Music as a postoperative pain management intervention. *Journal of PeriAnesthesia Nursing, 34*(3), 662–666.

Tjeertes, E., Hoeks, S., Beks S., et al. (2015). Obesity—a risk factor for postoperative complications in general surgery? *BMC Anesthesiology, 112*(15), 1–7.

Thomas, J. S., Maple, I., Williams, N., et al. (2019). Preoperative risk assessment to guide prophylaxis and reduce the incidence of postoperative nausea and vomiting. *Journal of PeriAnesthesia Nursing, 34*(1), 74–85.

Wishart, S. M. (2019). Decreasing the incidence of postoperative urinary retention and incontinence with total joint replacement patients after spinal anesthesia in the postanesthesia care unit: A quality improvement project. *Journal of PeriAnesthesia Nursing, 34*(5), 1040–1046. Retrieved on 8/16/19 at: www.jopan.org/article/S1089-9472(19)30081-4/fulltext.

Wolfe, R. C. (2018). Multimodal analgesia in the perioperative setting. *Journal of PeriAnesthesia Nursing, 33*(4), 563–569.

*Wortham, T. C., Rice, A. N., Gupta, D. K., et al. (2019). Implementation of an obstructive sleep apnea protocol in the postanesthesia care unit for patients undergoing spinal fusion surgery. *Journal of PeriAnesthesia Nursing, 34*(4), 739–748.

Resources

American Academy of Ambulatory Care Nursing (AAACN), www.aaacn.org

American Society of Anesthesiologists (ASA), www.asahq.org

American Society of PeriAnesthesia Nurses (ASPAN), www.aspan.org

Association of PeriOperative Registered Nurses (AORN), www.aorn.org

Malignant Hyperthermia Association of the United States (MHAUS), www.mhaus.org

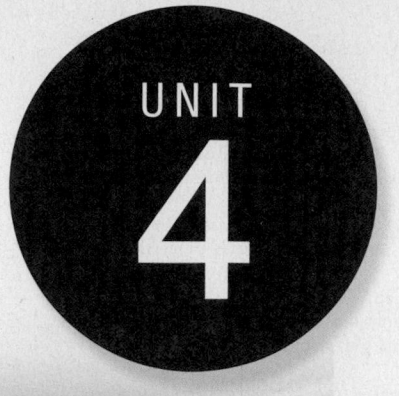

UNIT 4

Gas Exchange and Respiratory Function

PROVIDING EVIDENCE-BASED CARE FOR A PATIENT WITH COVID-19

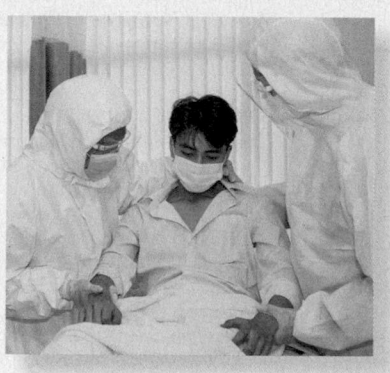

The medical unit where you work has just been designated to exclusively admit patients with coronavirus 2019 (COVID-19). A 35-year-old male admitted to the unit has a history of asthma and hypertension that are both normally well controlled with medication. His temperature is 39°C (101.4°F), he has a cough and tests positive for COVID-19. The nurse manager asks you to develop an evidence-based plan of care that can be individualized for this patient and used as a template for other patients admitted to your unit with COVID-19.

QSEN Competency Focus: Evidence-Based Practice (EBP)

The complexities inherent in today's health care system challenge nurses to demonstrate integration of specific interdisciplinary core competencies. These competencies are aimed at ensuring the delivery of safe, quality patient care (Institute of Medicine, 2003). The Quality and Safety Education for Nurses project (Cronenwett, Sherwood, Barnsteiner, et al., 2007; QSEN, 2020) provides a framework for the knowledge, skills, and attitudes (KSAs) required for nurses to demonstrate competency in these key areas, which include *patient-centered care*, *interdisciplinary teamwork and collaboration*, *evidence-based practice*, *quality improvement*, *safety*, and *informatics.*

Evidence-Based Practice Definition: Integrate best current evidence with clinical expertise and patient/family preferences and values for delivery of optimal health care.

SELECT PRE-LICENSURE KSAs	APPLICATION AND REFLECTION
Knowledge	
Differentiate clinical opinion from research and evidence summaries	Identify the pathophysiologic basis for why patients with asthma and hypertension are at higher risk for COVID-19. What is the strength of the evidence for an evidence-based plan of care for this patient?
Skills	
Locate evidence reports related to clinical practice topics and guidelines	What strategies would you use to search for and then identify appropriate evidence for developing an evidence-based plan of care for this patient? What resources might you mobilize for this patient so he can become educated on the best practices to prevent the spread of COVID-19 while he is in the hospital and upon discharge?
Attitudes	
Value the concept of EBP as integral to determining best clinical practice	Reflect on your attitudes toward using EBP for patients with COVID-19. Do you tend to think that infection is inevitable in patients with risk factors?

Cronenwett, L., Sherwood, G., Barnsteiner, J., et al. (2007). Quality and safety education for nurses. *Nursing Outlook*, *55*(3), 122–131; Institute of Medicine. (2003). *Health professions education: A bridge to quality.* Washington, DC: National Academies Press; QSEN Institute. (2020). *QSEN Competencies: Definitions and pre-licensure KSAs; Evidence based practice.* Retrieved on 8/15/2020 at: qsen.org/competencies/pre-licensure-ksas/ #evidence-based_practice

LEARNING OUTCOMES

On completion of this chapter, the learner will be able to:

1. Describe the structures and functions of the upper and lower respiratory tracts and concepts of ventilation, diffusion, perfusion, and ventilation–perfusion imbalances.
2. Explain and demonstrate proper techniques utilized to perform a comprehensive respiratory assessment.
3. Discriminate between normal and abnormal assessment findings of the respiratory system identified by inspection, palpation, percussion, and auscultation.
4. Recognize and evaluate the major symptoms of respiratory dysfunction by applying concepts from the patient's health history and physical assessment findings.
5. Identify the diagnostic tests used to evaluate respiratory function and related nursing implications.

NURSING CONCEPTS

Assessment   Oxygenation   Perfusion

GLOSSARY

apnea: temporary cessation of breathing

bronchophony: abnormal increase in clarity of transmitted voice sounds heard when auscultating the lungs

bronchoscopy: direct examination of the larynx, trachea, and bronchi using an endoscope

cilia: short, fine hairs that provide a constant whipping motion that serves to propel mucus and foreign substances away from the lung toward the larynx

compliance: measure of the force required to expand or inflate the lungs

crackles: nonmusical, discontinuous popping sounds during inspiration caused by delayed reopening of the airways heard on chest auscultation

dyspnea: subjective experience that describes an uncomfortable or painful breathing sensation when either at rest or while walking or climbing stairs; also commonly referred to as shortness of breath

egophony: abnormal change in tone of voice that is heard when auscultating the lungs

fremitus: vibrations of speech felt as tremors of the chest wall during palpation

hemoptysis: expectoration of blood from the respiratory tract

hypoxemia: decrease in arterial oxygen tension in the blood

hypoxia: decrease in oxygen supply to the tissues and cells

obstructive sleep apnea: temporary absence of breathing during sleep secondary to transient upper airway obstruction

orthopnea: shortness of breath when lying flat; relieved by sitting or standing

oxygen saturation: percentage of hemoglobin that is bound to oxygen

physiologic dead space: portion of the tracheobronchial tree that does not participate in gas exchange

pulmonary diffusion: exchange of gas molecules (oxygen and carbon dioxide) from areas of high concentration to areas of low concentration

pulmonary perfusion: blood flow through the pulmonary vasculature

respiration: gas exchange between atmospheric air and the blood and between the blood and cells of the body

rhonchi: deep, low-pitched snoring sound associated with partial airway obstruction, heard on chest auscultation

stridor: continuous, high-pitched, musical sound heard on inspiration, best heard over the neck; may be heard without use of a stethoscope, secondary to upper airway obstruction

tachypnea: abnormally rapid respirations

tidal volume: volume of air inspired and expired with each breath during normal breathing

ventilation: movement of air in and out of the airways

wheezes: continuous musical sounds associated with airway narrowing or partial obstruction

whispered pectoriloquy: whispered sounds heard loudly and clearly upon thoracic auscultation

Disorders of the respiratory system are common and are encountered by nurses in every setting, from the community to the intensive care unit. Expert assessment skills must be developed and used to provide the best care for patients with acute and chronic respiratory problems. Alterations in respiratory status have been identified as important predictors of clinical deterioration in hospitalized patients (Institute for Healthcare Improvement [IHI], 2019). To differentiate between normal and abnormal assessment findings and recognize subtle changes that may negatively impact patient outcomes, nurses require an understanding of respiratory function and the significance of abnormal diagnostic test results.

Anatomic and Physiologic Overview

The respiratory system is composed of the upper and lower respiratory tracts. Together, the two tracts are responsible for **ventilation** (movement of air in and out of the airways). The upper respiratory tract, known as the upper airway, warms and filters inspired air so that the lower respiratory tract (the lungs) can accomplish gas exchange or diffusion. Gas exchange involves delivering oxygen to the tissues through the bloodstream and expelling waste gases, such as carbon dioxide, during expiration. The respiratory system depends on the cardiovascular system for perfusion, or blood flow through the pulmonary system (Norris, 2019).

Anatomy of the Respiratory System

Upper Respiratory Tract

Upper airway structures consist of the nose; paranasal sinuses; pharynx, tonsils, and adenoids; larynx; and trachea.

Nose

The nose serves as a passageway for air to pass to and from the lungs. It filters impurities and humidifies and warms the air as it is inhaled. The nose is composed of an external and an internal portion. The external portion protrudes from the face and is supported by the nasal bones and cartilage. The anterior nares (nostrils) are the external openings of the nasal cavities.

The internal portion of the nose is a hollow cavity separated into the right and left nasal cavities by a narrow vertical divider, the septum. Each nasal cavity is divided into three passageways by the projection of the turbinates from the lateral walls. The turbinate bones are also called *conchae* (the name suggested by their shell-like appearance). Because of their curves, these bones increase the mucous membrane surface of the nasal passages and slightly obstruct the air flowing through them (Fig. 17-1).

Air entering the nostrils is deflected upward to the roof of the nose, and it follows a circuitous route before it reaches the nasopharynx. It comes into contact with a large surface of moist, warm, highly vascular, ciliated mucous membrane (called *nasal mucosa*) that traps practically all of the dust and organisms in the inhaled air. The air is moistened, warmed to body temperature, and brought into contact with sensitive nerves. Some of these nerves detect odors; others provoke sneezing to expel irritating dust. Mucus, secreted continuously by goblet cells, covers the surface of the nasal mucosa and is moved back to the nasopharynx by the action of the **cilia** (short, fine hairs).

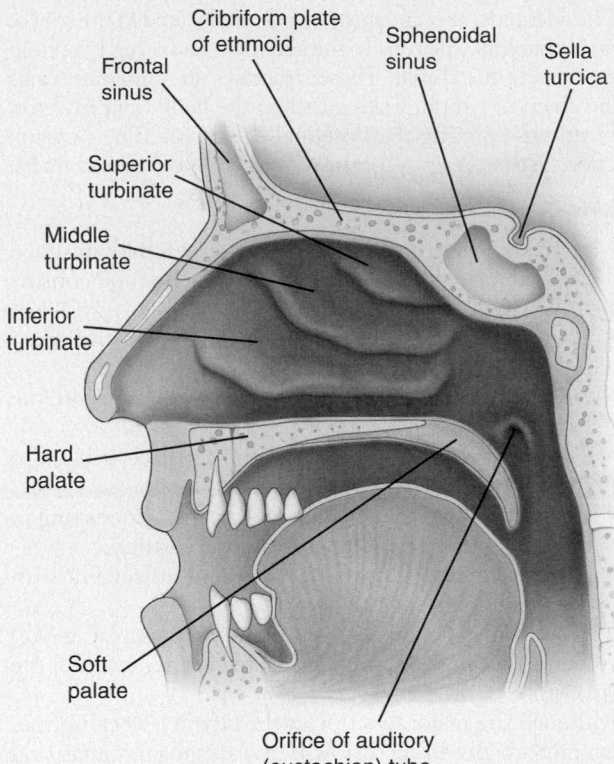

Figure 17-1 • Cross-section of nasal cavity.

Paranasal Sinuses

The paranasal sinuses include four pairs of bony cavities that are lined with nasal mucosa and ciliated pseudostratified columnar epithelium. These airspaces are connected by a series of ducts that drain into the nasal cavity. The sinuses are named by their location: frontal, ethmoid, sphenoid, and maxillary (Fig. 17-2). A prominent function of the sinuses is to serve as a resonating chamber in speech. The sinuses are a common site of infection.

Pharynx, Tonsils, and Adenoids

The pharynx, or throat, is a tubelike structure that connects the nasal and oral cavities to the larynx. It is divided into three regions: nasal, oral, and laryngeal. The nasopharynx is located posterior to the nose and above the soft palate. The oropharynx houses the faucial, or palatine, tonsils. The laryngopharynx extends from the hyoid bone to the cricoid cartilage. The epiglottis forms the entrance to the larynx.

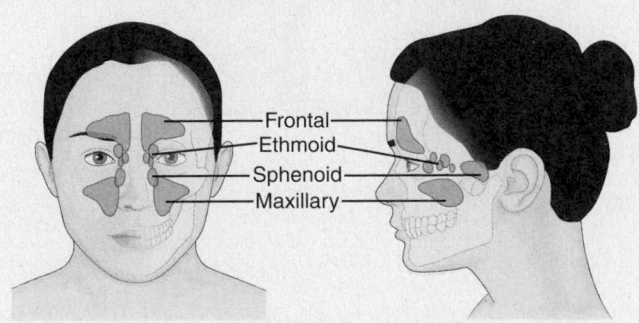

Figure 17-2 • The paranasal sinuses.

The adenoids, or pharyngeal tonsils, are located in the roof of the nasopharynx. The tonsils, the adenoids, and other lymphoid tissue encircle the throat. These structures are important links in the chain of lymph nodes guarding the body from invasion by organisms entering the nose and the throat. The pharynx functions as a passageway for the respiratory and digestive tracts.

Larynx

The larynx, or voice box, is a cartilaginous epithelium-lined organ that connects the pharynx and the trachea and consists of the following:

- *Epiglottis:* a valve flap of cartilage that covers the opening to the larynx during swallowing
- *Glottis:* the opening between the vocal cords in the larynx
- *Thyroid cartilage:* the largest of the cartilage structures; part of it forms the Adam's apple
- *Cricoid cartilage:* the only complete cartilaginous ring in the larynx (located below the thyroid cartilage)
- *Arytenoid cartilages:* used in vocal cord movement with the thyroid cartilage
- *Vocal cords:* ligaments controlled by muscular movements that produce sounds; located in the lumen of the larynx

Although the major function of the larynx is vocalization, it also protects the lower airway from foreign substances and facilitates coughing; it is, therefore, sometimes referred to as the "watchdog of the lungs" (Norris, 2019).

Trachea

The trachea, or windpipe, is composed of smooth muscle with C-shaped rings of cartilage at regular intervals. The cartilaginous rings are incomplete on the posterior surface and give firmness to the wall of the trachea, preventing it from collapsing. The trachea serves as the passage between the larynx and the right and left main stem bronchi, which enter the lungs through an opening called the *hilus.*

Lower Respiratory Tract

The lower respiratory tract consists of the lungs, which contain the bronchial and alveolar structures needed for gas exchange.

Lungs

The lungs are paired elastic structures enclosed in the thoracic cage, which is an airtight chamber with distensible walls (Fig. 17-3). Each lung is divided into lobes. The right lung has upper, middle, and lower lobes, whereas the left lung consists of upper and lower lobes (Fig. 17-4). Each lobe is further subdivided into two to five segments separated by fissures, which are extensions of the pleura.

Pleura

The lungs and wall of the thoracic cavity are lined with a serous membrane called the *pleura.* The visceral pleura covers the lungs; the parietal pleura lines the thoracic cavity, lateral wall of the mediastinum, diaphragm, and inner aspects of the

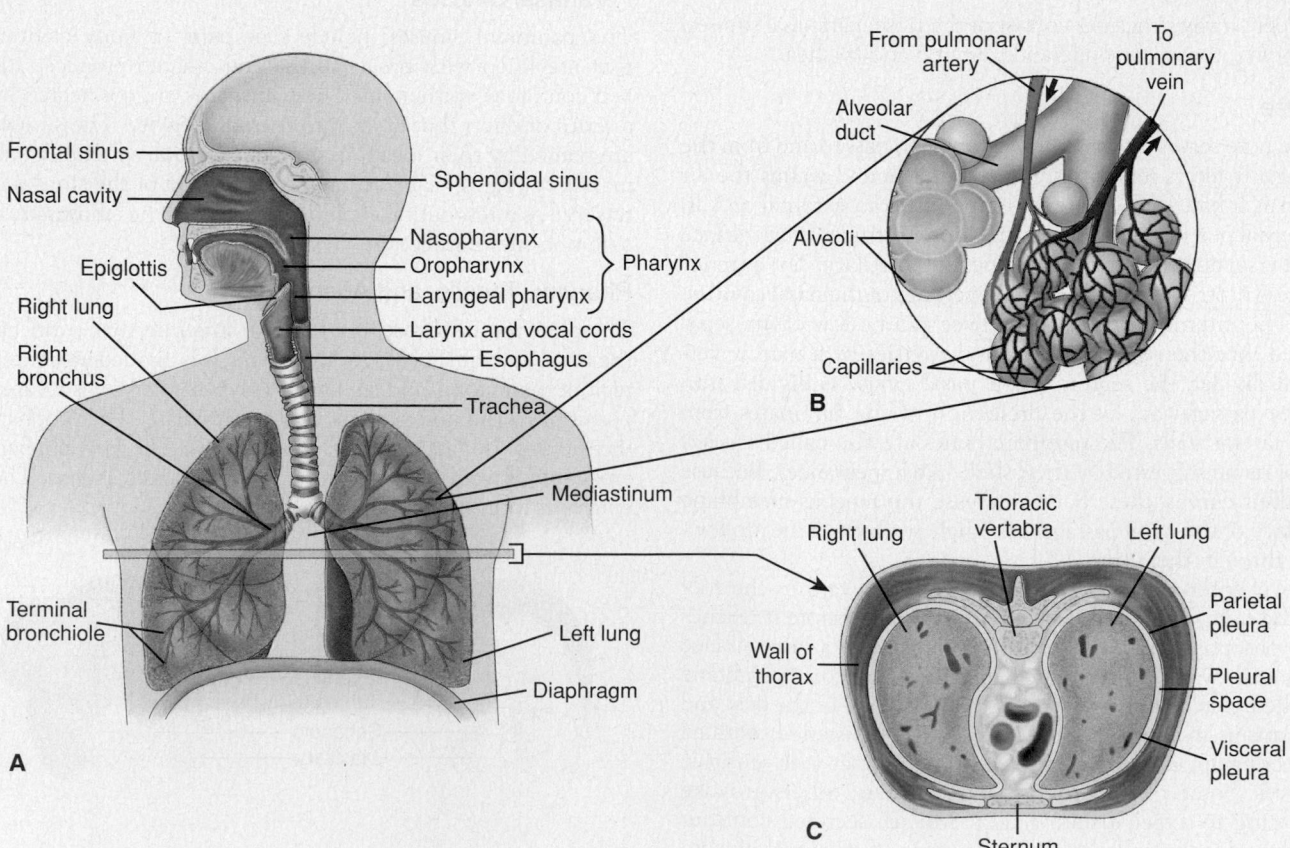

Figure 17-3 • The respiratory system. A. Upper respiratory structures and the structures of the thorax. **B.** Alveoli. **C.** A horizontal cross-section of the lungs.

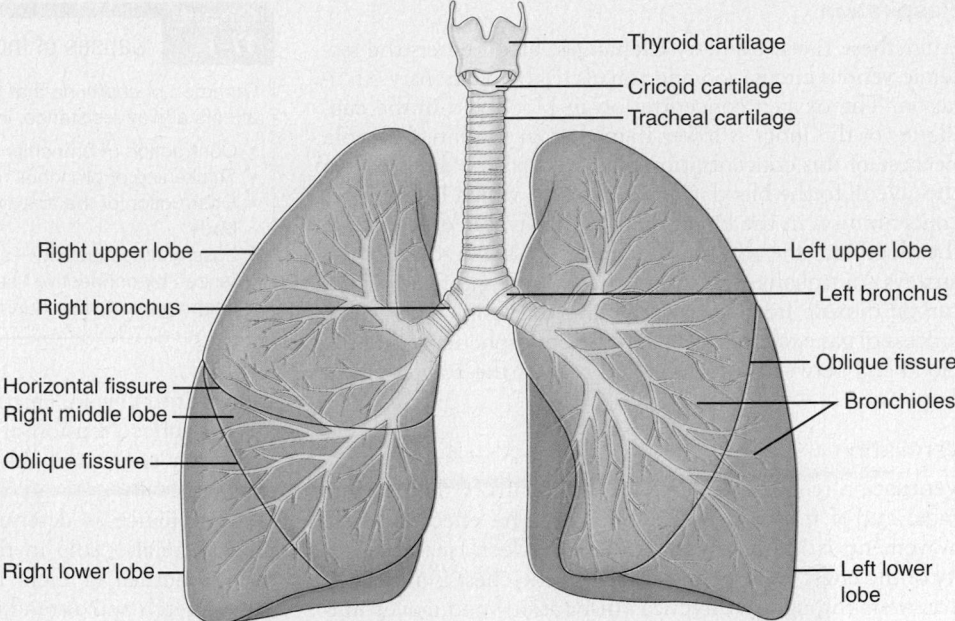

Figure 17-4 • Anterior view of the lungs. The lungs consist of five lobes. The right lung has three lobes (upper, middle, lower); the left has two (upper and lower). The lobes are further subdivided by fissures. The bronchial tree, another lung structure, inflates with air to fill the lobes.

Labels on figure: Thyroid cartilage; Cricoid cartilage; Tracheal cartilage; Right upper lobe; Left upper lobe; Right bronchus; Left bronchus; Oblique fissure; Bronchioles; Horizontal fissure; Right middle lobe; Oblique fissure; Right lower lobe; Left lower lobe

ribs. The visceral and parietal pleura and the small amount of pleural fluid between these two membranes serve to lubricate the thorax and the lungs and permit smooth motion of the lungs within the thoracic cavity during inspiration and expiration.

Mediastinum

The mediastinum is in the middle of the thorax, between the pleural sacs that contain the two lungs. It extends from the sternum to the vertebral column and contains all of the thoracic tissue outside the lungs (heart, thymus, the aorta and vena cava, and esophagus).

Bronchi and Bronchioles

There are several divisions of the bronchi within each lobe of the lung. First are the lobar bronchi (three in the right lung and two in the left lung). Lobar bronchi divide into segmental bronchi (10 on the right and 8 on the left); these structures facilitate effective postural drainage in the patient. Segmental bronchi then divide into subsegmental bronchi. These bronchi are surrounded by connective tissue that contains arteries, lymphatics, and nerves.

The subsegmental bronchi then branch into bronchioles, which have no cartilage in their walls. Their patency depends entirely on the elastic recoil of the surrounding smooth muscle and on the alveolar pressure. The bronchioles contain submucosal glands, which produce mucus that covers the inside lining of the airways. The bronchi and bronchioles are also lined with cells that have surfaces covered with cilia. These cilia create a constant whipping motion that propels mucus and foreign substances away from the lungs toward the larynx.

The bronchioles branch into terminal bronchioles, which do not have mucous glands or cilia. Terminal bronchioles become respiratory bronchioles, which are considered to be the transitional passageways between the conducting airways and the gas exchange airways. Up to this point, the conducting airways contain about 150 mL of air in the tracheobronchial tree that does not participate in gas exchange, known as **physiologic**

dead space. The respiratory bronchioles then lead into alveolar ducts and sacs and then alveoli (see Fig. 17-3). Oxygen and carbon dioxide exchange takes place in the alveoli.

Alveoli

The lung is made up of about 300 million alveoli, constituting a total surface area between 50 and 100 m² (Norris, 2019). There are three types of alveolar cells. Type I and type II cells make up the alveolar epithelium. Type I cells account for 95% of the alveolar surface area and serve as a barrier between the air and the alveolar surface; type II cells account for only 5% of this area but are responsible for producing type I cells and surfactant. Surfactant reduces surface tension, thereby improving overall lung function. Alveolar macrophages, the third type of alveolar cells, are phagocytic cells that ingest foreign matter and, as a result, provide an important defense mechanism.

Function of the Respiratory System

The cells of the body derive the energy they need from the oxidation of carbohydrates, fats, and proteins. This process requires oxygen. Vital tissues, like the brain and the heart, cannot survive long without a continuous supply of oxygen. As a result of oxidation, carbon dioxide is produced and must be removed from the cells to prevent the buildup of acid waste products. The respiratory system performs this function by facilitating life-sustaining processes such as oxygen transport, respiration, ventilation, and gas exchange.

Oxygen Transport

Oxygen is supplied to, and carbon dioxide is removed from, cells by way of the circulating blood through the thin walls of the capillaries. Oxygen diffuses from the capillary through the capillary wall to the interstitial fluid. At this point, it diffuses through the membrane of tissue cells, where it is used by mitochondria for cellular respiration. The movement of carbon dioxide occurs by diffusion in the opposite direction—from cell to blood.

Respiration

After these tissue capillary exchanges, blood enters the systemic venous circulation and travels to the pulmonary circulation. The oxygen concentration in blood within the capillaries of the lungs is lower than that in the lungs' alveoli. Because of this concentration gradient, oxygen diffuses from the alveoli to the blood. Carbon dioxide, which has a higher concentration in the blood than in the alveoli, diffuses from the blood into the alveoli. Movement of air in and out of the airways continually replenishes the oxygen and removes the carbon dioxide from the airways and the lungs. This whole process of gas exchange between the atmospheric air and the blood and between the blood and cells of the body is called **respiration**.

Ventilation

Ventilation requires movement of the walls of the thoracic cage and of its floor, the diaphragm. The effect of these movements is alternately to increase and decrease the capacity of the chest. When the capacity of the chest is increased, air enters through the trachea (inspiration) and moves into the bronchi, bronchioles, and alveoli, and inflates the lungs. When the chest wall and the diaphragm return to their previous positions (expiration), the lungs recoil and force the air out through the bronchi and the trachea. Inspiration occurs during the first third of the respiratory cycle; expiration occurs during the latter two thirds. The inspiratory phase of respiration normally requires energy; the expiratory phase is normally passive, requiring very little energy. Physical factors that govern airflow in and out of the lungs are collectively referred to as the mechanics of ventilation and include air pressure variances, resistance to airflow, and lung compliance.

Air Pressure Variances

Air flows from a region of higher pressure to a region of lower pressure. During inspiration, movements of the diaphragm and intercostal muscles enlarge the thoracic cavity and thereby lower the pressure inside the thorax to a level below that of atmospheric pressure. As a result, air is drawn through the trachea and the bronchi into the alveoli. During expiration, the diaphragm relaxes and the lungs recoil, resulting in a decrease in the size of the thoracic cavity. The alveolar pressure then exceeds atmospheric pressure, and air flows from the lungs into the atmosphere.

Airway Resistance

Resistance is determined by the radius, or size of the airway through which the air is flowing, as well as by lung volumes and airflow velocity. Any process that changes the bronchial diameter or width affects airway resistance and alters the rate of airflow for a given pressure gradient during respiration (Chart 17-1). With increased resistance, greater-than-normal respiratory effort is required to achieve normal levels of ventilation.

Compliance

Compliance is the elasticity and expandability of the lungs and thoracic structures. Compliance allows the lung volume to increase when the difference in pressure between the atmosphere and the thoracic cavity (pressure gradient)

Chart 17-1 **Causes of Increased Airway Resistance**

Common phenomena that may alter bronchial diameter, which affects airway resistance, include the following:

- Contraction of bronchial smooth muscle—as in asthma
- Thickening of bronchial mucosa—as in chronic bronchitis
- Obstruction of the airway—by mucus, a tumor, or a foreign body
- Loss of lung elasticity—as in emphysema, which is characterized by connective tissue encircling the airways, thereby keeping them open during both inspiration and expiration

---

causes air to flow in. Factors that determine lung compliance are the surface tension of the alveoli, the connective tissue and water content of the lungs, and the compliance of the thoracic cavity.

Compliance is determined by examining the volume–pressure relationship in the lungs and the thorax. Compliance is normal (1 L/cm H_2O) if the lungs and the thorax easily stretch and distend when pressure is applied. Increased compliance occurs if the lungs have lost their elastic recoil and become overdistended (e.g., in emphysema). Decreased compliance occurs if the lungs and the thorax are "stiff." Conditions associated with decreased compliance include severe obesity, pneumothorax, hemothorax, pleural effusion, pulmonary edema, atelectasis, pulmonary fibrosis, and acute respiratory distress syndrome (ARDS). Lungs with decreased compliance require greater-than-normal energy expenditure by the patient to achieve normal levels of ventilation.

Lung Volumes and Capacities

Lung function, which reflects the mechanics of ventilation, is viewed in terms of lung volumes and lung capacities. Lung volumes are categorized as tidal volume, inspiratory reserve volume, expiratory reserve volume, and residual volume. Lung capacity is evaluated in terms of vital capacity, inspiratory capacity, functional residual capacity, and total lung capacity. These terms are explained in Table 17-1.

Pulmonary Diffusion and Perfusion

Pulmonary diffusion is the process by which oxygen and carbon dioxide are exchanged from areas of high concentration to areas of low concentration at the air–blood interface. The alveolar–capillary membrane is ideal for diffusion because of its thinness and large surface area. In the normal healthy adult, oxygen and carbon dioxide travel across the alveolar–capillary membrane without difficulty as a result of differences in gas concentrations in the alveoli and capillaries.

Pulmonary perfusion is the actual blood flow through the pulmonary vasculature. The blood is pumped into the lungs by the right ventricle through the pulmonary artery. The pulmonary artery divides into the right and left branches to supply both lungs. Normally, about 2% of the blood pumped by the right ventricle does not perfuse the alveolar capillaries. This shunted blood drains into the left side of the heart without participating in alveolar gas exchange. Bronchial arteries extending from the thoracic aorta also support perfusion but do not participate in gas exchange, further diluting oxygenated blood exiting through the pulmonary vein (Norris, 2019).

TABLE 17-1	Lung Volumes and Lung Capacities			
Term	Symbol	Description	Normal Value[a]	Significance
Lung Volumes				
Tidal volume	VT or TV	The volume of air inhaled and exhaled with each breath	500 mL or 5–10 mL/kg	The tidal volume may not vary, even with severe disease.
Inspiratory reserve volume	IRV	The maximum volume of air that can be inhaled after a normal inhalation	3000 mL	
Expiratory reserve volume	ERV	The maximum volume of air that can be exhaled forcibly after a normal exhalation	1100 mL	Expiratory reserve volume is decreased with restrictive conditions, such as obesity, ascites, pregnancy.
Residual volume	RV	The volume of air remaining in the lungs after a maximum exhalation	1200 mL	Residual volume may be increased with obstructive disease.
Lung Capacities				
Vital capacity	VC	The maximum volume of air exhaled from the point of maximum inspiration: VC = TV + IRV + ERV	4600 mL	A decrease in vital capacity may be found in neuromuscular disease, generalized fatigue, atelectasis, pulmonary edema, COPD, and obesity.
Inspiratory capacity	IC	The maximum volume of air inhaled after normal expiration: IC = TV + IRV	3500 mL	A decrease in inspiratory capacity may indicate restrictive disease. It may also be decreased in obesity.
Functional residual capacity	FRC	The volume of air remaining in the lungs after a normal expiration: FRC = ERV + RV	2300 mL	Functional residual capacity may be increased with COPD and decreased in ARDS and obesity.
Total lung capacity	TLC	The volume of air in the lungs after a maximum inspiration TLC = TV + IRV + ERV + RV	5800 mL	Total lung capacity may be decreased with restrictive disease such as atelectasis and pneumonia and increased in COPD.

[a]Values for healthy men; women are 20–25% less.
ARDS, acute respiratory distress syndrome; COPD, chronic obstructive pulmonary disease.
Adapted from West, J. B., & Luks, A. M. (2016). *West's respiratory physiology: The essentials* (10th ed.). Philadelphia, PA: Wolters Kluwer Health Lippincott Williams & Wilkins.

The pulmonary circulation is considered a low-pressure system because the systolic blood pressure in the pulmonary artery is 20 to 30 mm Hg and the diastolic pressure is 5 to 15 mm Hg. Because of these low pressures, the pulmonary vasculature normally can vary its capacity to accommodate the blood flow it receives. However, when a person is in an upright position, the pulmonary artery pressure is not great enough to supply blood to the apex of the lung against the force of gravity. Thus, when a person is upright, the lung may be considered to be divided into three sections: an upper part with poor blood supply, a lower part with maximal blood supply, and a section between the two with an intermediate supply of blood. When a person who is lying down turns to one side, more blood passes to the dependent lung.

Perfusion is also influenced by alveolar pressure. The pulmonary capillaries are sandwiched between adjacent alveoli. If the alveolar pressure is sufficiently high, the capillaries are squeezed. Depending on the pressure, some capillaries completely collapse, whereas others narrow.

Pulmonary artery pressure, gravity, and alveolar pressure determine the patterns of perfusion. In lung disease, these factors vary, and the perfusion of the lung may become abnormal.

Ventilation and Perfusion Balance and Imbalance

Adequate gas exchange depends on an adequate ventilation–perfusion ($\dot{V}/\dot{Q}$) ratio. In different areas of the lung, the $\dot{V}/\dot{Q}$ ratio varies. Airway blockages, local changes in compliance, and gravity may alter ventilation. Alterations in perfusion may occur with a change in the pulmonary artery pressure, alveolar pressure, or gravity.

$\dot{V}/\dot{Q}$ imbalance occurs as a result of inadequate ventilation, inadequate perfusion, or both. There are four possible $\dot{V}/\dot{Q}$ states in the lung: normal $\dot{V}/\dot{Q}$ ratio, low $\dot{V}/\dot{Q}$ ratio (shunt), high $\dot{V}/\dot{Q}$ ratio (dead space), and absence of ventilation and perfusion (silent unit) (Chart 17-2). $\dot{V}/\dot{Q}$ imbalance causes shunting of blood, resulting in **hypoxia** (low level of cellular oxygen). Shunting appears to be the main cause of hypoxia after thoracic or abdominal surgery and most types of respiratory failure. Severe hypoxia results when the amount of shunting exceeds 20%. Supplemental oxygen may eliminate hypoxia, depending on the type of $\dot{V}/\dot{Q}$ imbalance.

Gas Exchange

Partial Pressure of Gases

The air we breathe is a gaseous mixture consisting mainly of nitrogen (78%), oxygen (21%), argon (1%), and trace amounts of other gases including carbon dioxide, methane, and helium, among other gases. The atmospheric pressure at sea level is about 760 mm Hg. Partial pressure is the pressure exerted by each type of gas in a mixture of gases. The partial pressure of a gas is proportional to the concentration of that gas in the mixture. The total pressure exerted by the gaseous mixture, whether in the atmosphere or in the lungs, is equal to the sum of the partial pressures. The partial pressure of nitrogen is approximately 596 mm Hg, oxygen is 152 mm Hg, and argon is 7.6 mm Hg. Chart 17-3 identifies and defines terms and abbreviations related to partial pressure of gases. However, the partial pressure of gases will be affected when the air is inhaled and humidified by the pulmonary tract. It is

Chart 17-2 Ventilation–Perfusion Ratios

Normal Ratio (A)

In the healthy lung, a given amount of blood passes an alveolus and is matched with an equal amount of gas **(A)**. The ratio is 1:1 (ventilation matches perfusion).

Low Ventilation–Perfusion Ratio: Shunts (B)

Low ventilation–perfusion states may be called *shunt-producing disorders*. When perfusion exceeds ventilation, a shunt exists **(B)**. Blood bypasses the alveoli without gas exchange occurring. This is seen with obstruction of the distal airways, such as with pneumonia, atelectasis, tumor, or a mucus plug.

High Ventilation–Perfusion Ratio: Dead Space (C)

When ventilation exceeds perfusion, dead space results **(C)**. The alveoli do not have an adequate blood supply for gas exchange to occur. This is characteristic of a variety of disorders, including pulmonary emboli, pulmonary infarction, and cardiogenic shock.

Silent Unit (D)

In the absence of both ventilation and perfusion or with limited ventilation and perfusion, a condition known as a silent unit occurs **(D)**. This is seen with pneumothorax and severe acute respiratory distress syndrome.

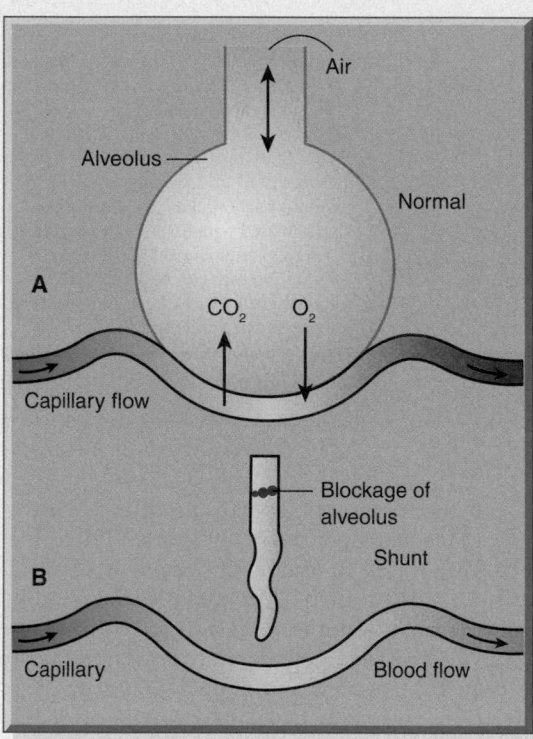

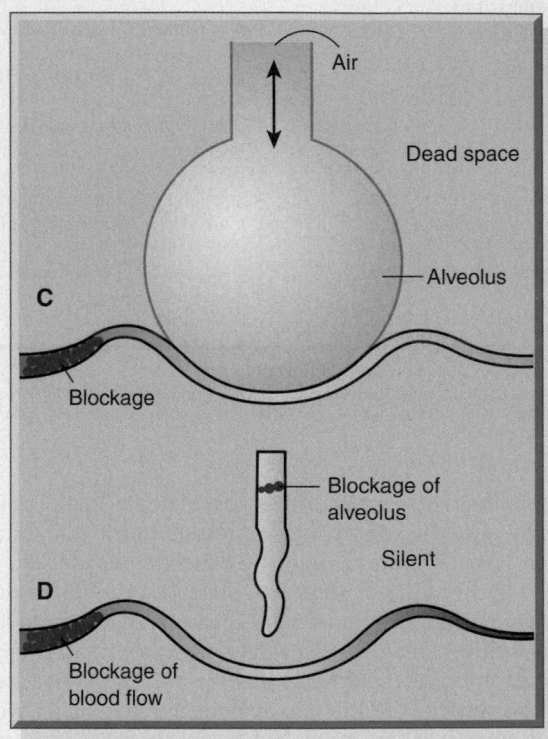

possible to calculate the partial pressure of gases, specifically oxygen, within the alveoli.

Once the air enters the trachea, it becomes fully saturated with water vapor, which displaces some of the other gases. Water vapor exerts a pressure of 45 mm Hg when it fully saturates a mixture of gases at the body temperature of 37°C (98.6°F). Nitrogen and oxygen are responsible for almost all of the remaining 715 mm Hg pressure. Once this mixture enters the alveoli, it is further diluted by carbon dioxide. In the alveoli, the water vapor continues to exert a pressure of 45 mm Hg. Under typical baseline conditions (i.e., without supplemental oxygen and at sea level), the partial pressure of alveolar oxygen (PAO_2) is approximately 100 mm Hg. This pressure ensures diffusion of oxygen across the alveolar–capillary membranes, and then eventually into the arterial blood and to red blood cells for transport to meet systemic oxygenation needs (Sharma, Hashmi, & Rawat, 2019).

When a gas is exposed to a liquid, the gas dissolves in the liquid until equilibrium is reached. The dissolved gas also exerts a partial pressure. At equilibrium, the partial pressure of the gas in the liquid is the same as the partial pressure of the gas in the gaseous mixture. Oxygenation of venous blood in the lung illustrates this point. In the lung, venous blood and alveolar oxygen are separated by a very thin alveolar membrane. Oxygen diffuses across this membrane to dissolve in the blood until

Chart 17-3 Partial Pressure Abbreviations

P = Pressure
PO_2 = Partial pressure of oxygen
PCO_2 = Partial pressure of carbon dioxide
PAO_2 = Partial pressure of alveolar oxygen
$PACO_2$ = Partial pressure of alveolar carbon dioxide
PaO_2 = Partial pressure of arterial oxygen
$PaCO_2$ = Partial pressure of arterial carbon dioxide
PvO_2 = Partial pressure of venous oxygen
$PvCO_2$ = Partial pressure of venous carbon dioxide
P_{50} = Partial pressure of oxygen when the hemoglobin is 50% saturated

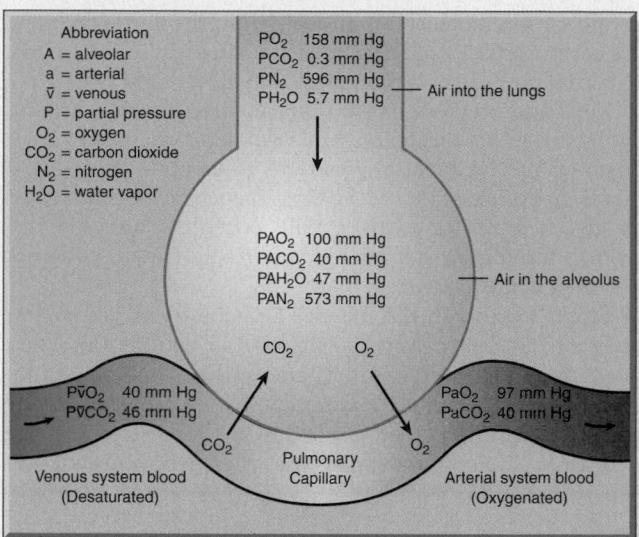

Figure 17-5 • Changes occur in the partial pressure of gases during respiration. These values vary as a result of the exchange of oxygen and carbon dioxide and the changes that occur in their partial pressures as venous blood flows through the lungs.

the partial pressure of oxygen in the blood is the same as that in the alveoli. However, because carbon dioxide is a by-product of oxidation in the cells, venous blood contains carbon dioxide at a higher partial pressure than that in the alveolar gas. In the lung, carbon dioxide diffuses out of venous blood into the alveolar gas. At equilibrium, the partial pressure of carbon dioxide in the blood and in alveolar gas is the same. The changes in partial pressure are shown in Figure 17-5.

Effects of Pressure on Oxygen Transport

Oxygen and carbon dioxide are transported simultaneously, either dissolved in blood or combined with hemoglobin in red blood cells. Each 100 mL of normal arterial blood carries 0.3 mL of oxygen physically dissolved in the plasma and 20 mL of oxygen in combination with hemoglobin. Large amounts of oxygen can be transported in the blood because oxygen combines easily with hemoglobin to form oxyhemoglobin:

$$O_2 + Hgb \leftrightarrow HgbO_2$$

The volume of oxygen physically dissolved in the plasma is measured by the partial pressure of oxygen in the arteries (PaO_2). The higher the PaO_2, the greater the amount of oxygen dissolved. For example, at a PaO_2 of 10 mm Hg, 0.03 mL of oxygen is dissolved in 100 mL of plasma. At PaO_2 of 20 mm Hg, twice this amount is dissolved in plasma, and at PaO_2 of 100 mm Hg, 10 times this amount is dissolved. Therefore, the amount of dissolved oxygen is directly proportional to the partial pressure, regardless of how high the oxygen pressure becomes.

The amount of oxygen that combines with hemoglobin depends on both the amount of hemoglobin in the blood and on PaO_2, although only up to a PaO_2 of about 150 mm Hg. This is measured as **oxygen saturation** (SaO_2), the percentage of the O_2 that could be carried if all the hemoglobin held the maximum possible amount of O_2. When the PaO_2 is 150 mm Hg, hemoglobin is 100% saturated and does not combine with any additional oxygen. When hemoglobin is 100%

saturated, 1 g of hemoglobin combines with 1.34 mL of oxygen. Therefore, in a person with 14 g/dL of hemoglobin, each 100 mL of blood contains about 19 mL of oxygen associated with hemoglobin. If the PaO_2 is less than 150 mm Hg, the percentage of hemoglobin saturated with oxygen decreases. For example, at a PaO_2 of 100 mm Hg (normal value), saturation is 97%; at a PaO_2 of 40 mm Hg, saturation is 70%.

Oxyhemoglobin Dissociation Curve

The oxyhemoglobin dissociation curve (Chart 17-4) shows the relationship between the partial pressure of oxygen (PaO_2) and the percentage of saturation of oxygen (SaO_2). The percentage of saturation can be affected by carbon dioxide, hydrogen ion concentration, temperature, and 2,3-diphosphoglycerate. An increase in these factors shifts the curve to the right, thus less oxygen is picked up in the lungs, but more oxygen is released to the tissues, if PaO_2 is unchanged. A decrease in these factors causes the curve to shift to the left, making the bond between oxygen and hemoglobin stronger. If the PaO_2 is still unchanged, more oxygen is picked up in the lungs, but less oxygen is given up to the tissues. The unusual shape of the oxyhemoglobin dissociation curve is a distinct advantage to the patient for two reasons:

1. If the PaO_2 decreases from 100 to 80 mm Hg as a result of lung disease or heart disease, the hemoglobin of the arterial blood remains almost maximally saturated (94%), and the tissues do not suffer from hypoxia.

Chart 17-4 **Oxyhemoglobin Dissociation Curve**

The oxyhemoglobin dissociation curve is marked to show three oxygen levels:

1. Normal levels—PaO_2 >70 mm Hg
2. Relatively safe levels—PaO_2 45–70 mm Hg
3. Dangerous levels—PaO_2 <40 mm Hg

The normal (middle) curve (N) shows that 75% saturation occurs at a PaO_2 of 40 mm Hg. If the curve shifts to the right (R), the same saturation (75%) occurs at the higher PaO_2 of 57 mm Hg. If the curve shifts to the left (L), 75% saturation occurs at a PaO_2 of 25 mm Hg.

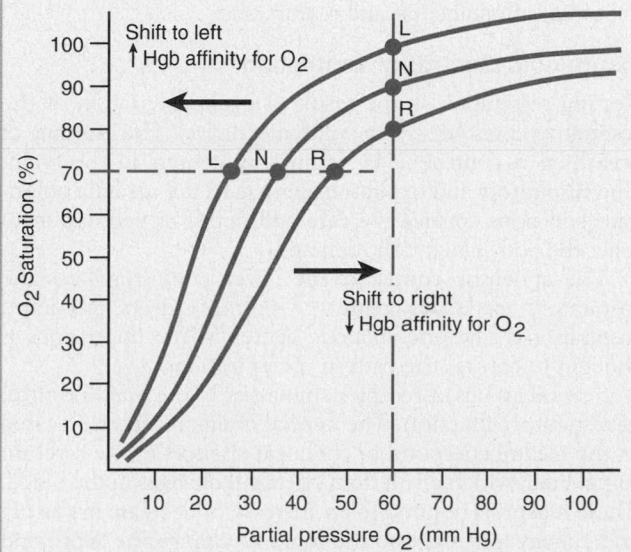

2. When the arterial blood passes into tissue capillaries and is exposed to the tissue tension of oxygen (about 40 mm Hg), hemoglobin gives up large quantities of oxygen for use by the tissues.

With a normal value for PaO_2 (80 to 100 mm Hg) and SaO_2 (95% to 98%), there is a 15% margin of excess oxygen available to the tissues. With a normal hemoglobin level of 15 mg/dL and a PaO_2 level of 40 mm Hg (SaO_2 75%), there is adequate oxygen available for the tissues but no reserve for physiologic stresses that increase tissue oxygen demand. If a serious incident occurs (e.g., bronchospasm, aspiration, hypotension, or cardiac arrhythmias) that reduces the intake of oxygen from the lungs, tissue hypoxia results.

An important consideration in the transport of oxygen is cardiac output, which determines the amount of oxygen delivered to the body and affects lung and tissue perfusion. If the cardiac output is normal (5 L/min), the amount of oxygen delivered to the body per minute is normal. Under normal conditions, only 250 mL of oxygen is used per minute, which is approximately 25% of available oxygen. The rest of the oxygen returns to the right side of the heart, and the PaO_2 of venous blood drops from 80 to 100 mm Hg to about 40 mm Hg. If cardiac output falls, however, the amount of oxygen delivered to the tissues also falls and may be inadequate to meet the body's needs.

Carbon Dioxide Transport

At the same time that oxygen diffuses from the blood into the tissues, carbon dioxide diffuses from tissue cells to blood and is transported to the lungs for excretion. The amount of carbon dioxide in transit is one of the major determinants of the acid–base balance of the body. Normally, only 6% of the venous carbon dioxide is removed in the lungs and enough remains in the arterial blood to exert a pressure of 40 mm Hg. Most of the carbon dioxide (90%) is carried by red blood cells; the small portion (5%) that remains dissolved in the plasma (partial pressure of carbon dioxide [PCO_2]) is the critical factor that determines carbon dioxide movement in or out of the blood.

Although the many processes involved in respiratory gas transport seem to occur in intermittent stages, the changes are rapid, simultaneous, and continuous.

Neurologic Control of Ventilation

Resting respiration is the result of cyclic excitation of the respiratory muscles by the phrenic nerve. The rhythm of breathing is controlled by respiratory centers in the brain. The inspiratory and expiratory centers in the medulla oblongata and pons control the rate and depth of ventilation to meet the body's metabolic demands.

The apneustic center in the lower pons stimulates the inspiratory medullary center to promote deep, prolonged inspirations. The pneumotaxic center in the upper pons is thought to control the pattern of respirations.

Several groups of receptor sites assist in the brain's control of respiratory function. The central chemoreceptors, located in the medulla, respond to chemical changes in the cerebrospinal fluid, which result from chemical changes in the blood. These receptors respond to an increase or decrease in the pH and convey a message to the lungs to change the depth and then the rate of ventilation to correct the imbalance. The peripheral chemoreceptors are located in the aortic arch and the carotid arteries and respond first to changes in PaO_2, then to partial pressure of carbon dioxide ($PaCO_2$) and pH.

Mechanoreceptors in the lung include stretch, irritant, and juxtacapillary receptors, and respond to changes in resistance by altering breathing patterns to support optimal lung function. For example, the Hering–Breuer reflex is activated by stretch receptors in the alveoli. When the lungs are distended, inspiration is inhibited; as a result, the lungs do not become overdistended.

Proprioceptors in the muscles and chest wall respond to body movements, causing an increase in ventilation. Thus, range-of-motion exercises in a patient who is immobile stimulate breathing. Finally, baroreceptors, also located in the aortic and carotid bodies, respond to an increase or decrease in arterial blood pressure and cause reflex hypoventilation or hyperventilation.

 Gerontologic Considerations

A gradual decline in respiratory function begins in early to middle adulthood and affects the structure and function of the respiratory system. The vital capacity of the lungs and the strength of the respiratory muscles peak between 20 and 25 years of age and decrease thereafter. With aging (40 years and older), changes occur in the alveoli that reduce the surface area available for the exchange of oxygen and carbon dioxide. At approximately 50 years of age, the alveoli begin to lose elasticity. A decrease in vital capacity occurs with the loss of chest wall mobility, which restricts the tidal flow of air. The amount of respiratory dead space increases with age. These changes result in a decreased diffusion capacity for oxygen with increasing age, producing lower oxygen levels in the arterial circulation. Older adults have a decreased ability to rapidly move air in and out of the lungs.

Gerontologic changes in the respiratory system are summarized in Table 17-2. Despite these changes, in the absence of chronic pulmonary disease, older adults are able to carry out activities of daily living, but they may have decreased tolerance for, and require additional rest after, prolonged or vigorous activity.

Assessment

Health History

The health history initially focuses on the patient's presenting problem and associated symptoms. In conducting the history, the nurse should explore the onset, location, duration, character, aggravating and alleviating factors, radiation (if relevant), and timing of the presenting problem and associated signs and symptoms. The nurse should also explore how these factors impact the patient's activities of daily living, usual work and family activities, and quality of life.

Common Symptoms

The major signs and symptoms of respiratory disease are dyspnea, cough, sputum production, chest pain, wheezing, and hemoptysis. During the health history, the nurse should also consider nonpulmonary diseases when evaluating symptoms, as these symptoms may occur with a variety of other illnesses.

| TABLE 17-2 | Age-Related Changes in the Respiratory System |
	Structural Changes	**Functional Changes**	**History and Physical Findings**
Defense Mechanisms (Respiratory and Nonrespiratory)	↓ Number of cilia and ↓ mucus ↓ Cough and gag reflex Loss of surface area of the capillary membrane Lack of a uniform or consistent ventilation and/or blood flow	↓ Protection against foreign particles ↓ Protection against aspiration ↓ Antibody response to antigens ↓ Response to hypoxia and hypercapnia (chemoreceptors)	↓ Cough reflex and mucus ↑ Infection rate History of respiratory infections, chronic obstructive pulmonary disease (COPD), pneumonia. Risk factors: smoking, environmental exposure, exposure to tuberculosis (TB)
Lung	↓ Size of airway ↑ Diameter of alveolar ducts ↑ Collagen of alveolar walls ↑ Thickness of alveolar membranes ↓ Elasticity of alveolar sacs	↑ Airway resistance ↑ Pulmonary compliance ↓ Expiratory flow rate ↓ Oxygen diffusion capacity ↑ Dead space Premature closure of airways ↑ Air trapping ↓ Expiratory flow rates Ventilation–perfusion mismatch ↓ Exercise capacity ↑ Anteroposterior (AP) diameter	Unchanged total lung capacity (TLC) ↑ Residual volume (RV) ↓ Inspiratory reserve volume (IRV) ↓ Expiratory reserve volume (ERV) ↓ Forced vital capacity (FVC) and vital capacity (VC) ↑ Functional residual capacity (FRC) ↓ PaO_2 ↑ CO_2
Chest Wall and Muscles	Calcification of intercostal cartilages Arthritis of costovertebral joints ↓ Continuity of diaphragm Osteoporotic changes ↓ Muscle mass Muscle atrophy	↑ Rigidity and stiffness of thoracic cage ↓ Respiratory muscle strength ↑ Work of breathing ↓ Capacity for exercise ↓ Peripheral chemosensitivity ↑ Risk for inspiratory muscle fatigue	Kyphosis, barrel chest Skeletal changes ↑ AP diameter Shortness of breath ↑ Abdominal and diaphragmatic breathing ↓ Maximum expiratory flow rates

↓, decreased; ↑, increased.

Adapted from Ramly, E., Kaafarani, H. M. A., & Velmahos, G. C. (2015). The effect of aging on pulmonary function: Implications for monitoring and support of the surgical and trauma patient. *Surgical Clinics of North America, 95*(1), 53–69.

Dyspnea

The official American Thoracic Society Statement (2012) defines **dyspnea** as a subjective feeling of discomfort while breathing; its causes may include multiple physiologic, psychological, environmental, or social factors (Parshall, Schwartzstein, Adams, et al., 2012). In general, acute diseases of the lungs produce a more severe grade of dyspnea than do chronic diseases. Sudden dyspnea in a healthy person may indicate pneumothorax (air in the pleural cavity), acute respiratory obstruction, allergic reaction, or myocardial infarction. In patients who are immobilized, sudden dyspnea may denote pulmonary embolism (PE). Dyspnea and **tachypnea** (abnormally rapid respirations) accompanied by progressive **hypoxemia** (low blood oxygen level) in a person who has recently experienced lung trauma, shock, cardiopulmonary bypass, or multiple blood transfusions may signal ARDS. **Orthopnea** (shortness of breath when lying flat, relieved by sitting or standing) may be found in patients with heart disease and occasionally in patients with chronic obstructive pulmonary disease (COPD); dyspnea with an expiratory wheeze occurs with COPD. Dyspnea associated with noisy breathing may result from a narrowing of the airway or localized obstruction of a major bronchus by a tumor or foreign body. The high-pitched sound heard (usually on inspiration) when someone is breathing through a partially blocked upper airway is called **stridor**. To help determine the cause of dyspnea, the nurse should ask the following questions:

- Is the shortness of breath related to other symptoms? Is a cough present?
- Was the onset of shortness of breath sudden or gradual?
- At what time of day or night does the shortness of breath occur?
- Is the shortness of breath worse when lying flat?
- How much exertion triggers shortness of breath? Does it occur with exercise? Climbing stairs? At rest?
- How severe is the shortness of breath? On a scale of 0 to 10, if 0 is not at all breathless and 10 is very breathless, how hard is it to breathe?

Because patients use a variety of terms to describe breathlessness, the nurse must explore what these terms mean to each patient. The use of a standardized tool to assess dyspnea, as part of the routine nursing assessment, can be beneficial (Fig. 17-6). It is especially important to assess the patient's rating of the intensity or distress of breathlessness, what breathing feels like, and its impact on the patient's general health, function, and quality of life (Baker, DeSanto-Madeya, & Banzett, 2017). See the Nursing Research Profile in Chart 17-5.

Cough

Cough is a reflex that protects the lungs from the accumulation of secretions or the inhalation of foreign bodies. Its presence or absence can be a diagnostic clue because some disorders cause coughing and others suppress it. The cough reflex may be impaired by weakness or paralysis of the respiratory muscles, prolonged inactivity, the presence of a nasogastric tube, or depressed function of the brain's medullary centers (e.g., anesthesia, brain disorders).

Cough results from irritation or inflammation of the mucous membranes anywhere in the respiratory tract and is associated with multiple pulmonary disorders. Mucus,

Dyspnea: How to score the dyspnea assessment. Ask patient once per shift <u>and</u> any change in patient status.
How much breathing discomfort (shortness of breath) do you have right now?

0	1	2	3	4	5	6	7	8	9	10		N/A
None			Mild		Moderate			Severe		Unbearable		Unable to respond

1. How much breathing discomfort (shortness of breath) do you have right now?

○	○	○	○	○	○	○	○	○	○	○	○
0	1	2	3	4	5	6	7	8	9	10	Unable to respond
None			Mild		Moderate			Severe		Unbearable	

2a. During the 24 hrs before you came to the hospital, what was the worst level of breathing discomfort (shortness of breath) you experienced?

○	○	○	○	○	○	○	○	○	○	○	○
0	1	2	3	4	5	6	7	8	9	10	Unable to respond
None			Mild		Moderate			Severe		Unbearable	

Note: If answer to 2a is 'None', questions 2b and 3 do not apply, and will not appear on the electronic form.

2b. What were you doing when you experienced your worst breathing discomfort?
○ Heavier activity   (e.g., mowing the lawn, raking leaves, walking uphill)
○ Moderate activity   (e.g., walking, making the bed)
○ Light activity   (e.g., eating, dressing, speaking, preparing lunch)
○ Resting   (e.g., sitting in a chair or lying in bed)

3. Has your shortness of breath gotten worse in the last week (before coming to the hospital)?

○	○	○
About the same	Worse	Much worse

Figure 17-6 • Dyspnea scale and patient's report of current and recent dyspnea. Reprinted from Baker, K. M., DeSanto-Madeya, S., & Banzett, R. B. (2017). Routine dyspnea assessment and documentation: Nurses experience yields wide acceptance. *BMC Nursing, 16*(3), 1–11. This article is distributed under the terms of the Creative Commons Attribution 4.0 International License (www.creativecommons.org/licenses/by/4.0), which permits unrestricted use, distribution, and reproduction in any medium.

pus, blood, or an airborne irritant, such as smoke or a gas, may stimulate the cough reflex. Common causes of cough include asthma, gastrointestinal reflux disease, infection, and side effects of medications, such as angiotensin-converting enzyme (ACE) inhibitors (Norris, 2019).

To help determine the cause of the cough, the nurse inquires about the onset and time of coughing. Coughing at night may indicate the onset of left-sided heart failure or bronchial asthma. A cough in the morning with sputum production may indicate bronchitis. A cough that worsens when the patient is supine suggests postnasal drip (rhinosinusitis). Coughing after food intake may indicate aspiration of material into the tracheobronchial tree or reflux. A cough of recent onset is usually from an acute infection.

The nurse assesses the character of the cough and associated symptoms. A dry, irritative cough is characteristic of an upper respiratory tract infection of viral origin, or it may be a side effect of ACE inhibitor therapy. An irritative, high-pitched cough can be caused by laryngotracheitis. A brassy cough is the result of a tracheal lesion, and a severe or changing cough may indicate bronchogenic carcinoma. Pleuritic chest pain that accompanies coughing may indicate pleural or chest wall (musculoskeletal) involvement. Violent coughing causes bronchial spasm, obstruction, and further irritation of the bronchi and may result in syncope (fainting).

 Concept Mastery Alert

A nurse interviewing a patient who says he has a dry, irritating cough that is not "bringing anything up" should ask whether he is taking ACE inhibitors.

A persistent cough may affect a patient's quality of life and may produce embarrassment, exhaustion, inability to sleep,

Chart 17-5

NURSING RESEARCH PROFILE
Dyspnea Assessment

Baker, K. M., DeSanto-Madeya, S., & Banzett, R. B. (2017). Routine dyspnea assessment and documentation: Nurses' experience yields wide acceptance. *BMC Nursing, 16*(3), 1–11.

Purpose

The study aims to explore nurses' approaches to dyspnea assessment, their perception of patient response, and their perception of the utility and burden of dyspnea measurement.

Design

This was a qualitative, descriptive study utilizing a three-part assessment of practice: a series of focus group interviews, a time-motion observation, and a randomized, anonymous online survey. A convenience sample of 63 nurses from six medical-surgical units participated in 12 half-hour focus group sessions. The focus group included questions about the process nurses used for assessment of dyspnea, views on the importance of dyspnea assessment and awareness, patients' abilities to rate and use a dyspnea scale, impact of routine assessment on workflow, and suggestions for improvement. Focus group sessions were conducted during regular work shifts and were recorded. Forty registered nurses representing 14 medical-surgical inpatient

units were randomly selected for participation in the time-motion study. For this observation, a clinical nurse specialist recorded the time nurses spent assessing and documenting pain and dyspnea during routine morning nursing assessment of patients. The online survey addressed issues raised during the focus group sessions. Seventy registered nurses, from 14 inpatient medical-surgical units, were randomly selected to complete the anonymous, online survey.

Findings

Nursing assessment of dyspnea and pain took less than 1 min. Overwhelmingly, most of the nurses surveyed (94%) reported understanding the importance of assessing dyspnea. They described assessment of dyspnea as "easy" or "very easy" to complete and that the utilization of an assessment tool enhanced awareness of dyspnea, improved workflow, and standardized documentation.

Nursing Implications

Findings from this study support the use of a standardized tool to assess dyspnea as part of routine nursing assessment of patients.

---

and pain. Therefore, the nurse should explore how a chronic cough impacts all aspects of the patient's life.

Sputum Production

Sputum production is the reaction of the lungs to any constantly recurring irritant and often results from persistent coughing. It may also be associated with a nasal discharge. The nature of the sputum is often indicative of its cause. A profuse amount of purulent sputum (thick and yellow, green, or rust colored) or a change in color of the sputum is a common sign of a bacterial infection. Thin, mucoid sputum frequently results from viral bronchitis. A gradual increase of sputum over time may occur with chronic bronchitis or bronchiectasis. Pink-tinged mucoid sputum suggests a lung tumor. Profuse, frothy, pink material, often welling up into the throat, may indicate pulmonary edema. Foul-smelling sputum and bad breath point to the presence of a lung abscess, bronchiectasis, or an infection caused by fusospirochetal or other anaerobic organisms.

Chest Pain

Chest pain or discomfort may be associated with pulmonary, cardiac, gastrointestinal, or musculoskeletal disease or anxiety. Chest pain associated with pulmonary conditions may be sharp, stabbing, and intermittent, or it may be dull, aching, and persistent. The pain usually is felt on the side where the pathologic process is located, although it may be referred elsewhere—for example, to the neck, back, or abdomen.

Chest pain may occur with pneumonia, pulmonary infarction, or pleurisy, or as a late symptom of bronchogenic carcinoma. In carcinoma, the pain may be dull and persistent because the cancer has invaded the chest wall, mediastinum, or spine.

Lung disease does not always cause thoracic pain because the lungs and the visceral pleura lack sensory nerves and are insensitive to pain stimuli. However, the parietal pleura have

a rich supply of sensory nerves that are stimulated by inflammation and stretching of the membrane. Pleuritic pain from irritation of the parietal pleura is sharp and seems to "catch" on inspiration; patients often describe it as being "like the stabbing of a knife." Patients are more comfortable when they lay on the affected side because this position splints the chest wall, limits expansion and contraction of the lung, and reduces the friction between the injured or diseased pleurae on that side. Pain associated with cough may be reduced manually by splinting the rib cage.

The nurse assesses the onset, quality, intensity, and radiation of pain and identifies and explores precipitating factors and their relationship to the patient's position. In addition, the nurse must assess the relationship of pain to the inspiratory and expiratory phases of respiration (see Chapter 9 for further discussion on assessment of pain).

Wheezing

Wheezing is a high-pitched, musical sound which is continuous, meaning it is heard on either expiration (asthma) or inspiration (bronchitis). It is often the major finding in a patient with bronchoconstriction or airway narrowing (see later discussion under Thoracic Auscultation).

Hemoptysis

Hemoptysis is the expectoration of blood from the respiratory tract. It can present as small to moderate blood-stained sputum to a large hemorrhage and always warrants further investigation. The onset of hemoptysis is usually sudden, and it may be intermittent or continuous. The most common causes are:

- Pulmonary infection
- Carcinoma of the lung
- Abnormalities of the heart or blood vessels
- Pulmonary artery or vein abnormalities
- PE or infarction

The nurse must determine the source of the bleeding, as the term *hemoptysis* is reserved for blood coming from the respiratory tract. Potential sources of bleeding include the gums, nasopharynx, lungs, or stomach. The nurse may be the only witness to the episode, and when evaluating the bleeding episode, the following points should be considered:

- Bloody sputum from the nose or the nasopharynx is usually preceded by considerable sniffing, with blood possibly appearing in the nose.
- Blood from the lung is usually bright red, frothy, and mixed with sputum. Initial symptoms include a tickling sensation in the throat, a salty taste, a burning or bubbling sensation in the chest, and perhaps chest pain, in which case, the patient tends to splint the bleeding side. This blood has an alkaline pH (greater than 7).
- Blood from the stomach is vomited rather than expectorated, may be mixed with food, and is usually much darker and often referred to as "coffee ground emesis." This blood has an acid pH (less than 7).

Past Health, Social, and Family History

In addition to the presenting problem and associated symptoms, the history should also focus on the patient's health, personal, and social history, and the family health history. Specific questions are asked about childhood illnesses, immunizations (including the most recent influenza and pneumonia vaccinations), medical conditions, injuries, hospitalizations, surgeries, allergies, and current medications (including over-the-counter medications and herbal remedies). Personal and social history addresses issues such as diet, exercise, sleep, recreational habits, and religion. Psychosocial factors that may affect the patient are also explored (Chart 17-6).

The nurse assesses for risk factors and genetic factors that may contribute to the patient's lung condition (Charts 17-7 and 17-8). Many lung disorders are related to or exacerbated by tobacco smoke; therefore, smoking history (including exposure to secondhand smoke) is also obtained. Smoking history is usually expressed in pack-years, which is the number of packs of cigarettes smoked per day times the number of years the patient has smoked. It is important to find out

---

Chart 17-6

ASSESSMENT

Assessing Psychosocial Factors Related to Respiratory Function and Disease

- What strategies does the patient use to cope with the signs, symptoms, and challenges associated with pulmonary disease?
- What effect has the pulmonary disease had on the patient's quality of life, goals, role within the family, and occupation?
- What changes has the pulmonary disease had on the patient's family and relationships with family members?
- Does the patient exhibit depression, anxiety, anger, hostility, dependency, withdrawal, isolation, avoidance, nonadherence, acceptance, or denial?
- What support systems does the patient use to cope with the illness?
- Are resources (relatives, friends, or community groups) available? Do the patient and the family use them effectively?

Chart 17-7

RISK FACTORS

Respiratory Disease

- Atypical immune responses in disease (e.g., asthma)
- Exposure to indoor pollutants (e.g., tobacco smoke, radon gas)
- Exposure to outdoor pollutants (e.g., smog, vehicle exhaust emissions, pollen)
- Genetic makeup
- Infection (e.g., influenza, pneumonia)
- Obesity
- Personal or family history of lung disease
- Smoking (e.g., cigarettes, e-cigarettes)

Adapted from American Lung Association. (2019). Protecting your lungs: Tips to keep your lungs healthy. Retrieved on 12/22/2019 at: www.lung.org/lung-health-and-diseases/protecting-your-lungs

---

whether the patient is still smoking or when the patient quit smoking. The nurse should also ask patients whether they use electronic nicotine delivery systems (ENDS) including e-cigarettes, e-pens, e-pipes, e-hookah, and e-cigars, or any other smokeless tobacco products. In 2016, the U.S. Food and Drug Administration (FDA) finalized a rule that extended its regulatory authority to all tobacco products, including e-cigarettes, cigars, hookah, and pipe tobacco. The new rule mandates health warnings on products, bans free samples, and restricts youth (those under the age of 18) access to newly regulated tobacco products. The FDA has not found ENDS to be safe or effective in helping smokers curb the habit, as previously marketed by some manufacturers. The FDA has approved five forms of nicotine replacement therapy including nicotine gum, nicotine skin patches, nicotine lozenges, nicotine oral inhaled products, and nicotine nasal spray (American Lung Association, 2020). The American Lung Association views ENDS as a public health threat and calls for additional research regarding the risks and long-term effects to better understand potential risks (American Lung Association, 2019). In January 2018, The National Academies of Sciences, Engineering, and Medicine released a report on the public health consequences of e-cigarettes. The report presented 47 conclusions from a review of 800 studies and concluded that using e-cigarettes causes health risks. E-cigarettes contain and emit a number of potentially toxic substances such as propylene glycol, acetaldehyde, acrolein, and formaldehyde, among others. Acrolein, also used as a weed killer, is known to cause acute lung injury, COPD, asthma, and lung cancer. Additionally, e-cigarette use is associated with an increased risk for cough, wheeze, and asthma exacerbations in adolescents (The National Academies of Sciences, Engineering, and Medicine, 2018). Differences in socioeconomic factors, rooted in race and ethnicity, may predispose certain groups to greater burdens related to lung disease and should also be considered (Chart 17-9).

If the patient is experiencing severe dyspnea, the nurse may need to modify the questions asked and the timing of the health history to avoid increasing the patient's breathlessness and anxiety. Once the history is complete, the nurse conducts a comprehensive assessment. Data obtained from both the history and the assessment guide the development of a nursing care plan and patient education.

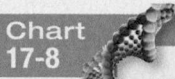

Chart 17-8 — GENETICS IN NURSING PRACTICE
Respiratory Disorders

Various conditions that affect gas exchange and respiratory function are influenced by genetic factors. Some are known to have a direct inherited pathway while others have a strong familial association, but the exact inheritance pattern is not entirely clear. The following are examples of respiratory disorders with a known or associated familial component:

- Asthma
- Cystic fibrosis
- Chronic obstructive pulmonary disease
- Alpha$_1$-antitrypsin deficiency
- Primary ciliary dyskinesia
- Pulmonary fibrosis
- Pulmonary hypertension
- Tuberous sclerosis

Nursing Assessments

Refer to Chapter 4, Chart 4-2: Genetics in Nursing Practice: Genetic Aspects of Health Assessment

Family History Assessment Specific to Genetic Respiratory Disorders

- Assess family history for three generations for family members with histories of respiratory impairment.
- Assess family history for individuals with early-onset chronic pulmonary disease and family history of hepatic disease in infants (clinical symptoms of alpha$_1$-antitrypsin deficiency).
- Inquire about family history of cystic fibrosis, an autosomal recessive inherited respiratory disorder.

Patient Assessment Specific to Genetic Respiratory Disorders

- Assess for symptoms such as changes in respiratory status and triggers that precede changes in respiratory function
- Frequency of respiratory tract infections or sinus infections
- Determine exposure to environmental risks (e.g., radon, asbestos) or occupational exposures (e.g., coal miner, sandblaster, painter)
- Determine presence of secondary risk factors (e.g., smoking or exposure or secondhand smoke)
- Assess for:
  - Clubbing of fingers
  - Skin color in general or the presence of white patches on the skin
  - Presence of angiofibromas or ungual fibromas (seen with primary ciliary dyskinesia)
- Assess for presence and frequency of:
  - Wheezing or coughing
  - Mucous production (frequency, amount, and characteristics of the mucous)
  - Mucosal edema
- Assess for multisystem effects (gastrointestinal disorders, pancreatic insufficiency, liver or kidney disorders)

Genetic Resources

American Lung Association, www.lung.org
Cystic Fibrosis Foundation, www.cff.org
COPD Foundation, www.copdfoundation.org
Primary Ciliary Dyskinesia, www.pcdfoundation.org
- See also Chapter 6, Chart 6-7: Components of Genetic Counseling

Physical Assessment of the Respiratory System

General Appearance

The patient's general appearance may give clues to respiratory status. In particular, the nurse inspects for clubbing of the fingers and notes skin color.

Clubbing of the Fingers

Clubbing of the fingers is a change in the normal nail bed. It appears as sponginess of the nail bed and loss of the nail bed angle (Fig. 17-7). It is a sign of lung disease that is found in patients with chronic hypoxic conditions, chronic lung infections, or malignancies of the lung. Clubbing can also be seen in congenital heart disease and other chronic infections or inflammatory conditions, such as endocarditis or inflammatory bowel disease (Hogan-Quigley, Palm, & Bickley, 2017).

Cyanosis

Cyanosis, a bluish coloring of the skin, is a very late indicator of hypoxia. The presence or absence of cyanosis is determined by the amount of unoxygenated hemoglobin in the blood. Cyanosis

Chart 17-9
Disparities in Pulmonary Health Related to Socioeconomics, Race, and Ethnicity: A Snapshot

- Individuals living in rural areas are more likely to use tobacco and be exposed to secondhand smoke at work and at home, to start smoking at a younger age, and to use more than 15 cigarettes daily, yet have less access to smoking cessation programs.
- Individuals with lower income and lower levels of education are more likely to use tobacco products.
- Adults living below the poverty level are more likely to experience severe asthma exacerbations, hospitalizations, and death.
- More Hispanics live and work in areas with greater levels of pollution, have higher prevalence rates of asthma than Caucasians, and yet are less likely to be diagnosed with asthma than all other racial and ethnic groups. Hispanics are less likely than non-Hispanic Whites to receive health insurance as a benefit from an employer.
- African American men are 37% more likely to get lung cancer than Caucasian men even though smoking rates between these two groups are comparable.
- American Indians/Alaska Natives and African Americans are at a higher risk of complications resulting from influenza and pneumonia.
- Death rates for African Americans are 55 percent higher for asthma than among Caucasians.
- Older African Americans and older Hispanics are less likely than older Caucasians to receive influenza vaccines (28% and 24% less, respectively) and pneumonia vaccines (37% and 46%, respectively).

Adapted from American Lung Association. Disparities in lung health series. Retrieved on 6/23/2019 at: www.lung.org/our-initiatives/research/lung-health-disparities

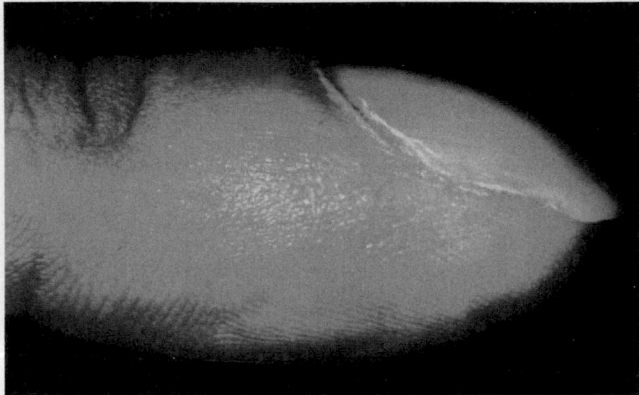

Figure 17-7 • Clubbed finger. In clubbing, the distal phalanx of each finger is rounded and bulbous. The nail plate is more convex, and the angle between the plate and the proximal nail fold increases to 180 degrees or more. The proximal nail fold, when palpated, feels spongy or floating. Among the many causes are chronic hypoxia and lung cancer.

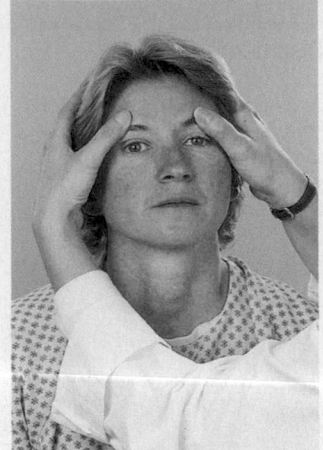 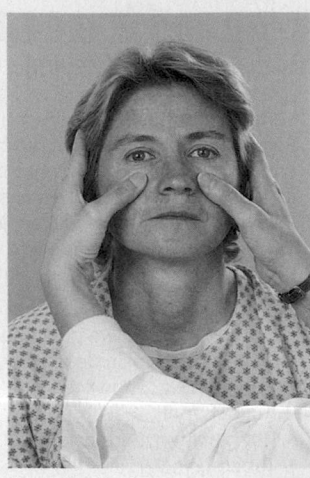

Figure 17-8 • Technique for palpating the frontal sinuses at left and the maxillary sinuses at right.

appears when there is at least 5 g/dL of unoxygenated hemoglobin. A patient with a hemoglobin level of 15 g/dL does not demonstrate cyanosis until 5 g/dL of that hemoglobin becomes unoxygenated, reducing the effective circulating hemoglobin to two thirds of the normal level.

A patient with anemia rarely manifests cyanosis, and a patient with polycythemia may appear cyanotic even if adequately oxygenated. Therefore, cyanosis is *not* a reliable sign of hypoxia.

Assessment of cyanosis is affected by room lighting, the patient's skin color, and the distance of the blood vessels from the surface of the skin. In the presence of a pulmonary condition, central cyanosis is assessed by observing the color of the tongue and lips. This indicates a decrease in oxygen tension in the blood. Peripheral cyanosis results from decreased blood flow to the body's periphery (fingers, toes, or earlobes), as in vasoconstriction from exposure to cold, and does not necessarily indicate a central systemic problem.

Upper Respiratory Structures

For a routine examination of the upper airway, only a simple light source, such as a penlight, is necessary. A more thorough examination requires the use of a nasal speculum.

Nose and Sinuses

The nurse inspects the external nose for lesions, asymmetry, or inflammation and then asks the patient to tilt the head backward. Gently pushing the tip of the nose upward, the nurse examines the internal structures of the nose, inspecting the mucosa for color, swelling, exudate, or bleeding. The nasal mucosa is normally redder than the oral mucosa. It may appear swollen and hyperemic if the patient has a common cold; however, in allergic rhinitis, the mucosa appears pale and swollen.

Next, the nurse inspects the septum for deviation, perforation, or bleeding. Most people have a slight degree of septal deviation; such deviation usually causes no symptoms. However, actual displacement of the cartilage into either the right or left side of the nose may produce nasal obstruction.

While the head is still tilted back, the nurse inspects the inferior and middle turbinates. In chronic rhinitis, nasal polyps may develop between the inferior and middle turbinates; they are distinguished by their gray appearance. Unlike the turbinates, they are gelatinous and freely movable.

Next, the nurse may palpate the frontal and maxillary sinuses for tenderness (Fig. 17-8). Using the thumbs, the nurse applies gentle pressure in an upward fashion at the supraorbital ridges (frontal sinuses) and in the cheek area adjacent to the nose (maxillary sinuses). Tenderness in either area suggests inflammation. The frontal and maxillary sinuses can be inspected by transillumination (passing a strong light through a bony area, such as the sinuses, to inspect the cavity; see Fig. 17-9). If the light fails to penetrate, the cavity likely contains fluid or pus.

Mouth and Pharynx

After the nasal inspection, the nurse assesses the mouth and the pharynx, instructing the patient to open the mouth wide and take a deep breath. Usually, this flattens the posterior tongue and briefly allows a full view of the anterior and posterior pillars, tonsils, uvula, and posterior pharynx (see Chapter 39,

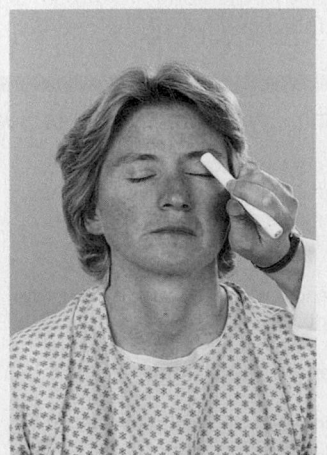 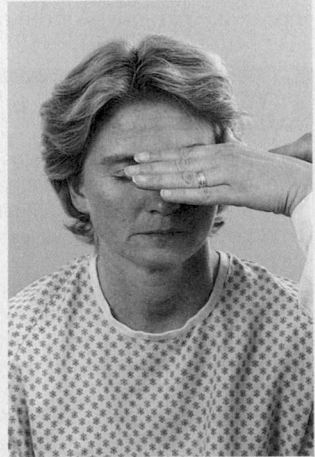

Figure 17-9 • At left, the nurse positions the light source for transillumination of the frontal sinus. At right, the nurse shields the patient's brow and shines the light. In normal conditions (a darkened room), the light should shine through the tissues and appear as a reddish glow (above the nurse's hand) over the sinus.

Fig. 39-2). The nurse inspects these structures for color, symmetry, and evidence of exudate, ulceration, or enlargement. If a tongue blade is needed to depress the tongue to visualize the pharynx, it is pressed firmly beyond the midpoint of the tongue to avoid a gagging response.

Trachea

Next, the position and mobility of the trachea are noted by direct palpation. This is performed by placing the thumb and the index finger of one hand on either side of the trachea just above the sternal notch. The trachea is highly sensitive and palpating too firmly may trigger a coughing or gagging response. The trachea is normally in the midline as it enters the thoracic inlet behind the sternum; however, it may be deviated by masses in the neck or the mediastinum. Pulmonary disorders such as a pneumothorax or pleural effusion may also displace the trachea.

Lower Respiratory Structures and Breathing

Assessment of the lower respiratory structures includes inspection, palpation, percussion, and auscultation of the thorax. The patient should be positioned as necessary prior to the assessment.

Positioning

To assess the posterior thorax and the lungs, the patient should be in a sitting position with arms crossed in front of the chest and hands placed on the opposite shoulders (Hogan-Quigley et al., 2017). This position separates the scapulae widely and exposes more lung area for assessment. If the patient is unable to sit, with the patient supine, the nurse should roll the patient from side to side to complete the posterior examination. To assess the anterior thorax and lungs, the patient should be either supine or sitting. The supine position allows easier displacement of the patient's breast tissue, improving the nurse's ability to perform the chest examination.

Thoracic Inspection

Inspection of the thorax provides information about the respiratory system, the musculoskeletal structure, and the patient's nutritional status. The nurse observes the skin over the thorax for color and turgor and for evidence of loss of subcutaneous tissue. It is important to note asymmetry, if present. In documenting or reporting the findings, anatomic landmarks are used as points of reference (Chart 17-10).

Chest Configuration

Normally, the ratio of the anteroposterior diameter to the lateral diameter is 1:2. However, there are four main deformities of the chest associated with respiratory disease that alter this relationship: barrel chest, funnel chest (pectus excavatum), pigeon chest (pectus carinatum), and kyphoscoliosis.

Barrel Chest. Barrel chest occurs as a result of overinflation of the lungs, which increases the anteroposterior diameter of the thorax. It occurs with aging and is a hallmark sign of emphysema and COPD. In a patient with emphysema, the ribs are more widely spaced and the intercostal spaces tend to bulge on expiration. The appearance of the patient with advanced emphysema is thus quite characteristic, allowing the nurse to detect its presence easily, even from a distance.

Funnel Chest (Pectus Excavatum). Funnel chest occurs when there is a depression in the lower portion of the sternum. This may compress the heart and great vessels, resulting in murmurs. Funnel chest may occur with rickets or Marfan syndrome.

Pigeon Chest (Pectus Carinatum). A pigeon chest occurs as a result of the anterior displacement of the sternum, which also increases the anteroposterior diameter. This may occur with rickets, Marfan syndrome, or severe kyphoscoliosis.

Kyphoscoliosis. Kyphoscoliosis is characterized by elevation of the scapula and a corresponding S-shaped spine. This deformity limits lung expansion within the thorax. It may occur with osteoporosis and other skeletal disorders that affect the thorax.

Breathing Patterns and Respiratory Rates

Observation of the rate, depth, and symmetry during respiration is a simple but important aspect of assessment. The normal adult who is at rest comfortably takes 12 to 20 breaths/min (Hogan-Quigley et al., 2017). Except for the occasional sigh, respirations are quiet with a regular rate, depth, and rhythm. The normal pattern associated with breathing is known as eupnea. Certain pathologic conditions may alter the rate and rhythm and are characteristic of certain disease states. For example, wheezing is commonly seen in the patient with asthma. Changes found during the act of breathing may be the first clinical sign that the patient's condition is deteriorating (IHI, 2019). The rate and depth of various patterns of respiration are presented in Table 17-3.

> **Concept Mastery Alert**
>
> There are subtle differences between Cheyne–Stokes and Biot's respiration patterns. Between regularly cycled periods of apnea, Cheyne–Stokes respirations demonstrate a regular pattern with the rate and depth of breathing increasing and then decreasing. In Biot's respiration, irregularly cycled periods of apnea are interspersed with cycles of normal rate and depth.

Temporary pauses of breathing, or **apnea,** may be noted. When episodes of apnea occur repeatedly during sleep, secondary to transient upper airway blockage, the condition is called **obstructive sleep apnea.** In thin people, it is quite normal to note a slight retraction of the intercostal spaces during quiet breathing. Bulging of the intercostal spaces during expiration implies obstruction of expiratory airflow, as in emphysema. Marked retraction on inspiration, particularly if asymmetric, implies blockage of a branch of the respiratory tree. Asymmetric bulging of the intercostal spaces, on either side of the thorax, is created by an increase in pressure within the hemithorax. This may be a result of air trapped under pressure within the pleural cavity, where it is not normally present (pneumothorax), or the pressure of fluid within the pleural space (pleural effusion).

Use of Accessory Muscles

In addition to breathing patterns and respiratory rates, the nurse should observe for the use of accessory muscles, such as the sternocleidomastoid, scalene, and trapezius muscles during inspiration, and the abdominal and internal intercostal

Chart 17-10 Locating Thoracic Landmarks

With respect to the thorax, location is defined both horizontally and vertically. With respect to the lungs, location is defined by lobe.

Horizontal Reference Points

Horizontally, thoracic locations are identified according to their proximity to the rib or the intercostal space under the examiner's fingers. On the anterior surface, identification of a specific rib is facilitated by first locating the angle of Louis. This is where the manubrium joins the body of the sternum in the midline. The second rib joins the sternum at this prominent landmark.

Other ribs may be identified by counting down from the second rib. The intercostal spaces are referred to in terms of the rib immediately above the intercostal space; for example, the fifth intercostal space is directly below the fifth rib.

Locating ribs on the posterior surface of the thorax is more difficult. The first step is to identify the spinous process. This is accomplished by finding the seventh cervical vertebra (*vertebra prominens*), which is the most prominent spinous process. When the neck is slightly flexed, the seventh cervical spinous process stands out. Other vertebrae are then identified by counting downward.

Vertical Reference Points

Several imaginary lines are used as vertical referents or landmarks to identify the location of thoracic findings. The *midsternal line* passes through the center of the sternum. The *midclavicular line* is an imaginary line that descends from the middle of the clavicle. The *point of maximal impulse* of the heart normally lies along this line on the left thorax.

When the arm is abducted from the body at 90 degrees, imaginary vertical lines may be drawn from the anterior axillary fold, from the middle of the axilla, and from the posterior axillary fold. These lines are called, respectively, the *anterior axillary line,* the *midaxillary line,* and the *posterior axillary line.* A line drawn vertically through the superior and inferior poles of the scapula is called the *scapular line,* and a line drawn down the center of the vertebral column is called the *vertebral line.* Using these landmarks, for example, the examiner communicates findings by referring to an area of dullness extending from the vertebral to the scapular line between the 7th and 10th ribs on the right.

Lobes of the Lungs

The lobes of the lung may be mapped on the surface of the chest wall in the following manner. The line between the upper and lower lobes on the left begins at the fourth thoracic spinous process posteriorly, proceeds around to cross the fifth rib in the midaxillary line, and meets the sixth rib at the sternum. This line on the right divides the right middle lobe from the right lower lobe. The line dividing the right upper lobe from the middle lobe is an incomplete one that begins at the fifth rib in the midaxillary line, where it intersects the line between the upper and lower lobes and traverses horizontally to the sternum. Thus, the upper lobes are dominant on the anterior surface of the thorax, and the lower lobes are dominant on the posterior surface. There is no presentation of the right middle lobe on the posterior surface of the chest.

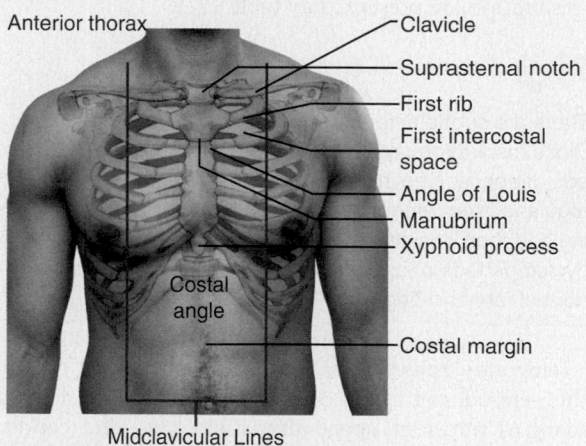

Anterior thorax — Clavicle — Suprasternal notch — First rib — First intercostal space — Angle of Louis — Manubrium — Xyphoid process — Costal angle — Costal margin — Midclavicular Lines

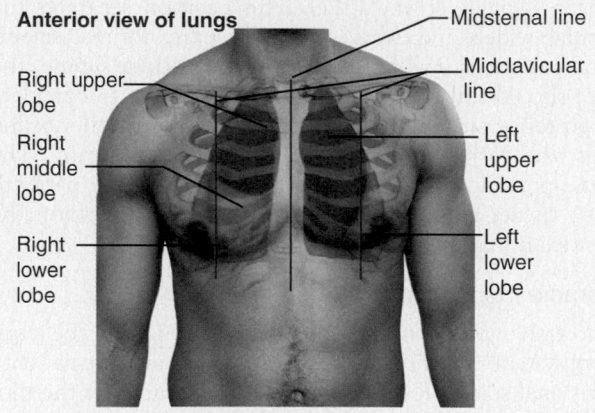

Anterior view of lungs — Midsternal line — Midclavicular line — Right upper lobe — Right middle lobe — Right lower lobe — Left upper lobe — Left lower lobe

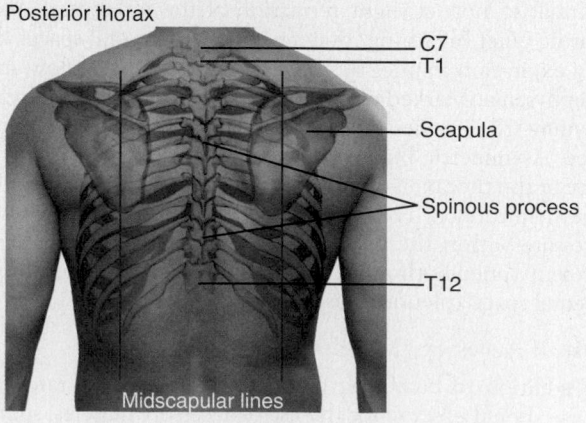

Posterior thorax — C7 — T1 — Scapula — Spinous process — T12 — Midscapular lines

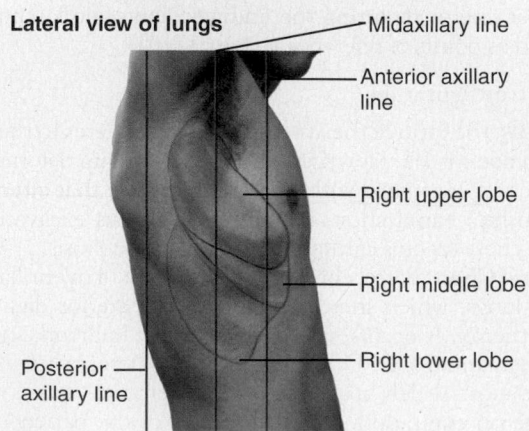

Lateral view of lungs — Midaxillary line — Anterior axillary line — Right upper lobe — Right middle lobe — Right lower lobe — Posterior axillary line

TABLE 17-3	Rates and Depths of Respiration
Type	**Description**
Eupnea 	Normal, breathing at 12–20 breaths/min
Bradypnea 	Slower than normal rate (<10 breaths/min), with normal depth and regular rhythm Associated with increased intracranial pressure, brain injury, and drug overdose
Tachypnea 	Rapid, shallow breathing >24 breaths/min Associated with pneumonia, pulmonary edema, metabolic acidosis, septicemia, severe pain, or rib fracture
Hypoventilation 	Shallow, irregular breathing
Hyperpnea	Increased depth of respirations, see also hyperventilation
Hyperventilation 	Increased rate and depth of breathing that results in decreased $PaCO_2$ level Inspiration and expiration nearly equal in duration Associated with exertion, anxiety, and metabolic acidosis Called *Kussmaul's respiration* if associated with diabetic ketoacidosis or untreated kidney failure
Apnea 	Period of cessation of breathing; time duration varies; apnea may occur briefly during other breathing disorders, such as with sleep apnea; life-threatening if sustained
Cheyne–Stokes 	Regular cycle where the rate and depth of breathing increase, then decrease until apnea (usually about 20 s) occurs Duration of apnea may vary and progressively lengthen; therefore, it is timed and reported. Associated with heart failure and damage to the respiratory center (drug induced, tumor, trauma)
Biot's respiration 	Periods of normal breathing (3–4 breaths), followed by a varying period of apnea (usually 10–60 s) Also called *ataxic breathing*; associated with complete irregularity Associated with respiratory depression resulting from drug overdose and brain injury, normally at the level of the medulla
Obstructive 	Prolonged expiratory phase of respiration Associated with airway narrowing and seen in asthma, chronic obstructive pulmonary disease, and bronchitis

Adapted from Hogan-Quigley, B., Palm, M. L., & Bickley, L. (2017). *Bates' nursing guide to physical examination and history taking* (2nd ed.). Philadelphia, PA: Wolters Kluwer Health Lippincott Williams & Wilkins.

muscles during expiration. These muscles provide additional support to assist the breathing effort during times of exertion as seen in exercise or certain disease states (Hogan-Quigley et al., 2017).

Thoracic Palpation

The nurse palpates the thorax for tenderness, masses, lesions, respiratory excursion, and vocal fremitus. If the patient has reported an area of pain or if lesions are apparent, the nurse performs direct palpation with the fingertips (for skin lesions and subcutaneous masses) or with the ball of the hand (for deeper masses or generalized flank or rib discomfort).

Respiratory Excursion

Respiratory excursion is an estimation of thoracic expansion and may disclose significant information about thoracic movement during breathing. The nurse assesses the patient for range and symmetry of excursion. For anterior assessment, the nurse places the thumbs along the costal margin of the chest wall and instructs the patient to inhale deeply.

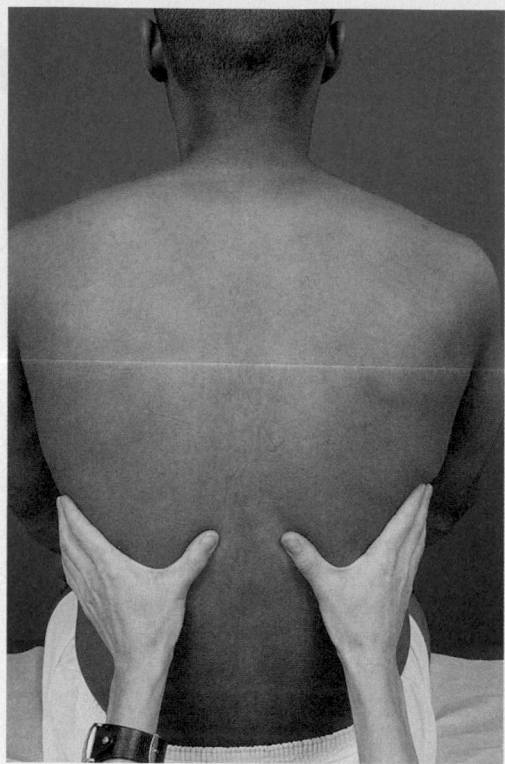

Figure 17-10 • Method for assessing posterior respiratory excursion. Place both hands posteriorly at the level of T9 or T10. Slide hands medially to pinch a small amount of skin between your thumbs. Observe for symmetry as the patient exhales fully following a deep inspiration.

The nurse observes movement of the thumbs during inspiration and expiration. This movement is normally symmetric (Hogan-Quigley et al., 2017).

Posterior assessment is performed by placing the thumbs adjacent to the spinal column at the level of the 10th rib (Fig. 17-10). The hands lightly grasp the lateral rib cage. Sliding the thumbs medially about 2.5 cm (1 inch) raises a small skin fold between the thumbs. The patient is instructed to take a full inspiration and to exhale fully. The nurse observes for normal flattening of the skin fold and feels the symmetric movement of the thorax.

Decreased chest excursion may be caused by chronic fibrotic disease. Asymmetric excursion may be due to splinting secondary to pleurisy, fractured ribs, trauma, or unilateral bronchial obstruction.

Tactile Fremitus

Tactile **fremitus** describes vibrations of the chest wall that result from speech detected on palpation. Normally, sounds generated by the larynx travel distally along the bronchial tree to set the chest wall in resonant motion. This is most pronounced with consonant sounds.

Normal fremitus varies on the basis of numerous factors. It is influenced by the thickness of the chest wall, especially muscle, and the subcutaneous tissue associated with obesity. It is also influenced by pitch; lower-pitched sounds travel better through the normal lung and produce greater vibration of the chest wall. Therefore, fremitus is more pronounced in men than in women because of the deeper male voice. Normally, fremitus is most pronounced where the large bronchi are closest to the chest wall, is more prominent on the right side, and is decreased or absent over the anterior chest wall which overlies the heart and great vessels (Hogan-Quigley et al., 2017).

The patient is asked to repeat "ninety-nine" or "one, one, one" as the nurse's hands move down the patient's thorax (Hogan-Quigley et al., 2017). The vibrations are detected with the palmar surfaces of the hands, or the ulnar aspect of the extended hands, on the thorax. The hand or hands are moved in sequence down the thorax. Corresponding areas of the thorax are compared (Fig. 17-11). Bony areas are not assessed.

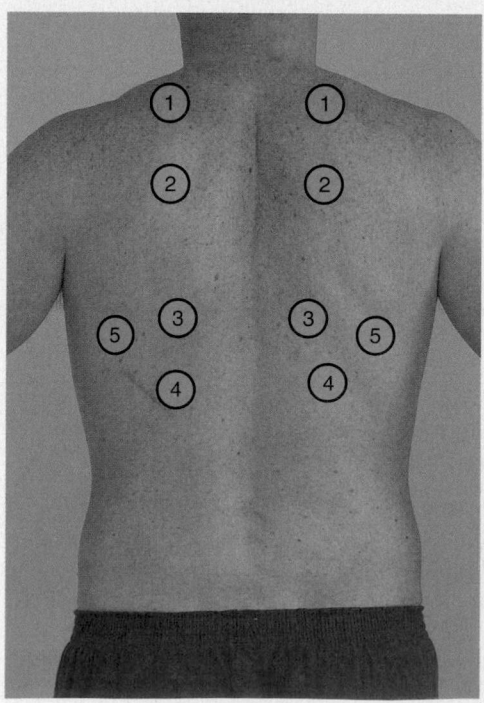
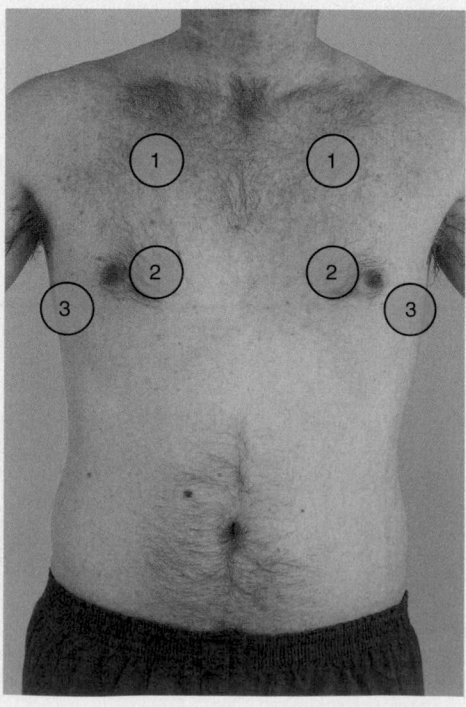

Figure 17-11 • Palpation sequence for tactile fremitus: posterior thorax (**left**) and anterior thorax (**right**).

TABLE 17-4	Characteristics of Percussion Sounds				
Sound	Relative Intensity	Relative Pitch	Relative Duration	Location Example	Examples
Flatness	Soft	High	Short	Thigh	Large pleural effusion
Dullness	Medium	Medium	Medium	Liver	Lobar pneumonia
Resonance	Loud	Low	Long	Normal lung	Simple chronic bronchitis
Hyperresonance	Very loud	Lower	Longer	None normally	Emphysema, pneumothorax
Tympany	Loud	High[a]	Medium	Gastric air bubble or puffed-out cheek	Large pneumothorax

[a]Distinguished mainly by its musical timbre.
Adapted from Hogan-Quigley, B., Palm, M. L., & Bickley, L. (2017). *Bates' nursing guide to physical examination and history taking* (2nd ed.). Philadelphia, PA: Wolters Kluwer Health Lippincott Williams & Wilkins.

Air does not conduct sound well; however, a solid substance such as tissue does, provided that it has elasticity and is not compressed. Therefore, an increase in solid tissue per unit volume of lung enhances fremitus, and an increase in air per unit volume of lung impedes sound. Patients with emphysema exhibit almost no tactile fremitus. A patient with consolidation of a lobe of the lung from pneumonia has increased tactile fremitus over that lobe.

Thoracic Percussion

Percussion produces audible and tactile vibration and allows the nurse to determine whether underlying tissues are filled with air, fluid, or solid material. Healthy lung tissue is resonant. Dullness over the lung occurs when air-filled lung tissue is replaced by fluid or solid tissue. Table 17-4 reviews percussion sounds and their characteristics. Percussion is also used to estimate the size and location of certain structures within the thorax (e.g., diaphragm, heart, liver).

Percussion usually begins with the posterior thorax. The nurse percusses across each shoulder top, locating the 5-cm width of resonance overlying the lung apices (Fig. 17-12). Then the nurse proceeds down the posterior thorax, percussing symmetric areas at intervals of 5 to 6 cm (2 to 2.5 inches). To perform percussion, the middle finger of the nondominant hand is firmly placed against the area of the chest wall to be percussed. The distal interphalangeal joint of this finger is struck with the tip of the middle finger of the dominant hand. This finger is partially flexed, and percussion occurs in a smooth, dartlike fashion. Bony structures (scapulae or ribs) are not percussed.

To perform percussion over the anterior chest, the nurse begins in the supraclavicular area and proceeds downward, from one intercostal space to the next. Dullness noted to the left of the sternum between the third and fifth intercostal spaces is a normal finding, because that is the location of the heart. Similarly, there is a normal span of liver dullness below the lung at the right costal margin (Hogan-Quigley et al., 2017).

Diaphragmatic Excursion

The normal resonance of the lung stops at the diaphragm. The position of the diaphragm is different during inspiration and expiration.

To assess the position and motion of the diaphragm, the nurse instructs the patient to take a deep breath and hold it while the maximal descent of the diaphragm is percussed.

The point at which the percussion note at the midscapular line changes from resonance to dullness is marked with a pen. The patient is then instructed to exhale fully and hold it while the nurse again percusses downward to the dullness of the diaphragm. This point is also marked. The distance between the two markings indicates the range of motion of the diaphragm.

Maximal excursion of the diaphragm may be as much as 8 to 10 cm (3 to 4 inches) in healthy, tall young men, but for most people, it is usually 5 to 7 cm (2 to 2.75 inches). Normally, the diaphragm is about 2 cm (0.75 inch) higher on the right because of the location of the liver. Decreased diaphragmatic excursion may occur with pleural effusion. Atelectasis, diaphragmatic paralysis, or pregnancy may account for a diaphragm that is positioned high in the thorax (Hogan-Quigley et al., 2017).

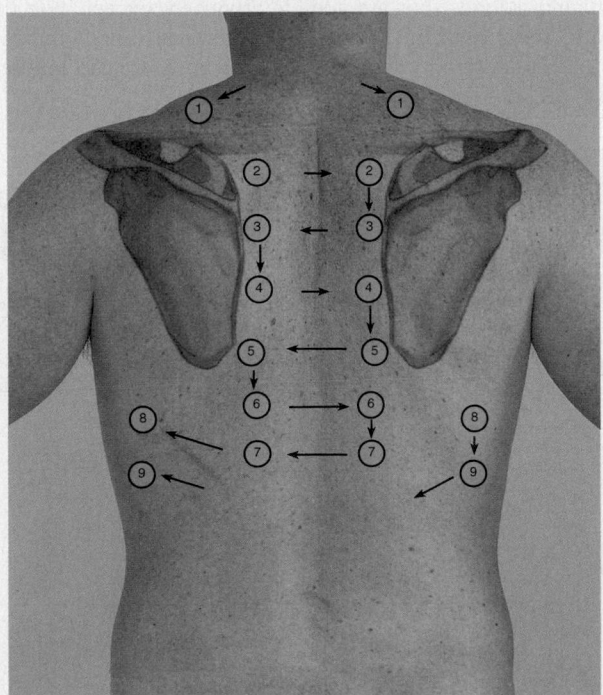

Figure 17-12 • Percussion of the posterior thorax. With the patient in a sitting position, symmetric areas of the lungs are percussed at 5-cm intervals. This progression starts at the apex of each lung and concludes with percussion of each lateral chest wall.

Thoracic Auscultation

Assessment concludes with auscultation of the anterior, posterior, and lateral thorax. Auscultation helps the nurse assess the flow of air through the bronchial tree and evaluate the presence of fluid or solid obstruction in the lung. The nurse auscultates for normal breath sounds, adventitious sounds, and voice sounds.

The nurse places the diaphragm of the stethoscope firmly against the bare skin of the chest wall as the patient breathes slowly and deeply through the mouth. Corresponding areas of the chest are auscultated in a systematic fashion from the apices to the bases and along midaxillary lines. The sequence of auscultation is similar to that used for percussion. The nurse may need to listen to two full inspirations and expirations at each anatomic location for valid interpretation of the sound heard. Repeated deep breaths may result in symptoms of hyperventilation (e.g., lightheadedness); this is avoided by having the patient rest and breathe normally periodically during the examination.

Breath Sounds

Normal breath sounds are distinguished by their location over a specific area of the lung and are identified as vesicular, bronchovesicular, and bronchial (tubular) breath sounds (Table 17-5).

The location, quality, and intensity of breath sounds are determined during auscultation. When airflow is decreased by bronchial obstruction (atelectasis) or when fluid (pleural effusion) or tissue (obesity) separates the air passages from the stethoscope, breath sounds are diminished or absent. For example, the breath sounds of the patient with emphysema are faint or often completely inaudible. When they are heard, the expiratory phase is prolonged. In the patient with obesity, breath sounds may be inaudible. Bronchial and bronchovesicular sounds that are audible anywhere except over the main bronchus in the lungs signify pathology, usually indicating consolidation in the lung (e.g., pneumonia, heart failure). This finding requires further evaluation.

Adventitious Sounds

An abnormal condition that affects the bronchial tree and alveoli may produce adventitious (additional) sounds. Some adventitious sounds are divided into two categories: **crackles,** or nonmusical, discontinuous sounds; and **wheezes,** or continuous musical sounds (Table 17-6). **Rhonchi,** a type of wheezing, are lower-pitched continuous sounds heard over the lungs in partial airway obstruction. Depending on their location and severity, wheezes and rhonchi may be heard with or without a stethoscope. The duration of the sound is the important distinction to make in identifying the sound as discontinuous or continuous. Friction rubs may be either discontinuous or continuous. Stridor is a continuous, high-pitched musical sound which is heard over the neck. This sound is caused by an interruption of airflow and indicates a narrowing of the upper respiratory tract. Stridor warrants emergent attention.

Voice Sounds

The sound heard through the stethoscope as the patient speaks is known as vocal resonance. The nurse should assess voice sounds when abnormal breath sounds are auscultated. The vibrations produced in the larynx are transmitted to the chest wall as they pass through the bronchi and alveolar tissue. Voice sounds are evaluated by having the patient repeat "ninety-nine" or "eee" while the nurse listens with the stethoscope in corresponding areas of the chest from the apices to the bases. With normal physiology, the sounds are faint and indistinct. Pathology that increases lung density, such as pneumonia and pulmonary edema, alters this normal physiologic response and may result in the following sounds:

- **Bronchophony** describes vocal resonance that is more intense and clearer than normal.
- **Egophony** describes voice sounds that are distorted. It is best appreciated by having the patient repeat the letter E. The distortion produced by consolidation transforms the sound into a clearly heard A rather than E.

TABLE 17-5	**Breath Sounds**			
	Duration of Sounds	Intensity of Expiratory Sound	Pitch of Expiratory Sound	Locations Where Heard Normally
Vesicular[a]	Inspiratory sounds last longer than expiratory ones.	Soft	Relatively low	Entire lung field except over the upper sternum and between the scapulae
Bronchovesicular	Inspiratory and expiratory sounds are about equal.	Intermediate	Intermediate	Often in the first and second interspaces anteriorly and between the scapulae (over the main bronchus)
Bronchial	Expiratory sounds last longer than inspiratory ones.	Loud	Relatively high	Over the manubrium, if heard at all
Tracheal	Inspiratory and expiratory sounds are about equal.	Very loud	Relatively high	Over the trachea in the neck

[a]The thickness of the bars indicates intensity of breath sounds: The steeper their incline, the higher the pitch of the sounds.
Adapted from Hogan-Quigley, B., Palm, M. L., & Bickley, L. (2017). *Bates' nursing guide to physical examination and history taking* (2nd ed.). Philadelphia, PA: Wolters Kluwer Health Lippincott Williams & Wilkins.

TABLE 17-6	Abnormal (Adventitious) Breath Sounds	
Breath Sound	**Description**	**Etiology**
Crackles		
Crackles in general	Nonmusical, discontinuous popping sounds that occur during inspiration (while usually heard on inspiration, they may also be heard on expiration); may or may not be cleared by coughing	Secondary to fluid in the airways or alveoli or to delayed opening of collapsed alveoli during inspiration Associated with heart failure and pulmonary fibrosis
Coarse crackles	Discontinuous popping sounds heard in early inspiration and throughout expiration; harsh, moist sound originating in the large bronchi; can be heard over any lung region; do not vary with body position	Associated with obstructive pulmonary disease
Fine crackles	Soft, high-pitched, discontinuous popping sounds heard in mid to late inspiration; sounds like hair rubbing together; originates in the alveoli, especially in dependent areas; may vary with body position	Associated with interstitial pneumonia, restrictive pulmonary disease (e.g., fibrosis); fine crackles in early inspiration are associated with bronchitis or pneumonia
Wheezes		
Wheezes in general	Continuous, musical, high-pitched, shrill sound usually heard on expiration but may be heard on inspiration depending on the cause	Associated with bronchial wall oscillation and narrowed airway diameter or partially obstructed airway Associated with chronic bronchitis or bronchiectasis
Rhonchi	Deep, lower-pitched rumbling sounds, snoring quality, heard primarily during expiration; may clear with coughing	Associated with secretions or tumor; variant of a wheeze; caused by air moving through narrowed tracheobronchial passages
Friction Rubs		
Pleural friction rub	Discontinuous, low-pitched, rubbing or grating sound, like two pieces of leather being rubbed together (sound imitated by rubbing thumb and finger together near the ear) Heard during inspiration and expiration May subside when patient holds breath; coughing will not clear sound Best heard in axillae and bases of lungs	Secondary to inflammation and loss of lubricating pleural fluid between the visceral and parietal pleurae
Other Breath Sounds		
Stridor	Continuous, high-pitched, musical sound, heard over the neck	Narrowing of the upper respiratory tract; immediate intervention is warranted

Adapted from Hogan-Quigley, B., Palm, M. L., & Bickley, L. (2017). *Bates' nursing guide to physical examination and history taking* (2nd ed.). Philadelphia, PA: Wolters Kluwer Health Lippincott Williams & Wilkins.

- **Whispered pectoriloquy** describes the ability to clearly and distinctly hear whispered sounds that should not normally be heard.

Whenever an abnormality is detected on examination, it should be evident using more than one assessment method. A change in tactile fremitus is more subtle and can be missed, but bronchophony can be noted loudly and clearly.

Interpreting Findings

The physical findings for the most common respiratory diseases are summarized in Table 17-7.

Assessment of Respiratory Function in the Patient Who Is Acutely or Critically Ill

Assessment of respiratory status is essential for the well-being of the patient who is acutely or critically ill. Often, such a patient is intubated and receiving mechanical ventilation. The nurse analyzes findings from the health history and assessment while considering laboratory and diagnostic test results. After checking the ventilator settings to make sure that they are set as prescribed and that alarms are always in the "on" position, the nurse must assess for patient–ventilator synchrony and for agitation, restlessness, and other signs of respiratory distress (nasal flaring, excessive use of intercostals and accessory muscles, uncoordinated movement of the chest and abdomen, and a report by the patient of shortness of breath). The nurse must note changes in the patient's vital signs and evidence of hemodynamic instability and report them to the primary provider, because they may indicate that the mechanical ventilation is ineffective or that the patient's status has deteriorated. It is important for the nurse to position the patient to promote adequate oxygenation and ventilation and to prevent potential complications. For example, the patient may need to be positioned with the head of bed elevated to prevent aspiration, especially if the patient is receiving enteral feedings. Alternatively, in patients with ARDS who are experiencing refractory hypoxemia, prone positioning is recommended (see Chapter 19). In addition, the patient's mental status should be assessed and compared to previous status. Lethargy and somnolence may be signs of increasing carbon dioxide levels and should not be considered insignificant, even if the patient is receiving sedation or analgesic agents.

Chest auscultation, percussion, and palpation are essential and routine parts of the evaluation of the patient who is critically ill, with or without mechanical ventilation. A recumbent patient must be turned to assess all lung fields. Dependent areas must be assessed for normal breath sounds and adventitious sounds. Failure to examine the dependent areas of the lungs can result in missing the findings associated with disorders such as atelectasis or pleural effusion.

TABLE 17-7	Assessment Findings in Common Respiratory Disorders

This table lists the typical changes seen in respiratory disorders. The changes described vary with the extent and severity of the disorder. Use the table for the direction of typical changes, not for absolute distinctions.

Condition	Percussion Note	Trachea	Breath Sounds	Adventitious Sounds	Tactile Fremitus and Transmitted Voice Sounds
Normal The tracheobronchial tree and alveoli are open; pleurae are thin and close together; mobility of the chest wall is unimpaired.	Resonant	Midline	Vesicular, except perhaps bronchovesicular and bronchial sounds over the large bronchi and trachea, respectively	None, except perhaps a few transient inspiratory crackles at the bases of the lungs	Normal
Chronic Bronchitis The bronchi are chronically inflamed and a productive cough is present. Airway obstruction may develop.	Resonant	Midline	Vesicular (normal)	None; or scattered coarse crackles in early inspiration and perhaps expiration; or wheezes or rhonchi	Normal
Left-Sided Heart Failure (Early) Increased pressure in the pulmonary veins causes congestion and interstitial edema (around the alveoli); bronchial mucosa may become edematous.	Resonant	Midline	Vesicular	Late inspiratory crackles in the dependent portions of the lungs; possibly wheezes	Normal
Lobar Pneumonia Alveoli fill with fluid or blood cells, as in pneumonia, pulmonary edema, or pulmonary hemorrhage.	Dull over the airless area	Midline	Bronchial over the involved area	Late inspiratory crackles over the involved area	Increased over the involved area, with bronchophony, egophony, and whispered pectoriloquy
Partial Lobar Obstruction Atelectasis When a plug in a mainstem bronchus (as from mucus or a foreign object) obstructs bronchial air flow, affected alveoli collapse and become airless.	Dull over the airless area	May be shifted toward involved side	Usually absent when bronchial plug persists. Exceptions include right upper lobe atelectasis, where adjacent tracheal sounds may be transmitted	None	Usually absent when the bronchial plug persists. In exceptions (e.g., right upper lobe atelectasis) may be increased
Pleural Effusion Fluid accumulates in the pleural space and separates air-filled lung from the chest wall, blocking the transmission breath sounds.	Dull to flat over the fluid	Shifted toward the unaffected side in a large effusion	Decreased to absent, but bronchial breath sounds may be heard near top of large effusion	None, except a possible pleural rub	Decreased to absent, but may be increased toward the top of a large effusion
Pneumothorax When air leaks into the pleural space, usually unilaterally, the lung recoils away from the chest wall. Pleural air blocks transmission of sound.	Hyperresonant or tympanitic over the pleural air	Shifted toward the unaffected side if tension pneumothorax	Decreased to absent over the pleural air	None, except a possible pleural rub	Decreased to absent over the pleural air
Chronic Obstructive Pulmonary Disease (COPD) Slowly progressive disorder in which the distal airspaces enlarge and lungs become hyperinflated. Chronic inflammation may precede or follow the development of COPD.	Diffusely hyperresonant	Midline	Decreased to absent with delayed expiration	None, or the crackles, wheezes, and rhonchi of associated chronic bronchitis	Decreased

TABLE 17-7	Assessment Findings in Common Respiratory Disorders (continued)				
Condition	Percussion Note	Trachea	Breath Sounds	Adventitious Sounds	Tactile Fremitus and Transmitted Voice Sounds
Asthma Widespread usually reversible airflow obstruction with bronchial hyper-responsiveness and underlying inflammation. During attacks, as air flow decreases lungs hyperinflate.	Resonant to diffusely hyperresonant	Midline	Often obscured by wheezes	Wheezes, possibly crackles	Decreased

Reprinted with permission from Hogan-Quigley, B., Palm, M. L., & Bickley, L. (2017). *Bates' nursing guide to physical examination and history taking table* (2nd ed., Table 13-8). Philadelphia, PA: Wolters Kluwer.

Tests of the patient's respiratory status are easily performed at the bedside by measuring the respiratory rate, end-tidal carbon dioxide (ETCO₂), tidal volume, minute ventilation, vital capacity, inspiratory force, and compliance. These tests are particularly important for patients who are at risk for pulmonary complications, including those who have undergone chest or abdominal surgery, have had prolonged anesthesia, or have preexisting pulmonary disease, and those who are older or have obesity. These tests are also used routinely for patients who are mechanically ventilated. Although some of these tests are performed by respiratory therapists, it is useful for nurses to understand the significance of these test results.

The patient whose chest expansion is limited by external restrictions such as obesity or abdominal distention, or who cannot breathe deeply because of postoperative pain, sedation, or drug overdose will inhale and exhale a low volume of air (referred to as low tidal volumes). Prolonged hypoventilation at low tidal volumes can produce alveolar collapse (atelectasis). Consequently, when the forced residual capacity decreases, compliance is reduced, and the patient must breathe faster to maintain the same degree of tissue oxygenation. These events can be exaggerated in patients who have preexisting pulmonary diseases; in older adult patients whose airways are less compliant because the small airways may collapse during expiration; or in patients with obesity or who have relatively low tidal volumes even when healthy. (More details of the assessment of the patient with various lung disorders are described in subsequent chapters in this unit.)

> ### Quality and Safety Nursing Alert
>
> *The nurse should not rely only on visual inspection of the rate and depth of a patient's respiratory excursions to determine the adequacy of ventilation. Respiratory excursions may appear normal or exaggerated due to an increased work of breathing, but the patient may actually be moving only enough air to ventilate the dead space. If there is any question regarding adequacy of ventilation, the nurse should use auscultation or pulse oximetry (or both) for additional assessment of respiratory status.*

Tidal Volume

The volume of each breath is referred to as the **tidal volume** (see Table 17-1 to review lung capacities and volumes). A spirometer is an instrument that can be used at the bedside to measure volumes. If the patient is breathing through an endotracheal (ET) tube or tracheostomy, the spirometer is directly attached to it and the exhaled volume is obtained from the reading on the gauge. In other patients, the spirometer is attached to a facemask or a mouthpiece positioned so that it is airtight, and the exhaled volume is measured.

The tidal volume may vary from breath to breath. To ensure that the measurement is reliable, it is important to measure the volumes of several breaths and to note the range of tidal volumes, together with the average tidal volume.

Minute Ventilation

Because respiratory rates and tidal volumes vary widely from breath to breath, these data alone are unreliable indicators of adequate ventilation. However, the tidal volume multiplied by the respiratory rate provides what is called *minute ventilation* or *minute volume*, the volume of air exchanged per minute. This value is useful in detecting respiratory failure. In practice, the minute volume is not calculated but is measured directly using a spirometer. In a patient receiving mechanical ventilation, minute volume is often monitored by the ventilator and can be viewed on the monitoring screen.

Minute ventilation may be decreased by a variety of conditions that result in hypoventilation. When the minute ventilation falls, alveolar ventilation in the lungs also decreases and the PaCO₂ increases.

Vital Capacity

Vital capacity is measured by having the patient take in a maximal breath and exhale fully through a spirometer. The normal value depends on the patient's age, gender, body build, and weight.

> ### Quality and Safety Nursing Alert
>
> *Most patients can generate a vital capacity twice the volume they normally breathe in and out (tidal volume). If the vital capacity is less than 10 mL/kg, the patient will be unable to sustain spontaneous ventilation and will require respiratory assistance.*

When the vital capacity is exhaled at a maximal flow rate, the forced vital capacity (FVC) is measured. Most patients can exhale at least 80% of their vital capacity in 1 second (forced expiratory volume in 1 second, or FEV₁) and almost all of it in 3 seconds (FEV₃). A reduction in FEV₁ suggests abnormal pulmonary airflow. If the patient's FEV_1 and FVC are proportionately reduced, maximal lung expansion is restricted in some way. If the reduction in FEV_1 greatly exceeds the reduction in FVC (FEV_1/FVC less than 85%), the patient may have some degree of airway obstruction.

Inspiratory Force

Inspiratory force evaluates the effort the patient is making during inspiration. It does not require patient cooperation and, therefore, is a useful measurement in the patient who is unconscious. The equipment needed for this measurement includes a manometer that measures negative pressure and adapters that are connected to an anesthesia mask or a cuffed ET tube. The manometer is attached, and the airway is completely occluded for 10 to 20 seconds while the inspiratory efforts of the patient are registered on the manometer. The normal inspiratory pressure is about 100 cm H_2O. If the negative pressure registered after 15 seconds of occluding the airway is less than about 25 cm H_2O, mechanical ventilation is usually required because the patient lacks sufficient muscle strength for deep breathing or effective coughing.

Diagnostic Evaluation

A wide range of diagnostic studies may be performed in patients with respiratory conditions. The nurse should educate the patient on the purpose of the studies, what to expect, and any possible side effects related to these examinations prior to testing. The nurse should note trends in results because they provide information about disease progression as well as the patient's response to therapy.

Pulmonary Function Tests

Pulmonary function tests (PFTs) are routinely used in patients with chronic respiratory disorders to aid diagnosis. They are performed to assess respiratory function and to determine the extent of dysfunction, response to therapy, and as screening tests in potentially hazardous industries, such as coal mining and those that involve exposure to asbestos and other noxious irritants. PFTs are also used prior to surgery to screen patients who are scheduled for thoracic and upper abdominal surgical procedures, patients who are obese, and symptomatic patients with a history suggesting high risk. Such tests include measurements of lung volumes, ventilatory function, and the mechanics of breathing, diffusion, and gas exchange.

PFTs generally are performed by a respiratory therapist using a spirometer that has a volume-collecting device attached to a recorder that demonstrates volume and time simultaneously. Several tests are carried out because no single measurement provides a complete picture of pulmonary function. The most frequently used PFTs are described in Table 17-8. Technology is available that allows for more complex assessment of pulmonary function. Methods include exercise tidal flow–volume loops, negative expiratory pressure, nitric oxide, forced oscillation, and diffusing capacity for helium or carbon monoxide. These assessment methods allow for detailed evaluation of expiratory flow limitations and airway inflammation (Pagana, Pagana, & Pagana, 2017).

PFT results are interpreted on the basis of the degree of deviation from normal, taking into consideration the patient's height, weight, age, gender, and ethnicity. Because there is a wide range of normal values, PFTs may not detect early localized changes. The patient with respiratory symptoms usually undergoes a complete diagnostic evaluation, even if the results of PFTs are "normal." Patients with respiratory disorders may be taught how to measure their peak flow rate (which reflects maximal expiratory flow) at home using a spirometer. This allows them to monitor the progress of therapy, to alter medications and other interventions as needed on the basis of caregiver guidelines, and to notify the primary

TABLE 17-8	Pulmonary Function Tests		
Term Used	**Symbol**	**Description**	**Remarks**
Forced vital capacity	FVC	Vital capacity performed with a maximally forced expiratory effort	Forced vital capacity is often reduced in chronic obstructive pulmonary disease because of air trapping
Forced expiratory volume (qualified by subscript indicating the time interval in seconds)	FEV_t (usually FEV_1)	Volume of air exhaled in the specified time during the performance of forced vital capacity; FEV_1 is volume exhaled in 1 s	A valuable clue to the severity of the expiratory airway obstruction
Ratio of timed forced expiratory volume to forced vital capacity	FEV_t/FVC%, usually FEV_1/FVC%	FEV_t expressed as a percentage of the forced vital capacity	Another way of expressing the presence or absence of airway obstruction
Forced expiratory flow	$FEF_{200-1200}$	Mean forced expiratory flow between 200 and 1200 mL of the FVC	An indicator of large airway obstruction
Forced midexpiratory flow	$FEF_{25-75\%}$	Mean forced expiratory flow during the middle half of the FVC	Slowed in small airway obstruction
Forced end-expiratory flow	$FEF_{75-85\%}$	Mean forced expiratory flow during the terminal portion of the FVC	Slowed in obstruction of smallest airways
Maximal voluntary ventilation	MVV	Volume of air expired in a specified period (12 s) during repetitive maximal effort	An important factor in exercise tolerance

Adapted from Fishbach, F. T., & Fishbach, M. A. (2018). *Fishbach's a manual of laboratory and diagnostic tests* (10th ed.). Philadelphia, PA: Wolters Kluwer.

provider if there is inadequate response to their own interventions. (Instructions for home care education are described in Chapter 20, which discusses asthma.)

Arterial Blood Gas Studies

Arterial blood gas (ABG) studies aid in assessing the ability of the lungs to provide adequate oxygen and remove carbon dioxide, which reflects ventilation, and the ability of the kidneys to reabsorb or excrete bicarbonate ions to maintain normal body pH, which reflects metabolic states. ABG levels are obtained through an arterial puncture at the radial, brachial, or femoral artery or through an indwelling arterial catheter. Pain (related to nerve injury or noxious stimulation), infection, hematoma, and hemorrhage are potential complications that may be associated with obtaining ABGs (Pagana et al., 2017) (see Chapter 10 for discussion of ABG analysis).

Venous Blood Gas Studies

Venous blood gas (VBG) studies provide additional data on oxygen delivery and consumption. VBG levels reflect the balance between the amount of oxygen used by tissues and organs and the amount of oxygen returning to the right side of the heart in the blood. VBG levels can be obtained by drawing blood from the venous circulation; this test is performed to provide an estimation of this balance when the ability to draw ABGs is not feasible. Mixed venous oxygen saturation ($S\bar{v}O_2$) levels, the most accurate indicator of this balance, can be obtained only from blood samples drawn from a pulmonary artery catheter. However, central venous oxygen saturation ($Sc\bar{v}O_2$) levels, which are measured using blood drawn from a central venous catheter placed in the superior vena cava, closely approximate $S\bar{v}O_2$ levels and are, therefore, useful as an alternative measure in patients without pulmonary artery catheters (Morton, Reck, & Headly, 2018).

Pulse Oximetry

Pulse oximetry, or SpO_2, is a noninvasive method of continuously monitoring the oxygen saturation of hemoglobin (SaO_2). Although pulse oximetry does not replace blood gas analysis, it is an effective tool to monitor for changes in SaO_2 and can easily be used in the home and various health care settings.

A probe or sensor is attached to the fingertip (Fig. 17-13), forehead, earlobe, or bridge of the nose. The sensor detects changes in oxygen saturation levels by monitoring light signals generated by the oximeter and reflected by blood pulsing through the tissue at the probe. Normal SpO_2 values are more than 95%. Values less than 90% indicate that the tissues are not receiving enough oxygen, in which case further evaluation is needed. Advantages of pulse oximetry include the ability to obtain rapid results and continuous data using a noninvasive technique. Limitations of pulse oximetry include its inability to detect significant hyperoxemia (excess levels of oxygen), and to measure PaO_2 and ventilation. In order to ensure accurate readings, the nurse should verify correct placement of the probe and decrease or eliminate excess motion (e.g., from patient shivering or movement of the extremity). Readings are unreliable in settings of hypothermia, hemodynamic instability, or low perfusion states (e.g.,

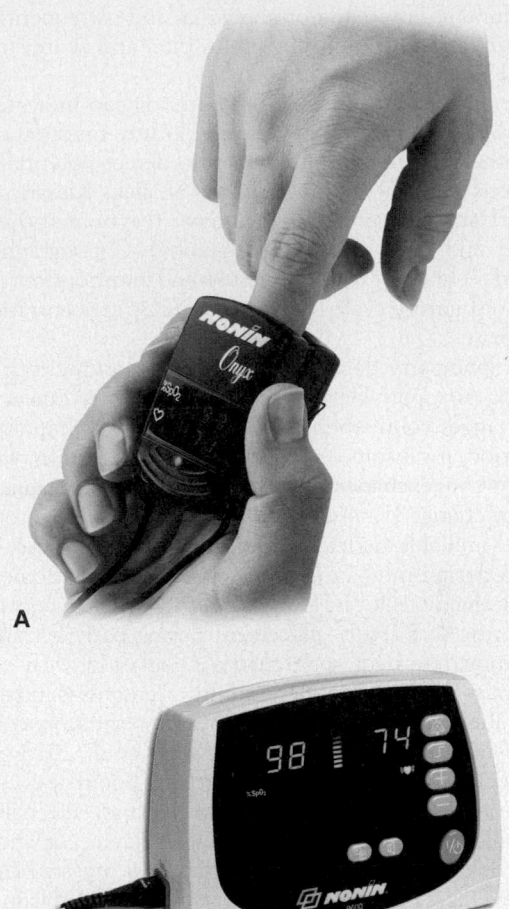

A

B

Figure 17-13 • Measuring blood oxygenation with pulse oximetry reduces the need for invasive procedures, such as drawing blood for analysis of oxygen levels. **A.** Self-contained digital fingertip pulse oximeter, which incorporates the sensor and the display into one unit. **B.** Tabletop model with sensor attached. Memory permits tracking heart rate and oxygen saturation over time.

shock, vasoconstriction, or decreased perfusion of the limb), and when a patient has dark skin or is wearing nail polish. In these situations, analysis of ABGs should be conducted, and when hyperoxemia is suspected, analysis of PaO_2 or $PaCO_2$ is required (Mechem, 2019).

End-Tidal Carbon Dioxide

End-tidal carbon dioxide ($ETCO_2$) monitoring is a noninvasive method of monitoring partial pressure of carbon dioxide (CO_2) at end exhalation. $ETCO_2$ monitoring is considered to be a reliable tool for detecting and monitoring life-threatening conditions because it provides immediate information about ventilation, perfusion, and metabolism by determining the concentration of CO_2. Changes in $ETCO_2$ and the concentration of CO_2 at the end of each breath can help to diagnose or indicate the severity of a disease or the outcome of a treatment. It is now part of the standard of care for all patients receiving general anesthesia, procedural sedation and/or analgesia, and is frequently part of routine monitoring in the prehospital and acute care settings (Krauss, Falk, & Ladde, 2018).

The application of $ETCO_2$ monitoring can indicate early respiratory depression and impaired airway function sooner than other devices, helping nurses to detect potential complications earlier (Aminiahidashti, Shafiee, Kiasari, et al., 2018). Data are reported as a number (capnometry) or as a number and a waveform (capnography). Capnography uses infrared technology to obtain results and monitors four phases of the respiratory cycle to depict the CO_2 concentrations of each phase.

A capnometry device, such as the colorimetric $ETCO_2$ detector, is a portable device which contains litmus paper that changes color when exposed to CO_2. An improper ET intubation, for instance with esophageal intubation, will not result in CO_2 exchange and thus the color of the litmus paper will not change (Krauss et al., 2018). $ETCO_2$ monitoring is the most reliable indicator that an ET tube is placed in the trachea during intubation (Krauss et al., 2018). Some additional indications for $ETCO_2$ monitoring include continuous monitoring of ET tube placement during patient transport, confirming return of spontaneous circulation with cardiopulmonary resuscitation, determining a prognosis in patients with trauma, and as an early indicator of respiratory compromise (Aminiahidashti et al., 2018; Krauss et al., 2018; Smallwood & Walsh, 2017). The clinician should use caution when interpreting results in patients who are mechanically ventilated with a bag or mask ventilation device, or who have received sodium bicarbonate, or who have ingested carbonated beverages or antacids, as any of these can result in false-positive results (Aminiahidashti et al., 2018).

Cultures

Throat, nasal, and nasopharyngeal cultures can identify pathogens responsible for respiratory infections, such as pharyngitis. Throat cultures are performed in adults with severe or ongoing sore throats accompanied by fever and lymph node enlargement and are most useful in detecting streptococcal infection. Rapid strep tests are now available that can provide results within 15 minutes, often replacing the need for throat cultures. Other sources of infection, such as *Staphylococcus aureus* or *Influenza*, are detected via nasal or nasopharyngeal cultures. Ideally, all cultures should be obtained prior to the initiation of antibiotic therapy. Results usually take between 48 and 72 hours, with preliminary reports available usually within 24 hours. Cultures may be repeated to assess a patient's response to therapy (Pagana et al., 2017).

Sputum Studies

Sputum is obtained for analysis to identify pathogenic organisms and to determine whether malignant cells are present. Periodic sputum examinations may be necessary for patients receiving antibiotics, corticosteroids, and immunosuppressive medications for prolonged periods because these agents are associated with opportunistic infections.

Sputum samples ideally are obtained early in the morning before the patient has had anything to eat or drink. The patient is instructed to clear the nose and the throat and rinse the mouth to decrease contamination of the sputum and not to simply spit saliva into the container. Rather, after taking a few deep breaths, the patient coughs deeply and expectorates sputum from the lungs into a sterile container.

If the patient cannot expel an adequate sputum sample following the above techniques, coughing can be induced by administering an aerosolized hypertonic solution via a nebulizer. Other methods of collecting sputum specimens include endotracheal or transtracheal aspiration or bronchoscopic removal. The nurse should label the specimen and send it to the laboratory as soon as possible to avoid contamination.

Imaging Studies

Imaging studies, including x-rays, computed tomography (CT), magnetic resonance imaging (MRI), and radioisotope or nuclear scanning may be part of any diagnostic workup, ranging from a determination of the extent of infection in sinusitis to tumor growth in cancer.

Chest X-Ray

Normal pulmonary tissue is radiolucent because it consists mostly of air and gases; therefore, densities produced by fluid, tumors, foreign bodies, and other pathologic conditions can be detected by x-ray examination. In the absence of symptoms, a chest x-ray may reveal an extensive pathologic process in the lungs. The routine chest x-ray consists of two views: the posteroanterior projection and the lateral projection. Chest x-rays are usually obtained after full inspiration because the lungs are best visualized when they are well aerated. In addition, the diaphragm is at its lowest level and the largest expanse of lung is visible. Patients, therefore, need to be able to take a deep breath and hold it without discomfort. Chest x-rays are contraindicated in pregnant women.

Nursing Interventions

The nurse should notify the patient that chest x-rays do not require fasting, nor typically cause pain. However, in order to best visualize the lungs, the patient must be able to take a deep breath and hold it without discomfort, while the technician takes the images. The patient will be positioned in a standing, sitting, or recumbent position, in order to obtain the appropriate view of the chest (posterior–anterior, lateral, oblique, or decubitus position). The patient will be asked to wear a gown, remove metal objects from the chest, such as necklaces, and may be given a lead shield to minimize radiation exposure to the thyroid gland, ovaries, or testicles (Pagana et al., 2017).

Computed Tomography

A CT of the chest is an imaging method in which the lungs, mediastinum, and vascular structures within the chest are scanned in successive layers by a narrow-beam x-ray. The images produced provide a cross-sectional view of the chest. Whereas a chest x-ray shows major contrasts between body densities such as bone, soft tissue, and air, a CT scan can distinguish fine tissue density. A CT scan may be used to define pulmonary nodules and small tumors adjacent to pleural surfaces that are not visible on routine chest x-rays and to demonstrate mediastinal abnormalities and hilar adenopathy, which are difficult to visualize with other techniques. Contrast agents are useful when evaluating the mediastinum and its contents, particularly its vasculature. CT with contrast agent is not suitable for patients with compromised kidney function, or those with an allergy to iodine dye or shellfish, or who are pregnant, claustrophobic, or have severe obesity. Patients taking metformin should withhold the dose the day of the test in order to prevent lactic acidosis from developing (Pagana et al., 2017; Thompson & Kabrhel, 2018).

Advancements in CT scanning technology, referred to as multidetection, spiral, or helical CT, enable the chest to be scanned quickly while generating an extensive number of images that can generate a three-dimensional analysis (Pagana et al., 2017).

Nursing Interventions

The nurse should inform patients preparing for CT scans that they will be required to remain supine and still for a short period, typically less than 30 minutes, while a body scanner surrounds them and takes multiple images. Patients typically do not experience claustrophobia during CT scanning but can be given antianxiety medications preprocedure if this is a concern. If contrast agent is required, patients will need to stay *nil per os* (NPO) for 4 hours prior to the examination. In this case, the nurse should also assess for allergies to iodine or shellfish (Pagana et al., 2017). Vital signs should be monitored and documented before, during, and after the scan especially if sedation or analgesia is administered.

Pulmonary Angiography

Pulmonary angiography is used to investigate congenital abnormalities of the pulmonary vascular tree, and less frequently PE, when less invasive tests are inconclusive. This study has primarily been replaced by CT scan of the chest. To visualize the pulmonary vessels, a radiopaque agent is injected through a catheter, which has been initially inserted into a vein (e.g., jugular, subclavian, brachial, or femoral vein) and then threaded into the pulmonary artery. Contraindications include allergy to the radiopaque agent, pregnancy, and bleeding abnormalities, whereas potential complications include acute kidney injury, acidosis, cardiac arrhythmias, and bleeding (Pagana et al., 2017).

CT pulmonary angiography (CTPA) combines pulmonary angiography and CT scan imaging. CTPA images the pulmonary arteries and is used primarily if treatment is required for a PE. This procedure typically takes no longer than 30 minutes to complete (Pagana et al., 2017). The patient lies in a supine position on an x-ray table. A catheter is placed in the femoral vein, advanced into the inferior vena cava and into the pulmonary artery. Contrast agent and fluoroscopy are utilized for visualization of the pulmonary vasculature when CTPA is performed. The same contraindications for CT with contrast agent apply to CTPA (Pagana et al., 2017; Thompson & Kabrhel, 2018).

Nursing Interventions

Prior to the angiography, the nurse should verify that informed consent has been obtained; assess for known allergies that may suggest allergies to radiopaque agent (e.g., iodine and shellfish); assess anticoagulation status and renal function; ensure that the patient has not eaten or had anything to drink preprocedurally as prescribed (normally for 4 hours); and administer preprocedure medications that may include antianxiety medications, secretion-reducing agents, and antihistamines (Pagana et al., 2017). The nurse should instruct patients that they may experience a warm flushing sensation or chest pain during the injection of the dye. If an arterial puncture is necessary, the affected extremity will need to be immobilized for a certain amount of time depending on the size of the sheath used and the type of arterial closure device employed. Introduction of the catheter into the right ventricle may trigger ventricular irritability. Therefore, during and after the procedure, the patient should be monitored for cardiac arrhythmias such as premature ventricular contractions (PVCs). Following the procedure, the nurse should closely monitor vital signs, level of consciousness, oxygen saturation, and the vascular access site for bleeding or hematoma, and perform frequent assessment of neurovascular status. It may be indicated to apply cold compresses to the puncture site to decrease swelling (Pagana et al., 2017).

Magnetic Resonance Imaging

MRI is similar to a CT scan except that magnetic fields and radiofrequency signals are used instead of radiation. MRI is able to better distinguish between normal and abnormal tissues than CT and, therefore, yields a much more detailed diagnostic image. MRI is used to characterize pulmonary nodules; to help stage bronchogenic carcinoma (assessment of chest wall invasion); and to evaluate inflammatory activity in interstitial lung disease, acute PE, and chronic thrombolytic pulmonary hypertension. Contraindications for MRI include severe obesity, claustrophobia, confusion and agitation, and having implanted metal or metal support devices that are considered unsafe (Pagana et al., 2017). Various labels and icons are used to indicate whether a medical device is safe or unsafe for use during MRI. Recent improvements in technology have contributed to the design of certain medical devices, such as infusion pumps and ventilators, deemed safe for the MRI room. The nurse should consult with specially trained MRI personnel to clarify the safety of various devices (Wells & Murphy, 2014). Gadolinium-based contrast agents used during MRI may potentially lead to nephrogenic systemic fibrosis in patients with reduced kidney function. Therefore, additional kidney function testing may be necessary, especially in adults older than 60 years of age (Pagana et al., 2017).

Nursing Interventions

Patients scheduled for MRI should be instructed to remove all metal items such as hearing aids, hair clips, and medication patches with metallic foil components (e.g., nicotine patches). Prior to the MRI, the nurse should assess for the presence of implanted metal devices, such as aneurysm clips or a cardiac implantable electronic device. Patients with any type of cardiac implantable electronic device need to be screened to determine if they can safely undergo MRI (Indik, Gimbel, Abe, et al., 2017).

The nurse should inform patients preparing for MRI that they will need to lie flat and remain still for between 30 and 90 minutes, while the table that they are on moves into a large tubular magnet. Patients should be notified that they will hear a loud humming or thumping noise. Earplugs are typically offered to patients to minimize this noise. Patients will be able to communicate with the MRI staff via a microphone and earphones. The nurse should clarify with the primary provider or the technologist if the prescribed test requires the use of a contrast agent or if the patient should remain NPO pre-examination. Patients who experience claustrophobia should be offered antianxiety medications preprocedure or be scheduled at a facility that uses an open MRI system (Pagana et al., 2017).

Fluoroscopic Studies

Fluoroscopy, which allows live x-ray images to be generated via a camera to a video screen, is used to assist with invasive procedures, such as a chest needle biopsy or transbronchial biopsy, that are performed to identify lesions. It also may be used to study the movement of the chest wall, mediastinum, heart, and diaphragm; to detect diaphragm paralysis; and to locate lung masses. The specific procedure performed under fluoroscopy will guide those respective nursing interventions (e.g., see nursing interventions described in the Lung Biopsy Procedures section).

Radioisotope Diagnostic Procedures (Lung Scans)

Several types of lung scans—$\dot{V}/\dot{Q}$ scan, gallium scan, and positron emission tomography (PET)—are performed to assess normal lung functioning, pulmonary vascular supply, and gas exchange. Pregnancy is a contraindication for these scans.

A $\dot{V}/\dot{Q}$ lung scan is performed by injecting a radioactive agent into a peripheral vein and then obtaining a scan of the chest to detect radiation. The isotope particles pass through the right side of the heart and are distributed into the lungs in proportion to the regional blood flow, making it possible to trace and measure blood perfusion through the lung. This procedure is used clinically to measure the integrity of the pulmonary vessels relative to blood flow and to evaluate blood flow abnormalities, as seen in PE. The imaging time is 20 to 40 minutes, during which the patient lies under the camera with a mask fitted over the nose and the mouth. This is followed by the ventilation component of the scan. The patient takes a deep breath of a mixture of oxygen and radioactive gas, which diffuses throughout the lungs. A scan is performed to detect ventilation abnormalities in patients who have regional differences in ventilation. It may be helpful in the diagnosis of bronchitis, asthma, inflammatory fibrosis, pneumonia, emphysema, and lung cancer. Ventilation without perfusion is seen with PE.

A gallium scan is a radioisotope lung scan used to detect inflammatory conditions, abscesses, adhesions, and the presence, location, and size of tumors. It is used to stage bronchogenic cancer and to document tumor regression after chemotherapy or radiation. Gallium is injected intravenously, and scans are obtained at intervals (e.g., 6, 24, and 48 hours) to evaluate gallium uptake by the pulmonary tissues.

PET is a radioisotope study with advanced diagnostic capabilities that is used to evaluate lung nodules for malignancy. PET can detect and display metabolic changes in tissue, distinguish normal tissue from diseased tissue (such as in cancer), differentiate viable from dead or dying tissue, and show regional blood flow. PET is more accurate in detecting malignancies than CT and has equivalent accuracy in detecting malignant nodules when compared with invasive procedures such as thoracoscopy. Images from PET scans are now being superimposed on CT and MRI images to enhance the accuracy of diagnosis (Pagana et al., 2017).

Nursing Interventions

For each of these nuclear scans, the nurse should educate the patient on what to expect. Intravenous access is required. Chest x-ray should be performed prior to a $\dot{V}/\dot{Q}$ scan. Patients should be told that $\dot{V}/\dot{Q}$ and gallium scans require only a small amount of radioisotopes; therefore, radiation safety measures are not indicated. Normally, the patient may eat or drink prior to $\dot{V}/\dot{Q}$ or gallium scans. Multiple factors can hinder the uptake of radioactive agents used for a PET scan. The nurse should instruct the patient to avoid caffeine, alcohol, and tobacco for 24 hours prior to the PET scan and abstain from food and fluids for 4 hours prior to the scan. Accurate results depend on an empty bladder; thus, a Foley catheter may be indicated. The nurse should encourage fluid intake postprocedure to facilitate the elimination of radioisotopes in the urine (Pagana et al., 2017).

Endoscopic Procedures

Endoscopic procedures include bronchoscopy, thoracoscopy, and thoracentesis.

Bronchoscopy

Bronchoscopy is the direct inspection and examination of the larynx, trachea, and bronchi through either a flexible fiberoptic bronchoscope or a rigid bronchoscope (Fig. 17-14). The fiberoptic scope is used more frequently in current practice.

Procedure

The purposes of diagnostic bronchoscopy are (1) to visualize tissues and determine the nature, location, and extent of the pathologic process; (2) to collect secretions for analysis and to obtain a tissue sample for diagnosis; (3) to determine whether a tumor can be resected surgically; and (4) to diagnose sources of hemoptysis.

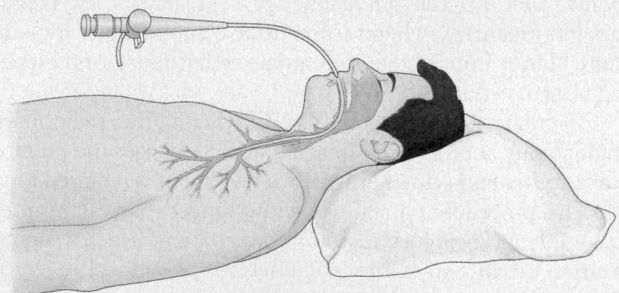

Fiberoptic bronchoscopy

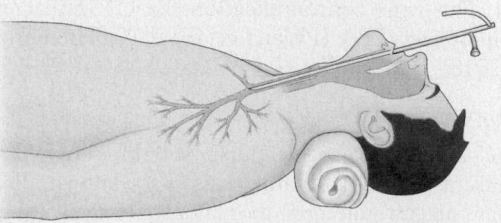

Rigid bronchoscopy

Figure 17-14 • Endoscopic bronchoscopy permits visualization of bronchial structures. The bronchoscope is advanced into bronchial structures orally. Bronchoscopy permits the clinician to not only diagnose but also treat various lung problems.

Therapeutic bronchoscopy is used to (1) remove foreign bodies or secretions from the tracheobronchial tree, (2) control bleeding, (3) treat postoperative atelectasis, (4) destroy and excise lesions, and (5) provide brachytherapy (endobronchial radiation therapy). It has also been used to insert stents to relieve airway obstruction that is caused by tumors or miscellaneous benign conditions or that occurs as a complication of lung transplantation.

The fiberoptic bronchoscope is a thin, flexible bronchoscope that can be directed into the segmental bronchi. Because of its small size, its flexibility, and its excellent optical system, it allows increased visualization of the peripheral airways and is ideal for diagnosing pulmonary lesions. Fiberoptic bronchoscopy allows biopsy of previously inaccessible tumors and can be performed at the bedside. It also can be performed through ET or tracheostomy tubes of patients on ventilators. Cytologic examinations can be performed without surgical intervention.

The rigid bronchoscope is a hollow metal tube with a light at its end. It is used mainly for removing foreign substances, investigating the source of massive hemoptysis, or performing endobronchial surgical procedures. Rigid bronchoscopy is performed in the operating room, not at the bedside.

Possible complications of bronchoscopy include a reaction to the local anesthetic, oversedation, prolonged fever, infection, aspiration, vasovagal response, laryngospasm, bronchospasm, hypoxemia, pneumothorax, and bleeding (Pagana et al., 2017).

Nursing Interventions

Before the procedure, the nurse should verify that informed consent has been obtained. Food and fluids are withheld for 4 to 8 hours before the test to reduce the risk of aspiration when the cough reflex is blocked by anesthesia. The patient must remove dentures and other oral prostheses. The nurse explains the procedure to the patient to reduce fear and decrease anxiety and then administers preoperative medications (usually atropine and a sedative or opioid) as prescribed to inhibit vagal stimulation (thereby guarding against bradycardia, arrhythmias, and hypotension), suppress the cough reflex, sedate the patient, and relieve anxiety.

> ► *Quality and Safety Nursing Alert*
>
> *Sedation given to patients with respiratory insufficiency may precipitate respiratory arrest.*

The examination is usually performed under local anesthesia or moderate sedation; however, general anesthesia may be used for rigid bronchoscopy. A topical anesthetic such as lidocaine is normally sprayed on the pharynx or dropped on the epiglottis and vocal cords and into the trachea to suppress the cough reflex and minimize discomfort.

After the procedure, the patient must take nothing by mouth until the cough reflex returns, because the preoperative sedation and local anesthesia impair the protective laryngeal reflex and swallowing. Once the patient demonstrates a cough reflex, the nurse may offer ice chips and eventually fluids. In the older adult patient, the nurse assesses for confusion and lethargy, which may be owing to the large doses of lidocaine given during the procedure. The nurse also monitors

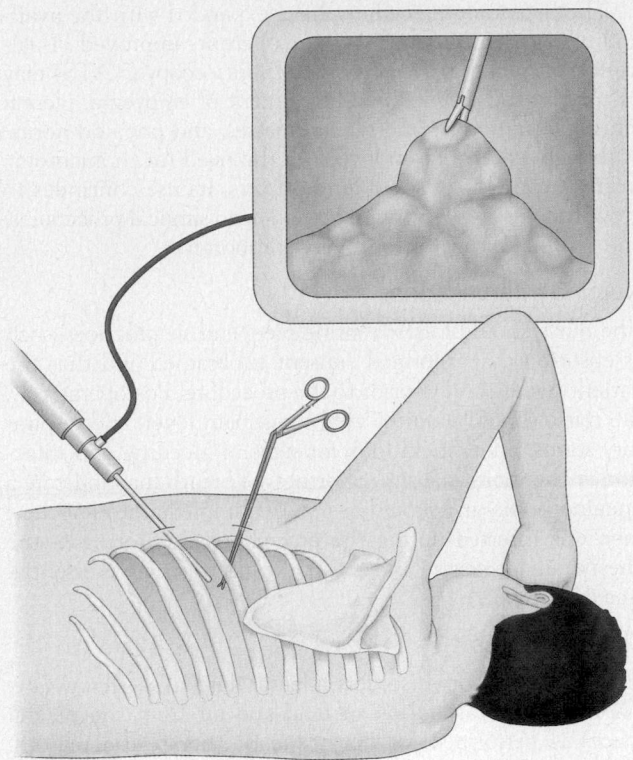

Figure 17-15 • Endoscopic thoracoscopy. Like bronchoscopy, thoracoscopy uses fiberoptic instruments and video cameras for visualizing thoracic structures. Unlike bronchoscopy, thoracoscopy usually requires the surgeon to make a small incision before inserting the endoscope. A combined diagnostic–treatment procedure, thoracoscopy includes excising tissue for biopsy.

the patient's respiratory status and observes for hypoxia, hypotension, tachycardia, arrhythmias, hemoptysis, and dyspnea. Any abnormality is reported promptly. A small amount of blood-tinged sputum and fever may be expected within the first 24 hours (Pagana et al., 2017). The patient is not discharged from the postanesthesia care unit (PACU) until adequate cough reflex and respiratory status are present. The nurse instructs the patient and caregivers to report any shortness of breath or bleeding immediately.

Thoracoscopy

Thoracoscopy is a diagnostic procedure in which the pleural cavity is examined with an endoscope and fluid and tissues can be obtained for analysis (Fig. 17-15).

Procedure

This procedure is performed in the operating room, normally under anesthesia. Small incisions are made into the pleural cavity in an intercostal space at the location indicated by clinical and diagnostic findings. The fiberoptic mediastinoscope is inserted into the pleural cavity, any fluid present is aspirated, and the pleural cavity is inspected through the instrument. After the procedure, a chest tube may be inserted to facilitate re-expansion of the lung.

Thoracoscopy is primarily indicated in the diagnostic evaluation and treatment of pleural effusions, pleural disease, and tumor staging. Biopsies of the lesions and resection of tissues can be performed under visualization for diagnosis.

Thoracoscopic procedures have expanded with the availability of video monitoring, which permits improved visualization of the lung. Video-assisted thoracoscopy (VATS) may be used in the diagnosis and treatment of empyema, pleural effusion, pulmonary and pleural masses, and pneumothorax. Although VATS does not replace the need for thoracotomy in the treatment of some lung cancers, its use continues to grow, because it is less invasive than open surgical procedures, and hospitalization and recovery are shorter.

Nursing Interventions

The nurse should follow routine preoperative practices, such as ensuring that informed consent is obtained and that the patient remains NPO prior to the procedure. Postoperatively, the nurse should monitor vital signs, pain level, and respiratory status, and should look for signs of bleeding and infection at the incisional site. Shortness of breath may indicate a pneumothorax and should be reported immediately. If a chest tube was inserted during the procedure, monitoring of the chest drainage system and chest tube insertion site is essential (see Chapter 19).

Thoracentesis

In some respiratory disorders, pleural fluid may accumulate. Thoracentesis (aspiration of fluid and air from the pleural space) is performed for diagnostic or therapeutic reasons. Purposes of the procedure include removal of fluid and, very rarely, air from the pleural cavity; aspiration of pleural fluid for analysis; pleural biopsy; and instillation of medication into the pleural space. Studies of pleural fluid include Gram stain culture and sensitivity, acid-fast staining and culture, differential cell count, cytology, pH, total protein, lactic dehydrogenase, glucose, amylase, triglycerides, and cancer markers such as carcinoembryonic antigen.

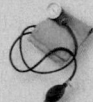 For the procedural guidelines for assisting with a thoracentesis, go to **thepoint.lww. com/Brunner15e**.

Biopsy

Biopsy—the excision of a small amount of tissue—may be performed to permit examination of cells from the upper and lower respiratory structures and adjacent lymph nodes. Local, topical, or moderate sedation, or general anesthesia, may be given, depending on the site and the procedure.

Pleural Biopsy

Pleural biopsy is accomplished by needle biopsy of the pleura, thoracoscopy, or pleuroscopy, a visual exploration through a fiberoptic pleuroscope inserted into the pleural space or through a thoracotomy. Pleural biopsy is performed when there is pleural exudate of undetermined origin or when there is a need to culture or stain the tissue to identify tuberculosis or fungi.

Lung Biopsy Procedures

Lung biopsy is performed to obtain tissue for examination when other diagnostic testing indicates potential interstitial lung disease, such as cancer, infection, or sarcoidosis. Several nonsurgical lung biopsy techniques are used because they yield accurate information with low morbidity: transbronchial brushing or needle aspiration, transbronchial lung biopsy, and percutaneous (through-the-skin) needle biopsy. Possible complications for all methods include pneumothorax, pulmonary hemorrhage, and empyema (Pagana et al., 2017).

Procedure

In transbronchial brushing, a fiberoptic bronchoscope is introduced into the bronchus under fluoroscopy. A small brush attached to the end of a flexible wire is inserted through the bronchoscope. Under direct visualization, the area under suspicion is brushed back and forth, causing cells to slough off and adhere to the brush. The catheter port of the bronchoscope may be used to irrigate the lung tissue with saline solution to secure material for additional studies. The brush is removed from the bronchoscope, and a slide is made for examination under the microscope. The brush may be cut off and sent to the pathology laboratory for analysis. This procedure is especially useful in the immunologically compromised patient.

In transbronchial needle aspiration, a catheter with a needle is inserted into the tissue through the bronchoscope and aspirated, whereas in transbronchial lung biopsy, biting or cutting forceps are introduced by a fiberoptic bronchoscope to excise the tissue.

In percutaneous needle biopsy, a cutting needle or a spinal-type needle is used to obtain a tissue specimen for histologic study under fluoroscopic or CT guidance. Analgesia may be given before the procedure. The skin over the biopsy site is cleansed and anesthetized and a small incision is made. The biopsy needle is inserted through the incision into the pleura with the patient holding their breath in midexpiration. The surgeon guides the needle into the periphery of the lesion and obtains a tissue sample from the mass.

Nursing Interventions

After the procedure, recovery and home care are similar to those for bronchoscopy and thoracoscopy. Nursing care involves monitoring the patient for complications such as shortness of breath, bleeding, or infection. In preparation for discharge, the patient and the family are instructed to report pain, shortness of breath, visible bleeding, redness of the biopsy site, or purulent drainage (pus) to the primary provider immediately. Patients who have undergone biopsy are often anxious because of the need for the biopsy and the potential findings; the nurse must consider this in providing postbiopsy care and patient education.

Lymph Node Biopsy

The scalene lymph nodes, which are enmeshed in the deep cervical pad of fat overlying the scalenus anterior muscle, drain the lungs and mediastinum and may show histologic changes from intrathoracic disease. If these nodes are palpable on physical examination, a scalene node biopsy may be performed. A biopsy of these nodes may be performed to detect spread of pulmonary disease to the lymph nodes and to establish a diagnosis or prognosis in such diseases as Hodgkin lymphoma, sarcoidosis, fungal disease, tuberculosis, and carcinoma.

Procedure

Mediastinoscopy is the endoscopic examination of the mediastinum for exploration and biopsy of mediastinal lymph nodes that drain the lungs; this examination does not require a thoracotomy. Biopsy is usually performed through a suprasternal incision. Mediastinoscopy is carried out to detect mediastinal involvement of pulmonary malignancy and to obtain tissue for diagnostic studies of other conditions (e.g., sarcoidosis).

An anterior mediastinotomy is thought to provide better exposure and diagnostic possibilities than a mediastinoscopy. An incision is made in the area of the second or third costal cartilage. The mediastinum is explored, and biopsies are performed on any lymph nodes found. Chest tube drainage is required after the procedure. Mediastinotomy is particularly valuable to determine whether a pulmonary lesion is resectable.

Nursing Interventions

Postprocedure care focuses on providing adequate oxygenation, monitoring for bleeding, and providing pain relief. The patient may be discharged a few hours after the chest drainage system is removed. The nurse should instruct the patient and the family about monitoring for changes in respiratory status, taking into consideration the impact of anxiety about the potential findings of the biopsy on their ability to remember those instructions.

CRITICAL THINKING EXERCISES

1 `ebp` You are caring for an 82-year-old male who was transferred to the medical-surgical unit from the postanesthesia care unit (PACU), status post appendectomy. The patient is currently alert to time, person, and place and his vital signs are as follows: temperature 37.5°C (99.0°F), HR 79 bpm, BP 125/74, RR 16 breaths/min, and SaO_2 96% on oxygen at 2 L/min via nasal cannula. The patient is receiving morphine via patient-controlled analgesia (PCA) for pain management. What changes in his assessment would indicate that he is at risk for developing respiratory depression? What evidence-based scales and diagnostic tests could help you to identify this potential complication?

2 `pq` A patient with a significant pulmonary history is admitted to the medical unit where you work with complaints of shortness of breath. He reports that he worked in the coal mines for 42 years and smokes cigarettes every day. As part of the history, he tells you, "For the past couple of days, I can't seem to catch my breath." He informs you that he coughs up "yellow stuff" throughout the day and it has been "thicker" than usual. What components of his assessment are most important for you to perform first?

REFERENCES

*Asterisk indicates nursing research.
**Double asterisk indicates classic reference.

Books

Hogan-Quigley, B., Palm, M. L., & Bickley, L. (2017). *Bates' nursing guide to physical examination and history taking* (2nd ed.). Philadelphia, PA: Wolters Kluwer.

Morton, P. G., Reck, K., & Headly, J. (2018). Patient assessment: Cardiovascular system. In P. G. Morton, & D. K. Fontaine (Eds.). *Critical care nursing: A holistic approach* (11th ed.). Philadelphia, PA: Wolters Kluwer.

Norris, T. L. (2019). *Porth's pathophysiology: Concepts of altered health states* (10th ed.). Philadelphia, PA: Wolters Kluwer.

Pagana, K. D., Pagana, T. J., & Pagana, T. N. (2017). *Mosby's diagnostic and laboratory test reference* (13th ed.). St. Louis, MO: Mosby Elsevier.

West, J. B., & Luks, A. M. (2016). *West's respiratory physiology: The essentials* (10th ed.). Philadelphia, PA: Wolters Kluwer Health Lippincott Williams & Wilkins.

Journals and Electronic Documents

American Lung Association. (2019). The impact of e-cigarettes on the lung. Retrieved on 12/19/2019 at: www.lung.org/stop-smoking/smoking-facts/impact-of-e-cigarettes-on-lung.html

American Lung Association. (2019). Tobacco: Statement on e-cigarettes. Retrieved on 6/26/2019 at: www.lung.org/our-initiatives/tobacco/oversight-and-regulation/statement-on-e-cigarettes.html

American Lung Association. (2020). Nicotine replacement therapy to help you quit tobacco. Retrieved on 12/16/20 at: www.cancer.org/healthy/stay-away-from-tobacco/guide-quitting-smoking/nicotine-replacement-therapy.html

Aminiahidashti, H., Shafiee, S., Kiasari, A. Z., et al. (2018). Applications of end-tidal carbon dioxide (ETCO2) monitoring in emergency department; a narrative review. Retrieved on 12/19/2019 at: www.ncbi.nlm.nih.gov/pmc/articles/PMC5827051

*Baker, K. M., DeSanto-Madeya, S., & Banzett, R. B. (2017). Routine dyspnea assessment and documentation: Nurses' experience yields wide acceptance. *BMC Nursing, 16*(3), 1–11.

Indik, J. H., Gimbel, J. R., Abe, H., et al. (2017). 2017 HRS consensus statement on magnetic resonance imaging and radiation exposure in patients with cardiovascular implantable electronic devices. *Heart Rhythm, 14*(7), e97–e153.

Institute for Healthcare Improvement (IHI). (2019). Early warning systems: Scorecards that save lives. Retrieved on 6/23/2019 at: www.ihi.org/resources/Pages/ImprovementStories/EarlyWarningSystemsScorecardsThatSaveLives.aspx

Krauss, B., Falk, J., & Ladde, J. (2018). Carbon dioxide monitoring (capnography). *UpToDate.* Retrieved on 12/20/2019 at: www.uptodate.com/contents/carbon-dioxide-monitoring-capnography

Mechem, C. C. (2019). Pulse oximetry. *UpToDate.* Retrieved on 12/20/2019 at: www.uptodate.com/contents/pulse-oximetry

**Parshall, M. B., Schwartzstein, R. M., Adams, L., et al. (2012). An official American Thoracic Society statement: Update on the mechanisms, assessment, and management of dyspnea. *American Journal of Respiratory and Critical Care Medicine, 185*(4), 435–452.

Ramly, E., Kaafarani, H. M. A., & Velmahos, G. C. (2015). The effect of aging on pulmonary function: Implications for monitoring and support of the surgical and trauma patient. *Surgical Clinics of North America, 95*(1), 53–69.

Sharma, S., Hashmi, M., & Rawat, D. (2019). Partial pressure of oxygen (PO2). *StatPearls.* Retrieved on 12/20/2019 at: www.ncbi.nlm.nih.gov/books/NBK493219

Smallwood, C., & Walsh, B. (2017). Noninvasive monitoring of oxygenation and ventilation. *Respiratory Care, 62*(6), 751–764.

The National Academies of Sciences, Engineering, and Medicine. (2018). *Public health consequences of e-cigarettes.* Washington, DC: The National Academies Press. Retrieved on 12/20/2019 at: www.nationalacademies.org/eCigHealthEffects

Thompson, B. T., & Kabrhel, C. (2018). Patient education. Pulmonary embolism (Beyond the Basics). In J. Finlay (Ed.). *UpToDate.* Retrieved on 6/26/2019 at: www.uptodate.com/contents/pulmonary-embolism-beyond-the-basics

Wells, J. L., & Murphy, P. S. (2014). Clearing the runway: An innovative approach to preparing the intensive care unit patient for a magnetic resonance imaging scan. *Journal of Radiology Nursing, 33*(3), 147–151.

Resources

American Association for Respiratory Care (AARC), www.aarc.org
American Lung Association, www.lung.org
American Thoracic Society, www.thoracic.org
Centers for Disease Control and Prevention (CDC), www.cdc.gov
Cystic Fibrosis Foundation, www.cff.org
National Heart, Lung, and Blood Institute, National Institutes of Health, www.nhlbi.nih.gov
U.S. Food and Drug Administration, www.fda.gov

18 Management of Patients with Upper Respiratory Tract Disorders

LEARNING OUTCOMES

On completion of this chapter, the learner will be able to:

1. Describe nursing management of patients with upper airway disorders and of patients with epistaxis.
2. Compare and contrast the upper respiratory tract infections according to cause, incidence, clinical manifestations, management, and the significance of preventive health care.
3. Use the nursing process as a framework for care of the patient with upper airway infection and the patient undergoing laryngectomy.

NURSING CONCEPTS

Infection

Oxygenation

GLOSSARY

alaryngeal communication: alternative modes of speaking that do not involve the normal larynx; used by patients whose larynx has been surgically removed

aphonia: impaired ability to use one's voice due to disease or injury to the larynx

apnea: cessation of breathing

dysphagia: difficulty swallowing

epistaxis: hemorrhage from the nose due to rupture of tiny, distended vessels in the mucous membrane of any area of the nose

herpes simplex: a cutaneous viral infection with painful vesicles and erosions on the tongue, palate, gingiva, buccal membranes, or lips (*synonym:* cold sore)

laryngectomy: surgical removal of all or part of the larynx and surrounding structures

laryngitis: inflammation of the larynx; may be caused by voice abuse, exposure to irritants, or infectious organisms

nuchal rigidity: stiffness of the neck or inability to bend the neck

pharyngitis: inflammation of the throat

rhinitis: inflammation of the mucous membranes of the nose

rhinitis medicamentosa: rebound nasal congestion commonly associated with overuse of over-the-counter nasal decongestants

rhinorrhea: drainage of a large amount of fluid from the nose

rhinosinusitis: inflammation of the nares and paranasal sinuses, including frontal, ethmoid, maxillary, and sphenoid sinuses; replaces the term *sinusitis*

tonsillitis: inflammation of the tonsils

xerostomia: dryness of the mouth

Upper respiratory tract disorders are those that involve the nose, paranasal sinuses, pharynx, larynx, trachea, or bronchi. Many of these conditions are relatively minor, and their effects are limited to mild and temporary discomfort and inconvenience for the patient. However, others are acute, severe, and life-threatening and may require permanent alterations in breathing and speaking. Therefore, the nurse must have expert assessment skills, an understanding of the wide variety of disorders that may affect the upper airway, and an awareness of the impact of these alterations on patients. Patient education is an important aspect of nursing care because many of these disorders are treated outside the hospital or at home by patients themselves. When caring for patients with acute, life-threatening disorders, the nurse needs highly developed assessment and clinical management skills, along with a focus on rehabilitation needs.

UPPER AIRWAY INFECTIONS

Upper airway infections (otherwise known as upper respiratory infections [URIs]) are the most common cause of illness and affect most people on occasion. Some infections are acute, with symptoms that last several days; others are chronic, with symptoms that may last for weeks or months or recur. A URI is often defined as an infection of the mucous membranes of the nose, sinuses, pharynx, upper trachea, or larynx (Pokorski, 2015).

The common cold is the most frequently occurring example of a URI. URIs occur when microorganisms such as viruses and bacteria are inhaled. There are many causative organisms, and people are susceptible throughout life. Viruses, the most common cause of URIs, affect the upper respiratory passages and lead to subsequent mucous membrane inflammation. URIs are the most common reason for seeking health care and for absences from school and work (Pokorski, 2015).

URIs affect the nasal cavity; ethmoidal air cells; and frontal, maxillary, and sphenoid sinuses; as well as the pharynx, larynx, and upper portion of the trachea. On average, adults typically develop two to four URIs per year because of the wide variety of respiratory viruses that circulate in the community (Weinberger, Cockrill, & Mandel, 2019). Although patients are rarely hospitalized for the treatment of URIs, nurses working in community settings or long-term care facilities may encounter patients who have these infections. It is important for nurses to recognize the signs and symptoms of URIs and provide appropriate care. Nurses in these settings also can influence patient outcomes through patient education. Special considerations with regard to URIs in older adults are summarized in Chart 18-1.

Rhinitis

Rhinitis is a group of disorders characterized by inflammation and irritation of the mucous membranes of the nose. These conditions can have a significant impact on quality of life and contribute to sinus, ear, and sleep problems and learning disorders. Rhinitis often coexists with other respiratory disorders, such as asthma. It affects between 10% and 30% of the population worldwide annually. Viral rhinitis, especially the common cold, affects approximately one billion individuals yearly (Meneghetti, 2018).

Rhinitis may be acute or chronic, and allergic or nonallergic. Allergic rhinitis is further classified as seasonal or perennial rhinitis and is commonly associated with exposure to airborne particles such as dust, dander, or plant pollens in people who are allergic to these substances. Seasonal rhinitis occurs during pollen seasons, and perennial rhinitis occurs throughout the year. See Chapter 33 for detailed descriptions of allergic disorders, including allergic rhinitis.

Pathophysiology

Rhinitis may be caused by a variety of factors, including changes in temperature or humidity; odors; infection; age; systemic disease; use of over-the-counter (OTC) and prescribed nasal decongestants; and the presence of a foreign body. Allergic rhinitis may occur with exposure to

---

Chart 18-1 — **Upper Respiratory Tract Disorders in Older Adults**

- Upper respiratory infections in older adults may have more serious consequences if patients have concurrent medical problems that compromise their respiratory or immune status.
- Influenza causes exacerbations of chronic obstructive pulmonary disease and reduced pulmonary function.
- Antihistamines and decongestants used to treat upper respiratory disorders must be used cautiously in older adults because of their side effects and potential interactions with other medications.
- The prevalence of nonallergic rhinosinusitis is greater among older adults than among adults of other age groups. Rhinosinusitis is the sixth most common chronic disease among older adults. With anticipated future growth in the older adult population, the need for endoscopic sinus surgery will increase. Older patients with nonallergic rhinosinusitis present with symptoms similar to those of younger adults and experience a similar degree of improvement and quality of life after endoscopic sinus surgery.
- The structure of the nose changes with aging; it lengthens and the tip droops from loss of cartilage. This can cause restriction in airflow and predispose older adult patients to geriatric rhinitis, characterized by increased thin, watery sinus drainage. These structural changes may also adversely affect the sense of smell.
- Laryngitis in older adults is common and may be secondary to gastroesophageal reflux disease (GERD). Older adults are more likely to have impaired esophageal peristalsis and a weaker esophageal sphincter. Treatment measures include sleeping with the head of the bed elevated and the use of medications such as histamine-2 receptor blockers (e.g., famotidine) or proton pump inhibitors (e.g., omeprazole).
- Age-related loss of muscle mass and thinning of the mucous membranes can cause structural changes in the larynx that may change characteristics of the voice. In general, the pitch of voice becomes higher in older adult men and lower in older adult women. The voice also "thins" (decreased projection) and may sound tremulous. These changes should be discriminated from signs that could indicate pathologic conditions.

Adapted from Eliopoulos, C. (2018). *Gerontological nursing* (9th ed.). Philadelphia, PA: Wolters Kluwer; Lehmann, A. E., Scangas, G. A., Sethi, R. K., et al. (2018). Impact of age on sinus surgery outcomes. *The Laryngoscope, 128*, 2681–2687; Valdes, C. J., & Tewfik, M. A. (2018). Rhinosinusitis and allergies in elderly patients. *Clinics in Geriatric Medicine, 34*(2), 217–231.

---

allergens such as foods (e.g., peanuts, walnuts, Brazil nuts, wheat, shellfish, soy, cow's milk, eggs), medications (e.g., penicillin, sulfa medications, aspirin), and particles in the indoor and outdoor environment (Chart 18-2). The most common cause of nonallergic rhinitis is the common cold (Peters, 2015).

Drug-induced rhinitis may occur with antihypertensive agents, such as angiotensin-converting enzyme (ACE) inhibitors and beta-blockers; "statins," such as atorvastatin and simvastatin; antidepressants and antipsychotics such as risperidone; aspirin; and some antianxiety medications (Comerford & Durkin, 2020). Figure 18-1 shows the pathologic processes involved in rhinitis and rhinosinusitis. Other causes of rhinovirus are identified in Table 18-1.

Chart 18-2 · Examples of Common Indoor and Outdoor Allergens

Common Indoor Allergens

- Dust mite feces
- Dog dander
- Cat dander
- Cockroach droppings
- Molds

Common Outdoor Allergens

- Trees (e.g., oak, elm, western red cedar, ash, birch, syca-more, maple, walnut, cypress)
- Weeds (e.g., ragweed, tumbleweed, sagebrush, pigweed, cockle weed, Russian thistle)
- Grasses (e.g., timothy, orchard, sweet vernal, bermuda, sour dock, redtop, bluegrass)
- Molds (*Alternaria, Cladosporium, Aspergillus*)

Adapted from Patel, B. (2017). Aeroallergens. Retrieved on 5/27/2019 at: www.emedicine.medscape.com/article/137911-overview

Clinical Manifestations

The signs and symptoms of rhinitis include **rhinorrhea** (excessive nasal drainage, runny nose); nasal congestion; nasal discharge (purulent with bacterial rhinitis); sneezing; and pruritus of the nose, roof of the mouth, throat, eyes, and ears. Headache may occur, particularly if rhinosinusitis is also present (see later discussion of rhinosinusitis). Nonallergic rhinitis can occur throughout the year.

TABLE 18-1 · Causes of Rhinosinusitis

Category	Causes
Vasomotor	Idiopathic Abuse of nasal decongestants (rhinitis medicamentosa) Psychological stimulation (anger, sexual arousal) Irritants (smoke, air pollution, exhaust fumes, cocaine)
Mechanical	Tumor Deviated septum Crusting Hypertrophied turbinates Foreign body Cerebrospinal fluid leak
Chronic inflammatory	Polyps (in cystic fibrosis) Sarcoidosis Wegener granulomatosis Midline granuloma
Infectious	Acute viral infection Acute or chronic rhinosinusitis Rare nasal infections (syphilis, tuberculosis)
Hormonal	Pregnancy Use of oral contraceptives Hypothyroidism

Adapted from Peters, A. (2015). Rhinosinusitis: Synopsis. Retrieved on 6/2/2019 at: www.worldallergy.org/professional/allergic_diseases_center/rhinosinusitis/sinusitis synopsis.php

Physiology/Pathophysiology

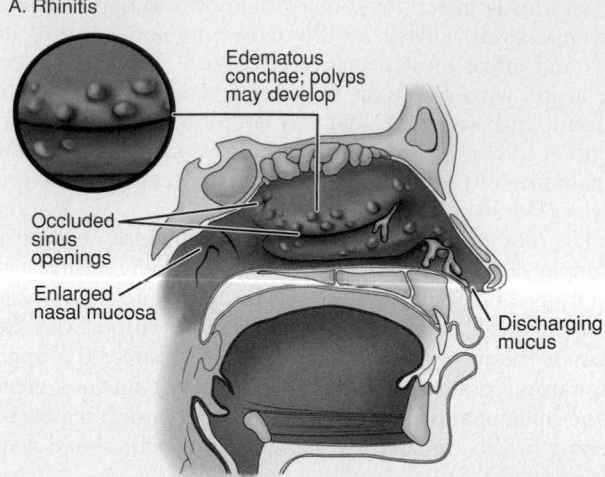

A. Rhinitis

Edematous conchae; polyps may develop

Occluded sinus openings

Enlarged nasal mucosa

Discharging mucus

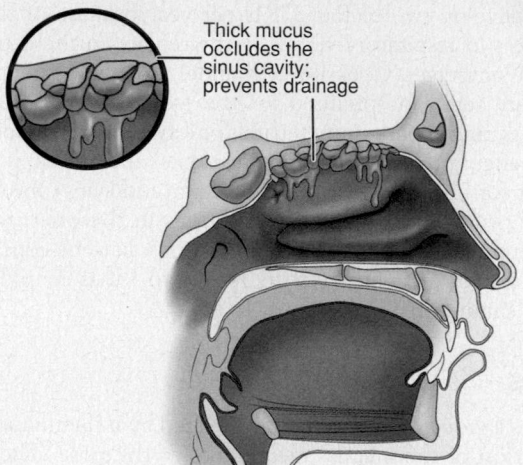

B. Rhinosinusitis

Thick mucus occludes the sinus cavity; prevents drainage

Figure 18-1 • Pathophysiologic processes in rhinitis and rhinosinusitis. Although pathophysiologic processes are similar in rhinitis and rhinosinusitis, they affect different structures. **A.** In rhinitis, the mucous membranes lining the nasal passages become inflamed, congested, and edematous. The swollen nasal conchae block the sinus openings, and mucus is discharged from the nostrils. **B.** Rhinosinusitis is also marked by inflammation and congestion, with thickened mucous secretions filling the sinus cavities and occluding the openings.

Medical Management

The management of rhinitis depends on the cause, which may be identified through the history and physical examination. The nurse asks the patient about recent symptoms as well as possible exposure to allergens in the home, environment, or workplace. If viral rhinitis is the cause, medications may be prescribed to relieve the symptoms. In allergic rhinitis, allergy tests may be performed to identify possible allergens. Depending on the severity of the allergy, desensitizing immunizations and corticosteroids may be required (see Chapter 33 for more details). If symptoms suggest a bacterial infection, an antimicrobial agent is used. Patients with nasal septal deformities or nasal polyps may be referred to an ear, nose, and throat specialist.

Pharmacologic Therapy

Medication therapy for allergic and nonallergic rhinitis focuses on symptom relief. Antihistamines and nasal sprays may be useful. Antihistamines remain the most common treatment and are given for sneezing, pruritus, and rhinorrhea. (Examples of commonly prescribed antihistamines are discussed in more detail in Chapter 33.) Brompheniramine/pseudoephedrine is an example of combination antihistamine/decongestant medications. Cromolyn, a mast cell stabilizer that inhibits the release of histamine and other chemicals, is also used in the treatment of rhinitis. Oral decongestant agents may be used for nasal obstruction. The use of saline nasal spray can act as a mild decongestant and can liquefy mucus to prevent crusting. Two inhalations of intranasal ipratropium can be given in each nostril two to three times per day for symptomatic relief of rhinorrhea. In addition, intranasal corticosteroids may be used for severe congestion, and ophthalmic agents (cromolyn ophthalmic solution 4%) may be used to relieve irritation, itching, and redness of the eyes. Appropriate allergy treatments may include leukotriene modifiers (e.g., montelukast, zafirlukast, zileuton), and immunoglobulin E modifiers (e.g., omalizumab), which are also components of asthma treatment guidelines (discussed further in Chapter 20). The choice of medications depends on the symptoms, adverse reactions, adherence factors, risk of drug interactions, and cost to the patient (Hauk, 2018).

Nursing Management

 Educating Patients About Self-Care

The nurse instructs the patient with allergic rhinitis to avoid or reduce exposure to allergens and irritants, such as dusts, molds, animals, fumes, odors, powders, sprays, and tobacco smoke. Patient education is essential when assisting the patient in the use of all medications. To prevent possible drug interactions, the patient is cautioned to read drug labels before taking any OTC medication.

The nurse instructs the patient about the importance of controlling the environment at home and at work. Saline nasal sprays or aerosols may be helpful in soothing mucous membranes, softening crusted secretions, and removing irritants. The nurse instructs the patient in correct administration of nasal medications. To achieve maximal relief, the patient is instructed to blow the nose before applying any medication into the nasal cavity. In addition, the patient is taught to keep the head upright; spray quickly and firmly into each nostril away from the nasal septum; and wait at least 1 minute before administering the second spray. The container should be cleaned after each use and should never be shared with other people to avoid cross-contamination.

In the case of infectious rhinitis, the nurse reviews hand hygiene technique with the patient as a measure to prevent transmission of organisms. This is especially important for those in contact with vulnerable populations such as the very young, older adults, or people who are immunosuppressed (e.g., patients with human immune deficiency virus [HIV] infection, those taking immunosuppressive medications).

In older adults and other high-risk populations, the nurse reviews the importance of receiving an influenza vaccination each year to achieve immunity before the beginning of the flu season.

Viral Rhinitis (Common Cold)

Viral rhinitis is the most frequent viral infection in the general population (Meneghetti, 2018). The term *common cold* often is used when referring to a URI that is self-limited and caused by a virus. The term *cold* refers to an infectious, acute inflammation of the mucous membranes of the nasal cavity characterized by nasal congestion, rhinorrhea, sneezing, sore throat, and general malaise. More broadly, the term refers to an acute URI, whereas terms such as *rhinitis, pharyngitis,* and *laryngitis* distinguish the sites of the symptoms. The term is also used when the causative virus is influenza (the flu). Colds are highly contagious because virus is shed for about 2 days before the symptoms appear and during the first part of the symptomatic phase.

Colds caused by rhinoviruses tend to occur in the early fall and spring. Other viruses tend to cause winter colds (Centers for Disease Control and Prevention [CDC], 2019). Seasonal changes in relative humidity may affect the prevalence of colds. The most common cold-causing viruses survive better when humidity is low, in the colder months of the year.

Colds are caused by as many as 200 different viruses. Rhinoviruses are the most likely causative organisms. Other viruses implicated in the common cold include coronavirus, adenovirus, respiratory syncytial virus, influenza virus, and parainfluenza virus. Each virus may have multiple strains; as a result, people are susceptible to colds throughout life (Buensalido, 2019b). Some virus strains may be particularly virulent, causing more severe manifestations than those implicated with common colds, such as the SARS-CoV-2 virion, which caused the COVID-19 pandemic. Development of a vaccine against the multiple strains of virus is almost impossible. Immunity after recovery is variable and depends on many factors, including a person's natural host resistance and the specific virus that caused the cold. Despite popular belief, cold temperatures and exposure to cold rainy weather do not increase the incidence or severity of the common cold.

Clinical Manifestations

Signs and symptoms of viral rhinitis may include low-grade fever, nasal congestion, rhinorrhea and nasal discharge, halitosis, sneezing, tearing watery eyes, "scratchy" or sore throat, general malaise, chills, and often headache and muscle aches. As the illness progresses, cough usually appears. In some people, the virus exacerbates **herpes simplex**, commonly called a *cold sore* (Chart 18-3).

The symptoms of viral rhinitis may last from 1 to 2 weeks. If severe systemic respiratory symptoms occur, it is no longer considered viral rhinitis but one of the other acute URIs. Allergic conditions can affect the nose, mimicking the symptoms of a cold.

Medical Management

Management consists of symptomatic therapy that includes adequate fluid intake, rest, prevention of chilling, and the use

Chart 18-3 Colds and Cold Sores (Herpes Simplex Virus)

Overview

Herpes labialis is an infection that is caused by herpes simplex virus type 1 (HSV-1). Herpes labialis is extremely contagious and can be spread through contaminated razors, towels, and dishes. It is activated by overexposure to sunlight or wind, colds, influenza and similar infections, heavy alcohol use, and physical or emotional stress.

Statistics

- Once the patient is infected with this virus, it can lie latent in the cells. The incubation period is between 2 and 12 d.
- Between 50% and 80% of Americans are infected by age 30 y, because HSV-1 is typically transmitted during childhood through nonsexual contact.
- Estimates suggest that 80% of people infected are asymptomatic.

Clinical Manifestations

- Herpes labialis is characterized by an eruption of small, painful blisters on the skin of the lips, mouth, gums, tongue, or the skin around the mouth. The blisters are commonly referred to as cold sores or fever blisters.
- Early symptoms of herpes labialis include burning, itching, and increased sensitivity or tingling sensation. These symptoms may occur several days before the appearance of lesions.
- Lesions appear as macules or papules, progressing to small blisters (vesicles) filled with clear, yellowish fluid. They are raised, red, and painful and can break and ooze. The lesions typically extend through the epidermis and penetrate into the underlying dermis, consistent with a partial-thickness wound.
- Eventually, yellow crusts slough over the lesions to reveal pink, healing skin.
- Typically, the virus is no longer detectable in the lesion or wound 5 d after the vesicle has developed.

Medical and Nursing Management

- Antiviral medications (e.g., acyclovir, valacyclovir) may be prescribed to minimize the symptoms and the duration or length of flare-up.
- Acetaminophen may be given for analgesia.
- Topical anesthetics such as lidocaine can help in the control of discomfort.
- Occlusive dressings have been shown to speed the healing process. Occlusive ointments with antiviral properties (e.g., docosanol) might be considered for lip and mucosal lesions.

Patient Education

- Patients should understand that the virus can be transmitted by people who are asymptomatic.
- Patients should seek treatment with antiviral medications and ointments when they are first experiencing symptoms (e.g., tingling, burning, or itching sensations) as early treatment with these drugs can result in a speedier recovery.
- Although herpes simplex virus type 2 (HSV-2) typically causes painful vesicular and ulcerative lesions in the genital and anal areas, HSV-1 may also cause genital herpes. Oral–genital contact can spread oral herpes to the genitals (and vice versa). People with active herpetic lesions should avoid oral sex.

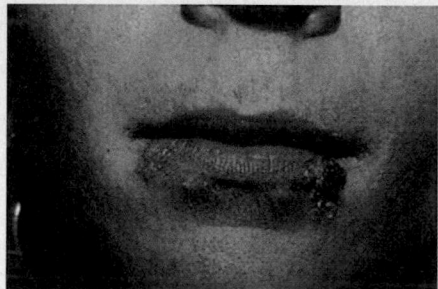

Photo reprinted with permission from Ayoade, F. (2018). Herpes simplex. Retrieved on 5/27/2019 at: www.emedicine.medscape.com/article/218580-overview

---

of expectorants as needed. Warm salt-water gargles soothe the sore throat, and nonsteroidal anti-inflammatory drugs (NSAIDs), such as aspirin or ibuprofen, relieve aches and pains. Antihistamines are used to relieve sneezing, rhinorrhea, and nasal congestion. Petroleum jelly can soothe irritated, chapped, and raw skin around the nares (Buensalido, 2019b).

Guaifenesin, an expectorant, is available without a prescription and is used to promote removal of secretions. Antimicrobial agents (antibiotics) should not be used, because they do not affect the virus or reduce the incidence of bacterial complications. In addition, their inappropriate use has been implicated in the development of organisms resistant to therapy.

Topical nasal decongestants (e.g., phenylephrine nasal and oxymetazoline nasal) should be used with caution. Topical therapy delivers medication directly to the nasal mucosa, and its overuse can produce **rhinitis medicamentosa**, or rebound rhinitis. Most patients treat the common cold with OTC medications that produce moderate clinical benefits, such as relief of symptoms.

In addition, alternative medicines (e.g., echinacea, zinc lozenges, and zinc nasal spray) are frequently used to treat the common cold; however, evidence regarding their effectiveness in shortening the symptomatic phase is limited (Mousa, 2017). The inhalation of steam or heated, humidified air has been a mainstay of home remedies to treat the common cold; however, the value of this therapy has not been demonstrated.

Nursing Management

 Educating Patients About Self-Care

Most viruses can be transmitted in several ways: direct contact with infected secretions, inhalation of large particles from others' coughing or sneezing, or inhalation of small particles (aerosol) that may be suspended in the air for up to an hour. Implementation of appropriate hand hygiene measures (see Chapter 66, Chart 66-1 for further information) remains the most effective measure to prevent transmission of organisms. The nurse educates the patient about how to break the chain of infection with appropriate hand hygiene and the use of tissues to avoid the spread of the virus with coughing and sneezing, and to cough or sneeze into the upper arm if tissues are not readily available. The nurse instructs the patient about methods to treat symptoms of the common cold and provides both verbal and written information to assist in the prevention and management of URIs.

Rhinosinusitis

Rhinosinusitis, formerly called *sinusitis*, is an inflammation of the paranasal sinuses and nasal cavity. The American Academy of Otolaryngology–Head and Neck Surgery Foundation (2018; Rosenfeld, Andes, Bhattacharyya, et al., 2015) recommends the use of the term *rhinosinusitis* because sinusitis is almost always accompanied by inflammation of the nasal mucosa. Rhinosinusitis affects about 35 million people in the United States each year and accounts for 16 million office visits (Brook, 2018a).

Uncomplicated rhinosinusitis occurs without extension of inflammation outside of the paranasal sinuses and nasal cavity. Rhinosinusitis is classified by duration of symptoms as acute (less than 4 weeks), subacute (4 to 12 weeks), and chronic (more than 12 weeks). Rhinosinusitis can be caused by a bacterial or viral infection.

Acute Rhinosinusitis

Acute rhinosinusitis is classified as acute bacterial rhinosinusitis (ABRS) or acute viral rhinosinusitis (AVRS). Recurrent acute rhinosinusitis is characterized by four or more acute episodes of ABRS per year (Patel & Hwang, 2019) and is discussed with chronic rhinosinusitis (CRS).

Pathophysiology

Acute rhinosinusitis usually follows a viral URI or cold, such as an unresolved viral or bacterial infection, or an exacerbation of allergic rhinitis. Normally, the sinus openings into the nasal passages are clear and infections resolve promptly. However, if their drainage is obstructed by a deviated septum or by hypertrophied turbinates, spurs, or nasal polyps or tumors, sinus infection may persist as a secondary infection or progress to an acute suppurative process (causing purulent discharge).

Nasal congestion, caused by inflammation, edema, and transudation of fluid secondary to URI, leads to obstruction of the sinus cavities (see Fig. 18-1). This provides an excellent medium for bacterial growth. Other conditions and activities that can block the normal flow of sinus secretions include abnormal structures of the nose, enlarged adenoids, diving and swimming, tooth infection, trauma to the nose, tumors, and the pressure of foreign objects. Some people are more prone to rhinosinusitis because exposure to environmental hazards such as paint, sawdust, and chemicals may result in chronic inflammation of the nasal passages.

Bacterial organisms account for more than 60% of the cases of acute rhinosinusitis. Typical pathogens include *Streptococcus pneumoniae, Haemophilus influenzae*, and less commonly *Staphylococcus aureus*, and *Moraxella catarrhalis* (Brook, 2018b). Biofilms, which consist of organized, heterogeneous communities of bacteria, have been found to be 10 to 1000 times more resistant to antibiotic treatment and more likely to contribute to host resistance when compared with other bacteria. They serve as bacterial reservoirs that can cause systemic illness when released into the circulation. Although antibiotics kill bacteria in the biofilm margin, cells deep in the biofilm are not affected, allowing for regrowth once antibiotic therapy has been discontinued. Pathogens in the upper respiratory tract that form biofilms include those species listed earlier as well as *Pseudomonas aeruginosa*.

Other organisms that are occasionally isolated include *Chlamydia pneumoniae, Streptococcus pyogenes*, viruses, and fungi (*Aspergillus fumigatus*). Fungal infections occur most often in patients who are immunosuppressed (Brook, 2018b). The most common organisms found with health care-associated (nosocomial) infections include *P. aeruginosa, Escherichia coli, Proteus mirabilis, Klebsiella pneumoniae*, and *Enterobacter* species, accounting for 60% of those cases (Brook, 2018b).

Clinical Manifestations

Symptoms of ABRS include purulent nasal drainage (anterior, posterior, or both) accompanied by nasal obstruction or a combination of facial pain, pressure, or a sense of fullness (referred to collectively as facial pain–pressure–fullness), or both (Rosenfeld et al., 2015; Sedaghat, 2017). The facial pain–pressure–fullness may involve the anterior face or the periorbital region. The patient may also report cloudy or colored nasal discharge congestion, blockage, or stuffiness as well as a localized or diffuse headache. Patients with ABRS may present with a high fever (i.e., 39°C [102°F] or higher). In addition, the occurrence of symptoms for 10 days or more after the initial onset of upper respiratory symptoms indicates ABRS (Brook, 2018a).

The symptoms of AVRS are similar to those of ABRS, except the patient does not present with a high fever, nor with the same intensity of symptoms (e.g., there tends to be an absence of facial pain–pressure–fullness), nor with symptoms that persist for as long a period of time. Symptoms of AVRS occur for fewer than 10 days after the onset of upper respiratory symptoms and do not worsen (Papadakis, McPhee, & Rabow, 2018).

Assessment and Diagnostic Findings

A careful history and physical examination are performed. The head and neck, particularly the nose, ears, teeth, sinuses, pharynx, and chest, are examined. There may be tenderness to palpation over the infected sinus area. The sinuses are percussed using the index finger, tapping lightly to determine whether the patient experiences pain. Although less frequently performed, transillumination of the affected area may reveal a decrease in the transmission of light with rhinosinusitis (see Chapter 17). Diagnostic imaging (x-ray, computed tomography [CT], magnetic resonance imaging [MRI]) is not recommended and generally not needed for the diagnosis of acute rhinosinusitis if the patient meets clinical diagnostic criteria (Aring & Chan, 2016; Rosenfeld et al., 2015). When a complication or alternative diagnosis is suspected, diagnostic imaging may be indicated to help identify inflammatory changes, bone destruction, and anatomic variations that can guide sinus surgery (if indicated).

To confirm the diagnosis of maxillary and frontal rhinosinusitis and identify the pathogen, sinus aspirates may be obtained. Flexible endoscopic culture techniques and swabbing of the sinuses have been used for this purpose (Papadakis et al., 2018).

Complications

If untreated, acute rhinosinusitis may lead to severe complications. Local complications include osteomyelitis and mucocele (cyst of the paranasal sinuses). Osteomyelitis requires prolonged antibiotic therapy and at times removal of necrotic bone. Intracranial complications, although rare, include cavernous sinus thrombosis, meningitis, brain abscess, ischemic brain infarction, and severe orbital cellulitis (Papadakis et al., 2018). Mucoceles may require surgical treatment to establish intranasal drainage or complete excision with ablation of the sinus cavity. Brain abscesses occur by direct spread and can be life-threatening. Frontal epidural abscesses are usually quiescent but can be detected by CT scan.

Medical Management

Treatment of acute rhinosinusitis depends on the cause; a 14-day course of antibiotics is prescribed for bacterial cases (Tewfik, 2018). The goals of treatment for acute rhinosinusitis are to shrink the nasal mucosa, relieve pain, and treat infection. Because of the inappropriate use of antibiotics for nonbacterial illness, including AVRS, and the resulting resistance that has occurred, oral antibiotics are only prescribed when there is sufficient empiric evidence that the patient has ABRS (e.g., high fever or symptoms that persist for at least 10 days or worsening symptoms following a viral respiratory illness).

Antibiotics should be given as soon as the diagnosis of ABRS is established. Amoxicillin or amoxicillin–clavulanic acid are the antibiotics of choice. For patients who are allergic to penicillin, doxycycline or respiratory quinolones such as levofloxacin or moxifloxacin can be prescribed (CDC, 2017). Other antibiotics prescribed previously to treat ABRS, including cephalosporins (e.g., cephalexin, cefuroxime, cefaclor, and cefixime), macrolides (e.g., clarithromycin and azithromycin), and trimethoprim–sulfamethoxazole are no longer recommended because they are not effective in treating antibiotic-resistant organisms that are now more commonly implicated in ABRS (Tewfik, 2018). Intranasal saline lavage is an effective adjunct therapy to antibiotics in that it may relieve symptoms, reduce inflammation, and help clear the passages of stagnant mucus. Neither decongestants nor antihistamines are recommended adjunctive medications for treating ABRS (Tewfik, 2018).

Treatment of AVRS typically involves nasal saline lavage and decongestants (guaifenesin/pseudoephedrine).

Decongestants or nasal saline sprays can increase patency of the ostiomeatal unit and improve drainage of the sinuses. Topical decongestants should not be used for longer than 3 or 4 days. Oral decongestants must be used cautiously in patients with hypertension. OTC antihistamines, such as diphenhydramine and cetirizine, and prescription antihistamines, such as fexofenadine, are used if an allergic component is suspected.

Intranasal corticosteroids have been shown to produce complete or marked improvement in acute symptoms of either bacterial or viral rhinosinusitis; however, they are only recommended for use in patients with a previous history of allergic rhinitis (Rosenfeld et al., 2015). Examples of intranasal corticosteroids, side effects, and contraindications are presented in Table 18-2.

Nursing Management

 Educating Patients About Self-Care

Patient education is an important aspect of nursing care for the patient with acute rhinosinusitis. The nurse instructs the patient about symptoms of complications that require immediate follow-up. Referral to the primary provider is indicated if periorbital edema and severe pain on palpation occur. The nurse instructs the patient about methods to promote drainage of the sinuses, including humidification of the air in the home and the use of warm compresses to relieve pressure. The patient is advised to avoid swimming, diving, and air travel during the acute infection. Patients using tobacco are instructed to immediately stop smoking or using any form of tobacco. Many patients use nasal sprays incorrectly, which can lead to several side effects that include nasal irritation, nasal burning, bad taste, and drainage in the throat or even **epistaxis** (hemorrhage from the nose). Therefore, if an intranasal corticosteroid is prescribed, it is important to instruct the patient about the correct use of prescribed nasal sprays through demonstration, explanation, and return demonstration to evaluate the patient's understanding of the correct method of administration. The nurse also educates the patient about the side effects of prescribed and OTC nasal sprays and about rhinitis medicamentosa (rebound congestion). Once the decongestant is discontinued, the nasal passages close and congestion results. Appropriate medications to use for pain relief include acetaminophen and NSAIDs such as ibuprofen,

TABLE 18-2	Select Nasal Corticosteroids and Common Side Effects	
Nasal Corticosteroids	**Side Effects**	**Contraindications (for All Nasal Corticosteroids)**
Beclomethasone	Nasal irritation, headache, nausea, lightheadedness, epistaxis, rhinorrhea, watering eyes, sneezing, dry nose and throat	Avoid in patients with recurrent epistaxis, glaucoma, and cataracts. Patients who have been exposed to measles/varicella or who have adrenal insufficiency should avoid these medications.
Budesonide	Epistaxis, pharyngitis, cough, nasal irritation, bronchospasm	
Mometasone	Headache, viral infection, pharyngitis, epistaxis, cough, dysmenorrhea, musculoskeletal pain, arthralgia	
Triamcinolone	Pharyngitis, epistaxis, cough, headache	

Adapted from Comerford, K. C., & Durkin, M. T. (Eds.). (2020). *Nursing2020 drug handbook*. Philadelphia, PA: Wolters Kluwer; Peters, A. (2015). Rhinosinusitis: Synopsis. Retrieved on 5/8/2019 at: www.worldallergy.org/professional/allergic_diseases_center/rhinosinusitis/sinusitissynopsis.php

naproxen sodium, and aspirin for adults older than 20 years as long as there are no contraindications to use.

The nurse tells patients with recurrent rhinosinusitis to begin decongestants, such as pseudoephedrine, at the first sign of rhinosinusitis. This promotes drainage and decreases the risk of bacterial infection. Patients should also check with their primary provider or pharmacist before using OTC medications because many cold medications can worsen symptoms or other health problems, specifically hypertension.

The nurse stresses the importance of following the recommended antibiotic regimen because a consistent blood level of the medication is critical to treat the infection. The nurse educates the patient about the early signs of a sinus infection and recommends preventive measures such as following healthy practices and avoiding contact with people with URIs.

The nurse explains to the patient that fever, severe headache, and **nuchal rigidity** (stiffness of the neck or inability to bend the neck) are signs of the potential complication of meningitis. Patients with chronic symptoms of rhinosinusitis who do not have marked improvement in 4 weeks with continuous medical treatment may be candidates for functional endoscopic sinus surgery (FESS, see later discussion) (Tajudeen & Kennedy, 2017).

> ▶ **Quality and Safety Nursing Alert**
>
> *Patients with nasotracheal and nasogastric tubes in place are at the risk for development of sinus infections (Brook, 2018a; Brook, 2018b). Thus, accurate assessment of patients with these tubes is critical. Removal of the nasotracheal or nasogastric tube as soon as the patient's condition permits allows the sinuses to drain, possibly avoiding septic complications.*

Chronic Rhinosinusitis and Recurrent Acute Rhinosinusitis

The prevalence of CRS is about 146 per 1000 population in the United States and occurs most commonly in young and middle-aged adults (Brook, 2018b). It is diagnosed when the patient has experienced 12 weeks or longer of two or more of the following symptoms: mucopurulent drainage, nasal obstruction, facial pain–pressure–fullness, or hyposmia (decreased sense of smell). It is estimated that in about 40% of patients, CRS is accompanied by nasal polyps (Rosenfeld et al., 2015). Recurrent acute rhinosinusitis is diagnosed when four or more episodes of ABRS occur per year with no signs or symptoms of rhinosinusitis between the episodes. The use of antibiotics in patients with recurrent acute rhinosinusitis is higher than in patients with CRS. Both CRS and recurrent acute rhinosinusitis affect quality of life as well as physical and social function (Hamilos, 2018).

Pathophysiology

Mechanical obstruction in the ostia of the frontal, maxillary, and anterior ethmoid sinuses (known collectively as the ostiomeatal complex) is the usual cause of CRS and recurrent acute rhinosinusitis. Obstruction prevents adequate drainage of the nasal passages, resulting in accumulation of secretions and an ideal medium for bacterial growth. Persistent blockage

in an adult may occur because of infection, allergy, or structural abnormalities. Other associated conditions and factors may include cystic fibrosis, ciliary dyskinesia, neoplastic disorders, gastroesophageal reflux disease, tobacco use, and environmental pollution (Brook, 2018a).

Both aerobic and anaerobic bacteria have been implicated in CRS and recurrent rhinosinusitis. Common aerobic bacteria include alpha-hemolytic streptococci, microaerophilic streptococci, and *S. aureus*. Common anaerobic bacteria include gram-negative bacilli, *Peptostreptococcus,* and *Fusobacterium*.

In addition, immunodeficiency should be considered in patients with CRS or acute recurrent rhinosinusitis. Acute fulminant/invasive rhinosinusitis is a life-threatening illness and is commonly attributed to *Aspergillus* in immunocompromised patients. Chronic fungal sinusitis also poses a risk. Chronic invasive fungal sinusitis occurs in immunocompromised patients along with fungus ball/mycetoma and allergic fungal sinusitis—the more common forms of chronic fungal sinusitis—which are considered noninvasive conditions in immunocompromised patients. The fungus ball is characterized by the presence of a noninvasive accumulation of a dense conglomeration of fungal hyphae in one sinus cavity, usually the maxillary sinus. The fungus generally remains contained in the fungus ball, which consists of mucopurulent cheesy or claylike materials within the sinus, but can become invasive when immunosuppression occurs, leading to encephalopathy (Ramadan, 2018). Symptoms include nasal stuffiness, nasal discharge, and facial pain. Vision loss, headache, and cranial nerve palsies have been identified in patients with a sphenoid sinus fungal ball (Ramadan, 2018).

Clinical Manifestations

Clinical manifestations of CRS include impaired mucociliary clearance and ventilation, cough (because the thick discharge constantly drips backward into the nasopharynx), chronic hoarseness, chronic headaches in the periorbital area, periorbital edema, and facial pain. As a result of chronic nasal congestion, the patient is usually required to breathe through the mouth. Snoring, sore throat, and, in some situations, adenoidal hypertrophy may also occur. Symptoms are generally most pronounced on awakening in the morning. Fatigue and nasal congestion are also common. Many patients experience a decrease in smell and taste and a sense of fullness in the ears.

Assessment and Diagnostic Findings

The health assessment focuses on onset and duration of symptoms. It addresses the quantity and quality of nasal discharge and cough, the presence of pain, factors that relieve or aggravate the pain, and allergies. It is essential to obtain any history of comorbid conditions, including asthma and history of tobacco use and smoking or use of electronic nicotine delivery systems (ENDS) including e-cigarettes, e-pens, e-pipes, e-hookah, and e-cigars. A history of fever, fatigue, previous episodes and treatments and previous response to therapies is also obtained.

In the physical assessment, the external nose is evaluated for any evidence of anatomic abnormality. A crooked-appearing external nose may imply septal deviation internally. The nasal mucous membranes are assessed for erythema, pallor, atrophy, edema, crusting, discharge, polyps, erosions, and septal perforations or deviations. Appropriate lighting improves visualization of the nasal cavity and should be used in every examination. Pain on examination of the teeth, with tapping with a tongue blade, suggests tooth infection (Bickley & Szilagyi, 2017).

Assessment of the posterior oropharynx may reveal purulent or mucoid discharge, which is indicative of an infection caused by CRS. The patient's eyes are examined for conjunctival erythema, tearing, photophobia, and edema of the lids. Additional assessment techniques include transillumination of the sinuses and palpation of the sinuses. The frontal and maxillary sinuses are palpated, and the patient is asked whether this produces tenderness. The pharynx is inspected for erythema and discharge and palpated for cervical node adenopathy (Hamilos, 2018).

Imaging studies such as x-ray, sinoscopy, ultrasound, CT scanning, and MRI may be used in the diagnosis of CRS. X-ray is an inexpensive and readily available tool to assess disorders of the paranasal sinuses. A CT scan of the paranasal sinuses can identify mucosal abnormalities, sinus ostial obstruction, anatomic variants, sinonasal polyposis, and neoplastic disease. In addition, nasal endoscopy allows for visualization of the posterior nasal cavity, nasopharynx, and sinus drainage pathways and can identify posterior septal deviation and polyps. Osseous destruction, extrasinus extension of the disease process, and local invasion suggest malignancy (Rosenfeld et al., 2015).

Complications

Complications of CRS, although uncommon, include severe orbital cellulitis, subperiosteal abscess, cavernous sinus thrombosis, meningitis, encephalitis, and ischemic infarction. CRS can lead to intracranial infection either by direct spread through bone or via venous channels, resulting in epidural abscess, subdural empyema, meningitis, and brain abscess. Clinical sequelae can include personality changes with frontal lobe abscesses, headache, symptoms of elevated intracranial pressure to include alterations of consciousness, visual changes, focal neurologic deficits, seizures, and, ultimately, coma and death.

Frontal rhinosinusitis can lead to osteomyelitis of the frontal bones. Patients typically present with headache, fever, and a characteristic doughy edema over the involved bone. Ethmoid rhinosinusitis may result in orbital cellulitis, which usually begins with edema of the eyelids and rapidly progresses to ptosis (droopy eyelid), proptosis (bulging eye), chemosis (edema of the bulbar conjunctiva), and diminished extraocular movements. Patients are usually febrile and acutely ill and require immediate attention, because pressure on the optic nerve can lead to loss of vision and spread of infection can lead to intracranial infection (Brook, 2018a). Cavernous sinus thrombophlebitis can result from extension of infection along venous channels from the orbit, ethmoid or frontal sinuses, or nose. Symptoms may include altered consciousness, lid edema, and proptosis, as well as third, fourth, and sixth cranial nerve palsies.

Medical Management

Medical management of CRS and recurrent acute rhinosinusitis is similar to that of acute rhinosinusitis. General measures include encouraging adequate hydration and recommending the use of OTC nasal saline sprays, antispasmodic agents such as acetaminophen or NSAIDs, and decongestants such as oxymetazoline and pseudoephedrine (Brook, 2018b; Tewfik, 2018). Patients are instructed to sleep with the head of the bed elevated and to avoid exposure to cigarette smoke and fumes. Patients are cautioned to avoid caffeine and alcohol, which can cause dehydration.

Prescribed antibiotics may include amoxicillin–clavulanic acid, erythromycin–sulfisoxazole, second- or third-generation cephalosporins such as cefuroxime or cefixime, or newer fluoroquinolones such as moxifloxacin (Brook, 2018b). The course of antibiotic treatment for CRS and recurrent ABRS is typically as long as 2 to 4 weeks to effectively eradicate the offending organism, and may be indicated for up to 12 months in some cases (Brook, 2018b). Corticosteroid nasal sprays such as fluticasone or beclomethasone may be indicated in patients with concomitant allergic rhinitis or nasal polyps. Patients with allergic rhinitis may also benefit from the addition of a mast cell stabilizer such as cromolyn. For patients with concomitant asthma, leukotriene inhibitors such as montelukast and zafirlukast may be used (Brook, 2018b).

Surgical Management

If standard medical therapy fails and symptoms persist, FESS may be indicated to correct structural deformities that obstruct the ostia (openings) of the sinuses. FESS is a minimally invasive surgical procedure that is associated with reduced postoperative discomfort and improvement in the patient's quality of life. In particular, FESS is associated with either complete or moderate relief of symptoms in more than 85% to 91% of patients (Patel, 2016). Some of the specific procedures performed include excising and cauterizing nasal polyps, correcting a deviated septum, incising and draining the sinuses, aerating the sinuses, and removing tumors. Computer-assisted or computer-guided surgery is used to increase the precision of the surgical procedure and to minimize complications. Antimicrobial agents are typically prescribed after surgery (Patel, 2016).

Surgical intervention is first-line treatment in acute invasive fungal rhinosinusitis to excise the fungus ball and necrotic tissue and drain the sinuses. Patients require aggressive surgical débridement and drainage as well as systemic antifungal medications (Ramadan, 2018).

Nursing Management

Patients usually perform care measures for rhinosinusitis at home; therefore, nursing management consists of good patient education.

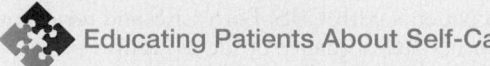 **Educating Patients About Self-Care**

Many people with sinus infections tend to blow their nose frequently and with force to clear their nasal passages. Doing so often increases the symptoms; therefore, the patient is instructed to blow the nose gently and to use tissue to remove the nasal drainage. Increasing fluid intake, applying local heat (hot wet packs), and elevating the head of the bed promote drainage of the sinuses. The nurse also instructs the patient about the importance of following the prescribed medication regimen. Instructions on the early signs of a sinus infection are provided, and preventive measures are reviewed. The nurse instructs the patient about signs and symptoms that require follow-up and provides these instructions verbally and in writing. Instructions in alternative formats (e.g., large font, patient's language) may be needed to increase the patient's understanding and adherence to the treatment plan. The nurse encourages the patient to follow up with their primary provider if symptoms persist (American Academy of Otolaryngology–Head and Neck Surgery Foundation, 2018).

> ### ◣ Quality and Safety Nursing Alert
>
> *URIs, specifically CRS and recurrent acute rhinosinusitis, may be linked to primary or secondary immune deficiency or treatment with immunosuppressive therapy (e.g., for cancer or organ transplantation). Typical symptoms may be blunted or absent due to immunosuppression. Immunocompromised patients are at the increased risk for acute or chronic fungal infections; these infections can progress rapidly and become life-threatening (Brook, 2018a; Brook, 2018b). Thus, assessment, early reporting of symptoms to the patient's primary provider, and immediate initiation of treatment are essential.*

Pharyngitis

Acute Pharyngitis

Acute **pharyngitis** is a sudden painful inflammation of the pharynx, the back portion of the throat that includes the posterior third of the tongue, soft palate, and tonsils. It is commonly referred to as a sore throat. In the United States, approximately 12 million health care visits are due to acute pharyngitis each year (Chow & Doron, 2018). Because of environmental exposure to viral agents and poorly ventilated rooms, the incidence of viral pharyngitis peaks during winter and early spring in regions that have warm summers and cold winters. Viral pharyngitis spreads easily in the droplets of coughs and sneezes, as well as from unclean hands that have been exposed to the contaminated fluids.

Pathophysiology

Viral infection causes most cases of acute pharyngitis. Responsible viruses include the adenovirus, influenza virus, Epstein–Barr virus, and herpes simplex virus. Bacterial infection accounts for the remainder of cases. Five percent to 15% of adults with pharyngitis have group A beta-hemolytic

streptococcus (GABHS), which is commonly referred to as group A streptococcus (GAS) or streptococcal pharyngitis. Streptococcal pharyngitis warrants the use of antibiotic treatment. When GAS causes acute pharyngitis, the condition is known as strep throat. The body responds by triggering an inflammatory response in the pharynx. This results in pain, fever, vasodilation, edema, and tissue damage, manifested by redness and swelling in the tonsillar pillars, uvula, and soft palate. A creamy exudate may be present in the tonsillar pillars (Fig. 18-2). Other organisms implicated in acute pharyngitis include groups B and G streptococci, *Neisseria gonorrhoeae*, *Mycoplasma pneumoniae*, *C. pneumoniae*, *Arcanobacterium haemolyticum*, and HIV (Chow & Doron, 2018).

Uncomplicated viral infections usually subside promptly, within 3 to 10 days after onset. However, pharyngitis caused by bacteria, such as GAS, is a more severe illness. If left untreated, the complications can be severe and life-threatening. Complications include rhinosinusitis, otitis media, peritonsillar abscess, mastoiditis, and cervical adenitis. In rare cases, the infection may lead to sepsis, pneumonia, meningitis, rheumatic fever, and glomerulonephritis (Buensalido, 2019a).

Clinical Manifestations

The signs and symptoms of acute pharyngitis include a fiery-red pharyngeal membrane and tonsils, lymphoid follicles that are swollen and flecked with white-purple exudate, enlarged and tender cervical lymph nodes, and no cough. Fever (higher than 38.3°C [101°F]) and malaise also may be present. Occasionally, patients with GAS pharyngitis exhibit vomiting, anorexia, and a scarlatina-form rash with urticaria known as scarlet fever.

People who have streptococcal pharyngitis suddenly develop a painful sore throat 1 to 5 days after being exposed to the streptococcus bacteria. They usually report malaise, fever (with or without chills), headache, myalgia, painful cervical adenopathy, and nausea. The tonsils appear swollen and erythematous, and they may or may not have an exudate. The roof of the mouth is often erythematous and may demonstrate petechiae. Bad breath is common.

Assessment and Diagnostic Findings

Accurate diagnosis of pharyngitis is essential to determine the cause (viral or bacterial) and to initiate treatment early. Rapid antigen detection testing (RADT) uses swabs that collect specimens from the posterior pharynx and tonsil. RADT is reported to be 90% to 95% sensitive, thus facilitating earlier

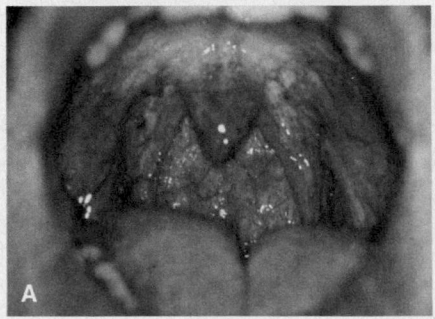 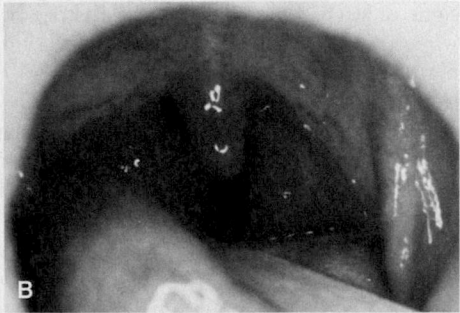

Figure 18-2 • Pharyngitis—inflammation without exudate. **A.** Redness and vascularity of the pillars and uvula are mild to moderate. **B.** Redness is diffuse and intense. Each patient would probably complain of a sore throat. Reprinted with permission from the Wellcome Trust, National Medical Slide Bank, London, UK.

treatment and earlier symptom improvement and reductions in pathogen transmission. Negative results should be confirmed by a throat culture (Acerra, 2018). In most communities, preliminary culture reports are available in 24 hours. Once a definitive diagnosis of GAS is made, administration of appropriate antibiotics hastens symptom resolution and reduces the transmission of the illness.

Medical Management

Viral pharyngitis is treated with supportive measures because antibiotics have no effect on the causal organism. Bacterial pharyngitis is treated with a variety of antimicrobial agents (Uyeki, Bernstein, Bradley, et al., 2018).

Pharmacologic Therapy

If the cause of pharyngitis is bacterial, penicillin is usually the treatment of choice. Penicillin V potassium given orally for 10 days is the regimen of choice. Penicillin injections are recommended only if there is a concern that the patient will not adhere to therapy (Papadakis et al., 2018).

For patients who are allergic to penicillin or have organisms that are resistant to erythromycin (one fifth of GAS and most *S. aureus* organisms are resistant to penicillin and erythromycin), cephalosporins and macrolides (clarithromycin and azithromycin) may be used. Once-daily azithromycin may be given for only 3 days due to its long half-life (Acerra, 2018). A 5- or 10-day course of cephalosporin may be prescribed. Five-day administration of cefpodoxime and cefuroxime has also been successful in producing bacteriologic cures.

Severe sore throats can also be relieved by analgesic medications. For example, aspirin or acetaminophen can be taken at 4- to 6-hour intervals; if required, acetaminophen with codeine can be taken three or four times daily. In severe cases, gargles with benzocaine may relieve symptoms.

Nutritional Therapy

A liquid or soft diet is provided during the acute stage of the disease, depending on the patient's appetite and the degree of discomfort that occurs with swallowing. Cool beverages, warm liquids, and flavored frozen desserts such as ice pops are often soothing. Occasionally, the throat is so sore that liquids cannot be taken in adequate amounts by mouth. In severe situations, intravenous (IV) fluids may be needed. Otherwise, the patient is encouraged to drink as much fluid as possible (at least 2 to 3 L/day).

Nursing Management

Nursing care for patients with viral pharyngitis focuses on symptomatic management. For patients who demonstrate signs of strep throat and have a history of rheumatic fever, who have scarlet fever, or who have symptoms suggesting peritonsillar abscess, nursing care focuses on prompt initiation and correct administration of prescribed antibiotic therapy. The nurse instructs the patient about signs and symptoms that warrant prompt contact with the primary provider. These include dyspnea, drooling, inability to swallow, and inability to fully open the mouth.

The nurse instructs the patient to stay in bed during the febrile stage of illness and to rest frequently once up and about. Used tissues should be disposed of properly to prevent the spread of infection. The nurse (or the patient or family member, if the patient is not hospitalized) should examine the skin once or twice daily for possible rash, because acute pharyngitis may precede some other communicable diseases (e.g., rubella).

Depending on the severity of the pharyngitis and the degree of pain, warm saline gargles or throat irrigations are used. The benefits of this treatment depend on the degree of heat that is applied. The nurse educates the patient about these procedures and about the recommended temperature of the solution, which should be high enough to be effective and as warm as the patient can tolerate, usually 40.6° to 43.3°C (105° to 110°F). Irrigating the throat may reduce spasm in the pharyngeal muscles and relieve soreness of the throat.

An ice collar also can relieve severe sore throats. Mouth care may promote the patient's comfort and prevent the development of fissures (cracking) of the lips and oral inflammation when bacterial infection is present. The nurse instructs the patient to resume activity gradually and to delay returning to work or school until after 24 hours of antibiotic therapy. A full course of antibiotic therapy is indicated in patients with strep infection because of the potential complications such as nephritis and rheumatic fever, which may have their onset 2 or 3 weeks after the pharyngitis has subsided. The nurse instructs the patient and family about the importance of taking the full course of antibiotic therapy and informs them about the symptoms to watch for that may indicate complications.

In addition, the nurse instructs the patient about preventive measures that include not sharing eating utensils, glasses, napkins, food, or towels; cleaning telephones after use; using a tissue to cough or sneeze; disposing of used tissues appropriately; coughing or sneezing into the upper arm if tissues are not readily available; and avoiding exposure to tobacco and secondhand smoke. The nurse also instructs the patient with pharyngitis, especially streptococcal pharyngitis, to replace their toothbrush with a new one.

Chronic Pharyngitis

Chronic pharyngitis is a persistent inflammation of the pharynx. It is common in adults who work in dusty surroundings, use their voice to excess, suffer from chronic cough, or habitually use alcohol and tobacco.

There are three types of chronic pharyngitis:
- Hypertrophic—characterized by general thickening and congestion of the pharyngeal mucous membrane
- Atrophic—probably a late stage of the first type (the membrane is thin, whitish, glistening, and at times wrinkled)
- Chronic granular—characterized by numerous swollen lymph follicles on the pharyngeal wall

Clinical Manifestations

Patients with chronic pharyngitis complain of a constant sense of irritation or fullness in the throat, mucus that collects in the throat and can be expelled by coughing, and difficulty swallowing. This is often associated with intermittent postnasal drip that causes minor irritation and inflammation of the pharynx. A sore throat that is worse with swallowing in the absence of pharyngitis suggests the possibility of thyroiditis, and patients with this symptom are referred for the evaluation of possible thyroiditis.

Medical Management

Treatment of chronic pharyngitis is based on relieving symptoms; avoiding exposure to irritants; and correcting any upper respiratory, pulmonary, gastrointestinal, or cardiac condition that might be responsible for a chronic cough.

Nasal congestion may be relieved by short-term use of nasal sprays or medications containing ephedrine sulfate or phenylephrine. For a patient with a history of allergy, one of the antihistamine decongestant medications, such as pseudoephedrine or brompheniramine/pseudoephedrine, is prescribed orally every 4 to 6 hours. Aspirin (for patients older than 20 years) or acetaminophen is recommended for its analgesic properties.

For adults with chronic pharyngitis, tonsillectomy may be offered as an option, although its effectiveness in reaping long-term improvement in symptoms has not been established (Burton, Glasziou, Chong, et al., 2014). For further information, see the Tonsillitis and Adenoiditis section.

Nursing Management

 Educating Patients About Self-Care

The nurse recommends avoidance of alcohol, tobacco, ENDS use, secondhand smoke, and exposure to cold or to environmental or occupational pollutants. The patient may minimize exposure to pollutants by wearing a disposable facemask, preferably an N95 mask, which can filter out 95% of small particles, including dusts and molds (National Institute for Occupational Safety and Health, 2018). The nurse encourages the patient to drink plenty of fluids. Gargling with warm saline solution may relieve throat discomfort. Lozenges keep the throat moistened (Stead, 2017).

Tonsillitis and Adenoiditis

The tonsils are composed of lymphatic tissue and are situated on each side of the oropharynx. The faucial or palatine tonsils and lingual tonsils are located behind the pillars of fauces and tongue, respectively. They frequently serve as the site of infection (**tonsillitis**). Acute tonsillitis can be confused with pharyngitis. Chronic tonsillitis is less common and may be mistaken for other disorders such as allergy, asthma, and rhinosinusitis.

The adenoids or pharyngeal tonsils consist of lymphatic tissue near the center of the posterior wall of the nasopharynx. Infection of the adenoids frequently accompanies acute tonsillitis. Frequently occurring bacterial pathogens include GABHS, the most common organism. The most common viral pathogen is Epstein–Barr virus, although cytomegalovirus may also cause tonsillitis and adenoiditis. Often thought of as a childhood disorder, tonsillitis can occur in adults.

Clinical Manifestations

The symptoms of tonsillitis include sore throat, fever, snoring, and difficulty swallowing. Enlarged adenoids may cause mouth breathing, earache, draining ears, frequent head colds, bronchitis, foul-smelling breath, voice impairment, and noisy respiration. Unusually enlarged adenoids fill the space behind the posterior nares, making it difficult for the air to travel from the nose to the throat and resulting in nasal obstruction. Infection can extend to the middle ears by way of the auditory (eustachian) tubes and may result in acute otitis media, which can lead to spontaneous rupture of the tympanic membranes (eardrums) and further extension of the infection into the mastoid cells, causing acute mastoiditis. The infection also may reside in the middle ear as a chronic, low-grade, smoldering process that eventually may cause permanent deafness.

Assessment and Diagnostic Findings

The diagnosis of acute tonsillitis is primarily clinical, with attention given to whether the illness is viral or bacterial in nature. As in acute pharyngitis, RADT is quick and convenient; however, it is less sensitive than the throat swab culture.

A thorough physical examination is performed and a careful history is obtained to rule out related or systemic conditions. The tonsillar site is cultured to determine the presence of bacterial infection. When cytomegalovirus infection is present, the differential diagnosis should include HIV, hepatitis A, and rubella. In adenoiditis, if recurrent episodes of suppurative otitis media result in hearing loss, comprehensive audiometric assessment is warranted (see Chapter 59).

Medical Management

Tonsillitis is treated with supportive measures that include increased fluid intake, antispasmodic agents, salt-water gargles, and rest. Bacterial infections are treated with penicillin (first-line therapy) or cephalosporins. Viral tonsillitis is not effectively treated with antibiotic therapy.

Tonsillectomy (with or without adenoidectomy) continues to be a commonly performed surgical procedure and remains the treatment of choice for patients with chronic tonsillitis (Shah, 2018). Adults who have undergone a tonsillectomy to treat recurrent streptococcal infections experience a decrease in the number of episodes of streptococcal or other throat infections or days with throat pain (Busaba & Doron, 2018).

Tonsillectomy is indicated if the patient has had repeated episodes of tonsillitis despite antibiotic therapy; hypertrophy of the tonsils and adenoids that could cause obstruction and obstructive sleep apnea (OSA); repeated attacks of purulent otitis media; and suspected hearing loss due to serous otitis media that has occurred in association with enlarged tonsils and adenoids. Indications for adenoidectomy include chronic nasal airway obstruction, chronic rhinorrhea, obstruction of the auditory tube with related ear infections, and abnormal speech. Surgery is also indicated if the patient has developed a peritonsillar abscess that occludes the pharynx, making swallowing difficult and endangering the patency of the airway (particularly during sleep). The presence of persistent tonsillar asymmetry should prompt an excisional biopsy to rule out lymphoma (Papadakis et al., 2018). Antibiotic therapy may be initiated for patients undergoing tonsillectomy or adenoidectomy. Therapy may include oral penicillin or a cephalosporin (e.g., cefdinir or moxifloxacin).

Nursing Management

Providing Postoperative Care

Continuous nursing observation is required in the immediate postoperative and recovery periods because of the risk of hemorrhage, which may also compromise the patient's airway (Drake & Carr, 2017). In the immediate postoperative period, the most comfortable position is prone, with the patient's head turned to the side to allow drainage from the mouth and pharynx. The nurse must not remove the oral airway until the patient's gag and swallowing reflexes have returned. The nurse applies an ice collar to the neck, and a basin and tissues are provided for the expectoration of blood and mucus.

Symptoms of postoperative complications include fever, throat pain, ear pain, and bleeding. Pain can be effectively controlled with analgesic medications. Postoperative bleeding may be seen as bright red blood if the patient expectorates it before swallowing it. If the patient swallows the blood, it becomes brown because of the action of the acidic gastric juice. If the patient vomits large amounts of dark blood or bright-red blood at frequent intervals, or if the pulse rate and temperature rise and the patient is restless, the nurse notifies the surgeon immediately. The nurse should have the following items ready for the examination of the surgical site for bleeding: a light, a mirror, gauze, curved hemostats, and a waste basin.

Occasionally, suture or ligation of a bleeding vessel is required. In such cases, the patient is taken to the operating room and given general anesthesia. After ligation, continuous nursing observation and postoperative care are required, as in the initial postoperative period. If there is no bleeding, water and ice chips may be given to the patient as soon as desired. The patient is instructed to refrain from too much talking and coughing, because these activities can produce throat pain (see Chapter 16 for further discussion of postoperative nursing care).

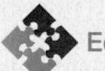 **Educating Patients About Self-Care**

Tonsillectomy and adenoidectomy are usually performed as outpatient surgery, and the patient is sent home from the recovery room once awake, oriented, and able to drink liquids and void. The patient and family must understand the signs and symptoms of hemorrhage. Bleeding may occur up to 8 days after surgery. The nurse instructs the patient about the use of liquid acetaminophen with or without codeine for pain control and explains that the pain will subside during the first 3 to 5 days. The nurse informs the patient about the need to take the full course of any prescribed antibiotic for the first postoperative week (Drake & Carr, 2017).

Alkaline mouthwashes and warm saline solutions are useful in coping with the thick mucus and halitosis that may be present after surgery. The nurse should explain to the patient that a sore throat, stiff neck, minor ear pain, and vomiting may occur in the first 24 hours. The patient should eat an adequate diet with soft foods, which are more easily swallowed than hard foods. The patient should avoid spicy, hot, acidic, or rough foods. Milk and milk products (ice cream and yogurt) may be restricted because they make removal of mucus more difficult for some patients. The nurse instructs the patient about the need to maintain good hydration. The

patient is advised to avoid vigorous toothbrushing or gargling because these activities can cause bleeding. The nurse encourages the use of a cool-mist vaporizer or humidifier in the home postoperatively. The patient should avoid smoking and heavy lifting or exertion for 10 days.

Peritonsillar Abscess

Peritonsillar abscess (also called *quinsy*) is the most common major suppurative complication of sore throat accounting for roughly 30% of soft tissue head and neck abscesses. It most commonly afflicts adults between the ages of 20 and 40 years, with the incidence roughly the same between men and women (Flores, 2018). This collection of purulent exudate between the tonsillar capsule and the surrounding tissues, including the soft palate, may develop after an acute tonsillar infection that progresses to a local cellulitis and abscess. Several bacteria are typically implicated in the pathogenesis of these abscesses, including *S. pyogenes*, *S. aureus*, *Neisseria* species, and *Corynebacterium* species (Flores, 2018; Shah, 2018). In more severe cases, the infection can spread over the palate and to the neck and chest. Edema can cause airway obstruction, which can be life-threatening and is a medical emergency. Peritonsillar abscess can be life-threatening with mediastinitis, intracranial abscess, and empyemas resulting from spread of infection. Early detection and aggressive management are essential (Flores, 2018).

Clinical Manifestations

The patient with a peritonsillar abscess is acutely ill with a severe sore throat, fever, trismus (inability to open the mouth), and drooling. Inflammation of the medial pterygoid muscle that lies lateral to the tonsil results in spasm, severe pain, and difficulty in opening the mouth fully. The pain may be so intense that the patient has difficulty swallowing saliva. The patient's breath often smells rancid. Other symptoms include a raspy voice, odynophagia (a severe sensation of burning, squeezing pain while swallowing), **dysphagia** (difficulty swallowing), and otalgia (pain in the ear). Odynophagia is caused by the inflammation of the superior constrictor muscle of the pharynx that forms the lateral wall of the tonsil. This causes pain on lateral movement of the head. The patient may also have tender and enlarged cervical lymph nodes. Examination of the oropharynx reveals erythema of the anterior pillar and soft palate as well as a purulent tonsil on the side of the peritonsillar abscess. The tonsil is pushed inferomedially, and the uvula is shifted contralaterally (Flores, 2018).

Assessment and Diagnostic Findings

Emergency department (ED) physicians frequently are the providers who diagnose patients with peritonsillar abscesses. When this occurs in the ED setting, the ED physician decides whether aspiration—an invasive procedure—should be carried out based on the patient's clinical picture. Intraoral ultrasound and transcutaneous cervical ultrasound are used in the diagnosis of peritonsillar cellulitis and abscesses (Gosselin, 2018).

Medical Management

Antimicrobial agents and corticosteroid therapy are used for the treatment of peritonsillar abscess. Antibiotics (usually penicillin) are extremely effective in controlling the infection, and if they are prescribed early in the course of the disease, the abscess may resolve without needing to be incised. However, if the abscess does not resolve, treatment choices include needle aspiration, incision and drainage under local or general anesthesia, and drainage of the abscess with simultaneous tonsillectomy. Following needle aspiration (discussed later) intramuscular administration of clindamycin can be used in the outpatient setting, thus reducing both antibiotic and hospital costs. The use of topical anesthetic agents and throat irrigations may be prescribed to promote comfort along with administration of prescribed analgesic agents (Flores, 2018).

Patients with complications require hospitalization for IV antibiotics, imaging studies, observation, and proper airway management. Rarely, the patient with a peritonsillar abscess presents with acute airway obstruction and requires immediate airway management. Procedures may include intubation, cricothyroidotomy, or tracheotomy (Flores, 2018).

Surgical Management

Needle aspiration may be preferred over a more extensive procedure due to its high efficacy, low cost, and patient tolerance. The mucous membrane over the swelling is first sprayed with a topical anesthetic and then injected with a local anesthetic. Single or repeated needle aspirations are performed to decompress the abscess. Alternatively, the abscess may be incised and drained (Flores, 2018). These procedures are performed best with the patient in the sitting position to make it easier to expectorate the pus and blood that accumulate in the pharynx. The patient experiences almost immediate relief. Incision and drainage is also an effective option but is more painful than needle aspiration.

Tonsillectomy is considered for patients who are poor candidates for needle aspiration or incision and drainage (Flores, 2018).

Nursing Management

If the patient requires intubation, cricothyroidotomy, or tracheotomy to treat airway obstruction, the nurse assists with the procedure and provides support to the patient before, during, and after the procedure. The nurse also assists with the needle aspiration when indicated.

The nurse encourages the patient to use prescribed topical anesthetic agents and assists with throat irrigations or the frequent use of mouthwashes or gargles, using saline or alkaline solutions at a temperature of 40.6° to 43.3°C (105° to 110°F). Gentle gargling after the procedure with a cool normal saline gargle may relieve discomfort. The patient must be upright and clearly expectorate forward. The nurse instructs the patient to gargle *gently* at intervals of 1 or 2 hours for 24 to 36 hours. Liquids that are cool or at room temperature are usually well tolerated. Adequate fluids must be provided to treat dehydration and prevent its recurrence.

The nurse also observes the patient for complications and instructs the patient about signs and symptoms of complications that require prompt attention by the patient's primary provider. At discharge, the nurse provides verbal and written instructions regarding foods to avoid, when to return to work, and the need to refrain from or cease smoking. The need for continuation of good oral hygiene is also reinforced.

Laryngitis

Laryngitis, an inflammation of the larynx, can occur as a result of voice abuse, exposure to dust, chemicals, smoke and other pollutants; or as part of a URI. It also may be caused by isolated infection involving only the vocal cords. Laryngitis can also be associated with gastroesophageal reflux (referred to as reflux laryngitis).

Laryngitis is very often caused by the pathogens that cause the common cold and pharyngitis; the most common cause is a virus, and laryngitis is often associated with allergic rhinitis or pharyngitis. Bacterial invasion may be secondary. The onset of infection may be associated with exposure to sudden temperature changes, dietary deficiencies, malnutrition, or an immunosuppressed state. Viral laryngitis is common in the winter and is easily transmitted to others.

Clinical Manifestations

Signs of acute laryngitis include hoarseness or **aphonia** (loss of voice) and severe cough. Chronic laryngitis is marked by persistent hoarseness. Other signs of acute laryngitis include sudden onset made worse by cold dry wind. The throat feels worse in the morning and improves when the patient is indoors in a warmer climate. At times, the patient presents with a dry cough and a dry, sore throat that worsens in the evening hours. If allergies are present, the uvula will be visibly edematous. Many patients also complain of a "tickle" in the throat that is made worse by cold air or cold liquids.

Medical Management

Management of acute laryngitis includes resting the voice, avoiding irritants (including smoking), resting, and inhaling cool steam or an aerosol. If the laryngitis is part of a more extensive respiratory infection caused by a bacterial organism or if it is severe, appropriate antibacterial therapy is instituted. The majority of patients recover with conservative treatment; however, laryngitis tends to be more severe in older adult patients and may be complicated by pneumonia.

For chronic laryngitis, the treatment includes resting the voice, eliminating any primary respiratory tract infection, eliminating smoking, and avoiding secondhand smoke. Corticosteroids, such as beclomethasone, may be given. These preparations have few systemic or long-lasting effects and may reduce local inflammatory reactions. Treatment of reflux laryngitis typically involves use of proton pump inhibitors such as omeprazole given once daily.

Nursing Management

The nurse instructs the patient to rest the voice and to maintain a well-humidified environment. If laryngeal secretions are present during acute episodes, expectorant agents are suggested, along with a daily fluid intake of 2 to 3 L to thin secretions. The nurse instructs the patient about the importance of taking prescribed medications, including proton pump inhibitors, and using continuous positive airway therapy at bedtime, if prescribed for OSA. In cases involving infection, the nurse informs the patient that the symptoms of laryngitis often extend a week to 10 days after completion of antibiotic therapy. The nurse instructs the patient about signs and symptoms that require contacting the primary provider. These signs and symptoms include loss of voice with sore throat that makes swallowing saliva difficult, hemoptysis, and noisy respirations. Continued hoarseness after voice rest or laryngitis that persists for longer than 5 days must be reported because of the possibility of malignancy.

NURSING PROCESS

The Patient with Upper Airway Infection

Assessment

A health history may reveal signs and symptoms of headache, sore throat, pain around the eyes and on either side of the nose, difficulty in swallowing, cough, hoarseness, fever, stuffiness, and generalized discomfort and fatigue. Determining when the symptoms began, what precipitated them, what if anything relieves them, and what aggravates them is part of the assessment. The nurse should also determine any history of allergy or the existence of a concomitant illness. Inspection may reveal swelling, lesions, or asymmetry of the nose as well as bleeding or discharge. The nurse inspects the nasal mucosa for abnormal findings such as increased redness, swelling, exudate, and nasal polyps, which may develop in chronic rhinitis. The mucosa of the nasal turbinates may also be swollen (boggy) and pale bluish-gray. The nurse palpates the frontal and maxillary sinuses for tenderness, which suggests inflammation and then inspects the throat by having the patient open the mouth wide and take a deep breath. Redness, asymmetry, or evidence of drainage, ulceration, or enlargement of the tonsils and pharynx is abnormal. Palpation of the neck lymph nodes for enlargement and tenderness is necessary.

Diagnosis

NURSING DIAGNOSES

Based on the assessment data, nursing diagnoses may include the following:

- Impaired airway clearance associated with excessive mucus production secondary to retained secretions and inflammation
- Acute pain associated with upper airway irritation secondary to an infection
- Impaired verbal communication associated with physiologic changes and upper airway irritation secondary to infection or swelling
- Hypovolaemia associated with decreased fluid intake and increased fluid loss secondary to diaphoresis associated with a fever
- Lack of knowledge regarding prevention of URIs, treatment regimen, surgical procedure, or postoperative self-care

COLLABORATIVE PROBLEMS/POTENTIAL COMPLICATIONS

Based on the assessment data, potential complications include:

- Sepsis
- Meningitis or brain abscess
- Peritonsillar abscess, otitis media, or rhinosinusitis

Planning and Goals

The major goals for the patient may include maintenance of a patent airway, relief of pain, maintenance of effective means of communication, normal hydration, knowledge of how to prevent upper airway infections, and absence of complications.

Nursing Interventions

MAINTAINING A PATENT AIRWAY

An accumulation of secretions can block the airway in patients with an upper airway infection. As a result, changes in the respiratory pattern occur and the work of breathing increases to compensate for the blockage. The nurse can implement several measures to loosen thick secretions or to keep the secretions moist so that they can be easily expectorated. Increasing fluid intake helps thin the mucus. The use of room vaporizers or steam inhalation also loosens secretions and reduces inflammation of the mucous membranes. To enhance drainage from the sinuses, the nurse instructs the patient about positioning; this depends on the location of the infection or inflammation. For example, drainage for rhinosinusitis or rhinitis is achieved in the upright position. In some conditions, topical or systemic medications, when prescribed, help relieve nasal or throat congestion.

PROMOTING COMFORT

URIs usually produce localized discomfort. In rhinosinusitis, pain may occur in the area of the sinuses, or a general headache may be produced. In pharyngitis, laryngitis, or tonsillitis, a sore throat occurs. The nurse encourages the patient to take antispasmodic agents, such as acetaminophen with codeine, as prescribed, to relieve this discomfort. A pain intensity rating scale (see Chapter 9) may be used to assess effectiveness of pain relief measures. Other helpful measures include topical anesthetic agents for symptomatic relief of herpes simplex blisters (see Chart 18-3) and sore throats, hot packs to relieve the congestion of rhinosinusitis and promote drainage, and warm water gargles or irrigations to relieve the pain of a sore throat. The nurse encourages rest to relieve the generalized discomfort and fever that accompany many upper airway conditions (especially rhinitis, pharyngitis, and laryngitis). For postoperative care after tonsillectomy and adenoidectomy, an ice collar may reduce swelling and decrease bleeding.

PROMOTING COMMUNICATION

Upper airway infections may result in hoarseness or loss of speech. The nurse instructs the patient to refrain from speaking as much as possible and, if possible, to communicate in writing instead. Additional strain on the vocal cords may delay full return of the voice. The nurse encourages the patient and family to use alternative forms of communication, such as a memo pad, bell, or a smartphone or other electronic devices to signal for assistance.

ENCOURAGING FLUID INTAKE

Upper airway infections lead to fluid loss. Sore throat, malaise, and fever may interfere with a patient's willingness to eat and drink. The nurse provides a list of easily ingested foods to increase caloric intake during the acute phase of illness. These include soups, gelatin, pudding, yogurt, cottage cheese, high-protein drinks, water, ice, and ice pops. The nurse encourages the patient to drink 2 to 3 L of fluid per day during the acute stage of airway infection, unless contraindicated, to thin the secretions and promote drainage. Liquids (hot or cold) may be soothing, depending on the disorder.

Promoting Home, Community-Based, and Transitional Care

Educating Patients About Self-Care. Prevention of most upper airway infections is challenging because of the many potential causes. But because most URIs are transmitted by hand-to-hand contact, the nurse educates the patient and family about techniques to minimize the spread of infection to others, including implementing hand hygiene measures. The nurse advises the patient to avoid exposure to people who are at the risk for serious illness if respiratory infection is transmitted (older adults, people who are immunosuppressed, and those with chronic health problems).

The nurse instructs patients and their families about strategies to relieve symptoms of URIs and reinforces the need to complete the treatment regimen, particularly when antibiotics are prescribed.

Continuing and Transitional Care. Referral for home, community-based, or transitional care is rare. However, it may be indicated for people whose health status was compromised before the onset of the respiratory infection and for those who cannot manage self-care without assistance. In such circumstances, the home health nurse assesses the patient's respiratory status and progress in recovery. The nurse may advise older adult patients and those at increased risk from a respiratory infection to consider annual influenza and pneumococcal vaccination. A follow-up appointment with the primary provider may be indicated for patients with compromised health status to ensure that the respiratory infection has resolved.

Monitoring and Managing Potential Complications

Although major complications of URIs are rare, the nurse must be aware of them and assess the patient for them. Because most patients with URIs are managed at home, patients and their families must be instructed to monitor for signs and symptoms and to seek immediate medical care if the patient's condition does not improve or if the patient's physical status appears to be worsening.

Sepsis or meningitis may occur in patients with compromised immune status or in those with an acute bacterial infection. The patient and caregiver are instructed to seek medical care if the patient's condition fails to improve within several days after the onset of symptoms, if unusual symptoms develop, or if the patient's condition deteriorates. They are instructed about signs and symptoms that require further attention: persistent or high fever, increasing shortness of breath, confusion, and increasing weakness and malaise. The patient with sepsis requires expert care to treat the infection, stabilize vital signs, and prevent or treat septic shock (see Chapter 11). Deterioration of the patient's condition necessitates intensive care measures (e.g., hemodynamic monitoring and administration of vasoactive medications, IV fluids, nutritional support, and corticosteroids) to monitor the patient's status and to support the patient's vital signs. High doses of antibiotics may be given to treat the causative organism. The nurse's role is to monitor the patient's vital signs, hemodynamic status, and laboratory values; administer needed treatment; alleviate the patient's physical discomfort; and provide explanations, education, and emotional support to the patient and family.

Peritonsillar abscess may develop after an acute infection of the tonsils. The patient requires treatment to drain the abscess and receives antibiotics for infection and topical anesthetic agents and throat irrigations to relieve pain and sore throat. Follow-up is necessary to ensure that the abscess resolves; tonsillectomy may be required. The nurse assists the patient in administering throat irrigations and instructs the patient and family about the importance of adhering to the prescribed treatment regimen and recommended follow-up appointments.

In some severe situations, peritonsillar abscess may progress to meningitis or brain abscess. The nurse assesses for changes in mental status ranging from subtle personality changes through drowsiness to coma, nuchal rigidity, and focal neurologic signs that signal increasing cerebral edema around the abscess (see Chapter 64). Seizures, typically tonic–clonic, occur in this setting. Intensive care measures are necessary. High doses of antibiotics may be used to treat the causative organism. The nurse's role is similar to caring for the patient with sepsis in an intensive care setting. The nurse monitors the patient's neurologic status and reports changes immediately.

Otitis media and rhinosinusitis may develop with URI. The patient and family are instructed about the signs and symptoms of otitis media and rhinosinusitis and about the importance of follow-up with the primary provider to ensure adequate evaluation and treatment of these conditions.

Evaluation

Expected patient outcomes may include the following:

1. Maintains a patent airway by managing secretions
   a. Reports decreased congestion
   b. Assumes best position to facilitate drainage of secretions
   c. Uses self-care measures appropriately and consistently to manage secretions during the acute phase of illness
2. Reports relief of pain and discomfort using pain intensity scale
   a. Uses comfort measures: antispasmodic agents, hot packs, gargles, rest
   b. Demonstrates adequate oral hygiene
3. Demonstrates ability to communicate needs, wants, level of comfort
4. Maintains adequate fluid and nutrition intake
5. Utilizes strategies to prevent upper airway infections and allergic reactions
   a. Demonstrates hand hygiene technique
   b. Identifies the value of the influenza vaccine
6. Demonstrates an adequate level of knowledge and performs self-care adequately
7. Becomes free of signs and symptoms of infection
   a. Exhibits normal vital signs (temperature, pulse, respiratory rate)
   b. Absence of purulent drainage
   c. Free of pain in ears, sinuses, and throat
   d. Absence of signs of inflammation
8. Absence of complications
   a. No signs of sepsis: fever, hypotension, deterioration of cognitive status
   b. Vital signs and hemodynamic status normal
   c. No evidence of neurologic involvement
   d. No signs of development of peritonsillar abscess
   e. Resolution of URI without development of otitis media or rhinosinusitis
   f. No signs and symptoms of brain abscess

OBSTRUCTION AND TRAUMA OF THE UPPER RESPIRATORY AIRWAY

Obstructive Sleep Apnea

OSA is a disorder characterized by recurrent episodes of upper airway obstruction and a reduction in ventilation. It is defined as **apnea** (cessation of breathing) during sleep usually caused by repetitive upper airway obstruction. The estimated prevalence of OSA is approximately 26% of adults between the ages of 30 and 70 years (Wickramasinghe, 2019). It is believed that between 4% and 9% of women and 9% and 24% of men in the United States have OSA, and that up to 90% are not diagnosed; these increased rates have been linked to the increase in rates of obesity (Wickramasinghe, 2019) (see Chapter 42). OSA interferes with people's ability to obtain adequate rest, thus affecting memory, learning, and decision making.

Risk factors for OSA include obesity, male gender, post-menopausal status in women, and advanced age. The major risk factor is obesity; a larger neck circumference and increased amounts of peripharyngeal fat narrow and compress the upper airway. Because OSA is often found in patients with hypertension, all adult patients with hypertension should be screened for OSA (Showalter & O'Keefe, 2019). Other associated factors include alterations in the upper airway, such as structural changes (e.g., tonsillar hypertrophy, abnormal posterior positioning of one or both jaws, and variations in craniofacial structures) that contribute to the collapsibility of the upper airway (Wickramasinghe, 2019).

Pathophysiology

The pharynx is a collapsible tube that can be compressed by the soft tissues and structures surrounding it. The tone of the muscles of the upper airway is reduced during sleep. Mechanical factors such as reduced diameter of the upper airway or dynamic changes in the upper airway during sleep may result in obstruction. These sleep-related changes may predispose to upper airway collapse when small amounts of negative pressure are generated during inspiration.

Repetitive apneic events result in hypoxia (decreased oxygen saturation) and hypercapnia (increased concentration of carbon dioxide), which triggers a sympathetic response. As a consequence, patients with OSA have a high prevalence of hypertension. In addition, OSA is associated with an increased risk of myocardial infarction and stroke, which may be mitigated with appropriate treatment (Wickramasinghe, 2019).

Clinical Manifestations

OSA is characterized by frequent and loud snoring with breathing cessation for 10 seconds or longer, for at least five episodes per hour, followed by awakening abruptly with a loud snort as the blood oxygen level drops. Patients with sleep apnea may have anywhere from five apneic episodes per hour to several hundred per night.

Classic signs and symptoms of OSA include the "3 S's"—namely, snoring, sleepiness, and significant-other report of sleep apnea episodes. Common signs and symptoms of OSA are presented in Chart 18-4. Symptoms typically progress with increases in weight and aging (Wickramasinghe, 2019). Patients

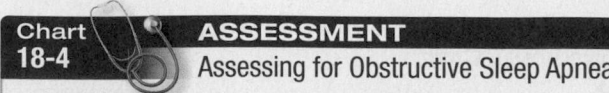

Chart 18-4 ASSESSMENT

Assessing for Obstructive Sleep Apnea

Be alert for the following signs and symptoms of obstructive sleep apnea:

- Excessive daytime sleepiness
- Frequent nocturnal awakening
- Insomnia
- Loud snoring
- Morning headaches
- Intellectual deterioration
- Personality changes, irritability
- Impotence
- Systemic hypertension
- Arrhythmias
- Pulmonary hypertension, cor pulmonale
- Polycythemia
- Enuresis

Adapted from Wickramasinghe, H. (2019). Obstructive sleep apnea. Retrieved on 5/27/2019 at: www.emedicine.medscape.com/article/295807-overview

are typically unaware of nocturnal upper airway obstruction during sleep. They frequently complain of insomnia, including difficulty in going to sleep, nighttime awakenings, and early morning awakenings with an inability to go back to sleep, as well as chronic fatigue and hypersomnolence (daytime sleepiness). When obtaining the health history, the nurse asks the patient about sleeping during normal activities such as eating or talking. Patients with this symptom are considered to have pathologic hypersomnolence (Wickramasinghe, 2019).

Assessment and Diagnostic Findings

The diagnosis of sleep apnea is based on clinical features plus a polysomnographic finding (i.e., sleep study), which is the definitive test for OSA. The test is an overnight study, performed in a specialized sleep disorders center, which continuously measures multiple physiologic signals while the patient sleeps. These signals are analyzed as they are related to stages of sleep; measures include those taken by electroencephalogram (EEG), electro-oculogram, and chin electromyogram (EMG). In addition, cardiac rhythms and arrhythmias are monitored with a single-lead electrocardiogram (ECG) and leg movements are recorded by an anterior tibialis EMG. Airflow at the nose and mouth is monitored using both a thermal sensor and a nasal pressure transducer, breathing effort is monitored using inductance plethysmography, and hemoglobin oxygen saturation is monitored by oximetry. The breathing pattern is analyzed for the presence of apneas and hypopneas. Characteristic findings consistent with OSA include apneic episodes occurring in the presence of respiratory muscle effort, clinically significant apneic episodes lasting 10 seconds or longer, and apneic episodes most prevalent during the rapid eye movement (REM) stage of sleep. Sleep disruption from automated patient arousal is usually seen at the termination of an episode of apnea (Wickramasinghe, 2019).

Medical Management

Patients usually seek medical treatment because their sleeping partners express concern or because they experience excessive sleepiness at inappropriate times or settings (e.g., while driving a car). A variety of treatments are used. Weight loss, avoidance of alcohol, positional therapy (using devices that prevent patients from sleeping on their backs), and oral appliances such as mandibular advancement devices (MADs) are the first steps (American Sleep Apnea Association, 2019; Joshi, 2018). When applied correctly, an MAD advances the mandible so that it is slightly anterior to the upper front teeth, preventing airway obstruction by the tongue and soft tissue during sleep. A randomized controlled trial that compared the effectiveness of these devices among patients with OSA with the more conventional therapy, continuous positive airway pressure (CPAP), found no difference in short-term outcomes between MAD and CPAP, including daytime sleepiness and quality of life, suggesting that MAD is as effective a treatment as CPAP in patients with mild-to-moderate OSA (Petri, Christensen, Svanholt, et al., 2019; Viscuso & Arena, 2016). In more severe cases involving hypoxemia and severe hypercapnia, the treatment includes CPAP or bilevel positive airway pressure (BiPAP) therapy with supplemental oxygen via nasal cannula. CPAP is used to prevent airway collapse, whereas BiPAP makes breathing easier and results in a lower average airway pressure (Patil, Ayappa, Caples, et al., 2019; the use of CPAP and BiPAP is discussed in more detail in Chapter 19).

Surgical Management

Surgical procedures also may be performed to correct OSA. Simple tonsillectomy may be effective for patients with larger tonsils when deemed clinically necessary, or when other options have failed or are refused by patients (Morgan, 2017). Uvulopalatopharyngoplasty is the resection of pharyngeal soft tissue and removal of approximately 15 mm of the free edge of the soft palate and uvula. Effective in about 50% of patients, it is more effective in eliminating snoring than apnea. Nasal septoplasty may be performed for gross anatomic nasal septal deformities. Maxillomandibular surgery may be performed to advance the maxilla and mandible forward in order to enlarge the posterior pharyngeal region (Morgan, 2017). Tracheostomy relieves upper airway obstruction but has numerous adverse effects, including speech difficulties and increased risk of infections. These procedures, as well as other maxillofacial surgeries, are reserved for patients with concomitant cardiovascular disease and life-threatening arrhythmias or severe disability who have not responded to conventional therapy (Papadakis et al., 2018).

Pharmacologic Therapy

Some medications are useful in managing symptoms associated with OSA. Modafinil is approved by the U.S. Food and Drug Administration (FDA) for use in patients who have residual daytime sleepiness despite optimal use of CPAP. The most improvement has been seen in patients who have taken modafinil at daily doses of 200 to 400 mg. Armodafinil is also now approved by the FDA for use in these patients. It is more potent than modafinil because it is pure R-modafinil, which is the most psychoactive compound of modafinil (Wickramasinghe, 2019). Protriptyline given at bedtime may increase the respiratory drive and improve upper airway muscle tone. Medroxyprogesterone acetate and acetazolamide might be prescribed for sleep apnea associated with chronic alveolar hypoventilation; however, their benefits have not been well established. The patient must understand that these medications are not a substitute for CPAP, BiPAP, or MAD. Administration of low-flow nasal oxygen at night can help relieve hypoxemia in some patients but has little effect on the frequency or severity of apnea.

Nursing Management

The patient with OSA may not recognize the potential consequences of the disorder. Therefore, the nurse explains the disorder in terms that are understandable to the patient and relates symptoms (daytime sleepiness) to the underlying disorder. The nurse also instructs the patient and family about treatments, including the correct and safe use of CPAP, BiPAP, MAD, and oxygen therapy, if prescribed. The nurse educates the patient about the risk of untreated OSA and the benefits of treatment approaches.

Epistaxis

Epistaxis, a hemorrhage from the nose, is caused by the rupture of tiny, distended vessels in the mucous membrane of any area of the nose. Rarely does epistaxis originate in the densely vascular tissue over the turbinates. Most commonly, the site is the anterior septum, where three major blood vessels enter the nasal cavity: (1) the anterior ethmoidal artery on the forward part of the roof (Kiesselbach plexus), (2) the sphenopalatine artery in the posterosuperior region, and (3) the internal maxillary branches (the plexus of veins located at the back of the lateral wall under the inferior turbinate).

Several risk factors are associated with epistaxis (Chart 18-5).

Medical Management

Management of epistaxis depends on its cause and the location of the bleeding site. A nasal speculum, penlight, or headlight may be used to identify the site of bleeding in the nasal cavity. Most nosebleeds originate from the anterior portion of the nose. Initial treatment may include applying direct pressure. The patient sits upright with the head tilted forward to prevent swallowing and aspiration of blood and is directed

---

Chart 18-5 **RISK FACTORS**
Epistaxis

- Local infections (vestibulitis, rhinitis, rhinosinusitis)
- Systemic infections (scarlet fever, malaria)
- Drying of nasal mucous membranes
- Nasal inhalation of corticosteroids (e.g., beclomethasone) or illicit drugs (e.g., cocaine)
- Trauma (digital trauma, blunt trauma, fracture, forceful nose blowing)
- Arteriosclerosis
- Hypertension
- Tumor (sinus or nasopharynx)
- Thrombocytopenia
- Use of aspirin
- Liver disease
- Rendu–Osler–Weber syndrome (hereditary hemorrhagic telangiectasia)

Adapted from Nguyen, Q. A. (2018). Epistaxis. Retrieved on 5/27/2019 at: www.emedicine.medscape.com/article/863220-overview

to pinch the soft outer portion of the nose against the midline septum for 5 or 10 minutes continuously. Application of nasal decongestants (phenylephrine, one or two sprays) to act as vasoconstrictors may be necessary. If these measures are unsuccessful in stopping the bleeding, the nose must be examined using good illumination and suction to determine the site of bleeding. Visible bleeding sites may be cauterized with silver nitrate or electrocautery (high-frequency electrical current). A supplemental patch of Surgicel or Gelfoam may be used (Papadakis et al., 2018).

Alternatively, a cotton tampon may be used to try to stop the bleeding. Suction may be used to remove excess blood and clots from the field of inspection. The search for the bleeding site should shift from the anteroinferior quadrant to the anterosuperior, then to the posterosuperior, and finally to the posteroinferior area. The field is kept clear by using suction and by shifting the cotton tampon.

If the origin of the bleeding cannot be identified, the nose may be packed with gauze impregnated with petrolatum jelly or antibiotic ointment; a topical anesthetic spray and decongestant agent may be used before the gauze packing is inserted, or a balloon-inflated catheter may be used (Fig. 18-3). Alternatively, a compressed nasal sponge may be used. Once the sponge becomes saturated with blood or is moistened with a small amount of saline, it will expand and produce tamponade to halt the bleeding. The packing may remain in place for 3 to 4 days if necessary to control bleeding (Nguyen, 2018). Antibiotics may be prescribed because of the risk of iatrogenic rhinosinusitis and sepsis.

Nursing Management

The nurse monitors the patient's vital signs, assists in the control of bleeding, and provides tissues and an emesis basin to

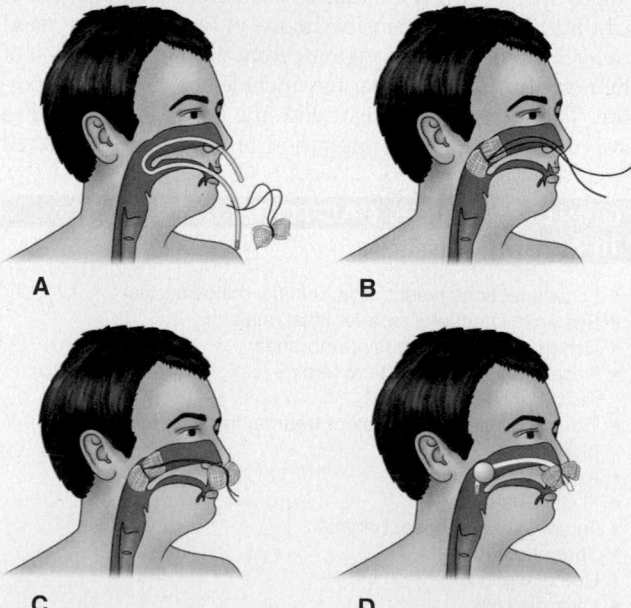

Figure 18-3 • Packing to control bleeding from the posterior nose. **A.** Catheter is inserted and packing is attached. **B.** Packing is drawn into position as the catheter is removed. **C.** Strip is tied over a bolster to hold the packing in place with an anterior pack installed "accordion pleat" style. **D.** Alternative method, using a balloon catheter instead of gauze packing.

allow the patient to expectorate any excess blood. It is common for patients to be anxious in response to a nosebleed. Blood loss on clothing and handkerchiefs can be frightening, and the nasal examination and treatment are uncomfortable. Assuring the patient in a calm, efficient manner that bleeding can be controlled can help reduce anxiety. The nurse continuously assesses the patient's airway and breathing as well as vital signs. On rare occasions, a patient with significant hemorrhage requires IV infusions of crystalloid solutions (normal saline) as well as cardiac and pulse oximetry monitoring.

 Educating Patients About Self-Care

Once the bleeding is controlled, the nurse instructs the patient to avoid vigorous exercise for several days and to avoid hot or spicy foods, tobacco use by smoking, or ENDS use, because this may cause vasodilation and increase the risk of rebleeding. Discharge education includes reviewing ways to prevent epistaxis: avoiding forceful nose blowing, straining, high altitudes, and nasal trauma (including nose picking). Adequate humidification may prevent drying of the nasal passages. The nurse explains how to apply direct pressure to the nose with the thumb and the index finger for 15 minutes in the case of a recurrent nosebleed. If recurrent bleeding cannot be stopped, the patient is instructed to seek additional medical attention.

Nasal Obstruction

The passage of air through the nostrils is frequently obstructed by a deviation of the nasal septum, hypertrophy of the turbinate bones, or the pressure of nasal polyps. Chronic nasal congestion forces the patient to breathe through the mouth, thus producing dryness of the oral mucosa and associated problems including persistent dry, cracked lips. Patients with chronic nasal congestion often suffer from sleep deprivation due to difficulty maintaining an adequate airway while lying flat and during sleep.

Persistent nasal obstruction also may lead to chronic infection of the nose and result in frequent episodes of nasopharyngitis. Frequently, the infection extends to the nasal sinuses. When rhinosinusitis develops and the drainage from these cavities is obstructed by deformity or swelling within the nose, pain is experienced in the region of the affected sinus.

Medical Management

The treatment of nasal obstruction requires the removal of the obstruction, followed by measures to treat whatever chronic infection exists. In many patients, an underlying allergy also requires treatment. Measures to reduce or alleviate nasal obstruction include nonsurgical as well as surgical techniques. Commonly used medications include nasal corticosteroids (see Table 18-2) as well as oral leukotriene inhibitors, such as montelukast. Treatment with nasal corticosteroids for 1 to 3 months is usually successful for the treatment of small polyps and may even reduce the need for surgical intervention. A short course of oral corticosteroids (6-day course of prednisone) may be beneficial in the treatment of nasal obstruction due to polyps (Papadakis et al., 2018). Additional medications may include antibiotics for the treatment of underlying infection or antihistamines for the management of allergies.

Hypertrophied turbinates may be treated by applying an astringent agent to shrink them.

A more aggressive approach in treating nasal obstruction caused by turbinate hypertrophy involves surgical reduction of the hypertrophy. Surgical procedures used to treat obstructive nasal conditions are collectively known as functional rhinoplasty. Technical advances with newer techniques provide a number of options for reconstruction and reshaping of the nose.

Nursing Management

When a surgical procedure is indicated, most often it is performed on an outpatient basis. The nurse explains the procedure to the patient. Postoperatively, the nurse elevates the head of the bed to promote drainage and to alleviate discomfort from edema. Frequent oral hygiene is encouraged to overcome dryness caused by breathing through the mouth. Before discharge from the outpatient or same-day surgical unit, the patient is instructed to avoid blowing the nose with force during the postoperative recovery period. The patient is also instructed about the signs and symptoms of bleeding and infection and when to contact the primary provider. The patient is provided with written postoperative instructions, including emergency phone numbers.

Fractures of the Nose

The location of the nose makes it susceptible to injury. Nasal fracture is the most common facial fracture and the most common fracture in the body (Becker, 2018). Fractures of the nose usually result from a direct assault. Nasal fractures may affect the ascending process of the maxilla and the septum. The torn mucous membrane results in a nosebleed. Complications include hematoma, infection, abscess, and avascular or septic necrosis. However, as a rule, serious consequences usually do not occur.

Clinical Manifestations

The signs and symptoms of a nasal fracture are pain, bleeding from the nose externally and internally into the pharynx, swelling of the soft tissues adjacent to the nose, periorbital ecchymosis, nasal obstruction, and deformity. The patient's nose may have an asymmetric appearance that may not be obvious until the edema subsides.

Assessment and Diagnostic Findings

The nose is examined internally to rule out the possibility that the injury may be complicated by a fracture of the nasal septum and a submucosal septal hematoma. Intranasal examination is performed in all cases to rule out septal hematoma (Papadakis et al., 2018). Because of the swelling and bleeding that occur with a nasal fracture, an accurate diagnosis can be made only after the swelling subsides.

Clear fluid draining from either nostril suggests a fracture of the cribriform plate with leakage of cerebrospinal fluid. Usually, careful inspection or palpation discloses any deviations of the bone or disruptions of the nasal cartilages. An x-ray may reveal displacement of the fractured bones and may help rule out extension of the fracture into the skull.

Medical Management

A nasal fracture very often produces bleeding from the nasal passage. As a rule, bleeding is controlled with the use of packing. Cold compresses are used to prevent or reduce edema. For the patient who has sustained enough trauma to break the nose or any facial bone, the emergency medical team must consider the possibility of a cervical spine fracture. Therefore, it is essential to ensure a patent airway and to rule out a cervical spine fracture (see Chapter 63). Uncomplicated nasal fractures may be treated initially with antibiotics, analgesic agents, and a decongestant nasal spray.

Treatment of nasal fractures is aimed at restoring nasal function and returning the appearance of the nose to baseline. The patient is referred to a specialist to evaluate the need to realign the bones. Although improved outcomes are obtained when reduction in the fracture is performed during the first 3 hours after the injury, this is often not possible because of the edema. If immediate reduction of the fracture is not possible, it is performed within 3 to 7 days. Timing is important when treating nasal fractures because further delay in treatment may result in problematic bone healing, which ultimately may require surgical intervention that includes rhinoplasty to reshape the external appearance of the nose (Becker, 2018). A septorhinoplasty is performed when the nasal septum needs to be repaired. In patients who develop a septal hematoma, the physician drains the hematoma through a small incision. A septal hematoma that is not drained can lead to permanent deformity of the nose.

Nursing Management

Immediately after the fracture, the nurse applies ice and encourages the patient to keep the head elevated. The nurse instructs the patient to apply ice packs to the nose to decrease swelling. The patient who experiences epistaxis is usually frightened and anxious and needs reassurance. The packing inserted to stop the bleeding may be uncomfortable and unpleasant, and obstruction of the nasal passages by the packing forces the patient to breathe through the mouth. This in turn causes the oral mucous membranes to become dry. Mouth rinses help to moisten the mucous membranes and to reduce the odor and taste of dried blood in the oropharynx and nasopharynx. The use of analgesic agents such as acetaminophen or NSAIDs (e.g., ibuprofen, naproxen) is encouraged. When removing the cotton pledgets, the nurse carefully inspects the mucosa for lacerations or a septal hematoma. The nurse instructs the patient to avoid sports activities for 6 weeks.

Laryngeal Obstruction

Obstruction of the larynx because of edema is a serious condition that may be fatal without swift, decisive intervention. The larynx is a stiff box that will not stretch. It contains a narrow space between the vocal cords (glottis), through which air must pass. Swelling of the laryngeal mucous membranes may close off the opening tightly, leading to life-threatening hypoxia or suffocation. Edema of the glottis occurs rarely in patients with acute laryngitis, occasionally in patients with urticaria, and more frequently in patients with severe inflammation of the throat, as in scarlet fever. It is an occasional cause of death in severe anaphylaxis (angioedema).

TABLE 18-3	Causes of Laryngeal Obstruction
Precipitating Event	**Mechanism of Obstruction**
History of allergies; exposure to medications, latex, foods (peanuts, tree nuts [e.g., walnuts, pecans]), bee stings	Anaphylaxis
Foreign body	Inhalation/ingestion of meat or other food items, coin, chewing gum, balloon fragments, drug packets (ingested to avoid criminal arrest)
Heavy alcohol consumption; heavy tobacco use	Obstruction from tumor
Family history of airway problems	Suggests angioedema (type I hypersensitivity reaction)
Use of angiotensin-converting enzyme inhibitor	Increased risk of angioedema of the mucous membranes
Recent throat pain or recent fever	Infectious process
History of surgery or previous tracheostomy	Possible subglottic stenosis

Adapted from Reardon, R. F., Mason, P. E., & Clinton, J. E. (2017). Basic airway management and decision-making. In J. D. Roberts (Ed.). *Roberts & Hedges' clinical procedures in emergency medicine* (7th ed.). Philadelphia, PA: Elsevier Saunders.

Hereditary angioedema is also characterized by episodes of life-threatening laryngeal edema. Laryngeal edema in people with hereditary angioedema can occur at any age, although young adults are at greatest risk (Reardon, Mason, & Clinton, 2017). Some causes of laryngeal obstruction appear in Table 18-3.

When foreign bodies are aspirated into the pharynx, the larynx, or the trachea a twofold problem occurs. First, they obstruct the air passages and cause difficulty in breathing, which may lead to asphyxia; later, they may be drawn farther down, entering the bronchi or a bronchial branch and causing symptoms of irritation, such as a croupy cough, expectoration of blood or mucus, or labored breathing.

Clinical Manifestations

The patient's clinical presentation and x-ray findings confirm the diagnosis of laryngeal obstruction. The patient may demonstrate lowered oxygen saturation; however, normal oxygen saturation should not be interpreted as a sign that the obstruction is not significant. The use of accessory muscles to maximize airflow may occur and is often manifested by retractions in the neck or abdomen during inspirations. Patients who demonstrate these symptoms are at an immediate risk of collapse, and respiratory support (i.e., mechanical ventilation or positive-pressure ventilation) is considered.

Assessment and Diagnostic Findings

A thorough history can be very useful in diagnosing and treating the patient with a laryngeal obstruction. However, emergency measures to secure the patient's airway should not be delayed to obtain a history or perform tests. If possible, the nurse obtains a history from the patient or family about heavy alcohol or tobacco consumption, ENDS use, current medications, history of airway problems, recent infections, pain or fever, dental pain or poor dentition, and any previous surgeries, radiation therapy, or trauma.

Medical Management

Medical management is based on the initial evaluation of the patient and the need to ensure a patent airway. If the airway is obstructed by a foreign body and signs of asphyxia are apparent, immediate treatment is necessary using principles from basic and advanced cardiopulmonary resuscitation (CPR). If all efforts are unsuccessful, an immediate tracheotomy is necessary (see Chapter 19 for further discussion). If the obstruction is caused by edema resulting from an allergic reaction, treatment may include immediate administration of subcutaneous epinephrine and a corticosteroid (see Chapter 33). Ice may be applied to the neck in an effort to reduce edema. Continuous pulse oximetry is essential in the patient who has experienced acute upper airway obstruction (Reardon et al., 2017).

Cancer of the Larynx

Cancer of the larynx accounts for approximately half of all head and neck cancers. The American Cancer Society (ACS, 2017) estimates that about 12,410 new cases and 3760 deaths occur annually, with a 5-year relative survival rate that ranges from 32% to 90%, depending on the location of the tumor and its stage at the time of diagnosis (ACS, 2017). Cancer of the larynx is most common in people older than 65 years and is four times more common in men (ACS, 2017) (Chart 18-6).

Chart 18-6 ⚠ **RISK FACTORS**
Laryngeal Cancer

Carcinogens

- Tobacco (smoke, smokeless, e-cigarettes, hookahs, second-hand smoke)
- Heavy alcohol consumption (defined as more than one drink daily)
- Combined effects of alcohol and tobacco
- Asbestos
- Paint fumes
- Wood dust
- Chemicals used in metalworking, petroleum, plastics, and textiles

Other Factors

- Nutritional deficiencies (vitamins)
- Genetic predisposition
- Age (higher incidence after 65 years of age)
- Gender (more common in men)
- Race (more prevalent in African Americans and Whites)
- Weakened immune system

Adapted from American Cancer Society (ACS). (2017). What are the risk factors for laryngeal and hypopharyngeal cancers? Retrieved on 5/27/2019 at: www.cancer.org/Cancer/LaryngealandHypopharyngealCancer/DetailedGuide/laryngeal-and-hypopharyngeal-cancer-risk-factors

Almost all malignant tumors of the larynx arise from the surface epithelium and are classified as squamous cell carcinoma. Approximately 55% of patients with laryngeal cancer present with involved lymph nodes at the time of diagnosis, with bilateral lesions present in 16% of patients (De Vita, Hellman, & Rosenberg, 2018). Recurrence occurs usually within the first 2 to 3 years after diagnosis. The presence of disease after 5 years is often secondary to a new primary malignancy. The incidence of distant metastasis with squamous cell carcinoma of the head and neck (including larynx cancer) is relatively low.

Clinical Manifestations

Hoarseness of more than 2 weeks' duration occurs in the patient with cancer in the glottic area because the tumor impedes the action of the vocal cords during speech. The voice may sound harsh, raspy, and lower in pitch. Affected voice sounds are not always early signs of subglottic or supraglottic cancer, however. The patient may complain of a persistent cough or sore throat and pain and burning in the throat, especially when consuming hot liquids or citrus juices. A lump may be felt in the neck. Later symptoms include dysphagia, dyspnea (difficulty breathing), unilateral nasal obstruction or discharge, persistent hoarseness, persistent ulceration, and foul breath. Cervical lymph adenopathy, unintentional weight loss, a general debilitated state, and pain radiating to the ear may occur with metastasis.

Assessment and Diagnostic Findings

An initial assessment includes a complete history and physical examination of the head and neck. This includes identification of risk factors, family history, and any underlying medical conditions. An indirect laryngoscopy, using a flexible endoscope, is initially performed in the otolaryngologist's office to visually evaluate the pharynx, larynx, and possible tumor. Mobility of the vocal cords is assessed; if normal movement is limited, the growth may affect muscle, other tissue, and even the airway. The lymph nodes of the neck and the thyroid gland are palpated for enlargement.

Diagnostic procedures that may be used include fine-needle aspiration (FNA) biopsy, a barium swallow, endoscopy, CT or MRI scan, and a positron emission tomography (PET) scan (ACS, 2017). FNA biopsy may be done as an initial screening procedure to obtain samples of any enlarged lymph nodes in the neck. A barium swallow may be done if the patient initially presents with a chief complaint of difficulty in swallowing, to outline any structural anomalies of the neck that could pinpoint a tumor. However, if a tumor of the larynx is suspected on an initial examination, a direct laryngoscopic examination is indicated. Laryngoscopy is performed under local or general anesthesia to evaluate all areas of the larynx. In some cases, intraoperative examination obtained by direct microscopic visualization and palpation of the vocal folds may yield a more accurate diagnosis. Samples of the suspicious tissue are obtained for analysis. It is uncommon that human papillomavirus (HPV) is implicated in laryngeal cancers, although it is frequently implicated in oropharyngeal and tonsillar cancers. Whether or not the tumor is positive for HPV does not have an effect on the course of treatment (ACS, 2017).

The classification, including stage of the tumor (i.e., size and histology of the tumor, presence and extent of cervical lymph node involvement) and location of the tumor serve as a basis for treatment. CT scanning and MRI are used to assess regional adenopathy and soft tissues and to stage and determine the extent of a tumor. MRI is also helpful in post-treatment follow-up to detect a recurrence. PET scanning may also be used to detect recurrence of the laryngeal tumor after treatment.

Medical Management

The goals of treatment of laryngeal cancer include cure; preservation of safe, effective swallowing; preservation of useful voice; and avoidance of permanent tracheostoma (Papadakis et al., 2018). Treatment options include surgery, radiation therapy, and adjuvant chemoradiation therapy. The prognosis depends on the tumor location (i.e., supraglottic, glottis, subglottic), as well as the tumor grade and stage (i.e., using the TNM system; see Chapter 12, Chart 12-3). The treatment plan also depends on whether the cancer is an initial diagnosis or a recurrence. In addition, before treatment begins, a complete dental examination is performed to rule out any oral disease. A consultation with a dental oncologist may be warranted. Any dental problems are resolved, if possible, before surgery and radiotherapy (ACS, 2017).

For patients with early-stage tumors (i.e., stages I and II) and lesions without lymph node involvement, external-beam radiation therapy or conservation surgery (i.e., less invasive surgery, such as vocal cord stripping or cordectomy) may be effective. Other indicated surgical procedures may include transoral endoscopic laser excision or partial **laryngectomy** (i.e., in this instance, removal of part of the larynx) (National Cancer Institute [NCI], 2019). Patients with stage III and IV tumors that are resectable may be advised to have either total laryngectomies with or without postoperative radiation therapy or radiation therapy with concurrent adjuvant chemotherapy (with single-agent cisplatin) and surgical resection aimed at preserving some of the larynx (i.e., organ preservation surgery). Patients with late-stage tumors that extend through cartilage and into soft tissues are generally advised to have total laryngectomies with postoperative radiation therapy (NCI, 2019).

Patients should be educated so that they carefully consider the various side effects and complications associated with the different treatment modalities. The presence of lymph node involvement in the neck can affect the outcome. Supraglottic tumors metastasize early and bilaterally even when there appears to be no lymph node involvement at the time of diagnosis. When the neck lymph nodes are involved, the treatment includes surgery, chemoradiation, or both (Papadakis et al., 2018).

Surgical Management

The overall goals for the patient undergoing surgical treatment include minimizing the effects of surgery on speech, swallowing, and breathing while maximizing the likelihood of a cure of the cancer. Several different curative procedures are available that can offer voice-sparing results while achieving a positive cure rate for the patient who has an early laryngeal carcinoma. Surgical options include vocal cord stripping, cordectomy, laser surgery, partial laryngectomy, or total laryngectomy (NCI, 2019).

Vocal Cord Stripping

Stripping of the vocal cord is used to treat dysplasia, hyperkeratosis, and leukoplakia and is often curative for these lesions. The procedure involves removal of the mucosa of the edge of the vocal cord, using an operating microscope. Early vocal cord lesions are initially treated with radiation therapy.

Cordectomy

Cordectomy, which is an excision of the vocal cord, is usually performed via transoral laser. This procedure is used for lesions limited to the middle third of the vocal cord. The resulting voice quality is related to the extent of tissue removed.

Laser Surgery

Laser microsurgery is well known to have several advantages for the treatment of early glottic cancers. Treatment and recovery are shorter, with fewer side effects, and treatment may be less costly than for other forms of therapy. Microelectrodes are useful for surgical resection of smaller laryngeal carcinomas. The carbon dioxide (CO_2) laser can be used for the treatment of many laryngeal tumors, with the exception of large vascular tumors. When compared with the results of other treatments for early laryngeal cancer, laser microsurgery is considered to be the method of choice based on patient outcomes (NCI, 2019).

Partial Laryngectomy

A partial laryngectomy (laryngofissure–thyrotomy) is often used for patients in the early stages of cancer in the glottic area when only one vocal cord is involved. The surgery is associated with a very high cure rate. It may also be performed for recurrence when high-dose radiation has failed. A portion of the larynx is removed, along with one vocal cord and the tumor; all other structures remain. The airway remains intact, and the patient is expected to have no difficulty swallowing. The voice quality may change, or the patient may sound hoarse.

Total Laryngectomy

Complete removal of the larynx (total laryngectomy) can provide a cure in most advanced laryngeal cancers, when the tumor extends beyond the vocal cords, or for cancer that recurs or persists after radiation therapy. In a total laryngectomy, the laryngeal structures are removed, including the hyoid bone, epiglottis, cricoid cartilage, and two or three rings of the trachea. The tongue, pharyngeal walls, and most of the trachea are preserved. A total laryngectomy results in permanent loss of the voice and a change in the airway, requiring a permanent tracheostomy (Fig. 18-4). Occasionally, patients continue to have a laryngectomy tube in the stoma. Laryngectomy tubes are similar in appearance to tracheostomy tubes; however, a laryngectomy tube can be distinguished from a tracheostomy tube because the patient is unable to speak or breathe when the laryngectomy tube is occluded. Patients who have a total laryngectomy require alternatives to normal speech; these may include a prosthetic device, such as a Blom–Singer valve, to speak without aspirating (see later discussion).

Surgery is more difficult when the lesion involves the midline structures or both vocal cords. With or without neck dissection, a total laryngectomy requires a permanent tracheal stoma because the larynx that provides the protective sphincter is no longer present. The tracheal stoma prevents

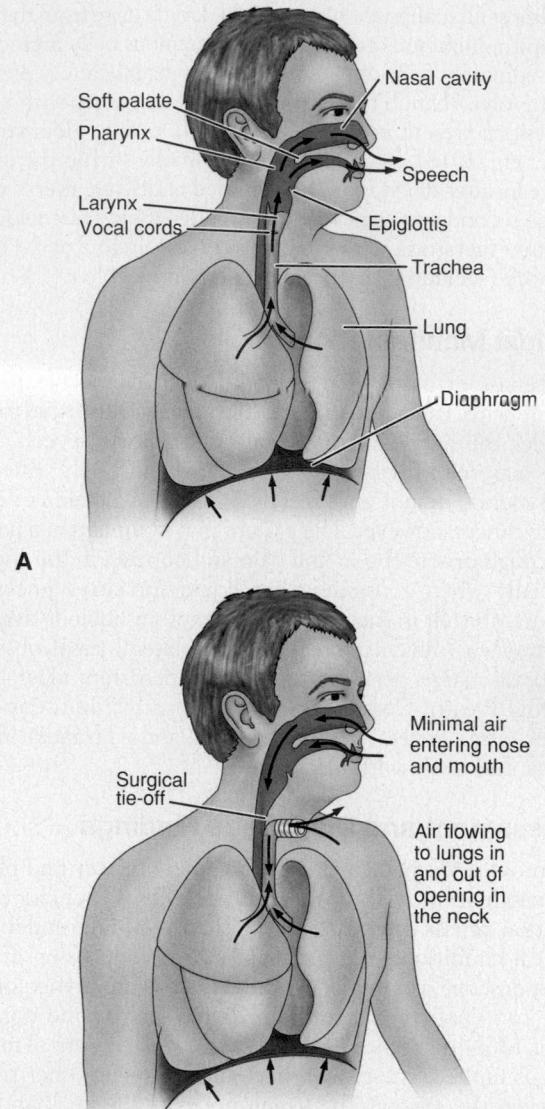

Figure 18-4 • Total laryngectomy produces a change in airflow for breathing and speaking. **A.** Normal airflow. **B.** Airflow after total laryngectomy.

the aspiration of food and fluid into the lower respiratory tract. The patient has no voice but has normal swallowing. A total laryngectomy changes the manner in which airflow is used for breathing and speaking, as depicted in Figure 18-4. The patient has significant loss of the natural voice and the need to breathe through a stoma (an opening) created in the lower neck. Complications that may occur include a salivary leak, wound infection from the development of a pharyngocutaneous fistula, stomal stenosis, and dysphagia secondary to esophageal stricture. In some cases, the patient may be a candidate for a near-total laryngectomy. In this situation, the patient would be a candidate for chemoradiation therapy regimens postoperatively. Voice preservation can be achieved in most cases and tends to be associated with overall improved quality of life (Adil, 2018). Advances in surgical techniques for treating laryngeal cancer may minimize the cosmetic and functional deficits previously seen with total laryngectomy. Some microlaryngeal surgery can be performed endoscopically.

Radiation Therapy

The goal of radiation therapy is to eradicate the cancer and preserve the function of the larynx. The decision to use radiation therapy is based on several factors, including the staging of the tumor and the patient's overall health status, lifestyle (including occupation), and personal preference. Excellent results have been achieved with radiation therapy in patients with early-stage glottic tumors when only one vocal cord is involved and there is normal mobility of the cord (i.e., with phonation), as well as in small supraglottic lesions. One of the benefits of radiation therapy is that patients retain a near-normal voice. A few may develop chondritis (inflammation of the cartilage) or stenosis; a small number may later require laryngectomy.

Radiation therapy may also be used preoperatively to reduce the tumor size. Radiation therapy is combined with surgery in advanced laryngeal cancer as adjunctive therapy to surgery or chemotherapy and as a palliative measure.

Complications from radiation therapy are a result of external radiation to the head and neck area, which may also include the parotid gland, which is responsible for mucus production. Symptoms may include acute mucositis, ulceration of the mucous membranes, pain, **xerostomia** (dry mouth), loss of taste, dysphasia, fatigue, and skin reactions. Later complications may include laryngeal necrosis, edema, and fibrosis (see Chapter 12).

Speech Therapy

The patient who undergoes a laryngectomy and the patient's family face potentially complex challenges, including significant changes in the ability to communicate. To minimize anxiety and frustration on the part of the patient and family, the loss or alteration of speech is discussed with them. To plan postoperative communication strategies and speech therapy, the speech therapist or pathologist conducts a preoperative evaluation (ACS, 2017). During this time, the nurse discusses with the patient and family the methods of communication that will be available in the immediate postoperative period. These include writing, lip speaking and reading, communication or word boards, or smartphones or other electronic devices. A system of communication is established with the patient, family, nurse, and primary provider and is implemented consistently after surgery.

In addition, a long-term postoperative communication plan for **alaryngeal communication** (modes of speaking not involving the normal larynx) is developed. The three most common techniques of alaryngeal communication are esophageal speech, artificial larynx (electric larynx), and tracheoesophageal puncture. Training in these techniques begins once medical clearance is obtained from the primary provider.

Esophageal Speech

The patient needs the ability to compress air into the esophagus and expel it, setting off a vibration of the pharyngeal esophageal segment for esophageal speech. The technique can be taught once the patient begins oral feedings, approximately 1 week after surgery. First, the patient learns to belch and is reminded to do so an hour after eating. Then, the technique is practiced repeatedly. Later, this conscious belching action is transformed into simple explosions of air from the esophagus for speech purposes. The speech therapist continues to work with the patient to make speech intelligible and as close to normal as possible. Because it takes a long time to become proficient, the success rate is low (ACS, 2017).

Artificial Larynx

If esophageal speech is not successful, or until the patient masters the technique, an electric larynx may be used for communication. This battery-powered apparatus projects sound into the oral cavity. When the mouth forms words (articulation), the sounds from the electric larynx become audible words. The voice that is produced sounds mechanical, and some words may be difficult to understand. The advantage is that the patient is able to communicate with relative ease while working to become proficient at either esophageal or tracheoesophageal puncture speech.

Tracheoesophageal Puncture

The third technique of alaryngeal speech is tracheoesophageal puncture (Fig. 18-5). This technique for voice restoration is simple and has few complications. It is associated with high phonation success, good phonation quality, and steady long-term results. This technique is the most widely used because the speech associated with it most resembles normal speech (the sound produced is a combination of esophageal speech and voice), and it is easily achieved either during the initial surgery to treat the tumor or at a later date (ACS, 2017). A valve is placed in the tracheal stoma to divert air into the esophagus and out the mouth. Once the puncture is surgically created and has healed, a voice prosthesis (Blom–Singer) is fitted over the puncture site. A speech therapist teaches the patient how to produce sounds. Moving the tongue and lips to form the sound into words produces speech as before. To prevent airway obstruction, the prosthesis is removed and cleaned when mucus builds up.

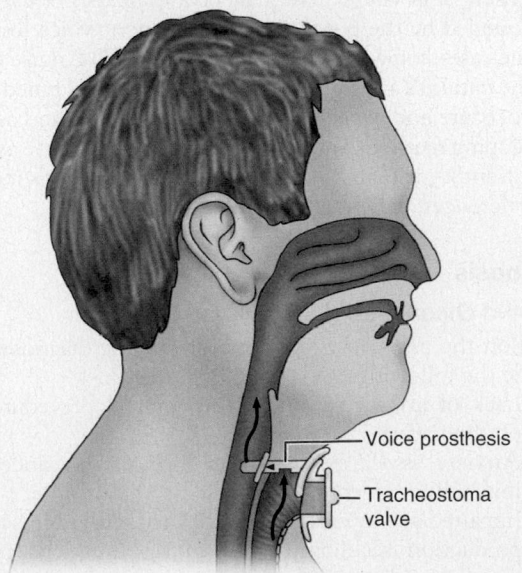

— Voice prosthesis

— Tracheostoma valve

Figure 18-5 • Schematic representation of tracheoesophageal puncture speech. Air travels from the lung through a puncture in the posterior wall of the trachea into the esophagus and out the mouth. A voice prosthesis is fitted over the puncture site.

NURSING PROCESS

The Patient Undergoing Laryngectomy

Assessment

The nurse obtains a health history and assesses the patient's physical, psychosocial, and spiritual domains. The health history focuses on the following symptoms: hoarseness, sore throat, dyspnea, dysphagia, and pain or burning in the throat. The physical assessment includes a thorough head and neck examination with an emphasis on the patient's airway. In addition, the neck and thyroid are palpated for swelling, nodularity, or adenopathy.

The nurse also assesses the patient's general state of nutrition, including height and weight and body mass index and reviews laboratory values that assist in determining the patient's nutritional status (albumin, protein, glucose, and electrolyte levels). If treatment includes surgery, the nurse must know the nature of the surgery to plan appropriate care. If the patient is expected to have no voice as a result of the surgical procedure, a preoperative evaluation by the speech therapist is essential. The patient's ability to hear, see, read, and write is assessed. Visual impairment and functional illiteracy may create additional problems with communication and may require creative approaches to ensure that the patient is able to communicate any needs. Because alcohol abuse is a risk factor for cancer of the larynx, the patient's pattern of alcohol intake must be assessed. Patients who are accustomed to daily consumption of alcohol are at the risk for delirium tremens (alcohol withdrawal syndrome) when alcohol intake is stopped suddenly. It is also not uncommon that patients are active smokers at the time of diagnosis; assessment of readiness for smoking cessation should be done, and nicotine replacements prescribed to avoid nicotine withdrawal, as indicated (NCI, 2019) (see Chapter 23: Promoting Cessation of Tobacco Use).

In addition, the nurse assesses the psychological status of the patient and family. The fear of a diagnosis of cancer is compounded by the possibility of permanent voice loss and, in some cases, some degree of disfigurement. The nurse evaluates the patient's and family's knowledge of the planned surgical procedure and expected postoperative course and assesses their coping methods and support systems. The nurse assesses the patient's spirituality needs based on the patient's individual preferences, beliefs, and culture.

Diagnosis

NURSING DIAGNOSES

Based on the assessment data, major nursing diagnoses may include the following:

- Lack of knowledge about the surgical procedure and postoperative course
- Anxiety associated with the diagnosis of cancer and impending surgery
- Impaired airway clearance associated with excess mucus production secondary to surgical alterations in the airway
- Impaired verbal communication associated with anatomic deficit secondary to removal of the larynx and to edema
- Impaired nutritional intake associated with inability to ingest food secondary to swallowing difficulties

- Disturbed body image and risk for chronic low self-esteem secondary to major neck surgery, change in appearance, and altered structure and function
- Impaired ability to manage regime associated with pain, weakness, fatigue, musculoskeletal impairment related to surgical procedure and postoperative course

COLLABORATIVE PROBLEMS/POTENTIAL COMPLICATIONS

Based on the assessment data, potential complications may include the following:

- Respiratory distress (hypoxia, airway obstruction, tracheal edema)
- Hemorrhage, infection, and wound breakdown
- Aspiration
- Tracheostomal stenosis

Planning and Goals

The major goals for the patient may include attainment of an adequate level of knowledge, reduction in anxiety, maintenance of a patent airway (patient is able to handle own secretions), effective use of alternative means of communication, attainment of optimal levels of nutrition and hydration, improvement in body image and self-esteem, improved self-care management, and absence of complications.

Nursing Interventions

 PROVIDING PREOPERATIVE PATIENT EDUCATION

The diagnosis of laryngeal cancer often produces misconceptions and fears. Many people assume that loss of speech and disfigurement are inevitable with this condition. Once the primary provider explains the diagnosis and discusses treatment options with the patient and family, the nurse clarifies any misconceptions by identifying the location of the larynx, its function, the nature of the planned surgical procedure, and its effect on speech. Further, the patient's ability to sing, laugh, and whistle will be lost. Informational materials (written and audiovisual) about the surgery are given to the patient and family for review and reinforcement. If a complete laryngectomy is planned, the patient must understand that the natural voice will be lost, but that special training can provide a means for communicating. The patient needs to know that until training is started, communication will be possible by using the call light, by writing, or by using a communication device. The interdisciplinary team conducts an initial assessment of the patient and family. In addition to the nurse and the primary provider, the team might include an advanced practice nurse (e.g., nurse practitioner), speech therapist, respiratory therapist, social worker, dietitian, and home health nurse. The services of a spiritual advisor are made available to the patient and family, as appropriate.

The nurse also reviews equipment and treatments for postoperative care with the patient and family, educates the patient about important coughing and deep breathing exercises, and helps the patient perform return demonstrations. The nurse clarifies the patient's role in the postoperative and rehabilitation periods. The family's needs must also be addressed because family members are often responsible for complex care of the patient in the home.

REDUCING ANXIETY

Because surgery of the larynx is performed most often for a malignant tumor, the patient may have many questions: Will the surgeon be able to remove all of the tumor? Is it cancer? Will I die? Will I choke? Will I suffocate? Will I ever speak again? What will I look like? Because of these and other questions, the psychological preparation of the patient is as important as the physical preparation.

Any patient undergoing surgery may have many fears. In laryngeal surgery, these fears may relate to the diagnosis of cancer and the possibility of permanent loss of the voice and disfigurement. The nurse provides the patient and family with opportunities to ask questions, verbalize feelings, and discuss perceptions. The nurse should address any questions and misconceptions the patient and family have. During the preoperative or postoperative period, a visit from someone who has had a laryngectomy may reassure the patient that people are available to assist and that rehabilitation is possible.

In the immediate postoperative period, the nurse attempts to build trust and reduce the patient's anxiety. Active listening provides an environment that promotes open communication and allows the patient to verbalize feelings. Clear instructions and explanations are given to the patient and family in a calm, reassuring manner. The nurse listens attentively, encourages the patient, and identifies and reduces environmental stressors. The nurse seeks to learn from the patient what activities promote feelings of comfort and assists the patient in such activities (e.g., listening to music, reading). Relaxation techniques such as guided imagery and meditation are often helpful. During episodes of severe anxiety, the nurse remains with the patient and includes them in decision making.

MAINTAINING A PATENT AIRWAY

The nurse helps maintain a patent airway by positioning the patient in the semi-Fowler or Fowler position after recovery from anesthesia. This position decreases surgical edema and promotes lung expansion. Observing the patient for restlessness, labored breathing, apprehension, and increased pulse rate helps identify possible respiratory or circulatory problems. The nurse assesses the patient's lung sounds and reports changes that may indicate impending complications. Medications that depress respiration, particularly opioids, should be used cautiously. However, adequate use of analgesic medications is essential for pain relief because postoperative pain can result in shallow breathing and an ineffective cough (see Chapter 9 for discussion of pain management). The nurse encourages the patient to turn, cough, and take deep breaths. If necessary, suctioning may be performed to remove secretions, but disruption of suture lines must be avoided. The nurse also encourages and assists the patient with early ambulation to prevent atelectasis, pneumonia, and venous thromboemboli formation (e.g., pulmonary embolism and deep vein thrombosis). Pulse oximetry is used to monitor the patient's oxygen saturation level.

If a total laryngectomy was performed, a laryngectomy tube will most likely be in place. In some instances a laryngectomy tube is not used; in others it is used temporarily; and in many it is used permanently. The laryngectomy tube, which is shorter than a tracheostomy tube but has a larger diameter, is the patient's only airway. The care of this tube is similar to that for a tracheostomy tube (see Chapter 19). The nurse changes the inner cannula (if present) every 8 h if it is disposable. Although nondisposable tubes are used infrequently, if one is used, the nurse cleans the inner cannula every 8 h or more often as needed. If a tracheostomy tube without an inner cannula is used, humidification and suctioning of this tube are essential to prevent formation of mucus plugs. If a T-shaped laryngectomy tube is used, both sides of the T-tube should be suctioned to prevent obstruction due to copious secretions. The nurse should also use secure tracheostomy ties to prevent tube dislodgement. The nurse cleans the stoma daily with soap and water or another prescribed solution and a soft cloth or gauze, taking care to prevent water and soap or solution from entering the stoma. If a non–oil-based antibiotic ointment is prescribed, it is applied around the stoma and suture line. If crusting appears around the stoma, the crusts are removed with sterile tweezers and additional ointment is applied.

Wound drains, inserted during surgery, may be in place to assist in removal of fluid and air from the surgical site. Suction also may be used, but cautiously, to avoid trauma to the surgical site and incision. The nurse observes, measures, and records drainage. When drainage is less than 30 mL/day for 2 consecutive days, the surgeon usually removes the drains.

Frequently, the patient coughs up large amounts of mucus through this opening. Because air passes directly into the trachea without being warmed and moistened by the upper respiratory mucosa, the tracheobronchial tree compensates by secreting excessive amounts of mucus. Therefore, the patient has frequent coughing episodes and may develop a brassy-sounding, mucus-producing cough. The nurse reassures the patient that these problems will diminish in time as the tracheobronchial mucosa adapts to the altered physiology.

After the patient coughs, the tracheostomy opening must be wiped clean and clear of mucus. A simple gauze dressing, washcloth, or even paper towel (because of its size and absorbency) worn below the tracheostomy may serve as a barrier to protect the clothing from the copious mucus that the patient may initially expel.

One of the most important factors in decreasing cough, mucus production, and crusting around the stoma is adequate humidification of the environment. Mechanical humidifiers and aerosol generators (nebulizers) increase the humidity and are important for the patient's comfort. The laryngectomy tube may be removed when the stoma is well healed, within 3 to 6 wk after surgery. The nurse educates the patient about how to clean and change the tube and remove secretions.

PROMOTING ALTERNATIVE COMMUNICATION METHODS

Establishing an effective means of communication is usually the ultimate goal in the rehabilitation of the laryngectomy patient. To understand and anticipate the patient's postoperative needs, the nurse works with the patient, speech therapist, and family to encourage the use of alternative communication methods. These means of communication are established preoperatively and must be used consistently by all personnel who come in contact with the patient postoperatively. The patient is now unable to use an intercom system. A call bell or hand bell must be placed within easy reach of the patient. In the immediate postoperative period, a handheld communication device like a Magic Slate, electronic tablet, notebook, or smartphone can be used. If the patient cannot write, a picture–word–phrase board or hand signals can be used. The nurse documents which hand is the patient's dominant hand (e.g., used for writing) so that the opposite arm can be used for IV infusions. (To ensure the patient's privacy, the nurse shreds notes used for communication.)

Writing everything or communicating through gestures can be very time-consuming and frustrating. The patient must be given adequate time to communicate their needs. The patient may become impatient and angry when not understood.

PROMOTING ADEQUATE NUTRITION AND HYDRATION

Postoperatively, the patient may not be permitted to eat or drink for at least 7 d (Suslu, 2016). Alternative sources of nutrition and hydration include IV fluids, enteral feedings through a nasogastric or gastrostomy tube, and parenteral nutrition (see Chapters 39 and 41).

When the patient is ready to start oral feedings, a swallow study (a video fluoroscopy radiology procedure) may be conducted to evaluate the patient's risk of aspiration. Once the patient is cleared for oral feedings, the nurse explains that thick liquids will be used first because they are easy to swallow. Different swallowing maneuvers are attempted with various food consistencies. Once the patient is cleared for food intake, the nurse stays with the patient during initial oral feedings and keeps a suction setup at the bedside for needed suctioning. The nurse instructs the patient to avoid sweet foods, which increase salivation and suppress the appetite. Solid foods are introduced as tolerated. The patient is instructed to rinse the mouth with warm water or mouthwash after oral feedings and to brush the teeth frequently.

Because taste and smell are so closely related, taste sensations are altered for a while after surgery because inhaled air passes directly into the trachea, bypassing the nose and the olfactory end organs. In time, however, the patient usually accommodates to this change and olfactory sensation adapts, often with return of interest in eating. The nurse observes the patient for any difficulty in swallowing, particularly when eating resumes, and reports its occurrence to the primary provider.

The patient's weight and laboratory data are monitored to ensure that nutritional and fluid intake are adequate. In addition, skin turgor and vital signs are assessed for signs of decreased fluid volume.

PROMOTING POSITIVE BODY IMAGE AND SELF-ESTEEM

Disfiguring surgery and an altered communication pattern are threats to a patient's body image and self-esteem. The reaction of family members and friends is a major concern for the patient. The nurse encourages the patient to express feelings about the changes brought about by surgery, particularly feelings related to fear, anger, depression, and isolation. Encouraging the use of previous effective coping strategies may be helpful. Referral to a support group, such as the International Association of Laryngectomees (IAL) and WebWhispers, and to resources available through the American Cancer Society may help the patient and family deal with the changes in their lives. Information about these support groups can be found in the Resources section at the end of the chapter.

PROMOTING EFFECTIVE HEALTH MANAGEMENT

A positive approach along with promotion of effective health management is important when caring for the patient. The patient should begin participating in effective health management activities as soon as possible. The nurse assesses the patient's readiness for decision making and encourages the patient to participate actively in performing care. Positive reinforcement is provided when the patient makes an effort in managing health effectively. The nurse needs to be a good listener and a support to the family, especially when explaining the tubes, dressings, and drains that are in place postoperatively.

MONITORING AND MANAGING POTENTIAL COMPLICATIONS

The potential complications after laryngectomy include respiratory distress and hypoxia, hemorrhage, infection, wound breakdown, aspiration, and tracheostomal stenosis.

Respiratory Distress and Hypoxia. The nurse monitors the patient for signs and symptoms of respiratory distress and hypoxia, particularly restlessness, irritation, agitation, confusion, tachypnea, the use of accessory muscles, and decreased oxygen saturation on pulse oximetry (SpO_2). Any change in respiratory status requires immediate intervention. Hypoxia may cause restlessness and an initial rise in blood pressure; this is followed by hypotension and somnolence. Cyanosis is a late sign of hypoxia. Obstruction needs to be ruled out immediately by suctioning and by having the patient cough and breathe deeply. Hypoxia and airway obstruction, if not treated immediately, are life-threatening.

Other nursing measures include repositioning of the patient to ensure an open airway and administering oxygen as prescribed. Oxygen is used with caution in patients with chronic obstructive pulmonary disease. The nurse should always be prepared for possible intubation and mechanical ventilation and must be knowledgeable about the hospital's emergency code protocols and skilled in the use of emergency equipment. The nurse must remain with the patient at all times during respiratory distress and initiate a call to the rapid response team as necessary.

Hemorrhage. Bleeding from the drains at the surgical site or with tracheal suctioning may signal the occurrence of hemorrhage. The nurse promptly notifies the surgeon of any active bleeding, which can occur at a variety of sites, including the surgical site, drains, and trachea. Rupture of the carotid artery is especially dangerous. Should this occur, the nurse must apply direct pressure over the artery, summon assistance, and provide emotional support to the patient until the vessel is ligated. The nurse monitors vital signs for changes, particularly increased pulse rate, decreased blood pressure, and rapid deep respirations. Cold, clammy, pale skin may indicate active bleeding. IV fluids and blood components may be given and other measures implemented to prevent or treat hemorrhagic shock. (Management of the patient with shock is discussed in detail in Chapter 11.)

Infection. The nurse monitors the patient for signs of postoperative infection. These include an increase in temperature and pulse, a change in the type of wound drainage, and increased areas of redness or tenderness at the surgical site. Other signs include purulent drainage, odor, and increased wound drainage. The nurse monitors the patient's white blood cell (WBC) count; a rise in WBCs may indicate the body's effort to combat infection. In older adult patients, infection can be present without an increase in the patient's WBC count; therefore, the nurse must monitor the patient for more subtle signs, such as lethargy, weakness, and decreased appetite. WBCs are suppressed in the patient with decreased immune function (e.g., patients receiving chemotherapy or radiation therapy); this predisposes the patient to a severe infection and sepsis. Antimicrobial (antibiotic) medications must be given as scheduled. All suspicious drainage is cultured, and the patient may be placed on the appropriate infection prevention precautions. Strategies are implemented to minimize the exposure of the patient to microorganisms and their spread to others. The nurse reports any significant change in the patient's status to the surgeon.

Wound Breakdown. Wound breakdown caused by infection, poor wound healing, development of a fistula, radiation therapy, or tumor growth can create a life-threatening emergency. The carotid artery, which is close to the stoma, may rupture from erosion if the wound does not heal properly. The nurse observes the stoma area for wound breakdown, hematoma, and bleeding and reports their occurrence to the surgeon. If wound breakdown occurs, the patient must be monitored carefully and identified as at high risk for carotid hemorrhage.

Aspiration. The patient who has undergone a laryngectomy is at the risk for aspiration and aspiration pneumonia due to depressed cough, the sedating effects of anesthetic and analgesic medications, alteration in the airway, impaired swallowing, and the administration of tube feedings. The nurse assesses for the presence of nausea and administers antiemetic medications, as prescribed. The nurse keeps a suction setup available in the hospital and instructs the family to do so at home for use if needed. Patients receiving tube feedings are positioned with the head of the bed at 30 degrees or higher during feedings and for 30 to 45 min after tube feedings. Patients receiving oral feedings are positioned with the head of the bed in an upright position for 30 to 45 min after feedings. For patients with a nasogastric or gastrostomy tube, the placement of the tube and residual gastric volume must be checked before each feeding. High amounts of residual volume (greater than 50% of previous intake) indicate delayed gastric emptying; this can lead to reflux and aspiration (Papadakis et al., 2018). Signs or symptoms of aspiration are reported to the primary provider immediately.

Tracheostomal Stenosis. Tracheostomal stenosis is an abnormal narrowing of the trachea or the tracheostomy stoma. Infection at the stoma site, excessive traction on the tracheostomy tube by the connecting tubing, and persistent high tracheostomy cuff pressure are risk factors for tracheostomal stenosis. The incidence of this condition varies widely, and it is often preventable. The nurse assesses the patient's stoma for signs and symptoms of infection and reports any evidence of this to the primary provider immediately. Tracheostomy care is performed routinely. The nurse assesses the connecting tubing (e.g., ventilation tubing) and secures the tubing to avoid excessive traction on the patient's tracheostomy. The nurse ensures that the tracheostomy cuff is deflated (for a patient with a cuffed tube) except for short periods, such as when the patient is eating or taking medications.

PROMOTING HOME, COMMUNITY-BASED, AND TRANSITIONAL CARE

Educating Patients About Self-Care. The nurse has an important role in the recovery and rehabilitation of the patient who has had a laryngectomy. To facilitate the patient's ability to manage self-care, discharge instruction begins as soon as the patient is able to participate. Nursing care and patient education in the hospital, outpatient setting, and rehabilitation or long-term care facility must take into consideration the many emotions, physical changes, and lifestyle changes experienced by the patient. In preparing the patient to go home, the nurse assesses the patient's readiness to learn and the level of knowledge about self-care management. The nurse also reassures the patient and family that most self-care management strategies can be mastered. The patient needs to learn a variety of self-care behaviors, including tracheostomy and stoma care, wound care, and oral hygiene. The nurse also instructs the patient about the need for adequate dietary intake, safe hygiene, and recreational activities.

Tracheostomy and Stoma Care. The nurse provides specific instructions to the patient and family about what to expect with a tracheostomy and its management. The nurse instructs the patient and caregiver how to perform suctioning and emergency measures and tracheostomy and stoma care. The nurse stresses the importance of humidification at home and instructs the family to obtain and set up a humidification system before the patient returns home.

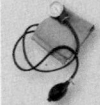

For the procedural guidelines for care of the patient with a tracheostomy tube, go to **thepoint.lww.com/Brunner15e**.

Hygiene and Safety Measures. The nurse instructs the patient and family about safety precautions that are needed because of the changes in structure and function resulting from the surgery. Special precautions are needed in the shower to prevent water from entering the stoma. Wearing a loose-fitting plastic bib over the tracheostomy or simply holding a hand over the opening is effective. Swimming is not recommended because a person with a laryngectomy can drown without submerging their face. Barbers and beauticians need to be alerted so that hair sprays, loose hair, and powder do not get near the stoma, because they can block or irritate the trachea and possibly cause infection. These self-care points are summarized in Chart 18-7.

The nurse educates the patient and caregiver about the signs and symptoms of infection and identifies indications that require contacting the primary provider after discharge. A discussion regarding cleanliness and infection control behaviors is essential. The nurse educates the patient and family to use hand hygiene before and after caring for the tracheostomy, to use tissues to remove mucus, and to dispose of soiled dressings and equipment properly. If the patient's surgery included cervical lymph node dissection, the nurse instructs the patient about how to perform exercises to strengthen the shoulder and neck muscles. A referral to a physical therapist might be helpful.

Recreation and exercise are important for the patient's well-being and quality of life, and all but very strenuous exercise

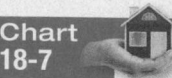

Chart 18-7 — HOME CARE CHECKLIST
The Patient with a Laryngectomy

At the completion of education, the patient and/or caregiver will be able to:

- Name the procedure that was performed and identify any permanent changes in anatomic structure or function as well as changes in ADLs, IADLs, communication, roles, relationships, and spirituality.
- State the name, dose, side effects, frequency, and schedule for all medications.
- Identify interventions and strategies (e.g., durable medical equipment, oxygen, nebulizer, humidifier) used in adapting to any permanent changes in structure or function.
- Describe ongoing postoperative therapeutic regimen, including stoma care, diet, and activities to perform (e.g., shoulder and neck exercises if a node dissection was performed) and to limit or avoid (e.g., swimming and contact sports).
  - Demonstrate tracheostomy care and tracheal suctioning to clear the airway and handle secretions.
  - Explain the rationale for maintaining adequate humidification with a humidifier or nebulizer.
  - Demonstrate how to clean the skin around the stoma and how to use ointments and tweezers to remove encrustations.
  - State the rationale for wearing a loose-fitting protective cloth at the stoma and covering the stoma when showering or bathing.
  - Discuss the need to avoid sprays, powders, particulates, and cold air from air-conditioning and the environment to prevent irritation of the airway.
  - Demonstrate safe technique in changing the laryngectomy/tracheostomy tube.

- Identify fluid and caloric needs.
- Describe mouth care and discuss its importance.
- Identify the signs and symptoms of wound infection and state what to do about them.
- Describe safety or emergency measures to implement in case of breathing difficulty or bleeding.
- State the rationale for wearing or carrying special medical identification and ways to obtain help in an emergency.
- Demonstrate alternative communication methods.
- Relate how to reach primary provider with questions or to report complications.
- State time and date of follow-up appointments.
- Obtain an annual influenza vaccine, and discuss vaccination against pneumonia with the primary provider.
- State understanding of community resources, support groups, and referrals (if any).
- Identify the need for health promotion (e.g., weight reduction, smoking cessation, and stress management), disease prevention, and screening activities.

Resources

In student resources for Chapter 19 at thepoint.lww.com/Brunner15e, see Procedural Guidelines: Care of the Patient with a Tracheostomy Tube and Procedural Guidelines: Performing Tracheal Suction.

ADL, activities of daily living; IADL, independent activities of daily living.

---

can be enjoyed safely. Avoidance of strenuous exercise and fatigue is important because the patient will have more difficulty speaking when tired, which can be discouraging. Additional safety points to address include the need for the patient to wear or carry medical identification, such as a bracelet or card, to alert medical personnel to the special requirements for resuscitation should this need arise. If resuscitation is needed, direct mouth-to-stoma ventilation should be performed. For home emergency situations, prerecorded emergency messages for police, the fire department, or other rescue services can be kept near the phone or programmed into smartphones or other electronic devices to be used quickly.

The nurse instructs and encourages the patient to perform oral care frequently to prevent halitosis and infection. If the patient is receiving radiation therapy, synthetic saliva may be required because of decreased saliva production. Patients receiving radiation therapy frequently report dry mouth, change in taste, lack of appetite, and mouth sores (Cullen, Baumler, Farrington, et al., 2018) (see the Nursing Research Profile in Chart 18-8). The nurse instructs the patient to drink water or sugar-free liquids throughout the day and to use a humidifier at home. Brushing the teeth or dentures and rinsing the mouth several times a day will assist in maintaining proper oral hygiene.

Continuing and Transitional Care. Referral for home, community-based, or transitional care is an important aspect of postoperative care for the patient who has had a laryngectomy and will assist the patient and family in the discharge home. The nurse assesses the patient's general health status and the ability of the patient and family to care for the stoma and tracheostomy. The surgical incisions, nutritional and respiratory status, and adequacy of pain management are also assessed. The nurse assesses for signs and symptoms of complications and the patient's and family's knowledge of signs and symptoms to be reported to the physician. During the home visit, the nurse identifies and addresses other learning needs and concerns of the patient and family, such as adaptation to physical, lifestyle, and functional changes, as well as the patient's progress with learning and using new communication strategies. The nurse assesses the patient's psychological status, reinforces previous instructions, and provides reassurance and support to the patient and family caregivers as needed.

The person who has had a laryngectomy should have regular physical examinations and seek advice concerning any problems related to recovery and rehabilitation. The nurse reminds the patient to participate in health promotion activities and health screening and about the importance of keeping scheduled appointments with the physician, speech therapist, and other health care providers.

Evaluation

Expected patient outcomes may include the following:

1. Demonstrates an adequate level of knowledge, verbalizing an understanding of the surgical procedure and performing self-care adequately

Chart 18-8	**NURSING RESEARCH PROFILE**

Mitigating the Effects of Radiation Therapy on the Oral Mucosa of Patients with Head and Neck Cancers

Cullen, L., Baumler, S., Farrington, M., et al. (2018). Oral care for head and neck cancer symptom management. *American Journal of Nursing, 118*(1), 24–34.

Purpose

Patients diagnosed with laryngeal and oropharyngeal cancer (head and neck cancer [HNC]) commonly receive radiation therapy on an outpatient basis. These patients often develop mucositis, which causes symptoms that include pain, difficulty swallowing, dry mouth, change in taste, lack of appetite, and mouth sores. An evidence-based practice intervention at a radiation oncology center in a large academic medical center in the Midwestern United States was designed to reduce the severity of oral mucositis in adults receiving radiation therapy for HNC.

Design

Study participants included adults with HNC who were receiving outpatient radiation therapy with or without concurrent chemotherapy. Twenty participants were recruited to the usual care group. The usual care group received extensive oral care preparation prior to radiation treatment. This included a visit with an oncologic dentist for a professional dental evaluation, fluoride treatments, the provision of oral care supplies, and tooth extraction if needed. Radiation treatment then proceeded as usual for 6 to 8 wk. These participants served as historical controls for the intervention group.

The 85 participants who were then recruited into the intervention group received the same care as those in the usual care group plus targeted education, a comprehensive oral care kit, and information on how to use the kit. The targeted education included a brochure from the U.S. Department of Health and Human Services, Head and Neck Radiation Treatment and Your Mouth, and a one-page additional insert, which was developed by the team. Nurses were integral throughout the study process in educating patients about the intervention.

Both clinicians and participants were surveyed at various intervals. Clinicians' (i.e., nurses, physicians, and radiation therapists) knowledge of oral care and correct use of oral care products, perceptions and attitudes about oral care, and behaviors and practices related to the documentation of patients' oral health and education were assessed. Participant feedback was obtained before radiation treatment, during weeks 4 to 5 of treatment, and 1 mo after treatment. The participants' questionnaires included sections that surveyed oral care practices (the frequency of care and products used), perceptions about oral care (feeling well prepared and the usefulness of oral care products), and oral mucositis symptoms.

Findings

The percentage of clinicians with correct responses to knowledge assessment items improved from 71% preimplementation to 80% postimplementation. The clinicians' mean scores on questions capturing their perceptions were higher postimplementation than preimplementation.

Feedback provided by patients during radiation treatment on weeks 4 to 5 demonstrated improvement in oral hygiene behaviors. More patients in the intervention group reported brushing at least daily, using Biotene toothpaste, performing oral rinses at least twice a day, and using lanolin lip balm, compared with those in the usual care group. Patients in the intervention group showed higher adherence with the targeted education and oral care kit intervention which led to a reduction of symptoms at weeks 4 to 5 of radiation treatment, when symptoms are expected to peak. The intervention group reported less severity than the usual care patients regarding the following symptoms: mouth and throat soreness, difficulty swallowing, difficulty eating, and difficulty talking. Furthermore, the intervention group reported less difficulty with xerostomia 1 mo after radiation was completed.

Nursing Implications

Mucositis is a frequent and distressing complication of radiation therapy in the treatment of patients with HNC. Nurses are key members of the treatment team and play many roles in caring for these patients, from assessing patients' symptoms to educating them on ways to reduce these symptoms. Findings from this study show that the distribution of standardized oral care kits and related educational materials can offer an effective way to meet patients' needs and reduce oral mucositis severity in adults treated with radiation therapy for HNC. The success of the project also highlights the key role nurses play in cancer symptom management, before radiation therapy begins, throughout the course of treatment, and in the months afterward.

---

2. Demonstrates less anxiety
   a. Expresses a sense of hope
   b. Is aware of available community organizations and agencies that provide patient education and support groups
   c. Participates in support group for people with a laryngectomy
3. Maintains a clear airway and handles own secretions; also demonstrates practical, safe, and correct technique for cleaning and changing the tracheostomy or laryngectomy tube
4. Acquires effective communication techniques
   a. Uses assistive devices and strategies for communication (Magic Slate, call bell, picture board, sign language, speech reading, handheld electronic devices, smartphones)
   b. Follows the recommendations of the speech therapist
   c. Demonstrates ability to communicate with new communication strategy
   d. Reports availability of prerecorded messages to summon emergency assistance by telephone
5. Maintains adequate nutrition and adequate fluid intake
6. Exhibits improved body image, self-esteem, and self-concept
   a. Expresses feelings and concerns
   b. Manages health effectively
   c. Accepts information about support group
7. Adheres to rehabilitation and home care program
   a. Practices recommended speech therapy
   b. Demonstrates proper methods for caring for stoma and laryngectomy or tracheostomy tube (if present)
   c. Verbalizes understanding of symptoms that require medical attention
   d. States safety measures to take in emergencies
   e. Performs oral hygiene as prescribed

8. Absence of complications
   a. Demonstrates a patent airway
   b. No bleeding from surgical site and minimal bleeding from drains; vital signs (blood pressure, temperature, pulse, respiratory rate) are normal
   c. No redness, tenderness, or purulent drainage at surgical site
   d. No wound breakdown
   e. Clear breath sounds; oxygen saturation level within acceptable range; chest x-ray clear
   f. No indications of infection, stenosis, or obstruction of tracheal stoma

CRITICAL THINKING EXERCISES

1 **pq** A 19-year-old college student presents to the student health center where you work as a staff nurse with complaints of a "stuffed up head," severe headache, green mucous when blowing her nose, and "teeth achiness." She reports a fever of 100.8 for the past 2 days. What further questions do you have regarding her symptoms? What is your priority focus for your physical examination? What diagnostic tests and treatments may you anticipate?

2 **ebp** You are attending a wedding shower when the bride's grandmother starts bleeding from her nose. You find out from her granddaughter that she has been receiving intravenous pembrolizumab for advanced lung cancer and had her last treatment 5 days ago. What is your priority focus for your nursing assessment? What types of interventions are indicated for epistaxis? What additional concerns do you have for this patient related to her immunotherapy regimen? Would you consider transport to an urgent care center or ED? Why or why not? What is the strength of the evidence that might guide your recommendations for follow-up for this older adult woman?

3 **ipc** You are working in a family practice clinic and are triaging a 58-year-old male who is complaining of weight loss, difficulty swallowing, sore throat, and hoarseness for the past month. He is worried about having cancer. What risk factors would you screen for in this patient? What type of referral do you expect to be made for this patient? Who else might need to be involved in his care?

REFERENCES

*Asterisk indicates nursing research.

Books

Bickley, L. S., & Szilagyi, P. G. (2017). *Bates' guide to physical examination and history taking* (12th ed.). Philadelphia, PA: Lippincott Williams & Wilkins.

Comerford, K. C., & Durkin, M. T. (Eds.). (2020). *Nursing2020 drug handbook*. Philadelphia, PA: Wolters Kluwer.

De Vita, V., Hellman, S., & Rosenberg, S. (Eds.). (2018). *Cancer: Principles and practice of oncology* (11th ed.). Philadelphia, PA: Lippincott Williams & Wilkins.

Eliopoulos, C. (2018). *Gerontological nursing* (9th ed.). Philadelphia, PA: Wolters Kluwer.

Papadakis, M., McPhee, S. J., & Rabow, M. (2018). *Current medical diagnosis and treatment* (57th ed.). New York: McGraw-Hill.

Pokorski, M. (2015). *Pulmonary infection*. New York: Springer Publishing Company.

Reardon, R. F., Mason, P. E., & Clinton, J. E. (2017). Basic airway management and decision-making. In J. D. Roberts (Ed.). *Roberts & Hedges' clinical procedures in emergency medicine* (7th ed.). Philadelphia, PA: Elsevier Saunders.

Weinberger, S., Cockrill, B., & Mandel, J. (2019). *Principles of pulmonary medicine* (7th ed.). Philadelphia, PA: Elsevier.

Journals and Electronic Documents

Acerra, J. (2018). Pharyngitis. Retrieved on 6/2/2019 at: www.emedicine.medscape.com/article/764304-overview

Adil, E. (2018). Total laryngectomy. Retrieved on 5/27/2019 at: www.emedicine.medscape.com/article/2051731-overview

American Academy of Otolaryngology–Head and Neck Surgery Foundation. (2018). Sinusitis. Retrieved on 5/27/2019 at: www.enthealth.org/conditions/sinusitis

American Cancer Society (ACS). (2017). What are the risk factors for laryngeal and hypopharyngeal cancers? Retrieved on 5/27/2019 at: www.cancer.org/Cancer/LaryngealandHypopharyngealCancer

American Sleep Apnea Association. (2019). Obstructive sleep apnea. Retrieved on 5/27/2019 at: www.sleepapnea.org/learn/sleep-apnea/obstructive-sleep-apnea.html

Aring, A., & Chan, M. (2016). Current concepts in adult acute rhinosinusitis. *American Family Physician*, 94(2), 97–105.

Ayoade, F. (2018). Herpes simplex. Retrieved on 5/27/2019 at: www.emedicine.medscape.com/article/218580-overview

Becker, D. (2018). Nasal and septal fractures. Retrieved on 5/27/2019 at: www.emedicine.medscape.com/article/878595-overview

Brook, I. (2018a). Acute sinusitis. Retrieved on 8/2/2019 at: www.emedicine.medscape.com/article/232670-overview

Brook, I. (2018b). Chronic sinusitis. Retrieved on 5/27/2019 at: www.emedicine.medscape.com/article/232791-overview

Buensalido, J. (2019a). Bacterial pharyngitis. Retrieved on 8/14/2019 at: www.emedicine.medscape.com/article/225243-overview#showall

Buensalido, J. (2019b). Rhinovirus (RV) infection (common cold). Retrieved on 8/4/2019 at: www.emedicine.medscape.com/article/227820-overview#a1

Burton, M. J., Glasziou, P. P., Chong, L. Y., et al. (2014). Tonsillectomy or adenotonsillectomy versus non-surgical treatment for chronic/recurrent acute tonsillitis (review). *The Cochrane Library*, 2014(11), 1–85.

Busaba, N., & Doron, S. (2018). Tonsillectomy in adults: Indications. Retrieved on 6/2/2019 at: www.uptodate.com/contents/tonsillectomy-in-adults-indications#!

Centers for Disease Control and Prevention (CDC). (2017). Antibiotic prescribing and use in doctor's offices. Adult treatment recommendations. Retrieved on 6/2/2019 at: www.cdc.gov/antibiotic-use/community/for-hcp/outpatient-hcp/adult-treatment-rec.html

Centers for Disease Control and Prevention (CDC). (2019). Common colds: Protect yourself and others. Retrieved on 5/27/2019 at: www.cdc.gov/Features/Rhinoviruses/index.html

Chow, A., & Doron, S. (2018). Evaluation of acute pharyngitis in adults. Retrieved on 6/2/2019 at: www.uptodate.com/contents/evaluation-of-acute-pharyngitis-in-adults

*Cullen, L., Baumler, S., Farrington, M., et al. (2018). Oral care for head and neck cancer symptom management. *American Journal of Nursing*, 118(1), 24–34.

Drake, A. F., & Carr, M. M. (2017). Tonsillectomy. Retrieved on 5/27/2019 at: www.reference.medscape.com/article/872119-overview

Flores, J. (2018). Peritonsillar abscess in emergency medicine. Retrieved on 5/27/2019 at: www.emedicine.medscape.com/article/764188-overview

Gosselin, B. (2018). Peritonsillar abscess. Retrieved on 6/2/2019 at: www.emedicine.medscape.com/article/194863-overview

Hamilos, D. (2018). Chronic rhinosinusitis: Clinical manifestations, pathophysiology, and diagnosis. Retrieved on 8/2/2019 at: www.uptodate.com/contents/chronic-rhinosinusitis-management

Hauk, L. (2018). Treatment of seasonal allergic rhinitis: A guideline from the AAAI/ACAAI Joint Task Force on Practice Parameters. *American Family Physician*, 97(11), 756–757.

Joshi, A. (2018). Oral appliances in snoring and obstructive sleep apnea. Retrieved on 6/9/2019 at: www.emedicine.medscape.com/article/869831-overview

Lehmann, A. E., Scangas, G. A., Sethi, R. K., et al. (2018). Impact of age on sinus surgery outcomes. *The Laryngoscope, 128,* 2681–2687.

Meneghetti, A. (2018). Upper respiratory tract infection. Retrieved on 6/2/2019 at: www.emedicine.medscape.com/article/302460-overview

Morgan, C. (2017). Surgical approach to snoring and sleep apnea. Retrieved on 5/27/2019 at: www.emedicine.medscape.com/article/868770-overview

Mousa, H. (2017). Prevention and treatment of influenza, influenza-like illness, and common cold by herbal, complementary, and natural therapies. *Journal of Evidence-Based Complementary and Alternative Medicine, 22*(1), 166–174.

National Cancer Institute (NCI). (2019). Laryngeal cancer treatment (PDQR). Retrieved on 5/27/2019 at: www.cancer.gov/types/head-and-neck/hp/adult/laryngeal-treatment-pdq

National Institute for Occupational Safety and Health. (2018). Pandemic planning: Recommended guidance for extended use and limited reuse of N95 filtering facepiece respirators in healthcare settings. Retrieved on 8/14/2019 at: www.cdc.gov/niosh/topics/hcwcontrols/recommendedguidanceextuse.html

Nguyen, Q. A. (2018). Epistaxis. Retrieved on 5/27/2019 at: www.emedicine.medscape.com/article/863220-overview

Patel, A. (2016). Functional endoscopic sinus surgery. Retrieved on 5/27/2019 at: www.emedicine.medscape.com/article/863420-overview

Patel, B. (2017). Aeroallergens. Retrieved on 5/27/2019 at: www.emedicine.medscape.com/article/137911-overview

Patel, Z., & Hwang, P. (2019). Uncomplicated acute sinusitis and rhinosinusitis in adults: Treatment. Retrieved on 8/2/2019 at: www.uptodate.com/contents/uncomplicated-acute-sinusitis-and-rhinosinusitis-in-adults-treatment

Patil, S., Ayappa, I., Caples, S., et al. (2019). Treatment of adult obstructive sleep apnea with positive airway pressure: An American Academy of Sleep Medicine clinical practice guideline. *Journal of Clinical Sleep Medicine, 15*(2), 335–343.

Peters, A. (2015). Rhinosinusitis: Synopsis. Retrieved on 6/2/2019 at: www.worldallergy.org/professional/allergic_diseases_center/rhinosinusitis/sinusitissynopsis.php

Petri, N., Christensen, J., Svanholt, P., et al. (2019). Mandibular advancement device therapy for obstructive sleep apnea: A prospective study on predictors of treatment success. *Sleep Medicine, 54,* 187–194.

Ramadan, H. (2018). Fungal sinusitis. Retrieved on 6/2/2019 at: www.emedicine.medscape.com/article/863062-overview

Rosenfeld, R. M., Andes, D., Bhattacharyya, M., et al. (2015). Clinical practice guideline update: Adult sinusitis executive summary. *Otolaryngology Head & Neck Surgery, 152*(4), 598–609.

Sedaghat, A. (2017). Chronic rhinosinusitis. *American Family Physician, 96*(8), 500–506.

Shah, U. K. (2018). Tonsillitis and peritonsillar abscess. Retrieved on 5/27/2019 at: www.emedicine.medscape.com/article/871977-overview

*Showalter, L., & O'Keefe, C. (2019). Implementation of an obstructive sleep apnea screening tool with hypertensive patients in the primary care clinic. *Journal of the American Association of Nurse Practitioners, 31*(3), 184–188.

Stead, W. (2017). Patient education: Sore throat in adults (beyond the basics). Retrieved on 6/2/2019 at: www.uptodate.com/contents/sore-throat-in-adults-beyond-the-basics

Suslu, N. (2016). Early oral feeding after total laryngectomy: Outcome of 602 patients in one cancer center. *Auris, Nasus Larynx, 43*(5), 546–550.

Tajudeen, B., & Kennedy, D. (2017). Thirty years of endoscopic sinus surgery: What have we learned? *World Journal of Otorhinolaryngology – Head and Neck Surgery, 3*(2), 115–121.

Tewfik, T. (2018). Medical treatment for acute sinusitis. Retrieved on 5/27/2019 at: www.emedicine.medscape.com/article/861646-overview

Uyeki, T., Bernstein, H., Bradley, J., et al. (2018). Clinical practice guidelines by the Infectious Diseases Society of America: 2018 update on diagnosis, treatment, chemoprophylaxis, and institutional outbreak management of seasonal influenza. *Clinical Infectious Diseases, 68*(10), e1–e47.

Valdes, C. J., & Tewfik, M. A. (2018). Rhinosinusitis and allergies in elderly patients. *Clinics in Geriatric Medicine, 34*(2), 217–231.

Viscuso, D., & Arena, O. (2016). Efficacy of mandibular advancement devices in the treatment of mild to moderate obstructive sleep apnea and the usefulness of sleep endoscopy. *Italian Journal of Dental Medicine, 1*(1–2016), 19–22.

Wickramasinghe, H. (2019). Obstructive sleep apnea. Retrieved on 5/27/2019 at: www.emedicine.medscape.com/article/295807-overview

Resources

American Academy of Allergy, Asthma & Immunology (AAAAI), www.aaaai.org

American Academy of Family Physicians, www.aafp.org/home.html

American Academy of Otolaryngology–Head and Neck Surgery, www.entnet.org

American Cancer Society (ACS), www.cancer.org

American Sleep Apnea Association (ASAA), www.sleepapnea.org

International Association of Laryngectomees (IAL), www.theial.com

National Cancer Institute (NCI), www.cancer.gov

National Comprehensive Cancer Network (NCCN), www.nccn.org

National Institute of Allergy and Infectious Diseases (NIAID), www.niaid.nih.gov

National Sleep Foundation, www.sleepfoundation.org

WebWhispers, www.webwhispers.org

Management of Patients with Chest and Lower Respiratory Tract Disorders

LEARNING OUTCOMES

On completion of this chapter, the learner will be able to:

1. Identify patients at risk for atelectasis and the nursing interventions related to its prevention and management.
2. Compare the various pulmonary infections with regard to causes, clinical manifestations, nursing management, complications, and prevention.
3. Identify the nursing care of a patient with an endotracheal tube, with mechanical ventilation, or with a tracheostomy.
4. Relate the therapeutic management of acute respiratory distress syndrome to the underlying pathophysiology of the syndrome.
5. Describe preventive measures appropriate for controlling and eliminating occupational lung disease.
6. Discuss the modes of therapy and related nursing management of patients with lung cancer.
7. Use the nursing process as a framework for care of the patient with pneumonia, receiving mechanical ventilation, or with a thoracotomy.
8. Describe the complications of chest trauma and their clinical manifestations and nursing management.
9. Explain the principles of chest drainage and the nursing responsibilities related to the care of the patient with a chest drainage system.

NURSING CONCEPTS

Infection

Oxygenation

GLOSSARY

acute lung injury: an umbrella term for hypoxemic respiratory failure; equivalent to mild acute respiratory distress syndrome (ARDS)

acute respiratory distress syndrome (ARDS): nonspecific pulmonary response to a variety of pulmonary and nonpulmonary insults to the lung; characterized by interstitial infiltrates, alveolar hemorrhage, atelectasis, refractory hypoxemia, and, with the exception of some patients with coronavirus disease 2019 (COVID-19) and ARDS, decreased compliance

airway pressure release ventilation (APRV): mode of mechanical ventilation that allows unrestricted, spontaneous breaths throughout the ventilatory cycle; on inspiration the patient receives a preset level of continuous positive airway pressure, and pressure is periodically released to aid expiration

aspiration: inhalation of either oropharyngeal or gastric contents into the lower airways

atelectasis: collapse or airless condition of the alveoli caused by hypoventilation, obstruction to the airways, or compression

bilevel positive airway pressure (BiPAP): noninvasive spontaneous breath mode of mechanical ventilation that allows for the separate control of inspiratory and expiratory pressures; given via a mask

central cyanosis: bluish discoloration of the skin or mucous membranes due to hemoglobin carrying reduced amounts of oxygen

chest drainage system: the use of a chest tube and closed drainage system to re-expand the lung and to remove excess air, fluid, or blood

consolidation: lung tissue that has become more solid in nature due to collapse of alveoli or infectious process (pneumonia)

continuous mandatory (volume or pressure) ventilation (CMV): also referred to as assist–control (A/C) ventilation; mode of mechanical ventilation in which the patient's breathing pattern may trigger the ventilator to deliver a preset tidal volume or set pressure; in the absence of spontaneous breathing, the machine delivers a controlled breath at a preset minimum rate and tidal volume or set pressure

continuous positive airway pressure (CPAP): positive pressure applied throughout the respiratory cycle to a spontaneously breathing patient to promote alveolar and airway stability and increase functional residual capacity;

may be given with endotracheal or tracheostomy tube or by mask

cor pulmonale: "heart of the lungs"; enlargement of the right ventricle from hypertrophy or dilation or as a secondary response to disorders that affect the lungs

empyema: accumulation of purulent material in the pleural space

endotracheal intubation: insertion of a breathing tube (type of artificial airway) through the nose or mouth into the trachea

fraction of inspired oxygen (FiO$_2$): concentration of oxygen delivered (e.g., 1.0 = 100% oxygen)

hemoptysis: the coughing up of blood from the lower respiratory tract

hemothorax: partial or complete collapse of the lung due to blood accumulating in the pleural space; may occur after surgery or trauma

hypoxemia: decrease in oxygen tension in the arterial blood

hypoxia: decrease in oxygen supply to the tissues and cells

incentive spirometry: method of deep breathing that provides visual feedback to help the patient inhale deeply and slowly and achieve maximum lung inflation

induration: an abnormally hard lesion or reaction, as in a positive tuberculin skin test

intermittent mandatory (volume or pressure) ventilation (IMV): mode of mechanical ventilation that provides a combination of mechanically assisted breaths at a preset volume or pressure and rate and spontaneous breaths

mechanical ventilator: a positive- or negative-pressure breathing device that supports ventilation and oxygenation

orthopnea: shortness of breath when reclining or in the supine position

pleural effusion: abnormal accumulation of fluid in the pleural space

pleural friction rub: localized grating or creaking sound caused by the rubbing together of inflamed parietal and visceral pleurae

pleural space: the area between the parietal and visceral pleurae; a potential space

pneumothorax: partial or complete collapse of the lung due to positive pressure in the pleural space

positive end-expiratory pressure (PEEP): positive pressure maintained at the end of exhalation (instead of a normal zero pressure) to increase functional residual capacity and open collapsed alveoli

pressure support ventilation (PSV): mode of mechanical ventilation in which preset positive pressure is delivered with spontaneous breaths to decrease work of breathing

proportional assist ventilation (PAV): mode of mechanical ventilation that provides partial ventilatory support in proportion to the patient's inspiratory efforts; decreases the work of breathing

purulent: consisting of, containing, or discharging pus

respiratory weaning: process of gradual, systematic withdrawal or removal of ventilator, breathing tube, and oxygen

restrictive lung disease: disease of the lung that causes a decrease in lung volumes

synchronized intermittent mandatory ventilation (SIMV): mode of mechanical ventilation in which the ventilator allows the patient to breathe spontaneously while providing a preset number of breaths to ensure adequate ventilation; ventilated breaths are synchronized with spontaneous breathing

tension pneumothorax: pneumothorax characterized by increasing positive pressure in the pleural space with each breath; this is an emergency situation, and the positive pressure needs to be decompressed or released immediately

thoracentesis: insertion of a needle or catheter into the pleural space to remove fluid that has accumulated and decrease pressure on the lung tissue; may also be used diagnostically to identify potential causes of a pleural effusion

thoracotomy: surgical opening into the chest cavity

tidal volume: volume of air inspired and expired with each breath

tracheostomy tube: indwelling tube inserted directly into the trachea to assist with ventilation

tracheotomy: surgical opening into the trachea

transbronchial: through the bronchial wall, as in a transbronchial lung biopsy

ventilation–perfusion ($\dot{V}/\dot{Q}$): refers to the ratio between ventilation and perfusion in the lung; matching of ventilation to perfusion optimizes gas exchange

---

Disorders affecting the chest and lower respiratory tract range from acute to chronic conditions. Many of these disorders are serious and often life-threatening. Patients with chest and lower respiratory tract disorders require care from nurses with astute assessment and clinical management skills as well as knowledge of evidence-based practice. Nurses must also understand the impact of the particular disorder on the patient's quality of life and ability to carry out activities of daily living. Patient and family education is an important nursing intervention in the management of all chest and lower respiratory tract disorders.

INFLAMMATORY AND INFECTIOUS PULMONARY DISORDERS

Inflammatory pulmonary disorders may include relatively common disorders such as atelectasis, as well as uncommon disorders such as aspiration and sarcoidosis. Infectious pulmonary disorders are responsible for much morbidity and mortality, and include diseases such as pneumonia and tuberculosis, as well as lung abscesses.

Atelectasis

Atelectasis refers to closure or collapse of alveoli and often is described in relation to chest x-ray findings and clinical signs and symptoms. Atelectasis is one of the most commonly encountered abnormalities seen on a chest x-ray (Stark, 2019). Atelectasis may be acute or chronic and may cover a broad range of pathophysiologic changes, from microatelectasis (which is not detectable on chest x-ray) to macroatelectasis with loss of segmental, lobar, or overall lung volume. The most commonly described is acute atelectasis, which occurs most often in the postoperative setting usually following thoracic and upper abdominal procedures or in people who are immobilized and have a shallow, monotonous breathing pattern (Conde & Adams, 2018; Smetana, 2018). Excess secretions or mucus plugs may also cause obstruction of airflow and result in atelectasis in an area of the lung. Atelectasis also is observed in patients with a chronic airway obstruction that impedes or blocks the flow of air to an area of the lung (e.g., obstructive atelectasis in the patient with lung cancer that is invading or compressing the airways). This type of atelectasis is more insidious and slower in onset (Conde & Adams, 2018; Stark, 2019).

Pathophysiology

Atelectasis may be described as either nonobstructive or obstructive. Nonobstructive atelectasis occurs in adults as a result of reduced ventilation. Obstructive atelectasis results from any blockage that impedes the passage of air to and from the alveoli, reducing alveolar ventilation (Stark, 2019). Obstructive atelectasis is the most common type and results from reabsorption of gas (trapped alveolar air is absorbed into the bloodstream); no additional air can enter into the alveoli

because of the blockage. As a result, the affected portion of the lung becomes airless and the alveoli collapse. Causes of atelectasis include foreign body, tumor or growth in an airway, altered breathing patterns, retained secretions, pain, alterations in small airway function, prolonged supine positioning, increased abdominal pressure, reduced lung volumes due to musculoskeletal or neurologic disorders, restrictive defects, and specific surgical procedures (e.g., upper abdominal, thoracic, or open heart surgery) (Conde & Adams, 2018).

Patients are at high risk for atelectasis postoperatively because of several factors. A monotonous, low tidal breathing pattern may cause small airway closure and alveolar collapse. This can result from the effects of anesthesia or analgesic agents, supine positioning, splinting of the chest wall because of pain, or abdominal distention. Secretion retention, airway obstruction, and an impaired cough reflex may also occur, or patients may be reluctant to cough because of pain (Conde & Adams, 2018). Figure 19-1 shows the mechanisms and consequences of acute atelectasis in postoperative patients.

Atelectasis resulting from bronchial obstruction by secretions may also occur in patients with impaired cough

Physiology/Pathophysiology

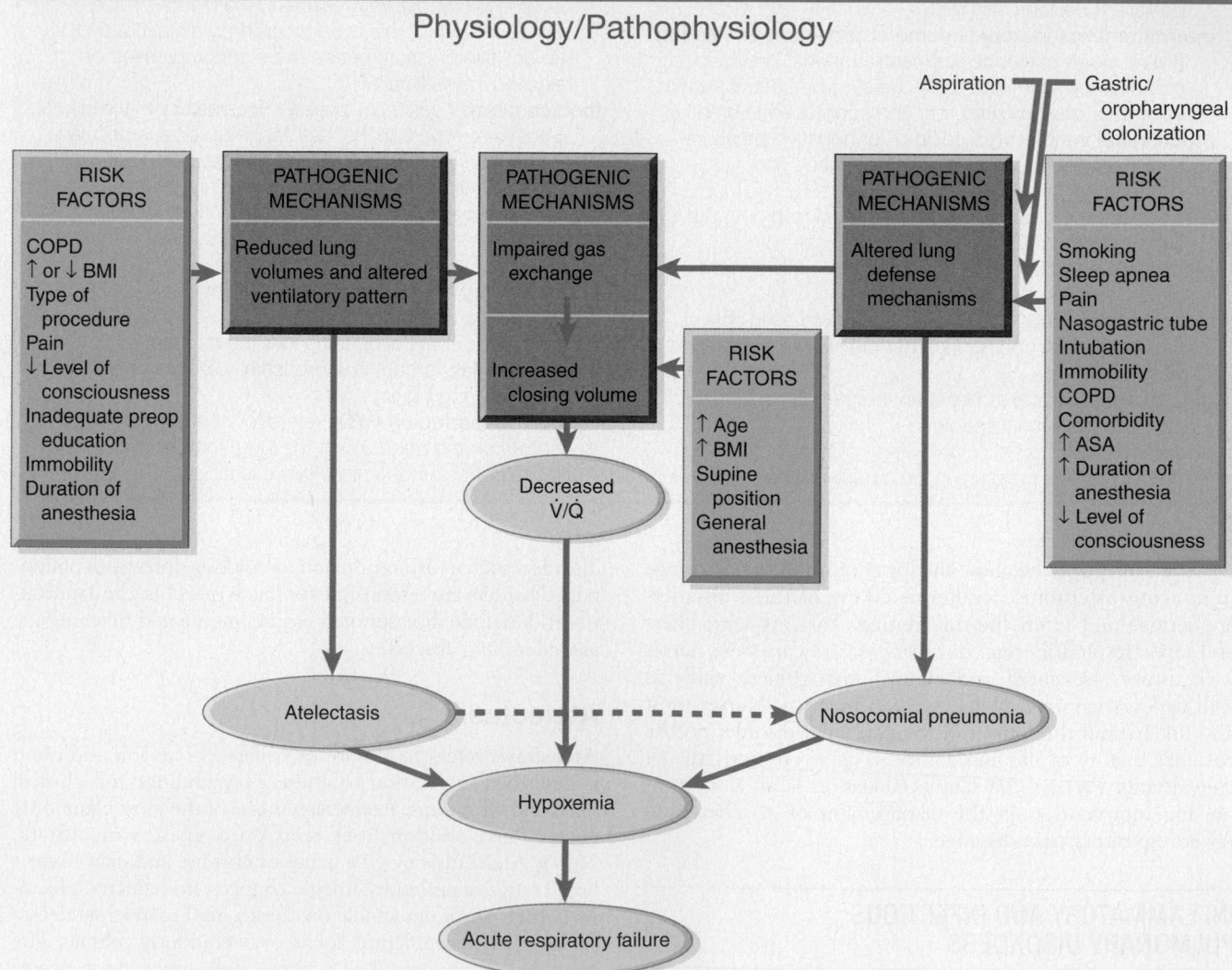

Figure 19-1 • Relationship of risk factors, pathogenic mechanisms, and consequences of acute atelectasis in the postoperative patient. ASA, acetylsalicylic acid; BMI, body mass index; COPD, chronic obstructive pulmonary disease; V̇/Q̇, ventilation–perfusion ratio.

mechanisms (e.g., musculoskeletal or neurologic disorders) as well as in those who are debilitated and confined to bed. In addition, atelectasis may develop because of excessive pressure on the lung tissue (i.e., compressive atelectasis), which restricts normal lung expansion on inspiration (Stark, 2019). Such pressure can be produced by a **pleural effusion** (fluid accumulating within the pleural space), a **pneumothorax** (air in the pleural space), or a **hemothorax** (blood in the pleural space). The **pleural space** is the area between the parietal and the visceral pleurae, and is normally a potential rather than an actual space. Pressure may also be produced by a pericardial effusion (pericardium distended with fluid), tumor growth within the thorax, or an elevated diaphragm.

Clinical Manifestations

The development of atelectasis usually is insidious. Signs and symptoms include increasing dyspnea (shortness of breath), cough, and sputum production.

In acute atelectasis involving a large amount of lung tissue (lobar atelectasis), marked respiratory distress may be observed. In addition to the previously mentioned signs and symptoms, tachycardia, tachypnea, pleural pain, and **central cyanosis** (a bluish skin hue that is a late sign of hypoxemia) may be anticipated. Patients characteristically have difficulty breathing in the supine position and are anxious.

In chronic atelectasis, signs and symptoms are similar to those of acute atelectasis. The chronic nature of the alveolar collapse predisposes patients to infection distal to the obstruction. Therefore, the signs and symptoms of a pulmonary infection also may be present.

Assessment and Diagnostic Findings

When clinically significant atelectasis develops, it is generally characterized by increased work of breathing and **hypoxemia** (i.e., a decrease in oxygen tension in the arterial blood). Decreased breath sounds and crackles are heard over the affected area. A chest x-ray may suggest a diagnosis of atelectasis before clinical symptoms appear; the x-ray may reveal patchy infiltrates or consolidated areas. Depending on the degree of hypoxemia, pulse oximetry (SpO_2) may demonstrate a low saturation of hemoglobin with oxygen (less than 90%) or a lower-than-normal partial pressure of arterial oxygen (PaO_2).

 Quality and Safety Nursing Alert

Tachypnea, dyspnea, and mild-to-moderate hypoxemia are hallmarks of the severity of atelectasis.

Prevention

Nursing measures to prevent atelectasis include frequent turning, early mobilization, and strategies to expand the lungs and to manage secretions. Voluntary deep-breathing maneuvers (at least every 2 hours) assist in preventing and treating atelectasis. The performance of these maneuvers requires the patient to be alert and cooperative. Patient education and reinforcement are key elements to the success of these interventions. The use of incentive spirometry or voluntary deep breathing enhances lung expansion, decreases the potential

for airway closure, and may generate a cough. **Incentive spirometry** is a method of deep breathing that provides visual feedback to encourage the patient to inhale slowly and deeply to maximize lung inflation and prevent or reduce atelectasis. The purpose of an incentive spirometer is to ensure that the volume of air inhaled is increased gradually as the patient takes deeper and deeper breaths.

Incentive spirometers are available in two types: volume or flow. In the volume type, the tidal volume is set using the manufacturer's instructions. The patient takes a deep breath through the mouthpiece, pauses at peak lung inflation, and then relaxes and exhales. Taking several normal breaths before attempting another with the incentive spirometer helps avoid fatigue. The volume is periodically increased as tolerated.

In the flow type, the volume is not preset. The spirometer contains a number of movable balls that are pushed up by the force of the breath and held suspended in the air while the patient inhales. The amount of air inhaled and the flow of the air are estimated by how long and how high the balls are suspended (see Chart 19-1).

Secretion management techniques include directed cough, suctioning, aerosol nebulizer treatments followed by chest physiotherapy (CPT; see Figs. 20-6 and 20-7 and further

---

Chart 19-1

PATIENT EDUCATION
Performing Incentive Spirometry

The inspired air helps inflate the lungs. The ball or weight in the spirometer rises in response to the intensity of the intake of air. The higher the ball rises, the deeper the breath.

The nurse instructs the patient to:

- Assume a semi-Fowler position or an upright position before initiating therapy.
- Use diaphragmatic breathing.
- Place the mouthpiece of the spirometer firmly in the mouth, breathe air in (inspire) slowly through the mouth, and hold the breath at the end of inspiration for about 3 seconds to maintain the ball/indicator between the lines. Exhale slowly through the mouthpiece.
- Cough during and after each session. Splint the incision when coughing postoperatively.
- Perform the procedure approximately 10 times in succession, repeating the 10 breaths with the spirometer each hour during waking hours.

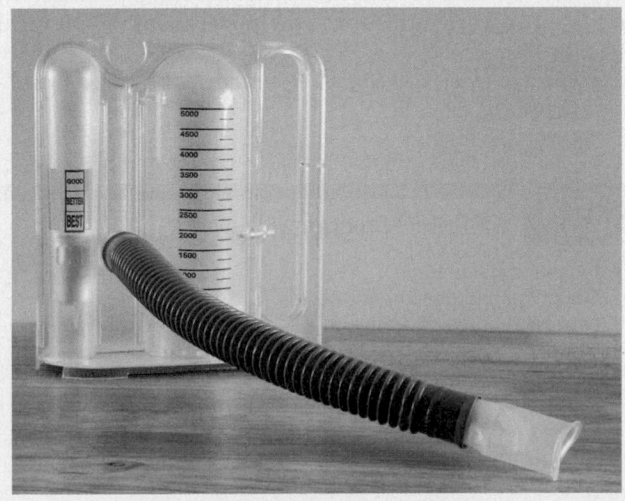

discussion of CPT principles in Chapter 20), and bronchoscopy. In some settings, a pressurized metered-dose inhaler (pMDI) is used to dispense a bronchodilator rather than an aerosolized, small-volume nebulizer (SVN) (see Chapter 20 for further discussion of pMDIs and SVNs). Chart 19-2 summarizes measures used to prevent atelectasis.

Management

The goal of the treatment is to improve ventilation and remove secretions. Strategies to prevent atelectasis, which include frequent turning, early ambulation, lung volume expansion maneuvers (e.g., deep-breathing exercises and incentive spirometry), and coughing, also serve as the first-line measures to minimize or treat atelectasis by improving ventilation. Multidisciplinary, evidence-based standardized intervention programs that incorporate ICOUGH[SM] (see Chart 19-3) can prevent atelectasis (Moore, Conway, Thomas, et al., 2017; Smetana, 2018).

In patients who do not respond to first-line measures or who cannot perform deep-breathing exercises, other treatments such as **positive end-expiratory pressure** (**PEEP**; a simple mask and one-way valve system that provides varying amounts of expiratory resistance, usually 10 to 15 cm H_2O), continuous positive airway breathing, or bronchoscopy may be used. Before initiating more complex, costly, and labor-intensive therapies, the nurse should ask several questions:

- Has the patient been given an adequate trial of deep-breathing exercises?

- Has the patient received adequate education, supervision, and coaching to carry out the deep-breathing exercises?
- Have other factors been evaluated that may impair ventilation or prevent a good patient effort (e.g., lack of turning, mobilization; excessive pain; excessive sedation)?

If the cause of atelectasis is bronchial obstruction from secretions, the secretions must be removed by coughing or suctioning to allow air to reenter that portion of the lung. CPT and postural drainage may also be used to mobilize secretions. SVN treatments with a bronchodilator may be used to assist patients in the expectoration of secretions. If respiratory care measures fail to remove the obstruction, a bronchoscopy is performed. Although bronchoscopy is an excellent measure to acutely remove secretions and increase ventilation, it is imperative for the nurse to assist the patient with maintaining the patency of the airways after bronchoscopy, using the traditional techniques of deep breathing, coughing, and suctioning. Severe or massive atelectasis may lead to acute respiratory failure, especially in patients with underlying lung disease. Endotracheal (ET) intubation and mechanical ventilation may be necessary.

If the cause of atelectasis is compression of lung tissue, the goal is to decrease the compression. With a large pleural effusion that is compressing lung tissue and causing alveolar collapse, treatment may include **thoracentesis** (removal of the fluid by needle aspiration) or insertion of a chest tube. The measures to increase lung expansion described previously also are used.

Management of chronic atelectasis focuses on removing the cause of the obstruction of the airways or the compression of the lung tissue. For example, bronchoscopy may be used to open an airway obstructed by lung cancer or a nonmalignant lesion, and the procedure may involve cryotherapy or laser therapy. If the atelectasis is a result of obstruction caused by lung cancer, an airway stent or radiation therapy to shrink a tumor may be used to open the airways and provide ventilation to the collapsed area. However, reopening the airways and reaerating the area of the lung may not be possible in patients who have experienced chronic, long-term collapse. In some cases, surgical management may be indicated.

Acute Tracheobronchitis

Acute tracheobronchitis, an acute inflammation of the mucous membranes of the trachea and the bronchial tree, often follows infection of the upper respiratory tract usually as a result of a viral infection (see Chapter 18). Patients with viral infections have decreased resistance and can readily develop a secondary bacterial infection. Adequate treatment of upper respiratory tract infection is one of the major factors in the prevention of acute tracheobronchitis.

Pathophysiology

In acute tracheobronchitis, the inflamed mucosa of the bronchi produces mucopurulent sputum, often in response to infection by *Streptococcus pneumoniae*, *Haemophilus influenzae*, or *Mycoplasma pneumoniae*. A fungal infection (e.g., *Aspergillus*) may also cause tracheobronchitis. A sputum culture is essential to identify the specific causative organism.

In addition to infection, inhalation of physical and chemical irritants, gases, or other air contaminants can also cause acute bronchial irritation (File, 2019a).

Clinical Manifestations

Initially, the patient has a dry, irritating cough and expectorates a scanty amount of mucoid sputum. The patient may report sternal soreness from coughing and have fever or chills, night sweats, headache, and general malaise. As the infection progresses, the patient may be short of breath, have noisy inspiration and expiration (inspiratory stridor and expiratory wheeze), and produce **purulent** (pus-filled) sputum. In severe tracheobronchitis, blood-streaked secretions may be expectorated as a result of the irritation of the mucosa of the airways.

Medical Management

Antibiotic treatment for an infection may be indicated depending on the symptoms, sputum purulence, and results of the sputum culture and sensitivity. Antihistamines usually are not prescribed, because they can cause excessive drying and make secretions more difficult to expectorate. Fluid intake is increased to thin viscous and tenacious secretions. Copious, purulent secretions that cannot be cleared by coughing place patients at risk for increasing airway obstruction and the development of more severe lower respiratory tract infections, such as pneumonia. Suctioning and bronchoscopy may be needed to remove secretions. Rarely, ET intubation may be necessary in cases of acute tracheobronchitis leading to acute respiratory failure, such as in patients who are severely debilitated or who have coexisting diseases that impair the respiratory system.

In most cases, treatment of tracheobronchitis is largely symptomatic. Increasing the vapor pressure (moisture content) in the air reduces airway irritation. Cool vapor therapy or steam inhalations may help relieve laryngeal and tracheal irritation. Moist heat to the chest may relieve the soreness and pain, and mild analgesics may be prescribed.

Nursing Management

Acute tracheobronchitis is usually treated in the home setting. A primary nursing function is to encourage bronchial hygiene, such as increased fluid intake and directed coughing to remove secretions. The nurse encourages and assists the patient to sit up frequently to cough effectively and to prevent retention of mucopurulent sputum. If the patient is taking antibiotics for an underlying bacterial infection, the need to complete the full course of antibiotics prescribed is emphasized. Fatigue is a consequence of tracheobronchitis; therefore, the nurse cautions the patient against overexertion, which can induce a relapse or exacerbation of the infection. The patient is advised to rest (File, 2019a).

Pneumonia

Pneumonia is an inflammation of the lung parenchyma caused by various microorganisms, including bacteria, mycobacteria, fungi, and viruses. *Pneumonitis* is a more general term that describes an inflammatory process in the lung tissue that may predispose or place the patient at risk for microbial invasion.

Chart 19-4

Classifications and Definitions of Pneumonias

- *Community-acquired pneumonia (CAP):* Pneumonia occurring in the community or ≤48 hours after hospital admission or institutionalization of patients who do not meet the criteria for health care–associated pneumonia (HCAP)
- *Health care–associated pneumonia (HCAP):* Pneumonia occurring in a nonhospitalized patient with extensive health care contact with one or more of the following:
  - Hospitalization for ≥2 days in an acute care facility within 90 days of infection
  - Residence in a nursing home or long-term care facility
  - Antibiotic therapy, chemotherapy, or wound care within 30 days of current infection
  - Hemodialysis treatment at a hospital or clinic
  - Home infusion therapy or home wound care
  - Family member with infection due to multidrug-resistant bacteria
- *Hospital-acquired pneumonia (HAP):* Pneumonia occurring ≥48 hours after hospital admission that did not appear to be incubating at the time of admission
- *Ventilator-associated pneumonia (VAP):* A type of HAP that develops ≥48 hours after endotracheal tube intubation

Adapted from Klompas, M., File, T. M., & Bond, S. (2019). Treatment of hospital-acquired, ventilator-associated and health-care-associated pneumonia in adults. *UpToDate.* Retrieved on 8/22/2019 at: www.uptodate.com/contents/treatment-of-hospital-acquired-ventilator-associated-and-healthcare-associated-pneumonia-in-adults

---

Pneumonia and influenza are the most common causes of death from infectious diseases in the United States. Pneumonia and influenza accounted for 55,672 deaths in the United States in 2017 (Centers for Disease Control and Prevention [CDC], 2017a). Together, these diseases were the eighth leading cause of death in the United States in 2017, accounting for 5.9% of all deaths (CDC, 2017a).

Classification

Pneumonia can be classified into four types: community-acquired pneumonia (CAP), health care–associated pneumonia (HCAP), hospital-acquired pneumonia (HAP), and ventilator-associated pneumonia (VAP) (American Thoracic Society & Infectious Diseases Society of America, 2005; Klompas, 2019a). HCAP was conceived as a specific category in order to identify patients at increased risk for multidrug-resistant organisms (MDRO) versus community-acquired organisms (Klompas, 2019a). Chart 19-4 describes the different classifications and definitions of pneumonias. Other subcategories of HCAPs are those in the immunocompromised host and aspiration pneumonia. There is overlap in how specific pneumonias are classified, because they may occur in differing settings. Risk factors associated for specific pathogens are shown in Chart 19-5.

Community-Acquired Pneumonia

CAP, a common infectious disease, occurs either in the community setting or within the first 48 hours after hospitalization or institutionalization. The need for hospitalization for CAP depends on the severity of the pneumonia. The causative pathogens for CAP by site of care are shown in

Chart 19-5 ⚠ RISK FACTORS
Pneumonia Based upon Pathogen Type

Risk Factors for Infection with Penicillin-Resistant and Drug-Resistant Pneumococci

- Age >65 years
- Alcoholism
- Beta-lactam therapy (e.g., cephalosporins) in past 3 months
- Immunosuppressive disorders
- Multiple medical comorbidities
- Exposure to a child in a day care facility

Risk Factors for Infection with Enteric Gram-Negative Bacteria

- Residency in a long-term care facility
- Underlying cardiopulmonary disease
- Multiple medical comorbidities
- Recent antibiotic therapy

Risk Factors for Infection with *Pseudomonas aeruginosa*

- Structural lung disease (e.g., bronchiectasis)
- Corticosteroid therapy
- Broad-spectrum antibiotic therapy (>7 days in the past month)
- Malnutrition

Adapted from Ramirez, J. A. (2019). Overview of community acquired pneumonia in adults. *UpToDate*. Retrieved on 9/23/2019 at: www.uptodate.com/contents/overview-of-community-acquired-pneumonia-in-adults

Table 19-1. The specific etiologic pathogen is identified in about 50% of cases. The rate of CAP increases with age, with 2000 per 100,000 adults 65 years of age and older hospitalized with CAP each year (Ramirez, 2019).

S. pneumoniae (pneumococcus) is the most common bacterial cause of CAP in people younger than 60 years without comorbidity and in those 60 years and older with comorbidity (Baer, 2019; Ramirez, 2019). *S. pneumoniae*, a gram-positive organism that resides naturally in the upper respiratory tract, colonizes the upper respiratory tract and can cause disseminated invasive infections, pneumonia and other lower respiratory tract infections, and upper respiratory tract infections such as otitis media and rhinosinusitis. It may occur as a lobar or bronchopneumonic form in patients of any age and may follow a recent respiratory illness.

H. influenzae causes a type of CAP that frequently affects older adults and those with comorbid illnesses (e.g., chronic obstructive pulmonary disease [COPD], alcoholism, diabetes). The presentation is indistinguishable from that of other forms of bacterial CAP and may be subacute, with cough or low-grade fever for weeks before diagnosis.

Mycoplasma pneumonia is caused by *M. pneumoniae*. Mycoplasma pneumonia is spread by infected respiratory droplets through person-to-person contact. Patients can be tested for mycoplasma antibodies. The inflammatory infiltrate is primarily interstitial rather than alveolar. It spreads throughout the entire respiratory tract, including the bronchioles, and has the characteristics of a bronchopneumonia. Earache and bullous myringitis are common. Impaired ventilation and diffusion may occur.

Viruses are the most common cause of pneumonia in infants and children. Until the advent of the coronavirus disease 2019 (COVID-19) pandemic, viruses were relatively uncommon causes of CAP in adults (see later discussion). Pre-COVID-19, cytomegalovirus was the most commonly implicated viral pathogen in adults with compromised immune systems, followed by herpes simplex virus, adenovirus, and respiratory syncytial virus. The acute stage of a viral respiratory infection occurs within the ciliated cells of the airways, followed by infiltration of the tracheobronchial tree. With pneumonia, the inflammatory process extends into the alveolar area, resulting in edema and exudation. The clinical signs and symptoms of a viral pneumonia are often difficult to distinguish from those of a bacterial pneumonia.

Health Care–Associated Pneumonia

An important distinction of HCAP is that the causative pathogens are often MDROs because of prior contact with a health care environment. Consequently, identifying this type of pneumonia in areas such as the emergency department is crucial. Because HCAP is often difficult to treat, initial antibiotic treatment must not be delayed. Initial antibiotic treatment of HCAP is often different from that for CAP due to the possibility of MDROs (Ramirez, 2019).

Hospital-Acquired Pneumonia

HAP develops 48 hours or more after hospitalization and does not appear to be incubating at the time of admission. VAP can be considered a subtype of HAP, as the only differentiating factor is the presence of an ET tube (see later discussion of VAP). Certain factors may predispose patients to HAP because of impaired host defenses (e.g., severe acute or chronic illness), a variety of comorbid conditions, supine positioning and aspiration, coma, malnutrition, prolonged hospitalization, hypotension, metabolic disorders. Hospitalized patients are also exposed to potential bacteria from other sources (e.g., respiratory therapy devices and equipment, transmission of pathogens by the hands of health care personnel). Numerous intervention-related factors also may play a role in the development of HAP (e.g., therapeutic agents leading to central nervous system depression with decreased ventilation, impaired removal of secretions, or potential

TABLE 19-1	Community-Acquired Pneumonia Microbial Causes by Site of Care[a]		
		Hospitalized Patients	
Outpatients	Non-ICU	ICU	
Streptococcus pneumoniae	*S. pneumoniae*	*S. pneumoniae*	
Mycoplasma pneumoniae	*M. pneumoniae*	*Staphylococcus aureus*	
Haemophilus influenzae	*Chlamydophila pneumoniae*	*Legionella*	
C. pneumoniae	*H. influenzae*	Gram-negative bacilli	
Respiratory viruses	*Legionella*	*H. influenzae*	

ICU, intensive care unit.
[a]Listed in descending order of frequency at each site.
Adapted from Klompas, M. (2019b). Treatment of hospital-acquired and ventilator-associated pneumonia in adults. *UpToDate*. Last updated: July 10, 2019. Retrieved on 9/23/2019 at: www.uptodate.com/contents/treatment-of-hospital-acquired-and-ventilator-associated-pneumonia-in-adults/print

aspiration; prolonged or complicated thoracoabdominal procedures, which may impair mucociliary function and cellular host defenses; ET intubation [VAP]; prolonged or inappropriate use of antibiotics; the use of nasogastric tubes). In addition, patients with compromised immune systems are at particular risk. HAP is associated with a high mortality rate, in part because of the virulence of the organisms, the resistance to antibiotics, and the patient's underlying disorder. It is the most common cause of death among all patients with hospital-acquired infections, with mortality rates up to 33% (Cunha, 2018; Klompas, 2019a).

The common organisms responsible for HAP include the *Enterobacter* species, *Escherichia coli, H. influenzae, Klebsiella pneumoniae, Pseudomonas aeruginosa, Acinetobacter* species, methicillin-sensitive or methicillin-resistant *Staphylococcus aureus* (MRSA), and *S. pneumoniae*. Most patients with HAP are colonized by multiple organisms. Pseudomonal pneumonia occurs in patients who are debilitated, those with altered mental status, and those with prolonged intubation or with tracheostomy. Staphylococcal pneumonia can occur through inhalation of the organism or spread through the hematogenous route. It is often accompanied by sepsis and positive blood cultures. Its mortality rate is high. Specific strains of staphylococci are resistant to many available antimicrobial agents; notable exceptions include vancomycin and linezolid (Klompas, 2019b). Overuse and misuse of antimicrobial agents are major risk factors for the emergence of these resistant pathogens. Because MRSA is highly virulent, steps must be taken to prevent its spread. Patients with MRSA are isolated in a private room, and contact precautions (gown, gloves, and antibacterial soap or alcohol-based hand rub) are used. The number of people in contact with affected patients is minimized, and appropriate precautions must be taken when transporting these patients within or between facilities.

The usual presentation of HAP is a new pulmonary infiltrate on chest x-ray combined with evidence of infection such as fever, respiratory symptoms, purulent sputum, or leukocytosis. Pneumonias from *Klebsiella* or other gram-negative organisms are characterized by the destruction of lung structure and alveolar walls, **consolidation** (tissue that solidifies as a result of collapsed alveoli or infectious process such as pneumonia), and sepsis. Older adult patients and those with alcoholism, chronic lung disease, or diabetes are at increased risk (Klompas, 2019a). Development of a cough or increased cough and sputum production are common presentations, along with low-grade fever and general malaise. In patients who are debilitated or dehydrated, sputum production may be minimal or absent. Pleural effusion, high fever, and tachycardia are common.

Ventilator-Associated Pneumonia

As noted previously, VAP can be thought of as a subtype of HAP; however, in such cases, the patient has been endotracheally intubated and has received mechanical ventilatory support for at least 48 hours (see later discussions on ET intubation and mechanical ventilation). VAP is a complication in as many as 27% of patient who require mechanical ventilation (Gamache, 2019). The incidence of VAP increases with the duration of mechanical ventilation and

---

> **Chart 19-6**
>
> ### Collaborative Practice Interventions to Prevent Ventilator-Associated Pneumonia
>
> Current best practices can include the implementation of specific evidence-based bundle interventions that, when used together (i.e., as a "bundle"), improve patient outcomes. This chart outlines specific parameters for the ventilator-bundled collaborative interventions that have been found to reduce ventilator-associated pneumonia (VAP).
>
> *What are the five key elements of the VAP bundle?*
>
> - Elevation of the head of the bed (30° to 45°)
> - Daily "sedation vacations" and assessment of readiness to extubate (see below)
> - Peptic ulcer disease prophylaxis
> - Deep venous thrombosis (DVT) prophylaxis (see below)
> - Daily oral care with chlorhexidine (0.12% oral rinses)
>
> *What is meant by daily "sedation vacations," and how does this tie into assessing readiness to extubate?*
>
> - Protocols should be developed so that sedative doses are purposely decreased at a time of the day when it is possible to assess the patient's neurologic readiness for extubation.
> - Vigilance must be employed during the time that sedative doses are lower to ensure that the patient does not self-extubate.
>
> *What effect does DVT prophylaxis have on preventing VAP?*
>
> - The exact relationship is unclear. However, when appropriate, evidence-based methods to ensure DVT prophylaxis are applied (see Chapter 26); then the rates of VAP also drop.
>
> Adapted from Institute for Healthcare Improvement. (2012). How-to guide: Prevent ventilator-associated pneumonia. Cambridge, MA: Institute for Healthcare Improvements. Retrieved on 3/6/2020 at: www.ihi.org/resources/Pages/Tools/HowtoGuidePreventVAP.aspx

the mortality rate is variable, depending upon the complexity of the underlying illness. The etiologic bacteriologic agents associated with VAP typically differ based on the timing of the occurrence of the infection relative to the start of mechanical ventilation. VAP occurring within 96 hours of the onset of mechanical ventilation is usually due to antibiotic-sensitive bacteria that colonize the patient prior to hospital admission, whereas VAP developing after 96 hours of ventilatory support is more often associated with MDROs. Prevention remains the key to reducing the burden of VAP (Klompas, File, & Bond, 2019; Timsit, Esaied, Neuville, et al., 2017). See Chart 19-6 for an overview of bundled interventions aimed at preventing VAP.

Pneumonia in the Immunocompromised Host

Due to advances in immunosuppressive therapy, prevalence of MDROs, and improvements in diagnostic studies, there is an increased incidence of pneumonia in patients who are immunocompromised. Common causative organisms include *Pneumocystis* pneumonia (PCP), fungal pneumonias, and *Mycobacterium tuberculosis*. The organism that causes PCP is now known as *Pneumocystis jiroveci* instead of *Pneumocystis carinii*. The acronym PCP still applies because it can be read "**P**neumo**c**ystis **p**neumonia."

Pneumonia in the immunocompromised host can occur with the use of corticosteroids or other immunosuppressive agents, chemotherapy, nutritional depletion, the use of broad-spectrum antimicrobial agents, acquired immune deficiency syndrome (AIDS), genetic immune disorders, and long-term advanced life support technology (mechanical ventilation). It is seen with increasing frequency because affected patients constitute a growing portion of the population; however, pneumonias that typically occur in people who are immunocompromised may also occur in those who are immunocompetent. Pneumonia carries a higher morbidity and mortality rate in patients who are immunocompromised than in those who are immunocompetent (Zhao & Shin, 2019). Patients with compromised immune systems commonly develop pneumonia from organisms of low virulence. In addition, increasing numbers of patients with impaired defenses develop HAP from gram-negative bacilli (*Klebsiella, Pseudomonas, E. coli,* Enterobacteriaceae, *Proteus, Serratia*) (Zhao & Shin, 2019).

Whether patients are immunocompromised or immunocompetent, the clinical presentation of pneumonia is similar. PCP has a subtle onset, with progressive dyspnea, fever, and a nonproductive cough.

Aspiration Pneumonia

Aspiration pneumonia refers to the pulmonary consequences resulting from entry of endogenous or exogenous substances into the lower airway. The most common form of aspiration pneumonia is bacterial infection from aspiration of bacteria that normally reside in the upper airways. Aspiration pneumonia may occur in the community or hospital setting. Common pathogens are anaerobes, *S. aureus, Streptococcus* species, and gram-negative bacilli (Bartlett, 2019a). Substances other than bacteria may be aspirated into the lung, such as gastric contents, exogenous chemical contents, or irritating gases. This type of aspiration or ingestion may impair the lung defenses, cause inflammatory changes, and lead to bacterial growth and a resulting pneumonia (see later discussion of aspiration).

Pathophysiology

Normally, the upper airway prevents potentially infectious particles from reaching the sterile lower respiratory tract. Pneumonia arises from normal flora present in patients whose resistance has been altered or from aspiration of flora present in the oropharynx; patients often have an acute or chronic underlying disease that impairs host defenses. Pneumonia may also result from bloodborne organisms that enter the pulmonary circulation and are trapped in the pulmonary capillary bed.

Pneumonia affects both ventilation and diffusion. An inflammatory reaction can occur in the alveoli, producing an exudate that interferes with the diffusion of oxygen and carbon dioxide. White blood cells, mostly neutrophils, also migrate into the alveoli and fill the normally air-filled spaces. Areas of the lung are not adequately ventilated because of secretions and mucosal edema that cause partial occlusion of the bronchi or alveoli, with a resultant decrease in alveolar oxygen tension. Bronchospasm may also occur in patients with reactive airway disease. Because of hypoventilation, a **ventilation–perfusion** ($\dot{V}/\dot{Q}$) mismatch occurs in the affected area of the lung. $\dot{V}/\dot{Q}$ refers to the ratio between ventilation and perfusion in the lung,

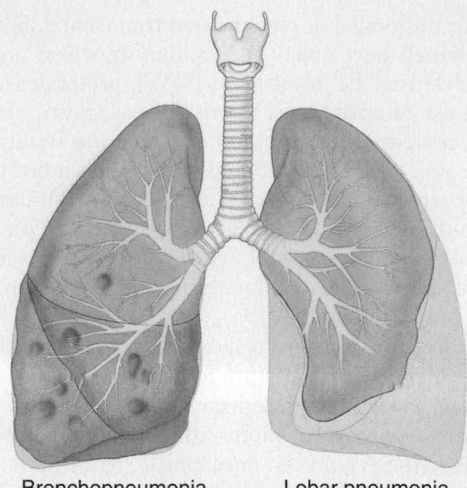

Bronchopneumonia   Lobar pneumonia

Figure 19-2 • Distribution of lung involvement in bronchial and lobar pneumonia. In bronchopneumonia (*left*), patchy areas of consolidation occur. In lobar pneumonia (*right*), an entire lobe is consolidated.

which is normally approximately 4 to 5, or 0.8; matching of ventilation to perfusion optimizes gas exchange. Venous blood entering the pulmonary circulation passes through the underventilated area and travels to the left side of the heart poorly oxygenated. The mixing of oxygenated and unoxygenated or poorly oxygenated blood eventually results in arterial hypoxemia.

If a substantial portion of one or more lobes is involved, the disease is referred to as lobar pneumonia. The term *bronchopneumonia* is used to describe pneumonia that is distributed in a patchy fashion, having originated in one or more localized areas within the bronchi and extending to the adjacent surrounding lung parenchyma. Bronchopneumonia is more common than lobar pneumonia (see Fig. 19-2).

Risk Factors

Being knowledgeable about the factors and circumstances that commonly predispose people to pneumonia helps identify patients at high risk for the disease (Bartlett, 2019a). Table 19-2 describes risk factors for pneumonia; additional risk factors are travel or exposure to certain environments and residence in a long-term care facility. Increasing numbers of patients who have compromised defenses against infections are susceptible to pneumonia. Some types of pneumonia, such as those caused by viral infections, occur in previously healthy people, often after a viral illness.

Pneumonia occurs in patients with certain underlying disorders such as heart failure, diabetes, alcoholism, COPD, and AIDS (Klompas, 2019a). Certain diseases also have been associated with specific pathogens. For example, staphylococcal pneumonia has been noted after epidemics of influenza, and patients with COPD are at increased risk for development of pneumonia caused by pneumococci or *H. influenzae*. In addition, cystic fibrosis is associated with respiratory infection caused by pseudomonal and staphylococcal organisms, and PCP has been associated with AIDS. Pneumonias occurring in hospitalized patients often involve organisms not usually found in CAP, including enteric gram-negative bacilli and *S. aureus*.

TABLE 19-2 Risk Factors and Preventive Measures for Pneumonia	
Risk Factor	**Preventive Measure**
Conditions that produce mucus or bronchial obstruction and interfere with normal lung drainage (e.g., cancer, cigarette smoking, chronic obstructive pulmonary disease)	Promote coughing and expectoration of secretions. Encourage smoking cessation
Patients who are immunosuppressed or neutropenic (low neutrophil count)	Initiate special precautions against infection
Smoking (cigarette smoke disrupts both mucociliary and macrophage activity)	Encourage smoking cessation
Prolonged immobility and shallow breathing pattern	Reposition frequently and promote lung expansion exercises and coughing. Initiate suctioning and chest physical therapy if indicated
Depressed cough reflex (due to medications, a debilitated state, or weak respiratory muscles); aspiration of foreign material into the lungs during a period of unconsciousness (head injury, anesthesia, depressed level of consciousness), or abnormal swallowing mechanism	Reposition frequently to prevent aspiration and administer medications judiciously, particularly those that increase risk for aspiration. Perform suctioning and chest physical therapy if indicated
Nothing-by-mouth (NPO) status; placement of nasogastric, orogastric, or endotracheal tube	Promote frequent oral hygiene. Minimize risk for aspiration by checking placement of tube and proper positioning of patient
Supine positioning in patients unable to protect their airway	Elevate head of bed at least 30 degrees
Antibiotic therapy (in people who are very ill, the oropharynx is likely to be colonized by gram-negative bacteria)	Monitor patients receiving antibiotic therapy for signs and symptoms of pneumonia
Alcohol intoxication (because alcohol suppresses the body's reflexes, may be associated with aspiration, and decreases white cell mobilization and tracheobronchial ciliary motion)	Encourage reduced or moderate alcohol intake (in case of alcohol stupor, position patient to prevent aspiration)
General anesthetic, sedative, or opioid preparations that promote respiratory depression, which causes a shallow breathing pattern and predisposes to the pooling of bronchial secretions and potential development of pneumonia	Observe the respiratory rate and depth during recovery from general anesthesia and before giving medications. If respiratory depression is apparent, withhold the medication and contact the primary provider
Advanced age, because of possible depressed cough and glottic reflexes and nutritional depletion	Promote frequent turning, early ambulation and mobilization, effective coughing, breathing exercises, and nutritious diet
Respiratory therapy with improperly cleaned equipment	Make sure that respiratory equipment is cleaned properly; participate in continuous quality improvement monitoring with the respiratory care department
Transmission of organisms from health care providers	Use strict hand hygiene and gloves. Implement health care provider education

Adapted from Ramirez, J. A. (2019). Overview of community acquired pneumonia in adults. *UpToDate*. Retrieved on 9/23/2019 at: www.uptodate.com/contents/overview-of-community-acquired-pneumonia-in-adults

Clinical Manifestations

Pneumonia varies in its signs and symptoms depending on the type, causal organism, and presence of underlying disease. However, it is not possible to diagnose a specific form or classification of pneumonia by clinical manifestations alone. The patient with streptococcal (pneumococcal) pneumonia usually has a sudden onset of chills, rapidly rising fever (38.5° to 40.5°C [101° to 105°F]), and pleuritic chest pain that is aggravated by deep breathing and coughing. The patient is severely ill, with marked tachypnea (25 to 45 breaths/min), accompanied by other signs of respiratory distress (e.g., shortness of breath and the use of accessory muscles in respiration) (Weinberger, Cockrill, & Mandel, 2019). A relative bradycardia (a pulse–temperature deficit in which the pulse is slower than that expected for a given temperature) may suggest viral infection, mycoplasma infection, or infection with a *Legionella* organism.

Some patients exhibit an upper respiratory tract infection (nasal congestion, sore throat), and the onset of symptoms of pneumonia is gradual and nonspecific. The predominant symptoms may be headache, low-grade fever, pleuritic pain, myalgia, rash, and pharyngitis. After a few days, mucoid or mucopurulent sputum is expectorated. In severe pneumonia, the cheeks are flushed and the lips and nail beds demonstrate central cyanosis (a late sign of hypoxemia).

The patient may exhibit **orthopnea** (shortness of breath when reclining or in the supine position), preferring to be propped up or sitting in bed leaning forward (orthopneic position) in an effort to achieve adequate gas exchange without coughing or breathing deeply. Appetite is poor, and the patient is diaphoretic and tires easily. Sputum is often purulent; however, this is not a reliable indicator of the etiologic agent. Rusty, blood-tinged sputum may be expectorated with streptococcal (pneumococcal), staphylococcal, and *Klebsiella* pneumonia.

Signs and symptoms of pneumonia may also depend on a patient's underlying condition. Different signs occur in patients with conditions such as cancer, and in those who are undergoing treatment with immunosuppressant medications, which decrease the resistance to infection. Such patients have fever, crackles, and physical findings that indicate consolidation of lung tissue, including increased tactile fremitus (vocal vibration detected on palpation), percussion dullness, bronchial breath sounds, egophony (when auscultated, the spoken "E" becomes a loud, nasal-sounding "A"), and whispered pectoriloquy (whispered sounds are easily auscultated through the chest wall). These changes occur because sound is transmitted better through solid or dense tissue (consolidation) than through normal air-filled tissue; these sounds are described in Chapter 17.

Purulent sputum or slight changes in respiratory symptoms may be the only sign of pneumonia in patients with COPD. Determining whether an increase in symptoms is an exacerbation of the underlying disease process or an additional infectious process may be difficult.

Assessment and Diagnostic Findings

The diagnosis of pneumonia is made by history (particularly of a recent respiratory tract infection), physical examination, chest x-ray, blood culture (bloodstream invasion [bacteremia] occurs frequently), and sputum examination. The sputum sample is obtained by having patients rinse the mouth with water to minimize contamination by normal oral flora, breathe deeply several times, cough deeply, and expectorate the raised sputum into a sterile container.

More invasive procedures may be used to collect specimens. Sputum may be obtained by nasotracheal or orotracheal suctioning with a sputum trap or by fiberoptic bronchoscopy (see Chapter 17). Bronchoscopy is often used in patients with acute severe infection, in patients with chronic or refractory infection, in patients with compromised immune systems when a diagnosis cannot be made from an expectorated or induced specimen, and in patients who are mechanically ventilated. Bronchoscopic techniques may include a protected brush specimen or bronchoalveolar lavage.

Unfolding Patient Stories: Kenneth Bronson • Part 1

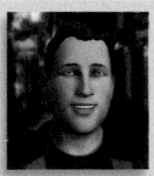

Kenneth Bronson, a 27-year-old man, has a history of fatigue, high fever, and a productive cough for a week and arrives in the emergency department with difficulty breathing. A chest x-ray reveals a right lower lobe pneumonia. What are the clinical manifestations and assessment findings associated with a right lower lobe pneumonia that the nurse should investigate when evaluating the patient? (Kenneth Bronson's story continues in Chapter 22.)

Care for Kenneth and other patients in a realistic virtual environment: *vSim for Nursing* (**thepoint.lww.com/vSimMedicalSurgical**). Practice documenting these patients' care in DocuCare (**thepoint.lww.com/DocuCareEHR**).

Prevention

Pneumococcal vaccination reduces the incidence of pneumonia, hospitalizations for cardiac conditions, and deaths in the older adult population. There are two types of pneumococcal vaccine recommended for adults: a pneumococcal conjugate vaccine (PCV13) and a pneumococcal polysaccharide vaccine (PPSV23) (CDC, 2017c).

PCV13 protects against 13 types of pneumococcal bacteria. PCV13 is recommended for all adults 65 years of age or older as well as adults 19 years or older with conditions that weaken the immune system, such as HIV infection, organ transplantation, leukemia, lymphoma, chronic kidney disease, and asplenism, or with cerebrospinal fluid leak or with cochlear implants (CDC, 2017b). PPSV23 is a newer vaccine and protects against 23 types of pneumococcal bacteria. It is recommended for all adults 65 years of age or older and for those adults 19 through 64 years of age who smoke cigarettes or who have chronic heart, lung, or liver disease, or alcoholism (CDC, 2017b). Most patients who have previously received PCV13 should receive PPSV23. In particular, all adults 65 years of age or older who previously received the PCV13 should receive the PPSV23 vaccine. For immunocompetent adults age 65 or older who have not received PCV13, a dose of PCV13 should be given followed by PPSV23 at least 1 year later. These two vaccines should not be co-administered (CDC, 2017b). As pneumococcal vaccination guidelines may change from year to year, it is important to consult the CDC web site for the most current recommendations. Other preventive measures are summarized in Table 19-2.

Medical Management

Medical management of patients with pneumonia includes prescribing appropriate antibiotics for bacterial pneumonias; assisting the patient to get adequate rest and hydration; and managing complications if they occur. In some patients, supplemental oxygenation may be prescribed.

Pharmacologic Therapy

The treatment of pneumonia includes administration of the appropriate antibiotic as determined by the results of a culture and sensitivity. However, the causative organism is not identified in half of CAP cases when therapy is initiated (File, 2019b). Guidelines are used to guide antibiotic choice; however, the resistance patterns, prevalence of causative organisms, patient risk factors, treatment setting (inpatient vs. outpatient), and costs and availability of newer antibiotic agents must all be considered. See Table 19-3 for the treatment of patients with pneumonia due to specific pathogens.

Inpatients should be switched from intravenous (IV) to oral therapy when they are hemodynamically stable, are improving clinically, are able to take medications/fluids by mouth, and have a normally functioning gastrointestinal tract. As soon as patients are clinically stable, have no medical problems, and have a safe environment for continued care, they should be discharged from the hospital. Clinical stability is defined as temperature less than or equal to 37.8°C (100°F), heart rate less than or equal to 100 bpm, respiratory

TABLE 19-3	Commonly Encountered Pneumonias			
Type (Causal Organism)	Epidemiology	Clinical Features	Treatment	Complications/ Comments
Community-Acquired Pneumonia				
Streptococcal pneumonia (*Streptococcus pneumoniae*)	Most prevalent in winter months More frequent occurrence in African Americans Incidence greatest in older adults and in patients with COPD, heart failure, alcoholism, asplenia, diabetes, and after influenza Leading infectious cause of illness worldwide among young children, people with underlying chronic health conditions, and older adults Mortality rate (in hospitalized adults with invasive disease): 14%	Abrupt onset, toxic appearance, pleuritic chest pain; usually involves ≥1 lobes Lobar infiltrate common on chest x-ray or bronchopneumonia pattern	Severity determines type of antibiotic and route (IV vs. oral) PCN sensitive: PCN, amoxicillin, ceftriaxone, cefotaxime, cefprozil or a macrolide PCN resistant: levofloxacin, moxifloxacin, vancomycin, or linezolid	Shock, pleural effusion, superinfections, pericarditis, and otitis media
Haemophilus influenzae (*Haemophilus influenzae*)	Incidence greatest in patients with alcoholism, older adults, patients in long-term care facilities and nursing homes, patients with diabetes or COPD, and children <5 yrs of age Accounts for 5–20% of community-acquired pneumonias Mortality rate: 30%	Frequently insidious onset associated with upper respiratory tract infection 2–6 wks before onset of illness; fever, chills, productive cough; usually involves ≥1 lobes Sepsis is common. Infiltrate, occasional bronchopneumonia pattern on chest x-ray	Severity determines type of antibiotic and route (IV vs. oral) doxycycline, third-generation cephalosporin (ceftriaxone) or a fluoroquinolone	Lung abscess, pleural effusion, meningitis, arthritis, pericarditis, epiglottitis
Legionnaires disease (*Legionella pneumophila*)	Highest occurrence in summer and fall May cause disease sporadically or as part of an epidemic Incidence greatest in middle-aged and older men, people who smoke, patients with chronic diseases, those receiving immunosuppressive therapy, and those in close proximity to excavation sites Accounts for 15% of community-acquired pneumonias Mortality rate: 15–50%	Flulike symptoms; high fevers, mental confusion, headache, pleuritic pain, myalgias, dyspnea, productive cough, hemoptysis, leukocytosis Bronchopneumonia, unilateral or bilateral disease, lobar consolidation	Severity determines type of antibiotic and route (IV vs. oral) Azithromycin, moxifloxacin, or a fluoroquinolone	Hypotension, shock, and acute kidney injury
Mycoplasma pneumoniae (*Mycoplasma pneumoniae*)	Increase in fall and winter Responsible for epidemics of respiratory illness Most common type of atypical pneumonia Accounts for 20% of community-acquired pneumonias; more common in children and young adults Mortality rate: <0.1%	Onset is usually insidious. Patients not usually as ill as in other pneumonias. Sore throat, nasal congestion, ear pain, headache, low-grade fever, pleuritic pain, myalgias, diarrhea, erythematous rash, pharyngitis. Interstitial infiltrates on chest x-ray	Severity determines type of antibiotic and route (IV vs. oral) Macrolides, combination drugs (macrolide plus ampicillin and sulbactam) or tetracyclines (doxycycline)	Aseptic meningitis, meningoencephalitis, transverse myelitis, cranial nerve palsies, pericarditis, myocarditis
Viral pneumonia (influenza viruses types A, B adenovirus, parainfluenza, cytomegalovirus, coronavirus, varicella-zoster)	Incidence greatest in winter months Epidemics occur every 2–3 yrs. Most common causative organisms in adults; other organisms in children (e.g., cytomegalovirus and respiratory syncytial virus) Accounts for 20% of community-acquired pneumonias	Patchy infiltrate, small pleural effusion on chest x-ray In most patients, influenza begins as an acute upper respiratory infection; others have bronchitis, pleurisy, and so on, and still others develop gastrointestinal symptoms	Treated symptomatically; treat in high-risk patients; oseltamivir or zanamivir (+ other agents depending upon dominant strain [type of virus]) Does not respond to treatment with currently available antimicrobials	Superimposed bacterial infection, bronchopneumonia

(continued on page 538)

TABLE 19-3	Commonly Encountered Pneumonias (continued)			
Type (Causal Organism)	Epidemiology	Clinical Features	Treatment	Complications/ Comments
Chlamydial pneumonia (*Chlamydophila pneumoniae*)	Reported mainly in college students, military recruits, and older adults May be a common cause of community-acquired pneumonia or observed in combination with other pathogens Mortality rate is low because the majority of cases are relatively mild. Older adults with coexistent infections, comorbidities, and reinfections may require hospitalization.	Hoarseness, fever, chills, pharyngitis, rhinitis, nonproductive cough, myalgias, arthralgias Single infiltrate on chest x-ray; pleural effusion possible	Macrolide or doxycycline	Reinfection and acute respiratory failure

Hospital-Acquired and Health Care–Associated Pneumonias

Pseudomonas pneumonia (*Pseudomonas aeruginosa*)	Incidence greatest in those with preexisting lung disease, cancer (particularly leukemia); those with homograft transplants, burns; people who are debilitated; and patients receiving antimicrobial therapy and treatments such as tracheostomy, suctioning, and in postoperative settings. Almost always of nosocomial origin Accounts for 15% of hospital-acquired pneumonias Mortality rate: 40–60%	Diffuse consolidation on chest x-ray; toxic appearance: fever, chills, productive cough, relative bradycardia, leukocytosis	Sensitivity tests guide choice and severity determines type of antibiotic and route (IV vs. oral): ceftazidime, ciprofloxacin, cefepime, aztreonam, imipenem/ cilastatin, meropenem, piperacillin, +/– an aminoglycoside	Lung cavitation; has capacity to invade blood vessels, causing hemorrhage and lung infarction; usually requires hospitalization
Staphylococcal pneumonia (*Staphylococcus aureus*)	Incidence greatest in immunocompromised patients, IV drug users, and as a complication of epidemic influenza Commonly nosocomial in origin Accounts for 10–30% of hospital-acquired pneumonias Mortality rate: 25–60% MRSA may also cause community-based infection	Severe hypoxemia, cyanosis, necrotizing infection. Sepsis is common	Severity determines type of antibiotic and route (IV vs. oral) MSSA: oxacillin or nafcillin MRSA or PCN allergy: vancomycin or linezolid	Pleural effusion/ pneumothorax, lung abscess, empyema, meningitis, endocarditis Frequently requires hospitalization. Treatment must be vigorous and prolonged because disease tends to destroy lung tissue
Klebsiella pneumonia (*Klebsiella pneumoniae* [Friedländer's bacillus-encapsulated gram-negative aerobic bacillus])	Incidence greatest in older adults; patients with alcoholism; patients with chronic disease, such as diabetes, heart failure, COPD; patients in chronic care facilities and nursing homes Accounts for 2–5% of community-acquired and 10–30% of hospital-acquired pneumonias Mortality rate: 40–50%	Tissue necrosis occurs rapidly. Toxic appearance: fever, cough, sputum production, bronchopneumonia, lung abscess. Lobar consolidation, bronchopneumonia pattern on chest x-ray	Severity determines type of antibiotic and route (IV vs. oral) Hospital acquired: cefepime, ceftazidime, imipenem, meropenem, or piperacillin/tazobactam plus an aminoglycoside or a fluoroquinolone; Community acquired: a levofloxacin plus ciprofloxacin or nitrofurantoin or nitrofurantoin macrocrystals	Multiple lung abscesses with cyst formation, empyema, pericarditis, pleural effusion; may be fulminating, progressing to fatal outcome

Pneumonia in the Immunocompromised Host

Pneumocystis pneumonia (*Pneumocystis jiroveci*)	Incidence greatest in patients with AIDS and patients receiving immunosuppressive therapy for cancer, organ transplantation, and other disorders Frequently seen with cytomegalovirus infection Mortality rate 15–20% in hospitalized patients and fatal if not treated	Pulmonary infiltrates on chest x-ray; nonproductive cough, fever, dyspnea	Severity determines type of antibiotic and route (IV vs. oral) Trimethoprim/ sulfamethoxazole	Respiratory failure

TABLE 19-3	Commonly Encountered Pneumonias (continued)			
Type (Causal Organism)	Epidemiology	Clinical Features	Treatment	Complications/Comments
Fungal pneumonia (*Aspergillus fumigatus*)	Incidence greatest in patients who are immunocompromised or neutropenic. Mortality rate: 15–20%	Cough, hemoptysis, infiltrates, fungus ball on chest x-ray	Severity determines type of antibiotic and route (IV vs. oral). Voriconazole; for invasive disease: amphotericin B or liposomal amphotericin B or caspofungin. Lobectomy for fungus ball	Dissemination to brain, myocardium, and thyroid gland
Tuberculosis (*Mycobacterium tuberculosis*)	Incidence increased in indigent, immigrant, and prison populations; people with AIDS; and people who are homeless. Mortality rate: <1% (depending on comorbidity)	Weight loss, fever, night sweats, cough, sputum production, hemoptysis, nonspecific infiltrate (lower lobe), hilar node enlargement, pleural effusion on chest x-ray	Isoniazid + rifampin + ethambutol + pyrazinamide (see section on TB and Table 19-4)	Reinfection and acute respiratory infection
Pneumonia from Aspiration				
Anaerobic bacteria (*S. pneumoniae, H. influenzae, S. aureus*)	Risk: reduced consciousness, dysphagia, disorders of upper GI tract; mechanical disruption of glottic closure (endotracheal tube, tracheostomy, nasogastric feeding)	Abrupt onset of dyspnea, low-grade fever, cough, predisposing condition for aspiration	Severity determines type of antibiotic and route (IV vs. oral). Clindamycin +/– a fluoroquinolone	Identification of potential aspirate is important for treatment

AIDS, acquired immune deficiency syndrome; COPD, chronic obstructive pulmonary disease; GI, gastrointestinal; IV, intravenous; MRSA, methicillin resistant *Staphylococcus aureus*; MSSA, methicillin-sensitive *Staphylococcus aureus*; PCN, penicillin; TB, tuberculosis.
Adapted from Gilbert, D. N., Chambers, H. F., Eliopoulos, G. M., et al. (2018). *The Sanford guide to antimicrobial therapy 2018* (48th ed.). Sperryville, VA: Antimicrobial Therapy, Inc.

rate less than or equal to 24 breaths/min, systolic blood pressure greater than or equal to 90 mm Hg, and oxygen saturation greater than or equal to 90%, with ability to maintain oral intake and normal (baseline) mental status.

In suspected HAP, treatment is usually initiated with a broad-spectrum IV antibiotic and may be monotherapy or combination therapy. For patients with no known multidrug resistance, monotherapy with ceftriaxone, ampicillin/sulbactam, levofloxacin, or ertapenem is used. With known multidrug resistance, a three-drug combination therapy may be used; this drug regimen may include an antipseudomonal cephalosporin or ceftazidime or antipseudomonal carbapenem or piperacillin/tazobactam plus antipseudomonal fluoroquinolone or aminoglycoside plus linezolid or vancomycin. The patient's status must be assessed 72 hours after the initiation of therapy, and antibiotics should be discontinued or modified based on the culture results. Of concern is the rampant rise in respiratory pathogens that are resistant to available antibiotics. Examples include vancomycin-resistant enterococcus (VRE), MRSA, and drug-resistant *S. pneumoniae*. Providers tend to prescribe antibiotics aggressively in the presence of suspected infection. Mechanisms to monitor and minimize the inappropriate use of antibiotics are in place. In response to antibiotic resistant organisms, the CDC recommends all acute care hospitals participate in an antibiotic stewardship program (CDC, 2019b). Antibiotic stewardship refers to a set of coordinated strategies to improve the use of antimicrobial medications with the goal of enhancing patient health outcomes, reducing resistance to antibiotics, and decreasing unnecessary costs (CDC, 2019a; Nathwani, Varghese, Stephens, et al., 2019). Education of

clinicians about the use of evidence-based guidelines in the treatment of respiratory infection is important, and some institutions have implemented algorithms to assist clinicians in choosing the appropriate antibiotics. Monitoring and surveillance of susceptibility patterns for pathogens are also important.

Other Therapeutic Regimens

Antibiotics are ineffective in viral upper respiratory tract infections and pneumonias, and their use may be associated with adverse effects. Antibiotics are indicated with a viral respiratory infection *only* if a secondary bacterial pneumonia, bronchitis, or rhinosinusitis is present. With the exception of the use of antimicrobial therapy, treatment of viral pneumonia is generally the same as that for bacterial pneumonia; however, different treatments have been used for the patient who develops pneumonia as a result of infection with the severe acute respiratory syndrome coronavirus 2 (SARS-CoV-2), the virion implicated in COVID-19 (Kim & Gandhi, 2020) (see later discussion).

Treatment of viral pneumonia is primarily supportive. Hydration is a necessary part of therapy, because fever and tachypnea may result in insensible fluid losses. Antipyretic agents may be used to treat headache and fever; antitussive medications may be used for the associated cough. Warm, moist inhalations are helpful in relieving bronchial irritation. Antihistamines may provide benefit with reduced sneezing and rhinorrhea. Nasal decongestants may also be used to treat symptoms and improve sleep; however, excessive use can cause rebound nasal congestion. Bed rest is prescribed until the infection shows signs of clearing. If hospitalized, the patient is observed carefully until the clinical condition improves.

If hypoxemia develops, oxygen is administered. Pulse oximetry or arterial blood gas analysis is used to determine the need for oxygen and to evaluate the effectiveness of the therapy. Arterial blood gases may be used to obtain a baseline measure of the patient's oxygenation and acid–base status; however, pulse oximetry is used to continuously monitor the patient's oxygen saturation and response to therapy. More aggressive respiratory support measures include administration of high concentrations of oxygen (**fraction of inspired oxygen [FiO_2]**, or the concentration of oxygen that is delivered), ET intubation, and mechanical ventilation. Different modes of mechanical ventilation may be required. Modes of mechanical ventilation are discussed later in this chapter.

 ### Gerontologic Considerations

Pneumonia in older adult patients may occur as a primary diagnosis or as a complication of a chronic disease. Pulmonary infections in older adults frequently are difficult to treat and result in a higher mortality rate than in younger people (Ramirez, 2019). General deterioration, weakness, abdominal symptoms, anorexia, confusion, tachycardia, and tachypnea may signal the onset of pneumonia. The diagnosis of pneumonia may be missed because the classic symptoms of cough, chest pain, sputum production, and fever may be absent or masked in older adult patients. In addition, the presence of some signs may be misleading. Abnormal breath sounds, for example, may be caused by microatelectasis that occurs as a result of decreased mobility, decreased lung volumes, or other respiratory function changes. Chest x-rays may be needed to differentiate chronic heart failure, which is often seen in older adults, from pneumonia as the cause of clinical signs and symptoms.

Supportive treatment includes hydration (with caution and with frequent assessment because of the risk of fluid overload in older adults); supplemental oxygen therapy; and assistance with deep breathing, coughing, frequent position changes, and early ambulation. All of these are particularly important in the care of older adult patients with pneumonia. To reduce or prevent serious complications of pneumonia in older adults, vaccination against pneumococcal and influenza infections is recommended.

 ### COVID-19 Considerations

SARS-CoV-2 is a community-acquired coronavirus whose primary pathologic evolution occurs within the respiratory system. Viral transmission is presumed to occur through direct person-to-person contact via respiratory droplets, although it is hypothesized that fomite transmission (i.e., transmission from inanimate surfaces that carry the virus) might be possible (Cascella, Rajnik, Cuomo, et al., 2020; Kim & Gandhi, 2020). SARS-CoV-2 enters host cells through ACE2 cellular surface receptors where it replicates; these ACE2 receptors are particularly abundant in type II alveolar and vascular endothelial cells within the pulmonary vascular circuit (see Chapter 27, Fig. 27-2 for an illustration of viral transmission and replication; see Chapter 66 for a discussion of risks of SAR-CoV-2).

At the time of this writing, although it is believed that some patients infected with SARS-CoV-2 may remain asymptomatic, others exhibit signs and symptoms consistent with a type of viral upper respiratory tract infection that may lead to viral pneumonia. Clinical manifestations consistent with mild COVID-19 may include fever, nonproductive cough, sore throat, fatigue, myalgias (muscle aches), nasal congestion, nausea, vomiting, diarrhea, anosmia (loss of smell), and ageusia (loss of taste) (Cascella et al., 2020; CDC, 2020). Data derived from epidemiologic studies in China, where the COVID-19 pandemic originated, suggest that approximately 81% of patients with COVID-19 have mild illness, with either mild viral pneumonia or no pneumonia (Wu & McGoogan, 2020).

Ideally, the diagnosis of COVID-19 is confirmed by patient self-administered bilateral nasal swabbing for viral antigen or nucleic acid. Self-swabbing minimizes risk of person-to-person transmission of respiratory droplets. The act of patient self-swabbing ideally should be observed by a health care provider to assure it is performed properly (CDC, 2020).

Most patients with known or suspected mild COVID-19 may be managed on an outpatient basis within their homes, which conserves hospital resources and diminishes likelihood of exposure to others, including health care workers (Kim & Gandhi, 2020). At the present time, no specific medications are prescribed to either treat COVID-19 or mitigate its effects in patients with mild disease who are managed at home. The therapeutic regimens that patients with mild COVID-19 are advised to follow mirror those for other viral respiratory illnesses. Patients are advised to rest, hydrate, take antipyretic agents (e.g., acetaminophen) and monitor their symptoms. However, given the virulence of SARS-CoV-2, these patients must be capable of maintaining self-quarantine/isolation at home until all of the following criteria are met (CDC, 2020):

- At least 72 hours have transpired since the patient had a fever and the patient has not taken any antipyretic agents during that timeframe;
- The patient reports an improvement in any respiratory manifestations of COVID-19; and
- At least 10 days have elapsed since the patient first noted clinical manifestations suggestive of COVID-19.

Clinicians and others in contact with patients with suspected or known COVID-19 should observe infection control and prevention measures and utilize appropriate personal protective equipment (PPE; CDC, 2020) (see Chapter 66 for further discussion).

Patients with moderate COVID-19 should be hospitalized so that they may be closely observed on an ongoing basis, because many of these patients may rapidly deteriorate to severe COVID-19 and respiratory failure. These patients have clear evidence of viral pneumonia that may be diagnosed based upon clinical examination, chest x-ray or CT scan findings but have SpO_2 levels >93% on room air, suggesting adequate oxygenation (Cascella et al., 2020; National Institutes of Health COVID-19 Treatment Guidelines Panel [NIH], 2020). These patients may or may not have dyspnea. Laboratory tests upon admission include a CBC with differential, a complete metabolic panel, creatine kinase (CK), lactate dehydrogenase (LDH), C-reactive protein (CRP), ferritin, and D-dimer. Notable findings may include leukopenia (low white blood cell count), lymphopenia (low lymphocyte count), and elevated CK, LDH, CRP, ferritin, and D-dimer levels (Cascella et al., 2020).

It appears at the present time that few patients with COVID-19 have a superinfection with bacterial pathogens (i.e., concomitant bacterial pneumonia); therefore, antibiotic agents are not routinely prescribed for the patient hospitalized to manage moderate COVID-19 pneumonia. However, if it is believed that the patient has a bacterial pneumonia or sepsis, then antibiotic agents indicated to treat CAP are prescribed (Kim & Gandhi, 2020; NIH, 2020) (see previous discussion). Most patients are prescribed anticoagulant agents as prophylaxis, as they have a higher risk of venous thromboembolism (VTE) (see Chapter 26 for further discussion of VTE). The typical agents prescribed are low-molecular-weight heparins (e.g., enoxaparin, dalteparin), administered twice daily (Kim & Gandhi, 2020).

Currently, there is insufficient evidence to support prescribing any antiviral or immunomodulating agents to manage patients with moderate COVID-19 pneumonia (NIH, 2020). If a patient must be prescribed an inhaled medication (e.g., to manage a preexisting chronic respiratory disease), then to the extent possible, that medication should be administered by a pMDI rather than an SVN, to minimize the likelihood of aerosolizing the patient's respiratory droplets into the ambient air. Ideally, patients hospitalized with moderate COVID-19 pneumonia should be placed in airborne infection isolation rooms, with limitations enforced so that clinicians enter only as necessary, wearing appropriate PPE (NIH, 2020) (see Chapter 66 for further discussion). For instance, the nurse caring for the patient might arrange activities so that assessments are performed and medications are administered at the same time (see Chart 19-7).

 The patient with severe COVID-19 pneumonia has SpO_2 ≤93% on room air with tachypnea and requires supplemental oxygen, perhaps with ET intubation and

---

Chart 19-7 — ETHICAL DILEMMA

Is It Ever Ethical to Refuse to Care for a Patient?

Case Scenario

You are a staff nurse in a medical intensive care unit (MICU). Within the past week, there has been a significantly increased incidence of patients infected with severe acute respiratory syndrome coronavirus 2 (SARS-CoV-2) in two counties that border the county where your hospital is located. Your nurse manager holds an emergency mandatory staff meeting, and informs all staff present that preparations are being made for the hospital to receive and treat a large volume of patients with coronavirus disease 2019 (COVID-19). The MICU where you work has been designated to exclusively treat these patients who are critically ill, while the surgical ICU (SICU) in the hospital will admit all patients who are critically ill but do not have COVID-19. The MICU nurse manager describes hospital administration's plans to manage the distribution and rationing of personal protective equipment (PPE) for MICU staff and identifies new policies that have been emergently put in place to guide their usage, conservation, and disposal. H.S., a MICU staff nurse who works with you, turns to you and says "I am not going to take care of patients with COVID-19! They can find another safer place for me to work in this hospital or I will quit. I did not sign up to be a nurse here to risk my life."

Discussion

Nurses who work in MICUs confront risks to their health on a continuing basis by being in contact with patients who have infectious diseases. Prior to the COVID-19 pandemic, most of these health risks to nurses were minimal. Most pathogens that caused infectious diseases in patients in MICUs could be effectively treated pharmacologically (e.g., with antibiotics) in people with healthy immune systems. Many patients in MICUs who were critically ill with these infectious diseases had comorbid disorders that hampered their immune responses; however, a healthy nurse who became exposed to the pathogen would likely not become infected. Yet if the nurse did become ill, the nurse could have expected an expedient recovery to health after treatment was instituted. The personal risk to the nurse changes dramatically during pandemics, when the nurse is confronted with a novel aggressive contagious pathogen that can cause life-threatening illness in the previously healthy person, without the benefit of clearly effective evidence-based treatment strategies.

Analysis

- Identify the ethical principles that are in conflict in this case (see Chapter 1, Chart 1-7). Should the principle of beneficence have preeminence during pandemics? Can the desire to do the greatest good for the greatest number of people ever be given greater moral credence than ensuring that individual rights are preserved?
- Assume that H.S. is a healthy 24-year-old woman without any known risk factors for COVID-19. Now assume she is 62 years old, with diabetes and hypertension, and that her 88-year-old mother resides with her. Do these factors make a difference in whether or not you would support her desire to not care for patients with COVID-19?
- Do you and H.S. have a professional obligation to care for patients with COVID-19 who are critically ill? Do you have the right to refuse to care for these patients? How might your viewpoint change, depending upon the availability or lack of availability of appropriate PPE? How would you evaluate the new policies put in place that guide the usage, conservation, and disposal of PPE in the MICU? What resources are available for you to evaluate the soundness of this policy, to ensure that you, H.S., and your MICU colleagues are not placed at undue risk? Identify professional resources that might help you to resolve this dilemma.

References

Binkley, C. E., & Kemp, D. S. (2020). Ethical rationing of personal protective equipment to minimize moral residue during the COVID-19 pandemic. *Journal of the American College of Surgeons, 230*(6), 1111–1113.

Kramer, J. B., Brown, D. E., & Kopar, P. K. (2020). Ethics in the time of coronavirus: Recommendations in the COVID-19 pandemic. *Journal of the American College of Surgeons, 230*(6), 1114–1118.

Morley, G., Grady, C., McCarthy, J., et al. (2020). COVID-19: Ethical challenges for nurses. *Hastings Center Report, 50*(3), 35–39.

Resources

See Chapter 1, Chart 1-10 for Steps of an Ethical Analysis and Ethics Resources.

The Centers for Disease Control and Prevention (CDC). (2020). Optimizing supply of PPE and other equipment during shortages. Retrieved on 8/6/2020 at: www.cdc.gov/coronavirus/2019-ncov/hcp/ppe-strategy/index.html

mechanical ventilation (see later discussions on ET intubation and mechanical ventilation). Chest x-ray findings typically show diffuse, bilateral, "ground-glass" opacities (Cascella et al., 2020). Some patients have severe dyspnea, while others report no dyspnea and have been referred to as the *happy hypoxemics* by Caputo, Strayer, and Levitan (2020). Reportedly, many patients deteriorate rapidly and without clear prodromal clinical indicators from moderate to severe disease (Cascella et al., 2020).

Although patients with severe COVID-19 pneumonia were nearly universally managed with ET intubation and mechanical ventilation during the first weeks of the pandemic, case fatality rates were reportedly much higher than anticipated (Caputo et al., 2020). That observation, along with actual or anticipated shortages of mechanical ventilators, led some providers to try managing patients with other strategies, including trials of placing nonintubated hospitalized patients with COVID-19 in the prone position at periodic intervals, along with administering high flow oxygen therapy. Although not universally effective, data from preliminary research suggest that periodic prone positioning with high flow oxygen therapy can prevent eventual ET intubation in some patients with severe COVID-19 pneumonia (Caputo et al., 2020).

At the present time, there are no immunomodulating agents that are recommended to treat severe COVID-19 pneumonia, although interleukin-6 (IL-6) antagonists (e.g., tocilizumab) are currently under investigation. IL-6 is believed to be a key cytokine responsible for propagating the haywire inflammatory response called cytokine release syndrome (CRS) or the "cytokine storm" that occurs in some patients with severe COVID-19 (NIH, 2020) (see Chapter 12 for further discussion of CRS). Another therapy that is under investigation and approved for emergency use is using convalescent plasma, which transfuses antibodies from patients recovered from COVID-19 into patients with severe disease (Kim & Gandhi, 2020).

It is recommended that the antiviral agent remdesivir be prescribed to treat patients with severe COVID-19 pneumonia as it has demonstrated promising results in clinical trials, notably improved recovery times and overall outcomes (Beigel, Tomashek, Dodd, et al., 2020; NIH, 2020; Wang, Zhang, Du, et al., 2020). Among patients with severe COVID-19 pneumonia, a frequent and serious complication is acute respiratory distress syndrome (ARDS), which is commonly managed with ET intubation and mechanical ventilation (see later discussion). Among patients with COVID-19 and ARDS, the mortality rate is reported at 50% (Anesi, 2020).

Complications

Shock and Respiratory Failure

Severe complications of pneumonia include hypotension and septic shock and respiratory failure (especially with gram-negative bacterial disease or with SARS-CoV-2 infection in older adult patients). These complications are encountered chiefly in patients who have received no specific treatment or inadequate or delayed treatment or in patients at risk for severe COVID-19. These complications are also encountered when the infecting organism is resistant to therapy, when a comorbid disease complicates the pneumonia, or when the patient is immune compromised. (See Chapter 11 for further discussion of management of the patient with septic shock.)

Pleural Effusion

A pleural effusion is an accumulation of pleural fluid in the pleural space (space between the parietal and visceral pleurae of the lung). A parapneumonic effusion is any pleural effusion associated with bacterial pneumonia, lung abscess, or bronchiectasis. After the pleural effusion is detected on a chest x-ray, a thoracentesis may be performed to remove the fluid, which is sent to the laboratory for analysis. There are three stages of parapneumonic pleural effusions based on pathogenesis: uncomplicated, complicated, and thoracic empyema. An **empyema** occurs when thick, purulent fluid accumulates within the pleural space, often with fibrin development and a loculated (walled-off) area where the infection is located (see later discussion). A chest tube may be inserted to treat pleural infection by establishing proper drainage of the empyema. Sterilization of the empyema cavity requires 4 to 6 weeks of antibiotics, and sometimes surgical management is required.

NURSING PROCESS

The Patient with Bacterial Pneumonia

Assessment

Nursing assessment is critical in detecting pneumonia. Fever, chills, or night sweats in a patient who also has respiratory symptoms should alert the nurse to the possibility of bacterial pneumonia. Respiratory assessment further identifies the clinical manifestations of pneumonia: pleuritic-type pain, fatigue, tachypnea, the use of accessory muscles for breathing, bradycardia or relative bradycardia, coughing, and purulent sputum. The nurse monitors the patient for the following: changes in temperature and pulse; amount, odor, and color of secretions; frequency and severity of cough; degree of tachypnea or shortness of breath; changes in physical assessment findings (primarily assessed by inspecting and auscultating the chest); and changes in the chest x-ray findings.

In addition, it is important to assess older adult patients for unusual behavior, altered mental status, dehydration, excessive fatigue, and concomitant heart failure.

Diagnosis

NURSING DIAGNOSES

Based on the assessment data, major nursing diagnoses may include the following:
- Impaired airway clearance associated with copious tracheobronchial secretions
- Fatigue and activity intolerance associated with impaired respiratory function
- Risk for hypovolaemia associated with fever and a rapid respiratory rate
- Impaired nutritional status
- Lack of knowledge about the treatment regimen and preventive measures

COLLABORATIVE PROBLEMS/POTENTIAL COMPLICATIONS

Based on the assessment data, collaborative problems or potential complications that may occur include the following:

- Continuing symptoms after initiation of therapy
- Sepsis and septic shock
- Respiratory failure
- Atelectasis
- Pleural effusion
- Delirium

Planning and Goals

The major goals may include improved airway patency, increased activity, maintenance of proper fluid volume, maintenance of adequate nutrition, an understanding of the treatment protocol and preventive measures, and absence of complications.

Nursing Interventions

IMPROVING AIRWAY PATENCY

Removing secretions is important because retained secretions interfere with gas exchange and may slow recovery. The nurse encourages hydration (2 to 3 L/day), because adequate hydration thins and loosens pulmonary secretions. Humidification may be used to loosen secretions and improve ventilation. A high-humidity facemask (using either compressed air or oxygen) delivers warm, humidified air to the tracheobronchial tree, helps liquefy secretions, and relieves tracheobronchial irritation. Coughing can be initiated either voluntarily or by reflex. Lung expansion maneuvers, such as deep breathing with an incentive spirometer, may induce a cough. To improve airway patency, the nurse encourages the patient to perform an effective, directed cough, which includes correct positioning, a deep inspiratory maneuver, glottic closure, contraction of the expiratory muscles against the closed glottis, sudden glottic opening, and an explosive expiration. In some cases, the nurse may assist the patient by placing both hands on the lower rib cage (either anterior or posterior) to focus the patient on a slow deep breath, and then manually assisting the patient by applying constant, external pressure during the expiratory phase.

CPT is important in loosening and mobilizing secretions (see Figs. 20-6 and 20-7 and further discussion in Chapter 20). Indications for CPT include sputum retention not responsive to spontaneous or directed cough, a history of pulmonary problems previously treated with chest physiotherapy, continued evidence of retained secretions (decreased or abnormal breath sounds, change in vital signs), abnormal chest x-ray findings consistent with atelectasis or infiltrates, and deterioration in oxygenation. The patient is placed in the proper position to drain the involved lung segments, then the chest is percussed and vibrated either manually or with a mechanical percussor. The nurse may consult the respiratory therapist for volume expansion protocols and secretion management protocols that help direct the respiratory care of the patient and match the patient's needs with appropriate treatment schedules.

After each position change, the nurse encourages the patient to breathe deeply and cough. If the patient is too weak to cough effectively, the nurse may need to remove the mucus by nasotracheal suctioning. It may take time for secretions to mobilize and move into the central airways for expectoration. Therefore, it is important for the nurse to monitor the patient for cough and sputum production after the completion of CPT.

The nurse also administers and titrates oxygen therapy as prescribed or via protocols. The effectiveness of oxygen therapy is monitored by improvement in clinical signs and symptoms, patient comfort, and adequate oxygenation values as measured by pulse oximetry or arterial blood gas analysis.

PROMOTING REST AND CONSERVING ENERGY

The nurse encourages the patient who is debilitated to rest and avoid overexertion and possible exacerbation of symptoms. The patient should assume a comfortable position to promote rest and breathing (e.g., semi-Fowler position) and should change positions frequently to enhance secretion clearance and pulmonary ventilation and perfusion. Outpatients must be instructed to avoid overexertion and to engage in only moderate activity during the initial phases of treatment.

PROMOTING FLUID INTAKE

The respiratory rate of patients with pneumonia increases because of the increased workload imposed by labored breathing and fever. An increased respiratory rate leads to an increase in insensible fluid loss during exhalation and can lead to dehydration. Therefore, unless contraindicated, increased fluid intake (at least 2 L/day) is encouraged. Hydration must be achieved more slowly and with careful monitoring in patients with preexisting conditions such as heart failure (see Chapter 25).

MAINTAINING NUTRITION

Many patients with shortness of breath and fatigue have a decreased appetite and consume only fluids. Fluids with electrolytes (commercially available drinks, such as Gatorade) may help provide fluid, calories, and electrolytes. Other nutritionally enriched drinks such as oral nutritional supplements may be used to supplement calories. Small, frequent meals may be advisable. In addition, IV fluids and nutrients may be given if necessary.

PROMOTING PATIENTS' KNOWLEDGE

The patient and family are educated about the cause of pneumonia, management of symptoms, signs and symptoms that should be reported to the primary provider or nurse, and the need for follow-up. The patient also needs information about factors (both patient risk factors and external factors) that may have contributed to the development of pneumonia and strategies to promote recovery and prevent recurrence. If the patient is hospitalized, they are instructed about the purpose and importance of management strategies that have been implemented and about the importance of adhering to them during and after the hospital stay. Explanations should be given simply and in language that the patient can understand. If possible, written instructions and information should be provided, and alternative formats should be provided for patients with hearing or vision loss, if necessary. Because of the severity of symptoms, the patient may require that instructions and explanations be repeated several times.

MONITORING AND MANAGING POTENTIAL COMPLICATIONS

Continuing Symptoms After Initiation of Therapy. The patient is observed for response to antibiotic therapy; patients usually begin to respond to treatment within 24 to 48 hours after antibiotic therapy is initiated. If the patient started taking antibiotics before evaluation by culture and sensitivity of the causative organisms, antibiotics may need to be changed once the results are available. The patient is monitored for changes in physical status (deterioration of condition or resolution of symptoms) and for persistent recurrent fever, which may be a result of medication allergy (signaled possibly by a rash); medication resistance or slow response (greater than 48 hours) of the susceptible organism to therapy; pleural effusion; or pneumonia caused by an unusual organism, such as *P. jiroveci* or *Aspergillus fumigatus*. Failure of the pneumonia to resolve or persistence of symptoms despite changes on the chest x-ray raises the suspicion of other underlying disorders, such as lung cancer. As described previously, lung cancers may invade or compress airways, causing an obstructive atelectasis that may lead to pneumonia.

In addition to monitoring for continuing symptoms of pneumonia, the nurse also monitors for other complications, such as septic shock and multiple organ dysfunction syndrome (MODS) and atelectasis, which may develop during the first few days of antibiotic treatment.

Shock and Respiratory Failure. The nurse assesses for signs and symptoms of septic shock and respiratory failure by evaluating the patient's vital signs, pulse oximetry values, and hemodynamic monitoring parameters. The nurse reports signs of deteriorating patient status and assists in administering IV fluids and medications prescribed to combat shock. Intubation and mechanical ventilation may be required if respiratory failure occurs. (Sepsis and septic shock are described in detail in Chapter 11, and care of the patient receiving mechanical ventilation is described later in this chapter.)

Pleural Effusion. If pleural effusion develops and thoracentesis is performed to remove fluid, the nurse assists in the procedure and explains it to the patient. After thoracentesis, the nurse monitors the patient for pneumothorax or recurrence of pleural effusion. If a chest tube needs to be inserted, the nurse monitors the patient's respiratory status (see discussion on chest tubes later in this chapter).

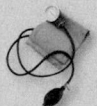 For the procedural guidelines for assisting the patient undergoing a thoracentesis, go to **thepoint.lww.com/Brunner15e**.

Delirium. A patient with pneumonia is assessed for delirium and other more subtle changes in cognitive status; this is especially true in the older adult. The Confusion Assessment Method (CAM) is a commonly used screening tool (see Chapter 8, Chart 8-7). Confusion, suggestive of delirium, and other changes in cognitive status resulting from pneumonia are poor prognostic signs (File, 2019b). Delirium may be related to hypoxemia, fever, dehydration, sleep deprivation, or developing sepsis. The patient's underlying comorbid conditions may also play a part in the development of confusion. Addressing and correcting underlying factors as well as ensuring patient safety are important nursing interventions.

PROMOTING HOME, COMMUNITY-BASED, AND TRANSITIONAL CARE

 Educating Patients About Self-Care. Depending on the severity of the pneumonia, treatment may occur in the hospital or in the outpatient setting. Patient education is crucial regardless of the setting, and the proper administration of antibiotics is important. In some instances, the patient may be treated initially with IV antibiotics as an inpatient and then discharged to continue the IV antibiotics at home. A seamless system of care must be maintained for the patient from hospital to home; this includes communication between the nurses caring for the patient in both settings.

If oral antibiotics are prescribed, the nurse educates the patient about their proper administration and potential side effects. The patient should be educated about symptoms that require contacting the primary provider: difficulty breathing, worsening cough, recurrent/increasing fever, and medication intolerance.

After the fever subsides, the patient may gradually increase activities. Fatigue and weakness may be prolonged after pneumonia, especially in older adults. The nurse encourages breathing exercises to promote secretion clearance and volume expansion. A patient who is being treated as an outpatient should be contacted by the health care team or instructed to contact the primary provider 24 to 48 hours after starting therapy. The patient is also instructed to return to the clinic or primary provider's office for a follow-up chest x-ray and physical examination. Often, improvement in chest x-ray findings lags behind improvement in clinical signs and symptoms.

The nurse encourages the patient who smokes to stop smoking. Smoking inhibits tracheobronchial ciliary action, which is the first line of defense of the lower respiratory tract. Smoking also irritates the mucous cells of the bronchi and inhibits the function of alveolar macrophage (scavenger) cells. The patient is instructed to avoid stress, fatigue, sudden changes in temperature, and excessive alcohol intake, all of which lower resistance to pneumonia. The nurse reviews with the patient the principles of adequate nutrition and rest, because one episode of pneumonia may make a patient susceptible to recurring respiratory tract infections.

Continuing and Transitional Care. Patients who are severely debilitated or who cannot care for themselves may require referral for home, transitional, or community-based care. During home visits, the nurse assesses the patient's physical status, monitors for complications, assesses the home environment, and reinforces previous education. The patient's adherence to the therapeutic regimen is evaluated (i.e., taking medications as prescribed; performing breathing exercises; consuming adequate fluid and dietary intake; and avoiding smoking, alcohol, and excessive activity). The nurse stresses to the patient and family the importance of monitoring for complications or exacerbation of the pneumonia. The patient is encouraged to obtain an influenza vaccination at the prescribed times, because influenza increases susceptibility to secondary bacterial pneumonia, especially that caused by staphylococci, *H. influenzae*, and *S. pneumoniae*. The patient also is urged to receive the pneumococcal vaccine(s) according to CDC recommendations (see previous discussion).

Evaluation

Expected patient outcomes may include the following:
1. Demonstrates improved airway patency, as evidenced by adequate oxygenation by pulse oximetry or arterial blood gas analysis, normal temperature, normal breath sounds, and effective coughing

2. Rests and conserves energy by limiting activities and remaining in bed while symptomatic and then slowly increasing activities
3. Maintains adequate hydration, as evidenced by an adequate fluid intake and urine output and normal skin turgor
4. Consumes adequate dietary intake, as evidenced by maintenance or increase in body weight without excess fluid gain
5. Verbalizes increased knowledge about management strategies
6. Adheres to management strategies
7. Exhibits no complications
   a. Exhibits acceptable vital signs, pulse oximetry, and arterial blood gas measurements
   b. Reports productive cough that diminishes over time
   c. Has absence of signs or symptoms of sepsis, septic shock, respiratory failure, or pleural effusion
   d. Remains oriented and aware of surroundings
8. Maintains or increases weight
9. Adheres to treatment protocol and prevention strategies

Aspiration

Aspiration is inhalation of foreign material (e.g., oropharyngeal or stomach contents) into the lungs. It is a serious complication that can cause pneumonia and result in the following clinical picture: tachycardia, dyspnea, central cyanosis, hypertension, hypotension, and potentially death. It can occur when the protective airway reflexes are decreased or absent due to a variety of factors (see Chart 19-8). Studies suggest that aspiration pneumonia accounts for 5% to 15% of CAP (Gamache, 2019).

Pathophysiology

The primary factors responsible for death and complications after aspiration are the volume and character of the aspirated contents. Aspiration pneumonia develops after inhalation of colonized oral or pharyngeal material. The pathologic process involves an acute inflammatory response to bacteria and bacterial products. Most commonly, the causative organisms

---

Chart 19-8 **RISK FACTORS**
Aspiration

- Seizure activity
- Brain injury
- Decreased level of consciousness from trauma, drug or alcohol intoxication, excessive sedation, or general anesthesia
- Flat body positioning
- Stroke
- Swallowing disorders
- Cardiac arrest

Adapted from American Association of Critical-Care Nurses. (2017b). AACN practice alert: Prevention of aspiration in adults. *Critical Care Nurse, 37*(3), 88; Bartlett, J. (2019a). Aspiration pneumonia in adults. *UpToDate.* Retrieved on 9/23/2019 at: www.uptodate.com/contents/aspiration-pneumonia-in-adults

---

in community-acquired aspiration pneumonia may include *S. aureus, S. pneumoniae, H. influenzae,* and *Enterobacter* species (Gamache, 2019).

A full stomach contains solid particles of food. If these are aspirated, the problem then becomes one of mechanical blockage of the airways and secondary infection. During periods of fasting, the stomach contains acidic gastric juice, which, if aspirated, can be very destructive to the alveoli and capillaries. Fecal contamination (more likely seen in intestinal obstruction) increases the likelihood of death, because the endotoxins produced by intestinal organisms may be absorbed systemically, or the thick proteinaceous material found in the intestinal contents may obstruct the airway, leading to atelectasis and secondary bacterial invasion.

Esophageal conditions may also be associated with aspiration pneumonia. These include dysphagia, esophageal strictures, neoplasm or diverticula, tracheoesophageal fistula, and gastroesophageal reflux disease.

Prevention

The risk of aspiration is indirectly related to the level of consciousness of the patient. Aspiration of small amounts of material from the buccal (oral) cavity is not uncommon, particularly during sleep; however, disease as a result of aspiration does not occur in healthy people because the material is cleared by the mucociliary tree and the macrophages. Witnessed aspiration of large volumes occurs occasionally; however, small-volume clinically silent aspiration is more common. Prevention is the primary goal when caring for patients at risk for aspiration (American Association of Critical Care Nurses [AACN], 2017b).

▶ *Quality and Safety Nursing Alert*

When a nonfunctioning nasogastric tube allows the gastric contents to accumulate in the stomach, a condition known as silent aspiration may result. Silent aspiration often occurs unobserved and may be more common than suspected. If untreated, massive inhalation of gastric contents develops in a period of several hours.

Compensating for Absent Reflexes

Aspiration may occur if the patient cannot adequately coordinate protective glottic, laryngeal, and cough reflexes. This hazard is increased if the patient has a distended abdomen, is supine, has the upper extremities immobilized in any manner, receives local anesthetic agents to the oropharyngeal or laryngeal area for diagnostic procedures, has been sedated, or has had long-term intubation. Clinical interventions are key to preventing aspiration (see Chart 19-9).

For patients with known swallowing dysfunction or those recently extubated following prolonged ET intubation, a swallowing screen is necessary. Patients deemed at risk are then assessed by a speech therapist. Besides positioning the patient semirecumbent or upright prior to eating, other helpful techniques may include suggesting a soft diet and encouraging the patient to take small bites. The patient should be instructed to keep the chin tucked and the head turned with repeated swallowing. Straws should not be used.

> **Chart 19-9** **Clinical Practices That Prevent Aspiration**
>
> - Maintain head-of-bed elevation at an angle of 30 to 45 degrees, unless contraindicated
> - Use sedatives as sparingly as possible
> - Before initiating enteral tube feeding, confirm the tip location
> - For patients receiving tube feedings, assess placement of the feeding tube at 4-hour intervals, assess for gastrointestinal residuals (<150 mL before next feeding) to the feedings at 4-hour intervals
> - For patients receiving tube feedings, avoid bolus feedings in those at risk for aspiration
> - Consult with primary provider about obtaining a swallowing evaluation before oral feedings are started for patients who were recently extubated but were previously intubated for >2 days
> - Maintain endotracheal cuff pressures at an appropriate level, and ensure that secretions are cleared from above the cuff before it is deflated.
>
> American Association of Critical Care Nurses (AACN). (2017b). AACN practice alert: Prevention of aspiration in adults. *Critical Care Nurse, 37*(3), 88.

When vomiting, people can normally protect their airway by sitting up or turning on the side and coordinating breathing, coughing, gag, and glottic reflexes. If these reflexes are active, an oral airway should not be inserted. If an airway is in place, it should be pulled out the moment the patient gags so as not to stimulate the pharyngeal gag reflex and promote vomiting and aspiration. Suctioning of oral secretions with a catheter should be performed with minimal pharyngeal stimulation.

For patients with an ET tube and feeding tube, the ET cuff pressure should be maintained at greater than 20 cm H_2O (but less than 30 cm H_2O to minimize injury) to prevent leakage of secretions from around the cuff into the lower respiratory tract. In addition, hypopharyngeal suctioning is recommended before the cuff is deflated (AACN, 2017a).

Assessing Feeding Tube Placement

Tube feedings must be given only when it is certain that the feeding tube is positioned correctly in the stomach. Many patients receive enteral feeding directly into the duodenum through a small-bore flexible feeding tube or surgically implanted tube. (See Chapter 39 for discussion of enteral tube feedings.)

Identifying Delayed Stomach Emptying

A full stomach can cause aspiration because of increased intragastric or extragastric pressure. The following may delay emptying of the stomach: intestinal obstruction; increased gastric secretions in gastroesophageal reflux disease; increased gastric secretions during anxiety, stress, or pain; and abdominal distention due to paralytic ileus, ascites, peritonitis, the use of opioids or sedatives, severe illness, or vaginal delivery. (See Chapter 39 for discussion of management of patients receiving gastric tube feedings.)

Managing Effects of Prolonged Intubation

Prolonged ET intubation or tracheostomy (see later discussions) can depress the laryngeal and glottic reflexes because of disuse. Patients with prolonged tracheostomies are encouraged to phonate and exercise their laryngeal muscles. For patients who have had long-term intubation or tracheostomies, it may be helpful to have a speech therapist experienced in swallowing disorders work with the patient to address swallowing problems, as noted previously.

Pulmonary Tuberculosis

Tuberculosis (TB) is an infectious disease that primarily affects the lung parenchyma. It also may be transmitted to other parts of the body, including the meninges, kidneys, bones, and lymph nodes. The primary infectious agent, M. *tuberculosis*, is an acid-fast aerobic rod that grows slowly and is sensitive to heat and ultraviolet light. *Mycobacterium bovis* and *Mycobacterium avium* have rarely been associated with the development of a TB infection.

TB is a worldwide public health problem that is closely associated with poverty, malnutrition, overcrowding, substandard housing, and inadequate health care. Mortality and morbidity rates continue to rise; M. *tuberculosis* infects an estimated one third of the world's population and remains the leading cause of death from infectious disease in the world. In 2017, 10 million people were sick with TB throughout the world, and there were 1.3 million TB-related deaths (CDC, 2018b).

In the United States, 9105 cases of TB were reported in 2017, which is a 2.3% decrease from 2016 (CDC, 2018b). Factors that prevent elimination of TB in the United States include the prevalence of TB among foreign-born residents, delays in detecting and reporting cases of TB, the lack of protection of contacts of people with infectious cases of TB, the presence of a substantial number of people with latent TB, and barriers to supporting clinical and public health expertise in this disease (CDC, 2018b).

Transmission and Risk Factors

TB spreads from person to person by airborne transmission. An infected person releases droplet nuclei (usually particles 1 to 5 mcm in diameter) through talking, coughing, sneezing, laughing, or singing. Larger droplets settle; smaller droplets remain suspended in the air and are inhaled by a susceptible person. Chart 19-10 lists risk factors for TB. Chart 19-11 summarizes the CDC's recommendations for the prevention of TB transmission in health care settings.

Pathophysiology

TB begins when a susceptible person inhales mycobacteria and becomes infected. The bacteria are transmitted through the airways to the alveoli, where they are deposited and begin to multiply. The bacilli also are transported via the lymph system and bloodstream to other parts of the body (kidneys, bones, cerebral cortex) and other areas of the lungs (upper lobes). The body's immune system responds by initiating an inflammatory reaction. Phagocytes (neutrophils and macrophages) engulf many of the bacteria, and TB-specific lymphocytes lyse (destroy) the bacilli and normal tissue. This tissue reaction results in the accumulation of exudate in the alveoli, causing bronchopneumonia. The initial infection usually occurs 2 to 10 weeks after exposure.

Granulomas, new tissue masses of live and dead bacilli, are surrounded by macrophages, which form a protective wall.

Chart 19-10 ⚠ RISK FACTORS
Tuberculosis

- Close contact with someone who has active TB. Inhalation of airborne nuclei from a person who is infected is proportional to the amount of time spent in the same air space, the proximity of the person, and the degree of ventilation.
- Immunocompromised status (e.g., those with HIV infection, cancer, transplanted organs, and prolonged high-dose corticosteroid therapy).
- Substance use disorder (individuals who use IV/injection drug or abuse alcohol).
- Any person without adequate health care (those experiencing homelessness; those who are impoverished; and racial–ethnic minorities, particularly children <15 years and young adults between ages 15 and 44 years).
- Preexisting medical conditions or special treatment (e.g., diabetes, chronic kidney disease, malnourishment, select malignancies, hemodialysis, transplanted organ, gastrectomy, and jejunoileal bypass).
- Immigration from or recent travel to countries with a high prevalence of TB (southeastern Asia, Africa, Latin America, Caribbean).
- Institutionalization (e.g., long-term care facilities, psychiatric institutions, prisons).
- Living in overcrowded, substandard housing.
- Being a health care worker performing high-risk activities: administration of aerosolized pentamidine and other medications, sputum induction procedures, bronchoscopy, suctioning, coughing procedures, caring for patients who are immune suppressed, home care with the high-risk population, and administering anesthesia and related procedures (e.g., intubation, suctioning).

TB, tuberculosis.
Adapted from Centers for Disease Control and Prevention (CDC). (2018b). *TB fact sheets-infection control and prevention; TB in specific populations*. Retrieved on 9/26/2019 at: www.cdc.gov/tb/statistics/default.htm

Chart 19-11
Centers for Disease Control and Prevention Recommendations for Preventing Transmission of Tuberculosis in Health Care Settings

1. Early identification and treatment of people with active TB
   a. Maintain a high index of suspicion for TB to identify cases rapidly.
   b. Promptly initiate effective multidrug anti-TB therapy based on clinical and drug-resistance surveillance data.
2. Prevention of spread of infectious droplet nuclei by source control methods and by reduction of microbial contamination of indoor air
   a. Initiate AFB isolation precautions immediately for all patients who are suspected or confirmed to have active TB and who may be infectious. AFB isolation precautions include the use of a private room with negative pressure in relation to surrounding areas and a minimum of six air exchanges per hour. Air from the room should be exhausted directly to the outside. The use of ultraviolet lamps or high-efficiency particulate air filters to supplement ventilation may be considered.
   b. People entering the AFB isolation room should use disposable particulate respirators that fit snugly around the face.
   c. Continue AFB isolation precautions until there is clinical evidence of reduced infectiousness (i.e., cough has substantially decreased and the number of organisms on sequential sputum smears is decreasing). If drug resistance is suspected or confirmed, continue AFB precautions until the sputum smear is negative for AFB.
   d. Use special precautions during cough-inducing procedures.
3. Surveillance for TB transmission
   a. Maintain surveillance for TB infection among health care workers (HCWs) by routine, periodic tuberculin skin testing. Recommend appropriate preventive therapy for HCWs when indicated.
   b. Maintain surveillance for TB cases among patients and HCWs.
   c. Promptly initiate contact investigation procedures among HCWs, patients, and visitors exposed to a patient with infectious TB who is untreated, or ineffectively treated, and for whom appropriate AFB procedures are not in place. Recommend appropriate therapy or preventive therapy for contacts with disease or TB infection without current disease. Therapeutic regimens should be chosen based on the clinical history and local drug-resistance surveillance data.

AFB, acid-fast bacilli; TB, tuberculosis.
Adapted from Centers for Disease Control and Prevention (CDC). (2018b). *TB fact sheets-infection control and prevention; TB in specific populations*. Retrieved on 9/26/2019 at: www.cdc.gov/tb/statistics/default.htm

They are then transformed to a fibrous tissue mass, the central portion of which is called a *Ghon tubercle*. The material (bacteria and macrophages) becomes necrotic, forming a cheesy mass. This mass may become calcified and form a collagenous scar. At this point, the bacteria become dormant, and there is no further progression of active disease.

After initial exposure and infection, active disease may develop because of a compromised or inadequate immune system response. Active disease also may occur with reinfection and activation of dormant bacteria. In this case, the *Ghon tubercle* ulcerates, releasing the cheesy material into the bronchi. The bacteria then become airborne, resulting in the further spread of the disease. Then, the ulcerated tubercle heals and forms scar tissue. This causes the infected lung to become more inflamed, resulting in the further development of bronchopneumonia and tubercle formation.

Unless this process is arrested, it spreads slowly downward to the hilum of the lungs and later extends to adjacent lobes. The process may be prolonged and is characterized by long remissions when the disease is arrested, followed by periods of renewed activity. Approximately 10% of people who are initially infected develop active disease (Pozniak, 2019). Some people develop reactivation TB (also called *adult-type progressive TB*). The reactivation of a dormant focus occurring during the primary infection is the cause.

Clinical Manifestations

The signs and symptoms of pulmonary TB are insidious. Most patients have a low-grade fever, cough, night sweats, fatigue, and weight loss. The cough may be nonproductive, or mucopurulent sputum may be expectorated. **Hemoptysis** (i.e., coughing up blood) also may occur. Both the systemic and the pulmonary symptoms are chronic and may have been present for weeks to months. Older adult patients usually present with less pronounced symptoms than younger patients.

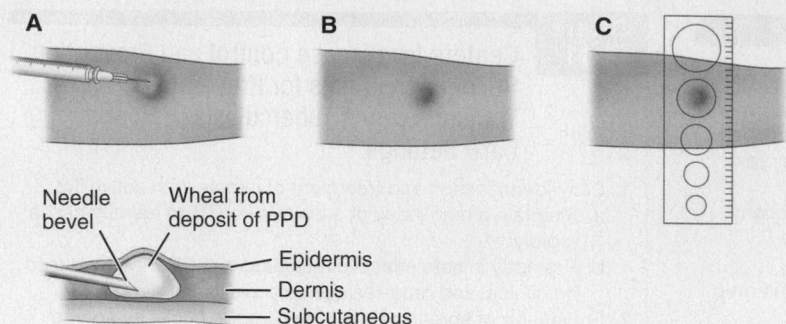

Figure 19-3 • The Mantoux test for tuberculosis. **A.** Correct technique for inserting the needle involves depositing the purified protein derivative (PPD) subcutaneously with the needle bevel facing upward. **B.** The reaction to the Mantoux test usually consists of a wheal, a hivelike, firm welt. **C.** To determine the extent of the reaction, the wheal is measured using a commercially prepared gauge. Interpretation of the Mantoux test is discussed in the text.

Extrapulmonary disease occurs in up to 20% of cases in the United States (Bernardo, 2019). In patients infected with HIV, extrapulmonary disease is more prevalent.

Assessment and Diagnostic Findings

Once a patient presents with a positive skin test, blood test, or sputum culture for acid-fast bacilli (AFB; see later discussion on these), additional assessments must be done. These tests include a complete history, physical examination, tuberculin skin test, chest x-ray, and drug susceptibility testing.

Clinical manifestations of fever, anorexia, weight loss, night sweats, fatigue, cough, and sputum production prompt a more thorough assessment of respiratory function—for example, assessing the lungs for consolidation by evaluating breath sounds (diminished, bronchial sounds; crackles), fremitus, and egophony. If the patient is infected with TB, the chest x-ray usually reveals lesions in the upper lobes. For all patients, the initial M. *tuberculosis* isolate should be tested for drug resistance. Drug susceptibility patterns should be repeated at 3 months for patients who do not respond to therapy (Sterling, 2019).

Tuberculin Skin Test

The Mantoux method is used to determine whether a person has been infected with the TB bacillus and is used widely in screening for latent M. *tuberculosis* infection. The Mantoux method is a standardized, intracutaneous injection procedure and should be performed only by those trained in its administration and reading. Tubercle bacillus extract (tuberculin), purified protein derivative (PPD), is injected into the intradermal layer of the inner aspect of the forearm, approximately 4 inches below the elbow (see Fig. 19-3). Intermediate-strength PPD, in a tuberculin syringe with a half-inch 26- or 27-gauge needle, is used. The needle, with the bevel facing up, is inserted beneath the skin. Then, 0.1 mL of PPD is injected, creating an elevation in the skin, a well-demarcated wheal 6 to 10 mm in diameter. The site, antigen name, strength, lot number, date, and time of the test are recorded. The test result is read 48 to 72 hours after injection. Tests read after 72 hours tend to underestimate the true size of **induration** (raised hard area or swelling). A delayed localized reaction indicates that the person is sensitive to tuberculin.

A reaction occurs when both induration and erythema (redness) are present. After the area is inspected for induration, it is lightly palpated across the injection site, from the area of normal skin to the margins of the induration. The diameter of the induration (not erythema) is measured in millimeters at its widest part (see Fig. 19-3), and the size of the induration is documented. Erythema without induration is not considered significant.

The size of the induration determines the significance of the reaction. A reaction of 0 to 4 mm is considered not significant. A reaction of 5 mm or greater may be significant in people who are considered to be at risk. It is defined as positive in patients who are HIV positive or have HIV risk factors and are of unknown HIV status, in those who are close contacts of someone with active TB, and in those who have chest x-ray results consistent with TB. An induration of 10 mm or greater is usually considered significant in people who have normal or mildly impaired immunity. A significant reaction indicates past exposure to M. *tuberculosis* or vaccination with bacille Calmette-Guérin (BCG) vaccine. The BCG vaccine is given to produce a greater resistance to development of TB. The BCG vaccine is used in Europe and Latin America but not routinely in the United States.

A significant (positive) reaction does not necessarily mean that active disease is present in the body. More than 90% of people who are tuberculin-significant reactors do not develop clinical TB (CDC, 2018b). However, all significant reactors are candidates for active TB. In general, the more intense the reaction, the greater the likelihood of an active infection. Additional testing is needed to determine if the person has latent TB infection or active TB.

A nonsignificant (negative) skin test means the person's immune system did not react to the test and that latent TB infection or TB disease is not likely. It does not exclude TB infection or disease, because patients who are immunosuppressed cannot develop an immune response that is adequate to produce a positive skin test. This is referred to as anergy.

QuantiFERON-TB Gold® Plus and T-SPOT®

There are two TB blood tests (called interferon–gamma release assays or IGRAs) available in the United States: the QuantiFERON-TB Gold® Plus (QFT-Plus) test and the T-SPOT®. TB blood tests are the preferred diagnostic tests for patients who have received the BCG vaccine and for patients who are not likely to return for a second appointment to look for a reaction to the tuberculin skin test. The results of both of these tests are available within 24 to 36 hours. A positive IGRA signifies that the patient has been infected with TB bacteria and additional tests are needed. A negative IGRA means that the patient's blood did not react to the test and a latent or active TB infection is not likely (CDC, 2019d; Theel, Hilgart, Breen-Lyles, et al., 2018).

Sputum Culture

A sputum specimen may be used to screen for TB. The presence of AFB on a sputum smear may indicate disease but does not confirm the diagnosis of TB because some AFB are not M. *tuberculosis*. A culture is done to confirm the diagnosis. For all patients, the initial M. *tuberculosis* isolate should be tested for drug resistance (Sterling, 2019).

 Gerontologic Considerations

TB may have atypical manifestations in older adult patients, whose symptoms may include unusual behavior and altered mental status, fever, anorexia, and weight loss. In many older adult patients, the tuberculin skin test produces no reaction (loss of immunologic memory) or delayed reactivity for up to 1 week (recall phenomenon). A second skin test is performed in 1 to 2 weeks. Older adults who live in long-term care facilities are at increased risk for primary and reactivated TB as compared to those in the community (Rajagopalan, 2016).

Medical Management

Pulmonary TB is treated primarily with anti-TB agents for 6 to 12 months. A prolonged treatment duration is necessary to ensure eradication of the organisms and to prevent relapse. The continuing and increasing resistance of M. *tuberculosis* to TB medications is a worldwide concern and challenge in TB therapy. Drug resistance must be considered when planning effective therapy, including the following:

- *Multidrug resistance (MDR TB):* Resistance to two agents, isoniazid and rifampin. The populations at greatest risk for multidrug resistance are those who are HIV positive, institutionalized, or homeless.
- *Extensively drug resistant (XDR TB):* Resistance to isoniazid and rifampin, in addition to any fluroquinolone, and at least one of three injectable second-line agents (i.e., amikacin, kanamycin, or capreomycin). The populations at greatest risk are those with HIV infection or other immunocompromised conditions (CDC, 2019d).

The increasing prevalence of drug resistance points out the need to begin TB treatment with four or more medications, to ensure completion of therapy, and to develop and evaluate new anti-TB medications.

In current TB therapy, four first-line medications are used (see Table 19-4): isoniazid, rifampin, pyrazinamide, and ethambutol. Combination medications, such as isoniazid and rifampin or isoniazid, pyrazinamide, and rifampin and

| TABLE 19-4 | First-Line Antituberculosis Medications for Active Disease |

Commonly Used Agents	Adult Daily Dosage[a]	Most Common Side Effects	Drug Interactions[b]	Nursing Considerations[a]
Isoniazid	5 mg/kg (300 mg maximum daily)	Peripheral neuritis, hepatic enzyme elevation, hepatitis, hypersensitivity	Phenytoin—synergistic Antabuse Alcohol	Bactericidal Pyridoxine is used as prophylaxis for neuritis. Monitor AST and ALT
Rifampin	10 mg/kg (600 mg maximum daily)	Hepatitis, febrile reaction, purpura (rare), nausea, vomiting	Rifampin increases metabolism of oral contraceptives, quinidine, corticosteroids, coumarin derivatives and methadone, digoxin, oral hypoglycemics. PAS may interfere with absorption of rifampin	Bactericidal Orange urine and other body secretions Discoloring of contact lenses Monitor AST and ALT
Rifabutin	5 mg/kg (300 mg maximum daily)		Avoid protease inhibitors	
Rifapentine	10 mg/kg (600 mg twice weekly)	Hepatotoxicity, thrombocytopenia		Orange-red coloration of body secretions, contact lenses, dentures Use with caution in older adults or in those with renal disease
Pyrazinamide	15–30 mg/kg (2 g maximum daily)[a]	Hyperuricemia, hepatotoxicity, skin rash, arthralgias, GI distress		Bactericidal Monitor uric acid, AST, and ALT
Ethambutol	15–25 mg/kg (1.6 g maximum daily dose)[a]	Optic neuritis (may lead to blindness; very rare at 15 mg/kg), skin rash		Bacteriostatic Use with caution with renal disease or when eye testing is not feasible. Monitor visual acuity, color, and discrimination[c]
Combinations: isoniazid + rifampin	150-mg and 300-mg caps (2 caps daily)			

ALT, alanine transaminase; AST, aspartate transaminase; GI, gastrointestinal; PAS, para-aminosalicylic acid.
[a]Check product labeling for detailed information on dose, contraindications, drug interactions, adverse reactions, and monitoring.
[b]Refer to current literature, particularly on rifampin, because it increases hepatic microenzymes and therefore interacts with many drugs.
[c]Initial examination should be performed at start of treatment.
Adapted from Gilbert, D. N., Chambers, H. F., Eliopoulos, G. M., et al. (2018). *The Sanford guide to antimicrobial therapy 2018* (48th ed.). Sperryville, VA: Antimicrobial Therapy, Inc.

medications given twice a week (e.g., rifapentine) are available to help improve patient adherence. However, these medications are more costly.

Multidrug-resistant TB is difficult to treat. Treatment is guided by sputum specimen culture and sensitivity testing as the patient typically is resistant to isoniazid and rifampin. The World Health Organization (WHO, 2019) recently published recommendations for treatment consisting of multiple medications to combat drug-resistant organisms. It is important to consult current recommendations for treatment (WHO, 2019).

Recommended treatment guidelines for newly diagnosed cases of pulmonary TB have two phases: an initial treatment phase and a continuation phase (CDC, 2019d). The initial phase consists of a multiple-medication regimen of isoniazid, rifampin, pyrazinamide, and ethambutol plus vitamin B_6 50 mg. All are taken once a day and are oral medications. This initial intensive-treatment regimen is given daily for 8 weeks, after which options for the continuation phase of treatment include isoniazid and rifampin or isoniazid and rifapentine. The continuation regimen lasts for an additional 4 or 7 months. The 4-month period is used for the large majority of patients. The 7-month period is recommended for patients with cavitary pulmonary TB whose sputum culture after the initial 2 months of treatment is positive, for those whose initial phase of treatment did not include pyrazinamide, and for those being treated once weekly with isoniazid and rifapentine whose sputum culture is positive at the end of the initial phase of treatment. People are considered noninfectious after 2 to 3 weeks of continuous medication therapy. The total number of doses taken, not simply the duration of treatment, more accurately determines whether a course of therapy has been completed (CDC, 2019d).

Isoniazid also may be used as a prophylactic (preventive) measure for people who are at risk for significant disease, including:

- Household family members of patients with active disease
- Patients with HIV infection who have a PPD test reaction with 5 mm of induration or more
- Patients with fibrotic lesions suggestive of old TB detected on a chest x-ray and a PPD reaction with 5 mm of induration or more
- Patients whose current PPD test results show a change from former test results, suggesting recent exposure to TB and possible infection (skin test converters)
- Patients who use IV/injection drugs who have PPD test results with 10 mm of induration or more
- Patients with high-risk comorbid conditions and a PPD result with 10 mm of induration or more

Other candidates for preventive isoniazid therapy are those 35 years or younger who have PPD test results with 10 mm of induration or more and one of the following criteria:

- Individuals who are foreign-born from countries with a high prevalence of TB
- Populations that are high-risk and medically underserved
- Patients living in institutions

Prophylactic isoniazid treatment involves taking daily doses for 6 to 12 months. Liver enzymes, blood urea nitrogen (BUN), and creatinine levels are monitored monthly. Sputum culture results are monitored for AFB to evaluate the effectiveness of treatment and the patient's adherence to the treatment regimen.

Nursing Management

Nursing management includes promoting airway clearance, advocating adherence to the treatment regimen, promoting activity and nutrition, and preventing transmission.

Promoting Airway Clearance

Copious secretions obstruct the airways in many patients with TB and interfere with adequate gas exchange. Increasing the fluid intake promotes systemic hydration and serves as an effective expectorant. The nurse instructs the patient about correct positioning to facilitate airway drainage, referred to as postural drainage (see Chapter 20). Postural drainage allows the force of gravity to assist in the removal of bronchial secretions.

Promoting Adherence to Treatment Regimen

Adherence to the prescribed treatment regimen is key in treating the disease and controlling the spread of infection. The multiple-medication regimen that the patient must follow can be quite complex. Understanding of the medications, schedule, and side effects is important. The nurse educates the patient that TB is a communicable disease and that taking medications is the most effective means of preventing transmission. The major reason treatment fails is that patients do not take their medications regularly and for the prescribed duration. This may be due to side effects or the complexity of the treatment regimen. Risk factors for nonadherence to the drug regimen include patients who have previously failed to complete the course of therapy; patients who are physically, emotionally, or mentally challenged; patients unable to pay for medication; patients actively abusing illicit substances; and patients who do not understand the importance of treatment (Reichman & Lardizabal, 2019).

The nurse educates the patient to take the medication either on an empty stomach or at least 1 hour before meals, because food interferes with medication absorption (although taking medications on an empty stomach frequently results in gastrointestinal upset). Patients taking isoniazid should avoid foods that contain tyramine and histamine (tuna, aged cheese, red wine, soy sauce, yeast extracts), because eating them while taking isoniazid may result in headache, flushing, hypotension, lightheadedness, palpitations, and diaphoresis. Patients should also avoid alcohol because of the high potential for hepatotoxic effects.

In addition, rifampin can alter the metabolism of certain other medications, making them less effective. These medications include beta-blockers, oral anticoagulants such as warfarin, digoxin, quinidine, corticosteroids, oral hypoglycemic agents, oral contraceptives, theophylline, and verapamil. This issue should be discussed with the primary provider and pharmacist so that medication dosages can be adjusted accordingly. The nurse informs the patient that rifampin may discolor contact lenses and that the patient may want to wear eyeglasses during treatment. The nurse monitors for other side effects of anti-TB medications, including hepatitis, neurologic changes (hearing loss, neuritis), and rash. Liver enzymes, BUN, and serum creatinine levels are monitored to detect changes in liver and kidney function. Sputum culture results are monitored for AFB to evaluate the effectiveness of the treatment regimen and adherence to therapy.

The nurse educates the patient about the risk of drug resistance if the medication regimen is not strictly and continuously followed. The nurse carefully monitors vital signs and observes for spikes in temperature or changes in the patient's clinical status. Caregivers of patients who are not hospitalized are taught to monitor the patient's temperature and respiratory status. Changes in the patient's respiratory status are reported to the primary provider.

For patients at risk for nonadherence, programs used in the community setting may include comprehensive case management and directly observed therapy (DOT). In case management, each patient with TB is assigned a case manager who coordinates all aspects of the patient's care. DOT consists of a health care provider or other responsible person who directly observes that the patient ingests the prescribed medications. Although successful, DOT is a resource intensive program (Herchline, 2020).

Promoting Activity and Adequate Nutrition

Patients with TB are often debilitated from prolonged chronic illness and impaired nutritional status. The nurse plans a progressive activity schedule that focuses on increasing activity tolerance and muscle strength. Anorexia, weight loss, and malnutrition are common in patients with TB. The patient's willingness to eat may be altered by fatigue from excessive coughing; sputum production; chest pain; generalized debilitated state; or cost, if the patient has few resources. Identifying facilities (e.g., shelters, soup kitchens, Meals on Wheels) that provide meals in the patient's neighborhood may increase the likelihood that the patient with limited resources and energy will have access to a more nutritious intake. A nutritional plan that allows for small, frequent meals may be required. Liquid nutritional supplements may assist in meeting basic caloric requirements.

Preventing Transmission of Tuberculosis Infection

To prevent transmission of TB to others, the nurse carefully educates the patient about important hygiene measures, including mouth care, covering the mouth and nose when coughing and sneezing, proper disposal of tissues, and hand hygiene. TB is a disease that must be reported to the health department so that people who have been in contact with the affected patient during the infectious stage can undergo screening and possible treatment, if indicated.

In addition to the risk of transmission of TB infection to other people, it can also be spread to other parts of the body of affected patients. Spread or dissemination of TB infection to nonpulmonary sites of the body is known as miliary TB. Miliary TB is seen in approximately 1.5% of all patients with TB (Lessnau, 2019). It is the result of invasion of the bloodstream by the tubercle bacillus. Usually, it results from late reactivation of a dormant infection in the lung or elsewhere. The origin of the bacilli that enter the bloodstream is either a chronic focus that has ulcerated into a blood vessel or multitudes of miliary tubercles lining the inner surface of the thoracic duct. The organisms migrate from these foci into the bloodstream, are carried throughout the body, and disseminate throughout all tissues, with tiny miliary tubercles developing in the lungs, spleen, liver, kidneys, meninges, and other organs.

The clinical course of miliary TB may vary from an acute, rapidly progressive infection with high fever to a slowly developing process with low-grade fever, anemia, and debilitation. At first, there may be no localizing signs except an enlarged spleen and a reduced number of leukocytes. However, within a few weeks, the chest x-ray reveals small densities scattered diffusely throughout both lung fields; these are the miliary tubercles, which gradually grow.

The possibility of spread to nonpulmonary sites in the body requires careful monitoring for this very serious form of TB. The nurse monitors vital signs and observes for spikes in temperature as well as changes in renal and cognitive function. Few physical signs may be elicited on physical examination of the chest, but at this stage, the patient has a severe cough and dyspnea. Treatment of miliary TB is the same as for pulmonary TB.

Lung Abscess

A lung abscess is a localized collection of pus caused by microbial infection (Kamangar, 2018). It is generally caused by aspiration of anaerobic bacteria. By definition, in a lung abscess, the chest x-ray demonstrates a cavity of at least 2 cm. Patients who are at risk for aspiration of foreign material and development of a lung abscess include those with impaired cough reflexes who cannot close the glottis and those with swallowing difficulties. Other patients at risk include those with central nervous system disorders (e.g., seizure, stroke), substance use disorder, esophageal disease, or compromised immune function; patients without teeth and those receiving nasogastric tube feedings; and patients with an altered state of consciousness due to anesthesia (Bartlett, 2019a).

Pathophysiology

Most lung abscesses are a complication of bacterial pneumonia or are caused by aspiration of oral anaerobes into the lung. Abscesses also may occur secondary to mechanical or functional obstruction of the bronchi by a tumor, foreign body, or bronchial stenosis, or from necrotizing pneumonias, TB, pulmonary embolism (PE), or chest trauma.

Most lung abscesses are found in areas of the lung that may be affected by aspiration. The site of the lung abscess is related to gravity and is determined by position. For patients who are confined to bed, the posterior segment of an upper lobe and the superior segment of the lower lobe are the most common areas. However, atypical presentations may occur, depending on the position of the patient when the aspiration occurred.

Initially, the cavity in the lung may or may not extend directly into a bronchus. Eventually, the abscess becomes surrounded, or encapsulated, by a wall of fibrous tissue. The necrotic process may extend until it reaches the lumen of a bronchus or the pleural space and establishes communication with the respiratory tract, the pleural cavity, or both. If the bronchus is involved, the purulent contents are expectorated continuously in the form of sputum. If the pleura is involved, the result is an empyema. A communication or connection between the bronchus and pleura is known as a bronchopleural fistula. The organisms frequently associated with lung abscesses are anaerobic; however, aerobic organisms may be involved as well. The organisms vary depending on the underlying predisposing factors (Kamangar, 2018).

Clinical Manifestations

The clinical manifestations of a lung abscess may vary from a mild productive cough to acute illness. Most patients have a fever and a productive cough with moderate to copious amounts of foul-smelling, sometimes bloody, sputum. The fever and cough may develop insidiously and may have been present for several weeks before diagnosis. Leukocytosis may be present. Pleurisy or dull chest pain, dyspnea, weakness, anorexia, and weight loss are common.

Assessment and Diagnostic Findings

Physical examination of the chest may reveal dullness on percussion and decreased or absent breath sounds with an intermittent **pleural friction rub** (grating or creaking sound) on auscultation. Crackles may be present. Confirmation of the diagnosis is made by chest x-ray, sputum culture, and, in some cases, fiberoptic bronchoscopy. The chest x-ray reveals an infiltrate with an air–fluid level. A computed tomography (CT) scan of the chest may be required to provide more detailed images of different cross-sectional areas of the lung.

Prevention

The following measures reduce the risk of lung abscess:
- Appropriate antibiotic therapy before any dental procedures in patients who must have teeth extracted while their gums and teeth are infected
- Adequate dental and oral hygiene, because anaerobic bacteria play a role in the pathogenesis of lung abscess
- Appropriate antimicrobial therapy for patients with pneumonia

Medical Management

The findings of the history, physical examination, chest x-ray, and sputum culture indicate the type of organism and the treatment required. Adequate drainage of the lung abscess may be achieved through postural drainage and chest physiotherapy. Patients should be assessed for an adequate cough. Some patients require insertion of a percutaneous chest catheter for long-term drainage of the abscess. Therapeutic use of bronchoscopy to drain an abscess is uncommon. A diet high in protein and calories is necessary, because chronic infection is associated with a catabolic state, necessitating increased intake of calories and protein to facilitate healing. Surgical intervention is rare, but pulmonary resection (lobectomy) is performed if massive hemoptysis occurs or if there is little or no response to medical management.

IV antimicrobial therapy depends on the results of the sputum culture and sensitivity and is given for an extended period. Standard treatment of an anaerobic lung infection is clindamycin, ampicillin-sulbactam, or carbapenem (Bartlett, 2019b). Large IV doses are usually required, because the antibiotic must penetrate the necrotic tissue and the fluid in the abscess. The duration of treatment with IV antibiotics is not well studied and remains controversial (Bartlett, 2019b). Treatment with IV antibiotics may continue for 3 weeks and longer, depending upon the clinical severity and organism involved. Improvement is demonstrated by normal temperature, decreased white blood cell count, and improvement on chest x-ray (resolution of surrounding infiltrate, reduction in cavity size, and absence of fluid). Once improvement is demonstrated, IV antibiotics are discontinued and oral administration of antibiotic therapy is continued for an additional 4 to 12 weeks and sometimes longer. If treatment is stopped too soon, a relapse may occur (Bartlett, 2019b).

Nursing Management

The nurse administers antibiotics and IV treatments as prescribed and monitors for adverse effects. CPT is initiated as prescribed to facilitate drainage of the abscess. The patient is educated on how to perform deep-breathing and coughing exercises to help expand the lungs. To ensure proper nutritional intake, the nurse encourages a diet that is high in protein and calories. The nurse also offers emotional support, because the abscess may take a long time to resolve.

Promoting Home, Community-Based, and Transitional Care

 Educating Patients About Self-Care

A patient who has had surgery may return home before the wound closes entirely or with a drain or tube in place. In these cases, the nurse educates the patient or caregivers about how to change the dressings to prevent skin excoriation and odor, how to monitor for signs and symptoms of infection, and how to care for and maintain the drain or tube. The nurse also reminds the patient to perform deep-breathing and coughing exercises every 2 hours during the day and shows caregivers how to perform chest percussion and postural drainage to facilitate expectoration of lung secretions.

Continuing and Transitional Care

A patient whose condition requires therapy at home may need referral for home, transitional, or community-based care. During home visits, the nurse assesses the patient's physical condition, nutritional status, and home environment, as well as the ability of the patient and family to carry out the therapeutic regimen. Patient education is reinforced, and nutritional counseling is provided with the goal of attaining and maintaining an optimal state of nutrition. To prevent relapses, the nurse emphasizes the importance of completing the antibiotic regimen and of following suggestions for rest and appropriate activity. If IV antibiotic therapy is to continue at home, the services of home health nurses may be arranged to initiate IV therapy and to evaluate its administration by the patient or family.

Although most outpatient IV therapy is given in the home setting, the patient may visit a nearby clinic or provider's office for this treatment. In some cases, patients with lung abscess may have ignored their health. Therefore, the nurse should use this opportunity to address health promotion strategies and health screening with the patient.

Sarcoidosis

Sarcoidosis is a type of interstitial lung disease that is also an inflammatory, multisystem, granulomatous disease of unknown etiology (King, 2019a). Although 90% of patients demonstrate thoracic involvement, any organ may be affected. Sarcoidosis usually presents between 20 and 40 years of age and is slightly more common in women than in men (Weinberger et al., 2019). In the United States, the disease is more common in African Americans, and the estimated prevalence is 10 to 20 per 100,000 people (King, 2019a).

Pathophysiology

Sarcoidosis is thought to be a hypersensitivity response to one or more exogenous agents (bacteria, fungi, virus, chemicals) in people with an inherited or acquired predisposition to the disorder. The hypersensitivity response and inflammation result in the formation of a noncaseating granuloma, which is a noninfectious organized collection of macrophages that appear as a nodule. In the lung, granuloma infiltration and fibrosis may occur, resulting in low lung compliance, impaired diffusing capacity, and reduced lung volumes (King, 2019a).

Clinical Manifestations

Hallmarks of sarcoidosis are its insidious onset and lack of prominent clinical signs or symptoms. The clinical picture depends on the systems affected. The lung is most commonly involved; signs and symptoms may include dyspnea, cough, hemoptysis, and congestion. Other signs include uveitis; joint pain; fever; and granulomatous lesions of the skin, liver, spleen, kidney, and central nervous system. With multisystem involvement, patients may also have fatigue, fever, anorexia, and weight loss. The granulomas may disappear or gradually convert to fibrous tissue.

Assessment and Diagnostic Findings

Chest x-rays and CT scans are used to assess pulmonary adenopathy. These may show hilar adenopathy and disseminated miliary and nodular lesions in the lungs. A mediastinoscopy or **transbronchial** biopsy (in which a tissue specimen is obtained through the bronchial wall) may be used to confirm the diagnosis. In rare cases, an open lung biopsy is performed. Diagnosis is confirmed by a biopsy that shows noncaseating granulomas. Pulmonary function test results are abnormal if there is restriction of lung function (reduction in total lung capacity). Arterial blood gas measurements may be normal or may show hypoxemia (reduced oxygen levels) and hypercapnia (increased carbon dioxide levels).

Medical Management

Many patients undergo remission without specific treatment. Corticosteroids may be beneficial because of their anti-inflammatory effects. Oral corticosteroids have been the most commonly used agents for the relief of symptoms and control of potentially disabling respiratory impairment from pulmonary sarcoidosis. Once begun, corticosteroid therapy is usually continued in tapering doses for 12 months, and longer if the patient has recurrence of symptoms and chest x-ray indications (i.e., continued pulmonary adenopathy) (King, 2019b). Corticosteroids (e.g., prednisone) have been shown to be useful in patients with ocular and myocardial involvement, skin involvement, extensive pulmonary disease that compromises pulmonary function, hepatic involvement, and hypercalcemia. However, it is not known if corticosteroids

alter the long-term course of the disease (King, 2019b). When there is inadequate response to prednisone or the dose cannot be decreased, an immune modulator may be added (e.g., methotrexate, azathioprine, leflunomide, mycophenolate). No single test monitors the progression or recurrence of sarcoidosis; multiple tests are used to monitor involved systems.

Nursing Management

The role of the nurse in the care of patients with sarcoidosis includes supporting the medical regimen and providing education and psychosocial support. Since treatment is aimed at reducing inflammation, patients should be educated on the effects and correct usage of corticosteroids. Patients should be instructed to notify their primary provider if symptoms do not improve or respiratory symptoms worsen. Sarcoidosis is a chronic illness warranting follow-ups at 3 to 6 month intervals to assess disease progression. Patients should be encouraged to contact the Foundation for Sarcoidosis Research to identify additional community resources that can be of assistance to them (see Resources section at the end of the chapter).

PLEURAL DISORDERS

Pleural disorders involve the membranes covering the lungs (visceral pleura) and the surface of the chest wall (parietal pleura) or disorders affecting the pleural space.

Pleurisy

Pleurisy (pleuritis) refers to inflammation of both layers of the pleurae (parietal and visceral). Pleurisy may develop in conjunction with pneumonia or an upper respiratory tract infection, TB, or collagen disease; after trauma to the chest, pulmonary infarction, or PE; in patients with primary or metastatic cancer; and after thoracotomy. The parietal pleura has nerve endings, and the visceral pleura does not. When the inflamed pleural membranes rub together during respiration (intensified on inspiration), the result is severe, sharp, knife-like pain.

Clinical Manifestations

The key characteristic of pleuritic pain is its relationship to respiratory movement. Taking a deep breath, coughing, or sneezing worsens the pain. Pleuritic pain is limited in distribution rather than diffuse; it usually occurs only on one side. The pain may become minimal or absent when the breath is held. It may be localized or radiate to the shoulder or abdomen. Later, as pleural fluid develops, the pain decreases (Weinberger et al., 2019).

Assessment and Diagnostic Findings

In the early period, when little fluid has accumulated, a pleural friction rub can be heard with the stethoscope, only to disappear later as more fluid accumulates and separates the inflamed pleural surfaces. Diagnostic tests may include chest x-rays, sputum analysis, thoracentesis to obtain a specimen of pleural fluid for examination, and, less commonly, a pleural biopsy.

Medical Management

The objectives of treatment are to discover the underlying condition causing the pleurisy and to relieve the pain. As the underlying disease (pneumonia, infection) is treated, the pleuritic inflammation usually resolves. At the same time, the patient must be monitored for signs and symptoms of pleural effusion, such as shortness of breath, pain, assumption of a position that decreases pain, and decreased chest wall excursion.

Prescribed analgesic agents and topical applications of heat or cold provide symptomatic relief. A nonsteroidal anti-inflammatory drug may provide pain relief while allowing the patient to take deep breaths and cough more effectively. If the pain is severe, an intercostal nerve block may be required (Weinberger et al., 2019).

Nursing Management

Because the patient has pain on inspiration, the nurse offers suggestions to enhance comfort, such as turning frequently onto the affected side to splint the chest wall and reduce the stretching of the pleurae. The nurse also educates the patient to use the hands or a pillow to splint the rib cage while coughing.

Pleural Effusion

Pleural effusion, a collection of fluid in the pleural space, is rarely a primary disease process; it is usually secondary to other diseases. Normally, the pleural space contains a small amount of fluid (5 to 15 mL), which acts as a lubricant that allows the pleural surfaces to move without friction (see Fig. 19-4). Pleural effusion may be a complication of heart failure, TB, pneumonia, pulmonary infections (particularly viral infections), nephrotic syndrome, connective tissue disease, PE, and neoplastic tumors. The most common malignancy associated with a pleural effusion is bronchogenic carcinoma.

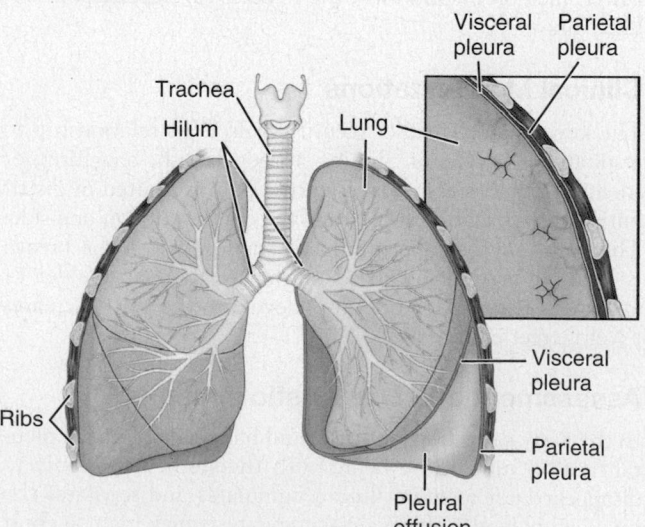

Figure 19-4 • In pleural effusion, an abnormal volume of fluid collects in the pleural space, causing pain and shortness of breath. Pleural effusion is usually secondary to other disease processes.

Pathophysiology

In certain disorders, fluid may accumulate in the pleural space to a point at which it becomes clinically evident. This almost always has pathologic significance. The effusion can be a relatively clear fluid, or it can be bloody or purulent. An effusion of clear fluid may be a transudate or an exudate. A transudate (filtrate of plasma that moves across intact capillary walls) occurs when factors influencing the formation and reabsorption of pleural fluid are altered, usually by imbalances in hydrostatic or oncotic pressures. The finding of a transudative effusion generally implies that the pleural membranes are not diseased. A transudative effusion most commonly results from heart failure. An exudate (extravasation of fluid into tissues or a cavity) usually results from inflammation by bacterial products or tumors involving the pleural surfaces (Heffner, 2019a).

Clinical Manifestations

Usually, the clinical manifestations are caused by the underlying disease. Pneumonia causes fever, chills, and pleuritic chest pain, whereas a malignant effusion may result in dyspnea, difficulty lying flat, and coughing. The severity of symptoms is determined by the size of the effusion, the speed of its formation, and the underlying lung disease. A large pleural effusion causes dyspnea. A small-to-moderate pleural effusion causes minimal or no dyspnea.

Assessment and Diagnostic Findings

Assessment of the area of the pleural effusion reveals decreased or absent breath sounds; decreased fremitus; and a dull, flat sound on percussion. In the case of an extremely large pleural effusion, the assessment reveals a patient in acute respiratory distress. Tracheal deviation away from the affected side may also be apparent.

Physical examination, chest x-ray, chest CT, and thoracentesis confirm the presence of fluid. In some instances, a lateral decubitus x-ray is obtained. For this x-ray, the patient lies on the affected side in a side-lying position. A pleural effusion can be diagnosed because this position allows for the "layering out" of the fluid, and an air–fluid line is visible.

Pleural fluid is analyzed by bacterial culture, Gram stain, AFB stain (for TB), red and white blood cell counts, chemistry studies (glucose, amylase, LDH, and protein), cytologic analysis for malignant cells, and pH. A pleural biopsy also may be performed as a diagnostic tool.

Medical Management

The objectives of treatment are to discover the underlying cause of the pleural effusion; to prevent reaccumulation of fluid; and to relieve discomfort, dyspnea, and respiratory compromise. Specific treatment is directed at the underlying cause (e.g., heart failure, pneumonia, cirrhosis). If the pleural fluid is an exudate, more extensive diagnostic procedures are performed to determine the cause. Treatment of the primary cause is then instituted.

Thoracentesis is performed to remove fluid, to obtain a specimen for analysis, and to relieve dyspnea and respiratory compromise (see Chapter 17). Thoracentesis may be performed under ultrasound guidance. Depending on the size of the pleural effusion, the patient may be treated by removing the fluid during the thoracentesis procedure or by inserting a chest tube connected to a water-seal drainage system or suction to evacuate the pleural space and re-expand the lung.

However, if the underlying cause is a malignancy, the effusion tends to recur within a few days or weeks. Repeated thoracenteses result in pain, depletion of protein and electrolytes, and sometimes pneumothorax. Once the pleural space is adequately drained, a chemical pleurodesis may be performed to obliterate the pleural space and prevent reaccumulation of fluid. Pleurodesis may be performed using either a thoracoscopic approach or a chest tube. A chemically irritating agent (e.g., talc or another chemical irritant) is instilled or aerosolized into the pleural space. With the chest tube approach, after the agent is instilled, the chest tube is clamped for 60 to 90 minutes and the patient is assisted to assume various positions to promote uniform distribution of the agent and to maximize its contact with the pleural surfaces (Heffner, 2019b). The tube is unclamped as prescribed, and chest drainage may be continued several days longer to prevent reaccumulation of fluid and to promote the formation of adhesions between the visceral and parietal pleurae.

Other treatments for pleural effusions caused by malignancy include surgical pleurectomy, insertion of a small catheter attached to a drainage bottle for outpatient management (e.g., PleurX® catheter), or implantation of a pleuroperitoneal shunt. A pleuroperitoneal shunt consists of two catheters connected by a pump chamber containing two one-way valves. Fluid moves from the pleural space to the pump chamber and then to the peritoneal cavity. The patient manually pumps on the reservoir daily to move fluid from the pleural space to the peritoneal space.

Nursing Management

The nurse's role in the care of a patient with a pleural effusion includes supporting the medical regimen. The nurse prepares and positions the patient for thoracentesis and offers support throughout the procedure. The nurse ensures the thoracentesis fluid amount is recorded and sent for appropriate laboratory testing. If a chest tube drainage and water-seal system is used, the system's function is monitored and the amount of drainage is recorded at prescribed intervals (see later discussion). Nursing care related to the underlying cause of the pleural effusion is specific to the underlying condition.

Patients with a pleural effusion secondary to a malignancy may have a chest tube inserted to instill talc (Bhatnagar, Piotrowska, Laskawiec-Szkonter, et al., 2019). Pain management is a priority, and the nurse helps the patient assume positions that are the least painful. However, frequent turning and movement are important to facilitate adequate spreading of the talc over the pleural surface. The nurse evaluates the patient's pain level and administers analgesic agents as prescribed and as needed.

If the patient is to be managed as an outpatient with a pleural catheter for drainage, the nurse educates the patient and family about management and care of the catheter and drainage system.

Empyema

An empyema is an accumulation of thick, purulent fluid within the pleural space, often with fibrin development and a loculated (walled-off) area where infection is located (Strange, 2019).

Pathophysiology

Most empyemas occur as complications of bacterial pneumonia or lung abscess. They also result from penetrating chest trauma, hematogenous infection of the pleural space, nonbacterial infections, and iatrogenic causes (after thoracic surgery or thoracentesis). At first the pleural fluid is thin, with a low leukocyte count, but it frequently progresses to a fibropurulent stage and, finally, to a stage where it encloses the lung within a thick exudative membrane (loculated empyema).

Clinical Manifestations

The patient is acutely ill and has signs and symptoms similar to those of an acute respiratory infection or pneumonia (fever, night sweats, pleural pain, cough, dyspnea, anorexia, weight loss). If the patient is immunocompromised, the symptoms may be vague. If the patient has received antimicrobial therapy, the clinical manifestations may be less obvious.

Assessment and Diagnostic Findings

Chest auscultation demonstrates decreased or absent breath sounds over the affected area, and there is dullness on chest percussion as well as decreased fremitus. The diagnosis is established by chest CT. Usually, a diagnostic thoracentesis is performed, often under ultrasound guidance.

Medical Management

The objectives of treatment are to drain the pleural cavity and to achieve complete expansion of the lung. The fluid is drained, and appropriate antibiotics (usually begun by the IV route) in large doses are prescribed based on the causative organism. Sterilization of the empyema cavity requires 4 to 6 weeks of antibiotics (Strange, 2019). Drainage of the pleural fluid depends on the stage of the disease and is accomplished by one of the following methods:

- Thoracentesis (needle aspiration) with a thin percutaneous catheter, if the volume is small and the fluid is not too purulent or too thick
- Tube thoracostomy (chest drainage using a large-diameter intercostal tube attached to water-seal drainage; see later discussion) with thrombolytic agents instilled through the chest tube in patients with loculated or complicated pleural effusions
- Open chest drainage via thoracotomy, including potential rib resection, to remove the thickened pleura, pus, and debris and to remove the underlying diseased pulmonary tissue

With long-standing inflammation, an exudate can form over the lung, trapping it and interfering with its normal expansion. This exudate must be removed surgically by decortication. The drainage tube is left in place until the pus-filled space is obliterated completely. The complete obliteration of the pleural space is monitored by serial chest x-rays, and the patient should be informed that treatment may be long term (weeks to months). Patients are frequently discharged from the hospital with a chest tube in place, with instructions to monitor fluid drainage at home.

Nursing Management

Resolution of empyema is a prolonged process. The nurse helps the patient cope with the condition and instructs the patient in lung-expanding breathing exercises to restore normal respiratory function. The nurse also provides care specific to the method of drainage of the pleural fluid (e.g., needle aspiration, closed chest drainage, rib resection, and drainage). When the patient is discharged home with a drainage tube or system in place, the nurse instructs the patient and family on care of the drainage system and drain site, measurement and observation of drainage, signs and symptoms of infection, and how and when to contact the primary provider (see later discussion).

 ACUTE RESPIRATORY FAILURE

Respiratory failure is a sudden and life-threatening deterioration of the gas exchange function of the lungs and indicates their failure to provide adequate oxygenation or ventilation for the blood. Acute respiratory failure is defined as hypoxemia (a decrease in arterial oxygen tension [PaO_2] to less than 60 mm Hg) and hypercapnia (an increase in arterial carbon dioxide tension [$PaCO_2$] to greater than 50 mm Hg), with acidosis (an arterial pH of less than 7.35) (Kaynar, 2018).

It is important to distinguish between acute and chronic respiratory failure. Chronic respiratory failure is defined as deterioration in the gas exchange function of the lungs that has developed insidiously or has persisted for a long period after an episode of acute respiratory failure. The absence of acute symptoms and the presence of a chronic respiratory acidosis suggest the chronicity of the respiratory failure. Two causes of chronic respiratory failure are COPD (discussed in Chapter 20) and neuromuscular diseases (discussed in Chapter 65). Patients with these disorders develop a tolerance to the gradually worsening hypoxemia and hypercapnia. However, patients with chronic respiratory failure can develop acute failure. For example, a patient with COPD may develop an exacerbation or infection that causes additional deterioration of gas exchange. The principles of management of acute versus chronic respiratory failure are different; the following discussion is limited to acute respiratory failure.

Pathophysiology

In acute respiratory failure, the ventilation or perfusion mechanisms in the lung are impaired. Some of the many ventilatory failure mechanisms leading to acute respiratory failure include impaired function of the central nervous system (e.g., drug overdose, head trauma, infection, hemorrhage, sleep apnea), neuromuscular dysfunction (e.g., myasthenia gravis, Guillain–Barré syndrome, amyotrophic lateral sclerosis, spinal cord trauma), musculoskeletal dysfunction (e.g., chest trauma, kyphoscoliosis, malnutrition), and pulmonary dysfunction (e.g., COPD, asthma, cystic fibrosis).

Oxygenation failure mechanisms leading to acute respiratory failure include pneumonia, ARDS, heart failure, COPD, PE, and **restrictive lung diseases** (diseases that cause decrease in lung volumes).

In the postoperative period, especially after major thoracic or abdominal surgery, inadequate ventilation and respiratory failure may occur because of several factors. During this period, for example, acute respiratory failure may be caused by the effects of anesthetic, analgesic, and sedative agents, which may depress respiration (as described earlier) or enhance the effects of opioids and lead to hypoventilation. Pain may interfere with deep breathing and coughing. A $\dot{V}/\dot{Q}$ mismatch is the usual cause of respiratory failure after major abdominal, cardiac, or thoracic surgery.

Clinical Manifestations

Early signs are those associated with impaired oxygenation and may include restlessness, fatigue, headache, dyspnea, air hunger, tachycardia, and increased blood pressure. As the hypoxemia progresses, more obvious signs may be present, including confusion, lethargy, tachycardia, tachypnea, central cyanosis, diaphoresis, and finally respiratory arrest. Physical findings are those of acute respiratory distress, including the use of accessory muscles, decreased breath sounds if the patient cannot adequately ventilate, and other findings related specifically to the underlying disease process and cause of acute respiratory failure.

Medical Management

The objectives of treatment are to correct the underlying cause and to restore adequate gas exchange in the lungs. ET intubation and mechanical ventilation may be required to maintain adequate ventilation and oxygenation while the underlying cause is corrected (see later discussion on ET intubation and mechanical ventilation).

Nursing Management

Nursing management of patients with acute respiratory failure includes assisting with intubation and maintaining mechanical ventilation. Patients are usually managed in the intensive care unit (ICU). The nurse assesses the patient's respiratory status by monitoring the level of responsiveness, arterial blood gases, pulse oximetry, and vital signs. In addition, the entire respiratory system is assessed and strategies to prevent complications (e.g., turning schedule, mouth care, skin care, and range of motion of extremities) are implemented. The nurse also assesses the patient's understanding of the management strategies that are used and initiates some form of communication to enable the patient to express concerns and needs to the health care team.

Finally, the problems that led to the acute respiratory failure are addressed. As the patient's status improves, the nurse assesses the patient's knowledge of the underlying disorder and provides education as appropriate to address the disorder.

Endotracheal Intubation

Endotracheal intubation involves passing an ET tube through the nose or mouth into the trachea (see Fig. 19-5). The oral route is preferred since oral intubation is associated with less trauma and lesser rates of infection; furthermore, the oral route can typically accommodate a larger diameter ET tube than may be passed when the nasal route is used. Intubation provides a patent airway when the patient is having respiratory distress that cannot be treated with simpler methods and is the method of choice in emergency care. ET intubation

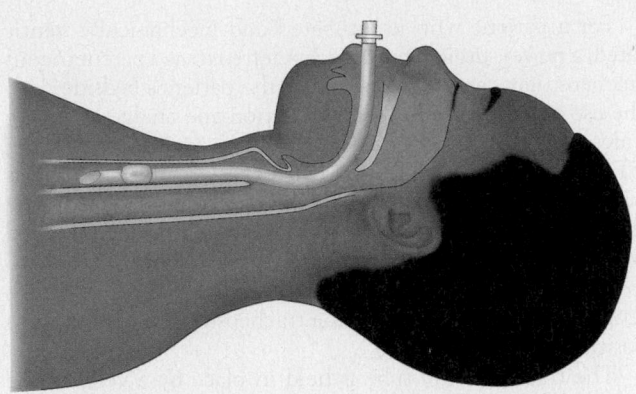

Figure 19-5 • Endotracheal tube in place. The tube has been inserted using the oral route. The cuff has been inflated to maintain the tube's position and to minimize the risk of aspiration.

is a means of providing an airway for patients who cannot maintain an adequate airway on their own (e.g., patients who are comatose and patients with upper airway obstruction), for patients needing mechanical ventilation, and for suctioning secretions from the pulmonary tree.

An ET tube usually is passed with the aid of a laryngoscope by specifically trained medical, nursing, or respiratory therapy personnel. Once the tube is inserted and positioned about 2 cm above the carina, a cuff at the distal end of the ET tube is inflated with the use of a pilot balloon. Inflation of the cuff prevents air from leaking around the outer part of the tube in order to minimize the possibility of aspiration and secure the tube. The position of the ET tube is verified by checking end-tidal carbon dioxide levels and confirmed with chest x-ray. Chart 19-12 discusses the nursing care of the patient with an ET tube.

Complications can occur from pressure exerted by the cuff on the tracheal wall. Cuff pressures should be maintained between 20 and 25 mm Hg (24 and 30 cm H_2O) because high cuff pressure can cause tracheal bleeding, ischemia, and pressure necrosis, whereas low cuff pressure can increase the risk of aspiration pneumonia. Routine deflation of the cuff is not recommended because of the increased risk of aspiration and **hypoxia** (i.e., decrease in oxygen supply to the tissues and cells) (Urden et al., 2018). Tracheobronchial secretions are suctioned through the tube. Warmed, humidified oxygen should always be introduced through the tube, whether the patient is breathing spontaneously or is receiving ventilatory support. ET intubation may be used for no longer than 14 to 21 days, by which time a tracheostomy must be considered to decrease irritation of and trauma to the tracheal lining, to reduce the incidence of vocal cord paralysis (secondary to laryngeal nerve damage), and to decrease the work of breathing (Wiegand, 2017).

ET and tracheostomy tubes have several disadvantages. The tubes cause discomfort. The cough reflex is depressed because glottis closure is hindered. Secretions tend to become thicker because the warming and humidifying effect of the upper respiratory tract has been bypassed. The swallowing reflexes (glottic, pharyngeal, and laryngeal reflexes) are depressed because of prolonged disuse and the mechanical trauma produced by the ET or tracheostomy tube, increasing the risk of aspiration as well as microaspiration and subsequent VAP (Urden et al., 2018). In addition, ulceration and stricture of the larynx or trachea may develop. Of great concern to the patient is the inability to talk and to communicate needs.

Tracheostomy

A **tracheotomy** is a surgical procedure in which an opening is made into the trachea. The indwelling tube inserted into the

---

Chart 19-12 Care of the Patient with an Endotracheal Tube

Immediately After Intubation

1. Check symmetry of chest expansion.
2. Auscultate breath sounds of anterior and lateral chest bilaterally.
3. Obtain capnography or end-tidal CO_2 as indicated.
4. Ensure chest x-ray obtained to verify proper tube placement.
5. Check cuff pressure every 6 to 8 hours.
6. Monitor for signs and symptoms of aspiration.
7. Ensure high humidity; a visible mist should appear in the T-piece or ventilator tubing.
8. Administer oxygen concentration as prescribed by the primary provider.
9. Secure the tube to the patient's face with tape, and mark the proximal end for position maintenance.
   a. Cut proximal end of tube if it is longer than 7.5 cm (3 inches) to prevent kinking.
   b. Insert an oral airway or mouth device if orally intubated to prevent the patient from biting and obstructing the tube.
10. Use sterile suction technique and airway care to prevent iatrogenic contamination and infection.
11. Continue to reposition patient every 2 hours and as needed to prevent atelectasis and to optimize lung expansion.
12. Provide oral hygiene and suction the oropharynx whenever necessary.

Extubation (Removal of Endotracheal Tube)

1. Explain procedure.
2. Have self-inflating bag and mask ready in case ventilatory assistance is required immediately after extubation.
3. Suction the tracheobronchial tree and oropharynx, remove tape, and then deflate the cuff.
4. Give 100% oxygen for a few breaths, then insert a new, sterile suction catheter inside tube.
5. Have the patient inhale. At peak inspiration, remove the tube, suctioning the airway through the tube as it is pulled out.

Note: In some hospitals, this procedure can be performed by respiratory therapists; in others, by nurses. Check hospital policy.

Care of Patient Following Extubation

1. Give heated humidity and oxygen by facemask and maintain the patient in a sitting or high-Fowler position.
2. Monitor respiratory rate and quality of chest excursions. Note stridor, color change, and change in mental alertness or behavior.
3. Monitor the patient's oxygen level using a pulse oximeter.
4. Keep patient NPO (nothing by mouth), or give only ice chips for next few hours.
5. Provide mouth care.
6. Educate the patient about how to perform coughing and deep-breathing exercises.

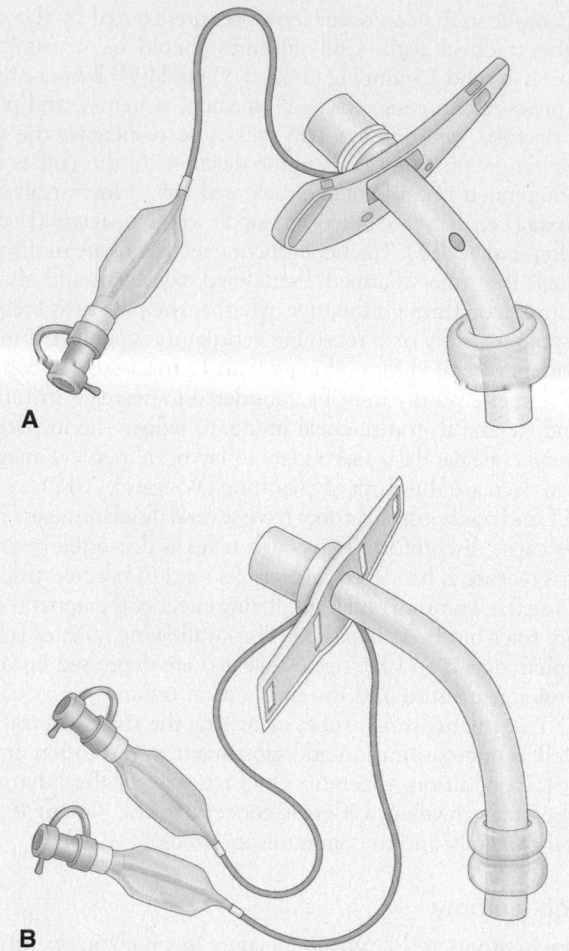

Figure 19-6 • Tracheostomy tubes. **A.** Fenestrated tube, which allows patient to talk. **B.** Double-cuffed tube. Inflating the two cuffs alternately can help prevent tracheal damage.

trachea is called a **tracheostomy tube** (see Fig. 19-6 for the different types of tracheostomy tubes). A tracheostomy (the stoma that is the product of the tracheotomy) may be either temporary or permanent.

A tracheotomy is used to maintain a patent airway, bypass an upper airway obstruction, facilitate removal of tracheobronchial secretions, permit the long-term use of mechanical ventilation, replace an ET tube, and prevent aspiration of oral or gastric secretions in the patient who is unconscious or paralyzed (by closing off the trachea from the esophagus). Many disease processes and emergency conditions make a tracheotomy necessary.

Tracheotomy

The tracheotomy procedure is usually performed in the operating room under general anesthesia, where the patient's ventilation can be well controlled and optimal aseptic technique can be maintained. A surgical opening is made between the second and third tracheal rings. After the trachea is exposed, a cuffed tracheostomy tube of an appropriate size is inserted. The cuff is an inflatable attachment to the tracheostomy tube that is designed to occlude the space between the tracheal walls and the tube, to permit effective mechanical ventilation, and to minimize the risk of aspiration.

For a patient who is intubated and mechanically ventilated, a newer surgical technique referred to as a percutaneous tracheostomy can be performed at the patient's bedside with the use of local anesthesia and sedation and analgesia. Using video-assisted guidance, a bronchoscope is passed down the ET tube. Following ET tube cuff deflation, the ET tube is withdrawn to the subglottic level. An opening is made in the skin between the second and third tracheal ring and enlarged with the use of dilators until the space is large enough to safely insert a tracheostomy tube. The ET tube and bronchoscope are then removed and the tracheostomy is secured into position (Lindman, 2018).

The tracheostomy tube is held in place by a velcro tube holder or twill tape ties fastened around the patient's neck. Usually, a square of sterile gauze is placed between the tube and the skin to absorb drainage and reduce the risk of infection.

Complications

Complications may occur early or late in the course of tracheostomy tube management. They may even occur years after the tube has been removed. Early complications include tube dislodgement, accidental decannulation, bleeding, pneumothorax, air embolism, aspiration, subcutaneous or mediastinal emphysema, recurrent laryngeal nerve damage, and posterior tracheal wall penetration. Long-term complications include airway obstruction from accumulation of secretions or protrusion of the cuff over the opening of the tube, infection, rupture of the innominate artery, dysphagia, tracheoesophageal fistula, tracheal dilation, tracheal ischemia, and necrosis. Tracheal stenosis may develop after the tube is removed. Chart 19-13 outlines measures nurses can take to prevent complications with use of ET and tracheostomy tubes.

Care of the Patient with an Endotracheal Tube or Tracheostomy

The patient requires continuous monitoring and assessment. The newly made opening must be kept patent by proper suctioning of secretions. After the vital signs are stable, the patient is placed in a semi-Fowler position to facilitate ventilation, promote drainage, minimize edema, and prevent strain on the suture lines. Analgesia and sedative agents must be given with caution because of the risk of suppressing the cough reflex.

Chart 19-13

Preventing Complications Associated with Endotracheal and Tracheostomy Tubes

- Administer adequate warmed humidity.
- Maintain cuff pressure at appropriate level.
- Suction as needed per assessment findings.
- Maintain skin integrity. Change tape and dressing as needed or per protocol.
- Auscultate lung sounds.
- Monitor for signs and symptoms of infection, including temperature and white blood cell count.
- Administer prescribed oxygen and monitor oxygen saturation.
- Monitor for cyanosis.
- Maintain adequate hydration of the patient.
- Use sterile technique when suctioning and performing tracheostomy care.

Major objectives of nursing care are to ensure a patent airway, monitor the patient's respiratory status, assess for complications, alleviate the patient's apprehension, and provide an effective means of communication. The nurse keeps paper and pencil or a Magic Slate® or a cellular device and the call light within the patient's reach at all times to ensure a means of communication.

For the procedural guidelines for nursing care of a patient with a tracheostomy tube, go to **thepoint.lww.com/Brunner15e**.

Suctioning the Tracheostomy or Endotracheal Tube

When a tracheostomy or ET tube is in place, it is usually necessary to suction the patient's secretions because of the decreased effectiveness of the cough mechanism. Tracheal suctioning is performed when adventitious breath sounds are detected or whenever secretions are obviously present. Unnecessary suctioning can initiate bronchospasm and cause mechanical trauma to the tracheal mucosa.

All equipment that comes into direct contact with the patient's lower airway must be sterile to prevent sepsis.

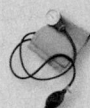

For the procedural guidelines for suctioning a patient with a tracheostomy tube, go to **thepoint.lww.com/Brunner15e**.

In patients who are mechanically ventilated (see later discussion), an in-line suction catheter may be used to allow rapid suction when needed and to minimize cross-contamination by airborne pathogens. An in-line suction device allows the patient to be suctioned without being disconnected from the ventilator circuit. In-line suctioning (also called *closed suctioning*) decreases hypoxemia, sustains PEEP, and can decrease patient anxiety associated with suctioning (Wiegand, 2017). Because in-line suctioning protects staff from patient secretions, it can be performed in most cases without using personal protective gear. A notable exception is when the patient has COVID-19, when PPE must be used.

Managing the Cuff

The cuff on an ET or tracheostomy tube should be inflated if the patient requires mechanical ventilation or is at high risk for aspiration. The pressure within the cuff should be the lowest possible pressure (20 to 25 mm Hg) that allows delivery of adequate tidal volumes and prevents pulmonary aspiration (Urden et al., 2018). Cuff pressure must be monitored by the respiratory therapist or nurse at least every 8 hours by attaching a handheld pressure gauge to the pilot balloon of the tube or by using the minimal leak volume or minimal occlusion volume technique.

Promoting Home, Community-Based, and Transitional Care

Educating Patients About Self-Care. If the patient is pending discharge to the home setting with a tracheostomy tube, the nurse should ensure that suction and other appropriate equipment is in place in the home prior to discharge. The nurse also educates the patient and family about daily care, including techniques to prevent infection, as well as measures to take in an emergency. The nurse provides the patient and family with a list of community contacts for education and support needs.

Continuing and Transitional Care. A referral for home, community-based, or transitional care is indicated for ongoing assessment of the patient and of the ability of the patient and family to provide appropriate and safe care. The nurse assesses the patient's and family's ability to cope with the physical changes and psychological issues associated with having a tracheostomy. Minimizing the amount of dust or particles in the air and providing adequate humidification may make it easier for the patient to breathe. Dust and particles in the air can be decreased by removing drapes and upholstered furniture; using air filters; and washing floors, dusting, and vacuuming frequently. The nurse identifies resources and makes referrals for appropriate services to assist the patient and family to manage the tracheostomy tube at home.

Mechanical Ventilation

Mechanical ventilation may be required to manage acute respiratory failure. It may also be indicated for a variety of other reasons including to: control the patient's respirations during surgery or treatment, oxygenate the blood when the patient's ventilatory efforts are inadequate, and rest the respiratory muscles. Many patients placed on a ventilator can breathe spontaneously, although the effort needed to do so may be exhausting.

A **mechanical ventilator** is a positive- or negative-pressure breathing device that can maintain ventilation and oxygen delivery for a prolonged period.

Indications

If a patient has evidence of respiratory failure or a compromised airway, ET intubation and mechanical ventilation are indicated. This clinical evidence may be corroborated by a continuous decrease in PaO_2, an increase in $PaCO_2$, and a persistent acidosis (decreased pH); however, if the patient's status appears emergent, then waiting for these laboratory results prior to ensuring these ventilator support measures is imprudent. Conditions such as thoracic or abdominal surgery, drug overdose, neuromuscular disorders, inhalation injury, COPD, multiple trauma, shock, multisystem failure, and coma may lead to respiratory failure and the need for mechanical ventilation. General indications for mechanical ventilation are displayed in Chart 19-14.

Classification of Ventilators

Mechanical ventilators were traditionally classified according to the method by which they supported ventilation. The two general categories are negative- and positive-pressure ventilators. Figure 19-7 displays commonly used positive-pressure ventilators. Negative-pressure ventilators (e.g., "iron lungs," chest cuirass) are older modes of ventilatory support that are rarely utilized today.

Positive-Pressure Ventilators

Positive-pressure ventilators inflate the lungs by exerting positive pressure on the airway, pushing air in, similar to a bellows mechanism, and forcing the alveoli to expand during inspiration. Expiration occurs passively. ET intubation

Indications for Mechanical Ventilation

Laboratory Values

PaO_2 <55 mm Hg
$PaCO_2$ >50 mm Hg and pH <7.32
Vital capacity <10 mL/kg
Negative inspiratory force <25 cm H_2O
FEV_1 <10 mL/kg

Clinical Manifestations

Apnea or bradypnea
Respiratory distress with confusion
Increased work of breathing not relieved by other interventions
Confusion with need for airway protection
Circulatory shock
Controlled hyperventilation (e.g., patient with a severe head injury)

Adapted from Amitai, A. (2018). Introduction to ventilator management. *Medscape.* Retrieved on 2/2/2020 at: emedicine.medscape.com/article/810126-overview

or tracheostomy is usually necessary. These ventilators are widely used in the hospital setting and are increasingly used in the home for patients with primary lung disease. Three types of positive-pressure ventilators are classified by the method of ending the inspiratory phase of respiration: volume-cycled, pressure-cycled, and high-frequency oscillatory support. The fourth type, noninvasive positive-pressure ventilation (NIPPV), does not require intubation (Wiegand, 2017).

Volume-Cycled Ventilators. Volume-cycled ventilators deliver a preset volume of air with each inspiration. Once this preset volume is delivered to the patient, the ventilator cycles off and exhalation occurs passively. From breath to breath, the volume of air delivered by the ventilator is relatively constant, ensuring consistent, adequate breaths despite varying airway pressures. A major disadvantage to using volume-cycled ventilators is that patients may experience barotrauma (trauma to the trachea or alveoli secondary to positive pressure) because the pressures required to deliver the breaths may be excessive. This trauma causes damage to the alveolar capillary membrane and air to leak into the surrounding tissues (Urden et al., 2018).

Pressure-Cycled Ventilators. When the pressure-cycled ventilator cycles on, it delivers a flow of air (inspiration) until it reaches a preset pressure, and then cycles off, and expiration occurs. The major limitation is the volume of air or oxygen can vary as the patient's airway resistance or compliance changes. As a result, the tidal volume delivered (i.e., volume of air inspired and expired with each breath) may be inconsistent, possibly compromising ventilation.

High-Frequency Oscillatory Support Ventilators. These types of ventilators deliver very high respiratory rates (i.e., 180 to 900 breaths/min) that are accompanied by very low tidal volumes and high airway pressures (hence the name *high-frequency oscillatory support*). These small pulses of oxygen-enriched air move down the center of the airways, allowing alveolar air to exit the lungs along the margins of the airways. This ventilatory mode is used to open the alveoli in situations characterized by closed small airways, such as atelectasis and ARDS and it is also thought to protect the lung from pressure injury (Wiegand, 2017).

Noninvasive Positive-Pressure Ventilation. NIPPV is a method of positive-pressure ventilation that can be given via facemasks that cover the nose and mouth, nasal masks, or other oral or nasal devices such as the nasal pillow (a small nasal cannula that seals around the nares to maintain the prescribed pressure). NIPPV eliminates the need for ET intubation or tracheostomy and decreases the risk of nosocomial infections such as pneumonia. The most comfortable mode for the patient is pressure-controlled ventilation with pressure support. This eases the work of breathing and enhances gas exchange. The ventilator can be set with a minimum backup rate for patients with periods of apnea.

Patients are candidates for NIPPV if they have acute or chronic respiratory failure, acute pulmonary edema, COPD, chronic heart failure, or a sleep-related breathing disorder. The technique also may be used at home to improve tissue oxygenation and to rest the respiratory muscles while patients sleep at night. NIPPV is contraindicated for those who have experienced respiratory arrest, serious arrhythmias, cognitive impairment, or head or facial trauma. NIPPV may also be used for obstructive sleep apnea, for patients at the end of life, and for those who do not want ET intubation but may need short- or long-term ventilatory support (Wiegand, 2017).

Continuous positive airway pressure (CPAP) provides positive pressure to the airways throughout the respiratory cycle. Although it can be used as an adjunct to mechanical ventilation with a cuffed ET tube or tracheostomy tube to open the alveoli, it is also used with a leak-proof mask to keep alveoli open, thereby preventing respiratory failure. CPAP is an effective treatment of obstructive sleep apnea because the positive pressure acts as a splint, keeping the upper airway and trachea open during sleep. To use CPAP, the patient must be breathing independently.

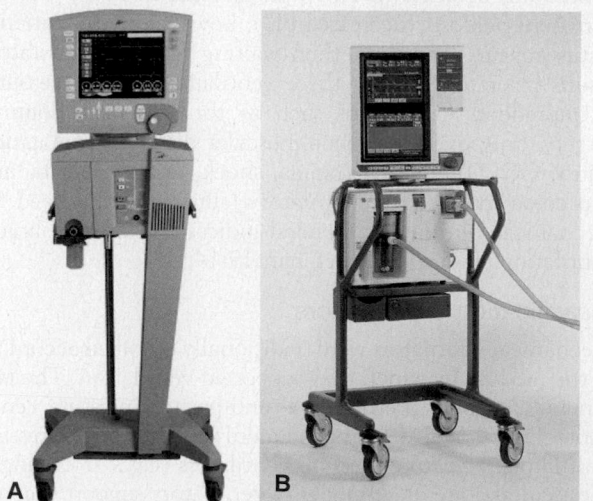

Figure 19-7 • Positive-pressure ventilators. **A.** The AVEA can be used to both ventilate and monitor neonatal, pediatric, and adult patients. It can also deliver noninvasive ventilation with Heliox to adult and pediatric patients. Courtesy of Vyaire Medical Inc., Yorba Linda, CA. **B.** The Puritan-Bennett 840 Ventilator System has volume, pressure, and mixed modes designed for adult, pediatric, and infant ventilation. Courtesy of Tyco Healthcare/Nellcor Puritan Bennett, Pleasanton, CA.

Bilevel positive airway pressure (BiPAP) ventilation offers independent control of inspiratory and expiratory pressures while providing pressure support ventilation (PSV). It delivers two levels of positive airway pressure provided via a nasal or oral mask, nasal pillow, or mouthpiece with a tight seal and a portable ventilator. Each inspiration can be initiated either by the patient or by the machine if it is programmed with a backup rate. The backup rate ensures that the patient receives a set number of breaths per minute. BiPAP is most often used for patients who require ventilatory assistance at night, such as those with severe COPD or sleep apnea. Tolerance is variable; BiPAP usually is most successful with patients who are highly motivated.

Ventilator Modes

Ventilator mode refers to how breaths are delivered to the patient. The most commonly used modes are controlled mechanical ventilation, continuous mandatory ventilation, also known as assist–control (A/C), intermittent mandatory ventilation (IMV), synchronized intermittent mandatory ventilation (SIMV), PSV, and airway pressure release ventilation (APRV) (see Fig. 19-8).

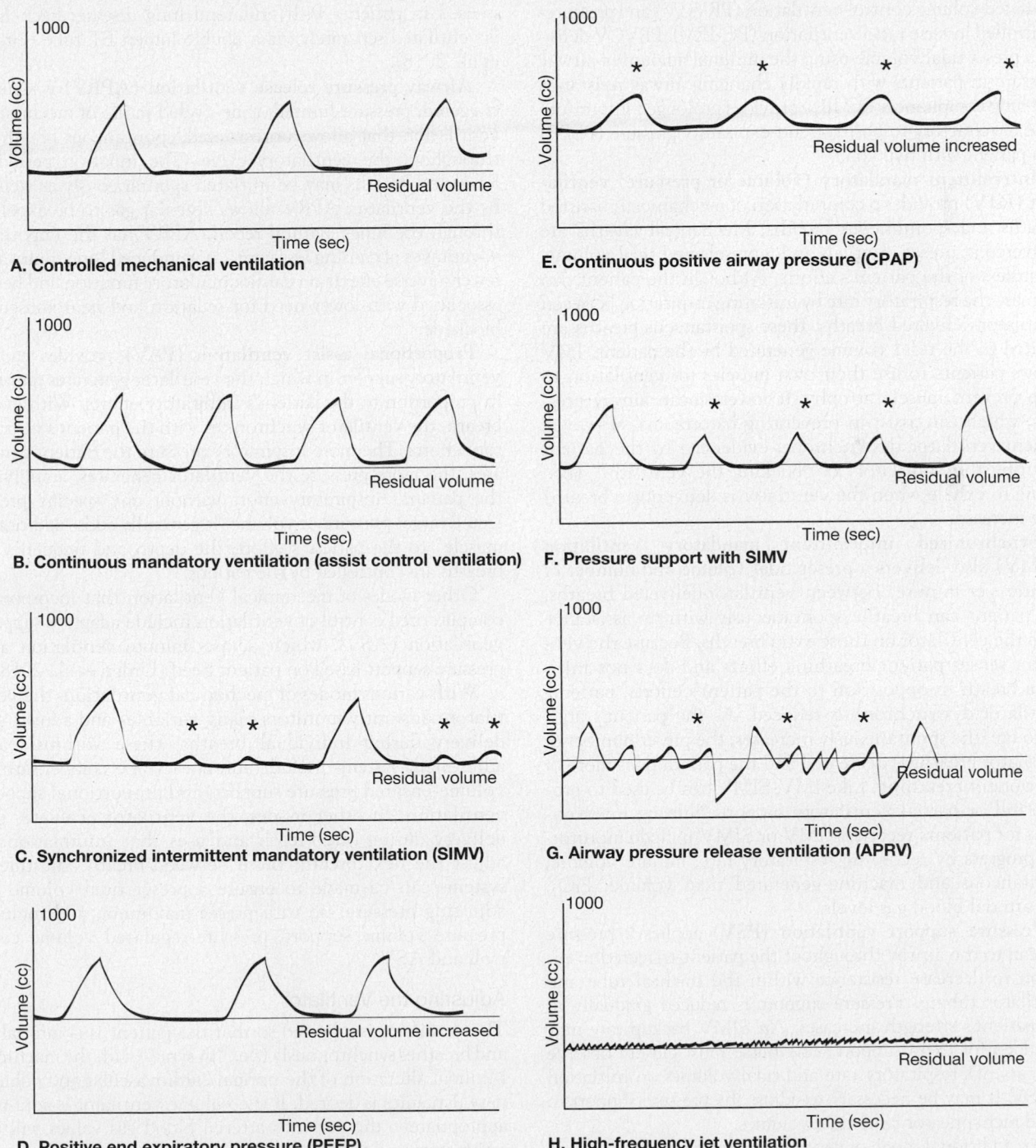

Figure 19-8 • Modes of mechanical ventilation with airflow waveforms. Inhalations marked with an asterisk (*) are spontaneous.

Controlled mechanical ventilation provides full ventilator support by delivering a preset tidal volume and respiratory rate. This mode of ventilation is indicated for patients who are apneic. In A/C ventilation, more commonly called **continuous mandatory (volume or pressure) ventilation (CMV)**, the ventilator delivers a preset tidal volume or pressure at a preset rate of respirations. However, if the patient initiates a breath between the machine's breaths, the ventilator delivers at the preset volume or pressure (assisted breath). Therefore, every breath is the preset volume or pressure, regardless of whether it is initiated by the patient or the ventilator. Two variations to CMV include: pressure-regulated volume control ventilation (PRVCV) and pressure-controlled inverse ratio ventilation (PC-IRV). PRVCV delivers a preset tidal volume using the minimal amount of airway pressure in patients with rapidly changing airway resistance and lung compliance. PC-IRV provides prolonged inspiratory time in refractory to positive end-expiratory pressure (PEEP) in a patient with hypoxia.

Intermittent mandatory (volume or pressure) ventilation (IMV) provides a combination of mechanically assisted breaths and spontaneous breaths. Mechanical breaths are delivered at preset intervals and a preselected tidal volume, regardless of the patient's efforts. Although the patient can increase the respiratory rate by initiating inspiration between ventilator-delivered breaths, these spontaneous breaths are limited to the tidal volume generated by the patient. IMV allows patients to use their own muscles for ventilation to help prevent muscle atrophy. It lowers mean airway pressure, which can assist in preventing barotrauma. However, patient-ventilator dyssynchrony, evidenced by the patient "fighting the ventilator" or "bucking the ventilator" (i.e., trying to exhale when the ventilator is delivering a breath) may increase.

Synchronized intermittent mandatory ventilation (SIMV) also delivers a preset tidal volume and number of breaths per minute. Between ventilator-delivered breaths, the patient can breathe spontaneously with no assistance from the ventilator on those extra breaths. Because the ventilator senses patient breathing efforts and does not initiate a breath in opposition to the patient's efforts, patient-ventilator dyssynchrony is reduced. As the patient's ability to breathe spontaneously increases, the preset number of ventilator breaths is decreased and the patient does more of the work of breathing. Like IMV, SIMV can be used to provide full or partial ventilatory support. Nursing interventions for patients receiving IMV or SIMV include monitoring progress by recording respiratory rate, minute volume, spontaneous and machine-generated tidal volume, FiO_2, and arterial blood gas levels.

Pressure support ventilation (PSV) applies a pressure plateau to the airway throughout the patient-triggered inspiration to decrease resistance within the tracheal tube and ventilator tubing. Pressure support is reduced gradually as the patient's strength increases. An SIMV backup rate may be added for extra support. The nurse must closely observe the patient's respiratory rate and tidal volumes on initiation of PSV. It may be necessary to adjust the pressure support to avoid tachypnea or large tidal volumes.

An additional mode of ventilation used to facilitate weaning is volume-assisted pressure support ventilation (VAPSV)

also referred to as pressure augmentation (PA). This mode of ventilation ensures the patient receives a minimum tidal volume with each pressure support breath.

A newer mode of ventilation which requires an esophageal catheter to monitor electrical activity of the diaphragm is neurally adjusted ventilatory assist (NAVA). This mode delivers assisted breaths in synchrony with the patient's own breath. The esophageal catheter monitors electrical activity of the diaphragm and signals the ventilator when to initiate a breath.

Another unique mode of ventilation used in special circumstances is independent lung ventilation (ILV). This mode is used in patients with unilateral lung disease. Each lung is ventilated separately via a double lumen ET tube (Urden et al., 2018).

Airway pressure release ventilation (APRV) is a time-triggered, pressure-limited, time-cycled mode of mechanical ventilation that allows unrestricted, spontaneous breathing throughout the ventilatory cycle. The inflation period is long, and breaths may be initiated spontaneously as well as by the ventilator. APRV allows alveolar gas to be expelled through the lungs' natural recoil. APRV has the important advantages of causing less ventilator-induced lung injury and fewer adverse effects on cardiocirculatory function and being associated with lower need for sedation and neuromuscular blockade.

Proportional assist ventilation (PAV) provides partial ventilatory support in which the ventilator generates pressure in proportion to the patient's inspiratory efforts. With every breath, the ventilator synchronizes with the patient's ventilatory efforts. The more inspiratory pressure the patient generates, the more pressure the ventilator generates, amplifying the patient's inspiratory effort without any specific preselected target pressure or volume. It generally adds "additional muscle" to the patient's effort; the depth and frequency of breaths are controlled by the patient.

Other modes of mechanical ventilation that incorporate computerized control of ventilation include adaptive support ventilation (ASV), which adjusts minute ventilation and pressure support based on patient need (Urden et al., 2018).

With various modes of mechanical ventilation, the ventilator constantly monitors many variables and adjusts gas delivery during individual breaths; these within-breath adjustment systems include automatic tube compensation, volume-ensured pressure support, and proportional support ventilation. In other modes, the ventilator evaluates gas delivery during one breath and uses that information to adjust the next breath; these between-breath adjustment systems can be made to ensure a preset tidal volume by adjusting pressure, up to a preset maximum, and include pressure volume support, pressure-regulated volume control, and ASV.

Adjusting the Ventilator

The ventilator is adjusted so that the patient is comfortable and breathes synchronously (i.e., "in sync") with the machine. Minimal alteration of the normal cardiovascular and pulmonary dynamics is desired. If the volume ventilator is adjusted appropriately, the patient's arterial blood gas values will be satisfactory and there will be little or no cardiovascular compromise. Chart 19-15 describes initial ventilator settings.

Chart 19-15	Initial Ventilator Settings

The following guide is an example of the steps involved in operating a mechanical ventilator. The nurse, in collaboration with the respiratory therapist, always reviews the manufacturer's instructions, which vary according to the equipment, before beginning mechanical ventilation.

1. Set the machine to deliver the tidal volume required (6 to 10 mL/kg) or (4 to 8 mL/kg for patients with ARDS).
2. Adjust the machine to deliver the lowest concentration of oxygen to maintain normal PaO_2 (greater than 60 mm Hg) or an SpO_2 level greater than 92%. This setting may be high initially but will gradually be reduced based on arterial blood gas (ABG) results.
3. Record peak inspiratory pressure.
4. Set mode (continuous mandatory ventilation [also known as assist–control], or synchronized intermittent mandatory ventilation) and rate as prescribed by the primary provider. (See the glossary for definitions of modes of mechanical ventilation.) Set positive end-expiratory pressure (PEEP) and pressure support if prescribed.
5. Set sigh settings (usually set at 1.5 times the tidal volume and ranging from 1 to 3 per hour), if applicable.
6. Adjust sensitivity so that the patient can trigger the ventilator with a minimal effort (usually 2 mm Hg negative inspiratory force).
7. Record minute volume and obtain ABGs to measure carbon dioxide partial pressure ($PaCO_2$), pH, and PaO_2 after 20 minutes of continuous mechanical ventilation.
8. Adjust setting (FiO_2 and rate) according to results of ABG analysis to provide normal values or those set by the primary provider.
9. If there is poor coordination between the breathing rhythms of the patient and the ventilator (i.e., patient-ventilator dyssynchrony), assess for hypoxia and manually ventilate on 100% oxygen with a resuscitation bag.

Adapted from Amitai, A. (2018). Introduction to ventilator management. *Medscape.* Retrieved on 2/2/2020 at: emedicine.medscape.com/article/810126-overview

NURSING PROCESS

The Patient Receiving Mechanical Ventilation

Nursing management of patients with acute respiratory failure includes assisting with intubation and maintaining mechanical ventilation. Furthermore, caring for a patient on mechanical ventilation has become an integral part of nursing care for many patients in critical care or general medical-surgical units, extended care facilities, and the home. Nurses, physicians, and respiratory therapists must understand each patient's specific pulmonary needs and work together to set realistic goals. Positive patient outcomes depend on an understanding of the principles of mechanical ventilation and the patient's care needs as well as open communication among members of the health care team about the goals of therapy, weaning plans, and the patient's tolerance of changes in ventilator settings.

Assessment

The nurse plays a vital role in assessing the patient's status and the functioning of the ventilator. In assessing the patient, the nurse evaluates the patient's physiologic status and how they are coping with mechanical ventilation. Physical assessment includes systematic assessment of all body systems, with an in-depth focus on the respiratory system. Respiratory assessment includes vital signs, respiratory rate and pattern, breath sounds, evaluation of spontaneous ventilatory effort, and potential evidence of hypoxia (e.g., skin color). Increased adventitious breath sounds may indicate a need for suctioning. The nurse maintains the patient's head of the bed so that it is elevated 30 degrees or higher unless contraindicated to prevent the risk of aspiration and VAP. The nurse verifies endotracheal tube position as applicable and evaluates the settings and functioning of the mechanical ventilator. Although the nurse may not be primarily responsible for adjusting the settings on the ventilator or measuring ventilator parameters (these are usually responsibilities of the respiratory therapist), the nurse is responsible for the patient and therefore needs to evaluate how the ventilator affects the patient's overall status.

When monitoring the ventilator, the nurse notes the following:

- Controlling mode (e.g., CMV ventilation and SIMV).
- Tidal volume and rate settings (tidal volume is usually set at 6 to 10 mL/kg [ideal body weight] or 4 to 8 mL/kg for the patient with ARDS [ideal body weight]; rate is usually set at 12 to 16 breaths/min).
- FiO_2 setting may be set between 21% and 100% to maintain an optimal PaO_2 level (e.g., greater than 60 mm Hg) or SpO_2 level greater than 92%.
- Peak inspiratory pressure (PIP) (normal is 15 to 20 cm H_2O; this increases if there is increased airway resistance or decreased compliance).
- Sensitivity (A 2 cm H_2O inspiratory force should trigger the ventilator).
- Inspiratory-to-expiratory ratio (usually 1:2 [1 second of inspiration to 2 seconds of expiration] unless inverse ratio is ordered).
- Minute volume (tidal volume × respiratory rate).
- Sigh settings (usually set at 1.5 times the tidal volume and ranging from 1 to 3 per hour), if applicable.
- Water in the tubing, disconnection or kinking of the tubing, which, if present, are corrected.
- Humidification (humidifier filled with water) and temperature.
- Alarms (turned on and functioning properly at all times per The Joint Commission [TJC] Alarm Safety Goal) (TJC, 2020).
- PEEP and pressure support level, if applicable.

As is true with any type of patient-sensitive life support equipment, mechanical ventilators have multiple alarms that are set to alert the health care team of potential patient problems. With the increased number of alarms and their high sensitivity to subtle changes, members of the health care team, including nurses, are at risk for experiencing alarm fatigue, which means that they may become desensitized to alarms and not respond to them with sufficient speed. According to the National Patient Safety Goals (TJC, 2020), measures must be instituted to prevent alarm fatigue.

Assessment also addresses the patient's neurologic status and effectiveness of coping with the need for assisted ventilation and the changes that accompany it. The nurse assesses the patient's comfort level and ability to communicate as well. Because weaning from mechanical ventilation requires adequate nutrition, it is important to assess the patient's gastrointestinal system and nutritional status.

Diagnosis

NURSING DIAGNOSES

Based on the assessment data, major nursing diagnoses may include:

- Impaired gas exchange associated with underlying illness, ventilator setting adjustments, or weaning
- Impaired airway clearance associated with increased mucus production associated with presence of the tube in trachea or continuous positive-pressure mechanical ventilation
- Risk for injury and infection associated with endotracheal intubation or tracheostomy
- Impaired mobility associated with ventilator dependency
- Impaired verbal communication associated with endotracheal tube or tracheostomy tube
- Difficulty coping associated with ventilator dependency

COLLABORATIVE PROBLEMS/POTENTIAL COMPLICATIONS

Based on the assessment data, potential complications may include the following (see Table 19-5):

- Ventilator problems (increase in peak airway pressure or decrease in pressure or loss of volume)
- Alterations in cardiac function
- Barotrauma and pneumothorax
- Pulmonary infection and sepsis (e.g., VAP; see Chart 19-6)
- Delirium and postintensive care syndrome

Planning and Goals

The major goals for the patient may include achievement of optimal gas exchange, maintenance of a patent airway, absence of injury or infection, attainment of optimal mobility, adjustment to nonverbal methods of communication, acquisition of successful coping measures, and absence of complications.

Nursing Interventions

Nursing care of the patient who is mechanically ventilated requires expert technical and interpersonal skills. Nursing interventions are similar regardless of the setting; however, the frequency of interventions and the stability of the patient vary from setting to setting. Nursing interventions for the patient who is mechanically ventilated are not uniquely different from those for patients with other pulmonary disorders, but astute nursing assessment and a therapeutic nurse–patient relationship are critical. The specific interventions used by the nurse are determined by the underlying disease process and the patient's response.

TABLE 19-5	Troubleshooting Problems with Mechanical Ventilation	
Problem	**Cause**	**Solution**
Ventilator Problems		
Increase in peak airway pressure	Coughing or plugged airway tube	Suction airway for secretions; empty condensation fluid from circuit.
	Patient-ventilator dyssynchrony	Adjust sensitivity; consider administering sedatives as prescribed
	Decreasing lung compliance	Manually ventilate patient. Assess for hypoxia or bronchospasm. Check arterial blood gas values. Sedate only if necessary.
	Tubing kinked	Check tubing; reposition patient; insert oral airway if necessary.
	Pneumothorax	Manually ventilate patient; notify primary provider.
	Atelectasis or bronchospasm	Clear secretions.
Decrease in pressure or loss of volume	Increase in compliance	None.
	Leak in ventilator or tubing; cuff on tube/humidifier not tight	Check entire ventilator circuit for patency. Correct leak.
Patient Problems		
Cardiovascular compromise	Decrease in venous return due to application of positive pressure to lungs	Assess for adequate volume status by measuring heart rate, blood pressure, central venous pressure, pulmonary capillary wedge pressure, and urine output; notify primary provider if values are abnormal.
Barotrauma/pneumothorax	Application of positive pressure to lungs; high mean airway pressures lead to alveolar rupture	Notify primary provider. Prepare patient for chest tube insertion. Avoid high pressure settings for patients with COPD, ARDS, or history of pneumothorax.
Pulmonary infection	Bypass of normal defense mechanisms; frequent breaks in ventilator circuit; decreased mobility; impaired cough reflex	Use strict aseptic technique. Provide frequent mouth care. Optimize nutritional status.

ARDS, acute respiratory distress syndrome; COPD, chronic obstructive pulmonary disease.

Two general nursing interventions that are important in the care of the patient who is mechanically ventilated are pulmonary auscultation and interpretation of arterial blood gas measurements. The nurse is often the first to note changes in physical assessment findings or significant trends in blood gases that signal the development of a serious problem (e.g., pneumothorax, tube displacement, pulmonary embolus).

ENHANCING GAS EXCHANGE

The purpose of mechanical ventilation is to optimize gas exchange by maintaining alveolar ventilation and oxygen delivery. The alteration in gas exchange may be caused by the underlying illness or by mechanical factors related to adjustment of the ventilator to the patient. The health care team, including the nurse, physician, and respiratory therapist, continually assesses the patient for adequate gas exchange, signs and symptoms of hypoxia, and response to treatment. Therefore, the nursing diagnosis of impaired gas exchange is, by its complex nature, multidisciplinary and collaborative. The team members must share goals and information freely. All other goals directly or indirectly relate to this primary goal.

Nursing interventions to promote optimal gas exchange include judicious administration of analgesic agents to relieve pain without suppressing the respiratory drive and frequent repositioning to diminish the pulmonary effects of immobility. The nurse also monitors for adequate fluid balance by assessing for the presence of peripheral edema, calculating daily intake and output, and monitoring daily weights. The nurse administers medications prescribed to control the primary disease and monitors for their side effects.

PROMOTING EFFECTIVE AIRWAY CLEARANCE

Continuous positive-pressure ventilation increases the production of secretions regardless of the patient's underlying condition. The nurse assesses for the presence of secretions by lung auscultation at least every 2 to 4 hours. Measures to clear the airway of secretions include suctioning, CPT, frequent position changes, and increased mobility as soon as possible. Frequency of suctioning should be determined by patient assessment. If excessive secretions are identified by inspection or auscultation techniques, suctioning should be performed. Sputum is not produced continuously or every 1 to 2 hours but as a response to a pathologic condition. Therefore, there is no rationale for routine suctioning of all patients every 1 to 2 hours. Although suctioning is used to aid in the clearance of secretions, it can damage the airway mucosa and impair cilia action.

The sigh mechanism on the ventilator may be adjusted to deliver at least 1 to 3 sighs per hour at 1.5 times the tidal volume if the patient is receiving A/C ventilation. Periodic sighs prevent atelectasis and the further retention of secretions. Because of the risk for hyperventilation and trauma to pulmonary tissue from excess ventilator pressure (barotrauma, pneumothorax), the sigh feature is not used frequently. If the SIMV mode is being used, the mandatory ventilations act as sighs because they are of greater volume than the patient's spontaneous breaths.

Humidification of the airway via the ventilator is maintained to help liquefy secretions so that they are more easily removed. Bronchodilators may be indicated to dilate the bronchioles in patients with acute lung injury or COPD and are classified as adrenergic or anticholinergic. Adrenergic bronchodilators (see Chapter 20, Table 20-4) are mostly inhaled and work by stimulating the beta-receptor sites, mimicking the effects of epinephrine in the body. The desired effect is smooth muscle relaxation, which dilates the constricted bronchial tubes. Anticholinergic bronchodilators (see Chapter 20, Table 20-4) produce airway relaxation by blocking cholinergic-induced bronchoconstriction. Patients receiving bronchodilator therapy of either type should be monitored for adverse effects, including dizziness, nausea, decreased oxygen saturation, hypokalemia, increased heart rate, and urine retention. Mucolytic agents (e.g., acetylcysteine) may also be indicated in these patients to liquefy secretions so that they are more easily mobilized. Nursing management of patients receiving mucolytic therapy includes assessment of an adequate cough reflex, sputum characteristics, and (in patients not receiving mechanical ventilation) improvement in incentive spirometry. Side effects include nausea, vomiting, bronchospasm, stomatitis (oral ulcers), urticaria, and rhinorrhea (runny nose) (Karch, 2020).

PREVENTING INJURY AND INFECTION

Maintaining the endotracheal or tracheostomy tube is an essential part of airway management. Cuff pressure is monitored every 8 hours to maintain the pressure at 20 to 25 mm Hg (Urden et al., 2018). The nurse assesses for the presence of a cuff leak at the same time. The nurse positions the ventilator tubing so that there is minimal pulling or distortion of the tube in the trachea, reducing the risk of trauma to the trachea. Unintentional or premature removal of the tube is a potentially life-threatening complication of endotracheal intubation. Removal of the tube is a frequent problem in intensive care units (ICUs) and occurs mainly during nursing care or by the patient. Nurses must instruct and remind patients and family members about the purpose of the tube and the dangers of removing it. Baseline and ongoing assessment of the patient and of the equipment ensures effective care. Providing comfort measures, including opioid analgesia and sedation, can improve the patient's tolerance of the endotracheal tube.

> ### ▶ Quality and Safety Nursing Alert
>
> *Inadvertent removal of an endotracheal tube can cause laryngeal swelling, hypoxemia, bradycardia, hypotension, and even death. Measures must be taken to prevent premature or inadvertent removal.*

To prevent tube removal by the patient, the nurse should explain to the patient and family the purpose of the tube, distract the patient through one-to-one interaction or with television, and maintain comfort measures. If the patient cannot move the arms and hands to the endotracheal tube, restraints are not needed. If the patient is alert, oriented, able to follow directions, and cooperative to the point that it is highly unlikely that they will remove the endotracheal tube, restraints are not needed. However, if the nurse determines there is a risk that the patient may try to remove the tube, the least invasive method of restraints (e.g., soft wrist restraints and hand mitts) may be appropriate as prescribed by the primary provider (check agency policy) (TJC, 2019). The rationale for use of restraints should be documented, and the patient's significant others should receive explanations why restraints are necessary. Close monitoring of the patient is essential to ensure safety and prevent harm.

Patients with an endotracheal or tracheostomy tube do not have the normal defenses of the upper airway. In addition, these patients frequently have multiple additional body system disturbances that lead to immune compromise. Tracheostomy care is performed at least every 8 hours, and more frequently if needed, because of the increased risk of infection. The ventilator circuit tubing and in-line suction tubing are replaced periodically, according to infection prevention guidelines, to decrease the risk of infection.

The nurse administers oral hygiene frequently because the oral cavity is a primary source of contamination of the lungs in the patient who is intubated. The presence of a nasogastric tube in the patient who is intubated can increase the risk of aspiration, leading to nosocomial pneumonia. The nurse positions the patient with the head elevated above the stomach as much as possible. Chart 19-6 provides an overview of strategies to prevent VAP.

PROMOTING OPTIMAL LEVEL OF MOBILITY

Being connected to a ventilator limits the patient's mobility. Immobility in patients who are mechanically ventilated is associated with decreases in muscle strength and increases length of hospital stay, as well as increased mortality rates (Hodgson, Capell, & Tipping, 2018). The nurse helps the patient whose condition has become stable to get out of bed and move to a chair as soon as possible. If the patient is unable to get out of bed, the nurse encourages performance of active range-of-motion exercises at least every 6 to 8 hours. If the patient cannot perform these exercises, the nurse performs passive range-of-motion exercises at least every 8 hours to prevent contractures and venous stasis.

PROMOTING OPTIMAL COMMUNICATION

It is important to develop alternative methods of communication for the patient who is receiving mechanical ventilation. The nurse assesses the patient's communication abilities to evaluate for limitations. Questions to consider when assessing the ability of the patient who is ventilator dependent to communicate include the following:

- Is the patient conscious and able to communicate? Can the patient nod or shake their head?
- Is the patient's mouth unobstructed by the tube so that words can be mouthed?
- Is the patient's dominant hand strong and available for writing? For example, if the patient is right handed, the IV line should be placed in the left arm if possible so that the right hand is free.
- Is the patient a candidate for a fenestrated tracheostomy tube or a one-way speaking valve (such as Passy-Muir valve® or Olympic Trach-Talk®) that permits talking?

Once the patient's limitations are known, the nurse offers several appropriate communication approaches: lip or speech reading (use single key words), pad and pencil or Magic Slate®, iPad® or tablet, communication board, gesturing, sign language, or electric larynx. The use of a "talking" or fenestrated tracheostomy tube or one-way valve may be suggested to the primary provider, which would allow the patient to talk while on the ventilator. The nurse makes sure that the patient's eyeglasses, hearing aid, sign interpreter, and language translator are available if needed to enhance the patient's ability to communicate.

Some communication methods may be frustrating to the patient, family, and nurse; these need to be identified and minimized. A speech therapist can assist in determining the most appropriate method.

PROMOTING COPING ABILITY

Dependence on a ventilator is frightening to both the patient and the family and disrupts even the most stable families. Encouraging the family to verbalize their feelings about the ventilator, the patient's condition, and the environment in general is beneficial. Explaining procedures every time they are performed helps reduce anxiety and familiarizes the patient with ventilator procedures. To restore a sense of control, the nurse encourages the patient to use alternative methods of communication in order to participate in decisions about care, schedules, and treatment when possible. The patient may become withdrawn or depressed while receiving mechanical ventilation, especially if its use is prolonged. To promote effective coping, the nurse informs the patient about progress when appropriate. It is important to provide diversions such as watching television, playing music, or taking a walk (if appropriate and possible). Stress reduction techniques (e.g., a back rub, relaxation measures) relieve tension and help the patient deal with anxieties and fears about both the condition and the dependence on the ventilator.

MONITORING AND MANAGING POTENTIAL COMPLICATIONS

Alterations in Cardiac Function. Alterations in cardiac output may occur as a result of positive-pressure ventilation. The positive intrathoracic pressure during inspiration compresses the heart and great vessels, thereby reducing venous return and cardiac output. This is usually corrected during exhalation when the positive pressure is off. The patient may have decreased cardiac output and resultant decreased tissue perfusion and oxygenation.

To evaluate cardiac function, the nurse first observes for signs and symptoms of hypoxia (restlessness, apprehension, confusion, tachycardia, tachypnea, pallor progressing to cyanosis, diaphoresis, transient hypertension, and decreased urine output). If a pulmonary artery catheter is in place, cardiac output, cardiac index, and other hemodynamic values can be used to assess the patient's status (see Chapter 21).

Barotrauma and Pneumothorax. Excessive positive pressure can cause lung damage, or barotrauma, which may result in a spontaneous pneumothorax, which may quickly develop into a tension pneumothorax, further compromising venous return, cardiac output, and blood pressure (see later discussion). The nurse considers any sudden changes in oxygen saturation or the onset of respiratory distress to be a life-threatening emergency requiring immediate action.

Pulmonary Infection. The patient is at high risk for infection, as described earlier. The nurse reports fever or a change in the color or odor of sputum to the primary provider for follow-up (see earlier discussion of VAP). Subglottic secretions may increase the patients' risk for the development of VAP. Patients expected to be intubated for longer than 72 hours may benefit from the use of an endotracheal tube with a subglottic suction port. This extra port that is connected to continuous suction (20 to 30 cm H_2O) allows for the removal of secretions above the cuff (Urden et al., 2018).

Delirium and Postintensive Care Syndrome. Patients who are critically ill are at risk for delirium during their time in the ICU. They are also at risk for cognitive impairment at a level consistent with mild dementia that may persist for months after they are discharged to the home setting. This critical illness-associated cognitive impairment is called postintensive care syndrome (PICS). The Awakening and Breathing Coordination, Delirium monitoring and management, Early mobility, Family engagement and empowerment (ABCDEF) bundle proposes an interdisciplinary process using evidence-based practice to manage delirium and weakness in the patient who is critically ill. It is believed that implementing this bundle can mitigate risks for delirium and possibly PICS. The goals of this bundle are to improve communication among members of the health care team, standardize care related to the assessment and use of sedation, provide nonpharmacologic interventions in the management of delirium, provide early exercise and ambulation, and incorporate family's concerns and participation in care planning (see Chart 19-16) (Marra, Ely, Pandharipande, et al., 2017).

Chart 19-16 The ABCDEF Bundle

The *A*wakening and *B*reathing *C*oordination, *D*elirium monitoring and management, *E*arly mobility, *F*amily engagement and empowerment bundle

Overview: Typically, patients on mechanical ventilators require some form of sedation or analgesia during their hospital stay. Recent studies suggest a correlation between the use of potent sedatives and analgesia and ICU-acquired delirium, oversedation, prolonged mechanical ventilation, and postintensive care syndrome (PICS).

Key components of each of the categories of the ABCDEF Bundle include:

1. *Awakening and spontaneous breathing trials*
   Using predefined criteria:
   - The nurse determines if it is safe to stop sedation.
   - If determined safe, the nurse will determine if patient tolerated the sedation interruption.
   - If the patient tolerated the interruption, the respiratory therapist will determine if the patient is a candidate for a breathing trial.
   - If the patient is a candidate for a breathing trial, the respiratory therapist and nurse will evaluate the patient's response.
2. *Monitoring and management of delirium*
   - The nurse assesses the patient at least every 2 to 4 hours using a sedation assessment scale (e.g., the CAM-ICU, see Chapter 11).
3. *Early Mobility*
   The nurse assesses the patient using the following criteria for mobility:
   - The patient is able to respond to verbal stimuli.
   - The patient is receiving less than 60% FiO_2 and less than 10 cm of PEEP.
   - The patient has no circulatory or central catheters or injuries that may contraindicate mobility.
4. *Family Engagement*
   - The nurse encourages engagement of family members and ensures unrestricted access for a designated family support person.

ICU, intensive care unit; PEEP, positive end-expiratory pressure.
Adapted from Shay, A. (2018). Optimizing the ABCDEF bundle. *American Nurse Today, 13*(7), 21–23.

PROMOTING HOME, COMMUNITY-BASED, AND TRANSITIONAL CARE

Increasingly, patients are being cared for in extended care facilities or at home while receiving mechanical ventilation, with a tracheostomy tube, or receiving oxygen therapy. Patients receiving home ventilator care usually have a chronic neuromuscular condition or COPD. Providing the opportunity for patients who are ventilator dependent to return home to live with their families in familiar surroundings can be a positive experience. The ultimate goal of home ventilator therapy is to enhance the patient's quality of life, not simply to support or prolong life.

Educating Patients About Self-Care. Caring for the patient with mechanical ventilator support at home can be accomplished successfully. A home or transitional care team consisting of the nurse, physician, respiratory therapist, social service or home care agency, and equipment supplier is needed. The home is evaluated to determine whether the electrical equipment needed can be operated safely. Chart 19-17 summarizes the basic assessment criteria needed for successful home care.

Once the decision to initiate mechanical ventilation at home is made, the nurse prepares the patient and family for home care. The nurse educates the patient and family about the ventilator, suctioning, tracheostomy care, signs of pulmonary infection, cuff inflation and deflation, and assessment of vital signs. Education begins in the hospital and continues at home. Nursing responsibilities include evaluating the patient's and family's understanding of the information presented.

The nurse educates the family about cardiopulmonary resuscitation, including mouth-to-tracheostomy tube (instead of mouth-to-mouth) breathing. The family is also instructed how to handle a power failure, which usually involves

---

Chart 19-17 Criteria for Successful Home Ventilator Care

The decision to proceed with home ventilation therapy is usually based on the following parameters.

Patient Criteria

- The patient has a chronic underlying pulmonary or neuromuscular disorder.
- The patient's clinical pulmonary status is stable.
- The patient is willing to go home on mechanical ventilation.

Home Criteria

- The home environment is conducive to care of the patient.
- The electrical facilities are adequate to operate all equipment safely.
- The home environment is controlled, without drafts in cold weather and with proper ventilation in warm weather.
- Space is available for cleaning and storing ventilator equipment.

Family Criteria

- Family members are competent, dependable, and willing to spend the time required for proper training as primary caregivers.
- Family members understand the diagnosis and prognosis.
- Family has sufficient financial and supportive resources and can obtain professional support if necessary.

Chart 19-18 **HOME CARE CHECKLIST**

Ventilator Care

At the completion of education, the patient and/or caregiver will be able to:

- Name the procedure that was performed, as indicated, and how the patient's present status impacts physiologic functioning, ADLs, IADLs, relationships, and spirituality.
- State the name, dose, side effects, frequency, and schedule for all medications.
- State what types of changes are needed (if any) to maintain a clean home environment and prevent infection.
- State how to contact the primary provider, the team of home care professionals overseeing care, respiratory vendor and obtain supplies.
- Complete CPR training program for caregivers.
- Identify a plan for operation of ventilator and other devices during a power outage or other emergency.
- State proper care of patient on ventilator:
  - Observe physical signs such as color, secretions, breathing pattern, and state of consciousness.
  - Perform physical care such as suctioning, postural drainage, and ambulation.
  - Observe the tidal volume and pressure manometer regularly. Intervene when they are abnormal (i.e., suction if airway pressure increases).
  - Provide a communication method for the patient (e.g., pad and pencil, electric larynx, talking tracheostomy tube, and sign language).
  - Monitor vital signs as directed.

- Use a predetermined signal to indicate when feeling short of breath or in distress.
- Care for and maintain equipment properly:
  - Check the ventilator settings twice each day and whenever the patient is removed from the ventilator.
  - Adjust the volume and pressure alarms if needed.
  - Fill humidifier as needed and check its level three times a day.
  - Empty water in tubing as needed.
  - Use a clean humidifier when circuitry is changed.
  - Keep exterior of ventilator clean and free of any objects.
  - Change external circuitry once a week or more often as indicated.
  - Report malfunction or strange noises immediately.
- Identify the contact details for support services for patients and their caregivers/families.

Resources

See Chapter 20, Figure 20-6 for additional information on postural drainage positions.

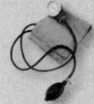

For the procedural guidelines for caring for a patient with a tracheostomy tube and performing tracheal suction, go to **thepoint.lww.com/Brunner15e.**

ADLs, activities of daily living; IADLs, instrumental activities of daily living.

---

converting the ventilator from an electrical power source to a battery power source. Conversion is automatic in most types of home ventilators and lasts approximately 1 hour. In addition, instructions are provided on the use of a manual self-inflation bag, should it be necessary. Chart 19-18 lists some of the patient's and family's responsibilities.

Continuing and Transitional Care. A home health or transitional care nurse monitors and evaluates how well the patient and family are adapting to providing care in the home. The nurse assesses the adequacy of the patient's ventilation and oxygenation as well as airway patency. The nurse addresses any unique adaptation problems that the patient may have and listens to the patient's and family's anxieties and frustrations, offering support and encouragement where possible. The nurse helps identify and contact community resources that may assist in home management of the patient with mechanical ventilation.

The technical aspects of the ventilator are managed by vendor follow-up. A respiratory therapist usually is assigned to the patient and makes home visits to evaluate the patient and perform a maintenance check of the ventilator as needed.

Transportation services are identified in case the patient requires transportation in an emergency. These arrangements must be made before an emergency arises.

Evaluation

Expected patient outcomes may include:

1. Exhibits adequate gas exchange, as evidenced by normal breath sounds, acceptable arterial blood gas levels, and vital signs

2. Demonstrates adequate ventilation with minimal mucus accumulation
3. Is free of injury or infection, as evidenced by normal temperature, white blood cell count, and clear sputum
4. Is mobile within limits of ability
   a. Gets out of bed to chair, bears weight, or ambulates as soon as possible
   b. Performs range-of-motion exercises every 6 to 8 hours
5. Communicates effectively through written messages, gestures, or other communication strategies
6. Copes effectively
   a. Verbalizes fears and concerns about condition and equipment
   b. Participates in decision making when possible
   c. Uses stress reduction techniques when necessary
7. Absence of complications
   a. Absence of cardiac compromise, as evidenced by stable vital signs and adequate urine output
   b. Absence of pneumothorax, as evidenced by bilateral chest excursion, normal chest x-ray, and adequate oxygenation
   c. Absence of pulmonary infection, as evidenced by normal temperature, clear pulmonary secretions, and negative sputum cultures
   d. Absence of delirium and of postintensive care syndrome, as evidenced by no patient-ventilator dyssynchrony, and being oriented to person, place, and time

Weaning the Patient from the Ventilator

Respiratory weaning, the process of withdrawing the patient from dependence on the ventilator, takes place in three stages: the patient is gradually removed from the ventilator, then from either the ET or tracheostomy tube, and finally from oxygen. Weaning from mechanical ventilation is performed at the earliest possible time consistent with patient safety. The decision must be made from a physiologic rather than a mechanical viewpoint. A thorough understanding of the patient's clinical status is required in making this decision. Weaning is started when the patient is physiologically and hemodynamically stable, demonstrates spontaneous breathing capability, recovering from the acute stage of medical and surgical problems, and when the cause of respiratory failure is sufficiently reversed (Wiegand, 2017). Chart 19-19 presents information about patient care during weaning from mechanical ventilation.

Successful weaning involves collaboration among the primary provider, respiratory therapist, and nurse. Each health care provider must understand the scope and function of other team members in relation to patient weaning to conserve the patient's strength, use resources efficiently, and maximize successful outcomes.

Criteria for Weaning

Careful assessment is required to determine whether the patient is ready to be removed from mechanical ventilation. If the patient is stable and showing signs of improvement or reversal of the disease or condition that caused the need for mechanical ventilation, weaning indices should be assessed (see Chart 19-19).

Stable vital signs and arterial blood gases are also important predictors of successful weaning. Once readiness has been determined, the nurse records baseline measurements of weaning indices to monitor progress.

Patient Preparation

To maximize the likelihood of success of weaning, the nurse must consider the patient as a whole, taking into account factors that impair the delivery of oxygen and elimination of carbon dioxide as well as those that increase oxygen demand (e.g., sepsis, seizures, thyroid imbalances) or decrease the patient's overall strength (e.g., inadequate nutrition, neuromuscular disease). Adequate psychological preparation is necessary before and during the weaning process.

Methods of Weaning

Successful weaning depends on the combination of adequate patient preparation, available equipment, and an interdisciplinary approach to solve patient problems (see Chart 19-19). All usual modes of ventilation can be used for weaning.

CPAP (also known as spontaneous mode ventilation in this context) allows the patient to breathe spontaneously while applying positive pressure throughout the respiratory cycle to keep the alveoli open and promote oxygenation. Providing CPAP during spontaneous breathing also offers the advantage of an alarm system and may reduce patient anxiety if the patient has been taught that the machine is keeping track of breathing. It also maintains lung volumes and improves the patient's oxygenation status. CPAP is often used in conjunction with PSV. Nurses should carefully assess

---

Chart 19-19

Care of the Patient Being Weaned from Mechanical Ventilation

1. Assess patient for weaning criteria:
   a. Vital capacity: 10 to 15 mL/kg
   b. Maximum inspiratory pressure (MIP) at least –20 cm H_2O
   c. Tidal volume: 7 to 9 mL/kg
   d. Minute ventilation: 6 L/min
   e. Rapid/shallow breathing index: Below 100 breaths/min/L; PaO_2 >60 mm Hg with FiO_2 <40%
2. Monitor activity level, assess dietary intake, and monitor results of laboratory tests of nutritional status. Reestablishing independent spontaneous ventilation can be physically exhausting. It is crucial that the patient have enough energy reserves to succeed.
3. Assess the patient's and family's understanding of the weaning process and address any concerns about the process. Explain that the patient may feel short of breath initially and provide encouragement as needed. Reassure the patient that they will be attended closely and that if the weaning attempt is not successful, it can be tried again later.
4. Implement the weaning method as prescribed (e.g., continuous positive airway pressure [CPAP] and T-piece).
5. Monitor vital signs, pulse oximetry, electrocardiogram, and respiratory pattern constantly for the first 20 to 30 minutes and every 5 minutes after that until weaning is complete. Monitoring the patient closely provides ongoing indications of success or failure.
6. Maintain a patent airway; monitor arterial blood gas levels and pulmonary function tests. Suction the airway as needed.
7. In collaboration with the primary provider, terminate the weaning process if adverse reactions occur. These include a heart rate increase of 20 bpm, systolic blood pressure increase of 20 mm Hg, a decrease in oxygen saturation to <90%, respiratory rate <8 or >20 breaths/min, ventricular arrhythmias, fatigue, panic, cyanosis, erratic or labored breathing, paradoxical chest movement.
8. If the weaning process continues, measure tidal volume and minute ventilation every 20 to 30 minutes; compare with the patient's desired values, which have been determined in collaboration with the primary provider.
9. Assess for psychological dependence if the physiologic parameters indicate that weaning is feasible and the patient still resists. Possible causes of psychological dependence include fear of dying and depression from chronic illness. It is important to address this issue before the next weaning attempt.

Adapted from Wiegand, D. J. L. (2017). *AACN procedure manual for critical care* (6th ed.). St. Louis, MO: Elsevier Saunders.

---

for tachypnea, tachycardia, reduced tidal volumes, decreasing oxygen saturations, and increasing carbon dioxide levels.

SIMV can also be used as a weaning method. The patient is placed on SIMV mode of ventilation and the rate is slowly decreased by 1 to 3 breaths/min until the patient is fully breathing on their own (Urden et al., 2018).

Furthermore, T-piece spontaneous breathing trials can also be used. When the patient can breathe spontaneously, weaning trials using a T-piece for the patient with an ET tube or tracheostomy mask for the patient with a tracheostomy tube (see Fig. 19-6) are normally conducted with the patient disconnected from the ventilator, receiving humidified oxygen only and performing all work of breathing. Because patients do not have to overcome the resistance of the ventilator, they may find this mode more comfortable, or they may become anxious as they breathe with no support from the ventilator. During these trial periods, the nurse monitors the patient closely and provides encouragement. This method of weaning is usually used when the patient is awake and alert, is breathing without difficulty, has good gag and cough reflexes, and is hemodynamically stable. During the weaning process, the patient is maintained on the same or a higher oxygen concentration than when receiving mechanical ventilation. While the patient is using the T-piece or tracheostomy mask, they are observed for signs and symptoms of hypoxia, increasing respiratory muscle fatigue, or systemic fatigue. These include restlessness, increased respiratory rate (greater than 35 breaths/min), the use of accessory muscles, tachycardia with premature ventricular contractions, and paradoxical chest movement (asynchronous breathing, chest contraction during inspiration and expansion during expiration). Fatigue or exhaustion is initially manifested by an increased respiratory rate associated with a gradual reduction in tidal volume; later there is a slowing of the respiratory rate.

If the patient appears to be tolerating the T-piece/tracheostomy mask trial, a second set of arterial blood gas measurements is drawn 20 minutes after the patient has been on spontaneous ventilation at a constant FiO_2 PSV. (Alveolar–arterial equilibration takes 15 to 20 minutes to occur.)

Signs of exhaustion and hypoxia correlated with deterioration in the blood gas measurements indicate the need for ventilatory support. The patient is placed back on the ventilator each time signs of fatigue or deterioration develop.

If clinically stable, the patient usually can be extubated within 2 or 3 hours after weaning and allowed spontaneous ventilation by means of a mask with humidified oxygen. Patients who have had prolonged ventilatory assistance usually require more gradual weaning; it may take days or even weeks. They are weaned primarily during the day and placed back on the ventilator at night to rest.

Because patients respond in different manners to weaning methods, there is no definitive way to assess which method is best. Regardless of the weaning method being used, ongoing assessment of respiratory status is essential to monitor patient progress.

Successful weaning from the ventilator is supplemented by intensive pulmonary care. The following methods are used: oxygen therapy; arterial blood gas evaluation; pulse oximetry; bronchodilator therapy; CPT; adequate nutrition, hydration, and humidification; blood pressure measurement; and incentive spirometry. Daily spontaneous breathing trials may be used to evaluate the patient's ability to breathe without ventilatory support. If the patient is receiving IV sedatives (e.g., propofol, dexmedetomidine), current guidelines recommend that the patient's sedative dose be decreased by 25% to 50% prior to weaning. In order to decrease agitation in patients who do not tolerate withdrawal of sedation, dexmedetomidine may be initiated for spontaneous breathing trials without causing significant respiratory depression (Devlin, Skrobik, Gélinas, et al., 2018; Urden et al., 2018). A patient may still have borderline pulmonary function and need vigorous supportive therapy before their respiratory status returns to a level that supports activities of daily living.

Removal of the Tracheostomy Tube

Removal of the tracheostomy tube is considered when the patient can breathe spontaneously; maintain an adequate airway by effectively coughing up secretions, swallow, and move the jaw. Secretion clearance and aspiration risks are assessed to determine whether active pharyngeal and laryngeal reflexes are intact.

Once the patient can clear secretions adequately, a trial period of mouth breathing or nose breathing is conducted. This can be accomplished by several methods. The first method requires changing to a smaller size tube to increase the resistance to airflow or plugging the tracheostomy tube (deflating the cuff first). The smaller tube is sometimes replaced by a cuffless tracheostomy tube, which allows the tube to be plugged at lengthening intervals to monitor patient progress. A second method involves changing to a fenestrated tube (a tube with an opening or window in its bend). This permits air to flow around and through the tube to the upper airway and enables talking. A third method involves switching to a smaller tracheostomy button (stoma button). A tracheostomy button is a plastic tube approximately 1 inch long that helps keep the windpipe open after the larger tracheostomy tube has been removed. Finally, when the patient demonstrates the ability to maintain a patent airway, the tube can be removed. An occlusive dressing is placed over the stoma, which heals in several days to weeks.

Weaning from Oxygen

The patient who has been successfully weaned from the ventilator, cuff, and tube and has adequate respiratory function is then weaned from oxygen. The FiO_2 is gradually reduced until the PaO_2 is in the range of 70 to 100 mm Hg while the patient is breathing room air. If the PaO_2 is less than 70 mm Hg on room air, supplemental oxygen is recommended. To be eligible for financial reimbursement from the Centers for Medicare and Medicaid Services (CMS) for in-home oxygen, the patient must have a PaO_2 at or less than 55 mm Hg while awake and at rest or arterial oxygen saturation at or below 88%, breathing room air (American Association of Respiratory Care, 2007; CMS, 1993).

Nutrition

Success in weaning the patient who is long-term ventilator dependent requires early and aggressive but judicious nutritional support. The respiratory muscles (diaphragm and especially intercostals) become weak or atrophied after just a few days of mechanical ventilation and may be catabolized for energy, especially if nutrition is inadequate. Compensation for inadequate nutrition must be undertaken with care; excessive intake can increase the production of carbon dioxide and the demand for oxygen and lead to prolonged ventilator dependence and difficulty in weaning. Because the metabolism of fat produces less carbon dioxide than the metabolism of carbohydrates, it was long presumed that a high-fat and limited carbohydrate diet would be most therapeutic; however, evidence-based findings do not support its efficacy (Seres, 2020). Adequate protein intake is important in increasing respiratory muscle strength. Protein intake should be approximately 25% of total daily kilocalories, or 1.2 to 1.5 g/kg/day. Daily nutrition should be closely monitored.

Soon after the patient is admitted, a consultation with a dietitian or nutrition support team should be arranged to plan the best form of nutritional replacement. Adequate nutrition may decrease the duration of mechanical ventilation and prevent other complications, especially sepsis. Sepsis can occur if bacteria enter the bloodstream and release toxins that, in turn, cause vasodilation and hypotension, fever, tachycardia, increased respiratory rate, and coma. Aggressive treatment of sepsis is essential to reverse this threat to survival and to promote weaning from the ventilator when the patient's condition improves.

Acute Respiratory Distress Syndrome

Acute respiratory distress syndrome (ARDS) can be thought of as a spectrum of disease, progressing from mild to moderate to its most severe, fulminant form. **Acute lung injury** is a term commonly used to describe mild ARDS. ARDS is a clinical syndrome characterized by a severe inflammatory process causing diffuse alveolar damage that results in sudden and progressive pulmonary edema, increasing bilateral infiltrates on chest x-ray, hypoxemia unresponsive to oxygen supplementation regardless of the amount of PEEP, and the absence of an elevated left atrial pressure (Siegel, 2019a). Patients often demonstrate reduced lung compliance. A wide range of factors are associated with the development of ARDS (see Chart 19-20), including direct injury to the lungs (e.g., smoke inhalation) or indirect insult to the lungs (e.g., shock). ARDS has been associated with a mortality rate ranging from 27% to 50%. Patients who survive the initial cause of ARDS may die later, commonly from HCAP or sepsis (Anesi, 2020; Siegel, 2019a).

> ### Quality and Safety Nursing Alert
>
> *Be alert for the development of acute lung injury in the patient population using e-cigarettes, also known as vaping. This syndrome is called e-cigarette or vaping associated acute lung injury (EVALI). According to the CDC (2019c), patients diagnosed with EVALI have been identified in most states.*

Pathophysiology

Inflammatory triggers initiate the release of cellular and chemical mediators, causing injury to the alveolar capillary membrane in addition to other structural damage to the lungs. Severe $\dot{V}/\dot{Q}$ mismatching occurs. Alveoli collapse because of the inflammatory infiltrate, blood, fluid, and surfactant dysfunction. Small airways are narrowed because of interstitial fluid and bronchial obstruction. Lung compliance may markedly decrease, resulting in decreased functional residual capacity and severe hypoxemia. The blood returning to the lung for gas exchange is pumped through the nonventilated, nonfunctioning areas of the lung, causing shunting. This means that blood is interfacing with nonfunctioning alveoli and gas exchange is markedly impaired, resulting in severe, refractory hypoxemia. Figure 19-9 shows the sequence of pathophysiologic events leading to ARDS.

Clinical Manifestations

Initially, ARDS closely resembles severe pulmonary edema. The acute phase of ARDS is marked by a rapid onset of severe dyspnea that usually occurs less than 72 hours after

---

Chart 19-20 · RISK FACTORS
Acute Respiratory Distress Syndrome

- Aspiration (gastric secretions, drowning, hydrocarbons)
- COVID-19 pneumonia
- Drug ingestion and overdose
- Fat or air embolism
- Hematologic disorders (disseminated intravascular coagulation, massive transfusions, cardiopulmonary bypass)
- Localized infection (bacterial, fungal, viral pneumonia)
- Major surgery
- Metabolic disorders (pancreatitis, uremia)
- Prolonged inhalation of high concentrations of oxygen, smoke, or corrosive substances
- Sepsis
- Shock (any cause)
- Trauma (pulmonary contusion, multiple fractures, head injury)

COVID-19, coronavirus disease 2019.
Adapted from Cascella, M., Rajnik, M., Cuomo, A., et al. (2020). Features, evaluation and treatment Coronavirus (COVID-19). *StatPearls*. Treasure Island, FL: StatPearls Publishing. Retrieved on 6/9/2020 at: www.ncbi.nlm.nih.gov/books/NBK554776/; Siegel, M. D. (2019a). Acute respiratory distress syndrome: Epidemiology, pathophysiology, pathology, and etiology in adults. *UpToDate*. Retrieved on 9/23/2019 at: www.uptodate.com/contents/acute-respiratory-distress-syndrome-epidemiology-pathophysiology-pathology-and-etiology-in-adults

---

Physiology/Pathophysiology

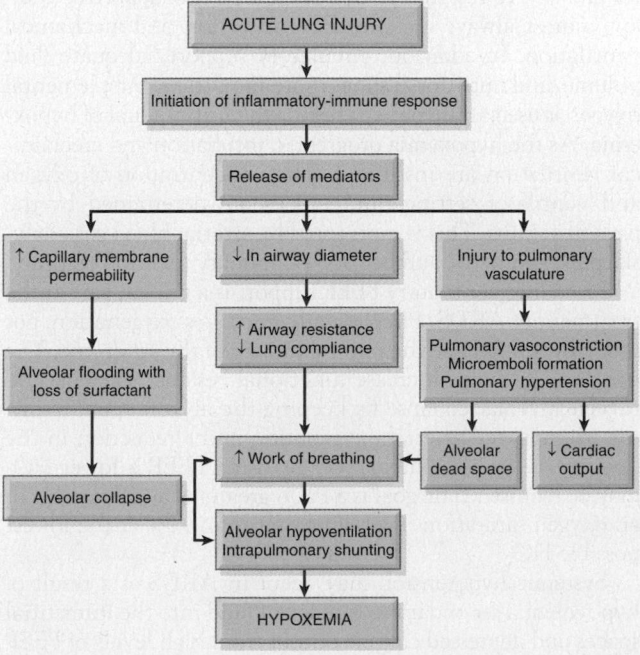

Figure 19-9 • Pathogenesis and pathophysiology of acute respiratory distress syndrome.

the precipitating event. Arterial hypoxemia that does not respond to supplemental oxygen is characteristic. ARDS is classified according to the severity of hypoxemia experienced by the patient as (Siegel, 2019a):

- mild ARDS, with arterial oxygen tension (PaO_2)/ fraction of inspired oxygen (FIO_2) > 200 mm Hg but ≤300 mm Hg,
- moderate ARDS, with PaO_2/FIO_2 > 100 mm Hg but ≤200 mm Hg, or
- severe ARDS, with PaO_2/FIO_2 ≤ 100 mm Hg.

Findings on chest x-ray are similar to those seen with cardiogenic pulmonary edema and are visible as bilateral infiltrates that quickly worsen. Mild ARDS progresses to fibrosing alveolitis with persistent, severe hypoxemia. The patient also has increased alveolar dead space (ventilation to alveoli but poor perfusion) and typically has decreased pulmonary compliance ("stiff lungs," which are difficult to ventilate). Clinically, the patient is thought to be in the recovery phase if the hypoxemia gradually resolves, the chest x-ray improves, and the lungs become more compliant.

Assessment and Diagnostic Findings

On physical examination, intercostal retractions and crackles may be present as the fluid begins to leak into the alveolar interstitial space. Common diagnostic tests performed in patients with potential ARDS include plasma brain natriuretic peptide (BNP) levels, echocardiography, and pulmonary artery catheterization. The BNP level is helpful in distinguishing ARDS from cardiogenic pulmonary edema. Transthoracic echocardiography may be used if the BNP is not conclusive.

Medical Management

The primary focus in the management of ARDS includes identification and treatment of the underlying condition. Aggressive, supportive care must be provided to compensate for the severe respiratory dysfunction. This supportive therapy almost always includes ET intubation and mechanical ventilation. In addition, circulatory support, adequate fluid volume, and nutritional support are important. Supplemental oxygen is used as the patient begins the initial spiral of hypoxemia. As the hypoxemia progresses, intubation and mechanical ventilation are instituted. The concentration of oxygen and ventilator settings and modes are determined by the patient's status. This is monitored by arterial blood gas analysis, pulse oximetry, and bedside pulmonary function testing.

Providing ventilatory PEEP support is a critical part of the treatment of ARDS. PEEP usually improves oxygenation, but it does not influence the natural history of the syndrome. The use of PEEP helps increase functional residual capacity and reverse alveolar collapse by keeping the alveoli open, resulting in improved arterial oxygenation and a reduction in the severity of the $\dot{V}/\dot{Q}$ imbalance. By using PEEP, a lower FIO_2 may be required. The goal is a PaO_2 greater than 60 mm Hg or an oxygen saturation level of greater than 90% at the lowest possible FIO_2.

Systemic hypotension may occur in ARDS as a result of hypovolemia secondary to leakage of fluid into the interstitial spaces and depressed cardiac output from high levels of PEEP therapy. Hypovolemia must be carefully treated without causing further overload. Inotropic or vasopressor agents may

be required. Additional supportive treatments may include prone positioning, sedation, paralysis, and nutritional support (Siegel, 2019b).

Pharmacologic Therapy

There is no specific pharmacologic treatment of ARDS except supportive care. Neuromuscular blocking agents, sedatives, and analgesics may be used to improve patient–ventilator synchronization and help to decrease severe hypoxemia (see later discussion in Ventilator Considerations section). Inhaled nitric oxide (an endogenous vasodilator) was thought to reduce $\dot{V}/\dot{Q}$ mismatch and improve oxygenation; however, findings from clinical trials have not shown an improvement in mortality rates between patients who did and did not receive nitric oxide (Harman, 2018).

Nutritional Therapy

Adequate nutritional support is vital in the treatment of ARDS. Patients with ARDS require 35 to 45 kcal/kg/day to meet caloric requirements. Enteral feeding is the first consideration; however, parenteral nutrition also may be required.

Nursing Management

General Measures

A patient with ARDS is critically ill and requires close monitoring in an ICU. Respiratory modalities used in this situation include oxygen administration, nebulizer therapy, CPT, ET intubation or tracheostomy, mechanical ventilation, suctioning, and bronchoscopy. Frequent assessment of the patient's status is necessary to evaluate the effectiveness of treatment.

In addition to supporting the medical plan of care, the nurse considers other needs of the patient. Positioning is important. The nurse turns the patient frequently to improve ventilation and perfusion in the lungs and enhance secretion drainage. However, the nurse must closely monitor the patient for deterioration in oxygenation with changes in position. Oxygenation in patients with ARDS is sometimes improved in the prone position; this seems to be particularly true for patients with COVID-19 and ARDS (see later discussion). This position may be evaluated for improvement in oxygenation and used in special circumstances. Devices and specialty beds are available to assist the nurse in placing the patient in a prone position.

The patient is extremely anxious and agitated because of the increasing hypoxemia and dyspnea. It is important to reduce the patient's anxiety because anxiety increases oxygen expenditure by preventing rest. Rest is essential to limit oxygen consumption and reduce oxygen needs.

Ventilator Considerations

Several considerations must be addressed for the patient intubated and receiving mechanical ventilation with PEEP. PEEP, which causes increased end-expiratory pressure, is an unnatural pattern of breathing and feels strange to the patient. The patient may be anxious, and patient-ventilator dyssynchrony may be the consequence. Nursing assessment is important to identify problems with ventilation that may be causing the anxiety reaction: tube blockage by kinking or retained secretions, other acute respiratory problems (e.g., pneumothorax and pain), a sudden decrease in the oxygen level, the level of dyspnea, or ventilator malfunction. In some cases, sedation may be required to decrease the patient's oxygen consumption, allow the ventilator to provide full support of ventilation, and decrease the patient's anxiety. Sedatives that may be prescribed are lorazepam, midazolam, dexmedetomidine, propofol, and short-acting barbiturates.

If the PEEP level cannot be maintained despite the use of sedatives, neuromuscular blocking agents (paralytic agents) may be given to paralyze the patient. Examples of these agents include pancuronium, vecuronium, atracurium, and rocuronium. The resulting paralysis allows the patient to be ventilated more easily. With paralysis, the patient appears to be unconscious; loses motor function; and cannot breathe, talk, or blink independently. However, the patient retains sensation and is awake and able to hear. The nurse must reassure the patient that the paralysis is a result of the medication and is temporary. Paralysis should be used for the shortest possible time and never without adequate sedation and pain management.

Peripheral nerve stimulators are used to assess nerve impulse transmissions at the neuromuscular junction of select skeletal muscles when neuromuscular blocking agents are used. A "train-of-four" test may be used to measure the level of neuromuscular blockade. With this test, four consecutive stimuli are delivered along the path of a nerve, and the response of the muscle is measured in order to evaluate whether or not stimuli are effectively blocked. Four equal muscle contractions, seen as "twitches," will result if there is no neuromuscular blockade. However, if neuromuscular blockade is present, there will be a loss of twitch height and number, which will indicate the degree of blockade. If all four stimulations result in an absence of twitches, it is estimated that 100% of the receptors are blocked (Wiegand, 2017).

The use of neuromuscular blocking agents has many dangers and side effects. The nurse must be sure the patient does not become disconnected from the ventilator, because respiratory muscles are paralyzed and the patient will be apneic. Consequently, the nurse ensures that the patient is closely monitored; all ventilator and patient alarms must be on at all times. Eye care is important as well, because the patient cannot blink, increasing the risk of corneal abrasions. Neuromuscular blockers predispose the patient to venous thromboembolism (VTE), muscle atrophy, foot drop, stress ulcers that may cause hemorrhage, and skin breakdown.

> ### ◤ Quality and Safety Nursing Alert
>
> Nursing assessment is essential to minimize the complications related to neuromuscular blockade. The patient may have discomfort or pain but cannot communicate these sensations. In addition, frequent oral care and suctioning may be needed.

Analgesia must be given concurrently with neuromuscular blocking agents (Saenz, 2019). The nurse must anticipate the patient's needs regarding pain and comfort. The nurse checks the patient's position to ensure it is comfortable without excessive pressure points and in normal alignment. Talking to and not about the patient while in the patient's presence is important.

In addition, the nurse must describe the purpose and effects of the neuromuscular blocking agents to the patient's family. If family members are unaware that these agents have been given, they may become distressed by the change in the patient's status.

COVID-19 Considerations

The most serious complication and most frequent cause of death among patients with COVID-19 is ARDS (Anesi, 2020). In China, where the SARS-CoV-2 virus first emerged, approximately one quarter of patients who were hospitalized in the early days of the pandemic required treatment in critical care units, the majority with respiratory failure and ARDS. Of these, 52.4% died secondary to complications of ARDS (Niederman, Richeldi, Chotirmall, et al., 2020; Wu & McGoogan, 2020).

The pathogenesis of ARDS in patients with COVID-19 pneumonia appears to have some differences from other cases of ARDS. In particular, although there is evidence of damage to epithelial cells within alveoli, epithelial cells within the pulmonary endothelium are not damaged, resulting in less exudative pathologic changes than with other types of ARDS. In terms of clinical manifestations, some patients with severe COVID-19 pneumonia do not voice complaints of dyspnea but nonetheless may deteriorate rapidly into respiratory failure. Furthermore, some patients with COVID-19 and ARDS who are mechanically ventilated do not exhibit the poor lung compliance that is a classic manifestation of typical ARDS. In addition, the onset of most non-COVID-19 cases of ARDS is typically one week or less from the time of the causative insult; however, the median time from onset of COVID-19 symptoms to ARDS is longer, at between 8 to 12 days (Li & Ma, 2020).

The same classification system used to diagnosis other cases of ARDS is used to classify patients with COVID-19 pneumonia with ARDS (i.e., as having mild, moderate, or severe ARDS) (Cascella et al., 2020). Many of the same strategies used to manage patients without COVID-19 who have ARDS apply to the patient with COVID-19 and ARDS. For instance, it is recommended that the patient with COVID-19 and ARDS who is mechanically ventilated receive low tidal volumes (i.e., 4 to 8 mL/kg ideal body weight). However, there are some specific differences in the recommended treatment of the adult with COVID-19 and ARDS who is mechanically ventilated, which include the following (Alhazzani, Moller, Arabi, et al., 2020; Anesi, 2020):

- PEEP > 5 cm H_2O should be delivered (although the patient should be closely monitored for barotrauma if the PEEP is >10 cm H_2O);
- Low dosages of intravenous corticosteroids (e.g., dexamethasone, methylprednisolone) may be prescribed;
- Nitric oxide should not be routinely prescribed; however, for patients with severe ARDS refractory to other treatments, nitric oxide might be tried;
- For the patient with moderate or severe ARDS, prone positioning for 12 to 16 hours daily is recommended, if feasible; and
- For the patient with moderate or severe ARDS, intermittent boluses of neuromuscular blocking agents are preferred over continuous infusions, unless there is persistent patient-ventilator dyssynchrony.

Other treatments recommended for patients with severe COVID-19 pneumonia should also be followed (see previous discussion on COVID-19 pneumonia).

It has been reported that more patients with COVID-19 and ARDS who are mechanically ventilated have neurologic impairment (e.g., delirium, encephalopathy) than other patients with ARDS who are mechanically ventilated. Therefore, sedative requirements for these patients are reportedly higher than for most other patients with ARDS (Anesi, 2020). These neurologic manifestations are that much more difficult to manage because family members and friends, who may be a source of solace to the patient who is agitated, are typically not permitted to visit. Furthermore, the nurse caring for these patients must also practice isolation precautions and minimize interactions with the patient, which can serve to make the patient feel more isolated and agitated.

PULMONARY VASCULAR DISORDERS

Pulmonary Edema (Noncardiogenic)

Pulmonary edema is defined as abnormal accumulation of fluid in the lung tissue, the alveolar space, or both. It is a severe, life-threatening condition. Pulmonary edema can be classified as cardiogenic or noncardiogenic (see Chapter 25 for further discussion of cardiogenic pulmonary edema). Noncardiogenic pulmonary edema occurs due to damage of the pulmonary capillary lining. It may be due to direct injury to the lung (e.g., chest trauma, aspiration, and smoke inhalation), hematogenous injury to the lung (e.g., sepsis, pancreatitis, multiple transfusions, cardiopulmonary bypass), or injury plus elevated hydrostatic pressures. Management of noncardiogenic pulmonary edema mirrors that of cardiogenic pulmonary edema; however, hypoxemia may persist despite high concentrations of supplemental oxygen, due to the intrapulmonary shunting of blood.

Pulmonary Hypertension

Pulmonary hypertension (PH) is characterized by elevated pulmonary arterial pressure greater than 25 mm Hg at rest and greater than 30 mm Hg with exercise and secondary right heart ventricular failure (Rubin & Hopkins, 2019). It may be suspected in a patient with dyspnea with exertion without other clinical manifestations. Unlike systemic blood pressure, the pulmonary pressures cannot be measured indirectly. In the absence of these measurements, clinical recognition becomes the only indicator of PH. However, PH is a condition that is often not clinically evident until late in its progression. Patients are classified by the World Health Organization (WHO) into five groups based upon the mechanism of PH (Rubin & Hopkins, 2019) (see Chart 19-21).

Pathophysiology

Conditions such as collagen vascular disease, congenital heart disease, anorexigens (specific appetite depressants), chronic use of stimulants, portal hypertension, and HIV infection increase the risk of PH in susceptible patients. Vascular injury occurs with endothelial dysfunction and vascular

---

Chart 19-21	Clinical Classification of Pulmonary Hypertension (PH)

Group 1: Pulmonary Arterial Hypertension (PAH)

- Sporadic idiopathic PAH
- Heritable idiopathic PAH
- Drug and toxin-induced PAH
- PAH due to diseases such as connective tissues disorders, HIV infection, portal hypertension, congenital heart disease

Group 2: PH due to left heart disease

- Systolic dysfunction
- Diastolic dysfunction
- Valvular heart disease

Group 3: PH due to chronic lung diseases and/or hypoxemia

- Chronic obstructive pulmonary disease
- Interstitial lung disease
- Mixed restrictive and obstructive lung disease
- Sleep disordered breathing

Group 4: Chronic thromboembolic pulmonary hypertension (CTEPH)

- Due to thromboembolic occlusion of the proximal or distal pulmonary vasculature

Group 5: PH with unclear multifactorial mechanisms

- Hematologic disorders
- Systemic disorders (e.g., sarcoidosis)
- Metabolic disorders

Adapted from Rubin, L., & Hopkins, W. (2019). Overview of pulmonary hypertension in adults. *UpToDate*. Retrieved on 8/22/2019 at: www.uptodate.com/contents/overview-of-pulmonary-hypertension-in-adults

---

smooth muscle dysfunction, which leads to disease progression (vascular smooth muscle hypertrophy, adventitial and intimal proliferation [thickening of the wall], and advanced vascular lesion formation). Normally, the pulmonary vascular bed can handle the blood volume delivered by the right ventricle. It has a low resistance to blood flow and compensates for increased blood volume by dilation of the vessels in the pulmonary circulation. However, if the pulmonary vascular bed is destroyed or obstructed, as in PH, the ability to handle whatever flow or volume of blood it receives is impaired, and the increased blood flow then increases the pulmonary artery pressure. As the pulmonary arterial pressure increases, the pulmonary vascular resistance also increases. Both pulmonary artery constriction (as in hypoxemia or hypercapnia) and a reduction of the pulmonary vascular bed (which occurs with PE) result in increased pulmonary vascular resistance and pressure. This increased workload affects right ventricular function. The myocardium ultimately cannot meet the increasing demands imposed on it, leading to right ventricular hypertrophy (enlargement and dilation) and failure. Passive hepatic congestion may also develop.

Clinical Manifestations

Dyspnea, the main symptom of PH, occurs at first with exertion and eventually at rest. Substernal chest pain also is common.

Other signs and symptoms include weakness, fatigue, syncope, occasional hemoptysis, and signs of right-sided heart failure (peripheral edema, ascites, distended neck veins, liver engorgement, crackles, heart murmur). Anorexia and abdominal pain in the right upper quadrant may also occur.

Assessment and Diagnostic Findings

Diagnostic testing is used to confirm that PH exists, determine its severity, and identify its causes. Initial diagnostic evaluation includes a history, physical examination, chest x-ray, pulmonary function studies, electrocardiogram (ECG), and echocardiogram. Echocardiography can be used to estimate the pulmonary artery systolic pressure and to assess right ventricular size, thickness, and function. It can also evaluate the right atrial size, left ventricular system, and diastolic function as well as valve function. Right heart catheterization is necessary to confirm the diagnosis of PH and to accurately assess the hemodynamic abnormalities. PH is confirmed with a mean pulmonary artery pressure greater than 25 mm Hg. If left heart disease is identified via echocardiography and correlates with the degree of estimated PH, then exercise testing and both a right and left heart catheterization may be done to determine the functional severity of the disease and the abnormalities in pressures (left heart filling, pulmonary vascular resistance, transpulmonary gradient) (Rubin & Hopkins, 2019).

Pulmonary function studies may be normal or show a slight decrease in vital capacity and lung compliance, with a mild decrease in the diffusing capacity. The PaO_2 also is decreased (hypoxemia). The ECG reveals right ventricular hypertrophy, right axis deviation, and tall peaked P waves in inferior leads; tall anterior R waves; and ST-segment depression, T-wave inversion, or both anteriorly. An echocardiogram can assess the progression of the disease and rule out other conditions with similar signs and symptoms. A $\dot{V}/\dot{Q}$ scan or pulmonary angiography detects defects in pulmonary vasculature, such as PE.

Medical Management

The primary goal of treatment is to manage the underlying condition related to PH if the cause is known. Recommendations regarding therapy are tailored to the patient's individual situation, functional New York Heart Association class, and specific needs (Rubin & Hopkins, 2019). All patients with PH should be considered for the following therapies: diuretics, oxygen, anticoagulation, digoxin, and exercise training. Diuretics and oxygen should be added as needed. Appropriate oxygen therapy reverses the vasoconstriction and reduces the PH in a relatively short time. Most patients with PH do not have hypoxemia at rest but require supplemental oxygen with exercise. Anticoagulation should be considered for patients at risk for intrapulmonary thrombosis. Digoxin may improve right ventricular ejection fraction in some patients and may help to control heart rate; however, patients must be monitored closely for potential complications (Rubin & Hopkins, 2019).

Pharmacologic Therapy

Recent advances in pharmacologic management and medication delivery options have offered more effective treatment regimens for patients affected with PH. Medications prescribed to treat PH include calcium channel blockers and specific pathogenetic therapies, including prostanoids, endothelin receptor antagonists, phosphodiesterase-5 inhibitors, and soluble guanylate cyclase stimulants. The choice of therapeutic agents is based on many facets, including the classification group status of the patient with PH (see Chart 19-21), as well as the cost and the patient's tolerance of the agents (Hopkins & Rubin, 2019). In addition, a vasoreactivity test may be done to identify which medication is best suited for the patient with PH; this is done during cardiac catheterization using vasodilating medications such as inhaled nitric oxide, adenosine, or prostacyclin. A positive vasoreactivity test occurs when there is a decrease of at least 10 mm Hg in the pulmonary artery pressure with an overall pressure that is less than 40 mm Hg in the presence of both an increased or unchanged cardiac output and a minimally decreased or unchanged systemic blood pressure (Hopkins & Rubin, 2019).

Patients with a positive vasoreactivity test and who do not have right-sided heart failure may be prescribed calcium channel blockers. Calcium channel blockers have a significant advantage over some medications taken to treat PH in that they may be taken orally and are generally less costly; however, because calcium channel blockers are indicated in only a small percentage of patients, other treatment options, including prostanoids, are often necessary (Hopkins & Rubin, 2019).

Prostanoids mimic the effect of the prostaglandin prostacyclin. Prostacyclin relaxes vascular smooth muscle by stimulating the production of cyclic 3′,5′-adenosine monophosphate (AMP) and inhibits the growth of smooth muscle cells. Prostanoids used to treat PH include epoprostenol, iloprost, treprostinil, and selexipag. Limitations of the prostanoids include their short half-life and variable patient responses to therapy (Hopkins & Rubin, 2019). IV epoprostenol was the first FDA-approved prostanoid and is the most widely studied advanced therapy for PH. Epoprostenol has a half-life of less than 3 minutes and must be continuously delivered through a permanently implanted central venous catheter using a portable infusion pump in order to maintain therapeutic effectiveness. Although a useful therapy, it requires extensive patient education and caregiver support. An advantage to iloprostis over epoprostenol is that it is an inhaled preparation; however, it needs to be administered six to nine times daily. The first formulations of treprostinil could only be taken parenterally; however, it has recently been approved in an inhaled formulation, and an oral preparation is under development. Parenteral trepostinil can be administered IV or subcutaneously, although the subcutaneous method causes severe pain at the injection site (Hopkins & Rubin, 2019). Selexipag is the newest FDA-approved prostanoid. It is available in tablet form administered in twice-daily doses, a clear advantage over-the-other prostanoids. However, it is a costly medication and not all insurance plans cover all of its costs (Pulmonary Hypertension Association Scientific Leadership Council, 2016).

Endothelin receptor antagonists bind to vascular endothelin-1 receptors, effectively blocking constriction of the pulmonary arteries, resulting in vasodilation. Endothelin receptor antagonists used to treat PH include bosentan, ambrisentan, and macitentan. These medications are available as oral preparations. A disadvantage to them is that they are hepatotoxic. Liver function must be monitored in patients using these agents.

The oral medications sildenafil, tadalafil, and vardenafil are potent, specific phosphodiesterase-5 inhibitors that degrade cyclic 3',5'-guanosine monophosphate (cGMP) and promotes pulmonary vasodilation. These drugs are also prescribed to treat erectile dysfunction (Hopkins & Rubin, 2019; Korokina, Zhernakova, Korokin, et al., 2018).

Soluble guanylate cyclase stimulants, which act on the nitrous oxide pathway, are currently undergoing clinical trials to target many cardiopulmonary diseases. Riociguat, a medication in this category, is newly FDA approved for use in PH. Riociguat, an oral preparation administered three times daily, is contraindicated in patients with liver or kidney disease (Tsai, Sung, & de Jesus Perez, 2016).

Surgical Management

Lung transplantation remains an option for a select group of patients with PH who are refractory to medical therapy. Bilateral lung or heart–lung transplantation is the procedure of choice. Atrial septostomy may be considered for select patients with severe disease (Hopkins & Rubin, 2019); this procedure results in shunting of blood from the right side of the heart to the left, decreasing the strain on the right side of the heart and maintaining left ventricular output.

Nursing Management

The major nursing goal is to identify patients at high risk for PH, such as those with COPD, PE, congenital heart disease, and mitral valve disease so that early treatment can commence. The nurse must be alert for signs and symptoms, administer oxygen therapy appropriately, and instruct the patient and family about the use of home oxygen therapy. In patients treated with some of the prostanoids, education about the need for central venous access (epoprostenol), subcutaneous infusion (treprostinil), proper administration and dosing of the medication, pain at the injection site, and potential severe side effects is extremely important. Emotional and psychosocial aspects of this disease must be addressed. It is important to provide contact details for support services for patients and families.

Pulmonary Heart Disease (Cor Pulmonale)

Cor pulmonale is a condition that results from PH, which causes the right side of the heart to enlarge because of the increased work required to pump blood against high resistance through the pulmonary vascular system. This causes right-sided heart failure (see Chapter 25 for further discussion of management of right-sided heart failure).

Pulmonary Embolism

PE refers to the obstruction of the pulmonary artery or one of its branches by a thrombus (or thrombi) that originates somewhere in the venous system or in the right side of the heart. Deep vein thrombosis (DVT), a related condition, refers to thrombus formation in the deep veins, usually in the calf or thigh, but sometimes in the arm, especially in patients with peripherally inserted central catheters. VTE is a term that includes both DVT and PE. (VTE and the medical and nursing management of patients with DVT and with PE are discussed in detail in Chapter 26.)

OCCUPATIONAL LUNG DISEASE: PNEUMOCONIOSES

Pneumoconiosis is a general term given to any lung disease caused by dusts that are breathed in and then deposited deep in the lungs causing damage. Pneumoconiosis is usually considered an occupational lung disease, and includes asbestosis, silicosis and coal workers' pneumoconiosis, also known as "Black Lung Disease" (American Lung Association [ALA], 2018a) (see Table 19-6). Pneumoconiosis refers to a non-neoplastic

TABLE 19-6	Occupational Lung Diseases: Pneumoconioses	
Disease (Source)	**Pathophysiology**	**Clinical Manifestations**
Silicosis (glass manufacturing, foundry work, stone cutting)	Inhaled silica dust produces nodular lesions in the lungs. Nodules enlarge and coalesce. Dense masses form on upper portion of lungs, resulting in loss of pulmonary volume. Fibrotic destruction of pulmonary tissue can lead to restrictive lung disease, emphysema, pulmonary hypertension, and cor pulmonale	*Acute silicosis:* dyspnea, fever, cough, weight loss *Chronic silicosis:* progressive symptoms indicative of hypoxemia, severe airflow obstruction, and right-sided heart failure
Asbestosis (shipbuilding, building demolition)	Inhaled asbestos fibers enter alveoli and are surrounded by fibrous tissue. Fibrous changes can also affect the pleura, which thicken and develop plaque. These changes lead to restrictive lung disease, with a decrease in lung volume, diminished exchange of oxygen and carbon dioxide, hypoxemia, cor pulmonale, and respiratory failure. It also increases risk of lung cancer, mesothelioma, and pleural effusion	Progressive dyspnea; persistent, dry cough; mild-to-moderate chest pain; anorexia; weight loss; malaise; clubbing of the fingers
Coal worker's pneumoconiosis	Encompasses a variety of lung diseases; is also known as black lung disease. Inhaled dusts that are mixtures of coal, kaolin, mica, and silica are deposited in the alveoli and respiratory bronchioles. When macrophages that engulf the dust can no longer be cleared, they aggregate and fibroblasts appear. The bronchioles and alveoli become clogged with dust, dying macrophages, and fibroblasts, leading to formation of coal macules. Fibrotic lesions develop and subsequently localized emphysema develops, with cor pulmonale and respiratory failure	Chronic cough, dyspnea, and expectoration of black or gray sputum, especially in coal workers who smoke and who have cavitation in the lungs

Adapted from American Lung Association (ALA). (2018a). Lung health & diseases: Pneumoconiosis. Retrieved on 10/4/2019 at: www.lung.org/lung-health-and-diseases/lung-disease-lookup/pneumoconiosis

alteration of the lung resulting from inhalation of mineral or inorganic dust (e.g., "dusty lung"). This alteration results in pulmonary fibrosis and parenchymal changes. Usually, extended exposure to irritating or toxic substances accounts for these changes, although severe single exposures may also lead to chronic lung disease. Occupational lung disease is the number one work-related illness in the United States based on its frequency, severity, and preventability (ALA, 2018a). Many people with early pneumoconiosis are asymptomatic, but advanced disease often is accompanied by disability and premature death.

Diseases of the lungs occur in numerous occupations as a result of exposure to several different types of agents, such as mineral dusts, metal dusts, biologic dusts, and toxic fumes. Smoking may compound the problem and may increase the risk of lung cancers in people exposed to the mineral asbestos and other potential carcinogens (ALA, 2018b). The effects of inhaling these materials depend on the composition of the substance, its concentration, its ability to initiate an immune response, its irritating properties, the duration of exposure, and the person's response or susceptibility to the irritant.

These diseases are not curable; however, they are preventable. Therefore, a major role for nurses, especially occupational health nurses, is that of advocate for employees. Nurses need to make every effort to promote measures to reduce the exposure of workers to industrial products. Strategies to control exposure should be identified and encouraged; these strategies include the use of protective devices (facemasks, hoods, industrial respirators) to minimize exposure and screening/monitoring of individuals at risk.

Key aspects of any assessment of patients with a potential occupational respiratory history include job and job activities, exposure levels, general hygiene, time frame of exposure, smoking history, effectiveness of respiratory protection used, and direct versus indirect exposures (Goldman, 2019). Specific information that should be obtained includes the following:

- Exposure to an agent known to cause an occupational disorder
- Length of time from exposure of agent to onset of symptoms
- Congruence of symptoms with those of known exposure-related disorder
- Lack of other more likely explanations of the signs and symptoms

More than one million workers are exposed to silica each year. Symptoms rarely develop in less than 5 years. Progression of the disease results in extreme shortness of breath, loss of appetite, chest pains, and potentially respiratory failure (ALA, 2018a). Asbestosis is progressive and causes severe scarring of the lung, which leads to fibrosis. The lungs become stiff, making it difficult to breathe or to oxygenate well. The disease may not evidence manifestations until 10 to 40 years after exposure (ALA, 2018a). Coal worker's pneumoconiosis is a collection of lung disease caused by exposure to inhaled dusts.

The nurse provides education about preventive measures to patients and their families, assesses patients for a history of exposure to environmental agents, and makes referrals so that pulmonary function can be evaluated and the patient can be treated early in the course of the disease. These diseases have no effective treatment because damage is irreversible. Supportive therapy is aimed at preventing infections and managing complications.

 Veterans Considerations

Many American veterans who served in Iraq and Afghanistan are experiencing respiratory disorders as a result of exposure to pollutants in situations such as sand storms and car bombings. Their illnesses can range from a new onset of asthma to constrictive bronchiolitis (Harrington, Schmidt, Szema, et al., 2017). These veterans could also have been exposed to organic contamination within the sand that could further irritate airways. When providing care to a veteran, it is important to assess exposure to airway irritants, particularly when the patient is complaining of chronic respiratory symptoms.

CHEST TUMORS

Tumors of the lung may be benign or malignant. A malignant chest tumor can be primary, arising within the lung, chest wall, or mediastinum or it can be a metastasis from a primary tumor site elsewhere in the body.

Lung Cancer (Bronchogenic Carcinoma)

Lung cancer is the leading cancer killer among men and women in the United States, with about 1 out of 4 cancer deaths from lung cancer; over 135,000 deaths were estimated in 2018 (Midthun, 2019). Each year, more people die of lung cancer than of colon, breast, and prostate cancers combined. Approximately 228,820 new cases of lung cancer are diagnosed annually; 13% of new cancers for men and women involve the lung or bronchus (American Cancer Society [ACS], 2019). In approximately 48.5% of patients with lung cancer, the disease has spread to regional lymphatics and other sites by the time of diagnosis. As a result, the long-term survival rate is low. Overall, the 5-year survival rate is 21.7% (ALA, 2020; Thomas & Gould, 2019).

Pathophysiology

The most common cause of lung cancer is inhaled carcinogens, most often cigarette smoke (>85%); other carcinogens include radon gas and occupational and environmental agents (ALA, 2020). Lung cancers arise from a single transformed epithelial cell in the tracheobronchial airways, in which the carcinogen binds to and damages the cell's DNA. This damage results in cellular changes, abnormal cell growth, and eventually a malignant cell. As the damaged DNA is passed on to daughter cells, the DNA undergoes further changes and becomes unstable. With the accumulation of genetic changes, the pulmonary epithelium undergoes malignant transformation from normal epithelium eventually to invasive carcinoma. Carcinoma tends to arise at sites of previous scarring in the lung (e.g., TB, fibrosis).

Classification and Staging

For purposes of staging and treatment, over 95% of lung cancers are classified into one of two major categories: small

TABLE 19-7	Five-Year Relative Survival Rates for Lung Cancer based on Surveillance, Epidemiology, End Results (SEER) Stage[a]
SEER Stage	**5-Year Relative Survival Rate (%)**
NSCLC	
Localized	60
Regional	33
Distant	6
All SEER stages combined	23
SCLC	
Localized	29
Regional	15
Distant	3
All SEER stages combined	6

[a]Data are for patients diagnosed between the years 2009 and 2015. The SEER database does not group patients by the TNM system; rather, SEER categorizes patients based upon whether or not cancer has spread to distant organs/tissues (*distant*), or to proximal tissues or lymph nodes (*regional*), or has not spread outside the lung (*localized*).

NSCLC, non-small cell lung cancer; SCLC, small cell lung cancer; TNM system, a tumor staging system promulgated by the American Joint Committee on Cancer that stages cancer based upon evidence of the size of the tumor (*T*), extent of lymph node involvement (*N*), and whether or not metastasis has occurred (*M*).

Adapted from American Cancer Society (ACS). (2019). Lung cancer survival rates. Last updated 10/1/2019. Retrieved on 10/4/2019 at: www.cancer.org/cancer/lung-cancer/detection-diagnosis-staging/survival-rates.html

cell lung cancer (SCLC) and non-small cell lung cancer (NSCLC). SCLC represents approximately 13% of tumors, and includes small cell and combined small cell cancers. NSCLC represents approximately 84% of tumors, and these are further classified by cell type, including squamous cell (20%), large cell (5%), adenocarcinoma (41%), and others, some of which cannot be classified (18%) (ACS, 2019; Midthun, 2019).

In terms of specific types of NSCLC, squamous cell cancer is usually more centrally located and arises more commonly in the segmental and subsegmental bronchi. Adenocarcinoma is the most prevalent carcinoma of the lung in both men and women; it occurs peripherally as peripheral masses or nodules and often metastasizes. Large cell carcinoma (also called *undifferentiated carcinoma*) is a fast-growing tumor that tends to arise peripherally. Bronchoalveolar cell cancer is found in the terminal bronchi and alveoli and is usually slower growing compared with other bronchogenic carcinomas.

In addition to classification according to cell type, lung cancers are staged using the TNM staging system. The stage of the tumor refers to the size of the tumor, its location, whether lymph nodes are involved, and whether the cancer has spread (ACS, 2019). NSCLC is staged as I to IV. Stage I is the earliest stage and has the highest cure rate, whereas stage IV designates metastatic spread. Survival rates for NSCLC are shown in Table 19-7. (Diagnostic tools and further information on staging are described in Chapter 12.)

Risk Factors

The National Comprehensive Cancer Network (NCCN; 2020) asserts that 85% to 90% of all lung cancer cases are caused by cigarette smoke, whether it is from voluntary or involuntary (secondhand) smoking. Other factors that have been associated with lung cancer include genetic predisposition, dietary deficits, and underlying respiratory diseases, such

as COPD and TB. Some familial predisposition to lung cancer exists. The incidence of lung cancer in close relatives of patients with lung cancer is two to three times higher than the general population, regardless of smoking status (ACS, 2019).

Tobacco Smoke

The risk of developing lung cancer is about 23 times higher in men who smoke and 13 times higher in women who smoke compared to individuals who have never smoked (ACS, 2019). Risk is determined by the pack-year history (number of packs of cigarettes used each day, multiplied by the number of years smoked), the age of initiation of smoking, the depth of inhalation, and the tar and nicotine levels in the cigarettes smoked. The younger a person is when they start smoking, the greater the risk of developing lung cancer. People who smoke and use smokeless products as a supplemental source of nicotine have an increased overall risk of lung cancer (ACS, 2019).

Almost all cases of SCLC are due to cigarette smoking. SCLC is rare in people who have never smoked. It is the most aggressive form of lung cancer, grows quickly, and usually starts in the airways in the center of the chest (ACS, 2019).

Electronic Nicotine Delivery Systems

Electronic nicotine delivery systems (ENDS) include e-cigarettes, e-pens, e-pipes, e-hookahs, and e-cigars. According to a 2018 survey of 44,000 high school adolescents, 37% of 12th graders self-reported use of e-cigarettes (NIH News in Health, 2019). The amounts of nicotine and other substances a person gets from each cartridge are also unclear and have been found to vary greatly even when comparing same brand cartridges from the same manufacturer. Since these ENDS products have only been available for about a decade, the link between their use and lung cancer is unclear at the present time (ACS, 2019).

Secondhand Smoke

Secondhand or involuntary smoking has been identified as a cause of lung cancer in people who do not smoke. People who are involuntarily exposed to tobacco smoke in a closed environment (house, automobile, building) have an increased risk of lung cancer when compared with unexposed individuals who do not smoke (CDC, 2018a; NCCN, 2020).

Environmental and Occupational Exposure

Various carcinogens have been identified in the atmosphere, including motor vehicle emissions and pollutants from refineries and manufacturing plants. Evidence suggests that the incidence of lung cancer is greater in urban areas as a result of the buildup of pollutants and motor vehicle emissions (ALA, 2018b).

Radon is a colorless, odorless gas found in soil and rocks. For many years, it has been associated with uranium mines, but it is now known to seep into homes through ground rock. High levels of radon have been associated with the development of lung cancer, especially when combined with cigarette smoking. Homeowners are advised to have radon levels checked in their houses and to arrange for special venting if the levels are high.

Chronic exposure to industrial carcinogens, such as arsenic, asbestos, mustard gas, chromates, coke oven fumes, nickel, oil, and radiation, has been associated with the development of lung cancer. Laws have been passed to control exposure to these carcinogens in the workplace.

Genetic Mutations

Genetic mutations can cause certain changes in the DNA of lung cells. These changes can lead to abnormal cell growth and, sometimes, cancer. Acquired mutations in lung cells often result from exposure to factors in the environment, such as cancer-causing chemicals in tobacco smoke (ACS, 2019). The most common genetic mutations occur in *EGFR* (the gene that produces epidermal growth factor receptor) and the *K-RAS* or *ALK* oncogenes. *EGFR* is abnormal in about 50% of all patients with lung cancer. Abnormalities in *K-RAS* or *ALK* oncogenes are thought to be important in the development of NSCLC (ACS, 2019).

Clinical Manifestations

Often, lung cancer develops insidiously and is asymptomatic until late in its course. The signs and symptoms depend on the location and size of the tumor, the degree of obstruction, and the existence of metastases to regional or distant sites.

The most frequent symptom of lung cancer is cough or change in a chronic cough. People frequently ignore this symptom and attribute it to smoking or a respiratory infection. The cough may start as a dry, persistent cough, without sputum production. When obstruction of airways occurs, the cough may become productive due to infection.

> ### ► *Quality and Safety Nursing Alert*
>
> *A cough that changes in character should arouse suspicion of lung cancer.*

Dyspnea is prominent in patients early in their disease. Causes of dyspnea may include tumor occlusion of the airway or lung parenchyma, pleural effusion, pneumonia, or complications of treatment. Hemoptysis or blood-tinged sputum may be expectorated. Chest or shoulder pain may indicate chest wall or pleural involvement by a tumor. Pain also is a late manifestation and may be related to metastasis to the bone.

In some patients, a recurring fever is an early symptom in response to a persistent infection in an area of pneumonitis distal to the tumor. In fact, cancer of the lung should be suspected in people with repeated unresolved upper respiratory tract infections. If the tumor spreads to adjacent structures and regional lymph nodes, the patient may present with chest pain and tightness, hoarseness (involving the recurrent laryngeal nerve), dysphagia, head and neck edema, and symptoms of pleural or pericardial effusion. The most common sites of metastases are lymph nodes, bone, brain, contralateral lung, adrenal glands, and liver (see Fig. 19-10). Nonspecific symptoms of weakness, anorexia, and weight loss also may be present (Eldridge, 2020).

Assessment and Diagnostic Findings

If pulmonary symptoms occur in individuals who currently smoke or who formerly smoked, or in people chronically

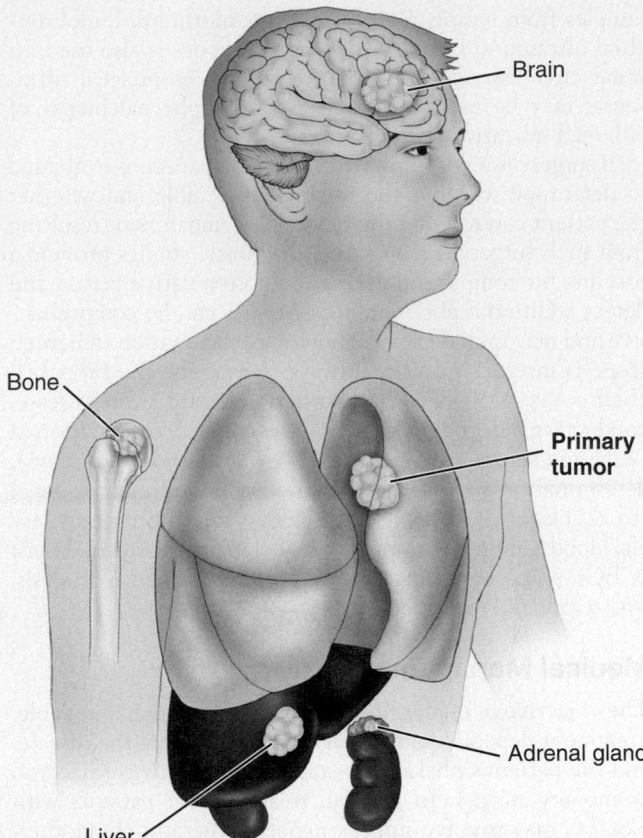

Figure 19-10 • Frequent sites of lung cancer metastasis.

exposed to secondhand smoke, cancer of the lung should be considered. A chest x-ray is performed to search for pulmonary density, a solitary pulmonary nodule (coin lesion), atelectasis, and infection. CT scans of the chest are used to identify small nodules not easily visualized on the chest x-ray and also to serially examine areas for lymphadenopathy. Additionally, the U.S. Preventive Services Task Force (USPSTF) recommends annual lung cancer screening using low dose CT (LDCT) for adults 55 to 80 years of age who have a 30 pack-year smoking history and either currently smoke or have quit smoking less than 15 years ago. Each pack-year is calculated based upon smoking one pack of cigarettes daily for 1 year; for instance, a 30 pack-year is defined as smoking one pack of cigarettes daily for 30 years, or 3 packs daily for 10 years (CDC, 2019e).

Fiberoptic bronchoscopy is commonly used to diagnose lung cancer; it provides a detailed study of the tracheobronchial tree and allows for brushings, washings, and biopsies of suspicious areas. For peripheral lesions not amenable to bronchoscopic biopsy, a transthoracic fine-needle aspiration may be performed under CT guidance to aspirate cells from a suspicious area.

A variety of scans may be used to assess for metastasis of the cancer. These may include bone scans, abdominal scans, positron emission tomography (PET) scans, and liver ultrasound. CT scan of the brain, magnetic resonance imaging (MRI), and other neurologic diagnostic procedures are used to detect central nervous system metastases. Mediastinoscopy or mediastinotomy may be used to obtain biopsy samples from lymph nodes in the mediastinum. Endobronchial ultrasound biopsy of mediastinal nodes is also used. In some circumstances, an endoscopy with esophageal ultrasound may be used to obtain a transesophageal biopsy of enlarged subcarinal lymph nodes.

If surgery is a potential treatment, the patient is evaluated to determine whether the tumor is resectable and whether the patient can tolerate the physiologic impairment resulting from such surgery. Preoperative diagnostic studies provide a baseline for comparison during the postoperative period and detect additional abnormalities. Studies can be comprehensive and may include a bronchoscopic examination (a lighted scope is inserted into the airways to examine the bronchi), chest x-ray, MRI, ECG (for arteriosclerotic heart disease, conduction defects), nutritional assessment, determination of BUN and serum creatinine levels (to assess renal function), determination of glucose tolerance or blood glucose level (to check for diabetes), serum electrolytes and protein levels, blood volume determinations, complete blood cell count (CBC), pulmonary function tests, arterial blood gas analysis, V̇/Q̇ scans, and exercise testing.

Medical Management

The objective of management is to provide a cure, if possible. Treatment depends on the cell type, the stage of the disease, and the patient's physiologic status (particularly cardiac and pulmonary status). In general, treatment for patients with NSCLC may involve surgery, radiation therapy, chemotherapy, immunotherapy—or a combination of these. Immunotherapy specifically targets patients' immune cells so that they are primed to more effectively kill cancer cells. Gene therapy using agents that target specific genetic mutations including *EGFR* mutations and *ALK* and *ROS1* rearrangements have shown promising results (Eldridge, 2020).

Treatment for patients with SCLC may include surgery (but only if the cancer is in one lung and there is no metastasis), radiation therapy, laser therapy to open airways blocked by tumor growth, and endoscopic stent placement (to open an airway). Although the cancer cells are small, they grow very quickly and create large tumors. These tumors often metastasize (spread) rapidly to other parts of the body, including the brain, liver, and bone. Typically, by the time a patient is diagnosed with SCLC, it is late in the course of the disease and metastasis has occurred.

Surgical Management: Thoracotomy

A **thoracotomy** (creation of a surgical opening into the thoracic cavity) may be performed to treat lung cancer. As noted previously, surgery is primarily used for patients with NSCLC, because SCLC grows rapidly and metastasizes early and extensively. Surgical resection is the preferred method of treating patients with localized NSCLCs without evidence of metastatic spread, and with adequate cardiopulmonary function. However, coronary artery disease, pulmonary insufficiency, and other comorbidities may contraindicate surgical intervention. The cure rate of surgical resection depends on the type and stage of the cancer. Several different types of lung resection may be performed (see Chart 19-22). The most common surgical procedure for a small, apparently curable tumor of the lung is lobectomy (removal of a lobe of the lung). In some cases, pneumonectomy (removal of an entire lung) may be required.

Nursing Management of the Patient Having a Thoracotomy

Patients are typically admitted on the day of surgery. The nurse in the outpatient surgical clinic setting is responsible for performing the preoperative assessment and education and for alleviating the anxiety experienced by the patient and family members by providing them with anticipatory guidance. Postoperatively, the patient may be managed by the nurse in the ICU. Successfully managing transitions in care for the patient from the ICU to other inpatient acute care settings (e.g., medical-surgical unit, step-down unit) to the outpatient setting is a key nursing responsibility.

 Educating the Patient Preoperatively

The nurse informs the patient about what to expect, from administration of anesthesia to thoracotomy, and the likely use of chest tubes and a drainage system in the postoperative period. The patient is also informed about the usual postoperative administration of oxygen to facilitate breathing and the possible use of a ventilator. It is essential to explain the importance of frequent turning to promote drainage of lung secretions. Instruction in the use of incentive spirometry begins before surgery to familiarize the patient with its correct use. The nurse educates the patient on the use of diaphragmatic and pursed-lip breathing, and the patient should begin practicing these techniques (see Chapter 20, Chart 20-5).

Because a coughing schedule is necessary in the postoperative period to promote the clearance or removal of secretions, the nurse instructs the patient in the technique of coughing and warns the patient that the coughing routine may be uncomfortable. The nurse educates the patient about how to splint the incision with the hands, a pillow, or a folded towel.

Encouraging the use of forced expiratory technique (FET) may be helpful for the patient with diminished expiratory flow rates or for the patient who refuses to cough because of severe pain. FET is the expulsion of air through an open glottis. This technique stimulates pulmonary expansion and assists in alveolar inflation (Kacmarek, Stoller, Heuer, et al., 2017). The nurse instructs the patient as follows:

- Take a deep diaphragmatic breath and exhale forcefully against the hand in a quick, distinct pant, or huff.
- Practice doing small huffs and progress to one strong huff during exhalation.

Patients should be informed preoperatively that blood and other fluids may be given, oxygen will be given, and vital signs will be checked often for several hours after surgery. If a chest tube is indicated (see later discussion on Chest Drainage Systems), the patient should be informed that it will drain the fluid and air that normally accumulate after chest surgery. The patient and family are informed that the patient may be admitted to the ICU for 1 to 2 days after surgery, that the patient may experience pain at the incision site, and that medication is available to relieve pain and discomfort.

Chart 19-22 Thoracic Surgeries and Procedures

Pneumonectomy

The removal of an entire lung, referred to as pneumonectomy, is performed chiefly for cancer when the lesion cannot be removed by a less extensive procedure. It also may be performed for lung abscesses, bronchiectasis, or extensive unilateral tuberculosis. The removal of the right lung is riskier than the removal of the left, because the right lung has a larger vascular bed and its removal imposes a greater physiologic burden.

A posterolateral or anterolateral thoracotomy incision is made, sometimes with resection of a rib. The pulmonary artery and the pulmonary veins are ligated and severed. The main bronchus is divided and the lung removed. The bronchial stump is stapled, and usually no drains are used because the accumulation of fluid in the empty hemithorax prevents mediastinal shift.

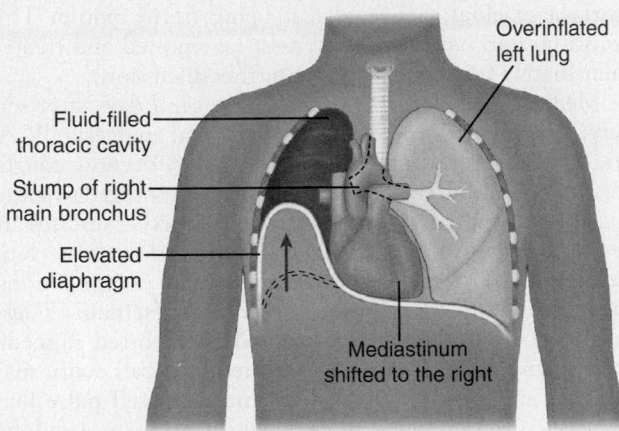

Pneumonectomy

Lobectomy

When the pathology is limited to one area of a lung, a lobectomy (removal of a lobe of a lung) is performed. Lobectomy, which is more common than pneumonectomy, may be carried out for bronchogenic carcinoma, giant emphysematous blebs or bullae, benign tumors, metastatic malignant tumors, bronchiectasis, and fungal infections.

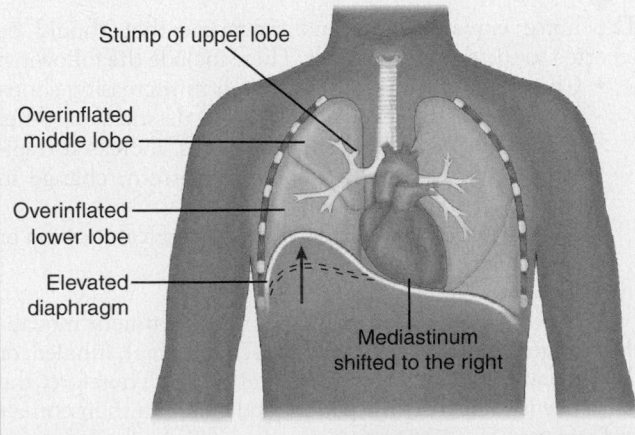

Lobectomy

The surgeon makes a thoracotomy incision. Its exact location depends on the lobe to be resected. When the pleural space is entered, the involved lung collapses and the lobar vessels and the bronchus are ligated and divided. After the lobe is removed, the remaining lobes of the lung are re-expanded. Usually, two chest catheters are inserted for drainage. The upper tube is for air removal; the lower one is for fluid drainage. Sometimes, only one catheter is needed. The chest tube is connected to a chest drainage apparatus for several days.

Segmentectomy (Segmental Resection)

Some lesions are located in only one segment of the lung. Bronchopulmonary segments are subdivisions of the lung that function as individual units. They are held together by delicate connective tissue. Disease processes may be limited to a single segment. Care is used to preserve as much healthy and functional lung tissue as possible, especially in patients who already have limited cardiopulmonary reserve. Single segments can be removed from any lobe; the right middle lobe, which has only two small segments, invariably is removed entirely. On the left side, corresponding to a middle lobe, is a "lingular" segment of the upper lobe. This can be removed as a single segment or by lingulectomy. This segment frequently is involved in bronchiectasis.

Wedge Resection

A wedge resection of a small, well-circumscribed lesion may be performed without regard to the location of the intersegmental planes. The pleural cavity usually is drained because of the possibility of an air or blood leak. This procedure is performed for diagnostic lung biopsy and for the excision of small peripheral nodules.

Bronchoplastic or Sleeve Resection

Bronchoplastic resection is a procedure in which only one lobar bronchus, together with a part of the right or left bronchus, is excised. The distal bronchus is reanastomosed to the proximal bronchus or trachea.

Lung Volume Reduction

Lung volume reduction is a surgical procedure involving the removal of 20% to 30% of a patient's lung through a midsternal incision or video thoracoscopy. The diseased lung tissue is identified on a lung perfusion scan. This surgery leads to significant improvements in dyspnea, exercise capacity, quality of life, and survival of a subgroup of people with end-stage emphysema.

Video Thoracoscopy

A video thoracoscopy is an endoscopic procedure that allows the surgeon to look into the thorax without making a large incision. The procedure is performed to obtain specimens of tissue for biopsy, to treat recurrent spontaneous pneumothorax, and to diagnose either pleural effusions or pleural masses. Thoracoscopy has also been found to be an effective diagnostic and therapeutic alternative for the treatment of mediastinal disorders. Some advantages of video thoracoscopy are rapid diagnosis and treatment of some conditions, a decrease in postoperative complications, and a shortened hospital stay.

Adapted from Urden, L. D., Stacy, K. M., & Lough, M. E. (2018). *Critical care nursing: Diagnosis and management* (8th ed.). St. Louis, MO: Elsevier Mosby.

The nurse listens to the patient and family to evaluate their feelings about the illness and proposed treatment. The nurse also determines the patient's motivation to return to normal or baseline function. The patient may reveal significant concerns: fear of hemorrhage because of bloody sputum, fear of discomfort from a chronic cough and chest pain, fear of ventilator dependence, or fear of death because of dyspnea and the underlying disease.

The nurse helps the patient to address fears and to cope with the stress of surgery by correcting any misconceptions, supporting the patient's decision to undergo surgery, and dealing honestly with questions about pain and discomfort and the patient's treatment. The management and control of pain begin before surgery, when the nurse informs the patient that many postoperative problems can be overcome by following certain routines related to deep breathing, coughing, turning, and moving. Nonopioid preemptive analgesic agents (e.g., acetaminophen and nonsteroidal anti-inflammatory drugs [NSAIDs]) may also be prescribed to help decrease the dose of postoperative opioid agents. This also helps to facilitate deep-breathing techniques and return to normal respiratory function. If patient-controlled analgesia (PCA) or patient-controlled epidural analgesia (PCEA) is to be used after surgery, the nurse instructs the patient in its use.

 ## Postoperative Management

After surgery, the vital signs are checked frequently. Oxygen is given by a mechanical ventilator, nasal cannula, or mask for as long as necessary. A reduction in lung capacity requires a period of physiologic adjustment, and fluids may be given at a low hourly rate to prevent fluid overload and pulmonary edema. After the patient has recovered from anesthesia and the vital signs have stabilized, the head of the bed may be elevated 30 to 45 degrees. Careful positioning of the patient is important. After pneumonectomy, a patient is usually turned every hour from the back to the operative side and should not be completely turned to the unoperated side. This allows the fluid left in the space to consolidate and prevents the remaining lung and the heart from shifting (mediastinal shift) toward the operative side. The patient with a lobectomy may be turned to either side, and a patient with a segmental resection usually is not turned onto the operative side unless the surgeon prescribes this position (see Chart 19-23: Plan of Nursing Care: Care of the Patient After Thoracotomy).

Complications after thoracic surgery are always possible and must be identified and managed early. The nurse monitors the patient at regular intervals for signs of respiratory distress or developing respiratory failure, arrhythmias, bronchopleural fistula, hemorrhage and shock, atelectasis, and incisional or pulmonary infection. Arrhythmias are often related to the effects of hypoxia or the surgical procedure. They are treated with antiarrhythmic medication and supportive therapy (see Chapter 22). Pulmonary infections or effusion, often preceded by atelectasis, may occur a few days into the postoperative course.

Pneumothorax may occur after thoracic surgery if there is an air leak from the surgical site to the pleural cavity or from the pleural cavity to the environment. Failure of the chest drainage system prevents return of negative pressure in the pleural cavity and results in pneumothorax. In the patient who is postoperative, pneumothorax is often accompanied by hemothorax. The nurse maintains the chest drainage system and monitors the patient for signs and symptoms of pneumothorax (see later discussions): increasing shortness of breath, tachycardia, increased respiratory rate, and increasing respiratory distress. Bronchopleural fistula is a serious but rare complication that prevents the return of negative intrathoracic pressure and lung re-expansion. Depending on its severity, it is treated with continued closed chest drainage and mechanical ventilation.

Hemorrhage and shock are managed by treating the underlying cause, whether by reoperation or by administration of blood products or fluids. Pulmonary edema from overinfusion of IV fluids is a significant danger. Early symptoms are dyspnea; crackles; tachycardia; and pink, frothy sputum. This constitutes an emergency and must be reported and treated immediately (see Chapter 25 for further discussion).

Medication for pain is needed for several days after surgery; it is usually a combination of epidural analgesia, PCA, and scheduled or as-needed oral analgesics. Because coughing can be painful, the patient should be encouraged to splint the chest as taught in the preoperative period. Exercises are resumed early in the postoperative period to facilitate lung ventilation. The nurse assesses for signs of complications, including cyanosis, dyspnea, and acute chest pain. These may indicate atelectasis and should be reported immediately. Increased temperature or white blood cell count may indicate an infection, and pallor and increased pulse may indicate internal hemorrhage. Dressings are assessed for fresh bleeding.

Promoting Home, Community-Based, and Transitional Care

The nurse educates the patient and family about postoperative care that will be continued in the community setting and at home.

 ### Educating Patients About Self-Care

The nurse explains signs and symptoms that should be reported to the primary provider. These include the following:

- Change in respiratory status, such as increasing shortness of breath, fever, increased restlessness or other changes in mental or cognitive status, increased respiratory rate, change in respiratory pattern, change in amount or color of sputum
- Bleeding or other drainage from the surgical incision or chest tube exit sites
- Increased chest pain

In addition, respiratory care and other treatment modalities (oxygen; incentive spirometry; CPT; and oral, inhaled, or IV medications) may be continued at home. Therefore, the nurse needs to instruct the patient and family in their correct and safe use.

The nurse emphasizes the importance of progressively increased activity. The patient is instructed to ambulate within limits and informed that return of strength is likely to be very gradual. Another important aspect of patient education addresses shoulder exercises. The patient is instructed to

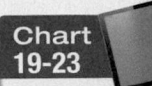

Chart 19-23

PLAN OF NURSING CARE
Care of the Patient After Thoracotomy

NURSING DIAGNOSIS: Impaired gas exchange associated with lung impairment and surgery
GOAL: Improvement of gas exchange and breathing

Nursing Interventions	Rationale	Expected Outcomes

1. Monitor pulmonary status as directed and as needed.
  a. Auscultate breath sounds.
  b. Check rate, depth, and pattern of respirations.
  c. Assess blood gases for signs of hypoxemia or CO_2 retention.
  d. Evaluate patient's color for cyanosis.
	1. Changes in pulmonary status indicate improvement or onset of complications.	• Lungs are clear on auscultation.
		• Respiratory rate is within acceptable range with no episodes of dyspnea.
		• Vital signs are stable.
		• Arrhythmias are not present or are treated effectively.
		• Demonstrates deep, controlled, effective breathing to allow maximal lung expansion.
		• Uses incentive spirometer every 2 hours while awake.
		• Demonstrates deep, effective coughing technique.
		• Lungs are expanded to capacity (evidenced by chest x-ray).

2. Monitor and record blood pressure, apical pulse, and temperature every 2 to 4 hours, and central venous pressure (if indicated) every 2 hours.	2. Vital signs aid in evaluating effect of surgery on cardiac status.	
3. Monitor continuous electrocardiogram for pattern and arrhythmias.	3. Arrhythmias (especially atrial fibrillation and atrial flutter) are more frequently seen after thoracic surgery. A patient with total pneumonectomy is especially prone to cardiac irregularity.	
4. Elevate head of bed 30° to 40° when patient is oriented and hemodynamic status is stable.	4. Maximum lung excursion is achieved when patient is as close to upright as possible.	
5. Encourage deep-breathing exercises and effective use of incentive spirometer.	5. Helps to achieve maximal lung inflation and to open closed airways	
6. Encourage and promote an effective cough routine to be performed every hour during first 24 hours.	6. Coughing is necessary to remove retained secretions.	

7. Assess and monitor the chest drainage system.[a]
  a. Assess for leaks and patency as needed (see procedural guidelines for setting up and managing chest drainage systems at thepoint.lww.com/Brunner15e).
  b. Monitor amount and character of drainage and document every 2 hours. Notify primary provider if drainage is ≥150 mL/h.
	7. System is used to eliminate any residual air or fluid after thoracotomy.	

NURSING DIAGNOSIS: Impaired airway clearance associated with lung impairment, anesthesia, and pain
GOAL: Improvement of airway clearance and achievement of a patent airway

Nursing Interventions	Rationale	Expected Outcomes
1. Maintain an open airway.	1. Provides for adequate ventilation and gas exchange.	• Airway is patent. • Coughs effectively. • Splints incision while coughing. • Sputum is clear or colorless. • Lungs are clear on auscultation.
2. Perform endotracheal suctioning until patient can cough effectively.	2. Endotracheal secretions are present in excessive amounts in patients who are post-thoracotomy due to trauma to the tracheobronchial tree during surgery, diminished lung ventilation, and cough reflex.	
3. Assess and medicate for pain. Encourage deep-breathing and coughing exercises. Help splint incision during coughing.	3. Helps to achieve maximal lung inflation and to open closed airways. Coughing is painful; incision needs to be supported.	
4. Monitor amount, viscosity, color, and odor of sputum. Notify primary provider if sputum is excessive or contains bright-red blood.	4. Changes in sputum suggest presence of infection or change in pulmonary status. Colorless sputum is not unusual; opacification or coloring of sputum may indicate dehydration or infection.	
5. Administer humidification and small-volume nebulizer therapy as prescribed.	5. Secretions must be moistened and thinned if they are to be raised from the chest with the least amount of effort.	
6. Perform postural drainage, percussion, and vibration as prescribed. Do not percuss or vibrate directly over operative site.	6. Chest physiotherapy uses gravity to help remove secretions from the lung.	
7. Auscultate both sides of chest to determine changes in breath sounds.	7. Indications for tracheal suctioning are determined by chest auscultation.	

(continued on page 584)

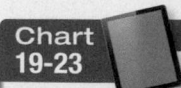

Chart 19-23 · PLAN OF NURSING CARE (continued)
Care of the Patient After Thoracotomy

NURSING DIAGNOSIS: Acute pain associated with incision, drainage tubes, and the surgical procedure
GOAL: Relief of pain and discomfort

Nursing Interventions	Rationale	Expected Outcomes
1. Evaluate location, character, quality, and severity of pain. Administer analgesic medication as prescribed and as needed. Observe for respiratory effect of opioid. Note if patient seems too somnolent to cough or if respirations are depressed.	1. Pain limits chest excursions and thereby decreases ventilation.	• Asks for pain medication but verbalizes that they expect some discomfort while deep breathing and coughing. • Verbalizes that they are comfortable and not in acute distress.

2. Maintain care postoperatively in positioning the patient.
  a. Place patient in semi-Fowler position.
  b. Patients with limited respiratory reserve may not be able to turn on unoperated side.
  c. Assist or turn patient every 2 hours.
	2. The patient who is comfortable and free of pain will be less likely to splint the chest while breathing. A semi-Fowler position permits residual air in the pleural space to rise to upper portion of pleural space and be removed via the upper chest catheter.	• No signs of incisional infection evident.

3. Assess incision area every 8 hours for redness, heat, induration, swelling, separation, and drainage.	3. These signs indicate possible infection.	
4. Request order for patient-controlled analgesia pump if appropriate for patient.	4. Encouraging patient control over frequency and dose improves comfort and adherence with treatment regimen.	

NURSING DIAGNOSIS: Anxiety associated with outcomes of surgery, pain, technology
GOAL: Reduction of anxiety to a manageable level

Nursing Interventions	Rationale	Expected Outcomes
1. Explain all procedures in understandable language.	1. Explaining what can be expected in understandable terms decreases anxiety and increases cooperation.	• States that anxiety is at a manageable level. • Participates with health care team in treatment regimen. • Uses appropriate coping skills (verbalization; pain relief strategies; the use of support systems such as family, clergy). • Demonstrates basic understanding of technology used in care.
2. Assess for pain and medicate, especially before potentially painful procedures.	2. Premedication before painful procedures or activities improves comfort and minimizes undue anxiety.	
3. Silence all *unnecessary* alarms on technology (monitors, ventilators).	3. *Unnecessary* alarms increase the risk of sensory overload and may increase anxiety. *Essential* alarms must be turned on at all times.	
4. Encourage and support patient while increasing activity level.	4. Positive reinforcement improves patient motivation and independence.	
5. Mobilize resources (family, clergy, social worker) to help patient cope with outcomes of surgery (diagnosis, change in functional abilities).	5. A multidisciplinary approach promotes the patient's strengths and coping mechanisms.	

NURSING DIAGNOSIS: Impaired mobility of the upper extremities associated with thoracic surgery
GOAL: Increased mobility of the affected shoulder and arm

Nursing Interventions	Rationale	Expected Outcomes

1. Assist patient with normal range of motion and function of shoulder and trunk.
  a. Educate about use of breathing exercises to mobilize thorax.
  b. Encourage skeletal exercises to promote abduction and mobilization of shoulder (see Chart 19-23).
  c. Assist out of bed to chair as soon as pulmonary and circulatory systems are stable (usually by evening of surgery).
	1. Necessary to regain normal mobility of arm and shoulder and to speed recovery and minimize discomfort	• Demonstrates arm and shoulder exercises and verbalizes intent to perform them on discharge.
		• Regains previous range of motion in shoulder and arm.

2. Encourage progressive activities according to level of fatigue.	2. Increases patient's use of affected shoulder and arm	

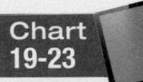

Chart 19-23	**PLAN OF NURSING CARE** (continued)
	Care of the Patient After Thoracotomy

NURSING DIAGNOSIS: Risk for hypovolaemia associated with the surgical procedure
GOAL: Maintenance of adequate fluid volume

Nursing Interventions	Rationale	Expected Outcomes

1. Monitor and record hourly intake and output. Urine output should be at least 0.5 mL/kg/h over 6 hours and at least 400 mL in 24 hours after surgery.
 	
2. Administer blood component therapy and parenteral fluids and diuretics as prescribed to restore and maintain fluid volume.
	1. Fluid management may be altered before, during, and after surgery, and patient's response to and need for fluid management must be assessed.
	
	2. Pulmonary edema due to transfusion or fluid overload is an ever-present threat; after pneumonectomy, the pulmonary vascular system has been greatly reduced.
		• Patient is adequately hydrated, as evidenced by:
		  • Urine output >0.5 mL/kg/h over 6 hours, and >400 mL in 24 hours
		  • Vital signs stable, heart rate, and central venous pressure approaching normal
		  • No excessive peripheral edema

NURSING DIAGNOSIS: Lack of knowledge of home care procedures
GOAL: Increased ability to carry out care procedures at home

Nursing Interventions	Rationale	Expected Outcomes
1. Encourage patient to practice arm and shoulder exercises 5 times daily at home. 2. Instruct patient to practice assuming a functionally erect position in front of a full-length mirror. 3. Instruct patient about home care (see Chart 19-25).	1. Exercise accelerates recovery of muscle function and reduces long-term pain and discomfort. 2. Practice will help restore normal posture. 3. Knowing what to expect facilitates recovery.	• Demonstrates arm and shoulder exercises. • Verbalizes need to try to assume an erect posture. • Verbalizes the importance of relieving discomfort, alternating walking and rest, performing breathing exercises, avoiding heavy lifting, avoiding undue fatigue, avoiding bronchial irritants, preventing colds or lung infections, getting influenza vaccine, keeping follow-up visits, and stopping smoking.

[a]A patient with a pneumonectomy usually does not have water-seal chest drainage because it is desirable that the pleural space fill with an effusion, which eventually obliterates this space. Some surgeons do use a modified water-seal system.

do these exercises five times daily (see Chart 19-24). Additional patient education is described in Chart 19-25.

Continuing and Transitional Care

Depending on the patient's physical status and the availability of family assistance, a referral for home, community-based, or transitional care may be indicated. The home health nurse assesses the patient's recovery from surgery, with special attention to respiratory status, the surgical incision, chest drainage, pain control, ambulation, and nutritional status. The patient's use of respiratory modalities is assessed to ensure that they are being used correctly and safely. In addition, the nurse assesses the patient's adherence to the postoperative treatment plan and identifies acute or late postoperative complications.

The recovery process may take longer than the patient had expected, and providing support to the patient is an important task for the nurse. Because of shorter hospital stays, follow-up appointments with the primary provider are essential. The nurse educates the patient about the importance of keeping follow-up appointments and completing laboratory tests as prescribed to assist the primary provider in evaluating recovery. The nurse provides continuous encouragement

and education to the patient and family during the process. As recovery progresses, the patient and family are reminded about the importance of participating in health promotion activities and recommended health screening.

Radiation Therapy

Radiation therapy may offer cure in a small percentage of patients with lung cancer. It is useful in controlling neoplasms that cannot be surgically resected but are responsive to radiation. Irradiation also may be used to reduce the size of a tumor, to make an inoperable tumor operable, or to relieve the pressure of the tumor on vital structures. It can reduce symptoms of spinal cord metastasis and superior vena caval compression. In addition, prophylactic brain irradiation is used in certain patients to treat microscopic metastases to the brain. Radiation therapy may help relieve cough, chest pain, dyspnea, hemoptysis, and bone and liver pain. Relief of symptoms may last from a few weeks to many months and is important in improving the quality of the remaining period of life. Stereotactic ablative radiotherapy (SABR) is a treatment option that delivers higher-than-typical doses of radiation directly to the tumor. This treatment is given over 1 to 5 days

Chart 19-24

PATIENT EDUCATION

Performing Arm and Shoulder Exercises

Arm and shoulder exercises are performed after thoracic surgery to restore movement, prevent painful stiffening of the shoulder, and improve muscle power. The nurse instructs the patient to perform these exercises as follows:

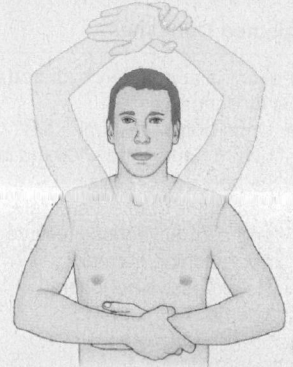

Hold hand of the affected side with the other hand, palms facing in. Raise the arms forward, upward, and then overhead, while taking a deep breath. Exhale while lowering the arms. Repeat five times.

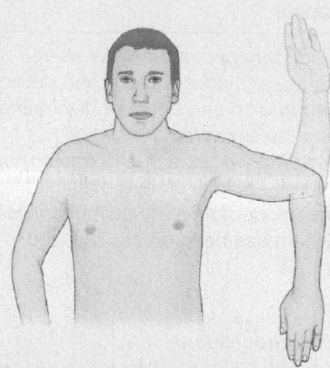

Raise arm sideward, upward, and downward in a waving motion

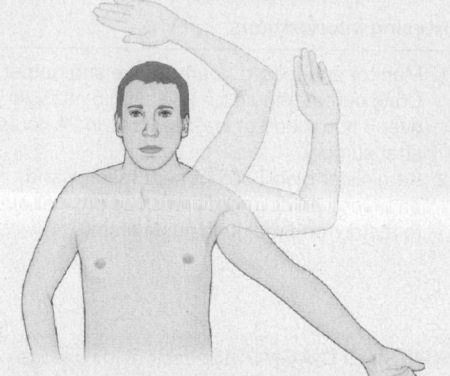

Place arm at side. Raise arm sideward, upward, and then overhead. Repeat five times. These exercises can also be performed while lying in bed.

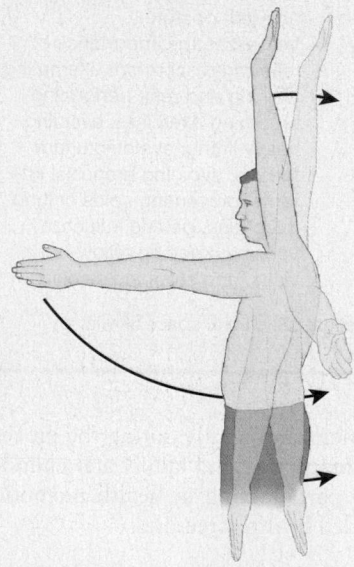

Extend the arm up and back, out to the side and back, down at the side, and back.

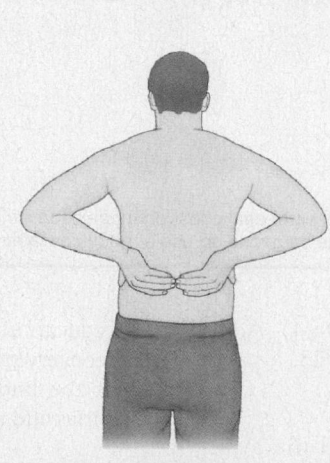

Place hands in small of back. Push elbows as far back as possible.

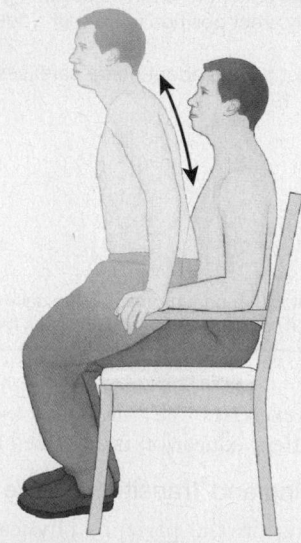

Sit erect in an armchair; place the hands on arms of the chair. Press down on hands, consciously pulling the abdomen in and stretching up from the waist. Inhale while raising the body until elbows are extended completely. Hold this position a moment, and begin exhaling while lowering the body slowly to the original position.

and is indicated for early stages of lung cancers in patients who either elect to not have surgery or are considered ineligible for surgery (ACS, 2019).

Radiation therapy usually is toxic to normal tissue within the radiation field, and this may lead to complications such as esophagitis, pneumonitis, and radiation lung fibrosis, although the incidence of these complications has decreased over time with improvements in delivery of radiation therapy (ACS, 2019). These complications may impair ventilatory and diffusion capacity and significantly reduce pulmonary reserve. The patient's nutritional status, psychological outlook, fatigue level, and signs of anemia and infection are monitored throughout the treatment (see Chapter 12 for management of the patient receiving radiation therapy).

Chart 19-25	HOME CARE CHECKLIST
	The Patient with a Thoracotomy

At the completion of education, the patient and/or caregiver will be able to:

- Name the procedure that was performed and identify any permanent changes in anatomic structure or function as well as changes in ADLs, IADLs, roles, relationships, and spirituality.
- State the name, dose, side effects, frequency, and schedule for all medications.
- Identify interventions and strategies (e.g., durable medical equipment, oxygen, and adaptive equipment) used in adapting to any permanent changes in structure or function.
- Describe ongoing postoperative therapeutic regimen, including diet and activities to perform (e.g., walking and breathing exercises) and to limit or avoid (e.g., lifting weights, driving a car, and contact sports).
  - Alternate walking and other activities with frequent rest periods, expecting weakness and fatigue for the first 3 weeks.
  - Walk at a moderate pace, gradually and persistently extending walking time and distance.
  - Perform arm and shoulder exercises as prescribed.
  - Perform breathing exercises several times daily for the first few weeks at home.
  - Avoid lifting >20 lb until complete healing has taken place; the chest muscles and incision may be weaker than normal for 3 to 6 months after surgery.
  - Use local heat and oral analgesia to relieve intercostal pain.

- Immediately stop any activity that causes undue fatigue, increased shortness of breath, or chest pain.
- Avoid bronchial irritants (smoke, fumes, air pollution, aerosol sprays).
- Avoid others with known colds or lung infections.
- Describe signs and symptoms of complications (e.g., increased shortness of breath, fever, restlessness, mental status changes, change in rate or pattern of respiration, increased pain, or bleeding from incision).
- Relate how to reach primary provider with questions or complications.
- State time and date of follow-up appointments.
- Obtain an annual influenza vaccine, and discuss vaccination against pneumonia with the primary provider.
- State understanding of community resources and referrals (if any).
- Identify the need for health promotion (e.g., weight reduction, smoking cessation, and stress management), disease prevention and screening activities

Resources

See Chapter 20, Chart 20-7 for additional information on oxygen therapy at home and Chart 19-23 for additional information on performing arm and shoulder exercises.

ADLs, activities of daily living; IADLs, instrumental activities of daily living.

Chemotherapy

Chemotherapy is used to alter tumor growth patterns, to treat distant metastases or small cell cancer of the lung, and as an adjunct to surgery or radiation therapy. Chemotherapy may provide relief, especially of pain, but it does not usually cure the disease or prolong life to any great degree. Chemotherapy is also accompanied by side effects. It is valuable in reducing pressure symptoms of lung cancer and in treating brain, spinal cord, and pericardial metastasis (see Chapter 12 for a discussion of chemotherapy for the patient with cancer).

The choice of agent depends on the growth of the tumor cell and the specific phase of the cell cycle that the medication affects. In combination with surgery, chemotherapy may be given before surgery (neoadjuvant therapy) or after surgery (adjuvant therapy). Specific guidelines are available for the treatment of differing stages of NSCLC and SCLC through the NCCN (2020).

Immunotherapy

Advances in immunotherapy have provided additional options for the treatment of advanced NSCLC and SCLC. Immunotherapy drugs referred to as checkpoint inhibitors are indicated for the treatment of unresectable stage III tumors in addition to lung cancers that have metastasized. These agents target programmed cell death proteins such as PD-1 or PD-L1 on T cells that prevent T cells from attacking other cells in the body. By blocking these PD proteins, the T cells are able to mount a better immune response against the tumor cells, more quickly and effectively killing them. Four checkpoint inhibitors are FDA-approved for use with lung cancer. The first three, pembrolizumab, nivolumab, and atezolizumab,

are approved for use in metastatic lung cancer (Hellman & West, 2020; Yang, Zhang, & Wang, 2019). In addition, pembrolizumab combined with chemotherapy may be used as a first-line treatment for metastatic NSCLC. Durvalumab is the only agent approved for nonoperable stage III NSCLC (Hellmann & West, 2020). Checkpoint inhibitors are delivered by IV infusion every 2, 3, or 4 weeks over several months or up to 1 year. They are generally well tolerated with few adverse effects, particularly as compared to chemotherapeutic agents. Side effects include fatigue, rashes, and diarrhea (ACS, 2019).

Palliative Care

Palliative care, concurrent with standard oncologic care for lung cancer, should be considered early in the course of illness for any patient with metastatic cancer or high symptom burden. In lung cancer, palliative therapy may include radiation therapy to shrink the tumor to provide pain relief, a variety of bronchoscopic interventions to open a narrowed bronchus or airway, and pain management and other comfort measures. Evaluation and referral for hospice care are important in planning for comfortable and dignified end-of-life care for the patient and family (see Chapter 13 for further discussion).

Complications

A variety of complications may occur as a result of treatment of lung cancer. Surgical resection may result in respiratory failure, particularly if the cardiopulmonary system is compromised before surgery. Surgical complications and prolonged mechanical ventilation are potential outcomes.

Despite advances in improved delivery of radiation therapy, complications may still ensue, including diminished cardiopulmonary function and other complications, such as pulmonary fibrosis, pericarditis, myelitis, and cor pulmonale (Benveniste, Gomez, Brett, et al., 2019). Chemotherapy, particularly in combination with radiation therapy, can cause pneumonitis. Pulmonary toxicity is a potential side effect of chemotherapy.

Nursing Management

Nursing care of patients with lung cancer is similar to that for other patients with cancer (see Chapter 12, Chart 12-6) and addresses the physiologic and psychological needs of the patient. The physiologic problems are primarily due to the respiratory manifestations of the disease. Nursing care includes strategies to ensure relief of pain and discomfort and to prevent complications.

Managing Symptoms

The nurse educates the patient and family about the potential side effects of the specific treatment and strategies to manage them. Strategies for managing such symptoms as dyspnea, fatigue, nausea and vomiting, and anorexia help the patient and family cope with therapeutic measures.

Relieving Breathing Problems

Airway clearance techniques are key to maintaining airway patency through the removal of excess secretions. This may be accomplished through deep-breathing exercises, chest physiotherapy, directed cough, suctioning, and in some instances bronchoscopy. Bronchodilator medications may be prescribed to promote bronchial dilation. As the tumor enlarges or spreads, it may compress a bronchus or involve a large area of lung tissue, resulting in an impaired breathing pattern and poor gas exchange. At some stage of the disease, supplemental oxygen will probably be necessary.

Nursing measures focus on decreasing dyspnea by encouraging the patient to assume positions that promote lung expansion and to perform breathing exercises for lung expansion and relaxation. Patient education about energy conservation and airway clearance techniques is also necessary. Many of the techniques used in pulmonary rehabilitation can be applied to patients with lung cancer. Depending on the severity of disease and the patient's wishes, a referral to a pulmonary rehabilitation program may be helpful in managing respiratory symptoms.

Reducing Fatigue

Fatigue is a devastating symptom that affects quality of life in patients with cancer. It is commonly experienced by patients with lung cancer and may be related to the disease itself, the cancer treatment and complications (e.g., anemia), sleep disturbances, pain and discomfort, hypoxemia, poor nutrition, or the psychological ramifications of the disease (e.g., anxiety and depression) (see Chapter 12 for nursing strategies to reduce fatigue).

Providing Psychological Support

Another important part of the nursing care of patients with lung cancer is provision of psychological support and identification of potential resources for the patient and family.

Often, the nurse must help the patient and family deal with the following:

- The poor prognosis and relatively rapid progression of this disease
- Informed decision making regarding the possible treatment options
- Methods to maintain the patient's quality of life during the course of this disease
- End-of-life treatment options

Oncology nurses are employed as *nurse navigators* in oncology practice settings to help patients and their families manage and coordinate the many challenging aspects of cancer care. Jeyathevan, Lemonde, and Cooper Brathwaite (2017) studied the effectiveness of the oncology nurse navigator role in helping patients and families deal with the complexities of a diagnosis of lung cancer (see Nursing Research Profile in Chart 19-26).

 Gerontologic Considerations

At the time of diagnosis of lung cancer, most patients are older than 65 years and have stage III or IV disease (Midthun, 2019). In older patients, the management of a cancer is complex and challenging. Although age is not a significant prognostic factor for overall survival and response to treatment of either NSCLC or SCLC, older patients have specific needs. The presence of comorbidities and the patient's cognitive, functional, nutritional, and social status are important issues to consider with the patient of advanced age. Depending on the comorbidities and functional status of older adult patients, chemotherapy agents, doses, and cycles may need to be adjusted to maintain quality of life.

Tumors of the Mediastinum

Tumors of the mediastinum include neurogenic tumors, tumors of the thymus, lymphomas, germ cell tumors, cysts, and mesenchymal tumors. These tumors may be malignant or benign. They are usually described in relation to location: anterior, middle, or posterior masses or tumors.

Clinical Manifestations

Nearly all symptoms of mediastinal tumors result from the pressure of the mass against important intrathoracic organs. Symptoms may include cough, wheezing, dyspnea, anterior chest or neck pain, bulging of the chest wall, heart palpitations, angina, other circulatory disturbances, central cyanosis, superior vena cava syndrome (i.e., swelling of the face, neck, and upper extremities), marked distention of the veins of the neck and the chest wall (evidence of the obstruction of large veins of the mediastinum by extravascular compression or intravascular invasion), and dysphagia and weight loss from pressure or invasion into the esophagus (Berry, 2019).

Assessment and Diagnostic Findings

Chest x-rays are the major method used initially to diagnose mediastinal tumors and cysts. A CT scan is the standard diagnostic test for the assessment of the mediastinum and surrounding structures. MRI, as well as PET, may be used in some circumstances (Berry, 2019).

Chart 19-26 NURSING RESEARCH PROFILE
The Role of the Oncology Nurse Navigator

Jeyathevan, G., Lemonde, M., & Cooper Brathwaite, A. (2017). The role of oncology nurse navigators in facilitating continuity of care within the diagnostic phase for adult patients with lung cancer. *Canadian Oncology Nursing Journal, 27*(1), 74–87.

Purpose

An emerging trend in the effective management of cancer care and treatment is the use of nurse navigators. The purpose of this phenomenologic qualitative research study was to explore the effectiveness of the oncology nurse navigator (ONN) in facilitating the care of the patient with lung cancer during the diagnostic period. Through the lens of both the ONN and the patient, the researchers explored the organizational and clinical component of the role and the impact on continuity of care and patient empowerment. This published report focused on continuity of care through the dimensions of informational, management, and relational continuity.

Design

A Bi-Dimensional Framework examining the organization and clinical role of the ONN guided this study. Using a phenomenologic approach, the "lived experience" of the patient and the ONN were explored. Purposive sampling yielded eight participants, four patients, and four ONNs. Criteria for patient participation in the study included: adults 18 years of age and older, symptoms suspicious of lung cancer, English speaking, and at least two prior contacts with the ONN. Criteria for nurse navigator participation in the study included: certification in oncology nursing, completion of courses specific to lung disease, and employed in the lung cancer diagnostic department as a nurse navigator. Semi-structured individual interviews were conducted with each participant; in addition, the ONNs participated in a focus group.

Findings

Five major themes emerged through an iterative process of thematic analysis from the perspective of the patient with lung cancer and the ONN. Themes identified included: patient focused care, needs assessment, shared decision making, accessibility, and eliminating barriers. These themes correspond to the continuity of care related to informational, management, and relational continuity.

Nursing Implications

Little is known about the impact of nurse navigators on the patient experience during the diagnostic and cancer treatment periods. This research provides empirical evidence on the importance of this role throughout the diagnostic period of cancer as perceived by both patients and ONNs. Patient-focused care was enhanced through the provision of timely, personalized information which aided in the patients' understanding of diagnostic tests and subsequent follow-up. Telephone needs assessment proved to be vital as the ONN explored not only medical symptoms and social aspects, but also included an assessment of cultural concerns prior to the patients' first visit to the cancer center. These interactions supported the theme of shared decision making; the participants felt empowered, rather than powerless, as the ONN involved them in their care. Empathy and therapeutic communication were expressed through the theme of accessibility. Participants acknowledged the "professional-personal" connection with the ONN. Through the trusting relationship that was formed, barriers were eliminated, and all aspects of care could be addressed during this phase of care. This research supports best practice standards for the role of the nurse navigator and provides a framework for continued study in other specialties of care.

Medical Management

If the tumor is malignant and has infiltrated the surrounding tissue and complete surgical removal is not feasible, radiation therapy, chemotherapy, or both are used.

Many mediastinal tumors are benign and operable. The location of the tumor (anterior, middle, or posterior compartment) in the mediastinum dictates the type of incision. The common incision used is a median sternotomy; however, a thoracotomy may be used, depending on the location of the tumor. Additional approaches include a bilateral anterior thoracotomy (clamshell incision) and video-assisted thoracoscopic surgery. The care is the same as for any patient undergoing thoracic surgery. Major complications include hemorrhage, injury to the phrenic or recurrent laryngeal nerve, and infection.

CHEST TRAUMA

Thoracic injuries occurred in over 194,622 patients and accounted for 22.58% of the types of trauma recently recorded in a national trauma database (American College of Surgeons, 2016). Four of the top 10 complications in trauma patients were related to the respiratory system: pneumonia, DVT/PE, unplanned extubation, and acute lung injury/ARDS (American College of Surgeons, 2016).

Major chest trauma may occur alone or in combination with multiple other injuries. Chest trauma is classified as either blunt or penetrating. Blunt chest trauma results from sudden compression or positive pressure inflicted to the chest wall. Penetrating trauma occurs when a foreign object penetrates the chest wall.

Blunt Trauma

Overall, blunt thoracic injuries are directly responsible for 20% to 25% of all trauma deaths (Mancini, 2018). Although blunt chest trauma is more common than penetrating trauma, it is often difficult to identify the extent of the damage because the symptoms may be generalized and vague. In addition, patients may not seek immediate medical attention, which may complicate the problem.

Pathophysiology

The most common causes of blunt chest trauma are motor vehicle crashes (trauma from steering wheel, seat belt), falls, and bicycle crashes (trauma from handlebars). Types of blunt chest trauma include chest wall fractures, dislocations, and barotraumas (including diaphragmatic injuries); injuries of the pleura, lungs, and aerodigestive tracts; and blunt injuries of the heart, great arteries, veins, and lymphatics (Mancini, 2018). Injuries to the chest are often life-threatening and result in one or more of the following pathologic states:

- Hypoxemia from disruption of the airway; injury to the lung parenchyma, rib cage, and respiratory musculature; massive hemorrhage; collapsed lung; and pneumothorax
- Hypovolemia from massive fluid loss from the great vessels, cardiac rupture, or hemothorax
- Cardiac failure from cardiac tamponade, cardiac contusion, or increased intrathoracic pressure

These pathologic states frequently result in impaired $\dot{V}/\dot{Q}$ leading to acute kidney injury, hypovolemic shock, and death.

Assessment and Diagnostic Findings

Because time is critical in treating chest trauma, the patient must be assessed immediately to determine the following: time elapsed since injury occurred, mechanism of injury, level of responsiveness, specific injuries, estimated blood loss, recent drug or alcohol use, and prehospital treatment. Initial assessment of thoracic injuries includes assessment of airway obstruction, tension pneumothorax, open pneumothorax, massive hemothorax, flail chest, and cardiac tamponade. These injuries are life-threatening and require immediate treatment. Secondary assessment includes assessment of simple pneumothorax, hemothorax, pulmonary contusion, traumatic aortic rupture, tracheobronchial disruption, esophageal perforation, traumatic diaphragmatic injury, and penetrating wounds to the mediastinum. Although listed as secondary, these injuries may be life-threatening as well.

The physical examination includes inspection of the airway, thorax, neck veins, and breathing difficulty. Specifics include assessing the rate and depth of breathing for abnormalities such as stridor, cyanosis, nasal flaring, the use of accessory muscles, drooling, and overt trauma to the face, mouth, or neck. The chest is assessed for symmetric movement, symmetry of breath sounds, open chest wounds, entrance or exit wounds, impaled objects, tracheal shift, distended neck veins, subcutaneous emphysema, and paradoxical chest wall motion. In addition, the chest wall is assessed for bruising, petechiae, lacerations, and burns. The vital signs and skin color are assessed for signs of shock. The thorax is palpated for tenderness and crepitus, and the position of the trachea is also assessed.

The initial diagnostic workup includes a chest x-ray, CT scan, complete blood count, clotting studies, type and crossmatch, electrolytes, oxygen saturation, arterial blood gas analysis, and ECG. The patient is completely undressed to avoid missing additional injuries that may complicate care. Many patients with injuries involving the chest have associated head and abdominal injuries that require attention. Ongoing assessment is essential to monitor the patient's response to treatment and to detect early signs of clinical deterioration.

Medical Management

The goals of treatment are to evaluate the patient's condition and to initiate aggressive resuscitation. An airway is immediately established with oxygen support and, in some cases, ET intubation and ventilatory support. Reestablishing fluid volume and negative intrapleural pressure and draining intrapleural fluid and blood are essential.

The potential for massive blood loss and exsanguination with blunt or penetrating chest injuries is high because of injury to the great blood vessels. Many patients die at the scene of the injury or are in shock by the time help arrives. Agitation and irrational and combative behavior are signs of decreased oxygen delivery to the cerebral cortex. Strategies to restore and maintain cardiopulmonary function include ensuring an adequate airway and ventilation; stabilizing and reestablishing chest wall integrity; occluding any opening into the chest (open pneumothorax); and draining or removing any air or fluid from the thorax to relieve pneumothorax, hemothorax, or cardiac tamponade. Hypovolemia and low cardiac output must be corrected. Many of these treatment efforts, along with the control of hemorrhage, are carried out simultaneously at the scene of the injury or in the emergency department. Depending on the success of efforts to control the hemorrhage in the emergency department, the patient may be taken immediately to the operating room. Principles of management are essentially those pertaining to care of the postoperative thoracic patient (Urden et al., 2018).

Sternal and Rib Fractures

Sternal fractures are most common in motor vehicle crashes with a direct blow to the sternum via the steering wheel. Rib fractures are the most common type of chest trauma with blunt chest injury (Mancini, 2018). Most rib fractures are benign and are treated conservatively; ribs 4 through 10 are most frequently involved. Fractures of the first three ribs are rare but can result in a high mortality rate because they are associated with laceration of the subclavian artery or vein. Fractures of the lower ribs are associated with injury to the spleen and liver, which may be lacerated by fragmented sections of the rib. Older adult patients with three or more rib fractures have been shown to have a fivefold increased mortality rate and a fourfold increased incidence of pneumonia (Mancini, 2018).

Clinical Manifestations

Patients with sternal fractures have anterior chest pain, overlying tenderness, ecchymosis, crepitus, swelling, and possible chest wall deformity. For patients with rib fractures, clinical manifestations are similar: severe pain, point tenderness, and muscle spasm over the area of the fracture that are aggravated by coughing, deep breathing, and movement. The area around the fracture may be bruised. To reduce the pain, the patient splints the chest by breathing in a shallow manner and avoids sighs, deep breaths, coughing, and movement. This reluctance to move or breathe deeply results in diminished ventilation, atelectasis (collapse of unaerated alveoli), pneumonitis, and hypoxemia. Respiratory insufficiency and failure can be the outcomes of such a cycle.

Assessment and Diagnostic Findings

The patient must be closely evaluated for underlying cardiac injuries. A crackling, grating sound in the thorax (subcutaneous crepitus) may be detected with auscultation. The diagnostic workup may include a chest x-ray, rib films of a specific area, ECG, continuous pulse oximetry, and arterial blood gas analysis.

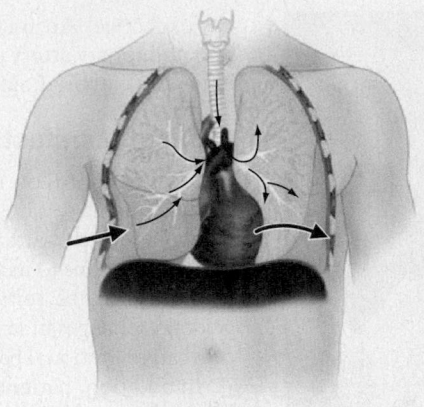
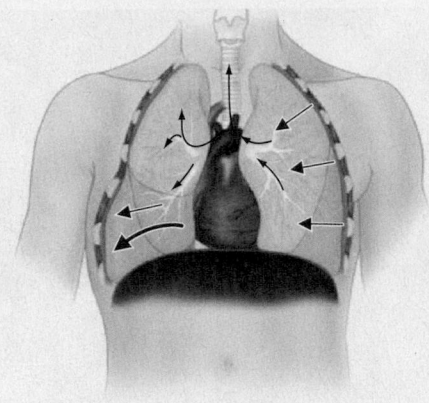

Figure 19-11 • Flail chest is caused by a free-floating segment of rib cage resulting from multiple rib fractures. **A.** Paradoxical movement on inspiration occurs when the flail rib segment is sucked inward and the mediastinal structures shift to the unaffected side. The amount of air drawn into the affected lung is reduced. **B.** On expiration, the flail segment bulges outward and the mediastinal structures shift back to the affected side.

A. Inspiration   B. Expiration

Medical Management

Medical management is directed toward relieving pain, avoiding excessive activity, and treating any associated injuries. Surgical fixation is rarely necessary unless fragments are grossly displaced and pose a potential for further injury.

The goals of treatment of rib fractures are to control pain and to detect and treat the injury. Sedation is used to relieve pain and to allow deep breathing and coughing. Care must be taken to avoid oversedation and suppression of respiratory drive. Alternative strategies to relieve pain include an intercostal nerve block and ice over the fracture site. A chest binder may be used as supportive treatment to provide stability to the chest wall and may decrease pain. The patient is instructed to apply the binder snugly enough to provide support, but not to impair respiratory excursion. Usually, the pain abates in 5 to 7 days, and discomfort can be relieved with epidural analgesia, PCA, or nonopioid analgesia. Most rib fractures heal in 3 to 6 weeks. The patient is monitored closely for signs and symptoms of associated injuries.

Flail Chest

Flail chest is frequently a complication of blunt chest trauma, which may occur from a steering wheel injury, motor vehicle crash involving a pedestrian or cyclist, a significant fall onto the chest, or an assault with a blunt weapon. The incidence of flail chest among patients with chest wall injury is 5% to 13% (Sarani, 2019). It occurs when three or more adjacent ribs (multiple contiguous ribs) are fractured at two or more sites, resulting in free-floating rib segments. It may also result as a combination fracture of ribs and costal cartilages or sternum. As a result, the chest wall loses stability, causing respiratory impairment and usually severe respiratory distress.

Pathophysiology

During inspiration, as the chest expands, the detached part of the rib segment (flail segment) moves in a paradoxical manner (pendelluft movement) in that it is pulled inward during inspiration, reducing the amount of air that can be drawn into the lungs. On expiration, because the intrathoracic pressure exceeds atmospheric pressure, the flail segment bulges outward, impairing the patient's ability to exhale. The mediastinum

then shifts back to the affected side (see Fig. 19-11). This paradoxical action results in increased dead space, a reduction in alveolar ventilation, and decreased compliance. Retained airway secretions and atelectasis frequently accompany flail chest. The patient has hypoxemia, and if gas exchange is greatly compromised, respiratory acidosis develops as a result of carbon dioxide retention. Hypotension, inadequate tissue perfusion, and metabolic acidosis often follow as the paradoxical motion of the mediastinum decreases cardiac output.

Medical Management

As with rib fracture, treatment of flail chest is usually supportive. Management includes providing ventilatory support, clearing secretions from the lungs, and controlling pain. Specific management depends on the degree of respiratory dysfunction. If only a small segment of the chest is involved, the objectives are to clear the airway through positioning, coughing, deep breathing, and suctioning to aid in the expansion of the lung, and to relieve pain by intercostal nerve blocks, high thoracic epidural blocks, or cautious use of IV opioids.

For mild-to-moderate flail chest injuries, the underlying pulmonary contusion is treated by monitoring fluid intake and appropriate fluid replacement while relieving chest pain. Pulmonary physiotherapy focusing on lung volume expansion and secretion management techniques is performed. The patient is closely monitored for further respiratory compromise.

For severe flail chest injuries, ET intubation and mechanical ventilation are required to provide internal pneumatic stabilization of the flail chest and to correct abnormalities in gas exchange. This helps to treat the underlying pulmonary contusion, serves to stabilize the thoracic cage to allow the fractures to heal, and improves alveolar ventilation and intrathoracic volume by decreasing the work of breathing. This treatment modality requires ET intubation and mechanical ventilator support. Differing modes of ventilation are used depending on the patient's underlying disease and specific needs.

Rib-specific plating systems may be used for three or more rib fractures or flail chest in order to achieve chest wall stabilization (CWS). These systems are inserted internally in the operating room, preferably within the first 72 hours of injury (see Fig. 19-12). The benefits of their use include decreased bleeding, less inflammation, and reduced chest wall deformities. Contraindications for CWS include traumatic brain injury and unstable spine fracture. With coexisting pulmonary

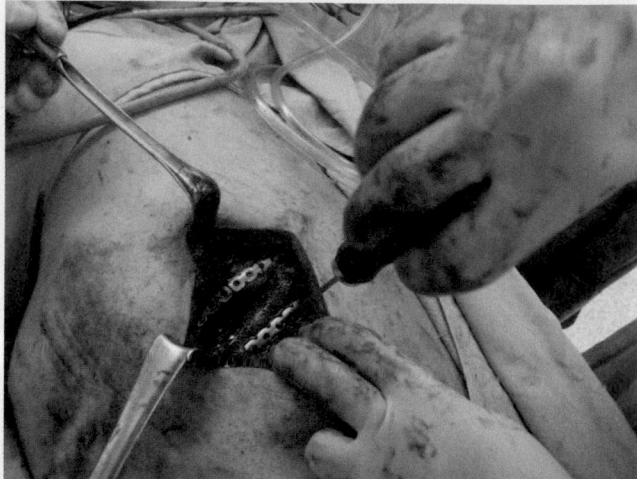

Figure 19-12 • Chest wall stabilization (CWS) plating system provides chest wall stability for multiple fractures or a flail chest. Reproduced from Moya, M., Nirula, R., & Biffl, W. (2017). Rib fixation: Who, What, When? *Trauma Surgery & Acute Care Open, 2*(1):e000059. Copyright © The American Association for the Surgery of Trauma with permission from BMJ Publishing Group Ltd. doi:10.1136/tsaco-2016-000059.

contusion the overall efficacy of CWS remains controversial (Milanez de Campos & White, 2018).

Regardless of the type of treatment, the patient is carefully monitored by serial chest x-rays, arterial blood gas analysis, pulse oximetry, and bedside pulmonary function monitoring. Pain management is key to successful treatment. PCA, intercostal nerve blocks, epidural analgesia, and intrapleural administration of opioids may be used to relieve or manage thoracic pain.

Pulmonary Contusion

Pulmonary contusion is a common thoracic injury and is frequently associated with flail chest. It is defined as damage to the lung tissues resulting in hemorrhage and localized edema. It is associated with chest trauma when there is rapid compression and decompression to the chest wall (i.e., blunt trauma). Pulmonary contusion represents a spectrum of lung injury characterized by the development of infiltrates and various degrees of respiratory dysfunction and sometimes respiratory failure. It is often cited as the most common potentially life-threatening chest injury; however, mortality is often attributed to other associated injuries. Pulmonary contusion may not be evident initially on examination but develops in the posttraumatic period; it may involve a small portion of one lung, a massive section of a lung, one entire lung, or both lungs. Depending on the extent of injury, this type of trauma may be associated with a mortality rate greater than 50% (Mancini, 2018).

Pathophysiology

The primary pathologic defect is an abnormal accumulation of fluid in the interstitial and intra-alveolar spaces. It is thought that injury to the lung parenchyma and its capillary network results in a leakage of serum protein and plasma. The leaking serum protein exerts an osmotic pressure that enhances loss of fluid from the capillaries. Blood, edema, and cellular debris (from cellular response to injury) enter the lung and accumulate in the bronchioles and alveoli, where they interfere with gas exchange. An increase in pulmonary vascular resistance and pulmonary artery pressure occurs. The patient has hypoxemia and carbon dioxide retention.

Clinical Manifestations

Pulmonary contusion may be mild, moderate, or severe. The clinical manifestations vary from decreased breath sounds, tachypnea, tachycardia, chest pain, hypoxemia, and blood-tinged secretions to more severe tachypnea, tachycardia, crackles, frank bleeding, severe hypoxemia (cyanosis), and respiratory acidosis. Changes in sensorium, including increased agitation or combative irrational behavior, may be signs of hypoxemia.

In addition, patients with moderate pulmonary contusion have a large amount of mucus, serum, and frank blood in the tracheobronchial tree; patients often have a constant cough but cannot clear the secretions. Patients with severe pulmonary contusion have signs and symptoms that mirror ARDS, which may include central cyanosis; agitation; combativeness; and productive cough with frothy, bloody secretions.

Assessment and Diagnostic Findings

The efficiency of gas exchange is determined by pulse oximetry and arterial blood gas measurements. Pulse oximetry is also used to measure oxygen saturation continuously. The initial chest x-ray may show no changes; changes may not appear for 1 or 2 days after the injury and appear as pulmonary infiltrates on chest x-ray.

Medical Management

Treatment priorities include maintaining the airway, providing adequate oxygenation, and controlling pain. In mild pulmonary contusion, adequate hydration via IV fluids and oral intake is important to mobilize secretions. However, fluid intake must be closely monitored to avoid hypervolemia. Volume expansion techniques, postural drainage, physiotherapy including coughing, and ET suctioning are used to remove the secretions. Pain is managed by intercostal nerve blocks or by opioids via PCA or other methods. Usually, antimicrobial therapy is given because the damaged lung is susceptible to infection. Supplemental oxygen is usually given by mask or cannula for 24 to 36 hours.

In patients with moderate pulmonary contusion, bronchoscopy may be required to remove secretions. Intubation and mechanical ventilation with PEEP may also be necessary to maintain the pressure and keep the lungs inflated. A nasogastric tube is inserted to relieve gastrointestinal distention.

In patients with severe contusion, who may develop respiratory failure, aggressive treatment with ET intubation and ventilatory support, diuretics, and fluid restriction may be necessary. Antimicrobial medications may be prescribed for the treatment of pulmonary infection. This is a common complication of pulmonary contusion (especially pneumonia in the contused segment) because the fluid and blood that extravasate into the alveolar and interstitial spaces serve as an excellent culture medium.

Penetrating Trauma

Any organ or structure within the chest is potentially susceptible to traumatic penetration. These organs include the chest wall, lung and pleura, tracheobronchial system, esophagus, diaphragm, and major thoracic blood vessels, as well as heart and other mediastinal structures. The clinical consequence of penetrating trauma to the chest depends on the mechanism of injury, location, associated injuries, and underlying illnesses (Shahani, 2017). Common injuries include pneumothorax and cardiac tamponade.

Medical Management

The objective of immediate management is to restore and maintain cardiopulmonary function. After an adequate airway is ensured and ventilation is established, examination for shock and intrathoracic and intra-abdominal injuries is necessary. The patient is undressed completely so that additional injuries are not missed (see Chapter 67 for discussion of primary and secondary survey). There is a high risk of associated intra-abdominal injuries with stab wounds below the level of the fifth anterior intercostal space. Death can result from exsanguinating hemorrhage or intra-abdominal sepsis.

The diagnostic workup includes a chest x-ray, chemistry profile, arterial blood gas analysis, pulse oximetry, and ECG. The patient's blood is typed and cross-matched in case blood transfusion is required. After the status of the peripheral pulses is assessed, a large-bore IV line is inserted. An indwelling catheter is inserted to monitor urinary output. A nasogastric tube is inserted and connected to low suction to prevent aspiration, minimize leakage of abdominal contents, and decompress the gastrointestinal tract.

Hemorrhagic shock is treated simultaneously with colloid solutions, crystalloids, or blood, as indicated by the patient's condition. Diagnostic procedures are carried out as dictated by the needs of the patient (e.g., CT scans of chest or abdomen, flat plate x-ray of the abdomen) (see Chapter 11).

A chest tube is inserted into the pleural space in most patients with penetrating wounds of the chest to achieve rapid and continuing re-expansion of the lungs. The insertion of the chest tube frequently results in a complete evacuation of the blood and air. The chest tube also allows early recognition of continuing intrathoracic bleeding, which would make surgical exploration necessary. If the patient has a penetrating wound of the heart or great vessels, the esophagus, or the tracheobronchial tree, surgical intervention is required.

Pneumothorax

Pneumothorax occurs when the parietal or visceral pleura is breached and the pleural space is exposed to positive atmospheric pressure. Normally, the pressure in the pleural space is negative or subatmospheric; this negative pressure is required to maintain lung inflation. When either pleura is breached, air enters the pleural space, and the lung or a portion of it collapses.

Types of Pneumothorax

Types of pneumothorax include simple, traumatic, and tension pneumothorax.

Simple Pneumothorax

A simple, or spontaneous, pneumothorax occurs when air enters the pleural space through a breach of either the parietal

or visceral pleura. Most commonly, this occurs as air enters the pleural space through the rupture of a bleb or a bronchopleural fistula. A spontaneous pneumothorax may occur in an apparently healthy person in the absence of trauma due to rupture of an air-filled bleb, or blister, on the surface of the lung, allowing air from the airways to enter the pleural cavity. It may be associated with diffuse interstitial lung disease and severe emphysema.

Traumatic Pneumothorax

A traumatic pneumothorax occurs when air escapes from a laceration in the lung itself and enters the pleural space or from a wound in the chest wall. It may result from blunt trauma (e.g., rib fractures), penetrating chest or abdominal trauma (e.g., stab wounds or gunshot wounds), or diaphragmatic tears. Traumatic pneumothorax may occur during invasive thoracic procedures (i.e., thoracentesis, transbronchial lung biopsy, and insertion of a subclavian line) in which the pleura is inadvertently punctured, or with barotrauma from mechanical ventilation.

A traumatic pneumothorax resulting from major injury to the chest is often accompanied by hemothorax (collection of blood in the pleural space resulting from torn intercostal vessels, lacerations of the great vessels, or lacerations of the lungs). Hemopneumothorax (both blood and air in the chest cavity) is also common after major trauma. Chest surgery can be classified as a traumatic pneumothorax as a result of the entry into the pleural space and the accumulation of air and fluid in the pleural space.

Open pneumothorax is one form of traumatic pneumothorax. It occurs when a wound in the chest wall is large enough to allow air to pass freely in and out of the thoracic cavity with each attempted respiration. Because the rush of air through the wound in the chest wall produces a sucking sound, such injuries are termed *sucking chest wounds*. In such patients, not only does the lung collapse, but the structures of the mediastinum (heart and great vessels) also shift toward the uninjured side with each inspiration and in the opposite direction with expiration. This is termed *mediastinal flutter* or *swing*, and it produces serious circulatory problems.

> ⚑ *Quality and Safety Nursing Alert*
>
> Traumatic open pneumothorax calls for emergency interventions. Stopping the flow of air through the opening in the chest wall is a lifesaving measure.

Tension Pneumothorax

A **tension pneumothorax** occurs when air is drawn into the pleural space from a lacerated lung or through a small opening or wound in the chest wall. It may be a complication of other types of pneumothorax. In contrast to open pneumothorax, the air that enters the chest cavity with each inspiration is trapped; it cannot be expelled during expiration through the air passages or the opening in the chest wall. In effect, a one-way valve or ball valve mechanism occurs where air enters the pleural space but cannot escape. With each breath, tension (positive pressure) is increased within the affected pleural space. This causes the lung to collapse and the heart, the great vessels, and the trachea to shift toward the unaffected

Open pneumothorax

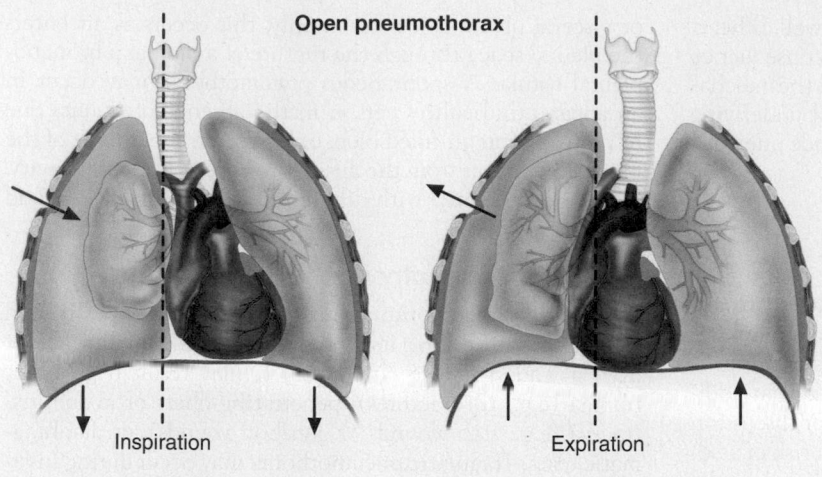

Inspiration   Expiration

Tension pneumothorax

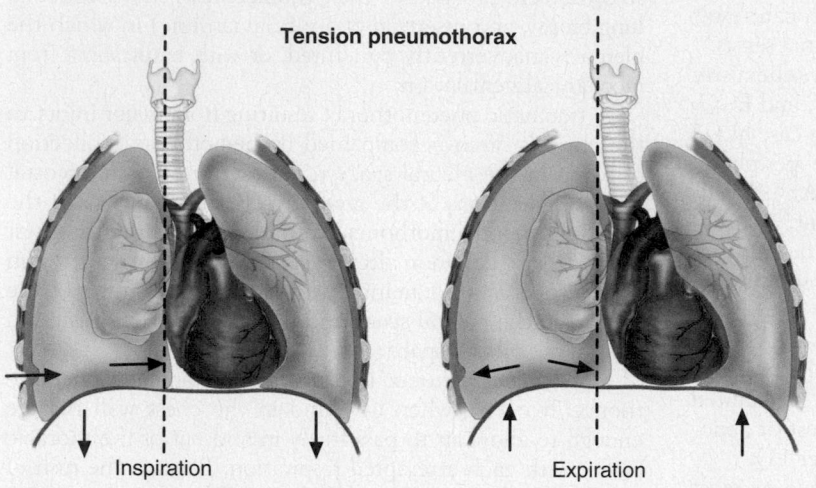

Inspiration   Expiration

Figure 19-13 • Open pneumothorax (**top**) and tension pneumothorax (**bottom**). In open pneumothorax, air enters the chest during inspiration and exits during expiration. A slight shift of the affected lung may occur because of a decrease in pressure as air moves out of the chest. In tension pneumothorax, air enters but cannot leave the chest. As the pressure increases, the heart and great vessels are compressed and the mediastinal structures are shifted toward the opposite side of the chest. The trachea is pushed from its normal midline position toward the opposite side of the chest, and the unaffected lung is compressed.

side of the chest (mediastinal shift). Both respiration and circulatory function are compromised because of the increased intrathoracic pressure, which decreases venous return to the heart, causing decreased cardiac output and impairment of peripheral circulation. In extreme cases, the pulse may be undetectable—this is known as pulseless electrical activity.

Clinical Manifestations

The signs and symptoms associated with pneumothorax depend on its size and cause. Pain is usually sudden and may be pleuritic. The patient may have only minimal respiratory distress with slight chest discomfort and tachypnea with a small simple or uncomplicated pneumothorax. If the pneumothorax is large and the lung collapses totally, acute respiratory distress occurs. The patient is anxious, has dyspnea and air hunger, has increased use of the accessory muscles, and may develop central cyanosis from severe hypoxemia.

In assessing the chest for any type of pneumothorax, the nurse assesses tracheal alignment, expansion of the chest, breath sounds, and percussion of the chest. In a simple pneumothorax, the trachea is midline, expansion of the chest is decreased, breath sounds may be diminished or absent, and percussion of the chest may reveal normal sounds or hyperresonance depending on the size of the pneumothorax. In a tension pneumothorax, the trachea is shifted away from the affected side, chest expansion may be decreased or fixed

in a hyperexpansion state, breath sounds are diminished or absent, and percussion to the affected side is hyperresonant. The clinical picture is one of air hunger, agitation, increasing hypoxemia, central cyanosis, hypotension, tachycardia, and profuse diaphoresis. Figure 19-13 compares open and tension pneumothorax.

Medical Management

Medical management of pneumothorax depends on its cause and severity. The goal of treatment is to evacuate the air or blood from the pleural space. A small chest tube (28 Fr) is inserted near the second intercostal space; this space is used because it is the thinnest part of the chest wall, minimizes the danger of contacting the thoracic nerve, and leaves a less visible scar. If a patient also has a hemothorax, a large-diameter chest tube (32 Fr or greater) is inserted, usually in the fourth or fifth intercostal space at the midaxillary line. The tube is directed posteriorly to drain the fluid and air. Once the chest tube or tubes are inserted and suction is applied (usually to 20 mm Hg suction), effective decompression of the pleural cavity (drainage of blood or air) occurs.

If an excessive amount of blood enters the chest tube in a relatively short period, an autotransfusion may be needed. This technique involves taking the patient's own blood that has been drained from the chest, filtering it, and then transfusing it back into the vascular system.

In such an emergency, anything may be used that is large enough to fill the chest wound—a towel, a handkerchief, or the heel of the hand. If conscious, the patient is instructed to inhale and strain against a closed glottis. This action assists in re-expanding the lung and ejecting the air from the thorax. In the hospital, the opening is plugged by sealing it with gauze impregnated with petrolatum. A pressure dressing is applied. Usually, a chest tube connected to water-seal drainage is inserted to remove air and fluid. Antibiotics usually are prescribed to combat infection from contamination.

The severity of open pneumothorax depends on the amount and rate of thoracic bleeding and the amount of air in the pleural space. The pleural cavity can be decompressed by thoracentesis or by chest tube drainage of the blood or air. The lung is then able to re-expand and resume the function of gas exchange. As a rule of thumb, thoracotomy is performed if more than 1500 mL of blood is aspirated initially by thoracentesis (or is the initial chest tube output) or if chest tube output continues at greater than 200 mL/h (Shahani, 2017). The urgency with which the blood must be removed is determined by the degree of respiratory compromise. An emergency thoracotomy may also be performed in the emergency department if a cardiovascular injury secondary to chest or penetrating trauma is suspected. The patient with a possible tension pneumothorax should immediately be given a high concentration of supplemental oxygen to treat the hypoxemia, and pulse oximetry should be used to monitor oxygen saturation. In an emergency situation, a tension pneumothorax can be decompressed or quickly converted to a simple pneumothorax by inserting a large-bore needle (14 gauge) at the second intercostal space, midclavicular line on the affected side. This relieves the pressure and vents the positive pressure to the external environment. A chest tube is then inserted and connected to suction to remove the remaining air and fluid, reestablish the negative pressure, and re-expand the lung. If the lung re-expands and air leakage from the lung parenchyma stops, further drainage may be unnecessary. If a prolonged air leak continues despite chest tube drainage to underwater seal, surgery may be necessary to close the leak.

Chest Drainage

Chest tubes and a closed drainage system are used to re-expand the involved lung and to remove excess air, fluid, and blood, and may be used in patients who have had a thoracotomy (see previous discussion). Chest drainage systems also are frequently indicated in the treatment of spontaneous pneumothorax and trauma resulting in pneumothorax. Table 19-8 describes and compares the main features of these systems.

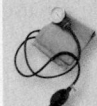 For the procedural guidelines for setting up and managing chest drainage systems, go to **thepoint.lww.com/Brunner15e**.

The normal breathing mechanism operates on the principle of negative pressure. The pressure in the chest cavity normally is lower than the pressure of the atmosphere, causing air to move into the lungs during inspiration. Whenever the chest is opened, there is a loss of negative pressure, which results in collapse of the lung. The collection of air, fluid, or other substances in the chest can compromise cardiopulmonary function and can also cause the lung to collapse. Pathologic substances that can collect in the pleural space include fibrin or clotted blood, liquids (serous fluids, blood, pus, chyle), and gases (air from the lung, tracheobronchial tree, or esophagus).

Chest tubes may be inserted to drain fluid or air from any of the three compartments of the thorax (the right and left pleural spaces and the mediastinum). The pleural space, located between the visceral and parietal pleura, normally contains 20 mL or less of fluid, which helps lubricate the visceral and parietal pleura (Norris, 2019).

There are two types of chest tubes: small-bore and large-bore catheters. Small-bore catheters (7 Fr to 12 Fr) have a one-way valve apparatus to prevent air from moving back into the chest. They can be inserted through a small skin incision. Large-bore catheters, which range in size up to 40 Fr, are usually connected to a chest drainage system to collect any

TABLE 19-8	Comparison of Chest Drainage Systems[a]	
Types of Chest Drainage Systems	**Description**	**Comments**
Traditional Water Seal Also referred to as wet suction	Has three chambers: a collection chamber, water-seal chamber (middle chamber), and wet suction control chamber	Requires that sterile fluid be instilled into water seal and suction chambers Has positive- and negative-pressure release valves Intermittent bubbling indicates that the system is functioning properly. Additional suction can be added by connecting system to a suction source.
Dry Suction Water Seal Also referred to as dry suction	Has three chambers: a collection chamber, water-seal chamber (middle chamber), and suction regulator dial	Requires that sterile fluid be instilled in water-seal chamber at 2-cm level No fluid-filled suction chamber Suction pressure is set with a suction regulator dial. Has positive- and negative-pressure release valves Has an indicator to signify that the suction pressure is adequate Quieter than traditional water-seal systems
Dry Suction Also referred to as one-way valve system	Has a one-way mechanical valve that allows air to leave the chest and prevents air from moving back into the chest	No need to fill suction chamber with fluid; thus, can be set up quickly in an emergency Works even if knocked over, making it ideal for patients who are ambulatory

[a]If no fluid drainage is expected, a drainage collection device may not be needed.

pleural fluid and monitor for air leaks. After the chest tube is positioned, it is sutured to the skin and connected to a drainage apparatus to remove the residual air and fluid from the pleural or mediastinal space. This results in the re-expansion of remaining lung tissue.

Chest Drainage Systems

Chest drainage systems have a suction source, a collection chamber for pleural drainage, and a mechanism to prevent air from reentering the chest with inhalation (see Fig. 19-14). Various types of chest drainage systems are available for use

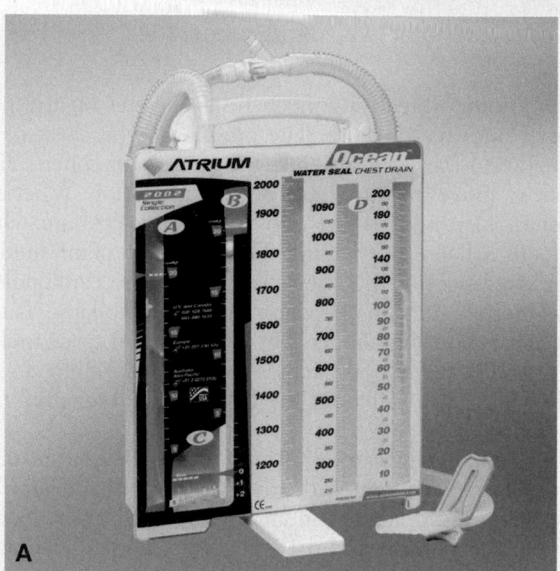

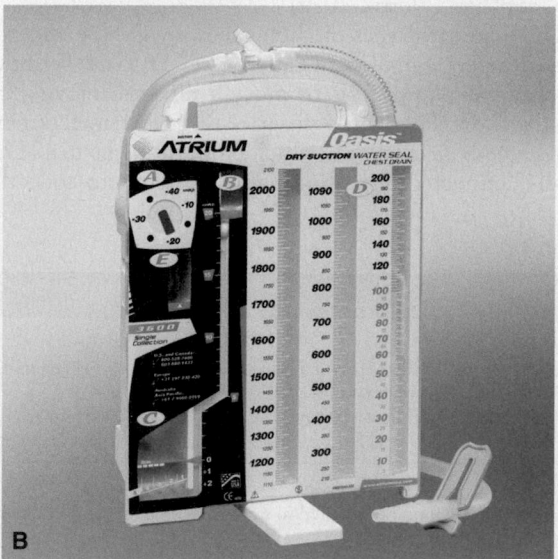

Figure 19-14 • Chest drainage systems. **A.** The Atrium Ocean is an example of a water-seal chest drain system composed of a drainage chamber and water-seal chamber. The suction control is determined by the height of the water column in that chamber (usually 20 cm). *A*, suction control chamber; *B*, water-seal chamber; *C*, air leak zone; *D*, collection chamber. **B.** The Atrium Oasis is an example of a dry suction water-seal system that uses a mechanical regulator for vacuum control, a water-seal chamber, and a drainage chamber. *A*, dry suction regulator; *B*, water-seal chamber; *C*, air leak monitor; *D*, collection chamber; *E*, suction monitor bellows. Photos used with permission from Atrium Medical Corporation, Hudson, NH.

in the removal of air and fluid from the pleural space and re-expansion of the lungs. Chest drainage systems come with either wet (water seal) or dry suction control. In wet suction systems, the amount of suction is determined by the amount of water instilled in the suction chamber. The amount of bubbling in the suction chamber indicates the strength of the suction. Wet systems use a water seal to prevent air from moving back into the chest on inspiration. Dry systems use a one-way valve and may have a suction control dial in place of the water. Both systems can operate by gravity drainage, without a suction source.

> ⚑ **Quality and Safety Nursing Alert**
>
> *When the wall vacuum is turned off, the drainage system must be open to the atmosphere so that intrapleural air can escape from the system. This can be done by detaching the tubing from the suction port to provide a vent.*

Water-Seal Systems

The traditional water-seal system (or wet suction) for chest drainage has three chambers: a collection chamber, a water-seal chamber, and a wet suction control chamber. The collection chamber acts as a reservoir for fluid draining from the chest tube. It is graduated to permit easy measurement of drainage. Suction may be added to create negative pressure and promote drainage of fluid and removal of air. The suction control chamber regulates the amount of negative pressure applied to the chest. The amount of suction is determined by the water level. It is usually set at 20 cm H_2O; adding more fluid results in more suction. After the suction is turned on, bubbling appears in the suction chamber. A positive-pressure valve is located at the top of the suction chamber that automatically opens with increases in positive pressure within the system. Air is automatically released through a positive-pressure relief valve if the suction tubing is inadvertently clamped or kinked.

The water-seal chamber has a one-way valve or water seal that prevents air from moving back into the chest when the patient inhales. There is an increase in the water level with inspiration and a return to the baseline level during exhalation; this is referred to as tidaling. Intermittent bubbling in the water-seal chamber is normal, but continuous bubbling can indicate an air leak. Bubbling and tidaling do not occur when the tube is placed in the mediastinal space; however, fluid may pulsate with the patient's heartbeat. If the chest tube is connected to gravity drainage only, suction is not used. The pressure is equal to the water seal only. Two-chamber chest drainage systems (water-seal chamber and collection chamber) are available for use with patients who need only gravity drainage.

The water level in the water-seal chamber reflects the negative pressure present in the intrathoracic cavity. A rise in the water level indicates negative pressure in the pleural or mediastinal space. Excessive negative pressure can cause trauma to tissue. Most chest drainage systems have an automatic means to prevent excessive negative pressure. By pressing and holding a manual high-negativity vent (usually located on the top of the chest drainage system) until the water level in the water-seal chamber returns to the 2-cm mark, excessive negative pressure is avoided, preventing damage to tissue.

Quality and Safety Nursing Alert

If the chest tube and drainage system become disconnected, air can enter the pleural space, producing a pneumothorax. To prevent pneumothorax if the chest tube is inadvertently disconnected from the drainage system, a temporary water seal can be established by immersing the chest tube's open end in a bottle of sterile water.

Dry Suction Water-Seal Systems

Dry suction water-seal systems, also referred to as dry suction, have a collection chamber for drainage, a water-seal chamber, and a dry suction control regulator. The water-seal chamber is filled with water to the 2-cm level. Bubbling in this area can indicate an air leak. The dry suction control regulator provides a dial that conveniently regulates vacuum to the chest drain. The system does not contain a suction control chamber filled with water. Without a water-filled suction chamber, the machine is quieter. However, if the container is knocked over, the water seal may be lost.

Once the tube is connected to the suction source, the regulator dial allows the desired level of suction to be set; the suction is increased until an indicator appears. The indicator has the same function as the bubbling in the traditional water-seal system—that is, it indicates that the vacuum is adequate to maintain the desired level of suction. Some drainage systems use a bellows (a chamber that can be expanded or contracted) or an orange-colored float device as an indicator of when the suction control regulator is set.

When the water in the water seal rises above the 2-cm level, intrathoracic pressure increases. Dry suction water-seal systems have a manual high-negativity vent located on top of the drain. The manual high-negativity vent is pressed until the indicator appears (either a float device or bellows) and the water level in the water seal returns to the desired level, indicating that the intrathoracic pressure is decreased.

 Quality and Safety Nursing Alert

The manual vent should not be used to lower the water level in the water seal when the patient is on gravity drainage (no suction) because intrathoracic pressure is equal to the pressure in the water seal.

Dry Suction Systems with a One-Way Valve

A third type of chest drainage system is dry suction with a one-way mechanical valve. This system has a collection chamber, a one-way mechanical valve, and a dry suction control chamber. The valve permits air and fluid to leave the chest but prevents their movement back into the pleural space. This model lacks a water-seal chamber and therefore can be set up quickly in emergency situations, and the dry control drain still works even if it is knocked over. This makes the dry suction systems useful for the patient who is ambulating or being transported. However, without the water-seal chamber, there is no way to tell by inspection whether the pressure in the chest has changed, even though an air leak indicator is present so that the system can be checked. If an air leak is suspected, 30 mL of water is injected into the air

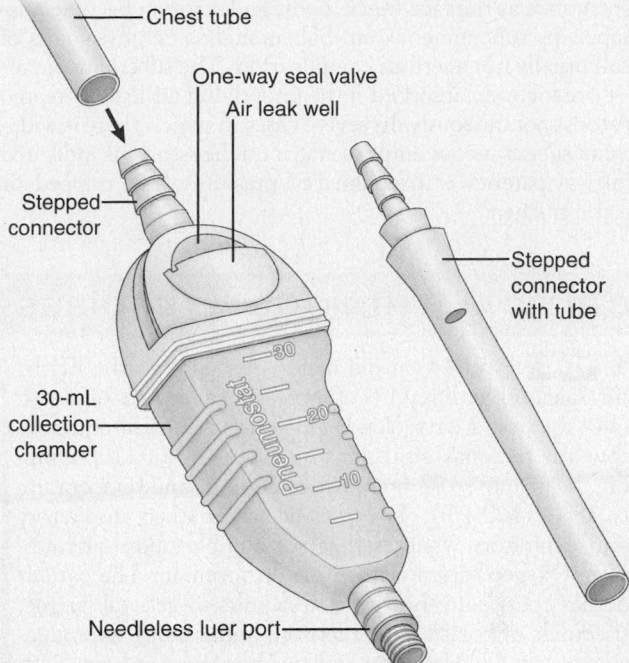

Figure 19-15 • One-way (Heimlich) valve, a disposable, single-use chest drainage system with 30-mL collection volume. Used when minimal volume of chest drainage is expected.

leak indicator or the container is tipped so that fluid enters the air leak detection chamber. Bubbles will appear if a leak is present.

If the chest tube has been inserted to re-expand a lung after pneumothorax, or if very little fluid drainage is expected, a one-way valve (Heimlich valve) may be connected to the chest tube. This valve may be attached to a collection bag (see Fig. 19-15) or covered with a sterile dressing if no drainage is expected.

Cardiac Tamponade

Cardiac tamponade is compression of the heart resulting from fluid or blood within the pericardial sac. It usually is caused by blunt or penetrating trauma to the chest. A penetrating wound of the heart is associated with a high mortality rate. Cardiac tamponade also may follow diagnostic cardiac catheterization, angiographic procedures, and pacemaker insertion, which can produce perforations of the heart and great vessels. Pericardial effusion with fluid compressing the heart also may develop from metastases to the pericardium from malignant tumors of the breast, lung, or mediastinum and may occur with lymphomas and leukemias, kidney injury, TB, and high-dose radiation to the chest (see Chapter 25 for a detailed discussion of cardiac tamponade).

Subcutaneous Emphysema

No matter what kind of chest trauma a patient has, when the lung or the air passages are injured, air may enter the tissue planes and pass for some distance under the skin (e.g., neck and chest). The tissues give a crackling sensation when palpated, and the subcutaneous air produces an alarming appearance as the face, neck, body, and scrotum become misshapen by subcutaneous air. Subcutaneous emphysema is of itself usually not a serious complication. The subcutaneous air is spontaneously absorbed if the underlying air leak is treated or stops spontaneously. In severe cases in which there is widespread subcutaneous emphysema, a tracheostomy is indicated if airway patency is threatened by pressure of the trapped air on the trachea.

CRITICAL THINKING EXERCISES

1 `ipc` An 84-year-old male is brought to the ED by his daughter with reports of increasing shortness of breath over the past 2 days. You begin your assessment and note that the patient's vital signs include a BP of 110/72 mm Hg, heart rate of 92 bpm, RR of 26/min, and temperature is 38°C (100.4°F). The patient has marked inspiratory and expiratory wheezes that are audible upon auscultation. Oxygen saturation is 92% on room air. The patient denies chest pain; however, he admits to general fatigue, shortness of breath with exertion, and a moist unproductive cough. The daughter explains he resides at home with her and is wheelchair dependent. His past medical history includes an occipital stroke, open reduction internal fixation (ORIF) of right and left hip following fractures, bilateral pulmonary emboli, and paroxysmal atrial fibrillation. The patient's daughter tells you that he has difficulty with dentition with frequent episodes of coughing while eating. The patient admits he stopped taking his prescribed warfarin 6 months ago since he experienced several falls. What are the potential causes of his respiratory problem and what nursing interventions are important? What interdisciplinary team members warrant consultation in the care of the patient?

2 `pq` A 26-year-old male arrives via Emergency Medical Services (EMS) to the ED following a motor vehicle crash (MVC). The patient is awake and alert; however, he complains of sharp pain in his chest that extends to his back, neck, and shoulders. You begin your assessment and note that the patient's vital signs include a BP of 90/42 mm Hg, heart rate of 101 bpm, and RR of 32/min. He is pale and dyspneic with an oxygen saturation of 89% on 4 L of O_2 via nasal cannula. Inspection of the chest wall reveals areas of ecchymoses over the right shoulder and right anterior chest wall. The emergency medical technician (EMT) reports the patient was the sole driver of the automobile and bystanders stated the driver swerved to avoid a deer and hit a telephone pole. The patient was wearing a seatbelt; however, the air bags did not deploy. Auscultation of the chest reveals an absence of lung sounds on the right side with diminished lung sounds on the left side. What are the possible respiratory conditions associated with the clinical presentation of this patient? Describe your priorities of care.

3 `ebp` An 18-year-old female is admitted to the ICU from the ED with a diagnosis of acute respiratory failure. She is endotracheally intubated and placed on mechanical ventilation. Her past medical history includes a fractured left ulnar at the age of 10 but is otherwise unremarkable. She denies drug use; however, she admits to use of e-cigarettes since the 10th grade. The intensivist suspects EVALI. Forty-eight hours following intubation, diffuse hazy opacities are noted on chest x-ray throughout all lung fields. What evidence is available associating the use of electronic nicotine delivery systems (ENDS) with acute lung injury? What strategies should you implement to prevent ventilator-associated pneumonia (VAP) in this patient? What is the evidence base for the strategies that you consider? How would you evaluate the strength of the evidence?

REFERENCES

*Asterisk indicates nursing research.
**Double asterisk indicates classic references.

Books

Cascella, M., Rajnik, M., Cuomo, A., et al. (2020). Features, evaluation, and treatment Coronavirus (COVID-19). *StatPearls*. Treasure Island, FL: *StatPearls* Publishing. Retrieved on 6/9/2020 at: www.ncbi.nlm.nih.gov/books/NBK554776/

Gilbert, D. N., Chambers, H. F., Eliopoulos, G. M., et al. (2018). *The Sanford guide to antimicrobial therapy 2018* (48th ed.). Sperryville, VA: Antimicrobial Therapy, Inc.

Kacmarek, R. M., Stoller, J. K., Heuer, A. J., et al. (2017). *Egan's fundamentals of respiratory care*. St. Louis, MO: Elsevier.

Karch, A. M. (2020). *Focus on nursing pharmacology* (8th ed.). Philadelphia, PA: LWW.

Norris, T. L. (2019). *Porth's pathophysiology: Concepts of altered health state* (10th ed.). Philadelphia, PA: Wolters Kluwer.

Urden, L. D., Stacy, K. M., & Lough, M. E. (2018). *Critical care nursing: Diagnosis and management* (8th ed.). St. Louis, MO: Elsevier Mosby.

Weinberger, S. E., Cockrill, B. A., & Mandel, J. (2019). *Principles of pulmonary medicine* (7th ed.). Philadelphia, PA: Elsevier Saunders.

Wiegand, D. J. L. (2017). *AACN procedure manual for critical care* (7th ed.). St. Louis, MO: Elsevier Saunders.

Journals and Electronic Documents

Alhazzani, W., Moller, M. H., Arabi, Y. M., et al. (2020). Surviving Sepsis Campaign: Guidelines on the management of critically ill adults with Coronavirus Disease 2019 (COVID-19). *Critical Care Medicine*, 48(6), e440–e469.

**American Association for Respiratory Care. (2007). Clinical practice guideline: Oxygen therapy in the home or alternate site health care facility. *Respiratory Care*, 52(1), 1063–1068.

American Association of Critical Care Nurses (AACN). (2017a). AACN practice alert: Prevention of ventilator-associated pneumonia in adults. *Critical Care Nurse*, 37(3), e22–e25.

American Association of Critical Care Nurses (AACN). (2017b). AACN practice alert: Prevention of aspiration in adults. *Critical Care Nurse*, 37(3), 88.

American Cancer Society (ACS). (2019). *Learn about cancer: Lung cancer*. Last updated October 1, 2019. Retrieved on 10/4/2019 at: www.cancer.org/cancer/lungcancer/index

American College of Surgeons. (2016). National trauma data bank 2016-annual report. Retrieved on 9/27/2019 at: www.facs.org/~/media/files/quality%20programs/trauma/ntdb/ntdb%20annual%20report%20 2016.ashx

American Lung Association (ALA). (2018a). Lung health and diseases: Pneumoconiosis. Retrieved on 10/4/2019 at: www.lung.org/lung-health-and-diseases/lung-disease-lookup/pneumoconiosis

American Lung Association (ALA). (2018b). The connection between lung cancer and outdoor air pollution. Retrieved on 1/12/2020 at: www.lung.org/about-us/blog/2016/06/lung-cancer-and-air-pollution.html

American Lung Association (ALA). (2020). State of lung cancer. Retrieved on 1/12/2020 at: www.lung.org/our-initiatives/research/monitoring-trends-in-lung-disease/state-of-lung-cancer/

**American Thoracic Society & Infectious Diseases Society of America. (2005). Guidelines for the management of adults with hospital-acquired, ventilator-associated, and healthcare-associated pneumonia. *American Journal of Respiratory and Critical Care Medicine, 171*(4), 388–416.

Amitai, A. (2018). Introduction to ventilator management. *Medscape*. Retrieved on 2/2/2020 at: emedicine.medscape.com/article/810126-overview

Anesi, G. (2020). Coronavirus disease 2019 (COVID-19): Critical care and airway management issues. *UpToDate*. Retrieved on 6/4/2020 at: www.uptodate.com/contents/coronavirus-disease-2019-covid-19-critical-care-and-airway-management-issues

Baer, S. (2019). Community-acquired pneumonia. *Medscape*. Retrieved on 9/23/2019 at: emedicine.medscape.com/article/234240-overview

Bartlett, J. (2019a). Aspiration pneumonia in adults. *UpToDate*. Retrieved on 9/23/2019 at: www.uptodate.com/contents/aspiration-pneumonia-in-adults

Bartlett, J. G. (2019b). Lung abscess in adults. *UpToDate*. Retrieved on 8/22/2019 at: www.uptodate.com/contents/lung-abscess

Beigel, J. H., Tomashek, K. M., Dodd, L. E.. (2020). Remdesivir for the treatment of covid-19: Preliminary report. *New England Journal of Medicine, 383*(10), 994 published online ahead-of-print on 5/22/2020. doi:10.1056/NEJMoa2007764

Benveniste, M. F., Gomez, D., Brett W., et al. (2019). Recognizing radiation therapy related complications in the chest. *Radiographics, 39*(2). doi.org/10.1148/rg.2019180061

Bernardo, J. (2019). Epidemiology and pathology of miliary and extra-pulmonary tuberculosis. *UpToDate*. Retrieved on 8/22/2019 at: www.uptodate.com/contents/epidemiology-and-pathology-of-miliary-and-extrapulmonary-tuberculosis

Berry, M. F. (2019). Approach to the adult patient with a mediastinal mass. *UpToDate*. Retrieved on 8/22/2019 at: www.uptodate.com/contents/evaluation-of-mediastinal-masses

Bhatnagar, R., Piotrowska, H. E. G., Laskawiec-Szkonter, M., et al. (2019). Effect of thoracoscopic talc poudrage vs talc slurry via chest tube on pleurodesis failure rate among patients with malignant pleural effusions: A randomized clinical trial. *JAMA, 323*(1), 60–69.

Binkley, C. E., & Kemp, D. S. (2020). Ethical rationing of personal protective equipment to minimize moral residue during the COVID-19 pandemic. *Journal of the American College of Surgeons, 230*(6), 1111–1113.

Boston University School of Medicine. (2019). ICOUGH^SM. Retrieved on 8/22/2019 at: www.bumc.bu.edu/surgery/quality-safety/i-cough

Caputo, N. D., Strayer, R. J., & Levitan, R. (2020). Early self-proning in awake, non-intubated patients in the emergency department: A single ED's experience during the COVID-19 pandemic. *Academic Emergency Medicine, 27*(6), 375–378.

Centers for Disease Control and Prevention (CDC). (2017a). FastStats pneumonia. Retrieved on 8/22/2019 at: www.cdc.gov/nchs/fastats/pneumonia.htm

Centers for Disease Control and Prevention (CDC). (2017b). Pneumococcal disease: Pneumococcal vaccination. Retrieved on 9/23/2019 at: www.cdc.gov/pneumococcal/vaccination.html

Centers for Disease Control and Prevention (CDC). (2017c). Vaccines and preventable diseases. Retrieved on 9/23/2019 at: www.cdc.gov/vaccines/vpd/pneumo/hcp/administering-vaccine.html

Centers for Disease Control and Prevention (CDC). (2018a). Health effects of secondhand smoke. Retrieved on 1/14/2020 at: www.cdc.gov/tobacco/data_statistics/fact_sheets/secondhand_smoke/health_effects/index.htm

Centers for Disease Control and Prevention (CDC). (2018b). TB fact sheets-infection control and prevention: TB in specific populations. Retrieved on 9/26/2019 at: www.cdc.gov/tb/statistics/default.htm

Centers for Disease Control and Prevention (CDC). (2019a). Antibiotic prescribing and use in hospitals and long-term care. Retrieved on 9/23/2019 at: www.cdc.gov/antibiotic-use/core-elements/hospital.html

Centers for Disease Control and Prevention (CDC). (2019b). Core elements of antibiotic stewardship. Retrieved on 9/23/2019 at: www.cdc.gov/antibiotic-use/core-elements/index.html

Centers for Disease Control and Prevention (CDC). (2019c). Outbreak of lung injury associated with the use of e-cigarette, or vaping, products.

Retrieved on 9/29/2019 at: www.cdc.gov/tobacco/basic_information/e-cigarettes/severe-lung-disease.html

Centers for Disease Control and Prevention (CDC). (2019d). Tuberculosis screening, testing, and treatment of U.S. health care personnel: Recommendations from the National Tuberculosis Controllers Association and CDC, 2019. Retrieved on 9/23/2019 at: www.cdc.gov/mmwr/volumes/68/wr/mm6819a3.htm?s_cid=mm6819a3_w

Centers for Disease Control and Prevention (CDC). (2019e). Who should be screened for lung cancer? Retrieved on 1/7/2020 at: www.cdc.gov/cancer/lung/basic_info/screening.htm

Centers for Disease Control and Prevention (CDC). (2020). Coronavirus disease. Retrieved on 6/9/2020 at: www.cdc.gov/coronavirus/2019-ncov/index.html

**Centers for Medicare and Medicaid Services. (1993). National coverage determination (NCD) for home use of oxygen (240.2). Retrieved on 2/5/2020 at: www.cms.gov/medicare-coverage-database/details/ncd-details.aspx?NCDId=169&ncdver=1&DocID=240.2

Conde, M. V., & Adams, S. G. (2018). Overview of the management of postoperative pulmonary complications. *UpToDate*. Retrieved on 8/22/2019 at: www.uptodate.com/contents/overview-of-the-management-of-postoperative-pulmonary-complications

Cunha, B. A. (2018). Hospital-acquired pneumonia (nosocomial pneumonia) and ventilator-associated pneumonia. *Medscape*. Available on 2/28/2020 at: emedicine.medscape.com/article/234753-overview#a1

Devlin, J., Skrobik, Y., Gélinas, C., et al. (2018). Clinical practice guidelines for the prevention and management of pain, agitation/sedation, delirium, immobility, and sleep disruption in adult patients in the ICU. *Critical Care Medicine, 46*(9), e825–e873.

Eldridge, L. (2020). An overview of lung cancer. *What is advanced lung cancer*. Retrieved on 1/27/2020 at: www.verywellhealth.com/lung-cancer-overview-4014694

File, T. M. (2019a). Acute bronchitis in adults. *UpToDate*. Retrieved on 8/22/2019 at: www.uptodate.com/contents/acute-bronchitis-in-adults

File, T. M. (2019b). Treatment of community-acquired pneumonia in adults who require hospitalization. *UpToDate*. Retrieved on 10/1/2019 at: www.uptodate.com/contents/treatment-of-community-acquired-pneumonia-in-adults-who-require-hospitalization

Gamache, J. (2019). What is ventilator associated pneumonia (VAP) and how common is it? *Medscape*. Retrieved on 10/1/2019 at: www.medscape.com/answers/300157-19059/what-is-ventilator-associated-pneumonia-vap-andhow-common-is-it

Goldman, R. H. (2019). Overview of occupational and environmental health. *UpToDate*. Retrieved on 9/23/2019 at: www.uptodate.com/contents/overview-of-occupational-and-environmental-health

Harman, E. M. (2018). Acute respiratory distress syndrome treatment and management. *Medscape*. Retrieved on 1/10/2020 at: emedicine.medscape.com/article/165139-treatment

Harrington, A. D., Schmidt, M. P., Szema, A. M., et al. (2017). The role of Iraqi dust in inducing lung injury in United States soldiers—An interdisciplinary study. *Geohealth, 1*(5), 237–246.

Heffner, J. E. (2019a). Diagnostic evaluation of pleural effusion in adults: Initial testing. *UpToDate*. Retrieved on 9/23/2019 at: www.uptodate.com/contents/diagnostic-evaluation-of-a-pleural-effusion-in-adults-initial-testing

Heffner, J. E. (2019b). Chemical pleurodesis. *UpToDate*. Retrieved on 9/23/2019 at: www.uptodate.com/contents/chemical-pleurodesis

Hellman, M., & West, H. (2020). Management of advanced non-small cell lung cancer lacking a driver mutation: Immunotherapy. *UpToDate*. Retrieved on 2/4/2020 at: www.uptodate.com/contents/management-of-advanced-non-small-cell-lung-cancer-lacking-a-driver-mutation-immunotherap

Herchline, T. (2020). Tuberculosis (TB). *Medscape*. Retrieved on 1/10/2020 at: emedicine.medscape.com/article/230802-overview

Hodgson, C. L., Capell, E., & Tipping, C. J. (2018). Early mobilization of patients in intensive care: Organization, communication and safety factors that influence translation into clinical practice. *Critical Care, 22*, 77. doi.org/10.1186/s13054-018-1998-9

Hopkins, W., & Rubin, L. (2019). Treatment of pulmonary hypertension (group 1) in adults: Pulmonary hypertension-specific therapy. *UpToDate*. Retrieved on 9/23/2019 at: www.uptodate.com/contents/treatment-of-pulmonary-hypertension-in-adults

**Institute for Healthcare Improvement (IHI). (2012). *How-to guide: Prevent ventilator-associated pneumonia*. Cambridge, MA: Institute for Healthcare Improvements. Retrieved on 3/6/2020 at: www.ihi.org/resources/Pages/Tools/HowtoGuidePreventVAP.aspx

*Jeyathevan, G., Lemonde, M., & Cooper Brathwaite, A. (2017). The role of oncology nurse navigators in facilitating continuity of care within the diagnostic phase for adult patients with lung cancer. *Canadian Oncology Nursing Journal, 27*(1), 74–87.

Kamangar, N. (2018). Lung abscess *Medscape*. Retrieved on 10/1/2019 at: emedicine.medscape.com/article/299425-overview

Kaynar, A. M. (2018). Respiratory failure treatment & management. *Medscape*. Retrieved on 10/1/2019 at: emedicine.medscape.com/article/167981-treatment

Kim, A. Y., & Gandhi, R. T. (2020). Coronavirus disease 2019 (COVID-19): Management in hospitalized adults. *UpToDate*. Retrieved on 6/4/2020 at: www.uptodate.com/contents/coronavirus-disease-2019-covid-19-management-in-hospitalized-adults

King, T. (2019a). Clinical manifestations and diagnosis of sarcoidosis. *UpToDate*, Retrieved on 9/23/2019 at: www.uptodate.com/contents/clinical-manifestations-and-diagnosis-of-pulmonary-sarcoidosis

King, T. (2019b). Treatment of pulmonary sarcoidosis: Initial therapy with glucocorticoids. *UpToDate*. Retrieved on 9/23/2019 at: www.uptodate.com/contents/treatment-of-pulmonary-sarcoidosis-with-glucocorticoids

Klompas, M. (2019a). Epidemiology, pathogenesis, microbiology, and diagnosis of hospital-acquired and ventilator-associated pneumonia in adults. *UpToDate*. Retrieved on 9/23/2019 at: www.uptodate.com/contents/epidemiology-pathogenesis-microbiology-and-diagnosis-of-hospital-acquired-and-ventilator-associated-pneumonia-in-adults

Klompas, M. (2019b). Treatment of hospital-acquired and ventilator-associated pneumonia in adults. *UpToDate*. Retrieved on 9/23/2019 at: www.uptodate.com/contents/treatment-of-hospital-acquired-and-ventilator-associated-pneumonia-in-adults/print

Klompas M., File T. M., & Bond S. (2019). Treatment of hospital-acquired and ventilator-associated pneumonia in adults. *UpToDate*. Retrieved on 8/22/2019 at: www.uptodate.com/contents/treatment-of-hospital-acquired-ventilator-associated-and-healthcare-associated-pneumonia-in-adults

Korokina L. V., Zhernakova N. I., Korokin M. V., et al. (2018). Principles of pharmacological correction of pulmonary arterial hypertension. *Research Results in Pharmacology, 4*(2), 59–76.

Kramer, J. B., Brown, D. E., & Kopar, P. K. (2020). Ethics in the time of coronavirus: Recommendations in the COVID-19 pandemic. *Journal of the American College of Surgeons, 230*(6), 1114–1118.

Lessnau, K. D. (2019). Miliary tuberculosis. *Medscape*. Retrieved on 1/20/2020 at: emedicine.medscape.com/article/221777-overview#a4

Li, X., & Ma, X. (2020). Acute respiratory failure in COVID-19: Is it "typical" ARDS? *Critical Care, 24*(1), 198. doi.org/10.1186/s13054-020-02911-9

Lindman, J. P. (2018). Tracheostomy. *Medscape*. Retrieved on 1/12/2020 at: emedicine.medscape.com/article/865068-overview

Mancini, M. C. (2018). Blunt chest trauma. *Medscape*. Retrieved on 9/23/2019 at: emedicine.medscape.com/article/428723-overview

Marra, A., Ely, E. W., Pandharipande, P. P., et al. (2017). The ABCDEF bundle in critical care. *Critical Care Clinics, 33*(2), 225–243.

Midthun, D. E. (2019). Clinical manifestations of lung cancer. *UpToDate*. Retrieved on 9/23/2019 at: www.uptodate.com/contents/overview-of-the-risk-factors-pathology-and-clinical-manifestations-of-lung-cancer

Milanez de Campos, J. R., & White, T. (2018). Chest wall stabilization in trauma patients: Why, when, and how? *Journal of Thoracic Disease, 10*(Suppl 8), S951–S962.

Moore, J. A., Conway, D. H., Thomas, N., et al. (2017). Impact of a perioperative quality improvement programme on postoperative pulmonary complications. *Anaesthesia, 72*(3), 317–327.

Morley, G., Grady, C., McCarthy, J., et al. (2020). COVID-19: Ethical challenges for nurses. *Hastings Center Report, 50*(3), 35–39.

Nathwani, D., Varghese, D., Stephens, J., et al. (2019). Value of hospital antimicrobial stewardship programs [ASPs]: A systematic review. *Antimicrobial Resistance & Infection Control, 8*, 35. doi:10.1186/s13756-019-0471-0

National Comprehensive Cancer Network (NCCN). (2020). NCCN clinical practice guideline version 3.2020: Non-small cell lung cancer. Retrieved on 3/8/2020 at: www.nccn.org/professionals/physician_gls/pdf/nscl.pdf

National Institutes of Health (NIH) COVID-19 Treatment Guidelines Panel. (2020). Coronavirus disease 2019 (COVID-19) treatment guidelines. Retrieved on 6/9/2020 at: www.covid19treatmentguidelines.nih.gov/

Niederman, M. S., Richeldi, L., Chotirmall, S. H., et al. (2020). Rising to the challenge of COVID-19: Advice for pulmonary and critical care

and an agenda for research. *American Journal of Respiratory and Critical Care Medicine, 201*(9), 1019–1022.

NIH News in Health. (2019). Vaping rises among teens. Retrieved on 2/1/2020 at: newsinhealth.nih.gov/2019/02/vaping-rises-among-teens

Pozniak, A. (2019). Clinical manifestations and complications of pulmonary tuberculosis. *UpToDate*. Retrieved on 9/23/2019 at: www.uptodate.com/contents/clinical-manifestations-and-complications-of-pulmonary-tuberculosis

Pulmonary Hypertension Association Scientific Leadership Council. (2016). Treatment fact sheet: Selexipag (Uptravi). Retrieved on 3/6/2020 at: phassociation.org/wp-content/uploads/2018/04/Patients-Treatment-Selexipag-4-12-18.pdf

Rajagopalan, S. (2016). Tuberculosis in older adults. *Clinics in Geriatric Medicine, 32*(3), 479–491.

Ramirez, J. A. (2019). Overview of community acquired pneumonia in adults. *UpToDate*. Retrieved on 9/23/2019 at: www.uptodate.com/contents/overview-of-community-acquired-pneumonia-in-adults

Reichman, L. E., & Lardizabal, A. (2019). Adherence to tuberculosis treatment. *UpToDate*. Retrieved on 9/23/2019 at: www.uptodate.com/contents/adherence-to-tuberculosis-treatment

Rubin, L., & Hopkins, W. (2019). Overview of pulmonary hypertension in adults. *UpToDate*. Retrieved on 8/22/2019 at: www.uptodate.com/contents/overview-of-pulmonary-hypertension-in-adults

Saenz, A. D. (2019). Peripheral nerve stimulator-train of four monitoring. *Medscape*. Retrieved on 9/27/2019 at: emedicine.medscape.com/article/2009530-overview

Sarani, B. (2019). Inpatient management of traumatic rib fractures. *UpToDate*. Retrieved on 1/23/2020 at: www.uptodate.com/contents/inpatient-management-of-traumatic-rib-fractures

Seres, D. (2020). Nutrition support in critically ill patients: An overview. *UpToDate*. Retrieved on 2/20/2020 at: www.uptodate.com/contents/nutrition-support-in-critically-ill-patients-an-overview

Shahani, R. (2017). Penetrating chest trauma. *Medscape*. Retrieved on 9/23/2019 at: emedicine.medscape.com/article/425698-overview

Shay, A. (2018). Optimizing the ABCDEF bundle. *American Nurse Today, 13*(7) 21–23.

Siegel, M. D. (2019a). Acute respiratory distress syndrome: Epidemiology, pathophysiology, pathology, and etiology in adults. *UpToDate*. Retrieved on 9/23/2019 at: www.uptodate.com/contents/acute-respiratory-distress-syndrome-epidemiology-pathophysiology-pathology-and-etiology-in-adults

Siegel, M. D. (2019b). Acute respiratory distress syndrome: Prognosis and outcomes in adults. *UpToDate*. Retrieved on 9/23/2019 at: www.uptodate.com/contents/acute-respiratory-distress-syndrome-prognosis-and-outcomes-in-adults

Smetana, G. W. (2018). Strategies to reduce postoperative pulmonary complications in adults. *UpToDate*. Retrieved on 8/22/2019 at: www.uptodate.com/contents/strategies-to-reduce-postoperative-pulmonary-complications

Stark, P. (2019). Atelectasis: Types and pathogenesis in adults. *UpToDate*. Retrieved on 8/22/2019 at: www.uptodate.com/contents/atelectasis-types-and-pathogenesis-in-adults

Sterling, T. R. (2019). Treatment of drug-susceptible pulmonary tuberculosis in HIV-uninfected adults. *UpToDate*. Retrieved on 9/27/2019 at: www.uptodate.com/contents/treatment-of-pulmonary-tuberculosis-in-hiv-uninfected-adults

Strange, C. (2019). Epidemiology, clinical presentation, and diagnostic evaluation of parapneumonic effusion and empyema in adults. *UpToDate*. Retrieved on 9/23/2019 at: www.uptodate.com/contents/parapneumonic-effusion-and-empyema-in-adults

Theel, E. S., Hilgart, H., Breen-Lyles, M., et al. (2018). Comparison of the QuantiFERON-TB Gold Plus and QuantiFERON-TB Gold In-Tube Interferon Gamma Release Assays in patients at risk for tuberculosis and in health care workers. *Journal of Clinical Microbiology, 56*(7), e00614–e00618.

The Joint Commission (TJC). (2019). Sentinel Event Alert 61: Managing the risks of direct oral anticoagulants. Retrieved on 10/4/2019 at: www.jointcommission.org/sentinel_event_alert_61_managing_the_risks_of_direct_oral_anticoagulants/

The Joint Commission (TJC). (2020). Hospital: 2021 National Patient Safety Goals. Retrieved on 1/10/2020 at: www.jointcommission.org/en/standards/national-patient-safety-goals/hospital-2020-national-patient-safety-goals

Thomas, K. W., & Gould, M. K. (2019). Overview of the initial evaluation, diagnosis, and staging of patient with suspected lung cancer.

UpToDate. Retrieved on 8/22/2019 at: www.uptodate.com/contents/overview-of-the-initial-evaluation-diagnosis-and-staging-of-patients-with-suspected-lung-cancer

Timsit, J. F., Esaied, W., Neuville, M., et al. (2017). Update on ventilator-associated pneumonia. *F1000Research*, 6, 2061. doi:10.12688/f1000

Tsai, H., Sung, Y. K., & de Jesus Perez, V. (2016). Recent advances in the management of pulmonary arterial hypertension. *F1000Research*, 5, 2755. doi:10.12688/f1000research.9739.1

Wang, Y., Zhang, D., Du, G., et al. (2020). Remdesivir in adults with severe COVID-19: A randomised, double-blind, placebo-controlled, multicentre trial. *Lancet*, 395(10236), 1569–1578 published online ahead-of-print on 4/29/2020. doi:10.1016/S0140-6736

World Health Organization (WHO). (2019). WHO consolidated guidelines on drug-resistant tuberculosis treatment. Retrieved on 10/1/2019 at: apps.who.int/iris/bitstream/handle/10665/311390/WHO-CDS-TB-2019.3-eng.pdf

Wu, Z., & McGoogan, J. M. (2020). Characteristics of and important lessons from the coronavirus disease 2019 (COVID-19) outbreak in China: Summary of a report of 72,314 cases from the Chinese Center for Disease Control and Prevention. *JAMA*, 323(13), 1239–1242.

Yang, S., Zhang, Z., & Wang, Q. (2019). Emerging therapies for small lung cancer. *Journal of Hematology & Oncology*, 12(47). doi.org/10.1186/s13045-019-0736-3

Zhao, J. B., & Shin, R. D. (2019). Pneumonia in immunocompromised patients. *Medscape*. Retrieved on 8/22/2019 at: emedicine.medscape.com/article/807846-overview

Resources

Agency for Healthcare Research and Quality (AHRQ), ahrq.gov
American Association for Respiratory Care (AARC), aarc.org
American Cancer Society, cancer.org
American College of Chest Physicians (ACCP), chestnet.org
American Lung Association, lung.org
American Thoracic Society (ATS), thoracic.org
Foundation for Sarcoidosis Research, www.stopsarcoidosis.org
National Cancer Institute (NCI), cancer.gov
Occupational Safety and Health Administration (OSHA), osha.gov
Pulmonary Hypertension Association (PHA), phassociation.org
Respiratory Nursing Society (RNS), respiratorynursingsociety.org

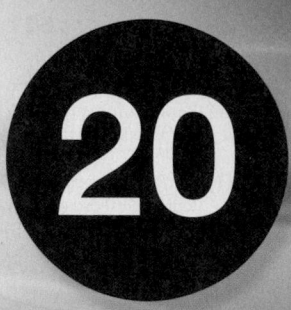

20 Management of Patients with Chronic Pulmonary Disease

LEARNING OUTCOMES

On completion of this chapter, the learner will be able to:

1. Describe the pathophysiology, clinical manifestations, treatment, and medical and nursing management of chronic pulmonary diseases, including chronic obstructive pulmonary disease, bronchiectasis, asthma, and cystic fibrosis.
2. Discuss the major risk factors for developing chronic obstructive pulmonary disease and nursing interventions to minimize or prevent these risk factors.
3. Use the nursing process as a framework for care of the patient with chronic obstructive pulmonary disease.
4. Develop an education plan for patients with chronic obstructive pulmonary disease.
5. Discuss nursing management of and patient education and transitions in care considerations for patients receiving oxygen therapy.
6. Describe asthma self-management strategies.

NURSING CONCEPT

Oxygenation

GLOSSARY

air trapping: incomplete emptying of alveoli during expiration due to loss of lung tissue elasticity (emphysema), bronchospasm (asthma), or airway obstruction

alpha$_1$-antitrypsin deficiency: genetic disorder resulting from deficiency of alpha$_1$-antitrypsin, a protective agent for the lung; increases patient's risk for developing panacinar emphysema even in the absence of smoking

asthma: a heterogeneous disease, usually characterized by chronic airway inflammation; defined by history of symptoms such as wheeze, shortness of breath, chest tightness, and cough that vary over time and in intensity

bronchiectasis: chronic, irreversible dilation of the bronchi and bronchioles that results from the destruction of muscles and elastic connective tissue; dilated airways become saccular and are a medium for chronic infection

chest percussion: manually cupping hands over the chest wall and using vibration to mobilize secretions by mechanically dislodging viscous or adherent secretions in the lungs

chest physiotherapy (CPT): therapy used to remove bronchial secretions, improve ventilation, and increase the efficiency of the respiratory muscles; types include postural drainage, chest percussion, and vibration, and breathing retraining

chronic bronchitis: a disease of the airways defined as the presence of cough and sputum production for at least a combined total of 3 months in each of 2 consecutive years

chronic obstructive pulmonary disease (COPD): disease state characterized by airflow limitation that is not fully reversible; sometimes referred to as chronic airway obstruction or chronic obstructive lung disease

desaturate: a precipitous drop in the saturation of hemoglobin with oxygen

dry-powder inhaler (DPI): a compact, portable inspiratory flow–driven inhaler that delivers dry-powder medications into the patient's lungs

emphysema: a disease of the airways characterized by destruction of the walls of overdistended alveoli

flutter valve: portable handheld mucous clearance device; consisting of a tube with an oscillating steel ball inside; upon expiration, high-frequency oscillations facilitate mucous expectoration

fraction of inspired oxygen (FiO$_2$): concentration of oxygen delivered (e.g., 1.0 equals to 100% oxygen)

hypoxemia: decrease in arterial oxygen tension in the blood

hypoxia: decrease in oxygen supply to the tissues and cells

polycythemia: increase in the red blood cell concentration in the blood; in COPD, the body attempts to improve oxygen-carrying capacity by producing increasing amounts of red blood cells

postural drainage: positioning the patient to allow drainage from all lobes of the lungs and airways

pressurized metered-dose inhaler (pMDI): a compact, portable patient-activated pressurized medication canister that provides aerosolized medication that the patient inhales into the lungs

small-volume nebulizer (SVN): a handheld generator-driven medication delivery system that provides aerosolized liquid medication that the patient inhales into the lungs

spirometry: pulmonary function tests that measure specific lung volumes (e.g., FEV_1, FVC) and rates (e.g.,

$FEF_{25\%-75\%}$); may be measured before and after bronchodilator administration

vibration: a type of massage given by quickly tapping the chest with the fingertips or alternating the fingers in a rhythmic manner, or by using a mechanical device to assist in mobilizing lung secretions

---

Chronic pulmonary disorders are a leading cause of morbidity and mortality in the United States. Nurses care for patients with chronic pulmonary disease across the spectrum of care, from outpatient and home care to emergency department (ED), critical care, and hospice settings. To care for these patients, nurses not only need to have astute assessment and clinical management skills, but they also need knowledge of how these disorders can affect quality of life. In addition, the nurse's knowledge of palliative and end-of-life care is important for applicable patients. Patient and family education is an important nursing intervention to enhance self-management in patients with any chronic pulmonary disorder.

Chronic Obstructive Pulmonary Disease

Chronic obstructive pulmonary disease (COPD) is a preventable and treatable slowly progressive respiratory disease of airflow obstruction involving the airways, pulmonary parenchyma, or both (Global Initiative for Chronic Obstructive Lung Disease [GOLD], 2019). The parenchyma includes any form of lung tissue, including bronchioles, bronchi, blood vessels, interstitium, and alveoli. The airflow limitation or obstruction in COPD is not fully reversible. Most patients with COPD present with overlapping signs and symptoms of emphysema and chronic bronchitis, which are two distinct disease processes.

COPD may include diseases that cause airflow obstruction (e.g., emphysema, chronic bronchitis) or any combination of these disorders. Other diseases such as cystic fibrosis (CF), bronchiectasis, and asthma are classified as chronic pulmonary disorders. Asthma is considered a distinct, separate disorder and is classified as an abnormal airway condition characterized primarily by reversible inflammation. COPD can coexist with asthma. Both of these diseases have the same major symptoms; however, symptoms are generally more variable in asthma than in COPD. This chapter discusses COPD as a disease and describes chronic bronchitis and emphysema as distinct disease states, providing a foundation for understanding the pathophysiology of COPD. Bronchiectasis, asthma, and CF are discussed separately.

While COPD and lower respiratory diseases are the fourth leading cause of death for people of all ages in the United States, they are the third leading cause of death for people ages 65 and over (Centers for Disease Control and Prevention [CDC], 2018a). In 2016, approximately 154,596 Americans died from COPD and lower respiratory diseases (CDC, 2017a). The CDC (2018b) reports that over 16 million Americans live with COPD. This number does not account for the millions of Americans who have COPD but are not diagnosed. Although the rate of hospitalizations for COPD is slowly decreasing, the Agency for Healthcare Research and Quality (AHRQ) reported in 2016 that there were still 501,849 hospitalizations

that had COPD as a primary diagnosis (AHRQ, 2016). The cost of individual hospital admissions for patients with COPD is approximately $6245 more per year than admissions for patients without COPD. COPD's economic burden goes beyond the direct medical costs. Patients with COPD were 60% more likely to call in sick to work and 2.6 times more likely to incur short-term disability than patients without COPD (Patel, Coutinho, Lunacsek, et al., 2018).

Pathophysiology

People with COPD commonly become symptomatic during the middle adult years, and the incidence of the disease increases with age. Although certain aspects of lung function normally decrease with age—for example, vital capacity and forced expiratory volume in 1 second (FEV_1)—COPD accentuates and accelerates these physiologic changes as described later. In COPD, the airflow limitation is both progressive and associated with the lungs' abnormal inflammatory response to noxious particles or gases. The inflammatory response occurs throughout the proximal and peripheral airways, lung parenchyma, and pulmonary vasculature (GOLD, 2019). Because of the chronic inflammation and the body's attempts to repair it, changes and narrowing occur in the airways. In the proximal airways (trachea and bronchi greater than 2 mm in diameter), changes include increased numbers of goblet cells and enlarged submucosal glands, both of which lead to hypersecretion of mucus. In the peripheral airways (bronchioles less than 2 mm diameter), inflammation causes thickening of the airway wall, peribronchial fibrosis, exudate in the airway, and overall airway narrowing (obstructive bronchiolitis). Over time, this ongoing injury-and-repair process causes scar tissue formation and narrowing of the airway lumen (GOLD, 2019). Inflammatory and structural changes also occur in the lung parenchyma (respiratory bronchioles and alveoli). Alveolar wall destruction leads to loss of alveolar attachments and a decrease in elastic recoil. Finally, the chronic inflammatory process affects the pulmonary vasculature and causes thickening of the lining of the vessel and hypertrophy of smooth muscle, which may lead to pulmonary hypertension (GOLD, 2019).

Processes related to imbalances of substances (proteinases and antiproteinases) in the lung may also contribute to airflow limitation. When activated by chronic inflammation, proteinases and other substances may be released, damaging the parenchyma of the lung. These parenchymal changes may also occur as a consequence of inflammation or environmental or genetic factors (e.g., alpha$_1$-antitrypsin deficiency).

Chronic Bronchitis

Chronic bronchitis, a disease of the airways, is defined as the presence of cough and sputum production for at least

Physiology/Pathophysiology

NORMAL BRONCHUS   CHRONIC BRONCHITIS

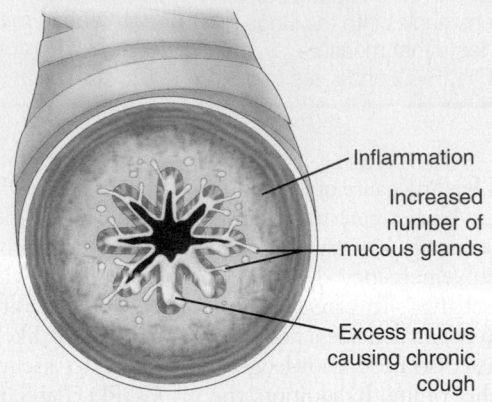

Smooth muscle

Open airway

Mucous gland

Inflammation

Increased number of mucous glands

Excess mucus causing chronic cough

Figure 20-1 • Pathophysiology of chronic bronchitis as compared to a normal bronchus. The bronchus in chronic bronchitis is narrowed and has impaired airflow due to multiple mechanisms: inflammation, excess mucus production, and potential smooth muscle constriction (bronchospasm).

3 months in each of 2 consecutive years. Although *chronic bronchitis* is a clinically and epidemiologically useful term, it does not reflect the major impact of airflow limitation on morbidity and mortality in COPD (GOLD, 2019). In many cases, smoke or other environmental pollutants irritate the airways, resulting in inflammation and hypersecretion of mucus. Constant irritation causes the mucus-secreting glands and goblet cells to increase in number, leading to increased mucus production. Mucus plugging of the airway reduces ciliary function. Bronchial walls also become thickened, further narrowing the bronchial lumen (Fig. 20-1). Alveoli adjacent to the bronchioles may become damaged and fibrosed, resulting in altered function of the alveolar macrophages. This is significant because the macrophages play an important role in destroying foreign particles, including bacteria. As a result, the patient becomes more susceptible to respiratory infection. A wide range of viral, bacterial, and mycoplasma infections can produce acute episodes of bronchitis. Exacerbations of chronic bronchitis are most likely to occur during the winter when viral and bacterial infections are more prevalent.

Emphysema

In **emphysema**, impaired oxygen and carbon dioxide exchange results from destruction of the walls of overdistended alveoli. *Emphysema* is a pathologic term that describes an abnormal distention of the airspaces beyond the terminal bronchioles and destruction of the walls of the alveoli (GOLD, 2019; Han, Dransfield, & Martinez, 2018). In addition, a chronic inflammatory response may induce disruption of the parenchymal tissues. This end-stage process progresses slowly for many years. As the walls of the alveoli are destroyed (a process accelerated by recurrent infections), the alveolar surface area in direct contact with the pulmonary capillaries continually decreases. This causes an increase in dead space (lung area where no gas exchange can occur) and impaired oxygen diffusion, which leads to hypoxemia. In the later stages of disease, carbon dioxide elimination is impaired, resulting in hypercapnia (increased carbon dioxide tension in arterial blood) leading to respiratory acidosis. As the alveolar walls continue to break down, the pulmonary capillary bed is reduced in size. Consequently, resistance to pulmonary blood flow is increased, forcing the right ventricle to maintain a

higher blood pressure in the pulmonary artery. Hypoxemia may further increase pulmonary artery pressures (pulmonary hypertension). Cor pulmonale, one of the complications of emphysema, is right-sided heart failure brought on by long-term high blood pressure in the pulmonary arteries. This high pressure in the pulmonary arteries and right ventricle lead to back up of blood in the venous system, resulting in dependent edema, distended neck veins, or pain in the region of the liver (see Chapter 25 for further discussion).

There are two main types of emphysema, based on the changes taking place in the lung (Fig. 20-2). Both types may occur in the same patient. In the panlobular (panacinar) type of emphysema, there is destruction of the respiratory bronchiole, alveolar duct, and alveolus. All airspaces within the

Physiology/Pathophysiology

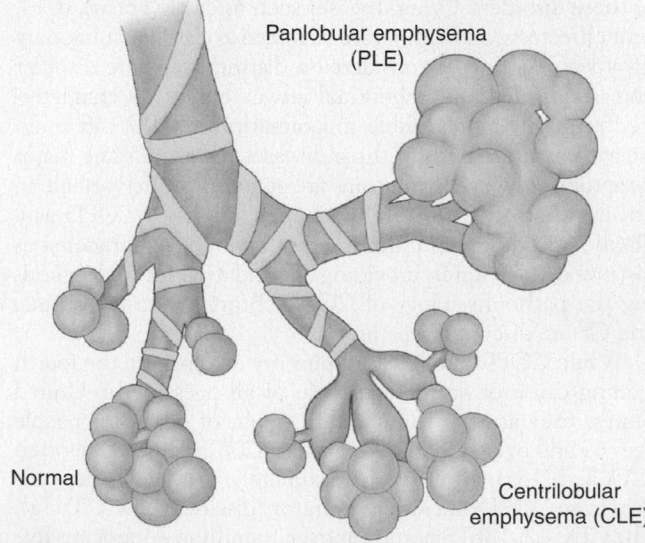

Panlobular emphysema (PLE)

Normal

Centrilobular emphysema (CLE)

Figure 20-2 • Changes in alveolar structure in centrilobular and panlobular emphysema. In panlobular emphysema, the bronchioles, alveolar ducts, and alveoli are destroyed, and the airspaces within the lobule are enlarged. In centrilobular emphysema, the pathologic changes occur in the lobule, whereas the peripheral portions of the acinus are preserved.

lobule are essentially enlarged, but there is little inflammatory disease. A hyperinflated (hyperexpanded) chest, marked dyspnea on exertion, and weight loss typically occur. To move air into and out of the lungs, negative pressure is required during inspiration, and an adequate level of positive pressure must be attained and maintained during expiration. Instead of being an involuntary passive act, expiration becomes active and requires muscular effort.

In the centrilobular (centroacinar) form, pathologic changes take place mainly in the center of the secondary lobule, preserving the peripheral portions of the acinus (i.e., the terminal airway unit where gas exchange occurs). Frequently, there is a derangement of ventilation–perfusion ratios, producing chronic hypoxemia, hypercapnia, **polycythemia** (i.e., an increase in red blood cells), and episodes of right-sided heart failure. This leads to central cyanosis and respiratory failure. The patient also develops peripheral edema.

Risk Factors

Risk factors for COPD include environmental exposures and host factors (Chart 20-1). The most important environmental risk factor for COPD worldwide is cigarette smoking. A dose–response relationship exists between the intensity of smoking (pack-year history) and the decline in pulmonary function. Other environmental risk factors include smoking other types of tobacco (e.g., pipes, cigars) and marijuana. Secondhand smoke also contributes to respiratory symptoms and COPD (GOLD, 2019). Smoking depresses the activity of scavenger cells and affects the respiratory tract's ciliary cleansing mechanism, which keeps breathing passages free of inhaled irritants, bacteria, and other foreign matter. When smoking damages this cleansing mechanism, airflow is obstructed and air becomes trapped behind the obstruction. The alveoli greatly distend, which diminishes lung capacity. Smoking also irritates the goblet cells and mucous glands, causing an increased accumulation of mucus, which in turn produces more irritation, infection, and damage to the lung (U.S. Department of Health & Human Services [HHS], 2014). In addition, carbon monoxide (a by-product of smoking) combines with hemoglobin to form carboxyhemoglobin. Hemoglobin that is bound by carboxyhemoglobin cannot carry oxygen efficiently. Cigarette smoking is the best studied COPD risk factor; however, it is not the only risk factor

---

Chart 20-1 ⚠	**RISK FACTORS** Chronic Obstructive Pulmonary Disease

- Exposure to tobacco smoke accounts for an estimated 80–90% of cases of chronic obstructive pulmonary disease
- Secondhand smoke
- Increased age
- Occupational exposure—dust, chemicals
- Indoor and outdoor air pollution
- Genetic abnormalities, including a deficiency of alpha$_1$-antitrypsin, an enzyme inhibitor that normally counteracts the destruction of lung tissue by certain other enzymes

Adapted from Global Initiative for Chronic Obstructive Lung Disease (GOLD). (2019). Global strategy for the diagnosis, management, and prevention of chronic obstructive pulmonary disease. Retrieved on 6/23/2019 at: www.goldcopd.org/wp-content/uploads/2018/11/GOLD-2019-v1.7-FINAL-14Nov2018-WMS.pdf

---

and studies have demonstrated nonsmokers may also develop chronic airflow obstruction.

Other environmental risk factors for COPD include prolonged and intense exposure to occupational dusts and chemicals, indoor air pollution, and outdoor air pollution (GOLD, 2019). Recent studies indicate that the use of electronic nicotine delivery systems (ENDS; e.g., e-cigarettes, e-pens, e-pipes, e-hookahs, e-cigars) could increase the risk for developing COPD, but additional research is needed to better understand how their use causes changes similar to COPD in the lungs (Canistro, Vivarelli, Cirillo, et al., 2017; Evans, Burton, & Schwartz, 2018; Larcombe, Janka, Mullins, et al., 2017). Smoke from ENDS has been shown to trigger lung changes (i.e., airway hyperreactivity and lung tissue destruction) that are normally associated with the development of COPD (Garcia-Arcos, Geraghty, Baumlin, et al., 2016). Further research demonstrated that different flavored e-cigarette fluids, aerosols, and solvents can produce different patterns of cytotoxicity (Behar, Wang, & Talbot, 2018). The Surgeon General reported that more than one third of adults ages 18 to 24 years of age had tried e-cigarettes (HHS, 2016). Young adults who have used e-cigarettes report being attracted to them due to perceptions of low harm, the flavorings/tastes of the product, and curiosity (HHS, 2016).

Host risk factors include a person's genetic makeup. One well-documented genetic risk factor is a deficiency of alpha$_1$-antitrypsin, an enzyme inhibitor that protects the lung parenchyma from injury. This deficiency may lead to lung and liver disease. Worldwide, **alpha$_1$-antitrypsin deficiency** impacts between 1/1500 and 1/3000 people with European ancestry (U.S. National Library of Medicine [NLM], 2019). This genetic risk is uncommon in people of Asian descent (NLM, 2019). Approximately 2% of people with COPD have been diagnosed with this deficiency (Stoller, Barnes, & Hollingsworth, 2018). This deficiency predisposes young people to rapid development of lobular emphysema, even in the absence of smoking. Among Caucasians, alpha$_1$-antitrypsin deficiency is one of the most common genetically linked lethal diseases. COPD may also result from gene–environment interactions (GOLD, 2019). People who are genetically susceptible are sensitive to environmental factors (e.g., smoking, air pollution, infectious agents, allergens) and eventually develop chronic obstructive symptoms. Carriers must be identified so that they can modify environmental risk factors to delay or prevent overt symptoms of disease. Genetic counseling should be offered. Alpha-protease inhibitor replacement therapy, which slows the progression of the disease, is available for patients with this genetic defect and for those with severe disease. However, this infusion therapy is costly and is required on an ongoing basis.

Other genetic risk factors may predispose a patient to COPD. Work is ongoing to identify specific variants of genes hypothesized to be involved in the development of COPD. These may include specific phenotypes to several chromosomal regions in families with multiple members developing early-onset COPD (see Chapter 17, Chart 17-8).

Age is often identified as a risk factor for COPD, but it is unclear whether healthy aging is an independent risk or whether the risk is related to cumulative exposures to risks over time (GOLD, 2019). There is a strong inverse relationship between COPD and lower socioeconomic status.

However, perhaps it is not the lower socioeconomic status but how the socioeconomic status places the person at risk for increased patterns of exposure (indoor and outdoor pollutants, crowding, poor nutrition, infections, and increased smoking).

Clinical Manifestations

Although the natural history of COPD is variable, it is generally a progressive disease characterized by three primary symptoms: chronic cough, sputum production, and dyspnea (GOLD, 2019). These symptoms often worsen over time. Chronic cough and sputum production often precede the development of airflow limitation by many years. However, not all people with cough and sputum production develop COPD. The cough may be intermittent and may be unproductive in some patients (GOLD, 2019). Dyspnea may be severe and interfere with the patient's activities and quality of life. It is usually progressive, worse with exercise, and persistent. As COPD progresses, dyspnea may occur at rest. Weight loss is common, because dyspnea interferes with eating and the work of breathing is energy depleting. As the work of breathing increases over time, the accessory muscles are recruited in an effort to breathe. Patients with COPD are at risk for respiratory insufficiency and respiratory infections or COPD exacerbation, which in turn increase the risk of acute and chronic respiratory failure.

In patients with COPD who have a primary emphysematous component, chronic hyperinflation leads to the "barrel chest" thorax configuration. This configuration results from a more fixed position of the ribs in the inspiratory position (due to hyperinflation) and from loss of lung elasticity (Fig. 20-3).

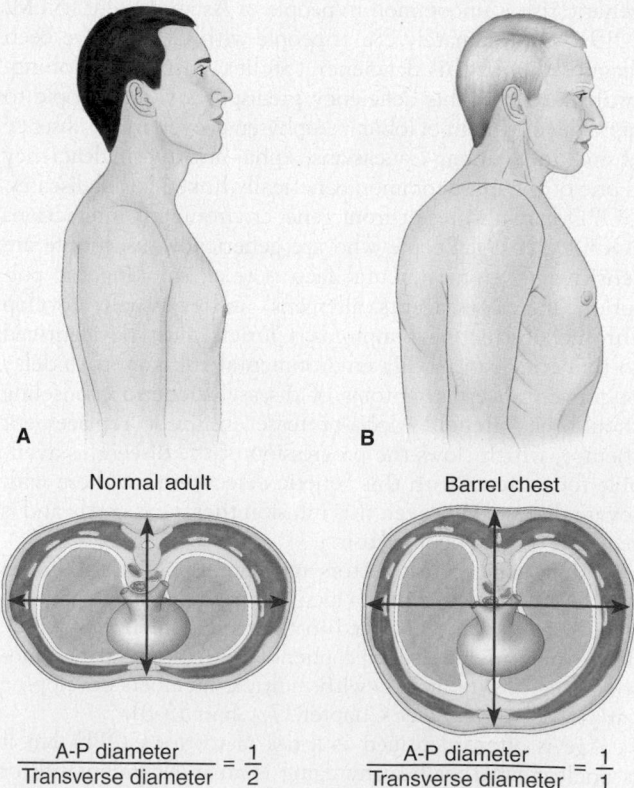

A Normal adult   **B** Barrel chest

$$\frac{\text{A-P diameter}}{\text{Transverse diameter}} = \frac{1}{2}$$

$$\frac{\text{A-P diameter}}{\text{Transverse diameter}} = \frac{1}{1}$$

Figure 20-3 • Characteristics of normal chest wall and chest wall in emphysema. **A.** The normal chest wall and its cross-section. **B.** The barrel-shaped chest of emphysema and its cross-section.

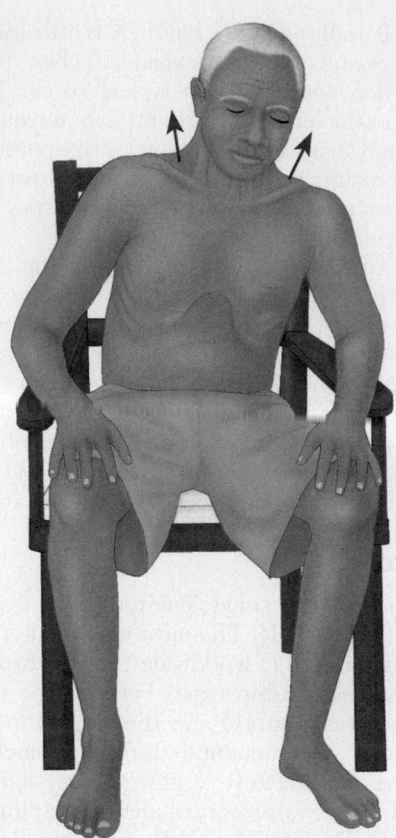

Figure 20-4 • Typical posture of a person with chronic obstructive pulmonary disease—primarily emphysema. The person tends to lean forward and uses the accessory muscles of respiration to breathe, forcing the shoulder girdle upward and causing the supraclavicular fossae to retract on inspiration.

Retraction of the supraclavicular fossae occurs on inspiration, causing the shoulders to heave upward (Fig. 20-4). In advanced emphysema, the abdominal muscles may also contract on inspiration.

There are systemic or extrapulmonary manifestations of COPD. These include musculoskeletal wasting (see Chapter 4 for discussion of nutrition assessment and Chapters 39 and 40 for discussion of nutrition therapy), metabolic disturbances, and depression (a frequent comorbidity that accompanies chronic debilitating illnesses). These clinical manifestations beyond the lungs must also be assessed and treated in order to decrease the morbidity and improve the quality of life of the patient with COPD. For example, research has indicated that depression, metabolic syndrome, and diabetes are frequent comorbidities of COPD (Raherison, Ouaalaya, Bernady, et al., 2018). It is speculated that measures to promote healthy eating and activity that may ameliorate metabolic syndrome, diabetes, and depression may also deter the development of COPD.

Assessment and Diagnostic Findings

The nurse obtains a thorough health history from patients with known or potential COPD. Chart 20-2 lists the key factors to assess for patients with known or suspected COPD. Pulmonary function studies are used to help confirm the diagnosis of COPD, determine disease severity, and monitor disease progression. **Spirometry** is used to evaluate

Chart 20-2 · ASSESSMENT

Assessing Patients with Chronic Obstructive Pulmonary Disease

Health History

- Has the patient been exposed to risk factors (see Chart 20-1)? If so, inquire about types, intensity, and duration of exposure; for instance:
  - How much exposure has the patient had to secondhand smoke?
  - Is there occupational exposure to smoke or other pollutants?
- Does the patient have a past medical history of respiratory diseases/problems, including asthma, allergy, sinusitis, nasal polyps, or respiratory infections?
- Does the patient have a family history of chronic obstructive pulmonary disease or other chronic respiratory diseases?
- How long has the patient had respiratory difficulty?
- What is the pattern of symptom development?
- Does exertion increase the dyspnea? What type of exertion?
- What are the limits of the patient's tolerance for exercise?
- At what times during the day does the patient complain most of fatigue and shortness of breath?
- Does the patient describe any discomfort or pain in any part of the body? If so, where does it occur, how intense is this pain, when does it occur, and does it interfere with activities of daily living? Is there any intervention that helps to alleviate the pain or discomfort?
- Which eating and sleeping habits have been affected?
- What is the impact of respiratory disease on quality of life?
- What does the patient know about the disease and their condition?
- What is the patient's smoking history?
- Does the patient have a history of using electronic nicotine delivery systems (ENDS) (e.g., vaping, e-cigarettes, e-pens, e-pipes, e-hookah, e-cigars)?
- What are the triggering events (e.g., exertion, strong odors, dust, exposure to animals)?

- Does the patient have a history of exacerbations or previous hospitalizations for respiratory problems?
- Are comorbidities present?
- How appropriate are current medical treatments?
- Does the patient have available social and family support?
- What is the potential for reducing risk factors (e.g., smoking cessation)?

Physical Assessment

- What position does the patient assume during the interview?
- What are the pulse and the respiratory rates?
- What is the character of respirations? Even and without effort? Other?
- Can the patient complete a sentence without having to take a breath?
- Does the patient contract the abdominal muscles during inspiration?
- Does the patient use accessory muscles of the shoulders and neck when breathing?
- Does the patient take a long time to exhale (prolonged expiration)?
- Is central cyanosis evident?
- Are the patient's neck veins distended?
- Does the patient have peripheral edema?
- Is the patient coughing?
- What are the color, amount, and consistency of the sputum?
- Is clubbing of the fingers present?
- What types of breath sounds (i.e., clear, diminished or distant, crackles, wheezes) are heard? Describe and document findings and locations.
- Are there any sensory deficits?
- Is there short- or long-term memory impairment?
- Is there increasing stupor?
- Is the patient apprehensive?

---

airflow obstruction, which is determined by the ratio of FEV_1 to forced vital capacity (FVC). Spirometric results are expressed as an absolute volume and as a percentage of the predicted value using appropriate normal values for gender, age, and height. With obstruction, the patient either has difficulty exhaling or cannot forcibly exhale air from the lungs, reducing the FEV_1. Spirometry is also used to determine reversibility of obstruction after the use of bronchodilators (GOLD, 2019). Spirometry is initially performed, the patient is given an inhaled bronchodilator treatment according to a standard protocol, and then spirometry is repeated. The patient demonstrates a degree of reversibility if the pulmonary function values improve after administration of the bronchodilator.

Arterial blood gas measurements may also be obtained to assess baseline oxygenation and gas exchange and are especially important in advanced COPD. A chest x-ray may be obtained to exclude alternative diagnoses. A computed tomography (CT) chest scan is not routinely obtained in the diagnosis of COPD, but a high-resolution CT scan may help in the differential diagnosis. Screening for alpha$_1$-antitrypsin deficiency is suggested for all adults who are symptomatic, especially for patients younger than 45 years. Screening in young adults is important for those with a family history of

COPD, particularly if they have a family history of blood relatives with alpha$_1$-antitrypsin deficiency or COPD that is primarily emphysematous in nature (Han et al., 2018).

COPD is classified into four grades depending on the severity measured by pulmonary function tests, as shown in Table 20-1 (GOLD, 2019). However, pulmonary function is not the only way to assess or classify COPD; pulmonary function is evaluated in conjunction with symptoms, health status impairment with COPD, and the potential for exacerbations. Factors that determine the clinical course and survival of patients with COPD include history of cigarette smoking, exposure to secondhand smoke, age, rate of decline of FEV_1, hypoxemia, pulmonary artery pressure, resting heart rate, weight loss, reversibility of airflow obstruction, and comorbidities.

In diagnosing COPD, several differential diagnoses must be ruled out. The primary differential diagnosis is asthma. It may be difficult to differentiate between a patient with COPD and one with chronic asthma. Other diseases that must be considered in the differential diagnosis include heart failure, bronchiectasis, tuberculosis, obliterative bronchiolitis, and diffuse panbronchiolitis (GOLD, 2019). Key factors in determining the diagnosis are the patient's history, severity of symptoms, and responsiveness to bronchodilators.

TABLE 20-1	Grades of Chronic Obstructive Pulmonary Disease	
Grade	**Severity**	**Pulmonary Function**
Grade I	Mild	FEV_1/FVC <70% FEV_1 ≥80% predicted
Grade II	Moderate	FEV_1/FVC <70% FEV_1 50–79% predicted
Grade III	Severe	FEV_1/FVC <70% FEV_1 30–49% predicted
Grade IV	Very severe	FEV_1/FVC <70% FEV_1 <30% predicted

FEV_1, forced expiratory volume in 1 s; FVC, forced vital capacity.
Adapted from Global Initiative for Chronic Obstructive Lung Disease (GOLD). (2019). Global strategy for the diagnosis, management, and prevention of chronic obstructive pulmonary disease. Retrieved on 06/23/2019 at: www.goldcopd.org/wp-content/uploads/2018/11/GOLD-2019-v1.7-FINAL-14Nov2018-WMS.pdf

Complications

Respiratory insufficiency and failure are major life-threatening complications of COPD. The acuity of the onset and the severity of respiratory failure depend on baseline pulmonary function, pulse oximetry or arterial blood gas values, comorbid conditions, and the severity of other complications of COPD. Respiratory insufficiency and failure may be chronic (with severe COPD) or acute (with severe bronchospasm or pneumonia in a patient with severe COPD). Acute respiratory insufficiency and failure may necessitate ventilatory support until other acute complications, such as infection, can be treated. (See Chapter 19 for the management of the patient requiring ventilatory support.) Other complications of COPD include pneumonia, chronic atelectasis, pneumothorax, and pulmonary arterial hypertension (cor pulmonale).

Medical Management

Therapeutic strategies for the patient with COPD include promoting smoking cessation as appropriate, providing supplemental oxygen therapy as indicated, prescribing medications, and managing exacerbations. Some patients may benefit from surgical interventions; whereas others with advanced COPD may benefit from palliative care.

Risk Reduction

For patients with stable disease, treatment aims to reduce risk and symptoms. The major risk factor associated with COPD is environmental exposure and it is modifiable. The most important environmental exposure is smoking. In 2017, over 34 million people in the United States reported that they were active smokers (CDC, 2018b). Smoking kills more than 480,000 people each year and costs the nation more than $300 billion in health care expenses and lost productivity annually (CDC, 2019a; CDC, 2019b). Smoking cessation is the single most cost-effective intervention to reduce the risk of developing COPD and to stop its progression (GOLD, 2019). However, smoking cessation is difficult to achieve and even more difficult to sustain in the long term. Factors associated with continued smoking vary among patients and may include the strength of the nicotine addiction, continued

exposure to smoking-associated stimuli (at work or in social settings), stress, depression, and habit.

Because multiple factors are associated with continued smoking, successful cessation often requires multiple strategies. Health care providers should promote cessation by explaining the risks of smoking and personalizing the "at-risk" message to the patient. After giving a strong warning about smoking, health care providers should work with the patient to set a definite "quit date." Referral to a smoking cessation program may be helpful. Follow-up within 3 to 5 days after the quit date to review progress and to address any problems is associated with an increased rate of success; this should be repeated as needed. Continued reinforcement with a modality that is individualized to the patient and the patient's lifestyle (e.g., telephone calls, texting, e-mail, or clinic visits) is beneficial. Relapses should be analyzed, and the patient and health care provider should jointly identify possible solutions to prevent future backsliding. It is important to emphasize successes rather than failures. Nicotine replacement—a first-line pharmacotherapy that reliably increases long-term smoking abstinence rates—comes in a variety of forms (gum, inhaler, nasal spray, transdermal patch, sublingual tablet, or lozenge). Bupropion SR and nortriptyline, both antidepressants, may also increase long-term quit rates. Other pharmacologic agents include the antihypertensive agent clonidine; however, its side effects limit its use. Varenicline, a nicotinic acetylcholine receptor partial agonist, may assist in smoking cessation (GOLD, 2019). Patients who are not appropriate candidates for such pharmacotherapy include those with medical contraindications, light smokers (fewer than 10 cigarettes per day), pregnant women, and adolescent smokers.

Smoking cessation can begin in a variety of health care settings—outpatient clinic, nursing center, pulmonary rehabilitation center, community, hospital, and in the home. Regardless of the setting, nurses have the opportunity to educate patients about the risks of smoking and the benefits of smoking cessation. Various materials, resources, and programs developed by several organizations (e.g., AHRQ, CDC, National Cancer Institute, American Lung Association, American Cancer Society) are available to assist with this effort.

General Principles of Oxygen Therapy

Oxygen therapy is the administration of oxygen at a concentration greater than that found in the environmental atmosphere. At sea level, the concentration of oxygen in room air is 21%. The goal of oxygen therapy is to provide adequate transport of oxygen in the blood while decreasing the work of breathing and reducing stress on the myocardium.

Oxygen transport to tissues depends on factors such as cardiac output, arterial oxygen content, concentration of hemoglobin, and metabolic requirements. These factors must be kept in mind when oxygen therapy is considered for use in all patients, regardless of underlying disorders.

Indications

A change in the patient's respiratory rate or pattern may be one of the earliest indicators of the need for oxygen therapy. These changes may result from hypoxemia or hypoxia. **Hypoxemia,** a decrease in the arterial oxygen tension in the blood, is manifested by changes in mental status (progressing through impaired judgment, agitation, disorientation, confusion, lethargy, and coma), dyspnea, increase in blood pressure, changes in heart rate, arrhythmias, central cyanosis (late sign), diaphoresis, and cool extremities. Hypoxemia usually leads to **hypoxia**, a decrease in oxygen supply to the tissues and cells that can also be caused by problems outside the respiratory system. Severe hypoxia can be life-threatening.

The signs and symptoms signaling the need for supplemental oxygen may depend on how suddenly this need develops. With rapidly developing hypoxia, changes occur in the central nervous system because the neurologic centers are very sensitive to oxygen deprivation. The clinical picture may resemble that of alcohol intoxication, with the patient exhibiting lack of coordination and impaired judgment. With longstanding hypoxia (as seen in patients with COPD as well as in patients with chronic heart failure), fatigue, drowsiness, apathy, inattentiveness, and delayed reaction time may occur. The need for oxygen is assessed by arterial blood gas analysis, pulse oximetry, and clinical evaluation.

Complications

Oxygen is a medication, and except in emergency situations it is given only when prescribed by a health care provider. As with other medications, the nurse administers oxygen with caution and carefully assesses its effects on each patient.

In general, a patient with any type of respiratory disorder is given oxygen therapy only to increase the partial pressure of arterial oxygen (PaO_2) back to the patient's normal baseline, which may vary from 60 to 95 mm Hg. In terms of the oxyhemoglobin dissociation curve (see Chapter 17), arterial hemoglobin at these levels is 80% to 98% saturated with oxygen; higher **fraction of inspired oxygen (FiO_2)** flow values add no further significant amounts of oxygen to the red blood cells or plasma. Instead of helping, increased amounts of oxygen may produce toxic effects on the lungs and central nervous system or may depress ventilation, which is a particularly lethal adverse effect in patients with COPD (see later discussion).

It is important to observe for subtle indicators of inadequate oxygenation when oxygen is given by any method. Therefore, the nurse assesses the patient frequently for confusion, restlessness progressing to lethargy, diaphoresis, pallor, tachycardia, tachypnea, and hypertension. Intermittent or continuous pulse oximetry is used to monitor oxygen levels.

Oxygen toxicity may occur when too high concentration of oxygen is given for an extended period (generally longer than 24 hours) (Kacmarek, Stoller, & Heuer, 2017). It is caused by overproduction of oxygen free radicals, which are by-products of cell metabolism. These free radicals then mediate a severe inflammatory response that can severely damage the alveolar capillary membrane leading to pulmonary edema and progressing to cell death. Clinical manifestations of oxygen toxicity causing lung damage are similar to acute respiratory distress syndrome (ARDS) (see Chapter 19).

Signs and symptoms of oxygen toxicity include substernal discomfort, paresthesias, dyspnea, restlessness, fatigue, malaise, progressive respiratory difficulty, refractory hypoxemia, alveolar atelectasis, and alveolar infiltrates evident on chest x-rays.

Using the lowest amount of oxygen needed to maintain an acceptable PaO_2 level and treating the underlying condition aids in the prevention of oxygen toxicity (Kacmarek et al., 2017).

An additional adverse effect of the administration of high concentrations of oxygen (greater than 50%) to patients who are sedated and breathing small tidal volumes of air (volume of air inspired and expired with each breath) is absorption atelectasis. Normally, 79% of room air is comprised of nitrogen. During inhalation, nitrogen, in addition to other gases, fills the alveoli and helps keep the alveoli open. With the administration of high concentrations of oxygen, nitrogen is diluted and replaced with oxygen. Oxygen in the alveoli is absorbed quickly into the bloodstream and not replaced rapidly enough in the alveoli to maintain patency. The alveoli collapse, causing atelectasis (Kacmarek et al., 2017).

Because oxygen supports combustion, there is always a danger of fire when it is used. It is important to post "No Smoking" signs when oxygen is in use. Oxygen therapy equipment is also a potential source of bacterial contamination; therefore, the nurse (or respiratory therapist) changes the tubing according to infection prevention policy, manufacturer's recommendations, and the type of oxygen delivery equipment.

 ## Gerontologic Considerations

The respiratory system changes throughout the aging process, and it is important for nurses to be aware of these changes when assessing older adult patients who are receiving oxygen therapy. As the respiratory muscles weaken and the large bronchi and alveoli become enlarged, the available surface area of the lungs decreases, resulting in reduced ventilation and respiratory gas exchange. The number of functional cilia is also reduced, decreasing ciliary action and the cough reflex. As a result of osteoporosis and calcification of the costal cartilages, chest wall compliance is decreased. Patients may display increased chest rigidity and respiratory rate and decreased PaO_2 and lung expansion. The older adult is at risk for aspiration and infection related to these changes. In addition, patient education regarding adequate nutrition is essential because appropriate dietary intake can help diminish the excess buildup of carbon dioxide and maintain optimal respiratory functioning (Meiner & Yeager, 2019).

Methods of Oxygen Administration

Oxygen is dispensed from a cylinder or a piped-in system. A reduction gauge is necessary to reduce the pressure to a working level, and a flow meter regulates the flow of oxygen in liters per minute (L/min). When oxygen is used at high flow rates, it should be moistened by passing it through a humidification system to prevent it from drying the mucous membranes of the respiratory tract.

The use of oxygen concentrators is another means of providing varying amounts of oxygen, especially in the home setting. These devices are relatively portable, easy to operate, and cost-effective but require more maintenance than tank or liquid systems. These models can deliver oxygen flows from 1 to 10 L/min and provide an FiO_2 of about 40% (Cairo, 2018).

Many different oxygen devices are used (Table 20-2). The amount of oxygen delivered is expressed as a percentage concentration (e.g., 70%). The appropriate form of oxygen therapy is best determined by arterial blood gas levels (see Chapter 10), which indicate the patient's oxygenation status.

(text continued on page 613)

TABLE 20-2	Oxygen Administration Devices				

Device	Suggested Flow Rate (L/min)	O₂ Percentage Setting	Advantages	Disadvantages
Low-Flow Systems				
Cannula (nasal and reservoir)	1–2 3–5 6	24–28 32–40 44	Lightweight, comfortable, inexpensive, continuous use with meals and activity	Easily dislodged, from nares, skin breakdown over ears or nares, nasal mucosal and/or pharyngeal mucosal drying, air swallowing, variable FiO₂
Nasal (oropharyngeal) catheter	1–6	24–44	Inexpensive, does not require a tracheostomy	Nasal mucosa irritation; catheter should be changed frequently to alternate nostril
Mask, simple	5–8	40–60	Simple to use, inexpensive	Poorly fitting, variable FiO₂, must remove to eat
Mask, partial rebreathing	8–11	50–75	Moderate O₂ concentration	Warm, poorly fitting, must remove to eat

TABLE 20-2	Oxygen Administration Devices (continued)				
Device	Suggested Flow Rate (L/min)	O$_2$ Percentage Setting	Advantages	Disadvantages
Mask, nonrebreathing	10–15	80–95	High O$_2$ concentration	Poorly fitting, must remove to eat

High-Flow Systems

Mask, Venturi	4–6 6–8	24, 26, 28 30, 35, 40	Provides low levels of supplemental O$_2$ Precise FiO$_2$, additional humidity available	Must remove to eat
Transtracheal oxygen catheter	¼–4	60–100	More comfortable than other high-flow systems, concealed by clothing, less oxygen liters per minute needed than nasal cannula	Requires frequent and regular cleaning, requires surgical intervention, with associated risk for surgical complications
Mask, aerosol	8–10	28–100	Good humidity, accurate FiO$_2$	Uncomfortable for some

(continued on page 612)

TABLE 20-2	Oxygen Administration Devices (continued)				
Device		Suggested Flow Rate (L/min)	O$_2$ Percentage Setting	Advantages	Disadvantages
Tracheostomy collar		8–10	28–100	Good humidity, comfortable, fairly accurate FiO$_2$	Requires surgery to place; needs cleaning and suctioning to maintain patency of airway
T-piece		8–10	28–100	Same as tracheostomy collar	Heavy with tubing; no need for surgery for placement
Face tent		8–10	28–100	Good humidity, fairly accurate FiO$_2$	Bulky and cumbersome
Oxygen-Conserving Devices					
Pulse dose (or demand)		10–40 mL/ breath		Deliver O$_2$ only on inspiration, conserve 50–75% of O$_2$ used	Must carefully evaluate function individually

Oxygen delivery systems are classified as low-flow systems (variable performance) or high-flow systems (fixed performance). Low-flow systems contribute partially to the inspired gas the patient breathes, which means that the patient breathes some room air along with the oxygen. These systems do not provide a constant or precise concentration of inspired oxygen. The amount of inspired oxygen changes as the patient's breathing changes. High-flow systems provide the total inspired air. A specific percentage of oxygen is delivered independent of the patient's breathing. High-flow systems are indicated for patients who require a constant and precise amount of oxygen (Cairo, 2018).

A nasal cannula is used when the patient requires a low to medium concentration of oxygen for which precise accuracy is not essential. This method allows the patient to move about in bed, talk, cough, and eat without interrupting oxygen flow. Although a nasal cannula can deliver up to 6 L/min, flow rates in excess of 4 L/min may lead to swallowing of air or may cause irritation and drying of the nasal and pharyngeal mucosa.

A reservoir cannula stores oxygen in a thin membrane during exhalation. When the patient's inspiration exceeds the flow rate into the cannula, the patient receives additional gas from the reservoir membrane. This reduces oxygen use because the patient can achieve adequate oxygenation with a lower flow rate than what would be used with a nasal cannula. The patient must exhale through the nose to reopen the reservoir. Any condition, such as pursed lipped breathing, that prevents nasal exhalation would limit the effectiveness of the device.

The nasal (oropharyngeal) catheter delivers low to moderate concentrations of oxygen and is rarely used. This method of delivering low-flow oxygen is usually reserved for use in special procedures, such as those that examine the patient's airways and lungs (bronchoscopy). When used during long procedures, the catheter should be changed frequently (e.g., every 8 hours), alternating nostrils to prevent nasal irritation and infection.

When oxygen is given via cannula or catheter, the percentage of oxygen reaching the lungs varies with the depth, rate, and technique of respirations. Anatomic occlusions in the nasal cavity, swollen nasal mucosa, and mouth breathing are examples of conditions that would alter the amount of gas the patient inhales.

Oxygen masks come in several forms. Each is used for different purposes (see Table 20-2). *Simple masks*, low-flow design, are used to administer low to moderate concentrations of oxygen. The body of the mask itself gathers and stores oxygen between breaths. The patient exhales directly through openings or ports in the body of the mask. If oxygen flow ceases, the patient can draw air in through these openings around the mask edges. Although widely used, these masks cannot be used for controlled oxygen concentrations and must be adjusted for proper fit. They should not press too tightly against the skin, because this can cause a sense of claustrophobia as well as skin breakdown; adjustable elastic bands are provided to ensure comfort and security.

Partial rebreathing masks have a reservoir bag that must remain inflated during both inspiration and expiration. The nurse adjusts the oxygen flow to ensure that the bag does not collapse during inhalation. A moderate concentration of oxygen can be delivered because both the mask and the bag serve as reservoirs for oxygen. Oxygen enters the mask through small-bore tubing that connects at the junction of the mask and bag. As the patient inhales, gas is drawn from the mask, from the bag, and potentially from room air through the exhalation ports. As the patient exhales, the first third of the exhalation fills the reservoir bag. This is mainly dead space and does not participate in gas exchange in the lungs. Therefore, it has a high oxygen concentration. The remainder of the exhaled gas is vented through the exhalation ports. The actual percentage of oxygen delivered is influenced by the patient's ventilatory pattern (Kacmarek et al., 2017).

Nonrebreathing masks are similar in design to partial rebreathing masks except that they have additional valves. A one-way valve located between the reservoir bag and the base of the mask allows gas from the reservoir bag to enter the mask on inhalation but prevents gas in the mask from flowing back into the reservoir bag during exhalation. One-way valves located at the exhalation ports prevent room air from entering the mask during inhalation. They also allow the patient's exhaled gases to exit the mask on exhalation. As with the partial rebreathing mask, it is important to adjust the oxygen flow so that the reservoir bag does not completely collapse on inspiration. In theory, if the nonrebreathing mask fits the patient snugly and both side exhalation ports have one-way valves, it is possible for the patient to receive 100% oxygen, making the nonrebreathing mask a high-flow oxygen system. However, because it is difficult to get an exact fit from the mask on every patient, and some nonrebreathing masks have only one one-way exhalation valves, it is almost impossible to ensure 100% oxygen delivery, making it a low-flow oxygen system.

The *Venturi mask* is the most reliable and accurate method for delivering precise concentrations of oxygen through noninvasive means. The mask is constructed in a way that allows a constant flow of room air blended with a fixed flow of oxygen. It is used primarily for patients with COPD because it can accurately provide appropriate levels of supplemental oxygen, thus avoiding the risk of suppressing the hypoxic drive.

The Venturi mask uses the Bernoulli principle of air entrainment (trapping the air like a vacuum), which provides a high airflow with controlled oxygen enrichment. For each liter of oxygen that passes through a jet orifice, a fixed proportion of room air is entrained. Varying the size of the jet orifice and adjusting the flow of oxygen can deliver a precise volume of oxygen. Excess gas leaves the mask through the two exhalation ports, carrying with it the exhaled carbon dioxide. This method allows a constant oxygen concentration to be inhaled regardless of the depth or rate of respiration.

The mask should fit snugly enough to prevent oxygen from flowing into the patient's eyes. The nurse checks the patient's skin for irritation. It is necessary to remove the mask so that the patient can eat, drink, and take medications, at which time supplemental oxygen is provided through a nasal cannula.

 Concept Mastery Alert

Oxygen delivery systems are classified as either low- or high-flow systems. Whereas a low-flow oxygen delivery system may imprecisely deliver high concentrations of oxygen (e.g., up to 100% via a nonrebreathing mask), the Venturi mask, which is a high-flow system, is specifically designed to deliver precise but lower concentrations of oxygen (less than 30% oxygen).

The *transtracheal oxygen catheter* requires minor surgery to insert a catheter through a small incision directly into the trachea. It is indicated for patients with chronic oxygen therapy needs. These catheters are more comfortable, less dependent on breathing patterns, and less obvious than other oxygen delivery methods. Because no oxygen is lost into the surrounding environment, the patient achieves adequate oxygenation at lower rates, making this method less expensive and more efficient.

Other oxygen devices include *aerosol masks, tracheostomy collars* (see Table 20-2), *T-pieces*, and *face tents*, all of which are used with aerosol devices (nebulizers) that can be adjusted for oxygen concentrations from 28% to 100% (0.28 to 1.00). If the gas mixture flow falls below patient demand, room air is pulled in, diluting the concentration. The aerosol mist must be available for the patient during the entire inspiratory phase.

Specific Considerations for the Patient with COPD Receiving Oxygen Therapy

Oxygen therapy can be given as long-term continuous therapy, during exercise, or to prevent acute dyspnea during an exacerbation (see later discussion). The goal of supplemental oxygen therapy in the patient with COPD is to increase the baseline resting partial pressure of arterial oxygen (PaO_2) to at least 60 mm Hg at sea level, which corresponds with an arterial oxygen saturation (SaO_2) of 90% (GOLD, 2019). Long-term oxygen therapy (more than 15 hours per day) has also been shown to improve quality of life, reduce pulmonary arterial pressure and dyspnea, and improve survival (GOLD, 2019). Long-term oxygen therapy is usually introduced in very severe COPD, and indications generally include a PaO_2 of 55 mm Hg or less or SaO_2 at or below 88% (GOLD, 2019). Other indications for long-term oxygen therapy include evidence of tissue hypoxia and organ damage such as cor pulmonale, secondary polycythemia, edema from right-sided heart failure, or impaired mental status (GOLD, 2019). For patients with exercise-induced hypoxemia, oxygen supplementation during exercise may improve dyspnea but will not diminish breathlessness in daily life (GOLD, 2019). Patients who are hypoxemic while awake are likely to be so during sleep. Therefore, nighttime oxygen therapy is recommended as well, and the prescription for oxygen therapy is for continuous, 24-hour use. Intermittent oxygen therapy is indicated for patients who **desaturate** (i.e., experience a precipitous drop in hemoglobin molecule saturation with oxygen) only during activities of daily living, exercise, or sleep.

The main objective in treating patients with hypoxemia and hypercapnia is to give sufficient oxygen to improve oxygenation. Patients with COPD who require oxygen may have respiratory failure that is caused primarily by a ventilation–perfusion mismatch. These patients respond to oxygen therapy and should be treated to keep the resting oxygen saturation at or above 90%, which is associated with a PaO_2 of 60 mm Hg or higher (GOLD, 2019). Nursing assessments of a patient with COPD on supplemental oxygen must include monitoring the respiratory rate and the oxygen saturation as measured by pulse oximetry (SpO_2) so that the patient has an adequate oxygen saturation (90%) on the lowest liter flow of oxygen (GOLD, 2019).

Administering too much oxygen can result in the retention of carbon dioxide. The high O_2 levels can then suppress

CO_2 chemoreceptors, which in turn would depress the respiratory drive and disrupt ventilation–perfusion balance (Kacmarek et al., 2017). The resulting increased O_2 tension in the alveoli causes a ventilation–perfusion mismatch that presents as hypercapnia. Monitoring and assessment are essential in the care of patients with COPD on supplemental oxygen due to complications of oxygen supplementation. Although pulse oximetry is helpful in assessing response to oxygen therapy, it does not assess $PaCO_2$ levels. A SaO_2 of 88% or less warrants further evaluation with arterial blood gas analysis (GOLD, 2019). The nurse must evaluate for other factors and medications which could further decrease the respiratory drive—neurologic impairment, fluid and electrolyte issues, and opioids or sedatives.

> **Quality and Safety Nursing Alert**
>
> Oxygen therapy is variable in patients with COPD; its aim in COPD is to achieve an acceptable oxygen level without a fall in the pH (increasing hypercapnia).

Pharmacologic Therapy

Medication regimens used to manage COPD are based on disease severity. For grade I (mild) COPD, a short-acting bronchodilator may be prescribed. For grade II or III (moderate or severe) COPD, a short-acting bronchodilator and regular treatment with one or more long-acting bronchodilators may be used. For grade III or IV (severe or very severe) COPD, medication therapy includes regular treatment with long-acting bronchodilators and/or inhaled corticosteroids (ICSs) for repeated exacerbations.

Bronchodilators

Bronchodilators are key for symptom management in stable COPD (GOLD, 2019). The choice of bronchodilator depends on availability and individual response in terms of symptom relief and side effects. Long-acting bronchodilators are more convenient for patients to use, and combining bronchodilators with different durations of action and different mechanisms may optimize symptom management (GOLD, 2019). Long-acting bronchodilators are typically used for maintenance treatment for long-term symptom control. Short-acting bronchodilators are usually used for acute management of symptomatic flairs. Even patients who do not show a significant response to a short-acting bronchodilator test may benefit symptomatically from long-term bronchodilator treatment.

Bronchodilators relieve bronchospasm by improving expiratory flow through widening of the airways and promoting lung emptying with each breath. These medications alter smooth muscle tone and reduce airway obstruction by allowing increased oxygen distribution throughout the lungs and improving alveolar ventilation. Although regular use of bronchodilators that act primarily on the airway smooth muscle does not modify the decline of function or the prognosis of COPD, their use is central in the management of COPD (GOLD, 2019). These agents can be delivered through a pressurized metered-dose inhaler (pMDI), a dry-powder inhaler (DPI), by a small-volume nebulizer (SVN), or via the oral route in pill or liquid form. Bronchodilators are often given regularly throughout the day as well as on an as-needed basis.

They may also be used prophylactically to prevent breathlessness by having the patient use them before participating in or completing an activity, such as eating or walking.

Several devices are available to deliver medication via the inhaled route. These may be categorized as pMDIs, DPIs, or SVNs, as noted previously (Cairo, 2018; Gregory, Elliott, & Dunne, 2013). The choice of an inhaler device will depend on availability, cost, prescribing provider, insurance coverage, and the skills and ability of the patient (GOLD, 2019). Key aspects of each are described in Table 20-3.

Both pMDIs and DPIs are small handheld devices that may be carried in a pocket or purse (Cairo, 2018; D'Urzo, Chapman, Donohue, et al., 2019). Attention to effective drug delivery and training in proper inhaler technique is essential when using a pMDI or DPI. A respiratory therapist is an excellent health care provider to consult on appropriate inhaler technique. **Pressurized metered-dose inhalers (pMDIs)** include conventional pMDIs or breath-actuated pMDIs; these may also feature spacer or valved-holding chambers (VHCs). They are pressurized devices that contain aerosolized powder of medications. A precise amount of medication is released with each activation of the pMDI canister. A spacer or VHC may also be indicated to enhance deposition of the medication in the lung and help the patient coordinate activation of the pMDI with inspiration. Spacers come in several designs, but all are attached to the pMDI and have a mouthpiece on the opposite end (Fig. 20-5).

All pMDIs are designed so that they require coordination between the patient's inspiration and the mechanics of the inhaler. In contrast, **dry-powder inhalers (DPIs)** (see Fig. 20-5) rely solely on the patient's inspiration for medication delivery. While DPIs still require the user to press a lever or button to dispense the medication, these inhalers do not require the coordination necessary to administer pMDIs.

Because of the significant relationship between poor inhaler technique and lack of symptom control, issues that could affect proper inhaler use must be considered when assessing the effectiveness of these medications (GOLD, 2019). Conditions such as decreased hand–inhalation coordination, insufficient hand strength, and the inability to generate a sufficient

TABLE 20-3	Aerosol Delivery Devices	
Devices/Drugs	**Optimal Technique**	**Therapeutic Issues**
Pressurized metered-dose inhaler (pMDI) Beta-2-adrenergic agonists Corticosteroids Anticholinergics	Actuation[a] during a slow (30 L/min or 3–5 s) deep inhalation, followed by 10-s breath-hold	Slow inhalation and coordination of actuation may be difficult for some patients. Patients may incorrectly stop inhalation at actuation. Deposition of 50–80% of actuated dose in the oropharynx. Mouth washing and spitting is effective in reducing the amount of drug swallowed and absorbed systemically
Breath-actuated pMDI Beta-2-adrenergic agonists	Tight seal around mouthpiece and slightly more rapid inhalation than standard pMDI (see above) followed by 10-s breath-hold	May be particularly useful for patients unable to coordinate inhalation and actuation. May also be useful for older patients. Patients may incorrectly stop inhalation at actuation. Cannot be used with currently available spacer/valved-holding chamber (VHC) devices
Spacer or VHC (*Note—this is an accessory to a pMDI*)	Slow (30 L/min or 3–5 s) deep inhalation, followed by 10-s breath-hold immediately following actuation. Actuate only once into spacer/VHC per inhalation. Rinse plastic VHCs once a month with low concentration of liquid household dishwashing detergent (1:5000 or 1–2 drops per cup of water) and let drip dry	Indicated for patients who have difficulty performing adequate pMDI technique. May be bulky. Simple tubes do not obviate coordinating actuation and inhalation. VHCs are preferred. Spacers or VHCs may increase delivery of inhalational corticosteroids to the lungs
Dry-powder inhaler (DPI) Beta-2-adrenergic agonists Corticosteroids Anticholinergics	Rapid (1–2 s) deep inhalation. Minimally effective inspiratory flow is device dependent	Dose is lost if patient exhales through device after actuating. Delivery may be greater or lesser than pMDIs, depending on device and technique. Delivery is more flow dependent in devices with highest internal resistance. Rapid inhalation promotes greater deposition in larger central airways. Mouth washing and spitting are effective in reducing amount of drug swallowed and absorbed systemically
Small-volume nebulizer (SVN) Beta-2-adrenergic agonists Corticosteroids Anticholinergics	Slow tidal breathing with occasional deep breaths. Tightly fitting facemask for those unable to use mouthpiece	Less dependent on patient's coordination and cooperation. May be expensive, time-consuming, and bulky; output depends on device and operating parameters (fill volume, driving gas flow); internebulizer and intranebulizer output variances are significant. The use of a facemask reduces delivery to lungs by 50%. Choice of delivery system depends on resources, availability, and clinical judgment of clinician caring for patient. There is potential for infections if device is not cleaned properly

[a]Actuation refers to release of dose of medication with inhalation.
Adapted from Cairo, J. M. (2018). *Mosby's respiratory care equipment* (10th ed.). St. Louis, MO: Elsevier Mosby.

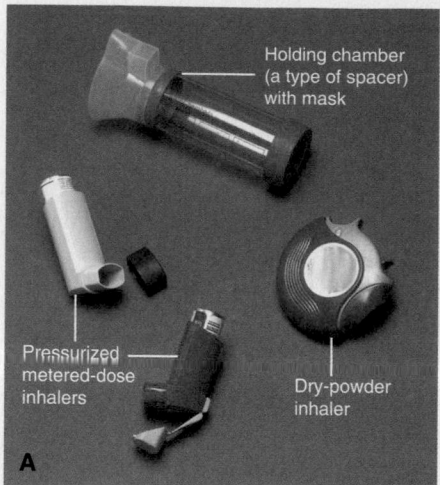

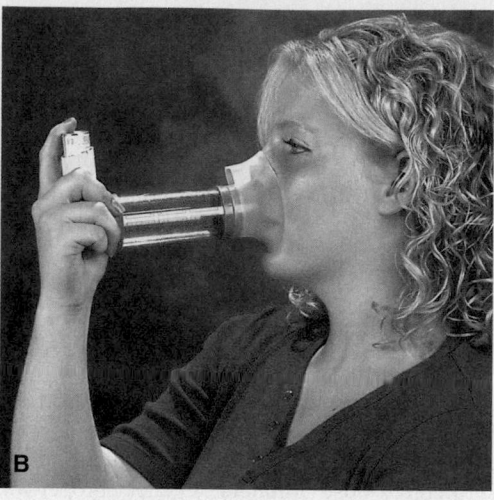

Figure 20-5 • **A.** Examples of pressurized metered dose inhalers (pMDIs) and spacers and a dry-powder inhaler (DPI). **B.** A pressurized metered-dose inhaler and spacer in use.

inspiratory flow could impair the delivery of the medication, and thus, impair symptom control (D'Urzo et al., 2019). For example, patients with decreased hand–inhalation coordination could fail to exhale prior to administering pMDIs, which would prevent them from inhaling the proper amount of the medication. While DPIs minimize the need for hand–inhalation coordination, patients with severe COPD may not have the ability to generate a sufficient inspiratory flow necessary to deliver the proper dose (D'Urzo et al., 2019).

The **small-volume nebulizer (SVN)** is a handheld apparatus that is easier to use than a pMDI or a DPI but lacks the convenience of these inhalers as it requires a power source in order to operate. Common SVNs include single-use pneumatic jet nebulizers with reservoir tubes, which are most commonly used in hospitals, and electronic nebulizers, which may be used in the home-based setting (Gregory et al., 2013). SVNs are commonly prescribed when patients are challenged with being able to administer their medications through either a pMDI or a DPI; some reasons why this might happen have been described previously (Cairo, 2018). The SVN may also be a preferred option to other inhalers because the nebulized particles in an SVN are smaller and can better penetrate the airways. Diaphragmatic breathing (see later discussion under "Breathing Retraining") is a helpful technique to prepare for proper use of the SVN.

Several classes of bronchodilators are used that include beta-adrenergic agonists, muscarinic antagonists (anticholinergics) and combination agents. Beta-adrenergic agonists include short-acting beta-2-adrenergic agonists (SABAs) and long-acting beta-2 adrenergic agonists (LABAs). The anticholinergic agents include short-acting muscarinic antagonists (SAMAs) and long-acting muscarinic antagonists (LAMAs) (GOLD, 2018; GOLD, 2019). ICSs may also be combined with bronchodilators. These medications may be used in combination to optimize bronchodilation. LABA bronchodilators are more convenient for patient use as compared to short-acting beta$_2$-agonist bronchodilators. Examples of these medications are described in Table 20-4.

Fixed dose combinations of LABAs and LAMAs have become the foundation for treating COPD (D'Urzo et al., 2019). Combining these classes of medications in one inhaler has synergistic effects, so that the dosages of each medication may be lesser than if they were each administered separately

(i.e., as monotherapy), without diminishing their effectiveness (GOLD, 2019). Furthermore, combination therapy is associated with less adverse reactions and promotes proper medication administration by avoiding the use of multiple inhaler devices (GOLD, 2019).

Corticosteroids

Although inhaled and systemic corticosteroids may improve the symptoms of COPD, they do not slow the decline in lung function. A short trial course of oral corticosteroids may be prescribed for patients to determine whether pulmonary function improves and symptoms decrease. Long-term treatment with oral corticosteroids is not recommended in COPD and can cause steroid myopathy, leading to muscle weakness, decreased ability to function, and, in advanced disease, respiratory failure (GOLD, 2019). ICSs are frequently prescribed in COPD.

Treatment of COPD with combination long-term beta$_2$-agonists plus corticosteroids in one inhaler may improve lung function (GOLD, 2018). Examples of these medications include formoterol/budesonide, vilanterol/fluticasone furoate, and salmeterol/fluticasone.

Other Medications

Other pharmacologic treatments that may be used in COPD include alpha$_1$-antitrypsin augmentation therapy, antibiotic agents, mucolytic agents, antitussive agents, vasodilators, and opioids. Vaccines are also effective in that they prevent exacerbations by thwarting respiratory infections. For instance, influenza vaccines can reduce serious illness and death in patients with COPD (GOLD, 2019). It is recommended that people limit their risk through influenza vaccination and smoking cessation. Pneumococcal vaccination also reduces the incidence of community-acquired pneumonia in the general older adult population (GOLD, 2019).

Management of Exacerbations

An exacerbation of COPD is defined as an event in the natural course of the disease characterized by acute changes (worsening) in the patient's respiratory symptoms beyond the normal day-to-day variations. An exacerbation also leads to change in medication (GOLD, 2019). During an exacerbation, there is increased dyspnea that is a result of amplified hyperinflation and air trapping (GOLD, 2019). Primary causes of an acute

TABLE 20-4 Common Types of Bronchodilator Medications for Chronic Obstructive Pulmonary Disease

Class/Drug	Method of Administration			Duration of Action[b]
	Inhaler[a]	Nebulizer	Oral	
Beta-2–Adrenergic Agonist Agents				
albuterol	X	X	X	SABA
levalbuterol	X	X		SABA
terbutaline	X			SABA
arformoterol	X			LABA
formoterol	X			LABA
salmeterol	X			LABA
indacaterol	X			LABA
olodaterol	X			LABA
Anticholinergic Agents				
ipratropium bromide	X	X		SAMA
tiotropium bromide	X			LAMA
umeclidinium	X			LAMA
Combination Short-Acting Beta-2–Adrenergic Agonist and Anticholinergic Agent				
salbutamol/ipratropium	X			SABA/SAMA
Inhaled Corticosteroids (ICSs)				
beclomethasone dipropionate	X	X		
budesonide	X	X		
fluticasone propionate	X	X		
Combination Inhaled Corticosteroids and Long-Acting Beta-2–Adrenergic Agonist				
budesonide/formoterol	X			ICS/LABA
mometasone/formoterol	X			ICS/LABA
fluticasone/salmeterol	X			ICS/LABA
fluticasone furoate/vilanterol	X			ICS/LABA

[a]Inhaler may include pressurized metered-dose inhaler (pMDI) or dry-powder inhaler (DPI).
[b]Short acting, 4–6 h; long acting, 12+ h.
ICS, inhaled corticosteroid; LABA, long-acting beta-2 adrenergic agonist; LAMA, long-acting muscarinic antagonist; SABA, short-acting beta-2 adrenergic agonist; SAMA, short-acting muscarinic antagonist.
Adapted from Global Initiative for Chronic Obstructive Lung Disease (GOLD). (2019). Global strategy for the diagnosis, management, and prevention of chronic obstructive pulmonary disease. Retrieved on 6/23/2019 at: www.goldcopd.org/wp-content/uploads/2018/11/GOLD-2019-v1.7-FINAL-14Nov2018-WMS.pdf

exacerbation are usually related to viral infections, particularly human rhinovirus (i.e., the common cold). However, bacterial infections and environmental factors have also been linked to the development of acute exacerbations (GOLD, 2019). Roflumilast may be used as a treatment to reduce the risk of exacerbations in patients with severe COPD associated with chronic bronchitis and a history of exacerbations. Roflumilast is a selective phosphodiesterase-4 (PDE4) inhibitor and is taken as a tablet once daily.

Treatment of an exacerbation requires identifying the primary cause (if possible) and administering the specific treatment. Optimization of bronchodilator medications is first-line therapy and involves identifying the best medication or combinations of medications taken on a regular schedule for a specific patient. Depending on the signs and symptoms, corticosteroids, antibiotic agents, oxygen therapy, and intensive respiratory interventions may also be used. The GOLD (2019) guidelines provide indications for assessment, hospital admission, and possible critical-care admission for patients with exacerbations of COPD. Indications for hospitalization include marked increase in intensity of symptoms, severe underlying COPD, onset of new physical signs (e.g., the use of accessory muscles, paradoxical chest wall movement, worsening or new onset of central cyanosis, peripheral edema, signs of right heart failure, reduced alertness), failure to respond to initial medical management, older age, and insufficient home support. Patients requiring hospitalization for

an exacerbation would exhibit severe dyspnea that does not respond adequately to initial therapy, confusion or lethargy, respiratory muscle fatigue, paradoxical chest wall movement, peripheral edema, worsening or new onset of central cyanosis, persistent or worsening hypoxemia, and the need for noninvasive or invasive assisted mechanical ventilation (GOLD, 2019). The outcome from an exacerbation of COPD is closely related to the development of respiratory acidosis, the presence of significant comorbidities, and the need for noninvasive or invasive positive pressure ventilatory support.

When the patient with an exacerbation of COPD arrives in an ED, the first line of treatment is supplemental oxygen therapy and rapid assessment to determine if the exacerbation is life-threatening (GOLD, 2019). A short-acting inhaled bronchodilator may be used to assess response to treatment. Oral or intravenous (IV) corticosteroids, in addition to bronchodilators, are recommended in the hospital management of a COPD exacerbation. The administration of antibiotics remains controversial, but in general, they should be administered when the patient has three cardinal symptoms of an exacerbation: increase in dyspnea, increase in sputum volume, and sputum purulence (GOLD, 2019).

Surgical Management

Surgical options might be appropriate for patients who do not demonstrate symptom improvement with nonsurgical therapies.

Bullectomy

A bullectomy is a surgical option for select patients with bullous emphysema. Bullae are enlarged airspaces that do not contribute to ventilation but occupy space in the thorax; these areas may be surgically excised. These bullae compress areas of the lung and may impair gas exchange. Bullectomy may help reduce dyspnea and improve lung function. It can be performed via a video-assisted thoracoscope or a limited thoracotomy incision (GOLD, 2019).

Lung Volume Reduction Surgery

Treatment options for patients with advanced or end-stage COPD (grade IV) with a primary emphysematous component are limited, although lung volume reduction surgery is a palliative surgical option. This includes patients with homogenous disease or disease that is focused in one area and not widespread throughout the lungs. Lung volume reduction surgery involves the removal of a portion of the diseased lung parenchyma. This reduces hyperinflation and allows the functional tissue to expand, resulting in improved elastic recoil of the lung and improved chest wall and diaphragmatic mechanics. This type of surgery does not cure the disease but may improve health status, exercise tolerance, and the patient's overall quality of life (GOLD, 2019).

Bronchoscopic lung volume reduction therapies are under investigation in clinical research protocols. These bronchoscopic procedures were developed to collapse areas of emphysematous lung and thus improve aeration of the functional lung tissue. Techniques include endobronchial placement of a one-way valve that allows air and mucus to exit the treated area but does not allow air to reenter. Another technique achieves biologic lung volume reduction through bronchoscopic instillation of nitinol coils into the airway of the hyperinflated lung tissue of patients with advanced emphysema. Because air can no longer enter the airway, the lung tissue beyond the sealed airway collapses over time. Patients receiving this procedure reported increased quality of life. However, there is insufficient evidence to determine the benefit–risk ratios, cost-effectiveness, and possible roles of these procedures in care of the patient with severe emphysema (GOLD, 2019).

Lung Transplantation

Lung transplantation is a viable option for definitive surgical treatment of severe COPD in select patients. It has been shown to improve quality of life and functional capacity in some patients with COPD. Limited not only by the shortage of donor organs, it is also a costly procedure with financial implications for months to years because of complications and the need for costly immunosuppressive medication regimens (GOLD, 2019).

Pulmonary Rehabilitation

Pulmonary rehabilitation, one of the most cost-effective treatment strategies, is a holistic intervention aimed at improving physical and psychological health of patients with COPD (GOLD, 2019). The primary goals of rehabilitation are to reduce symptoms, improve quality of life, and increase physical and emotional participation in everyday activities (GOLD, 2019). The benefits of this therapy include improvement of exercise capacity, reduction in the perceived intensity of breathlessness, improvement in health-related quality of life, reduction in the number of hospitalizations and days in the hospital, and reduction in the anxiety and depression associated with COPD (GOLD, 2019). Pulmonary rehabilitation services are multidisciplinary and include assessment, education, smoking cessation, physical reconditioning, nutritional counseling, skills training, and psychological support. Patients are taught methods to alleviate symptoms. Breathing exercises, as well as retraining and exercise programs, are used to improve functional status.

Pulmonary rehabilitation is appropriate for most patients with COPD, particularly those with moderate or severe COPD (GOLD, 2019). Optimum benefits are achieved in programs that are 6 to 8 weeks in length (GOLD, 2019). Programs vary in duration and may be conducted in inpatient, outpatient, or home settings. Program selection depends on the patient's physical, functional, and psychosocial status; insurance coverage; availability of programs; and preference. Pulmonary rehabilitation may also be used therapeutically in other disorders besides COPD, including asthma, CF, lung cancer, interstitial lung disease, thoracic surgery, and lung transplantation. Despite their proven efficacy, comprehensive programs for patients with moderate to severe COPD are covered by Medicare only for those who meet specific criteria.

 Patient Education

Nurses play a key role in identifying potential candidates for pulmonary rehabilitation and in facilitating and reinforcing the material learned in the rehabilitation program. Not all patients have access to a formal rehabilitation program. However, nurses can be instrumental in educating patients and families as well as facilitating specific services, such as respiratory therapy education, physical therapy for exercise and breathing retraining, occupational therapy for conserving energy during activities of daily living, and nutritional counseling. Patient education is a major component of pulmonary rehabilitation and includes a broad variety of topics. (See Chart 20-3, Nursing Research Profile: Managing Anxiety among Patients with Advanced COPD.)

Depending on the length and setting of the educational program, topics may include normal anatomy and physiology of the lung, pathophysiology and changes with COPD, medications and home oxygen therapy, nutrition, respiratory therapy treatments, symptom alleviation, smoking cessation, sexuality and COPD, coping with chronic disease, communicating with the health care team, and planning for the future (advance directives, living wills, informed decision making about health care alternatives). Education, including that relating to smoking cessation, should be incorporated into all aspects of care for COPD and in many settings (primary providers' offices, clinics, hospitals, home and community health care settings, and comprehensive rehabilitation programs).

Nutritional Therapy

Nutritional assessment and counseling are important for patients with COPD. Nutritional status is reflected in severity of symptoms, degree of disability, and prognosis. Significant weight loss is often a major problem; however, excessive weight can also be problematic, although it occurs less often. Most patients with COPD have difficulty gaining and maintaining weight. A thorough assessment of caloric needs and

Chart 20-3

NURSING RESEARCH PROFILE

Managing Anxiety among Patients with Advanced COPD

Bove, D. G., Midtgaard, G., Kaldan, D., et al. (2017). Home-based COPD psychoeducation: A qualitative study of the patients' experiences. *Journal of Psychosomatic Research, 98*, 71–77.

Purpose

This study was a nested posttrial qualitative study conducted in the context of a randomized controlled trial (RCT), *Efficacy of a Minimal Home-Based Psychoeducative Intervention in Patients with Advanced COPD*. Quantitative results from the RCT found that the nurse-led home-based intervention significantly reduced anxiety and increased mastery of dyspneic symptoms in patients with advanced COPD. The purpose of this qualitative study was to explore whether patients with advanced COPD who received this intervention found the intervention meaningful and applicable to their everyday lives.

Design

This qualitative study utilized the Interpretive Description methodology and collected data from 20 participants enrolled in the RCT. The participants accepted an invitation for the qualitative interview and signed informed consent to participate in the study. With one exception, all participants were interviewed at home. Interviews were conducted by researchers who did not previously meet the participants. All interviews were recorded and transcribed for data analysis.

Findings

Transcribed interviews revealed three main themes: (1) Making anxiety visible makes it manageable and provides relief; (2) Anxiety management is about getting control of cognitions; and (3) Being alone with anxiety and dyspnea. The first theme centered on recognition of anxiety as an aspect of COPD; nonetheless, participants expressed difficulty in talking about anxiety with relatives. Some participants felt that their spouses were annoyed when they talked about anxiety and dyspnea. They validated the usefulness of patient education materials that gave legitimacy to the problems they struggled with on a daily basis. The second theme focused on anxiety management and revealed that participants believed they had to deal with their anxiety privately. The behavioral cognitive intervention gave them the freedom to verbalize their thoughts and worries, especially thoughts of death and the dying process. The third theme revolved around feelings of isolation associated with anxiety and dyspnea. Participants verbalized that the psychoeducation intervention helped them establish a sense of control and self-preservation despite feeling alone during acute episodes.

Nursing Implications

This study validated that the nurse-led psychoeducation intervention that decreased anxiety and improved dyspneic symptoms among patients with advanced COPD also had the favorable effect of being perceived as meaningful and helpful to these participants. Participants in this study felt better equipped to manage their anxiety and dyspnea after having received the intervention, and found it valuable. They expressed relief that the intervention was focused upon their anxieties. These findings illustrate the importance of acknowledging and assessing anxiety during dyspneic episodes among patients with COPD. Legitimizing the anxiety experienced by patients with advanced COPD can establish a solid foundation for providing education to them and their spouses on the disease process and help them understand what to expect as the disease progresses. Increasing their knowledge on COPD and disease management will help them feel a sense of control that in turn could help diminish feelings of anxiety. Moreover, including family members in patient education could diminish feelings of isolation, which in turn will help decrease anxiety and ultimately improve disease management.

---

counseling about meal planning and supplementation is part of the rehabilitation process. Continual monitoring of weight and interventions as necessary are important parts of the care of patients with COPD.

Palliative Care

Palliative care is integral for the patient with advanced COPD. Unfortunately, palliative care is often not considered until the disease is far advanced. The overall goals of palliative care are to manage symptoms and improve the quality of life for patients and families with advanced disease (GOLD, 2019). Areas addressed in palliative care include effective and empathetic communication with patients and families; close attention to pain, dyspnea, panic, anxiety, depression and other symptoms; psychosocial, spiritual and bereavement support; and coordination of the wide range of medical and social services required with this disease (GOLD, 2019). Palliative, hospice care, and end-of-life care are fundamental components of treatment for patients with advanced COPD (GOLD, 2019) (see Chapter 13).

Nursing Management

An overview of the nursing care of the patient with COPD is provided in Chart 20-4. Additional nursing considerations with regard to assessing the patient with COPD and promoting optimal nursing and collaborative outcomes are specified as follows.

Assessing the Patient

Assessment involves obtaining information about current symptoms as well as previous disease manifestations. See Chart 20-2 for sample questions that may be used to obtain a clear history of the disease process. In addition to the history, the nurse reviews the results of diagnostic tests.

Achieving Airway Clearance

Bronchospasm, which occurs in many pulmonary diseases, reduces the caliber of the small bronchi and may cause dyspnea, static secretions, and infection. Bronchospasm can sometimes be detected on auscultation with a stethoscope when wheezing or diminished breath sounds are heard. Increased mucus production, along with decreased mucociliary action, contributes to further reduction in the caliber of the bronchi and results in decreased airflow and decreased gas exchange. This is further aggravated by the loss of lung elasticity that occurs with COPD (GOLD, 2019). These changes in the airway require that the nurse monitor the patient for dyspnea and hypoxemia. The relief

(text continued on page 624)

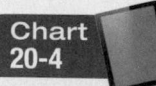

PLAN OF NURSING CARE
Chart 20-4
Care of the Patient with Chronic Obstructive Pulmonary Disease

NURSING DIAGNOSIS: Impaired gas exchange and impaired airway clearance due to chronic inhalation of toxins
GOAL: Improvement in gas exchange

Nursing Interventions	Rationale	Expected Outcomes

1. Evaluate current smoking status, educate regarding smoking cessation, and facilitate efforts to quit.
  a. Evaluate current smoking habits of patient and family.
  b. Educate regarding hazards of smoking and relationship to COPD.
  c. Evaluate previous smoking cessation attempts.
  d. Provide educational materials.
  e. Refer to a smoking cessation program or resource.
2. Evaluate current exposure to occupational toxins or pollutants and indoor/outdoor pollution.
  a. Emphasize primary prevention to occupational exposures. This is best achieved by elimination or reduction in exposures in the workplace.
  b. Educate regarding types of indoor and outdoor air pollution (e.g., biomass fuel burned for cooking and heating in poorly ventilated buildings, outdoor air pollution).
  c. Advise patient to monitor public announcements regarding air quality.
	1. Smoking causes permanent damage to the lungs and diminishes the lungs' protective mechanisms. Airflow is obstructed, secretions are increased, and lung capacity is reduced. Continued smoking increases morbidity and mortality in COPD and is also a risk factor for lung cancer.
	
	2. Chronic inhalation of both indoor and outdoor toxins causes damage to the airways and impairs gas exchange.
		• Identifies the hazards of cigarette smoking
		• Identifies resources for smoking cessation, if appropriate
		• Enrolls in smoking cessation program, if appropriate
		• Reports success in stopping smoking
		• Verbalizes types of inhaled toxins
		• Minimizes or eliminates exposures
		• Monitors public announcements regarding air quality and minimizes or eliminates exposures during episodes of severe pollution

NURSING DIAGNOSIS: Impaired gas exchange associated with ventilation–perfusion inequality
GOAL: Improvement in gas exchange

Nursing Interventions	Rationale	Expected Outcomes

1. Administer bronchodilators as prescribed.
  a. Inhalation is the preferred route.
  b. Observe for side effects: tachycardia, arrhythmias, central nervous system excitation, nausea, and vomiting.
  c. Assess for correct technique of pressurized metered-dose inhaler (pMDI), dry-powder inhaler (DPI), or small-volume nebulizer (SVN) administration.
2. Evaluate effectiveness of pMDI, DPI, or SVN treatments.
  a. Assess for decreased shortness of breath, decreased wheezing or crackles, loosened secretions, and decreased anxiety.
  b. Ensure that treatment is given before meals to avoid nausea and to reduce fatigue that accompanies eating.
3. Instruct and encourage patient in diaphragmatic breathing and effective coughing.
	1. Bronchodilators dilate the airways. The medication dosage is carefully adjusted for each patient, in accordance with clinical response.
	
	2. Combining medication with aerosolized bronchodilators is typically used to control bronchoconstriction in an acute exacerbation. Generally, however, the pMDI with spacer is the preferred route (less cost and time to treatment).
	
	3. These techniques improve ventilation by opening airways to facilitate clearing the airways of sputum. Gas exchange is improved, and fatigue is minimized.
		• Verbalizes need for bronchodilators and for taking them as prescribed
		• Evidences minimal side effects; heart rate near normal, absence of arrhythmias, normal mentation
		• Reports a decrease in dyspnea
		• Shows an improved expiratory flow rate
		• Uses and cleans respiratory therapy equipment as applicable
		• Demonstrates diaphragmatic breathing and coughing
		• Uses oxygen equipment appropriately when indicated
		• Evidences improved arterial blood gases or pulse oximetry
		• Demonstrates correct technique for use of pMDI, DPI, or SVN

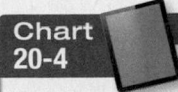

Chart 20-4

PLAN OF NURSING CARE (continued)
Care of the Patient with Chronic Obstructive Pulmonary Disease

Nursing Interventions	Rationale	Expected Outcomes
4. Administer oxygen by the method prescribed. a. Explain rationale and importance to patient. b. Evaluate effectiveness; observe for signs of hypoxemia. Notify primary provider if restlessness, anxiety, somnolence, cyanosis, or tachycardia is present. c. Analyze arterial blood gases and compare with baseline values. When arterial puncture is performed and a blood sample is obtained, hold puncture site for 5 minutes to prevent arterial bleeding and development of ecchymoses. d. Initiate pulse oximetry to monitor oxygen saturation. e. Explain that no smoking is permitted by patient or visitors while oxygen is in use.	4. Oxygen will correct the hypoxemia. Careful observation of the liter flow or the percentage given and its effect on the patient is important. These patients generally require low-flow oxygen rates of 1–2 L/min. Monitor and titrate to achieve desired PaO_2. Periodic arterial blood gases and pulse oximetry help evaluate adequacy of oxygenation. Smoking may render pulse oximetry inaccurate because the carbon monoxide from cigarette smoke also saturates hemoglobin.	

NURSING DIAGNOSIS: Impaired airway clearance associated with bronchoconstriction, increased mucus production, ineffective cough, bronchopulmonary infection, and other complications
GOAL: Achievement of airway clearance

Nursing Interventions	Rationale	Expected Outcomes
1. Adequately hydrate the patient. 2. Instruct in and encourage the use of diaphragmatic breathing and coughing techniques. 3. Assist in administering pMDI, DPI, or SVN. 4. If indicated, perform postural drainage with percussion and vibration in the morning and at night as prescribed. 5. Instruct patient to avoid bronchial irritants such as cigarette smoke, aerosols, extremes of temperature, and fumes. 6. Educate about early signs of infection that are to be reported to the primary provider immediately: a. Increased sputum production b. Change in color of sputum c. Increased thickness of sputum d. Increased shortness of breath, tightness in chest, or fatigue e. Increased coughing f. Fever or chills 7. Administer antibiotics as prescribed. 8. Encourage patient to be immunized against influenza and *Streptococcus pneumoniae*.	1. Systemic hydration keeps secretions moist and easier to expectorate. Fluids must be given with caution if right- or left-sided heart failure is present. 2. These techniques help to improve ventilation and mobilize secretions without causing breathlessness and fatigue. 3. This ensures adequate delivery of medication to the airways. 4. This uses gravity to help raise secretions so they can be more easily expectorated or suctioned. 5. Bronchial irritants cause bronchoconstriction and increased mucus production, which then interfere with airway clearance. 6. Minor respiratory infections that are of no consequence to the person with normal lungs can produce fatal disturbances in the lungs of the person with COPD. Early recognition is crucial. 7. Antibiotics may be prescribed to prevent or treat infection. 8. Patients with respiratory conditions are prone to respiratory infections and are encouraged to be immunized.	• Verbalizes need to drink fluids • Demonstrates diaphragmatic breathing and coughing • Performs postural drainage correctly • Coughing is minimized • Does not smoke • Verbalizes that pollens, fumes, gases, dusts, and extremes of temperature and humidity are irritants to be avoided • Identifies signs of early infection • Is free of infection (no fever, no change in sputum, lessening of dyspnea) • Verbalizes need to notify primary provider at the earliest sign of infection • Verbalizes need to stay away from crowds or people with colds in flu season • Discusses flu and pneumonia vaccines with clinician to help prevent infection

(continued on page 622)

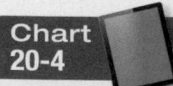

Chart 20-4

PLAN OF NURSING CARE (continued)

Care of the Patient with Chronic Obstructive Pulmonary Disease

NURSING DIAGNOSIS: Impaired breathing associated with shortness of breath, mucus, bronchoconstriction, and airway irritants

GOAL: Improvement in breathing pattern

Nursing Interventions	Rationale	Expected Outcomes
1. Instruct patient in diaphragmatic and pursed-lip breathing.	1. This helps patient prolong expiration time and decreases air trapping. With these techniques, patient will breathe more efficiently and effectively.	• Practices pursed-lip and diaphragmatic breathing and uses them when short of breath and with activity • Shows signs of decreased respiratory effort and paces activities
2. Encourage alternating activity with rest periods. Encourage patient to make some decisions (bath, shaving) about care based on tolerance level.	2. Pacing activities permits patient to perform activities without excessive distress.	• Uses inspiratory muscle trainer as prescribed
3. Encourage the use of an inspiratory muscle trainer if prescribed.	3. This strengthens and conditions the respiratory muscles.	

NURSING DIAGNOSIS: Impaired ability to manage regime associated with fatigue secondary to increased work of breathing and insufficient ventilation and oxygenation

GOAL: Independence in health management activities

Nursing Interventions	Rationale	Expected Outcomes
1. Educate patient to coordinate diaphragmatic breathing with activity (e.g., walking, bending).	1. This will encourage the patient to be more active and to avoid excessive fatigue or dyspnea during activity.	• Uses controlled breathing while bathing, bending, and walking • Paces activities of daily living to alternate with rest periods to reduce fatigue and dyspnea
2. Encourage patient to begin to bathe self, dress self, walk, and drink fluids. Discuss energy conservation measures.	2. As condition resolves, patient will be able to do more but needs to be encouraged to avoid increasing dependence.	• Describes energy conservation strategies • Performs same self-care activities as before
3. Educate patient about postural drainage if appropriate.	3. This encourages patient to become involved in own care and prepares patient to manage at home.	• Performs postural drainage correctly

NURSING DIAGNOSIS: Activity intolerance due to fatigue, hypoxemia, and impaired breathing

GOAL: Improvement in activity tolerance

Nursing Interventions	Rationale	Expected Outcomes
1. Support patient in establishing a regular regimen of exercise using treadmill and exercise bicycle, walking, or other appropriate exercises, such as mall walking. a. Assess the patient's current level of functioning, and develop exercise plan based on baseline functional status. b. Suggest consultation with a physical therapist or pulmonary rehabilitation program to determine an exercise program specific to the patient's capability. Have portable oxygen unit available if oxygen is prescribed for exercise.	1. Muscles that are deconditioned consume more oxygen and place an additional burden on the lungs. Through regular, graded exercise, these muscle groups become more conditioned, and the patient can do more without getting as short of breath. Graded exercise breaks the cycle of debilitation.	• Performs activities with less shortness of breath • Verbalizes need to exercise daily and demonstrates an exercise plan to be carried out at home • Walks and gradually increases walking time and distance to improve physical condition • Exercises both upper and lower body muscle groups

NURSING DIAGNOSIS: Difficulty coping associated with reduced socialization, anxiety, depression, lower activity level, and the inability to work

GOAL: Attainment of an optimal level of coping

Nursing Interventions	Rationale	Expected Outcomes
1. Help the patient develop realistic goals.	1. Developing realistic goals will promote a sense of hope and accomplishment rather than defeat and hopelessness.	• Expresses interest in the future • Participates in the discharge plan • Discusses activities or methods that can be performed to ease shortness of breath
2. Encourage activity to level of symptom tolerance.	2. Activity reduces tension and decreases degree of dyspnea as patient becomes conditioned.	• Uses relaxation techniques appropriately • Expresses interest in a pulmonary rehabilitation program

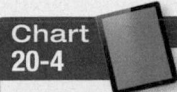

Chart 20-4

PLAN OF NURSING CARE (continued)

Care of the Patient with Chronic Obstructive Pulmonary Disease

Nursing Interventions	Rationale	Expected Outcomes
3. Educate the patient about relaxation techniques or provide a relaxation recording on audiotape, CD, or digital audio available on smartphones or tablets. 4. Enroll patient in pulmonary rehabilitation program where available.	3. Relaxation reduces stress, anxiety, and dyspnea and helps patient to cope with disability. 4. Pulmonary rehabilitation programs have been shown to promote a subjective improvement in a patient's status and self-esteem as well as increased exercise tolerance and decreased hospitalizations.	

NURSING DIAGNOSIS: Lack of knowledge about self-management to be performed at home
GOAL: Adherence to therapeutic program and home care

Nursing Interventions	Rationale	Expected Outcomes

1. Help patient identify/develop short- and long-term goals.
  a. Educate the patient about disease, medications, procedures, and how and when to seek help.
  b. Refer patient to pulmonary rehabilitation.
2. Give strong message to stop smoking. Discuss smoking cessation strategies. Provide information about resource groups (e.g., SmokEnders, American Cancer Society, American Lung Association).
	1. Patient needs to be a partner in developing the plan of care and needs to know what to expect. Education about COPD is one of the most important aspects of care; it will prepare the patient to live and cope with the COPD and improve quality of life.
	2. Smoking causes permanent damage to the lung and diminishes the lungs' protective mechanisms. Airflow is obstructed, and lung capacity is reduced. Smoking increases morbidity and mortality and is also a risk factor for lung cancer.
		• Understands disease and what affects it
		• Verbalizes the need to preserve existing lung function by adhering to the prescribed program
		• Understands purposes and proper administration of medications
		• Stops smoking or enrolls in a smoking cessation program
		• Identifies when and whom to call for assistance

COLLABORATIVE PROBLEM: Atelectasis
GOAL: Absence of atelectasis on x-ray and physical examination

Nursing Interventions	Rationale	Expected Outcomes
1. Monitor respiratory status, including rate and pattern of respirations, breath sounds, signs and symptoms of respiratory distress, and pulse oximetry. 2. Instruct in and encourage diaphragmatic breathing and effective coughing techniques. 3. Promote the use of lung expansion techniques (e.g., deep breathing exercises, incentive spirometry) as prescribed.	1. A change in respiratory status, including tachypnea, dyspnea, and diminished or absent breath sounds, may indicate atelectasis. 2. These techniques improve ventilation and lung expansion and ideally improve gas exchange. 3. Deep breathing exercises and incentive spirometry promote maximal lung expansion.	• Normal (baseline for patient) respiratory rate and pattern • Normal breath sounds for patient • Demonstrates diaphragmatic breathing and effective coughing • Performs deep breathing exercises, incentive spirometry as prescribed • Pulse oximetry ≥90%

COLLABORATIVE PROBLEM: Pneumothorax
GOAL: Absence of signs and symptoms of pneumothorax

Nursing Interventions	Rationale	Expected Outcomes
1. Monitor respiratory status, including rate and pattern of respirations, symmetry of chest wall movement, breath sounds, signs and symptoms of respiratory distress, and pulse oximetry. 2. Assess pulse. 3. Assess for chest pain and precipitating factors. 4. Palpate for tracheal deviation/shift away from the affected side.	1. Dyspnea, tachypnea, tachycardia, acute pleuritic chest pain, tracheal deviation away from the affected side, absence of breath sounds on the affected side, and decreased tactile fremitus may indicate pneumothorax. 2. Tachycardia is associated with pneumothorax and anxiety. 3. Pain may accompany pneumothorax. 4. Early detection of pneumothorax and prompt intervention will prevent other serious complications.	• Normal respiratory rate and pattern for patient • Normal breath sounds bilaterally • Normal pulse for patient • Normal tactile fremitus • Absence of pain • Tracheal position is midline • Pulse oximetry ≥90% • Maintains normal oxygen saturation and arterial blood gas measurements • Exhibits no hypoxemia and hypercapnia (or returns to baseline values) • Absence of pain

(continued on page 624)

Chart 20-4

PLAN OF NURSING CARE (continued)

Care of the Patient with Chronic Obstructive Pulmonary Disease

Nursing Interventions	Rationale	Expected Outcomes
5. Monitor pulse oximetry and, if indicated, arterial blood gases.	5. Recognition of deterioration in respiratory function will prevent serious complications.	• Symmetric chest wall movement • Lungs fully expanded bilaterally on chest x-ray
6. Administer supplemental oxygen therapy, as indicated.	6. Oxygen will correct hypoxemia; administer it with caution.	
7. Administer analgesic agents, as indicated, for chest pain.	7. Pain interferes with deep breathing, resulting in decreased lung expansion.	
8. Assist with chest tube insertion and use pleural drainage system, as prescribed.	8. Removal of air from the pleural space will re-expand the lung.	

COLLABORATIVE PROBLEM: Respiratory failure

GOAL: Absence of signs and symptoms of respiratory failure; no evidence of respiratory failure on laboratory tests

Nursing Interventions	Rationale	Expected Outcomes
1. Monitor respiratory status, including rate and pattern of respirations, breath sounds, and signs and symptoms of acute respiratory distress.	1. Early recognition of deterioration in respiratory function will avert further complications, such as respiratory failure, severe hypoxemia, and hypercapnia.	• Normal respiratory rate and pattern for patient with no acute distress • Recognizes symptoms of hypoxemia and hypercapnia • Maintains normal arterial blood gases/pulse oximetry or returns to baseline values
2. Monitor pulse oximetry and arterial blood gases.	2. Recognition of changes in oxygenation and acid–base balance will guide in correcting and preventing complications.	
3. Administer supplemental oxygen and initiate mechanisms for mechanical ventilation, as prescribed.	3. Acute respiratory failure is a medical emergency. Hypoxemia is a hallmark sign. Administration of oxygen therapy and mechanical ventilation (if indicated) are critical to survival.	

COLLABORATIVE PROBLEM: Pulmonary arterial hypertension

GOAL: Absence of evidence of pulmonary arterial hypertension on physical examination or laboratory tests

Nursing Interventions	Rationale	Expected Outcomes
1. Monitor respiratory status, including rate and pattern of respirations, breath sounds, pulse oximetry, and signs and symptoms of acute respiratory distress.	1. Dyspnea is the primary symptom of pulmonary arterial hypertension. Other symptoms include fatigue, angina, near-syncope, edema, and palpitations.	• Normal respiratory rate and pattern for patient • Exhibits no signs and symptoms of right-sided failure • Maintains baseline pulse oximetry values and arterial blood gases
2. Assess for signs and symptoms of right-sided heart failure, including peripheral edema, ascites, distended neck veins, crackles, and heart murmur.	2. Right-sided heart failure is a common clinical manifestation of pulmonary arterial hypertension due to increased right ventricular workload.	
3. Administer oxygen therapy, as prescribed.	3. Continuous oxygen therapy is a major component of management of pulmonary arterial hypertension; it prevents hypoxemia, thereby reducing pulmonary vascular constriction (resistance) secondary to hypoxemia.	

of bronchospasm is confirmed by measuring improvement in expiratory flow rates and volumes (the force of expiration, how long it takes to exhale, and the amount of air exhaled) as well as by assessing the dyspnea and making sure that it has lessened.

Diminishing the quantity and viscosity of sputum can clear the airway and improve pulmonary ventilation and gas exchange. All pulmonary irritants should be eliminated or reduced, particularly cigarette smoke, which is the most persistent source of pulmonary irritation. The nurse instructs the patient in directed or controlled coughing, which is more effective and reduces the fatigue associated with undirected forceful coughing. Directed coughing consists of a slow,

maximal inspiration followed by breath-holding for several seconds and then two or three coughs. "Huff" coughing may also be effective. The technique consists of one or two forced exhalations (huffs) from low to medium lung volumes with the glottis open.

Chest physiotherapy (CPT), increased fluid intake, and bland aerosol mists (with normal saline solution or water) may be useful for some patients with COPD. The use of these measures must be based on the response and tolerance of each patient. **Chest physiotherapy (CPT)** includes postural drainage, chest percussion and vibration, and breathing retraining. The goals of CPT are consistent with improved airway clearance as they are to remove bronchial secretions, improve ventilation, and increase the efficiency of the respiratory muscles.

Postural Drainage (Segmented Bronchial Drainage)

Postural drainage allows the force of gravity to assist in the removal of bronchial secretions. The secretions drain from

the affected bronchioles into the bronchi and trachea and are removed by coughing or suctioning. Because the patient usually sits in an upright position, secretions are likely to accumulate in the lower parts of the lungs. Several other positions (Fig. 20-6) are used so that the force of gravity helps move secretions from the smaller bronchial airways to the main

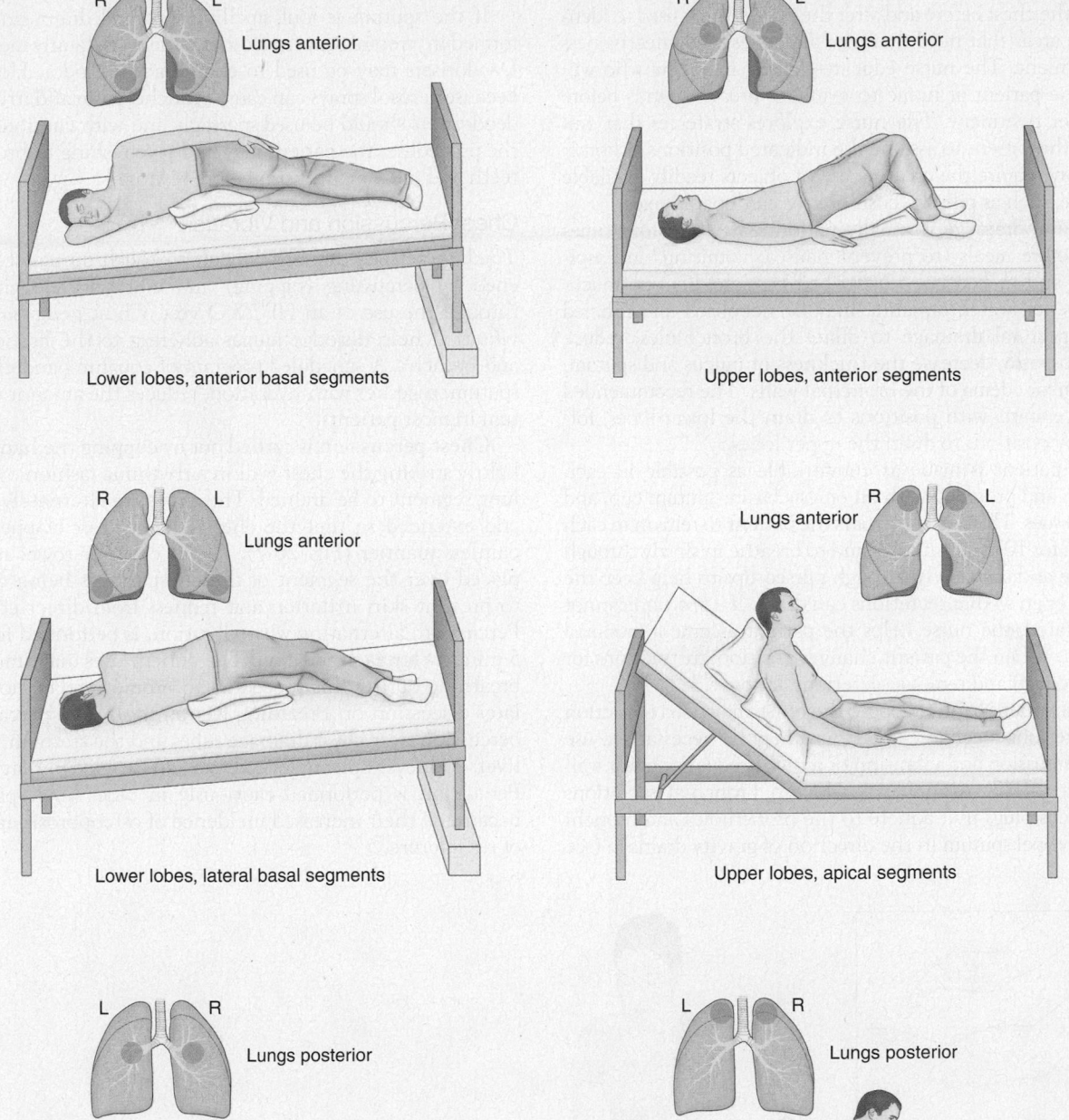

Figure 20-6 • Postural drainage positions and the areas of lung drained by each position.

bronchi and trachea. Each position contributes to effective drainage of a different lobe of the lungs; lower and middle lobe bronchi drain more effectively when the head is down, whereas the upper lobe bronchi drain more effectively when the head is up. The secretions then are removed by coughing.

The nurse should keep in mind the medical diagnosis, the lung lobes or segments involved, the cardiac status, and any structural deformities of the chest wall and spine. Auscultation of the chest before and after the procedure is used to identify the areas that need drainage and assess the effectiveness of treatment. The nurse educates family members who will assist the patient at home to evaluate breath sounds before and after treatment. The nurse explores strategies that will enable the patient to assume the indicated positions at home. This may require the creative use of objects readily available at home, such as pillows, cushions, or cardboard boxes.

Postural drainage is usually performed two to four times daily, before meals (to prevent nausea, vomiting, and aspiration) and at bedtime. Prescribed bronchodilators, mucolytic agents, water, or saline may be nebulized and inhaled before postural drainage to dilate the bronchioles, reduce bronchospasm, decrease the thickness of mucus and sputum, and combat edema of the bronchial walls. The recommended sequence starts with positions to drain the lower lobes, followed by positions to drain the upper lobes.

The patient is made as comfortable as possible in each position and provided with an emesis basin, sputum cup, and paper tissues. The nurse instructs the patient to remain in each position for 10 to 15 minutes and to breathe in slowly through the nose and out slowly through pursed lips to help keep the airways open so that secretions can drain. If a position cannot be tolerated, the nurse helps the patient assume a modified position. When the patient changes position, instructions for how to cough and remove secretions are provided.

If the patient cannot cough, the nurse may need to suction the secretions mechanically. It also may be necessary to use chest percussion and vibration or a high-frequency chest wall oscillation (HFCWO) vest to loosen bronchial secretions and mucus plugs that adhere to the bronchioles and bronchi and to propel sputum in the direction of gravity drainage (see later discussion). If suctioning is required at home, the nurse instructs caregivers in safe suctioning technique and care of the suctioning equipment.

After the procedure, the nurse or family caregivers note the amount, color, viscosity, and character of the expelled sputum. The nurse evaluates the patient's skin color and pulse the first few times the procedure is performed. It may be necessary to administer oxygen during postural drainage.

If the sputum is foul smelling, postural drainage is performed in a room away from other patients or family members. Deodorizers may be used to counteract the odor. However, because aerosol sprays can cause bronchospasm and irritation, deodorizers should be used sparingly and with caution. After the procedure, the patient may find it refreshing to brush the teeth and use a mouthwash before resting.

Chest Percussion and Vibration

Thick secretions that are difficult to cough up may be loosened by percussing (tapping) and vibrating the chest or through the use of an HFCWO vest. Chest percussion and vibration help dislodge mucus adhering to the bronchioles and bronchi. A scheduled program of coughing and clearing sputum, together with hydration, reduces the amount of sputum in most patients.

Chest percussion is carried out by cupping the hands and lightly striking the chest wall in a rhythmic fashion over the lung segment to be drained. The wrists are alternately flexed and extended so that the chest is cupped or clapped in a painless manner (Fig. 20-7). A soft cloth or towel may be placed over the segment of the chest that is being cupped to prevent skin irritation and redness from direct contact. Percussion, alternating with vibration, is performed for 3 to 5 minutes for each position. The patient uses diaphragmatic breathing during this procedure to promote relaxation (see later discussion on Breathing Retraining). As a precaution, percussion over chest drainage tubes and the sternum, spine, liver, kidneys, spleen, or breasts (in women) is avoided. Percussion is performed cautiously in older adult patients because of their increased incidence of osteoporosis and risk of rib fracture.

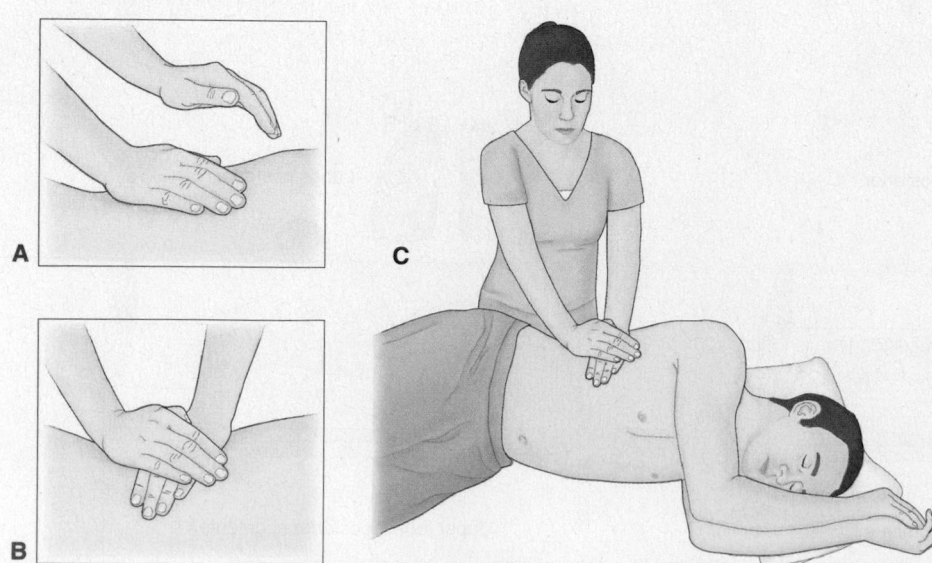

Figure 20-7 • Percussion and vibration. **A.** Proper hand position for percussion. **B.** Proper hand position for vibration. **C.** Proper technique for vibration. The wrists and elbows remain stiff; the vibrating motion is produced by the shoulder muscles.

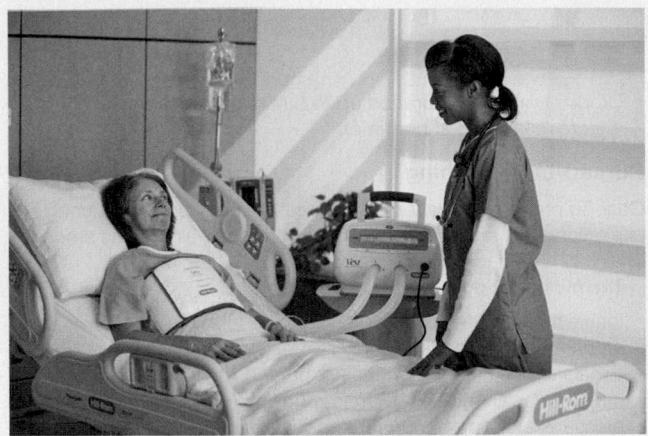

Figure 20-8 • High-frequency chest wall oscillation (HFCWO) vest. © 2013 Hill-Rom Services, Inc. Reprinted with permission—all rights reserved.

Vibration is the technique of applying manual compression and tremor to the chest wall during the exhalation phase of respiration (see Fig. 20-7). This helps increase the velocity of the air expired from the small airways, thus freeing mucus. After three or four vibrations, the patient is encouraged to cough, contracting the abdominal muscles to increase the effectiveness of the cough.

The number of times the percussion and coughing cycle is repeated depends on the patient's tolerance and clinical response. The nurse evaluates breath sounds before and after application of these techniques.

An inflatable HFCWO vest (Fig. 20-8) may be used to provide chest therapy. The vest uses air pulses to compress the chest wall 8 to 18 times/sec, causing secretions to detach from the airway wall and enabling the patient to expel them by coughing. Patients prescribed vest therapy are generally more satisfied with this mode of treatment delivery than patients who receive manual CPT. Furthermore, research suggests that the vest is equally effective to manual CPT; however, the mode of therapy selected should consider the patient's specific needs and preferences (Hanlon, 2015; Powner, Nesmith, Kirkpatrick, et al., 2019). Technologic advances to the HFCWO vest include portable versions, the AffloVest® and Monarch®, which allow users to move about freely during therapy, thus improving patient adherence and satisfaction. In addition, CPT may also be delivered using specialized beds. These beds feature programmable mattresses that deliver vibropercussion and may rotate the upper torso up to 45 degrees to help mobilize pulmonary secretions.

To increase the effectiveness of coughing, a flutter valve may be used, which is especially useful for patients who have CF (see later discussion). The **flutter valve** looks like a pipe but has a cap covering the bowl, which contains a steel ball. When the patient exhales actively into the device, movement of the ball causes pressure oscillations, thereby decreasing viscosity of the mucus, facilitating mucous clearance (Fig. 20-9).

When performing CPT, the nurse ensures that the patient is comfortable, is not wearing restrictive clothing, and has not just eaten. The nurse gives medication for pain, as prescribed, before applying the techniques of percussion and vibration, splints any incision, and provides pillows for support as needed. The positions are varied, but focus is placed on the affected areas. On completion of the treatment, the nurse assists the patient to assume a comfortable position.

If an HFCWO vest is being used, the patient may assume whatever position is most comfortable and may even continue to perform light activity during therapy, such as household chores (e.g., folding laundry) or engaging in hobbies (e.g., playing the guitar). The patient does not need to assume specific positions for the vest to be effective.

Treatment should be stopped if any of the following occur: increased pain, increased shortness of breath, weakness, lightheadedness, or hemoptysis. Therapy is indicated until the patient has normal respirations, can mobilize secretions, and has normal breath sounds, and until the chest x-ray findings are normal.

Nursing management of the patient using flutter valve therapy includes ensuring that the patient assumes the proper position, educating the patient on the technique for using the flutter valve, and setting realistic goals for the patient.

Improving Breathing Patterns

The breathing pattern of most people with COPD is shallow, rapid, and inefficient; the more severe the disease, the more inefficient the breathing pattern. Impaired breathing patterns and shortness of breath are due to the modified respiratory mechanics of the chest wall and lung resulting from **air trapping** (i.e., incomplete emptying of alveoli during expiration), ineffective diaphragmatic movement, airway obstruction, the metabolic cost of breathing, and stress. Breathing retraining may help improve breathing patterns. Training in diaphragmatic breathing reduces the respiratory rate, increases alveolar ventilation, and sometimes helps expel as much air as possible during expiration. Pursed-lip breathing helps slow expiration, prevent collapse of small airways, and control the rate and depth of respiration. It also promotes relaxation, which allows patients to gain control of dyspnea and reduce feelings of panic.

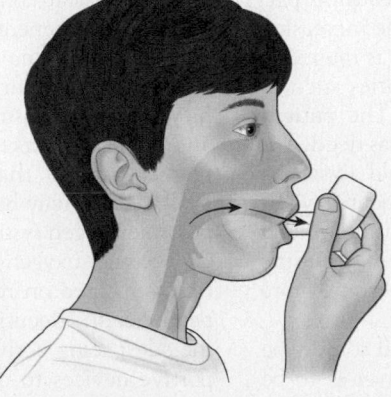
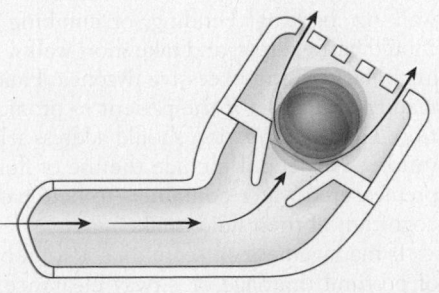

Figure 20-9 • The flutter valve is a handheld pipe-shaped device with a mouthpiece on one end, a perforated cover on the other end, and a steel ball on the inside. When the patient expires through this device, positive end pressure is enhanced, thus helping to clear respiratory secretions.

Chart 20-5

PATIENT EDUCATION
Breathing Exercises

General Instructions

The nurse instructs the patient to:

- Breathe slowly and rhythmically to exhale completely and empty the lungs completely.
- Inhale through the nose to filter, humidify, and warm the air before it enters the lungs.
- Breathe more slowly by prolonging the exhalation time when feeling out of breath.
- Keep the air moist with a humidifier.

Diaphragmatic Breathing

Goal: To use and strengthen the diaphragm during breathing
The nurse instructs the patient to:

- Place one hand on the abdomen (just below the ribs) and the other hand on the middle of the chest to increase the awareness of the position of the diaphragm and its function in breathing.
- Breathe in slowly and deeply through the nose, letting the abdomen protrude as far as possible.
- Breathe out through pursed lips while tightening (contracting) the abdominal muscles.
- Press firmly inward and upward on the abdomen while breathing out.
- Repeat for 1 min; follow with a rest period of 2 min.

- Gradually increase duration up to 5 min, several times a day (before meals and at bedtime).

Pursed-Lip Breathing

Goal: To prolong exhalation and increase airway pressure during expiration, thus reducing the amount of trapped air and the amount of airway resistance
The nurse instructs the patient to:

- Inhale through the nose while slowly counting to 3—the amount of time needed to say "Smell a rose."
- Exhale slowly and evenly against pursed lips while tightening the abdominal muscles. (Pursing the lips increases intratracheal pressure; exhaling through the mouth offers less resistance to expired air.)
- Count to 7 slowly while prolonging expiration through pursed lips—the length of time to say "Blow out the candle."
- While sitting in a chair:
  Fold arms over the abdomen.
  Inhale through the nose while counting to 3 slowly.
  Bend forward and exhale slowly through pursed lips while counting to 7 slowly.
- While walking:
  Inhale while walking two steps.
  Exhale through pursed lips while walking four or five steps.

Breathing Retraining

Breathing retraining consists of exercises and breathing practices that are designed to achieve more efficient and controlled ventilation and to decrease the work of breathing. These exercises promote maximal alveolar inflation and muscle relaxation; relieve anxiety; eliminate ineffective, uncoordinated patterns of respiratory muscle activity; and slow the respiratory rate (Kacmarek et al., 2017). Slow, relaxed, rhythmic breathing also helps to control the anxiety that occurs with dyspnea. Specific breathing exercises include diaphragmatic and pursed-lip breathing (Chart 20-5).

Diaphragmatic breathing can become automatic with sufficient practice and concentration. Pursed-lip breathing, which improves oxygen transport, helps induce a slow, deep breathing pattern and assists the patient to control breathing, even during periods of stress. Breathing exercises should be practiced in several positions because air distribution and pulmonary circulation vary with the position of the chest.

Promoting Self-Care

As gas exchange, airway clearance, and the breathing pattern improve, the patient is encouraged to assume increasing participation in self-care activities. The patient is taught to coordinate diaphragmatic breathing with activities such as walking, bathing, bending, or climbing stairs. The patient should bathe, dress, and take short walks, resting as needed to avoid fatigue and excessive dyspnea. Fluids should always be readily available for the patient to promote adequate hydration. Patient education should address self-regulation of fluid intake. This could include the use of fluid diaries and using premeasured water containers to help patients become more cognizant of their fluid intake.

If management of secretions is a problem and some type of postural drainage or airway clearance maneuver is to be performed at home, the nurse or respiratory therapist instructs and supervises the patient before discharge or in an outpatient setting.

Improving Activity Tolerance

People with COPD have decreased exercise tolerance during specific periods of the day, especially in the morning on arising, because bronchial secretions have collected in the lungs during the night while the patient was lying down. The patient may have difficulty bathing or dressing and may become fatigued. Activities that require the arms to be supported above the level of the thorax may produce fatigue or respiratory distress but may be tolerated better after the patient has been up and moving around for an hour or more. The nurse can help the patient reduce these limitations by planning self-care activities and determining the best times for bathing, dressing, and other daily activities.

Patients with COPD of all grades may benefit from exercise training programs. These benefits may include increased exercise tolerance and decreased dyspnea and fatigue (GOLD, 2019). Physical conditioning techniques include breathing exercises and general exercises intended to conserve energy and increase pulmonary ventilation. Graded exercises and physical conditioning programs using treadmills, stationary bicycles, and measured level walks can improve symptoms and increase work capacity and exercise tolerance. Any physical activity that can be performed regularly is helpful. Walking aids may be beneficial (GOLD, 2019). Lightweight portable oxygen systems are available for ambulatory patients who require oxygen therapy during physical activity. Education is focused on rehabilitative therapies to promote independence in executing activities of daily living. These may include pacing activities throughout the day or using supportive devices to decrease energy expenditure. The nurse evaluates the patient's activity tolerance and limitations and uses education strategies to promote independent activities of daily living. Other health care professionals (rehabilitation therapist, occupational therapist, physical therapist) may be consulted as additional resources.

Encouraging Effective Coping

Any factor that interferes with normal breathing quite naturally induces anxiety, depression, and changes in behavior. Constant shortness of breath and fatigue may make the patient irritable and apprehensive to the point of panic. Restricted activity (and reversal of family roles due to loss of employment), the frustration of having to work to breathe, and the realization that the disease is prolonged and unrelenting may cause the patient to become angry, depressed, and anxious. Sexual function may be compromised, which also diminishes self-esteem. The nurse should provide education and support to spouses or significant others and families, because the caregiver role in end-stage COPD can be challenging.

Monitoring and Managing Potential Complications

The nurse must assess for various complications of COPD, such as life-threatening respiratory insufficiency and failure, as well as respiratory infection and chronic atelectasis, which may increase the risk of respiratory failure. The nurse monitors for cognitive changes (personality and behavioral changes, memory impairment), increasing dyspnea, tachypnea, and tachycardia, which may indicate increasing hypoxemia and impending respiratory failure.

The nurse monitors pulse oximetry values to assess the patient's need for oxygen and administers supplemental oxygen as prescribed. The nurse also instructs the patient about signs and symptoms of respiratory infection that may worsen hypoxemia and reports changes in the patient's physical and cognitive status to the primary provider.

Bronchopulmonary infections must be controlled to diminish inflammatory edema and to permit recovery of normal ciliary action. Minor respiratory infections that are of no consequence to people with normal lungs can be life-threatening to people with COPD. Infection compromises lung function and is a common cause of respiratory failure in people with COPD. In COPD, infection may be accompanied by subtle changes. The nurse instructs the patient to report any signs of infection, such as a fever or change in sputum color, character, consistency, or amount. Any worsening of symptoms (increased tightness of the chest, increased dyspnea, fatigue) also suggests pneumonia and must be reported. Viral infections are hazardous to the patient because they are often followed by pneumonia caused by bacterial organisms, such as *Streptococcus pneumoniae*, *Moraxella catarrhalis*, and *Haemophilus influenzae* (Bartlett & Sethi, 2018).

To prevent pneumonia, the nurse encourages the patient with COPD to be immunized against influenza and pneumococcal pneumonia, because the patient is prone to respiratory infection. In addition, because each patient reacts differently to external exposures (significant air pollution, high or low temperatures, high humidity, strong smells), the nurse must assess the patient's actual and potential triggers that cause bronchospasm so that avoidance or a treatment plan can be established.

Pneumothorax is a potential complication of COPD and can be life-threatening in patients with COPD who have minimal pulmonary reserve. Patients with severe emphysematous changes can develop large bullae, which may rupture and cause a pneumothorax. Development of a pneumothorax may be spontaneous or related to an activity such as severe coughing or large intrathoracic pressure changes. If a rapid onset of shortness of breath occurs, the nurse should quickly evaluate the patient for potential pneumothorax by assessing the symmetry of chest movement, differences in breath sounds, and a decrease in pulse oximetry.

Over time, pulmonary hypertension may occur as a result of chronic hypoxemia, which causes the pulmonary arteries to constrict and leads to this complication. Pulmonary hypertension may be prevented by maintaining adequate oxygenation through an adequate hemoglobin level, improved ventilation–perfusion of the lungs, or continuous administration of supplemental oxygen (if needed).

Promoting Home, Community-Based, and Transitional Care

Referral for home, community-based, or transitional care is important. These referrals assess the patient's home environment in relation to their physical and psychological status and the patient's ability to adhere to a prescribed therapeutic regimen. These assessments include evaluating the patient's ability to cope with changes in lifestyle and physical status so that their medical management can be tailored to their specific needs. Once home care is set up, the visits provide an opportunity to reinforce the information and activities learned in the inpatient or outpatient pulmonary rehabilitation program and to have the patient and family demonstrate correct administration of medications and oxygen, if indicated, and performance of exercises. If the patient does not have access to a formal pulmonary rehabilitation program, the nurse provides the education and breathing retraining necessary to optimize the patient's functional status.

Educating Patients About Self-Care

When providing education about self-management, the nurse must assess the knowledge of patients and family members about self-care and the therapeutic regimen. The nurse should also consider whether they are comfortable with this knowledge. Familiarity with potential side effects of prescribed medications is essential. In addition, patients and family members need to learn the early signs and symptoms of infection and other complications so that they seek appropriate health care promptly. Nurses are key in promoting smoking cessation and educating patients about its importance. Patients diagnosed with COPD who continue to smoke must be encouraged and assisted to quit.

A major area of patient education involves setting and accepting realistic short-term and long-range goals. If the COPD is mild (e.g., grade I), the objectives of treatment are to increase exercise tolerance and prevent further loss of pulmonary function. If the COPD is severe (e.g., grade III), the objectives are to preserve current pulmonary function and relieve symptoms as much as possible. It is important to plan and share the goals and expectations of treatment with the patient. Both the patient and the care provider need patience to achieve these goals.

Chart 20-6 PATIENT EDUCATION
Use of Pressurized Metered-Dose Inhaler (pMDI)

The nurse instructs the patient to:

- Remove the cap and hold the inhaler upright.
- Shake the inhaler.
- Sit upright or stand upright. Breathe out slowly and all the way.
- Use one of two techniques: open- or closed-mouth technique.
  - *Open-mouth technique*
  - Place the pMDI 2 finger widths away from lips.
  - With mouth open and tongue flat, tilt outlet of the pMDI so that it is pointed toward the upper back of the mouth.
  - Actuate the pMDI and begin to breathe in slowly. Breathe slowly and deeply through the mouth and try to hold breath for 10 s.
  - *Closed-mouth technique*
  - Place the pMDI between the teeth and make sure the tongue is flat under the mouthpiece and does not block pMDI.
  - Seal lips around mouthpiece and actuate the pMDI. Breathe in slowly through the mouth and try to hold breath for 10 s.
- Repeat puffs as directed, allowing 1 min between puffs. There is no need to wait for other medications.
- Apply the cap to the pMDI for storage.
- After inhalation, rinse mouth with water when using a corticosteroid-containing pMDI.

The pMDI mouthpiece should be cleaned on a regular basis as should the nozzle of the canister based on the manufacturer's recommendations. As there are many types of inhalers, it is important to follow the manufacturer's instructions for use and care of the inhaler.

Adapted from Cairo, J. M. (2018). *Mosby's respiratory care equipment* (10th ed.). St. Louis, MO: Elsevier Mosby.

The nurse instructs the patient to avoid extremes of heat and cold. Heat increases the body temperature, thereby raising oxygen requirements, and cold tends to promote bronchospasm. Air pollutants such as fumes, smoke, dust, and even talcum, lint, and aerosol sprays may initiate bronchospasm. High altitudes aggravate hypoxemia.

A patient with COPD should adopt a lifestyle of moderate activity, ideally in a climate with minimal shifts in temperature and humidity. As much as possible, the patient should avoid emotional disturbances and stressful situations that might trigger a coughing episode. Self-management also includes getting sufficient rest and sleep. The medication regimen can be quite complex; patients receiving aerosol medications by a pMDI or other type of inhaler may be particularly challenged. The nurse must review educational information and have the patient demonstrate correct pMDI use before discharge, during follow-up visits to a caregiver's office or clinic, and during home visits (Chart 20-6).

Smoking cessation goes hand in hand with lifestyle changes, and reinforcing the patient's efforts is a key nursing activity. Smoking cessation is the single most important therapeutic intervention for patients with COPD. There are many strategies, including prevention, cessation with or without oral or topical patch medications, and behavior modification techniques.

At times, the patient will need oxygen at home. The nurse instructs the patient or family in the methods for administering oxygen safely and informs the patient and family that oxygen is available in gas, liquid, and concentrated forms. The gas and liquid forms come in portable devices so that the patient can leave home while receiving oxygen therapy. Humidity must be provided while oxygen is used (except with portable devices) to counteract the dry, irritating effects of compressed oxygen on the airway (Chart 20-7). To help the patient adhere to the oxygen prescription, the nurse explains

Chart 20-7 HOME CARE CHECKLIST
Oxygen Therapy

At the completion of education, the patient and/or caregiver will be able to:

- State proper care of and administration of oxygen to patient.
- State primary provider's prescription for oxygen and the manner in which it is to be used.
- Indicate when a humidifier should be used.
- Identify signs and symptoms indicating the need for change in oxygen therapy.
- Describe precautions and safety measures to be used when oxygen is in use:
  - Know NOT to smoke or be around people who are smoking while using oxygen.
  - Post "No Smoking—Oxygen in Use" signs on doors.
  - Notify local fire department and electric company of oxygen use in home.
  - Never use paint thinners, cleaning fluids, gasoline, aerosol sprays, and other flammable materials while using oxygen.
  - Keep all methods of oxygen delivery at least 15 feet away from matches, candles, gas stove, or other source of flame, and 5 feet away from television, radio, and other appliances.
  - Keep oxygen tank out of direct sunlight.
  - When traveling in automobile, place oxygen tank on floor behind front seat.

- If traveling by airplane, notify air carrier of need for oxygen at least 2 wks in advance.
- State how and when to place an order for more oxygen.
- Maintain and use equipment properly:
  - Identify when a portable oxygen delivery device should be used.
  - Demonstrate safe and appropriate use of and how to change from one oxygen delivery system to another (e.g., from oxygen concentrator to portable oxygen delivery).
  - Demonstrate correct adjustment of prescribed flow rate.
  - Describe how to clean and when to replace oxygen tubing.
  - Identify causes of malfunction of equipment and when to call for the replacement of equipment.
  - Describe the importance of determining that all electrical outlets are working properly.

Resources

See Chapter 2, Chart 2-6 for additional information related to durable medical equipment, adaptive equipment, and mobility skills.

the proper flow rate and required number of hours for oxygen use as well as the dangers of arbitrary changes in flow rate or duration of therapy. The nurse also reassures the patient that oxygen is not "addictive" and explains the need for regular evaluations of blood oxygenation by pulse oximetry or arterial blood gas analysis.

Numerous educational materials are available to assist nurses in educating patients with COPD (see Resources at the end of the chapter).

Continuing and Transitional Care

Home visits by a nurse or respiratory therapist may be arranged based on the patient's status and needs. It is important to assess the patient's home environment, the patient's physical and psychological status, and the need for further education. The nurse reinforces educational points on how to use oxygen safely and effectively, including fire safety tips. To maintain a consistent quality of care and to maximize the patient's financial reimbursement for home oxygen therapy, the nurse ensures that the prescription given by the primary provider includes the diagnosis, the prescribed oxygen flow, and conditions for use (e.g., continuous use, nighttime use only). Because oxygen is a medication, the nurse reminds the patient receiving long-term oxygen therapy and the family about the importance of keeping follow-up appointments with the patient's primary provider. The patient is instructed to see the primary provider every 6 months or more often, if indicated. Arterial blood gas measurements and laboratory tests are repeated annually or more often if the patient's condition changes.

The nurse directs patients to community resources, such as pulmonary rehabilitation programs and smoking cessation programs, to help improve patients' ability to cope with their chronic condition and the therapeutic regimen and to provide a sense of worth, hope, and well-being. In addition, the nurse reminds the patient and family about the importance of participating in general health promotion activities and health screening.

Patients with COPD have indicated that information about their end-of-life needs is limited. Areas to discuss regarding end-of-life care may include symptom management, quality of life, satisfaction with care, information/communication, use of care professionals, use of differing care facilities, hospital admission, and place of death. It is crucial that patients know what to expect as the disease progresses. In addition, they should have information about their role in decisions regarding aggressiveness of care near the end of life and access to specialists who may help them and their families. As the disease course progresses, a holistic assessment of physical and psychological needs should be undertaken at each hospitalization, clinic visit, or home visit. This helps gauge the patient's assessment of the progression of the disease and its impact on quality of life and guides planning for future interventions and management (see Chapter 13 for additional information).

Bronchiectasis

Bronchiectasis is a chronic, irreversible dilation of the bronchi and bronchioles that results from destruction of muscles and elastic connective tissue. Numerous factors can induce or contribute to the development of bronchiectasis. Some of these include recurrent respiratory infections, CF, rheumatic and other systemic diseases, primary ciliary dysfunction, tuberculosis, or immune deficiency disorders (Barker, King, & Hollingsworth, 2019). Between 340,000 and 522,000 adults were living with non-CF bronchiectasis in 2013, estimates show (Weycker, Hansen, & Seifer, 2017). The increased prevalence of bronchiectasis, with an annual growth rate of 8% since 2001, may be attributed to advances in the technology for diagnosing the disease (GOLD, 2019). Bronchiectasis, a disease process separate from COPD, is often a comorbidity with COPD (GOLD, 2019). Bronchiectasis and sinusitis are the major respiratory manifestations of CF (discussed later in this chapter) (Barker et al., 2019).

Pathophysiology

The inflammatory process associated with pulmonary infections damages the bronchial wall, causing a loss of its supporting structure and resulting in thick sputum that ultimately obstructs the bronchi. The walls become permanently distended and distorted, impairing mucociliary clearance. In saccular bronchiectasis, each dilated peribronchial tube amounts to a lung abscess, the exudate of which drains freely through the bronchus. Bronchiectasis is usually localized, affecting a segment or lobe of a lung, most frequently the lower lobes.

The retention of secretions and subsequent obstruction ultimately cause the alveoli distal to the obstruction to collapse (atelectasis). Inflammatory scarring or fibrosis replaces functioning lung tissue. In time, the patient develops respiratory insufficiency with reduced vital capacity, decreased ventilation, and an increased ratio of residual volume to total lung capacity. There is impairment in the match of ventilation to perfusion (ventilation–perfusion imbalance) and hypoxemia.

Clinical Manifestations

Characteristic symptoms of bronchiectasis include chronic cough and the production of purulent sputum in copious amounts. Many patients with this disease have hemoptysis. Clubbing of the fingers is also common because of respiratory insufficiency. Patients usually have repeated episodes of pulmonary infection.

Assessment and Diagnostic Findings

Bronchiectasis is not readily diagnosed because the symptoms can be mistaken for those of chronic bronchitis. A definite sign is a prolonged history of productive, chronic cough, with sputum consistently negative for tubercle bacilli. The diagnosis is established by a CT scan, which reveals bronchial dilation. The advent of high-resolution CT scanning makes it possible to diagnose this disease during its earlier stages.

Medical Management

Treatment objectives are to promote bronchial drainage, to clear excessive secretions from the affected portion of the lungs, and to prevent or control infection and inflammation. Chest physiotherapy (CPT; see previous discussion) is essential for promoting airway drainage. Sometimes, mucopurulent sputum must be removed by bronchoscopy. Smoking cessation is important, because smoking impairs bronchial drainage by paralyzing ciliary action, increasing bronchial secretions, and causing inflammation of the mucous membranes, resulting in hyperplasia of the mucous glands.

Antibiotics are the cornerstone therapy for management of a bronchiectatic exacerbation. Antimicrobial therapy choice is based on the results of sensitivity studies on organisms cultured from sputum; however, empiric coverage (i.e., broad-spectrum antibiotics that are effective in treating commonly implicated pathogens) is often prescribed initially, pending results of sputum cultures. The most commonly implicated pathogens include *H. influenzae, M. catarrhalis, Staphylococcus aureus,* and *Pseudomonas aeruginosa* (Barker, Stoller, King, et al., 2018). Because infection with *P. aeruginosa* is associated with a greater rate of lung function deterioration, more aggressive oral or IV antibiotic therapy may be used for a longer duration. For patients with recurrent exacerbations (usually two or more during the past year), a low dose macrolide antibiotic may be used as preventative, ongoing therapy (Barker et al., 2018). In addition, patients should be vaccinated against influenza and pneumococcal pneumonia.

Secretion management is an issue for patients with bronchiectasis. Nebulized mucolytics may help to clear airway secretions. These drugs promote expectoration by breaking down the mucus blocking the airways. The administration of nebulized hypertonic saline also improves airway clearance by decreasing the viscosity of the mucus and improving the ability of secretions to move out of the airways. Bronchodilators might be prescribed to help open up the airways, thus enhancing the ability of the other medications (e.g., mucolytics, hypertonic saline) to mobilize secretions. These agents also allow a better passageway for the secretions to move through. Bronchodilators are typically administered at the beginning of each pulmonary treatment. Ensuring adequate hydration and employing CPT may also be of help in loosening and thinning secretions (Barker et al., 2018).

Surgical intervention, although used infrequently, may be indicated for patients who continue to expectorate large amounts of sputum and have repeated bouts of pneumonia and hemoptysis despite adherence to treatment regimens. The disease must involve only one or two areas of the lung that can be removed without producing respiratory insufficiency. The goals of surgical treatment are to conserve normal pulmonary tissue and to avoid infectious complications. Diseased tissue is removed, provided that postoperative lung function will be adequate. It may be necessary to remove a segment of a lobe (segmental resection), a lobe (lobectomy), or, rarely, an entire lung (pneumonectomy). Segmental resection is the removal of an anatomic subdivision of a pulmonary lobe. In select cases, video-assisted surgery (VATS) segmentectomy or lobectomy may be performed, which is associated with fewer complications and decreased length of stay. The chief advantage is that only diseased tissue is removed, and healthy lung tissue is conserved.

The surgery is preceded by a period of careful preparation. The objective is to obtain a dry (free of infection) tracheobronchial tree to prevent complications (atelectasis, pneumonia, bronchopleural fistula, and empyema). This is accomplished by postural drainage or, depending on the location, by direct suction through a bronchoscope. A course of antibacterial therapy may be prescribed. After

surgery, care is the same as for any patient who has undergone chest surgery.

Nursing Management

Nursing management focuses on alleviating symptoms and helping patients clear pulmonary secretions. Patient education targets eliminating smoking and other factors that increase the production of mucus and hamper its removal. Patients and families are taught to perform postural drainage and to avoid exposure to people with upper respiratory or other infections. If the patient experiences fatigue and dyspnea, they are informed about strategies to conserve energy while maintaining as active a lifestyle as possible. The patient is educated about the early signs of respiratory infection and the progression of the disorder so that appropriate treatment can be implemented promptly. The presence of a large amount of mucus may decrease the patient's appetite and result in an inadequate dietary intake; therefore, the patient's nutritional status is assessed and strategies are implemented to ensure an adequate diet.

Asthma

Asthma is a heterogeneous disease, usually characterized by chronic airway inflammation (Global Initiative for Asthma [GINA], 2019a). This chronic inflammatory disease of the airways causes airway hyperresponsiveness, mucosal edema, and mucus production. This inflammation ultimately leads to recurrent episodes of asthma symptoms: cough, chest tightness, wheezing, and dyspnea (Fig. 20-10). In the United States, asthma affects approximately 19 million adults and accounted for approximately 3564 deaths in 2017 (CDC, 2017b; Kochanek, Murphy, Xu, et al., 2019). Of these adults, 35.2% have intermittent severity and 64.8% have persistent severity of asthma symptoms (CDC, 2015). Nearly 10% of all ED visits are related to asthma (CDC, 2018c). Although

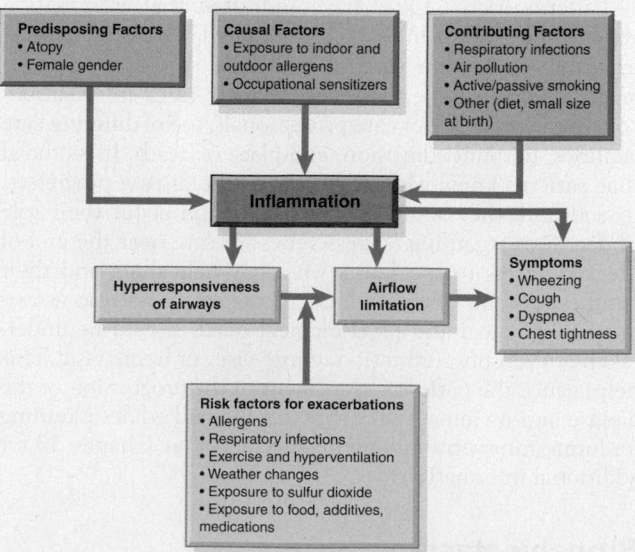

Figure 20-10 • Pathophysiology of asthma. Adapted from materials developed for the Global Initiative for Asthma (2019). Global strategy for asthma management and prevention. Available at: www.ginasthma.org

asthma is the most common chronic disease of childhood, it can occur at any age. For most patients, asthma is a disruptive disease, affecting school and work attendance, occupational choices, physical activity, and general quality of life.

Twenty-one percent of patients with asthma smoke, even though cigarette smoke is known to trigger an attack, while nearly 17% of people without asthma smoke (CDC, 2015). Asthma–COPD overlap refers to patients who have clinical presentations of both conditions (Papi, Brightling, Pedersen, et al., 2018). Smokers are at higher risk for having asthma–COPD overlap (Papi et al., 2018).

Despite increased knowledge regarding the pathology of asthma and the development of improved medications and management plans, the death rate from the disease continues to rise. Ethnic and racial disparities affect morbidity and mortality in asthma, particularly for African American and Hispanic/Latino American urban populations (Sullivan, Ghushchyan, Kavati, et al., 2019). Contributing to these disparities are epidemiologic considerations and risk factors that include genetic and molecular aspects; inner-city environments; limited community assets; health care access/delivery/ and quality; and insufficient health insurance coverage.

Unlike other obstructive lung diseases, asthma is largely reversible, either spontaneously or with treatment. Patients with asthma may experience symptom-free periods alternating with acute exacerbations that last from minutes to hours or days.

Allergy is the strongest predisposing factor for asthma. Chronic exposure to airway irritants or allergens also increases the risk of asthma. Common allergens can be seasonal (e.g., grass, tree, weed pollens) or perennial (e.g., mold, dust, roaches, animal dander). Common triggers for asthma symptoms and exacerbations include airway irritants (e.g., air pollutants, cold, heat, weather changes, strong odors or perfumes, smoke, occupational exposure), foods (e.g., shellfish, nuts), exercise, stress, hormonal factors, medications, viral respiratory tract infections, and gastroesophageal reflux. Most people who have asthma are sensitive to a variety of triggers.

Pathophysiology

The underlying pathology in asthma is reversible diffuse airway inflammation that leads to long-term airway narrowing. This narrowing, which is exacerbated by various changes in the airway, includes bronchoconstriction, airway edema, airway hyperresponsiveness, and airway remodeling (Papi et al., 2018). The interaction of these factors determines the clinical manifestations and severity of asthma (GINA, 2019a). Over the course of a lifetime, the impact of increasing pathophysiologic changes and environmental susceptibility lead to an irreversible disease process.

Asthma is a complex disease process that involves numerous inflammatory and structural cells as well as mediators that lead to the disorder's effects. Mast cells, macrophages, T lymphocytes, neutrophils, and eosinophils all play a key role in the inflammation of asthma. When activated, mast cells release several chemicals called *mediators*. These chemicals, which include histamine, bradykinin, prostanoids, cytokines, leukotrienes, and other mediators, perpetuate the inflammatory response, causing increased blood flow, vasoconstriction, fluid leak from the vasculature, attraction of white blood cells to the area, mucus secretion, and bronchoconstriction (Kacmarek et al., 2017; McCance & Huether, 2019).

During acute exacerbations of asthma, bronchial smooth muscle contraction or bronchoconstriction occurs quickly to narrow the airway in response to an exposure. Acute bronchoconstriction due to allergens results from an immunoglobulin E (IgE)-dependent release of mediators from mast cells; these mediators include histamine, tryptase, leukotrienes, and prostaglandins that directly contract the airway. In addition, alpha- and beta-2–adrenergic receptors of the sympathetic nervous system located in the bronchi play a role. When the alpha-adrenergic receptors are stimulated, bronchoconstriction occurs. The balance between alpha- and beta-2–adrenergic receptors is controlled primarily by cyclic 3′,5′-adenosine monophosphate (cyclic AMP). Beta-2–adrenergic stimulation results in increased levels of cyclic AMP, which inhibits the release of chemical mediators and causes bronchodilation.

As asthma becomes more persistent, the inflammation progresses and other factors may be involved in airflow limitation. These include airway edema, mucus hypersecretion, and the formation of mucus plugs. In addition, airway "remodeling" (i.e., structural changes) may occur in response to chronic inflammation, causing further airway narrowing.

Clinical Manifestations

The three most common symptoms of asthma are cough, dyspnea, and wheezing. In some instances, cough may be the only symptom. An asthma attack often occurs at night or early in the morning, possibly because of circadian variations that influence airway receptor thresholds.

An asthma exacerbation may begin abruptly but most frequently is preceded by increasing symptoms over the previous few days. There is cough, with or without mucus production. At times, the mucus is so tightly wedged in the narrowed airway that the patient cannot cough it up. There may be generalized wheezing (the sound of airflow through narrowed airways), first on expiration and then possibly during inspiration as well. Generalized chest tightness and dyspnea occur. Expiration requires effort and becomes prolonged. As the exacerbation progresses, diaphoresis, tachycardia, and a widened pulse pressure may occur along with hypoxemia and central cyanosis (a late sign of poor oxygenation). Severe, life-threatening hypoxemia can occur in asthma but is relatively uncommon. The hypoxemia is secondary to a ventilation–perfusion mismatch and readily responds to supplemental oxygenation.

Symptoms of exercise-induced asthma include maximal symptoms during exercise, absence of nocturnal symptoms, and sometimes only a description of a "choking" sensation during exercise.

Assessment and Diagnostic Findings

To establish the diagnosis, the clinician must determine that episodic symptoms of airflow obstruction are present, airflow is at least partially reversible, and other causes have been excluded. A positive family history and environmental factors, including seasonal changes, high pollen counts, mold, pet dander, climate changes (particularly cold air), and air pollution, are primarily associated with asthma. In addition, asthma is associated with a variety of foods, compounds, and occupation-related chemicals. Comorbid conditions that may accompany asthma include viral infections, gastroesophageal reflux disease, drug-induced asthma, and allergic bronchopulmonary aspergillosis. Other possible allergic reactions that may accompany asthma include eczema, rashes, and temporary edema. Questions in the assessment that may help to evaluate the patient's asthma control include:

- Have your symptoms awakened you at night or in the early morning?
- Have you needed your quick-acting relief medication more than usual?
- Have you needed unscheduled care for your asthma—a call to the primary provider's office, office visit, ED?
- Have your symptoms impacted your normal activities at school/work/sports?

During acute episodes, sputum and blood tests may disclose eosinophilia (elevated levels of eosinophils). Serum levels of IgE may be elevated if allergy is present. Arterial blood gas analysis and pulse oximetry reveal hypoxemia during acute attacks. Initially, hypocapnia and respiratory alkalosis are present. As the patient's condition worsens and they become more fatigued, the $PaCO_2$ may increase. Because carbon dioxide is 20 times more diffusible than oxygen, it is rare for $PaCO_2$ to be normal or elevated in a person who is breathing very rapidly.

 Quality and Safety Nursing Alert

Normal $PaCO_2$ during an asthma attack may be a signal of impending respiratory failure.

During an exacerbation, the FEV_1 and FVC are markedly decreased but improve with bronchodilator administration (demonstrating reversibility). Pulmonary function is usually normal between exacerbations. The occurrence of a severe, continuous reaction is referred to as status asthmaticus and is considered life-threatening (see later discussion).

Asthma severity is considered in the selection of the initial type, amount, and schedule of treatments (GINA, 2019a). Disease severity is classified by current impairment and future risk of adverse events. Impairment is defined by the following factors: nighttime awakenings, the need for short-acting bronchodilators for symptom relief, work/school days missed, ability to engage in normal activities, and quality of life. Lung function is evaluated by spirometry. Assessment of risk of future adverse events is evaluated by numbers of exacerbations, the need for ED care or hospitalizations in the past year, demographic data (gender, ethnicity, nonuse of prescribed ICS therapy, existing smoking), psychosocial factors and attitudes, and beliefs about taking medication (GINA, 2019a).

Prevention

Patients with recurrent asthma should undergo testing to identify the substances that precipitate the symptoms. Possible causes are dust, dust mites, roaches, certain types of cloth, pets, horses, detergents, soaps, certain foods, molds, and pollens. If the attacks are seasonal, pollens can be strongly suspected. Patients are instructed to avoid the causative agents whenever possible. Knowledge is the key to quality asthma care. Evaluation of impairment and risk are primary methods that help ensure control.

Occupational asthma refers to asthma induced by exposure in the work environment to dusts, vapors, or fumes, with or without a preexisting diagnosis of asthma. An estimated 5% to 20% of new asthma cases in the United States are related to workplace exposures (GINA, 2019a). Work-related asthma should be part of the differential diagnosis of every case of adult-onset asthma. A detailed work history evaluation is key to identifying occupational asthma. Immediate treatment is aimed at removing or decreasing the exposure in the patient's environment and following the patient on an ongoing basis. Standard asthma medications may be prescribed to minimize bronchoconstriction and airway inflammation. In certain cases, patients may be impaired or disabled from the disease. Compensation systems are in place to protect a worker, however, these systems are often slow and complex to navigate.

Complications

Complications of asthma may include status asthmaticus, respiratory failure, pneumonia, and atelectasis. Airway obstruction, particularly during acute asthmatic episodes, often results in hypoxemia, requiring the administration of oxygen and the monitoring of pulse oximetry and arterial blood gases. Fluids are given because people with asthma are frequently dehydrated from diaphoresis and insensible fluid loss with hyperventilation.

Medical Management

Primary treatment focuses on preventing impairment of lung function, minimizing symptoms, and preventing exacerbations (Papi et al., 2018). GINA (2019a) recommendations are based on the concept of severity and control of asthma along with the domains of reducing impairment and reducing risk as keys to improving care. Asthma control is assessed by symptom management and future risk of adverse outcomes (GOLD, 2019). In an acute situation, symptom control includes using immediate intervention to diminish bronchoconstriction, which prevents increased anxiety resulting from progressive dyspnea. Uncontrolled anxiety could aggravate the situation and ultimately worsen dyspnea. Poor symptom control increases the risk of exacerbations (GINA, 2019a).

Pharmacologic Therapy

There are two general classes of asthma medications: quick-relief medications for immediate treatment of asthma symptoms and exacerbations and long-acting medications to achieve and maintain control of persistent asthma (Tables 20-5 and 20-6). Because the underlying pathology of asthma is inflammation, control of persistent asthma is accomplished primarily with regular use of anti-inflammatory medications. The route of choice for administration of these medications is a pMDI or other type of inhaler, because it allows for localized administration within the lungs (see Chart 20-6 and Table 20-3).

Quick-Relief Medications

Short-acting beta-2–adrenergic agonists (SABAs) (e.g., albuterol, levalbuterol, pirbuterol) are the medications of choice for relief of acute symptoms and prevention of exercise-induced asthma. They are used to relax smooth muscle.

Anticholinergics (e.g., ipratropium) inhibit muscarinic cholinergic receptors and reduce intrinsic vagal tone of the

(text continued on page 639)

TABLE 20-5	Quick-Relief Medications for Treatment of Asthma		
Medication	**Indications/Mechanisms**	**Potential Adverse Effects**	**Nursing Considerations**
Inhaled Short-Acting Beta-2 Adrenergic Agonists albuterol levalbuterol HFA metaproterenol sulfate	*Indications* Relief of acute symptoms; quick-relief medication Preventive treatment for exercise-induced bronchospasm *Mechanisms* Bronchodilation; binds to the beta-2 adrenergic receptor, producing smooth muscle relaxation and decreased bronchoconstriction	Tachycardia, muscle tremor, hypokalemia, increased lactic acid, headache, and hyperglycemia. Inhaled route causes few systematic adverse effects. Patients with preexisting cardiovascular disease, especially older adults, may have adverse cardiovascular reactions with inhaled therapy Lack of effect or need for regular use indicates inadequate asthma control	Instruct patient in correct use of inhaled agents and how to evaluate amount of remaining medication in pressurized metered-dose inhaler. Recommend periodic cleaning of device. Inform patient about possible adverse effects and need to inform primary provider about increased use of medication to control symptoms.
Anticholinergics ipratropium	*Indications* Relief of acute bronchospasm *Mechanisms* Bronchodilation; inhibition of muscarinic cholinergic receptors Reduction in vagal tone of airways May decrease mucous gland secretion	Dryness of mouth and respiratory secretions; may cause increased wheezing in some patients Does not block exercise-induced bronchospasm Is not effective in long-term control of asthma	Instruct patient in correct use of inhaled agents. Ensure adequate fluid intake. Assess patient for hypersensitivity to atropine, soybeans, peanuts; glaucoma; prostatic hypertrophy.
Corticosteroids *Systemic* methylprednisolone prednisolone prednisone	*Indications* For short-term (3–10 d) "burst;" to gain prompt control of inadequately controlled persistent asthma For moderate or severe exacerbations to prevent progression of exacerbation, reverse inflammation, speed recovery, and reduce rate of relapse *Mechanisms* Anti-inflammatory; block reaction to allergen and reduce hyperresponsiveness; inhibit cytokine production, adhesion protein activation, and inflammatory cell migration and activation; reverses beta-2 receptor downregulation	Blood glucose abnormalities, increased appetite, fluid retention, weight gain, mood alteration, hypertension, peptic ulcer, insomnia Consideration must be given to comorbidities that may be worsened by systemic corticosteroids	Explain to patient that action is often rapid in onset, although resolution of symptoms may take 3–10 d. Instruct patient about possible side effects and the importance of taking the medication as prescribed. If the patient is taking multiple doses a day, administering the last dose prior to 2 PM (when possible) may help to prevent sleep disturbances.

HFA, hydrofluoroalkane.
Adapted from Global Initiative for Asthma (GINA) (2019b). Pocket guide for asthma management. Retrieved on 7/01/2019 at: www.ginasthma.org/wp-content/uploads/2019/04/GINA-2019-main-Pocket-Guide-wms.pdf

TABLE 20-6	Long-Term Medications for Treatment of Asthma (Controller Medications)			
Medication	**Dosage Information**	**Indications/Mechanisms**	**Potential Adverse Effects**	**Nursing Considerations**
Inhaled Corticosteroids beclomethasone dipropionate budesonide ciclesonide flunisolide fluticasone mometasone furoate		*Indications* Long-term prevention of symptoms; suppression, control, and reversal of inflammation Reduce need for oral corticosteroid *Mechanisms* Anti-inflammatory; block late reaction to allergen and reduce airway hyperresponsiveness Inhibit cytokine production, adhesion protein activation, and inflammatory cell migration and activation; reverse beta-2 receptor downregulation; inhibit microvascular leakage	Cough, dysphonia, oral thrush (candidiasis), headache In high doses, systemic effects may occur (e.g., adrenal suppression, osteoporosis, skin thinning, easy bruising)	Instruct patient in correct use of pMDI and use of spacer/holding chamber devices. Instruct patient to rinse mouth after inhalation to reduce local side effects.

(continued on page 636)

TABLE 20-6	Long-Term Medications for Treatment of Asthma (Controller Medications) (continued)			
Medication	**Dosage Information**	**Indications/Mechanisms**	**Potential Adverse Effects**	**Nursing Considerations**
Systemic Corticosteroids methylprednisolone prednisolone prednisone		*Indications* For prevention of symptoms in severe persistent asthma: suppression, control, and reversal of inflammation *Mechanisms* Same as inhaled corticosteroids	*Long-Term Use*: adrenal axis suppression, growth suppression, dermal thinning, hypertension, diabetes, Cushing's syndrome, cataracts, muscle weakness, and, in rare instances, impaired immune function, insomnia Consideration should be given to comorbidities that could be worsened by systemic corticosteroids	Instruct patient about possible side effects and the importance of taking the medication as prescribed (usually a single dose in the morning daily or on an alternate-day schedule, which may produce less adrenal suppression). If the patient is taking multiple doses a day, administering the last dose prior to 2 PM (when possible) may help to prevent sleep disturbances.
Long-Acting Beta-2 Adrenergic Agonists *Inhaled* salmeterol formoterol		*Indications* Long-term prevention of symptoms, added to ICS Prevention of exercise-induced bronchospasm *Mechanisms* Bronchodilation; smooth muscle relaxation following adenylate cyclase activation and increase in cAMP, producing functional antagonism of bronchoconstriction Compared to SABA, salmeterol (but not formoterol) has slower onset of action (15–30 min). Both salmeterol and formoterol have longer duration (>12 h) compared to SABA	Should *not* be used to treat acute symptoms or exacerbations Decreased protection against exercise-induced bronchospasm may occur with regular use Tachycardia, muscle tremor, hypokalemia, ECG changes with overdose. A diminished bronchoprotective effect may occur within 1 wk of chronic therapy. Potential risk of uncommon, severe, life-threatening, or fatal exacerbation	Reinforce to patient that these medications should *not* be used to treat acute asthma symptoms or exacerbations. Instruct patient about correct use of pMDI or aerolizer inhaler.
Oral albuterol sustained release			Inhaled route is preferred to oral route because LABAs are longer acting and have fewer side effects than oral sustained-release agents	
Phosphodiesterase Inhibitors theophylline sustained-release tablets and capsules		*Indications* Long-term control and prevention of symptoms in mild persistent asthma or as adjunctive with ICS, in moderate or persistent asthma *Mechanisms* Bronchodilation; smooth muscle relaxation from phosphodiesterase inhibition and possibly adenosine antagonism May affect eosinophilic infiltration into bronchial mucosa as well as decreased T-lymphocyte numbers in epithelium Increases diaphragm contractility and mucociliary clearance	Dose-related acute toxicities include tachycardia, nausea and vomiting, tachyarrhythmias (SVT), central nervous system stimulation, headache, seizures, hematemesis, hyperglycemia, and hypokalemia Adverse effects at usual therapeutic doses include insomnia, gastric upset, aggravation of ulcer or reflux, and difficulty in urination in older males who have prostatism Not generally recommended for exacerbations. There is minimal evidence for added benefit to optimal doses of SABA	Maintain steady-state serum concentrations between 5 and 15 mcg/mL. Be aware that absorption and metabolism may be affected by numerous factors that can produce significant changes in steady-state serum theophylline concentrations. Instruct patient to discontinue if toxicity occurs. Serum concentration monitoring is mandatory. Inform patient about the importance of blood tests to monitor serum concentration. Instruct patient to check with primary provider before taking any new medication.

TABLE 20-6	Long-Term Medications for Treatment of Asthma (Controller Medications) (continued)			
Medication	**Dosage Information**	**Indications/Mechanisms**	**Potential Adverse Effects**	**Nursing Considerations**
Combined Medication (Corticosteroid/Long-Acting Beta-2 Adrenergic Agonist)				
fluticasone/ salmeterol	Lowest dose of DPI or HFA used for patients whose asthma is not controlled on low- to medium-dose ICS. Higher doses of DPI or HFA used for patients whose asthma is not controlled on medium- to high-dose ICS	*DPI* 100 mcg/50 mcg 250 mcg/50 mcg 500 mcg/50 mcg *HFA* 45 mcg/21 mcg 115 mcg/21 mcg 230 mcg/21 mcg		
budesonide/ formoterol fluticasone furoate/vilanterol mometasone/ formoterol	Lower dose used for patients who have asthma not controlled on low- to medium-dose ICS. Higher dose used for patients who have asthma not controlled on medium- to high-dose ICS. Used if asthma not controlled on long-term asthma control medication.	*HFA pMDI* 80 mcg/4.5 mcg 160 mcg/4.5 mcg 100 mcg/25 mcg 200 mcg/25 mcg 100 mcg/5 mcg 200 mcg/5 mcg	Do not use with other long-acting beta-agonist drugs	
Leukotriene Modifiers *Leukotriene Receptor Antagonists* montelukast Available in tablets and granules		*Mechanism* Selective competitive inhibitor of CysLT1 receptor *Indications* Long-term control and prevention of symptoms in mild persistent asthma for patients ≥1 year of age May also be used with ICS as combination therapy in moderate persistent asthma	May attenuate EIB in some patients, but less effective than ICS therapy LTRA + LABA should not be used as a substitute for ICS + LABA. Headache, dizziness, upper respiratory infections, pharyngitis, sinusitis	Instruct patient to take at least 1 h before meals or 2 h after meals.
zafirlukast Available in tablets		Long-term control and prevention of symptoms in mild persistent asthma; may also be used with ICS as combination therapy in moderate persistent asthma	Cases of reversible hepatitis have been reported along with rare cases of irreversible hepatic failure resulting in death and liver transplantation	Inform patient that zafirlukast can inhibit the metabolism of warfarin. INRs should be monitored if patient is taking both zafirlukast and montelukast. Instruct patients to discontinue use if they experience signs and symptoms of liver dysfunction (right upper quadrant pain, pruritus, lethargy, jaundice, nausea), and to notify their primary provider.
5-Lipoxygenase Inhibitor zileuton		*Mechanism* Inhibits the production of leukotrienes from arachidonic acid, both LTB and the cysteinyl leukotrienes *Indications* Long-term control and prevention of symptoms in mild persistent asthma for patients May be used with ICS as combination therapy in moderate persistent asthma in patients	Elevation of liver enzymes has been reported. Limited case reports of reversible hepatitis and hyperbilirubinemia	Inform patient that zileuton can inhibit the metabolism of warfarin and theophylline. Therefore, the doses of these medications should be monitored accordingly. Educate patient about the importance of monitoring medication levels and tests of liver function.

(continued on page 638)

TABLE 20-6	Long-Term Medications for Treatment of Asthma (Controller Medications) (continued)			
Medication	**Dosage Information**	**Indications/Mechanisms**	**Potential Adverse Effects**	**Nursing Considerations**
Immunomodulators *IgE-Inhibiting IgG monoclonal antibody* omalizumab Given by subcutaneous injection	Dose is given either every 2 or 4 wks and depends on the patient's body weight and IgE level before therapy A maximum of 150 mg can be given in 1 injection Medication needs to be stored under refrigeration at 2°–8°C (35.6°–46.4°F)	*Indications* Long-term control and prevention of symptoms with moderate or severe persistent allergic asthma inadequately controlled with ICS *Mechanisms* Monoclonal antibody that binds to circulating IgE, preventing it from binding to the high-affinity receptors on basophils and mast cells Decreases mast cell mediator release from allergen exposure	Anaphylaxis has been reported in 0.2% of treated patients Pain, bruising, and skin reactions (itching, redness, stinging) at injection sites It is unknown if patients will develop significant antibody titers to the drug with long-term administration	Monitor patients for allergic reactions or anaphylaxis following administration. Be prepared to initiate emergency treatment if anaphylaxis occurs. Instruct patient about signs and symptoms that indicate allergic reaction and immediate action to take. Remind patient to continue to take other medications prescribed for treatment of asthma.
Interleukin-5 Receptor (IL-5R) Antagonists mepolizumab reslizumab benralizumab Mepolizumab and benralizumab are given by subcutaneous injection. Reslizumab is given by intravenous infusion.		*Indications* Long-term control and prevention of symptoms in patients with severe persistent asthma of eosinophilic phenotype. Mepolizumab and beralizumab are approved for adolescents and adults ≥12 years of age, and reslizumab is approved for adults ≥18 years of age *Mechanisms* Monoclonal antibodies that decrease production and survival of eosinophils by binding to and inhibiting IL-5R. However, the specific mechanism in which these agents exert their effects in asthma has not been definitively established		Ensure the patient understands appropriate administration technique to minimize administration and dosing errors and to optimize patient safety. Note that dose and frequency of administration of biologics may be influenced by various factors such as weight, blood work, or the need for titration. Education is key to adherence and it is important to confirm patient knowledge and understanding.
Interleukin-4 (Receptor Alpha (IL-4Rα) Antagonist dupilumab Given by subcutaneous injection		*Indications* Long-term control and prevention of symptoms in adolescents and adults ≥12 years of age with moderate or severe asthma of eosinophilic phenotype or oral corticosteroid dependent asthma *Mechanisms* Monoclonal antibody that binds to IL-4Rα, a receptor present on various cell types and mediators involved in the inflammatory response, that inhibits **IL-4 and IL-13** cytokine-induced inflammatory responses. However, the specific mechanism in which dupilumab exerts its effects in asthma has not been definitively established		

cyclic AMP, cyclic 3′,5′-adenosine monophosphate; CysLT1, cysteinyl leukotriene receptor 1; DPI, dry-powder inhaler; ECG, electrocardiogram; EIB, exercise-induced bronchospasm; HFA, hydrofluoroalkane; ICS, inhaled corticosteroid; IgE, immunoglobulin E; IgG, immunoglobulin G; INR, international normalized ratio; LABA, long-acting beta-2 adrenergic agonist; LTB, leukotriene B; LTRA, leukotriene receptor antagonist; pMDI, pressurized metered-dose inhaler; SABA, short-acting beta-2 adrenergic agonist; SVT, supraventricular tachycardia.

Adapted from Ferguson, G. T., Stoller, J. K., & Hollingsworth, H. (2019). Management of severe, chronic, obstructive pulmonary disease. *UpToDate.* Retrieved on 7/30/2019 at: www.uptodate.com/contents/management-of-stable-chronic-obstructive-pulmonary-disease; Global Initiative for Asthma (GINA). (2019b). Pocket guide for asthma management. Retrieved on 7/01/2019 at: www.ginasthma.org/wp-content/uploads/2019/04/GINA-2019-main-Pocket-Guide-wms.pdf; Wenzel, S., Bochner, B. S., & Hollingsworth, H. (2019). Treatment of severe asthma in adolescents and adults. *UpToDate.* Retrieved on 7/30/2019 at: www.uptodate.com/contents/treatment-of-severe-asthma-in-adolescents-and-adults

airway. These may be used in patients who do not tolerate short-acting beta-2–adrenergic agonists.

The combination medication ipratropium bromide and albuterol sulfate is used for quick relief of asthma symptoms and acute exacerbations. This medication is administered using a small-volume nebulizer (SVN; discussed previously).

Long-Acting Control Medications

Corticosteroids are the most potent and effective anti-inflammatory medications currently available. They are broadly effective in alleviating symptoms, improving airway function, and decreasing peak flow variability. Initially, an inhaled form is used. All patients should rinse their mouth with water (and should not swallow the rinse) after administration of ICSs to prevent thrush, a common complication associated with the use of these drugs. However, those who lack the coordination to ensure proper administration technique should use a spacer. This will reduce medication deposition within the mouth and further reduce the risk of thrush. A systemic preparation may be used to gain rapid control of the disease; to manage severe, persistent asthma; to treat moderate to severe exacerbations; to accelerate recovery; and to prevent recurrence.

Long-acting beta-2 adrenergic agonists (LABAs) are used with anti-inflammatory medications to control asthma symptoms, particularly those that occur during the night. These agents are also effective in the prevention of exercise-induced asthma. LABAs are not indicated for immediate relief of symptoms. Salmeterol and formoterol have duration of bronchodilation of at least 12 hours. They are used with other medications in long-term control of asthma.

Leukotriene modifiers (inhibitors), or *antileukotrienes*, are a class of medications that include montelukast, zafirlukast, and zileuton. Leukotrienes, which are synthesized from membrane phospholipids through a cascade of enzymes, are potent bronchoconstrictors that also dilate blood vessels and alter permeability. Leukotriene inhibitors act either by interfering with leukotriene synthesis or by blocking the receptors where leukotrienes exert their action. They may provide an alternative to ICSs for mild persistent asthma, or they may be added to a regimen of ICSs in more severe asthma to attain further control.

Phosphodiesterase inhibitors cause bronchodilation and act as mild anti-inflammatory agents by influencing epinephrine release. Theophylline is used as an add-on agent and in conjunction with inhaled steroids; however, it is not as effective in treating asthma as the medications previously discussed. Theophylline should be used with reservation because it has the potential to cause many drug interactions and its higher risk of side effects (GOLD, 2019).

Immunomodulators prevent binding of IgE to the high-affinity receptors of basophils and mast cells. The U.S. Food and Drug Administration (FDA) approved five biologic immunomodulators for the treatment of asthma (omalizumab, mepolizumab, reslizumab, benralizumab, and dupilumab) and several others are in development. Medications in this class are add-on treatments used when patients experience poor symptom control on high-dose inhaled corticosteroids with a LABA (ICS-LABA). These immunomodulators are monoclonal antibodies that are derived from biologic sources and are therefore sometimes referred to as biologics. They help with symptom control by interfering with the inflammatory response that is associated with acute asthmatic episodes (Krings, McGregor, Bacharier, et al., 2019). Cost and patient preference for route of administration must be considered when adding on this treatment (GOLD, 2019). Biologics are either administered subcutaneously or intravenously.

Management of Exacerbations

Asthma exacerbations are best managed by early treatment and education, including the use of written action plans as part of any overall effort to educate patients about self-management techniques, especially those with moderate or severe persistent asthma or with a history of severe exacerbations (GINA, 2019a). GINA (2019a) recommends using an ICS treatment for the prevention of exacerbations in adults. Short-acting beta-2–adrenergic agonist medications are used at the time of the exacerbation for prompt relief of airflow obstruction. Systemic corticosteroids may be necessary to decrease airway inflammation in patients who fail to respond to inhaled beta-adrenergic medications. In some patients, oxygen supplementation may be required to relieve hypoxemia associated with moderate to severe exacerbations. In addition, response to treatment may be monitored by serial measurements of lung function. Patients with persistent symptoms and/or exacerbations may benefit from routinely using ICS-LABA to improve symptom management and prevent the occurrence of exacerbations.

Evidence from clinical trials suggests that antibiotic therapy, whether given routinely or when suspicion of bacterial infection is low, is not beneficial for asthma exacerbations (GINA, 2019a). Antibiotics may be appropriate in the treatment of acute asthma exacerbations in patients who have symptoms of a respiratory infection (e.g., fever and purulent sputum, evidence of pneumonia, suspected bacterial sinusitis).

Despite insufficient data supporting or refuting the benefits of using a written asthma action plan as compared to medical management alone, it is recommended to use a written asthma action plan to educate patients about self-management (Fig. 20-11). Plans can be based on either symptoms or peak flow measurements. They should focus on daily management as well as the recognition and handling of worsening symptoms. Patient self-management and early recognition of problems lead to more efficient communication with health care providers about asthma exacerbations (GINA, 2019a).

Peak Flow Monitoring

Peak flow meters measure the highest airflow during a forced expiration (Fig. 20-12). Daily peak flow monitoring is recommended for patients who meet one or more of the following criteria: have moderate or severe persistent asthma, have poor perception of changes in airflow or worsening symptoms, have unexplained response to environmental or occupational exposures, or at the discretion of the clinician and patient (GINA, 2019a). Peak flow monitoring helps measure asthma severity and, when added to symptom monitoring, indicates the current degree of asthma control.

The patient is instructed in the proper technique (Chart 20-8), particularly about using maximal effort; peak flows are monitored for 2 or 3 weeks after receipt of optimal asthma therapy. Then, the patient's "personal best" value is measured. The green (80% to 100% of personal best), yellow (60% to 80%), and red (less than 60%) zones are determined, and

Asthma Action Plan

For: _____ Doctor: _____ Date: _____
Doctor's Phone Number _____ Hospital/Emergency Department Phone Number _____

GREEN ZONE

Doing Well

- No cough, wheeze, chest tightness, or shortness of breath during the day or night
- Can do usual activites

And, if a peak flow meter is used,
Peak flow: more than _____
(80% or more of my best peak flow)
My best peak flow is: _____

Take these long-term-control medicines each day (include an anti-inflammatory).

Medicine	How much to take	When to take it
_____	_____	_____
_____	_____	_____

Identify and avoid and control the things that make your asthma worse, like (list here):
_____ _____
_____ _____

Before exercise, if prescribed, take: ☐ 2 or ☐ 4 puffs _____ 5 to 60 minutes before exercise

YELLOW ZONE

Asthma Is Getting Worse

- Cough, wheeze, chest tightness, or shortness of breath, or
- Waking at night due to asthma, or
- Can do some, but not all, usual activites

-Or-

Peak flow: _____ to _____
(50% to 79% of my best peak flow)

First Add: quick-relief medicine—and keep taking your GREEN ZONE medicine.

_____ ☐ 2 or ☐ 4 puffs, every 20 minutes for up to 1 hour
(short-acting beta₂-agonist) ☐ Nebulizer, once

If applicable, remove yourself from the thing that made your asthma worse.

Second If your symptoms (and peak flow, if used) return to GREEN ZONE after 1 hour of above treatment:
Continue monitoring to be sure you stay in the green zone.

-Or-

If your symptoms (and peak flow, if used) do not return to GREEN ZONE after 1 hour of above treatment:
☐ Take: _____ ☐ 2 or ☐ 4 puffs or ☐ Nebulizer
(short-acting beta₂-agonist)
☐ Add: _____ mg per day For _____ (3-10) days
(oral corticosteroid)
☐ Call the doctor: _____, ☐ before/☐ within _____ hours after taking the oral corticosteroid.
(phone)

RED ZONE

Medical Alert!

- Very short of breath, or
- Quick-relief medicines have not helped, or
- Cannot do usual activites, or
- Symptoms are same or get worse after 24 hours in Yellow Zone

-Or-

Peak flow: less than _____
(50% of my best peak flow)

Take this medicine:

☐ _____ ☐ 4 or ☐ 6 puffs or ☐ Nebulizer
(short-acting beta₂-agonist)
☐ _____ mg
(oral corticosteroid)

Then call your doctor NOW. Go to the hospital or call an ambulance if:
- You are still in the red zone after 15 minutes AND
- You have not reached your doctor.

DANGER SIGNS
- **Trouble walking and talking due to shortness of breath**
- **Lips or fingernails are blue**

- **Take** ☐4 or ☐6 puffs of your quick-relief medicine AND
- **Go to the hospital or call for an ambulance** _____ NOW!
(phone)

Figure 20-11 • Asthma action plan. Adapted from National Heart, Lung, and Blood Institute (NHLBI). (2012). Asthma care quick reference: Diagnosing and managing asthma. NIH Publication No. 12–5075. Revised September 2012.

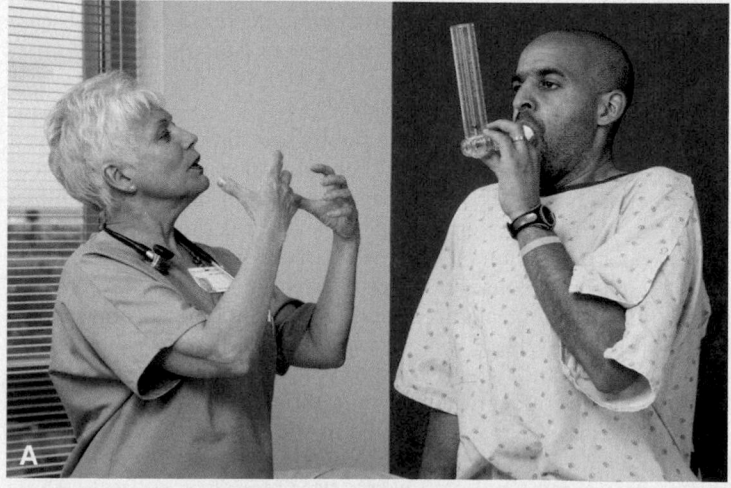
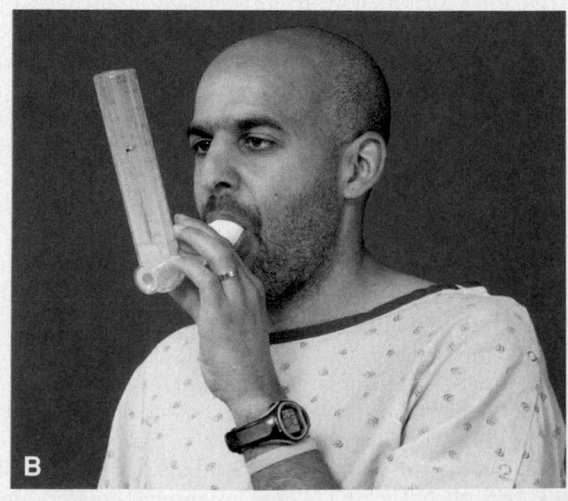

Figure 20-12 • Peak flow meters measure the highest volume of airflow during a forced expiration. The patient takes a deep breath and places lips around the mouthpiece (**A**), and then exhales hard and fast (**B**). Volume may be measured in color-coded zones: the green zone signifies 80% to 100% of personal best; yellow, 60% to 80%; and red, less than 60%. If peak flow falls below the red zone, the patient should take the appropriate actions prescribed by the patient's primary provider.

Chart 20-8 HOME CARE CHECKLIST
Use of Peak Flow Meter in Asthma Management

At the completion of education, the patient and/or caregiver will be able to:

- Describe the rationale for using a peak flow meter in asthma management.
- Explain how peak flow monitoring is used along with symptoms to determine severity of asthma.
- Demonstrate steps for using the peak flow meter correctly.
  1. Move the indicator to the bottom of the numbered scale.
  2. Stand up.
  3. Take a deep breath, and fill the lungs completely.
  4. Place mouthpiece in mouth, and close lips around mouthpiece. (Do not put tongue inside opening.)
  5. Blow out hard and fast with a single blow.

6. Record the number achieved on the indicator. If patient coughs or a mistake is made in the process, do it again.
7. Repeat steps 1–5 two more times, and write the highest number in the asthma diary.
- Explain how to determine the "personal best" peak flow reading.
- Describe the significance of the color zones for peak flow monitoring.
- Demonstrate how to clean the peak flow meter.
- Discuss how and when to contact the primary provider about changes or decreases in peak flow values.

---

specific actions are delineated for each zone, enabling the patient to monitor and manipulate their own therapy after careful instruction (GINA, 2019a).

GINA (2019a) recommends that peak flow monitoring be considered an adjunct to asthma management for patients with moderate to severe persistent asthma. Peak flow monitoring plans may enhance communication between the patient and health care providers and may increase the patient's awareness of disease status and control.

Nursing Management

The immediate nursing care of patients with asthma depends on the severity of symptoms. The patient may be treated successfully as an outpatient if asthma symptoms are relatively mild or may require hospitalization and intensive care if symptoms are acute and severe. The patient and family are often frightened and anxious because of the patient's dyspnea. Therefore, a calm approach is an important aspect of care. The nurse assesses the patient's respiratory status by monitoring the severity of symptoms, breath sounds, peak flow, pulse oximetry, and vital signs.

The nurse generally performs the following interventions:
- Obtains a history of allergic reactions to medications before administering medications.
- Identifies medications the patient is taking.
- Administers medications as prescribed and monitors the patient's responses to those medications. These medications may include an antibiotic if the patient has an underlying respiratory infection.
- Administers fluids if the patient is dehydrated.

If the patient requires intubation because of acute respiratory failure, the nurse assists with the intubation procedure, continues close monitoring of the patient, and keeps the patient and family informed about procedures. (See Chapter 19 for discussion of intubation and mechanical ventilation.)

Promoting Home, Community-Based, and Transitional Care

Implementation of basic asthma management principles at the community level is a major challenge. Strategies include education of health care providers, establishment of programs for asthma education (for patients and providers), the use of outpatient follow-up care for patients, and a focus on chronic management versus acute episodic care. Nurses are pivotal to achievement of these objectives.

 ### Educating Patients About Self-Care

Patient education is a critical component of care for patients with asthma. Multiple inhalers, different types of inhalers, antiallergy therapy, antireflux medications, and avoidance measures are essential for long-term control. This complex therapy requires a partnership between the patient and the health care providers to determine the desired outcomes and to formulate a plan to achieve those outcomes. The patient then carries out daily therapy as part of self-care management, with input and guidance by their health care providers. Before a partnership can be established, the patient must understand the following:
- Nature of asthma as a chronic inflammatory disease
- Definitions of inflammation and bronchoconstriction
- Purpose and action of each medication
- Triggers to avoid and how to avoid them
- Proper inhalation technique
- How to perform peak flow monitoring (see Chart 20-8)
- How to implement an asthma action plan (see Fig. 20-11)
- When to seek assistance, and how to do so

An assortment of excellent educational materials is available from the National Heart, Lung, and Blood Institute and other sources (see Resources section at the end of the chapter). The nurse should obtain current educational materials for the patient based on the patient's diagnosis, causative factors, educational level, and cultural background. If a patient has a coexisting sensory impairment (i.e., vision loss or hearing impairment), materials should be provided in an alternative format.

Continuing and Transitional Care

Nurses who have contact with patients with asthma in any setting use the opportunity to assess the patient's respiratory status and ability to manage self-care to prevent serious exacerbations. Nurses emphasize adherence to the prescribed therapy, preventive measures, and the need to keep follow-up appointments with health care providers. Home visits to assess the home environment for allergens may be indicated for patients with recurrent exacerbations. Nurses refer patients to community support groups. In addition, nurses remind patients and families about the importance of health promotion strategies and recommended health screening.

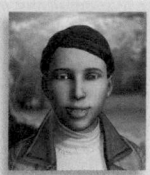

Jennifer Hoffman is a 33-year-old woman diagnosed with asthma in childhood. She has come to the clinic multiple times over the last 2 mo complaining of continued symptoms. Her asthma action plan was adjusted by her primary provider last month. What measures can the nurse take to determine areas needing education reinforcement? How can the nurse ensure that Jennifer is accurately following the prescribed asthma regimen and monitoring medication effectiveness? (Jennifer Hoffman's story continues in Chapter 33.)

Care for Jennifer and other patients in a realistic virtual environment: **vSim** *for Nursing* (**thepoint.lww. com/vSimMedicalSurgical**). Practice documenting these patients' care in DocuCare (**thepoint.lww.com/ DocuCareEHR**).

 ## Status Asthmaticus

An asthma exacerbation can range from mild to severe with potential respiratory arrest (GINA, 2019a). The term *status asthmaticus* is sometimes used to describe rapid onset, severe, and persistent asthma that does not respond to conventional therapy. The attacks can occur with little or no warning and can progress rapidly to asphyxiation. Infection, anxiety, inhaler abuse, dehydration, increased adrenergic blockage, and non-specific irritants may contribute to these episodes. An acute episode may be precipitated by hypersensitivity to medications, such as aspirin, beta-blockers, and nonsteroidal anti-inflammatory drugs (NSAIDs) (American Academy of Allergy, Asthma & Immunology [AAAAI], 2019; GOLD, 2019).

Pathophysiology

The basic characteristics of asthma (inflammation of bronchial mucosa, constriction of the bronchiolar smooth muscle, and thickened secretions) decrease the diameter of the bronchi and occur in status asthmaticus. The most common scenario is severe bronchospasm, with mucus plugging leading to asphyxia. A ventilation–perfusion abnormality results in hypoxemia. There is a reduced PaO_2 and initial respiratory alkalosis, with a decreased $PaCO_2$ and an increased pH. As status asthmaticus worsens, the $PaCO_2$ increases and the pH decreases, reflecting respiratory acidosis.

Clinical Manifestations

The clinical manifestations are the same as those seen in severe asthma; signs and symptoms include labored breathing, prolonged exhalation, distended neck veins, and wheezing. However, the extent of wheezing does not indicate the severity of the attack. As the obstruction worsens, the wheezing may disappear; this is frequently a sign of impending respiratory failure.

Assessment and Diagnostic Findings

The severity of an exacerbation may be evaluated by a general assessment of the patient (degree of breathlessness, ability to talk, positioning of patient, level of alertness or cognitive function), physical assessment (respiratory rate, the use of accessory muscles, presence of central cyanosis, auscultatory findings, pulse, and pulsus paradoxus), and laboratory evaluation (peak expiratory flow after a bronchodilator, PaO_2 and $PaCO_2$, and pulse oximetry). Pulmonary function studies are the most accurate means of assessing an acute, severe airway obstruction, though not practical to obtain during this type of an emergent situation. Arterial blood gas measurement and/ or pulse oximetry are obtained if the patient cannot perform pulmonary function maneuvers because of severe obstruction or fatigue, or if the patient does not respond to treatment. Respiratory alkalosis (low $PaCO_2$) is the most common early finding in patients with an ongoing asthma exacerbation and is due to hyperventilation. At this early stage, relatively fewer acinar units (i.e., pulmonary alveolar units where gas exchange occurs) are obstructed/constricted compared to those that are functional, and hyperventilation occurs as part of the sympathetic response.

 Quality and Safety Nursing Alert

In status asthmaticus, increasing $PaCO_2$ (to normal levels or levels indicating respiratory acidosis) is a danger sign signifying impending respiratory failure.

Medical Management

Close monitoring of the patient and objective reevaluation for response to therapy are key in status asthmaticus. In the emergency setting, the patient is treated initially with a short-acting beta-2–adrenergic agonist and subsequently a short course of systemic corticosteroids, especially if the patient does not respond to the short-acting beta-2–adrenergic agonist. Corticosteroids are critical in the therapy of status asthmaticus and are used to decrease the intense airway inflammation and swelling. Inhaled short-acting beta-2–adrenergic agonists provide the most rapid relief from bronchospasm. A pMDI, with or without a spacer, may be used for administering the medications. However, more commonly, short-acting bronchodilators will be given via an SVN. A mouthpiece or facemask can be used and the bronchodilator is continuously given to the patient. The patient does not have to work to coordinate the breathing pattern, which can otherwise cause additional anxiety in this acute situation. The patient requires supplemental oxygen and IV fluids for hydration. Oxygen therapy is initiated to treat dyspnea, central cyanosis, and hypoxemia. High-flow supplemental oxygen is best delivered using a partial or complete non-rebreathing mask. Sedatives are contraindicated. Magnesium sulfate, a calcium antagonist, may be given to induce smooth muscle relaxation; the magnesium can relax smooth muscle and hence cause bronchodilation by competing with calcium at calcium-mediated smooth muscle–binding sites. IV magnesium sulfate is not recommended for routine use in asthma exacerbations; however, when given as a single 2-g infusion over 20 minutes, it may be helpful in treating patients who present with severely compromised pulmonary function, who have not responded to initial therapy, and with persistent hypoxemia (GINA, 2019a). Adverse effects of magnesium sulfate may include facial warmth, flushing, tingling, nausea, central nervous system depression, respiratory depression, and hypotension.

If there is no response to repeated treatments, hospitalization is required. Other criteria for hospitalization include poor pulmonary function test results and deteriorating blood gas levels (respiratory acidosis), which may indicate that the patient is tiring and will require mechanical ventilation. Most patients do not need mechanical ventilation, but it is used for patients in respiratory failure, for those who tire and are too fatigued by the attempt to breathe, and for those whose condition does not respond to initial treatment.

For a very select group of patients with uncontrolled severe asthma, bronchial thermoplasty may be considered. Bronchial thermoplasty is the first nondrug therapy for the treatment of severe, uncontrolled asthma. It consists of controlled radiofrequency heating of the central airways through a bronchoscope. The thermal energy reduces the amount of smooth muscle involved in bronchospasm and potentially decreases the severity and frequency of symptoms. This therapy is invasive and relatively new; therefore, only select centers have the ability to perform this procedure, and it should only be considered in a select group of patients (GINA, 2019a).

Death from asthma is associated with several risk factors, including the following (GINA, 2019a):

- Past history of severe exacerbation (e.g., intubation or intensive care unit admission)
- Hospitalizations or emergency care visits for asthma within the past year
- Currently or having recently stopped using oral corticosteroids
- Not using ICSs
- Overuse of SABAs
- Concurrent psychiatric disease or psychosocial problems
- Poor adherence to written asthma action plan
- Poor adherence to medication regimen
- Presence of a food allergy

Nursing Management

The main focus of nursing management is to actively assess the airway and the patient's response to treatment. The nurse should be prepared for the next intervention if the patient does not respond to treatment.

The nurse vigilantly monitors the patient for the first 12 to 24 hours, or until the severe exacerbation resolves. The nurse also assesses the patient's skin turgor for signs of dehydration. Fluid intake is essential to combat dehydration, to loosen secretions, and to facilitate expectoration. Nurses administer IV fluids as prescribed, up to 3 to 4 L/day, unless contraindicated. Blood pressure and cardiac rhythm should be monitored continuously during the acute phase and until the patient stabilizes and responds to therapy. The patient's energy needs to be conserved, and his or her room should be quiet and free of respiratory irritants, including flowers, tobacco smoke, perfumes, or odors of cleaning agents. Nonallergenic pillows should be used. An asthma attack may also be precipitated or aggravated by exposure to latex if the patient has a latex allergy; therefore, this type of hypersensitivity must be identified and latex-free products used, as warranted.

Once the exacerbation is resolved, the factors that precipitated the exacerbation should be identified and strategies for their future avoidance implemented. In addition, the patient's medication plan should be reviewed.

Cystic Fibrosis

CF is the most common fatal autosomal recessive disease among Caucasians. It is less frequently found among Hispanic, Asian, and African Americans. A person must inherit a defective copy of the CF gene (one from each parent) to have CF. Each year, 1000 new cases of CF are diagnosed, and more than 75% of patients are diagnosed by 2 years of age (Cystic Fibrosis Foundation [CFF], 2019a). In 2010, over 50% of people with CF in the United States were diagnosed with newborn screening (Heltshe, Cogen, Ramos, et al., 2017). Approximately 30,000 children and adults in the United States have CF and half are over the age of 18. CF was once a fatal childhood disease; however, the median expected survival age is now 37 (National Institutes of Health, 2018). Furthermore, survival age is projected to rise to 57 years if the survival rate continues to improve 1.8% per year (Heltshe et al., 2017). The improved survival rate is due to advances in medical management and procedures such as lung transplantation. Now that the median survival age has increased to 37 years for patients with CF, issues that were not present in past generations have arisen. These issues include antibiotic resistance and the desire for patients with CF to have their own biologic children.

Although most patients are diagnosed by 2 years of age, this disease may not be diagnosed until later in life (CFF, 2019b). Respiratory symptoms are frequently the major manifestation of CF when it is diagnosed later in life. These patients will not demonstrate the classic symptoms of CF, which may potentially cause a diagnostic dilemma.

Pathophysiology

CF is caused by mutations or dysfunction in the protein cystic fibrosis transmembrane conductance regulator (CFTR), which normally transports chloride ions across epithelial cell membranes. Gene mutations affect transport of these ions, leading to CF, which is characterized by thick, viscous secretions in the lungs, pancreas, liver, intestine, and reproductive tract as well as increased salt content in sweat gland secretions. The most common mutation is ΔF508; however, researchers have identified more than 1700 mutations of the disease (CFF, 2019a). The numerous mutations of the CFTR gene create multiple variations in the presentation and progression of the disease.

The ability to detect the common mutations of this gene allows for routine screening for CF and the detection of carriers of the disease. Genetic counseling is an important part of health care for couples at risk (see Chapter 6). People who are heterozygous for CF (i.e., have one defective gene and one normal gene) do not have the disease but can be carriers and pass the defective gene on to their children. If both parents are carriers, their risk of having a child with CF is one in four (25%) with each pregnancy. Any biologic offspring of a patient with CF will have CF. Genetic testing should be offered to adults with a positive family history of CF and to partners of people with CF who are planning a pregnancy or seeking prenatal counseling. The hallmark pathology of CF is bronchial mucus plugging, inflammation, and eventual bronchiectasis. Commonly, the bronchiectasis begins in the upper lobes and progresses to involve all lobes.

Clinical Manifestations

The pulmonary manifestations of CF include a productive cough, wheezing, hyperinflation of the lung fields on chest x-ray, and pulmonary function test results consistent with obstructive disease of the airways. Chronic respiratory inflammation and infection are caused by impaired mucus clearance. Colonization of the airways with pathogenic bacteria usually occurs early in life. *S. aureus* and *H. influenzae* are common organisms during early childhood. As the disease progresses, *P. aeruginosa* is ultimately isolated from the sputum of most patients (Simon, Mallory, & Hoppin, 2019b). Upper respiratory manifestations of the disease include sinusitis and nasal polyps. Pulmonary complications of CF are the primary cause of morbidity and mortality in the United States (Simon, Mallory, & Hoppin, 2019a).

Nonpulmonary manifestations include gastrointestinal problems (e.g., pancreatic insufficiency, recurrent abdominal pain, biliary cirrhosis, vitamin deficiencies, recurrent pancreatitis, weight loss), CF-related diabetes, and genitourinary problems (male and female infertility). (See Chapter 44 for a discussion of pancreatitis.)

Assessment and Diagnostic Findings

The diagnosis of CF requires a clinical picture consistent with the CF phenotype and laboratory evidence of CFTR dysfunction. Key assessment findings in adults include (Katkin, Mallory, & Hoppin, 2019):

- Chronic sinopulmonary disease as manifested by chronic cough and sputum production, persistent infection consistent with typical CF pathogens, and x-ray evidence of bronchiectasis and chronic sinusitis, often with nasal polyps
- Gastrointestinal tract and nutritional abnormalities (pancreatic insufficiency, recurrent pancreatitis, biliary cirrhosis and portal hypertension, CF-related diabetes)
- Male urogenital problems as manifested by congenital bilateral absence of the vas deferens; reduced female fertility

Medical Management

CF requires both acute and chronic therapy. Cornerstones of treatment include multimodal antibiotic regimens, airway clearance measures, bronchodilators, CFTR modulators, nutritional support, and exercise (Simon et al., 2019a). Multimodal antibiotic regimens use different types of antibiotics and routes (oral, inhaled, and IV) to help control, suppress, and treat exacerbation of bacterial infections. Airway clearance measures entail the use of the mucolytics (e.g., dornase alfa; see later discussion), inhaled hypertonic saline, and various pulmonary techniques that promote mucus expectoration.

Because chronic infection (viral and bacterial) of the airways occurs in CF, control of infections is essential to treatment. It is best to prevent viral infections. Administering viral influenza vaccinations is essential for CF patients. Due to the increased risk of viral influenza, some CF patients may benefit from prophylactic treatment with a neuraminidase inhibitor (e.g., zanamivir, oseltamivir) (Simon et al., 2019a).

Bacterial infection requires aggressive therapy to improve airway clearance and the use of antibiotics based on results of sputum cultures. The majority of patients are colonized with *P. aeruginosa*; however, *S. aureus*, methicillin-resistant *Staphylococcus aureus*, and *Burkholderia cepacia* complex are examples of other commonly found pathogens (Simon et al., 2019b).

Chronic infection with *P. aeruginosa* is an independent risk factor for accelerated loss of lung function and decreased survival (Simon et al., 2019b). *P. aeruginosa* is also common in CF exacerbations and new strains may develop with recurring infections leading to different antibiotic-resistance profiles (Simon et al., 2019b). As CF patients are living longer and experiencing more exacerbations, antibiotic resistance is becoming a serious concern and can affect life expectancy.

B. cepacia complex consists of different species of bacteria. Infection with *B. cepacia* complex, in general, is associated with poor outcomes in CF patients as a result of the bacteria's inherent antibiotic resistance. Infection with this complex may prevent a CF patient from becoming a lung transplant candidate (Hachem, 2019).

Routine cultures of respiratory secretions are used to identify organisms and guide antibiotic selection. Two IV antibiotics have been typically prescribed to treat a severe exacerbation of *P. aeruginosa*. Tobramycin, along with piperacillin-tazobactam, a third-generation cephalosporin (e.g., ceftizoxime, ceftazidime), a carbapenem (e.g., meropenem, aztreonam) may be prescribed (Simon et al., 2019b). Three newer combination medications, ceftazidime and avibactam, meropenem and vaborbactam, and ceftolozane and tazobactam, unite commonly known antibiotics with a beta-lactamase inhibitor to counteract bacterial resistance. Dosing of antibiotics is determined on a case-by-case basis; some patients may require higher doses or an extended IV infusion. When methicillin-resistant *S. aureus* accompanies *P. aeruginosa*, vancomycin is administered in addition to dual IV antibiotic therapy (Simon et al., 2019b). Careful monitoring is always required to minimize any side effects of the antibiotics.

Maintenance oral antibiotic therapies are sometimes employed to help suppress infections caused by other common bacteria such as methicillin-sensitive *S. aureus*. These infections vary across patients and require individualized patient care. The antibiotic regimens used vary depending on the specific organism grown and severity of infection.

Inhaled antibiotics are mainly used to treat *P. aeruginosa*. Tobramycin is the first-line inhaled antibiotic choice but aztreonam can be used as an alternative treatment. Typically, these antibiotics are used on a 28-day on and 28-day off regimen. Patients with deteriorating lung function or recurrent exacerbations may use these antibiotics by rotating courses of inhaled tobramycin and aztreonam without implementing a 28-day off period (Simon, Mallory, & Hoppin, 2019c). Although there is no general consensus on the use of inhaled colistimethate sodium, this drug can be used with patients who do not respond well with the other inhaled antibiotics (Simon et al., 2019c).

Various pulmonary techniques are used to promote airway clearance through the expectoration of secretions. Examples include CPT with manual postural drainage; HFCWO; autogenic drainage (a combination of breathing techniques at different lung volume levels to move the secretions to where they can be huff-coughed out); and other devices that assist in airway clearance, such as masks that generate positive expiratory pressure (PEP masks) and flutter valves (devices that provide an oscillatory expiratory pressure pattern with PEP and assist with expectoration of secretions). It is important to assure that the patient is properly positioned when using the flutter valve and that the patient uses proper technique with this treatment.

Dornase alfa is a nebulized medication given to degrade the large amount of deoxyribonucleic acid (DNA) that accumulates within CF mucus. This agent helps decrease the viscosity of the sputum and promotes expectoration of secretions. It is recommended for patients with moderate to severe disease (severity of lung disease classification is based on predicted FEV_1 percentage). In addition, inhaled hypertonic saline may be used in the chronic treatment of CF. Inhalations increase hydration of the airway surface liquid in patients with CF and improve airway clearance.

Nebulized and IV antibiotics or a combination may be used to treat chronic colonization of the lung. Nebulization provides high intrapulmonary drug concentrations and minimal systemic absorption. Inhaled tobramycin or aztreonam have been shown to decrease the frequency of pulmonary exacerbations. Acute infections are treated with a variety of IV antibiotics. Such infections remain a major cause of mortality related to pulmonary exacerbations in adults with CF.

Other therapeutic measures may be necessary as well. Anti-inflammatory agents may be used to treat inflammatory response in the airways. There is insufficient evidence for the use of routine inhaled or oral corticosteroids (Simon et al., 2019b). IV corticosteroids are used during acute exacerbations and only for those patients with asthmalike symptoms (Simon et al., 2019b). Inhaled bronchodilators (e.g., salmeterol, tiotropium bromide) may be used in patients who have a significant bronchoconstrictive component; this is confirmed by spirometry before and after therapy is instituted (Simon et al., 2019c).

Pancreatic exocrine insufficiency occurs frequently in people with CF and requires oral pancreatic enzyme supplementation with meals (Katkin, Baker, & Baker, 2019). Given the fat malabsorption in CF and increased caloric needs due to the work of breathing, nutritional counseling and weight monitoring are extremely important. Supplements of fat-soluble vitamins A, D, E, and K are also used.

CFTR modulators are a class of drugs that help prevent the progression of CF (Simon et al., 2019c). These agents are novel in that they aim to address the cause of CF as opposed to treating symptoms. There are two classes of modulators used in treating CF: potentiators (help salt and water flow through the CFTR protein channel at the cell surface) and correctors (help the CFTR protein to form the right 3D shape so that it is able to move to the cell surface). The selection of the CFTR modulator depends on the patient's specific CFTR mutation and the patient's age (Simon et al., 2019a).

Ivacaftor, a potentiator, improves salt and water movement across the membrane (thus improving hydration and clearing of mucus from the airways). The drug does not correct the gene mutation; it only helps in the movement of salt and water across the membrane. Monotherapy of ivacaftor is approved for patients with CF who are 6 months of age and older (Simon et al., 2019c).

Although corrector drugs (e.g., lumacaftor, tezacaftor) help the CFTR protein reach the cell surface, they do not diminish CF symptoms because the proteins that do reach the cell surface are unable to improve the flow of salt and water across the cell membrane. This is why lumacaftor and tezacaftor are used in combination with ivacaftor. Combined, these drugs can modestly improve lung function and reduce CF exacerbations (Simon et al., 2019c). Lumacaftor-ivacaftor

is approved for patients 2 years of age and older, but is only recommended for treating patients age 2 to 5. Tezacaftor-ivacaftor is the preferred treatment for patients 6 years of age and older because it produces fewer side effects and drug–drug interactions than lumacaftor-ivacaftor (Simon et al., 2019c).

Currently, a triple combination of tezacaftor-ivacaftor with an additional CFTR corrector is being investigated for treating various CFTR mutations. One such medication, elexacaftor-tezacaftor-ivacaftor, completed phase 3 clinical trials and is being reviewed by the FDA to treat patients with CF age 12 years and older. This drug improves ΔF508 CFTR protein processing, trafficking, and function (Simon et al., 2019c). The goal of these new modulators is to improve the functionality of the CFTR and restore chloride transport at the cellular level, thus decreasing symptoms and complications related to the disease. These positive effects include less viscous mucus production, decreased exacerbation frequency, and improved nutrient absorption.

As the pulmonary deterioration advances, supplemental oxygen is used to treat the progressive hypoxemia that occurs with CF. It helps correct the hypoxemia and may minimize the complications seen with chronic hypoxemia (pulmonary hypertension). Lung transplantation is an option for a small, select population of patients with CF. A double-lung transplantation technique is used because of chronic infection of both lungs in end-stage CF. Because there is a long waiting list for lung transplants, many patients die while waiting for suitable lungs for transplantation.

Nursing Management

Nursing management is crucial to the interdisciplinary approach required for care of adults with CF. Nursing care includes helping patients manage pulmonary symptoms and prevent complications. Specific measures include strategies that promote removal of pulmonary secretions, CPT (including postural drainage, chest percussion, and vibration), and breathing exercises (which are implemented and taught to the patient and family when the patient is very young). The patient is reminded of the need to reduce risk factors associated with respiratory infections (e.g., exposure to crowds or to people with known infections). In addition, the patient is taught the early signs and symptoms of respiratory infection and disease progression that indicate the need to notify a primary provider.

The nurse emphasizes the importance of an adequate fluid and dietary intake to promote removal of secretions and to ensure an adequate nutritional status. Because CF is a lifelong disorder, patients often have learned to modify their daily activities to accommodate their symptoms and treatment modalities. As the disease progresses, periodic reassessment of the home environment may be warranted to identify modifications required to address changes in the patient's needs, increasing dyspnea and fatigue, and nonpulmonary symptoms.

As with any chronic disease, palliative care and end-of-life issues and concerns need to be addressed with the patient when warranted. For the patient whose disease is progressing and who is developing increasing hypoxemia, preferences for end-of-life care should be discussed, documented, and honored (see Chapter 13). Patients and family members require support as they face a shortened lifespan and an uncertain future (Tomaszek, Debska, Cepuch, et al., 2019).

CRITICAL THINKING EXERCISES

1 `ipc` A 55-year-old man presented to the ED with complaints of acute shortness of breath and difficulty breathing. SpO_2 on admission to the ED was 85% on room air. His admitting diagnosis was acute exacerbation of COPD. He was admitted to a general medicine unit, and arrived to his room on 4 L of O_2 via nasal cannula. During his admission assessment, the patient tells you that he works in the coal mines and his shift supervisor had to bring him to the hospital. He also states that he has a long history of smoking 1 to 2 packs of cigarettes per day and his attempts to quit have been unsuccessful. While conducting the assessment, you note that the patient has a productive cough and is becoming confused to time. What is your priority as you admit this patient? What information would you provide the primary provider? What tests might be ordered to help further evaluate the patient's condition? What information would you need to ask the patient to plan for a home discharge? What health care team members would you consult to plan for a home discharge?

2 `pq` A 20-year-old male with a history of asthma presents to the ED with severe shortness of breath and dyspnea at rest. He said he had a cold last week and was coughing up clear sputum. This morning he began expectorating yellow sputum and became increasingly short of breath. He used his rescue inhaler with little relief. Before he came to the ED, he used his rescue inhaler every half hour. Upon presentation to ED triage, his SpO_2 was 90% on room air, but is now 84% on room air. Physical examination reveals tachycardia at 136 bpm, cyanotic lips, and tachypnea at 30 breaths/min with signs of accessory muscle use. When asked about his asthma medications, he admits he only uses his prescribed daily inhaler once a day because it is too expensive. He also stated his primary provider gave him a breathing machine for medicine but he did not know how to use it. What is your priority of care? What evidence-based medical and nursing interventions would improve the patient's respiratory status? What educational needs does this patient have?

3 `ebp` A 25-year-old woman is hospitalized for CF. She was admitted for elevated temperature and weight loss. At the time of admission, she was not using oxygen therapy at home. She was working full-time in a department store prior to this exacerbation. She told the social worker yesterday that she is afraid she will have to quit her job and will lose her health insurance. Her husband, who is unemployed, is also dependent on her for health insurance. Today, she is unable to eat due to the severe dyspnea. Physical assessment reveals SpO_2 of 87% on 2 L of O_2 via nasal cannula, bilateral crackles with severely diminished breath sounds on the right, and expectoration of thick yellow sputum. What evidence-based interventions might be used to alleviate her CF symptoms? Identify the criteria used to evaluate the strength of the evidence for these practices.

REFERENCES

*Asterisk indicates nursing research.

Books

Cairo, J. M. (2018). *Mosby's respiratory care equipment* (10th ed.). St. Louis, MO: Elsevier Mosby.

Kacmarek, R. M., Stoller, J. K., & Heuer, A. J. (2017). *Egan's fundamentals of respiratory care* (11th ed.). St. Louis, MO: Elsevier.

McCance, K. L., & Huether, S. E. (2019). *Pathophysiology: The biologic basis for disease in adults and children* (5th ed.). St. Louis, MO: Elsevier.

Meiner, S. E., & Yeager, J. J. (2019). *Gerontologic nursing* (6th ed.). St. Louis, MO: Elsevier Mosby.

U.S. Department of Health & Human Services (HHS). (2014). *The health consequences of smoking—50 years of progress: A report of the Surgeon General*. Atlanta, GA: U.S. Department of Health & Human Services, Centers for Disease Control and Prevention, National Center for Chronic Disease Prevention and Health Promotion, Office on Smoking and Health.

U.S. Department of Health & Human Services (HHS). (2016). *E-cigarette use among youth and young adults. A report of the Surgeon General*. Atlanta, GA: U.S. Department of Health & Human Services, Centers for Disease Control and Prevention, National Center for Chronic Disease Prevention and Health Promotion, Office on Smoking and Health.

Journals and Electronic Documents

Agency for Healthcare Research and Quality (AHRQ). (2016). *Principle rank order of ICD-10-CM codes (ICD10) principle diagnosis by number* [Data file]. Retrieved on 7/19/2019 at: www.hcupnet.ahrq.gov/#setup

American Academy of Allergy, Asthma & Immunology (AAAAI). (2019). Asthma triggers and management. Retrieved on 7/19/2019 at: www.aaaai.org/conditions-and-treatments/library/asthma-library/asthma-triggers-and-management

Barker, A. F., King, T. E., & Hollingsworth, H. H. (2019). Treatment of bronchiectasis in adults. *UpToDate*. Retrieved on 10/26/2019 at: www.uptodate.com/contents/treatment-of-bronchiectasis-in-adults

Barker, A. F., Stoller, J. K., King, T. E., et al. (2018). Clinical manifestations and diagnosis of bronchiectasis in adults. *UpToDate*. Retrieved on 7/26/2019 at: www.uptodate.com/contents/clinical-manifestations-and-diagnosis-of-bronchiectasis-in-adults

Bartlett, J. G., & Sethi, S. (2018). Management of infection in exacerbations of chronic obstructive pulmonary disease. *UpToDate*. Retrieved on 11/18/2019 at: www.uptodate.com/contents/management-of-infection-in-exacerbations-of-chronic-obstructive-pulmonary-disease

Behar, R. Z., Wang, Y., & Talbot, P. (2018). Comparing the cytotoxicity of electronic cigarette fluids, aerosols, and solvents. *Tobacco Control*, 27(3), 325–333.

*Bove, D. G., Midtgaard, G., Kaldan, D., et al. (2017). Home-based COPD psychoeducation: A qualitative study of the patients' experiences. *Journal of Psychosomatic Research*, 98, 71–77.

Canistro, D., Vivarelli, F., Cirillo, S., et al. (2017). E-cigarettes induce toxicological effects that can raise the cancer risk. *Scientific Reports*, 7(1), 1–9.

Centers for Disease Control and Prevention (CDC). (2015). Asthma: Data, statistics, and surveillance. Retrieved on 7/19/2019 at: www.cdc.gov/asthma/asthmadata.htm

Centers for Disease Control and Prevention (CDC). (2017a). Chronic obstructive pulmonary disease (COPD): Includes: Chronic bronchitis and emphysema. Retrieved on 6/23/2019 at: www.cdc.gov/nchs/fastats/copd.htm

Centers for Disease Control and Prevention (CDC). (2017b). Summary health statistics: National Health Interview Survey, 2017. Retrieved on 7/13/2019 at: ftp.cdc.gov/pub/Health_Statistics/NCHS/NHIS/SHS/2017_SHS_Table_A-2.pdf

Centers for Disease Control and Prevention (CDC). (2018a). Health, United States, 2017—data finder. Retrieved on 6/23/2019 at: www.cdc.gov/nchs/hus/contents2017.htm?search=Chronic_lower_respiratory_diseases

Centers for Disease Control and Prevention (CDC). (2018b). Current cigarette smoking among adults—United States, 2017. *Morbidity and Mortality Weekly Report*, 67(44), 1225–1232.

Centers for Disease Control and Prevention (CDC). (2018c). QuickStats: Percentage of all emergency department (ED) visits made by patients with asthma, by sex and age group. *Morbidity and Mortality Weekly Report*, 67(167), 1225–1232.

Centers for Disease Control and Prevention (CDC). (2019a). Fast facts: Diseases and death. Retrieved on 6/30/2019 at: www.cdc.gov/tobacco/data_statistics/fact_sheets/fast_facts/index.htm

Centers for Disease Control and Prevention (CDC). (2019b). Economic trends in tobacco. Retrieved on 6/30/2019 at: www.cdc.gov/tobacco/data_statistics/fact_sheets/economics/econ_facts/index.htm

Cystic Fibrosis Foundation (CFF). (2019a). About cystic fibrosis. Retrieved on 7/25/2019 at: www.cff.org/What-is-CF/About-Cystic-Fibrosis

Cystic Fibrosis Foundation (CFF). (2019b). Late diagnosis. Retrieved on 7/25/2019 at: www.cysticfibrosis.ca/about-cf/living-with-cystic-fibrosis/adults/late-diagnosis

D'Urzo, A., Chapman, K. R., Donohue, J. F., et al. (2019). Inhaler devices for delivery of LABA/LAMA fixed-dose combinations in patients with COPD. *Pulmonary Therapy*, 5(1), 23–41.

Evans, C. M., Burton, F., & Schwartz, M. D. (2018). E-cigarettes: Mucus measurements make marks. *American Journal of Respiratory and Critical Care Medicine*, 197(4), 420–422.

Ferguson, G. T., Stoller, J. K., & Hollingsworth, H. (2019). Management of severe, chronic, obstructive pulmonary disease. *UpToDate*. Retrieved on 7/30/2019 at: www.uptodate.com/contents/management-of-stable-chronic-obstructive-pulmonary-disease

Garcia-Arcos, I., Geraghty, P., Baumlin, N., et al. (2016). Chronic electronic cigarette exposure in mice induces features of COPD in a nicotine-dependent manner. *Thorax*, 71(12), 1119–1129.

Global Initiative for Asthma (GINA). (2019a). Global strategy for asthma management and prevention. Retrieved on 7/01/2019 at: www.ginasthma.org/wp-content/uploads/2019/06/GINA-2019-main-report-June-2019-wms.pdf

Global Initiative for Asthma (GINA). (2019b). Pocket guide for asthma management. Retrieved on 7/01/2019 at: www.ginasthma.org/wp-content/uploads/2019/04/GINA-2019-main-Pocket-Guide-wms.pdf

Global Initiative for Chronic Obstructive Lung Disease (GOLD). (2018). Pocket guide to COPD diagnosis, management, and prevention: A guide for health care professionals, 2018 report. Retrieved on 7/11/2019 at: www.goldcopd.org/wp-content/uploads/2018/02/WMS-GOLD-2018-Feb-Final-to-print-v2.pdf

Global Initiative for Chronic Obstructive Lung Disease (GOLD). (2019). Global strategy for the diagnosis, management, and prevention of chronic obstructive pulmonary disease, 2019 report. Retrieved on 6/23/2019 at: www.goldcopd.org/wp-content/uploads/2018/11/GOLD-2019-v1.7-FINAL-14Nov2018-WMS.pdf

Gregory, K. L., Elliott, D., & Dunne, P. (2013). Guide to aerosol delivery devices for physicians, nurses, pharmacists, and other health care professionals. Retrieved on 8/6/2019 at: www.aarc.org/wp-content/uploads/2014/08/aerosol_guide_pro.pdf

Hachem, R. (2019). Lung transplantation: General guidelines for recipient selection. *UpToDate*. Retrieved on 10/06/2019 at: www.uptodate.com/contents/lung-transplantation-general-guidelines-for-recipient

Han, M. K., Dransfield, M. T., & Martinez, F. J. (2018). Chronic obstructive pulmonary disease: Definition, clinical manifestations, diagnosis, and staging. *UpToDate*. Retrieved on 7/26/2019 at: www.uptodate.com/contents/chronic-obstructive-pulmonary-disease-definition-clinical-manifestations-diagnosis-and-staging

Hanlon, P. (2015). Secretion and airway clearance: Techniques and devices offer a range of treatment options. *RT: The Journal for Respiratory Care Practitioners*, 28(8), 11–14.

Heltshe, S. L., Cogen, J., Ramos, K. J., et al. (2017). Cystic fibrosis: The dawn of a new therapeutic era. *American Journal of Respiratory and Critical Care Medicine*, 195(8), 979–984.

Katkin, J. P., Baker, R. D., & Baker, S. S. (2019). Cystic fibrosis: Assessment and management of pancreatic insufficiency. *UpToDate*. Retrieved on 7/25/2019 at: www.uptodate.com/contents/cystic-fibrosis-assessment-and-management-of-pancreatic-insufficiency

Katkin, J. P., Mallory, G. B., & Hoppin, A. G. (2019). Cystic fibrosis: Clinical manifestations and diagnosis. *UpToDate*. Retrieved on 7/25/2019 at: www.uptodate.com/contents/cystic-fibrosis-clinical-manifestations-and-diagnosis

Kochanek, K. D., Murphy, S. L., Xu, J., et al. (2019). Deaths: Final data for 2017. *National Vital Statistics Reports*, 68(9). Retrieved on 7/13/2019 at: www.cdc.gov/nchs/data/nvsr/nvsr68/nvsr68_09-508.pdf

Krings, J. G., McGregor, M. C., Bacharier, L. B., et al. (2019). Biologics for severe asthma: Treatment-specific effects are important in choosing a specific agent. *Journal of Allergy and Clinical Immunology in Practice*, 7(5), 1379–1392.

Larcombe A. N., Janka, M. A., Mullins, B. J., et al. (2017). The effects of electronic cigarette aerosol exposure on inflammation and lung function in mice. *American Journal of Physiology-Lung Cellular and Molecular Physiology*, 313(1), L67–L79.

National Institutes of Health. (2018). Medline Plus medical encyclopedia: Cystic fibrosis. Retrieved on 7/19/2019 at: www.medlineplus.gov/ency/article/000107.htm

Papi, A., Brightling, C., Pedersen, S., et al. (2018). Asthma. *The Lancet*, 391(10122), 783–800.

Patel, J. G., Coutinho, A. D., Lunacsek, O. E., et al. (2018). COPD affects worker productivity and health care costs. *International Journal of COPD*, 13, 2301–2311.

Powner, J., Nesmith, A., Kirkpatrick, D. P., et al. (2019). Employment of an algorithm of care including chest physiotherapy results in reduced hospitalizations and stability of lung function in bronchiectasis. *BMC Pulmonary Medicine*, 19(82). doi:10.1186/s12890-019-0844-4

Raherison, C., Ouaalaya, E., Bernady, A., et al. (2018). Comorbidities and COPD severity in a clinic-based cohort. *BMC Pulmonary Medicine*, 18(117), doi:10.1186/s12890-018-0684-7

Simon, R. H., Mallory, G. B., & Hoppin, A. G. (2019a). Cystic fibrosis: Overview of the treatment of lung disease. *UpToDate*. Retrieved on 7/26/2019 at: www.uptodate.com/contents/cystic-fibrosis-overview-of-the-treatment-of-lung-disease

Simon, R. H., Mallory, G. B., & Hoppin, A. G. (2019b). Cystic fibrosis: Treatment of acute pulmonary exacerbations. *UpToDate*. Retrieved on 7/26/2019 at: www.uptodate.com/contents/cystic-fibrosis-treatment-of-acute-pulmonary-exacerbations

Simon, R. H., Mallory, G. B., & Hoppin, A. G. (2019c). Cystic fibrosis: Treatment with CFTR modulators. *UpToDate*. Retrieved on 7/26/2019 at: www.uptodate.com/contents/cystic-fibrosis-treatment-with-cftr-modulators

Stoller, J. K., Barnes, P. J., & Hollingsworth, H. H. (2018). Clinical manifestations, diagnosis, and natural history of alpha-1 antitrypsin deficiency. *UpToDate*. Retrieved on 7/01/2019 at: www.uptodate.com/contents/clinical-manifestations-diagnosis-and-natural-history-of-alpha-1-antitrypsin-deficiency

Sullivan, P. W., Ghushchyan, V., Kavati, A., et al. (2019). Health disparities among children with asthma in the United States by place of residence. *Journal of Allergy and Clinical Immunology in Practice*, 7(1), 148–155.

Tomaszek, L., Debska, G., Cepuch, G., et al. (2019). Evaluation of quality of life predictors in adolescents and young adults with cystic fibrosis. *Heart and Lung*, 49(2), 159–165.

U.S. National Library of Medicine (NLM). (2019). Genetics Home Reference. Alpha-1 antitrypsin deficiency. Retrieved on 7/3/2019 at: www.ghr.nlm.nih.gov/condition/alpha-1-antitrypsin-deficiency#statistics

Wenzel, S., Bochner, B. S., & Hollingsworth, H. (2019). Treatment of severe asthma in adolescents and adults. *UpToDate*. Retrieved on 7/30/2019 at: www.uptodate.com/contents/treatment-of-severe-asthma-in-adolescents-and-adults

Weycker, D., Hansen, G. L., & Seifer, F. D. (2017). Prevalence and incidence of noncystic fibrosis bronchiectasis among US adults in 2013. *Chronic Respiratory Diseases*, 14(4), 377–384.

Resources

Agency for Healthcare Research and Quality (AHRQ), www.ahrq.gov
Alpha-1 Foundation, www.alpha1.org
American Academy of Allergy, Asthma & Immunology (AAAAI), www.aaaai.org
American Association for Respiratory Care (AARC), www.aarc.org
American Association of Cardiovascular and Pulmonary Rehabilitation (AACVPR), www.aacvpr.org
American Cancer Society, www.cancer.org
American College of Chest Physicians (ACCP), www.chestnet.org
American Lung Association, www.lung.org
American Thoracic Society (ATS), www.thoracic.org
Centers for Disease Control and Prevention (CDC), www.cdc.gov
COPD Foundation, www.copdfoundation.org
Cystic Fibrosis Foundation, www.cff.org
National Heart, Lung, and Blood Institute (NHLBI), www.nhlbi.nih.gov
SmokEnders, www.smokenders.org
U.S. Department of Health & Human Services (HHS), www.hhs.gov or healthfinder.gov

Cardiovascular and Circulatory Function

USING TECHNOLOGY TO PREVENT MEDICATION ERRORS

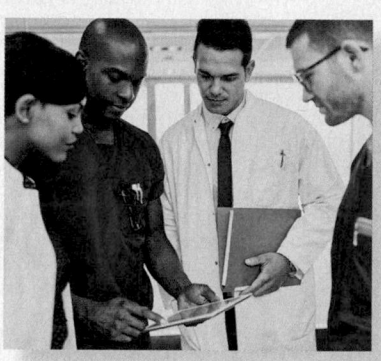

An 85-year-old male presents to the emergency department with complaints of substernal chest pressure rated 9 on a 0–10 pain scale with pain radiating to his left arm. Other signs and symptoms include nausea, dizziness, shortness of breath (SOB), diaphoresis, and a feeling of "something bad is happening to me."

He is emergently sent for cardiac catheterization; a 90% distal and 85% proximal stenosis of the right coronary artery was detected. He subsequently underwent a percutaneous coronary intervention with balloon angioplasty and placement of stents. Once recovered from anesthesia he is admitted to the cardiac step-down unit where you work. When receiving report you notice in the electronic health record (EHR) that the patient should have received the first dose of two medications in the cardiac catheterization lab following the procedure. However, these medications were not administered as prescribed and you notify the interventional cardiologist about this error.

QSEN Competency Focus: Informatics

The complexities inherent in today's health care system challenge nurses to demonstrate integration of specific interdisciplinary core competencies. These competencies are aimed at ensuring the delivery of safe, quality patient care (Institute of Medicine, 2003). The Quality and Safety Education for Nurses project (Cronenwett, Sherwood, Barnsteiner, et al., 2007; QSEN, 2020) provides a framework for the knowledge, skills, and attitudes (KSAs) required for nurses to demonstrate competency in these key areas, which include *patient-centered care*, *interdisciplinary teamwork and collaboration*, *evidence-based practice*, *quality improvement*, *safety*, and *informatics.*

Informatics Definition: Use information and technology to communicate, manage knowledge, mitigate error, and support decision-making.

SELECT PRE-LICENSURE KSAs	APPLICATION AND REFLECTION
Knowledge	
Explain why information and technology skills are essential for safe patient care	Describe how the use of the EHR and other technology can relay information to the nurse to prevent medication errors.
Skills	
Apply technology and information management tools to support safe processes of care	Describe the type of training needed to navigate the EHR efficiently. Identify how you can utilize technology to ensure effective communication, manage medication administration, and prevent errors.
Attitudes	
Value technologies that support clinical decision-making, error prevention, and care coordination	Reflect on how you value technologies that support clinical decision-making, error prevention, and care coordination. Do these values have the potential to create barriers to effective use of technology to prevent errors in your workplace?

Cronenwett, L., Sherwood, G., Barnsteiner, J., et al. (2007). Quality and safety education for nurses. *Nursing Outlook, 55*(3), 122–131; Institute of Medicine. (2003). *Health professions education: A bridge to quality*. Washington, DC: National Academies Press; QSEN Institute. (2020). *QSEN competencies: Definitions and pre-licensure KSAs; Informatics*. Retrieved on 8/15/2020 at: qsen.org/competencies/pre-licensure-ksas/#informatics

21 Assessment of Cardiovascular Function

LEARNING OUTCOMES

On completion of this chapter, the learner will be able to:

1. Describe the structure and function of the cardiovascular system as well as associated cardiac risk factors.
2. Explain and demonstrate the proper techniques to perform a comprehensive cardiovascular assessment.
3. Discriminate between normal and abnormal assessment findings identified by inspection, palpation, percussion, and auscultation of the cardiovascular system.

4. Recognize and evaluate the major manifestations of cardiovascular dysfunction by applying information from the patient's health history and physical assessment findings.
5. Identify diagnostic tests and methods of hemodynamic monitoring (e.g., central venous pressure, pulmonary artery pressure, arterial pressure monitoring) of the cardiovascular system and related nursing implications.

NURSING CONCEPT

Perfusion

GLOSSARY

acute coronary syndrome: a constellation of signs and symptoms due to the rupture of atherosclerotic plaque and resultant partial or complete thrombosis within a diseased coronary artery

afterload: the amount of resistance to ejection of blood from the ventricle

apical impulse: impulse normally palpated at the fifth intercostal space, left midclavicular line; caused by contraction of the left ventricle (*synonym:* point of maximal impulse)

atrioventricular (AV) node: secondary pacemaker of the heart, located in the right atrial wall near the tricuspid valve

baroreceptors: nerve fibers located in the aortic arch and carotid arteries that are responsible for control of the blood pressure

cardiac catheterization: an invasive procedure used to measure cardiac chamber pressures and assess patency of the coronary arteries

cardiac conduction system: specialized heart cells strategically located throughout the heart that are responsible for methodically generating and coordinating the transmission of electrical impulses to the myocardial cells

cardiac output: amount of blood pumped by each ventricle in liters per minute

cardiac stress test: a test used to evaluate the functioning of the heart during a period of increased oxygen demand; test may be initiated by exercise or medications

contractility: ability of the cardiac muscle to shorten in response to an electrical impulse

depolarization: electrical activation of a cell caused by the influx of sodium into the cell while potassium exits the cell

diastole: period of ventricular relaxation resulting in ventricular filling

ejection fraction: percentage of the end-diastolic blood volume ejected from the ventricle with each heartbeat

hemodynamic monitoring: the use of pressure monitoring devices to directly measure cardiovascular function

hypertension: blood pressure that is persistently greater than 130/80 mm Hg

hypotension: a decrease in blood pressure to less than 90/60 mm Hg that compromises systemic perfusion

murmurs: sounds created by abnormal, turbulent flow of blood in the heart

myocardial ischemia: condition in which heart muscle cells receive less oxygen than needed

myocardium: muscle layer of the heart responsible for the pumping action of the heart

normal heart sounds: sounds produced when the valves close; normal heart sounds are S_1 (atrioventricular valves) and S_2 (semilunar valves)

opening snaps: abnormal diastolic sounds generated during opening of rigid atrioventricular valve leaflets

orthostatic hypotension: a significant drop in blood pressure (20 mm Hg systolic or more or 10 mm Hg diastolic or more) after an upright posture is assumed

preload: degree of stretch of the cardiac muscle fibers at the end of diastole

pulmonary vascular resistance: resistance to blood flow out of the right ventricle created by the pulmonary circulatory system

pulse deficit: the difference between the apical and radial pulse rates

radioisotopes: unstable atoms that give off small amounts of energy in the form of gamma rays as they decay; used in cardiac nuclear medicine studies

repolarization: return of the cell to resting state, caused by reentry of potassium into the cell while sodium exits the cell

S_1: the first heart sound produced by closure of the atrioventricular (mitral and tricuspid) valves

S_2: the second heart sound produced by closure of the semilunar (aortic and pulmonic) valves

S_3: an abnormal heart sound detected early in diastole as resistance is met to blood entering either ventricle; most often due to volume overload associated with heart failure

S_4: an abnormal heart sound detected late in diastole as resistance is met to blood entering either ventricle during atrial contraction; most often caused by hypertrophy of the ventricle

sinoatrial (SA) node: primary pacemaker of the heart, located in the right atrium

stroke volume: amount of blood ejected from one of the ventricles per heartbeat

summation gallop: abnormal sounds created by the presence of an S_3 and S_4 during periods of tachycardia

systemic vascular resistance: resistance to blood flow out of the left ventricle created by the systemic circulatory system

systole: period of ventricular contraction resulting in ejection of blood from the ventricles into the pulmonary artery and aorta

systolic click: abnormal systolic sound created by the opening of a calcified aortic or pulmonic valve during ventricular contraction

telemetry: the process of continuous electrocardiographic monitoring by the transmission of radio waves from a battery-operated transmitter worn by the patient

---

Nearly half, or 121.5 million, of American adults have one or more types of cardiovascular disease (CVD), including hypertension, coronary artery disease (CAD), heart failure (HF), and stroke (American Heart Association [AHA], 2019). Because of the increased prevalence of CVD, nurses practicing in any setting across the continuum of care, whether in the home, office, hospital, long-term care facility, or rehabilitation facility, must be able to assess the cardiovascular system. Key components of assessment include a health history, physical assessment, and monitoring of a variety of laboratory and diagnostic test results. This assessment provides the information necessary to identify nursing diagnoses, formulate an individualized plan of care, evaluate the response of the patient to the care provided, and revise the plan as needed.

Anatomic and Physiologic Overview

An understanding of the structure and function of the heart in health and in disease is essential to develop cardiovascular assessment skills.

Anatomy of the Heart

The heart is a hollow, muscular organ located in the center of the thorax, where it occupies the space between the lungs (mediastinum) and rests on the diaphragm. It weighs approximately 300 g (10.6 oz); the weight and size of the heart are influenced by age, gender, body weight, extent of physical exercise and conditioning, and heart disease. The heart pumps blood to the tissues, supplying them with oxygen and other nutrients.

The heart is composed of three layers (Fig. 21-1). The inner layer, or endocardium, consists of endothelial tissue and lines the inside of the heart and valves. The middle layer, or **myocardium**, is made up of muscle fibers and is responsible for the pumping action. The exterior layer of the heart is called the *epicardium*.

The heart is encased in a thin, fibrous sac called the *pericardium*, which is composed of two layers. Adhering to the epicardium is the visceral pericardium. Enveloping the visceral pericardium is the parietal pericardium, a tough fibrous tissue that attaches to the great vessels, diaphragm, sternum, and vertebral column and supports the heart in the mediastinum. The space between these two layers (pericardial space) is normally filled with about 20 mL of fluid, which lubricates the surface of the heart and reduces friction during systole.

Heart Chambers

The pumping action of the heart is accomplished by the rhythmic relaxation and contraction of the muscular walls of its two top chambers (atria) and two bottom chambers (ventricles). During the relaxation phase, called **diastole**, all four chambers relax simultaneously, which allows the ventricles to fill in preparation for contraction. Diastole is commonly referred to as the period of ventricular filling. **Systole** refers to the events in the heart during contraction of the atria and the ventricles. Unlike diastole, atrial and ventricular systoles are not simultaneous events. Atrial systole occurs first, just at the end of diastole, followed by ventricular systole. This synchronization allows the ventricles to fill completely prior to ejection of blood from these chambers.

The right side of the heart, made up of the right atrium and right ventricle, distributes venous blood (deoxygenated blood) to the lungs via the pulmonary artery (pulmonary circulation) for oxygenation. The pulmonary artery is the only artery in the body that carries deoxygenated blood. The right atrium receives venous blood returning to the heart from the superior vena cava (head, neck, and upper extremities), inferior vena cava (trunk and lower extremities), and coronary sinus (coronary circulation). The left side of the heart, composed of the left atrium and left ventricle, distributes oxygenated blood to the remainder of the body via the aorta (systemic circulation). The left atrium receives oxygenated blood

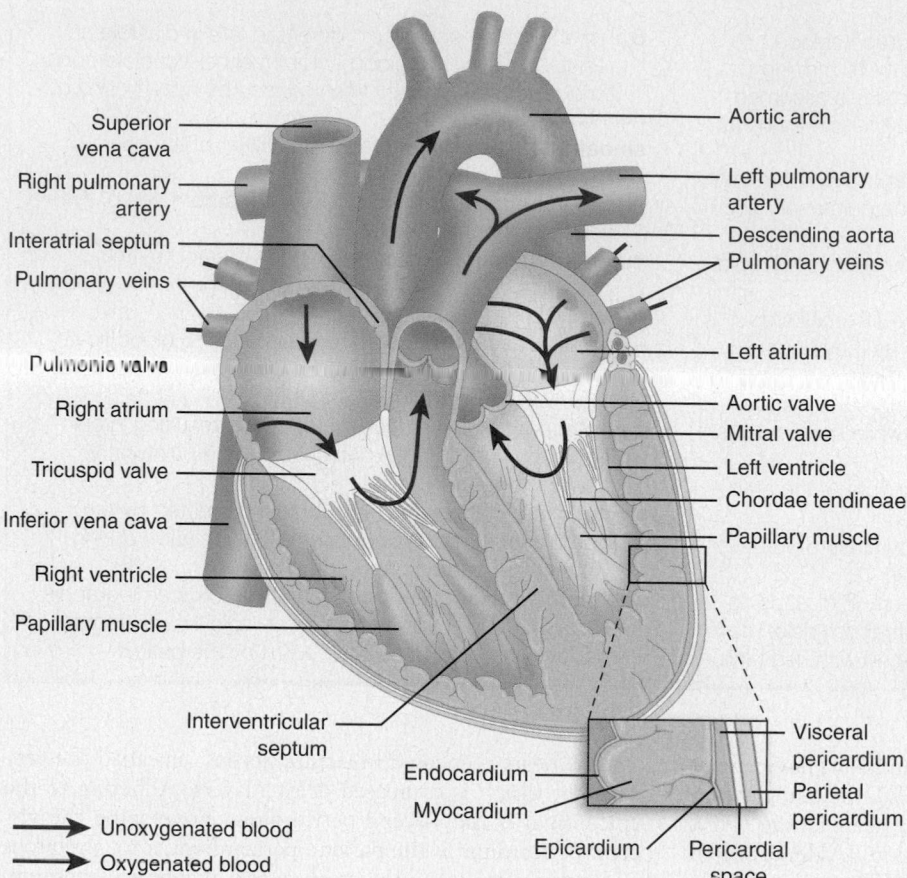

Superior
vena cava

Right pulmonary
artery

Interatrial septum

Pulmonary veins

Pulmonic valve

Right atrium

Tricuspid valve

Inferior vena cava

Right ventricle

Papillary muscle

Interventricular
septum

Endocardium

Myocardium

Epicardium

Pericardial
space

Aortic arch

Left pulmonary
artery

Descending aorta

Pulmonary veins

Left atrium

Aortic valve

Mitral valve

Left ventricle

Chordae tendineae

Papillary muscle

Visceral
pericardium

Parietal
pericardium

→ Unoxygenated blood

→ Oxygenated blood

Figure 21-1 • Structure of the heart.
Arrows show course of blood flow
through the heart chambers.

from the pulmonary circulation via four pulmonary veins. The flow of blood through the four heart chambers is shown in Figure 21-1.

The varying thicknesses of the atrial and ventricular walls are due to the workload required by each chamber. The myocardial layer of both atria is much thinner than that of the ventricles because there is little resistance as blood flows out of the atria and into the ventricles during diastole. In contrast, the ventricular walls are much thicker than the atrial walls. During ventricular systole, the right and left ventricles must overcome resistance to blood flow from the pulmonary and systemic circulatory systems, respectively. The left ventricle is two to three times more muscular than the right ventricle. It must overcome high aortic and arterial pressures, whereas the right ventricle contracts against a low-pressure system within the pulmonary arteries and capillaries (Pappano & Weir, 2019). Figure 21-2 identifies the pressures in each of these areas.

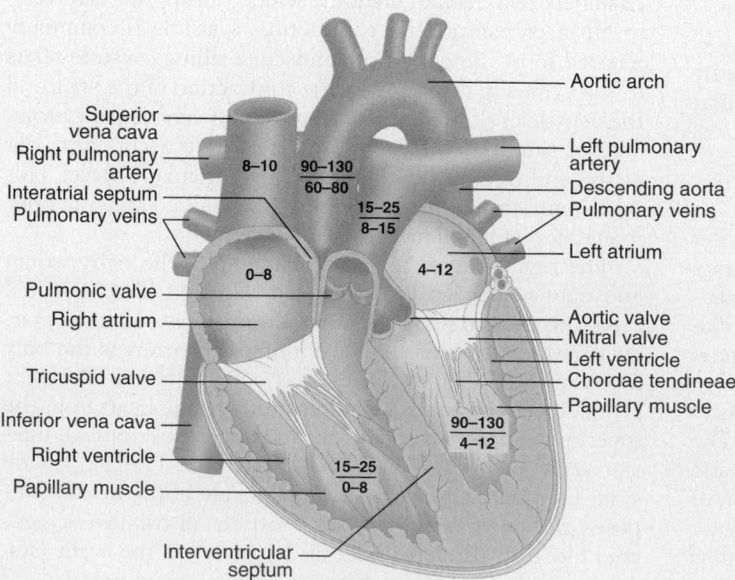

Superior
vena cava

Right pulmonary
artery

Interatrial septum

Pulmonary veins

Pulmonic valve

Right atrium

Tricuspid valve

Inferior vena cava

Right ventricle

Papillary muscle

Interventricular
septum

8–10

90–130
60–80

15–25
8–15

0–8

4–12

90–130
4–12

15–25
0–8

Aortic arch

Left pulmonary
artery

Descending aorta

Pulmonary veins

Left atrium

Aortic valve

Mitral valve

Left ventricle

Chordae tendineae

Papillary muscle

Figure 21-2 • Great vessel and chamber pressures. Pressures are identified in millimeters of mercury (mm Hg) as mean pressure or systolic over diastolic pressure.

The heart lies in a rotated position within the chest cavity. The right ventricle lies anteriorly (just beneath the sternum), and the left ventricle is situated posteriorly. As a result of this close proximity to the chest wall, the pulsation created during normal ventricular contraction, called the **apical impulse** (also called the *point of maximal impulse* [PMI]), is easily detected. In the normal heart, the PMI is located at the intersection of the midclavicular line of the left chest wall and the fifth intercostal space (Bickley, 2017).

Heart Valves

The four valves in the heart permit blood to flow in only one direction. The valves, which are composed of thin leaflets of fibrous tissue, open and close in response to the movement of blood and pressure changes within the chambers. There are two types of valves: atrioventricular (AV) and semilunar.

Atrioventricular Valves

The AV valves separate the atria from the ventricles. The tricuspid valve, so named because it is composed of three cusps or leaflets, separates the right atrium from the right ventricle. The mitral or bicuspid (two cusps) valve lies between the left atrium and the left ventricle (see Fig. 21-1).

During diastole, the tricuspid and mitral valves are open, allowing the blood in the atria to flow freely into the relaxed ventricles. As ventricular systole begins, the ventricles contract and blood flows upward into the cusps of the tricuspid and mitral valves, causing them to close. As the pressure against these valves increases, two additional structures, the papillary muscles and the chordae tendineae, maintain valve closure. The papillary muscles, located on the sides of the ventricular walls, are connected to the valve leaflets by the chordae tendineae, which are thin fibrous bands. During ventricular systole, contraction of the papillary muscles causes the chordae tendineae to become taut, keeping the valve leaflets approximated and closed. This action prevents backflow of blood into the atria (regurgitation) as blood is ejected out into the pulmonary artery and aorta.

Semilunar Valves

The two semilunar valves are composed of three leaflets, which are shaped like half-moons. The valve between the right ventricle and the pulmonary artery is called the *pulmonic valve*. The valve between the left ventricle and the aorta is called the *aortic valve*. The semilunar valves are closed during diastole. At this point, the pressure in the pulmonary artery and aorta decreases, causing blood to flow back toward the semilunar valves. This action fills the cusps with blood and closes the valves. The semilunar valves are forced open during ventricular systole as blood is ejected from the right and left ventricles into the pulmonary artery and aorta, respectively.

Coronary Arteries

The left and right coronary arteries and their branches supply arterial blood to the heart. These arteries originate from the aorta just above the aortic valve leaflets. Unlike other arteries, the coronary arteries are perfused during diastole. With a normal heart rate of 60 to 80 bpm, there is ample time during diastole for myocardial perfusion. However, as heart rate increases, diastolic time is shortened, which may not allow adequate time for myocardial perfusion. As a result, patients are at risk for **myocardial ischemia** (inadequate oxygen supply) during tachycardia (heart rate greater than 100 bpm), especially patients with CAD.

The left coronary artery has three branches. The artery from the point of origin to the first major branch is called the *left main coronary artery*. Two branches arise from the left main coronary artery: the left anterior descending artery, which courses down the anterior wall of the heart, and the circumflex artery, which circles around to the lateral left wall of the heart.

The right side of the heart is supplied by the *right coronary artery*, which travels to the inferior wall of the heart. The posterior wall of the heart receives its blood supply by an additional branch from the right coronary artery called the *posterior descending artery* (see Chapter 23, Fig. 23-2).

Superficial to the coronary arteries are the coronary veins. Venous blood from these veins returns to the heart primarily through the coronary sinus, which is located posteriorly in the right atrium.

Myocardium

The myocardium is the middle, muscular layer of the atrial and ventricular walls. It is composed of specialized cells called *myocytes*, which form an interconnected network of muscle fibers. These fibers encircle the heart in a figure-of-eight pattern, forming a spiral from the base (top) of the heart to the apex (bottom). During contraction, this muscular configuration facilitates a twisting and compressive movement of the heart that begins in the atria and moves to the ventricles. The sequential and rhythmic pattern of contraction, followed by relaxation of the muscle fibers, maximizes the volume of blood ejected with each contraction. This cyclical pattern of myocardial contraction is controlled by the conduction system.

Function of the Heart

Cardiac Electrophysiology

The **cardiac conduction system** generates and transmits electrical impulses that stimulate contraction of the myocardium. Under normal circumstances, the conduction system first stimulates contraction of the atria and then the ventricles. The synchronization of the atrial and ventricular events allows the ventricles to fill completely before ventricular ejection, thereby maximizing cardiac output. Three physiologic characteristics of two types of specialized electrical cells, the nodal cells and the Purkinje cells, provide this synchronization:

- *Automaticity:* ability to initiate an electrical impulse
- *Excitability:* ability to respond to an electrical impulse
- *Conductivity:* ability to transmit an electrical impulse from one cell to another

Both the **sinoatrial (SA) node** (the primary pacemaker of the heart) and the **atrioventricular (AV) node** (the secondary pacemaker of the heart) are composed of nodal cells. The SA node is located at the junction of the superior vena cava and the right atrium (Fig. 21-3). The SA node in a normal resting adult heart has an inherent firing rate of 60 to 100 impulses per minute; however, the rate changes in response to the metabolic demands of the body (Weber & Kelley, 2018).

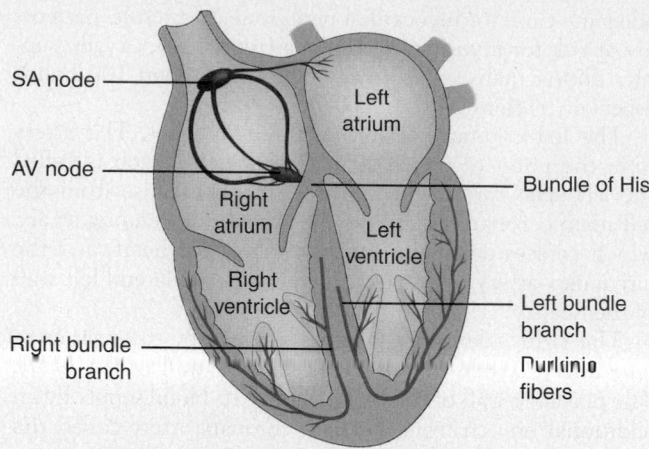

Figure 21-3 • Cardiac conduction system. AV, atrioventricular; SA, sinoatrial.

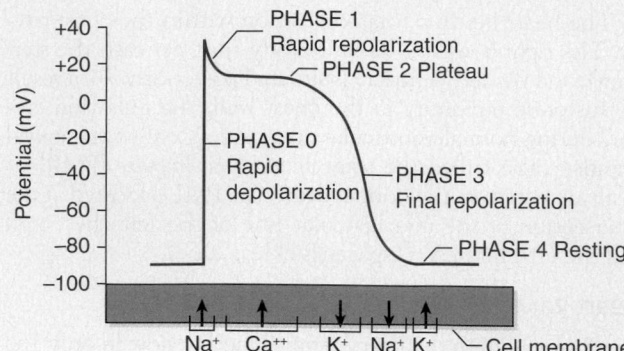

Figure 21-4 • Cardiac action potential of a fast-response Purkinje fiber. The *arrows* indicate the approximate time and direction of movement of each ion influencing membrane potential. Ca^{++} movement out of the cell is not well defined but is thought to occur during phase 4.

The electrical impulses initiated by the SA node are conducted along the myocardial cells of the atria via specialized tracts called *internodal pathways*. The impulses cause electrical stimulation and subsequent contraction of the atria. The impulses are then conducted to the AV node, which is located in the right atrial wall near the tricuspid valve (see Fig. 21-3). The AV node coordinates the incoming electrical impulses from the atria and after a slight delay (allowing the atria time to contract and complete ventricular filling) relays the impulse to the ventricles.

Initially, the impulse is conducted through a bundle of specialized conducting tissue, referred to as the bundle of His, which then divides into the right bundle branch (conducting impulses to the right ventricle) and the left bundle branch (conducting impulses to the left ventricle). To transmit impulses to the left ventricle—the largest chamber of the heart—the left bundle branch divides into the left anterior and left posterior bundle branches. Impulses travel through the bundle branches to reach the terminal point in the conduction system, called the *Purkinje fibers*. These fibers are composed of Purkinje cells that rapidly conduct impulses throughout the thick walls of the ventricles. This action stimulates the ventricular myocardial cells to contract (Weber & Kelley, 2018).

The heart rate is determined by the myocardial cells with the fastest inherent firing rate. Under normal circumstances, the SA node has the highest inherent rate (60 to 100 impulses per minute), the AV node has the second-highest inherent rate (40 to 60 impulses per minute), and the ventricular pacemaker sites have the lowest inherent rate (30 to 40 impulses per minute) (Wesley, 2017). If the SA node malfunctions, the AV node generally takes over the pacemaker function of the heart at its inherently lower rate. Should both the SA and the AV nodes fail in their pacemaker function, a pacemaker site in the ventricle will fire at its inherent bradycardic rate of 30 to 40 impulses per minute.

Cardiac Action Potential

The nodal and Purkinje cells (electrical cells) generate and transmit impulses across the heart, stimulating the cardiac myocytes (working cells) to contract. Stimulation of the myocytes occurs due to the exchange of electrically charged particles, called *ions*, across channels located in the cell membrane. The channels regulate the movement and speed of specific ions—namely, sodium, potassium, and calcium—as they enter and exit the cell. Sodium rapidly enters into the cell through sodium-fast channels, in contrast to calcium, which enters the cell through calcium-slow channels. In the resting or polarized state, sodium is the primary extracellular ion, whereas potassium is the primary intracellular ion. This difference in ion concentration means that the inside of the cell has a negative charge compared with the positive charge on the outside. The relationship changes during cellular stimulation, when sodium or calcium crosses the cell membrane into the cell and potassium ions exit into the extracellular space. This exchange of ions creates a positively charged intracellular space and a negatively charged extracellular space that characterizes the period known as **depolarization**. Once depolarization is complete, the exchange of ions reverts to its resting state; this period is known as **repolarization**. The repeated cycle of depolarization and repolarization is called the *cardiac action potential*.

As shown in Figure 21-4, the cardiac action potential has five phases:

- *Phase 0:* Cellular depolarization is initiated as positive ions influx into the cell. During this phase, the atrial and ventricular myocytes rapidly depolarize as sodium moves into the cells through sodium-fast channels. The myocytes have a fast-response action potential. In contrast, the cells of the SA and AV node depolarize when calcium enters these cells through calcium-slow channels. These cells have a slow-response action potential.
- *Phase 1:* Early cellular repolarization begins during this phase as potassium exits the intracellular space.
- *Phase 2:* This phase is called the *plateau phase* because the rate of repolarization slows. Calcium ions enter the intracellular space.
- *Phase 3:* This phase marks the completion of repolarization and return of the cell to its resting state.
- *Phase 4:* This phase is considered the resting phase before the next depolarization.

Refractory Periods

Myocardial cells must completely repolarize before they can depolarize again. During the repolarization process, the cells are in a refractory period. There are two phases of the refractory period: the effective (or absolute) refractory period and the relative refractory period. During the effective refractory period, the cell is completely unresponsive to any electrical stimulus; it is incapable of initiating an early depolarization. The effective refractory period corresponds with the time in phase 0 to the middle of phase 3 of the action potential. The relative refractory period corresponds with the short time at the end of phase 3. During the relative refractory period, if an electrical stimulus is stronger than normal, the cell may depolarize prematurely. Early depolarizations of the atrium or ventricle cause premature contractions, placing the patient at risk for arrhythmias. Premature ventricular contractions in certain situations, such as the presence of myocardial ischemia, are of concern because these early ventricular depolarizations can trigger life-threatening arrhythmias, including ventricular tachycardia or ventricular fibrillation. Several circumstances make the heart more susceptible to early depolarization during the relative refractory period, thus increasing the risk for serious arrhythmias. (These arrhythmias and others are discussed in detail in Chapter 22.)

Cardiac Hemodynamics

An important determinant of blood flow in the cardiovascular system is the principle that fluid flows from a region of higher pressure to one of lower pressure (see Fig. 21-2). The pressures responsible for blood flow in the normal circulation are generated during systole and diastole.

Cardiac Cycle

The cardiac cycle refers to the events that occur in the heart from the beginning of one heartbeat to the next. The number of cardiac cycles completed in a minute depends on the heart rate. Each cardiac cycle has three major sequential events: diastole, atrial systole, and ventricular systole. These events cause blood to flow through the heart due to changes in chamber pressures and valvular function during diastole and systole. During diastole, all four heart chambers are relaxed. As a result, the AV valves are open and the semilunar valves are closed. Pressures in all of the chambers are the lowest during diastole, which facilitates ventricular filling. Venous blood returns to the right atrium from the superior and inferior vena cava, then into the right ventricle. On the left side, oxygenated blood returns from the lungs via the four pulmonary veins into the left atrium and ventricle.

Toward the end of this diastolic period, atrial systole occurs as the atrial muscles contract in response to an electrical impulse initiated by the SA node. Atrial systole increases the pressure inside the atria, ejecting the remaining blood into the ventricles. Atrial systole augments ventricular blood volume by 15% to 25% and is sometimes referred to as the atrial kick (Wesley, 2017). At this point, ventricular systole begins in response to propagation of the electrical impulse that began in the SA node some milliseconds earlier.

Beginning with ventricular systole, the pressure inside the ventricles rapidly increases, forcing the AV valves to close. As a result, blood ceases to flow from the atria into the ventricles, and regurgitation (backflow) of blood into the atria is prevented. The rapid increase in pressure inside the right and left ventricles forces the pulmonic and aortic valves to open, and blood is ejected into the pulmonary artery and aorta, respectively. The exit of blood is at first rapid; then, as the pressure

in each ventricle and its corresponding artery equalizes, the flow of blood gradually decreases. At the end of systole, pressure within the right and left ventricles rapidly decreases. As a result, pulmonary arterial and aortic pressures decrease, causing closure of the semilunar valves. These events mark the onset of diastole, and the cardiac cycle is repeated.

Chamber pressures can be measured with the use of special monitoring catheters and equipment. This technique is called **hemodynamic monitoring.** Methods of hemodynamic monitoring are covered in more detail at the end of this chapter.

Cardiac Output

Cardiac output refers to the total amount of blood ejected by one of the ventricles in liters per minute. The cardiac output in a resting adult is 4 to 6 L/min but varies greatly depending on the metabolic needs of the body. Cardiac output is computed by multiplying the stroke volume by the heart rate. **Stroke volume** is the amount of blood ejected from one of the ventricles per heartbeat. The average resting stroke volume is about 60 to 130 mL (Wiegand, 2017).

Effect of Heart Rate on Cardiac Output

The cardiac output responds to changes in the metabolic demands of the tissues associated with stress, physical exercise, and illness. To compensate for these added demands, the cardiac output is enhanced by increases in both stroke volume and heart rate. Changes in heart rate are due to inhibition or stimulation of the SA node mediated by the parasympathetic and sympathetic divisions of the autonomic nervous system. The balance between these two reflex control systems normally determines the heart rate. Branches of the parasympathetic nervous system travel to the SA node by the vagus nerve. Stimulation of the vagus nerve slows the heart rate. The sympathetic nervous system increases heart rate by innervation of the beta-1 receptor sites located within the SA node. The heart rate is increased by the sympathetic nervous system through an increased level of circulating catecholamines (secreted by the adrenal gland) and by excess thyroid hormone, which produces a catecholamine-like effect.

In addition, the heart rate is affected by central nervous system and baroreceptor activity. **Baroreceptors** are specialized nerve cells located in the aortic arch and in both right and left internal carotid arteries (at the point of bifurcation from the common carotid arteries). The baroreceptors are sensitive to changes in blood pressure (BP). During hypertension (significant elevations in BP), these cells increase their rate of discharge, transmitting impulses to the cerebral medulla. This action initiates parasympathetic activity and inhibits sympathetic response, lowering the heart rate and the BP. The opposite is true during hypotension (low BP). Decreased baroreceptor stimulation during periods of hypotension prompts a decrease in parasympathetic activity and enhances sympathetic responses. These compensatory mechanisms attempt to elevate the BP through vasoconstriction and increased heart rate.

Effect of Stroke Volume on Cardiac Output

Stroke volume is primarily determined by three factors: preload, afterload, and contractility.

Preload refers to the degree of stretch of the ventricular cardiac muscle fibers at the end of diastole. The end of diastole is the period when filling volume in the ventricles is the highest and the degree of stretch on the muscle fibers is the greatest. The volume of blood within the ventricle at the end of diastole determines preload, which directly affects stroke volume. Therefore, preload is commonly referred to as left ventricular end-diastolic pressure. As the volume of blood returning to the heart increases, muscle fiber stretch also increases (increased preload), resulting in stronger contraction and a greater stroke volume. This relationship, referred to as the Frank–Starling (or Starling) law of the heart, is maintained until the physiologic limit of the muscle is reached.

The Frank–Starling law is based on the fact that, within limits, the greater the initial length or stretch of the sarcomeres (cardiac muscle cells), the greater the degree of shortening that occurs. This result is caused by increased interaction between the thick and thin filaments within the cardiac muscle cells. Preload is decreased by a reduction in the volume of blood returning to the ventricles. Diuresis, venodilating agents (e.g., nitrates), excessive loss of blood, or dehydration (excessive loss of body fluids from vomiting, diarrhea, or diaphoresis) reduce preload. Preload is increased by increasing the return of circulating blood volume to the ventricles. Controlling the loss of blood or body fluids and replacing fluids (i.e., blood transfusions and intravenous [IV] fluid administration) are examples of ways to increase preload.

Afterload, or resistance to ejection of blood from the ventricle, is the second determinant of stroke volume. The resistance of the systemic BP to left ventricular ejection is called **systemic vascular resistance.** The resistance of the pulmonary BP to right ventricular ejection is called **pulmonary vascular resistance.** There is an inverse relationship between afterload and stroke volume. For example, afterload is increased by arterial vasoconstriction, which leads to decreased stroke volume. The opposite is true with arterial vasodilation, in which case afterload is reduced because there is less resistance to ejection, and stroke volume increases.

Contractility refers to the force generated by the contracting myocardium. Contractility is enhanced by circulating catecholamines, sympathetic neuronal activity, and certain medications (e.g., digoxin, dopamine, or dobutamine). Increased contractility results in increased stroke volume. Contractility is depressed by hypoxemia, acidosis, and certain medications (e.g., beta-adrenergic–blocking agents such as metoprolol).

The heart can achieve an increase in stroke volume (e.g., during exercise) if preload is increased (through increased venous return), if contractility is increased (through sympathetic nervous system discharge), and if afterload is decreased (through peripheral vasodilation with decreased aortic pressure).

The percentage of the end-diastolic blood volume that is ejected with each heartbeat is called the **ejection fraction.** The ejection fraction of the normal left ventricle is 55% to 65% (Wiegand, 2017). The right ventricular ejection fraction is rarely measured. The ejection fraction is used as a measure of myocardial contractility. An ejection fraction of less than 40% indicates that the patient has decreased left ventricular function and likely requires treatment of HF (refer to Chapter 25 for further discussion).

Gerontologic Considerations

Changes in cardiac structure and function occur with age. A loss of function of the cells throughout the conduction system leads to a slower heart rate. The size of the heart increases due to hypertrophy (thickening of the heart walls), which reduces the volume of blood that the chambers can hold. Hypertrophy also changes the structure of the myocardium, reducing the strength of contraction. Both of these changes negatively affect cardiac output. The valves, due to stiffening, no longer close properly. The resulting backflow of blood creates heart murmurs, a common finding in older adults (Bickley, 2017; Pappano & Weir, 2019).

As a result of these age-related changes, the cardiovascular system takes longer to compensate from increased metabolic demands due to stress, exercise, or illness. In these situations, older adults may become symptomatic with fatigue, shortness of breath, or palpitations and present with new physical examination findings (Bickley, 2017; Zipes, Libby, Bonow, et al., 2019). The structural and functional changes with aging and associated history and physical examination findings are summarized in Table 21-1.

Gender Considerations

Structural differences between the hearts of men and women have significant implications. The heart of a woman tends to be smaller than that of a man. The coronary arteries of a woman are also narrower in diameter than a man's arteries. When atherosclerosis occurs, these differences make procedures such as cardiac catheterization and angioplasty technically more difficult.

Women typically develop CAD 10 years later than men, as women have the benefit of the cardioprotective effects of the female hormone estrogen. The three major effects of estrogen are (1) an increase in high-density lipoprotein (HDL) that transports cholesterol out of arteries; (2) a reduction in low-density lipoprotein (LDL) that deposits cholesterol in the artery; and (3) dilation of the blood vessels, which enhance blood flow to the heart. As testosterone increases and estrogen decreases, women who are postmenopausal have a greater risk of CAD, CVD, and HF (Zhao, Guallar, Ouyang, et al., 2018). Hormone therapy (HT) is not recommended for routine prevention of CAD in women who are postmenopausal, although there are possible benefits to cardiovascular health if HT is initiated soon after the initiation of menopause (Keck & Taylor, 2018).

Assessment of the Cardiovascular System

The frequency and extent of the nursing assessment of cardiovascular function are based on several factors, including the severity of the patient's symptoms, the presence of risk factors, the practice setting, and the purpose of the assessment. Although the key components of the cardiovascular assessment remain the same, the assessment priorities vary according to patient needs. For example, an emergency department (ED) nurse performs a rapid and focused assessment of a patient in which **acute coronary syndrome** (ACS), signs and symptoms caused by ruptured atheromatous plaque in a diseased coronary artery, is suspected. Diagnosis and

TABLE 21-1	Age-Related Changes of the Cardiac System		
Cardiovascular Structure	**Structural Changes**	**Functional Changes**	**History and Physical Findings**
Atria	↑ Size of left atrium Thickening of the endocardium	↑ Atrial irritability	Irregular heart rhythm from atrial arrhythmias
Left ventricle	Endocardial fibrosis Myocardial hypertrophy (thickening) Infiltration of fat into myocardium	Left ventricle stiff and less compliant Progressive decline in cardiac output ↑ Risk for ventricular arrhythmias Prolonged systole	Fatigue ↓ Exercise tolerance Signs and symptoms of heart failure or ventricular arrhythmias Point of maximal impulse palpated lateral to the midclavicular line ↓ Intensity S_1, S_2; split S_2 S_4 may be present
Valves	Thickening and rigidity of AV valves Calcification of aortic valve	Abnormal blood flow across valves during cardiac cycle	Murmurs may be present Thrill may be palpated if significant murmur is present
Conduction system	Connective tissue collects in SA node, AV node, and bundle branches ↓ Number of SA node cells ↓ Number of AV, bundle of His, and right and left bundle branch cells	Slower SA node rate of impulse discharge Slowed conduction across AV node and ventricular conduction system	Bradycardia Heart block ECG changes consistent with slowed conduction (↑ PR interval, widened QRS complex)
Sympathetic nervous system	↓ Response to beta-adrenergic stimulation	↓ Adaptive response to exercise: contractility and heart rate slower to respond to exercise demands Heart rate takes more time to return to baseline	Fatigue Diminished exercise tolerance ↓ Ability to respond to stress
Aorta and arteries	Stiffening of vasculature ↓ Elasticity and widening of aorta Elongation of aorta, displacing the brachiocephalic artery upward	Left ventricular hypertrophy	Progressive increase in systolic BP; slight ↑ in diastolic BP Widening pulse pressure Pulsation visible above right clavicle
Baroreceptor response	↓ Sensitivity of baroreceptors in the carotid artery and aorta to transient episodes of hypertension and hypotension	Baroreceptors unable to regulate heart rate and vascular tone, causing slow response to postural changes in body position	Postural BP changes and reports of feeling dizzy, fainting when moving from lying to sitting or standing position

AV, atrioventricular; BP, blood pressure; ECG, electrocardiographic; SA, sinoatrial.
Adapted from Bickley, L. S. (2017). *Bates' guide to physical examination and history taking* (12th ed.). Philadelphia, PA: Lippincott Williams & Wilkins.

treatment must be started immediately, which includes an electrocardiogram (ECG) within 10 minutes of arrival to the ED (Yiadom, Baugh, McWade, et al., 2017). The physical assessment is ongoing and concentrates on evaluating the patient for ACS complications, such as a myocardial infarction (MI), arrhythmias, and HF, and determining the effectiveness of medical treatment.

Health History

The patient's ability to recognize cardiac symptoms and to know what to do when they occur is essential for effective self-care management. All too often, a patient's new symptoms or those of progressing cardiac dysfunction go unrecognized, resulting in lifesaving treatment delays. Research findings suggest that ethnic and socioeconomic factors can lead to patient-related delays (Iacoe, Ratner, Wong, et al., 2018). Women, African Americans, and older patients are reported to delay seeking treatment when they have had MIs (Zipes et al., 2019). Socioeconomic factors such as poverty, high health care costs, lack of insurance, transportation, and proximity to a health care provider or hospital can also lead to delays in care. Patients may also lack knowledge

about ACS symptoms, or experience denial, fear, or uncertainty about what to do when having chest pain. Some women have the misperception that the risk for cardiac disease is only linked to weight. A female patient who is embarrassed from the social stigma of being overweight may not see a health care provider, or could be reluctant to disclose important cardiac symptoms (Merz, Andersen, Sprague, et al., 2017). Therefore, during the health history, the nurse determines if the patient and involved family members are able to recognize symptoms of an acute cardiac problem, such as ACS or HF, and seek timely treatment of these symptoms. Responses to this level of inquiry will help the nurse individualize the plan for patient and family education.

Common Symptoms

The signs and symptoms experienced by people with CVD are related to arrhythmias and conduction problems (see Chapter 22); CAD (see Chapter 23); structural, infectious, and inflammatory disorders of the heart (see Chapter 24); and complications of CAD such as HF and cardiogenic shock (see Chapters 11 and 25). These disorders have many signs and symptoms in common; therefore, the nurse must be skillful at recognizing these signs and symptoms so that patients are given timely and often lifesaving care.

The following are the most common signs and symptoms of CVD, with related medical diagnoses in parentheses:

- Chest pain or discomfort (angina pectoris, ACS, arrhythmias, valvular heart disease)
- Pain or discomfort in other areas of upper body, including one or both arms, back, neck, jaw, or stomach (ACS)
- Shortness of breath or dyspnea (ACS, cardiogenic shock, HF, valvular heart disease)
- Peripheral edema, weight gain, abdominal distention due to enlarged spleen and liver or ascites (HF)
- Palpitations (tachycardia from a variety of causes, including ACS, caffeine or other stimulants, electrolyte imbalances, stress, valvular heart disease, ventricular aneurysms)
- Unusual fatigue, sometimes referred to as vital exhaustion (an early warning symptom of ACS, HF, or valvular heart disease, characterized by feeling unusually tired or fatigued, irritable, and dejected)
- Dizziness, syncope, or changes in level of consciousness (cardiogenic shock, cerebrovascular disorders, arrhythmias, hypotension, orthostatic hypotension, vasovagal episode)

Symptoms of ACS can differ between men and women. Chest pain and discomfort related to ACS can occur in both men and women. However, women may experience more atypical or nonspecific symptoms such as chest pain at rest; pain in the jaw, arm, neck, shoulder, middle back, or epigastrium; nausea; vomiting; syncope; sweating; anxiety; and fatigue (Lichtman, Leifheit, Safdar, et al., 2018; Merz et al., 2017).

Chest Pain

Chest pain and chest discomfort are common symptoms that may be caused by a number of cardiac and noncardiac problems. Table 21-2 summarizes the characteristics and patterns of common causes of chest pain or discomfort. To differentiate among these causes of pain, the nurse asks the patient to identify the quantity (0 = no pain to 10 = worst pain), location, and quality of pain. The nurse assesses for radiation of the pain to other areas of the body and determines if associated signs and symptoms are present, such as diaphoresis or nausea. It is important to identify the events that precipitate the onset of symptoms, the duration of the symptoms, and measures that aggravate or relieve the symptoms.

The nurse keeps the following important points in mind when assessing patients reporting chest pain or discomfort:

- The location of chest symptoms is not well correlated with the cause of the pain. For example, substernal chest pain can result from a number of causes as outlined in Table 21-2.
- The severity or duration of chest pain or discomfort does not predict the seriousness of its cause. For example, when asked to rate pain using a 0 to 10 scale, patients experiencing esophageal spasm may rate their chest pain as a 10. In contrast, patients having an acute MI, which is a potentially life-threatening event, may report having moderate pain rated as a 4 to 6 on the pain scale.
- More than one clinical cardiac condition may occur simultaneously. During an MI, patients may report chest pain from myocardial ischemia, shortness of breath from HF, and palpitations from arrhythmias. Both HF and arrhythmias can be complications of an acute MI. (See Chapter 23 for discussion of clinical manifestations of ACS, including MI.)

Past Health, Family, and Social History

The health history provides an opportunity for the nurse to assess patients' understanding of their personal risk factors for peripheral vascular, cerebrovascular, and CAD and any measures that they are taking to modify these risks. Some risk factors, such as increasing age, male gender, and heredity, including race are not modifiable. However, there are a number of risk factors, such as smoking, hypertension, high cholesterol, diabetes, obesity, and physical inactivity that can be modified by lifestyle changes or medications (Arnett, Blumenthal, Albert, et al., 2019). Online tools from the AHA and the American College of Cardiology (ACC) can be used to screen a person's risk for CVD, including risk for having an MI or stroke (ACC, 2019; AHA, 2018; see Resources at the end of this chapter for a link to these tools).

In an effort to determine how patients perceive their current health status, the nurse asks the following questions:

- How is your health? Have you noticed any changes from last year? From 5 years ago?
- Do you have a cardiologist or primary provider? How often do you go for checkups?
- What health concerns do you have?
- Do you have a family history of genetic disorders that place you at risk for CVD (Chart 21-1)?
- What are your risk factors for CAD (see Chapter 23, Chart 23-1)?
- What do you do to stay healthy and take care of your heart?

Patients who do not understand the connection between risk factors and CAD may be unwilling to make recommended lifestyle changes or manage their illness effectively. In contrast, patients who have this understanding may be more motivated to alter their lifestyle to avoid the risk of future cardiac events. The AHA published lifestyle management guidelines that identify interventions and treatment goals for each of these risk factors (Arnett et al., 2019). Chapter 23 provides an overview of this information.

Medications

Nurses collaborate with other health care providers, including pharmacists, to obtain a complete list of the patient's medications, including dose and frequency. Vitamins, herbals, and other over-the-counter medications are included on this list. During this aspect of the health assessment, the nurse asks the following questions to ensure that the patient is safely and effectively taking the prescribed medications.

- What are the names and doses of your medications?
- What is the purpose of each of these medications?
- How and when are these medications taken? Do you ever skip a dose or forget to take them?
- Are there any special precautions associated with any of these medications?
- What symptoms or problems do you need to report to your primary provider?

TABLE 21-2	Assessing Chest Pain				
Location	**Character**	**Duration**	**Precipitating Events and Aggravating Factors**	**Alleviating Factors**

Angina Pectoris, ACS (unstable angina, MI)

Usual distribution of pain with myocardial ischemia

Jaw

Epigastrium

Right side   Back

Less common sites of pain with myocardial ischemia

	Character	Duration	Precipitating Events and Aggravating Factors	Alleviating Factors
	Angina: Uncomfortable pressure, squeezing, or fullness in substernal chest area. Can radiate across chest to the medial aspect of one or both arms and hands, jaw, shoulders, upper back, or epigastrium. Radiation to arms and hands, described as numbness, tingling, or aching	*Angina:* 5–15 min	*Angina:* Physical exertion, emotional upset, eating large meal, or exposure to extremes in temperature	*Angina:* Rest, nitroglycerin, oxygen
	ACS: Same as angina pectoris. Pain or discomfort ranges from mild to severe. Associated with shortness of breath, diaphoresis, palpitations, unusual fatigue, and nausea or vomiting	ACS: >15 min	ACS: Emotional upset or unusual physical exertion occurring within 24 h of symptom onset. Can occur at rest or while asleep	ACS: Morphine, reperfusion of coronary artery with thrombolytic (fibrinolytic) agent or percutaneous coronary intervention
Pericarditis	Sharp, severe substernal or epigastric pain. Can radiate to neck, arms, and back. Associated symptoms include fever, malaise, dyspnea, cough, nausea, dizziness, and palpitations	Intermittent	Sudden onset. Pain increases with inspiration, swallowing, coughing, and rotation of trunk	Sitting upright, analgesia, anti-inflammatory medications
Pulmonary Disorders (pneumonia, pulmonary embolism)	Sharp, severe substernal or epigastric pain arising from inferior portion of pleura (referred to as pleuritic pain). Patient may be able to localize the pain	≥30 min	Follows an infectious or noninfectious process (MI, cardiac surgery, cancer, immune disorders, uremia). Pleuritic pain increases with inspiration, coughing, movement, and supine positioning. Occurs in conjunction with community- or hospital-acquired lung infections (pneumonia) or venous thromboembolism (pulmonary embolism)	Treatment of underlying cause

(continued on page 660)

TABLE 21-2 Assessing Chest Pain (continued)

Location	Character	Duration	Precipitating Events and Aggravating Factors	Alleviating Factors
Esophageal Disorders (hiatal hernia, reflux esophagitis or spasm)	Substernal pain described as sharp, burning, or heavy Often mimics angina Can radiate to neck, arm, or shoulders	5–60 min	Recumbency, cold liquids, exercise	Food or antacid Nitroglycerin
Anxiety and Panic Disorders	Pain described as stabbing to dull ache Associated with diaphoresis, palpitations, shortness of breath, tingling of hands or mouth, feeling of unreality, or fear of losing control	>30 min	Can occur at any time including during sleep Can be associated with a specific trigger	Removal of stimulus, relaxation, medications to treat anxiety or underlying disorder
Musculoskeletal Disorders (costochondritis)	Sharp or stabbing pain localized in anterior chest Most often unilateral Can radiate across chest to epigastrium or back	Hours to days	Most often follows respiratory tract infection with significant coughing, vigorous exercise, or posttrauma Some cases are idiopathic. Exacerbated by deep inspiration, coughing, sneezing, and movement of upper torso or arms	Rest, ice, or heat Analgesic or anti-inflammatory medications

ACS, acute coronary syndrome; MI, myocardial infarction.

Adapted from Bickley, L. S. (2017). *Bates' guide to physical examination and history taking* (12th ed.). Philadelphia, PA: Lippincott Williams & Wilkins; Rushton, S., & Carman, M. J. (2018). Chest pain: If it is not the heart, what is it? *Nursing Clinics of North America, 53*(3), 421–431; Zipes, D. P., Libby, P., Bonow, R. O., et al. (2019). *Braunwald's heart disease: A textbook of cardiovascular medicine* (11th ed.). Philadelphia, PA: Elsevier.

Patients recovering from ACS, including coronary stent placement or coronary artery bypass graft (CABG), are commonly prescribed dual antiplatelet therapy (DAPT). DAPT means that two antiplatelet drugs are prescribed for the patient. Aspirin, an OTC antiplatelet medication, is often prescribed for life. In addition, a second antiplatelet P2Y12 inhibitor medication (clopidogrel, prasugrel, or ticagrelor) is prescribed for 1 to 12 months, depending upon a variety of factors, including the patient's diagnosis and the type of procedure done (see Chapter 23 for further discussion of ACS treatment and pharmacologic management) (Levine, Bates, Bittl, et al., 2016). During a careful medication history, the nurse reinforces the necessity for adherence to the medication regimen.

Nutrition

Dietary modifications, exercise, weight loss, and careful monitoring are important strategies for managing three major cardiovascular risk factors: hyperlipidemia, hypertension, and diabetes. Diets that are restricted in sodium, fat, cholesterol,

Chart 21-1 GENETICS IN NURSING PRACTICE

Cardiovascular Disorders

Several cardiovascular disorders are associated with genetic abnormalities. Some examples are:

- Arrhythmogenic right ventricular dysplasia (ARVD)
- Brugada syndrome
- Familial hypercholesterolemia
- Hypertrophic cardiomyopathy
- Long QT syndrome
  - Jervell and Lange-Nielsen syndrome (autosomal recessive form)
  - Romano–Ward syndrome (autosomal dominant form)

Genetic connective tissue disorders that impact the cardiovascular system:

- Ehlers–Danlos syndrome
- Loeys–Dietz syndrome
- Marfan syndrome

Genetic blood disorders that can impair the function of the cardiovascular system:

- Factor V Leiden
- Hemochromatosis
- Sickle cell disease

Nursing Assessments

Refer to Chapter 4, Chart 4-2: Genetics in Nursing Practice: Genetic Aspects of Health Assessment

Family History Assessment Specific to Cardiovascular Disorders

- Assess all patients with cardiovascular symptoms for coronary artery disease, regardless of age.
- Inquire about a family history of sudden death or unexplained death.
- Ask about other family members with biochemical or neuro-muscular conditions (e.g., hemochromatosis or muscular dystrophy).

Patient Assessment Specific to Cardiovascular Disorders

- Assess for signs and symptoms of hyperlipidemias (xanthomas, corneal arcus, or abdominal pain of unexplained origin).
- Obtain an electrocardiogram and an echocardiogram.
- Assess for muscular weakness.
- Assess for episodes of shortness of breath, dizziness, or palpitations.
- Review laboratory data for abnormal values.
- Gather dietary history.
- Assess for secondary risk factors (e.g., diet, smoking, overweight, high stress, alcohol use).

Genetics Resources

American Heart Association, www.heart.org

Familial Hypercholesterolemia Foundation, www.thefhfoundation.org

Hypertrophic Cardiomyopathy Association, www.4hcm.org

Sudden Arrhythmia Death Syndromes, www.sads.org

See Chapter 6, Chart 6-7 for additional components of genetic counseling.

---

or calories are commonly prescribed. The nurse obtains the following information:

- The patient's current height and weight (to determine body mass index [BMI]); waist measurement; BP; and any laboratory test results such as blood glucose, glycosylated hemoglobin (diabetes), total blood cholesterol, HDL and LDL levels, and triglyceride levels (hyperlipidemia)
- How often the patient self-monitors BP, blood glucose, and weight as appropriate to the medical diagnoses
- The patient's level of awareness regarding their target goals for each of the risk factors and any problems achieving or maintaining these goals
- What the patient normally eats and drinks in a typical day and any food preferences (including cultural or ethnic preferences)
- Eating habits (canned or commercially prepared foods vs. fresh foods, restaurant meals vs. home cooking, assessing for high-sodium foods, dietary intake of fats)
- Who shops for groceries and prepares meals

Elimination

Typical bowel and bladder habits need to be identified. Nocturia (awakening at night to urinate) is common in patients with HF. Fluid collected in gravity-dependent tissues (extremities) during the day (i.e., edema) redistributes into the circulatory system once the patient is recumbent at night. The increased circulatory volume is excreted by the kidneys (increased urine production).

When straining during defecation, the patient bears down (the Valsalva maneuver), which momentarily increases pressure on the baroreceptors. This triggers a vagal response, causing the heart rate to slow and resulting in syncope in some patients. Straining during urination can produce the same response.

Because many cardiac medications can cause gastrointestinal side effects or bleeding, the nurse asks about bloating, diarrhea, constipation, stomach upset, heartburn, loss of appetite, nausea, and vomiting. Screening for bloody urine or stools should be done for patients taking antiplatelet medications (aspirin, clopidogrel, prasugrel, ticagrelor), platelet aggregation inhibitors (abciximab, eptifibatide, tirofiban), or anticoagulants (low-molecular-weight heparins such as dalteparin or enoxaparin; heparin; or oral anticoagulants such as warfarin, rivaroxaban, or apixaban).

Activity and Exercise

Changes in the patient's activity tolerance are often gradual and may go unnoticed. The nurse determines if there are recent changes by comparing the patient's current activity level with that performed in the past 6 to 12 months. New symptoms or a change in the usual symptoms during activity is a significant finding. Activity-induced angina or shortness of breath may indicate CAD. These CAD-related symptoms occur when myocardial ischemia is present, due to an inadequate arterial blood supply to the myocardium, in the setting of increased demand (e.g., exercise, stress, or anemia). Patients experiencing these kinds of symptoms need to seek medical attention. Fatigue, associated with a low left ventricular ejection fraction (less than 40%) and certain medications (e.g., beta-adrenergic–blocking agents), can result in activity intolerance. Patients with fatigue may benefit from having their medications adjusted and learning energy conservation techniques.

Additional areas to explore include the presence of architectural barriers in the home (stairs, multilevel home); the patient's participation in cardiac rehabilitation; and his or her current exercise pattern including intensity, duration, and frequency.

Sleep and Rest

Clues to worsening cardiac disease, especially HF, can be revealed by sleep-related events. Patients with worsening HF often experience *orthopnea*, a term used to indicate the need to sit upright or stand to avoid feeling short of breath. Patients experiencing orthopnea will report that they need to sleep upright in a chair or add extra pillows to their bed. Sudden awakening with shortness of breath, called *paroxysmal nocturnal dyspnea*, is an additional symptom of worsening HF. This nighttime symptom is caused by the reabsorption of fluid from dependent areas of the body (arms and legs) back into the circulatory system within hours of lying in bed. This sudden fluid shift increases preload and places increased demand on the heart of patients with HF, causing sudden pulmonary congestion.

Sleep-disordered breathing (SDB) is an abnormal respiratory pattern due to intermittent episodes of upper airway obstruction causing apnea and hypopnea (shallow respirations) during sleep. These abnormal sleep events cause intermittent hypoxemia, sympathetic nervous system activation, and increased intrathoracic pressure that puts mechanical stress on the heart and large artery walls. SDB impacts the length and quality of sleep. Short sleep duration (less than 7 hours per night) and poor sleep quality (interrupted sleep) are associated with the cardiovascular risks of hypertension, atherosclerosis, CAD, and stroke (Domínguez, Fuster, Fernández-Alvira, et al., 2019). Untreated SDB is also linked to HF and arrhythmias. Obstructive sleep apnea (OSA) is a type of SDB that is treated by the use of continuous positive airway pressure (CPAP), although many patients have difficulty with CPAP adherance. Other treatment options include weight loss, positional therapy, mandibular advancement devices (MADs), oral appliances, or surgery (Won, Mohsenin, & Kryger, 2018; see Chapter 18 for further discussion of OSA, including risks).

During the health history, the nurse assesses for SDB by asking patients at risk if they snore loudly, have frequent bouts of awaking from sleep, awaken with a headache, or experience hypersomnolence (severe daytime sleepiness). For patients with a diagnosis of SDB or OSA, the nurse determines if the patient has been prescribed a CPAP, MAD, or oral appliance, and the frequency of its use. Patients who are being admitted to the hospital or going for an ambulatory surgical procedure should be instructed to bring their sleep aid devices with them.

Self-Perception and Self-Concept

Self-perception and self-concept are both related to the cognitive and emotional processes that people use to formulate their beliefs and feelings about themselves. Having a chronic cardiac illness, such as HF, or experiencing an acute cardiac event, such as an MI, can alter a person's self-perception and self-concept. Patients' beliefs and feelings about their health are key determinants of adherence to self-care recommendations and recovery after an acute cardiac event. To reduce the risk of future cardiovascular-related health problems, patients are asked to make difficult lifestyle changes, such as quitting smoking. Patients who have misperceptions about the health consequences of their illness are at risk for nonadherence to these recommended lifestyle changes. The health history is used to discover how patients perceive their health by asking questions that may include the following:

- What is your cardiac condition?
- How has this illness changed your feelings about your health?
- What do you think caused this illness?
- What consequences do you think this illness will have on your physical activity, work, social relationships, and role in your family?
- How much of an influence do you think you have on controlling this illness?

The patient's responses to these questions can guide the nurse in planning interventions to ensure that the patient is prepared to manage the illness and that adequate services are in place to support the patient's recovery and self-care needs.

Roles and Relationships

Patients with CVD are being managed with complex medical regimens and sophisticated technology, such as implantable cardioverter defibrillators (ICDs) and left ventricular assist devices. Hospital stays for cardiac disorders have shortened. Many invasive diagnostic cardiac procedures, such as cardiac catheterization, are being performed in the ambulatory setting. Support from family members helps to lessen the patient's burden of managing self-care for cardiac illnesses. Social support is closely linked to patient depression and CVD outcomes. Patients who are depressed and who have poor social support have an increased risk of poor cardiac outcomes (Kim, Kang, Bae, et al., 2019).

To assess patients' roles in their families and their relationships, both components of social support, the nurse asks each patient: Who do you live with? Who is your primary caregiver at home? Who helps you manage your health? The nurse also assesses for any significant effects that the cardiac illness has had on the patient's role in the family. Are there adequate finances and health insurance? The answers to these questions help the nurse determine if consultation with social services or others is necessary to tailor the plan of care to meet the patient's self-care needs.

Sexuality and Reproduction

Sexual dysfunction affects twice as many people with CVD compared with the general population. Depression, anxiety, erectile dysfunction, and major cardiac events such as an MI are common reasons that patients report decreased sexual activity. Patients and their partners are concerned about the effects of physical exertion on the heart and if the activity may cause another heart attack, sudden death, or untoward symptoms such as angina, dyspnea, or palpitations. Couples

Chart 21-2 — NURSING RESEARCH PROFILE

Depression, Self-Efficacy, and Physical Activity among Patients with Coronary Artery Disease

Siow, E., Leung, D. Y., Wong, E. M., et al. (2018). Do depressive symptoms moderate the effects of exercise self-efficacy on physical activity among patients with coronary heart disease? *Journal of Cardiovascular Nursing, 33*(4), e26–e34.

Purpose

Physical activity and exercise can reduce cardiac complications in patients with coronary artery disease (CAD). Patients with higher levels of self-efficacy are more likely to start and maintain an exercise program. Patients with CAD are also at risk for developing depression, which can lead to isolation and low activity levels. Therefore, the purpose of this study was to examine the relationship between the symptoms of depression, exercise self-efficacy, and physical activity among patients with CAD. The nurse researchers also explored if depression could impact the relationship between exercise self-efficacy and physical activity in this population.

Design

A cross-sectional, exploratory study was conducted with adult participants with CAD who were hospitalized in an emergency medicine or general medical unit. This study was performed at two hospitals in Hong Kong. The nurse researchers conducted a survey interview with 149 participants before discharge from the hospital. Participants completed a survey with questions about their socioeconomic status, current level of physical activity, self-efficacy about exercise, and symptoms of depression. Participants were then asked about their physical activity using the Godin–Shephard Leisure-Time Physical Activity questionnaire, about exercise self-efficacy using the Self-Efficacy for Exercise scale, and about depression using the Centre for Epidemiological Studies-Depression tool. Other information such as body mass index (BMI), medical diagnosis, and how many times participants were admitted to the hospital was obtained from the hospital records.

Findings

Most participants in this study were older adults with a mean age of 73 ±13 years, were male, married, living with family, and had a lower socioeconomic status. Approximately 50% of this sample had a normal BMI, and over half did some level of exercise. Participants with greater exercise self-efficacy were more likely to engage in physical activity. However, this relationship was stronger among participants with symptoms of depression. Participants who were depressed reported lower levels of self-efficacy and engaging in less physical activity.

Nursing Implications

The results of this study demonstrate the importance of assessing self-efficacy, physical activity, and depression among patients with CAD. It is important to intervene and educate patients about lifestyle changes that improve exercise self-efficacy. Improving this level of confidence can help patients who are depressed start or increase their level of physical activity, which may improve cardiovascular health.

---

often lack adequate information about the physical demands related to sexual activity, which is considered a low-intensity exercise. The nurse can help patients by initiating discussions about sexuality and encouraging them to discuss problems with their primary provider or cardiologist. The exercise and counseling provided in cardiac rehabilitation programs may also improve sexual activity (Boothby, Dada, Rabi, et al., 2018).

A reproductive history is necessary for women of childbearing age, particularly those with seriously compromised cardiac function. The reproductive history includes information about previous pregnancies, plans for future pregnancies, oral contraceptive use (especially in women older than 35 years who smoke), menopausal status, and the use of HT. Women who have a history of preeclampsia during pregnancy, preterm labor, or giving birth to an infant that was small for gestational age have a higher risk for developing CVD (Lane-Cordova, Khan, Grobman, et al., 2019).

Coping and Stress Tolerance

Anxiety, depression, and stress are known to influence both the development of and recovery from CAD and HF. Depression is twice as prevalent in women compared to men and has a negative impact on quality of life and overall prognosis. Patients who are depressed are more likely to be readmitted to the hospital after having a heart attack. The risk of depression is lower if the patient has relationship and work stability, a higher educational level, a healthy lifestyle, and the absence of comorbidities such as diabetes. Although the association between depression and CAD is not completely understood, biologic factors (e.g., platelet abnormalities, inflammatory responses, insulin resistance), lifestyle factors (e.g., diet, exercise, smoking), and behavioral factors (e.g., substance abuse, unemployment, social isolation) contribute to this link. Patients who are depressed are less motivated to adhere to follow-up appointments, take prescribed medications, or make recommended lifestyle changes such as smoking cessation, losing weight, exercising, or participating in cardiac rehabilitation (Jha, Qamar, Vaduganathan, et al., 2019; Vaccarino, Badimon, Bremner, et al., 2019; Yuan, Fang, Liu, et al., 2019). See Chart 21-2 for a Nursing Research Profile on depression, self-efficacy, and physical activity.

Patients with CAD or HF should be assessed for depression. Patients who have depression exhibit common signs and symptoms, such as feelings of worthlessness or guilt, problems falling asleep or staying asleep, having little interest or pleasure in doing things that they usually enjoy, having difficulty concentrating, restlessness, and recent changes in appetite or weight. The Patient Health Questionnaire (PHQ-2) is a two-question self-reported patient assessment tool recommended by the AHA. The nurse asks the patient:

- *Do you have little interest or pleasure in doing things over the last 2 weeks?*
- *Are you feeling down, depressed or hopeless over the last 2 weeks?*

The nurse scores the patient's responses to each question by assigning 0 for "not at all," 1 for "several days," 2 for "more than half the days," or 3 for "nearly every day." The PHQ-2 score ranges from 0 to 6. Patients with a positive score greater than or equal to 3 complete a focused screening called the PHQ-9 and are referred to their primary providers for further evaluation (Jha et al., 2019).

Stress initiates a variety of responses, including increased levels of catecholamines and cortisol, and has been strongly linked to cardiovascular events, such as an MI. Therefore, patients need to be assessed for sources of stress; the nurse asks about recent or ongoing stressors, previous coping styles and effectiveness, and the patient's perception of their current mood and coping ability. A widely used tool used to measure life stress is the Social Readjustment Rating Scale (Homes & Rahe, 1967). Examples of items on this scale include death of a spouse, divorce, and change in responsibilities at work. Each item is assigned a score of 11 to 100. Patients identify the items that happened to them in the previous year. Patients with a score less than 150 have a slight risk for future illness, whereas a score of 150 to 299 indicates a moderate risk. A score of 300 or higher indicates a high risk for future illness. Consultation with a psychiatric advanced practice nurse, psychologist, psychiatrist, or social worker is indicated for patients who are anxious or depressed or for patients who are having difficulty coping with their cardiac illness.

Physical Assessment

Physical assessment is conducted to confirm information obtained from the health history, to establish the patient's current or baseline condition, and, in subsequent assessments, to evaluate the patient's response to treatment. Once the initial physical assessment is completed, the frequency of future assessments is determined by the purpose of the encounter and the patient's condition. For example, a focused cardiac assessment may be performed each time the patient is seen in the outpatient setting, whereas patients in the acute care setting may require a more extensive assessment at least every 8 hours. During the physical assessment, the nurse evaluates the cardiovascular system for any deviations from normal with regard to the following (examples of abnormalities are in parentheses):

- The heart as a pump (reduced pulse pressure, displaced PMI from fifth intercostal space midclavicular line, gallop sounds, murmurs)
- Atrial and ventricular filling volumes and pressures (elevated jugular venous distention, peripheral edema, ascites, crackles, postural changes in BP)
- Cardiac output (reduced pulse pressure, hypotension, tachycardia, reduced urine output, lethargy, or disorientation)
- Compensatory mechanisms (peripheral vasoconstriction, tachycardia)

General Appearance

This part of the assessment evaluates the patient's level of consciousness (alert, lethargic, stuporous, comatose) and mental status (oriented to person, place, time; coherence). Changes in level of consciousness and mental status may be attributed to inadequate perfusion of the brain from a compromised cardiac output or thromboembolic event (stroke). Patients are observed for signs of distress, which include pain or discomfort, shortness of breath, or anxiety.

The nurse notes the size of the patient (normal, overweight, underweight, or cachectic). The patient's height and weight are measured to calculate BMI, as well as the waist circumference (see Chapter 4). These measures are used to determine if obesity (BMI greater than 30 kg/m²) and abdominal fat (males: waist greater than 40 inches; females: waist greater than 35 inches) are placing the patient at risk for CAD.

Assessment of the Skin and Extremities

Examination of the skin includes all body surfaces, starting with the head and finishing with the lower extremities. Skin color, temperature, and texture are assessed for acute and chronic problems with arterial or venous circulation. Table 21-3 summarizes common skin and extremity assessment findings in patients with CVD. The most noteworthy changes include the following:

- Signs and symptoms of acute obstruction of arterial blood flow in the extremities, referred to as the six Ps, are pain, pallor, pulselessness, paresthesia, poikilothermia (coldness), and paralysis. During the first few hours after invasive cardiac procedures (e.g., cardiac catheterization, percutaneous coronary intervention [PCI], or cardiac electrophysiology testing), affected extremities should be assessed frequently for these acute vascular changes.
- Major blood vessels of the arms and legs may be used for catheter insertion. During these procedures, systemic anticoagulation with heparin is necessary, and bruising or small hematomas may occur at the catheter access site. However, large hematomas are a serious complication that can compromise circulating blood volume and cardiac output. Patients who have undergone these procedures must have catheter access sites frequently observed until hemostasis is adequately achieved.
- Edema of the feet, ankles, or legs is called *peripheral edema*. Edema can be observed in the sacral area of patients on bed rest. The nurse assesses the patient for edema by using the thumb to place firm pressure over the dorsum of each foot, behind each medial malleolus, over the shins or sacral area for 5 seconds. *Pitting edema* is the term used to describe an indentation in the skin created by this pressure (see Chapter 25, Fig. 25-2). The degree of pitting edema relies on the clinician's judgment of depth of edema and time the indentation remains after release of pressure. Pitting edema is graded as absent (0) or as present on a scale from trace (1+ ≤0.25 inch) to severe (4+ ≥1 inch) (Urden, Stacy, & Lough, 2017). It is important that clinicians use a consistent scale in order to ensure reliable clinical measurements and management. Peripheral edema is a common finding in patients with HF and peripheral vascular diseases, such as deep vein thrombosis or chronic venous insufficiency.
- Prolonged capillary refill time indicates inadequate arterial perfusion to the extremities. To test capillary refill time, the nurse compresses the nail bed briefly to occlude perfusion and the nail bed blanches. Then, the nurse releases pressure and determines the time it takes to restore perfusion. Normally, reperfusion occurs within 2 seconds, as evidenced by the return of color to the nail bed. Prolonged capillary refill time indicates compromised arterial perfusion, a problem associated with cardiogenic shock and HF.
- Clubbing of the fingers and toes indicates chronic hemoglobin desaturation and is associated with congenital heart disease.

TABLE 21-3	Common Assessment Findings Associated with Cardiovascular Disease
Assessment Findings	**Associated Causes and Conditions**
Clubbing of the fingers or toes (thickening of the skin under the fingers or toes)	Chronic hemoglobin desaturation most often due to congenital heart disease, advanced pulmonary diseases
Cool/cold skin and diaphoresis	Low cardiac output (e.g., cardiogenic shock, acute myocardial infarction) causing sympathetic nervous system stimulation with resultant vasoconstriction
Cold, pain, pallor of the fingertips or toes	Intermittent arteriolar vasoconstriction (Raynaud disease). Skin may change in color from white, blue, and red accompanied by numbness, tingling, and burning pain
Cyanosis, central (a bluish tinge observed in the tongue and buccal mucosa)	Serious cardiac disorders (pulmonary edema, cardiogenic shock, congenital heart disease) result in venous blood passing through the pulmonary circulation without being oxygenated
Cyanosis, peripheral (a bluish tinge, most often of the nails and skin of the nose, lips, earlobes, and extremities)	Peripheral vasoconstriction, allowing more time for the hemoglobin molecules to become desaturated. It can be caused by exposure to cold environment, anxiety, or ↓ cardiac output
Ecchymosis or bruising (a purplish-blue color fading to green, yellow, or brown)	Blood leaking outside of the blood vessels. Excessive bruising is a risk for patients on anticoagulants or platelet-inhibiting medications
Edema, lower extremities (collection of fluid in the interstitial spaces of the tissues)	Heart failure and vascular problems (PAD, chronic venous insufficiency, deep vein thrombosis, thrombophlebitis)
Hematoma (localized collection of clotted blood in the tissue)	Bleeding after catheter removal/tissue injury in patients on anticoagulant/antithrombotic agents
Pallor (↓ skin color in fingernails, lips, oral mucosa, and lower extremities)	Anemia or ↓ arterial perfusion. Suspect PAD if feet develop pallor after elevating legs 60 degrees from a supine position
Rubor (a reddish-blue discoloration of the legs, seen within 20 s to 2 min after placing in a dependent position)	Filling of dilated capillaries with deoxygenated blood, indicative of PAD
Ulcers, feet and ankles: Superficial, irregular ulcers at medial malleolus. Red to yellow granulation tissue	Rupture of small skin capillaries from chronic venous insufficiency
Ulcers, feet and ankles: Painful, deep, round ulcers on feet or from exposure to pressure. Pale to black wound base	Prolonged ischemia to tissues due to PAD. Can lead to gangrene
Thinning of skin around a cardiac implantable electronic device	Erosion of the device through the skin
Xanthelasma (yellowish, raised plaques observed along nasal portion of eyelids)	Elevated cholesterol levels (hypercholesterolemia)

PAD, peripheral arterial disease.
Adapted from Bickley, L. S. (2017). *Bates' guide to physical examination and history taking* (12th ed.). Philadelphia, PA: Lippincott Williams & Wilkins.

- Hair loss, brittle nails, dry or scaling skin, atrophy of the skin, skin color changes, and ulcerations are indicative of chronically reduced oxygen and nutrient supply to the skin observed in patients with arterial or venous insufficiency (see Chapter 26 for a complete description of these conditions) (Weber & Kelley, 2018).

Blood Pressure

Systemic arterial BP is the pressure exerted on the walls of the arteries during ventricular systole and diastole. It is affected by factors such as cardiac output; distention of the arteries; and the volume, velocity, and viscosity of the blood. A normal adult BP is considered a systolic BP less than 120 mm Hg over a diastolic BP less than 80 mm Hg. High BP, called **hypertension,** is defined in two stages and is based upon BP taken on at least two instances. Stage 1 hypertension is a systolic BP between 130 and 139 mm Hg or a diastolic BP between 80 and 89 mm Hg. Stage 2 hypertension is a systolic BP over 140 mm Hg or a diastolic over 90 mm Hg (Whelton, Carey, Aronow, et al., 2018). **Hypotension** refers to an abnormally low systolic and diastolic BP that can result in lightheadedness or fainting. (See Chapter 27 for additional definitions, measurement, and management.)

Pulse Pressure

The difference between the systolic and the diastolic pressures is called the *pulse pressure.* A normal pulse pressure is 40 mm Hg. A narrow pulse pressure (e.g., BP of 92/74 mm Hg and pulse pressure of 18 mm Hg) occurs when there is vasoconstriction that is compensating for a low stroke volume and ejection velocity (shock, HF, hypovolemia, mitral regurgitation) or obstruction to blood flow during systole (mitral or aortic stenosis). This compensation allows for adequate organ perfusion. A wide pulse pressure (e.g., BP of 88/38 mm Hg and pulse pressure of 50 mm Hg) is associated with conditions that elevate the stroke volume (anxiety, exercise, bradycardia), or cause vasodilation (fever, septic shock). Abnormal pulse pressures require further cardiovascular assessment (Urden et al., 2017).

Orthostatic (Postural) Blood Pressure Changes

There is a gravitational redistribution of approximately 500 mL of blood into the lower extremities immediately upon standing. This venous pooling reduces blood return to the heart, compromising preload that ultimately reduces stroke volume and cardiac output. As a consequence, the autonomic nervous system is activated. The sympathetic nervous system increases heart rate and enhances peripheral vasoconstriction, whereas parasympathetic activity of the heart via the vagus nerve is decreased. This stabilization occurs within 1 minute (Ricci, De Caterina, & Fedorowski, 2015).

Normal postural responses that occur when a person moves from a lying to a standing position include (1) a heart rate increase of 5 to 20 bpm above the resting rate; (2) an unchanged systolic pressure, or a slight decrease of up to 10 mm Hg; and (3) a slight increase of 5 mm Hg in diastolic pressure.

Orthostatic (postural) hypotension is a sustained decrease of at least 20 mm Hg in systolic BP or 10 mm Hg in diastolic BP within 3 minutes of moving from a lying or sitting to a standing position. It is usually accompanied by dizziness, lightheadedness, or syncope. The risk of orthostatic hypotension increases with age and is associated with fall risk (Ricci et al., 2015).

Orthostatic hypotension in patients with CVD is most often due to a significant reduction in preload, which compromises cardiac output. Reduced preload, which is reflective of intravascular volume depletion, is caused by dehydration from overdiuresis, bleeding (due to antiplatelet or anticoagulant medications or post intravascular procedures), or medications that dilate the blood vessels (e.g., nitrates and antispasmodic agents). In these situations, the usual mechanisms needed to maintain cardiac output (increased heart rate and peripheral vasoconstriction) cannot compensate for the significant loss in intravascular volume. As a result, the BP drops and heart rate increases with changes from lying or sitting to upright positions (Chart 21-3).

The following is an example of BP and heart rate measurements in a patient with orthostatic hypotension:

Supine: BP 120/70 mm Hg, heart rate 70 bpm
Sitting: BP 100/55 mm Hg, heart rate 90 bpm
Standing: BP 98/52 mm Hg, heart rate 94 bpm

Arterial Pulses

The arteries are palpated to evaluate the pulse rate, rhythm, amplitude, contour, and obstruction to blood flow.

Pulse Rate

The normal pulse rate varies from a low of 50 bpm in healthy, athletic young adults to rates well in excess of 100 bpm after exercise or during times of excitement. Anxiety can raise

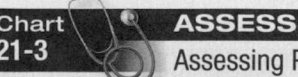

Chart 21-3	**ASSESSMENT** Assessing Patients for Orthostatic Hypotension

The following steps are recommended when assessing patients for orthostatic hypotension:

- Position the patient supine for 10 minutes before taking the initial blood pressure (BP) and heart rate measurements.
- Reposition the patient to a sitting position with legs in the dependent position, wait 2 minutes, then reassess both BP and heart rate measurements.
- If the patient is symptom free or has no significant decreases in systolic or diastolic BP, assist the patient into a standing position, obtain measurements immediately, and recheck in 2 minutes; continue measurements every 2 minutes for a total of 10 minutes to rule out orthostatic hypotension.
- Return the patient to a supine position if orthostatic hypotension is detected or if the patient becomes symptomatic.
- Document heart rate and BP measured in each position (e.g., supine, sitting, standing) and any signs or symptoms that accompany the postural changes.

Adapted from Momeyer, M. A., & Mion, L. C. (2018). Orthostatic hypotension: An often overlooked risk factor for falls. *Geriatric Nursing, 39*(4), 483–486; Urden, L. D., Stacy, K. M., & Lough, M. E. (2017). *Critical care nursing: Diagnosis and management* (8th ed.). St. Louis, MO: Elsevier Mosby.

the pulse rate during the physical examination. If the rate is higher than expected, the nurse should reassess the pulse near the end of the physical examination, when the patient may be more relaxed.

Pulse Rhythm

The rhythm of the pulse is normally regular. Minor variations in regularity of the pulse may occur with respirations. The pulse rate may increase during inhalation and slow during exhalation due to changes in blood flow to the heart during the respiratory cycle. This phenomenon, called *sinus arrhythmia*, occurs most commonly in children and young adults.

For the initial cardiac examination, or if the pulse rhythm is irregular, the heart rate should be counted by auscultating the apical pulse, located at the PMI, for a full minute while simultaneously palpating the radial pulse. Any discrepancy between contractions heard and pulses felt is noted. Disturbances of rhythm (arrhythmias) often result in a **pulse deficit,** which is a difference between the apical and radial pulse rates. Pulse deficits commonly occur with atrial fibrillation, atrial flutter, and premature ventricular contractions. These arrhythmias stimulate the ventricles to contact prematurely, before diastole is finished. As a result, these early ventricular contractions produce a smaller stroke volume, which can be heard during auscultation but do not produce a palpable pulse (see Chapter 22 for a detailed discussion of these arrhythmias).

Pulse Amplitude

The pulse amplitude, indicative of the BP in the artery, is used to assess peripheral arterial circulation. The nurse assesses pulse amplitude bilaterally and describes and records the amplitude of each artery. The simplest method characterizes the pulse as absent, diminished, normal, or bounding. Scales are also used to rate the strength of the pulse. The following is an example of a 0 to 4 scale:

0: Not palpable or absent

+1: Diminished—weak, thready pulse; difficult to palpate; obliterated with pressure

+2: Normal—cannot be obliterated

+3: Moderately increased—easy to palpate, full pulse; cannot be obliterated

+4: Markedly increased—strong, bounding pulse; may be abnormal

The numerical classification is subjective; therefore, when documenting the pulse amplitude, specify location of the artery and scale range (e.g., "left radial +3/+4") (Weber & Kelley, 2018).

If the pulse is absent or difficult to palpate, the nurse can use a continuous wave Doppler. This portable ultrasound device has a transducer that is placed over the artery. The transducer emits and receives ultrasound beams. Rhythmic changes are heard as blood cells flow through patent arteries, whereas obstruction to blood flow is evidenced by no changes in sound. (Ultrasound techniques are discussed in more detail in Chapter 26.)

Pulse Contour

The contour of the pulse conveys important information. In patients with stenosis of the aortic valve, the valve opening is narrowed, reducing the amount of blood ejected into the aorta. The pulse pressure is narrow, and the pulse feels feeble. In aortic insufficiency, the aortic valve does not close completely, allowing blood to flow back from the aorta into the left ventricle. The rise of the pulse wave is abrupt and strong, and its fall is precipitous—a "collapsing" or "water hammer" pulse. The true contour of the pulse is best appreciated by palpating over the carotid artery rather than the distal radial artery, because the dramatic characteristics of the pulse wave may be distorted when the pulse is transmitted to smaller vessels.

Palpation of Arterial Pulses

To assess peripheral circulation, the nurse locates and evaluates all arterial pulses. Arterial pulses are palpated at points where the arteries are near the skin surface and are easily compressed against bones or firm musculature. Pulses are detected over the right and left temporal, common carotid, brachial, radial, femoral, popliteal, dorsalis pedis, and posterior tibial arteries (see Chapter 26, Fig. 26-2). A reliable assessment of the pulses depends on accurate identification of the location of the artery and careful palpation of the area. Light palpation is essential; firm finger pressure can obliterate the temporal, dorsalis pedis, and posterior tibial pulses and confuse the examiner. In approximately 10% of patients, the dorsalis pedis pulses are not palpable (Sidawy & Perler, 2019). In such circumstances, both are usually absent and the posterior tibial arteries alone provide adequate blood supply to the feet. Arteries in the extremities are often palpated simultaneously to facilitate comparison of quality.

> ### ▶ *Quality and Safety Nursing Alert*
>
> *Do not simultaneously palpate both the temporal and carotid arteries, because it is possible to decrease the blood flow to the brain.*

Jugular Venous Pulsations

Right-sided heart function can be estimated by observing the pulsations of the jugular veins of the neck, which reflects central venous pressure (CVP). CVP is the pressure in the right atria or the right ventricle at the end of diastole. If the internal jugular pulsations are difficult to see, pulsations of the external jugular veins may be noted. These veins are more superficial and are visible just above the clavicles, adjacent to the sternocleidomastoid muscles.

In patients with euvolemia (normal blood volume), the jugular veins are normally visible in the supine position with the head of the bed elevated to 30 degrees (Bickley, 2017). Obvious distention of the veins with the patient's head elevated 45 to 90 degrees indicates an abnormal increase in CVP. This abnormality is observed in patients with right-sided HF, due to hypervolemia, pulmonary hypertension, and pulmonary stenosis; less commonly with obstruction of blood flow in the superior vena cava; and rarely with acute massive pulmonary embolism.

Heart Inspection and Palpation

The heart is examined by inspection, palpation, and auscultation of the precordium or anterior chest wall that covers the heart and lower thorax. A systematic approach is used to examine the precordium in the following six areas. Figure 21-5 identifies these important landmarks:

1. *Aortic area*—second intercostal space to the right of the sternum. To determine the correct intercostal space, the nurse first finds the angle of Louis by locating the bony ridge near the top of the sternum, at the junction of the sternum and the manubrium. From this angle, the second intercostal space is located by sliding one finger to the left or right of the sternum. Subsequent intercostal spaces are located from this reference point by palpating down the rib cage.

2. *Pulmonic area*—second intercostal space to the left of the sternum

3. *Erb point*—third intercostal space to the left of the sternum

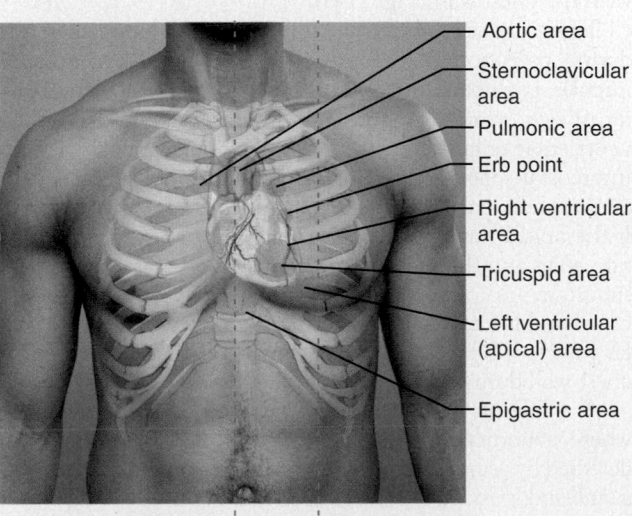

Midsternum   Midclavicular line

Figure 21-5 • Areas of the precordium to be assessed when evaluating heart function.

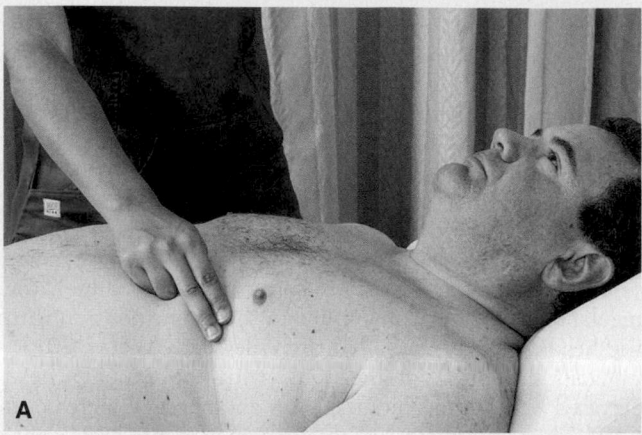
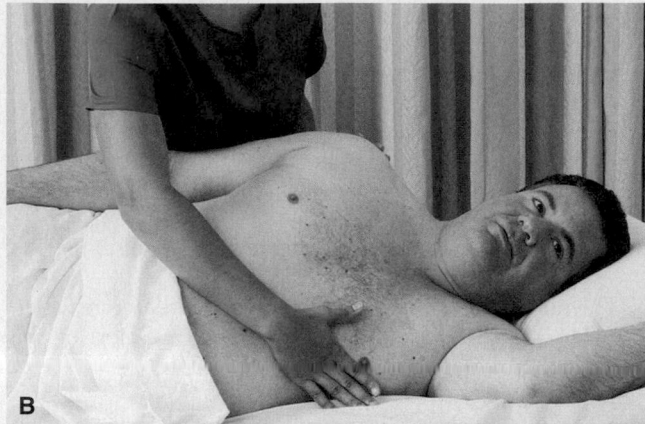

Figure 21-6 • Palpating the apical impulse. **A.** Remain on the patient's right side, and ask the patient to remain supine. Use the finger pads to palpate the apical impulse in the mitral area (fifth intercostal space at the midclavicular line). **B.** You may ask the patient to roll to the left side to better feel the impulse using the palmar surfaces of your hand. Photos used with permission from Weber, J. R., & Kelley, J. H. (2018). *Health assessment in nursing* (6th ed.). Philadelphia, PA: Lippincott Williams & Wilkins.

4. *Tricuspid area*—fourth and fifth intercostal spaces to the left of the sternum
5. *Mitral (apical) area*—left fifth intercostal space at the midclavicular line
6. *Epigastric area*—below the xiphoid process

For most of the examination, the patient lies supine, with the head of the bed or the examination table slightly elevated. A right-handed examiner stands at the right side of the patient, a left-handed examiner at the left side.

Each area of the precordium is inspected for pulsations and is then palpated. An apical impulse is a normal finding observed in young patients and adults who have thin chest walls.

The apical impulse may be felt as a light pulsation, 1 to 2 cm in diameter. It is felt at the onset of the first heart sound and lasts for only half of ventricular systole (see the next section for a discussion of heart sounds). The nurse uses the palm of the hand to locate the apical impulse initially and the finger pads to assess its size and quality. Palpation of the apical pulse may be facilitated by repositioning the patient to the left lateral position, which puts the heart in closer contact with the chest wall (Fig. 21-6).

There are several abnormalities that the nurse may find during palpation of the precordium. Normally, the apical impulse is palpable in only one intercostal space; palpability in two or more adjacent intercostal spaces indicates left ventricular enlargement. An apical impulse below the fifth intercostal space or lateral to the midclavicular line usually denotes left ventricular enlargement from left ventricular HF. If the apical impulse can be palpated in two distinctly separate areas and the pulsation movements are paradoxical (not simultaneous), a ventricular aneurysm may be suspected. A broad and forceful apical impulse is known as a left ventricular heave or lift because it appears to lift the hand from the chest wall during palpation.

A vibration or purring sensation may be felt over areas where abnormal, turbulent blood flow is present. It is best detected by using the palm of the hand. This vibration is called a *thrill* and is associated with a loud murmur. Depending on the location of the thrill, it may be indicative of serious valvular heart disease; an atrial or ventricular septal defect (abnormal opening); or stenosis of a large artery, such as the carotid artery.

Heart Auscultation

A stethoscope is used to auscultate each of the locations identified in Figure 21-5, with the exception of the epigastric area. The purpose of cardiac auscultation is to determine heart rate and rhythm and evaluate heart sounds. The apical area is auscultated for 1 minute to determine the apical pulse rate and the regularity of the heartbeat. Normal and abnormal heart sounds detected during auscultation are described next.

Normal Heart Sounds

Normal heart sounds, referred to as S_1 and S_2, are produced by closure of the AV valves and the semilunar valves, respectively. The period between S_1 and S_2 corresponds with ventricular systole (Fig. 21-7). When the heart rate is within the normal range, systole is much shorter than the period between S_2 and S_1 (diastole). However, as the heart rate increases, diastole shortens.

Normally, S_1 and S_2 are the only sounds heard during the cardiac cycle (Bickley, 2017).

S_1—First Heart Sound

Tricuspid and mitral valve closure creates the first heart sound (S_1). The word "lub" is used to replicate its sound. S_1 is usually heard the loudest at the apical area. S_1 is easily identifiable and serves as the point of reference for the remainder of the cardiac cycle.

The intensity of S_1 increases during tachycardias or with mitral stenosis. In these circumstances, the AV valves are wide open during ventricular contraction. The accentuated S_1 occurs as the AV valves close with greater force than normal. Similarly, arrhythmias can vary the intensity of S_1 from beat to beat due to lack of synchronized atrial and ventricular contraction.

S_2—Second Heart Sound

Closure of the pulmonic and aortic valves produces the second heart sound (S_2), commonly referred to as the "dub" sound. The aortic component of S_2 is heard the loudest over the aortic and pulmonic areas. However, the pulmonic component of S_2 is a softer sound and is heard best over the pulmonic area.

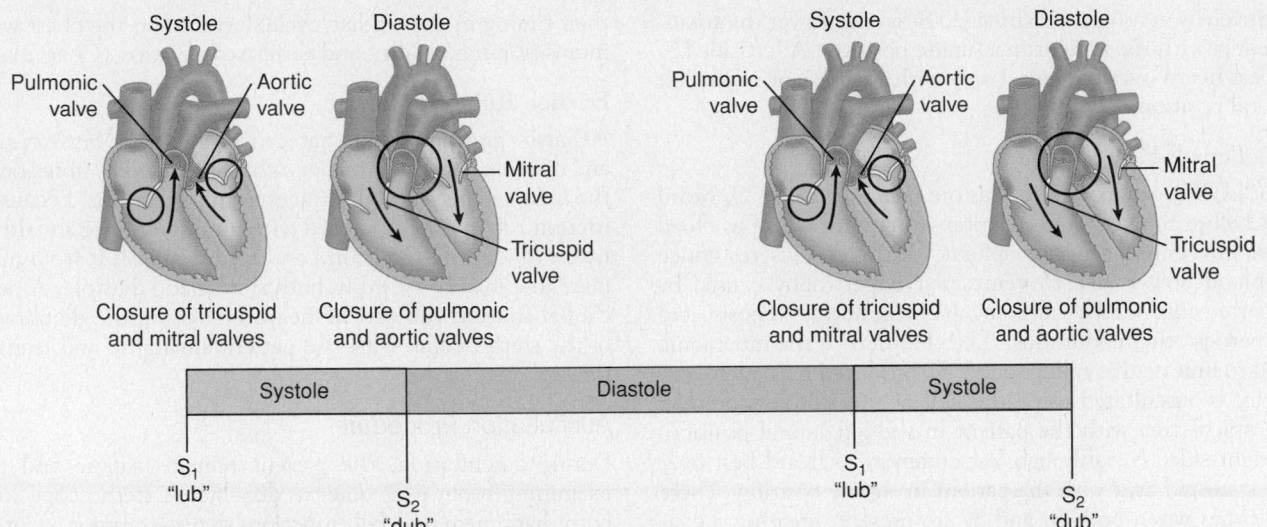

Figure 21-7 • Normal heart sounds. The first heart sound (S_1) is produced by closure of the mitral and tricuspid valves ("lub"). The second heart sound (S_2) is produced by closure of the aortic and pulmonic valves ("dub"). *Arrows* represent the direction of blood flow.

Although these valves close almost simultaneously, the pulmonic valve lags slightly behind the aortic valve. In some individuals, it is possible to distinguish between the closure of the aortic and pulmonic valves. When this situation occurs, the patient is said to have a split S_2. Normal physiologic splitting of S_2 is accentuated on inspiration and disappears on expiration. During inspiration, there is a decrease in intrathoracic pressure and subsequent increase in venous return to the right atrium and ventricle. The right ventricle takes a little longer to eject this extra volume, which causes the pulmonic valve to close a little later than normal. Splitting of S_2 that remains constant during inspiration and expiration is an abnormal finding. Abnormal splitting of the second heart sound can be caused by a variety of disease states (valvular heart disease, septal defects, bundle branch blocks). Splitting of S_2 is best heard over the pulmonic area.

Abnormal Heart Sounds

Abnormal sounds develop during systole or diastole when structural or functional heart problems are present. These sounds are called S_3 or S_4 gallops, opening snaps, systolic clicks, and murmurs. S_3 and S_4 gallop sounds are heard during diastole. These sounds are created by the vibration of the ventricle and surrounding structures as blood meets resistance during ventricular filling. The term *gallop* evolved from the cadence that is produced by the addition of a third or fourth heart sound, similar to the sound of a galloping horse. Gallop sounds are very low-frequency sounds and are heard with the bell of the stethoscope placed very lightly against the chest.

S_3—Third Heart Sound

An S_3 ("DUB") is heard early in diastole during the period of rapid ventricular filling as blood flows from the atrium into a noncompliant ventricle. It is heard immediately after S_2. "Lub-dub-DUB" is used to imitate the abnormal sound of a beating heart when an S_3 is present. It represents a normal finding in children and adults up to 35 or 40 years of age. In these cases, it is referred to as a physiologic S_3 (Fig. 21-8). In older adults, an S_3 is a significant finding, suggesting HF. It is best heard with the bell of the stethoscope. If the right

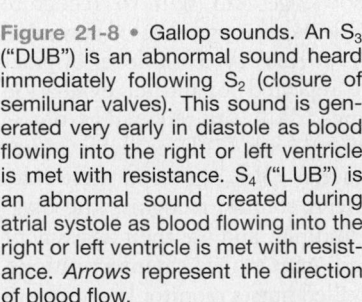

Figure 21-8 • Gallop sounds. An S_3 ("DUB") is an abnormal sound heard immediately following S_2 (closure of semilunar valves). This sound is generated very early in diastole as blood flowing into the right or left ventricle is met with resistance. S_4 ("LUB") is an abnormal sound created during atrial systole as blood flowing into the right or left ventricle is met with resistance. *Arrows* represent the direction of blood flow.

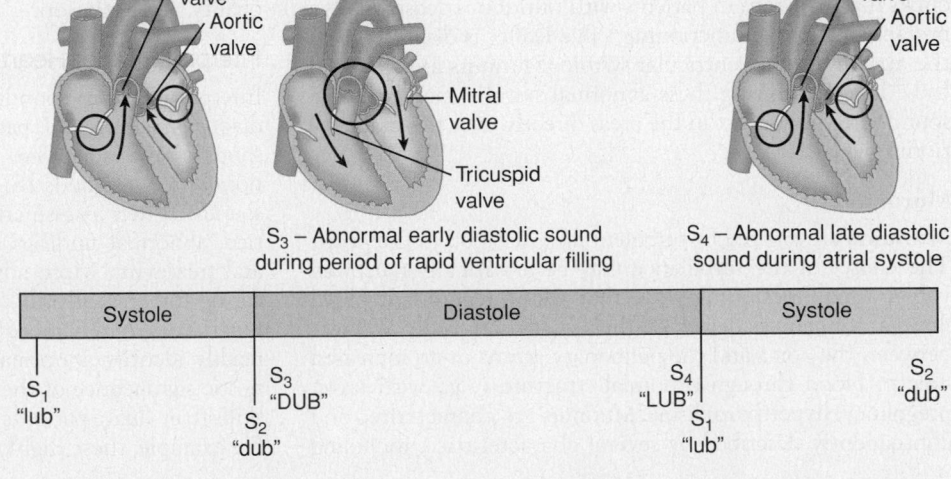

S_3 – Abnormal early diastolic sound during period of rapid ventricular filling

S_4 – Abnormal late diastolic sound during atrial systole

ventricle is involved, a right-sided S_3 is heard over the tricuspid area with the patient in a supine position. A left-sided S_3 is best heard over the apical area with the patient in the left lateral position.

S_4—Fourth Heart Sound

S_4 ("LUB") occurs late in diastole (see Fig. 21-8). S_4 heard just before S_1 is generated during atrial contraction as blood forcefully enters a noncompliant ventricle. This resistance to blood flow is due to ventricular hypertrophy caused by hypertension, CAD, cardiomyopathies, aortic stenosis, and numerous other conditions. "LUB lub-dub" is the mnemonic used to imitate this gallop sound. S_4, produced in the left ventricle, is auscultated using the bell of the stethoscope over the apical area with the patient in the left lateral position. A right-sided S_4, although less common, is heard best over the tricuspid area with the patient in supine position. There are times when both S_3 and S_4 are present, creating a quadruple rhythm, which sounds like "LUB lub-dub DUB." During tachycardia, all four sounds combine into a loud sound, referred to as a **summation gallop**.

Opening Snaps and Systolic Clicks

Normally, no sound is produced when valves open. However, diseased valve leaflets create abnormal sounds as they open during diastole or systole. **Opening snaps** are abnormal diastolic sounds heard during opening of an AV valve. For example, mitral stenosis can cause an opening snap, which is an unusually high-pitched sound very early in diastole. This sound is caused by high pressure in the left atrium that abruptly displaces or "snaps" open a rigid valve leaflet. Timing helps to distinguish an opening snap from the other gallop sounds. It occurs too long after S_2 to be mistaken for a split S_2 and too early in diastole to be mistaken for an S_3. The high-pitched, snapping quality of the sound is another way to differentiate an opening snap from an S_3. Hearing a murmur or the sound of turbulent blood flow is expected following the opening snap. An opening snap is heard best using the diaphragm of the stethoscope placed medial to the apical area and along the lower left sternal border.

In a similar manner, stenosis of one of the semilunar valves creates a short, high-pitched sound in early systole, immediately after S_1. This sound, called a **systolic click**, is the result of the opening of a rigid and calcified aortic or pulmonic valve during ventricular contraction. Mid to late systolic clicks may be heard in patients with mitral or tricuspid valve prolapse as the malfunctioning valve leaflet is displaced into the atrium during ventricular systole. Murmurs are expected to be heard following these abnormal systolic sounds. These sounds are the loudest in the areas directly over the malfunctioning valve.

Murmurs

Murmurs are created by turbulent flow of blood in the heart. The causes of the turbulence may be a critically narrowed valve, a malfunctioning valve that allows regurgitant blood flow, a congenital defect of the ventricular wall, a defect between the aorta and the pulmonary artery, or an increased flow of blood through a normal structure (e.g., with fever, pregnancy, hyperthyroidism). Murmurs are characterized and consequently described by several characteristics, including

their timing in the cardiac cycle, location on the chest wall, intensity, pitch, quality, and pattern of radiation (Chart 21-4).

Friction Rub

A harsh, grating sound that can be heard in both systole and diastole is called a *friction rub*. It is caused by abrasion of the inflamed pericardial surfaces from pericarditis. Because a friction rub may be confused with a murmur, care should be taken to identify the sound and to distinguish it from murmurs that may be heard in both systole and diastole. A pericardial friction rub can be heard best using the diaphragm of the stethoscope, with the patient sitting up and leaning forward.

Auscultation Procedure

During auscultation, the patient remains supine and the examining room is as quiet as possible. A stethoscope with both diaphragm and bell functions is necessary for accurate auscultation of the heart.

Using the diaphragm of the stethoscope, the examiner starts at the apical area and progresses upward along the left sternal border to the pulmonic and aortic areas. Alternatively, the examiner may begin the examination at the aortic and pulmonic areas and progress downward to the apex of the heart. Initially, S_1 is identified and evaluated with respect to its intensity and splitting. Next, S_2 is identified, and its intensity and any splitting are noted. After concentrating on S_1 and S_2, the examiner listens for extra sounds in systole and then in diastole.

Sometimes it helps to ask the following questions: Do I hear snapping or clicking sounds? Do I hear any high-pitched blowing sounds? Is this sound in systole, or diastole, or both? The examiner again proceeds to move the stethoscope to all of the designated areas of the precordium, listening carefully for these sounds. Finally, the patient is turned on the left side and the stethoscope is placed on the apical area, where an S_3, an S_4, and a mitral murmur are more readily detected.

Once an abnormality is heard, the entire chest surface is reexamined to determine the exact location of the sound and its radiation. The patient may be concerned about the prolonged examination and must be supported and reassured. The auscultatory findings, particularly murmurs, are documented by identifying the following characteristics (see Chart 21-4): location on chest wall, timing, intensity, pitch, quality, and radiation.

Interpretation of Heart Sounds

Interpreting heart sounds requires detailed knowledge of cardiac physiology and pathophysiology. However, all nurses should have adequate knowledge and skill to recognize normal heart sounds (S_1, S_2) and the presence of abnormal sounds. When assessment is at this very basic level of practice, abnormal findings are reported for further evaluation and treatment. More advanced skills are required of nurses caring for critically ill patients with CVD or those nurses functioning in advanced practice roles. Nurses in these roles readily identify abnormal heart sounds, recognize the diagnostic significance of their findings, and use their assessment skills to evaluate patients' responses to medical interventions. For example, these highly skilled nurses monitor heart sounds

Chart 21-4 Characteristics of Heart Murmurs

Heart murmurs are described in terms of location, timing, intensity, pitch, quality, and radiation. These characteristics provide information needed to determine the cause of the murmur and its clinical significance.

Location

Pinpointing the location of the murmur helps to determine the underlying structures that are involved in generating the abnormal sounds. The locations described in Figure 21-5 are used to identify where the loudest sounds are detected. The description should include the exact location from which the sound emanates, such as the location of the intercostal space and other important landmarks (right or left sternal border; midsternal, midclavicular, anterior axillary, or midaxillary lines). For example, a ventricular septal defect can be located at the left sternal border in the third and fourth intercostal spaces.

Timing

A murmur is described in terms of when it occurs during the cardiac cycle (systole or diastole). Murmurs are further differentiated by identifying exactly when during systole or diastole they are heard. A skilled clinician can detect that the murmur is occurring during early, mid, or late systole or diastole. Some murmurs have sounds that occur in both systole and diastole.

Intensity

A grading system is used to describe the intensity or loudness of a murmur.

Grade 1: Very faint and difficult for the inexperienced clinician to hear

Grade 2: Quiet but readily perceived by the experienced primary provider

Grade 3: Moderately loud

Grade 4: Loud and may be associated with a thrill

Grade 5: Very loud; heard when stethoscope is partially off the chest; associated with a thrill

Grade 6: Extremely loud; detected with the stethoscope off the chest; associated with a thrill

Pitch

Pitch describes the sound frequency, identified as high, medium, or low pitched. High-pitched murmurs are heard best with the stethoscope's diaphragm, whereas low-pitched sounds are detected using the bell of the stethoscope placed lightly on the chest wall.

Quality

Quality describes the sound that the murmur resembles. Murmurs can produce a rumbling, blowing, whistling, harsh, or musical sound. For example, murmurs caused by mitral or tricuspid regurgitation have a blowing quality, whereas mitral stenosis generates a rumbling sound.

Radiation

Radiation refers to the transmission of the murmur from the point of maximal intensity to other areas in the upper chest. The examiner determines if radiation is present by listening carefully to areas of the heart adjacent to the point where the murmur is the loudest. If radiation is present, the exact location is described. A murmur associated with aortic stenosis, for example, can radiate into the neck, down the left sternal border, and into the apical area.

Adapted from Bickley, L. S. (2017). *Bates' guide to physical examination and history taking* (12th ed.). Philadelphia, PA: Lippincott Williams & Wilkins.

---

in patients with HF to detect the resolution of an S₃ after treatment with a diuretic.

Assessment of Other Systems

Lungs

The details of respiratory assessment are described in Chapter 17. Findings frequently exhibited by patients with cardiac disorders include the following:

Hemoptysis: Pink, frothy sputum is indicative of acute pulmonary edema.

Cough: A dry, hacking cough from irritation of small airways is common in patients with pulmonary congestion from HF.

Crackles: HF or atelectasis associated with bed rest, splinting from ischemic pain, or the effects of analgesic, sedative, or anesthetic agents often results in the development of crackles. Typically, crackles are first noted at the bases (because of gravity's effect on fluid accumulation and decreased ventilation of basilar tissue), but they may progress to all portions of the lung fields.

Wheezes: Compression of the small airways by interstitial pulmonary edema may cause wheezing. Beta-adrenergic–blocking agents (beta-blockers), particularly noncardioselective beta-adrenergic–blocking agents such as propranolol, may cause airway narrowing, especially in patients with underlying pulmonary disease.

Abdomen

For the patient with CVD, several components of the abdominal examination are relevant:

Abdominal distention: A protuberant abdomen with bulging flanks indicates ascites. Ascites develops in patients with right ventricular or biventricular HF (both right- and left-sided HF). In the failing right heart, abnormally high chamber pressures impede the return of venous blood. As a result, the liver and spleen become engorged with excessive venous blood (hepatosplenomegaly). As pressure in the portal system rises, fluid shifts from the vascular bed into the abdominal cavity. Ascitic fluid, found in the dependent or lowest points in the abdomen, will shift with position changes.

Hepatojugular reflux: This test is performed when right ventricular or biventricular HF is suspected. The patient is positioned so that the jugular venous pulse is visible in the lower part of the neck. While observing the jugular venous pulse, firm pressure is applied over the right upper quadrant of the abdomen for 30 to 60 seconds. An increase of 1 cm or more in jugular venous pressure is indicative of a positive hepatojugular reflux. This positive test aids in confirming the diagnosis of HF.

Bladder distention: Urine output is an important indicator of cardiac function. Reduced urine output may indicate inadequate renal perfusion or a less serious problem such as one caused by urinary retention. When urine output is decreased, the patient must be assessed for a distended bladder or difficulty voiding. The bladder may be assessed with an ultrasound scanner (see Chapter 47, Fig. 47-8) or the suprapubic area palpated for an oval mass and percussed for dullness, indicative of a full bladder.

 Gerontologic Considerations

When performing a cardiovascular examination on an older patient, the nurse may note such differences as more readily palpable peripheral pulses because of decreased elasticity of the arteries and a loss of adjacent connective tissue. Palpation of the precordium in older adults is affected by the changes in the shape of the chest. For example, a cardiac impulse may not be palpable in patients with chronic obstructive pulmonary disease, because these patients usually have an increased anterior–posterior chest diameter. Kyphoscoliosis, a spinal deformity that occurs in many older adult patients, may move the cardiac apex downward so that palpation of the apical impulse is obscured.

Hypertension affects 46% of adults. The prevalence increases with age and is also impacted by race and ethnicity. The risk of a middle-age adult developing hypertension is over 90% for African Americans and Hispanic/Latino Americans. Untreated hypertension is associated with significant cardiovascular morbidity and mortality, including stroke (Whelton et al., 2018). Isolated systolic hypertension is of concern in adults over 55 year of age, and occurs because of stiffening of the vasculature and a decrease in vascular elasticity due to the aging process (Zipes et al., 2019). Another common BP problem in the older adult is orthostatic hypotension, which is a result of impaired baroreceptor function necessary to regulate BP. Other factors that heighten the risk for orthostatic hypotension include prolonged bed rest, dehydration, and many cardiovascular medications (e.g., beta-blockers, angiotensin-converting enzyme inhibitors, angiotensin receptor blockers, diuretics, nitrates).

An S_4 that is associated with hypertension is common in older adults. It is thought to be due to a decrease in compliance of the left ventricle. The S_2 is usually split. At least 60% of older patients have murmurs, the most common being a soft systolic ejection murmur resulting from sclerotic changes of the aortic leaflets (Bickley, 2017) (see Table 21-1).

Diagnostic Evaluation

A wide range of diagnostic studies may be performed in patients with cardiovascular conditions. The nurse should educate the patient on the purpose, what to expect, and any possible side effects related to these examinations prior to testing. The nurse should note trends in results because they provide information about disease progression as well as the patient's response to therapy.

Laboratory Tests

Samples of the patient's blood are sent to the laboratory for the following reasons:

- To screen for risk factors associated with CAD
- To establish baseline values before initiating other diagnostic tests, procedures, or therapeutic interventions
- To monitor response to therapeutic interventions
- To assess for abnormalities in the blood that affect prognosis

Normal values for laboratory tests may vary depending on the laboratory and the health care institution. This variation is due to the differences in equipment and methods of measurement across organizations.

Cardiac Biomarker Analysis

The diagnosis of MI is made by evaluating the history and physical examination, the 12-lead ECG, and the results of laboratory tests that measure serum cardiac biomarkers. Myocardial cells that become necrotic from prolonged ischemia or trauma release specific enzymes (creatine kinase [CK]), CK isoenzymes (CK-MB), and proteins (myoglobin, troponin T, and troponin I). These substances leak into the interstitial spaces of the myocardium and are carried by the lymphatic system into general circulation. As a result, abnormally high levels of these substances can be detected in serum blood samples. (See Chapter 23 for further discussion of cardiac biomarker analysis.)

Blood Chemistry, Hematology, and Coagulation Studies

Table 21-4 provides information about some common serum laboratory tests and the implications for patients with CVD. Discussion of lipid, brain (B-type) natriuretic peptide (BNP), C-reactive protein (CRP), and homocysteine measurements follows.

Lipid Profile

Cholesterol, triglycerides, and lipoproteins are measured to evaluate a person's risk of developing CAD, especially if there is a family history of premature heart disease, or to diagnose a specific lipoprotein abnormality. Cholesterol and triglycerides are transported in the blood by combining with plasma proteins to form lipoproteins called LDL and HDL. Although cholesterol levels remain relatively constant over 24 hours, the blood specimen for the lipid profile should be obtained after a 12-hour fast.

Cholesterol Levels

Cholesterol is a lipid required for hormone synthesis and cell membrane formation. It is found in large quantities in brain and nerve tissue. Two major sources of cholesterol are diet (animal products) and the liver, where cholesterol is synthesized. Factors that contribute to variations in cholesterol levels include age, gender, diet, exercise patterns, genetics, menopause, tobacco use, and stress levels. Total cholesterol level is calculated by adding the HDL, LDL, and 20% of the triglyceride level.

High cholesterol levels increase the risk of CVD regardless of the patient's age. Lifestyle changes are recommended to lower cholesterol levels. After determining a person's 10-year risk for atherosclerotic vascular disease, medication is prescribed if necessary. Statins, a class of cholesterol-lowering medications, are often prescribed. Other nonstatins may be added to medication management to further reduce cholesterol; these include ezetimibe, bile acid sequestrants, and PCSK9 inhibitors (Grundy, Stone, Bailey, et al., 2019) (see Chapter 23 for more details).

TABLE 21-4	Common Serum Laboratory Tests and Implications for Patients with Cardiovascular Disease
Laboratory Test Reference Range	**Implications**

Blood Chemistries

Blood urea nitrogen (BUN): 8–20 mg/dL	BUN and creatinine are end products of protein metabolism excreted by the kidneys. Elevated BUN reflects reduced renal perfusion from decreased cardiac output or intravascular fluid volume deficit as a result of diuretic therapy or dehydration.
Calcium (Ca^{++}): 8.8–10.4 mg/dL	Calcium is necessary for blood coagulability, neuromuscular activity, and automaticity of the nodal cells (sinus and atrioventricular nodes). *Hypocalcemia:* Decreased calcium levels slow nodal function and impair myocardial contractility. The latter effect increases the risk for heart failure. *Hypercalcemia:* Increased calcium levels can occur with the administration of thiazide diuretics because these medications reduce renal excretion of calcium. Hypercalcemia potentiates digitalis toxicity, causes increased myocardial contractility, and increases the risk for varying degrees of heart block and sudden death from ventricular fibrillation.
Creatinine *Male:* 0.6–1.2 mg/dL *Female:* 0.4–1.0 mg/dL	Both BUN and creatinine are used to assess renal function, although creatinine is a more sensitive measure. Renal impairment is detected by an increase in both BUN and creatinine. A normal creatinine level and an elevated BUN suggest an intravascular fluid volume deficit.
Magnesium (Mg^{++}): 1.8–2.6 mg/dL	Magnesium is necessary for the absorption of calcium, maintenance of potassium stores, and metabolism of adenosine triphosphate. It plays a major role in protein and carbohydrate synthesis and muscular contraction. *Hypomagnesemia:* Decreased magnesium levels are due to enhanced renal excretion of magnesium from the use of diuretic or digitalis therapy. Low magnesium levels predispose patients to atrial or ventricular tachycardias. *Hypermagnesemia:* Increased magnesium levels are commonly caused by the use of cathartics or antacids containing magnesium. Increased magnesium levels depress contractility and excitability of the myocardium, causing heart block and, if severe, asystole.
Potassium (K$^+$): 3.5–5 mEq/L	Potassium has a major role in cardiac electrophysiologic function. *Hypokalemia:* Decreased potassium levels due to administration of potassium-excreting diuretics can cause many forms of arrhythmias, including life-threatening ventricular tachycardia or ventricular fibrillation, and predispose patients taking digitalis preparations to digitalis toxicity. *Hyperkalemia:* Increased potassium levels can result from an increased intake of potassium (e.g., foods high in potassium or potassium supplements), decreased renal excretion of potassium, the use of potassium-sparing diuretics (e.g., spironolactone), or the use of angiotensin-converting enzyme inhibitors that inhibit aldosterone function. Serious consequences of hyperkalemia include heart block, asystole, and life-threatening ventricular arrhythmias.
Sodium (Na$^+$): 135–145 mEq/L	Low or high serum sodium levels do not directly affect cardiac function. *Hyponatremia:* Decreased sodium levels indicate fluid excess and can be caused by heart failure or administration of thiazide diuretics. *Hypernatremia:* Increased sodium levels indicate fluid deficits and can result from decreased water intake or loss of water through excessive sweating or diarrhea.

Coagulation Studies

	Injury to a vessel wall or tissue initiates the formation of a thrombus. This injury activates the coagulation cascade, the complex interactions among phospholipids, calcium, and clotting factors that convert prothrombin to thrombin. The coagulation cascade has two pathways: the intrinsic and extrinsic pathways. Coagulation studies are routinely performed before invasive procedures, such as cardiac catheterization, electrophysiology testing, and cardiac surgery.
Activated partial thromboplastin time (aPTT) *Lower limit of normal:* 21–35 s	aPTT measures the activity of the intrinsic pathway and is used to assess the effects of unfractionated heparin. A therapeutic range is 1.5–2.5 times baseline values. Adjustment of heparin dose is required for aPTT <50 s (↑ dose) or >100 s (↓ dose).
Prothrombin time (PT) *Lower limit of normal:* 11–13 s	PT measures the extrinsic pathway activity and is used to monitor the level of anticoagulation with warfarin.
International normalized ratio (INR): 0.8–1.2	The INR, reported with the PT, provides a standard method for reporting PT levels and eliminates the variation of PT results from different laboratories. The INR, rather than the PT alone, is used to monitor the effectiveness of warfarin. The therapeutic range for INR is 2–3.5, although specific ranges vary based on diagnosis.

Hematologic Studies

Complete blood count (CBC)	The CBC identifies the total number of white and red blood cells and platelets, and measures hemoglobin and hematocrit. The CBC is carefully monitored in patients with cardiovascular disease.
Hematocrit *Male:* 42–52% *Female:* 36–48% Hemoglobin *Male:* 14–17.4 g/dL *Female:* 12–16 g/dL	The hematocrit represents the percentage of red blood cells found in 100 mL of whole blood. The red blood cells contain hemoglobin, which transports oxygen to the cells. Low hemoglobin and hematocrit levels have serious consequences for patients with cardiovascular disease, such as more frequent angina episodes or acute myocardial infarction.
Platelets: 140,000–400,000/mm^3	Platelets are the first line of protection against bleeding. Once activated by blood vessel wall injury or rupture of atherosclerotic plaque, platelets undergo chemical changes that form a thrombus. Several medications inhibit platelet function, including aspirin, clopidogrel, and intravenous glycoprotein IIb/IIIa inhibitors (abciximab, eptifibatide, and tirofiban). When these medications are given, it is essential to monitor for thrombocytopenia (low platelet counts).
White blood cell (WBC) count: 4500–11,000/mm^3	WBC counts are monitored in patients who are immunocompromised, including patients with heart transplants or in situations where there is concern for infection (e.g., after invasive procedures or surgery).

Adapted from Fischbach, F. T., & Fischbach, M. A. (2018). *A manual of laboratory and diagnostic tests* (10th ed.). Philadelphia, PA: Wolters Kluwer; Urden, L. D., Stacy, K. M., & Lough, M. E. (2017). *Critical care nursing: Diagnosis and management* (8th ed.). St. Louis, MO: Elsevier Mosby.

LDL is the primary transporter of cholesterol and triglycerides into the cell. One harmful effect of LDL is the deposition of these substances in the walls of arterial vessels. HDL has a protective action because it transports cholesterol away from the tissue and cells of the arterial wall to the liver for excretion (Grundy et al., 2019).

Triglycerides

Triglycerides, composed of free fatty acids and glycerol, are stored in the adipose tissue and are a source of energy. Triglyceride levels increase after meals and are affected by stress. Diabetes, alcohol use, and obesity can elevate triglyceride levels. These levels have a direct correlation with LDL and an inverse one with HDL.

Brain (B-Type) Natriuretic Peptide

BNP is a neurohormone that helps regulate BP and fluid volume. It is primarily secreted from the ventricles in response to increased preload with resulting elevated ventricular pressure. The level of BNP in the blood increases as the ventricular walls expand from increased pressure, making it a helpful diagnostic, monitoring, and prognostic tool in the setting of HF. Because this serum laboratory test can be quickly obtained, BNP levels are useful for prompt diagnosis of HF in settings such as the ED. Elevations in BNP can occur from a number of other conditions such as pulmonary embolus, MI, and ventricular hypertrophy. Therefore, the primary provider correlates BNP levels with abnormal physical assessment findings and other diagnostic tests before making a definitive diagnosis of HF. A BNP level greater than 100 pg/mL is suggestive of HF.

C-Reactive Protein

CRP is a protein produced by the liver in response to systemic inflammation. Inflammation is thought to play a role in the development and progression of atherosclerosis. The high-sensitivity CRP (hs-CRP) test is used as an adjunct to other tests to predict CVD risk. People with high hs-CRP levels (3 mg/L or greater) may be at greatest risk for CVD compared to people with moderate (1 to 3 mg/L) or low (less than 1 mg/L) hs-CRP levels (Sidawy & Perler, 2019).

Homocysteine

Homocysteine, an amino acid, is linked to the development of atherosclerosis because it can damage the endothelial lining of arteries and promote thrombus formation. Therefore, an elevated blood level of homocysteine is thought to indicate a high risk for CAD, stroke, and peripheral vascular disease, although it is not an independent predictor of CAD. Genetic factors and a diet low in folate, vitamin B_6, and vitamin B_{12} are associated with elevated homocysteine levels. A 12-hour fast is necessary before drawing a blood sample for an accurate serum measurement. Test results are interpreted as optimal (less than 12 mcmol/L), borderline (12 to 15 mcmol/L), and high risk (greater than 15 mcmol/L) (Zipes et al., 2019).

Chest X-Ray and Fluoroscopy

A chest x-ray is obtained to determine the size, contour, and position of the heart. It reveals cardiac and pericardial calcifications and demonstrates physiologic alterations in the pulmonary circulation. Although it does not help diagnose acute MI, it can help diagnose some complications (e.g., HF). Correct placement of pacemakers and pulmonary artery catheters is also confirmed by chest x-ray.

Fluoroscopy is an x-ray imaging technique that allows visualization of the heart on a screen. It shows cardiac and vascular pulsations and unusual cardiac contours. This technique uses a movable x-ray source, which makes it a useful aid for positioning transvenous pacing electrodes and for guiding the insertion of arterial and venous catheters during cardiac catheterization and other cardiac procedures.

Electrocardiography

The ECG is a graphic representation of the electrical currents of the heart. The ECG is obtained by placing disposable electrodes in standard positions on the skin of the chest wall and extremities. Recordings of the electrical current flowing between two electrodes are made on graph paper or displayed on a monitor. Several different recordings can be obtained by using a variety of electrode combinations, called *leads*. Simply stated, a lead is a specific view of the electrical activity of heart. The standard ECG is composed of 12 leads or 12 different views, although it is possible to record 15 or 18 leads.

The 12-lead ECG is used to diagnose arrhythmias, conduction abnormalities, and chamber enlargement, as well as myocardial ischemia, injury, or infarction. It can also suggest cardiac effects of electrolyte disturbances (high or low calcium and potassium levels) and the effects of antiarrhythmic medications. A 15-lead ECG adds three additional chest leads across the right precordium and is used for early diagnosis of right ventricular and left posterior (ventricular) infarction. The 18-lead ECG adds three posterior leads to the 15-lead ECG and is useful for early detection of myocardial ischemia and injury. To enhance interpretation of the ECG, the patient's age, gender, BP, height, weight, symptoms, and medications (especially digitalis and antiarrhythmic agents) are noted on the ECG requisition. (See Chapter 22 for a more detailed discussion of ECG.)

Continuous Electrocardiographic Monitoring

Continuous ECG monitoring is the standard of care for patients who are at high risk for arrhythmias. This form of cardiac monitoring detects abnormalities in heart rate and rhythm. Many systems have the capacity to monitor for changes in ST segments, which are used to identify the presence of myocardial ischemia or injury (see Chapter 23). Two types of continuous ECG monitoring techniques are used in health care settings: hardwire cardiac monitoring, found in EDs, critical care units, and progressive care units; and telemetry, found in general nursing care units or outpatient cardiac rehabilitation programs. Hardwire cardiac monitoring and telemetry systems vary in sophistication; however, most systems have the following features in common:

- Monitor more than one ECG lead simultaneously.
- Monitor ST segments (ST-segment depression is a marker of myocardial ischemia; ST-segment elevation provides evidence of an evolving MI).
- Provide graded visual and audible alarms (based on priority, asystole merits the highest grade of alarm).
- Interpret and store alarms.

- Trend data over time.
- Print a copy of rhythms from one or more specific ECG leads over a set time (called a *rhythm strip*).
- Save electronic copies of cardiac rhythms into the electronic health record (EHR).

> ### ◢ *Quality and Safety Nursing Alert*
>
> *Patients placed on continuous ECG monitoring must be informed of its purpose and cautioned that it does not detect shortness of breath, chest pain, or other ACS symptoms. Thus, patients are instructed to report new or worsening symptoms immediately.*

 ## Hardwire Cardiac Monitoring

Hardwire cardiac monitoring is used to continuously observe the heart for arrhythmias and conduction disorders using one or two ECG leads. A real-time ECG is displayed on a bedside monitor and at a central monitoring station. In critical care units, additional components can be added to the bedside monitor to continuously monitor hemodynamic parameters (noninvasive BP, arterial pressures, pulmonary artery pressures), respiratory parameters (respiratory rate, oxygen saturation), and ST segments for myocardial ischemia. The nurse must know the specific indication for each patient's ECG monitoring.

Telemetry

In addition to hardwire cardiac monitoring, the ECG can be continuously observed by **telemetry**—the transmission of radio waves from a battery-operated transmitter to a central bank of monitors. The primary benefit of using telemetry is that the system is wireless, which allows patients to ambulate while one or two ECG leads are monitored. The patient has electrodes placed on the chest with a lead cable that connects to the transmitter. The transmitter can be placed in a disposable pouch and worn around the neck, or simply secured to the patient's clothing. Most transmitter batteries are changed every 24 to 48 hours.

Lead Systems

The number of electrodes needed for hardwire cardiac monitoring and telemetry is dictated by the lead system used in the clinical setting. Electrodes need to be securely and correctly placed on the chest wall to accurately capture arrhythmias (Sandau, Funk, Auerbach, et al., 2017). Chart 21-5 provides helpful hints on how to apply these electrodes. There are three-, four-, or five-lead systems available for ECG monitoring. The type of lead system used determines the number of lead options for monitoring. For example, the five-lead system provides up to seven different lead selections. Unlike the other two systems, the five-lead system can monitor the activity of the anterior wall of the left ventricle. Figure 21-9 presents diagrams of electrode placement.

The two ECG leads most often selected for continuous ECG monitoring are leads II and V_1. Lead II provides the best visualization of atrial depolarization (represented by the P wave). Lead V_1 best records ventricular depolarization and is most helpful when monitoring for certain arrhythmias (e.g., premature ventricular contractions, tachycardias,

---

> ### Chart 21-5 Applying Electrodes
>
> The monitoring system requires an adequate electrical signal to analyze the patient's cardiac rhythm. Proper use of this technology includes the correct application of electrodes to reduce false alarms on the cardiac monitor. When applying electrodes, the recommendations below should be followed to optimize skin adherence and conduction of the heart's electrical current:
>
> - Débride the skin surface of dead cells with soap and water; dry well using a wash cloth or gauze.
> - Clip (do not shave) hair from around the electrode site, if needed.
> - Connect the electrodes to the lead wires prior to placing them on the chest (connecting lead wires when electrodes are in place may be uncomfortable for some patients).
> - Peel the backing off the electrode, and check to make sure the center is moist with electrode gel.
> - Locate the appropriate lead placement, and apply the electrode to the skin, securing it in place with light pressure.
> - Change the electrodes every 24 hours, examine the skin for irritation, and apply the electrodes to different locations.
> - If the patient is sensitive to the electrodes, use hypoallergenic electrodes.
>
> Adapted from Jepsen, S., Sendelbach, S., Ruppel, H., et al. (2018). AACN Practice Alert: Managing alarms in acute care across the life span: Electrocardiography and pulse oximetry. *Critical Care Nurse, 38*(2), e16–e20.

bundle branch blocks) (see Chapter 22). In addition to proper lead and electrode placement, it is important for the nurse to review and customize alarm settings for each patient to reduce false alarms and alarm fatigue (Jepsen, Sendelbach, Ruppel, et al., 2018).

Ambulatory Electrocardiography

Ambulatory electrocardiography is a form of continuous or intermittent ECG home monitoring. It is used for longer-term monitoring, since some arrhythmias occur intermittently and

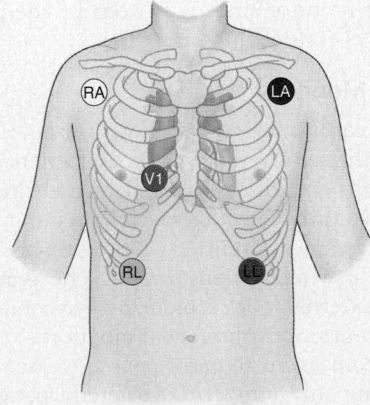

RA – Right arm (white)
LA – Left arm (black)
RL – Right leg (green)
LL – Left leg (red)
V_1 – Chest or precordium (brown)

Figure 21-9 • Electrode placement used in continuous electrocardiographic monitoring for three-lead system, placement on RA, LA, and LL; four-lead system, placement on RA, LA, RL, and LL; five-lead system, placement on RA, LA, RL, LL, and V_1.

are difficult to capture with a 12-lead ECG in the office setting. This monitoring can help to identify the etiology of chest pain, syncope or palpitation caused by arrhythmias, detect episodes of myocardial ischemia, evaluate effectiveness of treatment of HF and arrhythmias, and evaluate the functioning of ICDs and pacemakers. Several types of devices are available and are worn either externally or implanted under the skin. The ECG is transmitted to a centralized monitoring station via telephone or wireless technology to a secure Web site (Sampson, 2019).

Continuous Monitors

Commonly called Holter monitors, these small portable recorders are connected to chest electrodes (number varies based on model used) that record all ECG activity using two or more leads onto a digital memory device. The patient usually wears the recorder for 24 to 48 hours. The patient is also asked to keep a diary to note the date and time of symptoms and activities. The diary is used by the primary provider to correlate symptoms with detected arrhythmias. Once monitoring is completed, the patient returns the device and diary to the primary provider's office. Data from the digital memory device are then uploaded into a computer for analysis, and rhythms that need further evaluation by the primary provider are identified. Therefore, Holter monitors do not provide real-time ECG recordings or analysis. The effectiveness of this form of monitoring is dependent upon the patient's adherence with wearing the monitor, keeping an accurate diary, and if an arrhythmia occurred during the monitoring period (Sampson, 2019; Urden et al., 2017).

A novel alternative to the use of the Holter monitor is ECG patch monitoring, which uses Bluetooth technology. An ECG patch with adhesive backing is placed over the left pectoral area, eliminating the need for multiple ECG electrodes, wires, and recorders. The patch is single use, waterproof, and easily concealed under clothing. The patient wears the patch for 7 to 14 days and then returns it to the manufacturer for analysis. This device can detect more arrhythmias compared to the Holter monitor since it is worn by the patient for a longer period of time (Sampson, 2019).

Intermittent Monitors

Intermittent cardiac event monitors are devices that can capture arrhythmias when the patient experiences symptoms such as palpitations, dizziness, or lightheadedness. Patients may need to record events for several days to a month. The recorded ECGs are transmitted to the primary provider by telephone or a wireless transmission. The symptom event monitor and external loop recorder are two common forms of external intermittent cardiac event monitors.

The symptom event monitor is used to record and store the ECG during only during times when the patient is experiencing symptoms. Patients activate the symptom event monitor by pressing a button for devices that are worn on the wrist or by placing a small handheld device over the chest.

The loop recorder, a small battery-operated device, can record and store short periods of ECG activity. The monitor is inserted under the skin or worn on a wrist band. Some loop recorders are programmed to detect bradycardia, tachycardia, and irregular rhythms and do not require patient interaction. Other loop recorders require the patient to activate

ECG recordings by pushing a button. The device records the patient's ECG for a predetermined time before and after the device activation. This is a preferred method over the symptom event monitor because it has more monitoring capabilities.

Real-time smart phone monitoring is a novel approach to cardiac event recording. The KardiaMobile® is a small device that connects to a smart phone app. The patient places two fingers on the device which generates a PDF file that can be sent electronically to the provider. Similarly, a patient can place a finger on the digital section of the Apple watch® to generate a rhythm strip. This rhythm is displayed on the watch face and a PDF file is sent to an app on the Apple iPhone® (Sampson, 2019).

Cardiac Implantable Electronic Devices

Cardiac implantable electronic devices include pacemakers and ICDs. These lifesaving devices are used to manage patients with serious cardiac illnesses. The technology available today allows for remote wireless monitoring of these devices to determine battery life, pacing parameters and therapies, and occurrence of serious atrial and ventricular arrhythmias. A transmitter, which is placed in the patient's home, sends device data to a secure data repository on a secure Web portal. A unique feature of these implantable devices is that they have programmable alerts that automatically detect and transmit arrhythmias without the need for patient interaction (see Chapter 22 for further discussion).

An implantable cardiac monitor such as the Reveal LINQ™ is another type of electronic device. This small device is implanted subcutaneously under the skin and has a battery life of 3 years. Recordings are triggered when an arrhythmia is detected by the device. Recordings are sent wirelessly via a home monitoring device for expert evaluation. Compared with event recorders described previously, this device offers advantages such as eliminating the patient's need to change electrodes and wear or carry the monitoring device. This type of monitoring is recommended for patients who have infrequent symptoms or require longer-term ECG monitoring (Sampson, 2019).

Nursing Interventions for Inpatient Cardiac Monitoring

A body of evidence indicates that most alarms occurring during inpatient ECG monitoring are false alarms. Nurses dealing with excessive alarms become desensitized to these sounds and develop alarm fatigue. Alarm fatigue delays response time or results in missed alarms. Several nursing interventions facilitate acquisition of accurate data, reduce risk of alarm fatigue, and ensure patient safety when using cardiac monitoring (Jepsen et al., 2018; Sandau et al., 2017).

To minimize false alarms, the ECG recordings must be free of artifact, which is an abnormal ECG pattern caused by muscular activity, patient movement, electrical interference, or lead cable or electrode malfunction. Artifact can mimic arrhythmias and cause unnecessary false alarms. Key to the elimination of artifact is using proper skin preparation before applying electrodes and changing the electrodes every 24 hours. During electrode changes, the skin should be assessed for allergic responses (itchy, reddened skin) to the adhesive or electrode gel. If present, the electrodes are replaced with hypoallergenic electrodes. Rotation of electrode placement on the skin will reduce the risk for skin breakdown (see Fig. 21-9).

Electrodes and lead connections need to be positioned correctly. Improper positioning can result in artifact that mimics ischemia or arrhythmias. Two leads should be selected that provide the best tracing for arrhythmia monitoring, which are usually lead II and the chest lead V_1. Electrical equipment in use around the patient should be inspected to be certain that it is functioning properly and has been recently checked by the medical engineering department per organization policy, because improperly functioning equipment may cause false alarms from artifact.

An effort should be made to individualize the ECG alarm parameters to meet the patient's monitoring needs. For example, if the patient has atrial fibrillation, it is appropriate to turn off the irregular heart rate alarm. Keeping it on will create unnecessary alarms, contributing to alarm fatigue. Similarly, the bradycardia and tachycardia alarms should be adjusted, slightly below or above the patient's underlying heart rate (Jepsen et al., 2018; Sandau et al., 2017).

The nurse's role is to respond to and correct all monitor alarms immediately. Inoperative (inop) monitoring alarms—used to communicate that electrodes have fallen off, that leads are loose, or that the system's battery power is low (e.g., telemetry)—are just as significant as arrhythmia alarms indicating that the patient is tachycardic, bradycardic, or experiencing another potentially life-threatening arrhythmia. Timely responses to all alarms can prevent serious consequences, including death.

Hospital-acquired infections can be transmitted through lead wire cables. This may be prevented by using disposable lead wire cables, or by keeping reusable cables and transmitter equipment clean, per organizational policy. A patient should never be connected to monitoring equipment that has not been thoroughly cleaned between patients. If a patient is scheduled for a device implant, such as a pacemaker, electrodes should not be placed over the planned incision site. Likewise, electrodes should never be placed over an incision, implanted device, open wounds, or inflamed skin.

Electrodes should be removed once monitoring is discontinued and skin cleansed to remove excess electrode gel and adhesive. Metal-containing electrodes must be removed before sending a patient for any magnetic resonance scan, including magnetic resonance angiography (MRA).

Telemetry transmitters and other monitoring equipment should be maintained according to the manufacturer's recommendations. Monitoring devices of any type should not be submerged in water. A monitoring device may break if dropped; therefore, it should be secured to the patient's gown or clothing.

Cardiac Stress Testing

Normally, the coronary arteries dilate to four times their usual diameter in response to increased metabolic demands for oxygen and nutrients. However, coronary arteries affected by atherosclerosis dilate less, compromising blood flow to the myocardium and causing ischemia. Therefore, abnormalities in cardiovascular function are more likely to be detected during times of increased oxygen demand, or "stress." The **cardiac stress test** procedures—the exercise stress test, pharmacologic stress test, and radionucleotide imaging studies—are noninvasive ways to evaluate if there is myocardial ischemia and higher myocardial oxygen requirement during these tests. Cardiac imaging is performed during the resting state and immediately after stress testing. The results can identify specific coronary artery lesions and ischemic areas of the heart (King, 2017). Since complications of stress testing can be life-threatening (MI, cardiac arrest, HF, and bradycardia and tachycardia with hemodynamic compromise), testing facilities must have staff and equipment ready to provide treatment, including advanced cardiac life support.

Exercise Stress Testing

Procedure

During an exercise stress test, the patient walks or runs on a treadmill (most common) or pedals a stationary bicycle. A protocol guides exercise intensity based upon the patient's age and heart rate goal (King, 2017). During the test, the following are monitored: two or more ECG leads for heart rate, rhythm, and ischemic changes; BP; skin temperature; physical appearance; perceived exertion; and symptoms, including chest pain, dyspnea, dizziness, leg cramping, and fatigue. The test is stopped when the target heart rate is achieved or if the patient experiences signs of myocardial ischemia. Abnormal findings include chest pain, ventricular arrhythmia, ST-segment depression, and lack of heart rate or BP elevation with exercise (King, 2017).

Nursing Interventions

In preparation for the exercise stress test, the patient is instructed to fast for several hours before the test and to avoid stimulants such as tobacco and caffeine. Medications may be taken with sips of water. The primary provider may instruct the patient to hold beta-blockers, calcium channel blockers, and digitalis for up to 48 hours before the stress test. Clothes and sneakers or rubber-soled shoes suitable for exercising are to be worn. The nurse prepares the patient for the stress test by describing how the stress test is performed, the type of monitoring equipment used, the rationale for insertion of an IV catheter, and what symptoms to report. The exercise method is reviewed, and patients are asked to put forth their best exercise effort. If the test is to be performed with echocardiography or radionuclide imaging (described in the next section), this information is reviewed as well. After the test, the patient is monitored for 10 to 15 minutes until vital signs and assessment findings return to normal. Once stable, patients may resume their usual activities.

Pharmacologic Stress Testing

Procedure

Patients who are cognitively impaired and unable to follow directions or physically disabled or deconditioned will not be able to achieve their target heart rate by exercising on a treadmill or bicycle. Vasodilating agents such as dipyridamole, adenosine, or regadenoson given as an IV infusion are used to mimic the effects of exercise by maximally dilating normal coronary arteries and identifying stenotic arteries that cannot vasodilate. The side effects of these agents are related to the vasodilating action and include chest pain, headache, flushing, nausea, heart block, and dyspnea. If necessary the effects of these drugs can be reversed with IV aminophylline. Adenosine has an extremely short half-life (less than 10 seconds), so any severe effects subside rapidly. These vasodilating medications are the agents used in conjunction with radionuclide imaging techniques. Patients undergoing pharmacologic stress tests must avoid xanthine derivatives including theophylline, aminophylline, and caffeine as they block the effects of the vasodilating agents.

Dobutamine is another option for use during a pharmacologic stress test. This medication is a synthetic sympathomimetic agent that increases heart rate, myocardial contractility, and BP, thereby increasing the metabolic demands of the heart. It is the agent of choice when echocardiography is used because of its effects on altering myocardial wall motion (due to enhanced contractility). Dobutamine is also used for patients who have bronchospasm or pulmonary disease and cannot tolerate having doses of theophylline withheld.

Nursing Interventions

In preparation for the pharmacologic stress test, the patient is instructed not to eat or drink anything for at least 3 hours before the test. The patient must also be told to refrain from eating any liquid or food that contain chocolate or caffeine for 24 hours and to avoid taking medications that contain caffeine. This restriction also includes caffeine-free coffee, tea, and carbonated beverages. If caffeine is ingested before a stress test using vasodilating agents, the test will have to be rescheduled. Patients taking aminophylline, theophylline, or dipyridamole are instructed to stop taking these medications for 24 to 48 hours before the test (if tolerated). The patient is informed about the transient sensations that may occur during infusion of the vasodilating agent, such as flushing or nausea, which will disappear quickly. The patient is instructed to report the occurrence of any other symptoms during the test to the cardiologist or nurse. The stress test may take about 1 hour, or up to 3 hours if imaging is performed.

Radionuclide Imaging

Radionuclide imaging studies are noninvasive tests that use radioisotopes to evaluate coronary artery perfusion, detect myocardial ischemia and infarction, and/or assess left ventricular function. **Radioisotopes** are unstable atoms that give off small amounts of energy in the form of gamma rays as they decay. When radioisotopes are injected into the bloodstream, the energy emitted can be detected by a gamma scintillation camera positioned over the body. These radioisotopes are called tracers.

Myocardial Perfusion Imaging

Myocardial perfusion imaging is performed using two types of techniques: single photon emission computed tomography (SPECT) or positron emission tomography (PET). It is commonly performed after an acute MI to determine if arterial perfusion to the heart is compromised during activity and to evaluate the extent of myocardial damage. It is also used to evaluate if myocardial ischemia from CAD is the cause of chest pain or other CAD-related symptoms.

These imaging techniques are performed in combination with stress testing to compare images obtained when the heart is resting to images of the heart in a stressed state resulting from exercise or medications. An area of the myocardium that shows no perfusion or reduced perfusion is said to have a "defect" present. Comparing resting images with images taken after the stress test helps differentiate ischemic myocardium from infarct-related myocardium. A defect that does not change in size before and after stress is called a fixed defect. Fixed defects indicate that there is no perfusion in that area of the myocardium, which is the case after an MI. Defects that appear or that get larger after the stress test images are taken indicate reduced perfusion to that area of the heart. Because the defect disappears with rest, it is called a reversible defect. Reversible defects constitute positive stress test findings. Typically, cardiac catheterization is recommended after a positive test result to determine the severity of obstructions to blood flow caused by CAD.

The patient undergoing myocardial perfusion imaging with stress testing should be prepared for the type of stressor to be used (exercise or medication) and provided with details of what to expect during imaging. The imaging is performed in two stages. Usually, the resting images are taken first. An IV is inserted to administer the radioisotope, and electrodes are placed on the chest to monitor the heart rate and rhythm. Women who are nursing, pregnant or think they are pregnant should not undergo myocardial perfusion imaging. The nurse alerts the primary provider if any of these conditions are present.

Single Photon Emission Computed Tomography

SPECT is widely available and is the most common technique of myocardial perfusion imaging. In addition, the ability of SPECT to detect myocardial ischemia is between 80% and 90% (King, 2017).

Procedure

SPECT is a painless, noninvasive procedure that involves the injection of the nuclear medicine radionucleotide (technetium-99m [^{99m}Tc]; rubidium-82) and imaging. During SPECT, patients are positioned supine on the table with their arms over their heads. The gamma camera circles around the chest area converting the signals from the traces into pictures of the heart. The procedure takes approximately 30 minutes. The second scan is repeated after an exercise or pharmacologic stress test.

Nursing Interventions

The nurse's primary role is to prepare the patient for SPECT and insert an IV catheter or assess an existing IV for patency and suitability. The IV is used to inject the tracer. The patient may be concerned about receiving a radioactive substance and needs to be reassured that these tracers are safe—the radiation exposure is similar to that of other diagnostic x-ray studies. No postprocedure radiation precautions are necessary.

Positron Emission Tomography

PET is another noninvasive procedure in which a radioactive tracer chemical is administered to the patient and images are obtained. These images generally have a higher resolution compared to SPECT. PET technology is expensive and is likely to be found at large or academic medical centers.

Procedure

During PET, tracers are given by injection; one compound is used to determine blood flow in the myocardium, and another determines the metabolic function. The PET camera provides detailed three-dimensional images of the distributed compounds. The viability of the myocardium is determined by comparing the extent of glucose metabolism in the myocardium to the degree of blood flow. For example, ischemic but viable tissue will show decreased blood flow and elevated metabolism. For a patient with this finding, revascularization through surgery or angioplasty will probably be indicated to improve heart function. Restrictions of food intake before the test vary among institutions, but because PET evaluates glucose metabolism, the patient's blood glucose level should be within the normal range before testing.

Nursing Interventions

The nurse instructs the patient to refrain from using alcohol and caffeine for 24 hours before undergoing PET because of the stimulating effects they may have on the heart. For patients with diabetes and who are taking insulin, the nurse needs to discuss insulin doses and food restrictions with the primary provider. The nurse assesses patients for fear of closed spaces or claustrophobia. Patients who have this condition are reassured that medications can be given to help them relax. The nurse also reassures patients that radiation exposure is at safe and acceptable levels, similar to those of other diagnostic x-ray studies.

To prepare the patient for PET, the nurse inserts an IV or assesses the existing IV catheter for patency and suitability, and then describes the procedure to the patient. The patient is positioned on a table with hands above the head. The table then slides into a donut-shaped scanner. While in the scanner, the patient must lie still so that clear images of the heart can be obtained. A baseline scan is performed, which takes about 30 minutes. Then a tracer is injected into the IV and the scan is repeated. The patient's glucose level is monitored throughout the procedure. The scan takes from 1 to 3 hours to complete.

Test of Ventricular Function and Wall Motion

Equilibrium radionuclide angiocardiography (ERNA), also known as multiple-gated acquisition (MUGA) scanning, is a common noninvasive technique that uses a conventional scintillation camera interfaced with a computer to record images of the heart during several hundred heartbeats. The computer processes the data and allows for sequential viewing of the functioning heart. The sequential images are analyzed to evaluate left ventricular function, wall motion, and ejection fraction.

The patient is reassured that there is no known radiation danger and is instructed to remain motionless during the scan.

Additional Imaging

Additional cardiac imaging techniques include computed tomography (CT) and MRA.

Computed Tomography

Procedure

Cardiac CT scanning is a form of cardiac imaging that uses x-rays to provide accurate cross-sectional "virtual" slices of specific areas of the heart and surrounding structures. Complex mathematical and computer algorithms are used to analyze the slices to create three-dimensional images. Multidetector CT (MDCT) is a fast form of CT scanning that takes multiple slices at the same time. This technology produces high-resolution clear images of cardiac anatomy (Liddy, Buckley, Kok, et al., 2018). Two types of cardiac CT scanning include coronary CT angiography and electron beam CT (EBCT) (for coronary calcium scoring).

Coronary CT angiography requires the use of an IV contrast agent to enhance the x-rays and improve visualization of cardiac structures. This test is used to evaluate coronary arteries for stenosis, the aorta for aneurysms or dissections, graft patency after coronary artery bypass grafting, pulmonary veins in patients with atrial fibrillation, and cardiac structures for congenital anomalies. Patients may receive beta-blockers prior to the scan to control heart rate and rhythm and reduce artifact. Another way to minimize artifact is to have patients hold their breath periodically throughout the scan. Coronary CT angiography is used with caution in patients with renal insufficiency. The contrast agent used during the CT scan is excreted through the kidneys; therefore, renal function should be assessed prior to the scan. It may be necessary to administer IV hydration before and after the scan to minimize the effect of the contrast on renal function. Patients will require premedication with corticosteroids and antihistamines if they experienced a reaction to a contrast agent in the past (Mervak, Cohan, Ellis, et al., 2017).

EBCT is used to calculate a coronary artery calcium score that is based on the amount of calcium deposits in the coronary arteries. This score is used to predict the likelihood of cardiac events, such as MI, or the need for a revascularization procedure in the future. Coronary artery calcium scoring is used for the evaluation of individuals without known CAD and offers limited incremental prognostic value for individuals with known CAD, such as those with stents and bypass grafts. Currently, EBCT is thought to be a reasonable test to consider in patients with low to intermediate risk for future CAD-related events. Results of the test may help to reclassify them to higher risk and thus intensify primary prevention measures (Arnett et al., 2019).

Nursing Interventions

The nurse provides details of the procedure to help prepare the patient for the test. Patients need to be prepared to hold their breath at certain times during the procedure, so it is important for the nurse to practice with the patient before going for CT scan. The patient is positioned on a table, and the scanner rotates around the table during the test. The procedure is noninvasive and painless. However, to obtain adequate images, the patient must lie completely still during the scanning process. An IV is necessary if contrast is to be used to enhance the images. The patient should be told to expect transient flushing, metallic taste, nausea, or bradycardia during the contrast infusion.

Magnetic Resonance Angiography

Procedure

MRA is a noninvasive, painless technique that is used to examine both the physiologic and anatomic properties of the heart. MRA uses a powerful magnetic field and computer-generated pictures to image the heart and great vessels. It is valuable in diagnosing diseases of the aorta, heart muscle, and pericardium, as well as congenital heart lesions. The application of this technique to the evaluation of coronary artery anatomy is limited because the quality of the images is distorted by respirations, the beating heart, and certain implanted devices (stents and surgical clips). In addition, this technique cannot adequately visualize the small distal coronary arteries as accurately as conventional angiography performed during a cardiac catheterization.

Nursing Interventions

Because of the magnetic field used during MRA, patients must be screened for contraindications for its use. Patients with any type of cardiac implantable electronic device need to be screened to see if it is safe for the patient to undergo the test (Indik, Gimbel, Abe, et al., 2017). MRA cannot be performed on patients who have metal plates, prosthetic joints, or other metallic implants that can become dislodged if exposed to MRA. Patients are instructed to remove any jewelry, watches, or other metal items (e.g., ECG leads). Transdermal patches that contain a heat-conducting aluminized layer (e.g., nitroglycerin, clonidine, fentanyl) must be removed before MRA to prevent burning of the skin.

During MRA, the patient is positioned supine on a table that is placed into an enclosed imager or tube containing the magnetic field. A patient who is claustrophobic may need to receive a mild sedative before undergoing an MRA. An intermittent clanking or thumping that can be annoying is generated by the magnetic coils, so the patient may be offered a headset to listen to music. The scanner is equipped with a microphone so that the patient can communicate with the staff. The patient is instructed to remain motionless during the scan.

Echocardiography

Transthoracic Echocardiography

Echocardiography is a noninvasive ultrasound test that is used to measure the ejection fraction and examine the size, shape, and motion of cardiac structures. It is particularly useful for diagnosing pericardial effusions; determining chamber size and the etiology of heart murmurs; evaluating the function of heart valves, including prosthetic heart valves; and evaluating ventricular wall motion.

Procedure

Echocardiography involves transmission of high-frequency sound waves into the heart through the chest wall and the recording of the return signals. With the traditional transthoracic approach, the ultrasound is generated by a handheld transducer applied to the front of the chest. The transducer picks up the echoes and converts them to electrical impulses that are recorded and displayed on a monitor. It creates sophisticated, spatially correct images of the heart. An ECG is recorded simultaneously to assist in interpretation of the echocardiogram.

With the use of Doppler techniques, an echocardiogram can also show the direction and velocity of the blood flow through the heart. These techniques are used to assess for "leaking valves," conditions referred to as valvular regurgitation, and will also detect abnormal blood flow between the septum of the left and right heart.

Echocardiography may be performed with an exercise or pharmacologic stress test. Images are obtained at rest and then immediately after the target heart rate is reached. Myocardial ischemia from decreased perfusion during stress causes abnormalities in ventricular wall motion and is easily detected by echocardiography. A stress test using echocardiography is considered positive if abnormalities in ventricular wall motion are detected during stress but not during rest. These findings are highly suggestive of CAD and require further evaluation, such as a cardiac catheterization.

Nursing Interventions

Before transthoracic echocardiography, the nurse informs the patient about the test, explaining that it is painless. Echocardiographic monitoring is performed while a transducer that emits sound waves is moved over the surface of the chest wall. Gel applied to the skin helps transmit the sound waves. Periodically, the patient is asked to turn onto the left side or hold a breath. The test takes about 30 to 45 minutes. If the patient is to undergo an exercise or pharmacologic stress test with echocardiography, information on stress testing is also reviewed with the patient.

Transesophageal Echocardiography

Procedure

A significant limitation of transthoracic echocardiography is the poor quality of the images produced. Ultrasound loses its clarity as it passes through tissue, lung, and bone. An alternative technique involves threading a small transducer through the mouth and into the esophagus. This technique, called *transesophageal echocardiography* (TEE), provides clearer images because ultrasound waves pass through less tissue. A topical anesthetic agent and sedation are used during TEE because of the discomfort associated with the positioning of the transducer in the esophagus (refer to Chapter 15 for further discussion of sedation for procedures). Once the patient is comfortable, the transducer is inserted into the mouth and the patient is asked to swallow several times until it is positioned in the esophagus.

The high-quality imaging obtained during TEE makes this technique an important first-line diagnostic tool for evaluating patients with many types of CVD, including HF, valvular heart disease, arrhythmias, and many other conditions that place the patient at risk for atrial or ventricular thrombi. Pharmacologic stress testing using dobutamine and TEE can also be performed. It is frequently used during cardiac surgery to continuously monitor the response of the heart to the surgical procedure (e.g., valve replacement or coronary artery bypass). Complications are uncommon during TEE; however, if they do occur, they are serious. These complications are caused by sedation and impaired swallowing resulting from the topical anesthesia (respiratory depression and aspiration) and by insertion and manipulation of the transducer into the esophagus and stomach (vasovagal response or esophageal perforation). The patient must be assessed before TEE for a history of dysphagia or radiation therapy to the chest, which increases the likelihood of complications.

Nursing Interventions

Prior to the test, the nurse provides preprocedure education and ensures that the patient has a clear understanding of what the test entails and why it is being performed, instructs the patient not to eat or drink anything for 6 hours prior to the study, and checks to make sure that informed consent has been obtained. The nurse also inserts an IV line or assesses an existing IV for patency and suitability and asks the patient to remove full or partial dentures. During the test, the nurse provides emotional support and monitors level of consciousness, BP, ECG, respiration, and oxygen saturation (SpO$_2$). During the recovery period, the patient must maintain bed rest with the head of the bed elevated to 45 degrees. Following the procedural sedation policy of the agency, the nurse monitors the patient for dyspnea and assesses vital signs, SpO$_2$, level of consciousness, and gag reflex as recommended. Food and oral fluids are withheld until the patient is fully alert and the effects of the topical anesthetic agent are reversed, usually 2 hours after the procedure; if the gag reflex is intact, the nurse begins feeding with sips of water, then advances to the preprocedure diet. Patients are informed that a sore throat may be present for the next 24 hours; they are instructed to report the presence of a persistent sore throat, shortness of breath, or difficulty swallowing to the medical staff. If the procedure is performed in an outpatient setting, a family member or friend must be available to transport the patient home from the test site.

Cardiac Catheterization

Cardiac catheterization is a common invasive procedure used to diagnose structural and functional diseases of the heart and great vessels. The results guide treatment decisions including the need for revascularization (PCI or CABG) and other interventions to manage structural defects of the valves or septum (see Chapter 23).

This procedure involves the percutaneous insertion of radiopaque catheters into a large vein and an artery. Fluoroscopy is used to guide the advancement of the catheters through the right and left heart, referred to as right and left heart catheterizations, respectively. In most situations, patients undergo both right and left heart catheterizations. However, right heart catheterization is performed without a left heart catheterization when patients only need myocardial biopsies or measurement of pulmonary artery pressures. Of note, left heart catheterization involves the use of a contrast agent. These agents are necessary to visualize patency of the coronary arteries and evaluate left ventricular function.

In preparation for the procedure, patients have blood tests performed to evaluate metabolic function (electrolytes and glucose) and renal function (blood urea nitrogen and creatinine level). Baseline coagulation studies (activated partial thromboplastin time [aPTT], international normalized ratio [INR], and prothrombin time [PT]) are obtained to guide dosing of anticoagulation during the procedure. Because bleeding and hematoma formation are procedural risks, a complete blood cell count (CBC; includes the hematocrit, hemoglobin, and platelets) is necessary to establish baseline values. Later these results are compared with postprocedure results to monitor for blood loss.

A health history is obtained to assess for previous reactions to a contrast agent and determine if the patient has any risk factors for contrast-induced nephropathy (CIN). This uncommon complication is a form of acute kidney injury that is usually reversible. Patients with chronic kidney disease or renal insufficiency, diabetes, HF, hypotension, dehydration, use of nephrotoxic medications, and advanced age are at risk for CIN. CIN is defined as an increase in the baseline serum creatinine by 25% or more or an absolute increase of 0.5 mg/dL within 48 to 72 hours after the administration of contrast (Urden et al., 2017). See Chapter 47, Chart 47-5 for further discussion of nursing care of patient undergoing imaging study with the use of a contrast agent.

During a cardiac catheterization, the patient has one or more IV catheters for administration of fluids, sedatives, heparin, and other medications. The patient is continuously monitored for chest pain or dyspnea and for changes in BP and ECG, which are indicative of myocardial ischemia, hemodynamic instability, or arrhythmias. Resuscitation equipment must be readily available, and staff must be prepared to provide advanced cardiac life support measures as necessary.

Postprocedure, patients remain on bed rest for 2 to 6 hours before they are permitted to ambulate. Variations in time to ambulation are related to the size of the catheters used during the procedure, the site of catheter insertion (femoral or radial artery), the patient's anticoagulation status, and other factors (e.g., advanced age, obesity, bleeding disorder). The use of a radial access site and smaller (4- or 6-Fr) arterial catheters are associated with shorter bed rest restrictions.

Cardiac catheterization may be performed in the ambulatory setting. Unless the results demonstrate the need for immediate treatment, patients are discharged home. Hospitalized patients undergoing cardiac catheterization for diagnostic and interventional purposes (PCI, valvuloplasty) are returned to their hospital rooms for recovery (see Chapter 23).

Right Heart Catheterization

Right heart catheterization usually precedes left heart catheterization. It is performed to assess the function of the right ventricle and tricuspid and pulmonary valves. The procedure involves the passage of a catheter from a brachial, internal jugular, or femoral vein into the right atrium, right ventricle, pulmonary artery, and pulmonary arterioles. Pressures and oxygen saturations from each of these areas are obtained and recorded. The pulmonary artery pressures are used to diagnose pulmonary hypertension. A biopsy of a small piece of myocardial tissue can also be obtained during a right heart catheterization. The results of the biopsy are used to diagnose the etiology of a cardiomyopathy (abnormality of myocardium) or heart transplant rejection. At the completion of the procedure, the venous catheter is removed and hemostasis of the affected vein is achieved using manual pressure. Although right heart catheterization is considered relatively safe, potential complications include arrhythmias (from contact of the catheter with the endocardium), venous spasm, infection at the insertion site, and right heart perforation.

Left Heart Catheterization

Prior to left heart catheterization, patients who have previously experienced a reaction to a contrast agent are premedicated with antihistamines (e.g., diphenhydramine) and corticosteroids (e.g., prednisone). Patients at risk for CIN receive pre- and postprocedure preventive strategies. IV saline hydration increases vascular volume, facilitates removal of contrast from the kidneys, and reduces the risk of CIN (Liu, Hong, Wang, et al., 2019).

Left heart catheterization is performed to evaluate the aortic arch and its major branches, patency of the coronary arteries, and the function of the left ventricle and mitral and aortic valves. Left heart catheterization is performed by retrograde catheterization of the left ventricle. In this approach, the interventional cardiologist usually inserts the catheter into the right radial or a femoral artery and advances it into the aorta and left ventricle. Potential complications include arrhythmias, MI, perforation of the left heart or great vessels, and systemic embolization.

During a left heart catheterization, angiography is performed. Angiography is an imaging technique that involves the injection of the contrast agent into the arterial catheter. The contrast agent is filmed as it passes through the chambers of the left heart, aortic arch, and its major arteries. Coronary angiography is another technique used to observe the coronary artery anatomy and evaluate the degree of stenosis from atherosclerosis. To perform this test, a catheter is positioned into one of the coronary arteries. Once in position, the contrast agent is injected directly into the artery and images are obtained. The procedure is then repeated using the opposite coronary artery. Ventriculography is also performed to evaluate the size and function of the left ventricle. For this test, a catheter is positioned in the left ventricle and a large amount of contrast agent (30 mL) is rapidly injected into the ventricle.

The manipulation of catheters in the coronary arteries and left ventricle as well as injection of the contrast agent can cause intermittent myocardial ischemia. Vigilant monitoring throughout left heart catheterization is needed to detect myocardial ischemia, which can trigger chest pain and life-threatening arrhythmias.

Once the procedure is completed, the arterial catheter is withdrawn. There are several options available to achieve arterial hemostasis, including applying manual pressure and hemostatic devices available from numerous vendors. For the radial artery, a compression device, such as the Terumo TR Band®, is positioned over the artery. It has a mechanism that is inflated with air to put pressure against the artery. It remains in place for about 2 hours. A radial approach and a compression device are both common practices and are associated with lower risks for bleeding and vascular complications, as well as a shorter time to ambulation postprocedure (Mason, Shah, Tamis-Holland, et al., 2018).

For the femoral approach, manual pressure may be used alone or in combination with mechanical compression devices such as the FemoStop™. Many types of percutaneously deployed vascular closure devices are also available. These devices are positioned at the femoral arterial puncture site after completion of the procedure. They deploy a saline-soaked gelatin sponge (QUICKSEAL), collagen (VasoSeal), sutures (Perclose ProGlide™), or a combination of both collagen and sutures (Angio-Seal). Other products that expedite arterial hemostasis include external patches (Syvek Patch, Clo-Sur P.A.D.). These products are placed over the puncture site as the catheter is removed and manual pressure is applied for 4 to 10 minutes. Once hemostasis is achieved, the patch is covered with a dressing that remains in place for 24 hours. The interventional cardiologist determines which closure device, if any, will be deployed based on the artery used to insert the catheter, patient's condition, device availability, and personal preference.

Major benefits of the vascular closure devices include reliable, immediate hemostasis and a shorter time on bed rest without a significant increase in bleeding or other complications. Rare complications associated with these devices include bleeding around the closure device, infection, and arterial obstruction.

Nursing Interventions

Nursing responsibilities before cardiac catheterization include:

- Instructing the patient to fast, usually for 8 to 12 hours, before the procedure.
- Informing the patient that if catheterization is to be performed as an outpatient procedure, a friend, family member, or other responsible person must transport the patient home.
- Informing the patient about the expected duration of the procedure and advising that it will involve lying on a hard table for less than 2 hours.
- Reassuring the patient that IV medications are given to maintain comfort.
- Informing the patient about sensations that will be experienced during the catheterization. Knowing what to expect can help the patient cope with the experience. The nurse explains that an occasional pounding sensation (palpitation) may be felt in the chest because of extra heartbeats that almost always occur, particularly when the catheter tip touches the endocardium. The patient may be asked to cough and to breathe deeply, especially after the injection of the contrast agent. Coughing may help disrupt an arrhythmia and clear the contrast agent from the arteries. Breathing deeply and holding the breath help lower the diaphragm for better visualization of heart structures. The injection of a contrast agent into either side of the heart may produce a flushed feeling throughout the body and a sensation similar to the need to void, which subsides in 1 minute or less.
- Encouraging the patient to express fears and anxieties. The nurse provides education and reassurance to reduce apprehension.

Nursing responsibilities after cardiac catheterization are guided by hospital policy and primary provider preferences and may include:

- Observing the catheter access site for bleeding or hematoma formation and assessing peripheral pulses in the affected extremity (dorsalis pedis and posterior tibial pulses in the lower extremity, radial pulse in the upper extremity) every 15 minutes for 1 hour, every 30 minutes for 1 hour, and hourly for 4 hours or until discharge. BP and heart rate are also assessed during these same time intervals.
- Evaluating temperature, color, and capillary refill of the affected extremity during these same time intervals. The patient is assessed for affected extremity pain, numbness, or tingling sensations that may indicate arterial insufficiency. The best technique to use is to

compare the examination findings between the affected and unaffected extremities. Any changes are reported promptly.

- Screening carefully for arrhythmias by observing the cardiac monitor or by assessing the apical and peripheral pulses for changes in rate and rhythm. A vasovagal reaction, consisting of bradycardia, hypotension, and nausea, can be precipitated by a distended bladder or by discomfort from manual pressure that is applied during removal of an arterial or venous catheter. The vasovagal response is reversed by promptly elevating the lower extremities above the level of the heart, infusing a bolus of IV fluid, and administering IV atropine to treat the bradycardia.

- Maintaining activity restrictions for 2 to 6 hours after the procedure. The determination of bed rest, chair activity, and time to commence ambulation is dependent upon location of arterial approach, size of the catheter used during the procedure, medications administered, and method used to maintain hemostasis. If manual pressure or a mechanical device was used during a femoral artery approach, the patient remains on bed rest for up to 6 hours with the affected leg straight and the head of the bed elevated no greater than 30 degrees. For comfort, the patient may be turned from side to side with the affected extremity straight. If a percutaneous vascular closure device or patch was deployed, the nurse checks local nursing care standards and anticipates that the patient will have fewer activity restrictions. If the radial closure device was used, the patient can sit up in a chair until the effects of sedation have dissipated, and early ambulation is encouraged. After the vascular closure device removal, a dressing is applied over the catheter access site. Patients can return to normal activities the day after the procedure but must avoid strenuous wrist activities for several days (Mason et al., 2018). Analgesic medication is given as prescribed for discomfort.

- Instructing the patient to report chest pain and bleeding or sudden discomfort from the catheter insertion sites promptly.

- Monitoring the patient for CIN by observing for elevations in serum creatinine levels. IV hydration is used to increase urinary output and flush the contrast agent from the urinary tract; accurate oral and IV intake and urinary output are recorded.

- Ensuring patient safety by instructing the patient to ask for help when getting out of bed the first time after the procedure. The patient is monitored for bleeding from the catheter access site and for orthostatic hypotension, indicated by complaints of dizziness or lightheadedness.

For patients being discharged from the hospital on the same day as the procedure, additional instructions are provided (Chart 21-6).

Electrophysiologic Testing

The electrophysiology study (EPS) is an invasive procedure that plays a major role in the diagnosis and management of serious arrhythmias. EPS may be indicated for patients with syncope, palpitations, or both, and for survivors of cardiac arrest from ventricular fibrillation (sudden cardiac death)

Chart 21-6

PATIENT EDUCATION

Self-Management After Cardiac Catheterization

After discharge from the hospital for cardiac catheterization, patients should follow these guidelines for self-care:

- *If the artery in your wrist artery was used:* Return to normal activities tomorrow. Strenuous activities of the wrist such as manual labor, tennis, or driving may be restricted for a few days per your provider's orders.
- *If the artery in your groin was used:* For the next 24 hours, do not bend at the waist, strain, or lift heavy objects.
- Do not submerge the puncture site in water. Avoid tub baths, but shower as desired.
- Talk with your primary provider about when you may return to work, drive, or resume strenuous activities.
- If bleeding occurs, sit (arm or wrist approach) or lie down (groin approach) and apply firm pressure to the puncture site for 10 minutes. Notify your primary provider as soon as possible and follow instructions. If there is a large amount of bleeding, call 911. Do not drive to the hospital.
- Call your primary provider if any of the following occur: swelling, new bruising or pain from your procedure puncture site, temperature of 101°F or more.
- If test results show that you have coronary artery disease, talk with your primary provider about options for treatment, including cardiac rehabilitation programs in your community.
- Talk with your primary provider about lifestyle changes to reduce your risk for further or future heart problems, such as quitting smoking, lowering your cholesterol level, initiating dietary changes, beginning an exercise program, cardiac rehabilitation, or losing weight.
- Your primary provider may prescribe one or more new medications depending on your risk factors (medications to lower your blood pressure or cholesterol; aspirin or clopidogrel to prevent blood clots). Take all of your medications as instructed. If you feel that any of them are causing side effects, call your primary provider immediately. Do not stop taking any medications before talking to your primary provider.

Adapted from Mason, P. J., Shah, B., Tamis-Holland, J. E., et al. (2018). An update on radial artery access and best practices for transradial coronary angiography and intervention in acute coronary syndrome: A scientific statement from the American Heart Association. *Circulation: Cardiovascular Interventions*. Retrieved on 5/14/2019 at: www.ahajournals.org/toc/circinterventions/11/9

(Kusumoto, Schoenfeld, Barrett, et al., 2019). EPS is used to distinguish atrial from ventricular tachycardias when the determination cannot be made from the 12-lead ECG; to evaluate how readily a life-threatening arrhythmia (e.g., ventricular tachycardia, ventricular fibrillation) can be induced; to evaluate AV node function; to evaluate the effectiveness of antiarrhythmic medications in suppressing the arrhythmia; or to determine the need for other therapeutic interventions, such as a cardiac implantable electronic device, or radiofrequency ablation. (See Chapter 22 for a detailed discussion of EPS.)

 ## Hemodynamic Monitoring

Critically ill patients require continuous assessment of their cardiovascular system to diagnose and manage their complex medical conditions. This type of assessment is achieved by the use of direct pressure monitoring systems, referred to as hemodynamic monitoring. Common forms include CVP, pulmonary artery pressure, and intra-arterial BP monitoring. Patients requiring hemodynamic monitoring are cared for in critical care units. Some progressive care units also admit stable patients with CVP, pulmonary artery catheters, or intra-arterial BP monitoring. To perform hemodynamic monitoring, a CVP, pulmonary artery, or arterial catheter is introduced into the appropriate blood vessel or heart chamber. It is connected to a pressure monitoring system that has several components, including:

- A disposable flush system, composed of IV normal saline solution, tubing, stopcocks, and a flush device, which provides continuous and manual flushing of the system.
- A pressure bag placed around the flush solution that is maintained at 300 mm Hg of pressure. The pressurized flush system delivers 3 to 5 mL of solution per hour through the catheter to prevent clotting and backflow of blood into the pressure monitoring system.
- A transducer to convert the pressure coming from the artery or heart chamber into an electrical signal.
- An amplifier or monitor, which increases the size of the electrical signal for display on an oscilloscope.

Nurses caring for patients who require hemodynamic monitoring receive training prior to using this sophisticated technology. The nurse helps ensure safe and effective care by adhering to the following guidelines:

- Ensuring that the system is set up and maintained properly. For example, the pressure monitoring system must be kept patent and free of air bubbles.
- Checking that the stopcock of the transducer is positioned at the level of the atrium before the system is used to obtain pressure measurements. This landmark is referred to as the phlebostatic axis (Fig. 21-10). The nurse uses a marker to identify this level on the chest wall, which provides a stable reference point for subsequent pressure readings.
- Establishing the zero reference point in order to ensure that the system is properly functioning at atmospheric pressure. This process is accomplished by placing the stopcock of the transducer at the phlebostatic axis, opening the transducer to air, and activating the zero function key on the bedside monitor. Measurements of CVP, BP, and pulmonary artery pressures can be made

with the head of the bed elevated up to 60 degrees; however, the system must be repositioned to the phlebostatic axis to ensure an accurate reading (Urden et al., 2017).

Complications from the use of hemodynamic monitoring systems are uncommon and can include pneumothorax, infection, and air embolism. The nurse observes for signs of pneumothorax during the insertion of catheters using a central venous approach (CVP and pulmonary artery catheters). The longer any of these catheters are left in place (after 72 to 96 hours), the greater the risk of infection. Air emboli can be introduced into the vascular system if the stopcocks attached to the pressure transducers are mishandled during blood drawing, administration of medications, or other procedures that require opening the system to air. Therefore, nurses handling this equipment must demonstrate competence prior to caring independently for a patient requiring hemodynamic monitoring.

Catheter-related bloodstream infections are the most common preventable complication associated with hemodynamic monitoring systems. The Centers for Disease Control and Prevention (CDC) has published comprehensive guidelines for the prevention of these infections (O'Grady, Alexander, Burns, et al., 2011; Talbot, Stone, Irwin, et al., 2017). To minimize the risk of infection, a group of evidence-based interventions, called a care *bundle*, should be implemented.

The CDC and Infusion Nursing Society have additional infection control guidelines that pertain to the ongoing care of these patients, including skin care, dressing changes, and line and connector care that are outlined in Table 21-5.

Central Venous Pressure Monitoring

CVP is a measurement of the pressure in the vena cava or right atrium. The pressure in the vena cava, right atrium, and right ventricle is equal at the end of diastole; thus, the CVP also reflects the filling pressure of the right ventricle (preload). The normal CVP is 2 to 6 mm Hg. It is measured by positioning a catheter in the vena cava or right atrium and connecting it to a pressure monitoring system. The CVP is most valuable when it is monitored over time and correlated with the patient's clinical status. A CVP greater than 6 mm Hg

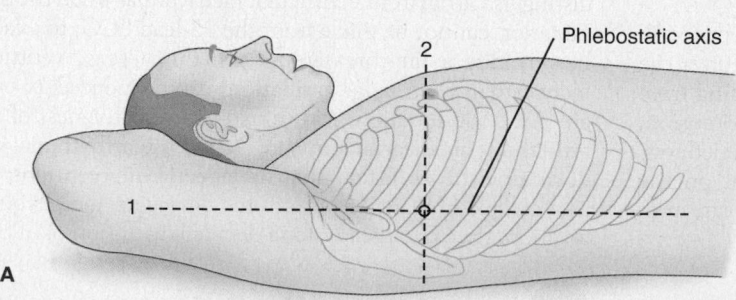
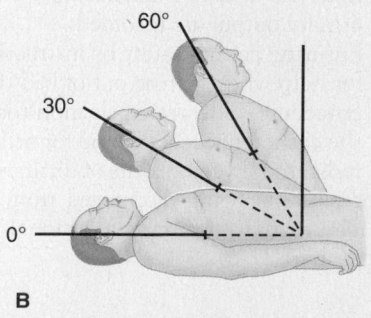

Figure 21-10 • A. The phlebostatic axis is the reference point for the atrium when the patient is positioned supine. It is the intersection of two lines on the chest wall: (*1*) the midaxillary line drawn between the anterior and posterior surfaces of the chest and (*2*) the line drawn through the fourth intercostal space. Its location is identified with a skin marker. The stopcock of the transducer used in hemodynamic monitoring is "leveled" at this mark prior to taking pressure measurements. **B.** Measurements can be taken with the head of the bed (HOB) elevated up to 60 degrees. Note the phlebostatic axis changes as the HOB is elevated; thus, the stopcock and transducer must be repositioned after each position change.

TABLE 21-5	Nursing Interventions to Prevent Intravascular Catheter-Related Bloodstream Infections	
Topic	**Intervention**
Hand hygiene	• Wash hands with soap and water or use alcohol-based hand rubs before and after contact with the catheter for any reason.
Dressing	• Wear clean or sterile gloves when changing the dressing. • Cleanse the skin during dressing changes with a >0.5% chlorhexidine preparation with alcohol. • Use a chlorhexidine-impregnated dressing at the catheter insertion site. Do not use topical antibiotic ointment or creams on insertion sites. • Dress the site with sterile gauze or sterile, transparent, semipermeable dressing to cover the catheter site. If the patient is diaphoretic or if the site is bleeding or oozing, use a gauze dressing until it is resolved. • Change gauze dressings every 2 d or transparent dressings at least every 7 d and whenever dressings become damp, loosened, or visibly soiled.
Catheter site	• Assess the site regularly—visually when changing the dressing or by palpation through an intact dressing. Remove the dressing for a thorough assessment if the patient has tenderness at the insertion site, fever without obvious source, or other signs of local or bloodstream infection.
Needleless catheter systems	• Change needleless connectors, administration sets, and pressure tubing per institutional policy, usually every 96 h. • Scrub ports, connectors, and hubs with alcohol, chlorhexidine/alcohol, or povidone–iodine before and after access. • Apply alcohol-impregnated caps to needless connectors between uses.
Bathing	• Clean the skin daily with a 2% chlorhexidine wash. • Do not submerge the catheter or catheter site in water. • Showering is permitted if the catheter and related tubing are placed in an impermeable cover.
Patient education	• Ask patients to report any new discomforts from the catheter site.

Adapted from Gorski, L. A., Hadaway, L., Hagle, M., et al. (2016). Infusion therapy standards of practice. *Journal of Infusion Nursing, 39*(1 Suppl.), S1–S159; O'Grady, N. P., Alexander, A., Burns, L., et al. (2011). 2017 Update of the guidelines for the prevention of intravascular catheter-related infections, 2011. Retrieved on 5/15/2019 at: www.cdc.gov/infectioncontrol/pdf/guidelines/bsi-guidelines-H.pdf; Talbot, T. R., Stone, E. C., Irwin, K., et al. (2017). 2017 Updated recommendations on the use of chlorhexidine-impregnated dressings for prevention of intravascular catheter-related infections. Retrieved on 5/15/ 2019 at: www.cdc.gov/infectioncontrol/pdf/guidelines/c-i-dressings-H.pdf

indicates an elevated right ventricular preload. There are many problems that can cause an elevated CVP, but the most common problem is hypervolemia (excessive fluid circulating in the body) or right-sided HF. In contrast, a low CVP (less than 2 mm Hg) indicates reduced right ventricular preload, which is most often from hypovolemia. Dehydration, excessive blood loss, vomiting or diarrhea, and overdiuresis can result in hypovolemia and a low CVP. This diagnosis can be substantiated when a rapid IV infusion of fluid causes the CVP to increase.

Before insertion of a CVP catheter, the site is prepared as recommended by the CDC (see Chapter 11, Chart 11-2). The preferred site is the subclavian vein; the femoral vein is generally avoided (O'Grady et al., 2011). A local anesthetic agent is used. During this sterile procedure, the physician threads a single-lumen or multilumen catheter through the vein into the vena cava just above or within the right atrium. Once the CVP catheter is inserted, it is secured and a dry sterile dressing is applied. Position of the catheter is confirmed by a chest x-ray.

Nursing Interventions

The frequency of CVP measurements is dictated by the patient's condition and the treatment plan. In addition to obtaining pressure readings, the CVP catheter is used for infusing IV fluids, administering IV medications, and drawing blood specimens. Nursing care of the patient with a CVP catheter follows central line and pressure tubing guidelines (see Table 21-5).

Pulmonary Artery Pressure Monitoring

Pulmonary artery pressure monitoring is used in critical care for assessing left ventricular function, diagnosing the etiology of shock, and evaluating the patient's response to medical interventions (e.g., fluid administration, vasoactive medications). A pulmonary artery catheter and a pressure monitoring system are used. A variety of catheters are available for cardiac pacing, oximetry, cardiac output measurement, or a combination of functions. Pulmonary artery catheters are balloon-tipped, flow-directed catheters that have distal and proximal lumens (Fig. 21-11). The distal lumen has a port that opens into the pulmonary artery. Once connected by its hub to the pressure monitoring system, it is used only to continuously measure pulmonary artery pressures. The proximal lumen has a port that opens into the right atrium. It is used to administer IV medications and fluids or to monitor right atrial pressures (i.e., CVP). Each catheter has a balloon inflation hub and valve. A syringe is connected to the hub, which is used to inflate or deflate the balloon with air (maximum 1.5-mL capacity). The valve opens and closes the balloon inflation lumen.

A pulmonary artery catheter with specialized capabilities has additional components. For example, the thermodilution catheter has three additional features that enable it to measure cardiac output: a thermistor connector attached to the cardiac output computer of the bedside monitor, a proximal injectate port used for injecting fluids when obtaining the cardiac output, and a thermistor (positioned near the distal port) (see Fig. 21-11).

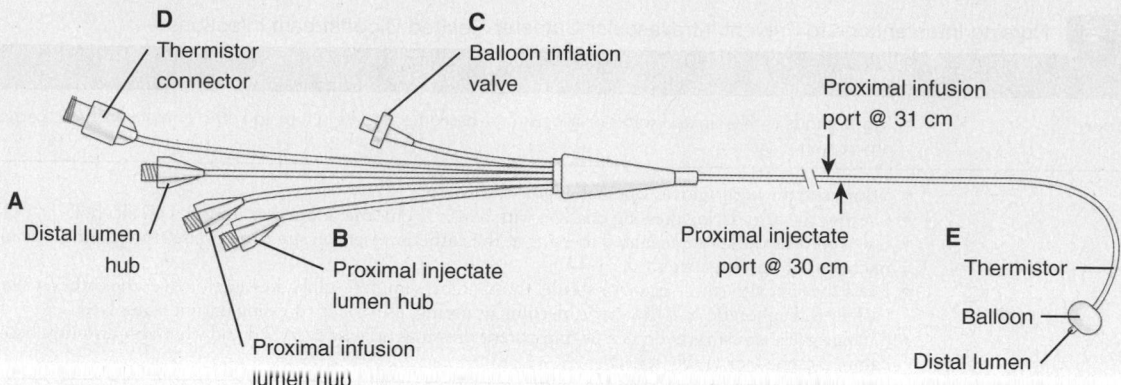

Figure 21-11 • The pulmonary artery catheter used for obtaining pressure measurements and cardiac output. **A.** The pressure monitoring system is connected to the distal lumen hub. **B.** Intravenous solutions are infused through the proximal infusion and injectate lumen hubs. **C.** An air-filled syringe connected to the balloon inflation valve is used for balloon inflation during catheter insertion and pulmonary artery wedge pressure measurements. **D.** To obtain cardiac output, the thermistor connector is inserted into the cardiac output component of the bedside cardiac monitor, and 5 to 10 mL of normal saline is injected in 4 seconds into the proximal injectate port. **E.** The thermistor located near the balloon is used to calculate the cardiac output. Redrawn courtesy of Baxter Healthcare Corporation, Edwards Critical Care Division, Santa Ana, California.

The pulmonary artery catheter, covered with a sterile sleeve, is inserted into a large vein, preferably the subclavian, through a sheath. As noted previously, the femoral vein is avoided; insertion techniques and protocols mirror those used for inserting a CVP catheter (see previous discussion) (O'Grady et al., 2011). The sheath is equipped with a side port for infusing IV fluids and medications. The catheter is then passed into the vena cava and right atrium. In the right atrium, the balloon tip is inflated, and the catheter is carried rapidly by the flow of blood through the tricuspid valve into the right ventricle, through the pulmonic valve, and into a branch of the pulmonary artery. When the catheter reaches the pulmonary artery, the balloon is deflated and the catheter is secured with sutures (Fig. 21-12). Fluoroscopy may be used during insertion to visualize the progression of the catheter through the right heart chambers to the pulmonary artery. This procedure can be performed in the operating room, in the cardiac catheterization laboratory, or at the bedside in the critical care unit. During insertion of the pulmonary artery catheter, the bedside monitor is observed for pressure and waveform changes, as well as arrhythmias, as the catheter progresses through the right heart to the pulmonary artery.

Once the catheter is in position, the following are measured: right atrial, pulmonary artery systolic, pulmonary artery diastolic, mean pulmonary artery, and pulmonary artery wedge pressures (see Fig. 21-2 for normal chamber pressures). Monitoring of the pulmonary artery diastolic and pulmonary artery wedge pressures is particularly important in critically ill patients because they are used to evaluate left ventricular filling pressures (i.e., left ventricular preload).

It is important to note that the pulmonary artery wedge pressure is achieved by inflating the balloon tip for a maximum of 15 seconds, which causes it to float more distally into a smaller portion of the pulmonary artery until it is wedged into position. This is an occlusive maneuver that impedes blood flow through that segment of the pulmonary artery. Therefore, the wedge pressure is measured immediately and the balloon deflated promptly to restore blood flow.

> ⚑ **Quality and Safety Nursing Alert**
>
> *After measuring the pulmonary artery wedge pressure, the nurse ensures that the balloon is deflated and that the catheter has returned to its normal position. This important intervention is verified by evaluating the return of the pulmonary artery systolic and diastolic waveform displayed on the bedside monitor.*

Nursing Interventions

Catheter site care is essentially the same as for a CVP catheter. Similar to CVP measurement, the transducer must be positioned at the phlebostatic axis to ensure accurate readings (see Fig. 21-10). Serious complications include pulmonary artery rupture, pulmonary thromboembolism, pulmonary infarction, catheter kinking, arrhythmias, and air embolism.

Intra-Arterial Blood Pressure Monitoring

Intra-arterial BP monitoring is used to obtain direct and continuous BP measurements in critically ill patients who have severe hypertension or hypotension. Arterial catheters are also useful when arterial blood gas measurements and blood samples need to be obtained frequently.

The radial artery is the usual site selected. However, placement of a catheter into the radial artery can further impede perfusion to an area that has poor circulation. As a result, the tissue distal to the cannulated artery can become ischemic or necrotic. Patients with diabetes, peripheral vascular disease, or hypotension, receiving IV vasopressors, or having had previous surgery are at highest risk for this complication. Before arterial line insertion, two tests may be considered to assess circulation; namely, a Doppler ultrasound or a modified Allen's test. A Doppler ultrasound assesses blood flow of the artery. The modified Allen's test assesses collateral circulation. To perform the Allen's test, the patient's hand is elevated and the patient is asked to make a fist. The nurse compresses the radial and ulnar arteries simultaneously, causing the hand to blanch. After the patient opens the fist, the nurse releases the pressure on the ulnar artery. If blood flow is restored (hand turns pink) within 7 seconds, the circulation

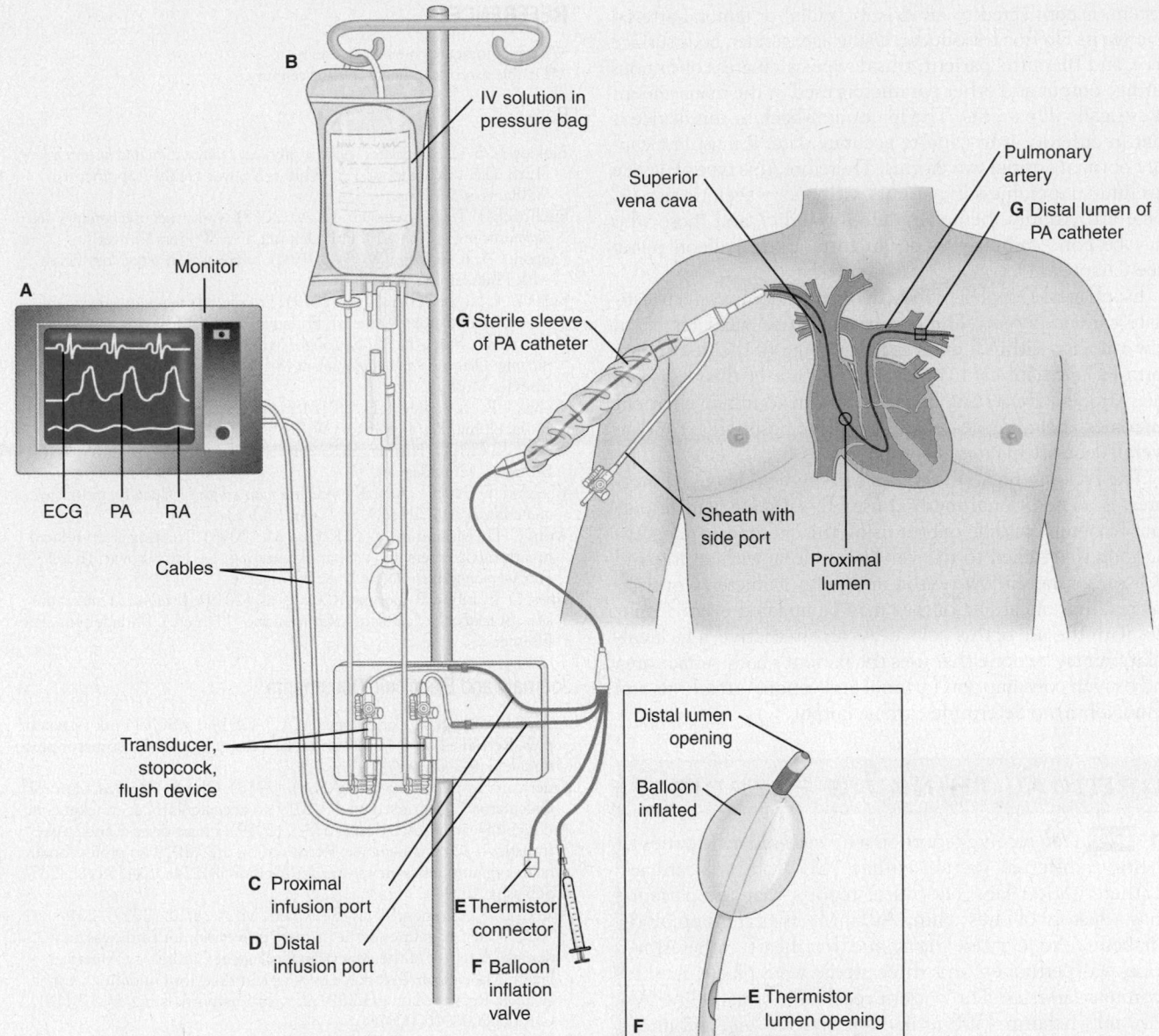

Figure 21-12 • Pulmonary artery (PA) catheter and pressure monitoring systems. Bedside monitor that connects with cables (**A**) to the pressure monitoring systems (includes intravenous [IV] solution in a pressure bag, IV tubing, and two transducers with stopcocks and flush devices) (**B**). This system connects to the proximal infusion port that opens in the right atria (**C**) and is used to infuse fluids or medications and monitor central venous pressures and the distal infusion port (**D**). This port opens in the PA and is used to monitor PA pressures. **E.** The thermistor connector is attached to the bedside cardiac monitor to obtain cardiac output. **F.** An air-filled syringe is attached to the balloon inflation valve during catheter insertion and measurement of PA wedge pressure. **G.** PA catheter positioned in the pulmonary artery. Note the sterile sleeve over the PA catheter. The PA catheter is threaded through the sheath until it reaches the desired position in the PA. The side port on the sheath is used to infuse medications or fluids. ECG, electrocardiogram; RA, right atrium.

to the hand may be adequate enough to tolerate placement of a radial artery catheter (Wiegand, 2017).

Nursing Interventions

Site preparation and care are the same as for CVP catheters. The catheter flush solution is normal saline, which is the same as for CVP and pulmonary artery catheters. A transducer is attached, and pressures are measured in millimeters of mercury (mm Hg). The nurse monitors the patient for complications, which include local obstruction with distal ischemia, external hemorrhage, massive ecchymosis, dissection, air embolism, blood loss, pain, arteriospasm, and infection.

Minimally Invasive Cardiac Output Monitoring Devices

Monitoring cardiac output using the pulmonary artery catheter has been the standard of practice in critical care since its inception over 50 years ago. Its use has diminished recently with the availability of new, less invasive devices. Several types of devices are commercially available. Selection of a specific device for clinical use is determined by availability, provider preferences, and the patient's clinical condition (Urden et al., 2017).

Pulse pressure analysis uses an arterial pressure waveform to continuously estimate the patient's stroke volume. One such device, the Edwards Lifesciences Vigileo monitoring system, is connected to an existing radial or femoral arterial line via its FloTrac transducer. Using age, gender, body surface area, and BP of the patient, this device calculates continuous cardiac output and other parameters used in the management of critically ill patients. The major drawback to this device is that in order for it to capture accurate data, it must first capture optimal arterial waveforms. Therefore, this type of device has limited usefulness in patients with poor waveform signals, some arrhythmias, hemodynamic instability, and those who may be concomitantly using an intra-aortic balloon pump (see Chapter 11).

Esophageal Doppler probes are used to noninvasively estimate cardiac output. The esophageal probe measures blood flow velocity within a cross-sectional area of the descending aorta to calculate cardiac output. The use of this device in the perioperative setting has been shown to improve patient outcomes, including decreased lengths of hospital stay and an overall decrease in rates of complications (Urden et al., 2017).

The Fick method, which uses carbon dioxide (CO_2) measures, is an additional method used to estimate cardiac output. To obtain cardiac output using this method, a rebreathing loop is attached to the ventilator along with an infrared CO_2 sensor, an airflow sensor, and pulse oximeter. Continuous readings of cardiac output may be updated every 3 minutes with the use of this device. As an alternative, a Fick calculation may be done that uses the patient's body surface area and oxygen consumption (arterial and venous saturations and hemoglobin) to determine cardiac output.

CRITICAL THINKING EXERCISES

1 `pa` You receive report on a 65-year-old male patient being transferred to the cardiac ICU from the cardiac catheterization lab. The nurse reports that the patient has a history of chest pain, ACS, MI, hypertension, and diabetes. An elective right and left heart catheterization was performed and three stents were placed in the coronary arteries. The patient received normal saline IV 250 mL, heparin 4500 units, fentanyl 100 mg, and midazolam 2 mg. A TR Band is in place over the right radial artery which must stay in place for 2 hours. The patient tolerated the procedure well. What are your top nursing priorities when the patient arrives to the unit? Discuss key nursing interventions after cardiac catheterization. Describe how the nursing care of a patient with radial access differs from a patient with femoral access. What education will you provide the patient concerning postprocedure care?

2 `ebp` You are assigned to care for a 48-year-old female patient with a pulmonary artery (PA) catheter. She has advanced heart failure and is on the transplant waiting list. What cardiac assessment findings do you expect to find? The charge nurse rounds and asks you if a care bundle has been implemented. What is a care bundle? How will you care for the pulmonary artery catheter to reduce the risk of catheter-related bloodstream infections? What is the strength of the evidence that guides these interventions?

REFERENCES

*Asterisk indicates nursing research.
**Double asterisk indicates classic reference.

Books

Bickley, L. S. (2017). *Bates' guide to physical examination and history taking* (12th ed.). Philadelphia, PA: Wolters Kluwer Health/Lippincott Williams & Wilkins.

Fischbach, F. T., & Fischbach, M. A. (2018). *A manual of laboratory and diagnostic tests* (10th ed.). Philadelphia, PA: Wolters Kluwer.

Pappano, A. J., & Weir, W. G. (2019). *Cardiovascular physiology* (11th ed.). Philadelphia, PA: Elsevier.

Sidawy, A. N., & Perler, B. A. (2019). *Rutherford's vascular surgery and endovascular therapy* (9th ed.). Philadelphia, PA: Elsevier.

Urden, L. D., Stacy, K. M., & Lough, M. E. (2017). *Critical care nursing: Diagnosis and management* (8th ed.). St. Louis, MO: Elsevier Mosby.

Weber, J. R., & Kelley, J. H. (2018). *Health assessment in nursing* (6th ed.). Philadelphia, PA: Lippincott Williams & Wilkins.

Wesley, K. (2017). *Huszar's ECG and 12-lead interpretation* (5th ed.). St. Louis, MO: Elsevier.

Wiegand, D. (2017). *AACN procedure manual for high acuity, progressive, and critical care* (7th ed.). St. Louis, MO: Elsevier.

Won, C. H., Mohsenin, V., & Kryger, M. (2018). Treating sleep-related breathing disorders. In A. Sharafkhaneh, & M. Hirshkowitz (Eds.). *Fatigue management*. New York: Springer.

Zipes, D. P., Libby, P., Bonow, R. O., et al. (2019). *Braunwald's heart disease: A textbook of cardiovascular medicine* (11th ed.). Philadelphia, PA: Elsevier.

Journals and Electronic Documents

American College of Cardiology (ACC). (2019). ASCVD risk estimator plus. Retrieved on 6/4/2019 at: tools.acc.org/ascvd-risk-estimator-plus/#!/calculate/estimate

American Heart Association (AHA). (2018). Check. Change. Control Calculator™. Retrieved on 4/3/2019 at: ccccalculator.ccctracker.com

American Heart Association (AHA). (2019). Heart disease and stroke statistics—2019 at-a-glance. Retrieved on 3/29/2019 at: professional. heart.org/en/science-news/-/media/22cf5db5b1a24b38a435fcecb42d588b.ashx

Arnett, D. K., Blumenthal, R. S., Albert, M. A., et al. (2019). 2019 ACC/AHA guideline on the primary prevention of cardiovascular disease: A report of the American College of Cardiology/American Heart Association Task Force on Clinical Practice Guidelines. *Circulation*. Retrieved on 4/3/2019 at: www.ahajournals.org/doi/10.1161/CIR.0000000000000678

Boothby, C. A., Dada, B. R., Rabi, D. M., et al. (2018). The effect of cardiac rehabilitation attendance on sexual activity outcomes in cardiovascular disease patients: A systematic review. *Canadian Journal of Cardiology, 34*(12), 1590–1599.

Domínguez, F., Fuster, V., Fernández-Alvira, J., et al. (2019). Association of sleep duration and quality with subclinical atherosclerosis. *Journal of the American College of Cardiology, 73*(2), 134–144.

Gorski, L. A., Hadaway, L., Hagle, M., et al. (2016). Infusion therapy standards of practice. *Journal of Infusion Nursing, 39*(1 Suppl.), S1–S159.

Grundy, S. M., Stone, N. J., Bailey, A. L., et al. (2019). 2018 AHA/ACC/AACVPR/AAPA/ABC/ACPM/ADA/AGS/APhA/ASPC/NLA/PCNA Guideline on the management of blood cholesterol: A report of the American College of Cardiology/American Heart Association Task Force on Clinical Practice Guidelines. *Journal of the American College of Cardiology, 73*(24), 3168–3209.

**Homes, T. H., & Rahe, R. H. (1967). The Social Readjustment Rating Scale. *Journal of Psychosomatic Research, 11*(2), 213–218.

*Iacoe, E., Ratner, P. A., Wong, S. T., et al. (2018). A cross-sectional study of ethnicity-based differences in treatment seeking for symptoms of acute coronary syndrome. *European Journal of Cardiovascular Nursing, 17*(4), 297–304.

Indik, J. H., Gimbel, J. R., Abe, H., et al. (2017). 2017 HRS consensus statement on magnetic resonance imaging and radiation exposure in patients with cardiovascular implantable electronic devices. *Heart Rhythm, 14*(7), e97–e153.

Jepsen, S., Sendelbach, S., Ruppel, H., et al. (2018). AACN Practice Alert: Managing alarms in acute care across the life span: Electrocardiography and pulse oximetry. *Critical Care Nurse, 38*(2), e16–e20.

Jha, M. K., Qamar, A., Vaduganathan, M., et al. (2019). Screening and management of depression in patients with cardiovascular disease: JACC state-of-the-art review. *Journal of the American College of Cardiology, 73*(14), 1827–1845.

*Keck, C., & Taylor, M. (2018). Emerging research on the implications of hormone replacement therapy on coronary heart disease. *Current Atherosclerosis Reports, 20*(57), 1–4.

Kim, J., Kang, H., Bae, K., et al. (2019). Social support deficit and depression treatment outcomes in patients with acute coronary syndrome: Findings from the EsDEPACS study. *The International Journal of Psychiatry in Medicine, 54*(1), 39–52.

King, J. E. (2017). Guidelines and implications for selecting preoperative cardiac stress tests. *The Journal for Nurse Practitioners, 13*(8), 505–511.

Kusumoto, F. M., Schoenfeld, M. H., Barrett, C., et al. (2019). 2018 ACC/AHA/HRS guideline on the evaluation and management of patients with bradycardia and cardiac conduction delay: A report of the American College of Cardiology/American Heart Association Task Force on Clinical Practice Guidelines and the Heart Rhythm Society. *Journal of the American College of Cardiology, 74*(7), e51–e156.

Lane-Cordova, A. D., Khan, S. S., Grobman, W. A., et al. (2019). Long-term cardiovascular risks associated with adverse pregnancy outcomes. *Journal of the American College of Cardiology, 73*(16), 2106–2116.

Levine, G. N., Bates, E. R., Bittl, J. A., et al. (2016). 2016 ACC/AHA guideline focused update on duration of dual antiplatelet therapy in patients with coronary artery disease: A report of the American College of Cardiology/American Heart Association Task Force on Clinical Practice Guidelines. *Journal of the American College of Cardiology, 68*(10), 1082–1115.

Lichtman, J. H., Leifheit, E. C., Safdar, B., et al. (2018). Sex differences in the presentation and perception of symptoms among young patients with myocardial infarction: Evidence from the VIRGO study (variation in recovery: role of gender on outcomes of young AMI patients). *Circulation, 137*(8), 781–790.

Liddy, S., Buckley, U., Kok, H. K., et al. (2018). Applications of cardiac computed tomography in electrophysiology intervention. *European Heart Journal Cardiovascular Imaging, 19*(3), 253–261.

Liu, Y., Hong, D., Wang, A. Y., et al. (2019). Effects of intravenous hydration on risk of contrast induced nephropathy and in-hospital mortality in STEMI patients undergoing primary percutaneous coronary intervention: A systematic review and meta-analysis of randomized controlled trials. *BMC Cardiovascular Disorders, 19*(87), 1–9.

Mason, P. J., Shah, B., Tamis-Holland, J. E., et al. (2018). An update on radial artery access and best practices for transradial coronary angiography and intervention in acute coronary syndrome: A scientific statement from the American Heart Association. *Circulation: Cardiovascular Interventions.* Retrieved on 5/4/2019 at: www.ahajournals.org/toc/circinterventions/11/9

Mervak, B. M., Cohan, R. H., Ellis, J. H., et al. (2017). Intravenous corticosteroid premedication administered 5 hours before CT compared with a traditional 13-hour oral regimen. *Radiology, 285*(2), 425–433.

Merz, C. N., Andersen, H., Sprague, E., et al. (2017). Knowledge, attitudes, and beliefs regarding cardiovascular disease in women: The women's heart alliance. *Journal of the American College of Cardiology, 70*(2), 123–132.

Momeyer, M. A., & Mion, L. C. (2018). Orthostatic hypotension: An often overlooked risk factor for falls. *Geriatric Nursing, 39*(4), 483–486.

O'Grady, N. P., Alexander, A., Burns, L., et al. (2011). 2017 Update of the guidelines for the prevention of intravascular catheter-related infections, 2011. Retrieved on 5/15/2019 at: www.cdc.gov/infectioncontrol/pdf/guidelines/bsi-guidelines-H.pdf

Ricci, F., De Caterina, R., & Fedorowski, A. (2015). Orthostatic hypotension: Epidemiology, prognosis, and treatment. *Journal of the American College of Cardiology, 66*(7), 848–860.

Rushton, S., & Carman, M. J. (2018). Chest pain: If it is not the heart, what is it? *Nursing Clinics of North America, 53*(3), 421–431.

Sampson, M. (2019). Ambulatory electrocardiography: Indications and devices. *British Journal of Cardiac Nursing, 14*(3), 114–121.

Sandau, K. E., Funk, M., Auerbach, A., et al. (2017). Update to practice standards for electrocardiographic monitoring in hospital settings: A scientific statement from the American Heart Association. *Circulation, 136*(19), e273–e344.

*Siow, E., Leung, D. Y., Wong, E. M., et al. (2018). Do depressive symptoms moderate the effects of exercise self-efficacy on physical activity among patients with coronary heart disease? *Journal of Cardiovascular Nursing, 33*(4), e26–e34.

Talbot, T. R., Stone, E. C., Irwin, K., et al. (2017). 2017 Updated recommendations on the use of chlorhexidine-impregnated dressings for prevention of intravascular catheter-related infections. Retrieved on 5/15/2019 at: www.cdc.gov/infectioncontrol/pdf/guidelines/c-i-dressings-H.pdf

Vaccarino, V., Badimon, L., Bremner, J. D., et al. (2019). Depression and coronary heart disease: 2018 ESC position paper of the working group of coronary pathophysiology and microcirculation developed under the auspices of the ESC Committee for Practice Guidelines. *European Heart Journal, 41*(17), 1687–1696.

Whelton, P. K., Carey, R. M., Aronow, W. S., et al. (2018). 2017 ACC/AHA/AAPA/ABC/ACPM/AGS/AphA/ASH/ASPC/NMA/PCNA Guideline for the prevention, detection, evaluation, and management of high blood pressure in adults. *Journal of the American College of Cardiology, 71*(19), e127–e248.

Yiadom, M. Y., Baugh, C. W., McWade, C. M., et al. (2017). Performance of emergency department screening criteria for an early ECG to identify ST-segment elevation myocardial infarction. *Journal of the American Heart Association, 6*(3), 1–11.

Yuan, M., Fang, Q., Liu, G., et al. (2019). Risk factors for post-acute coronary syndrome depression: A meta-analysis of observational studies. *Journal of Cardiovascular Nursing, 34*(1), 60–70.

Zhao, D., Guallar, E., & Ouyang, P., et al. (2018). Endogenous sex hormones and incident cardiovascular disease in post-menopausal women. *Journal of the American College of Cardiology, 71*(22), 2555–2566.

Resources

American Association of Critical Care Nurses (AACN), www.aacn.org

American College of Cardiology (ACC), www.acc.org

American College of Cardiology (ACC) (2019). ASCVD risk estimator plus, tools.acc.org/ascvd-risk-estimator-plus/#!/calculate/estimate

American Heart Association (AHA), www.heart.org

American Heart Association (AHA), 2018 Prevention Guidelines Tool CV Risk Calculator, static.heart.org/riskcalc/app/index.html#!/baseline-risk

American Heart Association (AHA) (2018). Check. Change. Control Calculator™, ccccalculator.ccctracker.com

National Institutes of Health (NIH), National Heart, Lung, and Blood Institute (NHLBI), www.nhlbi.nih.gov

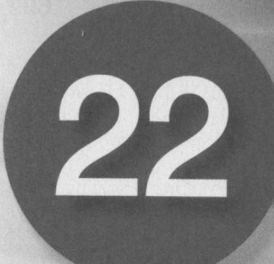

22

Management of Patients with Arrhythmias and Conduction Problems

LEARNING OUTCOMES

On completion of this chapter, the learner will be able to:

1. Correlate the components of the normal electrocardiogram with physiologic events of the heart.
2. Define the electrocardiogram as a waveform that represents the cardiac electrical event in relation to the lead (placement of electrodes).
3. Analyze elements of an electrocardiographic rhythm strip: ventricular and atrial rate, ventricular and atrial rhythm, QRS complex and shape, QRS duration, P wave and shape, PR interval, and P:QRS ratio.

4. Identify the electrocardiographic criteria, causes and management of arrhythmias, and use the nursing process as a framework for care of the patient with an arrhythmia, including conduction disturbances.
5. Compare the different types of pacemakers, their uses, possible complications, and nursing implications.
6. Describe the key points of using a defibrillator; identify the purpose of an implantable cardioverter defibrillator, the types available, and the nursing implications.
7. Describe the nursing management of patients with implantable cardiac devices.

NURSING CONCEPT

Perfusion

GLOSSARY

ablation: purposeful destruction of heart muscle cells, usually in an attempt to correct or eliminate an arrhythmia

arrhythmia: disorder of the formation or conduction (or both) of the electrical impulse within the heart, altering the heart rate, heart rhythm, or both and potentially causing altered blood flow (also referred to as dysrhythmia)

artifact: distorted, irrelevant, and extraneous electrocardiographic (ECG) waveforms

automaticity: ability of the cardiac cells to initiate an electrical impulse

cardiac resynchronization therapy (CRT): biventricular pacing used to correct interventricular, intraventricular, and atrioventricular conduction disturbances that occur in patients with heart failure

cardioversion: electrical current given in synchrony with the patient's own QRS complex to stop an arrhythmia

chronotropy: rate of impulse formation

conduction: transmission of electrical impulses from one cell to another

defibrillation: electrical current given to stop an arrhythmia, not synchronized with the patient's QRS complex

depolarization: process by which cardiac muscle cells change from a more negatively charged to a more positively charged intracellular state

dromotropy: conduction velocity

electrocardiogram (ECG): a record of a test that graphically measures the electrical activity of the heart, including each phase of the cardiac cycle

implantable cardioverter defibrillator (ICD): a device implanted into the chest wall to treat arrhythmias

inotropy: force of myocardial contraction

P wave: the part of an ECG that reflects conduction of an electrical impulse through the atrium; atrial depolarization

paroxysmal: arrhythmia that has a sudden onset and terminates spontaneously; usually of short duration, but may recur

PP interval: the duration between the beginning of one P wave and the beginning of the next P wave; used to calculate atrial rate and rhythm

PR interval: the part of an ECG that reflects conduction of an electrical impulse from the sinoatrial node through the atrioventricular node

QRS complex: the part of an ECG that reflects conduction of an electrical impulse through the ventricles; ventricular depolarization

QT interval: the part of an ECG that reflects the time from ventricular depolarization through repolarization

repolarization: process by which cardiac muscle cells return to a more negatively charged intracellular condition, their resting state

RR interval: the duration between the beginning of one QRS complex and the beginning of the next QRS complex; used to calculate ventricular rate and rhythm

sinus rhythm: electrical activity of the heart initiated by the sinoatrial node

ST segment: the part of an ECG that reflects the end of the QRS complex to the beginning of the T wave

T wave: the part of an ECG that reflects repolarization of the ventricles

TP interval: the part of an ECG that reflects the time between the end of the T wave and the beginning of the next P wave; used to identify the isoelectric line

U wave: the part of an ECG that may reflect Purkinje fiber repolarization; usually, it is not seen unless a patient's serum potassium level is low

It is essential for the heart to have a regular rate and rhythm to perform efficiently as a pump to circulate oxygenated blood and other life-sustaining nutrients to all of the body's tissues and organs (including the heart itself). With an irregular or erratic rhythm, the heart is considered to be arrhythmic (also called *dysrhythmic*). This is a potentially dangerous condition.

Nurses may encounter patients with arrhythmias in all health care settings, including primary care settings, skilled nursing facilities, rehabilitation settings, hospitals, and the home health care setting. Some arrhythmias are acute and others chronic; some require emergent interventions, while others may not. Because patients with arrhythmias are frequently encountered in many different types of settings, nurses must be able to identify and provide appropriate first-line treatment of arrhythmias.

ARRHYTHMIAS

Arrhythmias are disorders of the formation or conduction (or both) of the electrical impulse within the heart. These disorders can cause disturbances of the heart rate, the heart rhythm, or both. Arrhythmias may initially be evidenced by the hemodynamic effect they cause (e.g., a change in conduction may change the pumping action of the heart and cause decreased blood pressure), and are diagnosed by analyzing the electrocardiographic (ECG) waveform. Their treatment is based on the frequency and severity of symptoms produced. Arrhythmias are named according to the site of origin of the electrical impulse and the mechanism of formation or conduction involved. For example, an impulse that originates in the sinoatrial (SA) node and at a slow rate is called *sinus bradycardia*.

Normal Electrical Conduction

The electrical impulse that stimulates and paces the cardiac muscle normally originates in the SA node, also called the *sinus node,* an area located near the superior vena cava in the right atrium. In the adult, the electrical impulse usually occurs at a rate of 60 to 100 times a minute. The electrical impulse quickly travels from the SA node through the atria to the atrioventricular (AV) node (see Fig. 22-1); this process is known as **conduction**. The electrical stimulation of the muscle cells of the atria causes them to contract. The structure of the AV node slows the electrical impulse, giving the atria time to contract and fill the ventricles with blood. This part of atrial contraction is frequently referred to as the atrial kick and accounts for nearly one third of the volume ejected during ventricular contraction (Fuster, Harrington, Narula, et al., 2017). The electrical impulse then travels very quickly

through the bundle of His to the right and left bundle branches and the Purkinje fibers, located in the ventricular muscle.

The electrical stimulation is called **depolarization**, and the mechanical contraction is called *systole*. Electrical relaxation is called **repolarization**, and mechanical relaxation is called *diastole*. The process from sinus node electrical impulse generation through ventricular repolarization completes the electromechanical circuit, and the cycle begins again. (See Chapter 21 for a more complete explanation of cardiac function.)

Influences on Heart Rate and Contractility

The heart rate is influenced by the autonomic nervous system, which consists of sympathetic and parasympathetic fibers. Sympathetic nerve fibers (also referred to as adrenergic fibers) are attached to the heart and arteries as well as several other areas in the body. Stimulation of the sympathetic system results in positive **chronotropy** (increased heart rate), positive **dromotropy** (increased AV conduction), and positive **inotropy** (increased force of myocardial contraction). Sympathetic stimulation also constricts peripheral blood vessels, therefore increasing blood pressure. Parasympathetic nerve fibers are also attached to the heart and arteries. Parasympathetic stimulation reduces the heart rate (negative chronotropy), AV conduction (negative dromotropy), and the force of atrial myocardial contraction. The decreased sympathetic stimulation results in dilation of arteries, thereby lowering blood pressure.

Manipulation of the autonomic nervous system may increase or decrease the incidence of arrhythmias. Increased sympathetic stimulation (e.g., caused by exercise, anxiety, fever, or administration of catecholamines such as dopamine, aminophylline, or dobutamine) may increase the incidence of arrhythmias. Decreased sympathetic stimulation (e.g., with rest, anxiety reduction methods such as therapeutic communication or meditation, or administration of beta-adrenergic blocking agents) may decrease the incidence of arrhythmias.

The Electrocardiogram

The electrical impulse that travels through the heart can be viewed by means of electrocardiography, the end product of which is an **electrocardiogram (ECG)**. Each phase of the cardiac cycle is reflected by specific waveforms on the screen of a cardiac monitor or on a strip of ECG graph paper.

Obtaining an Electrocardiogram

An ECG is obtained by placing electrodes on the body at specific areas. Biomonitoring electrodes come in various

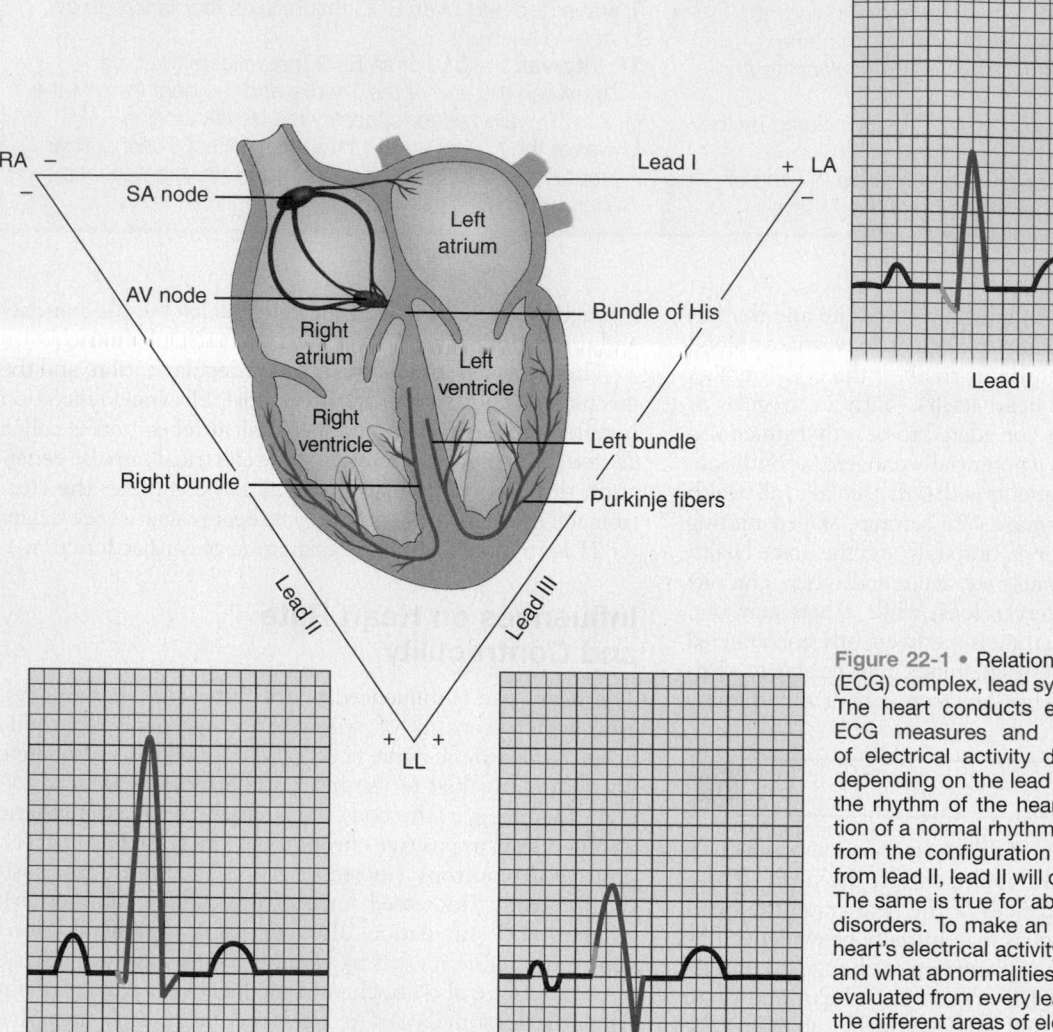

Figure 22-1 • Relationship of electrocardiographic (ECG) complex, lead system, and electrical impulse. The heart conducts electrical activity, which the ECG measures and shows. The configurations of electrical activity displayed on the ECG vary depending on the lead (or view) of the ECG and on the rhythm of the heart. Therefore, the configuration of a normal rhythm tracing from lead I will differ from the configuration of a normal rhythm tracing from lead II, lead II will differ from lead III, and so on. The same is true for abnormal rhythms and cardiac disorders. To make an accurate assessment of the heart's electrical activity or to identify where, when, and what abnormalities occur, the ECG needs to be evaluated from every lead, not just from lead II. Here the different areas of electrical activity are identified by color. RA, right arm; LA, left arm; SA, sinoatrial; AV, atrioventricular; LL, left leg.

shapes and sizes, but all have two components: (1) an adhesive substance that attaches to the skin to secure the electrode in place and (2) a substance that reduces the skin's electrical impedance, facilitating the transfer of ions from the tissue to electrons in the electrode, enhancing conductivity. Gently abrading the skin with a clean dry gauze pad or sandpaper edge of the electrode helps to expose the inner conductive layer of epidermis, which will reduce skin impedance. Although cleansing the skin with alcohol removes any oily residue from the skin, it also increases the skin's electrical impedance and hinders detection of the cardiac electrical signal. Washing the area with soap and water prior to electrode placement is recommended. If the amount of chest hair prevents the electrode from having good contact with the skin, the hair may need to be clipped (Sendelbach & Jepsen, 2018; see Chapter 21, Chart 21-5: Applying Electrodes). Poor electrode adhesion will cause significant **artifact** (distorted, irrelevant, and extraneous ECG waveforms), which may distort capturing an accurate ECG waveform.

The number and placement site of the electrodes depend on the type of ECG being obtained. Most continuous monitors use 2 to 5 electrodes, usually placed on the limbs and the chest. These electrodes create an imaginary line, called a *lead,* which serves as a reference point from which the electrical activity is viewed. A lead is like an eye of a camera—it has a narrow peripheral field of vision, looking only at the electrical activity directly in front of it. Therefore, the ECG waveforms that appear on the ECG paper and cardiac monitor represent the electrical impulse in relation to the lead (see Fig. 22-1). A change in the waveform can be caused by a change in the electrical impulse (where it originates or how it is conducted) or by a change in the lead. Electrodes are attached to cable wires, which are connected to one of the following:

- An ECG machine placed at the patient's side for an immediate recording (standard 12-lead ECG)
- A cardiac monitor at the patient's bedside for continuous reading; this kind of monitoring, usually called *hardwire monitoring,* is used in intensive care units
- A small box that the patient carries and that continuously transmits the ECG information by radiowaves to a central monitor located elsewhere (called *telemetry*)
- A small, lightweight tape recorder–like machine (called *continuous ECG monitoring,* which might include a

Holter monitor or a *patch monitor*) that the patient wears for a prescribed period of time and that continuously records the ECG, which is later viewed and analyzed with a scanner
- A very small device inserted under the skin or worn externally on a wrist band (called *intermittent monitoring* using a *looped recorder*) can perform ECG monitoring on demand whenever a patient is symptomatic (see Chapter 21 for further discussion of ECG monitoring systems)

A patient may undergo an electrophysiology study (EPS) in which electrodes are placed inside the heart in order to obtain an intracardiac ECG. This is used not only to diagnose the arrhythmia but also to determine the most effective treatment plan. However, because an EPS is invasive, it is performed in the hospital and may require that the patient be admitted (see later discussion).

During open heart surgery, temporary pacemaker wires may be lightly sutured to the epicardium and brought through the chest wall. These wires may be used not only for temporary pacing but also, when connected to the V lead cable, to obtain an atrial ECG, which can be helpful in the differential diagnosis of tachyarrhythmias (see Chapter 23 for further discussion).

The placement of electrodes for monitoring varies with the type of technology, the purpose of monitoring, and the protocols used in the health care facility. For a standard 12-lead ECG, 10 electrodes (6 on the chest and 4 on the limbs) are placed on the body (see Fig. 22-2). To prevent interference from the electrical activity of skeletal muscle, the limb electrodes are placed on areas that are not bony and that do not have significant movement. The limb electrodes provide the first six leads: leads I, II, III, aVR (augmented voltage right arm), aVL (augmented voltage left arm), and aVF (augmented voltage left leg/foot). The 6 chest electrodes are applied to the chest at very specific areas. The chest electrodes provide the V or precordial leads, V_1 through V_6. To locate the fourth intercostal space and the placement of V_1, the sternal angle and then the sternal notch, which is about 1 or 2 inches below the sternal angle, are located. When the fingers are moved to the patient's immediate right, the second rib can be palpated. The second intercostal space is the indentation felt just below the second rib. Locating the specific intercostal space is critical for the correct placement of each chest electrode. Errors in diagnosis can occur if electrodes are incorrectly placed. Sometimes, when a patient in the hospital needs to be monitored more closely for ECG changes, the chest electrodes are left in place to ensure the same placement for follow-up 12-lead ECGs.

A standard 12-lead ECG reflects the electrical activity primarily in the left ventricle. Placement of additional electrodes for other leads may be needed to obtain more complete information. For example, in patients with suspected right-sided heart damage, right-sided precordial leads are required to evaluate the right ventricle (see Fig. 22-2).

Components of the Electrocardiogram

The ECG waveform reflects the function of the heart's conduction system in relation to the specific lead. The ECG offers important information about the electrical activity of

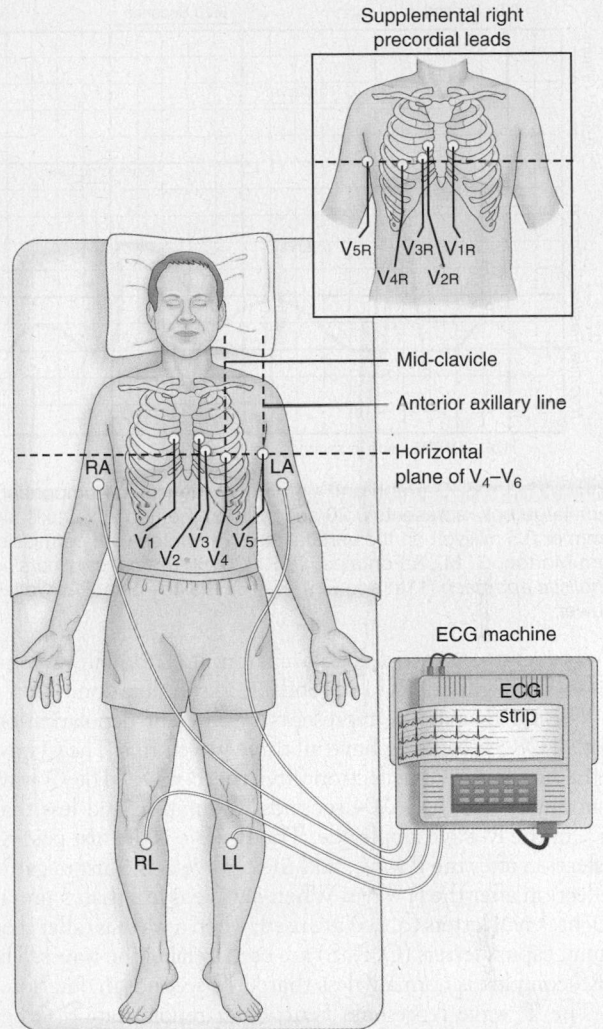

Figure 22-2 • ECG electrode placement. The standard left precordial leads are V_1—fourth intercostal space, right sternal border; V_2—fourth intercostal space, left sternal border; V_3—diagonally between V_2 and V_4; V_4—fifth intercostal space, left midclavicular line; V_5—same level as V_4, anterior axillary line; V_6 (not illustrated)—same level as V_4 and V_5, midaxillary line. The right precordial leads, placed across the right side of the chest, are the mirror opposite of the left leads. RA, right arm; LA, left arm; RL, right leg; LL, left leg.

the heart and is useful in diagnosing arrhythmias. ECG waveforms are printed on graph paper that is divided by vertical and horizontal lines at standard intervals (see Fig. 22-3). Time and rate are measured on the horizontal axis of the graph, and amplitude or voltage is measured on the vertical axis. When an ECG waveform moves toward the top of the paper, it is called a *positive deflection*. When it moves toward the bottom of the paper, it is called a *negative deflection*. When reviewing an ECG, each waveform should be examined and compared with the others.

Waves, Complexes, and Intervals

The ECG is composed of waveforms (including the P wave, the QRS complex, the T wave, and possibly a U wave) and of segments and intervals (including the PR interval, the ST segment, and the QT interval) (see Fig. 22-3).

The **P wave** represents the electrical impulse starting in the SA node and spreading through the atria. Therefore, the

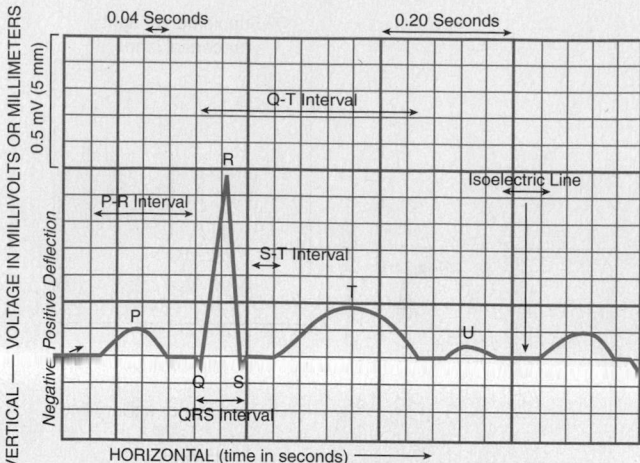

Figure 22-3 • ECG graph and commonly measured components. Each large box represents 0.20 seconds on the horizontal axis and 5 mm or 0.5 millivolt on the vertical axis. Reprinted with permission from Morton, G. M., & Fontaine, D. K. (2018). *Critical care nursing: A holistic approach* (11th ed., Fig. 17–16). Philadelphia, PA: Wolters Kluwer.

P wave represents atrial depolarization. It is normally 2.5 mm or less in height and 0.11 seconds or less in duration.

The **QRS complex** represents ventricular depolarization. Not all QRS complexes have all three waveforms. The Q wave is the first negative deflection after the P wave. The Q wave is normally less than 0.04 seconds in duration and less than 25% of the R-wave amplitude. The R wave is the first positive deflection after the P wave, and the S wave is the first negative deflection after the R wave. When a wave is less than 5 mm in height, small letters (q, r, s) are used; when a wave is taller than 5 mm, capital letters (Q, R, S) are used to label the waves. The QRS complex is normally less than 0.12 seconds in duration.

The **T wave** represents ventricular repolarization (when the cells regain a negative charge; also called the *resting state*). It follows the QRS complex and is usually the same direction (deflection) as the QRS complex. Atrial repolarization also occurs but is not visible on the ECG because it occurs at the same time as ventricular depolarization (i.e., the QRS).

The **U wave** is thought to represent repolarization of the Purkinje fibers; although this wave is rare, it sometimes appears in patients with hypokalemia (low potassium levels), hypertension, or heart disease. If present, the U wave follows the T wave and is usually smaller than the P wave. If larger in amplitude, it may be mistaken for an extra P wave.

The **PR interval** is measured from the beginning of the P wave to the beginning of the QRS complex and represents the time needed for sinus node stimulation, atrial depolarization, and conduction through the AV node before ventricular depolarization. In adults, the PR interval normally ranges from 0.12 to 0.20 seconds in duration.

The **ST segment,** which represents early ventricular repolarization, lasts from the end of the QRS complex to the beginning of the T wave. The beginning of the ST segment is usually identified by a change in the thickness or angle of the terminal portion of the QRS complex. The end of the ST segment may be more difficult to identify because it merges into the T wave. The ST segment is normally isoelectric (see later discussion of TP interval). It is analyzed to identify whether it is above or below the isoelectric line, which may be, among other signs and symptoms, a sign of cardiac ischemia (see Chapter 23).

The **QT interval**, which represents the total time for ventricular depolarization and repolarization, is measured from the beginning of the QRS complex to the end of the T wave. The QT interval varies with heart rate, gender, and age; therefore, the measured interval may be corrected (QT$_c$) for these variables through specific calculations. The QT$_c$ may be automatically calculated by the ECG technology, or a nurse may manually calculate or use a resource that contains a chart of these calculations. The QT interval is usually 0.32 to 0.40 seconds in duration if the heart rate is 65 to 95 bpm. Many medications commonly given in the hospital can cause prolongation of the QT interval (QT$_c$), placing the patient at risk for a lethal ventricular arrhythmia called *torsades de pointes*.

The **TP interval** is measured from the end of the T wave to the beginning of the next P wave—an isoelectric period (see Fig. 22-3). When no electrical activity is detected, the line on the graph remains flat; this is called the *isoelectric line*. The ST segment is compared with the TP interval to detect ST segment changes. The PR segment is sometimes used to determine the isoelectric line. However, because the PR segment sometimes is altered due to ischemic conditions, the TP interval is the preferred reference for the isoelectric line.

The **PP interval** is measured from the beginning of one P wave to the beginning of the next P wave. The PP interval is used to determine atrial rate and rhythm. The **RR interval** is measured from one QRS complex to the next QRS complex. The RR interval is used to determine ventricular rate and rhythm (see later discussion).

Analyzing the Electrocardiogram Rhythm Strip

The ECG rhythm strip must be analyzed in a systematic manner to determine the patient's cardiac rate and rhythm, and to detect arrhythmias and conduction disorders, as well as evidence of myocardial ischemia, injury, and infarction.

Determining Heart Rate from the Electrocardiogram

Heart rate can be obtained from the ECG rhythm strip by several methods. A 1-minute rhythm strip contains 300 large boxes and 1500 small boxes. Therefore, an easy and accurate method of determining heart rate with a regular rhythm is to count the number of small boxes within an RR interval and divide 1500 by that number. If, for example, there are 10 small boxes between two R waves, the heart rate is 1500/10, or 150 bpm; if there are 25 small boxes, the heart rate is 1500/25, or 60 bpm (see Fig. 22-4).

An alternative but less accurate method for estimating heart rate, which is usually used when the rhythm is irregular, is to count the number of RR intervals in 6 seconds and multiply that number by 10. The top of the ECG paper is usually marked at 3-second intervals, which is 15 large boxes horizontally. The RR intervals are counted, rather than QRS complexes, because a computed heart rate based on the latter might be inaccurately high.

The same methods may be used for determining atrial rate, using the PP interval instead of the RR interval.

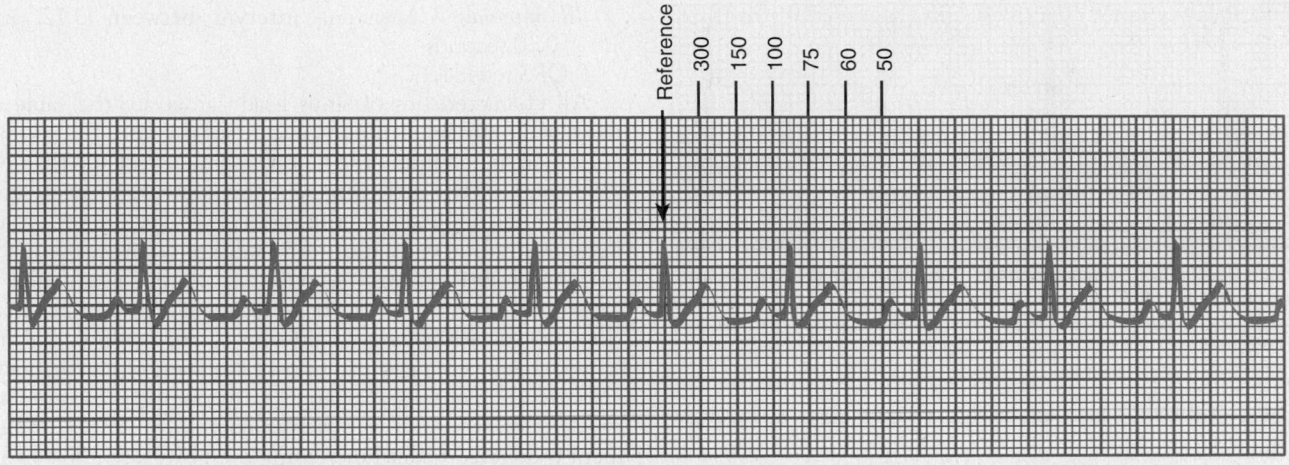

Figure 22-4 • Method for estimating heart rate. The number of small boxes in the RR interval is 17.5; divide this by 1500, and the heart rate is approximately 86 bpm. Reprinted with permission from Morton, G. M., & Fontaine, D. K. (2018). *Critical care nursing. A holistic approach* (11th ed., Fig. 17–18 (bottom portion)). Philadelphia, PA: Wolters Kluwer.

Determining Heart Rhythm from the Electrocardiogram

The rhythm is often identified at the same time the rate is determined. Chart 22-1 provides an example of a method that can be used to analyze the patient's rhythm. The RR interval is used to determine ventricular rhythm and the PP interval to determine atrial rhythm. If the intervals are the same or if the difference between the intervals is less than 0.8 seconds throughout the strip, the rhythm is called *regular*. If the intervals are different, the rhythm is called *irregular*.

Once the rhythm has been analyzed, the findings are compared with and matched to the ECG criteria for arrhythmias to determine a diagnosis. It is important for the nurse not only to identify the arrhythmia, but also to assess the patient to determine the physiologic effect of the arrhythmia and identify possible causes. Treatment of an arrhythmia is based on

clinical evaluation of the patient with identification of the arrhythmia's etiology and physiologic effect, not on its presence on ECG alone.

Most cardiac monitoring has functionality that includes the ability to continuously monitor the rhythm and alert health care personnel with an auditory and visual alarm when a clinically significant change in the rhythm occurs. However, a high rate of triggered, clinically insignificant alarms may lead to alarm fatigue, which has been linked to nurses ignoring, disabling, or silencing alarms (Sendelbach & Jepsen, 2018)—putting patients at increased risk of adverse events.

> ▶ *Quality and Safety Nursing Alert*
>
> *It is vital that the nurse assesses the cause(s) of a cardiac monitor's alarm and then adjusts the alarm default settings and individualizes the alarm parameter limits and levels. The assessment should also include an evaluation and discussion with the primary provider to validate that the patient needs to remain on continuous cardiac monitoring.*

Normal Sinus Rhythm

Electrical conduction that begins in the SA node generates a **sinus rhythm.** Normal sinus rhythm occurs when the electrical impulse starts at a regular rate and rhythm in the SA node and travels through the normal conduction pathway. Normal sinus rhythm has the following characteristics (see Fig. 22-5):

Ventricular and atrial rate: 60 to 100 bpm in the adult

Ventricular and atrial rhythm: Regular

QRS shape and duration: Usually normal, but may be regularly abnormal

P wave: Normal and consistent shape; always in front of the QRS

PR interval: Consistent interval between 0.12 and 0.20 seconds

P:QRS ratio: 1:1

Normal sinus rhythm is generally indicative of good cardiovascular health. However, an increase of 10 bpm or more in the resting heart rate increases the risk for sudden cardiac death, atrial fibrillation, heart failure, coronary artery disease,

---

Chart 22-1

Interpreting Arrhythmias: Systematic Analysis of the Electrocardiogram

When examining an electrocardiogram (ECG) rhythm strip to learn more about a patient's arrhythmia:

1. Determine the ventricular rate.
2. Determine the ventricular rhythm.
3. Determine the QRS duration.
4. Determine whether the QRS duration is consistent throughout the strip. If not, identify other duration.
5. Identify the QRS shape; if not consistent, then identify other shapes.
6. Identify P waves; is there a P in front of every QRS?
7. Identify the P-wave shape; identify whether it is consistent or not.
8. Determine the atrial rate.
9. Determine the atrial rhythm.
10. Determine each PR interval.
11. Determine if the PR intervals are consistent, irregular but with a pattern to the irregularity, or just irregular.
12. Determine how many P waves for each QRS (P:QRS ratio).

In many cases, the nurse may use a checklist and document the findings next to the appropriate ECG criterion.

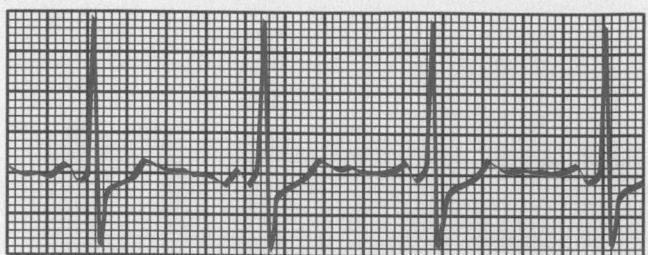

Figure 22-5 • Normal sinus rhythm. Reprinted with permission from Morton, G. M., & Fontaine, D. K. (2018). *Critical care nursing: A holistic approach* (11th ed., Fig. 17–19A). Philadelphia, PA: Wolters Kluwer.

stroke, and cardiovascular disease (Aune, Sen, ó'Hartaigh, et al., 2017).

 ## Types of Arrhythmias

Arrhythmias include sinus, atrial, junctional, and ventricular arrhythmias and their various subcategories, as well as conduction abnormalities.

Sinus Node Arrhythmias

Sinus node arrhythmias originate in the SA node; these include sinus bradycardia, sinus tachycardia, and sinus arrhythmia.

Sinus Bradycardia

Sinus bradycardia occurs when the SA node creates an impulse at a slower-than-normal rate. Causes include lower metabolic needs (e.g., sleep, athletic training, hypothyroidism), vagal stimulation (e.g., from vomiting, suctioning, severe pain), medications (e.g., calcium channel blockers [e.g., nifedipine, amiodarone], beta-blockers [e.g., metoprolol]), idiopathic sinus node dysfunction, increased intracranial pressure, and coronary artery disease, especially myocardial infarction (MI) of the inferior wall. Unstable and symptomatic bradycardia is frequently due to hypoxemia. Other possible causes include acute altered mental status (e.g., delirium) and acute decompensated heart failure (Fuster et al., 2017). Sinus bradycardia has the following characteristics (see Fig. 22-6):

Ventricular and atrial rate: Less than 60 bpm in the adult
Ventricular and atrial rhythm: Regular
QRS shape and duration: Usually normal, but may be regularly abnormal
P wave: Normal and consistent shape; always in front of the QRS

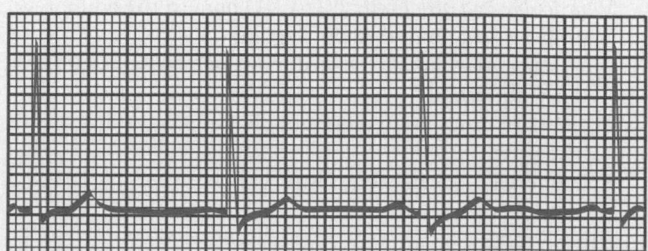

Figure 22-6 • Sinus bradycardia. Reprinted with permission from Morton, G. M., & Fontaine, D. K. (2018). *Critical care nursing: A holistic approach* (11th ed., Fig. 17–19C). Philadelphia, PA: Wolters Kluwer.

PR interval: Consistent interval between 0.12 and 0.20 seconds
P:QRS ratio: 1:1

All characteristics of sinus bradycardia are the same as those of normal sinus rhythm, except for the rate. The patient is assessed to determine the hemodynamic effect and the possible cause of the arrhythmia. If the decrease in heart rate results from stimulation of the vagus nerve, such as with bearing down during defecation or vomiting, attempts are made to prevent further vagal stimulation. If the bradycardia is caused by a medication such as a beta-blocker, the medication may be withheld. If the slow heart rate causes significant hemodynamic changes resulting in shortness of breath, acute alteration of mental status, angina, hypotension, ST-segment changes, or premature ventricular complexes (PVCs), treatment is directed toward increasing the heart rate. Slow heart rate may be due to sinus node dysfunction (previously known as *sick sinus syndrome*), which has a number of risk factors including increased body mass index, presence of right and left bundle branch block, history of a major cardiovascular event, increased age, and hypertension (Jackson, Rathakrishnan, Campbell, et al., 2017). *Tachy-brady syndrome* is the term used when bradycardia alternates with tachycardia.

Medical Management

Management depends on the cause and symptoms. Resolving the causative factors may be the only treatment needed. If the bradycardia produces signs and symptoms of clinical instability (e.g., acute alteration in mental status, chest discomfort, or hypotension), 0.5 mg of atropine may be given rapidly as an intravenous (IV) bolus and repeated every 3 to 5 minutes until a maximum dosage of 3 mg is given. Rarely, if the bradycardia is unresponsive to atropine, emergency transcutaneous pacing can be instituted, or medications, such as dopamine, isoproterenol, or epinephrine, are given (Kusumoto, Schoenfeld, Barrett, et al., 2019; see later discussion).

Sinus Tachycardia

Sinus tachycardia occurs when the sinus node creates an impulse at a faster-than-normal rate. Causes may include the following:

- Physiologic or psychological stress (e.g., acute blood loss, anemia, shock, hypervolemia, hypovolemia, heart failure, pain, hypermetabolic states, fever, exercise, anxiety)
- Medications that stimulate the sympathetic response (e.g., catecholamines, aminophylline, atropine), stimulants (e.g., caffeine, nicotine), and illicit drugs (e.g., amphetamines, cocaine, ecstasy)
- Enhanced automaticity of the SA node and/or excessive sympathetic tone with reduced parasympathetic tone that is out of proportion to physiologic demands, a condition called *inappropriate sinus tachycardia*
- Autonomic dysfunction, which results in a type of sinus tachycardia referred to as postural orthostatic tachycardia syndrome (POTS). POTS is characterized by tachycardia without hypotension, and by presyncopal symptoms such as palpitations, lightheadedness, weakness, and blurred vision, which occur with sudden posture changes

Sinus tachycardia has the following characteristics (see Fig. 22-7):

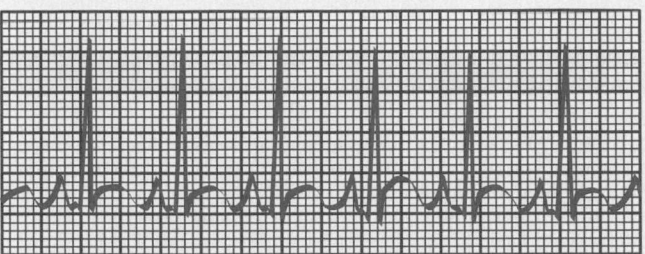

Figure 22-7 • Sinus tachycardia. Reprinted with permission from Morton, G. M., & Fontaine, D. K. (2018). *Critical care nursing: A holistic approach* (11th ed., Fig. 17–19B). Philadelphia, PA: Wolters Kluwer.

Ventricular and atrial rate: Greater than 100 bpm in the adult, but usually less than 120 bpm

Ventricular and atrial rhythm: Regular

QRS shape and duration: Usually normal, but may be regularly abnormal

P wave: Normal and consistent shape; always in front of the QRS, but may be buried in the preceding T wave

PR interval: Consistent interval between 0.12 and 0.20 seconds

P:QRS ratio: 1:1

All aspects of sinus tachycardia are the same as those of normal sinus rhythm, except for the rate. Sinus tachycardia does not start or end suddenly (i.e., it is nonparoxysmal). As the heart rate increases, the diastolic filling time decreases, possibly resulting in reduced cardiac output and subsequent symptoms of syncope (fainting) and low blood pressure. If the rapid rate persists and the heart cannot compensate for the decreased ventricular filling, the patient may develop acute pulmonary edema.

Medical Management

Medical management of sinus tachycardia is determined by the severity of symptoms and directed at identifying and abolishing its cause. Vagal maneuvers, such as carotid sinus massage, gagging, bearing down against a closed glottis (as if having a bowel movement), forceful and sustained coughing, and applying a cold stimulus to the face (such as applying an ice-cold wet towel to the face), or administration of adenosine should be considered to interrupt the tachycardia. If the tachycardia is persistent and causing hemodynamic instability (e.g., acute alteration in mental status, chest discomfort, hypotension), synchronized **cardioversion** (i.e., electrical current given in synchrony with the patient's own QRS complex to stop an arrhythmia) is the treatment of choice, if vagal maneuvers and adenosine are unsuccessful or not feasible (see later discussion). IV beta-blockers (Class II antiarrhythmic) and calcium channel blockers (Class IV antiarrhythmic) (see Table 22-1) may also be considered in treating hemodynamically stable sinus tachycardia, although synchronized cardioversion may be used if medications are ineffective or contradicted (Page, Joglar, Caldwell, et al., 2016). Catheter ablation (see later discussion) of the SA node may be used in cases of persistent inappropriate sinus tachycardia unresponsive to other treatments. Treatment for POTS often involves a combination of approaches, with treatment targeted at the underlying problem. For example, patients with hypovolemia may be advised to increase their fluid and sodium intake, or use salt tablets if necessary.

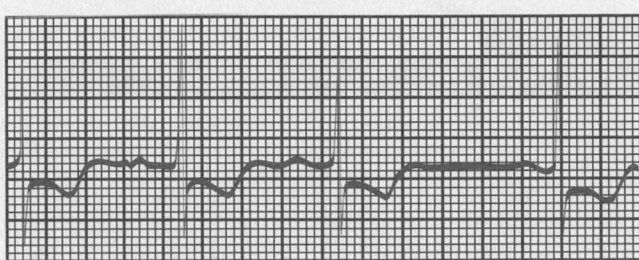

Figure 22-8 • Sinus arrhythmia. Note irregular RR and PP intervals. Reprinted with permission from Morton, G. M., & Fontaine, D. K. (2018). *Critical care nursing: A holistic approach* (11th ed., Fig. 17–19D). Philadelphia, PA: Wolters Kluwer.

Sinus Arrhythmia

Sinus arrhythmia occurs when the sinus node creates an impulse at an irregular rhythm; the rate usually increases with inspiration and decreases with expiration. Nonrespiratory causes include heart disease and valvular disease, but these are rare. Sinus arrhythmia has the following characteristics (see Fig. 22-8):

Ventricular and atrial rate: 60 to 100 bpm in the adult

Ventricular and atrial rhythm: Irregular

QRS shape and duration: Usually normal, but may be regularly abnormal

P wave: Normal and consistent shape; always in front of the QRS

PR interval: Consistent interval between 0.12 and 0.20 seconds

P:QRS ratio: 1:1

Medical Management

Sinus arrhythmia does not cause any significant hemodynamic effect and therefore is not typically treated.

Atrial Arrhythmias

Atrial arrhythmias originate from foci within the atria and not the SA node. These include aberrancies such as premature atrial complexes (PACs) as well as atrial fibrillation and atrial flutter.

Premature Atrial Complex

A PAC is a single ECG complex that occurs when an electrical impulse starts in the atrium before the next normal impulse of the sinus node. The PAC may be caused by caffeine, alcohol, nicotine, stretched atrial myocardium (e.g., as in hypervolemia), anxiety, hypokalemia (low potassium level), hypermetabolic states (e.g., with pregnancy), or atrial ischemia, injury, or infarction. PACs are often seen with sinus tachycardia. PACs have the following characteristics (see Fig. 22-9):

Ventricular and atrial rate: Depends on the underlying rhythm (e.g., sinus tachycardia)

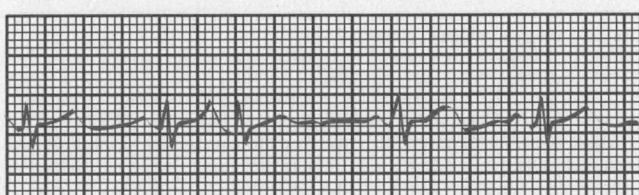

Figure 22-9 • Premature atrial complex (PAC). Reprinted with permission from Morton, G. M., & Fontaine, D. K. (2018). *Critical care nursing: A holistic approach* (11th ed., Fig. 17–22A). Philadelphia, PA: Wolters Kluwer.

TABLE 22-1 Summary of Antiarrhythmic Medications[a]

Class[a]	Action	Drug Names	Side Effects	Nursing Interventions
IA	Moderate depression of depolarization; prolongs repolarization Treats and prevents atrial and ventricular arrhythmias	quinidine, procainamide, disopyramide	Decreased cardiac contractility Prolonged QRS, QT Proarrhythmic Hypotension with IV administration Diarrhea with quinidine, constipation with disopyramide Cinchonism with quinidine Lupuslike syndrome with procainamide Anticholinergic effects: dry mouth, urinary hesitancy with disopyramide	Observe for HF. Monitor BP with IV administration. Monitor QRS duration for increase >50% from baseline. Monitor for prolonged QT. Monitor N-acetyl procainamide (NAPA) laboratory values during procainamide therapy. If given for atrial fibrillation, ensure that the patient has been pretreated with a medication to control AV conduction.
IB	Minimal depression of depolarization; shortened repolarization Treats ventricular arrhythmias	lidocaine, mexiletine	CNS changes (e.g., confusion, lethargy) Bradycardia GI distress Tremors	Monitor for CNS changes and tremors. Discuss with the primary provider decreasing lidocaine dose in older adult patients and patients with cardiac/liver dysfunction.
IC	Marked depression of depolarization; little effect on repolarization Treats atrial and ventricular arrhythmias	flecainide, propafenone	Proarrhythmic HF Dizziness, visual disturbances, dyspnea	Decrease dose with renal dysfunction and strict vegetarian diets. Avoid use in patients with structural heart disease (e.g., coronary artery disease and heart failure).
II	Decreases automaticity and conduction Treats atrial and ventricular arrhythmias	acebutolol[c], atenolol, bisoprolol/HCTZ, esmolol[c], labetalol, metoprolol, nadolol, propranolol[c], sotalol (also has class III actions)[c], timolol	Bradycardia, AV block Decreased contractility Bronchospasm Nausea Asymptomatic and symptomatic hypotension Masks hypoglycemia and thyrotoxicosis CNS disturbances (e.g., confusion, dizziness, fatigue, depression)	Monitor heart rate, PR interval, signs and symptoms of HF, especially in those also taking calcium channel blockers. Monitor blood glucose level in patients with type 2 diabetes. Caution the patient about abrupt withdrawal to avoid tachycardia, hypertension, and myocardial ischemia.
III	Prolongs repolarization Amiodarone treats and prevents ventricular and atrial arrhythmias, especially in patients with ventricular dysfunction. Dofetilide and ibutilide treat and prevent atrial arrhythmias.	amiodarone, dofetilide, dronedarone, ibutilide	Pulmonary toxicity (amiodarone) Corneal microdeposits (amiodarone) Photosensitivity (amiodarone) Bradycardia Hypotension, especially with IV administration Polymorphic ventricular arrhythmias (rare with amiodarone) Nausea and vomiting Potentiates digoxin (amiodarone) See beta-blockers above (sotalol).	Make sure that the patient is sent for baseline pulmonary function tests (amiodarone). Closely monitor the patient. Assess for contraindications prior to administration. Monitor QT duration. Continuous ECG monitoring with initiation of dofetilide and ibutilide. Monitor renal function.
IV	Blocks calcium channel Treats and prevents paroxysmal atrial arrhythmias[b]	verapamil, diltiazem	Bradycardia, AV blocks Hypotension with IV administration HF, peripheral edema Constipation, dizziness, headache, nausea	Monitor heart rate, PR interval. Monitor blood pressure closely with IV administration. Monitor for signs and symptoms of HF. Do not crush sustained-release medications.

[a]Based on Vaughan–Williams classification.
[b]There are other calcium channel blockers, but they are not approved or used for arrhythmias.
[c]Beta-blocker with labeled use for arrhythmias.
AV, atrioventricular; BP, blood pressure; CNS, central nervous system; ECG, electrocardiogram; GI, gastrointestinal; HCTZ, hydrochlorothiazide; HF, heart failure; IV, intravenous.
Adapted from the American Society of Health System Pharmacists. (2019). *AHFS drug information*. Bethesda, MD: Author; Fuster, V., Harrington, R. A., Narula, J., et al. (Eds.). (2017). *Hurst's the heart* (13th ed.). New York: McGraw-Hill; Al-Khatib, S. M., Stevenson, W. G., Ackerman, M. J., et al. (2018). 2017 AHA/ACC/HRS guideline for management of patients with ventricular arrhythmias and the prevention of sudden cardiac death: A report of the American College of Cardiology/American Heart Association Task Force on clinical practice guidelines and the Heart Rhythm Society. *Circulation, 138*(13), e272–e391.

Ventricular and atrial rhythm: Irregular due to early P waves, creating a PP interval that is shorter than the others. This is sometimes followed by a longer-than-normal PP interval, but one that is less than twice the normal PP interval. This type of interval is called a *noncompensatory pause*

QRS shape and duration: The QRS that follows the early P wave is usually normal, but it may be abnormal (aberrantly conducted PAC). It may even be absent (blocked PAC)

P wave: An early and different P wave may be seen or may be hidden in the T wave; other P waves in the strip are consistent

PR interval: The early P wave has a shorter-than-normal PR interval, but still between 0.12 and 0.20 seconds

P:QRS ratio: Usually 1:1

PACs are common in normal hearts. The patient may say, "My heart skipped a beat." A pulse deficit (a difference between the apical and radial pulse rate) may exist.

Medical Management

If PACs are infrequent; no treatment is necessary. If they are frequent (more than six per minute), this may herald a worsening disease state or the onset of more serious arrhythmias, such as atrial fibrillation. Medical management is directed toward treating the underlying cause (e.g., reduction of caffeine intake, correction of hypokalemia).

Atrial Fibrillation

Atrial fibrillation is a very common arrhythmia; between 2.7 and 6.1 million Americans are living with atrial fibrillation (Centers for Disease Control and Prevention [CDC], 2017). Atrial fibrillation is a serious public health concern because it is associated with aging, and the older adult population is increasing in the United States (Chen, Chung, Allen, et al., 2018). Atrial fibrillation can result from diverse pathophysiologic etiologies and risks (see Chart 22-2).

Atrial fibrillation results from abnormal impulse formation that occurs when structural or electrophysiologic abnormalities alter the atrial tissue causing a rapid, disorganized, and uncoordinated twitching of the atrial musculature (January, Wann, Alpert, et al., 2014; January, Wann, Calkins, et al., 2019). Both the extrinsic (central) and intrinsic cardiac autonomic nervous systems (CANS) are thought to play an important role in the initiation and continuance of atrial fibrillation (Qin, Zeng, & Liu, 2019). Separate from the extrinsic (central) nervous system, which includes the brain and spinal cord, the CANS consists of a highly interconnected network of autonomic ganglia and nerve cell bodies embedded within the epicardium, largely within the atrial myocardium and great vessels (pulmonary veins). Hyperactive autonomic ganglia in the CANS are thought to play a critical role in atrial fibrillation, resulting in impulses that are initiated from the pulmonary veins and conducted through to the AV node. The ventricular rate of response depends on the conduction of atrial impulses through the AV node, presence of accessory electrical conduction pathways, and therapeutic effect of medications.

Lack of consistency in describing patterns or types of atrial fibrillation has led to the use of numerous labels, such

as **paroxysmal** (i.e., sudden onset with spontaneous termination), persistent, and permanent. The recommended classification system is noted in Chart 22-3. The use of the term "chronic atrial fibrillation" is no longer included in the classification system, due to a lack of consensus on what constitutes chronicity (January et al., 2014, 2019).

Chart 22-2 ⚠ **RISK FACTORS**
Atrial Fibrillation

- Increasing age
- Hypertension
- Diabetes
- Obesity
- Valvular heart disease
- Heart failure
- Obstructive sleep apnea
- Alcohol abuse
- Hyperthyroidism
- Myocardial infarction
- Smoking
- Exercise
- Cardiothoracic surgery
- Increased pulse pressure
- European ancestry
- Family history

Adapted from January, C. T., Wann, L. S., Alpert, J. S., et al. (2014). 2014 AHA/ACC/HRS guideline for the management of patients with atrial fibrillation: A report of the ACC/AHA Task Force on practice guidelines and the Heart Rhythm Society. *Circulation, 130*(23), e199–e267; January, C. T., Wann, L. S., Calkins, H., et al. (2019). 2019 AHA/ACC/HRS focused update of the 2014 AHA/ACC/HRS guideline for the management of patients with atrial fibrillation: A Report of the American College of Cardiology/American Heart Association Task Force on Clinical Practice Guidelines and the Heart Rhythm Society in Collaboration With the Society of Thoracic Surgeons. *Circulation, 140*(2), e125–e151.

Chart 22-3 **Atrial Fibrillation Classification System**

Type	Description
Paroxysmal	Sudden onset with termination that occurs spontaneously or after an intervention; lasts ≤7 days, but may recur
Persistent	Continuous, lasting >7 days
Long-standing persistent	Continuous, lasting >12 months
Permanent	Persistent, but decision has been made not to restore or maintain sinus rhythm
Nonvalvular	Absence of moderate-to-severe mitral stenosis or mechanical heart valve

Adapted from January, C. T., Wann, L. S., Alpert, J. S., et al. (2014). 2014 AHA/ACC/HRS guideline for the management of patients with atrial fibrillation: A report of the ACC/AHA Task Force on practice guidelines and the Heart Rhythm Society. *Circulation, 130*(23), e199–e267; January, C. T., Wann, L. S., Calkins, H., et al. (2019). 2019 AHA/ACC/HRS Focused Update of the 2014 AHA/ACC/HRS Guideline for the Management of Patients With Atrial Fibrillation: A Report of the American College of Cardiology/American Heart Association Task Force on Clinical Practice Guidelines and the Heart Rhythm Society in Collaboration With the Society of Thoracic Surgeons. *Circulation, 140*(2), e125–e151.

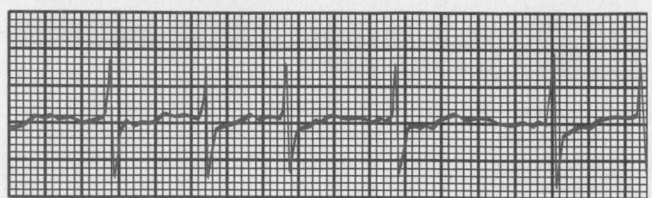

Figure 22-10 • Atrial fibrillation. Reprinted with permission from Morton, G. M., & Fontaine, D. K. (2018). *Critical care nursing: A holistic approach* (11th ed., Fig. 17–22D). Philadelphia, PA: Wolters Kluwer.

Atrial fibrillation has the following characteristics (Fig. 22-10):

Ventricular and atrial rate: Atrial rate is 300 to 600 bpm; ventricular rate is usually 120 to 200 bpm in untreated atrial fibrillation

Ventricular and atrial rhythm: Highly irregular

QRS shape and duration: Usually normal, but may be abnormal

P wave: No discernible P waves; irregular undulating waves that vary in amplitude and shape are seen and referred to as fibrillatory or f waves

PR interval: Cannot be measured

P:QRS ratio: Many:1

Patients with atrial fibrillation are at increased risk of heart failure, myocardial ischemia, and embolic events such as stroke (January et al., 2014, 2019). A rapid and irregular ventricular response reduces the time for ventricular filling, resulting in a smaller stroke volume. Because atrial fibrillation causes a loss in AV synchrony (the atria and ventricles contract at different times), the atrial kick (the last part of diastole and ventricular filling, which accounts for 25% to 30% of the cardiac output) is also lost. As a consequence, although some patients with atrial fibrillation are asymptomatic, others experience palpitations and clinical manifestations of heart failure (e.g., shortness of breath, hypotension, dyspnea on exertion, fatigue; see Chapter 25). In addition, a high ventricular rate of response during atrial fibrillation (greater than 80 bpm) can eventually lead to mitral valve dysfunction, mitral regurgitation, intraventricular conduction delays, and dilated ventricular cardiomyopathy.

Patients with atrial fibrillation may exhibit a pulse deficit—a numeric difference between apical and radial pulse rates. The shorter time in diastole reduces the time available for coronary artery perfusion, thereby increasing the risk of myocardial ischemia with the onset of anginal symptoms (see Chapter 23). Decreasing the ventricular rate may avoid and correct these effects.

The erratic nature of atrial contraction, alterations in ventricular ejection, and atrial myocardial dysfunction promote the formation of thrombi, especially within the left atrium, increasing the risk of an embolic event. The origin of embolisms resulting in stroke for patients with nonvalvular atrial fibrillation is most often the left atrial appendage (LAA) (Schellinger, Tsivgoulis, Steiner, et al., 2018). A therapeutic approach to addressing the role of the LAA in atrial fibrillation, left atrial appendage occlusion (LAAO), is discussed later in this chapter.

Assessment and Diagnostic Findings

The clinical evaluation of atrial fibrillation should include a history and physical examination that identifies the onset and nature of signs and symptoms, including their frequency, duration and any precipitating factors, and any response to medications. Whether or not the patient has a known history of heart disease or other risks is identified (see Chart 22-2). A 12-lead ECG is performed to verify the atrial fibrillation rhythm, as well as to identify the presence (or absence) of left ventricular (LV) hypertrophy, bundle branch block, prior myocardial ischemia, or other arrhythmias. The RR, QRS, and QT intervals are analyzed to verify the effectiveness of any prescribed antiarrhythmic medications (January et al., 2014, 2019). A transesophageal echocardiogram (TEE) can identify the presence of valvular heart disease, provide information about LV and right ventricular (RV) size and function, RV pressures (to identify pulmonary hypertension, which may exist concomitant with atrial fibrillation), LV hypertrophy, and presence of left atrial thrombi (January et al., 2014, 2019).

Blood tests to screen for diseases that are known risks for atrial fibrillation (see Chart 22-2), including thyroid, renal, and hepatic function, are assessed in the patient with a new onset of atrial fibrillation, as well as when the ventricular rate is difficult to control (January et al., 2014, 2019). Additional tests may include a chest x-ray (to evaluate pulmonary vasculature in a patient suspected of having pulmonary hypertension), exercise stress test (to exclude myocardial ischemia or reproduce exercise-induced atrial fibrillation), Holter or event monitoring (see Chapter 21), and an EPS (January et al., 2014, 2019; see later discussion).

Medical Management

Treatment of atrial fibrillation depends on the cause, pattern, and duration of the arrhythmia, the ventricular response rate, as well as the presence of structural or valvular heart disease and other cardiac conditions such as coronary artery disease or heart failure. Strategies for both rhythm control (i.e., conversion to sinus rhythm) and rate control are dependent on shared clinical decision making between the patient and primary provider. In some cases, atrial fibrillation spontaneously converts to sinus rhythm within 24 to 48 hours and without treatment. However, in instances where atrial fibrillation is concomitant with significant other morbid conditions (e.g., severe heart failure), the atrial fibrillation may be classified as "permanent," meaning that the patient and primary provider have made a joint decision to stop further attempts to restore or maintain sinus rhythm. Therefore, management of atrial fibrillation may not only be different in different patients, but it also may change over time for any one patient.

Medical management revolves around preventing embolic events such as stroke with anticoagulant medications, controlling the ventricular rate of response with antiarrhythmic agents, and treating the arrhythmia as indicated so that it is converted to a sinus rhythm (i.e., *cardioversion*).

Pharmacologic Therapy

Antithrombotic Medications. Antithrombotic drugs may include anticoagulants and antiplatelet drugs. Oral antithrombotic therapy is indicated for most patients with nonvalvular atrial fibrillation (e.g., absence of mechanical heart valve) because it reduces the risk of stroke (January et al., 2014, 2019). Atrial fibrillation guidelines recommend use of a scoring system to assist in assessment of stroke risk. Antithrombotic therapy is then selected based on risk factors outlined in the mnemonic $CHA_2DS_2\text{-}VAS_C$ (see Chart 22-4)

Chart 22-4	**Stroke Risk Assessment for the Patient with Atrial Fibrillation: The CHA_2DS_2-VAS_C Scoring System**	

	Risk Factor	Points
C	Congestive Heart Failure (left ventricular systolic dysfunction)	1
H	Hypertension (BP >130/80 mm Hg)	1
A_2	Age ≥75 years	2
D	Diabetes	1
S_2	Prior Stroke/TIA/Thromboembolism	2
V	Vascular disease (i.e., prior MI, PAD, or aortic plaque)	1
A	Age 65–74 years	1
S_c	Sex category (female gender)	1

MI, myocardial infarction; PAD, peripheral artery disease, TIA; transient ischemic attack.

Adapted from January, C. T., Wann, L. S., Alpert, J. S., et al. (2014). 2014 AHA/ACC/HRS guideline for the management of patients with atrial fibrillation: A report of the ACC/AHA Task Force on practice guidelines and the Heart Rhythm Society. *Circulation, 130*(23), e199–e267; January, C. T., Wann, L. S., Calkins, H., et al. (2019). 2019 AHA/ACC/HRS Focused Update of the 2014 AHA/ACC/HRS Guideline for the Management of Patients With Atrial Fibrillation: A Report of the American College of Cardiology/American Heart Association Task Force on Clinical Practice Guidelines and the Heart Rhythm Society in Collaboration With the Society of Thoracic Surgeons. *Circulation, 140*(2), e125–e151.

with each risk factor assigned points tallied for a total score that indicates an overall risk of stroke (January et al., 2014, 2019).

According to pharmacologic treatment guidelines (January et al., 2014, 2019):

- Patients with nonvalvular atrial fibrillation with a CHA_2DS_2-VAS_C score of zero may choose the option of no antithrombotic therapy.
- Patients with nonvalvular atrial fibrillation with a CHA_2DS_2-VAS_C score of one may choose no antithrombotic therapy, treatment with an oral anticoagulant, or aspirin.
- Patients with nonvalvular atrial fibrillation with a CHA_2DS_2-VAS_C score of 2 or higher for men and 3 or higher for women may choose warfarin, or a direct thrombin inhibitor (e.g., dabigatran), or a Factor Xa inhibitor (e.g., rivaroxaban, apixaban, edoxaban).

Patients with atrial fibrillation with valvular heart disease or bioprosthetic heart valves may be prescribed warfarin, or a direct-acting oral anticoagulant, or a Factor Xa inhibitor (Malik, Yandrapalli, Aronow, et al., 2019). For patients with mechanical heart valves, warfarin is recommended (January et al., 2014, 2019). If immediate or short-term anticoagulation is necessary, the patient may be placed on IV or low–molecular-weight heparin until warfarin therapy can be started and the international normalized ratio (INR) level reaches a therapeutic range consistent with antithrombosis, usually defined as an INR between 2.0 and 3.0 (see Chapter 26 for further discussion).

Medication selection for all patients with atrial fibrillation depends upon stroke and bleeding risks as well as patient preferences and values (January et al., 2014, 2019). For instance, treatment with warfarin will require weekly INR testing during initiation of therapy, as well as ongoing monitoring (see Chapter 26 for further discussion). Home monitoring of therapy is an option for some patients. Direct-acting oral anticoagulants and Factor Xa inhibitors require baseline assessment of hemoglobin and hematocrit, as well as liver and renal function, along with INR. Advantages of these medications include fewer drug–drug interactions and dietary limitations, as well as the elimination of frequent INR testing.

Medications that Control the Heart Rate. A strategy to control the ventricular rate of response so that the resting heart rate is less than 80 bpm is recommended in order to manage symptoms of atrial fibrillation (January et al., 2014, 2019). To decrease the ventricular rate in patients with paroxysmal, persistent, or permanent atrial fibrillation, a beta-blocker (Class II antiarrhythmic, see Table 22-1) or non-dihydropyridine calcium channel blocker (Class IV antiarrhythmic, see Table 22-1) is generally recommended (January et al., 2014, 2019).

Medications that Convert the Heart Rhythm or Prevent Atrial Fibrillation. For patients with atrial fibrillation lasting 48 hours or longer, anticoagulation is recommended prior to attempts to restore sinus rhythm, which may be achieved through pharmacologic or electrical cardioversion (January et al., 2014, 2019). In the absence of therapeutic anticoagulation, TEE may be performed prior to cardioversion to identify left atrial thrombus formation, including in the LAA (January et al., 2014, 2019). If no thrombus is identified, cardioversion can proceed.

Medications that may be given to achieve pharmacologic cardioversion to sinus rhythm include flecainide, dofetilide, propafenone, amiodarone, and IV ibutilide (January et al., 2014, 2019). These medications are most effective if given within 7 days of the onset of atrial fibrillation. It is recommended that patients who were prescribed dofetilide be hospitalized so that the QT interval and renal function both may be monitored. Despite a degree of risk, dofetilide is a preferred medication because it is highly effective at converting atrial fibrillation to sinus rhythm, has fewer drug-to-drug interactions, and is better tolerated by patients than other medications. Some patients with recurrent atrial fibrillation may be prescribed flecainide to self-administer at home, an approach referred to as "pill in the pocket" (January et al., 2014, 2019).

Preoperative administration of beta-blockers (see Table 22-1) has resulted in a significant reduction in atrial fibrillation after cardiac surgery (Burrage, Low, Campbell, et al., 2019). Cholesterol-lowering drugs such as the HMG-CoA reductase inhibitors (also called statins; see Chapter 23, Table 23-1) may also be prescribed to prevent new-onset atrial fibrillation following cardiac surgery (Burrage et al., 2019).

If symptomatic, paroxysmal atrial fibrillation is refractory to at least one Class I or Class III antiarrhythmic medication (see Table 22-1), and rhythm control is desired, catheter ablation may be indicated (January et al., 2014, 2019; see later discussion).

Electrical Cardioversion for Atrial Fibrillation

Electrical cardioversion is indicated for patients with atrial fibrillation who are hemodynamically unstable (e.g., acute alteration in mental status, chest discomfort, hypotension) and do not respond to medications (January et al., 2014, 2019). Flecainide, propafenone, amiodarone, dofetilide, or sotalol may be given prior to cardioversion to enhance the success of cardioversion and maintain sinus rhythm (January et al., 2014, 2019).

> ◤ **Quality and Safety Nursing Alert**
>
> *The patient with atrial fibrillation is at high risk for thrombus formation. When electrical cardioversion is indicated, the nurse may anticipate that a transesophageal echocardiogram may be performed to evaluate for possible atrial thrombi.*

Because atrial function may be impaired for several weeks after cardioversion, antithrombotic therapy (e.g., warfarin) is indicated for at least 4 weeks after the procedure (January et al., 2014, 2019). Repeated attempts at electrical cardioversion may be made, following administration of an antiarrhythmic medication (see later discussion on Electrical Cardioversion).

Cardiac Rhythm Therapies

Atrial fibrillation that does not respond to medications or electrical cardioversion may be treated by cardiac rhythm therapies, including catheter ablation, maze or mini-maze procedure, or convergent procedure.

Catheter Ablation Therapy

Catheter **ablation** destroys specific cells that are the cause of a tachyarrhythmia. Catheter ablation is performed most often today for atrial fibrillation, although it may also be useful in treating atrioventricular nodal reentry tachycardia (AVNRT) and recurrent ventricular tachycardia (VT) (see later discussion of these arrhythmias).

Atrial fibrillation is associated with intrinsic cardiac autonomic nervous system activity to the pulmonary veins. Ablation involves a procedure similar to a cardiac catheterization (see Chapter 21); however, in this instance, a special catheter is advanced at or near the origin of the arrhythmia, where high-frequency, low-energy sound waves are passed through the catheter, causing thermal injury, localized cell destruction, and scarring. The tissue damage is more specific to the arrhythmic tissue, with less trauma to the surrounding cardiac tissue. Ablation may also be accomplished using a special catheter to apply extremely cold temperature to destroy selected cardiac cells, called *cryoablation*. The goal of each of these ablation procedures is to eliminate the arrhythmia, by preventing the ectopic activity arising from the pulmonary veins from reaching the atria, thereby stopping fibrillation (Weber, Sagerer-Gerhardt, & Heinze, 2017).

An EPS (see later discussion) may be performed to induce the arrhythmia prior to the catheter ablation. During the ablation procedure, defibrillation pads, an automatic blood pressure cuff, and a pulse oximeter are used. The patient is usually given moderate sedation (see Chapter 15) and IV heparin to reduce the risk of periprocedural thromboembolism. Immediately postablation, the patient is monitored for another 30 to 60 minutes and then retested to ensure that the arrhythmia does not recur. Successful ablation is achieved when the arrhythmia cannot be induced. Major risks of catheter ablation include pericardial effusion and tamponade, phrenic nerve injury, stroke, hematoma, retroperitoneal bleeding, pulmonary vein stenosis, and atrioesophageal fistulas (Canpolat, Kocyigit, & Aytemir, 2017).

Nursing Management. Postprocedural care on a step-down unit for the patient who has had ablation is similar to the nursing management of a patient who has had a cardiac catheterization (see Chapter 21); the patient is monitored closely to ensure recovery from sedation. Postprocedural nursing interventions include frequent monitoring for arrhythmias and for signs and symptoms of a stroke and vascular access site complications.

Because of the prolonged time required for the procedure as well as the time needed in bed to obtain hemostasis at the vascular access site, it is not unusual for the patient to have back discomfort. In addition to administering any pain medications, the nurse may help to alleviate this pain by placing rolled towels under the patient's knees and waist.

Maze and Mini-Maze Procedures

The maze procedure is an open heart surgical procedure for refractory atrial fibrillation. Small transmural incisions are made throughout the atria. The resulting formation of scar tissue prevents reentry conduction of the aberrant electrical impulse. Because the procedure requires significant time and cardiopulmonary bypass, its use is reserved only for those patients undergoing cardiac surgery for another reason (e.g., coronary artery bypass; January et al., 2014, 2019). Some patients may need a permanent pacemaker after this surgery because of subsequent injury to the SA node.

A modification of the maze procedure, minimally invasive maze surgery, or mini-maze, may be performed by making small incisions between the ribs, through which video-guided instruments are inserted. The pulmonary veins are encircled with surgical incisions within the left atrium. This surgery eliminates the need for opening the sternum, heart–lung bypass, and the use of cardioplegia (see Chapter 23 for further discussion of cardiac surgery). This results in a shorter recovery time and a lower risk of infection (January et al., 2014, 2019).

Convergent Procedure

The convergent procedure utilizes a hybrid approach to ablation, requiring the skills of both a cardiothoracic surgeon and an electrophysiologist, a cardiologist with specialized training. This procedure is associated with lower rates of arrhythmia recurrence than catheter ablation, but more complications within 30 days of the procedure (e.g., infections, bleeding) (Jan, Zizek, Gersak, et al., 2018). The surgeon creates a few small incisions in the abdomen so that a special catheter that allows visualization can be inserted through the diaphragm and toward the posterior wall of the heart. The surgeon performs ablation of the epicardial wall in the area around the pulmonary veins and the electrophysiologist performs ablation around the endocardial area of the pulmonary veins. Because of the incisions, the patient usually has a 3-day hospital length of stay (Elrod, 2014). The patient may experience mild dull chest pain caused by the resulting inflammation from the ablation that usually resolves within a few days (Elrod, 2014). This pain is usually alleviated by treatment with acetaminophen as needed. In addition, if the phrenic nerve was affected, the patient may experience shortness of breath that may take days to weeks to resolve (Elrod, 2014).

Left Atrial Appendage Occlusion

LAAO is an alternative to antithrombotic medications for stroke prevention in patients with nonvalvular atrial fibrillation (Masoudi, Calkins, Kavinsky, et al., 2015). As noted previously, the LAA is the area where the majority of stroke-causing blood clots form in patients with nonvalvular atrial fibrillation. However, concerns about the risk of long-term anticoagulant use and the risk of bleeding can complicate effective management (Ojo, Yandrapalli, Veseli, et al., 2020).

Candidates for LAAO include those patients with increased risk of stroke based on $CHA_2DS_2\text{-}VAS_C$ scores of

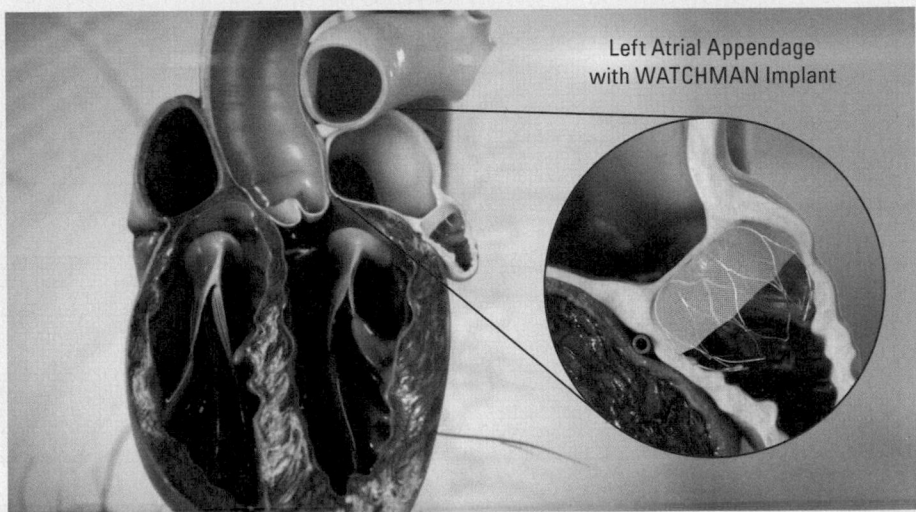

Left Atrial Appendage
with WATCHMAN Implant

Figure 22-11 • The WATCHMAN device in place over the left atrial appendage.

one or higher (see Chart 22-4) and those patients seeking a nonpharmacologic alternative to treatment (Masoudi et al., 2015). Commonly used is the WATCHMAN, a device typically inserted while the patient is under general anesthesia. Similar to a percutaneous coronary intervention (PCI) procedure (see Chapter 23), a small incision is made in the femoral area and a catheter is then inserted that guides the device into position. The parachute-shaped device is threaded through to the opening of the LAA, sealing it off and preventing it from releasing clots (see Fig. 22-11).

Patients typically stay in the hospital overnight after placement of a WATCHMAN device. The nursing management of patients who received this device is similar to that of patients post cardiac catheterization (see Chapter 21). Patients are prescribed aspirin and warfarin post procedure; approximately 6 weeks post procedure, they should return to the cardiology clinic for a TEE to confirm that the device has effectively occluded the LAA. If LAAO has occurred, then the patient may stop taking warfarin and is prescribed clopidogrel, an antiplatelet medication. After 6 months, the patient may stop taking clopidogrel but must continue taking daily aspirin indefinitely (Carlson & Doshi, 2017).

Wolff-Parkinson-White Syndrome

In the patient with atrial fibrillation, if the QRS is wide and the ventricular rhythm is very fast and irregular, an accessory pathway should be suspected. An accessory pathway is typically congenital tissue between the atria, bundle of His, AV node, Purkinje fibers, or ventricular myocardium. This anomaly is known as Wolff-Parkinson-White (WPW) syndrome. Electrical cardioversion is the treatment of choice for atrial fibrillation in the presence of WPW syndrome that causes hemodynamic instability. Medications that block AV conduction (e.g., digoxin, diltiazem, verapamil) should be avoided in WPW because they can increase the ventricular rate. If the patient is hemodynamically stable, procainamide, propafenone, flecainide, or amiodarone are recommended to restore sinus rhythm (January et al., 2014, 2019). Catheter ablation is performed for long-term management (see previous discussion).

Atrial Flutter

Atrial flutter occurs because of a conduction defect in the atrium and causes a rapid, regular atrial impulse at a rate

between 250 and 400 bpm. Because the atrial rate is faster than the AV node can conduct, not all atrial impulses are conducted into the ventricle, causing a therapeutic block at the AV node. This is an important feature of this arrhythmia. If all atrial impulses were conducted to the ventricle, the ventricular rate would also be 250 to 400 bpm, which would result in ventricular fibrillation, a life-threatening arrhythmia. Atrial flutter risk factors mirror those for atrial fibrillation (Fuster et al., 2017; see Chart 22-2).

Atrial flutter has the following characteristics (see Fig. 22-12):

Ventricular and atrial rate: Atrial rate ranges between 250 and 400 bpm; ventricular rate usually ranges between 75 and 150 bpm

Ventricular and atrial rhythm: The atrial rhythm is regular; the ventricular rhythm is usually regular but may be irregular because of a change in the AV conduction

QRS shape and duration: Usually normal, but may be abnormal or absent

P wave: Saw-toothed shape; these waves are referred to as F waves

PR interval: Multiple F waves may make it difficult to determine the PR interval

P:QRS ratio: 2:1, 3:1, or 4:1

Medical Management

Atrial flutter can cause serious signs and symptoms, such as chest pain, shortness of breath, and low blood pressure. Medical management involves the use of vagal maneuvers (see previous discussion under Sinus Tachycardia) or a trial administration of adenosine, which causes sympathetic block and slowing of conduction through the AV node. This may terminate the tachycardia; optimally, it will facilitate

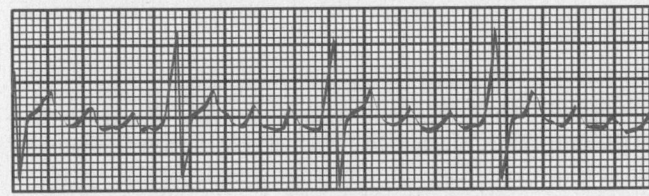

Figure 22-12 • Atrial flutter. Reprinted with permission from Morton, G. M., & Fontaine, D. K. (2018). *Critical care nursing: A holistic approach* (11th ed., Fig. 17–22C). Philadelphia, PA: Wolters Kluwer.

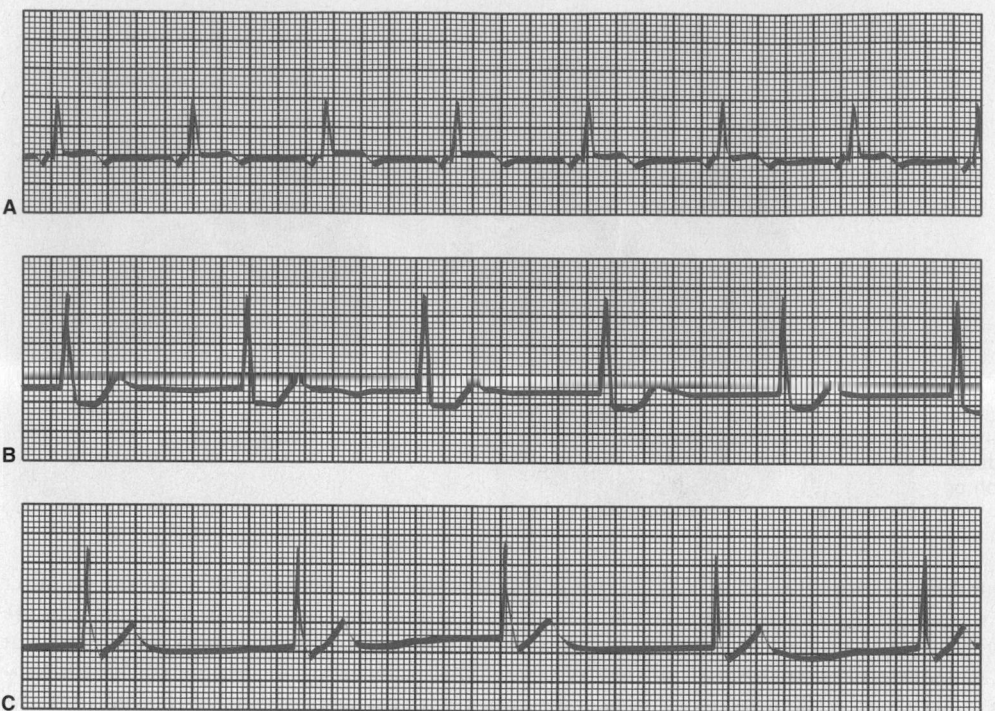

Figure 22-10 • Various types of junctional rhythms. **A.** Note that the inverted P wave appears before the normal QRS complex. **B.** Note that the inverted P wave is buried inside the QRS complex. **C.** Note that the inverted P wave follows the QRS complex. Reprinted with permission from Morton, G. M., & Fontaine, D. K. (2018). *Critical care nursing: A holistic approach* (11th ed., Fig. 17–23A, B, and C). Philadelphia, PA: Wolters Kluwer.

visualization of flutter waves for diagnostic purposes. Adenosine is given IV by rapid administration, and immediately followed by a 20-mL saline flush and elevation of the arm with the IV line to promote rapid circulation of the medication.

Atrial flutter is treated with antithrombotic therapy, rate control, and rhythm control in the same manner as atrial fibrillation (January et al., 2014, 2019). Electrical cardioversion is often successful in converting atrial flutter to sinus rhythm (see later discussion).

Junctional Arrhythmias

Junctional arrhythmias originate within AV nodal tissue, and may include premature junctional complexes, junctional rhythms, nonparoxysmal junctional tachycardia, and AV nodal reentry tachycardia.

Premature Junctional Complex

A premature junctional complex is an impulse that starts in the AV nodal area before the next normal sinus impulse reaches the AV node. Premature junctional complexes are less common than PACs. Causes include digitalis toxicity, heart failure, and coronary artery disease. The ECG criteria for premature junctional complex are the same as for PACs, except for the P wave and the PR interval. The P wave may be absent, may follow the QRS, or may occur before the QRS but with a PR interval of less than 0.12 seconds. This arrhythmia rarely produces significant symptoms. Treatment for frequent premature junctional complexes is the same as for frequent PACs.

Junctional Rhythm

Junctional or idionodal rhythm occurs when the AV node, instead of the sinus node, becomes the pacemaker of the heart. When the sinus node slows (e.g., from increased vagal tone) or when the impulse cannot be conducted through the AV node (e.g., because of complete heart block), the AV node automatically discharges

an impulse. Junctional rhythm not caused by complete heart block has the following characteristics (see Fig. 22-13):

Ventricular and atrial rate: Ventricular rate 40 to 60 bpm; atrial rate also 40 to 60 bpm if P waves are discernible

Ventricular and atrial rhythm: Regular

QRS shape and duration: Usually normal, but may be abnormal

P wave: May be absent, after the QRS complex, or before the QRS; may be inverted, especially in lead II

PR interval: If the P wave is in front of the QRS, the PR interval is less than 0.12 seconds

P:QRS ratio: 1:1 or 0:1

Medical Management

Junctional rhythm may produce signs and symptoms of reduced cardiac output. If this occurs, the treatment is the same as for sinus bradycardia. Emergency pacing may be needed (see later discussion under Pacemaker Therapy).

Nonparoxysmal Junctional Tachycardia

Junctional tachycardia is caused by enhanced automaticity in the junctional area, resulting in a rhythm similar to junctional rhythm, except at a rate of 70 to 120 bpm. Although this rhythm generally does not have any detrimental hemodynamic effect, it may indicate a serious underlying condition, such as digitalis toxicity, myocardial ischemia, hypokalemia, or chronic obstructive pulmonary disease.

Atrioventricular Nodal Reentry Tachycardia

AVNRT is a common arrhythmia that occurs when an impulse is conducted to an area in the AV node that causes the impulse to be rerouted back into the same area over and over again at a very fast rate. Each time the impulse is conducted through this area, it is also conducted down into the ventricles, causing a fast ventricular rate. AVNRT that has an abrupt onset and an abrupt cessation with a QRS of normal duration has frequently been called *paroxysmal atrial tachycardia (PAT)* and

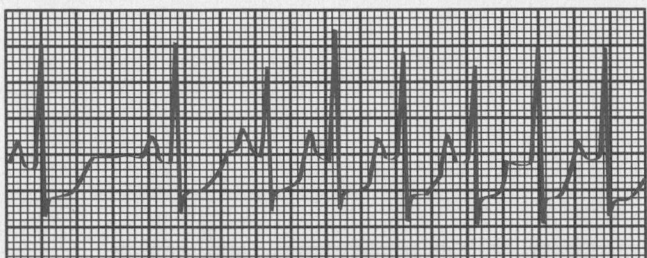

Figure 22-14 • Atrioventricular nodal reentry tachycardia (AVNRT), also called paroxysmal atrial tachycardia (PAT), and paroxysmal supraventricular tachycardia (PSVT). Reprinted with permission from Morton, G. M., & Fontaine, D. K. (2018). *Critical care nursing: A holistic approach* (11th ed., Fig. 17–22B). Philadelphia, PA: Wolters Kluwer.

also *paroxysmal supraventricular tachycardia (PSVT)*. AVNRT also occurs when the duration of the QRS complex is 0.12 seconds or greater and a block in the bundle branch is known to be present. This arrhythmia may last for seconds or several hours. Factors associated with the development of AVNRT include caffeine, nicotine, hypoxemia, and stress. Underlying pathologies include coronary artery disease and cardiomyopathy; however, it occurs more often in females and not in association with underlying structural heart disease. AVNRT has the following characteristics (see Fig. 22-14):

Ventricular and atrial rate: Atrial rate usually 150 to 250 bpm; ventricular rate usually 120 to 200 bpm

Ventricular and atrial rhythm: Regular; sudden onset and termination of the tachycardia

QRS shape and duration: Usually normal, but may be abnormal

P wave: Usually very difficult to discern

PR interval: If the P wave is in front of the QRS, the PR interval is less than 0.12 seconds

P:QRS ratio: 1:1, 2:1

Clinical symptoms vary with the rate and duration of the tachycardia and the patient's underlying condition. The tachycardia usually is of short duration, resulting only in palpitations. A fast rate may also reduce cardiac output, resulting in significant signs and symptoms such as restlessness, chest pain, shortness of breath, pallor, hypotension, and loss of consciousness.

Medical Management

Because AVNRT is generally a benign arrhythmia, the goal of medical management is to alleviate symptoms and improve quality of life. Patients who become significantly symptomatic and require emergency department visits to terminate the rhythm may want to initiate therapy immediately. However, those with minimum symptoms with an AVRNT that terminates spontaneously or with minimal treatment may choose just to be monitored and self-treat.

The aim of therapy is to break the reentry of the impulse. Catheter ablation is the initial treatment of choice and is used to eliminate the area that permits the rerouting of the impulse that causes the tachycardia (Katritsis, 2018; see previous discussion of Atrial Fibrillation: Catheter Ablation Therapy). Vagal maneuvers (see previous discussion under Sinus Tachycardia) may be used to interrupt AVNRT. These techniques increase parasympathetic stimulation, causing slower conduction through the AV node and blocking the reentry of the rerouted impulse. Some patients use some of these methods to terminate the episode on their own. Because of the risk of a cerebral embolic event,

carotid sinus massage, which may be performed by physicians, is contraindicated in patients with carotid artery disease.

Pharmacologic Therapy

If the vagal maneuvers are ineffective, the patient may then receive a bolus of adenosine to correct the rhythm; this is usually effective in terminating AVNRT. Because the effect of adenosine is so short, AVNRT may recur; the first dose may be followed with two additional doses. If the vagal maneuvers and adenosine are ineffective, IV non-dihydropyridine calcium channel blockers (e.g., verapamil), IV beta-blockers or IV digoxin may be considered (Hafeez & Armstrong, 2019). If the patient is unstable or does not respond to the medications, electrical cardioversion is the treatment of choice (see later discussion).

If P waves cannot be identified, the rhythm may be called supraventricular tachycardia (SVT), or PSVT if it has an abrupt onset, until the underlying rhythm and resulting diagnosis is determined. SVT and PSVT indicate only that the rhythm is not VT. SVT could be atrial fibrillation, atrial flutter, or AVNRT, among others. Vagal maneuvers and adenosine may be used to convert the rhythm or at least slow conduction in the AV node to allow visualization of the P waves.

Ventricular Arrhythmias

Ventricular arrhythmias originate from foci within the ventricles; these may include premature ventricular complexes, VT, ventricular fibrillation, and idioventricular rhythms. Technically, ventricular asystole is characterized by an absence of rhythm formation.

Premature Ventricular Complex

A PVC is an impulse that starts in a ventricle and is conducted through the ventricles before the next normal sinus impulse. PVCs can occur in healthy people, especially with intake of caffeine, nicotine, or alcohol. PVCs may be caused by cardiac ischemia or infarction, increased workload on the heart (e.g., heart failure and tachycardia), digitalis toxicity, hypoxia, acidosis, or electrolyte imbalances, especially hypokalemia.

In a rhythm referred to as bigeminy, every other complex is a PVC. In trigeminy, every third complex is a PVC, and in quadrigeminy, every fourth complex is a PVC. PVCs have the following characteristics (see Fig. 22-15):

Ventricular and atrial rate: Depends on the underlying rhythm (e.g., sinus rhythm)

Ventricular and atrial rhythm: Irregular due to early QRS, creating one RR interval that is shorter than the others. The PP interval may be regular, indicating that the PVC did not depolarize the sinus node

QRS shape and duration: Duration is 0.12 seconds or longer; shape is bizarre and abnormal. When these bizarrely shaped, widened QRS complexes resemble each other, they are called unifocal. When they have at least two different morphologic appearances, they are called multifocal

P wave: Visibility of the P wave depends on the timing of the PVC; may be absent (hidden in the QRS or T wave) or in front of the QRS. If the P wave follows the QRS, the shape of the P wave may be different

PR interval: If the P wave is in front of the QRS, the PR interval is less than 0.12 seconds

P:QRS ratio: 0:1; 1:1

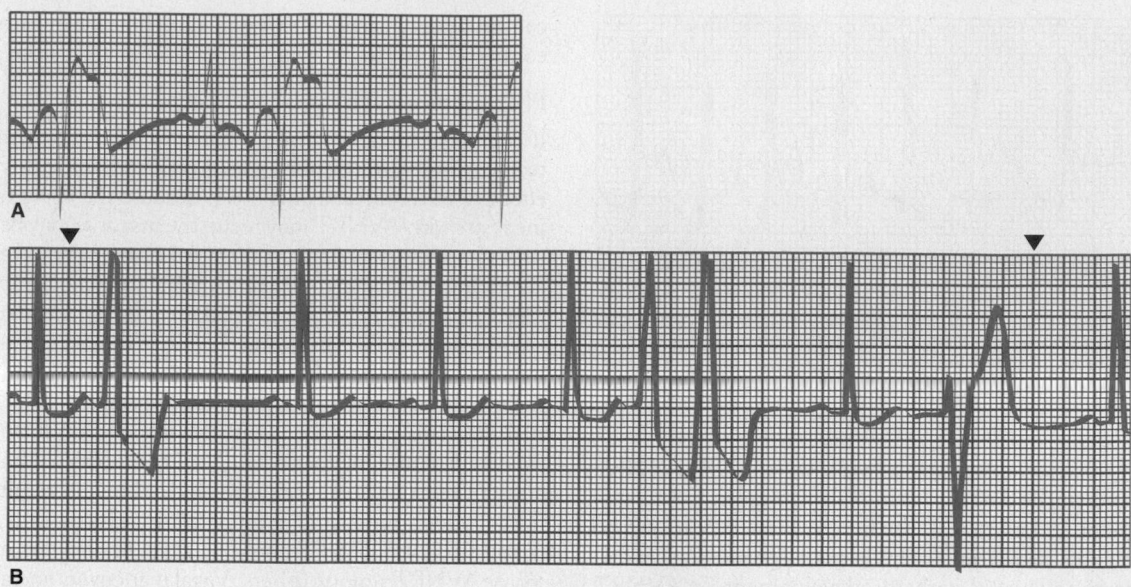

Figure 22-15 • Premature ventricular complexes (PVCs). **A.** Ventricular bigeminy that is unifocal; note that every other beat is a PVC, with the same morphologic appearance. **B.** Multifocal PVCs; note that there are at least two different appearing PVCs. Reprinted with permission from Morton, G. M., & Fontaine, D. K. (2018). *Critical care nursing: A holistic approach* (11th ed., Fig. 17–25B and C). Philadelphia, PA: Wolters Kluwer.

The patient may feel nothing or may say that the heart "skipped a beat." The effect of a PVC depends on its timing in the cardiac cycle and how much blood was in the ventricles when they contracted. Initial treatment is aimed at correcting the cause.

Medical Management

PVCs are a common occurrence and may increase in frequency with age (Al-khatib, Stevenson, Ackerman, et al., 2018). PVCs that are frequent and persistent may be treated with amiodarone or beta-blockers, but long-term pharmacotherapy for PVCs is not usually indicated. PVCs are not considered a warning for ensuing VT. However, studies have shown an association of PVCs with adverse outcomes; therefore, patients may need to be evaluated for underlying causes (e.g., ischemic heart disease and LV dysfunction) (Al-khatib et al., 2018).

Unfolding Patient Stories: Kenneth Bronson • Part 2

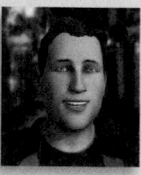

Recall from Chapter 19 **Kenneth Bronson**, who came to the emergency department with difficulty breathing after a week of flu-like symptoms, productive cough, and high fever. He was diagnosed with a right lower lobe pneumonia. Sinus tachycardia with occasional unifocal premature ventricular contractions (PVCs) is seen on the cardiac monitor. What are potential causes for the tachycardia and PVCs that the nurse should investigate when considering his age of 27 years, symptoms experienced over the last week, and the clinical manifestations associated with his diagnosis?

Care for Kenneth and other patients in a realistic virtual environment: **vSim** *for Nursing* (**thepoint.lww.com/vSimMedicalSurgical**). Practice documenting these patients' care in DocuCare (**thepoint.lww.com/DocuCareEHR**).

Ventricular Tachycardia

VT is defined as three or more PVCs in a row, occurring at a rate exceeding 100 bpm. The causes are similar to those of PVC. Patients with larger MIs and lower ejection fractions are at higher risk of lethal VT. VT is an emergency because the patient is nearly always unresponsive and pulseless. VT has the following characteristics (see Fig. 22-16):

Ventricular and atrial rate: Ventricular rate is 100 to 200 bpm; atrial rate depends on the underlying rhythm (e.g., sinus rhythm)

Ventricular and atrial rhythm: Usually regular; atrial rhythm may also be regular

QRS shape and duration: Duration is 0.12 seconds or more; bizarre, abnormal shape

P wave: Very difficult to detect, so the atrial rate and rhythm may be indeterminable

PR interval: Very irregular, if P waves are seen

P:QRS ratio: Difficult to determine, but if P waves are apparent, there are usually more QRS complexes than P waves

The patient's tolerance or lack of tolerance for this rapid rhythm depends on the ventricular rate and severity of ventricular dysfunction.

Medical Management

Several factors determine the initial treatment, including the following: identifying the rhythm as monomorphic (having a consistent QRS shape and rate) or polymorphic (having varying QRS shapes and rhythms), determining the existence of a prolonged QT interval before the initiation of VT, any comorbidities, and ascertaining the patient's heart function (normal or decreased). If the patient is stable, continuing the assessment, especially obtaining a 12-lead ECG, may be the only action necessary.

The patient may need antiarrhythmic medications, antitachycardia pacing, or direct cardioversion or defibrillation. Procainamide, amiodarone, sotalol, and lidocaine are all

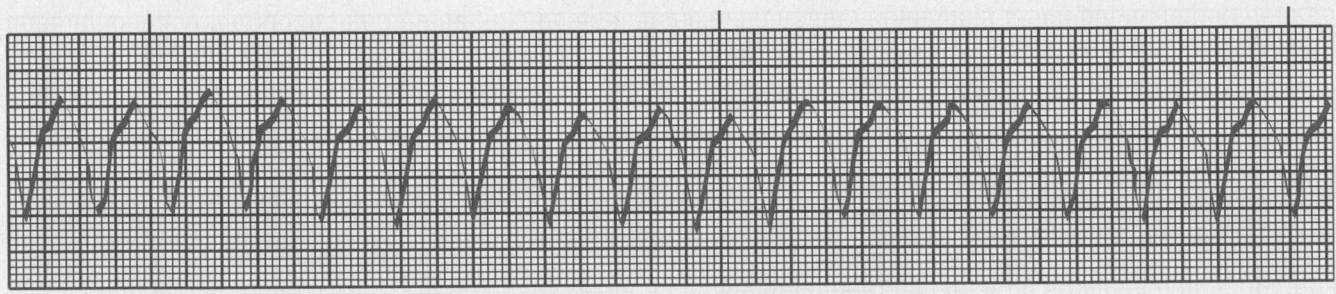

Figure 22-16 • Ventricular tachycardia. Reprinted with permission from Huff, J. (2002). *ECG Workout* (4th ed., p. 197). Philadelphia, PA: Lippincott, Williams & Wilkins.

antiarrhythmic medications that may be considered based upon type of VT (e.g., monomorphic or polymorphic), clinical presentation, and patient comorbidities (e.g., impaired cardiac function, acute MI).

Cardioversion is the treatment of choice for monophasic VT in a patient who is symptomatic. **Defibrillation**, which uses an electrical current given to stop the arrhythmia that is not set to synchronize with the patient's QRS complex, is the treatment of choice for pulseless VT. Any type of VT in a patient who is unconscious and without a pulse is treated in the same manner as ventricular fibrillation: immediate defibrillation is the action of choice (see later discussion on Cardioversion and Defibrillation).

For long-term management, patients with an ejection fraction less than 35% should be considered for an implantable cardioverter defibrillator (ICD) (see later discussion). Those with an ejection fraction greater than 35% may be managed with antiarrhythmic medication.

Torsades de pointes is a polymorphic VT preceded by a prolonged QT interval, which could be congenital or acquired. Common causes include central nervous system disease; certain medications (e.g., ciprofloxacin, erythromycin, haloperidol, lithium, methadone); or low levels of potassium, calcium, or magnesium. Congenital QT prolongation is another cause. Because this rhythm is likely to cause the patient to deteriorate and become pulseless, immediate treatment is required and includes correction of any electrolyte imbalance, such as administration of IV magnesium, and with IV isoproterenol or pacing if associated with bradycardia (Link, Berkow, Kudenchuk, et al., 2015; Soar, Donnino, Maconochie, et al., 2018).

 Ventricular Fibrillation

The most common arrhythmia in patients with cardiac arrest is ventricular fibrillation, which is a rapid, disorganized ventricular rhythm that causes ineffective quivering of the ventricles. No atrial activity is seen on the ECG. The most common cause of ventricular fibrillation is coronary artery disease and resulting acute MI. Other causes include untreated or unsuccessfully treated VT, cardiomyopathy, valvular heart disease, several proarrhythmic medications, acid–base and electrolyte

abnormalities, and electrical shock. Another cause is Brugada syndrome, in which the patient (frequently of Asian descent) has a structurally normal heart, few or no risk factors for coronary artery disease, and a family history of sudden cardiac death (Pappone & Santinelli, 2019). Ventricular fibrillation has the following characteristics (see Fig. 22-17):

Ventricular rate: Greater than 300 bpm

Ventricular rhythm: Extremely irregular, without a specific pattern

QRS shape and duration: Irregular, undulating waves with changing amplitudes. There are no recognizable QRS complexes

Medical Management

Ventricular fibrillation is always characterized by the absence of an audible heartbeat, a palpable pulse, and respirations. Because there is no coordinated cardiac activity, cardiac arrest and death are imminent if the arrhythmia is not corrected. Early defibrillation is critical to survival, with administration of immediate bystander cardiopulmonary resuscitation (CPR) until defibrillation is available. For refractory ventricular fibrillation, administration of amiodarone and epinephrine may facilitate the return of a spontaneous pulse after defibrillation (Link et al., 2015; see Chapter 25 for further discussion on interventions during Cardiac Arrest).

Idioventricular Rhythm

Idioventricular rhythm, also called *ventricular escape rhythm*, occurs when the impulse starts in the conduction system below the AV node. When the sinus node fails to create an impulse (e.g., from increased vagal tone) or when the impulse is created but cannot be conducted through the AV node (e.g., due to complete AV block), the Purkinje fibers automatically discharge an impulse. When idioventricular rhythm is not caused by AV block, it has the following characteristics (see Fig. 22-18):

Ventricular rate: Between 20 and 40 bpm; if the rate exceeds 40 bpm, the rhythm is known as accelerated idioventricular rhythm

Ventricular rhythm: Regular

QRS shape and duration: Bizarre, abnormal shape; duration is 0.12 seconds or more

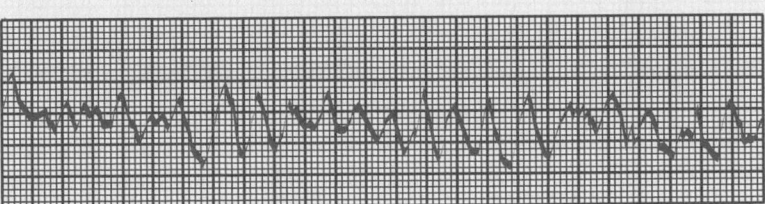

Figure 22-17 • Ventricular fibrillation. Reprinted with permission from Morton, G. M., & Fontaine, D. K. (2018). *Critical Care Nursing: A Holistic Approach* (11th ed., Fig. 17–27C). Philadelphia, PA: Wolters Kluwer.

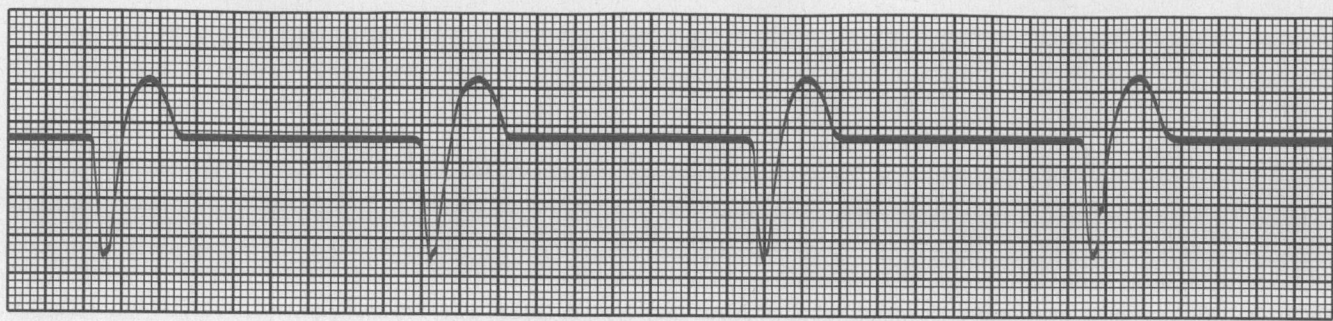

Figure 22-18 • Idioventricular rhythm.

Medical Management

Idioventricular rhythm commonly causes the patient to lose consciousness and experience other signs and symptoms of reduced cardiac output. In such cases, the treatment is the same as for asystole and pulseless electrical activity (PEA) (see Chapter 25) if the patient is in cardiac arrest or for bradycardia if the patient is not in cardiac arrest. Interventions include identifying the underlying cause; administering IV epinephrine, atropine, and vasopressor medications; and initiating emergency transcutaneous pacing. In some cases, idioventricular rhythm may cause no symptoms of reduced cardiac output.

Ventricular Asystole

Commonly called *flatline*, ventricular asystole is characterized by absent QRS complexes confirmed in two different leads, although P waves may be apparent for a short duration. There is no heartbeat, no palpable pulse, and no respiration. Without immediate treatment, ventricular asystole is fatal.

Medical Management

Ventricular asystole is treated the same as PEA, focusing on high-quality CPR with minimal interruptions and identifying underlying and contributing factors. The key to successful treatment is a rapid assessment to identify a possible cause, which is known as the Hs and Ts: hypoxia, hypovolemia, hydrogen ion (acid–base imbalance), hypo- or hyperglycemia, hypo- or hyperkalemia, hypothermia, trauma, toxins, tamponade (cardiac), tension pneumothorax, or thrombus (coronary or pulmonary) (Link et al., 2015). After the initiation of CPR, intubation and establishment of IV access are the next recommended actions, with no or minimal interruptions in chest compressions (see Chapter 25).

Conduction Abnormalities

When assessing the rhythm strip, the underlying rhythm is first identified (e.g., sinus rhythm, sinus arrhythmia). Then, the PR interval is assessed for the possibility of an AV block. AV blocks occur when the conduction of the impulse through the AV node or bundle of His area is decreased or stopped. These blocks can be caused by medications (e.g., digitalis, calcium channel blockers, beta-blockers), Lyme disease, myocardial ischemia and infarction, hypothyroidism, or activities that cause an increase in vagal tone (Kusumoto et al., 2019). If the AV block is caused by increased vagal tone (e.g., long-term athletic training, sleep, coughing, suctioning, pressure above the eyes or on large vessels, anal stimulation), it is commonly accompanied by sinus bradycardia. AV block may be temporary and resolve on its own, or it may be permanent and require permanent pacing.

The clinical signs and symptoms of a heart block vary with the resulting ventricular rate and the severity of any underlying disease processes. Whereas first-degree AV block rarely causes any hemodynamic effect, the other blocks may result in decreased heart rate, causing a decrease in perfusion to vital organs, such as the brain, heart, kidneys, lungs, and skin. A patient with third-degree AV block caused by digitalis toxicity may be stable; another patient with the same rhythm caused by acute MI may be unstable. Health care providers must always keep in mind the need to treat the patient, not the rhythm. The treatment is based on the hemodynamic effect of the rhythm.

First-Degree Atrioventricular Block

First-degree AV block occurs when all the atrial impulses are conducted through the AV node into the ventricles at a rate slower than normal. This conduction disorder has the following characteristics (see Fig. 22-19):

Ventricular and atrial rate: Depends on the underlying rhythm

Ventricular and atrial rhythm: Depends on the underlying rhythm

QRS shape and duration: Usually normal, but may be abnormal

P wave: In front of the QRS complex; shows sinus rhythm, regular shape

PR interval: Greater than 0.20 seconds; PR interval measurement is constant.

P:QRS ratio: 1:1

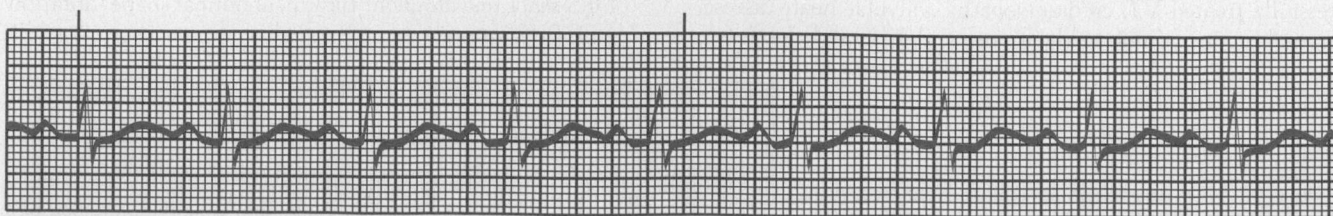

Figure 22-19 • First-degree atrioventricular block. Note that the PR interval is constant but greater than 0.20 seconds. Reprinted with permission from Huff, J. (2002). *ECG Workout* (4th ed., p. 150). Philadelphia, PA: Lippincott, Williams & Wilkins.

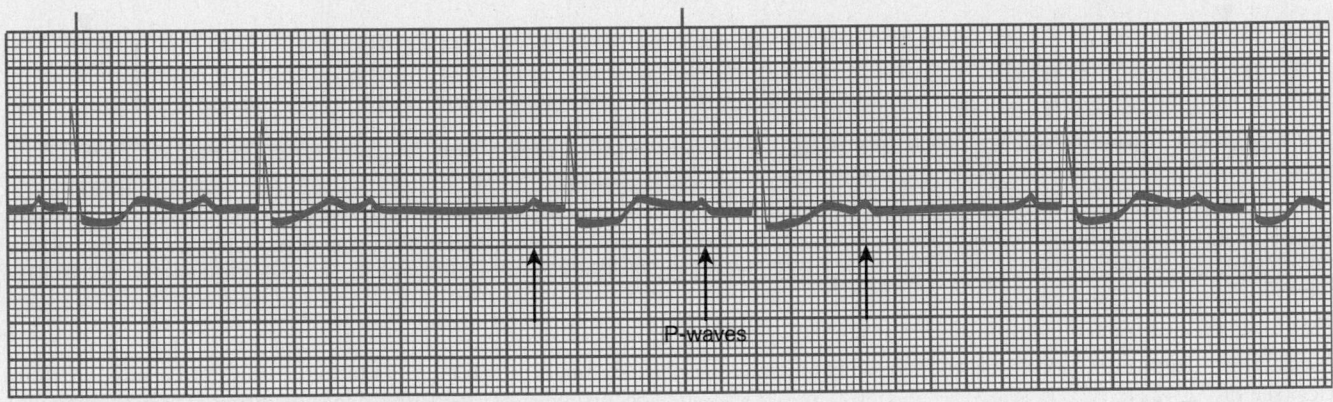

P-waves

Figure 22-20 • Second-degree atrioventricular block, type I. Note progressively longer PR durations until there is a nonconducted P wave. Reprinted with permission from Huff, J. (2017). *ECG Workout: Exercises in Arrhythmia Interpretation* (7th ed., Fig. 8-20). Philadelphia, PA: Wolters Kluwer.

Second-Degree Atrioventricular Block, Type I (Wenckebach)

Second-degree AV block, type I, occurs when there is a repeating pattern in which all but one of a series of atrial impulses are conducted through the AV node into the ventricles (e.g., every four of five atrial impulses are conducted). Each atrial impulse takes a longer time for conduction than the one before, until one impulse is fully blocked. Because the AV node is not depolarized by the blocked atrial impulse, the AV node has time to fully repolarize so that the next atrial impulse can be conducted within the shortest amount of time. Second-degree AV block, type I, has the following characteristics (see Fig. 22-20):

Ventricular and atrial rate: Depends on the underlying rhythm, but the ventricular rate is lower than the atrial rate

Ventricular and atrial rhythm: The PP interval is regular if the patient has an underlying normal sinus rhythm; the RR interval characteristically reflects a pattern of change. Starting from the RR that is the longest, the RR interval gradually shortens until there is another long RR interval

QRS shape and duration: Usually normal, but may be abnormal

P wave: In front of the QRS complex; shape depends on underlying rhythm.

PR interval: The PR interval becomes longer with each succeeding ECG complex until there is a P wave not followed by a QRS. The changes in the PR interval are repeated between each "dropped" QRS, creating a pattern in the irregular PR interval measurements

P:QRS ratio: 3:2, 4:3, 5:4, and so forth

Second-Degree Atrioventricular Block, Type II

Second-degree AV block, type II, occurs when only some of the atrial impulses are conducted through the AV node into the ventricles. Second-degree AV block, type II, has the following characteristics (see Fig. 22-21):

Ventricular and atrial rate: Depends on the underlying rhythm, but the ventricular rate is lower than the atrial rate

Ventricular and atrial rhythm: The PP interval is regular if the patient has an underlying normal sinus rhythm. The RR interval is usually regular but may be irregular, depending on the P:QRS ratio

QRS shape and duration: Usually abnormal, but may be normal

P wave: In front of the QRS complex; shape depends on underlying rhythm

PR interval: The PR interval is constant for those P waves just before QRS complexes

P:QRS ratio: 2:1, 3:1, 4:1, 5:1, and so forth

Third-Degree Atrioventricular Block

Third-degree AV block occurs when no atrial impulse is conducted through the AV node into the ventricles. In third-degree AV block, two impulses stimulate the heart: one stimulates the ventricles, represented by the QRS complex, and one stimulates the atria, represented by the P wave. P waves may be seen, but the atrial electrical activity is not conducted down into the ventricles to initiate the QRS complex, the ventricular electrical activity. Having two impulses stimulate the heart results in a condition referred to as AV dissociation, which may also occur during VT. Complete

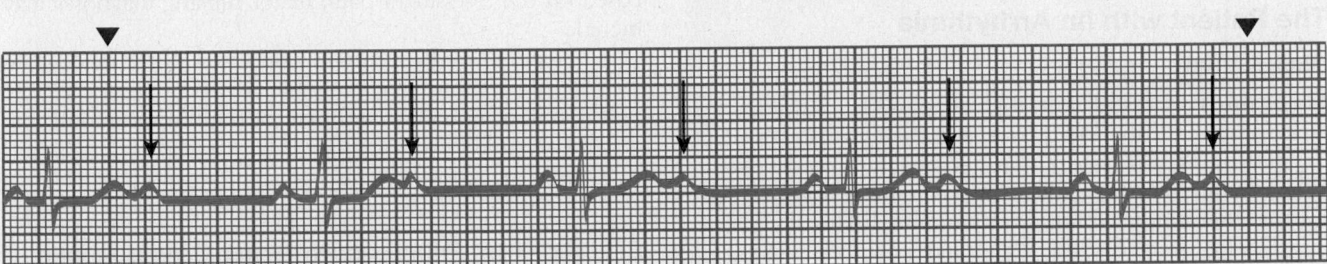

Figure 22-21 • Second-degree atrioventricular block, type II. Note constant PR interval and presence of more P waves than QRS complexes. Reprinted with permission from Morton, G. M., & Fontaine, D. K. (2018). *Critical care nursing: A holistic approach* (11th ed., Fig. 17–29C). Philadelphia, PA: Wolters Kluwer.

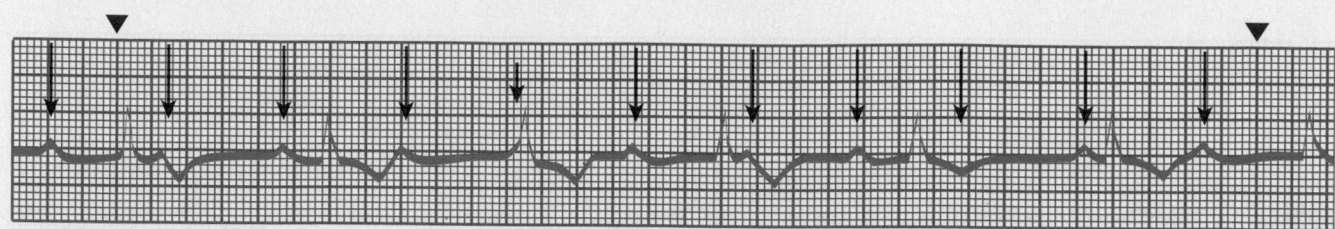

Figure 22-22 • Third-degree atrioventricular block; devoid relationship between P waves and QRS complexes. Reprinted with permission from Morton, G. M., & Fontaine, D. K. (2018). *Critical care nursing: A holistic approach* (11th ed., Fig. 17–29D). Philadelphia, PA: Wolters Kluwer.

block (third-degree AV block) has the following characteristics (see Fig. 22-22):

Ventricular and atrial rate: Depends on the escape rhythm (idionodal or idioventricular) and underlying atrial rhythm, but the ventricular rate is lower than the atrial rate

Ventricular and atrial rhythm: The PP interval is regular and the RR interval is regular, but the PP interval is not equal to the RR interval

QRS shape and duration: Depends on the escape rhythm; with junctional rhythm, QRS shape and duration are usually normal; with idioventricular rhythm, QRS shape and duration are usually abnormal

P wave: Depends on underlying rhythm

PR interval: Very irregular

P:QRS ratio: More P waves than QRS complexes

Medical Management of Conduction Abnormalities

Based on the cause of the AV block and the stability of the patient, treatment is directed toward increasing the heart rate to maintain a normal cardiac output. If the patient is stable and has no symptoms, no treatment may be indicated or it may simply consist of decreasing or eliminating the cause (e.g., withholding the medication or treatment). If the causal medication is necessary for treating other conditions and no effective alternative is available, pacemaker implantation may be indicated. The initial treatment of choice is an IV bolus of atropine, although it is not effective in second-degree AV block, type II, or third-degree AV block. If the patient does not respond to atropine, has advanced AV block, or has had an acute MI, temporary transcutaneous pacing may be started. If the patient has no pulse, treatment is the same as for ventricular asystole (Link et al., 2015; Soar et al., 2018). A permanent pacemaker may be necessary if the block persists (see later discussion).

NURSING PROCESS

The Patient with an Arrhythmia

Assessment

Major areas of assessment include possible causes of the arrhythmia, contributing factors, and the arrhythmia's effect on the heart's ability to pump an adequate blood volume. When cardiac output is reduced, the amount of oxygen reaching the tissues and vital organs is diminished. This diminished oxygenation produces the signs and symptoms associated with arrhythmias. If these signs and symptoms are severe or if they occur frequently, the patient may experience significant distress and disruption of daily life.

A health history is obtained to identify any previous occurrences of decreased cardiac output, such as syncope, lightheadedness, dizziness, fatigue, chest discomfort, and palpitations. Possible causes of the arrhythmia (e.g., heart disease, chronic obstructive pulmonary disease) need to be identified. All medications, prescribed and over-the-counter (including herbs and nutritional supplements), as well as the route of administration, are reviewed. If a patient is taking an antiarrhythmic medication, assessment for treatment adherence, side effects, adverse reactions, and potential contraindications is necessary. For example, some medications (e.g., digoxin) can cause arrhythmias. Laboratory results are reviewed to assess levels of medications as well as factors that could contribute to the arrhythmia (e.g., anemia). A thorough psychosocial assessment is performed to identify the possible effects of the arrhythmia, the patient's perception and understanding of the arrhythmia and its treatment, and whether anxiety is a significant contributing factor.

The nurse conducts a physical assessment to confirm the data obtained from the history and to observe for signs of diminished cardiac output during the arrhythmic event, especially changes in level of consciousness. The nurse assesses the patient's skin, which may be pale and cool. Signs of fluid retention, such as neck vein distention and crackles and wheezes auscultated in the lungs, may be detected. The rate and rhythm of apical and peripheral pulses are also assessed, and any pulse deficit is noted. The nurse auscultates for extra heart sounds (especially S_3 and S_4) and for heart murmurs, measures blood pressure, and determines pulse pressures. A declining pulse pressure indicates reduced cardiac output. One assessment may not disclose significant changes in cardiac output; therefore, the nurse compares multiple assessment findings over time, especially those that occur with and without the arrhythmia.

Diagnosis

NURSING DIAGNOSES

Based on the assessment data, major nursing diagnoses may include:

- Impaired cardiac output associated with inadequate ventricular filling or altered heart rate
- Anxiety associated with fear of the unknown outcome of altered health state
- Lack of knowledge about the arrhythmia and its treatment

COLLABORATIVE PROBLEMS/POTENTIAL COMPLICATIONS

Potential complications may include the following:

- Cardiac arrest (see Chapter 25)
- Heart failure (see Chapter 25)

- Thromboembolic event, especially with atrial fibrillation (see Chapter 26)

Planning and Goals

The major goals for the patient may include eliminating or decreasing the occurrence of the arrhythmia (by decreasing contributory factors) to maintain cardiac output; verbalizing reduction in anxiety; verbalizing an understanding about the arrhythmia, tests used to diagnose the problem, and its treatment; and developing or maintaining self-management skills.

Nursing Interventions

MONITORING AND MANAGING THE ARRHYTHMIA TO MAINTAIN CARDIAC OUTPUT

The nurse evaluates the patient's blood pressure, pulse rate and rhythm, rate and depth of respirations, and breath sounds on an ongoing basis to determine the arrhythmia's hemodynamic effect. The nurse also asks the patient about possible symptoms of the arrhythmia (e.g., episodes of lightheadedness, dizziness, or fainting) as part of the ongoing assessment. If a patient with an arrhythmia is hospitalized, the nurse may obtain a 12-lead ECG, continuously monitor the patient, and analyze rhythm strips to track the arrhythmia.

Control of the occurrence or the effect of the arrhythmia, or both, is often achieved with antiarrhythmic medications. The nurse assesses and observes for the benefits and adverse effects of each medication. The nurse, in collaboration with the primary provider, also manages medication administration carefully so that a constant serum level of the medication is maintained. The nurse may also conduct a 6-minute walk test as prescribed, which is used to identify the patient's ventricular rate in response to exercise. The patient is asked to walk for 6 minutes, covering as much distance as possible (Chen, Chen, Lu, et al., 2018). The nurse monitors the patient for symptoms. At the end, the nurse records the distance covered and the pre- and postexercise heart rate as well as the patient's response.

The nurse assesses for factors that contribute to the arrhythmia (e.g., oxygen deficits, acid–base and electrolyte imbalances, caffeine, or nonadherence to the medication regimen). The nurse also monitors for ECG changes (e.g., widening of the QRS, prolongation of the QT interval, increased heart rate) that increase the risk of an arrhythmic event.

REDUCING ANXIETY

When the patient experiences episodes of arrhythmia, the nurse stays with the patient and provides assurance of safety and security while maintaining a calm and reassuring attitude. This assists in reducing anxiety (reducing the sympathetic response) and fosters a trusting relationship with the patient. The nurse seeks the patient's view of the events and discusses the emotional response to the arrhythmia, encouraging verbalization of feelings and fears, providing supportive or empathetic statements, and assisting the patient to recognize feelings of anxiety, anger, or sadness. The nurse emphasizes successes with the patient to promote a sense of self-management of the arrhythmia. For example, if a patient is experiencing episodes of arrhythmia and a medication is given that begins to reduce the incidence of the arrhythmia, the nurse communicates that information to the patient and explores the patient's response to this information. In addition, the nurse can help the patient develop a system to identify possible causative, influencing, and alleviating factors (e.g., keeping a diary). The nursing goal is to maximize the patient's control and to make the episode less threatening.

PROMOTING HOME, COMMUNITY-BASED, AND TRANSITIONAL CARE

Educating Patients About Self-Care. When educating patients about arrhythmias, the nurse first assesses the patient's understanding, clarifies misinformation, and then shares needed information in terms that are understandable and in a manner that is not frightening or threatening. The nurse clearly explains the etiology of the arrhythmia and treatment options to the patient and family. If necessary, the nurse explains the importance of maintaining therapeutic serum levels of antiarrhythmic medications so that the patient understands why medications should be taken regularly each day and the importance of regular blood testing. If the medication has the potential to alter the heart rate, the patient should be taught how to take their pulse before each dose and to notify the primary provider if the pulse is abnormal. In addition, the relationship between an arrhythmia and cardiac output is explained so that the patient recognizes symptoms of the arrhythmia and the rationale for the treatment regimen. If the patient is prescribed an anticoagulant medication, patient education points about taking anticoagulant medications are summarized in Chapter 26, Chart 26-10. The patient and family need to be educated about measures to take to decrease the risk of recurrence of the arrhythmia. If the patient has a potentially lethal arrhythmia, the nurse establishes with the patient and family a plan of action to take in case of an emergency and, if appropriate, encourages a family member to obtain CPR training.

The patient and family should also be educated about potential risks of the arrhythmia and their signs and symptoms. For example, the patient with atrial fibrillation should be educated about the possibility of an embolic event.

Continuing and Transitional Care. A referral for home, community-based, or transitional care usually is not necessary for the patient with an arrhythmia unless the patient is hemodynamically unstable and has significant symptoms of decreased cardiac output. Home, community-based, or transitional care may be warranted if the patient has significant comorbidities, socioeconomic issues, or limited self-management skills that could increase the risk of nonadherence to the therapeutic regimen. A referral may also be indicated if the patient has had an electronic device implanted recently.

Evaluation

Expected patient outcomes may include:
1. Maintains cardiac output
   a. Demonstrates heart rate, blood pressure, respiratory rate, and level of consciousness within normal ranges
   b. Demonstrates no or decreased episodes of arrhythmia
2. Experiences reduced anxiety
   a. Expresses a positive attitude about living with the arrhythmia
   b. Expresses confidence in ability to take appropriate actions in an emergency

3. Expresses understanding of the arrhythmia and its treatment
   a. Explains the arrhythmia and its effects
   b. Describes the medication regimen and its rationale
   c. Explains the need to maintain a therapeutic serum level of the medication
   d. Describes a plan to eliminate or limit factors that contribute to the arrhythmia
   e. States actions to take in the event of an emergency

ADJUNCT MODALITIES AND MANAGEMENT

Arrhythmia treatments depend on whether the disorder is acute or chronic, as well as on the cause of the arrhythmia and its actual or potential hemodynamic effects.

Acute arrhythmias may be treated with medications or with external electrical therapy (emergency defibrillation, cardioversion, or pacing). Many antiarrhythmic medications are used to treat atrial and ventricular tachyarrhythmias (see Table 22-1). The choice of medication depends on the specific arrhythmia and its duration, the presence of structural heart disease (e.g., heart failure), and the patient's response to previous treatment. The nurse is responsible for monitoring and documenting the patient's responses to the medication and for ensuring that the patient has the knowledge and ability to manage the medication regimen.

If medications alone are ineffective in eliminating or decreasing the arrhythmia, certain adjunct mechanical therapies are available. The most common therapies are elective cardioversion and defibrillation for acute tachyarrhythmia, and implantable electronic devices for bradycardias (pacemakers) and chronic tachyarrhythmias (ICDs). Surgical treatments, although less common, are also available. The nurse is responsible for assessing the patient's understanding of and response to mechanical therapy, as well as the patient's self-management abilities. The nurse explains that the purpose of the device is to help the patient lead a life that is as active and productive as possible.

Cardioversion and Defibrillation

Cardioversion and defibrillation are used to treat tachyarrhythmias by delivering an electrical current that depolarizes a critical mass of myocardial cells. When the cells repolarize, the SA node is usually able to recapture its role as the heart's pacemaker.

 Concept Mastery Alert

One major difference between cardioversion and defibrillation is the timing of the delivery of electrical current. In cardioversion, the delivery of the electrical current is synchronized with the patient's electrical events; in defibrillation, the delivery of the current is immediate and unsynchronized.

The same type of device, called a *defibrillator*, is used for both cardioversion and defibrillation. The electrical voltage required to defibrillate the heart is usually greater than that required for cardioversion and may cause more myocardial

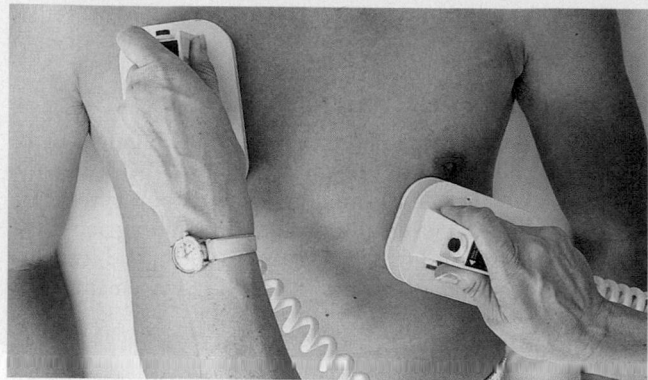

Figure 22-23 • Standard paddle placement for defibrillation.

damage. Only biphasic types of defibrillators are now manufactured; these deliver an electrical charge from one paddle that then automatically redirects its charge back to the originating paddle. Because the delivery of the electrical charge varies among devices, the manufacturer's recommended dose should be followed for the first and subsequent defibrillations (Link et al., 2015; Soar et al., 2018).

The electrical current may be delivered externally through the skin with the use of paddles or with conductor pads. The paddles or pads may be placed on the front of the chest (standard placement) (see Fig. 22-23), or one pad may be placed on the front of the chest and the other pad placed under the patient's back just left of the spine (anteroposterior placement) (see Fig. 22-24).

Defibrillator multifunction conductor pads contain a conductive medium and are connected to the defibrillator to allow for hands-off defibrillation. This method reduces the risk of touching the patient during the procedure and increases electrical safety. Automated external defibrillators (AEDs), which are now found in many public areas, use this type of delivery for the electrical current.

▶ *Quality and Safety Nursing Alert*

When using paddles, the appropriate conductant is applied between the paddles and the patient's skin. Any other type of conductant, such as ultrasound gel, should not be substituted.

Whether using pads or paddles, the nurse must observe two safety measures. First, good contact must be maintained between the pads or paddles and the patient's skin (with a

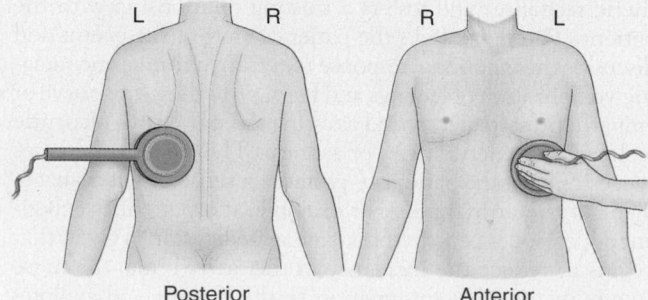

Figure 22-24 • Anteroposterior paddle placement for defibrillation.

Chart 22-5 Assisting with External Defibrillation or Cardioversion

When assisting with external defibrillation or cardioversion, the nurse should remember these key points:

- Multifunction conductor pads or paddles are used, with a conducting medium between the paddles and the skin in the proper locations. The conducting medium is available as a sheet, gel, or paste. Gels or pastes with poor electrical conductivity (e.g., ultrasound gel) should not be used.
- Paddles or pads should be placed so that they do not touch the patient's clothing or bed linen and are not near medication patches or in the direct flow of oxygen.
- Women with large breasts should have the left pad or paddle placed underneath or lateral to the left breast.
- During cardioversion, the monitor leads must be attached to the patient in order to set the defibrillator to the synchronized mode ("in sync"). If defibrillating, the defibrillator must *not* be in the synchronized mode (most machines default to the "not-sync" mode).
- When using paddles, 20–25 lb of pressure must be used in order to ensure good skin contact.
- When using a manual discharge device, it must not be charged until it is ready to shock; then thumbs and fingers must be kept off the discharge buttons until paddles or pads are on the chest and ready to deliver the electrical charge.
- When it is time to defibrillate, whomever is delivering the charge should announce, "charging to (number of joules)" prior to discharging.

- "Clear!" must be called three times before discharging: As "Clear" is called the first time, the discharger must visually check that they are not touching the patient, bed, or equipment; as "Clear" is called the second time, the discharger must visually check that no one else is touching the bed, the patient, or equipment, including the endotracheal tube or adjuncts; and as "Clear" is called the third time, the discharger must perform a final visual check to ensure that everyone is clear of the patient and anything touching the patient.
- The delivered energy and resulting rhythm are recorded.
- Cardiopulmonary resuscitation (CPR) is immediately resumed after the defibrillation charge is delivered, if appropriate, starting with chest compressions.
- If CPR is necessary, after five cycles (about 2 minutes) of CPR, the cardiac rhythm is checked again and another shock is delivered, if warranted. A vasoactive or antiarrhythmic medication is given as soon as possible after the rhythm check to facilitate a positive response to defibrillation.
- After the event is complete, the skin under the pads or paddles is inspected for burns; if any are detected, the primary provider or a wound care nurse is consulted about appropriate treatment.
- The defibrillator is plugged back into an outlet, and supplies are restocked as needed.

Adapted from Link, M. S., Berkow, L. C., Kudenchuk, P. J., et al. (2015). Part 7: Adult advanced cardiovascular life support: 2015 American Heart Association guidelines update for cardiopulmonary resuscitation and emergency cardiovascular care. *Circulation, 132*(18 supp 2), S444–S464; Soar, J., Donnino, M. W., Maconochie, I., et al. (2018). 2018 International consensus on cardiopulmonary resuscitation and emergency cardiovascular care science with treatment recommendations summary. *Resuscitation, 133*, 194–206.

conductive medium between them) to prevent electrical current from leaking through the air (arcing) when the defibrillator is discharged. Second, no one is to be in contact with the patient or with anything that is touching the patient when the defibrillator is discharged, to minimize the chance that electrical current is conducted to anyone other than the patient. Chart 22-5 provides a review of nursing responsibility when a patient is cardioverted or defibrillated.

Electrical Cardioversion

Electrical cardioversion involves the delivery of a "timed" electrical current to terminate a tachyarrhythmia. In cardioversion, the defibrillator is set to synchronize with the ECG on a cardiac monitor so that the electrical impulse discharges during ventricular depolarization (QRS complex). The synchronization prevents the discharge from occurring during the vulnerable period of repolarization (T wave), which could result in VT or ventricular fibrillation. The ECG monitor connected to the external defibrillator usually displays a mark or line that indicates sensing of a QRS complex. Sometimes the lead and the electrodes must be changed for the monitor to recognize the patient's QRS complex. When the synchronizer is on, no electrical current is delivered if the defibrillator does not discern a QRS complex. Therefore, it is important to ensure that the patient is connected to the monitor and to select a lead (not "paddles") that has the most appropriate sensing of the QRS. Because there may be a short delay until recognition of the QRS, the discharge buttons of an external

manual defibrillator must be held down until the shock has been delivered. In most monitors, the synchronization mode must be reactivated if the initial cardioversion was ineffective and another cardioversion is needed (i.e., the device defaults to unsynchronized defibrillation mode).

If the cardioversion is elective and the arrhythmia has lasted longer than 48 hours, anticoagulation for a few weeks before cardioversion may be indicated (January et al., 2014, 2019). Digoxin is usually withheld for 48 hours before cardioversion to ensure the resumption of sinus rhythm with normal conduction. The patient is instructed not to eat or drink for at least 4 hours before the procedure. Gel-covered paddles or conductor pads are positioned anteroposteriorly (front and back) for cardioversion. Before cardioversion, the patient receives moderate sedation IV as well as an analgesic medication or anesthesia. Respiration is then supported with supplemental oxygen delivered by a bag-valve mask device with suction equipment readily available. Although patients rarely require intubation, equipment is nearby in case it is needed. The amount of voltage used varies from 50 to 360 joules, depending on the defibrillator's technology, the type and duration of the arrhythmia, and the size and hemodynamic status of the patient (Link et al., 2015; Soar et al., 2018).

Indications of a successful response are conversion to sinus rhythm, adequate peripheral pulses, and adequate blood pressure. Because of the sedation, airway patency must be maintained and the patient's state of consciousness assessed. Vital signs and oxygen saturation are monitored and recorded until the patient is stable and recovered from sedation and analgesic medications or anesthesia. ECG monitoring is required during and after cardioversion (Link et al., 2015; Soar et al., 2018).

Defibrillation

Defibrillation is used in emergency situations as the treatment of choice for ventricular fibrillation and pulseless VT, the most common cause of abrupt loss of cardiac function and sudden cardiac death. Defibrillation is not used for patients who are conscious or have a pulse. The energy setting for the initial and subsequent shocks using a monophasic defibrillator should be set at 360 joules (Link et al., 2015; Soar et al., 2018). The energy setting for the initial shock using a biphasic defibrillator may be set at 150 to 200 joules, with the same or an increasing dose with subsequent shocks (Link et al., 2015; Soar et al., 2018). The sooner defibrillation is used, the better the survival rate (Hedge & Gnugnoli, 2019). Several studies have demonstrated that early defibrillation performed by lay people in a community setting can increase the survival rate (Hedge & Gnugnoli, 2019). If immediate CPR is provided and defibrillation is performed within 5 minutes, more adults in ventricular fibrillation may survive with intact neurologic function (Link et al., 2015; Soar et al., 2018). The availability and the use of AEDs in public places can shorten the interval from collapse to rhythm recognition and defibrillation, which can significantly improve survival out of the hospital (Hedge & Gnugnoli, 2019).

Epinephrine is given after initial unsuccessful defibrillation to make it easier to convert the arrhythmia to a normal rhythm with the next defibrillation. This medication may also increase cerebral and coronary artery blood flow. Antiarrhythmic medications such as amiodarone, lidocaine, or magnesium may be given if ventricular arrhythmia persists (see Table 22-1). This treatment with continuous CPR, medication administration, and defibrillation continues until a stable rhythm resumes or until it is determined that the patient cannot be revived.

Electrophysiology Studies

An EPS is an invasive procedure used to evaluate and treat various chronic arrhythmias that have caused cardiac arrest or significant symptoms. It also is indicated for patients with symptoms that suggest an arrhythmia that has gone undetected and undiagnosed by other methods. Because an EPS is invasive, it is performed in the hospital and may require that the patient be admitted. An EPS is used to do the following:

- Identify the impulse formation and propagation through the cardiac electrical conduction system
- Assess the function or dysfunction of the SA and AV nodal areas
- Identify the location (called *mapping*) and mechanism of the arrhythmogenic foci (the exact site where the arrhythmia originates)
- Assess the effectiveness of antiarrhythmic medications and devices for the patient with an arrhythmia
- Treat certain arrhythmias through the destruction of the causative cells (ablation)

An EPS procedure is a type of cardiac catheterization that is performed in a specially equipped cardiac catheterization laboratory by an electrophysiologist, assisted by other EPS laboratory personnel. The patient is conscious but lightly sedated. Usually, one or more catheters are inserted into the groin, neck, or antecubital fossa. The electrodes are positioned within the heart at specific locations—for instance, in the right atrium near the sinus node, in the coronary sinus, near the tricuspid valve, and at the apex of the right ventricle. The number and placement of electrodes depend on the type of study being conducted. These electrodes allow the electrical signal to be recorded from within the heart (intracardiogram).

The electrodes also allow the electrophysiologist to introduce a pacing stimulus to the intracardiac area at a precisely timed interval and rate, thereby stimulating the area (programmed stimulation). An area of the heart may be paced at a rate much faster than the normal rate of **automaticity**, the rate at which impulses are spontaneously formed (e.g., in the sinus node). This allows the pacemaker to become an artificial focus of automaticity and to assume control (overdrive suppression). Then, the pacemaker is stopped suddenly, and the time it takes for the sinus node to resume control is assessed. A prolonged time indicates dysfunction of the sinus node.

One of the main purposes of programmed stimulation is to assess the ability of the area surrounding the electrode to cause a reentry arrhythmia. One or a series of premature impulses is delivered to an area in an attempt to cause the tachyarrhythmia. Because the precise location of the suspected area and the specific timing of the pacing needed are unknown, the electrophysiologist uses many different techniques to cause the arrhythmia during the study. If the arrhythmia can be reproduced by programmed stimulation, it is called *inducible*. Once an arrhythmia is induced, a treatment plan is determined and implemented. If, on the follow-up EPS, the tachyarrhythmia cannot be induced, then the treatment is determined to be effective. Different medications may be given and combined with cardiac implantable electronic devices to determine the most effective treatment to suppress the arrhythmia.

Patient care, patient education, and associated complications of an EPS are similar to those associated with cardiac catheterization (see Chapter 21). The study is usually about 2 hours in length; however, if the electrophysiologist conducts not only a diagnostic procedure but also treatment, the study can take up to 6 hours. During the procedure, patients benefit from a calm, reassuring approach.

Patients who are to undergo an EPS may be anxious about the procedure and its outcome. A detailed discussion involving the patient, the family, and the electrophysiologist usually occurs to ensure that the patient can give informed consent and to reduce the patient's anxiety about the procedure. Before the procedure, the nurse educates the patient about the EPS and its usual duration, the environment where the procedure is performed, and what to expect. Although an EPS is not painful, it does cause discomfort and can be tiring. It may also cause feelings that were experienced when the arrhythmia occurred in the past. In addition, patients are educated about what will be expected of them (e.g., lying very still during the procedure, reporting symptoms or concerns).

The patient should also know that the arrhythmia may occur during the procedure. It often stops on its own; if it does not, treatment is given to restore the patient's normal rhythm. The arrhythmia may have to be terminated using cardioversion or defibrillation, but this is performed under more controlled circumstances than if performed in an emergency.

Postprocedural care is similar to that for cardiac catheterization, including restriction of activity to promote hemostasis at the insertion site (see Chapter 21). To identify any complications and to ensure healing, the patient's vital signs and the appearance of the insertion site are assessed frequently. Because an artery is not always used, there is a lower incidence of vascular complications than with other catheterization procedures (Zipes, Libby, Bonow, et al., 2018).

Pacemaker Therapy

A pacemaker is an electronic device that provides electrical stimuli to the heart muscle. Pacemakers are usually used when a patient has a permanent or temporary slower-than-normal impulse formation, or a symptomatic AV or ventricular conduction disturbance. They may also be used to control some tachyarrhythmias that do not respond to medication. Biventricular (both ventricles) pacing, also called **cardiac resynchronization therapy (CRT)**, may be used to treat advanced heart failure. Pacemaker technology also may be used in conjunction with an ICD.

Pacemakers can be permanent or temporary. Temporary pacemakers are used to support patients until they improve or receive a permanent pacemaker (e.g., after acute MI or during open heart surgery). Temporary pacemakers are used only in hospital settings.

Pacemaker Design and Types

Pacemakers consist of two components: an electronic pulse generator and pacemaker electrodes, which are located on leads or wires. The generator contains the circuitry and batteries that determine the rate (measured in beats per minute) and the strength or output (measured in milliamperes [mA]) of the electrical stimulus delivered to the heart. The generator also has circuitry that can detect the intracardiac electrical activity to cause an appropriate response; this component of pacing is called *sensitivity* and is measured in millivolts (mV). Sensitivity is set at the level that the intracardiac electrical activity must exceed to be sensed by the device. Leads, which carry the impulse created by the generator to the heart, can be threaded by fluoroscopy through a major vein into the heart, usually the right atrium and ventricle (endocardial leads), or they can be lightly sutured onto the outside of the heart and brought through the chest wall during open heart surgery (epicardial wires). These epicardial pacemakers are typically temporary and are removed by a gentle tug a few days after surgery. The endocardial leads may be temporarily placed with catheters through a vein (usually the femoral, subclavian, or internal jugular vein [transvenous wires]), usually guided by fluoroscopy. The leads may also be part of a specialized pulmonary artery catheter (see Chapter 21). However, obtaining a pulmonary artery wedge pressure may cause the leads to move out of pacing position. The endocardial and epicardial wires are connected to a temporary generator, which is about the size of a cellular phone. The energy source for a temporary generator is a common household battery. Monitoring for pacemaker malfunctioning and battery failure is a nursing responsibility.

The endocardial leads also may be placed permanently, passed into the heart through the subclavian, axillary, or cephalic vein, and connected to a permanent generator.

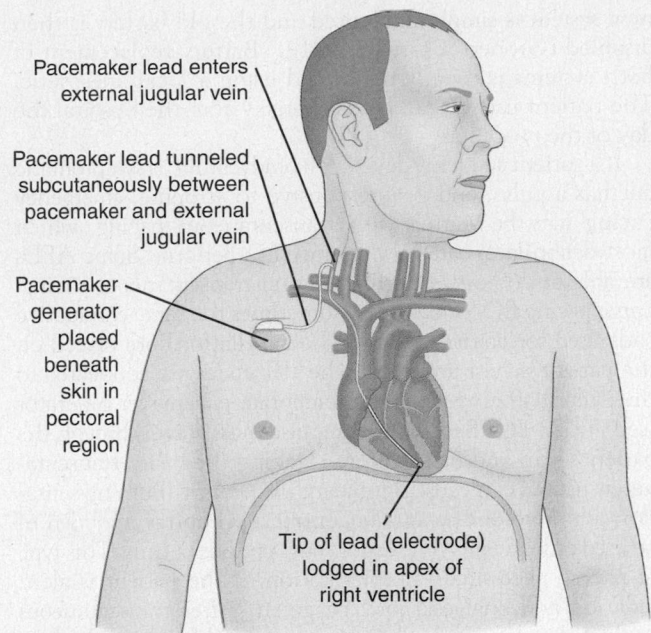

Figure 22-25 • Implanted transvenous pacing lead (with electrode) and pacemaker generator.

Labels on figure:
Pacemaker lead enters external jugular vein
Pacemaker lead tunneled subcutaneously between pacemaker and external jugular vein
Pacemaker generator placed beneath skin in pectoral region
Tip of lead (electrode) lodged in apex of right ventricle

These types of pacemakers are sometimes also called transvenous pacemakers. Most current leads have a fixation mechanism (e.g., a screw) at the end of the lead that allows precise positioning and avoidance of dislodgement. The permanent generator, which often weighs less than 1 ounce and is the size of a pack of chewing gum, is usually implanted in a subcutaneous pocket created in the pectoral region, below the clavicle in men, or behind the breast in women (see Fig. 22-25). This procedure usually takes about 1 hour, and it is performed in a cardiac catheterization laboratory using a local anesthetic and moderate sedation. Close monitoring of the respiratory status is needed until the patient is fully awake.

Leadless pacemakers, a newer type of permanent pacemaker, are 90% smaller than transvenous pacemakers. They feature a self-contained, single-unit pulse generator and electrode that is inserted transvenously directly into the right ventricle (Groner & Grippe, 2019; Hayes, 2018).

Permanent pacemaker generators are insulated to protect against body moisture and warmth and have filters that protect them from electrical interference from most household devices, motors, and appliances. Lithium cells are most commonly used; they last approximately 5 to 15 years, depending on the type of pacemaker, how it is programmed, and how often it is used. Most pacemakers have an elective replacement indicator (ERI), which is a signal that indicates when the battery is approaching depletion. The pacemaker continues to function for several months after the appearance of ERI to ensure that there is adequate time for a battery replacement. Although some batteries are rechargeable, most are not. Because the battery is permanently sealed in the pacemaker, the entire generator must be replaced. To replace a failing generator of a transvenous pacemaker, the leads are disconnected, the old generator is removed, and a new generator is reconnected to the existing leads and reimplanted in the already existing subcutaneous pocket. Sometimes the leads are also replaced. When leadless pacemaker batteries signal that they must be replaced, a new system is simply implanted and the old battery is then disabled (Groner & Grippe, 2019). Battery replacement of both systems is usually performed using a local anesthetic. The patient usually can be discharged from the hospital the day of the procedure.

If a patient suddenly develops a bradycardia, is symptomatic but has a pulse, and is unresponsive to atropine, emergency pacing may be started with transcutaneous pacing, which most defibrillators are now equipped to perform. Some AEDs are able to do both defibrillation and transcutaneous pacing. Large pacing ECG electrodes (sometimes the same conductive pads used for cardioversion and defibrillation) are placed on the patient's chest and back. The electrodes are connected to the defibrillator, which is the temporary pacemaker generator (see Fig. 22-26). Because the impulse must travel through the patient's skin and tissue before reaching the heart, transcutaneous pacing can cause significant discomfort (burning sensation and involuntary muscle contraction) and is intended to be used only in emergencies for short periods of time. This type of pacing necessitates hospitalization. If the patient is alert, sedation and analgesia may be given. After transcutaneous pacing, the skin under the electrode should be inspected for erythema and burns. Transcutaneous pacing is not indicated for pulseless bradycardia (Link et al., 2015; Soar et al., 2018).

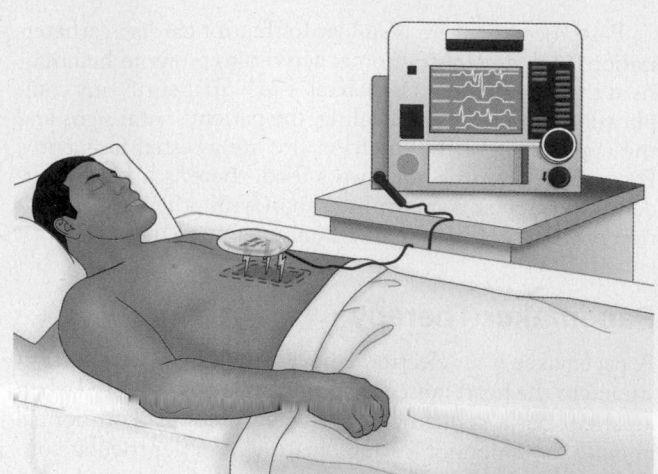

Figure 22-26 • Transcutaneous pacemaker with electrode pads connected to the anterior and posterior chest walls.

Pacemaker Generator Functions

Because of the sophistication and wide use of pacemakers, a universal code has been adopted to provide a means of safe communication about their function. The coding is referred to as the NASPE-BPEG code because it is sanctioned by the North American Society of Pacing and Electrophysiology and the British Pacing and Electrophysiology Group. The complete code consists of five letters; the fourth and fifth letters are used only with permanent pacemakers (Bernstein, Daubert, Fletcher, et al., 2002; Mulpuru, Madhavan, McLeod, et al., 2017; Tracy, Epstein, Darbar, et al., 2012; see Chart 22-6).

Chart 22-6

North American Society of Pacing and Electrophysiology and the British Pacing and Electrophysiology Group Code (NASPE-BPEG Code) for Pacemaker Generator Function

- The first letter of the code identifies the chamber or chambers being paced (i.e., the chamber containing a pacing electrode). The letter characters for this code are A (atrium), V (ventricle), or D (dual, meaning both A and V).
- The second letter identifies the chamber or chambers being sensed by the pacemaker generator. Information from the electrode within the chamber is sent to the generator for interpretation and action by the generator. The letter characters are A (atrium), V (ventricle), D (dual), and O (indicating that the sensing function is turned off).
- The third letter of the code describes the type of response that will be made by the pacemaker to what is sensed. The letter characters used to describe this response are I (inhibited), T (triggered), D (dual—inhibited and triggered), and O (none). Inhibited response means that the response of the pacemaker is controlled by the activity of the patient's heart—that is, when the patient's heart beats, the pacemaker does not function, but when the heart does not beat, the pacemaker does function. In contrast, a triggered response means that the pacemaker responds (paces the heart) when it senses intrinsic heart activity.
- The fourth letter of the code is related to a permanent generator's ability to vary the heart rate. This ability is available in most current pacemakers. The possible letters are O, indicating no rate responsiveness, or R, indicating that the generator

has rate modulation (i.e., the pacemaker has the ability to automatically adjust the pacing rate from moment to moment based on parameters, such as QT interval, physical activity, acid–base changes, body temperature, rate and depth of respirations, or oxygen saturation). A pacemaker with rate-responsive ability is capable of improving cardiac output during times of increased cardiac demand, such as exercise and decreasing the incidence of atrial fibrillation. All contemporary pacemakers have some type of sensor system that enables them to provide rate-adaptive pacing.

- The fifth letter of the code has two different indications: (1) that the permanent generator has multisite pacing capability with the letters A (atrium), V (ventricle), D (dual), and O (none); or (2) that the pacemaker has an antitachycardia function.
- Commonly, only the first three letters are used for a pacing code. An example of an NASPE-BPEG code is DVI:
  D: Both the atrium and the ventricle have a pacing electrode in place.
  V: The pacemaker is sensing the activity of the ventricle only.
  I: The pacemaker's stimulating effect is inhibited by ventricular activity—in other words, it does not create an impulse when the pacemaker senses that the patient's ventricle is active.

Adapted from Bernstein, A. D., Daubert, J-C., Fletcher, R. D., et al. (2002). The revised NASPE/BPEG generic code for antibradycardia, adaptive-rate, and multisite pacing. North American Society of Pacing and Electrophysiology/British Pacing and Electrophysiology Group. *Pacing and Clinical Electrophysiology, 25*(2), 260–264; Gillis, A. M., Russo, A. M., Ellenbogen, K. A., et al. (2012). HRS/ACCF expert consensus statement on pacemaker device and mode selection. *Journal of American College of Cardiology, 60*(7), 682–703; Mulpuru, S. K., Madhavan, M., McLeod, C. J., et al. (2017). Cardiac pacemakers: Function, troubleshooting, and management: Part 1 of a 2-Part Series. *Journal of the American College of Cardiology, 69*(2), 189–210.

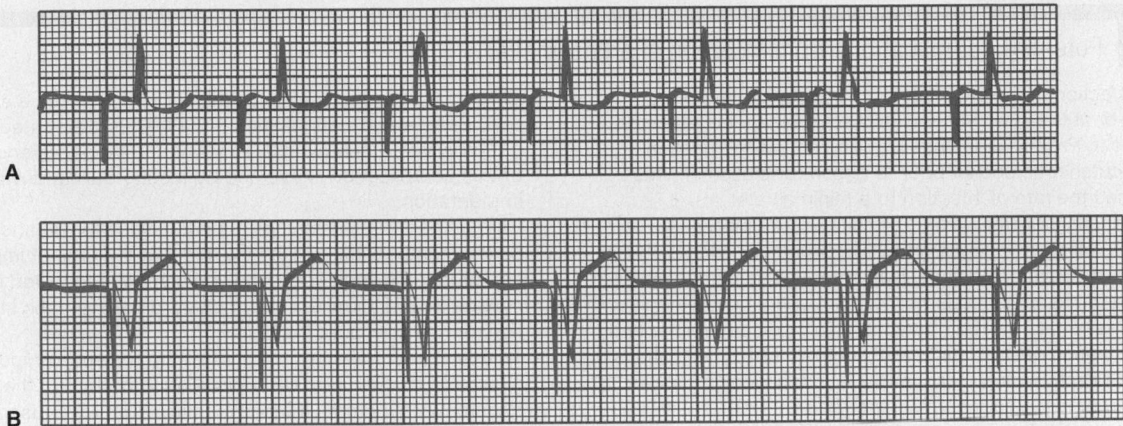

Figure 22-27 • Pacemaker capture. **A.** Atrial pacemaker; note that each vertical pacemaker spike is followed by a P wave. **B.** Ventricular pacemaker; note that each vertical pacemaker spike is followed by a QRS complex. Reprinted with permission from Morton, G. M., & Fontaine, D. K. (2018). *Critical care nursing: A holistic approach* (11th ed., Fig. 18–34A and B). Philadelphia, PA: Wolters Kluwer.

The pacemaker paces the atrium and then the ventricle when no ventricular activity is sensed for a period of time (the time is individually programmed into the pacemaker for each patient). A straight vertical line usually can be seen on the ECG when pacing is initiated. The line that represents pacing is called a *pacemaker spike*. The appropriate ECG complex should immediately follow the pacing spike; therefore, a P wave should follow an atrial pacing spike (see Fig. 22-27A) and a QRS complex should follow a ventricular pacing spike (see Fig. 22-27B). Because the impulse starts in a different place than the patient's normal rhythm, the QRS complex or P wave that responds to pacing looks different from the patient's normal ECG complex. *Capture* is a term used to denote that the appropriate complex followed the pacing spike.

The type of pacemaker generator and the settings selected depend on the patient's arrhythmia, underlying cardiac function, and age. Pacemakers are generally set to sense and respond to intrinsic activity, which is called *on-demand pacing*. If the pacemaker is set to pace but not to sense, it is called a *fixed* or *asynchronous pacemaker*; this is written in pacing code as AOO or VOO. The pacemaker paces at a constant rate, independent of the patient's intrinsic rhythm. VOO pacing may indicate battery failure.

VVI (V, paces the ventricle; V, senses ventricular activity; I, paces only if the ventricles do not depolarize) pacing causes loss of AV synchrony and atrial kick, which may cause a decrease in cardiac output and an increase in atrial distention and venous congestion. Pacemaker syndrome, causing symptoms such as chest discomfort, shortness of breath, fatigue, activity intolerance, and orthostatic hypotension, is most common with VVI pacing (Mulpuru et al., 2017; Tracy et al., 2012). Atrial pacing and dual-chamber (right atrial and RV) pacing have been found to reduce the incidence of atrial fibrillation, ventricular dysfunction, and heart failure (Mulpuru et al., 2017; Tracy et al., 2012).

Single-chamber atrial pacing (AAI) or dual-chamber pacing (DDD) is recommended over VVI in patients with sinus node dysfunction, the most common cause of bradycardias requiring a pacemaker, and a functioning AV node (Mulpuru et al., 2017; Tracy et al., 2012). AAI pacing ensures synchrony between atrial and ventricular stimulation (and therefore contraction), as long as the patient has no conduction disturbances in the AV node. Dual-chamber pacemakers are recommended as the treatment for patients with AV conduction disturbances (Mulpuru et al., 2017; Tracy et al., 2012).

Synchronized biventricular pacing, also called *cardiac resynchronization therapy (CRT)*, is associated with improved mortality rates in patients with heart failure and in patients with left bundle branch block (Agrawal, 2018). Synchronized biventricular pacing features three leads: one for the right atrium; one for the right ventricle; and one for the left ventricle, usually placed in the left lateral wall. This therapy improves cardiac function, resulting in decreased heart failure symptoms and an improved quality of life. Biventricular pacing may be used with an ICD (Agrawal, 2018).

Complications of Pacemaker Use

Complications associated with pacemakers relate to their presence within the body and improper functioning (see Chart 22-7). In the initial hours after a temporary or permanent pacemaker is inserted, the most common complication is dislodgment of the pacing electrode. Minimizing patient activity can help prevent this complication. If a temporary electrode is in place, the extremity through which the catheter has been advanced is immobilized. With a permanent pacemaker, the patient is instructed initially to restrict activity on the side of the implantation.

Leadless pacemakers are associated with fewer complications than transvenous pacemakers, including fewer infections, hematomas, lead dislodgement, and lead fracture. However, they provide only single-chamber RV pacing and do not feature concomitant defibrillator capabilities, limiting their usefulness (Groner & Grippe, 2019; Hayes, 2018).

The ECG is monitored very carefully to detect pacemaker malfunction. Improper pacemaker function, which can arise from failure in one or more components of the pacing system, is outlined in Table 22-2. The following data should be noted on the patient's record: model of pacemaker, type of generator, date and time of insertion, location of pulse generator, stimulation threshold, and pacer settings (e.g., rate, energy output [mA], sensitivity [mV], and duration of interval between atrial and ventricular impulses [AV delay]). This information is important for identifying normal pacemaker function and diagnosing pacemaker malfunction.

Chart 22-7 Potential Complications from Insertion of a Pacemaker

- Local infection at the entry site of the leads for temporary pacing, or at the subcutaneous site for permanent generator placement. Prophylactic antibiotic and antibiotic irrigation of the subcutaneous pocket prior to generator placement has decreased the rate of infection to a minimal rate.
- Pneumothorax or hemothorax. The risk is reduced if cephalic vein cut down, contrast venography, or ultrasound guidance is utilized.
- Bleeding and hematoma at the lead entry sites for temporary pacing, or at the subcutaneous site for permanent generator placement. This usually can be managed with cold compresses and discontinuation of antiplatelet and antithrombotic medications.
- Ventricular ectopy and tachycardia from irritation of the ventricular wall by the endocardial electrode.
- Movement or dislocation of the lead placed transvenously (perforation of the myocardium).

- Phrenic nerve, diaphragmatic (hiccupping may be a sign), or skeletal muscle stimulation if the lead is dislocated or if the delivered energy (mA) is set high. The occurrence of this complication is avoided by testing during device implantation.
- Cardiac perforation resulting in pericardial effusion and, rarely, cardiac tamponade, which may occur at the time of implantation or months later. This condition can be recognized by the change in QRS complex morphology, diaphragmatic stimulation, or hemodynamic instability.
- Twiddler syndrome may occur when the patient manipulates the generator, causing lead dislodgement or fracture of the lead.
- Pacemaker syndrome (hemodynamic instability caused by ventricular pacing and the loss of AV synchrony).

Adapted from Link, M. S., Berkow, L. C., Kudenchuk, P. J., et al. (2015). Part 7: Adult advanced cardiovascular life support: 2015 American Heart Association guidelines update for cardiopulmonary resuscitation and emergency cardiovascular care. *Circulation, 132*(18 suppl 2), S444–S464; Mulpuru, S. K., Madhavan, M., McLeod, C. J., et al. (2017). Cardiac pacemakers: Function, troubleshooting, and management: Part 1 of a 2-Part Series. *Journal of the American College of Cardiology, 69*(2), 189–210; Soar, J., Donnino, M. W., Maconochie, I., et al. (2018). 2018 International consensus on cardiopulmonary resuscitation and emergency cardiovascular care science with treatment recommendations summary. *Resuscitation, 133,* 194–206; Tracy, C. M., Epstein, A. E., Darbar, D., et al. (2012). ACCF/AHA/HRS focused update of the 2008 guidelines for device-based therapy of cardiac rhythm abnormalities: A report of the American College of Cardiology Foundation/American Heart Association Task Force on Practice Guidelines. *Journal of the American College of Cardiology, 60*(14), 1297–1313.

A patient experiencing pacemaker malfunction may develop bradycardia as well as signs and symptoms of decreased cardiac output (e.g., diaphoresis, orthostatic hypotension, syncope). The degree to which these symptoms become apparent depends on the severity of the malfunction, the patient's level of dependency on the pacemaker, and the patient's underlying condition. Pacemaker malfunction is diagnosed by analyzing the ECG. Manipulating the

TABLE 22-2 Assessing Pacemaker Malfunction

Problem	Possible Cause	Nursing Considerations
Loss of capture—complex does *not* follow pacing spike	Inadequate stimulus Lead dislodgement Lead wire fracture Catheter malposition Battery depletion Electronic insulation break Medication change Myocardial ischemia	Check security of all connections; increase milliamperage. Reposition extremity; turn patient to left side. Change battery. Change generator.
Undersensing—pacing spike occurs at preset interval despite the patient's intrinsic rhythm	Sensitivity too high Electrical interference (e.g., by a magnet) Faulty generator	Decrease sensitivity. Eliminate interference. Replace generator.
Oversensing—loss of pacing artifact; pacing does not occur at preset interval despite the lack of intrinsic rhythm	Sensitivity too low Electrical interference Battery depletion Change in medication	Increase sensitivity. Eliminate interference. Change battery.
Loss of pacing—total absence of pacing spikes	Oversensing Battery depletion Loose or disconnected wires Perforation	Change battery. Check security of all connections. Apply magnet over permanent generator. Obtain 12-lead ECG and portable chest x-ray. Assess for murmur. Contact physician.
Change in pacing QRS shape	Septal perforation	Obtain 12-lead ECG and portable chest x-ray. Assess for murmur. Contact physician.
Rhythmic diaphragmatic or chest wall twitching or hiccupping	Output too high Myocardial wall perforation	Decrease milliamperage. Turn pacer off. Contact physician at once. Monitor closely for decreased cardiac output.

ECG, electrocardiogram.
Adapted from Mulpuru, S. K., Madhavan, M., McLeod, C. J., et al. (2017). Cardiac pacemakers: Function, troubleshooting, and management: Part 1 of a 2-Part Series. *Journal of the American College of Cardiology, 69*(2), 189–210.

electrodes, changing the generator's settings, or replacing the pacemaker generator or leads (or both) may be necessary.

Inhibition of permanent pacemakers or reversion to asynchronous fixed rate pacing can occur with exposure to strong electromagnetic fields (electromagnetic interference [EMI]). However, pacemaker technology allows patients to safely use most household electronic appliances and devices (e.g., microwave ovens, electric tools). Gas-powered engines should be turned off before working on them. Objects that contain magnets (e.g., the earpiece of a phone, large stereo speakers, jewelry) should not be near the generator for longer than a few seconds. Patients are advised to place digital cellular phones at least 6 to 12 inches away from (or on the side opposite of) the pacemaker generator and not to carry them in a shirt pocket. Large electromagnetic fields, such as those produced by magnetic resonance imaging (MRI), radio and television transmitter towers and lines, transmission power lines (not the distribution lines that bring electricity into a home), and electrical substations may cause EMI. Patients should be cautioned to avoid such situations or to simply move farther away from the area if they experience dizziness or a feeling of rapid or irregular heartbeats (palpitations). Welding and the use of a chain saw should be avoided. If such tools are used, precautionary steps such as limiting the welding current to a 60- to 130-ampere range or using electric rather than gasoline-powered chain saws are advised.

In addition, the metal of the pacemaker generator may trigger store and library antitheft devices as well as airport and building security alarms; however, these alarm systems generally do not interfere with the pacemaker function. Patients should walk through them quickly and avoid standing in or near these devices for prolonged periods of time. The hand-held screening devices used in airports may interfere with the pacemaker. Patients should be advised to ask security personnel to perform a hand search instead of using the handheld screening device. Patients also should be educated to wear or carry medical identification to alert personnel to the presence of the pacemaker.

Pacemaker Surveillance

Remote monitoring technology is now routinely embedded in the pacemaker so that it replaces the need for frequent in-person follow-up cardiologist visits; this is also associated with improved survival (Costa, Yeung, Gilbert, et al., 2018). Remote monitoring systems in use include transtelephonic monitoring (use of an analog phone with transmission through a landline), inductive monitoring (use of a wand with transmission through a landline or a cellular connection), and remote wandless monitoring (use of wandless transmitter through radiofrequency) (Madhavan, Mulpuru, McLeod, et al., 2017). Remote monitoring allows pertinent information, such as ECG data, to be transmitted to the primary provider at the cardiology clinic. In addition, the pacemaker rate and other data concerning pacemaker function (e.g., generator setting, battery status, sensing function, lead integrity, pacing data, such as number of pacing events) are obtained and evaluated by the cardiologist. This simplifies the diagnosis of a failing generator, reassures the patient, and improves management when the patient is physically remote from pacemaker testing facilities. A follow-up schedule is variable, and is dependent upon the patient's needs and the pacemaker in use; the system is setup for maintenance checks on an annual basis.

Implantable Cardioverter Defibrillator

The **implantable cardioverter defibrillator (ICD)** is an electronic device that detects and terminates life-threatening episodes of tachycardia or fibrillation, especially those that are ventricular in origin. Patients at high risk of VT or ventricular fibrillation and who would benefit from an ICD are those who have survived sudden cardiac death, which usually is caused by ventricular fibrillation, or have experienced spontaneous, symptomatic VT (syncope secondary to VT) not due to a reversible cause (called a *secondary prevention intervention*). Patients with coronary artery disease who are 40 days postacute MI with moderate to severe LV dysfunction (ejection fraction less than or equal to 35%) are at risk of sudden cardiac death and therefore an ICD is indicated (called a *primary prevention intervention*). An ICD implantation is also recommended in patients who have been diagnosed with nonischemic dilated cardiomyopathy for at least 9 months and have functional NYHA Class II or III heart failure (Wilkoff, Fauchier, Stiles, et al., 2015) (see Chapter 25, Table 25-1) (Al-khatib et al., 2018; Ganz, 2019).

Because there may be a waiting period for ICD implantation, especially those postacute MI, patients who are at risk for sudden cardiac death may be prescribed a wearable vest-like automated defibrillator, which works just like an AED in that a shock is delivered less than a minute after a life-threatening rhythm is detected (National Heart, Lung, and Blood Institute [NHLBI], 2019; see Fig. 22-28). Prior to the delivery of the shock, the vest vibrates and issues an alarm to announce that a shock is imminent. The vest weighs about a pound, is worn under the patient's clothing, and is attached

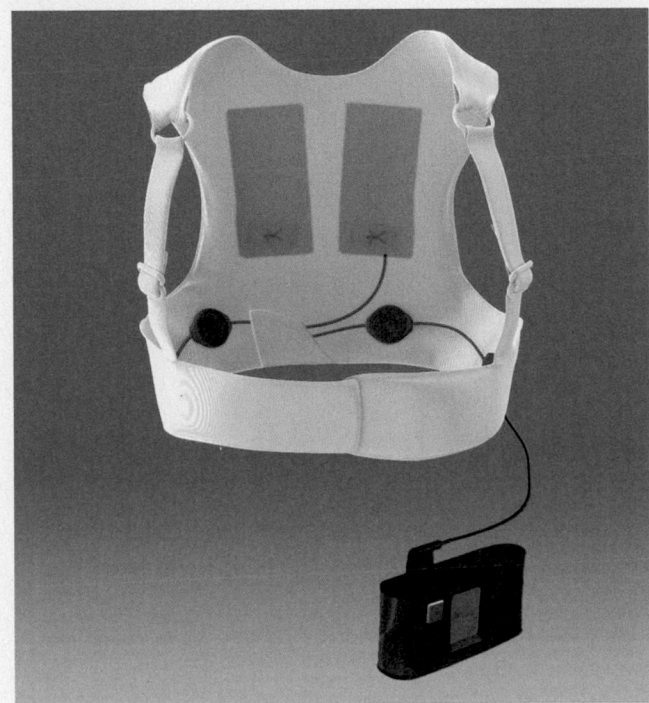

Figure 22-28 • The wearable cardioverter defibrillator vest. Courtesy of ZOLL LifeVest.

to a monitor with a battery that is worn in a holster or on a shoulder strap. The monitor automatically downloads information once a day, usually in the middle of the night. The vest must be worn at all times, even if the patient is admitted to the hospital and placed on an ECG monitor, and removed only when showering or bathing. The battery needs to be changed every day. Education is provided to the patient by the device manufacturer. However, the nurse should assess the patient's understanding of the education provided and explore any issues that may prevent the patient from wearing it.

An ICD has a generator about the size of a pack of chewing gum that is implanted in a subcutaneous pocket, usually in the upper chest wall. An ICD also has at least an RV lead that is implanted transvenously and can sense intrinsic electrical activity and deliver an electrical impulse. The implantation procedure, postimplantation care, and length of hospital stay are much like those for insertion of a pacemaker (see Fig. 22-29).

ICDs are designed to respond to two criteria: a rate that exceeds a predetermined level and a change in the isoelectric line segments. When an arrhythmia occurs, rate sensors require a set duration of time to sense the arrhythmia. Then, the device automatically charges; after a second "look" confirms the arrhythmia, it delivers the programmed charge through the lead to the heart. The time from arrhythmia detection to electrical discharge depends on the charging time, which depends on the programmed energy level (Zipes et al., 2018). However, in an ICD that has the capability of providing atrial therapies, the device can be programmed to be activated by the patient, giving the patient time to activate the charge at a time and place of their choosing. The life of the lithium battery is about 9 years but varies depending on the use of the ICD. ICD surveillance is similar to that of the pacemaker; however, it includes stored endocardial ECGs as well as information about the number and frequency of shocks that have been delivered.

Antiarrhythmic medication may be given with this technology to minimize the occurrence of a tachyarrhythmia and to reduce the frequency of ICD discharge.

Several types of devices are available. ICD, the generic name, is used as the abbreviation for these various devices. Each device offers a different delivery sequence, but all are capable of delivering high-energy (high-intensity) defibrillation to treat a tachycardia (atrial or ventricular).

Some ICDs can respond with (1) antitachycardia pacing, in which the device delivers electrical impulses at a fast rate in an attempt to disrupt the tachycardia, (2) low-energy (low-intensity) cardioversion, or (3) defibrillation; others may use all three techniques. Pacing is used to terminate tachycardias caused by a conduction disturbance called *reentry*, which is repetitive restimulation of the heart by the same impulse. An impulse or a series of impulses is delivered to the heart by the device at a fast rate to collide with and stop the heart's reentry conduction impulses, and therefore to stop the tachycardia. Typically, ICDs also have pacemaker capability if the patient develops bradycardia, which sometimes occurs after treatment of the tachycardia. Usually, the mode is VVI.

The subcutaneous ICD is a more recently introduced therapeutic alternative to the conventional ICD. The main advantage to subcutaneous defibrillators is that the complications associated with vascular access are avoided. Patients without pacing indications, or antitachycardia pacing, or cardiac resynchronization are best candidates for this technology (Sideris, Archontakis, Gatzoulis, et al., 2017).

Which device is used and how it is programmed depend on the patient's arrhythmia(s). The device may be programmed differently for different arrhythmias (e.g., ventricular fibrillation, VT with a fast ventricular rate, and VT with a slow ventricular rate). As with pacemakers, there is an NASPE-BPEG code for communicating the functions of the ICDs (Bernstein et al., 2002; Wilkoff et al., 2015). The first letter represents the chamber or chambers shocked (O, none; A, atrium; V, ventricle; D, both atrium and ventricle). The second letter represents the chamber that can be antitachycardia paced (O, A, V, D, meaning the same as the first letter). The third letter indicates the method used by the generator to detect a tachycardia (E, electrogram; H, hemodynamics). The last letter represents the chambers that have antibradycardia pacing (O, A, V, D, meaning the same as the first and second letters of the ICD code).

Complications of ICD implantation are similar to those associated with pacemaker insertion. The primary potential complication is surgery-related infection; its risk increases with battery or lead replacement. A few complications are associated with the technical aspects of the equipment, like those of pacemakers, such as premature battery depletion and dislodged or fractured leads. Inappropriate delivery of ICD therapy, usually due to oversensing or atrial and sinus tachycardias with a rapid ventricular rate response, is the most frequent long-term complication. This requires reprogramming of the device.

Nursing Management

After a permanent electronic device (pacemaker or ICD) is inserted, the patient's heart rate and rhythm are monitored by ECG. The device's settings are noted and compared with the ECG recordings to assess the device's function. For example, pacemaker malfunction is detected by examining the

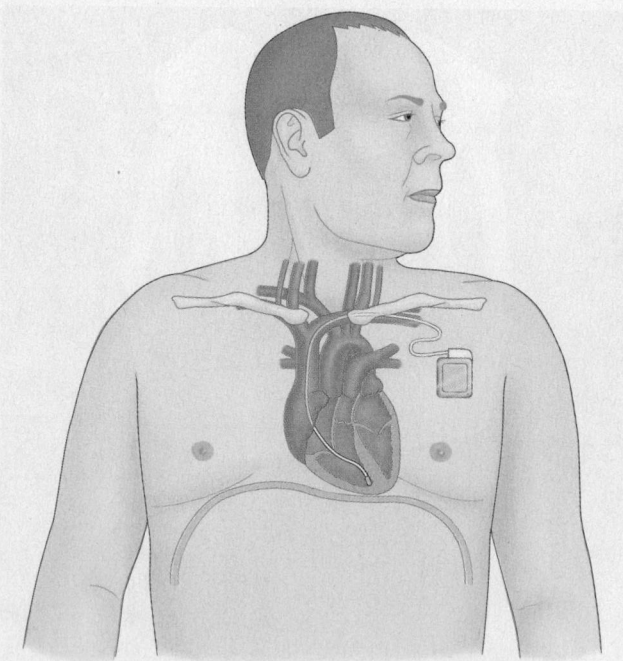

Figure 22-29 • The implantable cardioverter defibrillator consists of a generator and a sensing/pacing/defibrillating electrode.

pacemaker spike and its relationship to the surrounding ECG complexes. In addition, cardiac output and hemodynamic stability are assessed to identify the patient's response to pacing and the adequacy of pacing. The appearance or increasing frequency of arrhythmia is observed and reported to the primary provider. If the patient has an ICD implanted and develops VT or ventricular fibrillation, the ECG should be recorded to note the time between the onset of the arrhythmia and the onset of the device's shock or antitachycardia pacing.

The incision site where the generator was implanted is observed for bleeding, hematoma formation, or infection, which may be evidenced by swelling, unusual tenderness, drainage, and increased warmth. The patient may complain of continuous throbbing or pain. These symptoms are reported to the primary provider.

A chest x-ray is usually taken after the procedure and prior to discharge to document the position of leads in addition to ensuring that the procedure did not cause a pneumothorax. It is necessary to assess the function of the device throughout its lifetime and especially after changes in the patient's medication regimen. For example, antiarrhythmic agents, beta-blockers, and diuretics may increase the pacing threshold, whereas corticosteroids and alpha-adrenergic agents may decrease the pacing threshold; the opposite effect occurs when the patient is taken off these medications.

The patient is also assessed for anxiety, depression, or anger, which may be symptoms of ineffective coping with the implantation. In addition, the level of knowledge and education needs of the patient and family and the history of adherence to the therapeutic regimen should be identified. It is especially important to include the family when providing education and support.

In the peri- and postoperative phases, the nurse carefully observes the patient's responses to the device and provides the patient and family with further education as needed. The nurse also assists the patient and family in addressing concerns and in making decisions about self-care and lifestyle changes necessitated by the arrhythmia and resulting device implantation.

Preventing Infection

The nurse changes the dressing as needed and inspects the insertion site for redness, swelling, soreness, or any unusual drainage. Any change in wound appearance, an increase in the patient's temperature, or an increase in the patient's white blood count should be reported to the primary provider.

Promoting Effective Coping

The patient treated with an electronic device experiences not only lifestyle and physical changes but also emotional changes (Palese, Cracina, Purino, et al., 2019; see Chart 22-8 Nursing Research Profile: Experiences of Patients Shocked by an Implantable Cardioverter Defibrillator). At different times during the healing process, the patient may feel angry, depressed, fearful, anxious, or a combination of these emotions. Although each patient uses individual coping strategies (e.g., humor, prayer, communication with a significant other) to manage emotional distress, some strategies may work better than others. Signs that may indicate ineffective coping include social isolation, increased or prolonged irritability or depression, and difficulty in relationships.

To promote effective coping strategies, the nurse must recognize both the patient's and family's perceptions of the

---

Chart 22-8 — NURSING RESEARCH PROFILE

Experiences of Patients Shocked by an Implantable Cardioverter Defibrillator

Palese, A., Cracina, A., Purino, M., et al. (2019). The experiences of patients electrically shocked by an implantable cardioverter defibrillator: Findings from a descriptive qualitative study. *Nursing in Critical Care.* Retrieved on 7/9/2019 at: doi.org/10.1111/nicc.12424

Purpose

Insertion rates for implantable cardioverter defibrillators (ICDs) have steadily risen. ICDs may be surgically implanted as a secondary preventive measure for survivors of ventricular arrhythmias or sudden cardiac death and as primary prevention for patients with preexisting select cardiac conditions. The ICD is proven to be effective in lowering mortality rates in sudden cardiac death; however, little has been explored regarding the patients' experiences as lived before, during, and after shocks from an ICD.

Design

This study used a descriptive qualitative design. A convenience sample of adult patients with ICDs who reported at least one shock during their first follow-up visit post ICD implantation were eligible to participate. All patients were followed by a cardiology department in an academic hospital located in northern Italy. A total of 50 participants consented to enroll in this study. Each participant went through semi-structured face-to-face audiorecorded interviews. Content analysis methodology was used to analyze the data.

Findings

The content analysis revealed four themes: *feeling surprised versus feeling altered by the changes inside me; living an intense,* *monodimensional experience versus living a multidimensional storm experience; facing the event alone versus being supported;* and *living a drama versus being used to it.* Most participants reported that they received shocks in their homes or in other community-based settings, many with family members present, and that they then presented to their local emergency department. Most participants could not recall the moments preceding the shocks, but did report feeling vague physical symptoms.

Nursing Implications

Findings from this study suggest that ICD shocks can have a profound effect on patients' physical and emotional health. Nurses need to be vigilant to recognize patients' educational needs. Furthermore, nurses need to tailor appropriate, supportive interventions to improve patients' experiences living with an ICD. In particular, nurses can assist patients with ICDs in identifying pre-shock prodromal physical symptoms so that the ICD may be reprogrammed if indicated, or so that the doses of antiarrhythmic medications might be better titrated to prevent arrhythmias. Moreover, most participants in this study received shocks outside the health care setting, and many of them were shocked in the presence of family members. Tailoring education programs to include significant others in identifying prodromal symptoms pre-shock and in seeking appropriate treatment post-shock may improve the quality of life of family members and patients with ICDs.

situation and their resulting emotional state and assist them to explore their reactions and feelings. Because of the unpredictable and possibly painful ICD discharge, patients with ICDs are most vulnerable to feelings of helplessness, leading to depression. The nurse can help the patient identify positive methods to deal with the actual or perceived limitations and manage any lifestyle changes needed. The nurse may help the patient identify changes (e.g., loss of ability to participate in contact sports), the emotional responses to the change (e.g., anger), and how the patient responds to that emotion (e.g., quickly becomes angry when talking with spouse). The nurse reassures the patient that these responses are normal and helps the patient identify realistic goals (e.g., develop interest in another activity) and develop a plan to attain these goals. The patient and family should be encouraged to talk about their experiences and emotions with each other and the health care team. The nurse may refer the patient and family to a hospital, community, or online support group. The nurse may also encourage the use of spiritual resources. Based on

the patient's interest, the nurse also may educate the patient about easy-to-use stress reduction techniques (e.g., deep-breathing exercises, relaxation) to facilitate coping. Instructing the patient about the ICD may help the patient cope with changes that occur as a result of device implantation.

Promoting Home, Community-Based, and Transitional Care

After device insertion, the patient's hospital stay is typically short (e.g., may be 1 day or less), and follow-up in an outpatient clinic, office, or device clinic is common. The patient's anxiety and feelings of vulnerability may interfere with the ability to learn information provided. The nurse needs to include caregivers in the education and provide printed materials for use by the patient and caregiver. The nurse establishes priorities for learning with the patient and caregiver. Education includes the importance of periodic device monitoring, promoting safety, surgical site care, and avoiding EMI (see Chart 22-9). In addition, the educational plan should include

---

Chart 22-9 — HOME CARE CHECKLIST
Educating the Patient with an Implantable Cardiac Device

At the completion of education, the patient and/or caregiver will be able to:

- State the impact of device implantation on physiologic functioning, ADLs, IADLs, self-image and roles, relationships (including sexuality), and spirituality.
- State changes in lifestyle (e.g., diet, activity, mobility/driving restrictions) necessary to maintain health.
- State the name, dose, side effects, frequency, and schedule for all medications.
- For patients with pacemakers, check pulse daily. Report *immediately* any sudden slowing or increasing of the pulse rate. This may indicate pacemaker malfunction.
- Avoid infection at the insertion site of the device:
  - Leave the incision uncovered and observe it daily for redness, increased swelling, and heat.
  - Take temperature at same time each day; report any increase.
  - Avoid wearing tight, restrictive clothing that may cause friction over the insertion site.
  - Initially avoid soaking in the tub and lotion, creams, or powders in the area of the device.
- Adhere to activity restrictions:
  - Restrict movement of arm until incision heals; do not raise arm above head for 2 wks.
  - Avoid heavy lifting for a few weeks.
  - Discuss safety of activities (e.g., driving) with a primary provider.
  - Recognize that although it may take up to 2–3 wks to resume normal activities, physical activity does not usually have to be curtailed, with the exception of contact sports.
- Electromagnetic interference: Understand the importance of the following:
  - Avoid large magnetic fields, such as those created by MRI, large motors, arc welding, and electrical substations. Magnetic fields may deactivate the device, negating its effect on an arrhythmia.
  - At security gates at airports, government buildings, or other secured areas, show identification card and request a hand (not handheld device) search. Obtain and carry a letter from the primary provider about this requirement.
  - Some electrical and small motor devices, as well as products that contain magnets (e.g., cellular phones), may interfere

- with the functioning of the cardiac device if the electrical device is placed very close to it. Avoid leaning directly over large electrical devices or motors, or ensure that contact is of brief duration; place cellular phone on opposite side of cardiac device.
  - Household appliances (e.g., microwave ovens) should not cause any concern.
- Describe precautions and safety measures to be used:
  - Describe what to do if symptoms occur, and notify the primary provider if any discharges seem unusual.
  - Maintain a log that records discharges of an ICD. Record events that precipitate the sensation of shock. This provides important data for the primary provider to use in readjusting the medical regimen.
  - Encourage family members to attend a cardiopulmonary resuscitation class.
  - Call 911 for emergency assistance if feeling of dizziness occurs.
  - Wear medical identification (e.g., MedicAlert) that includes primary provider information.
  - Avoid frightening family or friends with unexpected shocks from an ICD, which will not harm them. Inform family and friends that in the event they are in contact with the patient when a shock is delivered, they may also feel the shock. It is especially important to warn sexual partners that this may occur.
  - Carry medical identification with the primary provider's name, type and model number of the device, manufacturer's name, and hospital where device was inserted.
- Identify community resources for peer and caregiver/family support.
- Adhere to appointments for follow-up care that are scheduled to monitor the electronic performance of the cardiac device. This is especially important during the first month after implantation and near the end of the battery life. Remember to take the log of ICD discharges to review with the primary provider.
- Identify the need for health promotion, disease prevention, and screening activities.

ADL, activities of daily living; IADL, instrumental activities of daily living; ICD, implantable cardioverter defibrillator.

information about activities that are safe and those that may be dangerous. The nurse discusses with the patient and family what they have to do when a shock is delivered. The nurse may facilitate CPR training for the family.

CRITICAL THINKING EXERCISES

1 **ebp** Your uncle, who has a history of alcohol abuse, calls to tell you that his primary provider told him that he has atrial fibrillation. He says that he has been prescribed warfarin and that he really doesn't want to take it because he heard that it is an ingredient in "rat poison." What is the strength of the evidence that supports your uncle's continued adherence to warfarin therapy? What are the risks involved should he decide that he will not take this drug as prescribed?

2 **pq** You work as a staff nurse on a surgical gynecology unit. A 55-year-old woman assigned to your care is one day post total abdominal hysterectomy. On your initial rounds, the patient is resting comfortably in bed with moderate pain, heart rate of 65 bpm, blood pressure of 120/70 mm Hg, and respiratory rate of 20 breaths per minute. Four hours later, you enter the patient's room and she is sleeping with a heart rate of 98 bpm, blood pressure of 110/60 mm Hg, and respiratory rate of 16 breaths per minute. What are the possible causes of this increase in heart rate? What are your assessment priorities?

3 **ipc** It is the start of the 12-hour day shift on the cardiovascular unit where you work. A 45-year-old patient who was admitted last evening with a MI is now suddenly experiencing frequent PVCs and a four-beat run of ventricular tachycardia. The patient has remained hemodynamically stable during these episodes. You are preparing for the morning huddle with team members that include unlicensed assistive personnel and attending health care providers. How will you facilitate this interprofessional discussion concerning your patient's PVCs and ventricular tachycardia?

REFERENCES

*Asterisk indicates nursing research.
**Double asterisk indicates classic reference, consensus statement, or guideline.

Books

American Society of Health System Pharmacists. (2019). *AHFS drug information*. Bethesda, MD: Author.
Fuster, V., Harrington, R. A., Narula, J., et al. (Eds.). (2017). *Hurst's the heart* (14th ed.). New York: McGraw-Hill.
Zipes, D. P., Libby, P., Bonow, R. O., et al. (2018). *Braunwald's heart disease: A textbook of cardiovascular medicine* (11th ed.). Philadelphia, PA: Elsevier.

Journals and Electronic Documents

Agrawal, A. (2018). Cardiac resynchronization therapy. *Medscape*. Retrieved on 12/4/2019 at: emedicine.medscape.com/article/1839506-overview#a1
Al-khatib, S. M., Stevenson, W. G., Ackerman, M. J., et al. (2018). 2017 AHA/ACC/HRS guideline for management of patients with ventricular arrhythmias and the prevention of sudden cardiac death: A report of the American College of Cardiology/American Heart Association Task Force on clinical practice guidelines and the Heart Rhythm Society. *Circulation, 138*(13), e272–e391.
Aune, D., Sen, A., ó'Hartaigh, B., et al. (2017). Resting heart rate and the risk of cardiovascular disease, total cancer, and all-cause mortality—A systematic review and dose–response meta-analysis of prospective studies. *Nutrition, Metabolism and Cardiovascular Diseases, 27*(6), 504–517.
**Bernstein, A. D., Daubert, J-C., Fletcher, R. D., et al. (2002). The revised NASPE/BPEG generic code for antibradycardia, adaptive-rate, and multisite pacing. North American Society of Pacing and Electrophysiology/British Pacing and Electrophysiology Group. *Pacing and Clinical Electrophysiology, 25*(2), 260–264.
Burrage, P. S., Low, Y. H., Campbell, N. G., et al. (2019). New onset atrial fibrillation in adult patients after cardiac surgery. *Critical Care Anesthesia, 9*(2), 174–193.
Canpolat, U., Kocyigit, D., & Aytemir, K. (2017). Complications of atrial fibrillation cryoablation. *Journal of Atrial Fibrillation, 10*(4), 1620.
Carlson, S. K., & Doshi, R. N. (2017). Termination of anticoagulation therapy at 45 days after concomitant atrial fibrillation catheter ablation and left atrial appendage occlusion resulting in device-related thrombosis and stroke. *HeartRhythm Case Reports, 3*(1), 18–21.
Centers for Disease Control and Prevention (CDC). (2017). Atrial fibrillation fact sheet. Division for Heart Disease and Stroke Prevention. Retrieved on 10/7/2019 at: www.cdc.gov/dhdsp/data_statistics/fact_sheets/fs_atrial_fibrillation.htm
Chen, L. Y., Chung, M. K., Allen, L. A., et al. (2018). Atrial fibrillation burden: Moving beyond atrial fibrillation as a binary entity: A scientific statement from the American Heart Association. *Circulation, 137*(20), e623–e644.
Chen, Y., Chen, K., Lu, K., et al. (2018). Validating the 6-minute walk test as an indicator of recovery in patients undergoing cardiac surgery. *Medicine, 97*(42), e12925.
Costa, V., Yeung, M. W., Gilbert, J., et al. (2018). Remote monitoring of implantable cardioverter-defibrillators, cardiac resynchronization therapy and permanent pacemakers: A health technology assessment. *Ontario Health Technology Assessments Series, 18*(7). Retrieved on 7/9/2019 at: www.ncbi.nlm.nih.gov/pubmed/30443279
Elrod, J. (2014). The convergent procedure: The CONVERGE IDE Clinical Trial. *EP Lab Digest, 14*(5), Retrieved on 12/4/2019 at: www.eplabdigest.com/articles/Convergent-Procedure-CONVERGE-IDE-Clinical-Trial
Ganz, L. I. (2019). Implantable cardioverter-defibrillators: Overview of indications, components, and functions. *UpToDate*. Retrieved on 12/4/2019 at: www.uptodate.com/contents/implantable-cardioverter-defibrillators-overview-of-indications-components-and-functions
**Gillis, A. M., Russo, A. M., Ellenbogen, K. A., et al. (2012). HRS/ACCF expert consensus statement on pacemaker device and mode selection. *Journal of the American College of Cardiology, 60*(7), 682–703.
Groner, A., & Grippe, K. (2019). The leadless pacemaker. *Journal of the American College of Cardiology, 32*, 48–50.
Hafeez Y., & Armstrong T. J. (2019). Atrioventricular nodal reentry tachycardia. *StatPearls*. Retrieved on 10/7/2019 at: www.ncbi.nlm.nih.gov/books/NBK499936/
Hayes, D. L. (2019). Permanent cardiac pacing: Overview of devices and indications. *UpToDate*. Retrieved on 12/4/2019 at: www.uptodate.com/contents/permanent-cardiac-pacing-overview-of-devices-and-indications
Hedge, S. A., & Gnugnoli, D. M. (2019). EMS public access to defibrillation. *Stat Pearls Publishing LLC*. Retrieved on 7/9/2019 at: www.ncbi.nlm.nih.gov/books/NBK539691/
Jackson, L. R., 2nd, Rathakrishnan, B., Campbell, K., et al. (2017). Sinus node dysfunction and atrial fibrillation: A reversible phenomenon? *Pacing and Clinical Electrophysiology, 40*(4), 442–450.
Jan, M., Zizek, D., Gersak, Z. M., et al. (2018). Comparison of treatment outcomes between convergent procedure and catheter ablation for paroxysmal atrial fibrillation evaluated with implantable loop recorder monitoring. *Journal of Cardiovascular Electrophysiology, 2018*(29), 1073–1080.
January, C. T., Wann, L. S., Alpert, J. S., et al. (2014). 2014 AHA/ACC/HRS guideline for the management of patients with atrial fibrillation: A report of the American College of Cardiology/American Heart Association Task Force on practice guidelines and the Heart Rhythm Society. *Circulation, 130*(23), e199–e267.
January, C. T., Wann, L. S., Calkins, H., et al. (2019). 2019 AHA/ACC/HRS focused update of the 2014 AHA/ACC/HRS Guideline for the

management of patients with atrial fibrillation: A Report of the American College of Cardiology/American Heart Association Task Force on Clinical Practice Guidelines and the Heart Rhythm Society in Collaboration With the Society of Thoracic Surgeons. *Circulation, 140*(2), e125–e151.

Katritsis, D. G. (2018). Catheter ablation of atrioventricular nodal reentrant tachycardia: Facts and fiction. *Arrhythmia & Electrophysiology Review, 7*(4), 230–231.

Kusumoto, F. M., Schoenfeld, M. H., Barrett, C., et al. (2019). 2018 ACC/AHA/HRS guideline on the evaluation and management of patients with bradycardia and cardiac conduction delay: A report of the American College of Cardiology/American Heart Association Task Force on clinical practice guidelines and the Heart Rhythm Society. *Circulation, 74*(7), e51–e156.

Link, M. S., Berkow, L. C., Kudenchuk, P. J., et al. (2015). Part 7: Adult advanced cardiovascular life support. 2015 American Heart Association guidelines update for cardiopulmonary resuscitation and emergency cardiovascular care. *Circulation, 132*(18 supp 2), S444–S464.

Madhavan, M., Mulpuru, S. K., McLeod, C. J., et al. (2017). Cardiac pacemakers: Function, troubleshooting, and management: Part 2 of a 2-Part Series. *Journal of the American College of Cardiology, 69*(2), 211–235.

Malik, A. H., Yandrapalli, S., Aronow, W. S., et al. (2019). Oral anticoagulants in atrial fibrillation with valvular heart disease and bioprosthetic heart valves. *Heart, 105*(18), 1432–1436.

Masoudi, F. A., Calkins, H., Kavinsky, C. J., et al. (2015). 2015 ACC/HRS/SCAI left atrial appendage occlusion device societal overview: A professional society overview from the American College of Cardiology, Heart Rhythm Society, and the Society for Cardiovascular Angiography and Interventions. *Catheterization & Cardiovascular Interventions, 86*(5), 791–807.

Mulpuru, S. K., Madhavan, M., McLeod, C. J., et al. (2017). Cardiac pacemakers: Function, troubleshooting, and management: Part 1 of a 2-Part Series. *Journal of the American College of Cardiology, 69*(2), 189–210.

National Heart, Lung, Blood Institute (NHLBI). (2019). Defibrillators. National Institutes of Health. Retrieved on 7/9/2019 at: www.nhlbi. nih.gov/health-topics/defibrillators

Ojo, A., Yandrapalli, S., Veseli, G., et al. (2020). Left atrial appendage occlusion in the management of stroke in patients with atrial fibrillation. *Cardiology in Review, 28*(1), 42–51.

Page, R. L., Joglar, J. A., Caldwell, M. A., et al. (2016). 2015 ACC/AHA/HRS guideline for the management of adult patients with supraventricular tachycardia. A Report of the American College of Cardiology/American Heart Association Task Force on Clinical Practice Guidelines and the Heart Rhythm Society. *Heart Rhythm, 13*(4), e136–e221.

*Palese, A., Cracina, A., Purino, M., et al. (2019). The experiences of patients electrically shocked by an implantable cardioverter defibrillator: Findings from a descriptive qualitative study. *Nursing in Critical Care.* Retrieved on 7/9/2019 at: doi.org/10.1111/nicc.12424

Pappone, C., & Santinelli, V. (2019). Brugada Syndrome: Progress in diagnosis and management. *Arrhythmia & Electrophysiology Review, 8*(1), 13–18.

Qin, M., Zeng, C., & Liu, X. (2019). The cardiac autonomic nervous system: A target for modulation of atrial fibrillation. *Clinical Cardiology, 42*(6), 644–652.

Schellinger, P. D., Tsivgoulis, G., Steiner, T., et al. (2018). Percutaneous left atrial appendage occlusion for the prevention of stroke in patients with atrial fibrillation: Review and critical appraisal. *Journal of Stroke, 20*(3), 281–291.

Sendelbach, S., & Jepsen, S. (2018). American Association of Critical Care Nurses practice alert: Managing alarms in acute care across the lifespan, electrocardiography and pulse oximetry. *Critical Care Nurse, 38*(2), e16–e20.

Sideris, S., Archontakis, S., Gatzoulis, K. A., et al. (2017). The subcutaneous ICD as an alternative to the conventional ICD system: Initial experience in Greece and a review of the literature. *Hellenic Journal of Cardiology, 58*(1), 4–16.

Soar, J., Donnino, M. W., Maconochie, I., et al. (2018). 2018 International consensus on cardiopulmonary resuscitation and emergency cardiovascular care science with treatment recommendations summary. *Resuscitation, 133*, 194–206.

**Tracy, C. M., Epstein, A. E., Darbar, D., et al. (2012). ACCF/AHA/HRS focused update of the 2008 guidelines for device-based therapy of cardiac rhythm abnormalities: A report of the American College of Cardiology Foundation/American Heart Association Task Force on practice guidelines. *Journal of the American College of Cardiology, 60*(14), 1297–1313.

Weber, H., Sagerer-Gerhardt, M., & Heinze, A. (2017). Laser catheter ablation of long lasting persistent atrial fibrillation: Long term results. *Journal of Atrial Fibrillation, 10*(2), 1588.

Wilkoff, B. L., Fauchier, L., Stiles, M. K., et al. (2016). 2015 HRS/EHRA/APHRS/SOLAECE expert consensus statement on optimal implantable cardioverter-defibrillator programming and testing. *Heart Rhythm, 13*(2), E50–E86.

Resources

American Association of Critical-Care Nurses, www.aacn.org
American Association of Heart Failure Nurses (AAHFN), www.aahfn.org
American College of Cardiology (ACC), www.acc.org
American Heart Association, National Center, www.heart.org
Heart Rhythm Society, www.hrsonline.org
National Institutes of Health, National Heart, Lung, Blood Institute, Health Information Center, www.nhlbi.nih.gov

23

Management of Patients with Coronary Vascular Disorders

LEARNING OUTCOMES

On completion of this chapter, the learner will be able to:

1. Describe the pathophysiology, clinical manifestations, and treatment of coronary vascular disorders including coronary atherosclerosis, angina pectoris, and myocardial infarction.
2. Use the nursing process as a framework for care of the patient with angina pectoris, with acute coronary syndrome, or who has undergone cardiac surgery.

3. Describe percutaneous coronary interventional and coronary artery revascularization procedures.
4. Identify the nursing care of a patient who has had a percutaneous coronary interventional procedure for treatment of coronary artery disease.

NURSING CONCEPT

Perfusion

GLOSSARY

acute coronary syndrome (ACS): signs and symptoms that indicate unstable angina or acute myocardial infarction

angina pectoris: chest pain brought about by myocardial ischemia

atheroma: fibrous cap composed of smooth muscle cells that forms over lipid deposits within arterial vessels and protrudes into the lumen of the vessel, narrowing the lumen and obstructing blood flow; also called *plaque*

atherosclerosis: abnormal accumulation of lipid deposits and fibrous tissue within arterial walls and the lumen

contractility: ability of the cardiac muscle to shorten in response to an electrical impulse

coronary artery bypass graft (CABG): a surgical procedure in which a blood vessel from another part of the body is grafted onto the occluded coronary artery below the occlusion in such a way that blood flow bypasses the blockage

high-density lipoprotein (HDL): a protein-bound lipid that transports cholesterol to the liver for excretion in the bile; composed of a higher proportion of protein to lipid than low-density lipoprotein; exerts a beneficial effect on the arterial wall

ischemia: insufficient tissue oxygenation

low-density lipoprotein (LDL): a protein-bound lipid that transports cholesterol to tissues in the body; composed of a lower proportion of protein to lipid than high-density lipoprotein; exerts a harmful effect on the arterial wall

metabolic syndrome: a cluster of metabolic abnormalities including insulin resistance, obesity, dyslipidemia, and hypertension that increase the risk of cardiovascular disease

myocardial infarction (MI): death of heart tissue caused by lack of oxygenated blood flow

percutaneous coronary intervention (PCI): a procedure in which a catheter is placed in a coronary artery, and one of several methods is employed to reduce blockage within the artery

percutaneous transluminal coronary angioplasty (PTCA): a type of percutaneous coronary intervention in which a balloon is inflated within a coronary artery to break an atheroma and open the vessel lumen, improving coronary artery blood flow

stent: a metal mesh that provides structural support to a coronary vessel, preventing its closure

sudden cardiac death: abrupt cessation of effective heart activity

thrombolytic: a pharmacologic agent that breaks down blood clots; alternatively referred to as a fibrinolytic

troponin: a cardiac muscle biomarker; measurement is used as an indicator of heart muscle injury

Cardiovascular disease is the leading cause of death in the United States for men and women of all racial and ethnic groups (Arnett, Blumenthal, Albert, et al., 2019). Research related to the identification of and treatment for cardiovascular disease includes all segments of the population affected by cardiac conditions, including women, children, and people of diverse racial and ethnic backgrounds. The results of ongoing research are used by nurses to identify specific prevention and treatment strategies in these populations.

Coronary Artery Disease

Coronary artery disease (CAD) is the most prevalent type of cardiovascular disease in adults. For this reason, nurses must recognize various manifestations of coronary artery conditions and evidence-based methods for assessing, preventing, and treating these disorders.

Coronary Atherosclerosis

The most common cause of cardiovascular disease in the United States is **atherosclerosis**, an abnormal accumulation of lipid, or fatty substances, and fibrous tissue in the lining of arterial blood vessel walls. These substances block and narrow the coronary vessels in a way that reduces blood flow to the myocardium. Atherosclerosis involves a repetitive inflammatory response to injury of the artery wall and subsequent alteration in the structural and biochemical properties of the arterial walls. New information that relates to the development of atherosclerosis has increased the understanding of treatment and prevention of this progressive and potentially life-threatening process.

Pathophysiology

The inflammatory response involved with the development of atherosclerosis begins with injury to the vascular endothelium and progresses over many years (Norris, 2019). The injury may be initiated by smoking or tobacco use, hypertension, hyperlipidemia, and other factors. The endothelium undergoes changes and stops producing the normal antithrombotic and vasodilating agents. The presence of inflammation attracts inflammatory cells, such as macrophages. The macrophages ingest lipids, becoming "foam cells" that transport the lipids into the arterial wall. Some of the lipid is deposited on the arterial wall, forming fatty streaks. Activated macrophages also release biochemical substances that can further damage the endothelium by contributing to the oxidation of low-density lipoprotein (LDL). The oxidized LDL is toxic to the endothelial cells and fuels progression of the atherosclerotic process (Norris, 2019).

Following the transport of lipid into the arterial wall, smooth muscle cells proliferate and form a fibrous cap over a core filled with lipid and inflammatory infiltrate. These deposits, called **atheromas**, or plaques, protrude into the lumen of the vessel, narrowing it and obstructing blood flow (see Fig. 23-1). Plaque may be stable or unstable, depending on the degree of inflammation and thickness of the fibrous cap. If the fibrous cap over the plaque is thick and the lipid pool remains relatively stable, it can resist the stress of blood flow and vessel movement. If the cap is thin and inflammation is ongoing, the lesion becomes

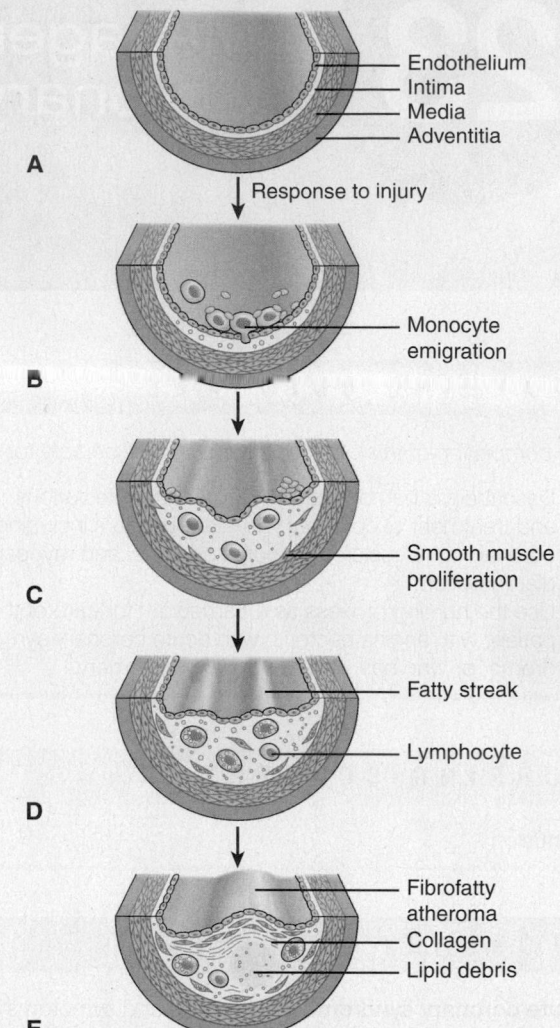

Figure 23-1 • A, B. Atherosclerosis begins as monocytes and lipids enter the intima of an injured vessel. Smooth muscle cells proliferate within the vessel wall (**C**), contributing to the development of fatty accumulations and atheroma (**D**). As the plaque enlarges, the vessel narrows and blood flow decreases (**E**). The plaque may rupture and a thrombus might form, obstructing blood flow.

what is called *vulnerable plaque*. At this point, the lipid core may grow, causing the fibrous plaque to rupture. A ruptured plaque attracts platelets and causes thrombus formation. A thrombus may then obstruct blood flow, leading to acute coronary syndrome (ACS), which may result in an acute **myocardial infarction (MI)**. When an MI occurs, a portion of the heart muscle no longer receives blood flow and becomes necrotic.

The anatomic structure of the coronary arteries makes them particularly susceptible to atherosclerosis. As Figure 23-2 shows, the three major coronary arteries have multiple branches. Atherosclerotic lesions most often form where the vessels branch and with turbulent blood flow, suggesting a hemodynamic component is involved in their formation (Norris, 2019). Although heart disease is most often caused by atherosclerosis of the coronary arteries, other phenomena may also decrease blood flow to the heart. Examples include vasospasm (sudden constriction or narrowing) of a coronary artery and profound hypotension.

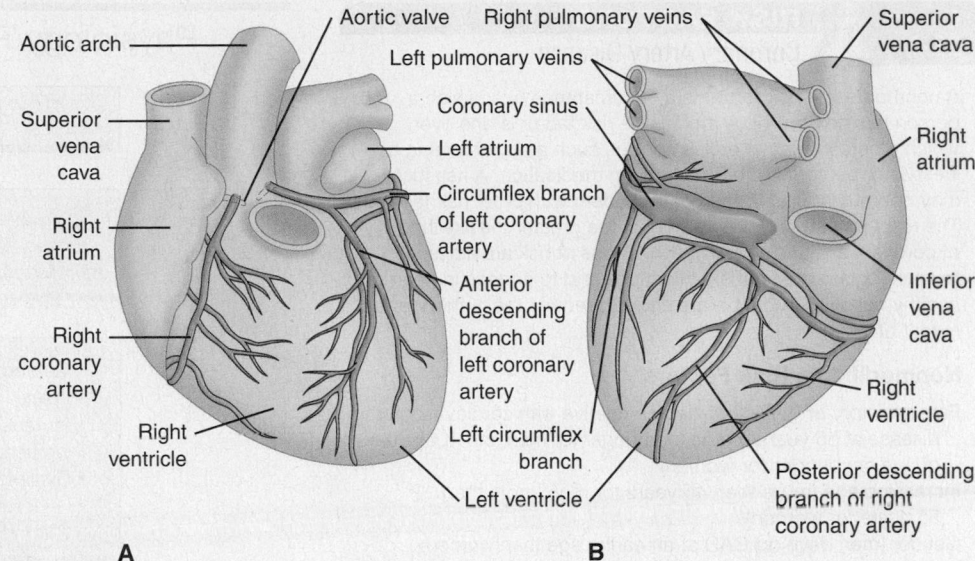

Figure 23-2 • The coronary arteries supply the heart muscle with oxygenated blood, adjusting the flow according to metabolic needs. **A.** Anterior view of the heart. **B.** Posterior view of heart.

Clinical Manifestations

CAD produces symptoms and complications according to the location and degree of narrowing of the arterial lumen, thrombus formation, and obstruction of blood flow to the myocardium. This impediment to blood flow is usually progressive, causing an inadequate blood supply that deprives the cardiac muscle cells of oxygen needed for their survival. The condition is known as **ischemia**. **Angina pectoris** refers to chest pain that is brought about by myocardial ischemia. Angina pectoris usually is caused by significant coronary atherosclerosis. If the decrease in blood supply is great enough, of long enough duration, or both, irreversible damage and death of myocardial cells may result. Over time, irreversibly damaged myocardium undergoes degeneration and is replaced by scar tissue, causing various degrees of myocardial dysfunction. Significant myocardial damage may result in persistently low cardiac output and heart failure where the heart cannot support the body's needs for blood. A decrease in blood supply from CAD may cause the heart to abruptly stop beating; this is known as **sudden cardiac death** (see Chapter 25 for further discussion on CPR).

The most common manifestation of myocardial ischemia is the onset of chest pain. However, the classic epidemiologic study of the people in Framingham, Massachusetts, showed that nearly 15% of men and women who had coronary events, which included unstable angina, MIs, or sudden cardiac death events, were totally asymptomatic prior to the coronary event (Kannel, 1986). Patients with myocardial ischemia may present to an emergency department (ED) or clinic with a variety of symptoms other than chest pain. Some complain of epigastric distress and pain that radiates to the jaw or left arm. Patients who are older or have a history of diabetes or heart failure may report shortness of breath. Many women have been found to have atypical symptoms, including indigestion, nausea, palpitations, and numbness (Davis, 2017). Prodromal symptoms may occur (e.g., angina a few hours to days before the acute episode), or a major cardiac event may be the first indication of coronary atherosclerosis.

Risk Factors

Epidemiologic studies point to several factors that increase the probability that a person will develop heart disease. Major risk factors are listed in Chart 23-1. Although many people with CAD have one or more risk factors, some do not have classic risk factors. Elevated **low-density lipoprotein (LDL)**, also known as bad cholesterol, is a well-known risk factor and the primary target of cholesterol-lowering therapy. People at the highest risk for having a cardiac event are those with known CAD or those with diabetes, peripheral arterial disease, abdominal aortic aneurysm, or carotid artery disease. The latter diseases are referred to as CAD risk equivalents, because patients with these diseases have the same risk for a cardiac event as patients with CAD. The likelihood of having a cardiac event is also affected by factors, such as age, gender, systolic blood pressure, smoking history, level of total cholesterol, and level of **high-density lipoprotein (HDL)**, also known as good cholesterol. The Framingham Risk Calculator is a tool commonly used to estimate the risk for having a cardiac event within the next 10 years (Grundy, Stone, Bailey, et al., 2018). This tool is designed for adults 20 years and older. The calculation is performed using the individual's risk factor data, including age, gender, total cholesterol, HDL, smoking status, systolic blood pressure, and need for antihypertensive medication.

In addition, a cluster of metabolic abnormalities known as **metabolic syndrome** has emerged as a major risk factor for cardiovascular disease (Grundy et al., 2018). A diagnosis of this syndrome is made when a patient has three of the following five risk factors:

- Enlarged waist circumference (greater than 35.4 inches in males, greater than 31.4 inches in females)
- Elevated triglycerides (greater than or equal to 175 mg/dL, or currently on drug treatment for elevated triglycerides)
- Reduced HDL (less than 40 mg/dL in males, less than 50 mg/dL in females, or currently on drug treatment for reduced HDL)
- Hypertension (systolic blood pressure greater than or equal to 130 mm Hg and/or diastolic blood pressure

Chart 23-1 — RISK FACTORS — Coronary Artery Disease

A nonmodifiable risk factor is a circumstance over which a person has no control. A modifiable risk factor is one over which a person may exercise control, such as by changing a lifestyle or personal habit or by using medication. A risk factor may operate independently or in tandem with other risk factors. The more risk factors a person has, the greater the likelihood of coronary artery disease (CAD). Those at risk are advised to seek regular medical examinations and to engage in heart-healthy behavior (a deliberate effort to reduce the number and extent of risks).

Nonmodifiable Risk Factors

Family history of CAD (first-degree relative with cardiovascular disease at 55 years of age or younger for men and at 65 years of age or younger for women)
Increasing age (more than 45 years for men; more than 55 years for women)
Gender (men develop CAD at an earlier age than women)
Race (higher incidence of heart disease in African Americans than in Caucasians)
History of premature menopause (before age 40) and history of pregnancy-associated disorders such as preeclampsia
Primary hypercholesterolemia (a genetic condition resulting in elevated LDL)

Modifiable Risk Factors

Hyperlipidemia
Tobacco use
Hypertension
Diabetes
Metabolic syndrome
Obesity
Physical inactivity
Chronic inflammatory conditions (e.g., rheumatoid arthritis, lupus, HIV/AIDS)
Chronic kidney disease

Adapted from Arnett, D. K., Blumenthal, R. S., Albert, M. A., et al. (2019). ACC/AHA Guideline on the Primary Prevention of Cardiovascular Disease. *Journal of the American College of Cardiology, 74*(10), e177–e232.

Physiology/Pathophysiology

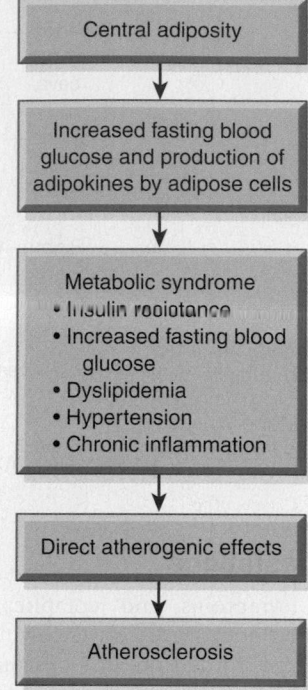

Figure 23-3 • Pathophysiology of cardiovascular disease in metabolic syndrome. Central adiposity plays a major role in the development of metabolic syndrome. Adipokines released from fat cells along with other hormones and metabolites are thought to contribute to the development of metabolic abnormalities. The eventual effect of these processes is the promotion of atherosclerosis.

determine overall cardiovascular risk, clinicians may view high sensitivity C-reactive protein (hs-CRP) test results together with other screening tools such as measurements of lipid levels.

Prevention

Four modifiable risk factors—cholesterol abnormalities, tobacco use, hypertension, and diabetes—are established risk factors for CAD and its complications. As a result, they receive much attention in health promotion programs.

Controlling Cholesterol Abnormalities

The association of a high blood cholesterol level with heart disease is well established, and the metabolism of fats is known to be an important contributor to the development of heart disease. Fats, which are insoluble in water, are encased in water-soluble lipoproteins that allow them to be transported within the circulatory system. The various lipoproteins are categorized by their protein content, which is measured in density. The density increases when more protein is present. Four elements of fat metabolism—total cholesterol, LDL, HDL, and triglycerides—are known to affect the development of heart disease. Cholesterol is processed by the gastrointestinal (GI) tract into lipoprotein globules called *chylomicrons*. These are reprocessed by the liver as lipoproteins (see Fig. 23-4). This is a physiologic process necessary for the formation of lipoprotein-based cell membranes and

greater than or equal to 80 mm Hg on an average of two to three measurements obtained on two to three separate occasions, or currently on antihypertensive drug treatment for a history of hypertension)
• Elevated fasting glucose (greater than or equal to 100 mg/dL on two separate occasions, or current drug treatment for elevated glucose)

Many people with type 2 diabetes fit this clinical picture. Theories suggest that in patients with obesity, excessive adipose tissue may secrete mediators that lead to metabolic changes. Adipokines (adipose tissue cytokines), free fatty acids, and other substances are known to modify insulin action and contribute to atherogenic changes in the cardiovascular system (see Fig. 23-3).

C-reactive protein (CRP) is known to be an inflammatory marker for cardiovascular risk, including acute coronary events and stroke. The liver produces CRP in response to a stimulus such as tissue injury, and high levels of this protein may occur in people with diabetes and those who are likely to have an acute coronary event (Norris, 2019). To

Physiology/Pathophysiology

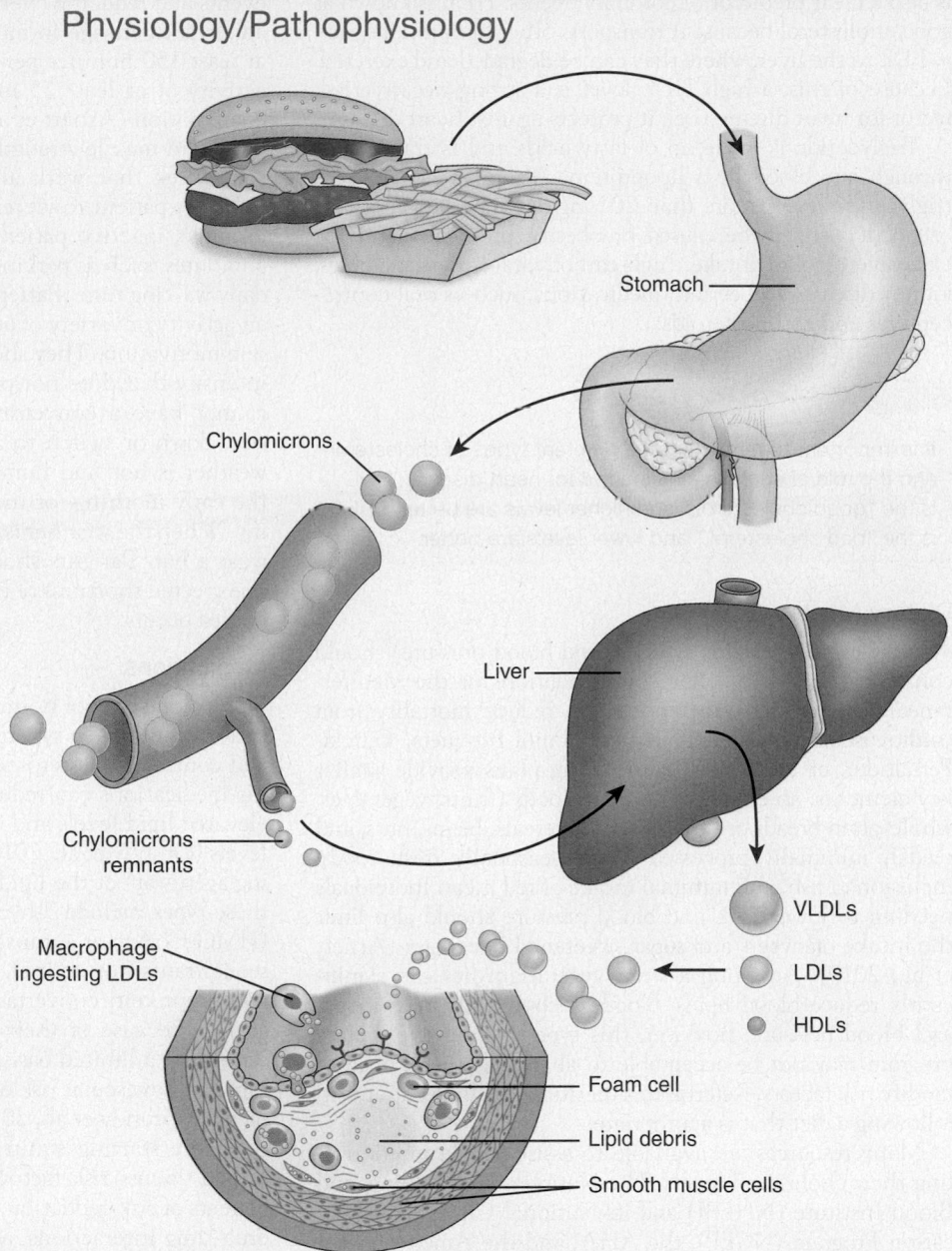

Figure 23-4 • Lipoproteins and the development of atherosclerosis. As dietary cholesterol and saturated fat are processed by the gastrointestinal tract, chylomicrons enter the blood. They are broken down into chylomicron remnants in the capillaries. The liver processes them into lipoproteins. When these are released into the circulation, excess low-density lipoproteins (LDLs) adhere to receptors on the intimal wall. Macrophages also ingest LDLs and transport them into the vessel wall, beginning the process of plaque formation. HDLs, high-density lipoproteins; VLDLs, very–low-density lipoproteins.

Labels in figure: Stomach; Chylomicrons; Liver; Chylomicrons remnants; Macrophage ingesting LDLs; VLDLs; LDLs; HDLs; Foam cell; Lipid debris; Smooth muscle cells

other important metabolic processes. When an excess of LDL is produced, LDL particles adhere to receptors in the arterial endothelium. Here, macrophages ingest them, contributing to plaque formation.

The American College of Cardiology and the American Heart Association (ACC/AHA) have developed clinical practice guidelines on the treatment of blood cholesterol to reduce cardiovascular risk in adults (Grundy et al., 2018). These guidelines address primary prevention (preventing the occurrence of CAD) and secondary prevention (preventing the progression of CAD). All adults 20 years and older should have a fasting lipid profile (total cholesterol, LDL, HDL, and triglycerides) performed at least once every 5 years, and more often if the profile is abnormal. Patients who have had an acute event (e.g., MI), a percutaneous coronary intervention (PCI), or a coronary artery bypass graft (CABG)

require assessment of their LDL cholesterol level within a few months of the event or procedure, because LDL levels may be low immediately after the acute event or procedure. Subsequently, lipids should be monitored every 4 to 12 weeks until the desired level is achieved and then every 3 to 12 months as needed (Grundy et al., 2018). A fasting lipid profile should demonstrate the following values (Stone, Robinson, Lichtenstein, et al., 2014):

- LDL cholesterol less than 100 mg/dL (less than 70 mg/dL for very high risk patients)
- Total cholesterol less than 200 mg/dL
- HDL cholesterol greater than 40 mg/dL for males and greater than 50 mg/dL for females
- Triglyceride less than 150 mg/dL

LDL is the target of current therapy because of its strong association with advancing CAD. The total cholesterol level is also a clear predictor of coronary events. HDL is known as good cholesterol because it transports other lipoproteins such as LDL to the liver, where they can be degraded and excreted. Because of this, a high HDL level is a strong negative risk factor for heart disease (i.e., it protects against heart disease).

Triglyceride is made up of fatty acids and is transported through the blood by a lipoprotein. Although an elevated triglyceride level (more than 200 mg/dL) may be genetic in origin, it also can be caused by obesity, physical inactivity, excessive alcohol intake, high-carbohydrate diets, diabetes, kidney disease, and certain medications, such as oral contraceptives and corticosteroids.

 Concept Mastery Alert

It is important to remember the different types of cholesterol and the role of each as a risk factor for heart disease. HDL is the "good cholesterol," and higher levels are better; LDL is the "bad cholesterol," and lower levels are better.

Dietary Measures

Adults who need to lower LDL (and blood pressure) should consider the AHA's diet recommendations or the Mediterranean diet, which are reported to reduce mortality from cardiovascular disease (Franquesa, Pujol-Busquets, García-Fernández, et al., 2019). Both eating plans provide similar key elements: an emphasis on plant foods (fruits, vegetables, whole-grain breads or other forms of cereals, beans, nuts, and seeds), minimally processed foods, seasonally fresh foods, inclusion of fish, and minimal intake of red meat. Individuals needing to lower LDL and blood pressure should also limit the intake of sweets and sugar sweetened beverages (Arnett et al., 2019). Adopting a strict vegetarian diet can significantly reduce blood lipids, blood glucose, body mass index, and blood pressure; however, this type of intensive dietary program may not be acceptable to all patients who need to modify risk factors. Referral to a dietitian can help patients in following a diet that is appropriate.

Many resources are available to assist people in controlling their cholesterol levels. The National Heart, Lung, and Blood Institute (NHLBI) and its National Cholesterol Education Program (NCEP), the AHA, and the American Diabetes Association (ADA), as well as CAD support groups and reliable Internet sources, are a few examples of the available resources (see Resources section at the end of this chapter). Cookbooks and recipes that include the nutritional contents of foods can be included as resources for patients. Dietary control has been made easier because food manufacturers are required to provide nutritional data on product labels. The label information of interest to a person attempting to eat a heart-healthy diet is as follows: serving size (expressed in household measures), amount of total fat per serving, amount of saturated fat and trans fat per serving, amount of cholesterol per serving, and amount of fiber per serving.

Physical Activity

Management of an elevated triglyceride level focuses on weight reduction and increased physical activity. Regular, moderate physical activity increases HDL levels and reduces triglyceride levels, decreasing the incidence of coronary events and reducing overall mortality risk. The goal for most adults is to engage in moderate-intensity aerobic activity of at least 150 minutes per week or vigorous-intensity aerobic activity of at least 75 minutes per week, or an equivalent combination (Arnett et al., 2019). In addition, adults should engage in muscle-strengthening activities on 2 or more days each week that work all major muscle groups. The nurse helps the patient to set realistic goals for physical activity. For example, inactive patients can start with activity that lasts 3 minutes, such as parking farther from a building to increase daily walking time. Patients should be instructed to engage in an activity or variety of activities that interest them to maintain motivation. They should also be taught to exercise to an intensity that does not preclude their ability to talk; if they cannot have a conversation while exercising, they should slow down or switch to a less intensive activity. When the weather is hot and humid, patients should exercise during the early morning, or indoors, and wear loose-fitting clothing. When the weather is cold, they should layer clothing and wear a hat. Patients should stop any activity if chest pain, unexpected shortness of breath, dizziness, lightheadedness, or nausea occurs.

Medications

If diet alone cannot normalize serum cholesterol levels, medications can have a synergistic effect with the prescribed diet and control cholesterol levels (see Table 23-1). Lipid-lowering medications can reduce CAD mortality in patients with elevated lipid levels and in at-risk patients with normal lipid levels (Grundy et al., 2018). The various types of lipid-lowering agents affect the lipid components somewhat differently; these types include 3-hydroxy-3-methylglutaryl coenzyme A (HMG-CoA) (or statins), fibric acids (or fibrates), bile acid sequestrants (or resins), cholesterol absorption inhibitors, and proprotein convertase subtilisin-kexin type 9 (PCSK9) agents. Because of their high cost, PCSK9 agents are prescribed on a limited basis, but may be considered for those at high cardiovascular risk or who have familial hypercholesterolemia (Grundy et al., 2018).

Before starting statin therapy, the provider and patient should discuss risk factors, adherence to a healthy lifestyle, benefits of risk-reduction, the potential of adverse effects and drug–drug interactions, as well as patient preferences for an individualized treatment plan (Grundy et al., 2018).

Promoting Cessation of Tobacco Use

Tobacco use contributes to the development and severity of CAD in at least three ways:

- Nicotinic acid in tobacco triggers the release of catecholamines, which raise the heart rate and blood pressure (Frandsen & Pennington, 2021). Nicotinic acid can also cause the coronary arteries to constrict. These effects lead to an increased risk of CAD and sudden cardiac death.
- Tobacco use can increase the oxidation of LDL, damaging the vascular endothelium (Lee, Ong, Zhou, et al., 2019). This increases platelet adhesion and leads to a higher probability of thrombus formation.
- Inhalation of smoke increases the blood carbon monoxide level and decreases the supply of oxygen to the myocardium (Frandsen & Pennington, 2021). Hemoglobin,

TABLE 23-1 Select Medications that Affect Lipoprotein Metabolism

Medications	Therapeutic Effects	Considerations
HMG-CoA Reductase Inhibitors (Statins)		
Atorvastatin Simvastatin Rosuvastatin	↓ Total cholesterol ↓ LDL ↑ HDL ↓ TGs Inhibit enzyme involved in lipid synthesis (HMG-CoA) Favorable effects on vascular endothelium, including anti-inflammatory and antithrombotic effects	Frequently given as initial therapy for significantly elevated cholesterol and LDL levels Myalgia and arthralgia are common adverse effects Myopathy and possible rhabdomyolysis are potential serious effects Monitor liver function tests Contraindicated in liver disease Check for drug interactions Indication for use now includes ACS and stroke Administer in evening
Fibric Acids (Fibrates)		
Fenofibrate Gemfibrozil	↑ HDL ↓ TGs ↓ Synthesis of TGs and other lipids	Adverse effects include diarrhea, flatulence, rash, myalgia Serious adverse effects include pancreatitis, hepatotoxicity, and rhabdomyolysis Contraindicated in severe kidney and liver disease Use with caution in patients who are also taking statins
Bile Acid Sequestrants		
Cholestyramine Colestipol Colesevelam	↓ LDL Slight ↑ HDL Oxidize cholesterol into bile acids, which ↓ fat absorption	Most often used as adjunct therapy when statins alone have not been effective in controlling lipid levels Side effects include constipation, abdominal pain, GI bleeding May decrease absorption of other drugs Taken before meals
Cholesterol Absorption Inhibitor		
Ezetimibe	↓ LDL Inhibits absorption of cholesterol in small intestine	Better tolerated than bile acid sequestrants Used in combination with other agents, such as statins Side effects include abdominal pain, arthralgia, myalgia Contraindicated in liver disease
Proprotein Convertase Subtilisin-Kexin Type 9 (PCSK9) Agents		
Alirocumab Evolocumab	Prolongs receptor activity to promote clearance of cholesterol ↓ LDL ↓ risk of MI and stroke ↓ need for stent or CABG	Only administered by subcutaneous injection via a pen device, one or two times per month as prescribed Side effects include rhinitis, sore throat, flulike symptoms, muscle pain, diarrhea, and redness, pain, or bruising at injection site

↓ decrease, ↑ increase; ACS, acute coronary syndrome; CABG, coronary artery bypass graft; GI, gastrointestinal; HDL, high-density lipoprotein; HMG-CoA, 3-hydroxy-3-methylglutaryl coenzyme A; LDL, low-density lipoprotein; MI, myocardial infarction; TGs, triglycerides.
Adapted from Frandsen, G., & Pennington, S. S. (2021). *Abrams' clinical drug therapy: Rationales for nursing practice* (12th ed.). Philadelphia, PA: Wolters Kluwer Health.

the oxygen-carrying component of blood, combines more readily with carbon monoxide than with oxygen. Myocardial ischemia and reduced contractility can result.

A person at increased risk for heart disease is encouraged to stop tobacco use through any means possible: educational programs, counseling, consistent motivation and reinforcement messages, support groups, and medications. Some people have found complementary therapies (e.g., acupuncture, guided imagery, hypnosis) to be helpful. People who stop smoking reduce their risk of heart disease within the first year, and the risk continues to decline as long as they refrain from smoking (Benjamin, Muntner, Alonso, et al., 2019).

The use of medications such as the nicotine patch, nicotine lozenges, nicotine gum, varenicline, or bupropion may assist with stopping the use of tobacco (Barua, Rigotti, Benowitz, et al., 2018). Products containing nicotine have some of the same effects as smoking: catecholamine release (increasing heart rate and blood pressure) and increased platelet adhesion. These medications should be used for a short time and at the lowest effective doses.

Exposure to others' smoke (passive or secondhand smoke) increases the risk for CAD by 25% to 30% and for stroke by 20% to 30% (Benjamin et al., 2019). Other forms of tobacco use are becoming increasingly common today. Use of electronic nicotine delivery systems (ENDS) including e-cigarettes, e-pens, e-pipes, e-hookah, and e-cigars has increased, particularly among adolescents and young adults. Specifically, e-cigarette use, which entails inhalation of a vaporized liquid that includes nicotine, solvents, and flavoring ("vaping"), has risen significantly in these groups. Use of cigarillos and other mass market cigars, hookahs, and water pipes are also on the rise. Short-term exposure to water pipe smoking is associated with an increase in systolic blood pressure and heart rate, but long-term effects remain unclear. The cardiovascular risks associated with e-cigarette use are not yet known (Benjamin et al., 2019).

Managing Hypertension

Hypertension is defined as systolic blood pressure measurements of greater than 130 mm Hg and/or diastolic blood pressure levels greater than 80 mm Hg. A single reading is not adequate to make a diagnosis. Averaging two or three measurements obtained on two to three different occasions will provide a more accurate measurement (Whelton, Carey,

Aronow, et al., 2018). The risk of cardiovascular disease increases as blood pressure increases, and current guidelines support treating hypertension with a goal of keeping the blood pressure under 130/80 for all adults (Whelton et al., 2018). Long-standing elevated blood pressure may result in increased stiffness of the vessel walls, leading to vessel injury and a resulting inflammatory response within the intima. Inflammatory mediators then lead to the release of growth-promoting factors that cause vessel hypertrophy and hyperresponsiveness. These changes result in acceleration and aggravation of atherosclerosis. Hypertension also increases the work of the left ventricle, which must pump harder to eject blood into the arteries. Over time, the increased workload causes the heart to enlarge and thicken (i.e., hypertrophy) and may eventually lead to heart failure.

Early detection of high blood pressure and adherence to a therapeutic regimen can prevent the serious consequences associated with untreated elevated blood pressure, including CAD. Intensive management of hypertension lowers the risk of cardiovascular events, including heart attack and stroke, and lowers the risk of death (Whelton et al., 2018; see Chapter 27 for a detailed discussion of hypertension).

Controlling Diabetes

Diabetes is known to accelerate the development of heart disease. Hyperglycemia fosters dyslipidemia, increased platelet aggregation, and altered red blood cell function, which can lead to thrombus formation. These metabolic alterations may impair endothelial cell–dependent vasodilation and smooth muscle function, promoting the development of atherosclerosis. Treatment with insulin, metformin, and other therapeutic interventions that lower plasma glucose levels can lead to improved endothelial function and patient outcomes. See Chapter 46 for a detailed discussion of diabetes.

Gender

Heart disease has long been recognized as a cause of morbidity and mortality in men, but it has not always been as readily recognized in women. Cardiovascular events in women occur an average of 10 years later in life than they do in men (Wada, Miyauchi, & Daida, 2019). Women tend to have a higher incidence of complications from cardiovascular disease and a higher mortality. In addition, women tend to not recognize the symptoms of CAD as early as men, and they wait longer to report their symptoms and seek medical assistance (Wada et al., 2019).

The age difference between women and men who were newly diagnosed with CAD was traditionally thought to be related to estrogen. Menopause is now recognized as a milestone in the aging process, during which risk factors tend to accumulate. Cardiovascular disease may be well developed by the time of menopause, and although hormone therapy (HT) (formerly referred to as hormone replacement therapy) for menopausal women was once promoted as preventive therapy for CAD, research does not support HT as an effective means of prevention. HT decreases menopausal symptoms and the risk of osteoporosis-related bone fractures; however, it also has been associated with an increased incidence of CAD, breast cancer, deep vein thrombosis, stroke, and pulmonary embolism. Current guidelines do not recommend HT for primary or secondary prevention of CAD (Wada et al., 2019; see Chapter 21 for further discussion).

In the past, women who possibly had coronary vascular events were less likely than men to be referred for coronary artery diagnostic procedures such as heart catheterization or treatment with invasive interventions (e.g., PCI). However, as a result of better education of health care professionals and the general public, gender differences now have less influence on diagnosis and treatment (Wada et al., 2019).

Unfolding Patient Stories: Carl Shapiro • Part 1

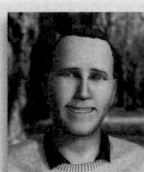

Carl Shapiro, who has a family history of atherosclerotic cardiovascular disease, is diagnosed with hypertension and hyperlipidemia during a routine visit to his primary provider. He is overweight, smokes a half pack of cigarettes per day, and describes his job as stressful. What questions can the nurse ask Carl Shapiro to help develop a plan for patient education? What topics are important for the nurse to address, and how can the information be presented? (Carl Shapiro's story continues in Chapter 67.)

Care for Carl and other patients in a realistic virtual environment: *vSim for Nursing* (thepoint.lww.com/vSimMedicalSurgical). Practice documenting these patients' care in DocuCare (thepoint.lww.com/DocuCareEHR).

Angina Pectoris

Angina pectoris is a clinical syndrome usually characterized by episodes or paroxysms of pain or pressure in the anterior chest. The cause is insufficient coronary blood flow, resulting in a decreased oxygen supply when there is increased myocardial demand for oxygen in response to physical exertion or emotional stress. In other words, the need for oxygen exceeds the supply.

Pathophysiology

Angina is usually caused by atherosclerotic disease and most often is associated with a significant obstruction of at least one major coronary artery. Normally, the myocardium extracts a large amount of oxygen from the coronary circulation to meet its continuous demands. When demand increases, flow through the coronary arteries needs to be increased. When there is a blockage in a coronary artery, flow cannot be increased and ischemia results. The types of angina are listed in Chart 23-2. Several factors are associated with typical anginal pain:

- Physical exertion, which precipitates an attack by increasing myocardial oxygen demand
- Exposure to cold, which causes vasoconstriction and elevated blood pressure, with increased oxygen demand
- Eating a heavy meal, which increases the blood flow to the mesenteric area for digestion, thereby reducing the blood supply available to the heart muscle; in a severely compromised heart, shunting of blood for digestion can be sufficient to induce anginal pain

- Stress or any emotion-provoking situation, causing the release of catecholamines, which increases blood pressure, heart rate, and myocardial workload

Unstable angina is not closely associated with these listed factors. It may occur at rest (see later discussion).

Clinical Manifestations

Ischemia of the heart muscle may produce pain or other symptoms, varying from mild indigestion to a choking or heavy sensation in the upper chest. The severity ranges from discomfort to agonizing pain. The pain may be accompanied by severe apprehension and a feeling of impending death. It is often felt deep in the chest behind the sternum (retrosternal area). Typically, the pain or discomfort is poorly localized and may radiate to the neck, jaw, shoulders, and inner aspects of the upper arms, usually the left arm. The patient often feels tightness or a heavy choking or strangling sensation that has a viselike, insistent quality. The patient with diabetes may not have severe pain with angina because autonomic neuropathy can blunt nociceptor transmission, dulling the perception of pain (Norris, 2019).

A feeling of weakness or numbness in the arms, wrists, and hands, as well as shortness of breath, pallor, diaphoresis, dizziness or lightheadedness, and nausea and vomiting, may accompany the pain. An important characteristic of angina is that it subsides with rest or administration of nitroglycerin. In many patients, anginal symptoms follow a stable, predictable pattern.

Unstable angina is characterized by attacks that increase in frequency and severity and are not relieved by rest and administration of nitroglycerin. Patients with unstable angina require medical intervention.

 Gerontologic Considerations

The older adult with angina may not exhibit a typical pain profile because of the diminished pain transmission that can occur with aging. Often the presenting symptom in older adults is dyspnea. Sometimes there are no symptoms ("silent" CAD), making recognition and diagnosis a clinical challenge. Older patients should be encouraged to recognize their chest pain–like symptom (e.g., weakness) as an indication that they should rest or take prescribed medications. Pharmacologic stress testing and cardiac catheterization may be used to diagnose CAD in older patients. Medications used to manage angina are given cautiously in older adults because they are associated with an increased risk of adverse reactions

(Frandsen & Pennington, 2021). Invasive procedures (e.g., PCI) that were once considered too risky in older adults are now being performed successfully, and many older adults benefit from symptom relief and longer survival (Lattuca, Kerneis, & Zeitouni, 2019).

Assessment and Diagnostic Findings

The diagnosis of angina begins with the patient's history related to the clinical manifestations of ischemia. A 12-lead electrocardiogram (ECG) may show changes indicative of ischemia, such as T-wave inversion, ST-segment elevation, or the development of an abnormal Q wave (Norris, 2019). Laboratory studies are performed; these generally include cardiac biomarker testing to rule out ACS (see later discussion). The patient may undergo an exercise or pharmacologic stress test in which the heart is monitored continuously by an ECG, echocardiogram, or both. The patient may also be referred for a nuclear scan or invasive procedure (e.g., cardiac catheterization, coronary angiography).

Medical Management

The objectives of the medical management of angina are to decrease the oxygen demand of the myocardium and to increase the oxygen supply. Medically, these objectives are met through pharmacologic therapy and control of risk factors. Alternatively, reperfusion procedures may be used to restore the blood supply to the myocardium. These include PCI procedures (e.g., percutaneous transluminal coronary angioplasty [PTCA] and intracoronary stents) and CABG (see later discussion).

Pharmacologic Therapy

Table 23-2 summarizes drug therapy.

Nitroglycerin

Nitrates are a standard treatment for angina pectoris. Nitroglycerin is a potent vasodilator that improves blood flow to the heart muscle and relieves pain. Nitroglycerin dilates primarily the veins and, to a lesser extent, the arteries. Dilation of the veins causes venous pooling of blood throughout the body. As a result, less blood returns to the heart, and filling pressure (preload) is reduced. If the patient is hypovolemic (does not have adequate circulating blood volume), the decrease in filling pressure can cause a significant decrease in cardiac output and blood pressure (Frandsen & Pennington, 2021).

Nitrates also relax the systemic arteriolar bed, lowering blood pressure and decreasing afterload. These effects decrease myocardial oxygen requirements, bringing about a more favorable balance between supply and demand.

Nitroglycerin may be given by several routes: sublingual tablet or spray, oral capsule, topical agent, and intravenous (IV) administration. Sublingual nitroglycerin is generally placed under the tongue or in the cheek (buccal pouch) and ideally alleviates the pain of ischemia within 3 minutes. Chart 23-3 provides more information on self-administration of sublingual nitroglycerin. Oral preparations and topical patches are used to provide sustained effects. A regimen in which the patches are applied in the morning and removed at bedtime allows for a nitrate-free period to prevent the development of tolerance.

TABLE 23-2	Select Medications Used to Treat Stable Angina
Medications	**Major Indications**
Nitrates Nitroglycerin	Short- and long-term reduction of myocardial oxygen consumption through selective vasodilation
Beta-Adrenergic Blocking Agents (Beta-Blockers) Metoprolol Atenolol	Reduction of myocardial oxygen consumption by blocking beta-adrenergic stimulation of the heart
Calcium Ion Antagonists (Calcium Channel Blockers) Amlodipine Diltiazem	Negative inotropic effects; indicated in patients not responsive to beta-blockers; used as primary treatment for vasospasm
Antiplatelet Medications Aspirin Clopidogrel Prasugrel Ticagrelor	Prevention of platelet aggregation

Anticoagulants
Heparin (unfractionated)
Low-molecular-weight heparins:
  Enoxaparin
  Dalteparin
	Prevention of thrombus formation

Adapted from Rousan, T. A., Mathew, S. T., & Thadani, U. (2017). Drug therapy for stable angina pectoris. *Drugs, 77*(3), 265–284.

A continuous or intermittent IV infusion of nitroglycerin may be given to the hospitalized patient with recurring signs and symptoms of ischemia or after a revascularization procedure. The rate of infusion is titrated to the patient's pain level and blood pressure. It usually is not given if the systolic blood pressure is less than 90 mm Hg. Generally, after the patient is symptom-free, the nitroglycerin may be switched to an oral or topical preparation within 24 hours. A common adverse effect of nitroglycerin is headache, which may limit the use of this drug in some patients.

Beta-Adrenergic Blocking Agents

Beta-blockers such as metoprolol reduce myocardial oxygen consumption by blocking beta-adrenergic sympathetic stimulation to the heart. The result is a reduction in heart rate, slowed conduction of impulses through the conduction system, decreased blood pressure, and reduced myocardial **contractility** (force of contraction). Because of these effects, beta-blockers balance the myocardial oxygen needs (demands) and the amount of oxygen available (supply). This helps control chest pain and delays the onset of ischemia during work or exercise. Beta-blockers reduce the incidence of recurrent angina, infarction, and cardiac mortality. The dose can be titrated to achieve a resting heart rate of 50 to 60 bpm (Frandsen & Pennington, 2021).

Cardiac side effects and possible contraindications include hypotension, bradycardia, advanced atrioventricular block, and acute heart failure. If a beta-blocker is given IV for an acute cardiac event, the ECG, blood pressure, and heart rate are monitored closely after the medication has been given.

Chart 23-3	PHARMACOLOGY Self-Administration of Nitroglycerin

Most patients with angina pectoris self-administer nitroglycerin on an as-needed basis. A key nursing role in such cases is educating patients about the medication and how to take it. Sublingual nitroglycerin comes in tablet and spray forms.

- Instruct the patient to make sure that the mouth is moist, the tongue is still, and saliva is not swallowed until the nitroglycerin tablet dissolves. If the pain is severe, the patient can crush the tablet between the teeth to hasten sublingual absorption.
- Advise the patient to carry the medication at all times as a precaution. However, because nitroglycerin is very unstable, it should be carried securely in its original container (e.g., capped dark glass bottle); tablets should never be removed and stored in metal or plastic pillboxes.
- Explain that nitroglycerin is volatile and is inactivated by heat, moisture, air, light, and time. Instruct the patient to renew the nitroglycerin supply every 6 months.
- Inform the patient that the medication should be taken in anticipation of any activity that may produce pain. Because nitroglycerin increases tolerance for exercise and stress when taken prophylactically (i.e., before angina-producing activity, such as exercise, stair-climbing, or sexual intercourse), it is best taken before pain develops.
- Recommend that the patient note how long it takes for the nitroglycerin to relieve the discomfort. Advise the patient that if pain persists after taking three sublingual tablets at 5-minute intervals, emergency medical services should be called.
- Discuss possible side effects of nitroglycerin, including flushing, throbbing headache, hypotension, and tachycardia.
- Advise the patient to sit down for a few minutes when taking nitroglycerin to avoid hypotension and syncope.

Adapted from Comerford, K. C., & Durkin, M. T. (Eds.) (2020). *Nursing2020 Drug Handbook*. Philadelphia, PA: Wolters Kluwer.

Side effects include depressed mood, fatigue, decreased libido, and dizziness. Patients taking beta-blockers are cautioned not to stop taking them abruptly, because angina may worsen, and MI may develop. Beta-blocker therapy should be decreased gradually over several days before being discontinued. Patients with diabetes who take beta-blockers are instructed to monitor their blood glucose levels as prescribed because beta-blockers can mask signs of hypoglycemia. Beta-blockers that are not cardioselective also affect the beta-adrenergic receptors in the bronchioles, causing bronchoconstriction, and therefore are contraindicated in patients with significant chronic pulmonary disorders, such as asthma.

Calcium Channel Blocking Agents

Calcium channel blockers have a variety of effects on the ischemic myocardium. These agents decrease sinoatrial node automaticity and atrioventricular node conduction, resulting in a slower heart rate and a decrease in the strength of myocardial contraction (negative inotropic effect). These effects decrease the workload of the heart. Calcium channel blockers also increase myocardial oxygen supply by dilating the smooth muscle wall of the coronary arterioles; they decrease myocardial oxygen demand by reducing systemic arterial pressure and the workload of the left ventricle (Frandsen & Pennington, 2021). The calcium channel blockers most commonly used are amlodipine and diltiazem. In addition to their use to treat angina, they are commonly prescribed for hypertension.

Hypotension may occur after the administration of any of the calcium channel blockers, particularly when administered IV. Other side effects may include atrioventricular block, bradycardia, and constipation.

Antiplatelet and Anticoagulant Medications

Antiplatelet medications are given to prevent platelet aggregation and subsequent thrombosis, which impedes blood flow through the coronary arteries.

Aspirin

Aspirin prevents platelet aggregation and reduces the incidence of MI and death in patients with CAD (Frandsen & Pennington, 2021). A 162- to 325-mg dose of aspirin should be given to the patient with a new diagnosis of angina and then continued with 81 to 325 mg daily. Patients should be advised to continue aspirin even if they concurrently take other analgesics such as acetaminophen. Because aspirin may cause GI upset and bleeding, the use of histamine-2 (H_2) blockers (e.g., famotidine) or proton pump inhibitors (e.g., omeprazole) should be considered concomitant with continued aspirin therapy (Ibanez, James, Agewall, et al., 2018).

Adenosine Diphosphate Receptor Antagonists ($P2Y_{12}$)

These medications act on different pathways than aspirin to block platelet activation. However, unlike aspirin, these agents may take a few days to achieve antiplatelet effects. Clopidogrel is commonly prescribed in addition to aspirin in patients at high risk for MI. Newer oral agents such as prasugrel and ticagrelor may be used in place of clopidogrel during coronary events and interventions (Frandsen & Pennington, 2021). Both carry the risk of bleeding from the GI tract or other sites.

Heparin

Unfractionated IV heparin prevents the formation of new blood clots (i.e., it is an anticoagulant). Treating patients with unstable angina with heparin reduces the occurrence of MI. If the patient's signs and symptoms indicate a significant risk for a cardiac event, the patient is hospitalized and may be given an IV bolus of heparin and started on a continuous infusion. The dose of heparin given is based on the results of the activated partial thromboplastin time (aPTT). Heparin therapy is usually considered therapeutic when the aPTT is 2 to 2.5 times the normal aPTT value.

A subcutaneous injection of low-molecular-weight heparin (LMWH; enoxaparin or dalteparin) may be used instead of IV unfractionated heparin to treat patients with unstable angina or non–ST-segment elevation myocardial infarction (NSTEMI) (Frandsen & Pennington, 2021). LMWH provides effective and stable anticoagulation, potentially reducing the risk of rebound ischemic events, and eliminating the need to monitor aPTT results. LMWHs may be beneficial before and during PCIs as well as for ACS.

Because unfractionated heparin and LMWH increase the risk of bleeding, the patient is monitored for signs and symptoms of external and internal bleeding, such as low blood pressure, increased heart rate, and decreased serum hemoglobin and hematocrit. The patient receiving heparin is placed on bleeding precautions, which include:

- Applying pressure to the site of any needle puncture for a longer time than usual

- Avoiding intramuscular (IM) injections
- Avoiding tissue injury and bruising from trauma or use of constrictive devices (e.g., continuous use of an automatic blood pressure cuff)

A decrease in platelet count or evidence of thrombosis may indicate heparin-induced thrombocytopenia (HIT), an antibody-mediated reaction to heparin that may result in thrombosis. Patients who have received heparin within the past 3 months and those who have been receiving unfractionated heparin for 4 to 14 days are at high risk for HIT (Frandsen & Pennington, 2021). As an alternative to LMWH and unfractionated heparin, argatroban, a direct antithrombotic agent might be prescribed (Frandsen & Pennington, 2021; see Chapter 29 for further discussion of HIT).

Glycoprotein IIb/IIIa Agents

IV administration of glycoprotein (GP) IIb/IIIa agents, such as abciximab or eptifibatide, is indicated for hospitalized patients with unstable angina and as adjunct therapy for PCI. These agents prevent platelet aggregation by blocking the GP IIb/IIIa receptors on the platelets, preventing adhesion of fibrinogen and other factors that crosslink platelets to each other and thus form intracoronary clots (Urden, Stacy, & Lough, 2019). As with heparin, bleeding is the major side effect, and bleeding precautions should be initiated.

Oxygen Administration

Oxygen therapy is usually initiated at the onset of chest pain in an attempt to increase the amount of oxygen delivered to the myocardium and to decrease pain. The therapeutic effectiveness of oxygen is determined by observing the rate and rhythm of respirations and the color of skin and mucous membranes. Blood oxygen saturation is monitored by pulse oximetry; the normal oxygen saturation (SpO_2) level is >95% on room air (Urden et al., 2019).

NURSING PROCESS

The Patient with Angina Pectoris

Assessment

The nurse gathers information about the patient's symptoms and activities, especially those that precede and precipitate attacks of angina pectoris. Appropriate questions are listed in Chart 23-4. The answers to these questions form the basis for designing an effective program of treatment and prevention. In addition to assessing angina pectoris or its equivalent, the nurse also assesses the patient's risk factors for CAD, the patient's response to angina, the patient's and family's understanding of the diagnosis, and adherence to the current treatment plan.

Diagnosis

NURSING DIAGNOSES

Based on the assessment data, major nursing diagnoses may include:

- Risk for impaired cardiac function
- Anxiety associated with cardiac symptoms and possible death
- Lack of knowledge about the underlying disease and methods for avoiding complications
- Able to perform self care

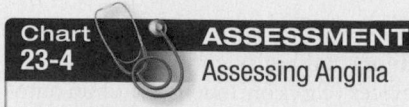

Chart 23-4

ASSESSMENT
Assessing Angina

Ask the following:

- "Where is the pain (or prodromal symptoms)? Can you point to it?"
- "Can you feel the pain anywhere else?"
- "How would you describe the pain?"
- "Is it like the pain you had before?"
- "Can you rate the pain on a 0–10 scale, with 10 being the most pain?"
- "When did the pain begin?"
- "How long does it last?"
- "What brings on the pain?"
- "What helps the pain go away?"
- "Do you have any other symptoms with the pain?"

COLLABORATIVE PROBLEMS/POTENTIAL COMPLICATIONS

Potential complications may include the following:

- ACS and/or MI (described later in this chapter)
- Arrhythmias and cardiac arrest (see Chapters 22 and 25)
- Heart failure (see Chapter 25)
- Cardiogenic shock (see Chapter 11)

Planning and Goals

Major patient goals include immediate and appropriate treatment when angina occurs, prevention of angina, reduction of anxiety, awareness of the disease process and understanding of the prescribed care, adherence to the self-care program, and absence of complications.

Nursing Interventions

TREATING ANGINA

If the patient reports pain (or cardiac ischemia is suggested by prodromal symptoms, which may include sensations of indigestion or nausea, choking, heaviness, weakness or numbness in the upper extremities, dyspnea, or dizziness), the nurse takes immediate action. The patient experiencing angina is directed to stop all activities and sit or rest in bed in a semi-Fowler position to reduce the oxygen requirements of the ischemic myocardium. The nurse assesses the patient's angina, asking questions to determine whether the angina is the same as the patient typically experiences. A change may indicate a worsening of the disease or a different cause. The nurse then continues to assess the patient, measuring vital signs and observing for signs of respiratory distress. If the patient is in the hospital, a 12-lead ECG is usually obtained and assessed for ST-segment and T-wave changes. If the patient has been placed on cardiac monitoring with continuous ST-segment monitoring, the ST segment is assessed for changes.

Nitroglycerin is given sublingually, and the patient's response is assessed (relief of chest pain and effect on blood pressure and heart rate). If the chest pain is unchanged or is lessened but still present, nitroglycerin administration is repeated up to three doses. Each time blood pressure, heart rate, and the ST segment (if the patient is on a monitor with ST-segment monitoring capability) are assessed. The nurse administers oxygen therapy if the patient's respiratory rate is increased or if the oxygen saturation level is decreased.

Oxygen is usually given at 2 L/min by nasal cannula, even without evidence of desaturation, although there is no current evidence of a positive effect on patient outcome. If the pain is significant and continues after these interventions, the patient is further evaluated for acute MI and may be transferred to a higher-acuity nursing unit (Ibanez et al., 2018).

REDUCING ANXIETY

Patients with angina often fear loss of their roles within society and the family. They may also fear that the pain (or the prodromal symptoms) may lead to an MI or death. Exploring the implications that the diagnosis has for the patient and providing information about the illness, its treatment, and methods of preventing its progression are important nursing interventions. Various stress reduction methods, such as guided imagery or music therapy, should be explored with the patient (Meghani, 2017). Addressing the spiritual needs of the patient and family may also assist in allaying anxieties and fears.

PREVENTING PAIN

The nurse reviews the assessment findings, identifies the level of activity that causes the patient's pain or prodromal symptoms, and plans the patient's activities accordingly. If the patient has pain frequently or with minimal activity, the nurse alternates the patient's activities with rest periods. Balancing activity and rest is an important aspect of the educational plan for the patient and family.

PROMOTING HOME, COMMUNITY-BASED, AND TRANSITIONAL CARE

Educating Patients About Self-Care. The program for educating the patient with angina is designed so that the patient and family understand the illness, identify the symptoms of myocardial ischemia, state the actions to take when symptoms develop, and discuss methods to prevent chest pain and the advancement of CAD. The goals of education are to reduce the frequency and severity of anginal attacks, to delay the progress of the underlying disease if possible, and to prevent complications. The factors outlined in Chart 23-5 are important in educating the patient with angina pectoris.

The self-care program is prepared in collaboration with the patient and family or friends. Activities should be planned to minimize the occurrence of anginal episodes. The patient needs to understand that any pain unrelieved within 15 minutes by the usual methods, including nitroglycerin (see Chart 23-3), should be treated at the closest ED; the patient should call 911 for assistance.

Continuing and Transitional Care. For patient with disability or special needs, arrangements are made for transitional, home, or community care when appropriate. A home health or transitional care nurse can assist the patient with scheduling and keeping follow-up appointments. The patient may need reminders about follow-up monitoring, including periodic laboratory testing. In addition, the home health nurse may monitor the patient's adherence to dietary restrictions and to prescribed antianginal medications, including nitroglycerin. If the patient has severe anginal symptoms, the nurse may assess the home environment and recommend modifications that diminish the occurrence of anginal episodes. For instance, if a patient cannot climb stairs without experiencing ischemia,

Chart 23-5	HOME CARE CHECKLIST
	Managing Angina Pectoris

At the completion of education, the patient and/or caregiver will be able to:

- State the impact of angina pectoris on physiologic functioning, ADLs, IADLs, roles, relationships, and spirituality.
- State changes in lifestyle (e.g., diet, activity) or home environment necessary to maintain health.
- Follow a diet low in saturated fat, high in fiber, and, if indicated, lower in calories.
- Reduce the probability of an episode of anginal pain by balancing rest with regular daily activities that do not produce chest discomfort, shortness of breath, or undue fatigue.
- Follow the prescribed exercise regimen.
  - Recognize that temperature extremes (particularly cold) may induce anginal pain; therefore, avoid exercise in temperature extremes.
- State the name, dose, side effects, frequency, and schedule for all medications
- Take medications, especially aspirin and beta-blockers, as prescribed.
- Carry nitroglycerin at all times; state when and how to use it; identify its side effects.

- Avoid using medications or any over-the-counter substances (e.g., diet pills, nasal decongestants) that can increase the heart rate and blood pressure without first discussing with the primary provider.
- Use appropriate resources for support during emotionally stressful times (e.g., counselor, nurse, clergy, primary provider).
- Stop smoking and the use of other forms of tobacco and avoid secondhand smoke (because smoking increases the heart rate, blood pressure, and blood carbon monoxide levels).
- Achieve and maintain normal blood pressure.
- Achieve and maintain normal blood glucose levels.
- State how to reach primary provider with questions or complications.
  - Report increase in symptoms to the primary provider.
  - State time and date of follow-up appointments and testing.
- Identify the need for health promotion (e.g., weight reduction, cessation of tobacco use, stress management), disease prevention, and screening activities.

ADLs, activities of daily living; IADLs, independent activities of daily living.

the home health nurse may help the patient plan daily activities that minimize stair-climbing.

Evaluation

Expected patient outcomes may include:

1. Reports that pain is relieved promptly
   a. Recognizes symptoms
   b. Takes immediate action
   c. Seeks medical assistance if pain persists or changes in quality
2. Reports decreased anxiety
   a. Expresses acceptance of diagnosis
   b. Expresses control over choices within medical regimen
   c. Does not exhibit signs and symptoms that indicate a high level of anxiety
3. Understands ways to avoid complications and is free of complications
   a. Describes the process of angina
   b. Explains reasons for measures to prevent complications
   c. Exhibits stable ECG
   d. Experiences no signs and symptoms of acute MI
4. Adheres to self-care program
   a. Takes medications as prescribed
   b. Keeps health care appointments
   c. Implements plan to reduce risk factors

Acute Coronary Syndrome and Myocardial Infarction

Acute coronary syndrome (ACS) is an emergent situation characterized by an acute onset of myocardial ischemia that results in myocardial death (i.e., MI) if definitive interventions do not occur promptly. (Although the terms *coronary occlusion*, *heart attack*, and *myocardial infarction* are used synonymously, the preferred term is *myocardial infarction*.) The spectrum of ACS includes unstable angina, NSTEMI, and ST-segment elevation myocardial infarction (STEMI).

Pathophysiology

In unstable angina, there is reduced blood flow in a coronary artery, often due to rupture of an atherosclerotic plaque. A clot begins to form on top of the coronary lesion, but the artery is not completely occluded. This is an acute situation that can result in chest pain and other symptoms that may be referred to as preinfarction angina because the patient will likely have an MI if prompt interventions do not occur.

In an MI, plaque rupture and subsequent thrombus formation result in complete occlusion of the artery, leading to ischemia and necrosis of the myocardium supplied by that artery. Vasospasm (sudden constriction or narrowing) of a coronary artery, decreased oxygen supply (e.g., from acute blood loss, anemia, or low blood pressure), and increased demand for oxygen (e.g., from a rapid heart rate, thyrotoxicosis, or ingestion of cocaine) are other causes of MI. In each case, a profound imbalance exists between myocardial oxygen supply and demand.

The area of infarction develops over minutes to hours. As the cells are deprived of oxygen, ischemia develops, cellular injury occurs, and the lack of oxygen results in infarction, or the death of cells. The expression "time is muscle" reflects the urgency of appropriate treatment to improve patient outcomes. Approximately every 40 seconds, an American will have an MI (Benjamin et al., 2019), and many of these people will die as a result. Early recognition and treatment of patients presenting with an MI will improve their chances of survival.

Various descriptions are used to further identify an MI: the type (NSTEMI, STEMI), the location of the injury to the ventricular wall (anterior, inferior, posterior, or lateral wall), and the point in time within the process of infarction (acute, evolving, or old). The differentiation between NSTEMI and STEMI is determined by diagnostic tests and is explained later in this chapter.

The 12-lead ECG identifies the type and location of the MI, and other ECG indicators, such as a Q wave, and patient history, identify the timing. Regardless of the location, the goals of medical therapy are to relieve symptoms, prevent or minimize myocardial tissue death, and prevent complications. The pathophysiology of CAD and the risk factors involved were discussed earlier in this chapter.

Clinical Manifestations

Chest pain that occurs suddenly and continues despite rest and medication is the presenting symptom in most patients with ACS. Some of these patients have prodromal symptoms or a previous diagnosis of CAD, but others report no previous symptoms. Patients may present with a combination of symptoms, including chest pain, shortness of breath, indigestion, nausea, and anxiety. They may have cool, pale, and moist skin. Their heart rate and respiratory rate may be faster than normal. These signs and symptoms, which are caused by stimulation of the sympathetic nervous system, may be present for only a short time or may persist. In many cases, the signs and symptoms of MI cannot be distinguished from those of unstable angina; hence, the evolution of the term *acute coronary syndrome*.

Assessment and Diagnostic Findings

The diagnosis of ACS is generally based on the presenting symptoms (see Chart 23-6); the 12-lead ECG and laboratory tests (e.g., serial cardiac biomarkers) are performed to clarify whether the patient has unstable angina, NSTEMI, or STEMI (Ibanez et al., 2018). The prognosis depends on the severity of coronary artery obstruction and the presence and extent of myocardial damage. Physical examination is always conducted, but the examination alone does not confirm the diagnosis.

Patient History

The patient history includes the description of the presenting symptom (e.g., pain), the history of previous cardiac and other illnesses, and the family history of heart disease. The history should also include information about the patient's risk factors for heart disease.

Electrocardiogram

The 12-lead ECG provides information that assists in ruling out or diagnosing an acute MI. It should be obtained within 10 minutes from the time a patient reports pain or arrives in the ED. By monitoring serial ECG changes over time, the location, evolution, and resolution of an MI can be identified and monitored.

The ECG changes that occur with an MI are seen in the leads that view the involved surface of the heart. The expected ECG changes are T-wave inversion, ST-segment elevation, and development of an abnormal Q wave (see Fig. 23-5). Because infarction evolves over time, the ECG also changes over time. The first ECG signs of an acute MI

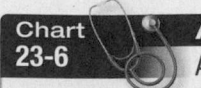

> **Chart 23-6**
>
> ### ASSESSMENT
> ### Assessing for Acute Coronary Syndrome or Acute Myocardial Infarction
>
> Be alert for the following signs and symptoms:
>
> **Cardiovascular**
>
> - Chest pain or discomfort not relieved by rest or nitroglycerin; palpitations. Heart sounds may include S_3, S_4, and new onset of a murmur.
> - Increased jugular venous distention may be seen if the myocardial infarction (MI) has caused heart failure.
> - Blood pressure may be elevated because of sympathetic stimulation or decreased because of decreased contractility, impending cardiogenic shock, or medications.
> - Irregular pulse may indicate atrial fibrillation.
> - In addition to ST-segment and T-wave changes, the electrocardiogram may show tachycardia, bradycardia, or other arrhythmias.
>
> **Respiratory**
>
> Shortness of breath, dyspnea, tachypnea, and crackles if MI has caused pulmonary congestion. Pulmonary edema may be present.
>
> **Gastrointestinal**
>
> Nausea, indigestion, and vomiting.
>
> **Genitourinary**
>
> Decreased urinary output may indicate cardiogenic shock.
>
> **Skin**
>
> Cool, clammy, diaphoretic, and pale appearance due to sympathetic stimulation may indicate cardiogenic shock.
>
> **Neurologic**
>
> Anxiety, restlessness, and lightheadedness may indicate increased sympathetic stimulation or a decrease in contractility and cerebral oxygenation. The same symptoms may also herald cardiogenic shock.
>
> **Psychological**
>
> Fear with feeling of impending doom, or denial that anything is wrong.

are usually seen in the T wave and ST segment (Urden et al., 2019). As the area of injury becomes ischemic, myocardial repolarization is altered and delayed, causing the T wave to invert. Myocardial injury also causes ST-segment changes. The ST segment is normally flat on the ECG tracing. The injured myocardial cells depolarize normally but repolarize more rapidly than normal cells, causing the ST segment to rise at least 1 mm above the isoelectric line (the area between the T wave and the next P wave is used as the reference for the isoelectric line). This change is measured 0.06 to 0.08 seconds after the end of the QRS—a point called the J point (Urden et al., 2019) (see Fig. 23-6). An elevation in the ST segment in two contiguous leads is a key diagnostic indicator for MI (i.e., STEMI).

The appearance of abnormal Q waves is another indication of MI. Q waves develop within 1 to 3 days because there is no depolarization current conducted from necrotic tissue (Urden et al., 2019). A new and significant Q wave is 0.04 seconds or longer and 25% of the R wave depth. An

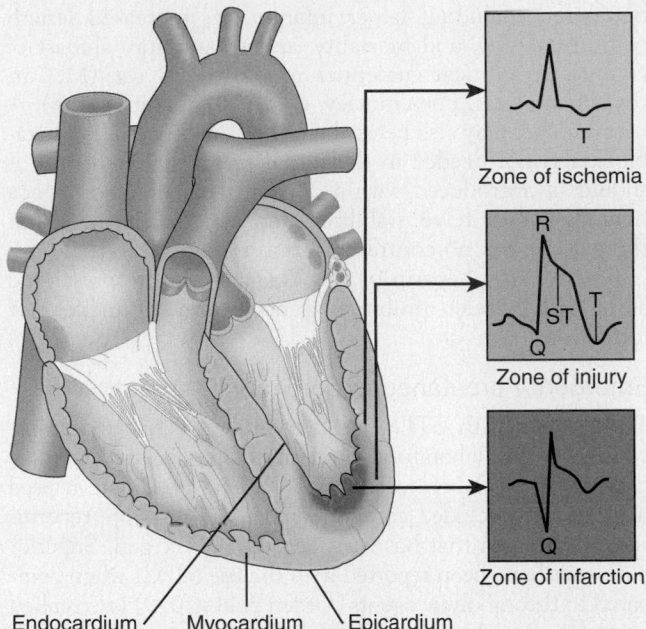

Figure 23-5 • Effects of ischemia, injury, and infarction on an electrocardiogram recording. Ischemia causes inversion of the T wave because of altered repolarization. Cardiac muscle injury causes elevation of the ST segment. Later, Q waves develop because of the absence of depolarization current from the necrotic tissue and opposing currents from other parts of the heart.

acute MI may also cause a significant decrease in the height of the R wave. During an acute MI, injury and ischemic changes are usually present. An abnormal Q wave may be present without ST-segment and T-wave changes, which indicates an old, not acute, MI. For some patients, there is no persistent ST elevation or other ECG changes; therefore, an NSTEMI is diagnosed by blood levels of cardiac biomarkers.

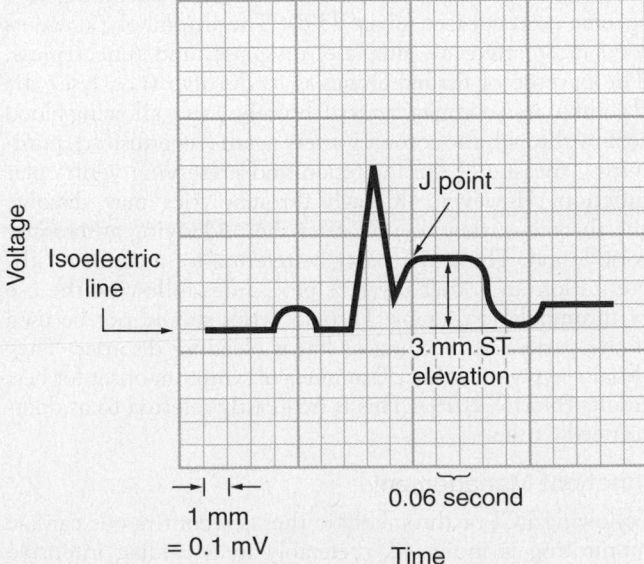

Figure 23-6 • Using the electrocardiogram to diagnose acute myocardial infarction (MI). (ST-segment elevation is measured 0.06 to 0.08 seconds after the J point. An elevation of more than 1 mm in contiguous leads is indicative of acute MI.)

Using the information presented, patients are diagnosed with one of the following forms of ACS:

- *Unstable angina:* The patient has clinical manifestations of coronary ischemia, but ECG and cardiac biomarkers show no evidence of acute MI.
- *STEMI:* The patient has ECG evidence of acute MI with characteristic changes in two contiguous leads on a 12-lead ECG. In this type of MI, there is a significant damage to the myocardium.
- *NSTEMI:* The patient has elevated cardiac biomarkers (e.g., troponin) but no definite ECG evidence of acute MI. In this type of MI, there may be less damage to the myocardium.

During recovery from an MI, the ST segment often is the first ECG indicator to return to normal. Q-wave alterations are usually permanent. An old STEMI is usually indicated by an abnormal Q wave or decreased height of the R wave without ST-segment and T-wave changes.

Echocardiogram

The echocardiogram is used to evaluate ventricular function. It may be used to assist in diagnosing an MI, especially when the ECG is nondiagnostic. The echocardiogram can detect hypokinetic and akinetic wall motion and can determine the ejection fraction (see Chapter 21).

Laboratory Tests

Cardiac enzymes and biomarkers, which include troponin, creatine kinase (CK), and myoglobin, are used to diagnose an acute MI. Cardiac biomarkers can be analyzed rapidly, expediting an accurate diagnosis. These tests are based on the release of cellular contents into the circulation when myocardial cells die.

Troponin

Troponin, a protein found in myocardial cells, regulates the myocardial contractile process. There are three isomers of troponin: C, I, and T. Troponins I and T are specific for cardiac muscle, and these biomarkers are currently recognized as reliable and critical markers of myocardial injury (Norris, 2019). An increase in the level of troponin in the serum can be detected within a few hours during acute MI. It remains elevated for a long period, often as long as 2 weeks, and it therefore can be used to detect recent myocardial damage. It should be noted that cardiac troponin levels may rise during inflammation and other forms of mechanical stress on the myocardium. These include sepsis, heart failure, and respiratory failure (Felker & Fudim, 2018).

Creatine Kinase and Its Isoenzymes

There are three CK isoenzymes: CK-MM (skeletal muscle), CK-MB (heart muscle), and CK-BB (brain tissue). CK-MB is the cardiac-specific isoenzyme; it is found mainly in cardiac cells and therefore increases when there has been damage to these cells. Elevated CK-MB is an indicator of acute MI; the level begins to increase within a few hours and peaks within 24 hours of an infarct.

Myoglobin

Myoglobin is a heme protein that helps transport oxygen. Like the CK-MB enzyme, myoglobin is found in cardiac and

Chart 23-7
Treatment Guidelines for Acute Myocardial Infarction

- Use rapid transit to the hospital.
- Obtain 12-lead electrocardiogram to be read within 10 minutes.
- Obtain laboratory blood specimens of cardiac biomarkers, including troponin.
- Obtain other diagnostics to clarify the diagnosis.
- Begin routine medical interventions:
  - Supplemental oxygen
  - Nitroglycerin
  - Morphine
  - Aspirin
  - Beta-blocker
  - Angiotensin-converting enzyme inhibitor within 24 hours
  - Anticoagulation with heparin and platelet inhibitors
  - Statin
- Evaluate for indications for reperfusion therapy:
  - Percutaneous coronary intervention
  - Thrombolytic therapy
- Continue therapy as indicated:
  - IV heparin, low-molecular-weight heparin, bivalirudin, or fondaparinux
  - Clopidogrel
  - Glycoprotein IIb/IIIa inhibitor
  - Bed rest for a minimum of 12–24 hours
  - Statin prescribed at discharge.

Adapted from Ibanez, B., James, S., Agewall, S., et al. (2018). 2017 ESC Guidelines for the management of acute myocardial infarction in patients presenting with ST-segment elevation. *European Heart Journal, 39*(2), 119–177.

skeletal muscle. The myoglobin level starts to increase within 1 to 3 hours and peaks within 12 hours after the onset of symptoms. An increase in myoglobin is not very specific in indicating an acute cardiac event; however, negative results can be used to rule out an acute MI.

Medical Management

The goals of medical management are to minimize myocardial damage, preserve myocardial function, and prevent complications. These goals are facilitated by the use of guidelines developed by the ACC and the AHA (see Chart 23-7).

The goal for treating patients with acute MI is to minimize myocardial damage by reducing myocardial oxygen demand and increasing oxygen supply with medications, oxygen administration, and bed rest. The resolution of pain and ECG changes indicate that demand and supply are in equilibrium; they may also indicate reperfusion. Visualization of blood flow through an open vessel in the catheterization laboratory is evidence of reperfusion.

Initial Management

The patient with suspected MI should immediately receive supplemental oxygen, aspirin, nitroglycerin, and morphine. Morphine is the drug of choice to reduce pain and anxiety. It also reduces preload and afterload, decreasing the work of the heart. The response to morphine is monitored carefully to assess for hypotension or decreased respiratory rate. Nurses should be aware that evolving research has suggested an association between morphine and potential adverse

outcomes, including larger infarct size, increased length of hospital stay, and mortality, and should stay abreast of changes to clinical guidelines impacting its use (McCarthy, Bhambhani, Pomerantsev, et al., 2018; Neto, 2018). A beta-blocker may also be used if arrhythmias occur. If a beta-blocker is not needed in the initial management period, it should be introduced within 24 hours of admission, once hemodynamics have stabilized and it is confirmed that the patient has no contraindications (Ibanez et al., 2018). Unfractionated heparin or LMWH may also be prescribed along with platelet-inhibiting agents to prevent further clot formation.

Emergent Percutaneous Coronary Intervention

The patient with STEMI is taken directly to the cardiac catheterization laboratory for an immediate PCI (if a cardiac catheterization laboratory is on site). The procedure is used to open the occluded coronary artery and promote reperfusion to the area that has been deprived of oxygen. Superior outcomes have been reported with the use of PCI when compared to thrombolytic agents (Urden et al., 2019) (also called *fibrinolytic* agents; see the Thrombolytics section). Thus, PCI is preferred as the initial treatment method for acute MI in all age groups (Urden et al., 2019). The procedure treats the underlying atherosclerotic lesion. Because the duration of oxygen deprivation determines the number of myocardial cells that die, the time from the patient's arrival in the ED to the time PCI is performed should be less than 60 minutes. This is frequently referred to as door-to-balloon time. A cardiac catheterization laboratory and staff must be available if an emergent PCI is to be performed within this short time. The nursing care related to PCI is presented later in this chapter.

Thrombolytics

Thrombolytic therapy is initiated when primary PCI is not available or the transport time to a PCI-capable hospital is too long. These agents are administered IV according to a specific protocol (see Chart 23-8). The thrombolytic agents used most often are alteplase, reteplase, and tenecteplase. The purpose of **thrombolytics** is to dissolve (i.e., lyse) the thrombus in a coronary artery (thrombolysis), allowing blood to flow through the coronary artery again (reperfusion), minimizing the size of the infarction and preserving ventricular function. However, although thrombolytics may dissolve the thrombus, they do not affect the underlying atherosclerotic lesion. The patient may be referred for a cardiac catheterization and other invasive procedures following the use of thrombolytic therapy. Thrombolytics should not be used if the patient is bleeding or has a bleeding disorder. They should be given within 30 minutes of symptom onset for best results (Norris, 2019). This is frequently referred to as door-to-needle time.

Inpatient Management

Following PCI or thrombolytic therapy, continuous cardiac monitoring is indicated, preferably in a cardiac intensive care unit (ICU). Continuing pharmacologic management includes aspirin, a beta-blocker, and an angiotensin-converting enzyme (ACE) inhibitor. ACE inhibitors prevent the conversion of angiotensin I to angiotensin II. In the

Chart 23-8   PHARMACOLOGY
Administration of Thrombolytic Therapy

Indications

- Chest pain lasting more than 20 minutes, unrelieved by nitroglycerin
- ST-segment elevation in at least two leads that face the same area of the heart
- Less than 12 hours from onset of pain

Absolute Contraindications

- Active bleeding
- Known bleeding disorder
- History of hemorrhagic stroke
- History of intracranial vessel malformation
- Recent major surgery or trauma
- Uncontrolled hypertension
- Pregnancy

Nursing Considerations

- Minimize the number of times the patient's skin is punctured.
- Avoid intramuscular injections.
- Draw blood for laboratory tests when starting the IV line.
- Start IV lines before thrombolytic therapy; designate one line to use for blood draws.
- Avoid continual use of noninvasive blood pressure cuff.
- Monitor for acute arrhythmias and hypotension.
- Monitor for reperfusion: resolution of angina or acute ST-segment changes.
- Check for signs and symptoms of bleeding: decrease in hematocrit and hemoglobin values, decrease in blood pressure, increase in heart rate, oozing or bulging at invasive procedure sites, back pain, muscle weakness, changes in level of consciousness, complaints of headache.
- Treat major bleeding by discontinuing thrombolytic therapy and any anticoagulants; apply direct pressure and notify the primary provider immediately.
- Treat minor bleeding by applying direct pressure if accessible and appropriate; continue to monitor.

Adapted from Urden, L. D., Stacy, K. M., & Lough, M. E. (2019). *Priorities in critical care nursing* (8th ed.). St. Louis, MO: Elsevier.

absence of angiotensin II, the blood pressure decreases and the kidneys excrete sodium and fluid (diuresis), decreasing the oxygen demand of the heart. The use of ACE inhibitors in patients after MI decreases mortality rates and prevents remodeling of myocardial cells that is associated with the onset of heart failure. Blood pressure, urine output, and serum sodium, potassium, and creatinine levels need to be monitored closely. If an ACE inhibitor is not suitable, an angiotensin receptor blocker (ARB) should be prescribed (Ibanez et al., 2018). Nicotine replacement therapy and tobacco cessation counseling should also be initiated for all tobacco users.

Cardiac Rehabilitation

After the patient with an MI is in a stable condition, an active rehabilitation program is initiated. Cardiac rehabilitation is an important continuing care program for patients with CAD that targets risk reduction by providing patient and family education, offering individual and group support, and encouraging physical activity and physical conditioning. The goals of rehabilitation for the patient who has had an MI are to extend life and improve the quality of life. The immediate objectives are to limit the effects and progression of atherosclerosis, return the patient to work and a pre-illness lifestyle, enhance the patient's psychosocial and vocational status, and prevent another cardiac event. Cardiac rehabilitation programs increase survival, reduce recurrent events and the need for interventional procedures, and improve quality of life (Dickins & Braun, 2017).

Physical conditioning is achieved gradually over time. Many times, patients will "overdo it" in an attempt to achieve their goals too rapidly. Patients are observed for chest pain, dyspnea, weakness, fatigue, and palpitations and are instructed to stop exercise if any of these occur. Patients may also be monitored for an increase in heart rate above the target heart rate, an increase in systolic or diastolic blood pressure of more than 20 mm Hg, a decrease in systolic blood pressure, onset or worsening of arrhythmias, or ST-segment changes on the ECG.

Cardiac rehabilitation programs are categorized into three phases (Dickins & Braun, 2017). Phase I begins with the diagnosis of atherosclerosis, which may occur when the patient is admitted to the hospital for ACS. Because of brief hospital lengths of stay, mobilization occurs early and patient education focuses on the essentials of self-care rather than instituting behavioral changes for risk reduction. Priorities for in-hospital education include the signs and symptoms that indicate the need to call 911 (seek emergency assistance), the medication regimen, rest–activity balance, and follow-up appointments with the primary provider. The patient is reassured that although CAD is a lifelong disease and must be treated as such, they can likely resume a normal life after an MI. The amount and type of activity recommended at discharge depend on the patient's age, his or her condition before the cardiac event, the extent of the disease, the course of the hospital stay, and the development of any complications.

Phase II occurs after the patient has been discharged. The patient attends sessions three times a week for 4 to 6 weeks but may continue for as long as 6 months. The outpatient program consists of supervised, often ECG-monitored, exercise training that is individualized. At each session, the patient is assessed for the effectiveness of and adherence to the treatment. To prevent complications and another hospitalization, the cardiac rehabilitation staff alerts the referring primary provider to any problems. Phase II cardiac rehabilitation also includes educational sessions for patients and families that are given by cardiologists, exercise physiologists, dietitians, nurses, and other health care professionals. These sessions may take place outside a traditional classroom setting. For instance, a dietitian may take a group of patients to a grocery store to examine labels and meat selections or to a restaurant to discuss menu offerings for a heart-healthy diet.

Phase III is a long-term outpatient program that focuses on maintaining cardiovascular stability and long-term conditioning. The patient is usually self-directed during this phase and does not require a supervised program, although it may be offered. The goals of each phase build on the accomplishments of the previous phase.

NURSING PROCESS

The Patient with Acute Coronary Syndrome

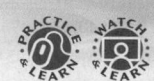

Assessment

One of the most important aspects of care of the patient with ACS is the assessment. It establishes the patient's baseline, identifies the patient's needs, and helps determine the priority of those needs. Systematic assessment includes a careful history, particularly as it relates to symptoms: chest pain or discomfort, dyspnea (difficulty breathing), palpitations, unusual fatigue, syncope (faintness), or other possible indicators of myocardial ischemia. Each symptom must be evaluated with regard to time, duration, and the factors that precipitate the symptom and relieve it, and in comparison with previous symptoms. A focused physical assessment is critical to detect complications and any change in patient status. Chart 23-6 identifies important assessments and possible findings.

Two IV lines are typically placed for any patient with ACS to ensure that access is available for administering emergency medications. Medications are administered IV to achieve rapid onset and to allow for timely adjustment. After the patient's condition stabilizes, IV lines may be changed to a saline lock to maintain IV access.

Diagnosis

NURSING DIAGNOSES

Based on the clinical manifestations, history, and diagnostic assessment data, major nursing diagnoses may include:

- Acute pain associated with increased myocardial oxygen demand and decreased myocardial oxygen supply
- Risk for impaired cardiac function associated with reduced coronary blood flow
- Risk for hypovolaemia
- Impaired peripheral tissue perfusion associated with impaired cardiac output from left ventricular dysfunction
- Anxiety associated with cardiac event and possible death
- Lack of knowledge about post-ACS self-care

COLLABORATIVE PROBLEMS/POTENTIAL COMPLICATIONS

Potential complications may include the following:

- Acute pulmonary edema (see Chapter 25)
- Heart failure (see Chapter 25)
- Cardiogenic shock (see Chapter 11)
- Arrhythmias and cardiac arrest (see Chapters 22 and 25)
- Pericardial effusion and cardiac tamponade (see Chapter 25)

Planning and Goals

The major goals for the patient include relief of pain or ischemic signs (e.g., ST-segment changes) and symptoms, prevention of myocardial damage, maintenance of effective respiratory function, maintenance or attainment of adequate tissue perfusion, reduced anxiety, adherence to the self-care program, and early recognition of complications. Care of the patient with ACS who has an uncomplicated MI is summarized in the Plan of Nursing Care (see Chart 23-9).

Nursing Interventions

RELIEVING PAIN AND OTHER SIGNS AND SYMPTOMS OF ISCHEMIA

Balancing myocardial oxygen supply with demand (e.g., as evidenced by the relief of chest pain) is the top priority in the care of the patient with an ACS. Although administering medications as described previously is required to accomplish this goal, nursing interventions are also important. Collaboration among the patient, nurse, and primary provider is critical in evaluating the patient's response to therapy and in altering the interventions accordingly.

Oxygen should be given along with medication therapy to assist with relief of symptoms. Administration of oxygen raises the circulating level of oxygen to reduce pain associated with low levels of myocardial oxygen. The route of administration (usually by nasal cannula) and the oxygen flow rate are documented. A flow rate of 2 to 4 L/min is usually adequate to maintain oxygen saturation levels of at least 95% unless chronic pulmonary disease is present.

Vital signs are assessed frequently as long as the patient is experiencing pain and other signs or symptoms of acute ischemia. Physical rest in bed with the head of the bed elevated or in a supportive chair helps decrease chest discomfort and dyspnea. Elevation of the head and torso is beneficial for the following reasons:

- Tidal volume improves because of reduced pressure from abdominal contents on the diaphragm and better lung expansion.
- Drainage of the upper lung lobes improves.
- Venous return to the heart (preload) decreases, reducing the work of the heart.

The pain associated with an acute MI reflects an imbalance in myocardial oxygen supply and demand or ineffective myocardial tissue perfusion. The pain also results in increases in heart rate, respiratory rate, and blood pressure. Promptly relieving the pain helps to reestablish this balance, thus decreasing the workload of the heart and minimizing damage to the myocardium. Relief of pain also helps to reduce the patient's anxiety level, which in turn reduces the sympathetic stress response, leading to a decrease in workload of the already stressed heart.

IMPROVING RESPIRATORY FUNCTION

Regular and careful assessment of respiratory function detects early signs of pulmonary complications. The nurse monitors fluid volume status to prevent fluid overload and encourages the patient to breathe deeply and change position frequently to maintain effective ventilation throughout the lungs. Pulse oximetry guides the use of oxygen therapy.

PROMOTING ADEQUATE TISSUE PERFUSION

Bed or chair rest during the initial phase of treatment helps reduce myocardial oxygen consumption. This limitation on mobility should remain until the patient is pain free and hemodynamically stable. Skin temperature and peripheral pulses must be checked frequently to monitor tissue perfusion.

REDUCING ANXIETY

Alleviating anxiety and decreasing fear are important nursing functions that reduce the sympathetic stress response. Less sympathetic stimulation decreases the workload of the

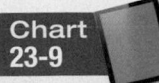

PLAN OF NURSING CARE

Chart 23-9

Care of the Patient with an Uncomplicated Myocardial Infarction

NURSING DIAGNOSIS: Risk for impaired cardiac function associated with reduced coronary blood flow
GOAL: Relief of chest pain/discomfort

Nursing Interventions	Rationale	Expected Outcomes

1. Initially assess, document, and report to the primary provider the following:
 	
a. The patient's description of chest discomfort, including location, intensity, radiation, duration, and factors that affect it; other symptoms such as nausea, diaphoresis, or complaints of unusual fatigue
b. The effect of coronary ischemia on perfusion to the heart (e.g., change in blood pressure, heart rhythm), to the brain (e.g., changes in level of consciousness), to the kidneys (e.g., decrease in urine output), and to the skin (e.g., color, temperature)
2. Obtain a 12-lead ECG recording during symptomatic events, as prescribed, to assess for ongoing ischemia.
3. Administer oxygen as prescribed.
 	
4. Administer medication therapy as prescribed and evaluate the patient's response continuously.
 	
5. Ensure physical rest: head of bed elevated to promote comfort; diet as tolerated; the use of bedside commode; the use of stool softener to prevent straining at stool. Provide a restful environment and allay fears and anxiety by being calm and supportive. Individualize visitation, based on patient response.
	1. These data assist in determining the cause and effect of the chest discomfort and provide a baseline with which post-therapy symptoms can be compared.
	a. There are many conditions associated with chest discomfort. There are characteristic clinical findings of ischemic pain and symptoms.
	
	b. Myocardial infarction (MI) decreases myocardial contractility and ventricular compliance and may produce arrhythmias. Cardiac output is reduced, resulting in reduced blood pressure and decreased organ perfusion.
	
	2. An ECG during symptoms may be useful in the diagnosis of ongoing ischemia.
	
	3. Oxygen therapy increases the oxygen supply to the myocardium.
	4. Medication therapy (nitroglycerin, morphine, beta-blocker, aspirin) is the first line of defense in preserving myocardial tissue.
	5. Physical rest reduces myocardial oxygen consumption. Fear and anxiety precipitate the stress response; this results in increased levels of endogenous catecholamines, which increase myocardial oxygen consumption.
		• Reports beginning relief of chest discomfort and symptoms
		• Appears comfortable and is free of pain and other signs or symptoms
		• Respiratory rate, cardiac rate, and blood pressure return to prediscomfort level
		• Skin warm and dry
		• Adequate cardiac output as evidenced by:
		  • Stable/improving electrocardiogram (ECG)
		  • Heart rate and rhythm
		  • Blood pressure
		  • Mentation
		  • Urine output
		  • Serum blood urea nitrogen (BUN) and creatinine
		  • Skin color and temperature
		• No adverse effects from medications

NURSING DIAGNOSIS: Risk for impaired cardiac function associated with left ventricular failure
GOAL: Absence of respiratory distress

Nursing Interventions	Rationale	Expected Outcomes
1. Initially, every 4 hours, and with chest discomfort or symptoms, assess, document, and report to the primary provider abnormal heart sounds (S_3 and S_4 gallop or new murmur), abnormal breath sounds (particularly crackles), decreased oxygenation, and activity intolerance.	1. These data are useful in diagnosing left ventricular failure. Diastolic filling sounds (S_3 and S_4) result from decreased left ventricular compliance associated with MI. Papillary muscle dysfunction (from infarction of the papillary muscle) can result in mitral regurgitation and a reduction in stroke volume. The presence of crackles (usually at the lung bases) may indicate pulmonary congestion from increased left heart pressures. The association of symptoms and activity can be used as a guide for activity prescription and a basis for patient education.	• No shortness of breath, dyspnea on exertion, orthopnea, or paroxysmal nocturnal dyspnea • Respiratory rate <20 breaths/min with physical activity and 16 breaths/min with rest • Skin color and temperature normal • SpO_2, PaO_2, and $PaCO_2$ within normal limits • Heart rate <100 bpm and >60 bpm, with blood pressure within patient's normal limits • Chest x-ray unchanged • Appears comfortable and rested

(continued on page 744)

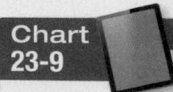

PLAN OF NURSING CARE (continued)

Chart 23-9

Care of the Patient with an Uncomplicated Myocardial Infarction

NURSING DIAGNOSIS: Impaired peripheral tissue perfusion associated with impaired cardiac output
GOAL: Maintenance/attainment of adequate tissue perfusion

Nursing Interventions	Rationale	Expected Outcomes
1. Initially, every 4 hours, and with chest discomfort, assess, document, and report to the primary provider the following: a. Hypotension b. Tachycardia and other arrhythmia c. Activity intolerance d. Mentation changes (use family input) e. Reduced urine output (<0.5 mL/kg/h) f. Cool, moist, cyanotic extremities, decreased peripheral pulses, prolonged capillary refill	1. These data are useful in determining a low cardiac output state.	• Blood pressure within the patient's normal range • Ideally, normal sinus rhythm without arrhythmia is maintained, or patient's baseline rhythm is maintained between 60 and 100 bpm without further arrhythmia. • Prescribed activity is well tolerated. • Remains alert and oriented and without cognitive or behavioral change • Appears comfortable • Urine output >0.5 mL/kg/h • Extremities warm and dry with normal color

NURSING DIAGNOSIS: Anxiety associated with cardiac event
GOAL: Reduction of anxiety

Nursing Interventions	Rationale	Expected Outcomes
1. Assess, document, and report to the primary provider the patient's and family's level of anxiety and coping mechanisms.	1. These data provide information about psychological well-being. Causes of anxiety are variable and individual, and may include acute illness, hospitalization, pain, disruption of activities of daily living at home and at work, changes in role and self-image due to illness, and financial concerns. Because anxious family members can transmit anxiety to the patient, the nurse must also identify strategies to reduce the family's fear and anxiety.	• Reports less anxiety • The patient and family discuss their anxieties and fears about illness and death. • The patient and family appear less anxious. • Appears restful, respiratory rate <16 breaths/min, heart rate <100 bpm without ectopic beats, blood pressure within patient's normal limits, skin warm and dry • Participates actively in a progressive rehabilitation program • Practices stress reduction techniques
2. Assess the need for spiritual counseling and refer as appropriate.	2. If a patient finds support in a religion, spiritual counseling may assist in reducing anxiety and fear.	
3. Assess the need for social service referral.	3. Social services can assist with posthospital care and financial concerns.	

NURSING DIAGNOSIS: Lack of knowledge about post-MI self-care
GOAL: Adheres to the home health care program; chooses lifestyle consistent with heart-healthy recommendations (see Chart 23-10).

---

heart, which may relieve pain and other signs and symptoms of ischemia.

The development of a trusting and caring relationship with the patient is critical in reducing anxiety. Providing information to the patient and family in an honest and supportive manner encourages the patient to be a partner in care and greatly assists in developing a positive relationship. Other interventions that can be used to reduce anxiety include ensuring a quiet environment, preventing interruptions that disturb sleep, and providing spiritual support consistent with the patient's beliefs. The nurse provides frequent opportunities for the patient to privately share concerns and fears. An atmosphere of acceptance helps the patient know that these concerns and fears are both realistic and normal. Alternative therapies such as pet therapy can help certain patients relax and reduce anxiety (Waite, Hamilton, & O'Brien, 2018). Many hospitals have developed infection control and safety procedures pertaining to the animals, their handlers, and the patients eligible for pet therapy.

MONITORING AND MANAGING POTENTIAL COMPLICATIONS

Complications that can occur after acute MI are caused by the damage that occurs to the myocardium and to the conduction system from reduced coronary blood flow. Because these complications can be life-threatening, close monitoring for and early identification of their signs and symptoms are critical (see Chart 23-9).

The nurse monitors the patient closely for changes in cardiac rate and rhythm, heart sounds, blood pressure, chest pain, respiratory status, urinary output, skin color and temperature, mental status, ECG changes, and laboratory values. Any changes in the patient's condition must be reported promptly to the primary provider and emergency measures instituted when necessary.

PROMOTING HOME, COMMUNITY-BASED, AND TRANSITIONAL CARE

Educating Patients About Self-Care. The most effective way to increase the probability that the patient will implement a self-care regimen after discharge is to identify the patient's priorities, provide adequate education about heart-healthy living, and facilitate the patient's involvement in a cardiac rehabilitation program (Ibanez et al., 2018). Patient participation in the development of an individualized program enhances the potential for an effective treatment plan (see Chart 23-10).

Continuing and Transitional Care. Depending on the patient's condition and the availability of family assistance, home, community-based, or transitional, care may be indicated. The nurse making a home visit can assist the patient with scheduling and keeping follow-up appointments and with adhering to the prescribed cardiac rehabilitation regimen. The patient may need reminders about follow-up monitoring, including periodic laboratory testing, as well as ongoing assessment of cardiac status. In addition, the home health nurse monitors the patient's adherence to dietary restrictions and to prescribed medications. If the patient is receiving home oxygen, the nurse ensures that the patient is using the oxygen as prescribed and that appropriate home safety measures are maintained. If the patient has evidence of heart failure secondary to an MI, appropriate home care guidelines for the patient with heart failure are followed (see Chapter 25).

Evaluation

Expected patient outcomes may include:
1. Experiences relief of angina
2. Has stable cardiac and respiratory status
3. Maintains adequate tissue perfusion
4. Exhibits decreased anxiety
5. Adheres to a self-care program
6. Has no complications

INVASIVE CORONARY ARTERY PROCEDURES

Methods to reperfuse ischemic myocardial tissue when patients are refractory to more conservative management methods include PCIs and CABG surgery, as noted previously. The following sections discuss specific indications for each of these and the nursing management of patients who are having either PCIs or CABGs.

Percutaneous Coronary Interventions

Invasive interventional procedures to treat CAD include PTCA and intracoronary stent implantation. These procedures are classified as **percutaneous coronary interventions (PCIs),** as they are performed through a skin puncture rather than a surgical incision.

Percutaneous Transluminal Coronary Angioplasty

In **percutaneous transluminal coronary angioplasty (PTCA),** a balloon-tipped catheter is used to open blocked

---

Chart 23-10 **HEALTH PROMOTION**

Promoting Health After Myocardial Infarction and Other Acute Coronary Syndromes

To extend and improve the quality of life, a patient who has had a myocardial infarction (MI) must make lifestyle adjustments to promote heart-healthy living. With this in mind, the nurse and patient develop a program to help achieve desired outcomes.

Making Lifestyle Modifications during Convalescence and Healing

Adaptation to an MI is an ongoing process and usually requires some modification of lifestyle. Educate patients to make the following specific modifications:

- Avoid any activity that produces chest pain, extreme dyspnea, or undue fatigue.
- Avoid extremes of heat and cold and walking against the wind.
- Lose weight, if indicated.
- Stop smoking and the use of tobacco; avoid secondhand smoke.
- Develop heart-healthy eating patterns and avoid large meals and hurrying while eating.
- Modify meals to align with the AHA dietary recommendations, the Mediterranean diet, or other recommended diets.
- Adhere to medical regimen, especially in taking medications.
- Follow recommendations that ensure that blood pressure and blood glucose are in control.
- Pursue activities that relieve and reduce stress.

Adopting an Activity Program

In addition, the patient needs to undertake a structured program of activity and exercise for long-term rehabilitation. Advise patients to:

- Engage in a regimen of physical conditioning with a gradual increase in activity duration and then a gradual increase in activity intensity.
- Enroll in a cardiac rehabilitation program.
- Walk daily, increasing distance and time as prescribed.
- Monitor pulse rate during physical activity.
- Avoid physical exercise immediately after a meal.
- Alternate activity with rest periods (some fatigue is normal and expected during convalescence).
- Participate in a daily program of exercise that develops into a program of regular exercise for a lifetime.

Managing Symptoms

The patient must learn to recognize and take appropriate action for recurrent symptoms. Make sure that patients know to do the following:

- Call 911 if chest pressure or pain (or prodromal symptoms) is not relieved in 15 minutes by taking 3 nitroglycerin tablets at 5-minute intervals.
- Contact the primary provider if any of the following occur: shortness of breath, fainting, slow or rapid heartbeat, swelling of feet and ankles.

coronary vessels and resolve ischemia. It is used in patients with angina and as an intervention for ACS. Catheter-based interventions can also be used to open blocked CABGs (see later discussion). The purpose of PTCA is to improve blood flow within a coronary artery by compressing the atheroma. The procedure is attempted when the interventional cardiologist determines that PTCA can improve blood flow to the myocardium.

PTCA is carried out in the cardiac catheterization laboratory. Hollow catheters called *sheaths* are inserted, usually in the femoral artery (and sometimes the radial artery), providing a conduit for other catheters. Catheters are then threaded through the femoral or radial artery, up through the aorta, and into the coronary arteries. Angiography is performed using injected radiopaque contrast agents (commonly called *dye*) to identify the location and extent of the blockage. A balloon-tipped dilation catheter is passed through the sheath and positioned over the lesion. The physician determines the catheter position by examining markers on the balloon that can be seen with fluoroscopy. When the catheter is properly positioned, the balloon is inflated with high pressure for several seconds and then deflated. The pressure compresses and often "cracks" the atheroma (see Fig. 23-7). The media and adventitia of the coronary artery are also stretched.

Several inflations with different balloon sizes may be required to achieve the goal, usually defined as an improvement in blood flow and a residual stenosis of less than 10% (Urden et al., 2019). Other measures of the success of PTCA are an increase in the artery's lumen and no clinically obvious arterial trauma. Because the blood supply to the coronary artery decreases while the balloon is inflated, the patient may complain of chest pain and the ECG may display ST-segment changes. Intracoronary stents are usually positioned in the

intima of the vessel to maintain patency of the artery after the balloon is withdrawn.

If thick, deep, or concentric calcification is present, the lesion may require the use of devices such as cutting, scoring, or high pressure balloons, rotational atherectomy, orbital atherectomy and excimer lasers to prepare the lesion for stenting (Shlofmitz, Shlofmitz, & Lee, 2019).

In addition to these approaches, intravascular lithotripsy (IVL) is currently being investigated to treat calcified artery blockages with sonic pressure waves in a similar way that is used to treat kidney stones. Pulsatile sonic pressure waves are used during balloon inflation to fracture both intimal and medial calcium in the artery wall but pass through the surrounding soft vascular tissue in a safe manner. This technology is approved for use in peripheral arteries at this time. Further studies are being done to assess their efficacy in coronary arteries (Riley, Corl, & Kereiakes, 2019).

Coronary Artery Stent

After PTCA, the area that has been treated may close off partially or completely—a process called *restenosis*. The intima of the coronary artery has been injured and responds by initiating an acute inflammatory process. This process may include release of mediators that leads to vasoconstriction, clotting, and scar tissue formation. A coronary artery stent may be placed to overcome these risks. A **stent** is a metal mesh that provides structural support to a vessel at risk of acute closure. The stent is initially positioned over the angioplasty balloon. When the balloon is inflated, the mesh expands and presses against the vessel wall, holding the artery open. The balloon is withdrawn, but the stent is left permanently in place within the artery (see Fig. 23-7). Eventually, endothelium covers the

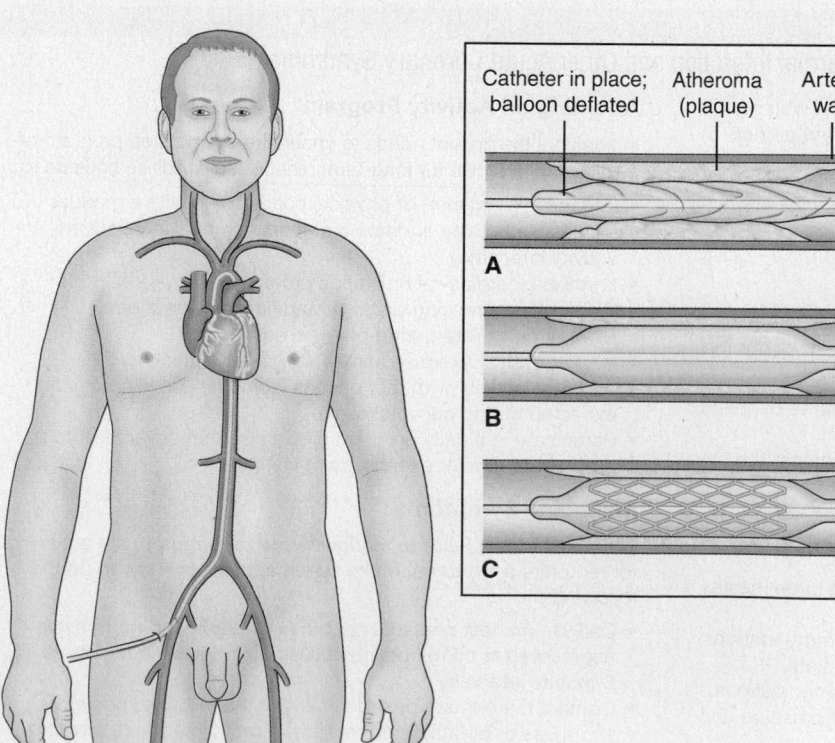

Figure 23-7 • Percutaneous transluminal coronary angioplasty. **A.** A balloon-tipped catheter is passed into the affected coronary artery and placed across the area of the atheroma (plaque). **B.** The balloon is then rapidly inflated and deflated with controlled pressure. **C.** A stent is placed to maintain patency of the artery, and the balloon is removed.

stent and it is incorporated into the vessel wall. The original stents do not contain medications and are known as bare metal stents. Some stents are coated with medications, such as sirolimus or paclitaxel, which may minimize the formation of thrombi or scar tissue within the coronary artery lesion. These drug-eluting stents (DES) have increased the success of PCI (Mishra, Edla, Tripathi, et al., 2019). Because of the risk of thrombus formation within the stent, the patient receives antiplatelet medications, usually aspirin and clopidogrel. Aspirin should be continued indefinitely and clopidogrel is continued for 1 year following stent placement (Urden et al., 2019).

Complications

Complications that can occur during a PCI procedure include coronary artery dissection, perforation, abrupt closure, or vasospasm. Additional complications include acute MI, serious arrhythmias (e.g., ventricular tachycardia), and cardiac arrest. Some of these complications may require emergency surgical treatment. Complications after the procedure may include abrupt closure of the coronary artery and a variety of vascular complications, such as bleeding at the insertion site, retroperitoneal bleeding, hematoma, and arterial occlusion (Urden et al., 2019). In addition, there is a risk of acute kidney injury from the contrast agent used during the procedure (see Table 23-3).

Postprocedure Care

Patient care is similar to that for a diagnostic cardiac catheterization (see Chapter 21). Patients who are not already hospitalized are admitted the day of the PCI. Those with no complications go home the same day. When the PCI is performed emergently to treat ACS, patients typically go to a critical care unit and stay in the hospital for a few days. During the PCI, patients receive IV heparin or a thrombin inhibitor (e.g., bivalirudin) and are monitored closely for signs of bleeding. Patients may also receive a GP IIb/IIIa agent (e.g., eptifibatide) for several hours following the PCI to prevent platelet aggregation and thrombus formation in the coronary artery (Urden et al., 2019). Hemostasis is achieved, and femoral sheaths may be removed at the end of the procedure by using a vascular closure device (e.g., Angio-Seal, VasoSeal) or a device that sutures the vessels. Hemostasis after sheath removal may also be achieved by direct manual pressure, a mechanical compression device (e.g., C-shaped clamp), or a pneumatic compression device (e.g., FemoStop).

Patients may return to the nursing unit with the large peripheral vascular access sheaths in place. The sheaths are then removed after blood studies (e.g., activated clotting time) indicate that the heparin is no longer active and the clotting time is within an acceptable range. This usually takes a few hours, depending on the amount of heparin given during the

TABLE 23-3 Complications After Percutaneous Coronary Interventions

Complication	Clinical Manifestations	Possible Causes	Nursing Actions
Myocardial ischemia	Chest pain Ischemic changes on ECG Arrhythmias	Thrombosis Restenosis of coronary artery	Administer oxygen and nitroglycerin. Obtain 12-lead ECG. Notify cardiologist.
Bleeding and hematoma formation	Continuation of bleeding from vascular access site Swelling at site Formation of hard lump Pain with leg movement Possible hypotension and tachycardia	Anticoagulant therapy Vascular trauma Inadequate hemostasis Leg movement	Keep patient on bed rest. Apply manual pressure over sheath insertion site. Outline hematoma with marking pen. Notify primary provider if bleeding continues.
Retroperitoneal hematoma	Back, flank, or abdominal pain Hypotension Tachycardia Restlessness, agitation	Arterial leak of blood into the retroperitoneal space	Notify primary provider. Stop anticoagulants. Administer IV fluids. Anticipate diagnostic testing (e.g., computed tomography scan). Prepare patient for intervention.
Arterial occlusion	Lost/weakened pulse distal to sheath insertion site Extremity cool, cyanotic, painful	Arterial thrombus or embolus	Notify primary provider. Anticipate intervention.
Pseudoaneurysm formation	Swelling at vascular access site Pulsatile mass, bruit	Vessel trauma during the procedure	Notify primary provider. Anticipate intervention.
Arteriovenous fistula formation	Swelling at vascular access site Pulsatile mass, bruit	Vessel trauma during the procedure	Notify primary provider. Anticipate intervention.
Acute kidney injury	Decreased urine output Elevated BUN, serum creatinine	Nephrotoxic contrast agent	Monitor urine output, BUN, creatinine, electrolytes. Provide adequate hydration. Administer renal protective agents (acetylcysteine) before and after procedure as prescribed.

BUN, blood urea nitrogen; ECG, electrocardiogram; IV, intravenous.
Adapted from Urden, L. D., Stacy, K. M., & Lough, M. E. (2019). *Priorities in critical care nursing* (8th ed.). St. Louis, MO: Elsevier.

procedure. The patient must remain flat in bed and keep the affected leg straight until the sheaths are removed and then for a few hours afterward to maintain hemostasis. Because immobility and bed rest may cause discomfort, treatment may include analgesics and sedation. Nonpharmacologic interventions include repositioning and heat application for back pain. Sheath removal and the application of pressure on the vessel insertion site may cause the heart rate to slow and the blood pressure to decrease (vasovagal response). A dose of IV atropine is usually given to treat this response.

Some patients with unstable lesions and at high risk for abrupt vessel closure are restarted on heparin after sheath removal, or they receive an IV infusion of a GP IIb/IIIa inhibitor. These patients are monitored closely and may have a delayed recovery period.

After hemostasis is achieved, a pressure dressing is applied to the site. Patients resume self-care and ambulate unassisted within a few hours of the procedure. The duration of immobilization depends on the size of the sheath inserted, the type of anticoagulant given, the method of hemostasis, the patient's condition, and the physician's preference. On the day after the procedure, the site is inspected and the dressing removed. The patient is instructed to monitor the site for bleeding or development of a hard mass indicative of hematoma.

Surgical Procedures: Coronary Artery Revascularization

Advances in diagnostics, medical management, and surgical and anesthesia techniques, as well as the care provided in critical care and surgical units, home care, and rehabilitation programs, have continued to make surgery an effective treatment option for patients with CAD. CAD has been treated by myocardial revascularization since the 1960s, and the most common CABG techniques have been performed for more than 40 years. **Coronary artery bypass graft (CABG)** is a surgical procedure in which a blood vessel is grafted to an occluded coronary artery so that blood can flow beyond the occlusion; it is also called a *bypass graft*.

The major indications for CABG are:

- Alleviation of angina that cannot be controlled with medication or PCI
- Treatment for left main coronary artery stenosis or multivessel CAD
- Prevention of and treatment for MI, arrhythmias, or heart failure
- Treatment for complications from an unsuccessful PCI

The recommendation for CABG is determined by a number of factors, including the number of diseased coronary vessels, the degree of left ventricular dysfunction, the presence of other health problems, the patient's symptoms, and any previous treatment. CABG and PCI have shown similar results in outcomes, such as MI rate, mortality, and improvement of angina post-intervention. However, the requirement of a second reperfusion intervention has been shown to be lower with CABG compared to PCI therapy (Gaudino, Spadaccio, & Taggart, 2019).

CABG is performed less frequently in women (Angraal, Khera, Wang, et al., 2018). Compared with men, women referred for this surgery tend to be older and have more comorbidities such as diabetes. In addition, they have a higher risk of surgical complications and increased mortality (Angraal et al., 2018). Although some women have good outcomes following CABG, men generally have a better rate of graft patency and symptom relief.

For a patient to be considered for CABG, the coronary arteries to be bypassed must have at least a 70% occlusion, or at least a 50% occlusion in the left main coronary artery (Urden et al., 2019). If significant blockage is not present, flow through the artery will compete with flow through the bypass, and circulation to the ischemic area of myocardium may not improve. The artery also must be patent beyond the area of blockage or the flow through the bypass will be impeded.

Current guidelines recommend use of the internal thoracic arteries (formerly called the internal mammary arteries) for CABG, because of their histologic characteristics and increased production of vasoactive molecules and anti-inflammatory cytokines which improve arterial patency. Recent studies demonstrate increased survival when using internal thoracic artery grafting. The left internal thoracic artery graft has been shown to have greater than 90% patency after 20 years and is the recommended conduit to use first (Gaudino et al., 2019). Arterial grafts are preferred to venous grafts because they do not develop atherosclerotic changes as quickly and remain patent longer. The surgeon leaves the proximal end of the thoracic artery intact and detaches the distal end of the artery from the chest wall. This end of the artery is then grafted to the coronary artery distal to the occlusion. The internal thoracic arteries may not be long enough to use for multiple bypasses. Because of this, many CABG procedures are performed with a combination of venous and arterial grafts.

A vein commonly used for CABG is the greater saphenous vein, followed by the lesser saphenous vein (see Fig. 23-8). The vein is removed from the leg and grafted to the ascending aorta and to the coronary artery distal to the lesion. Traditionally, a skin incision was made over the length of vein

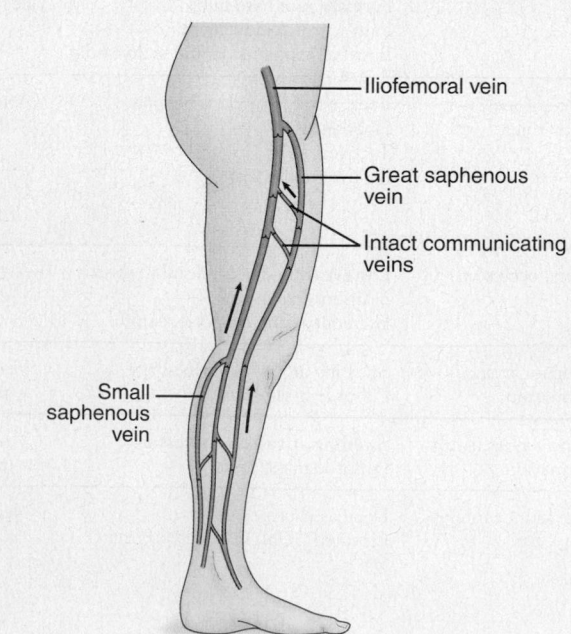

Iliofemoral vein

Great saphenous vein

Intact communicating veins

Small saphenous vein

Figure 23-8 • The greater and lesser saphenous veins are commonly used in bypass graft procedures.

segment, but new techniques allow small leg incisions. Endovascular methods of vein harvesting have reduced complications such as infection and wound dehiscence, which are associated with longer leg incisions (Gaudino et al., 2019). Lower extremity edema continues to be a common adverse effect of vein removal. The degree of edema varies and usually diminishes over time. The patency of vein grafts can be limited. Within 5 to 10 years, atherosclerotic changes often develop in saphenous vein grafts.

Traditional Coronary Artery Bypass Graft

CABG procedures are performed with the patient under general anesthesia. In the traditional CABG procedure, the surgeon performs a median sternotomy and connects the patient to the cardiopulmonary bypass (CPB) machine. Next, a blood vessel from another part of the patient's body (e.g., saphenous vein, left internal thoracic artery) is grafted distal to the coronary artery lesion, bypassing the obstruction (see Fig. 23-9). CPB is then discontinued, chest tubes and epicardial pacing wires are placed, and the incision is closed. The patient is then admitted to a critical care unit.

Cardiopulmonary Bypass

Many cardiac surgical procedures are possible because of CPB (i.e., extracorporeal circulation). The procedure mechanically circulates and oxygenates blood for the body while bypassing the heart and lungs. CPB maintains perfusion to body organs and tissues and allows the surgeon to complete the anastomoses in a motionless, bloodless surgical field.

CPB is accomplished by placing a cannula in the right atrium, vena cava, or femoral vein to withdraw blood from the body. The cannula is connected to tubing filled with an isotonic crystalloid solution. Venous blood removed from the body by the cannula is filtered, oxygenated, cooled or warmed by the machine, and then returned to the body. The cannula used to return the oxygenated blood is usually inserted in the ascending aorta, or it may be inserted in the femoral artery (see Fig. 23-10). The heart is stopped by the injection of a potassium-rich cardioplegia solution into the coronary

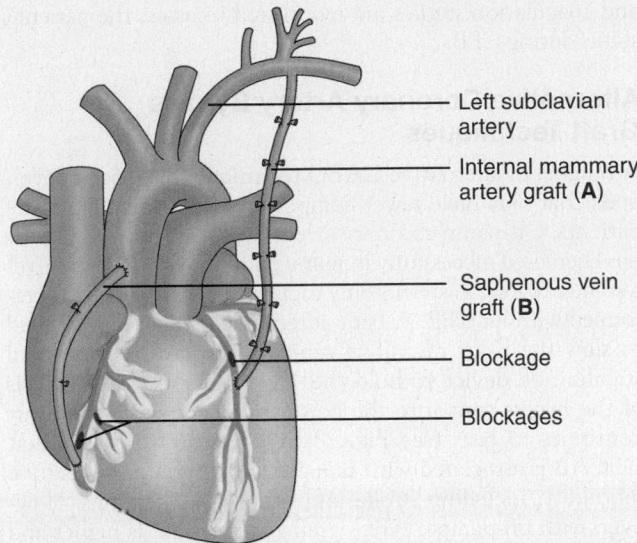

Figure 23-9 • Coronary artery bypass grafts. One or more procedures may be performed using various veins and arteries. **A.** Left internal thoracic artery (formerly called the left internal mammary artery), used frequently because of its functional longevity. **B.** Saphenous vein, also used as bypass graft.

arteries. The patient receives heparin to prevent clotting and thrombus formation in the bypass circuit when blood comes in contact with the surfaces of the tubing. At the end of the procedure when the patient is disconnected from the bypass machine, protamine sulfate is given to reverse the effects of heparin.

During the procedure, hypothermia is maintained at a temperature of about 28°C (82.4°F) (Urden et al., 2019). The blood is cooled during CPB and returned to the body. The cooled blood slows the body's basal metabolic rate, thereby decreasing the demand for oxygen. Cooled blood usually has a higher viscosity, but the crystalloid solution used to prime the bypass tubing dilutes the blood. When the surgical procedure is completed, the blood is rewarmed as it passes through the CPB circuit. Urine output, arterial blood gases, electrolytes,

Figure 23-10 • The cardiopulmonary bypass system, in which cannulas are placed through the right atrium into the superior and inferior vena cavae to divert blood from the body and into the bypass system. The pump system creates a vacuum, pulling blood into the venous reservoir. The blood is cleared of air bubbles, clots, and particulates by the filter and then is passed through the oxygenator, releasing carbon dioxide and obtaining oxygen. Next, the blood is pulled to the pump and pushed out to the heat exchanger, where its temperature is regulated. The blood is then returned to the body via the ascending aorta.

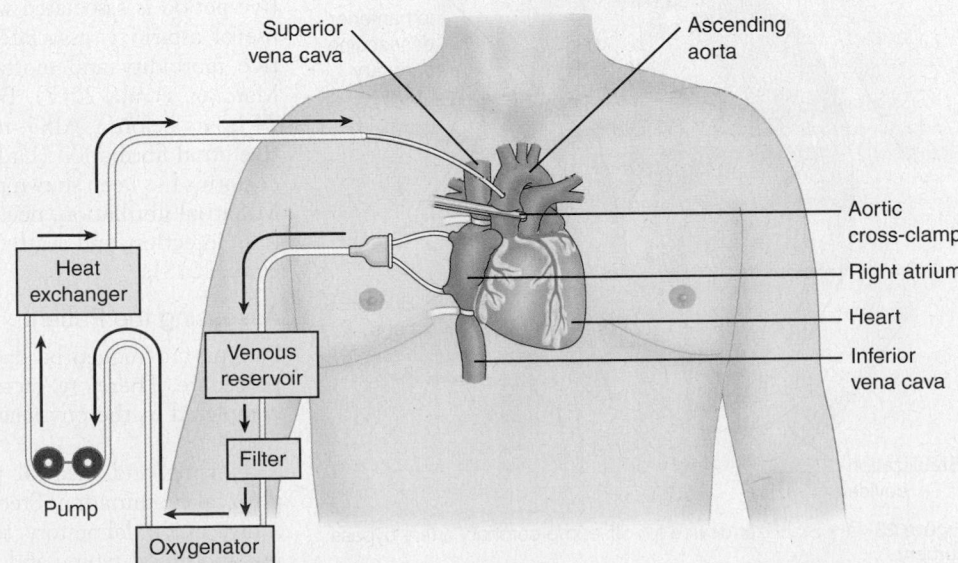

and coagulation studies are monitored to assess the patient's status during CPB.

Alternative Coronary Artery Bypass Graft Techniques

A number of alternative CABG techniques have been developed that may have fewer complications for some groups of patients. Off-pump coronary artery bypass (OPCAB) surgery has been used successfully in many patients. OPCAB involves a standard median sternotomy incision, but the surgery is performed without CPB. A beta-adrenergic blocker may be used to slow the heart rate. The surgeon also uses a myocardial stabilization device to hold the site still for the anastomosis of the bypass graft into the coronary artery while the heart continues to beat (see Fig. 23-11). Research suggests that OPCAB is associated with reduced short-term postoperative morbidity, including stroke and other complications. However, with on-pump CABG, graft patency rate is higher and long-term mortality may be lower (Gaudino et al., 2019).

Minimally invasive surgical techniques that eliminate median sternotomy have also been developed. These endoscopic techniques use smaller incisions via a right or left thoracotomy approach and a robotic system to place bypass grafts. The patient may or may not require CPB (Snyder, 2018). Minimally invasive heart surgery may be considered an acceptable alternative to conventional CABG for select patients, such as those who do not require bypass grafts to several vessels. It is most commonly used to bypass occlusions in the left anterior descending artery (Snyder, 2018). It has allowed patients to recover earlier, require fewer blood transfusions, experience fewer respiratory complications, and be less likely to experience acute kidney injury (Urden et al., 2019).

The most important criterion when deciding whether a patient needs a CABG or a PCI is the predicted surgical mortality, which takes into consideration the patient's individual characteristics, the anatomic complexity of the coronary lesions, and the ability to achieve revascularization. The cardiac surgeon will assess the following factors to determine risk and the ability to revascularize: clinical history (age, sex, diabetes, hypertension, left ventricular function, arrhythmias), previous cardiovascular events (previous cardiovascular surgery, PCI, MI, or stroke), and disease complexity (number of diseased vessels, concomitant valve disease). In some cases, CABG may still be recommended over PCI for only one lesion to achieve better revascularization (Gaudino et al., 2019).

Complications of Coronary Artery Bypass Graft

CABG may result in complications such as hemorrhage, arrhythmias, and MI (see Table 23-4). The patient may require interventions for more than one complication at a time. Collaboration among nurses, physicians, pharmacists, respiratory therapists, and dietitians is necessary to achieve the desired patient outcomes. Although most patients improve symptomatically following surgery, CABG is not a cure for CAD, and angina, exercise intolerance, or other symptoms experienced before CABG may recur. Medications required before surgery may need to be continued. Lifestyle modifications recommended before surgery remain important to treat the underlying CAD and for the continued viability of the newly implanted grafts.

Nursing Management

Cardiac surgery patients have many of the same needs and require the same perioperative care as other surgical patients (see Unit 3), as well as some special needs.

Preoperative Management

Comprehensive preoperative medical management prevents complications and improves outcomes. This is particularly important because patients undergoing CABG surgery tend to be older and often have multiple comorbidities. The use of aspirin, beta-blockers, and statins during the preoperative period is associated with better outcomes. Preoperative use of aspirin is associated with a reduction in perioperative morbidity and mortality (Aboul-Hassan, Stankowski, Marczak, et al., 2017). Beta-blockers, when given at least 24 hours before CABG, reduce the incidence of postoperative atrial fibrillation (Urden et al., 2019). Perioperative use of statins has been shown to reduce the rates of postoperative MI, atrial fibrillation, neurologic dysfunction, renal dysfunction, infection, and death (Katsiki, Triposkiadis, Giannoukas, et al., 2018).

Assessing the Patient

Patients are frequently admitted to the hospital the day of the procedure. Therefore, most of the preoperative evaluation is completed in the physician's office and during preadmission testing.

Nursing and medical personnel perform a history and physical examination. Preoperative testing consists of a chest x-ray; ECG; laboratory tests, including coagulation studies; and blood typing and cross-matching. The preoperative

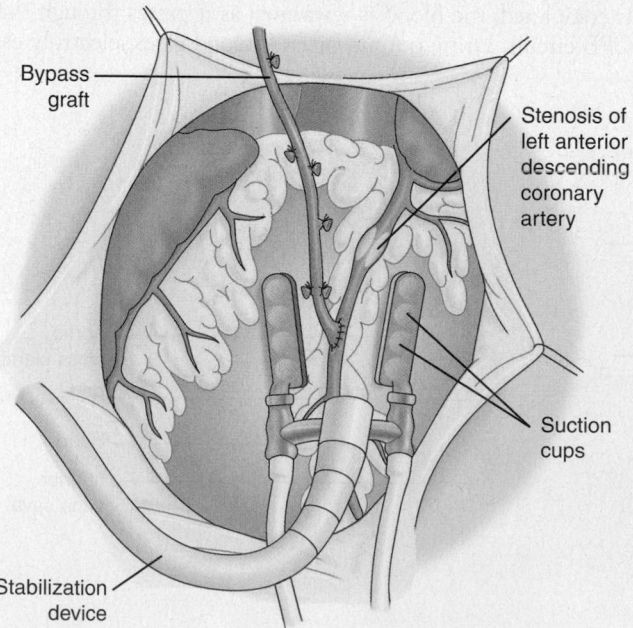

Figure 23-11 • Stabilizer device for off-pump coronary artery bypass surgery.

Bypass graft

Stenosis of left anterior descending coronary artery

Suction cups

Stabilization device

TABLE 23-4 Potential Complications of Cardiac Surgery

Complication	Cause	Assessment and Management
Cardiac Complications		
Hypovolemia (most common cause of decreased cardiac output after cardiac surgery)	Net loss of blood and intravascular volume Vasodilation due to postoperative rewarming Intravascular fluid loss to the interstitial spaces because surgery and anesthesia increase capillary permeability	Arterial hypotension, tachycardia, low CVP, and low PAWP are often seen. Fluid replacement may be prescribed. Replacement fluids include colloid (albumin), packed red blood cells, or crystalloid solution (normal saline, lactated Ringer's solution).
Persistent bleeding	Cardiopulmonary bypass causes platelet dysfunction, and hypothermia alters clotting mechanisms. Surgical trauma causes tissues and blood vessels to ooze bloody drainage. Intraoperative anticoagulant (heparin) therapy. Postoperative coagulopathy may also result from liver dysfunction and depletion of clotting components.	Accurate measurement of wound bleeding and chest tube blood is essential. Drainage should not exceed 200 mL/h for the first 4–6 h. Drainage should decrease and stop within a few days, while progressing from serosanguinous to serous. Serial hemoglobin, hematocrit, and coagulation studies guide therapy. Administration of blood products: packed red blood cells, fresh frozen plasma, platelet concentrate, recombinant factor VII Protamine sulfate may be given to neutralize unfractionated heparin. Administration of desmopressin acetate (DDAVP) to enhance platelet function If bleeding persists, the patient may return to the operating room.
Cardiac tamponade	Fluid and clots accumulate in the pericardial sac, which compress the heart, preventing blood from filling the ventricles.	Signs and symptoms include arterial hypotension, tachycardia, decreased urine output, and ↑ CVP. Arterial pressure waveform may show pulsus paradoxus (decrease of >10 mm Hg systolic blood pressure during inspiration). The chest drainage system is checked to eliminate possible kinks or obstructions in the tubing. Chest x-ray may show a widening mediastinum. Bedside echocardiogram may be done to confirm tamponade. Emergency medical management is required; may include return to surgery.
Fluid overload	IV fluids and blood products increase circulating volume.	High CVP and pulmonary artery pressures, as well as crackles, indicate fluid overload. Diuretics are prescribed, and the rate of IV fluid administration is reduced. Alternative treatments include continuous renal replacement therapy and dialysis.
Hypothermia	Low body temperature leads to vasoconstriction, shivering, and arterial hypertension.	Patient is rewarmed gradually after surgery, decreasing vasoconstriction.
Hypertension	Results from postoperative vasoconstriction. It may stretch suture lines and cause postoperative bleeding. The condition is usually transient.	Vasodilators (nitroglycerin, nitroprusside) may be used to treat hypertension. Administer cautiously to avoid hypotension.
Tachyarrhythmias	Increased heart rate is common with perioperative volume changes. Rapid atrial fibrillation commonly occurs during the first few days postoperatively.	If a tachyarrhythmia is the primary problem, the heart rhythm is assessed and medications (e.g., amiodarone, diltiazem) may be prescribed. Antiarrhythmic agents (e.g., beta-blockers) are often given before coronary artery bypass graft to minimize the risk. Cardioversion and defibrillation are alternatives for symptomatic tachyarrhythmias.
Bradycardias	Decreased heart rate due to surgical trauma and edema affecting the cardiac conduction system	Many postoperative patients have temporary pacer wires that can be attached to an external pacemaker to stimulate the heart to beat faster. Less commonly, atropine or other medications may be used to increase heart rate.
Cardiac failure	Myocardial contractility may be decreased perioperatively.	The nurse observes for and reports signs of heart failure, including hypotension, ↑ CVP, ↑ PAWP, venous distention; labored respirations; and edema. Medical management includes diuretics and IV inotropic agents.
MI (may occur intraoperatively or postoperatively)	Portion of the cardiac muscle dies; therefore, contractility decreases. Impaired ventricular wall motion further decreases cardiac output. Symptoms may be masked by the postoperative surgical discomfort or the anesthesia–analgesia regimen.	Careful assessment to determine the type of pain the patient is experiencing; MI is suspected if the mean blood pressure is low with normal preload. Serial electrocardiograms and cardiac biomarkers assist in making the diagnosis (alterations may be due to the surgical intervention).

(continued on page 752)

TABLE 23-4	Potential Complications of Cardiac Surgery (continued)	
Complication	**Cause**	**Assessment and Management**
Pulmonary Complications		
Impaired gas exchange	During and after anesthesia, patients require mechanical assistance to breathe. Anesthetic agents stimulate production of mucus, and chest incision pain may decrease the effectiveness of ventilation. Potential for postoperative atelectasis	Pulmonary complications are detected during assessment of breath sounds, oxygen saturation levels, arterial blood gases, and ventilator readings. Extended periods of mechanical ventilation may be required while complications are treated.
Neurologic Complications		
Neurologic changes; stroke	Thrombi and emboli may cause cerebral infarction, and neurologic signs may be evident when patients recover from anesthesia.	Inability to follow simple commands within 6 h of recovery from anesthesia, weakness on one side of body or other neurologic changes may indicate stroke. Patients who are older or who have renal or hepatic failure may take longer to recover from anesthesia.
Kidney Injury and Electrolyte Imbalance		
Acute kidney injury	May result from hypoperfusion of the kidneys or from injury to the renal tubules by nephrotoxic drugs	May respond to diuretics or may require continuous renal replacement therapy or dialysis. Fluids, electrolytes, and urine output are monitored frequently. May result in chronic kidney disease and require ongoing dialysis.
Electrolyte imbalance	Postoperative imbalances in potassium, magnesium, sodium, calcium, and blood glucose are related to surgical losses, metabolic changes, and the administration of medications and IV fluids.	Monitor electrolytes and basic metabolic studies frequently. Implement treatment to correct electrolyte imbalance promptly (see Chart 23-11).
Other Complications		
Hepatic failure	Surgery and anesthesia stress the liver. Most common in patients with cirrhosis, hepatitis, or prolonged right-sided heart failure.	The use of medications metabolized by the liver must be minimized. Bilirubin and albumin levels are monitored, and nutritional support is provided.
Infection	Surgery and anesthesia alter the patient's immune system. Multiple invasive devices used to monitor and support the patient's recovery may serve as a source of infection.	Monitor for signs of possible infection: body temperature, white blood cell and differential counts, incision and puncture sites, urine (clarity, color, and odor), bilateral breath sounds, sputum (color, odor, amount). Antibiotic therapy may be instituted or modified as necessary. Continuous insulin infusion to maintain blood glucose concentrations to ≤180 mg/dL while avoiding hypoglycemia may reduce the incidence of deep sternal wound infections. Invasive devices are discontinued as soon as they are no longer required. Institutional protocols for maintaining and replacing invasive lines and devices are followed to minimize the risk of infection.

↑, increased; CVP, central venous pressure; IV, intravenous; MI, myocardial infarction; PAWP, pulmonary artery wedge pressure.
Adapted from Urden, L. D., Stacy, K. M., & Lough, M. E. (2019). *Priorities in critical care nursing* (8th ed.). St. Louis, MO: Elsevier.

history and health assessment should be thorough and well documented because they provide a basis for postoperative comparison. The nurse assesses the patient for disorders that could complicate or affect the postoperative course, such as diabetes, hypertension, and lung disease.

The health assessment focuses on obtaining baseline physiologic, psychological, and social information. Cognitive status is carefully assessed, as patients with impaired cognitive status will need more assistance after surgery and may require subacute care prior to returning home. Older adults are at a high risk for suffering adverse cognitive outcomes following cardiac surgery (Jones, Matalanis, Mårtensson, et al., 2019). The patient's and family's education needs are identified and addressed. Of particular importance are the patient's usual functional level, coping mechanisms, and available support systems. These factors affect the patient's postoperative course, discharge plans, and rehabilitation.

The status of the cardiovascular system is determined by reviewing the patient's symptoms, including past and present experiences with chest pain, palpitations, dyspnea, intermittent claudication (leg pain that occurs with walking), and peripheral edema. The patient's history of major illnesses; previous surgeries; medication; and the use of illicit and over-the-counter drugs, herbal supplements, alcohol, and tobacco is also obtained. Particular attention is paid to blood glucose control in patients with diabetes because there is a higher incidence of postoperative complications when glycemic control is poor (Gordon, Lauver, & Buck, 2018).

The psychosocial assessment and the assessment of the patient's and family's learning needs are also important. Anticipation of cardiac surgery is a source of great stress to the patient and family, and patients with high anxiety levels have poorer outcomes (Ramesh, Nayak, Pai, et al., 2017). However, some anxiety is expected, and the work of worrying can help patients identify priorities and find coping strategies that help them face the threat of surgery. Questions may be asked to obtain the following information:

- Knowledge and understanding of the surgical procedure, postoperative course, and recovery
- Fears and concerns regarding the surgery and future health status
- Coping mechanisms helpful to the patient
- Support systems available during and following hospitalization

Reducing Fear and Anxiety

The nurse gives the patient and family time and opportunity to express their fears. Topics of concern may be pain, changes in body image, fear of the unknown, and fear of disability or death. It may be helpful to describe the sensations that the patient can expect, including the preoperative sedation, surgical anesthesia, and postoperative pain management. The nurse reassures the patient that the fear of pain is normal, that some pain will be experienced, that medication to relieve pain will be provided, and that the patient will be closely monitored. In addition, the nurse instructs the patient to request analgesic medication before the pain becomes severe. If the patient has concerns about scarring from surgery, the nurse encourages them to discuss this issue and corrects any misconceptions. The patient and family may want to discuss their fear of the patient dying. After the fear is expressed, the nurse can assure the patient and family that this fear is normal and further explore their feelings. For patients with extreme anxiety or fear and for whom emotional support and education are not successful, antianxiety medication such as lorazepam may be helpful.

Monitoring and Managing Potential Complications

Angina may occur because of increased stress and anxiety related to the forthcoming surgery. The patient who develops angina usually responds to typical therapy for angina, most commonly nitroglycerin. Some patients require oxygen and IV nitroglycerin infusions. Physiologically unstable patients may require preoperative management in a critical care unit.

 ## Providing Patient Education

Prior to surgery, patients and their families are given specific instructions. This includes information on how the patient should take or stop specific medications, including anticoagulant agents, antihypertensive medications, and medications that control diabetes. The patient is instructed to shower with an antiseptic solution such as chlorhexidine gluconate and to apply mupirocin calcium 2% ointment to each nostril to help reduce the risk of surgical site infections (Reiser, Scherag, Forstner, et al., 2017). Cardiac surgical infections are often caused by *Staphylococcus aureus* which is found in the nasal passages. Studies have shown that decolonizing the nasal passage preoperatively is effective in reducing sternal wound infections associated with cardiac surgery (Lemaignen, Armand-Lefevre, Birgand, et al., 2018) (see Chapter 14 for further discussion of preoperative preparation).

Education also includes information about the hospitalization and surgery. The nurse informs the patient and family about the equipment, tubes, and lines that will be present after surgery and their purposes. They should expect monitors, several IV lines, chest tubes, and a urinary catheter. Explaining the purpose and the approximate time that these devices will be in place helps reassure the patient. Most patients remain intubated and on mechanical ventilation for several hours after surgery. It is important for patients to know that this will prevent them from talking, and the nurse should reassure them that the staff will be able to assist them with other means of communication.

The nurse takes care to answer the patient's questions about postoperative care and procedures. After the nurse explains deep breathing and coughing, the use of the incentive spirometer, and foot exercises, the nurse practices these procedures with the patient. The benefit of early and frequent ambulation is discussed. The family's questions at this time usually focus on the length of the surgery, who will discuss the results of the procedure with them after surgery, where to wait during the surgery, the visiting procedures for the critical care unit, and how they can support the patient before surgery and in the critical care unit.

Intraoperative Management

The perioperative nurse performs assessments and prepares the patient as described in Chapters 14 and 15. In addition to assisting with the surgical procedure, perioperative nurses are responsible for the comfort and safety of the patient.

Possible intraoperative complications include low cardiac output, arrhythmias, hemorrhage, MI, organ failure from shock, and thromboembolic events including stroke (Urden et al., 2019). Astute intraoperative nursing assessment is critical to prevent, detect, and initiate prompt intervention for these complications. Before the chest incision is closed, chest tubes are inserted to evacuate air and drainage from the mediastinum and the thorax.

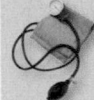 For the procedural guideline for setup and management of chest drainage systems, go to **thepoint.lww.com/Brunner15e.**

Temporary epicardial pacemaker electrodes may be implanted on the surface of the right atrium and the right ventricle. These epicardial electrodes can be connected to an external pacemaker if the patient has persistent bradycardia perioperatively (see Chapter 22 for a discussion of pacemakers).

Postoperative Nursing Management

Initial postoperative care focuses on achieving or maintaining hemodynamic stability and recovery from general anesthesia. Care may be provided in the postanesthesia care unit (PACU) or ICU. The immediate postoperative period for the patient who has undergone cardiac surgery presents many challenges to the health care team. All efforts are made to facilitate the transition from the operating room to the ICU or PACU with minimal risk. Specific information about the surgical procedure and important factors about postoperative management are communicated by the surgical team and anesthesia personnel to the critical care or PACU nurse, who then assumes responsibility for the patient's care. Figure 23-12 presents an overview of the many aspects of postoperative care of the cardiac surgical patient.

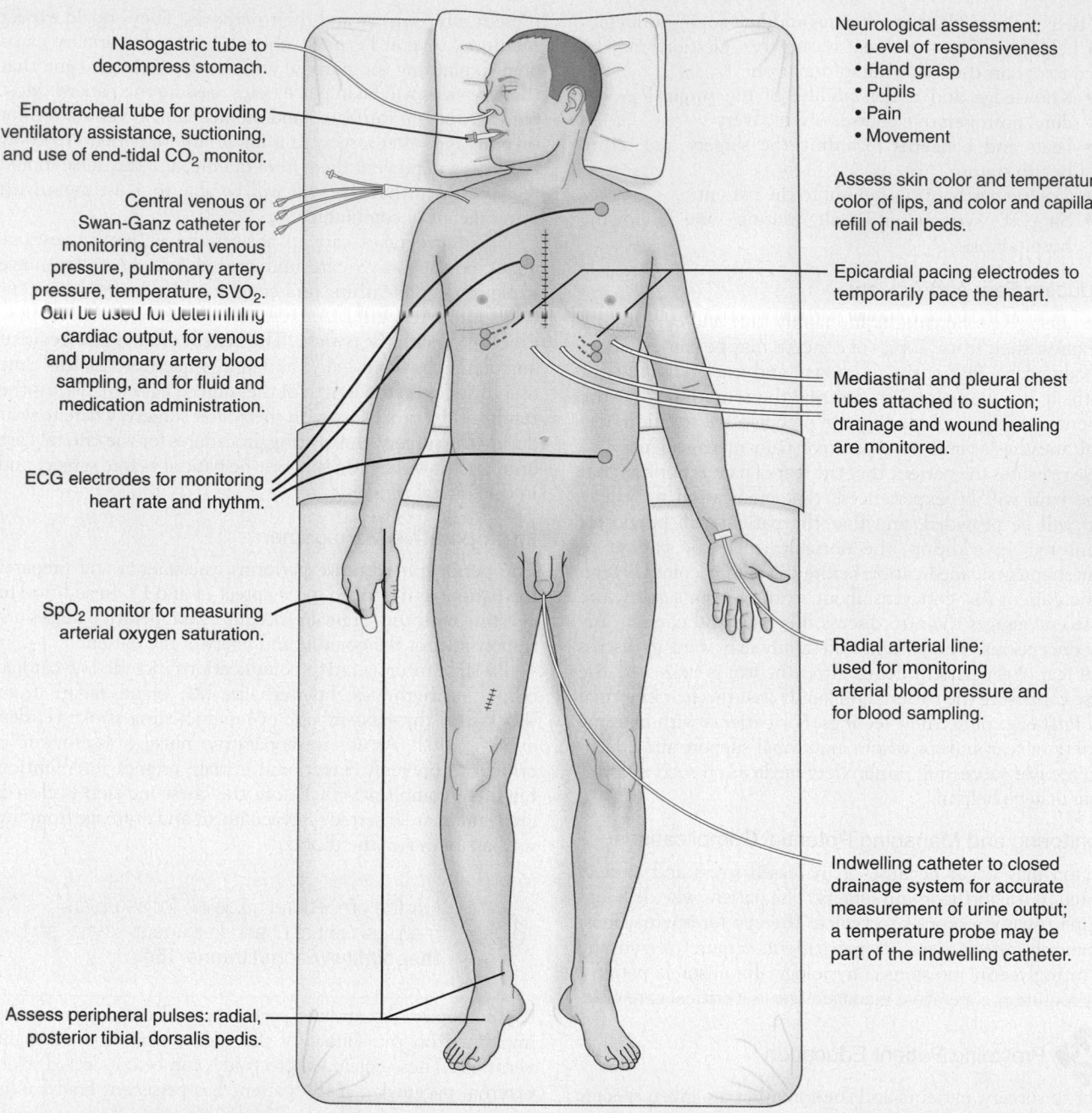

Nasogastric tube to decompress stomach.

Endotracheal tube for providing ventilatory assistance, suctioning, and use of end-tidal CO_2 monitor.

Central venous or Swan-Ganz catheter for monitoring central venous pressure, pulmonary artery pressure, temperature, SVO_2. Can be used for determining cardiac output, for venous and pulmonary artery blood sampling, and for fluid and medication administration.

ECG electrodes for monitoring heart rate and rhythm.

SpO₂ monitor for measuring arterial oxygen saturation.

Assess peripheral pulses: radial, posterior tibial, dorsalis pedis.

Neurological assessment:
• Level of responsiveness
• Hand grasp
• Pupils
• Pain
• Movement

Assess skin color and temperature, color of lips, and color and capillary refill of nail beds.

Epicardial pacing electrodes to temporarily pace the heart.

Mediastinal and pleural chest tubes attached to suction; drainage and wound healing are monitored.

Radial arterial line; used for monitoring arterial blood pressure and for blood sampling.

Indwelling catheter to closed drainage system for accurate measurement of urine output; a temperature probe may be part of the indwelling catheter.

Figure 23-12 • Postoperative care of the patient who has undergone cardiac surgery requires the nurse to be proficient in interpreting hemodynamics, correlating physical assessment data with laboratory results, sequencing interventions, and evaluating progress toward desired outcomes.

After the patient's cardiac status and respiratory status are stable, the patient is transferred to a surgical progressive care unit with telemetry. Care in both the ICU and progressive care unit focuses on monitoring of cardiopulmonary status, pain management, wound care, progressive activity, and nutrition. Education about medications and risk factor modification is emphasized.

A typical plan of postoperative nursing care is presented in Chart 23-11.

Assessing the Patient

When the patient is admitted to the critical care unit or PACU, nursing and medical personnel perform a complete assessment of all systems at least every 4 hours. It is necessary to assess the following parameters:

Neurologic status: level of responsiveness, pupil size and reaction to light, facial symmetry, movement of the extremities, and hand grip strength

Cardiac status: heart rate and rhythm, heart sounds, pacemaker status, arterial blood pressure, central venous pressure (CVP); in select patients, hemodynamic parameters: pulmonary artery pressure, pulmonary artery wedge pressure (PAWP), cardiac output and index, systemic and pulmonary vascular resistance, mixed venous oxygen saturation ($Sv–O_2$). A pulmonary artery catheter is often used to monitor these

(text continued on page 759)

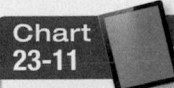

Chart 23-11

PLAN OF NURSING CARE
Care of the Patient After Cardiac Surgery

NURSING DIAGNOSIS: Impaired cardiac output associated with blood loss and compromised myocardial function
GOAL: Restoration of cardiac output to maintain organ and tissue perfusion

Nursing Interventions	Rationale	Expected Outcomes

1. Monitor cardiovascular status. Serial readings of blood pressure, other hemodynamic parameters, and cardiac rhythm and rate are obtained, recorded, and correlated with the patient's overall condition.	1. Effectiveness of cardiac output is evaluated by continuous monitoring.	• The following parameters are within the patient's normal ranges:
		  • Arterial pressure
		  • Central venous pressure (CVP)
		  • Pulmonary artery pressures
		  • Pulmonary artery wedge pressure (PAWP)
		  • Heart sounds
		  • Pulmonary and systemic vascular resistance
		  • Cardiac output and cardiac index
		  • Peripheral pulses
		  • Cardiac rate and rhythm
		  • Cardiac biomarkers
		  • Urine output
		  • Skin and mucosal color
		  • Skin temperature

a. Assess arterial blood pressure every 15 minutes until stable; then arterial or cuff blood pressure every 1–4 hours × 24 hours; then every 8–12 hours until hospital discharge.	a. Blood pressure is one of the most important physiologic parameters to monitor; vasoconstriction after cardiopulmonary bypass may require treatment with an IV vasodilator.	
b. Auscultate for heart sounds and rhythm.	b. Auscultation provides evidence of pericarditis (precordial rub), arrhythmias.	
c. Assess peripheral pulses (pedal, tibial, radial).	c. Presence or absence and quality of pulses provide data about cardiac output as well as obstructive lesions.	
d. Monitor hemodynamic parameters to assess cardiac output, volume status, and vascular tone.	d. Rising CVP and PAWP may indicate congestive heart failure or pulmonary edema. Low pressures may indicate need for volume replacement.	• <200 mL/h of drainage through chest tubes during first 4–6 hours • Vital signs stable • CVP and other hemodynamic parameters within normal limits • Urinary output within normal limits • Skin color normal • Respirations unlabored, clear breath sounds • Pain limited to incision
e. Watch for trends in hemodynamics, and note that mechanical ventilation may alter hemodynamics.	e. Trends are more important than isolated readings. Mechanical ventilation increases intrathoracic pressure.	
f. Monitor electrocardiogram (ECG) pattern for cardiac arrhythmias and ischemic changes.	f. Arrhythmias may occur with coronary ischemia, hypoxia, bleeding, and acid–base or electrolyte disturbances. ST-segment changes may indicate myocardial ischemia. Pacemaker capture and antiarrhythmic medications are used to maintain heart rate and rhythm and to support blood pressure.	
g. Assess cardiac biomarker results.	g. Elevations may indicate myocardial infarction.	
h. Measure urine output every ½ to 1 hour at first, then with vital signs.	h. Urine output <0.5 mL/kg/h indicates decreased renal perfusion and may reflect decreased cardiac output.	
i. Observe buccal mucosa, nail beds, lips, earlobes, and extremities.	i. Duskiness and cyanosis may indicate decreased cardiac output.	
j. Assess skin; note temperature and color.	j. Cool moist skin indicates vasoconstriction and decreased cardiac output.	
2. Observe for persistent bleeding: excessive chest tube drainage of blood; hypotension; low CVP; tachycardia. Prepare to administer blood products, IV fluids.	2. Bleeding can result from surgical trauma to tissues, anticoagulant medications, and clotting defects.	
3. Observe for cardiac tamponade: hypotension; rising CVP and PAWP, pulsus paradoxus; jugular vein distention; decreasing urinary output. Check for diminished amount of blood in chest drainage collection system. Prepare for reoperation.	3. Cardiac tamponade results from bleeding into the pericardial sac or accumulation of fluid in the sac, which compresses the heart and prevents adequate filling of the ventricles. Decrease in chest drainage may indicate that fluid and clots are accumulating in the pericardial sac.	
4. Observe for signs of cardiac failure. Prepare to administer diuretics, IV inotropic agents.	4. Cardiac failure results from decreased pumping action of the heart; can cause deficient perfusion to vital organs.	

(continued on page 756)

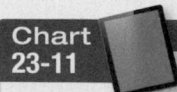

Chart 23-11

PLAN OF NURSING CARE (continued)

Care of the Patient After Cardiac Surgery

NURSING DIAGNOSIS: Impaired gas exchange associated with chest surgery
GOAL: Adequate gas exchange

Nursing Interventions	Rationale	Expected Outcomes
1. Maintain mechanical ventilation until the patient is able to breathe independently.	1. Ventilatory support is used to decrease work of the heart, to maintain effective ventilation, and to provide an airway in the event of complications.	• Airway patent • Arterial blood gases (ABGs) within normal range • Endotracheal tube correctly placed, as evidenced by x-ray • Breath sounds clear bilaterally
2. Monitor ABGs, tidal volume, peak inspiratory pressure, and extubation parameters.	2. ABGs and ventilator parameters indicate effectiveness of ventilator and changes that need to be made to improve gas exchange.	• Ventilator synchronous with respirations • Breath sounds clear after suctioning/coughing
3. Auscultate chest for breath sounds.	3. Crackles indicate pulmonary congestion; decreased or absent breath sounds may indicate pneumothorax, hemothorax, dislodgement of tube.	• Nail beds and mucous membranes pink • Mental acuity consistent with amount of sedatives and analgesics received
4. Sedate patient adequately, as prescribed, and monitor respiratory rate and depth.	4. Sedation helps the patient to tolerate the endotracheal tube and to cope with mechanical ventilation.	• Oriented to person; able to respond "yes" and "no" appropriately • Able to be weaned successfully from ventilator
5. Suction tracheobronchial secretions as needed, using strict aseptic technique.	5. Retention of secretions leads to hypoxia and possible infection.	
6. Assist in weaning and endotracheal tube removal.	6. Extubation decreases risk of pulmonary infections and enhances ability of patient to communicate.	
7. After extubation, promote deep breathing, coughing, and turning. Encourage the use of the incentive spirometer and compliance with breathing treatments. Instruct about incisional splinting with a "cough pillow" to decrease discomfort.	7. Aids in keeping airway patent, preventing atelectasis, and facilitating lung expansion	

NURSING DIAGNOSIS: Risk for hypovolaemia or hypervolaemia and electrolyte imbalance associated with alterations in blood volume
GOAL: Fluid and electrolyte balance

Nursing Interventions	Rationale	Expected Outcomes
1. Monitor fluid and electrolyte balance.	1. Adequate circulating blood volume is necessary for optimal cellular activity; fluid and electrolyte imbalance can occur after surgery.	• Fluid intake and output balanced • Hemodynamic assessment parameters negative for fluid overload or hypovolemia
a. Accurately document intake and output; record urine volume every half hour to 4 hours while in critical care unit; then every 8–12 hours while hospitalized.	a. Provides a method to determine positive or negative fluid balance and fluid requirements	• Normal blood pressure with position changes • Absence of arrhythmia • Stable weight • Arterial blood pH 7.35–7.45
b. Assess blood pressure, hemodynamic parameters, weight, electrolytes, hematocrit, jugular venous pressure, breath sounds, urinary output, and nasogastric tube drainage.	b. Provides information about state of hydration	• Serum potassium 3.5–5.0 mEq/L (3.5–5.0 mmol/L) • Serum magnesium 1.8–2.6 mg/dL (0.74–1.07 mmol/L) • Serum sodium 135–145 mEq/L (135–145 mmol/L)
c. Measure postoperative chest drainage; cessation of drainage may indicate kinked or blocked chest tube. Ensure patency and integrity of the drainage system.	c. Excessive blood loss from chest cavity can cause hypovolemia.	• Serum calcium 8.8–10.4 mg/dL (2.2–2.6 mmol/L) • Serum glucose ≤180 mg/dL
d. Weigh daily and correlate with intake and output.	d. Indicator of fluid balance	

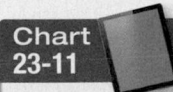

PLAN OF NURSING CARE (continued)
Care of the Patient After Cardiac Surgery

Chart 23-11

Nursing Interventions	Rationale	Expected Outcomes
2. Be alert to changes in serum electrolyte levels. a. Hypokalemia (low potassium) *Effects:* Arrhythmias: premature ventricular contractions, ventricular tachycardia. Observe for specific ECG changes. Administer IV potassium replacement as prescribed. b. Hyperkalemia (high potassium) *Effects:* ECG changes, tall peaked T waves, wide QRS, bradycardia. Be prepared to administer diuretic or an ion-exchange resin (sodium polystyrene sulfonate); or IV insulin and glucose. c. Monitor serum magnesium, sodium, and calcium. d. Hyperglycemia (high blood glucose) *Effects:* Increased urine output, thirst, impaired healing. Administer insulin as prescribed.	2. A specific concentration of electrolytes is necessary in both extracellular and intracellular body fluids to sustain life. a. *Causes:* Inadequate intake, diuretics, vomiting, excessive nasogastric drainage, perioperative stress response b. *Causes:* Increased intake, hemolysis from cardiopulmonary bypass/mechanical assist devices, acidosis, renal insufficiency. The resin binds potassium and promotes intestinal excretion of it. Insulin assists the cells with glucose and potassium absorption. c. Low levels of magnesium are associated with arrhythmias. Low levels of sodium are associated with weakness and neurologic symptoms. Low levels of calcium can lead to arrhythmias and muscle spasm. d. *Cause:* Stress response to surgery. Affects both patients with diabetes and those without diabetes.	

NURSING DIAGNOSIS: Risk for acute confusion associated with alteration in sleep–wake cycle, impaired metabolic functioning, use of multiple medications
GOAL: Prevention of acute confusion/postcardiotomy delirium

Nursing Interventions	Rationale	Expected Outcomes
1. Use measures to prevent postcardiotomy delirium: a. Explain all procedures and the need for patient cooperation. b. Plan nursing care to provide for periods of uninterrupted sleep with patient's normal day–night pattern. c. Promote continuity of care. d. Orient to time and place frequently. Encourage family to visit. e. Assess for medications that may contribute to delirium. 2. Observe for perceptual distortions, hallucinations, disorientation, and paranoid delusions.	1. Postcardiotomy delirium may result from alterations in sleep–wake cycle, impaired metabolic functioning, and use of multiple medications. Normally, sleep cycles are at least 50 minutes long. The first cycle may be as long as 90–120 minutes and then shorten during successive cycles. Sleep deprivation results when the sleep cycles are interrupted or are inadequate in number. 2. Delirium can indicate a serious medical condition such as hypoxia, acid–base imbalance, metabolic abnormalities, and cerebral infarction.	• Cooperates with procedures • Sleeps for long, uninterrupted intervals • Oriented to person, place, time • Experiences no perceptual distortions, hallucinations, disorientation, delusions

NURSING DIAGNOSIS: Acute pain associated with surgical trauma and pleural irritation caused by chest tubes
GOAL: Relief of pain

Nursing Interventions	Rationale	Expected Outcomes
1. Record nature, type, location, intensity, and duration of pain. 2. Encourage routine pain medication dosing for the first 24–72 hours, and observe for side effects of lethargy, hypotension, tachycardia, respiratory depression.	1. Pain and anxiety increase pulse rate, oxygen consumption, and cardiac workload. 2. Analgesia promotes rest, decreases oxygen consumption caused by pain, and aids patient in performing deep-breathing and coughing exercises; pain medication is more effective when taken before pain is severe.	• States pain is decreasing in severity • Restlessness decreased • Vital signs stable • Participates in deep-breathing and coughing exercises • Verbalizes fewer complaints of pain each day • Positions self; participates in care activities • Gradually increases activity

(continued on page 758)

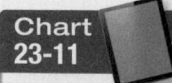

Chart 23-11

PLAN OF NURSING CARE (continued)
Care of the Patient After Cardiac Surgery

NURSING DIAGNOSIS: Risk for impaired cardiac function associated with alterations in afterload that may compromise renal perfusion
GOAL: Maintenance of adequate cardiac output and renal perfusion

Nursing Interventions	Rationale	Expected Outcomes
1. Assess renal function: a. Measure urine output every half hour to 4 hours in critical care, then every 8–12 hours until hospital discharge. b. Monitor and report lab results: BUN, serum creatinine, serum electrolytes. 2. Prepare to administer rapid-acting diuretics or inotropic drugs (e.g., dobutamine). 3. Prepare patient for dialysis or continuous renal replacement therapy if indicated.	1. Renal injury can be caused by deficient perfusion, hemolysis, low cardiac output, and the use of vasopressor agents to increase blood pressure. a. <0.5 mL/kg/h indicates decreased renal function. b. These tests indicate the kidneys' ability to excrete waste products. 2. These agents promote renal function and increase cardiac output and renal blood flow. 3. Provides patient with the opportunity to ask questions and prepare for the procedure	• Urine output consistent with fluid intake; >0.5 mL/kg/h • Urine specific gravity 1.005–1.030 • Blood urea nitrogen (BUN), creatinine, electrolytes within normal limits

NURSING DIAGNOSIS: Impaired thermoregulation associated with infection or postpericardiotomy syndrome
GOAL: Maintenance of normal body temperature

Nursing Interventions	Rationale	Expected Outcomes
1. Assess temperature every hour. 2. Use aseptic technique when changing dressings, suctioning endotracheal tube; maintain closed systems for all IV and arterial lines and for indwelling urinary catheter. 3. Observe for symptoms of postpericardiotomy syndrome. 4. Obtain cultures and other lab work (CBC, ESR); administer antibiotic agents as prescribed. 5. Administer anti-inflammatory agents as directed.	1. Fever can indicate infectious or inflammatory process. 2. Decreases risk of infection 3. Occurs in 10% of patients after cardiac surgery. 4. Antibiotic agents treat documented infection. 5. Anti-inflammatory agents relieve symptoms of inflammation.	• Normal body temperature • Incisions are free of infection and are healing. • Absence of symptoms of postpericardiotomy syndrome: fever, malaise, pericardial effusion, pericardial friction rub, arthralgia

NURSING DIAGNOSIS: Lack of knowledge about self-care activities
GOAL: Ability to perform self-care activities

Nursing Interventions	Rationale	Expected Outcomes
1. Develop education plan for patient and family. Provide specific instructions for the following: • Diet and daily weights • Activity progression • Exercise • Deep breathing, coughing, lung expansion exercises • Temperature and pulse monitoring • Medication regimen • Incision care • Access to the emergency medical system 2. Provide verbal and written instructions; provide several education sessions for reinforcement and answering questions. 3. Involve family in education sessions. 4. Provide contact information for surgeon and cardiologist and instructions about follow-up visit with surgeon. 5. Make appropriate referrals: home care agency, cardiac rehabilitation program, community support groups.	1. Each patient has unique learning needs. 2. Repetition promotes learning by allowing for questions and clarification of misinformation. 3. Family members responsible for home care are usually anxious and require adequate time for learning. 4. Arrangements for contacts with health care personnel help to allay anxieties. 5. Learning, recovery, and lifestyle changes continue after discharge from the hospital.	• Patient and family members explain and comply with therapeutic regimen. • Patient and family members identify necessary lifestyle changes. • Has copy of discharge instructions (in the patient's primary language and at appropriate reading level; has an alternate format if indicated) • Keeps follow-up appointments

parameters. Alternatively, minimally invasive monitoring of stroke volume, systemic vascular resistance, and cardiac output are calculated through pressures obtained in the arterial line (e.g., Vigileo monitor with FloTrac sensor). (See Chapter 21 for a detailed description of hemodynamic monitoring.)

Respiratory status: chest movement, breath sounds, ventilator settings (e.g., rate, tidal volume, oxygen concentration, mode such as assist-control, positive end-expiratory pressure, pressure support), respiratory rate, peak inspiratory pressure, percutaneous oxygen saturation (SpO_2), end-tidal carbon dioxide (CO_2), pleural chest tube drainage, arterial blood gases. (See Chapters 17 and 19 for detailed descriptions of respiratory assessment and ventilatory management, respectively.)

Peripheral vascular status: peripheral pulses; color of skin, nail beds, mucosa, lips, and earlobes; skin temperature; edema; condition of dressings and invasive lines

Renal function: urinary output; serum creatinine and electrolytes

Fluid and electrolyte status: strict intake and output, including all IV fluids and blood products, output from all drainage tubes; clinical and laboratory indicators of imbalance

Pain: nature, type, location, and duration; apprehension; response to analgesics

Assessment also includes checking all equipment and tubes to ensure that they are functioning properly: endotracheal tube, ventilator, end-tidal CO_2 monitor, SpO_2 monitor, pulmonary artery catheter, $Sv-O_2$ monitor, arterial and IV lines, IV infusion devices and tubing, cardiac monitor, pacemaker, chest tubes, and urinary drainage system.

As the patient regains consciousness and progresses through the postoperative period, the nurse also assesses indicators of psychological and emotional status. The patient may exhibit behavior that reflects denial or depression or may experience postoperative delirium. Characteristic signs of delirium include transient perceptual illusions, visual and auditory hallucinations, disorientation, and paranoid delusions. Patients who have delirium after cardiac surgery have poorer outcomes than do similar patients without this complication (Jones et al., 2019).

The family's needs also must be assessed. The nurse ascertains how family members are coping with the situation; determines their psychological, emotional, and spiritual needs; and finds out whether they are receiving adequate information about the patient's condition.

Monitoring for Complications

The patient is continuously assessed for impending complications (see Table 23-4). The nurse and the surgical team function collaboratively to prevent complications, to identify early signs and symptoms of complications, and to institute measures to reverse their progression.

Decreased Cardiac Output

A decrease in cardiac output is always a threat to the patient who has had cardiac surgery, and it can have a variety of causes. Preload alterations occur when too little blood volume returns to the heart as a result of persistent bleeding and hypovolemia. Excessive postoperative bleeding can lead to decreased intravascular volume, hypotension, and low cardiac output. Bleeding problems are common after cardiac surgery because of the effects of CPB, trauma from the surgery,

and anticoagulation. Preload can also decrease if there is a collection of fluid and blood in the pericardium (cardiac tamponade), which impedes cardiac filling. Cardiac output is also altered if too much volume returns to the heart, causing fluid overload.

Afterload alterations occur when the arteries are constricted as a result of postoperative hypertension or hypothermia, increasing the workload of the heart. Heart rate alterations from bradycardia, tachycardia, and arrhythmias can lead to decreased cardiac output, and contractility can be altered in cardiac failure, MI, electrolyte imbalances, and hypoxia.

Fluid Volume and Electrolyte Imbalance

Fluid and electrolyte imbalance may occur after cardiac surgery. Nursing assessment for these complications includes monitoring of intake and output, weight, hemodynamic parameters, hematocrit levels, neck vein distention, edema, breath sounds (e.g., fine crackles, wheezing), and electrolyte levels. The nurse reports changes in serum electrolytes promptly so that treatment can be instituted. Especially important are dangerously high or dangerously low levels of potassium, magnesium, sodium, and calcium. Elevated blood glucose levels are common in the postoperative period. Administration of IV insulin is recommended in patients both with and without diabetes to achieve the glycemic control necessary to promote wound healing, decrease infection, and improve survival after surgery (Gordon et al., 2018). Implementing an insulin infusion protocol that targets moderate glycemic control has been demonstrated as effective in treating acute hyperglycemia following cardiac surgery while also decreasing the incidence of hypoglycemia (Gordon et al., 2018).

Impaired Gas Exchange

Impaired gas exchange is another possible complication after cardiac surgery. All body tissues require an adequate supply of oxygen for survival. To achieve this after surgery, an endotracheal tube with ventilator assistance may be used for hours to days. The assisted ventilation is continued until the patient's blood gas values are acceptable and the patient demonstrates the ability to breathe independently. Patients who are stable after surgery may be extubated as early as 2 to 4 hours after surgery, which reduces their discomfort and anxiety and facilitates patient–nurse communication.

While receiving mechanical ventilation, the patient is continuously assessed for signs of impaired gas exchange: restlessness, anxiety, cyanosis of mucous membranes and peripheral tissues, tachycardia, and fighting the ventilator. Breath sounds are assessed often to detect pulmonary congestion and monitor lung expansion. Arterial blood gases, SpO_2, and end-tidal CO_2 are assessed for decreased oxygen and increased CO_2. Following extubation, aggressive pulmonary interventions such as turning, coughing, deep breathing, and early ambulation are necessary to prevent atelectasis and pneumonia.

Impaired Cerebral Circulation

Hypoperfusion or microemboli during or following cardiac surgery may produce injury to the brain. Brain function depends on a continuous supply of oxygenated blood. The brain does not have the capacity to store oxygen and must rely on adequate continuous perfusion by the heart. The nurse observes the patient for signs and symptoms of cerebral hypoxia: restlessness, confusion, dyspnea, hypotension, and cyanosis. An assessment of the patient's neurologic status includes the level of consciousness, response to verbal commands and painful stimuli, pupil size and reaction to light, facial symmetry, movement of the extremities, and hand grip strength. The nurse documents any indication of a change in status and reports abnormal findings to the surgeon because they may signal the onset of a complication such as a stroke.

Maintaining Cardiac Output

Ongoing evaluation of the patient's cardiac status continues as the nurse monitors the effectiveness of cardiac output through clinical observations and routine measurements: serial readings of blood pressure, heart rate, CVP, arterial pressure, and pulmonary artery pressures.

Renal function is related to cardiac function, as blood pressure and cardiac output drive glomerular filtration; therefore, urinary output is measured and recorded. Urine output less than 0.5 mL/kg/h may indicate a decrease in cardiac output or inadequate fluid volume.

Body tissues depend on adequate cardiac output to provide a continuous supply of oxygenated blood to meet the changing demands of the organs and body systems. Because the buccal mucosa, nail beds, lips, and earlobes are sites with rich capillary beds, they are observed for cyanosis or duskiness as possible signs of reduced cardiac output. Distention of the neck veins when the head of the bed is elevated to 30 degrees or more may signal right-sided heart failure.

Arrhythmias may develop due to decreased perfusion to or irritation of the myocardium from surgery. The most common arrhythmias encountered during the postoperative period are atrial fibrillation, bradycardias, tachycardias, and ectopic beats (Urden et al., 2019). Continuous observation of the cardiac monitor for arrhythmias is essential.

The nurse reports any indications of decreased cardiac output promptly. The assessment data are used to determine the cause of the problem. After a diagnosis has been made, the primary provider and the nurse work collaboratively to restore cardiac output and prevent further complications. When indicated, blood components; fluids; and antiarrhythmics, diuretics, vasodilators, or vasopressors are prescribed. If additional interventions are necessary, such as the placement of an intra-aortic balloon pump, the patient and family are prepared for the procedure.

Promoting Adequate Gas Exchange

To ensure adequate gas exchange, the patency of the endotracheal tube is assessed and maintained. The tube must be secured to prevent it from slipping out or down into the right mainstem bronchus. Suctioning is necessary when crackles or coughing is present.

 For the procedural guideline for performing tracheal suction, go to **thepoint.lww.com/Brunner15e.**

Arterial blood gas determinations are compared with baseline data, and changes are reported to the primary provider promptly.

When the patient's hemodynamic parameters stabilize, body position is changed every 1 to 2 hours. Frequent changes of patient position provide for optimal pulmonary ventilation and perfusion, allowing the lungs to expand more fully.

Physical assessment and arterial blood gas results guide the process of weaning the patient from the ventilator. The nurse assists with the weaning process and eventually with the removal of the endotracheal tube. After extubation, the nurse encourages deep breathing and coughing at least every 1 to 2 hours to clear secretions, open the alveolar sacs, and promote effective ventilation. See Chapter 19 for discussion of weaning the patient from the ventilator.

Maintaining Fluid and Electrolyte Balance

To promote fluid and electrolyte balance, the nurse carefully assesses the intake and output to determine positive or negative fluid balance. It is necessary to record all fluid intake, including IV, nasogastric tube, and oral fluids, as well as all output, including urine, nasogastric drainage, and chest drainage.

Hemodynamic parameters (e.g., blood pressure, CVP, cardiac output) are correlated with intake, output, and weight to determine the adequacy of hydration and cardiac output. Serum electrolytes are monitored, and the patient is observed for signs of potassium, magnesium, sodium, or calcium imbalance (see Chapter 10).

Indications of dehydration, fluid overload, or electrolyte imbalance are reported promptly, and the primary provider and nurse work collaboratively to restore fluid and electrolyte balance and monitor the patient's response to therapies.

Minimizing Confusion

Some patients exhibit abnormal behaviors and acute confusion that occur with varying intensity and duration. The risk of delirium is high in patients who have undergone cardiac surgery and increases with patients' age (Jones et al., 2019; Smulter, Lingehall, Gustafson, et al., 2019; see the Nursing Research Profile in Chart 23-12). Clinical manifestations of postoperative delirium include restlessness, agitation, visual and auditory hallucinations, and paranoia. The delirium typically appears after a 2- to 5-day stay in an ICU. Patients are assessed for this problem with tools such as the Confusion Assessment Method for the ICU (CAM-ICU) (Price, Garvan, Hizel, et al., 2017) (see Chapter 8, Chart 8-7, for discussion of CAM). The CAMU-ICU scale assesses for key indicators of delirium such as disorganized thinking and inattention. When this testing is positive, further assessment of the patient's physiologic and psychological status is required. Presumed causes of postoperative delirium include anxiety, sleep deprivation, increased sensory input, medications, and physiologic problems such as hypoxemia and metabolic imbalance (Blair, Mehmood, Rudnick, et al., 2019). Treatment includes correction of identified physiologic problems such as metabolic and electrolyte imbalances. In addition, behavioral interventions are used (e.g., frequent reorientation). Sedative medications such as haloperidol were once thought to reduce agitation and improve survival, but recent studies note that use of haloperidol causes oversedation and does not reliably treat or prevent delirium (Blair et al., 2019). The delirium often resolves after the patient is transferred from the unit, but nonetheless can be associated with negative outcomes including cognitive and

Chart 23-12 NURSING RESEARCH PROFILE
Use of a Postoperative Delirium Screening Scale in Older Adults After Cardiac Surgery

Smulter, N., Lingehall, H. C., Gustafson, Y., et al. (2019). The use of a screening scale improves the recognition of delirium in older patients after cardiac surgery: A retrospective observational study. *Journal of Clinical Nursing, 28*(11-12), 2309–2318.

Purpose

Postoperative delirium (POD) is a frequent occurrence in older patients undergoing cardiac surgery. However, it is often not recognized by health care providers and therefore may go undiagnosed. The purpose of this study was to assess whether the use of a delirium screening tool by nurses postoperatively will improve the recognition and diagnosis of POD.

Design

This study was a retrospective observational analysis. Seventy eight patients aged 70 and older who had cardiac surgery were diagnosed with POD. Nurses used the Nursing Delirium Screening Scale (Nu-DESC) to screen for delirium symptoms. This scale uses five items to assess for delirium: disorientation, inappropriate behavior, inappropriate communication, illusions and hallucinations, and psychomotor retardation. Each item is graded from 0 to 2 with a maximum score of 10. A Nu-DESC score of 2 or greater is thought to indicate the presence of delirium. The screening was conducted three times daily, beginning post-op day 1 through discharge.

Data describing the incidence and nature of POD from the clinical database and discharge summaries were retrospectively collected. This information was compared to the results of symptom screening using the Nu-DESC.

Findings

POD was correctly identified in 41 of 78 (52.6%) patients. "Inappropriate behavior" was the most common descriptor used by nurses and physicians within discharge summaries. Terminology like "confused," "aggressive/restless," and "disoriented" were commonly used to describe delirium symptoms. The cause and specific treatment of delirium was not addressed within the discharge summaries

Screening using the Nu-DESC identified 56 of 78 (72%) patients with POD. Use of the Nu-DESC showed greater sensitivity in identifying symptoms of delirium than the information documented within the discharge summaries and database.

Nursing Implications

Delirium is a serious complication that is underdiagnosed in patients after cardiac surgery and, when present, not well documented. Use of a validated screening scale, such as the Nu-DESC, can improve the ability of nurses to recognize delirium in postoperative patients.

---

functional decline, longer lengths of hospital stay, and higher mortality (Delaney, Hammond, & Litton, 2018).

For all postoperative patients, basic comfort measures are used in conjunction with prescribed analgesics and sedatives to promote rest. Invasive lines and tubes are discontinued as soon as possible. Patient care is coordinated to provide undisturbed periods of rest. As the patient's condition stabilizes and the patient is disturbed less frequently for monitoring and therapeutic procedures, rest periods can be extended. Uninterrupted sleep is provided as much as possible, especially during the patient's normal hours of sleep.

Careful explanations of all procedures and of the patient's role in facilitating them help keep the patient positively involved throughout the postoperative course. Continuity of care is desirable; a familiar face and a nursing staff with a consistent approach help the patient feel safe. The patient's family should be welcomed at the bedside. A well-designed and individualized plan of nursing care can assist the nursing team in coordinating its efforts for the emotional well-being of the patient.

Relieving Pain

Patients who have had cardiac surgery may have pain in the peri-incisional area or throughout the chest, shoulders, and back. Pain results from trauma to the chest wall and irritation of the pleura by the chest tubes as well as incisional pain from peripheral vein or artery graft harvest sites.

The nurse assesses patients for verbal and nonverbal indicators of pain and records the nature, type, location, and duration of the pain. To reduce the amount of pain, the nurse encourages the patient to accept medication on a regular basis. The addition of adjunctive pain relievers (anti-inflammatory agents, muscle relaxants) to opioids decreases the amount of opioids required for pain relief and increases patient comfort. Patients report the most pain during coughing, turning, and moving. Physical support of the incision with a folded bath blanket or small pillow during deep breathing and coughing helps minimize pain. The patient should then be able to participate in respiratory exercises and to progressively increase self-care. Patient comfort improves after removal of the chest tubes.

Pain produces distress, which may stimulate the central nervous system to release catecholamines, resulting in constriction of the arterioles and increased heart rate. This can cause increased afterload and decreased cardiac output. Opioids alleviate pain and induce sleep and feelings of well-being, which reduce the metabolic rate and oxygen demands. After the administration of opioids, it is necessary to document observations indicating relief of apprehension and pain in the patient's record. The nurse observes the patient for any adverse effects of opioids, including respiratory depression, hypotension, constipation, ileus, or urinary retention. If respiratory depression occurs, an opioid antagonist (e.g., naloxone) may be required (see Chapter 9 for further discussion of nonpharmacologic pain interventions).

Maintaining Adequate Tissue Perfusion

The nurse routinely palpates peripheral pulses (e.g., pedal, tibial, femoral, radial, brachial) to assess for arterial obstruction. If a pulse is absent in any extremity, the cause may be prior catheterization of that extremity, chronic peripheral vascular disease, or a thromboembolic obstruction. The nurse immediately reports newly identified absence of any pulse.

Thromboembolic events can result from vascular injury, dislodgment of a clot from a damaged valve, loosening of mural thrombi, or coagulation problems. Air embolism can result from CPB or central venous cannulation. Symptoms of embolization vary according to site. The usual embolic sites are the lungs, coronary arteries, mesentery, spleen, extremities, kidneys, and brain. The patient is observed for the onset of the following:

- Acute onset of chest pain and respiratory distress, as occur in pulmonary embolus or MI
- Abdominal or back pain, as occur in mesenteric emboli
- Pain, cessation of pulses, blanching, numbness, or coldness in an extremity
- One-sided weakness and pupillary changes, as occur in stroke

The nurse promptly reports any of these symptoms.

Venous stasis, which can cause venous thromboembolism (e.g., deep vein thrombosis, pulmonary embolism), may occur after surgery. It can be prevented by using the following measures:

- Apply sequential pneumatic compression devices as prescribed.
- Discourage crossing of legs.
- Avoid elevating the knees on the bed.
- Omit pillows in the popliteal space.
- Begin passive exercises followed by active exercises to promote circulation and prevent venous stasis.

Inadequate renal perfusion can occur as a complication of cardiac surgery. One possible cause is low cardiac output. Trauma to blood cells during CPB can cause hemolysis of red blood cells, which then occlude the renal glomeruli. The use of vasopressor agents to increase blood pressure may constrict the renal arterioles and reduce blood flow to the kidneys.

Nursing management includes accurate measurement of urine output. An output less than 0.5 mL/kg/h may indicate hypovolemia or renal insufficiency. The primary provider may prescribe fluids to increase cardiac output and renal blood flow, or IV diuretics may be given to increase urine output. The nurse should be aware of the patient's blood urea nitrogen, serum creatinine, glomerular filtration rate, and serum electrolyte levels. The nurse should report abnormal levels promptly, because it may be necessary to adjust fluids and the dose or type of medication given. If efforts to maintain renal perfusion are ineffective, the patient may require continuous renal replacement therapy or dialysis (see Chapter 48).

Maintaining Normal Body Temperature

Patients are usually hypothermic when admitted to the critical care unit following the cardiac surgical procedure. Because induced hypothermia from CPB and anesthesia lower the patient's core temperature, the patient must be gradually warmed to a normal temperature. This is accomplished partially by the patient's own basal metabolic processes and often with the assistance of heated air blanket systems. While the patient is hypothermic, shivering and hypertension are common. Lowering the blood pressure with a vasodilator such as nitroprusside may be necessary. These problems typically resolve as warming occurs.

After cardiac surgery, the patient is at risk for developing elevated body temperature as a result of tissue inflammation or infection. The inflammatory/immune response to surgery includes the release of cytokines that cause fever (Norris, 2019). The resultant increase in metabolic rate increases tissue oxygen demands and increases cardiac workload. Antipyretics and other measures are used to lower body temperature.

Common sites of postoperative infection include the lungs, urinary tract, incisions, and intravascular catheters. Meticulous care is used to prevent contamination at the sites of catheter and tube insertions. Aseptic technique is used when changing dressings and when providing endotracheal tube and catheter care. Clearance of pulmonary secretions is accomplished by frequent repositioning of the patient, suctioning, and chest physical therapy, as well as educating and encouraging the patient to breathe deeply and cough. All invasive lines and tubes are discontinued as soon as possible after surgery to avoid infection.

Postpericardiotomy syndrome may occur in patients who undergo cardiac surgery. The syndrome is characterized by fever, pericardial pain, pleural pain, dyspnea, pericardial effusion, pericardial friction rub, and arthralgia. These signs and symptoms may occur days to weeks after surgery, often after the patient has been discharged from the hospital.

Postpericardiotomy syndrome must be differentiated from other postoperative complications (e.g., infection, incisional pain, MI, pulmonary embolus, bacterial endocarditis, pneumonia, atelectasis). Treatment depends on the severity of the signs and symptoms. Use of colchicine and anti-inflammatory agents may produce an improvement in symptoms (Lehto, Kiviniemi, Gunn, et al., 2018).

Promoting Home, Community-Based, and Transitional Care

Educating Patients About Self-Care

Depending on the type of surgery and postoperative progress, the patient may be discharged from the hospital 3 to 5 days after surgery. Following recovery from the surgery, patients can expect fewer symptoms from CAD and an improved quality of life. CABG has been shown to increase the lifespan of high-risk patients, including those with left main artery blockages and left ventricular dysfunction with multivessel blockages (Urden et al., 2019).

Although the patient may be eager to return home, the patient and family usually are apprehensive about this transition. Family members often express the fear that they are not capable of caring for the patient at home or that they are unprepared to handle complications that may occur.

The nurse helps the patient and family set realistic, achievable goals. An education plan that meets the patient's individual needs is developed with the patient and family. Specific instructions are provided about incision care; signs and symptoms of infection; diet; activity progression and exercise; deep breathing, incentive spirometry, and tobacco use cessation; weight and temperature monitoring; the medication regimen; and follow-up visits with home health nurses, the rehabilitation personnel, the surgeon, and the cardiologist or internist.

Some patients have difficulty learning and retaining information after cardiac surgery. The patient may experience recent memory loss, short attention span, difficulty with simple math, poor handwriting, and visual disturbances. Patients

Chart 23-13	**HOME CARE CHECKLIST**
	Discharge After Cardiac Surgery

At the completion of education, the patient and/or caregiver will be able to:

- Name the procedure that was performed and identify any permanent changes in anatomic structure or function as well as changes in ADLs, IADLs, roles, relationships, and spirituality.
- Identify interventions and strategies (e.g., durable medical equipment, adaptive equipment) used in recovery period.
- Describe ongoing postoperative therapeutic regimen, including diet and activities to perform (e.g., walking and breathing exercises) and to limit or avoid (e.g., lifting weights, driving a car, contact sports).
- State the name, dose, side effects, frequency, and schedule for all medications.
- State how to obtain medical supplies and carry out dressing changes, wound care, and other prescribed regimens.

- Identify durable medical equipment needs, proper usage, and maintenance necessary for safe utilization.
- Describe signs and symptoms of complications.
- State time and date of follow-up appointments.
- Relate how to reach the primary provider with questions or complications.
- Identify community resources for peer and caregiver/family support:
  - Identify sources of support (e.g., friends, relatives, faith community)
  - Identify contact information of support groups for people and their caregivers/families
- Identify the need for health promotion (e.g., weight reduction, cessation of tobacco use, stress management), disease prevention, and screening activities

ADLs, activities of daily living; IADLs, independent activities of daily living.

---

with these difficulties often become frustrated when they try to resume normal activities. The patient and family are reassured that the difficulty is almost always temporary and will subside, usually in 6 to 8 weeks. In the meantime, instructions are given to the patient at a slower pace than normal, and a family member assumes responsibility for making sure that the prescribed regimen is followed.

Continuing and Transitional Care

Arrangements are made for home, community-based, or transitional care when appropriate. Because the hospital stay is relatively short, it is particularly important for the nurse to assess the patient's and family's ability to manage care in the home. The nurse making a home visit continues the education process (see Chart 23-13), monitors vital signs and incisions, assesses for signs and symptoms of complications, and provides support for the patient and family. Additional interventions may include dressing changes, diet counseling, and tobacco use cessation strategies. Patients and families need to know that cardiac surgery did not cure the patient's underlying heart disease process. Lifestyle changes for risk factor reduction are essential, and medications taken before surgery to control problems such as blood pressure and hyperlipidemia will still be necessary.

The nurse encourages the patient to contact the surgeon, cardiologist, or office nurse with problems or questions. This provides the patient and family with reassurance that professional support is available. The patient is expected to have at least one follow-up visit with the surgeon.

Education does not end at the time of discharge from the hospital, transitional, or home health care. Many patients and families benefit from supportive programs, including cardiac rehabilitation. These programs provide monitored exercise; instructions about diet and stress reduction; information about resuming work, driving, and sex; assistance with tobacco use cessation; and support groups for patients and families. Hospital or community-based support groups provide information as well as an opportunity for families to share experiences.

CRITICAL THINKING EXERCISES

1 ipc You have been assigned to care for a 64-year-old woman who was admitted last night complaining of fatigue and mild shortness of breath. She tells you that she does not understand why the doctors are so concerned about her heart. She states, "there is nothing wrong with my heart. I am just tired. What's all the fuss about?" What education would you provide to the patient about women and heart disease? What clinical manifestations can indicate heart disease in women? What laboratory and diagnostic studies would you expect to be done for this patient? Which members of the interprofessional team would you want to involve in her care?

2 pq You are assigned to care for a 56-year-old man who is scheduled for a drug eluting stent today. You receive report from the cardiac catheter lab nurse that the patient tolerated the procedure well, is currently stable, and will be returning shortly to your unit. How will you prioritize care for this patient once he returns to his room? What assessments will you do first? What complications is he most at risk of developing and how will you know if they are occurring? What patient education should be initiated and when?

3 ebp You have been asked to provide an educational in-service to a group of nursing students on how to care for a patient presenting with a myocardial infarction (MI). One of the students asks you to explain how you determine if the patient is having an NSTEMI or a STEMI. How do you respond? According to evidence-based guidelines, what medications are used in the initial management of patients with an acute MI? According to these guidelines, under what conditions would a patient receive thrombolytic therapy rather than undergo a percutaneous coronary intervention?

REFERENCES

*Asterisk indicates nursing research.
**Double asterisk indicates classic reference.

Books

Comerford, K. C., & Durkin, M. T. (Eds.) (2020). *Nursing2020 drug handbook*. Philadelphia, PA: Wolters Kluwer.

Frandsen, G., & Pennington, S. S. (2021). *Abrams' clinical drug therapy: Rationales for nursing practice* (12th ed.). Philadelphia, PA: Wolters Kluwer Health.

Norris, T. L. (2019). *Porth's pathophysiology: Concepts of altered health states* (10th ed.). Philadelphia, PA: Wolters Kluwer.

Snyder, M. (2018). Cardiac surgery. In P. G. Morton, & D. K. Fontaine (Eds.). *Critical care nursing: A holistic approach* (11th ed.). Philadelphia, PA: Wolters Kluwer.

Urden, L. D., Stacy, K. M., & Lough, M. E. (2019). *Priorities in critical care nursing* (8th ed.). St. Louis, MO: Elsevier.

Journals and Electronic Documents

Aboul-Hassan, S. S., Stankowski, T., Marczak, J., et al. (2017). The use of preoperative aspirin in cardiac surgery: A systematic review and meta-analysis. *Journal of Cardiac Surgery*, 32(12), 758–774.

Angraal, S., Khera, R., Wang, Y., et al. (2018). Sex and race differences in the utilization and outcomes of coronary artery bypass grafting among Medicare beneficiaries, 1999–2014. *Journal of the American Heart Association*, 7(14), e009014.

Arnett, D. K., Blumenthal, R. S., Albert, M. A., et al. (2019). ACC/AHA guideline on the primary prevention of cardiovascular disease. *Journal of the American College of Cardiology*, 74(10), e177–e232.

Barua, R. S., Rigotti, N. A., Benowitz, N. L., et al. (2018). 2018 ACC expert consensus decision pathway on tobacco cessation treatment. *Journal of the American College of Cardiology*, 72(25), 3332–3365.

Benjamin, E. J., Muntner, P., Alonso, A., et al. (2019). Heart disease and stroke statistics-2019 update: A report from the American Heart Association. *Circulation*, 139(10), e56–e66.

Blair G. J., Mehmood, T., Rudnick, M., et al. (2019). Nonpharmacologic and medication minimization strategies for the prevention and treatment of ICU delirium: A narrative review, *Journal of Intensive Care Medicine*, 34(3), 183–190.

*Davis, L. L. (2017). A qualitative study of symptom experiences of women with acute coronary syndrome. *Journal of Cardiovascular Nursing*, 32(5), 488–495.

Delaney, A., Hammond, N., & Litton, E. (2018). Preventing delirium in the intensive care unit. *Journal of the American Medical Association*, 319(7), 659–660.

Dickins, K. A., & Braun, L. T. (2017). Promotion of physical activity and cardiac rehabilitation for the management of cardiovascular disease. *The Journal for Nurse Practitioners*, 13(1), 47–53.

Felker, G. M., & Fudim, M. (2018). Unraveling the mystery of troponin elevation in heart failure. *Journal of the American College of Cardiology* (JACC), 71(25), 2917–2918.

Franquesa, M., Pujol-Busquets, G., García-Fernández, E., et al. (2019). Mediterranean diet and cardiodiabesity: A systematic review through evidence-based answers to key clinical questions. *Nutrients*, 11(3), 655.

Gaudino, M. F. L., Spadaccio, C., & Taggart, D. P. (2019). State-of-the-art coronary artery bypass grafting: Patient selection, graft selection, and optimizing outcomes. *Interventional Cardiology Clinics*, 8(2), 173–198.

*Gordon, J. M., Lauver, L. S., & Buck, H. G. (2018). Strict versus liberal insulin therapy in the cardiac surgery patient: An evidence-based practice development, implementation and evaluation project. *Applied Nursing Research*, 39, 265–269.

Grundy, S. M., Stone, N. J., Bailey, A. L., et al. (2018). AHA/ACC/AACVPR/AAPA/ABC/ACPM/ADA/AGS/APhA/ ASPC/NLA/PCNA Guideline on the Management of Blood Cholesterol. *Journal of the American College of Cardiology*, 73(24), e285–e350.

Ibanez, B., James, S., Agewall, S., et al. (2018). 2017 ESC Guidelines for the management of acute myocardial infarction in patients presenting with ST-segment elevation: The Task Force for the management of acute myocardial infarction in patients presenting with ST-segment elevation of the European Society of Cardiology (ESC), *European Heart Journal*, 39(2), 119–177.

Jones, D., Matalanis, G., Mårtensson, J., et al. (2019). Predictors and outcomes of cardiac surgery-associated delirium: A single centre retrospective cohort study. *Heart, Lung & Circulation*, 28(3), 455–463.

**Kannel, W. B. (1986). Silent myocardial ischemia and infarction: Insights from the Framingham Study. *Cardiology Clinics*, 4(4), 583–591.

Katsiki, N., Triposkiadis, F., Giannoukas, A. D., et al. (2018). Statin loading in cardiovascular surgery: Never too early to treat. *Current Opinion in Cardiology*, 33(4), 436–443.

Lattuca, B., Kerneis, M., Zeitouni, M., et al. (2019). Elderly patients with ST-segment elevation myocardial infarction: A patient-centered approach. *Drugs & Aging*, 36(6), 531–539.

Lee, W. H., Ong, S.-G., Zhou, Y., et al. (2019). Modeling cardiovascular risks of e-cigarettes with human-induced pluripotent stem cell-derived endothelial cells. *Journal of the American College of Cardiology*, 73(21), 2722–2737.

Lehto, J., Kiviniemi, T., Gunn, J., et al. (2018). Occurrence of postpericardiotomy syndrome: Association with operation type and postoperative mortality after open-heart operations. *Journal of the American Heart Association*, 7(22), 1–8.

Lemaignen, A., Armand-Lefevre, L., Birgand, G., et al. (2018). Thirteen-year experience with universal Staphylococcus aureus nasal decolonization prior to cardiac surgery: A quasi-experimental study. *Journal of Hospital Infection*, 100(3), 322–328.

McCarthy, C. P., Bhambhani, V., Pomerantsev, E., et al. (2018). In-hospital outcomes in invasively managed acute myocardial infarction patients who receive morphine. *Journal of Interventional Cardiology*, 31(2), 150–158.

Meghani, N. (2017). Part II: The effects of aromatherapy and guided imagery for the symptom management of anxiety, pain, and insomnia in critically ill patients: An integrative review of current literature. *Dimensions of Critical Care Nursing*, 36(6), 334–348.

Mishra, A., Edla, S., Tripathi, B., et al. (2019). Comparison of outcomes with drug eluting versus bare metal stent in very elderly population. *Journal of the American College of Cardiology* (suppl 1), 73(9), 240.

Neto, J. N. A. (2018). Morphine, oxygen, nitrates, and mortality reducing pharmacological treatment for acute coronary syndrome: An evidence-based review. *Cureus*, 10(1), e2114. Retrieved on 9/10/19 at: www.ncbi.nlm.nih.gov/pmc/articles/PMC5866121/pdf/cureus-0010-00000002114.pdf.

Price, C. C., Garvan, C., Hizel, L. P., et al. (2017). Delayed recall and working memory MMSE domains predict delirium following cardiac surgery. *Journal of Alzheimer's Disease*, 59(3), 1027–1035.

Ramesh, C., Nayak, B. S., Pai, V. B., et al. (2017). Effect of preoperative education on postoperative outcomes among patients undergoing cardiac surgery: A systematic review and meta-analysis. *Journal of PeriAnesthesia Nursing*, 32(6), 518–529.

Reiser, M., Scherag, A., Forstner, C., et al. (2017). Effect of pre-operative octenidine nasal ointment and showering on surgical site infections in patients undergoing cardiac surgery. *Journal of Hospital Infection*, 95(2), 137–143.

Riley, R. F., Corl, J. D., & Kereiakes, D. J. (2019). Intravascular lithotripsy-assisted Impella insertion: A case report. *Catheter Cardiovascular Interventions*, 93(7), 1–3.

Rousan, T. A., Mathew, S. T., & Thadani, U. (2017). Drug therapy for stable angina pectoris. *Drugs*, 77(3), 265–284.

Shlofmitz, E., Shlofmitz, R., & Lee, M. S. (2019). Orbital atherectomy: A comprehensive review. *Interventional Cardiology Clinics*, 8(2), 161–171.

*Smulter, N., Lingehall, H. C., Gustafson, Y., et al. (2019). The use of a screening scale improves the recognition of delirium in older patients after cardiac surgery: A retrospective observational study. *Journal of Clinical Nursing*, 28(11–12), 2309–2318.

Stone, N. J., Robinson, J. G., Lichtenstein, A. H., et al. (2014). Treatment of blood cholesterol to reduce atherosclerotic cardiovascular disease risk in adults: Synopsis of the 2013 American College of Cardiology/American Heart Association Cholesterol Guideline. *Annals of Internal Medicine*, 160(5), 339–343.

Wada, H., Miyauchi, K., & Daida, H. (2019). Gender differences in the clinical features and outcomes of patients with coronary artery disease. *Expert Review of Cardiovascular Therapy*, 17(2), 123–133.

Waite, T. C., Hamilton, L., & O'Brien, W. (2018). A meta-analysis of animal assisted interventions targeting pain, anxiety and distress in medical settings. *Complementary Therapies in Clinical Practice*, 33, 49–55.

Whelton, P. K., Carey, R. M., Aronow, W. S., et al. (2018). 2017ACC/AHA/AAPA/ABC/ACPM/AGS/APhA/ASH/ASPC/NMA/PCNA guideline for the prevention, detection, evaluation, and management of high blood pressure in adults: A report of the American College of Cardiology/American Heart Association Task Force on Clinical Practice Guidelines. *Journal of the American College of Cardiology*, 71(19), 123–248.

Resources

American Diabetes Association, www.diabetes.org/
American Heart Association, www.heart.org
Framingham Heart Study, www.framinghamheartstudy.org
National Heart, Lung, and Blood Institute, https://www.nhlbi.nih.gov/

Management of Patients with Structural, Infectious, and Inflammatory Cardiac Disorders

LEARNING OUTCOMES

On completion of this chapter, the learner will be able to:

1. Define valvular disorders of the heart and describe the pathophysiology, clinical manifestations, as well as the medical and nursing management of patients with mitral and aortic disorders.
2. Differentiate between the different types of cardiac valve repair and replacement procedures used to treat valvular problems and the care needed by patients who undergo these procedures.
3. Identify the pathophysiology, clinical manifestations, as well as the medical and nursing management of patients with cardiomyopathies.
4. Describe the pathophysiology, clinical manifestations, as well as the medical and nursing management of patients with infections of the heart.
5. Use the nursing process as a framework for care of the patient with a cardiomyopathy or the patient with pericarditis.

NURSING CONCEPTS

Infection   Inflammation   Perfusion

GLOSSARY

annuloplasty: repair of a cardiac valve's outer ring

aortic valve: semilunar valve located between the left ventricle and aorta

autograft: heart valve replacement made from the patient's own heart valve (e.g., pulmonic valve excised and used as an aortic valve)

bioprosthesis: heart valve replacement made of tissue from an animal heart valve (*synonym:* heterograft)

cardiomyopathy: disease of the heart muscle

chordae tendineae: nondistensible fibrous strands connecting papillary muscles to atrioventricular (mitral, tricuspid) valve leaflets

commissurotomy: splitting or separating fused cardiac valve leaflets

ejection fraction: percentage of the end-diastolic blood volume ejected from the ventricle with each heartbeat

homograft: heart valve replacement made from a human heart valve (*synonym:* allograft)

leaflet repair: repair of a cardiac valve's movable "flaps" (leaflets)

mitral valve: atrioventricular valve located between the left atrium and left ventricle

orthotopic transplantation: the recipient's heart is removed and a donor heart is grafted into the same site

prolapse: (of a valve): stretching of an atrioventricular heart valve leaflet into the atrium during systole

pulmonic valve: semilunar valve located between the right ventricle and pulmonary artery

regurgitation: backward flow of blood through a heart valve (*synonym:* insufficiency)

stenosis: narrowing or obstruction of a cardiac valve's orifice

total artificial heart: mechanical device used to aid a failing heart, replacing the right and left ventricles

tricuspid valve: atrioventricular valve located between the right atrium and right ventricle

valve replacement: insertion of either a mechanical prosthetic valve or a bioprosthetic, homograft, or autograft tissue valve at the site of a malfunctioning heart valve to restore normal blood flow through the heart

valvuloplasty: repair of a stenosed or regurgitant cardiac valve by commissurotomy, annuloplasty, or leaflet repair (or a combination of procedures)

ventricular assist device: mechanical device used to aid a failing right or left ventricle

Structural, infectious, and inflammatory disorders of the heart present many challenges for the patient, family, and health care team. Various mechanisms, heart valve disorders, cardiomyopathies, and infectious diseases of the heart alter cardiac output. Treatments for these disorders may be noninvasive or invasive. Noninvasive treatments often consist of medication therapy, diet changes, and activity modification. Invasive treatments include valve repair or replacement, ventricular assist devices (VADs), total artificial hearts (TAHs), cardiac transplantation, or other surgical procedures. Nurses have an integral role in the care of patients with structural, infectious, and inflammatory cardiac conditions.

VALVULAR DISORDERS

Valves of the heart control blood flow through the heart into the pulmonary artery and aorta by opening and closing in response to blood pressure changes during the cardiac cycle (systole, or heart contraction, and diastole, or relaxation of the heart).

Atrioventricular valves separate the atria from the ventricles and include the **tricuspid valve**, which separates the right atrium from the right ventricle, and the **mitral valve**, which separates the left atrium from the left ventricle. The tricuspid valve has three leaflets; the mitral valve has two. Both valves have **chordae tendineae**, which are nondistensible fibrous strands that anchor valve leaflets to papillary muscles of the ventricles.

Semilunar valves are located between the ventricles and their corresponding arteries. The **pulmonic valve** lies between the right ventricle and the pulmonary artery; the **aortic valve** lies between the left ventricle and the aorta. Figure 24-1 shows valves in the closed position (also refer to Chapter 21, Fig. 21-1 to review the structure of a normal heart).

When any heart valve does not close or open properly, blood flow is affected. When valves do not close completely, blood flows backward through the valve, a condition called **regurgitation** (also referred to as insufficiency). When valves do not open completely, a condition called **stenosis**, blood flow through the valve is reduced.

Regurgitation and stenosis may affect any heart valve. The mitral valve may also **prolapse** (i.e., stretching of the valve leaflet into the atrium during systole). For patients without symptoms, heart valve conditions may be monitored without treatment. If a patient has symptoms related to a valve disorder, treatment is based on the severity of symptoms, and patients may need to make lifestyle changes, take

medications, or undergo repair or replacement of the valve. Disorders of the mitral and aortic valve typically cause more symptoms, require treatment, and cause more complications than disorders of the tricuspid and pulmonic valves. Regurgitation and stenosis may occur at the same time in the same or different valves (Fig. 24-2).

Mitral Valve Prolapse

Mitral valve prolapse is a deformity that usually produces no symptoms. Rarely, it progresses and can result in sudden death (Han, Ha, Teh, et al., 2018; Nalliah, Mahajan, Elliott, et al., 2019). This condition occurs in up to 2.5% of the general

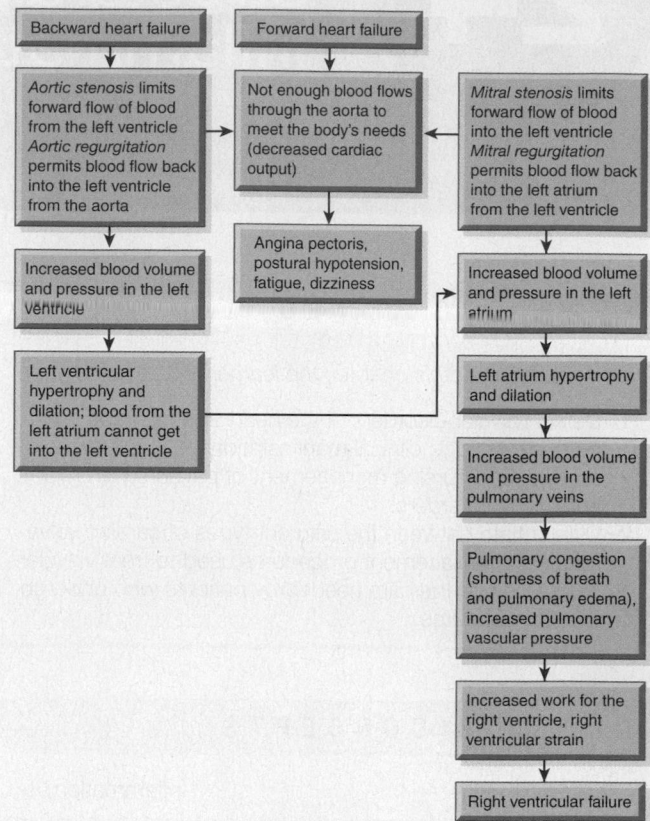

Physiology/Pathophysiology

Figure 24-2 • Pathophysiology. Left-sided heart failure as a result of aortic and mitral valvular heart disease and development of right ventricular failure.

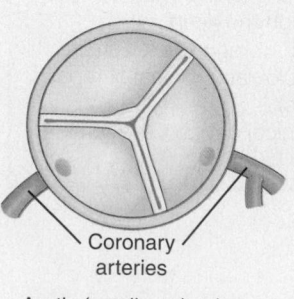

Coronary arteries

Aortic (semilunar) valve

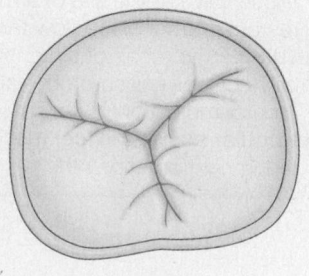

Tricuspid valve

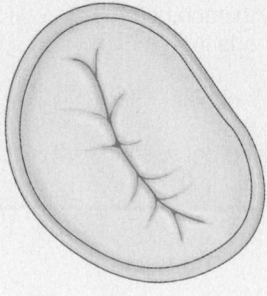

Mitral valve

Figure 24-1 • Valves of the heart (aortic or semilunar, tricuspid, and mitral) in closed positions.

population and twice as frequently in women as in men (Han et al., 2018). In most cases, there is no clear cause, but it has been associated with inherited connective tissue disorders, causing enlargement of one or both of the mitral valve leaflets (Asher, Chen, & Kallish, 2018; Wozniak-Mielczarek, Sabiniewicz, Drezek-Nojowicz, et al., 2019). The annulus often dilates; chordae tendineae and papillary muscles may elongate or rupture.

Pathophysiology

In mitral valve prolapse, a portion of one or both mitral valve leaflets balloons back into the atrium during systole. Rarely, ballooning stretches the leaflet to the point that the valve does not remain closed during systole. Blood then regurgitates from the left ventricle back into the left atrium. Although uncommon, mitral valve prolapse can result in mitral regurgitation, which can cause heart enlargement, atrial fibrillation, pulmonary hypertension, or heart failure (Ma, Igata, Strachan, et al., 2019).

Clinical Manifestations

Most people with mitral valve prolapse never have symptoms. A small number of patients will have fatigue, shortness of breath, lightheadedness, dizziness, syncope, palpitations, chest pain, or anxiety. To date, there has been no consensus about the cause of symptoms. Patients may report fatigue, regardless of activity level and amount of rest or sleep, as well as shortness of breath, palpitations, and chest pain (Althunayyan, Petersen, Lloyd, et al., 2019).

Assessment and Diagnostic Findings

Often, the first and only sign of mitral valve prolapse is an extra heart sound, referred to as a mitral click. A systolic click is an early sign that a valve leaflet is ballooning into the left atrium. In addition to the mitral click, a murmur of mitral regurgitation may be heard if the valve opens during systole and blood flows back into the left atrium. If mitral regurgitation exists, a patient may experience signs and symptoms of heart failure (see Chapter 25). Echocardiography is used to diagnose and monitor progression of mitral valve prolapse (Han et al., 2018).

Medical Management

Medical management is directed at controlling symptoms. If a patient who reports palpitations is found to have an arrhythmia, the patient may be advised to eliminate caffeine and alcohol from the diet and to stop the use of tobacco products as well as electronic nicotine delivery systems (ENDS), including e-cigarettes, e-pens, e-pipes, e-hookah, and e-cigars. Most patients do not require medication, but some are prescribed antiarrhythmic medications (see Chapter 22, Table 22-1). Prophylactic antibiotics are not recommended prior to dental or invasive procedures (Nishimura, Otto, Bonow, et al., 2017).

Patients who have chest pain related to mitral valve prolapse rarely require medical therapies, such as nitrates, calcium channel blockers, or beta-blockers. Heart failure, if present, is treated as it would be for any other case of heart failure (see Chapter 25). Patients with severe mitral regurgitation and symptomatic heart failure may require mitral valve repair or replacement (discussed later in this chapter).

Nursing Management

The nurse educates the patient about the diagnosis and the possibility that the condition is hereditary. First-degree relatives (e.g., parents, siblings) may be advised to have screening cardiac evaluations or echocardiograms. Because most patients with mitral valve prolapse are asymptomatic, the nurse explains the need to inform the patient's primary provider about any symptoms that may develop. The nurse encourages the patient to read product labels, particularly on over-the-counter products such as cough medicine, because these products may contain alcohol, caffeine, ephedrine, and epinephrine, which may produce arrhythmias and other symptoms. The nurse also explores diet, activity, sleep, and other lifestyle factors that may correlate with symptoms. (Treatment of arrhythmias, chest pain, heart failure, or other complications of mitral valve prolapse is described in Chapters 22 and 25.) Women diagnosed with mitral valve prolapse without mitral regurgitation or other complications may complete pregnancies without close cardiac monitoring and can safely proceed with vaginal deliveries (Yuan & Yan, 2016).

Mitral Regurgitation

Mitral regurgitation is a condition in which blood flows from the left ventricle back into the left atrium during systole. Often, the edges of mitral valve leaflets do not close completely during systole because leaflets and chordae tendineae have thickened and become fibrotic, resulting in abnormal contraction. Mitral regurgitation may be chronic or, less commonly, acute. The most common causes of mitral valve regurgitation in developed countries are degenerative changes of the mitral valve (including mitral valve prolapse) and ischemia of the left ventricle (Harb & Griffin, 2017). The most common cause in developing countries is rheumatic heart disease and its sequelae (Negi, Mahajan, Rana, et al., 2018).

Other conditions that lead to chronic mitral regurgitation include pathologic myxomatous changes, which enlarge and stretch the left atrium and ventricle, causing leaflets and chordae tendineae to stretch or rupture (Harb & Griffin, 2017). Infective endocarditis may cause acute mitral regurgitation through leaflet perforation, or scarring following an infection that may cause retraction of leaflets or chordae tendineae (Watanabe, 2019). Collagen vascular diseases (e.g., systemic lupus erythematosus), cardiomyopathy, and ischemic heart disease may result in changes in the left ventricle, causing papillary muscles, chordae tendineae, or leaflets to stretch, shorten, or rupture. These conditions are often referred to as functional, or secondary, mitral regurgitation (Dziadzko, Dziadzko, Medina-Inojosa, et al., 2019).

Pathophysiology

Mitral regurgitation may result from problems with one or more leaflets, chordae tendineae, the annulus, or the papillary muscles. A mitral valve leaflet may shorten or tear, and chordae tendineae may elongate, shorten, or tear. The annulus may be stretched by heart enlargement, as in functional mitral regurgitation, or it may be deformed by calcification. A papillary muscle may rupture, stretch, or be pulled out of position by changes in the ventricular wall (e.g., scar from a myocardial infarction, ventricular dilation). Papillary muscles may be unable to contract because of ischemia, a condition referred to as ischemic mitral regurgitation. Regardless of the cause, the effect is backward blood flow into the atrium during systole.

In this disorder, each beat of the left ventricle pushes blood backward into the left atrium, adding to blood flowing in from the lungs. This excess blood causes the left atrium to stretch and eventually thicken, or hypertrophy, then dilate. Over time, blood coming in from the ventricle prevents blood flow from the lungs into the atrium. As a result, the lungs become congested, eventually adding extra strain to the right ventricle. During diastole, the increased blood volume from the atrium fills the ventricle. The volume overload causes ventricular hypertrophy. Eventually, the ventricle dilates, and systolic heart failure develops.

Clinical Manifestations

Chronic mitral regurgitation is often asymptomatic, but acute mitral regurgitation (e.g., resulting from a myocardial infarction) usually manifests as severe and sudden congestive heart failure (Harb & Griffin, 2017). Dyspnea, fatigue, and weakness are the most common symptoms. Palpitations, shortness of breath on exertion, and cough from pulmonary congestion also occur.

Assessment and Diagnostic Findings

The systolic murmur of mitral regurgitation is a blowing sound best heard at the apex. The murmur may radiate to the left axilla (Harb & Griffin, 2017). The pulse may be regular, or it may be irregular because of extrasystolic beats or atrial fibrillation. Echocardiography is used to diagnose and monitor progression of this disorder (Nishimura et al., 2017).

Medical Management

Patients with mitral regurgitation who develop pulmonary congestion are managed with medications used for heart failure. Patients with mitral regurgitation and heart failure benefit from afterload reduction (arterial dilation) by treatment with angiotensin-converting enzyme (ACE) inhibitors (e.g., captopril, lisinopril) or angiotensin receptor blockers (ARBs) (e.g., losartan, valsartan), direct arterial dilators (e.g., hydralazine), and beta-blockers (e.g., carvedilol, metoprolol) (see Chapter 25, Table 25-3). Symptoms of heart failure also are an indication to consider surgical intervention by mitral **valvuloplasty** (i.e., surgical repair of the valve) or **valve replacement** (replacement of the dysfunctional valve with either a mechanical valve or a type of tissue valve; discussed later in this chapter) (Nishimura et al., 2017).

Mitral Stenosis

Mitral stenosis results in reduced blood flow from the left atrium into the left ventricle. It is usually caused by rheumatic endocarditis, which progressively thickens mitral valve leaflets and chordae tendineae, causing the leaflets to fuse together (Negi et al., 2018). Eventually, the mitral valve orifice narrows and progressively obstructs blood flow into the ventricle.

Pathophysiology

Normally, the mitral valve orifice is as wide as the diameter of three fingers. In severe mitral stenosis, the orifice narrows to the width of a pencil. Because of increased resistance through the narrowed valve orifice, the left atrium is less able to push blood into the left ventricle. This results in increased residual blood volume in the left atrium, which over time causes left atrial hypertrophy and dilation. Decreased blood flow into the left ventricle leads to reduced ventricular filling and decreased cardiac output. A stenotic valve fails to protect pulmonary veins from backward flow of blood from the atrium, resulting in congestion of the pulmonary circulation. The right ventricle must then contract against abnormally high pulmonary arterial pressure and is subjected to excessive strain. Over time, the right ventricle hypertrophies, enlarges, and eventually fails. If the heart rate increases, diastole is shortened; thus, the amount of time for forward flow of blood decreases, and more blood backs into the pulmonary veins. Therefore, as the heart rate increases, cardiac output further decreases, and pulmonary pressures increase.

Clinical Manifestations

Often, the first symptom of mitral stenosis is dyspnea on exertion (DOE) caused by pulmonary venous hypertension. Symptoms do not usually develop until after the valve opening is reduced by one third to one half its usual size (Harb & Griffin, 2017). Patients may experience progressive fatigue and decreased exercise tolerance because of low cardiac output. An enlarged left atrium may create pressure on the left bronchial tree, resulting in a dry cough or wheezing. In cases of severe mitral stenosis with significant pulmonary congestion, patients may expectorate blood (i.e., hemoptysis) or experience palpitations, orthopnea, paroxysmal nocturnal dyspnea (PND), or repeated respiratory infections. Increased blood volume and pressure cause the left atrium to dilate, hypertrophy, and become electrically unstable, which may result in patients developing atrial arrhythmias (Negi et al., 2018).

Assessment and Diagnostic Findings

Patients with mitral stenosis will have a low-pitched, rumbling diastolic murmur, best heard at the apex. Patients may have a weak and irregular pulse if they develop atrial fibrillation and may have signs or symptoms of heart failure (Nishimura et al., 2017). Echocardiography is used to diagnose and quantify the severity of mitral stenosis. Electrocardiography (ECG), exercise testing, and cardiac catheterization with angiography may be used to help determine the severity of mitral stenosis.

Prevention

Since rheumatic heart disease may result in mitral stenosis, prevention is aimed at decreasing the risk of contracting and providing early treatment for bacterial infections (see prevention of endocarditis later in this chapter). Prevention of acute rheumatic fever depends on effective antibiotic treatment of group A streptococcal infection (Nishimura et al., 2017). Antibiotic prophylaxis for recurrent rheumatic fever with rheumatic carditis may require 10 or more years of antibiotic coverage (e.g., penicillin G intramuscularly every 4 weeks, penicillin V orally twice daily, sulfadiazine orally daily, or erythromycin orally twice daily) (Szczygielska, Hernik, Kolodziejczyk, et al., 2018).

Medical Management

Congestive heart failure is treated as described in Chapter 25. Patients with severe left atrial dilation in mitral stenosis may benefit from anticoagulant medications to decrease the risk of developing atrial thrombi. If atrial fibrillation develops, cardioversion may be attempted to restore normal sinus rhythm. If unsuccessful, the ventricular rate is controlled with beta-blockers, digoxin, or calcium channel blockers; furthermore, patients will require anticoagulation for thromboembolism prevention (January, Wann, Calkins, et al., 2019). Patients with severe mitral stenosis are advised to avoid strenuous activities, competitive sports, and pregnancy, all of which increase heart rate (Nishimura et al., 2017). Surgical intervention consists of valvuloplasty, usually a **commissurotomy** (i.e., splitting or separating leaflets) to open the fused commissure of the valve. The *commissure* is the site where valve leaflets meet. Percutaneous transluminal valvuloplasty or valve replacement may be performed.

Aortic Regurgitation

Aortic regurgitation is backward flow of blood into the left ventricle from the aorta during diastole. It may be caused by a congenital valve abnormality (e.g., a bicuspid aortic valve), inflammatory lesions that deform aortic valve leaflets, or dilation of the aorta, preventing complete closure of the aortic valve. Chronic or acute aortic regurgitation may also be caused by infections such as rheumatic endocarditis or syphilis, or by a dissecting aortic aneurysm resulting in dilation or tearing of the ascending aorta, blunt chest trauma, or deterioration of a surgically replaced aortic valve (Akinseye, Pathak, & Ibebuogu, 2018; Nishimura et al., 2017).

Pathophysiology

During diastole, blood is normally delivered into the left atrium from the aorta. In aortic regurgitation, blood flows back into the left ventricle, which will dilate to accommodate increased blood volume. Over time, the left ventricle hypertrophies to expel more blood with above-normal force, thus increasing systolic blood pressure. Arteries attempt to compensate for higher pressures by reflex vasodilation; peripheral arterioles relax, reducing peripheral resistance and diastolic blood pressure.

Clinical Manifestations

Aortic regurgitation, also called aortic insufficiency, develops without symptoms in most patients. Some patients are aware of a pounding or forceful heartbeat, especially in the head or neck. Patients who develop left ventricular hypertrophy may have visible or palpable arterial pulsations at the carotid or temporal arteries due to increased force and blood volume. As aortic regurgitation worsens, DOE and fatigue follow; there may eventually be signs and symptoms of progressive left ventricular failure including increased shortness of breath, orthopnea, or PND (Akinseye et al., 2018).

Assessment and Diagnostic Findings

A high-pitched, blowing diastolic murmur is heard at the third or fourth intercostal space at the left sternal border. The difference between systolic and diastolic pressures (i.e., the pulse pressure) may be widened in patients with aortic regurgitation. One characteristic sign is the water hammer (Corrigan's) pulse, in which the pulse strikes a palpating finger with a quick, sharp stroke and then collapses (Pabba & Boudi, 2019). The diagnosis may be confirmed by echocardiography (preferably transesophageal), cardiac magnetic resonance imaging (MRI), or cardiac catheterization. Patients with symptoms usually have echocardiograms every 6 months, and those without symptoms have echocardiograms every 2 to 5 years (Nishimura et al., 2017).

Prevention

Prevention of aortic regurgitation is primarily based on prevention of and treatment for bacterial infections (see prevention of endocarditis later in this chapter). The same strategies aimed at preventing acute and recurrent rheumatic fever previously described for the patient with mitral stenosis apply to patients with aortic regurgitation.

Medical Management

A patient who is symptomatic or has developed a significant decrease in left ventricular function is advised to avoid physical exertion, competitive sports, and isometric exercise until the valve has been replaced (Gati, Malhotra, & Sharma, 2019). If arrhythmias and heart failure occur, they are treated as described in Chapters 22 and 25. Controlling high blood pressure in patients with aortic regurgitation can improve forward blood flow through the heart. ACE inhibitors and dihydropyridine calcium channel blockers may be recommended for management of hypertension; these are effective at reducing afterload. Beta-blockers are less commonly used, due to concern that a lower heart rate may actually increase blood pressure through negative chronotropic effects (Akinseye et al., 2018). Patients who are symptomatic should be instructed to restrict sodium intake to prevent volume overload and will require valve replacement (Nishimura, Otto, Bonow, et al., 2014).

The treatment of choice is aortic valve replacement or valvuloplasty (described later), preferably performed before left ventricular failure occurs. Surgery is recommended for any patient with significant left ventricular dilation, regardless of the presence or absence of symptoms (Nishimura et al., 2014). Surgery is also recommended for any patient who is symptomatic (Flint, Wunderlich, Shmueli, et al., 2019).

Aortic Stenosis

Aortic valve stenosis is narrowing of the orifice between the left ventricle and aorta. In adults, stenosis is usually caused by degenerative calcification. Calcification may be caused by proliferative and inflammatory changes that occur in response to years of normal mechanical stress, similar to changes that occur in atherosclerotic cardiovascular disease (Joseph, Naqvi, Giri, et al., 2017). Congenital leaflet malformations or an abnormal number of leaflets (i.e., one or two rather than three) are less common causes. Rheumatic endocarditis may cause adhesions or fusion of the commissures and valve ring, stiffening of the cusps, and calcific nodules on the cusps.

Pathophysiology

Typically, aortic stenosis progresses gradually over several years to several decades. As the valve orifice narrows, the left ventricle overcomes obstruction by contracting more slowly and more forcibly. Obstruction to left ventricular outflow increases pressure on the left ventricle, so the ventricular wall hypertrophies. When these compensatory mechanisms are insufficient to allow for normal heart function, clinical signs and symptoms of heart failure will develop (Joseph et al., 2017).

Clinical Manifestations

Many patients with aortic stenosis are asymptomatic. Often, the first symptom to appear is DOE, caused by increased pulmonary venous pressure due to a dilating left ventricle. Over time, left ventricular failure may occur, causing orthopnea, PND, and pulmonary edema. Reduced blood flow to the brain may cause dizziness, and in more severe aortic stenosis, syncope. Patients may also report angina pectoris, which is caused by limited blood flow into the coronary arteries, decreased time in diastole to allow for myocardial perfusion, and simultaneously increased oxygen demand of the hypertrophied left ventricle. Blood pressure is usually normal but may be low. In the setting of decreased blood flow, there may be a low pulse pressure (30 mm Hg or less).

Assessment and Diagnostic Findings

On physical examination, a loud, harsh systolic murmur is heard over the aortic area (i.e., right second intercostal space) and may radiate to the carotid arteries and apex of the left ventricle. The murmur may be described as low pitched, crescendo–decrescendo, rough, rasping, and vibrating (Libby, Zipes, Bonow, et al., 2018). An S_4 sound may be heard (see Chapter 21 for discussion of heart sounds). By having the patient lean forward during auscultation and palpation, especially during exhalation, the murmur may be accentuated. There may also be a palpable vibration extending from the base of the heart (second intercostal space next to the sternum and above the suprasternal notch) and up along the carotid arteries. The vibration is caused by turbulent blood flow across the narrowed valve orifice.

Cardiac imaging is used to diagnose and monitor the progression of aortic stenosis. This may consist of echocardiography, cardiac MRI, or computed tomography (CT) scanning (Lindman, Dweck, Lancellotti, et al., 2019). Patients with symptoms usually have echocardiograms every 6 to 12 months, and those without symptoms have echocardiograms every 2 to 5 years, depending on how severely the orifice is narrowed (Lindman et al., 2019; Nishimura et al., 2014). Left ventricular hypertrophy may be seen on a 12-lead ECG or an echocardiogram. Once aortic stenosis has progressed sufficiently to consider surgical intervention, left-sided heart catheterization is needed to measure the severity of the valvular abnormality and to evaluate the coronary arteries. Pressure measurements are taken from the left ventricle and base of the aorta. The systolic pressure in the left ventricle is considerably higher than that in the aorta during systole. Graded exercise studies (stress tests) to assess exercise capacity are performed with caution for patients with severe aortic stenosis due to the high risk of inducing ventricular tachycardia or fibrillation, and should not be performed on symptomatic patients (Joseph et al., 2017).

Prevention

Prevention of aortic stenosis is primarily focused on controlling risk factors for proliferative and inflammatory responses—namely, through treating diabetes, hypertension, hypercholesterolemia, and elevated triglycerides, and avoiding tobacco products and ENDS (see prevention of endocarditis later in this chapter).

Medical Management

Medications are prescribed to treat arrhythmias or left ventricular failure (see Chapters 22 and 25). Definitive treatment for aortic stenosis is replacement of the aortic valve, which may be done surgically or nonsurgically. Nonsurgical valve replacement, known as transcatheter aortic valve replacement (TAVR), is described in more detail later in this chapter. Patients who are symptomatic and are not candidates for valve replacement may benefit from one- or two-balloon percutaneous valvuloplasty procedures, which can provide symptom relief (Sandhu, Krishnamoorthy, Afif, et al., 2017).

Nursing Management: Valvular Heart Disorders

The nurse educates the patient with valvular heart disease about the diagnosis, progressive nature of the disease, and treatment plan. The patient is instructed to report new symptoms or changes in symptoms to the primary provider. The nurse also educates the patient that an infectious pathogen, usually a bacterium, can adhere to a diseased heart valve more readily than to a normal valve. Once attached to the valve, the infectious agent multiplies, resulting in endocarditis and further damage to the valve. In addition, the nurse educates the patient about how to minimize the risk of developing infective endocarditis (discussed later in this chapter).

The nurse measures the patient's heart rate, blood pressure, and respiratory rate, compares these results with previous data, and notes any changes. Heart and lung sounds are auscultated, and peripheral pulses palpated. The nurse assesses the patient with valvular heart disease for the following:

- Signs and symptoms of heart failure, such as fatigue, DOE, decreased activity tolerance, an increase in coughing, hemoptysis, multiple respiratory infections, orthopnea, and PND (see Chapter 25)
- Arrhythmias, by palpating the patient's pulse for strength and rhythm (i.e., regular or irregular) and asking whether the patient has experienced palpitations or felt forceful heartbeats (see Chapter 22)
- Symptoms such as dizziness, syncope, increased weakness, or angina pectoris (see Chapter 23)

The nurse collaborates with the patient to develop a medication schedule and provides education about the name, dosage, actions, adverse effects, and any drug–drug or drug–food interactions of prescribed medications for heart failure, arrhythmias, angina pectoris, or other symptoms. Specific precautions are emphasized, such as the risk to patients with aortic stenosis who experience angina pectoris and take nitroglycerin. The venous dilation that results from nitroglycerin use decreases blood return to the heart, thus decreasing cardiac output and increasing the risk of syncope and decreased coronary artery blood flow. The nurse educates the patient about the importance of attempting to relieve the symptoms of angina with rest and relaxation before taking nitroglycerin and to anticipate potential adverse effects.

For patients with heart failure, the nurse provides education on taking a daily weight and reporting sudden weight gain, as defined by the primary provider. The nurse may assist the patient with planning activity and rest periods to allow symptom relief while preventing deconditioning or loss of function. Care of patients treated with valvuloplasty or surgical valve replacement is described later in this chapter.

SURGICAL MANAGEMENT: VALVE REPAIR AND REPLACEMENT PROCEDURES

Valvuloplasty

Repair, rather than replacement, of a cardiac valve is referred to as valvuloplasty. The recommended procedure for valvuloplasty will depend on the cause and type of valve dysfunction. Repair may be made to commissures between the leaflets in a procedure known as commissurotomy, to the annulus of the valve by **annuloplasty** (i.e., specifically, repair of the cardiac valve's outer ring), or to leaflets. Transesophageal echocardiogram (TEE) is usually performed at the conclusion of a valvuloplasty to evaluate the effectiveness of the procedure.

Some valvuloplasty procedures are open-heart surgeries, which are performed under general anesthesia and usually use cardiopulmonary bypass. However, there are now several valvuloplasty procedures which utilize nonsurgical, or percutaneous, techniques; these do not require general anesthesia or cardiopulmonary bypass and can be performed in a cardiac catheterization laboratory or hybrid room. A hybrid room is an operating room with imaging capability (e.g., fluoroscopy, CT, MRI) and interventional devices for open, minimally invasive, image-guided and catheter-based procedures. Percutaneous partial cardiopulmonary bypass is used in some cardiac catheterization laboratories and hybrid rooms. (Cardiopulmonary bypass is described in Chapter 23.)

Commissurotomy

Valve leaflets may adhere to one another and close the commissure (i.e., stenosis). Less commonly, leaflets adhere to one another in a manner which creates stenosis as well as regurgitation, or backward blood flow. A commissurotomy is performed to separate the fused leaflets.

Closed Commissurotomy/Balloon Valvuloplasty

Commissurotomy is usually used for mitral valve stenosis. The preferred method is percutaneous transvenous mitral commissurotomy, which may be used for patients with congenital mitral stenosis, severe calcified mitral stenosis, left atrial thrombus, moderate to severe coexisting mitral regurgitation, or in patients with coexisting moderate to severe

tricuspid regurgitation who would also benefit from tricuspid valve repair (Nishimura et al., 2014).

Most often used for mitral and aortic valve stenosis, balloon valvuloplasty is less commonly used to treat tricuspid and pulmonic valve stenosis. With more widely available percutaneous valve repair and replacement procedures, balloon valvuloplasty is becoming a less common procedure in the United States (Kumar, Paniagua, Hira, et al., 2016). Balloon valvuloplasty may still be used for mitral valve stenosis in younger patients, and for patients with complex medical conditions that place them at high risk for complications of more extensive surgical procedures. The procedure is contraindicated for patients with left atrial or ventricular thrombus, severe aortic root dilation, significant mitral valve regurgitation, and severe valvular calcification (Nishimura et al., 2014).

Balloon valvuloplasty (Fig. 24-3) is performed in a cardiac catheterization laboratory. The patient may receive light or moderate sedation and a local anesthetic. Mitral balloon valvuloplasty involves advancing one or two catheters into the right atrium, through the atrial septum into the left atrium, across the mitral valve, and into the left ventricle. A guidewire is placed through each catheter, and the original catheter is removed. Most often a specially designed balloon catheter is placed over the guidewire and positioned with the balloon across the mitral valve. The balloon has three sections with progressively greater resistance to inflation. The balloon first expands in the ventricle to help position the catheter at the valve. The second section of the balloon expands above the valve, holding the catheter across the valve. Finally, the middle section of the balloon expands in the valve orifice

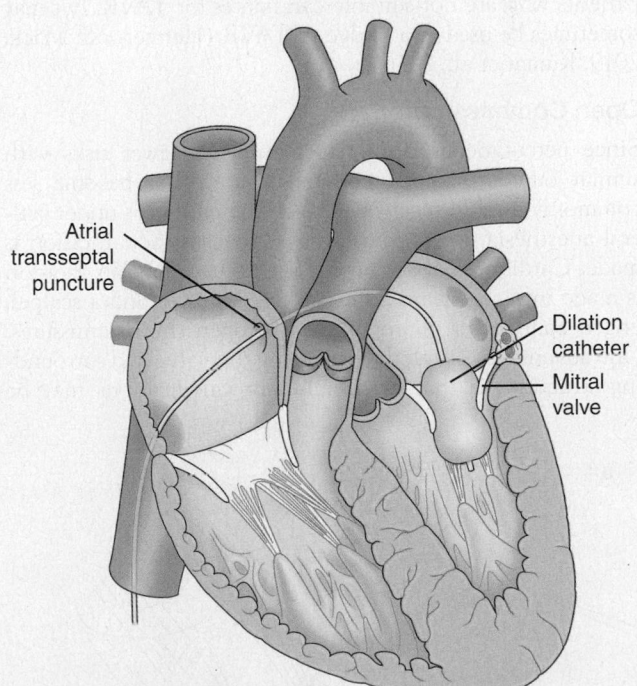

Figure 24-3 • Balloon valvuloplasty. Cross-section of heart illustrating the dilation catheter placed through an atrial transseptal puncture and across the mitral valve. The Inoue-Balloon inflates in three stages: first below the valve, then above, and finally in the valve orifice (this diagram shows the first two sections inflated).

opening the commissures. Alternately, two balloons are used. Guidewires may be advanced into the aorta to stabilize the balloons' positions. These single-section balloons are inflated simultaneously and expand their entire length. The advantage of two balloons is that each is smaller than the one large balloon, making smaller atrial septal defects. As the two balloons are inflated, they usually do not completely occlude the valve, thereby permitting some forward flow of blood during the inflation period. Balloons are inflated with a dilute angiographic solution for 10 to 30 seconds. Multiple inflations usually are required to achieve the desired results (Hermann & Mack, 2019).

All patients will have some degree of mitral regurgitation following mitral balloon valvuloplasty. Other possible complications include bleeding from the catheter insertion sites, emboli resulting in complications such as strokes, and, rarely, left-to-right atrial shunts through the atrial septal defect created during the procedure.

Aortic balloon valvuloplasty is usually performed by introducing a catheter through the aorta, across the aortic valve, and into the left ventricle; less commonly, it may be performed by passing the balloon or balloons through the atrial septum. The one- or two-balloon technique can be used for treating aortic stenosis. Balloons are inflated for 15 to 60 seconds, and inflation is usually repeated multiple times. Possible complications include aortic regurgitation, emboli, ventricular perforation, rupture of the aortic valve annulus, ventricular arrhythmia, mitral valve damage, and bleeding from the catheter insertion sites. The aortic valve procedure is not as effective as the mitral valve procedure, and the rate of restenosis is approximately 50% in the first 6 months after the procedure. It is usually used for palliation of symptoms in patients who are not suitable candidates for TAVR, but may sometimes be used as a bridge to TAVR (Hermann & Mack, 2019; Kumar et al., 2016).

Open Commissurotomy

Since percutaneous commissurotomy has fewer risks with similar outcomes, open commissurotomy has become less commonly used in recent decades. The patient is under general anesthesia, and a midsternal or left thoracic incision is made. Cardiopulmonary bypass is initiated, and an incision is made into the heart. The valve is exposed, and a scalpel, finger, balloon, or dilator is used to open the commissures. One advantage of directly visualizing the valve and surrounding structures is that a thrombus or calcifications may be removed. Chordae or papillary muscles may also be inspected and surgically repaired as necessary.

Annuloplasty

The junction at which valve leaflets connect to the heart wall is an annulus. Annuloplasty refers to repair of the valve annulus, resulting in narrowing of the valve orifice. It is used for valvular regurgitation. For the mitral valve, there may be damage or rupture of the chordae tendineae resulting in severe mitral regurgitation, which is an indication for urgent valve repair by annuloplasty with resuspension of the chordae tendineae. General anesthesia and cardiopulmonary bypass are required for most annuloplasties.

There are two annuloplasty techniques. One technique uses an annuloplasty ring (Fig. 24-4), which may be rigid/semirigid or flexible. Leaflets of the valve are sutured to a ring, creating an annulus of the desired size. When the ring is in place, tension created by moving blood and the contracting heart is borne by the ring rather than by the valve or a suture line, thereby preventing progressive regurgitation.

A second technique to tighten the annulus involves folding elongated tissue over onto itself in leaflets or tacking leaflets to the atrium or each other with sutures. Because the valve's leaflets and suture lines are subjected to direct forces of the blood and heart muscle movement, the repair may degenerate more quickly than one using an annuloplasty ring (Maisano, Skantharaja, Denti, et al., 2019).

Leaflet Repair

Damage to cardiac valve leaflets may result from stretching, shortening, or tearing. **Leaflet repair** for elongated, ballooning, or other excess tissue leaflets is achieved by removing the extra tissue. Elongated tissue may be tucked and sutured, a technique called plication. A wedge of tissue may be cut from the middle of the leaflet and the gap sutured closed (i.e., leaflet resection) (Fig. 24-5). After short chordae are released, leaflets often unfurl and resume their normal function, allowing the valve to close during systole. A leaflet may be extended by suturing a piece of pericardium to it. A pericardial or synthetic patch may be used to repair holes in the leaflets.

Valve Replacement

Valve replacement is preferred for patients with valves with anatomy which decreases the chance of success with repair;

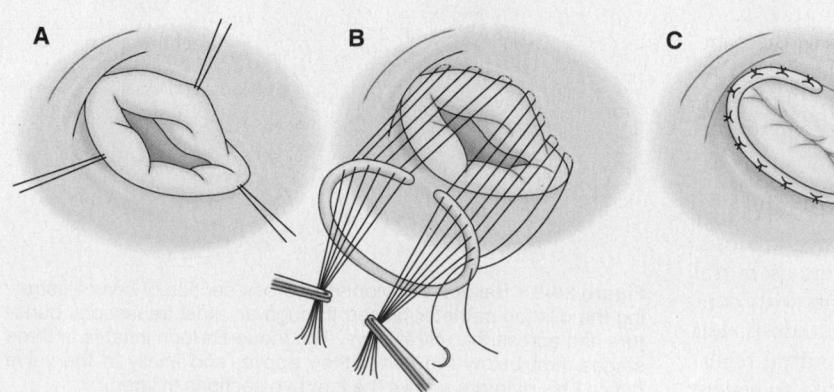
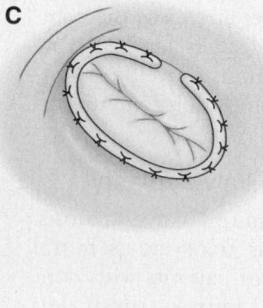

Figure 24-4 • Annuloplasty ring insertion. **A.** Mitral valve regurgitation; leaflets do not close. **B.** Insertion of an annuloplasty ring. **C.** Completed valvuloplasty; leaflets close.

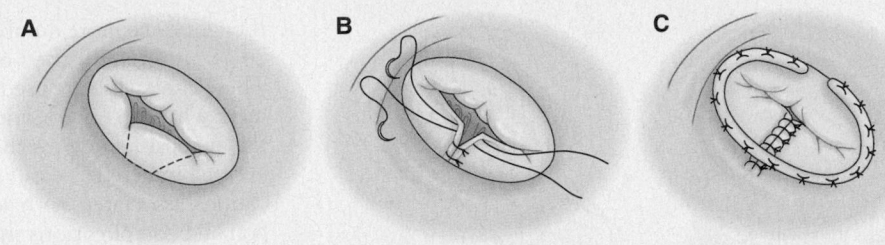

Figure 24-5 • Valve leaflet resection and repair with a ring annuloplasty. **A.** Mitral valve regurgitation; the section indicated by *dashed lines* is excised. **B.** Approximation of edges and suturing. **C.** Completed valvuloplasty, leaflet repair, and annuloplasty ring.

this includes valves that have extensive calcification, or with severely fibrotic or fused leaflets, chordae tendineae, or papillary muscles. Ideally, a multidisciplinary team (e.g., cardiologists, cardiac thoracic surgeons, structural valve interventionalists, anesthesiologists, nurses) will work together with the patient to determine candidacy for surgical versus more minimally invasive replacement (Nishimura et al., 2014). General anesthesia and cardiopulmonary bypass are used for surgical valve replacements. The standard surgical procedure is performed through a median sternotomy (i.e., incision through the sternum), although the mitral valve may be approached through a right thoracotomy incision.

Mitral and aortic valve replacements may be performed with minimally invasive techniques that do not involve cutting through the length of the sternum. Instead, a 2- to 4-inch incision is made in only the upper or lower half of the sternum or between ribs, or performed percutaneously. Some minimally invasive procedures are robot assisted; surgical instruments are connected to a robot, and the surgeon, watching a video display, uses a joystick to control the robot and surgical instruments. With these procedures, patients have lower rates of bleeding, pain, infection, and scarring, and shorter length of stay in the hospital (Nishimura et al., 2014).

After the valve is visualized, leaflets of the aortic or pulmonic valve are removed, but some or all of the mitral valve structures (leaflets, chordae, and papillary muscles) are left in place to help maintain the shape and function of the left ventricle after mitral valve replacement. Sutures are placed around the annulus and then through the valve prosthesis. The replacement valve is slid down the suture into position

and tied into place (Fig. 24-6). The patient is weaned from cardiopulmonary bypass, the quality of the surgical repair is often assessed with color flow Doppler TEE, and then surgery is completed.

TAVR, a minimally invasive aortic valve replacement procedure, may be performed in a catheterization laboratory or hybrid room. It does not involve cardiopulmonary bypass or sternotomy. TAVR was traditionally used only for patients who could not safely undergo surgical valve replacement, but more recently has been recommended for patients who have intermediate or even low risk (Nishimura et al., 2017). With the patient under general anesthesia, a balloon valvuloplasty is performed. Then, a bioprosthetic (tissue) replacement valve (Fig. 24-7A,B) attached to a catheter is inserted percutaneously, positioned at the aortic valve, and implanted. The MitraClip has been approved as a transcatheter procedure to treat degenerative forms of mitral regurgitation. This procedure is currently used primarily in patients with severe symptomatic mitral regurgitation and high surgical risk, but increasingly is considered even for lower-risk patients. The procedure creates a mechanical bridge between two leaflets and has demonstrated decreased regurgitant flow, resulting in fewer symptoms, and decreased rates of hospitalization for heart failure (Dahl & Ailawadi, 2018).

In patients requiring valve replacement or repair, the heart had gradually adjusted to the pathology; surgery abruptly "corrects" the way blood flows through the heart and may result in complications related to the sudden changes in intracardiac pressures. All prosthetic valve replacements create a degree of stenosis when they are implanted in the heart. Usually, the

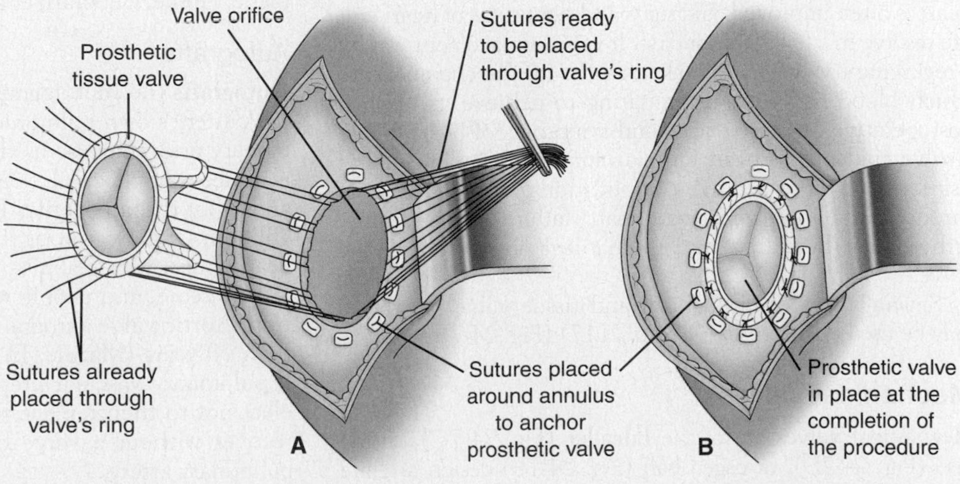

Figure 24-6 • Valve replacement. **A.** The native valve is trimmed, and the prosthetic valve is sutured in place. **B.** Once all sutures are placed through the ring, the surgeon slides the prosthetic valve down the sutures and into the natural orifice. Sutures are then tied off and trimmed.

Valve orifice

Prosthetic tissue valve

Sutures ready to be placed through valve's ring

Sutures already placed through valve's ring

Sutures placed around annulus to anchor prosthetic valve

Prosthetic valve in place at the completion of the procedure

A   **B**

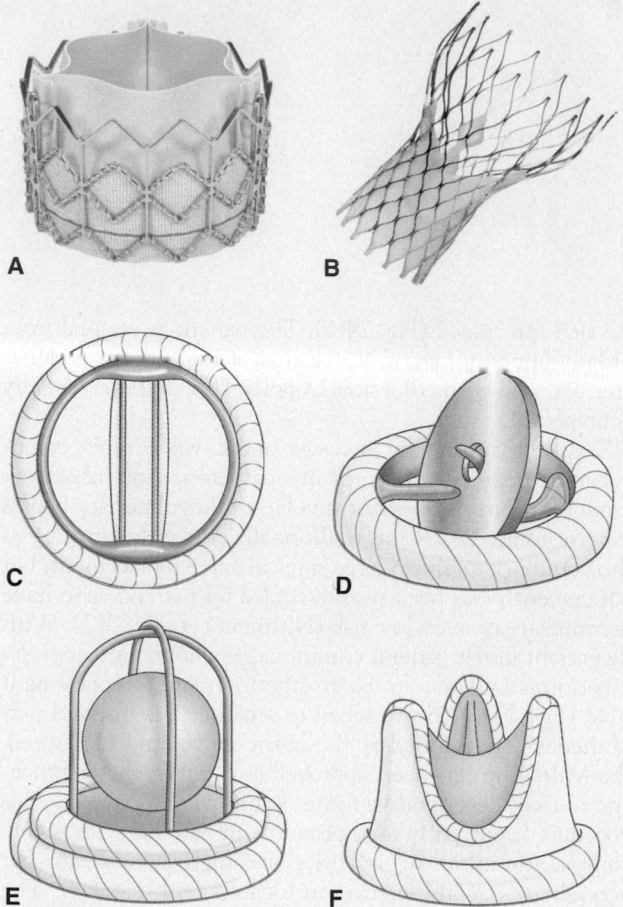

Figure 24-7 • Common mechanical and tissue valve replacements. A. Transcatheter aortic valve (Edwards SAPIEN transcatheter heart valve, tissue). Used with the permission of Edwards Lifesciences LLC, Irvine, CA; Edwards SAPIEN and SAPIEN are trademarks of Edwards Lifesciences Corporation. **B.** Transcatheter aortic valve (Medtronic The CoreValve® system, tissue). Used with the permission of Medtronic. The CoreValve System® CoreValve is a registered trademark of Medtronic CV Luxembourg S.A.R.L.). **C.** Bileaflet (St. Jude, mechanical). **D.** Tilting disc valve (Medtronic-Hall, mechanical). **E.** Caged ball valve (Starr-Edwards, mechanical). **F.** Porcine bioprosthesis valve (Carpenter-Edwards, tissue).

stenosis is mild and does not affect heart function. If valve replacement was for a stenotic valve, blood flow through the heart is often improved, and signs and symptoms of heart failure resolve in a few hours or days. If valve replacement was for a regurgitant valve, it may take months for the chamber into which blood had been regurgitating to achieve its optimal postoperative function. Signs and symptoms of heart failure resolve gradually as heart function improves. Patients are at risk for many postoperative complications, such as bleeding, thromboembolism, infection, heart failure, hypertension, arrhythmias, hemolysis, and mechanical obstruction of the valve.

Several types of mechanical and tissue valve prostheses may be used (Chikwe & Castillo, 2017) (Fig. 24-7).

Mechanical Valves

Mechanical valves are of the bileaflet (Fig. 24-7C), tilting disc (Fig. 24-7D), or caged ball (Fig. 24-7E) design and are thought to be more durable than tissue prosthetic valves (Fig. 24-7F); therefore, they often are used for younger patients. These valves also are used for patients requiring valve replacement who also have kidney injury, hypercalcemia, endocarditis, or sepsis, since mechanical valves do not deteriorate or become infected as easily as tissue valves. Significant complications associated with mechanical valves are thromboemboli and complications that can be associated with long-term use of required anticoagulants (see Chapter 26 for further discussion).

Tissue Valves

There are three types of tissue valves: bioprostheses, homografts, and autografts. Tissue valves are less likely than mechanical valves to generate thromboemboli, and long-term anticoagulation is not required. Tissue valves are not as durable as mechanical valves and require replacement more rapidly (Chikwe & Castillo, 2017; Nishimura et al., 2014).

Bioprostheses

Bioprostheses are valves made from animal tissues (i.e., heterografts) used for aortic, mitral, and tricuspid valve replacement. They are not thrombogenic; therefore, patients do not need long-term anticoagulation therapy. They are used for women of childbearing age to avoid potential complications of long-term anticoagulation associated with menses, placental transfer to a fetus, and delivery of a child. They also are considered for patients older than 70 years and others who cannot tolerate long-term anticoagulation. Most bioprostheses are from pigs (porcine), but some are from cows (bovine) or horses (equine). They may be stented or nonstented. Viability is 7 to 15 years.

Homografts

Homografts, also called allografts (i.e., human valves), are obtained from cadaver tissue donations and are used for aortic and pulmonic valve replacement. The aortic valve and a portion of aorta or the pulmonic valve and a portion of pulmonary artery are harvested and stored cryogenically. Homografts are not always available and are very expensive. They last for about 10 to 15 years and are typically used in younger patients who require replacement of the valve root (Tudorache, Horke, Cebotari, et al., 2016).

Autografts

Autografts (i.e., autologous valves) are obtained by excising the patient's own pulmonic valve and a portion of the pulmonary artery for use as the aortic valve. Anticoagulation is unnecessary because the valve is the patient's own tissue and is not thrombogenic. The autograft is an alternative for children (it may grow as the child grows), women of childbearing age, young adults, patients with a history of peptic ulcer disease, and people who cannot tolerate anticoagulation. Aortic valve autografts have remained viable for more than 20 years (Mazine, El-Hamamsy, Verma, et al., 2018). If pulmonary vascular pressures are normal, some surgeons elect not to then replace the pulmonic valve. Patients can recover without a valve between the right ventricle and pulmonary artery.

However, most aortic valve autograft procedures are double valve replacement procedures with a homograft pulmonic valve replacement also performed. If there is recurrent valve dysfunction after this procedure, patients may undergo further corrective surgery, often in the form of a reversal of the original homograft. In patients who are older and for whom this may no longer be an option, replacement with a prosthetic valve may be considered (Hussain, Majdalany, Dunn, et al., 2018).

 ## Nursing Management: Valvuloplasty and Valve Replacement

The nurse assists the patient and family to prepare for the procedure, reinforces and supplements explanations provided by the primary provider, and provides psychosocial support. (See Chapters 14 through 16 for care of the surgical patient.)

Patients who have undergone percutaneous balloon valvuloplasty with or without percutaneous valve replacement may be admitted to a telemetry unit or intensive care unit (ICU). The nurse assesses for signs and symptoms of heart failure and emboli (see Chapter 25), auscultates the chest for changes in heart sounds at least every 4 hours, and provides the patient with the same care as for postprocedure cardiac catheterization or percutaneous transluminal coronary angioplasty (see Chapter 23). After undergoing percutaneous balloon valvuloplasty, the patient usually remains in the hospital for 24 to 48 hours.

Patients who have undergone surgical valvuloplasty or valve replacements are admitted to the ICU. Care focuses on recovery from anesthesia and hemodynamic stability. Vital signs are assessed every 5 to 15 minutes and as needed until the patient recovers from anesthesia or sedation, and then are assessed according to unit protocol. Intravenous (IV) medications may be used to increase or decrease blood pressure, to treat arrhythmias, to increase or decrease heart rate; and, their effects are monitored. Medications are gradually decreased until they are no longer required, or the patient takes the needed medication by another route (e.g., oral, topical). Patient assessments are conducted every 1 to 4 hours and as needed, with attention to neurologic, respiratory, and cardiovascular systems (see Chapter 23, Chart 23-11).

After the patient has recovered from anesthesia and sedation, is hemodynamically stable without the use IV medications, and has stable physical assessment parameters, they are usually transferred to a telemetry unit, typically within 24 to 72 hours of surgery. Nursing care continues as for most postoperative patients, including wound care and patient education regarding diet, activity, medications, and self-care. The patient usually is discharged from the hospital in 3 to 7 days.

The nurse educates the patient about anticoagulant therapy, explaining the need for frequent follow-up appointments and blood laboratory studies. Patients who take warfarin have individualized target international normalized ratios, usually between 2 and 3.5 for mitral valve replacement and 1.8 and 2.2 for aortic valve replacement. Patients who have been treated with an annuloplasty ring or a tissue valve replacement usually require anticoagulation for only

3 months unless there are other risk factors such as atrial fibrillation or a history of thromboembolism. Aspirin is prescribed with warfarin for patients with bioprostheses or at high risk for embolic events (e.g., history of embolic event or having two or more preexisting conditions: diabetes, hypertension, coronary artery disease, congestive heart failure, older than 75 years) (Nishimura et al., 2014). The nurse provides education about all prescribed medications, including the name of medication, dosage, actions, prescribed schedule, potential adverse effects, and any drug–drug or drug–food interactions.

Patients with a mechanical valve prosthesis (including annuloplasty rings and other prosthetic materials used in valvuloplasty) require education to prevent infective endocarditis. Patients may be at risk for infective endocarditis, caused by bacteria entering the bloodstream and adhering to abnormal valve structures or prosthetic devices. The nurse educates the patient about how to minimize the risk of developing infective endocarditis (see prevention of endocarditis later in this chapter).

Transitional, home health, office, or clinic nurses help reinforce all new information and self-care instructions with patients and families for 4 to 8 weeks after the procedure (Chart 24-1). An echocardiogram may be performed 3 to 4 weeks after hospital discharge to further evaluate the effects and results of surgery. The echocardiogram also provides a baseline for future comparison if cardiac symptoms or complications develop. Echocardiograms usually are repeated every 1 to 2 years.

Cardiomyopathy

Cardiomyopathy is disease of the heart muscle that is associated with cardiac dysfunction. It is classified according to the structural and functional abnormalities of the heart muscle: dilated cardiomyopathy (DCM), hypertrophic cardiomyopathy (HCM), restrictive cardiomyopathy (RCM), arrhythmogenic right ventricular cardiomyopathy/dysplasia (ARVC/D), and unclassified cardiomyopathy (Elliott, Andersson, Arbustini, et al., 2008). A patient may have pathology representing more than one of these classifications, such as a patient with HCM with restrictive physiology. *Ischemic cardiomyopathy* is a term frequently used to describe an enlarged heart caused by coronary artery disease, which is usually accompanied by heart failure (see Chapter 25). In 2006, the American Heart Association proposed a set of Contemporary Classifications for cardiomyopathies, which continues to be in widespread use. Under this classification system, cardiomyopathies are divided into two major groups based on predominant organ involvement. These include *primary cardiomyopathies* (genetic, nongenetic, and acquired), which are focused primarily on the heart muscle, and *secondary cardiomyopathies*, which show myocardial involvement secondary to the influence of a vast list of disease processes that include, but are not limited to, amyloidosis, Fabry disease, sarcoidosis, and scleroderma (Maron, Towbin, Thiene, et al., 2006). This chapter focuses on the primary cardiomyopathies.

Pathophysiology

The pathophysiology of all cardiomyopathies is a series of events that culminate in impaired cardiac output. Decreased

Chart 24-1 HOME CARE CHECKLIST
Discharge After Valve Replacement

At the completion of education, the patient and/or caregiver will be able to:

- Name the procedure that was performed, any complications that occurred, and identify any permanent changes in anatomic structure or function as well as changes in ADLs, IADLs, roles, relationships, and spirituality.
- Identify interventions and strategies (e.g., durable medical equipment, adaptive equipment) used in recovery period.
- Describe ongoing postoperative therapeutic regimen, including diet and activities to perform (e.g., walking and breathing exercises) and to limit or avoid (e.g., lifting weights, driving a car, contact sports).
- State the name, dose, side effects, frequency, and schedule for all medications, including anticoagulant.
  - Identify the need to take anticoagulant for prescribed length of time
  - Take anticoagulant at same time each day
  - Keep appointments for laboratory tests, if indicated
  - Avoid injury that can cause bleeding
  - Report signs that could suggest occult bleeding to primary provider (e.g., bleeding gums, petechiae formation, tarry stools)
- State how to obtain medical supplies and carry out dressing changes, wound care, and other prescribed regimens.
- Identify durable medical equipment needs, proper usage, and maintenance necessary for safe utilization.

- Describe signs and symptoms of complications, including infective endocarditis, if at risk.
  - Report fevers, chills, clusters of petechiae, malaise, and weight loss to primary provider
- Engage in activities aimed at preventing infective endocarditis, as indicated:
  - Notify all health care providers of surgery and possible need for antibiotic prophylaxis preprocedure, if endorsed by primary provider
  - Practice good oral hygiene, including brushing, flossing, and regular appointments with dental hygienist
- State time and date of follow-up appointments.
- Relate how to reach the primary provider with questions or complications.
- Identify community resources for peer and caregiver/family support:
  - Identify sources of support (e.g., friends, relatives, faith community)
  - Identify the contact details for support services for patients and their caregivers/families
- Identify the need for health promotion (e.g., weight reduction, smoking cessation, stress management), disease prevention, and screening activities

ADL, activities of daily living; IADL, independent activities of daily living.

---

stroke volume stimulates the sympathetic nervous system and the renin–angiotensin–aldosterone response, resulting in increased systemic vascular resistance and increased sodium and fluid retention, which place an increased workload on the heart. Often, the decrease in cardiac output can be seen on echocardiogram as a decrease in **ejection fraction**, expressed as a percentage of the end-diastolic blood volume ejected from the ventricle with each heartbeat. These alterations can lead to heart failure (see Chapter 25).

 Concept Mastery Alert

Sodium is the major electrolyte involved with cardiomyopathy. Cardiomyopathy often leads to heart failure, which develops, in part, from fluid overload. Fluid overload is often associated with elevated sodium intake.

Dilated Cardiomyopathy

DCM is the most common form of cardiomyopathy, with a general prevalence of between 1 in 250 and 1 in 2500 (Merlo, Cannata, Gobbo, et al., 2018). DCM is distinguished by significant dilation of the ventricles without simultaneous hypertrophy and systolic dysfunction (Fig. 24-8). The ventricles have elevated systolic and diastolic volumes but a decreased ejection fraction.

Microscopic examination of the muscle tissue shows diminished contractile elements (actin and myosin filaments) of the muscle fibers and diffuse necrosis of myocardial cells. The result is poor systolic function. The structural changes decrease the amount of blood ejected from

the ventricle with systole, increasing the amount of blood remaining in the ventricle after contraction. Less blood is then able to enter the ventricle during diastole, increasing end-diastolic pressure and eventually increasing pulmonary and systemic venous pressures. Altered valve function, usually regurgitation, can result from an enlarged stretched ventricle. Poor blood flow through the ventricle may also cause ventricular or atrial thrombi, which may embolize to other locations in the body.

More than 75 conditions and diseases may cause DCM, including pregnancy, hypertension, heavy alcohol intake, viral infection (e.g., influenza), chemotherapeutic medications (e.g., daunorubicin, doxorubicin), thyrotoxicosis, myxedema, persistent tachycardia, and Chagas disease. When the causative factor cannot be identified, the diagnosis is idiopathic DCM which accounts for 20% to 30% of nonischemic DCM cases (McNally & Mestroni, 2017; Merlo et al., 2018). Familial DCM accounts for approximately 30% to 50% of all DCM cases and approximately 40% of familial DCM cases have a definitive genetic etiology (McNally & Mestroni, 2017). An elucidation of family history by the nurse is therefore a very important component of the assessment process. Early diagnosis and treatment can prevent or delay significant symptoms and sudden death from DCM.

Hypertrophic Cardiomyopathy

The estimated prevalence of HCM is 0.16% to 0.29% of the adult population (Marian & Braunwald, 2017). HCM is an autosomal dominant genetic disorder that leads to increased heart muscle size and mass, especially along the septum

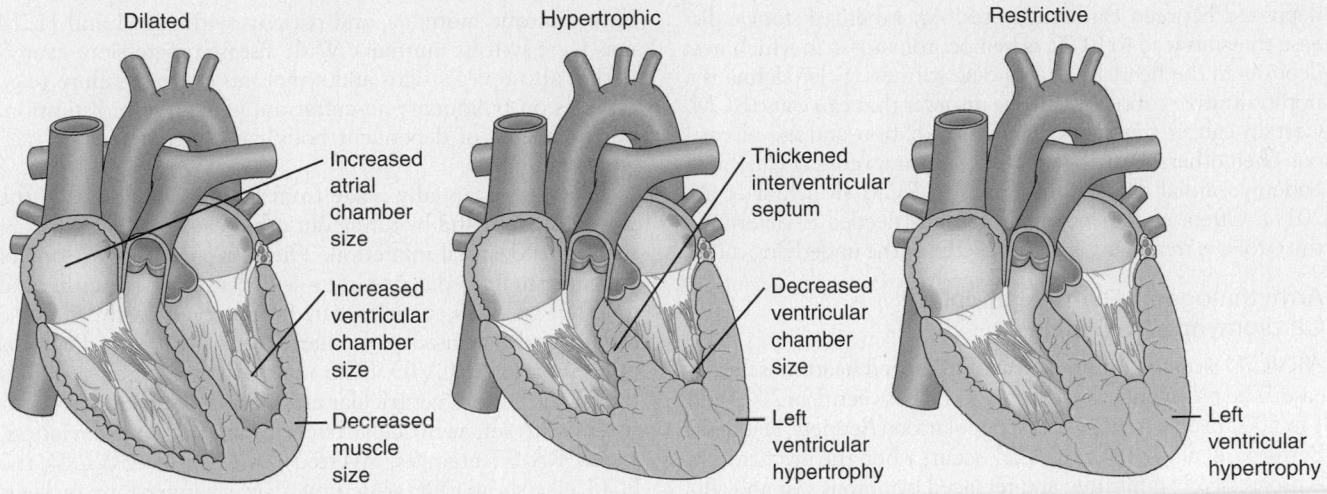

Figure 24-8 • Cardiomyopathies that lead to congestive heart failure. Adapted from Anatomical Chart Company. (2010). *Atlas of pathophysiology* (3rd ed.). Ambler, PA: Lippincott Williams & Wilkins.

(see Fig. 24-8) but can involve other areas of the heart. The phenotypic expression of the disease is age dependent. HCM is the leading cause of sudden death in adolescents and young adults, particularly in athletes (Marian & Braunwald, 2017). 12-lead ECGs, physical examinations, and echocardiograms are used to screen for the disease.

Patients with a suspected diagnosis of HCM should undergo genetic testing; if negative, the diagnosis is not completely ruled out. If genetic testing is positive for known HCM genetic mutations, first-degree relatives should also be tested for the genetic mutation found in the patient. In patients that have positive genetic testing, but are asymptomatic for cardiomyopathy, annual screening with an ECG, physical examination and echocardiogram should be done, as the likelihood of clinical progression increases with increasing age. The phenotype typically manifests sometime between adolescence and the fifth decade of life (Marian & Braunwald, 2017).

Cardiac muscle cells normally lie parallel to and end to end with each other. The hypertrophied cardiac muscle cells are disorganized, oblique, and perpendicular to each other, decreasing the effectiveness of contractions. In HCM, the coronary arteriole walls are thickened, which decrease the internal diameter of the arterioles. The narrow arterioles restrict the blood supply to the myocardium, causing numerous small areas of ischemia and necrosis. The necrotic areas of the myocardium ultimately fibrose and scar, further impeding ventricular contraction and possibly increasing the risk of arrhythmias such as ventricular tachycardia and ventricular fibrillation (see Chapter 22).

Increased thickness of the heart muscle reduces the size of the ventricular cavities and causes the ventricles to take a longer time to relax after systole. During the first part of diastole, it is more difficult for the ventricles to fill with blood. The atrial contraction at the end of diastole becomes critical for ventricular filling and systolic contraction.

HCM can lead to obstruction of the left ventricular outflow tract (LVOT) if there is systolic anterior motion of the mitral valve that abuts the mitral valve against the hypertrophied septum during systole (Marian & Braunwald, 2017; Nishimura, Seggewiss, & Schaff, 2017). LVOT obstruction is a dynamic process that is dependent on both the volume of blood in the left ventricle as well as the ability of the myocytes to contract. Approximately one third of patients with HCM have LVOT obstruction at rest that worsens with provocation, another one third do not have obstruction at rest, but can get obstruction with provocation (e.g., exercise or the Valsalva maneuver), and roughly one third of patients have no LVOT obstruction even with provocation (Marian & Braunwald, 2017). Obstruction of the LVOT can lead to syncope, ventricular arrhythmias, dyspnea, and heart failure. The presence of a systolic ejection murmur can be indicative of LVOT, and echocardiography is then indicated to confirm its presence. Hydration, beta-blockers, calcium channel blockers, and lifestyle modification can be used to minimize LVOT obstruction. In particular, patients should avoid activities that can cause rapid alterations to preload (e.g., hot tubs, saunas, prolonged hot showers) (Nishimura et al., 2017). However, patients that do not respond to medical therapy should be considered for surgical myectomy or alcohol septal ablation to decrease the size of the hypertrophied septum and thereby eliminate LVOT obstruction.

Restrictive Cardiomyopathy

RCM is the least common type of cardiomyopathy (Muchtar, Blauwet, & Gertz, 2017; Pereira, Grogan, & Dec, 2018). RCM is characterized by diastolic dysfunction caused by rigid ventricular walls that impair diastolic filling and ventricular stretch (see Fig. 24-8). A rigid ventricle alters the curve in the Frank–Starling law (see Chapter 21) and leads to the rapid rise of filling pressures despite only small increases in blood volume. However, chamber size and systolic function are usually normal. Arrhythmias and conduction disturbances are common. Signs and symptoms are similar to constrictive pericarditis (see later discussion) and include dyspnea, nonproductive cough, and chest pain. Echocardiography may be useful in differentiating between these two conditions.

Generally, RCM is either due to an inherited or acquired disease that may be systemic. There are four general categories for the causes of RCM: infiltrative disease, storage disease, noninfiltrative, and endomyocardial.

An example of an infiltrative disease that may cause RCM is amyloidosis, in which amyloid, a misfolded protein, is deposited between cardiomyocytes. An inherited storage disease that can lead to RCM is hemochromatosis, in which iron deposits in the heart lead to cardiac stiffness. Scleroderma is a noninfiltrative connective tissue disorder that can cause RCM. Certain cancer treatments, such as radiation and use of various chemotherapeutic agents (e.g., anthracyclines) can cause endomyocardial damage that leads to RCM (Muchtar et al., 2017). Often, endomyocardial biopsy is needed to determine the etiology; treatment is then directed at the underlying cause.

Arrhythmogenic Right Ventricular Cardiomyopathy/Dysplasia

ARVC/D is an uncommon form of inherited heart muscle disease. The prevalence is estimated to be between 1 in 2000 and 1 in 5000 people in the general population (Bennett, Haqqani, Berruezo, et al., 2019). ARVC/D occurs when the myocardium is progressively infiltrated and replaced by fibrous scar and adipose tissue. Infiltration of fibrous and adipose tissue leads to ventricle dilatation, poor contractility, and arrhythmias.

Initially, only localized areas of the right ventricle are affected, but as the disease progresses, the entire heart is affected. Because of this typical pathologic progression, there is a move to change the name of this cardiomyopathy to a more general term of arrhythmogenic cardiomyopathy (ACM) to recognize the left ventricular involvement (Bennett et al., 2019).

In patients with ARVC/D, palpitations or syncope may develop between 15 and 40 years of age. Sudden cardiac death may also be the first presentation. Diagnosis is made based on the ECG, echocardiogram, cardiac MRI, and family history. Since this is a genetic disorder, patients that are diagnosed are referred to a genetic counselor for testing. However, genetic testing can be negative in up to 50% of patients (Bennett et al., 2019). If a genetic mutation is identified, first-degree relatives of the patient should undergo genetic testing. Patients affected by arrhythmias may benefit from having an implantable cardioverter defibrillator (ICD) placed (see Chapter 22).

Unclassified Cardiomyopathies

Unclassified cardiomyopathies are different from or have characteristics of more than one of the previously described types and are caused by fibroelastosis, noncompacted myocardium, systolic dysfunction with minimal dilation, and mitochondrial diseases. Examples of unclassified cardiomyopathies can include left ventricular noncompaction and stress-induced (Takotsubo) cardiomyopathy (Elliott et al., 2008).

Clinical Manifestations

Patients with cardiomyopathy may remain stable and without symptoms for many years. As the disease progresses, so do the symptoms. Frequently, dilated or restrictive cardiomyopathy is first diagnosed when the patient presents with signs and symptoms of heart failure (e.g., DOE, fatigue, PND, cough [especially with exertion or at night], orthopnea, peripheral edema, early satiety, nausea; see Chapter 25). The patient also may experience chest pain, palpitations, dizziness, nausea, and syncope with exertion.

Assessment and Diagnostic Findings

Physical examination at early stages may reveal tachycardia and extra heart sounds (e.g., S_3, S_4). Patients with DCM may have diastolic murmurs, and patients with DCM and HCM may have systolic murmurs. With disease progression, examination also reveals signs and symptoms of heart failure (e.g., crackles on pulmonary auscultation, jugular vein distention, pitting edema of dependent body parts, hepatomegaly [i.e., enlarged liver]).

Diagnosis is usually made from findings disclosed by the patient history and by ruling out other causes of heart failure such as myocardial infarction. The echocardiogram is one of the most helpful diagnostic tools because the structure and function of the ventricles can be observed easily. Cardiac MRI may also be used, particularly to assist with the diagnosis of HCM and ARCV/D. ECG may demonstrate arrhythmias (atrial fibrillation, ventricular arrhythmias) and changes consistent with left ventricular hypertrophy (left axis deviation, wide QRS, ST changes, inverted T waves). In ARVC/D, the ECG may show QRS widening, T-wave inversions in leads V_1–V_4, and ventricular ectopy. Additionally, there is often a small epsilon wave at the end of the QRS (Bennett et al., 2019). The chest x-ray reveals heart enlargement and possibly pulmonary congestion. Cardiac catheterization, coronary CT, or stress testing is often used to rule out coronary artery disease as a causative factor. Endomyocardial biopsy may be performed to analyze myocardial cells, particularly in RCM.

Medical Management

Medical management is directed toward identifying and managing possible underlying or precipitating causes; correcting the heart failure with medications, a low sodium diet, and an exercise/rest regimen (see Chapter 25); and controlling arrhythmias with antiarrhythmic medications and possibly with an implanted electronic device, such as an ICD (see Chapter 22). If the patient has signs and symptoms of congestion, fluid intake may be limited to 2 L each day. However, patients with HCM should avoid dehydration and may need beta-blockers to maintain cardiac output and minimize the risk of LVOT obstruction during systole. Anticoagulants are no longer routinely prescribed.

For some patients with DCM, biventricular pacing (also known as cardiac resynchronization therapy or CRT) increases the ejection fraction and reverses some of the structural changes in the myocardium (see Chapter 22).

As noted previously, some forms of cardiomyopathy are inherited/genetic. Any family history of cardiomyopathy should be noted when the nurse is taking a family health history. In appropriate cases, the patient should be referred to a genetic counselor for testing. If genetic mutations are found, it is recommended that first-degree relatives also be tested. Unfortunately, there are currently some problems with patients receiving insurance reimbursement for genetic testing in the United States.

Surgical Management

When heart failure progresses and medical treatment is no longer effective, surgical intervention, including heart transplantation, is considered. However, because of the limited number of organ donors, many patients die waiting for transplantation. In some cases, a VAD is implanted to support the failing heart until a suitable donor heart becomes available (see later discussion).

Left Ventricular Outflow Tract Surgery

When patients with HCM and LVOT obstruction become symptomatic despite optimal medical therapy or cannot tolerate medical therapy, surgery is considered. The most common procedure done is a myectomy (sometimes referred to as a myotomy–myectomy or the Morrow procedure), in which some of the heart tissue is excised. Septal tissue approximately 1 cm wide and deep is cut from the enlarged septum below the aortic valve. The length of septum removed typically extends to the papillary muscles. Possible complications include complete heart block and subsequent pacemaker dependence, ventricular septal defects, or failure to adequately alleviate the obstruction. Surgical mortality rates are reportedly between less than 1% and as high as 16% (Nishimura et al., 2017).

Heart Transplantation

Because of advances in surgical techniques and immunosuppressive therapies, heart transplantation is now a therapeutic option for patients with end-stage heart disease. Cyclosporine and tacrolimus are some of the more common immunosuppressants that decrease the body's rejection of foreign proteins, such as transplanted organs. Unfortunately, these drugs also decrease the body's ability to resist infections and increase the risk of various cancers, and a satisfactory balance must be achieved between suppressing rejection and avoiding infection. In 2017, there were 3273 heart transplants performed in the United States (Scientific Registry of Transplant Recipients, 2017).

Cardiomyopathy, ischemic heart disease, valvular disease, rejection of previously transplanted hearts, and congenital heart disease are the most common indications for transplantation. Typical candidates have severe symptoms uncontrolled by medical therapy, no other surgical options, and a prognosis of less than 1 to 2 years to live. A multidisciplinary team screens the candidate before recommending the transplantation procedure. The person's age, pulmonary status, other chronic health conditions, psychosocial status, family support, infections, history of other transplantations, adherence to therapeutic regimens, and current health status are considered. The United Network for Organ Sharing (UNOS), a national organization that is regulated by the U.S. government, is charged with maintaining organ transplant waiting lists and allocating donor organs. When a donor heart becomes available, UNOS generates a list of potential recipients on the basis of ABO blood group compatibility, the body sizes of the donor and the potential recipient, age, severity of illness, length of time on the waiting list, and the geographic locations of the donor and potential recipient (Organ Procurement and Transplant Network [OPTN], 2019). Some patients are candidates for more than one organ transplant (e.g., heart–lung, heart–kidney, heart–liver).

Orthotopic transplantation is the most common surgical procedure for cardiac transplantation. Some surgeons prefer to remove the recipient's heart but leave a portion of the recipient's atria (with the vena cava and pulmonary veins) in place, which is known as the biatrial technique. However, this technique has been modified to a more common approach called the *bicaval technique*. This technique includes removal of the recipient's heart, and the implantation of the donor heart with intact atria at the vena cava and pulmonary veins (Fig. 24-9) (Kittleson, Patel, &

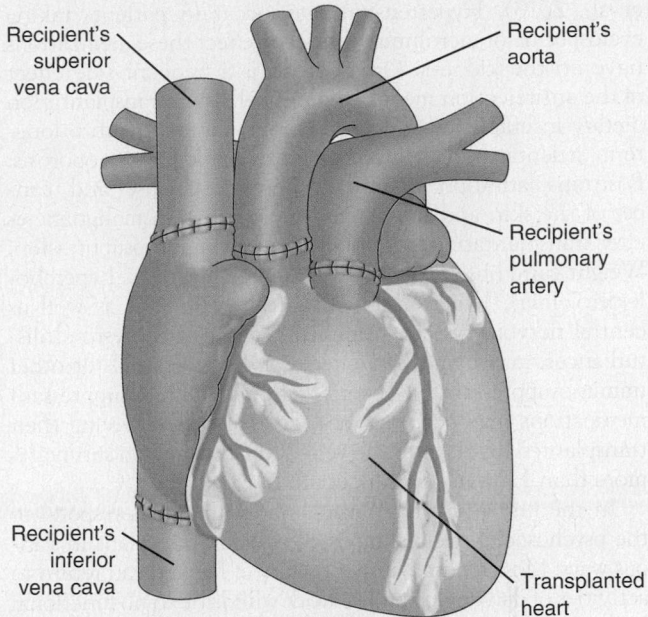

Figure 24-9 • Orthotopic method of heart transplantation.

Kobashigawa, 2017). This newer approach is associated with decreased AV valve regurgitation, arrhythmias, and conduction abnormalities.

Patients who have had heart transplantations are constantly balancing the risk of rejection with the risk of infection and diseases such as cancer. They must adhere to a complex regimen of diet, medications, activity, follow-up laboratory studies, biopsies of the transplanted heart (to diagnose rejection), and clinic visits. There are three classes of medications that are prescribed for a transplant patient to help minimize rejection: corticosteroids (e.g., prednisone), calcineurin inhibitors (tacrolimus, cyclosporine), and antiproliferative agents (mycophenolate mofetil, azathioprine, or sirolimus).

The transplanted heart has no nerve connections (i.e., denervated heart) to the recipient's body, so the sympathetic and vagus nerves do not affect the transplanted heart. The resting rate of the transplanted heart is approximately 90 to 110 bpm, but it increases gradually if catecholamines are in the circulation. Patients must gradually increase and decrease their exercise (i.e., extended warm-up and cool-down periods), because 20 to 30 minutes may be required to achieve the desired heart rate. Atropine does not increase the heart rate of transplanted hearts, and digoxin does not decrease the heart rate in atrial fibrillation. Additionally, many patients who have had heart transplantations do not experience angina with ischemia and may present with congestive heart failure, silent myocardial infarction, or sudden death without a prior history of coronary artery disease (Kittleson et al., 2017).

In addition to rejection and infection, complications may include accelerated atherosclerosis of the coronary arteries (i.e., cardiac allograft vasculopathy, accelerated graft atherosclerosis, transplant coronary artery disease). Both immunologic and nonimmunologic factors cause arterial injury and inflammation of the coronary arteries. The arterial smooth muscle proliferates, and there is hyperplasia of the coronary artery intima, accelerating atherosclerosis along the entire length of the coronary arteries (Stehlik, Kobashigawa, Hunt, et al., 2018). Hypertension may occur in patients taking cyclosporine or tacrolimus due to the effect these medications have on the kidneys. Osteoporosis is a frequent side effect of the antirejection medications as well as pretransplantation dietary insufficiency and medications. Patients with a long-term sedentary lifestyle are at greater risk for osteoporosis. Posttransplantation lymphoproliferative disease and cancer of the skin and lips are the most common malignancies after transplantation, possibly caused by immunosuppression. Weight gain, obesity, diabetes, dyslipidemias (e.g., hypercholesterolemia), hypertension, and kidney failure, as well as central nervous system, respiratory, and gastrointestinal disturbances, may be adverse effects of corticosteroids or other immunosuppressants. Toxicity from immunosuppressant medications may occur as well. For patients receiving their transplanted hearts after the year 2000, the median survival is more than 12 years (Stehlik et al., 2018).

In the first year after transplantation, patients respond to the psychosocial stresses imposed by organ transplant in various ways. Most report a higher quality of life and can return to activities of daily living and to work with little to no functional limitations (Stehlik et al., 2018). Some have significant feelings of indebtedness to the donor, or experience guilt that someone had to die for them to be able to live, which can negatively affect their adherence to the medical regimen (Shemesh, Peles-Bortz, Peled, et al., 2017) (see Chart 24-2 Nursing Research Profile: Factors Affecting Nonadherence After Heart Transplant).

Mechanical Assist Devices and Total Artificial Hearts

The use of cardiopulmonary bypass in cardiovascular surgery and the possibility of performing heart transplantation in patients with end-stage cardiac disease, as well as the desire for a treatment option for patients who are not transplant candidates, have increased the need for mechanical assist devices. Patients who cannot be weaned from cardiopulmonary bypass

and patients in cardiogenic shock may benefit from a period of mechanical heart assistance. The most commonly used device is the intra-aortic balloon pump (see Chapter 11). This pump decreases the work of the heart during contraction but does not perform the actual work of the heart.

Ventricular Assist Devices

More complex devices that perform some or all of the pumping function for the heart are now being used. These more sophisticated **ventricular assist devices** can circulate as much blood per minute as the heart, if not more (Fig. 24-10). There are short- and long-term devices available, depending on the indication. Each VAD is used to support one ventricle, although in some instances, two VAD pumps may be used for biventricular support. Additionally, some VADs can be combined with an oxygenator; the combination is called *extracorporeal membrane oxygenation (ECMO)*. The oxygenator–VAD combination is used for the patient whose heart cannot pump adequate blood through the body or when the lungs fail to oxygenate the blood despite supplemental oxygen or ventilation.

VADs may be external, internal (i.e., implanted) with an external power source, or completely internal, and they may generate a pulsatile or continuous blood flow. There are four types of VADs: pneumatic, electric or electromagnetic, axial flow, and centrifugal. Pneumatic VADs are external or implanted pulsatile devices with a flexible reservoir housed in a rigid exterior. The reservoir usually fills with blood drained from the atrium or ventricle. The device then forces pressurized air into the rigid housing, compressing the reservoir and returning the blood to the circulation, usually into the aorta. Electric or electromagnetic VADs are similar to pneumatic VADs, but instead of using pressurized air to return the blood to the circulation, one or more flat metal plates are pushed against the reservoir. Generally, pulsatile VADs have been replaced by the newer generation of axial and centrifugal pumps. The axial and centrifugal pumps have lower rates of pump thrombus

---

Chart 24-2

NURSING RESEARCH PROFILE

Factors Affecting Nonadherence After Heart Transplant

Shemesh, Y., Peles-Bortz, A., Peled, Y., et al. (2017). Feelings of indebtedness and guilt toward donor and immunosuppressive medication adherence among heart transplant (HTx) patients, as assessed in a cross-sectional study with the Basel Assessment of Adherence to Immunosuppressive Medications Scale (BAASIS). *Clinical Transplantation, 31*(10). doi:10.1111/ctr.13053

Purpose

The purpose of this study was to assess immunosuppression medication adherence among patients who had heart transplants and to test if adherence was affected by feelings of indebtedness and guilt toward the donor.

Design

This was a descriptive correlational study with a cross-sectional design. It utilized a convenience sample consisting of 102 patients who had heart transplants and who engaged in outpatient follow-up at the Sheba Medical Center in Israel. Participants were 76.5% male, 65.3% were born in Israel, and had a mean age of 56.66 y at the time of the study. The five-item BAASIS survey was used to assess adherence in the past 4 wks as it related to timing of medication intake, self-altering the prescribed dosage, and stopping or missing medication doses. Feelings of guilt and

indebtedness were assessed with two survey questions via a Likert scale. Medical record review was also utilized. Data were evaluated using a variety of statistical analyses, which included *t*-tests, correlation analyses, and logistic regression analysis.

Findings

Sixty-four percent of participants reported nonadherence with immunosuppression within the previous 4 wks. Age, time since transplant, and feelings of guilt were statistically associated with variance in adherence. An increase in age was associated with an increase in adherence, whereas an increase in time since transplant and feelings of guilt were associated with an increase in nonadherence.

Nursing Implications

Nonadherence to immunosuppression is associated with an increase in morbidity and mortality among patients with heart transplants. Nurses should assess patients' adherence to immunosuppression and be aware of the various factors that may influence adherence. Understanding what can contribute to nonadherence, such as feelings of guilt, enables the nurse to attempt to alleviate those feelings and thereby improve patient adherence and transplant outcomes.

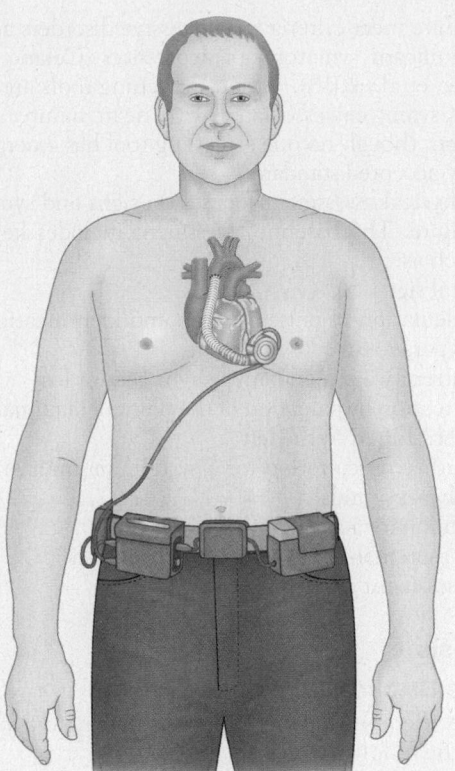

Figure 24-10 • Left ventricular assist device. Reproduced with permission of Medtronic.

formation and are of smaller device sizes. Axial flow VADs use a rotary mechanism (an impeller) to create nonpulsatile blood flow. The impeller spins rapidly within the VAD, creating a vacuum that pulls blood into the VAD and then pushes the blood out into the systemic circulation—the process is similar to a fan spinning in a tunnel, pulling air in one end of the tunnel and pushing it out the other. Centrifugal VADs are nonpulsatile devices that consist of a single moving impeller that is suspended in the pump housing by a combination of magnetic and hydrodynamic forces. The impeller rotates and pulls blood into the pump housing and ejects the blood out to the systemic circulation (Kittleson et al., 2017).

VADs may be used as (1) a "bridge to recovery" for patients who require temporary assistance for reversible ventricular failure, (2) a "bridge to transplant" for patients with end-stage heart failure until a donor organ becomes available for transplant, and (3) "destination therapy" for patients with end-stage heart failure who are not candidates for or decline heart transplantation and have the VAD implanted for permanent use (Kittleson et al., 2017). As patients spend an increased length of time on the transplant list and more VADs are being implanted, destination therapy now accounts for 50% of patients on mechanical circulatory support (Han, Acker, & Atluri, 2018). Thus, the volume of patients with VADs in the community is rapidly expanding and it is important that first responders and other providers are familiar with the basics of VAD management and equipment (Cook, Colvin, Francis, et al., 2017). In some instances, the patient may request deactivation of the VAD, which may cause ethical controversy (Chart 24-3).

Chart 24-3 ETHICAL DILEMMA

Can an Adult with a Left Ventricular Assist Device (LVAD) Have the LVAD Deactivated?

Case Scenario

You work on a cardiac intensive care unit (CICU) and are assigned to care for J.J., a 75-year-old man with an extensive cardiac history who received a left ventricular assist device (LVAD) 10 mo ago. When the device was implanted, J.J. knew the treatment was a destination therapy (i.e., a final treatment option) since he was not a candidate for a heart transplant. The goal was to improve his quality of life. However, this is now his 12th hospitalization since the LVAD was activated, and J.J. now questions the purported benefit of the LVAD. During morning rounds with the cardiologist, J.J. tells you, the cardiologist, his wife, and adult daughter that he feels that the quality of his life is poor and not going to improve. He pointedly asks the cardiologist to deactivate the device, saying that he realizes this will lead to his death. J.J. is mentally competent (i.e., possesses the mental capacity to understand the ramifications of his request). J.J.'s family, the cardiologist, and you are all stakeholders in this decision and each of you express reluctance at honoring his request.

Discussion

Many ethical dilemmas are inherent in this scenario. Although the LVAD is internally implanted, the control switch to deactivate the device is external. Some bioethicists argue that since the device has an external component, deactivating the device is similar to withdrawing treatment, which is ethical. Others argue that it becomes an integrated body part once it is implanted; therefore, to remove it is consistent with euthanasia. There is an obligation to respect J.J.'s autonomy and self-determination, especially since he has the capacity to make these decisions (i.e., he is mentally competent). Yet, there is a "slippery slope" at play here in terms of the principle of nonmaleficence.

Analysis

- Identify the ethical principles that are in conflict in this case (see Chapter 1, Chart 1-7). Which principle do you think should have preeminence as you work to resolve the conflicting emotions between J.J., his family, and the health care team?
- What arguments would you offer *in favor of* removal of the LVAD?
- What arguments would you offer *against* removal of the LVAD?
- Do you believe deactivation of an LVAD is the same as withdrawal of other life-sustaining treatments (e.g., extubation)? Do you believe deactivation of an LVAD constitutes euthanasia?
- Assume that J.J. is determined competent to make this decision and the deactivation is scheduled. Discuss the implications of this procedure on the stakeholders including you, the cardiologist, and the patient's wife and daughter. Do you have the right to refuse to participate in the procedure? Identify what resources might be of help to you as you grapple with making the best decision for all stakeholders.

References

Shinall, M. C. (2018). The evolving moral landscape of palliative care. *Health Affairs, 37*(4), 670–673.

Slavin, S. D., Allen, L. A., McIlvennan, C. K., et al. (2020). Left ventricular assist device withdrawal: Ethical, psychological, and logistical challenges. *Journal of Palliative Medicine, 23*(4), 456–458.

Resources

See Chapter 1, Chart 1-10 for Steps of an Ethical Analysis and Ethics Resources.

Total Artificial Hearts

Total artificial hearts are designed to replace both ventricles. Only one TAH has been approved by the U.S. Food and Drug Administration (FDA) as a bridge to transplant, the SynCardia TAH, and it requires the removal of the patient's heart for implant. Although there has been some short-term success, the long-term results have been disappointing. Researchers hope to develop a device that can be permanently implanted and will eliminate the need for donated human heart transplantation for end-stage cardiac disease. The CARMAT TAH is undergoing early clinical trials in Europe; it features biocompatible materials (Ewald, Milano, & Rogers, 2019).

Complications of VADs and TAHs include bleeding disorders, hemorrhage, thromboemboli, hemolysis, infection, kidney injury, right-sided heart failure, multisystem failure, and mechanical failure. Nursing care of patients with these mechanical assist devices focuses on assessment for and minimization of these complications as well as providing emotional support and education about the device and the underlying cardiac disease.

NURSING PROCESS

The Patient with Cardiomyopathy

Assessment

Nursing assessment for the patient with cardiomyopathy begins with a detailed history of the presenting signs and symptoms. The nurse identifies possible etiologic factors, such as heavy alcohol intake, recent illness or pregnancy, family history of sudden death or history of the disease in immediate family members. If the patient reports chest pain, a thorough review of the pain, including its precipitating factors, is warranted. The review of systems includes the presence of orthopnea, PND, and syncope or dyspnea with exertion. The number of pillows needed to sleep, usual weight, any weight change, and limitations on activities of daily living are assessed. The American College of Cardiology and American Heart Association Stages of Heart Failure classification is utilized to help identify disease progression, and the New York Heart Association Functional Classification for heart failure is determined based on the severity of the patient's symptoms (see Chapter 25, Tables 25-1 and 25-2). The patient's usual diet is evaluated to determine the need to reduce sodium intake, optimize nutrition, or supplement with vitamins.

Because of the chronicity of cardiomyopathy, the nurse conducts a careful psychosocial history, exploring the impact of the disease on the patient's role within the family and community. Identification of perceived stressors helps the patient and the health care team to implement activities that relieve anxiety associated with changes in health status. Very early on, the patient's support systems are identified, and members are encouraged to become involved in the patient's care and therapeutic regimen. The assessment addresses the effect the diagnosis has had on the patient and members of their support system and the patient's emotional status. Findings from a recent meta-analysis suggest that 19% of patients with heart failure meet criteria for depressive disorders and 21.5% have significant symptoms of depression (Celano, Villegas, Albanese, et al., 2018). Various screening tools are available to assess symptoms associated with heart failure, including depression, though no one screening tool has emerged as the generally accepted standard.

The physical assessment focuses on signs and symptoms of heart failure. The baseline assessment includes key components such as:

- Vital signs
- Calculation of pulse pressure and identification of pulsus paradoxus
- Current weight and any weight gain or loss
- Detection by palpation of the point of maximal impulse, often shifted to the left
- Cardiac auscultation for a systolic murmur and S_3 and S_4 heart sounds
- Pulmonary auscultation for crackles
- Measurement of jugular vein distention
- Assessment of edema and its severity

Diagnosis

NURSING DIAGNOSES

Based on the assessment data, major nursing diagnoses may include the following:

- Impaired cardiac output associated with structural disorders caused by cardiomyopathy or to arrhythmia from the disease process and medical treatments
- Risk for impaired cardiac function, ineffective tissue perfusion, and impaired peripheral tissue perfusion associated with decreased peripheral blood flow (resulting from impaired cardiac output)
- Impaired gas exchange associated with pulmonary congestion caused by myocardial failure (resulting from impaired cardiac output)
- Activity intolerance associated with impaired cardiac output or excessive fluid volume, or both
- Anxiety associated with the change in health status and in role functioning
- Powerlessness associated with disease process
- Able to perform self care associated with medication and diet therapies

COLLABORATIVE PROBLEMS/POTENTIAL COMPLICATIONS

Potential complications may include the following:

- Heart failure
- Ventricular arrhythmias
- Atrial arrhythmias
- Cardiac conduction defects
- Pulmonary or cerebral embolism
- Valvular dysfunction

These complications are discussed earlier in this chapter and in Chapters 22 and 25.

Planning and Goals

The major goals for patients include improvement or maintenance of cardiac output, increased activity tolerance, reduction of anxiety, effective management of the self-care program, increased sense of power with decision making, and absence of complications.

Nursing Interventions

IMPROVING CARDIAC OUTPUT AND PERIPHERAL BLOOD FLOW

During a symptomatic episode, rest is indicated. Many patients with DCM find that sitting up with their legs down is more comfortable than lying down in a bed. This position is helpful in pooling venous blood in the periphery and reducing preload. Assessing the patient's oxygen saturation at rest and during activity may assist with determining a need for supplemental oxygen. Oxygen usually is given through a nasal cannula when indicated.

Ensuring that medications are taken as prescribed is important to preserving adequate cardiac output. The nurse may assist the patient with planning a schedule for taking medications and identifying methods to remember to follow it, such as associating the time to take a medication with an activity (e.g., eating a meal, brushing teeth) or obtaining a pillbox.

It is also important to ensure that the patient receives or chooses food selections that are appropriate for a low sodium diet. One way to monitor a patient's response to treatment is to determine the patient's weight every day and identify any significant change. Another indication of the effect of treatment involves assessment of shortness of breath after activity and comparison to before treatment, as well as a change in the number of pillows needed to comfortably sleep. Patients with low cardiac output may need assistance keeping warm and frequently changing position to stimulate circulation and reduce the possibility of skin breakdown.

INCREASING ACTIVITY TOLERANCE AND IMPROVING GAS EXCHANGE

The nurse plans the patient's activities so that they occur in cycles, alternating rest with activity periods. This benefits the patient's physiologic status, and it helps educate the patient about the need for planned cycles of rest and activity. For example, after taking a bath or shower, the patient should plan to sit and read a newspaper or engage in other relaxing activities. Suggesting that the patient sit while chopping vegetables, drying their hair, or shaving helps the patient learn to balance rest with activity. The nurse also makes sure that the patient recognizes the symptoms indicating the need for rest and actions to take when the symptoms occur. Patients with HCM, ARVC/D, or RCM must avoid strenuous activity, isometric exercises, and competitive sports.

REDUCING ANXIETY

Spiritual, psychological, and emotional support may be indicated for patients, families, and significant others. Interventions are directed toward eradicating or alleviating perceived stressors. Patients receive appropriate information about cardiomyopathy and self-management activities. It is important to provide an atmosphere in which patients feel free to verbalize concerns and receive assurance that their concerns are legitimate. If the patient is awaiting transplantation or facing death, it is necessary to allow time to discuss these issues. Providing the patient with realistic hope helps reduce anxiety while they await a donor heart. The nurse helps the patient, family, and significant others with anticipatory grieving.

DECREASING THE SENSE OF POWERLESSNESS

Patients often go through a grieving process when cardiomyopathy is diagnosed. The patient is assisted in identifying the things in life that they have lost (e.g., foods that the patient enjoyed eating but are high in sodium, the ability to engage in an active lifestyle, the ability to play sports, the ability to lift grandchildren) and their emotional responses to the loss (e.g., anger, feelings of sadness). The nurse assists the patient in identifying the amount of control that they still have over life, such as making food choices, managing medications, and working with the patient's primary provider to achieve the best possible outcomes. A diary in which the patient records food selections and weight may help with understanding the relationship between sodium intake and weight gain and give patients a sense of control over their disease. Some patients can manage a self-titrating diuretic regimen in which they adjust the dose of diuretic to their symptoms.

PROMOTING HOME, COMMUNITY-BASED, AND TRANSITIONAL CARE

Educating Patients About Self-Care. A key part of the plan of nursing care involves educating patients about the medication regimen, symptom monitoring, and symptom management (Chart 24-4). The nurse plays an integral role as the patient learns to balance lifestyle and work while accomplishing therapeutic activities. Helping patients cope with their disease status helps them adjust their lifestyles and implement a self-care program at home. Attainment of a goal, no matter how small, also promotes the patient's sense of well-being.

Continuing and Transitional Care. The nurse reinforces previous education and performs ongoing assessment of the patient's symptoms and progress. The nurse also assists the patient and family to adjust to lifestyle changes. Patients are taught to read nutrition labels, to maintain a record of daily weights and symptoms, and to organize daily activities to increase activity tolerance. In addition, the nurse assesses the patient's response to recommendations about diet and fluid intake and to the medication regimen and stresses the signs and symptoms that should be reported to the primary provider. Because of the risk of arrhythmia, it may be necessary to educate the patient's family about cardiopulmonary resuscitation and the use of an automated external defibrillator (see Chapter 25). Women are often advised to avoid pregnancy, but each case is assessed individually. The nurse assesses the psychosocial needs of the patient and family on an ongoing basis. There may be concerns and fears about the prognosis, changes in lifestyle, effects of medications, and the possibility of others in the family having the same condition; these concerns often increase the patient's anxiety and interfere with effective coping strategies. Establishing trust is vital to the nurse's relationship with patients who are chronically ill and with these patients' families. This is particularly significant when the nurse is involved with a patient and family in discussions about end-of-life decisions. Patients who have significant symptoms of heart failure or other complications of cardiomyopathy may benefit from transitional or home care.

Evaluation

Expected patient outcomes may include:
1. Maintains or improves cardiac function
   a. Exhibits heart and respiratory rates within normal limits

---

Chart 24-4

HOME CARE CHECKLIST

The Patient with Cardiomyopathy

At the completion of education, the patient and/or caregiver will be able to:

- State the impact of cardiomyopathy on physiologic functioning, ADLs, IADLs, roles, relationships, and spirituality.
- Identify interventions and strategies (e.g., durable medical equipment, adaptive equipment) used in adapting to any permanent or temporary changes in structure or function.
- State the name, dose, side effects, frequency, and schedule for all medications.
- Take or administer medications daily, exactly as prescribed.
- Monitor effects of medication such as changes in breathing and edema.
- Know signs and symptoms of arrhythmia formation (e.g., lightheadedness, dizziness, orthostatic hypotension, racing heartbeats, diaphoresis, confusion):
  - Identify how to initiate emergency response.
  - Demonstrate skill set in cardiopulmonary resuscitation.
  - Demonstrate use of an automated external defibrillator.
- Weigh self daily at the same time with same clothes.
- Restrict sodium intake to no more than 2 g/day:
  - Adapt diet by examining nutrition labels to check sodium content per serving.
  - Avoid canned or processed foods, eating fresh or frozen foods.
  - Consult the written diet plan and the list of permitted and restricted foods.
  - Avoid salt use.
  - Avoid excesses in eating and drinking.
- Participate in prescribed activity program:
  - Participate in a daily exercise program, with walking and other activities, provided they do not cause unusual fatigue or dyspnea.

- Conserve energy by balancing activity with rest periods.
- Avoid strenuous activity, isometric exercises, and competitive sports.
- Develop methods to manage and prevent stress:
  - Avoid tobacco.
  - Avoid alcohol.
  - Engage in social and diversional activities.
- Identify community resources for peer and caregiver/family support:
  - Identify sources of support (e.g., friends, relatives, faith community).
  - Identify the contact details for support services for patients and their caregivers/families.
  - State meeting locations and times.
- Report immediately to the primary provider or clinic any of the following:
  - Gain in weight of 2–3 lb (0.9–1.4 kg) in 1 d, or 5 lb (2.3 kg) in 1 wk
  - Unusual shortness of breath with activity or at rest
  - Increased swelling of ankles, feet, or abdomen
  - Persistent cough
  - Loss of appetite
  - Development of restless sleep; increase in number of pillows needed to sleep
  - Profound fatigue
- State how to reach primary provider with questions or complications.
- State time and date of follow-up appointments and diagnostic tests.
- Identify the need for health promotion, disease prevention, and screening activities.

ADL, activities of daily living; IADL, independent activities of daily living.

---

b. Reports decreased dyspnea and increased comfort; maintains or improves gas exchange

c. Reports no weight gain; appropriate weight for height

d. Maintains or improves peripheral blood flow

2. Maintains or increases activity tolerance
   a. Carries out activities of daily living (e.g., brushes teeth, feeds self)
   b. Reports increased tolerance to activity

3. Is less anxious
   a. Discusses prognosis freely
   b. Verbalizes fears and concerns
   c. Participates in support groups if appropriate
   d. Demonstrates appropriate coping mechanisms

4. Decreases sense of powerlessness
   a. Identifies emotional response to diagnosis
   b. Discusses control that they have

5. Effectively manages self-care program
   a. Takes medications according to prescribed schedule
   b. Modifies diet to accommodate sodium and fluid recommendations
   c. Modifies lifestyle to accommodate activity and rest behavior recommendations
   d. Identifies signs and symptoms to be reported to health care professionals

INFECTIOUS DISEASES OF THE HEART

Any of the heart's three layers may be affected by an infectious process. Infections are named for the layer of the heart most involved in the infectious process: infective endocarditis (endocardium), myocarditis (myocardium), and pericarditis (pericardium) (see Chapter 21, Fig. 21-1). Rheumatic endocarditis is a unique infective endocarditis syndrome. Diagnosis of infection is made primarily on the basis of the patient's symptoms and echocardiography. Ideal management for all infectious diseases is prevention. IV antibiotics usually are necessary once an infection has developed in the heart.

Rheumatic Endocarditis

Acute rheumatic fever, which occurs most often in school-age children, may develop after an episode of group A beta-hemolytic streptococcal pharyngitis (Chart 24-5). Patients with rheumatic fever may develop rheumatic heart disease as evidenced by a new heart murmur, cardiomegaly, pericarditis, and heart failure. Prompt and effective treatment of "strep" throat with antibiotics can prevent development of rheumatic fever. Streptococcus is spread by direct contact with oral or respiratory secretions. Although bacteria are the causative agents, malnutrition, overcrowding, poor hygiene,

Chart 24-5	Rheumatic Fever

Rheumatic fever is a preventable disease. Diagnosing and effectively treating streptococcal pharyngitis can prevent rheumatic fever and, therefore, rheumatic heart disease. Signs and symptoms of streptococcal pharyngitis include:

- Sore throat that can start very quickly
- Pain when swallowing
- Fever
- Red and swollen tonsils, sometimes with white patches or streaks of pus
- Petechiae (tiny, red spots) on the roof of the mouth (the soft or hard palate)
- Swollen lymph nodes in the front of the neck

If signs and symptoms of streptococcal pharyngitis are present, a rapid strep test is necessary to make an accurate diagnosis. If the test is negative but strep throat is still suspected, then a throat culture can be done. For adults, it is usually not necessary to do a throat culture following a negative rapid strep test. Adults are generally not at risk for getting rheumatic fever following a strep throat infection. All patients with a positive rapid strep test or throat cultures positive for streptococcal pharyngitis must adhere to the prescribed antibiotic treatment. Penicillin or amoxicillin are typical first-line antibiotics used. Completing the course of prescribed antibiotics minimizes the risk of developing rheumatic fever (and subsequent rheumatic heart disease).

Adapted from Centers for Disease Control and Prevention (CDC). (2018). *Strep throat: All you need to know.* Retrieved on 12/3/2019 at: www.cdc.gov/groupastrep/diseases-public/strep-throat.html

Chart 24-6	⚠ RISK FACTORS Infective Endocarditis

- Prosthetic cardiac valves or prosthetic material used for cardiac valve repair
- Implanted cardiac devices (e.g., pacemaker, implanted cardioverter defibrillator)
- History of bacterial endocarditis (even without heart disease)
- Congenital heart disease:
  - Unrepaired cyanotic disease, including patients with palliative shunts and conduits
  - Repaired with prosthetic material or device either by surgery or catheter intervention during the first 6 mo after the procedure
  - Repaired with residual defects at the site or adjacent to the site of a prosthetic patch or device
- Cardiac transplant recipients with valvulopathy
- IV drug abuse
- Body piercing (especially oral, nasal, and nipple), branding, and tattooing
- Hemodialysis

Adapted from Nishimura, R. A., Otto, C. M., Bonow, R. O., et al. (2014). 2014 AHA/ACC guidelines for the management of patients with valvular heart disease. *Journal of the American College of Cardiology, 63*(22), e57–e185.

and lower socioeconomic status may predispose individuals to rheumatic fever. The incidence of rheumatic fever in developed countries has decreased and it is now primarily a disease of the developing world (Cannon, Roberts, Milne, et al., 2017). As noted earlier in the chapter, rheumatic heart disease may lead to mitral valve stenosis or regurgitation that remains an issue in adulthood. Further information about rheumatic fever and rheumatic endocarditis can be found in pediatric nursing books.

Infective Endocarditis

Infective endocarditis is a microbial infection of the endothelial surface of the heart. The disease is rare, but it has a high mortality rate; approximately 14% to 22% of patients die during their hospital stay, and up to 40% of patients die within 1 year of diagnosis (Kaura, Byrne, Fife, et al., 2017). It usually develops in older adults, or in people with prosthetic heart valves or cardiac devices. Staphylococcal endocarditis infections of valves in the right side of the heart are common among adults who use illicit IV drugs (Baddour, Wilson, Bayer, et al., 2015). Hospital-acquired infective endocarditis occurs most often in patients with debilitating disease or indwelling catheters and in patients who are receiving hemodialysis or prolonged IV fluid or antibiotic therapy (Chart 24-6).

Pathophysiology

A deformity or injury of the endocardium leads to accumulation of fibrin and platelets (clot formation) on the endocardium. Infectious organisms, usually staphylococci or streptococci, invade the clot and endocardial lesion. Infection most frequently results in platelets, fibrin, blood cells, and microorganisms that cluster as vegetations on the endocardium. Vegetations may embolize to other vessels throughout the body. As the clot on the endocardium continues to expand, the infecting organism is covered by new clot and concealed from the body's normal defenses. Infection may erode through the endocardium into underlying structures (e.g., valve leaflets), causing tears or other deformities of valve leaflets, dehiscence of prosthetic valves, deformity of chordae tendineae, or mural abscesses.

Clinical Manifestations

Onset of infective endocarditis usually is insidious. Signs and symptoms develop from toxic effects of the infection, destruction of heart valves, and embolization of fragments of vegetative growths on the endocardium. Primary presenting symptoms of infective endocarditis are fever and a heart murmur. Fever may be intermittent or absent, especially in patients who are receiving antibiotics or corticosteroids, in older adults, and in those who have heart failure or kidney injury. A heart murmur may be absent initially but develops in 85% of patients (Karchmer, 2018). Murmurs that worsen over time may indicate progressive damage and extension of the infectious vegetation (Baddour et al., 2015).

In addition to fever and heart murmur, clusters of petechiae may be found on the body. Small, painful nodules (Osler nodes) may be present in pads of fingers or toes. Irregular, red or purple, painless flat macules (Janeway lesions) may be present on palms, fingers, hands, soles, and toes. Hemorrhages with pale centers (Roth spots) caused by emboli may be observed in fundi of the eyes. Splinter hemorrhages (i.e., reddish-brown lines and streaks) may be seen under the proximal half of fingernails and toenails. Petechiae may appear in conjunctiva and mucous membranes.

Systemic embolization occurs in 22% to 50% of patients. It can occur at any time and may even be a presenting symptom. Up to 65% of emboli target the central nervous system and the majority of those are to the middle cerebral artery, effectively causing an embolic stroke. Metastatic foci of infection can also occur from embolization; for example, patients may develop a splenic abscess that requires splenectomy (Baddour et al., 2015).

Heart failure is the most frequent complication of infective endocarditis and may result from perforation of a valve leaflet, rupture of chordae, blood flow obstruction due to vegetations, or intracardiac shunts from dehiscence of prosthetic valves. It indicates a poor prognosis with medical therapy alone and is an indication for surgery (Alpert & Klotz, 2017).

Assessment and Diagnostic Findings

Although characteristics described previously may indicate infective endocarditis, signs and symptoms may indicate other diseases as well. Vague complaints of malaise, anorexia, weight loss, cough, and back and joint pain may be mistaken for influenza. Virulence of the causative organism usually correlates with the speed and degree of symptom development. A definitive diagnosis is made when a microorganism is found in two separate blood cultures and there is evidence of vegetation on imaging of the heart (e.g., echocardiogram). At least two sets of blood cultures (with each set including one aerobic and one anaerobic culture) drawn from different venipuncture sites over a 24-hour period (each set at least 2 hours apart), should be obtained before administration of any antibiotics (Karchmer, 2018). Negative blood cultures do not definitely rule out infective endocarditis. Patients may have elevated white blood cell (WBC) counts. In addition, patients may be anemic, have a positive rheumatoid factor, and an elevated erythrocyte sedimentation rate (ESR) or C-reactive protein.

Echocardiography may assist in diagnosis by demonstrating a mass on a valve, prosthetic valve, or supporting structures and by identifying vegetations, abscesses, new prosthetic valve dehiscence, or new regurgitation. An echocardiogram may reveal development of heart failure. TEE may provide additional data when transthoracic imaging is nondiagnostic; this method of echocardiography is superior in assessing vegetations and perivalvular complications (Karchmer, 2018).

Prevention

Antibiotic prophylaxis had been traditionally recommended in patients at high risk (e.g., those with previous infective endocarditis, prosthetic heart valves, patients with heart transplant and valve regurgitation, some patients with congenital heart disease) before and sometimes after dental procedures that involved manipulation of gingival tissue or periapical area of teeth or perforation of oral mucosa. Antibiotic prophylaxis was also indicated for patients at high risk having procedures which involved the airway, and procedures which involved manipulation of infected tissue (e.g., wound débridement). The latest U.S. guidelines assert that prophylaxis in patients at high risk is reasonable but admit that the data are mixed regarding whether prophylaxis really decreases rates of infective endocarditis (Nishimura et al., 2017).

Patients at high risk should practice good oral hygiene. Poor dental hygiene can lead to bacteremia, particularly in the setting of a dental procedure. Severity of oral inflammation and infection is a significant factor in the incidence and degree of bacteremia. Regular professional oral care combined with personal oral care may reduce the risk of bacteremia. Recommended ongoing personal oral care includes using a manual or electronic toothbrush, dental floss, and other plaque removing devices (Nishimura et al., 2017).

Any patient at risk with a fever of more than 7 days' duration should report that finding to a primary provider; patients should not self-medicate with antibiotics or stop taking them before the prescribed dosage has been completed (Nishimura et al., 2017).

Increased vigilance is also required in patients with IV catheters and during invasive procedures. To minimize the risk of infection, nurses must ensure meticulous hand hygiene, site preparation, and aseptic technique during insertion and maintenance procedures. All catheters, tubes, drains, and other devices are removed as soon as they are no longer needed or no longer function.

Medical Management

The objective of treatment is to eradicate invading organisms through adequate doses of an appropriate antibiotic. Antibiotic therapy usually is given intravenously for 2 to 6 weeks. Parenteral therapy is given in doses that produce a high serum concentration for a significant period to ensure eradication of the dormant bacteria within dense vegetations. This therapy is often delivered in the patient's home and is monitored by a home health nurse. Serum levels of the antibiotic and blood cultures are monitored to gauge effectiveness of therapy. If there is insufficient bactericidal activity, increased dosages of the antibiotic are prescribed or a different antibiotic is used. After adequate antibiotic therapy is initiated, the infective organism is usually eliminated. The patient should begin to feel better, regain an appetite, and have less fatigue. During this time, patients require psychosocial support because although they feel well, they may find themselves confined to the hospital or home with restrictive IV therapy.

Surgical Management

Surgical intervention may be required if the patient develops heart failure or an intracardiac abscess, or the patient has recurrent systemic embolizations, or the infection does not respond to medications. Surgical interventions include valve repair and replacement, débridement of vegetations, débridement and closure of an abscess, and closure of a fistula. Surgical valve replacement greatly improves the prognosis for patients with severe symptoms from damaged heart valves. Most patients who have prosthetic valve endocarditis require repeat valve replacement (Alpert & Klotz, 2017).

Nursing Management

The nurse monitors the patient's temperature at regular intervals, because the course of fever is one indication of treatment effectiveness. However, febrile reactions also may occur as a result of medication. The nurse administers antibiotic, antifungal, or antiviral medication as prescribed and educates the patient to take them as prescribed. Timing of antimicrobial medication administration is critical to maintain therapeutic drug levels. Fever often increases fatigue; rest periods should be planned and activities spaced to provide rest between activities. Good infection control and prevention practices include appropriate hand hygiene by both patients and caregivers. Nonsteroidal anti-inflammatory drugs (NSAIDs) may be prescribed as antipyretics or to decrease the discomfort of fever. Patients may be more comfortable with a light layer of linens and exposure of their skin to air. They may be cooled with a fan, tepid water baths, or cloth compresses; if shivering or piloerection occurs, these interventions should be discontinued due to increased oxygen consumption and potential to further increase of body temperature.

Heart sounds are assessed. A new or worsening murmur may indicate dehiscence of a prosthetic valve, rupture of an abscess, or injury to valve leaflets or chordae tendineae (Baddour et al., 2015). The nurse monitors for signs and symptoms of systemic embolization, or, for patients with right-sided heart endocarditis, for signs and symptoms of pulmonary infarction and infiltrates. In addition, the nurse assesses signs and symptoms of organ damage such as stroke, meningitis, heart failure, myocardial infarction, glomerulonephritis, and splenomegaly.

Patient care is directed toward management of infection. Long-term IV antimicrobial therapy often is necessary; therefore, many patients have peripherally inserted central catheters or other long-term IV access. All invasive lines and wounds must be assessed daily for redness, tenderness, warmth, swelling, drainage, or other signs of infection. The patient and family are educated about activity restrictions, medications, and signs and symptoms of infection. Patients with infective endocarditis are at high risk for another episode of infective endocarditis. If the patient has undergone surgical treatment, the nurse provides postoperative care and instructions (see Chapters 16 and 23).

As appropriate, the home health nurse supervises and monitors IV antibiotic therapy delivered in the home setting and educates the patient and family about prevention and health promotion. The nurse provides the patient and family with emotional support and facilitates coping strategies during the prolonged course of infection and antibiotic treatment.

Myocarditis

Myocarditis, an inflammatory process involving the myocardium, can cause heart dilation, thrombi on the heart wall (mural thrombi), infiltration of circulating blood cells around the coronary vessels and between the muscle fibers, and degeneration of the muscle fibers themselves. Mortality varies with the severity of symptoms. Most patients with mild symptoms recover completely; however, some patients develop cardiomyopathy and heart failure.

Pathophysiology

Myocarditis usually results from an infectious source, be it viral (e.g., coxsackieviruses A and B, human immune deficiency virus, influenza A), bacterial, rickettsial, fungal, parasitic, metazoal, protozoal (e.g., Chagas disease), or spirochetal. It also may be immune related, occurring after acute systemic infections such as rheumatic fever, or it may be related to an autoimmune disorder. It may also result from an inflammatory reaction to toxins such as pharmacologic agents used in the treatment of other diseases (Arbustini, Agozzino, Favalli, et al., 2017). It may begin in one small area of the myocardium and then spread throughout the myocardium. The degree of myocardial inflammation and necrosis determines the degree of interstitial collagen and elastin destruction. The greater the destruction, the greater is the hemodynamic effect and resulting signs and symptoms. It is thought that DCM and HCM are latent manifestations of myocarditis.

Clinical Manifestations

The symptoms of acute myocarditis depend on the type of infection, the degree of myocardial damage, and the capacity of the myocardium to recover. Patients may be asymptomatic, with an infection that resolves on its own. However, they may develop mild to moderate symptoms and seek medical attention, often reporting fatigue and dyspnea, syncope, palpitations, and occasional discomfort in the chest and upper abdomen. The most common symptoms are flulike. Patients may also sustain sudden cardiac death or quickly develop severe congestive heart failure in fulminant myocarditis.

Assessment and Diagnostic Findings

Assessment of the patient may reveal no detectable abnormalities; as a result, the illness can go undiagnosed. Patients may be tachycardic or may report chest pain. An endomyocardial biopsy can provide the definitive diagnosis (Arbustini et al., 2017), but cardiac MRI is being used more often as a diagnostic tool because of its noninvasive approach (Lakdawala, Stevenson, & Loscalzo, 2018). With contrast, cardiac MRI may be diagnostic and can guide clinicians to sites for endomyocardial biopsies, which may be also indicated to find an organism or its genome, an immune process, or a radiation reaction causing the myocarditis. Patients without any abnormal heart structure (at least initially) may suddenly develop arrhythmias or ST–T-wave changes. If the patient has structural heart abnormalities (e.g., systolic dysfunction), a clinical assessment may disclose cardiac enlargement, faint heart sounds (especially S_1), pericardial friction rub, a gallop rhythm, or a systolic murmur. The WBC count, C-reactive protein, leukocyte count, and ESR may be elevated.

Medical Management

Patients are given specific treatment for the underlying cause if it is known (e.g., penicillin for hemolytic streptococci) and are placed on bed rest to decrease cardiac workload. Bed rest also helps decrease myocardial damage and the complications of myocarditis. In young patients with myocarditis, activities, especially athletics, should be limited for a 6-month period or at least until heart size and function have returned to normal. Physical activity is increased slowly, and the patient is instructed to report any symptoms that occur with increasing activity, such as a rapidly beating heart. If heart failure or arrhythmia develops, management is essentially the same as for all causes of heart failure and arrhythmias (see Chapters 25 and 22, respectively). Although they are known for their anti-inflammatory effects, NSAIDs should not be used for pain control; they have been implicated in increased cardiac injury and viral replication in animal studies (Lakdawala et al., 2018).

Nursing Management

The nurse assesses for resolution of tachycardia, fever, and any other clinical manifestations. The cardiovascular assessment focuses on signs and symptoms of heart failure and arrhythmias. Patients with arrhythmias should have continuous cardiac monitoring with personnel and equipment readily available to treat life-threatening arrhythmias.

 Quality and Safety Nursing Alert

Patients with myocarditis are sensitive to digitalis. Nurses must closely monitor these patients for digitalis toxicity, which is evidenced by a new onset of arrhythmia, anorexia, nausea, vomiting, headache, and malaise. The primary provider should be notified immediately if this is suspected.

Anti-embolism stockings and passive and active exercises should be used because embolization from venous thrombosis and mural thrombi can occur, especially in patients on bed rest. In some patients, pharmacologic prophylaxis may also be indicated (see Chapter 26).

Pericarditis

Pericarditis refers to an inflammation of the pericardium, which is the membranous sac enveloping the heart. It accounts for 5% of emergency room visits for chest pain (Adler, Charron, Imazio, et al., 2015; Imazio, Gaita, & LeWinter, 2015). Classification of pericarditis may be acute, chronic, or recurrent. The etiology of pericarditis can be infectious or noninfectious (Imazio & Gaita, 2015). For example, pericarditis may occur after pericardiectomy (opening of the pericardium) following cardiac surgery. Pericarditis also may occur 10 days to 2 months after acute myocardial infarction (Dressler syndrome).

Pathophysiology

Causes underlying or associated with pericarditis are listed in Chart 24-7. The inflammatory process of pericarditis may lead to an accumulation of fluid in the pericardial sac (pericardial effusion) and increased pressure on the heart, leading to cardiac tamponade (see Chapter 25). Frequent or prolonged episodes of pericarditis also may lead to thickening and decreased elasticity of the pericardium, or scarring may fuse the visceral and parietal pericardium. These conditions restrict the heart's ability to fill with blood (constrictive pericarditis). The pericardium may become calcified, further restricting ventricular expansion during ventricular filling (diastole). With less filling, the ventricles pump less blood, leading to decreased cardiac output and signs and symptoms of heart failure. Restricted diastolic filling may result in increased systemic venous pressure, causing peripheral edema and hepatic failure.

Clinical Manifestations

Pericarditis may be asymptomatic. The most characteristic symptom of pericarditis is chest pain, although pain also may be located beneath the clavicle, in the neck, or in the left trapezius (scapula) region. Pain or discomfort usually remains fairly constant, but it may worsen with deep inspiration and when lying down or turning. The most characteristic clinical manifestation

Chart 24-7 — Causes of Pericarditis

- Idiopathic or nonspecific causes
- Infection:
  - Viral: most commonly infectious cause (e.g., enteroviruses, herpes viruses, adenoviruses, parvoviruses)
  - Bacterial: rare (but if bacterial cause, most commonly *Mycobacterium tuberculosis* is implicated)
  - Fungal: rare (e.g., *Histoplasma, Aspergillus, Candida*)
  - Parasitic: rare (e.g., *Echinococcus, Toxoplasma*)
- Autoimmune disorders (e.g., systemic lupus erythematosus, rheumatic fever, rheumatoid arthritis, polyarteritis, sarcoidosis, scleroderma)
- Immune-mediated drug reactions:
  - Lupuslike reaction
  - Antineoplastic drugs
  - Hypersensitivity eosinophilia
- Disorders of adjacent structures (e.g., myocardial infarction, dissecting aneurysm, pneumonia)
- Neoplastic disease:
  - Metastasis from lung or breast cancer
  - Primary neoplasms (e.g., mesothelioma)
- Radiation therapy of chest and upper torso (peak occurrence 5–9 mo after treatment)
- Intentional or unintentional chest trauma (e.g., chest injury, cardiac surgery, cardiac catheterization, implantation of pacemaker, or implantation of a cardiac implantable electronic device)
- Metabolic:
  - Uremia
  - Anorexia
  - Myxedema

Adapted from Miranda, W. R., Imazio, M., Greason, K. L., et al. (2017). Pericardial diseases. In V. Fuster, R. A. Harrington, J. Narula, et al. (Eds.). *Hurst's the heart* (14th ed.). New York: McGraw-Hill.

of pericarditis is a creaky or scratchy friction rub heard most clearly at the left lower sternal border. Other signs may include a mild fever, increased WBC count, anemia, and an elevated ESR or C-reactive protein level. Patients may have a nonproductive cough or hiccup. Dyspnea, as well as respiratory splinting because of pain upon inspiration, and other signs and symptoms of heart failure may occur as a result of pericardial compression due to constrictive pericarditis or cardiac tamponade. The heart rate may increase to maintain cardiac output.

Assessment and Diagnostic Findings

The diagnosis most often is made on the basis of history, signs, and symptoms. An echocardiogram may detect inflammation, pericardial effusion or tamponade, and heart failure. It may help confirm the diagnosis and may be used to guide pericardiocentesis (needle or catheter drainage of the pericardium). TEE may be useful in diagnosis but may underestimate the extent of pericardial effusions. CT imaging may be the best diagnostic tool for determining size, shape, and location of pericardial effusions and may be used to guide pericardiocentesis. Cardiac MRI may assist with detection of inflammation and adhesions. Occasionally, a video-assisted pericardioscope-guided biopsy of the pericardium or epicardium is performed to obtain tissue samples for culture and microscopic examination. Because the pericardial sac surrounds the heart, a 12-lead

ECG may show concave ST elevations in many, if not all, leads (with no reciprocal changes) and may show depressed PR segments or atrial arrhythmias (Imazio & Gaita, 2015).

Medical Management

Objectives of pericarditis management are to determine the cause, administer therapy for treatment and symptom relief, and detect signs and symptoms of cardiac tamponade. When cardiac output is impaired, the patient is placed on bed rest until fever, chest pain, and friction rub have subsided.

Analgesic medications and NSAIDs such as aspirin, indomethacin, or ibuprofen may be prescribed for pain relief during the acute phase. Corticosteroids (e.g., prednisone) can be used as an alternative when NSAIDs are contraindicated (e.g., kidney disease). Colchicine may be prescribed if the pericarditis is severe as an additive therapy to NSAIDs (Adler et al., 2015).

Pericardiocentesis, a procedure in which some pericardial fluid is removed, rarely is necessary. It may be performed to assist in identification of the cause or relieve symptoms, especially if there are signs and symptoms of heart failure or tamponade. Pericardial fluid is cultured if bacterial, tubercular, or fungal disease is suspected; a sample is sent for cytology if neoplastic disease is suspected. A pericardial window, a small opening made in the pericardium, may be performed to allow continuous drainage into the chest cavity. Surgical removal of tough encasing pericardium (pericardiectomy) may be necessary to release both ventricles from constrictive and restrictive inflammation and scarring.

Nursing Management

Patients with acute pericarditis require pain management with antispasmodic agents, assistance with positioning, and psychological support. Patients with chest pain often benefit from education and reassurance that the pain is not due to a heart attack. Pain may be relieved with a forward-leaning or sitting position. To minimize complications, the nurse helps the patient with activity restrictions until pain and fever subside. As the patient's condition improves, the nurse encourages gradual increases of activity. However, if pain, fever, or friction rub recurs, activity restrictions must be resumed. The nurse educates the patient and family about a healthy lifestyle to enhance the patient's immune system.

Nurses caring for patients with pericarditis must be alert to signs and symptoms of cardiac tamponade (see Chapter 25). The nurse monitors the patient for heart failure. Patients with hemodynamic instability or pulmonary congestion are treated as if they had heart failure (see Chapter 25).

NURSING PROCESS

The Patient with Pericarditis

Assessment

The primary symptom of pericarditis is pain, which is assessed by evaluating the patient in various positions. The nurse tries to identify whether pain is influenced by respiratory movements, while holding an inhaled breath or holding an exhaled breath; by flexion, extension, or rotation of the spine, including the neck; by movements of shoulders and arms; by coughing; or by swallowing. Recognizing events that precipitate or intensify pain may help establish a diagnosis and differentiate pain of pericarditis from pain of myocardial infarction.

When pericardial surfaces lose their lubricating fluid because of inflammation, a pericardial friction rub occurs. The rub is audible on auscultation and is synchronous with the heartbeat. However, it may be elusive and difficult to detect.

> ### ▶ *Quality and Safety Nursing Alert*
>
> *A pericardial friction rub is diagnostic of pericarditis. It is a creaky or scratchy sound and is louder at the end of exhalation. Nurses should monitor for pericardial friction rub by placing the diaphragm of the stethoscope tightly against the patient's thorax and auscultating the left sternal edge in the fourth intercostal space, which is the site where the pericardium comes into closest contact with the left chest wall. The rub may be heard best when a patient is sitting and leaning forward.*

If there is difficulty in distinguishing a pericardial friction rub from a pleural friction rub, the patient is asked to hold their breath; a pericardial friction rub will continue to be heard.

The patient's temperature is monitored frequently. Pericarditis may cause an abrupt onset of fever in a patient who has been afebrile.

Diagnosis

NURSING DIAGNOSES

Based on the assessment data, the major nursing diagnoses may be:

- Acute pain associated with inflammation of the pericardium
- Lack of knowledge of diagnosis and therapeutic self-care management

COLLABORATIVE PROBLEMS/POTENTIAL COMPLICATIONS

Potential complications may include the following:

- Pericardial effusion
- Cardiac tamponade

Planning and Goals

The patient's major goals may include relief of pain and absence of complications.

Nursing Interventions

RELIEVING PAIN

Relief of pain is achieved by rest. Because sitting upright and leaning forward is the posture that tends to relieve pain, chair rest may be more comfortable. The nurse instructs the patient to restrict activity until pain subsides. As chest pain and friction rub abate, activities of daily living may be resumed gradually. If the patient is taking antispasmodic agents, antibiotics, or corticosteroids for pericarditis, responses to these medications are monitored and recorded. Patients taking NSAIDs or colchicine are assessed for gastrointestinal adverse effects. If chest pain and friction rub recur, bed rest or chair rest is resumed.

ENHANCING KNOWLEDGE ABOUT PERICARDITIS AND SELF-CARE MANAGEMENT

There are a multitude of possible causes for pericarditis (see Chart 24-7). Some of these are life-threatening (e.g., metastatic cancers) while others are not; regardless, the patient is likely to be fearful and anxious because they are experiencing chest pain. Educating the patient about the cause of the pericarditis, and medications prescribed to treat it (e.g., NSAIDs), and methods to improve breathing patterns and alleviate pain (e.g., sitting up and leaning forward upon a pillow) can allay anxieties. The patient should verbalize when it is appropriate to follow up with the primary provider (i.e., for routine follow ups, with relapse of symptoms, with symptoms suggestive of cardiac tamponade, including lightheadedness, orthostasis and tachycardia [see following]).

MONITORING AND MANAGING POTENTIAL COMPLICATIONS

Abnormal accumulation of fluid between the pericardial linings (i.e., in the pericardial sac) is called *pericardial effusion*. Most patients have no effects or symptoms. However, enough fluid can accumulate to constrict the myocardium, impairing ventricular filling and the myocardium's ability to pump, a condition known as *cardiac tamponade* (discussed below) (Imazio et al., 2015). Failure to identify and treat this problem can lead to death.

Signs and symptoms of cardiac tamponade may begin with the patient reporting shortness of breath, chest tightness, or dizziness. The nurse may observe that the patient is becoming progressively more restless. Assessment of blood pressure may reveal a decrease of 10 mm Hg or more in systolic blood pressure during inspiration (pulsus paradoxus). Usually, the systolic pressure decreases and the diastolic pressure remains stable; hence, the pulse pressure narrows. The patient usually has tachycardia, and ECG voltage may be decreased or QRS complexes may alternate in height (electrical alternans). Heart sounds may progress from distant to imperceptible. Blood continues to return to the heart from the periphery but cannot flow into the heart to be pumped back into the circulation. The patient develops jugular vein distention and other signs of rising central venous pressure. The Beck triad (hypotension, muffled heart sounds, and an elevated jugular venous pressure) is a useful diagnostic parameter of severe tamponade.

In such situations, the nurse notifies the primary provider immediately and prepares to assist with diagnostic echocardiography and pericardiocentesis (see Chapter 25). The nurse stays with the patient and continues to assess and record signs and symptoms while intervening to decrease patient anxiety.

PROMOTING HOME, COMMUNITY-BASED, AND TRANSITIONAL CARE

Because patients, their family members, and health care providers tend to focus on the most obvious needs and issues related to pericarditis, the nurse reminds them about the importance of continuing health promotion and screening practices. The nurse educates patients who have not been involved in these practices in the past about their importance and refers them to appropriate health care providers.

Evaluation

Expected patient outcomes may include:
1. Freedom from pain
   a. Performs activities of daily living without pain, fatigue, or shortness of breath
   b. Temperature returns to normal range
   c. Exhibits no pericardial friction rub
2. Effectively manages self-care
   a. Identifies cause(s) of pericarditis and rationale for prescribed therapeutic regimen
   b. Follows-up with primary provider for ongoing appointments and as needed
3. Absence of complications
   a. Sustains blood pressure in normal range
   b. Heart sounds strong and can be auscultated
   c. Absence of jugular vein distention

CRITICAL THINKING EXERCISES

1 **ebp** A 67-year-old woman presents to the emergency department (ED) where you work as a staff nurse with reports of fevers, malaise, and painful nodules on the pads of her fingers. Upon review of her medical history, the patient reports an aortic valve replacement (prosthetic) as a child, but no other significant medical or surgical history. Based on the history and physical examination findings, the primary provider thinks that the patient may have infective endocarditis and prescribes antibiotics. What should you ensure happens before the antibiotics are given? What are the care priorities for this patient?

2 **ipc** A 57-year-old man presents to the cardiology clinic where you work with a complaint of ankle swelling and trouble breathing when he walks more than 20 feet. The cardiologist does an echocardiogram and diagnoses the patient with cardiomyopathy. The patient expresses anxiety about what this means. Based on what you know about cardiomyopathy, what would you focus on when educating this patient? What are the key roles of other members of the health care team in appropriately assisting the patient in managing a new diagnosis of cardiomyopathy?

3 **pq** A 47-year-old woman with HCM presents to the ED where you work after fainting. It is the middle of summer and the primary provider thinks the patient was dehydrated. Explain the pathophysiology of why dehydration in a patient with HCM might precipitate a syncopal episode. Describe your prioritized focused assessment of this patient in the ED.

REFERENCES

*Asterisk indicates nursing research.
**Double asterisk indicates classic reference.

Books

Alpert, J. S., & Klotz, S. A. (2017). Infective endocarditis. In V. Fuster, R. A. Harrington, J. Narula, et al. (Eds.). *Hurst's the heart* (14th ed.). New York: McGraw-Hill.

Arbustini, E., Agozzino, M., Favalli, V., et al. (2017). Myocarditis. In V. Fuster, R. A. Harrington, J. Narula, et al. (Eds.). *Hurst's the heart* (14th ed.). New York: McGraw-Hill.

Chikwe, J., & Castillo, J. G. (2017). Prosthetic heart valves. In V. Fuster, R. A. Harrington, J. Narula, et al. (Eds.). *Hurst's the heart* (14th ed.). New York: McGraw-Hill.

Dahl, J., & Ailawadi, G. (2018). Percutaneous mitral valve repair techniques. In F. W. Sellke & M. Ruel (Eds.). *Atlas of cardiac surgical techniques* (2nd ed., pp. 364–383). Philadelphia, PA: Elsevier.

Ewald, G. A., Milano, C. A., & Rogers, J. G. (2019). Circulatory assist devices in heart failure. In G. M. Felker & D. L. Mann (Eds.). *Heart failure: A companion to Braunwald's heart disease* (4th ed.). Philadelphia, PA: Elsevier.

Hermann, H. C., & Mack, M. J. (2019). Transcatheter therapies for valvular heart disease. In R. O. Bonow, D. L. Mann, G. F. Tomaselli, et al. (Eds.). *Braunwald's heart disease: A textbook of cardiovascular medicine* (11th ed., pp. 1464–1482). Philadelphia, PA: Elsevier.

Karchmer, A. W. (2018). Infective endocarditis. In J. L. Jameson, A. S. Fauci, D. L. Kasper, et al. (Eds.). *Harrison's principles of internal medicine* (20th ed.). New York: McGraw-Hill.

Kittleson, M., Patel, J., & Kobashigawa, J. (2017). Cardiac transplantation. In V. Fuster, R. Harrington, J. Narula, et al. (Eds.). *Hurst's the heart* (14th ed.). New York: McGraw-Hill.

Lakdawala, N. K., Stevenson, L. W., & Loscalzo, J. (2018). Cardiomyopathy and myocarditis. In J. L. Jameson, A. S. Fauci, D. L. Kasper, et al. (Eds.). *Harrison's principles of internal medicine* (20th ed.). New York: McGraw-Hill.

Libby, P., Zipes, D. P., Bonow, R. O., et al. (2018). *Braunwald's heart disease: A textbook of cardiovascular medicine* (11th ed., Vol. 2). The Netherlands: Elsevier.

Miranda, W. R., Imazio, M., Greason, K. L., et al. (2017). Pericardial diseases. In V. Fuster, R. A. Harrington, J. Narula, et al. (Eds.). *Hurst's the heart* (14th ed.). New York: McGraw-Hill.

Journals and Electronic Documents

Adler, Y., Charron, P., Imazio, M., et al. (2015). 2015 ESC Guidelines for the diagnosis and management of pericardial diseases: The Task Force for the Diagnosis and Management of Pericardial Diseases of the European Society of Cardiology (ESC) Endorsed by: The European Association for Cardio-Thoracic Surgery (EACTS). *European Heart Journal, 36*(42), 2921–2964.

Akinseye, O. A., Pathak, A., & Ibebuogu, U. N. (2018). Aortic valve regurgitation: A comprehensive review. *Current Problems Cardiology, 43*(8), 315–334.

Althunayyan, A., Petersen, S. E., Lloyd, G., et al. (2019). Mitral valve prolapse. *Expert Review of Cardiovascular Therapy, 17*(1), 43–51.

Asher, S. B., Chen, R., & Kallish, S. (2018). Mitral valve prolapse and aortic root dilation in adults with hypermobile Ehlers-Danlos syndrome and related disorders. *American Journal of Medical Genetics. Part A, 176*(9), 1838–1844.

Baddour, L. M., Wilson, W. R., Bayer, A. S., et al. (2015). Infective endocarditis in adults: Diagnosis, antimicrobial therapy, and management of complications: A scientific statement for healthcare professionals from the American Heart Association. *Circulation, 132*(15), 1435–1486.

Bennett, R. G., Haqqani, H. M., Berruezo, A., et al. (2019). Arrhythmogenic cardiomyopathy in 2018–2019: ARVC/ALVC or both? *Heart, Lung and Circulation, 28*(1), 164–177.

Cannon, J., Roberts, K., Milne, C., et al. (2017). Rheumatic heart disease severity, progression and outcomes: A multi-state model. *Journal of the American Heart Association, 6*(3). Retrieved on 7/14/2019 at: www.ahajournals.org/doi/10.1161/JAHA.116.003498

Celano, C. M., Villegas, A. C., Albanese, A. M., et al. (2018). Depression and anxiety in heart failure: A review. *Harvard Review of Psychiatry, 26*(4), 175–184.

Centers for Disease Control and Prevention (CDC). (2018). Strep throat: All you need to know. Retrieved on 12/3/2019 at: www.cdc.gov/groupastrep/diseases-public/strep-throat.html?CDC_AA_refVal=https%3A%2F%2Fwww.cdc.gov%2Ffeatures%2Fstrepthroat%2Findex.html

Cook, J. L., Colvin, M., Francis, G. S., et al. (2017). Recommendations for the use of mechanical circulatory support: Ambulatory and community patient care: A scientific statement from the American Heart Association. *Circulation, 135*(25), e1145–e1158.

Dziadzko, V., Dziadzko, M., Medina-Inojosa, J. R., et al. (2019). Causes and mechanisms of isolated mitral regurgitation in the community: Clinical context and outcome. *European Heart Journal, 40*(27), 2194–2202.

**Elliott, P., Andersson, B., Arbustini, E., et al. (2008). Classification of the cardiomyopathies: A position statement from the European Society Of Cardiology Working Group on Myocardial and Pericardial Diseases. *European Heart Journal, 29*(2), 270–276.

Flint, N., Wunderlich, N. C., Shmueli, H., et al. (2019). Aortic regurgitation. *Current Cardiol Reports, 21*(7), 65. doi:10.1007/s11886-019-1144-6

Gati, S., Malhotra, A., & Sharma, S. (2019). Exercise recommendations in patients with valvular heart disease. *Heart, 105*(2), 106–110.

Han, H. C., Ha, F. J., Teh, A. W., et al. (2018). Mitral valve prolapse and sudden cardiac death: A systematic review. *Journal of the American Heart Association, 7*(23), e010584.

Han, J. J., Acker, M. A., & Atluri, P. (2018). Left ventricular assist devices. *Circulation, 138*(24), 2841–2851.

Harb, S. C., & Griffin, B. P. (2017). Mitral valve disease: A comprehensive review. *Current Cardiology Reports, 19*(8), 73.

Hussain, S. T., Majdalany, D. S., Dunn, A., et al. (2018). Early and midterm results of autograft rescue by Ross reversal: A one-valve disease need not become a two-valve disease. *The Journal of Thoracic and Cardiovascular Surgery, 155*(2), 562–577.

Imazio, M., & Gaita, F. (2015). Diagnosis and treatment of pericarditis. *Heart, 101*(14), 1159–1168.

Imazio, M., Gaita, F., & LeWinter, M. (2015). Evaluation and treatment of pericarditis: A systematic review. *Journal of the American Medical Association, 314*(14), 1498–1506.

January, C. T., Wann, L. S., Calkins, H., et al. (2019). 2019 AHA/ACC/HRS focused update of the 2014 AHA/ACC/HRS guideline for the management of patients with atrial fibrillation: A report of the American College of Cardiology/American Heart Association task force on clinical practice guidelines and the Heart Rhythm Society. *Heart Rhythm.* Retrieved on 7/14/2019 at: www.heartrhythmjournal.com/article/S1547-5271(19)30037-2/pdf

Joseph, J., Naqvi, S. Y., Giri, J., et al. (2017). Aortic stenosis: Pathophysiology, diagnosis, and therapy. *The American Journal of Medicine, 130*(3), 253–263.

Kaura, A., Byrne, J., Fife, A., et al. (2017). Inception of the 'endocarditis team' is associated with improved survival in patients with infective endocarditis who are managed medically: Findings from a before-and-after study. *Open Heart, 4*(2), e000699.

Kumar, A., Paniagua, D., Hira, R. S., et al. (2016). Balloon aortic valvuloplasty in the transcatheter aortic valve replacement era. *Journal of Invasive Cardiology, 28*(8), 341–348.

Lindman, B. R., Dweck, M. R., Lancellotti, P., et al. (2019). Management of asymptomatic severe aortic stenosis: Evolving concepts in timing of valve replacement. *JACC Cardiovascular Imaging, 13*(2 Pt 1), 481–493.

Ma, J. I., Igata, S., Strachan, M., et al. (2019). Predictive factors for progression of mitral regurgitation in asymptomatic patients with mitral valve prolapse. *American Journal of Cardiology, 123*(8), 1309–1313.

Maisano, F., Skantharaja, R., Denti, P., et al. (2019). Mitral annuloplasty. Multimedia manual of cardio-thoracic surgery. Retrieved on 7/14/2019 at: www.mmcts.org/tutorial/763#references

Marian, A. J., & Braunwald, E. (2017). Hypertrophic cardiomyopathy: Genetics, pathogenesis, clinical manifestations, diagnosis, and therapy. *Circulation Research, 121*(7), 749–770.

**Maron, B. J., Towbin, J. A., Thiene, G., et al. (2006). Contemporary definitions and classification of the cardiomyopathies: An American Heart Association scientific statement from the Council on Clinical Cardiology, Heart Failure and Transplantation Committee; Quality of Care and Outcomes Research and Functional Genomics and Translational Biology Interdisciplinary Working Groups; and Council on Epidemiology and Prevention. *Circulation, 113*(14), 1807–1816.

Mazine, A., El-Hamamsy, I., Verma, S., et al. (2018). Ross procedure in adults for cardiologists and cardiac surgeons: JACC State-of-the-Art Review. *Journal of the American College of Cardiology, 72*(22), 2761–2777.

McNally, E. M., & Mestroni, L. (2017). Dilated cardiomyopathy: Genetic determinants and mechanisms. *Circulation Research, 121*(7), 731–748.

Merlo, M., Cannata, A., Gobbo, M., et al. (2018). Evolving concepts in dilated cardiomyopathy. *European Journal of Heart Failure, 20*(2), 228–239.

Muchtar, E., Blauwet, L. A., & Gertz, M. A. (2017). Restrictive cardiomyopathy: Genetics, pathogenesis, clinical manifestations, diagnosis, and therapy. *Circulation Research, 121*(7), 819–837.

Nalliah, C. J., Mahajan, R., Elliott, A. D., et al. (2019). Mitral valve prolapse and sudden cardiac death: A systematic review and meta-analysis. *Heart, 105*(2), 144–151.

Negi, P. C., Mahajan, K., Rana, V., et al. (2018). Clinical characteristics, complications, and treatment practices in patients with RHD: 6-year results from HP-RHD Registry. *Global Heart, 13*(4), 267–274.

Nishimura, R. A., Otto, C. M., Bonow, R. O., et al. (2014). 2014 AHA/ACC guideline for the management of patients with valvular heart disease: A report of the American College of Cardiology/American Heart Association Task Force on Practice Guidelines. *The Journal of Thoracic and Cardiovascular Surgery, 148*(1), e1–e132.

Nishimura, R. A., Otto, C. M., Bonow, R. O., et al. (2017). 2017 AHA/ACC focused update of the 2014 AHA/ACC guideline for the management of patients with valvular heart disease: A report of the American College of Cardiology/American Heart Association Task Force on Clinical Practice Guidelines. *Journal of the American College of Cardiology, 70*(2), 252–289.

Nishimura, R. A., Seggewiss, H., & Schaff, H. V. (2017). Hypertrophic obstructive cardiomyopathy: Surgical myectomy and septal ablation. *Circulation Research, 121*(7), 771–783.

Organ Procurement and Transplant Network (OPTN). (2019). Donor matching system. Retrieved on 12/2/2019 at: https://optn.transplant.hrsa.gov/learn/about-transplantation/donor-matching-system

Pabba, K., & Boudi, F. (2019). Water hammer pulse. In *StatPearls*. Treasure Island, FL: StatPearls Publishing. Retrieved on 9/24/2019 at: www.statpearls.com/sp/al/31306

Pereira, N. L., Grogan, M., & Dec, G. W. (2018). Spectrum of restrictive and infiltrative cardiomyopathies: Part 1 of a 2-part series. *Journal of the American College of Cardiology, 71*(10), 1130–1148.

Sandhu, K., Krishnamoorthy, S., Afif, A., et al. (2017). Balloon aortic valvuloplasty in contemporary practice. *Journal of Interventional Cardiology, 30*(3), 212–216.

Scientific Registry of Transplant Recipients. (2017). *OPTN/SRTR 2017 Annual Data Report: Heart*. Health Resources and Services Administration, Department of Health and Human Services. Retrieved on 7/13/2019 at: https://srtr.transplant.hrsa.gov/annual_reports/2017/Heart.aspx

*Shemesh, Y., Peles-Bortz, A., Peled, Y., et al. (2017). Feelings of indebtedness and guilt toward donor and immunosuppressive medication adherence among heart transplant (HTx) patients, as assessed in a cross-sectional study with the Basel Assessment of Adherence to Immunosuppressive Medications Scale (BAASIS). *Clinical Transplantation, 31*(10). doi:10.1111/ctr.13053

Shinall, M. C. (2018). The evolving moral landscape of palliative care. *Health Affairs, 37*(4), 670–673.

Slavin, S. D., Allen, L. A., McIlvennan, C. K., et al. (2020). Left ventricular assist device withdrawal: Ethical, psychological, and logistical challenges. *Journal of Palliative Medicine, 23*(4), 456–458.

Stehlik, J., Kobashigawa, J., Hunt, S. A., et al. (2018). Honoring 50 years of clinical heart transplantation in circulation: In-depth state-of-the-art review. *Circulation, 137*(1), 71–87.

Szczygielska, I., Hernik, E., Kolodziejczyk, B., et al. (2018). Rheumatic fever—new diagnostic criteria. *Reumatologia, 56*(1), 37–41.

Tudorache, I., Horke, A., Cebotari, S., et al. (2016). Decellularized aortic homografts for aortic valve and aorta ascendens replacement. *European Journal of Cardio-Thoracic Surgery, 50*(1), 89–97.

Watanabe, N. (2019). Acute mitral regurgitation. *Heart, 105*(9), 671–677.

Wozniak-Mielczarek, L., Sabiniewicz, R., Drezek-Nojowicz, M., et al. (2019). Differences in cardiovascular manifestation of Marfan Syndrome between children and adults. *Pediatric Cardiology, 40*(2), 393–403.

Yuan, S. M., & Yan, S. L. (2016). Mitral valve prolapse in pregnancy. *Brazilian Journal of Cardiovascular Surgery, 31*(2), 158–162.

Resources

American Heart Association, National Center, www.heart.org
Cardiomyopathy UK, www.cardiomyopathy.org
MyLVAD, www.mylvad.com

LEARNING OUTCOMES

On completion of this chapter, the learner will be able to:

1. Recognize the etiology, pathophysiology, and clinical manifestations of the different classifications of heart failure.
2. Describe the medical management, including recommended pharmacologic treatments, for patients with heart failure.
3. Use the nursing process as a framework for care of the patient with heart failure.
4. Identify additional heart disease disorders and medical and nursing management of patients with complications from heart disease.

NURSING CONCEPT

Perfusion

GLOSSARY

anuria: urine output of less than 50 mL/24 h

ascites: an accumulation of serous fluid in the peritoneal cavity

cardiac resynchronization therapy (CRT): a treatment for heart failure in which a device paces both ventricles to synchronize contractions

congestive heart failure (CHF): a fluid overload condition (congestion) associated with heart failure

diastolic heart failure: the inability of the left ventricle of the heart to fill and pump sufficiently; term used to define a type of heart failure (*synonym:* Heart Failure with preserved Ejection Fraction [HFpEF])

ejection fraction (EF): percentage of blood volume in the ventricles at the end of diastole that is ejected during systole; a measurement of contractility

heart failure (HF): a clinical syndrome resulting from structural or functional cardiac disorders that impair the ability of a ventricle to fill or eject blood

Heart Failure with midrange Ejection Fraction (HFmrEF): clinical heart failure syndrome with left ventricular ejection fraction that is 40% to 49%

Heart Failure with preserved Ejection Fraction (HFpEF): clinical heart failure syndrome with left ventricular ejection fraction greater than or equal to 50% (*synonym:* diastolic heart failure)

Heart Failure with reduced Ejection Fraction (HFrEF): clinical heart failure syndrome with left ventricular ejection fraction less than or equal to 40% (*synonym:* systolic heart failure)

left-sided heart failure: inability of the left ventricle to fill or eject sufficient blood into the systemic circulation (*synonym:* left ventricular failure)

oliguria: diminished urine output; less than 0.5 mL/kg/h over at least 6 hours, or less than 400 mL in 24 hours

orthopnea: shortness of breath when lying flat

paroxysmal nocturnal dyspnea (PND): shortness of breath that occurs suddenly during sleep

pericardiocentesis: procedure that involves aspiration of fluid from the pericardial sac

pericardiotomy: surgically created opening of the pericardium

pulmonary edema: pathologic accumulation of fluid in the interstitial spaces and alveoli of the lungs causing severe respiratory distress

pulseless electrical activity (PEA): condition in which electrical activity is present on an electrocardiogram, but there is not a physiologically adequate pulse or blood pressure

pulsus paradoxus: systolic blood pressure that is more than 10 mm Hg lower during inhalation than during exhalation; difference is normally less than 10 mm Hg

right-sided heart failure: inability of the right ventricle to fill or eject sufficient blood into the pulmonary circulation (*synonym:* right ventricular failure)

systolic heart failure: inability of the heart to pump sufficiently because of an alteration in the ability of the heart to contract; term used to describe a type of heart failure (*synonym:* Heart Failure with reduced Ejection Fraction [HFrEF])

Cardiovascular disease is the leading cause of death in the United States (Centers for Disease Control and Prevention [CDC], 2017). Because of advancements in diagnostic and screening procedures, greater recognition of the importance of diligent self-care practices, and new discoveries in pharmacotherapies, it is now possible for a person diagnosed with heart disease to continue to live with a high quality of life years after being diagnosed. Despite this progress, heart disease remains a chronic and often progressive condition, associated with serious comorbidities, such as heart failure (Benjamin, Muntner, Alonso, et al., 2019). This chapter presents the complications most often associated with heart disease, including the medical management and nursing processes for managing patients with complications of cardiovascular disease.

HEART FAILURE

Heart failure (HF) is a clinical syndrome resulting from structural or functional cardiac disorders so that the heart is unable to pump enough blood to meet the body's metabolic demands or needs (American Heart Association [AHA], 2019a). The term *heart failure* indicates myocardial disease in which impaired contraction of the heart (systolic dysfunction) or filling of the heart (diastolic dysfunction) may cause pulmonary or systemic congestion. Some cases of HF are reversible, depending on the cause. Most often, HF is a chronic, progressive condition that is managed with lifestyle changes and medications to prevent episodes of acute decompensated heart failure. These episodes are characterized by increased symptoms of respiratory distress, decreased cardiac output (CO), and poor perfusion. These episodes are also associated with increased hospitalizations, increased health care costs, and decreased quality of life (Benjamin et al., 2019).

Approximately six million people in the United States have HF, and 870,000 new cases are diagnosed each year (AHA, 2019a). As more people live longer with chronic heart diseases, HF has become an epidemic that challenges the country's health care resources. HF is the most common reason for hospitalization of people older than 65 years and is the second most common reason for visits to a provider's office. Emergency department (ED) visits and hospital readmissions for this disorder are very common, despite efforts to prevent rehospitalizations. Over 20% of patients discharged after treatment for HF are readmitted to the hospital within 30 days, and nearly 50% are readmitted to the hospital within 6 months (O'Connor, 2017). The estimated economic burden caused by HF in the United States is more than $30 billion annually in direct and indirect costs and is expected to continue to increase over time (CDC, 2017).

HF is more prevalent among African Americans and Hispanics than among Caucasians. The risk for having HF increases with advancing age. For adults over 60 years of age, HF is more prevalent among men than women (Benjamin et al., 2019). As typical for other major cardiovascular diseases and disorders, cigarette smoking, obesity, poorly managed diabetes, and metabolic syndrome are all risks for HF (Benjamin et al., 2019). The onset of HF is typically a morbid consequence of another disease or disorder, including coronary artery disease (CAD), hypertension, cardiomyopathy,

valvular disorders, and renal dysfunction with volume overload (McCance, Huether, Brashers, et al., 2019).

Atherosclerosis of the coronary arteries is a primary cause of HF, and CAD is found in the majority of patients with HF. Ischemia causes myocardial dysfunction because it deprives heart cells of oxygen and causes cellular damage. Myocardial infarction (MI) causes focal heart muscle necrosis, the death of myocardial cells, and a loss of contractility; the extent of the infarction correlates with the severity of HF. Revascularization of the coronary artery by a percutaneous coronary intervention (PCI) or by coronary artery bypass surgery (coronary artery bypass graft [CABG]) may improve myocardial oxygenation and ventricular function and prevent more extensive myocardial necrosis that can lead to HF (see Chapter 23).

Systemic or pulmonary hypertension increases afterload (resistance to ejection), increasing the cardiac workload and leading to the hypertrophy of myocardial muscle fibers. This can be considered a compensatory mechanism because it initially increases contractility. However, sustained hypertension eventually leads to changes that impair the heart's ability to fill properly during diastole, and the hypertrophied ventricles may dilate and fail (Norris, 2019; Yancy, Jessup, Bozkurt, et al., 2017).

Cardiomyopathy is a disease of the myocardium. The various types of cardiomyopathy lead to HF and arrhythmias. Dilated cardiomyopathy (DCM), the most common type of cardiomyopathy, causes diffuse myocyte necrosis and fibrosis, and commonly leads to progressive HF (Norris, 2019). DCM can be idiopathic (unknown cause), or it can result from an inflammatory process, such as myocarditis, or from a cytotoxic agent, such as alcohol or certain antineoplastic drugs. Usually, HF due to cardiomyopathy is chronic and progressive. However, cardiomyopathy and HF may resolve following removal of the causative agent. Genetic testing may be recommended for idiopathic cardiomyopathy (van der Meer, Gaggin, & Dec, 2019) (see Chapter 24).

Valvular heart disease is also a cause of HF. The valves ensure that blood flows in one direction. With valvular dysfunction, it becomes increasingly difficult for blood to move forward, increasing pressure within the heart and increasing cardiac workload, leading to HF (see Chapter 24).

Several systemic conditions, including progressive kidney failure, contribute to the development and severity of HF. Nearly 30% of patients with chronic HF also have chronic kidney disease (Benjamin et al., 2019). In addition, cardiac arrhythmias such as atrial fibrillation may either cause or result from HF; in both instances, the altered electrical stimulation impairs myocardial contraction and decreases the overall efficiency of myocardial function. Other factors, such as hypoxia, acidosis, and electrolyte abnormalities, can worsen myocardial function (Yancy et al., 2017).

Pathophysiology

Regardless of the etiology, the pathophysiology of HF results in similar changes and clinical manifestations. Significant myocardial dysfunction usually occurs before the patient experiences signs and symptoms of HF such as shortness of breath, edema, or fatigue.

As HF develops, the body activates neurohormonal compensatory mechanisms. These mechanisms represent the body's attempt to cope with the HF and are responsible for the signs and symptoms that develop (Norris, 2019). Understanding these mechanisms is important because the treatment for HF is aimed at correcting them and relieving symptoms.

The most common type of HF is systolic HF, also called Heart Failure with reduced Ejection Fraction (HFrEF; see later discussion in Assessment and Diagnostic Findings). **Systolic heart failure** results in decreased blood ejected from the ventricle. The decreased blood flow is sensed by baroreceptors in the aortic and carotid bodies, and the sympathetic nervous system is then stimulated to release epinephrine and norepinephrine (Fig. 25-1). The purpose of this initial response is to increase heart rate and contractility and support the failing myocardium, but the continued response has multiple negative effects. Sympathetic stimulation causes vasoconstriction in the skin, gastrointestinal tract, and kidneys. A decrease in renal perfusion due to low CO and vasoconstriction then causes the release of renin by the kidneys. Renin converts the plasma protein angiotensinogen to angiotensin

I, which then circulates to the lungs. Angiotensin-converting enzyme (ACE) in the lumen of pulmonary blood vessels converts angiotensin I to angiotensin II, a potent vasoconstrictor, which then increases the blood pressure and afterload. Angiotensin II also stimulates the release of aldosterone from the adrenal cortex, resulting in sodium and fluid retention by the renal tubules and an increase in blood volume. These mechanisms lead to the fluid volume overload commonly seen in HF. Angiotensin, aldosterone, and other neurohormones (e.g., endothelin) lead to an increase in preload and afterload, which increases stress on the ventricular wall, causing an increase in cardiac workload. A counterregulatory mechanism is attempted through the release of natriuretic peptides. Atrial natriuretic peptide (ANP) and B-type natriuretic peptide (BNP; brain type) are released from the overdistended cardiac chambers. These substances promote vasodilation and diuresis. However, their effect is usually not strong enough to overcome the negative effects of the other mechanisms (Norris, 2019).

Physiology/Pathophysiology

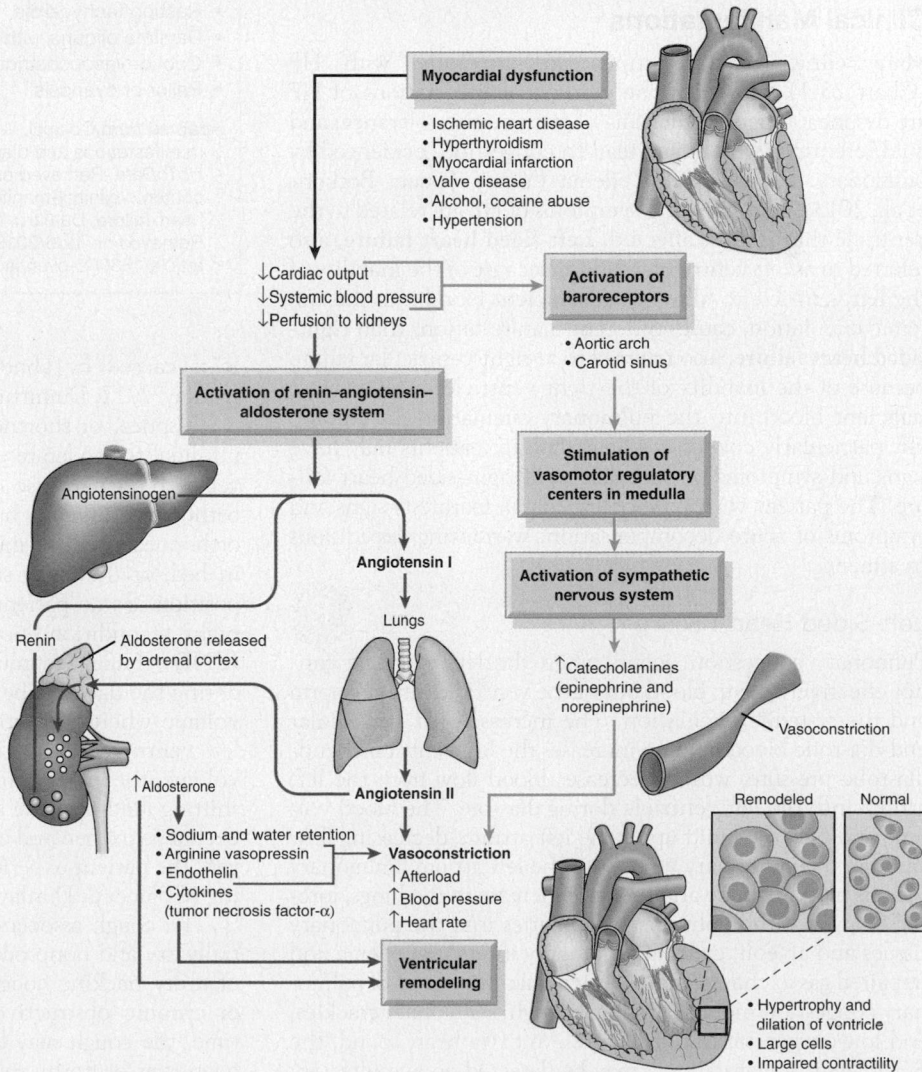

Figure 25-1 • The pathophysiology of heart failure. A decrease in cardiac output activates multiple neurohormonal mechanisms that ultimately result in the signs and symptoms of heart failure.

As the heart's workload increases, contractility of the myocardial muscle fibers decreases. Decreased contractility results in an increase in end-diastolic blood volume in the ventricle, stretching the myocardial muscle fibers and increasing the size of the ventricle (ventricular dilation). The heart compensates for the increased workload by increasing the thickness of the heart muscle (ventricular hypertrophy). Hypertrophy results in abnormal changes in the structure and function of myocardial cells, a process known as ventricular remodeling. Under the influence of neurohormones (e.g., angiotensin II), enlarged myocardial cells become dysfunctional and die early (a process called *apoptosis*), leaving the other, functional myocardial cells struggling to maintain CO.

As cardiac cells die and the heart muscle becomes fibrotic, **diastolic heart failure**, also called Heart Failure with preserved Ejection Fraction (HFpEF) (see later discussion in Assessment and Diagnostic Findings), can develop, leading to further dysfunction. A stiff ventricle resists filling, and less blood in the ventricles causes a further decrease in CO. All of these compensatory mechanisms of HF have been referred to as the "vicious cycle of heart failure" because low CO leads to multiple mechanisms that make the heart work harder, worsening the HF.

Clinical Manifestations

Many clinical manifestations are associated with HF (Chart 25-1). However, the cardinal manifestations of HF are dyspnea; fatigue, which may limit exercise tolerance; and fluid retention, which may lead to congestion, evidenced by pulmonary and peripheral edema (Yancy, Jessup, Bozkurt, et al., 2013). The signs and symptoms of HF are related to the ventricle that is most affected. **Left-sided heart failure**, also referred to as left ventricular failure because of the inability of the left ventricle to fill or eject sufficient blood into the systemic circulation, causes different manifestations than **right-sided heart failure**, also referred to as right ventricular failure because of the inability of the right ventricle to fill or eject sufficient blood into the pulmonary circulation. In chronic HF, particularly congestive heart failure, patients may have signs and symptoms of both left- and right-sided heart failure. The patient with pulmonary edema manifests signs and symptoms of acute decompensation, warranting expeditious treatment.

Left-Sided Heart Failure

Pulmonary congestion occurs when the left ventricle cannot effectively pump blood out of the ventricle into the aorta and the systemic circulation. The increased left ventricular end-diastolic blood volume increases the left ventricular end-diastolic pressure, which decreases blood flow from the left atrium into the left ventricle during diastole. The blood volume and pressure build up in the left atrium, decreasing flow through the pulmonary veins into the left atrium. Pulmonary venous blood volume and pressure increase in the lungs, forcing fluid from the pulmonary capillaries into the pulmonary tissues and alveoli, causing pulmonary interstitial edema and impaired gas exchange. The clinical manifestations of pulmonary congestion include dyspnea, cough, pulmonary crackles, and low oxygen saturation levels. An extra heart sound, the S$_3$, or "ventricular gallop," may be detected on auscultation.

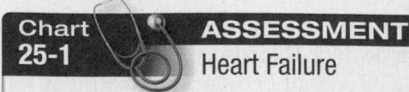

Chart 25-1 **ASSESSMENT**
Heart Failure

Be alert for the following signs and symptoms:

Congestion
- Dyspnea
- Orthopnea
- Paroxysmal nocturnal dyspnea
- Cough (recumbent or exertional)
- Pulmonary crackles that do not clear with cough
- Weight gain (rapid)
- Dependent edema
- Abdominal bloating or discomfort
- Ascites
- Jugular venous distention
- Sleep disturbance (anxiety or air hunger)
- Fatigue

Poor Perfusion/Low Cardiac Output
- Decreased exercise tolerance
- Muscle wasting or weakness
- Anorexia or nausea
- Unexplained weight loss
- Lightheadedness or dizziness
- Unexplained confusion or altered mental status
- Resting tachycardia
- Daytime oliguria with recumbent nocturia
- Cool or vasoconstricted extremities
- Pallor or cyanosis

Adapted from Colucci, W. S., & Dunlay, S. M. (2017). Clinical manifestations and diagnosis of advanced heart failure. *UpToDate*. Retrieved on 12/6/2019 at: www.uptodate.com/contents/clinical-manifestations-and-diagnosis-of-advanced-heart-failure; Dumitru, I. (2018). Heart failure. *Medscape*. Retrieved on 12/6/2019 at: www.emedicine.medscape.com/article/163062-overview

It is caused by abnormal ventricular filling (Colucci & Dunlay, 2017; Dumitru, 2018).

Dyspnea, or shortness of breath, may be precipitated by minimal to moderate activity (dyspnea on exertion [DOE]), yet dyspnea may also occur at rest. The patient may report **orthopnea**, difficulty breathing when lying flat. Patients with orthopnea may use multiple pillows to prop themselves up in bed, or they may sleep sitting up or in a high, reclined position. Some patients have sudden attacks of dyspnea at night, a condition known as **paroxysmal nocturnal dyspnea (PND)**. Fluid accumulating in the dependent extremities during the day may be reabsorbed into the circulating blood volume when the patient lies down. Because the impaired left ventricle cannot eject the increased circulating blood volume, the pressure in the pulmonary circulation increases, shifting fluid into the alveoli. The fluid-filled alveoli cannot exchange oxygen and carbon dioxide. Without sufficient oxygen, the patient experiences dyspnea and has difficulty sleeping (Colucci & Dunlay, 2017; Dumitru, 2018).

The cough associated with left ventricular failure is initially dry and nonproductive. Most often, patients complain of a dry hacking cough that may be mislabeled as asthma or chronic obstructive pulmonary disease (COPD). Over time, the cough may begin to accumulate secretions. Large quantities of frothy sputum, sometimes pink or tan, may be produced, indicating acute decompensated HF and pulmonary edema (Colucci & Dunlay, 2017; Dumitru, 2018).

Adventitious breath sounds may be heard in various areas of the lungs. Usually, bibasilar crackles that do not clear with coughing are detected in the early phase of left ventricular failure. As the failure worsens and pulmonary congestion increases, crackles may be auscultated throughout the lung fields. At this point, oxygen saturation may decrease.

In addition to pulmonary manifestations, the decreased amount of blood ejected from the left ventricle can lead to inadequate tissue perfusion. The diminished CO has widespread manifestations because not enough blood reaches all of the tissues and organs (low perfusion) to provide the necessary oxygen. The decrease in stroke volume (SV) can also stimulate the sympathetic nervous system to release catecholamines, which further impedes perfusion to many organs, including the kidneys.

As reduced CO and catecholamines decrease blood flow to the kidneys, urine output drops. Renal perfusion pressure falls, and the renin–angiotensin–aldosterone system is stimulated to increase blood pressure and intravascular volume. While the patient sleeps, the cardiac workload decreases, improving renal perfusion. This may cause **nocturia** (i.e., frequent urination at night) (Colucci & Dunlay, 2017; Dumitru, 2018).

As HF progresses, decreased output from the left ventricle may cause other symptoms. Decreased gastrointestinal perfusion causes altered digestion. Decreased brain perfusion causes dizziness, lightheadedness, confusion, restlessness, and anxiety due to decreased oxygenation and blood flow. As anxiety increases, so does dyspnea, increasing anxiety and creating a vicious cycle. Stimulation of the sympathetic system also causes the peripheral blood vessels to constrict, so the skin appears pale or ashen and feels cool and clammy.

A decrease in SV causes the sympathetic nervous system to increase the heart rate (tachycardia), often causing the patient to complain of palpitations. The peripheral pulses become weak. Without adequate CO, the body cannot respond to increased energy demands, and the patient becomes easily fatigued and has decreased activity tolerance. Fatigue also results from the increased energy expended in breathing and the insomnia that results from respiratory distress, coughing, and nocturia (Colucci & Dunlay, 2017; Dumitru, 2018).

Right-Sided Heart Failure

When the right ventricle fails, congestion in the peripheral tissues and the viscera predominates. This occurs because the right side of the heart cannot eject blood effectively and cannot accommodate all of the blood that normally returns to it from the venous circulation. Increased venous pressure leads to jugular venous distention (JVD) and increased capillary hydrostatic pressure throughout the venous system. Systemic clinical manifestations include dependent edema (edema of the lower extremities), **hepatomegaly** (enlargement of the liver), **ascites** (accumulation of fluid in the peritoneal cavity), and weight gain due to retention of fluid. Edema usually affects the feet and ankles and worsens when the patient stands or sits for a long period. The edema may decrease when the patient elevates the legs. Edema can gradually progress up

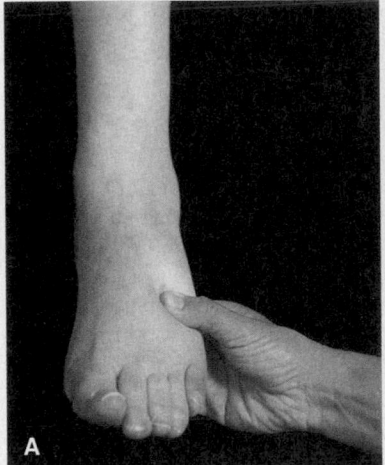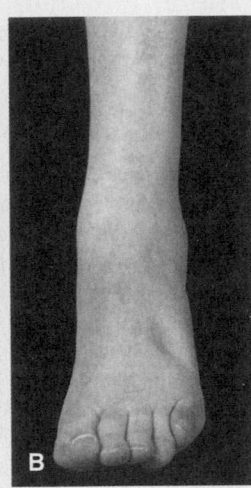

Figure 25-2 • Example of pitting edema. **A.** The nurse applies pressure to an area near the ankle. **B.** When the pressure is released, an indentation remains in the edematous tissue. Reprinted with permission from Bickley, L. S. (2017). *Bates' guide to physical examination and history taking* (12th ed.). Philadelphia, PA: Lippincott Williams & Wilkins.

the legs and thighs and eventually into the external genitalia and lower trunk. Ascites is evidenced by increased abdominal girth and may accompany lower body edema or may be the only edema present. Sacral edema is common in patients who are on bed rest, because the sacral area is dependent. Pitting edema, in which indentations in the skin remain after even slight compression with the fingertips (Fig. 25-2), is generally obvious after retention of at least 4.5 kg (10 lb) of fluid (4.5 L).

Hepatomegaly and tenderness in the right upper quadrant of the abdomen result from venous engorgement of the liver. The increased pressure may interfere with the liver's ability to function (secondary liver dysfunction). As hepatic dysfunction progresses, increased pressure within the portal vessels may force fluid into the abdominal cavity, causing ascites. Ascites may increase pressure on the stomach and intestines and cause gastrointestinal distress. Hepatomegaly may also increase pressure on the diaphragm, causing respiratory distress.

Anorexia (loss of appetite), nausea, or abdominal pain may result from the venous engorgement and venous stasis within the abdominal organs. The generalized weakness that accompanies right-sided HF results from reduced CO and impaired circulation (Colucci & Dunlay, 2017; Dumitru, 2018).

Congestive Heart Failure

Right-sided heart failure can sometimes occur as a result of left-sided failure. The failure of these dual mechanisms is sometimes referred to as **congestive heart failure**. When the left ventricle fails, increased fluid pressure is transferred back through the lungs, leading to damage of the right side of the heart. When the right side loses pumping power, the blood backs up in the body's venous system. This may cause swelling or congestion in the legs, ankles, and swelling within the abdomen such as the GI tract and liver. Increased venous pressure may also lead to JVD and increased capillary hydrostatic pressure throughout the venous system. Edema may be present in the periphery as well as within the pulmonary vascular bed. Without appropriate treatment, this may progress to pulmonary edema.

 ## Pulmonary Edema

Pulmonary edema is an acute event, reflecting a breakdown of physiologic compensatory mechanisms; hence, it is sometimes referred to as acute decompensated heart failure. It can occur following acute MI or as an exacerbation of chronic HF. When the left ventricle begins to fail, blood backs up into the pulmonary circulation, causing pulmonary interstitial edema. This may occur quickly in some patients, a condition sometimes called *flash pulmonary edema*. Pulmonary edema can also develop slowly, especially when it is caused by noncardiac disorders such as kidney injury and other conditions that cause fluid overload. The left ventricle cannot handle the volume overload, and blood volume and pressure build up in the left atrium. The rapid increase in atrial pressure results in an acute increase in pulmonary venous pressure, which produces an increase in hydrostatic pressure that forces fluid out of the pulmonary capillaries and into the interstitial spaces and alveoli (Norris, 2019).

As a result of decreased cerebral oxygenation, the patient may become increasingly restless and anxious. Along with a sudden onset of breathlessness and a sense of suffocation, the patient may be tachypneic with low oxygen saturation levels. The skin and mucous membranes may be pale to cyanotic, and the hands may be cool and clammy. Tachycardia and JVD may be present. Incessant coughing may occur, producing increasing quantities of foamy sputum. The patient may become progressively confused. The situation demands emergent action before oxygenation and perfusion levels become critical.

Assessment and Diagnostic Findings

For many years, the severity of HF was classified solely according to the patient's symptoms, using the New York Heart Association (NYHA) classification of HF. This classification system, which is still in widespread use, is described in Table 25-1. The American College of Cardiology and the American Heart Association (ACC/AHA) have developed another HF classification system (Yancy et al., 2013). This system, described in Table 25-2, takes into consideration the natural history and progressive nature of HF. The ACC/AHA periodically issues evidence-based guidelines for patients with HF or at high-risk of having HF, using this classification system as a framework for treatment (Yancy et al., 2013; Yancy, Jessup, Bozkurt, et al., 2016; Yancy et al., 2017).

HF may go undetected until the patient presents with signs and symptoms of pulmonary and peripheral edema. Some of the physical signs that suggest HF may also occur with other diseases, such as kidney injury and COPD; therefore, diagnostic testing is essential to confirm a diagnosis of HF.

Assessment of ventricular function is an essential part of the initial diagnostic workup. An echocardiogram is performed to determine the ejection fraction (EF), identify anatomic features such as structural abnormalities and valve malfunction, and confirm the diagnosis of HF. The **ejection fraction** is a measure of ventricular contractility; it is the percentage of the end-diastolic blood volume that is ejected

TABLE 25-1	New York Heart Association (NYHA) Classification of Heart Failure
Classification	**Signs and Symptoms**
I	No limitation of physical activity Ordinary activity does not cause undue fatigue, palpitation, or dyspnea.
II	Slight limitation of physical activity Comfortable at rest, but ordinary physical activity causes fatigue, palpitation, or dyspnea.
III	Marked limitation of physical activity Comfortable at rest, but less than ordinary activity causes fatigue, palpitation, or dyspnea.
IV	Unable to carry out any physical activity without discomfort Symptoms of cardiac insufficiency at rest If any physical activity is undertaken, discomfort is increased.

Adapted from Yancy, C. W., Jessup, M., Bozkurt, B., et al. (2013). 2013 ACCF/AHA Guideline for the management of heart failure. A report of the American College of Cardiology Foundation/American Heart Association Task Force on Practice Guidelines. *Circulation, 128*(16), e240–e327.

with each heartbeat. An expected EF is 55% to 65% of the ventricular volume; the ventricle does not completely empty between contractions (Wiegand, 2017).

There are two recognized main types of left-sided HF, with a third, emerging category. In **heart failure with reduced ejection fraction (HFrEF)**, or systolic heart failure, the left ventricle loses the ability to contract effectively, manifesting as EFs of less than 40%, reflecting decreased CO and pump failure (Yancy et al., 2017).

Heart failure with preserved ejection fraction (HFpEF), or diastolic heart failure, is diagnosed when the left ventricular function measures greater than or equal to 50%, yet the ventricle loses its ability to relax due to myocardial stiffness. Because of the noncompliance of the ventricular wall, the chamber is unable to fill at normal capacity during the relaxation phase of diastole (Yancy et al., 2017).

Heart failure with midrange ejection fraction (HFmrEF) is a third and emerging classification category, with EFs typically between 40% and 49% (van der Meer et al., 2019).

Diagnosing a patient with HFpEF is more challenging than diagnosing a patient with HFrEF, because the diagnosis of HFpEF is a *diagnosis of exclusion*. That is, it is made by excluding other potential noncardiac causes suggestive of HF. The incidence of HFpEF is increasing and is becoming more commonplace among older adult women with a history of hypertension; indeed, hypertension is the most common underlying cause of HFpEF. Comorbid conditions such as obesity, CAD, diabetes, atrial fibrillation, and hyperlipidemia are also common in patients with HFpEF (Yancy et al., 2013).

In addition to the echocardiogram, a chest x-ray and a 12-lead electrocardiogram (ECG) are obtained to assist in the diagnosis. Laboratory studies usually performed during the initial workup include serum electrolytes, blood urea nitrogen (BUN), creatinine, liver function tests, thyroid-stimulating hormone, complete blood count (CBC), BNP, and routine urinalysis. The results of these laboratory studies assist in determining the underlying cause and can also

TABLE 25-2	American College of Cardiology and American Heart Association (ACC/AHA) Classification of Heart Failure		
Classification	**Criteria**	**Patient Characteristics**	**Treatment Recommendations for Appropriate Patients**
Stage A	Patients at high risk for developing left ventricular dysfunction but without structural heart disease or symptoms of HF	Hypertension Atherosclerotic disease Diabetes Metabolic syndrome	Heart healthy lifestyle Risk factor control of hypertension, lipids, diabetes, obesity
Stage B	Patients with left ventricular dysfunction or structural heart disease who have not developed symptoms of HF	History of myocardial infarction Left ventricular hypertrophy Low ejection fraction	Implement stage A recommendations, plus: • ACE inhibitor, or ARB, or ARNI for low EF or history of MI • Beta-blocker • Statin
Stage C	Patients with left ventricular dysfunction or structural heart disease with current or prior symptoms of heart disease	Shortness of breath Fatigue Decreased exercise tolerance	Implement stage A and B recommendations, plus: • Diuretics • Aldosterone antagonist • Sodium restriction • Implantable defibrillator • Cardiac resynchronization therapy
Stage D	Patients with refractory end-stage HF requiring specialized interventions	Symptoms despite maximal medical therapy Recurrent hospitalizations	Implement stage A, B, and C recommendations, plus: • Fluid restriction • End-of-life care • Extraordinary measures: • Inotropes • Cardiac transplantation • Mechanical support

ACE, angiotensin-converting enzyme; ARB, angiotensin receptor blocker; ARNI, angiotensin receptor-neprilysin inhibitor, EF, ejection fraction; HF, heart failure; MI, myocardial infarction.

Adapted from Yancy, C. W., Jessup, M., Bozkurt, B., et al. (2013). 2013 ACCF/AHA guideline for the diagnosis and management of heart failure: A report of the American College of Cardiology Foundation/American Heart Association Task Force on Practice Guidelines. *Circulation, 128*(16), e240–e327; Yancy, C. W., Jessup, M., Bozkurt, B., et al. (2016). ACC/AHA/HFSA focused update on new pharmacological therapy for heart failure: An update of the 2013 ACCF/AHA guideline for the management of heart failure: A report of the American College of Cardiology Foundation/American Heart Association Task Force on Clinical Practice Guidelines and the Heart Failure Society of America. *Circulation, 134*(13), e282–e293.

be used to establish a baseline to assess effects of treatment. The BNP level is a key diagnostic indicator of HF; high levels are a sign of high cardiac filling pressure and can aid in both the diagnosis and management of HF; in particular, rising levels may suggest an acute exacerbation of HF (Yancy et al., 2013). BNP levels are best used for diagnostic purposes when there is a baseline measurement and a measurement obtained at the time of treatment (e.g., hospital discharge) to help in determining a posttreatment prognosis (Yancy et al., 2017).

Medical Management

The prognosis for patients with HF has improved with the use of evidence-based protocols for patient management. Specific interventions are based on the stage of HF (Yancy et al., 2013; Yancy et al., 2016; Yancy et al., 2017). The management goals of HF include the following (Cyrille & Patel, 2017):

- Improvement of cardiac function with optimal pharmacologic management
- Reduction of symptoms and improvement of functional status
- Stabilization of patient condition and lowering of the risk of hospitalization
- Delay of the progression of HF and extension of life expectancy
- Promotion of a lifestyle conducive to cardiac health

Treatment options vary according to the severity of the patient's condition, comorbidities, and cause of the HF, and may include oral and intravenous (IV) medications, lifestyle modifications, supplemental oxygen, and surgical interventions, including implantation of cardiac devices, and cardiac transplantation (see Chapter 24).

Managing the patient with HF begins with providing comprehensive education and counseling to the patient and family. The patient and family must understand the nature of HF and the importance of their participation in the treatment regimen, including side and adverse effects of pharmacologic therapies. Lifestyle recommendations include restriction of dietary sodium; avoidance of smoking, including secondhand smoke; avoidance of excessive fluid and alcohol intake; weight reduction when indicated; and regular exercise. The patient must also know how to recognize signs and symptoms that need to be reported to the primary provider.

Pharmacologic Therapy

Several types of medications are routinely prescribed for patients with HF. The cornerstone of therapy for patients with HFrEF (systolic HF), which is the most common type of HF, includes a diuretic, an angiotensin system blocker, and a beta-blocker (Table 25-3). Many of these medications, particularly angiotensin system blockers and beta-blockers, improve symptoms and extend survival. Others, such as diuretics, improve symptoms but may not affect survival

TABLE 25-3	Select Medications Used to Treat Heart Failure	
Medication	**Therapeutic Effects**	**Key Nursing Considerations**
Diuretics		
Loop diuretics: furosemide	↓ Fluid volume overload ↓ Signs and symptoms of HF	Observe for electrolyte abnormalities, renal dysfunction, diuretic resistance, and ↓ BP. Carefully monitor I&O and daily weight (see Chart 25-2).
Thiazide diuretics: metolazone hydrochlorothiazide		
Aldosterone antagonists: spironolactone	Improves HF symptoms in advanced HF	Observe for ↑ serum K⁺, ↓ serum Na⁺.
Angiotensin System Blockers		
ACE Inhibitors: lisinopril enalapril	↓ BP and ↓ afterload Relieves signs and symptoms of HF Prevents progression of HF	Observe for symptomatic ↓ BP, ↑ serum K⁺, cough, and worsening renal function.
ARBs: valsartan losartan	↓ BP and ↓ afterload Relieves signs and symptoms of HF Prevents progression of HF	Observe for symptomatic ↓ BP, ↑ serum K⁺, and worsening renal function.
ARNI: sacubitril-valsartan	↓ BP and ↓ afterload ↓ Fluid volume overload ↓ Signs and symptoms of HF Prevents progression of HF	Observe for symptomatic ↓ BP, ↑ serum K⁺, cough, dizziness, and renal failure.
Beta-Adrenergic–Blocking Agents (Beta-Blockers)		
carvedilol bisoprolol metoprolol	Dilates blood vessels and ↓ afterload ↓ Signs and symptoms of HF Improves exercise capacity	Observe for ↓ heart rate, symptomatic ↓ BP, dizziness, and fatigue.
Ivabradine	Decreases rate of conduction through the SA node	Observe for ↓ heart rate, symptomatic ↓ BP, dizziness, and fatigue.
Hydralazine-isosorbide dinitrate	Dilates blood vessels ↓ BP and ↓ afterload	Observe for symptomatic ↓ BP.
Digitalis digoxin	Improves cardiac contractility ↓ Signs and symptoms of HF	Observe for ↓ heart rate and digitalis toxicity.

ACE, angiotensin-converting enzyme; ARB, angiotensin receptor blocker; ARNI, angiotensin receptor-neprilysin inhibitor; BP, blood pressure; ↓, decreases; HF, heart failure; ↑, increases; I&O, input and output; K⁺, potassium; Na⁺, sodium; SA, sinoatrial.
Adapted from Burchum, J. R., & Rosenthal, L. D. (2019). *Lehne's pharmacology for nursing care* (9th ed.). St. Louis, MO: Elsevier.

(Meyer, 2019b). The patient with HFpEF (diastolic HF) may be prescribed a diuretic, most commonly an aldosterone antagonist (see Table 25-3), and may also be prescribed an angiotensin system blocker and/or a beta-blocker and find symptomatic relief; however, these drugs are not necessarily associated with improved survival in those patients (Borlaug & Colucci, 2019). Target doses for these medications and alternative medications for treating heart failure are identified in the ACC/AHA guidelines. Nurses, primary providers, and pharmacists work collaboratively toward achieving effective dosing of these medications (Yancy et al., 2013; Yancy et al., 2016; Yancy et al., 2017).

Diuretics

Diuretics are prescribed to remove excess extracellular fluid by increasing diuresis in patients with signs and symptoms of fluid overload. ACC/AHA guidelines advocate using the smallest dose of diuretic necessary to control fluid volume (Yancy et al., 2013). The type and dose of diuretic prescribed depend on clinical signs and symptoms and renal function. Careful patient monitoring and dose adjustments are necessary to balance the effectiveness of these medications with the side effects (Chart 25-2). Loop, thiazide, and aldosterone-blocking diuretics may be prescribed; these medications differ

in their site of action in the kidney and their effects on renal electrolyte excretion and reabsorption.

Loop diuretics, such as furosemide, inhibit sodium and chloride reabsorption mainly in the ascending loop of Henle. Patients with HF and with severe volume overload are generally treated with a loop diuretic first (Burchum & Rosenthal, 2019). *Thiazide diuretics,* such as metolazone, inhibit sodium and chloride reabsorption in the early distal tubules. Both of these classes of diuretics increase potassium excretion; therefore, patients treated with these medications must have their serum potassium levels closely monitored. Diuretics can also lead to orthostatic hypotension and kidney injury. Both a loop and a thiazide diuretic may be used in patients with severe HF who are unresponsive to a single diuretic. The need for diuretics can be decreased if the patient avoids excessive fluid intake (e.g., more than 2000 mL/day) and adheres to a low sodium diet (e.g., no more than 2 g/day).

Aldosterone antagonists, such as spironolactone, are potassium-sparing diuretics that block the effects of aldosterone in the distal tubule and collecting duct (Yancy et al., 2016). As noted previously, they are frequently prescribed for patients with HFpEF. Serum creatinine and potassium levels are monitored frequently (e.g., within the first week and then

Chart 25-2 PHARMACOLOGY
Administering and Monitoring Diuretic Therapy

When nursing care involves diuretic therapy for conditions such as heart failure, the nurse needs to administer the medication and monitor the patient's response carefully, as follows:

- Prior to administration of the diuretic, check laboratory results for electrolyte depletion, especially potassium, sodium, and magnesium.
- Prior to administration of the diuretic, check for signs and symptoms of volume depletion, such as orthostatic hypotension, lightheadedness, and dizziness.
- Administer the diuretic at a time conducive to the patient's lifestyle—for example, early in the day to avoid nocturia.
- Monitor urine output during the hours after administration, and analyze intake, output, and daily weights to assess response.
- Monitor blood pressure for orthostatic changes.
- Continue to monitor serum electrolytes for depletion. Replace potassium with increased oral intake of food rich in potassium or potassium supplements. Replace magnesium as needed.
- Monitor for hyperkalemia in patients receiving potassium-sparing diuretics.
- Continue to assess for signs of volume depletion.
- Monitor creatinine for increased levels indicative of diuretic-induced renal dysfunction.
- Monitor for elevated uric acid level and signs and symptoms of gout.
- Assess lungs sounds and edema to evaluate response to therapy.
- Monitor for adverse reactions such as arrhythmias.
- Assist patients to manage urinary frequency and urgency associated with diuretic therapy.

Adapted from Burchum, J. R., & Rosenthal, L. D. (2019). *Lehne's pharmacology for nursing care* (10th ed.). St. Louis, MO: Elsevier.

every 4 weeks) when spironolactone is first given. These drugs are not prescribed for patients with an elevated serum creatinine.

Loop diuretics are administered IV for exacerbations of HF when rapid diuresis is necessary, as when pulmonary edema is present (see later discussion). Diuretics improve the patient's symptoms, provided that renal function is adequate. As HF progresses, cardiorenal syndrome may develop or worsen. Cardiorenal syndrome is a type of prerenal acute kidney injury characterized by a disruption in adequate blood flow to the kidneys. Patients with this syndrome are resistant to diuretics and may require other interventions to deal with congestive signs and symptoms.

Angiotensin System Blockers

Angiotensin system blockers include classes of medications such as the ACE inhibitors, angiotensin receptor blockers (ARBs), and angiotensin receptor-neprilysin inhibitors (ARNIs).

Angiotensin-Converting Enzyme Inhibitors

ACE inhibitors, such as lisinopril, have been found to relieve clinical manifestations of HF and significantly decrease mortality and morbidity in patients with HFrEF. Specifically, they slow the progression of HF, improve exercise tolerance,

and decrease the number of hospitalizations in patients with HFrEF (Yancy et al., 2013; Yancy et al., 2017). ACE inhibitors are also appropriate for hypertension management in patients with HFpEF (Yancy et al., 2017). Available as oral and IV medications, ACE inhibitors promote vasodilation and diuresis, ultimately decreasing both afterload and preload. Vasodilation reduces resistance to left ventricular ejection of blood, diminishing the heart's workload and improving ventricular emptying. ACE inhibitors decrease the secretion of aldosterone, a hormone that causes the kidneys to retain sodium and water. ACE inhibitors also promote renal excretion of sodium and fluid (while retaining potassium), thereby reducing left ventricular filling pressure and decreasing pulmonary congestion. These agents are also recommended for prevention of HF in patients at risk due to vascular disease and diabetes (Yancy et al., 2013; Yancy et al., 2017).

Patients receiving ACE inhibitors are monitored for hypotension, hyperkalemia (increased potassium in the blood), and alterations in renal function, especially if they are also receiving diuretics. Because ACE inhibitors cause the kidneys to retain potassium, the patient who is also receiving a loop diuretic or a thiazide diuretic may not need to take oral potassium supplements. However, the patient receiving a potassium-sparing diuretic, such as an aldosterone antagonist, which does not cause potassium loss with diuresis, must be carefully monitored for hyperkalemia. ACE inhibitors may be discontinued if the potassium level remains greater than 5.5 mEq/L or if the serum creatinine rises.

An adverse effect of ACE inhibitors includes a dry, persistent cough that may not respond to cough suppressants due to the inhibition of the enzyme kininase, which inactivates bradykinin. The nurse should carefully assess any cough in a patient taking an ACE inhibitor, as this symptom can also indicate a worsening of ventricular function and failure. In less than 1% of patients, ACE inhibitors may cause an allergic reaction accompanied by angioedema. This reaction tends to occur more frequently in African Americans and women (Yancy et al., 2016; Yancy et al., 2017). If angioedema affects the oropharyngeal area and impairs breathing, the ACE inhibitor must be stopped immediately and appropriate emergency care must be provided.

If the patient cannot continue taking an ACE inhibitor because of development of cough, an elevated creatinine level, or hyperkalemia, an ARB, an ARNI, or a combination of hydralazine and isosorbide dinitrate is prescribed (see Table 25-3).

Angiotensin Receptor Blockers

Whereas ACE inhibitors block the conversion of angiotensin I to angiotensin II, ARBs, such as valsartan, block the vasoconstricting effects of angiotensin II at the angiotensin II receptors. ARBs are commonly prescribed as an alternative to ACE inhibitors, as they are associated with reduced morbidity and mortality in patients with HFrEF and can provide symptomatic relief in patients with HFpEF who are intolerant of ACE inhibitors (Yancy et al., 2013; Yancy et al., 2017). ARBs do not inhibit kininase; therefore, ARBs are not associated with the bothersome cough that occurs with some patients prescribed an ACE inhibitor.

Angiotensin Receptor-Neprilysin Inhibitors

An ARNI combines an ARB with a neprilysin inhibitor. Neprilysin is an enzyme that breaks down natriuretic peptides. Participants with HFrEF enrolled in clinical trials who were prescribed an ARNI demonstrated a significant reduction in cardiovascular death or hospitalization as compared with participants prescribed an ACE inhibitor (Meyer, 2019b). Based on these findings, updated ACC/AHA guidelines advocate prescribing an ARNI as first-line angiotensin system blocker therapy for most patients with symptomatic HFrEF. However, an ARNI is reportedly a costlier option than most ACE inhibitors and ARBs, which may preclude its practical use. For patients unable to take an ARNI, an ACE inhibitor or ARB is a good alternative. An ARNI should not be administered concurrently or within 36 hours of an ACE inhibitor as concomitant dosing with both agents is associated with angioedema (Yancy et al., 2016; Yancy et al., 2017). Adverse effects associated with use of an ARNI are similar to those associated with ACE inhibitor or ARB use; therefore, the nurse should assess for hypotension, renal insufficiency, and angioedema in patients taking an ARNI (Yancy et al., 2016; Yancy et al., 2017). The first U.S. Food and Drug Administration (FDA) approved ARNI for use in patients with HF is sacubitril-valsartan.

Beta-Blockers

Beta-blockers block the adverse effects of the sympathetic nervous system. They relax blood vessels, lower blood pressure, decrease afterload, and decrease cardiac workload. Beta-blockers, such as carvedilol, have been found to improve functional status and reduce mortality and morbidity in patients with HF (Burchum & Rosenthal, 2019). In addition, beta-blockers have been recommended for patients with asymptomatic HFrEF to prevent progression and the onset of symptoms of HF, even if patients do not have a history of MI. The therapeutic effects of these drugs may not be seen for several weeks or even months (Yancy et al., 2013, Yancy et al., 2017).

Beta-blockers can produce a number of side effects, including dizziness, hypotension, bradycardia, fatigue, and depression. Side effects are most common in the initial few weeks of treatment. Because of the potential for side effects, beta-blockers are started at a low dose. The dose is titrated up slowly (every few weeks), with close monitoring after each dosage increase. Nurses educate patients about potential symptoms during the early phase of treatment and stress that adjustment to the drug may take several weeks. Nurses must also provide support to patients going through this symptom-provoking phase of treatment. Because beta-blockade can cause bronchiole constriction, these drugs are used with caution in patients with a history of bronchospastic diseases such as asthma.

Ivabradine

Ivabradine is a new agent that is a hyperpolarization-activated cyclic nucleotide channel blocker. It is a medication with unique electrophysiologic effects, characterized by its negative chronotropic effect on the sinoatrial node, thereby decreasing the heart rate without targeting the neurohormonal system. It is indicated as an adjunct agent to beta-blockers in patients with symptomatic HFrEF and with high resting heart rates of at least 70 bpm (Koruth, Lala, Pinney, et al., 2017). It may also be beneficial for patients with HFrEF who cannot tolerate beta-blockers (Yancy et al., 2017). Adverse effects of ivabradine include bradycardia resulting in dizziness and fatigue; it is also associated with an increased risk of atrial fibrillation (Koruth et al., 2017).

Hydralazine and Isosorbide Dinitrate

A combination of hydralazine and isosorbide dinitrate may be an alternative medication for patients who cannot take any of the three angiotensin system blockers (i.e., ACE inhibitor, ARB, and ARNI), so long as the patient's systolic BP is at least 90 mm Hg. Nitrates (e.g., isosorbide dinitrate) cause venous dilation, which reduces the amount of blood return to the heart and lowers preload. Hydralazine lowers systemic vascular resistance and left ventricular afterload. Hydralazine-isosorbide dinitrate is associated with decreased hospitalizations and improved survival in patients with HFrEF; however, these improvements are not as robust as those associated with angiotensin system blockers (Meyer, 2019b; Yancy et al., 2017). Adverse effects may include hypotension, and rarely, a lupus-type reaction (Meyer, 2019b).

Digitalis

For many years, digitalis (i.e., digoxin) was considered an essential agent for the treatment of HF. With the introduction of newer medications, it is not prescribed as often. Digoxin increases the force of myocardial contraction and slows conduction through the atrioventricular node. It improves contractility, increasing left ventricular output. Although the use of digoxin does not result in decreased mortality rates among patients with HFrEF, it can be effective in decreasing the symptoms of HF and may help prevent hospitalization (Yancy et al., 2013). Patients with renal dysfunction and older patients should receive smaller doses of digoxin, as it is excreted through the kidneys.

A key concern associated with digoxin therapy is digitalis toxicity. Clinical manifestations of toxicity include anorexia, nausea, visual disturbances, confusion, and bradycardia. The serum potassium level is monitored because the effect of digoxin is enhanced in the presence of hypokalemia and digoxin toxicity may occur. A serum digoxin level is obtained if the patient's renal function changes or there are symptoms of toxicity.

 ### Intravenous Infusions

IV inotropes (e.g., dopamine, dobutamine, milrinone) increase the force of myocardial contraction; as such, they may be indicated for hospitalized patients with pulmonary edema (i.e., acute decompensated HF). These agents are used for patients who do not respond to routine pharmacologic therapy and are reserved for patients with severe ventricular dysfunction, low blood pressure, or impaired perfusion and evidence of significantly depressed CO, with or without congestion. They are used with caution, as some studies have associated their use with increased mortality (Malotte, Saguros, & Groninger, 2018; Yancy et al., 2013). Patients usually require admission to the intensive care unit (ICU) and may also have hemodynamic monitoring with a pulmonary artery catheter or alternative technology (see Chapter 21). Hemodynamic data are used to assess cardiac function and volume status and to guide therapy with inotropes, vasodilators, and diuretics (Urden, Stacy, & Lough, 2018). Patients with end-stage HF who cannot be weaned from IV inotropes may be candidates for continuous therapy at home (Malotte et al., 2018).

Dopamine

Dopamine is a vasopressor given to increase BP and myocardial contractility. Given at low doses, a dopamine infusion may be helpful as an adjunct therapy along with loop diuretics in improving diuresis, preserving renal function, and improving renal blood flow (Yancy et al., 2013).

Dobutamine

Dobutamine is given to patients with significant left ventricular dysfunction and hypoperfusion. A catecholamine, dobutamine stimulates the beta-1 adrenergic receptors. Its major action is to increase cardiac contractility and renal perfusion to enhance urine output. However, it also increases the heart rate and can precipitate ectopic beats and tachyarrhythmias (Burchum & Rosenthal, 2019).

Milrinone

Milrinone is a phosphodiesterase inhibitor that leads to an increase in intracellular calcium within myocardial cells, increasing their contractility (Ayres & Maani, 2019). This agent also promotes vasodilation, resulting in decreased preload and afterload and reduced cardiac workload. Milrinone is administered IV to patients with severe HF, including patients who are waiting for heart transplantation (see Chapter 24). Because the drug causes vasodilation, the patient's blood pressure is monitored prior to administration; if the patient is hypovolemic, the blood pressure could drop quickly. The major side effects are hypotension and increased ventricular arrhythmias. Blood pressure and ECG are monitored closely during and following infusions of milrinone.

Vasodilators

Intravenous vasodilators such as IV nitroglycerin, nitroprusside, or nesiritide may enhance symptom relief for acutely decompensated HF (Yancy et al., 2013). Their use is contraindicated in patients who are hypotensive. Blood pressure is continually assessed in patients receiving IV vasodilator infusions.

Adjunct Medications for Heart Failure

The importance of ensuring that patients with hypertension take prescribed antihypertensive agents as prescribed is of paramount importance (see Chapter 27 for further discussion of antihypertensive medications). Target blood pressures should be less than 130/80 mm Hg. Maintaining BPs at these levels is associated with reduced likelihood of morbid progression to symptomatic HF in patients who are asymptomatic. It is also associated with improved morbidity in patients who are symptomatic with both HFrEF and HFpEF (Yancy et al., 2017).

Anemia is independently associated with HF disease severity, and iron deficiency appears to be uniquely associated with reduced exercise capacity. IV iron repletion in patients with HF may improve functional capacity and quality of life; however, there is mixed evidence to support the use of oral iron supplementation. Erythropoietin-stimulating agents, such as darbepoetin alfa, are not recommended in patients with both HF and anemia as a risk of thromboembolic events associated with their use has been observed during clinical trials (Yancy et al., 2017).

Anticoagulants may be prescribed, especially if the patient has a history of atrial fibrillation or a thromboembolic event. Antiarrhythmic drugs such as amiodarone may be prescribed for patients with arrhythmias, along with an evaluation for device therapy with an implantable cardioverter defibrillator (ICD) (see Chapter 22). Medications to manage hyperlipidemia (e.g., statins) are also routinely prescribed, in tandem with guidance on nutritional therapy (see following section). It is recommended that patients with HF avoid nonsteroidal anti-inflammatory drugs (NSAIDs) such as ibuprofen because the risk of decreased renal perfusion is higher, especially in older adults (Schwartz, Schmader, Hanlon, et al., 2018).

Adjunct Therapies for Heart Failure

Additional therapies that may be indicated in the treatment of patients with HF include nutritional therapy, supplemental oxygen, management of sleep disorders, and procedural or surgical interventions.

Nutritional Therapy

Following a low sodium (no more than 2 g/day) diet and avoiding excessive fluid intake are usually recommended, although studies differ regarding the effectiveness of sodium restriction (Yancy et al., 2013). Decreasing dietary sodium reduces fluid retention and the symptoms of peripheral and pulmonary congestion. The purpose of sodium restriction is to decrease the amount of circulating blood volume, which decreases myocardial work. A balance should be achieved between the patient's ability to adhere to the diet and the recommended guidelines.

Nutritional supplements, such as vitamins and antioxidants, are not recommended for patients with HF as no benefits are associated with their use. Omega-3 polyunsaturated fatty acid (PUFA) supplementation is associated with decreased fatal cardiovascular events and is recommended for patients with either HFrEF or HFpEF, unless contraindicated (Yancy et al., 2013).

Any change in eating patterns should consider good nutrition as well as the patient's likes, dislikes, and cultural food patterns. Patient adherence is important because dietary indiscretions may result in exacerbations of HF symptoms. However, behavioral changes in eating patterns are difficult for many patients to achieve.

Supplemental Oxygen

Oxygen therapy may become necessary as HF progresses based on the degree of pulmonary congestion and resulting hypoxia. Some patients require supplemental oxygen only during periods of activity (see Chapter 20 for further discussion of oxygen delivery systems).

Management of Sleep Disorders

Sleep disorders, including sleep apnea, are common in patients with HF. It is estimated that 61% of patients with HF have either central or obstructive sleep apnea (OSA). A formal sleep study should be performed. Continuous positive airway pressure (CPAP) might be recommended if results from the sleep study suggest OSA (see Chapter 18). CPAP has been shown to improve sleep quality, reduce apneic episodes and excessive daytime sleepiness, and improve nocturnal oxygenation in patients with OSA and HF (Yancy et al., 2017).

Procedural and Surgical Interventions

A number of procedures and surgical approaches may benefit patients with HF. If the patient has underlying CAD, coronary artery revascularization with PCI or coronary artery bypass surgery (see Chapter 23) may be considered. Ventricular function may improve in some patients when coronary flow is increased.

Patients with HF are at high risk for arrhythmias, and sudden cardiac death is common among patients with advanced HF. In patients with severe left ventricular dysfunction and the possibility of life-threatening arrhythmias, placement of an ICD can prevent sudden cardiac death and extend survival (see Chapter 22). Candidates for an ICD include those with an EF less than 35%, including those with and without a history of ventricular arrhythmias (Yancy et al., 2013).

Patients with HF who do not improve with standard therapy may benefit from **cardiac resynchronization therapy (CRT)**. CRT involves the use of a biventricular pacemaker to treat electrical conduction defects and to synchronize ventricular contractions. A prolonged QRS duration on ECG indicates left bundle branch block, which is a type of delayed conduction that is frequently seen in patients with HF. This problem results in asynchronous conduction and contraction of the right and left ventricles, which can further decrease EF (Yancy et al., 2013). The use of a pacing device with leads placed in the right atrium, right ventricle, and left ventricular cardiac vein can synchronize the contractions of the right and left ventricles (Fig. 25-3). This intervention improves CO, optimizes myocardial energy consumption, reduces mitral regurgitation, and slows the ventricular remodeling process. For patients with a CRT, improvement of left ventricular EF is associated with reduced rates of ventricular arrhythmias. There are combination devices available for patients who require CRT and an ICD (Gulati & Udelson, 2018). See Chapter 22 for further discussion of care of patients with pacemakers, CRT, and ICDs.

Ultrafiltration is an alternative intervention for patients with severe fluid overload. It is reserved for patients with advanced HF who are resistant to diuretic therapy (Yancy et al., 2013). A dual-lumen central IV catheter is placed, and the patient's blood is circulated through a small bedside filtration machine. Liters of excess fluid and plasma are removed slowly from the patient's intravascular circulating volume over a number of hours. The patient's output of filtration fluid, blood pressure, and hemoglobin (analyzed for hemoconcentration) are monitored as indicators of volume status.

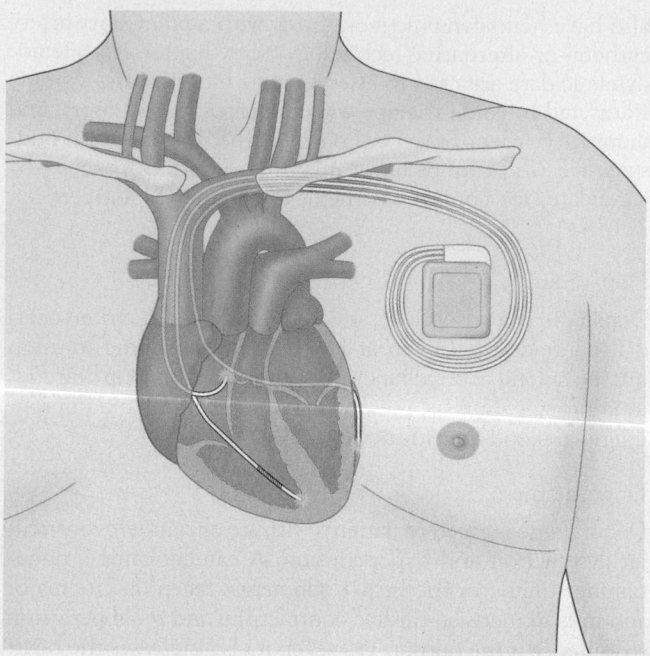

Figure 25-3 • Cardiac resynchronization therapy. To pace both ventricles, pacemaker leads are placed in the right atrium and right ventricle; a third lead is threaded through the coronary sinus into a lateral vein on the wall of the left ventricle.

Research on ultrafiltration is ongoing, and targets comparisons of its efficacy to diuretics and the optimal fluid removal target (Costanzo, 2019).

For some patients with end-stage HF, cardiac transplantation is one of the few options for long-term survival. Patients with ACC/AHA stage D HF who may be eligible are referred for consideration of transplantation. Some of these patients require mechanical circulatory assistance with an implanted ventricular assist device as a bridge therapy to cardiac transplantation. A left ventricular assist device may also be implanted as *destination therapy* (permanent therapy) for select patients (Yancy et al., 2013).

 Gerontologic Considerations

Several normal age-related changes increase the frequency of HF: increased systolic blood pressure, increased ventricular wall thickness, and increased myocardial fibrosis. There are a number of reasons that older adults may need to be hospitalized with HF (Albert, Barnason, Deswal, et al., 2015). Older adults may not always detect or accurately interpret common symptoms of HF such as shortness of breath, or they may have atypical symptoms such as weakness and somnolence. Decreased renal function can make the older patient resistant to diuretics and more sensitive to changes in volume. The administration of diuretics to older men requires nursing surveillance for bladder distention caused by urethral obstruction from an enlarged prostate gland. The bladder may be assessed with an ultrasound scanner or the suprapubic area palpated for an oval mass and percussed for dullness, indicative of bladder fullness. Urinary frequency and urgency may be particularly stressful to older patients, as many have arthritis and limited mobility.

NURSING PROCESS

The Patient with Heart Failure

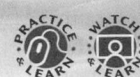

Despite advances in treatment of HF, morbidity and mortality remain high. Nurses have a major impact on outcomes for patients with HF, especially in the areas of patient education and monitoring.

Assessment

Nursing assessment for the patient with HF focuses on observing for effectiveness of therapy and for the patient's ability to understand and implement self-care management strategies. Signs and symptoms of worsening HF are analyzed and reported to the patient's provider so that therapy can be adjusted. The nurse also explores the patient's emotional response to the diagnosis of HF, because it is a chronic and often progressive condition that is commonly associated with depression and other psychosocial issues (Jiang, Shorey, Seah, et al., 2018).

Health History

The health history focuses on the signs and symptoms of HF, such as dyspnea, fatigue, and edema. Sleep disturbances, particularly sleep suddenly interrupted by shortness of breath, may be reported. Patients are asked about the number of pillows needed for sleep, edema, abdominal symptoms, altered mental status, activities of daily living, and the activities that cause fatigue. Nurses need to be aware of the variety of clinical manifestations that may indicate worsening HF and assess the patient accordingly. While obtaining the patient's history, the nurse assesses the patient's understanding of HF, self-care management strategies, and the patient's ability and willingness to adhere to those strategies.

Physical Examination

The patient is observed for restlessness and anxiety that might suggest hypoxia from pulmonary congestion. The patient's level of consciousness is also evaluated for any changes, as low CO can decrease the flow of oxygen to the brain.

The rate and depth of respirations are assessed along with the effort required for breathing. The lungs are auscultated to detect crackles and wheezes (Meyer, 2019a). Crackles are produced by the sudden opening of edematous narrowed airways and alveoli. They may be heard at the end of inspiration and are not cleared with coughing. Wheezing may also be heard in some patients who have bronchospasm along with pulmonary congestion.

The blood pressure is carefully evaluated, because patients with HF may present with hypotension or hypertension. Patients may be assessed for orthostatic hypotension, especially if they report lightheadedness, dizziness, or syncope. The heart is auscultated for an S_3 heart sound, which is an early sign that increased blood volume fills the ventricle with each beat. Heart rate and rhythm are also documented, and patients are often placed on continuous ECG monitoring in the hospital setting. When the heart rate is rapid or very slow, the CO decreases and potentially worsens the HF. JVD is assessed with the patient sitting at a 45-degree angle; distention greater than 4 cm above the sternal angle is considered abnormal and indicative of right ventricular failure (Bickley, 2017). This is an estimate, not a precise measurement, of high central venous pressure.

The nurse assesses peripheral pulses and rates their volume on a scale from 0 (not palpable) to 3+ (bounding). The skin is also assessed for color and temperature. With significant decreases in SV, there is a decrease in perfusion to the periphery, decreasing the volume of pulses and causing the skin to feel cool and appear pale or cyanotic. The feet and lower legs are examined for edema; if the patient is supine in bed, the sacrum and back are also assessed for edema. The upper extremities may also become edematous in some patients. Edema is typically rated on a scale from 0 (no edema) to 4+ (severe pitting edema).

The abdomen is examined for tenderness and hepatomegaly. The presence of firmness, distention, and possible ascites is noted. The liver may be assessed for hepatojugular reflux. The patient is asked to breathe normally while manual pressure is applied over the right upper quadrant of the abdomen for 30–60 s. If neck vein distention increases more than 1 cm, the finding is positive for increased venous pressure.

If the patient is hospitalized, the nurse measures urinary output and evaluates it in terms of diuretic use. Intake and output records are rigorously maintained and analyzed. It is important to track whether the patient has excreted excessive volume (i.e., negative fluid balance is generally the goal). The intake and output is then compared with changes in weight. Although diuresis is expected, the patient with HF must also be monitored for **oliguria** (diminished urine output, less than 0.5 mL/kg/h for at least 6 h or <400 mL/24 h) or **anuria** (urine output of less than 50 mL/24 h) because of the risk of renal dysfunction.

The patient is weighed daily in the hospital or at home, at the same time of day, with the same type of clothing, and on the same scale. If there is a significant change in weight (i.e., 2–3-lb increase in a day or 5-lb increase in a wk), the primary provider is notified and medications are adjusted (e.g., the diuretic dose is increased).

Diagnosis

NURSING DIAGNOSES

Based on the assessment data, major nursing diagnoses may include the following:

- Activity intolerance associated with decreased CO
- Hypervolaemia associated with the HF syndrome
- Anxiety associated with clinical manifestations of HF
- Powerlessness associated with chronic illness and hospitalizations
- Impaired family ability to manage regime

COLLABORATIVE PROBLEMS/POTENTIAL COMPLICATIONS

Potential complications may include the following:

- Pulmonary edema
- Hypotension, poor perfusion, and cardiogenic shock (see Chapter 11)
- Arrhythmias (see Chapter 22)
- Thromboembolism (see Chapter 26)
- Pericardial effusion (see later discussion in this chapter)

Planning and Goals

Major goals for the patient may include promoting activity and reducing fatigue, relieving fluid overload symptoms, decreasing anxiety or increasing the patient's ability to manage anxiety, encouraging the patient to verbalize their ability to make decisions and influence outcomes, and educating the patient and family about health management.

Nursing Interventions

Nursing interventions revolve around promoting the patient's activity tolerance, managing the patient's fluid volume status, assisting the patient so that anxiety is relieved, helping to minimize any feelings of powerlessness that the patient might experience, and assisting the patient and family members to effectively manage the patient's health. In addition, nursing interventions must be attuned to prevent and manage acute complications that can be experienced by patients with HF.

PROMOTING ACTIVITY TOLERANCE

Reduced physical activity caused by HF symptoms leads to physical deconditioning that worsens the patient's symptoms and exercise tolerance. Prolonged inactivity, which may be self-imposed, should be avoided because of its deconditioning effects and risks, such as pressure injuries (especially in edematous patients) and venous thromboembolism. An acute illness that exacerbates HF symptoms or requires hospitalization may be an indication for temporary bed rest. Otherwise, some type of physical activity every day should be encouraged. A typical program for a patient with HF might include a daily walking regimen, with the duration increased over a 6-wk period. The primary provider, nurse, and patient collaborate to develop a schedule that promotes pacing and prioritization of activities. The schedule should alternate activities with periods of rest and avoid having two significant energy-consuming activities occur on the same day or in immediate succession. Before undertaking physical activity, the patient should be given guidelines similar to those noted in Chart 25-3. Because some patients may be severely debilitated, they may need to limit physical activities to only 3–5 min at a time, one to four times per day. The patient should

---

Chart 25-3 **HEALTH PROMOTION**

An Exercise Program for Patients with Heart Failure

Before undertaking physical activity, the patient should be given the following guidelines:

- Talk with your primary provider for specific exercise program recommendations.
- Begin with low-impact activities such as walking.
- Start with warm-up activity followed by sessions that gradually build up to about 30 min.
- Follow your exercise period with cool-down activities.
- Avoid performing physical activities outside in extreme hot, cold, or humid weather.
- Wait 2 h after eating a meal before performing the physical activity.
- Ensure that you are able to talk during the physical activity; if you cannot do so, decrease the intensity of activity.
- Stop the activity if severe shortness of breath, pain, or dizziness develops.

Adapted from Piña, I. L. (2019). Cardiac rehabilitation in patients with heart failure. *UpToDate*. Retrieved on 9/11/2019 at: www.uptodate.com/contents/cardiac-rehabilitation-in-patients-with-heart-failure

---

increase the duration of the activity, then the frequency, before increasing the intensity of the activity (Piña, 2019).

Barriers to performing activities are identified, and methods of adjusting an activity are discussed. For example, vegetables can be chopped or peeled while sitting at the kitchen table rather than standing at the kitchen counter. Small, frequent meals decrease the amount of energy needed for digestion while providing adequate nutrition. The nurse helps the patient identify peak and low periods of energy, planning energy-consuming activities for peak periods. For example, the patient may prepare the meals for the entire day in the morning. Pacing and prioritizing activities help maintain the patient's energy to promote participation in regular physical activity.

The patient's response to activities needs to be monitored. If the patient is hospitalized, vital signs and oxygen saturation levels are monitored before, during, and immediately after an activity to identify whether they are within the desired range. Heart rate should return to baseline within 3 min following the activity. If the patient is at home, the degree of fatigue felt after the activity can be used to assess the response. If the patient tolerates the activity, short- and long-term goals can be developed to gradually increase the intensity, duration, and frequency of activity.

Adherence to exercise training is essential if the patient is to benefit from it, but it may be difficult for patients with other comorbid conditions (e.g., arthritis, anemia, cardiomyopathy, obesity, chronic kidney disease, chronic obstructive pulmonary disease) and those who have had HF for a longer time (Cattadori, Segurini, Picozzi, et al., 2018). Referral to a cardiac rehabilitation program may be indicated, especially for patients newly diagnosed with HF (Piña, 2019). A supervised program may also benefit those who need a structured environment, significant educational support, regular encouragement, and interpersonal contact.

MANAGING FLUID VOLUME

Patients with severe HF may receive IV diuretic therapy; however, patients with less severe symptoms are typically prescribed oral diuretics. Oral diuretics should be given early in the morning so that diuresis does not interfere with the patient's nighttime rest. Discussing the timing of medication administration is especially important for older patients who may have urinary urgency or incontinence. A single dose of a diuretic may cause the patient to excrete a large volume of fluid shortly after its administration.

The patient's fluid status is monitored closely by auscultating the lungs, monitoring daily body weight, and assisting the patient to adhere to a low sodium diet by reading food labels and avoiding high sodium foods such as canned, processed, and convenience foods (Chart 25-4). Weight gain in a patient with HF almost always reflects fluid retention. If the diet includes fluid restriction, the nurse can assist the patient to plan fluid intake throughout the day while respecting the patient's dietary preferences. If the patient is receiving IV fluids and medications, the amount of fluid needs to be monitored closely, and the primary provider or pharmacist can be consulted about the possibility of maximizing the amount of medication in the same volume of IV fluid (e.g., double concentrating to decrease the fluid volume given).

The patient is positioned or taught how to assume a position that facilitates breathing. The number of pillows may

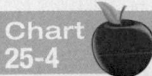

HEALTH PROMOTION
Facts About Dietary Sodium

Although the major source of sodium in the average American diet is salt, many types of natural foods contain varying amounts of sodium. Even if no salt is added in cooking and if salty foods are avoided, the daily diet will still contain about 2000 mg of sodium. Fresh fruits and vegetables are low in sodium and should be encouraged.

Additives in Food

In general, food prepared at home is lower in sodium than restaurant or processed foods. Added food substances (additives), such as sodium alginate, which improves food texture, sodium benzoate, which acts as a preservative, and disodium phosphate, which improves cooking quality in certain foods, increase the sodium intake when included in the daily diet. Therefore, patients on low sodium diets should be advised to check labels carefully for words such as "salt" or "sodium," especially on canned foods. For example, without looking at the sodium content per serving found on the nutrition labels, when given a choice between a serving of potato chips and a cup of canned cream of mushroom soup, most would think that soup is lower in sodium. However, when the labels are examined, the lower sodium choice is found to be the chips. Although potato chips are *not* recommended in a low sodium diet, this example illustrates that it is important to read food labels to determine both sodium content and serving size.

Nonfood Sodium Sources

Sodium is contained in municipal water. Water softeners also increase the sodium content of drinking water. Patients on sodium-restricted diets should be cautioned against using nonprescription medications such as antacids, cough syrups, and laxatives. Salt substitutes may be allowed, but it is recognized that they are high in potassium. Over-the-counter medications should not be used without first consulting the patient's primary provider.

Promoting Dietary Adherence

If patients find food unpalatable because of the dietary sodium restrictions and/or the taste disturbances caused by the medications, they may refuse to eat or to follow the dietary regimen. For this reason, severe sodium restrictions should be avoided, and diuretic medication should be balanced with the patient's ability to restrict dietary sodium. A variety of flavorings, such as lemon juice, vinegar, and herbs, may be used to improve the taste of the food and facilitate acceptance of the diet. It is important to consider the patient's food preferences. Diet counseling and educational handouts can be geared toward a patient–family-centered approach and with cultural practices considered.

Adapted from American Heart Association (AHA). (2016). Shaking the salt habit. Retrieved on 10/24/2019 at: www.heart.org/HEARTORG/Conditions/HighBloodPressure/PreventionTreatmentofHighBloodPressure/Shaking-the-Salt-Habit_UCM_303241_Article.jsp#.Vzy9eNe3BK8

be increased, the head of the bed may be elevated, or the patient may sit in a recliner. In these positions, the venous return to the heart (preload) is reduced, pulmonary congestion is reduced, and pressure on the diaphragm is minimized. The lower arms can be supported with pillows to eliminate the fatigue caused by the pull of the patient's weight on the shoulder muscles. If the patient is experiencing acute decompensation, positioning them upright, preferably with the legs dangling over the side of the bed, has the immediate effect of decreasing venous return, decreasing right ventricular stroke volume, and decreasing lung congestion.

Because decreased circulation in edematous areas increases the risk of pressure injuries, the nurse assesses for skin breakdown and institutes preventive measures. Positioning to avoid pressure and frequent changes of position help prevent pressure injuries.

CONTROLLING ANXIETY

Patients with HF may exhibit signs and symptoms of anxiety. In addition to psychosocial sources of anxiety, the physiologic compensatory mechanisms include activation of neurohormones including catecholamines. Complex medical interventions, such as implantation of an ICD can provoke anxiety in patients and families. These sources of anxiety include living with the threat of shocks, role changes, and concerns about the patient's ability to carry out activities of daily living. The patient's anxiety may intensify at night and interfere with sleep. Emotional stress further stimulates the sympathetic nervous system, causing vasoconstriction, elevated arterial pressure, and increased heart rate. This sympathetic response increases cardiac workload.

When the patient exhibits anxiety, the nurse takes steps to promote physical comfort and provide psychological support. As mentioned previously, the patient may be more comfortable sitting in a recliner. Oxygen may be given during an acute event to diminish the work of breathing and increase the patient's comfort. In many cases, a family member's presence provides reassurance. Patients with HF rely on their families for many aspects of care; therefore, nurses should assess the needs of family caregivers and provide support to them (Hodson, Peacock, & Holtslander, 2019).

Along with reassurance, the nurse can begin educating the patient and family about techniques for controlling anxiety and avoiding anxiety-provoking situations. This includes how to identify factors that contribute to anxiety and how to use relaxation techniques to control anxious feelings. As the patient's anxiety decreases, cardiac function may improve and symptoms of HF may decrease.

 Quality and Safety Nursing Alert

When patients with HF are delirious, confused, or anxious, restraints should be avoided. Restraints are likely to be resisted, and resistance inevitably increases the cardiac workload.

MINIMIZING POWERLESSNESS

Patients with HF may feel overwhelmed with their diagnosis and treatment regimen, leading to feelings of powerlessness. Contributing factors may include lack of knowledge and lack of opportunity to make decisions, particularly if health care providers or family members do not encourage the patient to participate in the treatment decision-making process.

Nurses should help patients recognize their choices, and that they can positively influence the outcomes of their diagnosis and treatment. Taking time to listen actively to patients encourages them to express their concerns and ask questions. Other strategies include providing the patient with decision making opportunities, such as when activities are to occur, or encouraging food and fluid choices consistent with the dietary restrictions. Encouragement is provided, progress is identified, and the patient is assisted to differentiate between factors that can and cannot be controlled.

In addition to feelings of powerlessness, patients with HF have a high incidence of depressive symptoms, which are associated with increased morbidity and mortality (Jiang et al., 2018). Because depressive symptoms are known to increase as the disease worsens, patients with HF need to be screened for depression so that it can be treated, hopefully maintaining the patient's functional status and quality of life.

ASSISTING PATIENTS AND FAMILIES TO EFFECTIVELY MANAGE HEALTH

Therapeutic regimens for HF are complex and require the patient and family to make significant lifestyle changes. An inability or unwillingness to adhere to dietary and pharmacologic recommendations can lead to episodes of acute decompensated HF and hospitalization. Nonadherence with prescribed diet and fluid restrictions and medications cause many hospital readmissions. Nursing research findings suggest that for some patients with HF who are taking more than one medication daily, the decision to not take HF medications as prescribed may actually reflect their efforts to best manage their personal health, and, therefore, may be a self-care strategy (see the Nursing Research Profile in Chart 25-5) (Meraz, 2020).

Nurses have a key role in managing episodes of acute decompensated HF and in developing a comprehensive education and discharge plan to prevent hospital readmissions and increase the patient's quality of life. Because of the high cost of hospitalization for HF, the Centers for Medicare & Medicaid Services (CMS) initiated a program that reduces reimbursement to hospitals with a high 30-d readmission rate (U.S. Department of Health and Human Services [HHS], 2019). Research continues to identify the most effective interventions that may decrease these rates. A number of evidence-based components are known to increase the effectiveness of a discharge plan for patients with HF, including providing them with comprehensive, patient-centered instructions, scheduling follow-up visits with their primary providers within 7 d of discharge, and following up by telephone within 3 d of discharge (Yancy et al., 2013; Yancy et al., 2016; Yancy et al., 2017).

MONITORING AND MANAGING POTENTIAL COMPLICATIONS

Because HF is a complex and progressive condition, patients are at risk for many complications, including acute decompensated HF and pulmonary edema; hypotension and cardiogenic shock (see Chapter 11); arrhythmias (see Chapter 22); thromboembolism formation (see Chapter 26); and pericardial effusion (see later discussion).

Pulmonary Edema. As described previously, pulmonary edema is associated with acute decompensated HF that can lead to acute respiratory failure and death. If it is recognized early, pulmonary edema may be alleviated by increasing dosages of diuretics and by implementing other interventions to decrease preload. For instance, placing the patient in an upright position with the feet and legs dependent

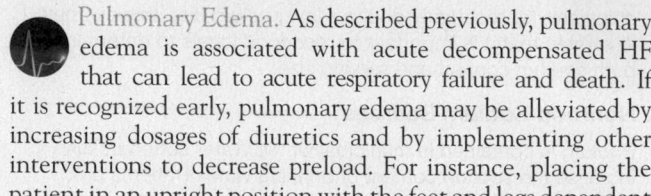

NURSING RESEARCH PROFILE

Chart 25-5

Medication Nonadherence or Self-Care?

Meraz, R. (2020). Medication nonadherence or self-care? Understanding the medication decision-making process and experiences of older adults with heart failure. *Journal of Cardiovascular Nursing, 35*(1), 26–34.

Purpose

It is estimated that over half of patients with heart failure do not take their medications as prescribed. The reasons why many patients with heart failure do not adhere to their prescribed medication regimen are elusive, particularly since nonadherence is associated with hospitalization and emergency department visits. Therefore, the purpose of this study was to discover why patients with heart failure might not take their heart failure medications as prescribed.

Design

This was a qualitative study that used narrative inquiry and storytelling to discover why community dwelling patients with heart failure might not adhere to their medication regimen. Eleven participants, all 65 y of age or older, volunteered to be interviewed. Each of these participants had to live independently in the community setting, had to take at least two medications daily to treat heart failure, and had to self-administer these medications in order to be eligible to participate in this study.

Findings

Results from participant interviews found that patients' nonadherence with the prescribed medication regimen was deliberate, and not because of forgetfulness. In all reported instances, it was not contingent upon financial constraints, either. Some participants stopped taking a medication while others adjusted the dosages. Participants' deliberate decisions to adjust their medication regimen tended to be made based on the belief that they knew their own bodies and needs best, and felt that they were best equipped to take care of their own needs. Others noted that at times it was too difficult to get in contact with their primary providers or nurses, and that their primary providers or nurses were too busy to discuss their medication regimen with them. Most noted that they researched online their medications' effects and felt competent to manage their medication dosage without necessarily consulting their providers. Paradoxically, participants did not view their decisions to self-adjust their prescribed medication regimens as consonant with nonadherence.

Nursing Implications

Patients with heart failure who are prescribed multiple medications to treat their heart failure may not view self-adjustment of their prescriptions as tantamount to nonadherence. It seems likely that these self-care/nonadherent practices place these patients at risk for hospitalization and morbid complications. Participants in this study noted that one key reason that they self-adjusted their medications was because their primary providers and nurses were "too busy" to talk to them about their medications. Nurses are in an ideal position to talk to patients with heart failure about their prescriptions, discover their concerns about their medications, help them find ways to problem-solve and manage side effects, and help them proactively engage in self-care so that they avoid hospitalization.

reduces left ventricular workload. The treatment regimen and the patient's understanding of and adherence to it are assessed. The long-range approach for preventing pulmonary edema must be directed at identifying and managing its precipitating factors.

Clinical management of a patient with acute pulmonary edema due to left ventricular failure is directed toward reducing volume overload, improving ventricular function, and increasing oxygenation. These goals are accomplished through a combination of oxygen and ventilatory support, IV medication, and nursing assessment and interventions.

The patient's airway and breathing are assessed to determine the severity of respiratory distress, along with vital signs. The patient is placed on pulse oximetry, a cardiac monitor, and IV access is confirmed or established for administration of medications. Laboratory tests are obtained, including arterial blood gases, electrolytes, BUN, and creatinine; other laboratory tests that may be indicated include a complete blood cell count (CBC), BNP, or a serum troponin-I. A chest x-ray or an ultrasound of the lungs may be obtained to confirm the extent of pulmonary edema (Meyer, 2019a).

Oxygen is given in concentrations adequate to relieve hypoxemia and dyspnea; a non-rebreathing mask may be used initially. If respiratory failure is severe or persists, noninvasive positive-pressure ventilation is the preferred mode of assisted ventilation (Colucci, 2019). For some patients, endotracheal (ET) intubation and mechanical ventilation are required. The ventilator can provide positive end-expiratory pressure (PEEP), which is effective in reducing venous return, decreasing fluid movement from the pulmonary capillaries to the alveoli, and improving oxygenation (see Chapter 19). Oxygenation is monitored by pulse oximetry and by measurement of arterial blood gases.

The patient who is experiencing pulmonary edema is likely going to be highly anxious, as are the patient's family members. As the ability to breathe decreases, the patient's fear and anxiety rise proportionately, making the condition more severe. Reassuring the patient and family and providing skillful anticipatory nursing care are integral parts of the therapy. Because the patient is in an unstable condition, the nurse must remain with the patient. The nurse gives the patient simple, concise information in a reassuring voice about what is being done to treat the condition and the expected results.

Vasodilators such as IV nitroglycerin or nitroprusside may enhance symptom relief in pulmonary edema, as previously described (Meyer, 2019a). Blood pressure is continually assessed in patients receiving IV vasodilator infusions.

Furosemide or another loop diuretic is given by IV push or as a continuous infusion to produce a rapid diuretic effect. The blood pressure is closely monitored as the urine output increases, because it is possible for the patient to become hypotensive as intravascular volume decreases. The patient receiving diuretic therapy may excrete a large volume of urine within minutes after a potent diuretic is given. A bedside commode may be used to decrease the energy required by the patient and to reduce the resultant increase in cardiac workload induced by getting on and off a bedpan. If necessary, in order to carefully monitor urine output, an indwelling urinary catheter may be inserted.

Once the patient is stable, they may transition to oral diuretics; intake and output, daily weights, serum electrolytes, and creatinine are carefully monitored.

Many potential problems associated with HF therapy relate to the use of diuretics. These problems require ongoing nursing assessment and collaborative intervention:

Excessive and repeated diuresis can lead to hypokalemia (i.e., potassium depletion). Signs include ventricular arrhythmias, hypotension, muscle weakness, and generalized weakness. In patients receiving digoxin, hypokalemia can lead to digitalis toxicity, which increases the likelihood of dangerous arrhythmias. Patients with HF may also develop low levels of magnesium, which can add to the risk of arrhythmias. Hyperkalemia may occur, especially with the use of ACE inhibitors, ARBs, or spironolactone. Hyperkalemia can also lead to profound bradycardia and other arrhythmias. Prolonged diuretic therapy may produce hyponatremia (deficiency of sodium in the blood), which can result in disorientation, weakness, muscle cramps, and anorexia. Volume depletion from excessive fluid loss may lead to dehydration and hypotension. ACE inhibitors and beta-blockers may contribute to the hypotension. Other problems associated with diuretics include increased serum creatinine (indicative of renal dysfunction) and hyperuricemia (excessive uric acid in the blood), which leads to gout.

PROMOTING HOME, COMMUNITY-BASED, AND TRANSITIONAL CARE

Facilitating an easy and smooth transition back into the community is of paramount importance for the patient living with HF. Community-based nursing interventions for patients with HF can improve health outcomes and health care value as evidenced by reduced hospital readmissions for up to 6 mo. Important nursing interventions that keep the patient with HF out of the hospital incorporate a multidisciplinary care planning approach (Jones, Bowles, Richard, et al., 2017).

Educating Patients About Self-Care. The nurse provides patient education and involves the patient and family in the therapeutic regimen to promote understanding and adherence to the plan. When the patient recognizes that the diagnosis of HF can be successfully managed with lifestyle changes and medications, recurrences of acute HF lessen, unnecessary hospitalizations decrease, and life expectancy increases. Nurses play a key role in educating patients and their families about medication management, a low sodium diet, moderate alcohol consumption, activity and exercise recommendations, smoking cessation, how to recognize the signs and symptoms of worsening HF, and when to contact the primary provider (Jones et al., 2017). Use of the teach-back technique to assess the patient's comprehension of the instructions can increase education effectiveness and prevent rehospitalization (Esquivel, White, Carroll, et al., 2018) (see Chapter 3 for further discussion of teach-back methods). In order for teach-back to be effective, the nurse must ensure adequate time is dedicated to ensuring that patient learning occurs (Esquivel et al., 2018). A basic home education plan for the patient with HF is presented in Chart 25-6. The patient should receive a written copy of the instructions.

The patient's readiness to learn and potential barriers to learning are assessed. Patients with HF may have temporary or ongoing cognitive impairment due to their illness or other factors, increasing the need to rely on an identified caretaker (Hodson et al., 2019). An effective treatment

Chart 25-6 HOME CARE CHECKLIST
The Patient with Heart Failure

At the completion of education, the patient and/or caregiver will be able to:

- Identify heart failure as a chronic disease that can be managed with medications and specific self-management behaviors.
- State the impact of heart failure on physiologic functioning, ADLs, IADLs, roles, relationships, and spirituality.
- State the name, dose, side effects, frequency, and schedule for all medications.
- Take or administer medications daily, exactly as prescribed.
- Monitor effects of medication such as changes in breathing and edema.
- Know signs and symptoms of orthostatic hypotension and how to prevent it.
- Weigh self daily at the same time, with same clothes.
- Restrict sodium intake to no more than 2 g/day:
  - Adapt diet by examining nutrition labels to check sodium content per serving.
  - Avoid canned or processed foods, eating fresh or frozen foods.
  - Consult the written diet plan and the list of permitted and restricted foods.
  - Avoid salt use.
  - Avoid excesses in eating and drinking.
- Participate in prescribed activity program:
  - Participate in a daily exercise program.
  - Increase walking and other activities gradually, provided they do not cause unusual fatigue or dyspnea.
  - Conserve energy by balancing activity with rest periods.
  - Avoid activity in extremes of heat and cold, which increase the work of the heart.

- Recognize that air-conditioning may be essential in a hot, humid environment.
- Develop methods to manage and prevent stress:
  - Avoid tobacco.
  - Avoid alcohol.
  - Engage in social and diversional activities.
- Identify community resources for peer and caregiver/family support:
  - Identify sources of support (e.g., friends, relatives, faith community).
  - Identify the contact details for support services for patients and their caregivers/families.
- Report immediately to the primary provider or clinic any of the following:
  - Gain in weight of 2–3 lb (0.9–1.4 kg) in 1 d, or 5 lb (2.3 kg) in 1 wk
  - Unusual shortness of breath with activity or at rest
  - Increased swelling of ankles, feet, or abdomen
  - Persistent cough
  - Loss of appetite
  - Development of restless sleep; increase in number of pillows needed to sleep
  - Profound fatigue
- State how to reach primary provider with questions or complications:
  - State time and date of follow-up appointments and diagnostic tests.
- Identify the need for health promotion, disease prevention, and screening activities.

ADLs, activities of daily living; IADLs, instrumental activities of daily living.

---

plan incorporates both the patient's goals and those of the health care providers. The nurse must consider cultural factors and adapt the education plan accordingly. Patients and families need to understand that effective HF management is influenced by choices made about treatment options and their ability to follow the treatment plan. They also need to be informed that health care providers are available to assist them in reaching their health care goals.

Continuing and Transitional Care. Successful management of HF requires adherence to a complex medical regimen that includes multiple lifestyle changes for most patients. Assistance may be provided through a number of options that optimize evidence-based recommendations for effective management of HF. Depending on the patient's physical status and the availability of family assistance, a home care referral or another type of disease management program may be indicated for a patient who has been hospitalized. Transitional care programs (hospital to home) that include telephone contact along with home visits have been shown to decrease rehospitalizations and increase patient quality of life (Cyrille & Patel, 2017; Jones et al., 2017). Home visits by nurses who are specially trained in managing patients with HF provide assessment and management tailored to specific individualized patient needs. Older patients and those who have long-standing heart disease with compromised physical stamina often require assistance with the transition to home after hospitalization for an acute episode of HF. The home

health nurse assesses the physical environment of the home and makes suggestions for adapting the home environment to meet the patient's activity limitations. If stairs are a concern, the patient can plan the day's activities so that stair-climbing is minimized; for some patients, a temporary bedroom may be set up on the main level of the home. The home health nurse works with the patient and family to maximize the benefits of these changes.

The home health nurse also reinforces and clarifies information about dietary changes and fluid restrictions, the need to monitor symptoms and daily body weight, and the importance of obtaining follow-up care with the primary provider's office or clinic. Assistance may be given in scheduling and keeping appointments as well. The patient is encouraged to gradually increase their self-care and responsibility for carrying out the therapeutic regimen.

Evidence-based HF guidelines also recommend patient referral to HF clinics, which provide intensive nursing management along with medical care in a collaborative model. Many of these clinics are managed by advanced practice nurses. Referral to an HF clinic gives the patient ready access to continuing education, professional nursing and medical staff, and timely adjustments to treatment regimens. HF clinics can also provide outpatient treatment (e.g., IV diuretics, laboratory monitoring) as an alternative to hospitalization. Because of the additional support and coordination of care, patients managed through HF clinics have fewer exacerbations of HF, fewer hospitalizations, decreased costs of medical care, and increased quality of life (Yancy, 2013).

Other disease management programs are carried out through telehealth, using telephones or computers to maintain contact with patients and to obtain patient data. This enables nurses and others to assess and manage patients on a frequent basis, without requiring patients to make frequent visits to health care providers. A variety of techniques ranging from simple telephone monitoring to sophisticated computer and video connections that monitor symptoms, daily weight, vital signs, heart sounds, and breath sounds may be used. Patient data may also include hemodynamics and other parameters transmitted from implantable devices. Studies have shown that telehealth management can decrease costs and hospitalizations for acute exacerbations of HF (Koehler, Koehler, Deckwart, et al., 2018).

End-of-Life Considerations. Because HF is a chronic and often progressive condition, patients and families need to consider issues related to the end-of-life and when palliative or hospice care should be considered (Cross, Kamal, Taylor, et al., 2019). Although the prognosis in patients with HF may be uncertain, issues often arise sooner or later related to the patient's thoughts and possible concerns about the use of complex treatment options (e.g., implantation of an ICD or a ventricular assist device [VAD]). VADs are an option for some patients with HF who have failed medical therapy and who are not candidates for cardiac transplantation. Discussions concerning the use of technology, preferences for end-of-life care, and advance directives should take place while the patient is able to participate and express preferences. For example, with the expanded use of ICDs in the HF population, patients with ICDs, their families, and their primary providers should receive instructions for ICD inactivation at the end-of-life to prevent inappropriate discharges. See Chapter 13 for further discussion of end-of-life care.

Evaluation

Expected patient outcomes may include:
1. Demonstrates tolerance for desired activity
    a. Describes adaptive methods for usual activities
    b. Schedules activities to conserve energy and reduce fatigue and dyspnea
    c. Maintains heart rate, blood pressure, respiratory rate, and pulse oximetry within the targeted range
2. Maintains fluid balance
    a. Exhibits decreased peripheral edema
    b. Verbalizes understanding of fluid intake and diuretic use
3. Decreased anxiety
    a. Avoids situations that produce stress
    b. Sleeps comfortably at night
    c. Reports decreased stress and anxiety
    d. Denies symptoms of depression
4. Makes sound decisions regarding care and treatment
    a. Demonstrates ability to influence outcomes
5. Patients and family members adhere to healthy regimen
    a. Performs and records daily weights
    b. Limits dietary sodium intake to no more than 2 g/day
    c. Takes medications as prescribed
    d. Reports symptoms of worsening HF
    e. Makes and keeps appointments for follow-up care

6. Exhibits no evidence of acute decompensation and pulmonary edema
7. Denies dyspnea
8. No apparent delirium or acute anxiety
9. Maintains fluid balance as noted previously
10. No evidence of electrolyte disturbances from diuretic therapy

COMPLICATIONS FROM HEART DISEASE

Cardiogenic Shock

Cardiogenic shock occurs when decreased CO leads to inadequate tissue perfusion and initiation of the shock syndrome. Cardiogenic shock most commonly occurs following acute MI when a large area of myocardium becomes ischemic and hypokinetic. It also can occur as a result of end-stage HF, cardiac tamponade, pulmonary embolism (PE), cardiomyopathy, and arrhythmias. Cardiogenic shock is a life-threatening condition with a high mortality rate. (See Chapter 11 for detailed information about the pathophysiology and management of cardiogenic shock.)

Thromboembolism

Patients with cardiovascular disorders are at risk for the development of arterial thromboemboli and venous thromboemboli (VTE). Intracardiac thrombi can form in patients with atrial fibrillation because the atria do not contract forcefully, resulting in slow and turbulent flow, and increasing the likelihood of thrombus formation. Mural thrombi can also form on ventricular walls when contractility is poor. Intracardiac thrombi can break off and travel through the circulation to other structures, including the brain, where they cause a stroke. Clots within the cardiac chambers can be detected by an echocardiogram and treated with anticoagulant agents, such as heparin and warfarin (see Chapter 26 for further discussion of assessment and treatment of VTEs; Table 26-2 discusses specific anticoagulant medications).

Decreased mobility and other factors in patients with cardiac disease also can lead to clot formation in the deep veins of the legs. Although signs and symptoms of deep vein thrombosis (DVT) can vary, patients may report leg pain and swelling and the leg may appear erythematous and feel warm. These clots can break off and travel through the inferior vena cava and through the right side of the heart into the pulmonary artery, where they can cause a pulmonary embolus (PE) (see Chapter 26 for further discussion of assessment and treatment of PE).

Pericardial Effusion and Cardiac Tamponade

Pericardial effusion (accumulation of fluid in the pericardial sac) may accompany advanced HF, pericarditis, metastatic carcinoma, cardiac surgery, or trauma. Normally, the pericardial sac contains about 20 mL of fluid, which is needed to decrease friction for the beating heart. An increase in pericardial fluid raises the pressure within the pericardial sac and compresses the heart. This has the following effects:

- Elevated pressure in all cardiac chambers
- Decreased venous return due to atrial compression
- Inability of the ventricles to distend and fill adequately

Pericardial fluid may build up slowly without causing noticeable symptoms until a large amount (1 to 2 L) accumulates (Hoit, 2019). However, a rapidly developing effusion (e.g., hemorrhage into the pericardial sac from chest trauma) can quickly stretch the pericardium to its maximum size and cause an acute problem. As pericardial fluid increases, pericardial pressure increases, reducing venous return to the heart and decreasing CO. This can result in cardiac tamponade, which causes low CO and obstructive shock.

Clinical Manifestations

The signs and symptoms of pericardial effusion can vary according to whether the problem develops quickly or slowly. In acute cardiac tamponade, the patient suddenly develops chest pain, tachypnea, and dyspnea. JVD results from poor right atrial filling and increased venous pressure. Hypotension occurs from low CO, and heart sounds are often muted. The subacute presentation of a pericardial effusion is less dramatic. The patient may report chest discomfort or a feeling of fullness. The feeling of pressure in the chest may result from stretching of the pericardial sac. These patients also develop dyspnea, JVD, and hypotension over time (Hoit, 2019). Patients with cardiac tamponade typically have tachycardia in response to low CO. In addition to hypotension, patients with cardiac tamponade may develop **pulsus paradoxus**, a systolic blood pressure that is markedly lower during inhalation. Also known as paradoxical pulse, this finding is characterized by an abnormal difference of at least 10 mm Hg in systolic pressure between the point that it is heard during exhalation and the point that it is heard during inhalation. This difference is caused by the variation in cardiac filling that occurs with changes in intrathoracic pressure during breathing. The cardinal signs of cardiac tamponade are illustrated in Figure 25-4.

Assessment and Diagnostic Findings

An echocardiogram is performed to confirm the diagnosis and quantify the amount of pericardial fluid. A chest x-ray may show an enlarged cardiac silhouette due to pericardial effusion. The ECG shows tachycardia and may also show low voltage (Hoit, 2019). See Chapter 22 for discussion of the significance of ECG abnormalities.

Medical Management

Acute management of cardiac tamponade may include a pericardiocentesis; whereas, recurrent effusions may be managed with a pericardiotomy.

Pericardiocentesis

If cardiac function becomes seriously impaired, **pericardiocentesis** (puncture of the pericardial sac to aspirate pericardial fluid) is performed. During this procedure, the patient is monitored by continuous ECG and frequent vital signs. Catheter pericardiocentesis is performed using echocardiography to guide placement of the drainage catheter (Hoit, 2019).

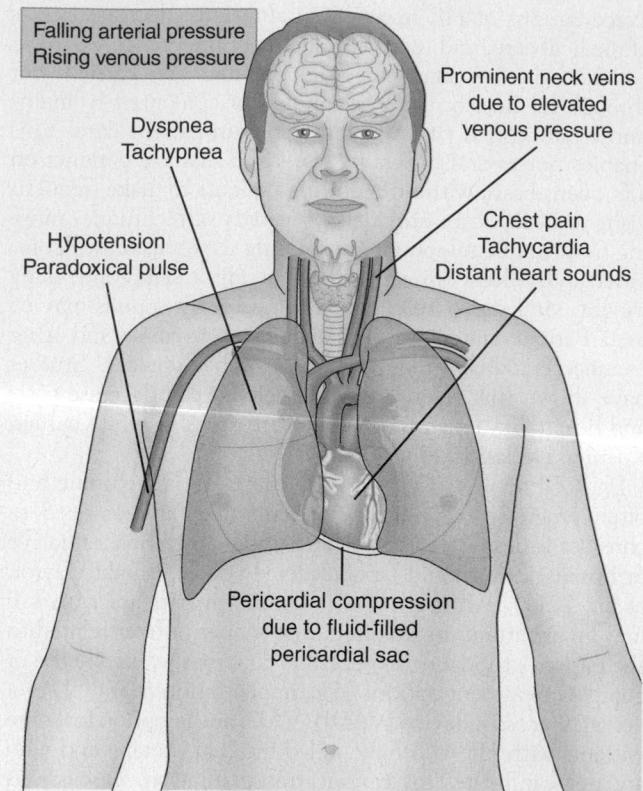

Figure 25-4 • Assessment findings in cardiac tamponade resulting from pericardial effusion include chest pain or fullness, dyspnea, tachypnea, jugular vein distention, hypotension, paradoxical pulse, tachycardia, and distant heart sounds.

A resulting decrease in central venous pressure and an associated increase in blood pressure after withdrawal of pericardial fluid indicate that the cardiac tamponade has been relieved. The patient almost always feels immediate relief. If there is a substantial amount of pericardial fluid aspirated, a small catheter may be left in place to drain recurrent accumulation of blood or fluid. Pericardial fluid is sent to the laboratory for examination for tumor cells, bacterial culture, chemical and serologic analysis, and differential blood cell count.

Complications of pericardiocentesis include coronary artery puncture, myocardial trauma, arrhythmias, pleural laceration, and gastric puncture. After pericardiocentesis, the patient's heart rhythm, blood pressure, venous pressure, and heart sounds are monitored frequently to detect possible recurrence of cardiac tamponade. A follow-up echocardiogram is also performed. If the effusion recurs, repeat aspiration is necessary. Cardiac tamponade may require treatment by open surgical drainage (pericardiotomy) (Hoit, 2019).

Pericardiotomy

Recurrent pericardial effusions, usually associated with neoplastic disease, may be treated by a **pericardiotomy** (pericardial window). Under general anesthesia, a portion of the pericardium is excised to permit the exudative pericardial fluid to drain into the lymphatic system. The nursing care following the procedure includes routine postsurgical care (see Chapter 16) in addition to observation for recurrent tamponade.

Cardiac Arrest

In cardiac arrest, the heart is unable to pump and circulate blood to the body's organs and tissues. It is often caused by an arrhythmia such as ventricular fibrillation, progressive brady-cardia, or asystole (i.e., absence of cardiac electrical activity and heart muscle contraction). Cardiac arrest can also occur when electrical activity is present on the ECG but cardiac contractions are ineffective, a condition called **pulseless electrical activity (PEA)**. PEA may be caused by a variety of problems such as profound hypovolemia (e.g., hemorrhage). Diagnoses that are commonly associated with cardiac arrest include MI, massive pulmonary emboli, hyperkalemia, hypo-thermia, severe hypoxia, and medication overdose. Rapid identification of these problems and prompt intervention can restore circulation in some patients.

Clinical Manifestations

In cardiac arrest, consciousness, pulse, and blood pressure are lost immediately. Breathing usually ceases, but ineffective respiratory gasping may occur. The pupils of the eyes begin dilating in less than a minute, and seizures may occur. Pallor and cyanosis are seen in the skin and mucous membranes. The risk of organ damage, including irreversible brain dam-age, and of death increases with every minute that passes. A patient's age and overall health determine their vulnerability to irreversible damage. As soon as possible, the diagnosis of cardiac arrest must be made and action taken immediately to restore circulation.

 Emergency Assessment and Management: Cardiopulmonary Resuscitation

Cardiopulmonary resuscitation (CPR) provides blood flow to vital organs until effective circulation can be reestablished. Following the recognition of unresponsiveness, a protocol for basic life support is initiated. The AHA Guidelines Update for Cardiopulmonary Resuscitation and Emergency Cardio-vascular Care direct the current protocols for CPR, medical emergency teams, postcardiac arrest care, and acute respira-tory compromise. The primary goal of resuscitation protocols is to save lives by preventing in-hospital cardiac arrest and optimizing outcomes (AHA, 2017).

The resuscitation process begins with the immediate assessment of the patient for breathing and consciousness, then a call for assistance, as CPR can be performed most effectively with the addition of more health care providers and equipment (e.g., defibrillator). The current resuscitation protocol recommends the following practices for CPR:

1. *Quick recognition of sudden cardiac arrest.* The patient is assessed for responsiveness and breathing.
2. *Activation of the Emergency Response System.* Within a medical facility, a call is made to alert the emergency response team. Outside of a medical facility, 911 is called to activate the Emergency Medical Service (EMS).
3. *Performance of high-quality CPR.* If there is no carotid pulse detected, chest compressions are initiated at a rate of 100 bpm.
4. *Rapid cardiac rhythm analysis and defibrillation* within 2 minutes for patients in ventricular fibrillation or pulseless ventricular tachycardia, followed by continu-ous chest compressions.

Rescue breathing is no longer recommended unless health care providers are present; if that is the case, it is then started after chest compressions. The airway is opened using a head-tilt/chin-lift maneuver, and any obvious material in the mouth or throat is removed. An oropharyngeal airway may be inserted if available to help maintain patency of the airway. Rescue ventilations are provided using a bag-valve mask or mouth-mask device. Oxygen is given at 100% dur-ing resuscitation to correct hypoxemia and improve tissue oxygenation.

Compressions are performed with the patient on a firm sur-face such as the floor or a cardiac board. The provider, facing the patient's side, places one hand in the center of the chest on the lower half of the sternum and positions the other hand on top of the first hand (Fig. 25-5). The chest is compressed 2 inches (approximately 5 cm) at a rate of 100 compressions/min. Complete recoil of the chest must be allowed between compressions to allow for cardiac filling. Interruptions in CPR to switch providers or check for a pulse are minimized (Panchal, Berg, Hirsch, et al., 2019). It is recommended pro-viders switch every 2 minutes due to the exertion of deliver-ing effective compressions.

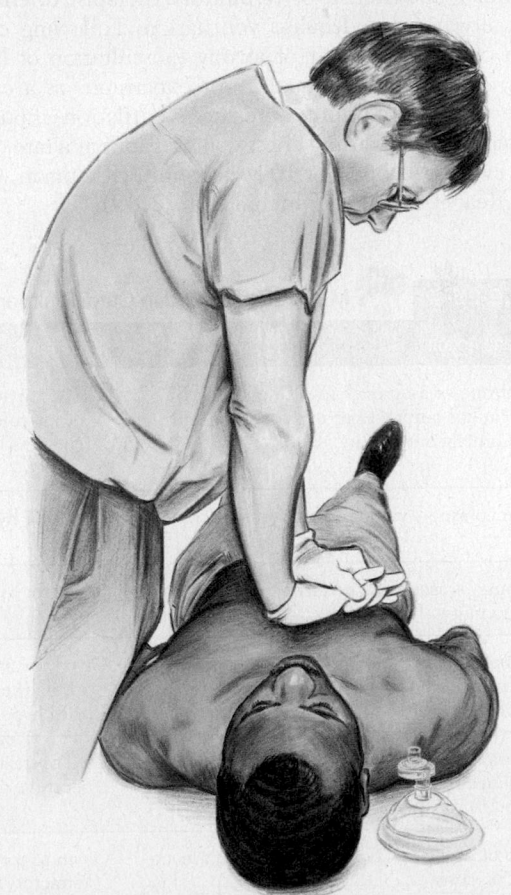

Figure 25-5 • Chest compressions in cardiopulmonary resuscitation are performed by placing the heel of one hand in the center of the chest over the sternum and the other hand on top of the first hand. Elbows are kept straight and body weight is used to apply forceful compressions to the lower sternum. The patient should be on a hard surface such as a cardiac board. Reprinted with permission from Field, J. M., Kudenchuk, P. J., O'Connor, R. E., et al. (2009). *The textbook of emergency cardiovascular care and CPR.* Philadelphia, PA: Lippincott Williams & Wilkins.

Defibrillation

As soon as a monitor/defibrillator is available, monitor electrodes are applied to the patient's chest and the heart rhythm is analyzed. When an automated external defibrillator (AED) is used, the device is turned on, the pads are applied to the patient's chest, and the rhythm is analyzed by the defibrillator to determine whether a shock is indicated. When the ECG shows ventricular fibrillation or pulseless ventricular tachycardia, immediate defibrillation is the treatment of choice.

The AHA (2017) recommends the first defibrillation to occur within 2 minutes of the first documented, pulseless rhythm. Survival time decreases for every minute that defibrillation is delayed. Following defibrillation, high-quality chest compressions are resumed immediately. Survival after cardiac arrest has been improved by extensive education of health care providers and by the use of AEDs.

Advanced Cardiovascular Life Support

During a resuscitation, an advanced airway (e.g., endotracheal tube, tracheal tube) may be placed by a primary provider, nurse anesthetist, or respiratory therapist to ensure a patent airway and adequate ventilation. Following confirmation of the placement of airway (auscultation of breath sounds, observation of equal chest expansion, or a carbon dioxide detector), positive-pressure ventilation should be delivered without pausing chest compressions at a rate of one breath every 6 seconds, or 10 breaths/min (Kleinman, Goldberger, Rea, et al., 2017; Panchal et al., 2019).

Specific subsequent advanced support interventions depend on the assessment of the patient's condition and response to therapy. For example, if asystole is detected on the monitor, CPR is continued while IV or intraosseous (IO) epinephrine is given. Additional medications (Table 25-4) may be indicated for the patient during and after resuscitation.

Each person on an effective Advanced Cardiac Life Support (ACLS) team, called a *CPR team* or sometimes a *code team,* has delineated roles. An efficient code team is characterized by individual members who are knowledgeable about their position and responsibilities. This ensures direct and clear lines of communication, effective team work, and a safe environment for the health care team and the patient (Panchal et al., 2019).

It is recommended practice to support family members of all patients who have had cardiac arrest and are undergoing resuscitation. In addition, there is clear support to have them present at the bedside if that is consonant with the patient's wishes. Written policies and procedures to support family presence during this time ought to be readily available for nurses and staff to easily access. Studies demonstrate family presence does not disrupt patient care, has no negative outcomes during the resuscitation event, and results in no adverse psychological effects (American Association of Critical-Care Nurses [AACN], 2016).

CPR is stopped when vital signs are detected or the patient responds. If the patient does not respond to interventions, the resuscitation effort may be stopped by the code team leader or other provider in charge of the resuscitation after options have been exhausted. Many factors are considered in the decision,

TABLE 25-4 Medications Used in Cardiopulmonary Resuscitation

Agent and Action	Indications	Nursing Considerations
Epinephrine—vasopressor used to optimize BP and cardiac output; improves perfusion and myocardial contractility	Given to patients in cardiac arrest caused by asystole, pulseless electrical activity, pulseless VT or VF	Administer 1 mg every 3–5 min by IV push or IO push. Follow peripheral IV administration with 20-mL saline flush and elevate extremity for 10–20 s.
Norepinephrine—vasopressor given to increase BP	Given for hypotension and shock	Administer 0.1–0.5 mcg/kg/min as IV infusion, preferably through a central line.
Dopamine—vasopressor given to increase BP and contractility	Given for hypotension and shock	Administer 5–10 mcg/kg/min as IV infusion, preferably through a central line.
Atropine—blocks parasympathetic action; increases SA node automaticity and AV conduction	Given to patients with symptomatic bradycardia (i.e., hemodynamically unstable with hypotension)	Administer 0.5-mg IV push; may repeat to dose of 3 mg, follow with saline flush.
Amiodarone—acts on sodium–potassium and calcium channels to prolong action potential and refractory period	Used to treat pulseless VT and VF unresponsive to shock delivery	Administer 300 mg IV; may give second dose of 150 mg in 3–5 min.
Sodium bicarbonate ($NaHCO_3$)—corrects metabolic acidosis	Given to correct metabolic acidosis that is refractory to standard advanced cardiac life support interventions (cardiopulmonary resuscitation, intubation, and respiratory management)	Administer initial dose of 1 mEq/kg IV/IO; then administer dose based on base deficit. Recognize that to prevent development of rebound metabolic alkalosis, complete correction of acidosis is not indicated.
Magnesium sulfate—promotes adequate functioning of cellular sodium–potassium pump	Given to patients with torsade de pointes, a type of VT	May administer 1–2 g diluted in 10 mL D_5W over 5–20 min.

AV, atrioventricular; BP, blood pressure; D_5W, dextrose 5% in water; IO, intraosseous; IV, intravenous; SA, sinoatrial; VF, ventricular fibrillation; VT, ventricular tachycardia.
Adapted from American Heart Association. (2019b). Part 7: Adult advanced cardiovascular life support. Resuscitation science: CPR and ECC guidelines. Retrieved on 12/9/2019 at: www.eccguidelines.heart.org/circulation/cpr-ecc-guidelines/part-7-adult-advanced-cardiovascular-life-support

such as the initiating arrhythmia, potential etiology, length of time for initiation of life support, the patient's response to treatment, and the patient's overall clinical status.

 Follow-Up Monitoring and Care

The care provided to the patient following resuscitation is another determinant of survival (AHA, 2017). A 12-lead ECG is performed to detect any new ST segment elevation or myocardial ischemia (see Chapter 23). Continuous ECG monitoring and frequent blood pressure assessments are essential until hemodynamic stability is established and blood pressure is kept in a range to support adequate perfusion. Factors that precipitated the arrest such as arrhythmias or electrolyte or metabolic imbalances are identified and treated.

Following resuscitation and the return of spontaneous circulation, patients who are comatose may benefit from targeted temperature management (TTM). With TTM, core body temperature is decreased to 32° and 36°C (89.6° to 96.8°F) for at least 24 hours. This induced hypothermia decreases the cerebral metabolic rate and need for oxygen. Similarly, hyperthermic conditions, such as fever, are avoided to reduce oxygen demands (Callaway, Donnino, Fink, et al., 2015).

Advances in cardiac care, such as new techniques for effective resuscitation and postresuscitation hypothermia, have improved outcomes for patients. Research studies demonstrate better neurologic recovery and overall survival for patients when the correct algorithms and team dynamics are used after cardiac arrest; there is hope for even better outcomes in the future.

CRITICAL THINKING EXERCISES

1 ipc After recently being discharged from the hospital with an episode of acute decompensated HFrEF, a 62-year-old man presents to the cardiology clinic where you work. You note that this was the third hospitalization for this patient within the past 6 months. The patient is a widower, lives alone in a two-story home without a bathroom or bedroom on the first floor, and has been receiving disability benefits for several years. Identify how you intend to further assess the patient. What questions will you ask him? Which community-based resources and health care team members could be mobilized to facilitate his transition from the hospital-based setting to the community setting so that he avoids continued rehospitalization?

2 ebp You are a nurse educator working in a home health agency. You are tasked with presenting an educational session on HF self-care strategies. Using knowledge of evidence-based practice guidelines, list the most important topics to cover. Consider gender differences, medications, dietary recommendations, and suggestions for exercise.

3 pq A 75-year-old woman with an acute MI is admitted to the unit where you work as a staff nurse. You assess the patient and find that she is developing a cough, an increasing respiratory rate (32 breaths/min), and pink-tinged sputum. The patient seems agitated and becomes disoriented; she asks you why she is in the hospital. You call the rapid response team, and the following are prescribed: chest x-ray, arterial blood gases and basic metabolic panel, furosemide 40 mg IV, oxygen per nasal cannula to maintain a saturation greater than 94%. Place your planned interventions in priority order and explain your rationale.

REFERENCES

*Asterisk indicates nursing research.
**Double asterisk indicates classic reference.

Books

Bickley, L. S. (2017). *Bates' guide to physical examination and history taking* (12th ed.). Philadelphia, PA: Lippincott Williams & Wilkins.

Burchum, J. R., & Rosenthal, L. D. (2019). *Lehne's pharmacology for nursing care* (10th ed.). St. Louis, MO: Elsevier.

McCance, K. L., Huether, S. E., Brashers, V. L., et al. (2019). *Pathophysiology: The biologic basis for disease in adults and children* (8th ed.). St. Louis, MO: Elsevier.

Norris, T. L. (2019). *Porth's pathophysiology* (10th ed.). Philadelphia, PA: Wolters Kluwer.

Urden, L. D., Stacy, K. M., & Lough, M. E. (2018). *Critical care nursing* (8th ed.). St. Louis, MO: Elsevier.

Wiegand, D. (2017). *AACN procedure manual for high acuity, progressive, and critical care* (7th ed.). St. Louis, MO: Elsevier.

Journals and Electronic Documents

Albert, N. M., Barnason, S., Deswal, A., et al. (2015). Transitions of care in heart failure: A scientific statement from the American Heart Association. *Circulation & Heart Failure, 8*(2), 384–409.

American Association of Critical-Care Nurses (AACN). (2016). AACN practice alert: Family presence during resuscitation and invasive procedures. *Critical Care Nurse, 36*(1), e11–e14.

American Heart Association (AHA). (2017). Get with the guidelines: Resuscitation fact sheet. Retrieved on 9/14/2019 at: www.heart.org/en/professional/quality-improvement/get-with-the-guidelines/get-with-the-guidelines-resuscitation/get-with-the-guidelines-resuscitation-overview

American Heart Association (AHA). (2019a). What is heart failure? Retrieved on 10/24/2019 at: www.heart.org/en/health-topics/heart-failure/what-is-heart-failure

American Heart Association (AHA). (2019b). Part 7: Adult advanced cardiovascular life support. Resuscitation science: CPR and ECC guidelines. Retrieved on 12/9/2019 at: www.eccguidelines.heart.org/circulation/cpr-ecc-guidelines/part-7-adult-advanced-cardiovascular-life-support

Ayres, J. K., & Maani, C. V. (2019). Milrinone. *StatPearls*. Retrieved on 10/24/2019 at: www.ncbi.nlm.nih.gov/books/NBK532943

Benjamin, E. J., Muntner, P., Alonso, A., et al. (2019). Heart disease and stroke statistics—2019 update. *Circulation, 139*(10), e56–e528.

Borlaug, B. A., & Colucci, W. S. (2019). Treatment and prognosis of heart failure with preserved ejection fraction. *UpToDate.* Retrieved on 12/6/2019 at: www.uptodate.com/contents/treatment-and-prognosis-of-heart-failure-with-preserved-ejection-fraction

Callaway, C. W., Donnino, M. W., Fink, E. L., et al. (2015). Part 8: Post-Cardiac Arrest Care: 2015 American Heart Association Guidelines update for cardiopulmonary resuscitation and emergency cardiovascular care. *Circulation, 132*, S465–S482.

Cattadori, G., Segurini, C., Picozzi, A., et al. (2018). Exercise and heart failure: An update. *ESC Heart Failure, 5*(2), 222–232.

Centers for Disease Control and Prevention (CDC). (2017). National Center for Health Statistics: Leading causes of death. Retrieved on 12/5/2019 at: www.cdc.gov/nchs/fastats/leading-causes-of-death.htm

Colucci, W. S. (2019). Treatment of acute decompensated heart failure: Components of therapy. *UpToDate.* Retrieved on 12/7/2019 at: www.uptodate.com/contents/treatment-of-acute-decompensated-heart-failure-components-of-therapy

Colucci, W. S., & Dunlay, S. M. (2017). Clinical manifestations and diagnosis of advanced heart failure. *UpToDate.* Retrieved on 12/6/2019 at: www.uptodate.com/contents/clinical-manifestations-and-diagnosis-of-advanced-heart-failure

Costanzo, M. R. (2019). Ultrafiltration in acute heart failure. *Cardiac Failure Review, 5*(1), 9–18.

Cross, S. H., Kamal, A. H., Taylor, D. H., et al. (2019). Hospice use among patients with heart failure. *Cardiac Failure Review, 5*(2), 93–98.

Cyrille, N. B., & Patel, S. R. (2017). Late in-hospital management of patients hospitalized with acute heart failure. *Progress in Cardiovascular Diseases, 60*(2), 198–204.

Dumitru, I. (2018). Heart failure. *Medscape.* Retrieved on 12/6/2019 at: www.emedicine.medscape.com/article/163062-overview

Esquivel, J., White, M., Carroll, M., et al. (2018). Teach-back is an effective strategy for educating older heart failure patients. *Circulation, 124*(suppl. 21), Abstract 10786.

Gulati, G., & Udelson, J. E. (2018). Heart failure with improved ejection fraction: Is it possible to escape one's past? *Journal of American Cardiology: Heart Failure, 6*(9), 725–733.

*Hodson, A. R., Peacock, S., & Holtslander, L. (2019). Family caregiving for persons with advanced heart failure: An integrative review. *Palliative and Supportive Care.* doi:10.1017/S1478951519000245

Hoit, B. D. (2019). Diagnosis and treatment of pericardial effusion. *UpToDate.* Retrieved on 9/11/2019 at: www.uptodate.com/contents/diagnosis-and-treatment-of-pericardial-effusion

*Jiang, Y., Shorey, S., Seah, B., et al. (2018). The effectiveness of psychological interventions on self-care, psychological and health outcomes in patients with chronic heart failure—A systematic review and meta-analysis. *International Journal of Nursing Studies, 78*, 16–25.

Jones, C. D., Bowles, K. H., Richard, A., et al. (2017). High-value home health care for patients with heart failure. *Circulation, 10*(5), 1–5.

Kleinman, M. E., Goldberger, Z. D., Rea, T., et al. (2017). American Heart Association focused update on adult basic life support and cardiopulmonary resuscitation quality an update to the American Heart Association guidelines for cardiopulmonary resuscitation and emergency cardiovascular care. *Circulation, 137*(1), e7–e13.

Koehler, F., Koehler, K., Deckwart, O., et al. (2018). Efficacy of telemedical interventional management in patients with heart failure (TIM-HF2): A randomised, controlled, parallel-group, unmasked trial. *The Lancet, 392*(10152), 1047–1057.

Koruth, J. S., Lala, A., Pinney, S., et al. (2017). The clinical use of ivabradine. *Journal of the American College of Cardiology, 70*(14), 1777–1784.

Malotte, K., Saguros, A., & Groninger, H. (2018). Continuous cardiac inotropes in patients with end-stage heart failure: An evolving experience. *Journal of Pain and Symptom Management, 55*(1), 159–163.

*Meraz, R. (2020). Medication nonadherence or self-care? Understanding the medication decision-making process and experiences of older adults with heart failure. *Journal of Cardiovascular Nursing, 35*(1), 26–34.

Meyer, T. E. (2019a). Approach to acute decompensated heart failure in adults. *UpToDate.* Retrieved on 10/22/2019 at: www.uptodate.com/contents/approach-to-acute-decompensated-heart-failure-in-adults

Meyer, T. E. (2019b). Initial pharmacologic therapy of heart failure with reduced ejection fraction in adults. *UpToDate.* Retrieved on 12/6/2019 at: www.uptodate.com/contents/overview-of-the-management-of-heart-failure-with-reduced-ejection-fraction-in-adults

O'Connor, C. M. (2017). High heart failure readmission rates: Is it the health system's fault? *Journal of the American College of Cardiology, 5*(5), 393.

Panchal, A. R., Berg, K. M., Hirsch, K. G., et al. (2019). 2019 American Heart Association focused update on advanced cardiovascular life support: Use of advanced airways, vasopressors, and extracorporeal cardiopulmonary resuscitation during cardiac arrest. *Circulation, 140*(24), e881–e894.

Piña, I. L. (2019). Cardiac rehabilitation in patients with heart failure. *UpToDate.* Retrieved on 9/11/2019 at: www.uptodate.com/contents/cardiac-rehabilitation-in-patients-with-heart-failure

Schwartz, J. B., Schmader, K. E., Hanlon, J. T., et al. (2018). Pharmocotherapy in older adults with cardiovascular disease: Report from an American College of Cardiology, American Geriatrics Society, and the National Institute on Aging workshop. *Journal of Geriatrics Society, 67*(2), 371–380.

U.S. Department of Health and Human Services (HHS). (2019). Hospital quality overview. Retrieved on 9/6/2019 at: www.cms.gov/Medicare/Medicare-Fee-for-Service-Payment/AcuteInpatientPPS/Readmissions-Reduction-Program.html

van der Meer, P., Gaggin, H. K., & Dec, G. W. (2019). ACC/AHA versus ESC guidelines on heart failure, JACC guideline comparison. *Journal of the American College of Cardiology, 73*(21), 2757–2768.

**Yancy, C. W., Jessup, M., Bozkurt, B., et al. (2013). 2013 ACCF/AHA Guideline for the management of heart failure. A report of the American College of Cardiology Foundation/American Heart Association Task Force on Practice Guidelines. *Circulation, 128*(16), e240–e327.

Yancy, C. W., Jessup, M., Bozkurt, B., et al. (2017). ACC/AHA/HFSA Focused Update of the 2013 ACCF/AHA Guideline for the Management of Heart Failure. A report of the American College of Cardiology/American Heart Association Task Force on Clinical Practice Guidelines and the Heart Failure Society of America. *Circulation, 136*(6), e137–e161.

Yancy, C. W., Jessup, M., Bozkurt, B., et al. (2016). ACC/AHA/HFSA focused update on new pharmacological therapy for heart failure: An update of the 2013 ACCF/AHA guideline for the management of heart failure: A report of the American College of Cardiology Foundation/American Heart Association Task Force on Clinical Practice Guidelines and the Heart Failure Society of America. *Circulation, 134*(13), e282–e293.

Resources

American Association of Heart Failure Nurses (AAHFN), www.aahfn.org
American College of Cardiology (ACC), www.acc.org
American Heart Association (AHA), www.heart.org
Heart Failure Society of America (HFSA), www.hfsa.org
National Heart, Lung, and Blood Institute, www.nhlbi.nih.gov

26

Assessment and Management of Patients with Vascular Disorders and Problems of Peripheral Circulation

On completion of this chapter, the learner will be able to:

1. Identify anatomic and physiologic factors that affect peripheral blood flow and tissue oxygenation.
2. Apply assessment parameters appropriate for determining the status of peripheral circulation.
3. Use the nursing process as a framework for care of the patient with arterial and venous disorders.
4. Compare the pathophysiology, clinical manifestations, management, and prevention of diseases of the arteries.
5. Describe the pathophysiology, clinical manifestations, management, and prevention of venous thromboembolism, venous insufficiency, leg ulcers, and varicose veins.
6. Describe the pathophysiology, clinical manifestations, and management of lymphatic disorders and cellulitis.

NURSING CONCEPTS

Assessment

Clotting

Functional Ability

Perfusion

GLOSSARY

anastomosis: junction of two vessels

aneurysm: a localized sac or dilation of an artery formed at a weak point in the vessel wall

angioplasty: an invasive procedure that uses a balloon-tipped catheter to dilate a stenotic area of a blood vessel

ankle-brachial index (ABI): ratio of the ankle systolic pressure to the brachial systolic pressure; an objective measurement of arterial disease that provides quantification of the degree of stenosis

arteriosclerosis: diffuse process whereby the muscle fibers and the endothelial lining of the walls of small arteries and arterioles thicken

atherectomy: an invasive procedure that uses a cutting device or laser to remove or reduce plaque in an artery

atherosclerosis: inflammatory process involving the accumulation of lipids, calcium, blood components, carbohydrates, and fibrous tissue on the intimal layer of a large- or medium-sized artery

bruit: sound produced by turbulent blood flow through an irregular, tortuous, stenotic, or dilated vessel

cyanosis: a bluish tint of the skin manifested when the amount of oxygenated hemoglobin contained in the blood is reduced

deep vein thrombosis (DVT): a blood clot or thrombus located within a deep vein that causes obstruction or occlusion

dissection: separation of the weakened elastic and fibromuscular elements in the medial layer of an artery

duplex ultrasonography: combines B-mode grayscale imaging of tissue, organs, and blood vessels with capabilities of estimating velocity changes by the use of a pulsed Doppler

embolus: a blood clot, fatty deposit, or air that travels through the blood, lodges in an artery or vein, and blocks flow

endovascular: a type of procedure that uses a puncture or small incision to place catheters inside a blood vessel to repair it or insert a device

intermittent claudication: a muscular, cramplike pain or fatigue in the extremities consistently reproduced with the same degree of exercise or activity and relieved by rest

ischemia: deficient blood supply

pulmonary embolism (PE): a blood clot or thrombus within a pulmonary artery that blocks or obstructs blood flow to the lungs

rest pain: persistent pain in the foot or digits when the patient is resting, indicating a severe degree of arterial insufficiency

rubor: reddish-blue discoloration of the extremities; indicative of severe peripheral arterial damage in vessels that remain dilated and unable to constrict

stenosis: narrowing or constriction of a blood vessel

thromboembolus: a blood clot that may become dislodged from the vessel where it originally formed

thrombus: a blood clot within an artery or a vein

venous thromboembolism (VTE): a blood clot that forms in the venous vasculature that may manifest as a DVT or a PE

Conditions of the vascular system include arterial disorders, venous disorders, lymphatic disorders, and cellulitis. These disorders may be seen in patients in both the inpatient and the outpatient setting. Nursing assessment and management depends on an understanding of the vascular system.

Anatomic and Physiologic Overview

Adequate perfusion ensures oxygenation and nourishment of body tissues, and it depends in part on a properly functioning cardiovascular system. Adequate blood flow depends on the efficiency of the heart as a pump, the patency and responsiveness of the blood vessels, and the adequacy of circulating blood volume. Nervous system activity, blood viscosity, and the metabolic needs of tissues influence the rate and adequacy of blood flow.

The vascular system consists of two interdependent systems. The right side of the heart pumps blood through the lungs to the pulmonary circulation, and the left side of the heart pumps blood to all other body tissues through the systemic circulation. The blood vessels in both systems channel the blood from the heart to the tissues and back to the heart (see Fig. 26-1). Contraction of the ventricles is the driving force that moves blood through the vascular system.

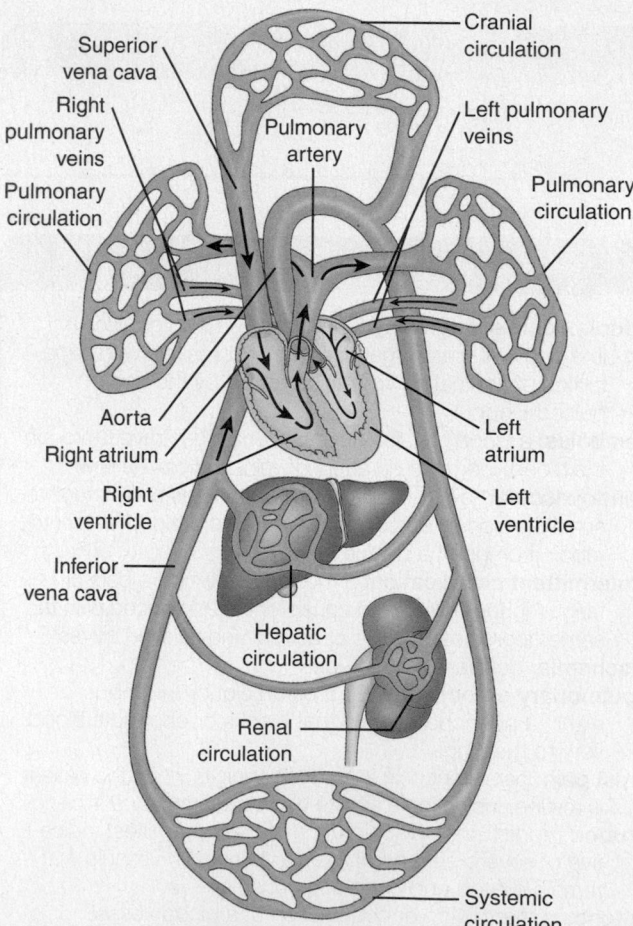

Figure 26-1 • Systemic and pulmonary circulation. Oxygen-rich blood from the pulmonary circulation is pumped from the left heart into the aorta and the systemic arteries to the capillaries, where the exchange of nutrients and waste products takes place. The deoxygenated blood returns to the right heart by way of the systemic veins and is pumped into the pulmonary circulation.

Arteries distribute oxygenated blood from the left side of the heart to the tissues, whereas the veins carry deoxygenated blood from the tissues to the right side of the heart. Capillary vessels located within the tissues connect the arterial and venous systems. These vessels permit the exchange of nutrients and metabolic wastes between the circulatory system and the tissues. Arterioles and venules immediately adjacent to the capillaries, together with the capillaries, make up the microcirculation.

The lymphatic system complements the function of the circulatory system. Lymphatic vessels transport lymph (a fluid similar to plasma) and tissue fluids (containing proteins, cells, and cellular debris) from the interstitial space to systemic veins. Lymphatic fluid empties into the subclavian and internal jugular veins.

Anatomy of the Vascular System

Arteries, arterioles, capillaries, veins, venules, and lymphatic vessels are the main structures that comprise the vascular system.

Arteries and Arterioles

Arteries are thick-walled structures that carry blood from the heart to the tissues. The aorta, which has a diameter of approximately 2.5 cm (1 inch) in the average-sized adult, gives rise to numerous branches, which continue to divide into progressively smaller arteries that are 4 mm (0.16 inches) in diameter. The vessels divide further, diminishing in size to approximately 30 mcm in diameter. These smallest arteries, called *arterioles*, are generally embedded within the tissues (Norris, 2019).

The walls of the arteries and arterioles are composed of three layers: the intima, an inner endothelial cell layer; the media, a middle layer of smooth muscle and elastic tissue; and the adventitia, an outer layer of connective tissue. The intima, a very thin layer, provides a smooth surface for contact with the flowing blood. The media makes up most of the vessel wall in the aorta and other large arteries of the body. This layer is composed chiefly of elastic and connective tissue fibers that give the vessels considerable strength and allow them to constrict and dilate to accommodate the blood ejected from the heart during each cardiac cycle (stroke volume) and maintain an even, steady flow of blood. The adventitia is a layer of connective tissue that anchors the vessel to its surroundings. There is much less elastic tissue in the smaller arteries and arterioles, and the media in these vessels is composed primarily of smooth muscle (Norris, 2019). Smooth muscle controls the diameter of the vessels by contracting and relaxing. Chemical, hormonal, and neuronal factors influence the activity of smooth muscle. Arterioles offer resistance to blood flow by altering their diameter and are often referred to as resistance vessels. Arterioles regulate the volume and pressure in the arterial system and the rate of blood flow to the capillaries. There is a large amount of smooth muscle in the media, and the walls of the arteries are relatively thick, accounting for approximately 25% of the total diameter of the artery.

The intima and the inner third of the smooth muscle layer of the media are in such close contact with the blood that the blood vessels receive their nourishment by direct diffusion. The adventitia and the outer media layers require their own blood supply to meet metabolic needs. The vasa vasorum is a network of small blood vessels that supplies blood and nutrients to the larger arteries.

Capillaries

The walls of the capillaries, which lack smooth muscle and adventitia, are composed of a single layer of endothelial cells. This thin-walled structure permits rapid and efficient transport of nutrients to the cells and removal of metabolic wastes. The diameter of capillaries ranges from 5 to 10 mcm; this means that red blood cells must alter their shape to pass through these vessels. Changes in a capillary's diameter are passive and are influenced by contractile changes in the blood vessels that carry blood to and from a capillary. The capillary's diameter also changes in response to chemical stimuli. In some tissues, a cuff of smooth muscle, called the *precapillary sphincter*, is located at the arteriolar end of the capillary and is responsible, along with the arteriole, for controlling capillary blood flow (Norris, 2019).

Some capillary beds, such as those in the fingertips, contain arteriovenous anastomoses, through which blood passes directly from the arterial to the venous system. These vessels are believed to regulate heat exchange between the body and the external environment.

The distribution of capillaries varies with the type of tissue. For example, skeletal tissue, which has high metabolic requirements, has a denser capillary network than cartilage, which has low metabolic needs.

Veins and Venules

Capillaries join to form larger vessels called *venules*, which join to form veins. The venous system is therefore structurally analogous to the arterial system; venules correspond to arterioles, veins to arteries, and the vena cava to the aorta. Analogous types of vessels in the arterial and venous systems have approximately the same diameters (see Fig. 26-1).

The walls of the veins, in contrast to those of the arteries, are thinner and considerably less muscular. In most veins, the wall makes up only 10% of the diameter, in contrast to 25% in most arteries. In veins, the walls are composed of three layers, like those of arteries; however, in veins, these layers are not as well defined.

The thin, less muscular structure of the vein wall allows these vessels to distend more than arteries. Greater distensibility and compliance permit large volumes of blood to remain in the veins under low pressure. For this reason, veins are referred to as capacitance vessels. Approximately 75% of total blood volume is contained in the veins. The sympathetic nervous system, which innervates the vein musculature, can stimulate venoconstriction (constriction of the veins), thereby reducing venous volume and increasing the volume of blood in the general circulation. Contraction of skeletal muscles in the extremities creates the primary pumping action to facilitate venous blood flow back to the heart (Norris, 2019).

Some veins, unlike arteries, are equipped with valves. In general, veins that transport blood against the force of gravity, as in the lower extremities, have one-way bicuspid valves that prevent blood from retrograde flow as it is propelled toward the heart. Valves are composed of endothelial leaflets, the competency of which depends on the integrity of the vein wall.

Lymphatic Vessels

The lymphatic vessels are a complex network of thin-walled vessels similar to the capillaries. This network collects lymphatic fluid from tissues and organs, and transports the fluid to the venous circulation. The lymphatic vessels converge into two main structures: the thoracic duct and the right lymphatic duct. These ducts empty into the junction of the subclavian and internal jugular veins. The right lymphatic duct conveys lymph primarily from the right side of the head, neck, thorax, and upper arms. The thoracic duct conveys lymph from the remainder of the body. Peripheral lymphatic vessels join larger lymph vessels and pass through regional lymph nodes before entering the venous circulation. The lymph nodes play an important role in filtering foreign particles.

The lymphatic vessels are permeable to large molecules and provide the only means by which interstitial proteins can return to the venous system. With muscular contraction, lymph vessels become distorted to create spaces between the endothelial cells, allowing protein and particles to enter. Muscular contraction of the lymphatic walls and surrounding tissues aids in propelling the lymph toward the venous drainage points (Norris, 2019).

Function of the Vascular System

Important functions of the vascular system include supplying the circulatory needs of tissue, maintaining blood flow and blood pressure, and providing capillary filtration and reabsorption, hemodynamic resistance, and other peripheral vascular regulating mechanisms.

Circulatory Needs of Tissues

The amount of blood flow needed by the body's tissues constantly changes. The percentage of blood flow received by individual organs or tissues is determined by the rate of tissue metabolism, the availability of oxygen, and the function of the tissue. When metabolic requirements increase, blood vessels dilate to increase the flow of oxygen and nutrients to the tissues. When metabolic needs decrease, vessels constrict and blood flow to the tissues decreases. Metabolic demands of tissues increase with physical activity or exercise, local heat application, fever, and infection. Reduced metabolic requirements of tissues accompany rest or decreased physical activity, local cold application, and cooling of the body. If the blood vessels fail to dilate in response to the need for increased blood flow, tissue **ischemia** (deficient blood supply to a body part) results. The mechanism by which blood vessels dilate and constrict to adjust for metabolic changes ensures that normal arterial pressure is maintained (Norris, 2019).

As blood passes through tissue capillaries, oxygen is removed and carbon dioxide is added. The amount of oxygen extracted by each type of tissue differs. For example, the myocardium tends to extract about 50% of the oxygen from arterial blood in one pass through its capillary bed, whereas the kidneys extract only about 7% of the oxygen from the blood that passes through them. The average amount of oxygen removed collectively by all of the body tissues is about 25%. This means that the blood in the vena cava contains about 25% less oxygen than aortic blood. This is known as the systemic arteriovenous oxygen difference (Norris, 2019). This difference becomes greater when less oxygen is delivered to the tissues than they need.

Blood Flow

Blood flow through the cardiovascular system always proceeds in the same direction: left side of the heart to the aorta, arteries, arterioles, capillaries, venules, veins, vena cava, and right side of the heart. This unidirectional flow is caused by a pressure difference that exists between the arterial and venous systems. Because arterial pressure (approximately 100 mm Hg) is greater than venous pressure (approximately 40 mm Hg) and fluid flows from an area of higher pressure to an area of lower pressure, blood flows from the arterial system to the venous system.

The pressure difference (ΔP) between the two ends of the vessel propels the blood. Impediments to blood flow exert an opposing force, which is known as resistance (R). The rate of blood flow is determined by dividing the pressure difference by the resistance:

$$\text{Flow rate} = \Delta P/R$$

This equation shows that when resistance increases, a greater pressure is required to maintain the same degree of flow (Norris, 2019). In the body, an increase in pressure is accomplished by an increase in the force of contraction of the heart. If arterial resistance is chronically elevated, the myocardium hypertrophies (enlarges) to sustain a greater contractile force.

In most long, smooth blood vessels, flow is laminar or streamlined, with blood in the center of the vessel moving slightly faster than the blood near the vessel walls. Laminar flow becomes turbulent when the blood flow rate increases, when blood viscosity increases, when the diameter of the vessel becomes greater than normal, or when segments of the vessel are narrowed or constricted (Norris, 2019). Turbulent blood flow creates an abnormal sound, called a **bruit,** which can be heard with a stethoscope.

Blood Pressure

Chapter 27 provides more information on the physiology and measurement of blood pressure.

Capillary Filtration and Reabsorption

Fluid exchange across the capillary wall is continuous. This fluid, which has the same composition as plasma without the proteins, forms the interstitial fluid. The equilibrium between hydrostatic and osmotic forces of the blood and interstitium, as well as capillary permeability, determines the amount and direction of fluid movement across the capillary. Hydrostatic force is a driving pressure that is generated by the blood pressure. Osmotic pressure is the pulling force created by plasma proteins. Normally, the hydrostatic pressure at the arterial end of the capillary is relatively high compared with that at the venous end. This high pressure at the arterial end of the capillaries tends to drive fluid out of the capillary and into the tissue space. Osmotic pressure tends to pull fluid back into the capillary from the tissue space, but this osmotic force cannot overcome the high hydrostatic pressure at the arterial end of the capillary. However, at the venous end of the capillary, the osmotic force predominates over the low hydrostatic pressure, and there is a net reabsorption of fluid from the tissue space back into the capillary (Norris, 2019).

Except for a very small amount, fluid that is filtered out at the arterial end of the capillary bed is reabsorbed at the venous end. The excess filtered fluid enters the lymphatic circulation. These processes of filtration, reabsorption, and lymph formation aid in maintaining tissue fluid volume and removing tissue waste and debris. Under normal conditions, capillary permeability remains constant.

Under certain abnormal conditions, the fluid filtered out of the capillaries may greatly exceed the amounts reabsorbed and carried away by the lymphatic vessels. This imbalance can result from damage to capillary walls and subsequent increased permeability, obstruction of lymphatic drainage, elevation of venous pressure, or a decrease in plasma protein osmotic force. Accumulation of excess interstitial fluid that results from these processes is called *edema.*

Hemodynamic Resistance

The most important factor that determines resistance in the vascular system is the vessel radius. Small changes in vessel radius lead to large changes in resistance. The predominant sites of change in the caliber or width of blood vessels, and therefore in resistance, are the arterioles and the precapillary sphincter. Peripheral vascular resistance is the opposition to blood flow provided by the blood vessels. This resistance is proportional to the viscosity or thickness of the blood and the length of the vessel and is influenced by the diameter of the vessels. Under normal conditions, blood viscosity and vessel length do not change significantly, and these factors do not usually play an important role in blood flow. However, a large increase in hematocrit may increase blood viscosity and reduce capillary blood flow.

Peripheral Vascular Regulating Mechanisms

Even at rest, the metabolic needs of body tissues are continuously changing. Therefore, an integrated and coordinated regulatory system is necessary so that blood flow to individual tissues is maintained in proportion to the needs of those tissues. This regulatory mechanism is complex and consists of central nervous system influences, circulating hormones and chemicals, and independent activity of the arterial wall itself.

Sympathetic (adrenergic) nervous system activity, mediated by the hypothalamus, is the most important factor in regulating the caliber and therefore the blood flow of peripheral blood vessels. All vessels are innervated by the sympathetic nervous system except the capillary and precapillary sphincters. Stimulation of the sympathetic nervous system causes vasoconstriction. The neurotransmitter responsible for sympathetic vasoconstriction is norepinephrine (Norris, 2019). Sympathetic activation occurs in response to physiologic and psychological stressors. Diminution of sympathetic activity by medications or sympathectomy results in vasodilation.

Other hormones affect peripheral vascular resistance. Epinephrine, released from the adrenal medulla, acts like norepinephrine in constricting peripheral blood vessels in most tissue beds. However, in low concentrations, epinephrine causes vasodilation in skeletal muscles, the heart, and the brain. Angiotensin I, which is formed from the interaction of renin (synthesized by the kidney) and angiotensinogen, a circulating serum protein, is then converted to angiotensin II by an enzyme secreted by the pulmonary vasculature, called *angiotensin-converting enzyme* (ACE). Angiotensin II is a potent vasoconstrictor, particularly of the arterioles. Although the amount of angiotensin II concentrated in the blood is usually small, its profound vasoconstrictive effects are important in certain abnormal states, such as heart failure and hypovolemia (Norris, 2019).

Alterations in local blood flow are influenced by various circulating substances that have vasoactive properties. Potent vasodilators include nitric oxide, prostacyclin, histamine, bradykinin, prostaglandin, and certain muscle metabolites. A reduction in available oxygen and nutrients and changes in local pH also affect local blood flow. Proinflammatory cytokines are substances liberated from platelets that aggregate at the site of damaged vessels, causing arteriolar vasoconstriction and continued platelet aggregation at the site of injury (Atherton, Sindone, De Pasquale, et al., 2018).

Pathophysiology of the Vascular System

Reduced blood flow through peripheral blood vessels characterizes all peripheral vascular diseases. The physiologic effects of altered blood flow depend on the extent to which tissue demands exceed the supply of oxygen and nutrients available. If tissue needs are high, even modestly reduced blood flow may be inadequate to maintain tissue integrity. Tissues become ischemic, malnourished, and ultimately die unless adequate blood flow is restored.

Pump Failure

Inadequate peripheral blood flow occurs when the heart's pumping action becomes inefficient. Heart failure with reduced left ventricular ejection fraction (HFrEF; also called systolic HF) causes an accumulation of blood in the lungs and a reduction in forward flow or cardiac output, which results in inadequate arterial blood flow to the tissues. Heart failure with preserved left ventricular ejection fraction (HFpEF; also called diastolic HF) causes systemic venous congestion and a reduction in forward flow (Atherton et al., 2018) (see Chapter 25).

Alterations in Blood and Lymphatic Vessels

Intact, patent, and responsive blood vessels are necessary to deliver adequate amounts of oxygen and nutrients to tissues and to remove metabolic wastes. Arteries can become damaged or obstructed as a result of atherosclerotic plaque, a **thromboembolus** (a blood clot that may become dislodged from the vessel from where it originally formed), chemical or mechanical trauma, infections or inflammatory processes, vasospastic disorders, and congenital malformations. A sudden arterial occlusion causes profound and often irreversible tissue ischemia and tissue death. When arterial occlusions develop gradually, there is less risk of sudden tissue death because collateral circulation may develop, giving that tissue the opportunity to adapt to gradually decreased blood flow.

Venous blood flow can be reduced by a thromboembolus obstructing the vein, by incompetent venous valves, or by a reduction in the effectiveness of the pumping action of surrounding muscles. Decreased venous blood flow results in increased venous pressure, a subsequent increase in capillary hydrostatic pressure, net filtration of fluid out of the capillaries into the interstitial space, and subsequent edema. Edematous tissues cannot receive adequate nutrition from the blood and consequently are more susceptible to breakdown, injury, and infection. Obstruction of lymphatic vessels also results in edema. Lymphatic vessels can become obstructed by a tumor or by damage from mechanical trauma or inflammatory processes.

Circulatory Insufficiency of the Extremities

Although many types of peripheral vascular diseases exist, most result in ischemia and produce some of the same symptoms: pain, skin changes, diminished pulses, and possible edema. The type and severity of symptoms depend in part on the type, stage, and extent of the disease process and on the speed with which the disorder develops. Table 26-1 highlights the distinguishing features of arterial and venous insufficiency. In this chapter, peripheral vascular disease is categorized as arterial, venous, or lymphatic.

 ## Gerontologic Considerations

Aging produces changes in the walls of the blood vessels that affect the transport of oxygen and nutrients to the tissues.

TABLE 26-1	Characteristics of Arterial and Venous Insufficiency and Resulting Ulcers	
Characteristic	**Arterial**	**Venous**
General Characteristics		
Pain	Intermittent claudication to sharp, unrelenting, constant	Aching, throbbing, cramping
Pulses	Diminished or absent	Present, but may be difficult to palpate through edema
Skin characteristics	Dependent rubor—with elevation pallor of foot; dry, shiny skin; cool-to-cold temperature; loss of hair over toes and dorsum of foot; nails thickened and ridged	Pigmentation in gaiter area (area of medial and lateral malleolus), skin thickened and tough, may be reddish blue, frequently with associated dermatitis
Ulcer Characteristics		
Location	Tip of toes, web spaces, heel or other pressure points if patient is immobile	Medial malleolus, lateral malleolus, or anterior tibial area
Pain	Very painful	Minimal pain to very painful
Depth of ulcer	Deep, often involving joint space	Superficial
Shape	Circular	Irregular border
Ulcer base	Pale to black and wet to dry gangrene	Granulation tissue—beefy red to yellow fibrinous in chronic long-term ulcer
Leg edema	Minimal unless extremity kept in dependent position constantly to relieve pain	Moderate to severe

Adapted from Ermer-Selton, J. (2016). Lower extremity assessment. In R. Bryant & D. Nix (Eds.). *Acute and chronic wounds: Current management* (5th ed.). St. Louis, MO: Elsevier.

The intima thickens as a result of cellular proliferation and fibrosis. Elastin fibers of the media become calcified, thin, and fragmented, and collagen accumulates in the intima and the media. These changes cause the vessels to stiffen, which results in increased peripheral resistance, impaired blood flow, and increased left ventricular workload causing hypertrophy, ischemia and HFrEF, and thrombosis along with hemorrhage in the microvessels in the brain and kidney (Atherton et al., 2018).

Assessment of the Vascular System

The nurse should perform a focused health history and physical assessment to establish a patient's baseline and identify alterations in the vascular system.

Health History

The nurse obtains an in-depth description from the patient with peripheral vascular disorders of any pain and its precipitating factors. A muscular, cramp-type pain, discomfort, or fatigue in the extremities consistently reproduced with the same degree of activity or exercise and relieved by rest is experienced by patients with peripheral arterial insufficiency. Referred to as **intermittent claudication,** this pain, discomfort, or fatigue is caused by the inability of the arterial system to provide adequate blood flow to the tissues in the face of increased demands for nutrients and oxygen during exercise. As the tissues are forced to complete the energy cycle without adequate nutrients and oxygen, muscle metabolites and lactic acid are produced. Pain is experienced as the metabolites aggravate the nerve endings of the surrounding tissue. Typically, about 50% of the arterial lumen or 75% of the cross-sectional area must be obstructed before intermittent claudication is experienced. When the patient rests and thereby decreases the metabolic needs of the muscles, the pain subsides. The progression of the arterial disease can be monitored by documenting the amount of exercise or the distance the patient can walk before the onset of pain. Distance is measured in blocks, feet, or meters. Persistent pain in the anterior portion of the foot (forefoot) when the patient is resting indicates a severe degree of arterial insufficiency and a critical state of ischemia. Known as **rest pain,** this discomfort is often worse at night and may interfere with sleep. This pain frequently requires that the extremity be lowered to a dependent position to improve perfusion to the distal tissues.

The site of arterial disease can be deduced from the location of claudication, because pain occurs in muscle groups distal to the diseased vessel. Calf pain may accompany reduced blood flow through the superficial femoral or popliteal artery, whereas pain in the hip or buttock may result from reduced blood flow in the abdominal aorta or the common iliac or hypogastric (also known as internal iliac) arteries.

Physical Assessment

A thorough assessment of the patient's skin color and temperature and the character or quality of the peripheral pulses is important in the diagnosis of arterial disorders.

Inspection of the Skin

Adequate blood flow warms the extremities and gives individuals with lighter skin tones a rosy coloring. Inadequate blood flow results in cool and pale extremities. In people with pigmented skin, the color changes are often more difficult to discriminate because of the darker skin tone. Further reduction of blood flow to these tissues, which occurs when the extremity is elevated, for example, results in pallor (a whiter or more blanched appearance). **Rubor,** a reddish-blue discoloration of the extremities, may be observed within 20 seconds to 2 minutes after the extremity is placed in the dependent position. Rubor suggests severe peripheral arterial damage in which vessels that cannot constrict remain dilated. Even with rubor, the extremity begins to turn pale with elevation. **Cyanosis,** a bluish tint of the skin, is manifested when the amount of oxygenated hemoglobin contained in the blood is reduced.

Additional changes resulting from a chronically reduced nutrient supply include loss of hair, brittle nails, dry or scaling skin, atrophy, and ulcerations. Edema may be apparent bilaterally or unilaterally and is related to the affected extremity's chronically dependent position because of rest pain. Gangrenous changes appear after prolonged, severe ischemia and represent tissue necrosis.

Palpation of Pulses

Determining the presence or absence, as well as the quality, of peripheral pulses is important in assessing the status of peripheral arterial circulation (see Fig. 26-2). Pulse assessment in an edematous extremity should be undertaken with caution. Palpation of pulses is subjective, and the nurse may mistake their own pulse for that of the patient. To prevent this, the nurse should use light touch and use more than just the index finger for palpation, because this finger has the strongest arterial pulsation of all the fingers. The thumb should not be used for the same reason. Absence of a pulse may indicate that the site of **stenosis** (narrowing or constriction) or occlusion is proximal to that level. Occlusive arterial disease impairs blood flow and can reduce or obliterate palpable pulsations in the extremities. Pulses should be palpated bilaterally and simultaneously, comparing both sides for symmetry in rate, rhythm, and quality.

Diagnostic Evaluation

The nurse should educate the patient on the purpose of the diagnostic studies, what to expect, and any possible side effects related to these examinations. Trends in results are noted because they provide information about disease progression as well as the patient's response to therapy. Various tests may be performed to identify and diagnose abnormalities that can affect the vascular structures (arteries, veins, and lymphatics).

Doppler Ultrasound Flow Studies

When pulses cannot be reliably palpated, a handheld continuous wave (CW) Doppler ultrasound device may be used to detect the blood flow. This handheld device emits a continuous signal through the patient's tissues. The signals are reflected by the moving blood cells and received by the device. The filtered-output Doppler signal is then transmitted to a loudspeaker or headphones, where it can be heard for interpretation as arterial or venous signals (Fischbach

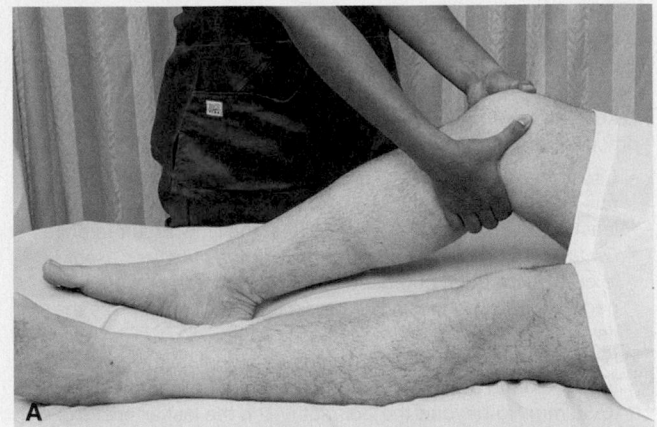

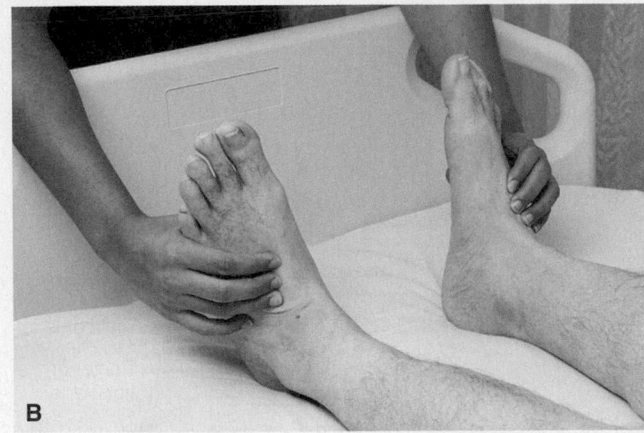

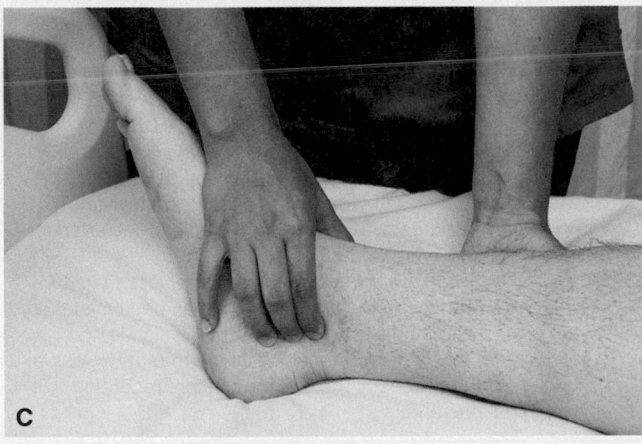

Figure 26-2 • Assessing peripheral pulses. **A.** Popliteal pulse. **B.** Dorsalis pedis pulse. **C.** Posterior tibial pulse. Reprinted with permission from Weber, J. R., & Kelley, J. H. (2018). *Health assessment in nursing* (6th ed.). Philadelphia, PA: Wolters Kluwer.

& Fischbach, 2018). The depth at which blood flow can be detected by Doppler is determined by the frequency (in megahertz [MHz]) it generates. The lower the frequency, the deeper the tissue penetration; a 5- to 10-MHz probe may be used to evaluate the peripheral arteries.

To evaluate the lower extremities, the patient is placed in the supine position with the head of the bed elevated 20 to 30 degrees; the legs are externally rotated, if possible, to permit adequate access to the medial malleolus. Acoustic water soluble gel is applied to the patient's skin to permit uniform transmission of the ultrasound wave. The tip of the Doppler transducer is positioned at a 45- to 60-degree angle over the expected location of the artery and angled slowly to identify arterial blood flow. Excessive pressure is avoided because severely diseased arteries can collapse with even minimal pressure.

The transducer can detect blood flow in advanced arterial disease states, especially if collateral circulation has developed; thus, identifying a signal indicates only the presence of blood flow. The patient's provider must be notified of the absence of a signal if one had been detected previously.

CW Doppler is more useful as a clinical tool when combined with ankle blood pressures, which are used to determine the **ankle-brachial index (ABI)** (see Fig. 26-3). The ABI is the ratio of the systolic blood pressure in the ankle to the systolic blood pressure in the arm (Zierler & Dawson, 2016). It is an objective indicator of arterial disease that allows the examiner to quantify the degree of stenosis. With increasing

degrees of arterial narrowing, there is a progressive decrease in systolic pressure distal to the involved sites.

The first step in determining the ABI is to have the patient rest in a supine position (not seated) for approximately 5 minutes. An appropriate-sized blood pressure cuff

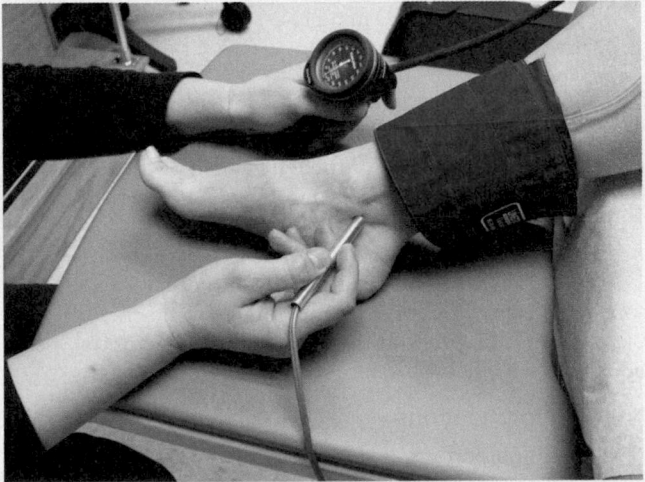

Figure 26-3 • Continuous wave Doppler ultrasound detects blood flow in peripheral vessels. Combined with computation of ankle or arm pressures, this diagnostic technique helps health care providers characterize the nature of peripheral vascular disease. Photograph courtesy of Kim Cantwell-Gab, MN, ACNP, ANP.

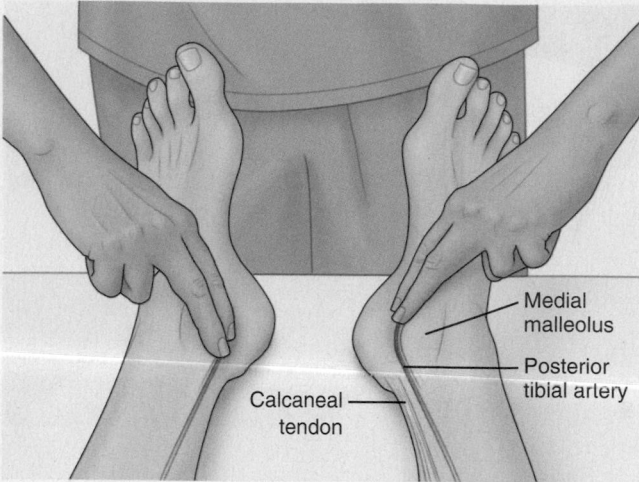

Figure 26-4 • Palpation of posterior tibial artery.

(typically, a 10-cm cuff for an average-sized adult) is applied to the patient's ankle above the malleolus. After identifying an arterial signal of the posterior tibial (see Fig. 26-4) and dorsalis pedis arteries, the systolic pressures, are obtained in both ankles, while listening to the Doppler signal of each artery. Diastolic pressures in the ankles cannot be measured with Doppler. If pressure in these arteries cannot be obtained, pressure can be measured in the peroneal artery, which can also be assessed at the ankle.

Doppler ultrasonography is used to measure brachial pressures in both arms. Both arms are evaluated because the patient may have an asymptomatic stenosis in the subclavian artery, causing brachial pressure on the affected side to be 15 to 20 mm Hg or more lower than systemic pressure. The abnormally low pressure should not be used for assessment.

To calculate the ABI, the highest systolic pressure for each ankle is divided by the higher of the two brachial systolic pressures (see Chart 26-1). The ABI can be computed for a patient with the following systolic pressures:

Right brachial: 160 mm Hg
Left brachial: 120 mm Hg
Right posterior tibial: 80 mm Hg
Right dorsalis pedis: 60 mm Hg
Left posterior tibial: 100 mm Hg
Left dorsalis pedis: 120 mm Hg

The highest systolic pressure for each ankle (80 mm Hg for the right, 120 mm Hg for the left) would be divided by the highest brachial pressure (160 mm Hg):

Right: 80/160 mm Hg = 0.50 ABI
Left: 120/160 mm Hg = 0.75 ABI

In general, systolic pressure in the ankle of a healthy person is the same or slightly higher than the brachial systolic pressure, resulting in an ABI of about 1.0 (no arterial insufficiency) (see Chart 26-2 for ABI pressure ranges).

Nursing Implications

Nurses should perform a baseline ABI on any patient with decreased pulses or any patient 65 years or older, especially patients with a history of diabetes or nicotine use (Gerhard-Herman, Gornik, Barrett, et al., 2016). Patients who undergo an arterial intervention or surgery should have ABIs performed per their institution's protocols. In addition, if there is

a change in the clinical status of a patient, such as a sudden cold or painful limb, an ABI should be performed.

Prior to the procedure, nurses should educate patients about the indications for ABI and what to expect. Patients should be instructed to avoid use of nicotine products or drinking caffeinated beverages for at least 2 hours prior to testing (if it is done on a nonurgent basis). There may be some discomfort involved when the cuffs are inflated.

Chart 26-1

Avoiding Common Errors in Obtaining the Ankle-Brachial Index

Take the following precautions to ensure an accurate ankle-brachial index (ABI) calculation:

- *Use correctly sized blood pressure (BP) cuffs.* To obtain accurate BP measurements, use a cuff with a bladder width at least 40% and length at least 80% of the limb circumference.
- *On the nursing plan of care, document the cuff sizes used* (e.g., "12-cm adult cuff used for brachial pressures; 10-cm pediatric cuff used for ankle pressures"). This minimizes the risk of shift-to-shift discrepancies in ABIs.
- *Use sufficient cuff inflation.* To ensure complete closure of the artery and the most accurate measurements, inflate cuff 20 to 30 mm Hg beyond the point at which the last arterial signal is detected.
- *Do not deflate cuff too rapidly.* Try to maintain a deflation rate of 2 to 4 mm Hg/s for patients without arrhythmias and 2 mm Hg/s or slower for patients with arrhythmias. Deflating the cuff more rapidly may miss the patient's highest pressure and result in recording an erroneous (low) BP measurement.
- *Suspect medial calcific sclerosis any time an ABI is 1.20 or greater or ankle pressure is more than 250 mm Hg.* Medial calcific sclerosis is associated with diabetes, chronic kidney disease, and hyperparathyroidism. It produces falsely elevated ankle pressures by hardening the media of the arteries, making the vessels noncompressible.
- *Be suspicious of arterial pressures recorded at less than 40 mm Hg.* This may mean the venous signal has been mistaken for the arterial signal. If the arterial pressure, which is normally 120 mm Hg, is measured at less than 40 mm Hg, ask a colleague to double-check the readings before recording this as an arterial pressure.

Chart 26-2

Range of Ankle-Brachial Index (ABI) Pressure and Ischemic Manifestations

ABI >1.40 is abnormal; indicates noncompressible arteries; requires further testing with a toe-brachial index (TBI)
ABI of 1.00 to 1.40 is normal
ABI of 0.91 to 0.99 is borderline
ABI of ≤0.90 is abnormal
ABI of 0.50 to 0.90 (i.e., moderate to mild insufficiency) is usually found in patients with claudication
ABI of <0.50 is found in patients with ischemic rest pain
ABI of ≤0.40 is found in patients with severe ischemia or tissue loss

Adapted from Gerhard-Herman, M., Gornik, H., Barrett, C., et al. (2016). AHA/ACC Guideline on the management of patients with lower extremity peripheral arterial disease: Executive summary. *Circulation, 134*(24), 1–208; Zierler, R. E., & Dawson, D. L. (Eds.). (2016). *Strandness's duplex scanning in vascular disorders* (5th ed.). Philadelphia, PA: Wolters Kluwer.

Exercise Testing

Exercise testing is used to determine how long a patient can walk and to measure the ankle systolic blood pressure in response to walking. The patient's brachial systolic blood pressure is obtained on each arm prior to treadmill walking. There are several exercise testing protocols; however, in most instances the patient walks on a treadmill at 1.5 mph with a 12% incline for a maximum of 5 minutes or walks with a gradual rise in speed and incline to the point of claudication. The exercise test can be modified to walking a set distance in a hallway. Most patients can complete the test unless they have significant arterial insufficiency, severe cardiac, pulmonary, or orthopedic problems, or a physical disability. A normal response is little or no drop in ankle systolic pressure after exercise. However, in a patient with true vascular claudication, the ankle pressure drops. Combining this hemodynamic information with the walking time helps to determine whether intervention is necessary. The nurse should reassure the patient that the treadmill test will not require running; rather, the test may require walking on a slight incline. In some instances cycling may be used to evaluate the patient's ability to walk.

Duplex Ultrasonography

Duplex ultrasonography involves B-mode grayscale imaging of the tissue, organs, and blood vessels (arterial and venous) and permits estimation of velocity changes by use of a pulsed Doppler (see Fig. 26-5). Color flow techniques, which can identify vessels, may be used to shorten the examination time. Duplex ultrasound may be used to determine the level and extent of venous disease as well as chronicity of the disease. Using B mode and Doppler, it is possible to image and assess blood flow, evaluate flow of the distal vessels, locate the disease (stenosis versus occlusion), and determine anatomic morphology and the hemodynamic significance of plaque causing stenosis. Duplex ultrasound findings help in planning treatment and monitoring its outcomes. The test is noninvasive and usually requires no patient preparation. Patients who undergo abdominal vascular duplex ultrasound, however, should be advised to not eat or drink (i.e., NPO status) for at least 6 hours prior to the examination to decrease production of bowel gas that can interfere with the examination. The equipment is portable, making it useful anywhere for initial diagnosis, screening, or follow-up evaluations.

Computed Tomography Scanning

Computed tomography (CT) scanning provides cross-sectional images of soft tissue and visualizes the area of volume changes to an extremity and the compartment where changes take place. CT scans of the abdomen are useful in assessing characteristics and monitoring changes within the aorta, such as an increasing aortic diameter indicating aneurysmal formation. CT of a lymphedematous arm or leg, for example, demonstrates a characteristic honeycomb pattern in the subcutaneous tissue. In multidetector-computed tomography (MDCT), a spiral CT scanner and rapid intravenous (IV) infusion of contrast agent are used to image very thin sections of the target area, and the results are configured in three dimensions so that the image can be rotated and viewed from multiple angles. The scanner's head moves circumferentially around the patient as the patient passes through the scanner, creating a series of overlapping images that are connected to one another in a continuous spiral. Scan times are short. However, the patient is exposed to x-rays, and a contrast agent is injected to visualize the blood vessels. The high volume of contrast agent injected into a peripheral vein may contraindicate the use of MDCT in children and patients with significantly impaired renal function (Gerhard-Herman et al., 2016).

Nursing Implications

Patients with impaired renal function scheduled for MDCT may require preprocedural treatment to prevent contrast-induced nephropathy. This may include oral or IV hydration 6 to 12 hours preprocedure or administration of sodium bicarbonate, which alkalinizes urine and protects against free radical damage. Studies do not support the use of oral and IV N-acetylcysteine for protection against contrast-induced nephropathy (Fähling, Seeliger, Patzak, et al., 2017). The nurse should encourage fluids and monitor the patient's urinary output post procedure, which should be at least 0.5 mL/kg/h. Contrast-induced acute kidney injury may occur within 48 to 96 hours post procedure; therefore, the nurse should follow up with the patient's primary provider if this occurs (see Chapter 48 for discussion of acute kidney injury). Patients who have known iodine or shellfish allergies may need premedication with steroids and histamine blockers.

Angiography

An arteriogram produced by angiography may be used to confirm the diagnosis of occlusive arterial disease when surgery or other interventions are considered. It involves injecting a radiopaque contrast agent directly into the arterial system to visualize the vessels. The location of a vascular obstruction or an **aneurysm** (abnormal dilation of a blood vessel) and the collateral circulation can be demonstrated. Typically, the patient experiences a temporary sensation of warmth as the contrast agent is injected, and local irritation may occur at the injection site. Infrequently, a patient may have an immediate or delayed allergic reaction to the iodine contained in the contrast agent. Manifestations include dyspnea, nausea and vomiting, sweating, tachycardia, and numbness of the extremities. Any reaction must be reported to the

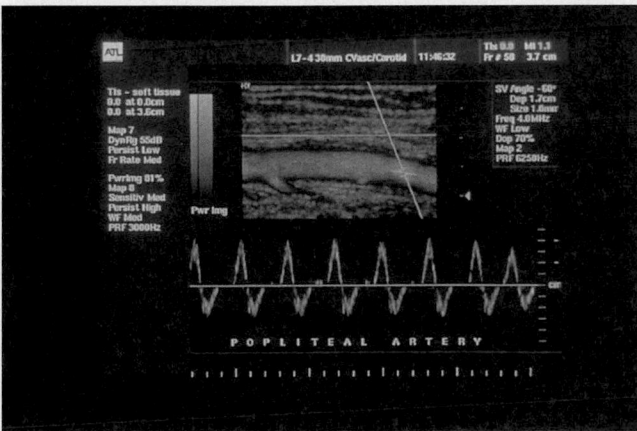

Figure 26-5 • Color flow duplex image of popliteal artery with normal triphasic Doppler flow.

interventionist at once; treatment may include the administration of epinephrine, antihistamines, or corticosteroids. Additional procedural risks include vessel injury, acute arterial occlusion, bleeding, or contrast nephropathy.

Magnetic Resonance Angiography

Magnetic resonance angiography (MRA) is performed with a standard magnetic resonance imaging (MRI) scanner and special software programmed to isolate the blood vessels. The resulting images can be rotated and viewed from multiple angles (Gerhard-Herman et al., 2016).

Nursing Implications

MRA is contraindicated in patients with metal implants. Prior to the MRA, the nurse should assess for the presence of any incompatible devices, such as aneurysm clips, old tattoos, which may contain trace elements (newer materials used in tattoos such as nitinol and titanium are MRI compatible), some medication patches, or a cardiac implantable electronic device. Patients with any type of cardiac implantable electronic device need to be screened to determine if they can safely undergo MRI (Indik, Gimbel, Abe, et al., 2017).

The nurse should educate the patient regarding what to expect during and after the procedure. The patient should be prepared to lie on a cold, hard table that slides into an enclosed small tube. The nurse should inform the patient that they will hear noises, including periodic banging and popping sounds. Patients with claustrophobia may be prescribed a sedative prior to the procedure. Patients should be instructed to close their eyes before entering the tube, and to keep them closed, as this may decrease claustrophobic symptoms. Patients should be reassured that they will be provided with a panic button to press if they feel a need to stop the procedure. MRA procedures require the use of IV contrast dye; therefore, nursing implications following MRA are the same as those for MDCT (discussed in CT section).

Contrast Phlebography (Venography)

Also known as venography, contrast phlebography involves injecting a radiopaque contrast agent into the venous system. If a **thrombus** (a blood clot within an artery or vein) exists, the x-ray image reveals an unfilled segment of vein in an otherwise completely filled vein. Injection of the contrast agent may cause brief but painful inflammation of the vein. This test is rarely performed, as duplex ultrasonography is considered the standard for diagnosing lower extremity venous thrombosis (Zierler & Dawson, 2016). The nurse should instruct the patient that they will receive contrast dye through a peripheral vein and will be monitored for 2 hours post venogram for access site oozing or hematoma. The guidelines for nursing care following venogram are the same as those for MDCT (see earlier discussion).

Lymphoscintigraphy

Lymphoscintigraphy involves injection of a radioactively labeled colloid subcutaneously in the second interdigital space. The extremity is then exercised to facilitate the uptake of the colloid by the lymphatic system, and serial images are obtained at preset intervals.

Nursing Implications

The nurse should educate the patient about what to expect. For instance, the blue dye typically used for this procedure may stain the injection site. If the patient has a lymphatic leak, as can occur with groin incisions, there may be blue drainage from the incision until the dye clears from the system, which may take several days.

ARTERIAL DISORDERS

Arterial disorders cause ischemia and tissue necrosis. These disorders may occur because of chronic progressive pathologic changes to the arterial vasculature (e.g., atherosclerotic changes) or an acute loss of blood flow to the tissues (e.g., aneurysm rupture).

Arteriosclerosis and Atherosclerosis

Arteriosclerosis (hardening of the arteries) is the most common disease of the arteries. It is a diffuse process whereby the muscle fibers and the endothelial lining of the walls of small arteries and arterioles become thickened. **Atherosclerosis** involves a different process, affecting the intima of large and medium-sized arteries. These changes consist of the accumulation of lipids, calcium, blood components, carbohydrates, and fibrous tissue on the intimal layer of the artery. These accumulations are referred to as atheromas or plaques.

Although the pathologic processes of arteriosclerosis and atherosclerosis differ, rarely does one occur without the other, and the terms are often used interchangeably. Atherosclerosis is a generalized disease of the arteries, and when it is present in the extremities, it is usually present elsewhere in the body.

Pathophysiology

The most common direct results of atherosclerosis in arteries include stenosis (narrowing) of the lumen, obstruction by thrombosis, aneurysm, ulceration, and rupture. Its indirect results are malnutrition and the subsequent fibrosis of the organs that the sclerotic arteries supply with blood. All actively functioning tissue cells require an abundant supply of nutrients and oxygen and are sensitive to any reduction in the supply of these nutrients. If such reductions are severe and permanent, the cells undergo ischemic necrosis (death of cells due to deficient blood flow) and are replaced by fibrous tissues, which require much less blood flow.

Atherosclerosis can develop in any part of the vascular system, but certain sites are more vulnerable, such as regions where arteries bifurcate or branch into smaller vessels, with males having more below-the-knee pathology than females (Jelani, Petrov, Martinez, et al., 2018). In the proximal lower extremity, these include the distal abdominal aorta, the common iliac arteries, the orifice of the superficial femoral and profunda femoris arteries, and the superficial femoral artery in the adductor canal, which is particularly narrow. Distal to the knee, atherosclerosis can occur anywhere along the course of the artery.

Although many theories exist about the development of atherosclerosis, no single theory explains the pathogenesis completely; however, tenets of several theories are

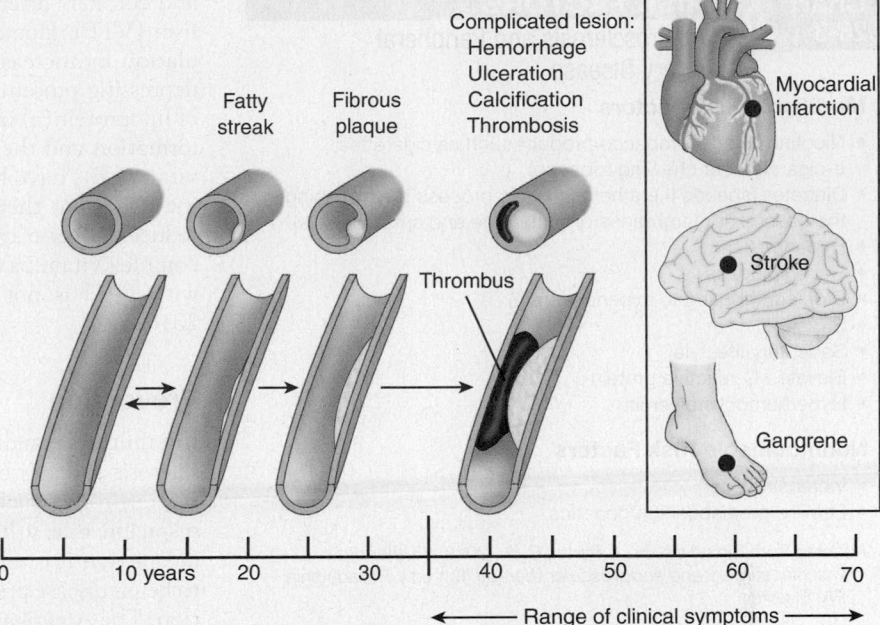

Figure 26-6 • Schematic concept of the progression of atherosclerosis. Fatty streaks are an early manifestation of atherosclerosis. Fatty streaks either regress or progress to fibrous plaques and eventually to atheroma. Atheromatous plaque may be complicated by hemorrhage, ulceration, calcification, or thrombosis leading to myocardial infarction, stroke, claudication, rest pain, or gangrene.

incorporated into the reaction-to-injury theory. According to this theory, vascular endothelial cell injury results from prolonged hemodynamic forces, such as shearing stresses and turbulent flow, irradiation, chemical exposure, or chronic hyperlipidemia. Injury to the endothelium increases the aggregation of platelets and monocytes at the site of the injury. Smooth muscle cells migrate and proliferate, allowing a matrix of collagen and elastic fibers to form (Norris, 2019).

Atherosclerotic lesions are of two types: fatty streaks and fibrous plaque.

- Fatty streaks are yellow and smooth, protrude slightly into the lumen of the artery, and are composed of lipids and elongated smooth muscle cells. These lesions have been found in the arteries of people of all ages, including infants. It is not clear whether fatty streaks predispose a person to the formation of fibrous plaques or whether they are reversible. They do not usually cause clinical symptoms.
- Fibrous plaques are composed of smooth muscle cells, collagen fibers, plasma components, and lipids. They are white to white-yellow and protrude to various degrees into the arterial lumen, sometimes completely obstructing it. These plaques are found predominantly in the abdominal aorta and the coronary, popliteal, and internal carotid arteries, and they are believed to be progressive lesions (see Fig. 26-6).

Gradual narrowing of the arterial lumen stimulates the development of collateral circulation (see Fig. 26-7). Collateral circulation arises from preexisting vessels that enlarge to reroute blood flow around a hemodynamically significant stenosis or occlusion. Collateral flow allows continued perfusion to the tissues, but it is often inadequate to meet increased metabolic demands, and ischemia results.

Risk Factors

Many risk factors are associated with atherosclerosis (see Chart 26-3). Although it is not entirely clear whether

modification of these risk factors prevents the development of cardiovascular disease, evidence indicates that it may slow the process.

The use of nicotine products may be one of the most important risk factors in the development of atherosclerotic lesions. Nicotine in tobacco decreases blood flow to the extremities and increases heart rate and blood pressure by stimulating the sympathetic nervous system, causing vasoconstriction (Quintella Farah, Silva Rigoni, de Almeida Correia, et al., 2019). It also increases the risk of clot formation by increasing the aggregation of platelets. Carbon monoxide, a toxin produced

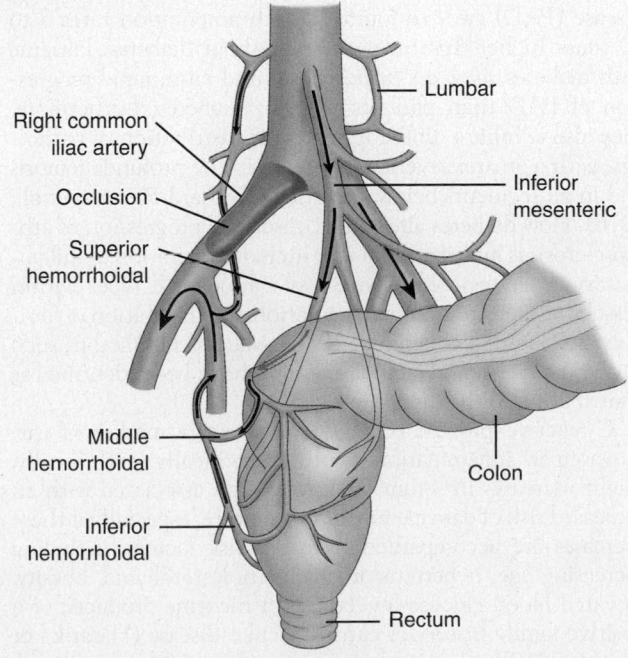

Figure 26-7 • Development of channels for collateral blood flow in response to occlusion of the right common iliac artery and the terminal aortic bifurcation.

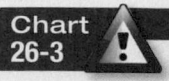

RISK FACTORS
Atherosclerosis and Peripheral Artery Disease

Chart 26-3

Modifiable Risk Factors

- Nicotine use (i.e., tobacco product such as cigarettes, e-cigarettes, or chewing tobacco)
- Diabetes (speeds the atherosclerotic process by thickening the basement membranes of both large and small vessels)
- Hypertension
- Hyperlipidemia
- Diet (contributing to hyperlipidemia)
- Stress
- Sedentary lifestyle
- Elevated C-reactive protein
- Hyperhomocysteinemia

Nonmodifiable Risk Factors

- Increasing age
- Familial predisposition/genetics

Adapted from Sidawy, A. N., & Perler, B. A. (2019). *Rutherford's vascular surgery and endovascular therapy* (9th ed.). Philadelphia, PA: Elsevier.

by burning tobacco, combines more readily with hemoglobin than oxygen, depriving the tissues of oxygen. There is evidence that smoking decreases high-density lipoprotein (HDL; good cholesterol) levels and alters the ratios between HDL and low-density lipoprotein (LDL; bad cholesterol), HDL and triglycerides, and HDL and total cholesterol levels (see Chapter 23 for discussion of HDL and LDL and their association with atherosclerosis). The amount of tobacco used—inhaled in traditional or e-cigarette form, or chewed—is directly related to the extent of the disease, and cessation of any type of nicotine product use reduces the risk (Jelani et al., 2018).

Diabetes increases the overall risk of peripheral artery disease (PAD) two- to fourfold, with amputation rates 5 to 10 times higher than in patients without diabetes. Patients with diabetes show an earlier onset and more rapid progression of PAD than patients without diabetes; furthermore, they also exhibit a different anatomic distribution of pathology, with a greater severity of disease in the profunda femoris and in all segments below the knee (Gerhard-Herman et al., 2016). How diabetes affects the onset and progression of atherosclerosis is multifactorial and includes incitation of inflammatory processes, derangement of various cell types within vessel walls, promotion of coagulation, and inhibition of fibrinolysis (Hazarika & Annex, 2017). Many other factors, such as obesity, stress, and lack of exercise, have been identified as contributing to the disease process.

C-reactive protein (CRP) is a sensitive marker of cardiovascular inflammation, both systemically and locally. Slight increases in serum CRP levels are associated with an increased risk of damage in the vasculature, especially if these increases are accompanied by other risk factors, including increasing age, hypertension, hypercholesterolemia, obesity, elevated blood glucose levels, use of nicotine products, or a positive family history of cardiovascular disease (Hazarika & Annex, 2017).

In some studies, hyperhomocysteinemia has been positively correlated with the risk of peripheral, cerebrovascular,

and coronary artery disease as well as venous thromboembolism (VTE). Homocysteine is a protein that promotes coagulation by increasing factor V and factor XI activity while depressing protein C activation and increasing the binding of lipoprotein(a) in fibrin. These processes increase thrombin formation and the propensity for thrombosis. Folic acid and vitamin B_{12} have been reported to reduce serum homocysteine levels but there are no data demonstrating this therapy reduces adverse cardiovascular events. Thus, the use of B complex vitamins to reduce cardiovascular disease in patients with PAD is not recommended (Gerhard-Herman et al., 2016).

Prevention

Intermittent claudication is a symptom of generalized atherosclerosis and may be a marker of atherosclerosis in other arterial territories, such as the coronary and carotid arteries. The suspicion that a high-fat diet contributes to atherosclerosis means that it is reasonable to measure serum cholesterol and to begin disease prevention efforts that include diet modification. The American Heart Association recommends reducing the amount of fat ingested, substituting unsaturated fats for saturated fats, and decreasing cholesterol intake to reduce the risk of cardiovascular disease.

Certain medications that supplement dietary modification and exercise are used to reduce blood lipid levels. Current evidence-based guidelines established by the American College of Cardiology and the American Heart Association (ACC/AHA) recommend 3-hydroxy-3-methylglutaryl coenzyme A (HMG-CoA) reductase inhibitors (statins) as first-line therapy in patients with PAD for secondary prevention and cardiovascular risk reduction (Conte, Bradbury, Kolh, et al., 2019). These statins may include medications such as atorvastatin, lovastatin, pitavastatin, pravastatin, simvastatin, fluvastatin, and rosuvastatin. Several other classes of medications used to reduce lipid levels include bile acid sequestrants (cholestyramine, colesevelam, colestipol), nicotinic acid (niacin), fibric acid inhibitors (gemfibrozil, fenofibrate), and cholesterol absorption inhibitors (ezetimibe). Patients receiving long-term therapy with these medications require close monitoring.

Hypertension, which may accelerate the rate at which atherosclerotic lesions form in high-pressure vessels, can lead to a stroke, ischemic renal disease, severe PAD, or coronary artery disease. Hypertension is a major risk factor for the development of PAD and may be a more significant risk factor for women than men based on research findings from the classic Framingham Heart Study and a similar study performed in Europe (Jelani et al., 2018). The majority of patients with hypertension require more than two antihypertensive agents to reach target blood pressure, and at least one third require more than three antihypertensive agents to achieve effective blood pressure control (Sidawy & Perler, 2019). See Chapter 27 for further discussion of hypertension.

Although no single risk factor has been identified as the primary contributor to the development of atherosclerotic cardiovascular disease, it is clear that the greater the number of risk factors, the greater the risk of atherosclerosis. Elimination of all controllable risk factors, particularly nicotine use, is strongly recommended.

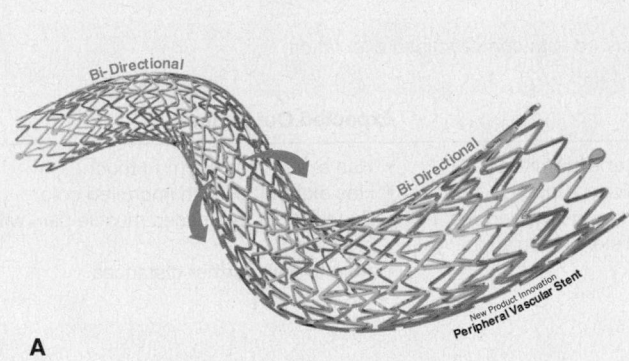
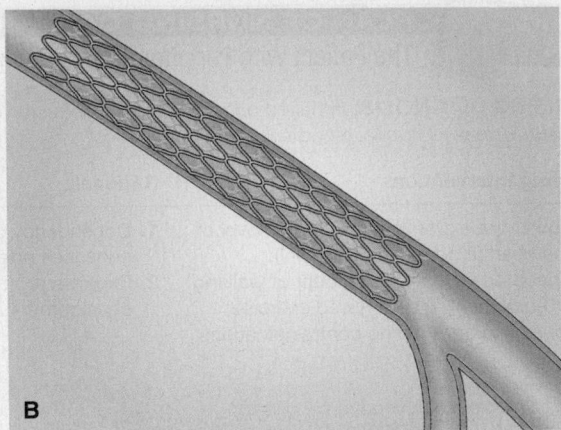

Figure 26-8 • A. Flexible stent. Used with permission from QualiMed Innovative Medizinprodukte GmbH, a Q3 Medical Company. **B.** Representation of a common iliac artery with a wall stent.

Clinical Manifestations

The clinical signs and symptoms resulting from atherosclerosis depend on the organ or tissue affected. Coronary atherosclerosis (heart disease), angina, and acute myocardial infarction are discussed in Chapter 23. Cerebrovascular diseases, including transient ischemic attacks and stroke, are discussed in Chapter 62. Atherosclerosis of the aorta, including aneurysm, and atherosclerotic lesions of the extremities are discussed later in this chapter. Renovascular disease (renal artery stenosis and end-stage kidney disease) is discussed in Chapter 48.

Medical Management

The management of atherosclerosis involves modification of risk factors, a controlled exercise program to improve circulation and functional capacity, medication therapy, and interventional or surgical procedures.

Surgical Management

Vascular surgical procedures are divided into two groups: inflow procedures, which improve blood supply from the aorta into the femoral artery, and outflow procedures, which provide blood supply to vessels below the femoral artery. Inflow surgical procedures are described with diseases of the aorta and outflow procedures with peripheral artery disease.

Endovascular Therapy

Endovascular therapies include various procedures that use a puncture or small incision to place catheters inside a blood vessel to repair it or insert a device and have replaced a large proportion of open surgical approaches to management. If an isolated lesion or lesions are identified on imaging, **angioplasty,** also called *percutaneous transluminal angioplasty* (PTA), or an atherectomy, may be performed. After the patient receives a local anesthetic agent, a balloon-tipped catheter is maneuvered across the area of stenosis. Although some clinicians theorize that PTA improves blood flow by overstretching (and thereby dilating) the elastic fibers of the nondiseased arterial segment, most believe that the procedure widens the arterial lumen by "cracking" and flattening the plaque against the vessel wall (see Chapter 23). An **atherectomy** reduces

the plaque buildup within an artery using a cutting device or laser. Complications from PTA and atherectomy include hematoma formation, **embolus** (blood clot, fatty deposit, or air that travels through the blood, lodges in an artery or vein, and blocks flow), **dissection** (separation of the intima) of the vessel, acute arterial occlusion, and bleeding. To decrease the risk of restenosis, stents (small mesh tubes made of nitinol, titanium, or stainless steel) may be inserted to support the walls of the artery and prevent collapse immediately after balloon deflation (see Fig. 26-8). A variety of stents and stent grafts may be used for short-segment stenoses. Complications associated with stent or stent graft use include distal embolization, dissection, and dislodgment. The advantage of angioplasty, atherectomy, stents, and stent grafts is a decreased length of hospital stay; many of the procedures are performed on an outpatient basis.

Nursing Management

An overview of the care of a patient with peripheral artery problems is provided in Chart 26-4.

Improving Peripheral Arterial Circulation

Arterial blood supply to a body part can be enhanced by positioning the body part below the level of the heart. For the lower extremities, this is accomplished by elevating the head of the patient's bed or by having the patient use a reclining chair or sit with the feet resting on the floor.

 Concept Mastery Alert

> For patients with PAD, blood flow to the lower extremities needs to be enhanced; therefore, the nurse encourages keeping the lower extremities in a neutral or dependent position. In contrast, for patients with venous insufficiency, blood return to the heart needs to be enhanced, so the lower extremities are elevated. Exercise promotes the development of collateral circulation (arterial) and activates the musculovenous pump (venous).

The nurse can assist the patient with walking or other moderate or graded isometric exercises that promote blood

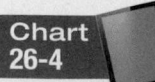

Chart 26-4 PLAN OF NURSING CARE
The Patient with Peripheral Vascular Problems

NURSING DIAGNOSIS: Impaired peripheral tissue perfusion associated with compromised circulation
GOAL: Increased arterial blood supply to extremities

Nursing Interventions	Rationale	Expected Outcomes
1. Lower the extremities below the level of the heart (if condition is arterial). 2. Encourage moderate amount of walking or enrollment in supervised exercise therapy program if no contraindications exist.	1. Dependency of lower extremities enhances arterial blood supply. 2. Exercise promotes blood flow and the development of collateral circulation.	• Has extremities warm to touch • Has extremities with improved color • Experiences decreased muscle pain with exercise • Able to walk further distances

GOAL: Decrease in venous congestion

Nursing Interventions	Rationale	Expected Outcomes
1. Elevate the extremities above the level of the heart (if condition is venous). 2. Discourage standing still or sitting for prolonged periods. 3. Encourage walking.	1. Elevation of extremities counteracts gravity, promotes venous return, and prevents venous stasis. 2. Prolonged standing still or sitting promotes venous stasis. 3. Walking promotes venous return by activating the "calf muscle pump."	• Elevates the extremities as prescribed • Has decreased edema of extremities • Avoids prolonged standing still or sitting • Gradually increases walking time daily

GOAL: Promotion of vasodilation and prevention of vascular compression

Nursing Interventions	Rationale	Expected Outcomes
1. Maintain warm temperature and avoid chilling. 2. Discourage use of nicotine products. 3. Counsel to avoid emotional upsets; encourage stress management. 4. Encourage avoidance of constrictive clothing and accessories. 5. Encourage avoidance of crossing the legs. 6. Administer vasodilator medications and adrenergic-blocking agents as prescribed, with appropriate nursing considerations.	1. Warmth promotes arterial flow by preventing vasoconstriction from chilling. 2. Nicotine in all tobacco products causes vasospasm, which impedes peripheral circulation. 3. Emotional stress causes peripheral vasoconstriction by stimulating the sympathetic nervous system. 4. Constrictive clothing and accessories impede circulation and promote venous stasis. 5. Crossing the legs causes compression of vessels with subsequent impediment of circulation, resulting in venous stasis. 6. Vasodilators relax smooth muscle; adrenergic-blocking agents block the response to sympathetic nerve impulses or circulating catecholamines.	• Protects extremities from cold • Avoids all nicotine products • Uses stress management to minimize emotional upset • Avoids constrictive clothing and accessories • Avoids crossing legs • Takes medication as prescribed

NURSING DIAGNOSIS: Chronic pain associated with impaired ability of peripheral vessels to supply tissues with oxygen
GOAL: Relief of pain

Nursing Interventions	Rationale	Expected Outcomes
1. Promote increased circulation through exercise (e.g., walking, upper extremity exercises, water aerobics, stationary cycling, supervised exercise therapy). 2. Administer analgesic agents as prescribed, with appropriate nursing considerations.	1. Enhancement of peripheral circulation increases the oxygen supplied to the muscle and decreases the accumulation of metabolites that cause muscle spasms. 2. Analgesic agents help reduce pain and allow the patient to participate in activities and exercises that promote circulation.	• Uses measures to increase arterial blood supply to extremities • Uses analgesic agents as prescribed

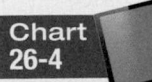

Chart 26-4   PLAN OF NURSING CARE (continued)
The Patient with Peripheral Vascular Problems

NURSING DIAGNOSIS: Risk for impaired skin integrity associated with compromised circulation
GOAL: Attainment/maintenance of tissue integrity

Nursing Interventions	Rationale	Expected Outcomes
1. Instruct in ways to avoid trauma to extremities.	1. Poorly nourished tissues are susceptible to trauma and microbial invasion; wound healing is delayed or inhibited due to poor tissue perfusion.	• Inspects skin daily for evidence of injury or ulceration • Avoids trauma and irritation to skin • Wears protective shoes • Adheres to meticulous hygiene regimen • Eats a healthy diet that contains adequate protein, zinc, and vitamins A and C
2. Encourage wearing protective shoes and padding for pressure points; wear new shoes for short period of time and then inspect feet for signs of injury.	2. Protective shoes and padding prevent foot injuries.	
3. Encourage meticulous hygiene: bathing with neutral soaps, applying lotions (avoiding application between toes), and carefully trimming nails; see podiatrist for nail care.	3. Neutral soaps and lotions prevent drying and cracking of skin; lotion application between toes increases moisture, which can lead to maceration of tissue.	
4. Use caution to avoid scratching or vigorous rubbing.	4. Scratching and rubbing can cause skin abrasions and microbial invasion.	
5. Promote good nutrition; adequate intake of vitamins A and C, protein, and zinc; and weight reduction, if the patient is overweight or has obesity.	5. Good nutrition promotes healing and prevents tissue breakdown.	

NURSING DIAGNOSIS: Lack of knowledge regarding self-care activities
GOAL: Adherence to the self-care program

Nursing Interventions	Rationale	Expected Outcomes
1. Include family/significant others in education.	1. Adherence to the self-care program is enhanced when the patient receives support from family and from appropriate self-help groups and agencies.	• Practices frequent position changes as prescribed • Practices postural exercises as prescribed • Takes medications as prescribed • Avoids vasoconstrictors • Uses measures to prevent trauma • Uses stress management • Accepts condition as chronic but amenable to therapies that will decrease symptoms
2. Provide written instructions about foot and leg care and exercise therapy program.	2. Written instructions serve as a reminder and reinforcement of information.	
3. Assist to obtain properly fitting clothing, shoes, and stockings.	3. Constrictive clothing and accessories impede circulation and promote venous stasis.	
4. Refer to self-help groups as indicated, such as smoking cessation clinics or stress management, weight management, and supervised exercise therapy programs.	4. Reducing risk factors may reduce symptoms or slow disease progression.	

flow and encourage the development of collateral circulation. The amount of exercise a patient can tolerate before the onset of pain is determined to provide a baseline for evaluation. The nurse instructs the patient to walk to the point of pain, rest until the pain subsides, and then resume walking so that endurance can be increased as collateral circulation develops. Pain can serve as a guide in determining the appropriate amount of exercise. The onset of pain indicates that the tissues are not receiving adequate oxygen, signaling the patient to rest. A supervised exercise therapy (SET) program should be prescribed for patients with claudication. SET can result in increased walking distance before the onset of claudication (Gerhard-Herman et al., 2016).

Before recommending any exercise program or SET, the patient's primary provider should be consulted. Conditions that worsen with exercise include leg ulcers, cellulitis, gangrene, or acute thrombotic occlusions.

Promoting Vasodilation and Preventing Vascular Compression

Arterial dilation increases blood flow to the extremities and is therefore a goal for patients with PAD. However, if the arteries are severely sclerosed, inelastic, or damaged, dilation is not possible. For this reason, measures to promote vasodilation, such as medications, endovascular interventions or surgery, may be only minimally effective.

Nursing interventions may involve applications of warmth to promote arterial flow and instructions to the patient to avoid exposure to cold temperatures, which causes vasoconstriction. Adequate clothing and warm temperatures protect the patient from chilling.

> ### ◤ Quality and Safety Nursing Alert
>
> *Patients are instructed to test the temperature of bath water and to avoid using hot-water bottles and heating pads on the extremities. It is safer to apply a hot-water bottle or a heating pad to the abdomen; this can cause reflex vasodilation in the extremities.*

In patients with vasospastic disorders (e.g., Raynaud's disease), heat may be applied directly to ischemic extremities using a warmed or electric blanket; however, the temperature of the heat source must not exceed body temperature. Even at low temperatures, trauma to the tissues can occur in ischemic extremities.

> ### ◤ Quality and Safety Nursing Alert
>
> *Excess heat may increase the metabolic rate of the extremities and the need for oxygen beyond that provided by the reduced arterial flow through the diseased artery. Heat must be used with great caution!*

Nicotine from any tobacco product causes vasospasm and can thereby dramatically reduce circulation to the extremities. Tobacco smoke also impairs transport and cellular use of oxygen and increases blood viscosity. Patients with arterial insufficiency who smoke, chew tobacco, or use electronic nicotine delivery systems (ENDS), including e-cigarettes, e-pens, e-pipes, e-hookah, and e-cigars, must be fully informed of the effects of nicotine on circulation and encouraged to stop.

Emotional stress can stimulate the sympathetic nervous system and cause peripheral vasoconstriction. Emotional stress can be minimized to some degree by avoiding stressful situations when possible or by consistently following a stress management program. Counseling services or use of alternative or complementary therapies (e.g., relaxation, yoga, aromatherapy, mindfulness) may be indicated for patients who cannot cope effectively with situational stressors.

Constrictive clothing and accessories such as tight socks or shoelaces may impede arterial circulation to the extremities and promote venous stasis and therefore should be avoided. Crossing the legs for more than 15 minutes at a time should be discouraged because it compresses vessels in the legs.

Relieving Pain

Frequently, the pain associated with peripheral arterial insufficiency is chronic, continuous, and disabling. It limits activities, affects work and life responsibilities, disturbs sleep, and alters the patient's sense of well-being. Patients may be depressed, irritable, and unable to exert the energy necessary to execute prescribed therapies, making pain relief even more difficult. Analgesic agents such as hydrocodone plus acetaminophen, oxycodone, oxycodone plus acetylsalicylic acid, or oxycodone plus acetaminophen may be helpful in reducing pain so that the patient can participate in therapies that can increase circulation and ultimately relieve pain more effectively. Particularly in older patients, these medications can be dangerous, contributing to delirium and falls. In all patients, issues of dependence need to be considered.

Maintaining Tissue Integrity

Poorly perfused tissues are susceptible to damage and infection. Patients with peripheral vascular disease and diabetes are at increased risk. When lesions develop, healing may be delayed or inhibited because of the poor blood supply to the area. Infected, nonhealing ulcerations of the extremities can be debilitating and may require prolonged and often expensive treatments. Amputation of an ischemic toe, forefoot or limb may eventually be necessary. Measures to prevent these complications must be a high priority and vigorously implemented. Centers of excellence for the prevention of amputation which involve a multidisciplinary, specialty team approach to management have become increasingly important for early intervention and surveillance.

Trauma to the extremities must be avoided. Advising the patient to wear sturdy, well-fitting shoes or slippers to prevent injury to the skin may be helpful, and recommending neutral soaps and body lotions may prevent drying and cracking of skin. However, the nurse should instruct the patient not to apply lotion between the toes, because the increased moisture can lead to maceration of the interdigital skin. Scratching and vigorous rubbing can abrade skin and create sites for microbial invasion; therefore, feet should be patted dry. Stockings should be clean and dry. Fingernails and toenails should be carefully trimmed straight across and sharp corners filed to follow the contour of the nail. If the nails cannot be trimmed safely, it is necessary to consult a podiatrist, who can also remove corns and calluses. Special shoe inserts may be needed to prevent calluses from recurring. Blisters, ingrown toenails, infection, or other problems should be reported to health care professionals for treatment and follow-up. Patients with diminished vision and those with disability that limits mobility of the arms or legs may require assistance in periodically examining the lower extremities for trauma or evidence of inflammation or infection.

Good nutrition promotes healing and prevents tissue breakdown and is therefore included in the plan for patients with peripheral vascular disease. Eating a diet that contains adequate protein and vitamins is necessary for patients with arterial insufficiency. Key nutrients, such as vitamin C and zinc, play specific roles in wound healing. However, a meta-analysis of randomized controlled trials found no evidence to support that supplementation with vitamins and antioxidants prevents vascular diseases (Sultan, Murarka, Jahangir, et al., 2017). Obesity strains the heart, increases venous congestion, and reduces circulation; therefore, a weight reduction plan may be necessary for patients who are overweight or have obesity. A diet low in fats and lipids is indicated for patients with atherosclerosis.

Gerontologic Considerations

In older adults, the symptoms of PAD may be more pronounced than in younger people. In older patients who are inactive, limb ischemia or gangrene may be the first sign of disease (Schorr, Treat-Jacobson, Lindquist, et al., 2017). See the Nursing Research Profile in Chart 26-5. These patients may have adjusted their lifestyle to accommodate the limitations imposed by the disease and may not walk far enough to develop symptoms of claudication due to other comorbid

Chart 26-5 · NURSING RESEARCH PROFILE

Understanding the Relationship Between Peripheral Artery Disease (PAD) Symptoms and Ischemia

Schorr, E. N., Treat-Jacobson, D., Lindquist, R. (2017). The relationship between peripheral artery disease symptomatology and ischemia. *Nursing Research, 66*(5), 378–387.

Purpose

Peripheral artery disease (PAD) impacts over eight million Americans and is associated with an increased risk for cardiovascular disease and mortality. It is typically identified when patients report claudication (i.e., aching, cramping pain, fatigue in calves with activity). However, less than 33% of individuals who have a diagnosis of PAD report classic claudication, potentially resulting in underdiagnosis of PAD. A better understanding of symptom presentation and changes in tissue oxygenation may enhance earlier detection and treatment of PAD. The aim of this study was to explore the range of symptoms (typical versus atypical, location, and description) that patients with PAD experience to better understand the relationship between symptom variation and calf muscle ischemia.

Design

This descriptive study explored symptoms during exercise testing and recovery in patients with a diagnosis of PAD. Individuals who were English speaking, 21 years of age or older, and met specific diagnostic criteria were recruited from a larger study. Participants with uncontrolled hypertension, angina or dyspnea on exercise testing, or vascular procedures performed within the last 3 months were excluded. Demographic and clinical data were collected. Ankle-brachial index (ABI) was used as a measure of disease severity. Participants exercised on a treadmill with a near-infrared spectroscopy device to measure calf muscle tissue saturation index (TSI). In addition, participants rated symptom intensity using a numerical rating scale (NRS) and provided self-report of symptom location and descriptors. Data were collected at three points (e.g., rest, exercise, recovery) during three successive treadmill tests. Descriptive statistics were generated and symptom variables and relevant demographic and clinical data (e.g., age, gender, race, ABI, diabetes, neuropathy) were

examined with the TSI measurements during exercise and recovery using multilevel modeling procedures.

Findings

Three successive episodes of treadmill testing with 40 participants resulted in 120 exercise tests. The majority of participants were Caucasian males (80%) with an average age of 68 years (SD 0.92). More than half (69.2%) of tests were stopped due to discomfort in the calf, with only 55% of participants reporting typical descriptors of claudication. TSI declined rapidly between the start of exercise and symptom onset. The lowest TSI was often reached before reported maximum discomfort. Changes in TSI were related to exercise time ($p < 0.001$), baseline TSI ($p < 0.001$), exercise rating ($p < 0.001$), and ABI ($p < 0.5$). In the recovery phase, TSI steadily increased as pain reduced; TSI was associated with recovery rating ($p < 0.001$) and ABI ($p < 0.03$).

Nursing Implications

Recognizing variations in symptom presentation (e.g., intensity, location, description) and associated ischemic changes in PAD is important in understanding individual patient experiences and tailoring education and treatment. Nurses should be aware that some patients with PAD may use terms such as *burn, pressure,* or *tight* to describe related discomfort and that patients may report discomfort in atypical locations, such as the foot. A better understanding of the full range of ischemic symptoms in PAD may prompt earlier diagnosis and facilitate risk factor modification and exercise therapy. Unlike other medical conditions, where the onset of pain indicates the potential of increasing tissue damage with ongoing activity, pain in PAD can be used as an indicator to adjust the exercise program to extend the person's walking distance. Exercise prescription can greatly reduce the progression of atherosclerosis, limiting not only distal disease but also coronary and cerebral disease. Although additional research is needed, nurses can consider these findings when planning care for patients with PAD to ensure they are providing appropriate education and encouraging safe exercise regimens.

---

conditions such as chronic obstructive pulmonary disease (COPD) or heart failure. Circulation is decreased, although this is not apparent to the patient until trauma occurs. At this point, gangrene develops when minimal arterial flow is impaired further by edema formation resulting from the traumatic event.

Intermittent claudication may occur after walking only one half to one block or after walking up a slight incline. Any prolonged pressure on the foot can cause pressure injuries that may become ulcerated, infected, or gangrenous. The outcomes of arterial insufficiency can include reduced mobility and activity as well as a loss of independence. Older adults with reduced mobility are less likely to remain in the community setting, have higher rates of hospitalizations, and experience a poorer quality of life. Those with cognitive impairment may also be unable to verbalize symptoms such as pain.

Promoting Home, Community-Based, and Transitional Care

The self-care program is planned with the patient so that activities that promote arterial and venous circulation,

relieve pain, and promote tissue integrity are acceptable. The patient and family are helped to understand the reasons for each aspect of the plan, the possible consequences of nonadherence, and the importance of keeping follow-up appointments. Long-term care of the feet and legs is of prime importance in the prevention of trauma, ulceration, and gangrene. Chart 26-6 provides detailed patient instructions for foot and leg care.

Peripheral Artery Disease

Arterial insufficiency of the extremities occurs most often in men and is a common cause of disability. The legs are most frequently affected; however, the upper extremities may be involved. The age of onset and the severity are influenced by the type and number of atherosclerotic risk factors (see Chart 26-3). In PAD, obstructive lesions are predominantly confined to segments of the arterial system extending from the aorta below the renal arteries to the popliteal artery (see Fig. 26-9). Distal occlusive disease is frequently seen in patients with diabetes and in older patients (Gerhard-Herman et al., 2016).

Chart 26-6 HOME CARE CHECKLIST

Foot and Leg Care in Peripheral Vascular Disease

At the completion of education, the patient and/or caregiver will be able to:

- Describe the rationale for proper foot and leg care in managing peripheral vascular disease.
- Demonstrate daily foot hygiene: Wash between toes with mild soap and lukewarm water, then rinse thoroughly and pat rather than rub dry.
- Recognize the dangers of thermal injury.
  - Wear clean, loose, soft cotton socks (they are comfortable, allow air to circulate, and absorb moisture).
  - In cold weather, wear extra socks in extra-large shoes.
  - Avoid heating pads, whirlpools, and hot tubs.
  - Avoid sunburn.
- Identify safety concerns.
  - Inspect feet daily with a mirror for redness, dryness, cuts, blisters, and so forth.
  - Always wear soft shoes or slippers when out of bed.
  - Trim nails straight across after showering.
  - Consult podiatrist to trim nails if vision is decreased and for care of corns, blisters, and ingrown nails.
  - Clear pathways in house to prevent injury.
  - Avoid wearing thong sandals.
  - Use lamb's wool or foam between toes if they overlap or rub each other.
- Demonstrate the use of comfort measures.
  - Wear leather shoes with an extra-depth toe box. Synthetic shoes do not allow air to circulate.

- If feet become dry and scaly, use cream or lotion with emollient. Never put cream or lotion between toes unless it has been prescribed.
- Avoid scratching or vigorous rubbing, which could cause abrasions.
- If feet perspire, especially between toes, use lamb's wool between toes to promote drying.
- Demonstrate strategies to decrease risk of constricting blood vessels.
  - Avoid circumferential compression around feet or legs—for example, by knee-high stockings or tight socks or constricting bandages.
  - Do not cross legs at knees.
  - Stop using all nicotine products (i.e., smoking or chewing) because nicotine causes vasoconstriction and vasospasm.
  - Participate in regular walking or supervised exercise therapy to stimulate circulation.
- Recognize when to seek medical attention.
  - Contact health care provider at the onset of skin breakdown such as abrasions, blisters, fungal infection (athlete's foot), or pain.
  - Do not use any medication on feet or legs unless prescribed.
  - Avoid using iodine, alcohol, corn/wart-removing compound, or adhesive products before checking with primary provider.
- State understanding of community resources and referrals (if any).

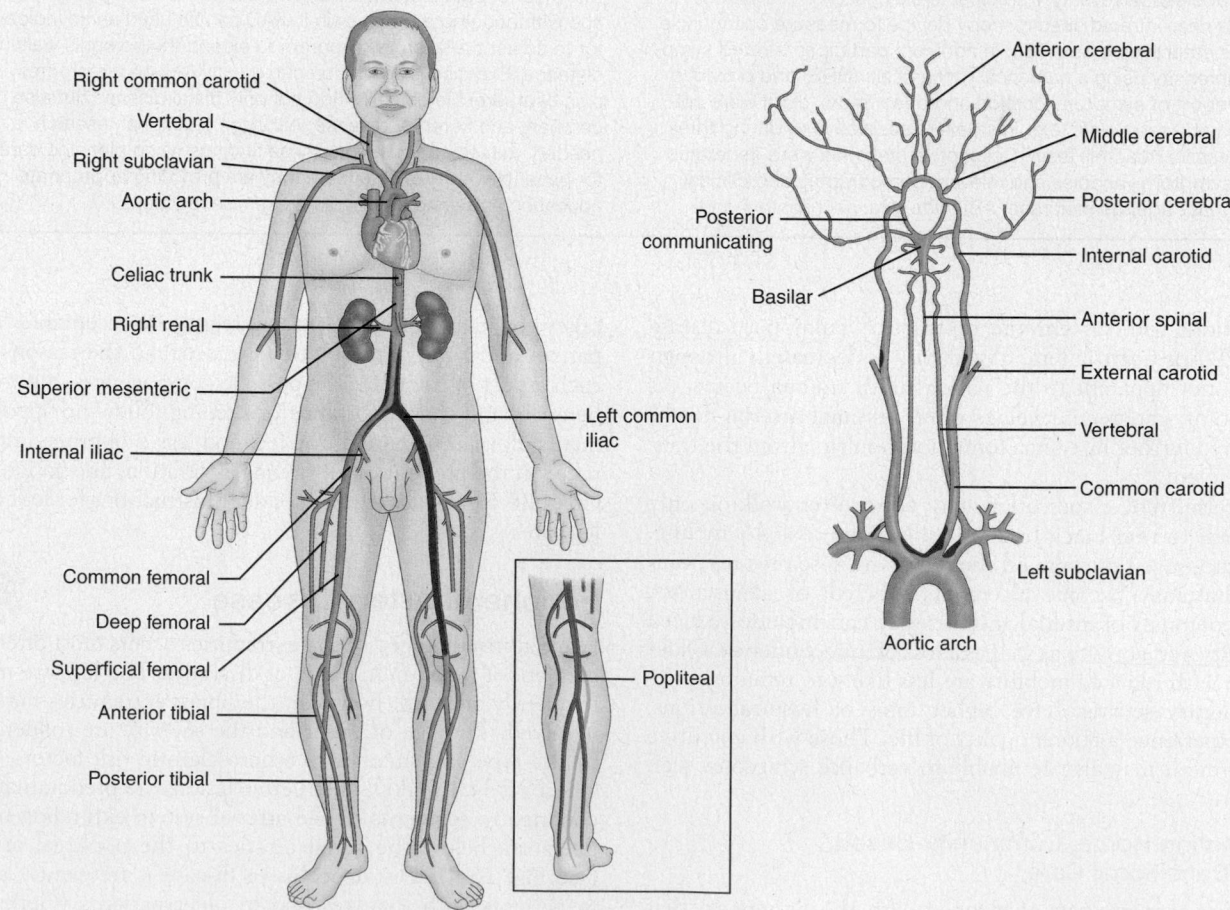

Figure 26-9 • Common sites of atherosclerotic obstruction in major arteries.

Clinical Manifestations

The hallmark symptom is intermittent claudication described as aching, cramping, or inducing fatigue or weakness that occurs with some degree of activity or exercise, which is relieved with rest. The pain commonly occurs in muscle groups distal to the area of stenosis or occlusion. As the disease progresses, the patient may have a decreased ability to walk the same distance as before or may notice increased pain with ambulation. When the arterial insufficiency becomes severe, the patient has rest pain. This pain is associated with critical ischemia of the distal extremity and is described as persistent, aching, or boring; it may be so excruciating that it is unrelieved by opioids and can be disabling. Ischemic rest pain is usually worse at night and often wakes the patient. Elevating the extremity or placing it in a horizontal position increases the pain, whereas placing the extremity in a dependent position reduces the pain. In an attempt to prevent or relieve the pain, some patients sleep with the affected leg hanging over the side of the bed or sleep in a reclining chair.

Assessment and Diagnostic Findings

A sensation of coldness or numbness in the extremities may accompany intermittent claudication and is a result of reduced arterial flow. The extremity is cool and pale when elevated or ruddy and cyanotic when placed in a dependent position. Skin and nail changes, ulceration, gangrene, and muscle atrophy may be evident. Bruits may be auscultated with a stethoscope. Peripheral pulses may be diminished or absent.

Examination of the peripheral pulses is an important part of assessing PAD. Unequal pulses between extremities or the absence of a normally palpable pulse is a sign of PAD.

The presence, location, and extent of PAD are determined by a careful history of the symptoms and by physical examination. The color and temperature of the extremity are noted and the pulses palpated. The nails may be thickened and opaque, and the skin may be shiny, atrophic, and dry, with sparse or absent hair. The assessment includes comparison of the right and left extremities.

The diagnosis of PAD may be made using CW Doppler and ABIs, treadmill testing for claudication, duplex ultrasonography, or other imaging studies described earlier in this chapter.

Medical Management

Generally, patients feel better and have fewer symptoms of claudication after they participate in a SET program. SET programs are covered by insurance for a specific number of sessions. Reimbursement requires that SET is administered under direct provider supervision. A provider (e.g., physician, nurse practitioner, clinical nurse specialist, physician assistant) must be immediately and physically available, although not necessarily physically present, while SET is provided. The person providing the program supervision must be trained in the optimal delivery of SET and in both basic life support and advanced cardiac life support techniques. Unsupervised walking exercise programs are attractive for many patients with PAD with limited access to a SET program. Two recent trials in patients with PAD had similar findings between the supervised and unsupervised groups, suggesting no greater therapeutic benefit for those who engage in supervised walking programs (McDermott, 2018). These findings suggest that home-based programs may be a viable and efficacious option for patients unable to participate in a structured, on-site, supervised exercise program. If a walking program is combined with weight reduction and cessation of nicotine use, patients often can further improve their activity tolerance. Patients should not be promised that their symptoms will be relieved if they stop nicotine use, however, because claudication may persist, and they may lose their motivation to stop using nicotine. In addition to these interventions, arm-ergometer exercise training effectively improves physical fitness, central cardiorespiratory function, and walking capacity in patients with claudication (Treat-Jacobson, McDermott, Beckman, et al., 2019).

Pharmacologic Therapy

Cilostazol is approved by the U.S. Food and Drug Administration (FDA) for the treatment of claudication. Cilostazol, a phosphodiesterase III inhibitor, is a direct vasodilator that inhibits platelet aggregation. Studies have shown it plays a role in decreasing intimal hyperplasia after angioplasty and stenting. Furthermore, patients prescribed cilostazol report improvement in maximal walking distance and pain-free walking distance within 4 to 6 weeks (Farkas, Járai, & Kolossváry, 2017). This agent is contraindicated in patients with a history of heart failure.

Antiplatelet agents, such as aspirin or clopidogrel, prevent the formation of thromboemboli which can lead to myocardial infarction and stroke and are recommended to treat patients with symptomatic PAD (Gerhard-Herman et al., 2016). Aspirin has been shown to reduce the risk of cardiovascular events (e.g., myocardial infarction, stroke, cardiovascular death) in patients with vascular disease; however, adverse events associated with aspirin use include gastrointestinal upset or bleeding (Gerhard-Herman et al., 2016).

Use of dual antiplatelet agents, such as aspirin and clopidogrel, in patients with symptomatic PAD has not been well established. However, dual antiplatelet agents may be effective and may be reasonable to reduce limb-threatening events after revascularization. Statins improve endothelial function in patients with PAD. Studies suggest that statins reduce severity of intermittent claudication and increase walking distance to the onset of claudication (Gerhard-Herman et al., 2016). These medications have beneficial effects on vascular inflammation, plaque stabilization, endothelial dysfunction, and thrombosis, and have been linked to decreased rates of repeat peripheral interventions, amputations, and major adverse cardiovascular events up to 3 years post procedure (Saxon, Safley, & Mena-Hurtado, 2020).

Endovascular Management

Endovascular interventions can include a balloon angioplasty, stent, stent graft, or an atherectomy. These revascularization procedures are less invasive than conventional surgery; their objective is to establish adequate inflow to the distal vessels. A meta-analysis reported that the efficacy and safety of all of these endovascular procedures are comparable to surgical interventions. Some stents that may be selected are drug eluting. Although costly, these are particularly efficacious in

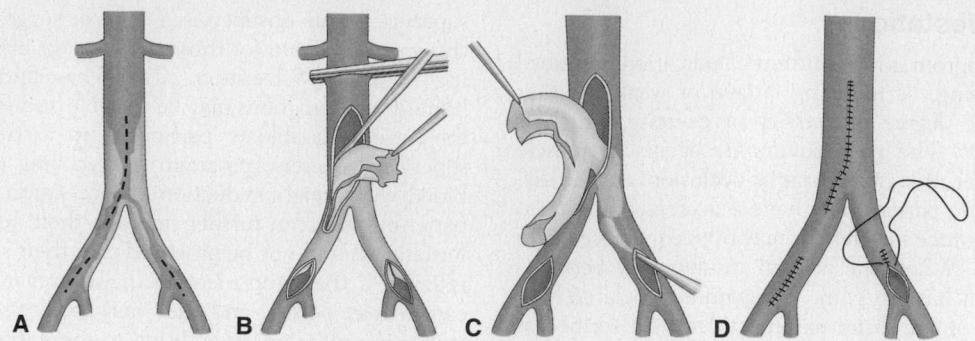

Figure 26-10 • In an aortoiliac endarterectomy, the vascular surgeon identifies the diseased area (**A**), clamps off the blood supply to the vessel (**B**), removes the plaque (**C**), and sutures the vessel shut (**D**), after which blood flow is restored. Adapted with permission from Sidawy, A. N., & Perler, B. A. (2019). *Rutherford's vascular surgery and endovascular therapy* (9th ed.). Philadelphia, PA: Elsevier.

patients who have recurrent disease. By releasing antiproliferative drugs, drug-eluting balloons and stents have been shown to reduce the risk of restenosis. Eligible candidates for drug-eluting stents must be able to take antiplatelet medications for at least 6 months post procedure (Sidawy & Perler, 2019).

Surgical Management

Surgery is reserved for the treatment of rest pain, severe and disabling claudication, or when the limb is at risk for amputation because of tissue necrosis. The choice of the surgical procedure depends on the degree, length, and location of the stenosis or occlusion and whether there are single or multiple lesions. Other important considerations are the overall health of the patient, the length of the procedure, and anesthesia required. If endarterectomy is performed, an incision is made into the artery and the atheromatous obstruction is removed (see Fig. 26-10).

Bypass grafts are performed to reroute the blood flow around the stenosis or occlusion. Before bypass grafting, the surgeon determines where the distal **anastomosis** (site where the vessels are surgically joined) will be placed. The distal outflow vessel must be at least 50% patent for the graft to remain open. If the atherosclerotic occlusion is below the inguinal ligament in the superficial femoral artery, the surgical procedure of choice is the femoral-to-popliteal graft. This procedure is further classified as above- and below-knee grafts, referring to the location of the distal anastomosis. Bypass grafts may be synthetic materials or autologous vein. Several synthetic materials are available for use as a peripheral bypass graft: woven or knitted Dacron or expanded polytetrafluoroethylene (PTFE). Cryopreserved saphenous veins and umbilical veins are also available. When using an autologous conduit (i.e., the patient's own veins), the vein is either grafted to the artery in situ (the vein remains in place with the valves stripped and the vein is anastomosed to the proximal and distal target arteries), or the vein is harvested, reversed, and anastomosed to the proximal and distal target arteries.

Lower leg or ankle vessels with occlusions may also require grafts. Occasionally, the popliteal artery is completely occluded and only collateral vessels maintain perfusion. The distal anastomosis may be made onto any of the tibial arteries (posterior tibial, anterior tibial, or peroneal arteries) or the dorsalis pedis or plantar artery. The distal anastomosis site is determined by the ease of exposure of the vessel in surgery and by which vessel provides the best flow to the distal limb. These grafts require the use of an autologous vein to ensure patency. The greater or lesser saphenous vein or a combination of one of the saphenous veins and an upper extremity vein such as the cephalic vein is used to provide the required length.

How long the graft remains patent is determined by several factors, including the size of the graft, graft location, and development of intimal hyperplasia at anastomosis sites (Sidawy & Perler, 2019). Infection of synthetic grafts may result in sepsis and almost always requires removal.

If a vein graft is the surgical choice, care must be taken in the operating room not to damage the vein after harvesting (removing the vein from the patient's body). The vein is occluded at one end and inflated with a heparinized solution to check for leakage and competency. The graft is then placed in a heparinized solution to keep it from becoming dry and brittle until use during the operative procedure.

For patients who cannot tolerate an extensive vascular surgical procedure, a palliative approach involving primary amputation rather than an endarterectomy or bypass may be considered (Conte et al., 2019).

Nursing Management

Nursing care for patients with PAD is reviewed in Chart 26-4. Nursing care for the patient who has had endovascular revascularization procedures mostly mirrors the care of patients who have had endovascular repair to aortic aneurysms (see later section). The patient who has had an endovascular procedure may be discharged home the day of the procedure, or by the following day.

Nursing Care of the Postoperative Patient

During the postoperative period, the nurse's care focuses on maintaining circulation, identifying and managing potential complications, and discharge planning.

Maintaining Circulation

The primary objective in the postoperative period is to maintain adequate circulation through the arterial repair. Pulses, Doppler assessment, color and temperature, capillary refill, and sensory and motor function of the affected extremity are checked and compared with those of the other extremity; these observations are recorded initially every 15 minutes and then at progressively longer intervals if the patient's status remains stable. Doppler evaluation of the vessels distal to the bypass graft should be performed, because it is more sensitive than palpation for pulses. The ABI is monitored at least once every 8 hours for the first 24 hours (not usually assessed with pedal artery bypasses due to the risk of compression of the anastomosis by the cuff) and then once each day until discharge; the typical hospital length of stay is 3 to 5 days. An adequate circulating blood volume should be established and maintained. Disappearance of a pulse that was present may indicate thrombotic occlusion of the graft; the surgeon is immediately notified.

Monitoring and Managing Potential Complications

Continuous monitoring of urine output, central venous pressure, mental status, and pulse rate and volume permits early recognition and treatment of fluid imbalances. Bleeding can result from the heparin given during surgery or from an anastomotic leak. A hematoma may form as well. The nurse should review the operative report to determine if the heparin was reversed (usually with protamine sulfate) in the operating room.

Leg crossing and prolonged extremity dependency are avoided to prevent thrombosis. Edema is a normal postoperative finding due to increased arterial flow; however, elevating the extremities and encouraging the patient to exercise the extremities while in bed reduces edema. Graduated compression or anti-embolism stockings may be prescribed for some patients, but care must be taken to avoid compressing distal vessel bypass grafts, inducing pressure injuries, and obscuring visualization of the extremity. Severe edema of the extremity, pain, and decreased sensation of toes or fingers can be an indication of compartment syndrome (see Chapter 37).

Promoting Home, Community-Based, and Transitional Care

Discharge planning includes assessing the patient's ability to manage activities of daily living (ADLs) independently. The nurse determines whether the patient has a network of family and friends to assist with ADLs. The patient is encouraged to make the lifestyle changes necessitated by the onset of disease, including pain management and modifications in diet, activity, and hygiene (skin care). The nurse ensures that the patient has the knowledge and ability to assess for any postoperative complications such as infection, occlusion of the artery or graft, and decreased blood flow. The nurse assists the patient in developing and implementing a plan to stop using tobacco products.

Upper Extremity Arterial Disease

Arterial stenosis and occlusions occur less frequently in the upper extremities (arms) than in the legs, and cause less severe symptoms because the collateral circulation is significantly better in the arms. The arms also have less muscle mass and are not subjected to the workload of the legs.

Clinical Manifestations

Stenosis and occlusions in the upper extremity result from atherosclerosis or trauma. The stenosis usually occurs at the origin of the vessel proximal to the vertebral artery, which results in the vertebral artery becoming the dominant vessel for blood flow. The patient typically complains of arm fatigue and pain with exercise (forearm claudication), inability to hold or grasp objects (e.g., combing hair, placing objects on shelves above the head), and occasionally difficulty driving.

The patient may develop a "subclavian steal" syndrome characterized by reverse flow in the vertebral and basilar arteries to provide blood flow to the arm. This syndrome may cause vertebrobasilar (cerebral) symptoms, including vertigo, ataxia, syncope, or bilateral visual changes.

Assessment and Diagnostic Findings

Findings on assessment include coolness and pallor of the affected extremity, decreased capillary refill, and a difference in arm blood pressures of more than 15 to 20 mm Hg (Zierler & Dawson, 2016). Noninvasive studies performed to evaluate upper extremity arterial occlusions include upper and forearm blood pressure determinations and duplex ultrasonography to identify the anatomic location of the lesion and to evaluate the hemodynamics of blood flow. Transcranial Doppler evaluation is performed to evaluate the intracranial circulation and to detect any siphoning of blood flow from the posterior circulation to provide blood flow to the affected arm. If an endovascular or surgical procedure is planned, a diagnostic arteriogram may be necessary.

Medical Management

If a short focal lesion is identified in an upper extremity artery, a PTA with possible stent or stent graft placement may be performed. If the lesion involves the subclavian artery with documented siphoning of blood flow from the intracranial circulation and an endovascular procedure is not possible, a surgical bypass may be performed.

Nursing Management

Nursing assessment involves bilateral comparison of upper arm blood pressures (obtained by stethoscope and Doppler), radial, ulnar, and brachial pulses, motor and sensory function, temperature, color changes, and capillary refill every 2 hours. Disappearance of a pulse or Doppler flow that had been present may indicate an acute occlusion of the vessel, and the primary provider is notified immediately.

After surgery or an endovascular procedure, the arm is kept at heart level or elevated, with the fingers at the highest level. Pulses are monitored with Doppler assessment of the arterial flow every hour for 2 hours and then every shift. Blood pressure (obtained by stethoscope and Doppler) is also assessed every hour for 4 hours and then every shift. Motor and sensory function, warmth, color, and capillary refill are monitored with each arterial flow (pulse) assessment.

> ▶ *Quality and Safety Nursing Alert*
>
> *Before surgery and for 24 hours after surgery, the patient's arm is kept at heart level and protected from cold, venous and arterial punctures, tape, pressure, and constrictive dressings.*

Discharge planning is similar to that for the patient with PAD. Chart 26-4 describes nursing care for patients with peripheral vascular disease.

Aortoiliac Disease

If collateral circulation has developed, patients with a stenosis or occlusion of the aortoiliac segment may be asymptomatic, or they may complain of buttock or low back discomfort associated with walking. Men may have erectile dysfunction or experience impotence. These patients may have decreased or absent femoral pulses.

Medical Management

The treatment of aortoiliac disease is essentially the same as that for atherosclerotic PAD. An endovascular procedure, such as bilateral common iliac stents, may be attempted if the aorta has a less than 50% diameter reduction (Gerhard-Herman et al., 2016). If there is significant aortic disease, the surgical procedure of choice is the aortoiliac graft. If possible, the distal graft is anastomosed to the iliac artery, and the entire surgical procedure is performed within the abdomen. If the iliac vessels are occluded, the distal anastomosis is made to the femoral arteries (aortobifemoral graft). A femoral–femoral crossover graft may also be needed to maintain circulation. Bifurcated woven or knitted Dacron grafts are preferred for this surgical procedure.

Nursing Management

Preprocedural or preoperative assessment, in addition to the standard parameters (see Chapter 14), includes evaluating the brachial, radial, ulnar, femoral, popliteal, posterior tibial, and dorsalis pedis pulses to establish a baseline for follow-up after arterial lines are placed and postoperatively. Patient education includes an overview of the procedure to be performed, the preparation for an endovascular procedure or surgery, and the anticipated postprocedural or postoperative plan of care. Sights, sounds, and sensations that the patient may experience are discussed.

Postprocedural endovascular care mirrors the care described for the patient who has had endovascular repair of an aortic aneurysm (see later discussion). Postoperative care includes monitoring for signs of thrombosis in arteries distal to the surgical site. The nurse assesses color and temperature of the extremity, capillary refill time, sensory and motor function, and pulses by palpation and Doppler initially every 15 minutes and then at progressively longer intervals if the patient's status remains stable. Any dusky or bluish discoloration, coldness, decrease in sensory or motor function, or decrease in pulse quality is reported immediately to the primary provider.

Postoperative care also includes monitoring urine output and ensuring that output is at least 0.5 mL/kg/h. Renal function may be impaired as a result of hypoperfusion from hypotension, ischemia to the renal arteries during the surgical procedure, hypovolemia, or embolization of the renal artery or renal parenchyma. Vital signs, pain, and intake and output are monitored with the pulse and extremity assessments. Results of laboratory tests are monitored and reported to the primary provider. Abdominal assessment for bowel sounds and paralytic ileus is performed at least every 8 hours. Bowel sounds may not return before the third postoperative day. The absence of bowel sounds, absence of flatus, and abdominal distention are indications of paralytic ileus. Manual manipulation of the bowel during surgery may have caused bruising, resulting in decreased peristalsis. Nasogastric suction may be necessary to decompress the bowel until peristalsis returns. A liquid bowel movement before the third postoperative day may indicate bowel ischemia, which may occur when the mesenteric blood supply (celiac, superior mesenteric, or inferior mesenteric arteries) is occluded. Ischemic bowel usually causes increased pain and a markedly elevated white blood cell count (20,000 to 30,000 cells/mm^3).

Aneurysms

An aneurysm is a localized sac or dilation formed at a weak point in the wall of the artery (see Fig. 26-11). It may be classified by its shape or form. The most common forms of aneurysms are saccular and fusiform. A saccular aneurysm projects from only one side of the vessel. If an entire arterial segment becomes dilated, a fusiform aneurysm develops. Very small aneurysms due to localized infection are called *mycotic aneurysms*.

Historically, the cause of abdominal aortic aneurysm, the most common type of degenerative aneurysm, has been attributed to atherosclerotic changes in the aorta. Other causes of

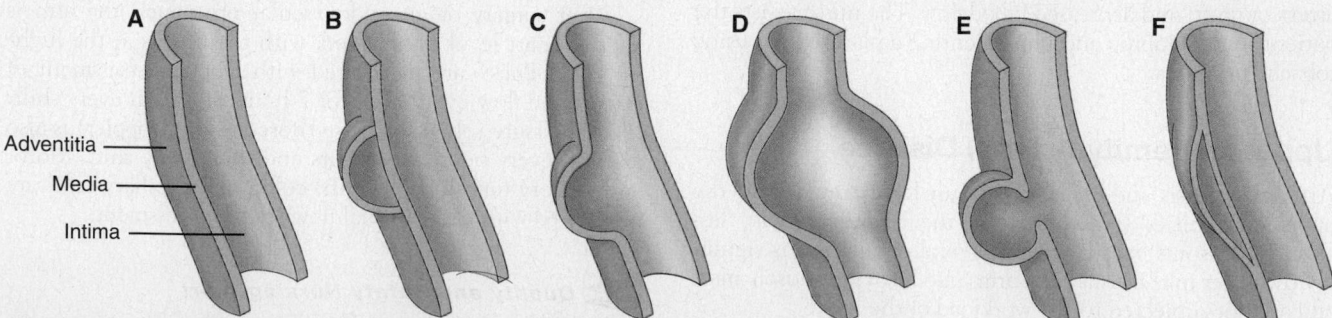

Figure 26-11 • Characteristics of arterial aneurysm. **A.** Normal artery. **B.** False aneurysm—actually a pulsating hematoma. The clot and connective tissue are outside the arterial wall. **C.** True aneurysm. One, two, or all three layers of the artery may be involved. **D.** Fusiform aneurysm—symmetric, spindle-shaped expansion of entire circumference of involved vessel. **E.** Saccular aneurysm—a bulbous protrusion of one side of the arterial wall. **F.** Dissecting aneurysm—this usually is a hematoma that splits the layers of the arterial wall. Adapted with permission from Sidawy, A. N., & Perler, B. A. (2019). *Rutherford's vascular surgery and endovascular therapy* (9th ed.). Philadelphia, PA: Elsevier.

Chart 26-7	Etiologic Classification of Arterial Aneurysms

Anastomotic (postarteriotomy) and graft aneurysms: Infection, arterial wall failure, suture failure, graft failure

Congenital: Primary connective tissue disorders (Marfan syndrome, Ehlers–Danlos syndrome) and other diseases (focal medial agenesis, tuberous sclerosis, Turner syndrome, Menkes syndrome)

Infectious (mycotic): Bacterial, fungal, spirochetal infections

Inflammatory (noninfectious): Associated with arteritis (Takayasu disease, giant cell arteritis, systemic lupus erythematosus, Behçet syndrome, Kawasaki disease) and periarterial inflammation (i.e., pancreatitis)

Mechanical (hemodynamic): Poststenotic and arteriovenous fistula and amputation related

Pregnancy-related degenerative: Nonspecific, inflammatory variant

Traumatic (pseudoaneurysms): Penetrating arterial injuries, blunt arterial injuries, pseudoaneurysms

Adapted from Sidawy, A. N., & Perler, B. A. (2019). *Rutherford's vascular surgery and endovascular therapy* (9th ed.). Philadelphia, PA: Elsevier.

aneurysm formation are listed in Chart 26-7. Aneurysms are potentially serious; if they are located in large vessels that rupture, this can lead to hemorrhage and death.

Thoracic Aortic Aneurysm

Approximately 70% of all cases of thoracic aortic aneurysm are caused by atherosclerosis. They occur most frequently in men between the ages of 50 and 70 years, and are estimated to affect 10 of every 100,000 older adults. The thoracic area is the most common site for a dissecting aneurysm. Thoracic aortic emergencies are associated with high morbidity and mortality rates, but with the emergence of endovascular aortic repair there is an improvement in the mortality rate; in particular, the mortality rate for patients treated at high-volume aortic centers can be as low as 4.8% (Harris, Olson, Panthofer, et al., 2019).

Clinical Manifestations

Symptoms vary and depend on how rapidly the aneurysm dilates and how the pulsating mass affects surrounding intrathoracic structures. Some patients are asymptomatic. In most cases, pain is the most prominent symptom. The pain is usually constant and boring but may occur only when the person is supine. Other conspicuous symptoms are dyspnea, the result of pressure of the aneurysm sac against the trachea, a main bronchus, or the lung itself; cough, frequently paroxysmal and with a brassy quality; hoarseness, stridor, or vocal weakness or aphonia (complete loss of the voice), resulting from pressure against the laryngeal nerve; and dysphagia (difficulty in swallowing) due to impingement on the esophagus by the aneurysm.

Assessment and Diagnostic Findings

When large veins in the chest are compressed by the aneurysm, the superficial veins of the chest, neck, or arms become dilated, and edematous areas on the chest wall and cyanosis are often evident. Pressure against the cervical sympathetic chain can result in unequal pupils. Diagnosis of a thoracic aortic aneurysm is principally made by chest x-ray, computed tomography angiography (CTA), MRA, or transesophageal echocardiography (TEE). CTAs are typically performed because they are widely available, can be completed rapidly, and can remove cardiac motion artifacts, enhancing their accuracy (Sidawy & Perler, 2019).

Medical Management

Treatment is based on whether the patient is symptomatic and whether the aneurysm is expanding in size, caused by an iatrogenic injury, contains a dissection, or involves branch vessels. General measures such as controlling blood pressure and correcting risk factors are helpful. For decades, beta-blockers (e.g., atenolol, metoprolol, carvedilol) have been the mainstay of medical treatment for aortic aneurysms; however, angiotensin receptor blockers (ARBs) (e.g., losartan, valsartan, irbesartan) may also retard aortic dilation (Rurali, Perrucci, Pilato, et al., 2018). It is also important to control blood pressure in patients with dissecting aneurysms. Preoperatively, the systolic pressure is maintained at approximately 90 to 120 mm Hg in order to maintain a mean arterial pressure at 65 to 75 mm Hg with a beta-blocker such as esmolol or metoprolol. Occasionally, antihypertensive agents such as hydralazine are used for this purpose. Sodium nitroprusside is the most established drug used for this purpose; it is given by continuous IV drip to emergently lower the blood pressure, as it has a rapid onset and short action of duration and is easily titrated (Sidawy & Perler, 2019). The goal of surgery is to repair the aneurysm and restore vascular continuity with a vascular graft. Intensive monitoring is required after this type of surgery, and the patient is cared for in the critical care unit.

Repair of thoracic aneurysms using endovascular grafts placed percutaneously in an interventional suite (e.g., interventional radiology, cardiac catheterization laboratory) or combined interventional suite and operating room (hybrid suite) may decrease postoperative recovery time and decrease complications compared with traditional surgical techniques. Thoracic endografts are made of PTFE material reinforced with nitinol or titanium stents. These endovascular grafts are inserted into the thoracic aorta via various vascular access routes, usually the brachial or femoral artery. Because a large surgical incision is not necessary to gain vascular access, the overall patient recovery time tends to be shorter than with open surgical repair. Despite the absence of aortic cross-clamping, there is still a 2% to 15% chance of spinal cord ischemia as a potential complication (Miranda, Sousa, & Mansilha, 2018). To decrease the chances of spinal cord ischemia and paraplegia, lumbar spinal drains are usually placed in patients undergoing an endovascular repair of thoracic aortic aneurysms. Cerebrospinal fluid drainage is performed to decrease the arterial to cerebral spinal fluid gradient, thereby improving spinal perfusion. What appears to be most important in preventing neurologic deficit is to maintain the cerebrospinal fluid pressure less than or equal to 10 mm Hg (14 cm H_2O) and to keep the mean arterial pressure greater than 90 mm Hg for the first 36 to 48 hours postoperatively (Scali, Kim, Kubilis, et al., 2018).

Abdominal Aortic Aneurysm

The most common cause of abdominal aortic aneurysm is atherosclerosis. This condition affects men two to six times more often than women, is two to three times more common in White versus Black men, and is most prevalent in patients older than 65 years of age (Sidawy & Perler, 2019). Most of these aneurysms occur below the renal arteries (infrarenal aneurysms). Untreated, the eventual outcome may be rupture and death.

Pathophysiology

All aneurysms involve a damaged media layer of the vessel. This may be caused by congenital weakness, trauma, or disease. After an aneurysm develops, it tends to enlarge. Risk factors include genetic predisposition, nicotine use, and hypertension; more than half of patients with aneurysms have hypertension.

Clinical Manifestations

Only about 40% of patients with abdominal aortic aneurysms have symptoms. Some patients complain that they can feel their heart beating in their abdomen when lying down, or they may say that they feel an abdominal mass or abdominal throbbing. If the abdominal aortic aneurysm is associated with thrombus, a major vessel may be occluded or smaller distal occlusions may result from emboli. Small cholesterol, platelet, or fibrin emboli may lodge in the interosseous or digital arteries, causing cyanosis and mottling of the toes (also referred to as trashing or trash toes).

Signs of impending rupture include severe back or abdominal pain, which may be persistent or intermittent. Abdominal pain is often localized in the middle or lower abdomen to the left of the midline. Low back pain may be present because of pressure of the aneurysm on the lumbar nerves. Indications that the abdominal aortic aneurysm may be leaking or rupturing include constant, intense back pain; falling blood pressure; and decreasing hematocrit. Rupture into the peritoneal cavity is rapidly fatal. A retroperitoneal rupture (contained rupture) of an aneurysm may result in hematomas in the scrotum, perineum, flank, or penis. Signs of heart failure or a loud bruit may suggest a rupture into the vena cava. If the aneurysm adheres to the adjacent vena cava, the vena cava may become damaged when rupture or leak of the aneurysm occurs. Rupture into the vena cava results in higher-pressure arterial blood entering the lower-pressure venous system and causing turbulence, which is heard as a bruit. The high blood pressure and increased blood volume returning to the right side of the heart from the vena cava may cause heart failure.

Assessment and Diagnostic Findings

The most important diagnostic indication of an abdominal aortic aneurysm is a pulsatile mass in the middle and upper abdomen. Most clinically significant aortic aneurysms are palpable during routine physical examination; however, the sensitivity depends on the size of the aneurysm, abdominal girth of the patient (i.e., more difficult to find in the patient with obesity), and the skill of the examiner (Sidawy & Perler, 2019). A systolic bruit may be heard over the mass. Duplex ultrasonography or CTA is used to determine the size, length, and location of the aneurysm. When the aneurysm is small, ultrasonography is conducted at 6-month intervals until the aneurysm reaches a size so that surgery to prevent rupture is of more benefit than the possible complications of a surgical procedure. Some aneurysms remain stable over many years of monitoring.

 Gerontologic Considerations

Most abdominal aortic aneurysms occur in patients between 60 and 90 years of age. Rupture is likely with coexisting hypertension and with aneurysms more than 6 cm wide. In most cases at this point, the chances of rupture are greater than the chances of death during surgical repair. If the older patient is considered at risk for complications related to surgery or anesthesia, the aneurysm is not repaired until it is at least 5.5 cm (2 inches) wide (Chaikof, Dalman, Eskandari, et al., 2018).

Medical Management

Medical management consists of pharmacologic, endovascular, and surgical interventions.

Pharmacologic Therapy

If the aneurysm is stable in size based on serial duplex ultrasound scans, the blood pressure is closely monitored over time, because there is an association between increased blood pressure and aneurysm rupture (Sidawy & Perler, 2019). Antihypertensive agents, including diuretics, beta-blockers, ACE inhibitors, ARBs, and calcium channel blockers, are frequently prescribed to maintain the patient's blood pressure within acceptable limits (see Chapter 27).

Endovascular and Surgical Management

An expanding or enlarging abdominal aortic aneurysm is likely to rupture. When an abdominal aortic aneurysm measured at least 5.5 cm (2 inches) wide or was enlarging, the standard treatment had been open surgical repair of the aneurysm by resecting the vessel and sewing a bypass graft in place. However, endovascular aortic repair has become a mainstay of therapy for treating an infrarenal abdominal aortic aneurysm and involves the transluminal placement and attachment of a sutureless aortic graft across the aneurysm (see Fig. 26-12). This procedure can be performed under local or regional anesthesia. Endovascular grafting of abdominal aortic aneurysms may be performed if the patient's abdominal aorta and iliac arteries are not extremely tortuous, small, calcified, or filled with thrombi. Results from multiple, prospective studies suggest comparable mortality rates among patients with aneurysms treated by endovascular grafting and those treated with surgical repair, with similar 5-year survival rates (Chaikof et al., 2018). Potential complications include bleeding, hematoma, or wound infection at the arterial insertion site; distal ischemia or embolization; dissection or perforation of the aorta; graft thrombosis or infection; break of the attachment system; graft migration; proximal or distal graft leaks; delayed rupture; and bowel ischemia.

Nursing Management

Before endovascular repair or surgery, nursing assessment is guided by anticipating rupture and recognizing that the

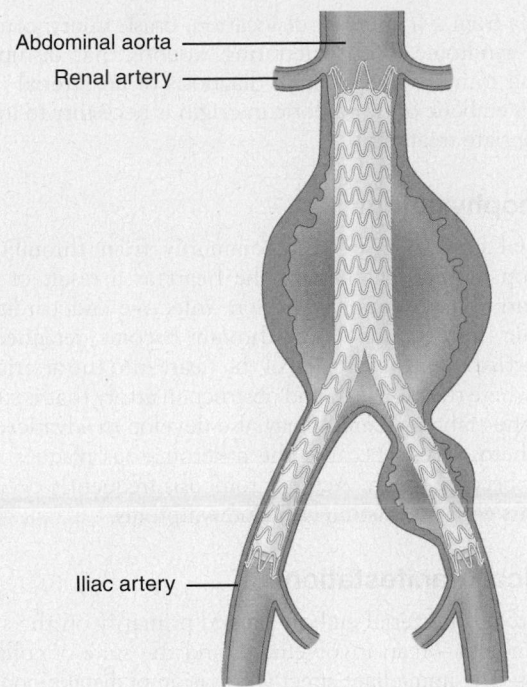

Figure 26-12 • Endograft repair of an abdominal aortic aneurysm.

(Labels on figure: Abdominal aorta, Renal artery, Iliac artery)

patient may have cardiovascular, cerebral, pulmonary, and renal impairment from atherosclerosis. The functional capacity of all organ systems should be assessed. Medical therapies designed to stabilize physiologic function should be promptly implemented. Hemorrhage that leads to shock is a serious adverse consequence that must be treated decisively (see Chapter 11).

The patient who has had an endovascular repair must lie supine for 6 hours; the head of the bed may be elevated up to 45 degrees after 2 hours. The patient needs to use a bedpan or urinal while on bed rest. Vital signs and Doppler assessment of peripheral pulses are performed initially every 15 minutes and then at progressively longer intervals if the patient's status remains stable. The access site (usually the femoral artery) is assessed when vital signs and pulses are monitored. The nurse assesses for bleeding and hematoma formation. Skin changes of the lower extremity, lumbar area, or buttocks that might indicate signs of embolization, such as extremely tender, irregularly shaped, cyanotic areas, as well as any changes in vital signs, pulse quality, bleeding, pulsation, swelling, pain, or hematoma, are immediately reported to the primary provider.

The patient's temperature should be monitored every 4 hours, and any signs of postimplantation syndrome should be reported. Postimplantation syndrome typically begins within 24 hours of stent graft placement and consists of a spontaneously occurring fever, leukocytosis, and occasionally, transient thrombocytopenia. This condition has been attributed to complex immunologic changes that occur because of manipulations with sheaths and catheters with the aortic lumen, although the exact etiology is unknown. The symptoms are thought to be related to the activation of cytokines (Martinelli, Di Girolamo, Belli, et al., 2019). They can be managed with a mild analgesic (e.g., acetaminophen) or an anti-inflammatory agent (e.g., ibuprofen) and usually subside within a week.

Because of the increased risk of hemorrhage, the primary provider is also notified of persistent coughing, sneezing, vomiting, or systolic blood pressure greater than 180 mm Hg. Most patients can resume their preprocedure diet and are encouraged to drink fluids. An IV infusion may be continued until the patient can drink normally. Fluids are important to maintain blood flow through the arterial repair site and to assist the kidneys with excreting IV contrast agents and other medications used during the procedure. Six hours after the procedure, the patient may be able to roll from side to side and may be able to ambulate with assistance to the bathroom. Once the patient can take adequate fluids orally, the IV infusion may be discontinued.

Postoperative care requires frequent monitoring of pulmonary, cardiovascular, renal, and neurologic status. Possible complications of surgery include arterial occlusion, hemorrhage, infection, ischemic bowel, kidney injury, and erectile dysfunction.

Other Aneurysms

Aneurysms may also arise in the peripheral vessels, most often as a result of atherosclerosis. These may involve such vessels as the subclavian artery, renal artery, femoral artery, or (most frequently) popliteal artery. Between 50% and 60% of popliteal aneurysms are bilateral; the true incidence is unknown but has been reported to be between 0.1% and 3% of the adult population and is associated with abdominal aortic aneurysms (Sidawy & Perler, 2019).

The aneurysm produces a pulsating mass and disturbs peripheral circulation distal to it. Pain and swelling develop because of pressure on adjacent nerves and veins. Diagnosis is made by duplex ultrasonography or CTA to determine the size, length, and extent of the aneurysm. Arteriography may be performed to evaluate the level of proximal and distal involvement. The major complication associated with popliteal artery aneurysms is not rupture but distal embolization (Sidawy & Perler, 2019). Surgical repair is performed with replacement grafts. As an alternative, endovascular repair using a stent graft or wall graft, which is a Dacron or PTFE graft with external structures made from a variety of materials (e.g., nitinol, titanium, stainless steel) may be selected for additional support.

Aortic Dissection

Occasionally, in an aorta diseased by arteriosclerosis, a tear develops in the intima or the media degenerates, resulting in a dissection (see Fig. 26-11). Aortic dissections are three times more common in men than in women, occur most commonly in the 50- to 70-year age group and are associated with hypertension (Sidawy & Perler, 2019).

Pathophysiology

Aortic dissections (separations) are commonly associated with poorly controlled hypertension, blunt chest trauma, and cocaine use. The profound increase in sympathetic response caused by cocaine use creates an increase in the force of left ventricular contraction that causes heightened shear forces upon the aortic wall leading to disruption of the intima

(Sidawy & Perler, 2019). Dissection is caused by rupture in the intimal layer. A rupture may occur through adventitia or into the lumen through the intima, allowing blood to reenter the main channel and resulting in chronic dissection (e.g., pseudoaneurysm) or occlusion of branches of the aorta.

As the separation progresses, the arteries branching from the involved area of the aorta shear and occlude. The tear occurs most commonly in the region of the aortic arch, with the highest mortality rate associated with ascending aortic dissection (Sidawy & Perler, 2019). The dissection of the aorta may progress backward in the direction of the heart, obstructing the openings to the coronary arteries or producing hemopericardium (effusion of blood into the pericardial sac) or aortic insufficiency, or it may extend in the opposite direction, causing occlusion of the arteries supplying the gastrointestinal tract, kidneys, spinal cord, and legs.

Clinical Manifestations

Onset of symptoms is usually sudden. Severe and persistent pain, described as tearing or ripping, may be reported. The pain is in the anterior chest or back and extends to the shoulders, epigastric area, or abdomen. Aortic dissection may be mistaken for an acute myocardial infarction, which confuses the clinical picture and initial treatment. Cardiovascular, neurologic, and gastrointestinal symptoms are responsible for other clinical manifestations, depending on the location and extent of the dissection. The patient may appear pale. Sweating and tachycardia may be detected. Blood pressure may be elevated or markedly different from one arm to the other if dissection involves the orifice of the subclavian artery on one side.

Assessment and Diagnostic Findings

Arteriography, multidetector-computed tomography angiography (MDCTA), TEE, duplex ultrasonography, and MRA, while limited in terms of expediency during an emergency situation, may aid in the diagnosis.

Medical Management

The medical or surgical treatment of an aortic dissection depends on the type of dissection present and follows the general principles outlined for the treatment of thoracic aortic aneurysms.

Nursing Management

A patient with an aortic dissection requires the same nursing care as a patient with an aortic aneurysm requiring intervention, as described earlier in this chapter. Nursing care as described in Chart 26-4 is also appropriate.

Arterial Embolism and Arterial Thrombosis

Acute vascular occlusion may be caused by an embolus or acute thrombosis. Acute arterial occlusions may result from iatrogenic injury, which can occur during insertion of invasive catheters such as those used for arteriography, PTA or stent placement, or an intra-aortic balloon pump, or it may occur as a result of illicit IV drug use. Other causes include trauma from a fracture or dislocation, crush injury, compartment syndrome, and penetrating wounds that disrupt the arterial intima. The accurate diagnosis of an arterial occlusion as embolic or thrombotic in origin is necessary to initiate appropriate treatment.

Pathophysiology

Arterial emboli arise most commonly from thrombi that develop in the chambers of the heart as a result of atrial fibrillation, myocardial infarction, infective endocarditis, or chronic heart failure. These thrombi become detached and are carried from the left side of the heart into the arterial system, where they lodge in and obstruct an artery that is smaller than the embolus. Emboli may also develop in advanced aortic atherosclerosis because the atheromatous plaques ulcerate or become rough. Acute thrombosis frequently occurs in patients with preexisting ischemic symptoms.

Clinical Manifestations

Symptoms of arterial emboli depend primarily on the size of the embolus, organ involvement, and the state of collateral vessels. The immediate effect is cessation of distal blood flow. The blockage can progress distal and proximal to the site of the obstruction. Secondary vasospasm can contribute to the ischemia. The embolus can fragment or break apart, resulting in occlusion of distal vessels. Emboli tend to lodge at arterial bifurcations and areas narrowed by atherosclerosis. Cerebral, mesenteric, renal, and coronary arteries are often involved in addition to the large arteries of the extremities.

The symptoms of acute arterial embolism in extremities with poor collateral flow are acute, severe pain, and a gradual loss of sensory and motor function. The six Ps associated with acute arterial embolism are pain, pallor, pulselessness, paresthesia, poikilothermia (coldness), and paralysis. Eventually, superficial veins may collapse because of decreased blood flow to the extremity. Because of ischemia, the part of the extremity distal to the occlusion is markedly colder and paler than the part proximal to the occlusion.

Arterial thrombosis can also acutely occlude an artery. A thrombosis is a slowly developing clot that usually occurs where the arterial wall has become damaged, generally as a result of atherosclerosis. Thrombi may also develop in an arterial aneurysm. The manifestations of an acute thrombotic arterial occlusion are similar to those described for an embolic occlusion. However, treatment is more difficult with a thrombus because the arterial occlusion has occurred in a degenerated vessel and requires more extensive reconstructive surgery to restore flow than is required with an embolic event (Sidawy & Perler, 2019).

Assessment and Diagnostic Findings

An arterial embolus is usually diagnosed on the basis of the sudden onset of symptoms and an apparent source for the embolus. Two-dimensional transthoracic echocardiography or transthoracic echocardiogram (TTE), chest x-ray, and electrocardiography (ECG) may reveal underlying cardiac disease. Noninvasive duplex and Doppler ultrasonography can determine the presence and extent of underlying atherosclerosis, and arteriography may be performed.

Medical Management

Management of arterial thrombosis depends on its cause. Management of acute embolic occlusion usually requires surgery because there is only a 4- to 6-hour window to restore blood flow before irreversible death of tissue. The event is acute with no collateral circulation developed, and the patient quickly moves through the list of six Ps to paralysis, the most advanced stage. Heparin therapy is initiated immediately to prevent further development of emboli and to prevent the extension of existing thrombi. Typically, an initial IV bolus of 60 to 80 U/kg body weight is given, followed by a continuous infusion of 12 to 18 U/kg/h until the patient undergoes an endovascular intervention or surgery (Comerford & Durkin, 2020; IBM Watson Health, 2020).

Endovascular Management

Emergency embolectomy is the procedure of choice if the involved extremity is viable (see Fig. 26-13). Arterial emboli are usually treated by insertion of an embolectomy catheter. The catheter is passed through an incision into the affected artery and extended through the embolus that is causing the arterial occlusion. The embolectomy catheter balloon is inflated with sterile saline solution, and the thrombus is extracted as the catheter is withdrawn. This procedure involves incising the vessel and removing the clot.

Percutaneous mechanical thrombectomy devices may also be used for the treatment of an acute thrombosis. All endovascular devices necessitate obtaining access to the patient's arterial system and inserting a catheter into the patient's artery to obtain access to the thrombus. The approach is similar to that used for angiograms, in that it is typically made through the groin to the femoral artery. In select cases, the radial or brachial artery can be accessed, allowing patients to be ambulatory post procedure. To qualify for this approach, the height of the patient is considered to ensure that the length of the catheter can reach the thrombus. Patients who are 5 feet 6 inches or shorter are potential candidates.

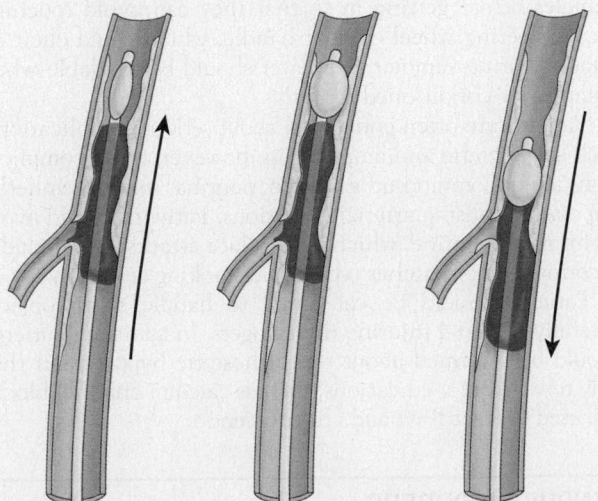

Figure 26-13 • Extraction of an embolus by a balloon-tipped embolectomy catheter. The deflated balloon-tipped catheter is advanced past the embolus, inflated, and then gently withdrawn, carrying the embolic material with it. Adapted with permission from Sidawy, A. N., & Perler, B. A. (2019). *Rutherford's vascular surgery and endovascular therapy* (9th ed.). Philadelphia, PA: Elsevier.

Some endovascular devices require that a small incision (cut-down) be made into the patient's artery. These devices may use a jet of fluid to disrupt the thrombus and then aspirate the particles; a rotating, sinusoidal-shaped wire that mixes a thrombolytic agent that simultaneously dissolves the clot; or high-frequency, low-energy ultrasound to dissolve an occlusive thrombus. Complications arising from the use of any endovascular device may include arterial dissection or distal artery embolization.

Pharmacologic Therapy

When the patient has adequate collateral circulation, treatment may include IV anticoagulation with heparin, which can prevent the thrombus from extending and reduce muscle necrosis. Intra-arterial thrombolytic medications are used to dissolve the embolus. Thrombolytic medications (e.g., tissue plasminogen activator [t-PA] and single-chain urokinase-type plasminogen activator) interact with plasminogen to generate plasmin which then breaks down fibrin clots. If t-PA is used for the treatment, heparin is usually given to prevent another thrombus from forming at the site of the lesion. The t-PA activates plasminogen on the thrombus, but it does not decrease the clotting factors as much as other thrombolytic therapies; therefore, patients receiving t-PA can make new thrombi more readily than if they receive other thrombolytics. Other thrombolytic medications are reteplase and tenecteplase (Millar & Laffan, 2017). Although these agents differ in their pharmacokinetics, they are given in a similar manner: A catheter is advanced under x-ray visualization to the clot, and the thrombolytic agent is infused.

Thrombolytic therapy should not be used when there are known contraindications to therapy or when the extremity cannot tolerate the several additional hours of ischemia that it takes for the agent to lyse (disintegrate) the clot. Contraindications to peripheral thrombolytic therapy include active internal bleeding, cerebrovascular hemorrhage, recent major surgery, uncontrolled hypertension, and pregnancy.

Nursing Management

Before an intervention or surgery, the patient remains on bed rest with the affected extremity level or slightly dependent (15 degrees). The affected extremity is kept at room temperature and protected from trauma. Heating and cooling pads are contraindicated because ischemic extremities are easily traumatized by alterations in temperature. If possible, tape and ECG electrodes should not be used on the extremity to protect from trauma. Pressure injury prevention through offloading the heel with a heel device and lifting the bedsheets using a bed cradle are important to protect the affected leg (European Pressure Ulcer Advisory Panel, National Pressure Injury Advisory Panel, Pan Pacific Pressure Injury Alliance [EPUAP/NPIAP/PPPIA], 2019).

If the patient is treated with thrombolytic therapy, the dose is based on the patient's weight. The patient is admitted to a critical care unit for continuous monitoring. Vital signs are taken initially every 15 minutes and then at progressively longer intervals if the patient's status remains stable. The patient is closely monitored for bleeding. The nurse minimizes the number of punctures for inserting IV lines and obtaining blood samples, avoids intramuscular injections, prevents any possible tissue trauma, and applies pressure at least twice as long as usual after any puncture is performed.

During the recovery phase, the nurse collaborates with the primary provider about the patient's appropriate activity level based on the patient's condition. Generally, every effort is made to encourage the patient to move the extremity to stimulate circulation and prevent stasis. Anticoagulant therapy may be continued postendovascular intervention to prevent thrombosis of the affected artery and to diminish the development of subsequent thrombi at the initiating site. The nurse assesses for evidence of local and systemic hemorrhage, including mental status changes, which can occur when anticoagulants are given. Pulses, Doppler signals, ABI, and motor and sensory function are assessed every hour for the first 24 hours, because significant changes may indicate reocclusion. Metabolic abnormalities, acute kidney injury, and compartment syndrome may be complications after an acute arterial occlusion.

Raynaud's Phenomenon and Other Acrosyndromes

Raynaud's phenomenon is a form of intermittent arteriolar vasoconstriction that results in coldness, pain, and pallor of the fingertips or toes. There are two forms of this disorder. Primary or idiopathic Raynaud's (Raynaud's disease) occurs in the absence of an underlying disease. Secondary Raynaud (Raynaud syndrome) occurs in association with an underlying disease, usually a connective tissue disorder, such as systemic lupus erythematosus, rheumatoid arthritis, or scleroderma; trauma; or obstructive arterial lesions. Symptoms may result from a defect in basal heat production that eventually decreases the ability of cutaneous vessels to dilate. Episodes may be triggered by emotional factors, stress, or by unusual sensitivity to cold. Raynaud's phenomenon is five times more common in women with the typical onset before age 30 (Dean, 2018). Acrocyanosis has been thought to be a variant of Raynaud's phenomenon because both are aggravated by cold and emotional stress and both present with blue discoloration of the fingers and hyperhidrosis (excessive sweating).

The prognosis for patients with Raynaud's phenomenon varies; some slowly improve, some become progressively worse, and others show no change. Raynaud symptoms may be mild so that treatment is not required. However, secondary Raynaud is characterized by vasospasm and fixed blood vessel obstructions that may lead to ischemia, ulceration, and gangrene. Acrocyanosis is a poorly understood phenomenon that may be benign and require little or no treatment, or the patient may have chronic pain and ulcerations.

Clinical Manifestations

The classic clinical picture of Raynaud reveals pallor brought on by sudden vasoconstriction. The skin then becomes cyanotic because of pooling of deoxygenated blood during vasospasm. As a result of hyperemia (exaggerated reflow) due to vasodilation, rubor is produced when oxygenated blood returns to the digits after the vasospasm stops. The characteristic sequence of color change of Raynaud's phenomenon is described as white, blue, and red. Numbness, tingling, and burning pain occur as the color changes. The manifestations tend to be bilateral and symmetric and may involve toes and fingers.

Acrocyanosis is differentiated from Raynaud by a relative persistence of skin color changes, symmetry, and an absence of the paroxysmal pallor that is found with Raynaud. Almost all patients with acrocyanosis have marked clamminess and hyperhidrosis of their hands and feet, which tend to worsen in warmer temperatures while the color changes improve. Finger color normalizes when the hands are transferred from the dependent to horizontal position (Dean, 2018).

Medical Management

Avoiding the particular stimulus (e.g., cold, nicotine) that provokes vasoconstriction is a primary factor in controlling Raynaud's phenomenon. Decongestants and other over-the-counter preparations containing sympathomimetics should be avoided. Calcium channel blockers (nifedipine, amlodipine) may be effective in relieving symptoms. Sympathectomy (interrupting the sympathetic nerves by removing the sympathetic ganglia, or blocking or dividing their branches) may help some patients.

Avoidance of exposure to cold and trauma and implementing measures to improve local circulation are the primary focus of treatment for acrocyanosis. Calcium channel blockers have not been effective in treating acrocyanosis (Belch, Carlizza, Carpentier, et al., 2017).

Nursing Management

The nurse instructs the patient with Raynaud or acrocyanosis to avoid situations that may be stressful or unsafe. Stress management strategies may be helpful. Exposure to cold must be minimized, and in areas where the fall and winter months are cold, the patient should wear layers of clothing when outdoors. Hats and gloves or mittens should be worn at all times when outside. Fabrics specially designed for cold climates (e.g., Thinsulate™) are recommended. Patients should wear gloves when accessing freezers. Patients should warm up their vehicles before getting in so that they can avoid touching a cold steering wheel or door handle, which could elicit an attack. During summer, a sweater should be available when entering air-conditioned rooms.

Patients are often concerned about serious complications, such as gangrene and amputation; however, these complications are uncommon unless the patient has another underlying disease causing arterial occlusions. Patients should avoid all forms of nicotine, which may induce attacks; this includes nicotine gum or patches used to aid smoking cessation.

Patients should be cautioned to handle sharp objects carefully to avoid injuring their fingers. In addition, patients should be informed about the orthostatic hypotension that may result from medications, such as calcium channel blockers, used to treat Raynaud's phenomenon.

VENOUS DISORDERS

Venous disorders cause a reduction in venous blood flow, which results in stasis of blood. This may then cause a host of pathologic changes, including coagulation defects, edema, tissue breakdown, and an increased susceptibility to infections.

Venous Thromboembolism

Deep vein thrombosis (DVT) and pulmonary embolism (PE) collectively make up the condition called **venous thromboembolism (VTE).** The annual incidence of VTE is estimated at 1 to 2 per 1000 population (Peñaloza-Martínez, Demelo-Rodríguez, Proietti, et al., 2018; Serhal & Barnes, 2019). The incidence of VTE is 10% to 20% in general medical patients and up to 80% in critically ill patients. VTE is frequently not diagnosed because DVT and PE are often clinically silent or asymptomatic. It is estimated that as many as 30% of patients hospitalized with VTE develop long-term postthrombotic complications. In surgical patients, most symptomatic thromboembolic complications occur after hospital discharge due to shorter lengths of stay (Stubbs, Assareh, Curnow, et al., 2018).

COVID-19 Considerations

An underlying cause of death in patients with severe coronavirus disease 2019 (COVID-19) has been linked to VTE or primary pulmonary thrombi. The majority of patients who are severely ill with COVID-19 have a markedly elevated D-dimer assay (blood test for evidence of blood clots) and a presumed prothrombotic state. Because of this, routine thromboprophylaxis of all hospitalized patients with COVID-19 is recommended regardless of their risk score (see later discussion) (Obi, Barnes, Wakefield, et al., 2020). The systemic inflammatory changes in the vascular system in patients with COVID-19 likely contribute to thrombosis, hemodynamic instability, and autonomic dysregulation. Early reports suggest long-term cardiovascular effects of COVID-19 may include accelerated atherosclerosis, VTE, arterial thromboembolic disease, and aortic aneurysm formation (Becker, 2020).

Pathophysiology

Superficial veins, such as the greater saphenous, short saphenous (also known as lesser saphenous), cephalic, basilic, and external jugular veins, are thick-walled muscular structures that lie just under the skin. In contrast, deep veins are thin walled and have less muscle in the media. Deep veins run parallel to arteries and bear the same names as the arteries. Deep and superficial veins have valves that permit unidirectional flow back to the heart. The valves lie at the base of a segment of vein that is expanded into a sinus. This arrangement enables the valves to open without coming into contact with the wall of the vein, thus permitting rapid closure when the blood starts to flow backward. Other types of veins are known as perforating veins. These veins have valves that allow one-way blood flow from the superficial venous system to the deep venous system.

Although the exact cause of VTE remains unclear, three factors, known as Virchow triad, are believed to play a significant role in its development: endothelial damage, venous stasis, and altered coagulation (see Chart 26-8). Damage to the intimal lining of blood vessels creates a site for clot formation. Direct trauma to the veins may occur with fractures or dislocation, diseases of the veins, and chemical irritation of the vein from IV medications or solutions. Venous stasis occurs when blood flow is reduced, as in heart failure or

Chart 26-8 ⚠	RISK FACTORS Deep Vein Thrombosis and Pulmonary Embolism

Endothelial Damage

- Central venous catheters
- Dialysis access catheters
- Local vein damage
- Pacing wires
- Repetitive motion injury
- Surgery
- Trauma

Venous Stasis

- Age (>65 years)
- Bed rest or immobilization
- Heart failure
- History of varicosities
- Obesity
- Spinal cord injury

Altered Coagulation

- Antiphospholipid antibody syndrome
- Antithrombin III deficiency
- Cancer
- Elevated factors II, VIII, IX, XI
- Factor V Leiden defect
- Hyperhomocysteinemia
- Oral contraceptive use
- Polycythemia
- Pregnancy
- Protein C deficiency
- Protein S deficiency
- Prothrombin G20210A defect
- Septicemia

Adapted from Patel, K., Fasanya, A., Yadam, S., et al. (2017). Pathogenesis and epidemiology of venous thromboembolic disease. *Critical Care Nursing Quarterly, 40*(3), 191–200.

shock; when veins are dilated, as an effect of some medication therapies; and when skeletal muscle contraction is reduced, as in immobility, paralysis of the extremities, or anesthesia. Altered coagulation occurs most commonly in patients for whom anticoagulant medications have been abruptly withdrawn. Oral contraceptive use, elevated CRP levels (Cauci, Francescato, Colannino, et al., 2020), and several blood dyscrasias (abnormalities) also can lead to hypercoagulability, with prevalence depending on the ethnicity of the patient. For example, factor V Leiden and prothrombin G20210A mutation is more prevalent in White persons, whereas antithrombin III deficiency, protein C deficiency, and protein S deficiency are found more commonly in patients of Southeast Asian descent (Sidawy & Perler, 2019). An increase in factor VIII concentrations is more common among African Americans (Folsom, Basu, Hong, et al., 2019). Pregnancy is also considered a hypercoagulable state, as it is accompanied by an increase in circulating clotting factors that may not return to baseline until longer than 6 weeks postpartum, increasing the risk of thrombosis. In addition, during pregnancy there is a 50% decrease in venous outflow due to hormonally decreased venous capacitance and reduced venous outflow due to compression from the uterus (Zheng, Chen, Fu, et al., 2019).

Deep Vein Thrombosis

Deep vein thrombosis (DVT) refers to thrombus formation in the deep veins, usually in the thigh or calf, but sometimes in the arm (e.g., patients with peripherally inserted central catheters).

Pathophysiology

Formation of a thrombus frequently accompanies phlebitis, which is an inflammation of the vein walls. When a thrombus develops initially in the veins as a result of stasis or hypercoagulability but without inflammation, the process is referred to as phlebothrombosis. Venous thrombosis can occur in any vein, but it occurs more often in the veins of the lower extremities. The superficial and deep veins of the extremities may be affected.

Upper extremity venous thrombosis accounts for 5% to 10% of all cases of DVT, but its incidence may be as high as 93% in the presence of central venous cannulation or upper extremity compression (Mintz & Levy, 2017). It typically involves more than one venous segment, with the subclavian vein the most frequently affected. In addition, upper extremity venous thrombosis is more common in patients with IV catheters or in patients with an underlying disease that causes hypercoagulability, such as cancer. Internal trauma to the vessels may result from pacemaker leads, chemotherapy ports, dialysis catheters, or parenteral nutrition lines. The lumen of the vein may be decreased as a result of the catheter or from external compression, such as by neoplasms or an extra cervical rib. Effort thrombosis, also known as Paget–Schroetter syndrome, of the upper extremity is caused by repetitive motion (e.g., as seen in competitive swimmers, tennis players, baseball players, weight lifters, or construction workers) that irritates the vessel wall, causing inflammation and subsequent thrombosis and is a manifestation of venous thoracic outlet syndrome where the veins becomes distorted and narrowed (Sidawy & Perler, 2019).

Venous thrombi are aggregates of platelets attached to the vein wall that have a tail-like appendage containing fibrin, white blood cells, and many red blood cells. The "tail" can grow or can propagate in the direction of blood flow as successive layers of the thrombus form. A propagating venous thrombosis is dangerous because parts of the thrombus can break off and occlude the pulmonary blood vessels. Fragmentation of the thrombus can occur spontaneously as it dissolves naturally, or it can occur with an elevated venous pressure, as may occur after standing suddenly or engaging in muscular activity after prolonged inactivity. After an episode of acute DVT, reestablishment of the lumen of the vessel, or recanalization, typically occurs. Lack of recanalization within the first 6 months after DVT appears to be an important predictor of postthrombotic syndrome, which is one complication of venous thrombosis (Sidawy & Perler, 2019) (see later discussion). Other complications of venous thrombosis are listed in Chart 26-9.

Clinical Manifestations

A major challenge in recognizing DVT is that the signs and symptoms are nonspecific. The exception is phlegmasia cerulea dolens (massive iliofemoral venous thrombosis), in which

---

> **Chart 26-9** Complications of Venous Thrombosis
>
> Chronic venous occlusion
> Pulmonary emboli from dislodged thrombi
> Valvular destruction:
>
> - Chronic venous insufficiency
> - Increased venous pressure
> - Varicosities
> - Venous ulcers
>
> Venous obstruction:
>
> - Edema
> - Fluid stasis
> - Increased distal pressure
> - Venous gangrene
>
> Adapted from Kahn, S. R., Galanaud, J. P., Vedantham, S., et al. (2016). Guidance for the prevention and treatment of the postthrombotic syndrome. *Journal of Thrombosis and Thrombolysis*, *41*(1), 144–153.

---

the entire extremity becomes massively swollen, tense, painful, and cool to the touch. The large DVT creates severe and sudden venous hypertension that leads to tissue ischemia with resultant translocation of fluid into the interstitial space. Venous gangrene occurs in 20% to 50% of cases and is associated with poor survival (Sidawy & Perler, 2019).

Deep Veins

Clinical manifestations of obstruction of the deep veins include edema and swelling of the extremity because the outflow of venous blood is inhibited. The affected extremity may feel warmer than the unaffected extremity, and the superficial veins may appear more prominent. Tenderness, which usually occurs later, is produced by inflammation of the vein wall and can be detected by gently palpating the affected extremity. In some cases, signs and symptoms of a PE are the first indication of DVT.

Superficial Veins

Thrombosis of superficial veins, or superficial thrombophlebitis, produces pain or tenderness, redness, and warmth in the involved area. The risk of the superficial venous thrombi becoming dislodged or fragmenting into emboli is very low because most of them dissolve spontaneously. This condition can be treated at home with bed rest, elevation of the leg, analgesic agents, and possibly, anti-inflammatory medication.

Assessment and Diagnostic Findings

Careful assessment is invaluable in detecting early signs of venous disorders of the lower extremities (see Chart 26-8). Diagnostic tests for VTE include laboratory and venous duplex studies. Laboratory tests are conducted to determine baseline levels and include complete blood count (CBC) and coagulation studies that include prothrombin time (PT), activated partial thromboplastin time (aPTT), and international normalized ratio (INR). If an underlying hypercoagulable state is suspected, additional laboratory testing may include CRP, factor V Leiden, prothrombin G20210A mutation, antithrombin III, protein C, and protein S (Fischbach & Fischbach, 2018). Duplex ultrasound findings may show veins that appear larger than normal with thrombus formation or veins that are incompressible and dilated. The thrombus may appear to be adherent to the vein wall or mobile with a thrombus tail.

Prevention

Patients with a prior history of VTE are at increased risk of a new episode; the rate of recurrence can be as high as 13.7% in men and 14.1% in women (Serhal & Barnes, 2019). VTE can be prevented, especially if patients who are considered at high risk are identified and preventive measures are instituted without delay. Preventive measures include encouragement of early ambulation and leg exercises, the application of graduated compression stockings, and the use of intermittent pneumatic compression devices (see later discussion). An additional method to prevent venous thrombosis in surgical patients is administration of subcutaneous unfractionated heparin or low-molecular-weight heparin (LMWH). Patients should be advised to make lifestyle changes as appropriate, which may include weight loss, smoking cessation, and regular exercise.

Medical Management

The objectives of treatment for DVT are to prevent the thrombus from extending and fragmenting (thus risking PE), recurrent thromboemboli, and postthrombotic syndrome (discussed later in the chapter) (Peñaloza-Martínez et al., 2018). Anticoagulant therapy involves the administration of a medication to delay the clotting time of blood, prevent the formation of a thrombus in postoperative patients, and forestall the extension of a thrombus after it has formed; it can be used to meet the treatment goals for DVT (Witt, Nieuwlaat, Clark, et al., 2018). However, anticoagulant agents cannot dissolve a thrombus that has already formed. Combining anticoagulation with mechanical thrombectomy and ultrasound-guided thrombolytic therapy may eliminate venous obstruction, maintain venous patency, and prevent postthrombotic syndrome by early removal of the thrombus (Kruger, Eikelboom, Douketis, et al., 2019).

Pharmacologic Therapy

Medications for preventing or reducing blood clotting within the vascular system are indicated in patients diagnosed with DVT. These medications are also indicated for patients with thrombophlebitis, recurrent embolus formation, persistent leg edema from heart failure, and in select patients who must be immobilized for a protracted time (e.g., older adults with hip fractures). The primary pharmacologic treatment for the prevention and management of DVT is anticoagulant therapy which consists of vitamin K antagonists (e.g., warfarin), indirect and direct thrombin inhibitors, and factor Xa inhibitors (see Table 26-2).

Endovascular Management

Endovascular management is necessary for DVT when anticoagulant or thrombolytic therapy is contraindicated, the danger of PE is extreme, or venous drainage is so severely compromised that permanent damage to the extremity is likely. A thrombectomy may be necessary. This mechanical method of clot removal may involve using intraluminal catheters with a balloon or other devices. Some of these spin to break the clot, and others use oscillation to break up the clot to facilitate removal. Ultrasound-assisted thrombolysis

may be another option. This intervention uses bursts or continuous high-frequency ultrasound waves emanating from the catheters to cause cavitation of the thrombus, making it more permeable to the thrombolytic agent (Kruger et al., 2019). A vena cava filter may be placed at the time of the thrombectomy or thrombolysis; this filter traps large emboli and prevents PE (see later discussion). Retrievable caval filters can be left in place and retrieved up to 6 months after placement. In patients with chronic iliac vein compression (e.g., as is seen in May–Thurner syndrome), balloon angioplasty with stent placement may successfully treat the patient's chronic leg symptoms (Ignatyev, Pokrovsky, & Gradusov, 2019).

Nursing Management

When performing the nursing assessment, key concerns include limb pain, a feeling of heaviness, functional impairment, ankle engorgement, and edema; increase in the surface temperature of the leg, particularly the calf or ankle; and areas of tenderness or superficial thrombosis (i.e., cordlike venous segment). The amount of swelling in the extremity can be determined by measuring the circumference of the affected extremity at various levels (i.e., thigh to ankle) with a tape measure and comparing one extremity with the other at the same level to determine size differences. If both extremities are swollen, a size difference may be difficult to detect. Homan sign (pain in the calf after the foot is sharply dorsiflexed) is *not* a reliable sign of DVT because it can be elicited in any painful condition of the calf and has no clinical value in assessment for DVT.

Assessing and Monitoring Anticoagulant Therapy

If the patient is receiving anticoagulant therapy, the nurse monitors laboratory values as indicated. The aPTT, PT, INR, ACT, hemoglobin and hematocrit values, platelet count, and fibrinogen levels can be affected, depending on the anticoagulant prescribed; baseline assessments before the initiation of therapy should be performed. Close observation is required to detect bleeding; if bleeding occurs, it must be reported immediately and anticoagulant therapy reversed or discontinued if appropriate (see Table 26-2).

Monitoring and Managing Potential Complications

Potential complications of anticoagulant therapy consist of bleeding, thrombocytopenia, and drug–drug interactions. The nurse should monitor for these potential complications, be familiar with medications approved to reverse effects of various anticoagulants, and educate patients and caregivers on ways to reduce these potential risks (see Table 26-2 and Chart 26-10).

Reducing Discomfort

Elevation of the affected extremity, graduated compression stockings (see later discussion), and analgesic agents for pain relief are adjuncts to therapy. They help improve circulation and increase comfort. Warm packs applied to the affected extremity reduce the discomfort associated with DVT.

Positioning the Body and Encouraging Exercise

When the patient is on bed rest, the feet and lower legs should be elevated periodically above the level of the heart. This

TABLE 26-2	Select Anticoagulant and Thrombolytic Agents Prescribed to Treat Venous Thromboemboli (VTE)		
Medication	**Mechanism of Action**	**Actions and Effects**	**Nursing Considerations**
Unfractionated Heparin			
Heparin	Binds to antithrombin; inactivates clotting factors XII, Xa; half-life of 60–90 min	Prevent extension of thrombus Prevent development of new thrombus	Can be administered subcutaneously or intermittently or continuous intravenously (IV); IV dosing is weight based Administer continuous IV infusions using an electronic infusion device Requires monitoring of aPTT and platelet count; monitor platelet counts for HIT Assess patient for bleeding Administer protamine sulfate for overdose or to reverse effects, as prescribed; monitor patient for hypotension and bradycardia if administered
Low-Molecular-Weight Heparin (LMWH)			
Dalteparin Enoxaparin	Inhibit factor Xa	Prevent extension of thrombus Prevent development of new thrombus	Can be administered subcutaneously once daily or twice a day Associated with fewer bleeding complications than unfractionated heparin Has lower risk of HIT Administer protamine sulfate for overdose or to reverse effects, as prescribed; monitor patient for hypotension and bradycardia if administered; protamine sulfate is less effective in reversing LMWH compared to unfractionated heparin Can be used in pregnancy if clearly indicated; however, patients should be monitored closely for bleeding
Oral Anticoagulant			
Warfarin	Vitamin K antagonist inhibits synthesis of vitamin K–dependent clotting factors: II, VII, IX, X Inhibits synthesis of vitamin K–dependent proteins: protein C and protein S	Has narrow therapeutic window Has slow onset of action Anticoagulant effect occurs 12–24 h after first dose Antithrombotic effect occurs 2–7 days after first dose	Administer once a day at the same time each day Requires routine monitoring of PT with goal of 1.5–2 times normal; and INR with goal of 2.0–3.0 Requires administration with heparin during drug initiation until desired anticoagulation is achieved Monitor for food and drug–drug interactions (see Chart 26-10) Assess patient for bleeding Administer vitamin K, fresh-frozen plasma, or prothrombin complex concentrate as prescribed for overdose or to reverse effects Requires periprocedural bridging (i.e., giving a short-acting anticoagulant, usually heparin or LMWH, if warfarin needs to be temporarily discontinued) Contraindicated in pregnancy
Factor Xa Inhibitor			
Fondaparinux	Selective inhibitor of factor Xa	Prevent DVT or PE in patients undergoing orthopedic surgery (e.g., hip or knee arthroplasty) Treatment of DVT or PE Excreted unchanged via kidneys Does not affect aPTT or ACT	Administer subcutaneously once daily Use with caution in patients with renal insufficiency Monitor creatinine Routine coagulation tests are not necessary
Oral Direct Factor Xa Inhibitor			
Rivaroxaban	Direct inhibitor of factor Xa	Fixed-dose regimen for treatment of DVT and PE Fixed-dose regimen to prevent recurrent DVT and PE Not indicated for patients with creatinine clearance less than 30 mL/min	Administer once or twice daily as prescribed based on indication Assess renal function Alter dose in individuals with obesity May require periprocedural bridging Administer andexanet alfa or activated charcoal as prescribed for overdose or to reverse effects
Apixaban		Fixed-dose regimen for treatment of DVT and PE Fixed-dose regimen to prevent recurrent DVT and PE Not indicated for patients with creatinine clearance less than 25 mL/min.	Administer twice a day Assess renal function Alter dose in patients 80 yrs of age or older and weight ≤60 kg Administer andexanet alfa or activated charcoal as prescribed for overdose or to reverse effects
Edoxaban		Fixed-dose regimen for treatment of DVT and PE	Administer once daily Assess renal function Alter dose for patients who weigh ≤60 kg
Betrixaban		Prevent DVT and PE in adults hospitalized for acute medical illness	Administer once daily Assess renal function No antidote available to reverse effects

TABLE 26-2	Select Anticoagulant and Thrombolytic Agents Prescribed to Treat Venous Thromboemboli (VTE) (continued)		
Medication	**Mechanism of Action**	**Actions and Effects**	**Nursing Considerations**
Direct Thrombin Inhibitor Argatroban Lepirudin	Reversibly binds to thrombin active site, inhibiting thrombin-mediated stimulation of coagulation factors	Prevention and treatment of thrombosis in patients with HIT or at risk for HIT during PCI	Administer as an IV bolus followed by a continuous infusion Assess hepatic function Monitor aPTT and ACT
Oral Direct Thrombin Inhibitor Dabigatran	Reversibly binds to thrombin active site, inhibiting thrombin-mediated stimulation of coagulation factors	Fixed-dose regimen for treatment of DVT Fixed-dose regimen to prevent recurrent DVT Not indicated for patients with creatinine clearance <30 mL/min	Administer twice a day Assess renal function Routine coagulation tests are not necessary; however if measured, aPTT levels may be prolonged 1.5–2 times normal Administer idarucizumab as prescribed to reverse effects
Thrombolytic Alteplase Reteplase Tenecteplase Urokinase	Binds to fibrin within the thrombus converting plasminogen to plasmin. Plasmin degrades fibrin, fibrinogen, and factors V, VIII, and XII.	Lyse and dissolve existing thrombus	Monitor lab values prior to initiation: CBC, platelets, aPTT; repeat during and post therapy Monitor for bleeding and hemorrhage Contraindicated with active bleeding

ACT, activated clotting time; aPTT, activated partial thromboplastin time; CBC, complete blood count; DVT, deep vein thrombosis; HIT, heparin-induced thrombocytopenia; INR, international normalized ratio; PCI, percutaneous coronary intervention; PE, pulmonary emboli; PT, prothrombin time; PTT, partial thromboplastin time.
Adapted from Cohen, A. T., Lip, G. Y., De Caterina, R., et al. (2018). State of play and future direction with NOACs: An expert consensus. *Vascular Pharmacology, 106*, 9–21; Comerford, K. C., & Durkin, M. T. (Eds.). (2020). *Nursing2020 Drug Handbook*. Philadelphia, PA: Wolters Kluwer; Kruger, P. C., Eikelboom, J. W., Douketis, J. D., et al. (2019). Deep vein thrombosis: Update on diagnosis and management. *Medical Journal of Australia, 210*(11), 516–524; Peñaloza-Martínez, E., Demelo-Rodríguez, P., Proietti, M., et al. (2018). Update on extended treatment for venous thromboembolism. *Annals of Medicine, 50*(8), 666–674; Serhal, M., & Barnes, G. D. (2019). Venous thromboembolism: A clinician update. *Vascular Medicine, 24*(2), 122–131.

position allows the superficial and tibial veins to empty rapidly and to remain collapsed. Active and passive leg exercises, particularly those involving calf muscles, should be performed to increase venous flow. Early ambulation is most effective in preventing venous stasis. The patient is encouraged to walk once anticoagulation therapy has been initiated and is advised that walking is better than standing or sitting for long periods. Once ambulatory, the patient is instructed to avoid sitting for more than an hour at a time. The goal is to walk at least 10 minutes every 1 to 2 hours. The patient

Chart 26-10 **PATIENT EDUCATION**
Taking Anticoagulant Medications

The nurse instructs the patient as follows:
• Take anticoagulation medication as prescribed.
• Do not stop taking your anticoagulation medication unless directed.
• If prescribed warfarin, take at the same time each day.
• Wear or carry identification indicating anticoagulant medication being taken.
• Keep all scheduled appointments for blood tests.
• Be aware that other medications may affect the action of the anticoagulant medication; if taking warfarin, consult with your health care provider before taking any of the following medications or supplements: vitamins, cold medicines, antihistamines, antibiotics, aspirin, laxatives, and anti-inflammatory agents, such as ibuprofen, and similar medications or herbal or nutritional supplements. Your primary provider should be contacted before taking any over-the-counter drugs.
• Avoid alcohol if taking warfarin because it may change the body's response to the warfarin. There are no interactions with the oral factor Xa inhibitors (e.g., rivaroxaban, apixaban, edoxaban) and alcohol.
• Avoid marked changes in eating habits, especially involving foods high in vitamin K, such as green leafy vegetables, which can reduce anticoagulation effectiveness if taking warfarin; dietary habits have no interactions with the oral factor Xa inhibitors.
• When seeking treatment from any health care provider, be sure to inform them that you are taking an anticoagulant medication.
• Contact your provider who manages your anticoagulation therapy before having dental work or surgery.
• Describe potential side effects of coagulation, such as bruising and bleeding, and identify ways to prevent bleeding.
  • Avoid the use of sharps (razors, knives, etc.) to prevent cuts; shave with an electric shaver.
  • Use a toothbrush with soft bristles to prevent gum injury.
  • Avoid contact sports or activities that may result in an injury that causes bleeding.
• If taking warfarin, report the following immediately to your primary provider:
  • Any bleeding—for example, cuts that do not stop bleeding
  • Bruises that enlarge, nosebleeds, or unusual bleeding from any part of the body
  • Reddish or brownish urine
  • Red or black bowel movements
• *For women:* Notify your primary provider and obstetrical provider if you suspect pregnancy.

is also instructed to perform active and passive leg exercises as frequently as necessary when they cannot ambulate, such as during long car, bus, train, and plane trips. In addition, deep breathing exercises are beneficial because they produce increased negative pressure in the thorax, which assists in emptying the large veins.

Promoting Home, Community-Based, and Transitional Care

In addition to instructing the patient on how to apply graduated compression stockings as indicated (see later discussion) and explaining the importance of elevating the legs and exercising adequately, the nurse provides education about the prescribed anticoagulant, its purpose, and the need to take the correct amount at the specific times, especially if warfarin is prescribed (see Chart 26-10). The patient should also be aware that if warfarin is prescribed, periodic blood tests are necessary to determine if a change in medication or dosage is required. If the patient fails to adhere to the therapeutic regimen, continuation of the medication therapy should be questioned. In patients with liver disease, the potential for bleeding may be exacerbated by anticoagulant therapy.

Pulmonary Embolism

Pulmonary embolism (PE) refers to the obstruction of the pulmonary artery or one of its branches by a thrombus (or thrombi) that originate(s) somewhere in the venous system or in the right side of the heart.

Pathophysiology

Most commonly, PE is due to a dislodged or fragmented DVT (see previous pathophysiology discussion in DVT). However, there are other types of emboli that may be implicated: air, fat, amniotic fluid, and septic (from bacterial invasion of the thrombus) (Norris, 2019).

A PE is described as an occlusion of the outflow tract of the main pulmonary artery or of the bifurcation of the pulmonary arteries. Multiple small emboli can lodge in the terminal pulmonary arterioles, producing multiple small infarctions of the lungs. A pulmonary infarction causes ischemic necrosis of part of the lung (Thompson & Kabrhel, 2020).

When a thrombus completely or partially obstructs a pulmonary artery or its branches, the alveolar dead space is increased. The area, although continuing to be ventilated, receives little or no blood flow. Therefore, gas exchange is impaired or absent in this area. In addition, various substances are released from the clot and surrounding area that cause regional blood vessels and bronchioles to constrict. This results in an increase in pulmonary vascular resistance—a reaction that compounds the ventilation–perfusion (V̇/Q̇) imbalance that ensues.

The hemodynamic consequences are increased pulmonary vascular resistance due to the regional vasoconstriction and reduced size of the pulmonary vascular bed. In severe instances, this may result in an increase in pulmonary arterial pressure and, in turn, an increase in right ventricular work to maintain pulmonary blood flow. When the work requirements of the right ventricle exceed its capacity, right ventricular failure occurs, leading to a decrease in cardiac output

followed by a decrease in systemic blood pressure and the development of shock (Norris, 2019).

Clinical Manifestations

Symptoms of PE depend on the size of the thrombus and the area of the pulmonary artery occluded by the thrombus; they may be nonspecific. Dyspnea is the most frequent symptom; the duration and intensity of the dyspnea depend on the extent of embolization. Chest pain is common and is usually sudden and pleuritic in origin; however, it may be substernal and may mimic angina (Thompson & Kabrhel, 2020). Other symptoms include anxiety, fever, tachycardia, apprehension, cough, diaphoresis, hemoptysis, and syncope. The most frequent sign is tachypnea (rapid respiratory rate) (De Palo, 2020).

In many instances, PE causes few signs and symptoms, whereas in other instances, it mimics various other cardiopulmonary disorders (e.g., pneumonia, heart failure). Obstruction of the pulmonary artery can result in pronounced dyspnea, sudden substernal pain, rapid and weak pulse, shock, syncope, and sudden death (Thompson & Kabrhel, 2020).

Assessment and Diagnostic Findings

Because the symptoms of PE can vary from few to severe, a diagnostic workup is performed to rule out other diseases. The initial diagnostic workup may include chest x-ray, ECG, pulse oximetry, arterial blood gas analysis, D-dimer assay and MDCTA or pulmonary arteriogram or V̇/Q̇ scan. The chest x-ray is usually normal but may show infiltrates, atelectasis, elevation of the diaphragm on the affected side, or a pleural effusion. The chest x-ray is most helpful in excluding other possible causes. In addition to sinus tachycardia, the most frequent ECG abnormality is nonspecific ST-T wave abnormalities. If an arterial blood gas analysis is performed, it may show hypoxemia and hypocapnia (from tachypnea); however, arterial blood gas measurements may be normal even in the presence of PE (De Palo, 2020).

MDCTA is the criterion standard for diagnosing PE. The MDCTA can be performed quickly and provides the advantage of high-quality visualization of the lung parenchyma (Weinberger, Cockrill, & Mandel, 2019). If MDCTA is not available, pulmonary angiography is considered a reasonable alternative diagnostic method (Ouellette, 2019). The pulmonary angiogram allows for direct visualization under fluoroscopy of the arterial obstruction and accurate assessment of the perfusion deficit. A specially trained team must be available to perform the procedure, in which a catheter is threaded through the vena cava to the right side of the heart to inject dye, similar to a cardiac catheterization.

The V̇/Q̇ scan continues to be used to diagnose PE, especially in facilities that do not use pulmonary angiography or do not have access to MDCTA. The V̇/Q̇ scan is minimally invasive and requires IV administration of a contrast agent. This scan evaluates different regions of the lung (upper, middle, lower) and allows comparisons of the percentage of V̇/Q̇ in each area. This test has a high sensitivity but is not as accurate as an MDCTA or pulmonary angiogram (De Palo, 2020).

Medical Management

Medical management of the patient with PE revolves around whether the patient is diagnosed with a hemodynamically unstable PE (also called a *massive PE*) or a stable PE. The patient with a hemodynamically unstable PE, which comprises a life-threatening emergency, may evidence hypotension, tachycardia, confusion, and cardiovascular collapse.

 ## Medical Management of Unstable Pulmonary Embolism

The immediate objective is to stabilize the cardiopulmonary system in the patient with a hemodynamically unstable PE. A sudden increase in pulmonary resistance increases the work of the right ventricle, which can cause acute right-sided heart failure with cardiogenic shock. Emergent measures are initiated to improve respiratory and cardiovascular status (see Chapter 11 for discussion of management of the patient in shock).

After emergency measures have been initiated, the treatment goal is to lyse (dissolve) the existing embolus and prevent new ones from forming. Thrombolytic therapy with t-PA or other agents such as reteplase (see Table 26-2) is used in treating unstable PE, particularly in patients who are severely compromised (e.g., those who are hypotensive and have significant hypoxemia despite oxygen supplementation) (Ouellette, 2019). Thrombolytic therapy lyses the thrombi or emboli quickly and restores hemodynamic functioning of the pulmonary circulation, thereby reducing pulmonary hypertension and improving perfusion, oxygenation, and cardiac output. However, the risk of bleeding is significant. Contraindications to thrombolytic therapy include having had a stroke within the past 2 months, other active intracranial processes, active bleeding, surgery within 10 days of the thrombotic event, recent labor and delivery, trauma, or severe hypertension. Consequently, thrombolytic agents are advocated only for PE affecting a significant area of blood flow to the lung and causing hemodynamic instability (Tapson & Weinberg, 2020).

Before thrombolytic therapy is started, INR, aPTT, hematocrit, and platelet counts are obtained. Any anticoagulant is stopped prior to administration of a thrombolytic agent. During therapy, all but essential invasive procedures are avoided because of potential bleeding. After the thrombolytic infusion is completed (which varies in duration according to the agent used), maintenance anticoagulation therapy is initiated.

A surgical embolectomy is rarely performed but may be indicated if there are contraindications to thrombolytic therapy. Embolectomy can be performed using catheters or surgically. Surgical removal must be performed by a cardiovascular surgical team with the patient on cardiopulmonary bypass (Ouellette, 2019).

For patients who have recurrent PE despite therapeutic anticoagulation, an inferior vena cava (IVC) filter may be inserted (Tapson, 2019). IVC filters are not recommended for the initial treatment of patients with PE and should not be used in patients receiving anticoagulants. The IVC filter provides a screen in the IVC, allowing blood to flow unobstructed while large emboli from the pelvis or lower extremities are blocked or fragmented before reaching the lung. Numerous devices have been developed since the introduction of the original Greenfield filter (see Fig. 26-14).

Medical Management of Stable Pulmonary Embolism

In patients with PE who do not demonstrate any cardiopulmonary instability (e.g., normotensive, no evidence of hypoxemia) immediate anticoagulation is indicated to

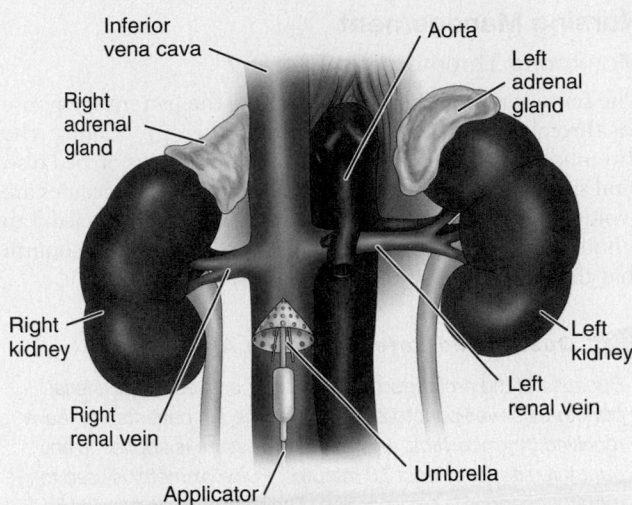

Figure 26-14 • An umbrella filter is in place in the inferior vena cava to prevent PE. The filter (compressed within an applicator catheter) is inserted through an incision in the right internal jugular vein. The applicator is withdrawn when the filter fixes itself to the wall of the inferior vena cava after ejection from the applicator.

prevent recurrence or extension of the thrombus and may continue for 10 days (Tapson, 2019). Long-term anticoagulation is also indicated up to 6 months following the PE and is critical in preventing recurrence of VTE. This duration may be extended indefinitely in patients who are at high risk for recurrence (Weinberger et al., 2019).

In patients with stable PE, the initial anticoagulant selected may include an LMWH (e.g., enoxaparin), unfractionated heparin, or a direct oral anticoagulant (DOAC), such as a direct thrombin inhibitor (e.g., dabigatran), or a factor Xa inhibitor (e.g., fondaparinux, rivaroxaban, apixaban, edoxaban) (Tapson & Weinberg, 2020) (see Table 26-2).

In select patients with PE who are hemodynamically stable, outpatient therapy can be started by administering the first dose in the emergency department or urgent care center and the remaining doses given at home. Although there are not specific selection criteria for outpatient treatment, the patient is usually at low risk of death, has no respiratory or hemodynamic compromise, does not require opioids for pain control, has no risk factors for bleeding, has no serious comorbid conditions, and has stable baseline mental status with a good understanding of the benefits and risks of treatment (Tapson, 2019). The ideal agent for outpatient administration is not empirically confirmed, although the DOACs are often prescribed.

Long-term treatment options include warfarin and the DOACs. An LMWH may also be selected but is usually not prescribed for long-term therapy since it is given via a subcutaneous injection. Warfarin dosing requires regular blood draws for INR monitoring and has a higher bleeding risk, but it has long been the standard of care prior to the development of DOACs. An antidote (vitamin K) is available if the INR is high and there is a risk of bleeding. Warfarin does have interactions with several medications (see Chart 26-10) and has dietary restrictions. DOACs do not require regular blood test monitoring; however, they are more costly than warfarin. The choice of warfarin versus a DOAC is dependent upon risk of bleeding, cost, presence of comorbidities, and provider preference (The Joint Commission [TJC], 2019).

Nursing Management

Monitoring Thrombolytic Therapy

The nurse is responsible for monitoring the patient's response to thrombolytic and anticoagulant therapy. During the thrombolytic infusion, while the patient remains on bed rest, vital signs are frequently assessed and invasive procedures are avoided. Tests to determine INR or aPTT are performed 3 to 4 hours after the thrombolytic infusion is started to confirm that the fibrinolytic systems have been activated.

> **Quality and Safety Nursing Alert**
>
> *Because of the prolonged clotting time, only essential arterial punctures or venipunctures are performed in patients who have received thrombolytics, and manual pressure is applied to any puncture site for at least 30 minutes. Pulse oximetry is used to monitor changes in oxygenation. The thrombolytic infusion is discontinued immediately if uncontrolled bleeding occurs.*

Managing Pain

Chest pain, if present, is usually pleuritic rather than cardiac in origin. A semi-Fowler position provides a more comfortable position for breathing. However, the nurse must continue to turn patients frequently and reposition them to improve V/Q. The nurse administers opioid analgesic agents as prescribed for severe pain.

Managing Oxygen Therapy

Careful attention is given to the proper use of oxygen. The patient must understand the need for continuous oxygen therapy. The nurse assesses the patient frequently for signs of hypoxemia and monitors the pulse oximetry values to evaluate the effectiveness of the oxygen therapy. Deep breathing and incentive spirometry are indicated for all patients to minimize or prevent atelectasis and improve ventilation (see Chapter 19 for discussion of incentive spirometry). Nebulizer therapy or percussion and postural drainage may be used for management of secretions.

Relieving Anxiety

The nurse encourages the patient who is stabilized to talk about any fears or concerns related to this frightening episode, answers the patient's and family's questions concisely and accurately, explains the therapy, and describes how to recognize untoward effects early.

Monitoring for Complications

When caring for a patient who has had PE, the nurse must be alert for the potential complication of cardiogenic shock or right ventricular failure subsequent to the effect of PE on the cardiovascular system. (Nursing activities for managing shock are found in Chapter 11; see Chapter 25 for nursing management of right ventricular failure.)

 Providing Postoperative Nursing Care

If the patient has undergone surgical embolectomy, the nurse measures the patient's pulmonary arterial pressure and urinary output. The nurse also assesses the insertion site of the arterial catheter for hematoma formation and infection. Maintaining the blood pressure at a level that supports perfusion of vital organs is crucial. To prevent peripheral venous stasis and edema of the lower extremities, the nurse elevates the foot of the bed and encourages isometric exercises, the use of intermittent pneumatic compression devices, and walking when the patient is permitted out of bed. Sitting for long periods is discouraged, because hip flexion compresses the large veins in the legs.

Promoting Home, Community-Based, and Transitional Care

 Educating Patients About Self-Care

Before hospital discharge and at follow-up visits to the clinic, the nurse educates the patient about preventing recurrence and reporting signs and symptoms. Patient education instructions, presented in Chart 26-11, are intended to help prevent recurrences and side effects of treatment.

Chart 26-11 **HOME CARE CHECKLIST**
Prevention of Recurrent Pulmonary Embolism

At the completion of education, the patient and/or caregiver will be able to:

- State the impact of pulmonary embolism (PE) on physiologic functioning, ADLs, IADLs, roles, relationships, and spirituality.
- State changes in lifestyle (e.g., diet, activity) necessary to restore health.
- State the name, dose, side effects, frequency, and schedule for all medications.
- Name the anticoagulant prescribed and describe relevant patient education related to taking anticoagulants described in Chart 26-10.
- Describe the importance of follow-up appointments with providers.
- Describe strategies to prevent recurrent deep venous thrombosis and pulmonary emboli:
  - Continue to wear anti-embolism stockings (compression hose) as long as directed.
  - Avoid sitting with legs crossed or sitting for prolonged periods of time.

- When traveling, change position regularly, walk occasionally, and do active exercises of moving the legs and ankles while sitting.
- Drink fluids, especially while traveling and in warm weather, to avoid hemoconcentration due to fluid deficit.
- Describe the signs and symptoms of lower extremity circulatory compromise and potential deep venous thrombosis: calf or leg pain, swelling, pedal edema.
- Describe the signs and symptoms of pulmonary compromise related to recurrent PE (e.g., dyspnea, chest pain, anxiety, fever, tachycardia, apprehension, cough, syncope, diaphoresis, hemoptysis).
- Describe how and when to contact the primary provider if symptoms of circulatory compromise or pulmonary compromise are identified.
- Identify the need for health promotion, disease prevention, and screening activities.

ADLs, activities of daily living; IADLs, instrumental activities of daily living.

Continuing and Transitional Care

During follow-up or home visits, the nurse monitors the patient's adherence to the prescribed management plan and reinforces previous instructions. The nurse also monitors the patient for residual effects of the PE and recovery. The patient is reminded about the importance of keeping follow-up appointments for coagulation tests, if indicated, and appointments with the primary provider.

Chronic Venous Insufficiency/ Postthrombotic Syndrome

Venous insufficiency results from obstruction of the venous valves in the legs or a reflux of blood through the valves. Superficial and deep leg veins can be involved. Resultant venous hypertension can occur whenever there has been a prolonged increase in venous pressure, such as occurs with DVT. Because the walls of veins are thinner and more elastic than the walls of arteries, they distend readily when venous pressure is consistently elevated. In this state, leaflets of the venous valves are stretched and prevented from closing completely, causing a backflow or reflux of blood in the veins. Duplex ultrasonography confirms the obstruction and identifies the level of valvular incompetence. Twenty percent to 50% of patients who have had a DVT develop deep vein incompetence leading to postthrombotic syndrome (Sidawy & Perler, 2019) (see Fig. 26-15).

Clinical Manifestations

Postthrombotic syndrome is characterized by chronic venous stasis, resulting in edema, altered pigmentation, pain, and stasis dermatitis. The patient may notice the symptoms less in the morning and more in the evening. Obstruction or poor calf muscle pumping in addition to valvular reflux must be present for the development of severe postthrombotic syndrome and stasis ulcers. Superficial veins may be dilated. The disorder is long-standing, difficult to treat, and often disabling (Kahn, Galanaud, Vedantham, et al., 2016).

Stasis ulcers develop as a result of the rupture of small skin veins and subsequent ulcerations. When these vessels rupture, red blood cells escape into surrounding tissues and then

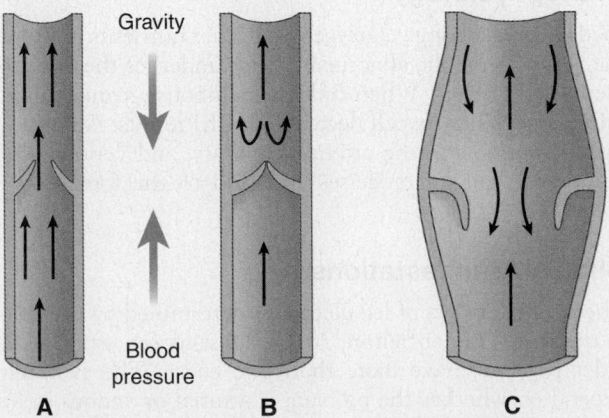

Figure 26-15 • Competent valves showing blood flow patterns when the valve is open (**A**) and closed (**B**), allowing blood to flow against gravity. **C.** With faulty or incompetent valves, the blood cannot move toward the heart.

degenerate, leaving a brownish discoloration of the tissues, called *hemosiderin staining.* The pigmentation and ulcerations usually occur in the lower part of the extremity, in the area of the medial malleolus of the ankle. The skin becomes dry, cracks, and itches; subcutaneous tissues fibrose and atrophy. The risk of injury and infection of the extremities is increased.

Complications

Venous ulceration is the most serious complication of chronic venous insufficiency and can be associated with other conditions affecting the circulation of the lower extremities. Cellulitis or dermatitis may complicate the care of chronic venous insufficiency and venous ulcerations.

Management

Management of the patient with venous insufficiency is directed at reducing venous stasis and preventing ulcerations. Extremities with venous insufficiency must be carefully protected from trauma; the skin is kept clean, dry, and soft. Signs of ulceration are immediately reported to the primary provider for treatment and follow-up. Measures that increase venous blood flow are antigravity activities, such as elevating the leg, and compression of superficial veins with graduated compression stockings and other compression therapies.

Elevating the legs decreases edema, promotes venous return, and provides symptomatic relief. The legs should be elevated frequently throughout the day (at least 15 to 20 minutes four times daily). At night, the patient should sleep with the foot of the bed elevated about 15 cm (6 inches). Prolonged sitting or standing in one position is detrimental; walking should be encouraged. When sitting, the patient should avoid placing pressure on the popliteal spaces, as occurs when crossing the legs or sitting with the legs dangling over the side of the bed. Constricting garments, especially socks that are tight at the top or that leave marks on the skin, should be avoided.

Compression of the legs with graduated compression stockings reduces the pooling of venous blood, enhances venous return to the heart, and is recommended for people with venous insufficiency.

Providing Compression Therapy

Stockings

Graduated compression stockings usually are prescribed for patients with venous disease as soon as possible after diagnosis (Bjork & Ehmann, 2019). The amount of pressure gradient is determined by the amount and severity of venous disease. For example, a pressure gradient of 20 to 30 mm Hg is prescribed for patients with asymptomatic varicose veins, whereas at least a pressure gradient of 30 to 40 mm Hg at the ankle is recommended for patients with venous stasis ulceration (Bjork & Ehmann, 2019). Compression stockings with at least 30 to 40 mm Hg pressure can be used during the 6 months post DVT to decrease symptoms and reduce the development of postthrombotic syndrome (Zierler & Dawson, 2016). These stockings should not be confused with anti-embolism stockings (i.e., thromboembolic deterrent [TED] stockings) that provide less compression (12 to 20 mm Hg at the ankle). Graduated compression stockings are designed to apply 100% of the prescribed pressure gradient at the ankle and then decrease along the length of the stocking, reducing the caliber of the superficial veins in the leg and increasing flow in the deep veins. Each stocking should fit so that pressure is greater at the foot and ankle and then gradually declines to a lesser pressure at the knee or groin. These stockings may be knee high, thigh high, or pantyhose. Several colors, fabrics, and styles are available to promote patient adherence. Stockings should be applied after the legs have been elevated for a period, when the amount of blood in the leg veins is at its lowest.

> ### ◤ Quality and Safety Nursing Alert
>
> *Any type of stocking can inadvertently become a tourniquet if applied incorrectly (i.e., rolled tightly at the top). In such instances, the stockings produce—rather than prevent— venous stasis. For ambulatory patients, graduated compression stockings can be removed at night and reapplied before the legs are lowered from the bed to the floor in the morning.*

When the stockings are off, the skin is inspected for signs of irritation, and the calves are examined for tenderness. Any skin changes or signs of tenderness are reported. Stockings are contraindicated in patients with severe PAD, epifascial arterial bypass, severe cardiac insufficiency, allergy to compression material, and severe diabetic neuropathy with sensory loss or microangiopathy (Rabe, Partsch, Morrison, et al., 2020).

 Gerontologic Considerations

Older patients have decreased strength and manual dexterity and may be unable to apply graduated compression stockings. If this is the case, a family member or friend should be taught to assist the patient to apply the stockings so that they do not cause excessive pressure on any part of the feet or legs. Frames and other devices have been designed to assist patients with applying stockings, and if there is any concern regarding patients' physical abilities, they should be referred to an occupational therapist who can provide examples of and training in the use of stocking assistance devices (Balcombe, Miller, & McGuiness, 2017).

External Compression Devices and Bandages

Short-stretch elastic bandages may be applied from the toes to the knee in a 50% spiral overlap. These bandages are available in a two-layer system, which includes an inner layer of soft padding. These bandages have extension indicators that are rectangular and become squares when extended correctly, which reduces the possibility of bandaging a leg too loosely or too tightly. Three- and four-layer systems are also available (e.g., Profore, Dyna-Care), but these may be used only once compared with the two-layer system, which can be used multiple times.

Other types of compression are available. The Unna boot, which consists of a paste bandage impregnated with zinc oxide, glycerin, gelatin, and sometimes calamine, is applied without tension in a circular fashion from the base of the toes to the tibial tuberosity with a 50% spiral overlap. The foot must remain dorsiflexed at a 90-degree angle to the leg, thus avoiding excess pressure or trauma to the anterior ankle area. Once the bandage dries, it provides a constant and consistent compression to the venous system. This type of compression

may remain in place for as long as 1 week, although it may be too heavy for patients who are too frail to tolerate. The Unna boot is more commonly used with venous insufficiency.

The CircAid, a nonelastic leg wrap with a series of overlapping, interlocking Velcro straps, augments the effect of muscle while the patient is walking. The CircAid is usually worn during the day. Patients may find the CircAid easier to apply and wear than the Unna boot because it is lighter, can be removed to shower, and is adjustable. However, its adjustability may also be problematic; if patients loosen the straps, the compression achieved may not be adequate.

Intermittent Pneumatic Compression Devices

Intermittent pneumatic compression devices can be used in conjunction with elastic bandages or graduated compression stockings to support venous circulation and prevent DVT. Compression devices consist of an electric controller that is attached by air hoses to either knee-high or thigh-high sleeves. The sleeves are divided into compartments, which sequentially fill to apply pressure to the ankle, calf, and thigh at variable pressures from 30 to 70 mm Hg. Intermittent pneumatic compression devices can increase blood velocity beyond that produced by elastic bandages or stockings. Intermittent pneumatic compression devices are prescribed for patients who are not physically able to apply compression bandages or wraps, or don a pair of stockings (Nicolaides, 2020). Nursing measures in caring for patients who use these devices include ensuring that sleeves are properly encircling the extremity and the prescribed pressures are set and not exceeded, assessing for patient comfort, and ensuring adherence to therapy.

Leg Ulcers

A leg ulcer is an excavation of the skin surface that occurs when inflamed necrotic tissue sloughs off. In the United States the most common lower extremity ulcerations have a venous etiology (estimated between 80% and 90%), with PAD the second leading cause. The coexistence of both venous and arterial disease is estimated to be present in 26% of patients with leg ulcers (Singer, Tassiopoulos, & Kirsner, 2017).

Pathophysiology

Inadequate exchange of oxygen and other nutrients in the tissue is the metabolic abnormality that underlies the development of leg ulcers. When cellular metabolism cannot maintain energy balance, cell necrosis (death) results. Alterations in blood vessels at the arterial, capillary, and venous levels may affect cellular processes and lead to the formation of ulcers.

Clinical Manifestations

The characteristics of leg ulcers are determined by the cause of the ulcer (Ermer-Selton, 2016). Most ulcers, especially in older patients, have more than one cause. The symptoms depend on whether the problem is arterial or venous in origin (see Table 26-1). The severity of the symptoms depends on the extent and duration of the vascular insufficiency. The ulcer itself appears as an open, inflamed sore. The area may be exuding or covered by eschar (dark, hard crust).

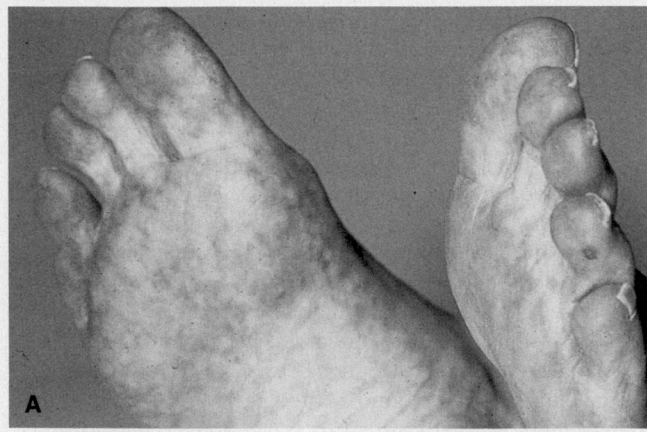

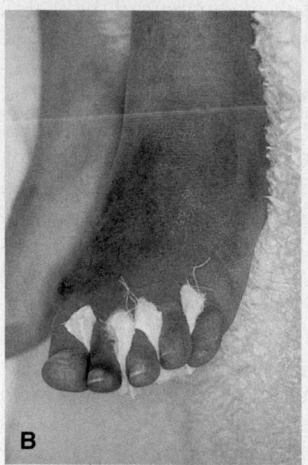
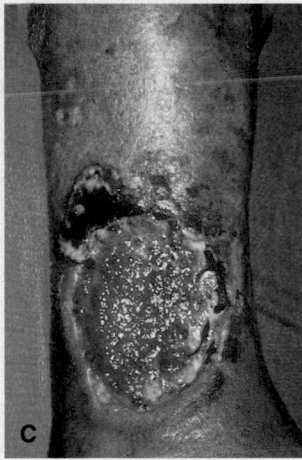

Figure 26-16 • **A.** Ulcers resulting from arterial emboli. **B.** Gangrene of the toes resulting from severe arterial ischemia. **C.** Ulcer from venous stasis.

Arterial Ulcers

Chronic arterial disease is characterized by intermittent claudication. The patient may also complain of digital or forefoot pain at rest. If the onset of arterial occlusion is acute, ischemic pain is unrelenting and rarely relieved even with opioids. Typically, arterial ulcers are small, circular, deep ulcerations on the tips of toes or in the web spaces between the toes. Ulcers often occur on the medial side of the hallux or lateral fifth toe and may be caused by a combination of ischemia and pressure (see Fig. 26-16).

Venous Ulcers

Chronic venous insufficiency is characterized by pain described as aching or heavy. The foot and ankle may be edematous. Ulcerations are in the area of the medial or lateral malleolus (gaiter area) and are typically large, superficial, and highly exudative. Venous hypertension causes extravasation of blood, which discolors the area (see Fig. 26-16). Studies report the average venous ulcer requires as long as 6 to 12 months to heal completely and in patients who do not adhere to compression therapy (see discussion later in the chapter), the recurrence rate is nearly 100% within 36 months (Nicolaides, 2020). Patients with neuropathy (e.g., a common occurrence in patients with diabetes) frequently have ulcerations on the side of the foot over the metatarsal

heads. These ulcers are painless and are described in further detail in Chapter 46.

Assessment and Diagnostic Findings

The cause of each ulcer needs to be identified so that appropriate therapy can be prescribed. The history of the condition is important in determining arterial or venous insufficiency. The pulses of the lower extremities (femoral, popliteal, posterior tibial, and dorsalis pedis) are carefully examined. More conclusive diagnostic aids include Doppler and duplex ultrasound studies, arteriography, and venography. Cultures of the ulcer bed may be necessary to determine whether an infection is contributing to tissue destruction.

Medical Management

Patients with ulcers can be effectively managed by advanced practice nurses or wound-ostomy-continence nurses in collaboration with the patients' primary provider. All ulcers have the potential to become infected.

Pharmacologic Therapy

Antiseptic agents, such as povidone–iodine, cadexomer iodine, and silver, inhibit growth and development of most microbes, are broad spectrum, generate relatively little antimicrobial resistance, and can be used for short periods of time. Once a wound is infected (e.g., erythema, induration, exudate, edema, wound breakdown, malodor), a systemic antibiotic is necessary (Swanson, Angel, Sussman, et al., 2016). The specific antibiotic agent selected is based on culture and sensitivity test results. Oral antibiotics usually are prescribed because topical antibiotics have not proven to be effective for leg ulcers and promote antimicrobial resistance (Swanson et al., 2016).

Pharmacologic therapy also is important in the management of wound-related pain.

Compression Therapy

After the circulatory status of the patient is assessed and an absolute ankle pressure of greater than 60 mm Hg and an ABI that exceeds 0.80 are confirmed, compression therapy can be used up to 40 mm Hg without impeding arterial perfusion (Singer et al., 2017). See the discussion on compression therapy in the Chronic Venous Insufficiency section.

Cleansing and Débridement

To promote healing, the wound bed is prepared by removing excessive wound exudate and nonviable tissue. The usual cleansing method is to flush the area with water or normal saline solution or clean it with a noncytotoxic wound-cleansing agent (Saf-Clens™, Biolex™, Restore™). If this is unsuccessful, therapeutic wound cleansing and/or débridement may be necessary (Swanson et al., 2016).

Therapeutic wound cleansing includes mechanical cleaning with a cleansing solution or gel such as:
- Polyhexamethylene biguanide (PHMB)
- Octenidine dihydrochloride
- Superoxidised solution with hypochlorous acid (HOCL) and sodium hypochlorite (NaOCL)
- Povidone–iodine

Many older antiseptics are no longer recommended due to the risk of tissue damage associated with their use. However, these agents may still be used for wound management in low-resource settings, where alternative, contemporary antiseptics are not always available. Solutions not recommended include:

- Hydrogen peroxide
- High-concentration sodium hypochlorite (EUSOL™, Milton, Dakin's solution)
- Chlorhexidine gluconate
- Chlorhexidine gluconate and cetrimide (Savlon™)
- High-concentration acetic acid
- Antibiotics for systemic administration
- High-concentration potassium permanganate

Débridement is the removal of nonviable tissue from wounds. Removing nonviable tissue is important, particularly for infection and biofilms (i.e., the microorganisms that grow on the surface of the wound). Biofilms have now been established as an important factor in wound healing and the need for serial débridement is important to disrupt the biofilm and allow the penetration of topical and systemic antimicrobial agent (Swanson et al., 2016).

Débridement can be accomplished by several different methods:

- Surgical débridement is the fastest method and can be performed by a primary provider under aseptic conditions using instruments to excise nonviable tissue. It is usually performed in the operating room with access to anesthesia and hemostasis.
- Conservative sharp wound débridement can be performed at the bedside or in a clinic by a primary provider, skilled advanced practice nurse or wound-ostomy-continence nurse in collaboration with the primary provider or advanced practice nurse. Instruments are used to remove loose, avascular, and insensate nonviable tissue and topical anesthetics may be used to manage procedural pain.
- Chemical débridement involves the application of chemical agents (e.g., cadexomer iodine, hypertonic saline) for the controlled removal of nonviable tissue. There may be some cytotoxic effects to healthy cells in the wound.
- Ultrasonic débridement uses ultrasonography to disrupt the attachment of the nonviable tissue.
- Hydrosurgical débridement uses a water-jet–powered wound débridement tool to cut nonviable tissue.
- Biologic débridement, or larval therapy, involves the deliberate infestation of disinfected fly larvae that secrete a proteolytic enzyme which liquifies and ingests nonviable tissues.
- Enzymatic débridement involves the application of ointments containing enzymes. The ointment is applied to the ulcer but not to surrounding skin. Most enzymatic ointments are covered with a secondary dressing that will not soak up the ointment. The enzymatic ointment is discontinued when the nonviable tissue has been débrided, and an appropriate wound dressing is applied.
- Autolytic débridement is achieved through the application of dressings that allow the lysozymes in wound exudate to naturally break down the nonviable tissue. These include calcium alginate dressings (e.g., Kaltostat™, Sorbsan™) or gelling fiber dressings (e.g., Aquacel

Hydrofiber™) and may be used for débridement when absorption of exudate is needed. These dressings are changed when the exudate seeps through the secondary dressing, or at least every 7 days. Calcium alginate dressings can be used on areas that are bleeding after débriding, because the material helps stop the bleeding. As the dry fibers absorb exudate, they become a gel that can be painlessly removed from the ulcer bed. Calcium alginate and gelling fiber dressings should not be used on dry or nonexudative wounds.

Nonselective débridement by applying and removing saline dressings of fine mesh gauze (wet to dry) are not recommended for vascular wounds because of the risk of removing viable tissue and wound-related pain. Preprocedural pain management is usually necessary.

Arterial insufficiency may result in gangrene of the toe(s), or digital gangrene, which is usually caused by trauma. The toe is stubbed and then turns black (see Fig. 26-16). Usually, patients with this problem are older people without adequate circulation. Débridement is contraindicated in these instances. Although the toe is gangrenous, it is dry. Managing dry gangrene is preferable to débriding the toe and causing an open wound that will not heal because of insufficient circulation. If the toe were to be amputated, the lack of adequate circulation would prevent healing and might make higher-level amputation necessary—a below- or an above-knee amputation. A higher-level amputation in an older adult could result in a loss of independence and possibly the need for institutional care. Dry gangrene of the toe in an older adult with poor circulation is usually left undisturbed. The nurse keeps the toe clean and dry, if it is stable, until it autoamputates or separates (without creating an open wound).

Topical Therapy

A variety of topical agents can be used in conjunction with cleansing and débridement to promote healing of leg ulcers. The goals of treatment are to remove nonviable tissue and biofilm, and keep the ulcer clean and moist while healing takes place. The treatment should not destroy developing tissue. For topical treatments to be successful, adequate nutrition must be maintained.

Wound Dressing

Semiocclusive or occlusive wound dressings prevent evaporative fluid loss from the wound and retain warmth; these factors favor healing. When determining the appropriate dressing to apply, the following should be considered: simplicity of application, frequency of required dressing changes, ability to absorb wound exudate, expense, and patient comfort (see Chapter 56 for further discussion of wound dressings).

Knowledge deficit, frustration, fear, anxiety, and depression can decrease the patient's and family's adherence with the prescribed therapy; therefore, patient and family education is necessary before beginning and throughout the wound care program.

Stimulated Healing

Tissue-engineered human skin equivalent (e.g., Apligraf™ [Graftskin™]) is a skin product cultured from human dermal fibroblasts and keratinocytes used in combination with therapeutic compression. When applied, it interacts with the patient's cells within the wound to stimulate the production of growth factors. Application is not difficult, no suturing is involved, and the procedure is painless. A dermal repair scaffold (e.g., PriMatrix™) is a bioactive and regenerative extracellular matrix that binds with the patient's own cells and growth factors. PriMatrix™ has been used successfully for tunneling wounds, as well as wounds with exposed tendon and bone, in which Apligraf™ cannot be used. Dermagraft™, which is a human fibroblast–derived dermal replacement, demonstrates efficacy similar to Apligraf™ (Nicolaides, 2020).

Hyperbaric Oxygenation

Hyperbaric oxygenation (HBO) may be beneficial as an adjunct treatment in patients with diabetes with no signs of wound healing after 30 days of standard wound treatment. HBO is accomplished by placing the patient into a chamber that increases barometric pressure while the patient is breathing 100% oxygen. Treatment regimens vary from 90 to 120 minutes once daily for 30 to 90 sessions. The process by which HBO is thought to work involves several mechanisms. The edema in the wound area is decreased because high oxygen tension facilitates vasoconstriction and enhances the ability of leukocytes to phagocytize and kill microbes. In addition, HBO is thought to increase diffusion of oxygen to the hypoxic wound, thereby enhancing epithelial migration and improving collagen production. The two most common adverse effects of HBO are middle-ear barotrauma and confinement anxiety. The benefit from this therapy on wound healing in patients without diabetes is unclear (Bonifant & Holloway, 2019).

Negative Pressure Wound Therapy

Research suggests that negative pressure wound therapy (NPWT) using vacuum-assisted closure (e.g., VAC™) devices decreases time to healing in complex wounds that have not healed in a 3-week period. Groin incisions, common in vascular surgery, may be complicated by wound dehiscence, lymphatic fistula, or infections in 5% to 10% of patients. NPWT has been found to be effective in treating patients who develop postoperative groin wound infections, decreasing hospital lengths of stay, rates of graft infection, and likelihood of limb loss (Apelqvist, Willy, Fagerdahl, et al., 2017). Patients who are ambulatory may be given small, portable NPWT devices, giving them the freedom to perform their ADLs (Harding, Chrysostomou, Mohamud, et al., 2017). Additional features such as instillation therapy (Veraflow™) are now available. This therapy facilitates cleansing via instillation of fluid followed by a negative pressure cycle. Research to evaluate the microbial load and changes in the bacterial spectrum in wounds while using a growing number of NPWT devices is ongoing (Kim, Applewhite, Dardano, et al., 2018).

NURSING PROCESS

The Patient with Leg Ulcers

Assessment

A focused nursing history and assessment are important. The extent and type of pain are carefully assessed, as are the appearance and temperature of the skin of both legs. The quality of all peripheral pulses is assessed, and the pulses in both legs are compared. The legs are checked for edema. If the extremity is edematous, the degree of edema is determined. Any limitation of mobility and activity that results from vascular insufficiency is identified. The patient's nutritional status is assessed, and a history of diabetes, collagen disease, or varicose veins is obtained.

Diagnosis

NURSING DIAGNOSES

Based on the assessment data, major nursing diagnoses may include:
- Impaired skin integrity associated with vascular insufficiency
- Impaired mobility associated with activity restrictions of the therapeutic regimen and pain
- Impaired nutritional status associated with increased need for nutrients that promote wound healing

COLLABORATIVE PROBLEMS/POTENTIAL COMPLICATIONS

Potential complications may include the following:
- Infection
- Gangrene

Planning and Goals

The major goals for the patient may include restoration of skin integrity, improved physical mobility, adequate nutrition, and absence of complications.

Nursing Interventions

Caring for these patients can be challenging, whether the patient is in the hospital, in a long-term care facility, or at home. Leg ulcers are often long term and disabling causing a substantial drain on the patient's physical, emotional, and economic resources.

RESTORING SKIN INTEGRITY

To promote wound healing, measures are used to keep the area clean. Cleansing requires very gentle handling, a neutral skin cleanser, and lukewarm water. Positioning of the legs depends on whether the ulcer is of arterial or venous origin. If there is arterial insufficiency, the patient should be referred for evaluation of vascular reconstruction. If there is venous insufficiency, dependent edema can be avoided by elevating the lower extremities and initiating graduated compression therapy. A decrease in edema promotes the exchange of cellular nutrients and waste products in the area of the ulcer, promoting healing.

Avoiding trauma to the lower extremities is imperative in promoting skin integrity. Heel suspension devices such as protective boots may be used (e.g., Rooke vascular boots, Prevalon); they are soft and provide warmth and protection from injury and displace tissue pressure to prevent pressure injury. If the patient is on bed rest or has reduced mobility, it is important to relieve pressure on the heels to prevent heel pressure injuries. When the patient is in bed, a bed cradle can be used to relieve pressure from bed linens and to prevent anything from touching the legs. When the patient is ambulatory, all obstacles are moved from the patient's path so that the patient's legs are not bumped. Heating pads, hot-water bottles, or hot baths are avoided, because they increase the oxygen demands and thus the blood flow demands of the already compromised tissue. The patient with diabetes and neuropathy has decreased sensation; therefore, heating pads may cause a burn without the patient noticing.

IMPROVING PHYSICAL MOBILITY

Generally, physical activity is initially restricted to promote wound healing. When infection resolves and healing begins, ambulation should resume gradually and progressively. Activity promotes arterial blood flow and venous return and is encouraged after the acute phase of the ulcer process. Until full activity is resumed, the patient is advised to move about when in bed, to turn from side to side frequently, and to exercise the upper extremities to maintain muscle tone and strength. Meanwhile, diversional activities are encouraged. Consultation with an occupational therapist and physical therapist may be helpful if prolonged immobility and inactivity are anticipated.

If pain limits the patient's activity, analgesic agents may be prescribed. The wound-related pain is typically chronic and often disabling. Analgesic agents may be taken before scheduled activities to help the patient participate more comfortably.

PROMOTING ADEQUATE NUTRITION

Nutritional deficiencies are common, requiring dietary alterations to remedy them. There is conflicting evidence that dietary supplementation aids in healing of ulcerations. Comorbidities that may contribute to ulceration may also cause ongoing inflammation, disuse atrophy, and other metabolic disturbances; these may have a greater effect on wound healing than nutritional intake. Further research is needed; however, eating a diet that is high in protein, vitamins C and A, iron, and zinc is encouraged to promote healing (Bonifant & Holloway, 2019). Particular consideration should be given to iron intake, because many patients are older adults who are at risk for iron deficiency anemia. After a dietary plan has been developed that meets the patient's nutritional needs and promotes healing, dietary instruction is provided to the patient and family.

PROMOTING HOME, COMMUNITY-BASED, AND TRANSITIONAL CARE

The self-care program is planned with the patient so that activities that promote arterial and venous circulation, relieve pain, and promote tissue integrity are encouraged. Reasons for each aspect of the program are explained to the patient and family. Leg ulcers are often chronic and difficult to heal; they frequently recur, even when the patient follows the plan of care. Long-term care of the feet and legs to promote healing of wounds and prevent recurrence of ulcerations is the primary goal. Leg ulcers increase the patient's risk of infection, may be painful, and may limit mobility, necessitating lifestyle changes. Participation of family members and home health care providers may be necessary for treatments such as dressing changes, reassessments, reinforcement of instruction, and evaluation of the effectiveness of the plan of care. Regular follow-up with a primary provider is necessary.

Evaluation

Expected patient outcomes may include:
1. Demonstrates restored skin integrity
   a. Exhibits absence of inflammation
   b. Exhibits absence of drainage
   c. Has negative wound culture
   d. Avoids trauma to the legs
2. Increases physical mobility
   a. Progresses gradually to optimal level of activity
   b. Reports that pain does not impede activity
3. Attains adequate nutrition
   a. Selects foods high in protein, vitamins C and A, iron, and zinc
   b. Discusses with family members dietary modifications that need to be made at home
   c. Plans, with the family, a diet that is nutritionally sound

Varicose Veins

Varicose veins (varicosities) are abnormally dilated, tortuous, superficial veins caused by incompetent venous valves (see Fig. 26-15). Most commonly, this condition occurs in the lower extremities, the saphenous veins, or the lower trunk, but it can occur elsewhere in the body, such as the esophagus (e.g., esophageal varices; see Chapter 43).

It is estimated that varicose veins occur in 23% of American adults, and if spider telangiectasias and reticular veins are included in these statistics, the prevalence increases to 80% of men and 85% of women (Sidawy & Perler, 2019). The condition is most common in people whose occupations require prolonged standing, such as salespeople, hairstylists, teachers, nurses and ancillary medical personnel, and construction workers. A hereditary weakness of the vein wall may contribute to the development of varicosities, and it commonly occurs in several members of the same family. Varicose veins are rare before puberty. Pregnancy may cause varicosities because of hormonal effects related to decreased venous outflow, increased pressure by the gravid uterus, and increased blood volume (Della Torre, Sutherland, & Digiovanni, 2019).

Pathophysiology

Varicose veins may be primary (without involvement of deep veins) or secondary (resulting from obstruction of deep veins). A reflux of venous blood results in venous stasis. If only the superficial veins are affected, the person may have no symptoms but may be concerned by the appearance of the veins.

Clinical Manifestations

Symptoms, if present, may include dull aches, muscle cramps, increased muscle fatigue in the lower legs, ankle edema, and a feeling of heaviness of the legs. Nocturnal cramps are common. When deep venous obstruction results in varicose veins, the patient may develop the signs and symptoms of chronic venous insufficiency: edema, pain, pigmentation, and ulcerations. Susceptibility to injury and infection is increased, thus increasing risk for ulceration.

Assessment and Diagnostic Findings

Diagnostic tests for varicose veins include the duplex ultrasound scan, which documents the anatomic site of reflux and provides a quantitative measure of the severity of valvular reflux. These scans are typically performed in a reverse Trendelenburg position or with the patient standing. Venography is now rarely performed due to the availability of ultrasound.

However, when it is used, it involves injecting a radiopaque contrast agent into the leg veins so that the vein anatomy can be visualized by x-ray studies during various leg movements. CT venography can be helpful, especially if the pelvic venous structures are involved.

Prevention and Medical Management

The patient should avoid activities that cause venous stasis, such as wearing socks that are too tight at the top or that leave marks on the skin, crossing the legs at the thighs, and sitting or standing for long periods. Changing position frequently, elevating the legs 3 to 6 inches higher than heart level when they are tired, and getting up to walk for several minutes of every hour promote circulation. The patient is encouraged to walk 30 minutes each day if there are no contraindications. Walking up the stairs rather than using the elevator or escalator is helpful, and swimming is good exercise.

Graduated compression stockings, especially knee-high stockings, are useful. The patient who is overweight should be encouraged to begin a weight reduction plan.

The most common treatment options for venous insufficiency and varicose veins are thermal ablation with radiofrequency and laser therapy, micro (stab) phlebectomy, and foam sclerotherapy. Surgical ligation and stripping are reserved for select cases not amenable to other treatment options.

Thermal Ablation

Thermal ablation is a nonsurgical approach using thermal energy. Radiofrequency ablation uses an electrical contact inside the vein. As the device is withdrawn, the vein is sealed. Laser ablation uses a laser fiber tip that seals the vein (decompressed). Topical gel may be used first to numb the skin along the course of the saphenous vein. To protect the surrounding tissue, several small punctures are made along the vein, and 100 to 200 mL of dilute lidocaine is delivered to the perivenous space using ultrasound guidance. The goal of this tumescent anesthesia (i.e., anesthesia that causes localized swelling) is to provide analgesia, thermal protection (the cuff of fluid surrounds the veins and accompanying nerves), and extrinsic compression of the vein (Poder, Fisette, Bédard, et al., 2018). The saphenous vein is entered percutaneously near the knee using ultrasound guidance. A catheter is introduced into the saphenous vein and advanced to the saphenofemoral junction. The device is then activated and withdrawn, sealing the vein. Bandages or graduated compression stockings are applied after the procedure. A simultaneous microphlebectomy of branch varicosities may be performed; this is associated with a lower incidence of thrombophlebitis. This is also associated with quality of life improvements such as decreased leg swelling, pain, skin changes and healing of ulcerations, because all symptomatic veins may be treated at one time (Berti-Hearn & Elliott, 2019).

Cyanoacrylate embolization is approved for the treatment of an incompetent greater saphenous vein. Cyanoacrylate adhesive has been used for the treatment of arteriovenous malformations and a modified cyanoacrylate adhesive was developed that has rapid polymerization on contact with blood and tissue, flexibility sufficient to tolerate dynamic movements in the legs without generation of symptoms or be perceptible by the patient, and has a high viscosity to decrease the risk of propagation or embolization into the deep veins (Sidawy & Perler, 2019). During this procedure, a sheath is placed into the greater saphenous vein (guided by ultrasound). A catheter is advanced to the proximal saphenous vein and injections of cyanoacrylate are given, followed by local compression, and then repeated injections with repeated compression until the entire length of the target vein segment is treated. Cyanoacrylate embolization has been associated with less procedural ecchymosis because heat is not needed during this procedure.

Microphlebectomy

If there are superficial varicose veins that are close to the surface, a microphlebectomy may be performed. This procedure involves removal of a superficial varicosity using anywhere from one to 20 small incisions. There can be extensive bruising and risk of infection with this procedure (Sidawy & Perler, 2019).

Sclerotherapy

Sclerotherapy involves injection of an irritating chemical into a vein to produce localized phlebitis and fibrosis, thereby obliterating the lumen of the vein. This treatment may be performed alone for small varicosities or may follow vein ablation, ligation, or stripping. Sclerotherapy is typically performed in a procedure room and does not require sedation. After the sclerosing agent is injected, graduated compression stockings are applied to the leg and are worn for approximately 1 week after the procedure. Ultrasound-guided foam sclerotherapy has been found to be more effective in achieving closure of the branch veins. It is also associated with decreased symptoms of leg aching, itching, and edema, less skin changes and ulcerations, and increased patient satisfaction (Berti-Hearn & Elliott, 2019). After sclerotherapy, walking is encouraged to activate the calf muscle pump and maintain blood flow in the leg.

Ligation and Stripping

Surgery for symptomatic varicose veins requires that the deep veins be patent and functional. The saphenous vein is ligated high in the groin, where the saphenous vein meets the femoral vein. In addition, the vein may be stripped (removed). After the vein is ligated, an incision is made 2 to 3 cm below the knee, and a metal or plastic wire is passed the full length of the vein to the point of ligation. The wire is then withdrawn, pulling (stripping) the vein as it is removed. Pressure and elevation minimize bleeding during surgery.

Nursing Management

Thermal ablation is performed in an outpatient or clinic setting. The patient is advised to maintain compression on the affected limb for at least 24 hours and then wear compression stockings while ambulatory for at least 1 week post procedure. Patients have no activity restrictions, but are advised to avoid strenuous exercise, such as weight lifting, bicycle riding, or swimming for 2 weeks. The patient is informed that bruising may occur along the course of the saphenous vein and that they may experience leg cramps for a few days and may find it difficult to straighten the knee for up to 1.5 weeks. Nonsteroidal anti-inflammatory medications such as ibuprofen and cool compresses are used as needed for pain.

Ligation and stripping can be performed in an outpatient setting, or the patient may be admitted to the hospital on the day of surgery and discharged the same or next day if a bilateral procedure is to be performed or the patient is at high risk for postoperative complications. If the procedure is performed in an outpatient setting, nursing measures are the same as if the patient were hospitalized. Bed rest is discouraged, and the patient is encouraged to ambulate as soon as sedation has worn off. The patient is instructed to walk every hour for 5 to 10 minutes while awake for the first 24 hours if they can tolerate the discomfort, and then to increase walking and activity as tolerated. Graduated compression stockings are worn continuously for about 1 week after vein stripping. The nurse assists the patient to perform exercises and move the legs. The foot of the bed should be elevated. Standing and sitting are discouraged.

Promoting Comfort and Understanding

Analgesic agents are prescribed to help the patient move the affected extremities more comfortably. Dressings are inspected for bleeding, particularly in the groin, where the risk of bleeding is greatest. The nurse is alert for reported sensations of "pins and needles." Hypersensitivity to touch in the involved extremity may indicate a temporary or permanent nerve injury resulting from surgery, because the saphenous vein and nerve are close to each other in the leg. Any of these signs or symptoms should be reported to the primary provider.

Usually, the patient may shower after 24 hours. A clean towel is used to gently pat dry, not rub, the incisions. Application of skin lotion is avoided until the incisions are completely healed to avoid infection. The patient is instructed to apply sunscreen to the incisional area prior to sun exposure; otherwise, hyperpigmentation of the incision, scarring, or both may occur.

If the patient has undergone sclerotherapy, a burning sensation in the injected leg may be experienced for 1 to 2 days. The nurse encourages the use of a mild analgesic medication as prescribed and walking to provide relief.

Promoting Home, Community-Based, and Transitional Care

Long-term venous compression is essential after discharge, and the patient needs to obtain adequate supplies of graduated compression stockings or elastic bandages. Exercise of the legs is necessary; the development of an individualized plan requires consultation with the patient and the health care team.

LYMPHATIC DISORDERS

The lymphatic system consists of a set of vessels that spread throughout most of the body, as described previously in this chapter. The fluid drained from the interstitial space by the lymphatic system is called *lymph*. The flow of lymph depends on the intrinsic contractions of the lymph vessels, the contraction of muscles, respiratory movements, and gravity. The lymphatic system of the abdominal cavity maintains a steady flow of chyle (digested fatty food) from the intestinal mucosa to the thoracic duct. In other parts of the body, the lymphatic system's function is regional; the lymphatic vessels of the head, for example, empty into clusters of lymph nodes located in the neck, and those of the extremities empty into nodes of the axillae and the groin.

Lymphangitis and Lymphadenitis

Lymphangitis is an acute inflammation of the lymphatic channels. It arises most commonly from a focal area of infection in an extremity. Usually, the infectious organism is a *hemolytic streptococcus*. The characteristic red streaks that extend up the arm or the leg from an infected wound outline the course of the lymphatic vessels as they drain.

The lymph nodes located along the course of the lymphatic channels also become enlarged, red, and tender; this is referred to as acute lymphadenitis. They can also become necrotic and form an abscess, called suppurative lymphadenitis. The nodes involved most often are those in the groin, axilla, or cervical region.

Because these infections are nearly always caused by organisms that are sensitive to antibiotics, it is unusual to see abscess formation. Recurrent episodes of lymphangitis are often associated with progressive lymphedema. After acute attacks, a graduated compression stocking should be worn on the affected extremity for several months to prevent long-term edema.

Lymphedema

Lymphedema may be primary (congenital malformations) or secondary (acquired obstructions). Tissue swelling occurs in the extremities because of an increased quantity of lymph that results from obstruction of lymphatic vessels. It is especially marked when the extremity is in a dependent position. Initially, the edema is soft and pitting. As the condition progresses, the edema becomes firm, nonpitting, and unresponsive to treatment. The most common type is congenital lymphedema, known as lymphedema praecox, which is caused by hypoplasia of the lymphatic system of the lower extremity. This disorder is usually seen in women and first appears before age 35 (Dayan, Ly, Kataru, et al., 2018).

The obstruction may be in the lymph nodes and the lymphatic vessels. Sometimes, it is seen in the arm after an axillary node dissection (e.g., for breast cancer) and in the leg in association with varicose veins or chronic thrombophlebitis. In the latter case, the lymphatic obstruction usually is caused by chronic lymphangitis. Lymphatic obstruction caused by a parasite (filaria) is most frequently seen in the tropics. When chronic swelling is present, there may be frequent bouts of acute infection characterized by high fever and chills and increased residual edema once the inflammation has resolved. These changes can lead to chronic fibrosis, thickening of the subcutaneous tissues, and hypertrophy of the skin. This specific type of lymphedema, in which chronic swelling of the extremity recedes only slightly with elevation, is referred to as elephantiasis. There are an estimated 120 million people in the world infected by lymph-dwelling filarial parasites; of these, 40 million have lymphedema and secondary infections, creating an enormous global burden (King, Suamani, Sanuku, et al., 2018).

Medical Management

The goal of therapy is to reduce and control the edema and prevent infection. Active and passive exercises assist in moving lymphatic fluid into the bloodstream. External compression devices milk the fluid proximally from the foot to the hip or from the hand to the axilla. When the patient is ambulatory, custom-fitted graduated compression stockings or sleeves are worn; those with the highest compression strength (exceeding 40 mm Hg) are suggested; however, many patients cannot tolerate these pressures. When the leg is affected, continuous bed rest with the leg elevated may aid in mobilizing the fluids but is not practical long term. Manual lymphatic drainage performed by specially trained therapists is designed to direct or shift the congested lymph through functioning lymphatics that have preserved drainage. Manual lymphatic drainage is performed with light touch (as opposed to deep massage) to the proximal then distal lymphatic channels. Manual lymphatic drainage is incorporated in a sequential treatment approach used in combination with multilayer compression bandages, stockings or wraps, exercises, skin care, pressure gradient sleeves, and pneumatic pumps, depending on the severity and stage of the lymphedema (Patullo & Rajagopalan, 2017).

Pharmacologic Therapy

As initial therapy, the diuretic furosemide may be prescribed to prevent fluid overload due to mobilization of extracellular fluid. Diuretics have also been used along with elevation of the leg and the use of graduated compression stockings or sleeves. The use of diuretics alone has little benefit because their main action is to limit capillary filtration by decreasing the circulating blood volume. If lymphangitis or cellulitis is present, antibiotic therapy is initiated. Lymphedema significantly increases the risk for cellulitis; therefore, the patient is taught to provide meticulous skin care and inspect the skin for evidence of infection.

Surgical Management

Surgery is performed if the edema is severe and uncontrolled by medical therapy, if mobility is severely compromised, or if infection persists. One surgical approach involves the excision of the affected subcutaneous tissue and fascia, with skin grafting to cover the defect. Another procedure involves the surgical relocation of superficial lymphatic vessels into the deep lymphatic system, also known as lymph node transfer, by means of a buried dermal flap to provide a conduit for lymphatic drainage (Pappalardo, Patel, & Cheng, 2018). Lymphaticovenous bypasses also are performed with anastomosing the end of the lymphatic vessels to the side of veins to reduce lymphatic flow in the limbs (Gallagher, Marulanda, & Gray, 2018).

Nursing Management

After surgery, antibiotics may be prescribed for 3 to 7 days (Pappalardo et al., 2018). Constant elevation of the affected extremity and observation for complications are essential. Complications may include flap necrosis, hematoma or abscess under the flap, and cellulitis. The nurse instructs the patient or caregiver to inspect the dressing daily. Unusual drainage or any inflammation around the wound margin suggests infection and should be reported to the surgeon. The patient is informed that there may be a loss of sensation in the surgical area. The patient is also instructed to avoid the application of heating pads or exposure to sun to prevent burns or trauma to the area.

CELLULITIS

Cellulitis is the most common infectious cause of limb swelling. Cellulitis can occur as a single isolated event or a series of recurrent events. It is sometimes misdiagnosed as recurrent thrombophlebitis or chronic venous insufficiency.

Pathophysiology

Cellulitis occurs when an entry point through broken skin allows microbes to enter and release their toxins in the subcutaneous tissues. The etiologic pathogen of cellulitis is typically either *Streptococcus* species or *Staphylococcus aureus* (Bystritsky & Chambers, 2018).

Clinical Manifestations

The onset of swelling, localized redness, warmth, and pain is frequently associated with systemic signs of fever, chills, and sweating. The redness may not be uniform and often skips areas and eventually develops a pitting "orange peel" appearance. Regional lymph nodes may also be tender and enlarged (Bystritsky & Chambers, 2018).

 Concept Mastery Alert

> Cellulitis needs to be differentiated from lymphangitis. With cellulitis, the swelling and redness is localized and anatomically nonspecific. With lymphangitis, characteristic red streaks appear denoting the outline of the lymphatic vessels that are affected.

Medical Management

Mild cases of cellulitis can be treated on an outpatient basis with oral antibiotic therapy. If the cellulitis is severe, the patient is treated with IV antibiotics. The key to preventing recurrent episodes of cellulitis lies in adequate antibiotic therapy for the initial event and in identifying the site of microbial entry. Cracks and fissures that occur in the skin between the toes must be examined as potential sites of microbial entry. Other locations include drug use injection sites, contusions, abrasions, ulceration, ingrown toenails, and hangnails. Prophylactic compression therapy to reduce the risk of recurrence may be indicated in some cases (Webb, Neeman, Bowden, et al., 2020).

Nursing Management

The patient is instructed to elevate the affected area 3 to 6 inches above heart level and apply cool packs to the site every 2 to 4 hours until the inflammation has resolved, and then transition to warm packs. Patients with sensory and circulatory deficits, such as those caused by diabetes and paralysis, should use caution when applying warm packs because burns may occur; it is advisable to use a thermometer or have a caregiver ensure that the temperature is not more than luke-warm. Education should focus on preventing a recurrent episode. The patient with peripheral vascular disease or diabetes should receive education or reinforcement about skin and foot care.

CRITICAL THINKING EXERCISES

1 `pq` A 27-year-old male with Marfan syndrome presents to the emergency department where you work complaining of a sudden onset of chest pain with dyspnea and left leg weakness. You are unable to palpate pulses in his left foot. The patient's laboratory findings indicate a decline in renal function. How would you triage and prioritize your initial nursing care for this patient? The provider orders an urgent CT angiogram, which reveals a dissection of the aorta and obstructed flow to the left kidney and left leg. What are the ongoing priorities for managing this patient's care?

2 `ebp` A 32-year-old woman presents to the primary care clinic where you work with leg pain. She has recently been on a long airplane flight and has had some unilateral leg swelling with calf tightness and pain. Her only medication is an oral contraceptive agent; she is generally healthy. What are her risk factors for venous thromboembolism (VTE)? What further diagnostic studies should be considered and what evidence-based practice recommendations will guide the management of her care? What pharmacologic options might be considered for anticoagulation and what therapies are indicated to manage her leg edema?

3 `ipc` A 70-year-old male presents to a preadmission center where you work to prepare for surgical repair of an abdominal aortic aneurysm. His aneurysm is 5.8 cm which is an increase of 1 cm in the last 6 months. His hypertension is well controlled, and he has had no further angina since coronary artery bypass grafts (CABGs) 2 years ago. He has good exercise tolerance and his weight is within a normal range. What preoperative assessments are required? The patient asks what he should do if he experiences increasing abdominal, back, or flank pain before surgery. How will you respond? How will the interprofessional team manage his postoperative care and coordinate a safe discharge?

REFERENCES

*Asterisk indicates nursing research.

Books

Comerford, K. C., & Durkin, M. T. (Eds.). (2020). *Nursing2020 drug handbook*. Philadelphia, PA: Wolters Kluwer.

Ermer-Selton, J. (2016). Lower extremity assessment. In R. Bryant & D. Nix (Eds.). *Acute and chronic wounds: Current management* (5th ed.). St. Louis, MO: Elsevier.

Fischbach, F. T., & Fischbach, M. A. (2018). *A manual of laboratory and diagnostic tests* (10th ed.). Philadelphia, PA: Wolters Kluwer.

Norris, T. L. (2019). *Porth's pathophysiology: Concepts of altered health states* (10th ed.). Philadelphia, PA: Wolters Kluwer.

Sidawy, A. N., & Perler, B. A. (2019). *Rutherford's vascular surgery and endovascular therapy* (9th ed.). Philadelphia, PA: Elsevier.

Weinberger, S. E., Cockrill, B. A., & Mandel, J. (2019). *Principles of pulmonary medicine* (7th ed.). Philadelphia, PA: Elsevier Saunders.

Zierler, R. E., & Dawson, D. L. (Eds.). (2016). *Strandness's duplex scanning in vascular disorders* (5th ed.). Philadelphia, PA: Wolters Kluwer.

Journals and Electronic Documents

Apelqvist, J., Willy, C., Fagerdahl, A. M., et al. (2017). EWMA Document: Negative pressure wound therapy. *Journal of Wound Care*, 26(Sup3), S1–S154.

Atherton, J. J., Sindone, A., De Pasquale, C. G., et al. (2018). National Heart Foundation of Australia and Cardiac Society of Australia and New Zealand: Guidelines for the prevention, detection, and management of heart failure in Australia 2018. *Heart, Lung and Circulation*, 27(10), 1123–1208.

Balcombe, L., Miller, C., & McGuiness, W. (2017). Approaches to the application and removal of compression therapy: A literature review. *British Journal of Community Nursing*, 22(Sup10), S6–S14.

Becker, R. C. (2020). Anticipating the long-term cardiovascular effects of COVID-19. *Journal of Thrombosis and Thrombolysis*, 50(3), 512–524.

Belch, J., Carlizza, A., Carpentier, P. H., et al. (2017). ESVM guidelines—the diagnosis and management of Raynaud's phenomenon. *VASA*, 46(6), 413–423.

Berti-Hearn, L., & Elliott, B. (2019). Chronic venous insufficiency: A review for nurses. *Nursing*, 49(12), 24–30.

Bjork, R., & Ehmann, S. (2019). S.T.R.I.D.E. professional guide to compression garment selection for the lower extremity. *Journal of Wound Care*, 28(Sup6a), 1–44.

Bonifant, H., & Holloway, S. (2019). A review of the effects of ageing on skin integrity and wound healing. *British Journal of Community Nursing*, 24(Sup3), S28–S33.

Bystritsky, R., & Chambers, H. (2018). Cellulitis and soft tissue infections. *Annals of Internal Medicine*, 168(3), ITC17–ITC32.

Cauci, S., Xodo, S., Buligan, C., et al. (2021). Oxidative stress is increased in combined oral contraceptives users and is positively associated with high-sensitivity C-reactive protein. *Molecules*, 26(4),1070.

Chaikof, E. L., Dalman, R. L., Eskandari, M. K., et al. (2018). The Society for Vascular Surgery practice guidelines on the care of patients with an abdominal aortic aneurysm. *Journal of Vascular Surgery*, 67(1), 2–77.e2.

Cohen, A. T., Lip, G. Y., De Caterina, R., et al. (2018). State of play and future direction with NOACs: An expert consensus. *Vascular Pharmacology*, 106, 9–21.

Conte, M. S., Bradbury, A. W., Kolh, P., et al. (2019). Global vascular guidelines on the management of chronic limb-threatening ischemia. *Journal of Vascular Surgery*, 69(6S), 3S–125S.e40.

Dayan, J. H., Ly, C. L., Kataru, R. P., et al. (2018). Lymphedema: Pathogenesis and novel therapies. *Annual Review of Medicine*, 69, 263–276.

Dean, S. M. (2018). Cutaneous manifestations of chronic vascular disease. *Progress in Cardiovascular Diseases*, 60(6), 567–579.

De Palo, V. (2020). Venous thromboembolism (VTE). *Medscape*. Retrieved on 7/21/2020 at: www.emedicine.medscape.com/article/1267714-overview

Della Torre, M., Sutherland, M. B., & Digiovanni, L. M. (2019). Pearls in clinical obstetrics: Challenges in anticoagulation in pregnancy. *Minerva Ginecologica*, 71(2), 125–132.

European Pressure Ulcer Advisory Panel, National Pressure Injury Advisory Panel, Pan Pacific Pressure Injury Alliance (EPUAP/NPIAP/PPPIA). (2019). Prevention and treatment of pressure ulcers/injuries: Clinical practice guideline: EPUAP/NPIAP/PPPIA. Retrieved on 4/4/2020 at: www.internationalguideline.com

Fähling, M., Seeliger, E., Patzak, A., et al. (2017). Understanding and preventing contrast-induced acute kidney injury. *Nature Reviews Nephrology*, 13(3), 169–180.

Farkas, K., Járai, Z., & Kolossváry, E. (2017). Cilostazol is effective and safe option for the treatment of intermittent claudication. Results of the NOCLAUD study. *Orvosi Hetilap, 158*(4), 123–128.

Folsom, A. R., Basu, S., Hong, CP., et al. (2019). Reasons for differences in the incidence of venous thromboembolism in Black versus white Americans. *The American Journal of Medicine, 132*(8), 970–976.

Gallagher, K., Marulanda, K., & Gray, S. (2018). Surgical intervention for lymphedema. *Surgical Oncology Clinics of North America, 27*(1), 195–215.

Gerhard-Herman, M., Gornik, H., Barrett, C., et al. (2016). AHA/ACC Guideline on the management of patients with lower extremity peripheral arterial disease: Executive summary. *Circulation, 134*(24), 1–208.

Harding, K., Chrysostomou, D., Mohamud, L., et al. (2017). The role of mechanically powered disposable negative pressure wound therapy (dNPWT) in practice. *Wounds International.* Retrieved on 9/7/2019 at: www.gdm-medical.nl/wp-content/uploads/2018/05/wi_international_consensus_paper_dnpwt.pdf

Harris, D. G., Olson, S. L., Panthofer, A. M., et al. (2019). A frailty-based risk score predicts morbidity and mortality after elective endovascular repair of descending thoracic aortic aneurysms. *Annals of Vascular Surgery, 67,* 90–99.

Hazarika, S., & Annex, B. H. (2017). Biomarkers and genetics in peripheral artery disease. *Clinical Chemistry, 63*(1), 236–244.

IBM Watson Health. (2020). IBM Micromedex®. Retrieved on 11/19/2020 at: www.micromedexsolutions.com/micromedex2/librarian/CS/4B61E3/ND_PR/evidencexpert/ND_P/evidencexpert/DUPLI-CATIONSHIELDSYNC/DC5D13/ND_PG/evidencexpert/ND_B/evidencexpert/ND_AppProduct/evidencexpert/ND_T/evidencexpert/PFActionId/evidencexpert.DoIntegratedSearch

Ignatyev, I. M., Pokrovsky, A., & Gradusov, E. (2019). Long-term results of endovascular treatment of chronic iliofemoral venous obstructive lesions. *Vascular and Endovascular Surgery, 53*(5), 373–378.

Indik, J. H., Gimbel, J. R., Abe, H., et al. (2017). 2017 HRS expert consensus statement on magnetic resonance imaging and radiation exposure in patients with cardiovascular implantable electronic devices. *Heart Rhythm, 14*(7), e97–e153.

Jelani, Q. U. A., Petrov, M., Martinez, S. C., et al. (2018). Peripheral arterial disease in women: An overview of risk factor profile, clinical features, and outcomes. *Current Atherosclerosis Reports, 20*(8), 40.

Kahn, S. R., Galanaud, J. P., Vedantham, S., et al. (2016). Guidance for the prevention and treatment of the post-thrombotic syndrome. *Journal of Thrombosis and Thrombolysis, 41*(1), 144–153.

Kim, P. J., Applewhite, A., Dardano, A. N., et al. (2018). Use of a novel foam dressing with negative pressure wound therapy and instillation: Recommendations and clinical experience. *Wounds: A Compendium of Clinical Research and Practice, 30*(3 suppl), S1–S17.

King, C. L., Suamani, J., Sanuku, N., et al. (2018). A trial of a triple-drug treatment for lymphatic filariasis. *New England Journal of Medicine, 379*(19), 1801–1810.

Kruger, P. C., Eikelboom, J. W., Douketis, J. D., et al. (2019). Deep vein thrombosis: Update on diagnosis and management. *Medical Journal of Australia, 210*(11), 516–524.

Martinelli, O., Di Girolamo, A., Belli, C., et al. (2019). Incidence of post-implantation syndrome with different endovascular aortic aneurysm repair modalities and devices and related etiopathogenetic implications. *Annals of Vascular Surgery, 63,* 155–161.

McDermott, M. M. (2018). Medical management of functional impairment in peripheral artery disease: A review. *Progress in Cardiovascular Diseases, 60*(6), 586–592.

Millar, C. M., & Laffan, M. A. (2017). Drug therapy in anticoagulation: Which drug for which patient? *Clinical Medicine (Lond), 17*(3), 233–244.

Mintz, A., & Levy, M. S. (2017). Upper extremity deep vein thrombosis. *American College of Cardiology.* Retrieved on 12/15/2020 at: www.acc.org/latest-in-cardiology/articles/2017/11/09/13/30/upper-extremity-deep-vein-thrombosis

Miranda, V., Sousa, J., & Mansilha, A. (2018). Spinal cord injury in endovascular thoracoabdominal aortic aneurysm repair: Prevalence, risk factors and preventive strategies. *International Angiology, 37*(2), 112–126.

Nicolaides, A. N. (2020). The most severe stage of chronic venous disease: An update on the management of patients with venous leg ulcers. *Advances in Therapy, 37*(Suppl 1), 19–24.

Obi, A. T., Barnes, G. D., Wakefield, T. W., et al. (2020). Practical diagnosis and treatment of suspected venous thromboembolism during COVID-19 pandemic. *Journal of Vascular Surgery: Venous and Lymphatic Disorders, 8*(4), 526–534.

Ouellette, D. R. (2019). Pulmonary embolism. *Medscape.* Retrieved on 10/17/2019 at: www.emedicine.medscape.com/article/300901-overview

Pappalardo, M., Patel, K., & Cheng, M. H. (2018). Vascularized lymph node transfer for treatment of extremity lymphedema: An overview of current controversies regarding donor sites, recipient sites and outcomes. *Journal of Surgical Oncology, 117*(7), 1420–1431.

Patel, K., Fasanya, A., Yadam, S., et al. (2017). Pathogenesis and epidemiology of venous thromboembolic disease. *Critical Care Nursing Quarterly, 40*(3), 191–200.

Patullo, L., & Rajagopalan, S. (2017). Successful outpatient management of lymphoedema and lymphorrhoea with wrap around compression: A case study. *Journal of Wound Care, 26*(3), 100–106.

Peñaloza-Martínez, E., Demelo-Rodríguez, P., Proietti, M., et al. (2018). Update on extended treatment for venous thromboembolism. *Annals of Medicine, 50*(8), 666–674.

Poder, T. G., Fisette, J. F., Bédard, S. K., et al. (2018). Is radiofrequency ablation of varicose veins a valuable option? A systematic review of the literature with a cost analysis. *Canadian Journal of Surgery, 61*(2), 128–138.

*Quintella Farah, B., Silva Rigoni, V. L., de Almeida Correia, M., et al. (2019). Influence of smoking on physical function, physical activity, and cardiovascular health parameters in patients with symptomatic peripheral arterial disease: A cross-sectional study. *Journal of Vascular Nursing, 37*(2), 106–112.

Rabe, E., Partsch, H., Morrison, N., et al. (2020). Risks and contraindications of medical compression treatment—A critical reappraisal. An international consensus statement. *Phlebology, 35*(7), 447–460.

Rurali, E., Perrucci, G. L., Pilato, C. A., et al. (2018). Precise therapy for thoracic aortic aneurysm in Marfan syndrome: A puzzle nearing its solution. *Progress in Cardiovascular Diseases, 61*(3–4), 328–335.

Saxon, J. T., Safley, D. M., Mena-Hurtado, C., et al. (2020). Adherence to guideline-recommended therapy-including supervised exercise therapy referral-across peripheral artery disease specialty clinics: Insights from the international PORTRAIT registry. *Journal of American Heart Association, 9*(3), e012541.

Scali, S. T., Kim, M., Kubilis, P., et al. (2018). Implementation of a bundled protocol significantly reduces risk of spinal cord ischemia after branched or fenestrated endovascular aortic repair. *Journal of Vascular Surgery, 67*(2), 409–423.e4.

*Schorr, E. N., Treat-Jacobson, D., & Lindquist, R. (2017). The relationship between peripheral artery disease symptomatology and ischemia. *Nursing Research, 66*(5), 378–387.

Serhal, M., & Barnes, G. D. (2019). Venous thromboembolism: A clinician update. *Vascular Medicine, 24*(2), 122–131.

Singer, A. J., Tassiopoulos, A., & Kirsner, R. S. (2017). Evaluation and management of lower-extremity ulcers. *New England Journal of Medicine, 377*(16), 1559–1567.

Stubbs, J. M., Assareh, H., Curnow, J., et al. (2018). Incidence of in-hospital and post-discharge diagnosed hospital-associated venous thromboembolism using linked administrative data. *Internal Medicine Journal, 48*(2), 157–165.

Sultan, S., Murarka, S., Jahangir, A., et al. (2017). Vitamins for cardiovascular diseases: Is the expense justified? *Cardiology in Review, 25*(6), 298–308.

Swanson, T., Angel, D., Sussman, G., et al. (2016). The International Wound Infection Institute (IWII) wound infection in clinical practice consensus document 2016 update. *Wound Practice & Research: Journal of the Australian Wound Management Association, 24*(4), 194–198.

Tapson, V. F. (2019). Overview of the treatment, prognosis, and follow-up of acute pulmonary embolism in adults. *UpToDate.* Retrieved on 9/22/2019 at: www.uptodate.com/contents/overview-of-the-treatment-prognosis-and-follow-up-of-acute-pulmonary-embolism-in-adults

Tapson, V. F., & Weinberg, A. S. (2020). Treatment, prognosis, and follow-up of acute pulmonary embolism in adults. *UpToDate.* Retrieved on 7/20/2020 at: www.uptodate.com/contents/treatment-prognosis-and-follow-up-of-acute-pulmonary-embolism-in-adults

The Joint Commission (TJC). (2019). Sentinel Event Alert 61: Managing the risks of direct oral anticoagulant. Retrieved on 10/4/2019 at: www.jointcommission.org/sentinel_event_alert_61_managing_the_risks_of_direct_oral_anticoagulants

Thompson, B. T., & Kabrhel, C. (2020). Overview of acute pulmonary embolism in adults. *UpToDate*. Retrieved on 7/20/2020 at: www.upto-date.com/contents/overview-of-acute-pulmonary-embolism-in-adults

Treat-Jacobson, D., McDermott, M. M., Beckman, J. A., et al. (2019). Implementation of supervised exercise therapy for patients with symptomatic peripheral artery disease: A science advisory from the American Heart Association. *Circulation, 140*(13), e700–e710.

Webb, E., Neeman, T., Bowden, F. J., et al. (2020). Compression therapy to prevent recurrent cellulitis of the leg. *New England Journal of Medicine, 383*(7), 630–639.

Witt, D. M., Nieuwlaat, R., Clark, N. P., et al. (2018). American Society of Hematology 2018 guidelines for management of venous thromboembolism: Optimal management of anticoagulation therapy. *Blood Advances, 2*(22), 3257–3291.

Zheng, J., Chen, Q., Fu, J., et al. (2019). Critical appraisal of international guidelines for the prevention and treatment of pregnancy-associated venous thromboembolism: A systematic review. *BMC Cardiovascular Disorders, 19*(1), 199.

Resources

American Heart Association (AHA), www.aha.org
American Venous Forum (AVF), www.veinforum.org
Society for Vascular Medicine (SVM), www.vascularmed.org
Society for Vascular Nursing (SVN), www.svnnet.org
Society for Vascular Surgery (SVS), www.vascularweb.org
Society for Vascular Ultrasound (SVU), www.svunet.org
Vascular Cures, www.vascularcures.org

LEARNING OUTCOMES

On completion of this chapter, the learner will be able to:

1. Compare and contrast normal blood pressure and various stages of hypertension.
2. Identify pathophysiologic processes implicated in the progression of hypertension.
3. Demonstrate the proper techniques to perform an assessment and discriminate between normal and abnormal findings identified in the patient with hypertension.
4. Discuss risk factors and treatment approaches for hypertension, including lifestyle modifications and medication therapy.
5. Use the nursing process as a framework for care of the patient with hypertension.
6. Describe hypertensive crises and their treatments.

NURSING CONCEPTS

Assessment
Perfusion

GLOSSARY

hypertensive emergency: an emergent situation in which blood pressure is severely elevated and there is evidence of actual or probable target organ damage

hypertensive urgency: an urgent situation in which blood pressure is severely elevated but there is no evidence of impending or progressive target organ damage

isolated systolic hypertension: a disorder most commonly seen in the older adult in which the systolic pressure is greater than 140 mm Hg and the diastolic pressure is less than 80 mm Hg

masked hypertension: blood pressure that is typically suggestive of a diagnosis of hypertension that is paradoxically normal in health care settings

primary hypertension: high blood pressure with no identifiable cause (*synonym:* essential hypertension)

rebound hypertension: blood pressure in a patient with hypertension that is controlled with medication and becomes abnormally high with the abrupt discontinuation of that medication

resistant hypertension: high blood pressure treated with three or more antihypertensive medications of different classes; one of these must be a diuretic agent

secondary hypertension: high blood pressure from an identified cause, such as chronic kidney disease

target organ damage: manifestations of pathophysiologic changes in various organs as a consequence of hypertension

white coat hypertension: blood pressure that increases to hypertensive readings in health care settings that is paradoxically within the normal ranges in other settings

---

Hypertension is the most common chronic disease among adults in the United States and in the world (Whelton, Carey, Aronow, et al., 2017). It is identified as the leading risk factor for premature death, disability, and overall disease burden worldwide because it may lead to cardiovascular disease (CVD), stroke, and chronic kidney disease (CKD) when not appropriately treated (Caillon, Paradis, & Schiffrin, 2019; DePalma, Himmelfarb, MacLaughlin, et al., 2018). The overall risk of developing these CVDs, strokes, and renal disorders is low among patients with blood pressures that are consistently stable around 115/75 mm Hg; however, each increase of 20 mm Hg in the systolic blood pressure (SBP) or 10 mm Hg increase in the diastolic blood pressure (DBP) doubles the risk of death from stroke or heart disease (Lee, Kim, Kang, et al., 2018). And yet, most patients with hypertension could lower their blood pressure through lifestyle changes (e.g., diet, exercise, medication adherence, smoking cessation) and lower these associated morbid risks (Whelton et al., 2017). This chapter presents an overview of hypertension and how it is defined and managed so that nurses may appropriately assess, monitor, educate, and intervene with patients with hypertension.

Hypertension

For many years, patients were diagnosed with hypertension if they had chronically elevated SBPs of 140 mm Hg or higher or DBPs of 90 mm Hg or higher. These parameters, which also specified that the diagnosis of hypertension must be based on an average of two or more accurate readings taken one to 4 weeks apart, were endorsed by the *Seventh Report of the Joint National Committee on prevention, detection, evaluation, and treatment of high blood pressure* (JNC 7) (Chobanian, Bakris, Black, et al., 2003), as well as the *Eighth Joint National Committee* (JNC 8) (James, Oparil, Carter, et al., 2014), and the *American Society of Hypertension* (ASH) and the *International Society of Hypertension* (ISH) (Weber, Schiffrin, White, et al., 2014). However, these parameters for diagnosing hypertension recently changed to less permissive parameters, and patients with average SBPs that are 130 mm Hg or higher or with average DBPs 80 mm Hg or higher may be diagnosed with hypertension, according to the *American College of Cardiology (ACC)/American Heart Association (AHA) Task Force* (Whelton et al., 2017).

The classification system for hypertension has been further revised by the ACC/AHA (Whelton et al., 2017) to include elevated, stage 1, and stage 2 categories, as displayed in Table 27-1. Table 27-1 compares this classification system to previous JNC 7 and JNC 8 guidelines classification systems, which are no longer followed (DePalma et al., 2018). The blood pressure categories emphasize the direct relationship between the SBP and DBP risks of morbidity, all-cause mortality, and specifically, cardiovascular mortality. Of particular note, the ACC/AHA guideline (Whelton et al., 2017) changed the previously labeled *prehypertension* category to *elevated blood pressure* category. The rationale for this change in terminology is to highlight the association between any elevated blood pressure and increased cardiovascular risk. The blood pressure readings should use the average of two or more valid, reproducible measurements obtained on more than two occasions, in most instances (see later discussion under Assessment and Diagnostic Findings).

The prevalence of hypertension among adults in the United States is substantially higher when the definition of the ACC/AHA guideline is used versus the JNC 7 or JNC 8 definition (46% vs. 32%) (Whelton et al., 2017). However, since nonpharmacologic treatment (i.e., lifestyle changes) is recommended for most adults whose blood pressures are within the elevated hypertension category, the newer guidelines that define hypertension have resulted in only a small increase in antihypertensive medication prescriptions, overall. Indeed, it has been asserted that the greatest benefit of the ACC/AHA (2017) guideline is its greater emphasis on lifestyle interventions, which include weight loss, healthy diet, physical exercise, reduced sodium intake, increased potassium intake, and decreased alcohol intake (Ioannidis, 2018).

The prevalence of hypertension increases as people age or have other cardiovascular risk factors. Of all adults with hypertension, it is estimated that 35.3% do not know that they have this disorder. Furthermore, approximately 45.4% of people with hypertension do not have their blood pressure under control (Benjamin, Muntner, Alonso, et al., 2019). The prevalence of hypertension varies by ethnicity and gender, and is estimated at approximately 48.2% among Caucasian men, 41.3% among Caucasian women, 58.6% among African American men, 56% among African American women, 47.4% among Hispanic men, 40.8% among Hispanic women, 46.4% among Asian American men, and 36.4% among Asian American women. The prevalence of hypertension among African Americans is among the highest in the world (Benjamin et al., 2019). Moreover, African Americans tend to develop hypertension at younger ages than Caucasian Americans (Spikes, Higgins, Quyyumi, et al., 2019). Chart 27-1 displays risk factors for hypertension.

Findings from the National Health and Nutrition Examination Survey (NHANES) have shown better hypertension control rates in women, in Caucasians than in African Americans and Hispanics, and in older versus younger patients. Additionally, adults of higher socioeconomic status have better control of their blood pressures compared to adults of lower socioeconomic status. Hypertension is most prevalent among adults 75 years of age and older, affecting 80% of men and 85.6% of women (Benjamin et al., 2019).

TABLE 27-1	Comparing Blood Pressure Classifications by Key Guidelines for Adults Age 18 and Older			
Systolic BP (mm Hg)		**Diastolic BP (mm Hg)**	**ACC/AHA (2017) Guideline**[a]	**JNC 7**[b] **and JNC 8**[c] **Guidelines**
<120	-and-	<80	Normal	Normal
120–129	-and-	<80	Elevated	Prehypertension
130–139	-or-	80–89	Stage 1 hypertension	Prehypertension
140–159	-or-	90–99	Stage 2 hypertension	Stage 1 hypertension
≥160	-or-	≥100	Stage 2 hypertension	Stage 2 hypertension

Note: For each guideline, if the patient's systolic and diastolic BPs fall into different categories, then the patient is classified according to the highest category.
BP, blood pressure.
Adapted from [a]Whelton, P. K., Carey, R. M., Aronow, W. S., et al. (2017). 2017 ACC/AHA/AAPA/ABC/ACPM/AGS/APhA/ASH/ ASPC/NMA/PCNA guideline for the prevention, detection, evaluation, and management of high blood pressure in adults: A report of the American College of Cardiology/American Heart Association Task Force on Clinical Practice Guidelines. *Hypertension, 71*(6), e13–e115; [b]Chobanian, A. V., Bakris, G. L., Black, H. R., et al; National High Blood Pressure Education Program Coordinating Committee (2003). Seventh Report of the Joint National Committee on prevention, detection, evaluation, and treatment of high blood pressure: The JNC 7 Report. *JAMA, 289*(19), 2560–2572; [c]James, P. A., Oparil, S., Carter, B. L., et al. (2014). 2014 evidence-based guideline for the management of high blood pressure in adults: Report from the panel members appointed to the Eighth Joint National Committee (JNC 8). *JAMA, 311*(5), 507–520.

Hypertension is categorized as either primary hypertension or secondary hypertension. **Primary hypertension** (also called *essential hypertension*) is diagnosed when there is no identifiable cause (Alexander, 2019). Approximately 90% to 95% of adults with hypertension have primary hypertension.

Secondary hypertension is defined as high blood pressure from an identifiable underlying cause. Between 5% and 10% of all adults with hypertension have secondary hypertension. Screening for secondary hypertension is indicated for new-onset, poorly controlled hypertension, in hypertension resistant to treatment with three or more drugs, with hypertension of an abrupt onset, or in patients younger than 30 years of age. In addition, a new diagnosis of hypertension with associated excessive target organ damage, such as cerebral vascular disease, retinopathy, left ventricular hypertrophy (LVH), heart failure with preserved ejection fraction, coronary artery disease, CKD, or peripheral arterial disease, could suggest secondary hypertension. Chart 27-2 displays some common underlying causes of secondary hypertension.

Pathophysiology

Blood pressure is the product of cardiac output multiplied by peripheral resistance. Cardiac output is the product of the heart rate multiplied by the stroke volume. Each time the heart contracts, pressure is transferred from the contraction of the myocardium to the blood and then pressure is exerted by the blood as it flows through the blood vessels.

Hypertension can result from increases in cardiac output, increases in peripheral resistance (constriction of the blood vessels), or both. Increases in cardiac output are often related to an expansion in vascular volume. Although no precise cause can be identified for most cases of hypertension, it is understood that hypertension is a multifactorial condition. Because hypertension can be a sign, it is most likely to have many causes, just as fever has many causes (Norris, 2019). For hypertension to occur there must be a change in one or more factors affecting peripheral resistance or cardiac output. In addition, there must also be a problem with the body's control systems that monitor or regulate pressure (Fig. 27-1).

Hypertension is thought to occur as a result of a complex interaction between behavioral–social–environmental risks and genetics (Zilbermint, Gaye, Berthon, et al., 2019). Behavioral–social–environmental risks may include dietary habits, including limited consumption of vegetables, fiber, fish fats, and potassium, and excessive intake of sodium; obesity; poor physical fitness; and excessive alcohol intake (Whelton et al., 2017).

Although single-gene mutations associated with hypertension have been identified, most types of hypertension are thought to be polygenic (i.e., mutations in more than one gene) (Whelton et al., 2017). The tendency to develop hypertension can be inherited; however, genetic profiles alone cannot predict who will and will not develop hypertension. The role of genetics in hypertension is complex and not fully understood at the present time.

To date, over 1000 genetic variants have been identified that may contribute to hypertension; however, collectively they explain only about 6% of the trait variance (Zilbermint et al., 2019).

Many physiologic precedents that can lead to hypertension have been identified (Caillon, Mian, Fraulob-Aquino, et al., 2017; Caillon et al., 2019; Norris, 2019):

- Increased sympathetic nervous system activity related to dysfunction of the autonomic nervous system

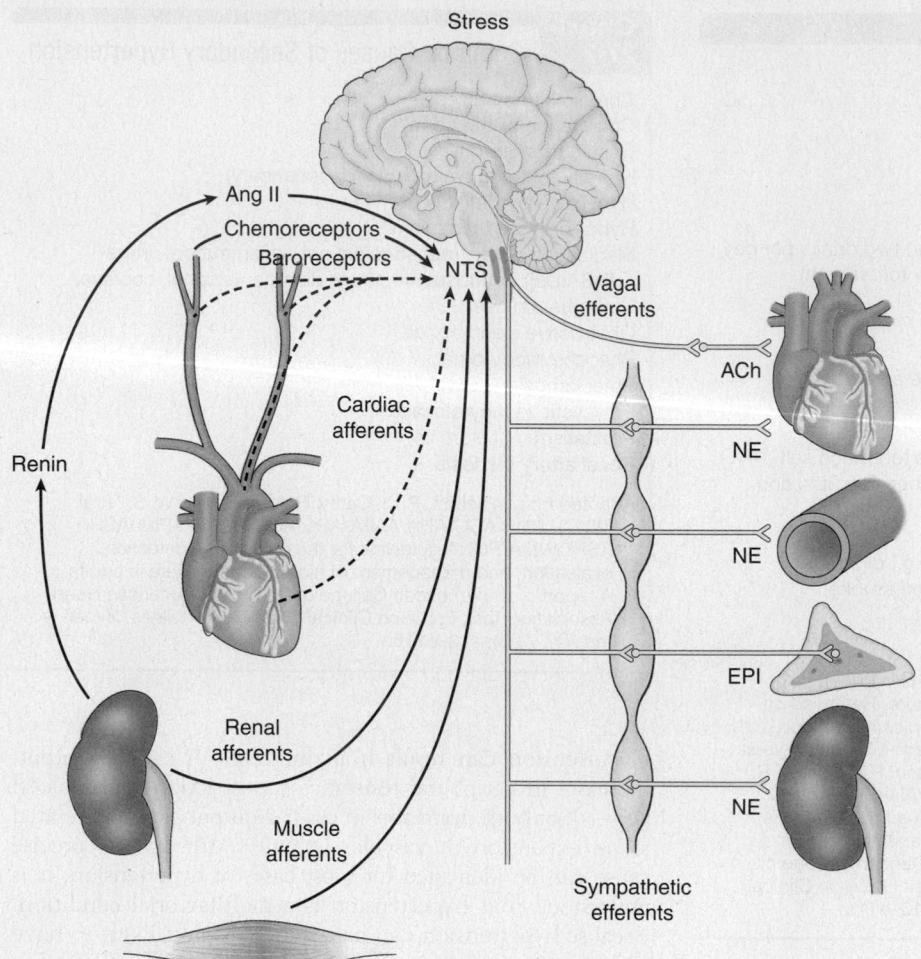

Figure 27-1 • Central and reflex mechanisms involved in the neural control of blood pressure. *Dotted arrows* represent inhibitory neural influences, and *solid arrows* represent excitatory neural influences on sympathetic outflow. ACH, acetylcholine; Ang II, angiotensin II; EPI, epinephrine; NE, norepinephrine; NTS, nucleus tractus solitarius. Adapted from Kaplan, N. M., & Victor, R. G. (2015). *Kaplan's clinical hypertension* (11th ed.). Philadelphia, PA: Lippincott Williams & Wilkins.

- Increased renal reabsorption of sodium, chloride, and water related to a genetic variation in the pathways by which the kidneys handle sodium
- Increased activity of the renin–angiotensin–aldosterone system, resulting in expansion of extracellular fluid volume and increased systemic vascular resistance
- Decreased vasodilation of the arterioles related to dysfunction of the vascular endothelium
- Resistance to insulin action, which may be a common factor linking hypertension, type 2 diabetes, hypertriglyceridemia, obesity, and glucose intolerance
- Activation of the innate and adaptive components of the immune response that contribute to vascular inflammation and dysfunction

 Gerontologic Considerations

Structural and functional changes in the heart, blood vessels, and kidneys contribute to increases in blood pressure that occur with aging. These changes include accumulation of atherosclerotic plaque, fragmentation of arterial elastins, increased collagen deposits, impaired vasodilation, and renal dysfunction. The result of these changes is decreased elasticity or stiffening of the major blood vessels, particularly the aorta, and volume expansion (Eliopoulos, 2018; Fajemiroye, da Cunha, Saavedra-Rodríguez, et al., 2018). Hence, both SBP and DBP increase linearly up to the sixth decade of life.

At that time, among most adults, DBP gradually decreases while SBP continues to rise. Thus, **isolated systolic hypertension** is the predominant form of hypertension in older people (Whelton et al., 2017). Results from randomized controlled studies have demonstrated that lowering blood pressure in older adults with isolated systolic hypertension is effective in reducing the incidence of adverse cardiovascular events and death (Whelton et al., 2017).

Clinical Manifestations

Physical examination may reveal no abnormalities other than elevated blood pressure. People with hypertension may be asymptomatic and remain so for many years. Hypertension is known as the "silent killer" because it typically has no warning signs or symptoms, and many people do not know they have it. However, when specific signs and symptoms appear, they usually indicate vascular damage, with specific manifestations related to the organs served by the involved vessels. These specific manifestations of pathophysiologic changes in various organs as a consequence of hypertension are referred to as **target organ damage**. Retinal changes such as hemorrhages, exudates (fluid accumulation), arteriolar narrowing, and cotton-wool spots (small infarctions) may occur. In severe hypertension, papilledema (swelling of the optic disc) may be seen (Weber & Kelley, 2018). Coronary artery disease with angina and myocardial infarction (MI) are common consequences of hypertension. LVH occurs in response to the increased workload placed on the ventricle as it contracts against higher systemic pressure. When heart damage is extensive, heart failure follows. Pathologic changes in the kidneys (indicated by increased blood urea nitrogen [BUN] and serum creatinine levels) may manifest as nocturia. Cerebrovascular involvement may lead to a transient ischemic attack (TIA) or stroke, manifested by alterations in vision or speech, dizziness, weakness, a sudden fall, or transient or permanent hemiplegia (paralysis on one side). Cerebral infarctions account for most of the strokes in patients with hypertension (Norris, 2019).

Assessment and Diagnostic Findings

The first step of diagnosis is an accurate blood pressure measurement (see Chart 27-3 for an overview of appropriate BP measurement equipment, instructions, and interpretation for both the patient and the clinician). It is important to use an average of at least two blood pressure readings on at least two occasions to confirm the diagnosis of hypertension for most patients. The notable exception is when a patient's average BP is greater than or equal to 160/100 mm Hg, confirmed by at least two accurate readings on one occasion (see later discussion) (Muntner, Shimbo, Carey, et al., 2019; Whelton et al., 2017).

Blood pressure measurement within a clinical setting is often not an accurate reading; therefore, home blood pressure measurement (HBPM) or ambulatory blood pressure measurement (ABPM) are considered more accurate reflections of the blood pressure status. HBPM and ABPM are used not only to confirm the diagnosis of hypertension in most cases, but also to evaluate whether success has been achieved with treatments, such as lifestyle modifications and prescription medications (see later discussion) (Whelton et al., 2017).

Utilizing HBPM and ABPM measurements have led to recognizing other manifestations of blood pressure. Examples of these alternative manifestations of hypertension include masked hypertension and white coat hypertension. Patients with **masked hypertension** exhibit elevated blood pressure at levels typically consistent with hypertension in settings outside the hospital or clinic, while their blood pressure is seemingly normal in health care settings. In contrast, patients with **white coat hypertension** have blood pressure readings that would suggest a diagnosis of hypertension when they are in health care settings (e.g., clinics), but are within the normal ranges in other settings. If untreated, the patient with masked hypertension can go on to experience adverse cardiovascular events (e.g., MI, strokes) and mortality. On the other hand, the patient with white coat hypertension may receive treatment that is not warranted (Cohen, Lotito, Trivedi, et al., 2019).

Chart 27-3 Measuring Blood Pressure

Equipment

For the Patient at Home
- Automatic or semiautomatic upper-arm electronic device with digital display of readings

For the Practitioner
- Preferably, a validated electronic oscillometric device; if not available, a recently calibrated aneroid sphygmomanometer
- Appropriately sized arm cuff

Instructions for the Patient

- Avoid eating, smoking, drinking caffeinated beverages, and physical activity for 30 min before blood pressure (BP) is measured.
- Empty bladder.
- Sit quietly for 5 min before the measurement.
- Sit comfortably, with back supported, with the forearm supported at heart level on a firm surface, with both feet on the ground; avoid talking while the measurement is being taken.

Instructions for the Practitioner

- Select the size of the cuff based on the size of the patient. (The cuff size should have a bladder width of at least 40% of limb circumference and length 80–100% of limb circumference.) Small adult cuffs are 12 cm wide and 22 cm long, average adult cuffs are 16 cm wide and 30 cm long, large adult cuffs are 16 cm wide and 36 cm long, and extra-large adult cuffs

are 16 cm wide and 42 cm long. Using a cuff that is too small will give a higher BP measurement, and using a cuff that is too large results in a lower BP measurement compared to one taken with a properly sized cuff.
- Wrap the cuff firmly around the arm. Center the cuff bladder directly over the brachial artery.
- Position the patient's arm at the level of the heart.
- If an aneroid sphygmomanometer is used, palpate the systolic pressure before auscultating. This technique helps to detect the presence of an auscultatory gap more readily.
- Ask the patient to sit quietly while the BP is measured, because the BP can increase when the patient is engaged in conversation.
- Initially, record BP results of both arms and take subsequent measurements from the arm with the higher BP. Normally, the BP should vary by no more than 5 mm Hg between arms.
- Take two readings 1–2 min apart and use the average of these measurements.
- Record the site where the BP was measured and the position of the patient (i.e., right arm).
- Inform the patient of their BP value and what it means. Emphasize the need for periodic reassessment, and encourage patients who measure BP at home to keep a written record of readings.

Interpretation

Assessment is based on the average of at least two readings. (If two readings differ by more than 5 mm Hg, additional readings are taken and an average reading is calculated from the results.)

Adapted from Muntner, P., Shimbo, D., Carey, R. M., et al. (2019). Measurement of blood pressure in humans: A scientific statement from the American Heart Association. *Hypertension, 73*(5), e35–e66; Padwal, R., Campbell, N. R. C., Schutte, A. E., et al. (2019). Optimizing observer performance of clinic blood pressure measurement: A position statement from the Lancet Commission on Hypertension Group. *Journal of Hypertension, 37*(9), 1737–1745.

A thorough health history and physical examination are necessary to ensure successful diagnosis and treatment. The onset of high blood pressure and the patient's health history can be used to determine whether the patient might have primary hypertension or secondary hypertension (see Chart 27-2).

Abnormal findings from the physical examination could suggest either target organ damage or secondary hypertension. The physical examination should include palpation of all peripheral pulses. Absent, weak, or delayed femoral pulses could suggest coarctation of the aorta or severe peripheral vascular disease. The neck should be examined for carotid bruits, distended veins, or an enlarged thyroid gland. The upper abdomen should be auscultated for the presence of a renal artery bruit that could be suggestive of renal artery stenosis. A careful cardiac examination is also needed to evaluate for signs of LVH. LVH signs include displacement of the apex, a sustained and enlarged apical impulse, and the presence of an S_4 cardiac sound (see Chapter 21) (Weber & Kelley, 2018).

Occasionally, signs of hypertension can be discovered during a fundoscopic eye examination manifested as hypertensive retinopathy (e.g., retinal hemorrhages, microaneurysms, cotton-wool spots, papilledema); these findings are associated with an increased cardiovascular risk (e.g., stroke). Acute or chronic ocular changes can be the initial finding in asymptomatic patients and typically require a referral to an ophthalmologist. Long-standing, untreated hypertension can cause heart failure, CKD (elevated BUN and creatinine), and increased risk for cerebrovascular disease (e.g., TIAs, strokes) (Weber & Kelley, 2018).

Laboratory tests are also performed to assess for possible target organ damage and to screen for primary hypertension or secondary hypertension. These typically include urinalysis, blood chemistry (i.e., analysis of sodium, potassium, creatinine, fasting glucose, cholesterol levels), and a 12-lead electrocardiogram. LVH can be assessed by echocardiography. Renal damage may be suggested by elevations in BUN and creatinine levels or by microalbuminuria or macroalbuminuria. Additional studies, such as creatinine clearance, renin level, urine tests, and 24-hour urine protein, may be performed. Optional testing may include uric acid and urine albumin to creatinine ratio (Whelton et al., 2017).

Medical Management

The goal of hypertension treatment is to prevent complications (i.e., target organ damage) and death by maintaining a blood pressure lower than 130/80 mm Hg. Findings from a systematic review and meta-analysis demonstrated that hypertension treatment that effectively achieves the aim of BP control to normal levels is associated with lower mortality and lower rates of CVD (Brunstrom & Carlberg, 2018). The optimal treatment plan is one that is inexpensive, simple, and causes the least possible disruption in the patient's life.

The ACC/AHA Guidelines (Whelton et al., 2017) have developed a series of recommendations for prevention, treatment, and management of hypertension. In addition, these guidelines specify that a diagnosis of hypertension must be made based on accurate blood pressure measurements (see Chart 27-3). As noted previously, an average of at least two blood pressure readings on at least two occasions should be used to confirm the diagnosis of hypertension for most patients. After having the BP measured to screen for hypertension, a patient not previously diagnosed with hypertension and with a normal BP (i.e., SBP less than 120 mm Hg and DBP less than 80 mm Hg) can be advised to have the BP reevaluated in 1 year. A patient without a prior diagnosis of hypertension with an elevated BP (i.e., SBP 120 to 129 mm Hg and DBP less than 80 mm Hg) should be advised to follow up with additional BP readings within 3 to 6 months. A patient with a BP that could be consistent with hypertension; that is, with an SBP greater than or equal to 130 mm Hg or a DBP greater than or equal to 80 mm Hg should follow-up with additional BP readings within 1 month's time to either confirm or rule out the diagnosis (Muntner et al., 2019; Whelton et al., 2017). So that patients with suspected white coat hypertension or masked hypertension may be accurately diagnosed, blood pressure readings should be based on HBPM or ABPM. Patients not instructed to follow up with additional BP readings to confirm a diagnosis of hypertension are patients with average BP readings greater than or equal to 160/100 mm Hg on one occasion; these patients are diagnosed with hypertension and begin treatment with antihypertensive medications (Muntner et al., 2019; Whelton et al., 2017).

All patients who report lifestyle choices that may put them at risk for hypertension should be counseled to adopt lifestyle changes, as appropriate. These lifestyle changes could include weight loss, dietary changes, physical activity modifications, decreased alcohol consumption, and smoking cessation (Table 27-2). In particular, the *Dietary Approach to Stop Hypertension* (DASH) diet has been one of the most effective diets in lowering BP; if used in conjunction with weight loss, this diet can lower SBP by 11 to 16 mm Hg (Campbell, 2017) (Table 27-3). In addition to this dietary advice, patients should be counseled to incorporate a low sodium (less than 2 g/day), high potassium (3500 to 5000 mg/day) diet; this dietary combination is more effective than following either a lone low sodium or high potassium diet (Perez & Chang, 2014). A high potassium diet must be avoided in patients with CKD, however.

Patients suspected to have secondary hypertension must be accurately screened and the disorder that caused the high blood pressure must be properly treated in order to bring the patient's blood pressure into normal parameters (see Chart 27-2). The recommended treatment for patients with elevated blood pressure but who are not diagnosed with hypertension is lifestyle changes, not antihypertensive medications, with follow-up in 3 to 6 months, as noted previously, to not only reevaluate the blood pressure but to see if it has responded positively to lifestyle modifications (Whelton et al., 2017).

The primary provider is advised by the ACC/AHA Guidelines (Whelton et al., 2017) to screen the patient diagnosed with Stage 1 hypertension for risk of having adverse cardiac events (e.g., stroke, MI) within the next 10 years by using the online *ASCVD Risk Estimator Plus*. This tool is published by the ACC and is free to use (links to this tool are provided in the Resources section at the end of this chapter). This tool screens patients based on factors that include blood pressure readings, age, gender, lipid panel results, use of medications, smoking status, and whether or not they have concomitant diabetes. The risk of having an adverse cardiac event is then determined as low, borderline, or high. Those patients

TABLE 27-2	Lifestyle Modifications to Prevent and Manage Hypertension[a]		
		Impact on SBP Reduction[b]	Impact on SBP Reduction[b]
Modification	Recommendation	Patients without Hypertension	Patients with Hypertension
Weight reduction	Maintain normal body weight (body mass index 18.5–24.9 kg/m²). Ideal body weight is best goal; but aim for at least 1 kg (2.2 lb) weight loss. Expect ~ 1 mm Hg SBP decrease per 1 kg reduction in weight.	–2–3 mm Hg	–5 mm Hg
Adopt DASH eating plan	Consume a diet rich in fruits, vegetables, and low-fat dairy products with a reduced content of saturated and total fat.	–3 mm Hg	–11 mm Hg
Dietary sodium reduction	Sodium <2 g/day is optimal goal; but aim for at least 1000 mg/day reduction. Check sodium amount on food labels.	–2–3 mm Hg	–5–6 mm Hg
Dietary potassium increase	Preferred potassium intake is 3500–5000 mg/day. Choose high potassium foods; check potassium amount on food labels.	–2 mm Hg	–4–5 mm Hg
Physical activity	Engage in: Regular aerobic physical activity such as brisk walking 90–150 min weekly	–2–4 mm Hg	–5–8 mm Hg
	Regular dynamic resistance training 90–150 min weekly	–2 mm Hg	–4 mm Hg
	Regular isometric resistance training at least three times weekly	–4 mm Hg	–5 mm Hg
Moderation of alcohol consumption	Limit consumption to ≤2 drinks (e.g., 24-oz beer, 10-oz wine, or 3-oz 80-proof whiskey) per day in most men and to ≤1 drink per day in women.	–3 mm Hg	–4 mm Hg

[a]For overall cardiovascular risk reduction, stop smoking.
[b]The effects of implementing these modifications are dose and time dependent and could be greater for some individuals.
DASH, dietary approaches to stop hypertension; SBP, systolic blood pressure.
Adapted from Whelton, P. K., Carey, R. M., Aronow, W. S., et al. (2017). 2017 ACC/AHA/AAPA/ABC/ACPM/AGS/APhA/ASH/ ASPC/NMA/PCNA guideline for the prevention, detection, evaluation, and management of high blood pressure in adults: A report of the American College of Cardiology/American Heart Association Task Force on Clinical Practice Guidelines. *Hypertension, 71*(6), e13–e115.

with a score of 10 or higher (consistent with mid-borderline risk) should be prescribed an antihypertensive medication, as should any patient diagnosed with stage 2 hypertension. All patients should be advised to institute relevant lifestyle changes, regardless of stage and use of antihypertensive medications.

Pharmacologic Therapy

Research findings have demonstrated that appropriately prescribing antihypertensive pharmacologic agents lowers BP, and reduces the risk of CVD, cerebrovascular disease, and

TABLE 27-3	The DASH (Dietary Approaches to Stop Hypertension) Diet
Food Group	Number of Servings Daily
Grains and grain products	7 or 8
Vegetables	4 or 5
Fruits	4 or 5
Low-fat or fat-free dairy foods	2 or 3
Lean meat, fish, and poultry	≤2
Nuts, seeds, and dry beans	4 or 5 servings weekly

Note: The diet is based on 2000 calories/day.
Adapted from U.S. Department of Health and Human Services. (2003). Your guide to lowering your blood pressure with DASH: DASH eating plan. Retrieved on 9/27//2019 at: www.nhlbi.nih.gov/health/public/heart/hbp/dash/new_dash/pdf

death (Whelton et al., 2017). Many classes of medications are available for hypertension management (Table 27-4). The medications that have been shown to prevent CVD are recommended as first-line agents for most patients. This first-line group includes thiazide or thiazide-type diuretics, angiotensin-converting enzyme (ACE) inhibitors, angiotensin receptor blockers (ARBs), and calcium channel blockers (CCBs). African American patients with hypertension and without heart failure or CKD should be prescribed either a thiazide diuretic or a CCB as a first-line agent (not an ACE inhibitor or an ARB). The recommended first-line antihypertensive agents for patients with select comorbid disorders or who are pregnant are displayed in Table 27-5.

Patients are first prescribed low doses of medication. If blood pressure does not fall to less than 130/80 mm Hg, the dose is increased gradually and additional medications are included as necessary to achieve control. The simplest treatment schedule possible is ideal as it promotes adherence to the regimen (e.g., one pill once each day, two or more agents combined into a single pill).

Resistant hypertension is diagnosed when a patient takes at least three antihypertensive medications from different classes (including a diuretic) and the blood pressure is still not controlled (i.e., not less than 130/80 mm Hg). A patient with controlled blood pressure but who requires at least four antihypertensive medications in order to maintain that control is also considered to have resistant hypertension (Whelton et al., 2017). Risk factors for resistant hypertension include older age, being African American, and having

(*text continued on page 875*)

TABLE 27-4	Oral Medication Therapy for Hypertension		
Medications	**Major Actions**	**Advantages and Contraindications**	**Effects and Nursing Considerations**
First-Line Antihypertensive Agents			
Thiazide or Thiazide-Type Diuretics chlorthalidone[a] hydrochlorothiazide indapamide metolazone [a]*preferred agent for its long half-life.*	Decrease of blood volume, renal blood flow, and cardiac output. Depletion of extracellular fluid. Negative sodium balance (from natriuresis), mild hypokalemia. Directly affect vascular smooth muscle.	Relatively inexpensive. Effective orally. Effective during long-term administration. Mild side effects. Enhance other antihypertensive medications. Counter sodium retention effects of other antihypertensive medications. *Contraindications:* Gout, known sensitivity to sulfonamide-derived medications, severely impaired kidney function, and history of hyponatremia.	Side effects include dry mouth, thirst, weakness, drowsiness, lethargy, muscle aches, muscular fatigue, tachycardia, GI disturbance. Orthostatic hypotension may be potentiated by alcohol, barbiturates, opioids, or hot weather. Because thiazides cause loss of sodium, potassium, and magnesium, and increase in uric acid and calcium, monitor for signs of electrolyte imbalance. Encourage intake of potassium-rich foods. *Gerontologic considerations:* Risk of orthostatic hypotension.
ACE Inhibitors benazepril captopril enalapril fosinopril lisinopril moexipril perindopril quinapril ramipril trandolapril	Inhibit conversion of angiotensin I to angiotensin II. Lower total peripheral resistance.	Angioedema is a rare but potentially life-threatening complication. *Contraindications:* Concomitant use of an ARB or a renin inhibitor or a potassium-sparing diuretic or potassium supplements; bilateral renal artery stenosis, pregnancy; history of angioedema with prior use of an ACE inhibitor.	Can cause hyperkalemia. Side effect can include cough. *Gerontologic considerations:* Require reduced dosages and the addition of loop diuretics when there is renal dysfunction. May cause upregulation of ACE2 receptors, making patients more susceptible to infection with SARS-CoV-2; however, may also mitigate deleterious effects of COVID-19.
Angiotensin Receptor Blockers azilsartan candesartan eprosartan irbesartan losartan olmesartan telmisartan valsartan	Block the effects of angiotensin II at the receptor. Reduce peripheral resistance.	Minimal side effects. *Contraindications:* Concomitant use of an ACE inhibitor or a renin inhibitor or a potassium-sparing diuretic or potassium supplements; bilateral renal artery stenosis; history of angioedema with prior use of an ARB; pregnancy, lactation, renovascular disease.	Monitor for hyperkalemia. Can be prescribed for patients with a history of angioedema from ACE inhibitor; however, must wait 6 wks to take after ACE inhibitor stopped. May cause upregulation of ACE2 receptors, making patients more susceptible to infection with SARS-CoV-2; however, may also mitigate deleterious effects of COVID-19.
Calcium Channel Blockers—Dihydropyridines amlodipine felodipine isradipine nicardipine SR nifedipine LA nisoldipine	Inhibit calcium ion influx across membranes. Vasodilatory effects on coronary arteries and peripheral arterioles. Decrease cardiac work and energy consumption, increase delivery of oxygen to myocardium.	Rapid action. Effective by oral or sublingual route. No tendency to slow SA nodal activity or prolong AV node conduction. Useful drug in treating isolated systolic hypertension. *Contraindication:* HFrEF (but can use amlodipine or felodipine, if necessary).	Can cause pedal edema, which is more common in women. Administer on empty stomach; recommend eating small, frequent meals if complaint of nausea. Use with caution in patients with diabetes. Muscle cramps, joint stiffness, sexual dysfunction may disappear if dose decreased. Report irregular heartbeat, constipation, shortness of breath, edema. May cause dizziness.
Calcium Channel Blockers—Nondihydropyridines diltiazem ER verapamil IR verapamil SR verapamil—delayed-onset ER	Inhibit calcium ion influx. Reduce cardiac afterload. Slow velocity of conduction of cardiac impulse.	Avoid concomitant dosing with beta-blockers. *Contraindications:* HFrEF; sinus node dysfunction, AV block.	Do not discontinue suddenly. Observe for hypotension. Report irregular heartbeat, dizziness, edema. Instruct on regular dental care because of potential gingivitis. Metabolized via cytochrome p450 system; therefore, many potential drug interactions.

TABLE 27-4	Oral Medication Therapy for Hypertension (continued)		
Medications	**Major Actions**	**Advantages and Contraindications**	**Effects and Nursing Considerations**
Second-Line Antihypertensive Agents			
Diuretics—Loop bumetanide furosemide torsemide	Volume depletion. Block reabsorption of sodium, chloride, and water in renal tubules.	Preferred diuretics for patients with symptomatic HF and for patients with moderate to severe CKD. *Contraindications*: Same as for thiazide diuretics.	Risk of volume and electrolyte depletion; monitor for hypokalemia. *Gerontologic considerations*: Risk for orthostatic hypotension.
Diuretics—Potassium-Sparing amiloride triamterene	Block sodium reabsorption. Act on distal tubule independently of aldosterone.	Not particularly effective antihypertensive drugs when prescribed as lone agents; can be effective when prescribed with a thiazide diuretic in patients with hypokalemia; causes potassium retention. *Contraindications*: Significant CKD, severe hepatic disease, hyperkalemia.	Drowsiness, lethargy, headache. Monitor for hyperkalemia if given with ACE inhibitor or ARB. Diarrhea and other GI symptoms—administer medication after meals.
Diuretics—Aldosterone Antagonists eplerenone spironolactone	Competitive inhibitors of aldosterone binding.	Indicated for patients with primary aldosteronism and resistant hypertension. *Contraindications*: Hyperkalemia and impaired renal function.	Drowsiness, lethargy, headache. Monitor for hyperkalemia if given with ACE inhibitor or ARB. Diarrhea and other GI symptoms—administer medication after meals. Avoid the use of potassium supplements or salt substitutes. Spironolactone may cause gynecomastia.
Beta-Blockers—Cardioselective atenolol betaxolol bisoprolol metoprolol tartrate metoprolol succinate	Selectively block the beta-1 adrenergic receptors of the sympathetic nervous system, slowing the heart rate and lowering the blood pressure.	Not recommended as first-line antihypertensive agents unless the patient has HF or CAD. Bisoprolol or metoprolol succinate preferred agents for patients with HFrEF. These agents are preferred over noncardioselective beta-blockers if patient has asthma, reactive airway disease, or COPD. *Contraindications*: Heart block, symptomatic bradycardia.	Avoid sudden discontinuation. Side effects may include insomnia, lassitude, weakness, fatigue and occasionally nausea, vomiting, and epigastric distress.
Beta-Blockers—Cardioselective and Vasodilatory nebivolol	Blocks beta-1 adrenergic receptors and induces nitric oxide vasodilation.	Similar to other beta-blockers with additional capacity for vasodilation. *Contraindications*: Similar to beta-blockers but with greater risk of severe bradycardia, heart block, cardiogenic shock, decompensated cardiac failure, sinus node dysfunction.	Avoid sudden discontinuation. Side-effect profile similar to other beta-blockers.
Beta-Blockers—Noncardioselective nadolol propranolol propranolol LA timolol	Nonselectively block the beta-adrenergic receptors of the sympathetic nervous system with intended effects of slowing the heart rate and lowering the blood pressure.	*Contraindications*: Asthma, reactive airway disease, COPD, heart block, symptomatic bradycardia.	Avoid sudden discontinuation. Side effects may include insomnia, lassitude, weakness, fatigue and occasionally nausea, vomiting, and epigastric distress.
Beta-Blockers—Intrinsic Sympathomimetic Activity acebutolol penbutolol pindolol	Block both beta-1 and beta-2 receptors. Also has antiarrhythmic activity by slowing atrioventricular conduction.	*Contraindications*: Avoid use in patients with HFrEF.	Avoid sudden discontinuation. Side-effect profile similar to other beta-blockers.

(continued on page 874)

TABLE 27-4	Oral Medication Therapy for Hypertension (continued)		
Medications	**Major Actions**	**Advantages and Contraindications**	**Effects and Nursing Considerations**
Beta-Blockers—Combined Alpha- and Beta-Receptor Blockers			
carvedilol carvedilol phosphate CR labetalol	Block alpha- and beta-adrenergic receptors. Cause peripheral dilation and decrease peripheral vascular resistance.	Carvedilol is a preferred agent for patient with HFrEF. *Contraindications:* Asthma, reactive airway disease, COPD, heart block, symptomatic bradycardia, cardiogenic shock, severe tachycardia.	Avoid sudden discontinuation. Side-effect profile similar to other beta-blockers.
Direct Renin Inhibitor			
Aliskiren	Blocks the conversion of angiotensinogen to angiotensin I by inhibiting the activity of the enzyme renin.	Cannot be given in combination with ACE inhibitors or ARBs. Very long acting. Contraindicated in pregnancy.	Monitor for hyperkalemia, especially for patients with CKD, or patients taking potassium supplements.
Alpha-1 Blockers			
doxazosin prazosin terazosin	Peripheral vasodilator acting directly on the blood vessel; action similar to direct vasodilators.	May be second-line agent in men with BPH. *Contraindication:* CAD.	Associated with orthostasis, especially in older adults.
Central Alpha₂-Agonists and Other Centrally Acting Drugs			
clonidine clonidine patch guanfacine methyldopa	clonidine: Exact mode of action is not understood, but acts through the central nervous system, apparently through centrally mediated alpha-adrenergic stimulation in the brain, producing blood pressure reduction. guanfacine: Stimulates central alpha₂-adrenergic receptors. methyldopa: Dopa decarboxylase inhibitor; displaces norepinephrine from storage sites.	Generally last-line agents—sometimes can be effective when other medications fail to lower blood pressure. Methyldopa may be drug of choice during pregnancy. *Contraindication:* Severe coronary artery disease.	Dry mouth, drowsiness, sedation, and occasional headaches and fatigue. Anorexia, malaise, and vomiting with mild disturbance of liver function have been reported. Rebound hypertension or hypertensive crisis is relatively common with withdrawal of clonidine; medication dosage should be tapered down when discontinuing clonidine and BP monitored carefully.
Direct Vasodilators			
hydralazine minoxidil	Direct vasodilatory action on smooth muscle of blood vessels, causing decreased peripheral vascular resistance.	Typically used in combination with other medications (diuretics, beta-blockers). Used also in pregnancy-induced hypertension. *Contraindications:* Angina or coronary disease, heart failure, hypersensitivity.	Sodium and fluid retention and reflex tachycardia are common effects; headache, flushing, and dyspnea may occur. Hydralazine may produce lupus erythematosus–like syndrome. Minoxidil may cause hirsutism.

ACE, angiotensin-converting enzyme; ARB, angiotensin receptor blocker; AV, atrioventricular; BP, blood pressure; BPH, benign prostatic hyperplasia; CAD, coronary artery disease; CKD, chronic kidney disease; COPD, chronic obstructive pulmonary disease; COVID-19, coronavirus disease 2019; CR, controlled release; ER, extended release; GI, gastrointestinal; HF, heart failure; HFrEF, heart failure with reduced ejection fraction; IR, intermediate release; LA, long acting; SA, sinoatrial; SARS-CoV-2, severe acute respiratory syndrome coronavirus 2; SR, sustained release.

Adapted from Comerford, K. C., & Durkin, M. T. (2020). *Nursing 2020 drug handbook.* Philadelphia, PA: Wolters Kluwer; Guo, J., Huang, Z., Lin, L., et al. (2020). Coronavirus disease 2019 (COVID-19) and cardiovascular disease: A viewpoint on the potential influence of angiotensin-converting enzyme inhibitors/angiotensin receptor blockers on onset and severity of severe acute respiratory syndrome coronavirus 2 infection. *Journal of the American Heart Association, 9,* e016219. doi:10.1161/JAHA.120.016219; Sommerstein, R., Kochen, M. M., Messerli, F. H., et al. (2020). Coronavirus disease 2019 (COVID-19): Do angiotensin-converting enzyme inhibitors/angiotensin receptor blockers have a biphasic effect? *Journal of the American Heart Association, 9,* e016509. doi:10.1161/JAHA.120.016509; Vaduganathan, M., Vardeny, O., Michel, T., et al. (2020). Renin-angiotensin-aldosterone system inhibitors in patients with COVID-19. *The New England Journal of Medicine, 382*(17), 1653–1659; Whelton, P. K., Carey, R. M., Aronow, W. S., et al. (2017). 2017 ACC/AHA/AAPA/ABC/ACPM/AGS/APhA/ASH/ ASPC/NMA/PCNA guideline for the prevention, detection, evaluation, and management of high blood pressure in adults: A report of the American College of Cardiology/American Heart Association Task Force on Clinical Practice Guidelines. *Hypertension, 71*(6), e13–e115.

TABLE 27-5	Oral Antihypertensive Medications for Patients with Select Comorbid Diseases or Who Are Pregnant	
Comorbid Disease or Special Patient Group	**First-Line Antihypertensive Agents**	**Second-Line Antihypertensive Agents Comments**
Stable coronary artery disease (e.g., myocardial infarction, angina) without heart failure	Beta-blockers, specifically carvedilol, metoprolol tartrate, metoprolol succinate, nadolol, bisoprolol, propranolol, or timolol; or ACE inhibitors; or ARBs.	Dihydropyridine calcium channel blockers may be prescribed if BP goal is not met and patient has continued angina. Dihydropyridine calcium channel blockers, thiazide diuretics, or aldosterone receptor antagonist diuretics may be prescribed if BP goal is not met.
Heart failure with reduced ejection fraction (HFrEF)	ACE inhibitors; ARBs; angiotensin receptor-neprilysin inhibitor (i.e., sacubitril-valsartan); aldosterone receptor antagonist diuretics; other diuretics; or beta-blockers, specifically carvedilol, metoprolol succinate, or bisoprolol.	Nondihydropyridine calcium channel blockers are NOT recommended. ACE inhibitors and ARBs should not be prescribed concomitantly.
Heart failure with preserved ejection fraction (HFpEF)	Diuretics should be prescribed to control hypertension when volume overload is present.	Nondihydropyridine calcium channel blockers are NOT recommended.
Chronic kidney disease (CKD) or kidney transplant	ACE inhibitors.	ARBs may be prescribed if patient is intolerant of ACE inhibitors. ACE inhibitors and ARBs should not be prescribed concomitantly.
Diabetes	Diuretics, calcium channel blockers, ACE inhibitors, or ARBs.	ACE inhibitors or ARBs are preferred if albuminuria is present.
History of atrial fibrillation	ARBs can prevent recurrence of atrial fibrillation and achieve BP control.	
Metabolic syndrome	The best first-line antihypertensive agent is not clear.	Caution with prescriptions of thiazide diuretics because they are associated with increased insulin resistance, dyslipidemia, increased uric acid and progression to diabetes.
Pregnancy	Stop ACE inhibitors, ARBs, and/or direct renin inhibitors due to teratogenic effects. Transition to methyldopa, nifedipine, and/or labetalol.	Beta-blockers or calcium channel blockers appear superior to other options for preventing preeclampsia.

ACE, angiotensin-converting enzyme; ARB, angiotensin receptor blocker; BP, blood pressure.
Adapted from DePalma, S. M., Himmelfarb, C. D., MacLaughlin, E. J., et al. (2018). Hypertension guideline update: A new guideline for a new era. *Journal of the American Academy of Physician Assistants*, *31*(6), 16–22; Whelton, P. K., Carey, R. M., Aronow, W. S., et al. (2017). 2017 ACC/AHA/AAPA/ABC/ACPM/AGS/APhA/ASH/ ASPC/NMA/ PCNA guideline for the prevention, detection, evaluation, and management of high blood pressure in adults: A report of the American College of Cardiology/American Heart Association Task Force on Clinical Practice Guidelines. *Hypertension*, *71*(6), e13–e115.

obesity, CKD, or diabetes. Treatment of patients with suspected resistant hypertension first revolves around ensuring that they are indeed adhering to their prescribed medication regimen, including ensuring that their finances do not preclude them from purchasing their prescriptions, that they understand the purpose of the medications, and that medication side effects are tolerable. Patients with suspected resistant hypertension should also be evaluated for possible secondary hypertension (Whelton et al., 2017).

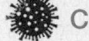 ### COVID-19 Considerations

The coronavirus disease 2019 (COVID-19) pandemic began in Wuhan, China, in late 2019. Since that time, several risks for both severe acute respiratory syndrome coronavirus 2 (SARS-CoV-2) infection and pathogenesis to coronavirus disease (COVID-19) have been posed. Epidemiologic findings from early data in China suggest that having a history of hypertension could be an important risk factor for becoming infected with SARS-CoV-2 as well as for being hospitalized to manage COVID-19 (Guo, Huang, Lin, et al., 2020;

Sommerstein, Kochen, Messerli, et al., 2020; Vaduganathan, Vardeny, Michel, et al., 2020; Yang, Tan, Zhou, et al., 2020).

Because it is a virus, the SARS-CoV-2 pathogen must replicate within host cells. SARS-CoV-2 gains entry into host cells through the ACE2 cellular surface receptors, which are key to regulating the renin–angiotensin–aldosterone system (Fig. 27-2). ACE2 converts angiotensin II to angiotensin 1–7. ACE2 receptors are particularly abundant in type II alveolar cells (also called type II pneumocytes), vascular endothelial cells, and central nervous system tissue cells.

Patients who take ACE inhibitors or ARBs to manage hypertension tend to have an upregulation of ACE2 receptors (i.e., an increase in numbers of ACE2 receptors). Therefore, it is hypothesized that having an abundance of ACE2 receptors makes individuals with hypertension who take these medications more susceptible to SARS-CoV-2 infection; this hypothesis seems to explain the prevalence of patients with hypertension who also have COVID-19. However, it has also been found that, once infected with SARS-CoV-2, host cells will then downregulate ACE2 receptors, interfering

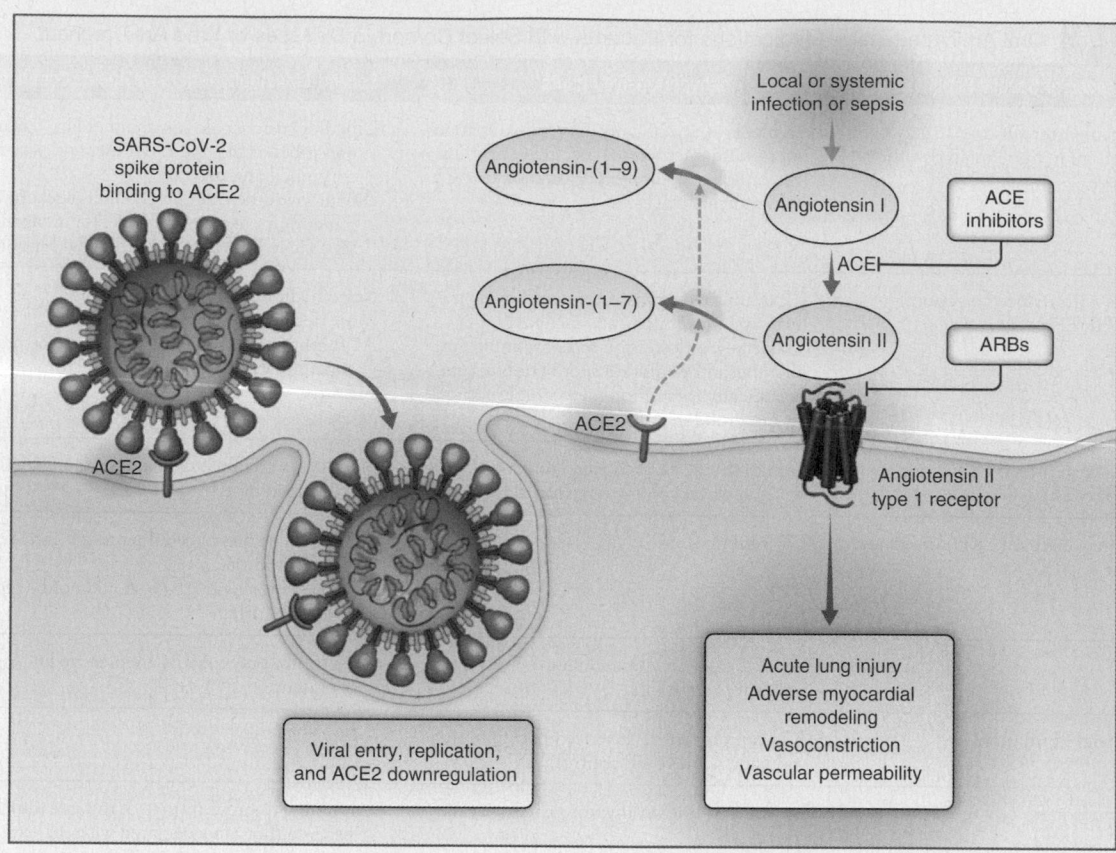

Figure 27-2 • Interaction between SARS-CoV-2 and the renin–angiotensin–aldosterone system. Shown is the initial entry of severe acute respiratory syndrome coronavirus 2 (SARS-CoV-2) into cells, primarily type II pneumocytes, after binding to its functional receptor, angiotensin-converting enzyme 2 (ACE2). After endocytosis of the viral complex, surface ACE2 is further downregulated, resulting in unopposed angiotensin II accumulation. Local activation of the renin–angiotensin–aldosterone system may mediate lung injury responses to viral insults. ACE, angiotensin-converting enzyme; ARB, angiotensin receptor blocker. Reprinted with permission from Vaduganathan, M., Vardeny, O., Michel, T., et al. (2020). Renin-angiotensin-aldosterone system inhibitors in patients with COVID-19. *The New England Journal of Medicine, 382*(17), 1653–1659.

with conversion of angiotensin II to angiotensin 1–7 (Vaduganathan et al., 2020). Angiotensin II and angiotensin 1–7 have opposing effects. While angiotensin II causes vasoconstriction, high blood pressure, thrombosis, fibrosis, and inflammation, angiotensin 1–7 causes vasodilation, lower blood pressure, antithrombosis, and anti-apoptosis, and has anti-inflammatory effects (Guo et al., 2020). Thus, once infected with SARS-CoV-2, patients who take ACE inhibitors or ARBs might have a protective advantage over patients who do not take these medications, as patients who take ACE inhibitors or ARBs theoretically should have more ACE2 receptors (Sommerstein et al., 2020).

Findings from a retrospective, single center study of patients hospitalized with COVID-19 in Wuhan, China, support the hypothesis that the use of ACE inhibitors or ARBs has a protective effect on patients with hypertension. In particular, patients with COVID-19 and hypertension who took these medications had significantly lower concentrations of C-reactive protein and procalcitonin (i.e., both are measures of inflammation) than patients with COVID-19 and hypertension who did not take these medications. In addition, fewer patients who took ACE inhibitors or ARBs were critically ill, and they had a lower mortality rate (Yang et al., 2020). Data to date supports continued use of both ACE inhibitors and ARBs in patients with hypertension during the

COVID-19 pandemic (Guo et al., 2020; Sommerstein et al., 2020; Vaduganathan et al., 2020).

 Gerontologic Considerations

The target blood pressure for all adults with hypertension is less than 130/80 mm Hg, regardless of age, including older adults (Whelton et al., 2017). There is a caveat, however, that community-dwelling, ambulatory older adults should be carefully monitored for adverse effects of prescribed antihypertensive medications, which can include falls, orthostatic hypotension, and reduced renal function. The usual adage for older adults commencing antihypertensive medications is to *start low and go slow*; that is, the medication regimen starts with a low medication dosage that is slowly increased over time as needed. For older adults with multiple comorbidities and limited life expectancy, advanced cognitive impairment, or who have had frequent falls, a less aggressive blood pressure target may be reasonable based on clinical judgment and patient preference (DePalma et al., 2018). Nonetheless, the *American College of Physicians (ACP)* and *American Academy of Family Physicians (AAFP)* recommend antihypertensive pharmacologic treatment of patients 60 years and older with a history of having had a stroke or a TIA to target SBP less than 140 mm Hg to reduce the risk of recurrent stroke (Qaseem, Wilt, Rich, et al., 2017).

NURSING PROCESS

The Patient with Hypertension

Assessment

Nurse-led hypertension management has demonstrated greater rates of blood pressure control than when nurses are not leading these management efforts (Himmelfarb, Commodore-Mensah, & Hill, 2016). In many health care settings, nurses provide the BP assessment, the education, and the counseling while actively engaging the patient to promote adherence to the treatment plan (Himmelfarb et al., 2016). Assessment includes BP assessment using the equipment, instructions, and interpretive guidelines displayed in Chart 27-3, and reviewing the patient's ambulatory or home blood pressure measurement technique and verifying its accuracy.

A complete history is obtained to assess for other cardiovascular risk factors and for signs and symptoms that indicate target organ damage (i.e., whether specific tissues are damaged by the elevated blood pressure). Manifestations of target organ damage may include angina; shortness of breath; alterations in speech, vision, or balance; nosebleeds; headaches; dizziness; or nocturia. The patient's partner may be helpful in identifying whether the patient may be experiencing obstructive sleep apnea (OSA), if the patient does not report being diagnosed or treated for OSA.

During the physical examination, the nurse must also pay specific attention to the rate, rhythm, and character of the apical and peripheral pulses to detect the effects of hypertension on the heart and blood vessels. A thorough assessment can yield valuable information about the extent to which the hypertension has affected the body and any other personal, social, or financial factors. For example, a patient's ability to adhere to an antihypertensive medication regimen may be influenced by the patient's financial resources to buy the medication and also by limited health insurance. Findings from research suggest that health beliefs, the presence of depressive symptoms, social support, and the presence of concomitant comorbidities might be associated with adherence to antihypertensive medication prescriptions (Spikes et al., 2019) (see the Nursing Research Profile in Chart 27-4).

Diagnosis

NURSING DIAGNOSES

Based on the assessment data, nursing diagnoses may include the following:

- Lack of knowledge regarding the relation between the treatment regimen and control of the disease process
- Impaired ability to manage regime as evidenced by difficulty adhering to prescribed regimen (e.g., lifestyle changes, antihypertensive medication prescriptions)

COLLABORATIVE PROBLEMS/POTENTIAL COMPLICATIONS

Potential complications may include the following:

- Left ventricular hypertrophy
- Myocardial infarction

Chart 27-4 · NURSING RESEARCH PROFILE

Medication Adherence among African Americans with Hypertension

Spikes, T., Higgins, M., Quyyumi, A., et al. (2019). The relationship among health beliefs, depressive symptoms, medication adherence, and social support in African Americans with hypertension. *Journal of Cardiovascular Nursing, 34*(1), 44–51.

Purpose

African American adults are disproportionately affected by hypertension. Not only is the prevalence of hypertension greater among African Americans than among Americans of other ethnic groups, African Americans tend to become hypertensive at earlier ages. They also tend to be at higher risk of having complications from hypertension earlier in life, including cardiovascular diseases such as strokes and heart failure, and chronic kidney disease. Evidence from previous research suggests that many African Americans hold different beliefs about the causes and consequences of hypertension than do patients with hypertension from other ethnic groups. These health beliefs are thought to affect adherence to prescribed antihypertensive medications. Furthermore, previous research suggests that depressive symptoms and social support may also affect adherence to prescribed medications. Therefore, the purpose of this study was to find associations between hypertension beliefs, depressive symptoms, social support, and medication adherence among African Americans with hypertension.

Design

This was a cross-sectional study that sampled African Americans with metabolic syndrome and hypertension managed with prescription antihypertensive medications (*N* = 120). Participants completed a series of surveys, including the medication taking subscale of the Hill-Bone Compliance to High Blood Pressure Therapy Scale, three select subscales of the Beliefs related to High Blood Pressure in African Americans Scale, the Beck Depression Index, and the Enhancing Recovery in Coronary Heart Disease Social Support Inventory.

Findings

Participants were mostly female (77%), with a mean age of 49.9 (±8.6) y. Slightly more than half of participants (54%) reported another comorbid condition in addition to having hypertension and metabolic syndrome. Approximately 37.5% of participants (*n* = 45) were deemed nonadherent to their prescribed antihypertensive regimen. Beliefs about high blood pressure, depressive symptoms, and social support were not found to correlate with antihypertensive medication adherence. However, participants with other comorbidities were found to have 2.63 times greater odds of adhering to their prescribed antihypertensive medications.

Nursing Implications

Findings from this study suggest that African Americans with hypertension may be more likely to adhere to their prescribed therapy if they have other comorbidities. The role of comorbidities among patients with hypertension needs to be further explored to determine how and why it might affect medication adherence. Nurses who manage the care of patients with hypertension should be cognizant that those without comorbidities might be at greater risk for nonadherence than those with multiple concomitant health disorders.

- Heart failure
- Cerebrovascular disease (TIA or stroke)
- Chronic kidney disease/end-stage renal disease
- Retinal hemorrhage

Planning and Goals

The major goals for the patient include understanding of the disease process and its treatment, participation in a self-care health management program, and absence of complications.

Nursing Interventions

The objective of nursing care for patients with hypertension focuses on lowering and controlling the blood pressure without adverse effects or undue cost. To achieve these goals, the nurse's role is to support and educate the patient about the treatment regimen, including making lifestyle changes, taking medications as prescribed, and scheduling regular follow-up appointments with the patient's primary provider to monitor progress or identify and treat any complications of disease or therapy.

INCREASING KNOWLEDGE

The patient needs to understand the disease process and how lifestyle changes and medications can control hypertension. The nurse needs to emphasize the concept of controlling hypertension rather than curing it. The nurse can encourage the patient to consult a dietitian to help develop a plan for improving nutrient intake or for weight loss. Explaining that it takes 2–3 mo for the taste buds to adapt to changes in salt intake may help the patient adjust to reduced salt intake and consider herbs and seasonings that add flavor without adding salt. The patient should be advised to limit alcohol intake, and tobacco and nicotine should be avoided because anyone with high blood pressure is already at risk for heart disease, and use of cigarettes and electronic nicotine delivery systems (ENDS) including e-cigarettes, e-pens, e-pipes, e-hookah, and e-cigars, amplifies this risk.

PROMOTING EFFECTIVE HEALTH MANAGEMENT

Deviating from the therapeutic health management program is a significant problem for people with hypertension and other chronic conditions requiring lifetime management. Blood pressure control is achieved by only 54% of patients (Whelton et al., 2017). Rates of blood pressure control are lowest among Mexican American men, at only 39% overall (Himmelfarb et al., 2016). Effective health management is more likely, however, when patients actively participate in self-care, including self-monitoring of blood pressure and diet, possibly because patients receive immediate feedback and have a greater sense of control. Nurse-led wellness programs that are tailored to the patients' behaviors and eating and exercise practices are more effective than generic programs. Patients with hypertension must make considerable effort to adhere to recommended lifestyle modifications (see Table 27-2) and to take regularly prescribed medications. The effort needed to follow the therapeutic plan may seem unreasonable to some, particularly when they have no symptoms without medications but do have side effects with medications. Continued education and encouragement are usually needed to enable patients to formulate an acceptable plan that helps them live with their hypertension and

adhere to the treatment plans. Compromises may have to be made about some aspects of therapy to achieve higher-priority goals.

The nurse can assist with behavior change by supporting patients in making small changes with each visit that moves them toward their goals. Another important factor is following up at each visit to see how the patient has progressed with the plans made at the prior visit. If the patient has had difficulty with the plan, the patient and nurse should work together to develop an alternative or modification that the patient believes will be more successful. Support groups for weight control, smoking cessation, and stress reduction may be beneficial for some patients; others can benefit from the support of family and friends. The nurse assists the patient to develop and adhere to an appropriate exercise regimen, because regular activity is a significant factor in reducing blood pressure (Himmelfarb et al., 2016).

PROMOTING HOME, COMMUNITY-BASED, AND TRANSITIONAL CARE

If asked to participate in a blood pressure screening program, the nurse should ensure that proper blood pressure measurement technique is being used (see Chart 27-3), that validated electronic devices are used or, if aneroid sphygmomanometers are used, that they are properly calibrated, and that provision has been made to provide follow-up for any person identified as having an elevated blood pressure level. Adequate time should also be allowed to educate each person screened about what the blood pressure numbers mean. Each person should be given a written record of their blood pressure at the screening.

Educating Patients About Self-Care. The therapeutic regimen is the responsibility of the patient in collaboration with the primary provider. The nurse can help the patient achieve blood pressure control through education about managing blood pressure (see earlier discussion), setting goal blood pressures, and providing assistance with social support. Involving family members in education programs enables them to support the patient's efforts to control hypertension. The American Heart Association and the National Heart, Lung, and Blood Institute both provide printed and electronic patient education materials (see Resources section).

Providing written information about the expected effects and side effects of medications is important. When side effects occur, patients need to understand the importance of reporting them and to whom they should be reported. Patients need to be informed that **rebound hypertension** can occur. This phenomenon is characterized by a pathologically high blood pressure exhibited by patients who suddenly stop taking prescribed antihypertensive medications. Thus, patients should be advised to have an adequate supply of medication, particularly when traveling and in case of emergencies such as natural disasters. If traveling by airplane, patients should pack the medication in their carry-on luggage. All patients should be informed that some medications, such as beta-blockers, might cause sexual dysfunction and that other medications are available if problems with sexual function or satisfaction occur. The nurse can encourage and educate patients to measure their blood pressure at home. This practice involves patients in their own care and emphasizes that failing to take medications may result in an identifiable rise in blood pressure. Patients need to know that blood pressure varies continuously and that the range within which their pressure varies should be monitored.

Gerontologic Considerations. Adherence to the therapeutic program may be more difficult for the older adult. The medication regimen may be difficult to remember, and the expense can be a challenge. Simplification of the medication regimen to treatment with a single antihypertensive medication, if possible, is helpful. Many older adults are taking other prescription and over-the-counter medications, and verifying that there are no medication interactions is important. As noted previously, community-dwelling, ambulatory older adults should be carefully monitored for adverse effects of prescribed antihypertensive medications, which can include falls, orthostatic hypotension, and reduced renal function (e.g., the nurse should assess patient's urinary output and weight for changes from baseline). Special care must be taken to ensure the older patient understands the medication regimen, can see and read the instructions, open the medication container, and can get the prescription refilled. The older adult's family or caregivers should be included in the educational program so that they understand the patient's needs, can encourage adherence to the treatment plan, and know when and whom to call if problems arise or further information is needed.

Continuing and Transitional Care. Regular follow-up care is imperative so that blood pressure control can be achieved. A history and physical examination should be completed at each clinic visit. The history should include all data pertaining to any potential problem, specifically medication-related problems such as orthostatic hypotension (experienced as dizziness or lightheadedness on standing). The patient should also bring a home blood pressure log and their own home blood pressure machine to verify accuracy and technique of home blood pressure monitor use. Patients and caregivers should also be given updated information at each visit on blood pressure medication, side effects, and important side effects to report immediately, such as low blood pressure or orthostatic hypotension. Low blood pressure readings can be due to impaired cardiovascular reflexes brought on by diuretics and other medication interactions.

Quality and Safety Nursing Alert

The patient and caregivers should be cautioned that antihypertensive medications might cause hypotension. Low blood pressure or orthostatic hypotension should be reported immediately. Older adults have impaired cardiovascular reflexes and thus are more sensitive to the extracellular volume depletion caused by diuretics and to the sympathetic inhibition caused by adrenergic antagonists. The nurse educates patients to change positions slowly when moving from a lying or sitting position to a standing position. The nurse also counsels older adult patients to use supportive devices such as hand rails and walkers as necessary to prevent falls that could result from dizziness.

MONITORING AND MANAGING POTENTIAL COMPLICATIONS

Target organ damage is a potential adverse effect of long standing or poorly controlled hypertension. When the patient returns for follow-up care, all body systems must be assessed to detect any evidence of vascular damage. An eye examination with an ophthalmoscope is particularly important because retinal blood vessel damage indicates similar damage elsewhere in the vascular system. The patient is questioned about blurred vision, spots in front of the eyes, and diminished visual acuity. The heart, nervous system, and kidneys are also carefully assessed. Any significant findings are promptly reported to determine whether additional diagnostic studies are required. Based on the findings, medications may be changed to improve blood pressure control.

Evaluation

Expected patient outcomes may include:

1. Reports knowledge of disease management sufficient to maintain adequate tissue perfusion
   a. Maintains blood pressure at less than 130/80 mm Hg with lifestyle modifications, medications, or both
   b. Demonstrates no symptoms of angina, palpitations, or vision changes
   c. Has stable BUN and serum creatinine levels
   d. Has palpable peripheral pulses
2. Effectively manages health program
   a. Adheres to the dietary regimen as prescribed: reduces calorie, sodium, and fat intake; increases fruit and vegetable intake
   b. Exercises regularly
   c. Takes medications as prescribed and reports any side effects
   d. Measures blood pressure routinely
   e. Abstains from tobacco, nicotine, and excessive alcohol intake
   f. Keeps follow-up appointments
3. Has no complications
   a. Reports no changes in vision
   b. Exhibits no retinal damage on vision testing
   c. Maintains pulse rate and rhythm and respiratory rate within normal ranges
   d. Reports no dyspnea or edema
   e. Maintains urine output consistent with intake
   f. Has renal function test results within normal range
   g. Demonstrates no motor, speech, or sensory deficits
   h. Reports no headaches, dizziness, weakness, changes in gait, or falls

Hypertensive Crises

Two classes of hypertensive crisis that require immediate intervention include hypertensive emergency and hypertensive urgency, which occur when the SBP exceeds 180 mm Hg or the DBP exceeds 120 mm Hg. Hypertensive emergencies and urgencies may occur in patients with secondary hypertension, and in those whose hypertension has been poorly controlled, whose hypertension has been undiagnosed, or in those who have abruptly discontinued their medications (i.e., rebound hypertension). Once the hypertensive crisis has been managed, a complete evaluation is performed to review the patient's ongoing treatment plan, and strategies to prevent the occurrence of subsequent hypertensive crises are implemented (Whelton et al., 2017).

Hypertensive Emergency

Hypertensive emergency is severe BP elevation (SBP greater than 180 mm Hg or DBP greater than 120 mm Hg) with new or worsening target organ damage. Some examples of target organ damage that may occur include hypertensive encephalopathy, ischemic stroke, MI, heart failure with pulmonary edema, dissecting aortic aneurysm, and renal failure. The 1-year mortality rate is more than 79% and median survival is 10.4 months if left untreated (Whelton et al., 2017). The patient needs to be admitted to the intensive care unit for continuous monitoring of BP and parenteral administration of an appropriate antihypertensive medication (Whelton et al., 2017).

A rapid and focused assessment is necessary to determine possible causes and target organ involvement. For patients with suspected aortic dissection, the management goal is to reduce the SBP to less than 120 mm Hg within the first hour of treatment (Fukui, 2018; Whelton et al., 2017). For those patients with suspected severe preeclampsia/eclampsia or pheochromocytoma crises, the management goal is to reduce the SBP to less than 140 mm Hg within the first hour of treatment (Lim, 2018; Whelton et al., 2017). The treatment management goal for other patients with hypertensive emergencies is to reduce the SBP by no more than 25% within the first hour of treatment, and then, if the patient is stable, to 160/100 mm Hg within the next 2 to 6 hours with an eventual goal of a normal, controlled blood pressure within 24 to 48 hours of when treatment commenced (Whelton et al., 2017). The antihypertensive medications of choice are those that have immediate onsets of action, and can include intravenous drugs such as nicardipine, clevidipine, labetalol, esmolol, nitroglycerin, and nitroprusside (Whelton et al., 2017). To date, there is a dearth of research findings that demonstrate the superiority of any antihypertensive medications in treating hypertensive emergencies (Whelton et al., 2017).

Hypertensive Urgency

Hypertensive urgency is severe BP elevation (SBP greater than 180 mm Hg or DBP greater than 120 mm Hg) in stable patients without target organ damage as evidenced based on clinical examination and results of laboratory studies. Many times, patients with a hypertensive urgency are nonadherent with antihypertensive therapy, resulting in rebound hypertension. The underlying reason for nonadherence should be explored (e.g., finances, anxiety, misunderstandings, miscommunication, drug side effects, or recreational drug use) and the team approach used and resources mobilized to prevent nonadherence from continuing or recurring. Restarting antihypertensive medication therapy or increasing dosages are indicated in treating these patients (Whelton et al., 2017).

Extremely close monitoring of the patient's blood pressure and cardiovascular status is required during treatment of hypertensive emergencies and urgencies (see Chapter 21 for discussion of cardiovascular assessment). The exact frequency of monitoring is a matter of clinical judgment and varies with the patient's condition. Taking vital signs every 5 minutes is appropriate if the blood pressure is changing rapidly; taking vital signs at 15- or 30-minute intervals in a more stable situation may be sufficient. A precipitous drop in blood pressure can occur that would require immediate action to restore blood pressure to an acceptable level.

CRITICAL THINKING EXERCISES

1 **pq** You are working as a nurse in a clinic that serves both an assisted living and a skilled nursing facility. One of your patients is an 80-year-old woman who is a new resident at the assisted living facility. When you take her blood pressure, you note that it is 110/70 mm Hg. While talking with her, you find that she reports episodes of dizziness and has fallen twice in the past 2 weeks. She tells you that she takes her medications as prescribed and has had no other concerns. What additional assessment data do you need to obtain? What is your priority plan of action?

2 **ipc** You are employed as an occupational health nurse in a manufacturing facility. A 32-year-old man who operates a forklift presents to be treated after injuring his forearm at work. During your assessment, he reports that he takes a beta-blocker for his hypertension and his blood pressure is 108/77 mm Hg. He also tells you that he is dedicated to staying healthy, has no underlying cardiac disease, and routinely exercises at the gym. He has noted that he cannot get his heart rate up no matter how long he works out and feels tired all the time. What further follow-up would you recommend and with whom?

3 **ebp** You are working in a clinic and a 50-year-old man presents for his annual examination. He takes no medications at present but reports that last year he was told that his blood pressure was elevated and that he needed to start taking an antihypertensive medication. He never filled that prescription because he had no symptoms and thought that if he had high blood pressure, he would feel bad. His blood pressure is 140/90 mm Hg and the rest of his examination is unremarkable. What education would you provide for him? What is the strength of the evidence that supports your education plan and follow-up with this patient?

REFERENCES

*Asterisk indicates nursing research.
**Double asterisk indicates classic reference.

Books

Comerford, K. C., & Durkin, M. T. (2020). *Nursing 2020 drug handbook.* Philadelphia, PA: Wolters Kluwer.
Eliopoulos, C. (2018). *Gerontological nursing* (9th ed.). Philadelphia, PA: Wolters Kluwer.
Norris, T. L. (2019). *Porth's pathophysiology: Concepts of altered health states* (10th ed.). Philadelphia, PA: Wolters Kluwer.
Weber, J. R., & Kelley, J. H. (2018). *Health assessment in nursing* (6th ed.). Philadelphia, PA: Wolters Kluwer.

Journals and Electronic Documents

Alexander, M. R. (2019). What is the difference between primary (essential) and secondary hypertension (high blood pressure)? Retrieved on 6/29/2019 at: www.medscape.com/answers/241381-7574/what-is-the-difference-between-primary-essential-and-secondary-hypertension-high-blood-pressure

American Heart Association (AHA). (2019). Know your risk factors for high blood pressure. Retrieved on 10/17/2019 at: www.heart.org/en/health-topics/high-blood-pressure/why-high-blood-pressure-is-a-silent-killer/know-your-risk-factors-for-high-blood-pressure

Benjamin, E. J., Muntner, P., Alonso, A., et al. (2019). Heart disease and stroke statistics—2019 update: A report from the American Heart Association. *Circulation, 139*(10), e56–e528.

Brunstrom, M., & Carlberg, B. (2018). Association of blood pressure lowering with mortality and cardiovascular disease across blood pressure levels. *JAMA Internal Medicine, 178*(1), 28–36.

Caillon, A., Mian, M. O. R., Fraulob-Aquino, J. C., et al. (2017). γδ T cells mediate angiotensin II-induced hypertension and vascular injury. *Circulation, 135*(22), 2155–2162.

Caillon, A., Paradis, P., & Schiffrin, E. L. (2019). Role of immune cells in hypertension. *British Journal of Pharmacology, 176*, 1818–1828.

Campbell, A. (2017). DASH eating plan: An eating pattern for diabetes management. *Diabetes Spectrum, 30*(2), 76–81.

**Chobanian, A. V., Bakris, G. L., Black, H. R., et al. (2003). National High Blood Pressure Education Program Coordinating Committee (2003). Seventh Report of the Joint National Committee on prevention, detection, evaluation, and treatment of high blood pressure: The JNC 7 Report. *JAMA, 289*(19), 2560–2572.

Cohen, J. B., Lotito, M. J., Trivedi, U. K., et al. (2019). Cardiovascular events and mortality in white coat hypertension: A systematic review and meta-analysis. *Annals of Internal Medicine, 170*(12), 853–862.

DePalma, S. M., Himmelfarb, C. D., MacLaughlin, E. J., et al. (2018). Hypertension guideline update: A new guideline for a new era. *Journal of the American Academy of Physician Assistants, 31*(6), 16–22.

Fajemiroye, J. O., da Cunha, L. C., Saavedra-Rodríguez, R., et al. (2018). Aging-induced biologic changes and cardiovascular diseases. *Biomed Research International, 2018* Jun 10. doi: 10.1155/2018/7156435

Fukui, T. (2018). Management of acute aortic dissection and thoracic aortic rupture. *Journal of Intensive Care, 6*, 15.

Guo, J., Huang, Z., Lin, L., et al. (2020). Coronavirus disease 2019 (COVID-19) and cardiovascular disease: A viewpoint on the potential influence of angiotensin-converting enzyme inhibitors/angiotensin receptor blockers on onset and severity of severe acute respiratory syndrome coronavirus 2 infection. *Journal of the American Heart Association, 9*, e016219.

Himmelfarb, C. D., Commodore-Mensah, Y., & Hill, M. N. (2016). Expanding the role of nurses to improve hypertension care and control globally. *Annals of Global Health, 82*(2), 243–253.

Ioannidis, J. P. A. (2018). Diagnosis and treatment of hypertension in the 2017 ACC/AHA guidelines and in the real world. *JAMA, 319*(2), 115–116.

**James, P. A., Oparil, S., Carter, B. L., et al. (2014). 2014 evidence-based guideline for the management of high blood pressure in adults: Report from the panel members appointed to the Eighth Joint National Committee (JNC 8). *JAMA, 311*(5), 507–520.

Lee, J. H., Kim, S. H., Kang, S. H., et al. (2018). Blood pressure control and cardiovascular outcomes: Real-world implications of the 2017 ACC/AHA Hypertension Guideline. *Scientific Reports, 8*(1), 13155.

Lim, K. H. (2018). Preeclampsia. *Medscape*. Retrieved on 2/3/2020 at: www.emedicine.medscape.com/article/1476919-overview

Muntner, P., Shimbo, D., Carey, R. M., et al. (2019). Measurement of blood pressure in humans: A scientific statement from the American Heart Association. *Hypertension, 73*(5), e35–e66.

Padwal, R., Campbell, N. R. C., Schutte, A. E., et al. (2019). Optimizing observer performance of clinic blood pressure measurement: A position statement from the Lancet Commission on Hypertension Group. *Journal of Hypertension, 37*(9), 1737–1745.

Perez, V., & Chang, E. T. (2014). Sodium-to-potassium ratio and blood pressure, hypertension and related factors. *Advances in Nutrition, 5*(6), 712–741.

Qaseem, A., Wilt, T. J., Rich, R., et al. (2017). Pharmacologic treatment of hypertension in adults aged 60 years or older to higher versus lower blood pressure targets: A clinical practice guideline from the American College of Physicians and the American Academy of Family Physicians. *Annals of Internal Medicine, 166*(6), 430–437.

Sommerstein, R., Kochen, M. M., Messerli, F. H., et al. (2020). Coronavirus disease 2019 (COVID-19): Do angiotensin-converting enzyme inhibitors/angiotensin receptor blockers have a biphasic effect? *Journal of the American Heart Association, 9*(7), e016509.

*Spikes, T., Higgins, M., Quyyumi, A., et al. (2019). The relationship among health beliefs, depressive symptom, medication adherence, and social support in African Americans with hypertension. *Journal of Cardiovascular Nursing, 34*(1), 44–51.

**U.S. Department of Health and Human Services (HHS). (2003). *Your guide to lowering your blood pressure with DASH: DASH eating plan*. Retrieved on 9/27/2019 at: www.nhlbi.nih.gov/health/public/heart/hbp/dash/new_dash/pdf

Vaduganathan, M., Vardeny, O., Michel, T., et al. (2020). Renin-angiotensin-aldosterone system inhibitors in patients with COVID-19. *The New England Journal of Medicine, 382*(17), 1653–1659.

Weber, M. A., Schiffrin, E. L., White, W. B., et al. (2014). Clinical practice guidelines for the management of hypertension in the community: A statement by the American Society of Hypertension and the International Society of Hypertension. *The Journal of Clinical Hypertension, 16*(1), 14–26.

Whelton, P. K., Carey, R. M., Aronow, W. S., et al. (2017). 2017 ACC/AHA/AAPA/ABC/ACPM/AGS/APhA/ASH/ ASPC/NMA/PCNA guideline for the prevention, detection, evaluation, and management of high blood pressure in adults: A report of the American College of Cardiology/American Heart Association Task Force on Clinical Practice Guidelines. *Hypertension, 71*(6), e13–e115.

Yang, G., Tan, Z., Zhou, L., et al. (2020). Effects of ARBs and ACEIs on virus infection, inflammatory status and clinical outcomes in COVID-19 patients with hypertension: A single center retrospective study. *Hypertension*. doi:10.1161/HYPERTENSIONAHA.120.15143

Zilbermint, M., Gaye, A., Berthon, A., et al. (2019). ARMC5 variants and risk of hypertension in blacks: MH-GRID Study. *Journal of the American Heart Association, 8*(14), e012508.

Resources

ACC ASCVD Risk Estimator Plus online application, www.tools.acc.org/ASCVD-Risk-Estimator-Plus/#!/calculate/estimate

American Heart Association, www.heart.org

International Society of Hypertension, www.ish-world.com/index.htm

National Heart, Lung, and Blood Institute, www.nhlbi.nih.gov

National Heart, Lung, and Blood Institute, In Brief: Your Guide to Lowering Your Blood Pressure with DASH, www.nhlbi.nih.gov/files/docs/public/heart/dash_brief.pdf

STRIDE BP, www.stridebp.org

World Health Organization (WHO), Cardiovascular Disease Information, www.who.int/health-topics/cardiovascular-diseases

UNIT
6

Hematologic Function

EVALUATING COMPLICATIONS OF CHEMOTHERAPY

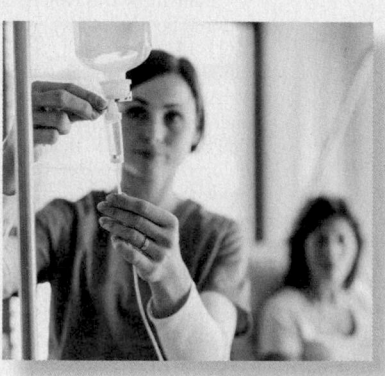

A 66-year-old woman is receiving a course of chemotherapy for non-Hodgkin lymphoma in the infusion center where you work. You note that upon arrival the patient is short of breath, her SpO_2 is 88% on room air, and her heart rate is regular at 104 bpm. Her chemotherapy infusion is placed on hold and laboratory tests reveal she has anemia. Upon initiation of chemotherapy, all patients receive education about strategies to help avoid complications such as anemia, bleeding, and infection. Earlier in the week another patient had their chemotherapy held due to an infection. You wonder if you should consider a different type of intervention aimed at decreasing complications of chemotherapy.

QSEN Competency Focus: Quality Improvement

The complexities inherent in today's health care system challenge nurses to demonstrate integration of specific interdisciplinary core competencies. These competencies are aimed at ensuring the delivery of safe, quality patient care (Institute of Medicine, 2003). The Quality and Safety Education for Nurses project (Cronenwett, Sherwood, Barnsteiner, et al., 2007; QSEN, 2020) provides a framework for the knowledge, skills, and attitudes (KSAs) required for nurses to demonstrate competency in these key areas, which include *patient-centered care*, *interdisciplinary teamwork and collaboration*, *evidence-based practice*, *quality improvement*, *safety*, and *informatics.*

Quality Improvement Definition: Use data to monitor the outcomes of care processes and use improvement methods to design and test changes to continuously improve the quality and safety of health care systems.

SELECT PRE-LICENSURE KSAs	APPLICATION AND REFLECTION
Knowledge	
Explain the importance of variation and measurement in assessing quality of care	How can you verify the observations made about increased complication rates among patients receiving chemotherapy? Identify the sources of data that could be accessed to demonstrate the need for a change in the processes of care.
Skills	
Use quality measures to understand performance	Specify the main objective that you hope to achieve with this population of patients receiving chemotherapy. Specify measurable, time-oriented expected outcomes. Might there be an opportunity for you to do a pilot test of change in the infusion center? If so, how would you go about designing this type of project? Who else from the infusion center team might you need to be involved in this type of project?
Attitudes	
Value measurement and its role in good patient care	Reflect on your attitudes toward patients with cancer receiving chemotherapy. Do you tend to think that anemia and infection are unavoidable in patients with cancer receiving treatment?

Cronenwett, L., Sherwood, G., Barnsteiner, J., et al. (2007). Quality and safety education for nurses. *Nursing Outlook*, *55*(3), 122–131; Institute of Medicine. (2003). *Health professions education: A bridge to quality*. Washington, DC: National Academies Press; QSEN Institute. (2020). *QSEN competencies: Definitions and pre-licensure KSAs; Quality improvement*. Retrieved on 8/15/2020 at: qsen.org/competencies/pre-licensure-ksas/#quality_improvement

28 Assessment of Hematologic Function and Treatment Modalities

GLOSSARY

anemia: decreased red blood cell (RBC) count

band cell: slightly immature neutrophil

blast cell: primitive white blood cell (WBC)

cytokines: proteins produced by leukocytes that are vital to regulation of hematopoiesis, apoptosis, and immune responses

differentiation: development of functions and characteristics that are different from those of the parent stem cell

erythrocyte: a cellular component of blood involved in the transport of oxygen and carbon dioxide (*synonym:* red blood cell [RBC])

erythropoiesis: process of the formation of RBCs

erythropoietin: hormone produced primarily by the kidney; necessary for erythropoiesis

fibrin: filamentous protein; basis of thrombus and blood clot

fibrinogen: protein converted into fibrin to form thrombus and clot

fibrinolysis: process of breakdown of fibrin clot

granulocyte: granulated WBC (i.e., neutrophil, eosinophil, basophil)

hematocrit: percentage of total blood volume consisting of RBCs

hematopoiesis: complex process of the formation and maturation of blood cells

hemoglobin: iron-containing protein of RBCs; delivers oxygen to tissues

hemostasis: intricate balance between clot formation and clot dissolution

leukocyte: one of several cellular components of blood involved in defense of the body; subtypes include neutrophils, eosinophils, basophils, monocytes, and lymphocytes (*synonym:* white blood cell [WBC])

leukopenia: less-than-normal amount of WBCs in circulation

lymphocyte: form of WBC involved in immune functions

lymphoid: pertaining to lymphocytes

macrophage: reticuloendothelial cells capable of phagocytosis

monocyte: large WBC that becomes a macrophage when it leaves the circulation and moves into body tissues

myeloid: pertaining to nonlymphoid blood cells that differentiate into RBCs, platelets, macrophages, mast cells, and various WBCs

myelopoiesis: formation and maturation of cells derived from myeloid stem cell

natural killer (NK) cells: lymphocytes that defend against microorganisms and malignant cells

neutrophil: fully mature WBC capable of phagocytosis; primary defense against bacterial infection

oxyhemoglobin: combined form of oxygen and hemoglobin; primarily found in arterial blood

phagocytosis: process of cellular ingestion and digestion of foreign bodies

plasma: liquid portion of blood

plasminogen: protein converted to plasmin to dissolve thrombi and clots

platelet: a cellular component of blood involved in blood coagulation (*synonym:* thrombocyte)

red blood cell (RBC): a cellular component of blood involved in the transport of oxygen and carbon dioxide (*synonym:* erythrocyte)

reticulocytes: slightly immature RBCs, usually only 1% of total circulating RBCs

reticuloendothelial system: complex system of cells throughout the body capable of phagocytosis

serum: portion of blood remaining after coagulation occurs

stem cell: primitive cell, capable of self-replication and differentiation into myeloid or lymphoid stem cell

stroma: component of the bone marrow not directly related to hematopoiesis but serves important supportive roles in this process

thrombocyte: a cellular component of blood involved in blood coagulation (*synonym:* platelet)

white blood cell (WBC): one of several cellular components of blood involved in defense of the body; subtypes include neutrophils, eosinophils, basophils, monocytes, and lymphocytes (*synonym:* leukocyte)

Unlike many other body systems, the hematologic system encompasses the entire human body. Patients with hematologic disorders often have significant abnormalities in blood tests but few or no symptoms. Therefore, the nurse must have a good understanding of the pathophysiology of the patient's condition and the ability to make a thorough assessment that relies heavily on the interpretation of laboratory tests. It is equally important for the nurse to anticipate potential patient needs and to target nursing interventions accordingly. Because it is so important to the understanding of most hematologic diseases, a basic appreciation of blood cells and bone marrow function is necessary.

Anatomic and Physiologic Overview

The hematologic system consists of the blood and the sites where blood is produced, including the bone marrow and the reticuloendothelial system (RES). Blood is a specialized organ that differs from other organs in that it exists in a fluid state. Blood is composed of plasma and various types of cells which account for 7% to 9% of total blood volume (Jouria, 2018). **Plasma** is the fluid portion of blood; it contains various proteins, such as albumin, globulin, **fibrinogen**, and other factors necessary for clotting, as well as electrolytes, waste products, and nutrients. About 55% of whole blood volume is plasma (American Society of Hematology, 2020).

Bone Marrow

The bone marrow is the site of hematopoiesis, or blood cell formation. In adults, blood cell formation is usually limited to the pelvis, ribs, vertebrae, and sternum. Marrow is one of the largest organs of the body, making up 4% to 5% of total body weight. It consists of islands of cellular components (red marrow) separated by fat (yellow marrow). As people age, the proportion of active marrow is gradually replaced by fat; however, in healthy adults, the fat can again be replaced by active marrow when more blood cell production is required. In adults with disease that causes marrow destruction, fibrosis, or scarring, the liver and spleen can also resume production of blood cells by a process known as extramedullary hematopoiesis.

The marrow is vascular. Within it are primitive cells called **stem cells**. The stem cells have the ability to self-replicate, thereby ensuring a continuous supply of stem cells throughout the life cycle. When stimulated to do so, stem cells can begin a process called **differentiation**, and develop into either **myeloid** or **lymphoid** stem cells (see Fig. 28-1). These stem cells are committed to produce specific types of blood cells.

Lymphoid stem cells produce either T or B **lymphocytes**, cells that have specific immune functions that will be described in more detail later. Myeloid stem cells differentiate into three broad cell types: erythrocytes, leukocytes, and platelets. Thus, with the exception of lymphocytes, all blood cells are derived from myeloid stem cells. A defect in a myeloid stem cell can cause problems with erythrocyte, leukocyte, and platelet production. In contrast, a defect in the lymphoid stem cell can cause problems with T or B lymphocytes, plasma cells (a more differentiated form of B lymphocyte), or natural killer (NK) (see Chapter 31 for additional information) (Wimberly, 2019).

The **stroma** of the marrow refers to all tissue within the marrow that is not directly involved in hematopoiesis. However, the stroma is important in an indirect manner, in that it produces the colony-stimulating factors needed for hematopoiesis. The yellow marrow is the largest component of the stroma. Other cells comprising the stroma include fibroblasts (reticular connective tissue), osteoclasts, osteoblasts (both needed for remodeling of skeletal bone), and endothelial cells.

Blood

The cellular component of blood consists of three primary cell types (see Table 28-1): **erythrocytes (red blood cells [RBCs], red cells), leukocytes (white blood cells [WBCs]),** and **thrombocytes (platelets)**. These cellular components of blood normally make up 40% to 45% of the blood volume (American Society of Hematology, 2020). Because most blood cells have a short lifespan, the need for the body to replenish its supply of cells is continuous; this process is termed **hematopoiesis**. The primary site for hematopoiesis is the bone marrow. During embryonic development and in other conditions, the liver and spleen may also be involved.

Under normal conditions, the adult bone marrow produces about 175 billion erythrocytes, 70 billion **neutrophils** (a mature type of WBC), and 175 billion platelets each day. When the body needs more blood cells, as in infection (when neutrophils are needed to fight the invading pathogen) or in bleeding (when more RBCs are required), the marrow increases its production of the cells required. Thus, under normal conditions, the marrow responds to increased demand and releases adequate numbers of cells into the circulation.

Blood makes up approximately 7% to 9% of the normal body weight and amounts to 5 to 6 L of volume for men and 4 to 5 L of volume for women (Nair, 2017). Circulating through the vascular system and serving as a link between body organs,

Physiology/Pathophysiology

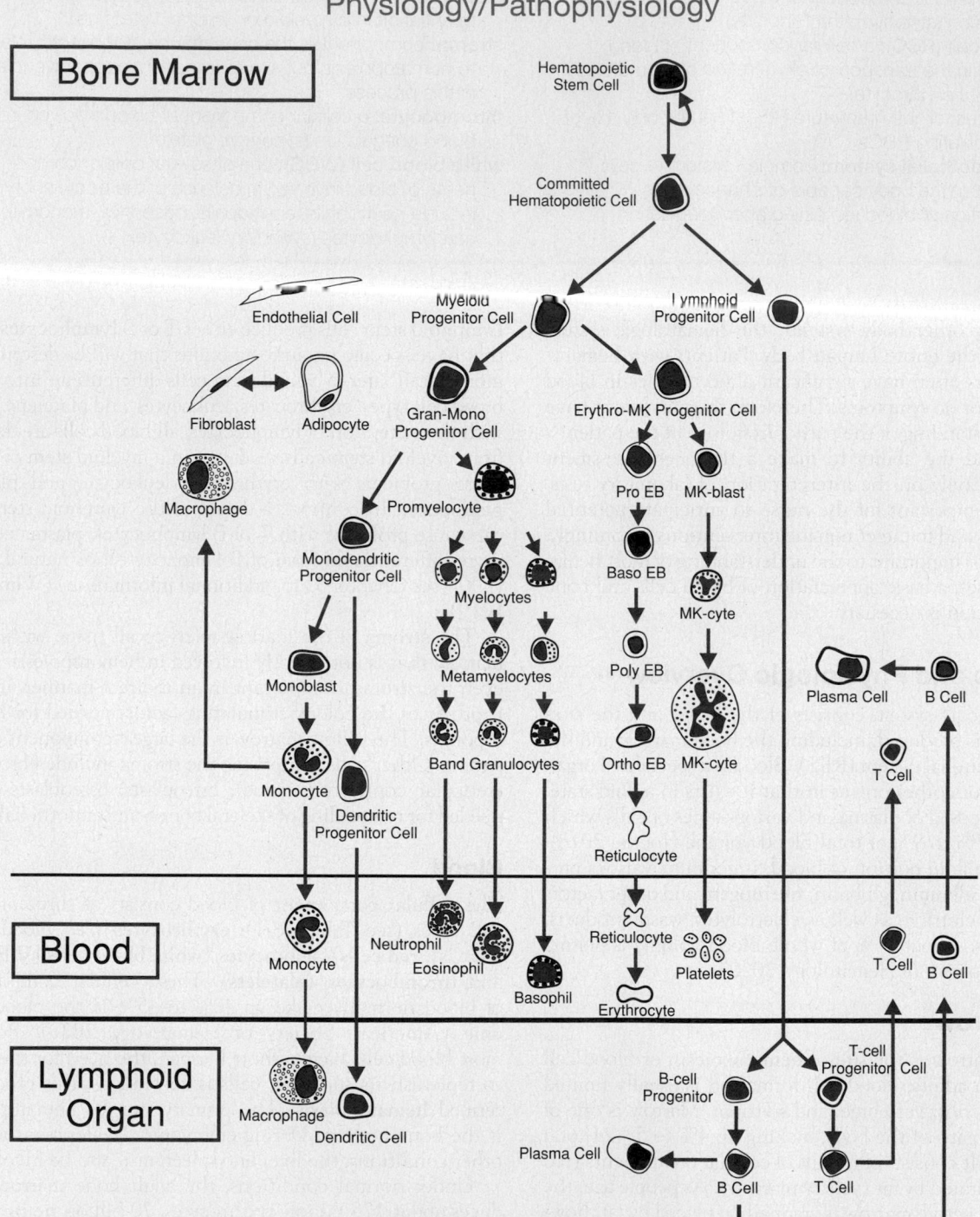

Figure 28-1 • Hematopoiesis and stromal stem cell differentiation. Uncommitted (pluripotent) stem cells can differentiate into myeloid or lymphoid stem cells. These stem cells then undergo a complex process of differentiation and maturation into normal cells that are released into the circulation. The myeloid stem cell is responsible not only for all nonlymphoid white blood cells but also for the production of red blood cells (RBCs) and platelets. Each step of the differentiation process depends in part on the presence of specific growth factors for each cell type. When the stem cells are dysfunctional, they may respond inadequately to the need for more cells, or they may respond excessively, and sometimes uncontrollably, as in leukemia. Reprinted with permission from Koury, M., Mahmud, N., & Rhodes, M. (2009). Origin and development of blood cells. In J. P. Greer, J. Foerster, G. M. Rodgers (Eds.). *Wintrobe's clinical hematology* (12th ed.). Philadelphia, PA: Lippincott Williams & Wilkins.

TABLE 28-1	Blood Cells
Cell Type	**Major Function**
WBC (Leukocyte)	Fights infection
Neutrophil	Essential in preventing or limiting bacterial infection via phagocytosis
Monocyte	Enters tissue as macrophage; highly phagocytic, especially against fungus; immune surveillance
Eosinophil	Involved in allergic reactions (neutralizes histamine); digests foreign proteins
Basophil	Contains histamine; integral part of hypersensitivity reactions
Lymphocyte	Integral component of immune system
T lymphocyte	Responsible for cell-mediated immunity; recognizes material as "foreign" (surveillance system)
B lymphocyte	Responsible for humoral immunity; many mature into plasma cells to form antibodies
Plasma cell	Secretes immunoglobulin (antibody); most mature form of B lymphocyte
RBC (Erythrocyte)	Carries hemoglobin to provide oxygen to tissues; average lifespan is 120 days
Platelet (Thrombocyte)	Fragment of megakaryocyte; provides basis for coagulation to occur; maintains hemostasis; average lifespan is 10 days

WBC, white blood cell; RBC, red blood cell.
Adapted from Norris, T. L. (2019). *Porth's pathophysiology: Concepts of altered health state* (10th ed.). Philadelphia, PA: Wolters Kluwer.

blood carries oxygen absorbed from the lungs and nutrients absorbed from the gastrointestinal (GI) tract to the body cells for cellular metabolism. Blood also carries hormones, antibodies, and other substances to their sites of action or use. In addition, blood carries waste products produced by cellular metabolism to the lungs, skin, liver, and kidneys, where they are transformed and eliminated from the body.

The danger that trauma can lead to excess blood loss always exists. To prevent this, an intricate clotting mechanism is activated when necessary to seal any leak in the blood vessels. Excessive clotting is equally dangerous, because it can obstruct blood flow to vital tissues. To prevent this, the body has a fibrinolytic mechanism that eventually dissolves clots (thrombi) formed within blood vessels. The balance between these two systems—clot (thrombus) formation and clot dissolution or **fibrinolysis**—is called **hemostasis**.

Erythrocytes (Red Blood Cells)

The normal erythrocyte is a biconcave disc that resembles a soft ball compressed between two fingers (see Fig. 28-2). It has a diameter of about 8 μm and is so flexible that it can pass easily through capillaries that may be as small as 2.8 μm in diameter. The membrane of the red cell is very thin so that gases, such as oxygen and carbon dioxide, can easily diffuse across it; the disc shape provides a large surface area that facilitates the absorption and release of oxygen molecules.

Mature erythrocytes consist primarily of **hemoglobin**, which contains iron and protein and makes up 95% of the cell mass. Mature erythrocytes have no nuclei, and they have many fewer metabolic enzymes than do most other cells. The presence of a large amount of hemoglobin enables the red cell to perform its principal function, which is the transport of oxygen between the lungs and tissues. Occasionally, the marrow releases slightly immature forms of erythrocytes, called **reticulocytes**, into the circulation. This occurs as a normal response to an increased demand for erythrocytes (as in bleeding) or in some disease states.

The oxygen-carrying hemoglobin molecule is made up of four subunits, each containing a heme portion attached to a globin chain. Iron is present in the heme component of the molecule. An important property of heme is its ability to bind to oxygen loosely and reversibly. Oxygen readily binds to hemoglobin in the lungs and is carried as **oxyhemoglobin** in arterial blood. Oxyhemoglobin is a brighter red than hemoglobin that does not contain oxygen (reduced hemoglobin); thus, arterial blood is a brighter red than venous blood. The oxygen readily dissociates (detaches) from hemoglobin in the tissues, where the oxygen is needed for cellular metabolism. In venous blood, hemoglobin combines with hydrogen ions produced by cellular metabolism and thus buffers excessive acid. Whole blood normally contains about 15 g of hemoglobin per 100 mL of blood (Fischbach & Fischbach, 2018).

Erythropoiesis

Erythroblasts arise from the primitive myeloid stem cells in bone marrow. The erythroblast is an immature nucleated cell that gradually loses its nucleus. At this stage, the cell is known as a reticulocyte. Further maturation into an erythrocyte entails the loss of the dark-staining material within the cell and slight shrinkage. The mature erythrocyte is then released into the circulation. Under conditions of rapid **erythropoiesis** (i.e., erythrocyte production), reticulocytes and other immature cells may be released prematurely into the circulation. This is often seen when the liver or spleen takes over as the site of erythropoiesis and more nucleated red cells appear within the circulation.

Differentiation of the primitive myeloid stem cell into an erythroblast is stimulated by **erythropoietin**, a hormone produced primarily by the kidney. If the kidney detects low levels of oxygen, as occurs when fewer red cells are available to bind oxygen (i.e., **anemia**), or with people living at high altitudes with lower atmospheric oxygen concentrations, erythropoietin levels increase. The increased erythropoietin then stimulates the marrow to increase the production of erythrocytes. The entire process of erythropoiesis occurs over 1 week (Wimberly, 2019). For normal erythrocyte production, the bone marrow also requires iron, vitamin B_{12}, folate, pyridoxine (vitamin B_6), protein, and other factors. A deficiency of these factors during erythropoiesis can result in decreased red cell production and anemia.

Iron Stores and Metabolism

The rate of iron absorption is regulated by the amount of iron already stored in the body and by the rate of erythrocyte production. Daily dietary iron requirements vary based on age, gender, and health status. For example, pregnant women require up to 30 mg of iron daily, while adult men require up

Blood smear

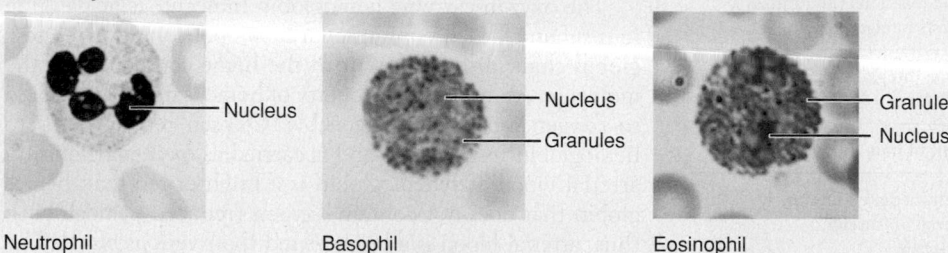

Note the clump of platelets

Granulocytes

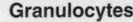

Neutrophil   Basophil   Eosinophil

Agranulocytes

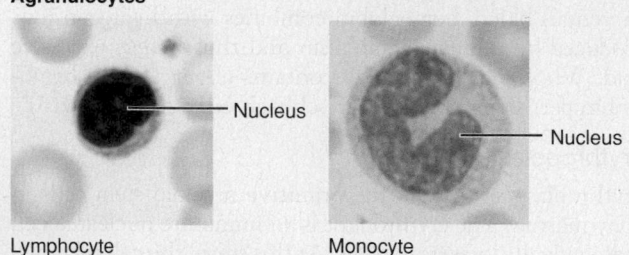

Lymphocyte   Monocyte

Figure 28-2 • Normal types of blood cells. Reprinted with permission from Cohen, B. J. (2005). *Memmler's the human body in health and disease* (10th ed.). Philadelphia, PA: Lippincott Williams & Wilkins.

to 12 mg and children up to 10 mg of iron daily (Trevithick, 2019). Additional amounts of iron, up to 2 mg daily, must be absorbed by women of childbearing age to replace that lost during menstruation. Total body iron content in the average adult is approximately 3 g, most of which is present in hemoglobin or in one of its breakdown products. Iron is stored as ferritin and when required, the iron is released into the plasma, binds to transferrin, and is transported into the membranes of the normoblasts (erythrocyte precursor cells) within the marrow, where it is incorporated into hemoglobin. Iron is lost in the feces, either in bile, blood, or mucosal cells from the intestine.

The normal findings for concentration of iron in blood can range from 50 to 250 μg/dL depending on age and gender (Fischbach & Fischbach, 2018). With iron deficiency, bone marrow iron stores are rapidly depleted; hemoglobin synthesis is depressed, and the erythrocytes produced by the marrow are small and low in hemoglobin. Iron deficiency in the adult generally indicates blood loss (e.g., from bleeding in the GI tract or heavy menstrual flow). Lack of dietary iron is rarely the sole cause of iron deficiency anemia in adults. The source of iron deficiency should be investigated promptly, because iron deficiency in an adult may be a sign of bleeding in the GI tract or colon cancer.

Vitamin B₁₂ and Folate Metabolism

Vitamin B_{12} and folate are required for the synthesis of deoxyribonucleic acid (DNA) in RBCs. Both vitamin B_{12} and folate

are derived from the diet. Folate is absorbed in the proximal small intestine, but only small amounts are stored within the body. If the diet is deficient in folate, stores within the body quickly become depleted. Because vitamin B_{12} is found only in foods of animal origin, strict vegetarians may ingest little vitamin B_{12}. Vitamin B_{12} combines with intrinsic factor produced in the stomach. The vitamin B_{12}–intrinsic factor complex is absorbed in the distal ileum. People who have had a partial or total gastrectomy may have limited amounts of intrinsic factor, and therefore the absorption of vitamin B_{12} may be diminished. The effects of either decreased absorption or decreased intake of vitamin B_{12} are not apparent for 2 to 4 years.

Vitamin B_{12} and folate deficiencies are characterized by the production of abnormally large erythrocytes called *megaloblasts*. Because these cells are abnormal, many are sequestered (trapped) while still in the bone marrow, and their rate of release is decreased. Some of these cells actually die in the marrow before they can be released into the circulation. This results in megaloblastic anemia.

Red Blood Cell Destruction

The average lifespan of a normal circulating erythrocyte is 120 days. Often, older erythrocytes lose elasticity and become trapped in small blood vessels and the spleen. These older erythrocytes are removed from the blood by the reticuloendothelial cells, particularly in the liver and the spleen. As the erythrocytes are destroyed, most of their hemoglobin is recycled. Some hemoglobin also breaks down to form bilirubin and is secreted in the bile. Most of the iron is recycled to form new hemoglobin molecules within the bone marrow; small amounts are lost daily in the feces and urine and monthly in menstrual flow.

Leukocytes (White Blood Cells)

Leukocytes are divided into two general categories: granulocytes and lymphocytes. In normal blood, the total leukocyte count is 4000 to 11,000 cells/mm^3. Of these, approximately 60% to 80% are granulocytes and 20% to 40% are lymphocytes. Both of these types of leukocytes primarily protect the body against infection and tissue injury.

Granulocytes

Granulocytes are defined by the presence of granules in the cytoplasm of the cell. Granulocytes are divided into three main subgroups—eosinophils, basophils, and neutrophils—that are characterized by the staining properties of these granules (see Fig. 28-2). Eosinophils have bright-red granules in their cytoplasm, whereas the granules in basophils stain deep blue. The third and most numerous cell in this class is the neutrophil, with granules that stain a pink to violet hue. Neutrophils are also called *polymorphonuclear neutrophils* (PMNs, or polys) or *segmented neutrophils* (segs).

The nucleus of the mature neutrophil has multiple lobes (usually two to five) that are connected by thin filaments of nuclear material, or a "segmented" nucleus; it is usually two times the size of an erythrocyte. The somewhat less mature granulocyte has a single-lobed, elongated nucleus and is called a **band cell**. Ordinarily, band cells account for only a small percentage of circulating granulocytes, although their percentage can increase greatly under conditions in which neutrophil production increases, such as infection. The increased number of band cells is sometimes called a left shift or shift to the left. (Traditionally, the diagram of neutrophil maturation showed the myeloid stem cell on the left with progressive maturation stages toward the right, ending with a fully mature neutrophil on the far right side. A shift to the left indicates that more immature cells are present in the blood than normal.)

Fully mature neutrophils result from the gradual differentiation of myeloid stem cells, specifically myeloid **blast cells** (i.e., immature white blood cells). The process, called **myelopoiesis**, is highly complex and depends on many factors. These factors, including specific **cytokines** (i.e., regulatory proteins produced by leukocytes) such as growth factors, are normally present within the marrow itself. As the blast cell matures, the cytoplasm of the cell changes in color (from blue to violet) and granules begin to form with the cytoplasm. The shape of the nucleus also changes. The entire process of maturation and differentiation takes about 10 days (see Fig. 28-1). Once the neutrophil is released into the circulation from the marrow, it stays there for only about 6 hours before it migrates into the body tissues to perform its function of **phagocytosis** (ingestion and digestion of foreign bodies, such as bacteria). Neutrophils die here within 1 to 2 days. The number of circulating granulocytes found in the healthy person is relatively constant; however, in infection, large numbers of these cells are rapidly released into the circulation.

Agranulocytes

Monocytes

Monocytes (also called *mononuclear leukocytes*) are leukocytes with a single-lobed nucleus and a granule-free cytoplasm—hence the term *agranulocyte* (see Fig. 28-2). In normal adult blood, monocytes account for approximately 5% of the total leukocytes. Monocytes are the largest of the leukocytes. Produced by the bone marrow, they remain in the circulation for a short time before entering the tissues and transforming into **macrophages**. Macrophages are particularly active in the spleen, liver, peritoneum, and alveoli; they remove debris from these areas and phagocytize bacteria within the tissues.

Lymphocytes

Mature **lymphocytes** are small cells with scanty cytoplasm (see Fig. 28-2). Immature lymphocytes are produced in the marrow from the lymphoid stem cells. A second major source of production for lymphocytes is the thymus. Cells derived from the thymus are known as T lymphocytes (or T cells); those derived from the marrow can also be T cells but are more commonly B lymphocytes (or B cells). Lymphocytes complete their differentiation and maturation primarily in the lymph nodes and in the lymphoid tissue of the intestine and spleen after exposure to a specific antigen. Mature lymphocytes are the principal cells of the immune system, producing antibodies and identifying other cells and organisms as "foreign." **Natural killer (NK) cells** serve an important role in the body's immune defense system. Like other lymphocytes, NK cells accumulate in the lymphoid tissues (especially spleen, lymph nodes, and tonsils), where they mature. When activated, they serve as potent killers of virus-infected and cancer cells. They also secrete cytokines to mobilize the T and B cells into action.

Function of Leukocytes

Leukocytes protect the body from invasion by bacteria and other foreign entities. The major function of neutrophils is phagocytosis. Neutrophils arrive at a given site within 1 hour after the onset of an inflammatory reaction and initiate phagocytosis, but they are short-lived. An influx of monocytes follows; these cells continue their phagocytic activities for long periods as macrophages. This process constitutes a second line of defense for the body against inflammation and infection. Although neutrophils can often work adequately against bacteria without the help of macrophages, macrophages are particularly effective against fungi and viruses. Macrophages also digest senescent (aging or aged) blood cells, primarily within the spleen.

The primary function of lymphocytes is to attack foreign material. One group of lymphocytes (T lymphocytes) kills foreign cells directly or releases lymphokines, substances that enhance the activity of phagocytic cells. T lymphocytes are responsible for delayed allergic reactions, rejection of foreign tissue (e.g., transplanted organs), and destruction of tumor cells. This process is known as *cellular immunity*. The other group of lymphocytes (B lymphocytes) is capable of differentiating into plasma cells. Plasma cells, in turn, produce antibodies called *immunoglobulins* (Igs), which are protein molecules that destroy foreign material by several mechanisms. This process is known as humoral immunity.

Eosinophils and basophils function in hypersensitivity reactions. Eosinophils are important in the phagocytosis of parasites. The increase in eosinophil levels in allergic states indicates that these cells are involved in the hypersensitivity reaction; they neutralize histamine. Basophils produce and store histamine as well as other substances involved in hypersensitivity reactions. The release of these substances provokes allergic reactions. See Chapter 31 for further information on the immune response.

Platelets (Thrombocytes)

Platelets, or thrombocytes, are not technically cells; rather, they are granular fragments of giant cells in the bone marrow called *megakaryocytes* (see Fig. 28-2). Platelet production in the marrow is regulated in part by the hormone thrombopoietin, which stimulates the production and differentiation of megakaryocytes from the myeloid stem cell. Each megakaryocyte has the capacity to produce approximately 2000 platelets; 80% of these platelets are active in the circulation and 20% are stored in the spleen (Ciesla, 2019a).

Platelets play an essential role in the control of bleeding. They circulate freely in the blood in an inactive state, where they nurture the endothelium of the blood vessels, maintaining the integrity of the vessel. When vascular injury occurs, platelets collect at the site and are activated. They adhere to the site of injury and to each other, forming a platelet plug that temporarily stops bleeding. Substances released from platelet granules activate coagulation factors in the blood plasma and initiate the formation of a stable clot composed of **fibrin**, a filamentous protein. Platelets have a normal lifespan of 7 to 10 days (Ciesla, 2019b).

Plasma and Plasma Proteins

After cellular elements are removed from blood, the remaining liquid portion is called *plasma*. More than 90% of plasma is water. The remainder consists primarily of plasma proteins; clotting factors (particularly fibrinogen); and small amounts of other substances, such as nutrients, enzymes, waste products, and gases. If plasma is allowed to clot, the remaining fluid is called **serum**. Serum has essentially the same composition as plasma, except that fibrinogen and several clotting factors have been removed during the clotting process.

Plasma proteins consist primarily of albumin and globulins. The globulins can be separated into three main fractions (alpha, beta, and gamma), each of which consists of distinct proteins that have different functions. Important proteins in the alpha and beta fractions are the transport globulins and the clotting factors that are made in the liver. The transport globulins carry various substances in bound form in the circulation. For example, thyroid-binding globulin carries thyroxin, and transferrin carries iron. The clotting factors, including fibrinogen, remain in an inactive form in the blood plasma until activated by the clotting cascade. The gamma-globulin fraction refers to the Igs, or antibodies. These proteins are produced by well-differentiated B lymphocytes and plasma cells. The actual fractionation of the globulins can be seen on a specific laboratory test (serum protein electrophoresis).

Albumin is particularly important for the maintenance of fluid balance within the vascular system. Capillary walls are impermeable to albumin, so its presence in the plasma creates an osmotic force that keeps fluid within the vascular space. Albumin, which is produced by the liver, has the capacity to bind to several substances that are transported in plasma (e.g., certain medications, bilirubin, and some hormones). People with impaired hepatic function may have low concentrations of albumin, with a resultant decrease in osmotic pressure and the development of edema.

Reticuloendothelial System (RES)

The **reticuloendothelial system (RES)** is composed of special tissue macrophages. When released from the marrow, monocytes spend a short time in the circulation (about 24 hours) and then enter the body tissues. Within the tissues, the monocytes continue to differentiate into macrophages, which can survive for months or years. Macrophages have a variety of important functions. They defend the body against foreign invaders (i.e., bacteria and other pathogens) via phagocytosis. They remove old or damaged cells from the circulation. They stimulate the inflammatory process and present antigens to the immune system (Banaski, 2019). Macrophages give rise to tissue histiocytes, phagocytic cells that are present in loose connective tissue. These include Kupffer cells of the liver, peritoneal macrophages, alveolar macrophages, and other components of the RES. Thus, the RES is a component of many other organs within the body, particularly the spleen, lymph nodes, lungs, and liver.

The spleen is the site of activity for most macrophages. Most of the spleen (75%) is made of red pulp; here, the blood enters the venous sinuses through capillaries that are surrounded by macrophages. Within the red pulp are tiny aggregates of white pulp, consisting of B and T lymphocytes. The spleen sequesters newly formed reticulocytes from the marrow, removing nuclear fragments and other materials (e.g., damaged or defective hemoglobin, iron) before the now fully mature erythrocyte returns to the circulation. If the spleen is enlarged, a greater number of red cells and platelets can be sequestered. The spleen is a major source of hematopoiesis in fetal life. It can resume hematopoiesis later in adulthood if necessary, particularly when marrow function is compromised (e.g., in bone marrow fibrosis). The spleen has important immunologic functions as well. It forms substances called *opsonins* that promote the phagocytosis of neutrophils; it also forms the antibody immunoglobulin M (IgM) after exposure to an antigen.

Hemostasis

Hemostasis is the process of preventing blood loss from intact vessels and of stopping bleeding from a severed vessel, which requires adequate numbers of functional platelets. Platelets nurture the endothelium and thereby maintain the structural integrity of the vessel wall. Two processes are involved in arresting bleeding: primary and secondary hemostasis (see Fig. 28-3).

In primary hemostasis, the severed blood vessel constricts. Circulating platelets aggregate at the site and adhere to the vessel and to one another. An unstable hemostatic plug is formed. For the coagulation process to be correctly activated, circulating inactive coagulation factors must be converted to active forms. This process occurs on the surface of the aggregated platelets at the site of vessel injury.

Physiology/Pathophysiology

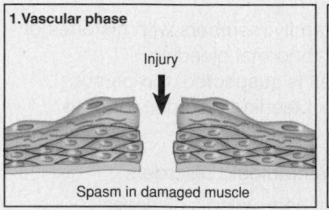

1. Vascular phase

Spasm in damaged muscle

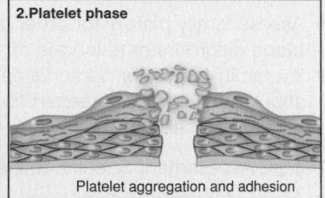

2. Platelet phase

Platelet aggregation and adhesion

3. Coagulation phase

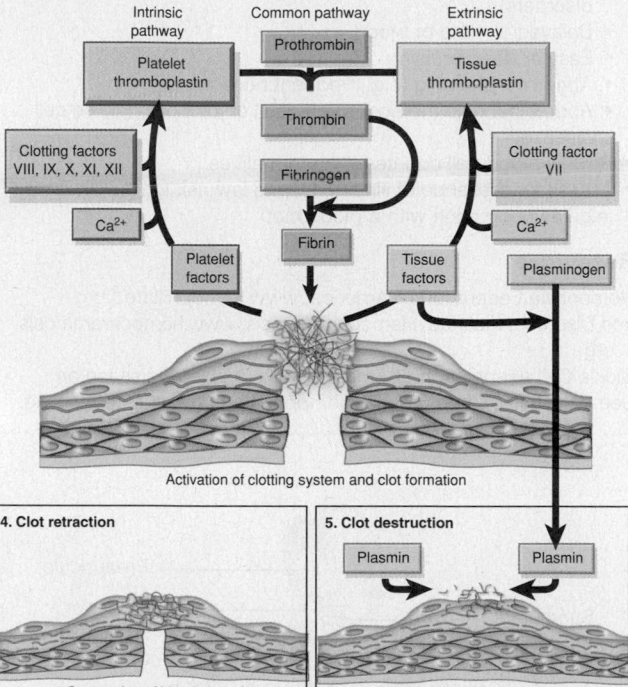

Activation of clotting system and clot formation

4. Clot retraction

Contraction of blood clot

5. Clot destruction

Plasmin

Plasmin

Enzymatic destruction of clot

Figure 28-3 • Hemostasis. When the endothelial surface of a blood vessel is injured, several processes occur. In primary hemostasis, platelets within the circulation are attracted to the exposed layer of collagen at the site of injury. They adhere to the site of injury, releasing factors that stimulate other platelets to aggregate at the site, forming an unstable platelet plug. In secondary hemostasis, based on the type of stimulus, one of two clotting pathways is initiated—the intrinsic or extrinsic pathway—and the clotting factors within that pathway are activated. The end result from either pathway is the conversion of prothrombin to thrombin. Thrombin is necessary for fibrinogen to be converted into fibrin, the stabilizing protein that anchors the fragile platelet plug to the site of injury to prevent further bleeding and permit the injured vessel or site to heal. Modified from www.irvingcrowley.com/cls/clotting.gif

The end result is the formation of fibrin, which reinforces the platelet plug and anchors it to the injury site. This process is referred to as secondary hemostasis. Blood coagulation is highly complex. It can be activated by the extrinsic pathway (also known as the tissue factor pathway) or the intrinsic pathway (also known as the contact activation pathway). Both pathways are needed for maintenance of normal hemostasis. Many factors are involved in the reaction cascade that forms fibrin. When tissue is injured, the extrinsic pathway is activated by the release of thromboplastin from the tissue. As the result of a series of reactions, prothrombin is converted to thrombin, which in turn catalyzes the conversion of fibrinogen

to fibrin. Clotting by the intrinsic or contact activation pathway is activated when the collagen that lines blood vessels is exposed. Clotting factors are activated sequentially until, as with the extrinsic pathway, fibrin is ultimately formed (Rockwell, 2019). The intrinsic pathway is slower, and this sequence is less often responsible for clotting in response to tissue injury. However, it is important if a noninjured vessel wall comes into contact with lipoproteins (e.g., atherosclerosis) or with bacteria, resulting in a clot that is formed for purposes other than protection from trauma or bleeding.

As the injured vessel is repaired and again covered with endothelial cells, the fibrin clot is no longer needed. The fibrin is digested via two systems: the plasma fibrinolytic system and the cellular fibrinolytic system. The protein **plasminogen** is required to lyse (break down) the fibrin. Plasminogen, which is present in all body fluids, circulates with fibrinogen and is therefore incorporated into the fibrin clot as it forms. When the clot is no longer needed (e.g., after an injured blood vessel has healed), the plasminogen is activated to form plasmin. Plasmin digests the fibrinogen and fibrin. The breakdown particles of the clot, called *fibrin degradation products*, are released into the circulation. Through this system, clots are dissolved as tissue is repaired, and the vascular system returns to its normal baseline state.

Gerontologic Considerations

In older adults, the bone marrow's ability to respond to the body's need for blood cells (erythrocytes, leukocytes, and platelets) may be decreased, resulting in **leukopenia** (a decreased number of circulating leukocytes) or anemia. This decreased ability is a result of many factors, including diminished production of the growth factors necessary for hematopoiesis by stromal cells within the marrow or a diminished response to the growth factors (in the case of erythropoietin). Over time, stem cells within the marrow acquire damage to their DNA, which compromises their function. T- and B-cell development is also decreased. This age-related decrease in immune system response due to diminished production and function of blood cells designed to protect the body is called immunosenescence (Yeager, 2019).

Assessment

Health History

A careful health history and physical assessment can provide important information related to a patient's known or potential hematologic diagnosis. Because many hematologic disorders are more prevalent in certain ethnic groups, assessments of ethnicity and family history are useful (see Chart 28-1). Similarly, obtaining a nutritional history and assessing the use of prescription and over-the-counter medications, as well as herbal supplements, are important to note, because several conditions can result from nutritional deficiencies, or from the use of certain herbs or medications. Careful attention to the onset of a symptom or finding (e.g., rapid vs. gradual; persistent vs. intermittent), its severity, and any contributing factors can further differentiate potential causes. Of equal importance is assessing the impact of these findings on the patient's functional ability, manifestations of distress, and coping mechanisms.

Chart 28-1 — GENETICS IN NURSING PRACTICE
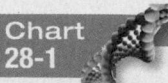

Hematologic Disorders

Hematologic disorders are marked by aberrations in the structure or function of the blood cells or the blood clotting mechanism. Some examples of genetic hematologic disorders are:

Autosomal Dominant:
- Factor V Leiden
- Familial hypercholesterolemia
- Hereditary angioedema
- Hereditary spherocytosis
- von Willebrand disease

Autosomal Recessive:
- Hemochromatosis
- Sickle cell disease
- Thalassemia

X-Linked:
- Hemophilia

Nursing Assessments

Refer to Chapter 4, Chart 4-2: Genetics in Nursing Practice: Genetic Aspects of Health Assessment

Family History Assessment Specific to Hematologic Disorders
- Collect family history information on maternal and paternal relatives from three generations of the family.

- Assess family history for other family members with histories of blood disorders or episodes of abnormal bleeding.
- If a family history or personal risk is suspected, the person should be carefully screened for bleeding disorders prior to surgical procedures.

Patient Assessment Specific to Hematologic Disorders
- Assess for specific symptoms of hematologic diseases:
  - Extreme fatigue (the most common symptom of hematologic disorders)
  - Delayed clotting of blood
  - Easy or deep bruising
  - Abnormal bleeding (e.g., frequent nosebleeds)
  - Abdominal pain (hemochromatosis) or joint pain (sickle cell disease)
- Review blood cell counts for abnormalities.
- Assess for presence of illness despite low risk for the illness (e.g., a young adult with a blood clot)

Resources

Hemophilia Federation of America, www.hemophiliafed.org
Iron Disorders Institute: Hemochromatosis, www.hemochromatosis.org
Sickle Cell Association of America, www.sicklecelldisease.org
See Chapter 6, Chart 6-7, for components of genetic counseling.

Physical Assessment

The physical assessment should be comprehensive and include careful attention to the skin, oral cavity, lymph nodes, and spleen (see Fig. 28-4). Table 28-2 highlights a general approach to the physical assessment findings in hematologic disorders (more specific findings are presented in Chapters 29 and 30).

Diagnostic Evaluation

Most hematologic diseases reflect a defect in the hematopoietic, hemostatic, or reticuloendothelial systems. The defect can be quantitative (e.g., increased or decreased production of cells), qualitative (e.g., the cells that are produced are defective in their expected functional capacity), or both. Initially, many hematologic conditions cause few symptoms, and extensive laboratory tests are often required to establish a diagnosis. For most hematologic conditions, continued monitoring via specific blood tests is required because it is very important to assess for changes in test results over time. In general, it is important to assess trends in test results because these trends help the clinician decide whether the patient is responding appropriately to interventions.

Hematologic Studies

The most common tests used are the complete blood count (CBC) and the peripheral blood smear. The CBC identifies the total number of blood cells (leukocytes, erythrocytes, and platelets) as well as the hemoglobin, **hematocrit** (percentage of blood volume consisting of erythrocytes), and RBC indices. Because cellular morphology (shape and appearance of the cells) is particularly important in accurately diagnosing most hematologic disorders, the blood cells involved must

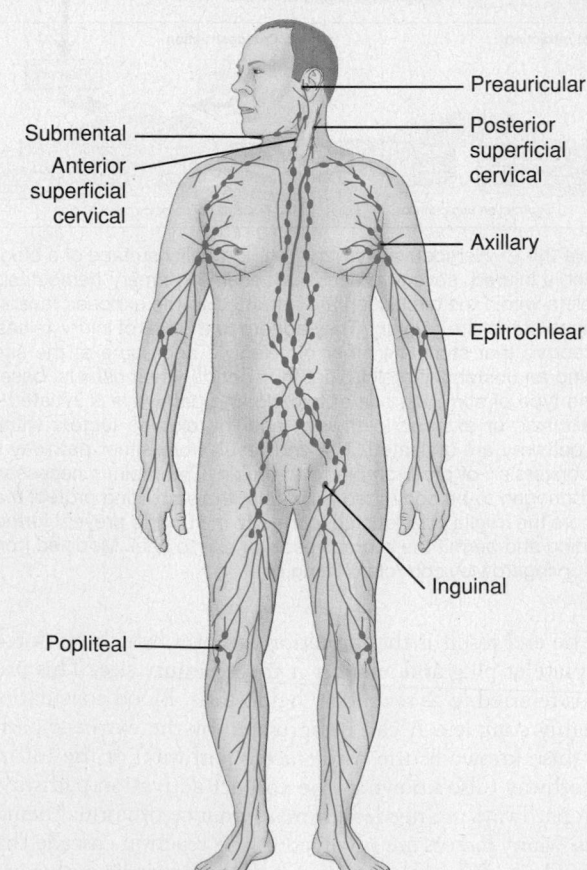

Figure 28-4 • Lymphatic system. Sites where lymph nodes are accessible for palpation. Developed by Thomas, M., & Morrow, K. (2011). Veterans Administration Palo Alto Health Care System.

TABLE 28-2 Health History and Physical Assessment in Hematologic Disorders[a]		
	Findings	**Potential Indications of Hematologic Disorder**
Health History	Prior episodes of bleeding (epistaxis, tooth, gum, hematuria, menorrhagia, hematochezia, gastrointestinal bleeding and/or ulcers)	Thrombocytopenia, coagulopathy, anemia
	Prior blood clots, pulmonary emboli, miscarriages	Thrombotic disorder
	Fatigue and weakness	Anemia, infection, malignancy, clonal disorders
	Dyspnea, particularly dyspnea on exertion, orthopnea, shortness of breath	Anemia, infection
	Prior radiation therapy (especially pelvic irradiation)	Anemia, pancytopenia, myelodysplastic syndrome, leukemia
	Prior chemotherapy	Myelodysplastic syndrome, leukemia
	Hobbies/occupational/military exposure history (especially benzene, Agent Orange)	Myelodysplastic syndrome, leukemia, myeloma, lymphoma
	Diet history	Anemia (due to vitamin B_{12}, folate, iron deficiency)
	Alcohol consumption	Anemia (effect on hematopoiesis, nutritional deficiency)
	Use of herbal supplements	Platelet dysfunction
	Concurrent medications	Neutropenia, anemia, hemolysis, thrombocytopenia
	Family history/ethnicity	Some hematologic disorders have a higher prevalence in certain ethnic groups and families (see Chart 28-1)
Physical Assessment		
Skin	Gray-tan or bronze skin color (especially genitalia, scars, exposed areas)	Hemochromatosis (primary or secondary)
	Ruddy complexion (face, conjunctiva, hands, feet)	Polycythemia
	Ecchymoses (i.e., bruises)	Thrombocytopenia, coagulopathy
	Petechiae (i.e., pinpoint hemorrhagic lesions, usually more prominent on trunk or anterior aspects of lower extremities)	Severe thrombocytopenia
	Rash	Variable; if pruritic, may indicate polycythemia, other non–hematologic-related disorders (see Chapter 56)
	Bleeding (including around vascular lines, tubes)	Thrombocytopenia, coagulopathy
	Conjunctival hemorrhage	Severe thrombocytopenia, coagulopathy
	Pallor, especially in mucous membranes (including conjunctiva), nail beds	Anemia
	Jaundice in mucous membranes (including conjunctiva), nail beds, palate	Hemolysis
Oral cavity	Petechiae in the buccal mucosa, gingiva, hard palate	Severe thrombocytopenia
	Ulceration of oral mucosa	Infection, leukemia
	Tongue: Smooth	Pernicious anemia
	Beefy red	Vitamin B_{12}/folate deficiency
	Enlarged	Amyloidosis
	Angular cheilosis (ulceration at corners of mouth)	Anemia
	Enlarged gums: hyperplasia	Leukemia
Lymph nodes	Enlarged size, firm and fixed vs. mobile and tender	Leukemia, lymphoma
Respiratory	Increased rate and depth of respirations; adventitious breath sounds	Anemia; infection
Cardiovascular	Distended neck veins, edema, chest pain on exertion, murmurs, gallops	Severe anemia
	Hypotension (below baseline)	Polycythemia
	Hypertension (above baseline)	
Genitourinary	Hematuria	Hemolysis, thrombocytopenia
	Proteinuria	Myeloma
Musculoskeletal	Rib/sternal tenderness to palpation	Leukemia, myeloma
	Back pain; tenderness to palpation over spine, loss of height, kyphosis	Myeloma
	Pain/swelling in knees, wrists, hands	Hemophilia, sickle cell disease
Abdominal	Enlarged spleen	Leukemia, myelofibrosis
	Enlarged liver	Myelofibrosis
	Stool positive for occult blood	Anemia, thrombocytopenia
Central nervous system	Cranial nerve dysfunction	Vitamin B_{12} deficiency
	Peripheral nerve dysfunction (especially sensory)	Vitamin B_{12} deficiency, amyloidosis, myeloma
	Visual changes, headache, alteration in mental status	Severe thrombocytopenia
Gynecologic	Menorrhagia	Thrombocytopenia, coagulopathy
Constitutional	Fever, chills, sweats, asthenia	Leukemia, lymphoma; infection

[a]Common findings (obtained via health history and physical assessment) that occur in patients with hematologic disorders. Note that signs and symptoms are not disease specific but are useful in guiding the nurse to establishing an etiology for the findings noted.

Adapted from Bickley, L. S. (2016). *Bates' guide to physical examination and history taking* (12th ed.). Philadelphia, PA: Lippincott Williams & Wilkins; Weber, J. W., & Kelley, J. (2018). *Health assessment in nursing* (6th ed.). Philadelphia, PA: Wolters Kluwer.

be examined. This process is referred to as the manual examination of the peripheral smear, which may be part of the CBC. In this test, a drop of blood is spread on a glass slide, stained, and examined under a microscope. The shape and size of the erythrocytes and platelets, as well as the actual appearance of the leukocytes, provide useful information in identifying hematologic conditions. Blood for the CBC is typically obtained by venipuncture (Fischbach & Fischbach, 2018).

Other common tests of coagulation are the prothrombin time (PT), typically replaced by the standardized test, international normalized ratio (INR), and the activated partial thromboplastin time (aPTT). The INR and aPTT serve as useful screening tools for evaluating a patient's clotting ability and monitoring the therapeutic effectiveness of anticoagulant medications. In both tests, specific reagents are mixed into the plasma sample, and the time taken to form a clot is measured. For these tests to be accurate, the test tube must be filled with the correct amount of the patient's blood; either excess or inadequate blood volume within the tube can render the results inaccurate.

Bone Marrow Aspiration and Biopsy

Bone marrow aspiration and biopsy are crucial when additional information is needed to assess how a patient's blood cells are being formed and to assess the quantity and quality of each type of cell produced within the marrow. Also, results of these tests can be used to document infection or tumor within the marrow. Other specialized tests can be performed on the marrow aspirate, such as cytogenetic analysis or immunophenotyping (i.e., identifying specific proteins expressed by cells), and are useful to identify certain malignant conditions and form a prognosis.

Normal bone marrow is in a semifluid state and can be aspirated through a special large needle. In adults, bone marrow is usually aspirated from the iliac crest and occasionally from the sternum. The bone marrow aspirate provides a sample of cells from the more fluid part of the bone marrow and may not be adequate for evaluating certain conditions, such as anemia. When more information is required, a bone marrow biopsy is performed, which examines a solid part of the bone marrow. Biopsy samples are taken from the posterior iliac crest; although occasionally, an anterior approach is required. A marrow biopsy shows the architecture of the bone marrow as well as its degree of cellularity.

Patient preparation includes a careful explanation of the procedure, which may be done at the patient's bedside (for a patient who is hospitalized) or in the outpatient setting. Some patients may be anxious, thus an anxiolytic agent may be prescribed. It is essential the physician or nurse explain the procedure, including risks, benefits and alternatives, and describe sensations the patient may experience. A signed informed consent is required for a bone marrow aspiration and biopsy.

Before aspiration, the skin is cleansed using aseptic technique. Next, a small area is anesthetized with a local anesthetic agent through the skin and subcutaneous tissue to the periosteum of the bone; it is not possible to anesthetize the bone itself. The bone marrow needle is introduced with a stylet in place. When the needle moves through the outer cortex of bone and enters the marrow cavity, the stylet is removed, and a syringe is attached. A small volume (5 mL) of blood and marrow is then aspirated. Patients typically feel a pressure sensation as the needle is advanced into position. The actual aspiration always causes sharp but brief pain, resulting from the suction exerted as the marrow is aspirated into the syringe. Taking deep breaths or using relaxation techniques often helps ease the discomfort (see Fig. 28-5).

A bone marrow biopsy is most often performed with a bone marrow aspiration and is called a bone marrow exam (Mayo Clinic, 2018a). The bone marrow aspirate is used to determine types and numbers of cells present in the bone marrow. The bone marrow biopsy consists of an actual tissue sample used to study the architecture of the bone marrow and confirm diagnoses (Wimberly, 2019). For a bone marrow biopsy, a special biopsy needle is used. Because these needles are large, the skin may be punctured first with a surgical blade to make a 3- to 4-mm incision. The biopsy needle is advanced well into the marrow cavity. When the needle is properly positioned, a portion of marrow is cored out. The patient feels a pressure sensation but should not feel actual pain. The nurse should assist the patient in maintaining a comfortable position and encourage relaxation and deep breathing throughout the procedure. The patient should be instructed to inform the physician if pain occurs so that an additional anesthetic agent can be given.

Potential complications of either bone marrow aspiration or biopsy include bleeding and infection. The risk of bleeding is somewhat increased if the patient's platelet count is low or if the patient has been taking a medication that alters platelet function (e.g., aspirin). After the marrow sample is obtained, pressure is applied to the site for several minutes. The site is then covered with a sterile dressing. Most patients have no discomfort after a bone marrow aspiration, but the site of a biopsy may ache for 1 or 2 days. Warm tub baths and a mild analgesic agent (e.g., acetaminophen) may be useful. Aspirin-containing analgesic agents should be avoided in the immediate postprocedure period because they can aggravate or potentiate bleeding. Also, no rigorous activity or exercise for 1 to 2 days is recommended (Mayo Clinic, 2018a).

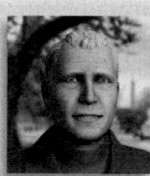

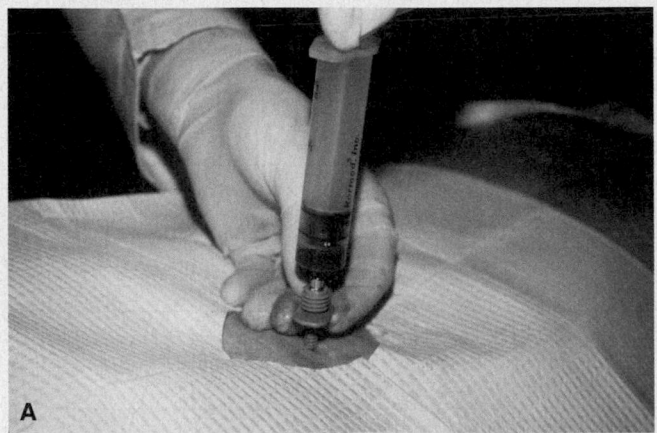

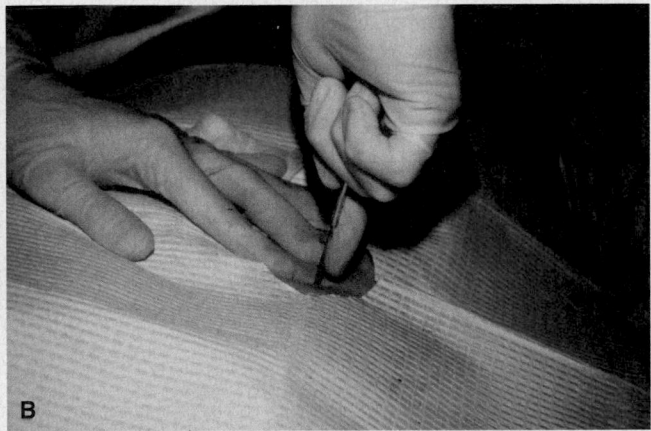

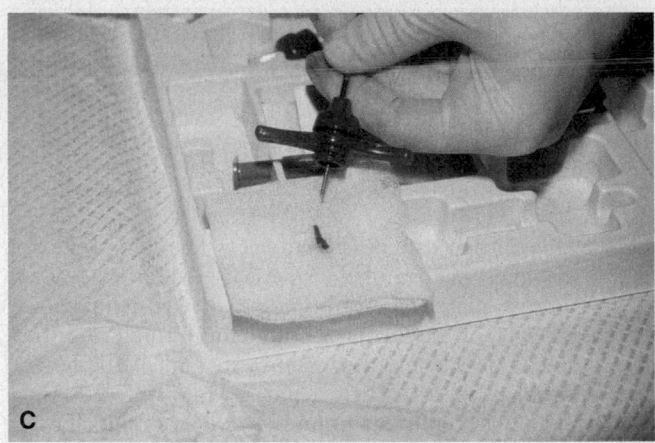

Figure 28-5 • Bone marrow aspiration procedure. The posterior superior iliac crest is the preferred site for bone marrow aspiration and biopsy because no vital organs or vessels are nearby. The patient is placed either in the lateral position with one leg flexed or in the prone position. The anterior iliac crest or sternum may also be used. Note that the sternum cannot be used for a marrow biopsy. **A.** Bone marrow aspiration. **B.** Inserting a Jamshidi biopsy needle. **C.** Dispensing the bone marrow core. Reprinted with permission from Farhi, D. C. (2009). *Pathology of bone marrow and blood cells* (2nd ed.). Philadelphia, PA: Lippincott Williams & Wilkins.

Therapeutic Approaches to Hematologic Disorders

Splenectomy

The surgical removal of the spleen, called splenectomy, is a possible treatment for some hematologic disorders. For example, an enlarged spleen may be the site of excessive destruction of blood cells. In addition, some patients with grossly enlarged spleens develop severe thrombocytopenia as a result of platelets being sequestered in the spleen. Splenectomy removes the "trap," and platelet counts may normalize over time.

Laparoscopic splenectomy is associated with decreased postoperative morbidity compared to open splenectomy. Acute risks associated with a splenectomy include hemorrhage, increased clotting, and injury to surrounding organs and tissues. Long-term risks post splenectomy includes greater likelihood to develop life-threatening infections. Patients should be vaccinated for pneumonia before undergoing splenectomy, if possible. The patient is instructed to seek prompt medical attention for even minor symptoms of infection. The Centers for Disease Control and Prevention (CDC, 2020) recommends patients without spleens receive vaccines for influenza, pneumonia, and meningococci. Also, if a patient has other conditions that increase risk of serious infection in addition to a history of splenectomy, they may need antibiotic prophylaxis (Mayo Clinic, 2018b).

Therapeutic Apheresis

Apheresis is a Greek word meaning "separation." In therapeutic apheresis (or pheresis), blood is taken from the patient and passed through a centrifuge, where a specific component is separated from the blood, removed (see Table 28-3), and the remaining blood is returned to the patient. The entire system is closed, so the risk of bacterial contamination is low. When platelets or leukocytes are removed, the decrease in these cells within the circulation is temporary. Platelet donors can have their platelets apheresed as often as every 14 days. Leukocytes can be obtained similarly, typically after the donor has received growth factors (granulocyte colony-stimulating factor, granulocyte-macrophage colony-stimulating factor) to stimulate the formation of additional leukocytes and thereby increase the leukocyte count. The use of these growth factors also stimulates the release of stem cells within the circulation. Apheresis is used to harvest these stem cells (typically over a period of several days) for use in peripheral blood stem cell transplant (Padmanabhan, Smith, Aqui, et al., 2019). Sometimes plasma is removed rather than blood cells, and this process is called plasmapheresis. Indications for plasmapheresis include obtaining plasma for transfusion and removing dangerous substances such as immune complexes and autoantibodies (Sarode, 2018).

Hematopoietic Stem Cell Transplantation

Hematopoietic stem cell transplantation (HSCT) is a therapeutic modality that offers the possibility of cure for some

TABLE 28-3   Types of Apheresis[a]

Procedure	Purpose	Examples of Clinical Use
Plateletpheresis	Remove platelets	Extreme thrombocytosis, essential thrombocythemia (temporary measure); single-donor platelet transfusion
Leukapheresis	Remove WBCs (can be specific to neutrophils or lymphocytes)	Extreme leukocytosis (e.g., AML, CML) (very temporary measure); harvest WBCs for transfusion
Erythrocytapheresis (RBC exchange)	Remove RBCs	RBC dyscrasias (e.g., sickle cell disease); RBCs replaced via transfusion
Plasmapheresis (plasma exchange)	Remove plasma proteins	Hyperviscosity syndromes; treatment for some renal and neurologic diseases (e.g., Goodpasture syndrome, TTP, Guillain–Barré, myasthenia gravis)
Stem cell harvest	Remove circulating stem cells	Transplantation (donor harvest or autologous)

[a]Therapeutic apheresis can be used to treat a wide variety of conditions. When it is used to treat a disease that causes an increase in a specific cell type with a short life in circulation (i.e., WBCs, platelets), the reduction in those cells is temporary. However, this temporary reduction permits a margin of safety while waiting for a longer-lasting treatment modality (e.g., chemotherapy) to take effect. Apheresis can also be used to obtain stem cells for transplantation, either from a matched donor (allogeneic) or from the patient (autologous).
AML, acute myeloid leukemia; CML, chronic myeloid leukemia; RBC, red blood cell; TTP, thrombotic thrombocytopenic purpura; WBCs, white blood cells.
Adapted from Padmanabhan, A., Smith, L., Aqui, N., et al. (2019). Guidelines on the use of therapeutic apheresis in clinical practice—evidence-based approach from the Writing Committee of the American Society for Apheresis: The eighth special issue. *Journal of Clinical Apheresis, 34*(3), 171–354.

patients with hematologic disorders such as severe aplastic anemia, some forms of leukemia, and thalassemia. It can also provide longer remission from disease even when cure is not possible, such as in multiple myeloma. Hematopoietic stem cells may be transplanted from either allogeneic or autologous donors. For most hematologic diseases, allogeneic transplant is more effective (Bazinet & Popradi, 2019); here, stem cells are obtained from a donor whose cells match those of the patient. In contrast, the patient's own stem cells are harvested and then used in autologous transplant. (See Chapter 12 for a detailed discussion of HSCT.)

Therapeutic Phlebotomy

Therapeutic phlebotomy is the removal of a certain amount of blood under controlled conditions. Patients with elevated hematocrits (e.g., those with polycythemia vera) or excessive iron absorption (e.g., hemochromatosis) can usually be managed by periodically removing 1 unit (about 500 mL) of whole blood. Over time, this process can produce iron deficiency, leaving the patient unable to produce as many erythrocytes. The actual procedure for therapeutic phlebotomy is similar to that for blood donation (see later discussion).

Blood Component Therapy

A single unit of whole blood contains 450 mL of blood and 50 mL of an anticoagulant, which can be processed and dispensed for administration. However, it is more appropriate, economical, and practical to separate that unit of whole blood into its primary components: erythrocytes, platelets, and plasma (leukocytes are rarely used; see later discussion).

Each component must be processed and stored differently to maximize the longevity of the viable cells and factors within it; thus, each individual blood component has a different storage life. Because the plasma is removed, a unit of packed red blood cells (PRBCs) is very concentrated (hematocrit approximately 70%) (Butterworth, Mackey, & Wasnick, 2018). PRBCs are stored at 4°C (39.2°F). With special

preservatives, they can be stored safely for up to 42 days before they must be discarded (American Red Cross, 2020a).

In contrast, platelets must be stored at room temperature because they cannot withstand cold temperatures, and they last for only 5 days before they must be discarded. To prevent clumping, platelets are gently agitated while stored. Plasma is immediately frozen to maintain the activity of the clotting factors within; it lasts for 1 year if it remains frozen. Alternatively, plasma can be further pooled and processed into blood derivatives, such as albumin, immune globulin, factor VIII, and factor IX. Table 28-4 describes each blood component and how it is commonly used.

Special Preparations

Factor VIII concentrate (antihemophilic factor) is a lyophilized, freeze-dried concentrate of pooled fractionated human plasma used in treating hemophilia A. Factor IX concentrate (prothrombin complex) is similarly prepared and contains factors II, VII, IX, and X. It is used primarily for the treatment of factor IX deficiency (hemophilia B). Factor IX concentrate is also useful in treating congenital factor VII and factor X deficiencies. Recombinant forms of factor VIII, such as Humate-P or Alphanate, are also useful. Because they contain von Willebrand factor, these agents are used in von Willebrand disease as well as in hemophilia A, particularly when patients develop factor VIII inhibitors.

Plasma albumin is a large protein molecule that usually stays within vessels and is a major contributor to plasma oncotic pressure. This protein is used to expand the blood volume of patients in hypovolemic shock and, rarely, to increase the concentration of circulating albumin in patients with hypoalbuminemia.

Immune globulin is a concentrated solution of the antibody immunoglobulin G (IgG), prepared from large pools of plasma. It contains very little immunoglobulin A (IgA) or IgM. Intravenous immunoglobulin (IVIG) is used in various clinical situations to replace inadequate amounts of IgG in patients who are at risk for recurrent bacterial infection

TABLE 28-4	Blood and Blood Components Commonly Used in Transfusion Therapy[a]	
Component	**Composition**	**Indications and Considerations**
Whole blood	Cells and plasma, hematocrit about 40%	Volume replacement and oxygen-carrying capacity; usually used only in significant bleeding (>25% blood volume lost)
PRBCs	RBCs with little plasma (hematocrit about 75%); some platelets and WBCs remain	↑ RBC mass; symptomatic anemia: • Platelets within the unit are not functional • WBCs within the unit may cause reaction and are not functional
Platelets—random	Platelets (5.5×10^{10} platelets/unit), plasma; some RBCs, WBCs	Bleeding due to severe ↓ platelets Prevent bleeding when platelets <5,000–10,000/mm^3 Survival ↓ in presence of fever, chills, infection Repeated treatment leads to ↓ survival due to alloimmunization
Platelets—single donor	Platelets (3×10^{11} platelets/unit) 1 unit is equivalent to 6–8 units of random platelets	Used for repeated treatment: • ↓ alloimmunization risk by limiting exposure to multiple donors
Plasma	Plasma; all coagulation factors Complement	Bleeding in patients with coagulation factor deficiencies; plasmapheresis
Granulocytes	Neutrophils (>1×10^{10}/unit); some lymphocytes, RBCs, and platelets will remain within the unit	Severe neutropenia in select patients; controversial
Lymphocytes	Lymphocytes (number varies)	Stimulate graft-vs.-host disease effect
Cryoprecipitate	Fibrinogen ≥150 mg/bag, AHF (VIII:C) 80–110 units/bag, von Willebrand factor; fibronectin	von Willebrand disease Hypofibrinogenemia Hemophilia A
AHF	Factor VIII	Hemophilia A
Factor IX concentrate	Factor IX	Hemophilia B (Christmas disease)
Factor IX complex	Factors II, VII, IX, X	Hereditary factor VII, IX, X deficiency; hemophilia A with factor VII inhibitors
Albumin	Albumin 5%, 25%	Hypoproteinemia; burns; volume expansion by 5% to ↑ blood volume; 25% leads to ↓ hematocrit
IV gamma-globulin	Immunoglobulin G antibodies	Hypogammaglobulinemia (in CLL, recurrent infections); ITP; primary immunodeficiency states
Antithrombin III concentrate (AT III)	AT III (trace amounts of other plasma proteins)	AT III deficiency with or at risk for thrombosis

[a]The composition of each type of blood component is described as well as the most common indications for using a given blood component. RBCs, platelets, and fresh-frozen plasma are the blood products most commonly used. When transfusing these blood products, it is important to realize that the individual product is always "contaminated" with very small amounts of other blood products (e.g., WBCs mixed in a unit of platelets). This contamination can cause some difficulties, particularly isosensitization, in certain patients.

↑, increased; ↓, decreased; AHF, antihemophilic factor; CLL, chronic lymphocytic leukemia; ITP, idiopathic thrombocytopenic purpura; IV, intravenous; PRBCs, packed red blood cells; RBCs, red blood cells; WBCs, white blood cells.

Adapted from American Red Cross. (2020b). How can one donation help multiple people? Retrieved on 1/15/2020 at: www.redcrossblood.org/faq.html#eligibility; Stowell, C. P. (2019). Transfusion medicine. In M. Laposata (Ed.). *Laboratory medicine: Diagnosis of disease in the clinical laboratory* (3rd ed., pp. 321–348). New York: McGraw-Hill.

(e.g., those with chronic lymphocytic leukemia, those receiving HSCT). It is also used in certain autoimmune disorders, such as idiopathic thrombocytopenic purpura (ITP). Albumin, antihemophilic factors, and IVIG, in contrast to all other fractions of human blood, cells, or plasma, can survive being subjected to heating at 60°C (140°F) for 10 hours to free them of the viral contaminants that may be present.

Procuring Blood and Blood Products

The process of procuring blood and blood products includes donation and processing.

Blood Donation

To protect both the donor and the recipients, all prospective donors are examined and interviewed before they are allowed to donate their blood. The intent of the interview is to assess the general health status of the donor and to identify risk factors that might harm a recipient of the donor's blood. There is no upper age limit to donation. The American Red Cross (2020c) requires that donors be in good health and meet specific eligibility criteria related to medications and vaccinations, medical conditions and treatments, travel outside the United States, lifestyle and life events, and so on. Detailed information about these criteria is available on the American Red Cross Web site (see the Resources section). Examples of these minimal requirements include (American Red Cross, 2020a, 2020d):

- Body weight should be at least 50 kg (110 lb) for a standard 450-mL donation.
- Donors must wait at least 8 weeks between whole blood (standard) donations.
- People younger than 17 years require parental consent in some states.
- The oral temperature should not exceed 37.5°C (99.6°F).
- The systolic arterial blood pressure should be 80 to 180 mm Hg, and the diastolic pressure should be 50 to 100 mm Hg.
- The hemoglobin level should be at least 12.5 g/dl
- The destinations of people who traveled outside the United States and Canada within the past 3 years are reviewed; a waiting period maybe required before a donation is accepted.
- Prospective donors who received a blood transfusion must wait 12 months before a donation is accepted.
- Men who have sexual relations with men must wait 3 months from their last sexual encounter before a donation is accepted.

The American Red Cross follows the U.S. Food and Drug Administration (FDA) policy for donors who are lesbian, gay, bisexual, transgender, or queer (LGBTQ) and provides support for these individuals through the American Red Cross LGBTQ+ Team Member Resource Group (see Resources section at the end of the chapter).

Directed Donation

At times, friends and family of a patient wish to donate blood for that person. These blood donations are referred to as directed donations. These donations are not any safer than those provided by random donors, because directed donors may not be as willing to identify themselves as having a history of any of the risk factors that disqualify a person from donating blood. Therefore, many blood centers no longer accept directed donations.

Standard Donation

Phlebotomy consists of venipuncture and blood withdrawal. Standard precautions are used. Donors are placed in a semirecumbent position. The skin over the antecubital fossa is carefully cleansed with an antiseptic preparation, a tourniquet is applied, and venipuncture is performed. Withdrawal of 450 mL of blood usually takes less than 15 minutes. After the needle is removed, donors are asked to hold the involved arm straight up, and firm pressure is applied with sterile gauze for 2 to 3 minutes. A firm bandage is then applied. The donor remains recumbent until they feel able to sit up, usually within a few minutes. Donors who experience weakness or faintness should rest for a longer period. The donor then receives food and fluids and is asked to remain another 15 minutes.

The donor is instructed to leave the dressing on and to avoid heavy lifting for several hours, to avoid smoking for 1 hour, to avoid drinking alcoholic beverages for 3 hours, to increase fluid intake for 2 days, and to eat healthy meals for at least 2 weeks. Specimens from the donated blood are tested to detect infections and to identify the specific blood type (see later discussion under Blood Processing).

Autologous Donation

A patient's own blood may be collected for future transfusion; this method is useful for many elective surgeries where the potential need for transfusion is high (e.g., orthopedic surgery). Preoperative donations are ideally collected 4 to 6 weeks before surgery. Iron supplements are prescribed during this period to prevent depletion of iron stores. Typically, 1 unit of blood is drawn each week; the number of units obtained varies with the type of surgical procedure to be performed (i.e., the amount of blood anticipated to be transfused). Phlebotomies are not performed within 72 hours of surgery. Individual blood components can also be collected.

The primary advantage of autologous transfusions is the prevention of viral infections from another person's blood. Other advantages include safe transfusion for patients with a history of transfusion reactions, prevention of alloimmunization, and avoidance of complications in patients with alloantibodies. It is the policy of the American Red Cross that autologous blood is transfused only to the donor. If the blood is not required, it is discarded. The blood is never returned to the general donor supply of blood products to be used by another person (American Red Cross, 2020a).

Needless autologous donation (i.e., performed when the likelihood of transfusion is small) is discouraged because it is expensive, takes time, and uses resources inappropriately. Moreover, in an emergency situation, the autologous units available may be inadequate, and the patient may still require additional units from the general donor supply. Furthermore, although autologous transfusion can eliminate the risk of viral contamination, the risk of bacterial contamination is the same as that in transfusion from random donors (Stowell, 2019).

Contraindications to donation of blood for autologous transfusion are acute infection, severely debilitating chronic disease, hemoglobin level less than 11 g/dL, unstable angina, and acute cardiovascular or cerebrovascular disease. A history of poorly controlled epilepsy may be considered a contraindication in some centers.

Intraoperative Blood Salvage

This transfusion method provides replacement for patients who cannot donate blood before surgery and for those undergoing vascular, orthopedic, or thoracic surgery. During a surgical procedure, blood lost into a sterile cavity (e.g., hip joint) is suctioned into a cell-saver machine. The whole blood or PRBCs are washed, often with saline solution; filtered; and then returned to the patient as an IV infusion. Salvaged blood cannot be stored, because bacteria cannot be completely removed from the blood and thus cannot be used when it is contaminated with bacteria. The use of intraoperative blood salvage has decreased the need for autologous blood donation but has not affected the need for allogeneic blood products (Sikorski, Rizkalla, Yang, et al., 2017).

Hemodilution

This transfusion method may be initiated before or after induction of anesthesia. About 1 to 2 units of blood are removed from the patient through a venous or arterial line and simultaneously replaced with a colloid or crystalloid solution. The blood obtained is then reinfused after surgery.

The advantage of this method is that the patient loses fewer erythrocytes during surgery, because the added IV solutions dilute the concentration of erythrocytes and lower the hematocrit. However, patients who are at risk for myocardial injury should not be further stressed by hemodilution. Hemodilution has been associated with adverse outcomes in patients having cardiopulmonary bypass; it has also been linked to tissue ischemia, particularly in the kidneys (Hare, Han, Leshchyshyn, et al., 2018).

Complications of Blood Donation

Excessive bleeding at the donor's venipuncture site is sometimes caused by a bleeding disorder but more often results from a technique error: laceration of the vein, excessive tourniquet pressure, or failure to apply enough pressure after the needle is withdrawn.

Fainting may occur after blood donation and may be related to emotional factors, a vasovagal reaction, or prolonged fasting before donation. Because of the loss of blood volume, hypotension and syncope may occur when the donor assumes an erect position (John, Theodora, Gloria, et al., 2017). A donor who appears pale or complains of faintness should immediately lie down or sit with the head lowered below the knees. The donor should be observed for another 30 minutes.

Anginal chest pain may be precipitated in patients with unsuspected coronary artery disease. Seizures can occur in donors with epilepsy, although the incidence is very low. Both angina and seizures require further medical evaluation and treatment.

Blood Processing

Samples of the unit of blood are always taken immediately after donation so that the blood can be typed and tested. Each donation is tested for antibodies to human immune deficiency virus (HIV) types 1 and 2, hepatitis B core antibody (anti-HBc), hepatitis C virus (HCV), human T-cell lymphotropic virus type I (anti-HTLV-I/II), hepatitis B surface antigen (HbsAG), and syphilis. Negative reactions are required for the blood to be used, and each unit of blood is labeled to certify the results. Nucleic acid amplification testing has increased the ability to detect the presence of HCV, HIV, and West Nile virus infections, because it directly tests for genomic nucleic acids of the viruses rather than for the presence of antibodies to the viruses. This testing significantly shortens the "window" of inability to detect HIV and HCV from a donated unit, further ensuring the safety of the blood; the risk of transmission of HIV or HCV is now estimated at 1 in 2 million units and 1 in 1.6 million units of blood donated, respectively (American Cancer Society, 2017). Blood is also screened for cytomegalovirus (CMV). If it tests positive for CMV, it can still be used, except in recipients who are negative for CMV and who are severely immunocompromised; any components are labeled as CMV positive.

Equally important is accurate determination of the blood type. More than 200 antigens have been identified on the surface of RBC membranes. Of these, the most important for safe transfusion are the ABO and Rh systems. The ABO system identifies which sugars are present on the membrane of a person's erythrocytes: A, B, both A and B, or neither A nor B (type O). To prevent a significant reaction, the same type of PRBCs should be transfused. Previously, it was thought that in an emergency situation in which the patient's blood type was not known, type O blood could be safely transfused. This practice is no longer recommended.

The Rh antigen (also referred to as D) is present on the surface of erythrocytes in 85% of the population (Rh positive). Those who lack the D antigen are referred to as being Rh negative. PRBCs are routinely tested for the D antigen as well as ABO. Patients should receive PRBCs with a compatible Rh type.

The majority of transfusion reactions are due to clerical errors, including mislabeling, inaccuracy transcribing orders and incorrect verification of product and patient. When these errors occur, the patient is transfused an incompatible unit of blood product (Stubbs, 2018). Reactions (other than those due to procedural error) are most frequently due to the presence of donor leukocytes within the blood component unit (PRBCs or platelets); the recipient may form antibodies to the antigens present on these leukocytes. PRBC components typically have 1 to 3×10^9 leukocytes remaining in each unit. Leukocytes from the blood product are frequently filtered to diminish the likelihood of developing reactions and refractoriness to transfusions, particularly in patients who have long-term transfusion needs. The process of leukocyte filtration renders the blood component "leukocyte poor" (i.e., leukopoor). Filtration can occur at the time the unit is collected from the donor and processed, which achieves better results but is more expensive, or at the time the blood component is transfused by attaching a leukocyte filter to the blood administration tubing. Many centers advocate routinely using leukopoor filtered blood components for people who have or are likely to develop long-term transfusion requirements.

When a patient is immunocompromised, as in the case following stem cell transplant, any donor lymphocytes must be removed from the blood components. In this situation, the blood component is exposed to low amounts of radiation (25 Gy) that kill any lymphocytes within the blood component. Irradiated blood products are highly effective in preventing transfusion-associated graft-versus-host disease, which is fatal in most cases. Irradiated blood products have a shorter shelf life.

Transfusion

Administration of blood and blood components requires knowledge of correct administration techniques and possible complications. It is very important to be familiar with the agency's policies and procedures for transfusion therapy.

Most blood transfusions are performed in the acute care setting, and sometimes must be done emergently. Patients with long-term transfusion requirements (i.e., patients who require transfusions on an ongoing, periodic basis) often can receive transfusions in other settings. Freestanding infusion centers, ambulatory care clinics, physicians' offices, and even patients' homes may be appropriate settings for transfusion. Typically, patients who need long-term transfusions but are otherwise stable physically are appropriate candidates for outpatient therapy. Verification and administration of the blood product are performed as in a hospital setting. Although most blood products can be transfused in the outpatient setting, the home is typically limited to transfusions of

PRBCs and factor components (e.g., factor VIII for patients with hemophilia).

Pretransfusion Assessment

Patient History

The patient history is an important component of the pretransfusion assessment to determine the history of previous transfusions as well as previous reactions to transfusion. The history should include the type of reaction, its manifestations, the interventions required, and whether any preventive interventions were used in subsequent transfusions. The nurse assesses the number of pregnancies a woman has had, because a high number can increase her risk of reaction due to antibodies developed from exposure to fetal circulation. Other concurrent health problems should be noted, with careful attention to cardiac, pulmonary, and vascular disease. Informed consent must be obtained preprocedure (see Chart 28-2).

Physical Assessment

A systematic physical assessment and measurement of baseline vital signs and fluid status are important before transfusing any blood product. The respiratory system should be assessed, including careful auscultation of the lungs and the patient's use of accessory muscles. Cardiac system assessment should include careful inspection for any edema as well as other signs of heart failure (e.g., jugular venous distention; see Chapter 25). The skin should be observed for rashes, petechiae, and ecchymoses. The sclera should be examined for icterus. In the event of a transfusion reaction, a comparison of findings can help differentiate between types of reactions.

Chart 28-2 **ETHICAL DILEMMA**
Can Surrogates Refuse Life-Saving Treatment?

Case Scenario

L.C. is a 34-year-old woman who was an unrestrained front-seat passenger in a motor vehicle crash 2 days ago. She sustained multiple trauma, including a fractured skull, traumatic brain injury, several fractured ribs, a pulmonary contusion, and a fractured right femur. After stabilization in the emergency department, she was admitted to the intensive care unit (ICU) endotracheally intubated and mechanically ventilated. You are a staff nurse in the ICU and have been assigned as L.C.'s nurse since her admission. You have come to know her family members, including her parents and her boyfriend, whom she has lived with for the past 10 months. During interdisciplinary rounds, L.C.'s trauma surgeon notes that her hemoglobin continues to drop since admission, and is now 7.7 g/dL; he asserts that she must receive blood transfusions. L.C.'s parents and her boyfriend are present during these rounds. L.C.'s parents tell the trauma surgeon that they are Jehovah's Witnesses, and that receiving blood transfusions is against their religious beliefs. L.C.'s boyfriend notes that she no longer adheres to the tenets of Jehovah's Witnesses and does not attend any religious meetings or services. L.C.'s parents become angry and tell her boyfriend that they are the ones to make decisions on L.C.'s behalf. L.C. does not have an advance directive or a power-of-attorney for health care.

Discussion

Whenever a patient lacks capacity to make their own health care decisions, those decisions are made by a legally identified surrogate. Had L.C. identified who that surrogate should be in a power-of-attorney for health care document, that person would have the rights and responsibilities to make those decisions. Since that document does not exist, and since L.C. does not have a spouse, her parents are her legal surrogates and authorized to make decisions on her behalf.

Had L.C. written an advance directive and specified whether or not she would wish to receive blood transfusions for life-threatening contingencies, that specification would be legally binding. For instance, had she noted in an advance directive that she would *not* wish to receive blood transfusions, even if that meant that she would die, that would be a legally binding decision, even if her parents wished for her to receive blood transfusions.

However, L.C.'s parents and her boyfriend disagree about what they believe L.C. would want to be done in this situation. Surrogates are charged with making decisions on behalf of patients who lack capacity. However, that charge is predicated on the belief that surrogates know which decision is consistent with what the patient would have wanted when the patient could have made a reasoned decision. It is noteworthy that L.C.'s parents insist that she not be transfused since it is against *their* religious beliefs. However, they do not note that their beliefs are also consistent with L.C.'s beliefs.

Analysis

- Describe the ethical principles that are in conflict in this case (see Chapter 1, Chart 1-7). Is it possible to preserve L.C.'s autonomy, given that she lacks capacity at this time, and given the conflict between her family members?
- There is a conflict between legal rights and moral decisions in this case. Are there situations where the decision that a legal surrogate makes for a patient who lacks capacity could and should be overturned?
- What if a family meeting is called to try to resolve the conflict between L.C.'s parents and her boyfriend, and her boyfriend is able to provide evidence that L.C. does not adhere to the tenets of the Jehovah's Witness faith? By contrast, what if her parents are able to provide evidence that L.C. has been faithfully attending Jehovah's Witnesses meetings for the past 10 months and that she has explicitly told her parents that she would not ever wish to have blood transfusions? Finally, what if L.C.'s parents and her boyfriend each express that none of them are certain what decision L.C. would make in this situation? Would the trauma surgeon be justified in then upholding the principle of beneficence and prescribe blood transfusions for L.C., despite her parents' objections? If those transfusions were prescribed, would you administer the blood transfusions or would you object?
- What resources might be mobilized to be of assistance to L.C.'s family and the health care team so that the decision that best respects L.C.'s wishes might be made?

References

Baumrucker, S. J., Stolick, M., Hutchinson, L., et al. (2019). Death or damnation: Surrogacy and religious beliefs. *American Journal of Hospice & Palliative Medicine, 36*(8), 740–745.

Resources

See Chapter 1, Chart 1-10, for Steps of an Ethical Analysis and Ethics Resources.

Patient Education

Reviewing the signs and symptoms of a transfusion reaction is crucial with all patients, including those who have and have not received a previous transfusion. Signs and symptoms of a reaction include fever, chills, respiratory distress, low back pain, nausea, pain at the IV site, or anything "unusual." Although a thorough review is very important, the nurse also reassures the patient that the blood is carefully tested against the patient's own blood (cross-matched) to diminish the likelihood of any untoward reaction. Similarly, the patient can be reassured about the very low possibility of contracting HIV from the transfusion; this fear persists among many people.

Transfusion Procedures

Methods for transfusing blood components and the role of the nurse in assessing patients before, during, and after these procedures are described in Charts 28-3 and 28-4.

Complications

Any patient who receives a blood transfusion is at risk for developing complications from the transfusion. Nursing management is directed toward preventing complications, promptly recognizing complications if they develop, and promptly initiating measures to control complications. Nurses assess patients' vital signs before, during, and after a blood transfusion is complete to screen for any adverse reactions; however, the optimal frequency for assessing these vital signs during the transfusion is not well established (Cortez-Gann, Gilmore, Foley, et al., 2017) (see the Nursing Research Profile in Chart 28-5). The following sections describe the most common or potentially severe transfusion-related complications.

Febrile Nonhemolytic Reaction

A febrile nonhemolytic reaction is caused by antibodies to donor leukocytes that remain in the unit of blood or blood

---

Chart 28-3

Transfusion of Packed Red Blood Cells

Preprocedure

1. Confirm that the transfusion has been prescribed.
2. Check that patient's blood has been typed and cross-matched.
3. Verify that patient has signed a written consent form per institution or agency policy and agrees to procedure.
4. Explain procedure to patient. Educate patient about signs and symptoms of transfusion reaction (itching, hives, swelling, shortness of breath, fever, chills).
5. Take patient's temperature, pulse, respiration, blood pressure, and assess fluid volume status (e.g., auscultate lungs, assess for jugular venous distention) to serve as a baseline for comparison during transfusion.
6. Note if signs of increased fluid overload present (e.g., heart failure, see Chapter 25), contact primary provider to discuss potential need for a prescription for diuretic, as warranted.
7. Use hand hygiene and wear gloves in accordance with standard precautions.
8. Use appropriately sized intravenous cannula for insertion in a peripheral vein.[a] Use special tubing that contains a blood filter to screen out fibrin clots and other particulate matter. Do not vent blood container.

Procedure

1. Obtain packed red blood cells (PRBCs) from the blood bank *after* the IV line is started. (Institution policy may limit release to only 1 unit at a time.)
2. Double-check labels with another nurse or physician to ensure that the ABO group and Rh type agree with the compatibility record. Check to see that number and type on donor blood label and on patient's medical record are correct. Confirm patient's identification by asking the patient's name and checking the identification wristband.
3. Check blood for gas bubbles and any unusual color or cloudiness. (Gas bubbles may indicate bacterial growth. Abnormal color or cloudiness may be a sign of hemolysis.)

4. Make sure that PRBC transfusion is initiated within 30 minutes after removal of PRBCs from blood bank refrigerator.
5. For the first 15 minutes, run the transfusion slowly—no faster than 5 mL/min. Observe patient carefully for adverse effects. If no adverse effects occur during the first 15 minutes, increase the flow rate unless patient is at high risk for circulatory overload.
6. Monitor closely for 15 to 30 minutes to detect signs of reaction. Monitor vital signs at regular intervals per institution or agency policy; compare results with baseline measurements. Increase frequency of measurements based on patient's condition. Observe patient frequently throughout the transfusion for any signs of adverse reaction, including restlessness, hives, nausea, vomiting, torso or back pain, shortness of breath, flushing, hematuria, fever, or chills. Should any adverse reaction occur, stop infusion immediately, notify primary provider, and follow the agency's transfusion reaction standard.
7. Note that administration time does not exceed 4 hours because of increased risk of bacterial proliferation.
8. Be alert for signs of adverse reactions: circulatory overload, sepsis, febrile reaction, allergic reaction, and acute hemolytic reaction.
9. Change blood tubing after every 2 units transfused to decrease chance of bacterial contamination.

Postprocedure

1. Obtain vital signs and breath sounds; compare with baseline measurements. If signs of increased fluid overload present (e.g., heart failure), consider obtaining prescription for diuretic as warranted.
2. Dispose of used materials properly.
3. Document procedure in patient's medical record, including patient assessment findings and tolerance to procedure.
4. Monitor patient for response to and effectiveness of procedure. If patient is at risk, monitor for at least 6 hours for signs of transfusion-associated circulatory overload (TACO); also monitor for signs of delayed hemolytic reaction.

Note: Never add medications to blood or blood products; if blood is too thick to run freely, normal saline may be added to the unit. If blood must be warmed, use an in-line blood warmer with a monitoring system.
[a]The size of the peripheral cannula used in a blood transfusion depends on two factors, size and integrity of the vein and desired speed for transfusion.
Adapted from Robinson, S., New, H., Shackleton, T., et al. (2018). The administration of blood components: A British Society for Haematology Guideline. *Transfusion Medicine, 28*(1), 3–21.

Chart 28-4 Transfusion of Platelets or Fresh-Frozen Plasma

Preprocedure

1. Confirm that the transfusion has been prescribed.
2. Verify that patient has signed a written consent form per institution or agency policy and agrees to procedure.
3. Explain procedure to patient. Educate patient about signs and symptoms of transfusion reaction (itching, hives, swelling, shortness of breath, fever, chills).
4. Take patient's temperature, pulse, respiration, blood pressure, and assess fluid status, and auscultate breath sounds to establish a baseline for comparison during transfusion.
5. Note if signs of increased fluid overload present (e.g., heart failure, see Chapter 25), contact primary provider to discuss potential need for a prescription for diuretic, as warranted; this is particularly important when plasma is also infused.
6. Use hand hygiene and wear gloves in accordance with standard precautions.
7. Use a 22-gauge or larger needle or catheter for placement in a large vein, if possible. Use appropriate tubing per institution policy (platelets often require different tubing from that used for other blood products).

Procedure

1. Obtain platelets or fresh-frozen plasma (FFP) from the blood bank (only *after* the IV line is started.)
2. Double-check labels with another nurse or physician to ensure that the ABO group matches the compatibility record (not usually necessary for platelets; here only if compatible platelets are ordered). Check to see that the number and type on donor blood label and on patient's medical record are correct. Confirm patient's identification by asking the patient's name and checking the identification wristband.
3. Check blood product for any unusual color or clumps (excessive redness indicates contamination with larger amounts of red blood cells).

4. Make sure that platelets or FFP units are given immediately after they are obtained.
5. Infuse each unit of FFP over 30 to 60 minutes per patient tolerance; be prepared to infuse at a significantly lower rate in the context of fluid overload. Infuse each unit of platelets as fast as patient can tolerate to diminish platelet clumping during administration. Observe patient carefully for adverse effects, especially circulatory overload. Decrease rate of infusion if necessary.
6. Observe patient closely throughout transfusion for any signs of adverse reaction, including restlessness, hives, nausea, vomiting, torso or back pain, shortness of breath, flushing, hematuria, fever, or chills. Should any adverse reaction occur, stop infusion immediately, notify primary provider, and follow the agency's transfusion reaction standard.
7. Monitor vital signs at the end of transfusion per institution policy; compare results with baseline measurements.
8. Flush line with saline after transfusion to remove blood component from tubing.

Postprocedure

1. Obtain vital signs and auscultate breath sounds; compare with baseline measurements. If signs of increased fluid overload present, consider obtaining prescription for diuretic, as warranted.
2. Dispose of used materials properly.
3. Document procedure in patient's medical record, including patient assessment findings and tolerance to procedure.
4. Monitor patient for response to and effectiveness of procedure. A platelet count may be ordered 1 hour after platelet transfusion to facilitate this evaluation.
5. If patient is at risk for transfusion-associated circulatory overload (TACO), monitor closely for 6 hours after transfusion if possible.

Note: FFP requires ABO but not Rh compatibility. Platelets are not typically cross-matched for ABO compatibility. Never add medications to blood or blood products.
Adapted from Robinson, S., New, H., Shackleton, T., et al. (2018). The administration of blood components: A British Society for Haematology Guideline. *Transfusion Medicine, 28*(1), 3–21.

---

component; it is the most common type of transfusion reaction (Stubbs, 2018). It occurs more frequently in patients who have had previous transfusions (exposure to multiple antigens from previous blood products) and in Rh-negative women who have borne Rh-positive children (exposure to an Rh-positive fetus raises antibody levels in the untreated mother).

The diagnosis of a febrile nonhemolytic reaction is made by excluding other potential causes, such as a hemolytic reaction or bacterial contamination of the blood product. The signs and symptoms of a febrile nonhemolytic transfusion reaction are chills (minimal to severe) followed by fever (more than 1°C elevation). The fever typically begins within 2 hours after the transfusion has begun. Although the reaction is not life threatening, the fever, and particularly the chills and muscle stiffness, can be frightening to the patient.

This reaction can be diminished, even prevented, by further depleting the blood component of donor leukocytes; this is accomplished by a leukocyte reduction filter. Antipyretic agents can be given to prevent fever; however, routine premedication is not advised because it can mask the beginning of a more serious transfusion reaction.

Acute Hemolytic Reaction

The most dangerous, and potentially life-threatening, type of transfusion reaction occurs when the donor blood is incompatible with that of the recipient (i.e., type II hypersensitivity reaction). Antibodies already present in the recipient's plasma rapidly combine with antigens on donor erythrocytes, and the erythrocytes are destroyed in the circulation (i.e., intravascular hemolysis). The most rapid hemolysis occurs in ABO incompatibility. Rh incompatibility often causes a less severe reaction. This reaction can occur after transfusion of as little as 10 mL of PRBCs. Although the overall incidence of such reactions is not high (1:20,000 to 1:40,000 units transfused) (Robinson, New, Shackleton, et al., 2018), they are largely preventable. The most common causes of acute hemolytic reaction are errors in blood component labeling, a type of clerical error, and errors in patient identification that result in the administration of an ABO-incompatible transfusion.

Symptoms consist of fever, chills, low back pain, nausea, chest tightness, dyspnea, and anxiety. As the erythrocytes are destroyed, the hemoglobin is released from the cells and excreted by the kidneys; therefore, hemoglobin appears in the urine (hemoglobinuria). Hypotension, bronchospasm,

Cortez-Gann, J., Gilmore, K. D., Foley, K. W., et al. (2017). Blood transfusion vital sign frequency: What does the evidence say? *MEDSURG Nursing, 26*(2), 89–92.

Chart 28-5 NURSING RESEARCH PROFILE
Blood Transfusions and Vital Sign Frequency

Purpose

Nurses are responsible for assuring patient safety during a blood transfusion through effective monitoring of vital signs. When and how often to take vital signs varies, based upon institutional protocols. There are no evidence-based research findings that provide direction regarding optimal timing and frequency of vital sign monitoring for patients who receive blood transfusions. Therefore, the purpose of this research was to discover the relationship between vital sign findings and blood transfusion-associated adverse events in order to find patterns suggestive of optimal vital sign timing and frequency for patients receiving blood transfusions.

Design

A retrospective descriptive study was conducted in a 921-bed hospital where approximately 77,800 units of blood products were transfused during 2008 through 2012. Of those patients transfused during this time, 116 experienced a blood transfusion reaction. Using a medical record data collection tool, information from these 116 patients was collected including demographics, type of blood product administered, transfusion start and stop times, vital signs before, during, and after transfusion, symptomatology and treatment protocol for the transfusion reaction, and patient outcomes.

Findings

Packed red blood cells were the most commonly transfused product. Of the 116 sampled patients who experienced a transfusion reaction, 67% were over 60 years of age. The most common changes among vital signs were an increase in temperature, blood pressure, and heart rate. Six of the 116 patients with transfusion reactions experienced severe life-threatening complications from the blood transfusion, but none died from them. The average time from the start of transfusion to an adverse reaction was approximately 92 minutes, with the quickest documented response occurring 5 minutes after initiation of the transfusion and the most delayed reaction taking place 2 hours and 30 minutes after the start of the transfusion.

Nursing Implications

Hospitals endorse different protocols that dictate when and how often nurses take vital signs for patients who receive blood products. While it is commonly believed that the most likely time for a patient to experience a transfusion reaction is within the first 15 minutes after the start of a transfusion, findings from this study established an average time to the reaction of 1.5 hours, with the most severe reaction occurring 2 hours after initiation of the transfusion. Only one severe reaction in this study occurred during the first 15 minutes of the transfusion period. Findings from this study suggest that nurses should take vital signs of patients receiving blood transfusions at periodic intervals during the entire timeframe that a patient receives a blood transfusion.

---

and vascular collapse may result. Diminished renal perfusion results in acute kidney injury, and disseminated intravascular coagulation may also occur. The reaction must be recognized promptly and the transfusion discontinued immediately (see the Nursing Management of Transfusion Reactions section).

Acute hemolytic transfusion reactions are preventable. Meticulous attention to detail in labeling blood samples and blood components and accurately identifying the recipient cannot be overemphasized. Bar coding methods can be useful safeguards in matching a patient's wristband with the label on the blood component; however, these methods are not fail proof and do not reduce the nurse's responsibility to ensure the correct blood component is transfused to the correct patient (Robinson et al., 2018).

Allergic Reaction

Some patients develop urticaria (hives) or generalized itching during a transfusion; the cause is thought to be a sensitivity reaction to a plasma protein within the blood component being transfused. Symptoms of an allergic reaction are urticaria, itching, and flushing. The reactions are usually mild and respond to antihistamines. If the symptoms resolve after administration of an antihistamine (e.g., diphenhydramine), the transfusion may be resumed. Rarely, the allergic reaction is severe, with bronchospasm, laryngeal edema, and shock. These reactions are managed with epinephrine, corticosteroids, and vasopressor support, if necessary.

Giving the patient antihistamines or corticosteroids before the transfusion may prevent future reactions. For severe reactions, future blood components are washed to remove any remaining plasma proteins. Leukocyte filters are not useful to prevent such reactions, because the offending plasma proteins can pass through the filter.

Transfusion-Associated Circulatory Overload (TACO)

If too much blood is infused too quickly, hypervolemia can occur. This condition, known as transfusion-associated circulatory overload (TACO), can be aggravated in patients who already have increased circulatory volume (e.g., those with heart failure, renal dysfunction, advanced age, acute myocardial infarction) (Carman, Uhlenbrock, & McClintock, 2018). A careful assessment for signs of circulatory overload or positive fluid status prior to initiating the transfusion is required, particularly in patients at risk for developing transfusion-related acute lung injury (TRALI) (see discussion below). PRBCs are safer to use than whole blood. If the administration rate is sufficiently slow, circulatory overload may be prevented. For patients who are at risk for, or already in, circulatory overload, diuretics are given prior to the transfusion or between units of PRBCs. Patients receiving fresh-frozen plasma or even platelets may also develop circulatory overload. The infusion rate of these blood components must also be titrated to the patient's tolerance. Rates of transfusion may need to decrease to less than 100 to 120 mL/h (Henneman, 2017).

Signs of circulatory overload include dyspnea, orthopnea, tachycardia, an increase in blood pressure, and sudden anxiety. Jugular vein distention, crackles at the base of the lungs, and hypoxemia will also develop. Pulmonary edema can quickly develop, as manifested by severe dyspnea and coughing of pink, frothy sputum.

If fluid overload is mild, the transfusion can often be continued after slowing the rate of infusion and administering diuretics. However, if the overload is severe, the patient is placed upright with the feet in a dependent position, the transfusion is discontinued, and the primary provider is notified. The IV line is kept patent with a very slow infusion of normal saline solution or a saline lock device to maintain access to the vein in case IV medications are necessary. Oxygen and morphine may be needed to treat severe dyspnea (see Chapter 25).

TACO can develop as late as 6 hours after transfusion (Henneman, 2017). Therefore, patients need close monitoring after the transfusion is completed, particularly those who are at higher risk for developing this complication (e.g., older adults, those with a positive fluid balance prior to transfusion, patients with renal dysfunction, patients with left ventricular dysfunction). Monitoring vital signs, auscultating breath sounds, and assessing for jugular venous distention should be included in patient monitoring.

Bacterial Contamination

The incidence of bacterial contamination of blood components is very low; however, administration of contaminated products puts the patient at great risk. Contamination can occur at any point during procurement or processing but often results from organisms on the donor's skin. Many bacteria cannot survive in the cold temperatures used to store PRBCs, but some organisms can. Platelets are at greater risk of contamination because they are stored at room temperature. In response to this, blood centers have developed rapid methods of culturing platelet units, thereby diminishing the risk of using a contaminated platelet unit for transfusion (CDC, 2019).

Preventive measures include meticulous care in the procurement and processing of blood components. When PRBCs or whole blood is transfused, it should be given within a 4-hour period, because warm room temperatures promote bacterial growth. A contaminated unit of blood product may appear normal, or it may have an abnormal color.

The signs of bacterial contamination are fever, chills, and hypotension. These manifestations may not occur until the transfusion is complete, and occasionally not until several hours after the transfusion. As soon as the reaction is recognized, any remaining transfusion is discontinued (see the Nursing Management of Transfusion Reactions section). If the condition is not treated immediately with fluids and broad-spectrum antibiotics, sepsis can occur. Sepsis is treated with IV fluids and antibiotics; corticosteroids and vasopressors are often also necessary (see Chapter 11).

Transfusion-Related Acute Lung Injury (TRALI)

TRALI is a potentially fatal, idiosyncratic reaction that is defined as the development of acute lung injury occurring within 6 hours after the blood transfusion. All blood components have been implicated in TRALI, including IVIG, cryoprecipitate, and stem cells. TRALI is the most common cause of transfusion-related death (Heering & Karakashian, 2017).

The underlying pathophysiologic mechanism for TRALI is unknown but is thought to involve specific human leukocyte antigen (HLA) or human neutrophil antigen (HNA) antibodies in the donor's plasma that react to the leukocytes in the recipient's blood. Occasionally, the reverse occurs, and antibodies present in the recipient's plasma agglutinate the antigens on the few remaining leukocytes in the blood component being transfused. Another theory suggests that an initial insult to the patient's vascular endothelium can predispose the neutrophils to aggregate at the injured endothelium. Various substances within the transfused blood component (lipids, cytokines) then activate these neutrophils. Each of these pathophysiologic mechanisms can contribute to the process. The end result of this process is interstitial and intra-alveolar edema, as well as extensive sequestration of WBCs within the pulmonary capillaries (Heering & Karakashian, 2017).

Onset is abrupt (usually within 6 hours of transfusion, often within 2 hours). Signs and symptoms include acute shortness of breath, hypoxia (arterial oxygen saturation [SaO_2] less than 90%; partial pressure of arterial oxygen [PaO_2] to fraction of inspired oxygen [FIO_2] ratio of less than 300), hypotension, fever, and eventual pulmonary edema. Diagnostic criteria include hypoxemia, bilateral pulmonary infiltrates (seen on chest x-ray), no evidence of cardiac cause for the pulmonary edema, and no other plausible alternative cause within 6 hours of completing transfusion. Aggressive supportive therapy (e.g., oxygen, intubation, fluid support) may prevent death. Immunologic therapy (e.g., corticosteroids) has not been shown to be effective in this setting; diuretics can worsen the situation (Raja, Rahul, Kumar, et al., 2019).

Although TRALI can occur with the transfusion of any blood component, it is more likely to occur when plasma and, to a lesser extent, platelets are transfused. One commonly used preventive strategy involves limiting the frequency and amount of blood products transfused. Another entails obtaining plasma and possibly platelets only from men because women who have been pregnant may have developed offending antibodies. A third strategy involves screening donors for the presence of these antibodies and discarding any plasma-containing blood products from those donors who screen positive. The efficacy of these approaches in preventing TRALI remains unclear (Otrock, Liu, & Grossman, 2017).

Delayed Hemolytic Reaction

Delayed hemolytic reactions usually occur within 14 days after transfusion, when the level of antibody has been increased to the extent that a reaction can occur (Siddon, Kenney, Hendrickson, et al., 2018). The hemolysis of the erythrocytes is extravascular via the RES and occurs gradually.

Signs and symptoms of a delayed hemolytic reaction are fever, anemia, increased bilirubin level, decreased or absent haptoglobin, and possibly jaundice. Rarely, there is hemoglobinuria. Generally, these reactions are not dangerous, but it is important to recognize them because subsequent transfusions with blood products containing these antibodies may cause a more severe hemolytic reaction. However, recognition is also difficult because the patient may not be in a health care setting to be tested for this reaction, and even if the patient is hospitalized, the reaction may be too mild to be recognized clinically. Because the amount of antibody present can be too low to detect, it is difficult to prevent delayed hemolytic reactions. Fortunately, the reaction is usually mild and requires no intervention (Siddon et al., 2018).

Disease Acquisition

Despite advances in donor screening and blood testing, certain diseases can still be transmitted by transfusion of blood components (see Chart 28-6).

Chart 28-6	Diseases Potentially Transmitted by Blood Transfusion

Hepatitis (Viral Hepatitis B, C)

- There is greater risk from pooled blood products and blood of paid donors than from volunteer donors.
- A screening test detects most hepatitis B and C.
- Transmittal risk for Hepatitis B is estimated at 1:350,000 donated units.

AIDS (HIV and HTLV)

- Donated blood is screened for antibodies to HIV.
- Transmittal risk is estimated at 1:1.5 million donated units.
- People with high-risk behaviors (multiple sex partners, anal sex, IV/injection drug use) and people with signs and symptoms that suggest AIDS should not donate blood.

Cytomegalovirus (CMV)

- Transmittal risk is greater for premature newborns with CMV antibody–negative mothers and for immunocompromised recipients who are CMV negative (e.g., those with acute leukemia, organ or tissue transplant recipients).
- Blood products rendered "leukocyte reduced" help reduce transmission of virus.

Graft-Versus-Host Disease (GVHD)

- GVHD occurs only in recipients who are severely immunocompromised (e.g., Hodgkin disease, bone marrow transplantation).
- Transfused lymphocytes engraft in recipient and attack host lymphocytes or body tissues; signs and symptoms are fever, diffuse reddened skin rash, nausea, vomiting, and diarrhea.
- Preventive measures include irradiating blood products to inactivate donor lymphocytes (no known radiation risks to transfusion recipient) and processing donor blood with leukocyte reduction filters.

Creutzfeldt–Jakob Disease (CJD)

- CJD is a rare, fatal disease that causes irreversible brain damage.
- There is no evidence of transmittal by transfusion.
- All blood donors must be screened for positive family history of CJD.
- Potential donors who spent a cumulative time of 5 years or more (January 1980 to present) in certain areas of Europe cannot donate blood; blood products from a donor who develops CJD are recalled.

AIDS, acquired immunodeficiency syndrome; HIV, human immunodeficiency virus; HTLV, human T-lymphotropic virus.
Adapted from Katz, L. M., & Dodd, R. Y. (2018). Transfusion-transmitted diseases. In B. H. Shaz, C. D. Hillyer, & M. R. Gil (Eds.). *Transfusion medicine and hemostasis: Clinical and laboratory aspects* (3rd ed.). Cambridge, MA: Elsevier.

Complications of Long-Term Transfusion Therapy

The complications that have been described represent a real risk to any patient any time a blood component is given. However, patients with long-term transfusion requirements (e.g., those with myelodysplastic syndrome, thalassemia, aplastic anemia, sickle cell disease) are at greater risk for infection transmission and for becoming more sensitized to donor antigens, simply because they are exposed to more units of blood and, consequently, more donors. A summary of complications associated with long-term transfusion therapy is given in Table 28-5.

Iron overload is a complication unique to people who have had long-term PRBC transfusions. One unit of PRBCs contains 250 mg of iron. Patients with long-term transfusion requirements can quickly acquire more iron than they

can use, leading to iron overload. Over time, the excess iron deposits in body tissues can cause organ damage, particularly in the liver, heart, testes, and pancreas. Promptly initiating a program of iron chelation therapy can prevent end-organ damage from iron toxicity (see Chapter 29, Hereditary Hemochromatosis, Nursing Management, and Chapter 30, Myelodysplastic Syndrome, Nursing Management).

Nursing Management of Transfusion Reactions

If a transfusion reaction is suspected, the transfusion must be stopped immediately, and the primary provider notified. A thorough patient assessment is crucial because many complications have similar signs and symptoms. The following

TABLE 28-5	Common Complications Resulting from Long-Term Packed Red Blood Cell Transfusion Therapy[a]	
Complication	**Manifestation**	**Management**
Infection	Hepatitis (B, C)	May immunize against hepatitis B; treat hepatitis C; monitor hepatic function
	CMV	WBC filters to protect against CMV
Iron overload	Heart failure	Prevent by chelation therapy
	Endocrine failure (diabetes, hypothyroidism, hypoparathyroidism, hypogonadism)	
Transfusion reaction	Sensitization	Diminish by RBC phenotyping, using WBC-filtered products
	Febrile reactions	Diminish by using WBC-filtered products

[a]Patients with long-term transfusion therapy requirements are at risk not only for the transfusion reactions discussed in the text but also for the complications noted in the table. In many cases, the use of WBC-filtered (i.e., leukocyte-poor) blood products is standard for patients who receive long-term packed RBC transfusion therapy. An aggressive chelation program initiated early in the course of therapy can prevent problems with iron overload.
CMV, cytomegalovirus; RBC, red blood cell; WBC, white blood cell.
Adapted from Carman, M., Uhlenbrock, J. S., & McClintock, S. M. (2018). CE: A review of current practice in transfusion therapy. *The American Journal of Nursing, 118*(5), 36–44.

steps are taken to determine the type and severity of the reaction:

- Stop the transfusion. Maintain the IV line with normal saline solution through new IV tubing, given at a slow rate.
- Assess the patient carefully. Compare the vital signs with baseline, including oxygen saturation. Assess the patient's respiratory status carefully. Note the presence of adventitious breath sounds; the use of accessory muscles; the extent of dyspnea; and changes in mental status, including anxiety and confusion. Note any chills, diaphoresis, jugular vein distention, and reports of back pain or urticaria.
- Notify the primary provider of the assessment findings and implement any treatments prescribed. Continue to monitor the patient's vital signs and respiratory, cardiovascular, and renal status.
- Notify the blood bank that a suspected transfusion reaction has occurred.
- Send the blood container and tubing to the blood bank for repeat typing and culture. The patient's identity

and blood component identifying tags and numbers are verified.

If a hemolytic transfusion reaction or bacterial infection is suspected, the nurse does the following:

- Obtains appropriate blood specimens from the patient.
- Collects a urine sample as soon as possible to detect hemoglobin in the urine.
- Documents the reaction according to the institution's policy.

Pharmacologic Alternatives to Blood Transfusions

Pharmacologic agents that stimulate the production of one or more types of blood cells by the marrow are commonly used (see Chart 28-7). Researchers continue to seek a blood substitute that is practical and safe. Manufacturing artificial blood is problematic, given the myriad functions of blood components. Currently, there are two types of products in development: hemoglobin-based oxygen carriers and perfluorocarbons

---

Chart 28-7 PHARMACOLOGY

Pharmacologic Alternatives to Blood Transfusions

Growth Factors

Recombinant technology has provided a means to produce hematopoietic growth factors necessary for the production of blood cells within the bone marrow. By increasing the body's production of blood cells, transfusions and complications resulting from diminished blood cells (e.g., infection from neutropenia) may be avoided. However, the successful use of growth factors requires functional bone marrow. Moreover, the safety of these products has been questioned, and the U.S. Food and Drug Administration is limiting their use in some patient populations.

Erythropoietin

Erythropoietin (epoetin alfa; darbopoietin) is an effective alternative treatment for patients with chronic anemia secondary to diminished levels of erythropoietin, as in chronic kidney disease. This medication stimulates erythropoiesis. It also has been used for patients who are anemic from chemotherapy or zidovudine (AZT) therapy and for those who have diseases involving bone marrow suppression, such as myelodysplastic syndrome (MDS). The use of erythropoietin can also enable a patient to donate several units of blood for future use (e.g., preoperative autologous donation). The medication can be administered IV or subcutaneously, although plasma levels are better sustained with the subcutaneous route. Side effects are rare, but erythropoietin can cause or exacerbate hypertension. If the anemia is corrected too quickly or is overcorrected, the elevated hematocrit can cause headache and, potentially, seizures. Thrombosis has been noted in some patients whose hemoglobins were raised to a high level; thus, it is recommended that a target hemoglobin level of less than 12 g/dL be used. These adverse effects are rare except for patients with renal failure. Serial complete blood counts (CBCs) must be performed to evaluate the response to the medication. The dose and frequency of administration are titrated to the hemoglobin level.

Granulocyte Colony-Stimulating Factor (G-CSF)

G-CSF (filgrastim) is a cytokine that stimulates the proliferation and differentiation of myeloid stem cells; a rapid increase in

neutrophils is seen within the circulation. G-CSF is effective in improving transient but severe neutropenia after chemotherapy or in some forms of MDS. It is particularly useful in preventing bacterial infections that would be likely to occur with neutropenia. G-CSF is given subcutaneously on a daily basis. The primary side effect is bone pain; this probably reflects the increase in hematopoiesis within the marrow. Serial CBCs should be performed to evaluate the response to the medication and to ensure that the rise in white blood cells is not excessive. The effect of G-CSF on myelopoiesis is short; the neutrophil count drops once the medication is stopped.

Granulocyte-Macrophage Colony-Stimulating Factor (GM-CSF)

GM-CSF (sargramostim) is a cytokine that is naturally produced by a variety of cells, including monocytes and endothelial cells. It works either directly or synergistically with other growth factors to stimulate myelopoiesis. GM-CSF is not as specific to neutrophils as is G-CSF; thus, an increase in erythroid (red blood cell) and megakaryocytic (platelet) production may also be seen. GM-CSF serves the same purpose as G-CSF. However, it may have a greater effect on macrophage function and therefore may be more useful against fungal infections, whereas G-CSF may be better used to fight bacterial infections. GM-CSF is also given subcutaneously. Side effects include bone pain, fevers, and myalgias.

Thrombopoietin

Thrombopoietin (TPO) is a cytokine that is necessary for the proliferation of megakaryocytes and subsequent platelet formation. Nonimmunogenic second-generation thrombopoietic growth factors (romiplostim; eltrombopag) are used for the treatment of idiopathic thrombocytopenic purpura. Eltrombopag is also approved for use in certain situations for patients with aplastic anemia and in patients requiring hepatitis C treatment that can cause significant thrombocytopenia.

Adapted from Hudgins, K., & Carter, E. (2019). Blood conservation: Exploring alternatives to blood transfusions. *Critical Care Nursing Quarterly, 42*(2), 187–191.

(which can dissolve gases and thus carry oxygen indirectly); none are approved for use in humans, to date (Adams, 2019).

CRITICAL THINKING EXERCISES

1 `pq` A 40-year-old female is receiving one unit of packed red blood cells after admission for trauma as a result of an automobile injury. She is alert and responsive but lost a large amount of blood and presented with a hematocrit of 28% and a hemoglobin of 10 mg/dL. The blood has been transfusing for approximately 15 minutes when the patient complains of a headache and feeling "achy." Her pulse is 96 bpm, respirations 20 per minute, blood pressure 128/76, and temperature 37.8°C (100.2°F). A nursing co-worker tells you this is a transfusion reaction, and you should stop the transfusion immediately. How would you respond to the nursing co-worker? What would you prioritize as the first three nursing actions most appropriate for this patient?

2 `ebp` You are a nurse working in a community health clinic and today during a vaccination health fair a 70-year-old male patient presents for varicella and Td/Tdap vaccines. You notice on his health history that he had a blood transfusion 2 months prior during a total hip replacement procedure. Based on this history, would you advise this patient to accept both vaccinations, varicella only, Td/Tdap only, or no vaccines? What is the strength of the evidence supporting the role of vaccinations in patients who have received blood transfusions? Which interprofessional resources and team members would you consult to help determine the best decision for this patient?

REFERENCES

*Asterisk indicates nursing research.

Books

Banaski, J. L. (2019). Inflammation and immunity. In J. Banaski & L. Copstead (Eds.). *Pathophysiology* (6th ed., pp. 158–193). St. Louis, MO: Elsevier.

Bickley, L. S. (2016). *Bates' guide to physical examination and history taking* (12th ed.). Philadelphia, PA: Lippincott Williams & Wilkins.

Butterworth, J. F., Mackey, D. C., & Wasnick, J. D. (2018). *Morgan & Mikhail's clinical anesthesiology* (6th ed.). Retrieved on 1/21/2020 at: accessmedicine.mhmedical.com/content.aspx?bookid=2444&sectionid=193557318

Ciesla, B. (2019a). Red blood cell production, function and relevant red blood cell morphology. In B. Ciesla (Ed.). *Hematology in practice* (3rd ed., pp. 31–45). Philadelphia, PA: F.A. Davis.

Ciesla, B. (2019b). Overview of hemostasis and platelet physiology. In B. Ciesla (Ed.). *Hematology in practice* (3rd ed., pp. 233–247). Philadelphia, PA: F.A. Davis.

Fischbach, F., & Fischbach, M. (2018). *A manual of laboratory and diagnostic tests* (10th ed.). Philadelphia, PA: Lippincott Williams & Wilkins.

Jouria, J. M. (2018). *Clinical applications of human anatomy and physiology for healthcare professionals.* Irvine: BrownWalker Press.

Katz, L. M., & Dodd, R. Y. (2018). Transfusion-transmitted diseases. In B. H. Shaz, C. D. Hillyer, & M. R. Gil (Eds.). *Transfusion medicine and hemostasis: Clinical and laboratory aspects* (3rd ed.). Cambridge, MA: Elsevier.

Nair, M. (2017). Circulatory system. In I. Peate & M. Nair (Eds.). *Fundamentals of anatomy and physiology: For nursing and healthcare students* (2nd ed., pp. 185–222). Malden, MA: Wiley-Blackwell.

Norris, T. L. (2019). *Porth's pathophysiology: Concepts of altered health state* (10th ed.). Philadelphia, PA: Wolters Kluwer.

Rockwell, C. (2019). Alterations in hemostasis and blood coagulation. In J. Banaski & L. Copstead (Eds.). *Pathophysiology* (6th ed., pp. 298–311). St. Louis, MO: Elsevier.

Stowell, C. P. (2019). Transfusion medicine. In M. Laposata (Ed.). *Laboratory medicine: Diagnosis of disease in the clinical laboratory* (3rd ed., pp. 321–348). New York: McGraw-Hill.

Stubbs, J. (2018). Blood transfusion. In M. Pacheco (Ed.). *Blood and blood disorders. Salem health Magill's medical guide (online edition)* (8th ed.). Retrieved on 1/21/2020 at: www.salempress.com/Magills-Medical-Guide.

Trevithick, S. G. (2019). Alterations in oxygen transport. In J. Banaski & L. Copstead (Eds.). *Pathophysiology* (6th ed., pp. 260–293). St. Louis, MO: Elsevier.

Weber, J. W., & Kelley, J. (2018). *Health assessment in nursing* (6th ed.). Philadelphia, PA: Wolters Kluwer.

Wimberly, P. (2019). Disorders of white blood cells and lymphoid tissues. In T. L. Norris (Ed.). *Porth's pathophysiology concepts of altered health states* (10th ed., pp. 664–683). Philadelphia, PA: Wolters Kluwer.

Yeager, J. (2019). Infection and inflammation. In S. E. Meiner & J. J. Yeager (Eds.). *Gerontologic nursing* (6th ed., pp. 231–238). St. Louis, MO: Elsevier.

Journals and Electronic Documents

Adams, J. (2019). The bizarre quest for artificial blood. *Science World, 76*(3), 8.

American Cancer Society. (2017). Possible risks of blood transfusions. Retrieved on 1/15/2020 at: www.cancer.org/treatment/treatments-and-side-effects/treatment-types/blood-transfusion-and-donation/how-blood-transfusions-are-done.html.

American Red Cross. (2020a). Frequently asked questions. Retrieved on 1/14/2020 at: www.redcrossblood.org/faq.html#eligibility

American Red Cross. (2020b). How can one donation help multiple people. Retrieved on 1/15/2020 at: www.redcrossblood.org/faq.html#eligibility

American Red Cross. (2020c). Requirements by donation type. Retrieved on 1/14/2020 at: www.redcrossblood.org/donate-blood/how-to-donate/eligibility-requirements.html.

American Red Cross. (2020d). LGBTQ+ Donors. Retrieved on 3/14/2020 at: www.redcrossblood.org/donate-blood/how-to-donate/eligibility-requirements/lgbtq-donors.html

American Society of Hematology. (2020). *Blood basics.* Washington, DC. Retrieved on 1/12/2020 at: www.hematology.org/Patients/Basics/

Baumrucker, S. J., Stolick, M., Hutchinson, L., et al. (2019). Death or damnation: Surrogacy and religious beliefs. *American Journal of Hospice & Palliative Medicine, 36*(8), 740–745.

Bazinet, A., & Popradi, G. (2019). A general practitioner's guide to hematopoietic stem-cell transplantation. *Current Oncology, 26*(3), 187–191.

Carman, M., Uhlenbrock, J. S., & McClintock, S. M. (2018). CE: A review of current practice in transfusion therapy. *The American Journal of Nursing, 118*(5), 36–44.

Centers for Disease Control and Prevention (CDC). (2019). Bacterial contamination of platelets. Retrieved on 1/15/2020 at: www.cdc.gov/bloodsafety/bbp/bacterial-contamination-of-platelets.html.

Centers for Disease Control and Prevention (CDC). (2020). Recommended adult immunization schedule by medical condition and other indications, United States, 2020. Retrieved on 3/14/2020 at: www.cdc.gov/vaccines/schedules/hcp/imz/adult-conditions.html

*Cortez-Gann, J., Gilmore, K. D., Foley, K. W., et al. (2017). Blood transfusion vital sign frequency: What does the evidence say? *MEDSURG Nursing, 26*(2), 89–92.

Hare, G. M. T., Han, K., Leshchyshyn, Y., et al. (2018). Potential biomarkers of tissue hypoxia during acute hemodilutional anemia in cardiac surgery: A prospective study to assess tissue hypoxia as a mechanism of organ injury. *Canadian Journal of Anaesthesia/Journal Canadien D'anesthesie, 65*(8), 901–913.

Heering, H. R. C., & Karakashian, A. R. B. (2017). Lung injury, acute, transfusion-related. *CINAHL Nursing Guide.* Retrieved on 1/14/2020 at: search.ebscohost.com/login.aspx?direct=true&AuthType=ip,shib&db=nup&AN=T703586&site=eds-live&custid=s9076023

Henneman, E. A. (2017). Transfusion-associated circulatory overload: Evidence-based strategies to prevent, identify, and manage a serious adverse event. *Critical Care Nurse, 37*(5), 58–66.

Hudgins, K., & Carter, E. (2019). Blood conservation: Exploring alternatives to blood transfusions. *Critical Care Nursing Quarterly, 42*(2), 187–191.

John, C. A., Theodora, U. E., Gloria, A. N., et al. (2017). Adverse reactions to blood donation: A descriptive study of 3520 blood donors in a Nigerian tertiary hospital. *Medical Journal of Dr. D.Y. Patil University, 10*(1), 36–40.

Mayo Clinic. (2018a). Bone marrow biopsy and aspiration. Retrieved on 1/21/2020 at: www.mayoclinic.org/tests-procedures/bone-marrow-biopsy/about/pac-20393117

Mayo Clinic. (2018b). Splenectomy. Retrieved on 1/21/2020 at: www.mayoclinic.org/tests-procedures/splenectomy/about/pac-20395066

Otrock, Z. K., Liu, C., & Grossman, B. J. (2017). Transfusion-related acute lung injury risk mitigation: An update. *Vox Sanguinis, 112*(8), 694–703.

Padmanabhan, A., Smith, L., Aqui, N., et al. (2019). Guidelines on the use of therapeutic apheresis in clinical practice—evidence-based approach from the Writing Committee of the American Society for Apheresis: The eighth special issue. *Journal of Clinical Apheresis, 34*(3), 171–354.

Raja, V. A., Rahul, C., Kumar, M. K., et al. (2019). Transfusion-related acute lung injury. *Journal of Clinical & Scientific Research, 7*(1), 24–29.

Robinson, S., New, H., Shackleton, T., et al. (2018). The administration of blood components: A British Society for Haematology Guideline. *Transfusion Medicine, 28*(1), 3–21.

Sarode, R. (2018). Therapeutic apheresis. Retrieved on 1/21/2020 at: www.merckmanuals.com/professional/hematology-and-oncology/transfusion-medicine/therapeutic-apheresis.

Siddon, A., Kenney, B., Hendrickson, J., et al. (2018). Delayed haemolytic and serologic transfusion reactions: Pathophysiology, treatment and prevention. *Current Opinion in Hematology, 25*(6), 459–467.

Sikorski, R. A., Rizkalla, N. A., Yang, W. W., et al. (2017). Autologous blood salvage in the era of patient blood management. *Vox Sanguinis, 112*(6), 499–510.

Resources

AABB (formerly known as the American Association of Blood Banks), www.aabb.org/Pages/default.aspx

American Cancer Society, www.cancer.org

American Red Cross, www.redcross.org

American Red Cross LGBTQ+ Team Member Resource Group, www.redcrossblood.org/donate-blood/how-to-donate/eligibility-requirements/lgbtq-donors.html

Blood and Marrow Transplant Information Network, www.bmtinfonet.org

Infusion Nurses Society, www.ins1.org

Myelodysplastic Syndromes Foundation, www.mds-foundation.org

National Cancer Institute, www.cancer.gov

National Hemophilia Foundation, www.hemophilia.org

National Marrow Donor Program, www.bethematch.org

Oncology Nursing Society (ONS), www.ons.org

LEARNING OUTCOMES

On completion of this chapter, the learner will be able to:

1. Differentiate between hypoproliferative and hemolytic anemias and compare the physiologic mechanisms, clinical manifestations, medical management, and nursing interventions for each.
2. Describe the processes involved in neutropenia and lymphopenia and the principles involved in medical and nursing management of patients with these disorders.
3. Specify the etiologies and the medical and nursing management of patients with secondary polycythemias and bleeding and thrombotic disorders.
4. Use the nursing process as a framework for care of the patient with anemia, with sickle cell disease, or with disseminated intravascular coagulation.

NURSING CONCEPTS

Cellular Regulation   Clotting   Perfusion

GLOSSARY

absolute neutrophil count (ANC): a calculation of the number of circulating neutrophils, derived from the total number of white blood cells (WBCs) and the percentage of neutrophils counted in a microscope's visual field

anemia: decreased red blood cell (RBC) count

aplasia: lack of cellular development (e.g., of cells within the bone marrow)

cytokines: proteins produced by leukocytes that are critical for regulation of hematopoiesis, apoptosis, and immune responses

erythrocyte: a cellular component of blood essential to the transport of oxygen and carbon dioxide (*synonym*: RBC)

erythroid cells: any cell that is or will become a mature RBC

erythropoietin: hormone produced primarily by the kidneys in response to cellular hypoxia that is necessary for erythropoiesis

haptoglobin: blood protein synthesized by the liver; binds free hemoglobin released from erythrocytes which is then removed by the reticuloendothelial system

hemolysis: destruction of RBCs with release of cellular components into the circulation; may occur within or outside the vasculature

hemosiderin: iron-containing pigment derived from the breakdown of hemoglobin

hypochromia: pallor within the RBCs caused by decreased hemoglobin content

leukemia: uncontrolled proliferation of WBCs

lymphopenia: a lymphocyte count less than 1500/mm^3

megaloblastic anemia: a type of anemia characterized by abnormally large, nucleated RBCs

microcytosis: smaller-than normal RBCs

neutropenia: lower-than-normal number of neutrophils

normochromic: normal RBC color, indicating normal amount of hemoglobin

normocytic: normal size of RBC

pancytopenia: abnormal decrease in WBCs, RBCs, and platelets

petechiae: tiny capillary hemorrhages

poikilocytosis: variation in shape of RBCs

polycythemia: excess RBCs

reticulocytes: slightly immature RBCs, usually 1% of total number of circulating RBCs

spherocytes: small, spherically shaped RBCs

thrombocytopenia: lower-than-normal platelet count

thrombocytosis: higher-than-normal platelet count

Hematologic disorders vary widely in their etiologies and manifestations. While some are malignant, most hematologic disorders are benign. Disease processes can be quite complex, so a comprehensive understanding of the processes involved is important so that nurses may effectively assess, intervene, monitor, and educate patients about their conditions.

ANEMIA

Anemia is a condition characterized by a lower-than-normal hemoglobin concentration. Fewer than the normal number of red blood cells (RBCs), also called **erythrocytes**, are present in the circulation. Subsequently, less oxygen reaches the tissues, causing a variety of signs and symptoms. Rather than a disease state, anemia is a sign of an underlying disorder. It is the most common of all hematologic conditions and is prevalent throughout the world (Bunn, 2017a; Nair, 2018).

Pathophysiology

Anemia is classified in several ways (see Table 29-1). Most often it is classified according to whether the decreased number of erythrocytes is associated with hypoproliferation (decreased production), hemolysis (increased destruction), or loss of cells through bleeding.

Hypoproliferative anemias occur when the bone marrow produces an inadequate number of erythrocytes. Decreased erythrocyte production results in a low or inappropriately normal **reticulocyte** (i.e., immature RBC) count. Causes of hypoproliferative anemia may include bone marrow damage from chemicals (e.g., benzene) or medication (e.g., chloramphenicol), lack of important factors that promote erythrocyte production such as **erythropoietin**, or lack of nutrients, including iron, vitamin B_{12} and folic acid.

In hemolytic anemias, premature destruction of erythrocytes results in the liberation of hemoglobin from the erythrocytes into the plasma; the released hemoglobin is converted in large part to bilirubin and, therefore, the bilirubin concentration rises. The increased erythrocyte destruction leads to tissue hypoxia, which in turn stimulates erythropoietin production. This increased production is reflected in an increased reticulocyte count as the bone marrow responds to the loss of erythrocytes. **Hemolysis** (destruction of RBCs with release of cellular components into the circulation) can result from an abnormality within the erythrocyte itself (e.g., sickle cell disease [SCD], glucose-6-phosphate dehydrogenase [G-6-PD] deficiency), within the plasma (e.g., immune hemolytic anemias), or from direct injury to the erythrocyte within the circulation (e.g., hemolysis caused by a mechanical heart valve). Chart 29-1 identifies causes of hemolytic anemias.

It is often possible to determine the cause of anemia in each patient based on the following factors:

- The ability of the bone marrow to respond to the decrease in erythrocytes by producing reticulocytes.
- The degree to which immature erythrocytes proliferate in the bone marrow and their ability to mature (as seen in a bone marrow biopsy).

TABLE 29-1	Classification of Anemias		
		Laboratory Findings	
Type of Anemia	**CBC**	**Other**	
Hypoproliferative (Resulting from Defective RBC Production)			
Iron deficiency (microcytic)	↓ MCV, ↓ reticulocytes	↓ Iron, % saturation, ferritin ↑ TIBC	
Vitamin B_{12} deficiency (megaloblastic)	↑ MCV	↓ Vitamin B_{12}	
Folate deficiency (megaloblastic)	↑ MCV	↓ Folate	
Decreased erythropoietin production (e.g., from chronic kidney disease)	Normal MCV	↓ Erythropoietin level ↑ Creatinine	
Cancer/inflammation	Normal MCV	↑ Ferritin, % saturation ↓ Iron, TIBC ↓ Erythropoietin level (usually)	
Bleeding (Resulting in RBC Loss)			
Bleeding from gastrointestinal tract, epistaxis (nosebleed), trauma, bleeding from genitourinary tract (e.g., menorrhagia)	↓ Hgb and Hct (*Note*: Hgb and Hct may be normal if measured soon after bleeding starts) ↓ MCV (normal MCV initially) ↑ Reticulocytes	↓ Iron, % saturation, ferritin (later)	
Hemolytic (Resulting from RBC Destruction)			
Altered erythropoiesis (sickle cell disease, thalassemia, other hemoglobinopathies)	↓ MCV ↑ Reticulocytes Fragmented RBCs (various shapes)		
Hypersplenism (hemolysis)	↑ MCV		
Drug-induced anemia	↑ Presence of spherocytes		
Autoimmune anemia	↑ Presence of spherocytes		
Mechanical heart valve–related anemia	Fragmented red cells		

↓, decreased; ↑, increased; %, percent; CBC, complete blood count; Hct, hematocrit; Hgb, hemoglobin; MCV, mean corpuscular volume; RBC, red blood cell; TIBC, total iron-binding capacity.

Adapted from Prchal, J. T. (2016a). Clinical manifestations and classification of erythrocyte disorders. In K. Kaushansky, M. A. Lichtman, J. T. Prchal, et al. (Eds.). *Williams hematology* (9th ed.). New York: McGraw-Hill Medical.

Chart 29-1 Causes of Hemolytic Anemias

Inherited Hemolytic Anemia

Sickle cell disease
Thalassemia

Red Blood Cell Membrane Abnormality

Acanthocytosis
Hereditary elliptocytosis
Hereditary spherocytosis
Stomatocytosis

Enzyme Deficiencies

Glucose-6-phosphate dehydrogenase deficiency

Acquired Hemolytic Anemia

Antibody Related

Autoimmune hemolytic anemia
Iso-antibody/transfusion reaction
Cold agglutinin disease

Not Antibody Related

Disseminated intravascular coagulation
Hypersplenism
Infection
   Bacterial
   Parasitic
Liver disease
Mechanical heart valve
Microangiopathic hemolytic anemia
Paroxysmal nocturnal hemoglobinuria
Toxins
Trauma
Uremia

- The presence or absence of end products of erythrocyte destruction in the circulation (e.g., increased bilirubin level, decreased haptoglobin level).

Clinical Manifestations

Several factors influence the development of symptoms associated with anemia. The severity of the anemia, the rapidity with which the anemia developed, the duration (chronicity) of the anemia, metabolic requirements of the patient, the presence of other conditions, such as cardiac or pulmonary disease, and complications or related features of the condition that produced the anemia are some of these factors.

In general, the more quickly the anemia develops, the more severe the symptoms (Bunn, 2017a). An otherwise healthy patient may be able to tolerate as much as a 50% reduction in hemoglobin over several months without pronounced symptoms or significant incapacity; however, a rapid loss of 30% of the hemoglobin over minutes may lead to profound vascular collapse in the same person. A patient who gradually becomes anemic, such as a woman experiencing heavy menses over several months with hemoglobin levels between 9 and 11 g/dL, may have few or no symptoms except for slight tachycardia on exertion or fatigue.

People who are more active or who have significant life demands are more likely to have symptoms than those who are more sedentary. Patients with hypothyroidism with decreased oxygen demands may be asymptomatic without tachycardia or dyspnea with a hemoglobin of 10 g/dL. Similarly, those with co-existing cardiac, vascular, or pulmonary disease may develop pronounced symptoms of anemia (e.g., dyspnea, chest pain, muscle pain, or cramping) with a higher hemoglobin level than those without concurrent health problems. Some anemias, such as SCD, or autoimmune diseases are often complicated by other abnormalities that do not result from the anemia but are inherent with the associated disease. Pain and other symptoms may overshadow those caused by the anemia.

Complications of severe anemia include heart failure, paresthesias, and delirium. Patients with underlying heart disease are more likely to have angina and symptoms associated with heart failure than those without heart disease. Complications of specific types of anemia are included in the description of each type.

Assessment and Diagnostic Findings

A number of studies are performed to determine the type and cause of the anemia. Initial evaluation includes hemoglobin, hematocrit, reticulocyte count, and RBC indices, including mean corpuscular volume (MCV), and red cell distribution width (RDW). Other studies may include iron studies (serum iron level, total iron-binding capacity [TIBC], percent saturation, and ferritin), serum vitamin B_{12}, folate levels, haptoglobin, and erythropoietin levels (Elder, Winland-Brown, & Porter, 2019; Nair, 2018). The remaining complete blood count (CBC) values are also useful in determining if the anemia is an isolated condition or associated with another hematologic condition such as **leukemia** (i.e., malignancy of the WBCs) or myelodysplastic syndrome (MDS). Bone marrow aspiration may be performed to asses for cellular abnormalities. Additional studies such as colonoscopy or upper endoscopy may be performed to determine if underlying conditions causing the anemia are present. Lesions in the gastrointestinal (GI) tract including ulcers, polyps, or tumors may be sources of blood loss.

Medical Management

Management of anemia is directed toward correcting or controlling the cause of the anemia; if the anemia is severe, the erythrocytes that are lost or destroyed may be replaced with a transfusion of packed red blood cells (PRBCs). Management of the various types of anemia is covered in the discussions that follow.

Gerontologic Considerations

Anemia is the most common hematologic condition affecting older adults, particularly those admitted to hospitals and in long-term care facilities. The overall prevalence of anemia is 17% in older adults, including approximately 10% of community-dwelling older adults, 45% of nursing homes residents, and 40% of those who are hospitalized. Most have mild anemia with hemoglobin level of 11 g/dL or higher, but even mild anemia may be associated with decreased functional ability and increased morbidity and mortality. Mild anemia in older adults is associated with decreased physical performance, decreased mobility, increased frailty, increased depression, increased risk of falls, and delirium (Lanier, Park, & Callahan, 2018). Studies have identified an association between anemia and cognitive decline. Older adults with anemia are more likely to have fatigue, dyspnea, and confusion because of reduced cardiac reserve and inability to respond with an increase in heart rate and increased cardiac output. Those with preexisting renal and cardiac disease and those who have had recent surgery are at increased risk for morbidity and mortality when anemic (Stauder, Valent, & Theurl, 2018).

NURSING PROCESS

The Patient with Anemia

Assessment

The health history and physical examination provide important data about the type of anemia involved, the extent and type of symptoms it produces, and the impact of the symptoms on the patient's life. Weakness, fatigue, and general malaise are common symptoms, and pallor of the skin and mucous membranes (conjunctivae, oral mucosa) are common signs (Fig. 29-1).

Jaundice, angular cheilitis (inflammation and fissures in the corners of the mouth), and brittle, concave, ridged nails may be associated with **megaloblastic anemia** (characterized by abnormally large, nucleated RBCs) or hemolytic anemia. The tongue may be sore and beefy red in megaloblastic anemia, and smooth and red with iron deficiency anemia. Patients with iron deficiency anemia often experience pica, a craving for ice, starch, or dirt (Cadet, 2018). Restless leg syndrome is also common among those with iron deficiency anemia (Van Wyk, 2018). The health history should include a medication history because some medications may depress bone marrow activity, induce hemolysis, interfere with folate metabolism, or cause GI irritation that leads to bleeding. An accurate social history should include alcohol intake, noting the amount consumed and the duration of alcohol use. Family history is also important since some types of anemia are inherited. The nurse should also inquire about athletic endeavors since extreme forms of exercise such as marathon running may influence erythropoiesis and erythrocyte survival (Leung, 2019).

A nutritional assessment is needed because it may indicate deficiencies in essential nutrients such as iron, vitamin B$_{12}$, and folate. People who follow strict vegetarian diets and do not supplement with vitamin B$_{12}$ are at risk for megaloblastic anemia. Older adults may also have decreased intake of foods rich in vitamin B$_{12}$ or folate.

Cardiac status should be assessed carefully. When hemoglobin levels are low, the heart attempts to compensate by pumping faster and harder to deliver more oxygen to hypoxic tissue. This increased cardiac workload can result in symptoms including tachycardia, palpitations, dizziness, orthopnea, and exertional dyspnea. Heart failure may eventually develop, evidenced by cardiomegaly (an enlarged heart), hepatomegaly (an enlarged liver), and peripheral edema.

GI assessment may reveal complaints of nausea, vomiting (with specific questions regarding the appearance of any emesis [e.g., looks like "coffee grounds"]), melena (dark stools), diarrhea, anorexia, and glossitis (inflammation of the tongue). Stool should be tested for occult blood. Women should be asked about their menstrual periods (e.g., excessive

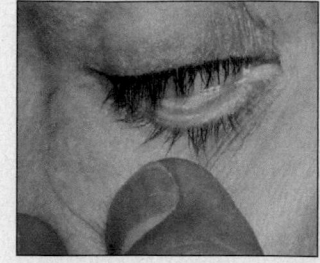
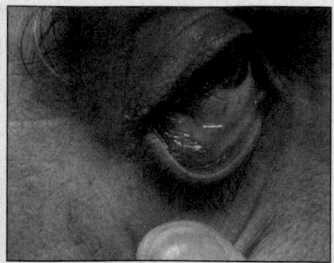
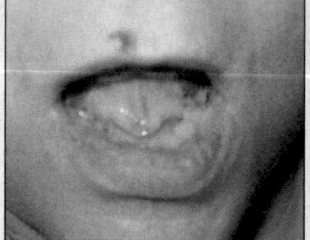
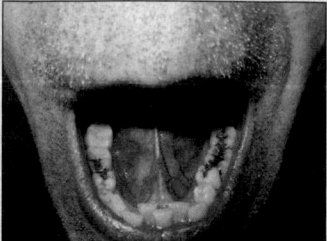
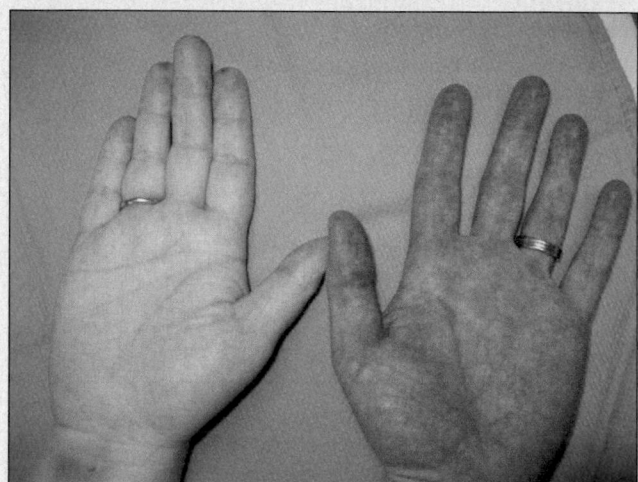

Figure 29-1 • Pallor seen in the patient with anemia. Reprinted with permission from Tkachuk, D. C., & Hirschman, J. V. (2007). *Wintrobe's atlas of clinical hematology* (Fig. 1.1, p. 9). Philadelphia, PA: Lippincott Williams & Wilkins.

flow, other vaginal bleeding) and the use of iron and vitamin supplements during pregnancy. Neurologic examination is important because pernicious anemia with vitamin B$_{12}$ deficiency affects the function of the central and peripheral nervous systems (see later discussion). Examination should include assessment for the presence and extent of peripheral numbness and paresthesia, ataxia, impaired coordination, and confusion. Delirium can sometimes result from other types of anemia, particularly in older adults. It is important to monitor relevant laboratory results over time and note any changes (see Chapter 28).

Diagnosis

NURSING DIAGNOSES

Based on assessment data, major nursing diagnoses may include:

- Fatigue associated with decreased hemoglobin and diminished oxygen-carrying capacity of the blood
- Impaired nutritional status associated with inadequate intake of essential nutrients

- Activity intolerance associated with inadequate hemoglobin and hematocrit
- Impaired ability to manage regime associated with prescribed therapy

COLLABORATIVE PROBLEMS/POTENTIAL COMPLICATIONS

Potential complications may include the following:

- Heart failure
- Paresthesias
- Confusion
- Injury associated with falls

Planning and Goals

The major goals for the patient with anemia include decreased fatigue, attainment or maintenance of adequate nutrition, attainment or maintenance of adequate tissue perfusion, effective management of prescribed treatment plan, and absence of complications.

Nursing Interventions

MANAGING FATIGUE

The most common symptom and complication of anemia is fatigue. Fatigue is often the symptom with the greatest negative impact on the patient's ability to function and subsequent quality of life. Fatigue is often described as overwhelming or oppressive. The sensation of fatigue may be severe even when the anemia is not severe enough to warrant transfusion. Fatigue may interfere with the patient's ability to engage in work as well as pleasurable activities with family and friends. Significant distress can stem from the inability to meet life's demands and responsibilities and the need to rely on others for assistance.

Nursing interventions can focus on assisting the patient to prioritize activities to establish a balance between activity and rest that is acceptable to the patient. Patients with chronic anemia will need assistance in establishing a program of activity and exercise to avoid deconditioning associated with inactivity. It is also important to assess for other conditions that may contribute to fatigue, such as pain, depression, and sleep disturbances.

MAINTAINING ADEQUATE NUTRITION

Inadequate intake of essential nutrients, including iron, vitamin B_{12}, folic acid and protein, can cause some forms of anemia. The symptoms associated with anemia (fatigue, anorexia) can interfere with maintaining adequate nutritional intake. A well-balanced diet should be encouraged. The nurse should advise the patient that alcohol can interfere with utilization of some essential nutrients and recommend limited alcohol intake (Stouten, Riedel, Droogendijk, et al., 2016). Dietary education involving family members when possible should be individualized to address specific needs and include cultural preferences for food preparation and selection (see Chapter 4). Dietary supplements (e.g., vitamins and iron) may be prescribed.

Equally important, the patient and family need to understand the role of nutritional supplements in the proper context. Some forms of anemia are not associated with nutritional deficiency. In some cases, excessive use of supplements will not improve the anemia and may be harmful. For example, patients with anemia who receive long-term transfusion therapy are at risk for iron overload from their transfusions. In this situation chelation therapy is implemented to reduce accumulation of excess iron (Murray, De Gelder, Pringle, et al., 2016; see Chapter 30 for discussion of chelation therapy). The use of oral iron supplements may exacerbate the situation.

MANAGING ACTIVITY INTOLERANCE

Patients with severe anemia, with acute blood loss from hemorrhage or severe hemolysis, may not tolerate decreased blood volume or reduced circulating erythrocytes. Lost volume can be replaced with transfusions or intravenous fluids based on symptoms and laboratory test results. Supplemental oxygen may be needed, especially if there is underlying cardiac or pulmonary disease. Monitoring the patient's vital signs and pulse oximetry, especially with activity, is an important nursing action. Medications, including antihypertensive drugs, may need to be adjusted or withheld based on the patient's vital signs.

PROMOTING EFFECTIVE MANAGEMENT OF PRESCRIBED THERAPY

Medications, including nutritional supplements, are frequently prescribed for patients with anemia. It is important that patients understand the purpose of these therapies, how to take them, and how to manage side effects of treatment. Nurses play an important role in promoting adherence to the prescribed plan by educating patients and family caregivers about ways to incorporate the therapeutic plan in daily activities. For example, side effects of oral iron supplements including GI distress may make adherence to treatment difficult for some patients and may contribute to some patients stopping treatment. Nurses can provide important education and support to assist patients to cope with side effects. Abrupt cessation of some medications, including high-dose steroids for treatment of hemolytic anemia, can have serious consequences for patients. The cost of some medications, such as hematologic growth factors, can be quite high. Patients requiring these medications may need assistance to find alternative ways to obtain the necessary medication. Nurses may need to collaborate with social workers or other health care team members to assist patients in meeting these needs.

MONITORING AND MANAGING POTENTIAL COMPLICATIONS

A significant complication of anemia is heart failure associated with chronic diminished blood volume and the heart's compensatory effort to increase cardiac output. Patients with anemia should be assessed for signs and symptoms of heart failure (see Chapter 25).

In megaloblastic anemias associated with folate or vitamin B_{12} deficiency, there is potential for neurologic complications. Neurologic assessment of patients with megaloblastic anemia should be performed. Patients may complain of paresthesias, often manifested by numbness and, as the anemia progresses, symptoms worsen and other signs become apparent. Position and vibration sense may be diminished. Difficulty maintaining balance and gait disturbances may occur. Mental status changes, beginning with confusion and progressing to more severe memory changes and delirium can occur with severe folate or vitamin B_{12} deficiency (Elder et al., 2019).

Evaluation

Expected patient outcomes may include:

1. Reports less fatigue
   a. Follows a graduated plan of rest, activity, and exercise
   b. Prioritizes activities
   c. Paces activities according to energy level

2. Attains and maintains adequate nutrition
   a. Eats a healthy diet
   b. Develops a meal plan that promotes optimal nutrition
   c. Maintains appropriate amounts of iron, vitamins, and protein from diet and supplements
   d. Adheres to nutritional supplements when prescribed
   e. Verbalizes understanding of rationale for using recommended nutritional supplements when prescribed
   f. Verbalizes understanding of rationale for avoiding nonrecommended nutritional supplements
3. Maintains appropriate activity level
   a. Vital signs will be within baseline for patient
   b. Pulse oximetry value within normal limits
4. Absence of complications
   a. Avoids or limits activities that trigger dyspnea, palpitations, dizziness, or tachycardia
   b. Uses rest and comfort measures to relieve dyspnea
   c. Has vital signs within baseline for patient
   d. Has no signs of increased fluid retention (e.g., peripheral edema, decreased urine output, neck vein distention)
   e. Remains oriented to time, place, and situation
   f. Verbalizes understanding of importance of serial CBC and other laboratory test measurements
   g. Maintains safe home environment; obtains and uses assistance as necessary

Hypoproliferative Anemias

The hypoproliferative anemias include iron deficiency anemia, anemias in renal disease, anemia of inflammation, aplastic anemia, and megaloblastic anemias.

Iron Deficiency Anemia

Iron deficiency anemia results when the intake of dietary iron is inadequate for synthesis of hemoglobin. The body is able to store about one fourth to one third of its iron requirements, and it is not until those stores are depleted that iron deficiency anemia develops. Iron deficiency anemia may occur when total body iron stores are adequate, but the amount of iron delivered to the erythroid precursors is inadequate. This is referred to as functional iron deficiency (Hashemi, Mashhadi, Mohammadi, et al., 2017). Iron deficiency anemia is the most common type of anemia in all age groups, and it is the most common form of anemia worldwide, affecting as many as one in eight people (Bunn & Heeney, 2017). It is especially prevalent in developing countries where iron stores may be chronically depleted because of lack of sources for iron-rich foods and from blood loss associated with intestinal parasites (Harper, Besa, & Conrad, 2019).

Iron deficiency anemia is also common among adults in the United States, with the most common cause being blood loss. Blood loss should always be considered as the cause of iron deficiency anemia until proven otherwise. The most common cause of this anemia in men and postmenopausal women is GI bleeding from ulcers, gastritis, tumors, or inflammatory bowel disease. The most common causes of iron deficiency anemia in premenopausal women are menorrhagia (i.e., excessive menstrual bleeding) and pregnancy with inadequate iron intake. Patients with chronic alcohol abuse and patients who take aspirin, steroids, or nonsteroidal anti-inflammatory drugs (NSAIDs) may have chronic blood loss from the GI tract, leading to iron loss and subsequent anemia. Other causes include iron malabsorption, as seen after gastrectomy or bariatric surgery, or from celiac disease and inflammatory bowel diseases (Harper et al., 2019).

Clinical Manifestations

Patients with iron deficiency primarily have symptoms of anemia. If the deficiency is severe or prolonged, they may also have a smooth, red tongue; brittle and ridged nails; and angular cheilosis. These signs subside after iron replacement therapy. The health history may be significant for multiple pregnancies, GI bleeding, and pica (Camaschella, 2019).

Assessment and Diagnostic Findings

The definitive method of establishing the diagnosis of iron deficiency anemia is bone marrow aspiration (see Chapter 28 for further discussion of bone marrow aspiration). The aspirate is stained to detect iron, which is at a low level or even absent. However, few patients with suspected iron deficiency anemia undergo bone marrow aspiration. In many patients, the diagnosis can be established with other tests, particularly in patients with a history of conditions that predispose them to this type of anemia.

A strong correlation exists between laboratory values that measure iron stores and hemoglobin levels. After iron stores are depleted (as reflected by low serum ferritin levels), the hemoglobin level falls. The diminished iron stores cause small erythrocytes to be produced by the marrow. Therefore, as the anemia progresses, the MCV, which measures the size of the erythrocytes, also decreases. Hematocrit and RBC levels are also low in relation to the hemoglobin level. Other laboratory tests that measure iron stores are useful but not as precise as ferritin levels. Typically, patients with iron deficiency anemia have a low serum iron level and an elevated TIBC, which measures the transport protein supplying the marrow with iron as needed (also referred to as transferrin) (Camaschella, 2019). However, other disease states, such as infection and inflammatory conditions, can also cause a low serum iron level and TIBC, as well as an elevated ferritin level. If these are suspected, measuring the soluble transferring receptor can aid in differentiating the cause of anemia. This test result will be increased in the setting of iron deficiency, but not in chronic inflammation (Camaschella, 2019).

Medical Management

Oral iron supplementation is often the primary mode of treatment for iron deficiency anemia. Several oral iron preparations, including ferrous sulfate, ferrous gluconate, and ferrous fumarate, are available. Ferric maltol, another oral preparation, was approved by the U.S. Food and Drug Administration (FDA) in 2019 for use in iron deficiency anemia in those with inflammatory bowel disease. After taking oral iron preparations, hemoglobin typically begins to increase within a few weeks and the anemia may be corrected within a few months. Replenishing iron stores takes several months so it

| Chart 29-2 | Parenteral Iron Formulations |

- Older formulations of parenteral iron had a high molecular weight and carried a significant risk for hypersensitivity reactions, including anaphylaxis. Newer formulations have a low molecular weight and a markedly lower risk for anaphylaxis.
- Ferric gluconate: Each 5 mL contains 62.5 mg of elemental iron; 125 mg is diluted in 100-mL normal saline and infused over 1 hour, or 5 mL undiluted is given as a slow IV push injection over 5 minutes. Although the likelihood of an allergic reaction is very low, a test dose is often given prior to the first infusion.
- Iron sucrose: Each 5 mL contains 100 mg of elemental iron; 100 to 200 g can be given, undiluted, as a slow IV push over 2 to 5 minutes. This procedure can be repeated as often as every 3 days for a cumulative dose of 1000 mg within a 2-week period.
- Ferumoxytol injection: The 17 mL vial is diluted in 50 to 200 mL of normal saline or 5% dextrose and water and infused over 15 minutes. Close observation for signs and symptoms of hypersensitivity reaction, including monitoring blood pressure and pulse, is recommended.

Adapted from Comerford, K. C., & Durkin, M. T. (2020). *Nursing 2020 drug handbook*. Philadelphia, PA: Wolters Kluwer.

| Chart 29-3 | **PATIENT EDUCATION** Taking Oral Iron Supplements |

The nurse instructs the patient to:

- Take iron on an empty stomach (1 hour before or 2 hours after a meal), preferably with orange juice or other source of vitamin C. Iron absorption is reduced by food, especially dairy products.
- Reduce gastrointestinal distress by using the following schedule when more than one tablet per day is prescribed: Take one tablet per day for the first few days, then increase to two tablets per day, then three tablets per day in divided doses. This allows gradual adjustment to the iron. If unable to tolerate oral supplements due to gastrointestinal distress despite using this intervention, a reduced amount of iron may be used rather than stopping it completely. Reduced doses will require that the treatment duration is extended to adequately replenish iron stores.
- Increase intake of foods rich in vitamin C to enhance iron absorption (citrus fruits and juices, strawberries, tomatoes, broccoli).
- Note that stool will be dark in color and often appear black.
- Eat foods high in fiber to reduce problems with constipation. A stool softener may be needed.
- Be aware that liquid iron preparations may stain the teeth. They may be taken through a straw or by placing the spoon at the back of the mouth. Rinse the mouth thoroughly after each dose.

is important that patients continue taking oral iron supplements for 6 to 12 months. If oral iron is poorly absorbed or poorly tolerated, or large amounts of supplemental iron are needed, intravenous (IV) iron may be given in repeated doses (see Chart 29-2). Initial evidence has shown that ferric maltol is not inferior to parenteral iron and may be an alternative for patients who cannot tolerate other oral preparations or do not wish to have parenteral iron; however, it is unknown whether use of ferric maltol will decrease demands for parenteral iron preparations (Harper et al., 2019).

Nursing Management

Preventive education is important for women who are menstruating and for those who are pregnant. Food sources rich in iron include organ meats (e.g., beef or calf's liver, chicken liver), other meats, beans (e.g., pinto, black, and garbanzo beans), leafy green vegetables, raisins, and molasses. Eating iron-rich foods with a source of vitamin C (e.g., orange juice) improves iron absorption.

The nurse assists the patient in selecting healthy diet options. Nutritional counseling can be provided for those who have an inadequate diet. Patients with history of strict vegetarian or other diets lacking in essential nutrients should be counseled about how to meet their dietary needs. The nurse also encourages the patient to continue the prescribed therapy for as long as needed to replenish iron stores even when fatigue and other symptoms have resolved.

Oral iron is best absorbed on an empty stomach, making it important for patients to be instructed to take the supplement approximately 1 hour before or 2 hours after meals. The least expensive, standard form of oral iron, ferrous sulfate, is tolerated by most patients. GI side effects, including constipation, cramping, nausea, and vomiting may result in difficulty adhering to the prescribed regimen. Decreasing the frequency of administration or taking iron supplements with food may reduce symptoms but will diminish iron

absorption, thus, it may take longer to replete iron stores. Taking iron with vitamin C can enhance absorption, but it may also increase the frequency of side effects (Heffernan, Evans, Holmes, et al., 2017). Some iron formulations have been designed to limit GI side effects by adding stool softeners to reduce constipation or sustained release formulations to reduce gastritis and nausea. However, enteric-coated tablets may be poorly absorbed. Slow release formulations are absorbed beyond the duodenum; however, the duodenum is the site where maximum iron absorption takes place (Auerbach & Adamson, 2016). Educational materials to assist patients with use of iron supplements are available (see Chart 29-3).

If taking iron on an empty stomach causes GI distress, the patient may need to take it with meals. However, this may reduce absorption by as much as 40%, therefore increasing the time needed to replenish iron stores. Antacids and dairy products should be avoided with iron as they can greatly diminish its absorption. Polysaccharide iron complex preparations are available. These reduce GI toxicity but are more expensive. Liquid forms of iron that cause less GI distress are also available. Oral iron replacement therapy may change the color of the stool but should not cause a false-positive result for occult blood on stool analysis.

IV supplementation may be used when the patient's iron stores are very low, if the patient cannot tolerate oral forms of iron, or both. The nurse must be aware of the type of parenteral formulation of iron ordered so that risk for anaphylaxis can be determined. High-molecular formulations are associated with a much higher risk for anaphylaxis and are seldom used. Administering a test dose of low-molecular formulations of iron dextran is recommended by many manufacturers. The nurse must assist the patient in understanding the need for repeated doses to replenish iron stores or to maintain iron stores in the setting of chronic blood loss, such as hemodialysis or chronic GI bleeding.

Anemias in Renal Disease

The degree of anemia in patients with chronic kidney disease (CKD) can vary greatly; however, in general, patients do not become severely anemic until the glomerular filtration rate (GFR) is less than 30 mL/min/1.73 m² (Fishbane & Spinowitz, 2018). The symptoms of anemia may be the most troubling of the patient's symptoms. In patients with CKD, anemia contributes to increased cardiac output, reduced oxygen utilization, decreased cognition and ability to concentrate, reduced immune responsiveness, and reduced libido. Anemia may be more severe in patients with both CKD and diabetes (Fishbane & Spinowitz, 2018). Anemia in patients with CKD is discussed in Chapter 48.

Anemia of Inflammation

Anemia of inflammation describes anemia associated with chronic diseases including inflammation, infection, and malignancy. This classification was previously known as anemia of chronic disease (Weiss, Ganz, & Goodnough, 2019). This classification also includes anemia of critical illness that can develop within days after the onset of serious illness, and the anemia associated with aging. Many chronic inflammatory diseases are associated with **normochromic**, **normocytic** anemia (i.e., RBCs are of normal color and size). These disorders include rheumatoid arthritis, chronic infections, and many cancers. It is important that the underlying condition be identified so that it can be treated appropriately.

The anemia of inflammation is usually mild to moderate and not progressive. The hemoglobin level does not usually fall below 9 g/dL and bone marrow samples have normal cellularity and normal stores of iron. Erythropoietin levels are low and iron use is blocked by **erythroid cells** (cells that are or will become mature RBCs). Erythrocyte survival may also be shortened.

Many patients with anemia of inflammation have few symptoms related to their anemia and do not require treatment. Treatment of the underlying disorder allows iron stored in the bone marrow to be utilized, promoting increased RBC production and facilitating the rise of hemoglobin levels. Iron supplementation is not beneficial for these patients.

 Gerontologic Considerations

Evidence suggests that inflammation may have a significant role in the development of anemia in older adults (Price, 2019). Higher-than-normal levels of inflammatory **cytokines** are found in older adults, and this pro-inflammatory state may predispose older adults to frailty. Frailty is manifested by weight loss, impaired mobility, generalized weakness, and loss of balance and is strongly associated with anemia of inflammation. Erythropoietin levels may not rise as expected in response to decreased hemoglobin (Price, 2019).

Aplastic Anemia

Aplastic anemia is a rare disease caused by a decrease in or damage to bone marrow stem cells, damage to the microenvironment within the bone marrow, and replacement of marrow with fat. Stem cell damage is caused by the body's T cells, which mediate an attack on the bone marrow resulting in **aplasia** (i.e., markedly reduced hematopoiesis). Therefore, in addition to severe anemia, significant **neutropenia** (i.e., lower-than-normal neutrophil count) and **thrombocytopenia** (i.e., lower-than-normal platelet count) also occur.

Pathophysiology

Aplastic anemia is a life-threatening condition associated with bone marrow failure evidenced by **pancytopenia** (i.e., anemia, neutropenia, and thrombocytopenia; lower-than-normal counts of erythrocytes, neutrophils, and platelets) (Peslak, Olson, & Babushok, 2017). It can be acquired, or in rare cases, congenital, but most cases are idiopathic (i.e., without apparent cause) (Young, 2018). It may also be associated with certain medications, chemicals, or radiation damage. Agents that have been associated with bone marrow aplasia include benzene and benzene derivatives (i.e., airplane glues, paint remover, dry cleaning solutions). Certain toxic materials, including inorganic arsenic, glycol ethers, plutonium, and radon, have also been suggested as possible causes (Young, 2018). Nonviral hepatitis may be a precipitating factor in about 10% of cases (Peslak et al., 2017).

Clinical Manifestations

The onset of symptoms of aplastic anemia is often insidious. Complications stemming from bone marrow failure may occur before the diagnosis is made. Typical complications include infection and symptoms of anemia, including fatigue, pallor, and dyspnea. Purpura (bruising) associated with thrombocytopenia may develop. Any combination of these signs and symptoms should prompt a CBC and hematologic evaluation. Lymphadenopathy and splenomegaly may also occur. Retinal hemorrhages are common.

Assessment and Diagnostic Findings

Aplastic anemia occurs in some situations when a medication or chemical is ingested in toxic amounts; however, it may occur even when medications are taken at the recommended dosage. This is known as an idiosyncratic reaction in those who are highly susceptible, possibly due to a genetic defect in the biotransformation of the medication or elimination process. The CBC reveals pancytopenia. Patients may have neutrophil counts less than 1,500/mm³, hemoglobins less than 10 g/dL, and platelet counts less than 50,000/mm³ (Segel & Lichtman, 2016). A bone marrow biopsy typically reveals an extremely hypoplastic or aplastic bone marrow (i.e., with few or no cells), often replaced with fat.

Medical Management

It is believed that aplastic anemia is an immune-mediated condition in which T lymphocytes attack hematopoietic stem cells with subsequent reduction in production of erythrocytes, leukocytes, and platelets. Aplastic anemia can be successfully treated in many cases. Patients under 60 years of age who are otherwise healthy can often be cured with a hematopoietic stem cell transplant (HSCT) from a compatible donor (see Chapter 12) (Young, 2018). In other situations, treatment with immunosuppressive therapy using antithymocyte globulin (ATG) and androgens or cyclosporine is useful in managing the disease (Young, 2018). ATG is a purified gamma-globulin solution that is obtained from rabbits or horses immunized with human T lymphocytes. Side effects of such therapy include fever and chills. There is risk for anaphylaxis with associated bronchospasm and hypotension requiring emergency treatment. Serum sickness, associated with rash, fever, arthralgias, and pruritus may occur in some patients but can be prevented or reduced in some cases with premedication with corticosteroids (Segel & Lichtman, 2016). Serum sickness resolves slowly, often over a few weeks when it occurs.

Immunosuppressive therapies prevent T cells from destroying stem cells. If relapse does occur, resuming the same immunosuppressive therapy may induce another remission but the response rate is usually reduced (Segel & Lichtman, 2016). Corticosteroids may be beneficial in the short-term; however, in aplastic anemia, long-term use is associated with bony abnormalities including aseptic necrosis and osteopenia.

Supportive therapies play a critical role in the management of aplastic anemia. All potentially offending medications should be discontinued. Transfusions with PRBCs and platelets are frequently required (see Chapter 28 for discussion of transfusions); however, judicious use of blood products is necessary, especially for patients who are candidates for bone marrow transplant because of the risk for alloimmunization (Peslak et al., 2017). Aggressive treatment of infections is necessary. Deaths associated with aplastic anemia are most often caused by bacterial or fungal infection and bleeding.

Prophylaxis against invasive fungal infection is needed for patients who are severely neutropenic. Patients who become lymphopenic after ATG require prophylaxis for pneumocystis pneumonia.

Nursing Management

Patients with aplastic anemia are at high risk for problems associated with deficiencies of erythrocytes, leukocytes, and platelets. Thorough assessment for signs of infection and bleeding are critical (see later sections on Neutropenia and Thrombocytopenia for specific interventions). Nursing care includes monitoring for side effects of therapy, including hypersensitivity reactions while administering ATG. Patients who require long-term cyclosporine therapy should be monitored for long-term effects, including renal and liver dysfunction, hypertension, pruritus, visual changes, tremor, and skin cancer. Education regarding drug–drug interactions between ATG and many other drugs is necessary. Patients should be informed that stopping immunosuppressive therapy abruptly is not recommended.

Megaloblastic Anemias

Anemias associated with vitamin B_{12} or folic acid deficiency cause the same bone marrow and peripheral blood changes because both are needed for normal DNA synthesis. The erythrocytes produced with these nutritional deficiencies are abnormally large, thus they are termed megaloblastic red blood cells. Other cells from the myeloid stem cell lines (nonlymphoid leukocytes and platelets) are also abnormal. Bone marrow analysis shows hyperplasia (an abnormal increase in the number of cells) and the precursor erythroid and myeloid cells are abnormally large and irregular in appearance. Many of these abnormal cells are destroyed within the bone marrow leading to an insufficient number of mature cells entering the peripheral blood. Over time, pancytopenia may develop. Cells that enter the circulation are often irregularly shaped; neutrophils are hypersegmented, and platelets may be abnormally large. Erythrocytes are abnormally shaped and shapes can vary greatly; this is known as **poikilocytosis**. Because erythrocytes are very large, the MCV is very high, often exceeding 110 fL. Megaloblastic anemias usually develop over months, allowing the body to compensate; thus, symptoms do not often occur until the anemia is severe (Green, 2016). In patients with light skin, the skin may develop a pale-yellow color resulting from simultaneous pallor and mild jaundice from red blood cell hemolysis.

Pathophysiology

The pathophysiologic mechanisms that undergird megaloblastic anemias are most commonly because of either a folic acid or vitamin B_{12} deficiency, as noted previously.

Folic Acid Deficiency

Folic acid is stored in the body as compounds known as folates. Folate stores are smaller than those of vitamin B_{12} and can be depleted within months if dietary intake of folate is deficient (Green, 2016). Folate is found in green vegetables and liver. Folate deficiency is rarely seen in patients who consume uncooked vegetables. Alcohol ingestion increases folic acid requirements and it is not uncommon for those with alcohol abuse disorder to have a diet deficient in folate and other nutrients. Folic acid requirements are also higher in those with liver disease, chronic hemolytic anemias, and in women who are pregnant because erythrocyte production is increased with these conditions. Small bowel diseases such as celiac disease may interfere with normal absorption of folic acid (Green, 2016).

Vitamin B_{12} Deficiency

Deficiency of vitamin B_{12} can occur in several ways. Inadequate dietary intake is unusual but sometimes can occur in people who follow a vegan diet and do not consume any meat or dairy products. Impaired absorption from the GI tract is more common, especially in older adults. Nearly 20% of older adults have low vitamin B_{12} levels; 5% to 10% have symptoms related to vitamin B_{12} deficiency (Langan & Goodbred, 2017). Vitamin B_{12} deficiency can occur in patients with disorders such as inflammatory bowel disease, or in patients who have had GI surgery such as ileal resection, bariatric surgery, or gastrectomy. Use of metformin for treatment of type 2 diabetes as well as chronic use of histamine blockers, antacids, and proton pump inhibitors to reduce gastric acid can also inhibit vitamin B_{12} absorption (Lanier et al., 2018).

Absence of intrinsic factor also impairs vitamin B_{12} absorption. When associated with lack of intrinsic factor, the anemia is referred to as pernicious anemia. Intrinsic factor is normally secreted by cells in the gastric mucosa; it binds to vitamin B_{12} and transports it to the ileum where it is absorbed. Without intrinsic factor, vitamin B_{12} taken orally cannot be absorbed and deficiency with associated anemia eventually results. Diseases of the pancreas and ileum may impair absorption even when adequate intrinsic factor and vitamin B_{12} are present. Pernicious anemia tends to run in families. It is typically a disease of adults, especially older adults. The body typically has large stores of vitamin B_{12} so years may pass before deficiency results in anemia. The body is able to compensate over time and the anemia is often severe before the patient becomes symptomatic. Because patients with pernicious anemia and low vitamin B_{12} levels have an increased incidence of gastric cancer they may benefit from screening for gastric cancer with endoscopy at regular intervals (Miranti, Stolzenberg-Solomon, Weinstein, et al., 2017).

Clinical Manifestations

Symptoms of folic acid and vitamin B_{12} deficiencies are similar, and the two anemias may coexist. However, the neurologic manifestations of vitamin B_{12} deficiency do not occur with folic acid deficiency, and they persist if vitamin B_{12} is not replaced. Therefore, careful distinction between the two anemias must be made.

After the body's stores of vitamin B_{12} are depleted, the patient may begin to show signs and symptoms of the anemia. However, because the onset and progression of the anemia are so gradual, the body can compensate well until the anemia is severe, so the typical manifestations of anemia (weakness, listlessness, fatigue) may not be apparent initially. The hematologic effects of vitamin B_{12} deficiency are accompanied by effects on other organ systems, particularly the GI tract and nervous system. Patients with pernicious anemia develop a smooth, sore, red tongue and mild diarrhea. They are extremely pale, particularly in the mucous membranes. They may become confused; more often, they have paresthesias in the extremities (particularly numbness and tingling in the feet and lower legs). They may have difficulty maintaining their balance because of damage to the spinal cord, and they also lose position sense (proprioception). These symptoms are progressive, although the course of illness may be marked by spontaneous partial remissions and exacerbations. Without treatment, heart failure associated with severe anemia may result, often leading to death several years after onset of symptoms (Leung, 2019).

Assessment and Diagnostic Findings

Serum levels of both folic acid and vitamin B_{12} are analyzed. Small amounts of folate can increase the serum folate level; therefore, measurement of the amount of folate within the red blood cells is a more sensitive test to determine true folate deficiency although it is not commonly performed.

The traditional method of determining the cause of vitamin B_{12} deficiency was the Schilling test, but in recent years this has been replaced by other testing methods. A vitamin B_{12} assay is usually the initial test performed but the reliability of the results is sometimes questionable, when vitamin B_{12} levels are not unequivocally low. Elevated methylmalonic acid and homocysteine levels are more sensitive for the diagnosis of vitamin B_{12} deficiency (Lanier et al., 2018). An intrinsic factor antibody test is often more useful in determining the presence of pernicious anemia. A positive test indicates that antibodies are present that interfere with the binding of the intrinsic factor–vitamin B_{12} complex to receptors in the ileum, preventing absorption. While not specific for only pernicious anemia, it is useful in helping arrive at the diagnosis.

Medical Management

Folate deficiency is easily treated in most cases by increasing the amount of folic acid in the diet and taking 1 mg of folic acid daily as a supplement. Folic acid can be given intramuscularly to those people with conditions associated with malabsorption. While many multivitamin supplements contain folic acid, the amount may not be enough to replace body stores completely. When folate deficiency is associated with alcohol abuse, supplementation should continue as long as the patient is consuming alcohol.

Vitamin B_{12} deficiency is treated with vitamin B_{12} replacement. People who follow a vegan diet can prevent or treat deficiency with oral supplements with vitamins or fortified soy milk. When deficiency is caused by impaired absorption or absence of intrinsic factor (i.e., pernicious anemia), replacement is typically given by monthly intramuscular injections. It is possible to treat patients with oral preparations in the absence of intrinsic factor but much larger doses are required. Intranasal sprays and gels are also available options to avoid the need for intramuscular injections.

As vitamin B_{12} is replaced, the reticulocyte count rises, often within 1 week, and within 4 to 8 weeks blood counts return to normal (Green, 2016). The tongue begins to feel better and appears less red after several days. Recovery from neurologic symptoms takes more time, and, if the neuropathy is severe, the patient may not fully recover. To prevent a recurrence of pernicious anemia, vitamin B_{12} supplementation must continue for life.

Nursing Management

Assessment of patients who have or are at risk for megaloblastic anemia includes inspection of the skin, tongue, and mucous membranes. Mild jaundice may be evident and is best seen in the sclera with natural lighting. Vitiligo and premature graying of the hair are frequently present in those with pernicious anemia. Careful neurologic assessment is important to identify neurologic complications. Assessment should include tests of position, vibration sense, and cognitive function. The nurse should pay close attention to the patient's gait and stability with ambulation. Safety is a concern when gait, coordination and position sense are affected. Physical and occupational therapy referrals may be needed to assist in obtaining assistive devices and making sure patients are instructed in their use. When sensation is impaired, patients should be instructed to avoid excessive heat and cold.

Mouth and tongue soreness may impair nutritional intake. The nurse may instruct the patient to choose soft bland foods that are less likely to cause further discomfort.

Promoting Home, Community-Based and Transitional Care

Education for patients with pernicious anemia must include the chronic nature of this condition and the necessity of monthly vitamin B_{12} injections or daily oral vitamin B_{12} supplements even when symptoms have resolved. Patients or a family caregiver can be taught to administer injections. The risk for gastric cancer is increased in patients with gastric atrophy associated with pernicious anemia making it important that patients understand the need for ongoing follow-up care and screening (see Chapter 40 for further discussion on gastric cancer).

Hemolytic Anemias

In hemolytic anemias, the erythrocytes have a shortened lifespan; thus, their number in the circulation is reduced. Fewer erythrocytes result in decreased available oxygen, causing hypoxia, which in turn stimulates an increase in erythropoietin release from the kidney. Erythropoietin then stimulates the bone marrow to compensate by producing new erythrocytes and releasing some of them into the circulation somewhat prematurely as reticulocytes. If the red cell destruction persists, the hemoglobin is broken down excessively; the majority of the heme is converted to bilirubin, conjugated in the liver, and excreted in the bile (Packman, 2016). Hemolytic anemias are far less common than other forms of anemia with approximately 5% of all anemias caused by hemolysis (Schick, 2019).

The mechanisms of erythrocyte breakdown vary, but common laboratory features are characteristic of hemolytic anemia. These include elevated reticulocyte count, increased fraction of indirect (unconjugated) bilirubin, and decreased **haptoglobin** (a binding protein for free hemoglobin) as additional hemoglobin is released from the cells. Anemia worsens if hemolysis persists and the bone marrow is unable to replace the destroyed cells.

Hemolytic anemia is associated with a variety of conditions. Inherited forms include SCD, thalassemias, G-6-PD deficiency, and hereditary spherocytosis. Acquired forms include immune hemolytic anemia, non–immune-mediated paroxysmal nocturnal hemoglobinuria, microangiopathic hemolytic anemia, heart valve–related hemolysis and anemias associated with hypersplenism.

Sickle Cell Disease

SCD is an autosomal recessive disorder caused by inheritance of the sickle hemoglobin (HbS) gene. It is associated with severe hemolytic anemia. The HbS gene results in production of a defective hemoglobin molecule that causes the erythrocyte to change shape when exposed to low oxygen tension. In some circumstances, even the oxygen level in venous blood can cause this change. The erythrocyte usually has a round, biconcave, pliable shape which in SCD can easily become rigid and sickle shaped (see Fig. 29-2). The long, rigid cells can subsequently adhere to the walls of small blood vessels where they accumulate, causing decreased blood flow to the tissues and organs in that region. When blood flow is severely reduced, ischemia or infarction of the tissue can cause severe pain, swelling, and fever referred to as a sickle cell crisis. Because the sickling process takes time, if the patient is exposed to adequate amounts of oxygen, the process can be reversed before the cell membranes become too rigid, allowing the erythrocytes to return to their normal shape. Sickle cell crises are intermittent and can be triggered by cold because of vasoconstriction that slows blood flow.

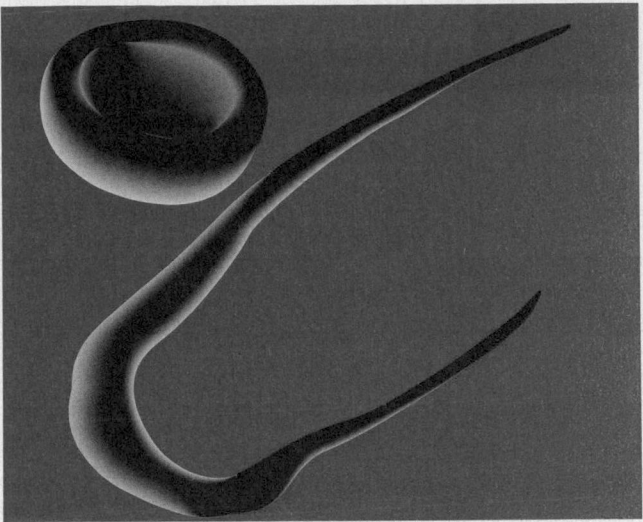

Figure 29-2 • A normal red blood cell (**upper left**) and a sickled red blood cell.

The HbS gene is inherited primarily in people of African descent. It may also be seen to a lesser degree in people of Middle Eastern and Mediterranean descent, and some tribal populations in India (Bunn, 2017b). Sickle cell anemia is the most severe form of SCD and is found in approximately 1 in 365 African Americans (National Heart Lung and Blood Institute, 2014). Other less severe forms of SCD include sickle cell hemoglobin C (SC) disease, sickle cell hemoglobin D (SD) disease, and sickle cell beta-thalassemia. Clinical presentation and treatment for these forms of the disease are the same as for sickle cell anemia.

The term sickle cell trait refers to the carrier state for SCD in which the patient has inherited a sickle gene from one parent and a normal gene from the other parent. Less than 50% of the hemoglobin within the erythrocytes is HbS. Those with sickle cell trait may be unaware that it is present unless severe hypoxia is experienced. Approximately 10% of African Americans have sickle cell trait (Bunn, 2017b). It is important that patients with sickle cell trait understand that if two people with sickle cell trait have children, the children have approximately one in four odds of inheriting two abnormal genes and will manifest SCD (see Chapter 6 for additional discussion of genetic diseases).

Clinical Manifestations

Symptoms of SCD vary and are not solely based on the amount of HbS present. Symptoms and complications are the result of chronic hemolysis and thrombosis. Sickled cells hemolyze rapidly and have a shortened lifespan. Anemia is typically present with hemoglobin values between 5 and 11 g/dL (Natrajan & Kutlar, 2016). Jaundice is often present. The bone marrow expands early in life to compensate for the resulting anemia, sometimes causing enlargement of the bones in the face and skull. Chronic anemia is often associated with tachycardia, cardiac murmurs, and cardiomegaly. Arrhythmias and heart failure may also occur, especially in adults.

Any organ can be affected by thrombosis, but those areas with slower circulation are frequently involved, including the lungs, spleen, and central nervous system (CNS). All tissues

TABLE 29-2	Complications in Sickle Cell Disease[a]		
Organ Involved	**Mechanisms**[a]	**Diagnostic Findings**	**Signs and Symptoms**
Spleen	Primary site of sickling → infarctions → ↓ phagocytic function of macrophages	Autosplenectomy; ↑ infection (especially pneumonia, osteomyelitis)	Abdominal pain; fever, other signs of infection
Lungs	Infection Infarction → ↑ pulmonary pressure → pulmonary hypertension	Pulmonary infiltrate ↑ sPLA$_2$[b]	Chest pain; dyspnea Chest pain; dyspnea
Central nervous system	Infarction	Stroke	Weakness; cognitive dysfunction, speech and swallowing dysfunction
Kidney	Sickling → damage to renal medulla	Hematuria; inability to concentrate urine; kidney injury	Dehydration
Heart	Anemia	Tachycardia; cardiomegaly → heart failure	Weakness, fatigue, dyspnea
Bone	↑ Erythroid production Infarction of bone	Widening of medullary spaces and cortical thinning Osteosclerosis → avascular necrosis	Ache, arthralgias Bone pain, especially hips
Liver	Hemolysis	Jaundice and gallstone formation; hepatomegaly	Abdominal pain
Skin and peripheral vasculature	↑ Viscosity/stasis → infarction → skin ulcers	Skin ulcers; ↓ wound healing	Pain
Eye	Infarction	Scarring, hemorrhage, retinal detachment	↓ Vision; blindness
Penis	Sickling → vascular thrombosis	Priapism → impotence	Pain, impotence

→, leading to; ↓, decreased; ↑, increased; sPLA$_2$, secretory phospholipase A$_2$.
[a]Problems encountered in sickle cell disease vary and are the result of a variety of mechanisms, as depicted in this table. Common physical findings and symptoms are also variable.
[b]Elevated sPLA$_2$ levels can predict impending acute chest syndrome (see text).
Adapted from Natrajan K., & Kutlar, A. (2016). Disorders of hemoglobin structure: Sickle cell anemia and related abnormalities. In K. Kaushansky, M. A. Lichtman, J. T. Prchal, et al. (Eds.). *Williams hematology* (9th ed.). New York: McGraw-Hill Medical.

and organs can be affected by thrombosis in the microcirculation caused by the sickling process leading to hypoxia and tissue damage and necrosis. Patients with SCD are particularly susceptible to infections, especially pneumonia and osteomyelitis. Additional complications of SCD include stroke, kidney injury, impotence, and pulmonary hypertension (see Table 29-2).

Sickle Cell Crisis

Three types of sickle cell crises affect adults. The most common is *acute vaso-occlusive crisis* (Kim, Brathwaite, & Kim, 2017). This very painful condition is the result of accumulation of erythrocytes and leukocytes in the microcirculation restricting blood flow to the tissue and causing hypoxia, inflammation, and necrosis. Substances released after tissue perfusion is restored include free radicals and free plasma hemoglobin, which cause oxidative damage to the blood vessel. As a result, the endothelial tissues in the vessel become dysfunctional (Bunn, 2017b). *Aplastic crisis* results from infection with the human parvovirus. The hemoglobin level falls rapidly and the marrow cannot compensate, as evidenced by an absence of reticulocytes (Natrajan & Kutlar, 2016). *Sequestration crisis* results when sickled cells are pooled in organs. In young children, the most common site of sequestration is the spleen; however, in many children with SCD over 10 years of age, the spleen has been infarcted and is no longer functional (Natrajan & Kutlar, 2016). In adults, the most common organs involved are the liver and the lungs.

Acute Chest Syndrome

Acute chest syndrome is a frequent complication in those hospitalized with SCD and is associated with significant morbidity and mortality. Acute chest syndrome is most frequently manifested by fever; respiratory distress that is manifested with tachypnea, cough and wheezing; and new infiltrates on the chest x-ray (Jain, Bakshi, & Krishnamurti, 2017). It is a common cause of death in young adults with SCD (Field, 2019). Infection with atypical bacteria including *Chlamydia pneumoniae* and *Mycoplasma pneumoniae* and viruses, including influenza, are often the cause. Other causes of acute chest syndrome include pulmonary thromboembolism, pulmonary fat embolism, bone marrow embolism, and pulmonary infarction. The patient's clinical condition can deteriorate very quickly leading to respiratory failure. Medical management includes blood transfusion, antibiotics, bronchodilators, inhaled nitric oxide, and when respiratory failure occurs, mechanical ventilation. Risk for acute chest syndrome can be reduced through immunization against influenza and pneumococcal pneumonia, and with use of incentive spirometry during vaso-occlusive crises, and with blood transfusion perioperatively (Jain et al., 2017). Prompt recognition and aggressive treatment can result in good outcomes for this potentially life-threatening condition.

Pulmonary Hypertension

Pulmonary hypertension is a common sequela of SCD and is a common cause of death (Natrajan & Kutlar, 2016). The onset of symptoms of pulmonary hypertension is insidious; diagnosis is difficult in the early stages and is usually delayed until irreversible damage occurs. Symptoms include fatigue, dyspnea on exertion, dizziness, chest pain, or syncope. Pulse oximetry is usually normal and breath sounds are often clear to auscultation until the condition is quite advanced. Pulmonary artery pressures are elevated above baseline but are generally lower than seen with idiopathic or hereditary pulmonary hypertension. Screening of patients with SCD with Doppler echocardiography may be helpful in identifying increased pulmonary artery pressure (Kling & Farber, 2019). High levels of the amino-terminal form of brain natriuretic peptide can be a biomarker for pulmonary hypertension in people with SCD and serve as a predictor of mortality (Kling & Farber, 2019). Computed tomography (CT) scan of the chest frequently reveals microvascular pulmonary occlusion and decreased lung perfusion while chest x-ray may appear normal.

Stroke

Stroke is a catastrophic consequence of SCD that affects approximately 10% of patients under 20 years of age (Natrajan & Kutlar, 2016). Ischemic stroke is most common, especially in young children and older adults, while hemorrhagic stroke is more common in young adults. The mechanisms vary but often result from decreased blood flow due to anemia, hemolysis, and increased hypoxic stress. Silent cerebral infarction occurs in about 40% of patients with SCD who have strokes, resulting in neurocognitive decline (Vichinsky, 2017). Medical management of stroke includes red blood cell transfusion to reduce the amount of hemoglobin S to less than 30% to reduce the risk of cerebral edema (George, 2019).

Reproductive Disorders

The adverse effects of SCD on sexual function have become more evident as patients with the disease are living longer. Hypogonadism with associated low testosterone levels, delayed puberty, low libido, erectile dysfunction, and infertility occur frequently in men with SCD (Huang & Muneyyirci-Delale, 2017). Episodes of priapism (prolonged penile erection, without sexual stimulation) also contribute to significant pain and decreased libido. Over time, repeated episodes lead to permanent damage and erectile dysfunction, thereby making priapism a medical emergency that needs early recognition and treatment to preserve normal sexual function (Field, Vemulakonda, DeBaun, et al., 2019). In addition to physical signs and symptoms, these problems can also lead to embarrassment and depression.

In young women, menarche may be delayed, but menstrual patterns are generally normal. Fertility problems in women are not well described. Contraception is important when hydroxyurea is used in SCD treatment because of its teratogenic effects. Concerns about infertility may be associated with poor adherence to hydroxyurea therapy. Although most pregnancies complicated by maternal SCD are likely to result in live births, these pregnancies are at increased risk of obstetrical and fetal complications, as well as medical complications of SCD (Vichinsky, 2018).

Assessment and Diagnostic Findings

The patient with sickle cell trait usually has a normal hemoglobin level, normal hematocrit, and normal blood smear. Conversely, the patient with SCD has a low hematocrit and sickled cells on the blood smear. The white blood cell count and platelet count are often elevated as a result of a chronic inflammatory state (Natrajan & Kutlar, 2016). Abnormal hemoglobin is identified by hemoglobin electrophoresis.

Medical Management

Patients with SCD are typically diagnosed in childhood, with anemia often occurring in infancy and crises beginning as early as 1 or 2 years of age. Some children die in the first few years of life as a result of infection; however, outcomes have improved considerably in recent years. Average life expectancy is lower than the general population, rarely exceeding the sixth decade (Field, 2019). Young adults often experience multiple, severe complications from their disease. A subgroup of patients experiences a decrease in symptoms and complications after age 30; however, at present there is no means to predict who will fall into this group. Death is most often caused by cardiac, lung, kidney, or neurologic complications, or from infection (Field, 2019).

Treatment of SCD is the focus of continued research. In addition to aggressive management of symptoms, including pain, and complications, there are a few primary treatment modalities.

Hematopoietic Stem Cell Transplant

HSCT may cure SCD. However, this treatment modality is available to only a small subset of affected patients, either due to a lack of compatible donors or due to severe organ damage (e.g., renal, liver, lung) that may be already present in the patient (see Chapter 12 for further discussion of HSCT).

Pharmacologic Therapy

For patients with SCD, hydroxyurea is a chemotherapeutic agent that is effective in increasing levels of fetal hemoglobin (i.e., hemoglobin F), which in turn decreases the formation of sickled cells. It is the only drug currently approved by the FDA for treatment of SCD. Studies have demonstrated that patients with SCD who received hydroxyurea experienced fewer episodes of painful crisis, had a lower incidence of acute chest syndrome, and needed fewer transfusions (Matte, Zorzi, & De Franceschi, 2019). Additional studies have shown a 40% decrease in mortality in patients receiving hydroxyurea (Natrajan & Kutlar, 2016). It is unknown whether hydroxyurea can prevent or reverse organ damage. Side effects of the drug include chronic lowering of the leukocyte count, teratogenesis, and potential for later development of a malignancy. Patients' response to the drug can vary widely. The incidence and severity of side effects are variable. Adherence to the prescribed treatment regimen may be difficult for some patients.

Patients with SCD often require daily folic acid supplements to maintain the amount needed for increased erythropoiesis to counteract the effects of hemolysis. Infections are common and should be treated promptly with the appropriate antibiotics. Pneumococcal pneumonia is common in children with SCD while in adults, *Staphylococcus aureus* infection is more common, involving bones and joints (Natrajan & Kutlar, 2016). Patients should be immunized against pneumococcal infection and receive annual influenza vaccines.

Acute chest syndrome is managed by prompt treatment with antibiotics. Incentive spirometry has been shown to significantly reduce the incidence of pulmonary complications. In severe cases, bronchoscopy may be needed to identify the source of acute chest syndrome symptoms. Hydration is important but must be monitored carefully to avoid fluid overload. Corticosteroids may also be helpful. Transfusion can reduce hypoxia. Pulmonary function should be monitored carefully to detect symptoms of pulmonary hypertension as soon as possible so that therapies, including hydroxyurea and HSCT, can be of the greatest benefit.

Transfusion Therapy

RBC transfusions have been shown to be highly effective in several situations: in an acute exacerbation of anemia (e.g., aplastic crisis, severe vaso-occlusive crisis), in the prevention of severe complications from anesthesia and surgery, in improving the response to infection (when it results in exacerbated anemia), in the case of acute chest syndrome and multiple organ dysfunction syndrome (MODS), and in thwarting the cerebral edema from a stroke. Transfusions are also effective in diminishing episodes of sickle cell crisis in pregnant women, although such transfusions do not improve fetal survival. Ongoing transfusion therapy may be effective in preventing or managing complications from SCD by keeping the HbS level to less than 30% (DeBaun, 2018).

Transfusions are not without risks, so it is important to consider the risks of complications versus benefits. Complications include difficulty with venous access, which necessitates placement of a vascular access device, and the concomitant risk for access site infection and thrombosis. Additional risks include other infections, particularly hepatitis; delayed hemolytic transfusion reactions; and iron overload that requires treatment with chelating agents.

Iron overload is very likely with long-term/ongoing transfusion therapy, causing deposition of iron in vital organs, including the liver, heart, pancreas, kidneys, and pituitary gland. It is sometimes difficult to distinguish organ damage associated with the disease process from damage associated with iron overload. Iron chelation therapy, aimed at keeping iron levels at near normal, reduces complications (see Chapter 30 for further discussion of chelation therapy) (Coates & Wood, 2017). An additional complication of transfusion therapy is increased blood viscosity without reduction in the concentration of hemoglobin S. Exchange transfusion, where some of the patient's blood is removed and replaced by RBC transfusion, may reduce the risk of increasing blood viscosity (Davis, Allard, Qureshi, et al., 2017). Additionally, repeated transfusions may result in development of multiple antibodies to other blood antigens, making cross matching increasingly difficult, and lead to increased risk for hemolytic transfusion reaction. This phenomenon is referred to as alloimmunization (Davis et al., 2017). Some patients who are alloimmunized have an increased risk of avascular necrosis, end-organ damage, and death (Holmes-Maybank, Martin, & Duckett, 2017). Hemolytic transfusion reaction may mimic the signs and symptoms of sickle cell crisis. A distinguishing feature of a hemolytic reaction versus sickle cell crisis is that the patient becomes more anemic after the transfusion than before. Close observation after hemolytic transfusion reaction is needed and further transfusion should be avoided until after the hemolytic process subsides. Patients are supported with corticosteroids, such as prednisone, intravenous immunoglobulins (IVIG) and erythropoietin alfa.

 For the procedural guidelines for managing immunoglobulin therapy, go to **thepoint.lww.com/Brunner15e**.

Supportive Therapy

Supportive care is essential for patients with SCD. Pain management is a significant problem. Acute pain is most often associated with vaso-occlusive crisis and is the frequent reason for hospitalization and emergency department visits in people with SCD. Pain may also be neuropathic in nature stemming from damage or inflammation of nerves as seen with avascular necrosis and leg ulcers (see Fig. 29-3). Chronic non-neuropathic pain may result from CNS dysfunction, including CNS sensitivity to peripheral afferent pain signals, or differences in psychosocial aspects of pain perception (Darbari & Brandow, 2017). Pain severity may interfere with ability to work, even when patients do seek assistance with pain management from health care providers.

The use of medications for acute pain relief is critical and should be appropriate for the etiology of the pain. Aspirin may be useful in patients with mild pain; it decreases inflammation and risk for potential thrombosis (because it inhibits platelet adhesion). NSAIDs are useful for moderate pain or in combination with opioid analgesics. While there is no risk of developing tolerance to NSAIDs there is a "ceiling effect" by which increased doses do not improve analgesia but increase the risk for adverse effects. NSAID use must be monitored carefully because of the risk for renal dysfunction and GI bleeding. Severe acute pain is most often treated with parenteral opioids (Okwerekwu & Skirvin, 2018). Patient-controlled analgesia is frequently used for this purpose in the acute care setting (see Chapter 9 for additional information on pain management). Neuropathic pain can be effectively managed with gabapentinoids, tricyclic antidepressants, and serotonin and norepinephrine reuptake inhibitors (Sharma & Brandow, 2019). With chronic pain management, the principal goal is to maximize functioning; pain may not be completely eliminated without sacrificing function. This concept

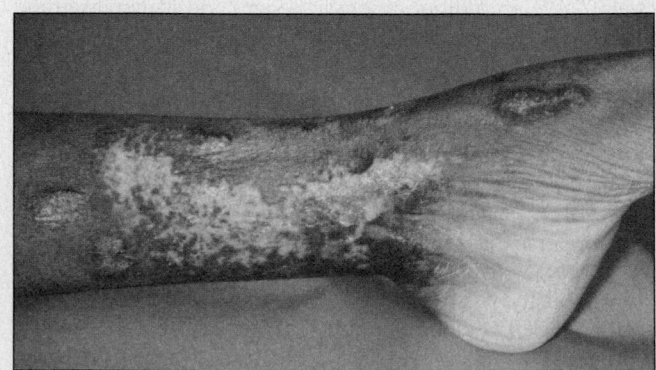

Figure 29-3 • Chronic skin ulcers seen in a patient with sickle cell anemia. Reprinted with permission from Tkachuk, D. C., & Hirschman, J. V. (2007). *Wintrobe's atlas of clinical hematology* (Fig. 1.71, p. 36). Philadelphia, PA: Lippincott Williams & Wilkins.

may be difficult for patients to understand and ongoing education and support is often needed. Nonpharmacologic pain management strategies are important in this setting. Such strategies include physical therapy including heat, massage and exercise; occupational therapy; cognitive and behavioral therapies, including distraction and relaxation techniques; and support groups (Okwerekwu & Skirvin, 2018).

Hydration is critical during a painful crisis. Oral hydration may be sufficient if the patient is able to maintain adequate intake. IV hydration may be needed if the patient is unable to consume 2 to 3 L of fluid during a crisis episode. Supplemental oxygen may also be needed.

Another significant problem for people with SCD is fatigue. Fatigue can interfere with ability to perform effectively at work and school and reduce quality of life. Its causes, as with pain, may be multifactorial. Fatigue may occur in response to hypoxia associated with low levels of normal hemoglobin and decreased capacity to carry oxygen with sickled cells. Endothelial cells in the blood vessels become inflamed as a result of hypoxia. Inflammatory cytokines are increased in patients with SCD resulting in reduced muscle strength and decreased exercise capacity, increased resting energy expenditure, and sleep disturbances, all exacerbating fatigue. Sleep disturbances and depression are common and contribute to fatigue (Ahmadi, Poormansouri, Beiranvand, et al., 2018).

Working with patients who have multiple episodes of severe pain and fatigue can be challenging. Health care providers must recognize that patients with SCD are confronted with lifelong experiences with severe pain and fatigue that impair physical and social functioning that may be associated with depression and helplessness. Patients without adequate sources of support may have more issues with coping.

NURSING PROCESS

The Patient with Sickle Cell Crisis

Assessment

The patient is asked to identify factors that precipitated previous crises and measures taken to prevent and manage crises. If a sickle cell crisis is suspected, the nurse needs to determine whether the pain currently experienced is the same as or different from the pain typically encountered in crisis. Pain levels should always be assessed (see Chapter 9). A similar assessment should be made of the patient's fatigue, including the impact of fatigue on the current lifestyle, quality of life, and the extent that the fatigue influences pain and interferes with sleep.

Because the sickling process can interrupt circulation in any organ or tissues, a thorough assessment of all body systems is needed. Particular attention should be placed on assessing pain, swelling, and fever. Careful examination of all joints for pain and swelling is necessary. The abdomen is assessed for pain and tenderness because of the possibility of splenic infarction.

The cardiovascular and respiratory systems must also be assessed carefully. These assessments include measurement of oxygen saturation, auscultation of breath sounds, and recognition of signs of cardiac failure, including the presence of dependent edema, increased size of the point of maximum impulse, and cardiomegaly (as seen on a chest x-ray). The patient is assessed for signs and symptoms of dehydration by a history of reduced fluid intake, and careful examination of mucous membranes, skin turgor, urine output, and serum creatinine and blood urea nitrogen levels.

A meticulous neurologic examination is essential to identify symptoms of cerebral hypoxia, but it is also important to recognize that evidence of ischemia may be present on magnetic resonance imaging (MRI) or Doppler studies before becoming evident on the physical examination. MRI or Doppler may be used for early diagnosis resulting in improved patient outcomes because therapy can be initiated promptly. Cognitive dysfunction is often present and may reflect reduced blood flow and oxygenation to the brain. Assessment for neurologic abnormalities is important in identifying silent cerebral ischemia or infarction.

Assessment for the presence of infectious processes is crucial as many patients with SCD are susceptible to infection. Special attention should be paid to examination of the chest, long bones, and femoral head because pneumonia and osteomyelitis are particularly common. Leg ulcers are common, frequently recurrent, occur in as many as 75% of adults with SCD, and may become infected and slow to heal (El Khatib & Hayek, 2016) (see Fig. 29-3).

The degree of anemia and ability of the bone marrow to replenish erythrocytes are assessed with hemoglobin level, hematocrit, and reticulocyte counts, and comparing these to baseline values. The patient's current and past history of medical care must also be obtained, particularly long-term transfusion therapy, hydroxyurea treatment, and prior treatment of infections.

Diagnosis

NURSING DIAGNOSES

Based on the assessment data, major nursing diagnoses may include:

- Acute pain, chronic pain, and fatigue associated with tissue hypoxia due to agglutination of sickled cells within blood vessels
- Risk for infection
- Risk for powerlessness associated with illness-induced helplessness
- Lack of knowledge regarding sickle cell crisis prevention

COLLABORATIVE PROBLEMS/POTENTIAL COMPLICATIONS

Potential complications may include the following:

- Hypoxia, ischemia, and poor wound healing leading to skin breakdown and ulcers
- Dehydration
- Cerebrovascular disease (stroke)
- Anemia
- Acute kidney injury and chronic kidney failure
- Heart failure, pulmonary hypertension, and acute chest syndrome
- Impotence and impaired fertility
- Cognitive dysfunction
- Poor adherence to therapy
- Mutual conflict and distrust between patient and health care providers due to poorly managed acute and chronic pain

Planning and Goals

The major goals for the patient are relief of pain, decreased incidence of crisis, enhanced sense of self-esteem and power, and absence of complications.

Nursing Interventions

MANAGING PAIN

Acute pain during a sickle cell crisis can be unpredictable and severe. The patient's subjective description of pain rating on a pain scale is useful in directing its treatment (see Chapter 9). Swollen joints should be supported and elevated until swelling subsides. Relaxation techniques, breathing exercises, yoga, and self-hypnosis may be helpful to some patients in coping with pain (DeBaun & Vichinsky, 2019). Following acute pain episodes, aggressive measures should be taken to preserve joint function. Physical therapy, whirlpool baths, and transcutaneous electrical nerve stimulation (TENS) are among modalities that may be used. While heat packs may be helpful, cold packs and ice should be avoided as cold may precipitate sickling (DeBaun & Vichinsky, 2019).

It is not unusual for patients to have difficulty coping with repeated episodes of acute pain and with chronic pain, making adherence to the prescribed treatment regimen difficult. Some patients with SCD develop substance use disorder although the incidence of substance abuse among people with SCD is not unlike that of patients with other chronic conditions (Natrajan & Kutlar, 2016). This can be a result of inadequate treatment of acute pain during episodes of crisis, which then leads to a lack of trust of the health care system and of health care providers. Research findings suggest that prompt treatment of pain during vaso-occlusive crises can improve patient satisfaction with care and also decrease patient length of stay or treatment times (Kim et al., 2017) (see Chart 29-4 Nursing Research

Profile: Acute Pain Management for Patients with Sickle Cell Disease).

MANAGING FATIGUE

Fatigue experienced with SCD may be acute or chronic. Assisting the patient to find a balance between activity and rest is important. Patients need to develop strategies to help cope with the demands on their lives while dealing with their fatigue. Maximizing nutrition, hydration, adequate sleep, and tissue perfusion can all help to minimize fatigue. Research is needed to better understand fatigue in this patient population and identify the most effective ways to relieve it. Although there are validated scales that have been used to quantify the extent of fatigue in patients with SCD, such as the PROMIS Fatigue short form®, standards for when to assess fatigue are currently lacking (Aslani, Georgios, & Maria, 2018; Hildenbrand, Quinn, Mara, et al., 2019).

PREVENTING AND MANAGING INFECTION

Nursing care focuses on monitoring patients for signs and symptoms of infection. Prescribed antibiotics should be administered as soon as possible. If oral antibiotics are prescribed at home, patients and caregivers must understand the importance of completing the entire course of antibiotics. Patients should be encouraged to seek immunizations per the latest guidelines (see Chapter 3, Table 3-3), particularly the pneumonia and influenza vaccines.

PROMOTING COPING SKILLS

SCD may cause patients to feel powerless and lacking in self-worth because of the health problems associated with repeated crises and chronic health conditions. These feelings can be exacerbated when pain and fatigue are not well controlled. Optimizing management of pain and fatigue are critical in helping patients to cope with their illness. Listening to and advocating for the needs of patients is important for building

---

Chart 29-4 · NURSING RESEARCH PROFILE

Acute Pain Management for Patients with Sickle Cell Disease

Kim, S., Brathwaite, R., & Kim, O. (2017). Evidence-based practice standard care for acute pain management in adults with sickle cell disease in an urgent care center. *Quality Management in Healthcare, 26*(2), 108–115.

Purpose

Vaso-occlusive episodes (VOEs) are the most common reason patients with sickle cell disease (SCD) seek emergency or urgent care services. Evidence-based guidelines specify that patients with SCD who seek urgent care for treatment of VOE should receive analgesics quickly. However, these guidelines are not followed by many clinicians, resulting in poorly managed pain in this patient population. The purpose of this study was to find whether implementing a VOE analgesic care algorithm in an urgent care (UC) center would decrease patient time to receipt of analgesics, improve patient satisfaction with care, and decrease length of treatment time.

Design

The setting for this study was an urban tertiary care UC center. Eligible participants were adults at least 18 years of age who sought care at the UC center for VOE from SCD. A Quality Improvement (QI) best practice VOE analgesic intervention was conducted with UC center staff so that all were educated to

follow the algorithm. Data were collected over 6 months. Time to administration of first analgesic medication for participants postintervention ($n = 63$) was compared with historical controls preintervention ($n = 61$), as were participant reports of satisfaction with care and their length of stay in the UC center.

Findings

The mean time to administration of analgesics decreased significantly from pre- to postintervention, from 92 minutes to 62 minutes ($p = 0.001$). Likewise, participant satisfaction with care improved from pre- to postintervention ($p = 0.002$) and mean time in the UC center decreased significantly from pre- to postintervention, from 283 minutes to 256 minutes ($p = 0.01$).

Nursing Implications

Findings from this study suggest that administering analgesics quicker to patients with SCD complicated with VOE not only mitigates their pain, but may also improve their satisfaction with care, and decrease their time in treatment. This may indirectly help to foster patient trust of the health care system and of providers. Nurses can leverage findings from this study to replicate this best practice algorithm and improve the care of patients with SCD complicated with VOE.

a therapeutic relationship based on mutual respect and trust. Nursing care that focuses on patients' strengths and not their deficits aids in promoting effective coping. Providing patients with opportunities to make decisions about their care can help foster autonomy and a sense of control. Supportive guidance can help patients understand the importance of adhering to their therapeutic regimen.

MINIMIZING KNOWLEDGE DEFICITS

Patients with SCD benefit greatly from understanding the circumstances that may precipitate a sickle cell crisis and the steps they can take to prevent or diminish the symptoms they may experience during a crisis. Keeping warm, reducing risks for infection, and maintaining adequate hydration can be effective in reducing the occurrence and severity of crises.

When hydroxyurea is prescribed for women of childbearing age, they should be informed that the drug can cause harm to an unborn fetus and advised that pregnancy should be avoided.

MONITORING AND MANAGING POTENTIAL COMPLICATIONS

Many of the measures for managing potential complications have already been described. Other measures follow.

Leg Ulcers. Leg ulcers require careful management and protection from trauma and contamination. Referral to a wound-ostomy-continence nurse or other wound care specialist may facilitate healing and promote prevention. If leg ulcers fail to heal, skin grafting may be needed (El Khatib & Hayek, 2016). Meticulous aseptic technique during wound care is needed to reduce risk for hospital-acquired wound infections.

Priapism and Impotence. Male patients may experience sudden, painful erection known as priapism. Initial management can include warm compresses or warm bath, and mild to moderate exercise, oral hydration, and masturbation with ejaculation (Field et al., 2019). If the priapism persists longer than 3 hours the patient should seek medical attention; treatment may consist of IV hydration, administration of analgesics, and possible aspiration of blood from the corpus carvernosa with or without injection of a sympathomimetic drug (Al-Qudah, 2016; Field et al., 2019). Repeated episodes of priapism may lead to extensive vascular damage resulting in impotence.

PROMOTING HOME, COMMUNITY-BASED, AND TRANSITIONAL CARE

Educating Patients About Self-Care. Because patients with SCD are typically diagnosed during childhood, their parents typically participate in the initial education. As the child ages, educational interventions prepare the child to assume more responsibility for self-care. Most families can learn about vascular access device management and chelation therapy. Nurses in outpatient facilities or home health nurses may need to provide follow-up care for patients with vascular access devices.

Continuing and Transitional Care. The illness trajectory of SCD is highly variable, often with unpredictable episodes of complications or crises. Care is frequently on an emergency basis, especially for some patients with pain management problems. All health care providers who offer services to patients with SCD and their families must communicate regularly with each other. Alternative methods of care delivery including day hospitals for acute symptom management and patient-centered medical homes, where multidisciplinary care is emphasized, are available in some regions. Nurses play an important role in serving as coordinators and facilitators of care by communicating with health care providers in a variety of settings to optimize the care of patients. Patient education about which parameters are important to monitor and how to monitor them is also a critical role for nurses. Making certain that patients understand when to seek urgent care for acute problems is essential.

Evaluation

Expected patient outcomes may include the following:
1. Control of pain and fatigue
   a. Uses analgesic agents appropriately to relieve pain
   b. Uses nonpharmacologic strategies to help relieve pain and fatigue, such as relaxation techniques, breathing exercises, and guided imagery
2. Absence of infection
   a. Is afebrile
   b. Maintains leukocyte count within normal baseline ($4500/mm^3$ to $11,000/mm^3$)
   c. Identifies importance of completing antibiotics as prescribed
   d. Demonstrates measures to prevent infection (i.e., obtains recommended immunizations)
3. Expresses improved sense of control
   a. Participates in goal setting, planning, and implementing daily activities
   b. Participates in making decisions about care
   c. Adheres to prescribed medical therapy
4. Increases knowledge about disease process
   a. Identifies situations and factors that can precipitate sickle cell crisis
   b. Describes lifestyle changes needed to prevent crisis
   c. Describes the importance of warmth, adequate hydration, and prevention of infection in preventing crisis
5. Absence of complications

Thalassemias

The thalassemias are a group of hereditary anemias characterized by **hypochromia** (an abnormal decrease in the hemoglobin content of erythrocytes), extreme **microcytosis** (smaller than normal size erythrocytes), hemolysis, and variable degrees of anemia. The thalassemias occur worldwide, but the highest prevalence is found in people of Mediterranean, African, and Southeast Asian ancestry (Weatherall, 2016).

Thalassemias are associated with impaired hemoglobin synthesis so that one or more globulin chains in the hemoglobin molecule are reduced. When this occurs, the imbalance in the configuration of the hemoglobin molecule causes it to precipitate in premature or mature erythrocytes. This increases the rigidity of erythrocytes, leading to premature cell destruction.

Thalassemias are classified into two major groups according to which hemoglobin chain is affected, alpha or beta. The alpha-thalassemias occur mainly in people of Southeast Asian and eastern Mediterranean descent (i.e., Middle Eastern), and the beta-thalassemias are most prevalent in those of African descent. Thalassemias are not limited to any geographic region because of extensive immigration (Weatherall, 2016). Symptoms of the alpha-thalassemias are typically less severe than those of beta-thalassemias. In alpha-thalassemias, erythrocytes are often quite microcytic but anemia, when present, is usually mild.

The severity of beta-thalassemia varies depending on the extent to which the hemoglobin chains are affected. Patients with mild forms have microcytosis and mild anemia. When untreated, severe beta-thalassemia (i.e., thalassemia major or Cooley's anemia) can be fatal within the first few years of life. HSCT offers a chance of cure. When this is not possible, treatment consists of PRBC transfusion and iron chelation therapy, as needed (Fibach & Rachmilewitz, 2017). Patient education for adolescents and young adults should include preconception counseling about the risk of thalassemia major in offspring (see Chapter 6 for discussion about genetic counseling and evaluation services).

Thalassemia major is characterized by severe anemia, profound hemolysis, and ineffective erythropoiesis. With early initiation of regular transfusions with PRBCs, growth and development through childhood is supported. Iron overload that can result from multiple transfusions can lead to organ dysfunction. Regular chelation therapy can reduce complications associated with iron overload and prolong life in those with thalassemia major. Long-term survivors of beta thalassemia may experience neurologic complications including cognitive dysfunction, peripheral neuropathy, and cerebrovascular disease (Fibach & Rachmilewitz, 2017).

Glucose-6-Phosphate Dehydrogenase Deficiency

The Glucose-6-Phosphate Dehydrogenase (G-6-PD) gene is responsible for the abnormality seen in this disorder. The gene produces an enzyme within the erythrocyte that is necessary to stabilize the cell membrane. Some patients produce an enzyme so defective that they have chronic hemolytic anemia; however, the most common type of defect only results in hemolysis when cells are under certain types of stress, associated with fever and certain types of medications. G-6-PD deficiency is one of the most common X-linked genetic blood disorders in the world, affecting more than 400 million people (see Chapter 6 for discussion of X-linked disorders). However, women may also develop the disease because one of the X chromosomes is inactivated in each cell of the female embryo; thus, a female who is heterozygous for the deficiency would have one half normal red blood cells and one half with the deficiency. While the deficient cells are at risk for hemolysis, symptoms are generally milder in affected women because normal cells are not subject to hemolysis. In the United States, African Americans and people of Mediterranean descent are most likely to be affected with G-6-PD (Anderle, Bancone, Domingo, et al., 2018). The type of deficiency found in person with Mediterranean ancestry is typically more severe than that in African Americans; it results in more hemolysis and sometimes life-threatening hemolytic anemia.

Oxidant drugs have hemolytic effects for people with G-6-PD deficiency, particularly some antibiotics including sulfadiazine, nitrofurantoin, trimethoprim-sulfamethoxazole, moxifloxacin, and chloramphenicol, as well as antimalarial agents including chloroquine, primaquine, and dapsone. Other medications associated with hemolysis include phenazopyridine, rasburicase, methylthioninium, tolonium chloride, tamsulosin, glyburide, nonsteroidal anti-inflammatory drugs, and the street drug amyl nitrate (van Solinge & van Wijk, 2016). A severe hemolytic episode can also occur in affected people after ingesting fava beans, menthol, tonic water, and some Chinese herbs.

Clinical Manifestations

Patients are typically asymptomatic and have normal hemoglobin levels and reticulocyte counts. However, within several days after exposure to an offending agent, pallor, jaundice, and hemoglobinuria develop. The reticulocyte count increases, and symptoms of hemolysis develop. Special stains of peripheral blood often show Heinz bodies (degraded hemoglobin) within the erythrocytes. Hemolysis may be mild and self-limited; however, in more severe cases, usually in the Mediterranean type of the disease, spontaneous recovery does not occur.

Assessment and Diagnostic Findings

The diagnosis is made by a screening test for the deficiency or by quantitative assay of G-6-PD.

Medical Management

Treatment requires discontinuation of the offending agent. Transfusion is not usually necessary unless severe hemolysis is present, as may be seen in the Mediterranean variety of G-6-PD deficiency.

Nursing Management

Patients should be educated about the disease and provided with a list of medications and other substances to be avoided. Patients with G-6-PD deficiency should always seek medical advice before taking any new medication or supplement. The G-6-PD Deficiency organization Web site (see Resources) is an excellent source of information. If hemolysis occurs, nursing interventions are the same as for hemolysis with other conditions. Patients should be advised to wear Medic-Alert bracelets that identify that they have G-6-PD deficiency. Genetic counseling may also be indicated (see Chapter 6).

Immune Hemolytic Anemias

Immune hemolytic anemias can result from exposure of erythrocytes to antibodies. Alloantibodies (antibodies against the host or "self") occur as a result of immunization of a person to foreign antigens (e.g., the immunization of an Rh-negative person with Rh-positive blood). Alloantibodies tend to be of the immunoglobulin G (IgG) type and cause immediate destruction of sensitized erythrocytes either within the blood vessels (intravascular) or the liver. Hemolysis and anemia associated with hemolytic transfusion reaction is an example of alloimmune hemolytic anemia.

Autoantibodies may develop for a number of reasons. In some circumstances, the person's immune system is dysfunctional and falsely identifies its own erythrocytes as foreign and produces antibodies against them. This may be seen in people with chronic lymphocytic leukemia (CLL) (see Chapter 30).

Another cause of autoimmune hemolytic anemia is a deficiency of suppressor lymphocytes, which normally prevents antibody production against the patient's own antigens. Erythrocytes are then sequestered in the spleen and destroyed by macrophages outside of blood vessels (extravascular hemolysis) (Phillips & Henderson, 2018).

Autoimmune hemolytic anemias may be classified based on the body temperature involved when the antibodies react with the RBC antigen. Warm-body antibodies are the most common (80%) and bind to erythrocytes most actively in warm-body conditions (37°C [98.6°F]); cold-body antibodies react in cold conditions (0°C [32°F]) (Packman, 2016). Autoimmune hemolytic anemia is associated with other disorders in most cases (e.g., medication exposure, lymphoma, CLL, other malignancies, collagen vascular diseases, autoimmune diseases, infection). In idiopathic autoimmune hemolytic states, the cause for antibody production is unknown. This primary form affects people of all ages and genders equally, while secondary forms occur more frequently in females and in people over the age of 45 years (Packman, 2016).

Clinical Manifestations

Clinical signs and symptoms vary and often reflect the severity of anemia. The hemolysis may range from very mild, with the patient's bone marrow able to compensate adequately with few or no symptoms, to severe, with life-threatening anemia. Most patients complain of fatigue and dizziness. Splenomegaly, with associated abdominal discomfort, is a common finding; hepatomegaly, lymphadenopathy, and jaundice are also frequently seen.

Assessment and Diagnostic Findings

Laboratory tests show a low hemoglobin level and hematocrit, usually associated with an elevated reticulocyte count. Erythrocytes appear abnormal; **spherocytes** (small, spherically shaped erythrocytes) are often seen on the peripheral blood smear. The serum bilirubin level is elevated, and if the hemolysis is severe, the haptoglobin level is low or absent. The Coombs test (also known as the direct antiglobulin test), which detects antibodies on the surface of the erythrocytes, is typically positive.

Medical Management

Any possible contributing medication should be immediately discontinued. Treatment most often consists of high doses of corticosteroids until hemolysis decreases; this is especially beneficial when treating warm-antibody–induced hemolysis (Packman, 2016). Corticosteroids have several actions including suppressing antibody production, reducing the affinity of antibodies for the erythrocytes, and reducing destruction of erythrocytes by macrophages in the spleen (Go, Winters, & Kay, 2017). If the hemoglobin levels return to normal, often within a few weeks, the corticosteroid dose can be gradually reduced, and in some cases be tapered and eventually discontinued. However, treatment with corticosteroids does not produce lasting effects. In severe cases, transfusions with PRBCs are needed to maintain adequate levels of hemoglobin until the hemolytic process can be reduced. The antibodies may react to donor cells, making careful typing and cross matching

essential. Transfusions are given slowly and cautiously with careful monitoring for transfusion reaction. Folic acid supplementation should be given when hemolysis is severe, because the bone marrow will attempt to compensate by increasing hematopoietic activity (Hill, Stamps, Massey, et al., 2017).

If corticosteroids do not result in remission, splenectomy (removal of the spleen) may be necessary to remove a major site of erythrocyte destruction. If neither corticosteroids nor splenectomy are successful, immunosuppressive medications may be given (Hill et al., 2017). Immunosuppressive drugs used include cyclophosphamide and azathioprine. Cyclophosphamide has a rapid onset of action but is associated with significant toxicity. Azathioprine has a slower onset of action but less toxicity. Danazol, a synthetic androgen, may be beneficial for some patients, especially when used in combination with corticosteroids. Immunosuppressive drugs and corticosteroids must be tapered slowly over several months to avoid a flare of the immune system leading to an exacerbation of hemolysis. Monoclonal antibodies, including rituximab, can be effective in some patients and may offer long-term control of symptoms (Hill et al., 2017).

> ◢ *Quality and Safety Nursing Alert*
>
> *Cross-matching blood when antibodies are present can be difficult. If imperfectly cross-matched PRBCs must be transfused, the nurse should begin the infusion very slowly (10 to 15 mL over 20 to 30 minutes) and monitor the patient very carefully for signs and symptoms of a hemolytic transfusion reaction.*

For patients with cold-antibody hemolytic anemia, no treatment may be needed, other than to advise the patient to keep warm. Relocation to a warmer climate may be advisable in some cases. In other situations, where hemolysis is more severe, more aggressive interventions as previously described may be needed.

Nursing Management

Patients may have difficulty understanding the complex nature of their illness and may need repeated explanations in terms they can understand. Patients who have had splenectomy should receive the pneumococcal pneumonia vaccine and annual influenza vaccine and be informed that they are permanently at increased risk for infection. Patients receiving long-term corticosteroid therapy, particularly those with diabetes or hypertension, need careful monitoring. They must understand the need for their medications and avoid abruptly discontinuing them. A written explanation and a tapering schedule should be provided, emphasizing adjustments based on hemoglobin levels. Similar information should be provided when immunosuppressive agents are used. Corticosteroid therapy is associated with risks and patients should be monitored frequently for complications (see Chapter 45, Table 45-3, Corticosteroid therapy and implications for nursing practice).

Hereditary Hemochromatosis

Hereditary hemochromatosis is a genetic condition characterized by excess iron absorption from the GI tract. Normally, the GI tract absorbs 1 to 2 mg of iron daily, but in those with hereditary hemochromatosis, this rate is significantly increased. The excess iron is deposited in various organs, especially the liver, skin, and pancreas; and less frequently, the heart, testes, and thyroid gland. Eventually, affected organs become dysfunctional. Although hereditary hemochromatosis is diagnosed in 1% to 6% of the U.S. population, the actual prevalence is unknown because it is not always recognized. The genetic defect associated with hemochromatosis is most commonly seen as a specific mutation (C282Y homozygosity) of the *HFE* gene. Despite the high prevalence of the genetic mutation, the actual expression of the disease is much lower; the reason for this discrepancy is not clear. The prevalence of hemochromatosis is lower in Asian Americans, African Americans, Latinos, and Pacific Islanders and higher in people of European descent (Kowdley, Brown, Ahn, et al., 2019). Women are less often affected than men because women lose iron through menses.

Clinical Manifestations

Tissue damage is seldom evident until middle age because the accumulation of iron in body organs occurs gradually. Symptoms of weakness, lethargy, arthralgia, and weight loss are common and occur earlier in the course of the disease. The skin may appear hyperpigmented or bronze in color from melanin deposits and **hemosiderin**, an iron-containing pigment. Cardiac arrhythmias and cardiomyopathy can occur, with resulting dyspnea and edema. Endocrine dysfunction can be manifested as hypothyroidism, diabetes, and hypogonadism with testicular atrophy, diminished libido, and impotence. Cirrhosis is common in later stages of the disease, shortens life expectancy, and is a risk factor for hepatocellular carcinoma (Kowdley et al., 2019).

Assessment and Diagnostic Findings

Diagnostic laboratory findings include an elevated serum ferritin and high serum transferrin saturation. CBC values are often normal. The definitive diagnostic test for hemochromatosis was formerly a liver biopsy but that test has been replaced by testing for the associated genetic mutation. While the prevalence of the genetic mutation is high (1 in 200 to 300 in persons of Northern European descent) few people with the gene will actually develop sufficient iron overload to cause symptoms and organ dysfunction (Bacon, 2019).

Medical Management

Therapy often involves the removal of excess iron with therapeutic phlebotomy (removal of whole blood via venipuncture). Each unit of blood removed results in a decrease of 200 to 250 mg of iron. Initial treatment typically involves weekly removal of one unit of whole blood. As the ferritin level decreases, the frequency of phlebotomy can be decreased. The goal is to maintain an iron saturation between 10% and 50% and a serum ferritin level of less than 100 mcg/L (Ganz, 2016). Evaluation of iron studies should be repeated regularly and phlebotomy resumed when the ferritin level rises. CBCs and iron panel tests should be performed at regular intervals during treatment to ensure that the patient is not becoming

anemic. If moderate anemia occurs, a delay in phlebotomy is often adequate to correct the problem. Aggressive removal of excess iron can prevent organ dysfunction and the complications associated with organ damage. Fatigue, skin pigmentation changes, and fibrosis are partially reversed by achieving and maintaining normal ferritin levels. Screening for hepatocellular carcinoma includes monitoring alpha-fetoprotein levels and serial abdominal ultrasounds (Kowdley et al., 2019).

Nursing Management

Patients with hemochromatosis frequently limit their iron intake; however, this is not typically effective as lone therapy. They should be advised to avoid taking additional iron supplements. Vitamin C supplementation should also be limited because it enhances iron absorption. Patients with hemochromatosis must be careful to avoid substances that might impair liver function including excessive alcohol ingestion. Other body systems should be monitored for evidence of organ dysfunction, particularly the endocrine and cardiac systems, so that appropriate interventions can be initiated without delay. Children of patients who are homozygous for the *HFE* gene mutation should be screened for the mutation. Patients who are heterozygous for the gene do not develop the disease but should be advised that they may transmit the gene to their children.

POLYCYTHEMIA

Polycythemia refers to an increased volume of RBCs. The term is used when the hematocrit is elevated (more than 55% in males and 50% in females). Dehydration can cause elevated hematocrit but not usually to the level seen with polycythemia. Polycythemia is classified as either primary or secondary. Primary polycythemia, also known as polycythemia vera, is a myeloproliferative neoplasm that is discussed in Chapter 30.

Secondary Polycythemia

Secondary polycythemia is caused by excessive production of erythropoietin. This may occur in response to a reduced amount of oxygen, which acts as a stimulus for production. Heavy smoking, obstructive sleep apnea (OSA), chronic obstructive pulmonary disease (COPD), severe heart disease, or conditions such as living at high altitudes or exposure to low levels of carbon monoxide may be responsible for increased erythropoietin production. Certain hemoglobinopathies (e.g., hemoglobin Chesapeake), in which the hemoglobin has a high affinity for oxygen, or genetic mutations that cause abnormally high erythropoietin levels may also increase erythropoiesis (Prchal, 2016b). Secondary polycythemia can also occur from certain neoplasms that stimulate erythropoietin production (e.g., renal cell carcinoma), excessive use of exogenous erythropoietin, and androgen use.

Management

When secondary polycythemia is mild, treatment may not be necessary. When treatment is necessary, however, it involves treating the primary condition. If the cause cannot be corrected (e.g., treatment of OSA or improving function with smoking cessation), therapeutic phlebotomy may be needed for symptom management and to reduce blood viscosity and volume. Therapeutic phlebotomy is not indicated when the cause for the elevated RBC count is an appropriate response to tissue hypoxia (Prchal, 2016b).

NEUTROPENIA

Neutropenia is defined as a neutrophil count less than 2,000/mm³. It is the result of decreased production of neutrophils or increased destruction of cells (see Chart 29-5). Neutrophils are essential in preventing and limiting bacterial infection. A patient with neutropenia is at increased risk for infection from both exogenous and endogenous sources (the GI tract and skin are common endogenous sources). The risk for infection is based not only on the severity of the neutropenia but also on its duration. The actual number of neutrophils, known as the **absolute neutrophil count (ANC)**, is determined by a simple mathematical calculation using information from the CBC and differential (see Chapter 12 for further discussion of the ANC). The risk for infection increases proportionately with a decrease in the neutrophil count. The risk is low when the ANC is greater than 1000/mm³, and high when less than 500/mm³ and greatest when less than 100/mm³ (Dale & Welte, 2016). The duration of neutropenia is another risk factor for developing infection as is the underlying etiology (see Chart 29-6).

Chart 29-5 — **Causes of Neutropenia**

Decreased Production of Neutrophils

- Aplastic anemia, due to medications or toxins
- Chemotherapy
- Metastatic cancer, lymphoma, leukemia
- Myelodysplastic syndromes
- Radiation therapy

Ineffective Granulocytopoiesis

- Megaloblastic anemia

Increased Destruction of Neutrophils

- Bacterial infections
- Hypersplenism
- Immunologic disorders (e.g., systemic lupus erythematosus)
- Medication induced[a]
- Viral disease (e.g., infectious hepatitis, mononucleosis)

[a]Formation of antibody to medication, leading to a rapid decrease in neutrophils.
Adapted from Dale, D. C., & Welte, K. (2016). Neutropenia and neutrophilia. In K. Kaushansky, M. A. Lichtman, J. T. Prchal, et al. (Eds.). *Williams hematology* (9th ed.). New York: McGraw-Hill Medical.

Clinical Manifestations

There are no definite symptoms of neutropenia until the patient develops an infection. A routine CBC with differential can reveal neutropenia before the onset of infection.

Chart 29-6 ⚠ **RISK FACTORS**
Development of Infection and Bleeding in Patients with Hematologic Disorders

Risk for Infection	Risk for Bleeding
• *Severity of neutropenia*: Risk for infection is proportional to severity of neutropenia.	• *Severity of thrombocytopenia:* Risk increases when platelet count decreases; usually not a significant risk until platelet count drops below 10,000/mm³, or less than 50,000/mm³ with trauma or when an invasion procedure is performed.
• *Duration of neutropenia:* Increased duration of neutropenia leads to increased risk for infection.	• *Duration of thrombocytopenia:* Risk increases when duration increases (e.g., risk is less when duration is transient as after chemotherapy than when duration is prolonged as with decreased cell production by bone marrow).
• *Nutritional status:* Decreased protein stores lead to decreased immune response and anergy.	
• *Deconditioning:* Decreased mobility leads to decreased respiratory effort, leading to increased pooling of secretions.	• *Sepsis:* Mechanism unclear; appears to cause increased platelet consumption.
• *Lymphocytopenia; disorders of lymphoid system (chronic lymphocytic leukemia, lymphoma, and myeloma)*: Decreased cell-mediated and humoral immunity.	• *Increased intracranial pressure:* Increased blood pressure leads to rupture of blood vessels.
• *Invasive procedures:* Breaks in skin integrity create increased opportunities for organisms to enter blood system.	• *Liver dysfunction:* Decreased synthesis of multiple clotting factors.
• *Hypogammaglobinemia:* Decreased antibody formation.	• *Renal dysfunction:* Decreased platelet function.
• *Poor hygiene:* Increased organisms on skin and mucous membranes, including perineum.	• *Dysproteinemia:* Protein coats surface of platelet, leading to decreased platelet function; protein causes increased blood viscosity, which leads to stretching of capillaries an increased risk for rupture and bleeding.
• *Poor dentition; mucositis:* Decreased endothelial integrity leads to increased opportunity for organisms to enter blood system.	• *Alcohol abuse:* Suppressive effect on bone marrow results in deceased platelet production and impaired platelet function; impaired liver function results in decreased production of clotting factors.
• *Antibiotic therapy*: Increased risk for superinfection, often fungal.	
• *Certain medications:* See text.	

Adapted from Dale, D. C., & Welte, K. (2016). Neutropenia and neutrophilia. In K. Kaushansky, M. A. Lichtman, J. T. Prchal, et al. (Eds.). *Williams hematology* (9th ed.). New York: McGraw-Hill Medical; Diz-Kucukkaya, R., & Lopez, J. (2016). Thrombocytopenia. In K. Kaushansky, M. A. Lichtman, J. T. Prchal, et al. (Eds.). *Williams hematology* (9th ed.). New York: McGraw-Hill Medical; Vasu, S., & Caligiuri, M. A. (2016). Lymphocytosis and lymphopenia. In K. Kaushansky, M. A. Lichtman, J. T. Prchal, et al. (Eds.). *Williams hematology* (9th ed.). New York: McGraw-Hill Medical.

◤ *Quality and Safety Nursing Alert*

*Patients with neutropenia do not always exhibit classic
signs of infection. Fever is the most common indicator
of infection, but is not always present, particularly if the
patient is taking corticosteroids or is an older adult.*

Medical Management

Treatment of neutropenia varies depending on its etiology.
If the neutropenia is medication induced, the offending
agent should be discontinued immediately whenever possible. Treatment of an underlying neoplasm can temporarily
make the neutropenia worse, but after bone marrow recovery,
treatment may improve it. Corticosteroids may be used if the
neutropenia is caused by an immunologic disorder. The use of
growth factors such as granulocyte colony-stimulating factor
or granulocyte-macrophage colony-stimulating factor can be
effective in increasing neutrophil production when the cause
is reduced cell production. Withholding or reducing the dose
of chemotherapy or radiation therapy may be necessary when
the neutropenia is caused by these cancer treatments; however, when treatment is potentially curative, administration
of growth factors is preferable so that the maximum antitumor effect of the cancer treatment can be achieved (Lyman,
2019).

If the neutropenia is associated with fever, it is assumed
that the patient has an infection. Cultures of blood, urine,
and sputum, as well as a chest x-ray are obtained. Broad-
spectrum antibiotics are initiated immediately after cultures
are obtained to ensure adequate treatment of infectious
organisms. After culture and sensitivity results are obtained,
the antibiotic regimen may be changed.

Nursing Management

Nurses in all settings can play a crucial role in assessing the
severity of neutropenia and in preventing and managing complications, which most often include infections. Knowledge
of risk factors for developing infection is an integral part of
nursing care, particularly for those who work with patients
who have cancer. Patient education is equally important,
particularly at the time of discharge from the hospital or in
the outpatient setting so that the patient can put an appropriate self-care plan into effect, including knowing when to
seek medical attention (see Chart 29-7). Patients at risk for
neutropenia should have blood drawn for a CBC with differential; the frequency is based on the suspected duration and
severity of the neutropenia. To assess the severity of neutropenia and risk for infection, nurses must assess the ANC (see
Chapter 12 for formula). Nursing interventions related to
neutropenia are delineated in Chapters 12 and 30.

LYMPHOPENIA

Lymphopenia is defined as a lymphocyte count less than
1500/mm³. It may occur as a result of exposure to ionizing
radiation, long-term use of corticosteroids, uremia, infections
(particularly viral infections), neoplasms (breast and lung cancer and advanced Hodgkin disease), and some protein-losing
enteropathies which may cause lymphocytes from the GI tract
to be lost (Vasu & Caligiuri, 2016). When lymphopenia is
mild, there are no serious sequelae, but when it is severe, it can
result in bacterial infections (due to reduced B lymphocytes)
or in opportunistic infections (due to reduced T lymphocytes).
T-lymphocyte depletion is frequently associated with viral
infections, including human immune deficiency virus (HIV).
Excessive or prolonged use of alcohol can also impair lymphocyte production; lymphocyte counts can improve when alcohol intake is discontinued (Vasu & Caligiuri, 2016).

BLEEDING DISORDERS

The failure of normal hemostatic mechanisms can result in
bleeding which may be severe. Bleeding is commonly provoked by trauma; however, in certain circumstances, it can
occur spontaneously. The causes of bleeding disorders can
be categorized based upon whether there is a deficiency of
platelets or a defect in the platelets, or based upon whether

---

Chart **HOME CARE CHECKLIST**
29-7 The Patient at Risk for Infection

At the completion of education, the patient and/or caregiver will be able to:

- State the impact of alterations in neutrophils, lymphocytes,
  immunoglobulins on physiologic functioning, ADLs, IADLs,
  roles, relationships, and spirituality.
- State changes in lifestyle (e.g., diet, activity) or home environ-
  ment necessary to decrease risk for infection.
  - Maintain good hand hygiene technique, oral hygiene, total
    body hygiene, and skin integrity.
  - Avoid cleaning birdcages and litter boxes; consider avoiding
    garden work (soil) and fresh flowers in stagnant water.
  - Maintain a high-calorie, high-protein diet, with fluid intake of
    3000 mL daily (unless fluids are restricted).
  - Avoid people with infections and crowds.
  - Perform deep breathing; use incentive spirometer every 4
    hours while awake if mobility is restricted.

- Provide adequate lubrication with gentle vaginal manipulation during penile-vaginal intercourse; avoid anal intercourse.
- Identify signs and symptoms of infection to report to the primary provider, such as fever; chills; wet or dry cough; breathing problems; white patches in the mouth; swollen glands;
  nausea; vomiting; persistent abdominal pain; persistent diarrhea; problems with urination or changes in the character of
  the urine; red, swollen, or draining wounds; sores or lesions on
  the body; persistent vaginal discharge with or without itching;
  and severe fatigue.
- Demonstrate how to monitor for signs of infection.
- Describe to whom, how, and when to report signs of
  infection.
- Describe appropriate actions to take should infection occur.

ADLs, activities of daily living; IADLs, instrumental activities of daily living.

there is an inherited or acquired coagulation factor abnormality, or based upon a defect in the vasculature. When the cause is platelet or coagulation factor abnormalities, bleeding can occur anywhere in the body. When the source is a vascular abnormality the site of bleeding is more localized. Some patients may have simultaneous defects in more than one hemostatic mechanism.

The bone marrow may be stimulated to increase platelet production. This can be a reactive response to significant bleeding, or a more general response to increased hematopoiesis, as in iron deficiency anemia. Sometimes an increase in platelets does not result from increased platelet production, but from a loss of platelet pooling in the spleen. The spleen typically holds about one third of circulating platelets at any time. If the spleen is absent (e.g., after splenectomy) the platelet reservoir is lost, and an abnormally high number of platelets enter the circulation. Eventually the rate of platelet production slows to reestablish a more normal platelet level.

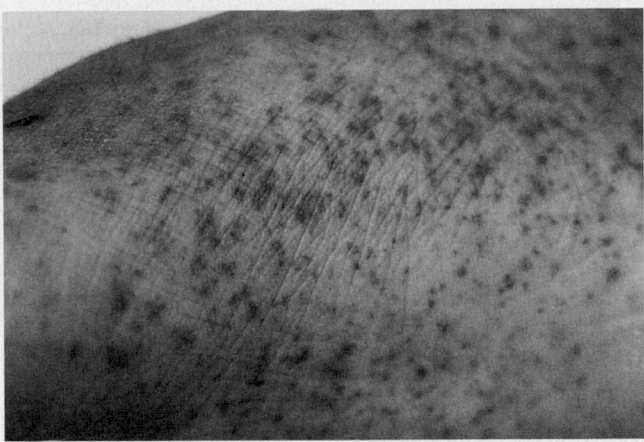

Figure 29-4 • Petechiae. Reprinted with permission from *Wintrobe's clinical hematology* (10th ed). (1999). Color plate 62.4. Philadelphia, PA: Lippincott Williams & Wilkins.

Clinical Manifestations

Signs and symptoms of bleeding disorders vary according to the type of defect. A careful history and physical examination can be useful in determining the source of the hemostatic defect. Abnormalities of the vascular system are sources of localized bleeding, usually into the skin. Because platelets are primarily responsible for stopping bleeding from small vessels, patients with decreased platelets develop **petechiae,** often in clusters. These lesions can be seen on the skin and mucous membranes and occur throughout the body (see Fig. 29-4). Bleeding from platelet disorders can be severe, but most often, bleeding from platelet disorders can be controlled when pressure is applied.

In contrast, coagulation factor defects do not tend to cause superficial bleeding because the primary hemostatic mechanisms are still intact. Instead, bleeding occurs deeper within the body (e.g., subcutaneous or intramuscular hematomas, hemorrhage into joint spaces). External bleeding diminishes very slowly when local pressure is applied; it frequently recurs several hours after pressure is removed. An example of this would be severe bleeding that occurs several hours after tooth extraction. Risk factors for bleeding are listed in Chart 29-6.

Medical Management

Management varies based on the underlying bleeding disorder. If bleeding is significant, transfusion of blood products may be indicated. The specific blood product used is determined by the underlying defect and the extent of blood loss. If fibrinolysis is excessive, hemostatic agents such as aminocaproic acid can be useful to inhibit the process, but this agent must be used cautiously because excessive inhibition of fibrinolysis can lead to thrombosis. A patient scheduled for an invasive procedure may need to have transfusions of select blood products to reduce risk for excessive bleeding.

Nursing Management

Patients who have bleeding disorders or who have the potential for development of such disorders as a result of disease or therapeutic agents must be educated to monitor themselves frequently and carefully for signs of bleeding (see Chart 29-8). They should understand the importance of avoiding activities that increase the risk for bleeding, such as contact sports. The skin should be examined for evidence of bleeding, including petechiae and ecchymoses (bruises) and the nose and gums

---

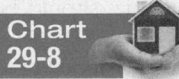

Chart 29-8 **HOME CARE CHECKLIST**
The Patient at Risk for Bleeding

At the completion of education, the patient and/or caregiver will be able to:

- Describe the source and function of platelets and clotting factors.
- State the impact of an alteration in platelets on physiologic functioning, ADLs, IADLs, roles, relationships, and spirituality.
- State changes in lifestyle (e.g., diet, activity) or home environment necessary to decrease risk of bleeding.
  - Avoid the use of suppositories, enemas, and tampons
  - Avoid constipation
  - Avoid vigorous sexual intercourse and anal sex
  - Avoid contact sports
  - Avoid or limit aggressive manual labor

- Use an electric razor for shaving and a soft-bristled toothbrush for teeth brushing
- Notify health care professional before having dental work or other invasive procedures
- Identify medications and other substances to avoid (e.g., aspirin-containing medications, alcohol).
- Identify signs and symptoms of bleeding.
- Demonstrate how to monitor for signs of bleeding.
- Describe to whom, how, and when to report signs of bleeding.
- Demonstrate appropriate actions to take should bleeding occur.

ADLs, activities of daily living; IADLs, instrumental activities of daily living.

TABLE 29-3	Causes and Management of Thrombocytopenia
Cause	**Management**
Decreased Platelet Production	
Hematologic malignancy; especially acute leukemia	Treat leukemia, platelet transfusion
MDS	Treat MDS, platelet transfusion
Bone marrow metastases from solid tumors	Treat solid tumor
Aplastic anemia	Treat underlying condition
Megaloblastic anemia	Treat underlying anemia
Toxins	Remove toxin
Medications (e.g., sulfa drugs, methotrexate)	Discontinue medication
Infection (especially sepsis, viral infections, tuberculosis, chronic hepatitis C)	Treat underlying infection
Chronic alcohol abuse	Refrain from alcohol, refer for substance use disorder
Chemotherapy	Delay or decrease dose, platelet transfusion
Chronic liver disease	Treat underlying disorder
Radiation (e.g., pelvic irradiation)	Platelet transfusion
Delayed engraftment after stem cell transplantation	Platelet transfusion
Increased Platelet Destruction	
Due to antibodies:	Treat underlying condition
ITP	
SLE	
Malignant lymphoma	
CLL	Treat CLL and/or treat as ITP
Medications	Discontinue medication
Due to infection: Bacteremia/sepsis; post-viral infection	Treat infection
Sequestration of platelets in spleen	If severe, splenectomy may be needed
Increased Platelet Consumption	
DIC	Treat underlying condition triggering DIC; refer to text for indicated treatments
Major bleeding	Transfusion support, surgery if appropriate
Severe pulmonary embolism/severe thrombosis	Treat clot
Intravascular devices (intra-aortic balloon pump, cardiac assist devices)	Transfusion support as needed
Extracorporeal circulation (hemofiltration, extracorporeal lung assist)	Transfusion support as needed

CLL, chronic lymphocytic leukemia; DIC, disseminated intravascular coagulation; ITP, idiopathic thrombocytic purpura; MDS, myelodysplastic syndrome; SLE, systemic lupus erythromatosus.

should also be examined for bleeding. When bleeding disorders are severe, patients who are hospitalized are monitored for bleeding by testing all drainage and excreta (feces, urine, emesis, and, gastric drainage) for obvious and occult blood.

Thrombocytopenia

Thrombocytopenia (low platelet level) can result from a variety of factors, including reduced production of platelets in the bone marrow, increased destruction of platelets, or increased consumption of platelets (e.g., the use of platelets for clot formation). Causes and treatments are summarized in Table 29-3.

Clinical Manifestations

Bleeding and petechiae rarely occur with platelet counts greater than 50,000/mm^3, but excessive bleeding can occur after surgery or other trauma. When platelet counts fall to 20,000/mm^3 or less, petechiae may occur. Additionally, nasal and gingival bleeding, excessive menstrual bleeding, and excessive bleeding from surgery or dental extractions can occur. Spontaneous and potentially fatal bleeding in the CNS or GI tract can occur when platelet counts fall to less than 5000/mm^3. If platelet function is abnormal as a result of disease (e.g., MDS) or medications (e.g., aspirin) the risk of bleeding may be much greater even when the platelet count is mildly reduced.

Assessment and Diagnostic Findings

Bone marrow aspiration and biopsy are used to identify platelet deficiency associated with decreased production. A number of genetic causes of thrombocytopenia have been identified. Autosomal dominant, autosomal recessive, and X-linked mutations are among such disorders. When platelet destruction is the cause of thrombocytopenia, the bone marrow shows increased megakaryocytes and normal or increased platelet production as the body attempts to compensate for the decreased platelets in the circulation. Screening for hepatitis B or C, which can cause thrombocytopenia, should be done.

An important cause to exclude is pseudothrombocytopenia. Platelets aggregate and clump in the presence of ethylenediaminetetraacetic acid (EDTA), the anticoagulant present in the tube used for CBC collection. This clumping can be seen 0.8% to 1.25% of the population. Manual examination of the peripheral smear can easily detect platelet clumping as the cause of thrombocytopenia. Redrawing the blood in a tube anticoagulated with citrate rather than EDTA, followed by rapid analysis of the platelet count can provide a more accurate count.

Medical Management

Secondary thrombocytopenia is usually managed with treatment of the underlying disease. If platelet production is impaired, platelet transfusion may be needed to increase the platelet count and stop bleeding or prevent spontaneous hemorrhage. If excessive platelet destruction occurs, transfused platelets may also be destroyed. The most common cause of increased platelet destruction is immune thrombocytopenic purpura (ITP) (see the following discussion). In some circumstances, splenectomy may be a therapeutic intervention, but it is not always feasible. For example, when an enlarged spleen is associated with portal hypertension related to cirrhosis, splenectomy may cause further issues with bleeding.

Nursing Management

When determining nursing interventions, the nurse considers the cause of the thrombocytopenia, the likely duration, and overall condition of the patient. Education is an important intervention to promote safety and should include fall prevention, particularly for older adults and those who are frail. Interventions for patients with secondary thrombocytopenia are the same as those for a patient with cancer who is at risk for bleeding (see Chapter 12).

Immune Thrombocytopenic Purpura

ITP is a condition that affects people of all ages but is most common in children and young women. This disorder is also referred to as idiopathic thrombocytopenic purpura, and immune thrombocytopenia. Primary ITP occurs as an isolated disorder while secondary ITP is associated with other disorders including autoimmune disorders (e.g., antiphospholipid antibody syndrome), viral infections (e.g., hepatitis C, HIV), and some drugs (e.g., cephalosporins, sulfonamides, furosemide). A platelet count less than 100,000/mm^3 with no explicable cause is the primary criterion for the diagnosis (Nomura, 2016).

Pathophysiology

Primary ITP is an acquired immune disorder characterized by thrombocytopenia that results from pathologic antiplatelet antibodies, impaired production of megakaryocytes, and T-cell–mediated destruction of platelets. Secondary ITP is associated with other underlying disorders, including autoimmune disease (systemic lupus erythematosus or rheumatoid arthritis), HIV infection, *Helicobacter pylori* infection, or underlying immune dysregulation syndromes, such as common variable immunodeficiency. The majority of adults with ITP (approximately 80%) have primary ITP. With both types of ITP, antiplatelet antibodies develop and bind to the patient's platelets. The antibody-bound platelets are then destroyed by the reticuloendothelial system (RES) and tissue macrophages. The body attempts to compensate for the platelet destruction by increasing platelet production within the bone marrow (Lambert & Gernsheimer, 2017).

Clinical Manifestations

ITP is often asymptomatic; the low platelet count frequently is an incidental finding. Platelet counts of less than 30,000/mm^3 are not uncommon. Common signs of thrombocytopenia include easy bruising, heavy menses, and petechiae on the extremities or trunk (see Fig. 29-4). Patients who experience only bruising and petechiae tend to have fewer complications from bleeding than those with bleeding from mucosal

surfaces, such as the GI tract and respiratory system (sometimes described as "wet purpura"). Patients with wet purpura have a greater risk of life-threatening bleeding which requires immediate aggressive treatment to reduce complications (Diz-Kucukkaya & Lopez, 2016). Severe thrombocytopenia, characterized by platelet count less than 20,000/mm^3, a prior history of minor bleeding episodes, and advanced age, is a risk factor for severe bleeding. Despite low platelet counts, platelets are typically immature yet very functional, with the ability to adhere to endothelial surfaces and each other. This may explain why spontaneous bleeding does not always occur. Treatment is not necessary unless bleeding becomes severe or if surgery or another invasive procedure is required (Diz-Kucukkaya & Lopez, 2016).

Assessment and Diagnostic Findings

A careful history and physical examination are essential to aid in excluding other causes of thrombocytopenia and identify sites of bleeding. Patients should be tested for hepatitis C and HIV, if not previously done to rule them out as potential causes. Bone marrow aspirate may reveal an increased number of megakaryocytes. The severity of the thrombocytopenia is highly variable.

H. pylori infection is associated with ITP, and treatment to eradicate the infection may improve the platelet count. The correlation between *H. pylori* infection and ITP is not clear; it is postulated that the presence of the *H. pylori* organism may stimulate an autoimmune reaction (Aljarad, Alhamid, Tarabishi, et al., 2018).

Medical Management

The primary goal of treatment is to achieve a platelet count high enough to maintain hemostasis. Because the risk for bleeding does not typically increase until the platelet count is less than 30,000/mm^3, a patient whose platelet count exceeds 30,000/mm^3 to 50,000/mm^3 may be carefully monitored without immediate intervention. However, if the platelet count is less than 30,000/mm^3 or if bleeding occurs, the goal is to improve the patient's platelet count and not to cure the disease. The decision to treat is made based upon the severity of bleeding (if any) and not solely on the platelet count. Potential treatment side effects, the patient's lifestyle, activity level, concurrent use of medications, and treatment preferences are also considered. A person with a sedentary lifestyle can tolerate a low platelet count more safely than a more active person; however, increasing age is also associated with increased risk for bleeding and mortality (Diz-Kucukkaya & Lopez, 2016).

Treatment for ITP usually involves several approaches. If the patient is taking a medication known to be associated with ITP (e.g., quinine, sulfa-containing drugs), then that medication should be discontinued. Transfusions are often ineffective because antiplatelet antibodies bind with transfused platelets, causing them to be destroyed. Platelet counts may drop even further after platelet transfusion. Thus, despite extremely low platelet counts, platelet transfusions may result in catastrophic bleeding in patients with wet purpura. Aminocaproic acid, a fibrinolytic enzyme inhibitor that slows the dissolution of blood clots, may be useful for patients with significant mucosal bleeding that is resistant to other treatments.

The mainstay of short-term therapy is the use of immunosuppressive agents. These agents block the binding receptors on macrophages to reduce platelet destruction. The American Society of Hematology recommends dexamethasone or prednisone in adults with newly diagnosed ITP as the types of corticosteroids that might be selected for initial therapy. Continuous long-term use of corticosteroids is not recommended because of the risk for side effects (Neunert, Terrell, Arnold, et al., 2019). Platelet counts typically begin to rise within a few days after initiating treatment with corticosteroids. The platelet count tends to decrease once the corticosteroid dose is tapered but may remain sufficiently adequate to prevent bleeding.

IVIG is commonly used to treat ITP. It renders its effect by binding to the receptors on macrophages. However, the need for high doses of IVIG and its high cost are disadvantages.

 For the procedural guidelines for managing immunoglobulin therapy, go to **thepoint.lww.com/Brunner15e**.

The effects of treatment are transient in most cases. Another approach to treatment of chronic ITP is the use of anti-D immunoglobulin in patients who are Rh (D) positive. The exact mechanism of action is unknown, but it is theorized that the anti-D binds to the patient's erythrocytes, which are in turn destroyed by the body's macrophages. The receptors in the RES may become flooded with sensitized erythrocytes, which then reduce the number of antibody-coated platelets. This then results in a transient reduction of hematocrit and an increased number of platelets in some patients with ITP (Neunert et al., 2019).

Eventually, the platelet count again declines and additional therapy is needed. Second-line treatment options should take the patient's individual needs and the potential treatment-related side effects into account.

Splenectomy is an alternative treatment and typically results in a sustained increase in platelets. Many patients can maintain a "safe" platelet count of more than 30,000/mm³ after splenectomy; however, many patients may have a recurrence of thrombocytopenia months or years later (Neunert et al., 2019). Patients who undergo splenectomy are permanently at risk for serious infection and should receive pneumococcal, influenzae, and meningococcal vaccines approximately 2 weeks prior to splenectomy, or 2 to 3 weeks postoperatively if splenectomy is performed emergently (Bonanni, Grazzini, Niccolai, et al., 2017) (see Chapter 19 for information on pneumonia vaccine).

Other management strategies include use of monoclonal antibodies, such as rituximab. Patients may have long lasting effects with increased platelet counts for up to 1 year after treatment. Unfortunately, when the response dwindles, platelets may fall to unsafe levels, making additional treatment necessary (Neunert et al., 2019).

Two thrombopoietin receptor agonists are available for treatment of refractory ITP. These include romiplostim and eltromopag. Romiplostim is given as a weekly subcutaneous injection and eltromopag is given orally. The response varies widely, and treatment must be continued indefinitely (Depré, Aboud, Ringel, et al., 2016).

Nursing Management

Nursing care includes a thorough assessment of the patient's lifestyle to determine risks for bleeding associated with activities. A careful medication history should also be obtained, including use of over-the-counter (OTC) medications, herbs, and nutritional supplements. The nurse must be alert to sulfa-containing medications and others that may interfere with platelet function (e.g., aspirin, NSAIDs). The nurse must assess for a history of recent viral illness and reports of headache, visual disturbances, and other symptoms that may indicate intracranial bleeding. Patients admitted to the hospital with wet purpura and low platelet counts should have neurologic assessment included with their vital sign measurements. Injections and rectal medications should be avoided. Rectal temperature measurements should also be avoided because they may cause trauma to the rectal mucosa and stimulate bleeding.

There is evidence that patients with ITP experience an increase in fatigue when compared to those without the disease that is not associated with the duration of the disease, corticosteroid use, bleeding, or low platelet counts (Diz-Kucukkaya & Lopez, 2016). Assessment of the extent of the patient's fatigue can be beneficial in helping the patient to identify coping strategies.

Patient and family education should address signs of exacerbation (e.g., petechiae and ecchymoses), how to contact appropriate health care personnel, the name and type of medications inducing ITP (if appropriate) current medical treatment (name of medications, side effects, tapering schedule, if indicated), frequency of monitoring for the platelet count, and follow-up appointments.

The patient should be instructed to avoid all agents that interfere with platelet function, including herbal therapies and OTC medications. The patient should avoid constipation, straining, and vigorous flossing of the teeth. Electric razors should be used for shaving and soft-bristled toothbrushes should be used for dental hygiene. Patients and their partners should be counseled to avoid vigorous sexual intercourse when platelet counts are low. Patients who are receiving long-term corticosteroids should understand that they are at increased risk for complications including osteoporosis, proximal muscle wasting, cataract formation, and dental caries (see Chapter 45, Table 45-3). Bone mineral density should be monitored, and patients may benefit from supplemental calcium, vitamin D, and bisphosphonate to reduce risk for significant bone disease.

Platelet Defects

Quantitative platelet defects (i.e., thrombocytopenia, thrombocytosis) are not uncommon, however qualitative defects may also occur. Despite normal platelet counts, when qualitative defects are present, platelets do not function normally. A platelet function analyzer is used to evaluate platelet function. This technique is valuable for rapid screening. Examination of platelet morphology with the peripheral blood smear in the laboratory can also identify possible qualitative defects. Platelet morphology is frequently hypogranular and pale and may also be larger than normal (Coutre, 2018).

Aspirin may induce a platelet disorder. Even small amounts of aspirin can reduce normal platelet aggregation and increase bleeding time for several days after ingestion. Although this

> **Chart 29-9**
>
> **PHARMACOLOGY**
>
> **Medications and Substances That Impair Platelet Function**
>
> **Medications**
>
> Angiotensin-converting enzyme inhibitors
> Angiotensin receptor blockers
> Antibiotics
> Beta-lactams
> Cephalosporins
> Penicillins
> Beta-blockers
> Calcium channel blockers
> Chemotherapeutic agents
> Mithramycin
> Vincristine
> Diuretics
> Ethacrynic acid
> Furosemide
> HMG-CoA reductase inhibitors (i.e., "statins")
> Atorvastatin
> Simvastatin
> Methylxanthines
> Aminophylline
> Theophylline
> Milrinone
> Misoprostol
> Nitrates
> Isosorbide
> Nitroglycerin
> Phosphodiesterase inhibitors
> Pentoxyfilline
> Sildanafil
> Tadalafil
> Protease inhibitors
>
> Ritonavir
> Tipranavir
> Phenytoin
> Selective serotonin reuptake inhibitors
> Fluoxetine
> Fluvoxamine
> Paroxetine
> Sertraline
> Tricyclic antidepressants
> Doxepin
> Imipramine
> Tyrosine kinase inhibitors
> Dasatinib
> Imatanib
> Valproic acid
>
> **Food and Food Additives**
>
> Caffeine
> Ethanol (Alcohol)
> Fish oils
> Garlic
> Ginger
> Grape juice
>
> **Over-the-Counter and Herbal Supplements**
>
> Ginkgo biloba
> Ginseng
> Saw palmetto
> Vitamin C
> Vitamin E
>
> Adapted from Comerford, K. C., & Durkin, M. T. (2020). *Nursing 2020 drug handbook.* Philadelphia, PA: Wolters Kluwer; Coutre, S. (2019). Congenital and acquired disorders of platelet function. *UpToDate.* Retrieved on 1/1/2020 at: www.uptodate.com/contents/congenital-and-acquired-disorders-of-platelet-function; Nagalla, S., & Bray, P. F. (2017). Hematology: Drug-induced platelet dysfunction. Cancer Therapy Advisor. Retrieved on 1/1/2020 at: www.cancertherapyadvisor.com/home/decision-support-in-medicine/hematology/drug-induced-platelet-dysfunction/

typically does not cause bleeding in most people, patients with thrombocytopenia and coagulation disorders such as hemophilia can experience significant bleeding after ingestion of aspirin, especially in conjunction with trauma and invasive procedures.

NSAIDs can also impair platelet function, but the effects are not as prolonged as with aspirin (4 days vs. 7 to 10 days). Other causes of platelet dysfunction include end-stage renal disease, MDS, multiple myeloma, cardiopulmonary bypass, herbal remedies, and other medications (see Chart 29-9).

Clinical Manifestations

Bleeding can range from mild to severe. The severity does not necessarily correlate with the platelet count or with tests that measure coagulation (prothrombin time [PT], activated partial thromboplastin time [aPTT]). However, results from these tests may be useful in determining the etiology of the bleeding disorder when abnormalities are present (Levi, Seligsohn, & Kaushansky, 2016). For example, an elevated PT in the setting of a normal aPTT and platelet count may suggest factor VII deficiency, whereas an elevated aPTT in the setting of a normal PT and platelet count is suggestive of von Willebrand disease (vWD) or hemophilia. Ecchymoses, particularly on the extremities, are frequently evident. Patients with platelet dysfunction are at increased risk for bleeding after trauma or invasive procedures (e.g., dental extraction, biopsy).

Medical Management

Platelet dysfunction that is associated with a medication requires stopping the medication when possible, especially when bleeding occurs. If platelet dysfunction is present, bleeding may be prevented by transfusion of platelets prior to an invasive procedure. Antifibrinolytic agents (e.g., aminocaproic acid) may be needed to prevent significant bleeding after procedures; desmopressin, a synthetic vasopressin analogue, can reduce the duration of bleeding and improve hemostasis for some patients (Levi et al., 2016).

Nursing Management

Patients with platelet dysfunction should be instructed to avoid substances that can interfere with platelet function. These include OTC medications such as aspirin and NSAIDs, as well as some herbal preparations, nutritional supplements, and alcohol. Patients should notify all health care providers, including dentists, of their underlying condition before undergoing any invasive procedure so that measures to reduce risk for bleeding can be implemented. Maintaining good oral hygiene is important to promote good dental health and reduce risk for gingival bleeding.

Inherited Bleeding Disorders

Two of the more commonplace inherited bleeding disorders include hemophilia and vWD. Each of these is discussed in the sections that follow.

Hemophilia

There are two forms of hemophilia: hemophilia A and hemophilia B. Both are clinically similar but are distinguishable by laboratory tests. Hemophilia A is caused by a genetic defect that results in deficient or defective factor VIII. Hemophilia B, also known as Christmas disease, is due to a genetic defect that causes a deficiency or defect in factor IX. Hemophilia is a relatively common disease, with hemophilia A occurring in 1 of every 5000 to 7000 births. Hemophilia A is five times more common than hemophilia B (Escobar & Key, 2016). Both hemophilia A and hemophilia B are inherited as X-linked traits, making both conditions much more common in males than in females. Females can be carriers of the gene but are typically asymptomatic. It is estimated that one third of cases result from spontaneous mutations rather than familial transmission (National Hemophilia Foundation, 2019).

The tendency for developing bleeding is the basis for the classification of hemophilia (Escobar & Key, 2016):

- Severe disease is defined by a plasma factor activity level of less than 1 IU/dL, or less than 1% normal factor VIII levels.
- Moderate disease reflects a level of 1 to 5 IU/dL or factor VIII level between 1% and 5% of normal.
- Mild disease reflects a level above 5 IU/dL or factor VIII level above 5%.

Hemophilia is often recognized in early childhood, usually in the toddler period. However, patients with mild hemophilia may not be diagnosed until they experience severe trauma or surgery.

Clinical Manifestations

Hemophilia is manifested by hemorrhages into various parts of the body; hemorrhages can be severe and can occur even with minimal trauma. The frequency and severity of bleeding depend on the degree of factor deficiency and the severity of the precipitating trauma. Those with mild factor deficiency rarely develop spontaneous bleeding; hemorrhage is usually associated with trauma. In contrast, spontaneous bleeding, including hemarthroses and hematomas, occur frequently in patients with severe factor deficiency (Escobar & Key, 2016).

About 75% of bleeding in patients with hemophilia occurs in the joints. Joints most frequently affected include the knees, elbows, ankles, shoulders, wrists, and hips. Pain is often noticed prior to the presence of swelling and limitations in movement. Recurrent joint hemorrhages can lead to joint arthropathy that causes ankylosis and chronic pain (see Fig. 29-5). Patients with severe factor deficiency may become disabled due to joint damage early in life. Bleeding may be superficial as hematomas or as deep hemorrhages into muscle and subcutaneous tissue. With severe factor VIII deficiency, hematomas can occur without trauma and extend into the

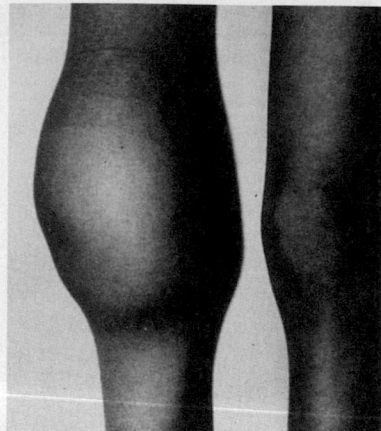

Figure 29-5 • Hemophilic arthropathy: Sequelae of recurrent joint bleeding. Reprinted with permission from *Wintrobe's clinical hematology* (10th ed). (1999). Color plate 68. Philadelphia, PA: Lippincott Williams & Wilkins.

surrounding tissue. Hematomas in the muscles, particularly in the extremities, may cause peripheral nerve compression with impaired sensation. Over time, nerve compression may lead to weakness and atrophy of the affected area.

Bleeding is not limited to joints and muscles. Dental procedures, including extractions, are associated with bleeding. Spontaneous hematuria and GI bleeding may also occur. Bleeding is also common in other mucous membranes, including the nasal passages and conjunctivae as well as soft tissue. Falls in adults are particularly dangerous. Intracranial and extracranial hemorrhages are the most serious sites of bleeding. Any head trauma requires immediate evaluation and treatment. Surgical procedures often result in excessive bleeding at the surgical site. Clot formation and wound healing are often poor.

Medical Management

Recombinant forms of factor VIII and IX concentrates are available and decrease the need for using plasma-derived factor concentrates and fresh-frozen plasma. Concentrates are used when patients are actively bleeding; it is important that treatment is initiated as soon as possible to reduce risk for bleeding complications. Factors should be administered prophylactically prior to traumatic procedures to prevent excessive bleeding (Escobar & Key, 2016). Children frequently receive prophylactic treatment three to four times per week to reduce risk for joint complications. The cost and challenges with adhering to the prescribed regimen may limit the effectiveness of this approach (Thornburg & Duncan, 2017). Initiating prophylactic treatment in adolescents and young adults can also lead to positive outcomes by reducing joint complications, pain, and disability and improving quality of life (Reding, 2018).

Development of neutralizing antibodies (inhibitors) to factor concentrates is a significant complication of factor replacement therapy. Up to 33% of patients with hemophilia A and 3% of patients with hemophilia B develop antibodies to factor concentrates (Reding, 2018). The presence of these inhibitors may be transient; however, the effects may be significant and lead to partial or complete refractoriness to factor replacement, leading to increased risk for bleeding. Ideally, antibody titers should remain low. It is important to identify rising antibody titers as soon as possible. To reduce the impact of inhibitors, inducing immune tolerance is critical. Immunosuppressive therapy in the form of corticosteroids, IVIG or cyclophosphamide may be used to remove inhibitors. Emicizumab is a new bispecific humanized monoclonal antibody that is effective in preventing bleeding in patients with hemophilia A. Initially indicated as effective therapy for patients with inhibitors, it is now also indicated for patients without inhibitors (Franchini, Marano, Pati, et al., 2019; Young, Liesner, Chang, et al., 2019). Patients with severe factor deficiency should be screened for antibodies, particularly prior to invasive procedures, so that appropriate therapy aimed at reducing risk for bleeding complications can be started. Other therapeutic options include administration of recombinant factor VIIa or activated prothrombin complex concentrates (Reding, 2018).

Aminocaproic acid inhibits fibrinolysis and subsequently stabilizes blood clots. It can be very effective as an adjunctive measure to treat mucosal bleeding after oral surgery. Desmopressin induces a significant but short-lived increase in factor VIII levels; the mechanism of this response is unclear. In patients with mild forms of hemophilia A, desmopressin is very useful and can significantly reduce the requirement for blood products (Mannucci, 2018).

Nursing Management

Most adult patients with hemophilia are diagnosed during childhood. They frequently need assistance in coping with the disease because it is chronic and imposes restrictions on their lifestyle. Additionally, the disease is inherited and can be passed to future generations. Helping patients cope with their condition, assisting them to identify positive aspects of their lives, and encouraging independence and self-sufficiency are important nursing activities. This must be balanced with promoting safety and preventing trauma that can result in acute bleeding. As patients mature, they can be encouraged to work through their feelings, progressing toward acceptance, and assuming greater responsibility for maintaining an optimal state of health.

Patients with mild factor deficiency may not be diagnosed until they reach adulthood if they do not have surgery or significant trauma during childhood. The nurse must provide these patients with extensive education to understand activity restrictions and self-care strategies to reduce risk for hemorrhage and complications associated with bleeding. Safety at home and at work should be emphasized.

Patients and family caregivers need to learn how to administer factor concentrate at home at the earliest signs of bleeding to minimize bleeding and reduce complications. Prophylactic factor replacement can be beneficial in reducing morbidity associated with repeated episodes of bleeding. This method requires factor administration several times a week, making adherence to the regimen difficult. Nurses can help patients and families understand the potential benefits of prophylactic therapy while helping them to minimize the disadvantages. Patients with hemophilia are also instructed to avoid agents that can interfere with platelet aggregation that can add additional risk for bleeding. Aspirin, NSAIDs, some herbal and nutritional supplements (e.g., nettle, chamomile, alfalfa), and alcohol should be avoided. Oral hygiene is an important measure to reduce gingival bleeding, and good dental health should be promoted to reduce the need for extractions over the long term. While application of pressure may be helpful

in controlling bleeding from minor injuries in patients with factor deficiency, it is inadequate in the presence of severe factor deficiency. Nasal packing for epistaxis should be avoided because bleeding often resumes when packing is removed. Splints and other orthopedic devices may be beneficial in supporting and immobilizing joints and muscles affected by hemorrhage. All injections should be avoided; invasive procedures (e.g., endoscopy, lumbar puncture) should be avoided or performed after administration of appropriate factor replacement. Patients with hemophilia should carry or wear medical identification (e.g., Medic-Alert bracelets). Additionally, patients and families should have a written emergency plan that includes measures to be taken in specific situations along with names and telephone numbers for emergency contacts.

During bleeding episodes, the extent of bleeding must be carefully assessed. Patients at risk for significant complications (e.g., bleeding into the respiratory tract or CNS) require close observation, specifically assessing for respiratory distress and altered levels of consciousness. Patients who have had recent surgery need careful monitoring to assess for bleeding from surgical sites. Frequent monitoring of vital signs, drains, and dressings is necessary to identify postoperative bleeding.

Significant pain requiring analgesics is often associated with hematomas and joint hemorrhage. Warm baths can be helpful in relieving pain, promoting relaxation, and improving mobility. During bleeding episodes, heat should be avoided because it may exacerbate bleeding; applications of cold are more efficacious.

Factor concentrates used since 1985 are free of viruses, including hepatitis C and HIV; however, patients treated prior to that time were exposed to these viruses (Escobar & Key, 2016). Patients who have acquired HIV and other viral infections may need assistance in coping with these additional diagnoses and the consequences of infection.

Genetic testing and counseling should be offered to female carriers so they can make informed decisions regarding childbearing and managing pregnancy (see Chapter 6).

Gerontologic Considerations

Advances in treatment have led to extended lifespans for patients with hemophilia, causing unique challenges for older patients with this disorder. Older adult patients with hemophilia are likely to have been managed with blood component transfusion and plasma-derived clotting factors prior to the advent of universal screening, at least early in life. For this reason, HIV and hepatitis B and C infections are not uncommon in this population; these infections carry significant risk for liver cancer and other liver diseases (Mannucci, 2019). Intracranial hemorrhage is the third most common cause of death after HIV and hepatitis and result from trauma. The likelihood of acquiring inhibitors increases with age.

Cardiovascular disease among adults with hemophilia can be difficult to manage. Antiplatelet therapy (including aspirin) can be challenging for patients with severe hemophilia. Stent placement and coronary artery bypass graft surgery are accompanied by significant risk but aggressive factor replacement therapy can make these therapeutic treatments possible (Kanellopoulou & Nomikou, 2018). Close collaboration and coordination of care with the patient's hematologist are required to improve outcomes.

Arthropathy is a major cause of morbidity in older patients with hemophilia and can result in reduced range of motion, impaired functioning, and chronic pain. However, quality of life can improve with arthroplasty and multidisciplinary rehabilitation tailored to address the special needs of older adults with hemophilia (Mannucci, 2019).

von Willebrand Disease

vWD is an inherited bleeding disorder characterized by a deficiency in von Willebrand factor (vWF), which is necessary for factor VIII activation. The disease is characterized primarily by mucosa-associated bleeding and bleeding following surgery and trauma. vWD is the most common inherited bleeding disorder, affecting up to 1% of the general population. It typically has an autosomal dominant inheritance pattern, affecting both genders equally (Rick, 2019). vWD is divided into types 1, 2, and 3. Type 1 accounts for 70% to 80% of cases, and is characterized by a quantitative deficiency of vWF. Type 2, accounting for approximately 20% of cases, is caused by dysfunctional vWF. Type 2 is further subdivided on the basis of certain phenotypic characteristics. Type 3 vWD is rare and accounts for fewer than 5% of cases. It is the most

severe form, and is caused by the absence of circulating vWF (Leebeek, & Eikenboom, 2016). Figure 29-6 illustrates the differences in clotting found with hemophilia and vWD.

Clinical Manifestations

Bleeding most often involves the mucous membranes. Nosebleeds, heavy menses, easy bruising, and prolonged bleeding from cuts and surgical sites are common. Soft tissue and joint hemorrhages are not seen often, unless the patient has type 3 vWD. As laboratory values fluctuate, so does bleeding. For example, postoperative bleeding may be minor with one procedure but significant with another (Rick, 2019).

Assessment and Diagnostic Findings

vWD may be suspected based upon a personal or family history of bleeding that may then be confirmed by laboratory evidence of abnormalities in vWF, factor VIII, or both. The diagnosis of vWD is based on measurements of vWF antigen; the level of vWF–dependent platelet adhesion, measured with the use of the vWF–ristocetin cofactor activity assay; and the coagulant activity of factor VIII. Type 3 vWD is diagnosed when vWF antigen is undetectable (or the level is less than

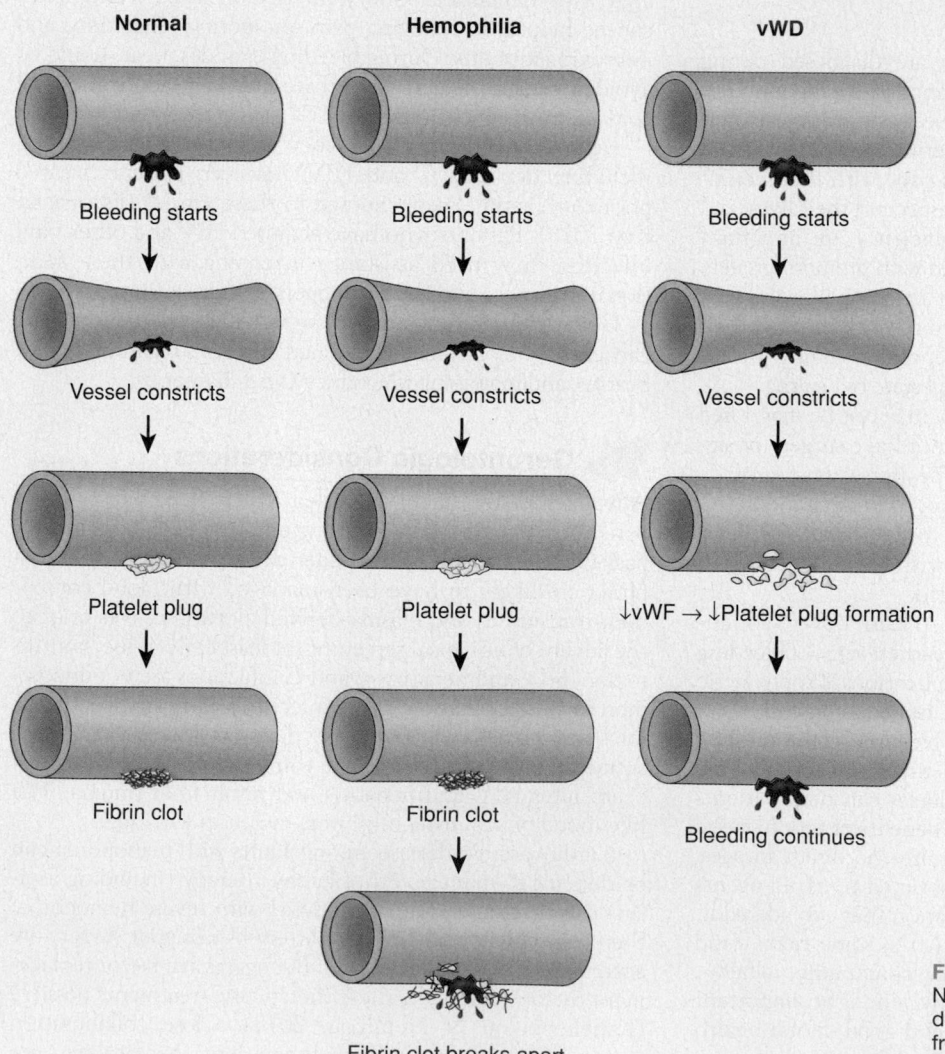

Figure 29-6 • Differences in bleeding. Normal, hemophilia, and von Willebrand disease (vWD). Reprinted with permission from Thomas, M., & Morrow, K. *Veterans Administration Palo Alto Health Care System*. Palo Alto: CA.

5 IU/dL). These results are variable with individual patients over time, making it important to review laboratory values over time and not rely on single measurements (Rick, 2019).

Management

The goal of treatment is to replace the deficient protein (e.g., vWF or factor VIII) at the time of spontaneous bleeding or prior to an invasive procedure to prevent subsequent bleeding. Desmopressin is often used to prevent bleeding associated with dental and surgical procedures or to manage mild bleeding after surgery in patients with mild vWD; it is often not effective in treating those with type 3 vWD (Leebeek, & Eikenboom, 2016). Desmopressin provides a transient increase in factor VIII coagulant activity and may also correct bleeding time. Desmopressin can be given as an IV infusion or intranasally. IV administration is preferred for invasive procedures, including surgery. Hyponatremia and seizures may occur after repeated doses; therefore, treatment longer than 3 consecutive days is not typically indicated.

Factor replacement concentrates of vWF and factor VIII are the treatments of choice for patients with type 3 vWD and most patients with type 2. The dosage and frequency of administration of these agents depend on the patient's factor VIII level and extent of bleeding. Treatment may be needed for up to 7 to 10 days after a surgical procedure and 3 to 4 days postpartum. In patients with type 3 vWD, prophylactic use of replacement agents is often successful in preventing or limiting spontaneous bleeding. Formation of antibodies to these agents is most likely to occur in patients with type 3 vWD receiving high doses.

Other agents are also effective in controlling bleeding. Aminocaproic acid is useful in managing mild mucosal bleeding because it inhibits dissolution of the thrombus at the site of bleeding. Topical agents that augment thrombin formation at the site of application help to achieve hemostasis in dental procedures. Estrogen-progesterone compounds may reduce bleeding associated with menses. Platelet transfusions are useful when there is significant bleeding. Cryoprecipitate, which is rich in vWF and factor VIII, typically is used only in emergencies due to risk for iatrogenic transmission of viruses. Herbs and medications that interfere with platelet function should be avoided (Leebeek & Eikenboom, 2016).

Acquired Bleeding Disorders

There are a plethora of acquired bleeding disorders. Common causes include liver disease, vitamin K deficiency, and heparin-induced thrombocytopenia (HIT).

Liver Disease

Excluding factor VIII, most blood coagulation factors are synthesized in the liver. Therefore, liver dysfunction (due to cirrhosis, hepatitis, and tumor) can lead to reduced amounts of the factors needed for coagulation and hemostasis (see Chapter 43). Prolongation of the PT may indicate severe hepatic dysfunction, unless associated with vitamin K deficiency. Patients may experience minor bleeding (e.g., ecchymoses) but are also at risk for significant bleeding, especially after surgery or trauma. Transfusion of fresh-frozen plasma may be needed to replace clotting factors and prevent or stop bleeding. Life-threatening hemorrhage associated with peptic ulcer or esophageal varices may occur. In the event of significant hemorrhage, transfusion of fresh-frozen plasma, PRBCs, and platelets is often necessary.

Vitamin K Deficiency

Vitamin K is an essential element for synthesis of many coagulation factors. Vitamin K deficiency is often seen in patients who are malnourished. Prolonged use of some antibiotics can reduce the intestinal flora that produce vitamin K, causing depletion of vitamin K stores. Correction of the deficiency can be achieved with oral or subcutaneous administration of vitamin K (phytonadione). Adequate synthesis of coagulation factors is reflected in normalization of the PT.

Heparin-Induced Thrombocytopenia

HIT is a serious complication of heparin-based therapy, a medication commonly prescribed for its anticoagulant effects (see Chapter 26 for description of indications for heparin). HIT involves the formation of antibodies against the heparin–platelet complex. HIT may occur in as many as 5% of patients receiving heparin (Brien, 2019). The type of heparin used, the duration of therapy (4 to 14 days), and surgery (especially if cardiopulmonary bypass is used) appear to be risk factors for developing HIT. Bovine heparin preparations are more likely to lead to HIT than porcine preparations; even low–molecular-weight heparins (LMWHs) carry risk for HIT. Neither the dose nor the route of administration of heparin is a risk factor. Women appear to be at higher risk and young adults are at low risk for developing this condition. A decline in the platelet count is the hallmark sign that most often develops 5 to 10 days after heparin therapy is initiated; therefore, monitoring the platelet count in patients receiving heparin therapy is essential. The platelet count can drop significantly, typically by 50% of the baseline over a period of 1 to 3 days. Autoantibodies develop that may activate platelets, causing thromboses. After patients with HIT are successfully managed, these autoantibodies typically disappear in 2 to 3 months.

Affected patients are at increased risk for thrombosis, either venous, arterial, or both, with thromboses that may manifest as deep vein thrombosis (DVT), acute coronary syndrome (ACS), stroke, or thrombosis to major vessels in an extremity, leading to amputation. Venous thromboembolism (VTE) is the most common manifestation of thrombosis secondary to HIT (i.e., DVT or pulmonary embolism [PE]) (Brien, 2019).

Treatment for HIT includes immediate cessation of heparin (including heparin-coated catheters) and initiation of another form of anticoagulation. If the heparin is discontinued without providing an alternative form of anticoagulation, the patient is at increased risk of developing new thrombi. Argatroban, a thrombin inhibitor, is an FDA-approved anticoagulant for the treatment of HIT. Oral anticoagulation with warfarin is contraindicated because it initially promotes thrombosis in the microvasculature by depletion of protein C. This can lead to tissue ischemia and gangrenous limbs, ultimately resulting in amputation if untreated (Arepally,

2017). Patients who develop thrombosis in the presence of HIT should receive anticoagulation for 3 to 6 months; in the absence of thrombosis, treatment may be shorter. Patients must be aware that the condition may be reactivated with re-exposure to heparin, even in small amounts, within 3 to 4 months of the diagnosis (Arepally, 2017).

 DISSEMINATED INTRAVASCULAR COAGULATION

Disseminated intravascular coagulation (DIC) is a systemic syndrome that is characterized by microthromboses and bleeding. DIC may be precipitated by sepsis, trauma, cancer, shock, abruptio placentae, allergic reactions, and other conditions. Most cases are associated with infection or malignancy (Levi & Seligsohn, 2016). The severity of DIC varies but it is potentially life-threatening.

Pathophysiology

Normal hemostatic mechanisms are altered in DIC. The inflammatory response generated by the underlying disease initiates the process of inflammation and coagulation within the vasculature. The normal anticoagulation pathways in the body are impaired, and fibrinolysis is suppressed allowing numerous small clots to form in the microcirculation. Coagulation time is initially normal; however, when platelets and clotting factors form microthrombi, coagulation fails. The result of these processes leads to both excessive clotting and bleeding (see Fig. 29-7).

The clinical manifestations of DIC are primarily reflected in compromised organ function or failure. Decline in organ function is usually a result of excessive clot formation (with resultant ischemia to all or part of the organ) or, less often, of bleeding. The excessive clotting triggers the fibrinolytic system to release fibrin degradation products, which are potent anticoagulants, furthering the bleeding. The bleeding is characterized by low platelet and fibrinogen levels; prolonged PT, aPTT, and thrombin time; and elevated fibrin degradation products and D-dimers.

The mortality rate can exceed 80% in patients who develop severe DIC with ischemic thrombosis, frank hemorrhage, and MODS. Identification of patients who are at risk for DIC and recognition of the early clinical manifestations of this syndrome can result in prompt medical intervention, which may improve the prognosis. However, the primary prognostic factor is the ability to treat the underlying condition that precipitated DIC (Levi & Seligsohn, 2016).

Clinical Manifestations

During the initial process of DIC, the patient may have no new symptoms—the only manifestation being a progressive decrease in the platelet count. As the thrombosis becomes more extensive, the patient exhibits signs and symptoms of thrombosis in the organs involved. Then, as the clotting factors and platelets are consumed to form these thrombi, bleeding occurs. Initially, the bleeding is subtle, but it can develop into frank hemorrhage. Signs and symptoms depend on the organs involved and are listed in Chart 29-10. Patients with

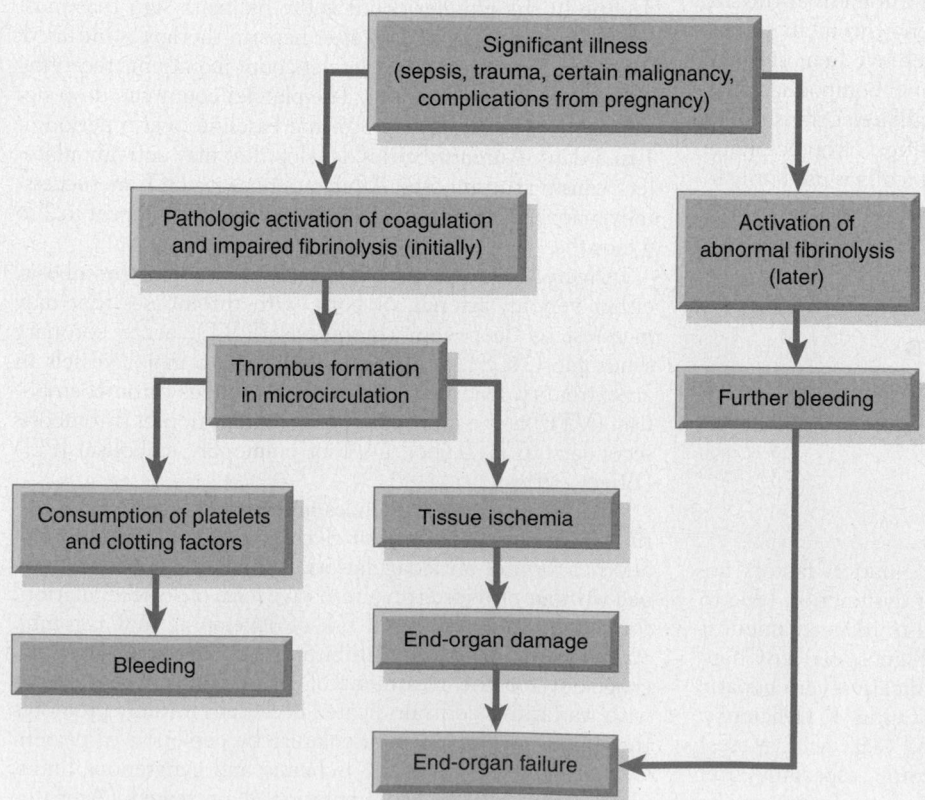

Figure 29-7 • Pathophysiology of disseminated intravascular coagulation.

Chart 29-10	**ASSESSMENT**

Assessing for Thrombosis and Bleeding in Disseminated Intravascular Coagulation

System	Signs and Symptoms of Microvascular Thrombosis	Signs and Symptoms of Microvascular and Frank Bleeding
Integumentary	↓ Temperature, sensation; ↑ pain; cyanosis in extremities, nose, earlobes; focal ischemia, superficial gangrene	Petechiae, including periorbital and oral mucosa; bleeding: gums, oozing from wounds, previous injection sites, around catheters (IVs, tracheostomies); epistaxis; diffuse ecchymoses; subcutaneous hemorrhage; joint pain
Circulatory	↓ Pulses; capillary filling time >3 seconds	Tachycardia
Respiratory	Hypoxia (secondary to clot in lung); dyspnea; chest pain with deep inspiration; ↓ breath sounds over areas of large embolism	High-pitched bronchial breath sounds; tachypnea; ↑ consolidation; signs and symptoms of acute respiratory distress syndrome
Gastrointestinal	Gastric pain; "heartburn"	Hematemesis (heme⊕ nasogastric output); melena (heme⊕ stools → tarry stools → bright-red blood from rectum); retroperitoneal bleeding (abdomen firm, distended, and tender to palpation; ↑ abdominal girth)
Renal	↓ Urine output; ↑ creatinine, ↑ blood urea nitrogen	Hematuria
Neurologic	↓ Alertness and orientation; ↓ pupillary reaction; ↓ response to commands; ↓ strength and mobility	Anxiety; restlessness; ↓ mentation, altered level of consciousness; headache; visual disturbances; conjunctival hemorrhage

↓, decreased; ↑, increased; heme⊕, positive for hemoglobin; IV, intravenous.
Note: Signs of microvascular thrombosis are the result of an inappropriate activation of the coagulation system, causing thrombotic occlusion of small vessels within all body organs. As the clotting factors and platelets are consumed, signs of microvascular bleeding appear. This bleeding can quickly worsen, becoming frank hemorrhage. Treatment must be aimed at the underlying disorder so that the stimulus for the syndrome is diminished or arrested.
Adapted from Levi, M., & Seligsohn, U. (2016). Disseminated intravascular coagulation. In K. Kaushansky, M. A. Lichtman, J. T. Prchal, et al. (Eds.). *Williams hematology* (9th ed.). New York: McGraw-Hill Medical.

frank DIC may exhibit bleeding from mucous membranes and venipuncture sites as well as the GI and urinary tracts. Bleeding may range from minimal, occult internal bleeding to copious bleeding from multiple orifices.

Assessment and Diagnostic Findings

The diagnosis of DIC is frequently made based on laboratory tests that demonstrate the consumption of platelets and clotting factors (see Table 29-4). Although each test is useful in establishing the diagnosis of DIC, the specificity of each individual test is lacking. The International Society

of Thrombosis and Haemostasis developed a highly sensitive and specific scoring system using platelet count, fibrin degradation products, PT, and fibrinogen level to diagnose DIC (Levi & Seligsohn, 2016) (see Table 29-5). Additionally, this system is useful in predicting the severity of the disease and subsequent mortality. Additional tests, such as thromboelastography, can be performed at the bedside and can effectively assess platelet function and fibrinolytic activity. Studies suggest that assessment of the status of the coagulation system at the bedside of critically ill patients is more useful than using conventional laboratory tests (Afzal & Syed, 2017).

TABLE 29-4 Laboratory Values Commonly Found in Disseminated Intravascular Coagulation[a]

Test	Function Evaluated	Normal Range	Changes in DIC
Platelet count	Platelet number	150,000–450,000/mm^3	↓
Prothrombin time (PT)	Extrinsic pathway	11–12.5 s	↑
Partial thromboplastin time (activated)(aPTT)	Intrinsic pathway	23–35 s	↑
Thrombin time (TT)	Clot formation	8–11 s	↑
Fibrinogen	Amount available for coagulation	170–340 mg/dL	↓
D-dimer	Local fibrinolysis	0–250 ng/mL	↑
Fibrin degradation products (FDPs)	Fibrinolysis	0–5 mcg/mL	↑
Euglobulin clot lysis	Fibrinolytic activity	≥2 h	≤1 h

[a]Because DIC is a dynamic condition, the laboratory values measured will change over time. Therefore, a progressive increase or decrease in a given laboratory value is likely to be more important than the actual value of a test at a single point in time.
↓, decreased; ↑, increased; DIC, disseminated intravascular coagulation.
Adapted from Fischbach, F. T., & Fischbach, M. A. (2018). *A manual of laboratory and diagnostic tests* (10th ed.). Philadelphia, PA: Wolters Kluwer.

TABLE 29-5	Scoring System for Disseminated Intravascular Coagulation			
Laboratory Test	**0**	**1**	**2**	**3**
Platelet count	>100,000/mm^3	>50,000/mm^3, <100,000/mm^3	<50,000/mm^3	
Fibrin degradation products	No increase		Moderate increase	Strong increase
Prothrombin time (upper limit of normal)	<3 s	>3 s, <6 s	>6 s	
Fibrinogen	>100 mg/dL	<100 mg/dL		

Note: 5 or more is compatible with overt disseminated intravascular coagulation.
Adapted from Taylor, F. B., Toh, C. H., Hoots, W. K., et al. (2007). Towards a definition, clinical and laboratory criteria, and a scoring system for DIC. *Journal of Thrombosis and Haemostasis, 5*(3), 445–659.

Medical Management

The most critical factor in managing DIC is treatment of the underlying cause; until the cause is controlled, DIC will continue. Correcting the secondary effects of tissue ischemia by increasing tissue oxygenation, replacing fluids, correcting electrolyte abnormalities, and administering vasopressor medications is also important. When serious hemorrhage is present, depleted coagulation factors and platelets are replaced to promote normal hemostasis and reduce bleeding. The extent of hemorrhage and need for any invasive procedure are important considerations in determining the decision to provide transfusion support. Cryoprecipitate is given to replace fibrinogen and factors V and VII (Levi & Seligsohn, 2016).

The use of a heparin infusion to interrupt the thrombosis process is a controversial treatment strategy. Heparin may inhibit the formation of microthrombi and allow improved tissue perfusion to vital organs. Traditionally, heparin has been used in patients with predominantly thrombotic manifestations or in those in whom blood component replacement failed to reduce hemorrhage or increased fibrinogen and other clotting levels. When bleeding is absent, LMWH can be used to prevent VTE, while therapeutic doses may be used when severe thrombosis is predominant. Normalization of plasma fibrinogen and diminished signs of bleeding serve as evidence of heparin's effectiveness. Fibrinolytic inhibitors, such as aminocaproic acid, are not routinely used as they block the lysis of fibrin that is necessary to preserve tissue perfusion. If bleeding is profuse and there is evidence of extensive fibrinolysis, fibrinolytic inhibitors are used along with continuous infusion of IV heparin (Levi & Seligsohn, 2016).

Recombinant forms of thrombomodulin were believed to inactivate thrombin, the main culprit in inciting the coagulopathy that undergirds DIC. However, a systematic review of clinical trials found no improvement in mortality rates with patients with DIC who were prescribed recombinant thrombomodulin (Murao & Yamakawa, 2019). All management strategies must be individualized to the specific patient, underlying cause of DIC, and response to interventions.

Nursing Management

Nurses need to identify patients at risk for DIC (see previous discussion on precipitating factors). It is important to assess patients frequently and thoroughly for signs and symptoms of thrombi and bleeding and monitor for progression of these signs (see Chart 29-10). Laboratory values must be monitored frequently to assess for trends over time as well as for changes in values.

Chart 29-11 describes care of the patient with DIC. Assessment and interventions should target potential sites of end-organ damage. As organs become ischemic from microthrombi, organ function diminishes; the kidneys, lungs, brain, and skin are particularly vulnerable. Lack of renal perfusion may result in acute tubular necrosis and kidney injury, sometimes requiring dialysis. Placement of a large-bore dialysis catheter is extremely hazardous for this patient population and should be accompanied by adequate platelet and plasma transfusions. Hepatic dysfunction is also relatively common, reflected in altered liver function tests, depleted albumin stores, and diminished synthesis of clotting factors. Respiratory function warrants careful monitoring and aggressive measures to diminish alveolar compromise. Suctioning should be performed as gently as possible to diminish the risk of additional bleeding. CNS involvement can be manifested as headache, visual changes, and alteration in level of consciousness.

SECONDARY THROMBOCYTOSIS

Increased platelet production is the primary mechanism of secondary or reactive **thrombocytosis**, characterized by an elevation in the platelet count. However, these elevations are rarely above 1 million/mm^3. This is in contrast to essential thrombocytosis which is a chronic myeloproliferative disease (see Chapter 30). In secondary thrombocytosis, platelet function and survival are typically normal; therefore, hemorrhage and thrombosis are rare (Kaushansky, 2016). A number of disorders are associated with a reactive increase in platelets, including infection, iron deficiency anemia, chronic inflammatory disorders, malignancy, acute hemorrhage, and splenectomy. Treatment is directed at the underlying disorder. When managed successfully, the platelet count often returns to normal.

THROMBOTIC DISORDERS

Several conditions can affect the balance of normal hemostasis, causing excessive thrombosis that can alter arterial or venous circulation. Arterial thrombosis is caused by platelet aggregation, while venous thrombosis is a result of accumulation of

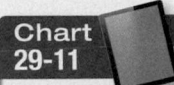

PLAN OF NURSING CARE

Chart 29-11

The Patient with Disseminated Intravascular Coagulation

NURSING DIAGNOSIS: Risk for hypovolaemia associated with bleeding
GOALS: Hemodynamic status maintained; urine output ≥0.5 mL/kg/h over 6 hours or <400 mL in 24 hours

Nursing Interventions	Rationale	Expected Outcomes
1. Avoid procedures/activities that can increase intracranial pressure (e.g., coughing, straining to have a bowel movement).	1. Prevents intracranial bleeding	• Level of consciousness (LOC) stable
2. Monitor vital signs closely, including neurologic checks: a. Monitor hemodynamics. b. Monitor abdominal girth. c. Monitor urine output.	2. Identifies signs of hemorrhage/shock as soon as possible	• Central venous pressure 5–12 cm H_2O, systolic blood pressure ≥70 mm Hg • Urine output ≥0.5 mL/kg/h • Decreased bleeding • Decreased oozing
3. Avoid medications that interfere with platelet function if possible (e.g., aspirin, nonsteroidal anti-inflammatory drugs, beta-lactam antibiotics).	3. Decreases problems with platelet aggregation and adhesion	• Decreased ecchymoses • Amenorrhea • Absence of oral and bronchial bleeding
4. Avoid rectal probes, rectal medications.	4. Decreases risk of rectal bleeding	• Oral mucosa clean, moist, intact
5. Avoid intramuscular injections.	5. Decreases risk of intramuscular bleeding	
6. Monitor amount of external bleeding carefully:	6.	
a. Monitor number of dressings, percentage of dressing saturated; time to saturate a dressing is more objective than "dressing saturated a moderate amount."	a. Provides accurate, objective assessment of extent of bleeding	
b. Assess suction output, all excreta for frank or occult blood.	b. Identifies presence of or quantifies extent of bleeding	
c. Monitor pad counts in women with vaginal bleeding.	c. Quantifies extent of bleeding	
d. Women may receive progesterone to prevent menses.	d. Decreases risk of bleeding from gynecologic source	
7. Use low pressure for any necessary suctioning.	7. Prevents excessive trauma that can cause additional bleeding	
8. Administer oral hygiene carefully. a. Avoid lemon-glycerin swabs, hydrogen peroxide, commercial mouthwashes. b. Use sponge-tipped swabs, salt/baking soda (bicarbonate of soda) mouth rinses.	8. Prevents excessive trauma that can cause bleeding. Glycerin and alcohol (in commercial mouthwashes) dry the mucosa, increasing risk for bleeding.	
9. Avoid dislodging any clots, including those around IV sites and injection sites.	9. Reduces risk for excessive bleeding from sites	

NURSING DIAGNOSIS: Risk for impaired skin integrity associated with ischemia or bleeding
GOALS: Skin integrity remains intact; oral mucosa remains intact

Nursing Interventions	Rationale	Expected Outcomes
1. Assess skin, with particular attention to bony prominences, skin folds.	1. Prompt identification of any area of risk for skin breakdown or showing early signs of breakdown can prompt early intervention and reduce complications.	• Skin integrity remains intact; skin is warm, and of normal color. • Oral mucosa is intact, pink, moist, without bleeding.
2. Reposition carefully; use pressure-reducing mattress.	2–4. Meticulous skin care and use of measures to prevent pressure on bony prominences decreases risk of skin trauma.	
3. Perform careful skin care every 2 hours, emphasizing dependent areas, all bony prominences, and perineum.		
4. Use lamb's wool between digits, around ears, as needed.		
5. Use prolonged pressure (at least 5 minutes) after injection or procedure when such measures must be performed.	5. Initial platelet plug is very unstable and can be easily dislodged, which can lead to increased bleeding.	
6. Perform oral hygiene carefully (see previous discussion).	6. Meticulous care is needed to decrease trauma, bleeding, and risk of infection.	

(continued on page 944)

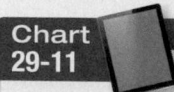

Chart 29-11

PLAN OF NURSING CARE (continued)
The Patient with Disseminated Intravascular Coagulation

NURSING DIAGNOSIS: Fluid imbalance associated with excessive blood and/or factor component replacement
GOALS: Absence of edema; absence of crackles; intake not greater than output

Nursing Interventions	Rationale	Expected Outcomes
1. Auscultate breath sounds every 2–4 hours. 2. Monitor extent of edema. 3. Monitor volume of IV fluids, blood products; decrease volume of IV medications if indicated. 4. Administer diuretics as prescribed.	1. Crackles can develop quickly. 2. Fluid may extend beyond intravascular space. 3. Helps prevent fluid overload 4. Decreases excess fluid volume	• Breath sounds clear • Absence of edema • Intake does not exceed output • Weight stable

NURSING DIAGNOSIS: Risk for injury associated with microthrombi
GOALS: Neurologic status remains intact; absence of hypoxemia; peripheral pulses remain intact; skin integrity remains intact; urine output remains ≥0.5 mL/kg/h over 6 hours and >400 mL in 24 hours

Nursing Interventions	Rationale	Expected Outcomes
1. Assess neurologic, pulmonary, integumentary systems. 2. Monitor response to heparin therapy. 3. Assess extent of bleeding. 4. Monitor fibrinogen levels. 5. Stop aminocaproic acid, if prescribed, if symptoms of thrombosis occur.	1. Initial signs of thrombosis may be subtle. 2. Assure anticoagulation effectiveness that may prevent formation of additional thromboses. 3. Objective measurements of all sites of bleeding are crucial to accurately assess extent of blood loss. 4. Response to heparin is most accurately reflected in fibrinogen level. 5. Aminocaproic acid should be used only in the setting of extensive hemorrhage not responding to replacement therapy.	• Arterial blood gases, O_2 saturation, pulse oximetry, LOC within normal limits • Breath sounds clear • Absence of edema • Intake does not exceed output • Weight stable

NURSING DIAGNOSIS: Anxiety associated with uncertain prognosis and risk for death
GOALS: Feelings identified/verbalized; realistic hope maintained

Nursing Interventions	Rationale	Expected Outcomes
1. Identify previous coping mechanisms, if possible; encourage patient to use them as appropriate. 2. Explain all procedures and their rationale in terms that the patient and family/significant others can understand. 3. Assist family in supporting patient. 4. Use services from behavioral health, chaplain as needed.	1. Identifying previous stressful situations can aid in recall of successful coping mechanisms. 2. Decreased knowledge and uncertainty can increase anxiety. 3. Family/significant others can be valuable in assisting the patient to use coping strategies and to maintain hope. 4. An interdisciplinary approach may be warranted, particularly when coping strategies are maladaptive or ineffective. The spiritual dimension of care may be especially important in a crisis.	• Previously used coping strategies are identified and utilized, to the extent the patient is able to do so. • Patient and family indicate understanding of procedures as situation permits.

LOC, level of consciousness.

platelets, red blood cells, and thrombin. Abnormalities that predispose a person to thrombotic events include decreased clotting inhibitors in the circulation, impaired liver function, lack of fibrinolytic enzymes, and vascular abnormalities that promote platelet aggregation. Thrombosis may also occur as the initial manifestation of an occult malignancy or as a complication of a previously diagnosed cancer. In some cases, more than one precipitating factor exists. There are several inherited or acquired disorders, including hyperhomocysteinemia, antithrombin (AT) deficiency, protein C deficiency, protein S deficiency, activated protein C (APC) resistance, and factor V Leiden deficiency that can predispose patients to repeated episodes of thrombosis. These are also referred to as hypercoagulable states or thrombophilia. Inherited disorders should prompt a referral for familial genetic testing. Genetic testing is not indicated with acquired disorders.

Thrombotic disorders require anticoagulation therapy; the duration of therapy varies with the location and extent of thrombosis, precipitating events (e.g., trauma, immobility), and any concurrent risk factors (e.g., use of oral contraceptives, obesity, tobacco use, integrity of blood vessels, previous thrombotic events; see Table 29-6). Conditions that

TABLE 29-6 ⚠	Risk Factors for Thrombosis	
Acquired	**Inherited**	**Mixed/Unknown**
Advanced age	Antithrombin	Activated
Antiphospholipid anti-	deficiency	protein C
body syndrome	Factor V Leiden	resistance
Atrial fibrillation	Factor XII deficiency	↑ Factor VII
Diabetes	Protein C deficiency	↑ Factor VIII
Drugs (e.g., cocaine,	Protein S deficiency	↑ Factor IX
ergot)	Prothrombin 20210[a]	↑ Factor XI
Estrogen therapy		↓ Fibrinolytic
Hypertension		activity
Inflammatory bowel		↑Homocysteine
disease		
Immobility		
Lupus anticoagulant		
Major surgery		
Myeloproliferative disease		
Nephrotic syndrome		
Obesity		
Paralysis		
Pregnancy/postpartum		
period		
Prior stroke		
Prior superficial vein		
thrombosis		
Smoking		
Trauma/fracture		
Vascular access devices		

Note: Risk factors for first, unprovoked venous thromboembolism. Note that the factor levels that are increased are procoagulant proteins.

↑, increased; ↓, decreased.

Adapted from Koupenova, M., Kehrel, B. E., Corkerey, H. A., & Freedman, J. E. (2016). Thrombosis and platelets: An update. *European Heart Journal, 38*(11), 785–791.

may result from thrombosis include ACS (see Chapter 23), ischemic stroke (see Chapter 62), and occlusive peripheral arterial disease (see Chapter 26). With some conditions, or with repeated thrombosis, lifelong anticoagulation may be required.

Hyperhomocysteinemia

Homocysteine is known to promote platelet aggregation. When hyperhomocysteinemia is present, the endothelial lining of blood vessels are denuded, which can lead to thrombus formation, specifically VTE (e.g., DVT, PE) and arterial thrombosis (e.g., ischemic stroke, ACS); however, the evidence available does not clearly identify homocysteine as a causal factor. Research suggests that the mechanisms through which hyperhomocysteinemia causes vascular disease are more complex than an increase in homocysteine alone (Ospina-Romero, Cannegieter, den Heijer, et al., 2018).

Hyperhomocysteinemia can be hereditary but may also occur as a result of folate deficiency, and to a lesser degree, deficiency of vitamins B_6 and B_{12}. These nutrients are cofactors in homocysteine metabolism. Additionally, for reasons that are unclear, older adults and those with kidney injury may also have elevated homocysteine levels without vitamin deficiency (Ostrakhovich & Tabibzadeh, 2019). While a fasting measurement of plasma homocysteine can be useful for screening in some cases, levels may be normal or slightly elevated in people with inherited hyperhomocysteinemia or those with vitamin B_6 deficiency. A more sensitive method

of measurement involves obtaining a second measurement 4 hours after consumption of methionine; hyperhomocysteinemia is found more often using this method. Supplemental use of folic acid, vitamin B_{12}, or vitamin B_6 has not been shown to be effective in reducing the recurrence of venous or arterial thromboemboli (Middeldorp & Coppens, 2016). Smoking is associated with reduced levels of vitamin B_6, vitamin B_{12}, and folate, making smoking cessation an important goal for patients with known hyperhomocysteinemia.

Antithrombin Deficiency

AT is a protein that inhibits thrombin and certain coagulation factors. It may also play a role in reducing inflammation within the endothelium of blood vessels. AT deficiency can be acquired by four mechanisms: accelerated consumption of AT (as in DIC); decreased synthesis of AT (as in hepatic dysfunction); increased excretion of AT (as in nephrotic syndrome); and medication induced (e.g., estrogens) (Bunn & Bauer, 2017). However, AT deficiency is most often an inherited condition that can lead to venous thrombosis, especially when AT levels are less than 60% of normal. The most common sites of thrombosis are the deep veins in the legs and within the mesentery. Recurrent thrombosis can occur, particularly as patients age. Patients with AT deficiency may exhibit heparin resistance and therefore require greater doses of heparin to achieve adequate anticoagulation. Patients with AT deficiency should encourage their family members to be tested for the condition.

Protein C Deficiency

Protein C is a vitamin K–dependent enzyme synthesized in the liver that, when activated, inhibits coagulation. When protein C levels are low, the risk for thrombosis increases and thrombosis may occur spontaneously. People with protein C deficiency are often asymptomatic until they reach adulthood; the risk for thrombosis then increases with age. A rare but important complication for patients with protein C deficiency receiving warfarin for anticoagulation is warfarin-induced skin necrosis. This condition is believed to be a result of progressive thrombosis of capillaries in the skin. The degree of necrosis can be quite extensive (Bunn & Bauer, 2017). Prompt recognition of the problem with immediate cessation of the warfarin, along with treatment with vitamin K, heparin, and fresh-frozen plasma infusions are needed to arrest the pathophysiologic process and reverse the effects of warfarin. Treatment with purified protein C concentrate may be necessary.

Protein S Deficiency

Protein S is another natural anticoagulant normally produced by the liver. APC requires protein S to inactivate certain clotting factors. When the level of protein S is deficient, this inactivation process is diminished and the risk of thrombosis increases. As with protein C deficiency, patients with protein S deficiency have a greater risk for recurrent venous thrombosis early in life, including risk for PE (Bunn & Bauer, 2017).

Thromboses frequently occur in axillary, mesenteric, and cerebral veins. Warfarin-induced skin necrosis is also possible with protein S deficiency. A number of conditions may lead to acquired protein S deficiency including pregnancy, DIC, liver disease, nephritic syndrome, HIV infection, and the use of L-asparaginase.

Activated Protein C Resistance and Factor V Leiden Mutation

APC resistance is a common condition that can occur with other hypercoagulable states. APC is an anticoagulant, and resistance to APC increases risk for venous thrombosis. A defect in the factor V gene has been identified in 90% of patients with APC resistance. This factor V Leiden mutation is the most common cause of inherited hypercoagulability in Caucasians; its incidence appears to be much lower in other ethnic groups (Bunn & Bauer, 2017; Middeldorp & Coppens, 2016). The risk of thrombosis significantly increases when factor V Leiden mutation is paired with other risk factors (e.g., increased age, use of oral contraceptives, hyperhomocysteinemia). People who are homozygous for factor V Leiden mutation are at extreme risk for thrombosis and therefore require lifelong anticoagulation. In contrast, those who are heterozygous for the mutation have a lower risk for developing a thrombus. The duration of anticoagulation is based on the coexistence of other risk factors for thrombus formation.

Antiphospholipid Antibody Syndrome

Antibodies to phospholipids are common causes of thrombophilia; up to 5% of the general population may have this disorder. These antibodies reduce levels of annexin V, a protein that binds to phospholipids and has anticoagulant activity. The most common of the antiphospholipid antibodies are lupus and anticardiolipin antibodies, or an antibody to beta-2 glycoprotein (Rand & Wolgast, 2016). Antiphospholipid antibody syndromes are classified as primary or secondary, with a reaction secondary to a preexisting autoimmune disease, with systemic lupus erythematosus being most frequently implicated. Primary antiphospholipid antibody syndrome is associated with a number of infections including hepatitis C, HIV, syphilis and malaria as well as certain medications (e.g., antibiotics, quinine, hydralazine, procainamide); a genetic predisposition to this syndrome has been postulated but has not been proven. Antiphospholipid antibodies are associated with multiple miscarriages and are strongly associated with stroke (Heuser & Branch, 2019). Most thromboses are venous, but arterial thrombosis is also possible in up to one third of patients with this syndrome. Recurrent thromboses tend to occur in the same fashion, with recurrent venous thrombosis after an initial venous presentation and recurrent arterial thromboses after an initial arterial thrombosis. Thrombi typically occur in large vessels. Therapy varies depending on the type of syndrome (e.g., secondary forms caused by autoimmune disorders may be treated with immunosuppressive therapy), history of prior thrombosis, and location of the thrombus (venous or arterial). Arterial thrombosis is often treated by adding low-dose aspirin to some form of heparin therapy (see later discussion).

Malignancy

Cancers, particularly stomach, pancreatic, lung, and ovarian cancers, are often associated with thrombophilia with significant risk for VTE. VTE contributes to morbidity and mortality of patients with cancer, with a fatal PE being three times more common in patients with cancer than in those without cancer. Patients with cancer have a five- to sevenfold increased risk of developing VTE, and those who develop VTE at diagnosis of cancer or within a year of diagnosis tend to have a significantly worse prognosis than patients with cancer without VTE. A diagnosis of VTE is a serious complication of cancer that adversely affects a patient's quality of life and reduces overall survival. Anticoagulation may be difficult to manage and thromboses can progress despite adequate doses of anticoagulants. LMWH may be more effective than warfarin in treating this group of patients (Razak, Jones, Bhandari, et al., 2018).

Medical Management

The primary treatment for thrombotic disorders is anticoagulation. However, when to treat and how long to treat with anticoagulant medications is controversial. Anticoagulation therapy is not without risk, with the most significant risk of bleeding. Anticoagulant medications used to treat a variety of thromboses are discussed in Chapter 26.

Nursing Management

Patients with thrombotic disorders should be counseled to avoid activities that lead to circulatory stasis (e.g., immobility, crossed legs). Exercise, especially ambulation, should be performed frequently throughout the day, especially during long trips by car or plane. Anti-embolism stockings may be prescribed and patients often need instruction in how to use them properly. Surgery increases risk for thrombosis significantly.

Medications that alter platelet aggregation, such as low-dose aspirin or clopidogrel, may be prescribed. Some patients require lifelong anticoagulation therapy.

Patients with thrombotic disorders, particularly those with thrombophilia, should be evaluated for concurrent risk factors for thrombosis and should avoid them whenever possible. For example, products containing tobacco and nicotine should be avoided, blood pressure should be controlled, and alcohol consumption limited. In some instances, younger patients with thrombophilia may not need prophylactic anticoagulation, but when concomitant risk factors (e.g., pregnancy), increasing age, or subsequent thrombotic events are present, prophylactic or long-term anticoagulation therapy may be needed. Being able to provide the health care provider with an accurate health history can be extremely useful and help in guiding the selection of the appropriate interventions. Patients need to be aware of risk factors for thrombosis and how they can be reduced or eliminated, such as avoiding tobacco, using alternative forms of contraception, avoiding immobility, and maintaining a healthy weight. Patients with hereditary disorders should encourage their siblings and children to be tested for the disorder.

When a patient with a thrombotic disorder is hospitalized, frequent assessment should be performed to promote early recognition of signs and symptoms of thrombus formation, particularly in the legs (DVT) and lungs (PE). Ambulation or range-of-motion exercises as well as anti-embolism stockings or sequential compression devices are used to decrease venous stasis.

CRITICAL THINKING EXERCISES

1 **pq** A 72-year-old man presents to the emergency department complaining of acute shortness of breath and chest pain. He reports increasing fatigue, exertional dyspnea, dull abdominal pain, and weight loss over the last few months. His CBC reveals a normal WBC count and platelet count; however, the hemoglobin is 7.2 mg/dL and the hematocrit is 22.3%. The MCV is reduced. Iron deficiency anemia is suspected. What are your priority interventions targeted at relieving the patient's symptoms? What other medical interventions do you anticipate might be prescribed? What additional laboratory tests do you anticipate for this patient?

2 **ipc** A 23-year-old female patient with sickle cell disease tells you during a routine office visit that she would like to become pregnant. Her condition has been well controlled with hydroxyurea. She takes ibuprofen on a regular basis for chronic pain. What additional information should you collect in the patient history? What challenges do you anticipate in caring for this patient? What other members of the interdisciplinary team do you think should be consulted to be part of the patient's prenatal care?

3 **ebp** Your 44-year-old female neighbor tells you that her brother has been "nagging her" to get tested for hemochromatosis since he was diagnosed with this disease a few months ago. Her brother has periodic therapeutic phlebotomies to treat his disease, and she feels her lifestyle is too busy to support these types of treatments. She tells you that she "feels fine" and wonders how likely it is that she has hemochromatosis, and if she does, whether treatment would be needed. What are the risks for hemochromatosis? If your neighbor does have hemochromatosis, what is the strength of the evidence for best treatment options for her?

REFERENCES

*Asterisk indicates nursing research.
**Double asterisk indicates classic reference.

Books

Bunn, H. F. (2017a). Overview of anemias. In J. C. Aster & H. F Bunn (Eds.). *Pathophysiology of blood disorders* (2nd ed.). New York: McGraw-Hill Medical.

Bunn, H. F. (2017b). Sickle cell disease. In J. C. Aster & H. F. Bunn (Eds.). *Pathophysiology of blood disorders* (2nd ed.). New York: McGraw-Hill Medical.

Bunn, H. F., & Bauer, K. A. (2017). Thrombotic disorders. In J. C. Aster & H. F. Bunn (Eds.). *Pathophysiology of blood disorders* (2nd ed.). New York: McGraw-Hill Medical.

Bunn, H. F., & Heeney, M. M. (2017). Iron homeostasis: Deficiency and overload. In J. C. Aster & H. F. Bunn (Eds.). *Pathophysiology of blood disorders* (2nd ed.). New York: McGraw-Hill Medical.

Comerford, K. C., & Durkin, M. T. (2020). *Nursing 2020 drug handbook.* Philadelphia, PA: Wolters Kluwer.

Dale, D. C., & Welte, K. (2016). Neutropenia and neutrophilia. In K. Kaushansky, M. A. Lichtman, J. T. Prchal, et al. (Eds.). *Williams hematology* (9th ed.). New York: McGraw-Hill Medical.

Diz-Kucukkaya, R., & Lopez, J. (2016). Thrombocytopenia. In K. Kaushansky, M. A. Lichtman, J. T. Prchal, et al. (Eds.). *Williams hematology* (9th ed.). New York: McGraw-Hill Medical.

Elder, J. D., Winland-Brown, J. E., & Porter, B. O. (2019). Hematologic disorders. In L. M. Dunphy, J. E. Winland-Brown, B. O. Porter, et al. (Eds.). *Primary care: The art and science of advance practice nursing—An interprofessional approach* (5th ed.). Philadelphia, PA: FA Davis.

Escobar, M. A., & Key, N. S. (2016). Hemophilia A and hemophilia B. In K. Kaushansky, M. A. Lichtman, J. T. Prchal, et al. (Eds.). *Williams hematology* (9th ed.). New York: McGraw-Hill Medical.

Fischbach, F. T., & Fischbach, M. A. (2018). *A manual of laboratory and diagnostic tests* (10th ed.). Philadelphia, PA: Wolters Kluwer.

Ganz, T. (2016). Iron deficiency and overload. In L. M. Dunphy, J. E. Winland-Brown, B. O. Porter, et al. (Eds.). *Primary care: The art and science of advance practice nursing—An interprofessional approach* (5th ed.). Philadelphia, PA: FA Davis.

Green, R. (2016). Folate, cobalamin, and megaloblastic anemias. In K. Kaushansky, M. A. Lichtman, J. T. Prchal, et al. (Eds.). *Williams hematology* (9th ed.). New York: McGraw-Hill Medical.

Heuser, C., & Branch, W. (2019). Diagnosis and management of antiphospholipid syndrome. In E. R. Norwitz, C. M. Zelop, D. A. Miller, et al. (Eds.). *Evidence-based obstetrics and gynecology.* Hoboken, NJ: Wiley Blackwell.

Kaushansky, K. (2016). Reactive thrombocytosis. In K. Kaushansky, M. A. Lichtman, J. T. Prchal, et al. (Eds.). *Williams hematology* (9th ed.). New York: McGraw-Hill Medical.

Levi, M., & Seligsohn, U. (2016). Disseminated intravascular coagulation. In K. Kaushansky, M. A. Lichtman, J. T. Prchal, et al. (Eds.). *Williams hematology* (9th ed.). New York: McGraw-Hill Medical.

Levi, M., Seligsohn, U., & Kaushansky, K. (2016). Classification, clinical manifestations, and evaluation of disorders of hemostasis. In K. Kaushansky, M. A. Lichtman, J. T. Prchal, et al. (Eds.). *Williams hematology* (9th ed.). New York: McGraw-Hill Medical.

Middeldorp, S., & Coppens, M. (2016). Hereditary thrombophilia. In K. Kaushansky, M. A. Lichtman, J. T. Prchal, et al. (Eds.). *Williams hematology* (9th ed.). New York: McGraw-Hill Medical.

Nair, M. (2018). The blood and associated disorders. In I. Peate (Ed.). *Fundamentals of applied pathophysiology* (3rd ed.). Hoboken, NJ: John Wiley & Sons.

Natrajan K., & Kutlar, A. (2016). Disorders of hemoglobin structure: Sickle cell anemia and related abnormalities. In K. Kaushansky, M. A. Lichtman, J. T. Prchal, et al. (Eds.). *Williams hematology* (9th ed.). New York: McGraw-Hill Medical.

Packman, C. H. (2016). Hemolytic anemia resulting from immune injury. In K. Kaushansky, M. A. Lichtman, J. T. Prchal, et al. (Eds.). *Williams hematology* (9th ed.). New York: McGraw-Hill Medical.

Prchal, J. T. (2016a). Clinical manifestations and classification of erythrocyte disorders. In K. Kaushansky, M. A. Lichtman, J. T. Prchal, et al. (Eds.). *Williams hematology* (9th ed.). New York: McGraw-Hill Medical.

Prchal, J. T. (2016b). Primary and secondary erythrocytoses. In K. Kaushansky, M. A. Lichtman, J. T. Prchal, et al. (Eds.). *Williams hematology* (9th ed.). New York: McGraw-Hill Medical.

Rand, J. H., & Wolgast, L. (2016). The antiphospholipid syndrome. In K. Kaushansky, M. A. Lichtman, J. T. Prchal, et al. (Eds.). *Williams hematology* (9th ed.). New York: McGraw-Hill Medical.

Segel, G. B., & Lichtman, M. A. (2016). Aplastic anemia: Acquired and inherited. In K. Kaushansky, M. A. Lichtman, J. T. Prchal, et al. (Eds.). *Williams hematology* (9th ed.). New York: McGraw-Hill Medical.

van Solinge, W. W., & van Wijk, R. (2016). Erythrocyte enzyme disorders. In K. Kaushansky, M. A. Lichtman, J. T. Prchal, et al. (Eds.). *Williams hematology* (9th ed.). New York: McGraw-Hill Medical.

Vasu, S., & Caligiuri, M. A. (2016). Lymphocytosis and lymphopenia. In K. Kaushansky, M. A. Lichtman, J. T. Prchal, et al. (Eds.). *Williams hematology* (9th ed.). New York: McGraw-Hill Medical.

Weatherall, D. J. (2016). The thalassemias: Disorders of globin synthesis. In K. Kaushansky, M. A. Lichtman, J. T. Prchal, et al. (Eds.). *Williams hematology* (9th ed.). New York: McGraw-Hill Medical.

Journals and Electronic Documents

Afzal, A., & Syed, N. M. (2017). Thromboelastography and thromboelastometry in patients with sepsis—A mini-review. *Journal of Anesthesia and Intensive Care Medicine, 3*(1), 555–603.

*Ahmadi, M., Poormansouri, S., Beiranvand, S., et al. (2018). Predictors and correlates of fatigue in sickle cell disease patients. *International Journal of Hematology-Oncology & Stem Cell Research, 12*(1), 69–76.

Aljarad, S., Alhamid, A., Tarabishi, A. S., et al. (2018). The impact of Helicobacter pylori eradication on platelet counts of adult patients with idiopathic thrombocytopenic purpura. *BMC Hematology, 18*(28).

Al-Qudah, H. S. (2016). Priapism treatment and management. *Medscape*. Retrieved on 9/20/2019 at: www.emedicine.medscape.com/article/437237-treatment

Anderle, A., Bancone, G., Domingo, G. J., et al. (2018). Point-of-care testing for G6PD deficiency: Opportunities for screening. *International Journal of Neonatal Screening, 4*(4), 34.

Arepally, G. M. (2017). Heparin-induced thrombocytopenia. *Blood, 129*(21), 2864–2872.

*Aslani, E., Georgios, L., & Maria, T. (2018). The measurement of fatigue in hemoglobinopathies: A systematic review of fatigue measures. *International Journal of Caring Science, 11*(31), 1970–1981.

Auerbach, M., & Adamson, J. W. (2016). How we diagnose and treat iron deficiency anemia. *American Journal of Hematology, 91*(1), 31–38.

Bacon, B. R. (2019). Clinical manifestations and diagnosis of hereditary hemochromatosis. *UpToDate*. Retrieved on 1/6/2020 at: www.uptodate.com/contents/clinical-manifestations-and-diagnosis-of-hereditary-hemochromatosis

Bonanni, P., Grazzini, M., Niccolai, G., et al. (2017). Recommended vaccinations for asplenic and hyposplenic adult patients. *Human Vaccines & Immunotherapeutics, 13*(2), 359–368.

Brien, L. (2019). Anticoagulant medications for the prevention and treatment of thromboembolism. *Advanced Critical Care, 30*(2), 126–137.

*Cadet, M. J. (2018). Iron deficiency anemia, a clinical case study. *MEDSURG Nursing, 27*(2), 108–120.

Camaschella, C. (2019). Iron deficiency. *Blood, 133*(1), 30–39.

Coates, T. D., & Wood, J. C. (2017). How we manage, overload in sickle cell patients. *British Journal of Haematology, 177*(5), 703–716.

Coutre, S. (2018). Congenital and acquired disorders of platelet function. *UpToDate*. Retrieved on 1/1/2020 at: www.uptodate.com/contents/congenital-and-acquired-disorders-of-platelet-function

Darbari, D. S., & Brandow, A. M. (2017). Pain-measurement tools in sickle cell disease: Where are we now? *Hematology American Society of Hematology Education Program, 2017*(1), 534–541.

Davis, B. A., Allard, S., Qureshi, A., et al. (2017). Guidelines on red cell transfusion in sickle cell disease. Part I: principles and laboratory aspects. *British Journal of Haematology, 178*(2), 179–191.

DeBaun, M. R. (2018). Red cell transfusion in sickle cell disease. *UpToDate*. Retrieved on 10/1/2019 at: www.uptodate.com/contents/red-blood-cell-transfusion-in-sickle-cell-disease

DeBaun, M. R., & Vichinsky, E. P. (2019). Vaso-occlusive pain management in sickle cell disease. *UpToDate*. Retrieved on 2/12/2020 at: www.uptodate.com/contents/vaso-occlusive-pain-management-in-sickle-cell-disease

Depré, F., Aboud, N., Ringel, F., et al. (2016). Thrombopoietin receptor agonists are often ineffective in immune thrombocytopenia and/or cause adverse reactions: Results from one hand. *Transfusion Medicine and Hemotherapy, 43*(5), 375–379.

El Khatib, A. M., & Hayek, S. N. (2016). Leg ulcers in sickle cell patients: Management challenges. *Chronic Wound Management and Research, 2016*(3), 157–161.

Fibach, E., & Rachmilewitz, E. A. (2017). Pathophysiology and treatment of patients with beta-thalassemia—an update. *F1000Research, 6*, 2156.

Field, J. J. (2019). Overview of management and prognosis of sickle cell disease. *UpToDate*. Retrieved on 10/1/2019 at: www.uptodate.com/contents/overview-of-the-management-and-prognosis-of-sickle-cell-disease

Field, J. J., Vemulakonda, V. M., DeBaun, M. R., et al. (2019). Priapism and erectile dysfunction in sickle cell disease. *UpToDate*. Retrieved on 10/1/2019 at: www.uptodate.com/contents/priapism-and-erectile-dysfunction-in-sickle-cell-disease

Fishbane, S., & Spinowitz, B. (2018). Update on anemia in ESRD and early stage CKD: Core curriculum 2018. *American Journal of Kidney Diseases, 71*(3), 423–435.

Franchini, M., Marano, G., Pati, I., et al. (2019). Emicizumab for the treatment of hemophilia A: A narrative review. *Blood Transfusion, 17*, 223–228.

George, A. (2019). Prevention of stroke (initial or recurrent) in sickle cell disease. *UpToDate*. Retrieved on 10/1/2019 at: www.uptodate.com/contents/prevention-of-stroke-initial-or-recurrent-in-sickle-cell-disease

Go, R. S., Winters, J. L., & Kay, N. E. (2017). How I treat autoimmune hemolytic anemia. *Blood, 129*(22), 2971–2979.

Harper, J. L., Besa, E. C., & Conrad, M. E. (2019). Iron deficiency anemia. *Medscape*. Retrieved on 10/1/2019 at: www.emedicine.medscape.com/article/202333-overview#a5

Hashemi, S. M., Mashhadi, M. A., Mohammadi, M., et al. (2017). *International Journal of Hematology Oncology and Stem Cell Research, 11*(3), 192–198.

Heffernan, A., Evans, C., Holmes, M., et al. (2017). The regulation of dietary iron bioavailability by vitamin C: A systematic review and meta-analysis. *Proceedings of the Nutrition Society Meeting*, July 10–12, 2017.

Hildenbrand, A. K., Quinn, C. T., Mara, C. A., et al. (2019). A preliminary investigation of the psychometric properties of PROMIS® scales in emerging adults with sickle cell disease. *Health Psychology, 38*(5), 386–390.

Hill, Q. A., Stamps, R., Massey, E., et al. (2017). The diagnosis and management of primary autoimmune haemolytic anaemia. *British Journal of Haematology, 17*(3), 395–411.

Holmes-Maybank, K. T., Martin, T. D., & Duckett, A. A. (2017). What are indications, complications of acute blood transfusions in sickle cell anemia? Key points additional reading. *The Hospitalist*. Retrieved on 2/11/2020 at: www.the-hospitalist.org/hospitalist/article/133618/hematology/what-are-indications-complications-acute-blood-transfusions

Huang, A. W., & Muneyyirci-Delale, O. (2017). Reproductive endocrine issues in men with sickle cell anemia. *Andrology, 5*(4), 679–690.

Jain, S., Bakshi, N., & Krishnamurti, L. (2017). Acute chest syndrome in children with sickle cell disease. *Pediatric Allergy, Immunology, and Pulmonology, 30*(4), 191–201.

Kanellopoulou, T., & Nomikou, E. (2018). Replacement therapy for coronary artery bypass surgery in patients with hemophilia A and B. *Journal of Cardiac Surgery, 33*(2), 76–82.

*Kim, S., Brathwaite, R., & Kim, O. (2017). Evidence-based practice standard care for acute pain management in adults with sickle cell disease in an urgent care center. *Quality Management in Healthcare, 26*(2), 108–115.

Kling, E. S., & Farber, H. W. (2019). Pulmonary hypertension associated with sickle cell disease. *UpToDate*. Retrieved on 10/1/2019 at: www.uptodate.com/contents/pulmonary-hypertension-associated-with-sickle-cell-disease

Koupenova, M., Kehrel, B. E., Corkerey, H. A., & Freedman, J. E. (2016). Thrombosis and platelets: An update. *European Heart Journal, 38*(11), 785–791.

Kowdley, K., Brown, K., Ahn, J., et al. (2019). ACG clinical guideline: Hereditary hemochromatosis. *American Journal of Gastroenterology, 114*(8), 1202–1218.

Lambert, M. P., & Gernsheimer, T. B. (2017). Clinical update in adult immune thrombocytopenia. *Blood, 129*(21), 2829–2835.

Langan, R. C., & Goodbred, A. J. (2017). Vitamin B12 deficiency: Recognition and management. *American Family Physician, 96*(6), 384–389.

Lanier, J. B., Park, J. B., & Callahan, R. C. (2018). Anemia in older adults. *American Family Physician, 98*(7), 437–442.

Leebeek, F. W., & Eikenboom, J. C. (2016). Von Willebrand's disease. *New England Journal of Medicine 375*(21), 2067–2080.

Leung, L. K. (2019). Approach to the adult with anemia. *UpToDate*. Retrieved on 10/1/2019 at: www.uptodate.com/contents/approach-to-the-adult-with-anemia

Lyman, G. (2019). Febrile neutropenia an ounce of prevention or a pound of cure. *Journal of Oncology Practice, 15*(1), 27–29.

Mannucci, P. M. (2018). Use of desmopressin in the treatment of hemophilia A: Towards a golden jubilee. *Haematologica, 103*(3), 379–381.

Mannucci, P. M. (2019). Aging with hemophilia: The challenge of appropriate drug prescription. *Mediterranean Journal of Hematology and Infectious Diseases, 11*(1), e2019056.

Matte, A., Zorzi, F., & De Franceschi, L. (2019). New therapeutic options for the treatment of sickle cell disease. *Mediterranean Journal of Hematology and Infectious Diseases, 11*(1), e2019002.

Miranti, E. H., Stolzenberg-Solomon, R., Weinstein, S., et al. (2017). Low vitamin B12 increases risk of gastric cancer: A prospective study of one-carbon metabolism nutrients and risk of upper intestinal tract cancer. *International Journal of Cancer, 141*(6), 1120–1129.

Murao, S., & Yamakawa, K. (2019). A systematic summary of systematic reviews on anticoagulant therapy in sepsis. *Journal of Clinical Medicine, 8*(11), 1869.

Murray, C., De Gelder, T., Pringle, N., et al. (2016). Management of iron overload in the Canadian hematology/oncology population: Implications for nursing practice. *Canadian Oncology Nursing Journal, 26*(1), 19–28.

Nagalla, S., & Bray, P. F. (2017). Hematology: Drug-induced platelet dysfunction. *Cancer Therapy Advisor.* Retrieved on 1/1/2020 at: www.cancertherapyadvisor.com/home/decision-support-in-medicine/hematology/drug-induced-platelet-dysfunction

National Heart Lung and Blood Institute. (2014). Evidence based management of sickle cell disease: Expert Panel Report. U.S. Department of Health and Human Services, National Institutes of Health. Retrieved on 2/11/2020 at: www.nhlbi.nih.gov/health-topics/evidence-based-management-sickle-cell-disease

National Hemophilia Foundation. (2019). Hemophilia A. Retrieved on 9/23/2019 at: www.hemophilia.org/Bleeding-Disorders/Types-of-Bleeding-Disorders/Hemophilia-A

Neunert, C., Terrell, D. R., Arnold, D. M., et al. (2019). American Society of Hematology 2019 guidelines for immune thrombocytopenia. *Blood Advances, 3*(23), 3829–3866.

Nomura S. (2016). Advances in diagnosis and treatments for immune thrombocytopenia. *Clinical Medicine Insights. Blood Disorders, 9,* 15–22.

Okwerekwu, I., & Skirvin, J. A. (2018). Sickle cell disease pain management. *U.S. Pharmacist.* Retrieved on 10/2/2019 at: www.uspharmacist.com/article/sickle-cell-disease-pain-management

Ospina-Romero, M., Cannegieter, S. C., den Heijer, M., et al. (2018). Hyperhomocysteinemia and risk for first venous thrombosis: The influence of (unmeasured) confounding indicators. *American Journal of Epidemiology, 18*(7), 1392–1400.

Ostrakhovich, E. A., & Tabibzadeh, S. (2019). Homocysteine and age related disorders. *Ageing Research Reviews, 49,* 144–164.

Peslak, S. A., Olson, T., & Babushok, D. V. (2017). Diagnosis and treatment of aplastic anemia. *Current Treatment Options in Oncology, 18*(12), 70.

Phillips, J., & Henderson, A. C. (2018). Hemolytic anemia: Evaluation and differential diagnosis. *American Family Physician, 98*(6), 354–361.

Price, E. A. (2019). Anemia in the older adult. *UpToDate.* Retrieved on 10/1/2019 at: www.uptodate.com/contents/anemia-in-the-older-adult .

Razak, N. B., Jones, G., Bhandari, M., et al. (2018). Cancer-associated thrombosis: An overview of mechanisms, risk factors, and treatment. *Cancers, 10*(10), 380.

Reding, M. T. (2018). Management insights for optimizing outcomes in the treatment of hemophilia. *Journal of Managed Care Medicine, 21*(4). Retrieved on 2/11/2020 at: www.jmcmpub.org/pdf/21-4-f8

Rick, M. E. (2019). Clinical presentation and diagnosis of von Willebrand disease. *UpToDate.* Retrieved on 1/6/2020 at: www.uptodate.com/contents/clinical-presentation-and-diagnosis-of-von-willebrand-disease

Schick, P. (2019). Hemolytic anemia. *Medscape.* Retrieved on 2/11/2020 at: www.emedicine.medscape.com/article/201066-overview

Sharma, D., & Brandow, A. M. (2019). Neuropathic pain in individuals with sickle cell disease. *Neuroscience Letters.* Retrieved on 10/2/2019 at: doi.org/10.1016/j.neulet.2019.134445.

Stauder, R., Valent, P., & Theurl, I. (2018). Anemia at older age: Etiologies, clinical implications, and management. *Blood, 131*(5), 505–514.

Stouten, K., Riedl, J., Droogendijk, J., et al. (2016). Prevalence of potential underlying aetiology of macrocytic anaemia in Dutch general practice. *BMC Family Practice, 17*(1), 113.

**Taylor, F. B., Toh, C. H., Hoots, W. K., et al. (2007). Towards a definition, clinical and laboratory criteria, and a scoring system for DIC. *Journal of Thrombosis and Haemostasis, 5*(3), 445–659.

Thornburg, C. D., & Duncan, N. A. (2017). Treatment adherence in hemophilia. *Patient Preference and Adherence, 2017*(11), 1677–1686.

Van Wyk, H. (2018). Iron supplementation. *Professional Nursing Today, 22*(4), 4–6.

Vichinsky, E. P. (2017). Overview of clinical manifestations of sickle cell disease. *UpToDate.* Retrieved on 10/1/2019 at: www.uptodate.com/contents/overview-of-the-clinical-manifestations-of-sickle-cell-disease

Vichinsky, E. P. (2018). Pregnancy in women with sickle cell disease. *UpToDate.* Retrieved on 10/2/2019 at: www.uptodate.com/contents/pregnancy-in-women-with-sickle-cell-disease

Weiss, G., Ganz, T., & Goodnough, L. T. (2019). Anemia of inflammation. *Blood, 133*(1), 40–50.

Young, G., Liesner, R., Chang, T., et al. (2019). A multicenter, open-label phase 3 study of emicizumab prophylaxis in children with hemophila A with inhibitors. *Blood, 134*(4), 2127–2138.

Young, N. S. (2018). Aplastic anemia. *New England Journal of Medicine, 379*(17), 1643–1656.

Resources

American Association of Blood Banks (AABB), www.aabb.org

American Hemochromatosis Society, www.americanhs.org

American Red Cross, www.redcross.org

American Society for Transplantation and Cellular Therapy, www.asbmt.org/home

Aplastic Anemia and MDS International Foundation, www.aamds.org

APS Foundation of America (antiphospholipid syndrome), www.apsfa.org

G6PD Deficiency, www.g6pd.org

National Heart, Lung, and Blood Institute, www.nhlbi.nih.gov

National Marrow Donor Program, www.bethematch.org

Platelet Disorder Support Association (PDSA), www.pdsa.org

Sickle Cell Disease Association of America (SCDAA), www.sicklecell-disease.org

30

Management of Patients with Hematologic Neoplasms

LEARNING OUTCOMES

On completion of this chapter, the learner will be able to:

1. Compare and contrast the different types of leukemias in terms of their incidence, physiologic alterations, clinical manifestations, complications, and medical and nursing management.
2. Use the nursing process as a framework for care of the patient with acute leukemia.
3. Explain the differences between the various myeloproliferative disorders in terms of their incidence, physiologic alterations, clinical manifestations, complications, and medical and nursing management.
4. Compare and contrast Hodgkin and non-Hodgkin lymphomas in terms of their incidence, physiologic alterations, clinical manifestations, complications, and medical and nursing management.
5. Discuss medical and nursing care of the patient with multiple myeloma.

NURSING CONCEPTS

Cellular Regulation

Clotting

GLOSSARY

absolute neutrophil count (ANC): a calculation of the number of circulating neutrophils, derived from the total white blood cells (WBCs) and the percentage of neutrophils counted in a microscope's visual field

angiogenesis: formation of new blood vessels

apoptosis: programmed cell death

blast cells: immature leukocytes

clone: proliferation from same cell of origin so that descendent cells are identical to the cell of origin

cytokines: proteins produced by leukocytes that are vital to regulation of hematopoiesis, apoptosis, and immune responses; also called *biochemical* or *inflammatory mediators*

erythrocyte sedimentation rate (ESR): laboratory test that measures the rate of settling of red blood cells (RBCs); elevation is indicative of inflammation; also called the *sed rate*

erythromelalgia: a burning, painful sensation and erythema in the fingers or toes

hematopoiesis: complex process of the formation and maturation of blood cells

indolent: when in reference to a neoplasm refers to a slow-growing cancer that often remains localized or causes few symptoms

leukemia: uncontrolled proliferation of WBCs, often immature

lymphadenopathy: enlargement of a lymph node or lymph nodes

lymphoid: pertaining to lymphocytes

myeloid: pertaining to nonlymphoid blood cells that differentiate into RBCs, platelets, macrophages, mast cells, and various WBCs

neutropenia: lower-than-normal number of neutrophils

pancytopenia: abnormal decrease in WBCs, RBCs, and platelets

petechiae: tiny capillary hemorrhages

phagocytosis: process of cellular ingestion and digestion of foreign bodies

reticulocytes: slightly immature RBCs, usually only 1% of total circulating RBCs

splenomegaly: enlargement of the spleen

stem cell: primitive cell, capable of self-replication and differentiation into myeloid or lymphoid stem cell

thrombocythemia: higher-than-normal platelet count that occurs without a known cause

thrombocytopenia: lower-than-normal platelet count

thrombocytosis: higher-than-normal platelet count that results because of a disease or disorder

Hematopoiesis is the process by which all blood cells develop, differentiate, and mature. This process starts with the hematopoietic stem cells (HSC) in the bone marrow. As these **stem cells** divide, they are delineated into one of two cell pathways, to become lymphoid or myeloid progenitor cells. The myeloid stem cells then differentiate into red blood cells, white blood cells (WBCs), and platelets, while the lymphoid stem cells differentiate into B and T lymphocytes. Normally, the differentiation of these progenitor cells is regulated according to the body's need. However, when the mechanisms that control the production of these cells is disrupted or impaired, the cells can proliferate uncontrollably, leading to the development of a hematologic malignancy. The pathophysiologic processes for the development of hematologic malignancies are complex. Understanding these processes and the rationale for treatments is important so that nurses may appropriately assess, monitor, educate, and intervene with patients with hematologic neoplasms.

Hematopoietic malignancies are classified by the specific blood cells involved. **Leukemia** is a neoplastic proliferation of a particular cell type (granulocytes, lymphocytes, or infrequently erythrocytes or megakaryocytes). This proliferation leads to an overcrowding in the bone marrow resulting in impaired hematopoietic cell function and can affect other organs in the body (i.e., lymph nodes, skin, and spleen) (Leukemia & Lymphoma Society, 2018b). The defect originates in the HSC, the myeloid, or the lymphoid stem cell. Lymphomas are neoplasms of lymphoid tissue, usually derived from B lymphocytes. Multiple myeloma is a malignancy of the most mature form of B lymphocyte—the plasma cell.

CLONAL STEM CELL DISORDERS

A key feature of hematologic malignancies is the increased proliferation of blood cells from an abnormal single HSC, known as clonal hematopoiesis. Despite this increase in proliferation, the clonal HSCs continue to differentiate, leading to increased myeloid cells, erythroid cells, and platelets in the peripheral blood as well as hyperplasia in the bone marrow (Leukemia & Lymphoma Society, 2018b). Figure 30-1 illustrates how hematopoietic malignancies develop and whether they are derived from the myeloid or lymphoid stem cells (Leukemia & Lymphoma Society, 2019f).

LEUKEMIA

The term *leukocytosis* refers to an increase of leukocytes (WBCs) in the circulation. Typically, only one specific cell type is increased. Because the proportions of several types of leukocytes (e.g., eosinophils, basophils, monocytes) are small, an increase in other types can be great enough to elevate the total leukocyte count, particularly the neutrophils or lymphocytes. Although leukocytosis can be a normal response to increased need (e.g., in acute infection), the elevation in leukocytes should decrease as the physiologic need decreases. A prolonged or progressively increasing elevation in leukocytes is abnormal and should be evaluated. A significant cause of persistent leukocytosis is a hematologic malignancy (i.e., leukemia).

The common feature of the leukemias is an unregulated proliferation of leukocytes in the bone marrow. In acute forms (or late stages of chronic forms), the proliferation of leukemic cells leaves little room for normal cell production. There can also be a proliferation of cells in the liver and spleen (extramedullary hematopoiesis). With acute forms, there can be infiltration of leukemic cells in other organs, such as the meninges, lymph nodes, gums, and skin. The cause of leukemia is not fully known, but exposure to radiation or chemicals, certain genetic disorders, and viral infections are known to be risk factors for certain types of leukemia. Bone marrow damage from pelvic radiation or certain types of chemotherapy drugs can cause acute leukemia, typically occurring years after treatment for another malignancy (Leukemia & Lymphoma Society, 2018b).

The leukemias are commonly classified according to the stem cell line involved, either **lymphoid** (referring to stem cells that produce lymphocytes) or **myeloid** (referring to stem cells that produce nonlymphoid blood cells). They are also classified as either acute or chronic, based on the time it takes for symptoms to evolve and the phase of cell development that is halted (i.e., with few leukocytes differentiating beyond that phase).

In acute leukemia, the onset of symptoms is abrupt, often occurring within a few weeks. Leukocyte development is halted at the blast phase, and thus most leukocytes are undifferentiated cells or blasts. Acute leukemia can progress rapidly, with death occurring within weeks to months without aggressive treatment.

In chronic leukemia, symptoms evolve over a period of months to years, and the majority of leukocytes produced are mature. Chronic leukemia progresses more slowly; the disease trajectory can extend for years.

Acute Myeloid Leukemia

Acute myeloid leukemia (AML) originates due to a series of genetic mutations in the myeloid HSC leading to clonal development of abnormal blast cells (National Comprehensive Cancer Network [NCCN], 2019a). As these **blast cells** (i.e., immature leukocytes) continue to proliferate, they crowd out normal bone marrow production resulting in anemia, **thrombocytopenia** (i.e., low platelet count), and either low or elevated WBC counts (rarely, the WBC may be within normal range). There is also impaired development of all myeloid cells: monocytes, granulocytes (i.e., neutrophils, basophils, eosinophils), erythrocytes, and platelets.

AML is the most common form of leukemia, as well as most common cause of death from all leukemias. AML can affect any age group. However, the incidence of this disease increases with age, with the median age at time of diagnosis being about 68 years (Leukemia & Lymphoma Society, 2019a). On an annual basis, AML accounts for approximately 1% of all cancer-related deaths (NCCN, 2019a).

The exact cause of AML is unclear, but there are several known risk factors. In addition to increasing age, males have a higher incidence than females. Other risks include having been exposed to chemicals such as benzene or pesticides or exposed to ionizing radiation; and a history of prior treatment with chemotherapeutic drugs,

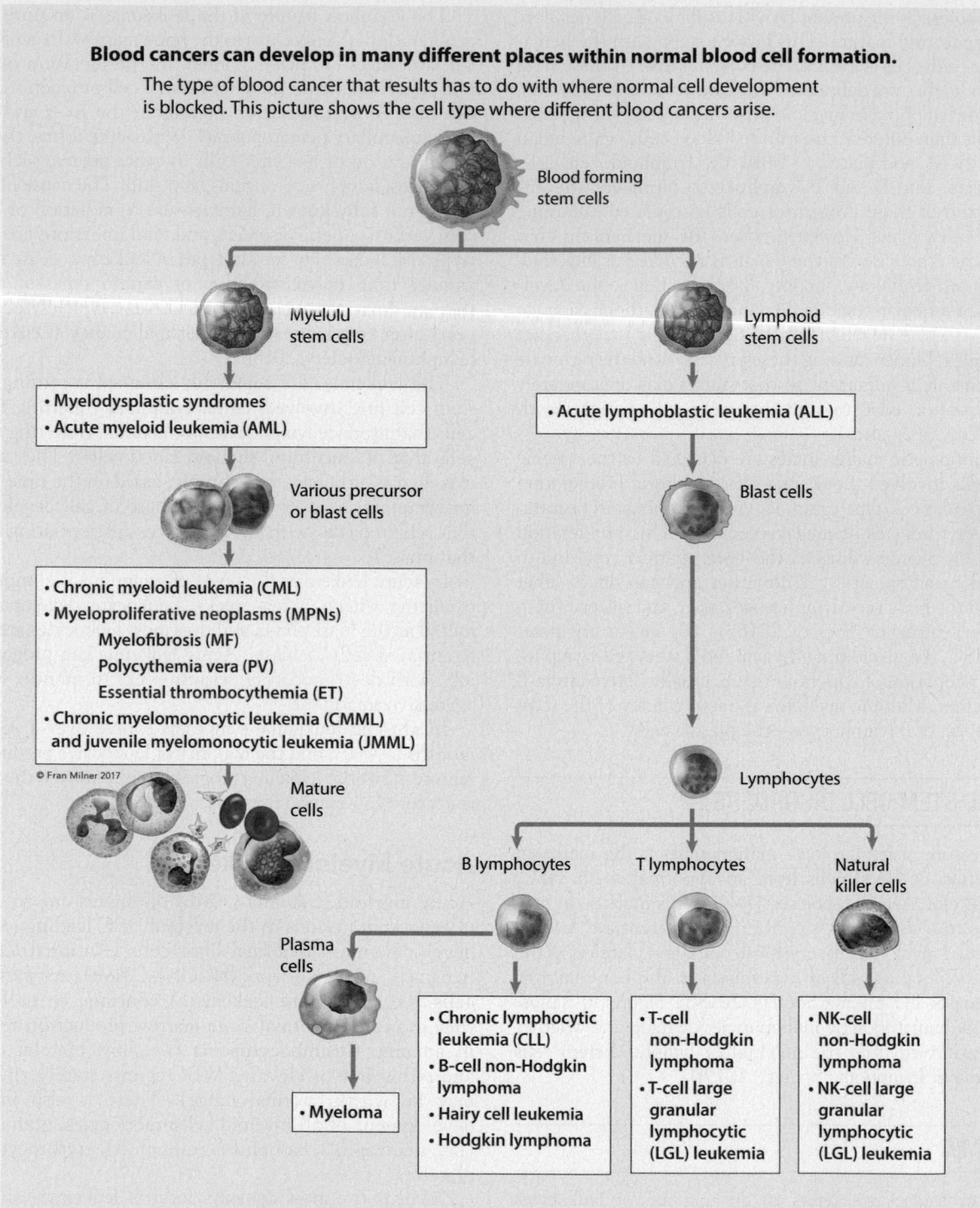

Blood cancers can develop in many different places within normal blood cell formation.

The type of blood cancer that results has to do with where normal cell development is blocked. This picture shows the cell type where different blood cancers arise.

Blood forming stem cells

Myeloid stem cells

Lymphoid stem cells

- Myelodysplastic syndromes
- Acute myeloid leukemia (AML)

- Acute lymphoblastic leukemia (ALL)

Various precursor or blast cells

Blast cells

- Chronic myeloid leukemia (CML)
- Myeloproliferative neoplasms (MPNs)
  Myelofibrosis (MF)
  Polycythemia vera (PV)
  Essential thrombocythemia (ET)
- Chronic myelomonocytic leukemia (CMML) and juvenile myelomonocytic leukemia (JMML)

© Fran Milner 2017

Mature cells

Lymphocytes

B lymphocytes

T lymphocytes

Natural killer cells

Plasma cells

- Chronic lymphocytic leukemia (CLL)
- B-cell non-Hodgkin lymphoma
- Hairy cell leukemia
- Hodgkin lymphoma

- T-cell non-Hodgkin lymphoma
- T-cell large granular lymphocytic (LGL) leukemia

- NK-cell non-Hodgkin lymphoma
- NK-cell large granular lymphocytic (LGL) leukemia

- Myeloma

Figure 30-1 • The development of myeloid and lymphoid neoplasms. Hematologic malignancies can occur when normal cell develop is inhibited. © Fran Milner 2017.

such as alkylating agents or topoisomerase inhibitors, tobacco smoking, other blood disorders (e.g., myeloproliferative diseases), and several genetic disorders (e.g., Down syndrome, Trisomy 8, or Fanconi anemia) (Leukemia & Lymphoma Society, 2019a).

The prognosis and survival rates are highly variable. Factors influencing a more positive outcome are younger age at diagnosis, more favorable cytogenetic alterations (which are strongly associated with younger age), and few concurrent (or mild) health problems. In contrast, patients with significant comorbidities, of older age, with cytogenetic features deemed to be adverse, or who are frail, are more likely to have a poor prognosis. AML evolving from a preexisting clonal myeloid disease or from prior cytotoxic therapy for another malignancy

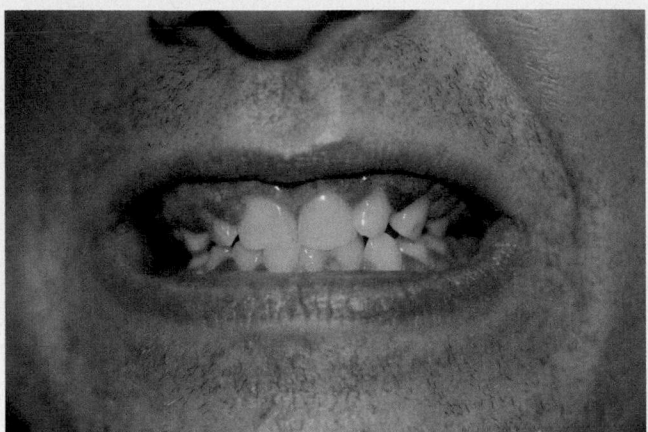

Figure 30-2 • Gingival infiltration of leukemic cells in a patient with acute myeloid leukemia. Reprinted with permission from Greer, J. P., Foerster, J., Rodgers, G. M., et al. (2009). *Wintrobe's clinical hematology* (12th ed., Fig. 72.8, p. 1680). Philadelphia, PA: Lippincott Williams & Wilkins.

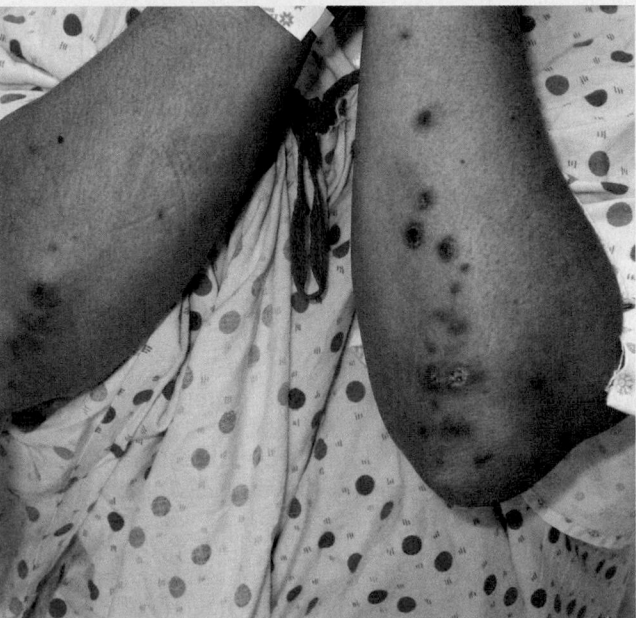

Figure 30-3 • Leukemia cutis. Infiltration of leukemic cells in skin on extensor surface of forearms. Reproduced with permission from Stedman's Medical Dictionary. Copyright 2008 Lippincott Williams & Wilkins.

or immune disease is associated with a poorer prognosis and less favorable outcomes (NCCN, 2019a).

Clinical Manifestations

AML often presents, initially, as nonspecific complaints that can abruptly occur or gradually worsen over time. The signs and symptoms result from inadequate production of normal blood cells, especially as the leukemic cells increasingly crowd out the bone marrow. Symptoms due to **neutropenia** (low neutrophil count) include fever and infection. Symptoms related to anemia include pallor, fatigue, weakness, dyspnea on exertion, and dizziness. Symptoms reflective of thrombocytopenia include ecchymoses (bruises), **petechiae** (pinpoint red or purple hemorrhagic spots on the skin), epistaxis (nosebleeds), and gingival bleeding. The proliferation of leukemic cells within organs leads to a variety of additional symptoms: pain from an enlarged liver or spleen, hyperplasia of the gums, and bone pain from expansion of marrow (see Fig. 30-2). Petechiae or ecchymoses are common on the skin (see Chapter 29, Fig. 29-4); occasionally, leukemic infiltrates are also seen (see Fig. 30-3). Leukemic cells can also infiltrate the gingiva or synovial spaces of joints. **Lymphadenopathy** (enlargement of lymph nodes) or **splenomegaly** (enlargement of the spleen) is rare. Fevers may occur and are not always due to infection.

Assessment and Diagnostic Findings

To confirm the diagnosis of AML, laboratory studies need to be performed. The complete blood count (CBC) commonly shows a decrease in both erythrocytes and platelets. Although the total leukocyte count can be low, normal, or high, the percentage of normal cells is usually vastly decreased. A bone marrow analysis shows an excess (more than 20%) of blast cells (Arber, Orazi, Hasserjian, et al., 2016); this is the hallmark of the diagnosis.

AML can be further classified into seven different subgroups, based on cytogenetics, histology, and morphology of the blasts, as well as the presence of genetic mutations. The actual prognosis varies somewhat between subgroups and with the extent of cytogenetic abnormalities and genetic mutations, yet the clinical course and treatment differ substantially with only one subtype. That is, patients with the specific AML subtype acute promyelocytic leukemia (APL, or AML-M3) have higher potential for fatal coagulopathies; however, the potential to cure this form of AML is high (NCCN, 2019a).

Medical Management

The overall objective of treatment for AML is to achieve complete remission of the disease, in which there is no residual leukemic cells in the bone marrow or peripheral blood. To obtain remission, chemotherapy treatment is administered in two parts: *induction* and *consolidation*. The choice of agents for induction therapy is based on the patient's age, physical status, and history of prior antineoplastic treatment. Induction therapy typically involves high doses of cytarabine and either daunorubicin, idarubicin, or mitoxantrone; etoposide is occasionally added to the regimen. Older patients (especially those older than 70 years) or those unable to tolerate standard therapy (in poor health) may receive lower-intensity therapy (using hypomethylating agents, low doses of cytarabine, or hydroxyurea), which may extend survival without a significant increase in toxicity beyond that of the underlying disease (NCCN, 2019a).

During induction therapy, chemotherapy not only destroys leukemic cells, but also healthy cells, requiring patients to be hospitalized for several weeks (typically 4 to 6 weeks) due to severe and potentially life-threatening side effects, such as neutropenia. For some patients, an **absolute neutrophil count (ANC**; a calculation of the number of circulating neutrophils, derived from the total WBCs and the percentage of neutrophils counted in a microscope's visual field) of zero is not uncommon (see Chapter 12 for formula used to calculate the ANC). Anemia, and severe thrombocytopenia (a platelet count of less than 5000/mm^3), is also common. During this time, the patient is typically very ill, with bacterial, fungal, and occasionally viral infections; bleeding; and severe mucositis, which cause pain, diarrhea, and an inability to maintain adequate nutrition. Management consists of administering blood products (packed red blood cells [PRBCs] and platelets) and promptly treating infections. The use of granulocytic growth factors, either granulocyte colony-stimulating factor (G-CSF; filgrastim) or granulocyte-macrophage colony-stimulating factor (GM-CSF; sargramostim), may be used during the induction phase only for patients who have a life-threatening infection in order to shorten the neutropenic period (NCCN, 2019a). Patients are discharged to home once blood counts recover and the risk of infection are diminished.

When the patient has recovered from the induction therapy (i.e., the neutrophil and platelet counts have returned to normal and any infection has resolved), consolidation therapy is given to eliminate any residual leukemic cells that are not clinically detectable and to reduce the chance for recurrence of leukemia. Multiple treatment cycles of various agents are used, usually containing some form of cytarabine. Frequently, the patient receives one cycle of treatment that is almost the same as, if not identical to, the induction treatment but at lower dosages.

Allogeneic stem cell transplant is the most common form of hematopoietic stem cell transplant (HSCT) used in the treatment of AML (see Chapter 12 for discussion of HSCT). HSCT is routinely done following induction and consolidation therapy. However, in certain instances (e.g., aggressive disease), HSCT may be performed following induction. The process of HSCT requires that patients begin by receiving high-dose, aggressive chemotherapy, sometimes in tandem with radiation therapy, to destroy the hematopoietic functioning in the bone marrow and to kill any residual leukemic cells. This process is called *conditioning therapy*. Then, the patient is given human leukocyte antigen (HLA-matched) donor stems cells via intravenous (IV) infusion to reestablish bone marrow functioning and to create a new immune system (Leukemia & Lymphoma Society, 2019a). The most appropriate use and timing of HSCT remain unclear. Patients with a poorer prognosis may benefit from early HSCT; those with a good prognosis may not ever require HSCT.

While most patients with AML achieve remission after these treatments, some patients have refractory or relapsed disease, even after aggressive therapy. Approximately 10% to 40% of patients do not obtain a complete remission following induction therapy (Leukemia & Lymphoma Society, 2019a). There are several other treatment options. The induction regimen might be repeated until remission or relapse occurs. Other approaches may include treatment with enasidenib, a cytarabine-based regimen, along with other agents (e.g., cladribine, fludarabine, mitoxantrone, etoposide); palliative care; or use of a hypomethylating agent (e.g., azacitidine or decitabine).

Supportive care may be the best treatment option to consider if the patient has significant comorbidity, such as extremely poor cardiac, pulmonary, renal, or hepatic function; is older and frail; or both. In such cases, the aggressive antileukemia therapy options previously described are not indicated; occasionally, hydroxyurea or hypomethylating agents such as azacitidine may be used briefly to control the increase of blast cells. The patient's symptoms may be mitigated with antimicrobial therapy and transfusions as needed. This treatment approach provides the patient with some additional time outside the hospital; however, death frequently occurs within months, typically from infection or bleeding (refer to Chapter 13 for a discussion of palliative and end-of-life care).

Complications

Complications of AML include bleeding and infection, which are the major causes of death. The risk of bleeding correlates with the level and duration of platelet deficiency. The low platelet count can cause ecchymoses and petechiae. Major hemorrhages also may develop when the platelet count drops to less than 10,000/mm^3. The most common bleeding sources include gastrointestinal (GI), pulmonary, vaginal, and intracranial. For undetermined reasons, fever and infection also increase the likelihood of bleeding. Disseminated intravascular coagulation (DIC) is common, particularly in patients with the APL subtype (NCCN, 2019a) (see Chapter 29 for further discussion of DIC). A very high WBC count (greater than 100,000/mm^3) can cause stasis within the cerebral or pulmonary circulation.

Because of the lack of mature and normal granulocytes that help fight infection, patients with leukemia are prone to infection. The likelihood of infection increases with the degree and duration of neutropenia; neutrophil counts that persist at less than 100/mm^3 dramatically increase the risk of systemic infections. While bacterial infections commonly occur in patients with AML who are neutropenic, the risk of developing a fungal infection also increases. Fungal infections remain difficult to treat; in many cases, patients are given antifungal agents prophylactically. Granulocytic growth factors, either granulocyte colony-stimulating factor (G-CSF; filgrastim) or granulocyte-macrophage colony-stimulating factor (GM-CSF) are used to stimulate the bone marrow to produce leukocytes, thereby shortening the period of neutropenia. These growth factors are not recommended for use in patients with APL, as differentiation syndrome (formerly known as retinoic acid syndrome), a life-threatening complication with symptoms such as unexplained fever, weight gain, hypotension, respiratory distress, and acute kidney injury can occur (NCCN, 2019a).

Massive leukemic cell destruction from chemotherapy results in the release of intracellular electrolytes and fluids into the systemic circulation. Increases in uric acid levels, potassium, and phosphate are seen; this process is referred to as tumor lysis syndrome (see Chapter 12 for further discussion of tumor lysis syndrome). The increased uric acid and phosphorus levels make the patient vulnerable to renal stone formation and renal colic, which can progress to acute kidney injury. Hyperkalemia and hypocalcemia can lead to cardiac arrhythmias; hypotension; neuromuscular effects such as muscle cramps, weakness, and spasm/tetany; and confusion; and seizures may also develop (Olsen, LeFebvre, & Brassil, 2019). Patients require a high fluid intake, and prophylaxis with allopurinol or rasburicase to prevent crystallization of uric acid and subsequent stone formation.

GI problems may result from the infiltration of abnormal leukocytes into the abdominal organs and from the toxicity of the chemotherapeutic agents. Anorexia, nausea, vomiting, diarrhea, and severe mucositis are common. Because of the profound myelosuppressive effects of chemotherapy, significant neutropenia and thrombocytopenia typically result in serious infection and increased risk of bleeding.

Nursing Management

Nursing management of the patient with acute leukemia, including AML, is presented at the end of the discussion of leukemia in this chapter.

Chronic Myeloid Leukemia

Chronic myeloid leukemia (CML) arises from a mutation in the myeloid stem cell. Normal myeloid cells continue to be produced, but there is a pathologic increase in the production of forms of blast cells. Therefore, a wide spectrum of cell types exists within the blood, from blast forms to mature neutrophils. Because there is an uncontrolled proliferation of cells, the marrow expands into the cavities of long bones, such as the femur, and cells are also formed in the liver and spleen (extramedullary hematopoiesis), resulting in enlargement of these organs that is sometimes painful.

CML results from a chromosomal translocation, where a section of deoxyribonucleic acid (DNA) is shifted from chromosome 22 to chromosome 9, forming what is known as a "fusion gene" that is abnormal. The specific fused gene found in all patients with CML is the *BCR-ABL* gene, which occurs when the *BCR* gene from chromosome 22 switches places with the *ABL* gene from chromosome 9 (Leukemia & Lymphoma Society, 2019b). Normally, the *ABL* gene signals the cells when to make tyrosine kinase; however, the abnormal *BCR-ABL* gene (known as the Philadelphia chromosome) signals cells to produce too many leukocytes and is responsible for converting normal cells into leukemic cells.

CML accounts for 15% of all new cases of leukemia (NCCN, 2019b). The average age of a patient at time of diagnosis is 67 years, but CML can occur at any age. Risk factors include increasing age, being male, having a history of smoking, and being exposed to high doses of radiation (e.g., atomic bomb survivors).

Clinical Manifestations

The clinical picture of CML varies, based upon phase of disease. There are three stages in CML that include chronic, accelerated, and blast crisis (Leukemia & Lymphoma Society, 2019b). During the chronic phase, patients have few symptoms, leukocytosis is detected by a CBC performed for some other reason, and complications from the disease itself are rare.

The accelerated phase can be insidious or rapid; it marks the process of evolution (or transformation) to the acute form of leukemia (blast crisis). In the accelerated phase of disease, blood counts begin to worsen, new chromosomal changes may be seen on analysis, and symptoms consistent with leukemia may start to appear, such as fatigue, anemia, splenomegaly, or dyspnea (NCCN, 2019b). The patient may complain of bone pain and may report fevers (without any obvious sign of infection) and weight loss.

Blast crisis or blast phase of CML is the most advanced phase. Patients in this phase exhibit signs and symptoms that are more like AML than a chronic disease. Some patients present with leukocytosis, with the WBC count exceeding 100,000/mm³ (NCCN, 2019b). Patients with extremely high leukocyte counts may be dyspneic or slightly confused because of decreased perfusion to the lungs and brain from leukostasis (the excessive volume of leukocytes inhibits blood flow through the capillaries). The patient may have an enlarged, tender spleen, and occasionally the liver may also be enlarged and tender. Some patients have insidious symptoms, such as malaise, anorexia, and weight loss. Lymphadenopathy is uncommon, but if present, indicates late disease and a poor prognosis (NCCN, 2019b).

Medical Management

The goal of treatment for CML is to control the disease, either by obtaining remission or by keeping the patient in the chronic phase for as long as possible. CML is not considered to be curable among older adults despite advances in understanding the pathophysiology of the disease and the advent of new agents. However, the use of tyrosine kinase inhibitors (TKIs) has significantly improved treatment and long-term survival for patients with CML (Leukemia & Lymphoma Society, 2019b). Medical management is based upon the patient's age, general health, calculation of risk-score (based upon stage of disease and prognosis), and phase of disease.

TKIs work by blocking the signals within the leukemic cells that express the *BCR-ABL* protein. This inhibition prevents a series of chemical reactions that cause the cells to grow and divide, thus inducing complete remission at the cellular level. The TKI imatinib mesylate is considered to be standard of care for patients with CML. Newer, alternative TKIs approved for first-line (primary) therapy for patients in the chronic phase of CML include dasatinib or nilotinib (NCCN, 2019b). Each of these TKIs has a different toxicity profile. For example, periorbital edema is common with long-term use of imatinib; dasatinib is very myelosuppressive, and its use carries a significant risk for pleural effusion and for causing a prolonged QT interval; and nilotinib has cardiotoxic effects. Other TKIs approved for second-line therapy (when patients do not respond satisfactorily to the first-line agents) are bosutinib and ponatinib. All TKIs are metabolized by the cytochrome P450 pathway, which means that drug-to-drug interactions are common. Drugs that may decrease the effects of the TKI are corticosteroids, antiseizure medications, antacids, and St. John's wort. Drugs that may increase the effects of the TKI include grapefruit juice, certain antibiotics (e.g., clarithromycin), and azole antifungals (e.g., clotrimazole, ketoconazole).

CML is a disease that can potentially be cured with allogeneic HSCT in otherwise healthy patients who are younger than 65 years. However, with the development of TKIs, the timing of transplant has come into question. Approximately 90% of patients who receive allogeneic HSCT during the chronic phase of CML are disease free for 5 years or more (Leukemia & Lymphoma Society, 2019b).

In the acute form of CML (blast crisis), treatment may resemble induction therapy for acute leukemia, using the same medications as for AML or acute lymphocytic leukemia (ALL; see later discussion). Patients whose disease evolves into a "lymphoid" blast crisis are more likely to be able to reenter a chronic phase after induction therapy. For those whose disease evolves into AML, therapy has been largely ineffective in achieving a second chronic phase. Life-threatening infections and bleeding occur frequently in this phase.

Nursing Management

Most TKIs are oral agents; therefore, their effectiveness is dependent upon the patient's ability and motivation to adhere to the prescribed treatment regimen. These drugs may cause side effects that the patient may find difficult to manage, such as fatigue, asthenia (weakness), pruritus (itching), headache, skin rash, and oropharyngeal pain. A study conducted in Germany of patients with CML treated on an outpatient basis revealed an adherence rate of 51% to oral TKIs (Hefner, Csef, & Kunzmann, 2017), which is consistent with prior studies. In this study, forgetting to take the drug or delays of 2 or more hours from the prescribed time were the most common reported reasons for decreased adherence. Another study examining challenges to oral agent adherence conducted by Gborogen and Polek (2018) reported that over half of nurse participants reported nonadherence to oral agents among their patients. Reasons for nonadherence ranged from patient forgetfulness to perceptions of inadequate support. It is extremely important for the nurse to educate the patient about the medication regimen, how to manage side effects, drug interactions, and safe handling (Olsen et al., 2019) (see Nursing Interventions in Table 30-1). The nurse should also monitor the patient for adverse signs and symptoms of therapy, such as decreased urinary output, changes in the electrocardiogram (ECG; TKIs can cause arrhythmias and prolonged QT intervals), and myelosuppression (e.g., fevers, chills, changes in the CBC).

Acute Lymphocytic Leukemia

ALL results from an uncontrolled proliferation of immature cells (lymphoblasts) derived from the lymphoid stem cell. The cell of origin is the precursor to the B lymphocyte in approximately 75% of ALL cases; T-lymphocyte ALL occurs in approximately 25% of cases. The *BCR-ABL* translocation (see previous discussion in CML section) is found in 20% of ALL blast cells (NCCN, 2019c). ALL can occur at any age, but 75% to 80% of all cases are found in children, with the median age at diagnosis being 15 years (NCCN, 2019c). Boys are affected more often than girls; the peak incidence is 4 years of age. After 15 years of age, it is relatively uncommon, until age 45 when the incidence again rises (Leukemia & Lymphoma Society, 2018a). For those over age 45, risk factors for ALL include older age (especially over 70 years), prior exposure to chemotherapy or radiation therapy, having certain genetic conditions (e.g., especially Down syndrome, also neurofibromatosis, Klinefelter syndrome, and Fanconi anemia) (NCCN, 2019c). In the last several decades, advances in understanding the pathophysiology and molecular genetics, as well as the incorporation of targeted therapy and HSCT, have resulted in improved cure rates and overall longer survival in patients with ALL.

Clinical Manifestations

For some patients with ALL, the clinical manifestations may be nonspecific while others have no symptoms initially. The disease is commonly found incidentally with routine laboratory studies or physical exam for another condition. At the time of diagnosis, the leukocyte counts may be either higher or lower than normal, with a high proportion of immature lymphoblasts. Immature lymphocytes proliferate in the marrow and impede the development of normal myeloid cells. As a result, normal hematopoiesis is inhibited, resulting in reduced numbers of granulocytes, erythrocytes, and platelets. Manifestations of leukemic cell infiltration into other organs are more common with ALL than with other forms of leukemia and include pain from an enlarged liver or spleen as well as bone pain. The central nervous system (CNS) is frequently

TABLE 30-1 ⚠ Risk Factors Associated with Lower Adherence to Oral Therapy for Chronic Myeloid Leukemia (CML)		
Risk Factor Category	**Risk Factor**	**Nursing Interventions**
Patient Characteristics	Lower education level (below high school) Higher self-report of functional status Low self-efficacy regarding medication administration[a] Taking medication independent of meals[a] Lack of knowledge regarding disease and treatment[a]	 Explore with patient perceived barriers related to medication administration Develop medication administration schedule with patient; use timer/watch alarm to alert patient when to take medication Provide relevant information in format understandable to patient
Social Characteristics	Living alone[a] Low levels of social support Low socioeconomic status	Evaluate need for phone follow-up, initiation of home care
Disease and Treatment Characteristics	Farther time from diagnosis Higher rates of treatment-related side effects[a] Higher number of cancer-related complications[a] Not participating in a clinical trial[a]	 Monitor patient closely for side effects Monitor patient closely for complications Provide patient with information on clinical trial enrollment eligibility as advisable

[a]Indicates risk factor amenable to nursing intervention.
Adapted from Gborogen, R., & Polek, C. (2018). Oral agents: Challenges with self-administered medication adherence in clinical trials. *Clinical Journal of Oncology Nursing*, 22(3), 333–339; Olsen, M., LeFebvre, K., & Brassil, K. (2019). *Chemotherapy and immunotherapy guidelines and recommendations for practice*. Pittsburgh, PA; Oncology Nursing Society.

a site for leukemic cells; thus, patients may exhibit cranial nerve palsies or headache and vomiting because of meningeal involvement. Other extranodal sites include the testes and breasts.

Medical Management

The goal of treatment is to obtain remission without excess toxicity and with a rapid hematologic recovery so that additional therapy can be given if needed. Because of the heterogeneity of the disease, treatment plans are based on genetic markers of the disease as well as risk factors of the patient, primarily age. Similar to treatment for AML, treatment for ALL can be grouped into induction, consolidation, and maintenance phases. Because ALL frequently invades the CNS, preventive intrathecal chemotherapy or, less frequently, cranial irradiation, are also a key part of the treatment plan (NCCN, 2019c).

Treatment protocols for ALL tend to be complex, using a wide variety of chemotherapeutic agents and complicated administration schedules. The expected outcome of treatment is complete remission. Despite its complexity, treatment can be provided in the outpatient setting in some circumstances until severe complications develop. TKIs (e.g., imatinib) are effective in patients with Philadelphia chromosome-positive ALL; these drugs can be used alone or in combination with conventional chemotherapy (Leukemia & Lymphoma Society, 2018a).

Lymphoid blast cells are typically very sensitive to corticosteroids and to vinca alkaloids; therefore, these medications are an integral part of the initial induction therapy (NCCN, 2019c). The corticosteroid dexamethasone is preferred to prednisone, as it is more toxic to lymphoid cells and has better CNS penetration. Typically, an anthracycline is included, sometimes with asparaginase. Once a patient is in remission, special testing (immunophenotyping, immunoglobulin gene rearrangements, T-cell receptor genes, molecular testing) is done to look for residual leukemic cells; these tests can detect as few as a single ALL cell among 10,000 to 100,000 normal cells. This minimal residual disease testing is useful as a prognostic indicator. Based on these results and the rapidity in which remission is achieved, a consolidation regimen ensues, using different combinations and dosages of the drugs used in induction therapy; the goal of consolidation is to improve outcomes in those patients at high risk for relapse. For patients with relapsed or refractory B-cell precursor ALL, agents such as blinatumomab or inotuzumab ozogamicin have been found to be effective (NCCN, 2019c).

Patients with ALL can experience some unique adverse effects from treatment. The use of corticosteroids to treat ALL increases the patient's susceptibility to infection; viral infections are common. Avascular necrosis can occur in patients treated with corticosteroid-based chemotherapy, as well as with transplantation. Patients treated with asparaginase are at increased risk for thrombosis. Hepatic toxicity is also common and may necessitate cessation of supportive drugs, such as proton pump inhibitors and certain antibacterial and antifungal drugs.

Allogeneic HSCT may be considered during initial remission if disease features and testing suggest the risk of relapse is high (NCCN, 2019c; Leukemia & Lymphoma Society, 2018a). The development of chimeric antigen receptor (CAR) T cells has significantly improved treatment outcomes and overall survival in patients with ALL (NCCN, 2019c). CAR-T therapy utilizes the patient's own immune system to fight disease; the patient's own T cells are collected, modified, and reinfused back into the patient. Treatment with CAR-T can serve as a bridge prior to transplant and has qualified patients for HSCT who were formerly ineligible. In the context of average-risk disease, HSCT may be postponed until the time of relapse, should it occur. HSCT can improve long-term disease-free survival; however, this potential benefit must be weighed with the risks associated with the procedure, including death and long-term morbid complications.

Nursing Management

Nursing management of the patient with acute leukemia, including ALL, is presented at the end of the leukemia section in this chapter.

Chronic Lymphocytic Leukemia

Chronic lymphocytic leukemia (CLL) is a common malignancy of older adults, and the most prevalent type of adult leukemia in the Western world (NCCN, 2019d). The average age at diagnosis is 71 years (Leukemia & Lymphoma Society, 2019c). CLL is rarely seen in Native Americans and infrequently among people of Asian descent. Unlike other forms of leukemia, a strong familial predisposition exists with CLL; the disease can occur in 10% of those with a first- or second-degree relative with the same diagnosis. Veterans of the Vietnam War who were exposed to Agent Orange may be at risk for developing this disease (see the following section), but there is no definitive link to other pesticides or exposure to chemicals. While many patients will have a normal life expectancy, others will have a very short life expectancy due to the aggressive nature of the disease.

 Veterans Considerations

Agent Orange was an herbicide used as a defoliant by the U.S. military in Vietnam from 1962 until 1975, when American involvement in the Vietnam War ended. Since that time, dioxin, a chemical used in Agent Orange, has been found to be carcinogenic. In particular, there is sufficient evidence that CLL, Hodgkin lymphoma, non-Hodgkin lymphomas (NHLs), and monoclonal gammopathy of undetermined significance (MGUS) are associated with Agent Orange exposure, while there is also evidence that suggests that Agent Orange exposure may be linked to multiple myeloma (American Cancer Society [ACS], 2020a). Approximately 3 million American veterans could have been exposed to the harmful effects of Agent Orange related to their military service in Vietnam. The U.S. Department of Veteran Affairs (VA) has administered an *Agent Orange Registry* since 1978. Qualified veterans who enroll in the registry are eligible for health care benefits and consultations. Those veterans who develop cancers secondary to exposure to Agent Orange may be eligible for VA disability benefits (see Resources for additional information for veterans exposed to Agent Orange) (ACS, 2020a).

Pathophysiology

CLL is typically derived from a malignant clone of B lymphocytes. A **clone** proliferates from a cell of origin so that descendent cells are identical to the cell of origin. In contrast to the acute forms of leukemia, most leukemic cells in CLL are fully mature. One possible mechanism that explains this oncogenesis is that these cells can escape **apoptosis** (programmed cell death), resulting in an excessive accumulation of the cells in the marrow and circulation. CLL is characterized by the progressive accumulation of leukemic cells in the bone marrow, blood, and lymphoid tissues (NCCN, 2019d).

Because the lymphocytes are small, they can easily travel through the small capillaries within the circulation, and the pulmonary and cerebral complications of leukocytosis seen with myeloid leukemias are not typically found in CLL. However, these cells often accumulate within the lymph nodes and spleen. When it takes less than 12 months for the absolute number of lymphocytes to double (lymphocyte doubling time), a more aggressive disease course may ensue.

Immunophenotyping of the circulating B cells is critical to establish the diagnosis by identifying the presence of a malignant clone of these cells; it is also used to gauge the prognosis (NCCN, 2019d). Other special cytogenetic and molecular analyses (e.g., fluorescence in situ hybridization [FISH]) are also used to guide prognosis and therapy. Beta-2 microglobulin, a protein found on the surface of lymphocytes, can be measured in the serum; an elevated level correlates with a more advanced clinical stage and poorer prognosis.

Autoimmune complications can occur at any stage, as either autoimmune hemolytic anemia or idiopathic thrombocytopenic purpura. In the autoimmune process, the reticuloendothelial system destroys the body's own erythrocytes or platelets. Patients with CLL also have a greater risk for developing other cancers. Approximately 2% to 10% of patients with CLL will experience transformation of their disease to a very aggressive lymphoma, known as Richter's transformation (NCCN, 2019d); this transformation results in markedly increased lymphadenopathy, splenomegaly, B symptoms (see Chart 30-1), and survival of only a few months despite

treatment. Second cancers typically involve the skin, colon, lung, breast, prostate, and kidney.

Clinical Manifestations

Many patients are asymptomatic and are diagnosed incidentally during routine physical examinations or during treatment for another disease. Lymphocytosis (an increased lymphocyte count) is always present. The erythrocyte and platelet counts may be normal or, in later stages of the illness, decreased. Lymphadenopathy is common; this can be severe and sometimes painful (see Fig. 30-4). Splenomegaly may also occur.

Patients with CLL can develop B symptoms (see Chart 30-1) which portends a worsening prognosis. T-cell function is impaired and may be the cause of tumor progression and increased susceptibility to second malignancies and infections. Life-threatening infections are particularly common with advanced disease, and account for over half of all deaths in this patient population. Viral infections, such as herpes zoster, can become widely disseminated. Defects in the complement system are also seen, which results in increased risk of developing infection with encapsulated organisms (e.g., *Haemophilus influenzae*). Patients should receive an annual comprehensive skin examination (as the incidence of skin cancer is higher in this group), and screening guidelines for other cancers should be followed, such as for breast, colorectal, lung, and prostate cancer (NCCN, 2019d) (see Chapter 12, Table 12-3, for cancer screening guidelines).

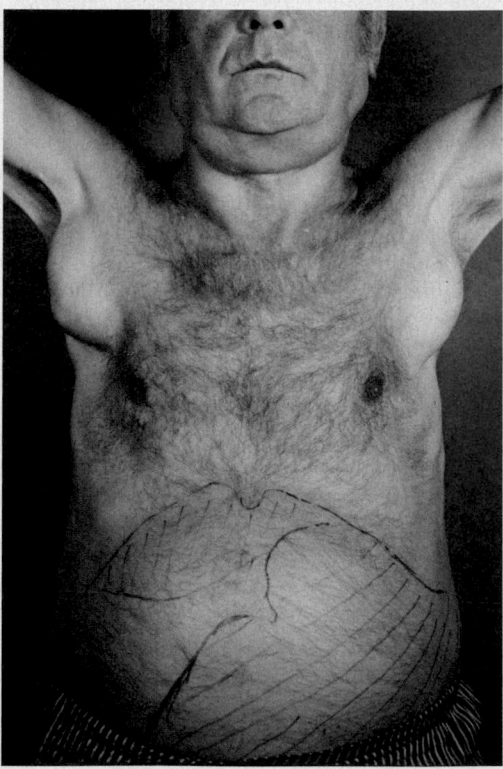

Figure 30-4 • Massive lymphadenopathy in a patient with chronic lymphocytic leukemia. Note the enlarged liver and spleen as well. Reprinted with permission from Tkachuk, D. C., & Hirschman, J. V. (2007). *Wintrobe's atlas of clinical hematology* (Fig. 5.1, p. 154). Philadelphia, PA: Lippincott Williams & Wilkins.

Chart 30-1 ⚠	**RISK FACTORS**
	B Symptoms

These symptoms include the following:

- Fever of at least 100.4° F (38°C) that may come and go over several weeks that is not explained by an underlying infection
- Drenching night sweats
- Unintentional loss of at least 10% body weight over the past 6 months

Overview: B symptoms:

- Are constitutional symptoms, meaning that they affect multiple systems
- Can manifest with many types of hematopoietic malignancies, including chronic lymphocytic leukemia (CLL), Hodgkin lymphoma, and non-Hodgkin lymphomas (NHLs)
- Are associated with worst prognoses in patients with CLL, Hodgkin lymphoma and NHL than in patients who do not report B symptoms

Adapted from Leukemia & Lymphoma Society. (2018c). Hodgkin lymphoma. Retrieved on 7/10/2019 at: www.lls.org/sites/default/files/file_assets/PS57_Hodgkin_Lymphoma2018.pdf

Medical Management

For patients with no symptoms at the time of diagnosis, the traditional "watch-and-wait" approach is often used until progression of disease is noted (which could be months to years). However, with the advent of newer treatment modalities (i.e., targeted therapies and immunotherapy), treatment may be initiated sooner in the illness trajectory (NCCN, 2019d). Additionally, clinical trials are ongoing to assess for an advantage in survival with newer agents. Various parameters are considered when treatment is selected, including the clinical stage of the disease, disease-associated symptoms, the functional status of the patient, genetic risk, and the extent and efficacy of any prior treatment. Functional status is a complex consideration; in this context, it incorporates the individual's life expectancy independent of CLL (due to other health problems), the ability to tolerate aggressive therapy (e.g., creatinine clearance is particularly important), and the ability to perform activities of daily living (Leukemia & Lymphoma Society, 2019c; NCCN, 2019d). Patients with good functional status can typically tolerate aggressive therapy and often achieve a lasting complete remission. In contrast, the objective of treatment in those with more impaired physical status focuses on controlling bothersome symptoms (e.g., drenching night sweats, painful lymphadenopathy).

Treatment for CLL is variable and can consist of a single immunotherapy agent administered in combination with chemotherapeutic agents, such as an immunotherapeutic antibody against the B-lymphocyte antigen CD20 (e.g., rituximab, ofatumumab, obinutuzumab) with chemotherapeutic agents (e.g., fludarabine, cyclophosphamide, bendamustine, chlorambucil) as initial therapy. The most commonly prescribed first-line chemotherapeutic agent is fludarabine. When the disease is accompanied by a deletion of the *TP53* gene or a mutation of this gene, TKIs such as ibrutinib or idelalisib may be used as either monotherapy or in combination with other agents (NCCN, 2019d). Depending upon the age of the patient (less than or greater than 65 years of age) and whether or not the patient has comorbidities, patients with relapsed or refractory disease may also receive newer agents such as venetoclax, duvelisib, or acalabrutinib (NCCN, 2019d).

The major side effect of fludarabine is prolonged bone marrow suppression, manifested by prolonged periods of neutropenia, lymphopenia, and thrombocytopenia, which puts patients at risk for such infections as *Pneumocystis jiroveci*, *Listeria*, mycobacteria, herpes viruses, and cytomegalovirus (CMV). The monoclonal antibody (MoAb) alemtuzumab is often used in combination with other chemotherapeutic agents when the disease is refractory to fludarabine, the patient has very poor prognostic markers, or it is necessary to eradicate residual disease after initial treatment. Alemtuzumab targets the CD52 antigen commonly found on CLL cells, and it is effective in clearing the marrow and circulation of these cells without affecting the stem cells. Because CD52 is present on both B and T lymphocytes, patients receiving alemtuzumab are at significant risk for infection; prophylactic use of antiviral agents and antibiotics (e.g., trimethoprim–sulfamethoxazole) is important and needs to continue for several months after treatment ends. CMV infection is also common with alemtuzumab, idelalisib, and duvelisib, and prophylaxis is important; among commonly prescribed antiviral agents, vancyclovir is more effective than acyclovir for treating CMV (NCCN, 2019d).

Patients receiving idelalisib or duvelisib have an increased risk of hepatotoxicity, severe diarrhea, colitis, and pneumonitis. TKIs have been found to increase the risk of cardiovascular toxicities, including hypertension, prolonged QT interval, left ventricular dysfunction, and heart failure (Olsen et al., 2019). Ongoing periodic assessment of the CBC, blood chemistries, ECG, blood pressure, and bowel habits are important parameters to monitor among patients taking these various agents.

Because of the older age of most patients with CLL, allogeneic HSCT may not be an option, particularly if significant comorbidities exist. However, allogeneic HSCT might be considered for some patients with *TP53* deletions or mutations who otherwise have a poor prognosis. Morbidity and mortality rates remain high (20%); thus, this treatment modality may be reserved for those patients with high-risk disease, younger age, and high degree of match from the donor (NCCN, 2019d).

Nursing Management

Virtually all patients with CLL have reduced levels of immunoglobulins, and bacterial infections are common, independent of treatment. IV treatment with immunoglobulin (IVIG) may be given to select patients with recurrent infection. While studies have not demonstrated improved survival, the rate of developing major infections is reduced (NCCN, 2019d). Patients with CLL should receive both pneumonia and flu vaccinations as indicated. Live vaccines should be avoided. The patient with CLL is at increased risk of a host of infections; nursing interventions focused on diminishing these risks are summarized in Chapter 12, Chart 12-6.

For the procedural guidelines for managing immunoglobulin therapy, go to **thepoint.lww.com/Brunner15e**.

NURSING PROCESS

The Patient with Acute Leukemia

Assessment

Although the clinical picture varies with the type of leukemia as well as with the treatment implemented, the health history may reveal a range of subtle symptoms reported by the patient before the problem is detectable on physical examination. If the patient is hospitalized, assessments should be performed daily, or more frequently as warranted. Because the physical findings may be subtle initially, a thorough, systematic assessment incorporating all body systems is essential. For example, a dry cough, mild dyspnea, and diminished breath sounds may indicate a pulmonary infection. However, the infection may not be seen initially on the chest x-ray; the absence of neutrophils delays the inflammatory response against the pulmonary infection, thus delaying radiographic changes. When serial assessments are performed, current findings are compared with previous findings to evaluate improvement or worsening. Specific body system assessments are delineated in the neutropenic and bleeding precautions found in Chapter 12, Chart 12-6.

The nurse also must closely monitor the results of laboratory studies, including tracking the leukocyte count, ANC, hematocrit, platelet, creatinine and electrolyte levels, and coagulation and hepatic function tests. Culture results need to be reported immediately so that appropriate antimicrobial therapy can begin or be modified.

Diagnosis

NURSING DIAGNOSES

Based on the assessment data, major nursing diagnoses may include:

- Risk for infection, haemorrhaging, or both
- Impaired oral mucous membrane integrity due to changes in epithelial lining of the GI tract from chemotherapy or prolonged use of antimicrobial medications
- Impaired nutritional status associated with hypermetabolic state, anorexia, mucositis, pain, and nausea
- Acute pain associated with mucositis, leukocyte infiltration of systemic tissues, fever, and infection
- Fatigue and activity intolerance associated with anemia, infection, inadequate nutrition, and deconditioning
- Fluid imbalance associated with renal dysfunction, diarrhea, bleeding, infection, increased metabolic rate, hypoproteinemia, and need for multiple intravenous medications and blood products
- Impaired ability to perform hygiene, impaired ability to dress, and impaired self toileting due to fatigue and malaise
- Anxiety and grief due to uncertainty about future, anticipatory loss, and altered role functioning
- Risk for spiritual distress
- Lack of knowledge about disease process, treatment, complication management, and self-care measures

COLLABORATIVE PROBLEMS/POTENTIAL COMPLICATIONS

Potential complications may include the following (see Chapter 12 for further discussion):

- Infection
- Bleeding/DIC
- Renal dysfunction
- Cardiac toxicity
- Infertility
- Tumor lysis syndrome

Planning and Goals

The major goals for the patient may include absence of complications and pain, attainment and maintenance of adequate nutrition, activity tolerance, ability to provide self-care and to cope with the diagnosis and prognosis, positive body image, and an understanding of the disease process and its treatment.

Nursing Interventions

PREVENTING OR MANAGING INFECTION AND BLEEDING

The nursing interventions related to diminishing the risk of infection and bleeding are delineated in Chapter 12, Chart 12-6.

MANAGING MUCOSITIS

Although emphasis is placed on the oral mucosa, the entire GI mucosa can be altered, not only by the effects of chemotherapy but also from prolonged administration of antibiotics. See Chapter 12 for assessment and management of mucositis.

IMPROVING NUTRITIONAL INTAKE

The disease process can increase the patient's metabolic rate and nutritional requirements. Nutritional intake is often reduced because of pain and discomfort associated with stomatitis. Encouraging or providing mouth care before and after meals and administering analgesic agents before eating can help increase intake. If oral anesthetic agents are used, the patient must be warned to chew with extreme care to avoid inadvertently biting the tongue or buccal mucosa.

Nausea should not interfere with nutritional intake, because appropriate antiemetic therapy is highly effective. However, nausea can result from antimicrobial therapy, so some antiemetic therapy may still be required after the chemotherapy has been completed.

Small, frequent feedings of foods that are soft in texture and moderate in temperature may be better tolerated. Low-microbial diets may be prescribed (avoiding uncooked fruits or vegetables and those without a peelable skin), although there is little evidence to support this intervention (Olsen et al., 2019). Nutritional supplements are frequently used. Daily body weight (as well as intake and output measurements) is useful in monitoring fluid status. Both calorie counts and more formal nutritional assessments are often useful. Parenteral nutrition may be required to maintain adequate nutrition.

EASING PAIN AND DISCOMFORT

Recurrent fevers are common in acute leukemia; at times, they are accompanied by shaking chills (rigors), which can be severe. Myalgias and arthralgias can result. Acetaminophen is typically given to decrease fever, but it also increases diaphoresis. Sponging with cool water may be useful, but cold water or ice packs should be avoided because the heat cannot dissipate from constricted blood vessels. Bedclothes need frequent changing as well. Gentle back and shoulder massage may provide comfort.

Mucositis can also cause significant discomfort. In addition to oral hygiene practices, patient-controlled analgesia can be effective in controlling the pain (see Chapter 9). With the exception of severe mucositis, less pain is associated with acute leukemia than with many other forms of cancer. However, the amount of psychological suffering that the patient endures can be immense. Patients often benefit from active listening and possible referral for professional counseling.

DECREASING FATIGUE AND ACTIVITY INTOLERANCE

Fatigue is a common and oppressive symptom. Nursing interventions should focus on assisting the patient to establish a balance between activity and rest. Patients with acute leukemia need to maintain some physical activity and exercise to prevent the deconditioning that results from inactivity. The use of a high-efficiency particulate air (HEPA) filter mask can permit the patient to ambulate outside the room despite severe neutropenia. Stationary bicycles may also be set up in the room; however, many patients lack the motivation or stamina to use them. At a minimum, patients should be encouraged to sit up in a chair while awake rather than staying in bed; even this simple activity can improve the patient's

NURSING RESEARCH PROFILE

Fatigue and Sleep Disturbances in Adults with Acute Leukemia

Bryant, A., Gosselin, T., Coffman, E., et al. (2018). Symptoms, mobility, and function, and quality of life in adults with acute leukemia during initial hospitalization. *Oncology Nursing Forum, 45*(5), 653–664.

Purpose

Patients newly diagnosed with acute leukemia require hospitalization, typically for 4 to 6 weeks, for managing aggressive induction therapy and its toxicities. These symptoms can greatly impact the patient's quality of life and ability to perform activities of daily living. The purpose of this study was to evaluate global, physical, and mental health symptoms in adults with newly diagnosed acute leukemia.

Design

This was a prospective, longitudinal study with a total of 49 adult participants, including 36 males and 13 females. Data were collected at time of hospitalization (baseline), then weekly until discharge from hospital. Evaluation tools for data included: the Patient-Reported Outcomes Measurement Information System (PROMIS) to determine several self-reported quality-of-life measures such as fatigue, anxiety, depression, pain, sleep disturbances, and global physical and mental health; the Functional Assessment of Cancer Therapy-Leukemia (FACT-Leu) to measure symptom concerns that are leukemic specific; Karnofsky Performance Status Scale (KPS) to measure function; and the Timed UP and Go Test (TUG) to measure physical mobility.

Findings

This study was the largest, to date, to evaluate the symptoms and quality of life of patients newly diagnosed with acute leukemia during hospitalization. All participants had one or more comorbidities, as well as a group mean body mass index of 30.8 (SD = 6.7), indicative of being overweight or having obesity, at time of hospitalization. No significant differences were seen in global mental health, pain, or KPS during hospitalization. There were significant decreases in fatigue ($p < 0.001$), anxiety ($p < 0.001$), depression ($p = 0.004$), and sleep disturbance ($p = 0.005$) from baseline to hospital discharge. Also significant were a decrease in leukemic symptoms ($p < 0.001$), indicating improved leukemic outcomes, which is the goal of therapy.

Nursing Implications

Nurses need to be aware of factors that can impact sleep in patients with cancer, both during and following treatment. As fatigue plays a major role in sleep disturbances, the nurse needs to assess for and develop strategies to address both concerns, especially while the patient is in the hospital. Poor sleep, fatigue, and pain can all contribute to the increased risk for falls, so safety issues should also be addressed with the patient and the patient's family. The nurse should encourage the patient to exercise and have some physical activity as part of the daily routine, to decrease fatigue while enhancing sleep. Additionally, the nurse should have a good understanding of the symptoms common to patients with leukemia and interventions to manage them as they occur.

---

tidal volume and enhance circulation. Physical therapy can also be beneficial. Patients with acute leukemia may require hospitalization for extensive nursing care (either during induction or consolidation therapy or during resultant complications); sleep deprivation frequently results. Nurses need to implement creative strategies that permit uninterrupted sleep for at least a few hours while still administering necessary medications on schedule (see Nursing Research Profile, Chart 30-2).

MAINTAINING FLUID AND ELECTROLYTE BALANCE

Febrile episodes, bleeding, and inadequate or overly aggressive fluid replacement can alter the patient's fluid status. Similarly, persistent diarrhea and vomiting that occur with certain chemotherapy and immunotherapy agents, and long-term use of certain antimicrobial agents can cause significant deficits in electrolytes. Intake and output need to be measured accurately, and daily weights should also be monitored. The patient should be assessed for signs of dehydration as well as fluid overload, with particular attention to pulmonary status and the development of dependent edema. Laboratory test results, particularly electrolytes, blood urea nitrogen, creatinine, and hematocrit, should be monitored and compared with previous results. Replacement of electrolytes, particularly potassium and magnesium, is commonly required. Patients receiving amphotericin or certain antibiotics are at increased risk for electrolyte depletion.

IMPROVING SELF-CARE: BATHING, DRESSING, AND TOILETING

Because hygiene measures are so important in this patient population, they must be performed by the nurse when the patient cannot do so. However, the patient should be encouraged to do as much as possible to preserve mobility and function as well as self-esteem. Patients may have negative feelings because they can no longer care for themselves. Empathetic listening is helpful, as is realistic reassurance that these deficits are temporary. As the patient recovers, the nurse assists them to resume more self-care. Patients are usually discharged from the hospital with a vascular access device (e.g., Hickman catheter, peripherally inserted central catheter [PICC]), and coordination with appropriate home care services is needed for catheter management.

MANAGING ANXIETY AND GRIEF

Being diagnosed with acute leukemia can be extremely frightening. In many instances, the need to begin treatment is emergent, and the patient has little time to process the fact that they have the illness before making decisions about therapy. Providing emotional support and discussing the uncertain future are crucial. The nurse also needs to assess how much information the patient wants to have regarding the illness, its treatment, and potential complications. This desire should be reassessed at intervals, because needs and interest in information change throughout the course of the disease and treatment. Priorities must be identified so that procedures, assessments, and self-care expectations are adequately explained even to those who do not wish extensive information.

Many patients exhibit depressive symptoms and begin to grieve for their losses, such as normal family functioning, professional roles and responsibilities, and social roles, as well as physical functioning. The nurse can assist the patient to identify the source of the grief and encourage them to allow time to adjust to the major life changes produced by the illness. Role restructuring, in both family and professional life, may be required. It is essential to encourage the patient to identify options and to take time in making important decisions.

The patient's physical condition can deteriorate quickly and it is not often easy to discern if the patient may recover or will die from complications. Providing emotional support to both the patient and the family is critical and equally as important as is rendering expert physical care.

Discharge from the hospital can also provoke anxiety. Although most patients are eager to go home, they may lack confidence in their ability to manage potential complications and to resume their normal activity. Close communication between nurses across care settings can reassure patients that they will not be abandoned.

Encouraging Spiritual Well-Being

Because acute leukemia is a serious, potentially life-threatening illness, the nurse may offer support to enhance the patient's spiritual well-being. The patient's spiritual and religious practices should be assessed and pastoral services offered. Throughout the patient's illness, the nurse assists the patient to maintain hope. However, that hope should be realistic and will certainly change over the course of the illness. For example, the patient may initially hope to be cured, but with repeated relapses and a change to hospice or palliative care, the same patient may hope for a quiet, dignified death. (Refer to Chapter 13 for a discussion of palliative and end-of-life care.)

Promoting Home, Community-Based, and Transitional Care

Educating Patients About Self-Care. Most patients cope better when they understand what is happening to them. Based on their health literacy level, and interest, educating the patient and family should begin with a focus on the disease (including some pathophysiology), its treatment, and certainly the resulting significant risk of infection and bleeding (see Chapter 29, Charts 29-7 and 29-8).

Although management of a vascular access device can be taught to most patients or family members, this care is typically performed by a home care agency or outpatient clinic nursing staff. Patients and family members do need basic education regarding management of the vascular access device, particularly with regard to prevention of infections.

Continuing and Transitional Care. For patients who are clinically stable but require parenteral antibiotics or blood products, these procedures are most often performed in an outpatient setting. Nurses in these settings must communicate regularly. They need to inform the patient about parameters that are important to monitor, how to monitor them, and to give the patient-specific instructions about when to seek care from the physician or other health care provider.

The patient and family need to have a clear understanding of the disease, the prognosis, and how to monitor for complications or recurrence. The nurse ensures that this information is provided. Should the patient no longer respond to therapy, it is important to respect the patient's choices about treatment and end-of-life care. Advance directives or other method should be used for patients to state their end-of-life preferences (see Chapter 13, Chart 13-5). In patients with acute leukemia, death typically occurs from infection or, less frequently, from bleeding. Family members need to have information about these complications and the measures to take should either occur. Many family members cannot cope with the care required when a patient begins to bleed actively. It is important to delineate alternatives to keeping the patient at home, such as inpatient hospice units.

Evaluation

Expected patient outcomes may include:
1. Shows no evidence of infection
2. Experiences no bleeding
3. Has intact oral mucous membranes
   a. Participates in oral hygiene regimen
   b. Reports no discomfort in mouth
4. Attains optimal level of nutrition
   a. Maintains weight with increased food and fluid intake
   b. Maintains adequate protein stores (e.g., albumin, prealbumin)
5. Reports satisfaction with pain and comfort levels
6. Has less fatigue and increased activity
7. Maintains fluid and electrolyte balance
8. Participates in self-care
9. Copes with anxiety and grief
   a. Discusses concerns and fears
   b. Uses stress management strategies appropriately
   c. Participates in decisions regarding end-of-life care
10. Reports sense of spiritual well-being
11. Absence of complications

MYELODYSPLASTIC SYNDROMES (MDSs)

The MDSs are a group of clonal disorders of the myeloid stem cell that cause dysplasia (abnormal development) in one or more types of cell lines. These disorders commonly result in cytopenias (low blood cell counts), with the tendency to develop into acute leukemia (Sockel & Platzbecker, 2018). A common feature of MDS is anemia due to dysplasia of the erythrocytes, although leukocytes (particularly neutrophils) and platelets can also be affected. Although the bone marrow is actually hypercellular, many of the cells within it die before being released into the circulation. Therefore, the actual number of cells in the circulation is typically lower than normal. In MDS, the affected cells do not function normally. The neutrophils have diminished ability to destroy bacteria by **phagocytosis** (cellular ingestion and digestion of foreign bodies); platelets are less able to aggregate and are less adhesive than usual. The result of these defects is an increased risk of infection and bleeding, even when the actual number of circulating cells may not be excessively low.

This disease is primarily seen in older adults (median age at diagnosis is 65 to 70 years), is idiopathic in nature due to HSC damage, and occurs more often in males than females (Montalban-Bravo & Garcia-Manero, 2017; Sockel & Platzbecker, 2018). In addition, about 10% to 15% of patients will develop MDS following exposure to alkylating agents, radiotherapy, or chemicals (e.g., benzene), and/or have an inherited genetic disorder, such as Fanconi anemia or trisomy 21 (Sockel & Platzbecker, 2018). Genetic syndromes account for about 50% of cases (e.g., Down syndrome, trisomy 8 syndrome, neurofibromatosis type 1) (Leukemia & Lymphoma Society, 2019d; NCCN, 2019e).

Clinical Manifestations

The manifestations of MDS can vary widely. Some patients are asymptomatic, with the illness being discovered incidentally when a CBC is performed for other purposes. Other patients have profound symptoms and complications from the illness. Because MDS tends to occur in older adults, other concurrent chronic health conditions may exacerbate symptoms associated with the disease. Fatigue is often present, with varying levels of intensity and frequency. Neutrophil dysfunction puts the patient at risk for recurrent pneumonias and other infections. Because platelet function can also be altered, bleeding can occur. These problems may persist in a fairly steady state for months, even years. Over time, the marrow may fail to provide enough cells despite support with transfusion or growth factors; this is called *bone marrow failure*. MDS may also progress over time; as the dysplasia evolves into a leukemic state, the complications increase in severity. However, it is important to note that the majority of patients with MDS succumb to complications from the disease itself or from other comorbidities, and not to those from acute leukemia (Leukemia & Lymphoma Society, 2019d).

Assessment and Diagnostic Findings

The CBC typically reveals a macrocytic anemia; leukocyte and platelet counts may be diminished as well. Other potential causes for cytopenia, which may include vitamin deficiencies, viral infection, GI bleeding, autoimmune disease, splenomegaly, and liver dysfunction, should be excluded. Serum erythropoietin levels may be variable and the **reticulocyte** count (immature RBCs) may be inappropriately low. The presence of blast cells on the CBC may be indicative of disease progression to acute leukemia. To help rule out other causes of anemia, other laboratory studies may include folate, serum vitamin B_{12}, ferritin, total iron-binding capacity (TIBC), iron, and thyroid-stimulating hormone (TSH).

The official diagnosis of MDS is based on the results of a bone marrow aspiration (to assess dysplasia) and biopsy (to assess characteristics of the affected cells). These tests help in determining prognosis, risk of leukemic transformation, and in some patients, the most effective therapy (Montalban-Bravo & Garcia-Manero, 2017); thus, the nurse must understand the risk stratification category of each patient. Those patients with low-risk disease have a much longer survival (as much as 10 years) compared with untreated patients with high-risk disease (where survival is usually less than 9 months) (NCCN, 2019e) (see Chapter 28 for discussion of bone marrow aspiration and biopsy).

Medical Management

Medical management strategies for MDS are based on risk stratification to determine stage of disease and prognosis. The most commonly used tool is the International Prognostic Scoring System (IPSS) that evaluates cytopenia, transfusion needs, percent of blast cells in the bone marrow, and cytogenetic characteristics (Montalban-Bravo & Garcia-Manero, 2017). Most patients with MDSs are diagnosed as having low-risk disease; for these patients, the objective of therapy is to maintain or restore quality of life, improve cytopenia, and decrease transfusion requirements. Some patients with mild symptoms may only require periodic monitoring of laboratory studies indicative of hematologic function (e.g., CBC, reticulocyte count, folate, ferritin, iron). Approximately two thirds of patients diagnosed as low risk have cytopenic-related complications at the time of diagnosis, however, and may require blood transfusions and/or an erythropoiesis-stimulating agent.

Patients who are at low to intermediate risk and transfusion dependent are typically treated with a hypomethylating agent (e.g., azacitidine, decitabine). These agents work by inhibiting the abnormal genes regulating methylation, promoting tumor suppression genes, and permitting myeloid differentiation within the bone marrow (NCCN, 2019e). Neither drug has been shown to modify the natural trajectory of low-risk MDS; therefore, hypomethylating agents are not typically used until erythroid-stimulating agents are no longer effective in controlling transfusion dependence (NCCN, 2019e). These agents can improve cytopenia, reduce transfusion requirements, reduce the likelihood of transformation to AML, and improve overall survival.

For the patient at high risk the goals of therapy are to delay leukemic transformation and prolong life expectancy (NCCN, 2019e; Sockel & Platzbecker, 2018). Allogeneic HSCT continues to be the only potential option of cure for MDS, but is not often a viable option for most patients, as many are of advanced age with significant comorbidities. Allogeneic HSCT is recommended for patients who have hypoplastic MDS, are younger, or those who have not responded satisfactorily to other treatment options (Montalban-Bravo & Garcia-Manero, 2017; NCCN, 2019e).

Lenalidomide (a thalidomide analog) is the standard of care for patients with the chromosomal abnormality deletion 5q, are considered low risk, and are not thrombocytopenic (NCCN, 2019e). Treatment with lenalidomide may cause neutropenia and thrombocytopenia, which may necessitate treatment delays or dose reduction (NCCN, 2019e). Other immunosuppressive therapies that have shown some efficacy in the treatment of MDS are antithymocyte globulin (ATG), with or without cyclosporine, and corticosteroids. These agents are used in a subset of patients with MDS who have weakened immune responses (e.g., have neutropenia) (Montalban-Bravo & Garcia-Manero, 2017).

Patients frequently need repeated transfusions (PRBCs, platelets, or both) throughout the illness trajectory to maintain adequate hemoglobin and platelet levels (termed *transfusion dependence*). Attempts to improve anemia and decrease RBC transfusion are often successful with the use of erythroid-stimulating agents (epoetin alfa or darbopoetin alfa). Higher-than-normal doses may be required to achieve an adequate improvement in hemoglobin. Adding myeloid growth factors such as G-CSF or GM-CSF can boost responsiveness to these agents (NCCN, 2019e). The median duration of response to this therapy is 2 years; transfusion requirements typically increase by this point.

Thrombocytopenia is a challenge to manage among patients with MDS. Severe thrombocytopenia is difficult to manage because patients can quickly develop refractoriness to platelet transfusions due to alloimmunization (Leukemia & Lymphoma Society, 2019d). Moreover, bleeding can develop even when the platelet level is not excessively low, due to poor platelet function. The cause of thrombocytopenia appears to be increased apoptosis and premature marrow destruction of the platelets prior to their release into the circulation (NCCN, 2019e). The recombinant thrombopoietin receptor agonists romiplostim and eltrombopag have been developed to stimulate the proliferation and differentiation of megakaryocytes into platelets within the bone marrow. Both drugs have demonstrated the ability to significantly raise platelet counts in this population, but their duration of action may not be long. Increased rates of marrow fibrosis and AML evolution seem to be ameliorated by discontinuing the drug, but additional study is needed (NCCN, 2019e).

Iron overload is another significant problem for patients with MDS, especially in patients who routinely receive PRBC transfusions (transfusion dependent). Surplus iron is deposited in cells within the reticuloendothelial system, and later in parenchymal organs (e.g., liver). While a true cause-and-effect has not yet been established, there is significant concern that patients with transfusion-dependent MDS are at high risk for developing cardiac disorders, particularly heart failure, as well as hepatic and endocrine dysfunction (NCCN, 2019e). Excess iron, and the resultant increased oxidative stress, is also associated with pancreatic dysfunction, the development of diabetes, increased rates of infection, and decreased hematopoiesis.

To prevent or reverse the complications of iron overload, iron chelation therapy is commonly implemented. Patients with preexisting liver disease, including cirrhosis, should not receive oral iron chelators. There are studies that have found that iron overload may play a role in increased mortality and morbidity in early-stage MDS due to hepatic, cardiac, and endocrine dysfunction (NCCN, 2019e). It is recommended that all patients with MDS who have regular transfusion needs have serum ferritin levels along with the number of PRBC transfusions routinely monitored to determine iron stores and possible overload. The ferritin level should be maintained at less than 1000 mcg/L. Iron is bound to the chelating agent and then excreted in the urine. Because chelation therapy removes only a small amount of iron with each treatment, patients with chronic iron overload from RBC transfusions need to continue chelation therapy as long as the iron overload exists. Oral iron chelation with deferasirox has replaced the need for the former standard therapy, which consisted of subcutaneous infusions of deferoxamine. However, adherence remains a challenge, largely due to toxicity associated with the drug.

Infection rates are high among patients with MDS, who frequently require hospitalization. Severe neutropenia, coexisting chronic obstructive pulmonary disease (COPD) or autoimmune disease, and history of other malignancy are associated with higher risk for developing infection, whereas the extent of thrombocytopenia, age, MDS therapy, or diabetes

are not (Leukemia & Lymphoma Society, 2019d; NCCN, 2019e). Pneumonia is the most common type of infection in this patient population; bacteria (both gram negative and gram positive) are the predominant pathogens.

The administration of myeloid growth factors alone may be useful in some patients with infections and severe neutropenia, but they are not typically used to prevent infection. Prophylactic antibiotics are not routinely used so that resistant organisms do not develop, but prompt initiation of antimicrobial therapy is crucial at the onset of infection to diminish the risk of increased mortality.

Nursing Management

Caring for patients with MDS can be challenging because the illness is unpredictable. As with other hematologic disorders, some patients (especially those with no symptoms) have difficulty perceiving that they have a serious illness that can place them at risk for life-threatening complications. At the other extreme, many patients have tremendous difficulty coping with the uncertain trajectory of the illness and fear that the illness will evolve into AML. Thus, it is important for patients to understand their unique risk of the disease transforming to AML and to recognize that, for most patients, MDS is a chronic illness. It is imperative that the nurse recognizes any concurrent health problems the patient may have. This knowledge will help the nurse better plan and manage the patient's care. For example, a patient with underlying heart failure or COPD may not tolerate anemia well, nor a more rapid rate of red blood cell transfusion.

Patients with MDS need extensive education about infection risk, measures to avoid it, signs and symptoms of developing infection, and appropriate actions to take should such symptoms occur. Education should also be provided regarding the risk of bleeding. Patients need to be encouraged to serve as their own health advocate, by informing other health care providers, including dentists, that they have MDS, and their risks for infection and bleeding. Patients with MDS who are hospitalized may require neutropenic precautions.

Fatigue is often a debilitating symptom for the patient with MDS and significantly interferes with quality of life. It can impair the patient's ability to function in the work or home setting and to engage in meaningful activities, and affect the patient's overall cognitive function (Leukemia & Lymphoma Society, 2019d; NCCN, 2019e). Patients may benefit from anticipatory guidance in learning how to live with this symptom, and creative strategies may be required.

Laboratory values need to be monitored closely to anticipate the need for transfusion and to determine response to treatment with growth factors. Patients with chronic transfusion requirements often benefit from the insertion of a vascular access device for this purpose. Those patients receiving chemotherapy need extensive education regarding treatment side effects (and how to manage them) and treatment schedules. Patients receiving growth factors need education about these medications, administration schedules, and side effects.

Chelation therapy is a process that is used to remove excess iron acquired from chronic transfusions. Side effects from oral chelators commonly include diarrhea and abdominal cramping. Educating the patient to take the medication in the evening prior to dinner and gradually increasing the dosage over time may diminish these side effects. Skin rash is usually mild and rarely warrants temporarily stopping the drug. Monitoring renal function is important as a rise in serum creatinine is common. The dosage should be reduced if the serum creatinine rises by more than one third of baseline. Patients with preexisting liver disease, including cirrhosis, should not receive oral iron chelators.

MYELOPROLIFERATIVE NEOPLASMS

Myeloproliferative neoplasms originate in the HSC and are characterized by clonal proliferation of one or more myeloid cell types (Arber et al., 2016; Spivak, 2018). These Philadelphia chromosome-negative myeloproliferative disorders include polycythemia vera, essential thrombocythemia, and primary myelofibrosis.

Polycythemia Vera

Polycythemia vera (sometimes called *P vera* or primary polycythemia) is the most common of the three Philadelphia chromosome-negative myeloproliferative disorders. In polycythemia vera the bone marrow is hypercellular, and the erythrocyte, leukocyte, and platelet counts in the peripheral blood are often elevated. Erythrocyte elevation predominates; the hematocrit can exceed 60% in some cases (Tefferi & Barbui, 2019). The median age at the onset is 60 years; median survival is typically 14 to 20 years (Fowlkes, Murray, Fulford, et al., 2018a; Tefferi & Barbui, 2019).

Clinical Manifestations

Clinical manifestations are variable. Some patients at the time of initial diagnosis may be asymptomatic (Spivak, 2018). If symptoms are present, they tend to be related to erythrocytosis, with or without leukocytosis and/or **thrombocytosis** (i.e., higher-than-normal platelet count that occurs from a disease or disorder; in this instance, the disease is polycythemia vera). This increase in blood cell mass increases blood viscosity leading to (Fowlkes et al., 2018b; Harrison, Koschmieder, Foltz, et al., 2017; Spivak, 2018):

- neurologic symptoms such as headache, dizziness, vision changes, and transient ischemic attacks (TIAs);
- abdominal symptoms such as early satiety, abdominal discomfort/pain (that can also be associated with splenomegaly);
- cardiovascular symptoms including ruddy complexion, angina, claudication, dyspnea, hypertension, and thrombophlebitis; and
- constitutional symptoms such as fatigue and night sweats.

Another common symptom is pruritus, which may be caused by histamine released from an increased number of basophils. **Erythromelalgia**, characterized by a burning, painful sensation, and erythema in the fingers or toes, may also occur. Uric acid may be elevated as well, resulting in gout and renal stones formation.

Assessment and Diagnostic Findings

Diagnosis is based upon the evaluation of clinical symptoms and laboratory findings as well as the presence of a mutation of the *JAK2* gene (Arber et al., 2016). Assessment should include palpation of the spleen, and finding if the patient has a history of thrombotic events or has ever received a blood transfusion or medications associated with causing erythrocytosis (e.g., recombinant erythropoietin), as well as assessment of cardiovascular risk factors (e.g., obesity, smoking, and poorly controlled hypertension, diabetes, or hyperlipidemia; see later discussion of thrombotic risks under Complications). Some patients with the *JAK2* mutation who do not meet the criteria for a diagnosis of polycythemia vera are identified as having "masked polycythemia vera" (McMullin, Harrison, Ali, et al., 2019; Spivak, 2018). These patients are more likely to transform to myelofibrosis (see later discussion) or AML and have a poorer overall rate of survival (McMullin et al., 2019; Spivak, 2018).

Complications

Patients with polycythemia vera are at increased risk for thromboses that may be either venous or arterial. Thrombosis can result in strokes or myocardial infarctions; thrombotic complications are the most common cause of death. Patients older than 60 years of age, those with a prior history of thrombosis, or those with an elevated platelet count (exceeding 1 million/mm^3) are at greater risk for developing thrombotic complications (Tefferi & Barbui, 2019). Patients with enlarged spleens are also at increased risk for thrombosis. Cardiovascular risk factors thought to increase thrombotic risk include obesity, smoking, and poorly controlled hypertension, diabetes, or hyperlipidemia (Barbui, Vannucchi, Carobbio, et al., 2017).

Bleeding may also be a complication of polycythemia vera and its treatment. The bleeding can be significant and can occur in the form of nosebleeds, ulcers, frank GI bleeding, hematuria, or intracranial hemorrhage. If the patient with polycythemia vera has a bleeding complication and is taking aspirin, the aspirin should be held until the bleeding is resolved (NCCN, 2019f).

Medical Management

The objectives of management are to reduce the risk of thrombosis without increasing the risk of bleeding, reduce the risk of evolution to myelofibrosis or AML, and ameliorate symptoms associated with the disease (McMullin et al., 2019) (see Table 30-2). Specific therapy is based on an established risk stratification. Patients less than age 60 and no prior history of thrombosis are considered "low risk"; those age 60 or older, or with a history of thrombosis, or both, are considered to be "high risk" (NCCN, 2019f).

Phlebotomy is considered the mainstay of therapy and is used to maintain the hematocrit level at less than 45% (Spivak, 2018) (see Fig. 30-5). It involves removing enough blood (initially 500 mL once or twice weekly) to reduce blood viscosity and to deplete iron stores, thereby rendering the patient iron deficient and consequently unable to continue to manufacture excessive RBCs. Low-dose aspirin prevents vascular thrombosis without increasing the risk of bleeding

TABLE 30-2	Common Constitutional Symptoms Associated with Myeloproliferative Neoplasms		

Symptoms vary between the three myeloproliferative neoplasms, both in frequency and severity. Nurses should assess these patients frequently for the presence of these symptoms and initiate appropriate measures to ameliorate them.

Symptom	P Vera (%)	ET (%)	Myelofibrosis (%)
Fatigue	85	84	94
Concentration	62	58	68
Early satiety	60	56	74
Night sweats	52	47	63
Pruritus	62	46	52
Abdominal discomfort	48	48	65
Bone pain	48	45	53
Weight loss	33	28	47
Fever	19	17	24

ET, essential thrombocythemia; P vera, polycythemia vera.
Adapted from Geyer, H. L., & Mesa, R. A. (2014). Therapy for myeloproliferative neoplasms: When, which agent, and how? *Hematology American Society of Hematology Education Program, 2014*(1), 277–286.

and is recommended for all patients with polycythemia vera, regardless of risk (Leukemia & Lymphoma Society, 2019e; NCCN, 2019f).

Cytoreductive therapy should be considered in patients at low risk who are symptomatic due to progressive splenomegaly, leukocytosis, thrombocytosis, or have poor tolerance to phlebotomy, or whose disease has progressed to myelofibrosis or AML (McMullin et al., 2019; NCCN, 2019f). In patients at high risk, cytoreductive therapy is considered first-line treatment and might be pursued in addition to or in place of phlebotomy. Hydroxyurea, also known as hydroxycarbamide,

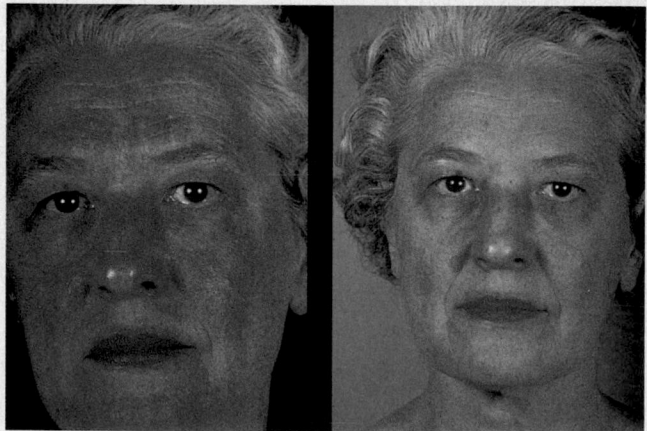

Figure 30-5 • Phlebotomy can markedly reduce the plethora seen in polycythemia vera. This is evidenced here by a marked reduction in facial rubor in a patient with polycythemia vera. Reprinted with permission from Turgeon, M. L. (2012). *Clinical hematology: Theory & procedures* (5th ed., Fig. 21.10, p. 373). Philadelphia, PA: Lippincott Williams & Wilkins.

can be used to suppress bone marrow function, thereby controlling blood counts. It has also been associated with preventing thrombotic complications (Tefferi & Barbui, 2019). Interferon-alfa is another first-line cytoreductive agent that can be selected; it is indicated in patients younger than 60 years of age, or in patients who are pregnant or intolerant of hydroxyurea (NCCN, 2019e). Interferon-alfa can also reduce splenomegaly, prevent thrombosis, and decrease pruritus. However, it may be difficult for patients to tolerate because of its side effects (e.g., flulike symptoms, depression); it is also very costly.

Ruxolitinib is a *JAK2* inhibitor; it is used in patients who are resistant or unable to tolerate hydroxyurea and for whom interferon-alfa is not indicated (e.g., patients older than 60 years of age). This drug has been shown to reduce splenomegaly, decrease symptoms, and improve quality of life (Fowlkes et al., 2018a; McMullin et al., 2019). Common side effects of ruxolitinib include dose-dependent anemia and thrombocytopenia.

Additional cytoreductive drugs, including busulfan, pipobroman, and anagrelide, have been shown to be effective in controlling blood counts; however, these agents have been linked to an increased risk for leukemic transformation and have significant side effects. These drugs are reserved for patients who are refractory to other cytoreductive agents or with limited life expectancy (McMullin et al., 2019).

Nursing Management

Fatigue is the most commonly reported symptom in patients with polycythemia vera. It is not always correlated to disease severity. The degree of fatigue may vary, but can become so debilitating that it impairs the patient's quality of life. There are many causes of fatigue, including a release of proinflammatory **cytokines** (proteins produced by leukocytes that are vital to regulation of hematopoiesis, apoptosis, and immune responses), impaired hematopoiesis, depression, inactivity, and the effects of certain medications (e.g., antihypertensive medications, antihistamines) (Fowlkes et al., 2018b; NCCN, 2019e). Management of fatigue can include pharmacologic agents (e.g., erythropoiesis-stimulating agents, antidepressant drugs, stimulants such as caffeine or amphetamines) and nonpharmacologic treatments (e.g., exercise, yoga, and optimizing sleep).

Another common symptom in patients is pruritus, described as strong itching, stinging, or burning. The exact etiology is not known but is thought to be related to proinflammatory cytokines. Pruritus can be triggered by contact with water of any temperature. Other causes include consuming alcohol or caffeine, having dry skin, experiencing changes in temperature, and sweating after exercise (Fowlkes et al., 2018b; Tefferi & Barbui, 2019). Antihistamines, emollient lotion, and selective serotonin reuptake inhibitors (SSRIs) are not particularly effective in controlling pruritus. Interferon-alfa and narrow band ultraviolet B phototherapy (which uses ultraviolet light for a prescribed length of time to decrease symptoms) may be used in severe cases. As the efficacy of pharmacologic strategies may not be optimal, it is important to individualize therapy and monitor for effectiveness. The nurse may recommend bathing in tepid water, avoiding vigorous toweling off after bathing, and using cocoa butter or oatmeal-based lotions.

Potentially life-threatening complications from the disease are thrombosis or hemorrhage. Risk factors for thrombotic complications, particularly a prior history of thrombosis, smoking, obesity, and poorly controlled hypertension, diabetes, and hyperlipidemia should be assessed, and patients should be encouraged to modify their cardiovascular risk factors. Adopting or maintaining a healthy lifestyle should be encouraged. Patients should be educated about the signs and symptoms of thrombosis. To reduce the likelihood of deep vein thrombosis (DVT), sedentary behavior, crossing the legs, and wearing tight or restrictive clothing (particularly stockings) should be discouraged. Patients with a history of significant bleeding are usually advised to avoid high-dose aspirin and aspirin-containing medications, because these medications alter platelet function. Minimizing alcohol intake should also be emphasized to further diminish the risk of bleeding. Patients should be counseled about the signs of bleeding. The patient needs to be instructed to avoid iron supplements, including those in over-the-counter multivitamin supplements, because the iron can further stimulate RBC production.

Essential Thrombocythemia

Essential thrombocythemia, also called primary thrombocythemia, is a rare, chronic, Philadelphia chromosome-negative myeloproliferative disorder characterized by an increased production of megakaryocytes. A marked increase in platelet production occurs, with the platelet count consistently greater than 450,000/mm³. The platelet count can exceed 1 to 2 million/mm³. Occasionally, the **thrombocythemia** (increase in platelets without a known cause) is accompanied by an increase in erythrocytes, leukocytes, or both; however, these cells are not increased to the extent they are in polycythemia vera or myelofibrosis (see later discussion).

The exact underlying cause of essential thrombocythemia is idiopathic (i.e., unknown). Approximately 50% to 60% of patients have the *JAK2* gene mutation, and 25% of patients have the *CALR* gene mutation (Fowlkes et al., 2018a; Tefferi & Barbui, 2019). This disease affects women twice as often as men and tends to occur later in life (median age at diagnosis is 65 to 70 years). Median survival is about 20 to 33 years (Haider, Gangat, Lasho, et al., 2016); overall survival does not differ from the general population. However, survival rates vary based upon the type of gene mutation present. For example, patients with the *CALR* mutation have fewer thrombotic events and higher survival rates compared to those with the *JAK2* mutation (Tefferi & Barbui, 2019).

Clinical Manifestations

Many patients with essential thrombocythemia are asymptomatic; the illness is frequently diagnosed as the result of an incidental finding of an elevated platelet count on a CBC. Symptoms occur most often when the platelet count exceeds 1 million/mm³; however, they do not always correlate with the extent to which the platelet count is elevated. When symptoms do occur, they primarily result from vascular occlusion. This occlusion can occur in large arterial vessels (cerebrovascular, coronary, or peripheral arteries) and deep

veins, as well as in the microcirculation; inflammation that may occur in the vascular endothelium may result in erythromelalgia. More common forms of venous thromboembolism (VTE), including DVT and pulmonary embolism (PE), can also occur.

One of the most common neurologic symptoms of essential thrombocythemia is headaches. Other neurologic manifestations that may be related to compromised blood flow include dizziness; lightheadedness; paresthesias; visual changes, such as diplopia; and TIAs (Fowlkes et al., 2018b; Harrison et al., 2017). Other symptoms can include tinnitus and chest pain.

Because the platelets can be dysfunctional, minor or major hemorrhage may occur. Bleeding is commonly limited to recurrent minor manifestations (e.g., ecchymoses, hematomas, epistaxis, gum bleeding), although significant GI bleeding and intracranial hemorrhage are both possible and considered major hemorrhagic events. Bleeding typically does not occur unless the platelet count exceeds 1.5 million/mm³. It results from a deficiency in von Willebrand factor as the platelet count increases (NCCN, 2019f).

Assessment and Diagnostic Findings

The diagnosis of essential thrombocythemia is made by ruling out other potential disorders—either other myeloproliferative disorders or underlying illnesses that cause a reactive or secondary thrombocytosis (see later discussion). Iron deficiency should be excluded, because a reactive increase in the platelet count often accompanies this deficiency. The diagnosis is typically based upon both an evaluation of clinical manifestations and laboratory findings. The CBC will show markedly enlarged and abnormal platelets, as well as a persistently elevated platelet count (greater than 450,000/mm³). A bone marrow examination (i.e., aspirate or biopsy) can help distinguish between true essential thrombocythemia and other myelofibrotic diseases (Tefferi & Barbui, 2019).

Complications

Complications include inappropriate formation of thrombi and hemorrhage. Patients with cardiovascular risk factors (e.g., obesity, smoking, and poorly controlled hypertension, diabetes, hyperlipidemia) are at higher risk for thrombotic complications (Tefferi & Barbui, 2019). Patients older than 60 years and those with a history of prior thrombosis are at higher risk for complications. Major bleeding tends to occur when the platelet count is very high (greater than 1.5 million/mm³) and there is a prior history of major bleeding. Cause of death in patients is often the result of thrombosis or major bleeding (collectively called thrombohemorrhagic events) or transformation to AML or myelofibrosis (Haider et al., 2016).

Medical Management

The goals of management are to minimize the risk of thrombohemorrhagic events and to control symptoms (see Table 30-2). Treatment for essential thrombocythemia is based upon a patient's risk stratification (NCCN, 2019f). Patients at low risk are less than 60 years of age, without the *JAK2* mutation, and without a prior history of thrombosis. Typical treatment for these patients includes ongoing monitoring for new thrombosis and acquired von Willebrand factor deficiency and disease-related major bleeding; management of cardiovascular risk factors (e.g., obesity, smoking, and poorly controlled hypertension, diabetes, or hyperlipidemia); and daily low-dose aspirin as long as the patient remains asymptomatic. Patients should be monitored every 3 to 6 months for signs and symptoms of disease progression. Patients at intermediate risk are those older than age 60, without the JAK2 mutation, and with no prior history of thrombosis. As long as the patient has not any thrombohemorrhagic events, the treatment remains the same as for low-risk patients.

A patient is deemed high risk when there is a history of thrombosis at any age or is age 60 or older or with the JAK2 mutation. Besides use of aspirin, treatment may also include prescribing hydroxyurea, interferon-alfa, or anagrelide (see previous discussion in polycythemia vera section), all of which are effective in decreasing platelet counts to a level below 400,000/mm³ and reducing risk for developing arterial thrombosis and hemorrhage. However, the side effects of these agents may be intolerable. As previously noted, anagrelide has been associated with disease progression to myelofibrosis or AML (McMullin et al., 2019).

Patients who develop arterial or venous thrombosis require additional treatment. Anticoagulant therapy may be useful for patients with active thrombosis (see Chapter 26 for further discussion of anticoagulation therapy) and platelet apheresis may be used in patients with acute life-threatening thrombosis or major bleeding (see Chapter 28, Table 28-3) (NCCN, 2019f).

Nursing Management

It is important to assess patients for a history of prior thrombohemorrhagic events, because these are the primary cause of morbidity and mortality. Patients with essential thrombocythemia should be educated on signs and symptoms of hemorrhage and thrombosis, particularly the neurologic manifestations, such as visual changes, numbness, tingling, and weakness. Patients should be encouraged about medication adherence and management of side effects. In particular, patients taking aspirin should be informed about the importance of taking this medication as well as the increased risk of bleeding. Those patients taking hydroxyurea should have their CBCs monitored regularly; the dosage is adjusted based on the platelet and WBC count. Patients taking interferon-alfa may be taught to self-administer the medication and how to manage its side effects.

Cardiovascular risk factors associated with thrombotic complications should be assessed, such as obesity, smoking, and poorly controlled hypertension, diabetes, or hyperlipidemia. Measures should be identified and encouraged to reduce these risks. Additionally, patients who are at risk for bleeding should be educated about medications (e.g., aspirin, nonsteroidal anti-inflammatory agents [NSAIDs]) and other substances (e.g., alcohol, certain herbal therapies) that can alter platelet function.

Primary Myelofibrosis

Primary myelofibrosis, also known as agnogenic myeloid metaplasia or myelofibrosis with myeloid metaplasia, is the rarest of the Philadelphia chromosome-negative myeloproliferative disorders; it arises from neoplastic transformation of an early HSC. This disease is characterized by bone marrow fibrosis or scarring, extramedullary hematopoiesis (typically involving the spleen or liver), leukocytosis, thrombocytosis, elevated lactic dehydrogenase (LDH), and anemia. Some patients have **pancytopenia** (i.e., diminished leukocyte, platelet, and erythrocyte counts). Patients with primary myelofibrosis have increased **angiogenesis** (formation of new blood vessels) within the marrow. Immature forms of blood cells, including nucleated RBCs and megakaryocyte fragments, are frequently found in the circulation.

The actual etiology for primary myelofibrosis is still unknown. As with polycythemia vera and essential thrombocythemia, mutations of the JAK2 or CALR gene are frequently seen; prognosis is worse in those without genetic mutations. Myelofibrosis may also be secondary in nature, evolving from polycythemia vera, or less frequently, from essential thrombocythemia. In these instances, the disease progression is then called *secondary myelofibrosis* (Harrison et al., 2017).

Primary myelofibrosis is a disease of the older adult, with a median age of diagnosis at approximately 65 to 70 years of age, and is more common in males (Leukemia & Lymphoma Society, 2019e). Another risk factor is exposure to chemicals (e.g., benzene). Average survival ranges from 2 to 14 years. Common causes of death are due to cardiovascular disease, liver failure, leukemic transformation, and consequences of marrow failure (e.g., infection or bleeding).

Approximately 90% of patients present at the time of diagnosis with splenomegaly, causing abdominal discomfort and early satiety. Many patients also experience constitutional symptoms such as fatigue, night sweats, and fever, as well as pruritus, bone pain, weight loss, cachexia, thrombosis, and bleeding (see Fig. 30-6) (Tefferi, 2018). Arterial or venous thrombosis can occur but is less frequent than that found in polycythemia vera or essential thrombocythemia. Anemia occurs due to impaired erythropoiesis.

Medical Management

The goals of therapy are based upon reducing the burden of disease (by decreasing symptoms and splenomegaly) and improving blood counts (NCCN, 2019f). Treatment is based upon a patient's risk stratification; risks are increased in patients older than 65 years of age, with WBC counts above 25,000/mm³, with hemoglobin levels less than 10 g/dL, with blast cells present in the peripheral blood, and with presence of constitutional symptoms (e.g., pruritus, night sweats, weight loss; see Table 30-2) (NCCN, 2019f).

For patients who are at low risk and asymptomatic, observation and monitoring every 3 to 6 months is recommended. Patients at intermediate risk may be started on the JAK2 inhibitor ruxolitinib if symptomatic (see previous discussion in Polycythemia Vera), or may be considered for allogeneic HSCT. HSCT is a useful treatment modality in younger, otherwise healthy patients; it is the only current therapy that can reverse the fibrosis within the marrow (NCCN, 2019f).

Splenectomy may be performed to control potential or actual complications of an enlarged spleen. However, a reactive thrombocytosis and leukocytosis can develop because

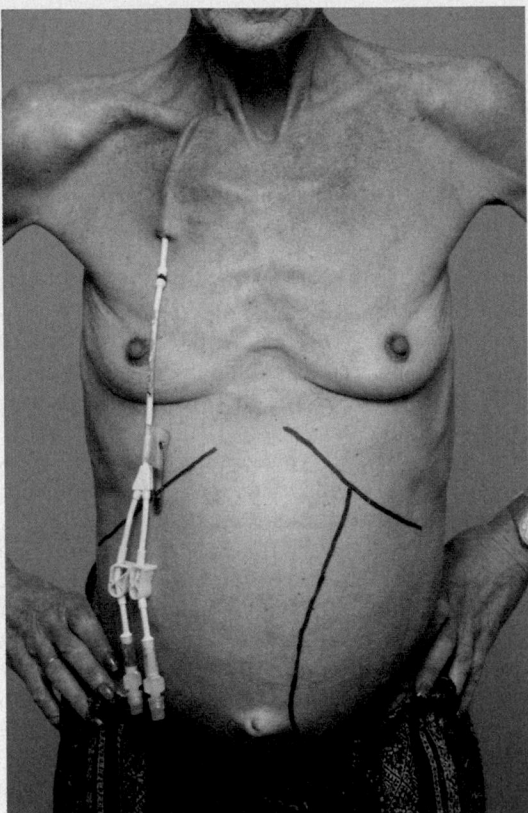

Figure 30-6 • Cachexia, severe wasting, and massively enlarged liver and spleen (hepatosplenomegaly) are seen in advanced myeloproliferative disorders, particularly myelofibrosis. (Note also the lack of adequate dressing over the patient's vascular access device.) Reprinted with permission from Tkachuk, D. C., & Hirschman, J. V. (2007). *Wintrobe's atlas of clinical hematology* (Fig. 4.1, p. 111). Philadelphia, PA: Lippincott Williams & Wilkins.

TABLE 30-3	Fatigue in Patients with Myeloproliferative Neoplasms

Self-reported strategies used to ameliorate fatigue by patients with myeloproliferative neoplasms. Data obtained from online surveys ($N = 1788$) gathered via myeloproliferative neoplasm Web sites.

Strategy	% Patients Reported Use
Setting priorities	75%
Postponing nonessential activities	74%
Exercise	73%
Naps	70%
Walking	66%
Socializing	65%
Nutrition	64%
Reading	62%
Scheduling activity during peak energy periods	62%
Pacing activities	58%
Structured daily routine	54%
Delegation	52%

Adapted from Scherber, R. M., Kosiorek, H. E., Senyak, Z., et al. (2016). Comprehensively understanding fatigue in patients with myeloproliferative neoplasms. *Cancer,* *122*(3), 477–485.

the platelets and leukocytes are no longer sequestered by the spleen and enter the circulation. Careful considerations of the advantages and disadvantages of a splenectomy should be discussed with the patient as the procedure is not without risk.

Anemia is most commonly managed with PRBC transfusions. Erythroid-stimulating agents (e.g., recombinant erythropoietin) may improve anemia to the extent that transfusion requirements are reduced. Other pharmacologic agents are used to diminish splenomegaly and improve blood counts. Hydroxyurea is often used to control high leukocyte and platelet counts and to reduce the size of the spleen. Angiogenic inhibitors such as thalidomide or pomalidomide may be useful in improving anemia and reducing an enlarged spleen.

Nursing Management

Splenomegaly can be profound in patients with myelofibrosis, with enlargement of the spleen that may extend to the pelvic rim. This condition is extremely uncomfortable and can severely limit nutritional intake. Analgesic agents are usually ineffective. Splenomegaly, coupled with the hypermetabolic state that ensues with having an active neoplasm, results in significant weight loss, muscle wasting, and weakness. Patients benefit from small, frequent meals of foods that are high in calories and protein. Fatigue has been reported in up to 94% of patients with primary myelofibrosis (Geyer & Mesa, 2014).

The nurse should educate patients about appropriate energy conservation methods. Table 30-3 identifies useful strategies at managing fatigue.

The patient needs to be educated about signs and symptoms of infection, bleeding, and thrombosis, as well as appropriate interventions if these occur. Ensuring that the patient takes steps to decrease cardiovascular risk factors associated with developing thrombosis (e.g., obesity, smoking, and poorly controlled hypertension, diabetes, or hyperlipidemia) is also important.

LYMPHOMA

The lymphomas are neoplasms of cells of lymphoid origin. These tumors usually start in lymph nodes but can involve lymphoid tissue in the spleen, GI tract (e.g., the wall of the stomach), liver, or bone marrow (see Chapter 31, Fig. 31-1). They are often classified according to the degree of cell differentiation and the origin of the predominant malignant cell. Lymphomas are broadly classified into two categories: Hodgkin lymphoma and NHL.

Hodgkin Lymphoma

Hodgkin lymphoma is a relatively rare malignancy that has a high cure rate. It is somewhat more common in males than in females and has two peaks of incidence: one from ages 15 to 34 and the other after 60 years of age (Leukemia & Lymphoma Society, 2018c). The cause of Hodgkin lymphoma is unknown. However, several risk factors have been identified, which include age, a history of viral infections (particularly the Epstein–Barr virus, human immune deficiency virus [HIV], or human herpesvirus 8 [HHV8]), having a family history, and being exposed to cytotoxic agents. Additionally, Hodgkin lymphoma is seen more commonly in patients receiving long-term immunosuppressive therapy (e.g., organ transplant recipients) and in veterans who were exposed to the herbicide Agent Orange (see Veterans Considerations section in CLL) (Leukemia & Lymphoma Society, 2018c). The 5-year survival rate for Hodgkin lymphoma is about 92% to 94% for localized/regional disease (stage I or II) and 78% for those with distant disease (stage IV) (ACS, 2019a).

Pathophysiology

Unlike other lymphomas, Hodgkin lymphoma is unicentric in origin, meaning that it initiates in a single node. The disease spreads by contiguous extension along the lymphatic system. The malignant cell of Hodgkin lymphoma is the Reed–Sternberg cell, a gigantic tumor cell that is morphologically unique and thought to be of immature lymphoid origin. These cells arise from the B lymphocyte. They may have more than one nucleus and often have an owl-like appearance (see Fig. 30-7). The presence of Reed–Sternberg cells is the pathologic hallmark and essential diagnostic criterion.

The World Health Organization (WHO) has classified Hodgkin lymphoma into five subtypes based on pathologic analyses that reflect the natural history of the disease and suggest the prognosis (NCCN, 2019g). Four of these subtypes of Hodgkin lymphoma are recognized as being consistent with classical disease (Leukemia & Lymphoma Society, 2018c; Spinner, Varma, & Advani, 2018):

- *Nodular sclerosis*: This is the most common form of Hodgkin lymphoma, accounting for about 70% of all cases. It is seen most often in the young; among these patients, the lymph node contains elements of fibrous (sclerotic) tissue; approximately 40% of patients have B

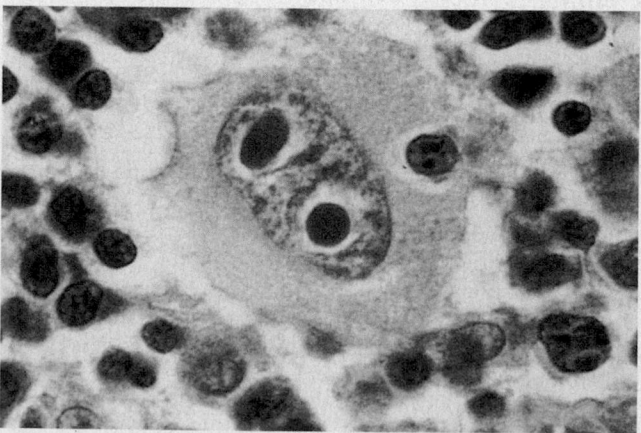

Figure 30-7 • Reed–Sternberg cell. Reed–Sternberg cells are large, abnormal lymphocytes that may contain more than one nucleus. These cells are found in Hodgkin lymphoma. Adapted with permission from Rubin, R., Strayer, D. S., & Rubin, E. (2011). *Rubin's pathology* (6th ed.). Philadelphia, PA: Lippincott Williams & Wilkins.

symptoms (see Chart 30-1). This type of Hodgkin lymphoma is highly curable.
- *Mixed cellularity*: This is the second most common form of Hodgkin lymphoma, accounting for 20% to 25% of all cases. This subtype is more common in older adults and in males; it is frequently seen in patients with HIV infection, and B symptoms are frequently reported.
- *Lymphocyte-depleted*: This form of Hodgkin lymphoma is rare; it is characterized by involved lymph node(s) with few normal lymphocytes but numerous Reed–Sternberg cells. B symptoms are commonly reported.
- *Lymphocyte-rich*: This type of Hodgkin lymphoma is also an uncommon form of the disease; the lymph node(s) has numerous normal lymphocytes and Reed–Sternberg cells and B symptoms are rare.
- *Nodular lymphocytes predominant Hodgkin lymphoma* (NLPHL): This is the lone type of Hodgkin lymphoma that is not considered of the classical type. In NLPHL there are few Reed–Sternberg cells; rather, there is a predominance of lymphocyte cells called "popcorn" cells. Furthermore, there is minimal involvement of the lymph nodes as compared to the subtypes that fall under the four classical Hodgkin types. NLPHL is seen more often in males than females and the age at diagnosis is more often between 30 and 50 years. Patients tend to present with peripheral adenopathy and with early-stage disease. NLPHL is slow growing and highly curable, but some patients can relapse while others can transform to an aggressive NHL (see later discussion).

Clinical Manifestations

Hodgkin lymphoma usually begins as an enlargement of one or more lymph nodes on one side of the neck. The individual nodes are painless and firm but not hard. The most common sites for lymphadenopathy are the cervical nodes. However, other nodes that can be affected include the supraclavicular and mediastinal nodes; involvement of the iliac or inguinal nodes or spleen is much less common (Leukemia & Lymphoma Society, 2018c). A mediastinal mass may be seen on chest x-ray; occasionally, the mass is large enough to compress the trachea and cause dyspnea. B symptoms, if present, are indicative of more advanced disease (see Chart 30-1). These symptoms are found in about 40% of patients with Hodgkin lymphoma and are used in determining stage and prognosis (NCCN, 2019g).

All organs are vulnerable to invasion by tumor cells. Clinical manifestations result from compression of organs by the tumor, such as cough and pulmonary effusion (from pulmonary infiltrates), jaundice (from hepatic involvement or bile duct obstruction), abdominal pain (from splenomegaly or retroperitoneal adenopathy), or bone pain (from skeletal involvement). A mild anemia is the most common hematologic finding. The leukocyte count may be elevated or decreased. The platelet count is typically normal, unless the tumor has invaded the bone marrow, suppressing hematopoiesis. Laboratory tests that may be assessed to detect disease activity include the serum copper level, which may be elevated, and the **erythrocyte sedimentation rate** (ESR). The ESR measures the rate of settling of RBCs; elevation is indicative of inflammation; it is also called the *sed rate*.

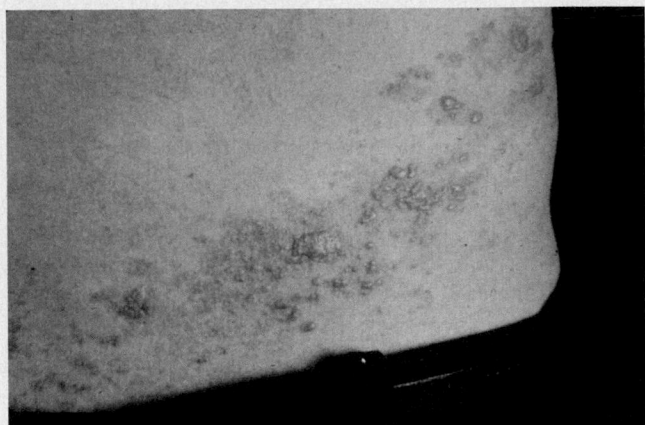

Figure 30-8 • Herpes zoster is a common complication in patients with lymphoproliferative disease, such as Hodgkin lymphoma here. Zoster infections are also common in patients on chronic steroid use for hematologic conditions and some chemotherapy regimens. Reprinted with permission from Tkachuk, D. C., & Hirschman, J. V. (2007). *Wintrobe's atlas of clinical hematology* (Fig. 5.152, p. 207). Philadelphia, PA: Lippincott Williams & Wilkins.

Other symptoms seen in patients with Hodgkin lymphoma are pruritus, which is common and can be extremely distressing, fatigue, decreased appetite, abdominal pain, splenomegaly, and although rare, occasional pain in affected lymph node after drinking alcohol (Leukemia & Lymphoma Society, 2018c). Patients may also have impaired cellular immunity, as evidenced by an absent or decreased reaction to skin sensitivity tests (i.e., Candida, mumps) and increased susceptibility to infections, particularly herpes zoster (see Fig. 30-8).

Assessment and Diagnostic Findings

Because many manifestations are similar to those occurring with infection, diagnostic studies are performed to rule out an infectious origin of the disease. The diagnosis is made by means of an excisional lymph node biopsy and the presence of Reed–Sternberg cells. Once the diagnosis is confirmed and the histologic type is established, it is necessary to assess the stage of the disease.

During the health history, the patient is assessed for any B symptoms (see Chart 30-1). Physical examination requires a careful, systematic evaluation of all palpable lymph node chains (see Chapter 28, Fig. 28-4), as well as the size of the spleen and liver. A chest x-ray and a computed tomography (CT) scan of the chest, abdomen, and pelvis are crucial to identify the extent of lymphadenopathy within these regions. A positron emission tomography (PET) scan is the most sensitive imaging test and is recommended for initial staging to help determine the extent of disease as well as later for evaluation of response to treatment (NCCN, 2019g). Laboratory tests include CBC with differential; serum electrolytes, blood urea nitrogen (BUN) and creatinine; ESR; liver and renal function studies; immunohistochemistry and cytogenetic evaluation; HIV testing; and hepatitis B and C testing. A multiple-gated acquisition (MUGA) scan and/or ECG should be performed prior to the start of therapy if the patient is to receive an anthracycline-based treatment regimen, as these chemotherapeutic agents are associated with adverse cardiovascular effects. Bone marrow biopsies are not routinely performed unless cytopenias are present and the PET scan is negative (NCCN, 2019g).

Medical Management

The goal in the treatment of Hodgkin lymphoma is cure, as the overall cure rate is about 90% (ACS, 2019a). Treatment is determined primarily by stage of disease, not histologic type, utilizing the Ann Arbor staging system (see Fig. 30-9).

Treatment guidelines for classical Hodgkin lymphoma (NCCN, 2019g) divide patients into groups. Patients with early disease (stage I-II) may receive one of the following combination chemotherapy regimens: ABVD (doxorubicin [trade name **A**driamycin], **b**leomycin, **v**inblastine, and **d**acarbazine) or Stanford V (doxorubicin, vinblastine, mechlorethamine, etoposide, vincristine, bleomycin, and prednisone)

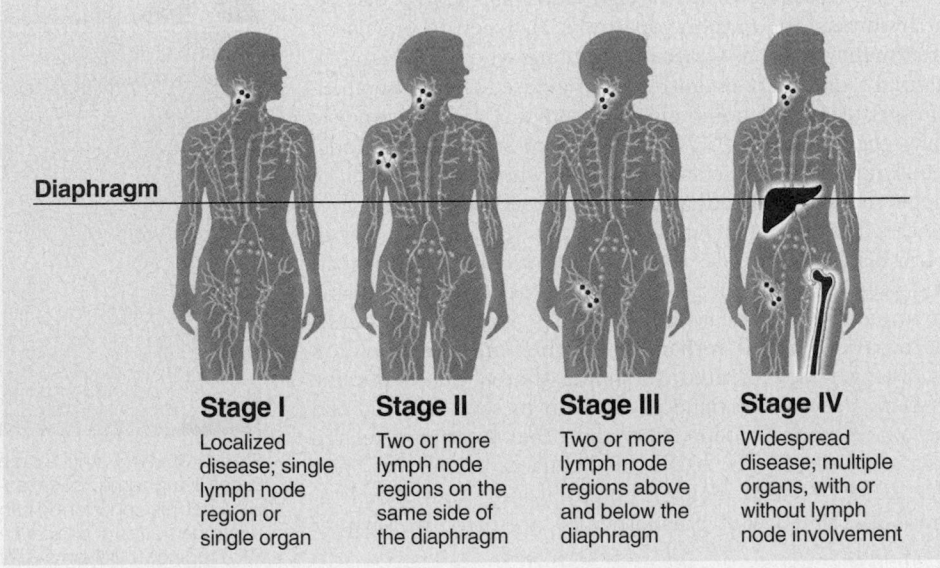

Figure 30-9 • Stages of Hodgkin lymphoma based upon the Ann Arbor staging system. Each category is subdivided and assigned to one of the following categories: Category A indicates no symptoms are present. Category B indicates the presence of B symptoms (see Chart 30-1). Category E indicates involvement of organs or tissues beyond the lymphatic system. Category S indicates involvement of the spleen. Image used with permission of The Leukemia & Lymphoma Society (Hodgkin Lymphoma, 2020).

Diaphragm

Stage I
Localized disease; single lymph node region or single organ

Stage II
Two or more lymph node regions on the same side of the diaphragm

Stage III
Two or more lymph node regions above and below the diaphragm

Stage IV
Widespread disease; multiple organs, with or without lymph node involvement

(see Chapter 12, Table 12-7, for further discussion of specific categories of chemotherapeutic/antineoplastic agents). Radiation therapy may or may not be included as part of the treatment regimen.

The standard treatment for patients with advanced disease (stages III to IV) and those with B symptoms is also ABVD chemotherapy, although these patients typically receive additional cycles of chemotherapy treatment. Other combinations of chemotherapy may be used; however, these options have more toxic effects.

When a patient has a suspected relapse of disease, a biopsy and a PET scan are performed to confirm the diagnosis and stage of disease. Treatment options for patients with refractory or relapsed disease include immunotherapeutic agents, such as a monoclonal antibody (MoAb) (e.g., everolimus, brentuximab), or a checkpoint inhibitor (e.g., nivolumab, pembrolizumab) (see discussion of MoAbs and checkpoint inhibitors in Chapter 12) (Leukemia & Lymphoma Society, 2018c; NCCN, 2019g).

Treatment for patients with NLPHL in the early stage of disease may include radiation therapy only. In a few instances (patients who are stage IA), observation rather than any therapy may be an option (Spinner et al., 2018). Patients with stage IB to IIB disease may receive ABVD, CHOP (cyclophosphamide, doxorubicin [also less commonly called hydroxydaunorubicin], vincristine [trade name of Oncovin], and prednisone), or CVP (cyclophosphamide, vincristine, and prednisone) regimens in combination with rituximab. Those with advanced stage disease are treated with these same regimens but with radiation therapy added.

Patients typically feel better following therapy. Late effects of treatment, which may occur months to years following treatment, include development of a secondary malignancy, or cardiovascular disease, hypothyroidism, and infertility (Leukemia & Lymphoma Society, 2018c; NCCN, 2019g). Secondary malignancies (most common are lung and breast) often develop more than 10 years following completion of therapy. This is especially true in females who received radiation therapy to the chest or axillary areas (NCCN, 2019g).

Cardiovascular disease (e.g., coronary artery disease, arrhythmias, and cardiomyopathy) is also seen 10 years post-treatment and tends to occur in patients who received mediastinal radiation or an anthracycline-based chemotherapeutic agent (e.g., daunorubicin, doxorubicin). Hypothyroidism may occur in about 50% of long-term survivors of Hodgkin lymphoma, particularly in those who received neck or upper mediastinal radiation (NCCN, 2019g). The use of some chemotherapy combinations can lead to infertility in both males and females. For instance, females of childbearing years may experience premature menopause following treatment with alkylating agents (e.g., cyclophosphamide, dacarbazine, mechlorethamine). Other organ dysfunction is also well documented, including that of the endocrine system. Persistent fatigue is common in survivors and can be exacerbated by depression and other treatment-related comorbidities (ACS, 2019a; Leukemia & Lymphoma Society, 2018c; NCCN, 2019g). Potential long-term complications associated with chemotherapy are listed in Chapter 12, Chart 12-4.

Nursing Management

The potential development of a second malignancy should be addressed with the patient when initial treatment decisions are made. However, patients need to be informed that Hodgkin lymphoma is often curable. The nurse should encourage patients to reduce factors that increase the risk of developing second cancers, such as use of tobacco and alcohol and exposure to environmental carcinogens and excessive sunlight. Screening for late effects of treatment, such as chemotherapy (see Chapter 12, Chart 12-4), is necessary. In addition, the nurse should provide education about relevant self-care strategies and disease management. See also the Nursing Management Section for Non-Hodgkin Lymphoma.

Non-Hodgkin Lymphomas

The NHLs are a heterogeneous group of cancers that originate from the neoplastic growth of lymphoid tissue. Similar to CLL, the neoplastic cells are thought to arise from a single clone of lymphocytes; however, in NHL, the cells may vary morphologically. In contrast to Hodgkin lymphoma, the lymphoid tissues involved are largely infiltrated with malignant cells. The spread of these malignant lymphoid cells occurs unpredictably; true localized disease is uncommon. Lymph nodes from multiple sites may be infiltrated, as may sites outside the lymphoid system (i.e., extranodal tissue; see Fig. 30-10).

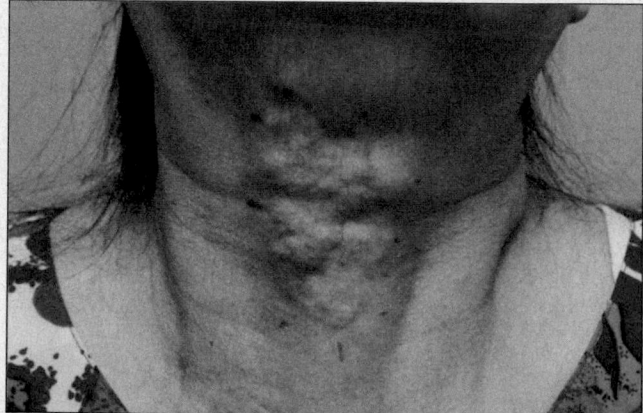
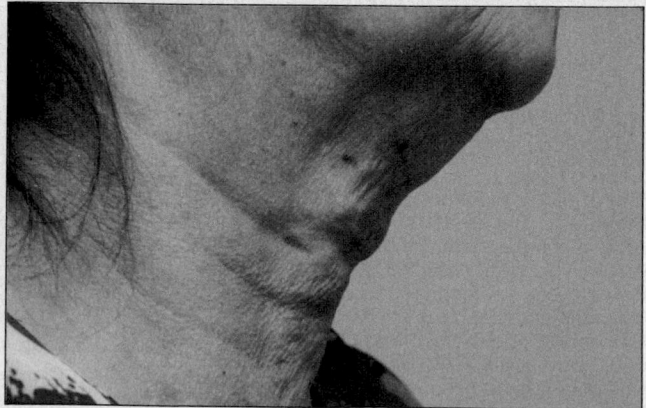

Figure 30-10 • Any extranodal location can be a site for diffuse B-cell lymphoma, such as the thyroid, as shown here. Reprinted with permission from Tkachuk, D. C., & Hirschman, J. V. (2007). *Wintrobe's atlas of clinical hematology* (Fig. 5.87, p. 183). Philadelphia, PA: Lippincott Williams & Wilkins.

TABLE 30-4	Select Types of Lymphomas
Indolent	**Aggressive**
Cutaneous T cell	Anaplastic large cell
Follicular	AIDS associated
Gastric MALT	Burkitt
Lymphoplasmacytic: Waldenstrom macroglobulinemia	Diffuse large B cell
Marginal zone B cell	Mantle cell
Small-cell lymphocytic	Peripheral T cell

AIDS, acquired immune deficiency syndrome; MALT, mucosa-associated lymphoid tissue.
Adapted from Leukemia & Lymphoma Society. (2016). NHL subtypes. Retrieved on 5/14/2020 at: www.lls.org/lymphoma/non-hodgkin-lymphoma/diagnosis/nhl-subtypes

Approximately 85% of NHLs involve malignant B-cell lymphocytes, with the remaining 15% involving T-cell lymphocytes or natural killer cells (NCCN, 2019h). NHL is the seventh most common type of cancer diagnosed in the United States, accounting for about 4% to 5% of all new cancer cases each year. It occurs more commonly in males (NCCN, 2019h). The incidence increases with each decade of life; the median age at diagnosis is 66 years (Leukemia & Lymphoma Society, 2018d). The natural course of the disease is variable and dependent upon the type of lymphoma. NHLs can be categorized as **indolent** (i.e., a slow-growing cancer that often remains localized or causes few symptoms) or aggressive (i.e., a fast-growing cancer that spreads rapidly and causes significant morbidity) (see Table 30-4). For example, the 5-year survival rate for diffuse large B-cell lymphoma is 72%; for follicular lymphoma it is about 90% (96% localized disease and 85% for distant disease) (ACS, 2019b).

Although no common etiologic factor has been identified, the incidence of NHL is increased in patients who have immune deficiencies or autoimmune disorders; had prior treatment for cancer; been an organ transplant recipient; had a history of viral infections (e.g., Epstein–Barr virus, HIV, HHV8); and been exposed to herbicides, pesticides, solvents, dyes, and defoliating agents, such as Agent Orange (see Veterans Considerations section in CLL) (ACS, 2019b).

Clinical Manifestations

Symptoms of NHL are highly variable, reflecting the diverse nature of the disease. Similar to Hodgkin lymphoma, NHL may start as a painless swelling in one or more lymph nodes in the neck, axillary region, or groin. If the lymphoma is indolent in nature, symptoms may be absent or very minor. Indolent disease accounts for about 40% of all NHL cases (Leukemia & Lymphoma Society, 2018d). However, the majority of patients are not diagnosed until the disease has progressed to a later stage, when they have become symptomatic. About one third of patients with NHL have B symptoms (see Chart 30-1) at the time of diagnosis (Leukemia & Lymphoma Society, 2018d).

Other symptoms depend upon enlarged lymph node site and size, which can compress organs, compromising function. For example, a mass in the mediastinum can cause cough, shortness of breath, and chest pain that may lead to cardiovascular or respiratory distress. An abdominal mass may compromise the bowel or ureters, leading to acute kidney injury or bowel obstruction. Splenomegaly can cause abdominal pain, nausea, early satiety, and weight loss.

Assessment and Diagnostic Findings

Similar to Hodgkin lymphoma, an incisional or excisional lymph node biopsy is required for immunophenotyping and cytogenetic analysis testing (NCCN, 2019h). The specific histopathologic type of the disease is used to differentiate the subtype of NHL; it also has important prognostic implications and is used to determine appropriate treatment (Leukemia & Lymphoma Society, 2018d). Flow cytometry is commonly performed to determine the specific antigen on the malignant cell. Another test that may be performed is fluorescence in situ hybridization (FISH), which analyzes the DNA and RNA of the biopsy or blood sample for chromosomal abnormalities.

Laboratory studies mirror those done for a patient with Hodgkin lymphoma (see that previous discussion). In addition, there may be testing for viruses (e.g., Epstein–Barr, HHV8, hepatitis B); polymerase chain reaction (PCR); CT scans of the chest, abdomen, and pelvis; PET scan; MUGA or ECG (if patient is to receive anthracycline-based regimen); and bone marrow biopsy and aspirate (if marrow involvement is suspected).

Although the stage of disease is important, often it is not an accurate predictor of prognosis. Two prognostic classification systems are used: the International Prognostic Index (IPI) and, for follicular lymphomas, the Follicular Lymphoma International Prognostic Index (FLIPI). Age, performance status, lactate dehydrogenase levels, stage of disease, and extranodal involvement are scored to determine risk of failure or death from disease (ACS, 2020b).

Medical Management

The goal of treatment for NHL is to obtain remission of disease by killing as many of the malignant cells as possible; in contrast, the goal is cure for Hodgkin lymphoma. Treatment for NHL is based upon the specific subtype of lymphoma and the stage of disease. Other factors that impact treatment decisions include the patient's age, functional status, laboratory values (especially renal, hepatic, and cardiac), comorbid conditions, and presence of extranodal involvement (i.e., presence of cancer cells outside of the lymph nodes) (Leukemia & Lymphoma Society, 2016). If the disease is indolent and localized, the treatment of choice may be radiation therapy alone. "Watchful waiting" may also be a choice for patients with an indolent form of NHL, such as stage I follicular lymphoma, who have no or few symptoms at time of diagnosis.

For aggressive subtypes of NHL, combination chemotherapy is typically indicated. One of the most common combinations is CHOP. A MoAb (e.g., rituximab, obinutuzumab) may be given along with the chemotherapy (NCCN, 2019h). Radiation therapy may or may not be added to the treatment regimen. In some cases, a MoAb may be conjugated with a radioactive isotope and used for treatment (e.g., ibritumomab tiuxetan). CNS involvement is common with some aggressive forms of NHL; in this situation, cranial radiation or intrathecal chemotherapy is used in addition to systemic chemotherapy.

When NHL has relapsed or is refractory to standard treatments, other single agent or combination chemotherapy regimens may be used. For instance, the ICE regimen (i.e., *i*fosfamide, *c*arboplatin, and *e*toposide) may be implemented; or agents such as bendamustine, brentuximab vedotin, romidepsin, or axicabtagene may be tried (NCCN, 2019h). Autologous HSCT (AuHSCT) is another treatment option for relapsed or refractory NHL, particularly in patients younger than 60 years (see Chapter 12 for further discussion of AuHSCT).

A rare but potentially life-threatening complication of chemotherapy is tumor lysis syndrome. Tumor lysis syndrome occurs when the intracellular content of the malignant cell breaks down and is released into the peripheral blood and typically occurs 12 to 72 hours after initiation of therapy (NCCN, 2019h). Patients with NHL at highest risk for the development of tumor lysis syndrome are those with large bulky disease and/or deemed to have high-risk or aggressive NHL (e.g., Burkitt's or diffuse large B-cell lymphoma [DLBCL]). See Chapter 12, Table 12-13, for a discussion of manifestations of and treatment for tumor lysis syndrome.

Reactivation of hepatitis B virus may be seen in patients with NHL who become immunosuppressed following chemotherapy. For example, hepatitis B reactivation can occur in patients treated with rituximab-containing regimens, even if the patient had tested negative for hepatitis B prior to start of treatment (Leukemia & Lymphoma Society, 2018d). Preemptive treatment is recommended, including antiviral therapy (i.e., lamivudine or entecavir) and close surveillance in patients at high risk.

Another rare but potentially life-threatening complication is progressive multifocal leukoencephalopathy, which may occur in patients with NHL who are severely immunocompromised and treated with chemotherapeutic agents (Leukemia & Lymphoma Society, 2018d; NCCN, 2019h). Symptoms include confusion, motor weakness or poor motor coordination, and visual and possibly speech changes. Currently, there is no effective treatment for this complication. The fatality rate is 90% and tends to occur within 2 months after the diagnosis is confirmed (NCCN, 2019h).

Nursing Management

Lymphoma is a highly complex constellation of diseases. When caring for patients with lymphoma, it is extremely important for the nurse to know the specific disease type, stage of disease, treatment history, and current treatment plan. Most of the care for patients with Hodgkin lymphoma or NHL takes place in the outpatient setting, unless complications occur (e.g., infection, respiratory compromise due to mediastinal mass). The most commonly used treatment methods are chemotherapy (often combined with a MoAb) and radiation therapy. Chemotherapy causes systemic side effects (e.g., myelosuppression, nausea, hair loss, risk of infection), whereas radiation therapy causes specific side effects

that are limited to the area being irradiated. For example, patients receiving abdominal radiation therapy may experience nausea and diarrhea but not hair loss. Regardless of the type of treatment, all patients may experience fatigue (see Chapter 12, Chart 12-6, Fatigue).

The risk of infection is significant for these patients, not only from treatment-related myelosuppression but also from the defective immune response that results from the disease itself. Patients need to be educated to minimize the risks of infection, to recognize signs of possible infection, and to contact their primary provider if such signs develop (see Chapter 12, Chart 12-6, Infection).

Many lymphomas can be cured with current treatments. However, as survival rates increase, the incidence of second malignancies, particularly AML or MDS, also increases. Therefore, survivors should be screened regularly for the development of second malignancies. Survivors of both Hodgkin lymphoma and NHL may be faced with managing persistent fatigue, depression, anxiety, and cardiac and pulmonary toxicity (ACS, 2019b). Therefore, survivors should be encouraged to have regular follow-up appointments and be screened for the signs and symptoms of possible secondary malignancies. Additionally, patients should be evaluated for cardiovascular and fertility concerns with each patient visit.

The ACS (2019b) developed health behavior recommendations for cancer survivors, which include avoiding or stopping smoking, maintaining a normal body weight, practicing good nutrition habits (i.e., consuming fruits and vegetables), and engaging in a minimum of 150 minutes of exercise per week. While many survivors do not adhere to these recommendations, those patients who do report higher health-related quality of life (ACS, 2019b).

MULTIPLE MYELOMA

Multiple myeloma is a malignant disease of the most mature form of B lymphocyte—the plasma cell. Plasma cells secrete immunoglobulins, which are proteins necessary for antibody production to fight infection. This disease accounts for approximately 1.8% of all cancers and about 17% of the hematologic malignancies in the United States (NCCN, 2019i). The etiology of multiple myeloma is not known, but risk factors are identified (see Chart 30-3). The incidence of multiple myeloma increases with age; the median age at diagnosis is approximately 70 years (NCCN, 2019i; Rajkumar, 2018). This disease, if left untreated, can lead to bone destruction and bone marrow failure. Due to the increased number of newer agents to fight multiple myeloma, survival of this disease has significantly improved in the last 5 years.

Pathophysiology

In multiple myeloma, the malignant plasma cells produce a specific immunoglobulin that is nonfunctional. Functional types of immunoglobulins are still produced by nonmalignant plasma cells, but in lower-than-normal quantities. The specific immunoglobulin secreted by the malignant plasma cells is referred to as the monoclonal protein, or M protein. Malignant plasma cells also secrete certain substances to stimulate angiogenesis to enhance the growth of these clusters of plasma

- Age: rarely occurs in those less than 35 years of age; risks increase with increasing age
- African Americans have twice the risk of Whites
- Exposure to radiation, petroleum products, benzenes, and Agent Orange
- Family history, particularly among first-degree relatives (e.g., siblings, parents)
- Men have slightly higher risks than women
- Overweight or obesity
- Plasma cell disease history:
  - Monoclonal gammopathy of undetermined significance (MGUS)
  - Plasmacytoma[a]

[a]Note: in rare instances, may precede multiple myeloma.
Adapted from American Cancer Society (ACS). (2018). Risk factors for multiple myeloma. Retrieved on 5/15/2020 at: www.cancer.org/cancer/multiple-myeloma/causes-risks-prevention/risk-factors.html; National Comprehensive Cancer Network (NCCN). (2019i). Clinical practice guidelines in oncology: Multiple myeloma. Version 2.2019. Retrieved on 7/10/2019 at: www.nccn.org/professional/physician_gls/pdf/myeloma.pdf; Rajkumar, S. (2018). Multiple myeloma: 2018 update on diagnosis, risk-stratification, and management. *American Journal of Hematology, 93*, 1091–1110.

cells. Occasionally, the malignant plasma cells infiltrate other tissue, in which case they are referred to as plasmacytomas. Plasmacytomas can occur in the sinuses, spinal cord, and soft tissues.

Multiple myeloma may evolve from a premalignant stage, known as monoclonal gammopathy of undetermined significance (MGUS) (NCCN, 2019i). Although patients with MGUS have the M protein in their blood, they generally do not have any signs and symptoms that are seen in multiple myeloma. Patients with MGUS are monitored for signs and symptoms indicative of disease progression to multiple myeloma. The rate of progression from MGUS to multiple myeloma is 0.5% to 1% per year (Rajkumar, 2018).

Clinical Manifestations

Clinical manifestations of multiple myeloma result not only from the malignant cells themselves, but also from the abnormal protein they produce. The classic clinical manifestations of multiple myeloma are referred to as the CRAB features, because they refer to the following:

- hyperCalcemia
- Renal dysfunction
- Anemia
- Bone destruction

Bone-related manifestations may be seen in up to 85% of patients with multiple myeloma (NCCN, 2019i). Bone pain (usually in the back or ribs) is considered to be a classic presenting symptom. Bone pain associated with multiple myeloma increases with movement and decreases with rest; patients may report that they have less pain on awakening but more during the day. In multiple myeloma, a substance secreted by the malignant plasma cells, osteoclast activating factor, and other substances, such as interleukin-6 (IL-6) stimulate osteoclasts, which break down bone matrix. In some cases, the bone breakdown or lysis can be severe

enough to cause vertebral collapse and fractures, including spinal fractures, which can impinge on the spinal cord and result in spinal cord compression (see Fig. 30-11). When vertebral collapse occurs, the patient's height is reduced and kyphosis (an excessive curvature of the spine) is common.

If the bone lysis is extensive, bone lesions result and excessive ionized calcium is lost from the bone and enters the serum; hypercalcemia may therefore develop and may be manifested by excessive thirst, dehydration, constipation, altered mental status, confusion, and perhaps coma.

> **Quality and Safety Nursing Alert**
>
> *Any older adult whose chief complaint is back pain and who has an elevated total protein level should be evaluated for possible multiple myeloma.*

Renal dysfunction occurs in 33% of patients at the time of diagnosis, while 50% will experience renal dysfunction at some point during the course of the disease (Chim, Kumar, Orlowski, et al., 2018; NCCN, 2019i). The etiology of renal dysfunction is multicausal and related to: myeloma kidney as the result of Bence–Jones proteins (i.e., myeloma infiltration of the kidneys) causing obstruction in the renal tubules; hypercalcemia as the result of bone matrix lysis; amyloid deposits which may lead to renal insufficiency and/or hydronephrosis; and hyperviscosity leading to renal tubule obstruction. Other causes of renal dysfunction in patients with multiple myeloma are infections, use of NSAIDs, and nephrotoxic agents (e.g., chemotherapy) to treat multiple myeloma (Faiman, Doss, Colson, et al., 2017).

As more malignant plasma cells are produced, the marrow has less space for erythrocyte production, and anemia may develop. If renal dysfunction is also present, anemia may also be caused by a diminished production of erythropoietin by the kidney. In the late stage of the disease, a reduced number of leukocytes and platelets may also be seen because the bone marrow is infiltrated by malignant plasma cells.

Assessment and Diagnostic Findings

All patients suspected of having multiple myeloma should have a CBC with differential, BUN, serum creatinine, creatinine clearance, serum electrolytes (especially calcium and albumin), LDH, and beta-2 microglobulin analyzed. Elevated BUN and creatinine may be indicative of renal dysfunction. The total protein level is frequently elevated because of the production of M protein. LDH and beta-2 microglobulin measure degree of tumor burden. In addition to these, a peripheral smear of the blood may reveal an abnormal stacking of RBCs (known as Rouleaux formation) due to elevated serum proteins (NCCN, 2019i). Serum protein electrophoresis or free light chain assay should be performed to detect the presence of M protein (see Fig. 30-12). This protein is elevated in patients with multiple myeloma and serves as a useful marker to monitor the extent of the disease and to gauge the patient's eventual response to therapy. Additionally, cytogenetic studies are performed to see if any of several chromosomal abnormalities typically found in patients with multiple myeloma are present. Radiographic evaluation (CT scan, MRI, and PET scan) should be performed to determine the presence of lytic bone lesions. Bone marrow aspiration

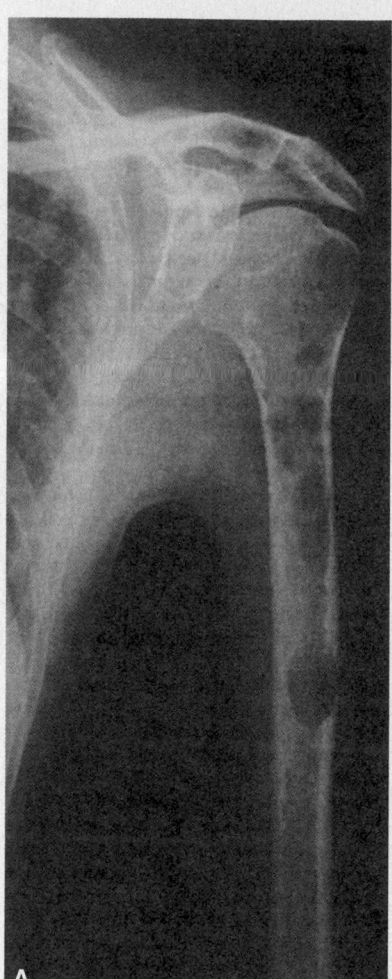

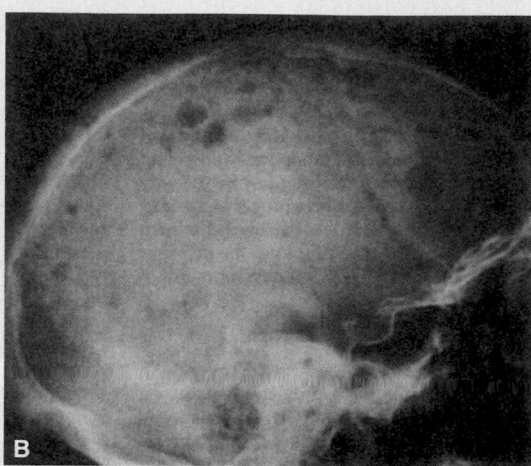

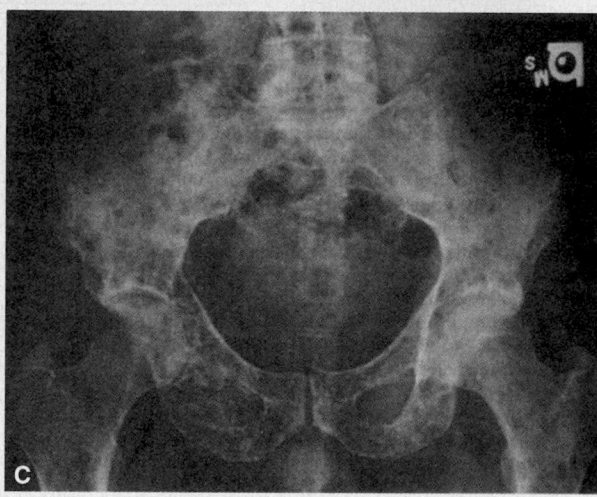

Figure 30-11 • Lytic lesions seen in the humerus and skull in patients with multiple myeloma. These lesions typically occur in the long bones, vertebrae, and skull. Long bones are susceptible to fracture when the lesion occurs near the surface of the bone; vertebrae are susceptible to collapse, resulting in loss of height and potential for spinal cord compression. Reprinted with permission from *Wintrobe's clinical hematology* (10th ed., p. 2640). Philadelphia, PA: Lippincott Williams & Wilkins.

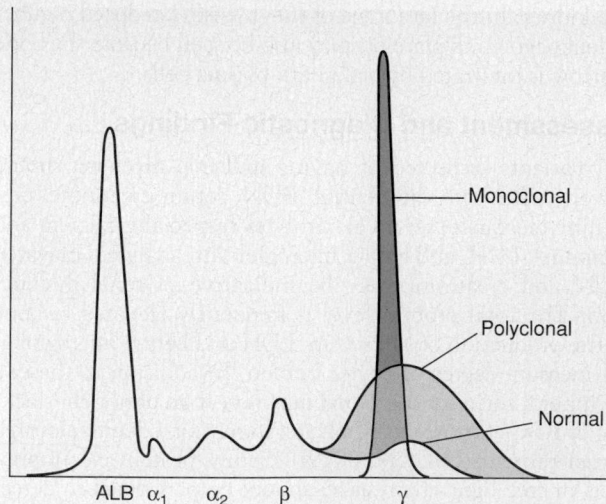

Figure 30-12 • Abnormal serum protein electrophoresis patterns contrasted with a normal pattern. Polyclonal peaks are characterized by a broad-based increase in immunoglobulin (Ig) by myriad reactive plasma cells and indicate a benign reactive process. In contrast, a narrow spike indicates homogeneity of the Ig secreted by a single clone of plasma cells. M spikes are seen in monoclonal gammopathies of undetermined significance or in plasma malignancies (myeloma, Waldenstrom macroglobulinemia). Reprinted with permission from Turgeon, M. (2012). *Clinical hematology theory & procedures* (5th ed., Fig. 20.7, p. 347). Philadelphia, PA: Lippincott Williams & Wilkins.

and biopsy are conducted to evaluate bone marrow plasma cell abnormalities.

Diagnosis and staging of multiple myeloma was traditionally based on the CRAB criteria, and included:

- hypercalcemia (>11.5 mg/dL)
- renal insufficiency (creatinine >2 mg/dL or creatinine clearance of less than 40 mL/min)
- anemia (hemoglobin less than 10 g/dL or 2 g/dL less than normal)
- the presence of bony lesions.

The International Myeloma Working Group (IMWG) recently revised the metrics used to define the disease to include specific biomarkers (clonal plasma cells on bone marrow biopsy of 60% or greater, involved/uninvolved serum free light chain ratio of 100 or greater, and/or more than one focal lesion on MRI that is at least 5 mm or greater in size) in addition to any one or more of the CRAB criteria (NCCN, 2019i; Rajkumar, 2018). This revision is believed to facilitate earlier diagnosis and implementation of treatment (NCCN, 2019i).

Medical Management

There is no cure for multiple myeloma; the aims of treatment are to reduce symptoms and to prolong disease progression. Therapy has changed substantively for multiple myeloma, and has resulted in impressive increases in duration of survival. Importantly, patients not only live longer, the new treatment modalities provide the opportunity for enhanced quality of life. Management of multiple myeloma depends upon whether the patient has smoldering (asymptomatic) or active (symptomatic) disease. Smoldering multiple myeloma is similar to MGUS as patients do not report any symptoms; however, there are higher levels of M protein than seen in MGUS and malignant plasma cells are present.

For most patients with smoldering multiple myeloma, observation with close surveillance for the possibility of transforming to symptomatic disease every 3 to 6 months is the standard of care (NCCN, 2019i; Rajkumar, 2018). Patients who present with symptomatic disease are evaluated for eligibility for an autologous HSCT (AuHSCT), based on age, presence of comorbidities, and risk stratification (Rajkumar, 2018).

Primary treatment for patients who are eligible for AuHSCT includes several cycles of a combination of different pharmacologic agents before stem cells are procured. These drugs all target the disease via different mechanisms than do conventional chemotherapeutic agents. Combinations of two or three drugs are commonly used with the goal of reducing the tumor burden as much as possible. These frequently include either one of the following two regimens (Rajkumar, 2018):

- Proteasome inhibitor–based bortezomib regimen, which commonly includes an immunomodulatory drug (e.g., lenalidomide, pomalidomide, or thalidomide) and the corticosteroid dexamethasone.
- MoAb-based daratumumab regimen, which commonly includes either an immunomodulatory drug (e.g., lenalidomide, pomalidomide, or thalidomide) or a proteasome inhibitor (e.g., bortezomib, carfilzomib, or ixazomib) and the corticosteroid dexamethasone.

Other agents that may be part of these regimens include doxorubicin, cyclophosphamide, cisplatin, or etoposide (see Table 30-5).

AuHSCT is considered to be the standard of care for patients with multiple myeloma following primary therapy (NCCN, 2019i), as it has demonstrated improved response rates, improved quality of life, and increased overall survival. AuHSCT may also be indicated in patients with relapsed and refractory multiple myeloma. Single AuHSCT and tandem AuHSCT (with two AuHSCT within a 6-month period) are possible options. Another option could be an allogeneic HSCT; however, this is considered an inferior option to AuHSCT as it is associated with increased morbidity and mortality (Rajkumar, 2018).

Lenalidomide is recommended as maintenance therapy for patients following an AuHSCT and after the initial 8 to 12 cycles of primary therapy for patients who have not received an HSCT. Bortezomib may be used as an alternative maintenance treatment in patients who are intermediate to high risk.

Patients who are not candidates for AuHSCT might be prescribed the three-drug, bortezomib-based regimen, as this regimen is associated with a better response rate. For older adults or frail patients, two-drug regimens may be given (e.g., lenalidomide and dexamethasone) (Rajkumar, 2018). The regimen for patients with renal dysfunction includes bortezomib, cyclophosphamide, and dexamethasone (NCCN, 2019i).

In addition to these agents, all patients with multiple myeloma should be prescribed a bisphosphonate, such as pamidronate or zoledronic acid (NCCN, 2019i). Bisphosphonates have been shown to strengthen bone by diminishing survival of osteoclasts, thus controlling bone pain and potentially preventing bone fractures. These agents are also effective in managing and preventing hypercalcemia by preventing excessive bone resorption. Some evidence suggests that bisphosphonates may activate an antimyeloma immune response, inducing myeloma cell death, acting synergistically with antineoplastic drugs, and enhancing immune surveillance (Faiman et al., 2017) (see Chapter 36, Table 36-1, for further discussion of bisphosphonates).

Complications

Infection is a potential complication of multiple myeloma and a frequent cause of morbidity and mortality. In contrast to other hematologic malignancies, the incidence of infection does not appear to be related to the extent of neutropenia in patients with multiple myeloma. Rather, the lack of adequate levels of normal immunoglobulins, as well as other alterations of the immune system, renders the patient at increased risk for developing infection, particularly due to *Streptococcus pneumoniae* or *H. influenzae*. Therapy for the disease also predisposes the patient for acquiring infections, particularly when corticosteroids are used in treating the disease; herpes zoster and *Pneumocystis* are common causative organisms in this context (NCCN, 2019i). Infection prophylaxis with antiviral agents and antibiotics (e.g., trimethoprim–sulfamethoxazole) is important to decrease infection risk.

When plasma cells secrete excessive amounts of immunoglobulin, the serum viscosity can increase. Hyperviscosity may be manifested by bleeding from the nose or mouth, headache, visual changes such as blurred vision or diplopia, paresthesias, or heart failure. The incidence of hyperviscosity is rare but does have the potential to be lethal. It is considered to be an oncologic emergency and as such, requires immediate intervention with aggressive hydration and plasmapheresis or therapeutic phlebotomy to reduce immunoglobulin and protein levels and to decrease symptoms (see Chapter 28, Table 28-3, for further discussion of plasmapheresis).

Neurologic complications can also occur. Spinal cord compression is the most common (see Chapter 12, Table 12-13, for discussion of manifestations and management of spinal cord compression), and other neurologic symptoms may be present, particularly peripheral neuropathy. Peripheral neuropathy may occur in as many as 75% of patients with multiple myeloma either due to infiltration of malignant plasma cells into the peripheral nerves or due to neurotoxic agents prescribed to treat the disease (e.g., bortezomib and thalidomide) (Faiman et al., 2017). Symptoms of peripheral neuropathy can range from mild discomfort to severe impairment and even paralysis and may lead to dose reduction or discontinuation of therapy.

VTE may occur in patients with myeloma; the incidence is thought to be as high as 10% (NCCN, 2019i). The risk increases substantially when high doses of corticosteroids and immumodulatory drugs (e.g., thalidomide, lenalidomide, or

TABLE 30-5 Select Pharmacologic Agents for Multiple Myeloma[a]

Medication	Adverse Effects	Nursing Considerations
CHEMOTHERAPY		
Alkylating Agents Mechanism of Action: Bond with DNA, RNA, and protein molecules leading to impaired DNA replication, RNA transcription, and cell functioning; all resulting in cell death; cell cycle nonspecific		
Cisplatin Cyclophosphamide	Alopecia Bone marrow suppression (e.g., anemia, leukopenia, thrombocytopenia) Electrolyte disturbances Hemorrhagic cystitis[b] Hypersensitivity reaction Nausea and vomiting Peripheral neuropathy Renal toxicity[c] Second cancers SIADH Stomatitis	Monitor blood counts, blood chemistries and creatinine Monitor hydration status; encourage 2–3 L of fluid intake daily May premedicate patient to avoid or minimize risk for hypersensitivity reaction (e.g., dexamethasone, diphenhydramine, famotidine) and/or with antiemetics
Antitumor Antibiotic (Anthracycline-Based) Mechanism of Action: Interfere with DNA synthesis by binding DNA; prevent RNA synthesis; cell cycle nonspecific		
Doxorubicin	Alopecia Bone marrow suppression (e.g., anemia, leukopenia, thrombocytopenia) Cardiotoxicity (e.g., cardiomyopathy, arrhythmias) Diarrhea Nausea and vomiting Red urine Stomatitis	Drug is a vesicant and should be administer via central venous access. Patients should have ECG, MUGA scan to evaluate cardiac function prior to initiation of treatment. Educate patient to understand that urine will be red in color as drug is excreted.
Topoisomerase II Inhibitor Mechanism of Action: Induce breaks in the DNA strand by binding to enzyme topoisomerase, preventing cells from dividing; specific to the S phase of the cell cycle		
Etoposide	Alopecia Anorexia Bone marrow suppression (e.g., anemia, leukopenia, thrombocytopenia) Diarrhea Hypotension Hypersensitivity reaction Nausea and vomiting Stomatitis	Monitor blood counts. Monitor vital signs (especially blood pressure) prior to, during, and following administration. May premedicate patient to avoid or minimize risk for hypersensitivity reaction (e.g., dexamethasone, diphenhydramine, famotidine) and/or with antiemetics
CORTICOSTEROID Mechanism of Action: Induce apoptosis in myeloma cells and markedly decrease bone pain		
Dexamethasone	Cataract formation Dental caries Fluid retention Immunosuppression Increased appetite, weight gain Insomnia Osteoporosis Peptic ulcers Pseudodiabetes Psychosis Venous thromboembolism	Monitor blood counts Monitor blood glucose levels Monitor intake and output, assess for peripheral edema Assess daily weights Assess stools for occult blood Educate patient on methods to decrease risk for infection (e.g., flu vaccine, antibiotic prophylaxis as indicated) Educate patient to follow-up with dental and eye examinations Risk for venous thromboembolism is increased in patients concomitantly taking immunomodulators
IMMUNOMODULATORS Mechanism of Action: Display broad antimyeloma effects by inhibiting angiogenesis and by mitigating the effects of the cytokines interleukin-6 and tumor necrosis factor (both support myeloma cell growth)		
Lenalidomide Pomalidomide Thalidomide	Arthralgia[d] Bone marrow suppression (e.g., anemia, leukopenia, thrombocytopenia)[d,e] Constipation[f] Fatigue, dizziness, sedation[f] Fetal birth defects Peripheral neuropathy[f] Rash, dry skin Venous thromboembolism	Pregnancy test prior to initial therapy; repeat every 4 wk in women of childbearing age Male patients should be educated to use strict methods of contraception Patients must be educated about the teratogenic effects of therapy Excreted by the kidneys; therefore, monitor renal function, including urine output and serum creatinine and urea nitrogen Patient may be prescribed antithrombotic prophylaxis (e.g., aspirin, DOAC, LMWH, warfarin) (see Chapter 26 for further discussion of these drugs and nursing interventions) Risk for venous thromboembolism is increased in patients concomitantly taking corticosteroids Monitor blood counts in patients taking lenalidomide and pomalidomide Assess for peripheral neuropathy in patients taking thalidomide (see Table 30-6)

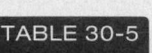

TABLE 30-5	Select Pharmacologic Agents for Multiple Myeloma[a] (continued)	
Medication	**Adverse Effects**	**Nursing Considerations**

MONOCLONAL ANTIBODIES

Mechanism of Action: Antibodies made from clonal immune cells that target specific antigens found on the surface of multiple myeloma cells; various agents target different antigenic receptors and therefore, adverse effects may differ

| Daratumumab | Back pain, arthralgia
Bone marrow suppression (e.g., anemia, leukopenia, thrombocytopenia)
Constipation or diarrhea
Fatigue
Herpes zoster reactivation
Hypersensitivity reaction: most common with first infusions; manifestations include dyspnea, bronchospasm, cough, rhinitis
Injection site reaction
Insomnia
Nausea and vomiting | May premedicate patient to avoid or minimize risk for hypersensitivity reaction (e.g., acetaminophen, diphenhydramine, methylprednisolone) and/or with antiemetics
Monitor blood counts.
Prophylactic antiviral agents may be considered in patients with history of herpes zoster.
Female patients should avoid becoming pregnant or breastfeeding while on drug, as risks to fetus are unknown |
| Elotuzumab | Anorexia
Bone marrow suppression (e.g., anemia, leukopenia, thrombocytopenia)
Bradycardia or tachycardia
Constipation or diarrhea
Fatigue
Hypersensitivity reaction: include dyspnea, bronchospasm, cough, rhinitis
Peripheral neuropathy | May premedicate patient to avoid or minimize risk for hypersensitivity reaction (e.g., acetaminophen, diphenhydramine, dexamethasone, famotidine)
Monitor blood counts
Assess for peripheral neuropathy (see Table 30-6) |

PROTEASOME INHIBITORS

Mechanism of Action: Proteasomes process and clear the excess mis/unfolded protein that accumulates within malignant plasma cells; inhibiting this process causes an excess accumulation of these proteins that results in apoptosis of malignant cells

| Bortezomib
Carfilzomib
Ixazomib | Bone marrow suppression (e.g., anemia, leukopenia, thrombocytopenia)
Cardiovascular events, such as heart failure, ischemia, arrhythmias (*more common with carfilzomib*)
Constipation or diarrhea
Fatigue
Fetal birth defects
Herpes zoster reactivation
Metabolized via the cytochrome P450 system[g]
Nausea and vomiting
Peripheral neuropathy (*more common with bortezomib*)
Renal dysfunction
Reversible posterior leukoencephalopathy syndrome (RPLS), evidenced by seizures, visual disturbances, delirium, and hypertension
Transient thrombocytopenia[h] | Monitor blood counts
Patients should have ECG, MUGA scan to evaluate cardiac function prior to initiation of treatment, particularly with carfilzomib.
Female patients should avoid becoming pregnant or breastfeeding.
Prophylactic antiviral agents may be considered in patients with history of herpes zoster
For patients prescribed bortezomib, advocate for SQ rather than IV administration, to diminish likelihood of peripheral neuropathy (see Table 30-6 for further discussion)
Monitor urine output and blood creatinine and urea nitrogen
If RPLS suspected, discontinue treatment and call primary provider
Monitor platelet counts in patients taking bortezomib; assess for signs of occult bleeding (e.g., black tarry stools, petechiae formation)
Monitor for drug-to-drug interactions in patients taking ixazomib
Ixazomib may be taken orally; administer at least 1 h prior to or 2 h post meal |

[a]Refer to Chapter 12 for additional nursing interventions to mitigate adverse effects of antineoplastic therapy.
[b]Specific to cyclophosphamide.
[c]Specific to cisplatin.
[d]Specific to lenalidomide.
[e]Specific to pomalidomide.
[f]Specific to thalidomide.
[g]Specific to ixazomib.
[h]Specific to bortezomib.
DOAC, direct oral anticoagulant; ECG, electrocardiogram; LMWH, low-molecular-weight heparin; MUGA, multiple-gated acquisition; SIADH, syndrome of inappropriate antidiuretic hormone.
Adapted from National Comprehensive Cancer Network (NCCN). (2019i). Clinical practice guidelines in oncology: Multiple myeloma. Version 2.2019. Retrieved on 7/10/2019 at: www.nccn.org/professional/physician_gls/pdf/myeloma.pdf; Olsen, M., LeFebvre, K., & Brassil, K. (2019). *Chemotherapy and immunotherapy guidelines and recommendations for practice.* Pittsburgh, PA: Oncology Nursing Society; Rajkumar, S. (2018). Multiple myeloma: 2018 update on diagnosis, risk-stratification, and management. *American Journal of Hematology, 93,* 1091–1110.

pomalidomide) are used to treat the disease (see Chapter 26 for further discussion of VTE management).

 Gerontologic Considerations

Historically, aggressive multiple myeloma therapy, particularly HSCT, was limited to patients younger than age 65, but this approach has changed. Patients older than age 65 who have excellent organ function (i.e., renal, hepatic, cardiopulmonary) and who have fewer comorbidities may tolerate more intense treatment, including AuHSCT (Faiman et al., 2017; NCCN, 2019i). Determining an older adult patient's ability to tolerate therapy *a priori* is important. In addition to chronologic age, organ function, and comorbidity, the ability to independently perform activities of daily living is another important factor. A comprehensive assessment of all these factors is useful to better determine the level of "fitness" in a given patient. Patients categorized as frail may develop more severe toxicity associated with therapy and consequently are more likely to discontinue that treatment.

The older adult patient may have different goals of care from that of younger patients. Effective symptom control, preserving cognitive function, and maintaining independence are often viewed as higher priority than survival in the older adult. Discussing these goals of care as well as the patient's physical and social needs can provide a more personalized approach to treating the older adult with multiple myeloma. Using lower doses of agents and focusing on side effect management are important treatment strategies. Side effects should be managed without additional medications to reduce the burden of polypharmacy. Incorporating the expertise of a palliative care clinician may be extremely beneficial, not only in devising an appropriate treatment plan, but also in managing symptoms and side effects more effectively.

Nursing Management

Pain management is very important in patients with multiple myeloma. NSAIDs can be very useful for mild pain or can be given in combination with opioid analgesics. Because NSAIDs can cause gastritis and renal dysfunction, renal function must be carefully monitored and patients assessed for GI complications; many patients are unable to use NSAIDs due to concurrent or newly developed renal insufficiency. Long-acting opioids are often prescribed to afford adequate pain relief.

Nursing care should focus on assessing for signs and symptoms of hypercalcemia. Common presenting symptoms include polyuria and GI problems (nausea, constipation, anorexia). Patients progressively become more dehydrated, with possible confusion and stupor as well as decreased renal function as the hypercalcemia worsens. Treatment for hypercalcemia includes aggressive hydration, bisphosphonates, and/or corticosteroids. See Chapter 12, Table 12-13, for a discussion of manifestations of and treatment for hypercalcemia.

Patient education should include methods to prevent and minimize the risk of infection, reportable signs and symptoms, medication side effects, and pain management. Any new complaint or worsening of pain requires immediate intervention. Another key nursing responsibility is to assess for and provide emotional/psychological support. Educating patients about effective coping skills to aid in dealing with multiple myeloma and its treatment is a key intervention.

Promoting Home, Community-Based, and Transitional Care

 Educating Patients About Self-Care

The patient needs to be educated about activity restrictions (e.g., lifting no more than 10 lb, the use of proper body mechanics) to reduce the risk of pathologic fracture. Braces are occasionally needed to support the spinal column, but may be uncomfortable and hamper adherence. Bisphosphonate therapy has markedly reduced the severity and extent of bone pain. However, patients need to understand the importance of comprehensive oral hygiene and good dental care to diminish the likelihood of developing osteonecrosis of the jaw that may arise from bisphosphonate therapy.

Renal function must be monitored closely. Kidney injury can become severe, and dialysis may be needed. Maintaining high urine output (3 L/day) can be very useful in preventing or limiting this complication, as is treating the underlying disease. The patient also needs to be educated about the signs and symptoms of hypercalcemia. While hypercalcemia usually occurs at the onset of the disease, it can also develop at the time of disease progression or when multiple myeloma becomes refractory to therapy. Maintaining mobility and hydration are important to diminish exacerbations of this complication.

Because antibody production is impaired, infections, particularly bacterial infections, are common and can be life-threatening. The patient needs education regarding appropriate infection prevention measures and should be advised to contact the primary provider immediately if fever or other signs and symptoms of infection develop. The patient should receive pneumococcal and influenza vaccines. Prophylactic antibiotics, such as trimethoprim–sulfamethoxazole, are often used, particularly when patients are treated with corticosteroid-containing regimens to prevent *Pneumocystis jirovecii* pneumonia (NCCN, 2019i). The antiviral agent acyclovir may be prescribed when patients are treated with bortezomib-based regimens to diminish the potential development of viral infection, such as herpes zoster. The patient must be educated about the indications for these prophylactic measures.

Continuing and Transitional Care

Many medications prescribed to treat multiple myeloma, particularly the immunomodulatory drugs (e.g., lenalidomide, thalidomide), are associated with higher risks of VTE formation, particularly when used concurrently with high doses of corticosteroids or erythropoietin. Other VTE risk factors include decreased mobility, obesity, prior thromboembolic events, diabetes, cardiac or renal disease, and the presence of a vascular access device (e.g., PICC). It is important to maintain mobility and to use strategies that enhance venous return (e.g., anti-embolism stockings, avoid crossing the legs). For patients without additional risk factors, VTE can be prevented by taking low-dose aspirin. Those patients with additional risk factors for developing VTE should receive anticoagulation therapy (see Chapter 26 for further discussion).

Peripheral neuropathy is a frequent issue for patients with multiple myeloma, affecting over 50% at the time of diagnosis (Faiman et al., 2017). It is particularly commonplace in patients who are prescribed thalidomide or bortezomib. Painful neuropathy can be quite disabling and may interfere with the patient's ability to perform normal activities of daily living (Olsen et al., 2019) (see Table 30-6). The nurse needs to carefully assess for symptoms related to peripheral neuropathy and make assessments of the home for safety. Sensation (touch, temperature, pain, vibration, proprioception), ankle reflexes, distal muscle strength, and blood pressure should be evaluated. Other risk factors for peripheral neuropathy (e.g., diabetes, vitamin deficiencies, viral infection, or excessive alcohol consumption) should be aggressively managed. Patients should be educated to report any symptoms of peripheral neuropathy and to not minimize such symptoms, because prompt cessation of therapy or reducing the dose can prevent the neuropathy from progressing. Resuming treatment with a lower dosage and at a longer interval between dosing may diminish the worsening of peripheral nerve

TABLE 30-6	Peripheral Neuropathy Associated with Multiple Myeloma	
Type of Neuropathy	**Manifestations**	**Nursing Interventions/Patient Education**
Sensory	Hypoesthesia	Warn patient to avoid extreme temperatures (e.g., bathwater)
		Inspect feet for trauma, potential infection
		Use loose-fitting stockings
	Paresthesia (tingling)	Gentle massage
		Gentle ROM exercises
	Hyperalgesia (pain)	Gentle massage (cocoa butter or menthol-based cream/lotion)
	Toes and fingers	Apply lidocaine 5% patch to affected area every 12 h
	Soles of feet/palms	Consider gabapentin, tricyclic antidepressants (e.g., amitriptyline)
Motor	Muscle cramps	Maximize hydration, ambulation (Quinine is not recommended)
	Tremor	
	↓ Strength in distal muscles	
	Gait disturbance	Encourage the use of appropriate footwear
	↓ Fine motor function (e.g., hand-writing, buttoning clothes)	Consider ambulatory aides (e.g., walker)
		Remove scatter rugs; perform a home safety evaluation
		PT referral
		OT referral (if severe limitations)
Autonomic Nervous System	Orthostatic hypotension	Warn patient to avoid abrupt position change
		Maximize hydration
		Consult with primary provider about adjusting antihypertensive medications, diuretics
	Bradycardia	Assess/warn patient for impact (fatigue, impairment in function)
		Consult with primary provider about adjusting drugs that cause bradycardia (e.g., calcium channel blockers, beta-blockers, alpha-/beta-adrenergic blockers, digoxin).
		Explore the use of activity to increase heart rate
	Sexual dysfunction	Explore alternative means of sexual activity beyond penile-vaginal intercourse
		Consult with primary provider about the use of erectile dysfunction medication
	Constipation	Maximize fluid intake, fiber
		Use stool softeners, laxatives

Note: Peripheral neuropathy can be classified into three main categories. Within each category, specific manifestations are delineated as well as relevant nursing interventions. If the neuropathy is related to multiple myeloma therapy, it is crucial to promptly stop the potentially offending medication. It is also important to reduce the impact from other predisposing factors. For example, diabetes should be well controlled and alcohol consumption reduced.
↓, decreased; OT, occupational therapy; PT, physical therapy; ROM, range of motion.
Adapted from Autissier, E. (2019). Chemotherapy-induced peripheral neuropathy. *Clinical Journal of Oncology Nursing, 23*(4), 405–410; Olsen, M., LeFebvre, K., & Brassil, K. (2019). *Chemotherapy and immunotherapy guidelines and recommendations for practice.* Pittsburgh, PA: Oncology Nursing Society.

damage. Recovery can occur over time, although it may be incomplete. Gabapentinoids (e.g., gabapentin, pregabalin), tricyclic antidepressants (e.g., amitriptyline, nortriptyline), and selective SSRIs (e.g., duloxetine) can be prescribed to diminish pain; opioids are fairly ineffective in this context.

As many drugs used in treating multiple myeloma are given orally, the nurse must ensure that the patient fully understands how to take the medication, manage side effects, and know what steps can be taken to diminish or mitigate adverse effects (see Table 30-6).

CRITICAL THINKING EXERCISES

1 **ipc** You work on an inpatient oncology unit and are assigned to care for a 47-year-old woman with AML who is a week and a half post induction therapy. The multidisciplinary team is now rounding on your patient and asks you for a brief report. What complications would you anticipate the patient could experience at this time? What key information do you think you should provide the multidisciplinary team? What aspects of multidisciplinary care do you identify?

2 **pg** You work in an outpatient infusion center and are assigned to provide a first treatment for a 74-year-old African American man who was recently diagnosed with multiple myeloma. What key assessment and laboratory studies would you focus on and why? Are there any comorbidities that could impact this patient's treatment?

3 **ebp** You are caring for a 57-year-old patient with diffuse large B-cell lymphoma who is not a candidate for autologous HSCT. The patient had only a partial response to consolidation therapy and is in the hospital to manage an infection. What do you anticipate are the best treatment options available for this patient? What are the possible adverse effects that you need to monitor? What evidence-based nursing interventions would you employ to manage this patient's care?

REFERENCES

*Asterisk indicates nursing research.

Books

Olsen, M., LeFebvre, K., & Brassil, K. (2019). *Chemotherapy and immunotherapy guidelines and recommendations for practice.* Pittsburgh, PA: Oncology Nursing Society.

Journals and Electronic Documents

American Cancer Society (ACS). (2018). Risk factors for multiple myeloma. Retrieved on 5/15/2020 at: www.cancer.org/cancer/multiple-myeloma/causes-risks-prevention/risk-factors.html

American Cancer Society (ACS). (2019a). Hodgkin lymphoma. Retrieved on 1/10/2020 at: www.cancer.org/cancer/hodgkin-lymphoma/detection-diagnosis-staging/survivssl-rates.html

American Cancer Society (ACS). (2019b). Non-Hodgkin lymphoma. Retrieved on 1/10/2020 at: www.cancer.org/cancer/non-hodgkin-lymphoma/about.html

American Cancer Society (ACS). (2020a). Agent Orange and cancer risk. Retrieved on 7/2/2020 at: www.cancer.org/cancer/cancer-causes/agent-orange-and-cancer.html#:~:text=International%20Agency%20for%20Research%20on,to%20be%20a%20human%20carcinogen.%E2%80%9D

American Cancer Society (ACS). (2020b). Survival rates and factors that affect prognosis (outlook) for non-Hodgkin lymphoma. Retrieved on 5/15/2020 at: www.cancer.org/cancer/non-hodgkin-lymphoma/detection-diagnosis-staging/factors-prognosis.html

Arber, D., Orazi, A., Hasserjian, R., et al. (2016). The 2016 revision to the World Health Organization classification of myeloid neoplasms and acute leukemia. *Blood, 127*(20), 2391–2405.

Autissier, E. (2019). Chemotherapy-induced peripheral neuropathy. *Clinical Journal of Oncology Nursing, 23*(4), 405–410.

Barbui, T., Vannucchi, A., Carobbio, A., et al. (2017). The effect of arterial hypertension on thrombosis in low-risk polycythemia vera. *American Journal of Hematology, 92*(1), E5–E6.

*Bryant, A., Gosselin, T., Coffman, E., et al. (2018). Symptoms, mobility, and function, and quality of life in adults with acute leukemia during initial hospitalization. *Oncology Nursing Forum, 45*(5), 653–664.

Chim, C., Kumar, S., Orlowski, R., et al. (2018). Management of relapsed and refractory multiple myeloma: Novel agents, antibodies, immunotherapies, and beyond. *Leukemia, 32*(2), 252–262.

Faiman, B., Doss, D., Colson, et al. (2017). Renal, GI, and peripheral nerves. *Clinical Journal of Oncology Nursing, 21*(5-suppl.), 19–36.

Fowlkes, S., Murray, C., Fulford, A., et al. (2018a). Myeloproliferative neoplasms (MPNs)—Part 1: An overview of the diagnosis and treatment of the "classical" MPNs. *Canadian Oncology Nursing Journal, 28*(4), 262–268.

Fowlkes, S., Murray, C., Fulford, A., et al. (2018b). Myeloproliferative neoplasms (MPNs)—Part 2: A nursing guide to managing the symptom burden of MPNs. *Canadian Oncology Nursing Journal, 28*(4), 276–284.

*Gborogen, R., & Polek, C. (2018). Oral agents: Challenges with self-administered medication adherence in clinical trials. *Clinical Journal of Oncology Nursing, 22*(3), 333–339.

Geyer, H. L., & Mesa, R. A. (2014). Therapy for myeloproliferative neoplasms: When, which agent, and how? *Hematology American Society of Hematology Education Program, 2014*(1), 277–286.

Haider, M., Gangat, N., Lasho, T., et al. (2016). Validation of the revised international prognostic score of thrombosis for essential thrombocytopenia (IPSET- thrombosis) in 585 Mayo Clinic patients. *American Journal of Hematology, 91*(4), 390–394.

Harrison, C., Koschmieder, S., Foltz, L., et al. (2017). The impact of myeloproliferative neoplasms (MPNs) on patient quality of life and productivity: Results from the international MPN Landmark survey. *Annals of Hematology, 96*(10), 1653–1665.

*Hefner, J., Csef, E., & Kunzmann, V. (2017). Adherence and coping strategies in outpatients with chronic myeloid leukemia receiving oral tyrosine kinase inhibitors. *Oncology Nursing Forum, 44*(6), E232–E240.

Leukemia & Lymphoma Society. (2016). NHL subtypes. Retrieved on 5/14/2020 at: www.lls.org/lymphoma/non-hodgkin-lymphoma/diagnosis/nhl-subtypes

Leukemia & Lymphoma Society. (2018a). Acute lymphocytic leukemia. Retrieved on 9/10/2019 at: www.lls.org/sites/default/files/file_assets/PS33__ALL_2018_FINAL.pdf

Leukemia & Lymphoma Society. (2018b). Updated data on blood cancers 2018–2019. Retrieved on 7/10/2019 at: www.lls.org/sites/default/files/file_assets/PS80_Facts_Book_2018-2019_FINAL.pdf

Leukemia & Lymphoma Society. (2018c). Hodgkin lymphoma. Retrieved on 7/10/2019 at: www.lls.org/sites/default/files/PS57_Hodgkin_Lymphoma2018.pdf

Leukemia & Lymphoma Society. (2018d). Non-Hodgkin lymphoma. Retrieved on 7/10/2019 at: www.lls.org/sites/default/files/file_assets/PS58_NHL_5.18FINAL.pdf

Leukemia & Lymphoma Society. (2019a). Acute myeloid leukemia. Retrieved on 9/10/2019 at: www.lls.org/sites/default/files/file_assets/PS32_AML_Booklet_2019_FINAL.pdf

Leukemia & Lymphoma Society. (2019b). Chronic myeloid leukemia. Retrieved on 9/10/2019 at: www.lls.org/sites/default/files/National/USA/Pdf/Publications/PS31_CML%20 Booklet_2019.pdf

Leukemia & Lymphoma Society. (2019c). Chronic lymphocytic leukemia. Retrieved on 9/10/2019 at: www.lls.org/sites/default/files/file_assets/PS34_CLL_Booklet_2019_FINAL.pdf

Leukemia & Lymphoma Society. (2019d). Myelodysplastic syndromes. Retrieved on 9/10/2019 at: www.lls.org/sites/default/files/file_assets/PS22_MDS_Book_2019_FINAL.pdf

Leukemia & Lymphoma Society. (2019e). Myeloproliferative neoplasms. Retrieved on 7/10/2019 at: www.lls.org/sites/default/files/National/USA/Pdf/Publications/MPNs_booklet_12_17_FINAL.pdf

Leukemia & Lymphoma Society. (2019f). Where do blood cancers develop? Retrieved on 2/3/2020 at: www.lls.org/sites/default/files/National/USA/Pdf/Publications/PS104_CancerOriginsChart_2019final.pdf

McMullin, M., Harrison, C., Ali, S., et al. (2019). A guideline for the diagnosis and management of polycythemia vera. A British Society for Haematology Guideline. *British Journal of Haematology, 184*(2), 176–191.

Montalban-Bravo, G., & Garcia-Manero, G. (2017). Myelodysplastic syndromes: 2018 update on diagnosis, risk-stratification, and management. *American Journal of Hematology, 93*(1), 129–147.

National Comprehensive Cancer Network (NCCN). (2019a). Clinical practice guidelines in oncology: Acute myeloid leukemia. Version 3.2019. Retrieved on 7/10/2019 at: www.nccn.org/professional/physician_gls/pdf/aml.pdf

National Comprehensive Cancer Network (NCCN). (2019b). Clinical practice guidelines in oncology: Chronic myeloid leukemia. Version 1.2019. Retrieved on 7/10/2019 at: www.nccn.org/professional/physician_gls/pdf/cml.pdf

National Comprehensive Cancer Network (NCCN). (2019c). Clinical practice guidelines in oncology: Acute lymphoblastic leukemia. Version 1.2019. Retrieved on 7/10/2019 at: www.nccn.org/professional/physician_gls/pdf/all.pdf

National Comprehensive Cancer Network (NCCN). (2019d). Clinical practice guidelines in oncology: Chronic lymphocytic leukemia/small lymphocytic lymphoma. Version 4.2019. Retrieved on 7/10/2019 at: www.nccn.org/professional/physician_gls/pdf/cll.pdf

National Comprehensive Cancer Network (NCCN). (2019e). Clinical practice guidelines in oncology: Myelodysplastic syndromes. Version 2.2019. Retrieved on 7/12/2019 at: www.nccn.org/professional/physician_gls/pdf/mds.pdf

National Comprehensive Cancer Network (NCCN). (2019f). Clinical practice guidelines in oncology: Myeloproliferative neoplasms. Version 2.2019. Retrieved on 7/12/2019 at: www.nccn.org/professional/physician_gls/pdf/mpn.pdf

National Comprehensive Cancer Network (NCCN). (2019g). Clinical practice guidelines in oncology: Hodgkin lymphoma. Version 2.2019. Retrieved on 7/10/2019 at: www.nccn.org/professional/physician_gls/pdf/hodgkin.pdf

National Comprehensive Cancer Network (NCCN). (2019h). Clinical practice guidelines in oncology: B-cell lymphomas. Version 2.2019. Retrieved on 7/10/2019 at: www.nccn.org/professional/physician_gls/pdf/b-cell lymphoma.pdf

National Comprehensive Cancer Network (NCCN). (2019i). Clinical practice guidelines in oncology: Multiple myeloma. Version 2.2019. Retrieved on 7/10/2019 at: www.nccn.org/professional/physician_gls/pdf/myeloma.pdf

Rajkumar, S. (2018). Multiple myeloma: 2018 update on diagnosis, risk-stratification, and management. *American Journal of Hematology, 93*, 1091–1110.

Scherber, R. M., Kosiorek, H. E., Senyak, Z., et al. (2016). Comprehensively understanding fatigue in patients with myeloproliferative neoplasms. *Cancer, 122*(3), 477–485.

Sockel, K., & Platzbecker, U. (2018). Current and future option for myelodysplastic syndromes: More than hypomethylating agents and lenalidomide. *Drugs, 78*(18), 1873–1885.

Spinner, M., Varma, G., & Advani, R. (2018). Modern principles in the management of nodular lymphocyte-predominant Hodgkin lymphoma. *British Journal of Haematology, 184*(1), 17–29.

Spivak, J. (2018). Polycythemia vera. *Current Treatment Options in Oncology, 19*(2), 12.

Tefferi, A. (2018). Primary myelofibrosis: 2019 update on diagnosis, risk-stratification and management. *American Journal of Hematology, 93*(12), 1551–1560.

Tefferi, A., & Barbui, T. (2019). Polycythemia vera and essential thrombocytopenia: 2019 update on diagnosis, risk-stratification, and management. *American Journal of Hematology*, 94(1), 133–143.

Resources

AABB (formerly known as the American Association of Blood Banks), www.aabb.org/Pages/default.aspx

American Cancer Society, www.cancer.org

American College of Surgeons Commission on Cancer, www.facs.org/quality-programs/cancer/coc

American Society for Transplantation and Cellular Therapy (ASTCT), www.astct.org/home

Aplastic Anemia & MDS International Foundation, www.aamds.org

Be The Match (Bone marrow transplantation network), www.bethematch.org

Blood and Marrow Transplant Information Network, www.bmtinfonet.org

Department of Veteran Affairs, information on Agent Orange, www.publichealth.va.gov/exposures/agentorange/benefits/health-care.asp

International Myeloma Foundation, www.myeloma.org

Leukemia & Lymphoma Society, www.lls.org

Lymphoma Research Foundation, lymphoma.org

Multinational Association of Supportive Care in Cancer, www.mascc.org

Myelodysplastic Syndromes Foundation (MDS Foundation), www.mds-foundation.org

National Cancer Institute, www.cancer.gov

National Comprehensive Cancer Network, www.nccn.org

National Heart, Lung, and Blood Institute, www.nhlbi.nih.gov

Oncology Nursing Society (ONS), www.ons.org

Immunologic Function

UTILIZING A TEAM APPROACH TO CARE FOR THE PATIENT WITH HIV

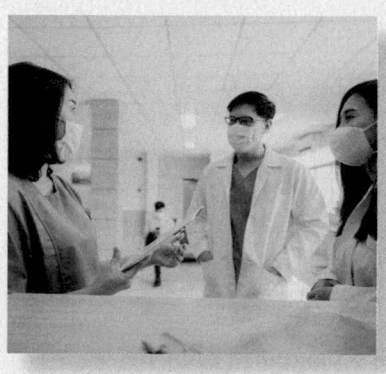

You are working in a community health center with an interdisciplinary team to provide care for patients with human immune deficiency virus (HIV). The team consists of a physician, nurse, pharmacist, social worker, mental health counselor, and a registered dietician. The team is discussing the interdisciplinary management plan for a 21-year-old Hispanic male who recently became positive for HIV infection. The goal is to develop strategies for him to treat his HIV infection and prevent progression to acquired immune deficiency syndrome (AIDS). How can you, as the sole nurse on the team, foster open communication, mutual respect, and shared decision-making within the team to achieve quality patient care?

QSEN Competency Focus: Teamwork and Collaboration

The complexities inherent in today's health care system challenge nurses to demonstrate integration of specific interdisciplinary core competencies. These competencies are aimed at ensuring the delivery of safe, quality patient care (Institute of Medicine, 2003). The Quality and Safety Education for Nurses project (Cronenwett, Sherwood, Barnsteiner, et al., 2007; QSEN, 2020) provides a framework for the knowledge, skills, and attitudes (KSAs) required for nurses to demonstrate competency in these key areas, which include *patient-centered care*, *interdisciplinary teamwork and collaboration*, *evidence-based practice*, *quality improvement*, *safety*, and *informatics.*

Teamwork and Collaboration Definition: Function effectively within nursing and interprofessional teams, fostering open communication, mutual respect, and shared decision-making to achieve quality patient care.

SELECT PRE-LICENSURE KSAs	APPLICATION AND REFLECTION
Knowledge	
Describe scopes of practice and roles of health care team members	Describe the various roles of the team in managing a patient with HIV. How does your role complement the other members of the team? Why does this patient require a variety of team members to facilitate his disease management?
Describe strategies for identifying and managing overlaps in team member roles and accountabilities	
Recognize contributions of other individuals and groups in helping patient/family achieve health goals	
Skills	
Demonstrate awareness of own strengths and limitations as a team member	Discuss how the team approaches the management of the laboratory findings for this patient who is newly diagnosed with HIV. Describe how each member can provide education to him regarding the antiretroviral medications and how they can be used to manage the abnormal laboratory results related to this disease process. Describe how the role of the team changes during the various phases of the disease process.
Initiate plan for self-development as a team member	
Attitudes	
Value teamwork and the relationships upon which it is based	After the members of the team meet with the patient, what are ways each member can advocate for this patient's needs? How can you ensure all team members are communicating and collaborating together as a team?
Value different styles of communication used by patients, families, and health care providers	

Cronenwett, L., Sherwood, G., Barnsteiner, J., et al. (2007). Quality and safety education for nurses. *Nursing Outlook, 55*(3), 122–131; Institute of Medicine. (2003). *Health professions education: A bridge to quality*. Washington, DC: National Academies Press; QSEN Institute. (2020). *QSEN competencies: Definitions and pre-licensure KSAs; Teamwork and collaboration*. Retrieved on 8/15/2020 at: qsen.org/competencies/pre-licensure-ksas/#teamwork_collaboration

31 Assessment of Immune Function

GLOSSARY

agglutination: clumping effect occurring when an antibody acts as a cross-link between two antigens

antibody: a protein substance developed by the body in response to and interacting with a specific antigen

antigen: substance that induces the production of antibodies

antigenic determinant: the specific area of an antigen that binds with an antibody-combining site and determines the specificity of the antigen–antibody reaction

apoptosis: programmed cell death that results from the digestion of deoxyribonucleic acid by end nucleases

B cells: cells that are important for producing a humoral immune response

cellular immune response: the immune system's third line of defense, involving the attack of pathogens by T cells

complement: series of enzymatic proteins in the serum that, when activated, destroy bacteria and other cells

cytokines: generic term for nonantibody proteins that act as intercellular mediators, as in the generation of immune response

cytotoxic T cells: lymphocytes that lyse cells infected with virus; also play a role in graft rejection

epitope: any component of an antigen molecule that functions as an antigenetic determinant by permitting the attachment of certain antibodies

genetic engineering: emerging technology designed to enable replacement of missing or defective genes

helper T cells: lymphocytes that attack foreign invaders (antigens) directly

humoral immune response: the immune system's second line of defense (*synonym:* antibody response)

immune response: the coordinated response of the components of the immune system to a foreign agent or organism

immune system: the collection of organs, cells, tissues, and molecules that mediate the immune response

immunity: the body's specific protective response to a foreign agent or organism; resistance to disease, specifically infectious diseases

immunopathology: study of diseases resulting in dysfunctions within the immune system

immunoregulation: complex system of checks and balances that regulates or controls immune responses

immunosenescence: the gradual deterioration of the immune system brought on by the aging process

interferons: proteins formed when cells are exposed to viral or foreign agents; capable of activating other components of the immune system

lymphokines: substances released by sensitized lymphocytes when they come in contact with specific antigens

memory cells: cells that are responsible for recognizing antigens from previous exposure and mounting an immune response

natural killer (NK) cells: lymphocytes that defend against microorganisms and malignant cells

null lymphocytes: lymphocytes that destroy antigens already coated with the antibody

---

opsonization: the coating of antigen–antibody molecules with a sticky substance to facilitate phagocytosis

phagocytic cells: cells that engulf, ingest, and destroy foreign bodies or toxins

phagocytic immune response: the immune system's first line of defense, involving white blood cells that have the ability to ingest foreign particles

stem cells: precursors of all blood cells; reside primarily in the bone marrow

suppressor T cells: lymphocytes that decrease B-cell activity to a level at which the immune system is compatible with life

T cells: cells that are important for producing a cellular immune response

---

Immunity is the body's specific protective response to a foreign agent or organism. The **immune system** functions as the body's defense mechanism against invasion and allows a rapid response to foreign substances in a specific manner. Genetic and cellular responses result. Any qualitative or quantitative change in the components of the immune system can produce profound effects on the integrity of the human organism. Immune function is affected by a variety of factors, such as central nervous system integrity, general physical and emotional status, medications, dietary patterns, and the stress of illness, trauma, or surgery. Immune memory is a property of the immune system that provides protection against harmful microbial agents despite the timing of re-exposure to the agent. Tolerance is the mechanism by which the immune system is programmed to eliminate foreign substances such as microbes, toxins, and cellular mutations but maintains the ability to accept self-antigens. Some credence is given to the concept of surveillance, in which the immune system is in a perpetual state of vigilance, screening and rejecting any invader that is recognized as foreign to the host. The term **immunopathology** refers to the study of diseases that result from dysfunctions within the immune system. Immune system dysfunctions can occur across the lifespan; many are genetically based, others are acquired. Disorders of the immune system may stem from excesses or deficiencies of immunocompetent cells, alterations in the function of these cells, immunologic attack on self-antigens, or inappropriate or exaggerated responses to specific antigens (Table 31-1).

Primary immunodeficiencies and acquired immune disorders affect large numbers of the population. Thus, nurses in many practice settings need to understand how the immune system functions as well as immunopathologic processes. In addition, knowledge about assessment and care of people with immunologic disorders enables nurses to make appropriate management decisions.

Anatomic and Physiologic Overview

Accurate assessment of immune function necessitates the nurse having a good working knowledge of the anatomy and physiology of the immune system.

Anatomy of the Immune System

The immune system is composed of an integrated collection of various cell types, each with a designated function in defending against infection and invasion by other organisms. Supporting this system are molecules that are responsible for the interactions, modulations, and regulation of the system. These molecules and cells participate in specific interactions with immunogenic **epitopes** (antigenic determinants) present on foreign materials, initiating a series of actions in a host, including the inflammatory response, the lysis of microbial agents, and the disposal of foreign toxins. The major components of the immune system include central and peripheral organs, tissues, and cells (Fig. 31-1).

Bone Marrow

The white blood cells (WBCs) involved in immunity are produced in the bone marrow (Fig. 31-2). Like other blood cells, lymphocytes are generated from **stem cells** (undifferentiated cells). There are two types of lymphocytes—**B cells**, also called B lymphocytes, and **T cells**, also called T lymphocytes (Fig. 31-3).

Lymphoid Tissues

The spleen, composed of red and white pulp, acts somewhat like a filter. The red pulp is the site where old and injured red blood cells (RBCs) are destroyed. The white pulp contains concentrations of lymphocytes. The lymph nodes, which are connected by lymph channels and capillaries, are distributed throughout the body. They remove foreign material from the lymph system before it enters the bloodstream. The lymph nodes also serve as centers for immune cell proliferation. The remaining lymphoid tissues contain immune cells that defend the body's mucosal surfaces against microorganisms (Klimov, 2019).

Function of the Immune System

The basic function of the immune system is to remove foreign antigens such as viruses and bacteria to maintain homeostasis. There are two general types of immunity: natural (innate) and acquired (adaptive). Natural immunity or

TABLE 31-1	Immune System Disorders
Disorder	**Description**
Autoimmunity	Normal protective immune response paradoxically turns against or attacks the body, leading to tissue damage
Hypersensitivity	Body produces inappropriate or exaggerated responses to specific antigens
Gammopathies	Overproduction of immunoglobulins
Immune deficiencies	
Primary	Deficiency results from improper development of immune cells or tissues; usually congenital or inherited
Secondary	Deficiency results from some interference with an already developed immune system; usually acquired later in life

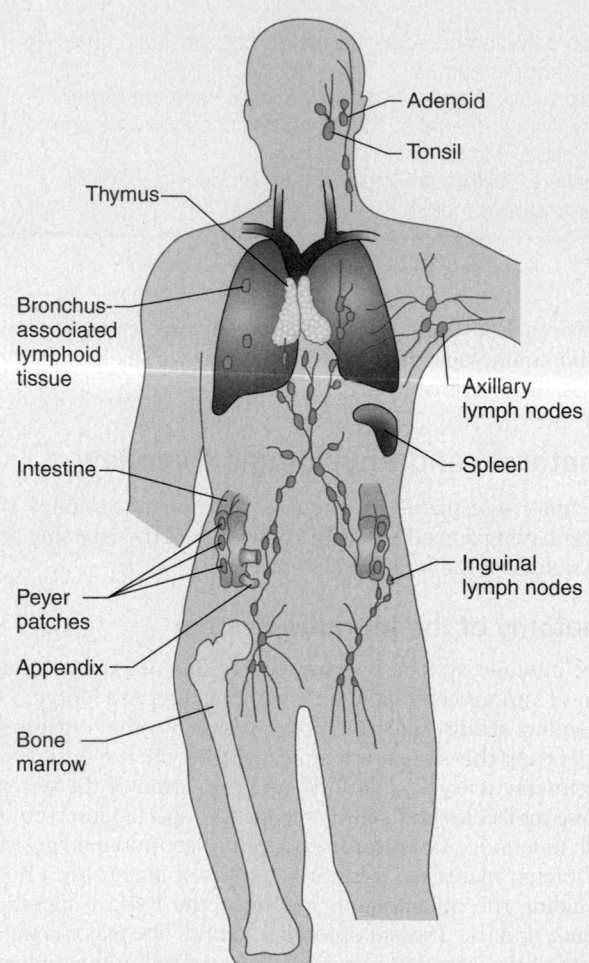

Figure 31-1 • Central and peripheral lymphoid organs, tissues, and cells. Reprinted with permission from Norris, T. L. (2019). *Porth's pathophysiology: Concepts of altered health states* (10th ed., Fig. 11.12, p. 296). Philadelphia, PA: Wolters Kluwer.

Physiology/Pathophysiology

Bone marrow

Lymphoblasts

Bone marrow maturation

Thymus

B lymphocytes

Regulator T cells

Effector T cells

Memory cells   Plasma cells

Helper T cells   Suppressor T cells

Cytotoxic T cells

Antibodies

Humoral response

Cellular (cell-mediated) response

Figure 31-2 • Development of cells of the immune system.

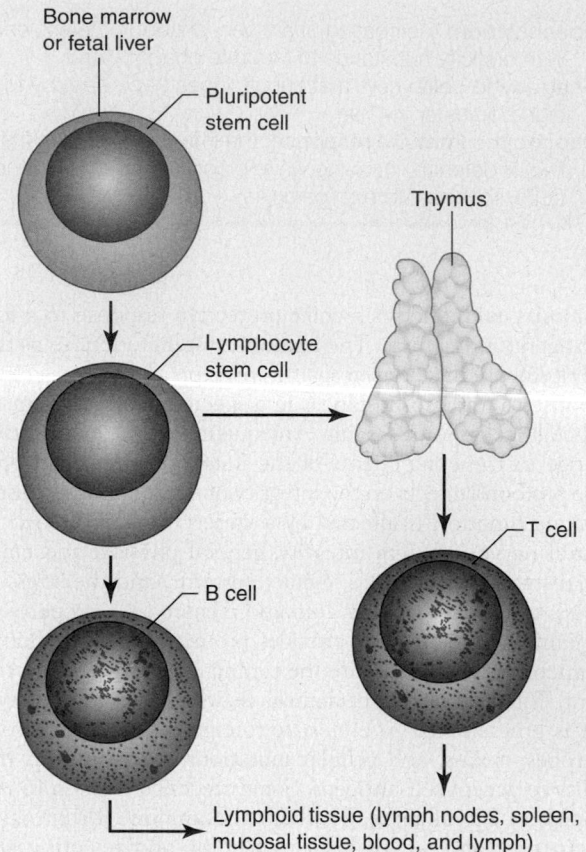

Figure 31-3 • Pathway for T- and B-cell differentiation. Reprinted with permission from Norris, T. L. (2019). *Porth's pathophysiology: Concepts of altered health states* (10th ed., Fig. 11.5, p. 288). Philadelphia, PA: Wolters Kluwer.

nonspecific immunity is present at birth. Acquired or specific immunity develops after birth. Each type of immunity has a distinct role in defending the body against harmful invaders, but the various components are usually interdependent (Klimov, 2019).

Natural Immunity

Natural immunity, which is nonspecific, provides a broad spectrum of defense against and resistance to infection. It is considered the first line of host defense following antigen exposure, because it protects the host without remembering prior contact with an infectious agent (Norris, 2019). Responses to a foreign invader are very similar from one encounter to the next, regardless of the number of times the invader is encountered. Natural (innate) immunity coordinates the initial response to pathogens through the production of cytokines and other effector molecules, which either activate cells for control of the pathogen (by elimination) or promote the development of the acquired **immune response**. The cells involved in this response are monocytes, macrophages, dendritic cells, **natural killer (NK) cells**, basophils, eosinophils, and granulocytes. The early events in this process are critical in determining the nature of the adaptive immune response. Natural immune mechanisms can be divided into two stages: immediate (generally occurring within minutes) and delayed (occurring within several days after exposure) (Norris, 2019).

White Blood Cell Action

The cellular response is the key to the effective initiation of the immune response. WBCs, or leukocytes, participate in both the natural and the acquired immune responses. Granular leukocytes, or granulocytes (so called because of granules in their cytoplasm), fight invasion by foreign bodies or toxins by releasing cell mediators, such as histamine, bradykinin, and prostaglandins, and by engulfing the foreign bodies or toxins. Granulocytes include neutrophils, eosinophils, and basophils.

Neutrophils (polymorphonuclear leukocytes) are the first cells to arrive at the site where inflammation occurs. Eosinophils and basophils, other types of granulocytes, increase in number during allergic reactions and stress responses. Nongranular leukocytes include monocytes or macrophages (referred to as histiocytes when they enter tissue spaces) and lymphocytes. Monocytes are the first to arrive on the scene and function as **phagocytic cells**, engulfing, ingesting, and destroying greater numbers and quantities of foreign bodies or toxins than granulocytes do. Lymphocytes, consisting of B cells and T cells, play major roles in humoral and cell-mediated immune responses. About 70% to 80% of lymphocytes in the blood are T cells, and about 10% to 15% are B cells (Haynes, Soderberg, & Fauci, 2018).

Inflammatory Response

The inflammatory response is a major function of the natural immune system that is elicited in response to tissue injury or invading organisms. Chemical mediators assist this response by minimizing blood loss, walling off the invading organism, activating phagocytes, and promoting formation of fibrous scar tissue and regeneration of injured tissue. The inflammatory response (discussed further in Chapter 5) is facilitated by physical and chemical barriers that are part of the human organism.

Physical and Chemical Barriers

Activation of the natural immunity response is enhanced by processes inherent in physical and chemical barriers. Physical surface barriers include intact skin, mucous membranes, and cilia of the respiratory tract, which prevent pathogens from gaining access to the body. The cilia of the respiratory tract, along with coughing and sneezing responses, filter and clear pathogens from the upper respiratory tract before they can invade the body further. Chemical barriers, such as mucus, acidic gastric secretions, enzymes in tears and saliva, and substances in sebaceous and sweat secretions, act in a nonspecific way to destroy invading bacteria and fungi. Viruses are countered by other means, such as interferon (see discussion later in chapter).

Immune Regulation

Regulation of the immune response involves balance and counterbalance. Dysfunction of the natural immune system can occur when the immune components are inactivated or when they remain active long after their effects are beneficial. A successful immune response eliminates the responsible antigen. If an immune response fails to develop and clear an antigen sufficiently, the host is considered immunocompromised or immunodeficient. If the response is overly robust or misdirected, allergies, asthma, or autoimmune disease results.

The immune system's recognition of one's own cells or tissues as "foreign" rather than as self is the basis of many autoimmune disorders (Norris, 2019). While the immune response is critical to the prevention of disease, it must be well controlled to curtail immunopathology. Most microbial infections induce an inflammatory response mediated by T cells and cytokines, which, in excess, can cause tissue damage (Haynes et al., 2018). Therefore, regulatory mechanisms must be in place to suppress or halt the immune response. This is mainly achieved by the production of cytokines and transformation of growth factor that inhibit macrophage activation. In some cases, T-cell activation is so acute that these mechanisms fail, and pathology develops. Ongoing research on **immunoregulation** holds the promise of preventing graft rejection and aiding the body in eliminating cancerous or infected cells (Chae & Bothwell, 2018; Romano, Fanelli, Albany, et al., 2019).

Although natural immunity can often effectively combat infections, many pathogenic microbes have evolved that resist natural immunity. Acquired immunity is necessary to defend against these resistant agents.

Acquired Immunity

Acquired (adaptive) immunity usually develops due to prior exposure to an antigen through immunization (vaccination) or by contracting a disease, both of which generate a protective immune response. Weeks or months after exposure to a disease or vaccine, the body produces an immune response that is sufficient to defend against the disease on re-exposure. In contrast to the rapid but nonspecific natural immune response, this form of immunity relies on the recognition of specific foreign antigens. The acquired immune response is broadly divided into two mechanisms: (1) the cell-mediated response, involving T-cell activation, and (2) effector mechanisms, involving B-cell maturation and production of antibodies (Haynes et al., 2018).

The two types of acquired immunity are known as active and passive and are interrelated. Active acquired immunity refers to immunologic defenses developed by the person's own body. This immunity typically lasts many years or even a lifetime. Passive acquired immunity is temporary immunity transmitted from a source outside the body that has developed immunity through previous disease or immunization. Examples include immunity resulting from the transfer of antibodies from the mother to an infant in utero or through breast-feeding or receiving injections of immune globulin. Active and passive acquired immunity involve humoral and cellular (cell-mediated) immunologic responses (described later).

Response to Invasion

When the body is invaded or attacked by bacteria, viruses, or other pathogens, it has three means of defense:

- The phagocytic immune response
- The humoral or antibody immune response
- The cellular immune response

The first line of defense, the **phagocytic immune response**, primarily involves the WBCs (granulocytes and macrophages), which ingest foreign particles and destroy the invading agent; eosinophils are only weakly phagocytic. Phagocytes also remove the body's own dying or dead cells. Cells in necrotic tissue that are dying release substances that trigger an inflammatory response. **Apoptosis**, or programmed cell death, is the body's way of destroying worn-out cells such as blood or skin cells or cells that need to be renewed (Norris, 2019).

A second protective response, the **humoral immune response** (*synonym:* antibody response), begins with the B lymphocytes, which can transform themselves into plasma cells that manufacture antibodies. An **antibody** is a protein substance developed by the body, transported in the bloodstream, and attempts to disable invaders. The third mechanism of defense, the **cellular immune response**, involves the T lymphocytes, which can turn into special cytotoxic (or killer) T cells that can attack the pathogens.

The structural part of the invading or attacking organism that is responsible for stimulating antibody production is called an **antigen** (or an immunogen). For example, an antigen can be a small patch of proteins on the outer surface of a microorganism. Not all antigens are naturally immunogenic; some must be coupled to other molecules to stimulate the immune response. A single bacterium or large molecule, such as a diphtheria or tetanus toxin, may have several antigens, or markers, on its surface, thus inducing the body to produce many different antibodies. Once produced, an antibody is released into the bloodstream and carried to the attacking organism. There, it combines with the antigen, binding with it like an interlocking piece of a jigsaw puzzle (Fig. 31-4). There are four well-defined stages in an immune response: recognition, proliferation, response, and effector (Fig. 31-5).

Recognition Stage

Recognition of antigens as foreign, or non-self, by the immune system is the initiating event in any immune response.

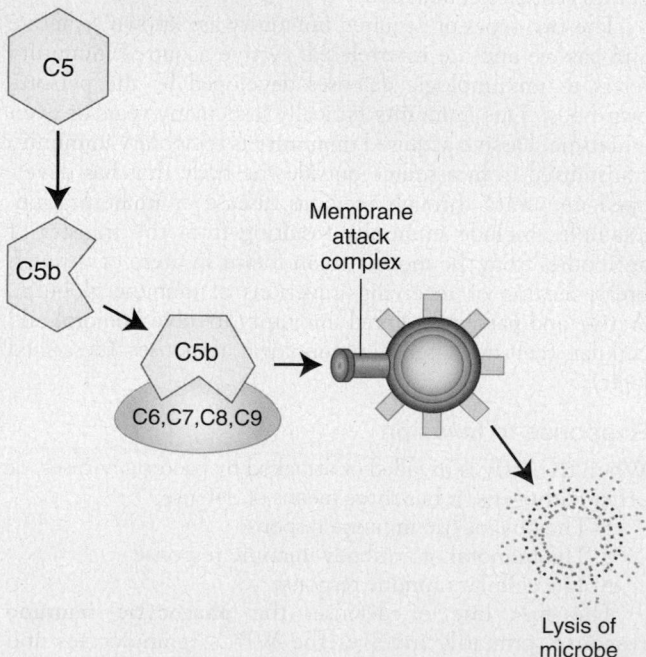

Figure 31-4 • Complement-mediated immune responses. Reprinted with permission from Norris, T. L. (2019). *Porth's pathophysiology: Concepts of altered health states* (10th ed., second figure in Understanding box, p. 286). Philadelphia, PA: Wolters Kluwer.

Recognition involves the use of lymph nodes and lymphocytes for surveillance. Lymph nodes are widely distributed internally throughout the body and in the circulating blood, as well as externally near the body's surfaces. They continuously discharge small lymphocytes into the bloodstream. These lymphocytes patrol the tissues and vessels that drain the areas served by that node. Lymphocytes recirculate from the blood to lymph nodes and from the lymph nodes back into the bloodstream in a continuous circuit. Lymphocytes and other cells have "microbial sensors" that identify molecules on microbes and other microorganisms. The interaction of these sensors with the offending agent sets off a cascade aimed at destroying the microbe. Invading organisms have pathogen-associated molecular patterns (PAMPs) contained in their cell membranes that are recognized by the immune system cells. Once the receptors on the immune cells reach the PAMPs, the immune response is triggered. Macrophages play an important role in helping the circulating lymphocytes process the antigens. Both macrophages and neutrophils have receptors for antibodies and complement; as a result, they coat microorganisms with antibodies, complement, or both, thereby enhancing phagocytosis (Norris, 2019).

In a streptococcal throat infection, for example, the streptococcal organism gains access to the mucous membranes of the throat. A circulating lymphocyte moving through the tissues of the throat comes in contact with the organism. The lymphocyte recognizes the antigens on the microbe as different (non-self) and the streptococcal organism as antigenic (foreign). This triggers the second stage of the immune response—proliferation.

Proliferation Stage

The circulating lymphocytes containing the antigenic message return to the nearest lymph node. Once in the node, these sensitized lymphocytes stimulate some of the resident T and B lymphocytes to enlarge, divide, and proliferate. T lymphocytes differentiate into cytotoxic (or killer) T cells, whereas B lymphocytes produce and release antibodies. Enlargement of the lymph nodes in the neck in conjunction with a sore throat is one example of the immune response.

Response Stage

In the response stage, the differentiated lymphocytes function in either a humoral or a cellular capacity. This stage begins with the production of antibodies by the B lymphocytes in response to a specific antigen. The cellular response stimulates the resident lymphocytes to become cells that attack microbes directly rather than through the action of antibodies. These transformed lymphocytes are known as cytotoxic (killer) T cells.

Viral antigens induce a cellular response. This response is manifested by the increasing number of T lymphocytes (lymphocytosis) seen in the blood tests of people with viral illnesses such as infectious mononucleosis. (Cellular immunity is discussed later in this chapter.) Most immune responses to antigens involve both humoral and cellular responses, although one usually predominates. For example, during transplant rejection, the cellular response involving T cells predominates, whereas in the bacterial pneumonias and sepsis, the humoral response involving B cells plays the dominant protective role (Chart 31-1).

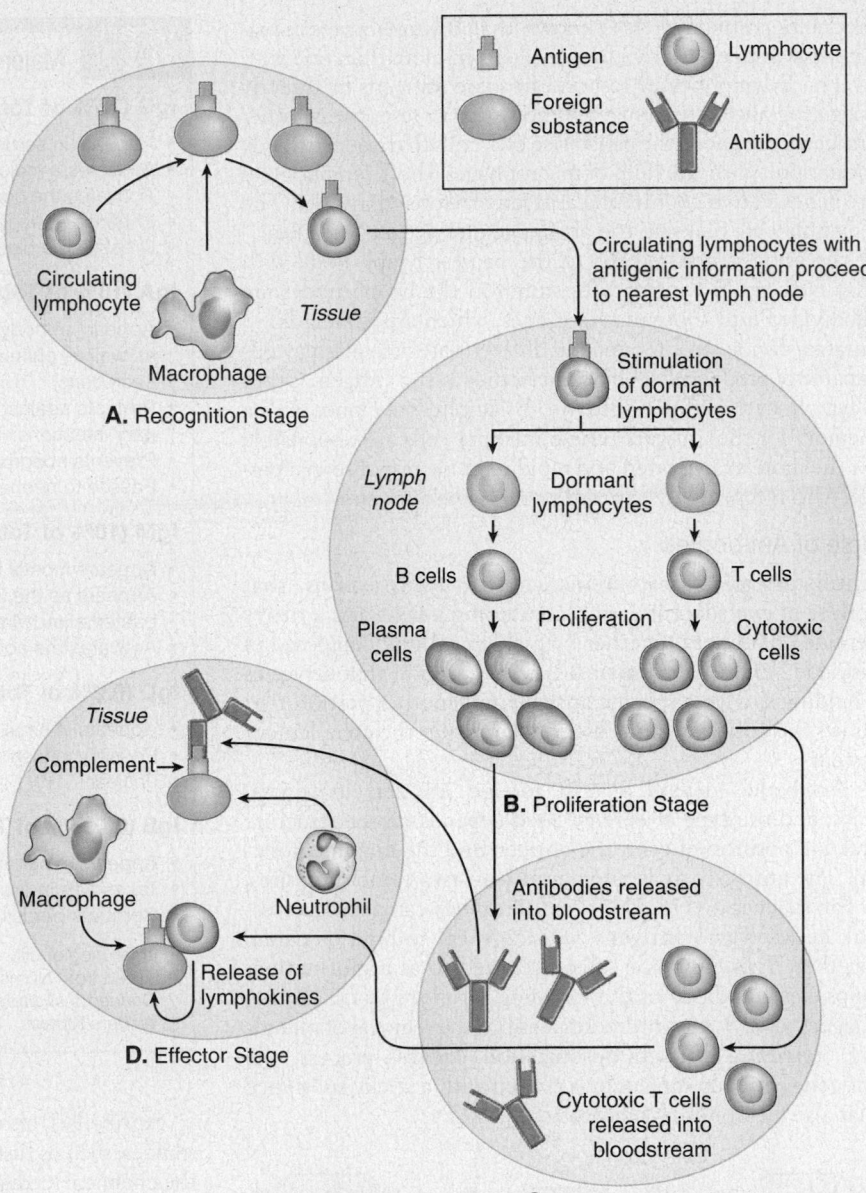

Figure 31-5 • Stages of the immune response. **A.** In the *recognition stage,* antigens are recognized by circulating lymphocytes and macrophages. **B.** In the *proliferation stage,* the dormant lymphocytes proliferate and differentiate into cytotoxic (killer) T cells or B cells responsible for formation and release of antibodies. **C.** In the *response stage,* the cytotoxic T cells and the B cells perform cellular and humoral functions, respectively. **D.** In the *effector stage,* antigens are destroyed or neutralized through the action of antibodies, complement, macrophages, and cytotoxic T cells.

Chart 31-1
Comparison of Humoral and Cellular Immune Responses

Humoral Responses (B Cells)

- Bacterial phagocytosis and lysis
- Anaphylaxis
- Allergic hay fever and asthma
- Immune complex disease
- Bacterial and some viral infections

Cellular Responses (T Cells)

- Transplant rejection
- Delayed hypersensitivity (tuberculin reaction)
- Graft-versus-host disease
- Tumor surveillance or destruction
- Intracellular infections
- Viral, fungal, and parasitic infections

Effector Stage

In the effector stage, either the antibody of the humoral response or the cytotoxic (killer) T cell of the cellular response reaches and connects with the antigen on the surface of the foreign invader. This action initiates activities involving an interplay of antibodies (humoral immunity), complement, and action by the cytotoxic T cells (cellular immunity).

Humoral Immune Response

The humoral response is characterized by the production of antibodies by B lymphocytes in response to a specific antigen. Following antibody production, the macrophages of natural immunity and the special T lymphocytes of cellular immunity are involved in antigen recognition.

Antigen Recognition

Several theories explain the mechanisms by which B lymphocytes recognize the invading antigen and respond by producing antibodies. It is known that B lymphocytes recognize and respond to invading antigens in more than one way.

The B lymphocytes respond to some antigens by directly triggering antibody formation; however, in response to other antigens, they need the assistance of T cells to trigger antibody formation. With the help of macrophages, the T lymphocytes are believed to recognize the antigen of a foreign invader. The T lymphocyte picks up the antigenic message, or "blueprint," of the antigen and returns to the nearest lymph node with that message. B lymphocytes stored in the lymph nodes are subdivided into thousands of clones, which are stimulated to enlarge, divide, proliferate, and differentiate into plasma cells capable of producing specific antibodies to the antigen. Other B lymphocytes differentiate into B-lymphocyte clones with a memory for the antigen. These memory cells are responsible for the more exaggerated and rapid immune response in a person who is repeatedly exposed to the same antigen.

Role of Antibodies

Antibodies are large proteins, called *immunoglobulins*, that consist of two subunits, each containing a light and a heavy peptide chain held together by a chemical link composed of disulfide bonds. Each subunit has one portion that serves as a binding site for a specific antigen and another portion that allows the antibody molecule to take part in the complement system.

Antibodies defend against foreign invaders in several ways, and the type of defense used depends on the structure and composition of both the antigen and the immunoglobulin. The antibody molecule has at least two combining sites, or Fab fragments (Fig. 31-6). One antibody can act as a crosslink between two antigens, causing them to bind or clump together. This clumping effect, referred to as **agglutination**, helps clear the body of the invading organism by facilitating phagocytosis. Some antibodies assist in the removal of offending organisms through **opsonization**. In this process, the antigen–antibody molecule is coated with a sticky substance that also facilitates phagocytosis.

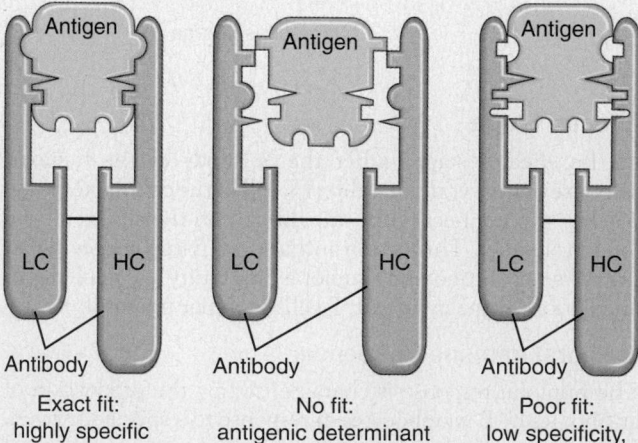

Figure 31-6 • Antigen–antibody binding. (**Left**) A highly specific antigen–antibody complex. (**Center**) No match and, therefore, no immune response. (**Right**) Poor fit or match with low specificity; antibody reacts to antigen with similar characteristics, producing cross-reactivity. HC, heavy chain; LC, light chain.

Chart 31-2 — Major Characteristics of the Immunoglobulins

IgG (75% of Total Immunoglobulin)

- Appears in serum and tissues (interstitial fluid)
- Assumes a major role in bloodborne and tissue infections
- Activates the complement system
- Enhances phagocytosis
- Crosses the placenta

IgA (15% of Total Immunoglobulin)

- Appears in body fluids (blood, saliva, tears, and breast milk, as well as pulmonary, gastrointestinal, prostatic, and vaginal secretions)
- Protects against respiratory, gastrointestinal, and genitourinary infections
- Prevents absorption of antigens from food
- Passes to neonate in breast milk for protection

IgM (10% of Total Immunoglobulin)

- Appears mostly in intravascular serum
- Appears as the first immunoglobulin produced in response to bacterial and viral infections
- Activates the complement system

IgD (0.2% of Total Immunoglobulin)

- Appears in small amounts in serum
- Possibly influences B-lymphocyte differentiation, but role is unclear

IgE (0.004% of Total Immunoglobulin)

- Appears in serum
- Takes part in allergic and some hypersensitivity reactions
- Combats parasitic infections

Ig, immunoglobulin.
Adapted from Norris, T. L. (2019). *Porth's pathophysiology: Concepts of altered health states* (10th ed.). Philadelphia, PA: Wolters Kluwer.

Antibodies also promote the release of vasoactive substances, such as histamine and slow-reacting substances, two of the chemical mediators of the inflammatory response. Antibodies do not function in isolation; rather, they mobilize other components of the immune system to defend against the invader.

The body can produce five different types of immunoglobulin (Ig). Each of the five types, or classes, is identified by a specific letter of the alphabet, IgA, IgD, IgE, IgG, and IgM. Classification is based on the chemical structure and biologic role of the individual immunoglobulin. Major characteristics of the immunoglobulins are summarized in Chart 31-2. The normal laboratory values for the three major Igs (IgA, IgG, and IgM) can be found in Appendix A on thePoint at thepoint.lww.com.

Antigen–Antibody Binding

The portion of the antigen involved in binding with the antibody is referred to as the **antigenic determinant**. The most efficient immunologic responses occur when the antibody and antigen fit like a lock and key. Poor fit can occur with an antibody that was produced in response to a different antigen. This phenomenon is known as cross-reactivity. For example, in acute rheumatic fever, the antibody produced against *Streptococcus pyogenes* in the upper respiratory tract may cross-react with the patient's heart tissue, leading to heart valve damage.

Cellular Immune Response

The T lymphocytes are primarily responsible for cellular immunity. Stem cells continuously migrate from the bone marrow to the thymus gland, where they develop into T cells. Despite the partial degeneration of the gland at puberty, T cells continue to develop in the thymus gland. Several types of T cells exist, each with designated roles in the defense against bacteria, viruses, fungi, parasites, and malignant cells. T cells attack foreign invaders directly rather than by producing antibodies.

Cellular reactions are initiated, with or without the assistance of macrophages, by the binding of an antigen to an antigen receptor located on the surface of a T cell. The T cells then carry the antigenic message, or blueprint, to the lymph nodes, where the production of other T cells is stimulated. Some T cells remain in the lymph nodes and retain a memory for the antigen. Other T cells migrate from the lymph nodes into the general circulatory system and ultimately to the tissues, where they remain until they bind with their respective antigens or die (Norris, 2019).

Types of T Lymphocytes

T cells include effector T cells, suppressor T cells, and memory T cells. The two major categories of effector T cells—helper T cells (also referred to as $CD4^+$ cells) and cytotoxic T cells (also referred to as $CD8^+$ cells)—participate in the destruction of foreign organisms. T cells interact closely with B cells, indicating that humoral and cellular immune responses are not separate, unrelated processes but rather are branches of the immune response that interact.

Helper T cells are activated on recognition of antigens and stimulate the rest of the immune system. When activated, helper T cells secrete **cytokines**, which attract and activate B cells, cytotoxic T cells, NK cells, macrophages, and other cells of the immune system. Cytokines are proteins produced by the cells of the immune system that determine the actions of the immune system cells. Separate subpopulations of helper T cells produce different types of cytokines and determine whether the immune response will be the production of antibodies or a cell-mediated immune response. Helper T cells also produce **lymphokines**, one category of cytokines (Table 31-2).

Cytotoxic T cells (killer T cells) attack the antigen directly by altering the cell membrane, causing cell lysis (disintegration), and releasing cytolytic enzymes and cytokines. Lymphokines can recruit, activate, and regulate other lymphocytes and WBCs. These cells then assist in destroying the invading organism. Delayed-type hypersensitivity is an example of an immune reaction that protects the body from antigens through the production and release of lymphokines (see later discussion).

Suppressor T cells have the ability to decrease B-cell production, thereby keeping the immune response at a level that is compatible with health (e.g., sufficient to fight infection adequately without attacking the body's healthy tissues). **Memory cells** are responsible for recognizing antigens from previous exposure and mounting an immune response (Table 31-3).

Null Lymphocytes and Natural Killer Cells

Null lymphocytes and NK cells are other lymphocytes that assist in combating organisms. These cells are distinct from B cells and T cells and lack the usual characteristics of those cells. **Null lymphocytes**, a subpopulation of lymphocytes, destroy antigens already coated with antibody. These cells have special receptor sites on their surface that allow them to connect with the end of antibodies; this is known as antibody-dependent, cell-mediated cytotoxicity.

NK cells are a class of lymphocytes that recognize infected and stressed cells and respond by killing these cells and by secreting macrophage-activating cytokine. The helper T cells contribute to the differentiation of null and NK cells.

Complement System

Circulating plasma proteins, known as **complement**, are made in the liver and activated when an antibody connects with its antigen. Complement plays an important role in the defense against microbes. Destruction of an invading or attacking organism or toxin is not achieved merely by the binding of the antibody and antigens; it also requires activation of complement, the arrival of killer T cells, or the attraction of macrophages. Complement has three major physiologic functions: defending the body against bacterial infection, bridging natural and acquired immunity, and disposing of immune complexes and the by-products associated with inflammation (Klimov, 2019).

The proteins that comprise complement interact sequentially with one another in a cascading effect. The complement cascade is important to modifying the effector arm of the immune system. Activation of complement allows important events, such as removal of infectious agents and initiation of the inflammatory response, to take place. These events involve active parts of the pathway that enhance chemotaxis of macrophages and granulocytes, alter blood vessel permeability, change blood vessel diameters, cause cells to lyse, alter blood clotting, and cause other points of modification. These macrophages and granulocytes continue the body's defense by devouring the antibody-coated microbes and by releasing bacterial products.

The complement cascade may be activated by any of three pathways: classic, lectin, and alternative. The classic pathway is triggered after antibodies bind to microbes or other antigens and is part of the humoral type of adaptive immunity. The lectin pathway is activated when a plasma protein (mannose-binding lectin) binds to terminal mannose residue on the surface glycoproteins of microbes. The alternative pathway is triggered when complement proteins are activated on microbial surfaces. This pathway is part of natural immunity.

Complement components, prostaglandins, leukotrienes, and other inflammatory mediators all contribute to the recruitment of inflammatory cells, as do chemokines, a group of cytokines. The activated neutrophils pass through the vessel walls to accumulate at the site of infection, where they phagocytize complement-coated microbes. This response is usually therapeutic and can be lifesaving if the cell attacked by the complement system is a true foreign invader. However, if that cell is part of the human organism, the result can be devastating disease and even death. Many autoimmune diseases and disorders characterized by chronic infection are thought to be caused in part by continued or chronic activation of complement, which in turn results in chronic inflammation.

TABLE 31-2	Cytokines of Innate and Adaptive Immunity	
Cytokines	**Source**	**Biologic Activity**
Interleukin-1 (IL-1)	Macrophages, endothelial cells, some epithelial cells	Wide variety of biologic effects; activates endothelium in inflammation; induces fever and acute-phase response; stimulates neutrophil production
Interleukin-2 (IL-2)	CD4+, CD8+ T cells	Growth factor for activated T cells; induces synthesis of other cytokines; activates cytotoxic T lymphocytes and NK cells
Interleukin-3 (IL-3)	CD4+ T cells	Growth factor for progenitor hematopoietic cells
Interleukin-4 (IL-4)	CD4+ T_H2 cells, mast cells	Promotes growth and survival of T, B, and mast cells; causes T_H2 cell differentiation; activates B cells and eosinophils and induces IgE-type responses
Interleukin-5 (IL-5)	CD4+ T_H2 cells	Induces eosinophil growth and development
Interleukin-6 (IL-6)	Macrophages, endothelial cells, T lymphocytes	Stimulates the liver to produce mediators of acute-phase inflammatory response; also induces proliferation of antibody-producing cells by the adaptive immune system
Interleukin-7 (IL-7)	Bone marrow stromal cells	Primary function in adaptive immunity; stimulates pre-B cells and thymocyte development and proliferation
Interleukin-8 (IL-8)	Macrophages, endothelial cells	Primary function in adaptive immunity; chemoattracts neutrophils and T lymphocytes; regulates lymphocyte homing and neutrophil infiltration
Interleukin-10 (IL-10)	Macrophages, some T-helper cells	Inhibitor of activated macrophages and dendritic cells; decreases inflammation by inhibiting T_H1 cells and release of interleukin-12 from macrophages
Interleukin-12 (IL-12)	Macrophages, dendritic cells	Enhances NK cell cytotoxicity in innate immunity; induces T_H1 cell differentiation in adaptive immunity
Type I interferons (IFN-α, IFN-β)	Macrophages, fibroblasts	Inhibit viral replication, activate NK cells, and increase expression of MHC-I molecules on virus-infected cells
Interferon-γ (IFN-γ)	NK cells, CD4+ and CD8+ T lymphocytes	Activates macrophages in both innate immune responses and adaptive cell–mediated immune responses; increases expression of MHC I and II and antigen processing and presentation
Tumor necrosis factor α (TNF-α)	Macrophages, T cells	Induces inflammation, fever, and acute-phase response; activates neutrophils and endothelial cells; kills cells through apoptosis
Chemokines	Macrophages, endothelial cells, T lymphocytes	Large family of structurally similar cytokines that stimulate leukocyte movement and regulate the migration of leukocytes from the blood to the tissues
Granulocyte–monocyte CSF (GM-CSF)	T cells, macrophages, endothelial cells, fibroblasts	Promotes neutrophil, eosinophil, and monocyte maturation and growth; activates mature granulocytes
Granulocyte CSF (G-CSF)	Macrophages, fibroblasts, endothelial cells	Promotes growth and maturation of neutrophils consumed in inflammatory reactions
Monocyte CSF (M-CSF)	Macrophages, activated T cells, endothelial cells	Promotes growth and maturation of mononuclear phagocytes

CSF, colony-stimulating factor; IgE, immunoglobulin E; MHC, major histocompatibility complex; NK, natural killer; T_H1, T-helper type 1; T_H2, T-helper type 2.
Adapted from Norris, T. L. (2019). *Porth's pathophysiology: Concepts of altered health states* (10th ed.). Philadelphia, PA: Lippincott Williams & Wilkins.

The RBCs and platelets have complement receptors and, as a result, play an important role in the clearance of immune complexes that consist of antigen, antibody, and components of the complement system (Norris, 2019).

Immunomodulators

Antimicrobial agents and vaccines have yielded considerable therapeutic success and the immune system usually works effectively; however, many infectious diseases remain difficult clinical challenges. Treatment success may be compromised by defects of the immune system; in this case, enhancement of the host immune response may be therapeutically beneficial. An immunomodulator (also known as a biologic response modifier) affects the host via direct or indirect effects on one or more components of the immunoregulatory network. Interferons, colony-stimulating factors, and monoclonal antibodies (MoAbs) are examples of agents used to help enhance the immune system (Davis & Ballas, 2017).

TABLE 31-3	Lymphocytes Involved in Immune Responses	
Type of Immune Response	**Cell Type**	**Function**
Humoral	B lymphocyte	Produces antibodies or immunoglobulins (IgA, IgD, IgE, IgG, IgM)
Cellular	T lymphocyte	
	Helper T	Attacks foreign invaders (antigens) directly
		Initiates and augments inflammatory response
	Helper T_1	Increases activated cytotoxic T cells
	Helper T_2	Increases B-cell (BG8) antibody production
	Suppressor T	Suppresses the immune response
	Memory T	Remembers contact with an antigen and on subsequent exposures mounts an immune response
	Cytotoxic T (killer T)	Lyses cells infected with virus; plays a role in graft rejection
Nonspecific	Non-T or non–B-lymphocyte null cell	Destroys antigens already coated with antibody
	Natural killer cell (granular lymphocyte)	Defends against microorganisms and some types of malignant cells; produces cytokines

Interferons

Interferon, one type of biologic response modifier, is a nonspecific viricidal protein that is naturally produced by the body and capable of activating other components of the immune system. Interferons continue to be investigated to determine their roles in the immune system and their potential therapeutic effects in disorders characterized by disturbed immune responses. These substances have antiviral and antitumor properties. In addition to responding to viral infection, interferons are produced by T lymphocytes, B lymphocytes, and macrophages in response to antigens. They are thought to modify the immune response by suppressing antibody production and cellular immunity. They also facilitate the cytolytic role of macrophages and NK cells. Interferons are used to treat immune-related disorders (e.g., multiple sclerosis) and chronic inflammatory conditions (e.g., chronic hepatitis). Research continues to evaluate the effectiveness of interferons in treating cancers (Makowska, Braunschweig, Denecke, et al., 2019) and acquired immunodeficiency syndrome.

Colony-Stimulating Factors

Colony-stimulating factors are a group of naturally occurring glycoprotein cytokines that regulate production, differentiation, survival, and activation of hematopoietic cells. Erythropoietin stimulates RBC production. Thrombopoietin plays a key regulatory role in the growth and differentiation of bone marrow cells. Interleukin-5 (IL-5) stimulates the growth and survival of eosinophils and basophils. Stem cell factor and IL-3 serve as stimuli for multiple hematopoietic cell lines. Granulocyte colony-stimulating factor, granulocyte–macrophage colony-stimulating factor, and macrophage colony-stimulating factor all serve as growth factors for specific cell lines. These cytokines have attracted considerable interest for their potential role in immunomodulation (Leleu, Gay, Flament, et al., 2017).

Monoclonal Antibodies

MoAbs have become available through technologic advances, enabling investigators to grow and produce targeted antibodies for specific pathologic organisms. This type of specificity allows MoAbs to destroy pathologic organisms and spare normal cells. The specificity of MoAbs depends on identifying key antigen proteins that are present on the surface of tumors, but not on normal tissues. When the MoAb attaches to the cell surface antigen, it blocks an important signal transduction pathway for communication between the malignant cells and the extracellular environment. The results may include an inability to initiate apoptosis, reproduce, or invade surrounding tissues (Pento, 2017; Singh, Tank, Dwiwedi, et al., 2018).

Advances in Immunology

Important developments in immunology revolve around advances in genetic engineering, use of stem cells, and immunotherapy treatments.

Genetic Engineering

One of the more remarkable evolving technologies is **genetic engineering**, which uses recombinant deoxyribonucleic acid (DNA) technology. Two facets of this technology exist. The first permits scientists to combine genes from one type of organism with genes of a second organism. This type of technology allows cells and microorganisms to manufacture proteins, monokines, and lymphokines, which can alter and enhance immune system function. The second facet of recombinant DNA technology involves gene therapy. If a specific gene is abnormal or missing, experimental recombinant DNA technology may be capable of restoring normal gene function. For example, a recombinant gene is inserted into a virus particle. When the virus particle splices its genes, the virus automatically inserts the missing gene and theoretically corrects the genetic anomaly. Extensive research into recombinant DNA technology and gene therapy is ongoing (Gonçalves & Paiva, 2017).

Stem Cells

Stem cells are capable of self-renewal and differentiation; they continually replenish the body's entire supply of both RBCs and WBCs. Some stem cells, described as totipotent cells, have tremendous capacity to self-renew and differentiate. Embryonic stem cells, described as pluripotent, give rise to numerous cell types that are able to form tissues. Research has shown that stem cells can restore an immune system that has been destroyed (Haynes et al., 2018). Stem cell transplantation has been carried out in humans with certain types of immune dysfunction, such as severe combined immuno-deficiency; clinical trials using stem cells are under way in patients with a variety of disorders having an autoimmune component, including systemic lupus erythematosus, rheumatoid arthritis, scleroderma, and multiple sclerosis. Research with embryonic stem cells has enabled investigators to make substantial gains in developmental biology, gene therapy, therapeutic tissue engineering, and the treatment of a variety of diseases (Haynes et al., 2018).

Cancer and Immunotherapy

It has long been understood that the immune system plays a role in fighting off malignancies. Recent advances in cancer treatment have sought to augment the body's natural antitumor activity and to shut down the pathways that allow malignancies to elude the immune system, which has led to the development of such treatments as MoAbs, cancer vaccines, immune adjuvants, immune checkpoint inhibitors, chimeric antigen receptor (CAR) T-cell therapy and cytokines. These immunotherapeutic treatments are designed to stimulate the patient's immune system to mount its own defense against the cancer and have revolutionized the treatment of many different cancer types. See Chapter 12 for a discussion on the use of immunotherapy in cancer (Gonçalves & Paiva, 2017; Ribas & Wolchok, 2018).

Assessment of the Immune System

An assessment of immune function begins during the health history and physical examination. Areas to be assessed include nutritional status; infections and immunizations; allergies; disorders and disease states, such as autoimmune disorders,

cancer, and chronic illnesses; surgeries; medications; and blood transfusions. In addition to inspection of general characteristics, palpation of the lymph nodes and examinations of the skin, mucous membranes, and respiratory, gastrointestinal, musculoskeletal, genitourinary, cardiovascular, and neurosensory systems are performed (Chart 31-3).

Health History

The history should note the patient's age along with information about past and present conditions and events that may provide clues to the status of the patient's immune system.

Gender

There are differences in the immune system functions of men and women. For example, many autoimmune diseases have a higher incidence in females than in males, a phenomenon believed to be correlated with sex hormones. In the past two decades, research has revealed that sex hormones are integral signaling modulators of the immune system. Sex hormones play definitive roles in lymphocyte maturation, activation, and synthesis of antibodies and cytokines. In autoimmune disease, expression of sex hormones is altered, and this change contributes to immune dysregulation (Rainville, Tsyglakova, & Hodes, 2018).

Gerontologic Considerations

Immunosenescence is the term for age-related changes in the immune system. These changes have been linked to the increased rates of illness and mortality in older adults (Tariq, Hazeldine, & Lord, 2017). Some of the changes that occur in immunosenescence include, but are not limited to, bone marrow defects, dysfunction of the thymus gland, and impaired lymphocytes. Cellular changes occur as the result of aging and

---

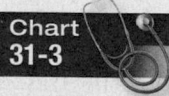

Chart 31-3

ASSESSMENT
Assessing for Immune Dysfunction

Be alert for the following signs and symptoms:

Respiratory System

- Changes in respiratory rate
- Cough (dry or productive)
- Abnormal lung sounds (wheezing, crackles, rhonchi)
- Rhinitis
- Hyperventilation
- Bronchospasm

Cardiovascular System

- Hypotension
- Tachycardia
- Arrhythmia
- Vasculitis
- Anemia

Gastrointestinal System

- Hepatosplenomegaly
- Colitis
- Vomiting
- Diarrhea

Genitourinary System

- Frequency and burning on urination
- Hematuria
- Discharge

Musculoskeletal System

- Joint mobility, edema, and pain

Skin

- Rashes
- Lesions
- Dermatitis
- Hematomas or purpura
- Edema or urticaria
- Inflammation
- Discharge

Neurosensory System

- Cognitive dysfunction
- Hearing loss
- Visual changes
- Headaches and migraines
- Ataxia
- Tetany

include impaired neutrophil function, decreased circulating macrophages, impaired dendritic cell function, and reduced T-cell activation. As the immune system undergoes age-associated alterations, its response to infections progressively deteriorates. The capacity for self-renewal of hematopoietic stem cells diminishes. There is a notable decline in the total number of phagocytes, coupled with an intrinsic reduction in their activity. The cytotoxicity of NK cells decreases, contributing to a decline in humoral immunity (Tariq et al., 2017). Inflammatory cytokines also tend to increase with age. Acquired immunity may be negatively affected as the efficacy of vaccines is frequently decreased in older adults (Smetana, Chlibek, Shaw, et al., 2018).

Older adults have an increased incidence of infections, autoimmune diseases, metabolic diseases, osteoporosis, and neurologic disorders (Eliopoulos, 2018; Tariq et al., 2017). The increased incidence of autoimmune diseases may be from a decreased ability of antibodies to differentiate between self and non-self. Failure of the surveillance system to recognize mutant or abnormal cells may also be responsible, in part, for the high incidence of cancer associated with increasing age.

Age-related changes in many body systems also contribute to impaired immunity (Table 31-4). For example, postmenopausal females are at a greater risk for urinary tract infections due to residual urine, urinary incontinence, and estrogen deficiency (Jung & Brubaker, 2019). Secondary changes, including malnutrition and poor circulation, as well as the breakdown of natural mechanical barriers such as the skin, place the aging immune system at even greater disadvantage against infection (Tariq et al., 2017).

The effects of the aging process and psychological stress interact, with the potential to negatively influence immune integrity (Gidron, 2019). Consequently, continual assessment of the physical and emotional status of older adults is imperative, because early recognition and management of factors influencing immune response may prevent or mitigate the high morbidity and mortality seen with illness in the older adult population.

Nutrition

Nutritional status is a key determinant of health. Traditionally, the relationship between infection and nutrition focused on the effect of nutrients on host defenses and the effect of infection on nutritional needs (Yaqoob, 2017). This has expanded in scope to encompass the role of specific nutrients in acquired immune function—the modulation of inflammatory processes and the virulence of the infectious agent itself (Lang & Aspinall, 2017). Iron and the immune system are linked in homeostasis and pathology, thus making it essential for maximum function (Martins, Almeida, Lima, et al., 2017). The list of nutrients affecting infection, immunity, inflammation, and cell injury has expanded from traditional proteins to several vitamins, multiple minerals, and, more recently, specific lipid components of the diet. The role of micronutrients and fatty acids on the response of cells and tissues to hypoxic and toxic damage has been recognized, suggesting that there is another dimension to the relationship. Deficiencies in micronutrients have been connected to impairment in various body functions, including immunity (Carr & Maggini, 2017; Mikkelsen & Apostolopoulos, 2018).

TABLE 31-4 Age-Related Changes in Immunologic Function

Body System	Changes	Consequences
Immune	Impaired function of B and T lymphocytes Failure of lymphocytes to recognize mutant or abnormal cells Decreased antibody production Failure of immune system to differentiate "self" from "non-self" Suppressed phagocytic immune response	Suppressed responses to pathogenic organisms with increased risk for infection Increased incidence of cancers Anergy (lack of response to antigens applied to the skin [allergens]) Increased incidence of autoimmune diseases Absence of typical signs and symptoms of infection and inflammation Dissemination of organisms usually destroyed or suppressed by phagocytes (e.g., reactivation or spread of tuberculosis)
Gastrointestinal	Decreased gastric secretions and motility Decreased phagocytosis by the liver's Kupffer cells Altered nutritional intake with inadequate protein intake	Proliferation of intestinal organisms resulting in gastroenteritis and diarrhea Increased incidence and severity of hepatitis B; increased incidence of liver abscesses Suppressed immune response
Urinary	Decreased kidney function and changes in lower urinary tract function (enlargement of prostate gland, neurogenic bladder); altered genitourinary tract flora	Urinary stasis and increased incidence of urinary tract infections
Pulmonary	Impaired ciliary action due to exposure to smoke and environmental toxins	Impaired clearance of pulmonary secretions; increased incidence of respiratory infections
Integumentary	Thinning of skin with less elasticity; loss of adipose tissue	Increased risk of skin injury, breakdown, and infection
Circulatory	Impaired microcirculation	Stasis and pressure injuries
Neurologic function	Decreased sensation and slowing of reflexes	Increased risk of injury, skin ulcers, abrasions, and burns

Adapted from Eliopoulos, C. (2018). *Gerontological nursing* (9th ed.). Philadelphia, PA: Wolters Kluwer.

Zinc deficiency in particular has been linked to the development of a number of diseases. Zinc plays an important role in homeostasis, immune function, and apoptosis, among other functions (Wessels, Maywald, & Rink, 2017).

The effects exerted by polyunsaturated fatty acids on immune system functions are under investigation. Studies suggest that these elements play a role in diminishing the incidence and severity of inflammatory disorders. Research suggests that diets high in olive oil are not as immunosuppressive as diets rich in fish oil. The contribution of immune modulation by lipids to the high risk of infectious complications associated with the use of parenteral nutrition is unclear (Raman, Almutairdi, Mulesa, et al., 2017).

Depletion of protein reserves results in atrophy of lymphoid tissues, depression of antibody response, reduction in the number of circulating T cells, and impaired phagocytic function. As a result, susceptibility to infection is greatly increased. During periods of infection or serious illness, nutritional requirements may be further altered, potentially contributing to depletion of protein, fatty acid, vitamin, and trace elements and causing even greater risk of impaired immune response and sepsis (Wischmeyer, 2018). Nutritional intake that supports a competent immune response plays an important role in reducing the incidence of infections (Shlisky, Bloom, Beaudreault, et al., 2017); patients whose nutritional status is compromised have a delayed postoperative recovery and often experience more severe infections and delayed wound healing. There is evidence that nutrition plays a role in the development of cancer and that diet and lifestyle can alter the risk of cancer development as well as other chronic diseases (Theodoratou, Timofeeva, Li, et al., 2017). The nurse must assume a proactive role in ensuring the best possible nutritional intake for all patients as a vital step in preventing disease and poor outcomes. The nurse must assess the patient's nutritional status, caloric intake, and quality of foods ingested (see Chapter 4 for further discussion of nutritional assessment).

Immunization

The patient is asked about childhood and adult immunizations, including vaccinations to provide protection against influenza, pneumococcal diseases, herpes zoster, pertussis, and the usual childhood diseases (e.g., measles, mumps). Education about the importance of adhering to the recommended schedule for adult vaccines should be initiated. See Chapter 3, Table 3-3: Select Health Promotion Screening for Adults for more information about adult immunizations.

Infection

A history of past and present infections and the dates and types of treatments, along with a history of any multiple persistent infections, fevers of unknown origin, lesions or sores, or any type of drainage, as well as the response to treatment, are obtained.

Known past or present exposure to tuberculosis is assessed, and the dates and results of any tuberculin tests (purified protein derivative [PPD] test) and chest x-rays are documented. Recent exposure to any infections, recent travel, and dates are elicited. The nurse must assess whether the patient has been exposed to any sexually transmitted infections (STIs) or bloodborne pathogens such as hepatitis B, C, and D viruses

and human immune deficiency virus (HIV). A history of STIs such as gonorrhea, syphilis, human papillomavirus infection, and chlamydia can alert the nurse that the patient may have been exposed to HIV or hepatitis. Herpes simplex virus infections have a significant impact on health, causing a wide range of diseases (e.g., oral and genital herpes).

Allergy

The patient is asked about any allergies, including types of allergens (e.g., pollens, dust, plants, cosmetics, food, medications, vaccines, latex), the symptoms experienced, and seasonal variations in occurrence or severity in the symptoms. A history of testing and treatments, including prescribed and over-the-counter medications that the patient has taken or is currently taking for these allergies and the effectiveness of the treatments, is obtained. All medication and food allergies are listed on paper records with an allergy alert sticker or within the patient's electronic health record (EHR) to make others aware of these allergies. Continued assessment for potential allergic reactions in the patient is vital. See Chapter 33 for more information on allergies.

Disorders and Diseases

Part of the focused immunologic assessment includes determining whether the patient has a history of autoimmune disorders, neoplasms, chronic illnesses, surgeries, or any recent major stressors that may place the patient at increased risk.

Autoimmune Disorders

Autoimmune disorders affect people of both genders of all ages, ethnicities, and social classes. Autoimmune disorders are a group of disorders that can affect almost any cell or tissue in the body (Norris, 2019). As mentioned previously, they tend to be more common in women because estrogen tends to enhance immunity. Androgen, on the other hand, tends to be immunosuppressive. Autoimmune diseases are a leading cause of death by disease in females of reproductive age.

The patient is asked about any autoimmune disorders, such as lupus erythematosus, rheumatoid arthritis, multiple sclerosis, or psoriasis. The onset, severity, remissions and exacerbations, functional limitations, treatments that the patient has received or is currently receiving, and effectiveness of the treatments are described. Certain autoimmune diseases appear to be genetically linked, so a family history of these is important (Generali, Ceribelli, Stazi, et al., 2017) (Chart 31-4).

Neoplastic Disease

If there is a history of cancer in the family, more information is obtained, including the type of cancer, age at onset, and relationship (maternal or paternal) of the patient to the affected family members. Dates and results of any cancer screening tests for the patient are documented.

A history of cancer in the patient is also obtained, along with the type of cancer, date of diagnosis, and treatment modalities used. Immunosuppression contributes to the development of cancers; however, cancer itself is immunosuppressive, as are many treatments for cancer. Large tumors can release antigens into the blood, and these antigens combine with circulating antibodies and prevent them from attacking the tumor cells. Furthermore, tumor cells may possess special

Chart 31-4 GENETICS IN NURSING PRACTICE

Immunologic Disorders

An immunologic disorder is a disorder of a person's immune system, which is a network of cells, tissues, and organs that work together to defend the body against attacks by foreign invaders such as bacteria, parasites, and fungi that can cause infection. A number of immunologic disorders have a known inheritance pattern, while others are noted to have a genetic abnormality that is influenced by environmental exposures. Therefore, the pattern of inheritance is unclear in some immunologic disorders. Examples of immunologic disorders caused by a genetic abnormality include:

- Adenosine deaminase deficiency (autosomal recessive)
- Alopecia areata
- Alopecia totalis
- Asthma
- Ataxia telangiectasia (autosomal recessive)
- Autoimmune polyglandular syndrome
- Bruton agammaglobulinemia (X-linked)
- Burkitt lymphoma
- Crohn's disease
- Diabetes, type 1
- DiGeorge syndrome (Autosomal dominant)
- Familial Mediterranean fever
- Job syndrome (autosomal dominant and recessive)
- Purine nucleoside phosphorylase deficiency (autosomal dominant)
- Severe combined immunodeficiency (primarily X-linked)
- Wiskott–Aldrich syndrome (X-linked)

Nursing Assessments

Refer to Chapter 4, Chart 4-2: Genetics in Nursing Practice: Genetic Aspects of Health Assessment

Family History Assessment Specific to Immunologic Disorders

- Collect a family history for both maternal and paternal relatives for three generations.
- Assess family history for other family members with histories of immunologic disorders.

- Obtain information about family members with a history of recurrent infections or illness.
- Recognize ethnic risk (non-Ashkenazi Jewish, Armenian, Arab, and Turkish are at greater risk for familial Mediterranean fever; Caucasians have a higher incidence of Crohn's disease)

Patient Assessment

- Assess for symptoms such as changes in respiratory status associated with asthma (e.g., wheezing, or airway hyperresponsiveness; mucosal edema; and mucus production).
- Gather information regarding immunizations and whether an altered response to any immunization has occurred.
- Assess for symptoms of Immunodeficiency disorders, such as unexplained weight gain or loss, skin rashes, changes in hair texture or distribution, joint or muscle pain, intolerance to cold, irregular menstrual periods, abdominal discomfort, or the presence of diarrhea.
- Identify pattern of sickness with regard to frequency of colds, respiratory infections, or history of illness that tends to linger.
- Obtain history of childhood illnesses and details of the illness experience.
- Assess for medical history of frequent or recurrent infections.
- Learn about susceptibility to infections, assess for patterns (frequency, length of illness, severity of symptoms), and recognize infections that would be atypical for age.
- Inquire about environmental exposures (e.g., smoke, chloroform, metal or dust particles, paint).
- Ask about exposure to other viruses such as Epstein–Barr or Influenza.

Resources

American Autoimmune Related Diseases Association, www.aarda.org
Genetic and Rare Diseases Information Center, www.rarediseases.info.nih.gov
See Chapter 6, Chart 6-7 for components of genetic counseling.

---

blocking factors that coat tumor cells and prevent their destruction by killer T lymphocytes. During the early development of tumors, the body may fail to recognize the tumor antigens as foreign and subsequently fail to initiate destruction of the malignant cells. Hematologic cancers, such as leukemia and lymphoma, are associated with altered production and function of WBCs and lymphocytes.

All treatments that the patient has received or is currently receiving, such as radiation, chemotherapy, and immunotherapy, are recorded in the health history. In addition, the nurse should elicit information related to complementary or alternative modalities that have been used and the response to these efforts. Radiation destroys lymphocytes and decreases the ability to mount an effective immune response. The size and extent of the irradiated area determine the extent of immunosuppression. Whole-body irradiation may leave the patient completely immunosuppressed. Chemotherapy and other cancer treatments also affect bone marrow function, destroying cells that contribute to an effective immune response and resulting in immunosuppression. Immunotherapy can cause inflammatory overreactions of the immune system that mimic autoimmune disorders (Kroschinsky, Stolzel, von Bonin, et al., 2017; Munro, 2019).

Chronic Illness and Surgery

The health assessment includes a history of chronic illness, particularly diabetes, renal disease, or chronic obstructive pulmonary disease (COPD). The onset and severity of illnesses, as well as treatment that the patient is receiving for the illness, are obtained. Chronic illness may contribute to immune system impairments in various ways. Kidney injury is associated with a deficiency in circulating lymphocytes. In addition, immune defenses may be altered by acidosis and uremic toxins. In diabetes, an increased incidence of infection has been associated with vascular insufficiency, neuropathy, and poor control of serum glucose levels. Recurrent respiratory tract infections are associated with COPD due to altered inspiratory and expiratory function and ineffective airway clearance. In addition, a history of organ transplantation or surgical removal of the spleen, lymph nodes, or thymus should be noted, because these conditions may place the patient at risk for impaired immune function (Bagatini, Cardoso, dos Santos, et al., 2017; Dionne, Dehority, Brett, et al., 2017).

Special Problems

Conditions such as burns and other forms of injury and infection may contribute to altered immune system function.

Major burns cause impaired skin integrity and compromise the body's first line of defense. Loss of large amounts of serum occurs with burn injuries and depletes the body of essential proteins, including immunoglobulins.

The physiologic and psychological stressors associated with surgery or injury stimulate cortisol release from the adrenal cortex; increased serum cortisol also contributes to suppression of normal immune responses. The immune system's inflammatory response to surgery is followed by an anti-inflammatory compensatory response, and it is thought that these responses may contribute to postoperative complications (Cerra, 2018).

Patients who have had an ischemic stroke or transient ischemic attack (TIA) are at risk for infection following the event. Evidence suggests that an acute stroke leads to immunosuppression and a subsequently high infection risk; infection is the leading cause of death following a stroke (Hoffmann, Harms, Ulm, et al., 2017). Stroke-induced immunosuppression is linked to the development of stroke-associated pneumonia, which is the most common infection seen in patients who have had a stroke (Liu, Chu, Chen, et al., 2018).

Medications and Blood Transfusions

A list of past and present medications is obtained. In large doses, antibiotics, corticosteroids, cytotoxic agents, salicylates, nonsteroidal anti-inflammatory drugs, and anesthetic agents can cause immune suppression (Table 31-5).

A history of blood transfusions is obtained; previous exposure to foreign antigens through transfusion may be associated with abnormal immune function. In addition, although the risk of HIV transmission through blood transfusion is extremely low in patients who received a transfusion after 1985 (when testing of blood for HIV was initiated in the United States), a small risk remains.

The patient is also asked about the use of herbal agents and over-the-counter medications. Because many herbal agents have not been subjected to rigorous testing, their effects have not been fully identified. It is important, therefore, to ask patients about their use of these substances, to document their use, and to educate patients about untoward effects that may alter immune responsiveness.

Lifestyle Factors

Personal lifestyle choices have an impact on the immune system. Poor nutritional intake, smoking (Qiu, Liang, Liu, et al., 2017), excessive consumption of alcohol (Rehm, Gmel, Gmel, et al., 2017), illicit drug use, and occupational or residential exposure to environmental radiation and pollutants have been associated with impaired immune function and are assessed in a detailed patient history. Although factors that

TABLE 31-5	Select Medications and Effects on the Immune System
Drug Classification (and Examples)	**Effects on the Immune System**
Antibiotics (in Large Doses)	**Bone Marrow Suppression**
ceftriaxone	Eosinophilia, hemolytic anemia, hypoprothrombinemia, neutropenia, thrombocytopenia
cefuroxime sodium	Eosinophilia, hemolytic anemia, hypoprothrombinemia, neutropenia, thrombocytopenia
chloramphenicol	Leukopenia, aplastic anemia
dactinomycin	Agranulocytosis, neutropenia
fluoroquinolones (ciprofloxacin, levofloxacin)	Hemolytic anemia, methemoglobinemia, eosinophilia, leukopenia, pancytopenia
gentamicin sulfate	Agranulocytosis, granulocytosis
macrolides (erythromycin, azithromycin, clarithromycin)	Neutropenia, leukopenia
penicillins	Agranulocytosis
streptomycin	Leukopenia, neutropenia, pancytopenia
vancomycin	Transient leucopenia
Antithyroid Drugs	
propylthiouracil	Agranulocytosis, leukopenia
Nonsteroidal Anti-Inflammatory Drugs (NSAIDs) (in Large Doses)	**Inhibit Prostaglandin Synthesis or Release**
aspirin	Agranulocytosis
COX-2 inhibitors (celecoxib)	Anemia, allergy, no other major adverse effects
ibuprofen	Leukopenia, neutropenia
indomethacin	Agranulocytosis, leukopenia
phenylbutazone	Pancytopenia, agranulocytosis, aplastic anemia
Adrenal Corticosteroids	**Immunosuppression**
prednisone	
Antineoplastic Agents (cytotoxic agents)	**Immunosuppression**
cyclophosphamide	Leukopenia, neutropenia
cisplatin	Leukopenia
cyclosporine	Leukopenia, inhibits T-lymphocyte function
Antimetabolites	**Immunosuppression**
pyrimidine antagonist	Leukopenia, eosinophilia
folic acid antagonist	Leukopenia, aplastic bone marrow
purine antagonist	Leukopenia, pancytopenia

COX, cyclo-oxygenase.
Adapted from Comerford, K. C., & Durkin, M. T. (Eds.). (2020). *Nursing 2020 drug handbook.* Philadelphia, PA: Wolters Kluwer.

are not consistent with a healthy lifestyle are predominately responsible for ineffective immune function, positive lifestyle factors can also negatively affect immune function and require assessment. For example, rigorous exercise or competitive exercise—usually considered a positive lifestyle factor—can be a physiologic stressor and cause negative effects on immune response (Aoi & Naito, 2019; Shaw, Merien, Braakhuis, et al., 2018).

Psychoneuroimmunologic Factors

The bidirectional pathway between the brain and immune system (the mind–body system) is referred to as psychoneuroimmunology. Patient assessment must also address psychoneuroimmunologic factors, such as stress and psychological illness, that may be influencing the patient's health. The immune response is regulated and modulated in part by neuroendocrine influences. Lymphocytes and macrophages have receptors that can respond to neurotransmitters and endocrine hormones. Lymphocytes can produce and secrete adrenocorticotropic hormone and endorphinlike compounds. Cells in the brain, especially in the hypothalamus, can recognize prostaglandins, interferons, and interleukins, as well as histamine and serotonin, all of which are released during the inflammatory process. Like all other biologic systems functioning to maintain homeostasis, the immune system is integrated with other psychophysiologic processes and is regulated and modulated by the brain. These relationships may have immunologic consequences (Lasselin, Schedlowski, Lekander, et al., 2019).

Growing evidence indicates that a measurable immune system response can be positively influenced by biobehavioral strategies such as relaxation, imagery techniques, biofeedback, humor, hypnosis, mindfulness-based strategies, and yoga (Park & Han, 2017; Pascoe, Thompson, & Ski, 2017; Reich, Lengacher, Klein, et al., 2017). Therefore, the assessment should address the patient's general psychological status and the patient's use of and response to these strategies. See the Nursing Research Profile in Chart 31-5.

Physical Assessment

During the physical examination (see Chart 31-3), the skin and mucous membranes are assessed for lesions, dermatitis, purpura (subcutaneous bleeding), urticaria, inflammation, or any discharge. Any signs of infection are noted. The patient's temperature is recorded, and the patient is observed for chills and sweating. The anterior and posterior cervical, supraclavicular, axillary, and inguinal lymph nodes are palpated for enlargement; if palpable nodes are detected, their location, size, consistency, and reports of tenderness on palpation are noted. Joints are assessed for tenderness, swelling, increased warmth, and limited range of motion. The patient's respiratory, cardiovascular, genitourinary, gastrointestinal, and neurosensory systems are evaluated for signs and symptoms indicative of immune dysfunction. Any functional limitations or disabilities the patient may have are also assessed.

Diagnostic Evaluation

A series of blood tests and skin tests, as well as bone marrow biopsy, may be performed to evaluate the patient's immune competence. Specific laboratory and diagnostic tests are discussed in greater detail along with individual disease processes in subsequent chapters in this unit. Select laboratory and diagnostic tests used to evaluate immune competence are summarized in Chart 31-6.

Nursing Management

The nurse needs to be aware that patients undergoing evaluation for possible immune system disorders experience not only physical pain and discomfort with certain types of diagnostic procedures but also many psychological reactions. It is the nurse's role to counsel, educate, and support patients throughout the diagnostic process. Many patients may be extremely anxious about the results of diagnostic tests and the

---

Chart 31-5 — NURSING RESEARCH PROFILE

Stress Reduction and Effect on Inflammatory Cytokines

Reich, R. R., Lengacher, C. A., Klein, T. W., et al. (2017). A randomized controlled trial of the effects of mindfulness-based stress reduction (MBSR[BC]) on levels of inflammatory biomarkers among recovering breast cancer survivors. *Biological Research for Nursing*, 19(4), 456–464.

Purpose

The purpose of this study was to evaluate the efficacy of the Mindfulness-Based Stress Reduction (Breast Cancer) (MBSR[BC]) program versus usual care in normalizing blood levels of proinflammatory cytokines among breast cancer survivors.

Design

This was a substudy of a large randomized controlled trial. A total of 322 participants were randomized to a 6-wk MBSR(BC) program or usual care. Blood samples, demographic data (age, race, and ethnicity), and clinical data (disease stage and treatments) were collected at baseline, 6 wks, and 12 wks. Plasma cytokines (IL-1β, IL-6, IL-10), tumor necrosis factor α (TNF-α), transforming growth factor β1, and soluble tumor necrosis factor receptor 1 (sTNFR1) were assayed. Linear mixed models were used to assess the cytokine levels across the three time points by group.

Findings

Three of the cytokines were not detectable and thus not analyzed further. For the remaining cytokines (TNF-α, IL-6, sTNFR1), TNFα and IL-6 increased during the follow-up period between 6 and 12 wks, but not during the MBSR(BC) training period (baseline to 6 wks). The sTNFR1 levels did not change across the 12-wk study period significantly. The s cytokines TNF-α and IL-6 may be markers for recovery.

Nursing Implications

Patients recovering from cancer treatment are at increased risk for infections and increased levels of psychological distress. Stress reducing activities and programs such as the 2 h per wk mindfulness program can be implemented in clinical practice as part of an interdisciplinary approach to cancer care. Nurses should advise patients that the programs may not take effect immediately; in fact, some of the increases in cytokine levels were not seen until 6 wks after the program ended.

Chart 31-6 Select Tests for Evaluating Immunologic Status

Various laboratory tests may be performed to assess immune system activity or dysfunction. The studies assess leukocytes and lymphocytes, humoral immunity, cellular immunity, phagocytic cell function, complement activity, hypersensitivity reactions, specific antigen–antibodies, or human immune deficiency virus infection.

Humoral (Antibody-Mediated) Immunity Tests

- B-cell quantification with monoclonal antibody
- In vivo immunoglobulin synthesis with T-cell subsets
- Specific antibody response
- Total serum globulins and individual immunoglobulins (electrophoresis, immunoelectrophoresis, single radial immunodiffusion, nephelometry, and isohemagglutinin techniques)

Cellular (Cell-Mediated) Immunity Tests

- Total lymphocyte count
- T-cell and T-cell subset quantification with monoclonal antibody
- Delayed hypersensitivity skin test
- Cytokine production
- Lymphocyte response to mitogens, antigens, and allogeneic cells
- Helper and suppressor T-cell functions

Adapted from Fischbach, F. T., & Fischbach, M. A. (2018). *A manual of laboratory and diagnostic tests* (10th ed.). Philadelphia, PA: Wolters Kluwer.

possible implications of those results for their future health, employment, and personal relationships. This is an ideal time for the nurse to provide counseling and education, should these interventions be warranted.

CRITICAL THINKING EXERCISES

1 **pq** You are caring for an 80-year-old woman who is admitted to a long-term care facility after having a stroke. What potential immunity-related complications do you need to be aware of for this patient? What are your priority nursing observations and assessments? Identify priorities for this patient's care given her recent stroke.

2 **ebp** A 40-year-old woman with melanoma is being treated with immunotherapy and is admitted to your hospital for treatment-related pneumonitis. She is prescribed high-dose corticosteroids for treatment of the pneumonitis. The patient has asked you to explain what is happening to her and why this has occurred. How will you educate her and her family about her current condition? Develop an evidence-based education plan for the patient and her family. Discuss the criteria used to assess the strength of the evidence for your education plan.

3 **ipe** A 35-year-old pregnant woman with systemic lupus erythematosus (SLE) presents with an acute flare-up of her symptoms. How might psychosocial and emotional factors impact her health? What interdisciplinary referrals would you anticipate for this patient's care?

REFERENCES

*Asterisk indicates nursing research.

Books

Aoi, W., & Naito, Y. (2019). Immune function, nutrition, and exercise. In D. Bagchi, S. Nair, & C. K. Sen (Eds.). *Nutrition and enhanced sports performance: Muscle building, endurance, and strength* (2nd ed.). Cambridge, MA: Elsevier.

Cerra, F. B. (2018). Tissue injury, nutrition, and immune function. In R. A. Forse (Ed.). *Diet, nutrition, and immunity*. Boca Raton, FL: CRC Press.

Comerford, K. C., & Durkin, M. T. (Eds.). (2020). *Nursing 2020 drug handbook*. Philadelphia, PA: Wolters Kluwer.

Eliopoulos, C. (2018). *Gerontological nursing* (9th ed.). Philadelphia, PA: Wolters Kluwer.

Fischbach, F. T., & Fischbach, M. A. (2018). *A manual of laboratory and diagnostic tests* (10th ed.). Philadelphia, PA: Wolters Kluwer.

Gidron, Y. (2019). Psychological aspects of ageing. In Y. Gidron (Ed.). *Behavioral medicine*. New York: Springer International Publishing.

Haynes, B. F., Soderberg, K. A., & Fauci, A. S. (2018). Introduction to the immune system. In J. L. Jameson, A. S. Fauci, D. L. Kasper, et al. (Eds.). *Harrison's principles of internal medicine* (20th ed.). New York: McGraw-Hill Education.

Klimov, V. V. (2019). *From basic to clinical immunology* (1st ed.). New York: Springer International Publishing.

Mikkelsen, K., & Apostolopoulos, V. (2018). B vitamins and aging. In J. Harris & V. Korolchuk (Eds.). *Biochemistry and cell biology of ageing: Part I biomedical science subcellular biochemistry*. Singapore: Springer.

Norris, T. L. (2019). *Porth's pathophysiology: Concepts of altered health states* (10th ed.). Philadelphia, PA: Wolters Kluwer.

Tariq, M. A., Hazeldine, J., & Lord, J. M. (2017). In V. Bueno, J. M. Lord, & T. A. Jackson (Eds.). *The ageing immune system and health*. New York: Springer International Publishing.

Journals and Electronic Documents

Bagatini, M. D., Cardoso, A. M., dos Santos, A. A., et al. (2017). Immune system and chronic disease. *Journal of Immunology Research*. Doi.org/10.1155/2017/4284327

Carr, A. C., & Maggini, S. (2017). Vitamin C and immune function. *Nutrients, 9*(11), E1211.

Chae, W. J., & Bothwell, A. L. M. (2018). Therapeutic potential of gene-modified regulatory T cells: From bench to bedside. *Frontiers in Immunology, 9*, 303.

Davis, B. P., & Ballas, Z. K. (2017). Biologic response modifiers: Indications, implications and insights. *Journal of Allergy and Clinical Immunology, 139*(5), 1445–1456.

Dionne, B., Dehority, W., Brett, M., et al. (2017). The asplenic patient: Post-insult immunocompetence, infection, and vaccination. *Surgical Infections, 18*(5), 267.

Generali, E., Ceribelli, A., Stazi, M. A., et al. (2017). Lessons learned from twins in autoimmune and chronic inflammatory diseases. *Journal of Autoimmunity, 83*, 51–61.

Gonçalves, G. A. R., & Paiva, R. de M. A. (2017). Gene therapy: Advances, challenges and perspectives. *Einstein (Sao Paolo), 15*(3), 369–375.

Hoffmann, S., Harms, H., Ulm, L., et al. (2017). Stroke-induced immunodepression and dysphagia independently predict stroke-associated pneumonia—The PREDICT study. *Journal of Cerebral Blood Flow and Metabolism, 37*(12), 3671–3682.

Jung, C., & Brubaker, L. (2019). The etiology and management of recurrent urinary tract infections in postmenopausal women. *Climacteric, 22*(3), 242–249.

Kroschinsky, F., Stolzel, F., von Bonin, S., et al. (2017). New drugs, new toxicities: Severe side effects of modern targeted and immunotherapy of cancer and their management. *Critical Care, 21*(89), 1–11.

Lang, P. O., & Aspinall, R. (2017). Vitamin D status and the host resistance to infections: What it is currently (not) understood. *Clinical Therapeutics, 39*(5), 930–945.

Lasselin, J., Schedlowski, M., Lekander, M., et al. (2019). Editorial: Clinical relevance of the immune-to-brain and brain-to-immune communications. *Frontiers in Behavioral Neuroscience, 12*, 336.

Leleu, X., Gay, F., Flament, A., et al. (2017). Incidence of neutropenia and use of granulocyte colony-stimulating factors in multiple myeloma: Is current clinical practice adequate? *Annals of Hematology, 97*(3), 387–400.

Liu, D. D., Chu, S. F., Chen, C., et al. (2018). Research progress in stroke-induced immunodepression syndrome (SIDS) and stroke-associated pneumonia (SAP). *Neurochemistry International, 114,* 42–54.

Makowska, A., Braunschweig, T., Denecke, B., et al. (2019). Interferon β and Anti-PD-1/PD-L1 checkpoint blockade cooperate in NK cell-mediated killing of nasopharyngeal carcinoma cells. *Translational Oncology, 12*(9), 1237–1256.

Martins, A. C., Almeida, J. I., Lima, I. S., et al. (2017). Iron metabolism and inflammatory response. *International Union of Biochemistry and Molecular Biology, 69*(6), 442–450.

Munro, N. (2019). Immunology and immunotherapy in critical care: An overview. *AACN Advanced Critical Care, 30*(2), 113–125.

Park, S. H., & Han, K. S. (2017). Blood pressure response to meditation and yoga: A systematic review and meta-analysis. *Journal of Alternative and Complementary Medicine, 23*(9), 685–695.

Pascoe, M. C., Thompson, D. R., & Ski, C. F. (2017). Yoga, mindfulness-based stress reduction and stress-related physiological measures: A meta-analysis. *Psychoneuroendocrinology, 86,* 152–168.

Pento, J. T. (2017). Monoclonal antibodies for the treatment of cancer. *Anticancer Research, 37*(11), 5935–5939.

Qiu, F., Liang, C. L., Liu, H., et al. (2017). Impacts of cigarette smoking on immune responsiveness: Up and down or upside down. *Oncotarget, 8*(1), 268–284.

Rainville, J. R., Tsyglakova, M., & Hodes, G. E. (2018). Deciphering sex differences in the immune system and depression. *Frontiers in Neuroendocrinology, 50,* 67–90.

Raman, M., Almutairdi, A., Mulesa, L., et al. (2017). Parenteral nutrition and lipids. *Nutrients, 9*(4), E388.

Rehm, J., Gmel, G. E., Gmel, G., et al. (2017). The relationship between different dimensions of alcohol use and the burden of disease—an update. *Addiction, 112*(6), 968–1001.

*Reich, R. R., Lengacher, C. A., Klein, T. W., et al. (2017). A randomized controlled trial of the effects of mindfulness-based stress reduction (MBSR[BC]) on levels of inflammatory biomarkers among recovering breast cancer survivors. *Biological Research for Nursing, 19*(4), 456–464.

Ribas, A., & Wolchok, J. D. (2018). Cancer immunotherapy using checkpoint blockade. *Science, 359*(6382), 1350–1355.

Romano, M., Fanelli, G., Albany, C. J., et al. (2019). Past, present, and future of regulatory T cell therapy in transplantation and autoimmunity. *Frontiers in Immunology, 10.* Doi.org/10.3389/fimmu.2019.00043

Shaw, D. M., Merien, F., Braakhuis, A., et al. (2018). T-cells and their cytokine production: The anti-inflammatory and immunosuppressive effects of strenuous exercise. *Cytokine, 104,* 136–142.

Shlisky, J., Bloom, D. E., Beaudreault, A. R., et al. (2017). Nutritional considerations for healthy aging and reduction in age-related chronic disease. *Advances in Nutrition, 8*(1), 17–26.

Singh, S., Tank, N. K., Dwivedi, P., et al. (2018). Monoclonal antibodies: A review. *Current Clinical Pharmacology, 13*(2), 85–99.

Smetana, J., Chlibek, R., Shaw, J., et al. (2018). Influenza vaccination in the elderly. *Human Vaccine and Immunotherapeutics, 14*(3), 540–549.

Theodoratou, E., Timofeeva, M., Li, X., et al. (2017). Nature, nurture, and cancer risks: Genetic and nutritional contributions to cancer. *Annual Review of Nutrition, 37,* 293–320.

Wessels, I., Maywald, M., & Rink, L. (2017). Zinc as a gatekeeper of immune function. *Nutrients, 9*(12), E1286.

Wischmeyer, P. E. (2018). Nutrition therapy in sepsis. *Critical Care Clinics, 34*(1), 107–125.

Yaqoob, P. (2017). Ageing alters the impact of nutrition on immune function. *Proceedings of the Nutrition Society, 76*(3), 347–351.

Resources

American Academy of Allergy, Asthma & Immunology, www.aaaai.org

American Cancer Society, www.cancer.org

Centers for Disease Control and Prevention, www.cdc.gov

National Institute of Allergy and Infectious Diseases, www.niaid.nih.gov

National Institutes of Health, Health Information, www.nih.gov/health/infoline.htm

National Institutes of Health, National Cancer Institute, www.cancer.gov

U.S. Department of Health & Human Services, www.hhs.gov

32

Management of Patients with Immune Deficiency Disorders

LEARNING OUTCOMES

On completion of this chapter, the learner will be able to:

1. Identify the pathophysiology, clinical manifestations, and nursing management of patients with primary immune deficiency disorders.
2. Describe the modes of transmission of human immune deficiency virus infection and prevention strategies.
3. Explain the pathophysiology associated with the clinical manifestations of human immune deficiency virus and

acquired immune deficiency syndrome and the purpose of antiretroviral therapy.
4. Use the nursing process as a framework for care of the patient with human immune deficiency virus/acquired immune deficiency syndrome.
5. Identify available resources for patients and support systems to promote self-management of immune deficiency disorders.

NURSING CONCEPTS

Family
Immunity

Infection
Nutrition

GLOSSARY

candidiasis: fungal infection, usually of skin or mucous membranes, caused by Candida species

enzyme immunoassay (EIA): a blood test that can determine the presence of antibodies to HIV in the blood or saliva; a variant of this test is called enzyme-linked immunosorbent assay (ELISA)

HIV-1: retrovirus isolated and recognized as the etiologic agent of HIV disease

HIV encephalopathy: clinical syndrome characterized by a progressive decline in cognitive, behavioral, and motor functions

immune reconstitution inflammatory syndrome (IRIS): a syndrome that results from rapid restoration of pathogen-specific immune responses to opportunistic infections

Kaposi sarcoma: malignancy that involves the epithelial layer of blood and lymphatic vessels

latent reservoir: the integrated HIV provirus within the CD4$^+$ T cell during the resting memory state; does not express viral proteins and is invisible to the immune system and antiviral medications

Mycobacterium avium complex (MAC): opportunistic infection caused by mycobacterial organisms that commonly causes a respiratory illness but can also infect other body systems

opportunistic infection: illness caused by various organisms, some of which typically do not cause disease in people with normal immune systems

peripheral neuropathy: disorder characterized by sensory loss, pain, muscle weakness, and wasting of muscles in the hands or legs and feet

Pneumocystis pneumonia (PCP): common opportunistic lung infection; pathogen implicated is *Pneumocystis jirovecii*

polymerase chain reaction (PCR): a sensitive laboratory technique that can detect and quantify HIV in a person's blood or lymph nodes

post-exposure prophylaxis (PEP): taking antiretroviral medicines as soon as possible, but no more than 72 hours (3 days) after possible HIV exposure; two to three drugs are usually prescribed which must be taken for 28 days

pre-exposure prophylaxis (PrEP): prevention method for HIV-negative people who are at high risk of HIV infection; involves taking a specific combination of HIV medicines daily; use with condoms and other prevention tools

primary immune deficiency diseases (PIDDs): rare, genetic disorders that impair the immune system

progressive multifocal leukoencephalopathy: opportunistic infection that infects brain tissue and causes damage to the brain and spinal cord

retrovirus: a virus that carries genetic material in ribonucleic acid (RNA) instead of DNA and contains reverse transcriptase

viral load test: measures the quantity of HIV RNA or DNA in the blood

viral set point: amount of virus present in the blood after the initial burst of viremia and the immune response that follows

wasting syndrome: involuntary weight loss consisting of both lean and fat body mass

The human immune system is complex and multidimensional. It works to protect against invasion by foreign substances, protect against the proliferation of neoplastic cells, and plays a key role in inflammation and healing. Patients with primary or secondary immune system disorders (Norris, 2019) require care from nurses who are knowledgeable about the pathophysiology, diagnostic procedures, and interventions that are used in the management of these disorders.

PRIMARY IMMUNE DEFICIENCIES DISEASES

The majority of **primary immune deficiency diseases (PIDDs)**, rare inherited disorders that impair the immune system, are commonly diagnosed in infancy, with a male-to-female ratio of 5 to 1. However, some PIDDs are not diagnosed until adolescence or early adulthood, when the gender distribution equalizes. Diagnosis at this stage frequently is confounded by frequent use of antibiotics that mask symptoms. Adults may present with clinical episodes of infectious diseases beyond the scope of normal immunocompetence, such as infections that are unusually persistent, recurrent, or resistant to treatment and that involve unexpected dissemination of disease or atypical pathogens. These rare inherited disorders not only lead to frequent infections, but also to increased risk of autoimmune disorders and malignancy (Hajjar, Guffey, Minard, et al., 2017).

Pathophysiology

There are more than 200 forms of PIDDs affecting about 500,000 people in the United States, and more than 270 different genes are associated with PIDDs. These rare genetic diseases prevent the body from developing normal immune responses resulting in a complex group of disorders with a wide array of clinical presentations. Many present during the first year of life and may be chronic, debilitating, and costly (National Institute of Allergy and Infectious Diseases [NIAID], 2019a).

Clinical Manifestations

Major signs and symptoms include multiple infections despite aggressive treatment, infections with unusual or opportunistic organisms, failure to thrive or poor growth, and a significant family history. Fatigue was reported in 18% of patients with PIDDs (Hajjar et al., 2017). See Table 32-1 for select PIDDs along with some of their clinical manifestations.

Assessment and Diagnostic Findings

There is often a considerable delay between the onset of symptoms and time of diagnosis of PIDDs. Because of the genetic origins of PIDDs, family history should be carefully assessed but epidemiologic data about specific infectious agents should be considered as well.

Laboratory tests are used to identify antibody deficiencies, cellular (T-cell) defects, neutrophil disorders, and complement deficiencies. A complete blood cell count with manual differential should always be analyzed first. Lymphopenia may indicate an immunologic abnormality; serum Ig levels (IgG, IgM, and IgA) and antibody responses to vaccines should be assessed to detect a humoral immune defect. Age-matched normal ranges need to be used since antibody levels change as the person ages (Fischbach & Fischbach, 2018).

Prevention

Live vaccines are contraindicated in patients with antibody deficiency disorders. The patient is incapable of generating antibodies and the live substance in the vaccine can cause disease. Family planning should be addressed in terms of future pregnancies; in some situations, prenatal in utero testing of a fetus can determine whether the infant will be affected.

Medical Management

A pattern of unusually frequent, opportunistic, or severe infections generates the possibility of a PIDD and initial testing or referral to an immunologist. Patients with neutropenia are at increased risk for developing severe infections despite substantial advances in supportive care. Epidemiologic shifts occur periodically and must be detected early because they influence prophylactic, empiric, and specific strategies for medical management. Attention to infection control practices is important, especially with the emergence of multidrug-resistant organisms.

Hematopoietic stem cell transplantation (HSCT) is a curative modality. The stem cells may be from embryos or adults. Toxicity and reduced efficacy are frequent limitations of HSCT. See Chapter 12 for further discussion of HSCT.

Another therapy involves the use of cells as vehicles for the delivery of genes or gene products. Gene therapy has had many adverse effects; the first studies in human participants revealed numerous toxicities with this therapy. Rapidly emerging new technologies allowing precise DNA targeting may prove to be a useful approach (McDermott & Murphy, 2019).

Pharmacologic Therapy

Pharmacologic treatment depends upon the type and severity of presenting infection and the particular PIDD diagnosis. Prophylactic drug treatment prevents some bacterial and

TABLE 32-1   Select Primary Immune Deficiency Disorders (PIDDs)

Disorder	Characteristics
Autoimmune lymphoproliferative syndrome (ALPS)	Unusually high numbers of lymphocytes accumulate in the lymph nodes, liver, and spleen leading to enlargement of those organs. Causes numerous autoimmune problems including low levels of red blood cells, platelets, and neutrophils that can increase the risk of infection and hemorrhage.
Autoimmune polyglandular syndrome type 1 (APS-1) (also called autoimmune polyendo-crinopathy-candidiasis-ectodermal dystrophy [APECED])	Causes a diverse range of symptoms, including autoimmunity against different types of organs and increased susceptibility to candidiasis, a fungal infection caused by *Candida* yeast.
CARD9 Deficiency and other syndromes of susceptibility to candidiasis	Results in susceptibility to fungal infections such as candidiasis; particularly susceptible to Candida infections of the central nervous system.
Chronic granulomatous disease (CGD)	May be caused by mutations in one of five different genes. Phagocytes are unable to kill certain bacteria and fungi resulting in increased susceptibility to infections.
Common variable immunodeficiency (CVID)	Caused by a variety of genetic abnormalities resulting in defective ability of immune cells to produce normal amounts of antibodies, resulting in frequent bacterial or viral infections of the upper airway, sinuses, and lungs.
Congenital neutropenia syndromes	Characterized by low levels of neutrophils from birth.
CTLA4 Deficiency	Autoimmunity, low levels of antibodies, and excessive numbers of lymphocytes which infiltrate the gut, lungs, bone marrow, central nervous system, kidneys resulting in recurrent infections.
DOCK8 Deficiency	Lower-than-normal numbers of immune cells, which have a diminished capacity to move through dense tissues like the skin leading to recurrent viral infections of the skin and respiratory system.
GATA2 Deficiency	Characterized by immune deficiency, lung disease, problems of the vascular and lymphatic systems, and myelodysplastic syndrome (a condition characterized by ineffective blood cell production).
Glycosylation disorders with immune deficiency	Defects in glycosylation, which refers to the attachment of sugars to proteins; can disrupt the immune system resulting in immune deficiency.
Hyper-immunoglobulin E syndrome (HIES)	A rare primary immune deficiency disease characterized by eczema, recurrent staphylococcal skin abscesses, recurrent lung infections, eosinophilia (a high number of eosinophils in the blood) and high serum levels of IgE.
Hyper-immunoglobulin M (hyper-IgM) syndromes	Immune system fails to produce normal IgA, IgG, and IgE antibodies but can produce normal or elevated IgM.
Interferon gamma, interleukin 12, interleukin 23 deficiencies	Interferon gamma, interleukin 12, and interleukin 23 are key signals that raise alert against bacteria and other infectious microbes; deficiencies result in susceptibility to infections caused by bacteria and viruses.
Leukocyte adhesion deficiency (LAD)	Phagocytes are unable to move to the site of an infection resulting in an inability to fight pathogens resulting in recurrent, life-threatening infections and poor wound healing.
PI3 Kinase disease	Genetic mutations overactivate an important immune signaling pathway causing a change reaction that disrupts the infection-fighting B and T cells resulting in a weakened immune system and frequent bacterial and viral infections.
PLCG2-associated antibody deficiency and immune dysregulation (PLAID)	Rare disorder with allergic response to cold (cold urticaria) as the most distinct symptom.
Severe combined immune deficiency (SCID)	Group of rare, life-threatening disorders caused by mutations in different genes involved in development and function of T and B cells; infants appear healthy at birth but are highly susceptible to severe infections.
Warts, hypogammaglobulinemia, infections, and myelokathexis syndrome (WHIMS)	Low levels of white blood cells, especially neutrophils, which predispose to frequent infections and persistent warts.
Wiskott–Aldrich syndrome (WAS)	Problems with B and T cells and platelets resulting in prolonged episodes of bleeding, recurrent bacterial and fungal infections and increased risk of cancers and autoimmune diseases.

Adapted from National Institute of Allergy and Infectious Diseases (NIAID). (2019a). Types of primary immune deficiency disorders. Retrieved on 10/13/1019 at: www.niaid.nih.gov/diseases-conditions/types-pidds

fungal infections but it must be used with caution because it has been implicated in the emergence of resistant organisms. The choices for empiric therapy include combination regimens and monotherapy. Specific choices depend on local factors (epidemiology, susceptibility/resistance patterns, availability, cost). Patients with antibody deficiencies receive regular Ig replacement therapy including both IV immunoglobulin (IVIG) and subcutaneous immunoglobulin (SCIG) to provide functional antibodies (Stonebraker, Hajjar, & Orange, 2018; Vitiello, Emmi, Silvestri, et al., 2019).

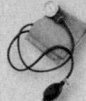 For the procedural guidelines for managing immunoglobulin therapy, go to **thepoint.lww.com/Brunner15e.**

Nursing Management

Many patients with PIDDs have comorbid autoimmune disorders, such as thyroid disease, rheumatoid arthritis, cytopenias, and inflammatory bowel disease. Many patients require immunosuppression to ensure engraftment of depleted bone marrow during transplantation procedures. For this reason, nursing care must be meticulous. Appropriate hand hygiene and infection prevention precautions are essential. See Chapter 66, Chart 66-1 for hand hygiene methods and Chart 66-2 for a summary of infection prevention precautions. Institutional policies and procedures related to infection prevention care must be followed scrupulously until definitive evidence demonstrates that precautions are unnecessary. Continual monitoring of the patient's condition is critical, so early signs of impending infection may be detected and treated before they seriously compromise the patient's status.

Patients and caregivers in the home are taught how to administer medications, including regular Ig replacement therapy, if prescribed. Instruction is provided to the patient and family about how to administer the therapy at home (see Chart 32-1). Nurses provide ongoing education and support for the patient and family.

ACQUIRED IMMUNE DEFICIENCY

Immune deficiency can be acquired due to medical treatment such as chemotherapy (see Chapter 12) or infection from pathogens such as human immune deficiency virus (HIV). Advances have been made in treating HIV infection and acquired immune deficiency syndrome (AIDS); however, AIDS remains a critical public health issue in communities across the United States and around the world. Prevention, early detection, and ongoing treatment remain important aspects of care for people living with HIV infection or AIDS, who are sometimes referred to as persons living with HIV/AIDS (PLWHA). The American Nurses Association (ANA) has issued a position statement in support of efforts to end HIV (ANA, 2019).

HIV Infection and AIDS

Since the disease now known as AIDS was first identified in 1981, remarkable progress has been made in improving the length and quality of life for PLWHA. During the first decade, progress was associated with the recognition and treatment, including prophylactic medications, of **opportunistic infections** (illnesses caused by various organisms, some of which usually do not cause disease in people with normal immune systems). The second decade witnessed progress in the development of highly active antiretroviral drug therapies (HAART) as well as continuing progress in the treatment of opportunistic infections. The third decade has focused on issues of preventing new infections, adherence to antiretroviral therapy (ART), development of second-generation combination medications that affect different stages of the viral life cycle, and continued need for an effective vaccine. The HIV antibody test, an **enzyme immunoassay** (**EIA**; or a variant of this test called *enzyme-linked immunosorbent assay* [ELISA]), became available in 1984, allowing early diagnosis of the infection before the onset of symptoms. Since then, HIV infection has been best managed as a chronic disease, most

---

Chart 32-1 **HOME CARE CHECKLIST**

Home Administration of Ig Replacement Therapy

At the completion of education, the patient and/or caregiver will be able to:

- State the impact of immune deficiency on physiologic functioning, ADLs, IADLs, roles, relationships, and spirituality.
- State what types of changes are needed (if any) to maintain a clean home environment and prevent infection.
- State how to contact the primary provider, the team of home care professionals overseeing care, and intravenous supply vendor.
- State how to obtain medical supplies and carry out dressing changes, IV access site care, and other prescribed regimens.
- Identify the benefits and expected outcome of regular Ig replacement therapy.
- State rationale for prophylactic use of acetaminophen and diphenhydramine before treatment begins.
- State the rationale for prehydration on the day before infusion.

- Demonstrate how to prepare regular Ig replacement therapy.
- Demonstrate how to administer regular Ig replacement therapy.
- Demonstrate how to clean and maintain IV equipment, as applicable.
- Identify side effects and adverse effects of regular Ig replacement therapy.
- Demonstrate how to monitor for adverse effects of regular Ig replacement therapy.
- Describe to whom, how, and when to report adverse effects of regular Ig replacement therapy.
- Describe appropriate actions to take for adverse effects.
- Verbalize understanding of emergency measures for anaphylactic shock.
- Describe time periods associated with possible development of adverse reactions

ADLs, activities of daily living; IADLs, instrumental activities of daily living.

appropriately in an outpatient care setting, whereas AIDS may involve acute conditions that require hospitalization.

Epidemiology

Since the first cases of AIDS were reported in the United States in 1981, surveillance case definitions for HIV infection and AIDS have undergone several revisions (in 1985, 1987, 1993, 2008, and 2014) in response to diagnostic advances. Criteria for a confirmed case of HIV infection can be met by either laboratory evidence or clinical evidence but laboratory evidence, usually obtained through blood tests, is preferred over clinical evidence (e.g., patient signs and symptoms). A case of HIV infection can be classified in one of five HIV infection stages (0, 1, 2, 3, or unknown). Stage 0 indicates early HIV infection, inferred from laboratory testing; stages 1, 2, and 3 are based on the CD4+ T-lymphocyte count; while cases with no information on CD4+ T-lymphocyte count or percentage are classified as stage unknown (Centers for Disease Control and Prevention [CDC], 2014). See Table 32-2 for further explanation of stages.

In July 2015, the Obama White House released the *National HIV/AIDS Strategy for the United States: Updated to 2020*. This document has four Strategic Goals, which include reducing new infections; increasing access to care and improving health outcomes for people living with HIV; reducing HIV-related health disparities and health inequities; and achieving a more coordinated national response to the HIV epidemic. The strategy is being updated by the Office of HIV/AIDS and Infectious Disease Policy (OHAIDP, 2019).

According to the CDC, 1,006,691 persons aged 13 years and older are living with HIV infection, and an additional 534,515 are living with AIDS in the United States (CDC, 2019a). From 2012 through 2016, the rate of diagnoses of HIV infection decreased, although the annual number of diagnoses remained stable as survival rates have increased. The incidence was 11.8 per 100,000 persons for 2017, with men accounting for 81% of all HIV infection diagnoses (CDC, 2019a). The incidence per 100,000 persons was 41.1 for Blacks/African Americans, followed by 16.1 for Hispanics/Latinos, and 12.6 for persons of multiple races. The highest rate (32.9%) was for persons aged 25 to 29 years, followed by 28.7% for persons aged 20 to 24 years. Male-to-male sexual contact (MSM) (70%, including 3% male-to-male sexual contact and injection drug use) and

TABLE 32-2	HIV Infection Stages 1, 2, and 3 Based on Age-Specific Laboratory Data					
	Age on Date of CD4+ T-lymphocyte Test					
	<1 yr		**1–5 yrs**		**≥6 yrs**	
Stage	**Cells/IL**	**%**	**Cells/IL**	**%**	**Cells/IL**	**%**
1	≥1500	≥34	≥1000	≥30	≥500	≥26
2	750–1499	26–33	500–999	22–29	200–499	14–25
3	<750	<26	<500	<22	<200	<14

If a stage-3-defining opportunistic illness has been diagnosed, then the stage is 3 regardless of CD4+ T-lymphocyte test.

Stage-3-Defining Opportunistic Illnesses in HIV Infection
Bacterial infections, multiple or recurrent (only among children aged less than 6 yrs)
Candidiasis of bronchi, trachea, or lungs
Candidiasis of esophagus
Cervical cancer, invasive (only in persons aged 6 yrs or older)
Coccidioidomycosis, disseminated or extrapulmonary
Cryptococcosis, extrapulmonary
Cryptosporidiosis, chronic intestinal (>1 mo duration)
Cytomegalovirus disease (other than liver, spleen, or nodes), onset at age >1 mo
Cytomegalovirus retinitis (with loss of vision)
Encephalopathy attributed to HIV
Herpes simplex: chronic ulcers (>1 mo duration) or bronchitis, pneumonitis, or esophagitis (onset at age >1 mo)
Histoplasmosis, disseminated or extrapulmonary Isosporiasis, chronic intestinal (>1 mo duration)
Kaposi sarcoma
Lymphoma, Burkitt (or equivalent term)
Lymphoma, immunoblastic (or equivalent term)
Lymphoma, primary, of brain
Mycobacterium avium complex or *Mycobacterium kansasii*, disseminated or extrapulmonary
Mycobacterium tuberculosis of any site, pulmonary (only in persons aged 6 yrs or older) disseminated, or extrapulmonary
Mycobacterium, other species or unidentified species, disseminated or extrapulmonary
Pneumocystis jirovecii (previously known as "*Pneumocystis carinii*") pneumonia (PCP)
Pneumonia, recurrent (only in persons aged 6 yrs or older)
Progressive multifocal leukoencephalopathy
Salmonella septicemia (recurrent)
Toxoplasmosis of brain, onset at age >1 mo
Wasting syndrome attributed to HIV

Adapted from Centers for Disease Control and Prevention (CDC). (2014). Revised surveillance case definition for HIV infection—United States, 2014. *MMWR. Recommendations and Reports: Morbidity and Mortality Weekly Report. Recommendations and Reports*, 63(RR-03), 1–10.

those attributed to heterosexual contact (24%) accounted for approximately 94% of diagnosed HIV infections. Rates within the United States were 16.1% in the South, 10.6% in the Northeast, 9.4% in the West, and 7.4% in the Midwest (CDC, 2019a). Data about infections in transgender persons were not collected.

According to the World Health Organization ([WHO], 2019), HIV through its morbid consequence of AIDS has claimed more than 32 million lives globally; in 2018, 770,000 people died from HIV-related causes. Globally, there were approximately 37.9 million people living with HIV at the end of 2018, with 1.7 million people becoming newly infected in 2018. The WHO African Region is the most affected region, with 25.7 million people living with HIV in 2018. The African region also accounts for almost two thirds of the global total of new HIV infections. Between 2000 and 2018, new HIV infections fell by 37%, and HIV-related deaths fell by 45% with 13.6 million lives saved due to patients receiving effective medication during that same period. The decrease in infection rates and deaths was the result of many efforts by national HIV programs supported by a range of funding partners (WHO, 2019).

HIV Transmission

Inflammation and breaks in the skin or mucosa result in the increased probability that an HIV exposure will lead to infection. Human immune deficiency virus type 1 (**HIV-1**) is transmitted in body fluids (blood, seminal fluid, vaginal secretions, amniotic fluid, and breast milk) that contain infected cells. Higher amounts of HIV and infected cells in the body fluid are associated with the probability that the exposure will result in infection. Mother-to-child transmission of HIV-1 may occur in utero, at the time of delivery, or through breastfeeding, but most perinatal infections are thought to occur during labor and delivery. HIV is not transmitted through casual contact (see Chart 32-2).

Blood and blood products can transmit HIV to recipients. However, the risk associated with transfusions has been virtually eliminated as a result of voluntary self-deferral, completion of a detailed health history, extensive testing, heat treatment of clotting factor concentrates, and more effective virus inactivation methods. Donated blood is tested for antibodies to HIV-1, human immune deficiency virus-2 (retrovirus identified in 1986 in patients with AIDS in Western Africa), and the p24 antigen; since 1999, additional testing has been performed.

Chart 32-2 ⚠️ **RISK FACTORS**
Risks Associated with HIV Infection

- Sharing infected injection drug use equipment
- Having sexual relations with infected persons (both genders)
- Infants born to mothers with HIV infection or who are breast-fed by HIV-infected mothers
- People who received organ transplants, HIV-infected blood, or blood products (especially between 1978 and 1985)

Adapted from Centers for Disease Control and Prevention (CDC). (2019a). HIV Surveillance Report, 2017. Retrieved on 10/21/2019 at: www.cdc.gov/hiv/library/reports/hiv-surveillance.html

---

 Gerontologic Considerations

According to the CDC, 91,127 persons between the ages of 60 and 64 years are living with HIV infection, and an additional 58,526 persons are living with AIDS. For persons aged 65 years and older, 82,046 persons are living with HIV infection and an additional 52,995 persons are living with AIDS (CDC, 2019a). Many were diagnosed with HIV in their younger years and are benefitting from effective treatment. However, thousands of older adults unknowingly become infected with HIV every year. Older adults are less likely than younger people to get tested. Thirty-five percent of persons aged 50 and older were diagnosed with late-stage infection or AIDS, indicating a failure to screen for HIV in this population. Although this rate is an improvement from 2011, when it was 42%, it is still high. Late diagnosis has an adverse impact on treatment effectiveness (CDC, 2019b). Medicare will pay for annual screenings up until age 65 but there needs to be a special indication (such as unprotected sex with an infected partner) for a person to be screened after that age in order for Medicare to cover the cost of testing (CDC, 2019a).

Persons are often embarrassed to share that they have engaged in activities associated with HIV infection and so might not disclose this to the health care provider. The provider needs to use other cues, such as the presence of other sexually transmitted diseases, and recommend HIV testing. Providers may bring societal age and gender biases to their perceptions of patient sexuality, which influence their communication about sexual health with older adult patients. For some providers, assumptions that discussions about sexual health will offend their patients, as well as their own discomfort with talking to older adults about sex, inhibit them from assessing risk factors that may indicate a need for HIV and STI testing.

Comorbidities in older persons with HIV/AIDS include type 2 diabetes; non-AIDS cancerous diseases; cardiovascular disease; osteoporosis; and depression (Guaraldi, Malagoli, Calcagno, et al., 2018). Due to the high number of chronic illnesses, polypharmacy along with drug interactions becomes a major clinical challenge. Loneliness has been defined as the distress that exists between actual and desired relationships and is different from the concept of aloneness or living alone. Loneliness was studied in older persons living with HIV/AIDS by Greene and colleagues, who found that 58% of the participants reported at least some loneliness. Compared to participants who did not report feeling lonely, those who did report loneliness were more likely to smoke, misuse alcohol, or use illicit drugs. They also reported less physical social supports in place, depressive symptoms, poor or fair health-related quality of life, and functional impairment in one or more Instrumental Activities of Daily Living (IADLs) (Greene, Hessol, Perissinotto, et al., 2018). Loneliness has been associated with increased mortality in the general population.

Prevention of HIV Infection

Nurses need to participate in efforts to prevent HIV infection by educating patients how to eliminate or reduce risks associated with HIV infection and AIDS, particularly in younger adults, in order to promote a healthy lifestyle and longevity (Eliopoulos, 2018). HIV is transmitted through the exchange of some infected body fluids (see Chart 32-2). While behavioral interventions such as encouraging the use of condoms are highly effective in reducing the transmission of HIV, the HIV-negative person must be motivated and have the freedom to choose to use the method. In some situations, however, that freedom is absent. For example, a lack of freedom exists in a discordant couple (those in which only one partner has HIV) if the husband refuses to use condoms and the wife's cultural and religious beliefs require sexual activity with her husband. In this context, **pre-exposure prophylaxis (PrEP)** might be appropriate. PrEP involves taking one pill containing two HIV medications (tenofovir disoproxil fumarate 300 mg and emtricitabine 200 mg) daily in order to avoid the risk of sexual HIV acquisition in adults and adolescents age 12 and older. HIV status should be checked every 3 months to be sure that the person has not become infected. The ultimate goal of PrEP is to reduce the acquisition of HIV infection with its resulting morbidity, mortality, and cost to individuals and society (CDC, 2019c). For persons taking ART as prescribed and achieving and maintaining viral suppression, there is no risk of transmitting HIV through sex. Since PrEP does not prevent other sexually transmitted infections, which are increasing (CDC, 2019d), it is important for couples to also use a condom.

 Preventive Education

Prevention of HIV infection is achieved through: (a) behavioral interventions have been effective in reducing the risk of

acquiring or transmitting HIV by ensuring that people have the information, motivation, and skills necessary to reduce their risk; (b) HIV testing, because most people change behaviors to protect their partners if they know they are infected with HIV; and (c) linkage to treatment and care, which enables individuals with HIV to live longer, healthier lives and reduce their risk of transmitting HIV (CDC, 2019e). The CDC (2019f), through the HIV/AIDS Prevention Research Synthesis Project, provides information about evidence-based behavioral interventions that can be used in a number of settings with targeted populations. Strategies to protect against infection are outlined in Chart 32-3. Other than abstinence, consistent and correct use of condoms (see Chart 32-4) is the only effective method to decrease the risk

---

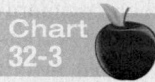

Chart 32-3 **HEALTH PROMOTION**

Protecting Against HIV Infection

All patients should be advised to:

- Abstain from exchanging sexual fluids (semen and vaginal fluid).
- Reduce the number of sexual partners to one.
- Always use latex condoms. If the patient is allergic to latex, nonlatex condoms should be used; however, they will not protect against HIV infection.
- Not reuse condoms.
- Avoid using cervical caps or diaphragms without using a condom as well.
- Always use dental dams for oral–genital or anal stimulation.
- Avoid anal intercourse, because this practice may injure tissues; if not possible, use lubricant—there are water and silicone-based products designed for anal sex.
- Avoid manual–anal intercourse ("fisting").
- Avoid sharing needles, razors, toothbrushes, sex toys, or blood-contaminated articles.
- Consider PrEP if regularly engage in high-risk behaviors.
- Use needle-exchange programs (as appropriate) and do not share drug-using equipment.

Patients who are HIV seropositive should also be advised to:

- Take ART regularly to achieve viral suppression.
- Inform previous, present, and prospective sexual and drug-using partners of their HIV-positive status. If the patient is concerned for their safety, advise the patient that many states have established mechanisms through the public health department in which professionals are available to notify exposed contacts.
- Avoid having unprotected sex with another HIV-seropositive person. Cross-infection with that person's HIV can increase the severity of infection.
- Not donate blood, plasma, body organs, or sperm.

ART, antiretroviral therapy; PrEP, pre-exposure prophylaxis.

Chart 32-4 **PATIENT EDUCATION**

The Correct Way to Use a Male Condom

The nurse instructs the patient to:

- Put on a new condom before any kind of sex.
- Hold the condom by the tip to squeeze out the air.

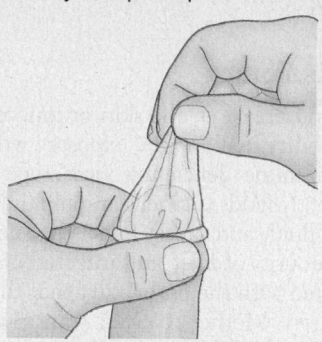

- Unroll the condom all the way over the erect penis.

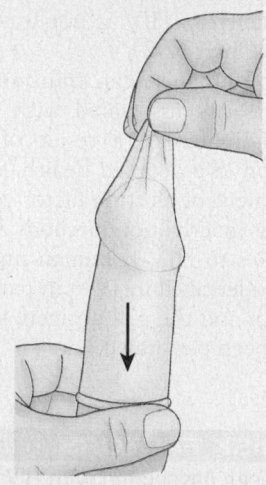

- Have sex.
- Hold the condom so it cannot come off the penis.
- Pull out.
- Use a new condom if you want to have sex again or if you want to have sex in a different place (e.g., in the anus and then in the vagina).

Note: Keep condoms cool and dry. Never use skin lotions, baby oil, petroleum jelly, or cold cream as lubricants; the oil in these products will cause the latex condom to break. Products made with water (such as K-Y jelly or glycerin) are safer to use.

of sexual transmission of HIV infection. When latex male condoms are used consistently and correctly during vaginal or anal intercourse, they are highly effective in preventing the sexual transmission of HIV. Nonlatex condoms made of natural materials such as lambskin are available for people with latex allergy but will not protect against HIV infection. A male condom should be used for oral contact with the penis, and a dental dam (a flat piece of latex used by dentists to isolate a tooth for treatment) or an altered condom can be used for oral contact with the vagina or rectum. Voluntary medical male circumcision (VMMC) is 50% to 60% effective at preventing the acquisition of HIV infection. This is a key intervention in generalized epidemic settings with high HIV prevalence and low male circumcision rates (Ensor, Davies, Rai, et al., 2019).

The polyurethane female condom, which is an effective contraceptive, provides a physical barrier that prevents exposure to genital secretions containing HIV, such as semen and vaginal fluid, and is inserted by the woman (see Chapter 50). Other safe and effective woman-controlled methods such as microbicides remain elusive although clinical trials continue globally. Microbicides are gels, films, or suppositories that can kill or neutralize viruses and bacteria; vaginal and rectal microbicides are being researched to see if they can prevent sexual transmission of HIV.

Total abstinence from addictive drugs might not be a realistic short-term goal. The harm reduction framework uses practical strategies and ideas aimed at reducing negative consequences associated with drug use. It is also a movement for social justice built on a belief in, and respect for, the rights of people who use drugs. Using a harm reduction framework, the nurse works with people who inject drugs to assist them to increase their healthy behaviors. Sharing of drug-use equipment is a high-risk behavior for a number of bloodborne infections and should be avoided. Syringe services programs are also referred to as syringe exchange programs and needle exchange programs. Although the services they provide may vary, they are community-based programs that provide access to sterile needles and syringes, facilitate safe disposal of used syringes, and provide and link to other important services and programs (CDC, 2019g). Therefore, under the harm reduction framework, participation in needle exchange programs is encouraged since they do not promote increased drug use; on the contrary, they have been found to decrease the incidence of bloodborne infections in people who inject drugs. Nurses should refer patients to accessible needle exchange programs whenever available.

Related Reproductive Education

Because HIV infection in women often occurs during the childbearing years, family planning issues need to be addressed. Attempts to achieve pregnancy by couples in which only one partner has HIV (known as discordant couples) expose the unaffected partner to the virus. Efforts at artificial insemination using processed semen from an HIV-infected partner continue. Studies are needed, because HIV has been found in the spermatozoa of patients with HIV infection, and it is possible that HIV can replicate in the male germ cell. Women considering pregnancy need to have accurate information about the risks of transmitting HIV infection to themselves, their partner, and their future children, and about the benefits

of taking ART to reduce perinatal HIV transmission. Results from the Evidence for Contraceptive Options and HIV Outcomes (ECHO) Trial Consortium found that, among African women seeking effective contraception and living in areas of high HIV incidence, there was no substantial difference in HIV risk among the methods evaluated (DMPA-IM, a copper IUD, and a levonorgestrel implant) and all methods were safe and highly effective (ECHO Trial Consortium, 2019). HIV-infected women in resource-rich settings should be instructed not to breast-feed their infants, because HIV is transmitted through breast milk.

Prevention in Lesbian, Gay, Bisexual, Transgender, and Queer Persons

Many health care providers are insufficiently prepared to meet the unique health needs of those who identify as lesbian, gay, bisexual, transgender, and queer (LGBTQ). Young gay men, in particular, are at higher risk for contracting HIV (CDC, 2019a). At the same time, these sexual and gender minorities experience significant challenges due to family rejection, lack of social support, stigma, isolation, minority stress, as well as abuse and harassment. Nurses need to be culturally competent in order to be effective in educating these unique populations about prevention methods (see Chapter 54).

Reducing the Risk of Transmission to Health Care Providers

Prevention of HIV and AIDS among health care providers involves the use of standard precautions to prevent exposure, using post-exposure prophylaxis when exposure does occur and hopefully, in the near future, the use of a vaccine.

Standard Precautions

Implementation of appropriate hand hygiene measures (see Chapter 66, Chart 66-1 for further information on hand hygiene methods) remains the most effective measure to prevent transmission of organisms. To reduce the risk of exposure of health care workers to HIV, the CDC developed standard precautions (see Chart 32-5; also see Chapter 66, Chart 66-2) which are designed to reduce the risk of transmission of pathogens. Standard precautions are used when working with all patients in all health care settings, regardless of their diagnosis or presumed infectious status.

Post-Exposure Prophylaxis for Health Care Providers

Post-exposure prophylaxis (PEP) includes taking antiretroviral medicines as soon as possible, but no more than 72 hours (3 days) after possible HIV exposure; three drugs are prescribed. Health care workers who are exposed to a needle stick involving HIV-infected blood in a health care setting have a 0.3% risk of becoming HIV infected; the risk of infection due to occupational exposure is very low (CDC, 2018a).

Occupational exposure is an urgent medical concern and should be managed immediately after possible exposure—the sooner the better; every hour counts (CDC, 2018a). The CDC suggests that these post-exposure guidelines be followed after occupational and other exposures such as sexual assault. Chart 32-6 provides the strategies and emphasizes the need for quick action. See the Resources section for the phone number for the Health Resources and Service

---

Chart 32-5 Recommendations for Standard Precautions

- **Hand hygiene:** Use after touching blood, body fluids, secretions, excretions, or contaminated items; immediately after removing gloves; and between patient contacts.
- **Personal protective equipment:**
  - *Gloves:* Use for touching blood, body fluids, secretions, excretions, and contaminated items, and for touching mucous membranes and nonintact skin.
  - *Gown:* Use during procedures and patient care activities when contact of clothing/exposed skin with blood or body fluids, secretions, and excretions is anticipated.
  - *Mask, eye protection (goggles), face shield[1]:* Use during procedures and patient care activities likely to generate splashes or sprays of blood, body fluids, and secretions, especially suctioning or endotracheal intubation.
- **Soiled patient care equipment:** Handle in a manner that prevents transfer of microorganisms to others and to the environment; wear gloves if visibly contaminated; and perform hand hygiene.
- **Environmental control:** Develop procedures for routine care, cleaning, and disinfection of environmental surfaces, especially frequently touched surfaces in patient care areas.
- **Textiles and laundry:** Handle in a manner that prevents transfer of microorganisms to others and to the environment.
- **Needles and other sharps:** Do not recap, bend, break, or hand manipulate used needles; if recapping is required, use a one-handed scoop technique only; use safety features when available; and place used sharps in a puncture-resistant container.
- **Patient resuscitation:** Use mouthpiece, resuscitation bag, and other ventilation devices to prevent contact with mouth and oral secretions.
- **Patient placement:** Prioritize for single-patient room if patient is at increased risk for transmission, is likely to contaminate the environment, does not maintain appropriate hygiene, or is at increased risk for acquiring infection or developing adverse outcome following infection.
- **Respiratory hygiene/cough etiquette** (source containment of infectious respiratory secretions in symptomatic patients, beginning at initial point of encounter, such as triage and reception areas in emergency departments and provider offices): Instruct symptomatic people to cover mouth and nose when sneezing or coughing, use tissues and dispose in no-touch receptacle, observe hand hygiene after soiling of hands with respiratory secretions, and wear surgical mask if tolerated.

[1]During aerosol-generating procedures on patients with suspected or proven infections transmitted by respiratory aerosols (e.g., severe acute respiratory syndrome), wear a fit-tested N95 or higher respirator in addition to gloves, gown, and face/eye protection.

Adapted from Centers for Disease Control and Prevention (CDC). (2018a). Updated U.S. Public Health Service guidelines for the management of occupational exposures to HIV and recommendations for postexposure prophylaxis. Retrieved on 10/27/2019 at: stacks.cdc.gov/view/cdc/20711

Chart 32-6 Post-HIV Exposure Prophylaxis for Health Care Providers

If you sustain an occupational exposure to HIV, take the following actions immediately:

- Alert your supervisor and initiate the occupational exposure reporting system used in the setting.
- Determine the HIV status of the exposure source (i.e., patient) when possible to guide appropriate use of HIV post-exposure prophylaxis (PEP). Use rapid-testing if the HIV status of the patient is unknown. Check laws in your state as you proceed to determine HIV status of the source patient.

Get counseling at the time of exposure and at follow-up appointments:

- Exposed health care providers (HCP) are advised to use precautions (e.g., use of barrier contraception and avoidance of blood or tissue donations, pregnancy, and, if possible, breast-feeding) to prevent secondary transmission, especially during the first 6 to 12 weeks after exposure.
- For exposures for which PEP is prescribed, HCPs are informed regarding the following:
  - Possible drug toxicities (e.g., rash and hypersensitivity reactions that could imitate acute HIV seroconversion and the need for monitoring)
  - Possible drug interactions
  - The need for adherence to PEP regimens

Undergo early reevaluation after exposure:

- Regardless of whether an HCP is taking PEP, reevaluation of exposed HCP within 72 hours after exposure is strongly recommended, as additional information about the exposure or the source patient may be available.

Follow up with HIV testing and appointments. At a minimum, this follow-up should include:

- HIV testing at baseline and at 6 weeks, 12 weeks, and 6 months after exposure; alternatively, if the HCP is certain that a fourth-generation combination HIV p24 antigen–HIV antibody test is being utilized, then HIV testing could be performed at baseline, 6 weeks after exposure, and 4 months after exposure
- Complete blood counts and renal and hepatic function tests (at baseline and 2 weeks after exposure; further testing may be indicated if abnormalities are detected)

Note: All HIV testing results should preferably be given to the exposed HCP during face-to-face appointments.

Adapted from Centers for Disease Control and Prevention (CDC). (2018a). Updated U.S. Public Health Service guidelines for the management of occupational exposures to HIV and recommendations for postexposure prophylaxis. Retrieved on 10/27/2019 at: stacks.cdc.gov/view/cdc/20711

Administration (HRSA) Post-exposure Prophylaxis Hotline which is answered by a health care provider.

Vaccination

In the face of a global pandemic, the search for an effective vaccine against the HIV remains an urgent priority. The first U.S. government-sponsored phase I trial of an HIV vaccine was launched in 1987 and intensive efforts worldwide using a variety of strategies continue (NIAID, 2019b).

Pathophysiology

Because HIV is an infectious disease, it is important to understand how HIV-1 integrates itself into a person's immune system and how the immune response plays a pivotal role in the course of HIV disease. This knowledge is also essential for understanding medication therapy and vaccine development. Viruses are intracellular parasites. HIV is in the subfamily of lentiviruses and is a **retrovirus** because it carries its genetic material in the form of ribonucleic acid (RNA) rather than deoxyribonucleic acid (DNA) (Norris, 2019).

Physiology/Pathophysiology

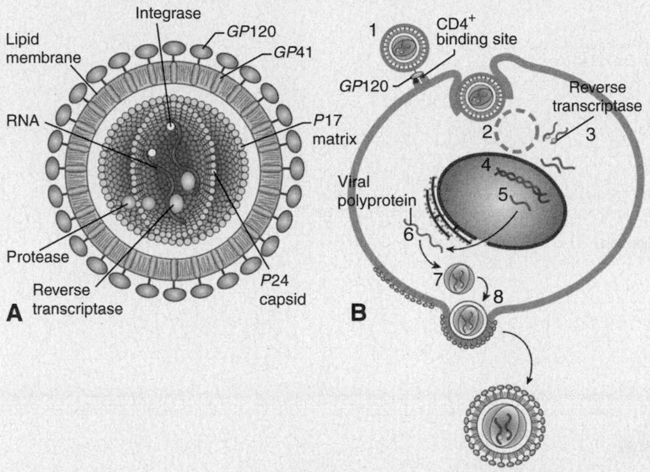

Figure 32-1 • Structure of HIV-1 virus. The virus surrounded by a lipid envelope. Reprinted with permission from Norris, T. L., & Lalchandani, R. (2019). *Porth's pathophysiology: Concepts of altered health states* (10th ed., Fig. 12.7 (left side)). Philadelphia, PA: Wolters Kluwer.

Two genetically different but closely related forms of HIV (HIV-1 and HIV-2) have been identified. Globally, it has been estimated that one to two million individuals have HIV-2, including people with HIV-1/HIV-2 dual infection. The course of illness is slower when infection is caused by HIV-2, which seems to be more common in Western Africa compared to HIV-1, which is more common in other regions of the globe (Panel, 2019). Blood tests may be used to screen for both forms of HIV. As shown in Figure 32-1, HIV consists of a viral core, containing viral RNA, which is surrounded by an envelope consisting of protruding glycoproteins.

All viruses target specific cells. HIV targets cells with $CD4^+$ receptors, which are expressed on the surface of T lymphocytes, monocytes, dendritic cells, and brain microglia. Mature T cells (T lymphocytes) are composed of two major subpopulations that are defined by cell surface receptors of $CD4^+$ or $CD8^+$. Approximately two thirds of peripheral blood T cells are $CD4^+$, and approximately one third is $CD8^+$. Most people have about 700 to 1000 $CD4^+$ cells/mm^3, but a level as low as 500 cells/mm^3 can be considered within normal limits.

The HIV life cycle is complex. Figure 32-2 illustrates the seven stages of the life cycle and the various classes of antiretroviral medications that target each specific stage (HIV Information, 2020; Norris, 2019).

In resting (nondividing) $CD4^+$ cells, HIV survives in a latent state as an integrated **provirus** that produces few or no viral particles. These resting $CD4^+$ T cells can be stimulated to produce new particles if something activates them, such as another infection. When a resting T cell that harbors this integrated DNA (also known as provirus) becomes activated against HIV or other microbes, the cell begins to produce new copies of both RNA and viral proteins. Consequently, whenever the infected $CD4^+$ cell is activated, HIV replication and budding occur, which can destroy the host cell. Newly formed HIV released into the blood can infect other $CD4^+$ cells.

HIV-1 mutates quickly, at a relatively constant rate, with about 1% of the virus's genetic material changing annually. HIV-1 exhibits substantial genetic diversity, and several different genotypes of HIV-1 exist throughout the world. There is a major group (group M), which consists of subtypes A through L, and a more diverse collection of outliers, which has been referred to as groups N and O. Subtype B HIV-1 viruses predominate in the Western world; this genetic variation is one of the major reasons why effective vaccine development has been such a challenge.

Stages of HIV Infection

There are five stages of HIV infection based on clinical history, physical examination, laboratory evidence (CDC, 2014), signs and symptoms, and associated infections and malignancies. See Table 32-2.

The period from infection with HIV to the development of HIV-specific antibodies is known as **primary infection or acute HIV infection** (previously known as the window period) and is part of stage 0 (CDC, 2014). Acute HIV infection is the interval between the appearance of detectable HIV RNA and the first detection of antibodies. Initially, persons test negative on the HIV antibody blood test, although they are not only infected, but also highly contagious because their viral loads are very high. About 40% to 80% of patients develop clinical symptoms of a nonspecific viral illness (e.g., fever, fatigue, or rash) lasting 1 to 2 weeks. After 2 to 3 weeks, antibodies to the glycoproteins of the HIV envelope can be detected in the sera of people infected with HIV, but most of these antibodies lack the ability to totally control the virus. By the time neutralizing antibodies can be detected, HIV-1 is firmly established in the host.

Primary or acute infection is characterized by high levels of viral replication, widespread dissemination of HIV throughout the body, and destruction of $CD4^+$ T cells, which leads to dramatic drops in $CD4^+$ T-cell counts (normally 500 to 1500 cells/mm^3 of blood). The host responds to the HIV infection through a $CD4^+$ T-cell response that causes other immune cells, such as $CD8^+$ lymphocytes, to increase their killing of infected, virus-producing cells. The body produces antibody molecules in an effort to contain the free HIV particles (outside cells) and assist in their removal. During this stage, the virus is widely disseminated in lymphoid tissue, and a **latent reservoir** within resting memory $CD4^+$ T cells is created.

During stage 1, the amount of virus in the body after the initial immune response subsides results in a **viral set point** which reflects an equilibrium between HIV levels and the immune response. Untreated, this set point can last for years and is inversely correlated with disease prognosis. The higher the viral set point, the poorer the prognosis. After the viral set point is reached, a chronic stage persists in which the immune system cannot eliminate the virus despite its best efforts. This set point varies greatly from patient to patient and dictates the subsequent rate of disease progression; on average, 8 to 10 years can pass before a major HIV-related complication develops. In this prolonged, chronic stage (stage 1), patients feel well and have few, if any, symptoms, which is why this stage had been referred to as asymptomatic. Apparent good health continues because $CD4^+$ T-cell levels remain high

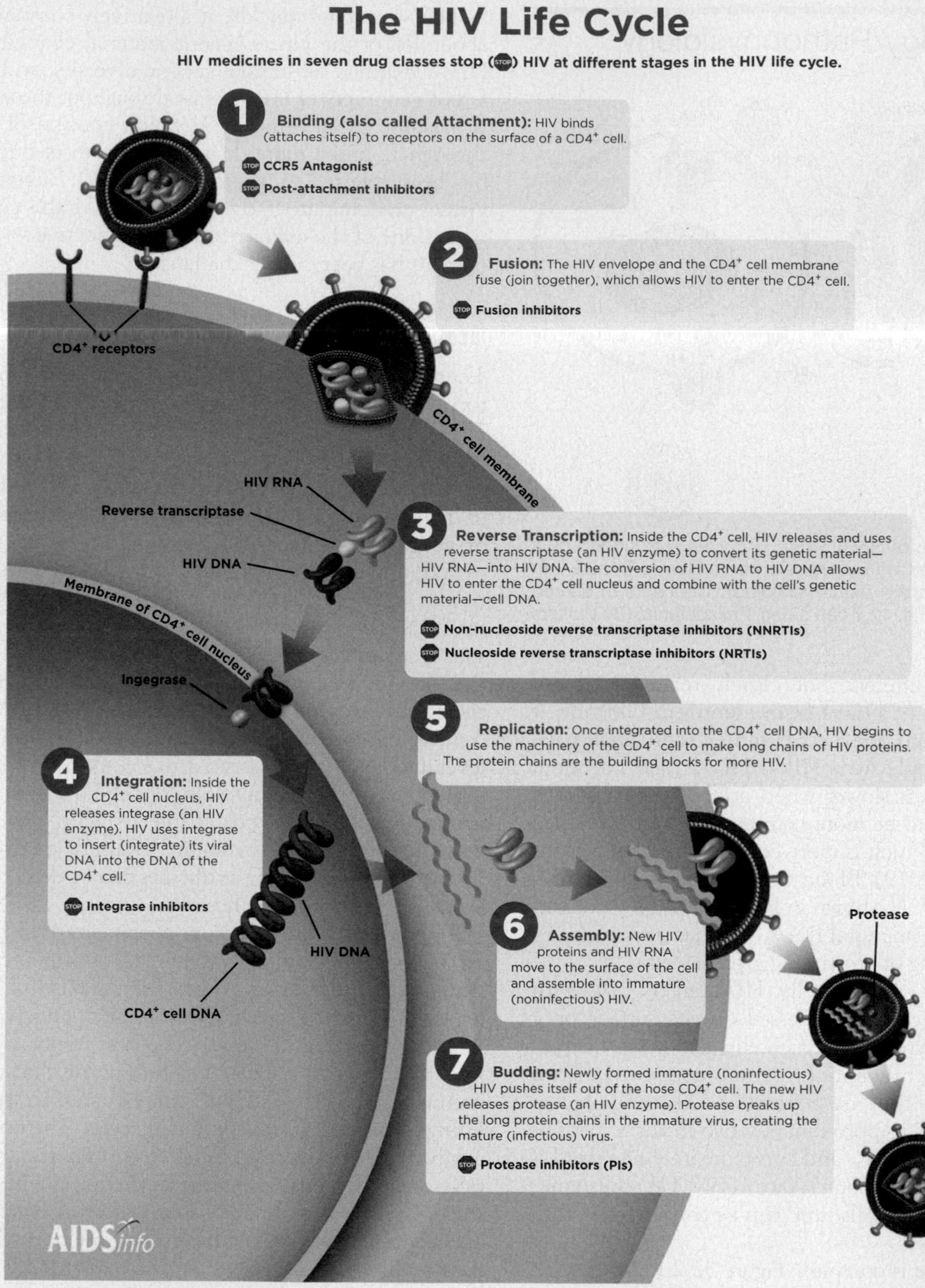

The HIV Life Cycle

HIV medicines in seven drug classes stop (🛑) HIV at different stages in the HIV life cycle.

1 **Binding (also called Attachment):** HIV binds (attaches itself) to receptors on the surface of a CD4⁺ cell.

🛑 **CCR5 Antagonist**
🛑 **Post-attachment inhibitors**

2 **Fusion:** The HIV envelope and the CD4⁺ cell membrane fuse (join together), which allows HIV to enter the CD4⁺ cell.

🛑 **Fusion inhibitors**

CD4⁺ receptors

CD4⁺ cell membrane

HIV RNA
Reverse transcriptase
HIV DNA

Membrane of CD4⁺ cell nucleus

3 **Reverse Transcription:** Inside the CD4⁺ cell, HIV releases and uses reverse transcriptase (an HIV enzyme) to convert its genetic material—HIV RNA—into HIV DNA. The conversion of HIV RNA to HIV DNA allows HIV to enter the CD4⁺ cell nucleus and combine with the cell's genetic material—cell DNA.

🛑 **Non-nucleoside reverse transcriptase inhibitors (NNRTIs)**
🛑 **Nucleoside reverse transcriptase inhibitors (NRTIs)**

Ingegrase

5 **Replication:** Once integrated into the CD4⁺ cell DNA, HIV begins to use the machinery of the CD4⁺ cell to make long chains of HIV proteins. The protein chains are the building blocks for more HIV.

4 **Integration:** Inside the CD4⁺ cell nucleus, HIV releases integrase (an HIV enzyme). HIV uses integrase to insert (integrate) its viral DNA into the DNA of the CD4⁺ cell.

🛑 **Integrase inhibitors**

HIV DNA

CD4⁺ cell DNA

Protease

6 **Assembly:** New HIV proteins and HIV RNA move to the surface of the cell and assemble into immature (noninfectious) HIV.

7 **Budding:** Newly formed immature (noninfectious) HIV pushes itself out of the hose CD4⁺ cell. The new HIV releases protease (an HIV enzyme). Protease breaks up the long protein chains in the immature virus, creating the mature (infectious) virus.

🛑 **Protease inhibitors (PIs)**

AIDSinfo

Figure 32-2 • The HIV life cycle. Adapted from HIV Information, 2020.

enough to preserve immune defensive responses, but, over time, the number of CD4⁺ T cells decrease.

Stage 2 occurs when CD4⁺ T-lymphocyte cells decrease to between 200 and 499 cells/mm³ and had previously been referred to as the symptomatic stage. Stage 3 is diagnosed when the count drops below 200 cells/mm³ and the person has AIDS. HIV disease progression is classified from less to more severe; once a case is classified into a surveillance severity stage, it cannot be reclassified into a less severe stage even if the CD4⁺ T lymphocytes increase, which often occurs when a person receives ART. A stage 3, AIDS, diagnosis has implications for services (e.g., disability benefits, housing, and

food stamps), because these programs are often linked to living with severe immune dysfunction.

Assessment and Diagnostic Findings in HIV Infection

During the first stage of HIV infection, the patient may have no symptoms or generalized signs and symptoms such as fatigue or skin rash. Patients who are in later stages of HIV infection may have a variety of symptoms related to their immunosuppressed state. The staging system requires laboratory evidence of HIV infection in order to diagnose HIV or AIDS (see Table 32-2).

HIV Tests

Several tests are used to diagnose HIV infection, and others are used to determine the stage and severity of the infection. A serologic testing algorithm for recent HIV seroconversion (STARHS) analyzes HIV-positive blood samples to determine whether an HIV infection is recent or has been ongoing. There are three types of HIV diagnostic tests: antibody tests, antigen/antibody tests, and nucleic acid (RNA) tests. Antibody tests detect antibodies, not HIV itself, while antigen and RNA tests directly detect HIV. The CDC recommends tests for HIV antigens and HIV nucleic acid because studies from high-risk populations found that antibody testing alone might miss a considerable percentage of HIV infections detectable by virologic tests, especially during stage 0.

Blood tests can detect HIV infection sooner after exposure compared to oral fluid tests because the level of antibody in blood is higher than it is in oral fluid. Likewise, antigen/antibody and RNA tests detect infection in blood before antibody tests. Some newer antigen/antibody laboratory tests can sometimes find HIV as soon as 3 weeks after exposure to the virus.

Follow-up testing is performed if the initial test result is positive to ensure a correct diagnosis. These tests include:
- antibody *differentiation tests*, which distinguishes HIV-1 from antibodies
- *HIV-1 nucleic acid tests*, which looks for the virus RNA directly

Table 32-3 identifies common blood tests used for screening.

Since negative perceptions and judgments associated with being HIV infected continue to persist, stigma remains one of the biggest social challenges (Glynn, Llabre, Lee, et al., 2019). When the result of the HIV antibody test is received, it is carefully explained to the patient in private (see Chart 32-7). All test results are confidential. Education and counseling about the test result and about preventing transmission are essential. The patient's psychological response to a positive test result may include feelings of panic, depression, and hopelessness. The social and interpersonal consequences of a positive test result can be devastating. The patient may lose their sexual partner, housing, and their job because of

disclosure. They may be subjected to physical abuse and, although illegal, experience discrimination in employment as well as social ostracism. For these reasons and others, patients who test positive may need ongoing counseling as well as referrals for social, financial, medical, and psychological support services. The HIV Care Continuum (CDC, 2019h) starts when patients receive their positive HIV blood test results. They must be connected to health care services to evaluate their stage of HIV infection and start treatment.

Patients whose test results are seronegative may develop a false sense of security, possibly resulting in continued high-risk behaviors or feelings that they are immune to the virus. These patients may need ongoing counseling to help modify high-risk behaviors and to encourage returns for repeated testing. Other patients may experience anxiety regarding the uncertainty of their status. In addition to screening for HIV, patients should be screened for other bloodborne coinfections such as hepatitis; other STIs such as syphilis; and other infections associated with T-cell immunity such as tuberculosis (TB). The rates of coinfection of hepatitis C and HIV are approximately 25% (Starbird, Hong, Sulkowski, et al., 2020).

Staging

Two surrogate markers are used routinely to assess immune function and level of HIV viremia: CD4$^+$ T-cell count (CD4$^+$ count) and plasma HIV RNA (viral load). CD4$^+$ count should be measured in all patients at entry into care. **Viral load tests** use target amplification methods to quantify HIV RNA or DNA levels in the plasma. Target amplification methods include reverse transcriptase–**polymerase chain reaction** (RT-PCR) and nucleic acid sequence–based amplification

TABLE 32-3 HIV Screening Blood Tests

Laboratory Test	Indications
HIV-1/HIV-2 immunoassay	Tests for both HIV-1 and HIV-2 antibodies
HIV/1-HIV-2 antigen/antibody combination immunoassay	Tests for both virus (antigen) and antibody for both HIV-1 and HIV-2
HIV-1 differentiation assay	Differentiates HIV-1 from HIV-2
HIV-1 nucleic acid amplification test	Tests directly for virus
HIV-1 p24 antigen	Tests directly for virus

HIV, human immune deficiency virus.
Adapted from Centers for Disease Control and Prevention. (2018b). Quick reference guide: Recommended laboratory HIV testing algorithm for serum or plasma specimens. Retrieved on 10/28/2019 at: stacks.cdc.gov/view/cdc/50872

(NAT). A widely used viral load test measures plasma HIV RNA levels. Currently, these tests are used to track viral load and response to treatment of HIV infection. RT-PCR is also used to detect HIV in high-risk seronegative people before antibodies are measurable, to confirm a positive EIA result, and to screen neonates. HIV culture or quantitative plasma culture and plasma viremia are additional tests that measure viral burden, but they are used infrequently. Viral load is a better predictor of the risk of HIV disease progression than the CD4+ count. The lower the viral load, the longer the time to AIDS diagnosis and the longer the survival time.

Treatment of HIV Infection

The U.S. Department of Health and Human Services Panel on Antiretroviral Guidelines for Adults and Adolescents (Panel) (2019) is composed of HIV specialists from across the country who regularly meet to review the latest scientific evidence. The CD4+ count serves as the major laboratory indicator of immune function and prophylaxis for opportunistic infections, and is the strongest predictor of subsequent disease progression and survival (Panel, 2019). New drugs offer strategies based on the interaction between the life cycle of HIV and the host response, improvements in potency and activity even against multidrug-resistant viruses, dosing convenience, and tolerability. Goals of ART treatment include: (1) reduce HIV-associated morbidity and prolong the duration and quality of survival, (2) restore and preserve immunologic function, (3) maximally and durably suppress plasma HIV viral load, and (4) prevent HIV transmission (Panel, 2019). HIV suppression with ART may also decrease inflammation and immune activation thought to contribute to higher rates of cardiovascular and other end-organ damage. ART is recommended for all HIV-infected patients regardless of their viral load or CD4+ count (Panel, 2019). Optimal viral suppression is defined generally as a viral load persistently below the level of detection (HIV RNA less than 20 to 75 copies/mL, depending on the assay used). Providers, in partnership with patients, make treatment decisions based on a number of factors, including whether the patient has already taken ART or is ART-naive and the willingness of the patient to adhere to the lifelong treatment regimen.

Achieving viral suppression requires the use of combination ART regimens that generally include three active drugs from two or more drug classes (Panel, 2019). Viral load suppression to below limits of assay detection usually occurs within the first 12 to 24 weeks of taking ART. Predictors of virologic reduction include: (1) low baseline viremia; (2) high potency of the ART regimen; (3) tolerability of the regimen; (4) convenience of the regimen; and (5) excellent adherence to the regimen.

More than 30 antiretroviral (ARV) drugs in seven classes are Food and Drug Administration (FDA)–approved for treatment of HIV infection. These seven classes target different stages of the HIV/host interaction. Examples include the nucleoside/nucleotide reverse transcriptase inhibitors (NRTIs) (stage 3), non-nucleoside reverse transcriptase inhibitors (NNRTIs) (stage 3), protease inhibitors (PIs) (stage 7), integrase strand transfer inhibitors (INSTIs) (stage 4), a fusion inhibitor (stage 2), a CCR5 antagonist (stage 1), and a CD4+ post-attachment inhibitor (stage 1) (see Fig. 32-2).

In addition, some drugs are used as pharmacokinetic enhancers (or boosters) to improve the effectiveness of other ARV drugs (Panel, 2019). The Panel (2019) provides clear directions regarding which medications should be prescribed for both ART-naive and experienced patients.

The CDC estimates that HIV has not yet been diagnosed in about 13% of the people living with HIV in the United States. After receiving an HIV diagnosis, about 75% of individuals are linked to care within 30 days, but only 57% of persons who receive an HIV diagnosis are retained in HIV care. It is estimated that only 55% of persons with diagnosed HIV are virally suppressed because of poor linkage to care and retention in care (Panel, 2019). Viral loads are often not suppressed because the patient is not adhering to the treatment plan. Psychosocial barriers such as depression and other mental illnesses, neurocognitive impairment, low health literacy, low levels of social support, stressful life events, high levels of alcohol consumption and active substance use, homelessness, poverty, nondisclosure of HIV serostatus, denial, stigma, and inconsistent access to medications affect adherence to ART. Failure to adopt practices that facilitate adherence, such as linking medication taking to daily activities or using a medication reminder system or a pill organizer, is also associated with treatment failure (Panel, 2019). Simplifying treatment regimens and decreasing the number of medications that must be taken each day also helps to increase patients' adherence to therapy. Although antiretroviral regimens have become less complex, side effects create barriers to adherence and inadequate dosing can lead to viral resistance. It is difficult to predict patients' adherence to medication regimens, but a positive relationship between the patient and health care provider is associated with better adherence (Hill, Golin, Pack, et al., 2020).

Chart 32-8 summarizes strategies that health care providers can encourage to promote treatment regimen adherence. Many real-time monitoring systems, such as electronic pill boxes, are under investigation as well as pharmacologic monitoring of blood and hair (Hill et al., 2020). Real-time monitoring has the potential to enhance ART intervention programs by providing objective information about medication taking behaviors. Every health care encounter should be used as an opportunity to briefly review the treatment regimen, identify any new issues, and reinforce successful behaviors.

Laboratory tests evaluate whether ART is effective for a specific patient. An adequate CD4+ response for most patients on ART is an increase in CD4+ count in the range of 50 to 150 mm^3 per year, generally with an accelerated response in the first 3 months (Panel, 2019). Viral load should be measured at baseline and on a regular basis thereafter because viral load is the most important indicator of response to ART.

Adverse effects associated with all HIV treatment regimens include hepatotoxicity, nephrotoxicity, and osteopenia, along with increased risk of cardiovascular disease and myocardial infarction (see Table 32-4). Many of the antiretroviral agents may cause fat redistribution syndrome and metabolic alterations such as dyslipidemia and insulin resistance, which put the patient at risk for early-onset heart disease and diabetes. The fat redistribution syndrome (lipodystrophy) consists of lipoatrophy (localized subcutaneous fat loss in the face, arms, legs, and buttocks) and lipohypertrophy (central visceral fat

(text continued on page 1020)

Chart 32-8 Promoting Adherence to ART

Strategies	Examples
Use a multidisciplinary team approach. Provide an accessible, trustworthy health care team.	• Nonjudgmental providers, nurses, social workers, pharmacists, and medication managers.
Strengthen early linkage to care and retention in care.	• Encourage health care team participation in linkage to and retention in care.
Assess patient readiness to start ART.	• Address specific concerns such as drug interactions between ART and hormones for transgender patients.
Evaluate patient's knowledge about HIV disease, prevention and treatment and, on the basis of the assessment, provide HIV-related information.	• Consider the patient's current knowledge base, provide information about HIV, including the natural history of the disease, HIV viral load and CD4$^+$ count and expected clinical outcomes according to these parameters, and therapeutic and prevention consequences of nonadherence.
Identify facilitators, potential barriers to adherence, and necessary medication management skills before starting ART medication.	• Assess patient's cognitive competence and any impairment. • Assess behavioral and psychosocial challenges including depression, mental illnesses, levels of social support, high levels of alcohol consumption and active substance use, nondisclosure of HIV serostatus and stigma. • Identify and address language and literacy barriers. • Assess beliefs, perceptions, and expectations about taking ART (e.g., impact on health, side effects, disclosure issues, consequences of nonadherence). • Ask about medication taking skills and foreseeable challenges with adherence (e.g., past difficulty keeping appointments, adverse effects from previous medications, issues managing other chronic medications, need for medication reminders and organizers). • Assess structural issues including unstable housing, lack of income, unpredictable daily schedule, lack of prescription drug coverage, lack of continuous access to medications.
Provide needed resources.	• Provide or refer for mental health and/or substance abuse treatment. • Provide resources to obtain prescription drug coverage, stable housing, social support, and income and food security. • Encourage use of valid Internet sites for health-related information.
Involve the patient in ARV regimen selection.	• Review regimen potency, potential side effects, dosing frequency, pill burden, storage requirements, food requirements, and consequences of nonadherence. • Assess daily activities and tailor regimen to predictable and routine daily events. • Use single tablet fixed-dose combination formulation. • Assess if cost/co-payment for drugs can affect access to medications and adherence.
Assess adherence at every clinic visit.	• Monitor viral load as a strong biologic measure of adherence. • Use a simple behavioral rating scale. • Employ a structured format that normalizes or assumes less-than-perfect adherence and minimizes socially desirable or "white coat adherence" responses. • Ensure that other members of the health care team also assess adherence.
Use positive reinforcement to foster adherence success.	• Inform patients of low or nondetectable levels of HIV viral load and increases in CD4$^+$ cell counts. • When needed, consider providing incentives and rewards for achieving high levels of adherence and treatment success.
Identify the type of and reasons for nonadherence.	• Failure to fill the prescription(s). • Failure to understand dosing instructions. • Complexity of regimen (e.g., pill burden, size, dosing schedule, food requirements). • Pill aversion. • Pill fatigue. • Adverse effects. • Inadequate understanding of drug resistance and its relationship to adherence. • Cost-related issues. • Depression, drug and alcohol use, homelessness, poverty. • Stigma. • Nondisclosure. • Other potential barriers.
Select from among available effective treatment adherence interventions.	• Use evidence-based interventions to promote adherence. • Use adherence-related tools to complement education and counseling interventions (e.g., pill boxes, dose planners, reminder devices). • Use community resources to support adherence (e.g., visiting nurses, community workers, family, peer advocates). • Use patient prescription assistance programs. • Use motivational interviews.

(continued on page 1018)

Chart 32-8 **Promoting Adherence to ART** (continued)

Strategies	Examples
Systematically monitor retention in care. On the basis of any problems identified through systematic monitoring, consider options to enhance retention in care given resources available.	• Record and follow up on missed visits. • Provide outreach for those patients who drop out of care. • Use peer or paraprofessional treatment navigators. • Employ incentives to encourage clinic attendance or recognize positive clinical outcomes resulting from good adherence. • Arrange for directly observed therapy (if feasible).

Adapted from Panel on Antiretroviral Guidelines for Adults and Adolescents (Panel). (2019). Guidelines for the use of antiretroviral agents in HIV-1-infected adults and adolescents. Department of Health and Human Services. Strategies to Improve Linkage to Care, Retention in Care, Adherence to Appointments, and Adherence to Antiretroviral Therapy (pp. 236–237).

TABLE 32-4 Select Antiretroviral Agents

Generic Name (Abbreviation) and Single-Tablet Combination Names (Italic)	Food Interactions	Adverse Effects
Nucleoside Reverse Transcriptase Inhibitors (NRTIs)		
Abacavir (ABC) *Trizivir* (ABC/ZDV/3TC) *Epzicom* (ABC/3TC) (ABC/3TC/DTG)	Take without regard to meals	Hypersensitivity reaction, which can be fatal; symptoms may include fever, rash, nausea, vomiting, diarrhea, abdominal pain, malaise or fatigue, loss of appetite, and respiratory symptoms such as sore throat, cough, shortness of breath.
Didanosine (ddI)	Take half hour before or 2 h after meals	Pancreatitis, peripheral neuropathy, retinal changes, nausea, diarrhea, lactic acidosis with fatty degeneration of the liver, insulin resistance/diabetes.
Emtricitabine (FTC) *Atripla* (FTC/EFV/TDF) *Biktarvy* (BIC/TAF/FTC) *Complera* (RPV/TDF/FTC) *Descovy* (TAF/FTC) *Genvoya* (EVG/c/TAF/FTC) *Odefsey* (RPV/TAF/FTC) *Symtuza* (DRV/c/TAF) *Stribild* (FTC/EVG/c/TDF) *Truvada* (FTC/TDF)	Take without regard to meals	Minimal toxicity; hyperpigmentation/skin discoloration. Severe acute exacerbation of hepatitis may occur in patients with HBV/HIV coinfection who discontinue FTC.
Lamivudine (3TC) *Cimduo* (TDF/3TC) *Combivir* (ZDV/3TC) *Epzicom* (ABC/3TC) *Temixys* (TDF/3TC) *Trizivir* (ABC/ZDV/3TC) *Delstrigo* (DOR/TDF/3TC) *Dovato* (DTG/3TC) *Symfi/Symfi LO* (EFV/TDF/3TC) *Triumeq* (DTG/ABC/3TC)	Take without regard to meals	Minimal toxicity. Severe acute exacerbation of hepatitis may occur in patients with HBV/HIV coinfection who discontinue 3TC.
Stavudine (d4T)	Take without regard to meals	Peripheral neuropathy; lipoatrophy; pancreatitis; lactic acidosis/severe hepatomegaly with hepatic steatosis (this is a rare, but potentially life-threatening, toxicity); hyperlipidemia; insulin resistance/diabetes mellitus; rapidly progressive ascending neuromuscular weakness (rare)
Tenofovir alafenamide (TAF) *Biktarvy* (BIC/TAF/FTC) *Descovy* (TAF/FTC) *Genvoya* (EVG/c/TAF/FTC) *Odefsey* (RPV/TAF/FTC) *Symtuza* (DRV/c/TAF/FTC)	Take without regard to meals	Renal insufficiency, Fanconi syndrome, and proximal renal tubulopathy are less likely to occur with TAF than with TDF. Osteomalacia and decrease in bone mineral density are less likely to occur with TAF than with TDF. Severe acute exacerbation of hepatitis may occur in patients with HBV/HIV coinfection who discontinue TAF. Diarrhea, nausea, headache
Tenofovir disoproxil fumarate (TDF) *Atripla* (EFV/TDF/FTC) *Cimduo* (TDF/3TC) *Complera* (RPV/TDF/FTC) *Delstrigo* (DOR/TDF/3TC) *Stribild* (EVG/c/TDF/FTC) *Symfi/Symfi Lo* (EFV/TDF/3TC) *Temixys* (TDF/3TC) *Truvada* (TDF/FTC)	Take without regard to meals	Renal insufficiency, Fanconi syndrome, proximal renal tubulopathy, osteomalacia, decrease in bone mineral density. Severe acute exacerbation of hepatitis may occur in patients with HBV/HIV coinfection who discontinue TDF. Asthenia, headache, diarrhea, nausea, vomiting, flatulence

TABLE 32-4 Select Antiretroviral Agents *(continued)*

Generic Name (Abbreviation) and Single-Tablet Combination Names (Italic)	Food Interactions	Adverse Effects
Zidovudine (AZT or ZDV) *Combivir* (3TC/AZT) *Trizivir* (ABC/3TC/AZT)	Take without regard to meals	Bone marrow suppression; macrocytic anemia or neutropenia; nausea, vomiting, headache, insomnia, asthenia, nail pigmentation; lactic acidosis/severe hepatomegaly with hepatic steatosis (this is a rare, but potentially life-threatening, toxicity). Hyperlipidemia; insulin resistance/diabetes mellitus; lipoatrophy; myopathy

Non-Nucleoside Reverse Transcriptase Inhibitors

Doravirine (DOR) *Delstrigo* (DOR/TDF/3TC)	Take without regard to meals	Nausea, dizziness, abnormal dreams
Efavirenz (EFV) *Atripla* (EFV/TDF/FTC) *Symfi/Symfi Lo* (EFV/TDF/3TC)	Take on empty stomach at bedtime	Rash; neuropsychiatric symptoms; serum transaminase elevations; hyperlipidemia; QT interval prolongation Use of EFV may lead to false-positive results with some cannabinoid and benzodiazepine screening assays.
Etravirine (ETR)	Take following a meal	Rash, including Stevens–Johnson syndrome; HSRs, characterized by rash, constitutional findings, and sometimes organ dysfunction (including hepatic failure), have been reported; nausea.
Nevirapine (NVP)	Take without regard to meals	Rash (reported in approximately 50% of cases), including Stevens–Johnson syndrome; symptomatic hepatitis, including fatal hepatic necrosis; symptomatic hepatitis occurs at a significantly higher frequency in ARV-naive female patients with pre-NVP CD4$^+$ counts >250 cells/mm^3 and in ARV-naive male patients with pre-NVP CD4$^+$ counts >400 cells/mm^3. NVP should not be initiated in these patients unless the benefit clearly outweighs the risk.
Rilpivirine (RPV) *Complera* (RPV/TDF/FTC) *Juluca* (DTG/RPV) *Odefsey* (RPV/TAF/FTC)	Take with a meal	Rash, depression, insomnia, headache, hepatotoxicity, QT interval prolongation

Protease Inhibitors

Atazanavir (ATV) *Evotaz* (ATV/c)	Take with food	Indirect hyperbilirubinemia; prolonged PR interval (some patients experience asymptomatic first-degree AV block); EKG changes; hyperglycemia; fat maldistribution; possible increased bleeding episodes in patients with hemophilia; Cholelithiasis; nephrolithiasis; renal insufficiency; serum transaminase elevations; hyperlipidemia (especially with RTV boosting); rash; hyperglycemia; fat maldistribution
Darunavir (DRV) *Prezcobix* (DRV/c)	Take with food	Rash: DRV has a higher allergy risk, Stevens–Johnson syndrome, toxic epidermal necrolysis, acute generalized exanthematous pustulosis, and erythema multiforme have been reported. Hepatotoxicity; diarrhea; nausea; headache; hyperlipidemia; serum transaminase elevation; hyperglycemia; fat maldistribution. An increase in serum creatinine may occur when DRV is administered with COBI.
Fosamprenavir (FPV)	Tablets may be taken with or without food	Rash has been reported in 12–19% of patients on FPV. FPV has an increased allergy risk. Diarrhea, nausea, vomiting, headache, hyperlipidemia, serum transaminase elevation, hyperglycemia, fat maldistribution, possible increase in the frequency of bleeding episodes in patients with hemophilia, nephrolithiasis.
Indinavir (IDV)	For upboosted IDV: Should be taken 1 h before or 2 h after meals; may take with skim milk or low-fat meal For RTV-boosted IDV: Can be taken with or without food Drink at least 48 oz of water daily	Nephrolithiasis, GI intolerance, nausea, hepatitis, indirect hyperbilirubinemia, hyperlipidemia, headache, asthenia, blurred vision, dizziness, rash, metallic taste, thrombocytopenia, alopecia, hemolytic anemia, hyperglycemia, fat maldistribution, possible increased bleeding episodes in patients with hemophilia.
Lopinavir + ritonavir (LPV/r)	Tablet: take without regard to meals Oral solution: take with food; contains 42% alcohol	GI intolerance, nausea, vomiting, diarrhea, asthenia, pancreatitis, hyperlipidemia (especially hypertriglyceridemia), elevated serum transaminase, hyperglycemia, insulin resistance/diabetes mellitus, fat maldistribution, possible increased bleeding episodes in patients with hemophilia, EKG changes.

(continued on page 1020)

TABLE 32-4 Select Antiretroviral Agents (continued)

Generic Name (Abbreviation) and Single-Tablet Combination Names (Italic)	Food Interactions	Adverse Effects
Nelfinavir (NFV)	Dissolve tablets in a small amount of water, mix admixture well, and consume immediately. Take with food	Diarrhea, hyperlipidemia, hyperglycemia, fat maldistribution, possible increased bleeding episodes in patients with hemophilia, serum transaminase elevation.
Ritonavir (RTV)	Take with food	GI intolerance, nausea, vomiting, diarrhea, paresthesias (circumoral and extremities), hyperlipidemia (especially hypertriglyceridemia), hepatitis, asthenia, taste perversion, hyperglycemia, fat maldistribution, possible increased bleeding in patients with hemophilia.
Saquinavir (SQV)	Take with meals or within 2 h after meal	GI intolerance, nausea, diarrhea, abdominal pain and dyspepsia, headache, hyperlipidemia, elevated transaminase enzymes, hyperglycemia, fat maldistribution, possible increased bleeding episodes in patients with hemophilia, EKG changes.
Tipranavir (TPV)	Take with food	Hepatotoxicity; clinical hepatitis (including hepatic decompensation and hepatitis-associated fatalities) has been reported. Skin rash. Rare cases of fatal and nonfatal intracranial hemorrhages have been reported. Hyperlipidemia, hyperglycemia, fat maldistribution. Possible increase in the frequency of bleeding episodes in patients with hemophilia.
Integrase Strand Transfer Inhibitors		
Dolutegravir (DTG) *Dovato* (DTG/3TC) *Juluca* (DTG/RPV) *Triumeq* (DTG/ABC/3TC)	Take without regard to meals	Insomnia, headache, depression and suicidal ideation (rare; usually occurs in patients with preexisting psychiatric conditions). Weight gain, hepatotoxicity. Preliminary data suggest an increased rate of neural tube defects in infants born to mothers who were taking DTG at the time of conception. Hypersensitivity reaction, including rash, constitutional symptoms, and organ dysfunction (including liver injury), have been reported.
Elvitegravir (EVG) *Stribild* (EVG/c/FTC/TDF)	Take with food	Nausea, diarrhea, depression and suicidal ideation (rare; usually occurs in patients with preexisting psychiatric conditions).
Raltegravir (RAL)	Take without regard to meals	Rash including Stevens–Johnson, hypersensitivity reaction and toxic epidermal necrolysis. Nausea, headache, diarrhea, pyrexia, CPK elevation, muscle weakness, rhabdomyolysis, insomnia. Depression and suicidal ideation (rare; usually occurs in patients with preexisting psychiatric conditions).
Fusion Inhibitor		
Enfuvirtide (T-20)	Injected	Local injection site reactions (e.g., pain, erythema, induration, nodules and cysts, pruritus, ecchymosis) in almost 100% of patients. Increased incidence of bacterial pneumonia. Hypersensitivity reaction can occur and rechallenge is not recommended.
CCR5 Antagonist		
Maraviroc (MVC)	Take without regard to meals; requires CCR5 tropism blood test before starting	Abdominal pain, cough, fever, dizziness, headache, orthostatic hypotension, nausea, bladder irritation; possible liver problems and cardiac events; an increased risk for some infections; a slight increase in cholesterol levels; orthostatic hypotension, especially in patients with severe renal insufficiency.
CD4 Post-Attachment Inhibitor		
Ibalizumab (IBA)	IV administration	Diarrhea, dizziness, nausea, rash

Adapted from Panel on Antiretroviral Guidelines for Adults and Adolescents (Panel). (2019). Guidelines for the use of antiretroviral agents in HIV-1-infected adults and adolescents. Department of Health and Human Services. Retrieved on 10/28/18 at: aidsinfo.nih.gov/contentfiles/lvguidelines/adultandadolescentgl.pdf

[lipomata] accumulation in the abdomen, although possibly in the breasts, dorsocervical region [buffalo hump], and within the muscle and liver). Facial wasting, characterized as a sinking of the cheeks, eyes, and temples caused by the loss of fat tissue under the skin, may be treated by injectable fillers such as poly-l-lactic acid (see Fig. 32-3). These changes can disturb the body image of people living with HIV/AIDS and may be a reason that they decline or stop ART.

ART Drug Resistance

Drug resistance is the ability of pathogens to withstand the effects of medications that should be toxic to them. There

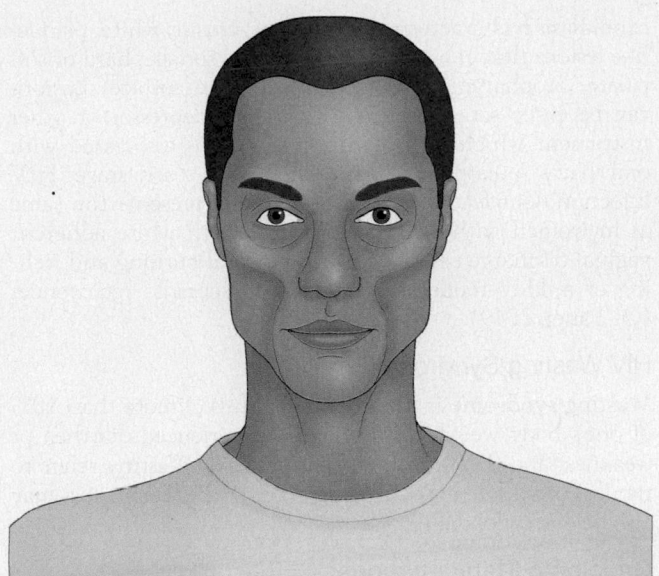

Figure 32-3 • Facial lipoatrophy.

are two major components of ART resistance: (1) transmission of drug-resistant HIV at the time of initial infection and (2) selective drug resistance in patients who are receiving nonsuppressive regimens. Genotypic and phenotypic resistance assays are used to assess viral strains and inform selection of treatment strategies. Genotypic assays detect drug-resistant mutations present in relevant viral genes while phenotypic assays measure the ability of a virus to grow in different concentrations of ART drugs. Resistance testing in persons who are chronically infected is recommended at the time of entry into HIV care. Although no definitive prospective data exist to support the choice of one type of resistance testing over another, genotypic testing is generally preferred because of lower cost, more rapid turnaround time, the assay's ability to detect mixtures of wild-type and resistant virus, and the relative ease of interpreting test results. If therapy is deferred, repeat testing soon before initiation of ART should be considered because the patient may have acquired drug-resistant virus (i.e., superinfection) (Panel, 2019).

Immune Reconstitution Inflammatory Syndrome

Immune reconstitution inflammatory syndrome (IRIS) results from rapid restoration of organism-specific immune responses to infections that cause either the deterioration of a treated infection or new presentation of a subclinical infection. This syndrome typically occurs during the initial months after beginning ART and is associated with a wide spectrum of organisms, most commonly mycobacteria, herpes viruses, and deep fungal infections. IRIS is characterized by fever, respiratory and/or abdominal symptoms, and worsening of the clinical manifestations of an opportunistic infection or the appearance of new manifestations. IRIS is treated with anti-inflammatory medications such as cortisone. The nurse should be alert to the possibility of IRIS, especially in the 3-month period after treatment with ART is initiated, because this syndrome is associated with significant morbidity and patients often require hospital admission.

Paradoxical tuberculosis-associated immune reconstitution inflammatory syndrome (TB-IRIS) is a serious complication

that arises during successful ART in patients with HIV-TB co-infection who are receiving TB treatment. In the majority of patients, TB-IRIS occurs within the first few weeks of ART but can occur much later. Patients with HIV-TB co-infection with low CD4$^+$ counts who start ART are at high risk of developing TB-IRIS. Although the immunopathogenesis of TB-IRIS is still not completely understood, the explosive restoration of T-cell function is believed to play a distinct role (Narendran, Oliveira-de-Souza, Vinhaes, et al., 2019).

Clinical Manifestations

Patients with HIV/AIDS experience a number of symptoms related to the disease, side effects of treatment, and other comorbidities, including pancreatitis, hepatitis, and cardiometabolic abnormalities. The clinical manifestations of HIV/AIDS are widespread and may involve virtually any organ system. Patients in stage 3 or AIDS (see Table 32-2) are severely immune depressed and can develop opportunistic infections. Nurses need to understand the causes, signs and symptoms, and interventions, including self-management strategies that can enhance the quality of life for patients throughout the different stages of the illness. Symptom assessment tools can be used to assess patients' symptom intensity and severity. PLWHA use a variety of self-management strategies to minimize common symptoms.

Respiratory Manifestations

Shortness of breath, dyspnea (labored breathing), cough, chest pain, and fever are associated with various opportunistic infections, such as those caused by *Pneumocystis jirovecii*, *Mycobacterium avium-intracellulare*, cytomegalovirus (CMV), and *Legionella* species.

Pneumocystis Pneumonia

***Pneumocystis* pneumonia (PCP)** is caused by *P. jirovecii* (formerly *P. carinii*) (Panel on Opportunistic Infections in Adults and Adolescents with HIV [OI-Panel], 2019) and is associated with CD4$^+$ T-lymphocyte (CD4$^+$) cell counts less than 200 cells/mm^3. The most common manifestations of PCP are subacute onset of progressive dyspnea, fever, nonproductive cough, and chest discomfort that worsens within days to weeks. In mild cases, pulmonary examination usually is normal at rest. With exertion, tachypnea, tachycardia, and diffuse dry (cellophane) rales may be auscultated. Fever is apparent in most cases and may be the predominant symptom. Hypoxemia is the most characteristic laboratory abnormality, along with elevated lactate dehydrogenase levels. Because clinical presentation, blood tests, and chest X-rays are not pathognomonic for PCP, and because the organism cannot be cultivated routinely, histopathologic or cytopathologic demonstration of organisms in tissue, bronchoalveolar lavage fluid, or induced sputum samples is required for a definitive diagnosis (OI-Panel, 2019).

Mycobacterium Avium Complex

***Mycobacterium avium* complex (MAC)** disease is a common opportunistic infection that typically occurs in patients with CD4$^+$ T-lymphocyte (CD4$^+$) cell counts less than 50 cells/mm^3. MAC is caused by infection with different types of mycobacterium: *Mycobacterium avium*, *Mycobacterium intracellulare*, or *Mycobacterium kansasii*. Early symptoms may be minimal and can precede detectable mycobacteremia by several weeks and include fever, night sweats, weight loss, fatigue, diarrhea, and abdominal pain. A confirmed diagnosis of disseminated MAC disease is based on compatible clinical signs and symptoms coupled with the isolation of MAC from cultures of blood, lymph node, bone marrow, or other normally sterile tissue or body fluids (OI-Panel, 2019).

Tuberculosis

The estimated annual risk of reactivation with TB among those with untreated HIV infection and latent TB infection is 3% to 16% and approximates the lifetime risk for individuals without HIV infection who have latent TB infection. TB disease can occur at any CD4+ T-lymphocyte (CD4+ cell) count, although the risk increases with progressive immune deficiency. Testing for latent TB at the time of HIV diagnosis should be routine, regardless of an individual's risk of TB exposure. Individuals with negative diagnostic tests for latent TB who have stage 3 HIV infection should be retested once their CD4+ count increases due to ART. Screening for symptoms (asking for cough of *any* duration) coupled with chest radiography is recommended to exclude TB disease in a patient with a positive skin test or interferon-gamma release assays. Latent TB in a person with HIV infection is treated with isoniazid, supplemented with pyridoxine to prevent peripheral neuropathy, for 9 months since it has proven efficacy, good tolerability, and infrequent severe toxicity (OI-Panel, 2019).

TB disease can develop in the lungs as well as in extrapulmonary sites such as the central nervous system (CNS), bone, pericardium, stomach, peritoneum, and scrotum and initial diagnostic testing is directed at the anatomic site of symptoms or signs, such as the lungs, lymph nodes, and cerebrospinal fluid. TB in individuals with advanced immune deficiency can be rapidly progressive and fatal if treatment is delayed and such patients often have smear-negative sputum specimens. Therefore, after collection of available specimens for culture and molecular diagnostic tests, empiric treatment for TB is warranted in patients with clinical and radiographic presentation suggestive of HIV-related TB. Treatment of suspected TB in individuals with HIV infection is the same as for those who are HIV uninfected and should include an initial four-drug combination of isoniazid, rifampin, pyrazinamide, and ethambutol (OI-Panel, 2019).

Gastrointestinal Manifestations

The gastrointestinal manifestations of HIV infection and AIDS include loss of appetite, nausea, vomiting, oral and esophageal candidiasis, and chronic diarrhea. Gastrointestinal symptoms may be related to the direct inflammatory effect of HIV on the cells lining the intestines. Some of the enteric pathogens that occur most frequently, identified by stool cultures or intestinal biopsy, are *Cryptosporidium muris*, *Salmonella* species, *Isospora belli*, *Giardia lamblia*, cytomegalovirus (CMV), *Clostridium difficile*, and *M. avium-intracellulare*. In patients with AIDS, the effects of diarrhea can be devastating in terms of profound weight loss (more than 10% of body weight), fluid and electrolyte imbalances, perianal skin excoriation, weakness, and inability to perform the usual activities of daily living.

Candidiasis

Oropharyngeal and esophageal **candidiasis** (fungal infections) are common in patients with HIV infection. Oropharyngeal candidiasis is characterized by painless, creamy white, plaque-like lesions that can occur on the buccal surface, hard or soft palate, oropharyngeal mucosa, or tongue surface. Lesions can be easily scraped off with a tongue depressor or other instrument which is in contrast to lesions associated with oral hairy leukoplakia. In women with early-stage HIV infection, *Candida* vulvovaginitis usually presents the same as in women without HIV infection, with white adherent vaginal discharge associated with mucosal burning and itching of mild-to-moderate severity and sporadic recurrences (OI-Panel, 2019).

HIV Wasting Syndrome

Wasting syndrome is the involuntary loss of more than 10% of one's body weight while having experienced diarrhea or weakness and fever for more than 30 days. Wasting refers to the loss of muscle mass, although part of the weight loss may also be due to loss of fat.

Oncologic Manifestations

Those with HIV/AIDS are at greater risk of developing certain cancers. These include **Kaposi sarcoma** (KS), lymphoma, and invasive cervical cancer. KS and lymphomas are discussed next. Cervical carcinoma is described later in the Gynecologic Manifestations section.

Kaposi Sarcoma

KS is caused by human herpesvirus-8 (HHV-8); affects eight times more men than women; and may spread through sexual contact. It involves the epithelial layer of blood and lymphatic vessels. AIDS-related KS exhibits a variable and aggressive course, ranging from localized cutaneous lesions to disseminated disease involving multiple organ systems. Cutaneous signs may be the first manifestation of HIV; they can appear anywhere on the body and are usually brownish pink to deep purple. They may be flat or raised and surrounded by ecchymosis (hemorrhagic patches) and edema (see Fig. 32-4). Rapid development of lesions involving large areas of skin is associated with extensive disfigurement and significant body image issues. The location and size of some lesions can lead

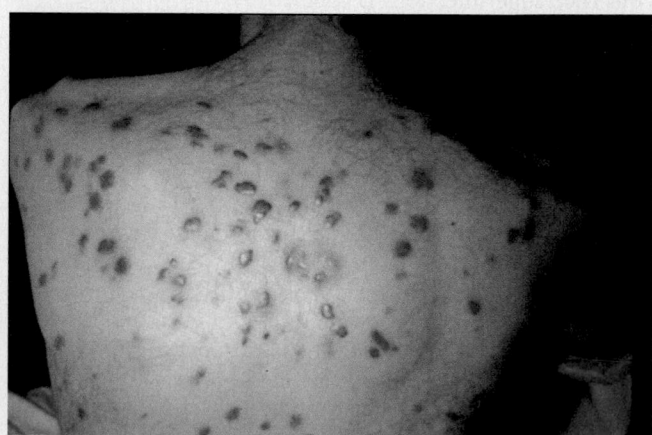

Figure 32-4 • Lesions of the AIDS-related Kaposi sarcoma. Whereas some patients may have lesions that remain flat, others experience extensively disseminated, raised lesions with edema. Reprinted with permission from DeVita, V. T., Jr., Hellman, S., & Rosenberg, S. (Eds.). (1993). *AIDS: Etiology, diagnosis, treatment, and prevention* (4th ed.). Philadelphia, PA: Lippincott Williams & Wilkins.

to venous stasis, lymphedema, and pain. Ulcerative lesions disrupt skin integrity and increase discomfort and susceptibility to infection. The most common sites of visceral involvement are the lymph nodes, gastrointestinal tract, and lungs. Involvement of internal organs may eventually lead to organ failure, hemorrhage, infection, and death.

Diagnosis of KS is confirmed by biopsy of suspected lesions. Prognosis depends on the extent of the tumor, the presence of other symptoms of HIV infection, and the CD4⁺ count. Death may result from tumor progression, but more often it results from other complications of HIV infection.

AIDS-Related Lymphomas

AIDS-related lymphomas include both Hodgkin lymphoma and non-Hodgkin lymphoma. Non-Hodgkin lymphoma is more common. AIDS-related lymphoma is usually aggressive; there are three main types: diffuse large B-cell; B-cell immunoblastic; and small noncleaved cell lymphoma. Symptoms include weight loss, night sweats, and fever. The complete blood count might be abnormal and a biopsy will confirm the diagnosis.

Neurologic Manifestations

HIV-related brain changes have profound effects on cognition, including motor function, executive function, attention, visual memory, and visuospatial function. Neurologic dysfunction results from direct effects of HIV on nervous system tissue, opportunistic infections, primary or metastatic neoplasm, cerebrovascular changes, metabolic encephalopathies, or complications secondary to therapy. Immune system response to HIV infection in the CNS includes inflammation, atrophy, demyelination, degeneration, and necrosis.

Subcortical Neurodegenerative Disease

Approximately 20% of those living with HIV infection are at risk for developing a subcortical neurodegenerative disease known as HIV-associated neurocognitive disorder (HAND) (Cummins, Waters, Aggar, et al., 2019). The signs of HAND can be subtle and include changes in language, memory, problem solving and slowing of psychomotor skills (Cummins et al., 2019). Early identification is important as HAND can be treated by changing ART medications.

Peripheral Neuropathy

Peripheral neuropathy is a common neurologic symptom at any stage of HIV infection. It may be a side effect of some ART drugs, and may occur in a variety of patterns, with distal sensory polyneuropathy or distal symmetric polyneuropathy the most frequently occurring type. It can lead to significant pain of feet and hands and functional impairment. Patients use a variety of physical and psychological self-management strategies to minimize this symptom.

HIV Encephalopathy

HIV encephalopathy was formerly referred to as AIDS dementia complex (see Chart 32-9). It is a clinical syndrome that is characterized by a progressive decline in cognitive, behavioral, and motor functions as a direct result of HIV infection. HIV has been found in the brain and cerebrospinal fluid (CSF) of patients with HIV encephalopathy. The

---

Chart 32-9	Care of the Patient with HIV Encephalopathy

Chronic Confusion

- Assess mental status and neurologic functioning.
- Monitor for medication interactions, infections, electrolyte imbalance, and depression.
- Frequently orient the patient to time, place, person, reality, and the environment.
- Use simple explanations.
- Instruct the patient to perform tasks in incremental steps.
- Provide memory aids (clocks and calendars).
- Provide memory aids for medication administration.
- Post activity schedule.
- Give positive feedback for appropriate behavior.
- Educate caretakers about orienting patient to time, place, person, reality, and the environment.
- Encourage the patient to designate a responsible person to assume power of attorney.

Disturbed Sensation

- Assess sensory impairment.
- Decrease number of stimuli in the patient's environment.
- Correct inaccurate perceptions.
- Provide reassurance and safety if the patient displays fear.
- Provide a secure and stable environment.
- Educate caregivers about recognizing inaccurate sensory perceptions.
- Provide caregivers techniques to correct inaccurate perceptions.
- Instruct the patient and caregivers to report any changes in the patient's vision to the patient's health care provider.

Risk for Injury

- Assess the patient's level of anxiety, confusion, or disorientation.
- Assess the patient for delusions or hallucinations.
- Remove potentially dangerous objects from the patient's environment.
- Structure the environment for safety (ensure adequate lighting, avoid clutter, provide bed rails if needed).
- Supervise smoking.
- Do not let the patient drive a car if confusion is present.
- Instruct the patient and caregiver in home safety.
- Provide assistance as needed for ambulation and in getting in and out of bed.
- Pad headboard and side rails if the patient has seizures.

Self-Care Deficits

- Encourage activities of daily living within the patient's level of ability.
- Encourage independence, but assist if the patient cannot perform an activity.
- Demonstrate any activity that the patient is having difficulty accomplishing.
- Monitor food and fluid intake.
- Weigh patient weekly.
- Encourage the patient to eat, and offer nutritious meals, snacks, and adequate fluids.
- If patient is incontinent, establish a routine toileting schedule.
- Educate caregivers about meeting the patient's self-care needs.

brain cells infected by HIV are predominantly the CD4⁺ cells of monocyte–macrophage lineage. HIV infection is thought to trigger the release of toxins or lymphokines that result in cellular dysfunction, inflammation, or interference with neurotransmitter function rather than cellular damage.

Signs and symptoms may be subtle and difficult to distinguish from fatigue, depression, or the adverse effects of treatment for infections and malignancies. Early manifestations include memory deficits, headache, difficulty concentrating, progressive confusion, psychomotor slowing, apathy, and ataxia. Later stages include global cognitive impairments, delay in verbal responses, a vacant stare, spastic paraparesis, hyperreflexia, psychosis, hallucinations, tremor, incontinence, seizures, mutism, and death.

Confirming the diagnosis of HIV encephalopathy can be difficult. Extensive neurologic evaluation includes a computed tomography scan, which may indicate diffuse cerebral atrophy and ventricular enlargement. Other tests that may detect abnormalities include magnetic resonance imaging, analysis of CSF through lumbar puncture, and brain biopsy.

Cryptococcus Neoformans

A fungal infection *Cryptococcus neoformans* is another common opportunistic infection among patients with AIDS, and it causes neurologic disease. Cryptococcal meningitis is characterized by symptoms such as fever, headache, malaise, stiff neck, nausea, vomiting, mental status changes, and seizures. Diagnosis is confirmed by CSF analysis.

Progressive Multifocal Leukoencephalopathy

Progressive multifocal leukoencephalopathy (PML) is a demyelinating CNS disorder that affects the oligodendroglia. Clinical manifestations often begin with mental confusion and rapidly progress to include blindness, aphasia, muscle weakness, paresis (partial or complete paralysis), and death. ART has greatly reduced the mortality associated with this disorder.

Other Neurologic Disorders

Other infections involving the nervous system include *Toxoplasma gondii*, CMV, and *Mycobacterium tuberculosis* infections.

Depressive Manifestations

Depression and apathy are neuropsychiatric complications of HIV infection. Estimates suggest that the prevalence of current depression is between 12% and 60% in persons with HIV/AIDS (Lu, Hsiao, Sheng, et al., 2018). Similarly, apathy, which refers to reduced, self-initiated, cognitive, emotional, and behavioral activity, is also commonly reported among those living with a diagnosis of HIV. Alcohol and cocaine use—both current and former—have been associated with depression and apathy in this population, and depression has been associated with less adherence with ART medications (Lu et al., 2018).

Integumentary Manifestations

Cutaneous manifestations are associated with HIV infection and the accompanying opportunistic infections and malignancies. KS (described earlier) and opportunistic infections such as herpes zoster and herpes simplex are associated with painful vesicles that disrupt skin integrity. Molluscum contagiosum is a viral infection characterized by deforming plaque formation. Seborrheic dermatitis is associated with an indurated, diffuse, scaly rash involving the scalp and face. Patients with AIDS may also exhibit a generalized folliculitis associated with dry, flaking skin or atopic dermatitis, such as eczema or psoriasis. Many patients treated with the antibacterial agent trimethoprim–sulfamethoxazole develop a drug-related rash that is pruritic with pinkish-red macules and papules (Panel, 2019). Patients with any of these rashes experience discomfort, have body image changes, and are at increased risk for infection from disrupted skin integrity.

Gynecologic Manifestations

Persistent, recurrent vaginal candidiasis may be the first sign of HIV infection in women. Past or present genital ulcers are a risk factor for the transmission of HIV infection. Women with HIV infection are more susceptible to genital ulcers and venereal warts and have increased rates of incidence and recurrence of these conditions. Ulcerative STIs such as chancroid, syphilis, and herpes are more severe in women with HIV infection. Human papillomavirus (HPV) causes venereal warts and is a risk factor for cervical intraepithelial neoplasia, a cellular change that is frequently a precursor to cervical cancer. Women who are HIV seropositive and have cervical carcinoma present at a more advanced stage of disease and have more persistent and recurrent disease and a shorter interval to recurrence and death than women without HIV infection.

Women with HIV are at increased risk for pelvic inflammatory disease, a reportable infection, and the associated inflammation may increase HIV transmission to the uninfected sexual partner. Moreover, women with HIV infection appear to have a higher incidence of menstrual abnormalities, including amenorrhea or bleeding between periods, than do women without HIV infection.

Medical Management

Treatment of Opportunistic Infections and Coinfection with Hepatitis C

Guidelines for the treatment of opportunistic infections should be consulted for the most current recommendations (OI-Panel, 2019). Although ART is highly effective in keeping the CD4⁺ cell count high, opportunistic infections continue to cause considerable morbidity and mortality for three main reasons: (1) many patients are unaware of their HIV infection and present with an opportunistic infection as the initial indicator of their disease, (2) some patients are aware of their HIV infection but do not take antiretroviral agents because of psychosocial or economic factors, and (3) others receive prescriptions for antiretroviral medications but fail to attain adequate virologic and immunologic response as a result of issues related to adherence, pharmacokinetics, or unexplained biologic factors.

Coinfection with hepatitis C requires careful medical management for the PLWHA. Hepatitis C is curable with an 8- to 12-week drug therapy in most patients. However, the medications for the treatment of hepatitis C interact with many ART medications and therefore need to be carefully managed to avoid interactions and maximize adherence (OI-Panel, 2019; Starbird et al., 2020).

Pneumocystis Pneumonia

Persons in stage 3 HIV infection should receive chemoprophylaxis to prevent PCP with trimethoprim–sulfamethoxazole if they have CD4$^+$ counts less than 200 cells/mm^3 or a history of oropharyngeal candidiasis (OI-Panel, 2019). Once the CD4$^+$ count improves, prophylaxis can be discontinued. When a person is diagnosed with PCP, trimethoprim–sulfamethoxazole is the treatment of choice, lowering the dose if there is abnormal renal function. Adjunctive corticosteroids are indicated as early as possible, preferentially within 72 hours after starting specific PCP therapy. Treatment duration is usually 21 days; rates of adverse reaction to trimethoprim–sulfamethoxazole are high including rash (30% to 55%) (including Stevens–Johnson syndrome), fever (30% to 40%), leukopenia (30% to 40%), hepatitis (20%), thrombocytopenia (15%), azotemia (1% to 5%), and hyperkalemia. Because long-term survival is possible for patients in whom ART is effective, individuals with AIDS and severe PCP should be given the option to choose mechanical ventilation and critical care management if their functional status is such that it would be appropriate, just as with patients without HIV infection. Paradoxical IRIS has been reported following PCP and starting ART (OI-Panel, 2019).

Mycobacterium Avium Complex

Initial treatment of MAC disease should consist of two or more antimycobacterial drugs to prevent or delay the emergence of resistance. Clarithromycin is the preferred first agent; however, azithromycin can be substituted for clarithromycin when drug interactions or intolerance to clarithromycin preclude its use. Ethambutol is the recommended second drug (OI-Panel, 2019).

Cryptococcal Meningitis

Cryptococcosis among patients with HIV infection most commonly occurs as a subacute meningitis or meningoencephalitis with fever, malaise, and headache. Treating cryptococcosis consists of three phases: induction, consolidation, and maintenance therapy. The preferred induction treatment for cryptococcal meningitis and other forms of extrapulmonary cryptococcosis is the IV lipid formulation of amphotericin B in combination with fluconazole. Serious potential adverse effects of amphotericin B include anaphylaxis, kidney and hepatic impairment, electrolyte imbalances, anemia, fever, and severe chills. After at least 2 weeks of successful induction therapy—defined as substantial clinical improvement and a negative CSF culture after repeat lumbar puncture—amphotericin B and flucytosine can be discontinued. Follow-up or consolidation therapy is then initiated with oral fluconazole daily which should continue for at least 8 weeks (OI-Panel, 2019).

Cytomegalovirus Retinitis

Retinitis caused by CMV is a leading cause of blindness in patients with AIDS. Oral valganciclovir, IV ganciclovir, IV ganciclovir followed by oral valganciclovir, IV foscarnet, IV cidofovir, and a ganciclovir intraocular implant coupled with valganciclovir are all effective treatments for CMV retinitis

(OI-Panel, 2019). All of these drugs have significant toxicities (bone marrow suppression, neutropenia, hepatitis, renal toxicity, seizures, etc.) and are used with caution.

Antidiarrheal Therapy

Although many forms of diarrhea respond to treatment, it is not unusual for this condition to recur and become a chronic problem for the patient with HIV infection. Therapy with octreotide acetate, a synthetic analogue of somatostatin, has been shown to effectively manage chronic severe diarrhea. High concentrations of somatostatin receptors have been found in the gastrointestinal tract and in other tissues. Somatostatin inhibits many physiologic functions, including gastrointestinal motility and intestinal secretion of water and electrolytes.

Chemotherapy

Kaposi Sarcoma

KS can be treated with local therapy, radiation therapy, chemotherapy, and biologic therapy depending upon the location of the lesions.

Lymphoma

There is no standard treatment for AIDS-related peripheral or systemic lymphoma. The treatment plan is adjusted for each patient and usually includes one or more of combination chemotherapy, high-dose chemotherapy and stem cell transplant.

Antidepressant Therapy

Treatment for depression in people with HIV infection involves cognitive behavioral therapy integrated with pharmacotherapy (Lu et al., 2018). If depressive symptoms are severe and of sufficient duration, treatment with antidepressants may be initiated. Antidepressants such as imipramine, desipramine, and fluoxetine may be used, because these medications also alleviate the fatigue and lethargy that are associated with depression. A psychostimulant such as methylphenidate may be used in low doses in patients with neuropsychiatric impairment. Electroconvulsive therapy may be an option for patients with severe depression who do not respond to pharmacologic interventions.

Nutrition Therapy

Alterations in lipid metabolism are associated with HIV infection and ART. Malnutrition increases the risk of infection and the incidence of opportunistic infections. Nutrition therapy should be part of the overall management plan and should be tailored to meet the nutritional needs of the patient, whether by oral diet, enteral tube feedings, or parenteral nutritional support, if needed. As with all patients, a healthy diet is essential for the patient with HIV infection. For all patients with AIDS who experience unexplained weight loss, calorie counts and weight monitoring should be obtained to evaluate nutritional status and initiate appropriate therapy. The goal is to maintain the ideal weight and, when necessary, to increase weight.

Appetite stimulants have been successfully used in patients with AIDS-related anorexia. Megestrol acetate, a synthetic oral progesterone preparation, promotes significant weight gain and inhibits cytokine IL-1 synthesis. In patients with

HIV infection, it increases body weight primarily by increasing body fat stores. Dronabinol, which is a synthetic tetrahydrocannabinol, the active ingredient in marijuana, has been used to relieve nausea and vomiting associated with cancer chemotherapy. After beginning dronabinol therapy, almost all patients with HIV infection experience a modest weight gain. The effects on body composition are unknown.

Oral supplements may be used when the diet is deficient in calories and protein. Ideally, oral supplements should be lactose free (people with HIV infection may be intolerant to lactose), high in calories and easily digestible protein, low in fat with the fat easily digestible, palatable, inexpensive, and tolerated without causing diarrhea. Nutritional supplements have been developed specifically for people with HIV infection and AIDS. Parenteral nutrition is the final option because of its prohibitive cost and associated risks, including possible infection.

Complementary, Alternative, and Integrative Health Therapies

People with HIV infection, along with many Americans, report the use of complementary, alternative, and integrative therapies. Combined with traditional therapies, these may improve the patient's overall well-being. However, there can be adverse drug–drug interactions between certain therapies (e.g., St. John's wort) and some ART.

Although there is insufficient research on the effects of complementary, alternative, and integrative therapies, a growing body of literature reports benefits for modalities involving nutrition, exercise, psychosocial treatment, and Chinese medicine. See Chapter 4 for further information on complementary, alternative, and integrative therapies.

Many patients who use these therapies do not report their use to their health care providers. To obtain a complete health history, the nurse should ask about the patient's use of complementary, alternative, and integrative therapies. Patients may need to be encouraged to report their use of these therapies to their primary provider. Problems may arise, for example, when patients are using complementary, alternative, and integrative therapies while participating in clinical drug trials; alternative therapies can have significant adverse side effects, making it difficult to assess the effects of the medications in the clinical trial. The nurse needs to become familiar with the potential adverse side effects of these therapies; if it is suspected that the therapy is causing side effects, the nurse needs to discuss this with the patient, the alternative therapy provider, and the primary provider. The nurse needs to view complementary, alternative, and integrative therapies with an open mind and try to understand the importance of this treatment to the patient. This approach will improve communication with the patient and reduce conflict.

Supportive Care

Patients who are weak and debilitated as a result of chronic illness associated with HIV infection and AIDS typically require many kinds of supportive care. Nutritional support may be as simple as providing assistance in obtaining or preparing meals. For patients with more advanced nutritional impairment resulting from decreased intake, wasting syndrome, or gastrointestinal malabsorption associated with diarrhea, parenteral feedings may be required. Imbalances that result from nausea, vomiting, and profuse diarrhea often necessitate IV fluid and electrolyte replacement.

Management of skin breakdown associated with KS, perianal skin excoriation, or immobility entails thorough and meticulous skin care that involves regular turning, cleansing, and applications of medicated ointments and dressings. To combat pain associated with skin breakdown, abdominal cramping, peripheral neuropathy, or KS, the nurse administers analgesic agents at regular intervals around the clock. Patients with a history of drug abuse will need to have tailored approaches for pain management. Relaxation and guided imagery may help reduce pain and anxiety.

Pulmonary symptoms, such as dyspnea and shortness of breath, may be related to opportunistic infections, KS, or fatigue. For patients with these symptoms, oxygen therapy, relaxation training, and energy conservation techniques may be effective. Patients with severe respiratory dysfunction may require mechanical ventilation. Before mechanical ventilation is instituted, the procedure is explained to the patient and the caregiver.

As noted previously, with the advent of ART, there are generally more positive outcomes than could be achieved years ago, and a patient mechanically ventilated has a reasonable likelihood of survival. However, if the patient decides to forego mechanical ventilation, those wishes must be followed. Ideally, the patient has prepared an advance directive identifying preferences for treatments and end-of-life care, including hospice care. If the patient has not identified preferences in advance, treatment options are described so that the patient can make informed decisions and have those wishes respected.

Nurses should anticipate that patients as well as family and friends will need support and time to share concerns. In some family systems, more than one person might be living with HIV/AIDS.

NURSING PROCESS

The Patient with HIV Infection

The nursing care of patients with HIV infection is complicated by many emotional, social, and ethical issues. The plan of care for the patient with AIDS (see Chart 32-10) is individualized to meet the needs of the patient. Care includes many of the interventions and concerns cited in the Supportive Care section.

Assessment

Nursing assessment includes identification of potential risk factors, including a history of risky sexual practices or IV/injection drug use. The patient's physical status and psychological status are assessed.

Nutritional status is assessed by obtaining a dietary history and identifying factors that may interfere with oral intake, such as anorexia, nausea, vomiting, oral pain, or difficulty swallowing. In addition, the patient's ability to purchase, prepare, and store food safely is assessed. Weight history (i.e., changes over time), anthropometric measurements, and blood urea nitrogen (BUN), serum protein, albumin, and transferrin levels provide objective measurements of nutritional status.

(text continued on page 1031)

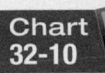

PLAN OF NURSING CARE

Chart 32-10

Care of the Patient with AIDS

NURSING DIAGNOSIS: Diarrhoae associated with enteric pathogens or HIV infection
GOAL: Resumption of usual bowel habits

Nursing Interventions	Rationale	Expected Outcomes

1. Assess patient's normal bowel habits.
2. Assess for diarrhea: frequent, loose stools; abdominal pain or cramping, volume of liquid stools, and exacerbating and alleviating factors.
3. Obtain stool cultures, and administer antimicrobial therapy as prescribed.
4. Initiate measures to reduce hyperactivity of bowel.
  a. Maintain food and fluid restrictions as prescribed. Suggest BRAT diet (*b*ananas, *r*ice, *a*pplesauce, *t*ea, and *t*oast).
  b. Discourage smoking and use of electronic nicotine delivery systems (ENDS) including e-cigarettes, e-pens, e-pipes, e-hookah, and e-cigars.
  c. Avoid bowel irritants such as fatty or fried foods, raw vegetables, and nuts. Offer small, frequent meals.
5. Administer anticholinergic antispasmodics and opioids or other medications as prescribed.
6. Maintain fluid intake of at least 3 L/day unless contraindicated.
	1. Provides baseline for evaluation.
	2. Detects changes in status, quantifies loss of fluid, and provides basis for nursing measures.
	
	3. Identifies pathogenic organism; therapy targets specific organism.
	4. Promotes bowel rest, which may decrease acute episodes.
	  a. Reduces stimulation of bowel.
	
	  b. Eliminates nicotine, which acts as bowel stimulant.
	
	  c. Prevents stimulation of bowel and abdominal distention and promotes adequate nutrition.
	5. Decreases intestinal spasms and motility.
	6. Prevents hypovolemia.
		• Exhibits return to normal bowel patterns
		• Reports decreasing episodes of diarrhea and abdominal cramping
		• Identifies and avoids foods that irritate the gastrointestinal tract
		• Takes appropriate therapy as prescribed
		• Exhibits normal stool cultures
		• Maintains adequate fluid intake
		• Maintains body weight and reports no additional weight loss
		• States rationale for avoiding smoking
		• Enrolls in program to stop smoking and using ENDS
		• Uses medication as prescribed
		• Maintains adequate fluid status
		• Exhibits normal skin turgor, moist mucous membranes, adequate urine output, and absence of excessive thirst

NURSING DIAGNOSIS: Risk for infection associated with immune deficiency
GOAL: Absence of infection

Nursing Interventions	Rationale	Expected Outcomes

1. Monitor for infection: fever, chills, and diaphoresis; cough; shortness of breath; oral pain or painful swallowing; creamy-white patches in oral cavity; urinary frequency, urgency, or dysuria; redness, swelling, or drainage from wounds; vesicular lesions on face, lips, or perianal area.
2. Educate patient or caregiver about need to report possible infection.
3. Monitor white blood cell (WBC) count and differential.
4. Obtain cultures of wound drainage, skin lesions, urine, stool, sputum, mouth, and blood as prescribed. Administer antimicrobial therapy as prescribed.
5. Instruct patient in ways to prevent infection.
  a. Clean kitchen and bathroom surfaces with disinfectants.
  b. Clean hands thoroughly after exposure to body fluids.
  c. Avoid exposure to others' body fluids or sharing eating utensils.
  d. Turn, cough, and deep breathe, especially when activity is decreased.
  e. Maintain cleanliness of perianal area.
  f. Avoid handling pet excreta or cleaning litter boxes, birdcages, or aquariums.
  g. Cook meat and eggs thoroughly.
6. Maintain aseptic technique when performing invasive procedures such as venipunctures, bladder catheterizations, and injections.
	1. Allows for early detection of infection, essential for prompt initiation of treatment. Repeated and prolonged infections contribute to patient's debilitation.
	
	2. Allows early detection of infection.
	
	3. Elevated WBC count possibly associated with infection.
	4. Assists in determining offending organism to initiate appropriate treatment.
	
	5. Minimizes exposure to infection and transmission of HIV infection to others.
	
	6. Prevents hospital-acquired infections.
		• Identifies reportable signs and symptoms of infection
		• Reports signs and symptoms of infection if present
		• Exhibits and reports absence of fever, chills, and diaphoresis
		• Exhibits normal (clear) breath sounds without adventitious breath sounds
		• Maintains weight
		• Reports adequate energy level without excessive fatigue
		• Reports absence of shortness of breath and cough
		• Exhibits pink, moist oral mucous membranes without fissures or lesions
		• Takes appropriate therapy as prescribed
		• Experiences no infection
		• States rationale for strategies to avoid infection
		• Modifies activities to reduce exposure to infection or infectious persons
		• Practices "safer sex"
		• Avoids sharing eating utensils and toothbrush
		• Exhibits normal body temperature
		• Uses recommended techniques to maintain cleanliness of skin, skin lesions, and perianal area
		• Has others handle pet excreta and cleanup
		• Uses recommended cooking techniques

(continued on page 1028)

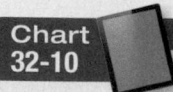

Chart 32-10

PLAN OF NURSING CARE (continued)
Care of the Patient with AIDS

NURSING DIAGNOSIS: Impaired airway clearance associated with *Pneumocystis* pneumonia, increased bronchial secretions, and decreased ability to cough associated with weakness and fatigue
GOAL: Improved airway clearance

Nursing Interventions	Rationale	Expected Outcomes
1. Assess and report signs and symptoms of altered respiratory status, tachypnea, the use of accessory muscles, cough, color and amount of sputum, abnormal breath sounds, dusky or cyanotic skin color, restlessness, confusion, or somnolence.	1. Indicates abnormal respiratory function.	• Maintains normal airway clearance: • Respiratory rate <20 breaths/min • Unlabored breathing without the use of accessory muscles and flaring nares (nostrils) • Skin color pink (without cyanosis) • Alert and aware of surroundings • Arterial blood gas values normal • Normal breath sounds without adventitious breath sounds
2. Obtain sputum sample for culture as prescribed. Administer antimicrobial therapy as prescribed.	2. Aids in identification of pathogenic organisms.	• Begins appropriate therapy • Takes medication as prescribed
3. Provide pulmonary care (cough, deep breathing, postural drainage, and vibration) every 2 to 4 hours.	3. Prevents stasis of secretions and promotes airway clearance.	• Reports improved breathing • Maintains clear airway
4. Assist patient in attaining semi- or high Fowler position.	4. Facilitates breathing and airway clearance.	• Coughs and takes deep breaths every 2 to 4 hours as recommended
5. Encourage adequate rest periods.	5. Maximizes energy expenditure and prevents excessive fatigue.	• Demonstrates appropriate positions and practices postural drainage every 2 to 4 hours
6. Initiate measures to decrease viscosity of secretions. a. Maintain fluid intake of at least 3 L/day unless contraindicated. b. Humidify inspired air as prescribed. c. Consult with primary provider concerning the use of mucolytic agents delivered through nebulizer or intermittent positive pressure breathing treatment.	6. Facilitates expectoration of secretions; prevents stasis of secretions.	• Reports reduced breathing difficulty when in semi- or high Fowler position • Practices energy-conserving strategies and alternates rest with activity • Demonstrates reduction in thickness (viscosity) of pulmonary secretions
7. Perform tracheal suctioning as needed.	7. Removes secretions if patient is unable to do so.	• Reports increased ease in coughing up sputum
8. Administer oxygen therapy as prescribed.	8. Increases availability of oxygen.	• Uses humidified air or oxygen as prescribed and indicated
9. Assist with endotracheal intubation; maintain ventilator settings as prescribed.	9. Maintains ventilation.	• Indicates need for assistance with removal of pulmonary secretions • Understands need for and cooperates with endotracheal intubation and the use of a mechanical ventilator • Verbalizes concerns about respiratory difficulty, intubation, and mechanical ventilation

NURSING DIAGNOSIS: Impaired nutritional intake associated with decreased oral intake
GOAL: Intake of nutrients sufficient to meet metabolic needs

Nursing Interventions	Rationale	Expected Outcomes
1. Assess nutritional status with height, weight, age; blood urea nitrogen, serum protein, albumin, transferrin, hemoglobin, and hematocrit levels; and cutaneous anergy.	1. Provides objective measurement of nutritional status.	• Identifies factors limiting oral intake, and uses resources to promote adequate dietary intake • Reports increased appetite
2. Obtain dietary history, including likes and dislikes and food intolerances.	2. Defines need for nutritional education; helps individualize interventions.	• States understanding of nutritional needs • Identifies ways to reduce factors that limit oral intake
3. Assess factors that interfere with oral intake.	3. Provides basis and directions for interventions.	• Rests before meals • Eats in pleasant, odor-free environment
4. Consult with dietitian to determine patient's nutritional needs.	4. Facilitates meal planning.	• Arranges meals to coincide with visitors' visits

Chart 32-10

PLAN OF NURSING CARE (continued)

Care of the Patient with AIDS

Nursing Interventions	Rationale	Expected Outcomes

5. Reduce factors limiting oral intake.
  a. Encourage patient to rest before meals
 	
  b. Plan meals so that they do not occur immediately after painful or unpleasant procedures.
  c. Encourage patient to eat meals with visitors or others when possible.
  d. Encourage patient to prepare simple meals or to obtain assistance with meal preparation if possible.
  e. Serve small, frequent meals: 6/day.
  f. Limit fluids 1 hour before meals and with meals.
6. Instruct patient in ways to supplement nutrition: consume protein-rich foods (meat, poultry, fish) and carbohydrates (pasta, fruit, breads).
7. Consult with primary provider and dietitian about alternative feeding (enteral or parenteral nutrition).
8. Consult with social worker or community liaison about financial assistance if patient cannot afford food.
	5. Addresses factors limiting intake.
	  a. Minimizes fatigue, which can decrease appetite.
	  b. Decreases noxious stimuli.
	
	  c. Limits social isolation.
	
	  d. Limits energy expenditure.
	
	  e. Prevents overwhelming patient.
	  f. Reduces satiety.
	
	6. Provides additional proteins and calories.
	
	7. Provides nutritional support if patient is unable to take sufficient amounts by mouth.
	8. Increases availability of resources and nutrition.
		• Reports increased dietary intake
		• Uses oral hygiene before meals
		• Takes analgesic agents before meals as prescribed
		• Identifies ways to increase protein and caloric intake
		• Identifies foods high in protein and calories
		• Consumes foods high in protein and calories
		• Reports decreased rate of weight loss
		• Maintains adequate caloric intake
		• States rationale for enteral or parenteral nutrition if needed
		• Demonstrates skill in preparing alternate sources of nutrition

NURSING DIAGNOSIS: Lack of knowledge associated with means of preventing HIV transmission
GOAL: Increased knowledge concerning means of preventing disease transmission

Nursing Interventions	Rationale	Expected Outcomes

1. Instruct patient, family, and friends about routes of transmission of HIV.
 	
2. Instruct patient, family, and friends about means of preventing transmission of HIV.
  a. Avoid sexual contact with multiple partners, and use precautions if sexual partner's HIV status is not certain.
 	
  b. Use condoms during sexual intercourse (vaginal, anal, oral–genital); avoid mouth contact with the penis, vagina, or rectum; avoid sexual practices that can cause cuts or tears in the lining of the rectum, vagina, or penis.
  c. Avoid sex with sex workers and others at high risk.
 	
  d. Do not use IV/injection drugs; if addicted and unable or unwilling to change behavior, use clean needles and syringes.
 	
  e. Women who may have been exposed to HIV through sexual or drug practices should consult with a primary provider before becoming pregnant; consider the use of antiretroviral agents if pregnant.
  f. Consider using PrEP
	1. Knowledge about disease transmission can help prevent spread of disease; may also alleviate fears.
	2. Reduces transmission risk.
	
	  a. The risk of infection increases with the number of sexual partners, male or female, and sexual contact with those who engage in high-risk behaviors.
	  b. Risk of HIV transmission is reduced.
	
	  c. Many sex workers are infected with HIV through sexual contact with multiple partners or IV/injection drug use.
	  d. Clean needles and syringes are the only way to prevent HIV transmission for those who continue to use drugs. Taking precautions is important for those who are antibody positive to prevent transmitting HIV.
	  e. HIV can be transmitted from mother to child in utero; the use of antiretroviral agents during pregnancy significantly reduces perinatal transmission of HIV.
	  f. Taking ART before engaging in high-risk activity seems to protect against infection.
		• Patient, family, and friends state means of transmission
		• Reports and demonstrates practices to reduce exposure of others to HIV
		• Demonstrates knowledge of safer sexual practices
		• Identifies means of preventing disease transmission
		• States that sexual partners are informed about patient's positive HIV status in blood
		• Avoids IV/injection drug use and sharing of drug equipment with others
		• Understands risks and benefits associated with PrEP

(continued on page 1030)

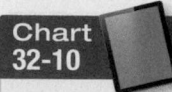

Chart 32-10   PLAN OF NURSING CARE (continued)
Care of the Patient with AIDS

NURSING DIAGNOSIS: Social isolation associated with stigma of the disease, withdrawal of support systems, isolation procedures, and fear of infecting others

GOAL: Decreased sense of social isolation

Nursing Interventions	Rationale	Expected Outcomes
1. Assess patient's usual patterns of social interaction.	1. Establishes basis for individualized interventions.	• Shares with others the need for valued social interaction
2. Observe for behaviors indicative of social isolation, such as decreased interaction with others, hostility, noncompliance, sad affect, and stated feelings of rejection or loneliness.	2. Promotes early detection of social isolation, which may be manifested in several ways.	• Demonstrates interest in events, activities, and communication • Verbalizes feelings and reactions to diagnosis, prognosis, and life changes
3. Provide instruction concerning modes of transmission of HIV.	3. Provides accurate information, corrects misconceptions, and alleviates anxiety.	• Identifies modes of transmission of HIV • States ways of preventing transmission of HIV to others while maintaining contact with valued friends and relatives
4. Assist patient to identify and explore resources for support and positive mechanisms for coping (e.g., contact with family, friends, AIDS task force).	4. Enables mobilization of resources and supports.	• Reveals HIV/AIDS diagnosis to others when appropriate • Identifies resources (i.e., family, friends, and support groups)
5. Allow time to be with patient other than for medications and procedures.	5. Promotes feelings of self-worth and provides social interaction.	• Uses resources when appropriate • Accepts offers of assistance and support
6. Encourage participation in diversional activities such as reading, television, or handcrafts.	6. Provides distraction.	• Reports decreased sense of isolation • Maintains contacts with those of importance to them • Develops or continues hobbies that effectively serve as diversion or distraction

COLLABORATIVE PROBLEMS: Opportunistic infections; impaired breathing; wasting syndrome and fluid and electrolyte imbalances; adverse reaction to medications

GOAL: Absence of complications

Nursing Interventions	Rationale	Expected Outcomes
Opportunistic Infections		
1. Monitor vital signs including temperature.	1. Changes in vital signs such as increases in pulse rate, respirations, blood pressure, and temperature may indicate infection.	• Exhibits stable vital signs • Experiences control of infection • Identifies signs and symptoms correctly and experiences no complications
2. Obtain laboratory specimens, and monitor test results.	2. Smears and cultures can identify causative agents such as bacteria, fungi, and protozoa, and sensitivity studies can identify antibiotics or other medications effective against the causative agent.	• Identifies signs and symptoms that are reportable to the primary provider • Takes medications as prescribed
3. Instruct the patient and caregiver about signs and symptoms of infection and the need to report them early.	3. Early recognition of symptoms facilitates prompt treatment and avoids extra complications.	
Impaired Breathing		
1. Monitor respiratory rate and pattern.	1. Rapid shallow breathing, diminished breath sounds, and shortness of breath may indicate respiratory failure resulting in hypoxia.	• Maintains stable respiratory rate and pattern within the normal limits • Exhibits no adventitious lung sounds; normal breath sounds
2. Auscultate the chest for breath sounds and abnormal lung sounds.	2. Crackles and wheezes may indicate fluid in the lungs, which disrupts respiratory function and alters the blood's oxygen-carrying capacity.	• Has stable pulse rate and blood pressure within normal limits, and exhibits no evidence of hypoxia • Oxygen saturation levels within acceptable range
3. Monitor pulse rate, blood pressure, and oxygen saturation levels.	3. Changes in pulse rate, blood pressure, and oxygen levels may indicate the development of respiratory or cardiac failure.	

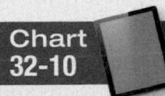

Chart 32-10

PLAN OF NURSING CARE (continued)
Care of the Patient with AIDS

Nursing Interventions	Rationale	Expected Outcomes
Wasting Syndrome and Fluid and Electrolyte Disturbances		
1. Monitor weight and laboratory values for nutritional status.	1. Weight loss, malnutrition, and anemia are common in HIV infection and increase risk of superinfection.	• Maintains stable weight • Eats a nutritious diet • Attains and maintains hemoglobin, hematocrit, and ferritin levels within normal limits • Sustains fluid and electrolyte balance within normal limits • Exhibits no signs and symptoms of dehydration
2. Monitor intake and output and laboratory values for fluid and electrolyte imbalance (potassium, sodium, calcium, phosphorus, magnesium, and zinc).	2. Chronic diarrhea, inadequate oral intake, vomiting, and profuse sweating deplete electrolytes. Small intestine inflammation may impair the absorption of fluids and electrolytes.	
3. Monitor for and report signs and symptoms of dehydration.	3. Fluid loss results in decreased circulating volume leading to tachycardia, dry skin and mucous membranes, poor skin turgor, elevated urine specific gravity, and thirst. Early detection allows early treatment.	
Reactions to Medications		
1. Monitor for medication interactions.	1. People with HIV infection receive many medications for HIV and for disease complications. Early detection of medication interactions is necessary to prevent complications.	• Experiences no serious side effects or complications from medications • Correctly describes medication regimen and complies with therapy, including adaptations in eating routines and type of food used with prescribed medications
2. Monitor for and promptly report side effects from antiretroviral agents.	2. Side effects from antiretroviral agents can be life-threatening. Serious side effects include anemia, pancreatitis, peripheral neuropathy, mental confusion, and persistent nausea and vomiting. Corrective measures need to be instituted.	
3. Instruct the patient and caregiver in the medication regimen.	3. Knowledge of the medication purpose, correct administration, side effects, and strategies to manage or prevent side effects promotes safety and greater compliance with treatment.	

The patient's level of knowledge about HIV infection, modes of disease transmission, and adherence to ART are evaluated. In addition, the level of knowledge of family (biologic and family of choice) and friends is assessed. The patient's psychological reaction to the diagnosis of HIV infection is important to explore. Reactions vary among patients and may include denial, anger, fear, shame, withdrawal from social interactions, and depressive symptoms (Lu et al., 2018). It is often helpful to gain an understanding of how the patient has dealt with illness and major life stresses in the past. The patient's resources for support are also identified.

Diagnosis

NURSING DIAGNOSES

Based on the assessment data, major nursing diagnoses may include the following:
- Impaired nutritional intake associated with decreased oral intake

- Social isolation associated with stigma of HIV infection, withdrawal of support systems, isolation procedures, and fear of infecting others
- Grief associated with changes in lifestyle and roles
- Lack of knowledge associated with HIV infection, means of preventing HIV transmission, ART, and self-management strategies

COLLABORATIVE PROBLEMS/POTENTIAL COMPLICATIONS

Possible complications may include the following:
- Adverse effects of medications
- Development of HAND
- Body image changes

Planning and Goals

Goals for the patient may include improved nutritional status, increased socialization, expression of grief, increased knowledge regarding disease prevention and self-care, and absence of complications.

Nursing Interventions

IMPROVING NUTRITIONAL STATUS

Nutritional status is assessed by monitoring weight; dietary intake; and serum albumin, BUN, protein, and transferrin levels. The patient is also assessed for factors that interfere with oral intake, such as anorexia and lactose intolerance. Based on the results of assessment, the nurse can implement specific measures to facilitate oral intake. The dietitian is consulted to determine the patient's nutritional requirements.

The patient is encouraged to eat foods that are easy to swallow and to avoid spicy or sticky food items and foods that are excessively hot or cold. Oral hygiene before and after meals is encouraged. The patient who is underweight is instructed about ways to enhance the nutritional value of meals. Adding eggs, butter, or fortified milk (milk to which powdered skim milk has been added to increase the caloric content) to gravies, soups, or milkshakes can provide additional calories and protein. High-calorie, nutritional foods such as puddings, powders, milkshakes, and nutritional supplements may also be useful.

DECREASING THE SENSE OF ISOLATION

People with HIV are at risk for double stigmatization. They have what society refers to as a "dreaded disease," and they may have a lifestyle that differs from what is considered acceptable by many people. The diagnosis might prompt disclosure about hidden lifestyles or behaviors to family, friends, coworkers, and health care providers. As a result, people with HIV infection may be overwhelmed with emotions such as anxiety, guilt, shame, and fear. They also may be faced with multiple losses, such as loss of financial security, normal roles and functions, self-esteem, privacy, ability to control bodily functions, ability to interact meaningfully with the environment, and sexual functioning as well as rejection by sexual partners, family, and friends. Some patients may harbor feelings of guilt because of their lifestyle or because they may have infected others in current or previous relationships. Other patients may feel anger toward sexual partners who transmitted the virus to them. Infection control measures used in the hospital or at home may further contribute to the patient's emotional isolation. Any or all of these stressors may cause the patient to withdraw both physically and emotionally from social contact.

Nurses are in a key position to provide an atmosphere of acceptance and understanding for people with HIV infection and their social networks. The patient's usual level of social interaction is assessed as early as possible to provide a baseline for monitoring changes in behaviors that suggest social isolation (e.g., decreased interaction with staff or family, hostility, nonadherence). Patients are encouraged to express feelings of isolation and loneliness, with the assurance that these feelings are not unique or abnormal.

Providing information about how to protect themselves and others may help patients avoid social isolation. Patients, family, and friends must be reassured that HIV is not spread through casual contact. Education of ancillary personnel, nurses, and physicians helps reduce factors that might contribute to patients' feelings of isolation.

COPING WITH GRIEF

The nurse can help the patient verbalize feelings and explore and identify resources for support and mechanisms for coping, especially when the patient is grieving anticipated losses. The patient is encouraged to maintain contact with family, friends, and coworkers and to use local or national support groups and hotlines. If possible, losses are identified and addressed. The patient is encouraged to continue usual activities whenever possible. Consultations with mental health counselors are useful for many patients and their families.

IMPROVING KNOWLEDGE OF HIV

The patient and family are educated about HIV infection, means of preventing HIV transmission, ART, and appropriate self-care measures. Information about the purpose of the medications, their correct administration, side effects, and strategies to manage or prevent side effects is provided.

MONITORING AND MANAGING POTENTIAL COMPLICATIONS

Side Effects of Medications. Adverse effects are of concern in patients who receive numerous medications for HIV infection. Many medications can cause severe toxic effects. Patients and their caregivers need to know which signs and symptoms of side/toxic effects should be reported immediately to their primary care provider (see Table 32-4).

In addition to medications used to treat HIV infection, other medications that may be required include opioids, tricyclic antidepressants, and NSAIDs for pain relief; medications for treatment of opportunistic and coinfections; antihistamines (diphenhydramine for relief of pruritus; acetaminophen or aspirin for management of fever; and antiemetic agents for control of nausea and vomiting). Concurrent use of these medications can cause many drug interactions, resulting in hepatic and hematologic abnormalities. Therefore, careful monitoring of laboratory test results is essential.

During each contact with the patient, the nurse not only asks about side effects, but also about how well the patient is adhering to the medication regimen. To promote adherence, the nurse should assist the patient to organize and plan the medication schedule. Individualized adherence plans should consider housing and social support issues, in addition to health indicators including possible drug–drug interactions. Self-reported adherence measures can distinguish clinically meaningful patterns of medication-taking behaviors; therefore, nurses should assess if patients can describe how they are taking their ART.

Research suggests that the development of effective self-management strategies leads to increased ART adherence (Schreiner, Perazzo, Currie, et al., 2019), PLWHA at risk for high treatment burden and subsequent nonadherence are those with multiple comorbidities and low social support (Schreiner et al., 2019). See the Nursing Research Profile in Chart 32-11.

Monitoring for HAND. Each contact with the patient is also an opportunity to assess for the presence of HAND. A baseline assessment and then an annual assessment for signs and symptoms are recommended (Cummins et al., 2019). Nurses also need to educate caregivers about signs and symptoms of this subtle disorder.

Body Image Changes. Body image changes often occur in patients with HIV and are an important collaborative problem. The nurse helps the patient verbalize feelings and explore and identify resources for support and mechanisms for coping with body image changes. Consultations with mental health counselors may be indicated for patients adjusting to body image changes.

Chart 32-11 NURSING RESEARCH PROFILE
Treatment Burden in People Living with HIV

Schreiner, N., Perazzo, J., Currie, J., et al. (2019). A descriptive, cross-sectional study examining treatment burden in people living with HIV. *Applied Nursing Research, 46*, 31–36.

Purpose

Successful HIV treatment associated with advances in ART has resulted in HIV being classified as a chronic condition. The purposes of this study were to: (1) describe persons living with HIV/AIDS (PLWHA) experiencing high levels of treatment burden who are at high risk for self-management nonadherence, and (2) test the relationship between known antecedent correlates (the number of chronic conditions, social capital, and age) of self-management and treatment burden in community dwelling sample of PLWHA while controlling for socio-demographics. As an indicator of social support, the relationship between social capital and treatment burden was tested.

Design

This was a descriptive, correlational, cross-sectional secondary analysis of a larger, multi-site study that examined physical activity patterns of PLWHA. Participants were ≥18 years of age and had confirmed HIV (HIV+ ELISA with confirmatory PCR or Western blot). An additional inclusion criterion was diagnosis of two or more chronic conditions identified in the patient's medical record. The Treatment Burden Questionnaire-13 (TBQ-13) was used to measure participant treatment burden. The TBQ-13 is a psychometrically tested instrument containing 13 items inquiring about burden associated with self-management tasks such as medication administration, self-monitoring of chronic conditions, or changes in diet. The TQB-13 asks the respondent to rank the level of burden for each question with responses ranging from 0-No Burden, to 10-Very High Burden, with summed scores ranging from 0 to 130 (higher scores indicating greater treatment burden). The Social Capital Measurement Tool was used to measure social resources.

Findings

Participants were on average 50 years of age; most were African American, male, Medicaid insured, and had a high school diploma. There was a mean of 3.63 (SD = 1.76) chronic conditions and the mean treatment burden score was 22.84 (SD = 24.57). Based on established cut-off points for low, medium, and high treatment burden, the sample experienced low levels of treatment burden, though there was wide variation in treatment burden scores. Approximately 60 PLWHA (58%) reported low treatment burden, 27 (26%) moderate treatment burden, and 16 (16%) high treatment burden. The number of comorbidities was positively associated with treatment burden, and social resources were negatively correlated with treatment burden.

Nursing Implications

Nurses need to be aware that there are potential benefits of treatment burden screening that may help to improve self-management adherence. These results can help inform nurses how to improve the self-management adherence in PLWHA who are affected by treatment burden in the clinical setting.

PROMOTING, HOME, COMMUNITY-BASED, AND TRANSITIONAL CARE

Educating Patients About Self-Care. Patients, families, and friends are educated about the routes of transmission of HIV. The nurse discusses precautions the patient can use to avoid transmitting HIV sexually (see Charts 32-2 and 32-3) or through sharing of body fluids, especially blood. Patients and their families or caregivers must receive instructions about how to prevent disease transmission, including hand hygiene techniques and methods for safely handling and disposing of items soiled with body fluids. Clear guidelines about avoiding and controlling infection, keeping regular health care appointments, symptom management, nutrition, rest, and exercise are necessary (see Chart 32-12). The importance of personal and environmental hygiene is emphasized. Caregivers are taught hand hygiene and appropriate infection prevention precautions (see Chapter 66, Charts 66-1 and 66-2). Kitchen and bathroom surfaces should be cleaned regularly with disinfectants to prevent growth of fungi and bacteria. Patients with pets are encouraged to have another person clean areas soiled by animals, such as birdcages and litter boxes. If this is not possible, patients should use gloves to clean the area and then wash their hands afterward. Patients are advised to avoid exposure to others who are sick or who have been recently vaccinated, especially with live vaccine. The importance of avoiding smoking, excessive alcohol, and over-the-counter and street drugs is emphasized. Patients who are HIV positive or who inject drugs are instructed not to donate blood. IV/injection drug users who are unwilling to stop using drugs are advised to avoid sharing drug equipment with others.

Caregivers in the home are taught how to administer medications. The medication regimens used for patients with HIV infection can be complex and expensive. Patients receiving combination therapies for the treatment of HIV infection require careful education about the importance of taking medications as prescribed and explanations and assistance in fitting the medication regimen into their lives (see Chart 32-8). If the patient requires enteral or parenteral nutrition, instruction is provided to the patient and family about how to administer nutritional therapies at home. Nurses provide ongoing education and support for the patient and family.

Continuing and Transitional Care. Many people with HIV remain in their community and continue their usual daily activities, whereas others can no longer work or maintain their independence. Families or caregivers may need assistance in providing supportive care. Many community-based organizations provide a variety of services for people living with HIV infection; nurses can help identify these services.

Home, community-based, transitional, and hospice nurses are in an excellent position to provide the support and guidance that is so often needed in the home setting. Home health nurses are key to the safe and effective administration of parenteral antibiotics, chemotherapy, and nutrition in the home.

During home visits, the nurse assesses the patient's physical and emotional status and home environment. The patient's adherence to the therapeutic regimen is assessed, and strategies are suggested to assist with adherence. The patient is assessed for progression of disease and for adverse side effects of medications. Previous education is reinforced, and the importance of keeping follow-up appointments is stressed.

Chart 32-12

HOME CARE CHECKLIST

Infection Prevention for the Patient with Immune Deficiency

At the completion of education, the patient and/or caregiver will be able to:

- State the impact of immune deficiency on physiologic functioning, ADLs, IADLs, roles, relationships, and spirituality.
- State changes in lifestyle (e.g., hygiene, activity) necessary to decrease risk for infection.
  - Maintain good hand hygiene technique before eating, after using the bathroom, and before and after performing health care procedures.
  - Maintain total body hygiene and foot care to prevent bacterial and fungal diseases.
  - Maintain skin integrity, using cream and emollients to prevent or manage dry, chafed, or cracked skin.
  - Maintain good oral hygiene and dental checkups.
  - Avoid people with infections, recent vaccinations, and crowds.
  - Perform deep breathing; use incentive spirometer every 4 hours while awake if mobility is restricted.
  - Provide adequate lubrication with gentle vaginal manipulation during sexual intercourse; avoid anal intercourse.
- State changes in home environment necessary to decrease risk for infection.
  - Avoid cleaning birdcages and litter boxes; consider avoiding garden work (soil) and fresh flowers in stagnant water.
  - Identify the rationale for frequent cleaning of kitchen and bathroom surfaces with disinfectant.

- Verbalize understanding of ways to maintain a nutritious diet and adequate calories and necessary changes to decrease risk of infection.
- State the reason for avoiding the eating of raw fruits and vegetables, cooking all foods thoroughly, and immediately refrigerating all leftover food.
- Identify rationale and benefits of avoiding alcohol, tobacco, and unprescribed medications.
- State the name, dose, side effects, frequency, and schedule for all medications.
- Verbalize ways to cope with stress successfully, plans for regular exercise, and rationale for obtaining adequate rest.
- Identify signs and symptoms of infection to report to the primary provider, such as fever; chills; wet or dry cough; breathing problems; white patches in the mouth; swollen glands; nausea; vomiting; persistent abdominal pain; persistent diarrhea; problems with urination or changes in the character of the urine; red, swollen, or draining wounds; sores or lesions on the body; persistent vaginal discharge with or without itching; and severe fatigue.
- Demonstrate how to monitor for signs of infection.
- Describe to whom, how, and when to report signs of infection.
- Describe appropriate actions to take should infection occur.

ADLs, activities of daily living; IADLs, instrumental activities of daily living.

Complex wound care or respiratory care may be required in the home. Patients and families are often unable to meet these skilled care needs without assistance. Nurses may refer patients to community programs that offer a range of services for patients, friends, and families, including help with housekeeping, hygiene, and meals; transportation and shopping; individual and group therapy; support for caregivers; telephone networks for the homebound; and legal and financial assistance. These services are typically provided by both professionals and nonprofessional volunteers. A social worker may be consulted to identify sources of financial support, if needed.

Home health and hospice nurses are increasingly called on to provide physical and emotional support to patients and families as patients with AIDS enter the terminal stages of disease. This support takes on special meaning when people with AIDS lose friends and when family members fear the disease or feel anger concerning the patient's lifestyle. The nurse encourages the patient and family to discuss end-of-life decisions and to ensure that care is consistent with those decisions, all comfort measures are employed, and the patient is treated with dignity at all times.

Evaluation

Expected patient outcomes may include:
1. Maintains adequate nutritional status
2. Experiences decreased sense of social isolation
3. Progresses through grieving process
4. Reports increased understanding of HIV infection, prevention of HIV transmission, and ART, and participates in self-management strategies as possible
5. Remains free of complications

Emotional and Ethical Concerns

Nurses in all settings are called on to provide care for patients with HIV infection. In doing so, they encounter not only the physical challenges of this epidemic but also emotional and ethical concerns. The concerns raised by health care professionals involve issues such as fear of infection, responsibility for giving care, values clarification, confidentiality, developmental stages of patients and caregivers, and poor prognostic outcomes.

Many patients with HIV infection have engaged in "stigmatized" behaviors. Because these behaviors challenge some traditional religious and moral values, nurses may feel reluctant to care for these patients. In addition, health care providers may still have fear and anxiety about disease transmission despite education concerning infection control and the low incidence of transmission to health care providers. Nurses are encouraged to examine their personal beliefs and to use the process of values clarification to approach controversial issues (see Chapter 1, Chart 1-10). The ANA's Code of Ethics for Nurses (ANA, 2015) provides guidance including the first provision which states, "The nurse practices with compassion and respect for the inherent dignity, worth, and unique attributes of every person" (p. 1).

Nurses are responsible for protecting the patient's right to privacy by safeguarding confidential information. Inadvertent disclosure of confidential patient information may result in personal, financial, and emotional hardships for the patient. The controversy surrounding confidentiality concerns the circumstances in which information may be disclosed to others (see Chart 32-13). Health care team members need accurate patient information to conduct assessment, planning, implementation, and evaluation of patient care. Failure to disclose HIV status could compromise the quality of patient care.

Chart 32-13 ETHICAL DILEMMA
What if Maintaining Confidentiality Results in Harm?

Case Scenario

You are a nurse employed on a *per diem* basis for a home health agency. A nursing professor whom you know has received funding to conduct a mixed methods research study on men in your community who are experiencing homelessness and living with being human immune deficiency virus (HIV) positive. She has funds to pay nurses with community health experience to gather data for her study, and you were solicited and received education to serve as one of her nurse data collectors. You are assigned to conduct interviews at a homeless shelter for veterans. Eligible participants must sign an informed consent prior to being interviewed; this informed consent was approved by an institutional review board (IRB) at the nursing professor's university and was also approved by the governance board of the homeless shelter for veterans. One day while you are conducting an interview with T.M., a 28-year-old man with a history of male prostitution and substance use disorder (SUD), he suddenly begins to cry softly and says to you "I am sorry.... I just feel life is no longer worth living. I need to end things and stop going on like this." After further validating the meaning of his words, you learn that T.M. has made a plan to commit suicide. The informed consent that T.M. has signed contains assurances that his name and any information that he shares will not be divulged to anyone outside of the research team. You are conflicted about whether or not you may share his suicidal intentions with anyone.

Discussion

It is standard practice that participants who enroll in research studies are guaranteed confidentiality of their identities. However, T.M. is a particularly vulnerable research participant because he is homeless and HIV positive. Interviewing a participant in a research study who is vulnerable can cause emotional distress that might cause harm. Ideally, this contingency should have been identified by the nursing professor and the IRB, and there should have been additional information in the informed consent that identified a behavioral health professional who could be contacted should participants experience distress. Furthermore, the clause in the informed consent that assured T.M. of the confidential nature of the interview should have specified that this confidentiality would need to be breached if it was determined that participant safety was compromised.

Analysis

- Describe the ethical principles that are in conflict in this case (see Chapter 1, Chart 1-7). Can the principle of nonmaleficence be considered the preeminent principle that guides your decision regarding next steps?
- Assume that the informed consent does not make any of the specifications previously noted to protect vulnerable participants. Would you feel obligated to relay these findings to the nursing professor who serves as the principal investigator of the research team? Would you feel obligated to relay these findings to the social worker at the homeless shelter? Now assume that the provisions to protect T.M. were indeed specified in the informed consent. Would that change whether or not you would notify either the nursing professor or the social worker?
- What resources might be mobilized to be of assistance to you as you navigate your role as a research assistant? What are your legal and ethical obligations? Do you have the right or the responsibility to contact the nursing professor's IRB?

References

Leyva-Moral, J. M., & Feijoo-Cid, M. (2017). Participants' safety versus confidentiality: A case study of HIV research. *Nursing Ethics, 24*(3), 376–380.

Resources

See Chapter 1, Chart 1-10, for Steps of an Ethical Analysis and Ethics Resources.

Sexual partners of patients infected with HIV should know about the potential for infection and the need to engage in safer sex practices, as well as the possible need for testing and health care. Nurses are advised to discuss concerns about confidentiality with nurse administrators and to consult professional nursing organizations such as the Association of Nurses in AIDS Care and legal experts in their state to identify the most appropriate course of action.

Education and provision of up-to-date information help to alleviate apprehension and prepare nurses to deliver safe, high-quality patient care. Interdisciplinary meetings allow participants to support one another and provide comprehensive patient care. Staff support groups give nurses an opportunity to solve problems and explore values and feelings about caring for patients with AIDS and their families; they also provide a forum for grieving. Other sources of support include nursing administrators, peers, and spiritual advisors.

CRITICAL THINKING EXERCISES

1 ebp Your patient is a 33-year-old transgender woman who has been diagnosed as HIV infected, stage 2. The patient tells you that they do not want to take ART because it is interfering with their self-managed hormone therapy. What is the evidence about the drug/drug interaction between ART and transitional hormone therapy? What strategies could you identify to promote adherence to ART regimen? What are the consequences of discontinuing ART?

2 pcc A 55-year-old male who uses injection drugs and is HIV infected comes to the clinic where you work. He tells you that he has been experiencing night sweats, late afternoon fevers, cough, and weight loss. Identify this patient's health priorities and state the next steps you will use to meet his identified needs and other health promotion needs.

3 ipc Your patient, a heterosexual woman who is HIV infected, tells you that she wants to have unprotected sexual relations with her male partner who is HIV negative. What preventive measures should you educate this patient about? What additional members of the health care team should be included in the care of this patient?

REFERENCES

*Asterisk indicates nursing research.

Books

American Nurses Association (ANA). (2015). *Code of ethics for nurses with interpretive statements.* Silver Spring, MD: Author.

American Nurses Association (ANA). (2016). Position statement on the nurse's role in ethics and human rights: Protecting and promoting individual worth, dignity, and human rights in practice settings. Retrieved on 10/27/2019 at: www.nursingworld.org/~4ad4a8/globalassets/docs/ana/nursesrole-ethicshumanrights-positionstatement.pdf

American Nurses Association (ANA). (2019). *Position statement: Prevention of and care for HIV and related conditions.* Silver Spring, MD: Author.

Comerford, K. C., & Durkin, M. T. (2020). *Nursing 2020 drug handbook.* Philadelphia, PA: Wolters Kluwer.

Eliopoulos, C. (2018). *Gerontological nursing* (9th ed.). Philadelphia, PA: Wolters-Kluwer.

Fischbach, F. T., & Fischbach, M. A. (2018). *Fischbach's manual of laboratory and diagnostic tests* (10th ed.). Philadelphia, PA: Wolters Kluwer.

Norris, T. (2019). *Porth's pathophysiology: Concepts of altered health status* (10th ed.). Philadelphia, PA: Wolters Kluwer.

Journals and Electronic Documents

*Centers for Disease Control and Prevention (CDC). (2014). Revised surveillance case definition for HIV infection—United States, 2014. *MMWR. Recommendations and Reports: Morbidity and Mortality Weekly Report. Recommendations and Reports,* 63(RR-03), 1–10.

Centers for Disease Control and Prevention (CDC). (2018a). Updated U.S. Public Health Service guidelines for the management of occupational exposures to HIV and recommendations for postexposure prophylaxis. Retrieved on 10/27/2019 at: npin.cdc.gov/publication/updated-us-public-health-service-guidelines-management-occupational-exposures-human

Centers for Disease Control and Prevention (CDC). (2018b). Quick reference guide: Recommended laboratory HIV testing algorithm for serum or plasma specimens. Retrieved on 10/28/2019 at: stacks.cdc.gov/view/cdc/50872

Centers for Disease Control and Prevention (CDC). (2019a). HIV Surveillance Report, 2017. Retrieved on 10/21/2019 at: www.cdc.gov/hiv/library/reports/hiv-surveillance.html

Centers for Disease Control and Prevention (CDC). (2019b). HIV and older Americans. Retrieved on 10/21/2019 at: www.cdc.gov/hiv/group/age/olderamericans/index.html

Centers for Disease Control and Prevention (CDC). (2019c). PrEP. Retrieved on 10/21/2019 at: www.cdc.gov/hiv/basics/prep.html

Centers for Disease Control and Prevention (CDC). (2019d). Sexually Transmitted Disease Surveillance 2018. Retrieved on 10/21/2019 at: www.cdc.gov/nchhstp/newsroom/2019/2018-STD-surveillance-report.html

Centers for Disease Control and Prevention (CDC). (2019e). CDC's HIV prevention progress in the United States. Retrieved on 10/21/2019 at: www.cdc.gov/hiv/dhap/progress/index.html

Centers for Disease Control and Prevention (CDC). (2019f). Compendium of evidence-based interventions and best practices for HIV prevention. Retrieved on 10/21/2019 at: www.cdc.gov/hiv/prevention/research/compendium/index.html

Centers for Disease Control and Prevention (CDC). (2019g). Syringe Services Programs (SSPs) FAQs. Retrieved on 10/27/2019 at: www.cdc.gov/ssp/syringe-services-programs-faq.html#reduce-infections

Centers for Disease Control and Prevention. (2019h). Understanding the HIV care continuum. Retrieved on 10/28/2019 at: www.cdc.gov/hiv/pdf/library/factsheets/cdc-hiv-care-continuum.pdf

*Cummins, D., Waters, D., Aggar, C., et al. (2019). Assessing risk of HIV-associated neurocognitive disorder. *Nursing Research,* 68(1), 22–28.

Ensor, S., Davies, B., Rai, T., et al. (2019). The effectiveness of demand creation interventions for voluntary male medical circumcision for HIV prevention in sub-Saharan Africa: A mixed methods systematic review. *Journal of The International AIDS Society,* 22(Suppl 4), e25299.

Evidence for Contraceptive Options and HIV Outcomes (ECHO) Trial Consortium. (2019). HIV incidence among women using intramuscular depot medroxyprogesterone acetate, a copper intrauterine device, or a levonorgestrel implant for contraception: A randomized, multicentre, open-label trial. *Lancet,* 394(10195), 303–313.

Glynn, T. R., Llabre, M. M., Lee, J. S., et al. (2019). Pathways to health: An examination of HIV-related stigma, life stressors, depression, and substance use. *International Journal of Behavioral Medicine,* 26(3), 286–296.

Greene, M., Hessol, N. A., Perissinotto, C., et al. (2018). Loneliness in older adults living with HIV. *AIDS and Behavior,* 22(5), 1475–1484.

Guaraldi, G., Malagoli, A., Calcagno, A., et al. (2018). The increasing burden and complexity of multi-morbidity and polypharmacy in geriatric HIV patients: A cross sectional study of people aged 65–74 years and more than 75 years. *BMC Geriatrics,* 18(1), 1–10.

Hajjar, J., Guffey, D., Minard, C. G., et al. (2017). Increased incidence of fatigue in patients with Primary Immunodeficiency Disorders: Prevalence and associations within the US Immunodeficiency Network Registry. *Journal of Clinical Immunology,* 37(2), 153–165.

Hill, L. M., Golin, C. E., Pack, A., et al. (2020). Using real-time adherence feedback to enhance communication about adherence to antiretroviral therapy: Patient and clinician perspectives. *Journal of the Association of Nurses in AIDS Care,* 31(1), 25–34.

HIV Information. (2020). The HIV life cycle. Retrieved on 10/13/2020 at: https://hivinfo.nih.gov/understanding-hiv/fact-sheets/hiv-life-cycle

Leyva-Moral, J. M., & Feijoo-Cid, M. (2017). Participants' safety versus confidentiality: A case study of HIV research. *Nursing Ethics,* 24(3), 376–380.

*Lu, H., Hsiao, F., Sheng, W., et al. (2018). Prevalence and predictors of depression among people living with HIV/AIDS: A national study. *Nursing Research,* 67(5), 379–386.

McDermott, D. H., & Murphy, P. M. (2019). WHIM syndrome: Immunopathogenesis, treatment and cure strategies. *Immunological Reviews,* 287(1), 91–102.

Narendran, G., Oliveira-de-Souza, D., Vinhaes, C. L., et al. (2019). Multifocal tuberculosis-associated immune reconstitution inflammatory syndrome—a case report of a complicated scenario. *BMC Infectious Diseases,* 19(1), 1–5.

National Institute of Allergy and Infectious Diseases (NIAID). (2019a). Primary immune deficiency diseases (PIDDs). Retrieved on 10/13/2019 at: www.niaid.nih.gov/diseases-conditions/primary-immune-deficiency-diseases-pidds

National Institute of Allergy and Infectious Diseases (NIAID). (2019b). HIV vaccine development. Retrieved on 10/27/2019 at: www.niaid.nih.gov/diseases-conditions/hiv-vaccine-development

Office of HIV/AIDS and Infectious Disease Policy (OHAIDP). (2019). Developing the Next National HIV/AIDS Strategy. Retrieved on 10/20/2019 at: www.hiv.gov/federal-response/national-hiv-aids-strategy/developing-the-next-nhas

Panel on Antiretroviral Guidelines for Adults and Adolescents (Panel). (2019). Guidelines for the use of antiretroviral agents in HIV-1-infected adults and adolescents. Department of Health and Human Services. Retrieved on 10/29/2019 at: clinicalinfo.hiv.gov/sites/default/files/inline-files/AdultandAdolescentGL.pdf

Panel on Opportunistic Infections in Adults and Adolescents with HIV (OI-Panel). (2019). Guidelines for the prevention and treatment of opportunistic infections in adults and adolescents with HIV: recommendations from the Centers for Disease Control and Prevention, the National Institutes of Health, and the HIV Medicine Association of the Infectious Diseases Society of America. Retrieved on 10/30/2019 at: aidsinfo.nih.gov/contentfiles/lvguidelines/adult_oi.pdf

*Schreiner, N., Perazzo, J., Currie, J., et al. (2019). A descriptive, cross-sectional study examining treatment burden in people living with HIV. *Applied Nursing Research: ANR,* 46, 31–36.

Starbird, L. E., Hong, H., Sulkowski, M. S., et al. (2020). Management of the patient with HIV/Hepatitis C drug interactions: A guide for nurses and nurse practitioners. *Journal of the Association of Nurses in AIDS Care,* 31(2), 241–248. doi:10.1097/JNC.0000000000000144

Stonebraker, J. S., Hajjar, J., & Orange, J. S. (2018). Latent therapeutic demand model for the immunoglobulin replacement therapy of primary immune deficiency disorders in the USA. *Vox Sanguinis.* doi:10.1111/vox.12651

Vitiello, G., Emmi, G., Silvestri, E., et al. (2019). Intravenous immunoglobulin therapy: A snapshot for the internist. *Internal and Emergency Medicine,* 14(7), 1041–1049.

World Health Organization. (2019). HIV/AIDS. Retrieved on 10/30/2019 at: www.who.int/en/news-room/fact-sheets/detail/hiv-aids

Resources

AIDS Community Research Initiative of America (ACRIA), www.acria.org

AIDS Education and Training Centers (AETCs) Program (regional, national, and international training opportunities), www.aidsetc.org

AIDSinfoglossary 9th edition (2018), clinicalinfo.hiv.gov/themes/custom/aidsinfo/documents/glossaryhivrelatedterms_english.pdf

AIDS vaccines, http://www.avac.org/prevention-option/aids-vaccines

Antiretroviral medication information websites: www.sfaf.org; hivinsite.ucsf.edu/; www.amfAR.org; www.natap.org; www.thebody.com

Centers for Disease Control and Prevention, HIV/AIDS Prevention Research Synthesis Project, http://www.cdc.gov/hiv/dhap/prb/prs/

Gay Men's Health Crisis Network (GMHC), www.gmhc.org

Harm Reduction Coalition, http://harmreduction.org/about-us/

Health Resources and Service Administration (HRSA), National Clinician's Post-exposure Prophylaxis Hotline (health care providers only), 1-888-448-4911

Health Resources and Service Administration (HRSA), National HIV Telephone Consultation Service, 1-800-933-3413

International AIDS Vaccine Initiative (AVI), www.iavi.org

International Partnership for Microbicides, www.ipmglobal.org

National Institutes of Health, HIV/AIDS Treatment, Prevention, and Research, www.aidsinfo.nih.gov

Office of Minority Health Resource Center, www.minorityhealth.hhs.gov/omh/browse.aspx?lvl=4&lvlid=21

POZ, *Health, Life, & HIV.* Published by Smart+Strong, 500 Fifth Avenue, Suite 320, New York, NY 10110, www.poz.com/

Prevention Access Campaign, www.preventionaccess.org

33

Assessment and Management of Patients with Allergic Disorders

LEARNING OUTCOMES

On completion of this chapter, the learner will be able to:

1. Describe the physiologic events involved with allergic reactions and types of hypersensitivity.
2. Use appropriate parameters for assessment of the status of patients with allergic disorders.
3. Identify the pathophysiology, clinical manifestations, and management of patients with allergic disorders.
4. Specify measures to prevent and manage anaphylaxis.
5. Use the nursing process as a framework for care of the patient with allergic rhinitis.

NURSING CONCEPTS

Cellular Regulation   Immunity   Infection

GLOSSARY

allergen: substance that causes manifestations of allergy

allergy: inappropriate and often harmful immune system response to substances that are normally harmless

anaphylaxis: rapid clinical response to an immediate immunologic reaction between a specific antigen and antibody

angioedema: condition characterized by urticaria and diffuse swelling of the deeper layers of the skin (*synonym:* angioneurotic edema)

antibody: protein substance developed by B cells in response to and interacting with a specific antigen

antigen: substance that the body identifies as a foreign invader; antigens induce the production of antibodies

antihistamine: medication that opposes the action of histamine

atopic dermatitis: type I hypersensitivity involving inflammation of the skin evidenced by itching, redness, and a variety of skin lesions

atopic march: a progression of allergic disease beginning with atopic dermatitis continuing to IgE-mediated food allergy, asthma, and allergic rhinitis

atopy: term often used to describe immunoglobulin E–mediated diseases (i.e., atopic dermatitis, asthma, and allergic rhinitis) with a genetic component

B cells: lymphocyte cells that are stimulated to produce antibodies

bradykinin: a substance that stimulates nerve fibers and causes pain

eosinophil: granular leukocyte

erythema: diffuse redness of the skin

hapten: incomplete antigen

histamine: substance in the body that causes increased gastric secretion, dilation of capillaries, and constriction of the bronchial smooth muscle

hypersensitivity: abnormal heightened reaction to a stimulus of any kind

immunoglobulins: a family of closely related proteins capable of acting as antibodies

leukotrienes: a group of chemical mediators that initiate the inflammatory response

mast cells: connective tissue cells that contain heparin and histamine in their granules

plasma cells: upon stimulation by antigen, B lymphocytes differentiate into plasma cells that secrete antibodies

prostaglandins: unsaturated fatty acids that have a wide assortment of biologic activity

serotonin: chemical mediator that acts as a potent vasoconstrictor and bronchoconstrictor

T cells: lymphocyte cells that participate in cellular immunity and assist in humoral (B-cell) immunity

urticaria: a round, reddened skin elevation or hives

Allergic disorders are common and are encountered by nurses in every setting, from the community to the intensive care unit. Expert management of patients with allergic disorders is integral to nursing regardless of the practice setting. This chapter covers general allergic assessment and management of various allergic disorders including anaphylaxis.

The human body is bombarded by a host of potential invaders—allergens as well as microbial organisms—that constantly threaten its defenses. These invaders are termed **antigens**. After penetrating the body's defenses, these antigens, if allowed to continue unimpeded, disrupt the body's enzyme systems and destroy its vital tissues. To protect against these antigens, the body is equipped with an elaborate defense system.

The epithelial cells that coat the skin and make up the lining of the respiratory, gastrointestinal, and genitourinary tracts provide the first line of defense against microbial invaders. The structure and continuity of these surfaces and their resistance to penetration are initial deterrents to antigens (Marshall, Warrington, Watson, et al., 2018).

One of the most effective defense mechanisms is the body's capacity to equip itself rapidly with antibodies specifically designed to combat each new invader—namely, specific protein antigens. Antibodies react with antigens in a variety of ways: (1) by coating the antigens' surfaces, (2) by neutralizing the antigens, and (3) by precipitating the antigens out of solution if they are dissolved. The antibodies prepare the antigens so that the phagocytic cells of the blood and the tissues can eliminate them. However, although this system is normally protective, in some cases the body produces inappropriate or exaggerated responses to specific antigens, and the result is an allergic or hypersensitivity disorder.

Physiologic Overview

An allergic reaction is a manifestation of tissue injury resulting from interaction between an antigen and an **antibody** (a protein substance developed by B cells in response to and interacting with a specific antigen) (Marshall et al., 2018). **Allergy** is an inappropriate and often harmful response of the immune system to normally harmless substances, called **allergens** (e.g., dust, weeds, pollen, dander). Chemical mediators released in allergic reactions may produce symptoms that range from mild to life-threatening.

In allergic reactions, the body encounters allergens that are types of antigens, usually proteins that the body's defenses recognize as foreign, and a series of events occurs in an attempt to render the invaders harmless, destroy them, and remove them from the body. There is a generalized white blood cell response to the entrance of antigens into the body. Specific types of white blood cells, called B lymphocytes (also called B cells), are specifically triggered by the presence of antigen. B lymphocytes differentiate into **plasma cells**, which then secrete antibodies that attack the antigen.

Specific antibodies develop in response to specific antigens. Antibodies combine with antigens in a special way, which has been likened to a lock and key. Antigens (the keys) fit only certain antibodies (the locks). Hence, the term *specificity* refers to the specific reaction of an antibody to an antigen. There are many variations and complexities in these patterns. In addition, antibodies have memory for the specific antigen, so that upon future exposure, the lock and key reaction occurs again (Actor, 2019).

Function of Immunoglobulins

Antibodies that are formed by plasma cells in response to an immunogenic stimulus constitute a group of serum proteins called **immunoglobulins**. Grouped into five classes (IgG, IgA, IgM, IgD, and IgE), immunoglobulins can be found in the lymph nodes, tonsils, appendix, and Peyer patches of the intestinal tract or circulating in the blood and lymph. These antibodies are capable of binding with a wide variety of antigens. Immunoglobulins of the IgE class are involved in allergic disorders and some parasitic infections. IgE-producing cells are located in the respiratory and intestinal mucosa. Two or more IgE molecules bind together to an allergen and trigger **mast cells** or basophils to release chemical mediators, such as histamine, serotonin, kinins, slow-reacting substances of anaphylaxis, and the neutrophil factor, which produces allergic skin reactions, asthma, and hay fever. **Atopy** refers to IgE-mediated diseases, such as allergic rhinitis, that have a genetic component (Actor, 2019). See Chapter 31 for more information on immunoglobulins.

Role of B Cells

B cells, or B lymphocytes, are programmed to produce one specific antibody. On encountering a specific antigen, B cells generate plasma cells, at the site of antibody production. The plasma cells secrete antibodies for the purpose of destroying and removing the antigens. B cells participate in humoral immunity (also called antibody-mediated immunity), which is one kind of adaptive immunity (Marshall et al., 2018).

Role of T Cells

There are different types of **T cells**, or T lymphocytes, that participate in cellular immunity (also called cell-mediated immunity), a type of adaptive immunity. T helper cells are specific types of T lymphocytes that assist B cells in the immune response. T cells secrete substances that direct the flow of cell activity and stimulate macrophages. Macrophages present the antigens to the T cells and initiate the immune response. They also digest antigens and assist in removing cells and other debris (Marshall et al., 2018).

Function of Antigens

Antigens are divided into two groups: complete protein antigens and low-molecular-weight substances. Complete protein antigens, such as animal dander, pollen, and horse serum, stimulate a complete humoral response. A humoral response is another name for a B lymphocyte–mediated response. See Chapter 31 for a discussion of humoral immunity. Low-molecular-weight substances, such as medications, function as **haptens** (incomplete antigens), binding to tissue or serum proteins to produce a carrier complex that initiates an antibody response. In an allergic reaction, the production of antibodies requires active communication between cells. When the allergen is absorbed through the respiratory tract, gastrointestinal tract, or skin, allergen sensitization occurs. In the humoral response, B cells mature into allergen-specific secreting plasma cells that synthesize and secrete antigen-specific antibodies (Marshall et al., 2018).

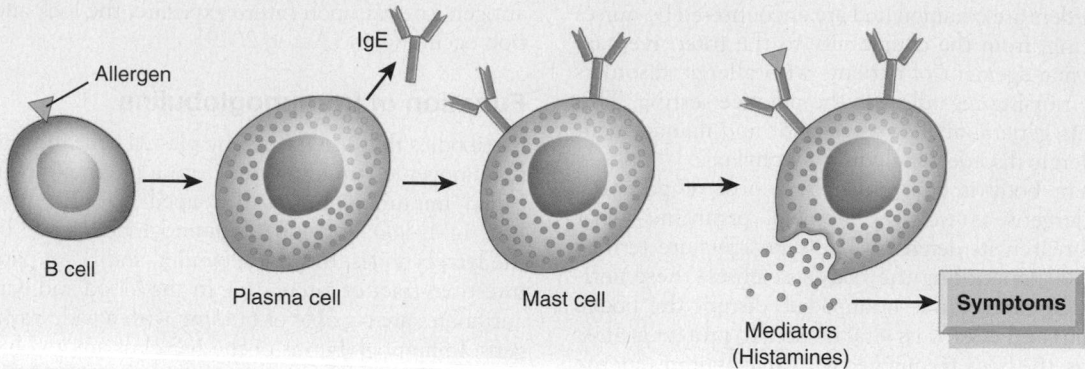

Figure 33-1 • Antigen stimulates activation of a B cell (B lymphocyte), which then transforms into a plasma cell that secretes immunoglobulins. Immunoglobulins stimulate mast cells to release histamine and other inflammatory mediators.

Function of Chemical Mediators

Mast cells, which are located in the skin, respiratory tract, and gastrointestinal tract, play a major role in IgE-mediated immediate hypersensitivity. When mast cells are stimulated by antigens, powerful chemical mediators, such as histamine, are released, causing a sequence of physiologic events that result in symptoms of immediate hypersensitivity (see Fig. 33-1). There are two types of chemical mediators: primary and secondary. Primary mediators are preformed and are found in mast cells or basophils. Secondary mediators are inactive precursors that are formed or released in response to primary mediators. Table 33-1 summarizes the actions of primary and secondary chemical mediators (Castells, 2017).

Primary Mediators

Histamine, eosinophil chemotactic factor of anaphylaxis, platelet-activating factor, and prostaglandins are primary chemical mediators in allergic responses.

Histamine

Histamine, which is released by mast cells, plays an important role in the immune response. It is the first chemical mediator to be released in immune and inflammatory responses. It is synthesized and stored in high concentrations in body tissues exposed to environmental substances. Histamine's effects peak 5 to 10 minutes after antigen contact and include the following: erythema; localized edema in the form of wheals; pruritus; contraction of bronchial smooth muscle, resulting in wheezing and bronchospasm; dilation of small venules and constriction of larger vessels; and increased secretion of gastric and mucosal cells, resulting in diarrhea. Histamine action results from stimulation of histamine-1 (H_1) and histamine-2 (H_2) receptors. H_1 receptors are found predominantly on bronchiolar and vascular smooth muscle cells; H_2 receptors are found on gastric parietal cells (Castells, 2017).

Certain medications are categorized by their action at these receptors. Diphenhydramine is an example of an **antihistamine**, a medication that displays an affinity for H_1

TABLE 33-1 Chemical Mediators of Hypersensitivity	
Mediators	**Action**
Primary Mediators	
Preformed and Found in Mast Cells or Basophils	
Histamine (preformed in mast cells)	Vasodilation
	Smooth muscle contraction, increased vascular permeability, increased mucus secretions
Eosinophil chemotactic factor of anaphylaxis (preformed in mast cells)	Attracts eosinophils
Platelet-activating factor (requires synthesis by mast cells, neutrophils, and macrophages)	Smooth muscle contraction
	Incites platelets to aggregate and release serotonin and histamine
Prostaglandins (chemically derived from arachidonic acid; require synthesis by cells)	D and F series → bronchoconstriction
	E series → bronchodilation
	D, E, and F series → vasodilation
Basophil kallikrein (preformed in mast cells)	Frees bradykinin, which causes bronchoconstriction, vasodilation, and nerve stimulation
Secondary Mediators	
Inactive Precursors Formed or Released in Response to Primary Mediators	
Bradykinin (derived from precursor kininogen)	Smooth muscle contraction, increased vascular permeability, stimulates pain receptors, increased mucus production
Serotonin (preformed in platelets)	Smooth muscle contraction, increased vascular permeability
Heparin (preformed in mast cells)	Anticoagulant
Leukotrienes (derived from arachidonic acid and activated by mast cell degranulation) C, D, and E or slow-reacting substance of anaphylaxis	Smooth muscle contraction, increased vascular permeability

Adapted from Norris, T. (2019). *Porth's pathophysiology: Concepts of altered health states* (10th ed.). Philadelphia, PA: Wolters Kluwer.

receptors. Cimetidine targets H_2 receptors to inhibit gastric secretions in peptic ulcer disease.

Eosinophil Chemotactic Factor of Anaphylaxis

Eosinophil chemotactic factor of anaphylaxis affects the movement of **eosinophils** (granular leukocytes) to the site of allergens. It is preformed in the mast cells and is released from disrupted mast cells.

Platelet-Activating Factor

Platelet-activating factor is responsible for initiating platelet aggregation and leukocyte infiltration at sites of immediate hypersensitivity reactions. It also causes vasodilation, bronchoconstriction, and increased vascular permeability (Castells, 2017).

Prostaglandins

Prostaglandins produce smooth muscle contraction as well as vasodilation and increased capillary permeability. They sensitize pain receptors and increase the pain associated with inflammation. In addition, prostaglandins induce inflammation and enhance the effects of mediators of inflammatory response. Local manifestations include erythema, heat, and edema (Castells, 2017).

Secondary Mediators

Leukotrines, bradykinin, and serotonin are all secondary chemical mediators.

Leukotrienes

Leukotrienes are chemical mediators that initiate the inflammatory response. Many manifestations of inflammation can be attributed in part to leukotrienes. In addition, leukotrienes cause smooth muscle contraction, bronchial constriction, mucus secretion in the airways, and the typical wheal-and-flare reactions of the skin. Compared with histamine, leukotrienes are 100 to 1000 times more potent in causing bronchospasm (Castells, 2017).

Bradykinin

Bradykinin is a substance that has the ability to cause increased vascular permeability, vasodilation, hypotension, and contraction of many types of smooth muscle, such as the bronchi. Increased permeability of the capillaries results in edema. Bradykinin stimulates nerve cell fibers and produces pain.

Serotonin

Serotonin is a chemical mediator that acts as a potent vasoconstrictor and causes contraction of bronchial smooth muscle.

Hypersensitivity

Although the immune system defends the host against infections and foreign antigens, immune responses can themselves cause tissue injury and disease. **Hypersensitivity** is an excessive or aberrant immune response to any type of stimulus (Actor, 2019). It usually does not occur with the first exposure to an allergen. Rather, the reaction follows a re-exposure after sensitization, or buildup of antibodies, in a predisposed person. Injurious or pathologic immune reactions are classed

as hypersensitivity reactions. To promote understanding of the immunopathogenesis of disease, hypersensitivity reactions have been classified into four specific types of reactions (see Fig. 33-2).

Anaphylactic (Type I) Hypersensitivity

The most severe hypersensitivity reaction is **anaphylaxis**. An unanticipated severe allergic reaction that is rapid in onset, anaphylaxis is characterized by edema in many tissues, including the larynx, and is often accompanied by hypotension, bronchospasm, and cardiovascular collapse in severe cases. Anaphylaxis is a severe type I hypersensitivity reaction, which is an immediate reaction beginning within minutes of exposure to an antigen. Primary chemical mediators are responsible for the symptoms of type I hypersensitivity because of their effects on the skin, lungs, and gastrointestinal tract. If chemical mediators continue to be released, a delayed reaction may occur and may last for up to 24 hours (Marshall et al., 2018).

Clinical symptoms are determined by the amount of the allergen, the amount of mediator released, the sensitivity of the target organ, and the route of allergen entry. Type I hypersensitivity reactions may include both local and systemic anaphylaxis (Actor, 2019).

Cytotoxic (Type II) Hypersensitivity

Type II, or cytotoxic hypersensitivity occurs when antibodies are directed against antigens on cells or basement membranes of tissues. This reaction can lead to cell lysis and tissue damage. Type II hypersensitivity reactions are associated with several disorders. The best example is a hemolytic transfusion reaction. For example, if a person with type A blood is mistakenly given type B blood, anti-B antibodies are triggered in the recipient that attack the infused type B blood cells and cause hemolysis (Actor, 2019).

Immune Complex (Type III) Hypersensitivity

Type III, or immune complex hypersensitivity, is a damaging inflammatory reaction caused by the insoluble immune complexes formed by antigens that bind to antibodies. These complexes are too large to be cleared from the circulation by phagocytic action. The immune complexes are deposited in tissues or vascular endothelium and trigger inflammation at different sites throughout the body. An example of this kind of hypersensitivity reaction occurs in rheumatoid arthritis. An unknown antigen triggers antibody formation, which then forms immune complexes that are deposited in the joints. Many autoimmune disorders are type III hypersensitivity reactions. In autoimmune reactions, such as systemic lupus erythematosus, patients form autoantibodies that form immune complexes that deposit in the lungs, skin, and kidney (Actor, 2019).

Delayed (Type IV) Hypersensitivity

Type IV, or delayed hypersensitivity, is a T cell–mediated immune reaction after exposure to an antigen. This immune reaction typically occurs 24 to 48 hours after exposure to an antigen. The prototypical type IV hypersensitivity reaction occurs in response to the subcutaneous injection of purified protein derivative (PPD) antigen from *Mycobacterium tuberculosis*. Patients who have had previous exposure or have

Type I

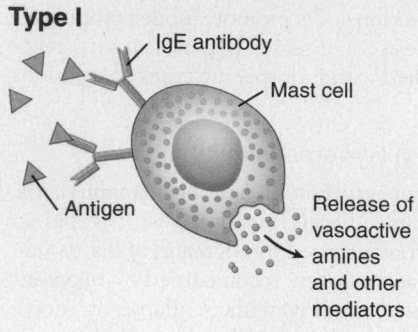

Type I. An anaphylactic reaction is characterized by vasodilation, increased capillary permeability, smooth muscle contraction, and eosinophilia. Systemic reactions may involve laryngeal stridor, angioedema, hypotension, and bronchial, GI, or uterine spasm; local reactions are characterized by hives. Examples of type I reactions include extrinsic asthma, allergic rhinitis, systemic anaphylaxis, and reactions to insect stings.

Type II

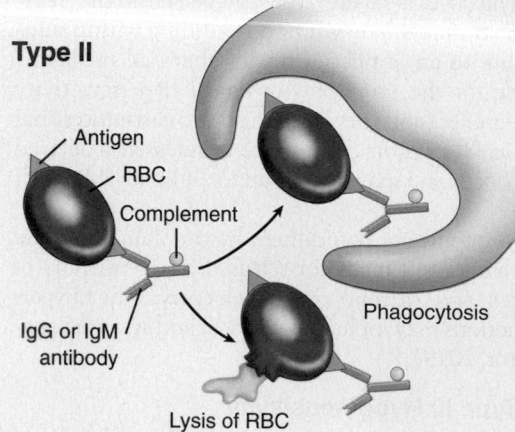

Type II. A cytotoxic reaction, which involves binding either the IgG or IgM antibody to a cell-bound antigen, may lead to eventual cell and tissue damage. The reaction is the result of mistaken identity when the system identifies a normal constituent of the body as foreign and activates the complement cascade. Examples of type II reactions are myasthenia gravis, Goodpasture syndrome, pernicious anemia, hemolytic disease of the newborn, transfusion reaction, and thrombocytopenia.

Type III

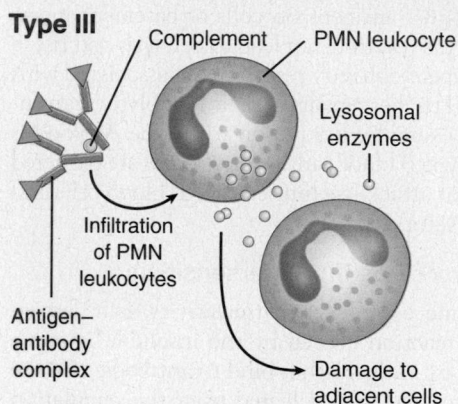

Type III. An immune complex reaction is marked by acute inflammation resulting from formation and deposition of immune complexes. The joints and kidneys are particularly susceptible to this kind of reaction, which is associated with systemic lupus erythematosus, serum sickness, nephritis, and rheumatoid arthritis. Some signs and symptoms include urticaria, joint pain, fever, rash, and adenopathy (swollen glands).

Type IV

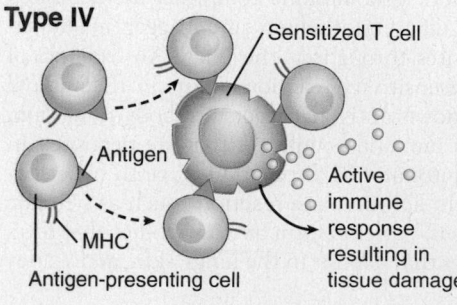

Type IV. A delayed, or cellular, reaction occurs 1 to 3 days after exposure to an antigen. The reaction, which results in tissue damage, involves activity by lymphokines, macrophages, and lysozymes. Erythema and itching are common; a few examples include contact dermatitis, graft-versus-host disease, Hashimoto's thyroiditis, and sarcoidosis.

Figure 33-2 • Four types of hypersensitivity reactions. GI, gastrointestinal; Ig, immunoglobulin; PMN, polymorphonuclear; RBC, red blood cell.

tuberculosis (TB) infection will demonstrate a reaction of erythema and induration due to sensitized T cells (Actor, 2019).

Assessment

A comprehensive allergy history and a thorough physical examination provide useful data for the diagnosis and management of allergic disorders. An allergy assessment form is useful for obtaining and organizing pertinent information (see Chart 33-1).

The degree of difficulty and discomfort experienced by the patient because of allergic symptoms and the degree of improvement in those symptoms with and without treatment are assessed and documented. The relationship of symptoms to exposure to possible allergens is noted.

Chart 33-1

ASSESSMENT

Allergy Assessment Form

Name _____ Age _____ Sex _____ Date _____

I. Chief complaint: _____

II. Present illness: _____

III. Collateral allergic symptoms: _____

Eyes: Pruritus _____   Burning _____   Lacrimation _____
          Swelling _____   Injection _____   Discharge _____

Ears: Pruritus _____   Fullness _____   Popping _____
          Frequent infections _____

Nose: Sneezing _____   Rhinorrhea _____   Obstruction _____
          Pruritus _____   Mouth breathing _____
          Purulent discharge _____

Throat: Soreness _____ Postnasal discharge _____
          Palatal pruritus _____ Mucus in the morning _____

Chest: Cough _____   Pain _____   Wheezing _____
          Sputum _____   Dyspnea _____
          Color _____   Rest _____
          Amount _____   Exertion _____

Skin: Dermatitis _____   Eczema _____   Urticaria _____

IV. Family allergies: _____

V. Previous allergic treatment or testing: _____
   Prior skin testing: _____

   Medications: Antihistamines   Improved _____   Unimproved _____
                  Bronchodilators   Improved _____   Unimproved _____
                  Nose drops   Improved _____   Unimproved _____
                  Hyposensitization   Improved _____   Unimproved _____
                      Duration _____
                      Antigens _____
                      Reactions _____
                  Antibiotics   Improved _____   Unimproved _____
                  Corticosteroids   Improved _____   Unimproved _____

VI. Physical agents and habits: _____

Bothered by:

Tobacco for _____ years   Alcohol _____   Air-conditioning _____
Cigarettes _____ packs/day   Heat _____   Muggy weather _____
Cigars _____ per day   Cold _____   Weather changes _____
Pipes _____ per day   Perfumes _____   Chemicals _____
Never smoked _____   Paints _____   Hair spray _____
Bothered by smoke _____   Insecticides _____   Newspapers _____
                                 Cosmetics _____   Latex _____

VII. When symptoms occur: _____
   Time and circumstances of 1st episode: _____
   Prior health: _____
   Course of illness over decades: progressing _____ regressing _____
   Time of year: _____ Exact dates: _____
       Perennial _____
       Seasonal _____
       Seasonally exacerbated _____
   Monthly variations (menses, occupation): _____
   Time of week (weekends vs. weekdays): _____
   Time of day or night: _____
   After insect stings: _____

VIII. Where symptoms occur: _____
   Living where at onset: _____
   Living where since onset: _____
   Effect of vacation or major geographic change: _____
   Symptoms better indoors or outdoors: _____
   Effect of school or work: _____
   Effect of staying elsewhere nearby: _____
   Effect of hospitalization: _____
   Effect of specific environments: _____
   Do symptoms occur around: _____
       old leaves _____ hay _____ lakeside _____ barns _____
       summer homes _____ damp basement _____ dry attic _____
       lawn mowing _____ animals _____ other _____

(continued on page 1044)

Chart 33-1

ASSESSMENT (continued)
Allergy Assessment Form

Do symptoms occur after eating:

cheese _____ mushrooms _____ beer _____ melons _____

bananas _____ fish _____ nuts _____ citrus fruits _____

other foods (list) _____

Home: city _____ rural _____

house _____ age _____

apartment _____ basement _____ damp _____ dry _____

heating system _____

vacuum cleaner system _____ use of HEPA filter _____

pets (how long) _____ dog _____ cat _____ other _____

Bedroom:	Type	Age	*Living room:*	Type	Age
Pillow	_____	_____	Rug	_____	_____
Mattress	_____	_____	Matting	_____	_____
Blankets	_____	_____	Furniture	_____	_____
Quilts	_____	_____			
Furniture	_____	_____			

Anywhere in home symptoms are worse: _____

IX. What does patient think makes symptoms worse? _____

X. Under what circumstances is patient free of symptoms? _____

XI. Summary and additional comments: _____

Diagnostic Evaluation

Diagnostic evaluation of the patient with allergic disorders commonly includes blood tests, smears of body secretions, skin tests, and the serum-specific IgE test (formerly known as radioallergosorbent test [RAST]). Results of laboratory blood studies provide supportive data for various diagnostic possibilities; however, they are not the major criteria for the diagnosis of allergic disease (Kowal & DuBuske, 2017).

Complete Blood Count with Differential

The white blood cell (WBC) count is usually within normal limits except when infection and inflammation are present along with an allergic disorder. Eosinophils, which are granular leukocytes, normally make up 2% to 5% of the total number of WBCs. They can be found in blood, sputum, and nasal secretions. A level greater than 5% to 10% is considered abnormal and may be found in patients with allergic disorders (Kowal & DuBuske, 2017).

Eosinophil Count

An actual count of eosinophils can be obtained from blood samples or smears of secretions. During symptomatic episodes, smears obtained from nasal secretions and sputum of patients with allergies usually reveal an increase in eosinophils, indicating an active allergic response (Kowal & DuBuske, 2017).

Total Serum Immunoglobulin E Levels

High total serum IgE levels support the diagnosis of allergic disease. In the majority of cases, the antibody typically responsible for an allergic reaction belongs to the IgE isotype. Patients with this disorder are said to have an IgE-mediated allergic disease (Kowal & DuBuske, 2017).

Skin Tests

Skin testing entails the intradermal injection or superficial application (epicutaneous) of solutions at several sites.

Depending on the suspected cause of allergic signs and symptoms, many different solutions may be applied at separate sites. These solutions contain individual antigens representing an assortment of allergens most likely to be implicated in the patient's disease. Positive (wheal-and-flare) reactions are clinically significant when correlated with the history, physical findings, and results of other laboratory tests. Skin testing is considered the most accurate confirmation of allergy (Kowal & DuBuske, 2016).

The results of skin tests complement the data obtained from the history. They indicate which of several antigens are most likely to provoke symptoms and indicate the intensity of the patient's sensitization. The dosage of the antigen (allergen) injected is also important. Most patients are hypersensitive to more than one allergen. Under testing conditions, they may not react (although they usually do) to the specific allergens that induce their attacks.

When there is doubt about the validity of the skin tests, a serum-specific IgE test or a provocative challenge test may be performed. If a skin test is indicated, there is a reasonable suspicion that a specific allergen is producing symptoms in a patient with allergies. However, several precautionary steps must be observed before skin testing with allergens is performed:

- Testing is not performed during periods of bronchospasm.
- Epicutaneous tests (scratch or prick tests) are performed before other testing methods, in an effort to minimize the risk of systemic reaction.
- Emergency equipment must be readily available to treat anaphylaxis.

Types of Skin Tests

The methods of skin testing include prick skin tests, scratch tests, and intradermal skin testing. After negative prick or scratch tests, intradermal skin testing is performed with allergens that are suggested by the patient's history to be problematic. The back is the most suitable area of the body for skin testing because it permits the performance of many tests. A multitest applicator with multiple test heads is commercially available for simultaneous administration of antigens by multiple punctures at different sites. Research suggests that use of a multi-prong applicator for allergy testing decreases patient discomfort and application time (Pestotnik & Krueger, 2018). A negative response on a skin test cannot be interpreted as an absence of sensitivity to an allergen. Such a response may occur with insufficient sensitivity of the test or with the use of an inappropriate allergen in testing. Therefore, it is essential to observe the patient undergoing skin testing for an allergic reaction even if the previous response was negative (Kowal & DuBuske, 2016).

Interpretation of Skin Test Results

Familiarity with and consistent use of a grading system are essential. The grading system used should be identified on a skin test record for later interpretation. A positive reaction, evidenced by the appearance of an urticarial wheal (round, reddened skin elevation) (see Fig. 33-3), localized **erythema** (diffuse redness) in the area of inoculation or contact, or pseudopodia (irregular projection at the end of a wheal) with associated erythema is considered indicative of sensitivity to the corresponding antigen. False-positive results may occur because of improper preparation or administration of allergen solutions (Kowal & DuBuske, 2016).

> ### ⚑ Quality and Safety Nursing Alert
>
> *Corticosteroids and antihistamines, including over-the-counter allergy medications, suppress skin test reactivity and should be stopped 48 to 96 hours before testing, depending on the duration of their activity. False-positive results may occur because of improper preparation or administration of allergen solutions.*

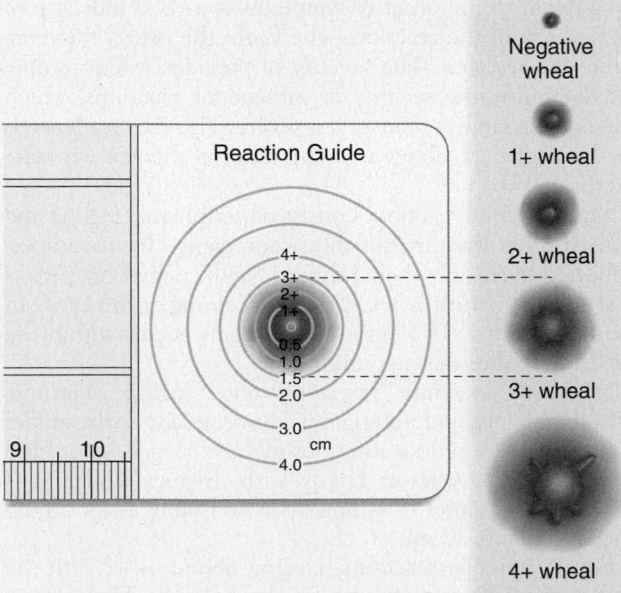

Figure 33-3 • Interpretation of reactions: Negative = wheal soft with minimal erythema; 1+ = wheal present (5 to 8 mm) with associated erythema; 2+ = wheal (7 to 10 mm) with associated erythema; 3+ = wheal (9 to 15 mm), slight pseudopodia possible with associated erythema; 4+ = wheal (12 mm+) with pseudopodia and diffuse erythema.

Positive or negative skin tests are interpreted in the context of a patient's history, clinical signs, and exposure to allergens. The following guidelines are used for the interpretation of skin test results:

- Skin tests are used most frequently with the diagnosis of allergic rhinitis.
- Negative test results are helpful in ruling out food allergy.
- Positive skin tests correlate highly with food allergy.

The use of skin tests to diagnose immediate hypersensitivity to medications is limited, because metabolites of medications, not the medications themselves, are usually responsible for causing hypersensitivity.

Provocative Testing

Provocative testing involves the direct administration of the suspected allergen to the sensitive tissue, such as the conjunctiva, nasal or bronchial mucosa, or gastrointestinal tract (by ingestion of the allergen), with observation of target organ response. This type of testing is helpful in identifying clinically significant allergens in patients who have a large number of positive tests. Major disadvantages of this type of testing are the limitation of one antigen per session and the risk of producing severe symptoms, particularly bronchospasm, in patients with asthma (Kowal & DuBuske, 2016).

Serum-Specific IgE Test

The serum-specific IgE test, formerly known as RAST, is an automated test performed on blood samples by a pathology laboratory. As the name suggests, it detects free antigen-specific IgE in serum as opposed to antigen-specific IgE bound to mast cells in the skin. The advantages of this test over other tests include decreased risk of systemic reaction, stability of antigens, and lack of dependence on skin reactivity modified by medications. The major disadvantages include limited allergen selection and reduced sensitivity compared with intradermal skin tests, lack of immediate results, and higher cost (Kowal & DuBuske, 2017).

ALLERGIC DISORDERS

There are two types of IgE-mediated allergic reactions: atopic and nonatopic disorders. Although the underlying immunologic reactions of the two types of disorders are the same, the predisposing factors and manifestations are different. Atopy is defined as the genetic predisposition to mount an IgE response to inhaled or ingested innocuous proteins. Atopic diseases consist of asthma, allergic rhinitis, and atopic dermatitis. All share a common pathogenesis, mediated by IgE, and are frequently present together in the same individual and in families. The nonatopic disorders lack the genetic component and organ specificity of the atopic disorders. Latex allergy (see later discussion) can present as an IgE-mediated anaphylaxis, type I reaction, or a type IV hypersensitivity referred to as contact dermatitis (Stokes & Casale, 2019).

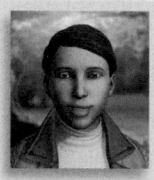
Anaphylaxis

Anaphylaxis is a clinical response to an immediate (type I hypersensitivity) immunologic reaction between a specific antigen and an antibody. The reaction results from a rapid release of IgE-mediated chemicals, which can induce a severe, life-threatening reaction (Actor, 2019).

Pathophysiology

Anaphylaxis is a type I IgE allergic reaction to an antigen, a foreign substance that has entered the body. It is caused by the cross-links of an allergen with allergen-specific IgE antibodies found on the surface membrane of mast cells and basophils, leading to cellular degranulation. The subsequent release of histamine and other bioactive mediators causes activation of platelets, eosinophils, and neutrophils. Histamine, prostaglandins, and inflammatory leukotrienes are potent vasoactive mediators that are implicated in the vascular permeability changes, flushing, **urticaria** (hives), angioedema, hypotension, and bronchoconstriction that characterize anaphylaxis. Smooth muscle spasm, bronchospasm, mucosal edema and inflammation, and increased capillary permeability result. Symptoms of anaphylaxis are sudden in onset and progress in severity over minutes to hours (Kemp, 2018).

Closely resembling anaphylaxis is an anaphylactoid reaction, which is caused by the release of mast cell and basophil mediators triggered by non–immunoglobulin E (IgE)-mediated events. This nonallergenic anaphylaxis reaction may occur with medications, food, exercise, or cytotoxic antibody transfusions. The reaction may be local or systemic. Local reactions usually involve urticaria and angioedema at the site of the antigen exposure. Although possibly severe, nonallergenic anaphylaxis reactions are rarely fatal. Systemic reactions occur within about 30 minutes after exposure and involve cardiovascular, respiratory, gastrointestinal, and integumentary organ systems. For the most part, the treatment of nonallergenic anaphylaxis reaction is identical to that of anaphylaxis (Campbell & Kelso, 2018).

Common causes of anaphylaxis are listed in Chart 33-2. Antibiotics and radiocontrast agents cause the most serious

Chart 33-2 Common Causes of Anaphylaxis

Foods

Peanuts, tree nuts (e.g., walnuts, pecans, cashews, almonds), shellfish (e.g., shrimp, lobster, crab), fish, milk, eggs, soy, wheat

Medications

Antibiotics, especially penicillin and sulfa antibiotics, allopurinol, radiocontrast agents, anesthetic agents (lidocaine, procaine), vaccines, hormones (insulin, vasopressin, adrenocorticotropic hormone), aspirin, nonsteroidal anti-inflammatory drugs

Other Pharmaceutical/Biologic Agents

Animal serums (tetanus antitoxin, snake venom antitoxin, rabies antitoxin), antigens used in skin testing

Insect Stings

Bees, wasps, hornets, yellow jackets, ants (including fire ants)

Latex

Medical and nonmedical products containing latex

---

anaphylactic reactions. Penicillin is the most common medication to cause anaphylaxis. Approximately 10% of the population report having an allergy to penicillin. However, less than 5% have clinically significant IgE or T cell–mediated penicillin allergy (Shenoy, Macy, Rowe, et al., 2019).

Clinical Manifestations

Anaphylactic reactions produce a clinical syndrome that affects multiple organ systems. Reactions may be categorized as mild, moderate, or severe. The time from the exposure to the antigen to the onset of symptoms is a good indicator of the severity of the reaction—the faster the onset, the more severe the reaction. The severity of previous reactions does not determine the severity of subsequent reactions, which could be the same or more or less severe. The severity depends on the degree of allergy and the dose of allergen exposure (Actor, 2019).

Mild systemic reactions consist of peripheral tingling and a sensation of warmth, possibly accompanied by a sensation of fullness in the mouth and throat. Nasal congestion, periorbital swelling, pruritus, sneezing, and tearing of the eyes can also be expected. The onset of symptoms begins within the first 2 hours after the exposure.

Moderate systemic reactions may include flushing, warmth, anxiety, and itching in addition to any of the milder symptoms. More serious reactions include bronchospasm and edema of the airways or larynx with dyspnea, cough, and wheezing. The onset of symptoms is the same as for a mild reaction (Kemp, 2018).

Severe systemic reactions have an abrupt onset with the same signs and symptoms described previously. These symptoms progress rapidly to bronchospasm, laryngeal edema, severe dyspnea, cyanosis, and hypotension. Dysphagia (difficulty swallowing), abdominal cramping, vomiting, diarrhea, and seizures can also occur. Cardiac arrest and coma may follow. Severe reactions are also referred to as anaphylactic shock (Marshall et al., 2018) (see Chapter 11).

Prevention

Strict avoidance of potential allergens is an important preventive measure for the patient at risk for anaphylaxis. Those at risk for anaphylaxis from insect stings should avoid areas populated by insects and should use appropriate clothing, insect repellent, and caution to avoid further stings.

If avoidance of exposure to allergens is impossible, an autoinjector system for epinephrine will be prescribed. The patient should be instructed to carry and administer epinephrine to prevent an anaphylactic reaction in the event of exposure to the allergen. People who are sensitive to insect bites and stings, those who have experienced food or medication reactions, and those who have experienced idiopathic or exercise-induced anaphylactic reactions should always carry an emergency kit that contains epinephrine. Autoinjection devices are commercially available for first aid and deliver premeasured doses of epinephrine (Comerford & Durkin, 2020). The autoinjector system requires no preparation, and the self-administration technique is not complicated. The patient must be given an opportunity to demonstrate the correct technique for use; a training device can be used for educating about the correct technique. Verbal and written information about the emergency kit, as well as strategies to avoid exposure to threatening allergens, must also be provided (Campbell & Kelso, 2018).

Screening for allergies before a medication is prescribed or first administered is an important preventive measure. A careful history of any sensitivity to suspected antigens must be obtained before administering any medication, particularly in parenteral form, because this route is associated with the most severe anaphylaxis. Nurses caring for patients in any setting (hospital, home, outpatient diagnostic testing sites, long-term care facilities) must assess patients' risks for anaphylactic reactions. Patients are asked about previous exposure to contrast agents used for diagnostic tests and any allergic reactions, as well as reactions to any medications, foods, insect stings, and latex. People who are predisposed to anaphylaxis should wear medical identification such as a bracelet or necklace, which identifies allergies to medications, food, and other substances.

People who are allergic to insect venom may require venom immunotherapy, which is used as a control measure and not a cure. The most common serious allergic reactions to insect stings are from the Hymenoptera family, which includes bees, ants, wasps, and yellow jackets (Warrell, 2019). Venom immunotherapy is an effective treatment for people with systemic reactions to an insect sting. It reduces the systemic reaction, reduces the risk of future large local reactions, and improves quality of life (Larsen, Broge, & Jacobi, 2016).

Patients with diabetes who are allergic to insulin and those who are allergic to penicillin may require desensitization. Desensitization is based on controlled anaphylaxis, with a gradual release of mediators. Patients who undergo desensitization are cautioned to avoid lapses in therapy, because this may lead to the reappearance of the allergic reaction when the use of the medication is resumed (Castells & Solensky, 2017).

Medical Management

Management depends on the severity of the reaction. Initially, respiratory and cardiovascular functions are evaluated. If the patient is in cardiac arrest, cardiopulmonary resuscitation (CPR) is instituted (Campbell & Kelso, 2018). Supplemental oxygen is provided during CPR or if the patient is cyanotic, dyspneic, or wheezing. Epinephrine, in a 1:1000 dilution, is given subcutaneously in the upper extremity or thigh and may be followed by a continuous intravenous infusion. Most adverse events associated with administration of epinephrine (i.e., adrenaline) occur when the dose is excessive or is given intravenously. Patients at risk for adverse effects include older patients and those with hypertension, arteriopathies, or known ischemic heart disease.

Antihistamines and corticosteroids should not be given in place of epinephrine. However, they may also be given as adjunct therapy (Campbell & Kelso, 2018).

Intravenous fluids (e.g., normal saline solution), volume expanders, and vasopressor agents are given to maintain blood pressure and normal hemodynamic status. In patients with episodes of bronchospasm or a history of bronchial asthma or chronic obstructive pulmonary disease, aminophylline and corticosteroids may also be given to improve airway patency and function. See Chapter 11 for management of anaphylactic shock.

Patients who have experienced anaphylactic reactions and received epinephrine should be transported to the local emergency department (ED) for observation and monitoring because of the risk for a "rebound" or delayed reaction 4 to 8 hours after the initial allergic reaction. However, the observation time should be individualized based on the severity of the anaphylaxis. Longer periods of observation should be considered for patients who ingested the allergen, required more than one dose of epinephrine, had hypotension or pharyngeal edema, or have a history of asthma (Lieberman, 2018).

Nursing Management

If a patient is experiencing an allergic response, the nurse assesses the patient for signs and symptoms of anaphylaxis. Airway, breathing pattern, and vital signs are assessed. The patient is observed for signs of increasing edema and respiratory distress. Prompt notification of the rapid response team, the provider, or both is required. Rapid initiation of emergency measures (e.g., intubation, administration of emergency medications, insertion of intravenous lines, fluid administration, and oxygen administration) is important to reduce the severity of the reaction and to restore cardiovascular function. The nurse documents the interventions used and the patient's vital signs and response to treatment (Campbell & Kelso, 2018).

The patient who has recovered from anaphylaxis needs to be educated about what occurred, how to avoid future exposure to antigens, and how to administer emergency medications to treat anaphylaxis. The nurse assesses the health literacy level of the patient and determines the best method of providing discharge instructions (Wilkin, 2020). See the Nursing Research Profile in Chart 33-3.

Patients who have experienced an anaphylactic reaction should receive a prescription for an autoinjectable epinephrine device. The nurse educates the patient and family in their use and has the patient and family return demonstrate correct administration (Moore, Kemp, & Kemp, 2015) (see Chart 33-4).

Chart 33-3 · NURSING RESEARCH PROFILE
Using Video Discharge Instructions

Wilkin, Z. L. (2020). Effects of video discharge instructions on patient understanding. *Advanced Emergency Nursing Journal, 42*(1), 71–78.

Purpose

Patients have difficulty understanding and retaining education at the time of discharge, particularly if instructions are given only in the form of printed materials. The purpose of this study was to evaluate the effects of using video discharge instructions on patient understanding of the education provided upon discharge from an emergency department (ED).

Design

This was a prospective, randomized, controlled trial that used a convenience sample of patients admitted to the ED. Participants were randomized to receive either standard discharge procedures, or standard discharge procedures plus video discharge instructions. Ten minutes after receiving one of the education methods, participants were tested with a 5-question multiple choice test.

Findings

Participants included 60 adults with a mean age of 37 years, and with a medical diagnosis of either upper respiratory infection, pharyngitis, or gastroenteritis. Thirty participants received the video discharge instructions, while the other 30 received the standard discharge procedure. There was a significant difference in knowledge level, with those receiving the video instructions having a higher level of knowledge (4.53 vs. 4, $p = 0.009$) on the multiple choice test.

Nursing Implications

This study provides evidence that video discharge instructions have the potential to increase the knowledge level of patients receiving discharge education. Nurses who work in busy settings, such as EDs, should consider developing supplemental materials to augment standard written discharge instructions to help increase patients' understanding and retention of important information.

Chart 33-4 · PATIENT EDUCATION
Self-Administration of Epinephrine

The nurse instructs the patient to:

1. After removing the autoinjector from its carrying tube, grasp the unit with the orange tip (injecting end) pointing downward. Form a fist around the unit with the orange tip down; with your other hand, remove the blue safety release cap.

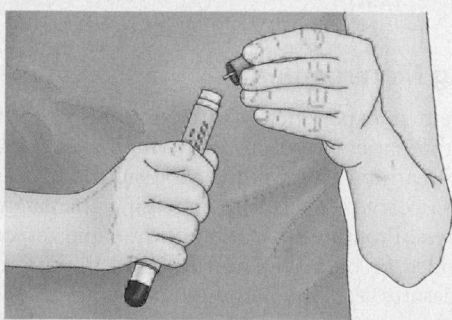

2. Hold the black tip near outer thigh. Swing and jab firmly into the outer thigh until a click is heard with the device perpendicular (90-degree angle) to the thigh. Do NOT inject into buttocks.

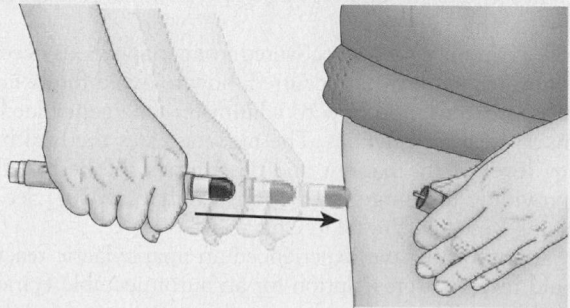

3. Hold firmly against the thigh for approximately 10 seconds. Remove the unit from the thigh, and gently massage the injection area for 10 seconds. Call 911 and seek immediate medical attention. Carefully place the used autoinjector unit, needle-end first, into the device storage tube without bending the needle. Screw on the storage tube completely, and take it with you to the hospital emergency room.

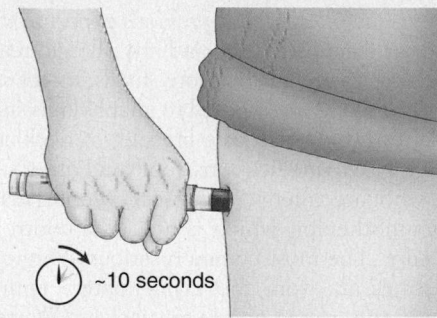

~10 seconds

Allergic Rhinitis

Allergic rhinitis (hay fever, seasonal allergic rhinitis) is the most common form of respiratory allergy, which is mediated by an immediate (type I hypersensitivity) immunologic reaction. In the United States approximately 20 million adults have allergic rhinitis (CDC, 2017). Early diagnosis and adequate treatment are essential to reduce complications and relieve symptoms.

Because allergic rhinitis is induced by airborne pollens or molds, it is characterized by the following seasonal occurrences (deShazo & Kemp, 2018a):

- Early spring—tree pollen
- Early summer—grass pollen
- Early fall—weed pollen (ragweed)

Each year, attacks begin and end at about the same time. Airborne mold spores require warm, damp weather. Although there is no rigid seasonal pattern, these spores appear in early spring, are rampant during the summer, then taper off and disappear by the first frost in areas that experience dramatic seasonal temperature variation. In temperate areas that do not experience freezing temperatures, these allergens, especially mold, can persist throughout the year.

Pathophysiology

Allergic rhinitis is caused by an allergen-specific IgE-mediated immunologic response. Sensitization most commonly begins by inhalation of antigen. IgE antibodies are stimulated and bind to mast cells in the respiratory mucosa, basophils in the peripheral blood, and eosinophils in the nasal and respiratory mucosa. Eosinophilia in the tissues is the key characteristic of allergic rhinitis. When IgE antibodies bind to mast cells there is histamine release. Histamine is the major mediator of allergic reactions in the nasal mucosa. Inflammation, tissue edema, vasodilation, and increased capillary permeability occur (deShazo & Kemp, 2017).

Clinical Manifestations

Symptoms include sneezing, rhinorrhea, nasal itching, conjunctivitis, and nasal obstruction. Postnasal drip, cough, itching of the eyes, and fatigue are often present. If symptoms are severe, allergic rhinitis may interfere with sleep, leisure, school, work, and overall quality of life. Allergic rhinitis is commonly associated with chronic sinusitis, atopic dermatitis (eczema), and asthma. Infraorbital edema and dilation of peripheral vessels (due to histamine) can cause darkening under the eyes, sometimes referred to as "allergic shiners." A horizontal nasal crease can develop from constant rubbing of the nose; commonly referred to as the "allergic salute." The nasal mucosa can exhibit a grayish hue. Clear rhinorrhea, tonsillar hyperplasia, and postnasal rhinorrhea may be visible on examination of the throat. Tympanic membranes can be retracted or serous fluid may accumulate in the middle ear. Some patients can suffer oral allergy syndrome (OAS) with itching and irritation of the hard and soft palate. Allergic rhinitis and sinusitis can trigger migraine headache in some patients (deShazo & Kemp, 2018a).

Assessment and Diagnostic Findings

Diagnosis of seasonal allergic rhinitis is mainly based on history and physical examination. Blood or laboratory testing is usually unnecessary. Diagnostic testing can be done with immediate hypersensitivity skin testing (skin prick testing). In sensitive patients, testing with select diagnostic solutions of tree, grass, or weed pollen, mold, house dust mites, and animal allergens results in a wheal-and-flare reaction at the skin test site within 20 minutes. IgE immunoassay can provide similar information to skin prick test. Nasal cytology can be performed to differentiate rhinitis due to allergy from that due to infection, although it is relatively nonspecific and insensitive (deShazo & Kemp, 2018a).

Medical Management

The goal of therapy is to provide relief from symptoms. Therapy may include one or all of the following interventions: avoidance therapy, pharmacologic therapy, and immunotherapy. Verbal instructions must be reinforced by written information. Knowledge of general concepts regarding assessment and therapy in allergic diseases is important so that the patient can learn to manage certain conditions as well as prevent severe reactions and illnesses.

Avoidance Therapy

In avoidance therapy, every attempt is made to remove the allergens that act as precipitating factors. Simple measures and environmental controls are often effective in decreasing symptoms. Examples include the use of air conditioners, air cleaners, humidifiers, and dehumidifiers; removal of dust-catching furnishings, carpets, and window coverings; removal of pets from the home or bedroom; the use of pillow and mattress covers that are impermeable to dust mites; and a smoke-free environment (Platts-Mills, 2019). Additional measures include changing clothing when coming in from outside, showering to wash allergens from hair and skin, and using an over-the-counter nasal irrigation device or saline nasal spray to reduce allergens in the nasal passages Because multiple allergens are often implicated, multiple measures to avoid exposure to allergens are often necessary. High-efficiency particulate air (HEPA) purifiers and vacuum cleaner filters may also be used to reduce allergens in the environment (Platts-Mills, 2019). Multiple avoidance strategies tailored to a person's risk factors can reduce the severity of symptoms, the number of work or school days missed because of symptoms, and the number of unscheduled health care visits for treatment. In many cases, it is impossible to avoid exposure to all environmental allergens, so pharmacologic therapy or immunotherapy is needed.

Pharmacologic Therapy

Many antihistamines, corticosteroid nasal sprays, adrenergic agents, mast cell stabilizers, nasal decongestant sprays, and corticosteroids are pharmacologic agents used in allergic rhinitis.

Antihistamines

First-generation antihistamines, which are readily absorbed, are most effective when administered orally at the first occurrence of symptoms because they prevent the development of new symptoms. Diphenhydramine is a common first-generation antihistamine available in over-the-counter (OTC) medications. Others include chlorpheniramine and hydroxyzine. First-generation antihistamines bind to histamine 1 receptors and can effectively relieve symptoms of hay fever, vasomotor rhinitis, urticaria (hives), and mild asthma. However, first-generation antihistamines cross the blood–brain barrier and cause significant sedation which impairs cognitive function and psychomotor performance. First-generation antihistamines can also have anticholinergic effects such as dry mouth, blurry vision, urinary hesitancy, and confusion. Due to their anticholinergic effects, first-generation antihistamines should be avoided in older adults (Fick, Semla, Steinman, et al., 2019). First-generation antihistamines have a limited role in the treatment of allergy due to their adverse effects (deShazo & Kemp, 2018b).

Second-generation (nonsedating H_1-receptor antagonists) are antihistamines that do not cross the blood–brain barrier to the same extent as first-generation antihistamines. They mainly bind to peripheral rather than central nervous system H_1 receptors, causing less sedation. Examples of these OTC medications are loratadine, cetirizine, and fexofenadine (Sanchez-Borges & Ansotegui, 2019). Contraindications, major side effects, nursing implications, and patient education for select H_1 antihistamines can be found in Table 33-2.

If H_1 antihistamines are not completely effective, H_2 antihistamines such as famotidine, which blocks the H_2 receptors found in the stomach, vascular smooth muscle, and elsewhere, can be added to the drug regimen. It is given twice a day with the same total dose as for gastroesophageal reflux. H_2 antihistamines do not relieve urticaria on their own, but can augment the effect of H_1 antihistamines (Randall & Hawkins, 2018).

Antihistamines may also be combined with decongestants to reduce the nasal congestion associated with allergies. Most combination products are available as OTC medications; examples are loratadine/pseudoephedrine and cetirizine/pseudoephedrine. Decongestants can cause an increase in blood pressure; therefore, patients with a history of hypertension should be cautioned about long-term use of any medication that contains decongestants (Randall & Hawkins, 2018). Decongestants are contraindicated in patients receiving monoamine oxidase inhibitor therapy and should be used with caution in patients with closed-angle glaucoma, cardiovascular or cerebrovascular disease, hyperthyroidism, or bladder neck obstruction.

Antihistamine nasal sprays azelastine and olopatadine are available by prescription. They not only reduce inflammation and decrease nasal congestion, but also have rapid onset of action and can be used "on demand" (deShazo & Kemp, 2018b).

Corticosteroid Nasal Spray

Corticosteroid nasal sprays are recognized as the most effective pharmacotherapy for allergic rhinitis. These anti-inflammatory agents work directly on the nasal mucosa but take a few hours to work. The patient should understand that maximal therapeutic effectiveness of these agents can take 1 to 2 weeks. They are recommended as the best single therapy for patients with mild to moderate or moderate to severe symptoms (Berger & Melizer, 2015).

Corticosteroid nasal sprays are derived from hydrocortisone and are divided into first-generation and second-generation

agents. Beclomethasone, flunisolide, triamcinolone, and budesonide are first-generation agents, whereas flucatisone, mometasone, and ciclesonide are second-generation agents (deShazo & Kemp, 2018b).

Corticosteroid nasal spray therapy should begin with the maximal dose for patient age. Once patient symptoms are adequately controlled, the dose can be reduced at 1-week intervals to the lowest effective dose that controls symptoms. Patients with severe symptoms usually need daily use of the nasal spray. Some patients may find relief of symptoms with use of the nasal spray every other day or as needed. Newer second-generation corticosteroid spray preparations act rapidly (within 3 to 12 hours), and as-needed use appears to be effective. This kind of treatment may be adequate in patients with episodic symptoms (deShazo & Kemp, 2018b).

Adverse effects of corticosteroid nasal sprays are mild and include drying of the nasal mucosa and burning and itching sensations caused by the vehicle used to administer the medication. Beclomethasone, budesonide, flunisolide, and triamcinolone are deactivated rapidly after absorption, so they do not achieve significant blood levels. Inhaled corticosteroids do not affect the immune system to the same degree as systemic corticosteroids (i.e., oral corticosteroids). Because corticosteroids are inhaled into the upper respiratory tract, tuberculosis or untreated bacterial infections of the lungs may become apparent and progress. Whenever possible, patients with tuberculosis or other bacterial infections of the lungs should avoid corticosteroid nasal sprays (deShazo & Kemp, 2018b).

The combination of an antihistamine and a corticosteroid nasal spray may be helpful for patients who do not obtain sufficient relief with one agent. A combination spray containing azelastine and fluticasone is available (deShazo & Kemp, 2018b).

Adrenergic Agents

Alpha-adrenergic agonist (also called sympathomimetic) medications, such as pseudoephedrine, can be used as decongestants in allergies. These agents activate alpha-adrenergic receptor sites on the smooth muscle causing vasoconstriction of the nasal mucosal blood vessels, reducing local blood flow, fluid exudation, and mucosal edema. Oral alpha-adrenergic medications have a systemic effect and are not recommended as first-line treatment of allergic rhinitis (Laccourreye, et al., 2015). Oral alpha-adrenergic agents are also available in combination with antihistamines (e.g., diphenhydramine and pseudoephredine fexofenadine and pseudoephedrine). Alpha-adrenergic topical nasal spray (e.g., oxymetazoline) is also available. Alpha-adrenergic agonist ophthalmic drops, such as tetrahydrozoline, are commonly used for allergic conjunctivitis as they vasoconstrict the blood vessels of the eye.

There are many potential side effects of oral alpha-adrenergic agonists. These include hypertension, arrhythmias, palpitations, central nervous system stimulation, irritability, tremor, and tachyphylaxis. Oral adrenergic agents are not first-line agents in allergy and have potential for cardiovascular and neurological adverse effects (deShazo & Kemp, 2018b). The topical preparations (i.e., drops and sprays) of alpha-adrenergic agonists cause fewer side effects than oral medications; however, the use of drops and sprays should

TABLE 33-2 Select H₁ Antihistamines

H₁ Antihistamine	Contraindications	Major Side Effects	Nursing Implications and Patient Education
First-Generation H₁ Antihistamines (Sedating)			
Diphenhydramine	Allergy to any antihistamines Third trimester of pregnancy Lactation Use cautiously with narrow-angle glaucoma, asthma, stenosing peptic ulcer, benign prostatic hyperplasia (BPH) or bladder neck obstruction, first and second trimester of pregnancy, older patients, hypertension	Drowsiness, confusion, dizziness, dry mouth, nausea, vomiting, photosensitivity, urinary retention	Administer with food if gastrointestinal (GI) upset occurs. Caution patients to avoid alcohol, driving, or engaging in any hazardous activities until central nervous system (CNS) response to medication is stabilized. Suggest sucking on sugarless lozenges or ice chips for relief of dry mouth. Encourage the use of sunscreen and hat while outdoors. Assess for urinary retention; monitor urinary output.
Chlorpheniramine	Allergy to any antihistamines Third trimester of pregnancy Lactation Use cautiously with narrow-angle glaucoma, asthma, stenosing peptic ulcer, BPH or bladder neck obstruction, first and second trimesters of pregnancy, older patients, hypertension	Drowsiness, sedation, and dizziness, although less than other sedating agents; confusion, dry mouth, nausea, vomiting, urinary retention, epigastric distress, thickening of bronchial secretions	Caution patients to avoid alcohol, driving, or engaging in any hazardous activities until CNS response to medication is stabilized. Suggest sucking on sugarless lozenges or ice chips for relief of dry mouth. Recommend the use of a humidifier.
Hydroxyzine	Allergy to hydroxyzine or cetirizine, pregnancy, lactation, hypertension	Drowsiness; dry mouth; involuntary motor activity, including tremor and seizures	Caution patients to avoid alcohol, driving, or engaging in any hazardous activities until CNS response to medication is stabilized. Suggest sucking on sugarless lozenges or ice chips for relief of dry mouth. Instruct patients to report tremors.
Second-Generation H₁ Antihistamines (Nonsedating)			
Cetirizine	Allergy to any antihistamines Narrow-angle glaucoma Asthma Stenosing peptic ulcer BPH or bladder neck obstruction Lactation Hypertension	Dry nasal mucosa, thickening of bronchial secretions	Can be taken without regard to meals. Instruct patients to use caution if driving or performing tasks that require alertness. Recommend the use of a humidifier.
Desloratadine	Allergy to loratadine Lactation Use cautiously with renal or hepatic impairment, pregnancy, hypertension	Somnolence, nervousness, dizziness, fatigue, dry mouth	Can be taken without regard to meals. Suggest sucking on sugarless lozenges or ice chips for relief of dry mouth. Recommend the use of a humidifier.
Loratadine	Allergy to any antihistamines Narrow-angle glaucoma Asthma Stenosing peptic ulcer BPH or bladder neck obstruction Hypertension	Headache, nervousness, dizziness, depression, edema, increased appetite	Instruct patients to take on empty stomach (1 h before or 2 h after meals or food). Instruct patients to avoid alcohol and to use caution if driving or performing tasks that require alertness. Suggest sucking on sugarless lozenges or ice chips for relief of dry mouth. Recommend the use of a humidifier.
Fexofenadine	Allergy to any antihistamines Pregnancy Lactation Use cautiously with hepatic or renal impairment, older patients, hypertension	Fatigue, drowsiness, GI upset	Should not be given within 15 min of ingestion of antacids. Instruct patients to use caution if driving or performing tasks that require alertness. Recommend the use of a humidifier.
Levocetirizine	Hypersensitivity to any antihistamines End-stage kidney disease Hemodialysis Use cautiously with pregnancy, lactation, older patients	Drowsiness, GI disturbance, headache	Can be taken without regard to meals. Instruct patients to use caution if driving or performing tasks that require alertness. Recommend the use of a humidifier.

Adapted from Comerford, K. C., & Durkin, M. T. (2020). *Nursing 2020 drug handbook.* Philadelphia, PA: Wolters Kluwer.

be limited to a few days to avoid rebound congestion, also referred to as rhinitis medicamentosa.

The Combat Methamphetamine Epidemic Act of 2005 banned OTC sales of medications that contain the ingredients pseudoephedrine, ephedrine, or phenylpropanolamine as these can be used to make methamphetamine, a highly addictive stimulant. Laws to enforce this act vary state by state. There is a legal age requirement to purchase these drugs and pharmacists must limit and keep records of the amount purchased. Some states require a prescription (U.S. Food and Drug Administration [FDA], 2017).

Mast Cell Stabilizers

Intranasal cromolyn sodium is a spray that acts by stabilizing the mast cell membrane, thus reducing the release of histamine and other mediators of the allergic response. In addition, it inhibits macrophages, eosinophils, monocytes, and platelets involved in the immune response. Cromolyn interrupts the physiologic response to nasal antigens, and it is used prophylactically (before the exposure to allergens) to prevent the onset of symptoms and to treat symptoms once they occur. It is also used therapeutically in chronic allergic rhinitis. This spray is as effective as antihistamines but is less effective than corticosteroid nasal sprays in the treatment of seasonal allergic rhinitis. It is best to use this agent 30 minutes prior to exposure to allergen. Frequent use is necessary to obtain an effect (1 to 2 nasal sprays 4 times per day). The patient must be informed that the beneficial effects of the medication may take a week or longer to manifest. The medication is of no benefit in the treatment of nonallergic rhinitis. Adverse effects (e.g., sneezing, local stinging and burning sensations) are usually mild (deShazo & Kemp, 2018b).

Nasal Decongestant Sprays

Nasal decongestant sprays include phenylephrine, oxymetazoline, and naphazoline. These agents vasoconstrict blood vessels in the nasal mucosa by blocking alpha-adrenergic receptors. Nasal decongestant sprays are not recommended as monotherapy. After using these agents for 3 to 7 days, reduced sensitivity of alpha-adrenergic receptors develops which can cause worsening nasal congestion. This effect of worsening nasal congestion often causes patients to overuse these agents with less and less therapeutic effect. This is termed rhinitis medicamentosa and can lead to increased need for the agent and eventual dependency (Wahid & Shermetaro, 2019).

The combination of a topical nasal decongestant and topical corticosteroid may effectively treat symptoms without causing rhinitis medicamentosa. Nasal decongestants are helpful when used just before air travel in patients who have difficulties with middle ear or sinus equilibration with flying or in patients who have problems with altitude changes (deShazo & Kemp, 2018b).

Corticosteroids

Oral and parenteral corticosteroids can be used when conventional therapy has failed and symptoms are severe and of short duration. They can control symptoms of allergic reactions such as hay fever, medication-induced allergies, and allergic reactions to insect stings. However, corticosteroids have a delayed onset of action and cannot be used for immediate relief of allergic symptoms. The agents are not effective as singular treatment for severe allergic reactions such as anaphylaxis (deShazo & Kemp, 2018b). Oral corticosteroids in the lowest dose to control symptoms for the shortest period of time may be prescribed if other agents fail. However, corticosteroids are usually avoided because of their side effects.

> ### ⚑ Quality and Safety Nursing Alert
>
> Patients who receive high-dose or long-term corticosteroid therapy must be cautioned not to stop taking the medication suddenly. Doses are tapered when discontinuing this medication to avoid adrenal insufficiency.

The patient should be cautioned about side effects, which include fluid retention, weight gain, hypertension, gastric irritation, glucose intolerance, osteoporosis, immunosuppression, and adrenal suppression. Further discussion of corticosteroids is provided in Chapter 45, Table 45-3.

Leukotriene Receptor Antagonists

Leukotrienes are inflammatory mediators that cause bronchospasm, vascular permeability, and activation of leukocytes. They are three to four times more potent than histamine in perpetuating inflammation in the upper respiratory tract (Castells, 2017). Leukotriene receptor antagonists (LTRAs), such as zafirlukast and montelukast, block the synthesis or action of leukotrienes and prevent the signs and symptoms associated with asthma (see Table 33-3). LTRAs are also used to counteract allergic rhinitis.

Montelukast efficacy has been compared to a second-generation antihistamine agent. In combination with a second-generation antihistamine such as loratadine, montelukast has shown to be more effective than montelukast alone. Adverse effects of montelukast include neuropsychiatric changes such as anxiety, depression, and insomnia. This agent may be not appropriate for patients with preexisting mood disorders (Badri & Takov, 2019).

Leukotriene receptor antagonists are for long-term use, and patients should be advised to take their medication daily. LTRAs are not effective as "rescue" medications. Patients take appropriate "rescue" medications for symptom exacerbation but continue to take the LTRA on a daily basis. Studies report that using an LTRA in conjunction with an inhaled corticosteroid is effective for mild persistent asthma (Chauchan, Jeyaraman, Singh Mann, et al., 2017).

Allergen Immunotherapy

Allergen immunotherapy (AIT) is primarily used to treat IgE-mediated diseases by injections of allergen extracts. Immunotherapy, also referred to as allergy vaccine therapy, involves the administration of gradually increasing quantities of specific allergens to the patient until a dose is reached that is effective in reducing disease severity from natural exposure. This is an effective treatment for 80% to 90% of certain allergens such as grass and pollen. This type of therapy provides

TABLE 33-3 Leukotriene Receptor Antagonists

Leukotriene Receptor Antagonist	Available Formulations	Frequency of Dosing
Zafirlukast	Tablets: 10 mg; 20 mg	Taken twice a day
Montelukast	Tablets: 10 mg Chewable tablets: 4 mg; 5 mg Granules: 4 mg/packet	Taken once a day in PM
Zileuton	Tablets: 600 mg extended release	Taken twice a day within 1 h after morning and evening meals

Chart 33-5 IMMUNOTHERAPY: Indications and Contraindications

Indications

- Allergic rhinitis, conjunctivitis, or allergic asthma
- History of a systemic reaction to Hymenoptera and specific immunoglobulin E antibodies to Hymenoptera venom
- Desire to avoid the long-term use, potential adverse effects, or costs of medications
- Lack of control of symptoms by avoidance measures or the use of medications

Contraindications

- The use of beta-blocker or angiotensin-converting enzyme inhibitor therapy, which may mask early signs of anaphylaxis
- Presence of significant pulmonary or cardiac disease or organ failure
- Inability of the patient to recognize or report signs and symptoms of a systemic reaction
- Nonadherence of the patient to other therapeutic regimens and nonlikelihood that the patient will adhere to the immunization schedule (often weekly for an indefinite period)
- Inability to monitor the patient for at least 30 minutes after administration of immunotherapy
- Absence of equipment or adequate personnel to respond to allergic reaction if one occurs

an adjunct to symptomatic pharmacologic therapy and can be used when avoidance of allergens is not possible. Specific immunotherapy has been used in the treatment of allergic disorders for many years. Goals of immunotherapy include reducing the level of circulating IgE, increasing the level of blocking antibody IgG, and reducing mediator cell sensitivity. Immunotherapy has been most effective for ragweed pollen, grass, tree pollen, cat dander, and house dust mite allergens (Akdis, 2018). Indications and contraindications for immunotherapy are presented in Chart 33-5.

Correlation of a positive skin test with a positive allergy history is an indication for immunotherapy if the allergen cannot be avoided. The benefit of immunotherapy has been fairly well established in instances of allergic rhinitis and bronchial asthma that are clearly due to sensitivity to one of the common pollens, molds, or household dust. Unlike antiallergy medication, allergen immunotherapy has the potential to alter the allergic disease course after 3 to 5 years of therapy. Because it may prevent the progression or development of asthma or multiple or additional allergies, it is also considered to be a potential preventive measure. The patient must understand what to expect and the importance of continuing therapy for several years before immunotherapy is accomplished. When skin tests are performed, the results are correlated with symptoms; treatment is based on the patient's needs rather than on the results of skin tests (Klimek, Pfaar, Bousquet, et al., 2017).

There are three methods of immunotherapy: subcutaneous immunotherapy (SCIT), sublingual immunotherapy (SLIT), and epicutaneous immunotherapy (EPIT).

Subcutaneous Immunotherapy

The most common method of treatment is SCIT, which consists of the serial injection of one or more antigens that are selected in each particular case on the basis of skin testing. This method provides a simple and efficient technique for targeting IgE antibodies to specific antigens. Specific treatment consists of injecting extracts of the allergens that cause symptoms in a particular patient. Injections begin with very small amounts and are gradually increased, usually at weekly intervals, until a maximum tolerated dose is attained. Although severe systemic reactions are rare, the risk of systemic and potentially fatal anaphylaxis exists. It tends to occur most frequently at the induction or "up-dosing" phase. Therefore, the patient must be monitored after administration of immunotherapy. Because of the risk of anaphylaxis, injections should not be given by a lay person or by the patient. The patient must remain in the office or clinic for at least 30 minutes after the injection and is observed for possible systemic symptoms. If a large, local swelling develops at the injection site, the next dose should not be increased, because this may be a warning sign of a possible systemic reaction (James & Bernstein, 2017).

Maintenance booster injections are given at 2- to 4-week intervals, frequently for a period of several years, before the maximum benefit is achieved, although some patients will note early improvement in their symptoms. Long-term benefit seems to be related to the cumulative dose of vaccine given over time (Nelson, 2018).

 Quality and Safety Nursing Alert

Because the injection of an allergen may induce systemic reactions, such injections are given only in a setting where epinephrine is immediately available (i.e., primary provider's office, clinic).

Sublingual Immunotherapy

SLIT has been reported to have a 30% to 40% reduction in reactions and rescue medication usage in seasonal allergic rhinitis. Administration of SLIT includes a buildup phase that is followed by a treatment plan of three times per week with a rapid dissolving tablet or liquid containing allergen extracts. Recent studies show comparable efficacy of SLIT with SCIT (Chaaban, Mansi, Tripple, et al., 2019; Durham & Penagos, 2016). Systemic side effects are rare but have been reported in patients who also report systemic reactions with SCIT. Side effects include irritation, minor swelling or itching inside the mouth, and stomach upset and nausea.

Epicutaneous Immunotherapy

EPIT is an investigational alternative allergen immunotherapy with delivery of the allergen to the epidermis. Because the epidermis is less vascular, it is theorized that there is reduced risk of systemic allergic side effect. Epicutaneous allergen patches are applied to the upper inner arm or interscapular region of the back. Doses are lower than those used in SCIT or SLIT. The allergen is soluble and absorbed into the skin. Adverse reactions include localized erythema, pruritus, and urticaria at the site of allergen patch. Studies of EPIT have shown modest results compared to placebo, and there has been a higher rate of treatment-related mild to moderate anaphylactic reactions. Long-term studies of EPIT are currently in progress for peanut allergies (Nowak-Wegrzyn, 2019).

Immunotherapy should not be initiated during pregnancy; for patients who have been receiving immunotherapy before pregnancy, the dosage should not be increased during pregnancy.

Therapeutic failure is evident when a patient does not experience a decrease of symptoms within 12 to 24 months, fails to develop increased tolerance to known allergens, and cannot decrease the use of medications to reduce symptoms. Potential causes of treatment failure include misdiagnosis of allergies, inadequate doses of allergen, newly developed allergies, and inadequate environmental controls (Akdis, 2018).

NURSING PROCESS

The Patient with Allergic Rhinitis

Assessment

The examination and history of the patient reveal sneezing, often in paroxysms; thin and watery nasal discharge; itching eyes and nose; lacrimation; and occasionally headache. The health history includes a personal or family history of allergy. The allergy assessment identifies the nature of antigens, seasonal changes in symptoms, and medication history. The nurse also obtains subjective data about how the patient feels just before symptoms become obvious, such as the occurrence of pruritus, breathing problems, and tingling sensations. In addition to these symptoms, hoarseness, wheezing, hives, rash, erythema, and edema are noted. Any relationship between emotional problems or stress and the triggering of allergy symptoms is assessed (Kakli & Riley, 2016).

Diagnosis

NURSING DIAGNOSES

Based on the assessment data, major nursing diagnoses may include:

- Impaired breathing associated with allergic reaction
- Lack of knowledge about allergy and the recommended modifications in lifestyle and self-care practices
- Difficulty coping with chronicity of condition and need for environmental modifications

COLLABORATIVE PROBLEMS/POTENTIAL COMPLICATIONS

Potential complications may include the following:

- Anaphylaxis
- Impaired breathing
- Nonadherence to the therapeutic regimen

Planning and Goals

The goals for the patient may include restoration of a breathing pattern that provides adequate ventilation, increased knowledge about the causes and control of allergic symptoms, improved coping with alterations and modifications, and absence of complications.

Nursing Interventions

IMPROVING BREATHING PATTERN

The patient is instructed and assisted to modify the environment to reduce the severity of allergic symptoms or to prevent their occurrence. The patient is also instructed to reduce exposure to people with upper respiratory tract infections. Adherence to medication schedules and other treatment regimens is encouraged and reinforced.

PROMOTING UNDERSTANDING OF ALLERGY AND ALLERGY CONTROL

Instruction includes strategies to minimize exposure to allergens and explanation about desensitization procedures and correct use of medications. The nurse informs and reminds the patient of the importance of keeping appointments for desensitization procedures, because dosages are usually adjusted on a weekly basis, and missed appointments may interfere with the dosage adjustment (Pitsios & Dietis, 2019).

Patients need to understand the difference between rescue medications for allergy exacerbation and seasonal flares (e.g., antihistamines) and medications used for allergy control throughout the year (e.g., inhaled corticosteroids, leukotriene modifiers). Patients also need to understand that medications for allergy exacerbation and seasonal flares should be used only when the allergy is apparent. Continued use of these medications when not required can result in tolerance; consequently, the medications will be ineffective when needed (Pitsios & Dietis, 2019; Scadding, 2017).

COPING WITH A CHRONIC DISORDER

Although allergic reactions are infrequently life-threatening, they require vigilance to avoid allergens and modification of the lifestyle or environment to prevent recurrence of symptoms. Allergic symptoms are often present year-round and create discomfort and inconvenience for the patient. Although patients may not feel ill during allergy seasons, they often do not feel well, either. The need to be alert for possible allergens in the environment may be tiresome, placing a burden on the patient's ability to lead a normal life. Stress related to these difficulties may in turn increase the frequency or severity of symptoms. To assist the patient in adjusting to these modifications, the nurse must have an appreciation of the difficulties encountered by the patient. The patient is encouraged to verbalize feelings and concerns in a supportive environment and to identify strategies to deal with them effectively (Scadding, 2017).

MONITORING AND MANAGING POTENTIAL COMPLICATIONS

Anaphylaxis and Impaired Breathing. Respiratory and cardiovascular functioning can be significantly altered during allergic reactions by the reaction itself or by the medications used to treat reactions. Anaphylaxis is an acute, systemic reaction that causes vasodilation and bronchiole constriction which can lead to hypotensive shock and asphyxiation. The respiratory status is evaluated by monitoring the respiratory rate and pattern and by assessing for breathing difficulties or abnormal lung sounds. The pulse rate and rhythm and blood pressure are monitored to assess cardiovascular status regularly or any time the patient reports symptoms such as itching or difficulty breathing. In the event of signs and symptoms suggestive of anaphylaxis, emergency medications and equipment must be available for immediate use. People with severe allergic reactions may be advised to carry an autoinjectable epinephrine device (Song & Lieberman, 2019). See Chapter 11 for treatment of anaphylactic shock.

Nonadherence to the Therapeutic Regimen. Knowledge about the treatment regimen does not ensure adherence.

Having the patient identify potential barriers and explore acceptable solutions for effective management of the condition (e.g., installing tile floors rather than carpet, not gardening in the spring) can increase adherence to the treatment regimen (Pitsios & Dietis, 2019).

PROMOTING HOME, COMMUNITY-BASED, AND TRANSITIONAL CARE

Educating Patients About Self-Care. The patient is instructed about strategies to minimize exposure to allergens, the actions and adverse effects of medications, and the correct use of medications. The patient should know the name, dose, frequency, actions, and side effects of all medications taken.

Instruction about strategies to control allergic symptoms is based on the needs of the patient as determined by the results of tests, the severity of symptoms, and the motivation of the patient and family to deal with the condition (Pitsios & Dietis, 2019). Suggestions for patients who are sensitive to dust and mold in the home are given in Chart 33-6.

If the patient is to undergo allergen immunotherapy (AIT), the nurse reinforces the primary provider's explanation regarding the purpose and procedure. Instructions are given regarding the series of injections, which usually are given initially every week and then at 2- to 4-week intervals. These instructions include remaining in the primary provider's office or the clinic for at least 30 minutes after the injection, so that emergency treatment can be given if the patient has a reaction; avoiding rubbing or scratching the injection site; and continuing with the series for the period of time required. In addition, the patient and family are instructed about emergency treatment of severe allergic symptoms (James & Bernstein, 2017).

Because antihistamines may produce drowsiness, the patient is cautioned about this and other side effects applicable to the medication. Operating machinery, driving a car, and performing activities that require intense concentration should be postponed. The patient is also informed about the dangers of drinking alcohol when taking antihistamines, because they tend to exaggerate the effects of alcohol.

The patient must be aware of the effects caused by overuse of the sympathomimetic agents in nose drops or sprays, because rhinitis medicamentosa may result. After topical application of the medication, a rebound period occurs in which the nasal mucous membranes become more edematous and congested than they were before the medication was used. Such a reaction encourages the use of more medication, and a cyclic pattern results. The topical agent must be discontinued immediately and completely to correct this problem (Wahid & Shermetaro, 2019).

Continuing and Transitional Care. Follow-up telephone calls to the patient are often reassuring to the patient and family and provide an opportunity for the nurse to answer any questions. The patient is reminded to keep follow-up appointments and informed about the importance of continuing with treatment. The importance of participating in health promotion activities and health screening is also emphasized.

Evaluation

Expected patient outcomes may include:

1. Exhibits a breathing pattern that provides adequate ventilation
   a. Demonstrates lungs clear on auscultation
   b. Exhibits absence of adventitious breath sounds (crackles, rhonchi, wheezing)
   c. Has a normal respiratory rate and pattern
   d. Reports no complaints of respiratory distress (shortness of breath, difficulty on inspiration or expiration)

Chart 33-6 HOME CARE CHECKLIST
Allergy Management

At the completion of education, the patient and/or caregiver will be able to:

- State the impact of environmental allergens (e.g., dust, molds, perfumes, foods) on physiologic functioning, ADLs, IADLs, roles, relationships, and spirituality.
- State changes in home environment necessary to minimize exposure to allergens.
  - Removing drapes, curtains, and venetian blinds and replacing them with pull shades; covering the mattress with a hypoallergenic cover that can be zipped; and removing rugs and replacing them with wood flooring or linoleum.
  - Reducing dust in the house as a whole by using steam or hot water for heating and using high-efficiency particulate air (HEPA) purifiers or air-conditioning.
  - Washing the floor and dusting and vacuuming daily, using clean filters, wearing a mask whenever cleaning is being done.
  - Replacing stuffed furniture with wood pieces that can easily be dusted.
  - Avoiding the use of tufted bedspreads, stuffed toys, and feather pillows and replacing them with washable cotton material.
  - Avoiding the use of any clothing that causes itching.

- Verbalize ways to reduce exposure to pollens or molds by identifying seasons of the year when pollen counts are high; wearing a mask at times of increased exposure (windy days and when grass is being cut); and avoiding contact with weeds, dry leaves, and freshly cut grass.
- State rationale for seeking air-conditioned areas at the height of the allergy season.
- State rationale for avoiding sprays and perfumes.
- State rationale for the use of hypoallergenic cosmetics.
- State rationale for taking prescribed medications as prescribed.
- Identify specific foods that may cause allergic symptoms and develop a list of foods to avoid (e.g., fish, nuts, eggs, chocolate).
- Verbalize ways to cope with stress successfully, plans for regular exercise, and rationale for obtaining adequate rest.
- State how to reach primary provider with questions or complications.
- State time and date of follow-up appointments, testing.
- Identify the need for health promotion, disease prevention, and screening activities.

ADLs, activities of daily living; IADLs, instrumental activities of daily living.

2. Demonstrates knowledge about allergy and strategies to control symptoms
   a. Identifies causative allergens, if known
   b. States methods of avoiding allergens and controlling indoor and outdoor precipitating factors
   c. Removes from the environment items that retain dust
   d. Wears a dampened mask if dust or mold may be a problem
   e. Avoids smoke-filled rooms and dust-filled or freshly sprayed areas
   f. Uses air-conditioning for a major part of the day when allergens are high
   g. Takes antihistamines as prescribed; participates in allergen immunotherapy program, if applicable
   h. Describes name, purpose, side effects, and method of administration of prescribed medications
   i. Identifies when to seek immediate medical attention for severe allergic responses
   j. Describes activities that are possible, including ways to participate in activities without activating the allergies
3. Adapts to the inconveniences of an allergy
   a. Relates the emotional aspects of the allergic response
   b. Demonstrates the use of measures to cope positively with allergy
4. Demonstrates absence of complications
   a. Exhibits vital signs within normal limits
   b. Reports no symptoms or episodes of anaphylaxis (urticaria, itching, peripheral tingling, fullness in the mouth and throat, flushing, difficulty swallowing, coughing, wheezing, or difficulty breathing)
   c. Demonstrates correct procedure to self-administer emergency medications to treat severe allergic reaction
   d. Correctly states medication names, dose and frequency of administration, and medication actions
   e. Correctly identifies side effects and untoward signs and symptoms to report to primary provider
   f. Discusses acceptable lifestyle changes and solutions for identified potential barriers to adherence to treatment and medication regimen

Contact Dermatitis

Contact dermatitis is an inflammatory reaction of the skin due to contact with an exogenous substance. There are two basic types of contact dermatitis: irritant contact dermatitis and allergic contact dermatitis (see Table 33-4). Irritant contact dermatitis is an inflammatory response of the skin to direct chemical damage that releases mediators predominantly from epidermal cells. Allergic contact dermatitis is a delayed (type 4) hypersensitivity reaction to exogenous contact antigens that involves activation of T cells (Litchman, Nair, & Atwater, 2019). Eighty percent of contact dermatitis is irritant type and 20% is allergic type (Fornacier & Noor, 2018). Most cases are caused by excessive exposure to or additive effects of irritants (e.g., soaps, detergents, metals, organic solvents, cosmetics). Skin sensitivity may develop after brief or prolonged periods of exposure, and the clinical picture may appear hours or weeks after the sensitized skin has been exposed.

Clinical Manifestations

Symptoms of acute contact dermatitis include itching, burning, erythema, skin lesions (vesicles and bullae), and oozing (Goldner & Fransway, 2018). The reaction is limited to the site of contact. Chronic contact dermatitis symptoms can include scaling, lichenification, thickening of the skin, and pigmentary changes. Secondary invasion by bacteria may develop in skin that is abraded by rubbing or scratching. Usually, there are no systemic symptoms unless the eruption is widespread.

Assessment and Diagnostic Findings

Determining allergens responsible requires a history, physical examination, and patch testing.

Assessment includes the date of onset and any identifiable relationship to work environment and skin care products. The location of the lesions, distribution of the dermatitis, absence of other etiologies, and the history of exposure aid in determining the condition (Goldner & Fransway, 2018). Patch testing and environmental history of exposure to contact allergens are required to verify the diagnosis. Patch testing

TABLE 33-4	Types, Testing, and Treatment of Contact Dermatitis			
Type	Etiology	Clinical Presentation	Diagnostic Testing	Treatment
Allergic	Results from contact of skin and allergenic substance; has a sensitization period of 10–14 days	Vasodilation and perivascular infiltrates on the dermis Intracellular edema Usually seen on dorsal aspects of hand	Patch testing (contraindicated in acute, widespread dermatitis)	Avoidance of offending material Aluminum acetate (Burow Solution, Domeboro Powder) or cool water compress Systemic corticosteroids (prednisone) for 7–10 days Topical corticosteroids for mild cases Oral antihistamines to relieve pruritus
Irritant	Results from contact with a substance that chemically or physically damages the skin on a nonimmunologic basis; occurs after first exposure to irritant or repeated exposures to milder irritants over an extended time	Dryness lasting days to months Vesiculation, fissures, cracks Hands and lower arms most common areas	Clinical picture Appropriate negative patch tests	Identification and removal of source of irritation Application of hydrophilic cream or petrolatum to soothe and protect Topical corticosteroids and compresses for weeping lesions Antibiotics for infection and oral antihistamines for pruritus

Adapted from Comerford, K. C., & Durkin, M. T. (2020). *Nursing 2020 drug handbook*. Philadelphia, PA: Wolters Kluwer.

is the standard test for identification of culprit allergens in persons with allergic contact dermatitis. The patch test most commonly used is the thin-layer rapid use epicutaneous (TRUE) test. An extended screening panel (North American screening series) has increased sensitivity. Researchers reported an extended screening panel identified an additional 10.8% of patients with positive tests that were negative to TRUE test allergens (Sundquist, Lang, & Pasha, 2019).

Atopic Dermatitis

Atopic dermatitis (commonly called eczema) is a chronic, inflammatory allergic skin disorder that is triggered by environmental factors in individuals who are genetically susceptible. This disorder affects 7% of adults in the United States (Weston & Howe, 2019). More than half of patients are also affected by asthma, allergic rhinitis, and food allergies.

Atopic dermatitis is a type I immediate hypersensitivity disorder involving IgE antibodies that causes dry, pruritic, hypersensitive skin. It often begins with small red pruritic papules that stimulate intense itching, leaving erythematous, excoriated areas of skin. This often triggers an "itch-scratch cycle" where rubbing or scratching the skin causes further irritation, redness, and skin breakdown. Skin thickening from chronic scratching (lichenification) and fissuring may develop over time. In many patients, lesions in different stages may be present at the same time (Weston & Howe, 2019). Atopic dermatitis in adults often occurs at the hands, wrists, elbows, knees, ankles, face, and neck.

Atopic dermatitis is due to a "leaky" skin barrier that allows water to leave the skin dried out and hypersensitive. Exposure of the hypersensitive skin to soaps, detergent, house dust mites, pollen, animal dander, and some bacteria break down the skin barrier (Weston & Howe, 2019).

Defective filaggrin (FLG) genes at chromosome 1q21.3 are common in persons with the disorder. Filaggrin is a protein produced by keratinocytes in the skin that is encoded by the FLG gene (Løset, Brown, Saunes, et al., 2019). Currently, there is ongoing investigation into the etiology of atopic dermatitis, including other genes involved in processing of filaggrin.

Nurses should be aware that atopic dermatitis is often linked to a process called the **atopic march** that refers to the natural history of allergic diseases as they begin in infancy and through childhood. Atopic march begins with atopic dermatitis and progresses to IgE-mediated food allergy, asthma, and allergic rhinitis. It is the result of interactions between susceptibility genes, the environment, defective function of the skin barrier, and immunologic responses (AAAAI, 2019a; Hill & Spergel, 2018).

The diagnosis of atopic dermatitis is based on the health history, morphology and distribution of skin lesions, and associated clinical signs. Laboratory testing, patch testing, and skin biopsy may be necessary if there is a need to rule out other skin conditions.

Medical Management

Treatment of patients with atopic dermatitis involves avoidance of irritative agents, use of anti-inflammatory topical agents, and moisturization of the skin. Patients should avoid potential triggers of atopic dermatitis, which include excessive bathing without subsequent moisturization, low humidity environments, animal dander, dust mites, xerosis (dry skin), overheating of skin, and exposure to solvents and detergents. Individuals are commonly hypersensitive to fragrances, perfumes, and contact allergens such as nickel.

Topical corticosteroids are the mainstay of treatment of atopic dermatitis. If mild OTC corticosteroids are not adequate, more potent corticosteroids such as fluocinoline 0.025%, triamcinolone, 0.1%, or betamethasone, 0.05% are prescribed. These agents should not be used on the face as they can cause skin atrophy. Topical calcineurin inhibitors, which are nonsteroidal immunomodulating agents (e.g., tacrolimus, pimecrolimus), are best for the facial area. Treatment of severe flare-ups of chronic disease can be treated with a short course of systemic corticosteroids (Weston & Howe, 2019).

Dupilumab is an interleukin (IL)-4 and IL-13 receptor-alpha antagonist that was approved by the FDA for the treatment of patients aged 12 years and older with moderate to severe atopic dermatitis not adequately controlled with topical prescription therapies (Spergel & Lio, 2019).

Colonization with *Staphylococcus aureus* occurs more frequently in individuals with atopic dermatitis than in the general population, and *S. aureus* is a common cause of secondary infection in these patients. The presence of purulence or honey-colored crusts suggests *S. aureus* infection. Antibiotic treatment is needed to eradicate infection (Spergel & Lio, 2019).

Nursing Management

Patients who experience atopic dermatitis and their families require assistance and support from the nurse to cope with the disorder. The symptoms are often disturbing to the patient and disruptive to the family. The appearance of the skin may affect the patient's self-esteem and their willingness to interact with others. Instructions and counseling about strategies to incorporate preventive measures and treatments into the lifestyle of the family may be helpful.

Skin hydration is a key component of treatment as atopic skin is low in moisture. Thick cream moisturizers and emollients that contain glycerol or urea should be used as these will keep the skin hydrated. A hydrating bath with mild soap followed by immediate emollient application is recommended, or a shower of short duration (Spergel & Lio, 2019).

Itching can be decreased by wearing cotton fabrics, washing clothes with a mild detergent, and humidifying dry heat in winter. Antihistamines such as diphenhydramine may be used as treatment, but since they are sedating, the patient can be advised that it is best to use them at bedtime.

The patient and family need to be aware of signs of secondary infection and of the need to seek treatment if infection occurs. The nurse also educates the patient and family about the side effects of medications used in treatment.

Drug Hypersensitivity

Drug hypersensitivity is the leading cause of fatal anaphylaxis, comprising 43% of deaths from anaphylaxis. All routes of administration are potentially fatal, but drugs given parenterally incur the greatest risk. Cutaneous rashes are among the most common reactions to medications and occur in approximately 2% to 3% of hospitalized patients (Habif, 2016).

A drug hypersensitivity reaction is defined by the time of appearance, possible mode of action (mechanism of immune stimulation), and resulting pathophysiology. According to the World Allergy Organization, immunologic drug reactions can be divided into immediate reactions (i.e., onset within 1 hour of exposure) and delayed reactions (onset after 1 hour), based on the timing of the appearance of symptoms (Tanno, Torres, Castells, et al., 2018).

IgE-mediated immediate type 1 hypersensitivity reactions to a drug occur within 1 hour of administration of the agent. Delayed hypersensitivity reactions occur after 1 hour; most occur after 6 hours or days of treatment. These reactions can also occur after the course of medication is finished. These reactions may be caused by several different mechanisms, but they are not IgE mediated. Types II, III, and IV immunologic reactions are all considered delayed reactions (Pichler, 2019).

A disorder known as drug rash with eosinophilia and systemic symptoms (DRESS) can occur after weeks of continuous treatment. Also known as "drug-induced hypersensitivity syndrome" (DiHS), it is characterized by fever, rash, and multiorgan involvement, and may or may not be associated with eosinophilia and lymphocytosis. Hepatitis and myocarditis can be part of DRESS. These reactions can persist for weeks to months, even after the medication is stopped (Mockenhaupt, 2019). Anticonvulsant agents (e.g., lamotrigine, phenytoin, phenobarbital) and allopurinol are the most frequently reported causes of DRESS (Mockenhaupt, 2019).

Anaphylaxis is the most severe presentation of an IgE-mediated drug reaction. Medications administered IV may cause symptoms in seconds to minutes, while the same drug administered orally may cause symptoms in 3 to 30 minutes if taken on an empty stomach, and in 10 to 60 minutes if taken with food. The agents that most commonly exhibit this type of reaction include the following (Pichler, 2019):

- Beta-lactam drugs (e.g., penicillins and cephalosporins)
- Neuromuscular blocking agents (e.g., pancuronium)
- Quinolones (e.g., ciprofloxacin)
- Platinum-containing chemotherapeutic agents (e.g., carboplatin)
- Foreign proteins such as monoclonal antibodies (e.g., rituximab)

Type II cytotoxic reactions involve antibody-mediated cell destruction. Type II reactions may arise when drugs bind to surfaces of certain cell types and act as antigens. Clinical manifestations include hemolytic anemia, thrombocytopenia, or neutropenia, since these are the cell types that are most often affected. The drugs most commonly implicated in hemolytic anemia are cephalosporins, penicillins, nonsteroidal anti-inflammatory drugs (NSAIDs), and quinine and quinidine. Drugs implicated in thrombocytopenia include heparin, abciximab, quinine and quinidine, sulfonamides, vancomycin, gold compounds, beta-lactam antibiotics, carbamazepine, and NSAIDs. Severe neutropenia due to type II drug reactions presents days to weeks after beginning the medication. Clinical manifestations include symptoms of infection, such as fever, stomatitis, pharyngitis, pneumonia, or sepsis. Propylthiouracil, amodiaquine, and flecainide can cause these reactions (Pichler, 2019).

Type III reactions are mediated by antigen–antibody complexes that deposit on basement membranes and usually present as serum sickness, vasculitis, or drug fever. Signs and symptoms take 1 or more weeks to develop after drug exposure, since significant quantities of antibody are needed to generate symptoms related to antigen–antibody complexes. These are uncommon reactions but are seen with antitoxins for rabies, botulism, and venoms, tetanus, hepatitis, and diphtheria vaccines (Pichler, 2019).

Type IV reactions involve activated T cells, which take time to develop. Type IV reactions usually take at least 48 to 72 hours and sometimes days to weeks to develop following exposure to the drug. Type IV reactions can vary from a nonurticarial, maculopapular rash (drug fever) to Stevens–Johnson syndrome and toxic epidermal necrolysis (see Chapter 56), or drug rash with eosinophilia and systemic symptoms, or DRESS/DiHS. Type IV reactions can appear after weeks of drug treatment (Pichler, 2019).

Medications are the most common agent responsible for approximately 90% of all drug rashes. Commonly prescribed medications (e.g., antibiotics, sulfonamides) are implicated in most cases (Samel & Chu, 2019).

Drug fever, which usually causes fever and rash, is associated with azathioprine, sulfasalazine, minocycline, trimethoprim-sulfamethoxazole, sirolimus, and tacrolimus (McDonald & Sexton, 2019). Contact dermatitis skin reactions can result from topical anesthetics such as benzocaine, topical antibiotics such as neomycin or bacitracin, and topic corticosteroids.

Symmetrical drug-related intertriginous and flexural exanthem (SDRIFE), formerly called baboon syndrome, is a distinctive drug eruption that typically develops within a few hours to days of drug exposure and presents with demarcated, V-shaped erythema in the gluteal/perianal or inguinal/perigenital areas, often with involvement of at least one other flexural area, such as the axillae, elbows, or knees. Aminopenicillins are a common trigger of SDRIFE (Bircher, 2018).

Acute generalized exanthematous pustulosis (AGEP) is a rare type of reaction characterized by superficial pustules, usually appearing within 24 hours after the administration of the culprit drug. Antimicrobial drugs (amoxicillin), antimalarials, and calcium channel blockers are the most frequently reported triggers of AGEP (Cho & Chu, 2017).

Stevens–Johnson syndrome and toxic epidermal necrolysis are severe reactions commonly triggered by medications. The disorder can evolve into extensive epidermal necrosis and become life-threatening. Mucous membranes are affected in over 90% of patients, usually at two or more distinct sites (ocular, oral, and genital). In some patients, an exanthematous eruption can be the heralding sign of Stevens–Johnson syndrome and toxic epidermal necrolysis. Fever, often exceeding 39°C (102.2°F), and influenzalike symptoms precede development of mucocutaneous lesions and erythematous macules with purpuric centers that evolve into blisters and bullae. Photophobia, conjunctival itching or burning, and pain on swallowing may be due to mucosal involvement. Malaise, myalgia, and arthralgia are present in most patients. The following agents are most commonly implicated in Stevens–Johnson syndrome and toxic epidermal necrolysis (High, 2019):

- Allopurinol
- Aromatic antiepileptic drugs and lamotrigine
- Antibacterial sulfonamides (including sulfasalazine)
- Nevirapine
- Oxicam NSAIDs

Some conventional and targeted anticancer drugs have been associated with these syndromes including thalidomide, capecitabine, afatinib, vemurafenib, tamoxifen, and immune checkpoint inhibitors ipilimumab, pembrolizumab, and nivolumab. Radiation treatment in combination with antiepileptic drugs (e.g., phenytoin, phenobarbital, carbamazepine) can trigger Stevens–Johnson syndrome and toxic epidermal necrolysis (High, 2019).

Pharmacogenetic studies suggest that there is a genetic predisposition to drug allergy. In some populations, individuals with HLA-B*1502, HLA-B*5801, or HLA-B*5701 have an increased risk of developing Stevens–Johnson syndrome and toxic epidermal necrolysis to aromatic anticonvulsants such as carbamazepine, allopurinol, cotrimoxazole, and abacavir, respectively (Bircher, 2018).

Pseudoallergic Drug Reactions

Pseudoallergic drug reactions are adverse drug reactions with signs and symptoms that mimic immunologic drug allergies, but no immunologic mechanisms are occurring. They are referred to as nonimmunologic hypersensitivity reactions or anaphylactoid reactions. It is unclear how certain drugs elicit pseudoallergic reactions. However, degranulation of mast cells occurs. Some affected patients have underlying dermographism which indicates an "instability" of their mast cells. In dermographism, when pressure is applied to the skin, the skin reddens for a prolonged time in the same pattern as the pressure was applied. The following drugs may cause a pseudoallergic drug reaction (Pichler, 2019):

- Radiocontrast agents
- Opioids (e.g., morphine and meperidine)
- NSAIDs (e.g., ibuprofen) and aspirin
- Vancomycin
- Local anesthetic agents (e.g., lidocaine, benzocaine)
- Chemotherapeutic agents (e.g., platinum-based drugs)

The patient should be educated about avoidance and provided with a written list of the generic and brand names of the causative agents to avoid in the future (Pichler, 2019).

Urticaria and Angioedema

Urticaria (hives) is a type I hypersensitive allergic reaction of the skin that is characterized by the sudden appearance of intensely pruritic pink or red discrete papules that progress to wheals of variable size. Urticarial lesions coalesce and evolve into large erythematous plaques (AAAAI, 2019b). This is a common condition with up to 20% of people having at least one episode of hives during their lifetime. Urticaria is most commonly instigated by infections, allergic reactions to food, insect stings, and medications (Asero, Tedeschi, Marzano, et al., 2017).

Acute urticaria evolves over a time span of minutes to hours and disappears by 24 hours; lesions can be in different stages over this time. Urticaria is considered acute if it has been present for less than 6 weeks. However, if urticaria occurs frequently and reoccurs daily for longer than 6 weeks, the condition is called chronic urticaria. In urticaria, mast cells and basophils within the skin are activated and release histamine and inflammatory mediators that cause vasodilation (AAAAI, 2019b).

Common causes of urticaria include allergic reactions to medications or contact allergens, foods, insect stings and bites; reactions to medications that cause nonallergic mast cell activation (e.g., opioids); latex allergy; transfusions; and NSAIDs. Physical urticarial syndromes are forms of chronic urticaria that are triggered by specific physical and environmental factors, such as cold exposure, sudden changes in body temperature, pressure or vibration against the skin, exercise, exposure to sunlight, or other stimuli (Asero, 2017). Serum sickness, a type III hypersensitivity reaction, commonly due to medication, can also cause urticaria. Serum sickness classically causes rash, fever, and polyarthralgias or polyarthritis, which begin 1 to 2 weeks after the first exposure to the responsible agent and resolve within a few weeks of discontinuation (Wener, 2018).

The diagnosis of urticaria can usually be made by health history and physical examination. Laboratory testing is usually not necessary.

Management of the condition includes eliminating the causative agent; avoiding the use of NSAIDs; and minimizing potential aggravators, including heat, stress, alcohol, and tight clothes. Treatment with second-generation H_1 antihistamine agents (e.g., cetirizine, fexofenadine, loratadine) is the mainstay of treatment. These agents are better tolerated as they have less sedating effects than first-generation H_1 antihistamines (e.g., diphenhydramine, chlorpheniramine, hydroxyzine). Doses of second-generation antihistamines may be increased as high as four times the standard dose (Khan, 2019a). Oral corticosteroids given in a decreasing dose schedule may be prescribed to relieve severe symptoms for a few days. About 50% of cases of chronic spontaneous urticaria will respond to treatment with antihistamines, as discussed above. For those patients who do not improve with antihistamines, 65% might respond to prescribed omalizumab. Omalizumab, a monoclonal antibody that acts against IgE antibodies, is injected under the skin every 2 to 4 weeks by a primary provider. Therapeutic effects can be seen within 3 to 6 months (AAAAI, 2019b; Stokes & Casale, 2018).

Angioedema is an allergic reaction that involves the infiltration of fluid in subcutaneous tissue and mucous membranes resulting in diffuse swelling. It is manifested by nonpruritic, brawny, widespread, nonpitting edema. Urticaria and angioedema often occur together (AAAAI, 2019b; Habif, 2016).

The regions most often involved in angioedema are the lips, eyelids, cheeks, hands, feet, genitalia, and tongue; the mucous membranes of the larynx, bronchi, and gastrointestinal tract may also be affected, particularly in the hereditary type (see discussion in the following section). On occasion, this reaction covers the entire back or large area of the body. Swellings may appear suddenly, in a few seconds or minutes, or slowly over 1 or 2 hours. It usually resolves within 24 hours. Angioedema is usually a benign and transient condition, although it can be life-threatening when severe angioedema of the larynx, upper airway, or tongue results in airway obstruction (Zuraw, 2019).

Two types of angioedema can be distinguished: mast cell–mediated, also called histaminergic angioedema, and bradykinin-mediated angioedema. Allergic reactions to foods, latex, certain drugs, or insect stings are common examples of mast cell–mediated angioedema. Histamine is the main inflammatory mediator and signs and symptoms include urticaria, flushing, generalized pruritus, bronchospasm, throat tightness, and/or hypotension. Patients may be experiencing anaphylaxis and should be treated immediately with epinephrine. Mast cell–mediated angioedema usually begins within minutes of exposure to the allergen, builds over a few hours, and resolves in 24 to 48 hours (Zuraw, 2019).

Alternatively, bradykinin-induced angioedema does not involve histamine and is not associated with urticaria, bronchospasm, or other symptoms of allergic reactions. Bradykinin is a potent vasodilator which also increases vasopermeability (Cicardi & Zuraw, 2018a). The fluid infiltration of the tissues usually develops over 24 to 36 hours and resolves within 2 to 4 days. The relationship between the trigger and the onset of symptoms is often not apparent. Angiotensin-converting enzyme inhibitors (e.g., captopril) are common causes of bradykinin-induced angioedema; swelling may appear within a week of starting the medication or after years of use (Zuraw, 2019).

Second-generation H_1 antihistamines and corticosteroids are the mainstay of treatment for mast cell–mediated angioedema. If angioedema is part of an anaphylactic reaction, intramuscular epinephrine is an important part of treatment (Guyer & Banerji, 2019).

Treatment of bradykinin-induced angioedema involves avoidance of drug, icatibant, C1 inhibitor concentrate, ecallantide, and possibly administration of fresh-frozen plasma. Antihistamines are ineffective (Cicardi & Zuraw, 2018b). Icatibant is a synthetic bradykinin beta-2-receptor antagonist. C1 inhibitor concentrate and exallantide inhibit kallikrein which is a protease involved in bradykinin production. Fresh-frozen plasma contains angiotensin-converting enzyme, and the administration of plasma is thought to degrade high levels of bradykinin (Guyer & Banerji, 2019).

Hereditary Angioedema

Hereditary angioedema (HAE) is a rare, potentially life-threatening, autosomal dominant genetic disorder. It is a bradykinin-mediated type of angioedema that is due to a lack of C1 inhibitor activity, a specific protein that takes part in kinin generation. Kinins are inflammatory mediators; bradykinin is one of these. C1INH usually plays a role in limiting bradykinin production, so when C1INH is deficient or dysfunctional, bradykinin production is relatively unchecked (AAAAI, 2019c).

There are two different types of HAE; HAE type I is due to C1 inhibitor (C1INH) deficiency, and type II is caused by C1INH dysfunction (Cicardi & Zuraw, 2018a).

Clinical Manifestations

HAE is commonly categorized as laryngeal, gastrointestinal, or cutaneous. Swelling of the skin is usually diffuse, nonpruritic, and not accompanied by urticaria. Attacks of swelling in patients with HAE generally involve the extremities, abdomen, genitourinary tract, face, oropharynx, or larynx and follow a stereotypical pattern in which the swelling worsens over 24 hours, peaks, and then slowly resolves over the following 48 hours. Gastrointestinal edema may cause abdominal pain severe enough to be incapacitating. Typically, attacks last 2 to 4 days and resolve without intervention; however, attacks can

occasionally affect the subcutaneous and submucosal tissues in the region of the upper airway and can be associated with respiratory obstruction and asphyxiation (Cicardi & Zuraw, 2018a).

Medical Management

Attacks usually subside within 2 to 4 days, but during this time the patient should be observed carefully for signs of laryngeal obstruction, which may necessitate tracheostomy as a lifesaving measure. Epinephrine, antihistamines, and corticosteroids are commonly administered in an attempt to relieve HAE; however, these are often ineffective. A trial of high doses of second-generation H_1 antihistamines for 1 month may be effective in some patients. If this proves unsuccessful, C1INH concentrate, derived from human plasma, recombinant human C1INH (rhC1INH, conestat alfa), icatibant, a synthetic bradykinin beta-2-receptor antagonist and ecallantide, a recombinant plasma kallikrein inhibitor are agents that are available (Cicardi & Zuraw, 2018b). Nurses need to be prepared to use different emergency approaches in the treatment of HAE and to have lifesaving equipment readily available.

Cold Urticaria

Cold urticaria is a type of physical urticaria. Physical urticarias are inducible urticarias that are stimulated by environmental triggers. Cold urticaria is the development of wheals (hives) or angioedema due to exposure to cold. Mast cells release histamine and inflammatory mediators are stimulated in response to skin contact with cold objects, cold fluids, or cold air. It is an IgE-mediated atopic immune reaction. Cold urticaria most commonly affects young adults as a self-limited disorder that occurs over a period of 5 to 6 years.

Clinical Manifestations

The patient feels a burning or pruritic sensation and the skin is erythematous due to activation of sensory nerves and vasodilation of arterioles. Most commonly it is a localized reaction in areas exposed to cold. However, extensive cold contact, such as swimming in cold water, may result in systemic reactions, ranging from generalized urticaria to anaphylaxis, with symptoms involving the respiratory, gastrointestinal, and/or cardiovascular systems. Oropharyngeal angioedema, which can cause suffocation and severe hypotension, has been observed in some persons with the disorder (Maurer, 2019).

Medical Management

Cold urticaria is diagnosed by cold stimulation testing. An ice cube within a thin plastic bag of cold water is applied to the volar aspect of the forearm for 1 to 5 minutes. A positive test results in development of urticaria at the site. The test is considered positive if the test site shows a palpable and clearly visible wheal-and-flare skin reaction upon rewarming. All patients with any form of cold urticaria should carry an autoinjectable epinephrine device for emergency use because hives can progress to anaphylaxis. Pretreatment with an antihistamine prior to predictable cold exposure is recommended, because clinical experience suggests that antihistamine pretreatment can prevent skin reactions and systemic reactions (Maurer, 2019). Patients with cold urticaria refractory to antihistamines can be treated with immunomodulator agents, such as omalizumab, certain antibiotics, leukotriene receptor antagonists, or cold desensitization therapy (Khan, 2019b).

Nursing Management

Prevention involves avoidance of cold stimuli. Patient education is needed about what environmental conditions can stimulate a reaction. For instance, patients should be instructed to expose a small section of the body to the water of a swimming pool prior to submerging the body in water. A wet suit can be used during swimming. Patients should understand that cold foods and beverages can stimulate oropharyngeal angioedema or anaphylaxis and should be avoided. Patients anticipating surgery may develop a reaction to the cold air within operating rooms and are instructed to alert surgical personnel that they have cold uriticaria and should be kept warm during any procedures. Cold intravenous solutions can also provoke a reaction (Singleton & Halverstam, 2016).

Food Allergy

Food allergy is an adverse reaction to certain foods due to immunologic mechanisms. Food allergies are categorized as either IgE-mediated or non–IgE-mediated allergies. IgE-mediated food allergy, a type I hypersensitivity reaction, occurs in about 5% of adults. IgE-mediated food allergy is more common and better understood than non–IgE-mediated food allergy (Commins, 2019). Recent studies show that within the population there are many with the misconception that they have a food allergy (19%) compared to persons with true immune-mediated food allergy (10%) (Gupta, Warren, & Smith, 2019).

Almost any food can cause an IgE-mediated allergic reaction. Allergic reactions can range from cutaneous urticaria to anaphylaxis. Fish and shellfish (e.g., lobster, shrimp, crab, clams, fin fish) as well as peanuts and tree nuts (e.g., cashew, walnut) are the two food groups that cause the majority of adult food allergies (Gupta et al., 2019). Other common foods causing allergy include cow's milk, eggs, soy, and wheat. Allergens are proteins and there is a danger that cross-reactivity can occur in foods containing similar proteins (AAAAI, 2018).

OAS, or pollen-food allergy syndrome (PFAS or PFS), is the most common form of IgE-mediated food allergy in adults. OAS often occurs in persons who are also allergic to pollen that causes seasonal allergic rhinitis. Raw fruits and vegetables often cause OAS but cooked fruit and vegetables do not (Burks, 2019).

Non–IgE-mediated food allergies present as more subacute and/or chronic symptoms that are typically isolated to the gastrointestinal tract and/or skin.

Clinical Manifestations

Acute urticaria and angioedema (swelling of the mouth, face, lips, tongue, and throat) are the most common clinical manifestations of food allergy. The reaction develops within minutes to hours after eating the offending food. The clinical symptoms may include wheezing, cough, laryngeal edema, and gastrointestinal symptoms (abdominal pain, nausea, cramps, vomiting, and diarrhea). Tree nuts and peanuts can cause the most severe allergic reactions evolving into anaphylaxis.

Assessment and Diagnostic Findings

Diagnosis of food allergy requires clinical history, physical examination, trial elimination diets, diet diaries, skin prick testing (SPT), and allergen-specific serum IgE immunoassay. A patch test is used if non–IgE-mediated food allergy is suspected. However, the standard is clinician-supervised oral food challenges to confirm or rule out the diagnosis. SPT is used to identify the source of symptoms and assists in identifying specific foods as causative agents. The patient is injected with a minute quantity of food antigen under the skin. Then the patient and primary provider wait to observe if hives and erythema arise within the 15 minute period. If the allergen triggers mast cells to release histamine, a localized wheal will be raised in the skin. A positive skin prick test for IgE-mediated food allergy is diagnosed when a wheal of 3 mm in diameter is raised within 15 minutes. A different kind of test, referred to as a 48-hour atopy patch test, is used for non–IgE-mediated food allergy. This is a topical application of food allergen that is applied to the small surface area of skin. This is a delayed reaction that requires 48 hours of observation (Andreae & Schreffler, 2019).

Medical Management

Therapy for food hypersensitivity includes avoidance of the food responsible for the hypersensitivity. Pharmacologic therapy is necessary for patients who cannot avoid exposure to offending foods and for patients with multiple food sensitivities not responsive to avoidance measures. Medication therapy involves the use of H_1 blockers, antihistamines, adrenergic agents, corticosteroids, and cromolyn sodium. All patients with food allergies, especially seafood and nuts, should have an autoinjectable epinephrine device prescribed. Another essential aspect of management is educating patients and family members about how to recognize and manage the early stages of an acute anaphylactic reaction.

Oral immunotherapy (OIT), or tolerance induction, is an increasingly used treatment. The patient ingests very small amounts of the allergen in increasing dosages over several months. OIT is not a curative treatment. The goal of OIT is to increase the threshold that triggers a reaction. OIT can be used to achieve desensitization or sustained unresponsiveness to a food allergen (AAAAI, 2018).

Initially, OIT has to be administered in a clinical setting equipped for treatment of potential anaphylaxis. Patients are generally started on a very small daily dose of the food (e.g., 3 to 6 mg of food protein) and advanced periodically (usually every 2 weeks) to a maintenance dose (e.g., 300 mg or, depending on the food and goals, 1 to 2 g of food protein daily) over several months (Nowak-Wegrzyn, 2019).

Peanut, egg, and milk OIT have been shown to desensitize approximately 60% to 80% of patients studied. OIT has not cured food allergy in these individuals; it has raised the patient's tolerance of the offending food. Most children outgrow their allergies to cow's milk, egg, soy and wheat, even if they have a history of a severe reaction. However, peanut, tree nuts, fish, and shellfish allergies tend to persist through adulthood (AAAAI, 2018).

Nursing Management

In addition to participating in management of the allergic reaction, the nurse focuses on preventing future exposure of the patient to the food allergen. The nurse should educate the patient about the signs of anaphylaxis and devise an action plan with the patient. If a severe allergic or anaphylactic reaction to food allergens has occurred, the nurse must instruct the patient and family about avoidance strategies to prevent its recurrence (see Chart 33-7). All patient allergies, including food allergies, should be noted on patient medical records, as dietary restrictions would be necessary in the case of hospitalization. Also, there may be risk of cross-reactivity with some medications containing similar substances. The patient also needs to understand how to select and specify preparation of restaurant food (Sicherer, 2019).

Latex Allergy

Latex allergy—the allergic reaction to the proteins in the saplike fluid of a rubber tree—has been implicated in rhinitis, conjunctivitis, contact dermatitis, urticaria, asthma, and anaphylaxis. The prevalence is estimated at 4% to 7% of the population, but this has been steadily declining because of the use of nonpowdered latex and latex-free gloves (Hamilton, 2017a).

The sap of the rubber tree (*Hevea brasiliensis*) contains 250 different polypeptides that can react with IgE. The polypeptides and proteins in natural rubber latex (Hevea proteins) or the various chemicals that are used in the manufacturing process are thought to be the source of the allergic reactions.

Those at risk include health care workers, patients who have undergone multiple surgeries, people working in factories that manufacture latex products, and patients with spina bifida. Patients with spina bifida are at risk because they have had multiple surgeries, multiple urinary catheterization procedures, and other treatments involving use of latex products (Hamilton, 2017a). Because food handlers, hairdressers, automobile mechanics, and police may wear latex gloves and use latex products, they are also at risk for latex allergy.

Increasingly, however, nonlatex gloves are being used in various occupational settings. Risk factors include occupational exposure to latex and atopic tendency in the affected person. Patients are at risk for anaphylactic reactions as a result of contact with latex during medical treatments, particularly surgical procedures (AAAAI, 2019d).

Persons with latex allergy are also prone to cross-reactions to pollen and some fruits; such as kiwis, bananas, pineapples, mangoes, passion fruit, avocados, and chestnuts (Hamilton, 2017a).

Routes of exposure to latex products can be cutaneous, percutaneous, mucosal, parenteral, or aerosol. The most frequent source of exposure is cutaneous, which usually involves the wearing of natural latex gloves. The powder used to facilitate putting on latex gloves can become a carrier of latex proteins from the gloves; when the gloves are put on or removed, the particles become airborne and can be inhaled or settle on skin, mucous membranes, or clothing (AAAAI, 2019d). Mucosal exposure can occur from the use of latex condoms, catheters, airways, and nipples. Parenteral exposure can occur from intravenous lines or hemodialysis equipment. In addition to latex-derived medical devices, many household items also contain latex. Examples of medical and household items containing latex and a list of alternative products are found in Table 33-5. It is estimated that more than 40,000 medical devices and nonmedical products contain latex (AAAAI, 2019d).

Clinical Manifestations

Many different types of reactions to latex are possible (see Table 33-6). Irritant contact dermatitis, a nonimmunologic response, may be caused by mechanical skin irritation or an alkaline pH associated with latex gloves. Common symptoms of irritant dermatitis include erythema and pruritus.

Delayed hypersensitivity to latex, a type IV reaction mediated by T cells, is localized to the area of exposure and is characterized by symptoms of contact dermatitis. These include vesicular skin lesions, papules, pruritus, edema, erythema, and crusting and thickening of the skin. These symptoms usually appear on the back of the hands 1 to 4 days postcontact. It is the most common allergic reaction to latex. Although usually not life-threatening, delayed hypersensitivity reactions often

TABLE 33-5   Select Products Containing Natural Rubber Latex and Latex-Free Alternatives

Products Containing Latex	Examples of Latex-Safe Alternatives[a]
Hospital Environment	
Ace bandage (brown)	Ace bandage, white all cotton
Adhesive bandages, Band-Aid dressing, Telfa	Cotton pads and plastic or silk tape, Active Strips (3M), DuoDERM
Anesthesia equipment	Neoprene anesthesia kit (King)
Blood pressure cuff, tubing, and bladder	Clean Cuff, single-use nylon or vinyl blood pressure cuffs or wrap with stockinette or apply over clothing
Catheters	All-silicone or vinyl catheters
Catheter leg bag straps	Velcro straps
Crutch axillary pads and hand grips, tips	Cover with cloth, tape
ECG pads	Baxter, Red Dot 3M ECG pads
Elastic compression stockings	Kendall SCD stockings with stockinette
Gloves	Derma Prene, neoprene, polymer, or vinyl gloves
IV catheters	Jelco, Deseret IV catheters
IV rubber injection ports	Cover Y-sites and ports; do not puncture. Use three-way stopcocks on plastic tubing
Levin tube	Salem sump tube
Medication vials	Remove rubber stopper
Penrose drains	Jackson-Pratt, Zimmer Hemovac drains
Prepackaged enema kits	Therevac, Fleet Ready-to-Use
Pulse oximeters	Noninoximeters
Resuscitation bags	Laerdal, Puritan Bennett, *certain* Ambu
Stethoscope tubing	PVC tubing; cover with latex-free stockinette
Suction tubing	PVC (Davol, Laerdal)
Syringes—single use (Monoject, BD)	Terumo syringes, Abbott PCA Abboject
Tapes	Dermicel, Micropore
Theraband	New Thera-band Exercisers, plastic tubing
Thermometer probes	Diatek probe covers
Tourniquets	X-Tourn straps (Avcor)
Home Environment	
Balloons	Mylar balloons
Condoms, diaphragms	Polyurethane products, Durex Avanti and Reality products (female condom)
Diapers, incontinence pads	Huggies, Always, *some* Attends
Feminine hygiene pads	Kimberly-Clark products
Wheelchair cushions	ROHO cushions, Sof Care bed/chair cushions

[a]Confirmation is essential to verify that all items are latex free before using, especially if risk of latex allergy is present.
ECG, electrocardiogram; IV, intravenous; PVC, polyvinyl chloride.
Adapted from Centers for Disease Control and Prevention (CDC). (2014). Latex allergy: A prevention guide. Retrieved on 12/2/2019 at: www.cdc.gov/niosh/docs/98-113/default.html; Mayo Foundation for Medical Education and Research. (2019). Diseases and conditions: Latex allergy. Retrieved on 12/2/2019 at: www.mayoclinic.org/diseases-conditions/latex-allergy/basics/definition/CON-20024233

require major changes in the patient's home and work environment to avoid further exposure (AAAAI, 2019d).

Latex allergy can also be an immediate hypersensitivity, type I allergic reaction, mediated by IgE. Localized itching, erythema, or local urticaria within 10 to 15 minutes after exposure to latex are often the initial symptoms (Hamilton, 2017a). Symptoms commonly include rhinitis, conjunctivitis, and nasal congestion. An asthma attack can be triggered. Severe anaphylaxis can occur, which includes generalized urticaria, angioedema, bronchospasm, and hypotension minutes after dermal or mucosal exposure to latex.

Assessment and Diagnostic Findings

The diagnosis of latex allergy is based on the history, physical examination, and diagnostic test results. Sensitization is detected by skin testing; serum-specific IgE, EIA, or ELISA; or the level of Hevea latex-specific IgE antibody in the serum. Testing for the chemicals found in the rubber production that makes latex is performed using the patch test. Skin patch testing is the preferred method for patients with contact allergies. The TRUE test and other skin tests should be performed only by primary providers who have expertise in their administration and interpretation and who have the necessary equipment available to treat local or systemic allergic reactions to the reagent (Hamilton, 2017a).

Medical Management

The best prevention strategy for latex allergy is the avoidance of latex-based products. A new, natural derivative from the desert plant guayule is now being used as a replacement for latex in many products. The predominant nonsterile, nonlatex examination gloves used in medical institutions today are made of nitrile, neoprene, vinyl, or synthetic polyisoprene rubber that is extracted from oil. Nonlatex condoms are available for contraception but these do not prevent transmission of HIV or other sexually transmitted infections (STIs). Persons allergic to latex should be cautioned to not blow up latex balloons or be in enclosed spaces where these are used, as these balloons are still used as decorations (AAAAI, 2019d).

Patients at risk for an anaphylactic reaction to latex should be instructed to carry auto-injectable epinephrine in case of a reaction (Hamilton, 2017b).

Patients should report their allergy prior to any medical, dental, gynecologic, or surgical procedure and request a latex-safe environment (Hamilton, 2017b).

TABLE 33-6	Types of Reactions to Latex		
Type of Reaction	**Cause**	**Signs/Symptoms**	**Treatment**
Irritant contact dermatitis	Damage to skin because of irritation and loss of epidermoid skin layer; not an allergic reaction. Can be caused by excessive use of soaps and cleansers, repeated handwashing, inadequate hand drying, mechanical irritation (e.g., sweating, rubbing inside powdered gloves), exposure to chemicals added during the manufacturing of gloves, and alkaline pH of powdered gloves. Reaction may occur with first exposure, is usually benign, and is not life-threatening.	*Acute:* Redness, edema, burning, discomfort, itching *Chronic:* Dry, thickened, cracked skin	Referral for diagnostic testing Avoidance of exposure to irritant Thorough washing and drying of hands Use of powder-free gloves with more frequent changes of gloves Changing glove types Use of water- or silicone-based moisturizing creams, lotions, or topical barrier agents Avoidance of oil- or petroleum-based skin agents with latex products, because they cause breakdown of the latex product
Allergic contact dermatitis	Delayed hypersensitivity (type IV) reaction. Usually affects only area in contact with latex; reaction is usually to chemical additives used in the manufacturing process rather than to latex itself. Cause of reaction is T-cell–mediated sensitization to additives of latex. Reaction is not life-threatening and is far more common than a type I reaction. Slow onset; occurs 18–24 h after exposure. Resolves within 3–4 days after exposure. More severe reactions may occur with subsequent exposures.	Pruritus, erythema, swelling, crusty thickened skin, blisters, other skin lesions	Referral for diagnosis (patch tests) and treatment Thorough washing and drying of hands Use of water- or silicone-based moisturizing creams, lotions, or topical barrier agents Avoidance of oil- or petroleum-based products unless they are latex compatible Avoidance of identified causative agent, because continued exposure to latex products in presence of breaks in skin may contribute to latex protein sensitization
Latex allergy	Type I IgE-mediated immediate hypersensitivity to plant proteins in natural rubber latex. In sensitized people, antilatex IgE antibody stimulates mast cell proliferation and basophil histamine release. Exposure can be through contact with the skin, mucous membranes, or internal tissues, or through inhalation of traces of powder from latex gloves. Severe reactions usually occur shortly after parenteral or mucous membrane exposure. People with any type I reaction to latex are at high risk for anaphylaxis. Local swelling, redness, edema, itching, and systemic reactions, including anaphylaxis, occur within minutes after exposure.	Rhinitis, flushing, conjunctivitis, urticaria, laryngeal edema, bronchospasm, asthma, severe vasodilation angioedema, anaphylaxis, cardiovascular collapse, death	Immediate treatment of reaction with epinephrine, fluids, vasopressors, and corticosteroids, and airway and ventilator support, with close monitoring for recurrence for the next 12–14 h Prompt referral for diagnostic evaluation Treatment and diagnostic evaluation in latex-free environment Assessment of all patients for symptoms of latex allergy Educating patients and family members about the disorder and the importance of preventing future reactions by avoiding latex (e.g., wearing medical identification, carrying and autoinjector of epinephrine)

IgE, immunoglobulin E.

Adapted from American Academy of Allergy, Asthma, and Immunology (AAAAI). (2019d). Latex Allergy. Retrieved on 7/7/2019 at: www.aaaai.org/conditions-and-treatments/library/allergy-library/latex-allergy

Nursing Management

The nurse can assume a pivotal role in the management of latex allergies in both patients and staff. All patients should be asked about latex allergy. Every time an invasive procedure must be performed, the nurse should consider the possibility of latex allergies. Nurses working in operating rooms, intensive care units, short procedure units, and EDs need to pay particular attention to latex allergy (Hamilton, 2017b). See Chapter 14, Figure 14-2, for a sample latex allergy assessment form.

Although the type I reaction is the most significant of the reactions to latex, care must be taken in the presence of irritant contact dermatitis and delayed hypersensitivity reaction to avoid further exposure of the person to latex. Patients with latex allergy are advised to notify their health care providers and to wear medical identification. Patients must become knowledgeable about what products contain latex and what products are safe, nonlatex alternatives. They must also become knowledgeable about signs and symptoms of latex allergy and emergency treatment and self-injection of epinephrine in case of allergic reaction (Hamilton, 2017b).

CRITICAL THINKING EXERCISES

1 **ipc** You are the nurse working in an outpatient walk-in clinic. A 28-year-old patient is newly diagnosed with allergic rhinitis. What nursing and interprofessional assessments are indicated? What interventions, including patient education, will you implement? What interprofessional referrals would be appropriate?

2 **ebp** A 44-year-old presents to the emergency department (ED) complaining of dyspnea after eating at a new restaurant. The patient states that this has happened two other times in the past and seems to be worse each time. What is the evidence for management of this patient? Describe the strength of the evidence and criteria used to assess its strength.

REFERENCES

*Asterisk indicates nursing research.

Books

Actor, J. K. (2019). *Introductory immunology* (2nd ed). Philadelphia, PA: Elsevier.

Comerford, K. C., & Durkin, M. T. (2020). *Nursing 2020 drug handbook.* Philadelphia, PA: Wolters Kluwer.

Habif, T. (2016). *Clinical dermatology a color guide to diagnosis and therapy* (6th ed.). St Louis, MO: Elsevier.

Norris, T. (2019). *Porth's pathophysiology: Concepts of altered health states* (10th ed.). Philadelphia, PA: Wolters Kluwer.

Journals and Electronic Documents

Akdis, M. (2018). Allergen immunotherapy for allergic disease: Therapeutic mechanisms. *UpToDate.* Retrieved on 6/21/2019 at: www.uptodate.com/contents/allergen-immunotherapy-for-allergic-disease-therapeutic-mechanisms

American Academy of Allergy, Asthma, and Immunology (AAAAI). (2018). Anaphylaxis. Retrieved on 6/26/19 at: www.aaaai.org/conditions-and-treatments/allergies/anaphylaxis

American Academy of Allergy, Asthma, and Immunology (AAAAI). (2019a). Atopic march definition. Retrieved on 6/24/2019 at: www.aaaai.org/conditions-and-treatments/conditions-dictionary/atopic-march

American Academy of Allergy, Asthma, and Immunology (AAAAI). (2019b). Hives (Urticaria) and Angioedema overview. Retrieved on 6/27/2019 at: www.aaaai.org/conditions-and-treatments/library/allergy-library/ hives (urticaria) and angioedema overview.

American Academy of Allergy, Asthma, and Immunology (AAAAI). (2019c). Understanding hereditary angioedema overview. Retrieved on 6/27/2019 at: www.aaaai.org/conditions-and-treatments/library/allergy-library/understanding-hereditary-angioedema

American Academy of Allergy, Asthma, and Immunology (AAAAI). (2019d). Latex Allergy. Retrieved on 7/7/2019 at: www.aaaai.org/conditions-and-treatments/library/allergy-library/latex-allergy

Andreae, D. A., & Schreffler, W. G. (2019). Future diagnostic tools for food allergy. *UpToDate.* Retrieved on 6/29/2019 at: www.uptodate.com/contents/future-diagnostic-tools-for-food-allergy

Asero, R., Tedeschi, A., Marzano, A.V., et al. (2017). Chronic urticaria: A focus on pathogenesis. *F1000Res, 11*(6),1095. doi: 10.12688/f1000research.11546.1. PMID: 28751972; PMCID: PMC5506533. Retrieved from: https://pubmed.ncbi.nlm.nih.gov/28751972/

Badri, T., & Takov, V. (2019). Montelukast. *STAT Pearls.* Retrieved on 10/15/2019 at: www.ncbi.nlm.nih.gov/books/NBK459301

Berger, W. E., & Meltzer, E. O. (2015). Intranasal spray medications for maintenance therapy of allergic rhinitis. *American Journal Rhinology & Allergy, 29*(4), 273–282.

Bircher, A. J. (2018). Exanthematous (maculopapular) drug eruption. *UpToDate.* Retrieved on 6/26/2019 at: www.uptodate.com/contents/exanthematous-maculopapular-drug-eruption

Burks, W. (2019). Clinical manifestations of food allergy: An overview. *UpToDate.* Retrieved on 10/15/2019 at: www.uptodate.com/contents/clinical-manifestations-of-food-allergy-an-overview

Campbell, R. L., & Kelso, J. M. (2018). Anaphylaxis: Emergency treatment. *UpToDate.* Retrieved on 10/13/2019 at: www.uptodate.com/contents/anaphylaxis-emergency-treatment

Castells, M. C. (2018). Mast cell-derived mediators. *UpToDate.* Retrieved on 6/20/2019 at: www.uptodate.com/contents/mast-cell-derived-mediators

Castells, M. C., & Solensky, R. (2017). Rapid drug desensitization for immediate hypersensitivity reactions. *UpToDate.* Retrieved on 6/26/2019 at: www.uptodate.com/contents/rapid-drug-desensitization-for-immediate-hypersensitivity-reactions

Centers for Disease Control and Prevention (CDC). (2014). Latex allergy: A prevention guide. Retrieved on 12/2/2019 at: www.cdc.gov/niosh/docs/98-113/default.html

Centers for Disease Control and Prevention (CDC)/National Center for Health Statistics. (2017). Allergies and Hay fever. Retrieved on 10/13/2019 at: www.cdc.gov/nchs/fastats/allergies.htm

Chaaban, M. R., Mansi, A., Tripple, J. W., et al. (2019). SCIT versus SLIT: Which one do you recommend, doc? *American Journal of Medical Sciences, 357*(5), 442–447.

Chauchan, B. F., Jeyaraman, M. M., Singh Mann, A., et al. (2017). Addition of anti-leukotriene agents to inhaled corticosteroids for adults and adolescents with persistent asthma. *Cochrane Database Systematic Reviews, 3,* CD010347.

Cho, Y. T., & Chu, C. Y. (2017). Treatments for severe cutaneous adverse reactions. *Journal of Immunological Research, 2017* (1503709). Retrieved on 10/15/2019 at: www.ncbi.nlm.nih.gov/pmc/articles/PMC5763067

Cicardi, M., & Zuraw, B. (2018a). Hereditary angioedema: Pathogenesis and diagnosis. *UpToDate.* Retrieved on 6/27/2019 at: www.uptodate.com/contents/hereditary-angioedema-pathogenesis-and-diagnosis

Cicardi, M., & Zuraw, B. (2018b). Hereditary angioedema: Treatment of acute attacks. *UpToDate.* Retrieved on 6/27/2019 at: www.uptodate.com/contents/hereditary-angioedema-treatment-of-acute-attacks

Commins, S. P. (2019). Food intolerance and food allergy in adults. An overview. *UpToDate.* Retrieved on 6/29/2019 at: www.uptodate.com/contents/food-intolerance-and-food-allergy-in-adults-an-overview

deShazo, R. D., & Kemp, S. F. (2017). Pathogenesis of allergic rhinitis (rhinosinusitis). *UpToDate.* Retrieved on 6/20/2019 at: www.uptodate.com/contents/pathogenesis-of-allergic-rhinitis

deShazo, R. D., & Kemp, S. F. (2018a). Allergic rhinitis: Clinical manifestations, epidemiology, and diagnosis. *UpToDate.* Retrieved on 6/20/2019 at: www.uptodate.com/contents/allergic-rhinitis-clinical-manifestations-epidemiology-and-diagnosis

deShazo, R. D., & Kemp, S. F. (2018b). Pharmacotherapy of allergic rhinitis. *UpToDate.* Retrieved on 6/20/2019 at: www.uptodate.com/contents/pharmacotherapy-of-allergic-rhinitis

Durham, S. R., & Penagos, M. (2016). Sublingual or subcutaneous immunotherapy for allergic rhinitis? *Journal of Allergy and Clinical Immunology, 137*(2), 339–349.

Fick, D. M., Semla, T. P., Steinman, M., et al. (2019). American Geriatrics Society 2019 updated AGS Beers Criteria® for potentially inappropriate medication use in older adults. *Journal of the American Geriatrics Society, 67*(4), 674–694.

Fornacier, L., & Noor, I. (2018). Contact dermatitis and patch testing for the allergist. *Annals of Allergy, Asthma, & Immunology, 120*(6), 592–598.

Goldner, R., & Fransway, A. F. (2018). Irritant contact dermatitis in adults. *UpToDate.* Retrieved on 6/24/2019 at: www.uptodate.com/contents/irritant-contact-dermatitis-in-adults

Gupta, R. S., Warren, C. M., & Smith, B. M. (2019). Prevalence and severity of food allergies among US adults. *Journal of the American Medical Association Network Open, 2*(1), e185630.

Guyer, A. C., & Banerji, A. (2019). ACE-inhibitor induced angioedema. *UpToDate.* Retrieved on 6/27/2019 at: www.uptodate.com/contents/ace-inhibitor-induced-angioedema

Hamilton, R. G. (2017a). Latex allergy: Epidemiology, clinical manifestations, and diagnosis. *UpToDate.* Retrieved on 7/8/2019 at: www.uptodate.com/contents/latex-allergy-epidemiology-clinical-manifestations-and-diagnosis

Hamilton, R. G. (2017b). Latex allergy: Management. *UpToDate.* Retrieved on 7/8/2019 at: www.uptodate.com/contents/latex-allergy-management

High, W. A. (2019). Stevens-Johnson syndrome and toxic epidermal necrolysis: Pathogenesis, clinical manifestations, and diagnosis. *UpToDate.* Retrieved on 10/15/2019 at: www.uptodate.com/contents/stevens-johnson-syndrome-and-toxic-epidermal-necrolysis-pathogenesis-clinical-manifestations-and-diagnosis

Hill, D. A., & Spergel, J. M. (2018). The atopic march: Critical evidence and clinical relevance. *Annals of Allergy, Asthma, & Immunology, 120*(2), 131–137.

James, C., & Bernstein, D. (2017). Allergen immunotherapy: An updated review of safety. *Current Opinion Allergy Clinical Immunology, 17*(1), 55–59.

Kakli, H. A., & Riley, T. D. (2016). Allergic rhinitis. *Primary Care, 43*(3), 465–475.

Kemp, S. F. (2018). Pathophysiology of anaphylaxis. *UpToDate.* Retrieved on 6/20/2019 at: www.uptodate.com/contents/pathophysiology-of-anaphylaxis

Khan, D. A. (2019a). Chronic spontaneous urticaria: Standard management and patient education. *UpToDate.* Retrieved on 6/27/2019 at: www.uptodate.com/contents/chronic-spontaneous-urticaria-standard-management-and-patient-eucation

Khan, D. A. (2019b). Chronic spontaneous urticaria: Treatment of refractory symptoms. *UpToDate.* Retrieved on 6/27/2019 at: www.uptodate.com/contents/chronic-spontaneous-urticaria-treatment-of-refractory-symptoms

Klimek, L., Pfaar, O., Bousquet, J., et al. (2017). Allergen immunotherapy in allergic rhinitis: Current use and future trends. *Expert Review Clinical Immunology, 13*(9), 897–906.

Kowal, K., & DuBuske, L. (2016). Overview of skin testing for allergic disease. *UpToDate*. Retrieved on 6/20/2019 at: www.uptodate.com./contents/overview-of-skin-testing-for-allergic-disease

Kowal, K., & DuBuske, L. (2017). Overview of in vitro allergy tests. *UpToDate*. Retrieved on 6/20/2019 at: www.uptodate.com/contents/overview-of-in-vitro-allergy-tests

Laccourreye, O., Werner, A., Giroud, J. P., et al. (2015). Benefits, limits, and danger of ephedrine and pseudoephedrine as nasal decongestants. *European Annals of Otorhinology and Head & Neck Disease, 132*(1), 31–34.

Larsen, J. N., Broge, L., & Jacobi, H. (2016). Allergy immunotherapy: The future of allergy treatment. *Drug Discovery Today, 21*(1), 26–37.

Lieberman, P. L. (2018). Biphasic and protracted anaphylaxis. *UpToDate*. Retrieved on 6/20/2019 at: www.uptodate.com/contents/biphasic-and-protracted-anaphylaxis

Litchman, G., Nair, P. A., & Atwater, A. R. (2019). Contact dermatitis. STAT Pearls. Treasure Island, Fla: STAT Pearls. Retrieved on 10/15/2019 at: www.ncbi.nlm.nih.gov/books/NBK459230

Løset, M., Brown, S. J., Saunes, M., et al. (2019). Genetics of atopic sermatitis: From DNA sequence to clinical relevance. *Dermatology, 235*(5), 355–364.

Marshall, J. S., Warrington, R., Watson, W., et al. (2018). An introduction to immunology and immunopathology. *Allergy, Asthma, and Clinical Immunology, 14*(Suppl 2), 49.

Maurer, M. (2019). Cold urticaria. *UpToDate*. Retrieved on 6/27/2019 at: www.uptodate.com/contents/cold-urticaria

McDonald, M., & Sexton, D. J. (2019). Drug fever. *UpToDate*. Retrieved on 10/15/2019 at: www.uptodate.com/contents/drug-fever

Mockenhaupt, M. (2019). Drug reaction with eosinophilia and systemic symptoms (DRESS). *UpToDate*. Retrieved on 10/14/2019 at: www.uptodate.com/contents/drug-reaction-with-eosinophilia-and-systemic-symptoms-dress

Moore, L. E., Kemp, A. M., Kemp, S. F. (2015). Recognition, treatment, and prevention of anaphylaxis. *Immunology and Allergy Clinics of North America, 35*(2), 363–374.

Nelson, H. (2018). SCIT: Standard schedules, administration techniques, adverse reactions, and monitoring. *UpToDate*. Retrieved on 6/21/2019 at: www.uptodate.com/contents/scit-standard-schedules-administration-techniques-adverse-reactions-and-monitoring

Nowak-Wegrzyn, A. (2019). Investigational therapies for food allergy: Immunotherapy and nonspecific therapies. *UpToDate*. Retrieved on 6/21/2019 at: www.uptodate.com/contents/investigational-therapies-for-food-allergy-immunotherapy-and-nonspecific-therapies

*Pestotnik, G., & Krueger, D. (2018). Comparing the discomfort and application time of allergy testing. *American Academy of Ambulatory Care Nurses Viewpoint, 40*(1), 4–8.

Pichler, W. J. (2019). Drug hypersensitivity: Classification and clinical features. *UpToDate*. Retrieved on 6/26/2019 at: www.uptodate.com/contents/drug-hypersensitivity-classification-and-clinical-features

Pitsios, C., & Dietis, N. (2019). Ways to increase adherence to allergen immunotherapy. *Current Medical and Research Opinion, 35*(6), 1027–1031.

Platts-Mills, T. A. (2019). Allergen avoidance in the treatment of asthma and allergic rhinitis. *UpToDate*. Retrieved on 6/21/2019 at: www.uptodate.com/contents/allergen-avoidance-in-the-treatment-of-asthma-and-allergic-rhinitis

Randall, K. L., & Hawkins, C. A. (2018). Antihistamines and allergy. *Australian Prescriber, 41*(2), 41–45.

Samel, A. D., & Chu, C. Y. (2019). Drug eruptions. *UpToDate*. Retrieved on 10/15/2019 at: www.uptodate.com/contents/drug-eruptions

Sanchez-Borges, M., & Ansotegui, I. J. (2019). Second-generation antihistamines: An update. *Current Opinion in Allergy & Clinical Immunology, 19*(4), 358–364.

Scadding, G. (2017). Rhinitis and rhinosinusitis: When to think allergy and what to do. *Practice Nursing, 28*(11), 472–480.

Shenoy, E. S., Macy, E., Rowe, T., et al. (2019). Evaluation and management of penicillin allergy: A review. *JAMA, 321*(2), 188–199.

Sicherer, S. H. (2019). Management of food allergy: Avoidance. *UpToDate*. Retrieved on 6/29/2019 at: www.uptodate.com/contents/management-of-food-allergy-avoidance

Singleton, R., & Halverstam, C. P. (2016). Diagnosis and management of cold urticaria. *Cutis, 97*(1), 59–62.

Song, T. T., & Lieberman, P. (2019). Who needs to carry an epinephrine autoinjector? *Cleveland Clinical Journal of Medicine, 86*(1), 66–72.

Spergel, J. M., & Lio, P. A. (2019). Management of severe atopic dermatitis (eczema) in children. *UpToDate*. Retrieved on 6/26/2019 at: www.uptodate.com/management-of-severe-atopic-dermatitis-eczema-in-children

Stokes, J., & Casale, T. B. (2018). Anti-IgE therapy. *UpToDate*. Retrieved on 6/27/2019 at: www.uptodate.com/contents/anti-ige-therapy

Stokes, J., & Casale, T. B. (2019). The relationship between Ig E and allergic disease. *UpToDate*. Retrieved on 6/20/2019 at: www.uptodate.com/contents/the-relationship-between-ige-and-allergic-disease

Sundquist, B. K., Lang, B., & Pasha, M. A. (2019). Experience in patch testing: A 6 year retrospective review from a single academic allergy practice. *Annals of Allergy, Asthma, & Immunology, 122*(5), 502–507.

Tanno, L. K., Torres, M. J., Castells, M., et al. (2018). What can we learn in drug allergy management from World Health Organization's international classifications? *Allergy, 73*(5), 987–992.

U.S. Federal Drug Administration (FDA). (2017). Legal requirements for the sale of drug products containing pseudoephedrine, ephedrine, and phenylpropanolamine. Retrieved on 6/23/2019 at: www.fda.gov/drugs/information-drug-class/legal-requirements-sale-and-purchase-drug-products-containing-pseudoephedrine-ephedrine-andphenylpropanolamine

Wahid, N. W. B., & Shermetaro, C. (2019). Rhinitis medicamentosa. STAT Pearls. Retrieved on 10/15/2019 at: www.ncbi.nlm.nih.gov/pubmed/30855902

Warrell, D. A. (2019). Venomous bites, stings, and poisoning: An update. *Infectious Disease Clinic of North America, 33*(1), 17–38.

Wener, M. H. (2018). Serum sickness and serum sickness-like reactions. *UpToDate*. Retrieved on 10/15/2019 at: www.uptodate.com/contents/serum-sickness-and-serum-sickness-like-reactions

Weston, W. L., & Howe, W. (2019). Atopic dermatitis (eczema): Pathogenesis, clinical manifestations, and diagnosis. *UpToDate*. Retrieved on 6/26/2019 at: www.uptodate.com/contents/atopic-dermatitis-eczema-pathogenesis-clinical-manifestations-and-diagnosis

*Wilkin, Z. L. (2020). Effects of video discharge instructions on patient understanding. *Advanced Emergency Nursing Journal, 42*(1), 71–78. www.aaaai.org/conditions-and-treatments/conditions-dictionary/hives

Zuraw, B. (2019). An overview of angioedema: Clinical features, diagnosis, and management. *UpToDate*. Retrieved on 10/15/2019 at: www.uptodate.com/contents/an-overview-of-angioedema-clinical-features-diagnosis-and-management

Resources

American Academy of Allergy, Asthma, and Immunology (AAAAI), www.aaaai.org

Asthma and Allergy Foundation of America (AAFA), www.aafa.org

Asthma and Allergy Foundation of America. (2021). Find a local support group. Retrieved from: https://www.aafa.org/aafa-affiliated-asthma-allergy-support-groups/

Food Allergy Research Education (FARE), www.foodallergy.org

Mayo Foundation for Medical Education and Research, www.mayoclinic.org

National Institute of Allergy and Infectious Diseases, www.niaid.nih.gov

Occupational Safety and Health Administration (OSHA), www.osha.gov

LEARNING OUTCOMES

On completion of this chapter, the learner will be able to:

1. Explain the pathophysiology of inflammatory rheumatic diseases and describe the assessment and diagnostic findings seen in patients with these disorders.
2. Use the nursing process as a framework for care of the patient with an inflammatory rheumatic disorder.
3. Devise an education plan for the patient with newly diagnosed inflammatory rheumatic disease.
4. Identify modifications in interventions to accommodate changes in patients' functional ability that may occur with disease progression.

NURSING CONCEPTS

Assessment	Comfort	Infection
Cellular Regulation	Immunity	Inflammation

GLOSSARY

arthritis: inflammation of a joint
cytokines: cell signaling proteins that are vital to regulation of hematopoiesis, apoptosis, and immune responses
exacerbation: period when disease symptoms occur or increase
pannus: proliferation of newly formed synovial tissue infiltrated with inflammatory cells
remission: period when disease symptoms are reduced or absent

rheumatic diseases: numerous disorders affecting skeletal muscles, bones, cartilage, ligaments, tendons, and joints
rheumatoid arthritis: a systemic autoimmune disease with symmetric arthritic manifestations and multiple extra-articular features
subchondral bone: bony plate that supports the articular cartilage
tophi: accumulation of crystalline deposits in articular surfaces, bones, soft tissue, and cartilage

The **rheumatic diseases** encompass autoimmune, degenerative, inflammatory, and systemic conditions that affect the joints, muscles, and soft tissues of the body. Rheumatic diseases most commonly manifest the clinical features of **arthritis** (inflammation of a joint) and pain. There are more than 100 types of rheumatic diseases. The problems caused by rheumatic diseases include limitations in mobility and activities of daily living, pain, fatigue, altered self-image, and sleep disturbances, as well as systemic effects that can lead to organ failure and death. An understanding of inflammatory rheumatic diseases and their effects on a patient's function and well-being is essential to developing an appropriate plan of nursing care.

Rheumatic Diseases

Rheumatic disease processes affect males and females of all ages and ethnic groups. Some disorders are more likely to occur at a particular time of life or to affect one gender more often than the other. In general, women are two to nine times more commonly affected by rheumatic diseases than men (Norris, 2019). Arthritis and other rheumatic diseases and the physical limitations that occur with them are becoming more prominent and a larger public health issue, which can be attributed to the increased number of older adults in the United States.

The onset of these conditions may be acute or insidious, with a course possibly marked by periods of **remission** (a period when disease symptoms are reduced or absent) and **exacerbation** (a period when symptoms occur or increase). Treatment can be simple, aimed at localized relief, or it can be complex, directed toward relief of systemic effects. Permanent changes and disability may result from these disorders.

Nurses need to understand the classification of rheumatic diseases. One system is to classify disease as either monoarticular (affecting a single joint) or polyarticular (affecting multiple joints). Another system is to classify the disease as either inflammatory or noninflammatory. This chapter focuses on inflammatory rheumatic diseases, while noninflammatory rheumatic diseases (i.e., osteoarthritis) are covered in Chapter 36. Conditions that may secondarily affect the musculoskeletal structure are also considered in disease classification.

Pathophysiology

Each of the inflammatory rheumatic diseases exhibits unique pathophysiologic features. Three distinct characteristics of pathophysiology include inflammation, autoimmunity, and degeneration.

Inflammation

Inflammation is a complex physiologic process mediated by the immune system that occurs in response to harmful stimuli like damaged cells or antigens, which may include pathogens (e.g., viruses, bacteria). Inflammation is meant to protect the body from insult by removing the triggering antigen or event. In response to a triggering episode, the antigen stimulus activates the body's immune system to form antibodies like monocytes and T lymphocytes (also referred to as T cells). Next, the immunoglobulin antibodies form immune complexes with antigens. Phagocytosis of the immune complexes is initiated, generating an inflammatory reaction (joint effusion, pain, and edema) (see Fig. 34-1). Phagocytosis produces chemicals such as leukotrienes and prostaglandins. Leukotrienes contribute to the inflammatory process by attracting other white blood cells to the area. Prostaglandins act as modifiers to inflammation. In some cases, they increase inflammation; in other cases, they decrease it. Leukotrienes and prostaglandins produce enzymes such

as collagenase that break down collagen, which is a vital part of a normal joint. The release of these enzymes in the joint causes edema and proliferation of synovial membrane. In patients with chronic inflammation, the immune response can deviate from normal. Instead of resolution of swelling and joint pain once the triggering event has subsided, **pannus** (proliferation of newly formed synovial tissue infiltrated with inflammatory cells) formation occurs. Destruction of the joint's cartilage and erosion of bone soon follow (Norris, 2019).

The immunologic inflammatory process begins when antigens are presented to T lymphocytes, leading to a proliferation of T and B cells. B cells (also referred to as plasma cells) are a source of antibody-forming cells. In response to specific antigens, plasma cells produce and release antibodies. Antibodies combine with corresponding antigens to form pairs, or immune complexes. The immune complexes build up and are deposited in synovial tissue or other organs in the body, triggering the inflammatory reaction that can ultimately damage the involved tissue (Norris, 2019).

Autoimmunity

A hallmark of inflammatory rheumatic diseases is autoimmunity, where the body mistakenly recognizes its own tissue as a foreign antigen. Autoimmunity leads to destruction of tissue via the same inflammatory process as discussed earlier, along with chronic and long-standing pain. Although focused in the joints, inflammation and autoimmunity also involve other areas. The blood vessels (vasculitis and arteritis), lungs, heart, and kidneys may be affected by the autoimmunity and inflammation. See Chapter 32 for more information on autoimmune disease. A large group of genes, called *human leukocyte antigen* (HLA) genes, has been linked to the immune

Physiology/Pathophysiology

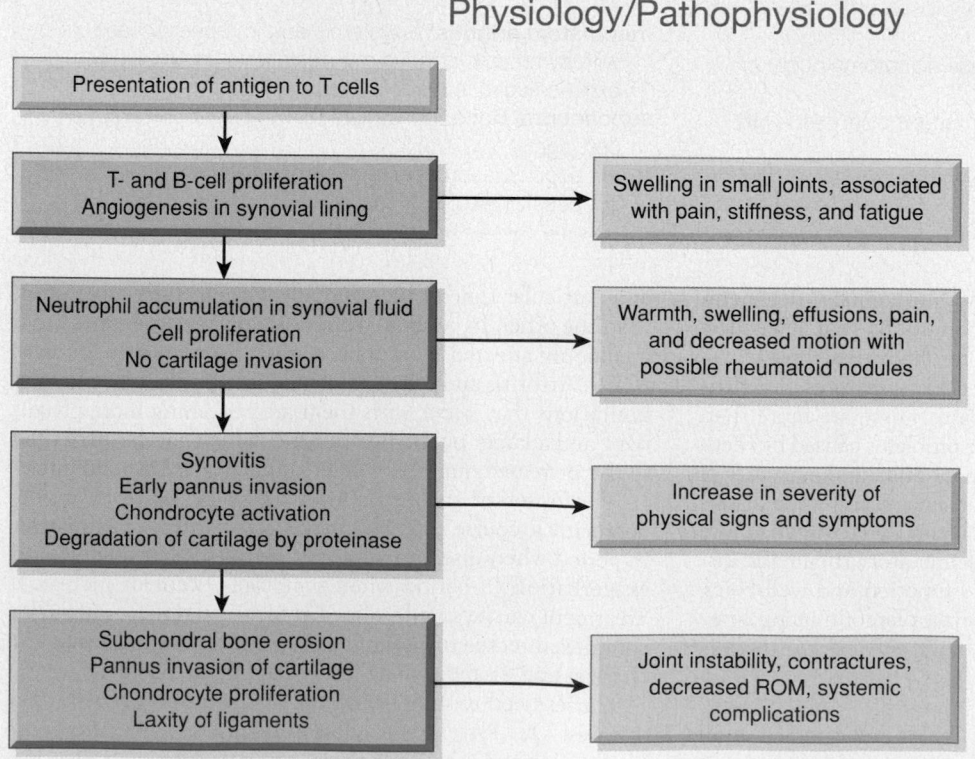

Figure 34-1 • Pathophysiology and associated physical signs of rheumatoid arthritis. ROM, range of motion.

response and the development of multiple rheumatic diseases (Norris, 2019).

Degeneration

In degenerative rheumatic diseases, inflammation also occurs, but as a secondary process. Although the cause of degeneration of the articular cartilage is poorly understood, the process is known to be metabolically active and therefore is more accurately called *degradation*. One theory of degradation is that genetic or hormonal influences, mechanical factors, and prior joint damage cause cartilage failure. Degradation of cartilage ensues, and increased mechanical stress on bone ends causes stiffening of bone tissue. Another theory is that bone stiffening occurs and results in increased mechanical stress on cartilage, which in turn initiates the processes of degradation. See Chapter 35 for more information on the structure and function of the articular system.

Clinical Manifestations

The most common symptom in the rheumatic diseases is pain. Other common symptoms include joint swelling, limited movement, stiffness, weakness, and fatigue.

Assessment and Diagnostic Findings

Assessment begins with a general health history, which includes the onset of symptoms and how they evolved, family history, past health history, and any other contributing factors. Because many of the rheumatic diseases are chronic conditions, the health history should also include information about the patient's perception of the problem, previous treatments and their effectiveness, the patient's support systems, and the patient's current knowledge base and the source of that information. A complete health history is followed by a complete physical assessment (see Chapter 4).

Assessment for rheumatic diseases combines the physical examination with a functional assessment (Eliopoulos, 2021). Inspection of the patient's general appearance occurs during the initial contact. Gait, posture, and general musculoskeletal size and structure are observed. Gross deformities and abnormalities in movement are noted. The symmetry, size, and contour of other connective tissues, such as the skin and adipose tissue, are also noted and recorded (Weber & Kelley, 2019). Chart 34-1 outlines the important areas for consideration during the physical assessment. The functional assessment is a combination of history (what the patient reports that they can and cannot do) and examination (observation of activities, in which the patient demonstrates what they can and cannot do, such as dressing and getting in and out of a chair). Observation also includes the adaptations and adjustments the patient may have made (sometimes without awareness)—for example, with shoulder or elbow involvement, the person may bend over to reach a fork rather than raising the fork to the mouth.

Laboratory Studies

In Table 34-1 common laboratory studies are listed with their corresponding normal ranges and significance. Many of the tests require special laboratory techniques and may not be performed in every health care facility. The primary provider determines which tests are necessary based on symptoms,

stage of disease, cost, and likely benefit. In some instances, tests are used to monitor the course of the disease.

Other Diagnostic Studies

Imaging studies commonly used for patients with rheumatic diseases include x-ray studies, computed tomography (CT) scans, magnetic resonance imaging (MRI) scans, and arthrography. See Chapter 35 for further information about these and other diagnostic studies.

Medical Management

The chronic nature of rheumatic conditions requires cooperation between the patient and the provider. Patient education regarding the disease process and treatment options is imperative to enable patients to make informed decisions regarding their care. Management of rheumatic diseases is based on a shared decision process between the provider and patient that takes into account the patient's values, preferences, and comorbidities (Singh, Saag, Bridges, et al., 2016).

Pharmacologic Therapy

Medications are used with the rheumatic diseases to manage symptoms, to control inflammation, and, in some instances, to modify the disease. Useful medications include the salicylates, nonsteroidal anti-inflammatory drugs (NSAIDs), and both biologic and nonbiologic disease-modifying antirheumatic drugs (DMARDs). As their name suggests, DMARDs have the ability to suppress the autoimmune response; alter disease progression; and stop or decrease further tissue damage on the joints, cartilage, and organs. DMARDs have been found to halt the progression of bone loss and destruction and can induce remission (Singh et al., 2016). Nonbiologic DMARDs are thought to reduce proinflammatory **cytokines** (cell signaling proteins vital to regulation of hematopoiesis, apoptosis, and immune responses) and increase anti-inflammatory cytokines. Biologic DMARDs, in contrast, have been specifically engineered to target a certain cell or molecule within the immune system to treat the specific rheumatic condition. Specific biologic DMARDs target tumor necrosis factor alpha (TNF-α), B cells, T cells, interleukin 1 (IL-1), and interleukin 6 (IL-6). Table 34-2 reviews select medications.

Controlling the inflammation related to the disease process helps manage pain, but this is often a delayed response. Nonopioid medications are often used for pain management, especially early in the treatment program, until other measures can be instituted.

Nonpharmacologic Pain Management

Nonpharmacologic methods of pain management are important. Heat applications are helpful in relieving pain, stiffness, and muscle spasm (Kapale, Vardharajulu, & Warude, 2017). Superficial heat may be applied in the form of warm tub baths or showers and warm moist compresses. Paraffin baths (dips), which offer concentrated heat, are helpful to patients with wrist and small-joint involvement. Maximum benefit is achieved within 20 minutes after application. More frequent use for shorter lengths of time is most beneficial. Therapeutic exercises can be carried out more comfortably and effectively after heat has been applied (Kapale et al., 2017).

(text continued on page 1073)

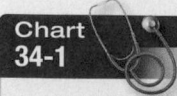

Chart 34-1

ASSESSMENT
Assessing for Rheumatic Disorders

In addition to the head-to-toe assessment or systems review, the following are important areas of consideration to be noted when performing the complete physical assessment of a patient with a known or suspected rheumatic disorder.

Manifestation	Significance
Skin (inquire and inspect)	
Rash, lesions	Associated with systemic lupus erythematosus (SLE) vasculitis, adverse effect of medication
Increased bruising	Associated with several rheumatic diseases and adverse effect of medication
Erythema	Sign of inflammation
Thinning	Adverse effect of medication
Warmth	Sign of inflammation
Photosensitivity	Associated with SLE, dermatomyositis, adverse effect of medication
Hair (inquire and inspect)	
Alopecia or thinning	Associated with rheumatic diseases or adverse effect of medication
Eye (inquire and inspect)	
Dryness, grittiness	Associated with Sjögren's syndrome (commonly occurring with rheumatoid arthritis [RA] and SLE)
Decreased acuity or blindness	Associated with temporal arteritis, medication complications
Cataracts	Adverse effect of medication
Decreased peripheral vision	Adverse effect of medication
Conjunctivitis, uveitis	Associated with ankylosing spondylitis and Reiter's syndrome
Ear (inquire)	
Tinnitus	Adverse effect of medication
Decreased acuity	Adverse effect of medication
Mouth (inquire and inspect)	
Buccal, sublingual lesions	Associated with vasculitis, dermatomyositis, adverse effect of medication
Altered sense of taste	Adverse effect of medication
Dryness	Associated with Sjögren's syndrome
Dysphagia	Associated with myositis
Difficulty chewing	Associated with decreased range of motion of jaw
Chest (inspect and inquire)	
Pleuritic pain	Associated with RA and SLE
Decreased chest expansion	Associated with ankylosing spondylitis
Activity intolerance (dyspnea)	Associated with pulmonary hypertension in scleroderma
Cardiovascular system (inquire, inspect, palpate)	
Blanching of fingers on exposure to cold	Associated with Raynaud's phenomenon
Peripheral pulses	Deficit may indicate vascular involvement or edema associated with medication effect or rheumatic diseases, especially SLE or scleroderma
Abdomen (inquire and palpate)	
Altered bowel habits	Associated with scleroderma, spondylosis, ulcerative colitis, decreased physical mobility, medication effect
Nausea, vomiting, bloating, and pain	Adverse effect of medication
Weight change (measure)	Associated with RA (decreased), adverse effect of medication (increased or decreased)
Genitalia (inquire and inspect)	
Dryness, itching	Associated with Sjögren's syndrome
Abnormal menses	Adverse effect of medication
Altered sexual performance	Fear of pain (or of pain caused by partner) and limitation of motion may affect sexual mobility
Hygiene	Poor hygiene may be related to limitations in activities of daily living
Urethritis, dysuria	Associated with ankylosing spondylitis and Reiter's syndrome
Lesions	Associated with vasculitis
Neurologic (inquire and inspect)	
Paresthesias of extremities; abnormal reflex pattern	Nerve compressions (e.g., carpal tunnel syndrome, spinal stenosis)
Headaches	Associated with temporal arteritis, adverse effect of medication
Musculoskeletal (inspect and palpate)	
Joint redness, warmth, swelling, tenderness, deformity—location of first joint involved, pattern of progression, symmetry, acute vs. chronic nature	Signs of inflammation
Joint range of motion	Decreased range of motion may indicate severity or progression of disease
Surrounding tissue findings	
Muscle atrophy, subcutaneous nodules, popliteal cyst	Extra-articular manifestations
Muscle strength (grip)	Muscle strength decreases with increased disease activity

Adapted from Weber, J. R., & Kelley, J. H. (2019). *Health assessment in nursing* (6th ed.). Philadelphia, PA: Wolters Kluwer.

TABLE 34-1	Common Blood Studies for Rheumatic Diseases	
Test	**Normal Value**	**Significance**
Serum		
Creatinine Metabolic waste excreted through the kidneys	Men: 0.6–1.2 mg/dL (71–106 mmol/L) Women: 0.4–1.0 mg/dL (36–90 mmol/L)	Increase may indicate kidney damage in SLE, scleroderma, and polyarteritis.
Erythrocyte Count Measures circulating erythrocytes	Men: 4,200,000–5,400,000/mm^3 (4.2–5.4 × 10^{12}/L) Women: 3,600,000–5,000,000/mm^3 (3.6–5.0 × 10^{12}/L)	Decrease can be seen in RA, SLE.
Erythrocyte Sedimentation Rate (ESR) Measures the rate at which RBCs settle out of unclotted blood in 1 hour	Westergren: Men under 50 yr: <15 mm/h Men over 50 yr: <20 mm/h Women under 50 yr: <20 mm/h Women over 50 yr: <30 mm/h	Increase is usually seen in inflammatory connective tissue diseases. An increase indicates rising inflammation, resulting in clustering of RBCs, which makes them heavier than normal. The higher the ESR, the greater the inflammatory activity.
Hematocrit Measures the size, capacity, and number of cells present in blood	Men: 42–52% Women: 36–48%	Decrease can be seen in chronic inflammation (anemia of chronic disease); also, blood loss through GI bleed.
White Blood Cell Count Measures circulating leukocytes	4,500–11,000 cells/mm^3	Decrease may be seen in SLE.
Uric Acid Measures level of uric acid in serum	Men: 3.4–7 mg/dL (202–416 μmol/L) Women: 2.4–6 mg/dL (143–357 μmol/L)	Increase is seen with gout. During acute flare, levels may be normal. After flare has subsided, levels will be elevated in gout.
Serum Immunology		
Antinuclear Antibody (ANA) Measures antibodies that react with a variety of nuclear antigens If antibodies are present, further testing determines the type of ANA circulating in the blood (anti-DNA, anti-RNP).	Negative Healthy adults may also have a positive ANA.	Positive test may be associated with SLE, RA, scleroderma, Raynaud's disease, Sjögren's syndrome, necrotizing arteritis. The higher the titer, the greater the inflammation. The pattern of immunofluorescence (speckled, homogeneous, or nucleolar) helps determine the diagnosis.
Anti-DNA, DNA Binding Titer measurement of antibody to double-stranded DNA	Negative	High titer is seen in SLE; increases in titer may indicate an increase in disease activity.
C-Reactive Protein (CRP) Shows presence of abnormal glycoprotein due to inflammatory process	<1 mg/dL (<10 mg/L)	A positive reading indicates active inflammation.
Immunoglobulin Electrophoresis Measures the values of immunoglobulins	IgA: 60–400 mg/dL (600–4000 mg/L) IgG: 700–1,500 mg/dL (7–15 g/L) IgM: 60–300 mg/dL (600–3000 mg/L)	Increased levels are found in people who have autoimmune disorders.
Rheumatoid Factor (RF) Determines the presence of abnormal antibodies seen in connective tissue disease	Negative	Positive titer >1:80 Present in 80% of those with RA Positive RF may also suggest SLE, Sjögren's syndrome, or mixed connective tissue disease. The higher the titer (number at right of colon), the greater the inflammation.
Tissue Typing		
HLA-B27 Antigen Measures presence of HLA antigens, which are used for tissue recognition	Negative	Found in 80–90% of those with ankylosing spondylitis and Reiter's syndrome

DNA, deoxyribonucleic acid; GI, gastrointestinal; HLA, human leukocyte antigen; IgA, immunoglobulin A; IgG, immunoglobulin G; IgM, immunoglobulin M; RA, rheumatoid arthritis; RBCs, red blood cells; RNP, ribonucleoprotein; SLE, system lupus erythematosus.
Adapted from Fischbach, F. T., & Fischbach, M. A. (2018). *A manual of laboratory and diagnostic tests* (10th ed.). Philadelphia, PA: Wolters Kluwer.

TABLE 34-2 Select Medications Used in Rheumatic Diseases

Medication	Action, Use, and Indication	Nursing Considerations
Salicylates *Acetylated:* aspirin *Nonacetylated:* choline trilisalicylate, salsalate, sodium salicylate	*Action:* Anti-inflammatory, analgesic, antipyretic Acetylated salicylates are platelet aggregation inhibitors	Administer with food, milk, antacids or large glass of water to reduce GI effects. Assess for tinnitus, gastric intolerance, GI bleeding, and purpura. Administer enteric coated or extended release whole, do not crush.
Nonsteroidal Anti-Inflammatory Drugs (NSAIDs) diclofenac, diflunisal, etodolac, ibuprofen, ketoprofen, meloxicam, nabumetone, naproxen, piroxicam, sulindac *COX-2 enzyme blockers:* celecoxib	*Action:* Anti-inflammatory, analgesic, antipyretic, platelet aggregation inhibitor Anti-inflammatory effect occurs 2–4 wk after initiation All NSAIDs are useful for short-term treatment of acute gout attack NSAIDs are an alternative to salicylates for first-line therapy in several rheumatic diseases *Action:* Inhibit only COX-2 enzymes, which are produced during inflammation, and spare COX-1 enzymes, which can be protective to the stomach	Administer NSAIDs with food. Monitor for GI, CNS, cardiovascular, renal, hematologic, and dermatologic adverse effects. Avoid salicylates; use acetaminophen for additional analgesia. Watch for possible confusion in older adults. Monitoring is the same as for other NSAIDs. Increased risk of cardiovascular events, including myocardial infarction and stroke. Appropriate for older adults and patients who are at high risk for gastric ulcers.
Disease-Modifying Antirheumatic Drugs (DMARDs) *Antimalarials:* hydroxychloroquine, chloroquine	*Action:* Anti-inflammatory, inhibit lysosomal enzymes Slow acting; onset may take 2–4 mo. May be used in conjunction with other DMARD therapy. Useful in RA and SLE.	May be administered concurrently with NSAIDs. Assess for visual changes, GI upset, skin rash, headaches, photosensitivity, bleaching of hair. Emphasize need for ophthalmologic examinations (every 6–12 mo).
Janus Kinase (JAK) inhibitors tofacitinibic, baricitinic	*Action:* Enters the cell and binds to the active JAK site, inhibits autophosphorylation and JAK activation that inhibits cytokine production. May be used in combination with methotrexate or other nonbiologic DMARDs. May also be used as monotherapy.	Administer twice a day (immediate release) or once daily (extended release). Do not administer with biologic DMARDs or potent immunosuppressants. Test for latent TB before initiation of therapy. Monitor liver enzymes routinely.
sulfasalazine	*Action:* Anti-inflammatory, reduces lymphocyte response, inhibits angiogenesis Useful in RA, seronegative spondyloarthropathies	Administer concurrently with NSAIDs. Do not use in patients with allergy to sulfa medications or salicylates. Emphasize adequate fluid intake. Assess for GI upset, skin rash, headache, liver abnormalities, anemia.
Immunosuppressives: methotrexate, azathioprine, cyclophosphamide	*Action:* Nonbiologic immune suppression, affect DNA synthesis and other cellular effects Have teratogenic potential; azathioprine and cyclophosphamide reserved for more aggressive or unresponsive disease Methotrexate is generally the first-line agent for RA treatment; also useful in SLE. Methotrexate may be given orally or by intramuscular or subcutaneous injection	Assess for bone marrow suppression, GI ulcerations, skin rashes, alopecia, bladder toxicity, increased infections. Monitor CBC, liver enzymes, creatinine at 6 wk after initiation, then every 2–3 mo or accordingly. Advise patient of contraceptive measures because of teratogenicity.
cyclosporine	*Action:* Nonbiologic immune suppression by inhibiting T lymphocytes Used for severe, progressive RA, unresponsive to other DMARDs Used in combination with methotrexate	Assess slow dose titration upward until response noted or toxicity occurs. Assess for toxic effects, such as bleeding gums, fluid retention, hair growth, tremors. Monitor blood pressure and renal function (creatinine) every 2 wk until stable.
Immunomodulators *Pyrimidine synthesis inhibitor:* leflunomide	*Action:* Nonbiologic with antiproliferative and anti-inflammatory effects; used in moderate to severe RA May be used alone or in combination with other DMARDs	Long half-life; requires loading dose followed by daily administration. Assess for diarrhea, hair loss, skin rash, mouth sores. Monitor liver function tests. Contraindicated in pregnancy and breast-feeding. Given orally.

TABLE 34-2 Select Medications Used in Rheumatic Diseases (continued)

Medication	Action, Use, and Indication	Nursing Considerations
TNF-blocking agents: adalimumab, certolizumabpegol, etanercept, infliximab, golimumab	*Action:* Biologic response modifier that binds to TNF, a cytokine involved in inflammatory and immune responses. Used in moderate to severe RA. Can be used alone or with methotrexate or other nonbiologic DMARDs. Adalimumab is given by subcutaneous injection every 2 wk, but may be used every week if efficacy not reached. Certolizumabpegol is given by subcutaneous injection every 2 wk. Etanercept is given by subcutaneous injection weekly. Infliximab is given intravenously over 2 h or more. Medication must be refrigerated. Golimumab is given by subcutaneous injection once a month. Golimumab SQ is a second alternative that is administered intravenously every 8 wk after initial 2 loading doses	Patient should be tested for tuberculosis before beginning this medication. Educate patient about subcutaneous self-injection. Monitor for injection site reactions. Educate patient about increased risk for infection and to withhold medication if fever occurs. Notify provider if any illness or infection occurs and medication is held.
T-cell costimulation modulator: abatacept	*Action:* Blocks one of the pathways needed to fully activate T cells, decreasing inflammatory and immunologic responses. Used in moderate to severe RA unresponsive to TNF inhibitors. Used with methotrexate or DMARDs other than TNF inhibitors or anakinra.	Administered IV initially, then transitions to subcutaneous dosage once weekly. Educate patient about subcutaneous self-injections given daily. Monitor for injection site reactions. Educate patient about increased risk of infection and to withhold medication if fever occurs. IV infusions are given every 4 wk over 30-min infusion.
B-cell production blocker: rituximab	*Action:* Binds to B-lymphocyte CD20 surface antigens. Used in refractory RA in patients with inadequate response to TNF antagonist. Given with methotrexate.	Rituximab is given as two 1000-mg doses via IV infusion separated by 2 wk. Given on wk 0 and 2, and then subsequent doses are infused 24 wk later or based on clinical diagnosis (commonly given every 6 mo). Premedicate with acetaminophen, antihistamine, and methylprednisolone 30 min prior to infusion of rituximab. Educate patient about increased risk of infection.
Human IL-1 receptor antagonist: anakinra	*Action:* Blocks IL-1 receptors, decreasing inflammatory and immunologic responses. Used in moderate to severe RA. Can be used alone or with methotrexate or DMARDs other than TNF-blocking agents	Given daily by subcutaneous injection. Educate patient about subcutaneous self-injections given daily. Medication must be refrigerated. Monitor for injection site reactions. Educate patient about increased risk of infection and to withhold medication if fever occurs.
Human IL-6 receptor antagonist: tocilizumab	*Action:* Binds to and inhibits IL-6 receptors, decreasing inflammatory and immunologic responses. Can be used alone or with methotrexate or in combination with other nonbiologic DMARDs	Administered IV every 4 wk. Educate patient about increased risk of infection.
Corticosteroids prednisone, prednisolone, hydrocortisone	*Action:* Anti-inflammatory. Used for shortest duration and at lowest dose possible to minimize adverse effects. Useful for unremitting RA, SLE, polymyalgia rheumatica, myositis, arteritis Fast acting; onset in days Intra-articular injections useful for joints unresponsive to NSAIDs	Assess for toxicity: Cataracts, GI irritation, hyperglycemia, hypertension, fractures, avascular necrosis, hirsutism, psychosis. Joints most amenable to injections include ankles, knees, hips, shoulders, and hands. Repeated injections can cause joint damage. Use caution in patients diagnosed with diabetes, due to effects causing elevation in blood sugar.

CBC, complete blood count; CNS, central nervous system; COX, cyclo-oxygenase; GI, gastrointestinal; IL-1, interleukin 1; IL-6, interleukin 6; IV, intravenous; RA, rheumatoid arthritis; SLE, systemic lupus erythematosus; TNF, tumor necrosis factor.
Adapted from Comerford, K. C., & Durkin, M. T. (2020). *Nursing 2020 drug handbook*. Philadelphia, PA: Wolters Kluwer; Mogul, A., Corsi, K., & McAuliffe, L. (2019). Baricitinic: The second FDA approved JAK inhibitor for the treatment of rheumatoid arthritis. *Annals of Pharmacotherapy, 53*(9), 947–953.

Devices such as braces, splints, and assistive devices for ambulation (e.g., canes, crutches, walkers) ease pain by limiting movement or stress from putting weight on painful joints. Acutely inflamed joints can be rested by applying splints to limit motion. Splints also support the joint to relieve spasm. Canes and crutches can relieve stress from inflamed and painful weight-bearing joints while promoting safe ambulation. Cervical collars may be used to support the weight of the head and limit cervical motion. A metatarsal bar or special pads may be put into the patient's shoes if foot pain or deformity is present. A combination of methods may be required, because different methods often work better at different times.

Exercise and Activity

The ongoing nature of most rheumatic diseases makes it important to maintain and, when possible, improve joint mobility and overall functional status. Appropriate programs of exercise have been shown to decrease pain and improve function (Eliopoulos, 2021). Changes in gait as well as joint limitations commonly require referral for rehabilitation

TABLE 34-3	Exercise to Promote Mobility		
Type of Exercise	**Purpose**	**Recommended Performance**	**Precautions**
Range of motion	Maintain flexibility and joint motion	Active or active/self-assisted at least daily	Reduce the number of repetitions when inflammation is present
Isometric exercise	Improve muscle tone, static endurance, and strength; prepare for dynamic and weight-bearing exercises	Perform at 70% of maximal voluntary contraction daily	Monitor blood pressure; isometric exercises may increase blood pressure and decrease blood flow to muscles
Dynamic exercise	Maintain or increase dynamic strength and endurance; increase muscle power; enhance synovial blood flow; promote strength of bone and cartilage	Start with repetitions against gravity and add progressive resistance; perform 2–3 days per week	May increase biomechanical stress on unstable or misaligned joints
Aerobic exercise	Improve cardiovascular fitness and endurance	Perform 3–5 days per week for 20–30 min of moderate-intensity exercise	Progress slowly as activity tolerance and fitness improve
Pool exercise	Water supports or resists movement; warm water may provide muscle relaxation	Provide buoyant medium for performance of dynamic or aerobic exercise	Heated swimming pool; deep water to minimize joint compression; non-slip footwear for safety and comfort. Receive appropriate education in a program designed for people with arthritis

Adapted from Kapale, P., Vardharajulu, G., & Warude, T. (2017). Effect of free exercise and rheumatoid arthritis. *Indian Journal of Physiotherapy and Occupational Therapy, 11*(3), 62–65.

therapy. An individualized exercise program is crucial to improve movement. Table 34-3 summarizes the exercises appropriate for patients with rheumatic diseases. Physical and occupational therapy programs and interventions are beneficial in improving physical activity and maintaining range of motion. Such interventions may include stretching exercises, muscle conditioning, aerobic exercise, massage, acupuncture, and chiropractic and osteopathic manipulation. Other strategies for decreasing pain include muscle relaxation techniques, imagery, self-hypnosis, and distraction. A mild analgesic agent may be suggested before exercise to improve pain during exercise. A weight reduction program may be recommended to relieve stress on painful joints for patients who are overweight. Any patient who experiences acute or prolonged pain associated with exercise should report the symptoms to their primary provider for evaluation.

The major challenge for the patient and the health care provider is the need to adjust all aspects of treatment according to the activity of the disease. Especially for the patient with an active diffuse connective tissue disease, such as rheumatoid arthritis (RA) or systemic lupus erythematosus (SLE), activity levels may vary from day to day and even within a single day.

Sleep

Short-term use of low-dose antidepressant medications, such as amitriptyline, may be prescribed to reestablish adequate sleep patterns and improve pain management (Comerford & Durkin, 2020). Patients need restful sleep so that they can cope with pain, minimize physical fatigue, and deal with the changes related to having a chronic disease. In patients with acute disease, sleep time is frequently reduced and fragmented by prolonged awakenings. Stiffness, depression, and medications may also compromise the quality of sleep and increase daytime fatigue. A sleep-inducing routine, medication, and comfort measures may help improve the quality of sleep.

Education about sleep hygiene strategies may help promote restorative sleep. These strategies include establishing a set time to sleep and a regular wake-up time, creating a quiet sleep environment with a comfortable room temperature, avoiding factors that interfere with sleep (e.g., the use of alcohol and caffeine), using relaxation exercises, and getting out of bed and engaging in another activity (e.g., reading) if unable to sleep.

Nursing Management

Much of the care of patients with arthritis involves self-management; thus, using a standardized assessment of self-management behaviors will help plan effective on-going care and treatment targets (Oh, Han, Kim, et al., 2018). The Nursing Research Profile in Chart 34-2 describes one such tool. Chart 34-3 details the nursing diagnoses, interventions, and expected outcomes for the patient with a rheumatic disorder.

 ### Gerontologic Considerations

The various rheumatic disease conditions in the older adult pose unique challenges. These challenges relate to disability, cognitive changes, comorbid conditions, and diagnosis. Musculoskeletal problems are the most frequently reported conditions in older adults (Eliopoulos, 2021) and will be seen more frequently by health professionals in the coming years along with associated disability, especially among frail older adults.

Comorbid conditions pose a unique challenge in diagnosing rheumatic disease in older adults because they have the potential to mask or alter presenting symptoms. The frequency, pattern of onset, clinical features, severity, and effects on function of the rheumatic disease in older patients needs to be assessed. One study reported that functional disability was correlated with disease state and thus must be addressed in planning care (Omma, Celik, Bes, et al., 2018). Additional medical conditions may take precedence over the rheumatic

Chart 34-2   NURSING RESEARCH PROFILE
Assessing Self-Management in Patients with Arthritis

Oh, H. S., Han, S. Y., Kim, S. H., et al. (2018). Development and validity testing of an arthritis self-management assessment tool. *Orthopaedic Nursing, 37*(1), 24–35.

Purpose

Self-management is central to arthritis treatment; yet, no instrument existed to measure arthritis self-management ability. Therefore, the purpose of this research was to develop and test the reliability and validity of a comprehensive tool to assess self-management in patients with arthritis.

Design

A nonexperimental correlational design was used for this study. Items for inclusion on the Arthritis Self-Management Assessment Tool (ASMAT) were generated using a chronic illness management model. Content validity of the initial 42 items were reviewed by a panel of experts and decreased to 32 items. The tool was then tested with 150 patients with arthritis in an outpatient setting. Factor analysis was used to test construct validity.

Findings

The mean age of participants was 52 years and approximately 60% were male. There were 32 items generated and tested in the final version of the ASMAT. The 32 items were validated and the scale was found to have 3 subscales: that of medical management tasks (10 items), behavioral management tasks (13 items), and psycho-emotional management tasks (9 items). Confirmatory factor analysis showed construct validity for the 32 item tool. Cronbach α levels showed the overall toll and the 3 subscales to be reliable.

Nursing Implications

Nurses are in a key position to assist patients with arthritis to self-manage their care. Performing an ASMAT helps evaluate the patient's self-management abilities and the effectiveness of self-management interventions. Early identification of barriers to adoption of self-management strategies can lead to improved symptom management, independence, and improved quality of life.

---

disease, causing it to become a secondary diagnosis and concern. Decreased vision and altered balance, often present in older adults, may be problematic if rheumatic disease in the lower extremities affects locomotion. The combination of decreased hearing and visual acuity, memory loss, and depression contributes to failure to follow the treatment regimen in older adult patients as well (Eliopoulos, 2021). Special techniques for promoting patient safety, self-management,

and strategies such as memory aids for medications may be necessary.

Behavioral clues such as gait patterns, guarding, and joint flexion may aid the nurse in assessing the patient's pain when cognitive impairment is present. Older adults, especially men, may also neglect to communicate their pain unless elicited by the provider. Pain, in general, in this population that is not *(text continued on page 1078)*

Chart 34-3   PLAN OF NURSING CARE
Care of the Patient with a Rheumatic Disorder

NURSING DIAGNOSIS: Acute and chronic pain associated with inflammation and increased disease activity, tissue damage, fatigue, or lowered tolerance level

GOAL: Improvement in comfort level; incorporation of pain management techniques into daily life

Nursing Interventions	Rationale	Expected Outcomes
1. Provide variety of comfort measures: a. Application of heat or cold b. Massage, position changes, rest c. Foam mattress, supportive pillow, splints d. Relaxation techniques, diversional activities	1. Pain may respond to nonpharmacologic interventions, such as exercise, relaxation, and thermal modalities.	• Identifies factors that exacerbate or influence pain response • Identifies and uses pain management strategies • Verbalizes decrease in pain • Reports signs and symptoms of side effects in timely manner to prevent additional problems • Verbalizes that pain is characteristic of rheumatic disease • Establishes realistic pain relief goals • Identifies changes in quality or intensity of pain
2. Administer anti-inflammatory, analgesic, and slow-acting antirheumatic medications as prescribed.	2. Pain of rheumatic disease responds to monotherapy or combination medication regimens.	
3. Individualize medication schedule to meet patient's need for pain management.	3. Previous pain experiences and management strategies may be different from those needed for persistent pain.	
4. Encourage verbalization of feelings about pain and chronicity of disease.	4. Verbalization promotes coping.	
5. Assess for subjective changes in pain.	5. The impact of pain on an individual's life often leads to misconceptions about pain and pain management techniques. The individual's description of pain is a more reliable indicator than objective measurements such as change in vital signs, body movement, and facial expression.	

(continued on page 1076)

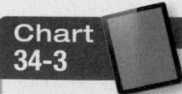

Chart 34-3 **PLAN OF NURSING CARE** (continued)
Care of the Patient with a Rheumatic Disorder

NURSING DIAGNOSIS: Fatigue associated with increased disease activity, pain, inadequate sleep/rest, deconditioning, inadequate nutrition, emotional stress, anxiety, and depressive symptoms
GOAL: Incorporates as part of daily activities strategies necessary to modify fatigue

Nursing Interventions	Rationale	Expected Outcomes

1. Provide education about fatigue.
 	
  a. Describe relationship of disease activity to fatigue.
  b. Describe comfort measures while providing them.
  c. Develop and encourage a sleep routine (warm bath and relaxation techniques that promote sleep).
  d. Explain importance of rest for relieving systematic, articular, and emotional stress.
  e. Explain how to use energy conservation techniques (pacing, delegating, setting priorities).
  f. Identify physical and emotional factors that can cause fatigue.
 	
2. Facilitate development of appropriate activity/rest schedule.
3. Encourage adherence to the treatment program.
4. Refer to and encourage a conditioning program.
 	
5. Encourage adequate nutrition, including source of iron from food and supplements.
	1. The patient's understanding of fatigue will affect their actions.
	  a. The amount of fatigue is directly related to the activity of the disease.
	  b. Relief of discomfort can relieve fatigue.
	
	  c. Effective bedtime routine promotes restorative sleep.
	
	  d. Different kinds of rest are needed to relieve fatigue and are based on patient's need and response.
	  e. A variety of measures can be used to conserve energy.
	
	  f. Awareness of the various causes of fatigue provides the basis for measures to modify the fatigue.
	
	2. Alternating rest and activity conserves energy while allowing most productivity.
	3. Overall control of disease activity can decrease the amount of fatigue.
	4. Deconditioning resulting from lack of mobility, understanding, and disease activity contributes to fatigue.
	5. A nutritious diet can help counteract fatigue.
		• Self-evaluates and monitors fatigue pattern
		• Verbalizes the relationship of fatigue to disease activity
		• Uses comfort measures as appropriate
		• Practices effective sleep hygiene and routine
		• Makes use of various assistive devices (splints, canes) and strategies (bed rest, relaxation techniques) to ease different kinds of fatigue
		• Incorporates time management strategies in daily activities
		• Uses appropriate measures to prevent physical and emotional fatigue
		• Has an established plan to ensure well-paced, therapeutic activity schedule
		• Adheres to therapeutic program
		• Follows a planned conditioning program
		• Consumes a nutritious diet consisting of the five major groups and recommended daily allowance of vitamins and minerals

NURSING DIAGNOSIS: Impaired mobility associated with decreased range of motion, muscle weakness, pain on movement, limited endurance, lack of or improper use of ambulatory devices
GOAL: Attains and maintains optimal functional mobility

Nursing Interventions	Rationale	Expected Outcomes

1. Encourage verbalization regarding limitations in mobility.
 	
2. Assess need for occupational or physical therapy consultation.
  a. Emphasize range of motion of affected joints.
  b. Promote the use of assistive ambulatory devices.
  c. Explain the use of safe footwear.
  d. Use individual appropriate positioning/posture.
3. Assist to identify environmental barriers.
 	
4. Encourage independence in mobility and assist as needed.
  a. Allow ample time for activity.
  b. Provide rest period after activity.
  c. Reinforce principles of pacing and work simplification.
5. Initiate referral to community health agency.
	1. Mobility is not necessarily related to deformity. Pain, stiffness, and fatigue may temporarily limit mobility. The degree of mobility is not synonymous with the degree of independence. Decreased mobility may influence a person's self-concept and lead to social isolation.
	2. Therapeutic exercises, proper footwear, and assistive equipment may improve mobility. Correct posture and positioning are necessary for maintaining optimal mobility.
	
	3. Furniture and architectural adaptations may enhance mobility.
	4. Changes in mobility may lead to a decrease in personal safety.
	
	5. The degree of mobility may be slow to improve or may not improve with intervention.
		• Identifies factors that interfere with mobility
		• Describes and uses measures to prevent loss of motion
		• Identifies environmental (home, school, work, community) barriers to optimal mobility
		• Uses appropriate techniques, assistive equipment, or both to aid mobility
		• Identifies community resources available to assist in managing decreased mobility

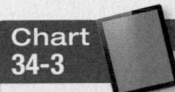

Chart 34-3

PLAN OF NURSING CARE (continued)

Care of the Patient with a Rheumatic Disorder

NURSING DIAGNOSIS: Able to perform self care associated with contractures, fatigue, or loss of motion
GOAL: Performs self-care activities independently or with the use of resources

Nursing Interventions	Rationale	Expected Outcomes
1. Assist patient to identify self-care deficits and factors that interfere with ability to perform self-care activities. 2. Develop a plan based on the patient's perceptions and priorities on how to establish and achieve goals to meet self-care needs, incorporating energy conservation, and work simplification concepts. a. Provide appropriate assistive devices. b. Reinforce correct and safe use of assistive devices. c. Allow patient to control timing of self-care activities. d. Explore with the patient different ways to perform difficult tasks or ways to enlist the help of someone else. 3. Consult with community health care agencies when individuals have attained a maximum level of self-care yet still have some deficits, especially regarding safety.	1. The ability to perform self-care activities is influenced by the disease activity and the accompanying pain, stiffness, fatigue, muscle weakness, loss of motion, and depression. 2. Assistive devices may enhance self-care abilities. Effective planning for changes must include the patient, who must accept and adopt the plan. 3. Individuals differ in ability and willingness to perform self-care activities. Changes in ability to care for self may lead to a decrease in personal safety.	• Identifies factors that interfere with the ability to perform self-care activities • Identifies alternative methods for meeting self-care needs • Uses alternative methods for meeting self-care needs • Identifies and uses other health care resources for meeting self-care needs

NURSING DIAGNOSIS: Disturbed body image associated with physical and psychological changes and dependency imposed by chronic illness
GOAL: Adapts to physical and psychological changes imposed by the rheumatic disease

Nursing Interventions	Rationale	Expected Outcomes
1. Help patient identify elements of control over disease symptoms and treatment. 2. Encourage patient's verbalization of feelings, perceptions, and fears. a. Help to assess present situation and identify problems.	1. The individual's self-concept may be altered by the disease or its treatment. 2. The individual's coping strategies reflect the strength of their self-concept.	• Verbalizes an awareness that changes taking place in self-concept are normal responses to rheumatic disease and other chronic illnesses • Identifies strategies to cope with altered self-concept

NURSING DIAGNOSIS: Difficulty coping associated with actual or perceived lifestyle or role changes
GOAL: Use of effective coping behaviors for dealing with actual or perceived limitations and role changes

Nursing Interventions	Rationale	Expected Outcomes
1. Identify areas of life affected by disease. Answer questions and dispel possible myths. a. Assist to identify past coping mechanisms. b. Assist to identify effective coping mechanisms. 2. Develop plan for managing symptoms and enlisting support of family and friends to promote daily function.	1. The effects of disease may be more or less manageable once identified and explored reasonably. 2. By taking action and involving others appropriately, patient develops or draws on coping skills and community support.	• Names functions and roles affected and not affected by disease process • Describes therapeutic regimen and states actions to take to improve, change, or accept a particular situation, function, or role

COLLABORATIVE PROBLEMS: Complications secondary to effects of medications
GOAL: Absence or resolution of complications

Nursing Interventions	Rationale	Expected Outcomes
1. Perform periodic clinical assessment and laboratory evaluation. 2. Provide education about correct self-administration, potential side effects, and importance of monitoring. 3. Counsel regarding methods to reduce side effects and manage symptoms. 4. Administer medications in modified doses as prescribed if complications occur.	1. Skillful assessment helps detect early symptoms of side effects of medications. 2. The patient needs accurate information about medications and potential side effects to avoid or manage them. 3. Appropriate identification and early intervention may minimize complications. 4. Modifications may help minimize side effects or other complications.	• Adheres to monitoring procedures and experiences minimal side effects • Takes medication as prescribed and lists potential side effects • Identifies strategies to reduce or manage side effects • Reports that side effects or complications have subsided

treated or undertreated may impact the quality of life for these patients, which can exacerbate all other medical conditions.

Pharmacologic therapy (including analgesic agents), exercise, postural assistance, modification of activities of daily living, and psychological support are useful components of a self-management program for the older adult (Oh et al., 2018).

Identifying the effects of the rheumatic disease on the patient's lifestyle, independence, and psychological status is important and can improve the quality of life for older adults. Depressed mood is routinely found in those suffering from chronic joint disease. The body image and self-esteem of the older adult with rheumatic disease, combined with underlying depression, may interfere with the use of assistive devices such as canes. The use of adaptive equipment such as long-handled reachers or tongs may be viewed by the older adult as evidence of aging rather than as a means of increasing independence.

Because most rheumatic diseases involve pain, especially with joints, some older adults may consider their symptoms as inevitable consequences of aging. In fact, many older adults expect and accept the immobility and self-care problems related to the rheumatic diseases and do not seek help, thinking that nothing can be done.

The older adult usually has a lifelong pattern of dealing with the stresses of daily life. Depending on the success of that pattern, the older adult can often maintain a positive attitude and self-esteem when faced with a rheumatic disease, especially if support is available. Previous stress management strategies are assessed. If these strategies have been effective, the patient is encouraged and supported in their use. If they were ineffective, the nurse assists the patient in identifying alternative strategies, encourages the use of new strategies, and assesses their effectiveness.

Pharmacologic treatment of rheumatic disease in older patients is more difficult than in younger patients. If therapeutic medications have an effect on the senses (hearing, cognition), this effect is intensified in the older adult. The cumulative effect of medications, in general, is accentuated because of the physiologic changes of aging. For example, decreased renal function in the older adult alters the metabolism of certain medications, such as NSAIDs. Older adults are more prone to side effects associated with the use of multiple-drug therapy.

Partly because of the more frequent contact of older adults with health care providers for a variety of health issues, overtreatment or inappropriate treatment is possible. Complaints of pain may be met with a prescription for analgesic agents rather than instructions for rest, the use of an assistive device, and local comfort measures such as heat or cold. Acetaminophen may be appropriate and worth trying before other medications that pose a greater chance of side effects. NSAIDs can be used; however, long-term use of NSAIDs can increase the risks of peptic ulcers, hemorrhage, and cardiovascular toxicity (Comerford & Durkin, 2020).

Intra-articular corticosteroid injections, with their usually rapid relief of symptoms, may be requested by the patient who is unaware of the consequences of too-frequent use of this treatment. In addition, exercise programs may not be instituted or may be ineffective because the patient expects results to occur quickly or fails to appreciate the effectiveness of a program of exercise. In fact, strength training is encouraged in the older adult with chronic diseases.

Diffuse Connective Tissue Diseases

Diffuse connective tissue disease refers to a group of systemic disorders that are chronic in nature and are characterized by diffuse inflammation and degeneration in the connective tissues. These disorders share similar clinical features and may affect some of the same organs. The characteristic clinical course is one of exacerbations and remissions. Although diffuse connective tissue diseases have unknown causes, they are thought to be the result of immunologic abnormalities. They include RA, SLE, Sjögren's syndrome, scleroderma, polymyositis, polymyalgia rheumatica (PMR), and giant cell arteritis (GCA).

Rheumatoid Arthritis

Rheumatoid arthritis is an autoimmune disease of unknown origin that affects 1% to 2% of the population worldwide, with females having a three times greater incidence than males. It may occur at any age but the onset commonly occurs between the third and sixth decade of life. The incidence of RA increases after the sixth decade of life (Norris, 2019). RA that occurs after the age of 65 is referred to as elderly onset RA (Norris, 2019). Additional risks that have been identified include family history, environmental influences such as diet or geographic location, nulliparity, as well as the modifiable factors of smoking and obesity (Mogul, Corsi, & McAuliffe, 2019).

Pathophysiology

The exact mechanism of action for the etiology of RA is unknown. Evidence points to a genetic predisposition and the development of immunologically mediated joint inflammation (Eliopoulos, 2021; Norris, 2019). An autoimmune reaction (see Fig. 34-1) occurs in the synovial tissue. RA synovium breaks down collagen, causing edema, proliferation of the synovial membrane, and ultimately pannus formation. Pannus destroys cartilage and erodes the bone. The consequence is the loss of articular surfaces and joint motion. Muscle fibers undergo degenerative changes. Tendon and ligament elasticity and contractile power are lost.

The RA inflammatory process has also been implicated in other disease processes (i.e., arteriosclerosis). It is hypothesized that the RA disease process somehow interferes with the production of high-density lipoprotein cholesterol, which is the form of cholesterol responsible for decreasing cellular lipids and, therefore, is considered antiatherosclerotic.

The nervous system is also affected by the RA inflammatory process. The synovial inflammation can compress the adjacent nerve, causing neuropathies and paresthesias. Axonal degeneration and neuronal demyelination are also possible due to the infiltration of polymorphonuclear leukocytes, eosinophils, and mononuclear cells, causing necrotizing or occlusive vasculitis (Norris, 2019).

Clinical Manifestations

The American College of Rheumatology and the European League Against Rheumatism have collaborated and established criteria for classifying RA. These criteria are based on a point system where a total score of 6 or greater is required for the diagnosis of RA. The scoring system is based on joint involvement (number of joints affected), serology (low positive or high positive rheumatoid factor [RF] or anti-citrullinated peptide antibody [ACPA]), abnormal results of the acute phase reactants (erythrocyte sedimentation rate [ESR] or C-reactive protein [CRP]), and duration of symptoms greater than 6 weeks. Patients diagnosed with RA who are excluded from these diagnostic criteria include: (1) patients who have one joint with synovitis that is not related to any other clinical disease and who also score at least 6 to 10 points on the scale, and (2) patients diagnosed with bony erosions on x-ray (Aletaha, Neogi, Silman, et al., 2010; Molano-Gonzalez, Olivares-Matinez, Anaya, et al., 2019).

The initial clinical manifestations of RA include symmetric joint pain and morning joint stiffness lasting longer than 1 hour. Over the course of the disease, clinical manifestations of RA vary, usually reflecting the stage and severity of the disease. Symmetric joint pain, swelling, warmth, erythema, and lack of function are classic symptoms. Palpation of the joints reveals spongy or boggy tissue. Often, fluid can be aspirated from the inflamed joint. Characteristically, the pattern of joint involvement begins in the small joints of the hands, wrists, and feet (Omma et al., 2018). As the disease progresses, the knees, shoulders, hips, elbows, ankles, cervical spine, and temporomandibular joints may be affected. The onset of symptoms is usually acute. Symptoms are usually bilateral and symmetric.

In the early stages of disease, even before the presentation of bony changes, limitation in function can occur when there is active inflammation in the joints. Joints that are hot, swollen, and painful are not easily moved. The patient tends to guard or protect these joints by immobilizing them. Immobilization for extended periods can lead to contractures, creating soft tissue deformity.

Deformities of the hands (e.g., ulnar deviation and swan neck deformity) and feet are common in RA (see Chapter 35, Fig. 35-6). The deformity may be caused by misalignment resulting from swelling, progressive joint destruction, or the subluxation (partial dislocation) that occurs when one bone slips over another and eliminates the joint space. Deformities of RA differ from those seen with osteoarthritis (OA), such as Heberden's and Bouchard's nodes (see Chapter 36).

RA is a systemic disease with multiple extra-articular features. Most common are fever, weight loss, fatigue, anemia, lymph node enlargement, and Raynaud's phenomenon (cold- and stress-induced vasospasm causing episodes of digital blanching or cyanosis). Rheumatoid nodules are common in patients with more advanced RA. These nodules are usually nontender and movable in the subcutaneous tissue. They usually appear over bony prominences such as the elbow, are varied in size, and can disappear spontaneously or progress to ulceration (Weber & Kelley, 2019; Young, 2019). Nodules occur only in people who have rheumatoid factor. Other extra-articular features include arteritis, neuropathy, pericarditis, splenomegaly, and Sjögren's syndrome (dry eyes and dry mucous membranes).

Assessment and Diagnostic Findings

Several assessment findings are associated with RA: rheumatoid nodules, joint inflammation detected on palpation, and certain laboratory findings. The history and physical examination focus on manifestations, such as bilateral and symmetric stiffness, tenderness, swelling, and temperature changes in the joints (Weber & Kelley, 2019). The patient is also assessed for extra-articular changes; these often include weight loss, sensory changes, lymph node enlargement, and fatigue. Symptoms and examination findings are often recorded using a disease activity score, a variety of which are in use, to evaluate disease activity, help guide treatment decisions, and monitor treatment efficacy (Mahmood, van Tuyl, Schoonmade, et al., 2019).

Rheumatoid factor is present in many patients with RA, but its presence alone is not diagnostic of RA, and its absence does not rule out the diagnosis. Antibodies to cyclic citrullinated peptide (anti-CCP) have a specificity of approximately 95% at detecting RA (Norris, 2019). The ESR and CRP tend to be significantly elevated in the acute phases of RA and are therefore useful in monitoring active disease and disease progression. The complete blood count (CBC) should be assessed to establish a baseline count especially prior to starting medications (Fischbach & Fischbach, 2018). Patients may exhibit anemia, and platelets may be elevated due to the inflammatory process. A tuberculin (TB) skin test should be done prior to the initiation of certain medications to rule out tuberculosis. In the event the patient has latent TB and has never been treated, the infection can be reactivated. The patient should also be assessed for hepatitis B and hepatitis C, which could impact treatment strategies if positive. If the client tests positive for hepatitis, the infection should be treated prior to starting medication. Liver and kidney monitoring are recommended for most DMARD therapy because it can cause elevation of the liver enzymes and can also affect kidney function.

X-ray, ultrasound, or both of the hands, wrists, and feet can be useful in establishing a baseline for joint evaluation, and assessing the joints for erosions and synovitis. Joint damage may occur within the first 6 to 12 months of diagnosis and should be followed as indicated. Plain x-ray is the most common radiographic study used to track disease progression as it is inexpensive, reliable, and reproducible (Mahmood et al., 2019). MRI can also be useful to detect small erosions that may not be visible on x-ray or ultrasound.

Medical Management

The goal of treatment at all phases of the RA disease process is to decrease joint pain and swelling, achieve clinical remission, decrease the likelihood of joint deformity, and minimize disability. Initial treatment delays have been implicated in greater long-term joint deformity. Aggressive and early treatment regimens are warranted. The use of a targeted pharmacologic treatment strategy is recommended to decrease RA disease activity (Singh et al., 2016).

Early Rheumatoid Arthritis

Once the diagnosis of RA is made, treatment should begin with either a nonbiologic or biologic DMARD. The goal of using DMARD therapy is preventing inflammation and joint damage.

Recommended treatment guidelines include beginning with the nonbiologic DMARDs (methotrexate is the preferred agent but leflunomide, sulfasalazine, or hydroxy-chloroquine are also used) biologics, or tofacitinibic within 3 months of disease onset. Care should be used with each of these medications by performing routine blood testing for liver and kidney function, along with monitoring the CBC for anemia. Dosage may need to be modified for patients with renal impairment (Comerford & Durkin, 2020).

Another treatment approach for RA is the use of biologic DMARDs. These agents have been specifically engineered to target the most prominent proinflammatory mediators in RA—TNF-α, B cells, T cells, IL-1, and IL-6 (see Table 34-2). Biologic DMARDs are the first targeted therapy for RA. Clinical evidence suggests that biologic DMARDs work more quickly and show a greater delay in radiologic disease progression when compared to nonbiologic DMARDs. The biologic DMARDs are more expensive and have fewer years of usage with the RA population. Therefore, they tend to be reserved for patients with persistent moderate to severe RA who have not responded adequately to synthetic DMARDs (Singh et al., 2016).

After initiating treatment with a DMARD, patients generally report a beneficial effect within 6 weeks and tolerate the medication relatively well. However, some patients may take longer to see improvement. Corticosteroids are recommended as a "bridge" in the early treatment but are not recommended for long-term therapy due to side effects (Singh et al., 2016).

A newer class of drugs, the Janus Kinase (JAK) inhibitors, bind to the active JAK enzyme sites, inhibiting autophosphorylation and thus inhibiting cytokine production and decreasing the immune response (Mogul et al., 2019). JAK inhibitors are used in combination with methotrexate or other nonbiologic DMARDs. They may also be used as monotherapy (Mogul et al., 2019; Singh et al., 2016).

NSAIDs and specifically the cyclo-oxygenase 2 (COX-2) enzyme blockers are used for pain and inflammation relief. NSAIDs, such as ibuprofen and naproxen, are commonly prescribed because of their low cost and analgesic properties. They must be used with caution, however, in long-term chronic diseases because of the possibility of gastric ulcers. Several COX-2 enzyme blockers have been approved for treatment of RA. Cyclo-oxygenase is an enzyme that is involved in the inflammatory process. COX-2 medications block the enzyme involved in inflammation (COX-2) while leaving intact the enzyme involved in protecting the stomach lining (COX-1). As a result, COX-2 enzyme blockers are less likely to cause gastric irritation and ulceration than other NSAIDs; however, they are associated with increased risk of cardiovascular disease and must be used with caution (Comerford & Durkin, 2020). The nurse should be aware that NSAIDs do not prevent erosions or alter disease progression and, consequently, are medications useful only for symptom relief (Singh et al., 2016).

Additional analgesia may be prescribed for periods of extreme pain. Opioid analgesic agents are avoided because of the potential for continuing need for pain relief. Nonpharmacologic pain management techniques (e.g., relaxation techniques, heat and cold applications) are taught.

Established Rheumatoid Arthritis

In patients with established RA, a formal program with occupational and physical therapy is prescribed to educate the patient about principles of pacing activities, work simplification, range of motion, and muscle-strengthening exercises. The patient is encouraged to participate actively in the management program. The medication program is reevaluated periodically, and appropriate changes are made if disease progression is occurring despite pharmacologic treatment. Additional agents may be added to enhance the disease-modifying effect of methotrexate. Combination therapy using one nonbiologic DMARD and one biologic DMARD is common (Singh et al., 2016).

For more established RA, reconstructive surgery and corticosteroids are often used. Reconstructive surgery is indicated when pain cannot be relieved by conservative measures and the threat of loss of independence is eminent. Surgical procedures include synovectomy (excision of the synovial membrane), tenorrhaphy (suturing of a tendon), arthrodesis (surgical fusion of the joint), surgical repair, and replacement of the joint. Surgery is not performed during exacerbations.

Systemic corticosteroids are used when the patient has unremitting inflammation and pain or needs a "bridging" medication while waiting for the slower DMARDs (e.g., methotrexate) to begin taking effect. Low-dose corticosteroid therapy is prescribed for the shortest time necessary to minimize side effects (Singh et al., 2016). Single large joints that are severely inflamed and fail to respond promptly to the measures outlined previously may be treated by local injection of a corticosteroid.

Topical analgesic agents such as capsaicin and methylsalicylate are often prescribed. Topical diclofenac sodium gel may help with joint pain in the hands and knees (Comerford & Durkin, 2020).

For most patients with RA, the emotional and possible financial burden of the disease can lead to depressive symptoms and sleep deprivation. The patient may require the short-term use of low-dose antidepressant medications, such as amitriptyline, paroxetine, or sertraline, to reestablish an adequate sleep pattern and manage depressive symptoms. Patients may benefit from referrals for talk therapy or group support.

Obesity Considerations

The prevalence of obesity is increasing in the general population and in patients with RA. One large study reported that the prevalence of obesity, diagnosed with a body mass index (BMI) of greater than or equal to 30 kg/m^2, was approximately 20% at diagnosis and increased each year (Nikiphorou, Norton, Young, et al., 2018). Furthermore, the presence of obesity adversely affected disease progression, function, and quality of life in patients with RA followed for 10 to 25 years (Nikiphorou et al., 2018). Management of obesity in the patient with RA is essential.

Certain medications (i.e., oral corticosteroids) used in RA treatment stimulate the appetite and, when combined with decreased activity, may lead to weight gain. In fact, one study reported that approximately half the increase in BMI within the first year of diagnosis with RA could be attributed to steroid use (Nikiphorou et al., 2018).

A dietician can counsel the patient about better food choices. Food selection should include the five major groups (grains, vegetables, fruits, dairy, and protein), with emphasis on foods high in vitamins, protein, and iron for tissue building and repair. Patients who are overweight or have obesity need to be counseled about eating a healthy, calorie-restricted diet.

Nursing Management

Nursing care of the patient with RA follows the basic plan of care presented earlier (see Chart 34-3). The most common issues for the patient with RA include pain, sleep disturbance, fatigue, altered mood, and limited mobility. The patient with newly diagnosed RA needs information about the disease to make daily self-management decisions and cope with having a chronic disease. Consultation with a dietician for assessment and assistance with appropriate food choices may be helpful.

Monitoring and Managing Potential Complications

Patients commonly have comorbid conditions such as cardiovascular disease that can lead to complications. It has been estimated that the primary cause of death for up to 40% of patients diagnosed with RA is cardiovascular disease. The cause of cardiovascular disease in these patients is thought to be due to elevated lipid values, chronic inflammation, dysfunction of the endothelium, and/or abnormal homocysteine levels (Norris, 2019).

Medications used for treating RA may cause serious and adverse effects. The primary provider bases the prescribed medication regimen on clinical findings and past medical history, and then, with the help of the nurse, monitors for side effects using periodic clinical assessments and laboratory testing. The nurse, who can be available for consultation between visits with the primary provider, works to help the patient recognize and deal with these side effects (see Table 34-2). Medication may need to be stopped or the dose reduced. If the patient experiences an increase in symptoms while the complication is being resolved or a new medication is being initiated, the nurse's counseling regarding symptom management may relieve potential anxiety and distress.

Promoting Home, Community-Based, and Transitional Care

 Educating Patients About Self-Care

Patient education is an essential aspect in nursing care of the patient with RA to enable the patient to maintain as much independence as possible, to take medications accurately and safely, and to use adaptive devices correctly (Oh et al., 2018). Patient education focuses on self-management related to the disorder, the therapeutic regimen prescribed to treat it, and the potential side effects of medications. Patients undergoing surgery need education as well. The nurse works with the patient and family on strategies to maintain independence, function, and safety in the home (see Chart 34-4).

The patient and family are encouraged to verbalize their concerns and ask questions. Because RA commonly affects young women, major concerns may be related to the effects of the disease on childbearing potential, caring for family, or work responsibilities. The patient with a chronic illness may seek a "cure" or have questions about alternative therapies. Research indicates that acupuncture is safe and may be beneficial for patients with RA (Chou & Chu, 2018). There is not enough evidence of the effectiveness of other complementary, alternative, and integrative health therapies, and more rigorous research is needed (Chou & Chu, 2018; Katz-Talmor, Katz, Porta-Katz, et al., 2018).

The nurse educates patients using topical analgesic agents to apply sparingly, avoid areas of open skin, and avoid contact with eyes and mucous membranes. Patients should also wash their hands carefully after application and assess for local skin irritation. Pain, fatigue, and depressive symptoms can interfere with the patient's ability to learn and should be addressed before the education is initiated. Various educational strategies may then be used, depending on the patient's previous knowledge base, interest level, degree of comfort, social or cultural influences, and readiness to learn. The nurse educates the patient about basic disease management and necessary adaptations in lifestyle. Some types of aerobic exercise and

---

Chart 34-4 HOME CARE CHECKLIST

The Patient with Rheumatoid Arthritis

At the completion of education, the patient and/or caregiver will be able to:

State the impact of rheumatoid arthritis on physiologic functioning, ADLs, IADLs, roles, relationships, and spirituality.

- State changes in lifestyle (e.g., diet, activity, rest) necessary to maintain health.
- State the name, dose, side effects, frequency, and schedule for all medications.
- Demonstrate accurate and safe self-administration of medications.
- Describe and demonstrate the use of pain management techniques.
- Demonstrate ability to perform ADLs independently or with assistive devices/adaptive equipment.
- Verbalize ways to cope with stress successfully, plans for regular, safe exercise, and rationale for obtaining adequate rest. Demonstrate a relaxation technique.

- Verbalize a dietary plan that includes maintaining or losing weight while maximizing vitamins, protein, and iron for tissue building and repair
- State how to reach primary provider with questions or complications
- State time and date of follow-up appointments, testing
- Identify the need for health promotion, disease prevention, and screening activities
- Identify community resources for peer and caregiver/family information and support:
  - Identify sources of support (e.g., friends, relatives, faith community)
  - Identify the contact details for support services for patients and their caregivers/families

ADLs, activities of daily living; IADLs, instrumental activities of daily living.

strength training should be discussed (Kapale et al., 2017). Because suppression of inflammation and autoimmune responses require the use of anti-inflammatory, disease-modifying antirheumatic, and immunosuppressive agents, the patient is taught about prescribed medications, including type, dosage, rationale, potential side effects, self-administration, and required monitoring procedures. If hospitalized, the patient is encouraged to practice new self-management skills with support from caregivers and significant others. The nurse then reinforces disease management skills during each patient contact. Barriers are assessed, and measures are taken to promote adherence to medications and the treatment program.

Continuing and Transitional Care

Depending on the severity of the disease and the patient's resources and supports, referral for home care may be warranted. For example, the patient who is an older adult or frail, has RA that limits function significantly, and lives alone may need referral for home care.

The impact of RA on everyday life is not always evident when the patient is seen in the hospital or in an ambulatory care setting. The increased frequency with which nurses see patients in the home provides opportunities for recognizing problems and implementing interventions aimed at improving the quality of life of patients with RA.

During home visits, the nurse has the opportunity to assess the home environment and its adequacy for patient safety and management of the disorder. Adherence to the treatment program can be more easily monitored in the home setting, where physical and social barriers to adherence are more readily identified. For example, a patient who also has diabetes and requires insulin may be unable to fill the syringe accurately or unable to administer the insulin because of impaired joint mobility. Appropriate adaptive equipment needed for increased independence is often identified more readily when the nurse sees how the patient functions in the home. Any barriers to adherence are identified, and appropriate referrals are made.

For patients at risk for impaired skin integrity, the home health nurse can closely monitor skin status and also educate, provide, or supervise the patient and family in preventive skin care measures. The nurse also assesses the patient's need for assistance in the home and supervises home health aides, who may meet many of the needs of the patient with RA. Referrals to physical and occupational therapists may be made as problems are identified and limitations increase. A home health nurse may visit the home to make sure that the patient can function as independently as possible despite mobility problems and can safely manage treatments, including pharmacotherapy. The patient and family should be informed about support services such as Meals on Wheels and local Arthritis Foundation chapters.

Because many of the medications used to suppress inflammation are injectable, the nurse may administer the medication to the patient or educate about self-injection. These frequent contacts allow the nurse to reinforce other disease management techniques.

The nurse also assesses the patient's physical and psychological status, adequacy of symptom management, and adherence to the management plan. Patients should know which type of rheumatic disease they have, not just that they have "arthritis" or "arthritis of the knee." The importance of attending follow-up appointments is emphasized to the patient and family, and they should be reminded about the importance of participating in other health promotion activities and health screening.

Systemic Lupus Erythematosus

SLE is an inflammatory, autoimmune disorder that affects nearly every organ in the body. The overall incidence of SLE is estimated to be 1.8 to 7.6 per 100,000 people (Centers for Disease Control and Prevention [CDC], 2018). It occurs 4 to 12 times more frequently in women than in men and occurs more often in African Americans, Hispanics/Latino Americans, Asians, and American Indians/Alaska Natives than among White Americans (CDC, 2018). In addition to SLE, other forms of adult lupus exist, including subacute cutaneous or discoid lupus erythematous, and drug-induced lupus (Aringer, Costenbader, Daikh, et al., 2019).

Pathophysiology

While the exact cause is not known, SLE starts with the body's immune system inaccurately recognizing one or more components of the cell's nucleus as foreign, seeing it as an antigen. The immune system starts to develop antibodies to the nuclear antigen. In particular, B cells begin to overproduce antibodies with the help of multiple cytokines such as B-lymphocyte stimulator (BLyS), which is overexpressed in SLE. The antibodies and antigens form antigen–antibody complexes and have the propensity to get trapped in the capillaries of visceral structures. The antibodies also act to destroy host cells. It is thought that those two mechanisms are responsible for the majority of the clinical manifestations of this disease process. The immunoregulatory disturbance is thought to be brought about by some combination of four distinct factors: genetic, immunologic, hormonal, and environmental (Norris, 2019).

Research into the genetic origins of SLE has thus far revealed that multiple genes are likely implicated in the development of SLE (Norris, 2019). The large majority of SLE cases, however, remain sporadic and unrelated to family medical history.

Given the high number of women with SLE compared with men, it is hypothesized that female sex hormones (estrogen) play a role in the predisposition to SLE. Estrogen may contribute to the body's response of overreacting to the body's own tissues.

Although genetics and hormones likely play a role in the predisposition of SLE, it is hypothesized that exogenous or environmental triggers are also implicated in the onset of the disease process. These triggers may include cigarette smoke, ultraviolet rays, exposure from sunlight and fluorescent light bulbs, medications (hydralazine, minocyline, or procainamide), viral infections, emotional stress, stress on the body (e.g., surgery, pregnancy), and silica dust exposure in the occupational setting (Norris, 2019).

Clinical Manifestations

SLE is an autoimmune, systemic disease that can affect any body system (Fig. 34-2). The disease process involves chronic

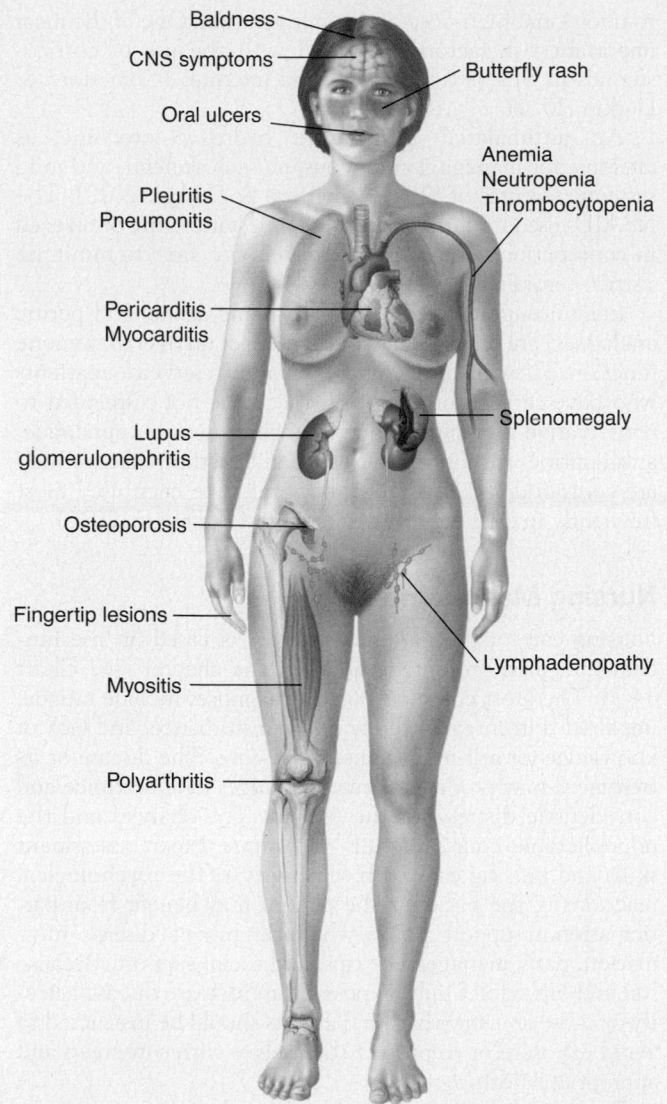

Baldness
CNS symptoms
Butterfly rash
Oral ulcers
Anemia
Neutropenia
Thrombocytopenia
Pleuritis
Pneumonitis
Pericarditis
Myocarditis
Splenomegaly
Lupus
glomerulonephritis
Osteoporosis
Fingertip lesions
Lymphadenopathy
Myositis
Polyarthritis

Figure 34-2 • Clinical manifestations of SLE. Reprinted with permission from Norris, T. L. (2019). *Porth's pathophysiology: Concepts of altered health states* (10th ed., Fig. 50.5). Philadelphia, PA: Wolters Kluwer.

states where symptoms are minimal or absent and acute flares where symptoms and lab results are elevated. Symptoms most often include fever, fatigue, skin rashes, as well as joint pain and swelling (Aringer et al., 2019; CDC, 2018). The mucocutaneous, musculoskeletal, renal, nervous, cardiovascular, and respiratory systems are most commonly involved. Less commonly affected are the gastrointestinal tract and liver as well as the ocular system.

Some type of cutaneous system manifestation is experienced in up to 85% of patients with SLE (Norris, 2019). Several skin manifestations may occur in patients with SLE, including subacute cutaneous lupus erythematosus, which involves papulosquamous or annular polycyclic lesions, and a discoid rash, which is a chronic rash with erythematous papules or plaques and scaling and can cause scarring and pigmentation changes (Aringer et al., 2019). In some cases, the only skin involvement may be a discoid rash. In some patients with SLE, the initial skin involvement is the precursor to more systemic involvement. The lesions often worsen during

exacerbations (flares) of the systemic disease and possibly are provoked by sunlight or artificial ultraviolet light (Norris, 2019). Oral ulcers, which may accompany skin lesions, may involve the buccal mucosa or the hard palate, occur in crops, and are often associated with exacerbations. Other cutaneous manifestations include splinter hemorrhages, alopecia, and Raynaud's phenomenon.

Joint pain and swelling occur in more than 90% of patients with SLE (Norris, 2019). Joint swelling, tenderness, and pain on movement are also common. Frequently, these are accompanied by morning stiffness.

The cardiac system is also commonly affected in SLE. Pericarditis is the most common cardiac manifestation (Norris, 2019). Patients may present with substernal chest pain that is aggravated by movement or inspiration. Symptoms can be acute and severe or last for weeks at a time. Other cardiac symptoms may involve myocarditis, hypertension, cardiac arrhythmias, and valvular incompetence.

Nephritis as a result of SLE, also referred to as lupus nephritis, occurs due to a buildup of antibodies and immune complexes that cause damage to the nephrons. Serum creatinine levels and urinalysis are used in screening for renal involvement. Early detection allows for prompt treatment so that renal damage can be prevented. Renal involvement may lead to hypertension, which also requires careful monitoring and management (see Chapter 27).

Central nervous system involvement is widespread, encompassing the entire range of neurologic disease. The varied and frequent neuropsychiatric presentations of SLE are now widely recognized and include psychosis, cognitive impairment, seizures, peripheral and cranial neuropathies, transverse myelitis, and strokes. These are generally demonstrated by subtle changes in behavior patterns or cognitive ability.

Assessment and Diagnostic Findings

Diagnosis of SLE is based on a complete history, physical examination, and blood tests. In addition to the general assessment performed for any patient with a rheumatic disease, assessment for known or suspected SLE has special features. The skin is inspected for erythematous rashes. Cutaneous erythematous plaques with an adherent scale may be observed on the scalp, face, or neck. Areas of hyperpigmentation or depigmentation may be noted, depending on the phase and type of disease. The patient should be questioned about skin changes (because these may be transitory) and specifically about sensitivity to sunlight or artificial ultraviolet light. The scalp should be inspected for alopecia and the mouth and throat for ulcerations reflecting gastrointestinal involvement.

Cardiovascular assessment includes auscultation for pericardial friction rub, possibly associated with myocarditis and accompanying pleural effusions. The pleural effusions and infiltrations, which reflect respiratory insufficiency, are demonstrated by abnormal lung sounds. Papular, erythematous, and purpuric lesions developing on the fingertips, elbows, toes, and extensor surfaces of the forearms or lateral sides of the hand that may become necrotic suggest vascular involvement.

Joint swelling, tenderness, warmth, pain on movement, stiffness, and edema may be detected on physical examination.

The joint involvement is often symmetric and similar to that found in RA.

The neurologic assessment is directed at identifying and describing any central nervous system changes. The patient and family members are asked about any behavioral changes, including manifestations of neurosis or psychosis. Signs of depression are noted, as are reports of seizures, chorea, or other central nervous system manifestations.

The antinuclear antibody (ANA) is positive in more than 95% of patients with SLE, indicating exceptional specificity (Aringer et al., 2019). Other laboratory tests include anti-DNA (antibody that develops against the patient's own DNA), anti-ds DNA (antibody against DNA that is highly specific to SLE, which helps differentiate it from drug-induced lupus), and anti-Sm (antibody against Sm, which is a specific protein found in the nucleus). Other blood work includes the CBC, which may reveal anemia, thrombocytopenia, leukocytosis, or leukopenia.

Medical Management

SLE can be life-threatening, but advances in its treatment have led to improved survival and reduced morbidity. Acute disease requires interventions directed at controlling increased disease activity or exacerbations that can involve any organ system. Disease activity is a composite of clinical and laboratory features that reflect active inflammation secondary to SLE. Management of the more chronic condition involves periodic monitoring and recognition of meaningful clinical changes requiring adjustments in therapy.

The goals of treatment include preventing progressive loss of organ function, reducing the likelihood of acute disease, minimizing disease-related disability, and preventing complications from therapy. Management of SLE involves regular monitoring to assess disease activity and therapeutic effectiveness.

Pharmacologic Therapy

The mainstay of SLE treatment is based on pain management and nonspecific immunosuppression. Therapy includes monoclonal antibodies, corticosteroids, antimalarial agents, NSAIDs, and immunosuppressive agents. Each of these medications has potentially serious side effects, including organ damage.

Belimumab is a monoclonal antibody that specifically recognizes and binds to BLyS. BLyS acts to stimulate B cells to produce antibodies against the body's own nuclei, which is an integral part of the disease process in SLE. Belimumab acts to render BLyS inactive, preventing it from binding to B-cell surfaces and stimulating B-cell activity. This action then halts the production of unnecessary antibodies and decreases disease activity in SLE. Live vaccines are contraindicated for 30 days before taking this medication (Comerford & Durkin, 2020). Rituximaub is an additional monoclonal antibody used in the treatment of SLE for its immune modulating effects (MacIsaac, Siddiqui, Jamula, et al., 2018).

Corticosteroids are another medication used topically for cutaneous manifestations, in low oral doses for minor disease activity, and in high doses for major disease activity. Intravenous (IV) administration of corticosteroids is an alternative to traditional high-dose oral administration. One of the most important risk factors associated with the use of corticosteroids in SLE is osteoporosis and fractures (Comerford & Durkin, 2020).

An antimalarial medication, hydroxychloroquine, is effective for managing cutaneous, musculoskeletal, and mild systemic features of SLE (Comerford & Durkin, 2020). The NSAIDs used for minor clinical manifestations are often used in conjunction with corticosteroids in an effort to minimize corticosteroid requirements.

Immunosuppressive agents (alkylating agents and purine analogues) are used because of their effect on overall immune function. These medications are generally reserved for patients who have serious forms of SLE that have not responded to conservative therapies. Examples include cyclophosphamide, azathioprine, mycophenolic acid, and methotrexate, which are contraindicated in pregnancy and have been used most frequently in SLE nephritis (Comerford & Durkin, 2020).

Nursing Management

Nursing care of the patient with SLE is based on the fundamental plan presented earlier in the chapter (see Chart 34-3). The most common nursing diagnoses include fatigue, impaired skin integrity, body image disturbance, and lack of knowledge for self-management decisions. The disease or its treatment may produce dramatic changes in appearance and considerable distress for the patient. The changes and the unpredictable course of SLE necessitate expert assessment skills and nursing care with sensitivity to the psychological reactions of the patient. The patient may benefit from participation in support groups, which can provide disease information, daily management tips, and social support. Because sun and ultraviolet light exposure can increase disease activity or cause an exacerbation, patients should be instructed to avoid exposure or to protect themselves with sunscreen and appropriate clothing.

Because of the increased risk of involvement of multiple organ systems, patients should understand the need for routine periodic screenings as well as health promotion activities. A dietary consultation may be indicated to ensure that the patient is knowledgeable about dietary recommendations, given the increased risk of cardiovascular disease, including hypertension and atherosclerosis.

In the healthy population, smoking and using electronic nicotine delivery systems (ENDS) including e-cigarettes, e-pens, e-pipes, e-hookah, and e-cigars clearly poses health risks. Smoking increases the incidence of respiratory infections, lung cancer, risk of coronary artery disease; increases blood pressure, which can worsen kidney function; inhibits liver function (which can also inhibit treatment medications from working appropriately, such as hydroxychloroquine); increases the risk for skin diseases; and increases the risk for osteoporosis. The health risks of ENDS use is under investigation. Patients diagnosed with SLE are at even higher risk of developing lung cancer and other rare cancers. Therefore, smoking cessation programs should be offered to all patients who report smoking habits (Montes, Mocarzel, Lanzieri, et al., 2016).

The nurse educates the patient about the importance of continuing prescribed medications and addresses the changes and potential side effects that are likely to occur with their use. The patient is reminded of the importance of monitoring because of the increased risk of systemic involvement, including renal and cardiovascular effects.

Because of the immunosuppression associated with systemic corticosteroid usage, the nurse must watch for signs and symptoms of infection, especially with patients who are acutely ill.

The nurse should also screen the patient for osteoporosis, because long-term use of corticosteroids increases the incidence of osteoporosis. Patients should have a bone mineral density test performed at diagnosis and prior to beginning steroid use to determine a baseline status and then every 2 years thereafter. Educating the patient regarding calcium and vitamin D supplementation daily is encouraged, along with the benefits of weight-bearing activities to support bone health.

Primary Sjögren's Syndrome

Primary Sjögren's syndrome is a rare systemic autoimmune disease that predominantly affects middle-aged women (Cornec, Devauchelle-Pensec, Mariette, et al., 2017).

Sjögren's syndrome often manifests in conjunction with other autoimmune diseases, most commonly autoimmune thyroid disease, RA, and SLE (MacIsaac et al., 2018; Molano-Gonzalez et al., 2019).

Pathophysiology

Primary Sjögren's is a multisystem disease characterized by lymphocytic infiltration leading to failure of the lacrimal and salivary glands (Cui, Li, Yin, et al., 2018).

Clinical Manifestations

The most common symptoms involve kerotoconjunctivitis sicca (dry eyes), xerostomia (dry mouth), pain, and fatigue (Cornec et al., 2017; Cui et al., 2018). Some patients will complain that their eyes feel "gritty," as if there is sand present. The patient's eyes will exhibit increased redness and lack of tearing. The mouth will have dry and sticky mucous membranes. The reduced saliva production may lead to difficulty swallowing.

Sjögren's syndrome can also exhibit symptoms in many other organ systems. Lesions may ulcerate and can be painful. Optic neuritis, trigeminal neuralgia, and sensory neuropathy may be present, with symptoms such as burning pain in the extremities, numbness, vertigo, arthralgia, and/or myalgia. Raynaud's phenomenon, which involves blood vessel spasms leading to decreased circulation to the toes, fingers, nose, and ears, may be reported. Patients experience symptoms of pain, fatigue, depression, and anxiety (Cui et al., 2018). Sleep disturbances are frequently reported and may be related to pain, fatigue, and depressive symptoms (Hackett, Gotts, Ellis, et al., 2017).

Assessment and Diagnostic Findings

The classification criteria for diagnosis of Sjögren's syndrome identify six distinct indices (Klippel, Stone, Crofford, et al., 2008):

- Ocular symptoms such as chronic dry eye (Kerotoconjunctivitis Sicca).

- Positive ocular tests (evaluating tear production, corneal, and conjunctival damage). Ocular testing may include Schemer tear test or Rose Bengal tests.
- Oral symptoms, dry mouth.
- Histopathology evaluation (of salivary glands). This will help differentiate the cause of dry mouth from other causes, such as infection, malignancy, stones, and sarcoidosis.
- Salivary gland involvement.

Laboratory tests include autoantibodies to ribonucleoprotein particles (Ro[SS-A] and/or La[SS-B]), which act as antigens in this disease process. Other laboratory indices are also useful in diagnosing Sjögren's syndrome. Rheumatoid factor is present in 50% to 70% of patients. ANA, circulating DNA (cDNA), anti-CCP, ACPA, and anticentromere antibody (ACA) are all potentially present in Sjögren's syndrome and in some cases may act as markers for disease activity (Molano-Gonzalez et al., 2019).

For vasculitis manifestations, a skin biopsy can yield useful information such as leukocytoclastic vasculitis found on histologic examination. If neurologic symptoms are present, nerve conduction studies, MRI, electroencephalograms, and cerebrospinal fluid testing may be used to aid in diagnosis and treatment planning.

Medical Management

There is no cure for Sjögren's syndrome, and treatment is aimed at symptom management and improving quality of life (Cornec et al., 2017; Cui et al., 2018; Hackett et al., 2017). Artificial tears, drops such as pilocarpine, and ocular ointments such as topical cyclosporine are used for dry eyes. Tears normally drain through the lacrimal puncta to the nose, which can render artificial tears ineffective. Therefore, punctum plugs may be a useful management tool. One systematic review reported that pilocarpine is highly effective in decreasing symptoms of dry mouth by increasing salivary flow (Hamad, Lodi, Porter, et al., 2018). Biotene oral rinse may also be useful for some patients. Additional suggestions include eating small frequent meals; omitting spicy, salty, and irritating food; and avoiding smoking (including ENDS), excessive alcohol use, and drugs with anticholinergic side effects. There is some evidence for the effectiveness of rituximab and interferone (Cornec et al., 2017; Hamad et al., 2018; MacIsaac et al., 2018). Patients need to be screened for depression and sleep disturbances, then appropriate referrals made when these comorbid conditions are present (Cui et al., 2018; Hackett et al., 2017).

Nursing Management

Nursing care is based on the fundamental plan of nursing care presented earlier (see Chart 34-3). The primary issues for the patient with Sjögren's syndrome are pain, fatigue, and inadequate knowledge of self-management techniques. The nurse is in the unique position to educate and reinforce the treatment regimen with the patient, especially involving the ocular treatments to avoid eye infections secondary to the dry eyes. The high prevalence of pain, fatigue, and depressive symptoms may interfere with the patient's ability to learn and engage in self-management techniques and should be addressed (Cui et al., 2018).

Scleroderma

Scleroderma is a rare autoimmune disease affecting the connective tissue of the skin, blood vessel walls, and internal organs. There are two general types: localized (affecting only the cutaneous system) or diffuse (routinely referred to as systemic sclerosis and affecting multiple organ systems). Similar to other autoimmune diseases, women are affected four times more than men, and the onset occurs typically between the ages of 25 and 50 years (Norris, 2019). Scleroderma has a variable course with remissions and exacerbations.

Pathophysiology

The pathogenesis is poorly understood. Scleroderma commonly begins with skin involvement. Mononuclear cells cluster on the skin and stimulate lymphokines to stimulate procollagen. Insoluble collagen is formed and accumulates excessively in the tissues (Norris, 2019). Initially, the inflammatory response causes edema, with a resulting taut, smooth, and shiny skin appearance. The skin then undergoes fibrotic changes, leading to loss of elasticity and movement. Eventually, the tissue degenerates and becomes nonfunctional. This chain of events, from inflammation to degeneration, also occurs in blood vessels, major organs, and body systems (Norris, 2019).

Clinical Manifestations

The skin and subcutaneous tissues become increasingly hard and rigid due to excess collagen and cannot be pinched up from the underlying structures. Wrinkles and lines are obliterated. The skin is dry because sweat secretion over the involved region is suppressed. The extremities stiffen and lose mobility. The condition spreads slowly; for years, these changes may remain localized in the hands and the feet. The face appears masklike, immobile, and expressionless, and the mouth becomes rigid; referred to as "stone facies" (Norris, 2019).

The changes within the body, although not visible directly, are vastly more important than the visible changes. The esophagus hardens, interfering with swallowing. The lungs become scarred, impeding respiration. Digestive disturbances occur because of sclerosing (hardening) of the intestinal mucosa. Vascular involvement of the kidneys leads to malignant hypertension and renal insufficiency. Cardiac disorders include pericarditis, heart block, and myocardial fibrosis (Norris, 2019).

The patient may manifest a variety of symptoms referred to as the CREST syndrome. CREST stands for calcinosis (calcium deposits in the tissues), Raynaud's phenomenon, esophageal dysmobility, sclerodactyly (scleroderma of the digits), and telangiectasia (capillary dilation that forms a vascular lesion) (Norris, 2019).

Assessment and Diagnostic Findings

Assessment focuses on the sclerotic changes in the skin, contractures in the fingers, and color changes or lesions in the fingertips. Assessment of systemic involvement requires a systems review with special attention to gastrointestinal, pulmonary, renal, and cardiac symptoms. Limitations in mobility and self-care activities should be assessed, along with the impact the disease has had (or will have) on body image.

There is no one conclusive diagnostic test used to diagnose scleroderma. Generally, the patient is diagnosed with the CREST type of scleroderma if they have four of the five symptoms in the syndrome (Norris, 2019).

Medical Management

Treatment of scleroderma is mainly symptomatic and supportive. No medication regimen is effective in modifying the disease process in scleroderma, but various medications are used to treat organ system involvement. The use of angiotensin-converting enzyme inhibitors when there is kidney involvement has led to a substantial decrease in mortality from hypertensive kidney disease (Norris, 2019).

All patients require counseling, during which realistic individual goals may be determined. Support measures include strategies to decrease pain and limit disability. A moderate exercise program is encouraged to prevent joint contractures. Patients are advised to avoid extreme temperatures and to use lotion to minimize skin dryness.

Nursing Management

Nursing care of the patient with scleroderma is based on the fundamental plan of nursing care presented earlier (see Chart 34-3). The primary nursing diagnoses are impaired skin integrity; self care deficits; impaired nutritional status; and disturbed body image. The patient with advanced disease may also have impaired gas exchange, impaired cardiac output, impaired swallowing, and constipation.

Providing meticulous skin care and preventing the effects of Raynaud's phenomenon are major nursing challenges. See Chapter 26 for further discussion of Raynaud's phenomenon.

Polymyositis

Polymyositis is a group of diseases that are termed *idiopathic inflammatory myopathies* (Klippel et al., 2008). They are rare chronic conditions, with an incidence estimated at 2 cases per 10,000 adults per year. Polymyositis is most commonly seen in women versus men (2:1) and usually seen between 40 and 50 years of age (Miller & Vleugels, 2019).

Pathophysiology

Polymyositis is classified as autoimmune because autoantibodies are present. However, these antibodies do not cause damage to muscle cells, indicating only an indirect role in tissue damage. The pathogenesis is multifactorial, including cellular and humoral immune mechanisms (Norris, 2019).

Clinical Manifestations

The onset may be very slow and insidious, with symptoms gradually worsening over weeks to months. Proximal muscle weakness is typically the first symptom. Muscle weakness is usually symmetric and diffuse. Common complaints include having difficulty rising from a chair, climbing steps, or holding up the head. Myalgia and muscle tenderness occur in 25% to 50% of patients. Dermatomyositis, a related condition, is most commonly identified by an erythematous smooth or scaly lesion found over the joint surface, which often occurs prior to symptoms of weakness in 50% to 60% of patients (Miller & Vleugels, 2019).

Assessment and Diagnostic Findings

A complete history and physical examination help exclude other muscle-related disorders. As with other diffuse connective tissue disorders, no single test confirms polymyositis. An electromyogram is performed to rule out degenerative muscle disease. A muscle biopsy may reveal inflammatory infiltrate in the tissue. Serum studies indicate increased muscle enzyme activity.

Medical Management

Corticosteroid therapy is the mainstay of medical management (Norris, 2019). IV immune globulin, plasmapheresis, lymphapheresis, and total-body irradiation have been used if there is no response to corticosteroids. The goal is to control inflammation and prevent long-term damage to muscles, joints, and internal organs (Norris, 2019). The antimalarial agent hydroxychloroquine may be effective for skin rashes. Physical therapy is initiated slowly, with range-of-motion exercises to maintain joint mobility, followed by gradual strengthening exercises (Klippel et al., 2008).

Nursing Management

Nursing care is based on the fundamental plan of nursing care presented earlier (see Chart 34-3). The primary nursing diagnoses for the patient with polymyositis are impaired mobility, fatigue, self care deficit, and lack of knowledge of self-management techniques.

Patients with polymyositis may have symptoms similar to those of other inflammatory diseases. However, proximal muscle weakness is characteristic, making activities such as combing the hair, reaching overhead, and using stairs difficult. Therefore, the use of assistive devices may be recommended, and referral to occupational or physical therapy may be warranted.

Polymyalgia Rheumatica and Giant Cell Arteritis

PMR involves stiffness of muscles and pain in the neck, shoulder, and pelvic girdle. GCA is a form of vasculitis affecting the medium-sized and large arteries of the body (Klippel et al., 2008). GCA is also sometimes referred to as temporal arteritis (Hill, Black, Nossent, et al., 2017). PMR and GCA represent a spectrum of one disease. Both primarily affect individuals older than 50 years and are associated with the same HLA haplotype genetic markers. PMR and GCA occur predominately in Caucasians and often in first-degree relatives. PMR has an annual incidence rate of 52 cases per 100,000 people older than 50 years. GCA varies by geographic location and has the highest incidence in Scandinavian countries. PMR is two to three times more common than GCA (Klippel et al., 2008).

Pathophysiology

The underlying mechanism of action involved with PMR and GCA is unknown. It is clear, however, that the immune system is abnormally activated in both disease processes with increases in circulating monocytes that produce IL-1 and IL-6. These circulating monocytes make the endothelial linings of blood vessels more vulnerable to vasculitis (Klippel et al., 2008). Immunoglobulin deposits in the walls of inflamed temporal arteries suggest that an autoimmune process is at work.

Clinical Manifestations

PMR is characterized by severe proximal muscle discomfort with mild joint swelling. Severe aching in the neck, shoulder, and pelvic muscles is common. Stiffness is noticeable most often in the morning and after periods of inactivity. This stiffness can become so severe that patients struggle putting on a coat or combing their hair. Systemic features include low-grade fever, weight loss, malaise, anorexia, and depression. Because PMR usually occurs in people 50 years and older, it may be confused with, or dismissed as, an inevitable consequence of aging.

GCA may cause headaches, changes in vision, and jaw claudication. These symptoms should be evaluated immediately because of the potential for blindness and stroke if left untreated (Hill et al., 2017). PMR and GCA have a self-limited course, lasting several months to several years (Klippel et al., 2008).

Assessment and Diagnostic Findings

Assessment focuses on musculoskeletal tenderness, weakness, and decreased function. Careful attention should be directed toward assessing the head (for changes in vision, headaches, and jaw claudication). An MRI scan may be used in the assessment of extra-articular synovitis in patients with PMR, regardless of symptoms.

Often, diagnosis is difficult because of the lack of specificity of tests. A markedly high ESR is a screening test but is not definitive. The CRP level and platelet count also provide valuable data. In fact, simultaneous elevation in the ESR and CRP has a sensitivity of 98.6% and a specificity of 75.7% in making the diagnosis of GCA when coupled with clinical findings (Seetharaman, 2019). Diagnosis of both GCA and PMR is more likely to be made by eliminating other potential diagnoses. The dramatic and immediate response to treatment with corticosteroids is considered by some to be diagnostic.

In the case of GCA, biopsy of the temporal artery is the definitive diagnostic tool (Seetharaman, 2019). High-resolution MRI is an alternative or adjunct to the traditional temporal artery biopsy.

Medical Management

The treatment for patients with PMR (without GCA) is moderate doses of corticosteroids. Longer durations of corticosteroid treatment are required with patients who have higher baseline inflammatory markers. Gradual tapering of the corticosteroid treatment should be monitored. NSAIDs are sometimes given in mild disease. The treatment for patients with

GCA is rapid initiation of and strict adherence to a regimen of corticosteroids. This is essential to avoid the complication of blindness (Hill et al., 2017). Aspirin is an adjunctive treatment may help reduce the risk of visual loss.

Nursing Management

Nursing care of the patient with PMR is based on the fundamental plan of nursing care presented earlier (see Chart 34-3). The most common nursing diagnoses are pain and lack of knowledge of medications.

A management concern is that the patient will take the prescribed medication, frequently corticosteroids, until symptoms improve and then discontinue the medication. The decision to discontinue the medication should be based on clinical and laboratory findings and the prescription. Nursing implications are related to helping the patient prevent and monitor adverse effects of medications (e.g., infections, diabetes, gastrointestinal problems, and depression) and adjust to those side effects that cannot be prevented (e.g., increased appetite and altered body image).

> ### ▶ Quality and Safety Nursing Alert
>
> *The nurse must emphasize to the patient the need for continued adherence to the prescribed medication regimen to avoid complications of GCA, such as blindness and stroke.*

The loss of bone mass with corticosteroid use increases the risk of osteoporosis in this already at-risk population. Interventions to promote bone health, such as adequate dietary calcium and vitamin D, measurement of bone mineral density, weight-bearing exercise, smoking and ENDS cessation, and reduction of alcohol consumption if indicated, should be emphasized.

Spondyloarthropathies

The spondyloarthropathies are another category of systemic inflammatory disorders of the skeleton. The spondyloarthropathies include ankylosing spondylitis (AS), reactive arthritis (formerly known as Reiter's syndrome), and psoriatic arthritis. Spondyloarthritis is also associated with inflammatory bowel diseases such as Crohn's disease (regional enteritis) and ulcerative colitis (Norris, 2019).

These rheumatic diseases share several clinical features. The inflammation tends to occur peripherally at the sites of attachment—at tendons, joint capsules, and ligaments. Periosteal inflammation may be present. Many patients have arthritis of the sacroiliac joints. The onset tends to occur during young adulthood, with the disease affecting men more often than women. There is a strong tendency for these conditions to occur in families. Frequently, the HLA-B27 genetic marker is found. In addition, more than one of these conditions can be found simultaneously in the same person or another family member (Norris, 2019).

As with other inflammatory conditions, patients with spondyloarthropathies have an increased risk for cardiovascular disease. These findings may be related to a state of chronic systemic inflammation and an increase in traditional cardiac risk factors, such as lack of exercise due to increased pain (Norris, 2019).

Ankylosing Spondylitis

AS is a chronic inflammatory disease of the spine. It is more prevalent in males than in females and is usually diagnosed in the second or third decade of life. The disease is also more severe in males, and significant systemic involvement is likely (Norris, 2019).

AS affects the cartilaginous joints of the spine and surrounding tissues, making them rigid, decreasing mobility, and leading to kyphosis (a stooped position). This kyphosis can, in turn, lead to decreased stability and balance. Back pain is the characteristic feature. The back pain can be so severe that it may mask symptoms of a cervical fracture, which can lead to neurologic problems if left untreated. Occasionally, the large synovial joints, such as the hips, knees, or shoulders, may be involved (Norris, 2019).

AS also exhibits systemic effects as the heart and lungs become constricted in the chest cavity (Norris, 2019). Another potential complication of AS is the risk of osteoporosis, which appears to be related to the inflammatory process as well as bone turnover and low vitamin D levels. Other complications involve atrioventricular conduction defects, aortic insufficiency, and pulmonary fibrosis. As the disease progresses, ankylosis (i.e., fixation or immobility) of the entire spine may occur, leading to respiratory compromise and further complications.

Reactive Arthritis (Reiter's Syndrome)

The disease process involved in reactive arthritis is called *reactive* because the arthritis occurs after an infection, primarily gastrointestinal or genitourinary (Norris, 2019). It mostly affects young adult males and is characterized primarily by urethritis, arthritis, and conjunctivitis. Dermatitis and ulcerations of the mouth and penis may also be present. Low back pain is common.

Psoriatic Arthritis

Psoriatic arthritis is an inflammatory arthritis associated with the skin disease psoriasis. Approximately 7% of people with psoriasis develop psoriatic arthritis (Norris, 2019). Psoriasis is the most common autoimmune disease in the United States, affecting 2% to 3% of the population. Psoriatic arthritis onset occurs between 30 and 50 years of age and affects equal numbers of men and women (Dewing, 2015). See Chapter 56 for more information on psoriasis.

Psoriatic arthritis is characterized by synovitis, polyarthritis, and spondylitis. Inflammatory back pain is a common symptom, which is differentiated from other back pain by symptoms of back pain presenting at a young age, pain improving with activity, and pain occurring at night. Radiographic evidence of asymmetrical sacroiliitis or spondylitis may also assist with diagnosing psoriatic arthritis (Dewing, 2015). Other sites of pain commonly seen in these patients are the Achilles tendon, plantar fascia, or tibial tuberosity areas. Pain in these areas is common from the inflammation that occurs at the entheses, where tendons and ligaments attach to the bone.

Medical Management

Medical management of spondyloarthropathies focuses on treating pain and maintaining mobility by suppressing inflammation. For the patient with AS, good body positioning and posture are essential so that if ankylosis does occur, the patient is in the most functional position. Maintaining range of motion with regular exercise and a muscle-strengthening program is especially important and has been linked with higher quality of life for patients.

Pharmacologic Management

NSAIDs are the first-line therapy for treating all spondylarthropathies. All chronic conditions (cardiac, renal, and gastrointestinal) should be taken into consideration when prescribing long-term NSAIDs. Methotrexate, sulfasalazine, and leflunomide may also be used; these drugs may help with skin and peripheral joint disease but may not prevent spinal changes. Corticosteroid injections may be used for periodic flares; however, oral and long-term use of steroids is not recommended due to the possibility of psoriatic skin flare when discontinuing use.

Disease remission is now the target for psoriatic arthritis (Mease & Coates, 2018). Anti-TNF medications that have been used effectively include etanercept, infliximab, adalimumab, golimumab, and certolizumabpegol. Additional agents include apremilast, which is a PDE4 inhibitor, and ustekinumab, an anti-IL12/anti-IL23 agent (Mease & Coates, 2018).

Surgical Management

With advanced AS and subsequent debilitating kyphosis, an osteotomy of the spine can be done. One study showed that an average correction of 45 degrees in the cervical spine was obtained and that quality of life also improved. Surgical management may also include total joint replacement (see Chapter 36).

Nursing Management

Major nursing interventions in the spondyloarthropathies are related to symptom management and maintenance of optimal functioning. Affected patients are primarily young men. Their major concerns are often related to prognosis and job modification, especially among those who perform physical work. Patients may also express concerns about leisure and recreational activities. Focusing on physical activity and staying active and maintaining good posture will help to prevent chronic changes that may lead to deformities. It is important to address psychological changes, such as depression and emotional stress, that can occur with the diagnosis and chronic nature of the disease. If symptoms are present, the primary provider should assess for emotional stress and treat as appropriate.

Metabolic and Endocrine Diseases Associated with Rheumatic Disorders

Metabolic and endocrine diseases may be associated with rheumatic disorders. These include biochemical abnormalities (amyloidosis and scurvy), endocrine diseases (diabetes and acromegaly), immune deficiency diseases (human immune deficiency virus infection, acquired immune deficiency syndrome), and some inherited disorders (hypermobility syndromes). However, the most common conditions are the crystal-induced arthropathies, in which crystals such as monosodium urate (gout) or calcium pyrophosphate (calcium pyrophosphate dihydrate disease or pseudogout) are deposited within joints and other tissues (Norris, 2019).

Gout

Gout is the most common form of inflammatory arthritis. More than 8.3 million Americans self-report the diagnosis of gout (CDC, 2019). The prevalence is reported to be about 3.9% and appears to be on the rise. Men are three to four times more likely to be diagnosed with gout than women. The incidence of gout increases with age, body mass index, alcohol consumption, hypertension, and diuretic use (CDC, 2019). Evidence links the consumption of fructose-rich beverages with the risk of gout for both men and women (CDC, 2019). Patients with gout have an increased risk of cardiovascular disease. Comorbid conditions such as hypertension, dyslipidemia, diabetes, osteoarthritis, kidney disease, and depression may be present in patients with gout (Lin, Zhang, & Ma, 2018; Norris, 2019).

Pathophysiology

Gout is caused by hyperuricemia (increased serum uric acid). Uric acid is a by-product of purine metabolism; purines are basic chemical compounds found in high concentrations in meat products. Urate levels are affected by diet, medications, overproduction in the body, and inadequate excretion by the kidneys. Hyperuricemia (serum concentration greater than 6.8 mg/dL) can, but does not always, cause urate crystal deposition. However, as uric acid levels increase, the risk becomes greater. The initial cause for the gout attack occurs when macrophages in the joint space phagocytize urate crystals. Through a series of immunologic steps, interleukin-1β is secreted, increasing the inflammation. This process is exacerbated by the presence of free fatty acids. Both alcohol and consumption of a large meal, especially with red meat, can lead to increases in free fatty acid concentrations; they also are implicated as triggers to acute gout attacks (Norris, 2019).

With repeated attacks, accumulations of sodium urate crystals, called tophi, are deposited in peripheral areas of the body, such as the great toe, the hands, and the ear. Renal uratelithiasis (kidney stones), with chronic kidney disease secondary to urate deposition, may develop.

Primary hyperuricemia may be caused by severe dieting or starvation, excessive intake of foods that are high in purines (shellfish, organ meats), or heredity. In secondary hyperuricemia, gout is a clinical feature secondary to any of a number of genetic or acquired processes, including conditions in which there is an increase in cell turnover (leukemia, multiple myeloma, some types of anemias, psoriasis) and an increase in cell breakdown. Altered renal tubular function, either as a major action or as an unintended side effect of certain pharmacologic agents (e.g., diuretics such as thiazides and furosemide), low-dose salicylates, or ethanol can contribute to uric acid underexcretion (Klippel et al., 2008). The finding of urate crystals in the synovial fluid of asymptomatic joints suggests that factors other than crystals may be related to the inflammatory reaction. Recovered monosodium urate crystals are coated with immunoglobulins that are mainly IgG. IgG enhances crystal phagocytosis, thereby demonstrating immunologic activity (Klippel et al., 2008).

Clinical Manifestations

Manifestations of the gout syndrome include acute gouty arthritis (recurrent attacks of severe articular and periarticular inflammation), **tophi** (crystalline deposits accumulating in articular tissue, osseous tissue, soft tissue, and cartilage), gouty nephropathy (renal impairment), and uric acid urinary calculi. Four stages of gout can be identified: asymptomatic hyperuricemia, acute gouty arthritis, intercritical gout, and chronic tophaceous gout (Neoai, Jansen, Dalbeth, et al., 2015). The subsequent development of gout is directly related to the duration and magnitude of the hyperuricemia. Therefore, the commitment to lifelong pharmacologic treatment of hyperuricemia is deferred until there is an initial attack of gout.

Acute arthritis is the most common early clinical manifestation. The metatarsophalangeal joint of the big toe is a commonly affected joint. The tarsal area, ankle, or knee may also be affected. Less commonly, the wrists, fingers, and elbows may be affected. Trauma, alcohol ingestion, dieting, medications, surgical stress, or illness may trigger the acute attack. The abrupt onset often occurs at night, awakening the patient with severe pain, redness, swelling, and warmth of the affected joint. Early attacks tend to subside spontaneously over 3 to 10 days without treatment. The attack is followed by a symptom-free period (the intercritical stage) until the next attack, which may not come for months or years. However, with time, attacks tend to occur more frequently, involve more joints, and last longer (Becker & Gaffo, 2019).

Tophi (seen in chronic tophaceous gout) are generally associated with more frequent and severe inflammatory episodes. Higher serum concentrations of uric acid are also associated with more extensive tophus formation. Tophi most commonly occur in the synovium, olecranon bursa, **subchondral bone** (bony plate that supports the articular cartilage), infrapatellar and Achilles tendons, and subcutaneous tissue on the extensor surface of the forearms and overlying joints. They have also been found in the aortic walls, heart valves, nasal and ear cartilage, eyelids, cornea, and sclera. Joint enlargement may cause a loss of joint motion. Uric acid deposits may cause renal stones and kidney damage.

Medical Management

Given that the incidence of gout increases with age, its management can be complicated by other medical conditions, medications, and age-related changes. A definitive diagnosis of gouty arthritis is established by polarized light microscopy of the synovial fluid of the involved joint. Uric acid crystals are seen within the polymorphonuclear leukocytes in the fluid during a disease flare up (CDC, 2019).

Acute attacks are managed with colchicine (oral or parenteral), an NSAID such as indomethacin, or a corticosteroid. Management of hyperuricemia, tophi, joint destruction, and renal disorders is usually initiated after the acute inflammatory process has subsided. Once the acute attack has subsided, uric acid lowering therapy should be considered. Xanthine oxidase inhibitors, such as allopurinol and febuxostat, are the agents of choice. Given the role of IL-1 in the pathogenesis of gout, some experts suggest that there may be a role for anakinra, an IL-1 receptor antagonist in the management of acute gout (Becker & Perez-Ruiz, 2019).

Management between gout attacks needs to include lifestyle changes such as avoiding purine-rich foods, weight loss, decreasing alcohol consumption, and avoiding certain medications. Uricosuric agents, such as probenecid, may be indicated in patients with frequent acute attacks. Uricosuric medications correct hyperuricemia and dissolve deposited urate. Corticosteroids may also be used in patients who have no response to other therapy. In patients with refractory chronic gout who are not controlled with the regimens mentioned earlier, pegloticase, a newer agent, has been shown to be effective in lowering uric acid levels (Becker & Perez-Ruiz, 2019). Specific treatment is based on the serum uric acid level, 24-hour urinary uric acid excretion, and renal function (see Table 34-4).

TABLE 34-4 Common Medications Used to Treat Gout

Medication	Actions and Use	Nursing Implications
colchicine	Lowers the deposition of uric acid and interferes with leukocyte infiltration, thus reducing inflammation; does not alter serum or urine levels of uric acid; used in acute and chronic management	*Acute management:* Administer when attack begins; dosage increased until pain is relieved or diarrhea develops, then stop medication *Chronic management:* Causes gastrointestinal upset in most patients.
probenecid	Uricosuric agent; inhibits renal reabsorption of urates and increases the urinary excretion of uric acid; prevents tophi formation	Be alert for nausea and rash.
allopurinol, febuxostat	Xanthine oxidase inhibitors; interrupt the breakdown of purines before uric acid is formed; inhibit xanthinoxidase because uric acid formation is blocked	Monitor for side effects, including bone marrow depression, nausea, vomiting, diarrhea, abdominal pain, or rash. Avoid starting medication or increasing dose if active flare present.

Adapted from Comerford, K. C., & Durkin, M. T. (2020). *Nursing 2020 drug handbook.* Philadelphia, PA: Wolters Kluwer.

Nursing Management

Research indicates that providers overestimate patient knowledge of gout and that patients prefer the use of both written and verbal materials (Abhishek & Doherty, 2018). Therefore, the nurse takes every opportunity to educate and reinforce knowledge of gout verbally and in writing. Severe dietary restriction is not necessary; however, the nurse encourages the patient to restrict consumption of foods high in purines, especially organ meats, and to limit alcohol intake. Maintenance of normal body weight should be encouraged. In an acute episode of gouty arthritis, pain management with prescribed medications is essential, along with avoidance of factors that increase pain and inflammation, such as trauma, stress, and alcohol. Medication adherence is critical but poor among patients prescribed urate lowering therapies (Scheepers, van Onna, Stehouwer, et al., 2018). The nurse reinforces the importance of taking prescribed medications. Between acute episodes, the patient feels well and may abandon medications and preventive behaviors, which may result in an acute attack. Acute attacks are most effectively treated if therapy begins early.

Fibromyalgia

Fibromyalgia is a chronic pain syndrome that involves chronic fatigue, generalized muscle aching, stiffness, sleep disturbances, and functional impairment. It is estimated to affect more than 5 million Americans, representing 2% to 5% of the general population, with women affected more than men. Between 25% and 65% of patients with fibromyalgia have other rheumatic conditions such as RA, SLE, and AS (CDC, 2017).

Pathophysiology

The amplified pain experienced by patients with fibromyalgia is thought to be neurogenic in origin. The central nervous system's ascending and descending pathways that regulate and moderate pain processing function abnormally, causing amplification of pain signals. Some describe this as if the "volume control setting" for pain were abnormally high. Therefore, stimulation that may not normally elicit pain, such as touch, may do so. In addition, there are a number of predisposing factors to pain, including anxiety, depression, physical trauma, emotional stress, sleep disorder, and viral infection (CDC, 2017; Melin, Svensson, & Thulesius, 2018).

Assessment and Diagnostic Findings

Since fibromyalgia is a diffuse syndrome, standard diagnostic testing is often not useful except to rule out other conditions that may be causing the pain. One study reported that two items, pain upon pinching the Achilles tendon using 4 kg of pressure for 4 seconds and an affirmative answer to the statement "I have a persistent deep aching all over my body," were the most useful in recognizing fibromyalgia (Jones, Aebischer, St John, et al., 2017). Positive responses to these screening items need to be followed by a comprehensive examination for confirmation of a diagnosis (Jones et al., 2017).

Medical Management

Treatment consists of attention to the specific symptoms reported by the patient. NSAIDs may be used to treat the diffuse muscle aching and stiffness. Tricyclic antidepressants such as amitriptyline and nortriptyline as well as sleep hygiene measures are used to improve or restore normal sleep patterns (CDC, 2017). Muscle relaxants such as cyclobenzaprine may also be used to help with relaxation and pain. Cognitive behavioral therapy is also useful in improving sleep and attentional dysfunction. In addition, serotonin norepinephrine reuptake inhibitors, such as duloxetine, venlafaxine, and milnacipran; selective serotonin reuptake inhibitors, including fluoxetine, paroxetine, and sertraline; as well as anticonvulsants such as gabapentin and pregabalin may be effective. Individualized programs of exercise are used to decrease muscle weakness and discomfort and to improve the general deconditioning that occurs in affected patients. There has been some promising research in complementary, alternative, and integrative health therapies, such as acupuncture (Kim, Kim, Lee, et al., 2019).

Nursing Management

Typically, patients with fibromyalgia have endured their symptoms for a long period of time. They may feel as if their symptoms have not been taken seriously. Nurses need to pay special attention to supporting these patients and providing encouragement as they begin their program of therapy. Patient support groups may be helpful (Melin et al., 2018). Careful listening to patients' descriptions of their concerns and symptoms is essential to help them make the changes that are necessary to improve their quality of life.

Miscellaneous Disorders

The last category in the classification of the rheumatic diseases is aptly labeled miscellaneous disorders because it contains a mix of disorders that are frequently associated with arthritis and other conditions. These include the direct consequences of trauma (including internal derangement and loose bodies of joints), pancreatic disease (related to avascular necrosis or osteonecrosis), sarcoidosis (a multisystem disorder particularly of the lymph nodes and lungs), and palindromic rheumatism (an uncommon variety of recurring and acute arthritis and periarthritis that in some may progress to RA but is characterized by symptom-free periods of days to months). Other conditions include villonodular synovitis, chronic active hepatitis, and drug-related rheumatic syndromes. The nursing interventions related to these varied conditions are specific to the multisystemic problems experienced by the patient. However, the musculoskeletal components should not be neglected or overlooked. Further information about these rare disorders can be found in specialty references.

CRITICAL THINKING EXERCISES

1 [QSEN] Your patient, a 52-year-old male with RA, is being discharged from the medical surgical unit where you work. He smokes 1 pack of cigarettes a day and drinks alcohol on occasion. He is 6'0" and weighs 240 lb. Identify the priorities, approach, and techniques you would use to provide discharge education to this patient. What lifestyle modifications are a priority for this patient?

2 **ipc** A 28-year-old patient who was recently diagnosed with SLE comes to the clinic where you work for a follow-up appointment. She tells you that she is planning to become pregnant soon. What additional members of the health care team should be included in the care of this patient given her childbearing plans?

3 **ebp** You are the nurse taking care of a woman newly diagnosed with fibromyalgia. What is the evidence for symptom management for this patient? What criteria would you use to assess the strength of the evidence? What is the evidence for complementary therapy options to improve her symptoms?

REFERENCES

*Asterisk indicates nursing research.
**Double asterisk indicates classic reference.

Books

Comerford, K. C., & Durkin, M. T. (2020). *Nursing 2020 drug handbook.* Philadelphia, PA: Wolters Kluwer.

Eliopoulos, C. (2021). *Gerontological nursing* (9th ed.). Philadelphia, PA: Wolters Kluwer.

Fischbach, F. T., & Fischbach, M. A. (2018). *A manual of laboratory and diagnostic tests* (10th ed.). Philadelphia, PA: Wolters Kluwer.

**Klippel, J. H., Stone, J. H., Crofford, L. J., et al. (Eds.). (2008). *Primer on the rheumatic diseases* (13th ed.). New York: Springer.

Norris, T. L. (2019). *Porth's pathophysiology: Concepts of altered health states* (10th ed.). Philadelphia, PA: Wolters Kluwer.

Weber, J. R., & Kelley, J. H. (2019). *Health assessment in nursing* (6th ed.). Philadelphia, PA: Wolters Kluwer.

Journals and Electronic Documents

Abhishek, A., & Doherty, M. (2018). Education and non-pharmacologic approaches for gout. *Rheumatology, 57,* i51–i58.

**Aletaha, D., Neogi, T., Silman, A. J., et al. (2010). 2010 Rheumatoid arthritis classification criteria: An American College of Rheumatology/ European League Against Rheumatism collaborative initiative. *Arthritis and Rheumatism, 62*(9), 2569–2581.

Aringer, M., Costenbader, K., Daikh, D., et al. (2019). 2019 European League Against Rheumatism/ American College of Rheumatology classification criteria for systemic lupus erythematosus. *Annals of Rheumatic Disorders, 78,* 1151–1159.

Becker, M. A., & Gaffo, A. L. (2019). Clinical manifestations and diagnosis of gout. *UpToDate.* Retrieved on 12/22/2019 at: www.uptodate.com/contents/search?search=Clinical+manifestations+and+diagnosis+of+gout&x=4&y=8

Becker, M. A., & Perez-Ruiz, F. (2019). Pharmacologic urate-lowering therapy and treatment of tophi. *UpToDate.* Retrieved on 12/22/2019 at: www.uptodate.com/contents/pharmacologic-urate-lowering-therapy-and-treatment-of-tophi-in-patients-withgout

Centers for Disease Control and Prevention (CDC). (2017). *Fibromyalgia.* Retrieved on 12/14/2019 at: www.cdc.gov/arthritis/basics/fibromyalgia.htm

Centers for Disease Control and Prevention (CDC). (2018). *Systemic lupus erythematous (SLE).* Retrieved on 12/4/2019 at: www.cdc.gov/lupus/facts/detailed.html

Centers for Disease Control and Prevention (CDC). (2019). *Gout.* Retrieved on 12/14/2019 at: www.cdc.gov/arthritis/basics/gout.htm

Chou, P., & Chu, H. (2018). Clinical efficacy of acupuncture on rheumatoid arthritis and associated mechanisms: A systematic review. *Evidence-Based Complementary and Alternative Medicine, 2018,* 1–21.

Cornec, D., Devauchelle-Pensec, V., Mariette, X., et al. (2017). Severe health-related quality of life impairment in active primary Sjögren's syndrome and patient-reported outcomes: Data from a large therapeutic trial. *Arthritis Care & Research, 69*(4), 528–535.

Cui, Y., Li, L., Yin, R., et al. (2018). Depression in primary Sjögren's syndrome: A systematic review and meta-analysis. *Psychology, Health & Medicine, 23*(2), 198–209.

Dewing, K. A. (2015). Management of patients with psoriatic arthritis. *The Nurse Practitioner, 40*(4), 40–46.

Hackett, K. L., Gotts, Z. M., Ellis, J., et al. (2017). An investigation into the prevalence of sleep disturbances in primary Sjögren's syndrome: A systematic review of the literature. *Rheumatology, 56*(4), 570–580.

Hamad, A. A., Lodi, G., Porter, S., et al. (2018). Interventions for dry mouth and hyposalivation in Sjögren's syndrome: A systematic review and meta-analysis. *Oral Diseases, 25,* 1027–1047.

Hill, C. L., Black, R. J., Nossent, J. C., et al. (2017). Risk of mortality in patients with giant cell arteritis: A systematic review and meta-analysis. *Seminars in Arthritis and Rheumatism, 46*(2017), 513–519.

*Jones, K. D., Aebischer, J. H., St John, A. W., et al. (2017). A simple screening test to recognize fibromyalgia in primary care patients with chronic pain. *Journal of Evaluation in Clinical Practice, 24*(1), 173–179.

Kapale, P., Vardharajulu, G., & Warude, T. (2017). Effect of free exercise and rheumatoid arthritis. *Indian Journal of Physiotherapy and Occupational Therapy, 11*(3), 62–65.

Katz-Talmor, D., Katz, I., Porta-Katz, B., et al. (2018). Cannabinoids for the treatment of rheumatic diseases—where do we stand? *Nature Reviews Rheumatology, 14*(2018), 488–497.

Kim, J., Kim, S., Lee H., et al. (2019). Comparing verum and sham acupuncture in fibromyalgia syndrome: A systematic review and meta-analysis. *Evidence-based Complementary and Alternative Medicine, 2019,* 1–13.

Lin, S., Zhang, H., & Ma, A. (2018). Association of gout and depression: A systematic review and meta-analysis. *Geriatric Psychiatry, 33.* 441–448.

MacIsaac, J., Siddiqui, R., Jamula, E., et al. (2018) Systematic review of rituximab for autoimmune diseases: A potential alternative to intravenous immune globulin. *Transfusion, 58,* 2729–2735.

Mahmood, S., van Tuyl, L., Schoonmade, L., et al. (2019). Systematic review of rheumatoid arthritis clinical studies: Suboptimal statistical analysis of radiological data. *Seminars in Arthritis and Rheumatism, 49*(2019), 218–221.

Mease, P. J., & Coates, L. C. (2018). Considerations for the definition of remission criteria in psoriatic arthritis. *Seminars in Arthritis and Rheumatism, 47*(2018), 786–796.

Melin, E. O., Svensson, R., & Thulesius, H. O. (2018). Psychoeducation against depression, anxiety, alexithymia and fibromyalgia: A pilot study in primary care for patients on sick leave. *Scandinavian Journal of Primary Health Care, 26*(2), 123–133.

Miller, M. L., & Vleugels, R. A. (2019). Clinical manifestations of dermatomyositis and polymyositis in adults. *UpToDate.* Retrieved on 12/22/2019 at: www.uptodate.com/contents/clinical-manifestations-of-dermatomyositis-and-polymyositis-in-adults

Mogul, A., Corsi, K., & McAuliffe, L. (2019). Baricitinic: The second FDA approved JAK inhibitor for the treatment of rheumatoid arthritis. *Annals of Pharmacotherapy, 53*(9), 947–953.

Molano-Gonzalez, N., Olivares-Matinez, E., Anaya, J. M., et al. (2019). Anti-citrullinated protein antibody and arthritis in Sjogren's syndrome: A systematic review and meta-analysis. *Scandinavian Journal of Rheumatology, 48*(2), 157–163.

Montes, R. A., Mocarzel, L. O., Lanzieri, P. G., et al. (2016). Smoking and its association with morbidity in systemic lupus erythematosus. *Arthritis and Rheumatology, 68*(2), 441–448.

Neoai, T., Jansen, T. A., Dalbeth, N., et al. (2015). 2105 Gout classification criteria: An American College of Rheumatology collaborative project. Retrieved on 12/22/2019 at: www.rheumatology.org/Practice-Quality/Clinical-Support/Criteria

Nikiphorou, E., Norton, S., Young, A., et al. (2018). The association of obesity with disease activity, functional ability and quality of life in early rheumatoid arthritis: Data from the Early Rheumatoid Arthritis Study/Early Rheumatoid Arthritis Network UK prospective cohorts. *Rheumatology, 57*(7), 1194–1202.

*Oh, H. S., Han, S. Y., Kim, S. H., et al. (2018). Development and validity testing of an arthritis self-management assessment tool. *Orthopaedic Nursing, 37*(1), 24–35.

Omma, A., Celik, S., Bes, C., et al. (2018). Short report: Correlates of functional ability with disease activity in elderly patients with rheumatoid arthritis. *Psychology Health & Medicine, 23*(5), 668–673.

Scheepers, L., van Onna, M., Stehouwer, C., et al. (2018). Medication adherence among patients with gout: A systematic review and meta-analysis. *Seminars in Arthritis and Rheumatism, 47*(2018), 689–702.

Seetharaman, M. (2019). Giant cell arteritis (temporal arteritis) workup. *Medscape.* Retrieved on 12/15/2019 at: emedicine.medscape.com/article/332483-workup

Singh, J. A., Saag, K. G., Bridges, S. L., et al. (2016). 2015 American College of Rheumatology guideline for treatment of rheumatoid arthritis. *Arthritis & Rheumatology, 68*(10), 1–26.

Young, T. (2019). Rheumatoid arthritis and its impact on ulceration and healing. *Wounds UK, 15*(4), 40–43.

Resources

American College of Rheumatology and Association of Rheumatology Health Professionals, www.rheumatology.org
American Fibromyalgia Syndrome Association (AFSA), www.afsafund.org
Arthritis Foundation, www.arthritis.org
Centers for Disease Control and Prevention, www.cdc.gov
Lupus Foundation of America, www.lupus.org
National Institute of Arthritis and Musculoskeletal and Skin Diseases, National Institutes of Health, www.niams.nih.gov
Scleroderma Foundation, www.scleroderma.org
Sjögren's Syndrome Foundation, www.sjogrens.org
Spondylitis Association of America, www.spondylitis.org

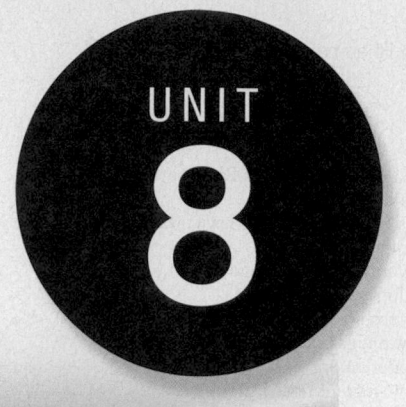

UNIT 8

Musculoskeletal Function

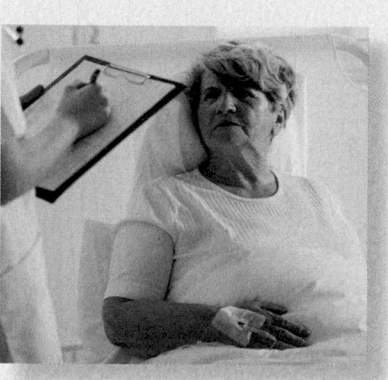

Case Study

IMPLEMENTING
EVIDENCE-BASED PRACTICE
IN PAIN MANAGEMENT

Y ou are a nurse working on an orthopedic unit caring for a 76-year-old female with osteoporosis who had fallen at home and underwent a right hip replacement. She is 2 days postoperative, recovering from her surgery without complications, and you are discussing plans for her transition to a skilled rehabilitation unit. However, the patient does not want to get out of bed and participate in physical or occupational therapy because she is in pain. Despite having spoken with the pain team, she states she does not want to take any medications that may cause her to become addicted. You need to develop an evidence-based plan of care that implements pharmacologic and nonpharmacologic strategies for pain management so the patient is able to participate in her physical and occupational therapies and thus help facilitate her recovery.

QSEN Competency Focus: Evidence-Based Practice (EBP)

The complexities inherent in today's health care system challenge nurses to demonstrate integration of specific interdisciplinary core competencies. These competencies are aimed at ensuring the delivery of safe, quality patient care (Institute of Medicine, 2003). The Quality and Safety Education for Nurses project (Cronenwett, Sherwood, Barnsteiner, et al., 2007; QSEN, 2020) provides a framework for the knowledge, skills, and attitudes (KSAs) required for nurses to demonstrate competency in these key areas, which include *patient-centered care*, *interdisciplinary teamwork and collaboration*, *evidence-based practice*, *quality improvement*, *safety*, and *informatics.*

Evidence-Based Practice Definition: Integrate best current evidence with clinical expertise and patient/family preferences and values for delivery of optimal health care.

SELECT PRE-LICENSURE KSAs	APPLICATION AND REFLECTION
Knowledge	
Explain the role of evidence in determining best clinical practice	Differentiate between evidence-based guidelines in managing acute postoperative pain verses chronic osteoporosis pain.
	Evidence-based practice guidelines include adherence to pharmacologic and nonpharmacologic interventions to promote recovery after surgery. How does managing the patient's pain reduce postoperative complications, including risk for blood clot, pneumonia, and gastric complications?
Skills	
Locate evidence reports related to clinical practice topics and guidelines	What additional strategies might you use to educate this patient on controlling acute postoperative pain? Differentiate between the various types of pain medications, including opioid and nonopioid analgesics, that are used to decrease pain.
	Evidence-based pain management includes the use of pain scales. Which scale would be the best to evaluate this patient's pain?
Attitudes	
Value the need for continuous improvement in clinical practice based on new knowledge	Reflect on your attitudes toward patients who are prescribed opioid medications postoperatively for pain control. Because this patient may have chronic pain due to her osteoporosis, how can your approach regarding acute and chronic pain management reflect evidence-based practice guidelines?

Cronenwett, L., Sherwood, G., Barnsteiner, J., et al. (2007). Quality and safety education for nurses. *Nursing Outlook, 55*(3), 122–131; Institute of Medicine. (2003). *Health professions education: A bridge to quality.* Washington, DC: National Academies Press; QSEN Institute. (2020). *QSEN Competencies: Definitions and pre-licensure KSAs: Evidence based practice.* Retrieved on 8/15/2020 at: qsen.org/competencies/pre-licensure-ksas/#evidence-based_practice

35 Assessment of Musculoskeletal Function

LEARNING OUTCOMES

On completion of this chapter, the learner will be able to:

1. Describe the basic structure and function of the musculoskeletal system.
2. Discuss the significance of the health history to the assessment of musculoskeletal health.
3. Recognize and evaluate the major manifestations of musculoskeletal dysfunction by applying concepts from the patient's health history and physical assessment findings.
4. Explain clinical indications, patient preparation, and other related nursing implications for common tests and procedures used to assess musculoskeletal function.

NURSING CONCEPTS

Assessment

Mobility

GLOSSARY

atonic: without tone; denervated muscle that atrophies

atrophy: decrease in the size of a muscle

bursa: fluid-filled sac found in connective tissue, usually in the area of joints

callus: cartilaginous/fibrous tissue at fracture site

cancellous bone: latticelike bone structure; trabecular bone

cartilage: tough, elastic, avascular tissue at ends of bone

clonus: rhythmic contractions of a muscle

contracture: abnormal shortening of muscle, joint, or both; fibrosis

cortical bone: compact bone

crepitus: grating or crackling sound or sensation; may occur with movement of ends of a broken bone or irregular joint surface

diaphysis: shaft of long bone

effusion: excess fluid in joint

endosteum: a thin, vascular membrane covering the marrow cavity of long bones and the spaces in cancellous bone

epiphysis: end of long bone

fascia: fibrous tissue that covers, supports, and separates muscles (*synonym:* epimysium)

fasciculation: involuntary twitch of muscle fibers

flaccid: limp; without muscle tone

hypertrophy: enlargement; increase in the size of a muscle

isometric contraction: muscle tension is increased without changing its length; there is no associated joint motion

isotonic contraction: muscle is shortened without a change in its tension; a joint is moved as a result

joint: area where bone ends meet; provides for motion and flexibility

joint capsule: fibrous tissue that encloses bone ends and other joint surfaces

kyphosis: increase in the convex curvature of the thoracic spine

lamellae: mature compact bone structures that form concentric rings of bone matrix; lamellar bone

ligament: ropelike bundles of collagen fibrils connecting bones

lordosis: increase in concave curvature of the lumbar spine

ossification: process in which minerals (calcium) are deposited in bone matrix

osteoblast: bone-forming cell

osteoclast: bone resorption cell

osteocyte: mature bone cell

osteogenesis: bone formation

osteon: microscopic functional bone unit

osteopenic: refers to a reduction in bone mass to below-normal levels

paresthesia: abnormal sensation (e.g., burning, tingling, numbness)

periosteum: fibrous connective tissue covering bone

remodeling: process that ensures bone maintenance through simultaneous bone resorption and formation

resorption: removal/destruction of tissue, such as bone
scoliosis: lateral curving of the spine
spastic: having greater-than-normal muscle tone
synovium: membrane in joint that secretes lubricating fluid

tendon: cord of fibrous tissue connecting muscle to bone
tone: normal tension (resistance to stretch) in resting muscle (*synonym:* tonus)
trabeculae: latticelike bone structure; cancellous bone

The musculoskeletal system is composed of the bones, joints, muscles, tendons, ligaments, and bursae of the body. The major functions of this system are to support and protect the body and foster movement of the extremities. The components of this system are highly integrated; therefore, disease in or injury to one component adversely affects the others. For instance, an infection in a joint (e.g., septic arthritis) causes degeneration of the articular surfaces of the bones within the joint and local muscle atrophy.

Musculoskeletal disorders and injuries directly affect the quality of life of individuals and are a leading cause of disability in the United States. The annual cost to treat these conditions is estimated to be over $980 billion for direct costs as well as indirect costs, such as lost wages from loss of work time (United States Bone and Joint Initiative [USBJI], 2018). Arthritis is the chief cause of musculoskeletal-related disability in the United States, with an estimated 54.4 million adults diagnosed with this disorder. Because the incidence of arthritis increases with age, the number of adults with arthritis is expected to increase to 78 million by 2040 (Centers for Disease Control and Prevention [CDC], 2019). Nurses in all practice areas may encounter patients with complaints about or impairment of the musculoskeletal system.

Anatomic and Physiologic Overview

The musculoskeletal system provides protection for vital organs, including the brain, heart, and lungs; serves as a framework to support body structures; and makes mobility possible. Muscles and tendons hold the bones together, and joints allow the body to move. They also move to produce heat that helps maintain body temperature. Movement facilitates the return of deoxygenated blood to the right side of the heart by massaging the venous vasculature. The musculoskeletal system serves as a reservoir for immature blood cells and essential minerals, including calcium, phosphorus, magnesium, and fluoride (Norris, 2019). More than 98% of total-body calcium is present in bone (National Institutes of Health [NIH], 2019a).

Structure and Function of the Skeletal System

There are 206 bones in the human body, divided into four categories classified by their shape: long, short, flat, and irregular. The long bones are found in the upper and lower extremities (e.g., the femur). Long bones are shaped like rods or shafts with rounded ends (Fig. 35-1). The shaft, known as the **diaphysis**, is primarily **cortical bone** (compact bone). The ends of the long bones, called **epiphyses**, are primarily **cancellous bone** (trabecular bone). During childhood and adolescence, there is a layer of cartilage known as the epiphyseal plate, or growth plate, that separates the epiphysis from the diaphysis. The epiphyseal plate nurtures and facilitates

longitudinal growth. The epiphyseal plate is calcified in adults. The ends of long bones are covered at the joints by articular **cartilage**, which is tough, elastic, and avascular tissue (Norris, 2019).

The short bones are the irregularly shaped bones located in the ankle and hand (e.g., metacarpals). The flat bones are located where extensive protection of underlying structures is needed (e.g., the sternum or skull). Finally, because of their shape, the irregular bones cannot be categorized in any other group and include bones such as the vertebrae and bones of the jaw.

The shape and construction of a specific bone are determined by its function and the forces exerted on it. Bones are constructed of cortical or cancellous bone tissue. Cortical bone exists in areas where support is needed, and cancellous bone is found where hematopoiesis and bone formation occur. For example, long bones are designed for weight bearing and movement and tend to be composed primarily of cortical bone, whereas flat bones, which are important sites of hematopoiesis and frequently protect vital organs, are made of cancellous bone layered between compact bone. Short bones consist of cancellous bone covered by a layer of cortical bone. Irregular bones have unique shapes related to their function. Generally, irregular bone structure is similar to that of flat bones (Norris, 2019).

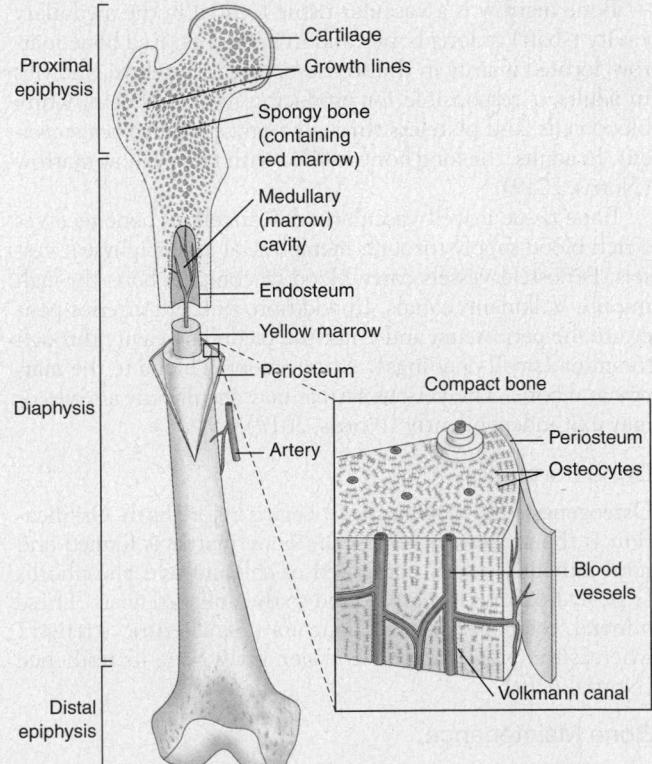

Figure 35-1 • Structure of a long bone; composition of compact bone.

Bone is composed of cells, protein matrix, and mineral deposits. The cells are of three basic types—osteoblasts, osteocytes, and osteoclasts. **Osteoblasts** function in bone formation by secreting bone matrix. The matrix consists of collagen and ground substances (glycoproteins and proteoglycans) that provide a framework in which inorganic mineral salts are deposited. These minerals are primarily composed of calcium and phosphorus. **Osteocytes** are mature bone cells involved in bone maintenance; they are located in lacunae (bone matrix units). **Osteoclasts**, located in shallow How-ship's lacunae (small pits in bones), are multinuclear cells involved in dissolving and resorbing bone. The microscopic functioning unit of mature cortical bone is the osteon, or haversian system. The center of the osteon—the haversian canal—contains a capillary. Around the capillary are circles of mineralized bone matrix called **lamellae**. Within the lamellae are lacunae that contain osteocytes. These are nourished through tiny structures called *canaliculi* (canals), which communicate with adjacent blood vessels within the haversian system. Lacunae in cancellous bone are layered in an irregular lattice network known as **trabeculae**. Red bone marrow fills the lattice network. Capillaries nourish the osteocytes located in the lacunae (Norris, 2019).

Covering the bone is a dense, fibrous membrane known as the **periosteum**. This membranous structure nourishes bone and facilitates its growth. The periosteum contains nerves, blood vessels, and lymphatics. It also provides for the attachment of tendons and ligaments (Norris, 2019).

The **endosteum** is a thin, vascular membrane that covers the marrow cavity of long bones and the spaces in cancellous bone. Osteoclasts, which dissolve bone matrix to maintain the marrow cavity, are located near the endosteum in How-ship's lacunae (Norris, 2019).

Bone marrow is a vascular tissue located in the medullary cavity (shaft) of long bones and in flat bones. Red bone marrow, located mainly in the sternum, ilium, vertebrae, and ribs in adults, is responsible for producing red blood cells, white blood cells, and platelets through a process called *hematopoiesis*. In adults, the long bone is filled with fatty, yellow marrow (Norris, 2019).

Bone tissue is well vascularized. Cancellous bone receives a rich blood supply through metaphyseal and epiphyseal vessels. Periosteal vessels carry blood to compact bone through minute Volkmann canals. In addition, nutrient arteries penetrate the periosteum and enter the medullary cavity through foramina (small openings). Arteries supply blood to the marrow and bone. The venous system may accompany arteries or may exit independently (Norris, 2019).

Bone Formation

Osteogenesis (bone formation) begins before birth. **Ossification** is the process by which the bone matrix is formed and hard mineral crystals composed of calcium and phosphorus (e.g., hydroxyapatite) are bound to the collagen fibers. These mineral components give bone its characteristic strength, whereas the proteinaceous collagen gives bone its resilience (Norris, 2019).

Bone Maintenance

Bone is a dynamic tissue in a constant state of turnover. Throughout the lifespan, a process known as bone **remodeling** occurs, in which old bone is removed and new bone is added to the skeleton (formation). During childhood and the teenage years, new bone is added faster than old bone is removed; therefore, bones become larger, heavier, and denser. This continues until peak bone mass is reached, typically by age 20 years. Remodeling maintains bone structure and function through simultaneous resorption and osteogenesis, and as a result, complete skeletal turnover occurs every 10 years (Norris, 2019).

The balance between bone **resorption** (removal or destruction) and formation is influenced by the following factors: physical activity; dietary intake of certain nutrients, especially calcium; and several hormones, including calcitriol (i.e., activated vitamin D), parathyroid hormone (PTH), calcitonin, thyroid hormone, cortisol, growth hormone, and the sex hormones estrogen and testosterone (Norris, 2019).

Physical activity, particularly weight-bearing activity, acts to stimulate bone formation and remodeling. Bones subjected to continued weight bearing tend to be thick and strong. Conversely, people who are unable to engage in regular weight-bearing activities, such as those on prolonged bed rest or those with some physical disabilities, have increased bone resorption from calcium loss, and their bones become **osteopenic** (reduced in terms of mass) and weak. These weakened bones may fracture easily (Meiner & Yeager, 2019).

Good dietary habits are integral to bone health. Daily intake of approximately 1000 to 1200 mg of calcium is essential to maintaining adult bone mass. Quality sources of calcium include low-fat milk, yogurt, and cheese. Foods with added calcium such as orange juice, cereals, and bread are also beneficial (NIH, 2019a). Vitamin D also plays a major role in calcium absorption and bone health. Young adults need a daily vitamin D intake of 600 IU, whereas adults 50 years and older require a daily intake of 800 to 1000 IU to ensure good bone health (NIH, 2019b). Dietary sources of vitamin D include vitamin D–fortified milk and cereals, egg yolks, saltwater fish, and liver.

Several hormones are vital in ensuring that calcium is properly absorbed and available for bone mineralization and matrix formation. Calcitriol functions to increase the amount of calcium in the blood by promoting absorption of calcium from the gastrointestinal tract. It also facilitates mineralization of osteoid tissue. A deficiency of vitamin D results in bone mineralization deficit, deformity, and fracture (Norris, 2019).

PTH and calcitonin are the major hormonal regulators of calcium homeostasis. PTH regulates the concentration of calcium in the blood, in part by promoting movement of calcium from the bone. In response to low calcium levels in the blood, increased levels of PTH prompt the mobilization of calcium, the demineralization of bone, and the formation of bone cysts. Calcitonin, secreted by the thyroid gland in response to elevated blood calcium levels, inhibits bone resorption and increases the deposit of calcium in bone (Norris, 2019).

Both thyroid hormone and cortisol have multiple systemic effects with specific effects on bones. Excessive thyroid hormone production in adults (e.g., Graves' disease) can result in increased bone resorption and decreased bone formation. Increased levels of cortisol have these same effects. Patients receiving long-term synthetic cortisol or corticosteroids (e.g., prednisone) are at increased risk for steroid-induced osteopenia and fractures.

Growth hormone has direct and indirect effects on skeletal growth and remodeling. It stimulates the liver and, to a lesser degree, the bones to produce insulinlike growth factor 1 (IGF-I), which accelerates bone modeling in children and adolescents. Growth hormone also directly stimulates skeletal growth in children and adolescents. It is believed that the low levels of both growth hormone and IGF-I that occur with aging may be partly responsible for decreased bone formation and resultant osteopenia (Norris, 2019).

The sex hormones testosterone and estrogen have important effects on bone remodeling. Estrogen stimulates osteoblasts and inhibits osteoclasts; therefore, bone formation is enhanced and resorption is inhibited. Testosterone has both direct and indirect effects on bone growth and formation. It directly causes skeletal growth in adolescence and has continued effects on skeletal muscle growth throughout the lifespan. Increased muscle mass results in greater weight-bearing stress on bones, resulting in increased bone formation. In addition, testosterone converts to estrogen in adipose tissue, providing an additional source of bone-preserving estrogen for aging men (Kennedy-Malone, Martin-Plank, & Duffy, 2019).

During the process of bone remodeling, osteoblasts produce a receptor for activated nuclear factor-kappa B ligand (RANKL) that binds to the receptor for activated nuclear factor-kappa B (RANK) present on the cell membranes of osteoclast precursors, causing them to differentiate and mature into osteoclasts, which causes bone resorption. Conversely, osteoblasts may produce osteoprotegerin (OPG), which blocks the effects of RANKL, thereby turning off the process of bone resorption. T cells that may become activated as a result of the inflammatory process may also produce RANKL, overriding the effects of OPG and causing continued bone resorption during times of stress and injury, which can lead to loss of bone matrix and fractures (Takeno, Kanazawa, Notsu, et al., 2018).

Blood supply to the bone also affects bone formation. With diminished blood supply or hyperemia (congestion), osteogenesis, and bone density decrease. Bone necrosis occurs when the bone is deprived of blood (Norris, 2019).

Bone Healing

Most fractures heal through a combination of intramembranous and endochondral ossification processes. When a bone is fractured, the bone begins a healing process to reestablish continuity and strength. The bone fragments are not patched together with scar tissue; instead, the bone regenerates itself.

Fracture healing occurs in the bone marrow, where endothelial cells rapidly differentiate into osteoblasts; in the bone cortex, where new osteons are formed; in the periosteum, where a hard **callus** (fibrous tissue) is formed through intramembranous ossification peripheral to the fracture, and where cartilage is formed through endochondral ossification adjacent to the fracture site; and in adjacent soft tissue, where a bridging callus forms that provides stability to the fractured bones (Norris, 2019).

When a fracture occurs, the body's response is similar to that after injury elsewhere in the body. The repair of a simple fracture occurs in essentially four stages. These include the following (Norris, 2019):

Stage I: Hematoma formation occurs during the first 1 to 2 days of the fracture. Bleeding into the injured tissue and local vasoconstriction occur, and a hematoma forms at the site of the fracture. Cytokines are released, initiating the fracture healing processes by causing replicating cells known as fibroblasts to proliferate, which in turn causes angiogenesis to occur (i.e., the growth of new blood vessels). Granulation tissue begins to form within the clot and becomes dense. At the same time, degranulated platelets and inflammatory cells release growth factor, which stimulates the generation of osteoclasts and osteoblasts.

Stage II: Inflammatory phase occurs with the formation of granulation tissue. Fibroblasts and osteoblasts migrate into the fractured site and begin the reconstruction of bone. The fibroblasts produce a fibrocartilaginous soft callus bridge that connects the bone fragments. Although tissue repair may reach maximum girth by the end of the second or third week, it is still not strong enough for weight bearing.

Stage III: Reparative phase usually begins during the third or fourth week of fracture healing and continues until a firm bony union is formed. During this stage, mature bone gradually replaces the fibrocartilaginous callus and the excess callus is gradually reabsorbed by the osteoclasts. During this stage, the fracture site feels immovable and appears aligned on x-ray. At this time, it is usually safe to remove a cast, if one is present.

Stage IV: Remodeling occurs as necrotic bone is removed by the osteoclasts. Compact bone replaces spongy bone around the periphery of the fracture. Although the final structure of the remodeled bone resembles the original unbroken bone, a thickened area on the surface of the bone may remain after healing. Remodeling may take months to years, depending on the extent of bone modification needed, the function of the bone, and the functional stresses on the bone.

Serial x-rays are used to monitor the progress of bone healing. The type of bone fractured, the adequacy of blood supply, the condition of the fracture fragments, the immobility of the fracture site, and the age and general health of the person influence the rate of fracture healing. Adequate immobilization is essential until there is x-ray evidence of bone formation with ossification (Norris, 2019).

When fractures are treated with internal or external fixation techniques, the bony fragments can be placed in direct contact. Primary bone healing occurs through cortical bone (haversian) remodeling. Little or no cartilaginous callus develops. Immature bone develops from the endosteum. There is an intensive regeneration of new osteons, which develop in the fracture line by a process similar to normal bone maintenance. Fracture strength is obtained when the new osteons have become established (Norris, 2019).

Structure and Function of the Articular System

The junction of two or more bones is called a **joint,** or articulation. There are three basic kinds of joints: synarthrosis, amphiarthrosis, and diarthrosis joints. Synarthrosis joints, also referred to as fibrous joints, are immovable because of fibrous tissue banding (e.g., the skull sutures). Amphiarthrosis joints, also referred to as cartilaginous joints, allow limited motion (e.g., the vertebral joints and the symphysis pubis). Diarthrosis joints, also referred to as synovial joints, are freely movable joints (Fig. 35-2).

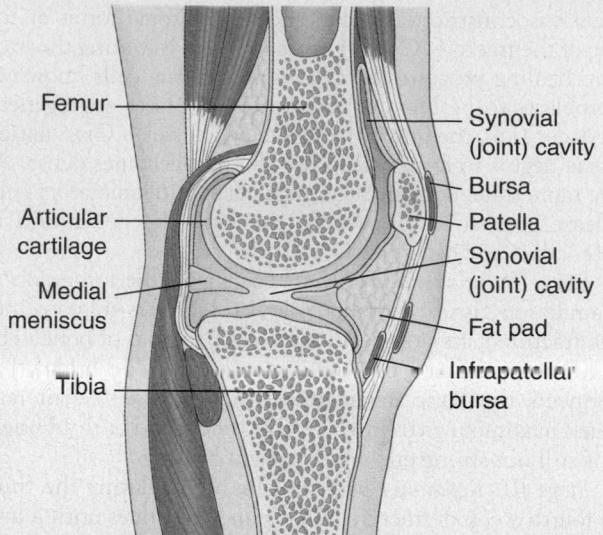

Femur
Articular cartilage
Medial meniscus
Tibia

Synovial (joint) cavity
Bursa
Patella
Synovial (joint) cavity
Fat pad
Infrapatellar bursa

Figure 35-2 • Hinge joint of the knee.

There are several types of diarthrosis joints:

- *Ball-and-socket joints* (e.g., the hip and the shoulder) permit full freedom of movement.
- *Hinge joints* permit bending in only one direction, either flexion or extension (e.g., the elbow and the knee).
- *Saddle joints* allow movement in two planes at right angles to each other. The joint at the base of the thumb is a saddle, biaxial joint.
- *Pivot joints* allow one bone to move around a central axis without displacement. An example of a pivot joint is the articulation between the radius and the ulna. They permit rotation for such activities as turning a doorknob.
- *Gliding joints* allow for limited movement in all directions and are represented by the joints of the carpal bones in the wrist.

The ends of the articulating bones of a typical movable joint are covered with smooth hyaline cartilage. A tough, fibrous sheath called the **joint capsule** surrounds the articulating bones. The capsule is lined with a membrane, the **synovium**, which secretes the lubricating and shock-absorbing synovial fluid into the joint capsule. Therefore, the bone surfaces are not in direct contact. In some synovial joints (e.g., the knee), fibrocartilage discs (e.g., medial meniscus) are located between the articular cartilage surfaces. These discs provide shock absorption (Bickley, 2017).

Ligaments (ropelike bundles of collagen fibrils) bind the articulating bones together. **Tendons** are cords of fibrous tissue that connect muscle to bone. Ligaments and tendons, which pass over the joint, provide joint stability. In some joints, interosseous ligaments (e.g., the cruciate ligaments of the knee) are found within the capsule and add anterior and posterior stability to the joint. Ligaments are pliable enough to allow movement of the joints; however, they can tear rather than stretch if they are subjected to excess stress (Norris, 2019).

A **bursa** is a sac filled with synovial fluid that cushions the movement of tendons, ligaments, and bones over bones or other joint structures. Bursae can be found in the joints of the elbow, shoulder, hip, and knee. They may become inflamed, causing discomfort, swelling, and limited movement in that area.

Structure and Function of the Skeletal Muscle System

Muscles are attached by tendons to bones, connective tissue, other muscles, soft tissue, or skin. The muscles of the body are composed of parallel groups of muscle cells (fasciculi) encased in fibrous tissue called **fascia** (epimysium). The more fasciculi contained in a muscle, the more precise the movements. Muscles vary in shape and size according to the activities for which they are responsible. Skeletal (striated) muscles are involved in body movement, posture, and heat-production functions. Muscles contract to bring the two points of attachment closer together, resulting in movement (Norris, 2019).

Skeletal Muscle Contraction

Each muscle cell (also referred to as a muscle fiber) contains myofibrils, which in turn are composed of a series of sarcomeres—the actual contractile units of skeletal muscle. Sarcomeres contain thick myosin and thin actin filaments.

Muscle cells contract in response to electrical stimulation delivered by an effector nerve cell at the motor end-plate. When stimulated, the muscle cell depolarizes and generates an action potential in a manner similar to that described for nerve cells. These action potentials propagate along the muscle cell membrane and lead to the release of calcium ions that are stored in a specialized organelle called *sarcoplasmic reticulum*. When there is a local increase in calcium ion concentration, the myosin and actin filaments slide across one another. Shortly after the muscle cell membrane is depolarized, it recovers its resting membrane voltage. Calcium is rapidly removed from the sarcomeres by active reaccumulation in the sarcoplasmic reticulum. When the calcium concentration in the sarcomere decreases, the myosin and actin filaments cease to interact, and the sarcomere returns to its original resting length (relaxation). Actin and myosin do not interact in the absence of calcium (Norris, 2019).

The contraction of muscle fibers can result in either isotonic or isometric contraction of the muscle. In **isometric contraction**, the length of the muscles remains constant but the force generated by the muscles is increased; an example of this is pushing against an immovable wall. **Isotonic contraction** is characterized by the shortening of the muscle without an increase in tension within the muscle; an example of this is flexing the forearm. In normal activities, many muscle movements are a combination of isometric and isotonic contraction. For example, during walking, isotonic contraction results in shortening of the leg, and isometric contraction causes the stiff leg to push against the floor.

Energy is consumed during muscle contraction and relaxation. The main source of energy for the muscle cells is adenosine triphosphate (ATP), which is generated through cellular oxidative metabolism. At low levels of activity (i.e., sedentary activity), the skeletal muscle synthesizes ATP from the oxidation of glucose to water and carbon dioxide. During periods of strenuous activity, when sufficient oxygen may not be available, glucose is metabolized primarily to lactic acid, an inefficient process compared with that of oxidative pathways. Stored muscle glycogen is used to supply glucose during periods of activity. Muscle fatigue is thought to be caused by depletion of glycogen and accumulation of lactic acid. As a result, the cycle of muscle contraction and relaxation cannot continue (Norris, 2019).

During muscle contraction, the energy released from ATP is not completely used. The excess energy is dissipated in the form of heat. During isometric contraction, almost all of the energy is released in the form of heat; during isotonic contraction, some of the energy is expended in mechanical work. In some situations (i.e., shivering), the need to generate heat is the main stimulus for muscle contraction.

The speed of the muscle contraction is variable. Myoglobulin is a hemoglobinlike protein pigment present in striated muscle cells that transports oxygen. Muscles containing large quantities of myoglobulin (red muscles) have been observed to contract slowly and powerfully (e.g., respiratory and postural muscles). Muscles containing little myoglobulin (white muscles) contract quickly (e.g., extraocular eye muscles). Most muscles contain both red and white muscle fibers (Norris, 2019).

Muscle Tone

Muscle **tone** (tonus) is produced by the maintenance of some of the muscle fibers in a contracted state. Muscle spindles, which are sense organs in the muscles, monitor muscle tone. Muscle tone is minimal during sleep and is increased when the person is anxious. A muscle that is limp and without tone is described as **flaccid**; a muscle with greater-than-normal tone is described as **spastic**. Typically, upper motor neuron lesions produce increased tone, whereas lower motor neuron lesions produce decreased tone. For example, in conditions characterized by upper motor neuron destruction (e.g., cerebral palsy), muscle becomes hypertonic and reflexes become hyperactive. In contrast, conditions characterized by lower motor neuron destruction (e.g., muscular dystrophy), denervated muscle becomes **atonic** (soft and flabby) and atrophies (Norris, 2019). See Chapter 60, Table 60-4, for a comparison of upper and lower motor function.

Muscle Actions

Muscle contraction produces movement. The body is able to perform a wide variety of movements as a result of the coordination of muscle groups (Fig. 35-3). The prime mover is the muscle that causes a particular motion. The muscles assisting the prime mover are known as synergists. The muscles causing movement opposite to that of the prime mover are known as antagonists. An antagonist must relax to allow the prime mover to contract, producing motion. For example, when contraction of the biceps causes flexion of the elbow joint, the biceps are the prime movers and the triceps are the antagonists. A person with muscle paralysis (i.e., loss of movement) may be able to retrain functioning muscles within the synergistic group to produce the needed movement. Muscles of the synergistic group then become the prime movers (Norris, 2019).

Exercise, Disuse, and Repair

Muscles need exercise to maintain function and strength. When a muscle repeatedly develops maximum or close to maximum tension over a long time, as in regular exercise with weights, the cross-sectional area of the muscle increases. This enlargement, known as **hypertrophy**, results from an increase in the size of individual muscle fibers without an increase in their number. Hypertrophy persists only if the exercise is continued. The opposite phenomenon occurs with disuse of muscle over a long period of time. Age and disuse cause loss of muscular function as fibrotic tissue replaces the contractile muscle tissue. The decrease in the size of a muscle is called **atrophy**. Bed rest and immobility cause loss of muscle mass and strength. When immobility is the result of a treatment modality (e.g., casting, traction, or bed rest), the patient can decrease the effects of immobility by isometric exercise of the muscles of the immobilized part. Quadriceps contraction exercises (tightening the muscles of the thigh) and gluteal setting exercises (tightening of the muscles of the buttocks) help maintain the larger muscle groups that are important in ambulation. Active and weight-resistance exercises of uninjured parts of the body maintain muscle strength. When muscles are injured, they need rest and immobilization until tissue repair occurs. The healed muscle then needs progressive exercise to resume its pre-injury strength and functional ability.

 Gerontologic Considerations

Multiple changes in the musculoskeletal system occur with aging (Table 35-1) and bring complaints of pain and joint limitations. There is a loss of height due to osteoporosis (abnormal excessive bone loss), kyphosis (forward curvature of the thoracic spine), thinned intervertebral discs, compressed vertebral bodies, and flexion of the knees and hips. Numerous metabolic changes, including menopausal withdrawal of estrogen and decreased activity, contribute to osteoporosis (National Osteoporosis Foundation [NOF], 2019). Women lose more bone mass than men. In addition, bones change in shape and have reduced strength. Fractures are common. Collagen structures are less able to absorb energy. Increased inactivity, diminished neuron stimulation, and nutritional deficiencies contribute to the loss of muscle strength. In addition, remote musculoskeletal problems for which the patient has compensated may become new problems with age-related changes. For example, people who have had polio and who have been able to function normally by using synergistic muscle groups may discover increasing incapacity because of a reduced compensatory ability. Older adults may suffer from chronic musculoskeletal disorders that limit mobility and interfere with their ability to perform self-care. This may lead older adults to depend on others for completion of their activities of daily living (ADLs); in turn, they may grieve over the loss of independence. In particular, musculoskeletal disorders of the hand and wrist are prevalent among older adults; and, the incidence of these disorders increases with increasing age (Leow, Teo, Low, et al., 2019) (see Nursing Research Profile: Hand Assessment of Older Adults in Chart 35-1). Despite a multitude of age-related musculoskeletal changes, the many effects of aging can be slowed if the body is kept healthy and active through positive lifestyle behaviors (Eliopoulos, 2018).

Assessment

The nursing assessment of the patient with musculoskeletal dysfunction includes a health history and physical examination that evaluate the effects of the musculoskeletal disorder on the patient.

(text continued on page 1104)

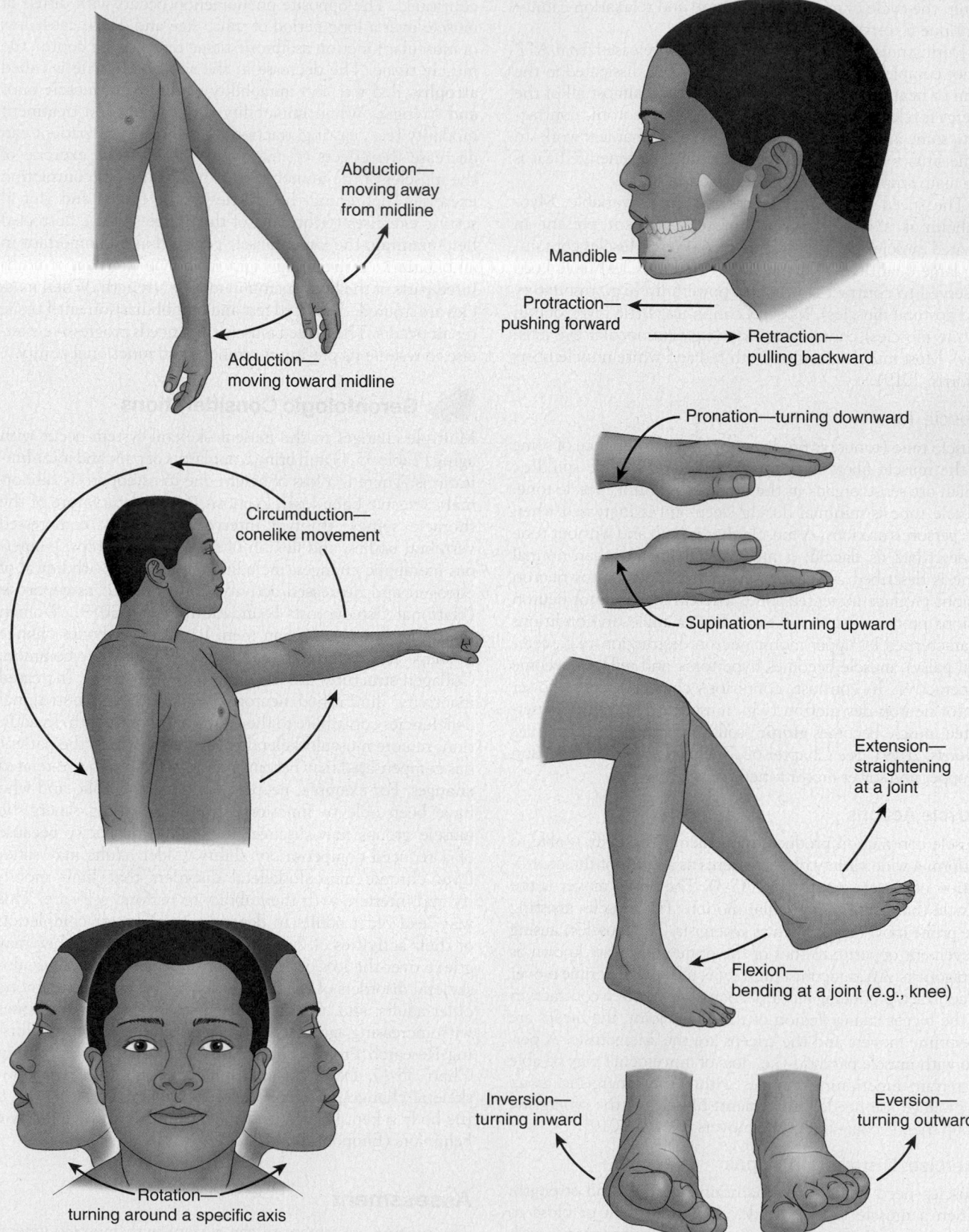

Abduction—moving away from midline

Adduction—moving toward midline

Mandible

Protraction—pushing forward

Retraction—pulling backward

Pronation—turning downward

Supination—turning upward

Circumduction—conelike movement

Extension—straightening at a joint

Flexion—bending at a joint (e.g., knee)

Inversion—turning inward

Eversion—turning outward

Rotation—turning around a specific axis

Figure 35-3 • Body movements produced by muscle contraction.

TABLE 35-1 Age-Related Changes of the Musculoskeletal System

Musculoskeletal System	Structural Changes	Functional Changes	History and Physical Findings
Bones	Gradual, progressive loss of bone mass after 30 y of age Vertebral collapse	Bones fragile and prone to fracture—vertebrae, hip, wrist	Loss of height Postural changes Kyphosis Loss of flexibility Flexion of hips and knees Back pain Osteoporosis Fracture
Muscles	Increase in collagen and resultant fibrosis Muscles atrophy (diminish in size); wasting Tendons less elastic	Loss of strength and flexibility Weakness Fatigue Stumbling Falls	Loss of strength Diminished agility Decreased endurance Prolonged response time (diminished reaction time) Diminished tone Broad base of support History of falls
Joints	Cartilage—progressive deterioration Thinning of intervertebral discs	Stiffness, reduced flexibility, and pain interfere with activities of daily living	Diminished range of motion Stiffness Loss of height
Ligaments	Lax ligaments (less-than-normal strength; weakness)	Postural joint abnormality Weakness	Joint pain on motion; resolves with rest Crepitus Joint swelling/enlargement Osteoarthritis (degenerative joint disease)

Chart 35-1 — NURSING RESEARCH PROFILE

Hand Assessment of Older Adults

Leow, M. Q., Teo, W., Low, T. L., et al. (2019). Hand assessment for elderly people in the community. *Orthopaedic Nursing, 38*(1), 25–30.

Purpose

Hand and wrist disorders are common, particularly among older adults. These disorders typically include osteoarthritis, trigger finger, and carpal tunnel syndrome. These conditions can cause significant pain, stiffness, numbness, and decreased range of motion in the affected extremity. Early treatment may mitigate the detrimental effects of these disorders; yet, treatment is uncommon until later, when there is a disruption in the patient's activities of daily living (ADLs). The purpose of this study was to evaluate the prevalence of these hand disorders among older adults in a community setting.

Design

This descriptive study solicited participation from older adults who frequented a neighborhood day center in Singapore. All eligible participants were independent in completing their ADLs. Demographic information, a brief health history, hand and wrist assessments, and grip and pinch strength were obtained from all participants. Questionnaires completed by participants included the 11-item QuickDASH questionnaire, a psychometrically validated tool for assessing functional ability of the upper extremities, and a numeric pain intensity scale score that assessed hand and wrist pain. Assessments were conducted specifically for participants who were experiencing symptoms associated with

osteoarthritis, trigger finger, and carpal tunnel syndrome. Fifty-five older adults participated in this study.

Findings

Participants (N = 55) ranged in age from 60 to 90 years with a mean age of 74 years. The majority of participants were female (n = 41). Nearly one third of participants presented with a hand condition (n = 17); 11 had osteoarthritis, one had trigger finger, three had carpal tunnel syndrome, and two had both trigger finger and carpal tunnel. Hand disorders were more prevalent in female participants than in males (39% in females, 7% in males). Of those with hand disorders, 34.5% reported difficulty in doing household chores, 21.8% had difficulty opening jars, and 21.8% reported difficulty participating in recreational activities that required arm, shoulder, or hand strength. This study found that participants who had an abnormal hand assessment finding did not seek medical attention until these conditions impacted their ADLs.

Nursing Implications

Findings from this study suggest that hand and wrist disorders are indeed commonplace among community-dwelling older adults; yet most study participants had not previously sought medical treatment for their disorders. Nurses may develop screening programs for hand and wrist disorders in older adults with the tools used in this study. Screening older adults for early-stage hand and wrist disorders can lead to timely and effective treatment that can preserve function and assist the older adult to maintain independence in ADLs.

Health History

An important aspect of a musculoskeletal assessment is the history of the present illness. Musculoskeletal disorders may be stable or progressive, characterized by symptom-free periods as well as fluctuations in symptoms. The health history therefore includes details about the onset, character, severity, location, duration, and frequency of symptoms and signs; associated complaints; precipitating, aggravating, and relieving factors; progression, remission, and exacerbation; and the presence or absence of similar symptoms among family members.

Common Symptoms

During the interview and physical assessment, the patient with a musculoskeletal disorder may report pain, tenderness, and altered sensations (Weber & Kelley, 2018).

Pain

Most patients with diseases and traumatic conditions or disorders of the muscles, bones, and joints experience pain. Bone pain is typically described as a dull, deep ache that is "boring" in nature. This pain is not typically related to movement and may interfere with sleep. Muscular pain is described as soreness or aching and is referred to as "muscle cramps." Fracture pain is sharp and piercing and is relieved by immobilization. Sharp pain may also result from bone infection with muscle spasm or pressure on a sensory nerve. Joint pain is felt around or in the joint and typically worsens with movement (Kennedy-Malone et al., 2019).

Rest relieves most musculoskeletal pain. Pain that increases with activity may indicate joint sprain, muscle strain, or compartment syndrome, whereas steadily increasing pain points to the progression of an infectious process (osteomyelitis), a malignant tumor, or neurovascular complications. Radiating pain occurs in conditions in which pressure is exerted on a nerve root (Kennedy-Malone et al., 2019).

The time of day that the pain occurs may be important to evaluate. Those experiencing pain with an inflammatory rheumatic disorder experience pain that is worse in the morning, especially upon waking. Tendonitis worsens during the early morning and eases by midday, whereas osteoarthritis worsens as the day progresses (Kennedy-Malone et al., 2019). Pain is variable, and its assessment and nursing management must be individualized.

The nurse assesses the patient's pain as described in Chapter 9. Specific assessments that the nurse should make regarding the pain include the following:

- Is the body in proper alignment?
- Are the joints symmetrical or are bony deformities present?
- Is there any inflammation or arthritis, swelling, warmth, tenderness, or redness?
- Is there pressure from traction, bed linens, a cast, or other appliances?
- Is there tension on the skin at a pin site?

The patient's pain and discomfort must be managed successfully. Not only is pain exhausting, but also, if prolonged, it can force the patient to become increasingly withdrawn and dependent on others as the musculoskeletal disorder continues.

Altered Sensations

Sensory disturbances are frequently associated with musculoskeletal problems. The patient may describe **paresthesias,** which are sensations of burning, tingling, or numbness. These sensations may be caused by pressure on nerves or by circulatory impairment. Soft tissue swelling or direct trauma to these structures can impair their function. The nurse assesses the neurovascular status of the involved musculoskeletal area.

Questions that the nurse should ask regarding altered sensations include the following:

- Is the patient experiencing abnormal sensations, such as burning, tingling, or numbness?
- If the abnormal sensation involves an extremity, how does this feeling compare to sensation in the unaffected extremity?
- When did the condition begin? Is it getting worse?
- Does the patient also have pain? (If the patient has pain, then the questions and assessments for pain discussed previously should be followed.)

Past Health, Social, and Family History

When assessing the musculoskeletal system, the nurse should gather pertinent data to include in the patient's health history, such as occupation (e.g., does the patient's work require physical activity or heavy lifting?), exercise patterns, alcohol consumption, tobacco use, and dietary intake (e.g., calcium, vitamin D). Concurrent health conditions (e.g., diabetes, heart disease, chronic obstructive pulmonary disease, infection, preexisting disability) and related problems (e.g., familial or genetic abnormalities; see Chart 35-2) need to be considered when developing and implementing the plan of care. Any previous history of trauma or injury to the musculoskeletal system or a history of falls should be included as well (Weber & Kelley, 2018).

The Fracture Risk Assessment Tool (FRAX®)

The Fracture Risk Assessment Tool (FRAX®) was developed in 2008 by a task force convened by the World Health Organization (WHO). It is a tool that predicts a patient's 10-year risk of fracturing a hip or other major bone, which includes the spine, forearm, or shoulder (NOF, 2019). The tool may be accessed online, where it automatically calculates a patient's odds of fracture. Data entered are validated risks for fracture, and include:

- age (risk increases with increasing age)
- gender (risk is higher in females)
- body mass index (risk is higher with lower body mass indices)
- history of a previous fracture
- parental history of hip fracture
- current cigarette smoker
- current use of a corticosteroid (e.g., prednisone)
- history of rheumatoid arthritis
- alcohol intake of 3 or more drinks per day
- history of secondary causes/risks for osteoporosis, which include any of the following:
  - type 1 diabetes
  - osteogenesis imperfecta
  - untreated long-standing hyperthyroidism
  - hypogonadism or premature menopause
  - chronic malnutrition or malabsorption syndromes
  - chronic liver disease

Chart 35-2 GENETICS IN NURSING PRACTICE
Musculoskeletal Disorders

Genetic musculoskeletal disorders vary in presentation and can tend to present at different points in time across the lifespan. Consideration must be given to other genetic disorders that will impact the musculoskeletal system. Some examples of inherited genetic musculoskeletal disorders include:

Autosomal Dominant:

- Achondroplasia
- Nail–Patella syndrome
- Osteogenesis imperfecta
- Polydactyly
- van der Woude syndrome

Autosomal Recessive:

- Tay-Sachs

Forms of Muscular Dystrophy:

- Becker muscular dystrophy
- Congenital muscular dystrophy
- Distal muscular dystrophy
- Duchenne muscular dystrophy (X-linked)
- Emery–Dreifuss muscular dystrophy (X-linked)
- Facioscapulohumeral muscular dystrophy (autosomal dominant)
- Limb–girdle muscular dystrophy (autosomal dominant and autosomal recessive forms)

Other genetic disorders that impact the musculoskeletal system:

- Amyotrophic lateral sclerosis (neurologic disorder)
- Ehlers–Danlos syndrome (connective tissue disorder)
- Marfan syndrome (connective tissue disorder)
- Spina bifida (neurologic disorder)
- Stickler syndrome (connective tissue disorder)

Nursing Assessments

See Chapter 4, Chart 4-2 for Genetics in Nursing Practice: Genetic Aspects of Health Assessment.

Family History Assessment Related to Genetic Musculoskeletal Disorders

- Assess for other similarly affected family members in the past three generations.
- Assess for the presence of other related genetic conditions (e.g., hematologic, cardiac, integumentary conditions).
- Determine the age at onset (e.g., fractures present at birth such as osteogenesis imperfecta, hip dislocation present at birth in DDH, or early-onset osteoporosis).

Patient Assessment Specific to Genetic Musculoskeletal Disorders

- Assess stature for general screening purposes (unusually short stature may be related to achondroplasia; unusually tall stature may be related to Marfan syndrome).
- Assess for disease-specific skeletal findings (e.g., pectus excavatum, scoliosis, long fingers [Marfan syndrome], osteoarthritis of the hip or waddling gait).
- Assessment findings that could indicate a genetic musculoskeletal disorder include:
  - Bone pain
  - Enlarged hands or feet
  - Excessive height, short stature, or decrease in height
  - Flat feet or highly arched feet
  - Frequency of bone-related injuries or unexplained fractures
  - Hypermobility of joints
  - Large or small head circumference
  - Protruding jaw or forehead
  - Unexplained changes in muscle tone (hypotonia)

Genetic Resources

The National Osteoporosis Foundation, www.nof.org
NIH Osteoporosis and Related Bone Diseases National Resource Center, www.niams.nih.gov/Health_Info/Bone
See Chapter 6, Chart 6-7 for components of genetic counseling.
DDH, developmental dysplasia of the hip(s)

An additional validated risk factor that may be entered into the FRAX® is the patient's bone mineral density (BMD), based on bone densitometry results, if those results are hip based (see later discussion). However, while entering BMD results in the FRAX® provides a more accurate fracture risk calculation, it is not necessary (Bickley, 2017). Thus, the FRAX® provides a good estimate of fracture risk in patients who may not have submitted to BMD testing. Patients who should be assessed for hip or major bone fracture risk include men and postmenopausal women over the age of 50, patients with known low BMD, and patients with known secondary causes/risks for osteoporosis. See Chapter 36 for further discussion of osteoporosis.

Physical Assessment

An examination of the musculoskeletal system ranges from a basic assessment of functional capabilities to sophisticated physical examination maneuvers that facilitate diagnosis of specific bone, muscle, and joint disorders. The extent of assessment depends on the patient's physical complaints, health history, and physical clues that warrant further exploration. The nursing assessment is primarily a functional evaluation, focusing on the patient's ability to perform ADLs.

Techniques of inspection and palpation are used to evaluate the patient's posture, gait, bone integrity, joint function, and muscle strength and size. In addition, assessing the skin and neurovascular status is an important part of a complete musculoskeletal assessment. The nurse should also understand and be able to perform correct assessment techniques on patients with musculoskeletal trauma. When specific symptoms or physical findings of musculoskeletal dysfunction are apparent, the nurse carefully documents the examination findings and shares the information with the primary provider, who may decide that a more extensive examination and a diagnostic evaluation are necessary.

Posture

The normal curvature of the spine is convex through the thoracic portion and concave through the cervical and lumbar portions. Common deformities of the spine include **kyphosis**, which is an increased forward curvature of the thoracic spine that causes a bowing or rounding of the back, leading to a hunchback or slouching posture. The second deformity of the spine is referred to as **lordosis**, or swayback, an exaggerated curvature of the lumbar spine. A third deformity is **scoliosis**, which is a lateral curving deviation of the spine (Fig. 35-4).

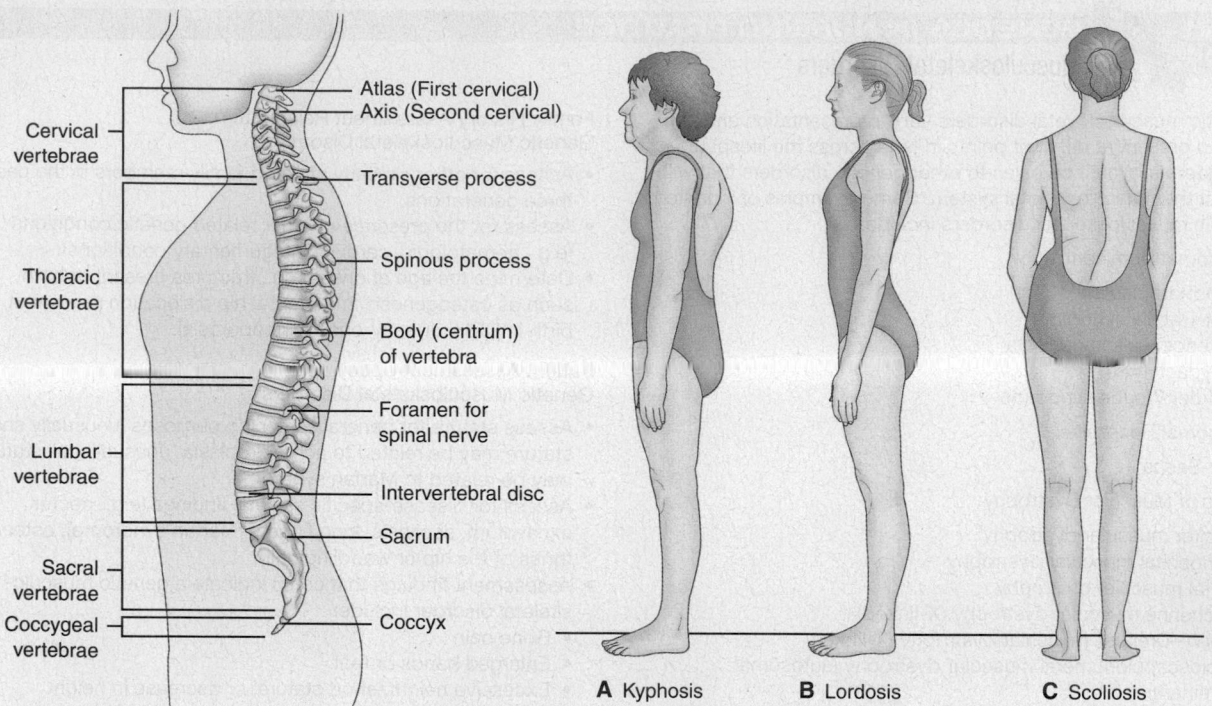

Figure 35-4 • A normal spine and three abnormalities. **A.** Kyphosis: an increased convexity or roundness of the spine's thoracic curve. **B.** Lordosis: swayback; exaggeration of the lumbar spine curve. **C.** Scoliosis: a lateral curvature of the spine.

Kyphosis can occur at any age and may be caused by degenerative diseases of the spine (e.g., arthritis or disc degeneration), fractures related to osteoporosis, and injury or trauma (Meiner & Yeager, 2019). It may also be seen in patients with other neuromuscular disease. Lordosis can affect people of any age. Common causes of lordosis include tight low back muscles, excessive visceral fat, and pregnancy as the woman adjusts her posture in response to changes in her center of gravity. Scoliosis may be congenital, idiopathic (without an identifiable cause), or the result of damage to the paraspinal muscles (e.g., muscular dystrophy).

During inspection of the spine, the entire back, buttocks, and legs are exposed. The examiner inspects the spinal curves and trunk symmetry from posterior and lateral views. Standing behind the patient, the examiner notes any differences in the height of the shoulders or iliac crests. Shoulder and hip symmetry, as well as the line of the vertebral column, is inspected with the patient erect and with the patient bending forward (flexion). Scoliosis is evidenced by an abnormal lateral curve in the spine; shoulders that are not level; an asymmetric waistline; and a prominent scapula, which is accentuated by bending forward. The examiner should then instruct the patient to bend backward (extension) with the examiner supporting the patient by placing hands on the posterior iliac spine (Weber & Kelley, 2018). Older adults experience a loss in height due to the loss of vertebral cartilage and osteoporosis-related vertebral compression fractures. Therefore, an adult's height should be measured during each health screening.

Gait

Gait is assessed by having the patient walk away from the examiner for a short distance. The examiner observes the patient's gait for smoothness and rhythm. Any unsteadiness or irregular movements (frequently noted in older adult

patients) are considered abnormal. A limping motion is most frequently caused by painful weight bearing. In such instances, the patient can usually pinpoint the area of discomfort, thus guiding further examination. If one extremity is shorter than another, a limp may also be observed as the patient's pelvis drops downward on the affected side with each step. The knee should be flexed during normal gait; therefore, limited joint motion may interrupt the smooth pattern of gait. Evaluation of the knee involves the joints, bones, ligaments, tendons, and cartilage, and may include tests for the anterior and collateral ligaments, medial and lateral ligaments, and medial meniscus (Weber & Kelley, 2018). In addition, a variety of neurologic conditions are associated with abnormal gait, such as a spastic hemiparesis gait (stroke), steppage gait (lower motor neuron disease), and shuffling gait (Parkinson's disease).

Bone Integrity

The bony skeleton is assessed for deformities and alignment. Symmetric parts of the body, such as extremities, are compared. Abnormal bony growths due to bone tumors may be observed. Shortened extremities, amputations, and body parts that are not in anatomic alignment are noted. Fracture findings may include abnormal angulation of long bones, motion at points other than joints, and **crepitus** (a grating or crackling sound or sensation) at the point of abnormal motion. Movement of fracture fragments must be minimized to avoid additional injury. The nurse should include the following observations (Weber & Kelley, 2018):

- If the affected part is an extremity, how does its overall appearance compare to the unaffected extremity?
- Can the patient move the affected part? If an extremity is involved, does each toe or finger have normal sensation and motion (flexion and extension), and is the skin warm or cool?

- What is the color of the part distal to the affected area? Is it pale? Dusky? Mottled? Cyanotic?
- Does rapid capillary refill occur? (The nurse can gently squeeze a nail until it blanches, then release the pressure. The amount of time for the color under the nail to return to normal is noted. Color normally returns within 3 seconds. The return of color is evidence of capillary refill.)
- Is a pulse distal to the affected area palpable? If the affected area is an extremity, how does the pulse compare to the pulse of the unaffected extremity?
- Is edema present?
- Is any constrictive device or clothing causing nerve or vascular compression?
- Does elevating the affected part or modifying its position affect the symptoms?

Joint Function

The articular system is evaluated by noting range of motion, deformity, stability, tenderness, and nodular formation. Range of motion is evaluated both actively (the joint is moved by the muscles surrounding the joint) and passively (the joint is moved by the examiner). The examiner is familiar with the normal range of motion of major joints. Precise measurement of range of motion can be made by a goniometer (a protractor designed for evaluating joint motion) (Bickley, 2017). Limited range of motion may be the result of skeletal deformity, joint pathology, or **contracture** (shortening of surrounding joint structures) of the surrounding muscles, tendons, and joint capsule. In older adult patients, limitations of range of motion associated with osteoarthritis may reduce their ability to perform ADLs (Eliopoulos, 2018).

If joint motion is compromised or the joint is painful, the joint is examined for **effusion** (excessive fluid within the capsule), swelling, and increased temperature that may reflect active inflammation. An effusion is suspected if the joint is swollen and the normal bony landmarks are obscured. The most common site for joint effusion is the knee. If large amounts of fluid are present in the joint spaces beneath the patella, it may be identified by assessing for the balloon sign and for ballottement of the knee (Fig. 35-5). If inflammation or fluid is suspected in a joint, consultation with a specialist (e.g., orthopedic surgeon or rheumatologist) is indicated.

Joint deformity may be caused by contracture, dislocation (complete separation of joint surfaces), subluxation (partial separation of articular surfaces), or disruption of structures

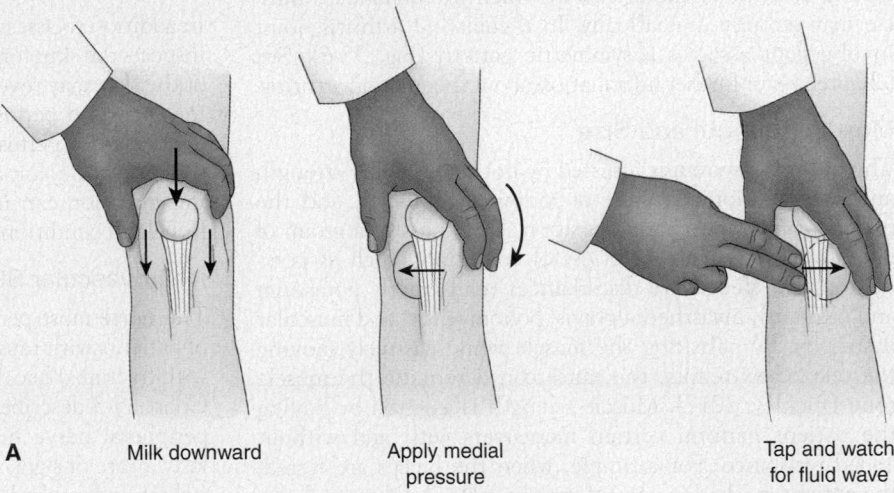

A   Milk downward   Apply medial pressure   Tap and watch for fluid wave

Figure 35-5 • Tests for detecting fluid in the knee. **A.** Technique for balloon sign. The medial and lateral aspects of the extended knee are milked firmly in a downward motion, which displaces any fluid downward. The examiner feels for any fluid entering the space directly inferior to the patella. When larger amounts of fluid are present, the subpatellar region feels as if it is "ballooning," and the balloon sign test is positive. **B.** Technique for ballottement sign. The medial and lateral aspects of the extended knee are milked firmly in a downward motion. The examiner pushes the patella toward the femur and observes for fluid return to the region superior to the patella. When larger amounts of fluid are present, the patella elevates, there is visible return of fluid to the region directly superior to the patella, and the ballottement test is positive. Photograph used with permission from Bickley, L. S. (2017). *Bates' guide to physical examination and history taking* (12th ed.). Philadelphia, PA: Lippincott Williams & Wilkins.

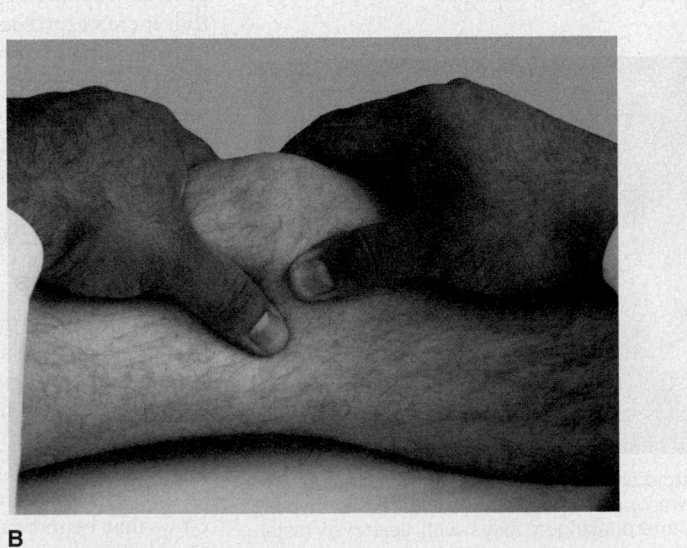

B

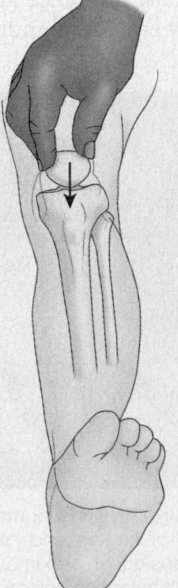

surrounding the joint. Weakness or disruption of joint-supporting structures may result in a weak joint that requires an external supporting appliance (e.g., brace).

Palpation of the joint while it is moved passively provides information about the integrity of the joint. Normally, the joint moves smoothly. A snap or crack may indicate that a ligament is slipping over a bony prominence. Slightly roughened surfaces, as in arthritic conditions, result in crepitus as the irregular joint surfaces move across one another (Bickley, 2017).

The tissues surrounding joints are examined for nodule formation. Rheumatoid arthritis, gout, and osteoarthritis may produce characteristic nodules. The subcutaneous nodules of rheumatoid arthritis are soft and occur within and along tendons that provide extensor function to the joints. The nodules of gout are hard and lie within and immediately adjacent to the joint capsule itself. They may rupture, exuding white uric acid crystals onto the skin surface. Osteoarthritic nodules are hard and painless and represent bony overgrowth that has resulted from the destruction of the cartilaginous surface of bone within the joint capsule. They are frequently seen in older adults (Bickley, 2017).

Often, the size of the joint is exaggerated by atrophy of the muscles proximal and distal to that joint. This is seen in rheumatoid arthritis of the knees, in which the quadriceps muscle may atrophy dramatically. In rheumatoid arthritis, joint involvement assumes a symmetric pattern (Fig. 35-6). See Chapter 34 for further information about rheumatoid arthritis.

Muscle Strength and Size

The muscular system is assessed by noting muscular strength and coordination, the size of individual muscles, and the patient's ability to change position. Weakness of a group of muscles may indicate a variety of conditions, such as polyneuropathy, electrolyte disturbances (particularly potassium and calcium), myasthenia gravis, poliomyelitis, and muscular dystrophy. By palpating the muscle while passively moving the relaxed extremity, the nurse can determine the muscle tone (Bickley, 2017). Muscle strength is assessed by having the patient perform certain maneuvers with and without added resistance. For example, when the biceps are tested, the patient is asked to extend the arm fully and then to flex it against resistance applied by the nurse. A simple handshake may provide an indication of grasp strength.

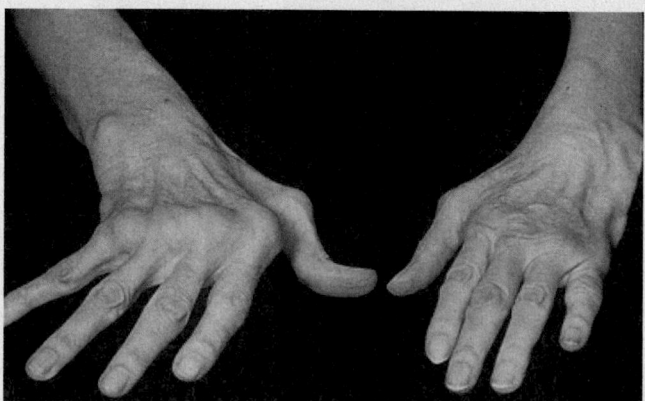

Figure 35-6 • Rheumatoid arthritis joint deformity with ulnar deviation of fingers and "swan neck" deformity of fingers (i.e., hyperextension of proximal interphalangeal joints with flexion of distal interphalangeal joints).

The nurse may elicit muscle **clonus** (rhythmic contractions of a muscle) in the ankle or wrist by sudden, forceful, sustained dorsiflexion of the foot or extension of the wrist. **Fasciculation** (involuntary twitching of muscle fiber groups) may be observed.

The nurse measures the girth of an extremity to monitor increased size due to exercise, edema, or bleeding into the muscle. Girth may decrease due to muscle atrophy. The unaffected extremity is measured and used as the reference standard for the affected extremity. Measurements are taken at the maximum circumference of the extremity. It is important that the measurements be taken at the same location on the extremity, and with the extremity in the same position, with the muscle at rest. Distance from a specific anatomic landmark (e.g., 10 cm below the medial aspect of the knee for measurement of the calf muscle) should be indicated in the patient's record so that subsequent measurements can be made at the same point. For ease of serial assessment, the nurse may indicate the point of measurement by marking the skin. Variations in size greater than 1 cm are considered significant (Bickley, 2017).

Skin

In addition to assessing the musculoskeletal system, the nurse inspects the skin for edema, temperature, and color. Palpation of the skin may reveal whether any areas are warmer, suggesting increased perfusion or inflammation, or cooler, suggesting decreased perfusion, and whether edema is present. Cuts, bruises, skin color, and evidence of decreased circulation or inflammation can influence nursing management of musculoskeletal conditions.

Neurovascular Status

The nurse must perform frequent neurovascular assessments of patients with musculoskeletal disorders (especially of those with fractures) because of the risk of tissue and nerve damage. Chart 35-3 describes methods the nurse may use to evaluate peripheral nerve function. The nurse needs to be particularly aware of signs and symptoms of compartment syndrome (which is described in detail later in this unit) when assessing the patient with a musculoskeletal injury. This neurovascular problem is caused by pressure within a muscle compartment that increases to such an extent that microcirculation diminishes, leading to nerve and muscle anoxia and necrosis. Function can be permanently lost if the anoxic situation continues for longer than 6 hours. Assessment of neurovascular status (Chart 35-4) is frequently referred to as assessment of CMS (circulation, motion, and sensation).

Diagnostic Evaluation

X-Ray Studies

Bone x-rays determine bone density, texture, erosion, and changes in bone relationships. X-ray study of the cortex of the bone reveals any widening, narrowing, or signs of irregularity. Joint x-rays reveal fluid, irregularity, spur formation, narrowing, and changes in the joint structure. Multiple x-rays, with multiple views (e.g., anterior, posterior, lateral), are needed for full assessment of the structure being examined. Serial x-rays may be indicated to determine the status of the healing process (Kennedy-Malone et al., 2019).

Chart 35-3 ASSESSMENT
Assessing for Peripheral Nerve Function

Assessment of peripheral nerve function has two key elements: evaluation of sensation and evaluation of motion. The nurse may perform one or all of the following during a musculoskeletal assessment.

Nerve	Test of Sensation	Test of Movement
Peroneal	Prick the skin midway between the great and second toe.	Ask the patient to dorsiflex the foot and extend the toes.
Tibial	Prick the medial and lateral surface of the sole.	Ask the patient to plantar flex toes and foot.
Radial	Prick the skin midway between the thumb and second finger.	Ask the patient to stretch out the thumb, then the wrist, and then the fingers at the metacarpal joints.
Ulnar	Prick the distal fat pad of the small finger.	Ask the patient to abduct all fingers.
Median	Prick the top or distal surface of the index finger.	Ask the patient to touch the thumb to the little finger. In addition, observe whether the patient can flex the wrist.

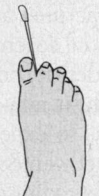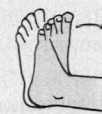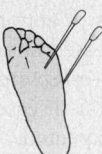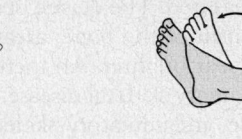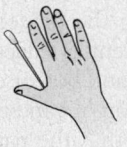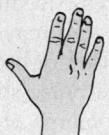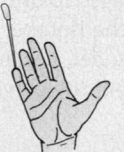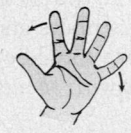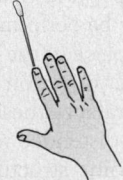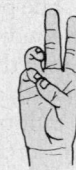

Adapted from Bickley, L. S. (2017). *Bates' guide to physical examination and history taking* (12th ed.). Philadelphia, PA: Wolters Kluwer; Weber, J., & Kelley, J. (2018). *Health assessment in nursing* (6th ed.). Philadelphia, PA: Lippincott Williams & Wilkins.

Chart 35-4 Indicators of Peripheral Neurovascular Dysfunction

Circulation

Color: Pale, cyanotic, or mottled
Temperature: Cool
Capillary refill: More than 3 s

Motion

Weakness
Paralysis

Sensation

Paresthesia
Unrelenting pain
Pain on passive stretch
Absence of feeling

Adapted from Bickley, L. S. (2017). *Bates' guide to physical examination and history taking* (12th ed.). Philadelphia, PA: Wolters Kluwer; Weber, J., & Kelley, J. (2018). *Health assessment in nursing* (6th ed.). Philadelphia, PA: Lippincott Williams & Wilkins.

Computed Tomography

A computed tomography (CT) scan, which may be performed with or without the use of oral or intravenous (IV) contrast agents, shows a more detailed cross-sectional image of the body. It may be used to visualize and assess tumors; injury to the soft tissue, ligaments, or tendons; and severe trauma to the chest, abdomen, pelvis, head, or spinal cord. It is also used to identify the location and extent of fractures in areas that are difficult to evaluate (e.g., acetabulum) and not visible on x-ray (Van Leeuwen & Bladh, 2019).

Magnetic Resonance Imaging

Magnetic resonance imaging (MRI) is a noninvasive imaging technique that uses magnetic fields and radio waves to create high-resolution pictures of bones and soft tissues. It can be used to visualize and assess torn muscles, ligaments, and cartilage; herniated discs; and a variety of hip or pelvic conditions. The patient does not experience any pain during the procedure. The MRI scanner is noisy, and it may take 30 to 90 minutes to complete the test. Because an electromagnet is used, patients with most metal implants (i.e., cochlear implants) or clips are not candidates for MRI (Van Leeuwen & Bladh, 2019).

> **Quality and Safety Nursing Alert**
>
> *Jewelry, hair clips, hearing aids, credit cards with magnetic strips, and other metal-containing objects must be removed before the MRI is performed; otherwise, they can become dangerous projectile objects or cause burns. Credit cards with magnetic strips may be erased, and nonremovable cochlear devices can become inoperable; therefore, their presence is a contraindication for MRI. In addition, transdermal patches (e.g., nicotine patch, nitroglycerin transdermal, scopolamine transdermal, clonidine transdermal) that have a thin layer of aluminized backing must be removed before MRI because they can cause burns. The primary provider should be notified before the patches are removed.*

To enhance visualization of anatomic structures, an IV contrast agent may be used. Patients who experience claustrophobia may be unable to tolerate the confinement of closed MRI equipment without sedation. Open MRI systems are available, but they use lower-intensity magnetic fields, which produce lower-quality images. Advantages of open MRI include increased patient comfort, reduced problems with claustrophobic reactions, and reduced noise.

Arthrography

Arthrography is used to identify the cause of any unexplained joint pain and progression of joint disease. A radiopaque contrast agent or air is injected into the joint cavity to visualize the joint structures, such as the ligaments, cartilage, tendons, and joint capsule. The joint is put through its range of motion to distribute the contrast agent while a series of x-rays are obtained. If a tear is present, the contrast agent leaks out of the joint and is evident on the x-ray image (Van Leeuwen & Bladh, 2019).

Bone Densitometry

Bone densitometry is used to evaluate BMD. This can be performed through the use of x-rays or ultrasound. The most common modalities used include dual-energy x-ray absorptiometry (DXA or DEXA), quantitative computed tomography (QCT), and quantitative ultrasound (QUS). DXA measures BMD and predicts fracture risk through accurate monitoring of bone density changes in patients with osteoporosis who are undergoing treatment. The density of bones in the spine, hip, and wrist may be calculated, as well as the total body. Peripheral dual-energy x-ray absorptiometry (pDXA) may be an alternative test that measures BMD of the forearm, finger, or heel, although its ability to project hip or spine fracture risk is less accurate than DXA (Felicilda-Reynaldo & Kenneally, 2019).

Bone density may vary among different skeletal areas; therefore, BMD results may be normal at one site but low at another. Because these tests only measure density at specific sites, they may miss abnormal findings in other skeletal areas. Thus, although the BMD of the heel can be used to diagnose and monitor osteoporosis, predicting bone fracture risk related to osteoporosis is best achieved through DXA of the hip and spine. Hence, DXA is the most commonly prescribed diagnostic test for determining BMD (Bickley, 2017; Van Leeuwen & Bladh, 2019). See Chapter 36 for a further discussion of osteoporosis risks.

Nursing Interventions

Before any of the imaging studies described previously (i.e., x-rays, CT scans, MRIs, arthrography, bone densitometry) are performed, the nurse prepares the patient. For all of these studies, the patient must lie still. During an MRI study, the patient may hear a knocking sound. In addition, the nurse assesses for conditions that may require special consideration during the study or that may be contraindications to the study (e.g., pregnancy; claustrophobia; inability to tolerate required positioning due to age, debility, or disability; metal implants). If contrast agents will be used for the CT scan, MRI, or arthrography, the patient is assessed for possible allergies (Van Leeuwen & Bladh, 2019).

The patient having an arthrogram may feel some discomfort or tingling during the procedure. After the arthrogram, a compression elastic bandage may be applied if prescribed, and the joint is usually rested for 12 hours. Strenuous activity should be avoided until approved by the primary provider. The nurse provides additional comfort measures (e.g., mild analgesia, ice) as appropriate and explains to the patient that it is normal to experience clicking or crackling in the joint for 24 to 48 hours after the procedure until the contrast agent or air is absorbed.

Bone Scan

A bone scan is performed to detect metastatic and primary bone tumors, osteomyelitis, some fractures, and aseptic necrosis, and to monitor the progression of degenerative bone diseases. A bone scan may accurately identify bone disease before it can be detected on x-ray; as such, it may diagnose a stress fracture in a patient who continues to experience pain after x-ray findings are negative (Van Leeuwen & Bladh, 2019). A bone scan requires the injection of a radioisotope through an IV line; the scan is performed 2 to 3 hours afterward. At this point, distribution and concentration of the isotope in the bone are measured. The degree of nuclide uptake is related to the metabolism of the bone; areas of abnormal bone formation will appear brighter. An increased uptake of the isotope is seen in primary skeletal disease (osteosarcoma), metastatic bone disease, inflammatory skeletal disease (osteomyelitis), and fractures that do not heal as expected.

Nursing Interventions

Prior to the bone scan, the nurse inquires about possible allergies to the radioisotope and assesses for any condition that would contraindicate performing the procedure (e.g., pregnancy, breast-feeding). The patient is educated about why the bone scan may be indicated and how it can assist in the identification of bone disease before it can be detected on an x-ray. The nurse should explain that the patient may experience moments of discomfort from the isotope (e.g., flushing, warmth) but provide reassurance that the radionuclide poses no radioactive hazard (Van Leeuwen & Bladh, 2019). In addition, the patient is encouraged to drink plenty of fluids to help distribute and eliminate the isotope. Before the scan, the patient should empty the bladder, because a full bladder interferes with accurate scanning of the pelvic bones.

Arthroscopy

Arthroscopy allows direct visualization of a joint through the use of a fiberoptic endoscope. Thus, it is a useful adjunct to diagnosing joint disorders. Biopsy and treatment of tears, defects, and disease processes may be performed through the arthroscope. The procedure takes place in the operating room under sterile conditions with either injection of a local anesthetic agent into the joint or general anesthesia. A large-bore needle is inserted, and the joint is distended with saline. The arthroscope is introduced, and joint structures, synovium, and articular surfaces are visualized. After the procedure, the puncture wound is closed with adhesive strips or sutures and covered with a sterile dressing. Complications are rare but may include infection, hemarthrosis, neurovascular compromise, thrombophlebitis, stiffness, effusion, adhesions, and delayed wound healing (Van Leeuwen & Bladh, 2019).

Nursing Interventions

After the arthroscopic procedure, the joint is wrapped with a compression dressing to control swelling. In addition, ice may be applied to control edema and enhance comfort. Frequently, the joint is kept extended and elevated to reduce swelling. The nurse monitors and documents the neurovascular status (see Chart 35-4). Analgesic agents are given as needed. The patient is instructed to avoid strenuous activity of the joint, and exercises must be approved by the primary provider. The patient and family are instructed to monitor for signs and symptoms of complications (e.g., fever, excessive bleeding, swelling, numbness, cool skin) and the importance of notifying the primary provider should any of these occur (Van Leeuwen & Bladh, 2019).

Arthrocentesis

Arthrocentesis (joint aspiration) is carried out to obtain synovial fluid for purposes of examination or to relieve pain due to effusion. Examination of synovial fluid is helpful in the diagnosis of septic arthritis and other inflammatory arthropathies and reveals the presence of hemarthrosis (bleeding into the joint cavity), which suggests trauma or a bleeding disorder. Normally, synovial fluid is clear, pale, straw colored, and scanty in volume. Using aseptic technique, the primary provider inserts a needle into the joint and aspirates fluid. Anti-inflammatory medications may be injected into the joint. A sterile dressing is applied after aspiration. There is a risk of infection after this procedure (Van Leeuwen & Bladh, 2019).

Nursing Interventions

The nurse should review the procedure with the patient and its indications. Hair may need to be removed from the site before the procedure. Pain may be a concern; telling the patient that antispasmodic agents may be given to alleviate discomfort during the procedure may help decrease anxiety. Ice may be prescribed for the first 24 to 48 hours postprocedure; the patient should be educated about why ice may be indicated (i.e., to diminish edema formation and pain). If antibiotics are prescribed postprocedure, the patient must be educated about their use and reminded to take medications as prescribed. The patient and family are educated about the possible signs and symptoms of complications, particularly infection and bleeding (e.g., fever, excessive bleeding, swelling, numbness, cool skin) and the importance of promptly notifying the primary provider if any of these occur (Van Leeuwen & Bladh, 2019).

Electromyography

Electromyography (EMG) provides information about the electrical potential of the muscles and the nerves leading to them. The test is performed to evaluate muscle weakness, pain, and disability. The purpose of the procedure is to determine any abnormality of function and to differentiate muscle and nerve problems. An EMG can be used to identify the extent of damage if nerve function does not return within 4 months of an injury. Needle electrodes are inserted into selected muscles, and responses to electrical stimuli are recorded on an oscilloscope. Warm compresses may relieve residual discomfort after the study.

Nursing Interventions

Before the patient undergoes an EMG, the nurse inquires if the patient is taking any anticoagulant medications and assesses for any active skin infection. If the patient is found to be taking an anticoagulant or has a skin infection, the primary provider is notified. An EMG is usually contraindicated in patients receiving anticoagulant therapy (e.g., warfarin) because the needle electrodes may cause bleeding within the muscle. EMG also may be contraindicated in patients with extensive skin infections due to the risk of spreading infection from the skin to the muscle. The nurse instructs the patient to avoid using any lotions or creams on the day of the test (Van Leeuwen & Bladh, 2019).

Biopsy

Biopsy may be performed to determine the structure and composition of bone marrow, bone, muscle, or synovium to help diagnose specific diseases. It involves excising a sample of tissue that can be analyzed microscopically to determine cell morphology and tissue abnormalities.

Nursing Interventions

The nurse educates the patient about the procedure and offers assurance that analgesic agents will be provided. The biopsy site is monitored for edema, bleeding, pain, hematoma formation, and infection. Ice is applied as prescribed to control bleeding and edema. In addition, antibiotics and analgesic agents are given as prescribed. The patient is instructed to report signs of redness, bleeding, or pain at the biopsy site as well as fever or chills to the primary provider (Van Leeuwen & Bladh, 2019).

Laboratory Studies

Examination of the patient's blood and urine is used to identify the presence and amount of chemicals and other substances. The results may indicate a primary musculoskeletal problem (e.g., Paget's disease of the bone), a developing complication (e.g., infection), the baseline for instituting therapy (e.g., anticoagulant therapy), or the response to therapy, as well as possible causes of bone loss. Before surgery, coagulation studies are performed to detect bleeding tendencies (because bone is vascular tissue).

Serum calcium levels are altered in patients with osteomalacia, parathyroid dysfunction, Paget's disease, metastatic bone tumors, or prolonged immobilization. Serum phosphorus levels are inversely related to calcium levels and are diminished in osteomalacia associated with malabsorption syndrome. Acid phosphatase is elevated in Paget's disease and metastatic cancer. Alkaline phosphatase (ALP) is elevated during early fracture healing and in diseases with increased osteoblastic activity (e.g., metastatic bone tumors). Bone metabolism may be evaluated through thyroid studies and determination of calcitonin, PTH, and vitamin D levels. Serum enzyme levels of creatine kinase and aspartate aminotransferase become elevated with muscle damage. Serum osteocalcin indicates the rate of bone turnover. Urine calcium levels increase with bone destruction (e.g., parathyroid dysfunction, metastatic bone tumors, multiple myeloma) (Van Leeuwen & Bladh, 2019).

Specific urine and serum biochemical markers can be used to provide information about the speed of bone resorption or bone formation, as well as to document the effects of therapeutic interventions prescribed for patients diagnosed with musculoskeletal disorders. These include urinary N-telopeptide of type 1 collagen (NTx) and deoxypyridinoline (Dpd), both of which reflect increased osteoclast activity and increased bone resorption. Conversely, elevated serum levels of bone-specific ALP, osteocalcin, and intact N-terminal propeptide of type 1 collagen (P1NP) reflect increased activity of osteoblasts and enhanced bone remodeling activity (NOF, 2019).

CRITICAL THINKING EXERCISES

1 `pq` You are a nurse working in an urgent care facility and are assigned to care for a 35-year-old man who fell while hiking. He is holding his left arm. You note a small laceration and a few abrasions to the arm as well as swelling and deformity. What are the priority interventions for this patient? What diagnostic test would most likely be indicated? What comfort measure should be provided until a diagnosis is confirmed?

2 `ebp` You are a faith community nurse and your parish has many older adult parishioners. You want to develop an educational program regarding healthy lifestyle choices and bone health. What are the current evidence-based recommendations to maintain bone health for older adults? What is the level of evidence that supports each of the recommendations and strategies for reducing musculoskeletal risk for the aging adult?

REFERENCES

*Asterisk indicates nursing research.

Books

Bickley, L. S. (2017). *Bates' guide to physical examination and history taking* (12th ed.). Philadelphia, PA: Wolters Kluwer.

Eliopoulos, C. (2018). *Gerontological nursing* (9th ed.). Philadelphia, PA: Wolters Kluwer.

Kennedy-Malone, L., Martin-Plank, L., & Duffy, E. (2019). *Advanced practice nursing in the care of older adults* (2nd ed.). Philadelphia, PA: F.A. Davis.

Meiner, S. E., & Yeager, J. J. (2019). *Gerontologic nursing* (6th ed.). St. Louis, MO: Elsevier.

Norris, T. (2019). *Porth's pathophysiology: Concepts of altered health states* (10th ed.). Philadelphia, PA: Wolters Kluwer.

Van Leeuwen, A., & Bladh, M. (2019). *Textbook of laboratory and diagnostic testing: Practical application of nursing process at the bedside*. Philadelphia, PA: F.A. Davis.

Weber, J., & Kelley, J. (2018). *Health assessment in nursing* (6th ed.). Philadelphia, PA: Lippincott Williams & Wilkins.

Journals and Electronic Documents

Centers for Disease Control and Prevention (CDC). (2019). *Arthritis: Addressing the nation's most common cause of disability*. Retrieved on 9/11/2019 at: www.cdc.gov/chronicdisease/resources/publications/aag/arthritis.htm

Felicilda-Reynaldo, R., & Kenneally, M. (2019). First-line medications for osteoporosis. *Medsurg Nursing, 28*(6), 381–386.

*Leow, M. Q., Teo, W., Low, T. L., et al. (2019). Hand assessment for elderly people in the community. *Orthopaedic Nursing, 38*(1), 25–30.

National Institutes of Health (NIH). (2019a). *Calcium: Fact sheet for health professionals*. Retrieved on 9/11/2019 at: www.ods.od.nih.gov/factsheets/Calcium-HealthProfessional

National Institutes of Health (NIH). (2019b). *Vitamin D: Fact sheet for health professionals*. Retrieved on 1/6/2020 at: www.ods.od.nih.gov/factsheets/VitaminD-HealthProfessional

National Osteoporosis Foundation (NOF). (2019). *Clinical exams*. Retrieved on 10/7/2019 at: www.nof.org/patients/diagnosis-information/clinical-exams

Takeno, A., Kanazawa, I., Notsu, M., et al. (2018). Glucose uptake inhibition decreases expressions of receptor activator of nuclear factor-kappa B ligand (RANKL) and osteocalcin in osteocytic MLO-Y4-A2 cells. *American Journal of Physiology, Endocrinology and Metabolism, 314*(2), E115–E123.

United States Bone and Joint Initiative (USBJI). (2018). *The burden of musculoskeletal diseases in the United States* (4th ed.). Rosemont, IL. Retrieved on 2/2/2020 at: www.boneandjointburden.org

Resources

American College of Sports Medicine (ACSM), www.acsm.org

International Osteoporosis Foundation (IOF), www.iofbonehealth.org

National Association of Orthopaedic Nurses (NAON), www.orthonurse.org

National Institute of Arthritis and Musculoskeletal and Skin Diseases, www.niams.nih.gov

National Osteoporosis Foundation, www.nof.org

World Health Organization (WHO) Collaborating Centre for Metabolic Bone Diseases: the fracture risk assessment tool (FRAX®), www.sheffield.ac.uk/FRAX/tool.aspx?country=9

36

Management of Patients with Musculoskeletal Disorders

NURSING CONCEPTS

Comfort   Inflammation   Mobility

GLOSSARY

abduction: movement away from the center or median line of the body
adduction: movement toward the center or median line of the body
arthroplasty: surgical replacement of a joint
avascular necrosis: death of tissue due to insufficient blood supply
bursitis: inflammation of a fluid-filled sac in a joint
contracture: abnormal shortening of muscle or fibrosis of joint structures
heterotopic ossification: misplaced formation of bone
involucrum: new bone growth around a sequestrum
osteolysis: lysis of bone from inflammatory reaction against polyethylene particulate debris
osteopenia: low bone mineral density

osteophyte: a bony outgrowth or protuberance; bone spur
osteoporosis: degenerative disease of the bone characterized by reduced mass, deterioration of matrix, and diminished architectural strength
osteotomy: surgical cutting of bone
radiculopathy: disease of a spinal nerve root, often resulting in pain and extreme sensitivity to touch
sciatica: inflammation of the sciatic nerve, resulting in pain and tenderness along the nerve through the thigh and leg
sequestrum: dead bone in abscess cavity
subchondral bone: bony plate that supports the articular cartilage
tendonitis: inflammation of muscle tendons

Musculoskeletal disorders, particularly impairment of the back, joints, and spine, are leading health problems and causes of disability. The functional and psychological limitations for the patient may be severe. Nurses should be cognizant of these limitations and the effects these disorders may have on these patients when providing care in inpatient and outpatient settings.

Low Back Pain

Most low back pain is caused by one of many musculoskeletal problems, including acute lumbosacral strain, unstable lumbosacral ligaments and weak muscles, intervertebral disc problems, and unequal leg length. Depression, smoking, alcohol abuse, obesity, and stress are frequent comorbidities (Ramanathan, Hibbert, Wiles, et al., 2018). Generally, back pain due to musculoskeletal disorders is aggravated by activity, whereas pain due to other conditions is not. Higher numbers of areas of pain are associated with a higher level of disability. Other nonmusculoskeletal causes of back pain, beyond the scope of this chapter, include kidney disorders, pelvic problems, retroperitoneal tumors, and abdominal aortic aneurysms.

Gerontologic Considerations

Older patients may experience back pain associated with osteoporotic vertebral fractures (see later discussion), osteoarthritis of the spine, and spinal stenosis. In addition, inactivity can have grave consequences on quality of life, progression of medical disease, energy level, and morbidity in older adults (Simon & Hicks, 2018).

Pathophysiology

The spinal column can be considered a rod constructed of rigid units (vertebrae) and flexible units (intervertebral discs) held together by complex facet joints, multiple ligaments, and paravertebral muscles. Its unique construction allows for flexibility while providing maximum protection for the spinal cord. The spinal curves absorb vertical shocks from running and jumping. The abdominal and thoracic muscles are important in lifting activities, working together to minimize stress on the spinal units. Disuse weakens these supporting muscular structures. Obesity, postural problems, structural problems, and overstretching of the spinal supports may result in back pain (McCance & Huether, 2019).

The intervertebral discs change in character as a person ages. A young person's discs are mainly fibrocartilage with a gelatinous matrix. Over time, the fibrocartilage becomes dense and irregularly shaped. Disc degeneration is a common cause of back pain. The lower lumbar discs, L4–5 and L5–S1, are subject to the greatest mechanical stress and the greatest degenerative changes. Disc protrusion or facet joint changes can cause pressure on nerve roots as they leave the spinal canal, which results in pain that radiates along the nerve (McCance & Huether, 2019). See Chapter 65 for discussion of the management of intervertebral disc disease.

Clinical Manifestations

The typical patient reports either acute back pain (lasting fewer than 3 months) or chronic back pain (3 months or longer without improvement) and fatigue. The patient may report pain radiating down the leg, which is known as **radiculopathy** (i.e., pain radiating from a diseased spinal nerve root) or **sciatica** (i.e., pain radiating from an inflamed sciatic nerve); presence of this symptom suggests nerve root involvement. The patient's gait, spinal mobility, reflexes, leg length, leg motor strength, and sensory perception may be affected. Physical examination may disclose paravertebral muscle spasm (greatly increased muscle tone of the back postural muscles) with a loss of the normal lumbar curve and possible spinal deformity.

Assessment and Diagnostic Findings

The initial evaluation of acute low back pain includes a focused history and physical examination, including observation of the patient, gait evaluation, and neurologic testing (see Chapter 35). The findings suggest either nonspecific

lumbar strain or potentially serious problems, such as a spinal fracture, cancer, infection, or rapidly progressing neurologic deficits. The presence of bruising, older age, and prolonged use of corticosteroid medications increases the risk of a fracture posttraumatic injury (Gironda, Nguyen, & Mosqueda, 2016). In addition, the nurse should be alert to the potential for older adult abuse.

Another potential cause of low back pain is *cauda equina syndrome*, which results from compression of the cauda equina, the bundle of spinal nerves that arise from the lower portion of the spinal cord. When these nerves become compressed, the patient will have signs and symptoms that include severe or progressive neurologic deficit, recent bowel or bladder dysfunction, and saddle anesthesia which is characterized by paresthesias in the perineal, inner thigh, or buttock region that may be asymmetrical (Qaseem, Wilt, McLean, et al., 2017). Cauda equina syndrome is a medical emergency requiring immediate referral to an emergency department so that the patient may receive expeditious treatment to relieve the underlying cause before nerve damage occurs (e.g., treatment can consist of surgical removal of vertebral fragments, decompression of a tumor mass).

The diagnostic procedures described in Chart 36-1 may be indicated for the patient with potentially serious or prolonged low back pain. Red flags that trigger prescribing these studies include suspected spinal infection, severe neurologic weakness, urinary or fecal incontinence, and a new onset of back pain in a patient with cancer (Qaseem et al., 2017). The nurse prepares the patient for these studies, provides the necessary support during the testing period, and monitors the patient for any adverse responses to the procedures.

Medical Management

Most back pain is self-limited and resolves within 4 to 6 weeks with analgesics, rest, and avoidance of strain. Based on initial

---

Chart 36-1 Diagnostic Procedures for Low Back Pain

X-ray of the spine: may demonstrate a fracture, dislocation, infection, osteoarthritis, or scoliosis

Bone scan and blood studies: may disclose infections, tumors, and bone marrow abnormalities

Computed tomography (CT) scan: useful in identifying underlying problems, such as obscure soft tissue lesions adjacent to the vertebral column and problems of vertebral discs

Magnetic resonance imaging (MRI) scan: permits visualization of the nature and location of spinal pathology

Electromyogram (EMG) and nerve conduction studies: used to evaluate spinal nerve root disorders (radiculopathies)

Myelogram: permits visualization of segments of the spinal cord that may have herniated or may be compressed (infrequently performed; indicated when MRI scan is contraindicated)

Ultrasound: useful in detecting tears in ligaments, muscles, tendons, and soft tissues in the back

Adapted from Fischbach, F. T., & Fischbach, M. A. (2018). *A manual of laboratory and diagnostic tests* (10th ed.). Philadelphia, PA: Wolters Kluwer; Wheeler, S. G., Wipf, J. E., Staiger, T. O., et al. (2019). Evaluation of low back pain in adults. *UpToDate.* Retrieved on 3/9/2020 at: www.uptodate.com/contents/evaluation-of-low-back-pain-in-adults

assessment findings indicating nonspecific back symptoms, the patient is reassured that the pain is not due to a serious condition and x-rays or other imaging modalities are not necessary (Qaseem et al., 2017). Management focuses on relief of discomfort, activity modification, and patient education. The presence of other medical problems and fear of pain complicates the picture and has higher cost, less favorable outcomes, and more long-term disability (Karasawa, Yamadada, Iseki, et al., 2019).

Nonprescription analgesics such as nonsteroidal anti-inflammatory drugs (NSAIDs) and short-term prescription muscle relaxants (e.g., cyclobenzaprine) are effective in relieving acute low back pain, but no one medication is considered superior to another (Michigan Quality Improvement Consortium [MQIC], 2018). Tricyclic antidepressants (e.g., amitriptyline) and the dual-action serotonin-norepinephrine reuptake inhibitors (e.g., duloxetine) or atypical anticonvulsant medications (e.g., gabapentin, which is prescribed for pain from radiculopathy) are used effectively in chronic low back pain. Opioid medications are indicated only short term (1 to 2 weeks) for acute moderate to severe cases of low back pain, except in older adults, those with kidney disease, or those who must avoid chronic NSAID exposure because of its adverse gastric effects. Systemic corticosteroids and acetaminophen are not effective in fully alleviating acute low back pain (Krebs, Gravely, Nugent, et al., 2018). For chronic pain, a reduction of pain by 30% less than baseline is the goal (Dupuis & Duff, 2019).

Effective nonpharmacologic interventions include thermal applications (hot or cold) and spinal manipulation (e.g., chiropractic therapy). Lumbar support belts are not recommended to treat acute low back pain but may be marginally effective devices for preventing low back pain in occupational health settings (MQIC, 2018). Orthopedic shoe inserts are not recommended for prevention but may help correct an underlying issue contributing to the problem (e.g., unequal leg length). Cognitive-behavioral therapy (e.g., biofeedback), exercise regimens, spinal manipulation, physical therapy, acupuncture, massage, and yoga are all effective nonpharmacologic interventions for treating chronic low back pain (Qaseem et al., 2017).

Most patients need to alter their activity patterns to avoid aggravating the pain. They should avoid twisting, bending, lifting, and reaching—all of which stress the back. The patient is taught to change position frequently. Sitting should be limited to 20 to 50 minutes based on level of comfort. Absolute bed rest is no longer recommended; typical activities of daily living (ADLs) should be resumed as soon as possible. A quick return to normal activities and a program of low-stress aerobic exercise are recommended (MQIC, 2018). Conditioning exercises for both back and trunk muscles are begun after about 2 weeks to help prevent recurrence of pain. Active motion activities such as walking have a beneficial impact on outcomes (Dupuis & Duff, 2019).

Nursing Management

The nurse asks the patient to describe the discomfort (e.g., location, severity, duration, characteristics, radiation, and weakness in the legs). Descriptions of how the pain occurred, such as with a specific action (e.g., opening a garage door) or with an activity in which weak muscles were overused (e.g., weekend gardening), and how the patient has dealt with the pain often suggest areas for intervention and patient education.

If back pain is a recurring problem, assessment about previous successful pain control methods helps in planning current management. Information about work and recreational activities helps identify areas for back health education. Because stress and anxiety can evoke muscle spasms and pain (Feinstein, Khalsa, Yeh, et al., 2018), the nurse assesses environmental variables, work situations, and family relationships. In addition, the nurse assesses the effect of chronic pain on the emotional well-being of the patient. Referral to a mental health professional for assessment and management of stressors contributing to the low back pain and related depression may be appropriate.

During the interview, the nurse observes the patient's posture, position changes, and gait. Often, the patient's movements are guarded, with the back kept as still as possible. The patient should be directed to a chair of standard seat height with arms for support. The patient may sit and stand in an unusual position, leaning away from the most painful side, and may need assistance when undressing for the physical examination.

On physical examination, the nurse assesses the spinal curve, any leg length discrepancy, and pelvic crest and shoulder symmetry. The nurse palpates the paraspinal muscles and notes spasm and tenderness. When the patient is in a prone position, the paraspinal muscles relax and any deformity caused by spasm can subside. The nurse asks the patient to bend forward and then laterally, noting any discomfort or limitations in movement. It is important to determine the effect of these limitations on ADLs. The nurse evaluates nerve involvement by assessing deep tendon reflexes, sensations (e.g., paresthesia), and muscle strength. Back and leg pain on straight-leg raising (with the patient supine, the patient's leg is lifted upward with the knee extended) suggests nerve root involvement.

The major nursing goals for patient management include relief of pain, improved physical mobility, the use of back-conserving techniques of body mechanics, improved self-esteem, and weight reduction (as necessary) (see Chart 36-2).

The nurse assesses the patient's response to analgesic agents. As the acute pain subsides, medication dosages are reduced. The nurse evaluates and notes the patient's response to various pain management modalities (see Chapter 9). The nurse cautions the patient with severe pain not to remain on bed rest because extended periods of inactivity are not effective and result in deconditioning. A medium to firm, nonsagging mattress (a bed board may be used) is recommended; there is no evidence to support the use of a firm mattress (Radwan, Fess, James, et al., 2015). Lumbar flexion is increased by elevating the head and thorax 30 degrees by using pillows or a foam wedge and slightly flexing the knees supported on a pillow. Alternatively, the patient can assume a lateral position with knees and hips flexed (curled position) with a pillow between the knees and legs and a pillow supporting the head (see Fig. 36-1). A prone position should be avoided because it accentuates lordosis. The nurse instructs the patient to get out of bed by rolling to one side and placing the legs down while pushing the torso up, keeping the back straight.

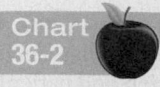

Chart 36-2

HEALTH PROMOTION

Strategies for Preventing Acute Low Back Pain

Prevention

- Weight reduction as needed
- Stress reduction
- Avoid high heels
- Walk daily and gradually increase the distance and pace of walking
- Avoid jumping and jarring activities
- Stretch to enhance flexibility. Do strengthening exercises

Body Mechanics

- Practice good posture
- Avoid twisting, lifting above waist level, and reaching up for any length of time
- Push objects rather than pull them
- Keep load close to your body when lifting
- Lift with the large leg muscles, not the back muscles
- Squat while keeping the back straight when it is necessary to pick something up off the floor
- Bend your knees and tighten abdominal muscles when lifting
- Avoid overreaching or a forward flexion position
- Use a wide base of support

Work Modifications

- Adjust height of chair using a footstool to position knees higher than hips
- Adjust height of work area to avoid stress on back
- Avoid bending, twisting, and lifting heavy objects
- Avoid prolonged standing and repetitive tasks
- Avoid work involving continuous vibrations
- Use lumbar support in straight back chair with arm rests
- When standing for any length of time, rest one foot on a small stool or box to relieve lumbar lordosis

As the patient achieves comfort, an exercise program is gradually initiated with low-stress aerobic exercises, such as short walks or swimming. The physical therapist designs an exercise program for the patient to reduce lordosis, increase flexibility, and reduce strain on the back. It may include hyperextension exercises to strengthen the paravertebral muscles, flexion exercises to increase back movement and strength, and isometric flexion exercises to strengthen trunk muscles. Each 30-minute daily exercise period begins and ends with muscle stretching and relaxation.

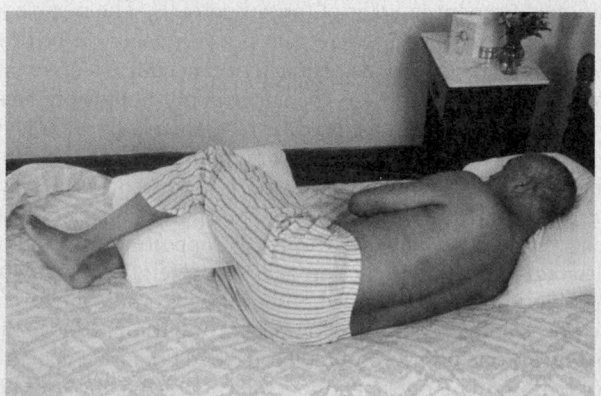

Figure 36-1 • Positioning to promote lumbar flexion. Photo by B. Proud.

The nurse encourages the patient to adhere to the prescribed exercise program. Some patients may find it difficult to do so for a long period. In these instances, alternating activities may help facilitate adherence to the regimen. Activities should not cause excessive lumbar strain or twisting, with avoidance of activities such as horseback riding and weight lifting.

Good body mechanics and posture are essential to avoid recurrence of back pain. The patient must be taught how to stand, sit, lie, and lift properly (see Fig. 36-2). Providing the patient with a list of suggestions helps in making these long-term changes (see Chart 36-2). The patient who wears high heels is encouraged to change to low heels with good arch support. The patient who is required to stand for long periods should shift weight frequently and rest one foot on a low stool, which decreases lumbar lordosis. Standing on a foot cushion made of foam or rubber can be helpful. The proper posture can be verified by looking in a mirror to see whether the chest is up, the abdomen is tucked in, and the shoulders are down and relaxed. Locking the knees when standing is avoided as well as bending forward for long periods.

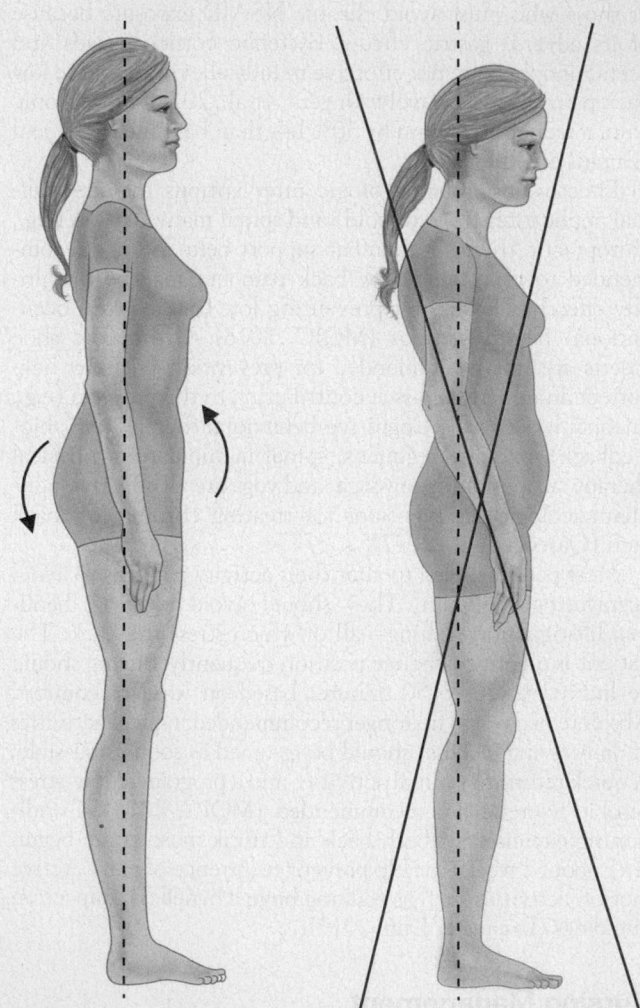

Figure 36-2 • Proper and improper standing postures. (*Left*) Abdominal muscles contracted, giving a feeling of upward pull, and gluteal muscles contracted, giving a downward pull. (*Right*) Slouch position, showing abdominal muscles relaxed and body out of proper alignment.

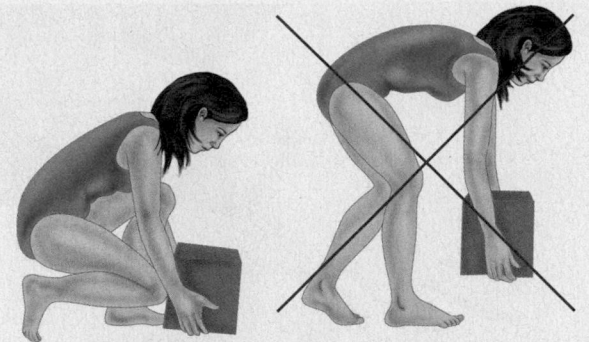

Figure 36-3 • Proper and improper lifting techniques. (**Left**) Correct position for lifting. This person is using the long and strong muscles of the arms and legs and holding the object so that the line of gravity falls within the base of support. (**Right**) Incorrect position for lifting. In this position, pull is exerted on the back muscles, and leaning causes the line of gravity to fall outside the base.

When sitting, the knees and hips should be flexed, with the knees in level with the hips or higher to minimize lordosis. The feet should be flat on the floor or supported on a raised surface. Patients should avoid sitting on stools or chairs that do not provide firm back support.

The nurse instructs the patient in the safe and correct way to lift objects—using the strong quadriceps muscles of the thighs, with minimal use of weak back muscles (see Fig. 36-3). With feet placed hip-width apart to provide a wide base of support, the patient should bend the knees, tighten the abdominal muscles, and lift the object close to the body with a smooth motion, avoiding twisting and jarring motions. The patient should avoid lifting more than one third of their ideal weight without help to prevent injury.

Role-related responsibilities may have to be modified with the onset of low back pain (e.g., carrying children). As recovery progresses, the patient may resume them. However, if these activities contributed to the development of low back pain, resuming them may lead to the development of chronic low back pain, with associated disability. If the patient experiences secondary gains associated with low back disability (e.g., workers' compensation, easier lifestyle or workload, increased emotional support), there is a risk that the patient will not fully resume work and family roles. Earlier return to work and lifestyle, even at a reduced level, have better outcomes than waiting for full recovery (Qaseem et al., 2017). Antidepressants and counseling may be needed to assist the person in resuming a full, productive life. Specialized back clinics use multidisciplinary approaches to help the patient with chronic pain resume role-related responsibilities; these approaches are especially beneficial for patients who experience fear and depression associated with chronic pain (Karasawa et al., 2019).

Obesity contributes to back strain by overtaxing the relatively weak back muscles in the absence of abdominal muscle support. Exercises are less effective and more difficult to perform when the patient is overweight. Weight reduction through diet modification is important to minimize recurrence of back pain. A sound nutritional plan that includes a change in eating habits and low-impact activities is vital. Noting achievement of weight reduction and providing positive reinforcement facilitate adherence. Back problems may or may not fully resolve as optimal weight is achieved (MQIC, 2018).

Common Upper Extremity Disorders

The structures in the upper extremities are frequently the sites of painful syndromes. This is especially true in occupational health settings, where many patient visits involve the shoulder, wrist, and hand.

Bursitis and Tendonitis

Bursitis and tendonitis are inflammatory conditions that commonly occur in the shoulder. Bursae are fluid-filled sacs that prevent friction between joint structures during joint activity and are painful when inflamed; **bursitis** is the consequence when these sacs become inflamed. Muscle tendon sheaths also become inflamed with repetitive stretching, causing **tendonitis**. The inflammation causes proliferation of synovial membrane and pannus formation, which restricts joint movement. Conservative treatment includes rest of the extremity, intermittent ice and heat to the joint, and NSAIDs to control the inflammation and pain. Newer therapies that include extracorporeal shock waves, pulsed magnetic fields, laser phototherapy, radiofrequency ablation, and stem cell therapies are touted to accelerate tendon healing, although further research is needed to determine their overall effectiveness (Cook & Young, 2020). There are no non–research-based sites for injection of cellular therapies that are registered with the Centers for Disease Control and Prevention (CDC) in the United States (Cook & Yong, 2020). The World Anti-Doping Agency (WADA) for sports allows autologous (self-donated) localized injections for soft tissue injuries, but IV infusions are prohibited (WADA, 2020). Arthroscopic synovectomy may be considered if shoulder pain and weakness persist. Corticosteroid injections remain more evidence based than most other interventions for short-term, rapid improvement, but are not always helpful in the long term (McAlindon, LaValley, Harvey, et al., 2017). Most tendon and bursal inflammatory problems are self-limiting; they go away on their own with or without therapy. The treatments are primarily aimed at pain relief, not cure.

Loose Bodies

Loose bodies ("joint mice") may occur in a joint space as a result of articular cartilage wear and bone erosion. These fragments can interfere with joint movement ("locking the joint"). Loose bodies are removed by arthroscopic surgery if they cause pain or mobility issues.

Impingement Syndrome

Impingement syndrome is a general term that describes impaired movement of the rotator cuff of the shoulder. Impingement usually occurs from repetitive overhead movement of the arm or from acute trauma resulting in irritation and eventual inflammation of the rotator cuff tendons or the subacromial bursa as they grate against the coracoacromial arch. Early manifestations of this syndrome are characterized by edema from hemorrhage of these structures, pain, shoulder tenderness, limited movement, muscle spasm, and eventual disuse atrophy. The process may progress to a partial or complete rotator cuff tear (see Chapter 37).

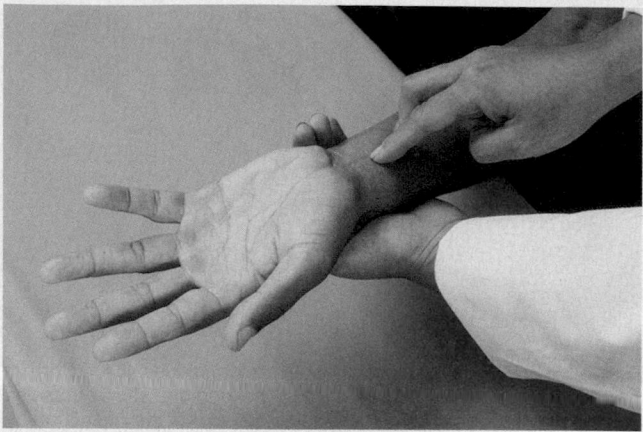

Figure 36-4 • Tinel sign may be elicited in patients with carpal tunnel syndrome by percussing lightly over the median nerve, located on the inner aspect of the wrist. If the patient reports tingling, numbness, and pain, the test for Tinel sign is considered positive. Reprinted with permission from Weber, J. W., & Kelley, J. (2018). *Health assessment in nursing* (6th ed.). Philadelphia, PA: Wolters Kluwer. Photo by B. Proud.

Medications used to treat early impingement syndrome include oral NSAIDs or intra-articular injections of corticosteroids. Application of superficial cold or heat may subjectively improve patients' symptoms; however, a therapeutic exercise program (see Chapter 37) is required to improve outcomes, including reduction of pain and improved shoulder function (see Chart 36-3).

Carpal Tunnel Syndrome

Carpal tunnel syndrome is an entrapment neuropathy that occurs when the median nerve at the wrist is compressed by a thickened flexor tendon sheath, skeletal encroachment, edema, or a soft tissue mass. It frequently occurs in women between 30 and 60 years of age. Women going through menopause or who are taking estrogen or birth control pills have the highest risk (Calandruccio & Thompson, 2018). While carpal tunnel syndrome is commonly caused by repetitive hand and wrist movements, it is also associated with rheumatoid arthritis (RA), diabetes, acromegaly, hyperthyroidism, or trauma (McCance & Huether, 2019). People employed in occupations that require frequent repetitive hand movements or flexing of the wrist, such as assembly line workers and hairdressers, and those exposed to vibration when doing tasks, such as construction workers and machinists, may be at increased risk for carpal tunnel syndrome (Calandruccio & Thompson, 2018).

The patient experiences pain, numbness, paresthesia, and, possibly, weakness along the median nerve distribution (thumb, index, and middle fingers). Night pain and/or fist clenching upon awakening is common. A positive Tinel sign helps identify patients requiring intervention (see Fig. 36-4).

Evidence-based treatment of acute carpal tunnel syndrome includes oral or intra-articular injections of corticosteroids, use of NSAIDs and acupuncture with and without electrical stimulation (attached to the needles). Application of splints to prevent hyperextension and prolonged flexion of the wrist is also effective; however, laser and ultrasound therapies are ineffective, as are prolotherapies, or the injection of substances (e.g., dextrose, lidocaine) purported to stimulate healing, diuretics, and vitamin B_6 (Calandruccio & Thompson, 2018). The risks of inhibiting the synthesis of reparative substrates like collagen can potentiate an increased risk for tendon rupture; therefore, long-term use of corticosteroids is not supported (McAlindon et al., 2017).

Traditional open nerve release or endoscopic laser surgery are the two most common surgical management options when nonsurgical treatments fail. Both of these procedures are performed under local anesthesia and involve making incisions into the affected wrist and cutting the carpal ligament so that the carpal tunnel is widened. Smaller incisions are made with the endoscopic laser procedure, resulting in less scar formation and a shorter recovery time than with the open method. Following either procedure, the patient wears a hand splint and limits hand use during healing. The patient may need assistance with personal care. Full recovery of motor and sensory function after either type of nerve release surgery may take several weeks or months.

Ganglion

A ganglion—a collection of neurologic gelatinous material near the tendon sheaths and joints—appears as a round, firm, cystic swelling, usually on the dorsum of the wrist. It frequently occurs in women younger than 50 years (McCance & Huether, 2019). The swelling is locally tender and may cause an aching pain. When a tendon sheath is involved, weakness of the finger occurs. Treatment may include aspiration, corticosteroid injection, or surgical excision. After treatment, a compression dressing and immobilization splint are used; however, a ganglion may recur after medical intervention (De Keyser, 2019).

Dupuytren Disease

Dupuytren disease results in a slowly progressive **contracture** (i.e., an abnormal shortening) of the palmar fascia that causes flexion of the fourth, fifth, and, sometimes, middle finger, rendering these fingers more or less useless (see Fig. 36-5). It is linked to an inherited autosomal dominant trait and occurs most frequently in men of Scandinavian or Celtic heritage who are older than 50 years (McCance & Huether, 2019). Dupuytren disease is also associated with arthritis, diabetes, gout, cigarette smoking, and alcoholism (Ball, Izadi, Verjee, et al., 2016). Starting as a nodule, it may or may not

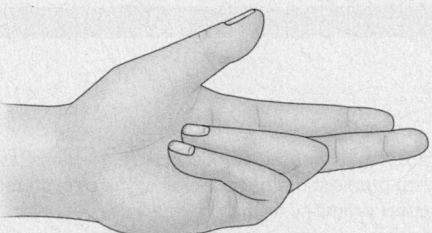

Figure 36-5 • Dupuytren contracture, a flexion deformity caused by an inherited trait, is a slowly progressive contracture of the palmar fascia, which severely impairs the function of the fourth, fifth, and, sometimes, middle finger.

progress, producing a contracture of the fingers and palmar skin changes. The patient may experience dull and aching discomfort, morning numbness, and stiffness in the affected fingers. This condition starts in one hand, but eventually both are affected. Finger-stretching exercises in early disease or intranodular injections of corticosteroids or collagenases may prevent contractures (Ball et al., 2016). With loss of movement, palmar and digital fasciotomies are performed to improve function.

Nursing Management of the Patient Undergoing Surgery of the Hand or Wrist

Surgery of the hand or wrist, unless related to major trauma, is generally an ambulatory procedure. Before surgery, the nurse assesses the patient's level and type of discomfort, as well as limitations in function, caused by the condition.

Hourly neurovascular assessment of the exposed fingers for the first 24 hours following surgery is essential for monitoring function of the nerves and perfusion. This is especially important if an intraoperative tourniquet technique was used, which is implicated in neurovascular deficits. The nurse compares the affected extremity with the unaffected extremity and the postoperative status with the documented preoperative status. The nurse asks the patient to describe sensations in the digits and has the patient demonstrate mobility, while enforcing limitations in movement prescribed by the patient's surgeon. With tendon repairs and nerve, vascular, or skin grafts, more extensive function is tested (see Chapter 35, Chart 35-3). Percutaneous pins may be used to hold bones in position. These pins serve as potential sites of infection. Patient education concerning aseptic wound and pin care may be necessary.

Dressings provide support but should be nonconstrictive. Intermittent use of ice packs to the surgical area during the first 24 to 48 hours may be prescribed to control edema. Unless contraindicated, active extension and flexion of the fingers to promote circulation are encouraged, even though movement is limited by the bulky dressing.

Generally, pain and discomfort can be controlled by the use of oral analgesic agents. Patient education concerning the risk of falls and impaired cognition is important. Pain out of proportion to what is expected, particularly if it is accompanied with compromised neurovascular functioning, needs to be evaluated as an indication of compartment syndrome (see Chapter 37). Pain may be related to surgery, edema, hematoma formation, or restrictive bandages. To control swelling that may increase the patient's discomfort, the nurse

instructs the patient to elevate the hand to heart level with pillows. If the patient is ambulatory, the arm is supported in a conventional sling with the hand elevated at heart level (see Chapter 37, Fig. 37-15).

During the first few days after surgery, independent self-care is impaired. The patient may need to arrange for assistance with feeding, bathing, dressing, and toileting. Within a few days, the patient develops skills in one-handed ADLs and is usually able to function with minimal help and assistive devices. The nurse encourages the patient to use the involved hand, unless contraindicated, within the limits of discomfort. As rehabilitation progresses, the patient resumes use of the limb. Physical or occupational therapy–directed exercises may be prescribed.

Promoting Home, Community-Based, and Transitional Care

 Educating Patients About Self-Care

After the patient has undergone surgery, the nurse instructs the patient how to monitor neurovascular status and the signs of complications that need to be reported to the surgeon (e.g., paresthesia, paralysis, uncontrolled pain, coolness of fingers, extreme swelling, excessive bleeding, purulent drainage, foul odor, fever). The nurse discusses prescribed medications and their side effects with the patient. In addition, the nurse instructs the patient how to elevate the extremity and to apply ice (if prescribed) to control swelling. The use of assistive devices is demonstrated if such devices would be helpful in promoting accomplishment of ADLs. For bathing, the nurse instructs the patient to keep the dressing dry by covering it with a secured plastic bag. Generally, the wound is not redressed until the patient's follow-up visit with the surgeon (see Chart 36-4). The nurse identifies any perceived barriers to being able to attend to this plan (such as childcare needs). The patient is referred to community-based resources as appropriate.

Common Foot Problems

Disorders of the foot may be caused by poorly fitting shoes, which distort normal anatomy while inducing deformity and pain. Dermatologic problems commonly affect the feet in the form of fungal infections and plantar warts. Several systemic diseases affect the feet. Patients with diabetes are prone to develop corns and peripheral neuropathies with diminished sensation, leading to diabetic ulcers at pressure points of the foot. Patients with peripheral vascular disease and arteriosclerosis complain of burning and itching feet, resulting in scratching and skin breakdown. Foot deformities may occur with RA. Obesity can cause a host of foot anomalies, including adult-onset pes planus (i.e., "fallen arches") and plantar fasciitis.

The discomforts of foot strain are treated with rest, elevation, physiotherapy, supportive taping, and orthotic devices (Luffy, Grosel, Thomas, et al., 2018). The patient must inspect the foot and skin under pads and orthotic devices for pressure and skin breakdown daily. If a "window" is cut into shoes to relieve pressure over a bony deformity, the skin must be monitored daily for breakdown from pressure exerted at the window area. Active foot exercises promote circulation and help strengthen the feet. Walking in properly fitting shoes is considered the ideal exercise.

Chart 36-4

HOME CARE CHECKLIST

Hand or Foot Surgery

At the completion of education, the patient and/or caregiver will be able to:

- Name the procedure that was performed and identify any permanent changes in anatomic structure or function as well as changes in ADLs, IADLs, roles, relationships, and spirituality.
- Identify modification of home environment, interventions, and strategies (e.g., durable medical equipment, adaptive equipment) used in safely adapting to changes in structure or function and promote effective recovery and rehabilitation.
- Describe ongoing postoperative therapeutic regimen, including diet and activities to perform (e.g., immobilization) and to limit or avoid (e.g., lifting weights, driving a car, contact sports).
  - Describe methods to prevent wound infection (e.g., keeping dressing clean and dry during activities of daily living).
  - Demonstrate how to assess neurovascular status.
  - Demonstrate control of edema by elevating extremity and applying ice intermittently if prescribed.
  - Observe prescribed weight-bearing, activity and exercise limits.
  - Demonstrate safe use of assistive devices, if appropriate.
  - Consume a healthy diet to promote healing.
- State the name, dose, side effects, frequency, and schedule for all prescribed therapeutic and prophylactic medications (e.g., antibiotics and analgesic agents).

- State indicators of wound infections (e.g., redness, swelling, tenderness, purulent drainage, fever, signs of systemic infection) to report promptly to the provider.
- State indicators of other potential complications to report promptly to the provider (e.g., uncontrolled swelling and pain; cool, pale fingers or toes; paresthesia; paralysis; purulent drainage; signs of deep vein thrombosis or pulmonary embolism).
- Relate how to reach the providers with questions or complications.
- Verbalize the need to keep appointment with surgeon for initial dressing change.
  - State time and date of follow-up appointments and testing.
- Identify the need for health promotion (e.g., weight reduction, smoking cessation, stress management), disease prevention and screening activities.

Resources

See Chapter 2, Chart 2-6 for additional information related to durable medical equipment, adaptive equipment, and mobility skills.

ADLs, activities of daily living; IADLs, instrumental activities of daily living.

Callus

A callus is a thickened area of the skin that has been exposed to persistent pressure or friction. Faulty foot mechanics usually precede the formation of a callus. Treatment consists of eliminating the underlying causes and having a painful callus treated by a podiatrist. A keratolytic ointment may be applied and a thin plastic cup worn over the heel if the callus is on this area. Felt padding with an adhesive backing is also used to prevent and relieve pressure. Prevention of the callus is best, with attention to well-fitting socks and shoes. Orthotic devices can be made to remove the pressure from bony protuberances, or the protuberance may be excised (van Netten, Sacco, Lavery, et al., 2020).

Corn

A corn is an area of hyperkeratosis (overgrowth of a horny layer of epidermis) produced by internal pressure (the underlying bone is prominent because of a congenital or acquired abnormality, commonly arthritis) or external pressure (ill-fitting shoes). The fifth toe is most frequently involved, but any toe may be involved.

Corns are treated by a podiatrist by soaking and scraping off the horny layer, by application of a protective shield or pad, or by surgical modification of the underlying offending osseous structure. Early intervention is required for patients with diabetes.

Soft corns are located between the toes and are kept soft by moisture. Treatment consists of drying the affected spaces and separating the affected toes with lamb's wool or gauze. A wider shoe and toe box may be helpful (Malhotra, Davda, & Singh, 2017).

Hammer Toe

Hammer toe is a flexion deformity of the interphalangeal joint, which may involve several toes (see Fig. 36-6A). Tight socks or shoes may push an overlying toe back into the line of the other toes. The toes usually are pulled upward, forcing the metatarsal joints (ball of the foot) downward. Corns develop on top of the toes, and tender calluses develop under the metatarsal area. Treatment consists of conservative measures: wearing open-toed sandals (unless the patient has diabetes) or shoes that conform to the shape of the foot with a round toe box, carrying out manipulative exercises, and protecting the protruding joints with pads. **Osteotomy** (surgical cutting of the bone) may be used to correct a resulting deformity. There is little evidence to support treatment of hammer toe when the patient does not report pain or other symptoms (Malhotra et al., 2017). Orthotics may help prevent hammer toe in people with high arches. Attention is required for patients with diabetes who may develop friction points, causing wounds.

Onychocryptosis

Onychocryptosis (ingrown toenail) is a condition in which the free edge of a nail plate penetrates the surrounding skin. A secondary infection or granulation tissue may develop. This painful condition is caused by improper self-treatment, external pressure (tight shoes or stockings), internal pressure (deformed toes, growth under the nail), trauma, or infection. Trimming the nails properly (clipping them straight across and filing the corners consistent with the contour of the toe) can prevent this problem. Active treatment consists of washing the foot twice a day and relieving the pain by decreasing the pressure of the nail plate on the surrounding soft tissue.

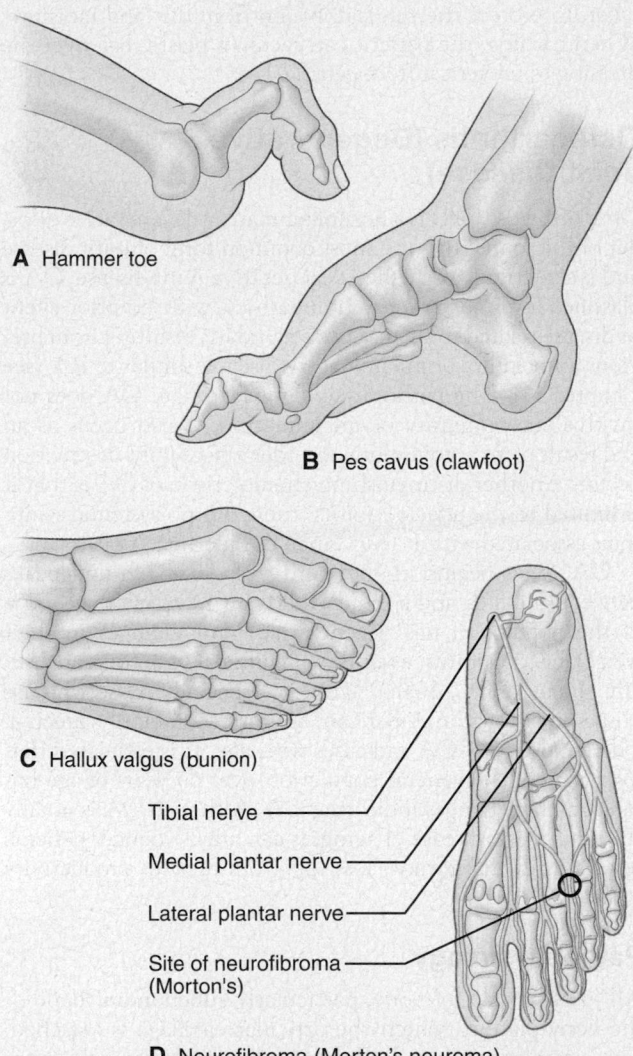

A Hammer toe

B Pes cavus (clawfoot)

C Hallux valgus (bunion)

Tibial nerve

Medial plantar nerve

Lateral plantar nerve

Site of neurofibroma
(Morton's)

D Neurofibroma (Morton's neuroma)

Figure 36-6 • Common foot deformities.

Warm, wet soaks help drain an infection. A toenail may need to be excised by the podiatrist or primary provider if there are recurrent infections (Malhotra et al., 2017).

Pes Cavus

Pes cavus (clawfoot) refers to a foot with an abnormally high arch and a fixed equines deformity of the forefoot (see Fig. 36-6B). The shortening of the foot and increased pressure produce calluses on the metatarsal area and on the dorsum of the foot. Charcot–Marie–Tooth disease (a peripheral neuromuscular disease associated with a familial degenerative disorder), diabetes, and progressive neurologic disorders are common causes (Alderson & Ghosh, 2019). Exercises are prescribed to manipulate the forefoot into dorsiflexion and relax the toes. Orthotic devices alleviate pain and can protect the foot. In severe cases, arthrodesis (fusion) is performed to reshape and stabilize the foot.

Hallux Valgus

Hallux valgus (bunion) is a deformity in which the great toe deviates laterally (see Fig. 36-6C). There is a marked prominence of the medial aspect of the first metatarsophalangeal joint. There is also osseous enlargement (exostosis) of the medial side of the first metatarsal head, over which a bursa may form (secondary to pressure and inflammation). Acute bursitis symptoms include a reddened area, edema, and tenderness.

Factors contributing to bunion formation include heredity, ill-fitting shoes, osteoarthritis, and the gradual lengthening and widening of the foot associated with aging. Treatment depends on the patient's age, the degree of deformity, and the severity of symptoms. In uncomplicated cases, wearing a shoe that conforms to the shape of the foot, or that is molded to the foot to prevent pressure on the protruding portions, may be the only treatment needed. Corticosteroid injections control acute inflammation. In advanced cases, surgical removal of the exostosis and toe realignment may be required to improve function, appearance, and symptoms. If surgery is required in an athlete, at least 3 months of rest is required before returning to play (Fournier, Saxena, & Maffuli, 2019).

Morton Neuroma

Morton neuroma (plantar digital neuroma, neurofibroma) is a swelling near the third (lateral) branch of the median plantar nerve (see Fig. 36-6D). Microscopically, digital artery changes cause an ischemia within the third intermetatarsal (web) space. The result is a throbbing, burning pain in the foot that is usually relieved with rest and massage.

Conservative treatment consists of inserting innersoles and metatarsal pads designed to spread the metatarsal heads and balance the foot posture. Local injections of a corticosteroid and a local anesthetic may provide relief. If these fail, surgical excision of the neuroma is necessary. Pain relief and loss of sensation are immediate and permanent with surgery. The risk of falls is increased because of the loss of all sensation (Matthews, Hum, Harding, et al., 2019).

Pes Planus

Pes planus (flatfoot) is a common disorder in which the longitudinal arch of the foot is diminished. It may be caused by congenital abnormalities or associated with bone or ligament injury, excessive weight, muscle fatigue, poorly fitting shoes, or arthritis. Signs and symptoms include a burning sensation, fatigue, clumsy gait, edema, and pain. Exercises to strengthen the muscles and to improve posture and walking habits are helpful (Unver, Erdem, & Akbas, 2019). Foot orthoses can give the foot additional support.

Plantar Fasciitis

Plantar fasciitis, an inflammation of the foot-supporting fascia, presents as an acute onset of heel pain experienced with the first steps in the morning. The pain is localized to the anterior medial aspect of the heel and diminishes with gentle stretching of the foot and Achilles tendon. Management includes stretching exercises, wearing shoes with support and cushioning to relieve pain, orthotic devices (e.g., heel cups, arch supports, night splints), and corticosteroid injections. Unresolved plantar fasciitis may progress to fascial tears at the heel and eventual development of heel spurs (Luffy et al., 2018).

Nursing Management of the Patient Undergoing Foot Surgery

Surgery of the foot may be necessary because of various conditions, including neuromas and foot deformities (bunion, hammer toe, clawfoot). Generally, foot surgery is performed on an outpatient basis. Before surgery, the nurse assesses the patient's gait and balance, as well as the neurovascular status of the foot. Additionally, the nurse considers the availability of assistance at home and the structural characteristics of the home in planning for care during the days after surgery.

Postoperative and home care follows the same principles as discussed earlier for hand surgery (see Chart 36-4). After surgery, neurovascular assessment of the exposed toes (every 1 to 2 hours for the first 24 hours) is essential to monitor the function of the nerves and the perfusion of the tissues. The nurse educates the patient and family about how to assess for edema and neurovascular status at home (circulation, motion, sensation). The affected foot is compared to the unaffected foot to determine differences in neurovascular function. Compromised neurovascular function can increase the patient's pain (see Chapter 35, Chart 35-4).

Pain experienced by patients who undergo foot surgery is related to inflammation and edema. Formation of a hematoma may contribute to the discomfort. To control the anticipated edema, the foot should be elevated on several pillows when the patient is sitting or lying. Support of the entire limb under the knee is preferable. Ice packs applied intermittently to the surgical area during the first 24 to 48 hours may be prescribed to control edema and provide some pain relief. As activity increases, the patient may find that dependent positioning of the foot is uncomfortable. Simply elevating the foot often relieves the discomfort. Oral analgesic agents may be used to control the pain. The nurse instructs the patient and family about appropriate use of these medications.

After surgery, the patient will have a bulky dressing on the foot, protected by a light cast or a special protective boot. Limits for weight bearing on the foot will be prescribed by the surgeon (Malhotra et al., 2017). Some patients are allowed to walk on the heel and progress to weight bearing as tolerated; other patients are restricted to non–weight-bearing activities. Assistive devices (e.g., crutches, walker) may be needed. The choice of the devices depends on the patient's general condition and balance and on the weight-bearing prescription. Safe use of the assistive devices must be ensured through adequate patient education and practice before discharge (see Chapter 2). Strategies to move around the house safely while using assistive devices are also discussed with the patient. As healing progresses, the patient gradually resumes ambulation within prescribed limits. The nurse emphasizes adherence to the therapeutic regimen.

The immobility of lower extremity surgery increases the risk of venous thromboembolism (VTE) development. See Chapter 26 for VTE risk assessment and treatment. Other postoperative complications may include limited range of motion, paresthesia, tendon injury, and recurrence of deformity. In addition, if percutaneous pins were used to hold bones in position, these pins may serve as potential sites of infection. Patient education concerning aseptic wound care and pin care may be necessary. See Chapter 37 for further discussion on pin care and infection prophylaxis. Care must be taken to protect the surgical wound from dirt and moisture. When bathing, the patient can secure a plastic bag over the dressing to prevent it from getting wet.

Osteoarthritis (Degenerative Joint Disease)

Osteoarthritis (OA) is a noninflammatory degenerative disorder of the joints. It is the most common form of joint disease and is sometimes also called degenerative joint disease. OA is classified as either primary (idiopathic), with no prior event or disease related to the OA, or secondary, resulting from previous joint injury or inflammatory disease, similar to RA (see Chapter 34). The pathophysiology of primary OA does not involve autoimmunity or inflammation. It can occur as an end result of an autoimmune disorder where joint destruction occurs. Another distinguishing characteristic of OA is that it is limited to the affected joints; there are no systemic symptoms associated with it (McCance & Huether, 2019).

OA often begins in the third decade of life and peaks between the fifth and sixth decades. By 40 years of age, 90% of the population has degenerative joint changes in their weight-bearing joints, even though clinical symptoms are usually absent (CDC, 2018). Women, especially those who are Hispanic or African American, are more commonly affected. The incidence of OA increases with age. It is estimated that over 85% of the general population over 65 years of age has radiographic changes indicating OA. Although OA is usually thought of as a disease of aging, it can affect younger patients resulting in significant loss of work-related productivity (CDC, 2018).

Pathophysiology

All joints consist of bone, particularly **subchondral bone** or the bony plate to which the articular cartilage is attached. This articular cartilage is a lubricated, smooth tissue that protects the bone from damage with physical activity. Between the articular cartilage of the bones forming the joint is a space (called the *joint space*) that allows for movement. To aid in fluidity, each joint contains synovial fluid to help lubricate and protect the joint's movement. With OA, the articular cartilage breaks down, leading to progressive damage to the underlying bone and eventual formation of **osteophytes** (bone spurs) that protrude into the joint space. The result is that the joint space is narrowed, leading to decreased joint movement and the potential for more damage. Consequently, the joint can progressively degenerate (see Fig. 36-7). Understanding of OA pathophysiology has been greatly expanded beyond what was previously thought of as simply "wear and tear" related to aging. The basic degenerative process in the joint exemplified in OA is presented in Figure 36-8. In addition to the degeneration, an infectious arthritis can occur. See later discussion of septic (infectious) arthritis.

Risk factors for the disease and its progression include older age, female gender, and obesity. In addition, certain occupations (e.g., those requiring laborious tasks); engaging in sport activities; and a history of previous injuries, muscle weakness, genetic predisposition, and certain diseases can also place patients at risk for joint destruction. The most prominent modifiable risk factor for OA is obesity. In fact, both quality

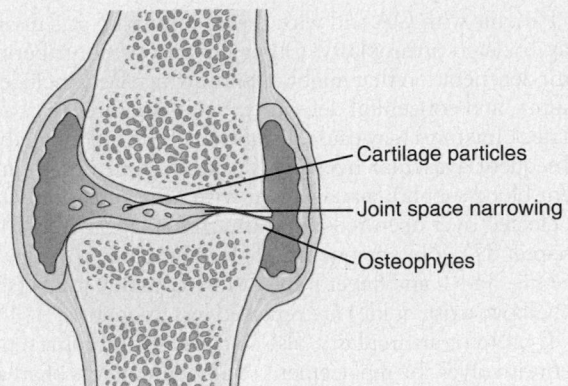

Figure 36-7 • Joint space narrowing and osteophytes (bone spurs) are characteristic of degenerative changes in joints.

Cartilage particles

Joint space narrowing

Osteophytes

and quantity of life are reduced with OA, especially when obesity and OA are combined. A program of diet and exercise can help minimize symptoms of OA in patients with obesity (CDC, 2018).

Clinical Manifestations

The main clinical manifestations of OA are pain, stiffness, and functional impairment. The joint pain is usually aggravated by movement or exercise and relieved by rest. If

Physiology/Pathophysiology

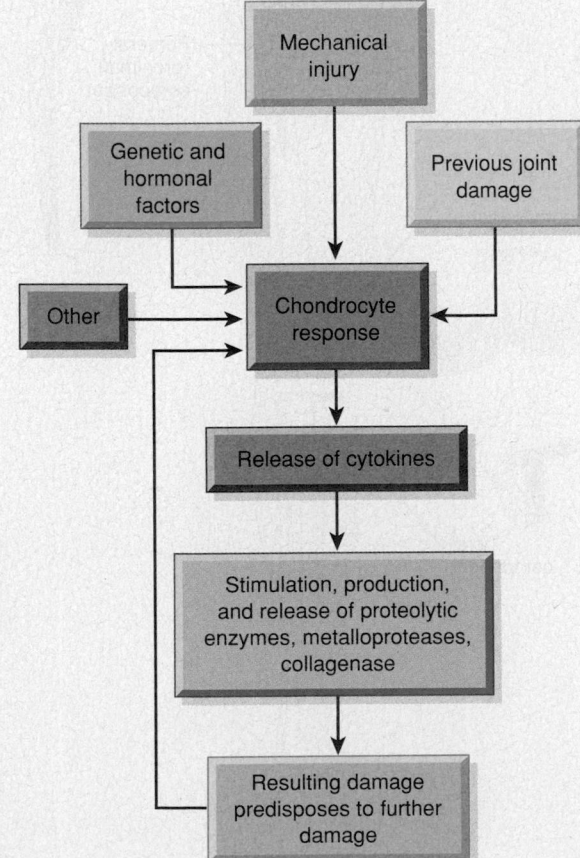

Figure 36-8 • Pathophysiology of osteoarthritis.

morning stiffness is present, it is usually brief, lasting less than 30 minutes. The onset is routinely insidious, progressing over multiple years.

On physical examination, the affected joint may be enlarged with a decreased range of motion. Although OA occurs most often in weight-bearing joints (hips, knees, cervical and lumbar spine), the proximal interphalangeal (PIP) and distal interphalangeal (DIP) joints are also often involved causing bony enlargements of the DIP (Heberden's nodes) and PIP (Bouchard's nodes) joints. Crepitus may be palpated, especially over the knee. Joint effusion, a sign of inflammation, is usually mild. No systemic manifestations are found.

Assessment and Diagnostic Findings

Blood tests and examination of joint fluid are not useful in the diagnosis of OA but are occasionally indicated to rule out an autoimmune cause for the joint pain, such as RA. X-rays may show a narrowing of the joint space; osteophyte formation; and dense, thickened subchondral bone (O'Neill & Felson, 2018).

Medical Management

The goals of management are to decrease pain and stiffness and to maintain or, when possible, improve joint mobility. Exercise, especially in the form of cardiovascular aerobic exercise and lower extremity strength training, has been found to prevent OA progression and decrease symptoms of OA. Along with exercise, weight loss, which in turn decreases excess load on the joint, can also be extremely beneficial. Occupational and physical therapy can help the patient adopt self-management strategies (Schmidt, 2018).

Wedged insoles, knee braces, and other modalities are being evaluated as possible therapies aimed at treating the abnormalities in biomechanics found in OA. The use of orthotic devices (e.g., splints, braces) and walking aids (e.g., canes) can improve pain and function by decreasing force on the affected joint (Schmidt, 2018). Patients with arthritis often use complementary, alternative, and integrative health therapies, such as massage, yoga, pulsed electromagnetic fields, transcutaneous electrical nerve stimulation (TENS), and music therapy. These therapies may also include herbal and dietary supplements, other special diets, acupuncture, acupressure, wearing copper bracelets or magnets, and participation in T'ai chi. Research is under way to determine the effectiveness of many of these treatments. To date, there is no definitive evidence showing their superiority to standard care; the American College of Rheumatology (ACR) has encouraged the use of these therapies only if they do not interfere with medications and are found to increase comfort, mobility, and function for patients (Kolasinski, Neogi, Hochberg, et al., 2020).

Pharmacologic Therapy

Pharmacologic management of OA is directed toward symptom management and pain control. Selection of medication is based on the patient's needs, the stage of disease, and the risk of side effects. Medications are used in conjunction with nonpharmacologic strategies. In most patients with OA, the initial analgesic therapy is acetaminophen. Some patients respond to the nonselective NSAIDs and COX-2 enzyme blockers; however, COX-2 enzyme blockers must be used with caution because of the associated risk of cardiovascular disease and little to no decrease in GI upset. Other medications that may be considered are nonopioids, such as tramadol, opioids in severe cases, and intra-articular corticosteroids (Cooper, Chapurlat, Al-Daghri, et al., 2019; Kolasinski et al., 2020). Topical analgesic agents such as capsaicin and methylsalicylate are also used. Topical diclofenac sodium gel has been FDA approved for the use of osteoarthritic joint pain in the hands and knees (Cooper et al., 2019; Kolasinski et al., 2020). Methotrexate and colchicine, typically prescribed for treating RA and gout, respectively, may also be considered for some patients with OA who are refractory to other treatments. The pathophysiologic antecedents of these diseases are similar to those in OA, and it is believed that may explain the effectiveness of these medications in some select patients with OA (Kolasinski et al., 2020; Raman, FitzGerald, & Murphy, 2018).

Other therapeutic approaches include glucosamine and chondroitin. Although it has been suggested that these substances modify cartilage structure, studies have not shown them to be effective (Kolasinski et al., 2020; Runhaar, Rozendaal, Middlekoop, et al., 2017). Viscosupplementation, the injection of gel-like substances (hyaluronates) into a joint (intra-articular), is thought to supplement the viscous properties of synovial fluid. These viscosupplements aim to prevent the loss of cartilage and repair chondral defects but lack strong evidence that support their use (Kolasinski et al., 2020; Raman, Henrontin, Chevalier, et al., 2018).

Nursing Management

Pain management and optimal functional ability are the major goals of nursing interventions. With those goals in mind, nursing management of the patient with OA includes pharmacologic and nonpharmacologic approaches as well as education. The patient's understanding of the disease process and symptom pattern is critical to the plan of care. Because patients with OA usually are older, they may have other health problems. Commonly they are overweight, and they may have a sedentary lifestyle. Weight loss and exercise are important approaches to lessen pain and disability. Canes or other assistive devices for ambulation should be considered, and any stigma about the use of these devices should be explored. Exercises such as walking should be begun in moderation and increased gradually. Patients should plan their daily exercise for a time when the pain is least severe or plan to use an analgesic agent, if appropriate, before exercising. Adequate pain management is important for the success of an exercise program. Open discussion regarding the use of complementary, alternative, and integrative health therapies is important to maintain safe and effective practices for patients looking for relief.

The Patient Undergoing Arthroplasty

In moderate to severe OA, when pain is severe or because of loss of function, surgical intervention may be used. The procedures most commonly used are osteotomy (to alter the distribution of weight within the joint) and arthroplasty. Joint **arthroplasty** refers to the surgical removal of an unhealthy joint and replacement of joint surfaces with metal or synthetic materials.

Patients with OA and with severe joint pain and disability may undergo arthroplasty. Other conditions contributing to joint degeneration that might require arthroplasty include RA, trauma, and congenital deformity. Some fractures (e.g., femoral neck fracture) may cause disruption of the blood supply and subsequent **avascular necrosis** (death of tissue due to insufficient blood supply); management with joint replacement may be elected over open reduction internal fixation (ORIF) (see Chapter 37). Joints frequently replaced include the hip, knee (see Fig. 36-9), and finger joints. More complex joints (shoulder, elbow, wrist, ankle) are replaced less frequently.

Total joint arthroplasty, also known as total joint replacement, involves the replacement of all components of an articulating joint. Most joint replacements consist of metal (e.g., stainless steel, cobalt-chromium, titanium) and high-density polyethylene components. In order to achieve fixation of components, the material can be cemented, cementless, or a hybrid of both of these materials. Cemented fixation uses a fast-curing bone cement (polymethylmethacrylate [PMMA]) to hold implants in place. Cementless fixation relies on new

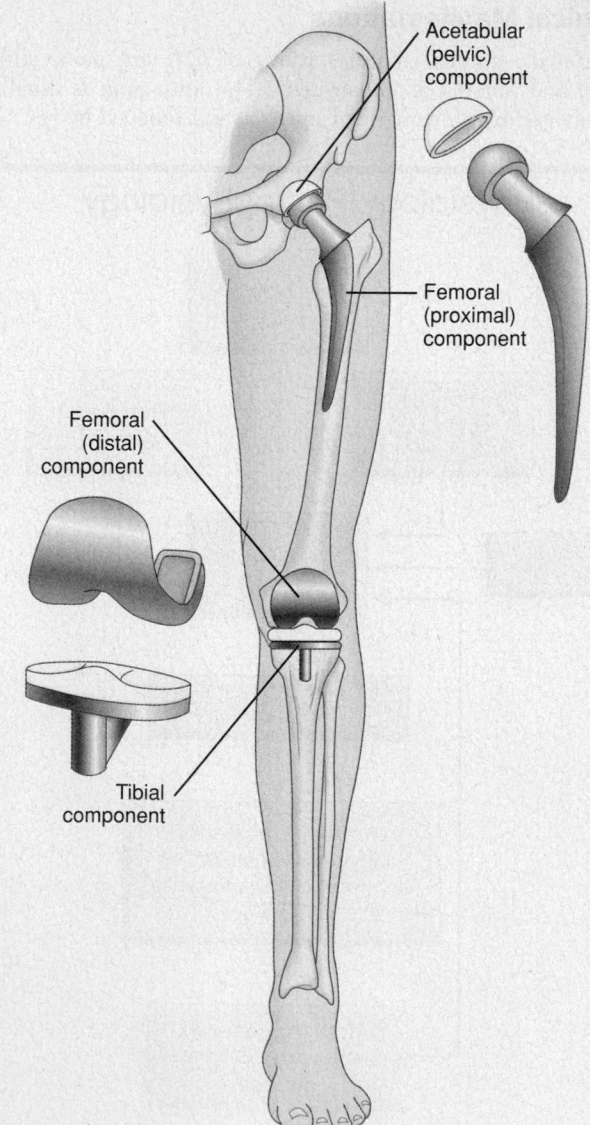

Figure 36-9 • Examples of Hip and Knee Replacement.

bone growing into the surface of the implant by using a press-fit, porous-coated prosthesis. There is also a hybrid fixation technique for total knee arthroplasty (TKA) where the femoral component is inserted without cement, and the tibial and patellar components are inserted with cement. Use of each of these materials and techniques have different benefits and risks. Current research evidence supports the use of either component fixation methods (cemented or cementless) because postoperative functional outcomes, rates of complications, and rates of reoperations are similar (Quinn, Murray, Pezold, et al., 2018). Identifying patient-specific factors that may inform the decision to utilize a particular fixation technique is important. Considerations include gender, age, diagnosis, weight and activity level as well as the presence of healthy bone with adequate blood supply. Issues of cost and cost-effectiveness should also be considered (Quinn et al., 2018).

With joint replacement, patients may expect pain relief, return of joint motion, and improved functional status and quality of life. The scope of these improvements depends in part on patients' preoperative soft tissue condition and general muscle strength. Serious complications seldom occur, and recent innovations in total joint replacement surgery have made this a safer and more routinely performed surgery. Rehabilitation with physical therapy that is initiated within the first 24 hours is associated with decreased hospital length of stay and improved balance and gait function (Quinn et al., 2018). In addition, minimally invasive surgical techniques, biomaterials, postoperative rehabilitation protocols, and multimodal analgesia strategies have led to earlier hospital discharge and quicker recovery (Lee, 2016). The American Joint Replacement Registry (AJRR) monitors the performance of devices and evaluates the cost-effectiveness of procedures. The data generated from the AJRR and other registries provide orthopedic researchers and practitioners with the information necessary to improve the quality of health care among patients in need of knee and hip replacement procedures (Dy, Bumpass, Makhni, et al., 2016). Annual reports are provided to hospital system members to facilitate quality improvement programs (American Academy of Orthopaedic Surgeons [AAOS], 2020).

Preoperative and Intraoperative Nursing Management

Preoperative and intraoperative assessment and management of the patient having arthroplasty are aimed at having the patient in optimal health for surgery (see Chapters 14 and 15). Risks for bleeding, VTE, infection, and pain are managed proactively.

Preventing and Managing Blood Loss

Until recently, acute postoperative anemia due to perioperative blood loss was a common occurrence in patients having total hip arthroplasty (THA) and TKA; allogeneic blood transfusions (i.e., blood transfused from a donor) were required in up to 50% of patients who had THA and TKA (Rasouli, Maltenfort, Erkocak, et al., 2016). Recent research findings suggest that rate has dropped significantly, to approximately 9% of patients who have THA and 4% for patients who have TKA (Bedard, Pugely, Lux, et al., 2017). This diminished demand for allogeneic blood transfusions is attributable to the following interventions

(Alexander & Frew, 2017; Loftus, Spratling, Stone, et al., 2016; Martin & Harris, 2020; Stalenhag & Sterner, 2019):

- Appropriate preoperative assessment and treatment of patients with anemia (i.e., low red blood cell counts) with pharmacologic agents, such as epoetin alfa or iron supplements
- Application of pneumatic tourniquets during orthopedic limb surgery (e.g., TKA), which not only minimizes bleeding but also helps maintain a clean surgical field
- Employment of intraoperative red blood cell salvage systems, as appropriate, during procedures when a large volume of blood is lost. This is effectively a type of autologous transfusion; that is, the patient's own blood is salvaged during the operative procedure and re-transfused back to the patient.
- Intraoperative administration of the antifibrinolytic agent tranexamic acid, which is thought to have significantly reduced overall blood loss and the need for blood transfusions in patients having THA or TKA.

Preventing Venous Thromboembolism

Patients having orthopedic surgery are particularly at risk for VTE, including deep vein thrombosis (DVT) and pulmonary embolism (PE). Therefore, factors that compound or further increase this risk are assessed preoperatively. Increasing age (older than age 40), obesity, taking prescription hormonal medications, preoperative leg edema, previous history of any VTE, and varicose veins increase the risk for postoperative DVT and PE (Menaka & Douketis, 2019). The use of medications that increase the risk of clotting, such as certain hormones and NSAIDs, may be discontinued a week before surgery. Prophylactic low-molecular-weight heparin (LMWH) or another anticoagulant agent may be prescribed prior to or after surgery (Quinn et al., 2018).

Assessing the neurovascular status of the extremity undergoing joint replacement is important, because postoperative assessment data are compared with preoperative assessment data to identify changes and any arterial impairment to the affected extremity. For example, an absent pulse postoperatively is of concern unless the pulse was also absent preoperatively. Nerve palsy could occur as a result of surgery.

Preventing Infection

Preoperative assessment of the patient for recent or active infections, including urinary tract infection, is necessary because of the risk for postoperative infection. Any infection presenting 2 to 4 weeks before planned surgery may result in postponement of surgery. Preoperative skin preparations, such as showers with antiseptic soap, are recommended the evening before and the morning of surgery. Scrubbing of the surgical site with a prescribed antiseptic soap the night before or on the morning of surgery decreases bacterial count on the skin and helps lower the chance of infection (Berrios-Torres, Umscheid, Bratzler, et al., 2017; Papas, Conguista, Scuderi, et al., 2018).

Research findings suggest that prophylactic broad-spectrum antibiotics given 60 minutes prior to skin incision and discontinued within 24 hours postoperatively are effective in preventing surgical site infections (De Francesco, Fu, Kalenberg, et al., 2019).

The use of antibiotic-loaded bone cement and preoperative nasal swabbing to screen for patients who are carriers of methicillin-resistant *Staphylococcus aureus* (MRSA) or methicillin-sensitive *Staphylococcus aureus* (MSSA) may help in further reducing postoperative infections; the effectiveness of these modalities is under research as is the use of dual antibiotic therapy (Villa, Pannu, Riesgo, et al., 2020). Culture of the joint during surgery may be important in identifying and treating subsequent infections.

Managing Pain

Assessment of the patient's pain preoperatively and any cultural and personal preferences are important components related to the control of pain following joint surgery. Assessing the patient's level of understanding of the surgery and explaining what to expect in the postoperative period (e.g., incentive spirometry, pain control methods, activity limits) can improve outcomes. Research findings suggest that patients who are supported and educated telephonically in the preoperative period report better quality of life and well-being postoperatively (Allsop, Fairhall, & Morphet, 2019) (see Nursing Research Profile in Chart 36-5). However, high anxiety and severe pain prior to surgery may have an impact on these outcomes (Jones, Al-Naseer, Bodger, et al., 2018) (see Chapter 9).

Total Hip Arthroplasty

THA is the replacement of a severely damaged hip with an artificial joint. Indications for this surgery include OA, as well as RA, femoral neck fractures (i.e., hip fracture; see Chapter 37), failure of previous reconstructive surgeries, such as a failed prosthesis with osteotomy, and conditions resulting from developmental dysplasia or Legg–Calvé–Perthes disease (avascular necrosis of the hip in childhood). A variety of total hip prostheses are available. Most consist of a metal femoral component topped by a spherical ball made of metal, ceramic, or plastic that is fitted into a plastic or metal acetabular socket (see Fig. 36-9).

The surgeon selects the prosthesis that is best suited to the individual patient, considering various factors including skeletal structure and activity level. The patient has irreversibly damaged hip joints, and the potential benefits, including improved quality of life, outweigh the surgical risks. With the advent of improved prosthetic materials and operative techniques, the life of the prosthesis has been extended, and today younger patients with severely damaged and painful hip joints are undergoing total hip replacement.

Nursing Management

The nurse must be aware of and monitor for specific potential complications associated with THA (Gabbert, Filson, Bodden, et al., 2019). Complications that may occur include dislocation of the hip prosthesis, excessive wound drainage, VTE, infection, and heel pressure injury (see Chart 36-6).

(text continued on page 1130)

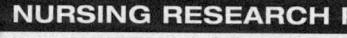

Chart 36-5 | **NURSING RESEARCH PROFILE**
Preoperative Telephone Support for Patients Having Total Knee Arthroplasty

Allsop, S., Fairhill, R., & Morphet, J. (2019). The impact of preoperative telephone support and education on symptoms of anxiety, depression, pain and quality of life post total knee replacement. *International Journal of Orthopaedic and Trauma Nursing, 34,* 21–27.

Purpose

Patients scheduled to have elective total knee arthroplasty (TKA) can experience anxiety and depression during the preoperative waiting period which may negatively impact postoperative outcomes. The purpose of this study was to determine whether preoperative patient support and education delivered via telephone would impact postoperative reports of quality of life (QOL), depression, anxiety and pain among patients having total knee replacement surgery.

Design

This mixed methods study explored the effects of a support intervention in a sample of participants (*N* = 18) who underwent unilateral total knee replacements. Pre-tests were administered up to 6 weeks prior to elective surgery in the clinic setting. Those with infections, malignancy, or repeat interventions were excluded. Baseline data included demographics and Patient Reported Outcomes Measures (PROMS) which assessed QOL, psychological distress, and pain; using scales previously validated in this population.

Two phone calls were made by the same researcher to address open- and closed-ended questions based on information considered essential for patients to understand before surgery. The researcher individualized content that was delivered to the participants in response to their unique questions and concerns. A thematic analysis was undertaken to identify patterns in responses. The PROMS scales were readministered 6 weeks after surgery, either during a clinic visit or by telephone.

Findings

Of the 18 enrolled participants, 16 completed the study. One third were men; 19% lived alone; half of the participants were under 65 years of age and 69% of them were not actively employed. Depression and anxiety (rated as high or very high) were reported by 31% of the patients preoperatively.

Participants' concerns related to the administrative processes of admission and discharge and the psychological processing of having a major surgery; some expressed fears of being awake with spinal anesthetic approaches. Participants voiced concerns about their caregivers, the potential for infection, and the wish to return home quickly. Many favorable comments were made concerning the positive impact of the program.

Fewer participants experienced anxiety and depression postsurgery; however, this change was not significant. There were significant improvements in QOL scores (*p* = 0.008) and pain scores (*p* < 0.001). However, compared to previous studies (most of which had longer duration of interventions and follow-up), the improvement in QOL, anxiety, and pain scores was not as substantial.

Nursing Implications

Findings from this study suggest that preoperative telephone support and education of patients scheduled for TKA can improve QOL and pain postoperatively. This study only spanned a 6-week postoperative period, potentially limiting the ability to capture change in study outcomes. This was a single site study which warrants replication in a greater number of facilities with greater attention to the optimal time period required to assess outcomes in this population. In addition, greater attention to more comprehensive psychological interventions preoperatively may also be required for better success in the long term.

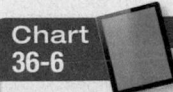

Chart 36-6

PLAN OF NURSING CARE
The Patient with a Total Hip Arthroplasty

NURSING DIAGNOSIS: Acute pain associated with total hip arthroplasty
GOAL: Relief of pain

Nursing Interventions	Rationale	Expected Outcomes
1. Assess patient for pain using a standard pain intensity scale.	1. Pain is expected after a surgical procedure because of the surgical trauma and tissue response. Muscle spasms occur after total hip replacements. Immobility causes discomfort at pressure points.	• Describes discomfort • Expresses confidence in efforts to control pain • States pain is reduced; pain intensity scores are decreasing • Appears comfortable and relaxed • Uses physical, psychological, and pharmacologic measures to reduce pain and discomfort
2. Ask patient to describe discomfort.	2. Pain characteristics may help to determine the cause of discomfort. Pain may be due to complications (hematoma, infection, dislocation). Pain is an individual experience—it means different things to different people.	
3. Acknowledge existence of pain; inform patient of available analgesic agents or muscle relaxants.	3. The nurse can reduce the stress experienced by patient by communicating concern and availability of assistance to help the patient deal with the pain.	
a. Use pain-modifying techniques. Administer analgesic agents as prescribed.	a. Patient will require parenteral opioids during the first 24–48 hours and then will progress to oral analgesic agents.	
b. Change position within prescribed limits.	b. The use of pillows to provide adequate support and relief of pressure on bony prominences assists in minimizing pain.	
c. Modify environment.	c. Interactions with others, distractions, and sensory overload or deprivation may affect pain experience.	
d. Notify primary provider about persistent pain.	d. Surgical intervention may be necessary if pain is due to hematoma or excessive edema.	
4. Evaluate and record discomfort and effectiveness of pain-modifying techniques.	4. Effectiveness of action is based on experience; data provide a baseline about pain experiences, pain management, and pain relief.	

NURSING DIAGNOSIS: Impaired mobility associated with positioning, weight bearing, and activity restrictions after total hip arthroplasty
GOAL: Achieves pain-free, functional, stable hip joint

Nursing Interventions	Rationale	Expected Outcomes
1. Maintain proper positioning of hip joint (abduction, neutral rotation, limited flexion).	1. Prevents dislocation of hip prosthesis.	• Maintains prescribed position • No heel pressure • Assists in position changes • Shows increased independence in transfers • Exercises hourly while awake • Participates in progressive ambulation program • Actively participates in exercise regimen • Uses ambulatory aids correctly and safely
2. Keep pressure off heel.	2. Prevents pressure injury on heel.	
3. Instruct and assist in position changes and transfers.	3. Encourages patient's active participation while preventing dislocation.	
4. Instruct and supervise isometric quadriceps and gluteal setting exercises.	4. Strengthens muscles needed for walking.	
5. In consultation with physical therapist, instruct and supervise progressive safe ambulation within limitations of weight-bearing prescription.	5. Amount of weight bearing depends on patient's condition and prosthesis; ambulatory aids are used to assist the patient with non–weight-bearing and partial weight-bearing ambulation.	
6. Offer encouragement and support exercise regimen.	6. Reconditioning exercises can be uncomfortable and fatiguing; encouragement helps patient comply with exercise program.	
7. Instruct and supervise safe use of ambulatory aids.	7. Prevents injury from unsafe use and prevents falls.	

(continued on page 1128)

Chart 36-6

PLAN OF NURSING CARE (continued)

The Patient with a Total Hip Arthroplasty

COLLABORATIVE PROBLEMS: Hemorrhage; neurovascular compromise; dislocation of prosthesis; venous thromboembolism; infection associated with surgery

GOAL: Absence of complications

Nursing Interventions	Rationale	Expected Outcomes
Hemorrhage		
1. Monitor vital signs, observing for shock.	1. Changes in pulse, blood pressure, and respirations may indicate development of shock. Blood loss and stress of surgery may contribute to development of shock.	• Vital signs stabilize within normal limits • Amount of drainage decreases • No bright-red bloody drainage • Hematology values are within normal limits
2. Note character and amount of drainage.	2. Within 48 hours, bloody drainage collected in portable suction device, if in use, should decrease to 25–30 mL per 8 hours. Excessive drainage (>250 mL in first 8 hours after surgery) and bright-red drainage may indicate active bleeding.	
3. Notify primary provider if patient develops shock or excessive bleeding, and prepare for administration of fluids, blood component therapy, and medications.	3. Corrective measures need to be instituted.	
4. Monitor hemoglobin and hematocrit values.	4. Anemia due to blood loss may develop. Blood replacement or iron supplementation may be needed.	
Neurovascular Dysfunction		
1. Assess affected extremity for color and temperature.	1. The skin becomes pale and feels cool with decreased tissue perfusion. Venous congestion may produce cyanosis.	• Color normal • Extremity warm • Normal capillary refill • Moderate edema and swelling; tissue not palpably tense • Pain controllable • No pain with passive dorsiflexion • Normal sensations • No paresthesia • Normal motor abilities • No paresis or paralysis • Pulses strong and equal
2. Assess toes for capillary refill response.	2. After compression of the nail, rapid return of pink color indicates good capillary perfusion.	
3. Assess extremity for edema and swelling. Report patient complaints of leg tightness.	3. The trauma of surgery will cause edema. Excessive swelling and hematoma formation can compromise circulation and function.	
4. Elevate lower extremity. Keep elevated extremity lower than hip when in chair.	4. Minimizes dependent edema. Hip is never flexed more than 90 degrees to prevent dislocation.	
5. Assess for deep, throbbing, unrelenting pain.	5. Surgical pain can be controlled with pharmacologic and nonpharmacologic interventions; pain due to neurovascular compromise typically does not respond to traditional postoperative pain management strategies.	
6. Assess for pain on passive flexion of foot.	6. With nerve ischemia, there will be pain on passive stretch. Additionally, pain or tenderness may indicate deep vein thrombosis.	
7. Assess for change in sensations and numbness.	7. Diminished pain and sensory function may indicate nerve damage. Sensation in web between great and second toe—peroneal nerve; sensation on sole of foot—tibial nerve.	
8. Assess ability to move foot and toes.	8. Dorsiflexion of ankle and extension of toes indicate function of peroneal nerve. Plantar flexion of ankle and flexion of toes indicate function of tibial nerve.	
9. Assess pedal pulses in both feet.	9. Indicator of extremity circulation.	
10. Notify surgeon if altered neurovascular status is noted.	10. Function of extremity needs to be preserved.	

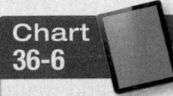

Chart 36-6

PLAN OF NURSING CARE (continued)
The Patient with a Total Hip Arthroplasty

Nursing Interventions	Rationale	Expected Outcomes
Dislocation of Prosthesis		
1. Position patient as prescribed.	1. Hip component positioning (femoral component in acetabular component) needs to be maintained.	• Prosthesis not dislocated • Adheres to recommendations to prevent dislocation
2. Use abductor splint or pillows to maintain position and to support extremity.	2. Keeps hip in abduction and in a neutral rotation to prevent dislocation.	
3. Support leg and place pillows between legs when patient is turning and side-lying; turn to the unaffected side.	3. Prevent dislocation.	
4. Avoid acute flexion of hip (head of bed ≤90 degrees).	4. Findings may indicate dislocation of prosthesis.	
5. Avoid crossing legs.	5. Joint dislocations compromise neurovascular status and future function of extremity.	
6. Assess for dislocation of prosthesis (extremity shortens, internally or externally rotated, severe hip pain, patient unable to move extremity).		
7. Notify surgeon of possible dislocation.		
Venous Thromboembolism		
1. Use anti-embolism stocking and sequential compression device as prescribed.	1. Aids in venous blood return and prevents stasis.	• Wears anti-embolism stocking; uses compression device • No skin breakdown • Pulses equal and strong • Skin temperature normal • No calf pain or tenderness • Changes position with assistance and supervision • Participates in exercise regimen • Well hydrated • No chest pain; lungs clear to auscultation; no evidence of pulmonary emboli
2. Remove stocking for 20 minutes twice a day and provide skin care.	2. Aids in venous blood return and prevents stasis.	
3. Assess popliteal, dorsalis pedis, and posterior tibial pulses.	3. Skin care is necessary to avoid breakdown. Extended removal of stocking defeats purpose of stocking.	
4. Assess skin temperature of legs.	4. Pulses indicate arterial perfusion of extremity.	
5. Assess for unilateral calf pain or tenderness every 8 hours.	5. Local inflammation will increase local skin temperature.	
6. Avoid pressure on popliteal blood vessels from equipment (e.g., abductor splint straps, sequential compression stockings) or pillows.	6. Pain or tenderness may indicate deep vein thrombosis.	
7. Change position and increase activity as prescribed.	7. Compression of blood vessels diminishes blood flow.	
8. Supervise ankle exercises hourly.	8. Activity promotes circulation and diminishes venous stasis.	
9. Monitor body temperature.	9. Muscle exercise promotes circulation.	
10. Encourage fluids.	10. Body temperature increases with inflammation.	
	11. Dehydration increases blood viscosity.	
Infection		
1. Monitor vital signs.	1. Temperature, pulse, and respirations increase in response to infection. (Magnitude of response may be minimal in older adults.)	• Vital signs normal • Well-approximated incision without drainage or excessive inflammatory response • Minimal discomfort; no hematoma • Tolerates antibiotics
2. Use aseptic technique for dressing changes and emptying of portable drainage.	2. Avoids introducing organisms.	
3. Assess wound appearance and character of drainage.	3. Red, swollen, draining incision is indicative of infection.	
4. Assess complaints of pain.	4. Pain may be due to wound hematoma–a possible locus of infection–that needs to be surgically evacuated.	
5. Administer prophylactic antibiotics if prescribed, and observe for side effects.	5. Infected prosthesis is avoided.	

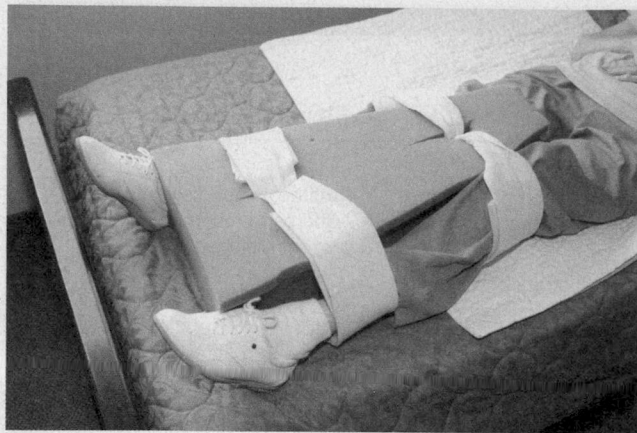

Figure 36-10 • An abduction pillow may be used after a total hip arthroplasty to prevent dislocation of the prosthesis.

The nurse also monitors for complications associated with immobility. Long-term complications include **heterotopic ossification** (formation of bone in the periprosthetic space), avascular necrosis, and loosening of the prosthesis.

Preventing Dislocation of the Hip Prosthesis

For patients undergoing a posterior or posterolateral approach for THA, maintenance of the femoral head component in the acetabular cup is essential. The risk for dislocation is more common with this approach and may occur when the hip is in full flexion, adducted (legs together), and internally rotated. Therefore, correct positioning is maintained at all times. The patient should be in a supine position with the head slightly elevated and the affected leg in a neutral position. The use of an abduction splint, a wedge pillow (see Fig. 36-10), or two or three pillows placed between the legs prevent adduction beyond the midline of the body. A cradle boot may be used to prevent leg rotation and to support the heel off the bed, preventing development of a pressure injury. When the nurse turns the patient in bed to the unaffected side, it is important to keep the operative hip in **abduction** (movement away from the center or median line of the body) (Gabbert et al., 2019). The patient should not be turned to the operative side, which could cause dislocation, unless specified by the surgeon.

The patient's hip is never flexed more than 90 degrees. When using a fracture bedpan, the nurse instructs the patient to flex the unaffected hip and to use the trapeze to lift the pelvis onto the pan. The patient is also reminded not to flex the affected hip.

Limited flexion is maintained during transfers and when sitting. When the patient is initially assisted out of bed, an abduction splint or pillows are kept between the legs. The nurse encourages the patient to keep the affected hip in extension, instructing the patient to pivot on the unaffected leg with assistance by the nurse, who protects the affected hip from **adduction** (movement toward the center or median line of the body), flexion, internal or external rotation, and excessive weight bearing.

High-seat (orthopedic) chairs with arm rests, semi-reclining chairs, and raised toilet seats are used to minimize hip joint flexion. When sitting, the patient's hips should be higher than the knees. The patient's affected leg should not be elevated when sitting. The patient may flex the knee.

The nurse educates the patient about protective positioning, which includes maintaining abduction and avoiding internal and external rotation, hyperextension, and acute flexion, as described previously. At no time should the patient cross the legs or bend at the waist past 90 degrees (e.g., to put on shoes and socks). Occupational therapists can provide the patient with devices to assist with dressing below the waist. Hip precautions for patients who had a posterior or posterolateral approach for THA should be enforced for 4 months or longer after surgery (see Chart 36-7). A patient who has had an anterior surgical approach may not need these precautions. Several studies have reported an anterolateral approach to THA results in a lower rate of dislocation than a posterior approach owing to its ease of access, superior visualization, and a predictable healing pattern. Using a less restrictive mobility protocol in these patients can lead to earlier and better resumption of ADL, earlier return to work, a shorter length of hospital stay, and improved patient satisfaction (Morris, Fornit, Marchoni, et al., 2018).

Dislocation may occur with positioning that exceeds the limits of the prosthesis. The nurse must monitor for signs and symptoms of dislocation of the prosthesis, which include:

- Increased pain at the surgical site, swelling, and immobilization
- Acute groin pain in the affected hip or increased discomfort
- Shortening of the affected extremity
- Abnormal external or internal rotation of the affected extremity
- Restricted ability or inability to move the leg
- Reported "popping" sensation in the hip

If any of these clinical manifestations occur, the nurse (or the patient, if at home) immediately notifies the surgeon, because the hip must be reduced and stabilized promptly so that the leg does not sustain circulatory and nerve damage. After closed reduction, the hip may be stabilized with Buck's traction or a brace to prevent recurrent dislocation (see Chapter 37, Fig. 37-11). As the muscles and joint capsule heal, the chance of dislocation diminishes. Stresses to the new hip joint should be avoided for the first 8 to 12 weeks, when the risk of dislocation is greatest (Gabbert et al., 2019).

Promoting Ambulation

Patients begin ambulation with the assistance of a walker or crutches within a day after surgery. The nurse and the physical therapist assist the patient in achieving the goal of independent ambulation. At first, the patient may be able to stand for only a brief period because of orthostatic hypotension. Specific weight-bearing limits on the prosthesis are based on the patient's condition, the procedure, and the fixation method. Weight bearing immediately after surgery may be limited to minimize micromotion of the prosthesis in the bone. As the patient is able to tolerate more activity, the nurse encourages transferring to a chair several times a day for short periods and walking for progressively greater distances.

Monitoring Wound Drainage

Fluid and blood accumulating at the surgical site, which could contribute to discomfort and provide a source for infection, may be drained with a closed suction portable suction device. The efficacy of using a wound drainage system is controversial,

---

Chart 36-7

PATIENT EDUCATION

Avoiding Hip Dislocation After Arthroplasty with Posterior or Posterolateral Approach

The nurse instructs the patient to:

Until the hip prosthesis stabilizes after hip replacement surgery, it is necessary to follow instructions for proper positioning so that the prosthesis remains in place. Dislocation of the hip is a serious complication of surgery that causes pain and loss of function and necessitates reduction under anesthesia to correct the dislocation. Desirable positions include abduction, neutral rotation, and flexion of less than 90 degrees. When you are seated, the knees should be lower than the hip.

The nurse notes the following methods for avoiding displacement:

- Keep the knees apart at all times.
- Put a pillow between the legs when sleeping.
- Never cross the legs when seated.
- Avoid bending forward when seated in a chair.
- Avoid bending forward to pick up an object on the floor.
- Use a high-seated chair and a raised toilet seat.
- Do not flex the hip to put on clothing such as pants, stockings, socks, or shoes. Positions to avoid after total hip replacement are shown in the illustrations.

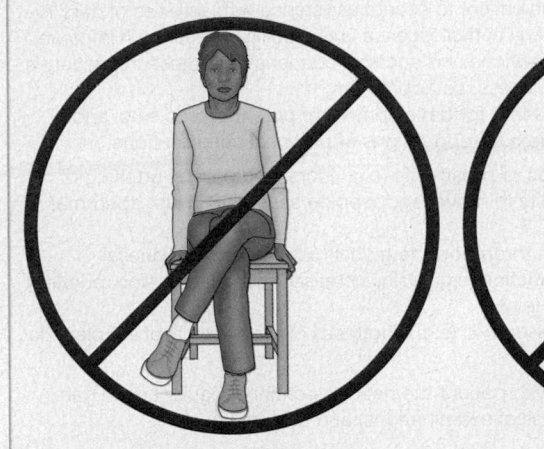

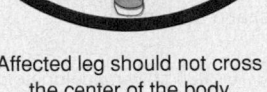

Affected leg should not cross the center of the body

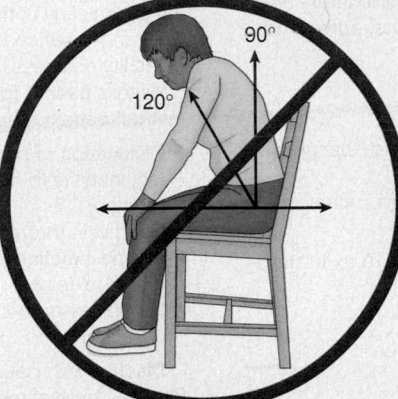

Hip should not bend more than 90 degrees

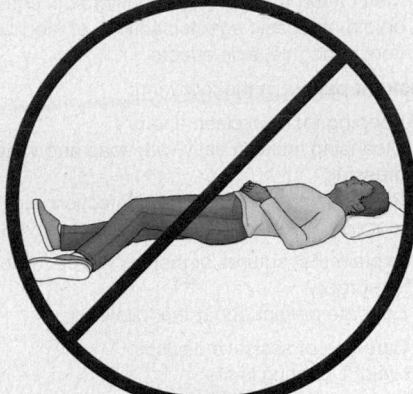

Affected leg should not turn inward

---

especially since the system can be a potential source for infection (Keeney, Austin, & Jevsevar, 2019; Mujagic, Hoffmann, Soysal, et al., 2019). In particular, drains that remain in place for longer than 24 hours create an increased risk for contamination and infection (Keeney et al., 2019; Mujagic et al., 2019). The nurse should monitor the amount of drainage and measure output each shift; the surgeon must be promptly notified of excessive or foul-smelling drainage. After the drain is removed, the drain tube site is cleaned with an antiseptic solution and a small gauze dressing is applied if there is oozing at the site (Gabbert et al., 2019).

Preventing Venous Thromboembolism

Without prophylaxis, DVT formation can develop within 7 to 14 days following surgery and lead to PE, which can be fatal. Early identification of the patient's VTE risk, ensuring that the patient receives the appropriate prophylaxis, instituting preventive measures, and monitoring the patient closely for clinical signs of the development of DVT and PE are key. However, the nurse should also be aware that VTE prevention may increase the postoperative risk for bleeding and stay alert for this potential complication (Erens & Walter, 2019).

Physical signs of DVT include pain and tenderness at or below the area of the clot, swelling or tightness of the affected leg, possibly with pitting edema, with either warmth or cooling, and skin discoloration; PE symptoms may include acute onset of dyspnea, tachycardia, confusion, and pleuritic chest pain (McCance & Huether, 2019).

Intermittent compression devices are applied either intraoperatively or immediately postoperatively; these devices must remain on the legs at all times, even when the patient is out of bed. Patients should be instructed to dorsi- and plantar flex the ankles and the toes 10 to 20 times every half hour while awake. In addition, patients who are post-THA should be mobilized as soon as possible to assist with decreasing venous stasis; even patients with epidural catheters should stand and ambulate when they are physically able (Erens & Walter, 2019).

Aspirin, LMWH and synthetic pentasaccharides (fondaparinux) can be used as prophylaxis for VTE. They typically are continued for up to 35 days following surgery based on surgeon preference and patient risk level (Menaka & Douketis, 2019) (see Chapter 26 for further discussion of VTE and VTE prophylaxis).

Preventing Infection

Infection—a serious complication of THA—may necessitate removal of the prosthesis. Patients who are older, poorly nourished, smoke cigarettes, or use corticosteroid medications and patients who have obesity, diabetes, RA, concurrent infections (e.g., urinary tract infection, dental abscess), carry MRSA, or have hematomas are at high risk for infection (Beam & Osmon, 2018). Use of two types of antibiotics is being investigated as a method to decrease MRSA infections both in THA and TKA (Villa et al., 2020).

Over time, one in five patients with THA will undergo revision of the prosthesis, most commonly because of aseptic

Chart 36-8 Providing Home Care After Total Hip Arthroplasty

Considerations

- Pain management
- Wound care
- Mobility
- Self-care (activities of daily living)
- Potential complications

Nursing Interventions

Discuss with patient the following methods to reduce pain:

- Periodic rest
- Distraction and relaxation techniques
- Medication therapy (e.g., nonsteroidal anti-inflammatory drugs, opioid analgesic agents): actions of medications, administration, schedule, side effects

Instruct patient in the following:

- Keeping incision clean and dry
- Cleansing incision daily with soap and water and changing the dressing
- Recognizing signs of wound infection (e.g., pain, increased redness, swelling, purulent drainage, fever)

Explain that sutures or staples will be removed 10 to 14 days after surgery.

Educate patient about the following:

- Safe use of assistive devices
- Weight-bearing limits
- How to change positions frequently

- Limitations on hip flexion and adduction (e.g., avoid acute flexion and crossing legs)
- How to stand without flexing hip acutely
- Avoidance of low-seated chairs and toilets
- Sleeping with pillow between legs to prevent adduction
- Gradual increase in activities and participation in prescribed exercise regimen
- Use of important medications such as warfarin and aspirin

Assess home environment for physical barriers.

Instruct patient to use elevated toilet seat and to use reachers to aid in dressing.

Encourage patient to accept assistance with activities of daily living during early convalescence until mobility and strength improve.

Arrange services and accommodations to address the patient's disability or illness, as appropriate.

Assess patient for development of potential problems, and instruct patient to report signs of potential complications:

- Dislocation of prosthesis (e.g., increased pain, shortening of leg, inability to move leg, popping sensation in hip, abnormal rotation)
- Deep vein thrombosis (e.g., calf pain, swelling, redness)
- Wound infection (e.g., pain, increased redness, swelling, purulent drainage, fever)
- Pulmonary emboli (e.g., shortness of breath, tachypnea, pleuritic chest pain)

Discuss with patient the need to continue regular health care (routine physical examinations) and screenings.

Adapted from Erens, G. A., Walter, B., & Crowley, M. (2020). Total hip arthroplasty. *UpToDate*. Retrieved on 3/16/2020 at: www.uptodate.com/contents/total-hip-arthroplasty

loosening, infection, instability, or a mechanical complication. Because these joint infections are difficult to treat, strategies for preventing infections should be implemented at various steps of the process of care. Strict hand hygiene and utilization of appropriate infection control practices can prevent transmission of infectious organisms. Appropriate antibiotic administration and discontinuation, as well as thorough patient education regarding subsequent antibiotic use are important.

Acute infections may occur within 3 months after surgery and are associated with progressive superficial infections or hematomas. Delayed surgical infections may appear 4 to 24 months after surgery and may cause return of discomfort in the hip. Routine use of antibiotic prophylaxis prior to dental procedures for patients with total joint prostheses remains controversial and is not recommended (Goff, Mangino, Glassman, et al., 2019). Antibiotic prophylaxis can still be prescribed for patients who are immunosuppressed.

Infections occurring more than 2 years after surgery are attributed to the spread of infection through the bloodstream from another site in the body. If an infection occurs, antibiotics are prescribed. Severe infections may require surgical débridement or removal of the prosthesis. (See sections on Septic Arthritis and Osteomyelitis later in this chapter.)

Promoting Home, Community-Based, and Transitional Care

Educating the Patient About Self-Care

Before the patient leaves the acute care setting, the nurse provides thorough education to promote continuity of the therapeutic regimen and active participation in the rehabilitation process (see Chart 36-8). The patient may be discharged to the home, a rehabilitation unit, a transitional care unit, or a long-term care facility. The nurse advises the patient of the importance of a daily exercise program in maintaining the functional motion of the hip joint and strengthening the abductor muscles of the hip, and reminds the patient that it will take time to strengthen and retrain the muscles.

Most patients benefit from physical therapy to regain mobility. Assistive devices (crutches, walker, or cane) may be used for a time. After sufficient muscle tone has developed to permit a normal gait without discomfort, these devices are not necessary. In general, by 3 months, the patient can resume routine ADLs. Stair climbing typically may resume within 3 to 6 weeks following surgery. Some discomfort with activity and at night is common for several weeks. Frequent walks, swimming, and the use of a high rocking chair are excellent for hip exercises.

Restrictions must be kept in mind when resuming sexual activity. Patients should be questioned about concerns and counseled on physical and functional aspects of sexual activity. Sexual activity can be resumed based upon the surgeon's recommendation (typically 3 to 6 months postoperatively). Attention to positioning and comfort may enhance the intimacy of the experience.

At no time during the first 4 months should the patient cross the legs or flex the hip more than 90 degrees. Assistive devices should be used for dressing, such as long-handled shoehorns or dressing sticks for putting on shoes and socks.

The patient should avoid low chairs and sitting for longer than 45 minutes at a time. These precautions minimize hip flexion and the risks of prosthetic dislocation, hip stiffness, and flexion contracture. Driving requires sufficient range of motion and muscle strength; most patients are given permission to drive 4 to 6 weeks postoperatively. Traveling long distances should be avoided unless frequent position changes are possible. Other activities to avoid include tub baths, jogging, lifting heavy loads, and excessive bending and twisting (e.g., lifting, shoveling snow, forceful turning). The surgeon may give the patient a card indicating that they have had a joint replacement; this card may be used to alert security personnel who use screening devices at airports or malls.

Continuing and Transitional Care

A nurse may assess the patient's home for potential problems and monitor wound healing (see Chart 36-9). The nurse, physical therapist, or occupational therapist assesses the home environment for physical barriers that may impede the patient's rehabilitation. In addition, the nurse or therapist may need to assist the patient in acquiring devices such as reachers and long-handled shoehorns or tongs to help with dressing, or a toilet seat extender to elevate the toilet seat. The home rehabilitation program came be done via telehealth (Eichler, Salzwedel, Rabe, et al., 2019). After successful surgery and rehabilitation, the patient can expect a hip joint that is free or almost free of pain, has good motion, is stable, and permits normal or near-normal ambulation and function.

 Gerontologic Considerations

The older adult patient who has had THA merits special postoperative care considerations. Early THA surgery for hip fractures (within 24 to 36 hours) is recommended for most patients once a medical assessment has been made and the patient's condition has been stabilized appropriately. If there are no contraindications (e.g., history of a bleeding disorder), these patients should receive LMWH for VTE prophylaxis; mechanical devices should be used for patients in whom anticoagulants and antiplatelet agents are contraindicated. Providing an appropriate postoperative analgesic regimen for older adults can be challenging in the presence of impaired cognition, medical comorbidities, and possible drug interactions. Consulting with a pain management specialist to specifically tailor the analgesic type and dose may be helpful (see Chapter 9).

All older adult patients who are post-THA should be placed on a higher-specification, foam pressure-relieving mattress rather than an air-bed hospital mattress (Morris et al., 2018). A major goal following surgery in this patient population is early mobilization, in an effort to prevent the complications associated with prolonged immobility and to return the patient to functional activity (Gabbert et al., 2019). Early assisted mobilization and ambulation on the day of surgery can decrease hospital length of stay, complications, and hospital costs and can prepare patients to care for themselves at home with a higher level of independent functioning. Patients who are assigned to restricted hip precautions have slower rehabilitation and return to usual ADLs (Morris et al., 2018) (see Chapter 37 for general discussion of the Postoperative Care of the Patient Undergoing Orthopedic Surgery). Research suggests that use of a telehealth connection to provide rehabilitation remotely has the same level of outcomes as traditional home physical therapy programs (Eichler et al., 2019). Patients who are assigned to restricted hip precautions have slower rehabilitation and return to usual ADLs (Morris et al., 2018).

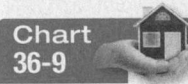

Chart 36-9

HOME CARE CHECKLIST

The Patient Who Has Had Orthopedic Surgery

At the completion of education, the patient and/or caregiver will be able to:

- Name the procedure that was performed and identify any permanent changes in anatomic structure or function as well as changes in ADLs, IADLs, roles, relationships, and spirituality.
- Identify modification of home environment, interventions, and strategies (e.g., durable medical equipment, adaptive equipment) used in safely adapting to changes in structure or function and promote effective recovery and rehabilitation.
- Describe ongoing postoperative therapeutic regimen, including diet and activities to perform (e.g., exercises) and to limit or avoid (e.g., lifting weights, driving a car, contact sports)
  - Consume a healthy diet to promote wound and bone healing.
  - Observe prescribed weight-bearing and activity limits.
  - Participate in prescribed exercise regimen to promote circulation and mobility.
  - Demonstrate safe use of mobility aid.
- State the name, dose, side effects, frequency, and schedule for all prescribed therapeutic and prophylactic medications (e.g., antibiotics, anticoagulants, analgesic agents).
- State how to obtain medical supplies and carry out dressing changes, wound care, and other prescribed regimens.

- State indicators of wound infections (e.g., redness, swelling, tenderness, purulent drainage, fever).
- State indicators of complications to report promptly to primary provider (e.g., uncontrolled swelling and pain; cool, pale fingers or toes; paresthesia; paralysis; purulent drainage; signs of systemic infection; signs of deep vein thrombosis or pulmonary embolism).
- State time and date of follow-up appointments and testing.
- Relate how to reach primary provider with questions or complications.
- State understanding of community resources and referrals as appropriate.
- Identify the need for health promotion (e.g., weight reduction, smoking cessation, stress management), disease prevention, and screening activities.

Resources

See Chapter 2, Chart 2-6 for additional information related to durable medical equipment, adaptive equipment, and mobility skills.

ADLs, activities of daily living; IADLs, instrumental activities of daily living.

Total Knee Arthroplasty

A TKA is considered for patients whose joint pain cannot be managed by nonsurgical treatment and who have severe pain and functional disability related to destruction of joint surfaces by OA, RA, or posttraumatic (osteonecrotic) arthritis. When activity and mobility severely prevent patients from participating in ADLs, TKA is a successful, cost-effective, low-risk therapy that offers significant pain relief and restores quality of life and function (Quinn et al., 2018). If the patient's ligaments have weakened, a fully constrained (hinged) or semi-constrained prosthesis may be used to provide joint stability. Selection of a nonconstrained prosthesis, characterized by components that are not linked, is dependent upon the patient having healthy and functional ligaments to provide joint stability (Quinn et al., 2018).

Nursing Management

Postoperatively, the knee is dressed with a compression bandage. Ice or cold packs may be applied to reduce postoperative swelling and bleeding. The nurse assesses the neurovascular status (movement, sensation, color, pulse, capillary refill) of the surgical extremity and compares it with the contralateral extremity every 2 to 4 hours. It is important to encourage active flexion of the foot every hour when the patient is awake. Postoperative efforts are directed at preventing complications (VTE, peroneal nerve palsy, infection, bleeding, limited range of motion).

Similar to hip surgery, a wound suction drain may be used to remove fluid accumulating in the joint. It is more likely to be used in patients with a body mass index (BMI) over 35 kg/m^2 (Keeney et al., 2019). If a drain is used, it is usually left in place for only 24 to 48 hours to reduce the risk of infection (Keeney et al., 2019). Antibiotics are given prophylactically and continued for 24 hours postoperatively. The color, type, and amount of drainage are documented, and any excessive drainage or change in characteristics of the drainage is promptly reported to the provider.

Research findings suggest that continuous passive motion devices (CPMs) have no influence on functional recovery, drainage, pain, or decreasing adverse outcomes in patient's post-TKA. However, they still may be used by some surgeons.

The physical therapist supervises exercises for strength and range of motion and educates the patient about how to use assistive devices based on weight-bearing restrictions. The goal is eventual flexion around 125 degrees to allow normal motion at the end of rehabilitation. If satisfactory flexion is not achieved, gentle manipulation of the knee joint under general anesthesia may be necessary about 2 weeks after surgery (Newman, Herschmiller, Attarian, et al., 2018).

Patients who are postoperative for TKA should mobilize and ambulate by the first postoperative day (Quinn et al., 2018). The patient's weight-bearing status is determined by the surgeon. The knee is usually protected with a knee immobilizer and is elevated when the patient sits in a chair. The typical requirements for discharge to home may include evidence of wound stability (e.g., no erythema, discharge, or redness), appropriate anticoagulation status by laboratory results (i.e., international normalized ratio [INR] between 1.5 and 2), progress toward physical therapy goals (e.g., appropriate use of walker), and satisfactory pain control with oral medications.

Acute rehabilitation usually takes about 1 to 2 weeks; length of time and discharge destination (e.g., home, acute rehabilitation unit) depend on the age and tolerance of the patient. If discharge is to home, the patient may undergo physical therapy on an outpatient basis. Total recovery takes 6 weeks or longer, especially for those older than 75 years. Late complications that may occur include **osteolysis** (polyethylene-induced breakdown infection), periprosthetic joint infections, and aseptic loosening of prosthetic components (Mar, Tan, Song, et al., 2019).

More than 82% of patients who have TKA will still have a functioning prosthesis 25 years after surgery (Evans, Walker, Evans, et al., 2019). TKA is a viable option for improving both disease-specific and generic health-related quality of life, especially pain and function, leading to positive patient satisfaction. Patients usually can achieve a pain-free, functional joint and participate more fully in life activities than before the surgery (Quinn et al., 2018). The nurse provides ongoing education and psychosocial support throughout the perioperative period to help facilitate these positive outcomes (see Chart 36-5).

Metabolic Bone Disorders

Osteoporosis

Osteoporosis is the most prevalent bone disease in the world. More than 1.5 million osteoporotic fractures occur every year. Fractures requiring hospitalization have risen significantly over the past two decades (International Osteoporosis Foundation [IOF], 2017). More than 10 million Americans have osteoporosis, and an additional 33.6 million have **osteopenia** (i.e., low bone mineral density [BMD])—the precursor to osteoporosis (IOF, 2017). The consequence of osteoporosis is bone fracture. It is projected that one of every three women and one of every five men over the age of 50 will have an osteoporosis-related fracture at some point in their lives (IOF, 2017).

Prevention

Peak adult bone mass is achieved between the ages of 18 and 25 years in both women and men and is affected by genetic factors, nutrition, physical activity, medications, endocrine status, and general health (IOF, 2017). Men typically develop larger, heavier bones than women; therefore, they manifest osteoporosis at more advanced ages.

Primary osteoporosis occurs in women after menopause (usually by age 51) but it is not merely a consequence of aging. Failure to develop optimal peak bone mass and low vitamin D levels contribute to the development of osteopenia without associated bone loss (Drezner, 2019). Early identification of at-risk teenagers and young adults, increased calcium and vitamin D intake, participation in regular weight-bearing exercise, and modification of lifestyle (e.g., reduced use of caffeine, tobacco products, carbonated soft drinks, and alcohol) are interventions that decrease the risk of fractures and associated disability later in life (Black, Cauley, Wagman, et al., 2017) (see Chart 36-10).

Secondary osteoporosis is the result of medications or diseases that affect bone metabolism. Men are more likely than women to have secondary causes of osteoporosis, including the use of corticosteroids (especially if they receive doses in

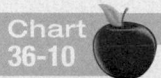

Chart 36-10 · HEALTH PROMOTION
Strategies for Preventing Osteoporosis

Adolescents and Young Adults

- Educate so that they can:
  - Characterize risk factors for osteoporosis.
  - Consume diet with adequate calcium (1000–1300 mg/day) and vitamin D.
  - Engage in weight-bearing exercise daily.
  - Identify calcium- and vitamin D–rich foods.
  - Modify lifestyle choices—avoid smoking, alcohol, caffeine, and carbonated beverages.

Women Who Are Menopausal and Postmenopausal (in addition to above)

- Educate so that they can:
  - Assess home environment for hazards contributing to falls.
  - Demonstrate good body mechanics.
  - Describe appropriate calcium supplements and pharmacologic agents to maintain and enhance bone mass.
  - Engage in exercise that improves balance to reduce risk of falls.
  - Review concurrent medical conditions and medications with primary provider to identify factors that contribute to bone mass loss.

Men (in addition to above)

- Educate so that they can:
  - Characterize risk factors associated with osteoporosis in men, including medications (e.g., corticosteroids, anticonvulsants, aluminum-containing antacids), chronic diseases (e.g., kidney, lung, gastrointestinal), and undiagnosed low testosterone levels.
  - Participate in screening for osteoporosis.
  - Talk with primary provider about the use of medications (e.g., alendronate) to enhance bone mass or to correct testosterone deficiency.

---

excess of 5 mg of prednisone daily for more than 3 months) and excessive alcohol intake. Specific disease states (e.g., celiac disease, hypogonadism) and medications such as anticonvulsants (e.g., phenytoin), thyroid replacement agents (e.g., levothyroxine), antiestrogens (e.g., medroxyprogesterone), androgen inhibitors (e.g., leuprolide), selective serotonin receptor inhibitors (SSRIs; e.g., fluoxetine) and proton pump inhibitors (e.g., esomeprazole) place patients at risk; these diseases and medications need to be identified and therapies instituted to halt the development of osteoporosis (Robinson, 2020). The degree of bone loss is related to the duration of medication therapy. When the drugs are discontinued or the metabolic problem is corrected, the progression is halted but restoration of lost bone mass may not occur.

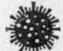

COVID-19 Considerations

An important source of vitamin D is through direct sunlight exposure. The National Osteoporosis Foundation (NOF) and IOF, in collaboration with other relevant stakeholders, have raised concerns that government initiated stay-at-home orders enacted in response to the coronavirus disease 2019 (COVID-19) pandemic may have reduced the amount of time adults were spending outside, potentially limiting exposure to sunlight (American Society for Bone and Mineral Research [ASBMR], 2020). Subsequently, a joint statement was published to reinforce the importance of vitamin D

to bone health and highlight current recommendations for vitamin D intake; these include that adults should obtain 15 to 30 minutes of direct skin exposure to sunlight daily, and, when they cannot meet this recommendation, they should consume between 400 to 1000 IU of vitamin D daily through diet or supplements (ASBMR, 2020). Research is ongoing to better understand the relationship between vitamin D and COVID-19 (ASBMR, 2020).

Gerontologic Considerations

The prevalence of osteoporosis in women older than 80 years is 50%. The average 75-year-old woman has lost 25% of her cortical bone and 40% of her trabecular bone. Most residents of long-term care facilities have a low BMD and are at risk for bone fracture. One third of all hip fractures occur among men, and men have a higher mortality rate than women after sustaining a hip fracture (Rapp, Büchele, Dreinhőfer, et al., 2019). It is estimated that the number of hip fractures and their associated costs will at least double by the year 2040 because of the projected aging of the U.S. population.

A fragility fracture is defined as one that occurs when a person falls from their natural height (or less) or with low velocity. Frequently, an underlying disease or metabolic alteration makes the bone more likely to fracture. Osteoporosis and osteopenia are the most frequently cited risks of fragility fractures. The aging of the population, the increased use of medications that contribute to falls risk, and a lack of caregivers contribute to the rising risk of fragility fractures. Inadequate staffing related to a worsening nursing shortage may result in gaps in care that increase the incidence of fragility fractures; decreased staffing may delay nursing assessments and follow-up and increase the likelihood that patients try to get up unsupervised, resulting in falls (Brent, Hommel, Maher, et al., 2018).

Routine vertebral fracture screenings are not recommended for older adults. However, 80% to 90% of these fractures can be seen incidentally on chest x-rays taken for other purposes. It is estimated that only one third of vertebral fractures are diagnosed. Vertebral fracture risk is five times higher among patients who have had prior fractures. Furthermore, 20% of women who are postmenopausal and have a vertebral fracture will have another one within 1 year (Pouresmaeili, Kamalidehghan, Kamerehei, et al., 2018). Nurses are the team members who frequently are first to uncover vertebral fractures by identifying a change in a patient's height during routine exams conducted in office or clinic settings.

Older adults absorb dietary calcium less efficiently and excrete it more readily through their kidneys. Women who are postmenopausal and older adults need to consume approximately 1200 mg of daily calcium. Quantities larger than this may place patients at heightened risk of renal calculi or cardiovascular disease (United States Preventive Services Task Force [USPSTF], 2018). Though bone density increases with calcium intake, the rate of fractures does not decrease in women who are postmenopausal and who routinely take calcium supplements (Bailey, Zou, Wallace, et al., 2020).

Pathophysiology

Osteoporosis is characterized by reduced bone mass, deterioration of bone matrix, and diminished bone architectural

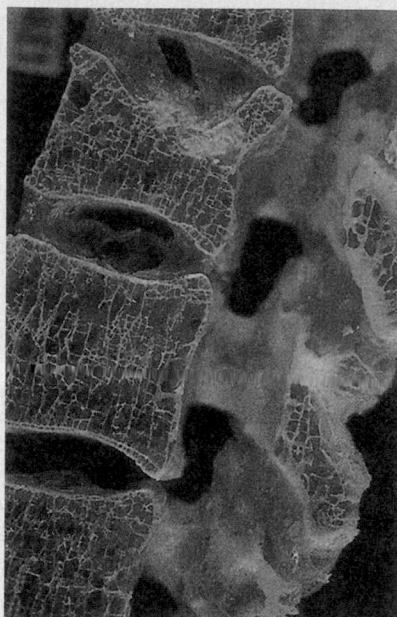

Figure 36-11 • Progressive osteoporotic bone loss and compression fractures. Reprinted with permission from Rubin, E., Gorstein, F., Schwarting, R., et al. (2004). *Pathology* (4th ed.). Philadelphia, PA: Wolters Kluwer.

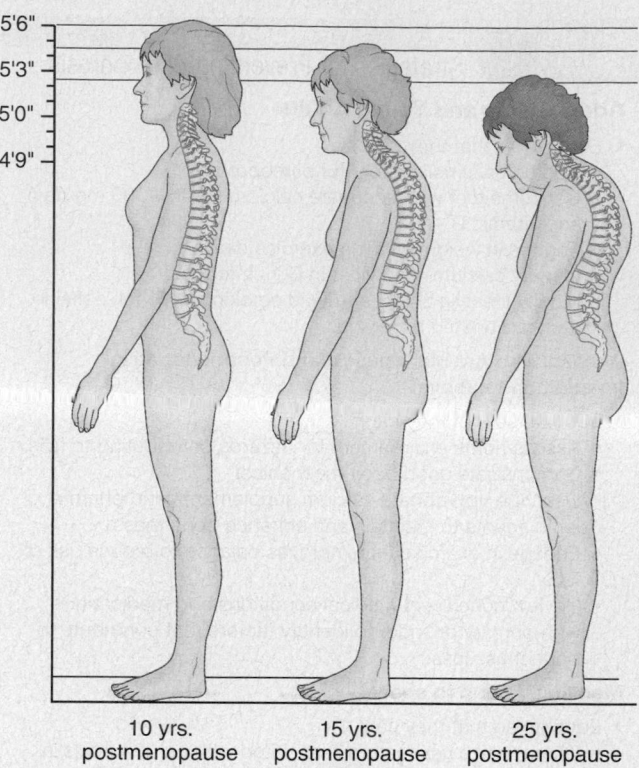

Figure 36-12 • Typical loss of height associated with osteoporosis and aging.

strength. Normal homeostatic bone turnover is altered; the rate of bone resorption that is maintained by osteoclasts is greater than the rate of bone formation that is maintained by osteoblasts, resulting in a reduced total bone mass. The bones become progressively porous, brittle, and fragile. They fracture easily under stresses that would not break normal bone. This occurs most commonly as compression fractures (see Fig. 36-11) of the thoracic and lumbar spine, hip fractures, and Colles fractures of the wrist. These fractures may be the first clinical manifestation of osteoporosis (Black et al., 2017).

The gradual collapse of a vertebra may be asymptomatic. With the development of kyphosis (i.e., Dowager hump), there is an associated loss of height (see Fig. 36-12). The postural changes result in relaxation of the abdominal muscles and a protruding abdomen. The deformity may also produce pulmonary insufficiency and increase the risk for falls related to balance issues.

Age-related loss begins soon after the peak bone mass is achieved (i.e., in the fourth decade). Calcitonin, which inhibits bone resorption and promotes bone formation, is decreased. Estrogen, which inhibits bone breakdown, also decreases with aging. On the other hand, parathyroid hormone (PTH) increases with aging, thus increasing bone turnover and resorption. The consequence of these changes is net loss of bone mass over time.

The withdrawal of estrogens at menopause or with oophorectomy causes an accelerated bone resorption within the first 5 years after cessation of menses. Most women lose 10% of their bone mass. More than half of all women older than 50 years show evidence of osteopenia (Black et al., 2017; MQIC, 2020).

Risk Factors

Small-framed women are at greatest risk for osteoporosis. In terms of ethnicity, Asian and Caucasian women are at highest risk. Although African American women tend to have higher mineral mass when younger, they are still at risk due to the prevalence of sickle cell and autoimmune diseases in this population. In addition, many African American women also have poor calcium intake due to lactose intolerance (National Institute of Arthritis and Musculoskeletal and Skin Diseases [NIAMSD], 2018). The use of aromatase inhibitors is an additional risk for women with breast cancer (Robinson, 2020).

Men have a greater peak bone mass and do not experience a sudden midlife estrogen reduction. As a result, osteoporosis occurs about one decade later, but one in four men still sustain an osteopenic fracture (Pouresmaeili et al., 2018). It is believed that both testosterone and estrogen are important in achieving and maintaining bone mass in men, although the risk profile for men is not as well established as it is for women (Pouresmaeili et al., 2018) (see Chart 36-11).

Nutritional factors contribute to the development of osteoporosis. A diet that includes adequate calories and nutrients needed to maintain bone, calcium, and vitamin D must be consumed. Patients who have had bariatric surgery are at increased risk for osteoporosis as the duodenum is bypassed, which is the primary site for absorption of calcium. Patients who have gastrointestinal (GI) diseases that cause malabsorption (e.g., celiac disease, alcoholism) may benefit from additional magnesium supplements (Rondanelli, Faliva, Gasparri, et al., 2019). However, in adults who follow a strict gluten free diet, magnesium supplements are currently not recommended.

Autoimmune diseases also contribute to poor bone health. Many of them are associated with nutritional deficiencies (e.g., celiac, autoimmune liver disease). Furthermore, many

- Alcohol intake of 3 or more drinks daily
- Corticosteroid prescription (e.g., prednisone) for longer than 3 months
- Current use of tobacco products
- Family history
- History of bone fracture during adulthood
- History of impaired glucose tolerance and diabetes
- History of rheumatoid disease
- Inactive or sedentary lifestyle
- Inadequate calcium and vitamin D intake
- Low body mass index
- Malabsorption disorders (e.g., eating disorder, celiac disease, bariatric surgery)
- Men older than 60 years of age
- Women who are postmenopausal

Adapted from Fasolino, T., & Whitright, T. (2015). A pilot study to identify modifiable and non-modifiable variables associated with osteopenia and osteoporosis in men. *Orthopaedic Nursing 34*(5), 289–293; International Osteoporosis Foundation. (2017). Retrieved on 3/7/2020 at: www.iofbonehealth.org/facts-statistics; Robinson, M. (2020). Drugs affecting the bones and joints. In T. Woo & M. Robinson (Eds.). *Pharmacotherapeutics for advanced practice prescribers* (5th ed.). Philadelphia, PA: F. A. Davis.

patients with autoimmune diseases are prescribed corticosteroid medications and, as a consequence of their disease processes, are relatively sedentary. These factors also can cause weak bones (Arase, Tsuruya, Hirose, et al., 2020).

Bone formation is enhanced by the stress of weight and muscle activity. When immobilized by casts, general inactivity, paralysis, or other disability, the bone is resorbed faster than it is formed, and osteoporosis results (McCance & Huether, 2019). Immobility contributes to the development of osteoporosis. Resistance and impact exercises are most beneficial in developing and maintaining bone mass.

Assessment and Diagnostic Findings

Osteoporosis may be undetectable on routine x-rays until there has been significant demineralization, resulting in radiolucency of the bones (Black et al., 2017). When the vertebrae collapse, causing compression fractures, the thoracic vertebrae become wedge shaped and the lumbar vertebrae become biconcave. Osteoporosis is diagnosed by dual-energy x-ray absorptiometry (DEXA), which provides information about BMD at the spine and hip (see Chapter 35). The DEXA scan data are analyzed and reported as T-scores (the number of standard deviations above or below the average BMD value for a 30-year-old healthy adult of the same sex).

Baseline DEXA testing is recommended for all women older than 65 years, for women who are postmenopausal older than 50 years with osteoporosis risk factors, and for all people who have had a fracture thought to occur as a consequence of osteoporosis (Black et al., 2017). BMD studies are also useful in assessing response to therapy and are recommended 3 months post any osteoporotic fracture. There is no evidence to support basic screening of men younger than 70 years of age or to determine the optimal time interval to repeat studies in either gender following a normal baseline report (USPSTF, 2019).

Female fracture risk can be estimated using the World Health Organization (WHO) Fracture Risk Assessment Tool (FRAX) (Cass, Shepard, Asirot, et al., 2016). These FRAX tables typically underestimate the bone loss risk in men. The Male Osteoporosis Risk Estimation Score (MORES) generates a more gender-specific evaluation than the standard FRAX score in men. Treatment for both genders is now reserved for those with a 10-year risk of more than 3% for hip fracture or 20% risk for other major fractures. Risk scores are based on BMD, personal and family history of fractures, BMI, gender, age, and secondary factors such as medication use, smoking, and history of rheumatoid disease. Impaired glucose tolerance and diabetes are now also recognized as additional risk factors (Robinson, 2020).

Laboratory studies (e.g., serum calcium, serum phosphate, serum alkaline phosphatase [ALP], urine calcium excretion, urinary hydroxyproline excretion, hematocrit, erythrocyte sedimentation rate [ESR]), and x-ray studies are used to exclude other possible disorders (e.g., multiple myeloma, osteomalacia, hyperparathyroidism, malignancy) that contribute to bone loss. In men, low testosterone levels may be part of the cause.

Medical Management

A diet rich in calcium and vitamin D throughout life, with an increased calcium intake during adolescence and the middle years, protects against skeletal demineralization. Such a diet includes three glasses of skimmed vitamin D–enriched milk or other foods high in calcium (e.g., cheese and other dairy products, steamed broccoli, canned salmon with bones) daily. A cup of milk or calcium-fortified orange juice contains about 300 mg of calcium. The recommended adequate intake level of calcium for men 50 to 70 years is 1000 mg daily, and for women aged 51 and older and men aged 71 and older is 1200 mg daily (USPSTF, 2018). Some researchers are challenging these levels as too low for patients with low baseline values, while others express concern of administering higher dosages, noting that they are associated with adverse events (e.g., renal calculi). The recommended vitamin D intake for most adults, which can be acquired from food or supplements, is between 400 and 1000 IU daily; however optimal vitamin D intake is influenced by a patient's age and sex (ASBMR, 2020).

Regular weight-bearing exercise promotes bone formation. Recommendations include 20 to 30 minutes of aerobic, bone-stressing exercise daily (e.g., not swimming). Weight training stimulates an increase in BMD. In addition, exercise improves balance, reducing the incidence of falls and fractures. Women who are postmenopausal and men aged 50 and older should be advised to avoid excessive intake of alcohol. Those who use tobacco products should be advised to quit. However, additional research is needed to better understand the relationship between smoking and bone health (Strozyk, Gress, & Brietling, 2018). Current guidelines recommend that hormone therapy with estrogen not be used for primary prevention of bone loss in women who are postmenopausal (USPSTF, 2017).

Pharmacologic Therapy

To ensure adequate calcium intake, a calcium supplement with vitamin D may be prescribed and taken with meals or with a beverage high in vitamin C to promote absorption. The recommended daily dose should be split and not taken as a single dose (Drezner, 2019). Common side effects of calcium supplements are abdominal distention and constipation. Calcium from foods is better absorbed, but calcium supplements may be necessary for patients who are lactose intolerant. Meta-analysis findings demonstrate that vitamin D taken alone is not effective in primary prevention of fractures. However, vitamin D plus calcium does reduce the risk of fractures in patients who are found to be vitamin D deficient by laboratory testing (USPSTF, 2018). Calcium and vitamin D should be taken as supplements to drugs prescribed to treat osteoporosis. These types of drugs include bisphosphonates, estrogen agonist/antagonists, and receptor activator of nuclear factor kappa-B ligand (RANKL) inhibitors (see Table 36-1). Salmon egg based PTH is no longer a therapy,

TABLE 36-1 Select Osteoporosis Medications

Medication	Therapeutic Effects and Indications	Key Nursing Considerations
Bisphosphonates	Inhibit osteoclasts, causing decreased bone loss and increased bone mass	Adequate calcium and vitamin D intake is needed to assure maximum effect; however, these supplements should not be taken at the same time as the bisphosphonates Side effects include gastrointestinal symptoms, including dyspepsia, nausea, flatulence, diarrhea, and constipation Adverse effects may include esophageal or gastric ulcers, osteonecrosis of the jaw, and atypical femur fractures; these effects may be mitigated by instituting a 1–2 yr drug-free holiday in patients with mild osteoporosis after 4–5 yrs of treatment, and in patients with higher fracture risk after 10 yrs of treatment
Alendronate Risedronate	• Treatment of osteoporosis in women who are postmenopausal • Treatment of osteoporosis in men, and in women and men taking corticosteroids	Administer PO, either daily or weekly Advise patient to take in AM on empty stomach with 250 mL of water while sitting upright and to remain upright for at least 30 min Effects of alendronate may be diminished in older adult patients who take proton pump inhibitors
Ibandronate	• Treatment of osteoporosis in women who are postmenopausal • IV dosing may be good option for patients either intolerant of PO bisphosphonates or nonadherent to prescribed therapy	May be given PO monthly or IV every 3 mo
Zoledronic acid	• Treatment of osteoporosis in women who are postmenopausal • Treatment of osteoporosis in men and in both men and women taking corticosteroids for at least 12 mo	Administer IV once yearly for osteoporosis treatment or once every 2 yrs for osteoporosis prevention This is the most potent bisphosphonate and is associated with acute kidney injury; therefore it is contraindicated in patients with creatinine clearances less than 35 mL/min or in patients with chronic kidney disease
Estrogen Agonist/Antagonist (formerly called selective estrogen receptor modulator [SERM]) Raloxifene	Promotes estrogenic effects on bone, preserving BMD, with concomitant antiestrogenic effects on the uterus and breasts • Prevention and treatment of osteoporosis in women who are postmenopausal, particularly those with breast cancer • May also reduce the risk of breast cancer in patients at risk	Administer PO once daily. May be given in tandem with calcium and vitamin D Side effects include hot flashes and leg cramps Adverse effects include VTE formation
RANKL Inhibitor Denosumab	Monoclonal antibody that increases BMD and reduces the porosity of cortical bone by inhibiting the effects of TNF on osteoclasts, inhibiting their activity • Treatment of osteoporosis in men and women who are postmenopausal at high risk of fracture; also indicated for women with osteoporosis and breast cancer receiving aromatase inhibitors and for men with osteoporosis and prostate cancer receiving gonadotropin-reducing hormones	Given once every 6 mo SQ Side effects include skin rashes Adverse effects include hypocalcemia, cellulitis, osteonecrosis of the jaw, and atypical femur fracture Note: when treatment with denosumab is stopped, loss of BMD can be rapid; other drugs should be started to mitigate this response
PTH Analogue Teriparatide	Synthetic parathyroid hormone which increases bone strength and density • Treatment of osteoporosis in men and women who are postmenopausal at high risk of fracture	Must be refrigerated Daily self-administered SQ injections for up to 2 yrs

BMD, bone mineral density; IV, intravenously; PO, orally; PTH, parathyroid hormone; SQ, subcutaneous; TNF, tissue necrosis factor; VTE, venous thromboembolism.
Adapted from International Osteoporosis Foundation. (2017). Retrieved on 3/7/2020 at: www.iofbonehealth.org/facts-statistics; Robinson, M. (2020). Drugs affecting the bones and joints. In T. Woo, & M. Robinson (Eds.). *Pharmacotherapeutics for advanced practice prescribers* (5th ed.). Philadelphia, PA: F. A. Davis.

but synthetic human PTH analogues are used in patients with advanced osteoporosis or who are treatment resistant (Robinson, 2020).

Bisphosphonate therapy is no longer recommended for patients who only have evidence of osteopenia without reaching the precise DEXA scores that define osteoporosis. These medications must be given on an empty stomach, only with water, and the person must sit upright for at least 30 minutes after ingestion. There are many gastric and esophageal risks, including gastritis, ulceration, and GI bleeding. Contradictions include previously known Barrett esophagus (see Chapter 39), low serum calcium levels, and pregnancy (Robinson, 2020). Atrial fibrillation has been reported after chronic use of these medications. Two rare side effects include osteonecrosis of the jaw (more likely with intravenous [IV] preparations of these medications) and subtrochanteric fractures. Concerns about these rare adverse effects must be addressed to ensure the patient will adhere to the therapeutic plan and take the medication (Robinson, 2020).

Fracture Management

Fractures of the hip that occur as a consequence of osteoporosis are managed surgically by joint replacement or by closed or open reduction with internal fixation (e.g., hip pinning) as described in Chapter 37. Management of Colles fractures is also described in Chapter 37.

Osteoporotic compression fractures of the vertebrae are managed conservatively. Patients with these findings should be referred to an osteoporosis specialist. Most patients who experience these fractures are asymptomatic and do not require acute care management; for those who experience pain, acute care management is indicated as outlined in the following Nursing Process section. Percutaneous vertebroplasty or kyphoplasty (injection of polymethylmethacrylate [PMMA] bone cement into the fractured vertebra, followed by inflation of a pressurized balloon to restore the shape of the affected vertebra) can provide rapid relief of acute pain and improve quality of life, but might contribute to other complications resulting from alterations in spinal mechanics. These procedures are contraindicated in the presence of infection, multiple old fractures, and certain coagulopathies. The use of vertebroplasty is highly contested in the medical literature (De Leacy, Chandra, Barr, et al., 2020).

NURSING PROCESS

The Patient with a Spontaneous Vertebral Fracture Related to Osteoporosis

Assessment

Recognition of risks and problems associated with osteoporosis form the basis for nursing assessment. The health history focuses on family history, previous fractures, dietary consumption of calcium, exercise patterns, onset of menopause, and the use of certain medications (e.g., corticosteroids), as well as alcohol, smoking, and caffeine intake. Any symptoms the patient is experiencing, such as back pain, constipation, or altered body image, are explored.

Physical examination may disclose localized pain, kyphosis of the thoracic spine, or shortened stature. Problems in mobility and breathing may exist as a result of changes in posture and weakened muscles.

Diagnosis

NURSING DIAGNOSES

Based on the assessment data, major nursing diagnoses may include the following:

- Lack of knowledge about the osteoporotic process and treatment regimen
- Acute pain associated with fracture and muscle spasm
- Risk for constipation associated with immobility or development of ileus (intestinal obstruction)
- Risk for injury: additional fractures associated with osteoporosis

Planning and Goals

The major goals for the patient may include knowledge about osteoporosis and the treatment regimen, relief of pain, improved bowel elimination, and absence of additional fractures.

Nursing Interventions

PROMOTING UNDERSTANDING OF OSTEOPOROSIS AND THE TREATMENT REGIMEN

Patient education focuses on factors influencing the development of osteoporosis, interventions to arrest or slow the process, and measures to relieve symptoms. The nurse emphasizes that people of any age need sufficient calcium, vitamin D, and weight-bearing exercise to slow the progression of osteoporosis (Drezner, 2019). Patient education related to medication therapy as described previously is important. Patients must understand that having one fracture increases the probability of sustaining another.

RELIEVING PAIN

Relief of back pain resulting from compression fracture may be accomplished by short periods of resting in bed in a supine or side-lying position. The mattress should be supportive. Knee flexion increases comfort by relaxing back muscles. Intermittent local heat and backrubs promote muscle relaxation. The nurse instructs the patient to move the trunk as a unit and to avoid twisting. When the patient is assisted out of bed, a trunk orthosis (e.g., lumbosacral corset) may be worn for temporary support and immobilization, although such a device is frequently uncomfortable and is poorly tolerated by many older adults. The patient gradually resumes activities as pain diminishes.

IMPROVING BOWEL ELIMINATION

Constipation is a problem related to immobility and medications. Early institution of a high-fiber diet, increased fluids, and the use of prescribed stool softeners help prevent or minimize constipation. If the vertebral collapse involves the T10–L2 vertebrae, the patient may develop a paralytic ileus. The nurse therefore monitors the patient's intake, bowel sounds, and bowel activity.

PREVENTING INJURY

Physical activity is essential to strengthen muscles, improve balance, prevent disuse atrophy, and retard progressive bone demineralization. Isometric exercises can strengthen trunk muscles. The nurse encourages walking, good body mechanics, and good posture. Daily weight-bearing activity, preferably outdoors in the sunshine to enhance the body's ability to produce vitamin D, is encouraged. Sudden bending, jarring, and strenuous lifting are avoided.

 Gerontologic Considerations. Older adults fall frequently as a result of environmental hazards, diminished senses and cardiovascular responses, and responses to medications. The patient and family need to be included in planning for care and preventive management regimens. For example, the home environment should be assessed for elimination of potential hazards (e.g., scatter rugs, cluttered rooms and stairwells, toys on the floor, pets underfoot). A safe environment can then be created (e.g., well-lighted staircases with secure handrails, grab bars in the bathroom, properly fitting footwear). Adequate nurse–patient ratios are also critical for fall prevention in inpatient settings (Brent et al., 2018).

Evaluation

Expected patient outcomes may include:
1. Acquires knowledge about osteoporosis and the treatment regimen
   a. States relationship of calcium and vitamin D intake and exercise to bone mass
   b. Consumes adequate dietary calcium and vitamin D
   c. Takes prescribed medications, following instructions for administration
   d. Increases level of exercise
   e. Adheres to prescribed screening and monitoring procedures
2. Achieves pain relief
   a. Experiences pain relief at rest
   b. Experiences minimal discomfort during ADLs
   c. Demonstrates diminished tenderness at fracture site
3. Demonstrates usual pattern of bowel elimination
   a. Has active bowel sounds
   b. Reports regular pattern of bowel movements
4. Experiences no new fractures
   a. Maintains good posture
   b. Uses good body mechanics
   c. Engages in weight-bearing exercises (walks daily)
   d. Creates a safe home environment
   e. Accepts assistance and supervision as needed

Osteomalacia

Osteomalacia is a metabolic bone disease characterized by inadequate mineralization of bone. As a result, the skeleton softens and weakens, causing pain, tenderness to touch, bowing of the bones, and pathologic fractures. On physical examination, skeletal deformities (spinal kyphosis and bowed legs) give patients an unusual appearance and a waddling gait. These patients may be uncomfortable with their appearance and are at risk for falls and pathologic fractures, particularly of the distal radius and the proximal femur (McCance & Huether, 2019).

Pathophysiology

The major defect in osteomalacia is a deficiency of activated vitamin D, which promotes calcium absorption from the GI tract and facilitates mineralization of bone. The supply of calcium and phosphate in the extracellular fluid is low and does not move to calcification sites in bones.

Osteomalacia may result from failed calcium absorption or from excessive loss of calcium from the body (e.g., kidney failure). GI disorders (e.g., celiac disease, chronic biliary tract obstruction, chronic pancreatitis, small bowel resection) in which fats are inadequately absorbed are likely to produce osteomalacia through loss of vitamin D (along with other fat-soluble vitamins) and calcium, the latter being excreted in the feces with fatty acids. In addition, liver and kidney diseases can produce a lack of vitamin D because these are the organs that convert vitamin D to its active form.

Severe renal insufficiency results in acidosis. The body uses available calcium to combat the acidosis, and PTH stimulates the release of skeletal calcium in an attempt to reestablish a physiologic pH. During this continual drain of skeletal calcium, bony fibrosis occurs, and bony cysts form. Chronic glomerulonephritis, obstructive uropathies, and heavy metal poisoning result in a reduced serum phosphate level and demineralization of bone.

Hyperparathyroidism leads to skeletal decalcification and thus to osteomalacia by increasing phosphate excretion in the urine. Prolonged use of anticonvulsant medication (e.g., phenytoin, phenobarbital) poses a risk of osteomalacia, as does insufficient vitamin D (dietary, sunlight).

Osteomalacia that results from malnutrition (deficiency in vitamin D often associated with poor intake of calcium) is a result of poverty, poor dietary habits, and lack of knowledge about nutrition. It occurs most frequently in parts of the world where vitamin D is not added to food, where dietary deficiencies exist, and where sunlight is rare (McCance & Huether, 2019).

Gerontologic Considerations

A nutritious diet is particularly important in older adults. Adequate intake of calcium and vitamin D is promoted. Because sunlight is necessary for synthesizing vitamin D, patients should be encouraged to spend 15 to 30 minutes each day in the sun, if not contraindicated and while avoiding sunburn (ASBMR, 2020). Prevention, identification, and management of osteomalacia in older adults are essential to reduce the incidence of fractures. When osteomalacia is combined with osteoporosis, the risk of fracture increases.

Assessment and Diagnostic Findings

On x-ray studies, generalized demineralization of bone is evident. Studies of the vertebrae may show a compression fracture with indistinct vertebral end plates. Laboratory studies show low serum calcium and phosphorus levels and a moderately elevated ALP. Urine excretion of calcium and creatinine is low. Bone biopsy demonstrates an increased amount of osteoid, a demineralized, cartilaginous bone matrix that is sometimes referred to as prebone.

Medical Management

Physical, psychological, and pharmaceutical measures are used to reduce the patient's discomfort and pain. If the underlying cause of osteomalacia is corrected, the disorder may resolve. If kidney disease prevents activation of absorbed vitamin D, then supplementation requires the activated form (calcitriol). If osteomalacia is caused by malabsorption, increased doses of vitamin D, along with supplemental calcium, are usually prescribed. Exposure to sunlight may be recommended; ultraviolet radiation transforms a cholesterol substance (7-dehydrocholesterol) present in the skin into vitamin D (McCance & Huether, 2019).

If osteomalacia is dietary in origin, the interventions are akin to those discussed previously in the discussion on osteoporosis. Long-term monitoring of the patient is appropriate to ensure stabilization or reversal of osteomalacia. Some persistent orthopedic deformities may need to be treated with braces or surgery (e.g., osteotomy may be performed to correct long bone deformity).

Paget Disease of the Bone

Paget disease (osteitis deformans) is a disorder of localized rapid bone turnover, most commonly affecting the skull, femur, tibia, pelvic bones, and vertebrae. The disease occurs in about 2% to 3% of the population older than 50 years. The incidence is slightly greater in aging men than in women. A family history has been noted, with siblings often developing the disease. The cause of Paget disease is not known (Ralston, Corral-Gudino, Cooper, et al., 2019).

Pathophysiology

In Paget disease, a primary proliferation of osteoclasts occurs, which induces bone resorption. This is followed by a compensatory increase in osteoblastic activity that replaces the bone. As bone turnover continues, a classic mosaic (disorganized) pattern of bone develops. Because the diseased bone is highly vascularized and structurally weak, pathologic fractures occur. Structural bowing of the legs causes malalignment of the hip, knee, and ankle joints, which contributes to the development of arthritis and back and joint pain (Cundy, 2017).

Clinical Manifestations

Paget disease is insidious. Some patients do not experience symptoms but only have skeletal deformity. The condition is most frequently identified on x-ray studies performed during a workup for another problem. Sclerotic changes and cortical thickening of the long bones occur.

In most patients, skeletal deformity involves the skull. The skull may thicken, and the patient may report that a hat no longer fits. In some cases, the cranium, but not the face, is enlarged. This gives the face a small, triangular appearance. Most patients with skull involvement have impaired hearing from cranial nerve compression and dysfunction. Other cranial nerves may also be similarly affected.

The femurs and tibiae tend to bow, producing a waddling gait. The spine is bent forward and is rigid; the chin rests on the chest. The thorax becomes immobile during respiration. The trunk is flexed on the legs to maintain balance and the arms are bent outward and forward, appearing long in relation to the shortened trunk (McCance & Huether, 2019).

Tenderness and warmth over bones may be noted due to increased bone vascularity. Patients with large, highly vascular lesions may develop high-output cardiac failure due to the increased vascular bed and metabolic demands (McCance & Huether, 2019). The pain is mild to moderate, deep, and aching. It increases with weight bearing. Pain and discomfort may precede skeletal deformities of Paget disease by years and are often wrongly attributed by the patient to old age or arthritis (Cundy, 2017).

Assessment and Diagnostic Findings

Elevated serum ALP concentration and urinary hydroxyproline excretion reflect increased osteoblastic activity. Higher values suggest more active disease. Patients with Paget disease have normal blood calcium levels. X-rays confirm the diagnosis of Paget disease by revealing local areas of demineralization and bone overgrowth in the characteristic mosaic patterns. Bone scans demonstrate the extent of the disease. Bone biopsy may aid in the differential diagnosis with other bone diseases (Cundy, 2017).

Medical Management

Pain usually responds to NSAIDs. Gait problems from bowing of the legs are managed with walking aids, shoe lifts, and physical therapy. Weight is controlled to reduce stress on weakened bones and misaligned joints. Patients who are asymptomatic may be managed with diets adequate in calcium and vitamin D and periodic monitoring.

Fractures, arthritis, and hearing loss are complications of Paget disease. Fractures are managed according to location. Healing occurs if fracture reduction, immobilization, and stability are adequate. Severe degenerative arthritis may require total joint replacement; however, the afflicted "soft" bones do not make ideal surgical sites and are thus prone to complications. Loss of hearing is managed with hearing aids and communication techniques used with people who have hearing impairments (e.g., speech reading, body language) (see Chapter 59).

Pharmacologic Therapy

Patients with moderate to severe disease may benefit from specific antiosteoclastic therapy. These medications reduce bone turnover, reverse the course of the disease, relieve pain, and improve mobility.

Bisphosphonates are the cornerstone of Paget therapy in that they stabilize the rapid bone turnover (Ralston et al., 2019). Their use may not suppress all Paget symptoms, but they reduce serum ALP and urinary hydroxyproline levels. See earlier discussion on bisphosphonates.

Plicamycin, a cytotoxic antibiotic, may be used to control the disease. This medication is reserved for severely affected patients with neurologic compromise and for those whose disease is resistant to other therapy. This medication has dramatic effects on pain reduction and on serum calcium, ALP, and urinary hydroxyproline levels; however, there are significant side effects. It is given by IV infusion; hepatic, kidney, and bone marrow function must be monitored during therapy. Clinical remissions may continue for months after the medication is discontinued.

Gerontologic Considerations

Because Paget disease tends to affect older adults, patients and their families and caregivers should be educated about how to compensate for altered musculoskeletal functioning with an emphasis on the risk of falls. The home environment is assessed for safety to prevent falls and to reduce the risk of fracture. Strategies for coping with a chronic health problem and its effect on quality of life need to be developed. If age-related hearing loss is exacerbated by Paget disease, alternative communication devices (e.g., text telephone, telecommunication device for the deaf) and home safety alarms may be indicated.

Musculoskeletal Infections

Osteomyelitis

Osteomyelitis is an infection of the bone that results in inflammation, necrosis, and formation of new bone. Osteomyelitis is classified as follows (McCance & Huether, 2019):

- Hematogenous osteomyelitis (i.e., due to bloodborne spread of infection)
- Contiguous-focus osteomyelitis, from contamination from bone surgery (especially with hardware insertion), open fracture, or traumatic injury (e.g., gunshot wound)
- Osteomyelitis with vascular insufficiency, seen most commonly among patients with diabetes and peripheral vascular disease, most commonly affecting the feet

Patients who are at high risk for osteomyelitis include older adults and those who are poorly nourished or obese. Other patients at risk include those with impaired immune systems, those with chronic illnesses (e.g., diabetes, RA), those receiving long-term corticosteroid therapy or immunosuppressive agents, and those who use illicit IV drugs (Lalani & Schmidt, 2019).

Postoperative surgical wound infections typically occur within 30 days after surgery. They are classified as incisional (superficial, located above the deep fascia layer) or deep (involving tissue beneath the deep fascia). If an implant has been used, deep postoperative infections may occur within a year. Osteomyelitis may become chronic and may affect the patient's quality of life.

Pathophysiology

More than 50% of bone infections are caused by *Staphylococcus aureus* and increasingly of the variety that is methicillin resistant (i.e., MRSA) (Lalani & Schmidt, 2019). Surgical site ink markers have been linked to infections by cross contamination between preoperative patients who use their markers; therefore, these items are now considered one patient or one-time use items (Driessche, 2012). Other pathogens include the gram-positive organisms *streptococci* and *enterococci*, followed by gram-negative bacteria, including *pseudomonas* (Lalani & Schmidt, 2019).

The initial response to infection is inflammation, increased vascularity, and edema. After 2 or 3 days, thrombosis of the local blood vessels occurs, resulting in ischemia with bone necrosis. The infection extends into the medullary cavity and under the periosteum and may spread into adjacent soft tissues and joints. Unless the infective process is treated promptly, a bone abscess forms. The resulting abscess cavity contains **sequestrum** (i.e., dead bone tissue), which does not easily liquefy and drain. Therefore, the cavity cannot collapse and heal, as it does in soft tissue abscesses. New bone growth, the **involucrum**, forms and surrounds the sequestrum. Although healing appears to take place, a chronically infected sequestrum remains and produces recurring abscesses throughout the patient's life. This is referred to as chronic osteomyelitis.

Clinical Manifestations

When the infection is bloodborne, the onset is usually sudden, occurring often with the clinical and laboratory manifestations of sepsis (e.g., chills, high fever, rapid pulse, general malaise). The systemic symptoms at first may overshadow the local signs. As the infection extends through the cortex of the bone, it involves the periosteum and the soft tissues. The infected area becomes painful, swollen, and extremely tender. The patient may describe a constant, pulsating pain that intensifies with movement as a result of the pressure of the collecting purulent material (i.e., pus). When osteomyelitis occurs from spread of adjacent infection or from direct contamination, there are no manifestations of sepsis. The surface area that lies over the infected bone is swollen, warm, painful, and tender to touch. The patient with chronic osteomyelitis presents with a nonhealing ulcer that overlies the infected bone with a connecting sinus that will intermittently and spontaneously drain pus (Lalani & Schmidt, 2019).

Diabetic osteomyelitis can occur without any external wounds. It may present as a nonhealing fracture. Microvascular and macrovascular pathophysiologic changes, along with an impaired immune response by patients with diabetes who have poor glycemic control can exacerbate the spread of infection from other sources. Any foot ulcer more than 2 cm in diameter is highly suspicious for osteomyelitis (Lalani & Schmidt, 2019).

Assessment and Diagnostic Findings

In acute osteomyelitis, early x-ray findings demonstrate soft tissue edema. In about 2 to 3 weeks, areas of periosteal elevation and bone necrosis are evident. Radioisotope bone scans and MRI help with early definitive diagnosis. Blood studies reveal leukocytosis and an elevated ESR. Wound and blood culture studies are performed, although they are only positive in 50% of cases. Therefore, treatment with antibiotics may be prescribed without isolating the organism and then refined after results are obtained. IV antibiotics and bone biopsies are preferably done prior to starting the antibiotics (Osmon & Tande, 2019).

With chronic osteomyelitis, large, irregular cavities, raised periosteum, sequestrum, or dense bone formations are seen on x-ray. Bone scans may be performed to identify areas of infection. The ESR and the WBC count are usually normal. Anemia, associated with chronic infection, may be evident. Cultures of blood specimens and drainage from the sinus tract are frequently unreliable for isolating the organisms involved. Bone cultures are aspirated through uninfected skin (Lalani & Schmidt, 2019).

Prevention

Prevention of osteomyelitis is the goal. Elective orthopedic surgery should be postponed if the patient has a current infection (e.g., urinary tract infection, sore throat that may suggest a *Streptococcal* infection). During surgery, careful attention is paid to the surgical environment. Prophylactic antibiotics, given to achieve adequate tissue levels at the time of surgery and for 24 hours after surgery, are helpful. Urinary catheters and drains are removed as soon as possible to decrease the incidence of hematogenous spread of infection.

Aseptic postoperative wound care reduces the incidence of superficial infections and osteomyelitis. Prompt management of soft tissue infections reduces extension of infection to the bone or hematogenous spread.

Medical Management

The initial goal of therapy is to control and halt the infective process. General supportive measures (e.g., hydration, diet high in vitamins and protein, correction of anemia) are instituted. The area affected with osteomyelitis is immobilized to decrease discomfort and to prevent pathologic fracture of the weakened bone.

Pharmacologic Therapy

Bone infections are more difficult to eradicate than soft tissue infections because bone is mostly avascular and less accessible to the body's natural immune response. Because there is decreased penetration by medications, antibiotic therapy is longer term than with other infections; typically, it continues for 6 to 12 weeks. After the infection appears to be controlled, the antibiotic may be given orally. However, there is little evidence to support optimal length of therapy (Li, Romach, Zabellas, et al., 2019).

Surgical Management

If the infection is chronic and does not respond to antibiotic therapy, surgical débridement is indicated. The infected bone is surgically exposed, the purulent and necrotic material is removed, and the area is irrigated with sterile saline solution. A sequestrectomy (removal of enough involucrum to enable the surgeon to remove the sequestrum) is performed. In many cases, sufficient bone is removed to convert a deep cavity into a shallow saucer (saucerization). All dead, infected bone and cartilage must be removed before permanent healing can occur. A closed suction irrigation system may be used to remove debris. Wound irrigation using sterile physiologic saline solution may be performed for extended periods if the debris remains. Typically, irrigation does not need to extend beyond a week.

The wound is either closed tightly to obliterate the dead space or packed and closed later by granulation or possibly by grafting. The débrided cavity may be packed with cancellous bone graft to stimulate healing. With a large defect, the cavity may be filled with a vascularized bone transfer or muscle flap (in which a muscle is moved from an adjacent area with blood supply intact). These microsurgery techniques enhance the blood supply. The improved blood supply facilitates bone healing and eradication of the infection. These surgical procedures may be staged over time to ensure healing. Because surgical débridement weakens the bone, internal fixation or external supportive devices may be needed to stabilize or support the bone to prevent pathologic fracture (Rüschenschmidt, Glombitza, Dahmen, et al., 2019). Original orthopedic hardware may need to be removed.

NURSING PROCESS

The Patient with Osteomyelitis

Assessment

The patient reports an acute onset of signs and symptoms (e.g., localized pain, edema, erythema, fever) or recurrent drainage of an infected sinus with associated pain, edema, and low-grade fever. The nurse assesses the patient for risk factors (e.g., older age, diabetes, long-term corticosteroid therapy) and for a history of previous injury, infection, or orthopedic surgery. The gait may be altered as the patient avoids pressure and movement of the area. In acute hematogenous osteomyelitis, the patient exhibits generalized weakness due to the systemic reaction to the infection.

Physical examination reveals an inflamed, markedly edematous, warm area that is tender. Purulent drainage may be noted. The patient has an elevated temperature. With chronic osteomyelitis, the temperature elevation may be minimal, occurring in the afternoon or evening.

Diagnosis

NURSING DIAGNOSES

Based on the assessment data, nursing diagnoses may include the following:
- Acute pain associated with inflammation and edema
- Impaired mobility associated with pain, use of immobilization devices, and weight-bearing limitations
- Risk for infection: bone abscess formation
- Lack of knowledge associated with the treatment regimen

Planning and Goals

The patient's goals may include relief of pain, improved physical mobility within therapeutic limitations, control and eradication of infection, and knowledge of the treatment regimen.

Nursing Interventions

RELIEVING PAIN

The affected part may be immobilized with a splint to decrease pain and muscle spasm. The nurse monitors the skin and neurovascular status of the affected extremity. The wounds are frequently very painful, and the extremity must be handled with great care and gentleness. Elevation reduces swelling and associated discomfort. Pain is controlled with prescribed analgesic agents and other pain-reducing techniques.

IMPROVING PHYSICAL MOBILITY

Treatment regimens restrict weight-bearing activity. The bone is weakened by the infective process and must be protected by avoidance of stress on the bone. The patient must understand the rationale for the activity restrictions. The joints above and below the affected part should be gently moved through their range of motion. The nurse encourages full participation in ADLs within the prescribed physical limitations to promote general well-being. Caution around external fixation devices is required (see Chapter 37 for discussion of external fixation devices).

CONTROLLING THE INFECTIOUS PROCESS

The nurse monitors the patient's response to antibiotic therapy and observes the IV access site for evidence of phlebitis, infection, or infiltration. With long-term, intensive antibiotic therapy, the patient is monitored for signs of superinfection (e.g., oral or vaginal candidiasis, loose or foul-smelling stools). The nurse carefully monitors for the development of additional sites that are painful or for sudden increases in body temperature.

If surgery is necessary, the nurse takes measures to ensure adequate circulation to the affected area (wound suction to prevent fluid accumulation, elevation of the area to promote venous drainage, avoidance of pressure on the grafted area), to maintain needed immobility, and to ensure the patient's adherence to weight-bearing restrictions. Dressings are changed using aseptic technique to promote healing and to prevent cross contamination.

PROMOTING HOME, COMMUNITY-BASED, AND TRANSITIONAL CARE

Educating Patients About Self-Care. The patient and family are educated about the importance of strictly adhering to the therapeutic regimen of antibiotics. Patients and families often need to learn to maintain and manage the IV access and IV administration equipment in the home. Education includes the medication name, dosage, frequency, administration rate, safe storage and handling, adverse reactions, and necessary laboratory monitoring. In addition, the nurse provides education on aseptic dressing and warm compression techniques.

Continuing and Transitional Care. The patient must be medically stable and physically able and motivated to adhere strictly to the therapeutic regimen of antibiotic therapy. The transitional care environment needs to be conducive to the promotion of health and to the requirements of the therapeutic regimen.

If warranted, the nurse completes a home assessment to determine the patient's and family's abilities regarding continuation of the therapeutic regimen. If the patient's support system is questionable or if the patient lives alone, a home health nurse may be needed to assist with IV administration of the antibiotics, monitoring for response to the treatment and evaluation of signs and symptoms of superinfections, and adverse drug reactions. This can also be done via telehealth (Eichler et al., 2019). The nurse stresses the importance of follow-up health care appointments (see Chart 36-12).

Evaluation

Expected patient outcomes may include:
1. Experiences pain relief
   a. Reports decreased pain at rest
   b. Experiences no tenderness at site of previous infection
   c. Experiences minimal discomfort with movement
2. Increases in safe physical mobility
   a. Participates in self-care activities within restrictions
   b. Maintains full function of unimpaired extremities
   c. Demonstrates safe use of immobilizing and assistive devices
   d. Modifies environment to promote safety and to avoid falls
3. Shows absence of infection
   a. Takes antibiotic as prescribed
   b. Reports normal temperature
   c. Exhibits no edema
   d. Reports absence of drainage
   e. Laboratory results indicate normal WBC count and ESR
   f. Wound cultures are negative

Chart 36-12 — HOME CARE CHECKLIST
The Patient with Osteomyelitis

At the completion of education, the patient and/or caregiver will be able to:

- State the impact of osteomyelitis on physiologic functioning, ADLs, IADLs, roles, relationships, and spirituality.
- Identify modification of home environment, interventions, and strategies (e.g., durable medical equipment, adaptive equipment) used in safely adapting to changes in structure or function and promote effective recovery and rehabilitation.
- State how to obtain medical supplies and carry out dressing changes, wound care, and other prescribed regimens.
- Describe ongoing postoperative therapeutic regimen, including diet and activities to perform (e.g., exercises) and to limit or avoid (e.g., lifting weights, driving a car, contact sports).
  - Consume a healthy diet to promote wound and bone healing.
  - Observe prescribed weight-bearing and activity limits.
  - Demonstrate proper wound care.
  - Demonstrate safe use of ambulatory aids and assistive devices.
- State the name, dose, side effects, frequency, and schedule for all medications.
  - Demonstrate accurate and safe administration of medications.
- When indicated, identify the benefits and expected outcomes of intravenous antibiotic therapy and IV access management.

- Demonstrate how to prepare, infuse, maintain, and clean IV access and equipment.
- Identify adverse effects of antibiotic therapy and actions to take for adverse effects.
- Describe to whom, how, and when to report adverse effects.
- Relieve pain with pharmacologic and nonpharmacologic interventions.
- State indicators of wound infections (e.g., redness, swelling, tenderness, purulent drainage, fever) and systemic infection (e.g., fever, chills, rapid pulse, general malaise) to report promptly to primary provider.
- Relate how to reach primary provider with questions or complications.
- State time and date of follow-up appointments and testing.
- Identify the need for health promotion (e.g., weight reduction, smoking cessation, stress management), disease prevention, and screening activities.

Resources

See Chapter 2, Chart 2-6 for additional information related to durable medical equipment, adaptive equipment, and mobility skills.

ADLs, activities of daily living; IADLs, instrumental activities of daily living; IV, intravenous.

4. Adheres to therapeutic plan
   a. Takes medications as prescribed
   b. Protects weakened bones
   c. Demonstrates proper wound care
   d. Reports signs and symptoms of complications promptly
   e. Consumes a healthy diet
   f. Keeps follow-up health care appointments

Septic (Infectious) Arthritis

Joints can become infected through spread of pathogens from other parts of the body (hematogenous spread) or directly through trauma, injection, or surgical instrumentation, causing septic arthritis. People at greatest risk include older adults, particularly those older than 80 years; people with comorbid conditions such as diabetes, RA, skin infection, or alcoholism; and people with a history of a joint replacement or other joint surgery or IV drug abuse. *S. aureus* is the most common cause of joint infections in all age groups, followed by other gram-positive bacteria, including streptococci. Gonococcal infection may cause septic arthritis through hematogenous spread. *Pseudomonas aeruginosa* is a commonly implicated pathogen in those who use illicit IV drugs (Goldenberg & Sexton, 2019).

Single knee or hip joints are most commonly infected in patients with septic arthritis, although up to 20% of cases involve more than one joint (i.e., polyarticular disease). Prompt recognition and treatment of an infected joint are important because accumulating purulent material may result in chondrolysis (destruction of hyaline cartilage), and continued hematogenous spread may lead to sepsis and death. See Chapter 11 for further discussion of sepsis. The overall mortality rate for single joint infections is about 11%, but it approaches 50% in patients with polyarticular disease or in those who are immunocompromised (Oh, Wurcel, Tybor, et al., 2018).

Clinical Manifestations

The patient with acute septic arthritis presents with a warm, painful, swollen joint with decreased range of motion. Systemic chills, fever, and leukocytosis are sometimes present. Fever may not occur in older patients. Although any joint may be infected, approximately half of all cases involve a knee (Goldenberg & Sexton, 2019).

Assessment and Diagnostic Findings

An assessment for the source and cause of infection is performed. Diagnostic studies include aspiration, examination, and culture of the synovial fluid. Computed tomography (CT) and MRI scans may reveal damage to the joint lining. Radioisotope scanning may be useful in localizing the infectious process. There may not be any external wound or reported recent trauma.

Medical Management

Prompt treatment is essential and may save the prosthesis for patients who have had joint replacement surgery or may prevent sepsis. Broad-spectrum IV antibiotics are started promptly and then changed to organism-specific antibiotics after culture results are available (Goldenberg & Sexton, 2019). The IV antibiotics are continued until symptoms resolve. The synovial fluid is aspirated and analyzed periodically for sterility and decrease in WBCs.

Aspiration of the joint with a needle to remove excessive joint fluid, exudate, and debris promotes comfort and decreases joint destruction caused by the action of proteolytic enzymes in the purulent fluid. Arthrotomy or arthroscopy is used to drain the joint and remove dead tissue (Oh et al., 2018).

The inflamed joint is supported and immobilized in a functional position by a splint that increases the patient's comfort. Analgesic agents are prescribed to relieve pain. The patient's nutrition and fluid status is monitored. Progressive range-of-motion exercises are prescribed as soon as the patient can begin movement without exacerbating symptoms of acute pain. If septic joints are treated promptly, recovery of normal function is expected. If the articular cartilage was damaged during the inflammatory reaction, joint fibrosis and diminished function may result. The patient is assessed periodically for recurrence over the next year.

Nursing Management

The nurse educates the patient and family about the septic arthritis physiologic process and explains the importance of supporting the affected joint, adhering to the prescribed antibiotic regimen, inspecting the skin under any splints that may be prescribed, and observing weight-bearing and activity restrictions. The patient must understand that recurrence of infection in the near and far future is possible and is educated about signs and symptoms to observe and report to the primary provider. The same interventions used for the patient with osteomyelitis are planned for the patient with septic arthritis. See previous discussion.

Bone Tumors

Neoplasms of the musculoskeletal system are of various types, including osteogenic, chondrogenic, fibrogenic, muscle (rhabdomyogenic), and marrow (reticulum) cell tumors as well as nerve, vascular and fatty cell tumors. They may be primary tumors or metastatic tumors from cancers elsewhere in the body (e.g., breast, lung, prostate, kidney).

Benign Bone Tumors

Benign tumors of the bone and soft tissue are more common than malignant primary bone tumors. Benign bone tumors generally are slow growing, well circumscribed, and encapsulated; present few symptoms; and are not a cause of death. Benign masses include osteochondroma, enchondroma, bone cysts, osteoid osteoma, rhabdomyoma, and fibroma. Some benign tumors have the potential to become malignant.

Osteochondroma is the most common benign bone tumor. It usually occurs as a large projection of bone at the end of long bones (at the knee or shoulder), developing during growth. It then becomes a static bony mass. In fewer than 1% of patients, the cartilage cap of the osteochondroma may undergo malignant transformation after trauma, and a chondrosarcoma or osteosarcoma may develop (Czerniak, 2016).

Bone cysts are expanding lesions within the bone. Aneurysmal (widening) bone cysts are seen in young adults, who present with a painful, palpable mass of the long bones, vertebrae, or flat bone. Unicameral (single cavity) bone cysts occur more often in the first two decades of life and cause mild discomfort and possible pathologic fractures of the upper humerus and femur, which may heal spontaneously.

An osteoid osteoma is a painful tumor that occurs in children and young adults. The neoplastic tissue is surrounded by reactive bone formation that can be identified by x-ray. Enchondroma is a common tumor of the hyaline cartilage that develops in the hand, femur, tibia, or humerus. Usually, the only symptom is a mild ache. Pathologic fractures may occur in both types of tumors.

Giant cell tumors (osteoclastomas) are benign for long periods but may invade local tissue and cause destruction. They occur in young adults and are soft and hemorrhagic. Eventually, giant cell tumors may undergo malignant transformation and metastasize (Czerniak, 2016).

Malignant Bone Tumors

Primary malignant musculoskeletal tumors are relatively rare and arise from connective and supportive tissue cells (sarcomas) or bone marrow elements (multiple myeloma; see Chapter 30). Malignant primary musculoskeletal tumors include osteosarcoma, chondrosarcoma, Ewing sarcoma, and fibrosarcoma. Soft tissue sarcomas include liposarcoma, fibrosarcoma of soft tissue, and rhabdomyosarcoma. Bone tumor metastasis to the lungs is common (Davis, James, & Saifuddin, 2015).

Osteosarcoma is the most common and most often fatal primary malignant bone tumor. Prognosis depends on whether the tumor has metastasized to the lungs at the time the patient seeks health care. It appears most frequently in children, adolescents and young adults (in bones that grow rapidly), in older adults with Paget disease of the bone, and in people with a prior history of radiation exposure. Clinical manifestations typically include localized bone pain that may be accompanied by a tender, palpable soft tissue mass. The primary lesion may involve any bone, but the most common sites are the distal femur, the proximal tibia, and the proximal humerus.

Malignant tumors of the hyaline cartilage are called *chondrosarcomas*. These tumors are the second most common primary malignant bone tumors affecting middle aged and older adults (Hornicek, 2019). They may grow and metastasize slowly or very fast, depending on the characteristics of the tumor cells involved (i.e., grade). Patients with low-grade chondrosarcomas tend to have a much better prognosis than those with high-grade chondrosarcomas. See Chapter 12 for a discussion of tumor grades. The usual tumor sites include the pelvis, femur, humerus, spine, scapula, and tibia. Metastasis to the lungs occurs in fewer than half of patients. These tumors may recur after excision.

Metastatic Bone Disease

Metastatic bone disease (secondary bone tumor) is more common than primary bone tumors (Mu, Shen, Liang, et al., 2018). Tumors arising from tissues elsewhere in the body may invade the bone and produce localized bone destruction (lytic lesions) or bone overgrowth (blastic lesions). The most common primary sites of tumors that metastasize to bone are the kidney, prostate, lung, breast, ovary, and thyroid (Mu et al., 2018). Metastatic tumors are most frequently found in the skull, spine, pelvis, femur, and humerus and often involve more than one bone (polyostotic).

Pathophysiology

A tumor in the bone causes the normal bone tissue to react by osteolytic response (bone destruction) or osteoblastic response (bone formation). Adjacent normal bone responds to the tumor by altering its normal pattern of remodeling. The bone's surface changes, and the contours enlarge in the tumor area.

Malignant bone tumors invade and destroy adjacent bone tissue (Mu et al., 2018). Benign bone tumors, in contrast, have a symmetric, controlled growth pattern and place pressure on adjacent bone tissue. Malignant bone tumors invade and weaken the structure of the bone until it can no longer withstand the stress of ordinary use; pathologic fracture commonly results.

Clinical Manifestations

Patients with metastatic bone tumor may have a wide range of associated clinical manifestations. They may be symptom free or have pain that ranges from mild and occasional to constant and severe, varying degrees of disability, and, at times, obvious bone growth. Weight loss, malaise, and fever may be present. The tumor may be diagnosed only after pathologic fractures occur or as an incidental finding.

With spinal metastasis, spinal cord compression may occur. It can progress rapidly or slowly. Neurologic deficits (e.g., progressive pain, weakness, gait abnormality, paresthesia, paraplegia, urinary retention, loss of bowel or bladder control) must be identified early and treated with decompression laminectomy to prevent permanent spinal cord injury.

Assessment and Diagnostic Findings

The differential diagnosis is based on the history, physical examination, and diagnostic studies, including CT, myelography, arteriography, MRI, biopsy, and biochemical assays of the blood and urine. General bone scans lack specificity. Positron emission tomography (PET) scans, although more expensive than other diagnostic tests, are assuming a larger role in whole body surveys after the initial diagnosis (Hornicek, 2019). PET scans generate images of the metabolic activity of cells and highlight metastatic bone disease when an increase uptake of radioactive substances is noted. A surgical or core needle biopsy is performed for histologic identification. Extreme care is taken during the biopsy to prevent seeding and resultant recurrence after excision of the tumor. Chest x-rays are performed to determine the presence of lung metastasis. Surgical staging of musculoskeletal tumors is based on tumor grade and site (intra- or extracompartmental), as well as on metastasis. Staging is used for planning treatment (see Chapter 12).

Serum ALP levels are frequently elevated with osteogenic sarcoma or bone metastasis. Hypercalcemia is also present with bone metastases from breast, lung, or kidney cancer.

Symptoms of hypercalcemia include muscle weakness, fatigue, anorexia, nausea, vomiting, polyuria, cardiac arrhythmias, seizures, and coma. Hypercalcemia must be identified and treated promptly.

During the diagnostic period, the nurse explains the diagnostic tests and provides psychological and emotional support to the patient and family. The nurse assesses coping behaviors and encourages the use of support systems. Because the terminology associated with benign and malignant growths sound similar, the nurse can clarify the meaning of these in terms of treatment and prognosis and may allay fears.

Medical Management

Primary Bone Tumors

The goal of primary bone tumor treatment is to destroy or remove the tumor rapidly. This may be accomplished by surgical excision, radiation therapy if the tumor is radiosensitive, and chemotherapy for possible micrometastases. Survival and quality of life are important considerations in procedures that attempt to save the involved extremity; however, surgical removal of the tumor may require amputation of the affected extremity, with the amputation extending well above the tumor to achieve local control of the primary lesion (see Chapter 37).

If possible, limb-sparing (salvage) procedures are used to remove the tumor and adjacent tissue. A customized prosthesis, total joint arthroplasty, or bone tissue from the patient (autograft) or from a cadaver donor (allograft) replaces the resected tissue. Soft tissue and blood vessels may need grafting because of the extent of the excision. Complications may include infection, loosening or dislocation of the prosthesis, allograft nonunion, fracture, devitalization of the skin and soft tissues, joint fibrosis, and recurrence of the tumor.

Because of the danger of metastasis with malignant bone tumors, chemotherapy is started before and continued after surgery in an effort to eradicate micrometastatic lesions. The goal of combined chemotherapy is greater therapeutic effect at a lower toxicity rate with reduced resistance to the medications. Soft tissue sarcomas are treated with radiation, limb-sparing excision, and adjuvant chemotherapy (see Chapter 12).

Secondary Bone Tumors

The treatment of advanced metastatic bone cancer is palliative. The therapeutic goal is to relieve the patient's pain and discomfort while promoting quality of life. If the bone is weakened, structural support and stabilization are needed to prevent pathologic fracture. Bones are strengthened by prophylactic internal fixation, arthroplasty, or PMMA (bone cement) reconstruction. Patients with metastatic disease are at higher risk than other patients for postoperative pulmonary congestion, hypoxemia, VTE, and hemorrhage.

Hematopoiesis is frequently disrupted by tumor invasion of the bone marrow or by treatment (chemotherapy, surgery, or radiation). Blood component therapy restores hematologic factors. Additional therapies may be used to treat the original cancer. Radiation, chemotherapy, and hormonal therapy may also be effective in promoting healing of osteolytic lesions (see Chapter 12). Bisphosphonates are effective in stabilizing bone and may prevent cancer spread, as are the RANKL drugs (see Table 36-1).

Nursing Management

The nurse asks the patient about the onset and course of symptoms. During the interview, the nurse assesses the patient's understanding of the disease process, how the patient and the family have been coping, and how the patient has managed the pain. Palpation of the mass is limited to decrease any potential seeding process. The mass size and associated soft tissue swelling, pain, and tenderness are noted. Assessment of the neurovascular status and range of motion of the extremity provides baseline data for future comparisons. Evaluation of the patient's mobility and ability to perform ADLs is also documented.

The nursing care of a patient who has undergone excision of a bone tumor is similar to that of other patients who have had skeletal surgery. Explanation of diagnostic tests, treatments (e.g., wound care), and expected results (e.g., decreased range of motion, numbness, change of body contours) helps the patient deal with the procedures and changes and adhere to the therapeutic regimen. The nurse can most effectively reinforce and clarify information provided by the surgeon by being present during these discussions.

Pain can result from multiple factors. Oncology-associated bone pain is recognized as difficult to control. Pain must be assessed accurately and managed with adequate interventions. External-beam radiation to involved metastatic sites may be used. Patients with multiple bony metastases may achieve pain control with systemically given "bone-seeking" isotopes (e.g., strontium 89). (See Chapter 9 for more information about pain management.)

Bone tumors weaken the bone to a point at which normal activities or even position changes can result in fracture. During nursing care, the affected extremities must be supported and handled gently. External supports (e.g., splints) may be used for additional protection. Surgery (e.g., open reduction with internal fixation, joint replacement) may be done in an attempt to prevent pathologic fracture. Prescribed weight-bearing restrictions must be followed. The nurse and physical therapist must educate the patient about using assistive devices safely and strengthening unaffected extremities.

The nurse encourages the patient and family to verbalize their fears, concerns, and feelings. They need to be supported as they deal with the impact of the malignant bone tumor. Referral to a psychiatric advanced practice nurse, psychologist, counselor, or spiritual advisor may be indicated for specific psychological help and emotional support.

Monitoring and Managing Potential Complications

Delayed Wound Healing

Wound healing may be delayed because of tissue trauma from surgery, previous radiation therapy, inadequate nutrition, or infection. The nurse minimizes pressure on the wound site to promote circulation to the tissues. An aseptic, nontraumatic wound dressing promotes healing. Monitoring and reporting of laboratory findings facilitate initiation of interventions to promote homeostasis and wound healing.

Repositioning the patient at frequent intervals reduces the incidence of skin breakdown and pressure injuries. Special therapeutic beds or mattresses may be needed to prevent skin breakdown and to promote wound healing after extensive surgical reconstruction and skin grafting.

Inadequate nutrition impairs healing as well. Antiemetic agents and relaxation techniques reduce the adverse GI effects of chemotherapy. Stomatitis is controlled with anesthetic or antifungal mouthwash (see Chapter 12). Adequate hydration is essential. Nutritional supplements or parenteral nutrition may be prescribed to achieve adequate nutrition.

Osteomyelitis and Wound Infections

Prophylactic antibiotics and strict aseptic dressing techniques are used to diminish the occurrence of osteomyelitis and wound infections. During healing, other infections (e.g., upper respiratory infections) need to be prevented so that healing efforts are not divided between the cancer and the new, acute process. If the patient is receiving chemotherapy, the nurse monitors the WBC count and instructs the patient to avoid contact with people who have colds or other infections.

Hypercalcemia

Hypercalcemia is a dangerous complication of bone cancer or any process involved with breakdown of bone. Symptoms include muscular weakness, incoordination, anorexia, nausea and vomiting, constipation, electrocardiographic changes (e.g., shortened QT interval and ST segment, bradycardia, heart blocks), and altered mental states (e.g., confusion, lethargy, psychotic behavior). Treatment includes hydration with IV administration of normal saline solution, diuresis, mobilization, and medications such as IV bisphosphonates (e.g., zoledronic acid). Because inactivity leads to additional loss of bone mass and increased calcium in the blood, the nurse assists the patient to increase activity and ambulation. Denosumab may be prescribed if the calcium levels are not responsive to the IV bisphosphonates (see Table 36-1). See Chapters 10 and 12 for further discussion of hypercalcemia and its management.

Promoting Home, Community-Based, and Transitional Care

 Educating Patients About Self-Care

Preparation for and coordination of continuing health care are begun early as a multidisciplinary effort. Patient education addresses medication, dressing changes, treatment regimens, and the importance of physical and occupational therapy programs. The nurse educates the patient about weight-bearing limitations and special handling to prevent pathologic fractures. The patient and family must be educated about the signs and symptoms of possible complications as well as resources available for continuing care (see Chart 36-13).

Continuing and Transitional Care

Arrangements may be made for home, community-based, or transitional care. A home visit allows the nurse to assess the patient's and family's abilities to meet the patient's needs and determine whether other services are needed. The nurse advises the patient to have telephone numbers readily available so that providers can be contacted in case concerns arise.

The nurse emphasizes the need for long-term health monitoring to ensure cure or to detect tumor recurrence or metastasis and the need for recommended health screening. If the patient has metastatic disease, end-of-life issues may need to be explored. Referrals for hospice and palliative care are made if appropriate.

Chart 36-13 **HOME CARE CHECKLIST**

The Patient with a Bone Tumor

At the completion of education, the patient and/or caregiver will be able to:

- State the impact of the bone tumor growth process and treatment on physiologic functioning, ADLs, IADLs, roles, relationships, and spirituality.
- Identify modification of home environment, interventions, and strategies (e.g., durable medical equipment, wound care/dressings, adaptive equipment, ADL assistance) used in safely adapting to changes in structure or function and promote effective recovery and rehabilitation.
- Describe ongoing therapeutic regimen, including diet and activities to perform (e.g., exercises) and to limit or avoid (e.g., lifting weights, driving a car, contact sports).
  - Consume a healthy diet to promote healing and health.
  - State weight-bearing and activity restrictions.
  - Support affected musculoskeletal area, position to decrease risk of skin breakdown.
  - Demonstrate safe use of ambulatory aids and assistive devices.
  - Engage in exercise that improves balance to reduce risk of falls.
- State the name, dose, side effects, frequency, and schedule for all prescribed therapeutic and prophylactic medications (e.g., antibiotics, analgesic agents).
- Control pain with pharmacologic and nonpharmacologic interventions.

- State indicators of complications to report promptly to the provider such as:
  - Wound infection/delayed wound healing (e.g., redness, swelling, tenderness, purulent drainage, fever).
  - Osteomyelitis (e.g., localized pain, edema, erythema, fever).
  - Hypercalcemia (e.g., muscular weakness, anorexia, decreased coordination, nausea, vomiting, constipation).
- Relate how to reach the primary provider with questions or complications.
- State time and date of follow-up appointments, therapy, and testing.
- Identify community resources for peer and caregiver/family support:
  - Identify sources of support (e.g., friends, relatives, faith community).
  - Identify the contact details for support services for patients and their caregivers/families.
- Identify the need for health promotion, disease prevention, and screening activities.

Resources

See Chapter 2, Chart 2-6 for additional information related to durable medical equipment, adaptive equipment, and mobility skills.

ADLs, activities of daily living; IADLs, instrumental activities of daily living.

CRITICAL THINKING EXERCISES

1 `ebp` A patient is being scheduled for a total knee arthroplasty. He shares with you that many years ago his mother had a total hip arthroplasty and experienced ongoing issues related to pain and infection. He is concerned that he may also experience postoperative complications. He asks you to explain to him common complications and how they can be prevented. What evidence-based practice guidelines support your patient education? Explain the strength of the evidence that supports various nursing interventions to prevent infection and venous thromboembolism and to promote improved physical mobility.

2 `pq` You work as a nurse at a college's student health center. A student presents to the health center after a very busy final exam schedule and end of semester paper writing session. She is a varsity basketball player and is having issues with grabbing the ball. In the past, she has had episodes where she "jammed" a finger playing basketball, but this has not occurred recently. She is complaining of severe wrist pain and numbness in her fingers. Describe the priority assessment process that you would follow when you examine her hands. What is the expected care for a possible carpel tunnel disorder and how would you prioritize nursing interventions?

3 `ipc` A patient with a history of profound deafness, poor nutritional habits, and a significantly increased body mass index is status post total knee arthroplasty. The patient lives on the second floor of an apartment building. Develop an interprofessional plan of care that addresses the patient's care needs, both during hospitalization and upon discharge.

REFERENCES

*Asterisk indicates nursing research.

Books

Czerniak, B. (2016). *Dorfman and Czerniak's bone tumors* (2nd ed.). Philadelphia, PA: WB Saunders.

Davis, A., James, S., & Saifuddin, A. (2015). Bone tumours (2): Malignant bone tumours. In A. Grainger & P. O'Connor (Eds.). *Grainger and Allison's diagnostic radiology: The musculoskeletal system*. New York: Elsevier.

Fischbach, F. T., & Fischbach, M. A. (2018). *A manual of laboratory and diagnostic tests* (10th ed.). Philadelphia, PA: Wolters Kluwer.

McCance, K., & Huether, S. (2019). *Pathophysiology: The biologic basis for disease in children & adults* (8th ed.). St. Louis, MO: Elsevier.

Robinson, M. (2020). Drugs affecting the bones and joints. In T. Woo & M. Robinson (Eds.). *Pharmacotherapeutics for advanced practice prescribers* (5th ed.). Philadelphia, PA: F. A. Davis.

Journals and Electronic Documents

Alderson, J., & Ghosh, P. (2019). Clinical reasoning: Pes cavus and neuropathy: Think beyond Charcot-Marie-Tooth disease. *Neurology*, 93(8), e823–e826.

Alexander, D. P., & Frew, N. (2017). Preoperative optimization of anaemia for primary total hip arthroplasty: A systematic review. *Hip International*, 27(6), 515–522.

*Allsop, S., Fairhall, R., & Morphet, J. (2019). The impact of pre-operative telephone support and education on symptoms of anxiety, depression, pain and quality of life post total knee replacement. *International Journal of Orthopaedic and Trauma Nursing*, 34, 21–27.

American Academy of Orthopaedic Surgeons (AAOS). (2020). The AAOS American joint replacement registry. Retrieved on 3/6/2020 at: www.aaos. org/registries/registry-program/american-joint-replacement-registry

American Society for Bone and Mineral Research (ASBMR). (2020). Joint guidance on vitamin D in the era of COVID-19 from the ASBMR, AACE, Endocrine Society, ECTS, NOF, and IOF. Retrieved on 7/10/2020 at: www.asbmr.org/ASBMRStatementsDetail/joint-guidance-on-vitamin-d-in-era-of-covid-19-fro

Arase, Y., Tsuruya, K., Hirose, S., et al. (2020). Efficacy and safety of 3- year denosumab therapy for osteoporosis in patients with autoimmune liver diseases. *Hepatology*, 71(2), 757–759.

Bailey, R., Zou, P., Wallace, T., et al. (2020). Calcium supplement use is associated with less bone mineral density loss, but does not lessen the risk of bone fracture across the menopausal transition: Data from the Study of Women's Health across the nation. *Journal of Bone and Mineral Research*, 4(1), 1–8.

Ball, C., Izadi, D., Verjee, L., et al. (2016). Systematic review of non-surgical treatments for early Dupuytren's disease. *BMC Musculoskeletal Disorders*, 17(1), 345–362.

Beam, E., & Osmon, D. (2018). Prosthetic joint infection. *Infectious Disease Clinics of North America*, 32(4), 843–859.

Bedard, N. A., Pugely, A. J., Lux, N. R., et al. (2017). Recent trends in blood utilization after primary hip and knee arthroplasty. *Journal of Arthroplasty*, 32(3), 724–727.

Berrios-Torres, S. I., Umscheid, C. A., Bratzler, D. W., et al. (2017). Centers for Disease Control and Prevention guideline for the prevention of surgical site infection, 2017. *JAMA Surgery*, 152(8), 784–791.

Black, D., Cauley, J., Wagman, R., et al. (2017). The ability of a single BMD and facture history assessment to predict fracture over 25 years in postmenopausal women. *Journal of Bone Mineral Research*, 33(3), 389–395.

Brent, L., Hommel, A., Maher, A., et al. (2018). Nursing care of fragility fracture patients. *Injury*, 49(8), 1409–1412.

Calandruccio, J., & Thompson, N. (2018). Carpel tunnel syndrome: Making evidence-based treatment decisions. *Orthopedic Clinics*, 49(2), 223–229.

Cass, A., Shepard, A., Asirot, R., et al. (2016). Comparison of the male osteoporosis risk estimation score (MORES) with FRAX in identifying men at risk for osteoporosis. *Annals of Family Medicine*, 26(4), 365–369.

Centers for Disease Control and Prevention (CDC). (2018). Osteoarthritis (OA). Retrieved on 11/24/2019 at: www.cdc.gov/arthritis/basics/osteoarthritis.htm

Cook, J., & Young, M. (2020). Biologic therapies for tendon and muscle injury. In P. Fricker (Ed.). *UpToDate*. Retrieved on 3/11/2020 at: www.uptodate.com/contents/Biologictherapies-for-tendon-and-muscle-injury

Cooper, C., Chapurlat, R., Al-Daghri, N., et al. (2019). Safety of oral non-selective non-steroidal anti-inflammatory drugs in osteoarthritis: What does the literature say? *Drugs & Aging*, 36(1), 15–24.

Cundy, T. (2017). Treating Paget's disease—Why and how much? *Journal of Bone and Mineral Research*, 32(6), 1163–1164.

De Francesco, C., Fu, M., Kalenberg, C., et al. (2019). Extended antibiotic prophylaxis may be linked to lower peri-prosthetic joint infection rates in high-risk patients: An evidence-based review. *HSS Journal*, 15(3), 297–301.

De Keyser, F. (2019). *Ganglion cysts of the wrist and hand*. UpToDate. Retrieved on 3/7/2020 at: www.uptodate.com/contents/ganglion-cysts-of-the-wrist-and-hand

De Leacy, R., Chandra, R., Barr, J., et al. (2020). The evidentiary basis of vertebral augmentation: A 2019 update. *Journal of Neurointerventional Surgery*, 12(5). Retrieved on 3/6/2020 at: www.jnis.bmj.com/content/early/2020/01/27/neurintsurg-2019-015026.info

Drezner, M. (2019). *Patient education: Vitamin D deficiency (beyond the basics)*. UpToDate. Retrieved on 3/7/2020 at: www.uptodate.com/contents/vitamin-d-deficiency-beyond-the-basics

Driessche, A. M. (2012). Surgical site markers: Potential source of infection. *Orthopaedic Nursing*, 31(6), 344–347.

Dupuis, M., & Duff, E. (2019). Chronic low back pain: Evidence informed management considerations for nurse practitioners. *The Journal for Nurse Practitioners*, 15(2019), 583–587.

Dy, C. J., Bumpass, D. B., Makhni, E. C., et al. (2016). The evolving role of clinical registries: Existing practices and opportunities for orthopaedic surgeons. *The Journal of Bone & Joint Surgery, 98*(2), e7.

Eichler, S., Salzwedel, A., Rabe, S., et al. (2019). The effectiveness of telerehabilitation as a supplement to rehabilitation in patients after total knee or hip replacement: randomized controlled trial. *Journal of Medical Internet Research Rehabilitation and Assistive Technologies, 6*(2), e14236. Retrieved on 3/7/2020 at: www.ncbi.nlm.nih.gov/pmc/articles/PMC6873150/pdf/rehab_v6i2e14236.pdf

Erens, G., & Walter, B. (2019). *Complications of total hip arthroplasty. UpToDate.* Retrieved on 3/7/2020 at: www.uptodate.com/contents/complications-of-total-hip-arthroplasty

Erens, G. A., & Walter, B., & Crowley, M. (2020). *Total hip arthroplasty. UpToDate.* Retrieved on 3/16/2020 at: www.uptodate.com/contents/total-hip-arthroplasty

Evans, J., Walker, R., Evans, J., et al. (2019). How long does a knee replacement last? A systematic review and meta-analysis of case series and national registry reports with more than 15 years of follow-up. *The Lancet, 393*(10172), 655–663.

Fasolino, T., & Whitright, T. (2015). A pilot study to identify modifiable and nonmodifiable variables associated with osteopenia and osteoporosis in men. *Orthopaedic Nursing, 34*(5), 289–293.

Feinstein, J., Khalsa, S., Yeh, H., et al. (2018). The elicitation of relaxation and interoceptive awareness using floatation therapy in individuals with high anxiety sensitivity. *Biological Psychiatry, 3*(6), 555–562.

Fournier, M., Saxena, A., & Maffuli, N. (2019). Hallus valgus surgery in the athlete: Current evidence. *Journal of Foot and Ankle Surgery, 58*(4), 641–643.

Gabbert, T., Filson, R., Bodden, J., et al. (2019). Summary: NAON's best practice guideline, total hip replacement (arthroplasty). *Orthopedic Nursing, 38*(1), 4–5.

Gironda, M., Nguyen, A., & Mosqueda, L. (2016). Is this broken bone because of abuse? Characteristics and comorbid diagnoses in older adults with fractures. *Journal of the American Geriatric Society, 64*(8), 1651–1655.

Goff, D., Mangino, J. E., Glassman, A. H., et al. (2020). Review of guidelines for dental antibiotic prophylaxis for prevention of endocarditis and prosthetic joint infections and need for dental stewardship. *Clinical Infectious Diseases, 71*(2), 455–462.

Goldenberg, D. L., & Sexton, D. J. (2019). *Septic arthritis in adults. UpToDate.* Retrieved on 11/24/2020 at: www.uptodate.com/contents/septic-arthritis-in-adults

Hornicek, F. (2019). *Bone tumors: Diagnosis and biopsy techniques. UpToDate.* Retrieved on 3/7/2020 at: www.uptodate.com/contents/bone-tumors-diagnosis-and-biopsy-techniques

International Osteoporosis Foundation (IOF). (2017). Facts and statistics about osteoporosis and its impact. Retrieved on 3/7/2020 at: www.iofbonehealth.org/facts-statistics

Jones, A., Al-Naseer, S., Bodger, O., et al. (2018). Does pre-operative anxiety and/or depression affect patient outcome after primary knee replacement arthroplasty? *Knee, 25*(6), 1238–1246.

Karasawa, Y., Yamadada, K., Iseki, M., et al. (2019). Association between change in self-efficacy and reduction in disability among patients with chronic pain. *PLoS One, 14*(4), e021504.

Keeney, B., Austin, D., & Jevsevar, D. (2019). Preoperative weight loss for morbidly obese patients undergoing total knee arthroplasty: Determining the necessary amount. *Journal of Bone and Joint Surgery, 101*(16), 1440–1450.

Kolasinski, S. L., Neogi, T., Hochber, M. C., et al. (2020). 2019 American College of Rheumatology/Arthritis Foundation guideline for the management of osteoarthritis of the hand, hip, and knee. *Arthritis Care & Research (Hoboken), 72*(2), 149–162.

Krebs, E., Gravely, A., Nugent, S., et al. (2018). Effect of opioid vs nonopioid medications on pain-related function in patients with chronic back pain or hip or knee osteoarthritis: The SPACE randomized clinical trial. *Journal of the American Medical Association, 319*(9), 872–882.

Lalani, T., & Schmidt, S. (2019). *Osteomyelitis in adults: Clinical manifestations and diagnosis. UpToDate.* Retrieved on 1/3/2020 at: www.uptodate.com/contents/-osteomyelitis-in-adults

Lee, G. C. (2016). What's new in adult reconstructive knee surgery. *Journal of Bone & Joint Surgery American, 98*(2), 156–165.

Li, H., Romach, I., Zabellas, R., et al. (2019). Oral versus intravenous antibiotics for bone and joint infection. *New England Journal of Medicine, 380*(5), 425–436.

Loftus, T. J., Spratling, L., Stone, B. A., et al. (2016). A patient blood management program in prosthetic joint arthroplasty decreases blood use and improves outcomes. *The Journal of Arthroplasty, 31*(1), 11–14.

Luffy, L., Grosel, J., Thomas, R., et al. (2018). Plantar fasciitis: A review of treatments. *Journal American Academy of Physician Assistants, 31*(1), 20–24.

Malhotra, K., Davda, K., & Singh, D. (2017). The pathology and management of lesser toe deformities. *EFFORT Open Review, 1*(11), 409–419. Retrieved on 1/3/2020 at: www.ncbi.nlm.nih.gov/pmc/articles/PMC5367573

Mar, W., Tan, I., Song, A., et al. (2019). Update on imaging of knee arthroplasties: Normal findings and hardware complications. *Seminars in Musculoskeletal Radiology, 23*(2), e20–e35.

Martin, G. M., & Harris, I. (2020). *Total knee arthroplasty. UpToDate.* Retrieved on 3/26/2020 at: www.uptodate.com/contents/search?search=total-knee-replacement-arthroplasty-beyond-the-basics

Matthews, B., Hum, C., Harding, M., et al. (2019). The effectiveness of non-surgical interventions for common plantar digital compressive neuropathy (Morton's Neuroma): A systematic review and meta-analysis. *Journal of Foot and Ankle Research, 12*(12), 1–21.

McAlindon, T., LaValley, M., Harvey, W., et al. (2017). Effects of intra-articular triamcinolone vs sale on knee cartilage volume and pain in patients with knee osteoarthritis. *Journal of the American Medical Association, 317*(19), 1967–1975.

Menaka P., & Douketis, J. (2019). *Prevention of venous thromboembolism in adult orthopedic surgical patients. UpToDate.* Retrieved on 1/3/2020 at: www.uptodate.com/contents/prevention-of-venous-thromboembolism-in-adult-orthopedic-surgical-patients/print#!

Michigan Quality Improvement Consortium (MQIC). (2018). Management of acute low back pain in adults. Retrieved on 1/3/2020 at: www.mqic.org/pdf/mquic_management_of_acute_low_back_pain_in_adults_cpg.pdf

Michigan Quality Improvement Consortium (MQIC). (2020). Management and prevention of osteoporosis. Retrieved on 1/24/2021 at: www.mqic.org/pdf/mqic_management_and_prevention_of_osteoporosis_cpg.pdf

Morris, M., Fornit, C., Marchoni, M., et al. (2018). Which factors are independent predictors of early recovery of mobility in the older adults' population after hip fracture. *Archives of Orthopaedic and Trauma Surgery, 138*(1), 35–41.

Mu, C-F., Shen, J., Liang, J., et al. (2018). Targeted drug delivery for tumor therapy inside the bone marrow. *Biomaterials, 155*, 191–202.

Mujagic, E., Hoffmann, H., Soysal, S., et al. (2019). Teaching in the operating room: A risk for surgical site infections. *American Journal of Surgery, 220*(2), 322–327.

National Institute of Arthritis and Musculoskeletal and Skin Diseases (NIAMSD). (2018). Osteoporosis and African American women. Retrieved on 1/3/2020 at: www.bones.nih.gov/health-info/bones/background/african-american-women.pdf

Newman, E. T., Herschmiller, T. A., Attarian, D. A., et al. (2018). Risk factors, outcomes and timing of manipulation under anesthesia after total knee arthroplasty. *The Journal of Arthroplasty, 33*(1), 245–249.

Oh, D., Wurcel, A., Tybor, D., et al. (2018). Increased mortality and reoperation rates after treatment for septic arthritis of the knee in people who inject drugs: Nationwide inpatient sample, 2000–2013. *Clinical Orthopedic and Related Research, 476*(8), 1557–1565.

O'Neill, T., & Felson, D. (2018). Mechanisms of osteoarthritis (OA) pain. *Current Osteoporosis Reports, 16*(5), 611–616.

Papas, P., Conguista, D., Scuderi, G., et al. (2018). A modern approach to preventing prosthetic joint infections. *Journal of Knee Surgery, 31*(7), 610–617.

Pouresmaeili, F., Kamalidehghan, B., Kamerehei, M., et al. (2018). A comprehensive overview on osteoporosis and its risk factors. *Therapeutics and Clinical Risk Management, 2018*(14), 2029–2049.

Qaseem, A., Wilt, T., McLean, R., et al. (2017). Non-invasive treatments for acute, subacute, and chronic low back pain; A clinical practice guideline from the American College of Physicians. *Annals of Internal Medicine, 166*(7), 514–530.

Quinn, R., Murray, J., Pezold, R., et al. (2018). Surgical management of osteoarthritis of the knee. *Journal of the American Academy of Orthopedic Surgeons, 26*(9), e191–e193.

Radwan, A., Fess, P., James, D., et al. (2015). Effect of different mattress designs on promoting sleep quality, pain reduction, and spinal alignment in adults with or without back pain; Systematic review of controlled trials. *Sleep Health, 1*(4), 257–267.

Ralston, S. H., Corral-Gudino, L., Cooper, C., et al. (2019). Diagnosis and management of Paget's disease of bone in adults: A clinical guideline. *Journal of Bone and Mineral Research, 34*(4), 579–604.

Raman, S., FitzGerald, U., & Murphy, J. M. (2018). Interplay of inflammatory mediators with epigenetics and cartilage modifications in osteoarthritis. *Frontiers in Bioengineering and Biotechnology, 6*(22), 1–9.

Raman, R., Henrontin, Y., Chevalier, X., et al. (2018). Decision algorithms for the retreatment with viscosupplementation in patients suffering from knee osteoarthritis: Recommendations from the EUROpean VIScosupplementation Consensus Group (EUROVISCO). *Cartilage, 9*(3), 263–275.

Ramanathan, S., Hibbert, P., Wiles, L., et al. (2018). What is the association between the presence of comorbidities and the appropriateness of care for low back? A population-based medical record review study. *BMC Musculoskeletal Disorders, 19*(391), 1–9.

Rapp, K., Büchele, G., Dreinhőfer, K., et al. (2019). Epidemiology of hip fractures: Systematic literature of German data and an overview of the international literature. *Z Gerontol Geriatr, 52*(1), 10–16.

Rasouli, M. R., Maltenfort, M. G., Erkocak, O. F., et al. (2016). Blood management after total joint arthroplasty in the United States: 19-year trend analysis. *Transfusion, 56*(5), 1112–1120.

Rondanelli, M., Faliva, M., Gasparri, C., et al. (2019). Micronutrients dietary supplementation advices for celiac patients on long-term gluten-free diet with good compliance. *Medicina (Kaunas), 55*(7), 337.

Runhaar, J., Rozendaal, R., Middlekoop, M., et al. (2017). Subgroup analysis of the effectiveness of oral glucosamine for knee and hip osteoarthrtitis. *Annals of Rheumatic Diseases, 76*(11), 1862–1869.

Rüschenschmidt, M., Glombitza, M., Dahmen, J., et al. (2019). External versus internal fixation for arthrodesis of chronic ankle joint infections—A comparative retrospective study. *Foot Ankle Surg, 26*(4), 398–404.

Schmidt, T. (2018). Approach to osteoarthritis management for the primary care provider. *Primary Care, 45*(2), 361–378.

Simon, C., & Hicks, G. (2018). Paradigm shift in geriatric low back pain management: Integrating influences, experiences, and consequences. *Physical Therapy, 98*(5), 434–446.

*Stalenhag, S., & Sterner, E. (2019). Factors that creates obstacles and opportunity for patient participation in orthopaedic nursing care. *European Wound Management Association Journal, 20*(1), 49–59.

Strozyk, D., Gress, T., & Brietling, L. (2018). Smoking and bone mineral density: comprehensive analysis of the third National Health and Nutrition Examination Survey (NHANES III). *Arch Osteoporos, 13*(1), 16.

United States Preventive Services Task Force (USPSTF). (2017). Hormone therapy for the primary prevention of chronic conditions in post-menopausal women. *Journal of the American Medical Association, 318*(22), 2224–2233.

United States Preventive Services Task Force (USPSTF). (2018). Final recommendation statement: Vitamin D, calcium, or combined supplementation for the primary prevention of fractures in community-dwelling adults. Retrieved on 11/27/2020 at: www.uspreventiveservicestaskforce.org/Page/Document/RecommendationStatementFinal/vitamin-d-calcium-or-combined-supplementation-for-the-primary-prevention-of-fractures-in-adults-preventive-medication

United States Preventive Services Task Force (USPSTF). (2019). Final recommendation statement: screening in osteoporosis to prevent fractures: screening. Retrieved on 1/3/2020 at: www.uspreventiveservicestaskforce.org/Page/Document/RecommendationStatementFinal/osteoporosis-screening1

Unver, B., Erdem, E., & Akbas, E. (2019). Effects of short-foot exercises on foot posture, pain, disability, and plantar pressure in pes planus. *Journal of Sport Rehabilitation, 29*(4), 436–440.

van Netten, J. J., Sacco, I. C. N., Lavery, L. A., et al. (2020). Treatment of modifiable risk factors for foot ulceration in persons with diabetes: A systematic review. *Diabetes Metabolism Research and Reviews, 36*(Suppl 1), e3271.

Villa, J. M., Pannu, T. S., Riesgo, A. M., et al. (2020). Dual antibiotic prophylaxis in total knee arthroplasty: Where do we stand? *Journal of Knee Surgery 33*(2), 100–105.

Wheeler, S. G., Wipf, J. E., Staiger, T. O., et al. (2019). Evaluation of low back pain in adults. *UpToDate.* Retrieved on 3/9/2020 at: www.uptodate.com/contents/evaluation-of-low-back-pain-in-adults

World Anti-Doping Agency. (2020). Retrieved on 3/6/2020 at: www.wada-ama.org/en

Resources

American Cancer Society, www.cancer.org

American Joint Replacement Registry, www.aaos.org/registries/registry-program/american-joint-replacement-registry

Arthritis Foundation, www.arthritis.org

National Cancer Institute, www.cancer.gov

National Institute of Arthritis and Musculoskeletal and Skin Diseases, www.niams.nih.gov

National Osteoporosis Foundation Bone Source®, www.nbha.org

National Osteoporosis Foundation, www.nof.org

The Paget Foundation, www.paget.org

Vitamin D Council, www.vitamindcouncil.org

World Anti-Doping Agency, www.wada-ama.org/en

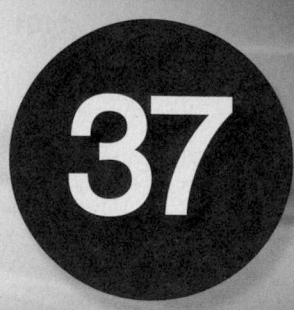

37 Management of Patients with Musculoskeletal Trauma

Unintentional injury is the third leading cause of death in the United States (Kochanek, Murphy, Xu, et al., 2019). Unintentional injuries are commonly called *accidents*; however, this term is considered inaccurate by trauma professionals. The term *accident* infers that there is no potential for prevention; yet, health care professionals understand that prevention plays a major role in decreasing the rate of unintentional injuries. The implementation of evidence-based primary prevention policies (e.g., mandatory use of seat belts for drivers and passengers in motor vehicles) may prevent many unintentional injuries from occurring.

Trauma is a frequent cause of musculoskeletal injury and is among the most common reasons for people to seek medical attention (Centers for Disease Control and Prevention [CDC], National Center for Health Statistics, 2017). Therefore, nurses who work in emergency departments (EDs), critical care units, and inpatient medical-surgical units frequently encounter patients who have experienced musculoskeletal trauma. The management of musculoskeletal injuries frequently includes the use of casts, splints, braces, traction, surgery, or a combination of these. Nursing care is planned to maximize the effectiveness of these treatment modalities and to prevent potential complications associated with each of the interventions. However, upon discharge from the hospital, many of these patients require extensive periods of rehabilitation and follow-up. Thus, nurses who work in rehabilitation centers, long-term care facilities, ambulatory surgery centers, occupational health settings, and primary care clinics may all care for patients with musculoskeletal injuries.

Contusions, Strains, and Sprains

A **contusion** is a soft tissue injury produced by blunt force, such as a blow, kick, or fall, causing small blood vessels to rupture and bleed into soft tissues (ecchymosis or bruising). A hematoma develops from bleeding at the site of impact, leaving a characteristic "black and blue" appearance. Contusions can be minor or severe, isolated or in conjunction with additional injuries (e.g., fracture). Local symptoms include pain, swelling, and discoloration. Contusions can limit joint range of motion (ROM) near the injury, and the injured muscle may feel weak and stiff (American Academy of Orthopedic Surgeons [AAOS], 2019a). Most contusions resolve in 1 to 2 weeks; severe contusions may take longer to heal.

A **strain** is an injury to a muscle or tendon from overuse, overstretching, or excessive stress; it is commonly known as a muscle pull (Babarinde, Ismail, & Schellack, 2018). Tendons are fibrous cords that attach muscle to a bone; strains often occur in tendons of the foot, leg (e.g., hamstring), and back. Strains can be categorized as acute or chronic and are graded along a continuum based on postinjury symptoms and loss of function. Acute strains can result from a single injurious incident; whereas, chronic strains result from repetitive injuries. Chronic strains can result from improper management of acute strains. Depending on the severity of muscle fiber damage, three degrees of strains can be classified (Babarinde et al., 2018):

- A **first-degree** strain is mild stretching of the muscle or tendon with no loss of ROM. Signs and symptoms may include the gradual onset of palpation-induced tenderness and mild muscle spasm.

- A **second-degree** strain involves moderate stretching and/or partial tearing of the muscle or tendon. Signs and symptoms include acute pain during the precipitating event, followed by tenderness at the site with increased pain with passive ROM (PROM), edema, significant muscle spasm, and ecchymosis.

- A **third-degree** strain is severe muscle or tendon stretching with rupturing and complete tearing of the involved tissue. Signs and symptoms include immediate pain described as tearing, snapping, or burning, muscle spasm, ecchymosis, edema, and loss of function. An x-ray should be obtained to rule out bone injury, because an avulsion fracture (in which a bone fragment is pulled away from the bone by a tendon) may be associated with a third-degree strain. X-rays do not reveal injuries to soft tissue or muscles, tendons, or ligaments, but magnetic resonance imaging (MRI) and ultrasound can identify tendon injury.

A **sprain** is an injury to the ligaments and tendons that surround a joint. It is caused by a twisting motion or hyperextension (forcible) of a joint (Babarinde et al., 2018). While tendons connect muscle to bone, ligaments connect bone to bone. The function of a ligament is to stabilize and support the body's joints while permitting mobility. An injured ligament causes joint instability, with the most vulnerable areas of the body being the ankles, knees, and wrists. The severity of a sprain is graded according to how badly the ligament has been damaged and whether or not the joint has been made unstable (Maughan, 2019):

- A Grade I sprain is stretching or slight tearing in some fibers of the ligament and mild, localized hematoma formation. Manifestations include mild pain, edema, and local tenderness.

- A Grade II sprain is more severe and involves partial tearing of the ligament. Manifestations include increased pain with motion, edema, tenderness, joint instability, ecchymosis, and partial loss of normal joint function.

- A Grade III sprain is a complete tear or rupture of the ligament. A Grade III sprain may also cause an avulsion of the bone. Symptoms include severe pain, edema, tenderness, ecchymosis, and abnormal joint motion.

Management

The treatment for contusions, strains, and sprains is guided by the severity of injury and the goal of protecting from further injury. Protection from further injury is accomplished through support of the affected area (e.g., sling, brace) and/or splinting, taping, or compression bandages. To control pain, bleeding, and inflammation, most contusions, strains, and sprains are managed with the **RICE** method, an acronym that refers to *r*est, *i*ce, *c*ompression, and *e*levation (AAOS, 2019a). Rest prevents additional injury and promotes healing. Intermittent application of cold or ice packs during the first 24 to 72 hours after injury produces vasoconstriction, which decreases bleeding, edema, and discomfort. Cold packs should not be in place for longer than 20 minutes at a time, and care must be taken to avoid skin and tissue damage from excessive cold (AAOS, 2019a). An elastic compression bandage controls bleeding, reduces edema, and provides support for the injured tissues. Elevation at or just above the level of the heart controls the swelling (AAOS, 2019a). If the sprain or strain is the most severe grade or degree, immobilization by a splint, brace, or cast may be necessary so that the joint will not lose its stability (see later discussions). Nonsteroidal anti-inflammatory drugs (NSAIDs) may be prescribed for pain management (AAOS, 2019a). The **neurovascular status**, a type of focused assessment of the neurologic (motor and sensory) and vascular function of the injured extremity, is monitored at frequent intervals (e.g., every 15 minutes for the first 1 to 2 hours after injury) and then at lesser intervals (e.g., every 30 minutes) until stable. Decreases in sensation or motion and increases in pain level should be documented and reported to the patient's primary provider immediately so that acute compartment syndrome can be prevented (see later discussion).

Joint Dislocations

A **dislocation** of a joint is a condition in which the articular surfaces of the distal and proximal bones that form the joint are no longer in anatomic alignment. A **subluxation** is a partial or incomplete dislocation and does not cause as much deformity as a complete dislocation. In complete dislocation, the bones are literally "out of joint." Acute traumatic dislocations are orthopedic emergencies because the associated joint structures, blood supply, and nerves are displaced and may be entrapped with extensive pressure on them. If a dislocation or subluxation is not reduced immediately, **avascular necrosis (AVN)** may develop. AVN of bone is caused by ischemia, which leads to necrosis or death of the bone cells.

Signs and symptoms of a traumatic dislocation include acute pain, change in or awkward positioning of the joint, and decreased ROM. Bilateral assessment will usually make apparent the abnormality in the affected joint. X-rays are usually taken to confirm the diagnosis and reveal any associated fracture (DeBerardino, 2018).

Medical Management

When a joint is dislocated, the main treatment priorities are to avoid neurovascular complications and reduce the joint as atraumatically as possible (DeBerardino, 2018). The affected joint needs to be immobilized at the scene and during transport to the hospital. Informed consent for the procedure is obtained and the dislocation is promptly reduced so that displaced parts are placed back in proper anatomic position to preserve joint function (see Chart 37-1). Analgesia, muscle relaxants, and possibly anesthesia are used to facilitate closed reduction. The joint is immobilized by splints, casts, or traction and is maintained in a stable position. Neurovascular status is assessed at a minimum of every 15 minutes until stable. After reduction, if the joint is stable, gentle, progressive, active and passive movement is begun to preserve ROM and restore strength. The joint is supported between exercise sessions.

Nursing Management

The focus of nursing care is on frequent assessment and evaluation of the injury, including complete neurovascular assessment with proper documentation and communication with the primary provider. The patient and family members are educated regarding proper exercises and activities as well as

danger signs and symptoms to look for, such as increasing pain (even with analgesic agents), numbness or tingling, and increased edema in the extremity. These signs and symptoms may indicate acute compartment syndrome; if acute compartment syndrome is not identified and communicated to the primary provider, it may lead to disability or loss of the extremity (see later discussion).

Injuries to the Tendons, Ligaments, and Menisci

Rotator Cuff Tears

A rotator cuff tear is a rip in a tendon that connects one of the rotator muscles to the humeral head. The rotator cuff stabilizes the humeral head and keeps the arm in the shoulder socket. The rotator cuff is composed of four muscles that come together as tendons (supraspinatus, infraspinatus, teres minor, and subscapularis) that cover the head of the humerus, helping to raise and rotate the arm (AAOS, 2019b).

Rotator cuff tears may result from acute or chronic stresses on the joint and from intrinsic (e.g., age-related) or extrinsic (e.g., overuse, fracture, etc.) factors. Physical examination should include bilateral evaluation of the joint. The patient complains of aching pain that is typically insidious in nature (unless related to an acute injury) and worsens with use. The patient will complain of tenderness to palpation and difficulty sleeping on the affected side and will exhibit decreased ROM and decreased strength. A thorough physical examination and imaging studies, including x-ray, MRI scan and musculoskeletal ultrasound, aid in confirming diagnosis and extent of injury (AAOS, 2019b; Simons, Dixon, & Kruse, 2019). Arthrography with MRI or computed tomography (CT) scan may be more sensitive for certain tears but is usually reserved for cases when a labral injury is suspected (Simons et al., 2019).

Treatment options depend upon several factors, including the duration of symptoms, hand dominance, the type of tear, and patient characteristics such as age, general health, and activity level. Initial conservative management consists primarily of physical therapy, injury surveillance, NSAIDs, rest with modification of activities, and corticosteroid injections into the shoulder joint (Simons et al., 2019). If conservative methods fail, surgical management is warranted. Multiple surgical approaches (e.g., open, mini-open, and arthroscopic) can be employed. Selection of surgical modality is based upon the factors discussed above and the surgeon's preference as there is limited evidence whether surgery provides clinically important benefits (Karjalainen, Jain, Heikkinen, et al., 2019). Postoperatively, the shoulder is immobilized with a **sling**, a supportive arm bandage, for 4 to 6 weeks; length of time of immobilization depends on the severity of injury. Physical therapy with shoulder exercises is begun as prescribed, and the patient is educated on how to perform the exercises at home. The course of rehabilitation is lengthy (e.g., 3 to 6 months); functionality post rehabilitation depends on the patient's commitment to the rehabilitation regimen (AAOS, 2019b).

Lateral and Medial Epicondylitis

Epicondylitis is a chronic, painful condition that is caused by excessive, repetitive extension, flexion, pronation, and

Chart 37-1 — ETHICAL DILEMMA
Does Informed Consent Always Uphold Autonomy?

Case Scenario

D.N. is a 27-year-old man brought by ambulance to the emergency department (ED) where you work as a staff nurse. You are his admitting nurse. Paramedics bring him to the trauma bay by stretcher; he is sitting upright, alert and fully oriented, breathing room air, and gripping his right elbow in flexion with his left hand, holding his right arm slightly away from his torso. The right arm has had a sling applied. As you approach him, you can hear him groaning and see that his forehead is diaphoretic. You see an obvious deformity at his right shoulder, which is slumped, and observe a bulge below his right clavicle, which is likely his dislocated right humeral head. The ED physician meets you and D.N. in the trauma bay and tells D.N. that he could send him to x-ray to confirm that his right shoulder is dislocated and to ensure he does not have any associated fractures; however, that will delay his treatment and fractures are very uncommon occurrences when shoulders dislocate in young men. The ED physician asks D.N. if he can attempt to correct his dislocation manually first, and that if that does not work, he will send him to x-ray. D.N. agrees that the ED physician may correct his dislocation; the physician begins to quickly note the risks associated with this manual procedure and procures an informed consent for D.N. to sign. D.N. blurts out "Oh for heaven's sakes just fix my shoulder!" as he scribbles a jumbled signature on the form with his nondominant left hand. The ED physician quickly and efficiently reduces the dislocated shoulder, and D.N. immediately sighs with relief and says "Oh thank you, doctor! You are a miracle worker!" After you send D.N. to radiology for a follow-up x-ray, the physician turns to you and says "What a crock about these consents. Was that patient really going to not consent to have me try to fix his shoulder? It is just useless paperwork that takes additional time, and that poor guy had to needlessly suffer those extra minutes while we got that paperwork signed!"

Discussion

Obtaining informed consent from a patient prior to any procedure that incurs any risk is a legal requirement. The informed consent must clearly identify what is going to be done and what adverse consequences may ensue from the procedure. The informed consent must meet a *professional standard* so that it includes information that most other health care professionals would disclose during the informed consent process. Furthermore, the informed consent must also meet the *reasonable patient standard,* meaning that information is shared that the patient needs to know in order to make a decision whether or not to have the procedure performed. The informed consent process is considered central to ensuring patient autonomy.

However, some bioethicists have asserted that patients who have had a traumatic injury many times do not remember information shared during the informed consent process. They counter that because of pain, fear, and anxiety, patients with trauma are not focused on the actual risks associated with treatments. Therefore, these bioethicists note that the informed consent process with patients with trauma is actually a sham process and fundamentally does little to preserve patient self-determination.

Analysis

- Describe the ethical principles that are in conflict in this case (see Chapter 1, Chart 1-7). In most instances, the principle of autonomy is considered preeminent. In this case, are the principles of beneficence or nonmaleficence of more importance?
- Think about what the ED physician said about the informed consent process for D.N. Were there any benefits to D.N. by upholding the informed consent process? What risks could D.N. have incurred if there had not been an informed consent process?
- What if D.N. does indeed have a fracture associated with his dislocated shoulder? What risks are there to the ED physician or to you had you not ensured an informed consent occurs?
- What resources might be mobilized to be of assistance to you, the ED physician, and to D.N. so that D.N.'s autonomy is upheld and he can be assured the best treatment options?

References

Bivens, M. (2020). The dishonesty of informed consent rituals. *The New England Journal of Medicine, 382*(12),1089–1091.

Lin, Y.-K., Liu, K.-T., Chen, C.-W., et al. (2019). How to effectively obtain informed consent in trauma patients: A systematic review. *BMC Medical Ethics, 20*(8), 1–15.

Resources

See Chapter 1, Chart 1-10, for Steps of an Ethical Analysis and Ethics Resources.

---

supination motions of the forearm. These motions result in inflammation (tendonitis) and minor tears in the tendons at the origin of the muscles on the lateral or medial epicondyles. Lateral epicondylitis (e.g., tennis elbow) is frequently identified in someone who repeatedly extends the wrist with supination of the forearm. Patients complain of pain and tenderness over the lateral epicondyle and in the proximal wrist extensor muscles (Cutts, Gangoo, Modi, et al., 2020). Medial epicondylitis (e.g., golfer's elbow) is consistent with repetitive wrist flexion and pronation of the forearm. Extreme tenderness occurs at the medial epicondyle and in the proximal wrist flexor muscles (Neeru, 2020). Lateral epicondylitis is seven times more common than its medial counterpart (Cutts et al., 2020).

To date, there is no universally accepted regimen of treatment (Cutts et al., 2020); however, some general principles can be considered. Rest and cessation of aggravating actions is the first-line treatment. Intermittent application of ice and administration of NSAIDs usually relieve the pain and inflammation. In some instances, the arm is immobilized in a molded splint for support and pain relief. Local injection of corticosteroids may be used for symptom management, but because of its degenerative effects on tendons, this treatment is traditionally reserved for patients with severe pain who do not respond to first-line treatment methods (Lenoir, Mares, & Carlier, 2019). Physical therapy and rehabilitation exercises are also considered first-line, nonsurgical treatments (Lai, Erickson, Mlynarek, et al., 2018). Multiple electrophysical modalities, such as transcutaneous electrical nerve stimulation (TENS), ultrasound, extracorporeal shock wave therapy (ESWT), and laser therapy, may provide limited benefit; however, more research is needed to validate their efficacy (Cutts et al., 2020). Surgical interventions are typically a last resort and can be considered in patients who have no response to nonoperative management, want faster symptom management, or have severe pain (Lenoir et al., 2019).

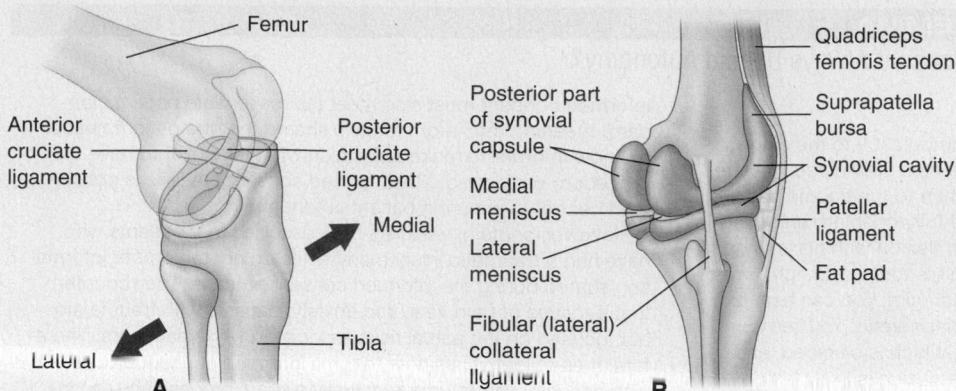

Figure 37-1 • Knee ligaments, tendons, and menisci. **A.** Anterolateral view. **B.** Posterolateral view.

Lateral and Medial Collateral Ligament Injury

Lateral and medial collateral ligaments (MCLs) of the knee (see Fig. 37-1) provide stability to the knee. Injury to these ligaments occurs when the foot is firmly planted and the knee is struck—either medially, causing stretching and tearing injury to the lateral collateral ligament (LCL), or laterally, causing stretching and tearing injury to the MCL. The patient experiences an acute onset of pain, joint tenderness, joint instability, and inability to walk without assistance.

Medical Management

Early management includes the RICE method, use of analgesics, and protection of the joint from further injury (Dexter, 2019). The joint is evaluated for fracture. Hemarthrosis (bleeding into the joint) may develop, contributing to the pain; should this occur, the joint fluid may be aspirated to relieve pressure.

Treatment depends on the severity of the injury. Conservative management includes weight bearing as tolerated and the use of a hinged-brace for support. Crutches may be indicated to assist ambulation until weight bearing can be tolerated. Exercises to strengthen the supportive muscles to the knee without straining the ligaments are beneficial. Severe MCL injuries are initially treated with non–weight-bearing status with progression to weight bearing as tolerated in a hinged-brace for a lengthy timeframe; the healing process may take 8 to 12 weeks. Severe LCL injuries with knee instability usually require surgical intervention, followed by bracing and physical therapy (Agranoff, 2019). A progressive rehabilitation program helps restore the function and strength of the knee. Rehabilitation occurs over many months, and the patient may need to wear a derotational brace while engaging in sports to prevent recurrence of injury.

Nursing Management

The nurse educates the patient about proper use of ambulatory devices, the healing process, and activity limitation to promote healing. Education addresses pain management, the use of analgesic agents, the use of a brace, wound care, cold therapy, signs and symptoms of possible complications (e.g., altered neurovascular status, infection, skin breakdown, venous thromboembolism [VTE]), and self-care (Dexter, 2019).

Cruciate Ligament Injury

The anterior cruciate ligament (ACL) and the posterior cruciate ligament (PCL) of the knee stabilize anterior and posterior motion of the tibia articulating with the femur (see Fig. 37-1A). These ligaments cross each other in the center of the knee. Injury occurs when the foot is firmly planted and the leg sustains direct force, either forward or backward. If the force is forward, the ACL suffers the impact from the force, whereas backward force places force on the PCL. The injured person may report feeling and hearing a "pop" in the knee with this injury. If the patient exhibits significant swelling of the joint within 2 hours after the injury, the ACL or PCL may be torn. A torn cruciate ligament produces pain, joint instability, and pain with weight bearing. Immediate postinjury management includes the RICE protocol, use of NSAIDs, and stabilization of the joint until it is evaluated for a fracture (Graham, 2019). Severe joint effusion and hemarthrosis may require joint aspiration and wrapping with an elastic compression dressing. Crutches may be needed to avoid weight bearing, especially if the knee is unstable (Friedberg, 2019).

Treatment depends on the severity of the injury, patient characteristics, and the effect of the injury on daily activities. Ligament injuries can be managed operatively or nonoperatively; most active, younger patients and high performing athletes opt for surgery due to the risk for reinjury and osteoarthritis (Friedberg, 2019). Older and less active patients, whose physical activity is community ambulation, tend to benefit from nonsurgical therapy (Graham, 2019). Surgical ACL or PCL reconstruction may be scheduled after near-normal joint ROM is achieved and includes tendon repair using a graft (e.g., autograft, allograft, or synthetic ligament; see later discussions). This is typically performed as ambulatory arthroscopic surgery, a procedure in which the surgeon uses an **arthroscope** to visualize and repair the damage. After surgery, the patient is instructed to control pain with oral analgesic medications and cryotherapy (e.g., a cooling pad incorporated in a dressing). The patient and family are educated about monitoring the neurovascular status of the leg, wound care, and signs of complications (e.g., infection, VTE) that need to be reported promptly to the surgeon (Cox, 2017). Exercises (ankle pumps, quadriceps sets, and hamstring sets) are encouraged during the early postoperative period. The patient must protect the graft by adhering to exercise restrictions. The physical therapist supervises progressive ROM and weight bearing (as permitted).

Meniscal Injuries

Within the knee are two semilunar (crescent-shaped) pads of fibrocartilages, called *menisci,* located on the right and left side of the proximal tibia, between the tibia and the femur (see Fig. 37-1B). These structures act as shock absorbers in the knee. Normally, little twisting movement is permitted in the knee joint. Forceful twisting of the knee or repetitive squatting and impact may result in either tearing or detachment of the cartilage from its attachment to the head of the tibia. The peripheral third of the menisci have a small amount of blood flow, which allows that portion to heal if torn.

These injuries leave loose cartilage in the knee joint that may slip between the femur and the tibia, preventing full extension of the leg. If this happens during walking or running, the patient often describes the leg as "giving way." The patient may hear or feel a click in the knee when walking, especially when extending the leg that is bearing weight. When the cartilage is attached to the front and back of the knee but torn loose laterally (bucket-handle tear), it may slide between the bones to lie between the condyles and prevent full flexion or extension. As a result, the knee "locks."

When a meniscus is torn, the synovial membrane secretes additional synovial fluid due to the irritation, and the knee becomes very edematous. Initial conservative management includes rest and immobilization of the knee, ice to the knee for 15 minutes every 4 to 6 hours, the use of crutches for support, anti-inflammatory agents, analgesic agents, and modification of activities to avoid those that cause the symptoms. Home exercises and physical therapy may be prescribed to increase strength in supporting muscles (e.g., quadriceps, hamstrings). Diagnosis is confirmed through MRI or arthroscopy; the approach to treatment depends on the patient's age, type of tear, associated mechanical symptoms (e.g., knee is locked, or motion is severely impaired) and the presence of persistent knee effusions (Cardone & Jacobs, 2019). Surgical options include a partial or total meniscectomy to repair the meniscal tissue. Open or arthroscopic surgery can be performed (Baker, Wolf, & Lubowitz, 2018). The most common complication is an effusion into the knee joint, which produces pain. To ensure independent home performance, the patient is instructed to continue quadriceps strengthening and progressive ROM exercises; neuromuscular electrical stimulation/biofeedback is also recommended (Logerstedt, Snyder-Mackler, Ritter, et al., 2018). There is a lack of consensus regarding the optimal postoperative time to return to activity; therefore, prescribed weight-bearing status can range from non–weight bearing for 4 to 6 weeks to full weight bearing in a "locked" (extension) knee brace (Spang, Nasr, Mohamadi, et al., 2018).

Rupture of the Achilles Tendon

The Achilles tendon is a tough band of fibrous tissue that attaches the soleus and gastrocnemius (e.g., calf) muscles to the calcaneus (e.g., heel bone). Injury to the Achilles tendon is often multifactorial; despite being the strongest and thickest tendon in the body, it is vulnerable to injury due to its limited blood supply and the high tensions placed upon it (Egger & Berkowitz, 2017). Rupture of the Achilles tendon most commonly occurs in active young to middle-aged adults with a predilection among males. The traumatic rupture of the Achilles tendon occurs with the "pushing off" or unexpected dorsiflexion of the foot and ankle (Karlsson Westin, Carmont, et al., 2019). Patients usually describe a "popping" sound or a "giving way" sensation in their posterior heel. Immediate pain is usually experienced but gradually subsides, leaving a patient with difficulty performing plantar flexion, and the inability to fully bear weight on the affected leg (Egger & Berkowitz, 2017).

Clinical examination is paramount in diagnosis; the ability to plantar flex is decreased and to dorsiflex is improved. MRI or ultrasound is indicated to determine the extent of the injury. The decision of surgical or nonsurgical treatment for Achilles tendon rupture is much debated and depends on the patient's comorbidities, goals, and preferences (Karlsson et al., 2019). Nonoperative modalities include cast immobilization for 2 to 8 weeks; there is some controversy regarding optimal time. After immobilization with the cast, a boot and functional brace with a heel lift is worn with increasing weight-bearing status. Progressive physical therapy to promote ankle ROM and strength is implemented as well. Operative treatment has typically been reserved for young, healthy athletes, because surgery was associated with fewer cases of re-rupture. After surgery, a cast may be initially used to immobilize the ankle joint; however, early functional rehabilitation has been shown to be superior to cast immobilization in terms of patient satisfaction and the time to return to prior employment and sporting activity (Zhao, Meng, Liu, et al., 2017). The total rehabilitation is approximately 6 weeks (Karlsson et al., 2019).

Fractures

A **fracture** is a complete or incomplete disruption in the continuity of bone structure and is defined according to its type and extent. Fractures occur when the bone is subjected to stress greater than it can absorb (Buckley & Page, 2018). Fractures may be caused by direct blows, crushing forces, sudden twisting motions, and extreme muscle contractions. When the bone is broken, adjacent structures are also affected, which may result in soft tissue edema, hemorrhage into the muscles and joints, joint dislocations, ruptured tendons, severed nerves, and damaged blood vessels. Body organs may be injured by the force that caused the fracture or by fracture fragments.

Types of Fractures

Fractures types are identified by the name of the injured bone and location (e.g., proximal, midshaft, distal) (Beutler & Titus, 2019). Fractures are also described according to the degree of break (e.g., a *greenstick fracture* refers to a partial break) or the character of any fractured bone fragments (e.g., a *comminuted fracture* has more than two fragments). Select specific types of fractures are displayed in Figure 37-2.

A *closed fracture* (simple fracture) is one that does not cause a break in the skin. An *open fracture* (compound, or complex, fracture) is one in which the skin or mucous membrane wound extends to the fractured bone. Open fractures are often classified using a modified system by Gustilo-Anderson which classifies the severity into three categories based on the extent

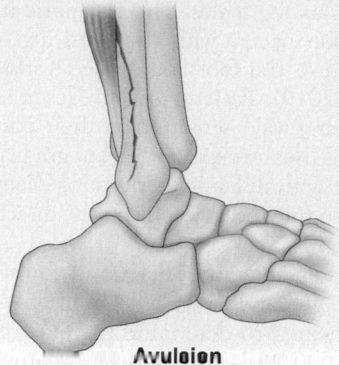

Avulsion
A fracture in which a fragment of bone has been pulled away by a tendon and its attachment

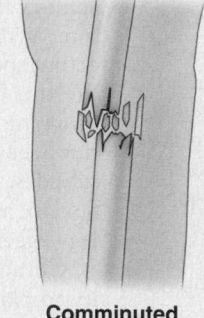

Comminuted
A fracture in which bone has splintered into several fragments

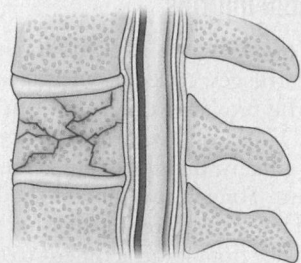

Compression
A fracture in which bone has been compressed (seen in vertebral fractures)

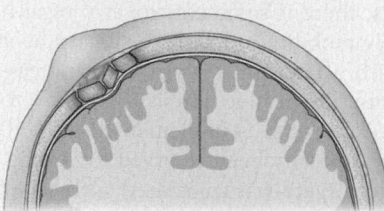

Depressed
A fracture in which fragments are driven inward (seen frequently in fractures of skull and facial bones)

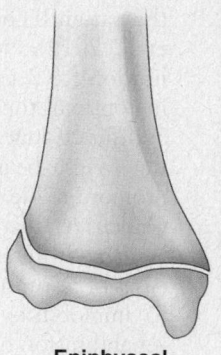

Epiphyseal
A fracture through the epiphysis

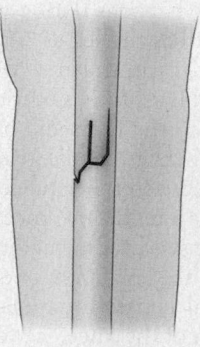

Greenstick
A fracture in which one side of a bone is broken and the other side is bent

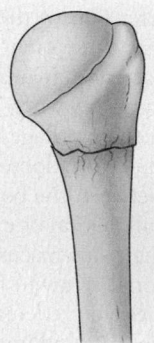

Impacted
A fracture in which a bone fragment is driven into another bone fragment

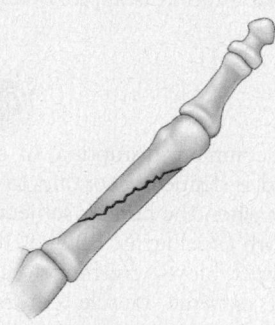

Oblique
A fracture occurring at an angle across the bone (less stable than a transverse fracture)

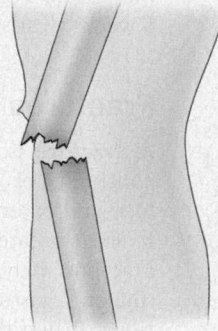

Open
A fracture in which damage also involves the skin or mucous membranes, also called a compound fracture

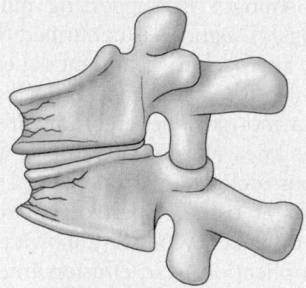

Pathologic
A fracture that occurs through an area of diseased bone (e.g., osteoporosis, bone cyst, Paget disease, bony metastasis, tumor); can occur without trauma or fall

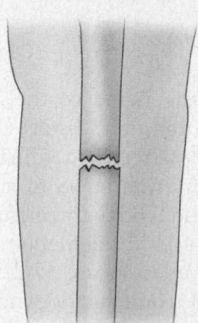

Simple
A fracture that remains contained, with no disruption of the skin integrity

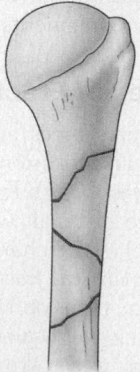

Spiral
A fracture that twists around the shaft of the bone

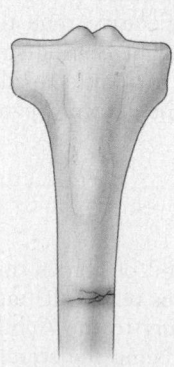

Stress
A fracture that results from repeated loading of bone and muscle

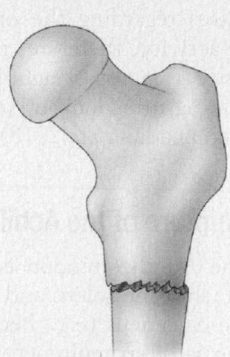

Transverse
A fracture that is straight across the bone shaft

Figure 37-2 • Specific types of fractures.

of soft-tissue injury and the size of the corresponding skin wounds (Elniel & Giannoudis, 2018):

- Type I is a clean wound less than 1 cm long and simple fracture pattern.
- Type II is a larger wound with minimal soft tissue damage and no flaps or avulsions.
- Type III (A, B, and C subtypes) is considered the most severe, highly contaminated, and has extensive soft tissue damage; it involves vascular injury or traumatic amputation.

An *intra-articular fracture* extends into the joint surface of a bone. Because each end of a long bone is cartilaginous, if the fracture is nondisplaced, x-rays will not always reveal the fracture because cartilage is nonradiopaque. MRI or arthroscopy will identify the fracture and confirm the diagnosis. The joint is stabilized and immobilized with a splint or cast, and no weight bearing is allowed until the fracture has healed. Because of the damage to articular cartilage, intra-articular fractures often lead to early posttraumatic osteoarthritis (Mittal & Mittal, 2019).

Clinical Manifestations

The clinical signs and symptoms of a fracture vary according to which bone is affected, the patient's health and age, and the severity of the injury (Whittle, 2017a). However, they often include acute pain, loss of function, deformity, shortening of the extremity, crepitus, localized edema and ecchymosis, muscle spasm, and tenderness (Iyer, 2019).

Pain

The pain is continuous and increases in severity until the bone fragments are immobilized. Immediately after a fracture, the injured area becomes numb and the surrounding muscles flaccid. The muscle spasms that accompany a fracture begin shortly thereafter, within a few to 30 minutes, and result in more intense pain than the patient reports at the time of injury. The muscle spasms can minimize further movement of the fracture fragments or can result in further bony fragmentation or malalignment (Norris, 2020).

Loss of Function

After a fracture, the extremity cannot function properly because normal function of the muscles depends on the integrity of the bones to which they are attached. Pain contributes to the loss of function. In addition, abnormal movement (false motion) may be present.

Deformity

Displacement, angulation, or rotation of the fragments in a fracture of the arm or leg causes a deformity that is detectable when the limb is compared with the uninjured extremity.

Shortening

In fractures of long bones, there is actual shortening of the extremity because of the compression of the fractured bone. Sometimes, muscle spasms can cause the distal and proximal site of the fracture to overlap, causing the extremity to shorten (Norris, 2020).

Crepitus

When the extremity is gently palpated, a crumbling sensation, called **crepitus,** can be felt or may be heard. It is caused by the rubbing of the bone fragments against each other.

Localized Edema and Ecchymosis

After a fracture, localized edema and ecchymosis occur as a result of trauma and bleeding into the tissues. These signs may not develop for several hours after the injury or may develop within an hour, depending on the severity of the fracture.

Emergency Management

Immediately after injury, if a fracture is suspected, the body part must be immobilized before the patient is moved. Adequate splinting is essential. Joints proximal and distal to the fracture also must be immobilized to prevent movement of fracture fragments. Immobilization of the long bones of the lower extremities may be accomplished by bandaging the legs together, with the unaffected extremity serving as a splint for the injured one. In an upper extremity injury, the arm may be bandaged to the chest, or an injured forearm may be placed in a sling. The neurovascular status distal to the injury should be assessed both before and after splinting to determine the adequacy of peripheral tissue perfusion and nerve function (Derby & Beutler, 2018).

With an open fracture, the wound is covered with a sterile dressing to achieve homeostasis as rapidly as possible at the injury site and to prevent contamination of deeper tissues (Buckley & Page, 2018). No attempt is made to reduce the fracture, even if one of the bone fragments is protruding through the wound. Splints are applied for immobilization.

In the ED, the patient is evaluated completely. The clothes are gently removed, first from the uninjured side of the body and then from the injured side. The patient's clothing may be cut away. The fractured extremity is moved as little as possible to avoid more damage.

Medical Management

Reduction

Fracture reduction refers to restoration of bone fragments to anatomic realignment and positioning with immobilization (Iyer, 2019). Either closed reduction or open reduction may be used to reduce a fracture. The specific method selected depends on the nature of the fracture; however, the underlying principles are the same. Usually, the primary provider reduces a fracture as soon as possible to prevent loss of elasticity from the tissues through infiltration by edema or hemorrhage. In most cases, fracture reduction becomes more difficult as the injury begins to heal (Buckley & Page, 2018).

Before fracture reduction and immobilization, the patient is prepared for the procedure; consent for the procedure is obtained, and an analgesic agent is given as prescribed. Regional anesthesia can also be very useful for pain control with fractures and dislocation reduction (Eiff, Hatch, & Higgins, 2020a). The injured extremity must be handled gently to avoid additional damage.

Closed Reduction

In most instances, closed reduction is accomplished by bringing the bone fragments into anatomic alignment through manipulation and manual traction. The extremity is held in the aligned position while a cast, splint, or other device is applied (see later discussion). Reduction under anesthesia with percutaneous pinning may also be used. The immobilizing device maintains the reduction and stabilizes the extremity for bone healing. X-rays are obtained after reduction to verify that the bone fragments are correctly aligned (Buckley & Page, 2018).

Traction (skin or skeletal) may be used until the patient is physiologically stable to undergo surgical fixation (see later discussion).

Open Reduction

Some fractures require open reduction. Through a surgical approach, the bone fragments are anatomically aligned. Internal fixation devices (e.g., metallic pins, wires, screws, plates, nails, or rods) may be used to hold the bone fragments in position until solid bone healing occurs (Iyer, 2019). These devices may be attached to the sides of bone, or they may be inserted through the bony fragments or directly into the medullary cavity of the bone (see Fig. 37-3). Internal fixation devices ensure firm approximation and fixation of the bony fragments (Buckley & Page, 2018). Open reduction internal fixation (ORIF) is a common orthopedic surgical procedure used to treat severe fractures.

Immobilization

After the fracture has been reduced, the bone fragments must be immobilized and maintained in proper position and alignment until union occurs. Immobilization may be accomplished by external or internal fixation. Methods of external fixation include bandages, casts, splints, continuous traction, and external fixators.

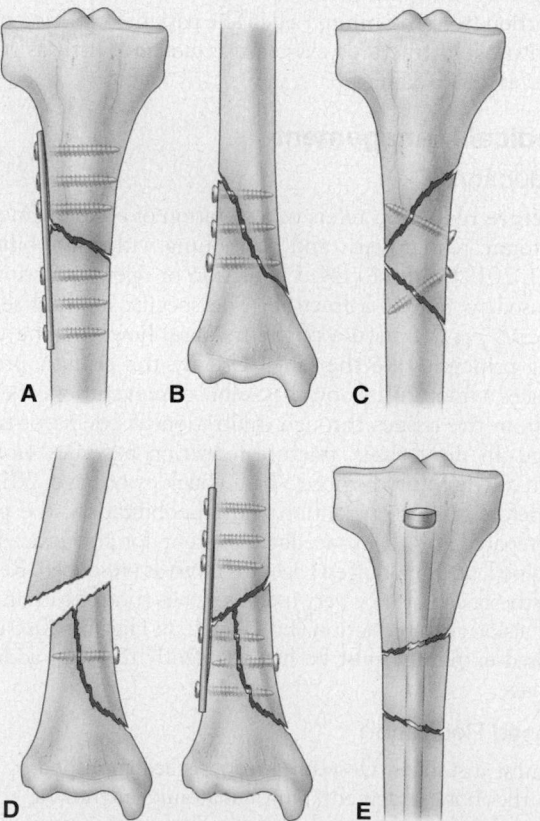

Figure 37-3 • Techniques of internal fixation. **A.** Plate and six screws for a transverse or short oblique fracture. **B.** Screws for a long oblique or spiral fracture. **C.** Screws for a long butterfly fragment. **D.** Plate and six screws for a short butterfly fragment. **E.** Medullary nail for a segmental fracture.

Maintaining and Restoring Function

Reduction and immobilization are maintained as prescribed to promote bone and soft tissue healing. Edema is controlled by elevating the injured extremity and applying ice as prescribed. Neurovascular status is monitored routinely, and the primary provider is notified immediately if signs of neurovascular compromise develop. Restlessness, anxiety, and discomfort are controlled with a variety of approaches, such as reassurance, position changes, and pain-relief strategies, including the use of analgesic medications. Isometric and muscle setting exercises are encouraged to minimize atrophy and to promote circulation. Participation in activities of daily living (ADLs) is encouraged to promote independent functioning and self-esteem. Gradual resumption of activities is promoted as prescribed. With internal fixation, the surgeon determines the amount of movement and weight-bearing stress the extremity can sustain and prescribes the level of activity (Buckley & Page, 2018). See later discussion for more information about caring for patients who have casts, are in traction, or are undergoing surgery for fractures.

Nursing Management

Patients with Closed Fractures

The patient with a closed fracture has no opening in the skin at the fracture site. The fractured bones may be nondisplaced or slightly displaced, but the skin is intact. The nurse educates the patient regarding the proper methods to control edema and pain (see Chart 37-2). It is important to educate about exercises to maintain the health of unaffected muscles and to increase the strength of muscles needed for transferring and for using assistive devices such as crutches, walkers, and special utensils. The patient is also educated to use assistive devices safely. Plans are made to help patients modify the home environment as needed and to ensure safety, such as removing floor rugs or anything that obstructs walking paths throughout the house. Patient education includes self-care, medication information, monitoring for potential complications, and the need for continuing health care supervision. Fracture healing and restoration of strength and mobility may take an average of 6 to 8 weeks, depending on the quality of the patient's bone tissue (Iyer, 2019).

Patients with Open Fractures

In an open fracture, there is a risk for **osteomyelitis** (i.e., infection of the bone), tetanus, and gas gangrene (see Chapter 36 for discussion of osteomyelitis). The objectives of management are to prevent infection of the wound, soft tissue, and bone, and to promote healing of bone and soft tissue. Intravenous (IV) antibiotics are given upon the patient's arrival in the hospital along with intramuscular (IM) tetanus toxoid as indicated (Howe, 2018).

Wound irrigation using a sterile isotonic saline solution and **débridement** (removal of tissues and foreign material) are initiated in the operating room as soon as possible. The wound is cultured, and bone grafting may be performed to fill in areas of bone defects. The fracture is carefully reduced and stabilized by external fixation (see later discussion), and the wound is usually left open. If there is any damage to blood vessels, soft tissue, muscles, nerves, or tendons, appropriate treatment is implemented.

Chart 37-2	**HOME CARE CHECKLIST**
	The Patient with a Closed Fracture

At the completion of education, the patient and/or caregiver will be able to:

- Name the procedure that was performed and identify any changes in anatomic structure or function as well as changes in ADLs, IADLs, roles, relationships, and spirituality.
- Identify modification of home environment, interventions, and strategies (e.g., durable medical equipment, adaptive equipment) used in safely promoting effective recovery and rehabilitation.
- Describe ongoing therapeutic regimen, including diet and activities to perform (e.g., exercises) and to limit or avoid (e.g., lifting weights, driving a car, contact sports).
  - Describe approaches to control swelling (e.g., elevate extremity to heart level).
  - Consume a healthy diet to promote bone healing.
  - Observe prescribed weight-bearing and activity limits.
  - Participate in prescribed exercise regimen to maintain the health of unaffected muscles and those muscles now needed for safe transfer, mobility, etc.
  - If indicated, demonstrate safe use of mobility aid, assistive device, immobilizing device and transfer technique.
- State the name, dose, side effects, frequency, and schedule for all prescribed therapeutic and prophylactic medications (e.g., antibiotics, analgesic agents).
- Control pain with pharmacologic and nonpharmacologic interventions.

- Report pain uncontrolled by elevation and analgesics (may be an indicator of impaired tissue perfusion or compartment syndrome).
- State indicators of complications to report promptly to primary provider (e.g., uncontrolled swelling and pain; cool, pale fingers or toes; paresthesia; paralysis; signs of local and systemic infection; signs of venous thromboembolism; problems with immobilization device).
- State possible complications of fractures (e.g., delayed union; nonunion; avascular necrosis; complex regional pain syndrome, formerly called *reflex sympathetic dystrophy syndrome;* heterotopic ossification).
- Describe gradual resumption of normal activities when medically cleared and discuss how to protect fracture site from undue stresses.
- Relate how to reach primary provider with questions or complications.
- State time and date of follow-up appointments, therapy, and testing.
- Identify the need for health promotion, disease prevention, and screening activities.

Resources

See Chapter 2, Chart 2-6, for additional information related to durable medical equipment, adaptive equipment, and mobility skills.

ADLs, activities of daily living; IADLs, instrumental activities of daily living.

With open fractures, primary wound closure is usually delayed, particularly with higher-grade fractures. Heavily contaminated wounds are left unsutured and treated with vacuum-assisted closures (VACs) to facilitate wound drainage. Wound irrigation and débridement may be repeated, removing infected and devitalized tissue and increasing vascularity in the region (Dunbar & Cannada, 2017).

The extremity is elevated to minimize edema. Neurovascular status must be assessed frequently. Temperature is monitored at regular intervals, and the patient is monitored for signs of infection. Bone grafting may be necessary to bridge bone defects and to stimulate bone healing (Dunbar & Cannada, 2017).

Unfolding Patient Stories: Marilyn Hughes • Part 1

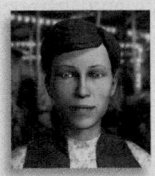

Marilyn Hughes, a 45-year-old female, was brought to the emergency department by her husband after a fall down icy stairs. She is complaining of severe left lower leg pain. She is wearing long pants and boots. What are priority assessments and interventions that the nurse should implement for a suspected lower leg fracture? (Marilyn Hughes' story continues in Chapter 60.)

Care for Marilyn and other patients in a realistic virtual environment: *vSim for Nursing* (**thepoint.lww.com/vSimMedicalSurgical**). Practice documenting these patients' care in DocuCare (**thepoint.lww.com/DocuCareEHR**).

Fracture Healing and Complications

Weeks to months are required for most fractures to heal. Many factors influence the timeframe of the healing process (see Chart 37-3). With a comminuted fracture, bone fragments must be properly aligned to attain the best healing possible. It is essential for the fractured bone to have blood supply to the area to facilitate the healing process. In general, fractures of flat bones (pelvis, sternum, and scapula) heal rapidly. A complex, comminuted fracture may heal slowly. Fractures at the ends of long bones, where the bone is more vascular and cancellous, heal more quickly than do fractures in areas where the bone is dense and less vascular (midshaft). Fractures typically heal more quickly in younger patients (Howe, 2018).

If fracture healing is disrupted, bone union may be delayed or stopped completely. Factors that can impair fracture healing include inadequate fracture immobilization, inadequate blood supply to the fracture site or adjacent tissue, multiple trauma, extensive bone loss, infection, poor adherence to prescribed restrictions (e.g., cigarette smoking and excessive alcohol use), malignancy, certain medications (e.g., corticosteroids), older age, and some disease processes (e.g., rheumatoid arthritis) (Howe, 2018).

Complications of fractures may be either acute or delayed. Early complications include shock, fat embolism, acute compartment syndrome, VTE (deep vein thrombosis [DVT], pulmonary embolism [PE]), disseminated intravascular coagulation (DIC) and infection (Iyer, 2019). Late complications include delayed union, malunion, nonunion, AVN of bone, complex regional pain syndrome (CRPS), and heterotopic ossification.

> **Chart
> 37-3** Factors That Inhibit Fracture Healing
>
> - Age >40 years
> - Avascular necrosis
> - Bone loss
> - Cigarette smoking
> - Comorbidities (e.g., diabetes, rheumatoid arthritis)
> - Corticosteroids, nonsteroidal anti-inflammatory drugs
> - Extensive local trauma
> - Inadequate immobilization
> - Infection
> - Local malignancy
> - Malalignment of the fracture fragments
> - Space or tissue between bone fragments
> - Weight bearing prior to approval
>
> Adapted from Buckley, R., & Page, J. L. (2018). General principles
> of fracture care. *Medscape.* Retrieved on 1/7/2020 at: emedicine.
> medscape.com/article/1270717-overview#a6; Norris, T. L. (2020).
> *Porth's essentials of pathophysiology* (5th ed.). Philadelphia, PA:
> Wolters Kluwer.

Early Complications

Shock

Hypovolemic or traumatic shock resulting from hemorrhage is more frequently noted in trauma patients with pelvic fractures and in patients with a displaced or open femoral fracture in which the femoral artery is torn by bone fragments. Treatment for shock consists of stabilizing the fracture to prevent further hemorrhage, restoring blood volume and circulation, relieving the patient's pain, providing proper immobilization, and protecting the patient from further injury and other complications (Iyer, 2019). See Chapter 11 for a discussion of shock.

Fat Embolism Syndrome

Fat embolism syndrome (FES) describes the clinical manifestations that occur when fat emboli enter circulation following orthopedic trauma, especially long bone (e.g., femur) and pelvic fractures. FES is more frequent in closed fractures than in open fractures (Weinhouse, 2019). At the time of fracture, fat globules may diffuse from the marrow into the vascular compartment. The fat globules (e.g., emboli) may occlude the small blood vessels that supply the lungs, brain, kidneys, and other organs. The onset of symptoms is rapid, typically within 24 to 72 hours of injury, but may occur up to a week after injury (Iyer, 2019). FES occurs more frequently in males than in females, with its highest incidence in those between the ages of 10 and 40 years.

Clinical Manifestations

The classic triad of clinical manifestations of FES includes hypoxemia, neurologic compromise, and a petechial rash (Weinhouse, 2019). The typical first manifestations are pulmonary and include hypoxia, tachypnea, and dyspnea accompanied by tachycardia, substernal chest pain, low-grade fever, crackles, and additional manifestations of respiratory failure. Chest x-ray may show evidence of acute respiratory distress syndrome (ARDS) or it may be normal. Petechial rash may develop 2 to 3 days after the onset of symptoms. This rash is secondary to dysfunction in the microcirculation and/or thrombocytopenia and is typically located in nondependent regions (e.g., chest, mucous membranes) of the body. There may be varying degrees of neurologic deficits that can include restlessness, agitation, seizures, focal deficits, and encephalopathy (Fukumoto & Fukumoto, 2018). There are no universal criteria for diagnosis of FES; diagnosis relies on clinical suspicion based upon the classic triad of symptoms and imaging findings (Uranslip, Muengtaweepongsa, Chanalithichai, et al., 2018).

 Quality and Safety Nursing Alert

Subtle personality changes, restlessness, irritability, or confusion in a patient who has sustained a fracture are indications for immediate arterial blood gas studies.

Prevention and Management

Prevention is the most important aspect of treatment; immediate immobilization of fractures, including early surgical fixation, minimal fracture manipulation, and adequate support for fractured bones during turning and positioning, and maintenance of fluid and electrolyte balance are measures that may reduce the incidence of fat emboli. There is no specific treatment for FES; the treatment is supportive. Fluid resuscitation, oxygenation, vasopressors, mechanical ventilation, and sometimes corticosteroids are used as supportive therapy (Weinhouse, 2019).

Acute Compartment Syndrome

An anatomic compartment is an area of the body encased by bone or fascia (e.g., the fibrous membrane that covers and separates muscles) that contains muscles, nerves, and blood vessels. The human body has 46 anatomic compartments, and 36 of these are located in the extremities (see Fig. 37-4). Acute compartment syndrome, a time-sensitive surgical emergency, is characterized by the elevation of pressure within an anatomic compartment that is above normal perfusion pressure. Acute compartment syndrome arises from an increase in compartment volume (e.g., from edema or bleeding), a decrease in compartment size (e.g., from a restrictive cast), or aspects of both. When the pressure within an affected compartment rises above normal, perfusion to the tissues is impaired, causing cell death, which may lead to tissue necrosis and permanent dysfunction (Papachristos & Giannoudis, 2018). The most common cause is fractures, with tibial fractures having the highest risk (Long, Koyfman, & Gottlieb, 2019). Acute compartment syndrome is most common among young adults, and although it may take up to 48 hours for symptoms to present, it typically has a rapid progression of symptoms and signs over a few hours after the initial injury or fracture repair (Stracciolini & Hammerberg, 2019).

Assessment and Diagnostic Findings

Frequent assessment of neurovascular function after a fracture is essential and focuses on the "five Ps": *p*ain, *p*allor, *p*ulselessness, *p*aresthesia, and *p*aralysis (Papachristos & Giannoudis, 2018). The patient with acute compartment syndrome typically presents with severe pain that is out of proportion to the injury, which is considered the cardinal symptom (Stracciolini & Hammerberg, 2019). Additionally, patients often describe this pain as deep and burning, and that it is unrelieved by

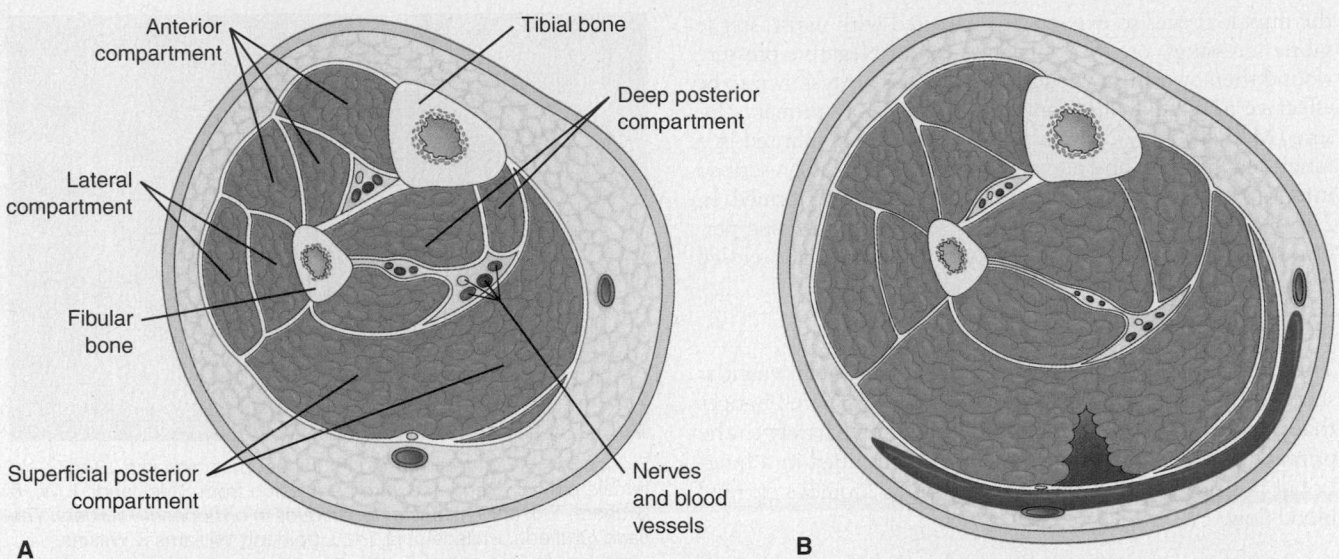

Figure 37-4 • **A.** Cross-section of normal lower leg with muscle compartments. **B.** Cross-section of lower leg with compartment syndrome.

medications. Exacerbation of pain on passive stretching of the muscles within the involved compartment is highly predictive (McMillan, Gardner, Schmidt, et al., 2019). With continued nerve ischemia and edema, the patient experiences diminished sensation followed by complete numbness. Motor weakness may occur as a late sign of nerve ischemia. Motion is evaluated by asking the patient to flex and extend the wrist or plantar flex and dorsiflex the foot. Paralysis (no movement) is a late finding after prolonged ischemia and is associated with neurovascular injury (McMillan et al., 2019).

Peripheral circulation is evaluated by assessing color, temperature, capillary refill time, edema, and pulses. Cyanotic nail beds suggest venous congestion. Pallor or dusky and cold digits, prolonged capillary refill time, and diminished pulses suggest impaired arterial perfusion. Edema may obscure the function of arterial pulsation, and Doppler ultrasonography may be used to verify a pulse. Pulselessness is a late sign (McMillan et al., 2019).

A prompt diagnosis of acute compartment syndrome is based on clinical suspicion and repeated clinical examinations of the "five Ps"; however, it is important to keep in mind that pain is a subjective measure and may only be detected in patients who are conscious (AAOS, 2018). As well, some of the clinical signs and symptoms may only present in the late stages of acute compartment syndrome (Stracciolini & Hammerberg, 2019). Palpation of the muscle, if possible, reveals it to be swollen and hard with the skin taut and shiny. The orthopedic surgeon may measure tissue pressure by inserting a tissue pressure-monitoring device, such as a handheld direct injection device (e.g., Stryker Intra-Compartmental Pressure Monitor), into the muscle compartment (normal pressure is 8 mm Hg or less) (see Fig. 37-5). Nerve and muscle tissues deteriorate as compartment pressure increases. Prolonged pressure of more than 30 mm Hg can result in irreversible changes (Long et al., 2019).

Medical Management

Prompt management of acute compartment syndrome is essential and includes relieving all external pressure on the compartment. The orthopedic surgeon needs to be notified immediately if neurovascular compromise is suspected. Delay in treatment may result in permanent nerve and muscle damage, necrosis, infection, rhabdomyolysis with acute kidney injury, and amputation (Stracciolini & Hammerberg, 2019).

If conservative measures do not restore tissue perfusion and relieve pain, a fasciotomy (surgical decompression with excision of the fascia) is considered the definitive treatment to relieve the constrictive muscle fascia (AAOS, 2018). After fasciotomy, the wound is not sutured but is left open to allow

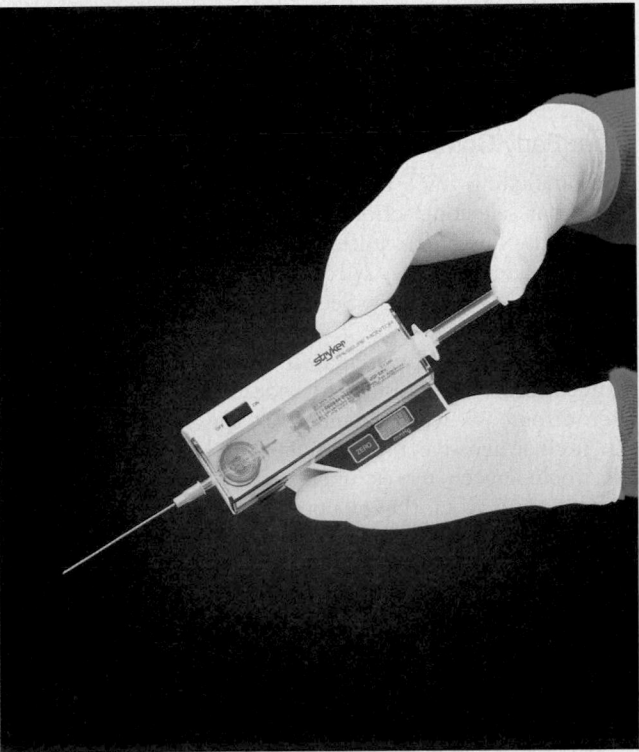

Figure 37-5 • The Stryker Intra-Compartmental Pressure Monitor. Reprinted with permission from Stryker Inc.

the muscle tissues to expand; it is covered with moist, sterile saline dressings or with artificial skin. Negative-pressure wound therapy using a vacuum dressing has been shown to be effective to remove fluids and decrease times to primary closure (Modrall, 2019). The affected arm or leg is splinted in a functional position and elevated to heart level and prescribed intermittent passive ROM exercises are usually performed. In 2 to 3 days, when the swelling has resolved and tissue perfusion has been restored, the wound is débrided and closed (possibly with skin grafts).

Nursing Management

The nurse should frequently assess pain and neurovascular status of the affected limb and report any negative changes that may suggest compartment syndrome immediately to the primary provider. The limb should be maintained in a functional position at the level of the heart to promote optimal blood flow.

> ### Quality and Safety Nursing Alert
>
> *Acute compartment syndrome is managed by maintaining the extremity at heart level (not above heart level) and removing constrictive dressings by opening and bivalving the cast or opening the splint, if one or the other is present.*

Pain management is essential and is accomplished with opioid analgesia, as prescribed. Careful assessment of intake and output and urinalysis could alert the nurse to the development of rhabdomyolysis (see Chapter 48).

Education is necessary for those patients discharged to home-based or community settings with fractures and casts and should include recognition of the unique characteristics of acute compartment syndrome (increasing, refractory pain and neurovascular manifestations) and instructions when to contact the primary provider for emergent follow-up.

Other Early Complications

VTE, including DVT and PE, are associated with reduced skeletal muscle contractions and bed rest. Patients with fractures of the lower extremities and pelvis are at high risk for VTE (Buckley & Page, 2018). PE may cause death several days to weeks after injury. See Chapter 26 for a discussion of VTE, PE, and DVT.

Disseminated intravascular coagulation (DIC) is a systemic disorder that results in widespread hemorrhage and microthrombosis with ischemia. Its causes are diverse and can include massive tissue trauma. Early manifestations of DIC include ecchymoses, unexpected bleeding after surgery and bleeding from the mucous membranes, venipuncture sites, and gastrointestinal and urinary tracts (Iyer, 2019). See Chapter 29 for discussion of treatment for DIC.

All open fractures are considered contaminated and are treated as soon as possible with copious irrigation, débridement, tetanus immunization/prophylaxis, and IV antibiotics (Schaller, 2018). Surgical internal fixation of fractures carries a risk of infection. The nurse must monitor and educate the patient regarding signs and symptoms of infection, including tenderness, pain, redness, swelling, local warmth, elevated temperature, and purulent drainage.

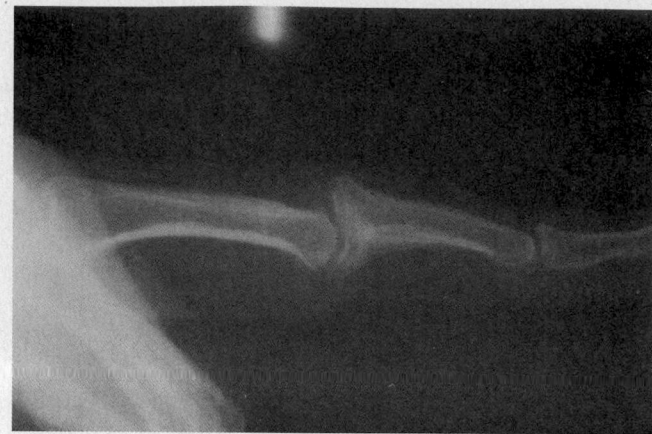

Figure 37-6 • Eight-month-old ring finger malunion in a 19-year-old female patient. Reprinted with permission from Strickland, J. W., & Graham, T. J. (2005). *Master techniques in orthopaedic surgery: The hand* (2nd ed.). Philadelphia, PA: Lippincott Williams & Wilkins.

Delayed Complications

Delayed Union, Nonunion, and Malunion

Delayed union occurs when healing does not occur within the expected timeframe for the location and type of fracture. Delayed union may be associated with distraction (pulling apart) of bone fragments, systemic or local infection, poor nutrition, or comorbidity (e.g., diabetes, autoimmune disease). The healing time is prolonged, but the fracture eventually heals (Nyary & Scammell, 2018). **Nonunion** is an incomplete healing of a fracture and results from failure of the ends of a fractured bone to unite, whereas **malunion** is the healing of a fractured bone in a malaligned (deformed) position (see Fig. 37-6). In both of these instances, the patient complains of persistent discomfort and abnormal movement at the fracture site. Nonunion occurs most commonly in tibial fractures, whereas malunion occurs most commonly in fractures of the hand (or fingers) (Howe, 2018). Factors contributing to delayed union, nonunion, and malunion are those associated with impaired bone healing (see Chart 37-3).

Medical Management

Impaired bone healing can be treated with nonsurgical and surgical interventions. Nonsurgical treatment modalities include low-intensity pulsed ultrasound and externally applied electrical bone growth stimulators (Osman, Gabr, & Haddad, 2019). Electrical stimulation techniques enhance the process of bone healing by exposure of osteoblasts to electromagnetic fields, which stimulate the secretion of growth factors (Bhavsar, Leppik, Oliveira, et al., 2019). In some cases, electrical bone stimulators can also be invasive: completely implanted or partially implanted in the form of pins to the site of impaired healing (see Fig. 37-7). Surgical interventions include bone grafts and internal and external fixation (Weinlein, 2017; Whittle, 2017b).

Grafted bone undergoes a reconstructive process that results in a gradual replacement of the graft with new bone. During surgery, the bone fragments are débrided and aligned, infection (if present) is removed, and a bone graft is placed in the bony defect. The bone graft may be an **autograft** (tissue, frequently from the iliac crest, harvested from the patient for their own use; also called autogenous), an **allograft** (tissue

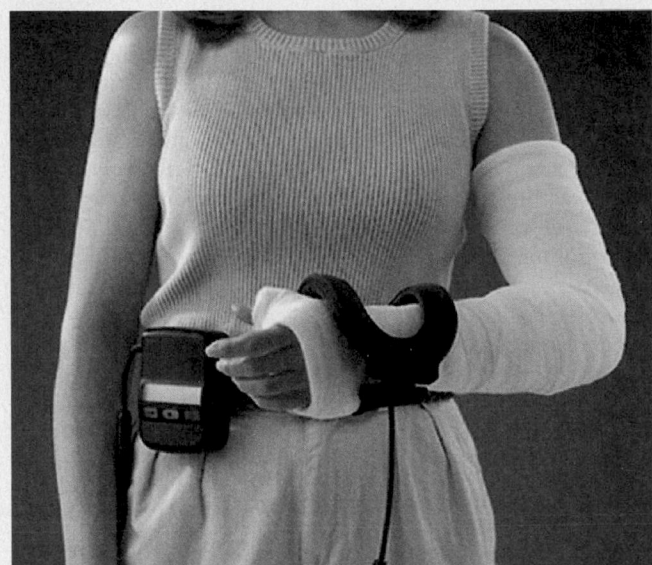

Figure 37-7 • Bone healing stimulator applied to the arm. Reprinted with permission from EBI Medical Systems, Parsippany, NJ.

harvested from a donor), or a bone graft substitute (Baldwin, Li, Auston, et al., 2019). The bone graft fills the bone gap and provides a lattice structure for invasion by bone cells and actively promotes bone growth. The type of bone selected for grafting depends on function—cortical bone is used for structural strength, cancellous bone for osteogenesis, and corticocancellous bone for strength and rapid incorporation (Baldwin et al., 2019). Free vascularized bone autografts are grafted with their own blood supply, allowing for primary fracture healing.

After grafting, immobilization and non–weight-bearing restrictions are required while the bone graft becomes incorporated and the fracture or defect heals, which may be confirmed on an x-ray (Whittle, 2017b). Depending on the type of bone grafted and the age of the patient, healing may take from 6 to 12 months or longer. Bone grafting complications include wound or graft infection, fracture of the graft, and nonunion. Specific problems associated with autografts include a limited quantity of bone available for harvest and harvest site pain that may persist for up to 2 years after harvest. Infrequent specific allograft complications include partial acceptance (lack of host and donor histocompatibility, which retards graft incorporation), graft rejection (rapid and complete resorption of the graft), and transmission of disease (rare) (Whittle, 2017b).

Nursing Management

The patient with a nonunion has experienced an extended time in fracture treatment and may become frustrated with prolonged therapy. The nurse provides emotional support and encouragement to the patient and encourages adherence to the treatment regimen. The orthopedic surgeon evaluates the progression of bone healing with periodic x-rays.

Nursing care for the patient with a bone graft includes providing pain management and monitoring the patient for possible complications. The nurse needs to reinforce educational information concerning the objectives of the bone graft, immobilization, non–weight-bearing regimen and

exercises, wound care, monitoring for signs of infection, and the importance of follow-up care with the orthopedic surgeon (Whittle, 2017b).

Nursing care for the patient using a bone growth stimulator focuses on patient education that addresses immobilization, weight-bearing restrictions, and correct use of the stimulator as prescribed (Mains, 2017).

Avascular Necrosis of Bone (AVN; Osteonecrosis)

AVN occurs when the bone loses its blood supply and dies; the process eventually leads to bony collapse and destruction of the associated joint. It may occur after a fracture with disruption of the blood supply to the distal area. It is also seen with prolonged high-dose corticosteroid therapy, exposure to radiation, sickle cell disease, rheumatoid arthritis, and other diseases; chronic alcohol use and cigarette smoking are other atraumatic etiologies (Graham, 2020). The process is often progressive, and the patient develops pain with movement that progresses to pain at rest. Diagnostics include history and physical examination with x-rays, CT scans, and bone scans. AVN of the hip is the most commonly affected site; the knee is the second most common site. The goal of treatment is to preserve the native joint for as long as possible and includes both conservative and surgical interventions (Graham, 2020). Nonoperative management includes activity modification, administration of analgesics, and partial weight bearing of the affected region. Joint preserving procedures are aimed at revascularizing the affected area by drilling the avascular segment or using a bone marrow graft. In extreme cases, it is advisable to remove the fragment and reconstruct the joint (Jones & Mont, 2018).

Complex Regional Pain Syndrome (CRPS)

CRPS is a complex and rare disorder characterized by regional pain in a limb that is disproportionate; it typically begins following a fracture, soft tissue injury, or surgery. Dysfunctional peripheral and central nervous system responses that mount an excessive response to the precipitating event (e.g., fracture, surgery) are thought to be the cause of the pain. Women are affected more often than men, and the average age of diagnosis is 40 years (National Institute of Neurological Disorders and Stroke [NINDS], 2017). Two subtypes of CRPS have been recognized: Type I (formerly called *reflex sympathetic dystrophy*) applies to patients with CRPS without evidence of peripheral nerve injury, and Type II (formerly called *causalgia*) refers to patients with nerve injury (Abdi, 2020).

Clinical manifestations of CRPS include severe burning pain, local edema, hyperesthesia, stiffness, discoloration, vasomotor skin changes (e.g., fluctuating warm, red, dry and cold, sweaty, cyanotic), and trophic changes that may include glossy, shiny skin, and changes in hair and nail growth. This syndrome is frequently chronic, with extension of symptoms to adjacent areas of the body. Dysfunction of the affected limb may also be manifested in CRPS. The diagnosis is made through the history and physical examination and ruling out other organic causes (NINDS, 2017).

Nursing Management

The primary objective of treatment is physical functional maintenance or recovery of physical function (Stanton-Hicks, 2018). Early effective pain relief is the focus of management. Pain may be controlled with analgesic agents. NSAIDs, topical anesthetics (e.g., lidocaine patches), corticosteroids, and opioids. Anticonvulsant agents (e.g., gabapentin) and antidepressant agents (e.g., amitriptyline) can be effective in treating neuropathic pain. Additional treatments may include sympathetic nerve blocks, neural stimulation, and intrathecal delivery of prescribed medications. Novel treatments under investigation include infusions of immunoglobulin (IVIG) and ketamine and the use of hyperbaric oxygen (Abdi, 2020). The nurse evaluates the effectiveness of these interventions and therapies (see Chapter 9) and helps the patient cope with CRPS manifestations through therapeutic listening, initiation of relaxation techniques and behavior modification, and referral for rehabilitation therapy. Rehabilitation initiated early can improve circulation to the affected area and maximize function. Depression and anxiety are often associated with severe pain disorders; therefore, the nurse should recommend a mental health referral as necessary (NINDS, 2017).

Quality and Safety Nursing Alert

The nurse avoids using the affected extremity for blood pressure measurements and venipuncture in the patient with CRPS.

Heterotopic Ossification

Heterotopic ossification refers to benign bone growth in an atypical location, such as in the soft tissue (Speed, 2019). Heterotopic ossification that is categorized as traumatic myositis ossificans usually develops in response to soft tissue trauma (e.g., contusion, sprain). It is characterized by pain and joint stiffness that causes decreased ROM. It typically occurs in young males after musculoskeletal sports injuries (Meyers, Lisiecki, Miller, et al., 2019). If significant ROM dysfunction persists, surgery may be indicated to remove the bone growth and restore function (Speed, 2019).

The Patient with a Cast, Splint, or Brace

The patient with musculoskeletal trauma typically requires immobilization at some point as part of the management plan. Casts, splints, and braces are external immobilizers that are frequently indicated to treat these injuries.

Casts

A **cast** is a rigid external immobilizing device that is molded to the contours of the body. The cast must fit the shape of the injured limb correctly to provide the best support possible (AAOS, 2019c). A cast is used to immobilize a reduced fracture, to correct or prevent a deformity (e.g., clubfoot, hip displacement), apply uniform pressure to underlying soft tissue, or support and stabilize weakened joints. Generally, casts permit mobilization of the patient while restricting movement of the affected body part.

Because of their ability to provide more complete immobilization, casting is the mainstay of treatment for many fractures as it provides a protected environment for bone healing to occur (Beutler & Titus, 2019). The most common casting

materials consist of fiberglass or plaster of Paris, as these are materials that can be molded. The choice of material depends on several factors, which include the condition being treated, availability, and costs. Maximal immobilization is achieved with casts that include the joints proximal and distal to the fracture site (Alexandre & Hodax, 2017). However, with some fractures, cast construction and molding may allow movement of a joint while immobilizing a fracture (e.g., three-point fixation in a patellar tendon weight-bearing cast).

Generally, casts can be divided into three main groups: arm casts, leg casts, and body or spica casts:

Short arm cast: Extends from below the elbow to the palmar crease, secured around the base of the thumb. If the thumb is included, it is known as a thumb spica or gauntlet cast.

Long arm cast: Extends from the axillary fold to the proximal palmar crease. The elbow usually is immobilized at a right angle.

Short leg cast: Extends from below the knee to the base of the toes. The foot is flexed at a right angle in a neutral position.

Long leg cast: Extends from the junction of the upper and middle third of the thigh to the base of the toes. The knee may be slightly flexed.

Walking boot: Also called an air or walking cast; protects and supports the foot, ankle or lower leg by controlling alignment and reducing movement; also supports the user's weight while walking.

Body cast: Encircles the trunk.

Shoulder spica cast: A body jacket that encloses the trunk, shoulder, and elbow.

Hip spica cast: Encloses the trunk and a lower extremity. A double hip spica cast includes both legs.

Figure 37-8 illustrates long arm and long leg casts and areas in which pressure problems commonly occur with these casts.

The application of a cast is a specialized skill, typically performed by orthopedic technologists. The skillset needed to apply and remove casts requires education, training, practice, and constant review of provider competence to ensure patients receive safe, high-quality care. Casts that are not properly applied or cared for may hinder healing and predispose patients to a number of complications (Adib-Hajbaghery & Mokhtari, 2018).

Fiberglass Casts

Fiberglass casts are composed of polyurethane resins that have the versatility of plaster but are lighter in weight, stronger, water resistant, and more durable than plaster. In addition, fiberglass casts facilitate radiographic imaging better than plaster (AAOS, 2019c) and have the benefit of reaching full rigidity within 30 minutes of application. Because they tend to be more difficult to contour and mold, fiberglass casts are more commonly used for simple fractures of the upper and lower extremities. They consist of an open-weave, nonabsorbent fabric that requires tepid water for activation. Heat is given off (an exothermic reaction) while the cast is applied. The heat given off during this reaction can be uncomfortable, and the nurse should prepare the patient for the sensation of increasing warmth so that the patient does not become alarmed. Fiberglass casts can cause thermal injury like plaster casts, but the risk is less (Beutler & Titus, 2019).

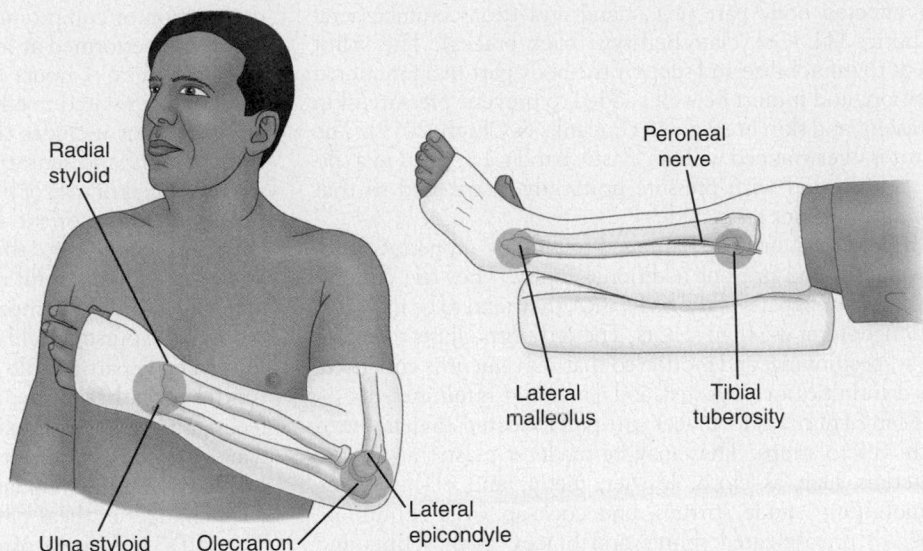

Figure 37-8 • Pressure areas in common types of casts. **Left.** Long arm cast. **Right.** Long leg cast.

Some fiberglass casts use a waterproof lining (Gore-Tex), which permits the patient to shower, swim, or engage in hydrotherapy (the use of water for treatment). When the cast is wet, the patient is instructed to remove excess water by blotting or patting the cast with a towel and making sure to drain the water out of it. The patient must understand that thorough drying is important to prevent skin breakdown, infection, or irritation; sweeping motions with a blow dryer on a cool or warm setting for approximately 1 hour can help to dry the cast inside and out (Mains, 2017). The best results are achieved with casts that can easily drain, such as short arm casts. Heels and elbows encased in wet casts may become macerated from the trapped water and therefore are associated with more skin breakdown.

Plaster Casts

Casts made of plaster of Paris are less costly and achieve a better mold than fiberglass casts; however, they are heavy, not water resistant, and can take up to 24 to 72 hours to dry postapplication. The exothermic reaction during cast application has the potential to cause serious burns (Szostakowski, Smitham, & Khan, 2017). Extra care should be taken when these types of casts are applied to older adults because their skin is more temperature sensitive than average adult skin. During the cast application process, clean, room temperature water should be used. Minimal layers of padding should be used. In addition, the cast should not be covered while it is drying because the heat generated by the chemical reaction cannot escape.

The time that it takes for a plaster cast to dry completely depends on its size, thickness, and location, as well as environmental drying conditions (Nemeth, Halanski, & Noonan, 2020). A freshly applied cast should be handled as little as possible to prevent denting and cracking (Mains, 2017). The wet plaster cast should be handled by only the palms so that indentations in the cast may be prevented; indentations can result in areas of pressure on the skin (Mains, 2017). The cast should be exposed to circulating air to dry and supported on a firm and smooth surface; it should not be placed on a metallic surface or one with sharp edges. If elevation is requested to reduce swelling, a cloth-covered pillow is preferred to

one covered in plastic, which could retain heat and prevent drying. A wet plaster cast feels damp, appears dull and gray, sounds dull on percussion, and smells musty. The cast is dry when it feels hard and firm, has a white and shiny appearance, is resonant to percussion, and odorless.

On occasion, the plaster cast may have rough edges, which can crumble and cause skin irritation. Petaling, or smoothing the rough edges of the cast, resolves this problem if the underlying stockinette does not cover the edges of the cast. To prevent skin breakdown, moleskin can be used over any rough area of the cast that may rub against the patient's skin.

Splints and Braces

Many injuries that were treated previously with casts may now be treated with other immobilization devices such as splints and braces. Application of a **splint** (i.e., a process called splinting) is usually more practical and common and is the preferred method of fracture immobilization in the acute care setting and for the initial treatment of fractures that eventually require casting (Beutler & Titus, 2019). Splints are often used for simple and stable fractures, sprains, tendon injuries, and other soft tissue injuries. They offer many advantages over casts in that they are faster and easier to apply; however, increased joint mobility and decreased patient adherence may be a concern (Eubanks & Chien, 2019). Splints are also noncircumferential and allow for natural swelling during the inflammatory phase of injury. Pressure-related complications (e.g., skin breakdown, necrosis, acute compartment syndrome) are more prevalent when soft tissue swelling occurs within a contained space (e.g., a circumferential cast). Splints are easily removed, facilitating inspection of the injury site. In addition, splints can be indicated to provide initial stability for fractures that are unstable while awaiting definitive care (Schub & Balderrama, 2017).

Contoured splints of plaster or pliable thermoplastic materials may be used for conditions that do not require rigid immobilization, for those in which swelling may be anticipated, and for those that require special skin care. Splints made of thermoplastics are warmed and molded to custom-fit the affected body part (e.g., hand and thoracolumbosacral orthotics [TLSOs], clamshell-type back braces). The splint needs to immobilize and support the body part in a functional position, and it must be well padded to prevent pressure, skin abrasion, and skin breakdown (Eubanks & Chien, 2019). The splint is overwrapped with an elastic bandage applied in a spiral fashion and with pressure uniformly distributed so that circulation is not restricted.

Braces (e.g., orthoses) are used to provide support, control movement, and prevent additional injury. They are custom-fitted to various parts of the body; thus, they tend to be indicated for longer-term use than splints. The orthotist adjusts the brace for fit, positioning, and motion so that movement is enhanced, any deformities are corrected, and discomfort is minimized.

Many splints and braces are prefabricated and fastened with Velcro straps. They may be made of plastic and other materials such as cloth, leather, metal, and elastic. Knee immobilizers, ankle stirrups, and cock-up wrist splints are types of prefabricated splints and braces. Both splints and braces may be either custom-made or standard "off the shelf." Splints and braces are generally less compliant and permit more motion at the injury site than casts, which can be a serious disadvantage in that underlying injuries are not as well stabilized (Schub & Balderrama, 2017).

Nursing Management

Before the cast, splint, or brace is applied, the nurse completes an assessment of the patient's general health, presenting signs and symptoms, emotional status, understanding of the need for the device, and condition of the body part to be immobilized (Schub & Balderrama, 2017). Physical assessment of the part to be immobilized must include a thorough assessment of the skin and neurovascular status, including the degree and location of swelling, bruising, and skin abrasions (Mains, 2017).

To promote healing, any skin lacerations and abrasions that may have occurred as a result of the trauma that caused the fracture must be treated before the cast, brace, or splint is applied. The nurse thoroughly cleanses the skin and treats it as prescribed. The patient may require a tetanus booster if the wound is dirty and if the last known booster was given more than 5 years ago. Sterile dressings are used to cover the injured skin. If the skin wounds are extensive, an alternative method (e.g., external fixator) may be chosen to immobilize the body part (AAOS, 2019c).

The nurse gives the patient or family information about the underlying pathologic condition and the purpose and expectations of the prescribed treatment regimen. This knowledge promotes the patient's active participation in and adherence to the treatment program.

The nurse prepares the patient for the application of the cast, splint, or brace by describing the anticipated sights, sounds, and sensations (e.g., heat from the hardening reaction of the fiberglass or plaster) that they may experience (Chinai, Walker, Rebesco, et al., 2019). Asking the patient and family what they know about the application and care of the cast can help determine opportunities for education. The patient needs to know what to expect during application and the reason the body part must be immobilized.

The main concern following the application of an immobilization device is assessment and prevention of neurovascular dysfunction or compromise of the affected extremity. Assessments are performed at least every hour for the first 24 hours and every 1 to 4 hours thereafter to prevent neurovascular compromise related to edema and/or the device. Neurovascular assessment includes the assessment of peripheral circulation, motion, and sensation of the affected extremity, assessing the fingers or toes of the affected extremity, and comparing them with those of the opposite extremity. When assessing peripheral circulation, the nurse must check peripheral pulses as well as capillary refill response (within 3 seconds), edema, and the color and temperature of the skin. While assessing motion, the nurse should note any weakness or paralysis of the injured body part. While assessing sensation, the nurse monitors for **paresthesia** (i.e., numbness or tingling) or absence of feeling in the affected extremity, which could indicate nerve damage (Schub & Balderrama, 2017).

Nurses must be vigilant in assessing for subtle neurovascular changes in these patients (Schub & Balderrama, 2017). The "5 Ps" indicative of symptoms of neurovascular compromise, described previously, including pain, pallor, pulselessness, paresthesia, and paralysis, are assessed (Papachristos & Giannoudis, 2018). Early recognition of diminished circulation and nerve function is essential to prevent loss of function. Swelling is a concern and can create excessive pressure under the cast (AAOS, 2019c). To augment the flow of fluid, the nurse elevates the extremity so that it is above the level of the heart during the first 24 to 48 hours postapplication to enhance arterial perfusion and control edema and notifies the primary provider at once if signs of compromised neurovascular status are present.

The nurse must carefully evaluate pain associated with the musculoskeletal condition, asking the patient to indicate the exact site and to describe the character and intensity of the pain using a pain rating scale (see Chapter 9). Pain associated with the underlying condition (e.g., fracture) is frequently controlled by immobilization. Pain due to edema that is associated with trauma, surgery, or bleeding into the tissues can frequently be controlled by elevation and, if prescribed, intermittent application of ice or cold packs (AAOS, 2019c). Ice bags (one third to one half full) or cold application devices are placed on each side of the cast, if prescribed, making sure not to indent or wet the cast. Unrelieved or pain out of proportion following cast application may indicate complications. Pain associated with acute compartment syndrome (see previous discussion) is relentless and is not controlled by modalities such as elevation, application of ice or cold, and usual dosages of analgesic agents. Severe burning pain over bony prominences, especially the heels, anterior ankles, and elbows, warns of an impending pressure injury (Chinai et al., 2019). This may also occur from too-tight elastic wraps used to hold splints in place.

> ▶ **Quality and Safety Nursing Alert**
>
> *The nurse must never ignore complaints of pain from the patient in a cast because of the possibility of problems, such as impaired tissue perfusion, acute compartment syndrome or pressure injury formation. A patient's unrelieved pain and increasing analgesic requirements must be reported immediately to the primary provider to avoid necrosis, neuromuscular damage, and possible paralysis.*

The nurse observes the patient for systemic signs of infection, which include an unpleasant odor from the cast, splint, or brace, and purulent drainage staining the cast. Infection is more common from an open wound, but the moist, warm environment of a splint or cast can be an ideal conduit for infection. Foul-smelling casts should be removed to prevent skin and wound infections (Nemeth et al., 2020). If the infection progresses, a fever may develop. The nurse must notify the primary provider if any of these signs occur.

Finally, some degree of joint stiffness is an inevitable complication of immobilization. Every joint that is not immobilized should be exercised and moved through its ROM to maintain function. The nurse encourages the patient to move all fingers or toes hourly when awake to stimulate circulation.

Monitoring and Managing Potential Complications

It is important to assess for potential complications resulting from casts, splints, and braces that can be serious and life-threatening, such as acute compartment syndrome, pressure injury formation, and disuse syndrome.

Acute Compartment Syndrome

Acute compartment syndrome—the most serious complication of casting and splinting—occurs when increased pressure within a confined space (e.g., cast, muscle compartment) compromises blood flow and tissue perfusion (Schub & Balderrama, 2017). Ischemia and potentially irreversible damage to the soft tissues within that space can occur within a few hours if action is not taken (see Fig. 37-4). A tight or rigid cast/splint that constricts a swollen limb is associated with this complication.

If the complication is due to a cast or tight splint, the splint may be loosened or removed and the cast univalved or bivalved (cut in half longitudinally, on one side or two parallel sides of the cast, respectively) to release constriction and allow for inspection of the skin (Nemeth et al., 2020). The nurse assists in maintaining limb alignment, and the extremity must then be elevated no higher than heart level to maintain arterial perfusion. If pressure is not relieved and circulation is not restored, an emergent surgical fasciotomy may be necessary to relieve the pressure within the muscle compartment. The nurse closely monitors the patient's response to conservative and surgical management of compartment syndrome. The nurse records frequent neurovascular responses and promptly reports changes to the primary provider.

Pressure Injuries

Casts or splints can put pressure on soft tissues, particularly if they are inappropriately applied, causing tissue anoxia and pressure injuries. Although the term pressure ulcer has been previously used, the European Pressure Ulcer Advisory Panel, National Pressure Ulcer Advisory Panel and Pan Pacific Pressure Injury Alliance (2019) currently considers pressure injury the best term to use, given that open ulceration does not always occur. Lower extremity sites most susceptible are the heel, malleoli, dorsum of the foot, head of the fibula, and anterior surface of the patella. The main pressure sites on the upper extremity are located at the medial epicondyle of the humerus and the ulnar styloid (see Fig. 37-8).

If pressure necrosis occurs, the patient typically reports a very painful "hot spot" and tightness under the cast. The cast may feel warmer in the affected area, suggesting underlying tissue erythema (Beutler & Titus, 2019). Drainage may stain the cast or splint and emit an unpleasant odor. Even if discomfort does not occur, there may still be extensive loss of tissue with skin breakdown and tissue necrosis. To assess for pressure injury development, the primary provider may univalve, bivalve, or cut an opening (window) in the cast to allow for inspection, access, and possible treatment (Szostakowski et al., 2017). A dressing may be applied over the exposed skin, and the cutout portion of the cast is replaced and held in place by an elastic compression dressing or tape. This prevents "window edema" from occurring, which is the swelling or bulging of the underlying soft tissue through the window opening.

Disuse Syndrome

Immobilization in a cast, splint, or brace can cause muscle atrophy and loss of strength, and can place patients at risk for disuse syndrome, which is the deterioration of body systems as a result of prescribed or unavoidable musculoskeletal inactivity. To prevent this, the nurse instructs the patient to tense or contract muscles (e.g., isometric muscle contraction) without moving the underlying bone (Arora, Erosa, & Danesh, 2019). Isometric exercises, such as instructing the patient with a leg or arm cast to splint or brace to "push down" the knee or to "make a fist," respectively, helps reduce muscle atrophy and maintain strength. Muscle setting exercises (e.g., quadriceps and gluteal setting exercises) are important in maintaining muscles essential for walking (see Chart 37-4). Isometric exercises should be performed hourly while the patient is awake.

Promoting Home, Community-Based, and Transitional Care

 Educating the Patient About Self-Care

Self-care deficits occur when a portion of the body is immobilized. The nurse encourages the patient to participate actively in personal care and to use assistive devices safely. The nurse

---

Chart 37-4 | **PATIENT EDUCATION**
Muscle Setting Exercises

The nurse instructs the patient to perform isometric contractions of the muscle to maintain muscle mass and strength and to prevent atrophy:

Quadriceps Setting Exercise
- Position patient supine with leg extended.
- Instruct patient to push knee back onto the mattress by contracting the anterior thigh muscles.
- Encourage patient to hold the position for 5 to 10 seconds.
- Let patient relax.
- Have patient repeat the exercise 10 times each hour when awake.

Gluteal Setting Exercise
- Position patient supine with legs extended, if possible.
- Instruct patient to contract the muscles of the buttocks.
- Encourage patient to hold the contraction for 5 to 10 seconds.
- Let the patient relax.
- Have patient repeat the exercise 10 times each hour when awake.

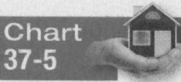

Chart 37-5 HOME CARE CHECKLIST
The Patient with a Cast, Splint, or Brace

At the completion of education, the patient and/or caregiver will be able to:

- State the impact of the musculoskeletal injury/disorder on physiologic functioning, ADLs, IADLs, roles, relationships, and spirituality.
- State rationale for use of cast, splint or brace and resulting changes in lifestyle (e.g., activity, exercise, rest) necessary to maintain health and safety.
  - Avoid excessive use of injured extremity.
  - Observe prescribed weight-bearing limits.
  - Demonstrate ability to transfer (e.g., from a bed to a chair) and/or safe use of mobility aid.
  - Demonstrate exercises to promote circulation and minimize disuse syndrome.
- State the name, dose, side effects, frequency, and schedule for all medications.
- Describe techniques to promote cast drying (e.g., do not cover cast; expose cast to circulating air; handle damp plaster cast with palms of hands; do not rest the cast on hard surfaces or sharp edges that can dent soft cast).
- Describe approaches to controlling swelling and pain (e.g., elevate immobilized extremity to heart level, apply ice bag intermittently if prescribed, take analgesic agents as prescribed).
- Report pain uncontrolled by elevating the immobilized limb and by analgesic agents (may be an indicator of impaired tissue perfusion—acute compartment syndrome or pressure injury).

- Verbalize care for minor skin irritations (e.g., for skin irritation from edge of cast, splint, or brace, pad rough edges with tape or moleskin; to relieve itching, blow cool air from hair dryer; do not insert foreign objects inside the cast, splint, or brace).
- Demonstrate ability to perform ADLs independently or with assistive devices/adaptive equipment.
- State indicators of complications to report promptly to primary provider (e.g., uncontrolled swelling and pain; cool, pale fingers or toes; paresthesia; paralysis; purulent drainage staining cast; signs of systemic infection; cast, splint, or brace breaks).
- State how to reach primary provider with questions or complications
  - State time and date of follow-up appointments and testing
- Identify the need for health promotion, disease prevention, and screening activities
- Describe care of extremity following cast, splint, or brace removal (e.g., skin care, gradual resumption of normal activities to protect limb from undue stresses, management of swelling).

Resources

See Chapter 2, Chart 2-6, for additional information related to durable medical equipment, adaptive equipment, and mobility skills.

ADLs, activities of daily living; IADLs, instrumental activities of daily living.

---

must assist the patient in identifying areas of self-care deficit and in developing strategies to achieve independence in ADLs (see Chart 37-5). Participating in self-care activities can have a positive effect on patient's knowledge and physical and psychological health (Khorais, Ebraheim, & Barakat, 2018). Patient and family education are also described in Chart 37-5.

Continuing and Transitional Care

For the patient with a cast that is ready for removal, the nurse should provide an explanation about what to expect, as the patient may be apprehensive about the procedure due to noise and vibration from the electric saw and fear of being cut (Mains, 2017). The cast saw uses an oscillating blade that vibrates but does not spin; thus, it cuts through the outer cast layer but does not penetrate deeply enough to injure the patient's skin. The cast will be cut in several places, usually along both sides of the cast. The cast is then spread and opened, and a special tool is used to lift it off. Scissors are used to cut through the protective padding and stockinette layers to ensure that the patient's skin will not be cut.

The formerly immobilized body part will be weak from disuse, stiff, and may appear atrophied. As the cast or splint is removed, the affected body part should be supported to prevent injury. The skin, which is usually dry and scaly from accumulated dead skin, is vulnerable to injury from scratching. The extremity is soaked in warm water to soften the skin; a warm washcloth may be used to loosen dead skin and an emollient lotion may be used as lubrication (Mains, 2017). The patient should be instructed to avoid rubbing and scratching the skin, because doing so can cause damage to newly exposed skin.

The nurse and physical therapist educate the patient to resume activities gradually within the prescribed therapeutic regimen. Exercises prescribed to help the patient restore muscle strength, joint motion, and flexibility are explained and demonstrated. Because the muscles are weak from disuse, the body part that has been immobilized cannot withstand normal stresses immediately. In addition, the patient should be instructed to control swelling by elevating the formerly immobilized body part, no higher than the heart, until normal muscle tone and use are reestablished (AAOS, 2019c).

Nursing Management of the Patient with an Immobilized Upper Extremity

The patient whose arm is immobilized must readjust to many routine tasks. The unaffected arm will assume all upper extremity activities. The nurse, in consultation with an occupational therapist, suggests devices designed to aid one-handed activities. The patient may experience fatigue due to modified activities and the weight of the cast, splint, or brace. Frequent rest periods are necessary.

To control swelling, the immobilized arm is elevated above heart level with a pillow. When the patient is lying down, the arm is elevated so that each joint is positioned higher than the preceding proximal joint (e.g., elbow higher than the shoulder, hand higher than the elbow).

A sling may be used when the patient ambulates. To prevent pressure on the cervical spinal nerves, the sling should distribute the supported weight over a large area of the shoulders and trunk, not just the back of the neck. The nurse encourages the patient to remove the arm from the sling and elevate it frequently.

Circulatory disturbances in the hand may become apparent with signs of cyanosis, swelling, and an inability to move the fingers. A missed acute compartment syndrome in the arm can result in a Volkmann ischemic contracture, which may lead to devastating impairment of motor function and sensibility (Rubinstein, Ahmed, & Vosbikian, 2018). Contracture of the fingers and wrist occurs as the result of obstructed arterial blood flow to the forearm and hand. The patient is unable to extend the fingers, describes abnormal sensation (e.g., unrelenting pain, pain on passive stretch), and exhibits signs of diminished circulation to the hand. Irreversible damage develops within a few hours if action is not taken. This serious complication can be prevented with nursing surveillance and proper care (Ferla, Ciravegna, Mariani, et al., 2019).

Nursing Management of the Patient with an Immobilized Lower Extremity

The application of a leg cast, splint, or brace imposes a degree of immobility on the patient. Casts may include short leg casts, extending to the knees, or long leg casts, extending to the groin. Hinged knee braces and immobilizers typically extend from ankle to groin.

The patient's leg must be supported on pillows to the level of the heart to control swelling. Cold therapy or ice packs should be applied as prescribed over the fracture site for 1 to 2 days. The patient is taught to elevate the immobilized leg when seated. The patient should also assume a recumbent position several times a day with the immobilized leg elevated to promote venous return and control swelling (Rasmussen, 2019). Gentle toe and ankle exercises that allow for isometric contraction of muscles beneath the cast have also been shown to increase venous return and diminish edema (AAOS, 2019c).

The nurse assesses circulation by observing the color, temperature, and capillary refill of the exposed toes. Nerve function is assessed by observing the patient's ability to move the toes and by asking about the sensations in the foot. Numbness, tingling, and burning may indicate peroneal nerve injury resulting from pressure at the head of the fibula.

 Quality and Safety Nursing Alert

Injury to the peroneal nerve as a result of pressure is a cause of footdrop (the inability to maintain the foot in a normally flexed position). Consequently, the patient drags the foot when ambulating.

The nurse and physical therapist instruct the patient how to transfer and ambulate safely with assistive devices (e.g., crutches, walker) (see Chapter 2). The gait to be used depends on whether the patient is permitted to bear weight. If weight bearing is allowed, the cast, splint, or brace is reinforced to withstand the body weight. A cast boot or shoe, which is worn over the casted foot, provides a broad, nonskid walking surface.

Nursing Management of the Patient with a Body or Spica Cast

Casts that encase the trunk of the body (body cast) and portions of one or two extremities (spica cast) require special nursing strategies. Body casts are used to immobilize the spine.

Hip spica casts are utilized to treat various fractures of the hip or femur or to correct or maintain the correction of hip deformities after reduction or surgery. These casts typically remain in place for 4 to 6 weeks (Nemeth et al., 2020). Shoulder spica casts are used for some humeral neck fractures.

Nursing responsibilities include preparing and positioning the patient, assisting with skin care and hygiene, and monitoring for complications. Explaining the casting procedure helps reduce the patient's apprehension about being encased in a large cast. The nurse reassures the patient that several people will provide care during the application, support for the injured area will be adequate, and care providers will be as gentle as possible. Patients immobilized in large casts may develop superior mesenteric artery syndrome, also known as cast syndrome, a rare condition characterized by compression of the third portion of the duodenum between the aorta and superior mesenteric artery (Karrer & Jones, 2018). A partial or complete obstruction of the duodenum can occur within days or weeks after the cast has been applied and includes psychological or physiologic manifestations. The psychological component is similar to a claustrophobic reaction. The patient exhibits an acute anxiety reaction characterized by behavioral changes and autonomic responses (e.g., increased respiratory rate, diaphoresis, dilated pupils, increased heart rate, elevated blood pressure). The nurse needs to recognize the anxiety reaction and provide an environment in which the patient feels secure. The administration of pain and antianxiety medications prior to the casting procedure may help to reduce this reaction.

With decreased physical activity, gastrointestinal motility decreases, and intestinal gases accumulate. Physiologic manifestations include abdominal distention and discomfort, nausea, and bilious vomiting, which can lead to food aversion, poor intake, malnourishment, and weight loss (Rai, Shah, Palliyil, et al., 2019). Eventually, increased abdominal pressure and ileus may occur. As with other instances of adynamic ileus, the patient is treated conservatively with decompression (nasogastric intubation connected to suction) and IV fluid therapy until gastrointestinal motility is restored. If conservative measures are ineffective, surgical intervention is warranted. Rarely, the abdominal distention can place added pressure on the superior mesenteric artery, reducing the blood supply to the bowel, which can result in gangrenous bowel. The descending aorta may also sustain pressure, as it may be compressed between the spine and pressure of abdominal distention, which results in ischemia. These complications can be severe, and the pressure needs to be relieved as soon as possible by cutting a window in the abdominal portion of the cast or bivalving the cast; these measures may be sufficient to prevent or relieve pressure on the duodenum.

 Quality and Safety Nursing Alert

The nurse monitors the patient in a large body cast for potential superior mesenteric artery syndrome, noting bowel sounds every 4 to 8 hours, and reports abdominal discomfort and distention, nausea, and vomiting to the primary provider.

Caring for a patient with a body or spica cast at home can be very stressful for the caregiver(s); therefore, it is essential that nurses provide appropriate support and discharge education. To minimize complications after the cast is applied, the nurse should give the patient a comprehensive discharge package that supplements home care instructions with visual training instructions, as well as provide telephone counseling after discharge (Schweich, 2019). Specifically, the nurse educates the family about how to care for the patient, including providing hygienic, cast and skin care, proper positioning, preventing complications, and recognizing symptoms that should be reported to the primary provider.

The Patient with an External Fixator

External fixator devices are used to manage fractures with large amounts of soft tissue damage. Complicated fractures of the humerus, forearm, femur, tibia, and pelvis are also managed with external skeletal fixators. They are also used to correct defects, treat nonunion, and lengthen limbs. Their use has increased in recent years with advances in orthopedic trauma care. The fixator provides skeletal stability for severe comminuted (crushed or splintered) fractures while permitting active treatment of extensive soft tissue damage (see Fig. 37-9).

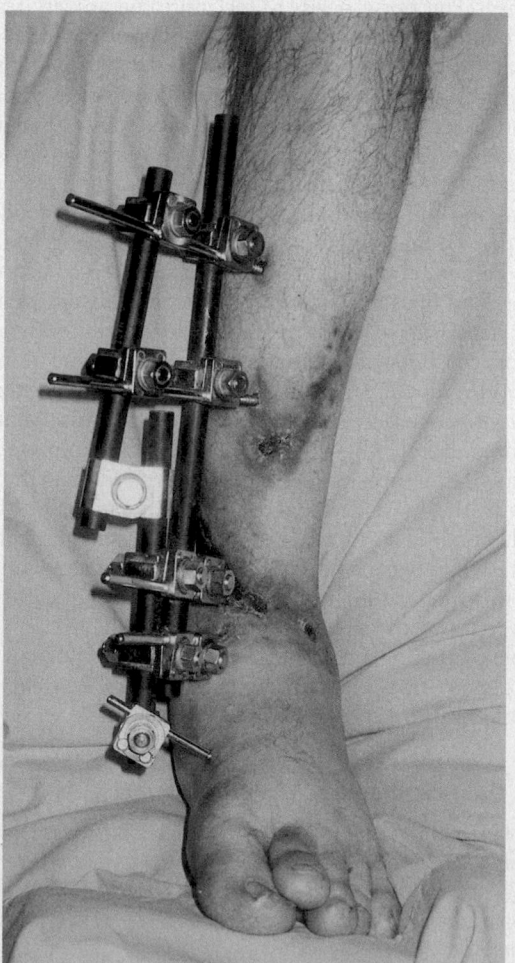

Figure 37-9 • External fixation device. Pins are inserted into bone. The fracture is reduced and aligned and then stabilized by attaching the pins to a rigid portable frame. The device facilitates treatment of soft tissue damaged in complex fractures.

External fixation is a technique that involves the surgical insertion of pins through the skin and soft tissues into and through the bone. A metal external frame is attached to these pins and is designed to hold the fracture in proper alignment to enable healing to occur (Kani, Porrino, & Chew, 2020). Advantages of external fixation, compared to other modes of treatment, include immediate fracture stabilization, minimization of blood loss (in comparison to internal fixation), increased patient comfort, improved wound care, promotion of early mobilization and weight bearing on the affected limb, and active exercise of adjacent uninvolved joints (AAOS, 2019d). The disadvantages are an increased risk for pin site loosening and infection, which can lead to osteomyelitis, septic arthritis, and progressive pain (Sayed, Mohammed, Mostafa, et al., 2019).

Management

Patients should be prepared psychologically for application of the external fixator, as they may be at risk for an altered body image related to the size and bulk of the apparatus. To promote acceptance of the device, patients should be given comprehensive information about the frame and reassurance that the discomfort associated with the device is minimal and that early mobility is anticipated (Walker, 2018); however, among patients who have had significant trauma, there may not be time to engage them in this type of preparation. Nurses should initiate open discussions to help patients describe their concerns about the apparatus and expectations about care.

After the external fixator is applied, the extremity is elevated to the level of the heart to reduce swelling, if appropriate. Any sharp points on the fixator or pins are covered with caps to prevent device-induced injuries. The nurse must be alert for potential problems caused by pressure from the device on the skin, nerves, or blood vessels and for the development of acute compartment syndrome. The nurse monitors the neurovascular status of the extremity every 2 to 4 hours and promptly reports changes to the primary provider (Hadeed, Werntz, & Varacallo, 2019). Because the pins are inserted externally, particular attention is focused on the pin sites for signs of inflammation and infection. The goal is to avoid osteomyelitis. The nurse assesses each pin site at least every 8 to 12 hours for redness, swelling, pain around the pin sites, warmth, and purulent drainage, because these are the most common indicators of pin site infections. In the first 48 to 72 hours postinsertion, some serous drainage, skin warmth, and mild redness at the pin sites are expected (Walker, 2018); these are expected to subside after 72 hours.

Currently, there is no consensus or research-based evidence to direct the best method for cleansing and dressing percutaneous pin sites to minimize infection rates and complications (Lobst, 2017). Additionally, there continues to be a lack of evidence regarding best management of crusting on pin sites (Georgiades, 2018). In the absence of such research, aseptic technique during pin insertion is advised (Gasiorowski, 2017), along with general strategies such as cleansing each pin site separately to avoid cross contamination with non-shedding material (e.g., gauze, cotton-tip swab) and using chlorhexidine 2 mg/mL solution once weekly. Chlorhexidine can be an allergen, however. Therefore, the patient should be monitored for manifestations of an allergic reaction, which

---

Chart 37-6 HOME CARE CHECKLIST
The Patient with an External Fixator

At the completion of education, the patient and/or caregiver will be able to:

- State the impact of the musculoskeletal injury/disorder on physiologic functioning, ADLs, IADLs, roles, relationships, and spirituality.
- State rationale for use of external fixation and resulting changes in lifestyle (e.g., activity, exercise, rest) necessary to maintain health and safety.
  - Avoid excessive use of injured extremity.
  - Observe prescribed weight-bearing limits.
  - Demonstrate ability to transfer (e.g., from a bed to a chair) and/or safe use of mobility aid.
  - Demonstrate exercises to promote circulation and minimize disuse syndrome.
- State signs of pin site infection (e.g., redness, tenderness, increased or purulent pin site drainage) to be reported promptly.
- Describe approaches to controlling swelling and pain (e.g., elevate extremity to heart level, take analgesic agents as prescribed).
- Verbalize plan to report pain uncontrolled by elevation and analgesic agents (may be an indicator of impaired tissue perfusion, acute compartment syndrome, or pin tract infection).

- State indicators of complications to report promptly to primary provider (e.g., uncontrolled swelling and pain; cool, pale fingers or toes; paresthesia; paralysis; purulent drainage; signs of systemic infection; loose fixator pins or clamps).
- State how to reach primary provider with questions or complications
  - State time and date of follow-up appointments and testing
- State the name, dose, side effects, frequency, and schedule for all medications.
- Identify the need for health promotion, disease prevention, and screening activities
- Describe care of extremity after fixator removal (e.g., gradual resumption of normal activities to protect limb from undue stresses).

Resources

See Chapter 2, Chart 2-6, for additional information related to durable medical equipment, adaptive equipment, and mobility skills.

ADLs, activities of daily living; IADLs, instrumental activities of daily living.

---

may include pruritus and/or contact dermatitis at the pin site, or, rarely in severe cases, angioedema and even anaphylactic shock (Campbell & Watt, 2020). Pin sites should be cleaned and dressed as prescribed unless there is copious drainage, the dressing becomes wet, or infection is suspected, in which case cleaning and dressing may be more frequent. If signs of an allergic reaction or infection are present or if the pins or clamps seem loose, the nurse notifies the primary provider.

> ### ▶ *Quality and Safety Nursing Alert*
>
> *The nurse never adjusts the clamps on the external fixator frame. It is the primary provider's responsibility to do so.*

If activity is restricted, the nurse encourages isometric exercises as tolerated to prevent complications of mobility (e.g., thrombus formation). When the swelling subsides, the nurse helps the patient become mobile within the prescribed weight-bearing limits (non–weight bearing to full weight bearing). Adherence to weight-bearing instructions minimizes the chance of loosening of the pins when stress is applied to the bone–pin interface. The external fixator may be removed once the soft tissue heals and there are no signs of infection. The fracture may require additional stabilization by a cast, molded orthosis, or internal fixation while healing.

Ilizarov fixation is a specialized type of external fixator consisting of numerous wires that penetrate the limb and are attached to a circular metal frame (Kani et al., 2020). This device is used to correct angulation and rotational defects, to treat nonunion (failure of bone fragments to heal), and to lengthen limbs. The device gently pulls apart the cortex of the bone and stimulates new growth through daily adjustment of the telescoping rods. The nurse must educate the patient about adjusting the telescoping rods and caring for

the pin sites and apparatus, because this fixator can be in place for many months. When discharge is anticipated, the nurse educates the patient or caregiver about how to perform pin site care according to the prescribed protocol (clean technique can be used at home) and to promptly report any signs of pin site inflammation, irritation, infection, or pin loosening (Sayed et al., 2019; Walker, 2018). The nurse also instructs the patient or family to monitor neurovascular status and report any changes promptly. The patient or family members are instructed to check the integrity of the fixator frame daily and to report loose pins or clamps. A physical therapy referral is helpful in educating the patient how to transfer, use ambulatory aids safely, and adjust to weight-bearing limits and altered gait patterns (see Chart 37-6).

The Patient in Traction

Traction uses a pulling force to promote and maintain alignment to an injured part of the body (Flynn, 2018). The goals of traction include decreasing muscle spasms and pain, realignment of bone fractures, and correcting or preventing deformities. The type of traction, amount of weight, and whether traction can be removed for nursing care must be determined to obtain its therapeutic effects.

At times, traction needs to be applied in more than one direction to achieve the desired line of pull. When this is done, one of the lines of pull counteracts the other. These lines of pull are known as the vectors of force. The actual resultant pulling force is somewhere between the two lines of pull (see Fig. 37-10). The effects of traction are evaluated with x-ray studies, and adjustments are made if necessary.

Traction is used primarily as a short-term intervention until other modalities, such as external or internal fixation, are possible (AAOS, 2019d). These operative techniques reduce the risk of disuse syndrome and minimize hospital

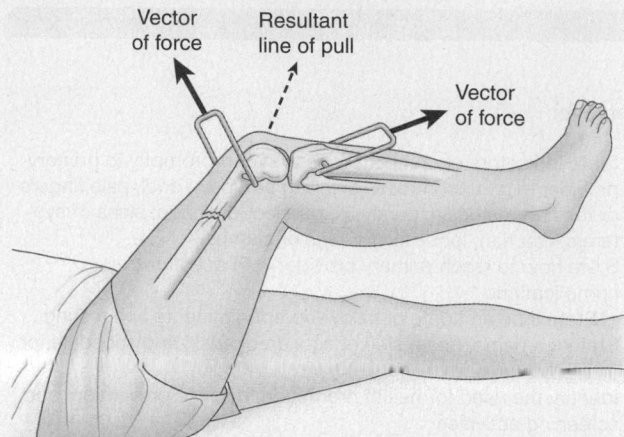

Figure 37-10 • Traction may be applied in different directions to achieve the desired therapeutic line of pull. Adjustments in applied forces may be prescribed over the course of treatment.

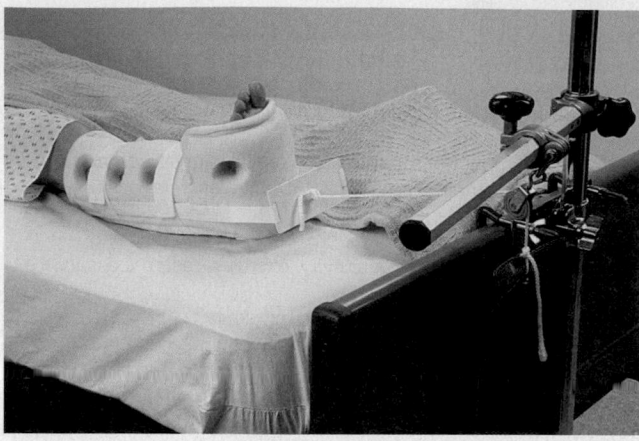

Figure 37-11 • Buck's extension traction. Lower extremity in unilateral Buck's extension traction is aligned in a foam boot and traction applied by the free-hanging weight. The Heelift® Traction Boot is shown here. Photo courtesy of DM Systems, Inc.

lengths of stay, often allowing the patient to be cared for in the home setting.

Principles of Effective Traction

Whenever traction is applied, countertraction must be used to achieve effective results. Countertraction is the force acting in the opposite direction. Usually, the patient's body weight and bed position adjustments supply the needed countertraction.

When caring for the patient in traction, the nurse should follow these additional principles:
- Traction must be continuous to be effective in reducing and immobilizing fractures.
- Skeletal traction is *never* interrupted.
- Weights are not removed unless intermittent traction is prescribed.
- Any factor that might reduce the effective pull or alter its resultant line of pull must be eliminated.
- The patient must be in good body alignment in the center of the bed when traction is applied.
- Ropes must be unobstructed.

- Weights must hang freely and not rest on the bed or floor.
- Knots in the rope or the footplate must not touch the pulley or the foot of the bed.

Types of Traction

The use of traction has decreased significantly due to advances in the surgical reduction of fractures, shortened lengths of hospital stay, and research that queries the effectiveness of its use (Biz, Fantoni, Crepaldi, et al., 2019). However, a basic working knowledge of the use of traction is necessary, because some orthopedic surgeons still prescribe traction for their patients (Santy-Tomlinson, 2017).

There are several types of traction. *Straight* or *running traction* applies the pulling force in a straight line with the body part resting on the bed. The countertraction is provided by the patient's body and movement can alter the traction provided. Buck's extension traction (discussed later; see Fig. 37-11) is an example of straight traction. *Balanced suspension traction* (see Fig. 37-12) supports the affected extremity off the bed

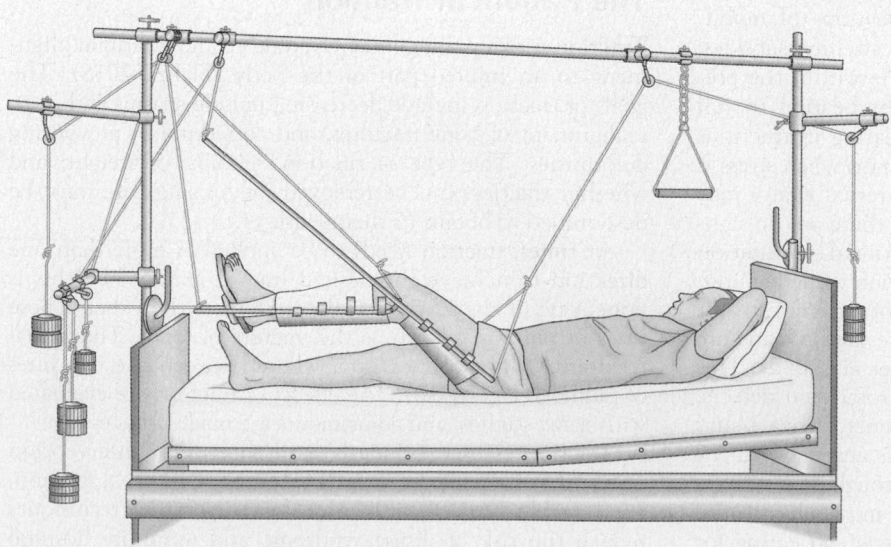

Figure 37-12 • Balanced suspension skeletal traction with Thomas leg splint. The patient can move vertically as long as the resultant line of pull is maintained. Note the use of overhead trapeze.

and allows for some patient movement without disruption of the line of pull. With this traction, the countertraction is produced by devices such as slings or splints.

Traction may be applied to the skin (*skin traction*) or directly to the bony skeleton (*skeletal traction*). The mode of application is determined by the purpose of the traction. Traction can be applied with the hands (*manual traction*). This is temporary traction that may be used when applying a cast, giving skin care under a Buck's extension foam boot, or adjusting the traction apparatus.

Skin Traction

Skin traction is not frequently used but it may be prescribed as a temporary measure to stabilize a fractured leg, control muscle spasms, and immobilize an area before surgery. The pulling force is applied by weights that are attached to the patient with Velcro, tape, straps, boots, or cuffs (Duperouzel, Gray, & Santy-Tomlinson, 2018). The amount of weight applied must not exceed the tolerance of the skin. No more than 2 to 3.5 kg (4.5 to 8 lb) of traction can be used on an extremity. Pelvic traction is usually limited to 4.5 to 9 kg (10 to 20 lb), depending on the weight of the patient. Buck's extension traction (applied to the lower leg) is the most common type of skin traction indicated for select adults with musculoskeletal injury.

Buck's Extension Traction

Buck's extension traction (unilateral or bilateral) is skin traction to the lower leg. The pull is exerted in one plane when partial or temporary immobilization is desired (see Fig. 37-11). It is used as a temporary measure to overcome muscle spasms and promote immobilization of hip fractures in adult patients waiting for more definitive treatment such as surgery. However, current data show no direct benefit; that is, there is no improvement in pain and better fracture reduction when Buck's traction is applied preoperatively in patients with hip fractures (Etxebarria-Foronda & Caeiro-Rey, 2018).

Before the traction is applied, the nurse inspects the skin for abrasions and circulatory disturbances. The skin and circulation must be in healthy condition to tolerate the traction. The extremity should be clean and dry before the foam boot or traction tape is applied.

To apply Buck's traction, the extremity is elevated and supported under the patient's heel and knee while the foam boot is placed under the leg, with the patient's heel in the heel of the boot. Next, the Velcro straps are secured around the leg. Traction tape that is overwrapped with an elastic bandage in a spiral fashion may be used instead of the boot. Excessive pressure is avoided over the malleolus and proximal fibula during application to prevent pressure injuries and nerve damage. The rope is then affixed to the spreader or footplate over a pulley fastened to the end of the bed and attaches the prescribed weight—usually approximately 2.25 to 3.5 kg (or more precisely 5 to 8 lb)—to the rope. The weight should hang freely, not touching parts of the bed or floor as this compromises the efficiency of the traction system (Duperouzel et al., 2018).

Nursing Interventions

To ensure effective skin traction, it is important to avoid wrinkling and slipping of the traction bandage and to maintain countertraction. Proper positioning must be maintained to keep the leg in a neutral position. To prevent bony fragments from moving against one another, the patient should not turn from side to side; however, the patient may shift position slightly with assistance.

Monitoring and Managing Potential Complications

The nurse monitors for complications of skin traction, which can include skin breakdown, nerve damage, and circulatory impairment.

Skin Breakdown

During the initial assessment, the nurse identifies sensitive, fragile skin (common in older adults). The nurse also inspects the skin area that is in contact with tape, foam, or shearing forces, at least every 8 hours, for signs of irritation or inflammation (Duperouzel et al., 2018). The nurse performs the following procedures to monitor and prevent skin breakdown:
- Removes the foam boots to inspect the skin, the ankle, and the Achilles tendon at least twice daily. A second person is needed to support the extremity during the inspection and skin care.
- Palpates the area of the traction tapes daily to detect underlying tenderness.
- Provides frequent repositioning to alleviate pressure and discomfort, because the patient who must remain in a supine position is at increased risk for development of a pressure injury.
- Uses advanced static mattresses or overlays rather than standard hospital foam or alternating-air/low-air-loss mattresses to reduce the risk of pressure injury formation (Kirman, 2018).

Nerve Damage

Skin traction can place pressure on peripheral nerves. Care must be taken to avoid pressure on the peroneal nerve at the point at which it passes around the neck of the fibula just below the knee when traction is applied to the lower extremity. Pressure at this point can cause footdrop. The nurse regularly questions the patient about sensation and asks the patient to move the toes and foot. The nurse should immediately investigate any complaint of a burning sensation under the traction bandage or boot. Dorsiflexion of the foot demonstrates function of the peroneal nerve. Weakness of dorsiflexion or foot movement and inversion of the foot might indicate pressure on the common peroneal nerve. Plantar flexion demonstrates function of the tibial nerve. In addition, the nurse should promptly report altered sensation or impaired motor function.

Circulatory Impairment

After skin traction is applied, the nurse assesses circulation of the foot within 15 to 30 minutes and then every 1 to 2 hours. Circulatory assessment consists of:
- Peripheral pulses, color, capillary refill, and temperature of the fingers or toes.
- Manifestations of DVT, which include unilateral calf tenderness, warmth, redness, and swelling.

The nurse also encourages the patient to perform active foot exercises every hour when awake.

Skeletal Traction

Skeletal traction is often used when continuous traction is desired to immobilize, position, and align a fracture of the femur, tibia, and cervical spine. It is used when traction is to be maintained for a significant amount of time, when skin traction is not possible, and when greater weight (11 to 18 kg [25 to 40 lb]) is needed to achieve the therapeutic effect. Skeletal traction involves passing a metal pin or wire (e.g., Steinmann pin, Kirschner wire) through the bone (e.g., proximal tibia or distal femur) under local anesthesia, avoiding nerves, blood vessels, muscles, tendons, and joints (Buckley & Page, 2018). Traction is then applied using ropes and weights attached to the end of the pin. Alternatively, skeletal traction may involve the application of tongs to the head that are fixed to the skull to immobilize cervical fractures (see Chapter 63).

The surgeon applies skeletal traction using surgical asepsis. The insertion site is prepared with a surgical scrub agent such as chlorhexidine solution. A local anesthetic agent is given at the insertion site and periosteum. The surgeon makes a small skin incision and drills the sterile pin or wire through the bone. The patient feels pressure during this procedure and possibly some pain when the periosteum is penetrated.

After insertion, the pin or wire is attached to the traction bow or caliper. The ends of the pin or wire are covered with caps to prevent injury to the patient or caregivers. The weights are attached to the pin or wire bow by a rope and pulley system that exerts the appropriate amount and direction of pull for effective traction (Biz et al., 2019). The weights applied initially must overcome the shortening spasms of the affected muscles. As the muscles relax, the traction weight is reduced to prevent fracture dislocation and to promote healing.

Often, skeletal traction is balanced traction, which supports the affected extremity, allows for some patient movement, and facilitates patient independence and nursing care while maintaining effective traction. The Thomas splint with a Pearson attachment is frequently used with skeletal traction for fractures of the femur (see Fig. 37-12). Because upward traction is required, an overbed frame is used (Gray & Santy-Tomlinson, 2018).

When skeletal traction is discontinued, the extremity is gently supported while the weights are removed. The pin is cut close to the skin and removed by the surgeon. Internal fixation, casts, or splints are then used to immobilize and support the healing bone.

Nursing Interventions

When skeletal traction is used, the nurse checks the traction apparatus to see that the ropes are in the wheel grooves of the pulleys, the ropes are not frayed, the weights hang freely, and the knots in the rope are tied securely. The nurse also evaluates the patient's position, making sure that the traction force is always in correct alignment with the leg, with the patient in the mid-line position (Gray & Santy-Tomlinson, 2018).

> ### ◤ *Quality and Safety Nursing Alert*
>
> *The nurse must never remove weights from skeletal traction unless a life-threatening situation occurs. Removal of the weights defeats their purpose and may result in injury to the patient.*

The nurse must maintain alignment of the patient's body in traction as prescribed to promote an effective line of pull (Gray & Santy-Tomlinson, 2018). The nurse positions the patient's foot to avoid footdrop (plantar flexion), inward rotation (inversion), and outward rotation (eversion). The patient's foot may be supported in a neutral position by orthopedic devices (e.g., foot supports).

If the patient reports severe pain from muscle spasm, the weights may be too heavy, or the patient may need realignment. Pain must be reported to the primary provider if body alignment fails to reduce discomfort. Opioid and nonopioid analgesics may be used to control pain. Muscle relaxants may be prescribed to relieve muscles spasms as needed.

Preventing Skin Breakdown

The patient's elbows frequently become sore, and nerve injury may occur if the patient repositions by pushing on the elbows. In addition, patients frequently push on the heel of the unaffected leg when they raise themselves. This digging of the heel into the mattress may injure the tissues. It is important to instruct patients not to use their heels or elbows to push themselves up in bed (El-saidy & Aboshehata, 2019). To encourage movement without using the elbows or heel, an assistive device called a **trapeze** can be suspended overhead within easy reach of the patient (see Fig. 37-12). The trapeze helps the patient move about in bed and move on and off the bedpan. Transparent film, hydrocolloid dressings, or skin sealants may also be applied to bony prominences (such as elbows) or critical areas to decrease the force of shearing and friction (Gaspar, Peralta, Marques, et al., 2019).

Specific pressure points are assessed for irritation and inflammation at least every 8 hours. Patients at high risk for skin breakdown (e.g., older adults, patients who are malnourished or who have impaired mobility or sensation) may need to be assessed more frequently (Mervis & Phillips, 2019). Areas that are particularly vulnerable to pressure caused by a traction apparatus applied to the lower extremity include the ischial tuberosity, popliteal space, Achilles tendon, and heel. If the patient is not permitted to turn on one side or the other, the nurse must make a special effort to provide back care and to keep the bed dry and free of crumbs and wrinkles. The patient can assist by holding the overhead trapeze and raising the hips off the bed. If the patient cannot do this, the nurse can push down on the mattress with one hand to relieve pressure on the back and bony prominences and to provide for some shifting of weight. Given the supine position that most patients with skeletal traction assume, the use of advanced static mattresses or overlays should be considered rather than foam or alternating-air/low-air-loss mattresses to reduce the risk of pressure injury (Serraes, Van Leen, Schols, et al., 2018). The patient's heel should be "off-loaded" and carefully placed on a pillow or heel suspension device to keep the heel from the bed's surface (Gray & Santy-Tomlinson, 2018).

For change of bed linens, the patient raises the torso while caregivers on both sides of the bed roll down and replace the upper mattress sheet. Then, as the patient raises the buttocks off the mattress, the sheets are slid under the buttocks. Finally, the lower section of the bed linens is replaced while the patient rests on the back. Sheets and blankets are placed over the patient in such a way that the traction is not disrupted.

Monitoring Neurovascular Status

The nurse evaluates the body part to be placed in traction and compares its neurovascular status (e.g., color, temperature, capillary refill, edema, pulses, ability to move, and sensations) to the unaffected extremity every hour for the first 24 hours after traction is applied and every 4 hours thereafter. The nurse instructs the patient to report any changes in sensation or movement immediately so that they can be promptly evaluated. VTE formation is a significant risk for the patient who is immobilized. The nurse encourages the patient to do active flexion–extension ankle exercises and isometric contraction of the calf muscles (calf-pumping exercises) 10 times an hour while awake to decrease venous stasis. In addition, anti-embolism stockings, compression devices, and anticoagulant therapy may be prescribed to help prevent thrombus formation.

 Quality and Safety Nursing Alert

The nurse must immediately investigate every report of discomfort expressed by the patient in traction. Prompt recognition of a developing neurovascular problem is essential so that corrective measures can be instituted quickly.

Providing Pin Site Care

The wound at the pin insertion site requires attention, and it is important to follow the facility's specific policy pertaining to skeletal pin care. The goal is to avoid infection and development of osteomyelitis (see Chapter 36). For the first 48 hours after insertion, the site is covered with a sterile absorbent nonstick dressing and a rolled gauze or Ace-type bandage. After this time, a loose cover dressing or no dressing is recommended (a bandage is necessary if the patient is exposed to airborne dust). Expert consensus-based recommendations for pin site care include the following (Walker, 2018):

- Pins located in areas with soft tissue are at greatest risk for infection.
- After the first 48 to 72 hours following skeletal pin placement, pin site care should be performed daily or weekly.
- Chlorhexidine 2 mg/mL solution is the most effective cleansing solution. If chlorhexidine is contraindicated (due to known hypersensitivity or skin reaction), saline solution should be used for cleansing.
- Strict hand hygiene before and after skeletal pin site care should always take place.

The nurse must inspect the pin sites at least every 12 hours for signs of hypersensitivity/allergic reaction (e.g., contact dermatitis, pruritus, urticaria, angioedema), irritation (e.g., normal changes that occur at the pin site after insertion) and infection. Signs of irritation may include redness, warmth, and serosanguineous drainage at the site, which tend to subside after 72 hours. Signs of infection may mirror those of reaction but also include the presence of purulent drainage, pain, pin loosening, tenting of skin at pin site, odor, and fever. Patient descriptions of their pin sites might be helpful as they are often the first to notice subtle changes in their symptoms and may be able to differentiate between different pin site states (Santy-Tomlinson, Jomeen, & Ersser, 2019).

Prophylactic broad-spectrum IV antibiotics may be given for 24 to 48 hours postinsertion to prevent infection; however, the evidence is confounding and there is no general consensus on the advisability of this practice (Walker, 2018). Minor infections may be readily treated with antibiotics, and infections that result in systemic manifestations may additionally warrant pin removal until the infection resolves.

Due to a lack of evidence-based research findings, controversy exists about skeletal pin care, showering, and the overall management of pin site crusts, which are the hardened plugs of exudate that adhere to and block the pin sites. Current evidence suggests that crusting at the pin site should be retained as long as the pin site remains uninfected as the retained crusts provides a natural barrier from the external environment, which can prevent bacterial contamination (Georgiades, 2018). The patient and family should be educated on the performance of any prescribed pin site care prior to discharge from the hospital and should be provided with written follow-up instructions that include the signs and symptoms of infection.

Promoting Exercise

Patient exercises, within the therapeutic limits of the traction, assist in maintaining muscle strength and tone, and in promoting circulation. Active exercises include pulling up on the trapeze, flexing and extending the feet, and range-of-motion and weight-resistance exercises for noninvolved joints. Isometric exercises of the immobilized extremity (quadriceps and gluteal setting exercises) are important for maintaining strength in major ambulatory muscles (see Chart 37-4). Without exercise, the patient will lose muscle mass and strength, and rehabilitation will be greatly prolonged.

Nursing Management of the Patient in Traction

Nursing management of the patient in traction includes assessing for and addressing anxiety, assisting with self-care, and monitoring for complications.

Assessing Anxiety

The nurse must consider the psychological and physiologic impact of the musculoskeletal problem, traction device, and immobility. Traction restricts mobility and independence. The equipment can look threatening, and its application can be frightening. Confusion, disorientation, and behavioral problems may develop in patients who are confined in a limited space for an extended time. Therefore, the nurse must assess and monitor the patient's anxiety level and psychological responses to traction.

Assisting with Self-Care

Initially, the patient may require assistance with self-care activities. The nurse helps the patient eat, bathe, dress, and toilet. Convenient arrangement of items such as the telephone, tissues, water, and assistive devices (e.g., reachers, overbed trapeze) may facilitate self-care. With resumption of self-care activities, the patient feels less dependent and less frustrated and experiences improved self-esteem. Because some assistance is required throughout the period of immobility, the nurse and the patient can creatively develop routines that maximize the patient's independence.

Monitoring and Managing Potential Complications

Immobility-related complications may include pressure injuries (see Chapter 56), atelectasis, pneumonia, constipation, loss of appetite, urinary stasis, urinary tract infections, and VTE formation. Early identification of preexisting or developing conditions facilitates prompt interventions to resolve them.

Atelectasis and Pneumonia

The nurse auscultates the patient's lungs every 4 to 8 hours to assess respiratory status and educates the patient about performing deep breathing and coughing exercises to aid in fully expanding the lungs and clearing pulmonary secretions. If the patient history and baseline assessment indicate that the patient is at risk for development of respiratory complications, specific therapies (e.g., the use of an incentive spirometer) may be indicated (see Chapter 19, Chart 19-1). If a respiratory complication develops, prompt institution of prescribed therapy is needed.

Constipation and Anorexia

Reduced gastrointestinal motility results in constipation and anorexia. A diet high in fiber and fluids may help stimulate gastric motility. If constipation develops, therapeutic measures may include stool softeners, laxatives, suppositories, and enemas. To improve the patient's appetite, the patient's food preferences are included, as appropriate, within the prescribed therapeutic diet.

Urinary Stasis and Infection

Incomplete emptying of the bladder related to positioning in bed can result in urinary stasis and infection. In addition, the patient may find the use of a bedpan uncomfortable and may limit fluids to minimize the frequency of urination. The nurse monitors the fluid intake and the character of the urine. Adequate hydration is important; therefore, the nurse instructs the patient to consume adequate amounts of fluid and to void every 3 to 4 hours. If the patient exhibits signs or symptoms of urinary tract infection (e.g., burning or pain on urination, hematuria), the nurse notifies the primary provider.

Venous Thromboembolism

Venous stasis that predisposes the patient to VTE occurs with immobility. The nurse educates the patient about how to perform ankle and foot exercises within the limits of the traction therapy every 1 to 2 hours when awake to prevent DVT. To increase adherence and promote the family's involvement with the patient's care, it is important to include the family members in any education and care decisions about VTE prevention (Health Services Advisory Group, 2019). The patient is encouraged to drink fluids to prevent dehydration and associated hemoconcentration, which contribute to stasis. The nurse monitors the patient for signs of DVT, including unilateral calf tenderness, warmth, redness, and swelling (increased calf circumference). The nurse promptly reports findings to the primary provider for evaluation and therapy.

During traction therapy, the nurse encourages the patient to exercise muscles and joints that are not in traction to prevent deterioration, deconditioning, and venous stasis. The physical therapist can design bed exercises that minimize loss of muscle strength. During the patient's exercise, the nurse ensures that traction forces are maintained and that the patient is properly positioned to prevent complications resulting from poor alignment.

Fractures of Specific Sites

Common sites of fractures include the clavicle, humeral neck, humeral shaft, elbow, proximal radius, radial and ulnar shafts, wrist, hand, pelvis, acetabulum, hips, femoral shaft, tibia and fibula, ribs, and thoracolumbar spine.

Clavicle

Fracture of the clavicle (collar bone) is a common injury that can result from a fall or a direct blow to the shoulder. The clavicle helps maintain the shoulder in the upward, outward, and backward position from the thorax. Therefore, when the clavicle is fractured, the patient assumes a protective position, slumping the shoulders and immobilizing the arm to prevent shoulder movements. The treatment goal is to align the shoulder in its normal position by means of closed reduction and immobilization. Surgical intervention is not typical but may be indicated if the fracture is located in the distal third of the clavicle or is severely displaced, which may result in neurovascular compromise or pneumothorax (Kleinhenz, 2019).

The majority of clavicle fractures occur in the middle third of the clavicle; clinical union (healing) takes 6 to 12 weeks in adults (Eiff, Hatch, & Higgins, 2020b). A clavicular strap, also called a *figure-eight bandage* (see Fig. 37-13), may be used

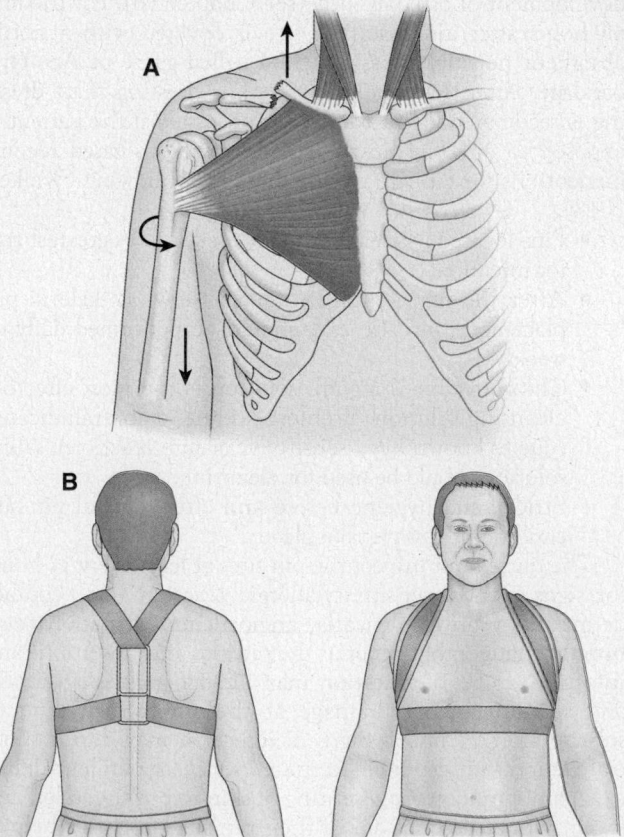

Figure 37-13 • Fracture of the clavicle. **A.** Anteroposterior view shows typical displacement in midclavicular fracture. **B.** Immobilization is accomplished with a clavicular strap.

to pull the shoulders back, reducing and immobilizing the fracture. The nurse monitors the circulation and nerve function of the affected arm and compares it with the unaffected arm to determine variations, which may indicate disturbances in neurovascular status. A sling may be used to support the arm and relieve pain. The patient may be permitted to use the arm for light activities as pain allows (Hatch, Clugston, & Taffee, 2019).

Fracture of the distal third of the clavicle, without displacement and ligament disruption, is treated with a sling and restricted motion of the arm. When a fracture in the distal third is accompanied by a disruption of the coracoclavicular ligament that connects the coracoid process of the scapula and the inferior surface of the clavicle, the bony fragments are frequently displaced. This type of injury may be treated surgically by ORIF.

Immobilization of the shoulder in the figure-eight bandage or arm sling should be continued until clinical union occurs (e.g., the fracture site is nontender and the patient can move the arm with little or no discomfort) (Hatch et al., 2019). The nurse cautions the patient not to elevate the arm above shoulder level until the fracture has healed but encourages the patient to exercise the elbow, wrist, and fingers as soon as possible. When prescribed, shoulder exercises are performed to obtain full shoulder motion (see Fig. 37-14). Contact sports or activities with potential for falling should be avoided for 1 to 2 months after healing is complete, and has been confirmed by clinical assessment and x-ray findings (Eiff et al., 2020b).

Complications of clavicular fractures are uncommon but can include neurovascular injuries (brachial plexus injury, subclavian vein or artery injury from a bony fragment, and thoracic outlet syndrome), pneumothorax, malunion, and nonunion (Hatch et al., 2019).

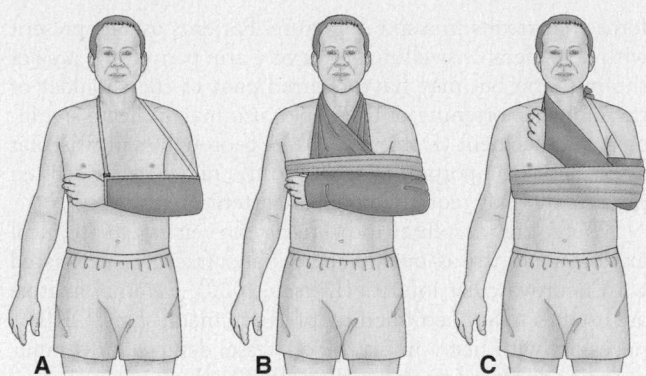

Figure 37-15 • Immobilizers for proximal humeral fractures. **A.** Commercial sling with immobilizing strap permits easy removal for hygiene and is comfortable on the neck. **B.** Conventional sling and swathe. **C.** Stockinette Velpeau and swathe are used when there is an unstable surgical neck component. This position relaxes the pectoralis major.

Humeral Neck

Fractures of the proximal humerus may occur through the neck of the humerus and are most often the result from a fall onto an outstretched hand. Most proximal humerus fractures occur in those older than 60 years of age and are more common in older women because of their greater risk of low bone density (Dorsey, 2020).

The patient presents with moderate to severe shoulder pain with the affected arm hanging limp at the side or supported by the uninjured hand. Neurovascular assessment of the extremity is essential to evaluate the full extent of injury and the possible involvement of the nerves and blood vessels of the arm.

The majority of proximal humerus fractures are impacted with little to no displacement and do not require surgical reduction. The arm is supported and immobilized by a sling and swathe splint that secures the supported arm to the trunk (see Fig. 37-15). Limitation of motion and stiffness of the shoulder occur with disuse. Therefore, pendulum exercises begin as soon as tolerated by the patient. In pendulum or circumduction exercises, the physical therapist instructs the patient to lean forward and allow the affected arm to hang in abduction and rotate. These fractures heal rapidly in about 6 to 10 weeks due to the large areas of cancellous bone (Dorsey, 2020). The goal of treatment is to restore as much function as possible; therefore, shoulder rehabilitation should begin as pain allows. Residual stiffness, aching, and some loss of shoulder motion ("frozen shoulder") and function may persist and is more likely to develop in patients who do not perform ROM exercises regularly during recovery (Bassett, 2019).

When a humeral neck fracture is significantly displaced, treatment consists of closed reduction with splinting, ORIF, hemiarthroplasty, and reverse shoulder arthroplasty. Exercises begin after an adequate period of immobilization (Bassett, 2019).

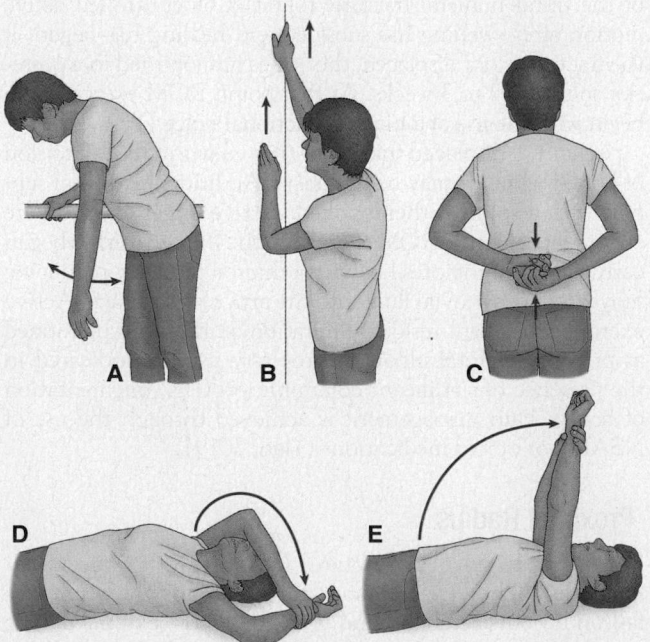

Figure 37-14 • Exercises that promote shoulder range of motion include pendulum exercise (**A**) and wall climbing (**B**). The unaffected arm is used to assist with internal rotation (**C**), external rotation(**D**), and elevation (**E**). In **C, D,** and **E,** the unaffected arm is used for power.

Humeral Shaft

Fractures of the midshaft of the humerus are most frequently caused by either a direct blow or trauma that results in a transverse, oblique, or comminuted fracture, or an indirect twisting force that results in a spiral fracture. Patients usually present with considerable swelling and severe arm pain in the area of the mid-arm but may have referred pain to the shoulder or the elbow; shortening of the upper arm may indicate significant displacement (Dorsey, 2020). A thorough neurovascular assessment is important as injury to the radial nerve is often present and may require immediate attention.

There are absolute indications for emergent surgical exploration such as open fractures and fractures associated with neurovascular injuries (Dorsey, 2020). External fixators are used to treat open fractures of the humeral shaft. ORIF is necessary with nerve injury, blood vessel damage, or comminuted or displaced fractures (Bassett, 2018).

However, most humeral midshaft fractures can be treated nonsurgically. Initial splinting is commonly done with a coaptation (*sugar tong*) splint. (A sugar tong splint is a U-shaped splint that looks like tongs used for sugar cubes.) The splint is placed around the medial and lateral arm to the elbow and up to the top of the shoulder. The splint supports the arm in 90 degrees of flexion at the elbow; a sling or collar and cuff support the forearm. The weight of the hanging arm and splints put traction on the fracture site.

The preferred definitive treatment for a humerus shaft fracture is functional bracing. A contoured thermoplastic sleeve is secured in place with interlocking fabric (Velcro) closures around the upper arm, immobilizing the reduced fracture. As swelling decreases, the sleeve is tightened, and uniform pressure and stability are applied to the fracture. The forearm is supported with a collar and cuff sling (see Fig. 37-16). Functional bracing allows active use of muscles, shoulder and elbow motion, and good approximation of fracture fragments. Pendulum shoulder exercises are performed as prescribed to provide active movement of the shoulder, thereby preventing a "frozen shoulder." Isometric exercises may be prescribed to prevent muscle atrophy. The callus that develops is substantial, and the sleeve can be discontinued in about 8 weeks.

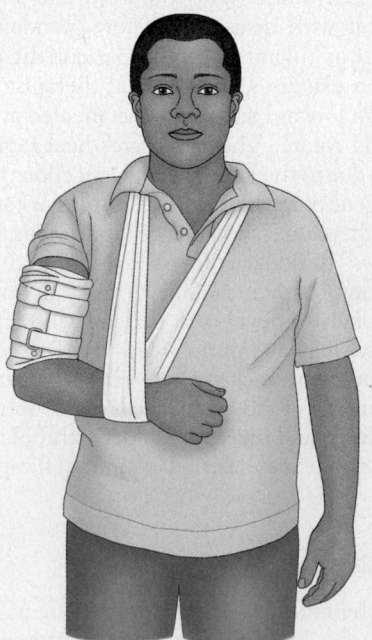

Figure 37-16 • Functional humeral brace with collar and cuff sling.

Complications that are seen with humeral shaft fractures include neurovascular compromise and nonunion because of decreased blood supply in that area.

Elbow

About 30% of adult elbow fractures involve the distal part of the humerus (Eiff, Hatch, & Higgins, 2020c) and are classified as supracondylar, single column (condyle), bicolumn and coronal shear fractures. Most fractures result from high-energy mechanisms such as motor vehicle crashes, falls directly on the elbow (in the extended or flexed position), or a direct blow. These fractures can be very painful and may result in injury to the brachial artery and median nerves (Yian, 2019).

A comprehensive examination of the neurovascular status of the affected extremity should be conducted. The patient is evaluated for paresthesia and signs of compromised circulation in the forearm and hand. The most serious complication of a supracondylar fracture of the humerus is Volkmann ischemia contracture (an acute compartment syndrome), which results from antecubital swelling or damage to the brachial artery and leads to contracture (shortening) of the forearm muscles. This more commonly occurs in children than in adults and will result in a "clawlike" appearance to the hand and wrist. The nurse needs to monitor the patient regularly for compromised neurovascular status with the "5 Ps"; marked swelling and induration of the forearm are other signs (Kare, 2019). Emergency fasciotomy with débridement of the muscle may be necessary to prevent progression to Volkmann contracture (Eiff et al., 2020c). Other potential complications are damage to the joint articular surfaces and hemarthrosis (e.g., blood in the joint), which may be treated by needle aspiration by the primary provider to relieve the pressure and pain.

The goal of therapy is prompt reduction and stabilization of the distal humeral fracture, followed by controlled active motion after swelling has subsided and healing has begun. If the fracture is not displaced, the arm is immobilized in a posterior splint for 2 to 3 weeks. At that point, ROM exercises can begin with the use of a hinged functional brace (Yian, 2019).

Usually, a displaced fracture is treated with ORIF. Excision of bone fragments may be necessary. Additional external support with a splint is then applied. Active finger exercises are encouraged. Gentle ROM exercise of the injured joint is begun early. Motion promotes healing of injured joints by producing movement of synovial fluid into the articular cartilage. Active exercise to prevent residual limitation of motion is performed as prescribed. Total elbow arthroplasty may be indicated in the presence of significant comminution (e.g., fragmentation of bone). Pain management is achieved through the use of NSAIDs or opioid medications (Yian, 2019).

Proximal Radius

Radial head and neck fractures are fractures of the proximal radius. They are common and are usually the result of a fall on an outstretched hand with the elbow extended. The patient presents with localized swelling over the lateral elbow, tenderness, and decreased motion; pain increases with passive rotation. If blood has collected in the elbow joint, it is aspirated to relieve pain and to allow early active elbow and forearm ROM exercises (Eiff et al., 2020c). Nondisplaced fractures are typically managed nonsurgically with a sling for comfort; elbow flexion and extension as tolerated out of the sling should begin as soon as tolerated, usually within the first few days after injury (Eiff et al., 2020c). If the fracture is displaced, surgery is typically indicated, with excision of or replacement of the radial head when necessary (Rabin, 2018).

Radial and Ulnar Shafts

Fractures of the distal radius are among the most common fractures and occur more frequently in children and adolescents but can occur in adults. The radius or the ulna may be fractured at any level. Frequently, displacement occurs when both bones are broken. The forearm serves an integral role in upper extremity function; therefore, the unique functions of pronation and supination must be preserved with proper anatomic alignment (Kakarala & Simons, 2019).

In adults, if the fragments are not displaced, the fracture is treated by closed reduction with immobilization in a bivalved long arm cast with the wrist in slight extension, the forearm in neutral rotation, and the elbow at 90 degrees (Michaudet, 2020). Circulation, motion, and sensation of the hand are assessed before and after the cast is applied. The arm is elevated to control edema. Frequent finger flexion and extension are encouraged to reduce edema. Active motion of the involved shoulder is essential. The reduction and alignment are monitored closely by x-rays at weekly intervals for the first 4 weeks to ensure proper alignment and then every 2 weeks until healing has occurred (usually 12 to 16 weeks). During the last 6 weeks, the arm may be in a functional forearm brace that allows exercise of the wrist and elbow. Lifting and twisting are avoided.

Displaced fractures of the radius and ulna require an ORIF, using a compression plate with screws, intramedullary nails, or rods. The arm is usually immobilized in a plaster splint or cast. Open and displaced fractures may be managed with external fixation devices. The arm is elevated to control swelling. Neurovascular status is assessed and documented. Elbow, wrist, and hand exercises are begun when prescribed by the primary provider.

Wrist

Fractures of the distal radius (Colles fracture) are common and are usually the result of a fall on an open, outstretched hand, with the wrist in extension. This fracture is frequently seen in older adults with osteoporotic bones that do not dissipate the energy of the fall; it can also occur in youth who are involved in sports who sustain a high-energy fall. The patient presents with a deformed wrist, pain, swelling, weakness, and limited finger ROM, and possibly reports of "tingling" in the affected hand. Tingling sensation may indicate injury to the median nerve (Nelson, 2018).

Treatment usually consists of closed reduction and immobilization with a sugar-tong splint until swelling resides. The splint is placed so that it extends from the palm around the elbow to the back of the hand just below the fingers. This splint should remain in place until the edema lessens and usually the splint is changed to a short arm cast in 2 to 3 weeks. For fractures with extensive comminution, ORIF, plating, percutaneous pinning, or external fixation is used to achieve

---

> ### Chart 37-7
> **PATIENT EDUCATION**
> ### Encouraging Exercise After Treatment for Wrist Fracture
>
> The nurse encourages active motion of the fingers and shoulder. The patient is instructed to perform the following exercises to reduce swelling and prevent stiffness:
>
> - Hold the hand at the level of the heart.
> - Move the fingers from full extension to flexion. Hold and release. Repeat at least 10 times every hour when awake.
> - Use the hand in functional activities.
> - Actively exercise the shoulder and elbow, including complete range-of-motion exercises of both joints.

and maintain reduction. Pain medication is given as prescribed to aid in pain control (Petron, 2018).

Active motion of the fingers and shoulder should begin promptly to reduce swelling and prevent stiffness (see Chart 37-7).

The fingers may swell due to diminished venous and lymphatic return. The nurse assesses the sensory function of the median nerve by pricking the distal aspect of the index finger. The motor function is assessed by the patient's ability to touch the thumb to the little finger. Diminished circulation and nerve function must be treated promptly (see previous discussion of acute compartment syndrome).

Hand

Fractures of the bones of the hand, phalanges and metacarpals, are a common injury of the skeletal system and a frequent reason that patients seek care in EDs (Muttath, Chung, & Ono, 2019). The most common type of metacarpal fracture in adults is referred to as boxer's fracture, which occurs when a closed fist bangs against a hard surface, fracturing the neck of the fifth finger. Falls and occupational injuries (e.g., machinery injuries, crushes) are the most common cause of phalangeal injury in adults (Lakshmanan, Damodaran, & Sher, 2018). When any of the bones of the hand are fractured, the objectives of treatment are to regain maximum function of the hand and minimize cosmetic deformities. X-rays are the diagnostic studies of choice (Muttath et al., 2019).

For a nondisplaced fracture of the phalanx (finger bone), the finger is splinted for 3 to 4 weeks to relieve pain and to protect the finger from further trauma. Splinting sometimes consists of "buddy taping" a fractured finger to an adjoining nonfractured finger. Serial x-rays may be done to monitor healing. Displaced fractures and open fractures may require ORIF, using wires or pins. If the fracture is open, or if a fingernail is avulsed, antibiotics may be prescribed (Basset, 2019).

The neurovascular status of the injured hand is evaluated and documented. Swelling is controlled by elevation of the hand. Functional use of the uninvolved portion of the hand is encouraged. Assistive devices might be recommended to aid the patient in performing ADLs until the hand has healed and functional status returns.

Pelvis

The sacrum, ilium, pubis, and ischium bones form the bony pelvis, which unites to form an anatomic ring in adults

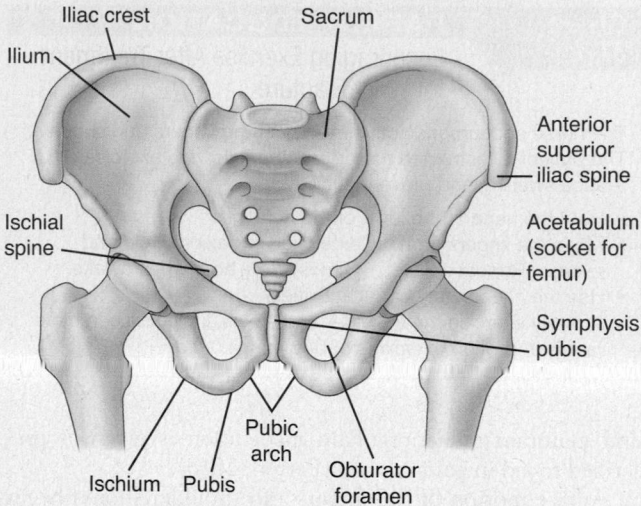

Figure 37-17 • Pelvic bones.

(see Fig. 37-17). Falls from a great height, motor vehicle and motorcycle crashes, vehicle versus pedestrian, and crush injuries can cause pelvic fractures. There is a high mortality rate associated with unstable pelvic fractures, second only to head injuries among trauma-related deaths; this is primarily related to hemorrhage, although pulmonary complications, fat emboli, thromboembolic complications, and infection are also implicated (Fiechtl, 2018). Management of severe, life-threatening pelvic fractures is coordinated with the trauma team.

Signs and symptoms of pelvic fracture may include ecchymosis; tenderness over the symphysis pubis, anterior iliac spines, iliac crest, sacrum, or coccyx; local edema; numbness or tingling of the pubis, genitals, and proximal thighs; inability to bear weight without discomfort; severe back pain (retroperitoneal bleed); alterations in neurovascular status of lower extremities (see later discussion of pedal pulse assessment); and clinical manifestations of shock (see Chapter 11). CT scanning of the pelvis helps determine the extent of injury by demonstrating sacroiliac joint disruption, soft tissue trauma, pelvic hematoma, and fractures. Neurovascular assessment of the lower extremities is completed to detect any injury to pelvic blood vessels and nerves. Assessment of underlying organs for injury is indicated especially in high-impact trauma (Eiff, Hatch, & Higgins, 2020d). Trauma to the ureters, urethra, rectum, vagina; abdominal vascular trauma to veins (more common) and arteries; and neurologic trauma, particularly spinal column and cord injury, should be assessed as potential concomitant injuries (Eiff et al., 2020d). See Chapter 67 for discussion of multi trauma and abdominal trauma.

Hemorrhage and shock are two of the most serious consequences that can occur. Bleeding arises mainly from the laceration of veins and arteries by bone fragments and possibly from a torn iliac artery. The peripheral pulses, especially the dorsalis pedis pulses of both lower extremities, are palpated; absence of a pulse may indicate a tear in the iliac artery or one of its branches. Abdominal CT may be performed to detect intra-abdominal hemorrhage. Excessive movement of the pelvis should be avoided, and the patient is handled gently so that bony fragments are not displaced, which may exacerbate bleeding and shock. Fluid replacement and analgesics are administered as needed. Exploratory laparotomy may be

performed to further visualize the peritoneum (Moore & Doty, 2017).

Assessment of adjacent structures must be completed when pelvic injury is suspected.

Numerous classification systems have been used to describe pelvic fractures in relation to anatomy, stability, and mechanism of injury. Some fractures of the pelvis do not disrupt the pelvic ring; others disrupt the ring, which may be rotationally or vertically unstable. The severity of pelvic fractures varies. Long-term complications of pelvic fractures include malunion, nonunion, DVTs, residual gait disturbances, back pain from ligament injury, and dyspareunia and erectile dysfunction (Eiff et al., 2020d).

Stable Pelvic Fractures

Stable fractures of the pelvis (see Fig. 37-18) include fracture of a single pubic or ischial ramus, fracture of ipsilateral pubic and ischial rami, fracture of the pelvic wing of the ilium (Duverney fracture), and fracture of the sacrum or coccyx. If injury results in only a slight widening of the pubic symphysis or the anterior sacroiliac joint and the pelvic ligaments are intact, the disrupted pubic symphysis is likely to heal spontaneously with conservative management. Most fractures of the pelvis heal rapidly because the pelvic bones are mostly cancellous bone, which has a rich blood supply.

Stable pelvic fractures can be treated with a few days of bed rest, analgesics, and progressive mobilization, depending on the level of patient discomfort, which can seriously hamper patient mobility. Fluids, dietary fiber, ankle and leg exercises, anti-embolism stockings to aid venous return, logrolling, deep breathing, early immobilization, and skin care reduce the risk of complications and increase the patient's comfort. The patient with a fractured sacrum is at risk for paralytic ileus; therefore, bowel sounds should be monitored.

The patient with a fracture of the coccyx experiences pain when sitting and when defecating. A donut ring cushion, sitz baths, and stool softeners to ease defecation are beneficial adjuncts to ease pain. As pain resolves, activity is gradually resumed with the use of assistive mobility devices. Early mobilization reduces problems related to immobility

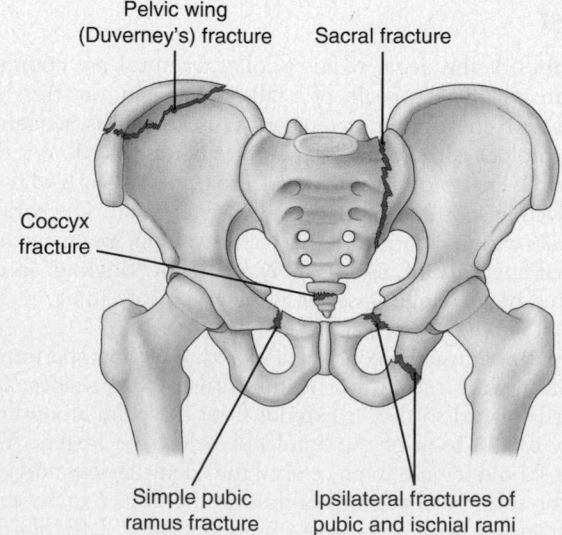

Figure 37-18 • Stable pelvic fractures.

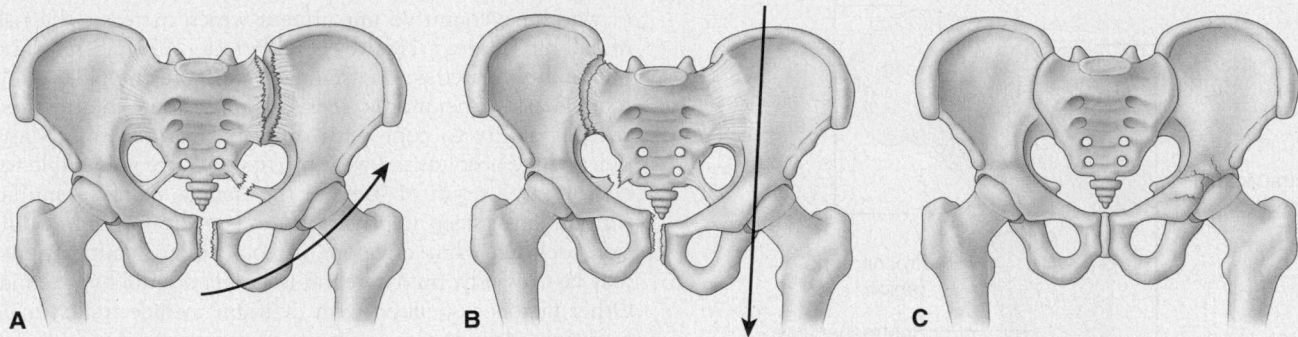

Figure 37-19 • Unstable pelvic fracture. **A.** Rotationally unstable fracture. The symphysis pubis is separated and the anterior sacroiliac, sacrotuberous, and sacrospinous ligaments are disrupted. **B.** Vertically unstable fracture. The hemipelvis is displaced anteriorly and posteriorly through the symphysis pubis, and the sacroiliac joint ligaments are disrupted. **C.** Undisplaced fracture of the acetabulum.

(Eiff et al., 2020d). Most patients should be managed with these conservative measures for at least 2 months until symptoms improve (Foye, 2020).

Unstable Pelvic Fractures

Unstable fractures of the pelvis (see Fig. 37-19) may result in rotational instability (e.g., the "open book" type, in which a separation occurs at the symphysis pubis with sacroiliac ligament disruption), vertical instability, or a combination of both. Lateral or anteroposterior compression of the pelvis produces rotationally unstable pelvic fractures. Vertically unstable pelvic fractures occur when force is exerted on the pelvis vertically, as may occur when the patient falls onto extended legs or is struck from above by a falling object. Vertical shear pelvic fractures involve the anterior and posterior pelvic ring with vertical displacement, usually through the sacroiliac joint. There is generally complete disruption of the posterior sacroiliac, sacrospinous, and sacrotuberous ligaments.

Trauma to soft-tissue, urethral, skeletal, neurovascular, and/or neurologic structures that are contiguous with the pelvis may also occur in unstable pelvic fractures as a result of high-energy mechanisms of injury (e.g., motor vehicle or motorcycle crashes, motor vehicles striking pedestrians, falls from great heights) (Russell & Jarrett, 2020). Immediate treatment in the ED for a patient with an unstable pelvic fracture includes stabilizing the pelvic bones and compressing bleeding vessels with a pelvic girdle, which is an external binding and stabilizing device. If major vessels are lacerated, the bleeding may be stopped through embolization using interventional radiology techniques prior to surgery. Because of the tremendous force necessary to cause an unstable pelvic fracture, hemorrhage and associated head injury are the most common causes of death within 24 hours post arrival to the hospital, and multiple organ dysfunction syndrome and sepsis resulting from infection are the main causes of death after that timeframe (Moore & Doty, 2017). See Chapter 11 for nursing management of the patient in shock. When the patient is hemodynamically stable, treatment generally involves external fixation or ORIF. These measures promote hemostasis, hemodynamic stability, comfort, and early mobilization.

Acetabulum

Acetabular fractures are a type of intra-articular fracture that require a very precise and delicate surgical reduction. The typical mechanism of injury is that an external force drives the femoral shaft into the hip joint, fracturing the acetabulum. This may be caused by high-speed motor vehicle crashes (e.g., knees driven into dashboard, pedals forcibly driven upward into legs) or from falls from heights (Thacker, Tejwani, & Thakkar, 2018). Treatment depends on the pattern of fracture. Stable, nondisplaced fractures may be managed with traction and protective weight bearing so that the affected foot is placed on the floor only for balance. Displaced and unstable acetabular fractures are treated either with closed reduction and skeletal traction or ORIF (Eiff et al., 2020d). Internal fixation permits early non–weight-bearing ambulation and ROM exercise. Complications seen with acetabular fractures include nerve damage, AVN, malunion, heterotopic ossification, and posttraumatic arthritis (Thacker et al., 2018).

Hip

Annually, more than 300,000 adults older than 65 years of age sustain a hip fracture requiring hospitalization; 95% of these result from falls (United Health Foundation, 2019). Hip fracture is a debilitating condition in older adults, particularly women (Veronese & Maggi, 2018). As the U.S. population ages, the annual number of hip fractures is expected to increase. The costs of treatment are high, due to long periods of hospitalization and subsequent rehabilitation. Contributing factors for falls and resultant hip fracture include weak quadriceps muscles, slowed reflexes, osteoporosis, poor vision, diminished balance, general frailty due to age, and conditions that produce decreased cerebral arterial perfusion and cognitive impairment (e.g., transient ischemic attacks, anemia, thromboemboli, cardiovascular disease). In addition to these factors, many medications may cause orthostasis and instability in the older adult. In recognition of this, the American Geriatrics Society periodically publicizes an updated list of *Potentially Inappropriate Medications* (PIM) for Older Adults, and a tool to evaluate medication use for problems in older adults, called the *Beers Criteria*. Medications that can cause orthostasis and instability in older adults, particularly if they take multiple medications (i.e., polypharmacy) include antihypertensive agents, diuretics, beta-blockers, sedatives and hypnotics, neuroleptics and antipsychotics, antidepressants, benzodiazepines, opioid analgesics, and NSAIDs (Fick, Semla, Steinman, et al., 2019; Ming & Zecevic, 2018).

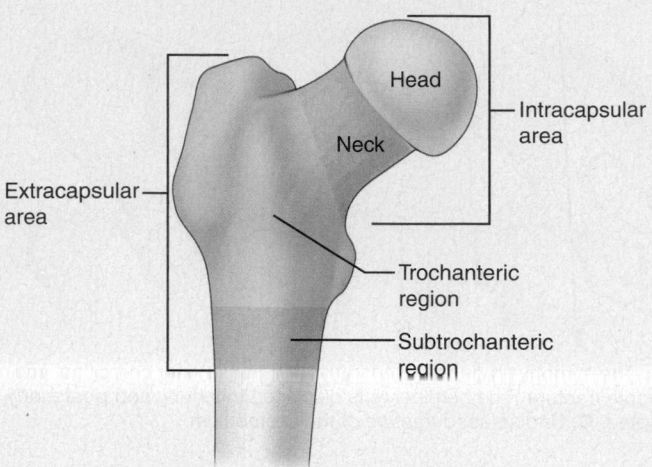

Figure 37-20 • Regions of the proximal femur.

Hip fractures are classified by anatomic location and fracture type. *Extracapsular fractures* (extending from the base of the femoral neck to the area just distal to the lesser trochanter) are fractures of the trochanteric, intertrochanteric, and subtrochanteric region. *Intracapsular fractures* are fractures of the femoral head and neck. Intrascapular fractures have a higher rate of nonunion or malunion and femoral neck fractures may damage the vascular system that supplies blood to the head and the neck of the femur, and the bone may become ischemic (Foster, 2020). For this reason, AVN is common in patients with femoral neck fractures (see Fig. 37-20). *Periprosthetic fractures* are fractures to the regions surrounding prosthetics joints which are increasing due to the growing number patients having previously had total joint replacements (Capone, Congia, Civinini, et al., 2017).

Clinical Manifestations

The patient with a hip fracture will have pain over the outer thigh or in the groin and limited ROM. There will be significant discomfort with any attempt to flex or rotate the hip (Bhatti & Ertl, 2019). With fractures of the femoral neck, the leg may be shortened, adducted, and externally rotated. With most fractures of the femoral neck, the patient cannot move the leg without a significant increase in pain. The patient is most comfortable with the leg slightly flexed in external rotation. Impacted intracapsular femoral neck fractures cause moderate discomfort (even with movement), may allow the patient to bear weight, and may not demonstrate obvious shortening or rotational changes. With extracapsular femoral fractures of the trochanteric or subtrochanteric region, the extremity is significantly shortened, externally rotated to a greater degree than intracapsular fractures, exhibits muscle spasm that resists positioning of the extremity in a neutral position, and has an associated area of ecchymosis. The diagnosis is confirmed by x-ray (Morrison & Siu, 2019).

 Gerontologic Considerations

Populations at higher risk of hip fracture include older adults (particularly women) who have decreased bone density and muscle mass and those with chronic conditions (e.g., endocrine and intestinal disorders) that lead to weakened bones

or who have cognitive impairment which increases the risk of falling (United Health Foundation, 2019). Stress and immobility related to the trauma predispose the older adult to atelectasis, pneumonia, sepsis, VTE, pressure injuries, and reduced ability to cope with other health problems. Many older adults hospitalized with hip fractures are vulnerable for delirium as a result of stress of the trauma, pain, unfamiliar surroundings, sleep deprivation, and medications. In addition, delirium that develops in some older adult patients may be caused by mild cerebral ischemia or mild hypoxemia. Other factors associated with delirium include frailty, malnutrition, dehydration, infectious processes, mood disturbances, and blood loss. In older patients with hip fractures who have dementia, the same factors that may cause delirium may exacerbate their dementia, further complicating recovery and increasing the risk for adverse outcomes (Mosk, Mus, Vroemen, et al., 2017).

To prevent complications, the nurse must assess the older patient for chronic conditions that require close monitoring. Examination of the legs may reveal edema due to heart failure or absence of peripheral pulses from peripheral vascular disease. Similarly, chronic respiratory problems may be present and may contribute to the possible development of atelectasis or pneumonia. Coughing and deep-breathing exercises are encouraged. Frequently, older adults take cardiac, antihypertensive, or respiratory medications that need to be continued. The patient's responses to these medications should be monitored.

Dehydration and poor nutrition may be present. At times, older adults who live alone cannot call for help at the time of injury. A day or two may pass before assistance is provided, and as a result, dehydration and debilitation occur. Nutritional status may have been poor prior to admission, so the nurse should monitor for complications of dehydration and malnutrition (e.g., pressure injuries, etc.). Screening for malnutrition and high-protein nutritional supplementation may be effective in improving outcomes in older adults with hip fractures and should be incorporated into the plan of care (Kramer, Blokhuis, Verdijk, et al., 2019).

Muscle weakness may have initially contributed to the fall and fracture. Bed rest and immobility cause an additional loss of muscle strength unless the nurse encourages the patient to move all joints except the involved hip and knee. Patients are encouraged to use their arms and the overhead trapeze to reposition themselves. This strengthens the arms and shoulders, which facilitates walking with assistive devices.

Medical Management

Surgery is indicated for most patients with hip fracture. Nonoperative management may be considered in some older patients with advanced comorbidities or cognitive impairment; certain types of fractures may be sufficiently stable to benefit from nonoperative treatment (Morrison & Sui, 2019). Buck's extension traction, a type of temporary skin traction, was traditionally applied because it was believed to reduce muscle spasm, to immobilize the extremity, and to relieve pain. However, skin traction is rarely used as a definitive therapy. It may be prescribed as a temporary measure until definitive therapy is achieved (Buckley & Page, 2018; Morrison & Siu, 2019). The goal of surgical treatment for

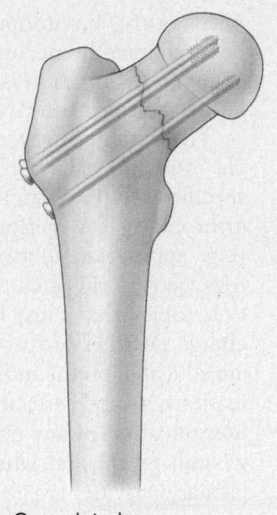

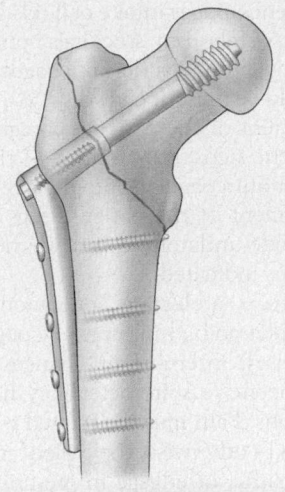

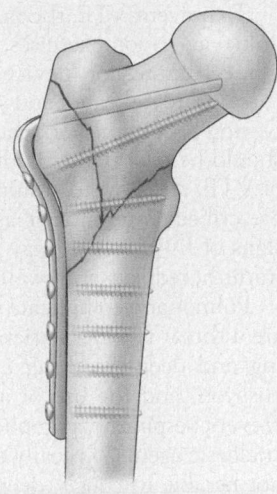

Cannulated screw fixation

Compression hip screw and side plate

Blade plate fixation

Figure 37-21 • Examples of internal fixation for hip fractures. Internal fixation is achieved through the use of screws and plates specifically designed for stability and fixation.

hip fractures is to obtain a satisfactory fixation so that the patient can be mobilized quickly and avoid secondary medical complications. Surgical treatment consists of open or closed reduction of the fracture and internal fixation, hemiarthroplasty (replacement of the femoral head with a prosthesis), or closed reduction with percutaneous stabilization for an intracapsular fracture. Surgical intervention is carried out as soon as possible after injury. The preoperative objective is to ensure that the patient is in as favorable a condition as possible for the surgery. Displaced femoral neck fractures are treated as emergencies, with reduction and internal fixation performed within 24 hours after fracture. The femoral head is often replaced with an orthopedic implant if there is complete disruption of blood flow to the femoral head, which may cause AVN (Lu & Uppal, 2019).

After general or spinal anesthesia, the hip fracture is reduced under fluoroscopic visualization. A stable fracture is usually fixed with nails, a nail and plate combination, multiple pins, or compression screw devices (see Fig. 37-21). The orthopedic surgeon determines the specific fixation device based on the fracture site or sites. Adequate reduction is important for fracture healing—the better the reduction, the better the healing.

Total hip arthroplasty (i.e., replacement of both the femoral head and acetabulum) or hemiarthroplasty (i.e., replacement of only the femoral head) (see Chapter 36) may be used in select patients with intracapsular fractures (Lu & Uppal, 2019).

Nursing Management

The immediate postoperative care for a patient with a hip fracture is similar to that for other patients undergoing major surgery (see Chapter 16). Attention is given to pain management, prevention of secondary medical problems, and early mobilization of the patient so that independent functioning can be restored.

During the first 24 to 48 hours, relief of pain and prevention of complications are important, and continuous neurovascular assessment is essential. The nurse encourages deep breathing and dorsiflexion and plantar flexion exercises every

1 to 2 hours. Thigh-high anti-embolism stockings or pneumatic compression devices are used, and anticoagulants are given as prescribed to prevent the formation of VTE. The nurse administers prescribed analgesic medications and monitors the patient's hydration, nutritional status, and urine output.

Repositioning the Patient

The most comfortable and safest way to turn the patient is to turn to the uninjured side. The standard method involves placing a pillow between the patient's legs to keep the affected leg in an abducted position. Proper alignment and supported abduction are maintained while turning (Hohler, 2018).

Promoting Exercise

The patient is encouraged to exercise as much as possible by means of the overbed trapeze. This device helps strengthen the arms and shoulders in preparation for protected ambulation (e.g., toe touch, partial weight bearing). On the first postoperative day, the patient transfers to a chair with assistance and begins assisted ambulation. The amount of weight bearing that can be permitted depends on the stability of the fracture reduction. The primary provider prescribes the degree of weight bearing. In general, hip flexion and internal rotation restrictions apply only if the patient has had a hemiarthroplasty or total arthroplasty (Kellam, 2020) (see Chapter 36). Physical therapists work with the patient on transfers, ambulation, and the safe use of assistive devices.

The patient can anticipate discharge to home or to an extended-care facility with the use of assistive devices (see Chapter 2). Some modifications in the home may be needed, such as installation of elevated toilet seats and grab bars.

Monitoring and Managing Potential Complications

Neurovascular complications may occur from direct injury or edema in the area that causes compression of nerves and blood vessels. With hip fracture, bleeding into the tissues and edema are expected. Monitoring and documenting the neurovascular status of the affected leg are vital.

To prevent VTE, the nurse encourages intake of fluids and ankle and foot exercises. Anti-embolism stockings, pneumatic compression devices, and prophylactic anticoagulant therapy are indicated and should be prescribed (Forsh, 2019). During hospitalization, the patient or the patient's caregiver should be educated regarding the signs, symptoms, and risks of VTE, and how to administer anticoagulant prophylaxis as prescribed. Intermittent assessment of the patient's legs for signs of DVT, which may include unilateral calf tenderness, warmth, redness, and swelling, is indicated.

Pulmonary complications (e.g., atelectasis, pneumonia) are a threat to older patients undergoing hip surgery. Coughing and deep-breathing exercises, intermittent changes of position, and the use of an incentive spirometer may help prevent respiratory complications. Pain must be treated with analgesic agents, typically opioids; otherwise, the patient may not be able to cough, deep breathe, or engage in prescribed activities. The nurse assesses breath sounds to detect adventitious or diminished sounds.

Skin breakdown is often seen in older patients with hip fracture. Blisters caused by tape are related to the tension of soft tissue edema under a nonelastic tape. An elastic hip wrap dressing or elastic tape applied in a vertical fashion may reduce the incidence of tape blisters. In addition, patients with hip fractures tend to remain in one position and may develop pressure injuries. Proper skin care, especially on the bony prominences, helps to relieve pressure. High-density foam mattress overlays may provide protection by distributing pressure evenly.

Loss of bladder control (incontinence or retention) may occur. If an indwelling catheter is inserted at the time of surgery, it usually is removed within 24 hours of surgery to avoid a hospital-acquired urinary tract infection (Morrison & Siu, 2020). If the patient does not void within 6 hours of catheter removal and/or is expressing symptoms of urinary retention (e.g., abdominal fullness, discomfort), a bladder scan should be performed to determine the volume of urine; intermittent catheterization may be indicated.

Delayed complications of hip fractures include infection, nonunion, and AVN of the femoral head (particularly with femoral neck fractures) (Bhatti & Ertl, 2019). Infection is suspected if the patient complains of constant pain in the hip and has an elevated erythrocyte sedimentation rate.

The nursing management of the older adult patient with a hip fracture is summarized in the Plan of Nursing Care (see Chart 37-8).

Promoting Home, Community-Based, and Transitional Care

 Educating the Patient About Self-Care

Most patients are discharged from the hospital to an inpatient rehabilitation facility. The patient and family members or caregivers are assessed for their readiness to commence activities that promote healing and mobility. The nurse collaborates with other members of the multidisciplinary physiotherapy team (e.g., physical therapist, occupational therapist) to gather baseline data on the patient's anticipated long-term care environment post discharge, whether that is home or a long-term care facility, such as a skilled nursing facility. The patient begins a rehabilitation routine geared to meet the needs of this environment. For instance, if the patient is to be discharged home, and there are stairs in the home, then a goal of rehabilitation is that the patient will be able to get up and down stairs before discharge.

The patient engages in regular exercises to improve muscle tone and balance. The safe use of ambulatory aids, any specific activity restrictions (e.g., hip precautions if total hip arthroplasty was performed), and fall prevention measures (e.g., appropriate footwear, proper lighting, removal of throw rugs, getting rid of clutter) are also vitally important education topics that must be adequately addressed prior to discharge (Walker & Revell, 2019). The patient and caregiver are educated on the indications for any newly prescribed medications, wound care, and the importance of proper nutrition. Identification of any potential complications (e.g., reddened wound, fever) and when and how to contact the patient's primary provider are also important to understand.

Continuing and Transitional Care

Referral for home, community-based, or transitional care is important to enable assessment of the patient's home environment and the adequacy of resources and support of caregivers. Home-based intensive physical therapy improves strength and gait for older adults with hip fractures; accommodations to the home may need to be made to ensure the patient's continuing care, safety, and mobility (Hohler, 2018). During follow-up home health or outpatient clinic visits, the nurse reevaluates the patient's healing process and the continued adequacy of resources and support of caregivers. Based upon these findings, modifications may need to be made. For instance, an older adult spouse may require assistance or respite care. Home health agencies, local area agencies on aging (for older adult patients), and faith community nursing organizations, may be tapped into to provide assistance within the home or with transporting the patient to follow-up outpatient appointments.

Osteoporosis screening of patients who have experienced hip fracture is important for prevention of future fractures. With dual-energy x-ray absorptiometry (DEXA) scan testing, the risk of additional fracture can be predicted. Specific patient education regarding dietary requirements, lifestyle changes, and weight-bearing exercise to promote bone health is needed. Adequate dietary or supplemental vitamin D and calcium supplements are also recommended (Conley, Adib, Adler, et al., 2020). Specific therapeutic interventions need to be initiated to slow bone loss and to build bone mineral density (see Chapter 36).

Femoral Shaft

The femur is the longest and strongest tubular bone in the body; it requires considerable force to break the shaft of a femur in adults. Most femoral fractures occur in young adults who have been involved in motor vehicle crashes or who have fallen from heights. Due to high-energy force, these patients frequently have associated multiple traumatic injuries (Asplund & Mezzanotte, 2019).

The patient presents with an edematous, deformed, painful thigh and cannot move the hip or the knee. The fracture may be transverse, oblique, spiral, or comminuted. Frequently, the

(text continued on page 1191)

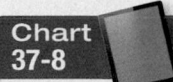

Chart 37-8

PLAN OF NURSING CARE
Care of the Older Adult Patient with a Fractured Hip

NURSING DIAGNOSIS: Acute pain associated with fracture, soft tissue damage, muscle spasm, and surgery
GOAL: Relief of pain

Nursing Interventions	Rationale	Expected Outcomes
1. Assess type and location of patient's pain whenever vital signs are obtained and as needed.	1. Pain is expected after fracture; soft tissue damage and muscle spasm contribute to discomfort; pain is subjective and is best evaluated on a pain scale of 0–10 and through description of characteristics and location, which are important for identifying cause of discomfort and for proposing interventions. Continuing pain may indicate development of neurovascular problems. Pain must be assessed periodically to gauge effectiveness of continuing analgesic therapy.	• Patient describes and rates pain on scale of 0–10. • Expresses confidence in efforts to control pain. • Expresses comfort with position changes. • Expresses comfort when leg is positioned and immobilized. • Minimizes movement of extremity before reduction and fixation. • Uses physical, psychological, and pharmacologic measures to reduce discomfort. • Describes acceptable pain level that does not interfere with ability to participate in rehabilitation activities within 24–48 hours after surgery. • Requests pain medications and uses pain-relief measures early in pain cycle. • Appears comfortable and relaxed. • Moves with increasing comfort as healing progresses.
2. Acknowledge existence of pain; inform patient of available analgesic agents and advocate for preemptive analgesia (e.g., prior to physical therapy); record patient's baseline discomfort.	2. Reduces stress experienced by the patient by communicating concern and availability of help in dealing with pain. Documentation provides baseline data.	
3. Handle the affected extremity gently, supporting it with hands or pillow.	3. Movement of bone fragments is painful; muscle spasms occur with movement; adequate support diminishes soft tissue tension.	
4. Apply Buck's traction if prescribed; advocate for its removal if pain worsens or is not improved; use trochanter roll.	4. Routine use of Buck's traction has not been proven to be effective.	
5. Use pain-modifying strategies.	5. Pain perception can be diminished by distraction and refocusing of attention.	
a. Modify the environment.	a. Interaction with others, distraction, and environmental stimuli may modify pain experiences.	
b. Administer prescribed analgesic agents preemptively and as needed.	b. Analgesics reduce the pain; muscle relaxants may be prescribed to decrease discomfort associated with muscle spasm.	
c. Encourage patient to use pain-relief measures to relieve pain.	c. Mild pain is easier to control than severe pain.	
d. Evaluate patient's response to medications and other pain reduction techniques.	d. Assessment of effectiveness of measures provides basis for future management interventions; early identification of adverse reactions is necessary for corrective measures and care plan modifications.	
e. Consult with primary provider if relief of pain is not obtained.	e. Change in treatment plan may be necessary.	
6. Position for comfort and function.	6. Alignment of body facilitates comfort; positioning for function diminishes stress on musculoskeletal system.	
7. Assist with frequent changes in position.	7. Change of position relieves pressure and associated discomfort.	

NURSING DIAGNOSIS: Impaired mobility associated with fractured hip
GOAL: Achieves pain-free, functional, stable hip

Nursing Interventions	Rationale	Expected Outcomes
1. Maintain neutral positioning of hip.	1. Prevents stress at the site of fixation.	• Patient engages in therapeutic positioning. • Uses pillow between legs when turning. • Assists in position changes; shows increased independence in transfers. • Exercises every 2 hours while awake.
2. Use trochanter roll; roll to uninjured side.	2. Minimizes external rotation.	
3. Place pillow between legs when turning.	3. Supports leg; prevents adduction.	
4. Instruct and assist in position changes and transfers.	4. Encourages patient's active participation while preventing stress on hip fixation.	
5. Instruct in and supervise isometric and quadriceps and gluteal setting exercises.	5. Strengthens muscles needed for walking.	
6. Encourage the use of trapeze.	6. Strengthens shoulder and arm muscles necessary for use of ambulatory aids.	

(continued on page 1188)

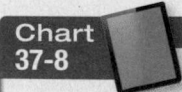

Chart 37-8

PLAN OF NURSING CARE (continued)

Care of the Older Adult Patient with a Fractured Hip

Nursing Interventions	Rationale	Expected Outcomes
7. In consultation with physical therapist, instruct in and supervise progressive safe ambulation within limitations of weight-bearing prescription.	7. Amount of weight bearing depends on the patient's condition, fracture stability, and fixation device; ambulatory aids are used to assist the patient with non–weight-bearing and partial–weight-bearing ambulation.	• Uses trapeze. • Participates in progressive ambulation program. • Actively participates in exercise regimen. • Uses ambulatory aids correctly and safely.
8. Offer encouragement and support exercise regimen.	8. Reconditioning exercises can be uncomfortable and fatiguing; encouragement helps patient adhere to the program.	
9. Instruct in and supervise safe use of ambulatory aids.	9. Prevents injury from unsafe use	

NURSING DIAGNOSIS: Risk for infection associated with surgical incision
GOAL: Maintains asepsis

Nursing Interventions	Rationale	Expected Outcomes
1. Monitor vital signs.	1. Temperature, pulse, and respiration increase in response to infection. (Magnitude of response may be minimal in older adult patients.)	• Patient maintains vital signs within normal range. • Exhibits well-approximated incision without drainage or excessive inflammatory response. • Relates minimal discomfort; demonstrates no hematoma. • Tolerates antibiotics if prescribed; exhibits no evidence of osteomyelitis.
2. Perform aseptic dressing changes.	2. Avoids introducing infectious organisms.	
3. Assess wound appearance and character of drainage.	3. Red, swollen, draining incision is indicative of infection.	
4. Assess report of pain.	4. Pain may be due to wound hematoma, a possible locus of infection, which needs to be surgically evacuated.	
5. Administer preoperative antibiotic as prescribed and postoperative antibiotics if prescribed, and observe for side effects.	5. Administration of 1–3 doses of perioperative antibiotics improves outcomes and reduces the risk of wound infection.	

NURSING DIAGNOSIS: Impaired urination associated with immobility
GOAL: Maintains normal urinary elimination patterns

Nursing Interventions	Rationale	Expected Outcomes
1. Monitor intake and output.	1. Adequate fluid intake ensures hydration; adequate urinary output minimizes urinary stasis.	• Intake and output are adequate; patient exhibits normal voiding patterns. • Demonstrates no evidence of urinary tract infection.
2. Avoid or minimize use of indwelling catheter.	2. Source of bladder infection.	
3. Use bladder scanner if available to confirm urinary stasis or postvoid residual (see Chapter 47, Fig. 47-8); perform intermittent catheterization for urinary retention as prescribed.	3. Empties bladder; reduces urinary tract infections	

NURSING DIAGNOSIS: Stress overload associated with injury, anticipated surgery, and dependence
GOAL: Uses effective coping mechanisms to modify stress

Nursing Interventions	Rationale	Expected Outcomes
1. Encourage patient to express concerns and to discuss the possible impact of fractured hip.	1. Verbalization helps patient deal with problems and feelings. Clarification of thoughts and feelings promotes problem solving.	• Patient describes feelings concerning fractured hip and implications for lifestyle. • Uses available resources and coping mechanisms; develops health promotion strategies. • Uses community resources as needed. • Participates in development of health care plan.
2. Support the use of coping mechanisms. Involve significant others and support services as needed.	2. Coping mechanisms modify disabling effects of stress; sharing concerns lessens the burden and facilitates necessary modification.	
3. Contact social services, if needed.	3. Anxiety may be related to financial or social problems; facilitates management of problems associated with continuing care.	
4. Explain anticipated treatment regimen and routines to facilitate positive attitude in relation to rehabilitation.	4. Understanding of plan of care helps to diminish fears of the unknown.	
5. Encourage patient to participate in planning.	5. Participating in care provides for some control of self and environment.	

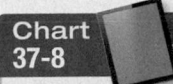

Chart 37-8

PLAN OF NURSING CARE (continued)

Care of the Older Adult Patient with a Fractured Hip

NURSING DIAGNOSIS: Risk for acute confusion associated with age, stress of trauma, unfamiliar surroundings, and medication therapy
GOAL: Remains oriented and participates in decision making

Nursing Interventions	Rationale	Expected Outcomes
1. Assess orientation status.	1. Evaluate presenting orientation of patient; confusion may result from stress of fracture, unfamiliar surroundings, coexisting systemic disease, cerebral ischemia, hypoxemia, or other factors. Baseline data are important for determining change.	• Patient establishes effective communication.
2. Interview family regarding patient's orientation and cognitive abilities before injury.	2. Provides data for evaluation of current findings.	• Demonstrates orientation to time, place, and person. • Participates in self-care activities.
3. Assess patient for auditory and visual deficits.	3. Diminished vision and auditory acuity frequently occur with aging; glasses and hearing aid may increase patient's ability to interact with environment.	• Remains mentally alert. • Does not exhibit episodes of confusion.
a. Assist patient with the use of sensory aids (e.g., glasses, hearing aid)	a. Aids must be in good working order and available for use.	
b. Control environmental distractors.	b. Facilitates communication	
4. Orient to and stabilize environment.	4.	
a. Use orientation activities and aids (e.g., clock, calendar, pictures, introduction of self).	a. Short-term memory may be faulty in the older adult; frequent reorientation helps.	
b. Minimize number of staff working with patient.	b. Consistency of caregivers promotes trust.	
5. Give simple explanations of procedures and plan of care.	5. Promotes understanding and active participation.	
6. Encourage participation in hygiene and nutritional activities.	6. Participation in routine activities promotes orientation and increases awareness of self.	
7. Provide for safety.	7. Mechanism for securing assistance is available to patient; independent activities based on faulty judgment may result in injury.	
a. Keep light on at night.		
b. Have call bell available.		
c. Provide prompt response to requests for assistance.		
8. Assess mental responses to medications, especially sedative and analgesic agents.	8. Older adults tend to be more sensitive to medications; abnormal responses (e.g., hallucinations, depression) may occur.	

COLLABORATIVE PROBLEMS: Hemorrhage; pulmonary complications; peripheral neurovascular dysfunction; venous thromboemboli; pressure injuries associated with surgery and immobility
GOAL: Absence of complications

Nursing Interventions	Rationale	Expected Outcomes
Hemorrhage		
1. Monitor vital signs, observing for shock.	1. Changes in pulse, blood pressure, and respirations may indicate development of shock; blood loss and stress may contribute to development of shock.	• Vital signs are stabilized within normal limits.
2. Consider preinjury blood pressure values and management of coexisting hypertension, if present.	2. Necessary for interpretation of current blood pressure determinations.	• Experiences no excessive or bright red drainage. • Exhibits stable postoperative hemoglobin and hematocrit values.
3. Note character and amount of drainage.	3. Excessive drainage and bright red drainage may indicate active bleeding.	
4. Notify primary provider if patient develops shock or excessive bleeding.	4. Corrective measures need to be instituted.	
5. Note hemoglobin and hematocrit values, and report decreases in values.	5. Anemia due to blood loss may develop; bleeding into tissues after hip fracture may be extensive; blood replacement may be needed.	

(continued on page 1190)

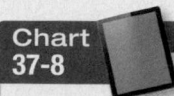

Chart 37-8

PLAN OF NURSING CARE (continued)
Care of the Older Adult Patient with a Fractured Hip

Nursing Interventions	Rationale	Expected Outcomes
Pulmonary Complications		
1. Assess respiratory status: respiratory rate, depth, and duration; breath sounds; sputum. Monitor temperature.	1. Anesthesia and bed rest diminish respiratory effort and cause pooling of respiratory secretions. Adventitious breath sounds, pain on respiration, shortness of breath, blood-tinged sputum, cough may indicate pulmonary dysfunction.	• Vital signs are stabilized within normal limits. • Patient has clear breath sounds. • Breath sounds are present in all fields.
2. Report adventitious and diminished breath sounds and elevated temperature.	2. Elevated temperature in the early postoperative period may be due to atelectasis or pneumonia.	• Exhibits no shortness of breath, chest pain, or elevated temperature.
3. Supervise deep-breathing and coughing exercises. Encourage the use of incentive spirometer if prescribed.	3. Deep-breathing and coughing exercises promote optimal ventilation. Coexisting respiratory conditions diminish lung expansion.	• Arterial oxygen saturation (SaO_2) on room air is within normal limits.
4. Administer oxygen as prescribed.	4. Reduced ventilatory efforts may diminish SaO_2 when patient is breathing room air.	• Performs respiratory exercises; uses incentive spirometer as instructed.
5. Turn and reposition patient at least every 2 hours. Mobilize patient (assist patient out of bed) as soon as possible.	5. Promotes optimal ventilation; diminishes pooling of respiratory secretions.	• Changes position frequently.
6. Ensure adequate hydration.	6. Liquefies respiratory secretions; facilitates expectoration.	• Consumes adequate fluids.
Peripheral Neurovascular Dysfunction		
1. Assess affected extremity for color and temperature.	1. The skin becomes pale and feels cool with decreased tissue perfusion. Venous congestion may cause cyanosis.	• Patient has normal color and the extremity is warm.
2. Assess toes for capillary refill response.	2. After compression of the nail, rapid return of pink color indicates good capillary perfusion.	• Demonstrates normal capillary refill response.
3. Assess affected extremity for edema and swelling.	3. The trauma of surgery will cause swelling; excessive swelling and hematoma formation can compromise circulation and function; edema may be due to coexisting cardiovascular disease.	• Exhibits moderate swelling; tissue not palpably tense. • States pain is tolerable.
4. Elevate affected extremity.	4. Minimizes dependent edema.	• Reports no pain with passive dorsiflexion.
5. Assess for deep, throbbing, unrelenting pain.	5. Surgical pain can be controlled; pain due to neurovascular compromise is refractory to treatment with analgesic medications.	• Reports normal sensations and no paresthesia.
6. Assess for pain on passive flexion of foot.	6. With nerve ischemia, there will be pain on passive stretch.	• Demonstrates normal motor abilities and no paresis or paralysis.
7. Assess for sensations and numbness.	7. Diminished pain and paresthesia may indicate nerve damage. Sensation in web between great and second toe—peroneal nerve; sensation on sole of foot—tibial nerve.	• Has strong and equal pulses bilaterally.
8. Assess ability to move foot and toes.	8. Dorsiflexion of ankle and extension of toes indicate function of peroneal nerve. Plantar flexion of ankle and flexion of toes indicate functioning of tibial nerve.	
9. Assess pedal pulses in both feet.	9. Indicates circulatory status of extremities.	
10. Notify primary provider of changes in neurovascular status.	10. Function of extremity needs to be preserved.	
Venous Thromboemboli		
1. Apply thigh-high anti-embolism stockings and/or sequential compression device as prescribed.	1. Compression aids venous blood return and prevents stasis.	• Wears thigh-high anti-embolism stockings. • Uses sequential compression device.
2. Remove stockings and/or sequential compression device for 20 minutes twice a day, and provide skin care.	2. Skin care is necessary to avoid skin breakdown. Extended removal of stocking or device defeats purpose.	• Experiences no more warmth than usual in skin areas.
3. Assess popliteal, dorsalis pedis, and posterior tibial pulses.	3. Pulses indicate arterial perfusion of extremity. With coexisting arteriosclerotic vascular disease, pulses may be diminished or absent.	• Exhibits no increase in calf circumference.
4. Assess skin temperature of legs.	4. Local inflammation increases local skin temperature.	• Demonstrates no evidence of calf tenderness, warmth, redness, or swelling.
5. Assess calf intermittently for tenderness, warmth, redness, and swelling.	5. Unilateral calf tenderness, warmth, redness, and swelling may indicate deep vein thrombosis.	• Changes position with assistance and supervision.

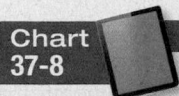

PLAN OF NURSING CARE (continued)
Care of the Older Adult Patient with a Fractured Hip

Nursing Interventions	Rationale	Expected Outcomes
6. Measure calf circumference daily.	6. Increased calf circumference indicates edema or altered perfusion.	• Participates in exercise regimen.
7. Avoid pressure on popliteal blood vessels from appliances or pillows.	7. Compression of blood vessels diminishes blood flow.	• Experiences no chest pain; has lungs clear to auscultation; presents no evidence of pulmonary emboli.
8. Change patient's position and increase activity as prescribed.	8. Activity promotes circulation and diminishes venous stasis.	• Exhibits no signs of dehydration; has normal hematocrit.
9. Supervise ankle exercises hourly while patient is awake.	9. Muscle exercise promotes circulation.	• Maintains normal body temperature.
10. Ensure adequate hydration.	10. Older adults may become dehydrated because of low fluid intake, resulting in hemoconcentration.	
11. Monitor body temperature.	11. Body temperature increases with inflammation (magnitude of response minimal in older adults).	

Pressure Injuries

1. Monitor condition of skin at pressure points (e.g., heels, sacrum, shoulders); inspect heels at least twice a day.	1. Older adults are more prone to skin breakdown at points of pressure because of diminished subcutaneous tissue.	• Patient exhibits no signs of skin breakdown.
2. Reposition patient at least every 2 hours. Avoid skin shearing.	2. Avoids prolonged pressure and trauma to the skin.	• Skin remains intact.
3. Administer skin care, especially to pressure points.	3. Immobility causes pressure at bony prominences; position changes relieve pressure.	• Repositions self frequently.
4. Use pressure redistribution mattress and other protective devices (e.g., heel protectors); support heel off the mattress.	4. Devices minimize pressure on skin at bony prominences.	• Uses protective devices.
5. Institute care according to protocol at first indication of potential skin breakdown.	5. Early interventions prevent tissue destruction and prolonged rehabilitation.	

patient develops shock, because the loss of 1 to 2.5 L of blood into the tissues is common with these fractures (Makhni, Makhni, Swartz, et al., 2017). Types of femoral fractures are illustrated in Figure 37-22.

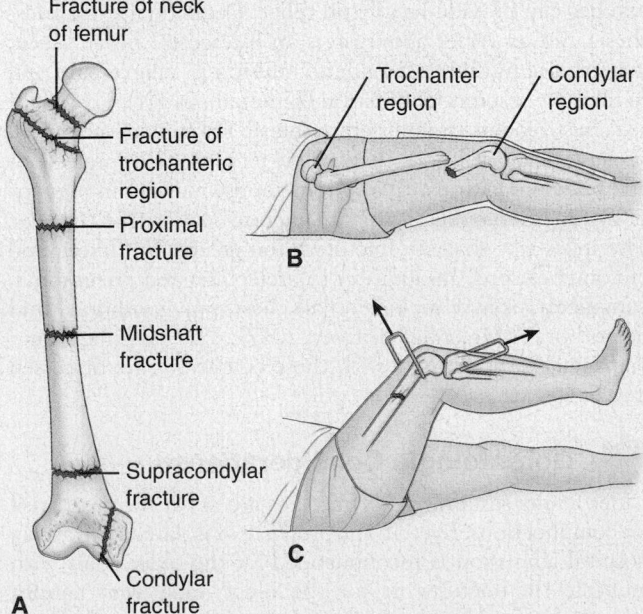

Figure 37-22 • A. Types of femoral fractures. **B.** Example of deformity on admission to hospital. **C.** Adequate reduction is achieved when additional wire is inserted in the lower femoral fragment and vertical lift is secured.

Assessment and Diagnostic Findings

Assessment includes checking the neurovascular status of the extremity, especially circulatory perfusion of the lower leg and foot (popliteal, posterior tibial, and pedal pulses and toe capillary refill time), and comparing with the unaffected leg. A Doppler ultrasound may be indicated to assess blood flow. X-rays are used to confirm the diagnosis and determine the extent of injury (Asplund & Mezzanotte, 2019). Dislocation of the hip and knee may accompany these fractures. Knee effusion suggests ligament damage and possible instability of the knee joint.

Management

Continued neurovascular monitoring and documentation are important. The fracture is immobilized so that additional soft tissue damage does not occur. Generally, skeletal traction (see Fig. 37-22B,C) or splinting is used to reduce the fracture to anatomic alignment which helps reduce pain and prevent hematoma formation (Keany & McKeever, 2019). IV opioid analgesic agents (e.g., morphine) are typically given to treat pain (Asplund & Mezzanotte, 2019).

Early fracture stabilization decreases morbidity and mortality; therefore, internal fixation usually is carried out as soon as the patient is physiologically stable. Intramedullary locking nail devices are typically used. Internal fixation permits early mobilization, which is associated with improved outcomes and recovery (Keany & McKeever, 2019).

Open femoral fractures require immediate and extensive irrigation and débridement in the operating suite (see previous discussion of treatment for open fractures). Tetanus toxoid (unless given within 5 years) and antibiotics with staphylococcal coverage and good tissue penetration are often administered. Depending on needs for continued débridement, intramedullary nailing may be delayed (Keany & McKeever, 2019).

Postoperatively, to preserve muscle strength, the patient is instructed to exercise the hip and the lower leg, foot, and toes on a regular basis. Active muscle movement enhances healing by increasing blood supply and electrical potentials at the fracture site. Prescribed weight-bearing limits are based on the type and location of the fracture and treatment approach. Physical therapy includes ROM and strengthening exercises, safe use of assistive devices, and gait training (Makhni et al., 2017).

A common complication after fracture of the femoral shaft is restriction of knee motion. Active and passive knee exercises begin as soon as possible, depending on the stability of the fracture and knee ligaments. Other complications in the immediate postoperative period can include hemorrhage, acute compartment syndrome, and neurovascular compromise. Long-term complications may include malrotation, malunion, delayed union, and nonunion (Keany & McKeever, 2019).

Tibia and Fibula

Fractures of the tibia and fibula often occur in association with each other and tend to result from a direct blow, falls with the foot in a flexed position, or a violent twisting motion. Most of these fractures tend to be more distal than proximal; distal fractures may extend into the ankle joint (e.g., distal fractures of the tibia that extend into the joint are collectively referred to as pilon fractures). The patient may present with severe pain, deformity or instability of the leg, obvious hematoma, swelling, and the inability to walk or bear weight on the leg (Norvell & Steele, 2017).

Assessment and Diagnostic Findings

The peroneal nerve is assessed; if damaged, the patient cannot dorsiflex the great toe and has diminished sensation in the first web space. The tibial artery is assessed for damage by evaluating pulses, skin temperature, and color and by testing the capillary refill response. The affected leg and ankle are compared with the unaffected leg and ankle. X-rays are indicated to determine the location, type, and extent of the fracture (Fields, 2020).

Management

Most closed, nondisplaced fractures that do not involve the ankle joint (e.g., extra-articular fractures) are treated with closed reduction and immobilization in a non–weight-bearing short leg cast or brace. The leg is elevated to control edema. Weight-bearing status varies and depends on the type of fracture. Activity decreases edema and increases circulation. Fracture healing, based upon clinical assessment and x-ray findings, takes about 10 to 14 weeks; it takes about 6 to 9 months until full function is restored (Eiff, Hatch, & Higgins, 2020e).

Displaced, open, or articular fractures may be treated with skeletal traction, internal fixation with intramedullary nails or plates and screws, or external fixation. External support may be used with internal fixation. Hip, foot, and knee exercises are encouraged within the limits of the immobilizing device. Partial weight bearing is begun when prescribed and is progressed as the fracture heals, which is dependent on the extent of injury (Eiff et al., 2020e).

As with any fracture, continued neurovascular evaluation is important. The development of acute compartment syndrome requires prompt recognition and communication to the primary provider. Other complications to monitor for include fat emboli, nonunion, delayed union, infection, impaired wound edge healing, long-term calf atrophy, sport limitation, and osteoarthritis (Fields, 2020).

Rib

Rib fractures are some of the most common thoracic injuries; they occur frequently in adults of all ages, typically from blunt trauma such as motor vehicle crashes or falls, and usually result in no impairment of function. They are typically diagnosed based on clinical presentation and confirmed with anteroposterior (AP) and lateral chest x-rays, CT scan (to rule out suspected thoracic or abdominal injury) or ultrasound (Eiff, Hatch, & Higgins, 2020f). Because these fractures cause pain with respiratory effort, the patient tends to decrease respiratory excursions and refrains from coughing. As a result, tracheobronchial secretions are not mobilized, aeration of the lung is diminished, and a predisposition to atelectasis and pneumonia results. The mainstay of treatment is pain control to decrease chest wall splinting and subsequent atelectasis. To help the patient cough and take deep breaths and use an incentive spirometer, the nurse may splint the chest with their hands, or may educate the patient on using a pillow to temporarily splint the affected site. Regularly scheduled analgesics such as acetaminophen in combination with an NSAID may be prescribed to provide analgesic relief. Topical anesthetic patches can provide local pain relief. Occasionally, an anesthesia care provider administers an intercostal nerve block, intrapleural infusion, or epidural infusion to relieve pain and to improve respiratory function (Eiff et al., 2020f).

Chest binders to immobilize the rib fracture are not used, because decreased chest expansion may result in atelectasis and pneumonia. Incentive spirometer use may aid in prevention of these complications. The fracture heals within 6 weeks. The more ribs that are fractured, the greater the likelihood of complications. In addition to atelectasis and pneumonia, complications may include a flail chest, pneumothorax, and hemothorax (Melendez & Doty, 2017). The assessment and management of patients with these conditions are discussed in Chapter 19.

Gerontologic Considerations

Older adults sustaining rib fractures are at an increased risk for complications. Even in the presence of isolated rib trauma, hospital admission is recommended for the older adult with multiple rib fractures or for the older adult who cannot effectively cough and mobilize sputum (Melendez & Doty, 2017). Careful monitoring of respiratory status and encouraging the patient to mobilize early, and, for the patient on bed rest, encouraging turning, coughing, and deep breathing and use of an incentive spirometer, can prevent respiratory complications.

Thoracolumbar Spine

Fractures of the thoracolumbar spine may involve the vertebral body, the laminae and articulating processes, and the spinous processes or transverse processes. The T12 to L2 area of the spine, called the *thoracolumbar junction*, is the second most commonly injured region of the spinal column; 90% of all thoracolumbar spine injuries occur at this junction. Fractures generally result from indirect trauma caused by excessive loading, sudden muscle contraction, or excessive motion beyond physiologic limits. Osteoporosis contributes to vertebral body collapse (compression fracture) and accounts for 50% to 70% of all thoracolumbar fractures (Kaji & Hockberger, 2018).

Stable spinal fractures are caused by flexion, extension, lateral bending, or vertical loading. The anterior structural column (vertebral bodies and discs) or the posterior structural column (neural arch, articular processes, ligaments) is disrupted. Unstable fractures occur with fracture dislocations and involve disruption of both anterior and posterior structural columns.

The patient with a spinal fracture presents with acute tenderness, swelling, paravertebral muscle spasm, and change in the normal curves or in the gap between spinous processes. Pain is greater with moving, coughing, or weight bearing. Thoracolumbar fractures can also present with lower extremity paresis, lower extremity or saddle anesthesia (i.e., loss of sensation to the perineum), or loss of bladder or rectal continence (Kaji & Hockberger, 2018). Immobilization is essential until initial assessments have determined if there is any spinal cord injury and whether the fracture is stable or unstable. X-rays are initially indicated to confirm the fracture(s), and CT scans or MRI studies are then indicated to precisely determine the extent of injury and spinal cord involvement (Vinas, 2018). If spinal cord injury with neurologic deficit does occur, it usually requires immediate surgery (laminectomy with spinal fusion) to decompress the spinal cord.

Stable spinal fractures are treated conservatively with limited bed rest. Analgesic medications are prescribed for pain relief. A spinal brace or plastic thoraco-lumbar-sacral orthosis is applied for support during progressive ambulation and resumption of activities (Kaji & Hockberger, 2018).

The patient with an unstable fracture is treated with bed rest, possibly with the use of a special turning device or bed to maintain spinal alignment. Within 24 hours after fracture, open reduction, decompression, and fixation with spinal fusion and instrument stabilization are usually accomplished. Neurologic status is monitored closely during the preoperative and postoperative periods. Postoperatively, the patient may be cared for on the turning device or in a bed with a firm mattress. Progressive ambulation is begun a few days after surgery, with the patient using a molded lumbar or thoracolumbar orthosis for approximately 3 months. Patient education emphasizes good posture, good body mechanics, and, after healing is sufficient, back-strengthening exercises. X-rays with flexion and extension views are taken to monitor the healing process at 6 weeks, 3 months, 6 months postoperatively; a CT scan can provide a clearer evaluation (Vinas, 2018). See Chapter 63 for discussion of spinal cord injury.

Sports-Related Musculoskeletal Injuries

Sports-related injuries are common. Table 37-1 displays common musculoskeletal sports injuries, their mechanisms of injury, assessment findings, and acute care management.

Management

Patients who have experienced sports-related musculoskeletal injuries are often highly motivated to return to their previous level of activity. Adherence to restriction of activities and gradual resumption of activities need to be reinforced. Injured athletes are at risk for reinjury and require follow-up and monitoring. With recurrence of symptoms, athletes need to diminish their level and intensity of activity to a comfortable level. The time required to recover from a sports-related injury can be as short as a few days or as long as 12 weeks, depending on the severity of the injury. The patient should be pain free with good ROM before returning to play (Norris, 2020).

Sports-related musculoskeletal injuries can often be prevented by using proper equipment and by effectively training and conditioning the body. Specific training needs to be tailored to the person and the sport. Stretching, maintaining hydration, and proper nutrition aid in injury prevention (Norris, 2020).

Occupation-Related Musculoskeletal Disorders

According to the U.S. Department of Labor, work-related musculoskeletal disorders (also called *ergonomic injuries*) are injuries or illnesses of the muscles, nerves, tendons, joints, cartilage, and spinal discs that occur because of exposure to work-related risks. In 2018, sprains, strains, or tears caused the highest incidence of days away from work among private industry workers in all occupations; soreness and pain accounted for the next highest incidence, with a smaller incidence related to fractures, cuts, lacerations, contusions, and bruises (U.S. Department of Labor, Bureau of Labor Statistics, 2019).

Occupation-Related Musculoskeletal Disorders in Nursing Personnel

Nurses working in all settings face workplace hazards performing their routines duties. The nursing profession is consistently ranked among the top 10 occupations that are most involved in occupation-related injuries and illnesses that result in lost days of work (Dressner & Kissinger, 2018). Nurses experience a higher-than-average incidence of musculoskeletal disorders that result from overexertion and strain due to heavy workloads and unsafe patient handling techniques. Organizations like the American Nurses Association (ANA) and the National Association of Orthopaedic Nurses (NAON) recognize the seriousness of work-related musculoskeletal disorders among nurses, and advocates for the implementation of evidence-based methods for safe patient handling and movement tasks whenever feasible (see Resources).

Amputation

Amputation is the removal of a body part by a surgical procedure or trauma. The majority of amputations are often consequences of vascular disease, especially from diabetes

TABLE 37-1 Common Musculoskeletal Sports Injuries

Anatomic Area	Mechanism of Injury	Assessment Findings	Sports Activity	Acute Management
Clavicle fracture	Fall on shoulder or outstretched arm Direct blow to the clavicle	Crepitus Holds arm closely to body Unable to raise affected arm above head Can feel movement of both ends of clavicle	Football Rugby Hockey Wrestling Gymnastics	Sling or shoulder immobilizer Ice NSAIDs
Dislocated shoulder	*Anterior:* Some combination of hyper-extension, external rotation, and abduction Anterior blow to shoulder *Posterior:* Fall on flexed and adducted arm Direct axial load to humerus	Pain Lack of motion May feel empty shoulder socket Uneven posture in comparison to other shoulder Affected arm appears longer Abduction limited	Rugby Hockey Wrestling Skiing	Closed reduction Immobilizer Pendulum exercises
Dislocated elbow	Falling on a hand with a flexed elbow Elbow overextended	Intense pain Edema Limited motion Deformity Ecchymosis	Football Gymnastics Squash Wrestling Cycling Skiing	Immobilization Ice ROM exercises
Wrist sprain or fracture	Falling on an outstretched arm	Pain Edema Ecchymosis Deformity Limited motion	Skating Hockey Wrestling Skiing Soccer Handball Horseback riding	Ice Elevation Immobilization Gentle ROM for 4–6 wks (for sprain only)
Knee sprain	Twisting injury that produces incomplete tear of ligaments and capsule around the joint	Pain Limited motion Edema Ecchymosis Tenderness over joint Joint appears stable	Basketball Football High jump	Ice Elevation Compression wrap Active ROM exercises Isometric exercises May immobilize
Knee strain	Sudden forced motion causing muscle to be stretched beyond normal capacity	Pain Limited motion Pain aggravated by activity	Soccer Swimming Skiing	Ice Elevation Rest Gradual return to activities
Meniscal tears of knee	Sharp, sudden pivot Direct blow to knee Forced internal rotation Wear from repetitive squatting or climbing Torsional weight-bearing force	Edema *Medial tear:* Pain occurs with hyperflexion, hyperextension, and turning in of knee with knee flexed. *Lateral tear:* Pain occurs with hyperflexion and hyper-extension and internal rotation of foot with knee flexed. *Displaced fragment:* Inability to extend knee; "locked" Positive McMurray sign[a]	Hockey Basketball Football	*Conservative:* RICE Exercising of quadriceps and hamstrings Resistive exercising NSAIDs Physical therapy *Surgical:* Arthroscopy
Ankle sprain	Foot is twisted, causing stretch-ing or tearing of ligaments.	Pain Edema Limited motion Ecchymosis	Tennis Basketball Football Skating	Immobilization in cast or brace Ice Elevation Rest
Ankle strain	Sudden forced motion, stretch-ing muscles beyond normal capacity	*Acute:* Severe pain *Chronic:* Achy pain	Running All ball sports	Immobilization in cast or brace Ice Elevation Rest
Ankle fracture	Inward turning on sole of foot and front of foot Supination with internal rotation Pronation with external rotation	Pain Edema Deformity Inability to bear weight	Contact sports Tennis Basketball	Ice Elevation Cast (4–6 wks) Surgery if fracture is displaced or unstable
Metatarsal stress fracture	Occurs with repeated loading of bone; often in an uncondi-tioned extremity	Forefoot pain that progressively worsens with activity Minimal or no forefoot swelling	Running Dance Skating	Rest Stop sports-related activity for 6 wks Ice Weight bearing as indicated

[a]McMurray sign—manipulation of tibia while knee flexed produces audible "click."
NSAIDs, nonsteroidal anti-inflammatory drugs; RICE, rest, ice, compression, elevation; ROM, range of motion.
Reprinted with permission from the National Association of Orthopedic Nurses (NAON). (2013). *Core curriculum for orthopaedic nursing* (7th ed.). Chicago, IL: NAON.

(see Chapters 26 and 46); trauma is the second most common indication. African Americans are at heightened risk of having amputations. Approximately 2 million individuals in the United States are living with some type of limb loss; by 2050, there will be an estimated 3.6 million (AAOS, 2019e).

An amputation is performed to control pain or disease process, to improve function, and to save or improve the patient's quality of life. If the health care team communicates a positive attitude, the patient adjusts to the amputation more readily and actively participates in the rehabilitative plan, learning how to modify activities and how to use assistive devices for ADLs and mobility.

Level of Amputation

The level of amputation is performed at the most distal point that will heal successfully and should take into account the ability of the patient to achieve a successful rehabilitation. The site and extent of amputation is determined by circulation in the area (and whether or not necrosis is present), the degree of tissue loss and viability of the tissues, functional usefulness (i.e., meets the requirements for the use of a prosthesis) and the presence of infection (Guest, Marshall, & Stansby, 2019).

The circulatory status of the limb is evaluated through physical examination and diagnostic studies. Muscle and skin perfusion are important for healing. Doppler flow studies with duplex ultrasound, segmental pressure determinations, and transcutaneous oxygen measurements of the limb are valuable diagnostic aids. Angiography is performed if revascularization is considered an option.

The objective of surgery is to conserve as much limb length as needed to preserve function and possibly to achieve a good prosthetic fit. Preservation of knee and elbow joints is desirable. Figure 37-23 shows the levels at which a limb may

be amputated. Most amputations involving limbs eventually can be fitted with a prosthesis.

The amputation of toes and portions of the foot can cause changes in gait and balance. A Syme amputation (modified ankle disarticulation amputation) is performed most frequently for extensive foot trauma and aims to produce a durable residual limb that can withstand full weight bearing. Below-knee amputation (BKA) is preferred to above-knee amputation (AKA) because of the importance of the knee joint and the energy requirements for walking. A knee **disarticulation** (e.g., amputation through the joint) is most successful with a young, active patient who can develop precise control of the prosthesis. When AKAs are performed, all possible length is preserved, muscles are stabilized and shaped, and hip contractures are prevented to maximize ambulatory potential (Guest et al., 2019). Most people who have a hip disarticulation amputation must rely on a wheelchair for mobility.

Upper limb amputations are performed with the goal of preserving maximal functional length. The prosthesis is fitted early to ensure maximum function.

A "staged" amputation may be used when gangrene and infection exist. Initially, a débriding amputation in the form of a guillotine amputation (i.e., transfemoral, transtibial) is performed to remove the infected and necrotic tissue. Once the infected limb is removed, systemic antibiotics are administered, and the wound is left open and allowed to drain. In a few days, after the infection has been controlled and the patient's condition has stabilized, a definitive amputation with skin closure is performed; a drain may be left in place (Kalapatapu, 2019).

Complications

Complications that may occur with amputation include hemorrhage, infection, skin breakdown, phantom limb pain, and joint contracture. Because major blood vessels have been severed, hemorrhage may occur. Infection is a risk with all surgical procedures. The risk of infection increases with contaminated wounds after traumatic amputation. Antibiotic prophylaxis prior to surgery is recommended. Skin irritation caused by the prosthesis may result in skin breakdown. **Phantom limb pain** (pain perceived in the amputated section) is caused by the severing of peripheral nerves. Joint contracture is caused by positioning and a protective flexion withdrawal pattern associated with pain and muscle imbalance (Kalapatapu, 2019). Associated comorbidities such as ischemic disease and psychological disorders such as depression and anxiety must also be monitored closely as they can contribute to further complications and chronic limb pain (Chung & Yoneda, 2020).

Medical Management

The objective of treatment is to achieve healing of the amputation wound, the result being a nontender residual limb with healthy skin for prosthetic use. Healing is enhanced by gentle handling of the residual limb, control of residual limb edema and pain, and the use of aseptic technique in wound care to avoid infection (Kalapatapu, 2019).

The primary postoperative dressings to support soft tissues, control pain and edema, and prevent joint contractures include nonremovable rigid dressings, removable rigid dressings, soft dressings (elastic and crepe), and weight-bearing

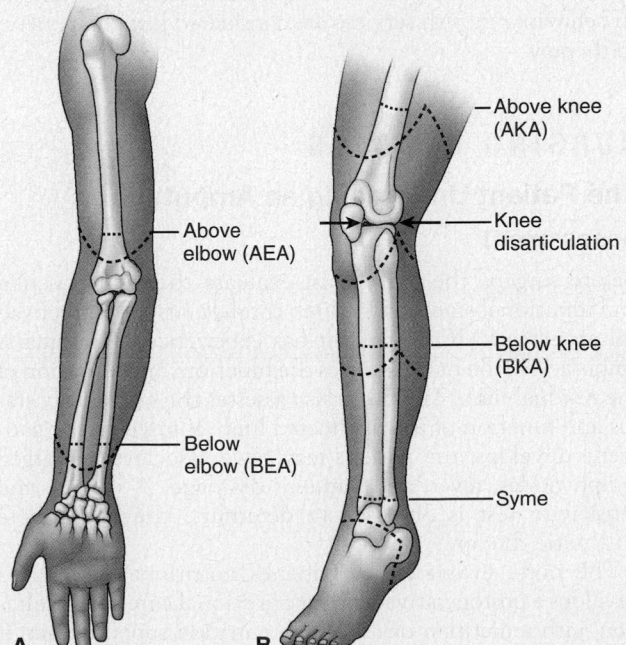

Figure 37-23 • Level of amputation is determined by circulatory adequacy, type of prosthesis, function of the part, and muscle balance. **A.** Level of amputation of upper limb. **B.** Level of amputation of lower limb.

immediate postoperative prostheses (Reichmann, Stevens, Rheinstein, et al., 2018).

The type of dressing used in patients with lower limb amputations varies. A reduction in edema, pain, contractures, healing time, time to prosthetic fitting, and injury due to falls has been shown for certain types of amputations (e.g., transtibial) with the use of removable rigid dressings as compared to soft dressings (Reichmann et al., 2018). However, a soft dressing with or without compression may be used if there is significant wound drainage, frequent inspection of the residual limb is required, and the patient has poor skin integrity (Kwah, Webb, Go, et al., 2019). An immobilizing splint may be incorporated in the soft dressing. Good clinical judgment over which dressing to use should consider the risks and benefits for each individual patient. A wound drain can be placed to remove excess blood and drainage from the surgical site (Schreiber, 2017). Staples or sutures maintain closure at the operative site and are typically removed approximately 3 weeks postoperatively.

Rehabilitation

The multidisciplinary rehabilitation team (patient, nurse, primary provider, social worker, physical therapist, occupational therapist, psychologist, prosthetist, vocational rehabilitation worker) helps the patient achieve the highest possible level of function and participation in life activities (see Fig. 37-24). Prosthetic clinics, amputee support programs, and peer visits (face-to-face, telephone, digital) for patients with a limb amputation facilitate the rehabilitation process, both physically and psychosocially (Reichmann & Bartman, 2018).

Patients who undergo amputation need support as they grieve the loss and change in body image. Their reactions can include anger, bitterness, and hostility. Psychological issues

(e.g., denial, anxiety, avoidance) may be influenced by the type of support the patient receives from the rehabilitation team, the effectiveness of pain management, and by how quickly ADLs and the use of the prosthesis are learned. Providing education about the full options and capabilities available with the various prosthetic devices, as well as the recovery of walking capacity, if appropriate, can give the patient a sense of control over the resulting disability and promote independence (Luza, Ferreira, Minsky, et al., 2019).

Patients undergoing amputation because of severe trauma are usually young and healthy. These patients heal rapidly and are physically able to participate in a vigorous rehabilitation program. Because the amputation is the result of an injury, the patient needs holistic multidisciplinary support from the beginning in order to accept the sudden change in body image and to deal with the stresses of hospitalization, long-term rehabilitation, and modification of lifestyle (Noblet, Lineham, Wiper, et al., 2019).

 Veterans Considerations

Within the past two decades, numerous U.S. military personnel have sustained conflict-related amputations from exposure to blasts from improvised explosive devices. The Department of Veterans Affairs/Department of Defense (VA/DoD) follows its own set of periodically updated evidence-based guidelines to ensure that veterans with amputations consistently receive quality care (VA/DoD, 2017). In addition, so that the complex needs of these young, previously healthy men and women may be met, the U.S. Army instituted both a specialized treatment center for patients with amputations and a database registry to facilitate long-term treatment and management. Treatment for these injured service members addresses not only physical rehabilitation needs, but also ways to optimize psychosocial functioning (VA/DoD, 2017). A multidisciplinary rehabilitation team with referral to behavioral health services are considered key components to therapy.

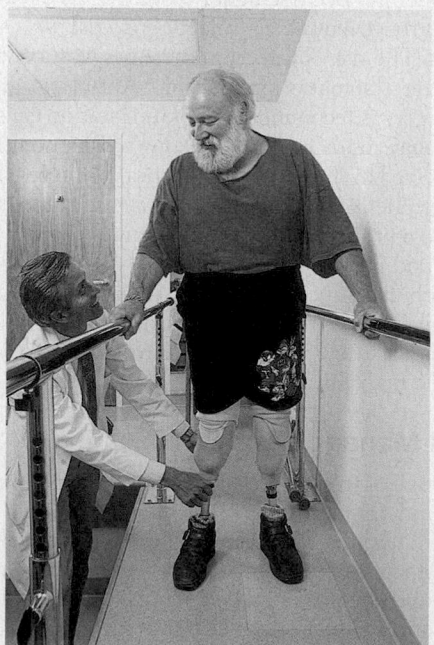

Figure 37-24 • Many patients with amputations receive prostheses soon after surgery and begin learning how to use them with the help and support of the rehabilitation team, which includes nurses, primary providers, physical therapists, and others.

NURSING PROCESS

The Patient Undergoing an Amputation

Assessment

Before surgery, the nurse must evaluate the neurovascular and functional status of the limb through history and physical assessment. If the patient has experienced a traumatic amputation, the nurse assesses the function and condition of the residual limb. The nurse also assesses the circulatory status and function of the unaffected limb. If infection or gangrene develops, the patient may have associated enlarged lymph nodes, fever, and purulent drainage. A culture and sensitivity test is obtained to determine the appropriate antibiotic therapy.

The nurse evaluates the patient's nutritional status and develops a postoperative plan for nutritional care in consultation with a dietitian or metabolic nutrition support team, if indicated. A diet with adequate protein and vitamins is essential to promote wound healing. Additional calories may be necessary due to the energy required for transfers and ADLs when using a prosthesis (Schreiber, 2017).

Any concurrent health problems (e.g., dehydration, anemia, cardiac insufficiency, chronic respiratory problems, diabetes) need to be identified and treated so that the patient is in the best possible condition to withstand the surgical procedure. The use of corticosteroids, anticoagulants, vasoconstrictors, or vasodilators may influence management and prolong or delay wound healing.

The nurse assesses the patient's psychological status. Evaluation of the patient's emotional reaction to amputation is important. Grief responses to permanent alterations in body image, function, and mobility are likely. Professional counseling and available support services can help the patient cope in the aftermath of amputation surgery.

Diagnosis

NURSING DIAGNOSES

Based on the assessment data, major nursing diagnoses may include the following:

- Acute pain associated with amputation
- Impaired skin integrity associated with surgical amputation
- Disturbed body image associated with amputation
- Grief and/or risk for dysfunctional grief associated with loss of body part and resulting disability
- Impaired ability to perform hygiene, impaired ability to dress, impaired self feeding, or impaired self toileting associated with amputation
- Impaired mobility associated with amputation

COLLABORATIVE PROBLEMS/POTENTIAL COMPLICATIONS

Potential complications may include the following:

- Hemorrhage
- Infection
- Skin breakdown

Planning and Goals

The major goals of the patient may include relief of pain, including phantom limb pain, wound healing, acceptance of altered body image, resolution of the grieving process, independence in self-care, restoration of physical mobility, and absence of complications.

Nursing Interventions

RELIEVING PAIN

Pain may be incisional or may be caused by inflammation, infection, pressure on a bony prominence, hematoma, or phantom limb pain. Muscle spasms may add to the patient's discomfort. Surgical pain can be effectively controlled with opioid analgesics that may be accompanied with evacuation of a hematoma or accumulated fluid. Changing the patient's position or placing a light sandbag on the residual limb to counteract the muscle spasm may improve the patient's level of comfort. Evaluation of the patient's pain and responses to interventions is an important component of pain management.

Many patients who have amputations begin to experience phantom limb pain soon after surgery. It is a complex pain condition that has been reported in 60% to 80% of patients with amputations (Hall, Abd-Elsayed, & Eldabe, 2019). The patient reports pain in the missing limb as if it were still present. The pain is described as if the amputated limb feels crushed, cramped, or twisted in an abnormal position; this pain is sometimes accompanied by numbness, tingling, or sensations of burning or electric shock. Phantom limb pain occurs intermittently and unpredictably; episodes of pain may last seconds or hours. When a patient describes phantom pains or sensations, the nurse acknowledges these feelings as real and encourages the patient to verbalize when in pain so that effective treatment may be given. Phantom limb pain typically diminishes over time for most patients, with episodes gradually becoming less frequent and of lesser duration; however, some patients continue to experience phantom limb pain as long as 2 years after the amputation.

The pathogenesis of the phantom limb pain phenomenon is believed to involve changes in both peripheral and central neuronal mechanisms. Disruption in neuronal pathways are thought to cause neuroplastic changes that in turn result in changes in cortical representation, or the proprioceptive, tactile, and visual image of body parts as perceived by the cerebral cortex (Hall et al., 2019). Preoperative epidural analgesia (preemptive analgesia) may reduce the incidence and severity of phantom limb pain over the long term (Guest et al., 2019). Perioperatively, the patient may be managed with acetaminophen, NSAIDs, anticonvulsants (gabapentin), opioids, and NMDA receptor antagonists (ketamine infusion). Epidural and perineural catheter analgesia may be used during and immediately after the operation (Hall et al., 2019). Opioid analgesics may be effective in relieving postoperative pain. In addition, beta-blockers may relieve dull, burning discomfort; anticonvulsants control stabbing and cramping pain; and tricyclic antidepressants may not only alleviate phantom limb pain but may also be prescribed to improve mood and coping ability. Therapies that may be used as adjuncts to pharmacologic treatments include mirror therapy (i.e., the patient views and moves the unaffected limb in a mirror that is in a box or blocking the view of the affected limb), massage, biofeedback, acupuncture, repositioning, TENS, guided imagery, virtual reality, and neuromodulation (Hall et al., 2019; Herrador Colmenero, Perez Marmol, Marti-Garcia, et al., 2018). The nurse monitors the effectiveness of these treatments and collaborates with the multidisciplinary team to advocate for optimal pain control. Successful pain management following amputation promotes positive patient outcomes and lowers the cost of care (VA/DoD, 2017).

PROMOTING WOUND HEALING

Following amputation, the incision should be examined daily for signs of infection. The residual limb must be handled gently and should be measured once every 8 to 12 hours postoperatively to assess for edema formation. Neurovascular assessments (including the most distal pulse, movement, sensation, skin temperature) are also performed at these intervals, and compared to the unaffected limb to ensure that there is adequate blood supply. The dressing is changed as prescribed and whenever soiled, using aseptic technique to prevent infection and possible osteomyelitis (Kalapatapu, 2019). Drains are maintained and can be discontinued when the volume in the drain reservoir is minimal.

If the rigid or soft dressing inadvertently comes off, the nurse must immediately wrap the residual limb with an elastic compression bandage. If this is not done, excessive edema will develop in a short time, resulting in a delay in rehabilitation. The nurse notifies the surgeon if the dressing comes off so that another one can be applied promptly.

Chart 37-9 — NURSING RESEARCH PROFILE
Patients' Postamputation Viewing of Selves in the Mirror

Freysteinson, W., Thomas, L., Sebastian-Deutsch, A., et al. (2017). A study of the amputee experience of viewing self in the mirror. *Rehabilitation Nursing, 37*(1), 22–32.

Purpose

Approximately two million individuals are living with the loss of a limb in the United States, and this incidence is expected to nearly double by 2050. The amputation of a limb is a traumatic event and affects an individual physically and psychologically. A visible disfigurement such as an amputation can lead to distortions in body image, depression, and low self-esteem as well as nonacceptance of a prosthesis in the rehabilitation phase. For a patient with an amputation, one of the most shocking and anxiety producing situations that can negatively impact the perception of body image is the mirror-viewing experience (viewing one's self in a mirror after the amputation of a limb). However, the research evidence addressing this topic is limited. The purpose of this study was to describe the experience of viewing of self in a mirror after an amputation and the perceptions of what nurses should know about clinical mirror interventions.

Design

A hermeneutic phenomenologic design was used. Snowball sampling was used to recruit 17 participants who consented to be in the study. In order to be included in the study, participants had to be at least 18 years of age, have an amputation of an upper or lower limb, and have an ability to speak, read, and understand English. Five focus groups of 3 to 6 participants, lasting approximately 60 to 90 minutes, were conducted in a research rehabilitative hospital setting. Key questions asked included: Describe an experience about one of the first times you saw yourself in a mirror after amputation; what were your feelings and emotions? What was your self-talk before/during/after looking in the mirror? How would you describe the journey of viewing self in the mirror

the first time to what it is like to view self in the mirror now, and what might each of the stages of this journey be called? The question which provided the most information about participant perceptions of potential mirror interventions was: What would you say is really important for health care providers to know about mirrors?

Findings

The interpretation of data revealed that the act of viewing self in a mirror at any time after an amputation had three key elements: decision, seeing self, and consent. The trajectory of mirror shock, mirror anguish, recognizing self, and accepting a new normal are key themes and adds to the existing literature. Reasons to decide to view self in the mirror included curiosity, appearance, care of incision or residual limb, and gait/posture assessment. The experience of viewing self in the mirror after an amputation changes over time, and each person's mirror trajectory begins when initially making the decision of viewing self in a mirror after the amputation. Participants recommend that the nurse facilitate the initial mirror viewing experience and use the mirror as a tool to assess for skin breakdown and to help correct gait and balance.

Nursing Implications

The viewing of self in the mirror after an amputation can be a very difficult and emotional experience. Nurses are in a unique position to show support and understanding of the situation by facilitating the initial mirror viewing of the patient's amputation in a proper and controlled setting. When nurses are present during the initial mirror viewing process, the patient realizes that they are not alone in this experience and that the nurse understands what they are going through. There appears to be a lack of mirrors in health care settings; therefore, it is recommended that rooms in private hospitals and rehabilitation facilities have more small and full-length mirrors.

Application of consistent pressure to the residual limb reduces edema formation and helps to shape the residual limb so that it may fit a prosthetic. The wound should be assessed to ensure that it is healing and that there are no signs of infection (e.g., redness, purulent drainage), which can also hamper optimal prosthetic fit. After the incision is healed and the limb is shaped appropriately, the patient is instructed how to care for the residual limb (VA/DoD, 2017).

ENHANCING BODY IMAGE

Amputation is a procedure that alters the patient's body image. The nurse who has established a trusting relationship with the patient is better able to communicate acceptance of the patient who has experienced an amputation. The nurse encourages the patient to look at, feel, and care for the residual limb. Nursing research findings suggest that the nurse be present with patients who view themselves in mirrors after an amputation (Freysteinson, Thomas, Sebastian-Deutsch, et al., 2017) (see Nursing Research Profile: Chart 37-9). It is important to identify the patient's strengths and resources to facilitate rehabilitation. The nurse helps the patient regain the previous level of independent functioning. The patient who is accepted as a whole person is more readily able to resume responsibility for self-care; self-concept improves, and body image changes are accepted. Even with highly motivated patients, this process may take months.

 Concept Mastery Alert

The nurse can provide the following interventions to foster a positive self-image: encouraging the patient to care for the residual limb, allowing the expression of grief, and promoting utilization of available resources.

HELPING THE PATIENT TO RESOLVE GRIEVING

The loss of a limb (or part of one) may come as a shock even if the patient was prepared preoperatively. The patient's behavior (e.g., crying, withdrawal, apathy, anger) and expressed feelings (e.g., depression, fear, helplessness) reveal how the patient is coping with the loss and working through the grieving process.

The nurse creates an accepting and supportive atmosphere in which the patient and family are encouraged to express and share their feelings and work through the grief process. The support from family and friends promotes the patient's acceptance of the loss. The nurse helps the patient deal with immediate needs and become oriented to realistic rehabilitation goals and future independent functioning. Psychological needs can be further addressed by mental health professionals; referrals for support services and spiritual advisors (e.g., pastoral care) may be appropriate (Myers, VanDamme, & Pasquina, 2018).

PROMOTING INDEPENDENT SELF-CARE

Amputation affects the patient's ability to provide adequate self-care. The patient is encouraged to be an active participant in self-care. The patient needs time to accomplish these tasks and must not be rushed. Practicing an activity with consistent, supportive supervision in a relaxed environment enables the patient to learn self-care skills. The patient and the nurse need to maintain positive attitudes and minimize fatigue and frustration during the learning process.

Independence in dressing, toileting, and bathing depends on balance, transfer abilities, and physiologic tolerance of the activities. The nurse works with the physical therapist and occupational therapist to educate and supervise the patient in these self-care activities.

The patient with an upper limb amputation has self-care deficits in feeding, bathing, and dressing. Assistance is provided only as needed; the nurse encourages the patient to learn to do these tasks, using assistive feeding and dressing aids when needed. The nurse, therapists, and prosthetist work with the patient to achieve maximum independence.

ASSISTING THE PATIENT TO ACHIEVE PHYSICAL MOBILITY

Assisting the Patient with a Lower Limb Amputation. Proper positioning of the residual limb prevents the development of hip or knee joint contracture in the patient with a lower limb amputation. The limb should be elevated for 24 hours after amputation to promote venous return and decrease edema (Schreiber, 2017). After this period, elevation, abduction, external rotation, and flexion of the lower limb are to be avoided. The patient is encouraged not to sit for long periods of time to prevent flexion contracture or with the affected extremity dangling or in a dependent position to prevent edema (Schreiber, 2017).

The residual limb should not be placed on a pillow because a flexion contracture of the hip may result. The nurse encourages the patient to turn from side to side and to assume a prone position, 20 to 30 minutes several times per day to stretch the flexor muscles and to prevent flexion contracture of the hip. The legs should remain close together to prevent an abduction deformity. The nurse encourages the patient to use assistive devices to more readily perform self-care activities and to identify what home modifications, if any, should be made to perform these activities in the home environment.

Postoperative ROM exercises are started early because contracture deformities develop rapidly. ROM exercises include hip and knee exercises for patients with BKAs and hip exercises for patients with AKAs. It is essential that the patient understands the importance of exercising the residual limb as well as the unaffected extremities for joint mobility and strengthening (Schreiber, 2017).

The upper limbs, trunk, and abdominal muscles are exercised and strengthened. The extensor muscles in the arm and the depressor muscles in the shoulder play an important part in crutch walking. The patient uses an overbed trapeze to change position and strengthen the biceps. The patient may flex and extend the arms while holding weights. Doing push-ups while seated strengthens the triceps muscles. Exercises (such as hyperextension of the residual limb), conducted under the supervision of the physical therapist, also aid in strengthening muscles as well as increasing circulation, reducing edema, and preventing atrophy.

Strength and endurance are assessed, and activities are increased gradually to prevent fatigue. As the patient progresses to independent use of the wheelchair, the use of ambulatory aids, or ambulation with a prosthesis, the nurse emphasizes safety considerations. Environmental barriers (e.g., steps, inclines, doors, throw rugs, wet surfaces) are identified, and methods of managing them are implemented. It is important to anticipate, identify, and manage problems associated with the use of the mobility aids. Proper education in using assistive devices will help prevent these problems.

Amputation of the leg changes the center of gravity; therefore, the patient may need to practice position changes (e.g., standing from sitting, standing on one foot). The patient is taught transfer techniques early and is reminded to maintain good posture when getting out of bed. A well-fitting shoe with a nonskid sole should be worn. During position changes, the patient should be guarded and stabilized with a transfer belt at the waist to prevent falling.

As soon as possible, the patient with a lower limb amputation is assisted to stand between parallel bars to allow extension of the temporary prosthesis to the floor with minimal weight bearing. How soon after surgery the patient is allowed to bear full body weight on the prosthesis depends on the patient's physical status and wound healing. As endurance increases and balance is achieved, ambulation is started with the use of parallel bars or crutches. The patient learns to use a normal gait, with the residual limb moving back and forth while walking with the crutches. To prevent a permanent flexion deformity from occurring, the residual limb should *not* be held up in a flexed position (Kalapatapu, 2019).

Assisting the Patient with an Upper Limb Amputation. Because a patient who has had an upper limb amputated uses both shoulders to operate the prosthesis, the muscles of both shoulders are exercised. A patient with an above-elbow amputation or shoulder disarticulation is likely to develop a postural abnormality caused by loss of the weight of the amputated limb. Postural exercises are helpful.

The patient with an upper limb amputation is taught how to carry out ADLs with one arm. The patient is started on one-handed self-care activities as soon as possible. The use of a temporary prosthesis is encouraged. The patient who learns to use the prosthesis soon after the amputation is less dependent on one-handed self-care activities.

The patient with an upper limb amputation may wear a cotton T-shirt to prevent contact between the skin and shoulder harness and to promote absorption of perspiration. The prosthetist advises about cleaning the washable portions of the harness. Periodically, the prosthesis is inspected for potential problems.

Preparing the Patient for a Prosthesis. The residual limb must be conditioned and shaped into a conical form to permit accurate fit, maximum comfort, and function of the prosthetic device. Elastic bandages, an elastic residual limb shrinker, or an air splint is used to condition and shape the residual limb. The nurse educates the patient or a member of the family about the correct method of bandaging.

Bandaging supports the soft tissue and minimizes the formation of edema while the residual limb is in a dependent position. The bandage is applied in such a manner that the remaining muscles required to operate the prosthesis are as firm as possible. An improperly applied elastic bandage contributes to circulatory problems and a poorly shaped residual limb.

Effective preprosthetic care is important to ensure proper fitting of the prosthesis. The major problems that can delay prosthetic fitting during this period are flexion deformities, nonshrinkage of the residual limb, and abduction deformities of the hip.

The primary provider usually prescribes activities to condition or "toughen" the residual limb in preparation for a prosthesis. The patient begins by pushing the residual limb into a soft pillow, then into a firmer pillow, and finally against a hard surface. The patient is taught to massage the residual limb to mobilize the surgical incision site, decrease tenderness, and improve vascularity. Massage is usually started once healing has occurred and is first performed by the physical therapist. Skin inspection and preventive care are taught; mirrors may be used to visualize the skin on the residual limb (Rossbach, 2017).

The prosthesis socket is custom-shaped to the residual limb by the prosthetist. Prostheses are designed for specific activity levels and patient abilities. Types of prostheses include those that are hydraulic, pneumatic, biofeedback controlled, myoelectrically controlled, and synchronized. Adjustments of the prosthetic socket are made by the prosthetist to accommodate the residual limb changes that occur during the first 6 months to 1 year after surgery.

Assisting the Patient Who Is Not a Candidate for a Prosthesis. Some patients with amputations are not candidates for a prosthesis due to preexisting factors (e.g., nonambulatory before amputation, dementia, AKA). If the use of a prosthesis is not possible, the patient is educated in safe use of a wheelchair to achieve independence. A special wheelchair designed for a patient who has had an amputation is recommended. Because of the decreased weight in the front, a regular wheelchair may tip backward when the patient sits in it. In wheelchairs designed for patients who have had amputations, the rear axle is set back about 5 cm (2 inches) to compensate for the change in weight distribution.

MONITORING AND MANAGING POTENTIAL COMPLICATIONS

After any surgery, efforts are made to reestablish homeostasis and to prevent complications related to surgery, anesthesia, and immobility. The nurse assesses body systems (e.g., respiratory, hematologic, gastrointestinal, genitourinary, skin) for problems associated with immobility (e.g., atelectasis, pneumonia, DVT, PE, anorexia, constipation, urinary stasis, pressure injuries).

Massive hemorrhage due to a loosened suture is a potentially life-threatening problem. The nurse monitors the patient for any signs or symptoms of bleeding and monitors the patient's vital signs and suction drainage.

◤ Quality and Safety Nursing Alert

Immediate postoperative bleeding may develop slowly or may take the form of massive hemorrhage resulting from a loosened suture. A large tourniquet should be in plain sight at the patient's bedside so that if severe bleeding occurs, it can be applied to the residual limb to control the hemorrhage. The nurse immediately notifies the surgeon in the event of excessive bleeding.

Infection is a common complication of amputation. Patients who have undergone traumatic amputation have contaminated wounds. The nurse administers prophylactic antibiotics as prescribed. The nurse must monitor the incision, dressing, and drainage for indications of infection (e.g., change in color, odor, or consistency of drainage; increasing discomfort). The nurse also assesses for systemic indicators of infection (e.g., elevated temperature, leukocytosis with an increase of more than 10% bands on the differential) and promptly reports indications of infection to the surgeon.

Skin breakdown may result from immobilization or pressure from various sources. The prosthesis may cause pressure areas to develop. The nurse and the patient assess for breaks in the skin. Careful skin hygiene is essential to prevent skin irritation, infection, and breakdown. The healed residual limb is washed and dried (gently) at least twice daily. The skin is inspected for persistent erythema, pressure areas, dermatitis, and blisters. If they are present, the prosthesis should not be worn until the complication is evaluated and treated in order to prevent further skin breakdown. Usually, a residual limb sock is worn to absorb perspiration and to prevent direct contact between the skin and the prosthetic socket. The sock is changed daily and must fit smoothly to prevent irritation caused by wrinkles. The socket of the prosthesis is washed with a mild detergent, rinsed, and dried thoroughly with a clean cloth. It must be thoroughly dry before the prosthesis is applied (Rossbach, 2017).

PROMOTING HOME, COMMUNITY-BASED, AND TRANSITIONAL CARE

Educating the Patient About Self-Care. Before the patient is discharged to home or to a rehabilitation facility, the patient and family are encouraged to become active participants in care. They participate in care of the skin, residual limb, and prosthesis as appropriate. The patient receives ongoing education and practice sessions to learn to transfer and to use mobility aids and other assistive devices safely. The nurse explains the signs and symptoms of complications that must be reported to the primary provider (see Chart 37-10).

Continuing and Transitional Care. After the patient has achieved physiologic homeostasis and has demonstrated achievement of major health care goals, rehabilitation continues either in a rehabilitation facility or at home. An inpatient rehabilitation facility may be indicated; these facilities have been shown to improve quality of life, ambulation and patient confidence, mobility, and prosthesis use with less associated pain (VA/DoD, 2017). In any case, continued support and evaluation by the home health nurse is essential.

The patient's home environment should be assessed prior to discharge. Modifications are made to ensure the patient's continuing care, safety, and mobility. An overnight or weekend experience at home may be tried to identify problems that were not identified on the assessment visit. Physical therapy and occupational therapy may continue in the home or on an outpatient basis. Transportation to continuing health care appointments must be arranged. The social service department of the hospital or the home health agency may be of great assistance in securing personal assistance and transportation services.

Chart 37-10

HOME CARE CHECKLIST
The Patient with an Amputation

At the completion of education, the patient and/or caregiver will be able to:

- Name the procedure that was performed and identify any permanent changes in anatomic structure or function as well as changes in ADLs, IADLs, roles, relationships, and spirituality.
- Identify modification of home environment, interventions, and strategies (e.g., durable medical equipment, adaptive equipment, ADL assistance), used in safely adapting to changes in structure or function and promote effective recovery and rehabilitation.
  - Identify professionals and community agencies to help with transition to home.
- Describe ongoing postoperative therapeutic regimen, including diet and activities to perform (e.g., exercises) and to limit or avoid (e.g., lifting weights, driving a car, contact sports).
  - Describe care of residual limb and conditioning for prosthesis.
  - Consume a healthy diet to promote wound healing.
  - Participate in rehabilitation program to regain functional independence, promote circulation, maintain the health of unaffected muscles and those muscles now needed for safe transfer, mobility, etc.
  - If indicated, demonstrate safe use of mobility aid, assistive device, and transfer technique.
  - Observe prescribed weight-bearing and activity limits.
- State the name, dose, side effects, frequency, and schedule for all prescribed therapeutic and prophylactic medications (e.g., antibiotics, anticoagulants, analgesic agents).

- State how to obtain medical supplies and carry out dressing changes, wound care, and other prescribed regimens.
- Describe approaches to controlling pain (e.g., take analgesics as prescribed; use nonpharmacologic interventions).
- State indicators of complications to report promptly to primary provider (e.g., uncontrolled pain; signs of local or systemic infection; residual limb skin breakdown).
- Relate how to reach primary provider with questions or complications.
- State time and date of follow-up appointments, therapy, and testing.
- Identify community resources for peer and caregiver/family support:
  - Identify sources of support (e.g., friends, relatives, faith community).
  - Identify the contact details for support services for patients and their caregivers/families.
- Identify the need for health promotion, disease prevention, and screening activities.

Resources

See Chapter 2, Chart 2-6, for additional information related to durable medical equipment, adaptive equipment, and mobility skills.

ADLs, activities of daily living; IADLs, instrumental activities of daily living.

During follow-up health visits, the nurse evaluates the patient's physical and psychosocial adjustment. Periodic preventive health assessments are necessary. An older adult spouse may not be able to provide the assistance required if needed at home. Modifications in the plan of care are made on the basis of such findings. Often, the patient and family find involvement in a postamputation support group and peer support programs to be of value; here, they can share problems, solutions, and resources (Reichmann & Bartman, 2018). Talking with those who have successfully dealt with a similar problem may help the patient develop a satisfactory solution.

Because patients and their family members and health care providers tend to focus on the most obvious needs and issues, the nurse reminds the patient and family about the importance of continuing health promotion and screening practices, such as regular physical examinations and diagnostic screening tests. Accessible facilities for screening, health care, and exercise are identified. Patients are instructed about their importance and are referred to appropriate health care providers.

Evaluation

Expected patient outcomes may include:

1. Experiences no pain, including phantom limb pain
   a. Appears relaxed
   b. Verbalizes comfort
   c. Uses measures to increase comfort and mitigate pain
   d. Participates in self-care and rehabilitative activities
   e. Reports diminished phantom sensations
2. Achieves wound healing
   a. Controls residual limb edema
   b. Exhibits healed, nontender, nonadherent scar
   c. Demonstrates residual limb care
3. Demonstrates improved body image and effective coping
   a. Acknowledges change in body image
   b. Participates in self-care activities
   c. Demonstrates increasing independence
   d. Projects self as a whole person
   e. Resumes role-related responsibilities
   f. Reestablishes social contacts
   g. Demonstrates confidence in abilities
4. Exhibits resolution of grieving
5. Expresses grief
6. Works through feelings with family, friends, and health care professionals
7. Focuses on future functioning
8. Utilizes available support
9. Achieves independent self-care
   a. Asks for assistance when needed
   b. Uses aids and assistive devices to facilitate self-care
   c. Verbalizes satisfaction with abilities to perform ADLs
10. Achieves maximum independent mobility
    a. Avoids positions contributing to contracture development
    b. Demonstrates full active ROM
    c. Maintains balance when sitting and transferring
    d. Increases strength and endurance

e. Demonstrates safe transferring technique
f. Achieves functional use of prosthesis
g. Overcomes environmental barriers to mobility
h. Uses community services and resources as needed
11. Exhibits absence of complications of hemorrhage, infection, or skin breakdown
   a. Does not experience excessive bleeding
   b. Maintains normal blood values
   c. Is free of local or systemic signs of infection
   d. Repositions self frequently
   e. Is free of pressure-related problems
   f. Reports any skin discomfort and irritations promptly

CRITICAL THINKING EXERCISES

1 `ebp` A 74-year-old woman was admitted to the hospital after she fell down a flight of stairs and fractured her right hip. She is now 48 hours postoperative after a right ORIF to that hip. She is moderately overweight and has a history of smoking. She has been reluctant to get out of bed to ambulate and complains that her intermittent compression devices are uncomfortable, and she does not want to wear them. What is the strength of the evidence that supports the use of compression devices postoperatively for patients who have had ORIF post-hip fractures? What are her risks if she does not wear these devices postoperatively? How will you respond to the patient's request to not wear these devices?

2 `ipc` You are caring for a 30-year-old female who was involved in a motor vehicle crash and had a traumatic amputation of her left upper extremity at the scene. She is 7 days postoperative and is now complaining of phantom limb sensation and severe pain in the missing limb. She describes the quality of the pain as crushing, burning, and "electric shock like" and it spreads from her missing fingers to the length of her arm. She is becoming anxious with the severity of the pain and does not understand what is happening to her. Describe the assessments and interventions as you prioritize care for this patient. Identify the multidisciplinary collaboration necessary to provide a comprehensive treatment plan for this patient to promote the best outcomes.

3 `qg` You have been assigned to care for a 36-year-old male admitted to the inpatient orthopedic unit following a motorcycle crash. He had an external fixation device applied 8 hours ago for a fracture of the left tibia. During shift report, the nurse reports that the patient has been complaining of throbbing pain and paresthesia in his left lower leg that has not been alleviated despite administration of prescription opioid pain medication. Upon your initial assessment, you note that the patient's left calf is very swollen, shiny, and taut. Describe the additional physical assessments that should be conducted for this patient. What is your priority nursing diagnosis and plan of care?

REFERENCES

*Asterisk indicates nursing research.

Books

Alexandre, V., & Hodax, J. D. (2017). Splinting and casting techniques. In J. Hodax, A. Eltorai, & A. Daniels (Eds.). *The orthopedic consult survival guide.* Cham, Switzerland: Springer International Publishing.

Arora, S., Erosa, S., & Danesh, H. (2019). Physical medicine and rehabilitation. In Y. Khelemsky, A. Malhotra, & K. Gritsenko (Eds.). *Academic pain medicine: A practical guide to rotations, fellowship, and beyond.* Cham, Switzerland: Springer International Publishing.

Chinai, S. A., Walker, L., Rebesco, M. R., et al. (2019). Immobilization. In D. Purcell, S. A. Chinai, B. R. Allen, & M. Davenport (Eds.). *Emergency orthopedics handbook.* Cham, Switzerland: Springer International Publishing.

Cox, P. (2017). Knee. In N. Connor (Ed.). *National Association of Orthopaedic Nurses: Orthopaedic surgery manual* (3rd ed.). Chicago, IL: National Association of Orthopaedic Nurses.

Dorsey, N. (2020). Humerus fractures. In M. P. Eiff, R. L. Hatch, & M. K. Higgins (Eds.). *Fracture management for primary care and emergency medicine* (4th ed.). Philadelphia, PA: Elsevier.

Eiff, M. P., Hatch, R. L., & Higgins, M. K. (2020a). General principles of fracture care. In M. P. Eiff, R. L. Hatch, & M. K. Higgins (Eds.). *Fracture management for primary care and emergency medicine* (4th ed.). Philadelphia, PA: Elsevier.

Eiff, M. P., Hatch, R. L., & Higgins, M. K. (2020b). Clavicle and scapula fractures. In M. P. Eiff, R. L. Hatch, & M. K. Higgins (Eds.). *Fracture management for primary care and emergency medicine* (4th ed.). Philadelphia, PA: Elsevier.

Eiff, M. P., Hatch, R. L., & Higgins, M. K. (2020c). Elbow fractures. In M. P. Eiff, R. L. Hatch, & M. K. Higgins (Eds.). *Fracture management for primary care and emergency medicine* (4th ed.). Philadelphia, PA: Elsevier.

Eiff, M. P., Hatch, R. L., & Higgins, M. K. (2020d). Femur and pelvis fractures. In M. P. Eiff, R. L. Hatch, & M. K. Higgins (Eds.). *Fracture management for primary care and emergency medicine* (4th ed.). Philadelphia, PA: Elsevier.

Eiff, M. P., Hatch, R. L., & Higgins, M. K. (2020e). Patellar, tibial, and fibular fractures. In M. P. Eiff, R. L. Hatch, & M. K. Higgins (Eds.). *Fracture management for primary care and emergency medicine* (4th ed.). Philadelphia, PA: Elsevier.

Eiff, M. P., Hatch, R. L., & Higgins, M. K. (2020f). Rib fractures. In M. P. Eiff, R. L. Hatch, & M. K. Higgins (Eds.). *Fracture management for primary care and emergency medicine* (4th ed.). Philadelphia, PA: Elsevier.

Eubanks, J. E., & Chien, G. C. (2019). Casting and splinting. In A. Abd-Elsayed (Ed.). *Pain.* Cham, Switzerland: Springer International Publishing.

Ferla, F., Ciravegna, A., Mariani, A., et al. (2019). Acute compartment syndrome. In P. Aseni, L. De Carlis, A. Mazzola, & A. M. Grande (Eds.). *Operative techniques and recent advances in acute care and emergency surgery.* Cham, Switzerland: Springer International Publishing.

Gasiorowski, K. (2017). External fixation. In N. Connor (Ed.). *National Association of Orthopaedic Nurses: Orthopaedic surgery manual* (3rd ed.). Chicago, IL: National Association of Orthopaedic Nurses.

Hadeed, A., Werntz, R. L., & Varacallo, M. (2019). External fixation principles and overview. In *StatPearls [Internet].* Treasure Island, FL: StatPearls Publishing.

Hall, N., Abd-Elsayed, A., & Eldabe, S. (2019). Phantom limb pain. In A. Abd-Elsayed (Ed.). *Pain.* Cham, Switzerland: Springer International Publishing.

Iyer, K. M. (2019). Anatomy of bone, fracture, and fracture healing. In K. M. Iyer & W. S. Khan (Eds.). *General principles of orthopedics and trauma.* Cham, Switzerland: Springer.

Karlsson, J., Westin, O., Carmont, M., et al. (2019). Achilles tendon ruptures. In G. L. Canata, P. d'Hooghe, K. J. Hunt, et al. (Eds.). *Sports injuries of the foot and ankle.* Berlin, Heidelberg: Springer.

Mains, C. (2017). Orthopaedic aspects of the operating room. In N. Connor (Ed.). *National Association of Orthopaedic Nurses: Orthopaedic surgery manual* (3rd ed.). Chicago, IL: National Association of Orthopaedic Nurses.

Makhni, M. C., Makhni, E. C., Swart, E. F., et al. (2017). Femoral shaft fracture. In: M. Makhni, E. Makhni, E. Swart, et al. (Eds.). *Orthopedic emergencies.* Cham, Switzerland: Springer International Publishing.

Michaudet, C. (2020). Radius and ulna fractures. In M. P. Eiff, R. L. Hatch, & M. K. Higgins (Eds.). *Fracture management for primary care and emergency medicine* (4th ed.). Philadelphia, PA: Elsevier.

Mittal, S., & Mittal, R. (2019). Intra-articular fractures: Principles of fixation. In M. N. Doran, J. Karlsson, J. Nyland, et al. (Eds.). *Intraarticular fractures.* Cham, Switzerland: Springer International Publishing.

Myers, K. P., VanDamme, T., & Pasquina, P. F. (2018). Rehabilitation of the blast injury casualty with amputation. In J. Galante, M. Martin, C. Rodriguez, et al. (Eds.). *Managing dismounted complex blast injuries in military & civilian settings.* Cham, Switzerland: Springer.

National Association of Orthopedic Nurses (NAON). (2013). *Core curriculum for orthopaedic nursing* (7th ed.). Chicago, IL: NAON.

Nemeth, B. A., Halanski, M. A., & Noonan, K. J. (2020). Cast and splint immobilization. In P. M. Waters, D. L. Skaggs, & J. M. Flynn (Eds.). *Rockwood and Wilkins' fractures in children.* Philadelphia, PA: Wolters Kluwer.

Norris, T. L. (2020). *Porth's essentials of pathophysiology* (5th ed.). Philadelphia, PA: Wolters Kluwer.

Osman, K., Gabr, A., & Haddad, F. S. (2019). Bone healing. In N. K. Paschos, & G. Bentley (Eds.). *General orthopaedics and basic science.* Cham, Switzerland: Springer International Publishing.

Stanton-Hicks, M. (2018). *Complex regional pain syndrome.* In J. Cheng & R. Rosenquist (Eds.). *Fundamentals of pain medicine.* Cham, Switzerland: Springer International Publishing.

Weinlein, J. C. (2017). Delayed union and nonunion of fractures. In F. M. Azar, J. H. Beaty, & S. T. Canale (Eds.). *Campbell's operative orthopedics* (13th ed.). Philadelphia, PA: Elsevier.

Whittle, A. P. (2017a). General principles of fracture management. In F. M. Azar, J. H. Beaty, & S. T. Canale (Eds.). *Campbell's operative orthopedics* (13th ed.). Philadelphia, PA: Elsevier.

Whittle, A. P. (2017b). Malunited fractures. In F. M. Azar, J. H. Beaty, & S. T. Canale (Eds.). *Campbell's operative orthopedics* (13th ed.). Philadelphia, PA: Elsevier.

Journals and Electronic Documents

Abdi, S. (2020). Complex regional pain syndrome in adults: Treatment, prognosis, and prevention. *UpToDate.* Retrieved on 1/13/2020 at: www.uptodate.com/contents/complex-regional-pain-syndrome-in-adults-treatment-prognosis-and-prevention

Adib-Hajbaghery, M., & Mokhtari, R. (2018). Quality of Care before, during, and after casting: A cross-sectional study. *Archives of Trauma Research, 7*(4), 155–160.

Agranoff, A. B. (2019). Medial collateral and lateral collateral ligament injury. *Medscape.* Retrieved on 1/9/2020 at: emedicine.medscape.com/article/307959-overview

American Academy of Orthopaedic Surgeons (AAOS). (2018). *Management of acute compartment syndrome clinical practice guideline.* Retrieved on 12/24/2019 at: www.aaos.org/globalassets/quality-and-practice-resources/dod/acs-cpg-final_approval-version-10-11-19.pdf

American Academy of Orthopaedic Surgeons (AAOS). (2019a). *Muscle contusion (bruise).* Retrieved on 12/14/2019 at: orthoinfo.aaos.org/en/diseases–conditions/muscle-contusion-bruise

American Academy of Orthopaedic Surgeons (AAOS). (2019b). *Management of rotator cuff injuries clinical practice guideline.* Retrieved on 12/23/2019 at: www.orthoguidelines.org/topic?id=1027

American Academy of Orthopaedic Surgeons (AAOS). (2019c). *Cast care.* Retrieved on 1/14/2020 at: orthoinfo.aaos.org/globalassets/pdfs/cast-care.pdf

American Academy of Orthopaedic Surgeons (AAOS). (2019d). *Internal fixation for fractures.* Retrieved on 1/29/2020 at: orthoinfo.aaos.org/en/treatment/internal-fixation-for-fractures/

American Academy of Orthopaedic Surgeons (AAOS). (2019e). *Clinical practice guideline for limb salvage and early amputation.* Retrieved on 2/22/2020 at: www.aaos.org/globalassets/quality-and-practice-resources/dod/lsa-cpg-final-draft-12-14-20.pdf

Asplund, C. A., & Mezzanotte, T. J. (2019). Midshaft femur fractures in adults. *UpToDate.* Retrieved on 2/18/2020 at: www.uptodate.com/contents/midshaft-femur-fractures-in-adults

Babarinde, O., Ismail, H., & Schellack, N. (2018). An overview of the management of muscle pain and injuries. *Professional Nursing Today, 22*(1), 14–23.

Baker, B., Wolf, B. T., & Lubowitz, J. H. (2018). Meniscus injuries. *Medscape.* Retrieved on 2/13/2020 at: emedicine.medscape.com/article/90661-overview

Baldwin, P., Li, D. J., Auston, D. A., et al. (2019). Autograft, allograft, and bone graft substitutes: Clinical evidence and indications for use in the setting of orthopaedic trauma surgery. *Journal of Orthopaedic Trauma, 33*(4), 203–213.

Bassett, R. (2018). Midshaft humeral fractures in adults. *UpToDate.* Retrieved on 2/11/2020 at: www.uptodate.com/contents/midshaft-humeral-fractures-in-adults

Bassett, R. (2019). Proximal humeral fractures in adults. *UpToDate.* Retrieved on 2/11/2020 at: www.uptodate.com/contents/proximal-humeral-fractures-in-adults

Beutler, A., & Titus, S. (2019). General principles of definitive fracture management. *UpToDate.* Retrieved on 1/7/2020 at: www.uptodate.com/contents/general-principles-of-definitive-fracture-management

Bhatti, N. S., & Ertl, J. P. (2019). Hip fracture. *Medscape.* Retrieved on 2/18/2020 at: emedicine.medscape.com/article/87043-overview

Bhavsar, M. B., Leppik, L., Oliveira, K. M. C., et al. (2019). Electrical stimulation–fracture treatment: New insights into the underlying mechanisms. *Bioelectronics in Medicine, 2*(1), 5–7.

Bivens, M. (2020). The dishonesty of informed consent rituals. *The New England Journal of Medicine, 382*(12),1089–1091.

Biz, C., Fantoni, I., Crepaldi, N., et al. (2019). Clinical practice and nursing management of pre-operative skin or skeletal traction for hip fractures in elderly patients: A cross-sectional three-institution study. *International Journal of Orthopaedic and Trauma Nursing, 32,* 32–40.

Buckley, R., & Page, J. L. (2018). General principles of fracture care. *Medscape.* Retrieved on 1/7/2020 at: emedicine.medscape.com/article/1270717-overview#a6

*Campbell, F., & Watt, E. (2020). An exploration of nursing practices related to care of orthopaedic external fixators (pin/wire sites) in the Australian context. *International Journal of Orthopaedic and Trauma Nursing, 36,* 100711.

Capone, A., Congia, S., Civinini, R., et al. (2017). Periprosthetic fractures: epidemiology and current treatment. *Clinical Cases in Mineral and Bone Metabolism, 14*(2), 189.

Cardone, D. A., & Jacobs, M. A. (2019). Meniscal injury of the knee. *UpToDate.* Retrieved on 12/14/2020 at: www.uptodate.com/contents/meniscal-injury-of-the-knee

Centers for Disease Control and Prevention, National Center for Health Statistics. (2017). *All injuries.* Retrieved on 11/14/2019 at: www.cdc.gov/nchs/fastats/injury.htm

Chung, K. C., & Yoneda, H. (2020). Upper extremity amputation. *UpToDate.* Retrieved on 6/20/2020 at: www.uptodate.com/contents/upper-extremity-amputation

Conley, R. B., Adib, G., Adler, R. A., et al. (2020). Secondary fracture prevention: Consensus clinical recommendations from a multistakeholder coalition. *Journal of Bone and Mineral Research, 35*(1), 36–52.

Cutts, S., Gangoo, S., Modi, N., et al. (2020). Tennis elbow: A clinical review article. *Journal of Orthopaedics, 17,* 203–207.

DeBerardino, T. (2018). BMJ practice alert: Joint dislocations. Retrieved on 12/12/2020 at: bestpractice.bmj.com/topics/en-us/583

Department of Veterans Affairs & Department of Defense (VA/DoD). (2017). VA/DoD Clinical practice guideline for rehabilitation of individuals with lower limb amputation. Retrieved on 2/10/2020 at: www.healthquality.va.gov/guidelines/Rehab/amp/VADoDLLACPG092817.pdf

Derby, R., & Beutler, A. (2018). General principles of acute fracture management. *UpToDate.* Retrieved on 1/9/2020 at: www.uptodate.com/contents/general-principles-of-acute-fracture-management

Dexter, W. W. (2019). Medial collateral ligament injury of the knee. *UpToDate.* Retrieved on 12/14/2020 at: www.uptodate.com/contents/medial-collateral-ligament-injury-of-the-knee

Dressner, M. A., & Kissinger, S. P. (2018). *Occupational injuries and illnesses among registered nurses.* Monthly Labor Review, U.S. Department of Labor, Bureau of Labor Statistics. Retrieved on 2/20/2020 at: doi.org/10.21916/mlr.2018.27

Dunbar, R. P., & Cannada, L. K. (2017). *Open fractures. OrthoInfo from the American Academy of Orthopaedic Surgeons (AAOS).* Retrieved on 1/3/2020 at: orthoinfo.aaos.org/en/diseases–conditions/open-fractures/

Duperouzel, W., Gray, B., & Santy-Tomlinson, J. (2018). The principles of traction and the application of lower limb skin traction. *International Journal of Orthopaedic and Trauma Nursing, 29,* 54–57.

Egger, A. C., & Berkowitz, M. J. (2017). Achilles tendon injuries. *Current Reviews in Musculoskeletal Medicine, 10*(1), 72–80.

Elniel, A. R., & Giannoudis, P. V. (2018). Open fractures of the lower extremity: Current management and clinical outcomes. *EFORT Open Reviews, 3*(5), 316–325.

El-saidy, T. M. K., & Aboshehata, O. K. (2019). Effect of skin care and bony prominence protectors on pressure ulcers among hospitalized bedridden patients. *American Journal of Nursing, 7*(6), 912–921.

Etxebarria-Foronda, I., & Caeiro-Rey, J. R. (2018). The usefulness of pre-operative traction in hip fracture. *Revista De Osteoporosis Y Metabolismo Mineral, 10*(2), 98–102.

European Pressure Ulcer Advisory Panel, National Pressure Injury Advisory Panel and Pan Pacific Pressure Injury Alliance. (2019). *Prevention and treatment of pressure ulcers/injuries: Clinical practice guideline. The international guideline* (3rd ed.). Emily Haesler (Ed.). Retrieved on 1/31/2020 at: www.internationalguideline.com

Fick, D. M., Semla, T. P., Steinman, M., et al. (2019). American Geriatrics Society 2019 updated AGS Beers Criteria® for potentially inappropriate medication use in older adults. *Journal of the American Geriatrics Society, 67*(4), 674–694.

Fiechtl, J. (2018). Pelvic trauma: Initial evaluation and management. *UpToDate.* Retrieved on 2/15/2020 at: www.uptodate.com/contents/pelvic-trauma-initial-evaluation-and-management?search=pelvis%20fracture&source=search_result&selectedTitle=2~116&usage_type=default&display_rank=2

Fields, K. (2020). Overview of tibial fractures in adults. *UpToDate.* Retrieved on 2/18/2020 at: www.uptodate.com/contents/overview-of-tibial-fractures-in-adults

Flynn, S. (2018). History of traction. *International Journal of Orthopaedic and Trauma Nursing, 28,* 4–7.

Forsh, D. A. (2019). Deep vein thrombosis prophylaxis in orthopedic surgery. *Medscape.* Retrieved on 1/18/2020 at: emedicine.medscape.com/article/1268573-overview

Foster, K. (2020). Overview of common hip fractures in adults. *UpToDate.* Retrieved on 2/18/2020 at: www.uptodate.com/contents/overview-of-common-hip-fractures-in-adults

Foye, P. (2019). Coccydynia. *UpToDate.* Retrieved on 2/16/2020 at: www.uptodate.com/contents/coccydynia-coccygodynia

*Freysteinson, W., Thomas, L., Sebastian-Deutsch, A., et al. (2017). A study of the amputee experience of viewing self in the mirror. *Rehabilitation Nursing, 42*(1), 22–32.

Friedberg, R. P. (2019). Anterior cruciate ligament injury. *UpToDate.* Retrieved on 12/7/2020 at: www.uptodate.com/contents/anterior-cruciate-ligament-injury

Fukumoto, L. E., & Fukumoto, K. D. (2018). Fat embolism syndrome. *Nursing Clinics, 53*(3), 335–347.

Gaspar, S., Peralta, M., Marques, A., et al. (2019). Effectiveness on hospital-acquired pressure ulcers prevention: A systematic review. *International Wound Journal, 16*(5), 1087–1102.

*Georgiades, D. S. (2018). A systematic integrative review of pin site crusts. *Orthopaedic Nursing, 37*(1), 36–42.

Graham, P. (2019). Tear of the anterior cruciate ligament. *Orthopaedic Nursing, 38*(1), 57–59.

Graham, P. (2020). Avascular necrosis and bone infarcts of the knee. *Orthopaedic Nursing, 39*(1), 59–61.

Gray, B., & Santy-Tomlinson, J. (2018). The Thomas' splint: Application and care. *International Journal of Orthopaedic and Trauma Nursing, 24,* 1–2.

Guest, F., Marshall, C., & Stansby, G. (2019). Amputation and rehabilitation. *Surgery (Oxford), 37*(2), 102–105.

Hatch, R. L., Clugston, J. R., & Taffee, R. (2019). Clavicle fractures. *UpToDate.* Retrieved on 2/10/2020 at: www.uptodate.com/contents/clavicle-fractures

Health Services Advisory Group. (2019). *Field guide: Venous thromboembolism.* Retrieved on 2/1/2020 at: www.hsag.com/contentassets/6c5869e24e55450b92d3625acbfaed1d/vtefieldguide508.pdf

Herrador Colmenero, L., Perez Marmol, J. M., Martí-García, C., et al. (2018). Effectiveness of mirror therapy, motor imagery, and virtual feedback on phantom limb pain following amputation: A systematic review. *Prosthetics and Orthotics International, 42*(3), 288–298.

*Hohler, S. E. (2018). Providing evidence-based practices for patients with hip fractures. *Nursing, 48*(6), 52–57.

Howe, A. S. (2018). General principles of fracture management: Early and late complications. *UpToDate.* Retrieved on 1/6/2020 at: www.uptodate.com/contents/general-principles-of-fracture-management-early-and-late-complications

Jones, L. C., & Mont, M. A. (2018). Osteonecrosis (avascular necrosis of the bone. *UpToDate.* Retrieved on 1/26/2020 at: www.uptodate.com/contents/osteonecrosis-avascular-necrosis-of-bone

Kaji, A., & Hockberger, R. S. (2018). Spinal column injuries in adults: Definitions, mechanisms, and radiographs. *UpToDate.* Retrieved on 2/19/2020 at: www.uptodate.com/contents/spinal-column-injuries-in-adults-definitions-mechanisms-and-radiographs

Kakarala, G., & Simons, A. W. (2019). Forearm fractures. *Medscape.* Retrieved on 2/16/2020 at: emedicine.medscape.com/article/1239187-overview#a1

Kalapatapu, V. (2019). Techniques for lower extremity amputation. *UpToDate.* Retrieved on 2/22/2020 at: www.uptodate.com/contents/techniques-for-lower-extremity-amputation

Kani, K. K., Porrino, J. A., & Chew, F. S. (2020). External fixators: Looking beyond the hardware maze. *Skeletal Radiology, 49*(3), 359–374.

Kare, J. A. (2019). Volkmann contracture. *Medscape.* Retrieved on 2/13/2020 at: emedicine.medscape.com/article/1270462-overview#a5

Karjalainen, T. V., Jain, N. B., Heikkinen, J., et al. (2019). Surgery for rotator cuff tears. *Cochrane Database of Systematic Reviews, 12*(12), CD013502.

Karrer, F. M., & Jones, S. A. (2018). Superior mesenteric artery (SMA) syndrome questions & answers. *Medscape.* Retrieved on 1/30/2020 at: emedicine.medscape.com/article/932220-overview

Keany, J. E., & McKeever, D. (2019). Femoral shaft fractures in emergency medicine treatment & management. *Medscape.* Retrieved on 2/18/2020 at: emedicine.medscape.com/article/821856 treatment

Kellam, J. F. (2020). Intertrochanteric hip fractures treatment & management. *Medscape.* Retrieved on 2/18/2020 at: emedicine.medscape.com/article/1247210-treatment#d17

*Khorais, A., Ebraheim, M., & Barakat, A. (2018). Self-care program: Quality of life and satisfaction among patients with external skeletal fixation. *IOSR Journal of Nursing and Health Science, 7*(4), 71–83.

Kirman, C. (2018). Pressure injuries (pressure ulcers) and wound care. *Medscape.* Retrieved on 2/8/2020 at: emedicine.medscape.com/article/190115-overview

Kleinhenz, B. P. (2019). Clavicle fractures. *Medscape.* Retrieved on 2/10/2020 at: emedicine.medscape.com/article/92429-overview

Kochanek, K. D., Murphy, S. L., Xu, J. Q., et al. (2019). Deaths: Final data for 2017. *National vital statistics reports, 68*(9). Hyattsville, MD: National Center for Health Statistics. Retrieved on 11/29/2020 at: www.cdc.gov/nchs/data/nvsr/nvsr68/nvsr68_09-508.pdf

Kramer, I. F., Blokhuis, T. J., Verdijk, L. B., et al. (2019). Perioperative nutritional supplementation and skeletal muscle mass in older hip-fracture patients. *Nutrition Reviews, 77*(4), 254–266.

Kwah, L. K., Webb, M. T., Goh, L., et al. (2019). Rigid dressings versus soft dressings for transtibial amputations. *Cochrane Database of Systematic Reviews, 6*(6), CD012427.

Lai, W. C., Erickson, B. J., Mlynarek, R. A., et al. (2018). Chronic lateral epicondylitis: Challenges and solutions. *Open Access Journal of Sports Medicine, 9,* 243–251.

Lakshmanan, P., Damodaran, P. R., & Sher, L. (2018). Malunion of hand fracture. *Medscape.* Retrieved on 2/14/2020 at: emedicine.medscape.com/article/1243899-workup

Lenoir, H., Mares, O., & Carlier, Y. (2019). Management of lateral epicondylitis. *Orthopaedics & Traumatology: Surgery & Research, 105*(8), S241–S246.

Lin, Y.-K., Liu, K.-T., Chen, C.-W., et al. (2019). How to effectively obtain informed consent in trauma patients: A systematic review. *BMC Medical Ethics, 20*(8), 1–15.

Lobst, C. A. (2017). Pin-track infection: Past, present and future. *Journal of Limb Lengthening and Reconstruction, 3*(2), 78–84.

Logerstedt, D. S., Snyder-Mackler, L., Ritter, R. C., et al. (2018). Knee pain and mobility impairments: Meniscal and articular cartilage lesions: Clinical practice guidelines linked to the international classification of functioning, disability, and health from the orthopaedic section of the American physical therapy association. *Journal of Orthopaedic & Sports Physical Therapy, 40*(6), A1–A35.

Long, B., Koyfman, A., & Gottlieb, M. (2019). Evaluation and management of acute compartment syndrome in the emergency department. *The Journal of Emergency Medicine, 56*(4), 386–397.

Lu, Y., & Uppal, H. S. (2019). Hip fractures: Relevant anatomy, classification, and biomechanics of fracture and fixation. *Geriatric Orthopaedic Surgery & Rehabilitation, 10,* 1–10.

Luza, L. P., Ferreira, E. G., Minsky, R. C., et al. (2019). Psychosocial and physical adjustments and prosthesis satisfaction in amputees: A systematic review of observational studies. *Disability and Rehabilitation: Assistive Technology, 2019,* 1–8.

Maughan, K. L. (2019). Ankle sprains. *UpToDate.* Retrieved on 12/12/2020 at: www.uptodate.com/contents/ankle-sprain

McMillan, T. E., Gardner, W. T., Schmidt, A. H., et al. (2019). Diagnosing acute compartment syndrome—where have we got to? *International Orthopaedics, 43*(11), 2429–2435.

Melendez, S. L., & Doty, C. I. (2017). Rib fracture. *Medscape.* Retrieved on 2/18/2020 at: emedicine.medscape.com/article/825981-overview

Mervis, J. S., & Phillips, T. J. (2019). Pressure ulcers: Pathophysiology, epidemiology, risk factors, and presentation. *Journal of the American Academy of Dermatology, 81*(4), 881–890.

Meyers, C., Lisiecki, J., Miller, S., et al. (2019). Heterotopic ossification: A comprehensive review. *JBMR Plus, 3*(4), e10172.

Ming, Y., & Zecevic, A. (2018). Medications & polypharmacy influence on recurrent fallers in community: A systematic review. *Canadian Geriatrics Journal, 21*(1), 14–25.

Modrall, J. G. (2019). Patient management following extremity fasciotomy. *UpToDate.* Retrieved on 1/29/2020 at: www.uptodate.com/contents/patient-management-following-extremity-fasciotomy

Moore, N., & Doty, C. I. (2017). Pelvic fracture in emergency medicine. *Medscape.* Retrieved on 2/15/2020 at: emedicine.medscape.com/article/825869-treatment#d2

Morrison, R. S., & Siu, A. L. (2019). Hip fracture in adults: Epidemiology and medical management. *UpToDate.* Retrieved on 2/18/2020 at: www.uptodate.com/contents/hip-fracture-in-adults-epidemiology-and-medical-management

Mosk, C. A., Mus, M., Vroemen, J. P., et al. (2017). Dementia and delirium, the outcomes in elderly hip fracture patients. *Clinical Interventions in Aging, 12,* 421–431.

Muttath, S., Chung, K., & Ono, A.S. (2019). Overview of finger, hand, and wrist fractures. *UpToDate.* Retrieved on 1/12/2020 at: www.uptodate.com/contents/overview-of-finger-hand-and-wrist-fractures

National Institute of Neurological Disorders and Stroke (NINDS). (2017). Complex regional pain syndrome fact sheet. Retrieved on 2/1/2020 at: www.ninds.nih.gov/disorders/patient-caregiver-education/fact-sheets/complex-regional-pain-syndrome-fact-sheet

Neeru, J. (2020). Elbow tendinopathy (tennis and golf elbow). *UpToDate.* Retrieved on 3/1/2020 at: www.uptodate.com/contents/elbow-tendinopathy-tennis-and-golf-elbow

Nelson, D. (2018). Distal radius fractures clinical presentation. *Medscape.* Retrieved on 2/14/2020 at: emedicine.medscape.com/article/1245884-clinical

Noblet, T., Lineham, B., Wiper, J., et al. (2019). Amputation in trauma—How to achieve a good result from lower extremity amputation irrespective of the level. *Current Trauma Reports, 5*(1), 69–78.

Norvell, J. G., & Steele, M. (2017). Tibia and fibula fracture in the ED. *Medscape.* Retrieved on 2/19/2020 at: emedicine.medscape.com/article/826304-overview

Nyary, T., & Scammell, B. E. (2018). Principles of bone and joint injuries and their healing. *Surgery (Oxford), 36*(1), 7–14.

Papachristos, I. V., & Giannoudis, P. V. (2018). Acute compartment syndrome of the extremities: An update. *Orthopaedics and Trauma, 32*(4), 223–228.

Petron, D. (2018). Distal radius fractures in adults. *UpToDate.* Retrieved on 2/14/2020 at: www.uptodate.com/contents/distal-radius-fractures-in-adults

Rabin, S. (2018). Radial head fractures. *Medscape.* Retrieved on 2/13/2020 at: emedicine.medscape.com/article/1240337-treatment#d10

Rai, R., Shah, S., Palliyil, N., et al. (2019). Superior mesenteric artery syndrome complicating spinal deformity correction surgery: A case report and review of the literature. *JBJS Case Connector, 9*(4), e0497.

Rasmussen, T. E. (2019). Severe lower extremity injury in the adult patient. *UpToDate.* Retrieved on 1/24/2020 at: www.uptodate.com/contents/severe-lower-extremity-injury-in-the-adult-patient

*Reichmann, J. P., & Bartman, K. R. (2018). An integrative review of peer support for patients undergoing major limb amputation. *Journal of Vascular Nursing, 36*(1), 34–39.

Reichmann, J. P., Stevens, P. M., Rheinstein, J., et al. (2018). Removable rigid dressings for postoperative management of transtibial amputations: A review of published evidence. *PM&R, 10*(5), 516–523.

Rossbach, P. (2017). *Care of your wounds after amputation surgery.* Retrieved on 2/22/2020 at: www.amputee-coalition.org/wp-content/uploads/2015/08/Care-of-Your-Wounds-After-Amputation-Surgery.pdf

Rubinstein, A. J., Ahmed, I. H., & Vosbikian, M. M. (2018). Hand compartment syndrome. *Hand Clinics, 34*(1), 41–52.

Russell, G. V., & Jarrett, C. A. (2020). Pelvic fractures. *Medscape.* Retrieved on 2/15/2020 at: emedicine.medscape.com/article/1247913-overview

Santy-Tomlinson, J. (2017). Traction survival skills. *International Journal of Orthopedic and Trauma Nursing, 24,* 1–2.

*Santy-Tomlinson, J., Jomeen, J., & Ersser, S. J. (2019). Patient-reported symptoms of 'calm', 'irritated' and 'infected' skeletal external fixator pin site wound states; a cross-sectional study. *International Journal of Orthopaedic and Trauma Nursing, 33,* 44–51.

*Sayed, M. A. E., Mohammed, M. A., Mostafa, K. M., et al. (2019). Effect of nursing management on pin site infection among incidence patients with external fixators. *Assiut Scientific Nursing Journal, 7*(16), 148–156.

Schaller, T. M. (2018). Open fractures. *Medscape.* Retrieved on 1/17/2020 at: emedicine.medscape.com/article/1269242-overview

Schreiber, M. L. (2017). Lower limb amputation: Postoperative nursing care and considerations. *Medsurg Nursing, 26*(4), 274.

Schub, E., & Balderrama, D. (2017). *Splints: Applying to an extremity.* In D. Pravikoff (Ed.). Nursing practice and skill. Glendale, CA: CINAHL Information Systems.

Schweich, P. (2019). Patient education: Casts and splint care (beyond the basics). *UpToDate.* Retrieved on 2/4/2020 at: www.uptodate.com/contents/cast-and-splint-care-beyond-the-basics

Serraes, B., Van Leen, M., Schols, J., et al. (2018). Prevention of pressure ulcers with a static air support surface: A systematic review. *International Wound Journal, 15*(4), 333–343.

Simons, S. M., Dixon, J. B., & Kruse, D. (2019). Presentation and diagnosis of rotator cuff tears. *UpToDate.* Retrieved on 12/23/2019 at: www.uptodate.com/contents/presentation-and-diagnosis-of-rotator-cuff-tears

Spang III, R. C., Nasr, M. C., Mohamadi, A., et al. (2018). Rehabilitation following meniscal repair: A systematic review. *BMJ Open Sport & Exercise Medicine, 4*(1), e000212.

Speed, J. (2019). Heterotopic ossification. *Medscape.* Retrieved on 1/21/2020 at: emedicine.medscape.com/article/327648-overview

Stracciolini, A., & Hammerberg, E. M. (2019). Acute compartment syndrome of the extremities. *UpToDate.* Retrieved on 1/27/2020 at: www.uptodate.com/contents/acute-compartment-syndrome-of-the-extremities

Szostakowski, B., Smitham, P., & Khan, W. S. (2017). Plaster of Paris—short history of casting and injured limb immobilization. *The Open Orthopaedics Journal, 11,* 291–296.

Thacker, M. M., Tejwani, N., & Thakkar, C. (2018). Acetabulum fractures. *Medscape.* Retrieved on 2/15/2020 at: emedicine.medscape.com/article/1246057-treatment#d14

United Health Foundation. (2019). *America's health rankings analysis of the Dartmouth atlas of health care, senior report, hip fractures.* Retrieved on 2/17/2020 at: www.americashealthrankings.org/explore/senior/measure/hip_fractures_sr/state/U.S

Uransilp, N., Muengtaweepongsa, S., Chanalithichai, N., et al. (2018). Fat embolism syndrome: A case report and review literature. *Case Reports in Medicine, 2018.*

U.S. Department of Labor, Bureau of Labor Statistics. (2019). *Employer-reported workplace injury and illness, 2018.* Retrieved on 2/17/2020 at: www.bls.gov/news.release/osh.nr0.htm

Veronese, N., & Maggi, S. (2018). Epidemiology and social costs of hip fracture. *Injury, 49*(8), 1458–1460.

Vinas, F. (2018). Lumbar spine fractures and dislocations. *Medscape.* Retrieved on 2/19/2020 at: emedicine.medscape.com/article/1264191-overview

Walker, J. (2018). Assessing and managing pin sites in patients with external fixators. *Nursing Times* [online], *114*(1), 18–21.

Walker, J., & Revell, R. (2019). Hip fracture 2: Nursing care from admission to secondary prevention. *Nursing Times* [online], *115*(2), 35–38.

Weinhouse, G. L. (2019). Fat embolism syndrome. *UpToDate.* Retrieved on 1/19/2020 at: www.uptodate.com/contents/fat-embolism-syndrome

Yian, E. (2019). Distal humerus fractures. *Medscape.* Retrieved on 2/12/2020 at: emedicine.medscape.com/article/1239515-treatment#d8

Zhao, J. G., Meng, X. H., Liu, L., et al. (2017). Early functional rehabilitation versus traditional immobilization for surgical Achilles tendon repair after acute rupture: A systematic review of overlapping meta-analyses. *Scientific Reports, 7*(1), 1–7.

Resources

American Academy of Orthopedic Surgeons (AAOS), www.aaos.org

American College of Sports Medicine (ACSM), www.acsm.org

American Nurses Association (ANA), Safe Patient Handling and Mobility, www.nursingworld.org/practice-policy/work-environment/health-safety/handle-with-care/

Amputee Coalition, www.amputee-coalition.org

National Amputation Foundation (NAF), www.nationalamputation.org

National Association of Orthopaedic Nurses (NAON), www.orthonurse.org

National Institute for Occupational Safety and Health (NIOSH), www.cdc.gov/niosh/index.htm

U.S. Department of Labor, Occupational Safety and Health Administration (OSHA), www.osha.gov

Wounded Warrior Project, www.woundedwarriorproject.org

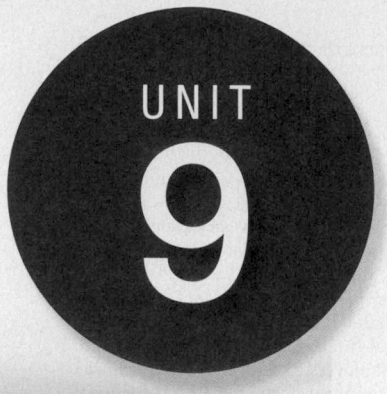

UNIT 9

Digestive and Gastrointestinal Function

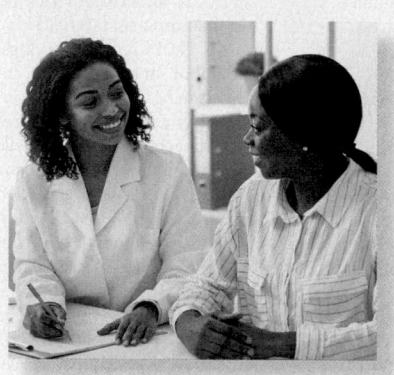

You are working in an outpatient clinic that has a high volume of patients with inflammatory bowel disease (IBD). You know that nutrition is an important focus for patients with IBD and that a low-residue, high-protein, high-calorie, and high-vitamin diet can help decrease symptoms such as diarrhea and weight loss. You recall several patients in the past few months who have presented with diarrhea and weight loss. For this reason, you report your observations to the nurse manager and suggest a quality improvement project for assessing the nutritional status of patients with IBD.

QSEN Competency Focus: Quality Improvement

The complexities inherent in today's health care system challenge nurses to demonstrate integration of specific interdisciplinary core competencies. These competencies are aimed at ensuring the delivery of safe, quality patient care (Institute of Medicine, 2003). The Quality and Safety Education for Nurses project (Cronenwett, Sherwood, Barnsteiner, et al., 2007; QSEN, 2020) provides a framework for the knowledge, skills, and attitudes (KSAs) required for nurses to demonstrate competency in these key areas, which include *patient-centered care*, *interdisciplinary teamwork and collaboration*, *evidence-based practice*, *quality improvement*, *safety*, and *informatics.*

Quality Improvement Definition: Use data to monitor the outcomes of care processes and use improvement methods to design and test changes to continuously improve the quality and safety of health care systems.

SELECT PRE-LICENSURE KSAs	APPLICATION AND REFLECTION
Knowledge	
Describe strategies for learning about the outcomes of care in the setting in which one is engaged in clinical practice	What strategies will you use to learn about the best indicators of nutritional status for patients with IBD?
Skills	
Seek information about outcomes of care for populations served in care setting Use quality measures to understand performance	After a review of the literature, you determine that frequent diarrhea and weight loss are important indicators of the nutritional status of patients with IBD. Identify the indicators that will need to be monitored, the frequency with which they will be monitored, and what type of interventions might be used to improve these indicators.
Attitudes	
Appreciate that continuous quality improvement is an essential part of the daily work of all health professionals	Reflect on how long it will take for this project to show an improvement in nutritional outcomes in these patients. Think about how the other members of the health care team can contribute to the project.

Cronenwett, L., Sherwood, G., Barnsteiner, J., et al. (2007). Quality and safety education for nurses. *Nursing Outlook*, *55*(3), 122–131; Institute of Medicine. (2003). *Health professions education: A bridge to quality*. Washington, DC: National Academies Press; QSEN Institute. (2020). *QSEN Competencies: Definitions and pre-licensure KSAs; Quality improvement*. Retrieved on 8/15/2020 at: qsen.org/competencies/pre-licensure-ksas/#quality_improvement

38 Assessment of Digestive and Gastrointestinal Function

LEARNING OUTCOMES

On completion of this chapter, the learner will be able to:

1. Describe the structure and function of the organs of the gastrointestinal tract.
2. Explain the mechanical and chemical processes involved in digesting and absorbing nutrients and eliminating waste products.
3. Discriminate between normal and abnormal assessment findings of the gastrointestinal system.

4. Recognize and evaluate the major symptoms of gastrointestinal dysfunction by applying the patient's health history and physical assessment findings.
5. Identify the diagnostic tests used to evaluate gastrointestinal tract function and related nursing implications.

NURSING CONCEPTS

Assessment

Elimination

GLOSSARY

absorption: phase of the digestive process that occurs when small molecules, vitamins, and minerals pass through the walls of the small and large intestine and into the bloodstream

amylase: an enzyme that aids in the digestion of starch

anus: last section of the gastrointestinal (GI) tract; outlet for waste products from the GI system

chyme: mixture of food with saliva, salivary enzymes, and gastric secretions that is produced as food passes through the mouth, esophagus, and stomach

digestion: phase of the digestive process that occurs when digestive enzymes and secretions mix with ingested food and when proteins, fats, and sugars are broken down into their component smaller molecules

dyspepsia: indigestion; upper abdominal discomfort associated with eating

elimination: phase of the digestive process that occurs after digestion and absorption, when waste products are evacuated from the body

esophagus: collapsible tube connecting the mouth to the stomach, through which food passes as it is ingested

hydrochloric acid: acid secreted by the glands in the stomach; mixes with chyme to break it down into absorbable molecules and to aid in the destruction of bacteria

ingestion: phase of the digestive process that occurs when food is taken into the GI tract via the mouth and esophagus

intrinsic factor: a gastric secretion that combines with vitamin B_{12} so that the vitamin can be absorbed

large intestine: the portion of the GI tract into which waste material from the small intestine passes as absorption continues and elimination begins; consists of several parts—ascending segment, transverse segment, descending segment, sigmoid colon, and rectum (*synonym:* colon)

lipase: an enzyme that aids in the digestion of fats

microbiome: the collective genome of all microbes in a microbiota

microbiota: the complement of microbes in a given environment

pepsin: a gastric enzyme that is important in protein digestion

small intestine: longest portion of the GI tract, consisting of three parts—duodenum, jejunum, and ileum—through which food mixed with all secretions and enzymes passes as it continues to be digested and begins to be absorbed into the bloodstream

stomach: distensible pouch into which the food bolus passes to be digested by gastric enzymes

trypsin: enzyme that aids in the digestion of protein

Abnormalities of the gastrointestinal (GI) tract are numerous and represent every type of major pathology that can affect other organ systems, including bleeding, perforation, obstruction, inflammation, and cancer. Congenital, inflammatory, infectious, traumatic, and neoplastic lesions have been encountered in every portion and at every site along the length of the GI tract. As with all other organ systems, the GI tract is subject to circulatory disturbances, faulty nervous system control, and aging.

Apart from the many organic diseases to which the GI tract is susceptible, many extrinsic factors can interfere with its normal function and produce symptoms. Stress and anxiety, for example, often find their chief expression in indigestion, anorexia, or motor disturbances of the intestines, sometimes producing constipation or diarrhea. In addition, factors such as fatigue and an inadequate or abruptly changed dietary intake can markedly affect the GI tract. When assessing and educating the patient, the nurse should consider the variety of mental and physical factors that affect the function of the GI tract.

Anatomic and Physiologic Overview

The GI tract is a pathway 7 to 7.9 m (23 to 26 feet) in length that extends from the mouth to the esophagus, stomach, small and large intestines, and rectum, to the terminal structure, the **anus** (Fig. 38-1). The **esophagus** is located in the mediastinum, anterior to the spine and posterior to the trachea

and heart. This hollow muscular tube, which is approximately 25 cm (10 inches) in length, passes through the diaphragm at an opening called the *diaphragmatic hiatus*.

The remaining portion of the GI tract is located within the peritoneal cavity. The **stomach** is situated in the left upper portion of the abdomen under the left lobe of the liver and the diaphragm, overlaying most of the pancreas (see Fig. 38-1). A hollow muscular organ with a capacity of approximately 1500 mL, the stomach stores food during eating, secretes digestive fluids, and propels the partially digested food, or chyme, into the small intestine. The gastroesophageal junction is the inlet to the stomach. The stomach has four anatomic regions: the cardia (entrance), fundus, body, and pylorus (outlet). Circular smooth muscle in the wall of the pylorus forms the pyloric sphincter and controls the opening between the stomach and the small intestine.

The **small intestine** is the longest segment of the GI tract, accounting for about two thirds of the total length. It folds back and forth on itself, providing approximately 70 m (230 feet) of surface area for secretion and **absorption,** the process by which nutrients enter the bloodstream through the intestinal walls. It has three sections: The most proximal section is the duodenum, the middle section is the jejunum, and the distal section is the ileum. The ileum terminates at the ileocecal valve. This valve, or sphincter, controls the flow of digested material from the ileum into the cecal portion of the large intestine and prevents reflux of bacteria into the small intestine. Attached to the cecum is the vermiform appendix, an appendage that has little or no physiologic function. Emptying into the duodenum at the ampulla of Vater is the common bile duct, which allows for the passage of both bile and pancreatic secretions.

The **large intestine** consists of an ascending segment on the right side of the abdomen, a transverse segment that extends from right to left in the upper abdomen, and a descending segment on the left side of the abdomen. The sigmoid colon, the rectum, and the anus complete the terminal portion of the large intestine. A network of striated muscle that forms both the internal and the external anal sphincters regulates the anal outlet.

The GI tract receives blood from arteries that originate along the entire length of the thoracic and abdominal aorta and veins that return blood from the digestive organs and the spleen. This portal venous system is composed of five large veins: the superior mesenteric, inferior mesenteric, gastric, splenic, and cystic veins, which eventually form the vena portae that enters the liver. Once in the liver, the blood is distributed throughout and collected into the hepatic veins that then terminate in the inferior vena cava. Of particular importance are the gastric artery and the superior and inferior mesenteric arteries. Oxygen and nutrients are supplied to the stomach by the gastric artery and to the intestine by the mesenteric arteries (Fig. 38-2). Venous blood is returned from the small intestine, cecum, and the ascending and transverse portions of the colon by the superior mesenteric vein, which corresponds with the distribution of the branches of the superior mesenteric artery. Blood flow to the GI tract is about 20% of the total cardiac output and increases significantly after eating.

Both the sympathetic and parasympathetic portions of the autonomic nervous system innervate the GI tract. In

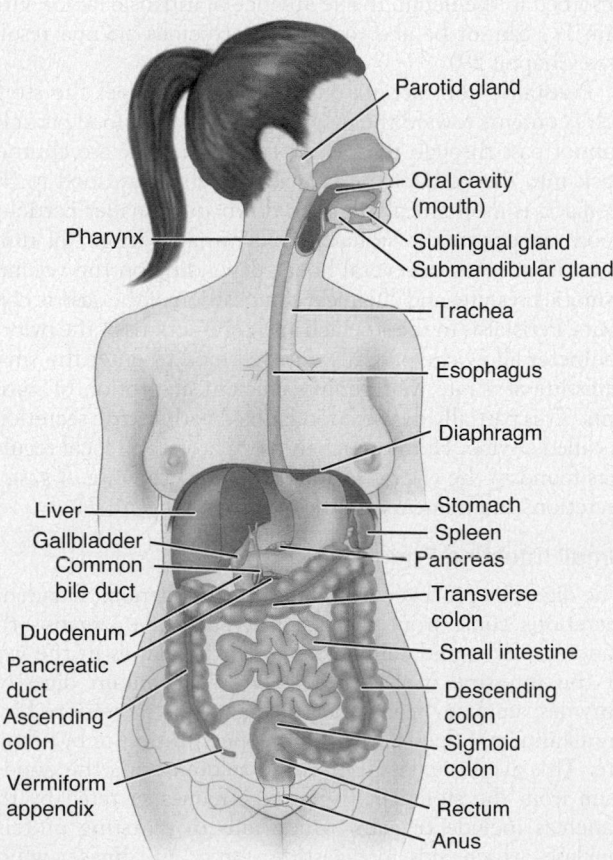

Figure 38-1 • Organs of the digestive system and associated structures.

Parotid gland
Oral cavity (mouth)
Sublingual gland
Submandibular gland
Trachea
Esophagus
Diaphragm
Stomach
Spleen
Pancreas
Transverse colon
Small intestine
Descending colon
Sigmoid colon
Rectum
Anus
Pharynx
Liver
Gallbladder
Common bile duct
Duodenum
Pancreatic duct
Ascending colon
Vermiform appendix

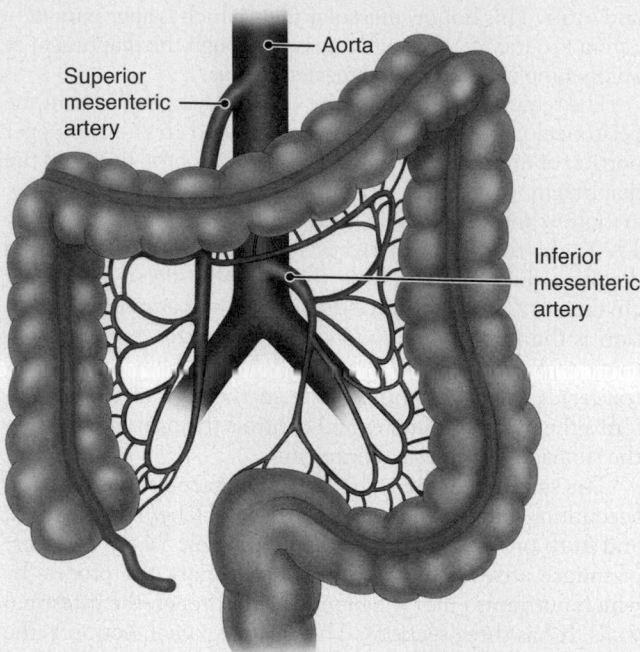

Figure 38-2 • Anatomy and blood supply of the large intestine.

general, sympathetic nerves exert an inhibitory effect on the GI tract, decreasing gastric secretion and motility and causing the sphincters and blood vessels to constrict. Parasympathetic nerve stimulation causes peristalsis and increases secretory activities. The sphincters relax under the influence of parasympathetic stimulation, except for the sphincter of the upper esophagus and the external anal sphincter, which are under voluntary control (Norris, 2019).

Function of the Digestive System

All cells of the body require nutrients. These nutrients are derived from the intake of food that contains proteins, fats, carbohydrates, vitamins, minerals, and cellulose fibers and other vegetable matter, some of which has no nutritional value. Major functions of the GI tract include:

- Breakdown of food particles into the molecular form for **digestion**
- Absorption into the bloodstream of small nutrient molecules produced by digestion
- **Elimination** of undigested unabsorbed foodstuffs and other waste products

After food is ingested, it is propelled through the GI tract, coming into contact with a wide variety of secretions that aid in its digestion, absorption, or elimination from the GI tract.

Chewing and Swallowing

The process of digestion begins with the act of chewing, in which food is broken down into small particles that can be swallowed and mixed with digestive enzymes. Eating—or even the sight, smell, or taste of food—can cause reflex salivation. Approximately 1.5 L of saliva is secreted daily from the parotid, the submaxillary, and the sublingual glands. Ptyalin, or salivary **amylase,** is an enzyme that begins the digestion of starches. Water and mucus, also contained in saliva, help lubricate the food as it is chewed, thereby facilitating swallowing.

Swallowing begins as a voluntary act that is regulated by the swallowing center in the medulla oblongata of the central nervous system (CNS). As a bolus of food is swallowed, the epiglottis moves to cover the tracheal opening and prevent aspiration of food into the lungs. Swallowing, which propels the bolus of food into the upper esophagus, thus ends as a reflex action. The smooth muscle in the wall of the esophagus contracts in a rhythmic sequence from the upper esophagus toward the stomach to propel the bolus of food along the tract. During this process of esophageal peristalsis, the lower esophageal sphincter relaxes and permits the bolus of food to enter the stomach. Subsequently, the lower esophageal sphincter closes tightly to prevent reflux of stomach contents into the esophagus.

Gastric Function

The stomach, which stores and mixes food with secretions, secretes a highly acidic fluid in response to the presence or anticipated **ingestion** of food. This fluid, which can total 2.4 L/day, can have a pH as low as 1 and derives its acidity from **hydrochloric acid** (HCl) secreted by the glands of the stomach. The function of this gastric secretion is twofold: to break down food into more absorbable components and to aid in the destruction of most ingested bacteria. **Pepsin,** an important enzyme for protein digestion, is the end product of the conversion of pepsinogen from the chief cells (Table 38-1). **Intrinsic factor,** also secreted by the gastric mucosa, combines with dietary vitamin B_{12} so that the vitamin can be absorbed in the ileum. In the absence of intrinsic factor, vitamin B_{12} cannot be absorbed, and pernicious anemia results (see Chapter 29).

Peristaltic contractions in the stomach propel the stomach's contents toward the pylorus. Because large food particles cannot pass through the pyloric sphincter, they are churned back into the body of the stomach. In this way, food in the stomach is mechanically broken down into smaller particles. Food remains in the stomach for a variable length of time, from 30 minutes to several hours, depending on the volume, osmotic pressure, and chemical composition of the gastric contents. Peristalsis in the stomach and contractions of the pyloric sphincter allow the partially digested food to enter the small intestine at a rate that permits efficient absorption of nutrients. This partially digested food mixed with gastric secretions is called **chyme.** Hormones, neuroregulators, and local regulators found in the gastric secretions control the rate of gastric secretions and influence gastric motility (Table 38-2).

Small Intestine Function

The digestive process continues in the duodenum. Duodenal secretions come from the accessory digestive organs—the pancreas, liver, and gallbladder—and the glands in the wall of the intestine itself. These secretions contain digestive enzymes: amylase, lipase, and bile. Pancreatic secretions have an alkaline pH due to their high concentration of bicarbonate. This alkalinity neutralizes the acid entering the duodenum from the stomach. Digestive enzymes secreted by the pancreas include **trypsin,** which aids in digesting protein; amylase, which aids in digesting starch; and **lipase,** which aids in digesting fats. These secretions drain into the pancreatic duct, which empties into the common bile duct at the ampulla of Vater. Bile, secreted by the liver and stored in the

TABLE 38-1 The Major Digestive Enzymes and Secretions

Enzyme/Secretion	Enzyme Source	Digestive Action
Enzymes That Digest Carbohydrates		
Ptyalin (salivary amylase)	Salivary glands	Starch→dextrin, maltose, glucose
Amylase	Pancreas and intestinal mucosa	Starch→dextrin, maltose, glucose
		Dextrin→maltose, glucose
Maltase	Intestinal mucosa	Maltose→glucose
Sucrase	Intestinal mucosa	Sucrose→glucose, fructose
Lactase	Intestinal mucosa	Lactose→glucose, galactose
Enzymes/Secretions That Digest Protein		
Pepsin	Gastric mucosa	Protein→polypeptides
Trypsin	Pancreas	Proteins and polypeptides→polypeptides, dipeptides, amino acids
Aminopeptidase	Intestinal mucosa	Polypeptides→dipeptides, amino acids
Dipeptidase	Intestinal mucosa	Dipeptides→amino acids
Hydrochloric acid	Gastric mucosa	Protein→polypeptides, amino acids
Enzymes/Secretions That Digest Fat (Triglyceride)		
Pharyngeal lipase	Pharynx mucosa	Triglycerides→fatty acids, diglycerides, monoglycerides
Steapsin	Gastric mucosa	Triglycerides→fatty acids, diglycerides, monoglycerides
Pancreatic lipase	Pancreas	Triglycerides→fatty acids, diglycerides, monoglycerides
Bile	Liver and gallbladder	Fat emulsification

→, converts to.

gallbladder, aids in emulsifying ingested fats, making them easier to digest and absorb. The sphincter of Oddi, found at the confluence of the common bile duct and duodenum, controls the flow of bile. Hormones, neuroregulators, and local regulators found in these intestinal secretions control the rate of intestinal secretions and also influence GI motility. Intestinal secretions total approximately 1 L/day of pancreatic juice, 0.5 L/day of bile, and 3 L/day of secretions from the glands of the small intestine. Tables 38-1 and 38-2 give further information about the actions of digestive enzymes and GI regulatory substances.

Two types of contractions occur regularly in the small intestine: segmentation contractions and intestinal peristalsis. *Segmentation contractions* produce mixing waves that move the intestinal contents back and forth in a churning motion. *Intestinal peristalsis* propels the contents of the small intestine toward the colon. Both movements are stimulated by the presence of chyme.

Food, ingested as fats, proteins, and carbohydrates, is broken down into absorbable particles (constituent nutrients) by the process of digestion. Carbohydrates are broken down into disaccharides (e.g., sucrose, maltose, galactose) and monosaccharides (e.g., glucose, fructose). Glucose is the major carbohydrate that tissue cells use as fuel. Proteins are a source of energy after they are broken down into amino acids and peptides. Ingested fats become monoglycerides and fatty acid through emulsification, which makes them smaller and easier to absorb. Chyme stays in the small intestine for

TABLE 38-2 The Major Gastrointestinal Regulatory Substances

Substance	Stimulus for Production	Target Tissue	Effect on Secretions	Effect on Motility
Neuroregulators				
Acetylcholine	Stomach distention, vagal and local nerves in the stomach	Gastric glands, other secretory glands, gastric and intestinal muscle	↑ Gastric acid	Generally increased
Norepinephrine	Stress, other various stimuli	Secretory glands, gastric and intestinal muscle	Generally inhibitory	Generally decreased; increased sphincter tone
Hormonal Regulators				
Gastrin	Vagal stimulation, calcium containing foods	Gastric glands, stomach antrum, duodenum	↑ Secretion of gastric acid and pepsinogen	Increased motility of stomach; stimulates smooth muscle contraction
Cholecystokinin	Protein digestion products, long-chain fatty acids, presence of chyme in duodenum	Gallbladder Pancreas Stomach	Release of bile into duodenum ↑ Production of enzyme-rich pancreatic secretions	Slows gastric emptying
Secretin	pH of chyme in duodenum (pH <3)	Pancreas Stomach	Inhibits gastrin and gastric acid secretion	Decreases GI motility
Local Regulator				
Histamine	Unclear; substances in food	Gastric glands	↑ Gastric acid production	

HCl, hydrochloric acid; ↑, increased.

Adapted from McCance, K. L., & Huether, S. E. (2019). *Pathophysiology: The biologic basis for disease in adults and children* (8th ed.). St. Louis, MO: Elsevier; Norris, T. L. (2019). *Porth's pathophysiology. Concepts of altered health states* (10th ed.). Philadelphia, PA: Wolters Kluwer.

3 to 6 hours, allowing for continued breakdown and absorption of nutrients.

Small, fingerlike projections called *villi* line the entire intestine and function to produce digestive enzymes as well as to absorb nutrients. Absorption is the major function of the small intestine. Vitamins and minerals are absorbed essentially unchanged. Absorption begins in the jejunum and is accomplished by active transport and diffusion across the intestinal wall into the circulation. Nutrients are absorbed at specific locations in the small intestine and duodenum, whereas fats, proteins, carbohydrates, sodium, and chloride are absorbed in the jejunum. Vitamin B_{12} and bile salts are absorbed in the ileum. Magnesium, phosphate, and potassium are absorbed throughout the small intestine.

Colonic Function

Within 4 hours after eating, residual waste material passes into the terminal ileum and slowly into the proximal portion of the right colon through the ileocecal valve. With each peristaltic wave of the small intestine, the valve opens briefly and permits some of the contents to pass into the colon.

Gut microbes (bacteria), a major component of the contents of the large intestine, assist in completing the breakdown of waste material, especially of undigested or unabsorbed proteins and bile salts. Two types of colonic secretions are added to the residual material: an electrolyte solution and mucus. The electrolyte solution is chiefly a bicarbonate solution that acts to neutralize the end products formed by the colonic bacterial action, whereas the mucus protects the colonic mucosa from the intraluminal contents and provides adherence for the fecal mass.

Slow, weak peristalsis moves the colonic contents along the tract. This slow transport allows for efficient reabsorption of water and electrolytes, which is the major function of the colon. Intermittent strong peristaltic waves propel the contents for considerable distances. This generally occurs after another meal is eaten, when intestine-stimulating hormones are released. The waste materials from a meal eventually reach and distend the rectum, usually in about 12 hours. As much as one fourth of the waste materials from a meal may still be in the rectum 3 days after the meal was ingested.

Waste Products of Digestion

Feces consist of undigested foodstuffs, inorganic materials, water, and bacteria. Fecal matter is about 75% fluid and 25% solid material (Norris, 2019). The composition is relatively unaffected by alterations in diet because a large portion of the fecal mass is of nondietary origin, derived from the secretions of the GI tract. The brown color of the feces results from the breakdown of bile by the intestinal bacteria. Chemicals formed by intestinal bacteria are responsible in large part for the fecal odor. Gases formed contain methane, hydrogen sulfide, and ammonia, among others. The GI tract normally contains approximately 150 mL of these gases, which are either absorbed into the portal circulation and detoxified by the liver or expelled from the rectum as flatus.

Elimination of stool begins with distention of the rectum, which initiates reflex contractions of the rectal musculature and relaxes the normally closed internal anal sphincter. The internal sphincter is controlled by the autonomic nervous system; the external sphincter is under the conscious control of the cerebral cortex. During defecation, the external anal sphincter voluntarily relaxes to allow colonic contents to be expelled. Normally, the external anal sphincter is maintained in a state of tonic contraction. Thus, defecation is seen to be a spinal reflex (involving the parasympathetic nerve fibers) that can be inhibited voluntarily by keeping the external anal sphincter closed. Contracting the abdominal muscles (straining) facilitates emptying of the colon. The average frequency of defecation in humans is once daily, but this varies among people.

Gut Microbiome

In addition to assisting in the breakdown of waste material, the gut **microbiota** (the complement of microbes in the GI tract) also has a role in vitamin synthesis and immune function, including protection against invading pathogens, regulatory influences on innate and adaptive immune responses, and inflammation. Colonization of the GI tract begins shortly after birth; the normal gut microbiota is established by 2 years of age. Several factors over time affect the composition of normal gut microbiota including genetics, diet, personal hygiene, infection, and vaccinations. The number and diversity of microbes within the gut change with aging and are influenced by diet, chronic disease, and medications. Additionally, administration of broad-spectrum antibiotics can disrupt the gut microbiota and lead to overgrowth of potentially pathogenic species (McCance & Huether, 2019; Norris, 2019).

The gut **microbiome,** the collective genome of the microbiota, protects the host against invasion by pathogenic organisms; it produces anti-inflammatory metabolites, destroys toxins, prevents colonization of pathogens, and provokes an immune response (McCance & Huether, 2019; Norris, 2019). The intestinal epithelium is the first line of defense against pathogenic microbes and microbial agents, as it contains innate immune cells such as macrophages, dendritic cells, granulocytes, and mast cells, and has a role in T-cell responses (Günther, 2018; Haller, 2018; Pezoldt, Yang, Zou, et al., 2018; Strowig, Thiemann, & Diefenbach, 2018). In addition, Peyer's patches (gut-associated lymph tissue) also have a role in antigen processing and immune defense (McCance & Huether, 2019). Collectively, the gut microbiome serves the roles of protection and defense.

Gerontologic Considerations

Although an increased prevalence of several common GI disorders occurs in the older adult population, aging per se appears to have minimal direct effect on most GI functions, in large part because of the functional reserve of the GI tract. Normal physiologic changes of the GI system that occur with aging are identified in Table 38-3. Careful assessment and monitoring of signs and symptoms related to these changes are imperative. Although irritable bowel symptoms decrease with aging, there seems to be an increase in many GI disorders of function and motility. Older adult patients frequently report dysphagia, anorexia, dyspepsia, and disorders of colonic function (Eliopoulos, 2018).

Assessment of the Gastrointestinal System

The nursing assessment of the GI system involves obtaining a focused health history and physical examination.

TABLE 38-3 — Age-Related Changes in the Gastrointestinal System

Structural Changes	Implications
Oral Cavity and Pharynx • Injury/loss or decay of teeth • Atrophy of taste buds • ↓ Saliva production • Reduced ptyalin and amylase in saliva	Difficulty chewing and swallowing
Esophagus • ↓ Motility and emptying • Weakened gag reflex • ↓ Resting pressure of lower esophageal sphincter	Reflux and heartburn
Stomach • Degeneration and atrophy of gastric mucosal surfaces with ↓ production of HCl • ↓ Secretion of gastric acids and most digestive enzymes • ↓ Gastric motility and emptying	Food intolerances, malabsorption, or ↓ vitamin B_{12} absorption
Small Intestine • Atrophy of muscle and mucosal surfaces • Thinning of villi and epithelial cells	↓ Motility and transit time, which lead to complaints of indigestion and constipation
Large Intestine • ↓ Mucus secretion • ↓ Elasticity of rectal wall • ↓ Tone of internal anal sphincter • Slower and duller nerve impulses in rectal area	↓ Motility and transit time, which lead to complaints of indigestion and constipation ↓ Absorption of nutrients (dextrose, fats, calcium, and iron) Fecal incontinence

↓, decreased; HCl, hydrochloric acid.
Adapted from Eliopoulos, C. (2018). *Gerontological nursing* (9th ed.). Philadelphia, PA: Wolters Kluwer.

Health History

A focused GI assessment begins with a complete history. Information about abdominal pain, dyspepsia, gas, nausea and vomiting, diarrhea, constipation, fecal incontinence, jaundice, and previous GI disease is obtained (Weber & Kelley, 2018).

Common Symptoms

Common GI symptoms that may lead patients to seek health care referrals include pain, dyspepsia, gas, nausea and vomiting, diarrhea, and constipation.

Pain

Pain can be a major symptom of GI disease; in particular, abdominal pain is a frequent presenting problem in general practice (Babakhanlou, 2018). The character, duration, pattern, frequency, location, distribution of referred abdominal pain (Fig. 38-3), and time of the pain can vary greatly depending on the underlying cause. Other factors such as meals, rest, activity, and defecation patterns may directly affect this pain (Weber & Kelley, 2018).

Dyspepsia

Dyspepsia—upper abdominal discomfort associated with eating (commonly called *indigestion*)—is the most common symptom of patients with GI dysfunction. Indigestion is an imprecise term that refers to a host of upper abdominal or epigastric symptoms such as pain, discomfort, fullness, bloating, early satiety, belching, heartburn, or regurgitation. Annually, dyspepsia affects approximately 25% of Americans (Longstreth & Lacy, 2019) while gastroesophageal reflux disease (GERD), which increases with age and manifests with dyspepsia (most frequently with heartburn), affects approximately 20% of adults in western cultures (Antunes & Curtis, 2019). Typically, fatty foods cause the most discomfort because they remain in the stomach for digestion longer than proteins or carbohydrates. Salads, coarse vegetables, and highly seasoned foods may also cause considerable GI distress. In some cases, health care providers make a distinction between gastroesophageal reflux (GER) and GERD; GERD is the more serious and longer-lasting condition (Mayo Clinic, 2019).

Intestinal Gas

The accumulation of gas in the GI tract may result in belching (expulsion of gas from the stomach through the mouth) or flatulence (expulsion of gas from the rectum). Usually, gases in the small intestine pass into the colon and are released as flatus. Patients often complain of bloating, distention, or feeling "full of gas" with excessive flatulence as a symptom of food intolerance or gallbladder disease.

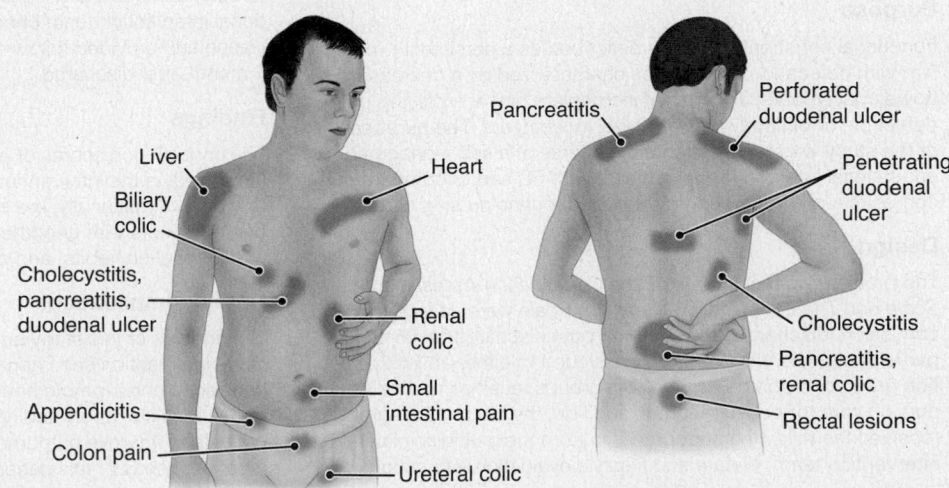

Figure 38-3 • Common sites of referred abdominal pain.

Nausea and Vomiting

Nausea is a vague, uncomfortable sensation of sickness or "queasiness" that may or may not be followed by vomiting. Distention of the duodenum or upper intestinal tract is a common cause of nausea; it may also be an early warning sign of a pathologic process. Nausea can be triggered by odors, activity, medications, or food intake. Vomiting is the forceful emptying of the stomach and intestinal contents through the mouth (McCance & Huether, 2019). The emesis, or vomitus, may vary in color and content and may contain undigested food particles, blood (hematemesis), or bilious material mixed with gastric juices. An acute onset of emesis that appears bright red or as coffee grounds is characteristic of a Mallory-Weiss tear (i.e., a laceration in the mucosal lining of the gastroesophageal junction) and indicates upper GI bleeding (Rich, 2018).

The causes of nausea and vomiting are many and may include visceral pain; motion or motion sickness; anxiety; several types of intestinal, vagal or sympathetic input including side effects of medications; and torsion or trauma of the ovaries, testes, uterus, bladder or kidney (McCance & Huether, 2019). Pathways for initiation of the vomiting reflex include medication therapy, metabolic abnormalities (chemoreceptor trigger zone), ingested toxins, chemotherapy, radiation therapy (vagal and splanchnic receptors), inner ear disorders, motion sickness (vestibular center), and anticipatory emesis (cerebral cortex) (Hainsworth, 2020).

Change in Bowel Habits and Stool Characteristics

Changes in bowel habits may signal colonic dysfunction or disease. Diarrhea, an abnormal increase in the frequency and liquidity of the stool or in daily stool weight or volume, commonly occurs when the contents move so rapidly through the intestine and colon that there is inadequate time for the GI secretions and oral contents to be absorbed. This physiologic function is typically associated with abdominal pain or cramping and nausea or vomiting. Constipation—a decrease in the frequency of stool, or stools that are hard, dry, and of smaller volume than typical—may be associated with anal discomfort and rectal bleeding, and is a frequent reason patients seek health care referrals (see the Nursing Research Profile in Chart 38-1) (Shen, Zhu, Jiang, et al., 2018). See Chapter 41 for further discussion of diarrhea and constipation.

The characteristics of the stool can vary greatly. Stool is normally light to dark brown; however, specific disease processes and ingestion of certain foods and medications may change the appearance of stool (Table 38-4). Blood in the stool can present in various ways and must be investigated. If blood is shed in sufficient quantities into the upper GI tract, it produces a tarry-black color (melena), whereas blood entering the lower portion of the GI tract or passing rapidly through it will appear bright or dark red. Lower rectal or anal bleeding is suspected if there is streaking of blood on the surface of the stool or if blood is noted on toilet tissue. Other common abnormalities in stool characteristics described by the patient may include:

- Bulky, greasy, foamy stools that are foul in odor and may or may not float
- Light gray or clay-colored stool, caused by a decrease or absence of conjugated bilirubin
- Stool with mucus threads or pus that may be visible on gross inspection of the stool
- Small, dry, rock-hard masses occasionally streaked with blood
- Loose, watery stool that may or may not be streaked with blood

Past Health, Family, and Social History

The nurse asks about the patient's normal toothbrushing and flossing routine; frequency of dental visits; awareness of any lesions or irritated areas in the mouth, tongue, or throat; recent history of sore throat or bloody sputum; discomfort

---

Chart 38-1	**NURSING RESEARCH PROFILE**
	Nurse-Led Educational Intervention for Patients with Functional Constipation

Shen, Q., Zhu, H., Jiang, G., et al. (2018). Nurse-led self-management educational intervention improves symptoms of patients with functional constipation. *Western Journal of Nursing Research, 40*(60), 874–888.

Purpose

Functional constipation (FC) is described as a persistent problem with defecation that may be characterized by a decrease in bowel movements, a feeling of incomplete bowel emptying post defection, or difficulty having bowel movements. The purpose of the study was to investigate the effects of a self-management educational intervention on patients with FC and to compare outcomes to a control group that received routine nursing care.

Design

The pretest/posttest scores of *The Constipation Assessment Scale* and *The Constipation Cognition Scale* were collected on admission, discharge, and 1-month post discharge for 66 eligible participants who were randomly assigned to either an intervention group or a control group. Both groups received routine nursing care for constipation. In addition, the intervention group received the following support: visits from the multidisciplinary intervention team, dietary and lifestyle evaluation, education, assistance in developing a self-management plan, timely consultations and weekly group meetings both inpatient and outpatient, and the option to include family members in sessions. Patients in the intervention group were also encouraged to maintain a diary to document food and lifestyle choices. Members of the educational intervention team checked the diaries daily during hospitalization and provided follow-up via a phone call 1 week and then 1 month after discharge.

Findings

The constipation scores of all clinical symptoms were lower (improved) in the intervention group at 1 month after discharge ($p < 0.05$). Additionally, the intervention group had a higher number of patients with good health habits, including diet, exercise, and defecation habits, and proper use of laxatives ($p < 0.05$).

Nursing Implications

The findings of this study suggest that a multifaceted educational intervention can improve clinical symptoms and adherence behaviors, and promote healthy lifestyle choices in patients with FC. Nurses can apply findings to better manage FC, educate patients to improve outcomes, and tailor interventions to best meet the needs of this patient population.

TABLE 38-4	Foods and Medications That Alter Stool Color
Altering Substance	Color
Leafy green vegetables, spinach, kale	Green
Beets, red gelatin, tomato soup, food coloring	Red
Bismuth, iron, black licorice	Black
Barium	Milky white

Adapted from McEvoy, G. E. (Ed.). (2020). *AHFS Drug Information*®. Bethesda, MD: American Society of Health-System Pharmacists. *STAT!Ref Online Electronic Medical Library*. Retrieved on 2/14/2020 at: www.ahfsdruginformation.com/ahfs-drug-information; Wedro, B. (2019). Stool color, changes in color, texture, and form. *MedicineNet*. Retrieved on 1/14/2020 at: www.medicinenet.com/stool_color_changes/article.htm

caused by certain foods; daily food intake; the use of alcohol and tobacco, including smokeless chewing tobacco; and the need to wear dentures or a partial plate. For information about denture care, see Chart 38-2.

Past and current medication use and any previous diagnostic studies, treatments, or surgery are noted. Current nutritional status is assessed via history; laboratory tests (complete metabolic panel including liver function studies, triglyceride, iron studies, and complete blood count [CBC]) are obtained. History of the use of tobacco and alcohol includes details about type, amount, length of use, and the date of discontinuation, if any. The nurse and patient discuss changes in appetite or eating patterns and any unexplained weight gain or loss over the past year. The nurse also asks questions about psychosocial, spiritual, or cultural factors that may be affecting the patient.

Physical Assessment

The physical examination includes assessment of the mouth, abdomen, and rectum and requires a good source of light, full exposure of the abdomen, warm hands with short fingernails, and a comfortable and relaxed patient with an empty bladder.

Oral Cavity Inspection and Palpation

Dentures should be removed to allow good visualization of the entire oral cavity.

Lips

The examination begins with inspection of the lips for moisture, hydration, color, texture, symmetry, and the presence of ulcerations or fissures. The lips should be moist, pink, smooth,

---

Chart 38-2 **HEALTH PROMOTION**

Denture Care

- Brush dentures twice a day.
- Clean well under partial dentures, where food particles tend to get caught.
- Consume nonsticky foods that have been cut into small pieces; chew slowly.
- Remove dentures at night and soak them in water or a denture product. Never put dentures in hot water, because they may warp.
- Rinse mouth with warm salt water in the morning, after meals, and at bedtime.
- See dentist regularly to assess and adjust fit.

---

and symmetric. The patient is instructed to open the mouth wide; a tongue blade is then inserted to expose the buccal mucosa for an assessment of color and lesions. Stensen duct of each parotid gland is visible as a small red dot in the buccal mucosa next to the upper molars.

Gums

The gums are inspected for inflammation, bleeding, retraction, and discoloration. The odor of the breath is also noted. The hard palate is examined for color and shape.

Tongue

The dorsum (back) of the tongue is inspected for texture, color, and lesions. A thin white coat and large, vallate papillae in a "V" formation on the distal portion of the dorsum of the tongue are normal findings. The patient is instructed to protrude the tongue and move it laterally. This provides the examiner with an opportunity to estimate the tongue's size as well as its symmetry and strength (to assess the integrity of the 12th cranial nerve [hypoglossal nerve]).

Further inspection of the ventral surface of the tongue and the floor of the mouth is accomplished by asking the patient to touch the roof of the mouth with the tip of the tongue. Any lesions of the mucosa or any abnormalities involving the frenulum or superficial veins on the undersurface of the tongue are assessed for location, size, color, and pain. This is a common area for oral cancer, which presents as a white or red plaque, lesions, ulcers, or nodules (Weber & Kelley, 2018).

A tongue blade is used to depress the tongue for adequate visualization of the pharynx. It is pressed firmly beyond the midpoint of the tongue; proper placement avoids a gagging response. The patient is told to tip the head back, open the mouth wide, take a deep breath, and say "ah." Often, this flattens the posterior tongue and briefly allows a full view of the tonsils, uvula, and posterior pharynx. These structures are inspected for color, symmetry, and evidence of exudate, ulceration, or enlargement. Normally, the uvula and soft palate rise symmetrically with a deep inspiration upon saying "ah"; this indicates an intact vagus nerve (10th cranial nerve).

A complete assessment of the oral cavity is essential because many disorders, such as cancer, diabetes, and immunosuppressive conditions resulting from medication therapy or acquired immunodeficiency syndrome, may be manifested by changes in the oral cavity, including stomatitis.

Abdominal Inspection, Auscultation, Percussion, and Palpation

The patient lies supine with knees flexed slightly for inspection, auscultation, percussion, and palpation of the abdomen. For the purposes of examination and documentation, the abdomen can be divided into either four quadrants or nine regions (Fig. 38-4).

Consistent use of one of these mapping methods results in a thorough evaluation of the abdomen and appropriate documentation. The four-quadrant method involves the use of an imaginary line drawn vertically from the sternum to the pubis through the umbilicus and a horizontal line drawn across the abdomen through the umbilicus. Inspection is performed first, noting skin changes, nodules, lesions, scarring, discolorations, inflammation, bruising, or striae. Lesions are of particular importance, because GI diseases

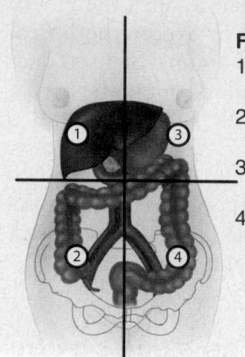

Four quadrants
1 - right upper quadrant (RUQ)
2 - right lower quadrant (RLQ)
3 - left upper quadrant (LUQ)
4 - left lower quadrant (LLQ)

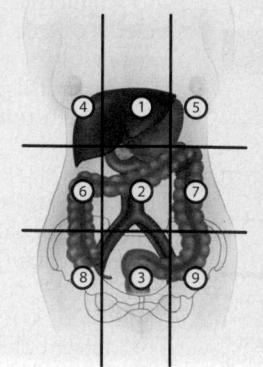

Nine regions
1 - epigastric region
2 - umbilical region
3 - hypogastric or suprapubic region
4 - right hypochondriac region
5 - left hypochondriac region
6 - right lumbar region
7 - left lumbar region
8 - right inguinal region
9 - left inguinal region

Figure 38-4 • Division of the abdomen into four quadrants or nine regions.

often produce skin changes. The contour and symmetry of the abdomen are noted, and any localized bulging, distention, or peristaltic waves are identified. Expected contours of the anterior abdominal wall can be described as flat, rounded, or scaphoid.

Auscultation always precedes percussion and palpation, because they may alter sounds. Auscultation is used to determine the character, location, and frequency of bowel sounds and to identify vascular sounds. Bowel sounds are assessed using the diaphragm of the stethoscope for soft clicks and gurgling sounds (Weber & Kelley, 2018). The frequency and character of the sounds are usually heard as clicks and gurgles that occur irregularly and range from 5 to 30 per minute. Bowel sounds are designated as normal, hyperactive, hypoactive, or absent. The nurse should auscultate for a minimum of 5 minutes; listening for at least 1 minute in each quadrant to confirm the absence of bowel sounds (Weber & Kelley, 2018). Using the bell of the stethoscope, any bruits in the aortic, renal, iliac, and femoral arteries are noted. Friction rubs are high pitched and can be heard over the liver and spleen during respiration. Borborygmus ("stomach growling") is heard as a loud prolonged gurgle.

Percussion is used to assess the size and density of the abdominal organs and to detect the presence of air-filled, fluid-filled, or solid masses. Percussion is used either independently or concurrently with palpation because it can validate palpation findings. All quadrants are percussed for overall tympani and dullness. Tympani is the sound that results from the presence of air in the stomach and small intestines; dullness is heard over organs and solid masses. The use of light palpation is appropriate for identifying areas of tenderness or muscular resistance, and deep palpation is used to identify masses. Testing for rebound tenderness is not performed by many examiners because it can cause severe pain; light percussion is used instead to produce a mild localized response when peritoneal irritation is present.

Rectal Inspection and Palpation

The final part of the examination is evaluation of the terminal portions of the GI tract, the rectum, perianal region, and anus. The anal canal is approximately 2.5 to 4 cm (1 to 1.6 inches) in length and opens into the perineum. Concentric rings of muscle, the internal and external sphincters, normally keep the anal canal securely closed. Gloves, water-soluble lubrication, a penlight, and drapes are necessary tools for the evaluation. Although the rectal examination is generally uncomfortable and often embarrassing for the patient, it is a mandatory part of every thorough examination. For women, the rectal examination may be part of the gynecologic examination. Positions for the rectal examination include knee-chest, left lateral with hips and knees flexed, or standing with hips flexed and upper body supported by the examination table. Most patients are comfortable on the right side with knees brought up to the chest. External examination includes inspection for lumps, rashes, inflammation, excoriation, tears, scars, pilonidal dimpling, and tufts of hair at the pilonidal area. The discovery of tenderness, inflammation, or both should alert the examiner to the possibility of a pilonidal cyst, perianal abscess, or anorectal fistula or fissure. The patient's buttocks are carefully spread and visually inspected until the patient has relaxed the external sphincter control. The patient is asked to bear down, thus allowing the ready appearance of fistulas, fissures, rectal prolapse, polyps, and internal hemorrhoids. Internal examination is performed with a gloved lubricated index finger inserted into the anal canal while the patient bears down. The tone of the sphincter is noted, as are any nodules or irregularities of the anal ring. Because this is an uncomfortable part of the examination for most patients, the patient is encouraged to focus on deep breathing and visualization of a pleasant setting during the brief examination.

Diagnostic Evaluation

GI diagnostic studies can confirm, rule out, stage, or diagnose various disease states, including cancer. After the diagnosis, time should be allotted for discussion with the patient, in addition to offering resource materials for information.

Many modalities are available for diagnostic assessment of the GI tract. The majority of these tests and procedures are performed on an outpatient basis in special settings designed for this purpose (e.g., endoscopy suite or GI laboratory). Preparation for many of these studies includes either a clear liquid or low residue diet, fasting, ingestion of a liquid bowel preparation, the use of laxatives or enemas, and ingestion or injection of a contrast agent or a radiopaque dye. These measures are poorly tolerated by some patients and are especially problematic in older adults or patients with comorbidities because bowel preparations can significantly alter the internal fluid and electrolyte balance. If further assessment or treatment is needed after any outpatient procedure, the patient may be admitted to the hospital.

Specific nursing interventions for each test are provided later in this chapter. General nursing interventions for the patient who is undergoing a GI diagnostic evaluation include:

- Establishing the need for more information
- Providing education to patients and families on the diagnostic test, and pre- and postprocedure restrictions and care
- Helping the patient cope with discomfort and alleviating anxiety
- Informing the primary provider of known medical conditions or abnormal laboratory values that may affect the procedure
- Assessing for adequate hydration before, during, and immediately after the procedure, and providing education about maintenance of hydration

Serum Laboratory Studies

Initial diagnostic tests begin with serum laboratory studies, including but not limited to CBC, complete metabolic panel, prothrombin time/partial thromboplastin time, triglycerides, liver function tests, amylase, and lipase; possibly, more specific studies may be indicated, such as carcinoembryonic antigen (CEA), cancer antigen (CA) 19-9, and alpha-fetoprotein, which are sensitive and specific for colorectal and hepatocellular carcinomas, respectively. CEA is a protein that is normally not detected in the blood of a healthy person; therefore, when detected it indicates that cancer is present, although not what type of cancer is present. CA 19-9 is also a protein that exists on the surface of certain cells and is shed by tumor cells, making it useful as a tumor marker to follow the course of the cancer. Tumor markers (e.g., mCEA and CA 19-9), along with other tests, are used in patients diagnosed with colorectal cancer to demonstrate the effectiveness of treatment or to provide an early warning that the cancer has returned (American Cancer Society [ACS], 2018).

Stool Tests

Basic examination of the stool includes inspecting the specimen for consistency, color, and occult (not visible) blood. Additional studies, including fecal urobilinogen, fecal fat, nitrogen, *Clostridium difficile*, fecal leukocytes, calculation of stool osmolar gap, parasites, pathogens, food residues, and other substances, require laboratory evaluation.

Stool samples are usually collected on a random basis unless a quantitative study (e.g., fecal fat, urobilinogen) is to be performed. Random specimens should be sent promptly to the laboratory for analysis; however, the quantitative 24- to 72-hour collections must be kept refrigerated until transported to the laboratory. Some stool collections require the patient to follow a specific diet or refrain from taking certain medications before the collection; patient education is important.

Guaiac-based fecal occult blood testing (gFOBT) is one of the most commonly performed stool tests. It can be useful in initial screening for several disorders, although it is used most frequently in early cancer detection programs. gFOBT can be performed at the bedside, in the laboratory, or at home. It is inexpensive, noninvasive, and carries minimal risk to the patient. However, it should not be performed when there is hemorrhoidal bleeding. Patients are advised to avoid ingesting red meats, aspirin, and nonsteroidal anti-inflammatory drugs for 72 hours prior to the study because it is thought that these factors are associated with false-positive results; likewise, patients are advised to avoid ingesting vitamin C from supplements or foods as it is believed that this is associated with false-negative results (ACS, 2019). A small amount of the specimen is applied to the guaiac-impregnated paper slide. If the test is performed at home, the patient mails the slide to the primary provider or the lab in an envelope provided for that purpose. The ACS (2019) recommends using the highly sensitive versions of this type of test (e.g., fecal immunochemical test [FIT], FIT-fecal DNA test) for screening.

The FIT reacts to the human hemoglobin protein. The stool sample can be obtained at home, and dietary or medication restrictions are not required prior to collecting the stool specimen. This test is less likely to react to bleeding from other areas of the digestive tract and is done annually (ACS, 2019).

FIT-fecal DNA testing can detect abnormal sections of DNA from cancer or polyp cells (ACS, 2019). The Centers for Medicare & Medicaid Services approved this test for reimbursement and recommends performing the test every 3 years (Rex, Boland, Dominitz, et al., 2017). The FIT-fecal DNA test does not require any dietary or medication restrictions and can detect neoplasia anywhere in the colon.

Breath Tests

The hydrogen breath test was developed to evaluate carbohydrate absorption, in addition to aiding in the diagnosis of bacterial overgrowth in the intestine and short-bowel syndrome. This test determines the amount of hydrogen expelled in the breath after it has been produced in the colon (on contact of galactose with fermenting bacteria) and absorbed into the blood.

Urea breath tests detect the presence of *Helicobacter pylori*, the bacteria that can live in the mucosal lining of the stomach and cause peptic ulcer disease. After the patient ingests a capsule of carbon-labeled urea, a breath sample is obtained 10 to 20 minutes later. Because *H. pylori* metabolizes urea rapidly, the labeled carbon is absorbed quickly; it can then be measured as carbon dioxide in the expired breath to determine whether *H. pylori* is present. Prior to urea breath testing, the patient is instructed to avoid antibiotics or bismuth subsalicylate for 1 month before the test; proton pump inhibitors for 2 weeks before the test; and cimetidine and famotidine for 24 hours before the test (HealthLinkBC, 2018). *H. pylori* also can be detected by assessing serum antibody levels without requiring medication therapy adjustments.

Abdominal Ultrasonography

Ultrasonography is a noninvasive diagnostic technique in which high-frequency sound waves are passed into internal body structures, and the ultrasonic echoes are recorded on an oscilloscope as they strike tissues of different densities. It is particularly useful in the detection of an enlarged gallbladder or pancreas, the presence of gallstones, an enlarged ovary, an ectopic pregnancy, or appendicitis. Ultrasonography can be limited by patient body type, bowel gas patterns, and operator experience (Babakhanlou, 2018).

Advantages of abdominal ultrasonography include an absence of ionizing radiation, no noticeable side effects, relatively low cost, and almost immediate results. It cannot be used to examine structures that lie behind bony tissue, because bone prevents sound waves from traveling into deeper structures. Gas and fluid in the abdomen or air in the lungs also prevent transmission of ultrasound. An ultrasound produces no ill effects. However, some patients, such as pregnant women, have concerns regarding the energy emitted by the probe.

Endoscopic ultrasonography (EUS) is a specialized enteroscopic procedure that aids in the diagnosis of GI disorders by providing direct imaging of a target area. A small high-frequency ultrasonic transducer is mounted at the tip of the fiberoptic scope, which displays images that are of higher-quality resolution and definition than regular ultrasound imaging. EUS may be used to evaluate submucosal lesions, specifically their location and depth of penetration. In addition, EUS may aid in the evaluation of Barrett esophagus, portal hypertension, chronic pancreatitis, suspected pancreatic neoplasm, biliary tract disease, and changes in the bowel wall due to ulcerative colitis. Intestinal gas, bone, and thick layers of adipose tissue that hamper conventional ultrasonography are not problems when EUS is used.

Nursing Interventions

The patient is instructed to fast for 8 to 12 hours before ultrasound testing to decrease the amount of gas in the bowel. If gallbladder studies are being performed, the patient should eat a fat-free meal the evening before the test. If barium studies are to be performed, they should be scheduled after ultrasonography; otherwise, the barium could interfere with the transmission of the sound waves. Patients who receive moderate sedation are observed for about 1 hour to assess for level of consciousness, orientation, and ability to ambulate. Patients treated on an outpatient basis are given instructions regarding diet, activity, and how to monitor for complications (National Institute of Diabetes and Digestive and Kidney Diseases [NIDDK], 2017).

Genetic Testing

Researchers have refined methods for genetics risk assessment, preclinical diagnosis, and prenatal diagnosis to identify people who are at risk for certain GI disorders (e.g., gastric cancer, lactose deficiency, inflammatory bowel disease, colon cancer) (Chart 38-3). People who are identified as being at risk for certain GI disorders may choose to have genetic counseling to learn about the disease and options for preventing and treating the disease, and to receive support in coping

---

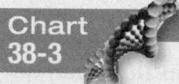

Chart 38-3

GENETICS IN NURSING PRACTICE

Digestive and Gastrointestinal Disorders

Several digestive and gastrointestinal disorders are associated with genetic abnormalities. Some examples include:

Autosomal dominant:

- Hereditary diffuse gastric cancer
- Hereditary non-polyposis colorectal cancer (Lynch syndrome)
- Hirschsprung disease (aganglionic megacolon)

Autosomal recessive:

- Glucose galactose malabsorption
- Glycogen storage disease (von Gierke disease)
- Pompe disease
- Zellweger syndrome

Inheritance pattern includes autosomal dominant and autosomal recessive:

- Familial adenomatous polyposis

X-linked:

- Fabry disease

Inheritance pattern is not distinct; however, there is a genetic predisposition for the disease:

- Crohn's disease
- Type 1 diabetes
- Celiac disease
- Pancreatic cancer

Other genetic disorders that will impact the digestive and gastrointestinal system:

- Cleft lip and/or palate
- Cystic fibrosis

Nursing Assessments

Refer to Chapter 4, Chart 4-2: Genetics in Nursing Practice: Genetic Aspects of Health Assessment

Family History Assessment Related to Digestive and Gastrointestinal Disorders

- Careful family history assessment for other family members with a similar condition (e.g., cleft lip/palate, pyloric stenosis).
- Assess for other family members in several generations with early-onset colorectal cancer.
- Inquire about other family members with inflammatory bowel disease.
- Assess family history for other cancers (e.g., endometrial, ovarian, kidney).

Patient Assessment Specific to Digestive and Gastrointestinal Disorders

- Ask about bowel pattern and color of stool.
- Assess if patient experiences episodes of abdominal cramping, diarrhea, or dehydration.
- Assess for unexplained weight loss.
- Identify intolerance to specific foods (e.g., gluten, high-fat foods, lactose).
- Assess for prior history of liver disorders.

Assess for presence of other clinical conditions:

- With clefting—congenital heart defect, other birth defects suggestive of a genetic syndrome.
- With familial adenomatous polyposis—congenital hypertrophy of retinal pigment epithelium.

Genetics Resources

Cancer.Net, www.cancer.net
Celiac Disease Foundation, www.celiac.org
Crohn's & Colitis Foundation, www.ccfa.org
See Chapter 6, Chart 6-7 for components of genetic counseling.

with the situation. Lynch syndrome is inherited in an autosomal dominant manner and is associated with colonic and extracolonic cancers; 3% of new cases of colon cancer are attributed to Lynch syndrome (Kohlmann & Gruber, 2018; Sinicrope, 2018). See Chapter 6 for further discussion of genetic counseling.

Imaging Studies

Numerous minimally invasive and noninvasive imaging studies, including x-ray and contrast studies, computed tomography (CT) scan, magnetic resonance imaging (MRI) scan, positron emission tomography (PET) scan, scintigraphy (radionuclide imaging), and virtual colonoscopy are available today.

Upper Gastrointestinal Tract Study

An upper GI fluoroscopy delineates the entire GI tract after the introduction of a contrast agent. A radiopaque liquid (e.g., barium sulfate) is commonly used; however, thin barium, diatrizoate sodium (Hypaque), and at times water are used due to their low associated risks. The GI series enables the examiner to detect or exclude anatomic or functional disorders of the upper GI organs or sphincters. It also aids in the diagnosis of ulcers, varices, tumors, regional enteritis, and malabsorption syndromes. The procedure may be extended to examine the duodenum and small bowel (small-bowel follow-through). As the barium descends into the stomach, the position, patency, and caliber of the esophagus are visualized, enabling the examiner to detect or exclude any anatomic or functional derangement of that organ. Fluoroscopic examination next extends to the stomach as its lumen fills with barium, allowing observation of stomach motility, thickness of the gastric wall, the mucosal pattern, patency of the pyloric valve, and the anatomy of the duodenum. Multiple x-ray images are obtained during the procedure, and additional images may be taken at intervals for up to 24 hours to evaluate the rate of gastric emptying. Small-bowel x-rays taken while the barium is passing through that area allow for observation of the motility of the small bowel. Obstructions, ileitis, and diverticula can also be detected.

Variations of the upper GI study include double-contrast studies and enteroclysis. The double-contrast method of examining the upper GI tract involves administration of a thick barium suspension to outline the stomach and esophageal wall, after which tablets that release carbon dioxide in the presence of water are given. This technique has the advantage of showing the esophagus and stomach in finer detail, permitting signs of early superficial neoplasms to be noted.

Enteroclysis is a very detailed, double-contrast study of the entire small intestine that involves the continuous infusion (through a duodenal tube) of 500 to 1000 mL of a thin barium sulfate suspension; after this, methylcellulose is infused through the tube. The barium and methylcellulose fill the intestinal loops and are observed continuously by fluoroscopy and viewed at frequent intervals as they progress through the jejunum and the ileum. Air may also be used, but methylcellulose is preferred as it is associated with enhanced visibility (Lampignano & Kendrick, 2018). This process (even with normal motility) can take up to 6 hours and can be quite uncomfortable for the patient. The procedure aids in the diagnosis of partial small-bowel obstructions or diverticula. After completion of the fluoroscopic component of the study, the patient may have a CT scan to assess for lesions or adhesions, and in this case an iodinated contrast media may be used (Lampignano & Kendrick, 2018).

Nursing Interventions

Instruction regarding dietary changes prior to the study may include a low residue or clear liquid diet, and nothing by mouth (*nil per os*; NPO) after midnight the night before the study. In addition, the patient is advised to not smoke or chew gum during the NPO period because these can increase gastric secretions and salivation (Lampignano & Kendrick, 2018). Polyethylene glycol (PEG)-based solutions are considered the most effective bowel cleansing preparatory agent; other agents include sodium phosphate, magnesium citrate, and preparations containing sodium picosulfate, citric acid, and magnesium oxide (Harrison & Hielkrem, 2016; Tan, Lin, Ma, et al., 2018). Typically, oral medications are withheld on the morning of the study and resumed that evening, but each patient's medication regimen should be evaluated on an individual basis. When a patient with insulin-dependent diabetes is NPO, their insulin requirements will need to be adjusted accordingly (see Chapter 46).

Follow-up care is provided after the upper GI procedure to ensure that the patient has eliminated most of the ingested barium. Fluids may be increased to facilitate evacuation of stool and barium.

Lower Gastrointestinal Tract Study

Visualization of the lower GI tract is obtained after rectal installation of barium. The barium enema can be used to detect the presence of polyps, tumors, or other lesions of the large intestine and demonstrate any anatomic abnormalities or malfunctioning of the bowel. After proper preparation and evacuation of the entire colon, each portion of the colon may be readily observed. The procedure usually takes about 15 to 30 minutes, during which time x-ray images are obtained.

Other means for visualizing the colon include double-contrast studies and a water-soluble contrast study. These tests are still occasionally used because they are relatively inexpensive and simple. A double-contrast or air-contrast barium enema involves the instillation of a thicker barium solution, followed by the instillation of air. The patient may feel some cramping or discomfort during this process. This test provides a contrast between the air-filled lumen and the barium-coated mucosa, allowing easier detection of smaller lesions. CT colonography has replaced double-contrast barium enema for nearly all indicated GI disorders (Rex et al., 2017) (see later discussion).

If active inflammatory disease, fistulas, or perforation of the colon is suspected, a water-soluble iodinated contrast agent (e.g., diatrizoic acid [Gastrografin]) can be used. The procedure is the same as for a barium enema, but the patient must first be assessed for allergy to iodine or contrast agent. The contrast agent is eliminated readily after the procedure, so there is no need for postprocedure laxatives. Diarrhea may occur in some patients until the contrast agent has been totally eliminated.

Nursing Interventions

Preparation of the patient includes emptying and cleansing the lower bowel. This often necessitates a low residue diet 1 to 2 days before the test, a clear liquid diet and a laxative the evening before, NPO after midnight, and cleansing enemas until returns are clear the following morning. The nurse makes sure that barium enemas are scheduled before any upper GI studies. If the patient has active inflammatory disease of the colon, enemas are contraindicated. Barium enemas also are contraindicated in patients with signs of perforation or obstruction; instead, a water-soluble contrast study may be performed. Active GI bleeding may prohibit the use of laxatives and enemas.

Postprocedural patient education includes information about increasing fluid intake, evaluating bowel movements for evacuation of barium, and noting increased number of bowel movements, because barium, due to its high osmolarity, may draw fluid into the bowel, thus increasing the intraluminal contents and resulting in greater output.

Computed Tomography

A CT scan provides cross-sectional images of abdominal organs and structures. Multiple x-ray images are taken from numerous angles, digitized in a computer, reconstructed, and then viewed on a computer monitor. As the sensitivity and specificity of CT scans have increased in recent years, so has their use. Volume CT scanners (i.e., helical or spiral scanning) provide more accurate reconstruction of patient data into alternate planes, require shorter scan times, and have less artifact when compared to single slice scanning (Lampignano & Kendrick, 2018). CT is a valuable tool for detecting and localizing many inflammatory conditions in the colon, such as appendicitis, diverticulitis, regional enteritis, and ulcerative colitis, as well as evaluating the abdomen for diseases of the liver, spleen, kidney, pancreas, and pelvic organs, and structural abnormalities of the abdominal wall. The CT procedure is completely painless, but radiation doses are considerable. A CT scan may be performed with or without oral or intravenous (IV) contrast, but the enhancement of the study is greater with the use of a contrast agent. In patients at risk for complications from use of contrast, the radiologist and provider must be in agreement that the scan is medically necessary and that the benefits outweigh the risks (Yale School of Medicine, 2019).

Nursing Interventions

Common risks from IV contrast agents include allergic reactions and contrast-induced nephropathy (CIN); therefore, patients must be screened for these risks (Hossain, Costanzo, Cosentino, et al., 2018). Any allergies to contrast agents, iodine, or shellfish, the patient's current serum creatinine level, and pregnancy status in females must be determined before administration of a contrast agent. Patients allergic to the contrast agent may be premedicated with a corticosteroid and antihistamine.

The most effective ways to prevent CIN include careful selection of patients, maintaining hydration status, using newer contrast agents, and avoiding nephrotoxic agents pre- and postprocedure (Hossain et al., 2018).

Magnetic Resonance Imaging

MRI is used in gastroenterology to supplement ultrasonography and CT. This noninvasive technique uses magnetic fields and radio waves to produce images of the area being studied. The use of oral contrast agents to enhance the image has increased the application of this technique for the diagnosis of GI diseases. It is useful in evaluating abdominal soft tissues as well as blood vessels, abscesses, fistulas, neoplasms, and other sources of bleeding.

The physiologic artifacts of heartbeat, respiration, and peristalsis may create a less-than-clear image; however, newer, fast-imaging MRI techniques help eliminate these physiologic motion artifacts. MRI is not totally safe for all people; having the patient complete a preprocedure MRI tool that screens for contraindications to MRI is required (Lampignano & Kendrick, 2018). Any ferromagnetic objects (metals that contain iron) can be attracted to the magnet and cause injury. Items that can be problematic or dangerous include jewelry, dental implants, paper clips, pens, keys, IV poles, clips on patient gowns, and oxygen tanks.

> ◤ *Quality and Safety Nursing Alert*
>
> *MRI is contraindicated in patients with any device containing metal because the magnetic field could cause malfunction. MRI is also contraindicated for patients with internal metal devices (e.g., aneurysm clips), intraocular metallic fragments, or cochlear implants. Foil-backed skin patches (e.g., nicotine, nitroglycerin, scopolamine, clonidine) should be removed before an MRI because of the risk of burns; however, the patient's primary provider should be consulted before the patch is removed to determine whether an alternate form of the medication should be provided.*

Nursing Interventions

Preprocedure patient education includes NPO status 6 to 8 hours before the study and removal of all jewelry and other metals. The patient and family are informed that the study may take 60 to 90 minutes; during this time, the technician will instruct the patient to take deep breaths at specific intervals. The close-fitting scanners used in many MRI facilities may induce feelings of claustrophobia, and the machine will make a knocking sound during the procedure. Patients may choose to wear a headset and listen to music or wear a blindfold during the procedure. Open MRIs that are less close fitting eliminate the claustrophobia that many patients experience; however, they produce lower-resolution images.

Positron Emission Tomography

PET scans produce images of the body by detecting the radiation emitted from radioactive substances. The radioactive substances are injected into the body IV and are usually tagged with radioactive isotopes of oxygen, nitrogen, carbon, or fluorine (Lampignano & Kendrick, 2018). These isotopes decay quickly, do not harm the body, have lower radiation levels than a typical x-ray or CT scan, and are eliminated in the urine or feces. The scanner essentially "captures" where the radioactive substances are in the body, transmits information to a scanner, and produces a scan with "hot spots" for evaluation by the radiologist or oncologist.

Scintigraphy

Scintigraphy (radionuclide testing) relies on the use of radioactive isotopes (i.e., technetium, iodine, indium) to reveal displaced anatomic structures, changes in organ size, and the presence of neoplasms or other focal lesions such as cysts or abscesses. Scintigraphic scanning is also used to measure the uptake of tagged red blood cells and leukocytes. Tagging of red blood cells and leukocytes by injection of a radionuclide is performed to define areas of inflammation, abscess, blood loss, or neoplasm. A sample of blood is removed, mixed with a radioactive substance, and reinjected into the patient. Abnormal concentrations of blood cells are then detected at 24- and 48-hour intervals. Tagged red cell studies are useful in determining the source of internal bleeding when all other studies have returned a negative result.

Gastrointestinal Motility Studies

Radionuclide testing also is used to assess gastric emptying and colonic transit time. During gastric emptying studies, the liquid and solid components of a meal (typically scrambled eggs) are tagged with radionuclide markers. After ingestion of the meal, the patient is positioned under a scintiscanner, which measures the rate of passage of the radioactive substance from the stomach (Parkman, 2018). This is useful in diagnosing disorders of gastric motility, diabetic gastroparesis, and dumping syndrome.

Colonic transit studies are used to evaluate colonic motility and obstructive defecation syndromes. The patient is given a capsule containing 20 radionuclide markers and instructed to follow a regular diet and usual daily activities. Abdominal x-rays are taken every 24 hours until all markers are passed. This process usually takes 4 to 5 days; in the presence of severe constipation it may take as long as 10 days. Patients with chronic diarrhea may be evaluated at 8-hour intervals. The amount of time that it takes for the radioactive material to move through the colon indicates colonic motility.

Endoscopic Procedures

Endoscopic procedures used in GI tract assessment include fibroscopy/esophagogastroduodenoscopy (EGD), colonoscopy, anoscopy, proctoscopy, sigmoidoscopy, small-bowel enteroscopy, and endoscopy through an ostomy.

Upper Gastrointestinal Fibroscopy/ Esophagogastroduodenoscopy

Fibroscopy of the upper GI tract allows direct visualization of the esophageal, gastric, and duodenal mucosa through a lighted endoscope (gastroscope) (Fig. 38-5). EGD is valuable when esophageal, gastric, or duodenal disorders or inflammatory, neoplastic, or infectious processes are suspected. This procedure also can be used to evaluate esophageal and gastric motility and to collect secretions and tissue specimens for further analysis.

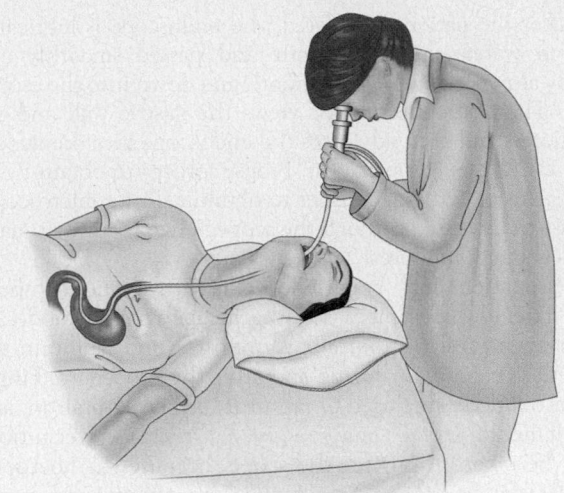

Figure 38-5 • Patient undergoing gastroscopy.

In EGD, the gastroenterologist views the GI tract through a viewing lens and can obtain images through the scope to document findings. Electronic video endoscopes also are available that attach directly to a video processor, converting the electronic signals into pictures that are projected on a screen. This allows larger and continuous viewing capabilities, as well as the simultaneous recording of the procedure.

PillCam ESO, or capsule endoscopy, requires that the patient swallows a capsule that travels by peristalsis through the small intestines. The capsule contains an oxide metal silicon chip video camera, which transmits digital images of the GI mucosa to a data recorder that is worn on the patient's waist. This technology is a diagnostic option for patients with esophageal diseases who cannot tolerate an EGD (Park, Cho, & Kim, 2018). Capsule colonoscopy is FDA approved for patients with previous incomplete colonoscopies, and for those who are not candidates for colonoscopies or sedation (Rex et al., 2017).

Endoscopic retrograde cholangiopancreatography (ERCP) uses the endoscope in combination with x-rays to view the bile ducts, pancreatic ducts, and gallbladder (MedlinePlus, 2019). The side-viewing flexible scopes are used to visualize the common bile duct and the pancreatic and hepatic ducts through the ampulla of Vater in the duodenum. ERCP is helpful in evaluating jaundice, pancreatitis, pancreatic tumors, common bile duct stones, and biliary tract disease. Current trends show an increase in ERCP use for therapeutic indications (sphincterotomy, stone removal, and biliary stenting), with a decline in its use for conventional diagnostic testing (Ahmed, Kanotra, Savani, et al., 2017). ERCP is described further in Chapter 44.

Upper GI fibroscopy also can be a therapeutic procedure when combined with other procedures. Therapeutic endoscopy can be used to remove common bile duct stones, dilate strictures, and treat gastric bleeding and esophageal varices. Laser-compatible scopes can be used to provide laser therapy for upper GI neoplasms. Sclerosing solutions can be injected through the scope in an attempt to control upper GI bleeding.

After the patient is sedated, the endoscope is lubricated with a water-soluble lubricant and passed smoothly and slowly along the back of the mouth and down into the esophagus. The gastroenterologist views the gastric wall and the sphincters and then advances the endoscope into the duodenum for further examination. Biopsy forceps to obtain tissue specimens or cytology brushes to obtain cells for microscopic study can be passed through the scope. The procedure usually takes about 30 minutes.

The patient may experience nausea, gagging, or choking. The use of topical anesthetic agents and moderate sedation makes it important to monitor and maintain the patient's oral airway during and after the procedure. Finger or ear oximeters are used to monitor oxygen saturation, and supplemental oxygen may be given if needed. Precautions must be taken to protect the scope, because the fiberoptic bundles can be broken if the scope is bent at an acute angle. The patient wears a mouth guard to keep from biting the scope.

Nursing Interventions

The patient should be NPO for 8 hours prior to the examination. Before the introduction of the endoscope, the patient is given a local anesthetic gargle or spray. Midazolam, a sedative that provides moderate sedation with loss of the gag reflex and relieves anxiety during the procedure, is given. Atropine may be given to reduce secretions, and glucagon may be given to relax smooth muscle. The patient is positioned in the left lateral position to facilitate clearance of pulmonary secretions and provide smooth entry of the scope.

After gastroscopy, assessment includes level of consciousness, vital signs, oxygen saturation, pain level, and monitoring for signs of perforation (i.e., pain, bleeding, unusual difficulty swallowing, rapidly elevated temperature). Temporary loss of the gag reflex is expected; after the patient's gag reflex has returned, lozenges, saline gargle, and oral analgesic agents may be offered to relieve minor throat discomfort. Patients who were sedated for the procedure must remain in bed until fully alert. After moderate sedation, the patient must be transported home with a family member or friend if the procedure was performed on an outpatient basis. Someone should stay with the patient until the morning after the procedure.

Because of sedation, many patients will not remember postprocedure instructions. For this reason, discharge and follow-up verbal and written instructions are provided to the person accompanying the patient home, as well as to the patient. In addition, many endoscopy suites have a program in which a nurse telephones the patient the morning after the procedure to find out if the patient has any concerns or questions related to the procedure.

Fiberoptic Colonoscopy

Historically, direct visualization of the bowel was the only means to evaluate the colon, but virtual colonoscopy (also known as CT colonography) is now available. Advantages include less risk for perforation when compared to colonoscopy; however, the need for bowel preparation is considered a disadvantage (Rex et al., 2017).

Direct visual inspection of the large intestine (anus, rectum, sigmoid, transcending and ascending colon) is possible by means of a flexible fiberoptic colonoscope (Fig. 38-6). These scopes have the same capabilities as those used for EGD but are larger in diameter and longer. Still and video recordings can be used to document the procedure and findings.

This procedure is used commonly as a diagnostic aid and screening device. It is most frequently used for cancer screening and for surveillance in patients with previous colon cancer or polyps. (See Chapter 12, Table 12-3 for details on the ACS's screening guidelines.) In addition, tissue biopsies can be obtained as needed, and polyps can be removed and evaluated. Other uses of colonoscopy include the evaluation of patients with diarrhea of unknown cause, occult bleeding, or anemia; further study of abnormalities detected on barium enema; and diagnosis, clarification, and determination of the extent of inflammatory or other bowel disease.

The procedure can be used to remove all visible polyps with a special snare and cautery through the colonoscope. Many colon cancers begin with adenomatous polyps of the colon; therefore, one goal of colonoscopic polypectomy is early detection and prevention of colorectal cancer. This procedure also can be used to treat areas of bleeding or stricture. The use of bipolar and unipolar coagulators and

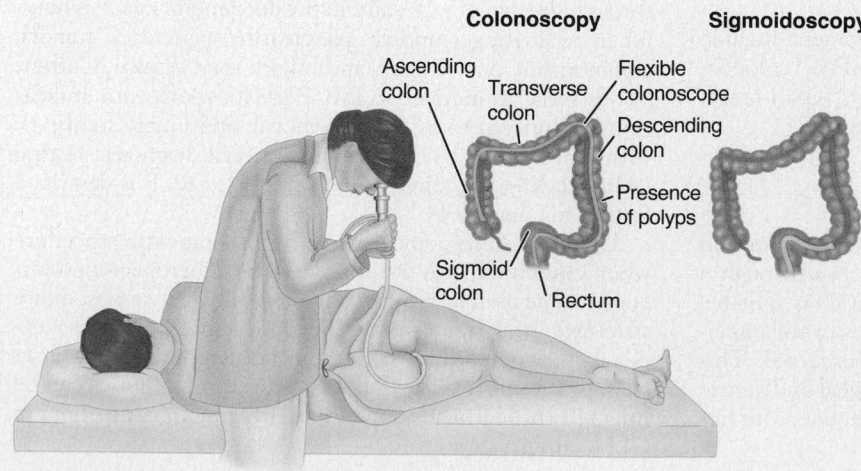

Colonoscopy

Ascending colon
Transverse colon
Flexible colonoscope
Descending colon
Presence of polyps
Sigmoid colon
Rectum

Sigmoidoscopy

Figure 38-6 • Colonoscopy and flexible fiberoptic sigmoidoscopy. For the colonoscopy, the flexible scope is passed through the rectum and sigmoid colon into the descending, transverse, and ascending colon. For the flexible fiberoptic sigmoidoscopy, the flexible scope is advanced past the proximal sigmoid and then into the descending colon.

heater probes, as well as injections of sclerosing agents or vasoconstrictors, is possible during this procedure. Laser-compatible scopes provide laser therapy for bleeding lesions or colonic neoplasms. Bowel decompression (removal of intestinal contents to prevent gas and fluid from distending the coils of the intestine) can also be completed during the procedure.

Colonoscopy is performed while the patient is lying on the left side with the legs drawn up toward the chest. The patient's position may be changed during the test to facilitate advancement of the scope. Biopsy forceps or a cytology brush may be passed through the scope to obtain specimens for histology and cytology examinations. Complications during and after the procedure can include cardiac arrhythmias and respiratory depression resulting from the medications given, vasovagal reactions, and circulatory overload or hypotension resulting from overhydration or underhydration during bowel preparation. The patient's cardiac and respiratory function and oxygen saturation are monitored continuously, with supplemental oxygen used as necessary. Typically, the procedure takes about 1 hour, and postprocedure discomfort results from instillation of air to expand the colon and insertion and movement of the scope during the procedure.

Capsule colonoscopy is another option for patients who cannot tolerate colonoscopy or for patients with incomplete colonoscopies. This minimally invasive test consists of an ingestible capsule with a two-sided camera (similar to the PillCam ESO). This test requires that the patient completes a more extensive bowel preparation than required for a colonoscopy; patients with a positive test then require a follow-up colonoscopy on a separate day (Rex et al., 2017).

Nursing Interventions

The success of colonoscopy depends on how well the colon is prepared (Tariq, Kamal, Sapkota, et al., 2019). Adequate colon cleansing provides optimal visualization and decreases the time needed for the procedure. Cleansing of the colon can be accomplished in various ways. The primary provider may prescribe a laxative for two nights before the examination and a Fleet or saline enema until the return is clear the morning of the test. However, more commonly, PEG electrolyte lavage solutions (GoLYTELY, CoLyte, and NuLYTELY) are used for effective cleansing of the bowel. Current preparations include either the nonsplit dose regimen, in which the entire solution is ingested the night before the procedure, or the split-dose regimen, in which half of the dose is ingested the night before and half is ingested the morning of the procedure, 3 hours prior to the scheduled test. Tariq et al. (2019) report improved bowel preparation and cleansing with the split prep.

Patient health history and comorbidities such as diabetes, chronic constipation, or history of opioid use, or problematic colonoscopies influence patient preparation. Preprocedure diet instructions include a clear liquid or a low residue diet starting the day before the procedure; diet type has not been shown to affect bowel preparation in patients ingesting the split preparations (Tariq et al., 2019). If necessary, the nurse can give the solution through a feeding tube if the patient cannot swallow. Patients with a colostomy can receive this same bowel preparation. The use of lavage solutions is contraindicated in patients with intestinal obstruction or inflammatory bowel disease.

A sodium phosphate tablet (OsmoPrep, Visicol) can be used for colon cleansing prior to colonoscopy. Dosing consists of 32 tablets: 20 tablets (4 tablets every 15 minutes) with 8 oz of any clear liquid (water, any clear carbonated beverage, or juice) on the evening prior to the examination, and 12 tablets (taken in the same manner) on the morning of the examination.

With the use of lavage solutions, bowel cleansing is fast (rectal effluent is clear in about 4 hours) and is tolerated fairly well by most patients. Side effects of the electrolyte solutions include nausea, bloating, cramps or abdominal fullness, fluid and electrolyte imbalance, and hypothermia (patients are often told to drink the preparation as cold as possible to make it more palatable). The side effects are especially problematic for older adults, and sometimes they have difficulty ingesting the required volume of solution. Monitoring older patients after a bowel preparation is especially important because their physiologic ability to compensate for fluid loss is diminished. Many older adults take multiple medications each day; therefore, the nurse's knowledge of their daily medication regimen can prompt assessment for and prevention of potential problems and early detection of physiologic changes.

Additionally, the nurse advises the patient with diabetes to consult with their primary provider about medication adjustment to prevent hyperglycemia or hypoglycemia resulting from the dietary modifications required in preparing for the test. The nurse also instructs all patients, especially older adults, to maintain adequate fluid, electrolyte, and caloric intake while undergoing bowel cleansing.

Special precautions must be taken for some patients. Implantable defibrillators and pacemakers are at high risk for malfunction if electrosurgical procedures (i.e., polypectomy) are performed in conjunction with colonoscopy. A cardiologist should be consulted before the test is performed for device management. These patients require careful cardiac monitoring during the procedure (American Society of Anesthesiology Taskforce, 2020; Neubauer, Wellman, Herzog-Niescery, et al., 2018).

Colonoscopy cannot be performed if there is a suspected or documented colon perforation, acute severe diverticulitis, or acute colitis. Patients with prosthetic heart valves or a history of endocarditis require prophylactic antibiotics before the procedure.

Informed consent is obtained by the practitioner before the patient is sedated. Before the examination, an opioid analgesic agent or sedative (e.g., midazolam) is given to provide moderate sedation and relieve anxiety during the procedure. Glucagon may be given, if needed, to relax the colonic musculature and to reduce spasm during the test. Patients who are older or debilitated may require a reduced dosage of the analgesic agent or sedative to decrease the risks of oversedation and cardiopulmonary complications.

During the procedure, the patient is monitored for changes in oxygen saturation, vital signs, color and temperature of the skin, level of consciousness, abdominal distention, vagal response, and pain intensity. After the procedure, patients are maintained on bed rest until fully alert. Some patients have abdominal cramps caused by increased peristalsis stimulated by the air insufflated into the bowel during the procedure.

Immediately after the test, the patient is monitored for signs and symptoms of bowel perforation (e.g., rectal bleeding, abdominal pain or distention, fever, focal peritoneal signs). Because of the amnesic effects of midazolam, the patient may be unable to recall verbal information and should receive written instructions. If the procedure is performed on an outpatient basis, someone must transport the patient home. After a therapeutic procedure, the nurse instructs the patient to report any bleeding to the primary provider.

Anoscopy, Proctoscopy, and Sigmoidoscopy

Endoscopic examination of the anus, rectum, and sigmoid and descending colon is used to evaluate chronic diarrhea, fecal incontinence, ischemic colitis, and lower GI hemorrhage and to observe for ulceration, fissures, abscesses, tumors, polyps, or other pathologic processes.

The flexible fiberoptic sigmoidoscope (see Fig. 38-6) permits the colon to be examined up to 40 to 50 cm (16 to 20 inches) from the anus, much more than the 25 cm (10 inches) that can be visualized with the rigid sigmoidoscope. It has many of the same capabilities as the scopes used for the upper GI study, including the use of still or video images to document findings.

For flexible scope procedures, the patient assumes a comfortable position on the left side with the right leg bent and placed anteriorly. It is important to keep the patient informed throughout the examination and to explain the sensations associated with it. Biopsies and polypectomies can be performed during this procedure. Biopsy is performed with small biting forceps introduced through the endoscope; one or more small pieces of tissue may be removed. If polyps are present, they may be removed with a wire snare, which is used to grasp the pedicle, or stalk. An electrocoagulating current is then used to sever the polyp and prevent bleeding. It is extremely important that all excised tissue be placed immediately in moist gauze or in an appropriate receptacle, labeled correctly, and delivered without delay to the pathology laboratory for examination.

Nursing Interventions

These examinations require only limited bowel preparation, including a warm tap water or Fleet enema until returns are clear. Dietary restrictions usually are not necessary, and sedation usually is not required. During the procedure, the nurse monitors vital signs, skin color and temperature, pain tolerance, and vagal response. After the procedure, the nurse monitors the patient for rectal bleeding and signs of intestinal perforation (i.e., fever, rectal drainage, abdominal distention, pain). On completion of the examination, the patient can resume regular activities and diet.

Small Bowel Studies

Several methods are available for visualization of the small intestine, including capsule endoscopy and double-balloon enteroscopy. Capsule endoscopy allows the noninvasive visualization of the mucosa throughout the entire small intestine. It is particularly useful in the evaluation of obscure GI bleeding. The technique consists of the patient swallowing a capsule embedded with a wireless miniature camera, a light source, and an image transmission system. The capsule is the size of a large vitamin pill. It is propelled through the intestine by peristalsis. Images are transmitted from the end of the capsule to a recording device worn by the patient. The capsule allows for inspection of the small intestine without patient discomfort (Yamamoto & Aabakken, 2019).

Double-balloon enteroscopy has made it possible to visualize the mucosa of the entire small bowel as well as carry out diagnostic and therapeutic interventions (Yamamoto & Aabakken, 2019). This endoscope is comprised of two balloons, one attached to the distal end of the scope and the other attached to the transparent overtube that slides over the endoscope. The endoscope is advanced alternately inflating and deflating the balloons; this causes telescoping of the small intestine onto the overtube. As a result of this telescoping, the endoscope can visualize much more of the small intestine than the length of the scope itself. The procedure takes between 1 and 3 hours and requires moderate sedation. Nursing interventions are similar to those for other endoscopic procedures.

Endoscopy through an Ostomy

Endoscopy through an ostomy stoma is useful for visualizing a segment of the small or large intestine and may be indicated to evaluate the anastomosis for recurrent disease, or to visualize and treat bleeding in a segment of the bowel. Nursing interventions are similar to those for other endoscopic procedures.

Manometry and Electrophysiologic Studies

Manometry and electrophysiologic studies are methods for evaluating patients with GI motility disorders. The manometry test measures changes in intraluminal pressures and the coordination of muscle activity in the GI tract with the pressures transmitted to a computer analyzer.

Esophageal manometry is used to detect motility disorders of the esophagus and the upper and lower esophageal sphincter. Also known as esophageal motility studies, these studies are very helpful in the diagnosis of achalasia (i.e., absence of peristalsis), diffuse esophageal spasm, scleroderma, and other esophageal motor disorders. The patient must refrain from eating or drinking for 8 to 12 hours before the test. Medications that could have a direct effect on motility (e.g., calcium channel blockers, anticholinergic agents, sedatives) are withheld for 24 to 48 hours. A pressure-sensitive catheter is inserted through the nose and is connected to a transducer and a video recorder. The patient then swallows small amounts of water while the resultant pressure changes are recorded. Evaluation of a patient for GERD typically includes esophageal manometry.

Gastroduodenal, small intestine, and colonic manometry procedures are used to evaluate delayed gastric emptying and gastric and intestinal motility disorders such as irritable bowel syndrome or atonic colon. This is often an ambulatory outpatient procedure lasting 24 to 72 hours. Anorectal manometry measures the resting tone of the internal anal sphincter and the contractibility of the external anal sphincter. It is helpful in evaluating patients with chronic constipation or fecal incontinence and is useful in biofeedback for the treatment of fecal incontinence. It can be performed in conjunction with rectal sensory functioning tests. Dibasic sodium (Phosphosoda) or a saline cleansing enema is given 1 hour before the test, and positioning for the test is either the prone or the lateral position.

Rectal sensory function studies are used to evaluate rectal sensory function and neuropathy. A catheter and balloon are passed into the rectum, with increasing balloon inflation until the patient feels distention. Then the tone and pressure of the rectum and anal sphincter are measured. The results are especially helpful in the evaluation of patients with chronic constipation, diarrhea, or incontinence.

Electrogastrography, an electrophysiologic study, also may be performed to assess gastric motility disturbances and can be useful in detecting motor or nerve dysfunction in the stomach. Electrodes are placed over the abdomen, and gastric electrical activity is recorded for up to 24 hours. Patients may exhibit rapid, slow, or irregular waveform activity.

Defecography measures anorectal function and is performed with very thick barium paste instilled into the rectum. Fluoroscopy is used to assess the function of the rectum and anal sphincter while the patient attempts to expel the barium. The test requires no preparation. The nurse educates the patient about what to expect during these procedures.

Gastric Analysis, Gastric Acid Stimulation Test, and pH Monitoring

Analysis of the gastric juice yields information about the secretory activity of the gastric mucosa and the presence or degree of gastric retention in patients thought to have pyloric or duodenal obstruction. It is also useful for diagnosing Zollinger-Ellison syndrome or atrophic gastritis.

The patient is NPO for 8 to 12 hours before the procedure. Any medications that affect gastric secretions are withheld for 24 to 48 hours before the test. Smoking is not allowed on the morning of the test because it increases gastric secretions. A small nasogastric tube with a catheter tip marked at various points is inserted through the nose. When the tube is at a point slightly less than 50 cm (21 inches), it should be within the stomach, lying along the greater curvature. Once in place, the tube is secured to the patient's cheek and the patient is placed in a semireclining position. The entire stomach contents are aspirated by gentle suction into a syringe, and gastric samples are collected every 15 minutes for the next hour.

Important diagnostic information to be gained from gastric analysis includes the ability of the mucosa to secrete HCl. This ability is altered in various disease states, including:

- *Pernicious anemia:* Patients with this disease secrete no acid under basal conditions or after stimulation.
- *Severe chronic atrophic gastritis or gastric cancer:* Patients with these diseases secrete little or no acid.
- *Gastric ulcer:* Patients with this disease secrete some acid.
- *Duodenal ulcers:* Patients with this disease usually secrete an excess amount of acid.

The gastric acid stimulation test usually is performed in conjunction with gastric analysis. Histamine or pentagastrin is given subcutaneously to stimulate gastric secretions. It is important to inform the patient that this injection may produce a flushed feeling. The nurse monitors the patient's blood pressure and pulse frequently to detect hypotension. Gastric specimens are collected after the injection every 15 minutes for 1 hour and are labeled to indicate the time of specimen collection after histamine injection. The volume and pH of the specimen are measured; in certain instances, cytologic study by the Papanicolaou technique may be used to determine the presence or absence of malignant cells.

Esophageal reflux of gastric acid may be diagnosed and evaluated by ambulatory pH monitoring (Triadafilopoulos, Zikos, Regalia, et al., 2018). The patient is NPO for 6 hours before the test. A sensor that measures pH is inserted and positioned via endoscopy. The sensor is then connected to an external recording device and is worn for 24 hours while the patient continues usual daily activities. The result is a computer analysis and graphic display of the results.

The Bravo pH monitoring system offers the advantage of pH monitoring of the esophagus without the transnasal catheter. The clinician, by means of endoscopy, attaches a capsule (approximately the size of a gel cap) to the patient's esophageal wall. Data related to pH are transmitted from the capsule to a pager-sized receiver that the patient wears. Data are collected for up to 96 hours and then downloaded and analyzed. The capsule spontaneously detaches from the esophagus in 7 to 10 days and then is passed through the patient's digestive system. The accuracy of this method of pH testing is greater than methods in which a catheter is used because the patient can eat normally and continue typical activities during the testing. The patient is evaluated for both acid reflux and nonacid reflux events (Medtronic, 2019).

Laparoscopy (Peritoneoscopy)

With the tremendous advances in minimally invasive surgery, diagnostic laparoscopy is efficient, cost-effective, and useful in the diagnosis of GI disease. After a pneumoperitoneum (injecting carbon dioxide into the peritoneal cavity to separate the intestines from the pelvic organs) is created, a small incision is made lateral to the umbilicus, allowing for the insertion of the fiberoptic laparoscope. This permits direct visualization of the organs and structures within the abdomen, permitting visualization and identification of any growths, anomalies, and inflammatory processes. In addition, biopsy samples can be taken from the structures and organs as necessary. This procedure can be used to evaluate peritoneal disease, chronic abdominal pain, abdominal masses, and gallbladder and liver disease. However, laparoscopy has not become an important diagnostic modality in patients with acute abdominal pain, because less invasive tools (e.g., CT and MRI scans) are readily available. Laparoscopy usually requires general anesthesia and sometimes requires that the stomach and bowel be decompressed. Gas (usually carbon dioxide) is insufflated into the peritoneal cavity to create a working space for visualization. One of the benefits of this procedure is that after visualization of a problem, excision (e.g., removal of the gallbladder) can then be performed at the same time, if appropriate.

CRITICAL THINKING EXERCISES

1 `pcq` You are caring for a 45-year-old woman recently admitted to the emergency department (ED) with new onset of right upper quadrant pain with radiation to the mid-upper back, accompanied by nausea and bloating. The symptoms began several hours after the patient ate lunch, which included several fatty foods. The patient's past medical history is unremarkable. Identify questions that you should ask when taking the patient's history. What are your priority assessments? What diagnostic tests would you expect? While in the ED, the patient reports that the pain has increased in intensity, and abdominal guarding and temperature elevation are noted. Given these new developments, what questions will you now ask and what are your priority assessments?

2 `ipc` A 50-year-old man presents to the ED with midsternal chest discomfort, nausea, and diaphoresis. He has a history of elevated cholesterol, which is managed with an oral medication. You recognize the symptoms of a potential cardiac or gastrointestinal condition. Given the urgency of the evolving situation, which members of the health care team do you anticipate will participate in the care of this patient? How can you best coordinate care to assure positive patient outcomes?

REFERENCES

*Asterisk indicates nursing research

Books

Antunes, C., & Curtis, S. A. (2019). Gastroesophageal reflux disease. *NCBI Bookshelf StatPearls*. Treasure Island, FL: StatPearls Publishing. Retrieved on 11/4/2019 at: www.ncbi.nlm.nih.gov/books/NBK441938

Eliopoulos, C. (2018). *Gerontological nursing* (9th ed.). Philadelphia, PA: Lippincott Williams & Wilkins.

Günther C. (2018). Microbiome and gut immunity: The epithelium. In D. Haller (Ed.). *The gut microbiome in health and disease*. New York: Springer. Retrieved on 2/16/2020 at: www.springer.com/gp/book/9783319905440

Hainsworth, J. D. (2020). Nausea and vomiting. In J. E. Niederhuber, J. O. Armitage, J. H. Doroshow, et al. (Eds.). *Abeloff's clinical oncology* (6th ed.). St. Louis, MO: Elsevier.

Haller, D. (2018). Intestinal microbiome in health and disease: Introduction. In D. Haller (Ed.). *The gut microbiome in health and disease*. New York: Springer. Retrieved on 2/16/2020 at: www.link.springer.com/chapter/10.1007/978-3-319-90545-7_1

Lampignano, J. P., & Kendrick, L. E. (2018). *Textbook of radiographic positioning and related anatomy* (9th ed.). St. Louis, MO: Elsevier.

McCance, K. L., & Huether, S. E. (2019). *Pathophysiology: The biologic basis for disease in adults and children* (8th ed.). St. Louis, MO: Elsevier.

McEvoy, G. E. (Ed.). (2020). *AHFS Drug Information®*. Bethesda, MD: American Society of Health-System Pharmacists. STAT!Ref Online Electronic Medical Library. Retrieved on 2/14/2020 at: www.ahfsdruginformation.com/ahfs-drug-information

Norris, T. L. (2019). *Porth's pathophysiology. Concepts of altered health states* (10th ed.). Philadelphia, PA: Wolters Kluwer.

Parkman, H. P. (2018). Gastric emptying studies. In E. Bardan & R. Shaker (Eds.). *Gastrointestinal motility disorders: A point of care clinical guide*. New York: Springer International Publishing.

Pezoldt, J., Yang, J., Zou, M., et al. (2018). Microbiome and gut immunity: T cells. In D. Haller (Ed.). *The gut microbiome in health and disease*.

New York: Springer. Retrieved on 2/16/2020 at: www.link.springer.com/chapter/10.1007%2F978-3-319-90545-7_9

Strowig, T., Thiemann, S., & Diefenbach, A. (2018). Microbiome and gut immunity: Innate immune cells. In D. Haller (Ed.). *The gut microbiome in health and disease*. New York: Springer. Retrieved on 2/17/2020 at: www.link.springer.com/chapter/10.1007/978-3-319-90545-7_8

Weber, J. R., & Kelley, J. H. (2018). *Health assessment in nursing* (6th ed.). Philadelphia, PA: Wolters Kluwer.

Journals and Electronic Documents

Ahmed, M., Kanotra, R., Savani, G. T., et al. (2017). Utilization trends in inpatient endoscopic retrograde cholangiopancreatography (ERCP): A cross-sectional US experience. *Endoscopy International Open, 5*(4), E261–E271.

American Cancer Society (ACS). (2018). Tests to diagnose and stage colorectal cancer. Retrieved on 10/29/2019 at: www.cancer.org/cancer/colon-rectal-cancer/detection-diagnosis-staging/how-diagnosed.html

American Cancer Society (ACS). (2019). Colorectal screening tests. Retrieved on 11/8/2019 at: www.cancer.org/cancer/colon-rectal-cancer/detection-diagnosis-staging/screening-tests-used.html

American Society of Anesthesiology Taskforce. (2020). Practice advisory for the perioperative management of patients with cardiac implantable electronic devices. *Anesthesiology, 132*(2), 225–252.

Babakhanlou, R. (2018). Upper abdominal pain. *InnovAiT, 11*(8), 428–434.

Harrison, N. M., & Hielkrem, M. C. (2016). Bowel cleansing before colonoscopy: Balancing efficacy, safety, cost and patient tolerance. *World Journal of Gastrointestinal Endoscopy, 8*(1), 4–12.

Health Link British Columbia (HealthLinkBC). (2018). Helicobacter pylori tests. Retrieved on 11/12/2019 at: www.healthlinkbc.ca/medical-tests/hw1531#hw1546

Hossain, M. A., Costanzo, E., Cosentino, J., et al. (2018). Contrast-induced nephropathy: Pathophysiology, risk factors, and prevention. *Saudi Journal of Kidney Diseases and Transplantation, 29*(1), 1–9.

Kohlmann, W., & Gruber, S. B. (2018). Lynch syndrome. In M. P. Adam, H. H. Ardinger, R. A. Pagon, et al. (Eds.). *GeneReviews® [Internet]*. Seattle, WA: University of Washington, Seattle; 1993–2019. Retrieved on 11/18/2019 at: www.ncbi.nlm.nih.gov/books/NBK1211

Longstreth, G. F., & Lacy, B. E. (2019). Functional dyspepsia in adults. *UpToDate*. Retrieved on 11/4/2019 at: www.uptodate.com/contents/functional-dyspepsia-in-adults

Mayo Clinic. (2019). Acid reflux and GERD: The same thing? Retrieved on 11/3/2019 at: www.mayoclinic.org/diseases-conditions/heartburn/expert-answers/heartburn-gerd/faq-20057894

MedlinePlus. (2019). ERCP. Retrieved on 11/20/2019 at: www.medlineplus.gov/ency/article/007479.htm

Medtronic. (2019). BRAVO™ Calibration-free reflux testing. Retrieved on 11/12/2019 at: www.medtronic.com/covidien/en-us/products/reflux-testing/bravo-reflux-testing-system.html#bravo-calibration-free-reflux-capsule

National Institute of Diabetes and Digestive and Kidney Diseases (NIDDK). (2017). Upper endoscopy. Retrieved on 11/20/2019 at: www.niddk.nih.gov/health-information/diagnostic-tests/upper-gi-endoscopy

Neubauer, H., Wellman, M., Herzog-Niescery, J., et al. (2018). Comparison of perioperative strategies in ICD patients: The perioperative ICD management study (PIM study). *Pacing Clinical Electrophysiology, 41*(11), 1536–1542.

Park, J., Cho, Y. K., & Kim, J. H. (2018). Current and future use of esophageal capsule endoscopy. *Clinical Endoscopy, 51*(4), 317–322.

Rex, D. K., Boland, R., Dominitz, J. A., et al. (2017). Colorectal cancer screening: Recommendations for physicians and patients from the U.S. Multi-Society Task Force on colorectal cancer. *Gastrointestinal Endoscopy, 86*(1), 18–33.

Rich, K. (2018). Overview of Mallory-Weis syndrome. *Journal of Vascular Nursing, 36*(2), 91–93.

*Shen, Q., Zhu, H., Jiang, G., et al. (2018). Nurse-led self-management educational intervention improves symptoms of patients with functional constipation. *Western Journal of Nursing Research, 40*(60), 874–888.

Sinicrope, F. A. (2018). Lynch syndrome–associated colorectal cancer. *New England Journal of Medicine, 379*(8), 764–773.

Tan, L., Lin, Z. C., Ma, S., et al. (2018). Bowel preparation for colonoscopy. *Cochrane Database of Systematic Reviews 11*. Retrieved on

11/21/2019 at: www.cochranelibrary.com/cdsr/doi/10.1002/14651858.
CD006330.pub3/full

Tariq, H., Kamal, M. U., Sapkota, B., et al. (2019). Evaluation of the
combined effect of factors influencing bowel preparation and adenoma
detection rates in patients undergoing colonoscopy. *BMJ Open Gastroenterology*, 6(10), 1–16.

Triadafilopoulos, G., Zikos, T., Regalia, K., et al. (2018). Use of esophageal pH monitoring to minimize proton-pump inhibitor utilization in
patients with gastroesophageal reflux symptoms. *Digestive Diseases and
Sciences*, 63(10), 2673–2680.

Wedro, B. (2019). Stool color, changes in color, texture, and form.
MedicineNet. Retrieved on 1/14/2020 at: www.medicinenet.com/stool_
color_changes/article.htm

Yale School of Medicine. (2019). Frequently asked questions about
contrast material usage. *Radiology & Biomedical Imaging*. Retrieved on
11/8/2019 at: www.medicine.yale.edu/diagnosticradiology/patientcare/
physicians/er/contrastquestions

Yamamoto, H., & Aabakken, L. (2019). Small-bowel endoscopy. *Endoscopy*,
51(5), 399–400.

Resources

American Cancer Society, www.cancer.org
American Society for Gastrointestinal Endoscopy (ASGE), www.asge.org
Society of Gastroenterology Nurses and Associates (SGNA),
www.sgna.org

39

Management of Patients with Oral and Esophageal Disorders

LEARNING OUTCOMES

On completion of this chapter, the learner will be able to:

1. Define the relationship of dental hygiene and dental problems to nutrition and disease.
2. Describe the nursing management of patients with abnormalities of the oral cavity, jaw, and salivary glands, including cancer of the oral cavity and disorders of the esophagus.

3. Describe the nursing management of the patient receiving enteral nutrition support.
4. Use the nursing process as a framework for care of the patient undergoing neck dissection, having a gastrostomy or jejunostomy feeding tube placed, or with noncancerous disorders of the esophagus.

NURSING CONCEPTS

Elimination

Nutrition

GLOSSARY

achalasia: absent or ineffective peristalsis (wavelike contraction) of the distal esophagus accompanied by failure of the esophageal sphincter to relax in response to swallowing

aspiration: inhalation of fluids or foods into the trachea and bronchial tree

dumping syndrome: physiologic response to rapid emptying of gastric contents into the small intestine; manifested by nausea, weakness, sweating, palpitations, syncope, and possibly diarrhea (*synonym:* vagotomy syndrome)

dysphagia: difficulty swallowing

dysplasia: bizarre cell growth resulting in cells that differ in size, shape, or arrangement from other cells of the same tissue type

enteral nutrition: nutritional formula feedings infused through a tube directly into the gastrointestinal tract

enteric: of or relating to the intestines

gastroesophageal reflux disease (GERD): disorder marked by backflow of gastric or duodenal contents into the esophagus that causes troublesome symptoms and mucosal injury to the esophagus

gastrostomy: surgical creation of an opening into the stomach for the purpose of administering fluids, nutrition formulas, and medications or for decompression and drainage of stomach contents

gingivitis: inflammation of the gums; change in color from pink to red, with associated swelling, bleeding, and sensitivity/tenderness

halitosis: foul odor from the oral cavity; in laypersons' terms, "bad breath"

hernia: protrusion of an organ or part of an organ through the wall of the cavity that normally contains it

jejunostomy: surgical creation of an opening into the jejunum for the purpose of administering fluids, nutrition formulas, and medications

lithotripsy: the use of shock waves to break up or disintegrate stones

odynophagia: pain on swallowing

osmolality: ionic concentration of fluid

parotitis: inflammation of the parotid gland

percutaneous endoscopic gastrostomy (PEG): a feeding tube inserted endoscopically into the stomach

periapical abscess: abscessed tooth

pyrosis: a burning sensation in the stomach and esophagus that moves up to the mouth; commonly called heartburn

sialadenitis: inflammation of the salivary glands

stoma: artificially created opening between a body cavity (e.g., stomach or intestine) and the body surface

stomatitis: inflammation of the oral mucosa

vagotomy syndrome: gastrointestinal symptoms that includes diarrhea and abdominal cramping, resulting from rapid gastric emptying (*synonym:* dumping syndrome)

xerostomia: dry mouth

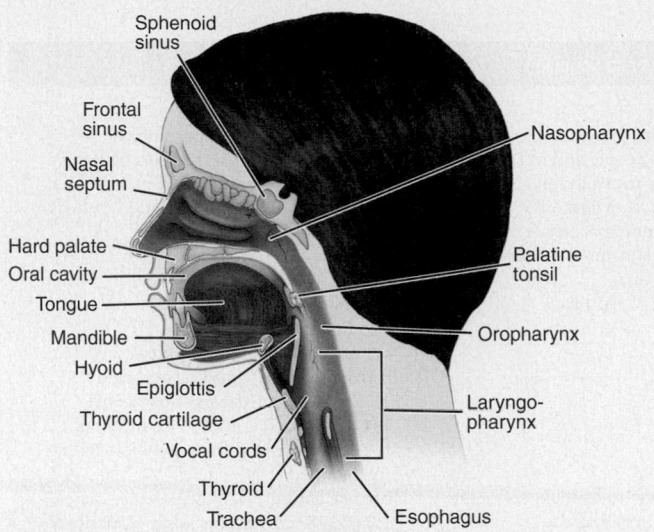

Figure 39-1 • Anatomy of the head and neck.

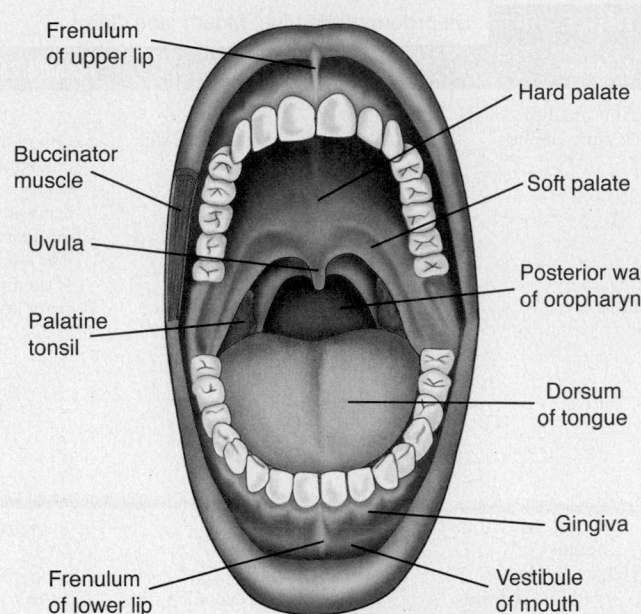

Figure 39-2 • Structures of the mouth, including the tongue and palate.

Because digestion normally begins in the mouth, adequate nutrition is related to good dental health and the general condition of the mouth. Any discomfort, abnormalities, or disease processes in the oral cavity can affect a person's nutritional status. Changes in the oral cavity can influence the type and amount of food ingested as well as the degree to which food particles are properly mixed with salivary enzymes. Disorders of the mouth or tongue can interfere with speech and thus affect communication and self-image. Esophageal problems related to swallowing can also adversely affect food and fluid intake, thereby jeopardizing general health and well-being. Given the close relationship between adequate nutritional intake and the structures of the upper gastrointestinal (GI) tract (lips, mouth, teeth, pharynx, esophagus), health education can help prevent disorders associated with these structures (see Fig. 39-1).

DISORDERS OF THE ORAL CAVITY

Oral health is a very important component of a person's physical and psychological sense of well-being. Periodontal disease, which encompasses both **gingivitis** (inflammation of the gums) and periodontitis (which involves the soft tissue and bone supporting the teeth), is the most common cause of tooth loss among adults (Office of the Surgeon General, 2003; U.S. Department of Health and Human Services [HHS], 2000). From 2011 to 2012, 44.7% of adults age 30 and older in the United States had periodontitis. When this prevalence is combined with the 2009 to 2010 data, there is a 45.9% prevalence of periodontitis, which means approximately 141 million adults ages 30 and older have diagnosed periodontitis. Severe periodontitis was diagnosed in 8.9% of adults ages 30 and older, but is most prevalent among adults ages 50 and older, males, Hispanic/Latino Americans (63.5%) and non-Hispanic/Latino African Americans (59.1%), those who didn't graduate high school, people living below 200% of the poverty level, and current smokers (Eke, Dye, Wei, et al., 2015). Current cigarette smoking, which increases the likelihood of periodontitis by at least 50%, remains a key modifiable risk factor for periodontitis at all severity levels (Eke, Wei, Thornton-Evans, et al., 2016). Periodontal disease can be connected to a variety of other systemic diseases, such as cardiovascular disease, diabetes, and rheumatoid disease (American Academy of Periodontology [AAP], 2021). Table 39-1 reviews common abnormalities of the oral cavity, their possible causes, and nursing considerations. Figure 39-2 illustrates structures of the oral cavity.

Dental Plaque and Caries

Tooth decay is an erosive process that begins with the action of bacteria on fermentable carbohydrates in the mouth, which produces acids that dissolve tooth enamel. Despite the fact tooth enamel is the hardest substance in the human body, caries and periodontal disease can still occur for several reasons. Contributing factors include nutrition, soft drink consumption, and genetic predisposition. In addition, the extent of damage to the teeth may be related to the following:

- Presence of dental plaque, which is a gluey, gelatinlike substance that adheres to the teeth
- Length of time acids are in contact with the teeth
- Strength of acids and the ability of the saliva to neutralize them
- Susceptibility of the teeth to decay

Dental decay begins with a small hole, usually in a fissure (a break in the tooth's enamel) or in an area that is hard to clean. Left unchecked, the decay extends into the dentin. Because dentin is not as hard as enamel, decay progresses more rapidly and in time, reaches the pulp of the tooth. The prevalence of dental caries in permanent teeth for adolescents ages 12 to 19 remains high at 56.8%, even though there is an increased use (48.1%) of sealants on permanent teeth in this age group. Adults ages 20 to 64 years have an 89.9% prevalence of dental caries in permanent teeth; however, only 26.1% of adults have untreated tooth decay in permanent teeth. Older

(text continued on page 1232)

TABLE 39-1	Disorders of the Lips, Mouth, and Gums		
Condition	**Signs and Symptoms**	**Possible Causes and Sequelae**	**Nursing Considerations**
Abnormalities of the Lips			
Actinic cheilitis	Irritation of lips associated with scaling, crusting, fissure; white hyperkeratosis (overgrowth of horny layer of epidermis) Considered a premalignant squamous cell skin cancer	Exposure to sun; more common in fair-skinned people and in those whose occupations involve sun exposure, such as farmers Chronic inflammatory lesion that may lead to squamous cell cancer of the lip	Educate patient on importance of protecting lips from the sun by using protective ointment such as sun block. Instruct patient to have a periodic checkup by primary provider.
Chancre	Reddened circumscribed lesion that ulcerates and becomes crusted	Primary lesion of syphilis	Use comfort measures such as cold soaks to lip, mouth care. Administer antibiotics as prescribed. Instruct patient regarding contagion. Use topical over-the-counter agents (e.g., Blistex, Carmex) or antiviral agents (e.g., acyclovir, penciclovir) as prescribed.
Contact dermatitis (i.e., allergic contact cheilitis)	Red area or rash; itching	Allergic reaction to lipstick, cosmetic ointments, or toothpaste	Instruct patient to avoid possible causes. Administer corticosteroids as prescribed.
Herpes simplex virus-1 (cold sore or fever blister)	Symptoms may be delayed up to 20 days after exposure; singular or clustered, irregular, painful vesicles throughout the oral cavity and lips that may rupture	An opportunistic infection; frequently seen in patients who are immunosuppressed May recur with menstruation, fever, or sun exposure	Use acyclovir ointment or systemic medications as prescribed. Administer analgesic agents as prescribed. Instruct patient to avoid irritating foods.
Abnormalities of the Mouth			
Aphthous stomatitis (canker sore) (Classified as *major* or *minor* depending upon size)	Shallow ulcer with a white or yellow center and typically a well-defined red border; seen on the inner side of the lip and cheek or on the tongue; it begins with a burning or tingling sensation and slight swelling; painful; usually lasts 7–10 days (*minor*) and heals without a scar	Immune-mediated inflammatory disorder associated with HIV infection Associated with emotional or mental stress, fatigue, hormonal factors, minor trauma (e.g., biting), allergies, acidic foods and juices, and dietary deficiencies May recur	Instruct the patient in comfort measures (e.g., saline rinses) and a soft or bland diet. Antibiotics or corticosteroids may be prescribed. Use over-the-counter benzocaine as indicated.
Candidiasis (moniliasis/thrush)	Cheesy white plaque that looks like milk curds; when rubbed off, it leaves an erythematous and often bleeding base	*Candida albicans* fungus; predisposing factors include diabetes, antibiotic therapy, and immunosuppression	Antifungal medications such as nystatin or clotrimazole may be prescribed as suspensions or troche; when used as a suspension, instruct the patient to swish vigorously for at least 1 min and then swallow. If these treatments fail, oral agents such as fluconazole may be prescribed.
Ewing sarcoma	Located most commonly on the mandible; initial symptoms include swelling, pain, paresthesia, and dental displacement	Cancer (most often the primary site) that is often initially mistaken for dental infection. Median age at onset is 14 yrs old	Most commonly treated with chemotherapy and surgery, followed by chemotherapy and radiation therapy.
Erythroplakia	Red, velvety, asymptomatic patch on the oral mucous membrane; most commonly located on the mouth floor, the ventral aspect of the tongue, and the soft palate	Nonspecific inflammation with a high risk of malignant transformation More frequently seen in older adults	
Kaposi sarcoma	Appears first on the oral mucosa as a red, purple, or blue lesion; may be singular or multiple; may be flat or raised Lesions can occur in other parts of the body: skin, lymph nodes, lungs, digestive tract	Cancer that develops from the cells that line the blood vessels and lymph system Associated with HIV infection (AIDS), men who are HIV negative and who have sex with men, organ transplantation, and geographic region (Africa, Mediterranean)	Instruct patient regarding side effects of planned treatment for HIV.
Leukoplakia	White patches; may be hyperkeratotic; usually in buccal mucosa; typically painless	Fewer than 2% are malignant, but may progress to cancer (premalignant) Common among tobacco users	Instruct patient to see the primary provider if leukoplakia persists >2 wks. Eliminate risk factors, such as cigarettes, smokeless tobacco.

TABLE 39-1	Disorders of the Lips, Mouth, and Gums (continued)		
Condition	**Signs and Symptoms**	**Possible Causes and Sequelae**	**Nursing Considerations**
Oral hairy leukoplakia	White patches with rough hairlike projections; typically found on lateral border of the tongue	Epstein–Barr virus-induced lesion Related to smoking and the use of tobacco Associated with HIV infection	Instruct patient to see the primary provider if condition persists >2 wks.
Lichen planus	Radiating white, lacelike striations on the tongue and buccal mucosa; often association with painful ulcerations and erythema	Chronic inflammatory condition of unknown cause Recurrences are common May lead to a malignant process	Apply topical corticosteroids such as fluocinolone acetonide gel. Avoid foods that irritate. Administer corticosteroids systemically or intralesionally as prescribed. Instruct the patient of need for follow-up if condition is chronic.
Nicotine stomatitis (smoker's patch)	Two stages—begins as a red stomatitis; over time, the tongue and mouth become covered with a creamy, thick, white mucous membrane, which may slough, leaving a beefy red base	Chronic irritation by tobacco	Cessation of tobacco use; if condition exists >2 wks, a primary provider should be consulted and a biopsy may be needed.
Stomatitis	Mild erythema and edema; severe forms include painful ulcerations, bleeding, and secondary infection	Inflammation of the mucous lining of the mouth Associated with chemotherapy; radiation therapy; severe drug allergy; myelosuppression (bone marrow depression)	Prophylactic mouth care, including brushing, flossing, and rinsing, for any patient receiving chemotherapy or radiation therapy. Educate patient about proper oral hygiene, including the use of a soft-bristled toothbrush and nonabrasive toothpaste; for painful ulcers, oral swabs with sponge-like applicators can be used in place of a toothbrush; avoid alcohol-based mouth rinses and hot or spicy foods. Apply topical anti-inflammatory, antibiotic, and anesthetic agents as prescribed.
Abnormalities of the Gums			
Gingivitis	Painful, inflamed, swollen gums; usually, the gums bleed in response to light contact	Reversible form of inflammation of the gingiva (i.e., mild form of periodontal disease) Associated with poor oral hygiene: food debris, bacterial plaque, and calculus (tartar) accumulate Gums may also swell in response to normal processes such as puberty and pregnancy, with certain medications (phenytoin, calcium channel blockers, cyclosporine), or with a deficiency in the immune system (i.e., AIDS) or nutritional status	Educate patient about proper oral hygiene; tooth-brushing, flossing, rinsing (i.e., chlorhexidine), dental appointments every 3–6 mo. Remove causal agents as appropriate—medications, smoking, dental appliances.
Herpetic gingivostomatitis	Burning sensation with the appearance of small vesicles 24–48 h later; vesicles may rupture, forming sore, shallow ulcers covered with a gray membrane	Herpes simplex viral infection Occurs most frequently in people who are immunosuppressed; may occur in other infectious processes such as streptococcal pneumonia, meningococcal meningitis, and malaria	Apply topical anesthetics as prescribed; may need opioids if pain is severe. Saline or 2–3% hydrogen peroxide irrigations Antiviral agents such as acyclovir may be prescribed. Educate patient about proper oral hygiene; see Chart 39-2.
Necrotizing gingivitis (trench mouth)	Gray-white pseudomembranous ulcerations affecting the edges of the gums, mucosa of the mouth, tonsils, and pharynx; halitosis; painful, bleeding gums; swallowing and talking are painful	Progressive, painful bacterial infection Related to poor oral hygiene, lack of access to dental care, inadequate rest, overwork, emotional stress, smoking, and poor nutrition	Irrigate with 2–3% hydrogen peroxide or normal saline solution. Avoid irritants such as smoking and spicy foods.
Periodontitis	Little discomfort at onset; may have bleeding, infection, gum recession, and loosening of teeth; later in the disease, tooth loss may occur	Deep, chronic inflammation of the gingiva May result from untreated gingivitis Poor or inadequate dental hygiene and inadequate diet contribute to development	Instruct patient in proper oral hygiene, chlorhexidine rinses. Instruct patient to consult a dentist or periodontist for antibiotic prescription, deep root scaling.

AIDS, acquired immune deficiency syndrome; HIV, human immune deficiency virus.
Adapted from American Cancer Society (ACS). (2021b). Kaposi sarcoma. Retrieved on 2/18/2021 at: www.cancer.org/cancer/kaposisarcoma/detailedguide/kaposi-sarcoma-what-is-kaposi-sarcoma; Lodi, G. (2020). Oral lesions. Retrieved on 2/18/2021 at: www.uptodate.com/contents/oral-lesions; Margaix- Muñoz, M., Bagán, J., & Poveda-Roda, R. (2017). Ewing sarcoma of the oral cavity. A review. *Journal of Clinical and Experimental Dentistry, 9*(2), 294–301; Mowad, C. (2019). Cheilitis. Retrieved on 2/18/2021 at: www.uptodate.com/contents/cheilitis; Silk, H. (2014). Disease of the mouth. *Primary Care: Clinics in Office Practice, 41*(1), 75–90.

Chart 39-1 Oral Conditions in the Older Adult

Many medications taken by older adults cause dry mouth, which is uncomfortable, impairs communication, and increases the risk of oral infection. These medications include the following:

- Antidepressant medications
- Antihypertensive medications
- Anti-inflammatory agents
- Diuretic agents

Poor dentition can exacerbate problems of aging, such as:

- Decreased food intake
- Increased susceptibility to systemic infection (from periodontal disease)
- Loss of appetite
- Social isolation
- Trauma to the oral cavity secondary to thinner, less vascular oral mucous membranes

Adapted from Eliopoulos, C. (2018). *Gerontological nursing* (9th ed.). Philadelphia, PA: Wolters Kluwer.

---

adults (65 years and older) present with a 96.2% prevalence of dental caries, with 15.9% of their tooth decay untreated (Centers for Disease Control and Prevention [CDC], 2019). Older adults are subject to decay from drug-induced or age-related oral dryness (see Chart 39-1).

Dentists can determine the extent of damage and the type of treatment needed using x-ray studies. Treatment for dental caries includes fillings, dental implants, or extraction, if necessary. In general, dental decay can occur in anyone.

Prevention

Measures used to prevent and control primary dental caries include applying fluoride varnish/gel (Marinho, Worthington, Walsh, et al., 2015), using fluoride toothpaste, use of silver diamine fluoride compounds (Donovan, Marzola, Murphy, et al., 2018), applying dental sealants (Twetman, 2015), and ensuring community water fluoridation (HHS, 2000; HHS Federal Panel on Community Water Fluoridation, 2015). Other recommendations include implementing daily oral hygiene practices, seeking routine professional dental treatment, refraining from smoking and excessive alcohol use, making good dietary choices, and managing related systemic diseases (HHS, 2019). The inability to afford dental care is associated with a decrease in the quality of life of adults ages 45 years and older (Naavaal, Griffin, & Jones, 2019), which must be considered when assisting patients in navigating health care systems.

Mouth Care

Healthy teeth must be cleaned several times a day. Brushing and flossing are particularly effective in mechanically breaking up the bacterial plaque that collects around teeth.

Mastication (chewing) and the normal flow of saliva also aid greatly in keeping the teeth clean. Because many ill patients do not consume adequate nutrients, they produce less saliva, which in turn reduces this natural tooth-cleaning process. The nurse may need to assume the responsibility for brushing the patient's teeth. Merely wiping the patient's mouth and teeth with a swab is ineffective. The most effective method is mechanical cleansing (brushing). If brushing is not possible, it is better to wipe the teeth with a gauze pad and then have the patient swish an antiseptic mouthwash several times before expectorating into an emesis basin. A soft-bristled toothbrush is more effective than a sponge or foam stick. Flossing should be performed daily. To prevent drying, the lips may be coated with a water-soluble gel.

Diet

Dental caries may be prevented by decreasing the amount of sugar and starch in the diet. Patients who snack should be encouraged to choose less cariogenic alternatives, such as fruits, vegetables, nuts, cheeses, or plain yogurt. Brushing after meals is recommended.

Fluoridation

Fluoridation of public water supplies has been found to decrease dental caries. Some areas of the country have natural fluoridation; other communities have added fluoride to public water supplies. As of 2014, 66.3% of Americans receive fluoridated water (CDC, 2020b). Studies suggest that by instituting a community water fluoridation program, tooth decay is reduced by 25% in both children and adults (CDC, 2018).

Fluoridation may also be achieved by having a dentist apply a concentrated gel or solution to the teeth; adding fluoride to home water supplies; using fluoridated toothpaste or mouth rinse; or using sodium fluoride tablets, drops, or lozenges.

Pit and Fissure Sealants

The occlusal surfaces of the teeth have pits and fissures—areas that are prone to caries. Some dentists apply a coating to fill and seal these areas on the primary and permanent molars to protect them from potential exposure to cariogenic processes. These sealants can last 36 to 48 months and significantly prevent tooth decay. The economic benefits of applying sealants, especially in high-risk groups, exceed the costs and provide solid evidence for their use (Donovan et al., 2018).

Dental Health and Disease

Studies are ongoing that show the link between oral health and chronic disease such as diabetes, heart disease, low birth weight, premature births, and stroke. It had long been posited that bacteria, specifically gram-negative bacteria, were the culprits that link periodontal disease to other systemic diseases, specifically coronary artery disease, including myocardial infarction and stroke. More recently, it was confirmed that these bacteria cause an inflammatory response that initiates an increase in inflammatory markers such as C-reactive protein, white blood cells, and fibrinogen. These markers are associated with an increased risk of cardiovascular disease. Data from short-term studies suggest that if periodontal disease is treated, systemic inflammation and endothelial dysfunction are reduced (Hegde & Awan, 2019). One study reported that thrombus aspirate and arterial blood taken from patients who had an ischemic stroke contained streptococcal bacteria. The most commonly identified *Streptococcus* species (found in 79% of the sample), *Streptococcus mitis*, is typically found in the mouth. Although a preliminary study, there is evidence that these oral bacteria may contribute to the progression of cardiovascular thrombotic events (Patrakka, Pienimäki, Tuomisto, et al., 2019).

The World Health Organization (WHO) Global Oral Health Programme (2019) espouses a global focus on oral health promotion and disease prevention, with an emphasis on policy and guideline development to support equitable implementation of evidence-based practices in global communities. The Programme supports an emphasis on addressing modifiable risk factors (e.g., diet, nutrition, tobacco, alcohol, and oral hygiene), water sanitation, and fluoride initiatives. Initiatives recognize the impact of social, economic, political, and cultural determinants of health, and seek to integrate the existing and emerging systems that address the burden and disability that stem from oral disease (WHO, 2019).

Periapical Abscess

A **periapical abscess**, more commonly referred to as an abscessed tooth, involves a collection of pus in the apical dental periosteum (fibrous membrane supporting the tooth structure) and the tissue surrounding the apex of the tooth (where it is suspended in the jaw bone). The abscess may be acute or chronic. An acute periapical abscess arises from an infection, usually secondary to dental caries. The infection of the dental pulp extends through the apical foramen of the tooth to form an abscess around the apex.

A chronic periodontal abscess occurs from a slowly progressive infectious process. In contrast to the acute form, a fully formed abscess may occur without the patient's knowledge. The infection eventually leads to a "blind dental abscess," which is actually a periapical granuloma. It may enlarge to as much as 1 cm in diameter. It is often discovered on x-ray images and is treated by extraction or root canal therapy, often with apicoectomy (excision of the apex of the tooth root).

Clinical Manifestations

The abscess produces a dull, gnawing, continuous pain, often with a surrounding cellulitis and swelling of the adjacent facial structures, temperature sensitivity, and mobility of the involved tooth. The gum opposite the apex of the tooth is usually swollen on the cheek side. Swelling and cellulitis of the facial structures may make it difficult for the patient to open the mouth. There may also be a systemic response, fever, and malaise.

Medical Management

In the early stages of an infection, a dentist or oral surgeon may perform a needle aspiration or drill an opening into the pulp chamber to relieve pressure and pain and to provide drainage. Drainage is provided by an incision through the gingiva down to the jawbone. Purulent material escapes under pressure. This procedure may be performed in a dentist's office, an outpatient surgery center, or a same-day surgery department. After the inflammatory reaction has subsided, the tooth may be extracted or root canal therapy performed. Antibiotics, in the presence of overt spreading infection, and analgesics may be prescribed (Robertson, Keys, Rautemaa-Richardon, et al., 2015).

Nursing Management

The patient is assessed for bleeding after treatment and is instructed to use a warm saline or warm water mouth rinse to keep the area clean. The patient is also instructed to take antibiotic and analgesic agents as prescribed, to advance from a liquid diet to a soft diet as tolerated, and to keep follow-up appointments.

DISORDERS OF THE JAW

Abnormal conditions affecting the mandible (jaw) and the temporomandibular joint (which connects the mandible to the temporal bone at the side of the head in front of the ear) include congenital malformation, fracture, chronic dislocation, cancer, and syndromes characterized by pain and limited motion. Temporomandibular disorders and jaw surgery, a treatment common in many structural abnormalities or cancer of the jaw, are presented in this section.

Temporomandibular Disorders

Temporomandibular disorders are categorized as follows (National Institute of Dental and Craniofacial Research [NIDCR], 2018):

- Myofascial pain—a discomfort in the muscles controlling jaw function and in neck and shoulder muscles
- Internal derangement of the joint—a dislocated jaw, a displaced disc, or an injured condyle
- Degenerative joint disease—rheumatoid arthritis or osteoarthritis in the jaw joint

Diagnosis and treatment of temporomandibular disorders remain somewhat ambiguous, but the condition is thought to affect about 10 million people in the United States (NIDCR, 2018). Misalignment of the joints in the jaw and other problems associated with the ligaments and muscles of mastication are thought to result in tissue damage and muscle tenderness. Suggested causes include arthritis of the jaw, head injury, trauma or injury to the jaw or joint, stress, and malocclusion, although research does not support malocclusion (misalignment of bite) or associated orthodonture as a cause (NIDCR, 2018).

Clinical Manifestations

Patients have jaw pain ranging from a dull ache to throbbing, debilitating pain that can radiate to the ears, teeth, neck muscles, and facial sinuses. They often have restricted jaw motion and locking of the jaw. There also may be a sudden change in the way the upper and lower teeth fit together. The patient may hear clicking, popping, and grating sounds when the mouth is opened, and chewing and swallowing may be difficult. Symptoms such as headaches, earaches, dizziness, and hearing problems may sometimes be related to temporomandibular disorders (Gauer & Semidey, 2015; NIDCR, 2018).

Assessment and Diagnostic Findings

Diagnosis is based on the patient's report of pain, limitations in range of motion, **dysphagia** (difficulty swallowing), difficulty chewing, difficulty with speech, or hearing difficulties. Magnetic resonance imaging (MRI) and other imaging studies are generally only used for severe or chronic symptoms.

Medical Management

Signs and symptoms improve over time for the majority of patients with temporomandibular joint disorders, with or without treatment. Conservative treatment is recommended

(NIDCR, 2018). Most patients improve with a combination of simple noninvasive therapies that may include: (1) patient education on self-care—eating soft foods, icing the jaw; (2) cognitive behavior modifications—stress reduction, sleep hygiene, avoidance of extreme mandibular movement, and elimination of habits such as chewing ice; (3) physical therapy—stretching and relaxing; (4) acupuncture—highly effective with six to eight 15- to 30-minute sessions; (5) psychosocial interventions; (6) analgesics—trial of nonsteroidal anti-inflammatory drugs (NSAIDs) and muscle relaxants initially; and (7) oral appliance therapy—splints (Gauer & Semidey, 2015; NIDCR, 2018).

Jaw Disorders Requiring Surgical Management

Correction of mandibular structural abnormalities may require surgery involving repositioning or reconstruction of the jaw. Simple fractures of the mandible without displacement, resulting from a blow to the chin, and planned surgical interventions, as in the correction of long or short jaw syndrome, may require wiring or surgery. Jaw reconstruction may be necessary in the aftermath of trauma from a severe injury or cancer, both of which can cause tissue and bone loss. Research supports screening for concussion (see Chapter 63) with mandibular fractures associated with high-force impacts (Sobin, Kopp, Walsh, et al., 2016). Cervical spine injury must be ruled out since 2% to 10% of patients with facial fractures (up to 20% with panfacial injuries) also have a spinal injury (Pickrell, Serebrakian, & Maricevich, 2017).

Mandibular fractures are usually closed fractures. In the acute trauma setting, surgery providers should assess the patient's perception of the bite ("bite feels normal") for malocclusion, the fracture site for fragment mobility, dentition for loose or infected teeth, and sensation in the lower lip for nerve damage. When the dentition is sufficient and the fracture is isolated, maxillomandibular fixation (MMF; wiring the jaw shut) is a viable option. However, open reduction, internal fixation (ORIF) with plate fixation (insertion of one or more metal plates and screws or arch bars into the bone to approximate and stabilize the bone) is the surgery of choice (Pickrell et al., 2017). Current research revolves around the use of various types and number of reconstruction plates and fixation devices, quality of life after specific instrumentation, approach used (ORIF or endoscopic-assisted), and device choice (van den Bergh, de Mol van Otterloo, van der Ploeg, et al., 2015). Bone grafting may be performed to replace structural defects using bones from the patient's own ilium, ribs, or cranial sites.

Nursing Management

If used, MMF generally requires a short period (7 to 10 days) of a liquid diet and oral rinses followed by rehabilitation and a soft diet. After ORIF, patients are typically on a liquid or soft diet for 4 to 6 weeks to allow for healing. The most common complications are infection that may progress to osteomyelitis (infection of the bone), alignment issues or hardware failure (requiring surgical repair or MMF), and wound dehiscence (Pickrell et al., 2017). Dietary counseling is provided to ensure adequate protein intake with supplementation as needed.

Oral care, including the use of medicated rinses, needs to be reinforced. To decrease the risk of complications, patients are advised to take prescribed medications and to abstain from smoking, use of electronic nicotine delivery systems (ENDS), including e-cigarettes, e-pens, e-pipes, e-hookah and e-cigars and use of alcohol and other substances. Regular follow-up with the surgeon is required to ensure healing is progressing.

DISORDERS OF THE SALIVARY GLANDS

The salivary glands consist of the parotid glands, one on each side of the face below the ear; the submandibular glands, located below the jawbone; the sublingual glands, in the floor of the mouth under the tongue; and the minor salivary glands in the lips, buccal mucosa, and the lining of the mouth and throat. About 1500 mL of saliva is produced daily and swallowed. The major functions of the salivary glands include lubrication, protection against harmful bacteria, and digestion.

Parotitis

Parotitis (inflammation of the parotid gland) is the most common inflammatory condition of the salivary glands. Inflammation of the parotid may be due to mumps (epidemic parotitis), a communicable disease caused by viral infection and most commonly affecting unvaccinated children (Grennan, 2019).

People who are older, acutely ill, or debilitated with decreased salivary flow from general dehydration or medications are at high risk for bacterial parotitis. The infecting organism, typically *Staphylococcus aureus*, travels from the mouth through the salivary duct. The onset of parotitis is sudden and associated with fever, chills, and other systemic signs of infection. The gland swells and becomes tense and tender. The patient feels pain in the ear, and swollen glands interfere with swallowing. The swelling increases rapidly, and the overlying skin soon becomes red and shiny.

Medical management includes maintaining adequate nutritional and fluid intake, good oral hygiene, applying cold packs, and discontinuing medications (e.g., tranquilizers, diuretic agents) that can diminish salivation. Antibiotic therapy is necessary for bacterial parotitis, and analgesics may be prescribed to control pain. If antibiotic therapy is not effective, the gland may need to be drained by a surgical procedure known as parotidectomy. This procedure may be necessary to treat chronic parotitis. The patient is advised to have any necessary dental work performed prior to surgery.

Sialadenitis

Sialadenitis (inflammation of the salivary glands) may be caused by dehydration, radiation therapy, stress, malnutrition, salivary gland calculi (stones; sialolithiasis), or improper oral hygiene. The inflammation is commonly associated with infection by *S. aureus*, which requires antibiotic therapy. In hospitalized or institutionalized patients, the infecting organism may be methicillin-resistant *S. aureus* (MRSA). Symptoms include pain, swelling, and purulent discharge. Massage, hydration, warm compresses, and sialagogues (substances that trigger saliva flow like hard candy or lemon juice) frequently cure the problem. Chronic sialadenitis is typically due to decreased salivary flow and may be treated with sialendscopy, an endoscopic procedure that allows for direct visualization of Stensen duct (diagnostic) and instillation of antibiotics, corticosteroids, or irrigation (treatment), particularly in adolescents with recurrent parotitis (Papadopoulou-Alataki, Dogantzis, Chatziavramidis, et al., 2019). Surgical drainage or excision of the gland and its duct are considered in cases of sialadenitis that are recurrent or refractory to antibiotics.

Salivary Calculus (Sialolithiasis)

Sialolithiasis, or salivary calculi (stones), occur in 80% of cases in the submandibular gland (Fabie, Kompelli, Naylor, et al., 2019). Calculi within the salivary gland itself may cause no symptoms unless infection arises; however, a calculus that obstructs the gland's duct causes swelling and sudden, local, and often colicky pain, which is abruptly relieved by a gush of saliva. On physical assessment, the gland is swollen and quite tender, the stone itself may be palpable, and may be visualized by ultrasound, noncontrast computed tomography (CT), or sialendoscopy.

Salivary calculi are formed mainly from calcium phosphate. If located within the gland, the calculi are irregular and vary in diameter from 1 to 35 mm. Sialendoscopy is considered the standard in the treatment of sialothiasis, but gland-preserving incisional approaches alone may also be used for palpable stones 6 mm or larger (Fabie et al., 2019). **Lithotripsy**, a procedure that uses shock waves to disintegrate the stone, may be used instead of surgical extraction for parotid stones and smaller submandibular stones. Lithotripsy requires no anesthesia, sedation, or analgesia. Side effects can include local hemorrhage and swelling. Gland removal may be necessary if symptoms and calculi recur repeatedly.

Neoplasms

Salivary gland neoplasms (tumors or growths) of almost any type may develop in the salivary gland. Malignant (cancerous) salivary gland neoplasms account for more than 0.5% of all malignancies and approximately 3% to 5% of head and neck cancers (National Cancer Institute [NCI], 2021d). Risk factors include prior exposure to ionizing radiation to the head and neck, older age, and specific carcinogens introduced in specific work environments (asbestos, plumbing, and woodworking). Most patients with a benign tumor present with painless swelling of the glands; patients with a malignancy tend to have neurologic symptoms (weakness or numbness of the facial nerve) and persistent facial pain (NCI, 2021d). Diagnosis is based on the health history, physical examination, and the results of fine-needle aspiration biopsy.

Early-stage salivary gland tumors are usually curable with surgery alone. Dissection is carefully performed to preserve the seventh cranial nerve (facial nerve). It may not be possible to safely dissect if the tumor is extensive. Complications from surgery may involve facial nerve dysfunction and Frey syndrome. Frey syndrome, also known as auriculotemporal syndrome, involves facial sweating and flushing in the general location of the (removed) parotid gland that occurs while eating. Frey syndrome may be successfully treated with botulinum toxin type A injections (NCI, 2021d). If the salivary gland tumor is malignant, radiation therapy may follow surgery. Radiation therapy alone may be a treatment choice for tumors thought to be localized or if there is risk of facial nerve damage from surgical intervention. Chemotherapy may be considered in late stages, but due to the many different subtypes of salivary gland cancer, tumor mapping, including immunohistochemistry and genomic profiling, should be used to optimize treatment (Lassche, van Boxtel, Ligtenberg, et al., 2019). Recurrent tumors usually are more aggressive than initial tumors.

CANCER OF THE ORAL CAVITY AND PHARYNX

Cancers of the oral cavity and pharynx, which can occur in any part of the mouth or throat, are curable if discovered early. Risk factors for cancer of the oral cavity and pharynx include any use of any form of tobacco or nicotine (cigarette, cigar, pipe, smokeless tobacco, ENDS), excessive use of alcohol, infection with human papillomavirus (HPV), and a history of previous head and neck cancer (NCI, 2021b). Oral cancers are often associated with the combined use of alcohol and tobacco—these substances have a synergistic carcinogenic effect. Patient education directed toward avoiding high-risk behaviors is critical to prevent oral cancers.

In the United States, approximately 53,000 new cases of oral cavity and oropharyngeal cancer occur annually, with an estimated 10,860 deaths. Men are diagnosed with oral and oropharyngeal cancer in almost 72% of diagnosed cases (Siegel, Miller, & Jemal, 2019). Despite a rise in rates associated with HPV over the past 10 years (0.8% rise each year), patients with cancer of the oral cavity and oropharynx have a relatively stable 5-year survival rate of 65.3% (NCI, 2021b; Siegel et al., 2019).

Pathophysiology

Malignancies of the oral cavity are usually squamous cell carcinomas (NCI, 2021c). Any area of the oropharynx can be a site of malignant growths, but the lips, the lateral aspects of the tongue, and the floor of the mouth are most commonly affected. High-risk HPV infection is associated with about 70% of oropharyngeal cancers. Vaccination against HPV shows promise in impacting rates of head and neck cancer. A study of young adults in the United Stated found oral HPV infections (including the two high-risk, cancer-causing types 16 and 18) were 88% lower among young adults who received at least one dose of the vaccine (NCI, 2017).

Clinical Manifestations

Many oral cancers produce few or no symptoms in the early stages. Later, the most frequent symptom is a painless sore or lesion that bleeds easily and does not heal. Oral cancer may also present as a red or white patch (leukoplakia) in the mouth or throat. A typical lesion in oral cancer is a painless indurated (hardened) ulcer with raised edges. Depending on the location (tonsil, base of the tongue, soft palate, or pharyngeal wall), the patient may report tenderness, difficulty in chewing, swallowing, or speaking, coughing of blood-tinged sputum, trismus (limited jaw range of motion), weight loss, a neck mass, or enlarged cervical lymph nodes (NCI, 2021c).

Assessment and Diagnostic Findings

Diagnostic evaluation consists of an oral examination as well as an assessment of the cervical lymph nodes to detect possible metastases. Positron emission tomography-computed tomography scan (PET-CT scan), MRI, endoscopy, laryngoscopy, and biopsy, including testing of HPV status may be used to detect and guide therapy (NCI, 2021c).

Human Papillomavirus Prevention

HPV vaccine is generally recommended for all children ages 11 or 12 (can be started at age 9), up to the age of 26 years for women and 21 years for men. Men who have sex with men, transgender men and women, and immunocompromised people, including those with human immune deficiency virus (HIV), may receive the vaccine up to 26 years of age (CDC, 2020a).

Medical Management

In patients diagnosed with oropharyngeal cancer, management varies with the nature of the lesion, the preference of the provider, and patient choice. Surgical resection and chemoradiation (CRT) are associated with improved survival for all adults over age 70, including those who are positive for HPV infection (Lu, Luu, Nguyen, et al., 2019).

In cancer of the lip, small lesions are usually excised liberally. Radiation therapy may be more appropriate for larger lesions involving more than one third of the lip because of superior cosmetic results. The choice depends on the extent of the lesion and what is necessary to cure the patient while preserving the best appearance. Tumors larger than 4 cm often recur.

In cancer of the tongue, treatment with radiation therapy and chemotherapy may preserve function and maintain quality of life. A combination of radioactive interstitial implants (surgical implantation of a radioactive source into the tissue adjacent to or at the tumor site) and external-beam radiation may be used. Total glossectomy (removal of the tongue) remains the principal treatment of advanced stage or cancers at the base of the tongue; long-term data on functional outcomes following these procedures are being studied (Han, Kuan, Mallen-St. Clair, et al., 2019).

Often, cancer of the oral cavity has metastasized through the extensive lymphatic channel in the neck region, requiring a neck dissection and reconstructive surgery of the oral cavity. Reconstructive techniques involve the use of the traditional pedicled (attached and tunneled) regional tissue flaps (graft of tissue with its own blood supply) or the current mainstay of free (cut and removed) tissue transfer most commonly obtained from the pectoralis major, vertical rectus abdominis myocutaneous, anterolateral thigh, fibula, or radial forearm. Laryngeal preservation is associated with better speech and verbal communication, but swallowing and aspiration issues remain common functional deficits with total glossectomy and free flap reconstruction (Han et al., 2019).

Nursing Management

The nurse assesses the patient's nutritional status preoperatively, and a dietary consultation may be necessary. The patient may require enteral (through the GI tract) or parenteral (intravenous [IV]) feedings before and after surgery to maintain adequate nutrition (see Chapter 41). The interprofessional team, including a registered dietician (RD), provides continual nutritional assessment and reevaluation.

Verbal communication may be impaired by radical surgery for oral cancer, especially if the larynx is removed. It is therefore vital to assess the patient's ability to communicate in writing before surgery. Pen and paper are provided postoperatively to patients who can use them to communicate. A communication board with commonly used words or pictures is obtained preoperatively and given after surgery to patients who cannot write so that they may point to needed items. Electronic devices, such as tablets or smartphones, may also be options for facilitating communication. The interprofessional team benefits from the input of a speech therapist, with physical and occupational therapists consulted as needed.

Postoperatively, the priority for the nurse is assessing for and maintaining a patent airway. The patient may be unable to manage oral secretions, making suctioning necessary. If grafting was part of the surgery, suctioning is performed with care to prevent damage to the graft. Nurses assess the graft postoperatively for viability. Although color should be assessed (white may indicate arterial occlusion, and blue mottling may indicate venous congestion), it can be difficult to assess the graft by looking into the mouth. A Doppler ultrasound device may be used to locate the pulse at the graft site and to assess tissue perfusion. Depending on the extent of the surgery, the patient may require a temporary or permanent tracheostomy after surgery (see Chapter 19).

NURSING MANAGEMENT OF THE PATIENT WITH DISORDERS OF THE ORAL CAVITY

The nurse caring for the patient with disorders of the oral cavity promotes mouth care, ensures adequate food and fluid intake, minimizes pain and discomfort, and prevents infection.

Promoting Mouth Care

Incidences of oral complications, such as infection, during cancer therapy may be decreased and less severe with the incorporation of professional oral care before and during cancer treatment. Guidelines, based on systematic review of the literature, support the implementation of multi-agent combination oral care protocols in patients undergoing head and neck chemotherapy and radiotherapy (radiation therapy) to prevent oral mucositis (OM), a painful inflammatory, typically ulcerative condition that is also referred to as **stomatitis**. Although there are limited data, experts recognize that using saline or sodium bicarbonate rinses increases oral clearance, promotes oral hygiene, and promotes patient comfort (Hong, Gueiros, Fulton, et al., 2019). The nurse facilitates the patient rinsing or irrigating with a solution of ½ to 1 teaspoon of baking soda (or ¼-teaspoon salt) in 8 oz of warm water. The nurse reinforces the need to perform oral care and provides such care to patients who cannot provide it for themselves. Chlorhexidine has been studied more rigorously than other rinses and is generally not recommended for the prevention of OM, specifically not for patients undergoing head and neck radiotherapy (Hong et al., 2019). There is continued debate about the efficacy of *magic mouthwash*, particularly for chemotherapy-induced OM. The recipe for the mouthwash varies and frequently involves out-of-pocket expense for the patient, but most commonly contains diphenhydramine, aluminum-magnesium hydroxide, and viscous lidocaine, with intended mechanism of action to both numb and protect the mouth. More research needs to be done on OM treatment and prevention (Uberoi, Brown, & Gupta, 2019a, 2019b).

Exciting developments regarding intra-oral photobiomodulation (PBM), specifically low-level laser therapy, show positive impact on the prevention of OM in patients with head and neck cancer undergoing radiotherapy with and without chemotherapy (Hong et al., 2019). If specific antimicrobial, antifungal, antibacterial, or antiviral agents are indicated (Maria, Eliopoulos, & Muanza, 2017), the nurse administers the prescribed medications and instructs the patient on how to administer the medications at home. The nurse monitors the patient's physical and psychological response to treatment.

Xerostomia (dryness of the mouth) is a frequent sequela of oral cancer, particularly when the salivary glands have been exposed to radiation or major surgery. It is also seen in patients who are receiving psychopharmacologic agents, taking multiple medications, or using drugs recreationally; in patients who have rheumatic diseases, eating disorders (Villa, Nordio, & Gohel, 2015) or HIV infection; and in patients who cannot close the mouth and, as a result, breathe through the mouth instead of the nose. Current recommendations to treat xerostomia include sipping water, using oral mucosal lubricants (saliva substitutes topically applied), incorporating the use of newer edible saliva substitutes such as oral moisturizing jelly (OMJ), and taking medications that stimulate saliva production (Nuchit, Lam-ubol, & Paemuang, 2020). The hope is that providing oral moisture increases swallowing ability, and ultimately improves nutritional status for these patients.

Ensuring Adequate Food and Fluid Intake

Determination of nutritional intake goals requires consideration of the patient's weight, age, and level of activity. A daily calorie count may be necessary to determine the exact quantity of food and fluid ingested. This intake should include enteral feedings, oral intake, and supplements. The frequency of intake; presence of symptoms such as oral discomfort/pain, dysphagia, nausea; increased or decreased saliva or mucous production; and changes in taste or smell all impact the typically diminishing food intake seen in these patients. The social aspects of eating, reasonable expectations for the timing and amount of intake, and the importance of supportive people are all important considerations. Recommendations to navigate this challenging time include involving a registered dietician or other health care professional with specific nutritional expertise (Sandmæl, Sand, Bye, et al., 2019). The goal is to help the patient attain and maintain desirable body weight and level of energy, as well as to promote the healing of tissue.

Supporting a Positive Self-Image

A patient who has a disfiguring oral condition or has undergone disfiguring surgery may experience an alteration in self-image.

The patient is encouraged to verbalize the perceived and actual change in body appearance and to realistically discuss changes or losses. The nurse offers support while the patient verbalizes fears and negative feelings (withdrawal, depressed mood, anger). The nurse listens attentively and determines the patient's needs and individualizes the plan of care.

The nurse should determine the patient's concerns about relationships with others. Referral to support groups, a psychiatric liaison nurse, a social worker, or a spiritual advisor may be useful in helping the patient cope with anxieties and fears. The patient's progress toward development of positive self-esteem is documented. The nurse should be alert to signs of effective and ineffective grieving and should document emotional changes. By providing acceptance and support, the nurse encourages the patient to verbalize feelings.

Minimizing Pain and Discomfort

Oral lesions can be painful. Strategies to reduce pain and discomfort include avoiding foods that are spicy, hot, or hard (e.g., pretzels, nuts). A soft or liquid diet may be preferred. The patient is instructed about mouth care, including the use of a soft toothbrush and any prescribed rinses or topical medications. The patient may require an analgesic agent such as viscous lidocaine or opioids, as prescribed. The nurse can reduce the patient's fear of pain by providing information about pain control methods.

Preventing Infection

Leukopenia (a decrease in white blood cells) may result from radiation, chemotherapy, acquired immune deficiency syndrome (AIDS), and some medications used to treat HIV infection. Leukopenia reduces defense mechanisms, increasing the risk of infections. Malnutrition, which is also common among these patients, may further decrease resistance to infection. If the patient has diabetes, the risk of infection is further increased.

Laboratory results should be evaluated frequently and the patient's temperature checked every 4 to 8 hours for an elevation that may indicate infection. Visitors who might transmit microorganisms are prohibited if the patient's immunologic system is depressed. Sensitive skin tissues are protected from trauma to maintain skin integrity and prevent infection. Aseptic technique is necessary when changing dressings. Desquamation (shedding of the epidermis) is a reaction to radiation therapy that can lead to a break in skin integrity and subsequent infection. Dry desquamation can be treated with topical lotions, but wet desquamation requires individualized treatment (see Chapter 12). Signs of wound infection (redness, swelling, drainage, tenderness) are reported to the primary provider. Antibiotics may be prescribed prophylactically.

Promoting Home, Community-Based, and Transitional Care

 Educating Patients About Self-Care

The patient who is recovering from treatment of an oral disorder is instructed about mouth care, nutrition, prevention of infection, and signs and symptoms of complications

At the completion of education, the patient and/or caregiver will be able to:

- State the impact of the oral disorder and treatment on communication and other physiologic functioning, ADLs, IADLs, body image, roles, relationships, and spirituality.
- Identify modification of home environment, interventions, and strategies (e.g., utilizing durable medical equipment, employing a home health aide) used in safely adapting to changes in structure or function and promote effective recovery and rehabilitation.
- Describe ongoing therapeutic regimen, including diet and activities to perform (e.g., oral care, suctioning) and to limit or avoid (e.g., oral foods if NPO).
  - Identify foods or therapies necessary to meet caloric needs and dietary needs (e.g., change in consistency, seasoning limitations, supplements, enteral or parenteral therapy).
  - Participate in prescribed therapy (e.g., speech therapy) to promote recovery and rehabilitation.
  - Demonstrate the use of suction equipment if indicated.

- Demonstrate use of humidification if indicated.
- Demonstrate effective oral hygiene.
- Demonstrate care of incision as appropriate.
- State the name, dose, side effects, frequency, and schedule for all medications.
  - Describe approaches to controlling pain (e.g., take analgesics as prescribed; use nonpharmacologic interventions).
- Identify possible complications and interventions.
- Relate how to reach primary provider with questions or complications.
- State time and date of follow-up medical/dental appointments, therapy, and testing.
- Identify sources of support (e.g., friends, relatives, faith community, cancer support, caregiver support).
- Identify the need for health promotion, disease prevention, and screening activities.

ADLs, activities of daily living; IADLs, instrumental activities of daily living; NPO, nothing by mouth.

(see Chart 39-2). Methods of preparing nutritious foods that are seasoned according to the patient's preference and at the preferred temperature are explained to the patient and family. For some patients, it may be more convenient (but also more expensive) to use commercial baby foods than to prepare liquid and soft diets. The patient who cannot take foods orally may receive enteral or parenteral nutrition; the nurse should demonstrate administration techniques and facilitate a return demonstration by the patient and/or caregiver(s).

For patients with oral cancer, instructions are provided in the use and care of any dentures. The importance of keeping dressings clean and the need for conscientious oral hygiene are emphasized.

Continuing and Transitional Care

The need for ongoing care in the home depends on the patient's condition. The patient, family members, and other health care team members responsible for home care (e.g., nurse, speech therapist, registered dietician/nutritionist, and psychologist) work together to prepare an individual plan of care.

If suctioning of the mouth or tracheostomy tube is required, the necessary equipment is obtained and the patient and caregivers are taught how to use it. Considerations include the control of odors and humidification of the home to keep secretions moist. The patient and caregivers are educated to assess for obstruction, hemorrhage, and infection, as well as what actions to take if they occur. The nurse may provide physical care, monitor for changes in the patient's physical status (e.g., skin integrity, nutritional status, respiratory function), and assess the adequacy of pain control measures. The nurse also assesses the patient's and family's ability to manage incisions, drains, and feeding tubes and the use of recommended strategies for communication. The ability of the patient and family to accept physical, psychological, and role changes is assessed and addressed.

Follow-up visits to the primary provider are important to monitor the patient's condition and to determine the need for modifications in treatment and general care. Because patients and their family members, as well as health care providers, tend to focus on the most obvious needs and issues, the nurse reminds the patient and family about the importance of continuing health promotion and screening practices and refers them to appropriate practitioners. The nurse also reinforces instructions in an effort to promote the patient's self-care and comfort.

NECK DISSECTION

Deaths from malignancies of the head and neck are primarily attributable to regional metastasis to the cervical lymph nodes in the neck and extra capsular spread, which is a specific characteristic of regional metastasis where the malignant tumor in the lymph node extends into the surrounding connective tissue (Stack & Moreno, 2019). Metastasis, both regional and distant, occurs by way of the lymphatics before the primary lesion has been treated. This regional metastasis is not amenable to surgical resection and responds poorly to chemotherapy and radiation therapy. The cervical lymph nodes are classified as anterior or posterior and divided into anatomic regions/nodal levels for classification (Grègoire, Ang, Budach, et al., 2014; Stack & Moreno, 2019) (see Fig. 39-3).

A radical neck dissection involves removal of all cervical lymph nodes from the mandible to the clavicle and removal of the sternocleidomastoid muscle, internal jugular vein, and spinal accessory nerve on one side of the neck. The associated complications include shoulder drop/dysfunction and poor cosmesis (visible neck depression). Because of the high mortality and known complications, a radical neck dissection is now only performed when the extent and growth pattern of the cancer require aggressive intervention. Modified radical neck dissection, which preserves one or more of the

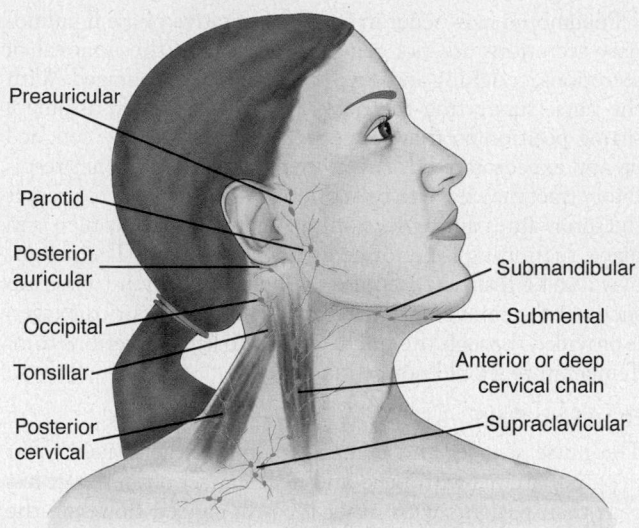

Preauricular

Parotid

Posterior auricular

Occipital

Tonsillar

Posterior cervical

Submandibular

Submental

Anterior or deep cervical chain

Supraclavicular

Figure 39-3 • Lymphatic drainage of the head and neck.

nonlymphatic structures (internal jugular vein, sternocleidomastoid muscle, and the spinal accessory nerve) is used more often. A selective neck dissection (in comparison to a radical neck dissection or modified radical neck dissection) preserves one or more of the lymph node groups that are typically removed in a radical neck dissection. The selective neck dissection is the treatment usually used in oral cavity cancer for patients who are infected with HPV (Sabatini & Chiocca, 2019; Stack & Moreno, 2019) (see Fig. 39-4).

Reconstructive techniques may be performed with a variety of grafts. A cutaneous flap (skin and subcutaneous tissue), such as the deltopectoral flap, may be used. A myocutaneous platysma flap (subcutaneous tissue, muscle, and skin) is a more frequently used graft; the pectoralis major muscle is usually used. For large grafts, a microvascular free flap may be used. This involves the transfer of muscle, skin, or bone with an artery and vein to the area of reconstruction, using microinstrumentation. Areas used for a free flap include the scapula, the radial area of the forearm, or the anterolateral thigh (Stack & Moreno, 2019).

NURSING PROCESS

The Patient Undergoing a Neck Dissection

Assessment

Preoperatively, the patient's physical and psychological preparation for major surgery is assessed, along with the patient's knowledge of the preoperative and postoperative procedures. Postoperatively, the patient is assessed for complications such as altered respiratory status, wound infection, and hemorrhage. As healing occurs, nutritional support is provided and neck range of motion is assessed to determine whether there has been a decrease in range of motion due to nerve or muscle damage.

Diagnosis

NURSING DIAGNOSES

Based on the assessment data, major nursing diagnoses may include the following:

- Lack of knowledge about preoperative and postoperative procedures
- Impaired airway clearance associated with obstruction by mucus, hemorrhage, or edema
- Acute pain associated with surgical incision
- Impaired tissue integrity secondary to surgery and grafting
- Impaired nutritional status associated with disease process or treatment
- Risk for situational low self-esteem associated with diagnosis or prognosis
- Risk for caregiver stress associated with physical and emotional effects of disease and related surgical procedure
- Impaired verbal communication secondary to surgical resection
- Impaired mobility secondary to nerve injury

COLLABORATIVE PROBLEMS/POTENTIAL COMPLICATIONS

Potential complications include the following (Stack & Moreno, 2019):

- Hemorrhage, including hematoma formation, and rupture ("blowout") of the internal jugular vein (IJV) or carotid artery
- Chyle leak, a lymphatic leak in the thoracic duct

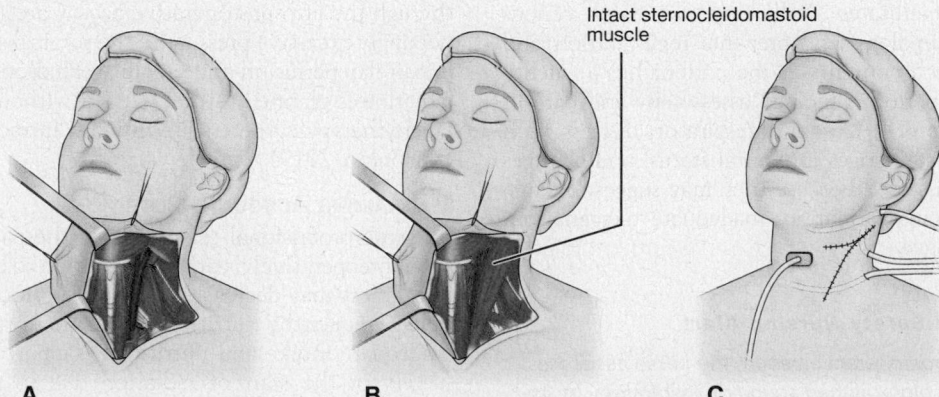

Intact sternocleidomastoid muscle

A   **B**   **C**

Figure 39-4 • A. A classic radical neck dissection in which the sternocleidomastoid and smaller muscles are removed. All tissue is removed, from the ramus of the jaw to the clavicle. The jugular vein has also been removed. **B.** The modified neck dissection is similar, but preserves the sternocleidomastoid muscle, internal jugular vein, and/or spinal accessory nerve. **C.** The wound is closed, and portable suction drainage tubes are in place.

- Neurologic complications, including stroke and nerve injury (spinal accessory, marginal mandibular, vagus, phrenic, hypoglossal, lingual, brachial plexus)

Planning and Goals

The major goals for the patient include increased knowledge of surgical procedure and treatment plan, maintenance of respiratory status, decreased pain, viability of the graft, maintenance of adequate intake of food and fluids, effective coping strategies (for patient and caregivers), effective communication, maintenance of shoulder and neck motion, and absence of complications.

Nursing Interventions

 PROVIDING PREOPERATIVE PATIENT EDUCATION

Before surgery, the patient should be informed about the nature and extent of the surgery and what to expect in the postoperative period. Preoperative education addresses interventions that cover the entire perioperative period. As part of the informed consent process, the patient should be made aware of the potential/actual risks and benefits of the procedure as well as other treatment options, and the projected outcome if the procedure is not done. The patient is encouraged to ask questions and to express concerns about the upcoming surgery and the expected results. During this exchange, the nurse has an opportunity to assess the patient's coping abilities, answer questions, and develop a plan for offering assistance. A sense of mutual understanding and rapport make the postoperative experience less traumatic for the patient. The patient's expressions of concern, anxieties, and fears guide the nurse in providing support postoperatively.

PROVIDING GENERAL POSTOPERATIVE CARE

The general postoperative nursing interventions are similar to those presented in Chapter 16 and are directed toward the identified nursing diagnoses and goals.

MAINTAINING AIRWAY CLEARANCE

After the endotracheal tube or airway has been removed and the effects of the anesthesia have worn off, the patient may be placed in the Fowler position to facilitate breathing and promote comfort. This position also increases lymphatic and venous drainage, facilitates swallowing, decreases venous pressure on the skin flaps, and prevents regurgitation and aspiration of stomach contents. If the patient has a tracheostomy, the nurse performs focused assessment and care of the stoma (see Chapter 19). Signs of respiratory distress, such as dyspnea, cyanosis, changes in mental status, and changes in vital signs, are assessed because they may suggest edema, hemorrhage/hematoma formation, inadequate oxygenation, or inadequate drainage.

 Quality and Safety Nursing Alert

In the immediate postoperative period, the nurse assesses for stridor (coarse, high-pitched sound on inspiration) by listening frequently over the trachea with a stethoscope. This finding must be reported immediately because it indicates obstruction of the airway.

Pneumonia may occur in the postoperative phase if pulmonary secretions are not removed. To aid in the removal of secretions, coughing and deep breathing are encouraged. With the nurse supporting the neck, the patient should assume a sitting position so that excessive secretions can be coughed up and expectorated. If this is ineffective, the patient's respiratory tract may have to be suctioned. Care is taken to protect the suture lines during suctioning. If a tracheostomy tube is in place, suctioning is performed through the tube. The patient may also be instructed on use of Yankauer suction (tonsil-tip suction) to remove oral secretions. Humidified air or oxygen is provided through the tracheostomy to keep secretions thin. Temperature should not be taken orally.

RELIEVING PAIN

The nurse assesses and manages pain and the patient's fear of pain. Patients with head and neck cancer often report less pain than patients with other types of cancer; however, the nurse needs to be aware that each person's pain experience is different. The nurse works with the patient to establish reasonable pain goals and creates an interprofessional plan to meet those mutually defined goals. Patient-controlled analgesia may be prescribed for postoperative pain management (see Chapters 9 and 16).

PROVIDING WOUND CARE

Wound drainage tubes are usually inserted during surgery to prevent the collection of fluid subcutaneously. The drainage tubes are connected to a portable suction device (e.g., Jackson-Pratt), and the container is emptied periodically. Between 80 and 120 mL of serosanguineous secretions may drain over the first 24 hours. Excessive drainage may be indicative of a chyle fistula or hemorrhage (see later discussion). Dressings are reinforced as needed and are observed for evidence of hemorrhage and constriction, which impair respiration and perfusion of the graft. A graft, if present, is assessed for color and temperature and for the presence of a pulse, if applicable, to determine viability. The graft should be pale pink and warm to the touch. The surgical incisions are also assessed for signs of infection (purulent, malodorous drainage), which are reported immediately. Prophylactic antibiotics may be prescribed in the early postoperative period. Aseptic technique is used when cleansing skin around the drains; dressings are changed as prescribed by the surgeon, usually on the second through the fifth postoperative days. Care should be taken to not apply excessive pressure to the surgical site in order to not impair flap perfusion and viability (Hudson & Carr, 2020). If radiation is planned (either with or without chemotherapy), brachytherapy catheters are inserted intraoperatively (Stack & Moreno, 2019).

MAINTAINING ADEQUATE NUTRITION

The interprofessional team assesses the patient's nutritional status preoperatively; early intervention to correct nutritional imbalances may decrease the risk of postoperative complications. Frequently, nutrition is less than optimal because of inadequate intake and nutritional support is required before surgery or the start of radiation due to the psychological stress of the cancer diagnosis, the location of the tumor(s), and diagnostic procedures. Prophylactic nutritional support using a tube feeding is common and may prevent weight loss, reduce fluid imbalances, decrease hospitalizations, and increase treatment tolerance (Sandmæl et al., 2019). Supplements that are nutritionally dense may help reestablish a positive nitrogen balance. They may be taken enterally by mouth, by a nasogastric (NG) feeding tube, or by a gastrostomy feeding tube (see later discussion).

The patient who can chew may take food by mouth; the patient's chewing ability determines whether some diet modification (e.g., soft, puréed, or liquid foods) is necessary. Food preferences should also be discussed with the patient. Oral care before eating may enhance the patient's appetite, and oral care after eating is important to prevent infection and dental caries.

SUPPORTING PATIENT SELF-ESTEEM AND THE NEEDS OF CAREGIVERS

Preoperatively, information about the planned surgery is given to the patient and family. Any questions are answered as accurately as possible. Postoperatively, psychological nursing interventions are aimed at supporting the patient who has had a change in body image or who has major concerns related to the prognosis. The patient may have difficulty communicating and may be concerned about having the ability to breathe and swallow normally. Head and neck cancer recovery is unique in that the patient's behavioral issues (e.g., HPV infection status, alcohol, smoking) often directly relate to the underlying cause of the cancer. The psychological adaptation required after a disfiguring surgery, and the social complications inherent in swallowing and speech are profound. The *patient–caregiver dyad* is often considered a single unit, which reinforces the need to consider both entities, as well as their interrelationship (Dri, Bressan, Cadorin, et al., 2019).

The person who has had extensive neck surgery often is sensitive about their appearance. This can occur when the operative area is covered by bulky dressings, when the incision line is visible, or later after healing has occurred and the appearance of the neck and possibly the lower face has been significantly altered. If the nurse accepts the patient's appearance and expresses a positive, optimistic attitude, the patient is more likely to be encouraged. The patient also needs an opportunity to express fears and concerns regarding the success of the surgery and the prognosis. The American Cancer Society (ACS) may be a resource to provide a volunteer who meets with the patient either preoperatively or postoperatively and shares their own experience about the diagnosis, treatment, and recovery. The Look Good Feel Better programs of the ACS provide information about clothing and cosmetics that can be used to improve body image and self-esteem (see the Resources section at the end of this chapter).

People with cancer of the head and neck frequently have used alcohol or tobacco before surgery; postoperatively, they are encouraged to abstain from these substances. Alternative methods of coping need to be explored. A referral to Alcoholics Anonymous, a smoking cessation program, and family counseling may be appropriate.

PROMOTING EFFECTIVE COMMUNICATION

Communication plans begin preoperatively, when the patient and family determine which method of communication will be the best postoperatively. Useful communication methods for the patient who has undergone a laryngectomy include dry-erase boards, writing materials, pictorial guides, computer aids, smart phones, tablets, and hand signals. During the postoperative period, the call bell must be readily accessible to the patient at all times. For the patient who is intubated and mechanically ventilated postoperatively, not being able to communicate well can result in anxiety, depression, and frustration, which can lead to prolonged stress and increased hospitalization (Koszalinski, Heidel, & McCarthy, 2020). (See the Nursing Research Profile in Chart 39-3.)

The nurse obtains a consultation with a speech-language pathologist. Alternative speech techniques, such as a voice prosthesis or esophageal speech, may be taught by a speech-language pathologist (see Chapter 18).

Chart 39-3 NURSING RESEARCH PROFILE

Envisioning a Positive Future: Patients Who Are Communication Vulnerable

Koszalinski, R. S., Heidel, R. E., & McCarthy, J. (2020). Difficulty envisioning a positive future: Secondary analyses in patients in intensive care who are communication vulnerable. *Nursing & Health Sciences, 22*(2), 374–380.

Purpose

This study explored the experience of patients who, for myriad reasons, find themselves unable to communicate in the intensive care unit (ICU) setting.

Design

This secondary analysis was based on an equivalent control group design. Data were analyzed with a mixed-effect analysis of variance (ANOVA; between and within groups), repeated measure to compare the control and treatment groups over time. The focus of this analysis was on considering the impact of a nurse-led electronic communication intervention, called *Speak for Myself Voice* (SFMV), on depression and anxiety. Data were collected using the Hospital Anxiety and Depression scale (HADS) from 36 participants in a trauma surgical ICU, neuro ICU, progressive care unit, medical ICU, and cardiovascular ICU at an academic medical center in rural Tennessee.

Findings

Although change was detected from preintervention to postintervention on several questions on the HADS, one item piqued the interest of the researchers: "I look forward with enjoyment to things." There was a statistically significant interaction ($p = 0.017$) from preintervention to postintervention. This indicates that patients who are mechanically ventilated or unable to communicate because of obstruction, trauma, or surgical resection (including head and neck procedures) may be silently suffering with depressive symptoms.

Nursing Implications

These results are supported by other studies in the literature. Nurses have the unique ability to make sure patients who are unable to communicate feel seen and heard. Intentional presence and honest interest in the patient as a person by the nurse opens the door to communication that extends beyond mere vocalizations and provides the patient comfort.

MAINTAINING PHYSICAL MOBILITY

Excision of the sternocleidomastoid muscle and spinal accessory nerve results in weakness at the shoulder that can cause shoulder drop, which is a forward curvature of the shoulder. Many problems can be avoided with a conscientious exercise program. These exercises are usually started in collaboration with a physical therapist after the drains have been removed and the neck incision is sufficiently healed. The purpose of the exercises depicted in Figure 39-5 is to promote maximal shoulder function and neck motion after surgery.

MONITORING AND MANAGING POTENTIAL COMPLICATIONS

Hemorrhage. Hemorrhage may occur from carotid artery rupture as a result of necrosis of the graft or damage to the artery itself from tumor or infection. This can result in frank bleeding or the formation of a hematoma. The following measures are indicated:

- Vital signs are assessed frequently (every 1 to 2 hours or every 15 minutes if the patient is critical). Once the patient is stabilized, assessment is performed every 4 hours. Tachycardia, tachypnea, and hypotension may indicate hemorrhage and impending hypovolemic

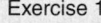

Exercise 1

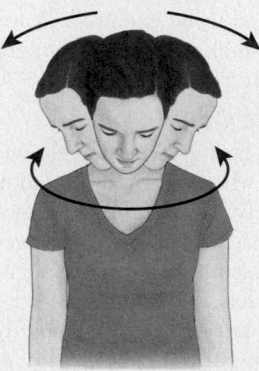

Gently turn head to each side and look as far as possible. Gently tip right ear toward right shoulder as far as possible. Repeat on left side. Move chin to chest and then lift head up and back.

Exercise 2

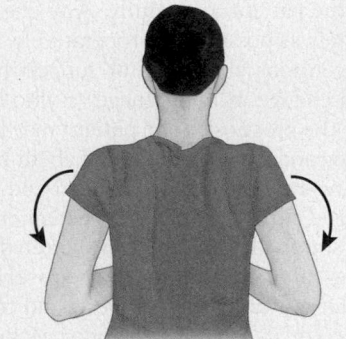

Place hands in front with elbows at right angles away from body. Rotate shoulders back, bringing elbows to side. Then relax whole body.

Exercise 3: Using the hand on the unaffected side, lean or hold onto a low table or chair.

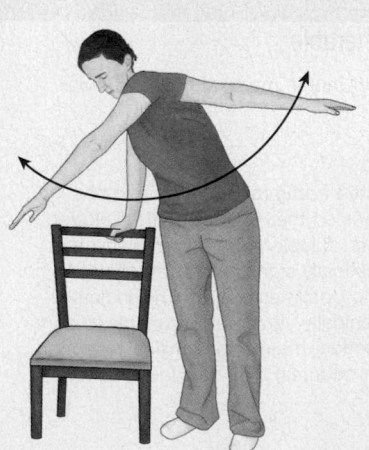

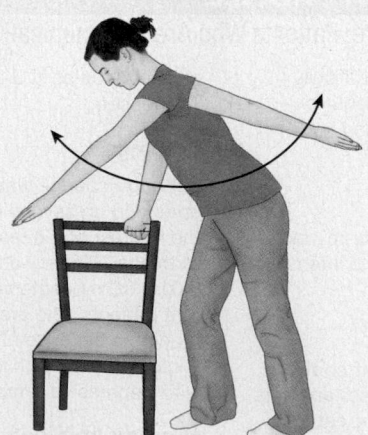

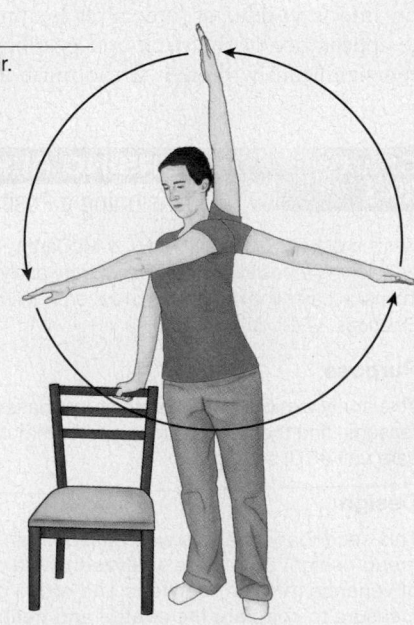

Bend body slightly at waist and swing shoulder and arm from left to right.

Swing shoulder and arm from front to back.

Swing shoulder and arm in a wide circle, gradually bringing arm above head.

Figure 39-5 • Three rehabilitation exercises after head and neck surgery. The objective is to regain maximum shoulder function and neck motion after neck surgery. Adapted from Exercise for radical neck surgery patients. Head and Neck Service, Department of Surgery, Memorial Hospital, New York, NY.

shock (see Chapter 11 for discussion of treatment of hypovolemic shock).

- The patient is instructed to avoid the Valsalva maneuver to prevent stress on the graft and carotid artery.
- Signs of impending rupture, such as high epigastric pain or discomfort, are reported.
- Dressings and wound drainage are observed for excessive bleeding.
- If hemorrhage occurs, assistance is summoned immediately.
- Hemorrhage requires the continuous firm application of pressure to the bleeding site or major associated vessel.
- The head of the patient's bed should be elevated at least 30 degrees to maintain airway patency and prevent aspiration.
- A controlled, calm manner allays the patient's anxiety.
- The surgeon is notified immediately, because a vascular or ligature tear requires surgical intervention.

Chyle Leak. A chyle leak (milklike, lymphatic fluid drainage from the thoracic duct into the thoracic cavity) may develop as a result of damage to the thoracic duct during surgery. Although not very common (3% to 5.7% of cases), this leak may be recognized during surgery (where it can be repaired immediately) or in the postoperative setting, especially when oral intake begins. If a chyle leak is suspected postoperatively, conservative measures to limit increases in intrathoracic pressure will reduce the flow of chyle fluid in the thoracic duct. Recommended interventions include initiating enteral feeding or supporting a low fat diet focused on the intake of small- and medium-chain fatty acids (chylous fluid is formed from long-chain fatty acids). Medium-chain triglycerides/fats, like those found in coconut oil, are metabolized in the liver into ketones to provide energy without the formation of chyle. Other interventions include fluid and electrolyte replacement, activity restriction, head of bed elevation, stool softeners (to prevent straining), and occasionally, pressure dressings.

Providers often prescribe octreotide, a synthetic analogue of the natural hormone somatostatin, that works primarily by inhibiting the release of gastrointestinal hormones that regulate digestion and absorption, thereby reducing lymph flow and decreasing the chyle flow (Rudrappa & Paul, 2019; Stack & Moreno, 2019).

Nerve Injury. Nerve injury can occur if the spinal accessory, marginal mandibular (branch of the facial nerve), vagus, phrenic, hypoglossal, lingual, or brachial plexus nerves are severed or injured during surgery. Because lower facial paralysis may occur as a result of injury to the facial nerve, this complication is observed for and reported. The patient with nerve damage may have difficulty swallowing liquids and food because of the partial lack of sensation of the glottis, impaired tongue movement, or vagus nerve injury. Speech therapy may be indicated to assist with the problems related to nerve injury. Shoulder dysfunction is most common in radical neck dissection and often requires extensive physical rehabilitation.

PROMOTING HOME, COMMUNITY-BASED, AND TRANSITIONAL CARE

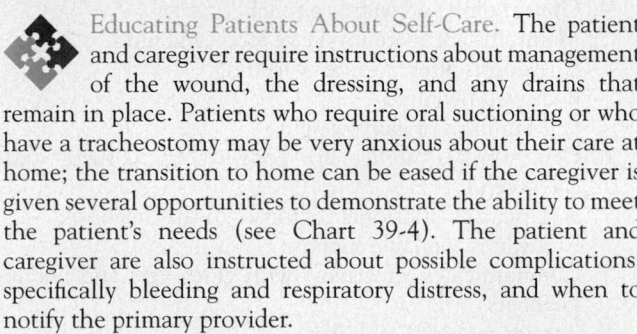

Educating Patients About Self-Care. The patient and caregiver require instructions about management of the wound, the dressing, and any drains that remain in place. Patients who require oral suctioning or who have a tracheostomy may be very anxious about their care at home; the transition to home can be eased if the caregiver is given several opportunities to demonstrate the ability to meet the patient's needs (see Chart 39-4). The patient and caregiver are also instructed about possible complications, specifically bleeding and respiratory distress, and when to notify the primary provider.

If the patient cannot take food by mouth, detailed instructions and demonstration of enteral or parenteral feedings will be required. Education in techniques of effective oral hygiene is also important.

Chart 39-4 **HOME CARE CHECKLIST**

The Patient Recovering from Neck Surgery

At the completion of education, the patient and/or caregiver will be able to:

- Name the procedure that was performed and identify any permanent changes in anatomic structure or function as well as changes in communication, ADLs, IADLs, roles, body image, relationships, and spirituality.
- Identify modification of home environment, interventions, and strategies (e.g., utilizing durable medical equipment, employing a home health aide) used in safely adapting to changes in structure or function and promote effective recovery and rehabilitation.
- Describe ongoing therapeutic regimen, including diet and activities to perform (e.g., oral care, suctioning) and to limit or avoid (e.g., lifting weights, driving a car, contact sports).
  - Identify foods or therapies necessary to meet caloric needs and dietary needs (e.g., change in consistency, seasoning limitations, supplements, enteral or parenteral therapy).
  - Participate in prescribed therapy (e.g., speech therapy, PT, OT) to promote recovery and rehabilitation.
  - Demonstrate the use of tracheostomy care and suctioning if indicated.

- Demonstrate use of humidification if indicated.
- Demonstrate effective oral hygiene.
- Demonstrate care of incision and drains.
- State the name, dose, side effects, frequency, and schedule for all medications.
- Describe approaches to controlling pain (e.g., take analgesics as prescribed; use nonpharmacologic interventions).
- Identify possible complications (e.g., bleeding, respiratory distress) and interventions.
- Relate how to reach primary provider with questions or complications.
- State time and date of follow-up medical/dental appointments, therapy, and testing.
- Identify sources of support (e.g., friends, relatives, faith community, cancer support, caregiver support).
- Identify the need for health promotion, disease prevention, and screening activities.

ADLs, activities of daily living; IADLs, instrumental activities of daily living; OT, occupational therapy; PT, physical therapy.

Continuing and Transitional Care. A referral for home, community-based, or transitional care may be necessary in the early period after discharge. The nurse assesses healing, ensures that feedings are being given properly, and monitors for any complications. The patient's adjustment to changes in physical appearance and status and ability to communicate and eat normally is also assessed. Physical and speech therapy also are likely to be continued at home.

The patient is given information regarding local support groups such as "New Voice Club," if indicated. The local chapter of the ACS may be contacted for information and equipment needed for the patient (see the Resources section).

Evaluation

Expected patient outcomes may include:
1. Exhibits increased knowledge of course of treatment
2. Demonstrates adequate respiratory exchange
   a. Lungs are clear to auscultation
   b. Breathes easily with no shortness of breath
   c. Demonstrates ability to use suction effectively
3. Verbalizes comfort and relief of pain
4. Graft is pink and warm to touch
5. Maintains adequate intake of foods and fluids
   a. Accepts altered route of feeding
   b. Is well hydrated
   c. Maintains or gains weight
6. Demonstrates ability to cope (both patient and caregivers)
   a. Discusses emotional responses to the diagnosis
   b. Utilizes available support
7. Communicates effectively with caregivers and family members
8. Attains maximal mobility
   a. Adheres to physical therapy exercises
   b. Attains maximal range of motion
9. Exhibits no complications
   a. Vital signs stable
   b. No excessive bleeding or discharge
   c. Able to move muscles of lower face and shoulders

DELIVERING NUTRITION ENTERALLY

Feeding via the **enteric** route infers that the intestines are receiving nutrients. Thus, delivering **enteral nutrition** refers to infusing nutritional formula feedings through a tube directly into the GI tract. The nurse plays a key role in ensuring that patients prescribed this therapy achieve nutritional balance sufficient to meet their metabolic needs.

Nursing Management

Administering Tube Feedings

Tube feedings are given to meet nutritional requirements when oral intake is inadequate or not possible and the GI tract is functional. The feedings are delivered to the stomach, duodenum, or proximal jejunum and help preserve GI integrity by preserving normal intestinal and hepatic metabolism. Tube feedings have several advantages over parenteral nutrition: they are lower in cost, safer, usually well tolerated by the

TABLE 39-2 Conditions That May Require Enteral Therapy

Condition or Need	Examples
Alcoholism, chronic depression, anorexia nervosa[a]	Chronic illness, psychiatric or neurologic disorder
Cancer therapy	Radiation, chemotherapy
Coma, semiconsciousness[a]	Stroke, head injury, neurologic disorder, neoplasm
Convalescent care	Surgery, injury, severe illness
Debilitation[a]	Disease or injury
Gastrointestinal problems	Fistula, short-bowel syndrome, mild pancreatitis, Crohn's disease, ulcerative colitis, nonspecific maldigestion or malabsorption
Hypermetabolic conditions	Burns, trauma, multiple fractures, sepsis, acquired immune deficiency syndrome, organ transplantation
Maxillofacial or cervical surgery	Disease or injury
Oropharyngeal or esophageal paralysis[a]	Disease or injury, neoplasm, inflammation, trauma, respiratory failure
Preoperative bowel preparation	After administration of larger-volume cathartics

[a]Because some patients with these conditions are at risk for regurgitating or vomiting and aspirating administered formula, each condition must be considered individually.

patient, and easier to use in extended care facilities and in the patient's home. When possible, the physiological-based preference is to *feed the gut*.

Nasoduodenal or nasojejunal feeding is indicated when the esophagus and stomach need to be bypassed or when the patient is at risk for **aspiration** (i.e., inhalation of fluids or foods into the trachea and bronchial tree). For tube feedings longer than 4 weeks, gastrostomy or jejunostomy tubes are preferred for administration of medications or nutrition. Indications for enteral nutrition are summarized in Table 39-2.

Osmolality

The **osmolality** of normal body fluids (i.e., concentration) is approximately 300 mOsm/kg. The body attempts to keep the osmolality of the contents of the stomach and intestines at this level. Osmolality is an important consideration for patients receiving tube feedings through the duodenum or jejunum because feeding formulas with a high osmolality may lead to undesirable effects. For example, when a concentrated solution of high osmolality entering the stomach is taken in quickly or in large amounts, the small intestines expand and water moves rapidly into the intestinal lumen from fluid surrounding the organs and the vascular compartment. The patient may have feelings of fullness, nausea, cramping, dizziness, diaphoresis, and osmotic diarrhea, collectively termed **dumping syndrome**. Dumping syndrome can lead to dehydration, hypotension, and tachycardia. Patients fed by the small intestinal route vary in the degree to which they tolerate the effects of high osmolality;

the nurse needs to be knowledgeable about the patient's formula and take steps to prevent this undesired effect. The small intestines may be able to adapt to a formula of high osmolality if it is initiated at a low hourly rate that is advanced slowly (Seres, 2019).

Formulas

The choice of formula to be delivered by tube feeding is influenced by the status of the GI tract and the nutritional needs of the patient. Formula characteristics that are considered include the chemical composition of the nutrient source (protein, carbohydrates, fat), caloric density, osmolality, fiber content, vitamins, minerals, electrolytes, and cost. Enteral formulas contain 70% to 85% free water and are not designed to meet total fluids needs (Seres, 2019). A wide variety of containers, delivery systems, and enteral pumps are available for use with tube feedings.

Various tube feeding formulas are available commercially. Polymeric formulas are the most common and are composed of protein (10% to 15%), carbohydrates (50% to 60%), and fats (30% to 35%). Standard polymeric formulas are undigested and require that the patient has relatively normal digestive function and absorptive capacity. Specialty formulas may be prescribed to treat disease-specific disorders (e.g., diabetes), organ-specific disorders (e.g., renal, pulmonary, or hepatic), sepsis, or trauma, or to support wound-healing or immune-modulation. Chemically defined or *predigested* formulas contain easier-to-absorb nutrients. Modular products contain only one major nutrient, such as protein, and are used to enhance commercially prepared products. Fiber, either premixed in or added to formulas, helps bulk the stool to decrease the occurrence of both diarrhea and constipation (McClave, Taylor, Martindale, et al., 2016).

Some feedings are given as supplements, and others are given to meet the patient's total nutritional needs. Registered dietitians (RD), registered dietitian nutritionists (RDN), and certified nutrition support clinicians collaborate with primary providers and nurses to determine the best formula for each patient. The volume of formula delivered varies depending on the caloric density of the formula and the energy needs of the patient. The overall goal is to achieve positive nitrogen balance and weight maintenance or gain without producing discomfort or diarrhea.

Administration Methods

The tube feeding method chosen depends on the location of the tube in the GI tract, patient tolerance, convenience, and cost. Large-bore (larger than 12-Fr) nasogastric (NG) tubes can be uncomfortable and their usefulness for tube feedings is limited; however, they may be used for administration of short-term feedings (Mueller, 2017). Small-bore (Dobhoff) tubes that are typically inserted into the jejunum with a guidewire and manufactured for tube feedings, are better tolerated for up to 6 weeks; however, they require diligent monitoring and frequent flushing to remain patent.

Bolus and intermittent drip tube feeding methods are practical and inexpensive options for the patient receiving tube feedings who resides at home or in a long-term care facility; however, these methods may be poorly tolerated in patients who are acutely ill. Bolus infusion requires dividing the total daily feeding volume into 4 to 6 feeds throughout the day. Boluses can be given into the stomach through a large (50-mL) syringe via gravity (see Fig. 39-6). The typical volume is 200 to 400 mL

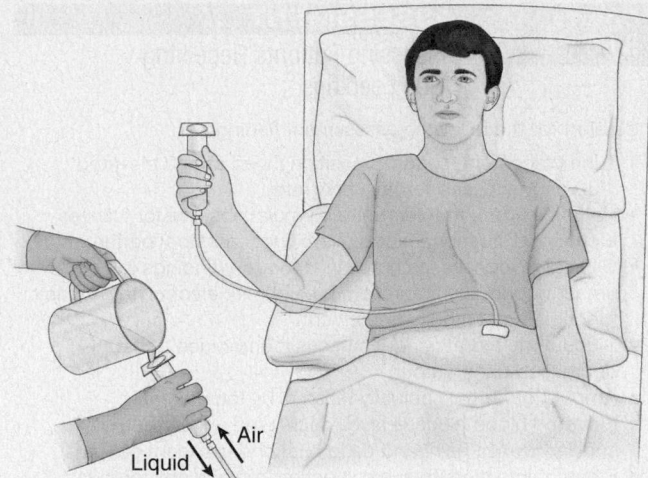

Figure 39-6 • Bolus gastrostomy feeding by gravity. Syringe is raised perpendicular to the abdomen so that feeding can enter by gravity.

of feeding over a 15- to 60-minute period, but these parameters should be outlined in the provider's prescription (Bischoff et al., 2020; Boullata et al., 2017). Bolus feedings can be delivered as quickly as the patient can tolerate them, but are initiated slowly, increasing the rate as tolerated. With gravity feedings, raising or lowering the syringe above the abdominal wall regulates the rate of flow. The amount and flow rate is often determined by the patient's reaction. If the patient feels full, it may be desirable to slow the delivery time or give smaller volumes more frequently. The intermittent gravity drip feeding method requires administering feedings over 30 minutes or longer at designated intervals by a reservoir enteral bag and tubing, with the flow rate regulated by a roller clamp or automated pump.

Continuous feeding is the delivery of feedings incrementally by a slow infusion over long periods. Slow drip feedings are recommended for patients who are critically ill, patients at high risk for aspiration, patients at risk for intolerance (e.g., patients with pancreatitis), and for small bowel feedings (Boullata, Carrera, Harvey, et al., 2017). Enteral feeding pumps control the delivery rate of the formula (see Fig. 39-7).

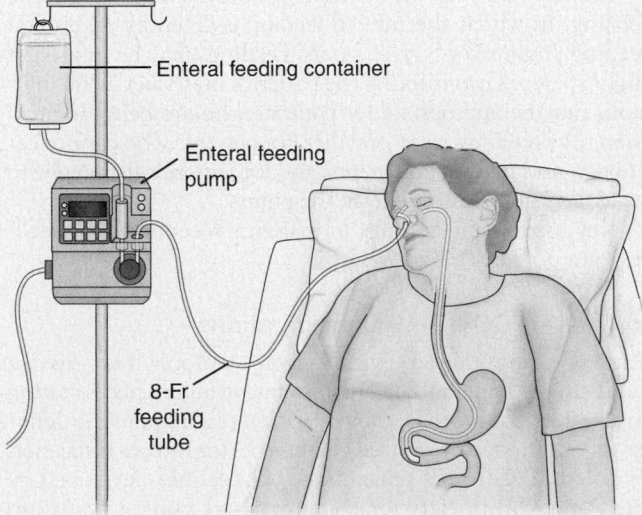

Figure 39-7 • Nasoenteric tube feeding by continuous controlled pump. The head of the bed should be elevated to prevent aspiration.

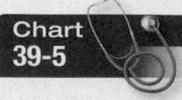

Chart 39-5

ASSESSMENT

Assessing Patients Receiving
Tube Feedings

Be alert for the following assessment findings:

- Tube placement, patient's position (head of bed elevated > 30 degrees), and formula flow rate
- Patient's ability to tolerate the formula; observe for fullness, bloating, distention, nausea, vomiting, and stool pattern
- Clinical responses, as noted in laboratory findings (blood urea nitrogen, serum protein, prealbumin, electrolytes, kidney function, hemoglobin, hematocrit)
- Signs of dehydration (dry mucous membranes, thirst, decreased urine output)
- Amount of formula actually taken in by the patient
- Elevated blood glucose level, decreased urinary output, sudden weight gain, and periorbital or dependent edema
- Signs of infection (to avoid infection, replace any formula given by an open system every 4 to 8 hours with fresh formula; change tube feeding container and tubing every 24 hours)
- Signs of complications (if suspected, check gastric residual volume before each feeding or, in the case of continuous feedings, every 4 hours; return the aspirate to the stomach)
- Intake and output
- Weekly weights
- Recommendations made on dietitian consult

Adapted from McClave, S. A., Taylor, B. E., Martindale, R. G., et al. (2016). Guidelines for the provision and assessment of nutrition support therapy in the adult critically ill patient: Society of Critical Care Medicine (SCCM) and American Society for Parenteral and Enteral Nutrition (ASPEN). *Journal of Parenteral and Enteral Nutrition, 40*(2), 159–211.

They allow for a constant flow rate and can infuse a viscous formula through a small-diameter feeding tube. However, they do not allow the patient as much flexibility as intermittent feedings. Portable lightweight enteral pumps are available for home use. In addition, feeding pumps have built-in alarms that signal when the bag is empty, the battery is low, or the tube is occluded. The patient and caregiver need to be aware of these alarms and know how to troubleshoot the pump.

An alternative to the continuous infusion method is cyclic feeding, in which the infused feeding is given by an enteral feeding pump over 8 to 18 hours. Feedings may be infused at night to avoid interrupting the patient's lifestyle. Cyclic infusions may be appropriate for patients who are being weaned from tube feedings to an oral diet, for patients who cannot eat enough and need supplements, and for patients at home who need daytime hours free from the pump.

Key assessment findings for patients receiving tube feedings are noted in Chart 39-5.

 COVID-19 Considerations

Patients hospitalized with severe coronavirus disease (COVID-19) pneumonia and respiratory failure necessitating intubation and mechanical ventilation may require the delivery of enteral nutrition (see Chapter 19 for further discussion of severe COVID-19 pneumonia). Guidelines developed by the American Society for Parenteral and Enteral Nutrition (ASPEN) stipulate that enteral nutrition should be initiated for these patients within 36 hours of admission to the

intensive care unit (Martindale, Patel, Taylor, et al., 2020). These guidelines should be implemented unless the decision has been made that the patient receives end-of-life palliative care. Large-bore nasogastric tubes are the preferred route of delivery; these can be placed rapidly and are less prone to clogging compared to small-bore nasoduodenal or nasojejunal feeding tube. Therefore, there is less risk of contamination for nurses and other providers responsible for inserting or manipulating the feeding tubes (Martindale et al., 2020).

However, inserting a nasogastric feeding tube still incurs risk. Placement of a nasogastric feeding tube can generate a cough, which can produce sputum; consequently, placing a nasogastric tube is considered an aerosol-generating procedure. When inserting a nasogastric tube in a patient with known or suspected COVID-19, whether for feeding or for decompression, the nurse should wear appropriate personal protective equipment (PPE) (see Chapter 66 for description of PPE) (Anderson, 2020). In addition, if possible, the patient's mouth should be covered with a mask during the procedure (Martindale et al., 2020). The feedings should be delivered as continuous rather than bolus infusions (Martindale et al., 2020).

Many patients with severe COVID-19 pneumonia who are intubated and mechanically ventilated experience an improvement in their respiratory status when they are placed in the prone position (see Chapter 19); however, if they are also receiving enteral nutrition, they are at greater risk for aspiration in this position. These patients should be placed in reverse Trendelenburg, with their heads elevated 10 to 25 degrees, to minimize this risk (Martindale et al., 2020). Some experts also advocate that feedings be held for 1 hour prior to the patient being moved into the prone position, to further reduce the risk of aspiration (Anderson, 2020; Arkin, Krishnan, & Chang, 2020).

Maintaining Feeding Equipment and Nutritional Balance

The temperature and volume of the feeding, the flow rate, and the patient's total fluid intake are important factors to consider when tube feedings are given. The schedule of tube feedings, including the correct quantity and frequency, is maintained. The nurse must carefully monitor the drip rate and avoid administering fluids too rapidly.

For patients receiving tube feedings, measuring gastric residual volumes (GRVs) by removing gastric contents with a large syringe at routine intervals has been a commonly prescribed practice. However, the usefulness of measuring GRVs has not been validated by research; furthermore, this practice may cause clogging of gastric tubes (Boullata et al., 2017). Previously, GRV in excess of 250 to 500 mL had been thought to indicate feeding intolerance. Other indicators of feeding tolerance that the nurse needs to consider include abdominal distention, patient reports of discomfort, vomiting, hypoactive bowel sounds, changes in passing flatus, and presence of diarrhea (McClave et al., 2016). The most recent guidelines for assessment and provision of nutrition in the patient who is critically ill, authored by the Society of Critical Care Medicine (SCCM) and the American Society for Parenteral and Enteral Nutrition (ASPEN), do not advocate using GRVs to monitor tolerance of enteral feedings (McClave et al., 2016). Research findings show that GRVs between 250 and 500 mL did not increase the incidence of vomiting, aspiration, or pneumonia (McClave et al., 2016). Although feedings should not routinely be held if residuals are 250 to 500 mL, measures to decrease the risk of aspiration should be implemented (Boullata et al., 2017; McClave et al., 2016). If agency protocols and policies include assessing GRV as part of routine care, research and guidelines support holding the feeding for 2 hours only if the GRV is greater than 500 mL (Boullata et al., 2017; McClave et al., 2016). Growing evidence supports moving away from routine assessment of GRVs (Seres, 2019).

Maintaining tube function is an ongoing responsibility of the nurse, patient, primary provider, and caregiver. To ensure patency and to decrease the chance of bacterial growth, sludge build-up, or occlusion of the tube, at least 30 mL of water flush is recommended for adults receiving tube feedings in each of the following instances (Bischoff, Austin, Boeykens, et al., 2020; Boullata et al., 2017):

- Before and after intermittent tube feeding
- Before and after medication administration (see later discussion)
- After checking for gastric residuals (if required by policy) and gastric pH
- Every 4 hours with continuous feedings
- When the tube feeding is discontinued or interrupted for any reason

Water used to flush these tubes must be recorded as fluid intake. Although distribution (i.e., tap) or drinking (i.e., distribution and bottled) water can be used for flushes, the likelihood of contamination with pathogens must be considered. Purified (contaminant free; distillation or ultrafiltration) or sterile (purified water free of microorganisms and pyrogens) should be used for medication preparation. The use of sterile water is considered best practice for patients who are immunocompromised and for reconstitution of powdered formula (Bischoff et al., 2020; Boullata et al., 2017).

Potential complications of enteral therapy are noted in Table 39-3.

Providing Medications by Tube

When different types of medications are prescribed, a bolus method is used for administration that is compatible with the medication's preparation. The feeding is paused, and the tube is flushed with at least 15 mL of water before and at least 15 mL of water after medication administration (30 mL total). Each medication should be prepared and administered separately, with a 15-mL flush provided between medications. When small-bore feeding tubes for continuous infusion are irrigated after administration of medications, a 20-mL or larger syringe is used because the pressure generated by smaller syringes could rupture the tube. Nursing judgment is required to individualize care; institutional protocols and pharmacist input should guide the primary provider's prescriptions regarding medication choices and route of delivery. Consideration needs to be given to preparations (tablets that can be crushed/dissolved; availability of elixirs), absorption (e.g., some medications bind to enteral feedings, location of distal end of tube in the stomach or jejunum), and the patient's fluid volume status (i.e., increased number of medications necessitates increases in the flush/water that is administered).

> ### ▶ Quality and Safety Nursing Alert
>
> *Administering medications through postpyloric enteric tubes may adversely affect their absorption; therefore, this should be avoided if possible. In addition, to avoid nutrient and drug interactions, medications should not be mixed with the feeding formulas.*

Maintaining Delivery Systems

Tube feeding formula is delivered to patients by either an open or a closed system. The open system is packaged as a liquid or a powder to be mixed with water that is either poured into a feeding container or given by a large syringe. The feeding container (which is hung on a pole) and the tubing used with the open system should be changed every 24 hours (Bischoff et al., 2020; Boullata et al., 2017). The open system can be used for bolus feedings, intermittent feedings, or continuous drip feedings and can be delivered by push (with a syringe and plunger), gravity (syringe with plunger removed or gravity bag with roller clamp), or pump. To avoid bacterial contamination, the formula hang time in the bag at room temperature should never exceed what the formula manufacturer recommends, which is usually no more than 4 to 8 hours. Closed delivery systems use a prefilled, sterile container of about 1 L of formula that is spiked with enteral tubing and allows a typical hang time of 24 hours at room temperature. The closed delivery system must always use a pump to control formula rate in order to avoid dispensing a large formula volume in a short period of time. Closed systems lower the risk of infection from bacterial contamination (Boullata et al., 2017).

Maintaining Normal Bowel Elimination Pattern

Patients receiving gastric or enteric tube feedings can experience diarrhea or constipation. Possible causes of diarrhea include:

- Intolerance to enteral nutrition, related to underlying disease
- Malnutrition: A decrease in the intestinal absorptive area can cause diarrhea
- Medication therapy:
  - Elixir-based medications—often contain sorbitol, which can act as a cathartic
  - Magnesium—acts as a cathartic
  - Antibiotics—thought to alter normal intestinal flora, allowing pathogenic bacteria to flourish
- *Clostridium difficile* (*C. difficile*) colitis: Can result after antibiotic use alters normal intestinal flora and promotes the abnormal growth of this potentially dangerous microbe; *C. difficile* colitis occurs most commonly in patients who are hospitalized (Read, Olson, & Calderwood, 2020)
- Zinc deficiency: Zinc is lost with diarrhea, and zinc deficiency can then cause continued diarrhea
- Concomitant lactose intolerance
- Concomitant hyperthyroidism
- Dumping syndrome: Formula is infused into the small intestine quickly or formula bypasses the stomach too readily into the small intestine and causes expansion of the intestinal wall. This leads to bloating, cramping, diarrhea, dizziness, diaphoresis, and weakness. Measures

TABLE 39-3	Potential Complications of Enteral Therapy		
		Select Nursing Interventions	
Complications	**Causes**	**Therapeutic**	**Preventive**
Gastrointestinal			
Constipation	Lack of fiber Inadequate fluid intake/dehydration Opioid use	Check fiber and water content; report findings.	Administer adequate amount of hydration as flushes. Consider cathartic.
Diarrhea	Hyperosmolar feedings Rapid infusion/bolus feedings Cold formula Medications, especially antibiotic therapy	Assess fluid balance and electrolyte levels; report findings. Implement changes in tube feeding formula or rate. Review medications.	Ensure appropriate rate of infusion and temperature of formula. Avoid multiple elixirs and prokinetic medications.
Gas/bloating/cramping	Air in tube Excess fiber	Notify primary provider if persistent.	Keep tubing free of air.
Nausea/vomiting	Change in formula or rate Inadequate gastric emptying	Review medications.	Check residuals; if ≥200 mL, reinstill and recheck; report if residual is consistently high.
Mechanical			
Aspiration pneumonia	Improper tube placement Vomiting with aspiration of tube feeding Flat in bed	Assess respiratory status and notify primary provider.	Implement reliable method for checking tube placement. Keep head of bed elevated 30 degrees.
Nasopharyngeal irritation	Tube position/improper taping Use of large tubes	Assess nasopharyngeal mucous membranes every 8 h.	Tape tube to prevent pressure on nares. Reposition tape.
Tube displacement	Excessive coughing/vomitus Tension on the tube or unsecured tube Tracheal suctioning Airway intubation	Stop feeding, and notify primary provider.	Check tube placement before administering feeding.
Tube obstruction	Inadequate flushing/formula rate Inadequate crushing of medications and flushing after administration	Follow policy for declogging feeding tubes (for the procedural guidelines for declogging a feeding tube, go to thepoint.lww.com/Brunner15e).	Obtain liquid medications when possible. Flush tube and crush medications adequately.
Metabolic			
Dehydration and azotemia (excessive urea in the blood)	Hyperosmolar feedings with insufficient fluid intake	Report signs and symptoms of dehydration. Implement changes in tube feeding formula, rate, or ratio to water.	Provide adequate hydration through flushes.
Hyperglycemia	Glucose intolerance High carbohydrate content of the feeding	Check blood glucose levels routinely. Dietary consult to reevaluate feeding regimen.	
Refeeding syndrome, caused by rapid shifts in intracellular and extracellular electrolytes	Inadequate nutritional intake for >2 wks/Anorexia Poorly controlled diabetes Cancer Short bowel syndrome/inflammatory bowel disease Older adult patient living alone Chronic infections	Monitor fluid balance, daily weight, electrolyte status, and metabolic/nutrition parameters	Initiate feedings at 25% of the estimated goal and advance slowly over 3–5 days with careful laboratory monitoring

Adapted from Blumenstein, I., Shastri, Y. H., & Stein, J. (2014). Gastroenteric tube feeding: Techniques, problems, and solutions. *World Journal of Gastroenterology, 20*(26), 8505–8524; Boullata, J. I., Carrera, A. L., Harvey, L., et al. (2017). ASPEN safe practices for enteral nutrition therapy. *Journal of Parenteral and Enteral Nutrition, 41*(1), 15–103.

for managing the GI symptoms associated with dumping syndrome are presented in Chart 39-6.

- Contamination of the formula and feeding equipment with diarrhea-causing pathogens (Boullata et al., 2017)

Possible causes of constipation include:

- Inadequate water intake: Tube feedings typically do not meet total fluid needs and additional water needs to be given.
- Administration of fiber-free tube feeding formulas
- Concomitant use of opioids

Maintaining Adequate Hydration

The nurse carefully monitors hydration because in many cases the patient cannot communicate the need for water. Water flushes are given every 4 hours and after feedings to prevent hypertonic dehydration. The feeding may be initially given as a continuous drip in order to help the patient develop tolerance, especially for hyperosmolar solutions. Key nursing interventions include observing for signs of dehydration (e.g., dry mucous membranes, thirst, decreased urine output); administering water routinely; and monitoring intake and output, residual volume, and fluid balance.

Promoting Coping Ability

The psychosocial goal of nursing care is to support and encourage the patient to accept physical changes and to convey hope that daily progressive improvement is possible. If the patient is having difficulty adjusting to the treatment, the

Chart 39-6	Preventing Dumping Syndrome

The following strategies may help prevent some of the uncomfortable signs and symptoms of dumping syndrome related to tube feeding:

- Slow the formula instillation rate to provide time for carbohydrates and electrolytes to be diluted.
- Administer feedings at room temperature, because temperature extremes stimulate peristalsis.
- Administer feeding by continuous drip (if tolerated) rather than by bolus, to prevent sudden distention of the intestine.
- Advise the patient to remain in semi-Fowler position for 1 hour after the feeding; this position prolongs intestinal transit time by decreasing the effect of gravity.
- Instill the minimal amount of water needed to flush the tubing before and after a feeding, because fluid given with a feeding increases intestinal transit time.

nurse intervenes by encouraging self-care within the parameters of the patient's activity level. In addition, the nurse reinforces an optimistic approach by identifying indicators of progress (daily weight trends, electrolyte balance, absence of nausea and diarrhea, improvement in plasma proteins).

Promoting Home, Community-Based, and Transitional Care

 Educating Patients About Self-Care

Patients who require long-term tube feedings may have had recent surgery, dysphagia due to a neuromuscular disease, head and neck cancer, radiation or other types of trauma to the throat, an obstruction of the upper GI tract, GI cancer and other malignancies, GI disease (including malabsorptive syndromes), or decreased level of consciousness. For a patient to be considered for tube feeding at home, the patient should:

- Be medically stable and successfully tolerating at least 60% to 70% of the feeding regimen
- Be capable of self-care or have a caregiver willing to assume the responsibility
- Have access to supplies and interest in learning how to administer tube feedings at home

Preparation of the patient for home administration of enteral feedings begins while the patient is still hospitalized. The nurse should educate the patient and caregiver while administering the feedings so that they can observe the mechanics and participate in the procedure, ask questions, and express any concerns. Before discharge, the nurse provides information about the equipment needed, formula purchase and storage, and administration of the feedings and water flushes (frequency, quantity, rate of instillation).

Family members who will be active in the patient's home care are encouraged to participate in education sessions. Available printed information about the equipment, the formula, and the procedure is reviewed. Arrangements are made to obtain the equipment and formula and have it ready for use before the patient's discharge.

Continuing and Transitional Care

Referral to home, community-based, or transitional care is important so that a nurse can supervise and provide support during the first tube feedings at home. Additional visits will depend on the skill and comfort of the patient or caregiver in administering the feedings. During all visits, the nurse monitors the patient's physical status (weight, hydration status, vital signs, activity level) and the ability of the patient and family to administer the tube feedings correctly and assess the enteral access device and site. Enteral access devices require periodic replacement, and the nurse should be sure that the patient and caregiver have the necessary information to set up these tube replacement appointments. In addition, the nurse assesses for any complications. The patient or caregiver is encouraged to record times and amounts of feedings and water flushes, bowel patterns, and any symptoms that occur. The nurse can review the record with the patient and caregiver during home visits.

Gastrostomy and Jejunostomy

A **gastrostomy** is a procedure in which an opening is created into the stomach either for the purpose of administering nutrition, fluids, and medications via a feeding tube, or for gastric decompression in patients with gastroparesis, gastroesophageal reflux disease, or intestinal obstruction. A gastrostomy is preferred over a nasally inserted tube to deliver enteral nutrition support longer than 4 to 6 weeks (Bischoff et al., 2020; Boullata et al., 2017). Gastrostomy is also preferred over nasogastric or orogastric feedings in the patient who is comatose because the gastroesophageal sphincter remains intact, making regurgitation and aspiration less likely. Placement involves creation of a **stoma**, an artificially created opening, that houses the tube.

Insertion of a **percutaneous endoscopic gastrostomy (PEG)** requires the services of a provider skilled in endoscopy, utilizes moderate sedation, and takes approximately 15 to 20 minutes. A lighted endoscope is inserted through the mouth into the stomach. Once in the stomach, the light indicates the location for hollow needle and guidewire insertion into the stomach. The wire is pulled back through the mouth, then the PEG tube itself is attached to the wire to guide the PEG tube as it moves into the mouth, down the esophagus, into the stomach, and out the incision in the abdominal wall. An internal fixation bolster, often called a *bumper*, is pulled snug against the stomach wall. An external retention disc/phalange sits close to the abdominal surface. The tension between the external and internal fixation bolsters keeps the tube in place (see Fig. 39-8A). A radiologically inserted gastrostomy tube (RIG) can be placed fluoroscopically by a skilled provider when an endoscope cannot be passed through a strictured or obstructed esophagus. The RIG is internally sutured and held in place by an internal balloon that is inflated with a small amount of water (Anderson, 2019; Thompson, 2017).

Feeding can be initiated via PEG tubes within several hours (≤4 hours) of placement. The stomal tract will take 30 to 90 days to mature, so replacement should not occur until at least 30 days after placement. Manufacturer guidelines should be followed for replacement of tubes, but deterioration or dysfunction, a ruptured balloon, stomal tract disruption, nonhealing ulcers, or fistula formation may accelerate this recommended time frame. With optimal care, tubes may last 1 to 2 years; however, most policies encourage preventative maintenance that includes elective changing of the balloon gastrostomy tube every 3 to 6 months (Boullata et al., 2017). An alternative to standard gastrostomy tubes that are bulky are

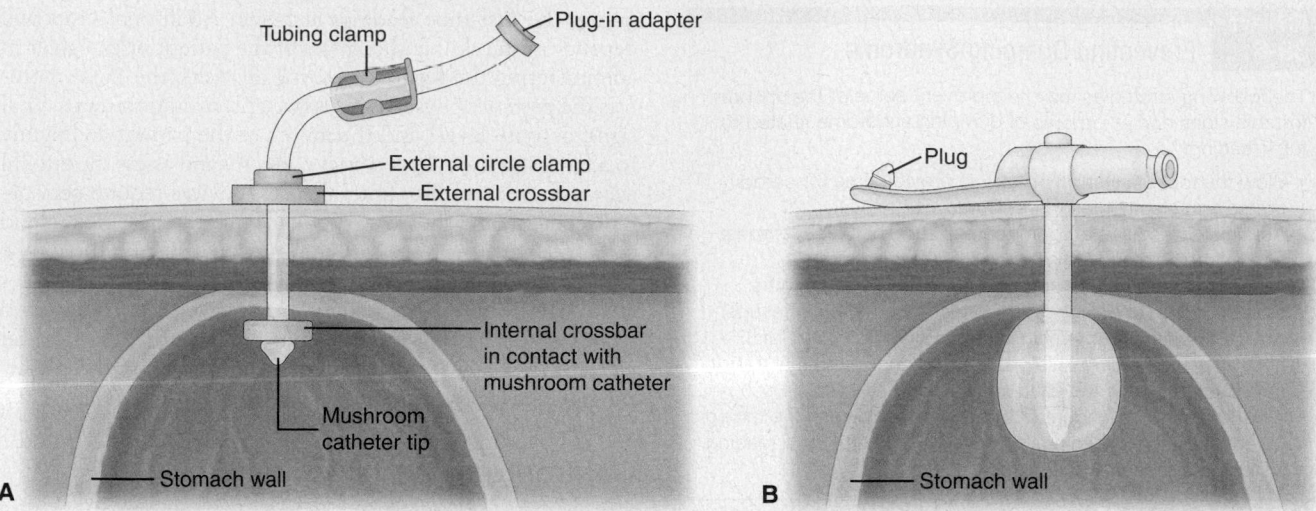

Figure 39-8 • A. A detail of the abdomen and the percutaneous endoscopic gastrostomy (PEG) tube showing catheter fixation. **B.** A detail of the abdomen and the nonobturated low-profile gastrostomy device showing balloon fixation.

low-profile gastrostomy devices (see Fig. 39-8B). Specific types of low-profile gastrostomy devices include the MIC-KEY or the Bard Button. These devices are flush with the skin, eliminate the possibility of inward tube migration, have antireflux valves to prevent gastric leakage, and do not require tape or other securement devices (Boullata et al., 2017). Patients requiring enteral nutrition support can conceal the feeding tube access site under their clothing. Low-profile gastrostomy devices require special connection tubing so they can be attached to the feeding container. Patients must be instructed to bring this connection tubing with them when traveling, going to the emergency department or hospital, or undergoing diagnostic procedures that require access into the GI tract.

A **jejunostomy** is a surgically, endoscopically (percutaneous gastrojejunostomy or jejunal; PEJ), or radiologically placed opening into the jejunum for the purpose of administering nutrition, fluids, and medications. A jejunostomy tube is indicated when the gastric route is not accessible, or to decrease aspiration risk when the stomach is not functioning adequately to process and empty food and fluids. These tubes either have an internal balloon or dacron cuff, or are sutured externally to secure them. Unlike the gastrostomy tubes, jejunostomy tubes should not be rotated and only last between 6 to 9 months (Anderson, 2019; Boullata et al., 2017). The small intestine can also be accessed by placing a jejunal extension tube through an existing gastrostomy tube and manipulating it through the pylorus into the small intestine endoscopically, fluoroscopically, or during a surgical procedure—this is referred to as a *gastrojejunostomy* tube.

NURSING PROCESS

The Patient with a Gastrostomy or Jejunostomy

Assessment

The focus of the preoperative assessment is to determine the patient's ability to understand and cooperate with the procedure. The nurse assesses the ability of both patient and family to adjust to a change in body image and to participate in self-care. There are multiple medical and ethical issues that the patient, the caregivers, and the primary provider should discuss together.

The purpose of the procedure and expected postoperative course should be explained. The patient needs to know that the feeding tube will bypass the mouth and esophagus so that liquid feedings can be given directly into the stomach or intestine. If the feeding tube is expected to be permanent, the patient should be made aware of this. If the procedure is being performed to relieve discomfort, prolonged vomiting, debilitation, or an inability to eat, the patient may find the feeding tube more acceptable.

In the postoperative period, the patient's fluid and nutritional needs are assessed to ensure proper intake and GI function. The nurse inspects the tube for proper maintenance and the incision for any drainage, skin breakdown, or signs of infection. As the nurse evaluates patients' responses to the change in body image and their understanding of the feeding methods, interventions are identified to help them cope with the tube and learn self-care measures.

Diagnosis

NURSING DIAGNOSES

Based on the assessment data, major nursing diagnoses may include the following:

- Impaired nutritional status
- Risk for infection associated with presence of wound and tube
- Risk for impaired skin integrity at tube insertion site
- Disturbed body image associated with presence of tube

COLLABORATIVE PROBLEMS/POTENTIAL COMPLICATIONS

Potential complications may include the following (Anderson, 2019):

- Wound infection, cellulitis, and leakage
- GI bleeding
- Premature dislodgement of the tube
- Tube obstruction/clogging

Planning and Goals

The major goals for the patient may include achieving nutritional requirements, preventing infection, maintaining skin integrity, adjusting to changes in body image, and preventing complications.

Nursing Interventions

MEETING NUTRITIONAL NEEDS

The first fluid nourishment is given soon after tube insertion and can consist of a sterile water or normal saline flush of at least 30 mL. Formula feeding can begin as prescribed, typically within 4 hours post tube insertion. The infusion rate or bolus amount given is gradually increased.

If the tube has been placed for gastric drainage, it can be connected to either low intermittent suction or to a gravity drainage bag. This drainage should be measured and recorded because it is a significant indicator of GI function. A decrease in the amount of drainage may indicate that the tube can be clamped for periods of time, allowing greater freedom of movement. High output can result in significant fluid and electrolyte losses.

PREVENTING INFECTION AND PROVIDING SKIN CARE

For the first week after insertion, interventions are focused on prevention of stomal tract infection and promotion of incisional healing. The insertion site should be kept clean and dry using aseptic wound care daily and/or a glycerin hydrogel or glycogel dressing. It is normal to see scant serous drainage at the site for a few days post insertion. After approximately 1 week, the site (including under the external disc, if one is present) can be cleansed twice a week with soap and water and left open to air. Skin at the exit site is evaluated daily for signs of breakdown, irritation, excoriation, and the presence of drainage, bleeding or hypertrophic tissue growth or scattered, raised red papules that could indicate a yeast or candidal infection. Candida may appear in warm moist areas of the body; the area beneath the gastric tube external retention bolster is a common location for it to develop and spread. The nurse encourages the patient and family members to participate in this evaluation and in hygiene activities. If gastric contents leak and irritate the skin at the stoma site, zinc oxide–based protectants may be used. After the first week of healing, buried bumper syndrome, a severe, but rare complication, can be prevented by rotating the gastric tube (not done with jejunostomy tubes) daily and moving the tube inward 2 to 10 cm at least once a week (Bischoff et al., 2020; Boullata et al., 2017).

ENHANCING BODY IMAGE

Eating is a major physiologic and social function, and the patient with a gastrostomy has experienced a major change in body image. The patient is also aware that gastrostomy as a therapeutic intervention is performed only in the presence of a major, chronic, or perhaps terminal illness. It is necessary to evaluate the existing family support system because adjustment takes time and is facilitated by family acceptance.

MONITORING AND MANAGING POTENTIAL COMPLICATIONS

During the postoperative course, the most common complications are wound infection or cellulitis at the exit site, bleeding, leakage, excessive tightness of external retention bolster, and dislodgement. Because many patients who receive tube feedings are debilitated and have compromised nutritional status, any signs of infection are promptly reported to the primary provider so that appropriate therapy can be instituted. Bleeding from the insertion site in the stomach can also occur and should be reported promptly. The nurse closely monitors the patient's vital signs and observes all operative site drainage, vomitus, and stool for evidence of bleeding. If an external retention bolster, tape, securement device, or sutures are present, they are evaluated for adequate tension and securement. Excessive tension of the external retention bolster can cause excruciating pain and will lead to skin breakdown and ulceration. The nurse should notify the primary provider if excessive pain occurs at the incision site post insertion.

Dislodgement of a recently inserted tube requires immediate attention because the tract can close within 4 to 6 hours if the tube is not replaced promptly. Aspiration is a potential risk with tube dislodgment, especially with nasally inserted tubes. The head of bed for the patient should be elevated to at least 30 degrees. Careful assessment of external tube markings that could suggest drift in placement, and of the patient for signs and symptoms of fullness or nausea that might lead to gastric reflux are important strategies that may prevent aspiration (Boullata et al., 2017).

Tube occlusion/clogging occurs in 23% to 35% of patients with feeding tubes and can lead to delays in feeding and medication administration (Boullata et al., 2017). Prevention is important and can be accomplished by administering adequate and frequent flushes as previously described. If a tube does become clogged, warm water may be instilled into the enteral nutrition device with a 30- to 60-mL syringe, followed by a gentle pulling and pushing on the plunger. If this method does not resolve the obstruction, an enzyme-containing commercially available declogging kit may be used or a combination of a pancreatic enzyme tablet and a bicarbonate tablet may be used (Boullata et al., 2017).

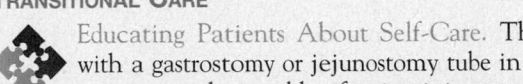

For the procedural guidelines for declogging a feeding tube, go to **thepoint.lww.com/ Brunner15e**.

PROMOTING HOME, COMMUNITY-BASED, AND TRANSITIONAL CARE

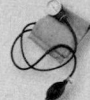

Educating Patients About Self-Care. The patient with a gastrostomy or jejunostomy tube in the home setting must be capable of maintaining patency of the tube or have a caregiver who can do so. The nurse assesses the patient's level of knowledge and interest in learning about the tube, as well as an ability to understand how to flush, provide site care, and administer feedings or facilitate decompression and drainage. Education is similar to that described earlier. To facilitate self-care, the nurse encourages the patient to participate in flushing the tube, administering medications and tube feedings during hospitalization, and establishing as normal a routine as possible.

Adapters are available that can be secured to the end of the tube to create a "Y" site for ease of flushing, suction, or medication delivery. The flushing equipment is cleaned with warm, soapy water and rinsed after each use. The tube can be marked at skin level to provide the patient with a baseline for later comparison. The patient or caregiver should be advised

---

Chart 39-7

HOME CARE CHECKLIST

The Patient Receiving Tube Feeding

At the completion of education, the patient and/or caregiver will be able to:

- Name the procedure that was performed and identify any permanent changes in anatomic structure or function as well as changes in ADLs, IADLs, roles, relationships, and spirituality.
- State what types of changes are needed (if any) to maintain a clean home environment and prevent infection.
- State how to contact the primary provider, the team of home care professionals overseeing care, and tube feeding supply vendor.
  - List emergency phone numbers.
- State how to obtain medical supplies and carry out dressing changes, site care, and other prescribed regimens.
- Demonstrate how to perform site care.
- Demonstrate how to prepare tube feeding.
- Demonstrate how to deliver tube feeding via prescribed method (e.g., bolus method, intermittent drip method, continuous feeding).
  - When indicated, demonstrate how to operate, disconnect, and clean the tube feeding pump.
  - When indicated, demonstrate tube maintenance functions.
    - Flush before and after bolus and intermittent feeding and medication administration

- Flush every 4 hours with continuous feeding
- Flush once daily if tube is not being used
- Demonstrate how to record all fluid intake and output.
- Identify a plan for operation of tube feeding pump during a power outage or other emergency.
- State the name, dose, side effects, frequency, and schedule for all medications.
- Demonstrate medication preparation and administration via bolus method, with flushing before, after and between medications.
- Identify possible tube feeding complications and interventions.
- Relate how to reach primary provider with questions or complications.
- State time and date of follow-up appointments and testing.
- State understanding of community resources and referrals (if any).
- Identify the need for health promotion (e.g., weight reduction, smoking cessation, stress management), disease prevention and screening activities.

ADLs, activities of daily living; IADLs, instrumental activities of daily living.

---

to monitor the tube's length and to notify the primary provider or home care nurse if the segment of the tube outside the body becomes shorter or longer.

Continuing and Transitional Care. Referral to home, community-based, or transitional care is important to ensure initial supervision and support for the patient and caregiver. The nurse assesses the patient's status and progress and evaluates the care of the tube and healing status of the tube insertion site. Further instruction and supervision in the home setting may be required to help the patient and caregiver adapt to a physical environment and equipment that are different from the hospital setting (see Chart 39-7). The nurse also reviews with the patient and caregiver what complications to report and assists the patient and family in establishing as normal a routine as possible.

Evaluation

Expected patient outcomes may include:

1. Achieves nutrition goals
   a. Attains weight goal
   b. Tolerates tube feeding prescription without nausea, emesis, cramping, abdominal pain, or feelings of early satiety
   c. Has acceptable bowel movements without constipation or large-volume liquid stools
   d. Has normal plasma protein, glucose, vitamin, and mineral levels
   e. Has normal electrolyte values
2. Is free of infection at enteral access site
   a. Is afebrile
   b. Has no induration, redness, pain, or purulent drainage
   c. Has no scattered papules indicative of a yeast infection
3. Has dry, intact skin surrounding enteral access site
   a. No evidence of excessive drainage or bleeding
   b. No skin breakdown or hypertrophic tissue growth

4. Adjusts to change in body image
   a. Is able to discuss expected changes
   b. Verbalizes concerns
5. Demonstrates skill in tube care
   a. Handles equipment competently
   b. Successfully maintains tube patency
   c. Keeps an accurate record of intake and output
   d. Demonstrates how to gently wash tube site daily and keep clean and dry
6. Avoids other complications
   a. Exhibits adequate wound healing
   b. Tube remains intact and is routinely replaced for the duration of therapy

DISORDERS OF THE ESOPHAGUS

The esophagus is a mucus-lined, muscular tube that carries food from the mouth to the stomach. It begins at the base of the pharynx and ends about 4 cm below the diaphragm. Its ability to transport food and fluid is facilitated by two sphincters. The upper esophageal sphincter, also called the *hypopharyngeal sphincter*, is located at the junction of the pharynx and the esophagus. The lower esophageal sphincter, also called the *gastroesophageal sphincter* or *cardiac sphincter*, is located at the junction of the esophagus and the stomach. An incompetent lower esophageal sphincter allows reflux (backward flow) of gastric contents. Because there is no serosal layer of the esophagus, if surgery is necessary, it is more difficult to perform suturing or anastomosis.

Disorders of the esophagus include motility disorders (achalasia, spasms), hiatal hernias, diverticula, perforation, foreign bodies, chemical burns, gastroesophageal reflux disease, Barrett esophagus (BE), benign tumors, and carcinoma.

Dysphagia, the most common symptom of esophageal disease, may vary from an uncomfortable feeling that a bolus of food is caught in the upper esophagus to acute **odynophagia** (pain on swallowing). Obstruction of food (solid and soft) and even liquids may occur anywhere along the esophagus. Often, the patient can indicate that the problem is located in the upper, middle, or lower third of the esophagus.

Achalasia

Achalasia is absent or ineffective peristalsis of the distal esophagus accompanied by failure of the esophageal sphincter to relax in response to swallowing. Narrowing of the esophagus just above the stomach results in a gradually increasing dilation of the esophagus in the upper chest. Achalasia is rare, may progress slowly, and occurs most often in people between ages 20 and 40 and ages 60 and 70 years (Swanström, 2019).

Clinical Manifestations

The main symptom is dysphagia, with the hallmark being difficulty with solid food. The patient has a sensation of food sticking in the lower portion of the esophagus. As the condition progresses, food is commonly regurgitated either spontaneously or intentionally by the patient to relieve the discomfort produced by prolonged distention of the esophagus by food that will not pass into the stomach. The patient may also report noncardiac chest or epigastric pain and **pyrosis** (heartburn) that may or may not be associated with eating. These symptoms mirror those of GERD, and patients are often misdiagnosed and treated for GERD (Swanström, 2019).

Assessment and Diagnostic Findings

X-ray studies show esophageal dilation above the narrowing at the lower gastroesophageal sphincter, which is called a *birds beak* deformity. Barium swallow, CT scan of the chest, and endoscopy may be used for diagnosis; however, high-resolution manometry, a process in which peristalsis, contraction amplitudes, and esophageal pressure is measured by a radiologist or gastroenterologist, confirms the diagnosis (Swanström, 2019).

Management

The patient is instructed to eat slowly and to drink fluids with meals. Injection of botulinum toxin into quadrants of the esophagus via endoscopy has been helpful because it inhibits the contraction of smooth muscle. However, because the benefits of these injections fade over time and there is a risk of submucosal fibrosis, botulinum toxin is only used in patients who cannot receive other definitive treatments (Swanström, 2019).

Achalasia may be treated conservatively by pneumatic dilation to stretch the narrowed area of the esophagus (see Fig. 39-9). Pneumatic dilation has a high success rate; however, typically two dilations are required and the long-term results are variable (Swanström, 2019). Although perforation is a potential complication, its incidence is low (see later discussion). The procedure can be painful; therefore, moderate sedation in the form of an analgesic or tranquilizer, or both, is given for the treatment.

Achalasia may be treated surgically by esophagomyotomy, called a Heller myotomy, which involves cutting the esophageal muscle fibers. A complete lower esophageal sphincter myotomy is usually performed laparoscopically, with or without a *fundoplication* (antireflux procedure that minimizes the incidence of GERD). A newer technique, an endoscopic myotomy (per-oral endoscopic myotomy [POEM]) provides an alternative procedure that has been adopted by many high-volume achalasia centers (Swanström, 2019).

Esophageal Spasm

The three types of esophageal spasm include jackhammer esophagus, diffuse esophageal spasm (DES), and type III

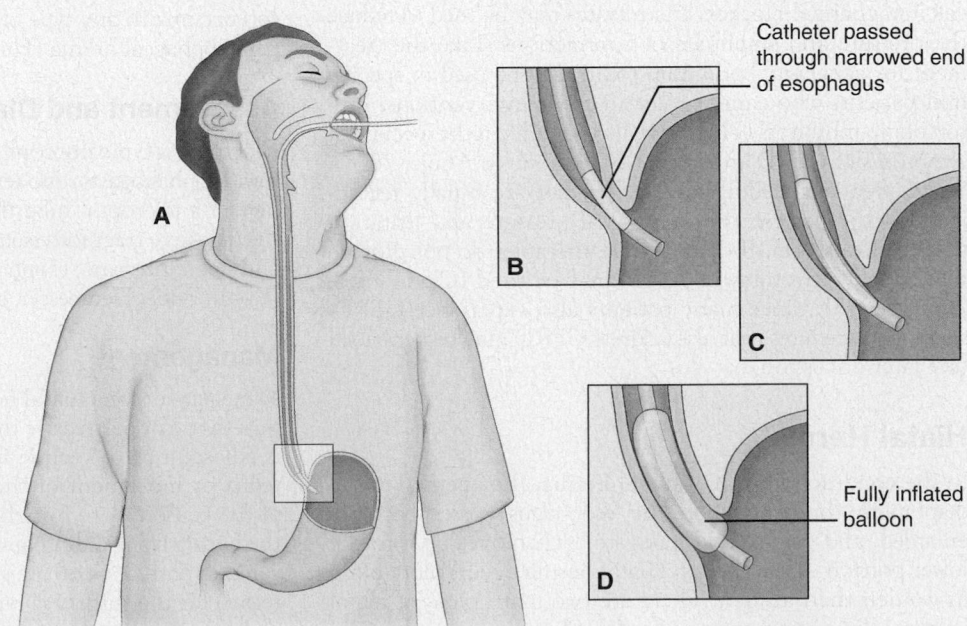

Figure 39-9 • Treatment of achalasia by pneumatic dilation. **A–C.** The dilator is passed, guided by a previously inserted guide wire. **D.** When the balloon is in proper position, it is distended by pressure sufficient to dilate the narrowed area of the esophagus.

Catheter passed through narrowed end of esophagus

Fully inflated balloon

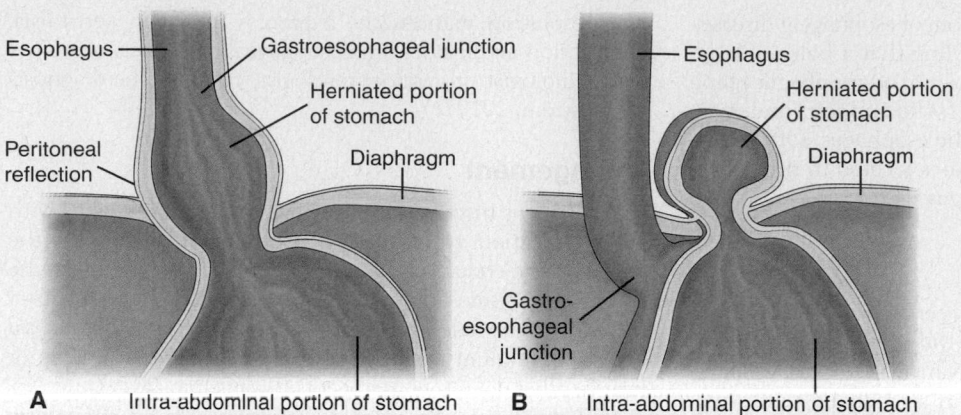

Figure 39-10 • A. Sliding esophageal hernia. The upper stomach and gastroesophageal junction have moved upward and slide in and out of the thorax. **B.** Paraesophageal hernia. All or part of the stomach pushes through the diaphragm next to the gastroesophageal junction.

(spastic) achalasia. In jackhammer esophagus, referred to as hypercontractile esophagus, spasms occur on more than 20% of swallows at a very high amplitude, duration, and length. In DES, the spasms are normal in amplitude but are premature/uncoordinated, move quickly, and occur at various places in the esophagus at once. Type III achalasia is characterized by lower esophageal sphincter obstruction with esophageal spasms (Clermont & Ahuja, 2018).

Clinical Manifestations

All three forms of esophageal spasm are characterized by dysphagia, pyrosis, regurgitation, and chest pain similar to that of coronary artery spasm.

Assessment and Diagnostic Findings

Esophageal manometry, which measures the motility and internal pressure of the esophagus, remains the standard test for irregular and high-amplitude spasms.

Management

In all three spastic disorders, smooth muscle relaxants such as calcium channel blockers and nitrates may be used to reduce the pressure and amplitude of contractions. Like the treatment for achalasia, botulinum toxin may be used in specific frail patients who cannot tolerate other interventions. Proton pump inhibitors (PPIs) may also be indicated, especially if symptoms of GERD are present (Clermont & Ahuja, 2018). Small, frequent feedings and a soft diet are usually recommended to decrease the esophageal pressure and irritation that lead to spasm. If conservative therapies do not provide relief, Heller myotomy or POEM may be tried (Clermont & Ahuja, 2018). Since many patients also experience GERD, surgical procedures that also address GERD may be beneficial (see later discussion).

Hiatal Hernia

In the condition known as hiatal **hernia**, the opening in the diaphragm through which the esophagus passes becomes enlarged, and part of the upper stomach moves up into the lower portion of the thorax. Hiatal hernia occurs more often in women than in men. There are two main types of hiatal hernias: sliding and paraesophageal. Sliding, or type I, hiatal hernia occurs when the upper stomach and the gastroesophageal junction are displaced upward and slide in and out of the thorax (see Fig. 39-10A). Between 90% and 95% of patients with esophageal hiatal hernia have a sliding hernia. A paraesophageal hernia occurs when all or part of the stomach pushes through the diaphragm beside the esophagus (see Fig. 39-10B). Paraesophageal hernias are further classified as types II, III, or IV, depending on the extent of herniation. Type IV has the greatest herniation, with other intra-abdominal viscera such as the colon, omentum, or small bowel present in the hernia sac that is displaced through the hiatus along with the stomach (Huerta, Plymale, Barrett, et al., 2019).

Clinical Manifestations

The patient with a sliding hernia may have pyrosis, regurgitation, and dysphagia, but many patients are asymptomatic. The patient may present with vague symptoms of intermittent epigastric pain or fullness after eating. Large hiatal hernias may lead to intolerance to food, nausea, and vomiting. Sliding hiatal hernias are commonly associated with GERD. Hemorrhage, obstruction, volvulus (bowel obstruction caused by a twist in the intestines and supporting mesentery), and strangulation can occur with any type of hernia but are more common with paraesophageal hernia (Huerta et al., 2019).

Assessment and Diagnostic Findings

Diagnosis is typically confirmed by x-ray studies; barium swallow; esophagogastroduodenoscopy (EGD), which is the passage of a fiberoptic tube through the mouth and throat into the digestive tract for visualization of the esophagus, stomach, and small intestine; esophageal manometry; or chest CT scan (Kohn, Price, Demeester, et al., 2013).

Management

Management for a hiatal hernia includes frequent, small feedings that can pass easily through the esophagus. The patient is advised not to recline for 1 hour after eating, to prevent reflux or movement of the hernia, and to elevate the head of the bed on 4- to 8-inch (10- to 20-cm) blocks to prevent the hernia from sliding upward. Surgical hernia repair is indicated in patients who are symptomatic, although the primary reason for the surgery is typically to relieve GERD symptoms and not repair the hernia. Current guidelines recommend a laparoscopic approach (Toupet or Nissen fundoplication procedures) (Huerta et al., 2019), with an open transabdominal or transthoracic approach reserved for patients with complications such as bleeding, dense adhesions, or injury to the spleen.

Up to 50% of patients may experience early postoperative dysphagia; therefore, the nurse advances the diet slowly from liquids to solids, while managing nausea and vomiting, tracking nutritional intake, and monitoring weight. The nurse also monitors for postoperative belching, vomiting, gagging, abdominal distention, and epigastric chest pain, which may indicate the need for surgical revision; these should be reported immediately to the primary provider. Surgical repair is often reserved for patients with more extreme cases that involve gastric outlet obstruction or suspected gastric strangulation, which may result in ischemia, necrosis, or perforation of the stomach (Kohn et al., 2013).

Diverticulum

An esophageal diverticulum is an out-pouching of mucosa and submucosa that protrudes through a weak portion of the musculature of the esophagus. Diverticula may occur in one of the three areas of the esophagus—pharyngoesophageal (upper), midesophageal (middle), or epiphrenic (lower).

The most common type of diverticulum is Zenker diverticulum (ZD). Located in the pharyngoesophageal area, ZD is caused by a dysfunctional sphincter that fails to open, which leads to increased pressure that forces the mucosa and submucosa to herniate through the esophageal musculature (called a pulsion diverticulum) (Smith, 2015) (see Fig. 39-11). It is usually seen in people older than 60 years of age.

Midesophageal diverticula are uncommon. Symptoms are less acute, and usually the condition does not require surgery. Epiphrenic diverticula are usually larger diverticula in the lower esophagus just above the diaphragm. They may be related to the improper functioning of the lower esophageal sphincter or to motor disorders of the esophagus. Intramural diverticulosis is the occurrence of numerous small diverticula associated with a stricture in the upper esophagus.

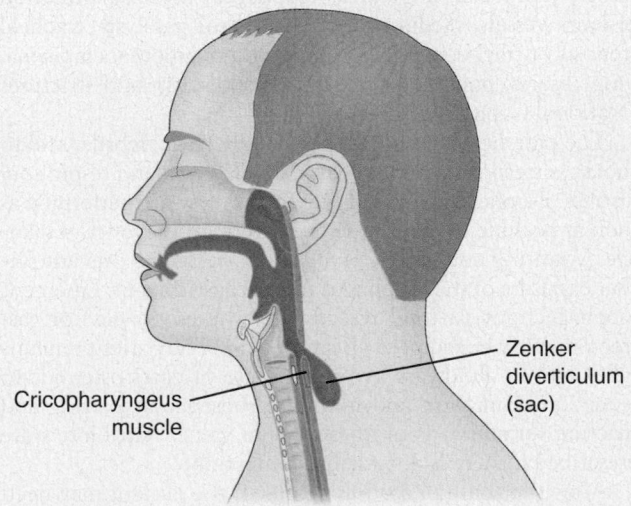

Figure 39-11 • Zenker diverticulum.

Clinical Manifestations

Symptoms experienced by the patient with a pharyngoesophageal pulsion diverticulum include dysphagia, fullness in the neck, belching, regurgitation of undigested food, and gurgling noises after eating. The diverticulum, or pouch, becomes filled with food or liquid. When the patient assumes a recumbent position, undigested food is regurgitated, and coughing may be caused by irritation of the trachea or aspiration. **Halitosis** (foul odor from the oral cavity) and a sour taste in the mouth are also common because of the decomposition of food retained in the diverticulum. Although less acute, dysphagia is the primary symptom in the other types of diverticula (Smith, 2015).

Assessment and Diagnostic Findings

A barium swallow may determine the exact nature and location of a diverticulum. Manometric studies may be performed for patients with epiphrenic diverticula to rule out a motor disorder. Esophagoscopy usually is contraindicated because of the danger of perforation of the diverticulum, with resulting mediastinitis (inflammation of the organs and tissues that separate the lungs). Blind insertion of an NG tube should be avoided.

Management

ZD can be treated by endoscopy (rigid or flexible) or open surgery. Endoscopic septotomy effectively treats ZD, with a recurrence rate of 11% to 30% of cases; POEM may be a better option as it is associated with a decreased risk of symptom recurrence (Gutierrez, Ichkhanian, Spadaccini, et al., 2019). If surgery is required, care is taken to avoid trauma to the common carotid artery and internal jugular veins. In addition to a diverticulectomy, a myotomy of the cricopharyngeal muscle is often performed to relieve spasticity of the musculature, which seems to contribute to a continuation of symptoms. An NG tube may be inserted at the time of surgery. Postoperatively, the nurse observes the incision for evidence of leakage from the esophagus and a developing fistula. Food and fluids are withheld until x-ray studies show no leakage at the surgical site. The diet begins with liquids and is progressed as tolerated.

Surgery is indicated for epiphrenic and midesophageal diverticula only if the symptoms are troublesome and becoming worse. Treatment consists of a diverticulectomy and long myotomy. Intramural diverticula usually regress after the esophageal stricture is dilated.

Perforation

Esophageal perforation is a surgical emergency. It may result from iatrogenic causes, such as endoscopy or intraoperative injury, or from spontaneous perforation associated with forceful vomiting or severe straining (Boerhaave syndrome), foreign-body ingestion, trauma, and malignancy. Immediate diagnosis and treatment are essential to minimize mortality. A delay of more than 24 hours is associated with higher mortality (20%) when compared to rapid recognition and treatment (7.4%). Perforation can occur at the cervical, thoracic, or abdominal portion of the esophagus (Olivero, 2019; Raymond, 2020).

Clinical Manifestations

The patient has excruciating retrosternal pain followed by dysphagia. Infection, fever, leukocytosis, and severe hypotension may be noted. In addition, mediastinal sepsis can occur with Boerhaave syndrome, which may be accompanied by pneumothorax and subcutaneous emphysema (see Chapter 19 for discussion of pneumothorax and subcutaneous emphysema).

Assessment and Diagnostic Findings

X-ray studies, fluoroscopy by either a barium swallow or esophagram (a noninvasive test), or a chest CT scan may be used to identify the site and scope of the injury.

Management

Esophageal perforation requires immediate treatment. Treatment includes having the patient remain NPO (*nil per os*; nothing by mouth), beginning IV fluid therapy, administering broad-spectrum antibiotics (ampicillin-sulbactam, piperacillin-tazobactam, or a carbapenem [e.g., imipenem]), considering the need for antifungal therapy (if the patient is immunosuppressed, has HIV infection, or shows no improvement with antibiotics), supportive monitoring and care (intensive care unit level-of-care often required), and evaluating and preparing the patient for surgery (Raymond, 2020). Surgical repair of the perforation site is performed in most cases, even if the diagnosis is made after 24 hours. If surgical repair of the perforation is not possible due to the clinical status of the patient, then drainage, diversion, stent placement, or an esophagostomy (removal of the esophagus) may be performed (Raymond, 2020).

Postoperative nutritional status is a major concern. The patient remains NPO for approximately 7 days, so enteral (e.g., jejunal feeding) or parenteral nutrition is started on postoperative day 2 or 3 (see Chapter 41 for further discussion of parenteral nutrition). The nurse uses water to moisten the patient's mouth for comfort measures only. A repeat esophagram is obtained on postoperative day 7 to verify there is no leak or ileus before the NG tube is removed and oral intake is permitted. It is common for broad-spectrum antibiotics to continue for 7 to 10 days postoperatively (Raymond, 2020).

Foreign Bodies

Many swallowed foreign bodies pass through the GI tract without the need for medical intervention. However, some swallowed foreign bodies (e.g., dentures, fish bones, pins, small batteries, items containing mercury or lead) may injure the esophagus or obstruct its lumen and must be removed. Pain and dysphagia may be present, and dyspnea may occur as a result of pressure on the trachea. The foreign body may be identified by x-ray. Perforation may have occurred (see earlier discussion).

> ▶ **Quality and Safety Nursing Alert**
>
> The nurse performs an initial and ongoing respiratory (airway-focused) assessment of a patient with a foreign body in the esophagus. Intubation may be required to protect the airway.

Glucagon, because of its relaxing effect on the esophageal muscle, may be injected IV (a 1-mg dose). A flexible endoscope and retrieval devices (e.g., forceps, graspers) may be used to remove the impacted food or object from the esophagus. Foreign bodies such as short-blunt objects, long objects, sharp-pointed objects, disc batteries, magnets, coins, or narcotic packets require special consideration (American Society for Gastrointestinal Endoscopy Standards of Practice Committee, 2011; Fung, Sweetser, Wong Kee Song, et al., 2019). Various devices can be used for endoscopic extraction (overtubes, forceps, snares, baskets, etc.) and dilation techniques can be used to facilitate the passage of foreign objects to the stomach. Decisions regarding the best course of action consider the likelihood of the object passing on its own (blunt, nontoxic objects), the patient's condition (airway maintenance), the length of time the obstruction has been present (typical intervention occurs within 24 hours), and the type of foreign object that is impacted. For example, ingested drug packets are not removed by endoscopy for fear of packet rupture; no intervention or surgical intervention are recommended in these cases. The endoscopic procedure usually is performed in the endoscopy suite or clinic by the gastroenterologist under moderate sedation (Fung et al., 2019).

Chemical Burns

Chemical burns of the esophagus occur most often when a patient, either intentionally (67%; typically adults) or unintentionally (33%; typically children), swallows a strong acid or base, with alkaline agents being the most common (Byard, 2015). The patient is often emotionally distraught as well as in acute physical pain. Chemical burns of the esophagus may also be caused by undissolved medications in the esophagus, or they may occur after swallowing of a battery, which may release a caustic alkaline. The National Capital Poison Center (2018) provides an algorithm for button battery ingestion and triage (see Resources section). An acute chemical burn of the esophagus may be accompanied by severe burns of the lips, mouth, and pharynx, with pain on swallowing. Breathing difficulties due to either edema of the throat or a collection of mucus in the pharynx may occur. The patient needs to be closely monitored for tracheoesophageal fistula, perforation of large vessels, mediastinitis, vocal cord paralysis, tracheal stenosis or tracheomalacia, aspiration pneumonia, empyema, lung abscess, pneumothorax, spondylodiscitis, and strictures (National Capital Poison Center, 2018).

The patient, who may be profoundly toxic, febrile, and in shock, is treated immediately for shock, pain, and respiratory distress. Esophagoscopy and barium swallow are performed as soon as possible to determine the extent and severity of damage. Vomiting and gastric lavage are avoided to prevent further exposure of the esophagus to the caustic agent. Emergent esophagectomy (a total resection of the esophagus) or gastrectomy may be required (Byard, 2015). The patient remains NPO and IV fluids are given. The use of corticosteroids to reduce inflammation and minimize subsequent scarring and stricture formation is of questionable value. Antibiotics are prescribed if there is documented infection.

After the acute phase has subsided, the patient may need nutritional support via enteral or parenteral feedings. The patient may require further treatment to prevent or manage strictures of the esophagus. Dilation may be sufficient, but may need to be repeated periodically (see previous discussion). For strictures that do not respond to dilation, surgical management may be necessary. Reconstruction may be accomplished by esophagectomy and colon interposition to replace the portion of esophagus removed. This surgery is quite complex and should be considered only when other options have failed.

Gastroesophageal Reflux Disease

Gastroesophageal reflux disease (GERD) is a fairly common disorder marked by backflow of gastric or duodenal contents into the esophagus that causes troublesome symptoms and/or mucosal injury to the esophagus. Excessive reflux may occur because of an incompetent lower esophageal sphincter, pyloric stenosis, hiatal hernia, or a motility disorder. The incidence of GERD seems to increase with aging and is seen in patients with irritable bowel syndrome and obstructive airway disorder exacerbations (e.g., asthma, COPD, cystic fibrosis) (Broers & Tack, 2017; Gabel, Galante, & Freedman, 2019), BE (see later discussion), peptic ulcer disease, and angina. GERD is associated with tobacco use, coffee drinking, alcohol consumption, and gastric infection with *Helicobacter pylori*.

Clinical Manifestations

Pyrosis (heartburn, specifically more commonly described as a burning sensation in the esophagus that is noncardiac in nature) and regurgitation are the hallmark symptoms, but patients may also experience dyspepsia (indigestion), dysphagia or odynophagia, hypersalivation, and esophagitis. GERD can result in dental erosion, ulcerations in the pharynx and esophagus, laryngeal damage, esophageal strictures, adenocarcinoma, and pulmonary complications (Kroch & Madanick, 2017; Patti, 2016).

Assessment and Diagnostic Findings

The patient's history aids in obtaining an accurate diagnosis. Diagnostic testing may include ambulatory pH monitoring, which is the gold standard for the diagnosis of GERD, or a PPI trial. Ambulatory pH monitoring involves transnasal catheter placement or endoscopic wireless capsule placement for approximately 24 hours. Endoscopy or barium swallow is used to evaluate damage to the esophageal mucosa and rule out strictures and hernias (Patti, 2016).

Management

Management begins with educating the patient to avoid situations that decrease lower esophageal sphincter pressure or cause esophageal irritation. Lifestyle modifications include tobacco cessation, limiting alcohol, weight loss, elevating the head of the bed, avoiding eating before bed, and altering the diet (Kroch & Madanick, 2017). See Table 39-4 for a list of medications commonly used to manage GERD.

If medical management is unsuccessful, surgical intervention may be necessary. Surgical management involves an open or laparoscopic Nissen fundoplication, which involves wrapping of a portion of the gastric fundus around the sphincter area of the esophagus (Huerta et al., 2019; Patti, 2016).

Barrett Esophagus

BE is a condition in which the lining of the esophageal mucosa is altered. It occurs predominantly in White men aged 50 or older, and occurs in association with family history of BE or esophageal adenocarcinoma (EAC), GERD, smoking, and obesity. The rate of BE was found to increase by 1.2% for each additional risk factor, indicating the additive effect of risk factors (Qumseya, Bukannan, Gendy, et al., 2019). BE is the only known precursor to EAC, one of the fastest rising cancers in Western populations (Qumseya et al., 2019). The 5-year survival rate for EAC does not exceed 20% (Iyer & Kaul, 2019; Qumseya et al., 2019).

Clinical Manifestations

The patient complains of symptoms of GERD, notably frequent heartburn. The patient may also complain of symptoms related to peptic ulcers or esophageal stricture, or both.

Assessment and Diagnostic Findings

An EGD provides screening in patients with multiple risk factors. This usually reveals an esophageal lining that is pink rather than pale white. Biopsies are performed, and BE is diagnosed when the squamous mucosa of the esophagus is replaced by columnar epithelium (columnar metaplasia) at least 1 cm above the gastric folds, and that area resembles that of the stomach or intestines (intestinal metaplasia) as evidenced by the presence of goblet cells (Iyer & Kaul, 2019).

Management

Monitoring varies depending on the extent of cell changes. When BE is caught and treated early, endoscopic ablation techniques have been shown to eliminate BE in up to 80% of patients, thereby preventing progression to **dysplasia**, the bizarre cell growth resulting in cells that differ in size, shape, or arrangement from other cells of the same tissue type. Such dysplasia is indicative of early EAC. Follow-up biopsies are recommended no sooner than 3 to 5 years after a biopsy shows no evidence of dysplasia (Iyer & Kaul, 2019; Sharma, Katzka, Gupta, et al., 2015). Treatment is individualized for each patient. Recommendations include surveillance with biopsies, the use of PPIs (see Table 39-4) to control reflux symptoms, followed by endoscopic resection and/or radiofrequency ablation (high-frequency heat/cold energy that kills surrounding cells and tissues) for progression of dysplasia (Iyer & Kaul, 2019; Sharma et al., 2015).

Benign Tumors of the Esophagus

Benign tumors are rare, but can arise anywhere along the esophagus. The most common lesion is a leiomyoma (tumor of the smooth muscle), which can occlude the lumen of the esophagus and cause dysphagia, pain, and pyrosis. Half of patients with benign tumors are asymptomatic and the other half present with multiple symptoms that have been present for a long period of time. The diagnosis may be made incidentally and is confirmed by endoscopy and needle biopsy. Due to the slow growth of most of these tumors, monitoring and minimally invasive techniques (endoscopic, thoracic, or laparoscopic resections) tend to be indicated rather than surgical resection (Ha, Regan, Cetindag, et al., 2015).

TABLE 39-4 Pharmacologic Management of GERD

Key Examples	Actions/Class	Key Nursing Considerations
Antacids/Acid neutralizing agents • Calcium carbonate • Aluminum hydroxide, magnesium hydroxide, and simethicone • Alginate	**Neutralize acid** *Therapeutic and Pharmacologic class—* Antacid	• Potential risk of gastric acid suppression is the loss of protective flora and an increased risk of infection, especially *Clostridium difficile*
Histamine-2 (H₂) receptor antagonists • Famotidine • Cimetidine	**Decrease gastric acid production** • *Therapeutic class*—Antiulcer drugs • *Pharmacologic class*—H₂-receptor antagonists	• Potential risk of gastric acid suppression is the loss of protective flora and an increased risk of infection, especially *Clostridium difficile* • For direct injection (IVP), dilute 2 mL (20 mg) with compatible solution to a total volume of either 5 or 10 mL; administer over at least 2 min • Monitor for QT-interval prolongation in patients with kidney injury
Prokinetic agents Metoclopramide	**Accelerate gastric emptying** *Therapeutic class*—GI stimulants *Pharmacologic class*—Dopamine antagonist	• May cause tardive dyskinesia • Typically used short term
Proton pump inhibitors (PPIs) **First-line drugs used** • Pantoprazole • Omeprazole • Esomeprazole • Lansoprazole • Rabeprazole • Dexlansoprazole	**Decrease gastric acid production** *Therapeutic class*—Antiulcer drugs *Pharmacologic class*—Proton pump inhibitors	• Potential risk of gastric acid suppression is the loss of protective flora and an increased risk of infection, especially *Clostridium difficile* • For a 2-min infusion (IVP), give the reconstituted vials (4 mg/mL) over at least 2 min • May increase the risk of hip fractures and interfere with some vitamin and mineral absorption (B₁₂, iron, magnesium) • Interact with commonly prescribed medications such as diuretics and clopidogrel
Reflux inhibitors Bethanechol chloride	**Stimulates parasympathetic** *Therapeutic and Pharmacologic class—* Cholinergic	• Primary use is for urinary retention • Do not use with possible GI obstruction or peptic ulcer
Surface agents/Alginate-based barriers Sucralfate	**Preserve mucosal barrier** *Therapeutic class*—Antiulcer drugs *Pharmacologic class*—GI protectants	• Give on an empty stomach—either one hour before or two hours after meals • Separate from doses of antacid by 30 min
Inhibitors of transient lower esophageal sphincter relaxations (TLESRs) Baclofen	**Reducing TLESRs to reduce reflux** *Therapeutic class*—Muscle relaxant *Pharmacologic class*—gamma-aminobutyric acid (GABA) agonist	• Only approved GABA-B agonist that that reduces TLESRs • Used when PPI therapy fails

GI, gastrointestinal; IVP, intravenous push.
Adapted from Kroch, D. A., & Madanick, R. D. (2017). Medical treatment of gastroesophageal reflux disease. *World Journal of Surgery, 41*(7), 1678–1684; Whalen, K. (2019). *Pharmacology* (7th ed.). Philadelphia, PA: Wolters Kluwer.

NURSING PROCESS

The Patient with a Noncancerous Disorder of the Esophagus

Assessment

Emergency disorders of the esophagus (perforation, chemical burns) usually occur in the home or away from medical help and require emergency medical care. The patient is treated for shock and respiratory distress and transported as quickly as possible to a health care facility. Foreign bodies in the esophagus do not pose an immediate threat to life unless pressure is exerted on the trachea, resulting in dyspnea or interfering with respiration, or unless there is leakage of caustic alkali from a battery or exposure to another corrosive agent.

For nonemergency symptoms, a complete health history may reveal the nature of the esophageal disorder. The nurse asks about the patient's appetite. Has it remained the same, increased, or decreased? Is there any discomfort with swallowing? If so, does it occur only with certain foods? Is it associated with pain? Does a change in position affect the discomfort? The patient is asked to describe the pain. Does anything aggravate it? Are there any other symptoms that occur regularly, such as regurgitation, nocturnal regurgitation, eructation (belching), pyrosis, substernal pressure, a sensation that food is sticking in the throat, a feeling of fullness after eating a small amount of food, nausea, vomiting, or weight loss? Are the symptoms aggravated by emotional upset? If the patient reports any of these symptoms, the nurse asks about when they occur, their relationship to eating, and factors that relieve or aggravate them (e.g., position change, belching, antacids, vomiting; Bickley, 2016).

This history also includes questions about past or present causative factors, such as infections and chemical, mechanical, or physical irritants; alcohol and tobacco use; and the amount of daily food intake. The nurse determines whether the patient appears emaciated and auscultates the patient's chest to assess for pulmonary complications (Bickley, 2016).

Diagnosis

NURSING DIAGNOSES

Based on the assessment data, nursing diagnoses may include the following:

- Impaired nutritional intake associated with difficulty swallowing
- Risk for aspiration associated with difficulty swallowing or tube feeding
- Acute pain associated with difficulty swallowing, ingestion of an abrasive agent, tumor, or frequent episodes of gastric reflux
- Lack of knowledge about the esophageal disorder, diagnostic studies, medical management, surgical intervention, and rehabilitation

Planning and Goals

The major goals for the patient may include attainment of adequate nutritional intake, avoidance of respiratory compromise from aspiration, relief of pain, and increased knowledge level.

Nursing Interventions

ENCOURAGING ADEQUATE NUTRITIONAL INTAKE

The patient is encouraged to eat slowly and to chew all food thoroughly so that it can pass easily into the stomach. Small, frequent feedings of nonirritating foods are recommended to promote digestion and to prevent tissue irritation. Sometimes liquid swallowed with food helps the food pass through the esophagus, but usually liquids should be consumed between meals. Food should be prepared in an appealing manner to help stimulate the appetite. Irritants such as tobacco and alcohol should be avoided. A baseline weight is obtained, and daily weights are recorded. The patient's intake of nutrients is assessed.

DECREASING RISK OF ASPIRATION

The patient who has difficulty swallowing or difficulty managing secretions should be kept in at least a semi-Fowler position to decrease the risk of aspiration. The patient is instructed in the use of oral suction to decrease the risk of aspiration further.

RELIEVING PAIN

Small, frequent feedings (6 to 8 per day) are recommended because large quantities of food overload the stomach and promote gastric reflux. The patient is advised to avoid any activities that increase pain and to remain upright for 1 to 4 hours after each meal to prevent reflux. The head of the bed should be placed on 4- to 8-inch (10- to 20-cm) blocks. Eating before bedtime is discouraged.

The patient is advised that excessive use of over-the-counter antacids can cause rebound acidity. Antacid use should be directed by the primary provider, who can recommend the daily, safe dose needed to neutralize gastric juices and prevent esophageal irritation. H_2-antagonists or PPIs (more commonly) are given as prescribed to decrease gastric acid irritation.

 PROVIDING PATIENT EDUCATION

The patient is prepared physically and psychologically for diagnostic tests, treatments, and possible surgery. Nursing interventions include reassuring the patient and explaining the procedures and their purposes. Some disorders of the esophagus evolve over time, whereas others are the result of trauma (e.g., chemical burns, perforation). In instances of trauma, the emotional and physical preparation for treatment is more difficult because of the short time available and the circumstances of the injury. Treatment interventions must be evaluated continually, and the patient is given sufficient information to participate in care and diagnostic tests. If endoscopic diagnostic methods are used, the patient is instructed regarding the moderate sedation that will be used during the procedure. If outpatient procedures are performed with the use of moderate sedation, someone must be available to drive the patient home after the procedure. If surgery is required, immediate and long-term evaluation is similar to that for a patient undergoing thoracic surgery.

PROMOTING HOME, COMMUNITY-BASED, AND TRANSITIONAL CARE

Educating Patients About Self-Care. The self-care required of the patient depends on the nature of the disorder and on the surgery or treatment measures used (e.g., diet, positioning, medications). If an ongoing condition exists, the nurse helps the patient plan for needed physical and psychological adjustments and for follow-up care (see Chart 39-8).

Special equipment, such as suction or enteral or parenteral feeding devices, may be required. The patient may need assistance in planning meals, using medications as prescribed, and resuming activities. Education about nutritional requirements and how to measure the adequacy of nutrition is important. Older adults and patients who are debilitated in particular often need assistance and education about ways they can adjust to their limitations and resume activities that are important to them.

Continuing and Transitional Care. Patients with chronic esophageal conditions require an individualized approach to their management at home. Foods may need to be prepared in a special way (blenderized foods, soft foods), and the patient may need to eat more frequently (e.g., 6 to 8 small servings per day). The medication schedule is adjusted to the patient's daily activities as much as possible. Analgesic medications and antacids can usually be taken as needed every 3 to 4 hours.

Postoperative home health care focuses on nutritional support, management of pain, and respiratory function. Some patients are discharged from the hospital with enteral feeding by means of a gastrostomy or jejunostomy tube, or parenteral nutrition. The patient and caregiver need specific instructions regarding management of the equipment and treatments. Home care visits by a nurse may be necessary to assess the patient and the caregiver's ability to provide the necessary care. A multidisciplinary team that includes a dietitian, a social worker, and family members is helpful. Hospice care and consideration of end-of-life issues are appropriate for some patients.

Chart 39-8

HOME CARE CHECKLIST

The Patient with an Esophageal Disorder

At the completion of education, the patient and/or caregiver will be able to:

- State the impact of the esophageal disorder and treatment on physiologic functioning, ADLs, IADLs, body image, roles, relationships, and spirituality.
- Identify modification of home environment, interventions, and strategies (e.g., utilizing durable medical equipment, employing a home health aide) used in safely adapting to changes in structure or function and promote effective recovery and rehabilitation.
- Describe ongoing therapeutic regimen, including diet and activities to perform (e.g., suctioning) and to limit or avoid (e.g., oral foods if NPO).
  - Identify foods or therapies necessary to meet caloric needs and dietary needs (e.g., change in consistency, seasoning limitations, supplements, enteral or parenteral therapy).
  - Participate in prescribed therapy (e.g., speech therapy) to promote recovery and rehabilitation.

- Demonstrate the use of suction equipment if indicated.
- Demonstrate care of incision if indicated.
- State the name, dose, side effects, frequency, and schedule for all medications.
  - Describe approaches to controlling pain (e.g., take analgesics as prescribed; use nonpharmacologic interventions).
- Identify possible complications (e.g., difficulty swallowing, pain, respiratory distress) and interventions.
- Relate how to reach primary provider with questions or complications.
- State time and date of follow-up medical appointments, therapy, and testing.
- Identify sources of support (e.g., friends, relatives, faith community, cancer support, caregiver support).
- Identify the need for health promotion, disease prevention, and screening activities.

ADLs, activities of daily living; IADLs, instrumental activities of daily living; NPO, nothing by mouth.

Evaluation

Expected patient outcomes may include:

1. Achieves an adequate nutritional intake
   a. Eats small, frequent meals
   b. Drinks small sips of water with small servings of food
   c. Avoids irritants (alcohol, tobacco, very hot beverages)
   d. Maintains optimal weight
2. Does not aspirate or develop pneumonia
   a. Maintains upright position during feeding
   b. Uses oral suction equipment effectively
3. Is free of pain or able to control pain within a tolerable level
   a. Avoids large meals and irritating foods
   b. Takes medications as prescribed and with adequate fluids (at least 4 oz), and remains upright for at least 10 minutes after taking medications
   c. Maintains an upright position after meals for 1 to 4 hours
   d. Reports that there is less eructation (belching) and chest pain
4. Increases knowledge level of esophageal condition, diagnostic tests, treatment, and prognosis
   a. States cause of condition
   b. Discusses rationale for medical or surgical management and diet or medication regimen
   c. Describes treatment program
   d. Practices preventive measures so that injuries are avoided

Cancer of the Esophagus

In the United States, there are about 18,440 newly diagnosed cases of carcinoma of the esophagus annually; of these, 14,350 are men and 4,090 are women. Adenocarcinoma is more common among Whites, and squamous cell carcinoma is more frequently seen in African Americans. In the 1960s

and 1970s, only about 5% of patients diagnosed with esophageal cancer survived at least 5 years. Today, survival rates are approximately 20% at the 5-year mark (ACS, 2021a).

Pathophysiology

Esophageal cancer can be of two cell types: adenocarcinoma and squamous cell carcinoma. The rate of adenocarcinoma is rapidly increasing in the United States as well as in other Western countries. It is found primarily in the distal esophagus and gastroesophageal junction (ACS, 2021a).

Risk factors for esophageal cancer include chronic esophageal irritation or GERD. In the United States, cancer of the esophagus has been associated with ingestion of alcohol and the use of tobacco. There is an apparent association between GERD and adenocarcinoma of the esophagus. Patients with BE (see previous discussion of risks) have a higher incidence of esophageal cancer (Iyer & Kaul, 2019; Sharma et al., 2015). Risk factors for squamous cell carcinoma of the esophagus include chronic ingestion of hot liquids or foods, nutritional deficiencies, poor oral hygiene, exposure to nitrosamines in the environment or food, cigarette smoking or chronic alcohol exposure (especially in Western cultures), and some esophageal medical conditions such as caustic injury.

Early stages of esophageal cancer are limited to the mucosa or submucosa; these stages of cancer have a 5-year survival rate of about 90% (Levine & Rubesin, 2012). In later stages, tumor cells of adenocarcinoma and of squamous cell carcinoma may spread beneath the esophageal mucosa or directly into, through, and beyond the muscle layers into the lymphatics. Obstruction of the esophagus is noted, with possible perforation into the mediastinum and erosion into the great vessels (Levine & Rubesin, 2012).

Clinical Manifestations

Many patients have an advanced ulcerated lesion of the esophagus before symptoms manifest. Symptoms include dysphagia, initially with solid foods and eventually with liquids;

a sensation of a mass in the throat; painful swallowing; substernal pain or fullness; and, later, regurgitation of undigested food with halitosis and hiccups. The patient first becomes aware of intermittent and increasing difficulty in swallowing. As the tumor grows and the obstruction becomes nearly complete, even liquids cannot pass into the stomach. Regurgitation of food and saliva occurs, hemorrhage may take place, and progressive loss of weight and strength occurs from inadequate nutrition. Later symptoms include substernal pain, persistent hiccup, respiratory difficulty, and halitosis.

The delay between the onset of early symptoms and the patient seeking medical advice is often 12 to 18 months. Any person having swallowing difficulties should be encouraged to consult the primary provider immediately.

Assessment and Diagnostic Findings

Several imaging techniques may provide useful diagnostic information. A CT scan of the chest and abdomen is beneficial for detecting any anatomic evidence of metastatic disease, especially of the lungs, liver, and kidney. A PET scan may also help detect metastasis. Endoscopic ultrasound is used to determine whether the cancer has spread to the lymph nodes and other mediastinal structures; it can also determine the size and invasiveness of the tumor. Exploratory laparoscopy is the best method for finding positive lymph nodes in patients with distal lesions (Cools-Lartigue, Molena, & Gerdes, 2018).

Future diagnostic techniques that may serve as predictors for dysplastic progression in patients with BE involve molecular markers. Some data have shown that a small percentage of people may have a genetic predisposition to esophageal cancer. Researchers have identified several biomarkers with strong potential to predict outcomes in esophageal cancer, but none of these biomarkers are currently recommended or clinically available (Iyer & Kaul, 2019). The usefulness of molecular markers in treating esophageal cancer continues to be researched.

Medical Management

If esophageal cancer is detected at an early stage, treatment goals may be directed toward cure; however, it is often detected in late stages, making relief of symptoms the only reasonable goal of therapy. Treatment may include surgery, radiation, chemotherapy, or a combination of these modalities, depending on the type of cancer cell, the extent of the disease, and the patient's condition. A standard treatment plan for a patient who is newly diagnosed with esophageal cancer will vary depending on the staging but may include: endoscopic resection, chemoradiation followed by surgery, chemotherapy followed by surgery, surgery alone, definitive chemoradiation, or palliative measures (NCI, 2021a).

Although minimally invasive surgery may be possible in some cases, standard surgical management includes esophagectomy with removal of the tumor plus a wide tumor-free margin of the esophagus and the lymph nodes in the area. Variations on the original esophagectomy preserve nerves, employ less invasive techniques, and target specific areas of the esophagus (Schlottmann, Molena, & Patti, 2018). The surgical approach may be through the neck, thorax and/or the abdomen, depending on the location of the tumor. When tumors occur in the cervical or upper thoracic area, and the

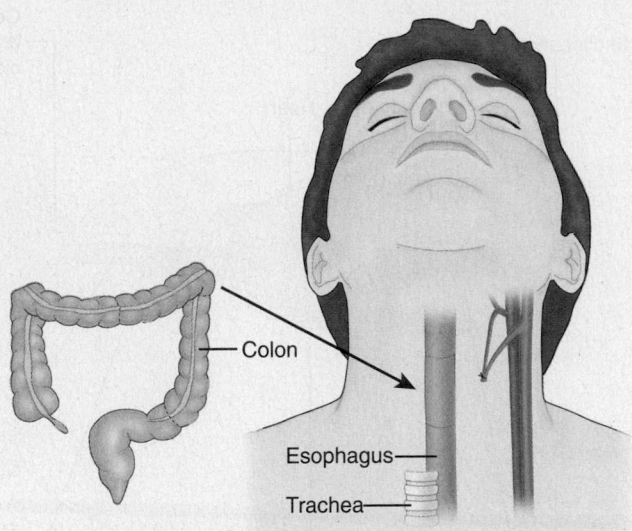

Figure 39-12 • Esophageal reconstruction with colonic interposition. A portion of the colon is grafted between the esophagus and pharynx to replace the abnormal portion of the esophagus. The vascular structures are also anastomosed.

stomach cannot be mobilized, pulled up, and anastomosed to the esophagus, esophageal continuity may be maintained by performing a colon graft transfer, in which the tumor is removed and the area is replaced with a portion of the colon (see Fig. 39-12). In many of these cases, a feeding tube is placed in the jejunum during surgery for feeding (Schlottman et al., 2018).

Tumors of the lower thoracic esophagus are more amenable to surgery than are tumors located higher in the esophagus. GI tract integrity is maintained by anastomosing the lower esophagus to the stomach (see Fig. 39-13).

Surgical resection of the esophagus has a relatively high mortality rate because of infection, pulmonary complications, or leakage through the anastomosis. Postoperatively, the patient has an NG tube in place that should not be manipulated. The patient remains NPO until x-ray studies that confirm that the anastomosis is free from an esophageal leak, there is no obstruction, and that there is no evidence of pulmonary aspiration.

Palliative treatment may be necessary to keep the esophagus open, to assist with nutrition, and to control saliva. Palliation may be accomplished with dilation of the esophagus, laser therapy, placement of an endoprosthesis (stent) via EGD, radiation, or chemotherapy.

Nursing Management

Preoperative nursing management is directed toward improving the patient's nutritional and physical status in preparation for surgery, radiation therapy, and/or chemotherapy. A program to promote weight gain based on a high-calorie and high-protein diet, in liquid or soft form, is provided if adequate food can be taken by mouth. If this is not possible, parenteral or enteral nutrition is initiated. Nutritional status is monitored throughout treatment. The patient is informed about the nature of the postoperative equipment that will be used, including that required for closed chest drainage, NG suction, parenteral fluid therapy, and gastric intubation.

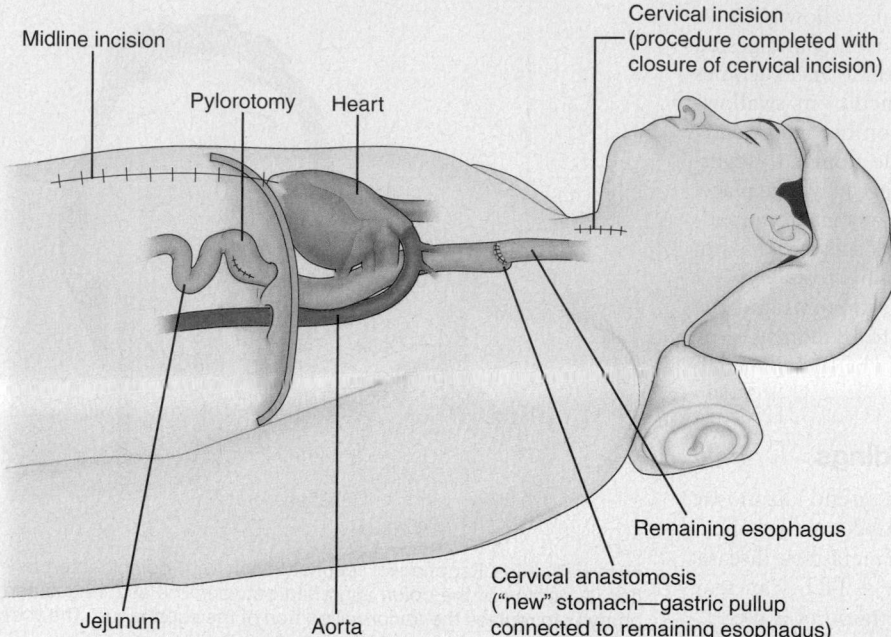

Midline incision

Pylorotomy   Heart

Cervical incision
(procedure completed with
closure of cervical incision)

Remaining esophagus

Cervical anastomosis
("new" stomach—gastric pullup
connected to remaining esophagus)

Jejunum   Aorta

Figure 39-13 • Transhiatal esophagectomy. Surgical removal of tumor of the lower esophagus with anastomosis of the remaining esophagus to the stomach. Redrawn from Heitmiller, R. F. (1999). Closed chest esophageal resection, 252–265. *Operative Techniques in Thoracic and Cardiovascular Surgery, 4*(3). © 1999, with permission from Elsevier. doi: 10.1016/S1522-2942(07)70121-6.

Immediate postoperative care is similar to that provided for patients undergoing thoracic surgery. It is not uncommon for patients to have a tracheostomy and be placed in an intensive care unit or step-down unit. After recovering from the effects of anesthesia, the patient is placed in a low Fowler position, and later in a Fowler position, to help prevent reflux of gastric secretions. The patient is observed carefully for regurgitation and dyspnea. A common postoperative complication is aspiration pneumonia (Brownlee & Ferguson, 2018). Therefore, the patient is placed on a vigorous pulmonary plan of care that includes incentive spirometry, sitting up in a chair, and, if necessary, nebulizer treatments. Chest physiotherapy is avoided due to the risk of aspiration. The patient's temperature is monitored to detect any elevation that may indicate aspiration or seepage of fluid through the operative site into the mediastinum, which would indicate an esophageal leak. Drainage from the cervical neck wound, usually saliva, is evidence of an early esophageal leak. Typically, no treatment other than maintaining NPO status and parenteral or enteral support is warranted. The patient is also monitored for a postoperative chylothorax (accumulation of chyle/lymphatic fluid in the pleural cavity), which would require pleural drainage (Brownlee & Ferguson, 2018; Rudrappa & Paul, 2019).

Cardiac complications include atrial fibrillation, which occurs due to irritation of the vagus nerve at the time of surgery. Typical medical management includes digitalization or the use of beta-blockers, calcium channel blockers, amiodarone, and/or cardioversion depending on the patient's hemodynamic status (Brownlee & Ferguson, 2018).

Esophageal anastomotic leak is managed by facilitating adequate drainage, initiating broad-spectrum antibiotics (often including antifungal agents), and optimizing nutrition via enteral or parenteral feeding (Brownlee & Ferguson, 2018). During surgery, an NG tube is inserted and taped in place. It is connected to low intermittent suction. The NG tube is not manipulated; if displacement occurs, it is not replaced because damage to the anastomosis may occur. The

NG tube is typically removed 5 days after surgery; before the patient is allowed to eat, a barium swallow is performed to assess for any anastomotic leak.

Once feeding begins, the nurse encourages the patient to swallow small sips of water. Eventually, the diet is advanced as tolerated to a soft, mechanical diet. When the patient can increase food and fluid intake to an adequate amount, parenteral fluids are discontinued. After each meal, the patient remains upright for at least 2 hours to allow the food to move through the GI tract. It is a challenge to encourage the patient to eat because the appetite is usually poor. Family involvement and home-cooked favorite foods may help the patient to eat. Antacids may help patients with gastric distress. Erythromycin, metoclopramide, or domperidone are useful in promoting gastric emptying (Brownlee & Ferguson, 2018).

If chemotherapy and radiation are part of the therapy, the patient's appetite will be further depressed, and esophagitis may occur, causing pain when food is eaten. Liquid supplements may be more easily tolerated. Surgical adjuncts to esophagectomy that address delayed gastric emptying (a major complication in 15% to 39% of patients after esophagectomy) may promote **vagotomy syndrome** (dumping syndrome), which can occur with each meal or approximately 20 minutes to 2 hours after eating (Zhang & Zhang, 2019). Vagotomy syndrome occurs due to interruption of vagal nerve fibers, which in turn causes an alteration in the storage function of the stomach and the pyloric emptying mechanism. As a result, large amounts of solids and liquids rapidly "dump" into the duodenum. The patient experiences severe abdominal cramping, followed by a liquid bowel movement that may or may not be associated with diaphoresis, rapid heart rate or rapid respirations, or both. It can be quite disabling but typically resolves without incident, and the patient is left feeling extremely tired. As the patient's recovery progresses and the patient begins to eat soft foods and remains in an upright position for 2 hours after eating, the frequency and severity of episodes decrease.

Often, in either the preoperative or the postoperative period, an obstructed or nearly obstructed esophagus causes difficulty with excess saliva, and drooling becomes a problem. Oral suction may be used if the patient cannot manage oral secretions, or a wick-type gauze may be placed at the corner of the mouth to direct secretions to a dressing or emesis basin. The possibility that the patient may aspirate saliva into the tracheobronchial tree and develop pneumonia is a concern.

When the patient is ready to go home, the family is instructed about how to promote nutrition, what observations to make, what measures to take if complications occur, how to keep the patient comfortable, and how to obtain needed physical and emotional support.

CRITICAL THINKING EXERCISES

1 **ebp** A 63-year-old female patient presents to a primary care clinic where you work reporting a slightly sore throat and a red patch on the side of her mouth that bleeds easily and simply will not heal. What questions should you ask? What are the primary risk factors for oral cancer? How should you frame assessment questions regarding actual and potential HPV exposure? What guidelines and evidence should inform this conversation?

2 **ipc** You are a nurse working on an inpatient oncology unit and have been assigned a postoperative patient who has had a classic, radical neck resection due to head and neck cancer. What nerve and muscular changes do you expect with this specific procedure? Based on this information, what are the key priority nursing interventions that will prevent short-term postoperative and long-term complications in this patient? What interprofessional consults should you plan to facilitate? What is the role of each of these interprofessional team members?

3 **pq** A patient diagnosed with stage III esophageal cancer undergoes the standard treatment of chemoradiation prior to an esophagostomy, and is admitted postoperatively to the surgical unit where you work. You notice on your first postoperative assessment that the NG tube that was placed in the OR has been pulled out 5 cm. What should you do *first*? What is the rationale for this NG tube? What are the risks (if any) with it being dislodged? For what other esophagostomy-specific postoperative complications should you monitor (*list four*)?

REFERENCES

*Asterisk indicates nursing research article.
**Double asterisk indicates classic reference.

Books

Bickley, L. S. (2016). *Bates' guide to physical examination and history taking* (12th ed.). Philadelphia, PA: Lippincott Williams & Wilkins.

Brownlee, A. R., & Ferguson, M. K. (2018). *Perioperative care and management of post-operative complications.* In F. Schlottmann, D. Molena, & M. G. Patti (Eds.). *Esophageal cancer: Diagnosis and treatment.* Cham, Switzerland: Springer International Publishing AG, part of Springer Nature 2018.

Cools-Lartigue, J., Molena, D., & Gerdes, H. (2018). *Staging of esophageal cancer: Implications for therapy.* In F. Schlottmann, D. Molena, & M. G. Patti (Eds.). *Esophageal cancer: Diagnosis and treatment.* Cham, Switzerland: Springer International Publishing AG, part of Springer Nature 2018.

Eliopoulos, C. (2018). *Gerontological nursing* (9th ed.). Philadelphia, PA: Wolters Kluwer.

Hudson, B., & Carr, E. (2020). Head and neck cancers. In J. M. Brandt (Ed.). *Core curriculum for oncology nursing* (6th ed.). St. Louis, MO: Elsevier Inc.

Levine, M. S., & Rubesin, S. E. (2012). Radiology of the pharynx and esophagus. In D. O. Castell & J. E. Richter (Eds.). *The esophagus* (5th ed.). Philadelphia, PA: Lippincott Williams & Wilkins.

Mueller, C. M. (Ed.). (2017). *The ASPEN adult nutrition support core curriculum* (3rd ed.). Silver Spring, MD: American Society for Parenteral and Enteral Nutrition.

Rudrappa, M., & Paul, M. (2019). *Chylothorax.* In *StatPearls* [Internet]. Treasure Island, FL: StatPearls Publishing. Retrieved on 2/20/2020 at: www.ncbi.nlm.nih.gov/books/NBK459206/

Schlottmann, F., Molena, D., & Patti, M. G. (Eds.). (2018). *Esophageal cancer: Diagnosis and treatment.* Cham, Switzerland: Springer International Publishing AG, part of Springer Nature 2018.

Stack, B. C., & Moreno, M. A. (2019). *Neck dissection.* New York: Thieme Medical Publishers, Incorporated.

Whalen, K. (2019). *Pharmacology* (7th ed.). Philadelphia, PA: Wolters Kluwer.

Journals and Electronic Documents

American Academy of Periodontology. (2021). *Periodontal disease fact sheet.* Retrieved on 2/18/2021 at: www.perio.org/newsroom/periodontal-disease-fact-sheet

American Cancer Society (ACS). (2021a). *About esophagus cancer.* Retrieved on 2/18/2021 at: www.cancer.org/content/dam/CRC/PDF/Public/8614.00.pdf

American Cancer Society (ACS). (2021b). *Kaposi sarcoma.* Retrieved on 2/18/2021 at: www.cancer.org/cancer/kaposisarcoma/detailedguide/kaposi-sarcoma-what-is-kaposi-sarcoma

**American Society for Gastrointestinal Endoscopy Standards of Practice Committee. (2011). Guideline: Management of ingested foreign bodies and food impactions. *Gastrointestinal Endoscopy, 73*(6), 1085–1091.

Anderson, L. (2019). Enteral feeding tubes: An overview of nursing care. *British Journal of Nursing, 28*(12), 748–754.

Anderson, L. (2020). Providing nutritional support for the patient with COVID-19. *British Journal of Nursing, 29*(8), 458–459.

Arkin, N., Krishnan, K., & Chang, M. G. (2020). Nutrition in critically ill patients with COVID-19: Challenges and special considerations. *Clinical Nutrition, 39*(2020), 2327–2328.

Bischoff, S. C., Austin, P., Boeykens, K., et al. (2020). ESPEN guideline on home enteral nutrition. *Clinical Nutrition, 39*(1), 5–22.

Blumenstein, I., Shastri, Y. H., & Stein, J. (2014). Gastroenteric tube feeding: Techniques, problems, and solutions. *World Journal of Gastroenterology, 20*(26), 8505–8524.

Boullata, J. I., Carrera, A. L., Harvey, L., et al. (2017). ASPEN safe practices for enteral nutrition therapy. *Journal of Parenteral and Enteral Nutrition, 41*(1), 15–103.

Broers, C., & Tack, J. (2017). Review article: Gastro-oesophageal reflux disease in asthma and chronic obstructive pulmonary disease. *Alimentary Pharmacology and Therapeutics, 47*(2), 176–191.

Byard, R. W. (2015). Caustic ingestion: A forensic overview. *Journal of Forensic Science, 60*(3), 812–815.

Centers for Disease Control and Prevention (CDC). (2020a). *HPV vaccine recommendations.* Retrieved on 2/18/2021 at: www.cdc.gov/vaccines/vpd/hpv/hcp/recommendations.html

Centers for Disease Control and Prevention (CDC). (2020b). 2014. *National water fluoridation statistics.* Retrieved on 2/18/2021 at: www.cdc.gov/fluoridation/statistics/2014stats.htm

Centers for Disease Control and Prevention (CDC). (2018). *Statement on the evidence supporting the safety and effectiveness of community water fluoridation.* Retrieved on 2/18/2021 at: www.cdc.gov/fluoridation/guidelines/cdc-statement-on-community-water-fluoridation.html

Centers for Disease Control and Prevention (CDC). (2019). *Oral health surveillance report, 2019.* Retrieved on 2/18/2021 at: www.cdc.gov/oral-health/publications/OHSR-2019-index.html

Clermont, M. P., & Ahuja, N. K. (2018). The relevance of spastic esophageal disorders as a diagnostic category. *Current Gastroenterology Reports*, 20(9), 42.

Donovan, T. E., Marzola, R., Murphy, K. R., et al. (2018). Annual review of selected scientific literature: A report of the Committee on Scientific Investigation of the American Academy of Restorative Dentistry. *Journal of Prosthetic Dentistry*, 120(6), 816–878.

*Dri, E., Bressan, V., Cadorin, L., et al. (2019). Providing care to a family member affected by head and neck cancer: A phenomenological study. *Supportive Care in Cancer*, 28, 2035–2036.

Eke, P. I., Dye, B. A., Wei, L., et al. (2015). Update on prevalence of periodontitis in adults in the United States: NHANES 2009-2012. *Journal of Periodontology*, 86(5), 611–622.

Eke, P. I., Wei, L., Thornton-Evans, G. O., et al. (2016). Risk indicators for periodontitis in US adults: NHANES 2009 to 2012. *Journal of Periodontology*, 87(10), 1174–1185.

Fabie, J. E., Kompelli, A. R., Naylor, T. M., et al. (2019). Gland-preserving surgery for salivary stones and the utility of sialendoscopes. *Head & Neck*, 41(5), 1320–1327.

Fung, B. M., Sweetser, S., Wong Kee Song, L. M., et al. (2019). Foreign object ingestion and esophageal food impaction: An update and review on endoscopic management. *World Journal of Gastrointestinal Endoscopy*, 11(3), 174–192.

Gabel, M. E., Galante, G. J., & Freedman, S. D. (2019). Gastrointestinal and hepatobiliary disease in cystic fibrosis. *Seminars in Respiratory and Critical Care Medicine*, 40(6), 825–841.

Gauer, R. L., & Semidey, M. J. (2015). Diagnosis and treatment of temporomandibular disorders. *American Family Physician*, 91(6), 378–386.

Grègoire, V., Ang, K., Budach, W., et al. (2014). Delineation of the neck node levels for head and neck tumors: A 2013 update. DAHANCA, EORTC, HKNPCSG, NCIC CTG, NCRI, RTOG, TROG consensus guidelines. *Radiotherapy and Oncology*, 110(1), 172–181.

Grennan, D. (2019). Mumps. *JAMA*, 322(10), 1022.

Gutierrez, O. I. B., Ichkhanian, Y., Spadaccini, M., et al. (2019). Zenker's diverticulum per-oral endoscopic myotomy techniques: Changing paradigms. *Gastroenterology*, 156(8), 2134–2135.

Ha, C., Regan, J., Cetindag, I. B., et al. (2015). Benign esophageal tumors. *Surgical Clinics of North America*, 95(3), 491–514.

Han, A. Y., Kuan, E. C., Mallen-St. Clair, J., et al. (2019). Total glossectomy with free flap reconstruction: Twenty-year experience at a tertiary medical center. *Laryngoscope*, 129(5), 1087–1092.

Hegde, R., & Awan, K. H. (2019). Effects of periodontal disease on systemic health. *Disease a Month*, 65(6), 185–192.

**Heitmiller, R. F. (1999). Closed chest esophageal resection. *Operative Techniques in Thoracic and Cardiovascular Surgery*, 4(3), 252–265.

Hong, C. H. L., Gueiros, L. A., Fulton, J. S., et al. (2019). Systematic review of basic oral care for the management of oral mucositis in cancer patients and clinical practice guidelines. *Supportive Care in Cancer*, 27(10), 3949–3967.

Huerta, C. T., Plymale, M., Barrett, P., et al. (2019). Long-term efficacy of laparoscopic Nissen versus Toupet fundoplication for the management of types III and IV hiatal hernias. *Surgical Endoscopy*, 33(9), 2895–2900.

Iyer, P. G., & Kaul, V. (2019). Barrett esophagus. *Mayo Clinical Proceedings*, 94(9), 1888–1901.

**Kohn, G. P., Price, R. R., Demeester, S. R., et al. (2013). *Guidelines for the management of hiatal hernia*. Retrieved on 11/20/2019 at: www.sages.org/publications/guidelines/guidelines-for-the-management-of-hiatal-hernia/

*Koszalinski, R. S., Heidel, R. E., & McCarthy, J. (2020). Difficulty envisioning a positive future: Secondary analyses in patients in intensive care who are communication vulnerable. *Nursing & Health Sciences*, 2019. doi: 10.1111/nhs.12664.

Kroch, D. A., & Madanick, R. D. (2017). Medical treatment of gastroesophageal reflux disease. *World Journal of Surgery*, 41(7), 1678–1684.

Lassche, G., van Boxtel, W., Ligtenberg, M. J. L., et al. (2019). Advances and challenges in precision medicine in salivary gland cancer. *Cancer Treatment Reviews*, 80, 101906.

Lodi, G. (2020). Oral lesions. Retrieved on 2/18/2021 at: www.uptodate.com/contents/oral-lesions

Lu, D. J., Luu, M., Nguyen, A. T., et al. (2019). Survival outcomes with concomitant chemoradiotherapy in older adults with oropharyngeal carcinoma in an era of increasing human papillomavirus (HPV) prevalence. *Oral Oncology*, 99, 104472. doi.org/10.1016/j.oraloncology.2019.104472

Margaix-Muñoz, M., Bagán, J., & Poveda-Roda, R. (2017). Ewing sarcoma of the oral cavity. A review. *Journal of Clinical and Experimental Dentistry*, 9(2), 294–301.

Maria, O. M., Eliopoulos, N., & Muanza, T. (2017). Radiation-induced oral mucositis. *Frontiers in Oncology*, 7, 89.

Marinho, V. C., Worthington, H. V., Walsh, T., et al. (2015). Fluoride gels for preventing dental caries in children and adolescents. *Cochrane Database of Systematic Reviews*, 15(6), CD002279.

Martindale, R., Patel, J. J., Taylor, B., et al. (2020). Nutrition therapy in the patient with COVID-19 disease requiring ICU care. Updated May 26, 2020. *ASPEN: Resources for Clinicians Caring for Patients with Coronavirus*. Retrieved on 2/18/2021 at: www.nutritioncare.org/uploadedFiles/Documents/Guidelines_and_Clinical_Resources/COVID19/Nutrition%20Therapy%20in%20the%20Patient%20with%20COVID-19%20Disease%20Requiring%20ICU%20Care_Updated%20May%2026.pdf

McClave, S. A., Taylor, B. E., Martindale, R. G., et al. (2016). Guidelines for the provision and assessment of nutrition support therapy in the adult critically ill patient: Society of Critical Care Medicine (SCCM) and American Society for Parenteral and Enteral Nutrition (ASPEN). *Journal of Parenteral and Enteral Nutrition*, 40(2), 159–211.

Mowad, C. (2019). Cheilitis. *UpToDate*. Retrieved on 2/18/2021 at: www.uptodate.com/contents/cheilitis

Naavaal, S., Griffin, S. O., & Jones, J. A. (2020). Impact of making dental care affordable on quality of life in adults aged 45 years and older. *Journal of Aging and Health*, 2019, 898264319857967. doi.org/10.1177/089826431985796

National Cancer Institute (NCI). (2017). HPV vaccination linked to decreased oral HPV infections. Retrieved on 2/18/2021 at: www.cancer.gov/news-events/cancer-currents-blog/2017/hpv-vaccine-oral-infection

National Cancer Institute (NCI). (2021a). *Esophageal cancer treatment (adult) (PDQ®)—Health professional version*. Retrieved on 2/18/2021 at: www.cancer.gov/types/esophageal/hp/esophageal-treatment-pdq

National Cancer Institute (NCI). (2021b). *Head and neck cancer (PDQ®)—Health professional version*. Retrieved on 2/18/2021 at: www.cancer.gov/types/head-and-neck/hp

National Cancer Institute (NCI). (2021c). *Oropharyngeal cancer treatment (adult) (PDQ®)—Health professional version*. Retrieved on 2/18/2021 at: www.cancer.gov/types/head-and-neck/hp/adult/oropharyngeal-treatment-pdq

National Cancer Institute (NCI). (2021d). *Salivary gland cancer treatment (adult) (PDQ®)—Health professional version*. Retrieved on 2/18/2021 at: www.cancer.gov/types/head-and-neck/hp/adult/salivary-gland-treatment-pdq

National Capital Poison Center. (2018). *National Capital Poison Center button battery ingestion triage and treatment guideline*. Retrieved on 2/18/2021 at: www.poison.org/battery/guideline

National Institute of Dental and Craniofacial Research (NIDCR). (2018). TMJ (temporomandibular joint and muscle disorders). Retrieved on 2/18/2021 at: www.nidcr.nih.gov/health-info/tmj/more-info

Nuchit, S., Lam-ubol, A., Paemuang, W., et al. (2020). Alleviation of dry mouth by saliva substitutes improved swallowing ability and clinical nutritional status of post-radiotherapy head and neck cancer patients: A randomized controlled trial. *Supportive Care in Cancer*, 2019. doi.org/10.1007/s00520-019-05132-1

**Office of the Surgeon General (US). (2003). *National call to action to promote oral health*. NIH Publication No. 03-5303. Rockville, MD: National Institute of Dental and Craniofacial Research (US). Retrieved on 11/16/2019 at: www.ncbi.nlm.nih.gov/books/NBK47472/

Olivero, R. (2019). Boerhaave syndrome: A rare postoperative condition. *Journal of the American Academy of Physician Assistants*, 32(8), 1–3.

Papadopoulou-Alataki, E., Dogantzis, P., Chatziavramidis, A., et al. (2019). Juvenile recurrent parotitis: The role of sialendoscopy. *International Journal of Inflammation*, 2019, 7278907.

Patrakka, O., Pienimäki, J-P., Tuomisto, S., et al. (2019). Oral bacterial signatures in cerebral thrombi of patients with acute ischemic stroke treated with thrombectomy. *Journal of the American Heart Association*, 8(11), e012330. doi: 10.1161/JAHA.119.012330

Patti, M. G. (2016). An evidence-based approach to the treatment of gastroesophageal reflux disease. *JAMA Surgery*, 151(1), 73–78.

Pickrell, B. B., Serebrakian, A. T., & Maricevich, R. S. (2017). Mandible fractures. *Seminars in Plastic Surgery*, 31(2), 100–107.

Qumseya, B. J., Bukannan, A., Gendy, S., et al. (2019). Systematic review and meta-analysis of prevalence and risk factors for Barrett's esophagus. *Gastrointestinal Endoscopy, 90*(5), 707–717.

Raymond, D. P. (2020). Surgical management of esophageal perforation. *UpToDate*. Retrieved on 2/18/2021 at: www.uptodate.com/contents/surgical-management-of-esophageal-perforation

Read, M. E., Olson, A. J., & Calderwood, M. S. (2020). Front-line education by infection preventionists helps reduce *Clostridioides difficile* infections. *American Journal of Infection Control, 48*(2), 227–229.

Robertson, D. P., Keys, W., Rautemaa-Richardon, R., et al. (2015). Management of severe acute dental infections. *The BMJ, 350*, h1300. doi.org/10.1136/bmj.h1300

Sabatini, M. E., & Chiocca, S. (2019). Human papillomavirus as a driver of head and neck cancers. *British Journal of Cancer, 122*(3), 306–314.

Sandmæl, J. A., Sand, K., Bye, A., et al. (2019). Nutritional experiences in head and neck cancer patients. *European Journal of Cancer Care, 28*(6), e13168. doi.org/10.1111/ecc.13168

Seres, D. (2019). Nutrition support in critically ill patients: Enteral nutrition. *UpToDate*. Retrieved on 2/18/2021 at: www.uptodate.com/contents/nutrition-support-in-critically-ill-patients-enteral-nutrition

Sharma, P., Katzka, D. A., Gupta, N., et al. (2015). Consensus statement: Quality indicators for the management of Barrett's esophagus, dysplasia, and esophageal adenocarcinoma: International consensus recommendations from the American Gastroenterological Association symposium. *Gastroenterology, 149*(6), 1599–1606.

Siegel, R. L., Miller, K. D., & Jemal, A. (2019). Cancer statistics, 2019. *CA: A Cancer Journal for Clinicians, 69*(1), 7–34.

Silk, H. (2014). Disease of the mouth. *Primary Care: Clinics in Office Practice, 41*(1), 75–90.

Smith, C. D. (2015). Esophageal strictures and diverticula. *Surgical Clinics of North America, 95*(3), 669–681.

Sobin, L., Kopp, R., Walsh, R., et al. (2016). Incidence of concussion in patients with isolated mandible fractures. *JAMA Facial Plastic Surgery, 18*(1), 15–18.

Swanström, L. L. (2019). Achalasia: Treatment, current status and future advances. *The Korean Journal of Internal Medicine, 34*(6), 1173–1180.

Thompson, R. (2017). Troubleshooting PEG feeding tubes in the community setting. *Journal of Community Nursing, 31*(2), 61–66.

Twetman, S. (2015). The evidence base for professional and self-care prevention—caries, erosion and sensitivity. *BMC Oral Health, 15*(Suppl 1), S4.

Uberoi, A. S., Brown, T. J., & Gupta, A. (2019a). Finding the magic in magic mouthwash—Reply. *JAMA Internal Medicine, 179*(5), 724–725.

Uberoi, A. S., Brown, T. J., & Gupta, A. (2019b). Magic mouthwash for oral mucositis: A teachable moment. *JAMA Internal Medicine, 179*(1), 104–105.

**U.S. Department of Health and Human Services (HHS). (2000). *Oral health in America: A report of the surgeon general. Executive summary*. Rockville, MD: U.S. Department of Health and Human Services, National Institutes of Dental and Craniofacial Research, National Institutes of Health. Retrieved on 11/13/2019 at: www.nidcr.nih.gov/sites/default/files/2017-10/hck1ocv.%40www.surgeon.fullrpt.pdf

U.S. Department of Health and Human Services (HHS). Federal Panel on Community Water Fluoridation. (2015). U.S. Public Health Service recommendation for fluoride concentration in drinking water for the prevention of dental carries. *Public Health Reports, 130*(4), 318–331.

U.S. Department of Health and Human Services (HHS). Office of Disease Prevention and Health Promotion. (2019). *Healthy People 2020: Oral health*. Retrieved on 11/15/2019 at: www.healthypeople.gov/2020/topics-objectives/topic/oral-health

van den Bergh, B., de Mol van Otterloo, J. J., van der Ploeg, T., et al. (2015). IMF-screws or arch bars as conservative treatment for mandibular condyle fractures: Quality of life aspects. *Journal of Cranio-Maxillo-Facial Surgery, 43*(7), 1004–1009.

Villa, A., Nordio, F., & Gohel, A. (2015). A risk prediction model for xerostomia: A retrospective cohort study. *Gerodontology, 33*(4), 562–568.

World Health Organization (WHO). (2019). *Strategies for oral disease prevention and health promotion*. Retrieved on 11/16/2019 at: www.who.int/oral_health/strategies/en/

Zhang, R., & Zhang, L. (2019). Management of delayed gastric conduit emptying after esophagectomy. *Journal of Thoracic Disease, 11*(1), 302–307.

Resources

Academy of General Dentistry (AGD), agd.org

American Cancer Society (ACS), cancer.org

American Cancer Society (ACS) Online Communities and Support, cancer.org/treatment/support-programs-and-services/online-communities.html

American Dental Association (ADA), ada.org/en/

Healthy People 2020, healthypeople.gov

Look Good Feel Better, lookgoodfeelbetter.org

National Capital Poison Center, Battery Ingestion Triage and Treatment Guideline, www.poison.org/battery/guideline

National Institute of Dental and Craniofacial Research (NIDCR), National Institutes of Health, nidcr.nih.gov

40 Management of Patients with Gastric and Duodenal Disorders

LEARNING OUTCOMES

On completion of this chapter, the learner will be able to:

1. Compare the etiology, pathophysiology, clinical manifestations, and management of acute gastritis, chronic gastritis, and peptic ulcer disease.
2. Use the nursing process as a framework for care of the patient with acute or chronic gastritis, or peptic ulcer.
3. Discuss the etiology, pathophysiology, clinical manifestations, and management of gastric cancer and tumors of the small intestine.
4. Use the nursing process as a framework for care of the patient with gastric cancer or tumors of the small intestine.

NURSING CONCEPT

Nutrition

GLOSSARY

achlorhydria: lack of hydrochloric acid in digestive secretions of the stomach

antrectomy: removal of the pyloric (antrum) portion of the stomach with anastomosis (surgical connection) either to the duodenum (gastroduodenostomy or Billroth I) or to the jejunum (gastrojejunostomy or Billroth II)

dumping syndrome: physiologic response to rapid emptying of gastric contents into the small intestines, manifested by nausea, weakness, sweating, palpitations, syncope, and diarrhea (*synonym:* vagotomy syndrome)

duodenum: first portion of the small intestine, between the stomach and the jejunum

dyspepsia: indigestion; upper abdominal discomfort associated with eating

gastric: refers to the stomach

gastric outlet obstruction: any condition that mechanically impedes normal gastric emptying; there is obstruction of the channel of the pylorus and duodenum through which the stomach empties; also called pyloric obstruction

gastritis: inflammation of the stomach

***Helicobacter pylori* (*H. pylori*):** a spiral-shaped gram-negative bacterium that colonizes the gastric mucosa; is involved in most cases of peptic ulcer disease

hematemesis: vomiting of blood

hematochezia: bright red, bloody stools

melena: tarry or black stools; indicative of occult blood in stools

omentum: fold of the peritoneum that surrounds the stomach and other organs of the abdomen

peritoneum: thin membrane that lines the inside of the wall of the abdomen and covers all of the abdominal organs

pyloroplasty: surgical procedure to increase the opening of the pyloric orifice

pylorus: opening between the stomach and the duodenum

pyrosis: a burning sensation in the stomach and esophagus that moves up to the mouth (*synonym:* heartburn)

serosa: thin membrane that covers the outer surface of the stomach; visceral peritoneum covering the outer surface of the stomach

steatorrhea: fatty stool; typically malodorous with an oily appearance and floats in water

stenosis: narrowing or tightening of an opening or passage in the body

A person's nutritional status depends not only on the type and amount of intake, but also on the functioning of the **gastric** (stomach) and intestinal portions of the gastrointestinal (GI) system. The scope of disorders that may affect a person's nutritional status is of particular note.

Given the prevalence of Americans who have gastric and duodenal disorders, nurses will encounter adults and older adults with these disorders in virtually every inpatient and outpatient clinical setting. This chapter describes disorders of the stomach and small intestine, their etiology, pathophysiology, clinical manifestations, management, and related nursing care.

Gastritis

Gastritis (inflammation of the gastric or stomach mucosa) is a common GI problem, accounting for approximately two million visits to outpatient clinics annually in the United States, with increasing prevalence occurring in adults older than 60 years of age (Wehbi, Dacha, Sarver, et al., 2019). It affects women and men about equally. Gastritis may be acute, lasting several hours to a few days, or chronic, resulting from repeated exposure to irritating agents or recurring episodes of acute gastritis.

Acute gastritis may be classified as erosive or nonerosive, based on pathologic manifestations present in the gastric mucosa (Wehbi et al., 2019). The erosive form of acute gastritis is most often caused by local irritants such as aspirin and other nonsteroidal anti-inflammatory drugs (NSAIDs) (e.g., ibuprofen); corticosteroids; alcohol consumption; and gastric radiation therapy (National Institute of Diabetes and Digestive and Kidney Diseases [NIDDK], 2020a; Norris, 2019; Wehbi et al., 2019). The nonerosive form of acute gastritis is most often caused by an infection with a spiral-shaped gram-negative bacterium, *Helicobacter pylori* (*H. pylori*) (Wehbi et al., 2019). It is estimated that 50% of individuals globally are infected with *H. pylori* (Santacroce & Bhutani, 2019).

A more severe form of acute gastritis is caused by the ingestion of strong acid or alkali, which may cause the mucosa to become gangrenous or to perforate (see Chapter 67). Scarring can occur, resulting in pyloric **stenosis** (narrowing or tightening) or obstruction. Acute gastritis also may develop in acute illnesses, especially when the patient has had major traumatic injuries, burns, severe infection, lack of perfusion to the stomach lining, or major surgery. This type of acute gastritis is often referred to as *stress-related gastritis or ulcer* (Clarke, Ferraro, Gbadehan, et al., 2020; Norris, 2019).

Chronic gastritis is often classified according to the underlying causative mechanism, which most often includes an infection with *H. pylori*. Chronic *H. pylori* gastritis is implicated in the development of peptic ulcers, gastric adenocarcinoma (cancer), and gastric mucosa–associated lymphoid tissue lymphoma (Akiva & Greenwald, 2019; Lloyd & Leiman, 2019). Chronic gastritis may also be caused by a chemical gastric injury (gastropathy) as the result of long-term drug therapy (e.g., aspirin and other NSAIDs) or reflux of duodenal contents into the stomach, which most often occurs after gastric surgery (e.g., gastrojejunostomy, gastroduodenostomy). Autoimmune disorders such as Hashimoto thyroiditis, Addison disease, and Graves disease are also associated with the development of chronic gastritis (see Chapter 45) (Akiva & Greenwald, 2019; Norris, 2019).

Pathophysiology

Gastritis is characterized by a disruption of the mucosal barrier that normally protects the stomach tissue from digestive juices (e.g., hydrochloric acid [HCl] and pepsin). The impaired mucosal barrier allows corrosive HCl, pepsin, and other irritating agents (e.g., alcohol, NSAIDs, *H. pylori*) to come in contact with the gastric mucosa, resulting in inflammation. In acute gastritis, this inflammation is usually transient and self-limiting in nature. Inflammation causes the gastric mucosa to become edematous and hyperemic (congested with fluid and blood) and to undergo superficial erosion (Fig. 40-1). Superficial ulceration may occur as

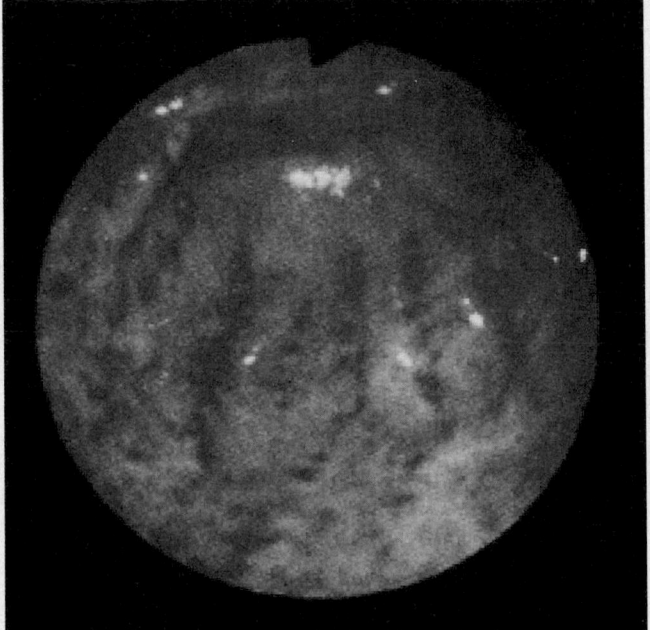
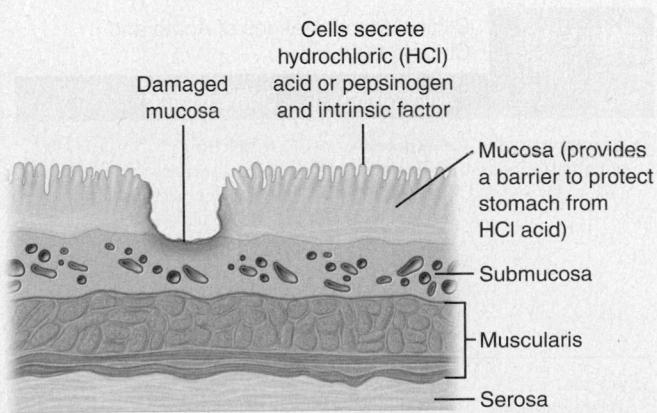

Figure 40-1 • Endoscopic view of erosive gastritis (**left**). Damage from irritants (**right**) results in increased intracellular pH, impaired enzyme function, disrupted cellular structures, ischemia, vascular stasis, and tissue death. Image at left reproduced with permission from Strayer, D. S., Saffitz, J. E., & Rubin, E. (2015). *Rubin's pathology: Mechanisms of human disease* (8th ed., Fig. 19-15). Philadelphia, PA: Lippincott Williams & Wilkins.

a result of erosive disease and may lead to hemorrhage. In chronic gastritis, persistent or repeated insults lead to chronic inflammatory changes, and eventually atrophy (or thinning) of the gastric tissue (Norris, 2019).

Clinical Manifestations

The patient with acute gastritis may have a rapid onset of symptoms, such as epigastric pain or discomfort, **dyspepsia** (indigestion; upper abdominal discomfort associated with eating), anorexia, hiccups, or nausea and vomiting, which can last from a few hours to a few days. Erosive gastritis may cause bleeding, which may manifest as blood in vomit or as **melena** (black, tarry stools; indicative of occult blood in stools) or **hematochezia** (bright red, bloody stools) (Wehbi et al., 2019).

The patient with chronic gastritis may complain of fatigue, **pyrosis** (a burning sensation in the stomach and esophagus that moves up to the mouth; heartburn) after eating, belching, a sour taste in the mouth, halitosis, early satiety, anorexia, or nausea and vomiting. Some patients may have only mild epigastric discomfort or report intolerance to spicy or fatty foods or slight pain that is relieved by eating (Akiva & Greenwald, 2019). Patients with chronic gastritis may not be able to absorb vitamin B_{12} because of diminished production of intrinsic factor by the stomach's parietal cells due to atrophy, which may lead to pernicious anemia (see Chapter 29) (Zayouna & Piper, 2018). Some patients with chronic gastritis have no symptoms (Marcus & Greenwald, 2019) (Table 40-1).

Assessment and Diagnostic Findings

The definitive diagnosis of gastritis is determined by an endoscopy and histologic examination of a tissue specimen obtained by biopsy (Akiva & Greenwald, 2019; Wehbi et al., 2019). A complete blood count (CBC) may be drawn to assess for anemia as a result of hemorrhage or pernicious anemia. Diagnostic measures for detecting *H. pylori* infection may be used and are discussed later in this chapter in the Peptic Ulcer Disease section.

TABLE 40-1	Clinical Manifestations of Acute and Chronic Gastritis	
	Acute Gastritis	**Chronic Gastritis**
Gastrointestinal Manifestations	• Anorexia • Epigastric pain (rapid onset) • Hematemesis • Hiccups • Melena or hematochezia • Nausea and vomiting	• Belching • Early satiety • Intolerance of spicy or fatty foods • Nausea and vomiting • Pyrosis • Sour taste in mouth • Vague epigastric discomfort relieved by eating
Systemic Manifestations	• Possible signs of shock	• Anemia • Fatigue

Adapted from Marcus, A. J., & Greenwald, D. (2019). Chronic gastritis. *Medscape.* Retrieved on 2/25/2020 at: www.emedicine.medscape.com/article/176156; Wehbi, M., Dacha, S., Sarver, G., et al. (2019). Acute gastritis. *Medscape.* Retrieved on 2/25/2020 at: www.emedicine.medscape.com/article/175909

Medical Management

The gastric mucosa is capable of repairing itself after an episode of acute gastritis. As a rule, the patient recovers in about 1 day, although the patient's appetite may be diminished for an additional 2 or 3 days. Acute gastritis is also managed by instructing the patient to refrain from alcohol and food until symptoms subside. When the patient can take nourishment by mouth, a nonirritating diet is recommended. If the symptoms persist, intravenous (IV) fluids may need to be given. If bleeding is present, management is similar to the procedures used to control upper GI tract hemorrhage discussed later in this chapter.

Therapy is supportive and may include nasogastric (NG) intubation, antacids, histamine-2 receptor antagonists (H_2 blockers) (e.g., famotidine, cimetidine), proton pump inhibitors (e.g., omeprazole, lansoprazole), and IV fluids (Wehbi et al., 2019). Fiberoptic endoscopy may be necessary. In extreme cases, emergency surgery may be required to remove gangrenous or perforated tissue. A gastric resection or a gastrojejunostomy (anastomosis of jejunum to stomach to detour around the pylorus) may be necessary to treat **gastric outlet obstruction,** also called *pyloric obstruction*, a narrowing of the pyloric orifice, which cannot be relieved by medical management.

Chronic gastritis is managed by modifying the patient's diet, promoting rest, reducing stress, recommending avoidance of alcohol and NSAIDs, and initiating medications that may include antacids, H_2 blockers, or proton pump inhibitors (Akiva & Greenwald, 2019). *H. pylori* may be treated with select drug combinations which typically include a proton pump inhibitor, antibiotics, and sometimes bismuth salts (Table 40-2).

Nursing Management

Reducing Anxiety

If the patient has ingested acids or alkalis, emergency measures may be necessary (see Chapter 67). The nurse offers supportive therapy to the patient and family during treatment and after the ingested acid or alkali has been neutralized or diluted. In some cases, the nurse may need to prepare the patient for additional diagnostic studies (endoscopies) or surgery. The patient may be anxious because of pain and planned treatment modalities. The nurse uses a calm approach to assess the patient and to answer all questions as completely as possible.

Promoting Optimal Nutrition

For acute gastritis, the nurse provides physical and emotional support and helps the patient manage the symptoms, which may include nausea, vomiting, and pyrosis. The patient should take no foods or fluids by mouth—possibly for a few days—until the acute symptoms subside, thus allowing the gastric mucosa to heal. If IV therapy is necessary, fluid intake and output are monitored, along with serum electrolyte values. After the symptoms subside, the nurse may offer the patient ice chips followed by clear liquids. Introducing solid food as soon as possible may provide adequate oral nutrition, decrease the need for IV therapy, and minimize irritation to the gastric mucosa. As food is introduced, the nurse evaluates and reports any symptoms that suggest a repeat episode of gastritis.

The nurse discourages the intake of caffeinated beverages, because caffeine is a central nervous system stimulant that

TABLE 40-2 Select Pharmacotherapy for Peptic Ulcer Disease and Gastritis

Pharmacologic Agent	Major Action	Key Nursing Considerations
Antibiotics		
Amoxicillin	A bactericidal antibiotic that assists with eradicating *H. pylori* bacteria in the gastric mucosa	• May cause abdominal pain and diarrhea • Should not be used in patients allergic to penicillin
Clarithromycin	Exerts bactericidal effects to eradicate *H. pylori* bacteria in the gastric mucosa	• May cause GI upset, headache, altered taste • Many drug–drug interactions (e.g., colchicine, lovastatin, warfarin); interacts with grapefruit juice
Metronidazole	A synthetic antibacterial and antiprotozoal agent that assists with eradicating *H. pylori* bacteria in the gastric mucosa when given with other antibiotics and proton pump inhibitors	• Should be given with meals to decrease GI upset; may cause anorexia and metallic taste • Patient should avoid alcohol; increases blood-thinning effects of warfarin
Tetracycline	Exerts bacteriostatic effects to eradicate *H. pylori* bacteria in the gastric mucosa	• May cause photosensitivity reaction; advise patient to use sunscreen • May cause GI upset • Must be used with caution in patients with renal or hepatic impairment • Milk or dairy products may reduce effectiveness
Antidiarrheal		
Bismuth subsalicylate	Suppresses *H. pylori* bacteria in the gastric mucosa and assists with healing of mucosal ulcers	• Given concurrently with antibiotics to eradicate *H. pylori* infection • Should be taken on empty stomach • May darken the bowel movements
H_2 Receptor Antagonists		
Cimetidine	Decreases amount of HCl produced by stomach by blocking action of histamine on histamine receptors of parietal cells in the stomach	• Least expensive of H_2 receptor antagonists • May cause confusion, agitation, or coma in older adults or those with renal or hepatic insufficiency • Long-term use may cause diarrhea, dizziness, and gynecomastia • Many drug–drug interactions (e.g., amiodarone, amitriptyline, benzodiazepines, metoprolol, nifedipine, phenytoin, warfarin)
Famotidine	Same as for cimetidine	• Best choice for patient who is critically ill because it is known to have the least risk of drug–drug interactions; does not alter liver metabolism • Prolonged half-life in patients with renal insufficiency • Short-term relief for GERD
Nizatidine	Same as for cimetidine	• Used for treatment of ulcers and GERD • Prolonged half-life in patients with renal insufficiency • May cause headache, dizziness, diarrhea, nausea/vomiting, GI upset, and urticaria
Proton Pump Inhibitors of Gastric Acid		
Esomeprazole	Decreases gastric acid secretion by slowing the H^+, K^+-ATPase pump on the surface of the parietal cells of the stomach	• Used mainly for treatment of duodenal ulcer disease and *H. pylori* infection • A delayed-release capsule that is to be swallowed whole and taken before meals
Lansoprazole	Same as for esomeprazole	• A delayed-release capsule that is to be swallowed whole and taken before meals
Omeprazole	Same as for esomeprazole	• A delayed-release capsule that is to be swallowed whole and taken before meals • May cause diarrhea, nausea, constipation, abdominal pain, vomiting, headache, or dizziness
Pantoprazole	Same as for esomeprazole	• A delayed-release tablet that is to be swallowed whole and taken before meals • May cause diarrhea and hyperglycemia, headache, abdominal pain, and abnormal liver function tests
Rabeprazole	Same as for esomeprazole	• A delayed-release tablet that is to be swallowed whole and taken without regard to meals; however, if used for duodenal ulcers give after meals and when used for *H. pylori* treatment, give with food. • May cause abdominal pain, diarrhea, nausea, and headache • Drug–drug interactions with digoxin, iron, and warfarin
Prostaglandin E_1 Analogue		
Misoprostol	Synthetic prostaglandin; protects the gastric mucosa from agents that cause ulcers; also increases mucus production and bicarbonate levels	• Used to prevent ulceration in patients using NSAIDs • Administer with food • May cause diarrhea and cramping (including uterine cramping) • Used mainly for the treatment of duodenal ulcers • Pregnancy category X (i.e., should not be taken by a pregnant woman as it can soften the cervix and result in miscarriage or premature labor.)
Sucralfate	Creates a viscous substance in the presence of gastric acid that forms a protective barrier, binding to the surface of the ulcer, and prevents digestion by pepsin	• Should be taken without food but with water 1 h prior to meals • Other medications should be taken 2 h before or after this medication • Many drug–drug interactions (e.g., digoxin, phenytoin, warfarin) • May cause constipation or nausea

CNS, central nervous system; GERD, gastroesophageal reflux disease; GI, gastrointestinal; H_2, histamine-2; HCl, hydrochloric acid; H^+, K^+-ATPase, hydrogen–potassium adenosine triphosphatase; NSAIDs, nonsteroidal anti-inflammatory drugs.
Adapted from Karch, A. M. (2018). *Lippincott nursing drug guide.* Philadelphia, PA: Lippincott Williams & Wilkins.

increases gastric activity and pepsin secretion. The nurse also discourages alcohol use. Discouraging cigarette smoking is important. The level of nicotine measured in gastric acid can be 10 times greater than arterial blood and 80 times greater than venous blood. Nicotine will increase secretion of gastric acid and will also interfere with the mucosal barrier in the GI tract (Berkowitz, Schultz, Salazar, et al., 2018). When appropriate, the nurse initiates and refers the patient for alcohol counseling and smoking cessation programs.

Promoting Fluid Balance

Daily fluid intake and output are monitored to detect early signs of dehydration (minimal fluid intake of 1.5 L/day, urine output of less than 1 mL/kg/h). If food and oral fluids are withheld, IV fluids (3 L/day) usually are prescribed and a record of fluid intake plus caloric value (1 L of 5% dextrose in water = 170 calories of carbohydrate) needs to be maintained. Electrolyte values (sodium, potassium, chloride) are assessed every 24 hours to detect any imbalance (see Chapter 10).

The nurse must always be alert to any indicators of hemorrhagic gastritis, which include **hematemesis** (vomiting of blood), tachycardia, and hypotension. All stools should be examined for the presence of frank or occult bleeding. If these occur, the primary provider should be notified, and the patient's vital signs are monitored as the patient's condition warrants. Guidelines for managing upper GI tract bleeding are discussed later in this chapter.

Relieving Pain

Measures to help relieve pain include instructing the patient to avoid foods and beverages that may irritate the gastric mucosa as well as the correct use of medications to relieve chronic gastritis. The nurse must regularly assess the patient's level of pain and the extent of comfort achieved through the use of medications and avoidance of irritating substances.

Promoting Home, Community-Based, and Transitional Care

 Educating Patients About Self-Care

The nurse evaluates the patient's knowledge about gastritis and develops an individualized education plan that includes information about stress management, diet, and medications (see Table 40-2). Dietary instructions take into account the patient's daily caloric needs as well as cultural aspects of food preferences and patterns of eating. The nurse and patient review foods and other substances to be avoided (e.g., spicy, irritating, or highly seasoned foods; caffeine; nicotine; alcohol). Consultation with a dietitian may be recommended (Chart 40-1).

Providing information about prescribed medications, which may include antacids, H_2 blockers, or proton pump inhibitors, may help the patient to better understand why these medications assist in recovery and prevent recurrence. The importance of completing the medication regimen as prescribed to eradicate *H. pylori* infection must be reinforced to the patient and caregiver (see later discussion).

Continuing and Transitional Care

The nurse reinforces previous education and conducts ongoing assessment of the patient's symptoms and progress. Patients with malabsorption of vitamin B_{12} need information about lifelong vitamin B_{12} injections; the nurse may instruct a family member or caregiver how to administer the injections or make arrangements for the patient to receive the injections from the primary provider. Finally, the nurse emphasizes the importance of keeping follow-up appointments with the primary provider.

Peptic Ulcer Disease

Peptic ulcer disease affects approximately 4.6 million Americans annually, with the peak onset between 30 and 60 years of age (Anand, 2020; Norris, 2019). A peptic ulcer may be referred to as a gastric, duodenal, or esophageal ulcer, depending on its location. A peptic ulcer is an excavation (hollowed-out area) that forms in the mucosa of the stomach, in the **pylorus** (the opening between the stomach and duodenum), in the **duodenum** (the first portion of the small intestine, between the stomach and the jejunum), or in the esophagus. Erosion of a circumscribed area of mucosa is the cause (Fig. 40-2). This erosion may extend as deeply as the muscle layers or through the muscle to the **peritoneum** (thin membrane that lines the inside of the wall of the abdomen) (Norris, 2019).

Peptic ulcers are more likely to occur in the duodenum than in the stomach. As a rule, they occur alone but they may

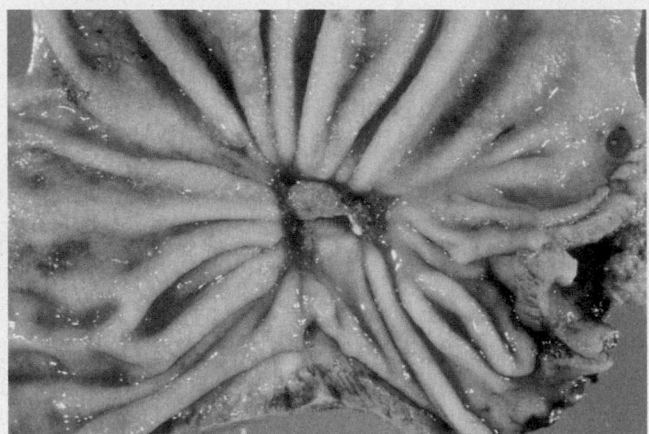

Figure 40-2 • Deep peptic ulcer. Reprinted with permission from Strayer, D. S., Saffitz, J. E., & Rubin, E. (2015). *Rubin's pathology: Mechanisms of human disease* (8th ed., Fig. 19-23). Philadelphia, PA: Lippincott Williams & Wilkins.

occur in multiples. Chronic gastric ulcers tend to occur in the lesser curvature of the stomach, near the pylorus. Esophageal ulcers occur as a result of the backward flow of HCl from the stomach into the esophagus (gastroesophageal reflux disease [GERD]).

Women have 8% to 11% and men have an 11% to 14% lifetime risk of developing peptic ulcers (Anand, 2020). The rates of peptic ulcer disease among middle-age men have diminished over the past several decades, whereas the rates among older adults have increased, particularly among women (Anand, 2020). Those who are 65 years and older present to both outpatient and inpatient settings for treatment of peptic ulcers more than any other age group. This trend may be explained, at least in part, by higher rates of NSAID use and *H. pylori* infections in older adult populations (Anand, 2020).

In the past, stress and anxiety were thought to be causes of peptic ulcers, but research has documented that most peptic ulcers result from infection with *H. pylori*, which may be acquired through ingestion of food and water. Person-to-person transmission of the bacteria also occurs through close contact and exposure to emesis. Although *H. pylori* infection is common in the United States, most infected people do not develop ulcers. It is not known why *H. pylori* infection does not cause ulcers in all people, but most likely the predisposition to ulcer formation depends on certain factors, such as the type of *H. pylori* and other as yet unknown factors (Anand, 2020; Norris, 2019; Santacroce & Bhutani, 2019).

The use of NSAIDs, such as ibuprofen and aspirin, represents a major risk factor for peptic ulcers. Studies report that both NSAIDs and *H. pylori* impair the protective gastric mucosa, and the failure of the GI tract to repair the mucosa may result in ulceration (Anand, 2020; Norris, 2019). It is believed that smoking and alcohol consumption may be risks, although the evidence is inconclusive (Anand, 2020; NIDDK, 2020c).

Familial tendency also may be a significant predisposing factor. People with blood type O are more susceptible to the development of peptic ulcers than are those with blood type A, B, or AB. There also is an association between peptic ulcer disease and chronic obstructive pulmonary disease, cirrhosis

of the liver, chronic kidney disease, and autoimmune disorders (Anand, 2020).

Peptic ulcer disease is also associated with Zollinger-Ellison syndrome (ZES). ZES is a rare condition in which benign or malignant tumors form in the pancreas and duodenum that secrete excessive amounts of the hormone gastrin (NIDDK, 2020d; Roy, 2019). The excessive amount of gastrin results in extreme gastric hyperacidity and severe peptic ulcer disease. While the exact cause of ZES is unknown, 25% to 30% of cases are linked to an inherited, genetic condition called multiple endocrine neoplasia, type 1 (MEN-1) (NIDDK, 2020b; Norris, 2019).

Pathophysiology

Peptic ulcers occur mainly in the gastroduodenal mucosa because this tissue cannot withstand the digestive action of gastric acid (HCl) and pepsin. The erosion is caused by the increased concentration or activity of acid–pepsin or by decreased resistance of the normally protective mucosal barrier. A damaged mucosa cannot secrete enough mucus to act as a barrier against normal digestive juices. Exposure of the mucosa to gastric acid (HCl), pepsin, and other irritating agents (e.g., NSAIDs or *H. pylori*) leads to inflammation, injury, and subsequent erosion of the mucosa. Patients with duodenal ulcers secrete more acid than normal, whereas patients with gastric ulcers tend to secrete normal or decreased levels of acid. When the mucosal barrier is impaired, even normal or decreased levels of HCl may result in the formation of peptic ulcers.

The use of NSAIDs inhibits prostaglandin synthesis, which is associated with a disruption of the normally protective mucosal barrier. Damage to the mucosal barrier also results in decreased resistance to bacteria, and thus infection from *H. pylori* bacteria may occur (Anand, 2020; Norris, 2019).

ZES is suspected when a patient has several peptic ulcers or an ulcer that is resistant to standard medical therapy. It is identified by the following: hypersecretion of gastrin, duodenal ulcers, and gastrinomas (islet cell tumors) in the pancreas or duodenum. More than 80% of gastrinomas are found in the "gastric triangle," which encompasses the cystic and common bile ducts, the second and third portions of the duodenum, and the junction of the head and body of the pancreas. Most gastrinomas tend to grow slowly; however, more than 50% of these tumors are malignant (Bonheur & Nachimuthu, 2019). The patient with ZES may experience epigastric pain, pyrosis, diarrhea, and **steatorrhea** (fatty stools). Patients with ZES associated with MEN-1 syndrome may have coexisting pituitary or parathyroid tumors. ZES-associated MEN-1 syndrome is diagnosed with hyperparathyroidism; therefore, patients may exhibit signs of hypercalcemia for several years before MEN-1 is diagnosed (NIDDK, 2020b).

Stress ulcer is the term given to the acute mucosal ulceration of the duodenal or gastric area that occurs after physiologically stressful events, such as burns, shock, sepsis, and multiple organ dysfunction syndrome (Clarke et al., 2020). Stress ulcers, which are clinically different from peptic ulcers, are most common in patients following significant burn injuries, traumatic brain injury, or who require mechanical ventilation. Stress ulcers are believed to be a result of ischemia to gastric mucosa and alterations in the mucosa barrier (Clarke et al., 2020; Norris, 2019). When the patient recovers, the lesions are reversed. This pattern is typical of stress ulceration.

Differences of opinion exist as to the actual cause of mucosal ulceration in stress ulcers. Usually, the ulceration results from a disruption of the normally protective mucosal barrier and decreased mucosal blood flow (ischemia). Mucosal ischemia results in the reflux of duodenal contents into the stomach, which increases exposure of the unprotected gastric mucosa to the digestive effects of gastric acid (HCl) and pepsin (Anand, 2020; Clarke et al., 2020; Norris, 2019). The combination of mucosal ischemia and increased gastric acid and pepsin exposure creates an ideal climate for ulceration.

Specific types of ulcers that result from stressful conditions include Curling ulcers and Cushing ulcers. Curling ulcer is frequently observed after extensive burn injuries and often involves the antrum of the stomach or the duodenum (Anand, 2020). Cushing ulcer is common in patients with a traumatic head injury, stroke, brain tumor, or following intracranial surgery. Cushing ulcer is thought to be caused by increased intracranial pressure, which results in overstimulation of the vagal nerve and an increased secretion of gastric acid (HCl) (Norris, 2019). Cushing ulcers are typically deep, single ulcerations and have increased risk of perforation (Anand, 2020).

Clinical Manifestations

Symptoms of peptic ulcer disease may last for a few days, weeks, or months and may disappear only to reappear, often without an identifiable cause. Many patients with peptic ulcers have no signs or symptoms. These *silent peptic ulcers* most commonly occur in older adults and those taking aspirin and other NSAIDs (Anand, 2020).

As a rule, the patient with an ulcer complains of dull, gnawing pain or a burning sensation in the mid epigastrium or the back. There are few clinical manifestations that differentiate gastric ulcers from duodenal ulcers; however, classically, the pain associated with gastric ulcers most commonly occurs immediately after eating, whereas the pain associated with duodenal ulcers most commonly occurs 2 to 3 hours after meals. In addition, approximately 50% to 80% of patients with duodenal ulcers awake with pain during the night, whereas 30% to 40% of patients with gastric ulcers voice this type of complaint. Patients with duodenal ulcers are more likely to express relief of pain after eating or after taking an antacid than patients with gastric ulcers (Anand, 2020).

Other nonspecific symptoms of either gastric ulcers or duodenal ulcers may include pyrosis, vomiting, constipation or diarrhea, and bleeding. These symptoms are often accompanied by sour eructation (burping), which is common when the patient's stomach is empty.

Although vomiting is rare in an uncomplicated peptic ulcer, it may be a symptom of a complication of an ulcer. It results from gastric outlet obstruction, caused by either muscular spasm of the pylorus or mechanical obstruction from scarring or acute swelling of the inflamed mucous membrane adjacent to the ulcer. Vomiting may or may not be preceded by nausea; usually, it follows a bout of severe pain and bloating, which is relieved by vomiting. Emesis may contain undigested food eaten many hours earlier. Constipation or diarrhea may occur, probably as a result of diet and medications.

The patient with bleeding peptic ulcers may present with evidence of GI bleeding, such as hematemesis or the passage of melena (Anand, 2020). Approximately 20% of patients with bleeding peptic ulcers do not experience abdominal pain at the time of diagnosis (Norris, 2019). Peptic ulcer perforation results in the sudden onset of signs and symptoms. The patient often reports severe, sharp upper abdominal pain, which may be referred to the shoulder; extreme abdominal tenderness; and nausea or vomiting. Hypotension and tachycardia may occur, indicating the onset of shock (Azer, 2018).

Assessment and Diagnostic Findings

A physical examination may reveal pain, epigastric tenderness, or abdominal distention. Upper endoscopy is the preferred diagnostic procedure because it allows direct visualization of inflammatory changes, ulcers, and lesions. Through endoscopy, a biopsy of the gastric mucosa and any suspicious lesions can be obtained. Endoscopy may reveal lesions that, because of their size or location, are not evident on x-ray studies. *H. pylori* infection may be determined by endoscopy and histologic examination of a tissue specimen obtained by biopsy, or a rapid urease test of the biopsy specimen. Other less invasive diagnostic measures for detecting *H. pylori* include serologic testing for antibodies against the *H. pylori* antigen, stool antigen test, and urea breath test (Anand, 2020).

The patient who has a bleeding peptic ulcer may require periodic CBCs to determine the extent of blood loss and whether or not blood transfusions are advisable (see Chapter 28). Stools may be tested periodically until they are negative for occult blood. Gastric secretory studies are of value in diagnosing ZES and **achlorhydria** (lack of HCl), hypochlorhydria (low levels of HCl), or hyperchlorhydria (high levels of HCl).

Medical Management

Once the diagnosis is established, the patient is informed that the condition can be managed. Recurrence may develop; however, peptic ulcers treated with antibiotics to eradicate *H. pylori* have a lower recurrence rate than those not treated with antibiotics. The goals are to eradicate *H. pylori* as indicated and to manage gastric acidity. Methods used include medications, lifestyle changes, and surgical intervention.

Pharmacologic Therapy

Currently, the most commonly used therapy for peptic ulcers is a combination of antibiotics, proton pump inhibitors, and sometimes bismuth salts that suppress or eradicate *H. pylori*. Recommended combination drug therapy is typically prescribed for 10 to 14 days and may include triple therapy with two antibiotics (e.g., metronidazole or amoxicillin and clarithromycin) plus a proton pump inhibitor (e.g., lansoprazole, omeprazole, or rabeprazole), or quadruple therapy with two antibiotics (metronidazole and tetracycline) plus a proton pump inhibitor and bismuth salts (Anand, 2020; Marcus & Greenwald, 2019). Research is currently being conducted to develop a vaccine against *H. pylori* (Liu, Zhong, Chen, et al., 2020).

H_2 blockers and proton pump inhibitors that reduce gastric acid secretion are used to treat ulcers not associated with *H. pylori* infection. Table 40-3 provides information about the medication regimens for peptic ulcer disease.

TABLE 40-3	Drug Regimens for Peptic Ulcer Disease	
Indications	**Drug Regimen**	**Nursing Considerations**
Ulcer healing	**H$_2$ receptor antagonist** Cimetidine 400 mg bid or 800 mg at bedtime Famotidine 20 mg bid or 40 mg at bedtime Nizatidine 150 mg bid or 300 mg at bedtime **PPIs:** Esomeprazole 40 mg daily Lansoprazole 30 mg daily Omeprazole 20 mg daily Pantoprazole 40 mg daily Rabeprazole 20 mg daily	Should be used for 6–8 wks for complete peptic ulcer healing; patients who are at high risk require a maintenance dose for 1 yr Should be used for 4–8 wks for complete peptic ulcer healing; patients who are at high risk require a maintenance dose for 1 yr
H. pylori infection	*Quadruple therapy* with bismuth subsalicylate 525 mg qid, plus tetracycline 500 mg qid, plus metronidazole 500 mg bid, plus a PPI daily for 10–14 days *Alternate therapy* with clarithromycin 500 mg bid, amoxicillin 1 g bid, metronidazole 500 mg bid, plus PPI for 10–14 days	Efficacy of therapy is approximately 85% qid dosing may decrease adherence to the regimen
Prophylactic therapy for NSAID ulcers	Peptic ulcer healing doses of PPIs (above) Misoprostol 100–200 mcg qid	Prevents recurrent ulceration in approximately 80–90% of patients; qid dosing may decrease adherence to the regimen Pregnancy category X (i.e., should not be taken by a pregnant woman as it can soften the cervix and result in miscarriage or premature labor.)

bid, two times a day; H$_2$, histamine-2; NSAID, nonsteroidal anti-inflammatory drug; PPIs, proton pump inhibitors; qid, four times a day.
Adapted from Anand, B. S. (2020). Peptic ulcer disease. *Medscape.* Retrieved on 4/29/2020 at: www.emedicine.medscape.com/article/181753

The patient is advised to adhere to and complete the medication regimen to ensure complete healing of the ulcer. The patient also is advised to avoid the use of NSAIDs. Because most patients become symptom free within a week, the nurse stresses to the patient the importance of following the prescribed regimen so that the healing process can continue uninterrupted and the return of chronic ulcer symptoms can be prevented. Maintenance dosages of H$_2$ blockers are usually recommended for 1 year.

For patients with ZES, hypersecretion of gastrin stimulates the release of gastric acid (HCl), which may be controlled with proton pump inhibitors. Octreotide, a medication that suppresses gastrin levels, also may be prescribed (Daniels, Khalili, Morano, et al., 2019). Patients with ZES will require periodic endoscopy to evaluate the effectiveness of medication therapy.

Patients at high risk for stress ulcers (e.g., patients who are mechanically ventilated for more than 48 hours) may be treated prophylactically with either H$_2$ blockers or proton pump inhibitors, and cytoprotective agents (e.g., misoprostol, sucralfate) because of the increased risk of upper GI tract hemorrhage (Clarke et al., 2020; Young, Bagshaw, Forbes, et al., 2020).

▶ *Quality and Safety Nursing Alert*

Misoprostol should not be taken by a pregnant woman as it can soften the cervix and result in miscarriage or premature labor. The nurse should be aware of this risk when caring for women of childbearing age.

Smoking Cessation

Smoking decreases the secretion of bicarbonate from the pancreas into the duodenum, resulting in increased acidity of the duodenum. Continued smoking is also associated with delayed healing of peptic ulcers (Berkowitz et al., 2018; Kennedy & Winter, 2017). Therefore, the patient is encouraged to stop smoking. Refer to Chapter 23 for information on how the nurse may promote cessation of tobacco use.

Dietary Modification

The intent of dietary modification for patients with peptic ulcers is to avoid oversecretion of acid and hypermotility in the GI tract. These can be minimized by avoiding extremes of temperature in food and beverages and overstimulation from the consumption of alcohol, coffee (including decaffeinated coffee, which also stimulates acid secretion), and other caffeinated beverages. In addition, an effort is made to neutralize acid by eating three regular meals a day. Small, frequent feedings are not necessary as long as an antacid or an H$_2$ blocker is taken. Diet compatibility becomes an individual matter: The patient eats foods that are tolerated and avoids those that produce pain.

Surgical Management

The introduction of antibiotics to eradicate *H. pylori* and of proton pump inhibitors as treatment for ulcers results in ulcer healing in approximately 85% to 90% of patients (Anand, 2020). However, surgery is usually recommended for patients with intractable ulcers (those failing to heal after 12 to 16 weeks of medical treatment), life-threatening hemorrhage, perforation, or obstruction and for those with ZES that is unresponsive to medications (Anand, 2020; Bonheur & Nachimuthu, 2019; Upchurch, 2019). Surgical procedures include vagotomy, with or without **pyloroplasty** (transecting nerves that stimulate acid secretion and opening the pylorus), and **antrectomy**, which is removal of the pyloric (antrum) portion of the stomach with anastomosis (surgical connection) to either the duodenum (gastroduodenostomy or Billroth I) or jejunum (gastrojejunostomy or Billroth II) (Table 40-4).

TABLE 40-4	Surgical Procedures for Peptic Ulcer Disease	
Operation	**Description**	**Adverse Effects**
Vagotomy Vagotomy	Severing of the vagus nerve. Decreases gastric acid by diminishing cholinergic stimulation to the parietal cells, making them less responsive to gastrin. May be performed via an open surgical approach or laparoscopy. May be performed to reduce gastric acid secretion. A drainage type of procedure (see pyloroplasty) is usually performed to assist with gastric emptying (because there is total denervation of the stomach).	Some patients experience problems with feeling of fullness, dumping syndrome, diarrhea, and gastritis.
Truncal vagotomy	Severs the right and left vagus nerves as they enter the stomach at the distal part of the esophagus; most commonly used to decrease acid secretions.	Some patients experience problems with feeling of fullness, dumping syndrome, diarrhea, or constipation.
Selective vagotomy	Severs vagal innervation to the stomach but maintains innervation to the rest of the abdominal organs.	Fewer associated adverse effects than with truncal vagotomy.
Proximal (parietal cell) gastric vagotomy without drainage	Denervates acid-secreting parietal cells but preserves vagal innervation to the gastric antrum and pylorus.	No associated dumping syndrome.
Pyloroplasty Pylorus—note longitudinal incision Vertical suture	Longitudinal incision is made into the pylorus and transversely sutured closed to enlarge the outlet and relax the muscle; usually accompanies truncal and selective vagotomies.	See adverse effects associated with truncal and selective vagotomies, as appropriate.
Antrectomy Billroth I (gastroduodenostomy) Fundus Body Antrectomy Duodenum Duodenal anastomosis	Removal of the lower portion of the antrum of the stomach (which contains the cells that secrete gastrin) as well as a small portion of the duodenum and pylorus. The remaining segment is anastomosed to the duodenum. May be performed in conjunction with a truncal vagotomy.	Patients may have problems with feeling of fullness, dumping syndrome, and diarrhea.

TABLE 40-4	Surgical Procedures for Peptic Ulcer Disease (continued)	
Operation	**Description**	**Adverse Effects**
Billroth II (gastrojejunostomy) Fundus, Jejunum, Body, Jejunal anastomosis	Removal of lower portion (antrum) of stomach with anastomosis to jejunum. *Dotted lines* show portion removed (antrectomy). A duodenal stump remains and is oversewn.	Patients frequently have associated dumping syndrome, anemia, weight loss, and malabsorption.

Surgery may be performed using a traditional open abdominal approach (requiring a long abdominal incision) or through the use of laparoscopy (only requiring small abdominal incisions). Laparoscopy is a type of minimally invasive surgery that involves the indirect visualization of the abdominal cavity through the use of a laparoscope (a thin flexible tube) attached to a camera. The laparoscope is placed into the abdomen through small "keyhole" incisions (0.5 to 1.5 cm in length). Laparoscopy has been associated with decreased postoperative bleeding, pain, infection, respiratory complications, and recovery time (Davenport, Ueland, Kumar, et al., 2019). The choice of using an open abdominal approach or laparoscopy is determined by the surgeon's preference and expertise as well as clinical factors, such as the patient's current health status; the presence of coexisting medical conditions; and a history of previous abdominal surgery.

Follow-Up Care

Recurrence of peptic ulcer disease within 1 year may be prevented with the prophylactic use of H_2 blockers taken at a reduced dose. Not all patients require maintenance therapy; it may be prescribed only for those with two or three recurrences per year, those who have had a complication such as bleeding or gastric outlet obstruction, or those for whom gastric surgery poses too high a risk. The likelihood of recurrence is reduced if the patient avoids smoking, coffee (including decaffeinated coffee) and other caffeinated beverages, alcohol, and ulcerogenic medications (e.g., NSAIDs).

NURSING PROCESS

The Patient with Peptic Ulcer Disease

Assessment

The nurse asks the patient to describe the pain, its pattern and whether or not it occurs predictably (e.g., after meals, during the night), and strategies used to relieve it (e.g., food, antacids).

If the patient reports a recent history of vomiting, the nurse determines how often emesis has occurred and notes important characteristics of the vomitus: Is it bright red, does it resemble coffee grounds, or is there undigested food from previous meals? Has the patient noted any bloody or tarry stools?

The nurse also asks the patient to list their usual food intake for a 72-h period. Lifestyle and other habits are a concern as well. For example, do they smoke cigarettes? If yes, how many? Do they use any type of electronic nicotine delivery systems (ENDS)? If yes, what type and how often? Does the patient ingest alcohol? If yes, how much and how often? Are NSAIDs used? Is there a family history of ulcer disease?

The nurse assesses the patient's vital signs and reports tachycardia and hypotension, which may indicate anemia from GI bleeding. The stool is tested for occult blood, and a physical examination, including palpation of the abdomen for localized tenderness, is performed.

Diagnosis

NURSING DIAGNOSES

Based on the assessment data, nursing diagnoses may include the following:
- Acute pain associated with the effect of gastric acid secretion on damaged tissue
- Anxiety associated with an acute illness
- Impaired nutritional intake associated with changes in diet

COLLABORATIVE PROBLEMS/POTENTIAL COMPLICATIONS

Potential complications may include the following:
- Hemorrhage
- Perforation
- Penetration
- Gastric outlet obstruction

Planning and Goals

The goals for the patient may include relief of pain, reduced anxiety, maintenance of nutritional requirements, and absence of complications.

Nursing Interventions

RELIEVING PAIN

Pain relief can be achieved with prescribed medications. The patient should avoid NSAIDs, aspirin in particular, as well as alcohol. In addition, meals should be eaten at regularly paced intervals in a relaxed setting. Medications prescribed to treat the peptic ulcer should provide relief of ulcer-associated pain. Some patients benefit from learning relaxation techniques to help manage stress and pain.

REDUCING ANXIETY

The nurse assesses the patient's level of anxiety. Explaining diagnostic tests and administering medications as scheduled help reduce anxiety. The nurse interacts with the patient in a relaxed manner; helps identify stressors; and explains various coping techniques and relaxation methods, such as biofeedback, hypnosis, or behavior modification. The patient's family is also encouraged to participate in care and to provide emotional support.

MAINTAINING OPTIMAL NUTRITIONAL STATUS

The nurse assesses the patient for malnutrition and weight loss. After recovery from an acute phase of peptic ulcer disease, the patient is advised about the importance of adhering to the medication regimen and dietary restrictions.

MONITORING AND MANAGING POTENTIAL COMPLICATIONS

Hemorrhage. Gastritis and hemorrhage from peptic ulcer are the two most common causes of upper GI tract bleeding (which may also occur with esophageal varices, as discussed in Chapter 43). Hemorrhage in patients with duodenal ulcers is associated with an approximately 5% mortality rate (Anand, 2020). Bleeding peptic ulcers account for 27% to 40% of all upper GI bleeds and it may be manifested by hematemesis or melena (Anand, 2020; Upchurch, 2019). The vomited blood can be bright red, or it can have a dark coffee grounds appearance from the oxidation of hemoglobin to methemoglobin. When the hemorrhage is large (2000 to 3000 mL), most of the blood is vomited. Because large quantities of blood may be lost quickly, immediate correction of blood loss may be required to prevent hemorrhagic shock. When the hemorrhage is small, much or all of the blood is passed in the stools, which appear tarry black because of the digested hemoglobin. Management depends on the amount of blood lost and the rate of bleeding.

The nurse assesses the patient for faintness or dizziness and nausea, which may precede or accompany bleeding. The nurse must monitor vital signs frequently and evaluate the patient for tachycardia, hypotension, and tachypnea. Other nursing interventions include monitoring the hemoglobin and hematocrit, testing the stool for gross or occult blood, and recording hourly urinary output to detect anuria or oliguria (absence of or decreased urine production).

Many times, the bleeding from a peptic ulcer stops spontaneously; however, the incidence of recurrent bleeding is high. Because bleeding can be fatal, the cause and severity of the hemorrhage must be identified quickly, and the blood loss treated to prevent hemorrhagic shock. The nurse monitors the patient carefully so that bleeding can be detected quickly. Patients suspected of having an ulcer who present with symptoms of acute GI bleeding should undergo evaluation with endoscopy within 12 h to confirm the diagnosis and allow targeted endoscopic interventions (Upchurch, 2019). These endoscopic interventions may include injecting the bleeding site with epinephrine or alcohol, or cauterizing the site, or clipping the ulcer, all in efforts to stop the bleeding (Anand, 2020; Upchurch, 2019). Arteriography with embolization may be needed if therapeutic endoscopy fails to control the bleeding (Spiliopoulos, Inchingolo, Lucatelli, et al., 2018). If bleeding cannot be managed by these methods, surgery may be indicated, in which the area of the ulcer is removed, or the bleeding vessels are ligated. Many patients also undergo procedures (e.g., vagotomy and pyloroplasty, gastrectomy) aimed at controlling the underlying cause of the ulcers (see Table 40-4).

For patients who are not candidates for surgery or for those with persistent, severe bleeding despite medical and endoscopic treatment, arteriography with embolization may be indicated (Spiliopoulos et al., 2018). Arteriography with embolization is more commonly referred to as *Transcatheter Arterial Embolization* (TAE). TAE is an interventional radiologic procedure in which a catheter is placed percutaneously (through the skin) into an artery (e.g., femoral or brachial artery) and is advanced under use of fluoroscopy to the site of the bleeding peptic ulcer. An embolic agent is then delivered via the catheter, which selectively occludes blood flow to the bleeding vessel(s), and thus stops bleeding of the peptic ulcer. Common embolic agents used include metallic coils (a small metal device) and ethylene vinyl alcohol copolymer (Loffroy, Midulla, Falvo, et al., 2018; Spiliopoulos et al., 2018).

The patient with GI bleeding may require treatment for hemorrhagic shock. If that is the case, then the collaborative treatment guidelines described in Chapter 11 must be followed (e.g., hemodynamic monitoring, IV line insertion for fluid resuscitation, blood component therapy). In addition, other related nursing and collaborative interventions may include inserting an NG tube to distinguish fresh blood from material resembling coffee grounds, to aid in the removal of clots and acid through administering a saline lavage, to prevent nausea and vomiting through suction decompression of gastric contents, and to provide a means of monitoring further bleeding.

Perforation and Penetration. Perforation is the erosion of the ulcer through the gastric **serosa** (thin membrane covering the outer surface of the stomach) into the peritoneal cavity without warning. It is an abdominal emergency and requires immediate surgery. Perforation occurs more commonly with duodenal ulcers than it does with gastric ulcers; however, in both cases, it is a very serious complication that can result in sepsis or multiorgan failure (Azer, 2018; Norris, 2019). Penetration is erosion of the ulcer through the gastric serosa into adjacent structures such as the pancreas, biliary tract, or gastrohepatic **omentum** (membranous fold of the peritoneum). Symptoms of penetration include back and epigastric pain not relieved by medications that were effective in the past. Like perforation, penetration usually requires surgical intervention.

Signs and symptoms of perforation include the following:

- Sudden, severe upper abdominal pain (persisting and increasing in intensity); pain may be referred to the shoulders, especially the right shoulder, because of irritation of the phrenic nerve in the diaphragm
- Vomiting
- Collapse (fainting)
- Extremely tender and rigid (boardlike) abdomen
- Hypotension and tachycardia, indicating shock

Because chemical peritonitis develops within a few hours of perforation and is followed by bacterial peritonitis, the perforation must be closed as quickly as possible and the abdominal cavity lavaged of stomach or intestinal contents. In some patients, it may be safe and advisable to perform surgery to treat the ulcer disease in addition to suturing the perforation.

During surgery and postoperatively, the stomach contents are drained by means of an NG tube. The nurse monitors fluid and electrolyte balance and assesses the patient for localized infection or peritonitis (increased temperature, abdominal pain, paralytic ileus, increased or absent bowel sounds, abdominal distention). Antibiotic therapy is given as prescribed.

Gastric Outlet Obstruction. Peptic ulcer disease is the leading benign (noncancerous) cause of gastric outlet obstruction (Castellanos & Podolsky, 2020). Gastric outlet obstruction occurs when the area distal to the pyloric sphincter becomes scarred and stenosed from spasm or edema or from scar tissue that forms when an ulcer alternately heals and breaks down. The patient may have nausea and vomiting, constipation, epigastric fullness, anorexia, and, later, weight loss.

In treating the patient with gastric outlet obstruction, the first consideration is to insert an NG tube to decompress the stomach. Confirmation that obstruction is the cause of the discomfort is accomplished by assessing the amount of fluid aspirated from the NG tube. A residual of more than 400 mL suggests obstruction. Usually, an upper GI study or endoscopy is performed to confirm gastric outlet obstruction. Decompression of the stomach and management of extracellular fluid volume and electrolyte balances may improve the patient's condition and avert the need for surgical intervention. Balloon dilation of the pylorus via endoscopy may be beneficial. If the obstruction is unrelieved by medical management, surgery (in the form of a vagotomy and antrectomy or gastrojejunostomy and vagotomy) may be required.

PROMOTING HOME, COMMUNITY-BASED, AND TRANSITIONAL CARE

Educating Patients About Self-Care. The nurse educates the patient about the factors that relieve and those that aggravate the condition. The nurse reviews information about medications to be taken at home, including name, dosage, frequency, and possible side effects, stressing the importance of continuing to take medications even after signs and symptoms have decreased or subsided (Chart 40-2). The patient is instructed to avoid medications and foods that exacerbate symptoms (e.g., NSAIDs, alcohol). If relevant, the nurse also informs the patient about the irritant effects of smoking on the ulcer and provides information about smoking cessation programs.

Continuing and Transitional Care. The nurse reinforces the importance of follow-up care; the need to report recurrence of symptoms; and the need for treating possible problems that occur after surgery, such as intolerance to specific foods. The patient and family are reminded of the importance of participating in health promotion activities and recommended health screening.

Evaluation

Expected patient outcomes may include:
1. Reports freedom from pain between meals and at night
2. Reports feeling less anxious
3. Maintains weight
4. Demonstrates knowledge of self-care activities
   a. Avoids irritating foods and beverages (alcohol) and medications such as NSAIDs, particularly aspirin
   b. Takes medications as prescribed
5. No evidence of complications (e.g., hemorrhage, perforation or penetration, gastric outlet obstruction)

Gastric Cancer

According to the American Cancer Society (ACS, 2020b), an estimated 27,000 Americans were expected to be diagnosed with gastric cancer in 2020, and an estimated 11,000 deaths from the disease were expected to occur that year. Gastric cancer is a more common diagnosis among older adults, with the mean age at diagnosis of 68 years (ACS, 2020b). Men have a higher incidence of gastric cancer than women. Hispanic Americans, African Americans, and Asian/Pacific

---

Chart 40-2 · HOME CARE CHECKLIST
The Patient with Peptic Ulcer Disease

At the completion of education, the patient and/or caregiver will be able to:

- State the impact of peptic ulcer disease on physiologic functioning, ADLs, IADLs, roles, relationships, and spirituality.
- Explain the importance of and necessity for adherence with prescribed medication regimen.
- Demonstrate methods of keeping track of the medication regimen and storage of the prescribed medications and use reminders such as beepers and/or pillboxes.
- State the name, dose, side effects, frequency, and schedule for all medications.
- Identify foods and other substances to avoid (e.g., food and drinks with extreme temperatures, coffee and other caffeinated beverages, alcohol, foods that were not tolerated in the past).
- Identify side effects and complications that should be reported to primary provider:

- Hemorrhage—cool skin, confusion, increased heart rate, labored breathing, blood in stool (either bright red or tarry black)
- Penetration and perforation—severe abdominal pain, rigid and tender abdomen, vomiting, elevated temperature, increased heart rate
- Gastric outlet obstruction—nausea and vomiting, distended abdomen, abdominal pain
- State how to reach primary provider with questions or complications.
- State time and date of follow-up appointments and testing.
- Identify the need for health promotion (e.g., cessation of use of tobacco products, stress management), disease prevention and screening activities.

ADLs, activities of daily living; IADLs, instrumental activities of daily living.

Islanders are at higher risk of developing gastric cancer than Caucasian Americans.

Worldwide, gastric cancer is the fifth most common cancer diagnosis, with the highest incidence in Eastern and Central Asia (e.g., Republic of Korea, Mongolia, and Japan) and Latin America (Rawla & Barsouk, 2019). Countries with high incidence of gastric cancer, such as Japan, have implemented mass screening programs, which resulted in earlier diagnosis (at a more curable stage of disease), and may have reduced the number of deaths from gastric cancer (ACS, 2020b).

Diet appears to be a significant risk factor for the development of gastric cancer. A diet high in smoked, salted, or pickled foods and low in fruits and vegetables may increase the risk of gastric cancer (ACS, 2020b). *H. pylori* infection is a major risk factor for the development of gastric cancer. Other factors related to the incidence of gastric cancer include gastritis, pernicious anemia, smoking, obesity, achlorhydria, gastric ulcers, previous partial gastrectomy (more than 20 years ago), and genetics (ACS, 2020b; National Cancer Institute [NCI], 2020).

The vast majority of gastric cancers are sporadic or occurring as a result of acquired, not inherited, gene mutations. However, it is understood that gastric cancers may have a familial component (e.g., blood type A and those with another first-degree relative [parent, sibling, or child] with gastric cancer) and are associated with inherited cancer predisposition syndromes (ACS, 2020b; Cabebe, 2020; NCI, 2020). Inherited cancer predisposition syndromes associated with increased risk of developing gastric cancer include hereditary diffuse gastric cancer, Lynch syndrome (i.e., hereditary nonpolyposis colorectal cancer), juvenile polyposis syndrome, familial adenomatosis polyposis, and Peutz–Jeghers syndrome (ACS, 2020b; Cabebe, 2020; NCI, 2020).

The prognosis for patients with gastric cancer is generally poor. The 5-year survival rate for all patients with gastric cancer is about 32% (NCI, 2020). One reason for the poor survival rate is that the diagnosis is usually made late because most patients are asymptomatic during the early stages of the disease. Most cases of gastric cancer are discovered only after the cancer has spread from the stomach to involve the lymph nodes or has metastasized to distant organs.

Pathophysiology

Ninety to 95% of gastric cancers are adenocarcinomas, which arise from the mucus-producing cells of the innermost lining of the stomach (ACS, 2020b). Gastric cancer begins with a lesion involving cells on the top layer of the stomach mucosa. The lesion then penetrates cells in the deeper layers of the mucosa, submucosa, and stomach wall. Eventually the lesion infiltrates the stomach wall and extends to organs or structures adjacent to the stomach. Lymph node involvement and metastasis tend to occur early due to the abundant lymphatic and vascular networks of the stomach. Common sites of metastasis include the liver, peritoneum, lungs, and brain (ACS, 2020b).

Clinical Manifestations

Gastric cancer is associated with few if any symptoms in the early stages of the disease (ACS, 2020b; Cabebe, 2020). Symptoms of early-stage disease may include pain that is relieved by antacids, resembling those of benign ulcers, and are seldom definitive. Symptoms of advanced disease are similar to those of peptic ulcer disease, such as dyspepsia, early satiety, weight loss, abdominal pain just above the umbilicus, loss or decrease in appetite, bloating after meals, and nausea or vomiting. Fatigue often occurs as a result of the cancer itself or blood loss from the lesion infiltrating the stomach or surrounding tissue (ACS, 2020b; Cabebe, 2020).

Assessment and Diagnostic Findings

The physical examination is usually not helpful in detecting the cancer because most early gastric tumors are not palpable. Advanced gastric cancer may be palpable as a mass. Ascites and hepatomegaly (enlarged liver) may be apparent if the cancer cells have metastasized to the liver. Palpable nodules around the umbilicus, called *Sister Mary Joseph's nodules*, are a sign of a GI malignancy, usually a gastric cancer (Cabebe, 2020).

Esophagogastroduodenoscopy for biopsy and cytologic washings is the diagnostic study of choice, and a barium x-ray examination of the upper GI tract may also be performed (ACS, 2020b; Cabebe, 2020; Li, Chung, & Mullen, 2019; Norris, 2019). Endoscopic ultrasound is an important tool to assess tumor depth and any lymph node involvement. Computed tomography (CT) scanning completes the diagnostic studies, particularly to assess for surgical resectability of the tumor before surgery is scheduled. CT scans of the chest, abdomen, and pelvis are valuable in staging gastric cancer.

A CBC may be used to evaluate for the presence of anemia. Assessment of tumor markers (blood analysis for antigens indicative of cancer), such as carcinoembryonic antigen (CEA), carbohydrate antigen (CA 19-9), and CA 50 are monitored to determine the effectiveness of treatment(s). Tumor marker values are usually elevated in the presence of gastric cancer before treatment and decrease if the tumor is responding to the treatment (Cabebe, 2020).

Medical Management

The treatment of gastric cancer is multimodal, often involving surgery, chemotherapy, targeted therapy, and radiation therapy. In general, the patient with a resectable tumor undergoes a surgical procedure to remove the tumor and appropriate lymph nodes. If the tumor can be removed while it is still localized to the stomach, the patient may be cured. In patients with a tumor that is not surgically resectable or those with advanced disease, cure is less likely. Treatment may include surgery to control the cancer growth or for the palliation of symptoms, chemotherapy, targeted therapy, and radiation therapy.

Surgical Management

A total gastrectomy may be performed for a resectable cancer in the midportion or body of the stomach. The entire stomach is removed along with the duodenum, the lower portion of the esophagus, supporting mesentery, and lymph nodes. Reconstruction of the GI tract is performed by anastomosing the end of the jejunum to the end of the esophagus, a procedure called an *esophagojejunostomy*. A radical partial (subtotal) gastrectomy is performed for a resectable tumor in the middle and distal portions of the stomach. A Billroth I or a Billroth II operation (see Table 40-4) is performed. The Billroth I involves a limited resection and offers a lower cure rate than the Billroth II. The Billroth II procedure is a wider resection that involves removing approximately 75% of the stomach and decreases the possibility of lymph node spread or metastatic recurrence. A proximal partial (subtotal) gastrectomy may be performed for a resectable tumor located in the proximal portion of the stomach or cardia. A total gastrectomy or an esophagogastrectomy is usually performed in place of this procedure to achieve a more extensive resection (Chisti & Willner, 2020; Norris, 2019).

Surgery may be also required to treat common complications of advanced gastric cancer, which may include gastric outlet obstruction, bleeding, and severe pain. Gastric perforation is an emergency situation requiring surgical intervention. A gastric resection may be the most effective palliative procedure for advanced gastric cancer. Palliative procedures such as gastric or esophageal bypass, gastrostomy, or jejunostomy may temporarily alleviate symptoms such as nausea and vomiting. Palliative rather than radical surgery may be performed if there is metastasis to other vital organs, such as the liver, or to achieve a better quality of life.

Complications of Gastric Surgery

The patient undergoing gastric surgery may experience complications, including hemorrhage, dumping syndrome, bile reflux, and gastric outlet obstruction. Postoperative bleeding from the surgical site is a common complication of gastric surgery. Bleeding may be severe (hemorrhage) and manifest as vomiting large amounts of bright red blood, which may result in hemorrhagic shock (see Chapter 11). The medical management and nursing care of the patient experiencing hemorrhage is discussed in the Peptic Ulcer Disease section of this chapter.

Dumping syndrome may occur as a result of any surgical procedure that involves the removal of a significant portion of the stomach or includes resection or removal of the pylorus (see Table 40-4). The rapid bolus of hypertonic food from the stomach to the small intestines draws extracellular fluid into the lumen of the intestines to dilute the high concentrations of electrolytes and sugars, which results in intestinal dilation, increased intestinal transit, hyperglycemia, and the rapid onset of GI and vasomotor symptoms (Kanth & Roy, 2019; NIDDK, 2019). It is estimated that 25% to 50% of all patients who have undergone gastric surgery experience at least some symptoms of dumping syndrome (Kanth & Roy, 2019). Early symptoms tend to occur within 10 to 30 minutes after a meal and often include early satiety, cramping abdominal pain, nausea, vomiting, and diarrhea. Vasomotor symptoms may manifest as a headache, flushing and feelings of warmth, diaphoresis, dizziness, palpations, drowsiness, faintness, or syncope. Early symptoms tend to resolve within 1 hour or with bowel evacuation (defecation) (NIDDK, 2019). Later, the rapid elevation in blood glucose is followed by the increased secretion of insulin, which results in hypoglycemia 2 to 3 hours after eating. Manifestations of hypoglycemia may include irritability, anxiety, shakiness, weakness, fatigue, diaphoresis, palpitations, and hunger. Dumping syndrome typically lasts for a few months after surgery, although in some patients, symptoms may persist on a long-term basis.

Bile reflux may occur with any gastric surgery that involves manipulation or removal of the pylorus, which acts as a barrier to prevent reflex of duodenal contents back into the stomach. Prolonged exposure of bile acid from the duodenum results in irritation and damage to the gastric mucosa, which may lead to gastritis, esophagitis, and possibly peptic ulcer formation. The patient with bile reflux may experience burning epigastric pain that may increase after meals. Vomiting usually does not provide relief from pain. Pharmacologic management of bile reflux includes the administration of proton pump inhibitors and ursodiol. Ursodiol changes the composition of bile, reducing acidity and promoting gastric healing (Kumar & Thompson, 2017; Li, Zhang, Yao, et al., 2020).

Gastric outlet obstruction may occur as a complication of gastric surgery. Postoperative gastric outlet obstruction may be caused by stenosis (narrowing) or stricture (scar tissue) formation at the surgical anastomosis site. Typical clinical manifestations and management of gastric outlet obstruction were previously discussed (see the Peptic Ulcer Disease section of this chapter).

Chemotherapy and Targeted Therapy

In instances where the gastric tumor is not resectable, treatment with chemotherapy may offer further control of the disease or palliation. Chemotherapy may also be used in addition to surgery as adjuvant treatment of gastric cancer. Chemotherapeutic agents often include fluorouracil, carboplatin, capecitabine, cisplatin, docetaxel, epirubicin, irinotecan, oxaliplatin, and paclitaxel. For improved tumor response rates, it is more common to administer combination chemotherapy, primarily fluorouracil-based therapy, with other agents (e.g., fluorouracil plus cisplatin or oxaliplatin) (ACS, 2020b; National Comprehensive Cancer Network [NCCN], 2020).

Targeted therapies have become an important addition to the treatment of advanced gastric cancers (NCCN, 2020). Trastuzumab (a recombinant humanized anti–HER-2 monoclonal antibody) prescribed in combination with fluorouracil or capecitabine and cisplatin has shown an improvement in survival of patients with advanced gastric cancer who are HER-2 positive (Miura, Sukawa, Hironaka, et al., 2018). Other targeted therapies are currently being investigated for the treatment of advanced gastric cancers. For example, ramucirumab is currently in clinical trial studies in combination with olaparib for tumors considered to be inoperable (NCI, 2020). Ramucirumab works by blocking VEGFR2, which reduces the blood supply to the tumor to decrease tumor growth (NCCN, 2020; Ramurcirumab, 2020) (Chart 40-3).

Radiation Therapy

Radiation therapy is primarily used for advanced gastric cancers to slow the rate of tumor growth or for the palliation of symptoms related to obstruction, bleeding, and significant pain (ACS, 2020b). Radiation therapy may also be used alone or along with chemotherapy before surgery to decrease the size of the tumor or after surgery to destroy any remaining cancer cells and to delay or prevent reoccurrence of the cancer (ACS, 2020b; NCCN, 2020). Common approaches to radiation therapy for gastric cancer include traditional external-beam radiation therapy or newer specialized approaches to

Chart 40-3 ETHICAL DILEMMA
Should Patients at the End-of-Life Be Enrolled in Clinical Trials?

Case Scenario

You are a nurse who works in an outpatient oncology treatment center. R.K. is a 68-year-old woman who was diagnosed with advanced gastric adenocarcinoma 13 months ago. She had a gastrectomy and peritonectomy last year, and finished six cycles of chemotherapy 2 months ago. Her most recent post-chemotherapy positron emission tomography (PET) scans reveal metastatic disease to her liver, lungs, and pelvis. The oncologist discusses her options with R.K. and her husband, and tells them that R.K. should make preparations for end of life. The oncologist tells them that R.K. can elect to receive palliative chemotherapy, which is associated with good quality of life and extended survival by 2 months in most patients like R.K. who take this option. Another option R.K. might pursue is to enroll in a phase I clinical trial with a novel immunotherapeutic agent. The oncologist is clear that the aim of this treatment would be not to extend R.K.'s life, but to test the safety of the new immunotherapy, and that any potential benefits could only be reaped by future patients with gastric cancer. R.K. and her husband decide to go home and discuss her options between themselves. A few days later, they return to the oncology center to tell the oncologist that they wish for R.K. to enroll in the clinical trial. After you finish checking them into an examination room in preparation to see the oncologist, R.K.'s husband turns to you with tears in his eyes and says "I want my wife to have the very best treatments possible. I will take any chance of a cure for her and this new drug might be the right ticket."

Discussion

Phase I of a clinical trial is one of the very earliest steps in testing a new therapy. This step in the research process aims to find if the new therapy is safe in humans. The effectiveness of the new therapy in treating a disease is not subject to testing at this early juncture. R.K.'s oncologist noted this during discussions with R.K. and her husband. However, it is not uncommon for patients and family members who face a life-threatening diagnosis to misunderstand the aims of an intervention or of enrolling in a research study, and falsely assume that there is indeed a therapeutic aim that does not exist. For this reason, most researchers who conduct clinical trials will give patients written information about the nature of the research to read at home and to give them time to digest and discuss their enrollment in the research study with their friends and family members so that they may make a fully informed decision.

Analysis

- Describe the ethical principles that are in conflict in this case (see Chapter 1, Chart 1-7). Do you believe that R.K. is making a well-informed decision should she go through with enrolling in the clinical trial?
- Is it just to not invite patients who are near end of life to participate in research? Is it morally defensible to offer a patient with a terminal diagnosis the option to enroll in a clinical trial when there is no clear potential benefit to them?
- What if R.K. turns to you, after her husband voices his hopes for a cure, and says "I agree with my husband and I will take any chance I can get!" On the other hand, what if she turns to you and says "My husband is having a difficult time letting go right now, and I am trying to do my best to support him. I want to do this because I want my death to have some meaning. I want to help future patients with my type of cancer."
- What resources might be mobilized to be of assistance to you and to R.K. and her husband so that they make the decision that is in R.K.'s best interests?

References

Comoretto, N., Larumbe, A., Arantzamendi, M., et al. (2017). Palliative care consultants' ethical concerns with advanced cancer patients participating in phase I clinical trials: A case study. *Progress in Palliative Care: Science and the Art of Caring, 25*(5), 230–234.

Resources

See Chapter 1, Chart 1-10 for Steps of an Ethical Analysis and Ethics Resources.

---

external-beam radiation therapy, such as three-dimensional conformal radiation therapy (3D-CRT), intraoperative radiotherapy, and intensity-modulated radiation therapy (IMRT). These specialized approaches to external radiation therapy precisely direct the radiation beam to the site of the tumor, thus limiting damage to the healthy surrounding tissue (ACS, 2020b; Cabebe, 2020).

Gerontologic Considerations

Gastric cancer mostly affects older adults. It is estimated that 6 of every 10 patients diagnosed with gastric cancer each year are 65 years old or older (ACS, 2020c). According to most recent Surveillance, Epidemiology, and End Results (SEER) data, 65.9% of all deaths from gastric cancer occur in patients 65 years old or older (NCI, 2020). Confusion, agitation, and restlessness may be the only symptoms seen in older adult patients, who may have no gastric symptoms until their tumors are well advanced. At this time, they present with reduced functional ability and other signs and symptoms of malignancy.

Surgery is more hazardous for the older adult, and the risk increases proportionately with increasing age. Nonetheless, gastric cancer should be treated with surgery in older patients. Patient education is important to prepare older patients with cancer for treatment, to help them manage adverse effects, and to face the challenges that cancer and aging present.

NURSING PROCESS

The Patient with Gastric Cancer

Assessment

The nurse obtains a dietary history from the patient, focusing on recent nutritional intake and status. Has the patient lost weight? If so, how much and over what period of time? Can the patient tolerate a full diet? If not, what foods can they eat? What other changes in eating habits have occurred? Does the patient have an appetite? Does the patient feel full after eating a small amount of food? Is the patient in pain? Do foods, antacids, or medications relieve the pain, make no difference, or worsen the pain? Is there a history of infection with *H. pylori*? Other health information to obtain includes the patient's tobacco use and alcohol history and family history (e.g., any first- or second-degree relatives with gastric or other cancer). A psychosocial assessment, including questions about social support, individual and family coping skills, and financial resources, helps the nurse plan for care in acute and community settings.

After the interview, the nurse performs a complete physical examination, carefully assesses the patient's abdomen for tenderness or masses, and palpates and percusses the abdomen to detect ascites.

Nursing Diagnosis

Based on the assessment data, major nursing diagnoses may include the following:

- Anxiety associated with the disease and anticipated treatment
- Impaired nutritional intake associated with early satiety or anorexia
- Acute pain associated with tumor mass
- Grief associated with the diagnosis of cancer
- Lack of knowledge regarding self-care activities

Planning and Goals

The major goals for the patient may include reduced anxiety, optimal nutrition, relief of pain, and adjustment to the diagnosis and anticipated lifestyle changes.

Nursing Interventions

REDUCING ANXIETY

A relaxed, nonthreatening atmosphere is provided so the patient can express fears, concerns, and possibly anger about the diagnosis and prognosis. The nurse encourages the family or significant other to support the patient, offering reassurance and supporting positive coping measures. The nurse educates the patient about any procedures and treatments so that the patient knows what to expect.

PROMOTING OPTIMAL NUTRITION

The nurse encourages the patient to eat small, frequent portions of nonirritating foods to decrease gastric irritation. Food supplements should be high in calories, as well as vitamins A and C and iron, to enhance tissue repair. Because the patient may develop dumping syndrome when enteral feeding resumes after gastric resection, the nurse explains ways to prevent and manage it and informs the patient that symptoms often resolve after several months. Management of dumping syndrome includes encouraging six small feedings daily that are low in carbohydrates and sugar and the consumption of fluids between meals rather than with meals. If a total gastrectomy is performed, injection of vitamin B_{12} will be required for life, because intrinsic factor, secreted by parietal cells in the stomach, binds to vitamin B_{12} so that it may be absorbed in the ileum. This deficiency in vitamin B_{12} metabolism can result in decreased production of red blood cells, or pernicious anemia. If the patient is unable to eat adequately prior to surgery to meet nutritional requirements, parenteral nutrition may be necessary. Weight loss is a common occurrence in the postoperative period following gastric surgery. Chemotherapy treatment can contribute to ongoing weight loss. Research suggests that a multidisciplinary approach is necessary to manage symptoms that may contribute to ongoing weight loss such as early satiety, dysphagia, reflux and regurgitation, and elimination

issues (Aoyama, Sato, Maezawa, et al., 2017; Grace, Shaw, Lalji, et al., 2018). The nurse monitors the IV therapy and nutritional status and records intake, output, and daily weights to ensure that the patient is maintaining or gaining weight. The nurse assesses for signs of dehydration (thirst, dry mucous membranes, poor skin turgor, tachycardia, decreased urine output) and reviews the results of daily laboratory studies to note any metabolic abnormalities (sodium, potassium, glucose, BUN). Antiemetic agents are given as prescribed.

RELIEVING PAIN

The nurse administers analgesic agents as prescribed. A continuous IV infusion of an opioid or a patient-controlled analgesia (PCA) pump set to infuse an opioid may be necessary to mitigate postoperative pain. The frequency, intensity, and duration of the pain are routinely assessed to determine the effectiveness of the analgesic agent. The nurse works with the patient to help manage pain by suggesting nonpharmacologic methods for pain relief, such as position changes, imagery, distraction, relaxation exercises (using relaxation apps and online videos), backrubs, massage, and periods of rest and relaxation. See Chapter 9 for further discussion of pain management.

PROVIDING PSYCHOSOCIAL SUPPORT

The nurse helps the patient express fears, concerns, and grief about the diagnosis. The nurse answers the patient's questions honestly and encourages the patient to participate in treatment decisions. Some patients mourn the loss of a body part and perceive their surgery as a type of mutilation. Some express disbelief and need time and support to accept the diagnosis (see the Nursing Research Profile in Chart 40-4 for more discussion).

The nurse offers emotional support and involves family members and significant others whenever possible. This includes recognizing mood swings and defense mechanisms (e.g., denial, rationalization, displacement, regression) and reassuring the patient, family members, and significant others that emotional responses are normal and expected. The services of clergy, psychiatric clinical nurse specialists, psychologists, social workers, and psychiatrists are made available, if needed. The nurse projects an empathetic attitude and spends time with the patient. Many patients may begin to participate in self-care activities after they have acknowledged their loss.

PROMOTING HOME, COMMUNITY-BASED, AND TRANSITIONAL CARE

Educating Patients About Self-Care. Self-care activities depend on the type of treatments used— surgery, chemotherapy, radiation, or palliative care. Patient and family education include information about diet and nutrition, treatment regimens, activity and lifestyle changes, pain management, and possible complications (Chart 40-5). Consultation with a dietitian is essential to determine how the patient's nutritional needs can best be met at home. The nurse instructs the patient or caregiver about administration of enteral or parenteral nutrition. If chemotherapy or radiation is prescribed, the nurse provides explanations to the patient and family about what to expect, including the length of treatments, the expected side effects (e.g., nausea, vomiting, anorexia, fatigue, neutropenia), and the need for transportation to appointments for treatment. Psychological counseling may also be helpful (see Chapter 12).

Chart 40-4 NURSING RESEARCH PROFILE

Understanding Uncertainty and Care Needs in Patients with Gastric Cancer

Lee, J. Y., Jang, Y., Kim, S., et al. (2020). Uncertainty and unmet care needs before and after surgery in patients with gastric cancer: A survey study. *Nursing & Health Sciences, 22*(2), 427–435.

Purpose

Patients diagnosed with cancer often experience uncertainty and a variety of other physical, psychological, emotional, and educational needs throughout their illness course. Little is known about unmet care needs across the illness trajectory in patients who have gastric cancer. Gastric cancer is frequently preceded by nonspecific symptoms that patients often attribute to less serious causes; symptom ambiguity at time of diagnosis may contribute to high levels of uncertainty. Varying symptom clusters and levels of symptom intensity and frequency after surgical intervention for gastric cancer may also increase uncertainty. Understanding how uncertainty and needs change over time may help improve the effectiveness of nursing interventions. The purpose of this study was to assess levels of uncertainty and unmet care needs before and after surgery in patients with gastric cancer.

Design

This was a descriptive study using a before and after design to evaluate uncertainty and unmet care needs at time of diagnosis and after gastrectomy in patients with a diagnosis of gastric cancer. Purposeful sampling was used to recruit participants 20 years of age or older with a new diagnosis of gastric cancer; patients receiving chemotherapy or with other types of cancer were excluded. Demographic and clinical data were collected at baseline. Uncertainty was measured using the *Uncertainty in Illness Scale* and unmet care needs were examined using the *Supportive Care Needs Survey-Short Form 34* at two time points; time 1 (day of admission after diagnosis) and time 2 (first post-operative outpatient follow-up). Both scales were translated to

Korean and validated. Data were analyzed using descriptive statistics and differences in uncertainty and unmet needs from time 1 to time 2 were examined using a dependent *t*-test.

Findings

Eighty-six participants with a mean age of 58.5 years completed the study; the majority were male (58.1%), married (83.7%), and educated at or above a high school level (74.4%). Most had a diagnosis of early gastric cancer (93%), with no family history of cancer (61.6%), or no cancer-related symptoms prior to their diagnosis (59.3%); the majority (81.4%) had sought out information about gastric cancer after their diagnosis. Patients reported moderate levels of uncertainty at time of diagnosis and after surgery; however, total uncertainty scores and the subscales of ambiguity, inconsistency, and unpredictability were significantly higher at time of diagnosis. Needs related to patient care support, psychological status, and health care system information (e.g., disease progression, testing, recovery, self-management) were also significantly higher at time of diagnosis compared to follow-up. However, physical needs (e.g., tiredness, pain, ability to do usual activities/work at home, and feeling unwell) were significantly higher at follow-up. Needs related to sexuality were low at both time points and there were no significant differences in scores from time of diagnosis to postoperative follow-up.

Nursing Implications

This study demonstrates that patients who have gastric cancer experience moderate levels of uncertainty related to symptoms, prognosis, and treatment duration that are higher at time of diagnosis. Patient care needs varied across the course of treatment, which suggests that nurses should perform ongoing assessments in various domains and individualize interventions based on patients' priority concerns.

Chart 40-5 HOME CARE CHECKLIST

The Patient with Gastric Cancer

At the completion of education, the patient and/or caregiver will be able to:

- State the impact of cancer and treatment on physiologic functioning, ADLs, IADLs, roles, relationships, and spirituality.
- Identify modification of home environment, interventions, and strategies (e.g., utilizing durable medical equipment, employing a home health aide) used in safely adapting to changes in structure or function and promote effective recovery and rehabilitation.
- Identify foods or therapies necessary to meet caloric needs and dietary needs (e.g., change in consistency, seasoning limitations or other dietary restrictions, supplements, enteral or parenteral therapy).
- Demonstrate safe management of enteral or parenteral feedings, if applicable.
- State the name, dose, side effects, frequency, and schedule for all medications.
- Describe approaches to controlling pain (e.g., take antispasmodic agents as prescribed; use nonpharmacologic interventions).
- When indicated, list possible side effects of chemotherapeutic agents and suggested management approaches.

- When indicated, list possible side effects of radiation therapy and suggested management approaches.
- Identify possible complications (e.g., infection, bleeding, obstruction, perforation or worsening pain or other symptoms) and interventions.
- Relate how to reach primary provider with questions or complications.
- State time and date of follow-up medical appointments, therapy, and testing.
- Identify sources of support (e.g., friends, relatives, faith community, cancer support, caregiver support).
- Identify the need for health promotion, disease prevention, and screening activities.
- Make decisions about end-of-life care as appropriate.

Resources

See Chapter 39, Chart 39-5 for additional information on The Patient Receiving Tube Feeding, and Chapter 41, Chart 41-7 The Patient Receiving Parenteral Nutrition.

ADLs, activities of daily living; IADLs, instrumental activities of daily living.

Continuing and Transitional Care. The need for ongoing care in the home depends on the patient's condition and treatment. The nurse reinforces nutritional counseling and supervises the administration of any enteral or parenteral feedings; the patient or caregiver must become skillful in administering the feedings and in detecting and preventing untoward effects or complications related to the feedings (see Chapter 39). The nurse instructs the patient or caregiver to record the patient's daily intake, output, and weight and explains strategies to manage pain, nausea, vomiting, or other symptoms. Education is provided on how to recognize and report signs and symptoms of complications that require immediate attention, such as bleeding, obstruction, perforation, or any symptoms that become progressively worse. The nurse must explain the chemotherapy or radiation therapy regimen and ensure that the patient and family or significant other understand the care that will be needed during and after treatments (see Chapter 12). Because the prognosis for gastric cancer is poor, the patient, family, or significant other may need assistance with decisions regarding end-of-life care; the nurse should provide support and make referrals as needed.

Evaluation

Expected patient outcomes may include the following:
1. Reports less anxiety
   a. Expresses fears and concerns about surgery
   b. Seeks emotional support
2. Attains optimal nutrition
   a. Eats small, frequent meals high in calories, iron, and vitamins A and C
   b. Adheres to enteral or parenteral nutrition as needed
3. Has decreased pain
4. Performs self-care activities and adjusts to lifestyle changes
   a. Resumes typical activities within 3 months
   b. Alternates periods of rest and activity
   c. Manages enteral feedings
5. Verbalizes knowledge of disease management
   a. Acknowledges disease process
   b. Reports control of symptoms
   c. Verbalizes fears and concerns about dying; involves family/caregiver in discussions
   d. Completes advance directives and other appropriate documents

Tumors of the Small Intestine

Benign or malignant tumors of the small intestine are rare. Approximately 64% of all tumors of the small intestines are malignant (Somasundar, Fisichella, & Espat, 2019). Malignant tumors of the small intestine account for only about 1% to 2% of all GI cancers (Somasundar et al., 2019); it was estimated that in 2020, approximately 11,000 new cases of cancer of the small intestine would be diagnosed in the United States (ACS, 2020a). Rates are higher among older adults (mean age at diagnosis of 60 years) and are also higher among African Americans and men (ACS, 2020c). Malignant tumors are often not discovered until they have metastasized to distant sites. Benign tumors may place patients at an increased risk for malignancy (Terry & Santora, 2019). The relative rarity of tumors of the small intestine, the diversity of tumor types (that may include adenocarcinomas, carcinoid tumors, lymphomas, or sarcomas), and the nonspecific nature of their manifestations complicate their diagnosis and treatment. Multiple factors, including preexisting GI disorders, can increase the risk of tumors in the small intestine and often contribute to advanced metastatic disease at the time of diagnosis. The lack of surveillance for multiple risk factors can contribute to a delay in treatment (Chen & Vaccaro, 2018; Somasundar et al., 2019).

Clinical Manifestations

Tumors of the small intestine often present insidiously with vague, nonspecific symptoms. Most benign tumors are discovered incidentally on an x-ray study, during surgery, or at autopsy. When the patient is symptomatic, benign tumors often present with intermittent pain. The next most common presentation is occult bleeding. Malignant tumors often result in symptoms that lead to their diagnosis, although these symptoms may reflect advanced disease. Most patients have sustained weight loss and may be malnourished at the time of diagnosis. Occult GI bleeding is less common than is found in patients with benign tumors, and complaints of pain are common. The patient also frequently presents with complaints of weakness, fatigue, nausea, vomiting, and intestinal obstruction (ACS, 2020a). Intestinal perforation is rare and associated with a poorer overall prognosis (ACS, 2020a; Somasundar et al., 2019). Clinical manifestations and management of the patient experiencing an intestinal obstruction and intestinal perforation are discussed in Chapter 41.

Assessment and Diagnostic Findings

A CBC may reveal a low hematocrit and hemoglobin level that is consistent with anemia if the patient has an occult source of GI bleeding. The bilirubin may also be elevated if tumor mass has caused biliary obstruction. CEA levels may also be elevated, consistent with a malignant mass.

An upper GI x-ray series with small bowel follow-through using oral water-insoluble contrast with frequent and detailed x-rays to follow the contrast through the small bowel is the traditional approach to diagnosis. A more sensitive examination is an enteroclysis, in which an NG tube is advanced into the small bowel to a position above the area in question; the area is then studied by single- and double-contrast techniques. Abdominal CT scan is used to determine the extent of disease (Somasundar et al., 2019).

Management

Benign tumors of the small intestine include adenomas, lipomas, hemangiomas, and hamartomas (a focal malformation that resembles a neoplasm, but unlike a neoplasm does not result in compression of adjacent tissue). These tumors may be treated endoscopically by excision/resection or electrocautery if the patient is symptomatic. Routine monitoring is recommended to assess for malignant transformation (Terry & Santora, 2019).

The most common primary malignant tumor of the small intestine is adenocarcinoma; the second and third portions of the duodenum are most often involved. These tumors may present with obstruction. If the tumor is located at the ampulla of Vater, obstructive jaundice is likely. Other rare malignant tumors of the small intestine include carcinoid tumors, lymphoma, and GI stromal tumors (Chen & Vaccaro, 2018; Terry & Santora, 2019). Abdominal surgery may be required to remove these rare tumors. Chemotherapy and radiation therapy are commonly part of the treatment regimen.

The nursing process related to the care of the patient with a tumor of the small intestine is similar to that of the patient with gastric cancer. Each patient requires specialized care, astute assessment for complications, prompt interventions, and individualized education for self-care.

CRITICAL THINKING EXERCISES

1 **ebp** A 65-year-old woman is diagnosed with a peptic ulcer after experiencing fatigue, epigastric pain associated with meals, and coffee ground emesis. She is started on treatment with omeprazole and sucralfate. The patient asks you if taking these medications will be successful in treating her ulcer. How would you respond to this patient? On what evidence do you base your response?

2 **pq** A 55-year-old female patient arrives in the emergency department with the onset of melena, abdominal pain, and weight loss of 18 lb. Upon admission, she is awake, alert, and oriented. Her pain level is 8 (on a 0 to 10 numeric pain scale). Her blood pressure is 90/60 mm Hg, heart rate is 126 bpm, respiratory rate is 16 breaths/min and regular, and temperature is 36.7°C (98.1°F). Her abdomen is hard and rigid and no bowel sounds are assessed upon auscultation. What is your first nursing action? Describe the priorities of care for this patient.

3 **ipc** You are caring for a 67-year-old man who was recently diagnosed with peptic ulcer disease and was admitted with melena. The dietitian met with the patient to discuss changes in his diet. Prior to discharge, you are reviewing a 7-day diet plan with the patient. Describe food selections that would necessitate follow-up with the dietitian prior to the patient's discharge.

REFERENCES

*Asterisk indicates nursing research.

Books

Karch, A. M. (2018). *Lippincott nursing drug guide*. Philadelphia, PA: Lippincott Williams & Wilkins.

Norris, T. L. (2019). *Porth's pathophysiology: Concepts of altered health states* (10th ed.). Philadelphia, PA: Wolters Kluwer.

Journals and Electronic Documents

Akiva, J. M., & Greenwald, D. (2019). Chronic gastritis. *Medscape*. Retrieved on 4/25/2020 at: www.emedicine.medscape.com/article/176156

American Cancer Society (ACS). (2020a). Small intestines cancer. Retrieved on 5/18/2020 at: www.cancer.org/cancer/small-intestine-cancer.html

American Cancer Society (ACS). (2020b). Stomach cancer. Retrieved on 5/18/2020 at: www.cancer.org/cancer/stomachcancer

American Cancer Society (ACS). (2020c). Cancer statistics center: Colorectum. Retrieved on 5/27/2020 at: www.cancerstatisticscenter.cancer.org/?_ga=2.55716267.1085099949.1590590345-2131236307.1590590345#!/cancer-site/Colorectum

Anand, B. S. (2020). Peptic ulcer disease. *Medscape*. Retrieved on 4/29/2020 at: www.emedicine.medscape.com/article/181753

Aoyama, T., Sato, T., Maezawa, Y., et al. (2017). Postoperative weight loss leads to poor survival through poor S-1 efficacy in patients with stage II/III gastric cancer. *International Journal of Clinical Oncology*, 22(3), 476–483.

Azer, S. A. (2018). Intestinal perforation clinical presentation. *Medscape*. Retrieved on 5/05/2020 at: www.emedicine.medscape.com/article/195537

Berkowitz, L., Schultz, B. M., Salazar, G. A., et al. (2018). Impact of cigarette smoking on the gastrointestinal tract inflammation: Opposing effects in Crohn's disease and ulcerative colitis. Retrieved on 4/27/2020 at: www.frontiersin.org/articles/10.3389/fimmu.2018.00074/full

Bonheur, J. L., & Nachimuthu, S. (2019). Gastrinoma. *Medscape*. Retrieved on 5/3/2020 at: www.emedicine.medscape.com/article/184332

Cabebe, E. W. (2020). Gastric cancer. *Medscape*. Retrieved on 5/18/2020 at: www.emedicine.medscape.com/article/278744

Castellanos, A. E., & Podolsky, E. R. (2020). Gastric outlet obstruction. *Medscape*. Retrieved on 5/5/2020 at: www.emedicine.medscape.com/article/190621

Chen, E. Y., & Vaccaro, G. M. (2018). Small bowel adenocarcinoma. *Clinics in Colon and Rectal Surgery*, 31(5), 267–277.

Chisti, M. M., & Willner, C. A. (2020). Gastric cancer treatment protocols. *Medscape*. Retrieved on 5/17/2020 at: www.emedicine.medscape.com/article/2005831

Clarke, R. C., Ferraro, R. M., Gbadehan, E., et al. (2020). Stress-induced gastritis. *Medscape*. Retrieved on 2/25/2020 at: www.emedicine.medscape.com/article/176319

Comoretto, N., Larumbe, A., Arantzamendi, M., et al. (2017). Palliative care consultants' ethical concerns with advanced cancer patients participating in phase I clinical trials: A case study. *Progress in Palliative Care: Science and the Art of Caring*, 25(5), 230–234.

Daniels, L. M., Khalili, M., Morano, W. F., et al. (2019). Case report: Optimal tumor cytoreduction and octreotide disease control in a patient with MEN-1 and Zollinger-Ellison syndrome—over a decade of follow-up. *World Journal of Surgical Oncology*, 17(213), 1–8.

Davenport, D. L., Ueland, W. R., Kumar, S., et al. (2019). A comparison of short-term outcomes between laparoscopic and open emergent repair of perforated peptic ulcers. *Surgical Endoscopy*, 33(3), 764–772.

Grace, E. M., Shaw, C., Lalji, A., et al. (2018). Nutritional status, the development and persistence of malnutrition and dietary intake in oesophagogastric cancer: A longitudinal cohort study. *Journal of Human Nutrition and Dietetics*, 31(6), 785–792.

Kanth, R., & Roy, P. K. (2019). Dumping syndrome. *Medscape*. Retrieved on 5/17/2020 at: www.emedicine.medscape.com/article/173594

Kennedy, N. D., & Winter, D. C. (2017). Impact of alcohol & smoking on the surgical management of gastrointestinal patients. *Best Practice & Research*, 31(5), 589–595.

Kumar, N., & Thompson, C. C. (2017). Remnant gastropathy due to bile reflux after Roux-en-Y gastric bypass: A unique cause of abdominal pain and successful treatment with ursodiol. *Surgical Endoscopy*, 31(12), 5399–5402.

*Lee, J. Y., Jang, Y., Kim, S., et al. (2020). Uncertainty and unmet care needs before and after surgery in patients with gastric cancer: A survey study. *Nursing & Health Sciences*, 22(2), 427–435.

Li, D., Zhang, J., Yao, W. Z., et al. (2020). The relationship between gastric cancer, its precancerous lesions and bile reflux: A retrospective study. *Journal of Digestive Diseases*, 21(4), 222–229.

Li, S. L., Chung, D. C., & Mullen, J. T. (2019). Screening high-risk populations for esophageal and gastric cancer. *Journal of Surgical Oncology*, 120(5), 831–846.

Liu, M., Zhong, Y., Chen, J., et al. (2020). Oral immunization of mice with a multivalent therapeutic subunit vaccine protects against Helicobacter pylori infection. *Vaccine*, 38(14), 3031–3041.

Lloyd, B. R., & Leiman, D. A. (2019). An updated approach to evaluation and treatment of Helicobacter pylori infection. *Southern Medical Journal*, 112(7), 392–398.

Loffroy, R., Midulla, M., Falvo, N., et al. (2018). Ethylene vinyl alcohol copolymer as first hemostatic liquid embolic agent for non-variceal upper gastrointestinal bleeding patients: Pros and cons. *Cardiovascular and Interventional Radiology*, 41(11), 1808–1809.

Marcus, A. J., & Greenwald, D. (2019). Chronic gastritis. *Medscape.* Retrieved on 2/25/2020 at: www.emedicine.medscape.com/article/176156

Miura, Y., Sukawa, Y., Hironaka, S., et al. (2018). Five-weekly S-1 plus cisplatin therapy combined with trastuzumab therapy in HER2-positive gastric cancer: A phase II trial and biomarker study. *Gastric Cancer, 21*, 84–95.

National Cancer Institute (NCI). (2020). Cancer stat facts: Stomach cancer. *SEER.* Retrieved on 5/27/2020 at: www.seer.cancer.gov/statfacts/html/stomach.html

National Comprehensive Cancer Network (NCCN). (2020). NCCN clinical guidelines version 2.2020 gastric cancer. Retrieved on 5/18/2020 at: www.nccn.org/professionals/physician_gls/pdf/gastric.pdf

National Institute of Diabetes and Digestive and Kidney Diseases (NIDDK). (2019). Dumping syndrome. *National Digestive Diseases Information Clearinghouse.* Retrieved on 6/27/2020 at: www.niddk.nih.gov/health-information/digestive-diseases/dumping-syndrome/definition-facts

National Institute of Diabetes and Digestive and Kidney Diseases (NIDDK). (2020a). Gastritis and gastropathy. *National Digestive Diseases Information Clearinghouse.* Retrieved on 02/25/2020 at: www.niddk.nih.gov/health-information/digestive-diseases/gastritis-gastropathy

National Institute of Diabetes and Digestive and Kidney Diseases (NIDDK). (2020b). Multiple endocrine neoplasia type 1. *National Digestive Diseases Information Clearinghouse.* Retrieved on 4/29/2020 at: www.niddk.nih.gov/health-information/endocrine-diseases/multiple-endocrine-neoplasia-type-1

National Institute of Diabetes and Digestive and Kidney Diseases (NIDDK). (2020c). Peptic ulcer (stomach ulcers). *National Digestive Diseases Information Clearinghouse.* Retrieved on 04/29/2020 at: www.niddk.nih.gov/health-information/digestive-diseases/peptic-ulcers-stomach-ulcers

National Institute of Diabetes and Digestive and Kidney Diseases (NIDDK). (2020d). Zollinger-Ellison syndrome. *National Digestive Diseases Information Clearinghouse.* Retrieved on 04/29/2020 at: www.niddk.nih.gov/health-information/digestive-diseases/zollinger-ellison-syndrome

Ramucirumab. (2020). *Medscape.* Retrieved on 5/18/2020 at: reference.medscape.com/drug/cyramza-ramucirumab-999926#0

Rawla, P., & Barsouk, A. (2019). Epidemiology of gastric cancer: Global trends, risk factors and prevention. *Gastroenterology Review, 14*(1), 26–38.

Roy, P. K. (2019). Zollinger-Ellison syndrome. *Medscape.* Retrieved on 4/29/2020 at: www.emedicine.medscape.com/article/183555-overview

Santacroce, L., & Bhutani, M. S. (2019). Helicobacter pylori infection. *Medscape.* Retrieved on 02/25/2020 at: www.emedicine.medscape.com/article/176938

Somasundar, P. S., Fisichella, P. M., & Espat, N. J. (2019). Malignant neoplasms of the small intestine. *Medscape.* Retrieved on 5/27/2020 at: www.emedicine.medscape.com/article/282684

Spiliopoulos, S., Inchingolo, R., Lucatelli, P., et al. (2018). Transcatheter arterial embolization for bleeding peptic ulcers: A multicenter study. *Cardiovascular and Interventional Radiology, 41*(9), 1333–1339.

Terry, S. M., & Santora, T. (2019). Benign neoplasm of the small intestines. *Medscape.* Retrieved on 5/27/2019 at: www.emedicine.medscape.com/article/189390

Upchurch, B. R. (2019). Upper gastrointestinal bleeding (UGIB). *Medscape.* Retrieved on 5/18/2020 at: www.emedicine.medscape.com/article/187857

Wehbi, M., Dacha, S., Sarver, G., et al. (2019). Acute gastritis. *Medscape.* Retrieved on 2/25/2020 at: www.emedicine.medscape.com/article/175909

Young, P. J., Bagshaw, S. M., Forbes, A. B., et al. (2020). Effect of stress ulcer prophylaxis with proton pump inhibitors vs histamine-2 receptor blockers on in-hospital mortality among ICU patients receiving invasive mechanical ventilation: The PEPTIC randomized clinical trial. *Journal of American Medical Association, 323*(7), 616–626.

Zayouna, N., & Piper, M. H. (2018). Atrophic gastritis. *Medscape.* Retrieved on 5/27/2020 at: www.emedicine.medscape.com/article/176036

Resources

American Cancer Society, www.cancer.org

American Gastroenterological Association (AGA), www.gastro.org

Centers for Disease Control and Prevention (CDC), www.cdc.gov

National Comprehensive Cancer Network (NCCN) Clinical Practice Guidelines, www.nccn.org

National Digestive Diseases Information Clearinghouse (NDDIC), www.digestive.niddk.nih.gov

Society of Gastroenterology Nurses and Associates, www.sgna.org

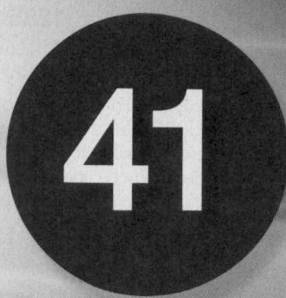

41

Management of Patients with Intestinal and Rectal Disorders

GLOSSARY

abscess: localized collection of purulent material surrounded by inflamed tissues

central venous access device (CVAD): a device designed and used for administration of sterile fluids, nutrition formulas, and medications into central veins

colostomy: surgical opening into the colon by means of a stoma to allow drainage of bowel contents; one type of fecal diversion

constipation: fewer than three bowel movements weekly or bowel movements that are hard, dry, small, or difficult to pass

diarrhea: an increased frequency of bowel movements or an increased amount of stool with altered consistency (i.e., increased liquidity) of stool

diverticulitis: inflammation of a diverticulum from obstruction by fecal matter resulting in abscess formation

diverticulosis: presence of several diverticula in the intestine

diverticulum: saclike out-pouching of the lining of the bowel protruding through the muscle of the intestinal wall

fecal incontinence: involuntary passage of feces

fissure: normal or abnormal fold, groove, or crack in body tissue

fistula: anatomically abnormal tract that arises between two internal organs or between an internal organ and the body surface

gastrocolic reflex: peristaltic movements of the large bowel occurring five to six times daily that are triggered by distention of the stomach

hemorrhoids: dilated portions of the anal veins

ileostomy: surgical opening into the ileum by means of a stoma to allow drainage of bowel contents; one type of fecal diversion

inflammatory bowel disease (IBD): group of chronic disorders (ulcerative colitis and Crohn's disease) that result in inflammation or ulceration (or both) of the bowel lining

irritable bowel syndrome (IBS): chronic functional disorder characterized by recurrent abdominal pain that affects frequency of defecation and consistency of stool; is associated with no specific structural or biochemical alterations

lipid injectable emulsion (ILE): an oil-in-water emulsion of oils, egg phospholipids, and glycerin (*synonym:* intravenous fat emulsion [IVFE] or lipid)

malabsorption: impaired transport across the mucosa

parenteral nutrition: method of supplying nutrients to the body by an intravenous route

peripherally inserted central catheter (PICC): a device inserted into a peripheral vein and designed and used for administration of sterile fluids, nutrition formulas, and medications into central veins

peritonitis: inflammation of the lining of the abdominal cavity

steatorrhea: excess of fatty wastes in the feces

tenesmus: ineffective and sometimes painful straining and urge to eliminate feces

total nutrient admixture (TNA): an admixture of lipid emulsions, proteins, carbohydrates, electrolytes, vitamins, trace minerals, and water

Between 60 and 70 million people in the United States are diagnosed with some type of disease of the gastrointestinal (GI) tract. These diseases account for more than 48.3 million office visits to health care facilities and clinics and approximately 21.7 million hospital admissions annually. GI diseases cost the American public more than $141.8 billion and account for approximately 246,000 deaths each year (National Institute of Diabetes and Digestive and Kidney Diseases [NIDDK], 2014b). The types of diseases and disorders that affect the lower GI tract are many and varied; examples include constipation, diarrhea, diverticulitis, and inflammatory bowel disease (IBD).

In all age groups, a fast-paced lifestyle, high levels of stress, irregular eating habits, insufficient intake of fiber and water, and lack of daily exercise contribute to GI disorders. There is a growing understanding of the biopsychosocial implications of GI disease. The mind and emotions can have a profound impact on the GI system. Nurses can influence these GI disorders by identifying behavior patterns that put patients at risk, by educating the public about prevention and management, and by helping those affected to improve their condition and prevent complications.

ABNORMALITIES OF FECAL ELIMINATION

Changes in patterns of fecal elimination are symptoms of functional disorders or diseases of the GI tract. The most common changes seen are constipation, diarrhea, and fecal incontinence.

Constipation

Constipation is defined as fewer than three bowel movements weekly or bowel movements that are hard, dry, small, or difficult to pass (Simren, Palsson, & Whitehead, 2017). Approximately 63 million Americans have chronic constipation, making it a very common GI disorder. People more likely to become constipated are women, particularly pregnant women, patients who recently had surgery, older adults, non-Caucasians, and people with a history of irritable bowel syndrome (NIDDK, 2018). Notably, constipation is a symptom and not a disease; however, constipation can indicate an underlying disease or motility disorder of the GI tract. Perceived constipation can also be an issue. This subjective problem occurs when a person's bowel elimination pattern is not consistent with what they consider normal (Dimidi, Cox, Grant, et al., 2019; Mari, Mahamid, Amara, et al., 2020).

Constipation can be caused by certain medications, such as anticholinergic agents, antidepressants, anticonvulsants, antispasmodics (muscle relaxants), calcium channel antagonists, diuretic agents, opioids, aluminum- and calcium-based antacids, and iron preparations. Other causes of constipation may include weakness, immobility, debility, fatigue, celiac

disease, and an inability to increase intra-abdominal pressure to facilitate the passage of stools, as may occur in patients with emphysema or spinal cord injury, for instance. Many people develop constipation because they do not take the time to defecate or ignore the urge to defecate. Constipation is also a result of dietary habits (i.e., low consumption of fiber and inadequate fluid intake), lack of regular exercise, and a stress-filled life (NIDDK, 2018). Fiber is particularly important to bowel health because it increases the bulk of stool, generally easing its passage. One of the most significant benefits of dietary fiber, most of which is derived from plant cell walls, is its fermentability, which affects the diversity of microbes in the GI tract and promotes good bowel wall health (Williams, Grant, Gidley, et al., 2017).

Pathophysiology

The pathophysiology of constipation is poorly understood, but it is thought to include interference with one of three major functions of the colon: mucosal transport (i.e., mucosal secretions facilitate the movement of colon contents), myoelectric activity (i.e., mixing of the rectal mass and propulsive actions), or the processes of defecation (e.g., pelvic floor dysfunction). There are four classes of constipation, based upon their underlying pathophysiologic mechanisms (Basson, 2019a):

- Functional constipation, which involves normal transit mechanisms of mucosal transport. This type of constipation is most common and can be successfully treated by increasing intake of fiber and fluids.
- Slow-transit constipation, which is caused by inherent disorders of the motor function of the colon (e.g., Hirschsprung disease), and is characterized by infrequent bowel movements.
- Defecatory disorders, which are caused by dysfunctional motor coordination between the pelvic floor and anal sphincter. Dyssynergic constipation is a common cause of chronic constipation and is caused by an inability to coordinate the abdominal, pelvic floor, and rectoanal muscles to defecate. *Anismus* is a term used to describe pelvic floor dysfunction and constipation. This can cause not only constipation but also fecal incontinence (see later discussion).
- Opioid-induced constipation, which includes new or worsening symptoms that occur when opioid therapy is initiated, changed, or increased and must include two or more symptoms of functional constipation (see later discussion).

The urge to defecate is stimulated normally by rectal distention that initiates a series of four actions: stimulation of the inhibitory rectoanal reflex, relaxation of the internal sphincter muscle, relaxation of the external sphincter muscle and muscles in the pelvic region, and increased intra-abdominal pressure. Interference with any of these processes can lead to constipation.

When the urge to defecate is ignored, the rectal mucous membrane and musculature become insensitive to the presence of fecal masses, and consequently a stronger stimulus is required to produce the necessary peristaltic rush for defecation. The initial effect of fecal retention is to produce irritability of the colon, which at this stage frequently goes into spasm, especially after meals, giving rise to colicky midabdominal or low abdominal pains. After several years of this process, the colon loses muscular tone and becomes essentially unresponsive to normal stimuli (similar to an overstretched balloon). Atony or decreased muscle tone occurs with aging. This may lead to constipation because the stool is retained for longer periods.

Clinical Manifestations

Clinical manifestations of constipation include fewer than three bowel movements per week; abdominal distention; abdominal pain and bloating; a sensation of incomplete evacuation; straining at stool; and the elimination of small-volume, lumpy, hard, dry stools. The patient may report **tenesmus** (i.e., ineffective and sometimes painful straining and urge to eliminate feces) or low back pain. Chronic constipation, often associated with psychological disorders, is the presence of these symptoms for at least 12 weeks during the previous year (Basson, 2019a).

Assessment and Diagnostic Findings

The diagnosis of constipation is based on the patient's history, physical examination, possibly the results of a barium enema or sigmoidoscopy, and stool testing for occult blood. These tests are used to determine whether this symptom results from spasm or narrowing of the bowel. Anorectal manometry (i.e., pressure studies such as a balloon expulsion test) may be performed to assess malfunction of the sphincter. Defecography and colonic transit studies can also assist in the diagnosis because they permit assessment of active anorectal function. X-ray, colonoscopy, and lower GI endoscopy can be used to evaluate the patient with constipation (Basson, 2019a).

As noted previously, the majority of patients with constipation have functional constipation. The Rome IV Diagnostic Criteria provide the framework to make this determination (Simren, Palsson, & Whitehead, 2017) (see Chart 41-1).

Secondary causes of constipation should be evaluated. Neurologic diseases that can impact bowel function include stroke, Parkinson's disease, diabetes, spinal cord injury, and traumatic brain injury. Other causes of secondary constipation include colonic obstruction, rectal or vaginal prolapse, effects of some medications, hemorrhoids, anal fissures, and diverticular disease. Diagnostic testing is usually indicated for patients who fail to respond to conservative treatment (e.g., increasing fluids, fiber, physical activity) after 3 to 6 months (Basson, 2019a).

Complications

Increased arterial pressure can occur with defecation. Straining at stool, which results in the Valsalva maneuver (i.e., forcibly exhaling with the glottis closed), has a striking effect on arterial blood pressure. During active straining, the flow of venous blood in the chest is temporarily impeded because of increased intrathoracic pressure. This pressure tends to collapse the large veins in the chest. The atria and the ventricles

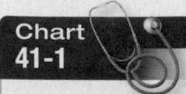

receive less blood, and consequently less blood is ejected by the left ventricle. Cardiac output is decreased, and there is a transient drop in arterial pressure, which may cause orthostasis, dizziness, or syncope (Norris, 2019).

Additional complications of constipation include fecal impaction, which may lead to fecal incontinence, **hemorrhoids** (dilated portions of anal veins), **fissures** (normal or abnormal folds, grooves, or cracks in body tissue), rectal prolapse, and megacolon (see later discussion of disorders of the anorectum, which includes hemorrhoids and fissures). Fecal impaction occurs when an accumulated mass of dry feces, called a *fecalith*, cannot be expelled. The mass may be palpable on digital examination, may produce pressure on the colonic mucosa that results in ulcer formation, most typically in the rectosigmoid colon, and may cause fecal incontinence, with seepage of liquid stools. Treatment can be embarrassing and also painful, because impaction removal usually involves digital dislodgement and enema administration. An ulcer also has the potential to perforate the colon wall, leading to **peritonitis** (i.e., inflammation of the lining of the abdominal cavity) (Basson, 2019a).

Hemorrhoids develop as a result of perianal vascular congestion caused by straining. Anal fissures may result from the passage of the hard stool through the anus, tearing the lining of the anal canal. The rectum may prolapse through the anal canal, causing seepage of mucus (NIDDK, 2018).

Megacolon is a dilated and atonic colon caused by a fecal mass that obstructs the passage of colon contents. Symptoms include constipation, liquid fecal incontinence, and abdominal distention. Megacolon can lead to perforation of the bowel and peritonitis (Norris, 2019).

 Gerontologic Considerations

Visits to primary providers for treatment of constipation are common in people 65 years and older. The most common complaint they voice is the need to strain at stool. The aging process inevitably generates changes in the colon; but the extent and physiologic implications for defecation remain unclear. The clinical situation is made more complex by ubiquitous factors among the aged (Eliopoulos, 2018). For instance, older adults who have loose-fitting dentures or have lost their teeth have difficulty chewing and frequently choose soft, processed foods that are low in fiber. Older adults tend to have decreased food intake, reduced mobility, and weak abdominal and pelvic muscles, and they are more likely to have multiple chronic illnesses requiring multiple medications (polypharmacy) that often cause constipation. Low-fiber convenience foods are widely used by people who have lost interest in eating. Some older adults reduce their fluid intake if they are not eating regular meals. Depression, weakness, and prolonged bed rest also contribute to constipation by decreasing intestinal motility and anal sphincter tone. Nerve impulses are dulled, and there is a decreased urge to defecate. Many older adults overuse laxatives in an attempt to have a daily bowel movement and become dependent on them. Chronic constipation profoundly impairs quality of life comparable to other conditions such as diabetes, rheumatoid arthritis, and osteoarthritis (Eliopoulos, 2018).

Medical Management

Treatment targets the underlying cause of constipation and prevention of recurrence. It includes education, exercise, bowel habit training, increased fiber and fluid intake, and judicious use of laxatives. Management may also include discontinuing laxative use or replacing medications that could cause or exacerbate constipation with other nonconstipating medications (Lacy, Mearin, Chang, et al., 2016). Patients can be educated to sit on the toilet with legs supported and to utilize the **gastrocolic reflex** (peristaltic movements of the large bowel occurring five to six times daily that are triggered by distention of the stomach) by attempting to defecate following a meal and a warm drink. Routine exercise to strengthen abdominal muscles is encouraged. Biofeedback is a technique that can be used to help patients learn to relax the sphincter mechanism to expel stool. Biofeedback is an effective therapy for patients with dyssynergic defecation and is considered first-line therapy once anorectal structural lesions have been excluded as the cause for constipation (Rao & Patcharatrakul, 2016; Rao, Valestin, Xiang, et al., 2018). Daily dietary intake of 25 to 30 g/day of fiber (soluble and bulk forming) is recommended, especially for the treatment of constipation in the older adult. It is important to add fiber to the diet slowly in order to avoid adverse effects such as abdominal cramping and bloating. Fiber is increased daily in 5 g increments, along with encouraging fluid intake (Mari et al., 2020). If laxative use is necessary, one of the following may be prescribed: bulk-forming agents (fiber laxatives), saline and osmotic agents, lubricants, stimulants, or emollient stool softeners. The physiologic action and patient education information related to these laxatives are presented in Table 41-1. Enemas and rectal suppositories are generally not recommended for treating constipation unless other medications have failed.

Nursing Management

The nurse elicits information about the onset and duration of constipation, current and past elimination patterns, the patient's expectation of normal bowel elimination, and lifestyle information (e.g., exercise and activity level, occupation, food and fluid intake, and stress level) during the health history interview. Past medical and surgical history, current medications, and laxative and enema use are important, as

is information about the sensation of rectal pressure or fullness, abdominal pain, excessive straining at defecation, and flatulence.

After the health history is obtained, the nurse sets specific goals for patient education (see Chart 41-2). Goals for the patient include restoring or maintaining a regular pattern of elimination by responding to the urge to defecate, ensuring adequate intake of fluids and high-fiber foods, learning about methods to avoid constipation, relieving anxiety about bowel elimination patterns, and avoiding complications.

Diarrhea

Diarrhea is an increased frequency of bowel movements (more than 3 per day) with altered consistency (i.e., increased liquidity) of stool. It can be associated with urgency, perianal discomfort, incontinence, nausea, or a combination of these factors (NIDDK, 2016b). Any condition that causes increased intestinal secretions, decreased mucosal absorption, or altered motility can produce diarrhea.

Diarrhea can be classified as acute, persistent, or chronic. Acute diarrhea is self-limiting, lasting 1 or 2 days; persistent diarrhea typically lasts between 2 and 4 weeks; and chronic diarrhea persists for more than 4 weeks and may return sporadically. Acute and persistent diarrheas are frequently caused by viral infections (e.g., norovirus). In addition, some drugs can cause acute or persistent diarrhea, including some antibiotics (e.g., erythromycin) and magnesium-containing antacids (e.g., magnesium hydroxide). Chronic diarrhea may be caused by adverse effects of chemotherapy, antiarrhythmic agents, antihypertensive agents, metabolic and endocrine disorders (e.g., diabetes, Addison disease, thyrotoxicosis), malabsorptive disorders (e.g., lactose intolerance, celiac disease), anal sphincter defect, Zollinger-Ellison syndrome, acquired immune deficiency syndrome (AIDS), and by parasitic or *Clostridium difficile* infections (NIDDK, 2016b).

TABLE 41-1 Select Laxative Medications

Classification/Medications	Action	Patient Education
Bulk Forming methylcellulose, psyllium, wheat dextrin	Polysaccharides and cellulose and wheat derivatives mix with intestinal fluids, swell, and stimulate peristalsis.	Take with 8-oz water and follow with 8-oz water; do not take dry. Report abdominal distention or unusual amount of flatulence.
Saline Agent magnesium hydroxide	Nonabsorbable magnesium ions alter stool consistency by drawing water into the intestines by osmosis; peristalsis is stimulated. Action occurs within 2 h.	Be aware that the liquid preparation is more effective than the tablet form. Note that only short-term use is recommended because of toxicity (central nervous system or neuromuscular depression, electrolyte imbalance). Do not take magnesium laxatives with renal insufficiency.
Lubricant mineral oil, glycerin suppository	Nonabsorbable hydrocarbons soften fecal matter by lubricating the intestinal mucosa; the passage of stool is facilitated. Action occurs within 6–8 h for mineral oil and within 30 min for glycerin suppository.	Do not take mineral oil with meals, because it can impair the absorption of fat-soluble vitamins and delay gastric emptying. Swallow carefully, because drops of oil that gain access to the pharynx can produce a lipid pneumonia. Insert glycerin suppositories fully and retain.
Stimulant bisacodyl, senna	Irritates the colonic epithelium by stimulating sensory nerve endings and increasing mucosal secretions and decreasing large intestinal water absorption. Action occurs within 6–8 h.	Be aware that catharsis may cause fluid and electrolyte imbalance, especially in the older adult. Do not swallow, crush, or chew tablets. Avoid milk or antacids within 1 h of taking medication, because the enteric coating may dissolve prematurely. Note that stimulant laxatives are *not* indicated for long-term use.
Emollient Stool Softener docusate	Hydrates the stool by its surfactant action on the colonic epithelium (increases the wetting efficiency of intestinal water); aqueous and fatty substances are mixed. Does *not* exert a laxative action.	Note that this can be used safely by patients who should avoid straining (cardiac patients, patients with anorectal disorders). Be aware that this will not evacuate hard stool because it is not a true laxative. Best for short-term use; decreased effectiveness with long-term use.
Osmotic Agent polyethylene glycol and electrolytes (sodium and potassium)	Attracts water and electrolytes, increasing intraluminal pressure, shorten colonic transit time, and increase bowel motility.	Polyethylene glycol-based agents originally used for bowel cleansing prior to colonoscopy; now available in powder-base daily dose, which is generally safe and effective. Monitor electrolyte levels with long-term use. Effects of long-term therapy not well known.
Chloride Channel Activator lubiprostone	Stimulates chloride channels in the colonic mucosa, causing passive passage of sodium and fluid into the colon.	Approved for opioid-induced constipation in people with chronic, non-cancer pain. Avoid pregnancy during treatment, keep in mind that it may cause increased flatulence and loose stools. Do not use for more than 4 wks.
Serotonin-4 Receptor Agonist prucalopride	Prokinetic, stimulates selective serotonin receptors in gastrointestinal tract, causing release of acetylcholine, stimulating gastrointestinal motility.	Approved for chronic idiopathic constipation. Selective action reduces cardiovascular adverse effects of other nonselective serotonin receptor agonists.

Adapted from Mari, A., Mahamid, M., Amara, H., et al. (2020). Chronic constipation in the elderly patient: Updates in evaluation and management. *Korean Journal of Family Medicine, 41*(3), 139–145. doi.org/10.4082/kjfm.18.0182

C. difficile is a gram-positive anaerobic organism and the most commonly identified bacterium in antibiotic-associated diarrhea (Mada & Alam, 2019). Approximately half a million patients are infected annually, causing 15,000 deaths. Antibiotic use, including penicillins, cephalosporins, fluoroquinalones, and clindamycin are known risk factors. More than half of patients admitted to the hospital will receive an antibiotic during their stay, and the Centers for Disease Control and Prevention (CDC) estimates that 30% to 50% of those antibiotics are either unnecessary or incorrectly prescribed (Mada & Alam, 2019). Other risk factors for *C. difficile* infection include advanced age, the use of proton pump inhibitors or chemotherapy, and a history of chronic liver disease, kidney disease, or malnutrition.

Pathophysiology

Acute and persistent diarrheas are classified as either noninflammatory (large-volume) or inflammatory (small-volume). Enteric pathogens that are noninvasive (e.g., *S. aureus, Giardia*) do not cause inflammation but secrete toxins that disrupt colonic fluid transport. They cause noninflammatory diarrhea, which is characterized by a large volume of loose, watery stools. Other pathogens that invade the intestinal mucosa and cause inflammatory changes typically result in smaller volumes of stool that is bloody (e.g., dysentery). Organisms implicated may include *Shigella, Salmonella,* and *Yersinia* species (Norris, 2019).

Types of chronic diarrhea include secretory, osmotic, malabsorptive, infectious, and exudative. Secretory diarrhea is usually high-volume diarrhea. Often associated with bacterial toxins and chemotherapeutic agents used to treat neoplasms, it is caused by increased production and secretion of water and electrolytes by the intestinal mucosa into the intestinal lumen. Osmotic diarrhea occurs when water is pulled into the intestines by the osmotic pressure of unabsorbed particles, slowing the reabsorption of water. It can be caused by lactase deficiency, pancreatic dysfunction, or intestinal hemorrhage. Malabsorptive diarrhea combines mechanical and biochemical actions, inhibiting effective absorption of nutrients. Low serum albumin levels lead to intestinal mucosa swelling and liquid stool. Infectious diarrhea results from infectious agents invading the intestinal mucosa. Exudative diarrhea is caused by changes in mucosal integrity, epithelial loss, or tissue destruction by radiation or chemotherapy. Diarrhea may also be caused by laxative misuse (Norris, 2019).

Clinical Manifestations

In addition to the increased frequency and fluid content of stools, the patient usually has abdominal cramps, distention, borborygmus (i.e., a rumbling noise caused by the movement of gas through the intestines), anorexia, and thirst. Painful spasmodic contractions of the anus and tenesmus may occur with defecation. Other symptoms depend on the cause and severity of the diarrhea but are related to dehydration and to fluid and electrolyte imbalances.

Voluminous, greasy stools suggest intestinal **malabsorption** (i.e., impaired transport across the mucosa), and the presence of blood, mucus, and pus in the stools suggests inflammatory enteritis or colitis. Oil droplets on the toilet water may be suggestive of pancreatic insufficiency. Nocturnal diarrhea may be a manifestation of diabetic neuropathy (NIDDK, 2016b; Weber & Kelley, 2018). The possibility of *C. difficile* infection should be considered in all patients with unexplained diarrhea who are taking or have recently taken antibiotics.

Assessment and Diagnostic Findings

When the cause of the diarrhea is not obvious, the following diagnostic tests may be performed: complete blood cell count (CBC); serum chemistries; urinalysis; routine stool examination; and stool examinations for infectious or parasitic organisms, bacterial toxins, blood, fat, electrolytes, and white blood cells. Endoscopy or barium enema may assist in identifying the cause.

Complications

The most common complication of diarrhea is dehydration. Dehydration with electrolyte loss (especially loss of potassium) may cause cardiac arrhythmias. Loss of bicarbonate with diarrhea can also lead to metabolic acidosis. Urinary output less than 0.5 mL/kg/h for 2 to 3 consecutive hours, muscle weakness, paresthesia, hypotension, anorexia, and drowsiness with a potassium level less than 3.5 mEq/L (3.5 mmol/L) must be reported. Chronic diarrhea can also result in skin care issues related to irritant dermatitis (NIDDK, 2016b). Cleansing with a wet wipe and applying barrier cream can prevent dermatitis.

Gerontologic Considerations

Older patients can become dehydrated quickly and develop hypokalemia (low potassium levels) as a result of diarrhea. The nurse observes for clinical manifestations of muscle weakness, arrhythmias, or decreased peristaltic motility that may lead to paralytic ileus. The older patient taking digitalis (e.g., digoxin) must be aware of how quickly dehydration and hypokalemia can occur with diarrhea. The nurse educates the patient to recognize the symptoms of hypokalemia, because low levels of potassium potentiate the action of digitalis, leading to digitalis toxicity (Eliopoulos, 2018).

The skin of an older person is more sensitive to excoriation due to decreased turgor and reduced subcutaneous fat layers. Gentle cleansing with a perineal cleansing solution (i.e., wet wiping method) and the use of a barrier cream or a liquid skin sealant will prevent or treat the excoriation (Eliopoulos, 2018).

Medical Management

Management is directed at controlling symptoms, preventing complications, and eliminating or treating the underlying disease. Until the definitive cause is discovered, infection control measures that restrict the transmission of infectious organisms (e.g., *C. difficile*–associated diarrhea) are warranted (see Chapter 66 for further discussion of *C. difficile* infection). Certain medications (e.g., antibiotics, anti-inflammatory agents) and antidiarrheal agents (e.g., loperamide, diphenoxylate with atropine) may be prescribed to reduce the severity of the diarrhea and treat the underlying disease. In most cases, loperamide is the medication of choice because it has fewer side effects than diphenoxylate with atropine. Findings from a systematic review supported the use of probiotics (live organisms given to a host) in some forms of diarrhea (Jones & Cantor, 2019). The specific organisms used were *Saccharomyces boulardii* (yeast) or lactic acid bacteria such as *Lactobacillus* and *Enterococcus lactic acid bacterium* species. Benefits include shortened duration of symptoms and early improvement of symptoms; there were no serious adverse effects reported (Jones & Cantor, 2019).

Nursing Management

The nurse assesses and monitors the characteristics and pattern of diarrhea. A health history should address the patient's medication therapy, medical and surgical history, and dietary patterns and intake. Reports of recent acute illness or recent travel to another geographic area are important. Assessment includes abdominal auscultation and palpation for tenderness. Inspection of the abdomen, mucous membranes, and skin is important to determine hydration status. Stool samples are obtained for testing. The perianal area should also be assessed for skin excoriation.

During an episode of diarrhea, the patient is encouraged to increase intake of liquids and foods low in bulk until the symptoms subside. When the patient is able to tolerate food intake, the patient should avoid caffeine, alcoholic beverages, dairy products, and fatty foods for several days (NIDDK, 2016b). Antidiarrheal medications such as diphenoxylate with atropine or loperamide may be taken as prescribed. Intravenous (IV) fluid therapy may be necessary for rapid rehydration in some patients, especially in older adults and in patients with preexisting GI conditions (e.g., IBD). It is important to monitor serum electrolyte levels closely. The nurse immediately reports evidence of arrhythmias or a change in a patient's level of consciousness.

The perianal area may become excoriated because diarrheal stool contains digestive enzymes that can irritate the skin. The patient should follow a perianal skin care routine to decrease irritation and excoriation (see Chapter 56).

Fecal Incontinence

Fecal incontinence or inadvertent bowel leakage describes the recurrent involuntary passage of stool from the rectum for at least 3 months. Factors that influence this disorder include the ability of the rectum to sense and accommodate stool, the amount and consistency of stool, the integrity of the anal sphincters and musculature, and rectal motility. Fecal incontinence is a widespread problem, affecting at least 7 out of 100 nonhospitalized adults and at least half of adults who reside in long-term care facilities (i.e., nursing homes) (NIDDK, 2017b). Fecal incontinence can have a substantially negative impact on quality of life (NIDDK, 2017b).

Pathophysiology

Fecal incontinence has many causes and risk factors and may be a symptom of an underlying condition. In general, it results from conditions that interrupt or disrupt the structure or function of the anorectal unit. Common causes include anal sphincter weakness, both traumatic (e.g., after surgical procedures involving the rectum) and nontraumatic (e.g., scleroderma); neuropathies, both peripheral (e.g., pudendal) and generalized (e.g., diabetes); disorders of the pelvic floor (e.g., rectal prolapse); inflammation (radiation proctitis, IBD); central nervous system disorders (e.g., dementia, stroke, spinal cord injury, multiple sclerosis); diarrhea; fecal impaction with overflow; and behavioral disorders. It is less commonly a long-term consequence of vaginal childbirth injuries than in years past, most likely because of improved delivery methods. It is more common with advancing age (i.e., weakness or loss of anal or rectal muscle tone) (Emmanuel, 2019; Rao, Bharucha, Chiaroni, et al., 2016).

Clinical Manifestations

Patients may have minor soiling, occasional urgency and loss of control, or complete incontinence. Patients may also experience poor control of flatus, diarrhea, or constipation. Passive incontinence occurs without warning; whereas, patients with urge incontinence have the sensation of the urge to defecate but cannot reach the toilet in time (Rao et al., 2016).

Assessment and Diagnostic Findings

Assessing the patient's medical history is helpful in identifying the most likely etiology. Diagnostic studies are necessary because the treatment of fecal incontinence depends on the cause. A rectal examination and an endoscopic examination such as a flexible sigmoidoscopy are performed to rule out tumors, inflammation, fissures, or impaction. Anorectal manometry, defecography, electromyography, anal endosonography, pelvic MRI scan, and transit studies may be helpful in identifying alterations in intestinal mucosa and muscle tone or in detecting other structural or functional problems (NIDDK, 2017b).

Medical Management

Medical management of fecal incontinence is directed at correcting the underlying cause. If fecal incontinence is related to diarrhea, the incontinence may disappear when diarrhea is successfully treated. Fecal incontinence secondary to a fecal impaction may cease after the impaction is removed and the rectum is cleansed. If the fecal incontinence is related to the use of contributory drugs (e.g., laxatives, antacids containing magnesium), the incontinence may improve or cease when the drug regimen is altered. When fecal incontinence is related to other disorders, treatments targeted at correcting the underlying disorder are initiated. Some patients benefit from the addition of psyllium as a fiber supplement. In addition, administering loperamide 30 minutes prior to meals can be an effective intervention in some patients. Biofeedback therapy with pelvic floor muscle training can be of assistance if the problem is decreased sensory awareness or sphincter control. Transanal irrigation and bowel training programs, including techniques to assist evacuation such as abdominal massage, Valsalva maneuver, and digital rectal stimulation can also be effective (Emmanuel, 2019; Rao et al., 2016). Sacral nerve stimulation, provided by implanting a subcutaneous stimulator that delivers low amplitude electrical stimulation to the sacral nerve, may be an option for some patients refractory to other interventions (Emmanuel, 2019). Surgical procedures include surgical reconstruction or repair of anal sphincter, artificial sphincter implantation, anal sphincter bulking by injection of synthetic agents, sacral nerve stimulation, or fecal diversion (Emmanuel, 2019).

Nursing Management

The nurse obtains a thorough health history, including information about previous surgical procedures, chronic illnesses, dietary patterns, bowel habits and problems, and current medication regimen. A bowel diary covering a 1- to 2-week period may be helpful in identifying elimination patterns and factors affecting bowel function (Emmanuel, 2019). Stool charts (e.g., Bristol Stool Form, see later discussion) may help with identifying frequency, volume, and consistency of the feces. The nurse also completes an examination of the rectal area. If a fecal impaction is noted, it must be removed before instituting any preventive therapies (Gump & Schmelzer, 2016; Taylor, Lynn, & Bartlett, 2019).

The nurse initiates a bowel training program that involves setting a schedule to establish bowel regularity. The goal is to help the patient achieve fecal continence. If this is not possible, the goal should be to manage the problem so the patient can have predictable, planned elimination. Sometimes it is necessary to use suppositories to stimulate the anal reflex. After the patient has achieved a regular schedule, the suppository can be discontinued. Biofeedback in conjunction with pelvic floor exercises can be used to help the patient improve sphincter contractility and rectal sensitivity. Bowel regulation also involves the therapeutic use of diet and fiber. Foods that thicken stool (e.g., applesauce) and fiber supplements help improve continence (Gump & Schmelzer, 2016). Conversely, foods that loosen stool (e.g., rhubarb, figs, prunes, plums) should be avoided. Some patients with fecal incontinence may benefit from the use of antidiarrheal medications (Gump & Schmelzer, 2016). Loperamide and diphenoxylate with atropine can be used; loperamide is the preferred medication because it does not cause central nervous system adverse effects (Comerford & Durkin, 2020; Rao et al., 2016).

Fecal incontinence can disrupt perineal skin integrity. Maintaining skin integrity is a priority, especially in the debilitated or older adult patient. Incontinence briefs or adult diapers, although helpful in containing the fecal material, permit increased skin contact with feces and may cause skin excoriation. In general, incontinence briefs are to be used only for brief periods of time. The nurse encourages and instructs about meticulous skin hygiene and uses perineal skin cleansers and skin protection products to protect perineal skin. Some patients may benefit from occasional use of foam anal plugs. However, many people find them unacceptable (Gump & Schmelzer, 2016).

Continence sometimes cannot be achieved, and the nurse assists the patient and family to accept and cope with this chronic situation. Patients with dementia may benefit from toileting assistance, including prompted or timed voiding and habit training, which is the setting of a regular time to go to the bathroom (e.g., after breakfast to have a bowel movement) (Gump & Schmelzer, 2016). The patient can use fecal incontinence devices, which include external collection devices and internal drainage systems. External devices are special rectal pouches (called *fecal incontinence collectors*) that are drainable. They are attached to a synthetic adhesive skin barrier specially designed to conform to the buttocks. Designed for patients with chronic, debilitating illnesses (e.g., in long-term care facilities) or acute illnesses, fecal management systems (e.g., Flexi-Seal Fecal Management System) can be used to eliminate fecal skin contact and are especially useful when there is extensive excoriation or skin breakdown. These systems, which consist of a tube with a low-pressure balloon that conforms to the internal rectal area, may be used for short-term management of liquid stools (no more than 4 consecutive weeks) (see Fig. 41-1).

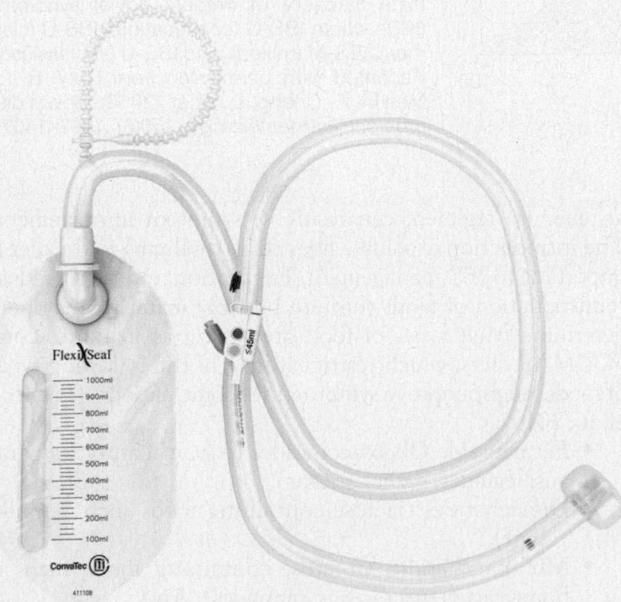

Figure 41-1 • Flexi-Seal Fecal Management System. Reprinted with permission from ConvaTec, Inc.

Irritable Bowel Syndrome (IBS)

Irritable bowel syndrome (IBS) is a chronic functional disorder characterized by recurrent abdominal pain associated with disordered bowel movements, which may include diarrhea, constipation, or both, without an identifiable cause (Lehrer, 2019; NIDDK, 2017c; Pacheco, Roizenblatt, Góis, et al., 2019). Global prevalence is estimated at 11%; its prevalence among American adults is estimated to be 12%. It is typically diagnosed in adults younger than 45 years of age (NIDDK, 2017c). Women are affected more often than men, with twice as many women diagnosed with IBS in the United States than men. A complex interplay of genetic, environmental, and psychosocial factors is thought to be associated with the onset of IBS. It is believed that some triggers can either herald the initial onset of IBS or exacerbate symptoms in those with diagnosed IBS; these may include chronic stress, sleep deprivation, neurohormonal deregulation, bacterial overgrowth, genetics, surgery, infections (e.g. *Giardia*), inflammation, and food intolerance (Pacheco et al., 2019).

Pathophysiology

IBS results from a functional disorder of intestinal motility. The change in motility may be related to neuroendocrine dysregulation, especially changes in serotonin signaling, infection, irritation, or a vascular or metabolic disturbance. The peristaltic waves are affected at specific segments of the intestine and in the intensity with which they propel the fecal matter forward. There is no evidence of inflammation or tissue changes in the intestinal mucosa (Norris, 2019).

Clinical Manifestations

Symptoms can vary widely, ranging in intensity and duration from mild and infrequent to severe and continuous. The main symptom is an alteration in bowel patterns: constipation (classified as IBS-C), diarrhea (classified as IBS-D), or a combination of both (classified as IBS-M for "mixed"). The few patients with IBS who do not fit any of these three categories of IBS-C, IBS-D, or IBS-M, are classified as IBS-U for "unclassified." Pain, bloating, and abdominal distention often accompany changes in bowel pattern. The abdominal pain is sometimes precipitated by eating and is frequently relieved by defecation. IBS frequently occurs concomitant with other GI disorders, including gastroesophageal reflux disease (GERD) and with a variety of non-GI functional disorders, including chronic fatigue syndrome, chronic pelvic pain, fibromyalgia, interstitial cystitis, migraine headaches, anxiety, and depression (NIDDK, 2017c).

Assessment and Diagnostic Findings

The Rome IV criteria define IBS as recurrent abdominal pain occurring at least once daily during the last 3 months, associated with two or more of the following (Lehrer, 2019):

- Abdominal pain related to defecation;
- Abdominal pain associated with a change in frequency of stool;
- Abdominal pain associated with a change in form/ appearance of stool.

Recording the quality and quantity of bowel movements in a stool diary such as the Bristol Stool Form Scale can be

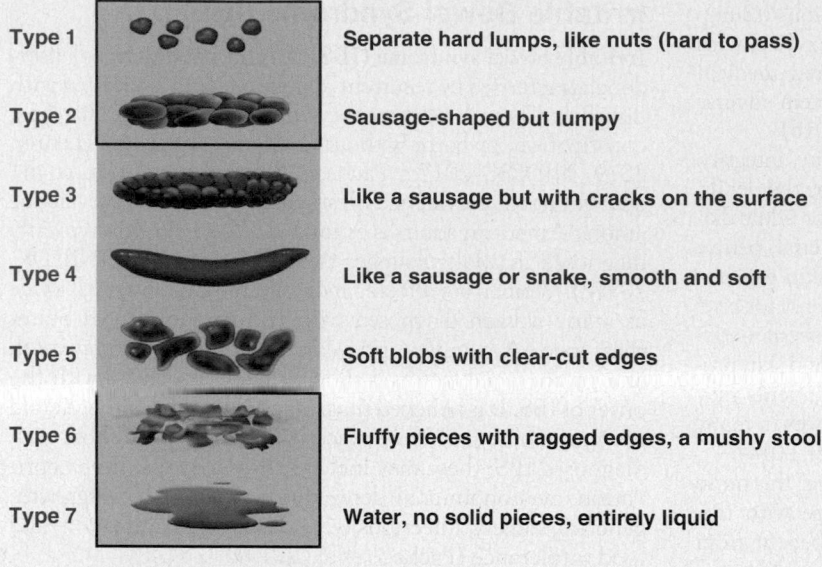

Type 1		Separate hard lumps, like nuts (hard to pass)
Type 2		Sausage-shaped but lumpy
Type 3		Like a sausage but with cracks on the surface
Type 4		Like a sausage or snake, smooth and soft
Type 5		Soft blobs with clear-cut edges
Type 6		Fluffy pieces with ragged edges, a mushy stool
Type 7		Water, no solid pieces, entirely liquid

A

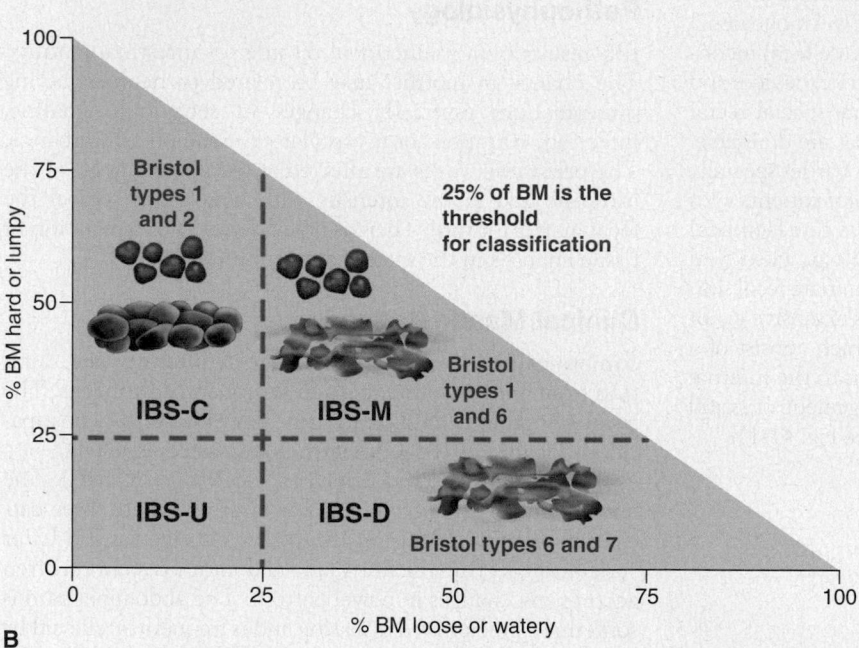

B

Figure 41-2 • **A.** The Bristol Stool Form Scale (BSFS) is used to evaluate bowel movement (BM) habit. **B.** Characteristics of stools as recorded on the BSFS are then used to determine category of irritable bowel syndrome (IBS), where IBS-C (constipation), IBS-D (diarrhea), IBS-M (mixed), and IBS-U (unclassified). Reprinted with permission from Lacy, B. E., Mearin, F., Chang, L., et al. (2016). Bowel disorders. *Gastroenterology*, *150*(6), 1393–1407.

useful in determining the category of IBS (Lacy et al., 2016) (see Fig. 41-2).

A definite diagnosis of IBS also necessitates testing to confirm the absence of structural or other disorders. Results from a CBC and C-reactive protein or fecal calprotectin can rule out IBD (see later discussion) for patients who may have IBS-D or IBS-M, as well as serologic tests for celiac disease (see later discussion). Stool studies and colonoscopy may be performed to rule out other colon diseases (e.g., colorectal cancer, colitis) (Lacy et al., 2016).

Medical Management

The goals of treatment are to relieve abdominal pain and control diarrhea or constipation. Lifestyle modification, including stress reduction, ensuring adequate sleep, and instituting an exercise regimen, can result in symptom improvement. The introduction of soluble fiber (e.g., psyllium) to the diet is important to IBS management. Restriction and then gradual reintroduction of foods that are possibly irritating may help determine what types of food are acting as irritants. Low-FODMAP diets, which restrict intake of the following types of foods, might improve symptoms for some patients (Pacheco et al., 2019):

- **F**ermentable **O**ligosaccharides (e.g., wheat, rye, asparagus, legumes, garlic, onions),
- **D**isaccharides (lactose-containing foods such as milk, yogurt),
- **M**onosaccharides (fructose-containing foods such as honey, agave nectar, figs, mangoes), **A**nd
- **P**olyols (e.g., blackberries, lychee, and low-calorie sweeteners)

For patients with IBS-D, antidiarrheal agents (e.g., loperamide) may be given to control the diarrhea and fecal urgency. Women with severe IBS-D that persists for more than 6 months that does not respond to other therapies may be prescribed alosetron, a highly selective 5-HT$_3$ antagonist that slows colonic motility. Other drugs that can mitigate IBS-D symptoms include rifaximin, a nonabsorbable oral antibiotic, and eluxadoline, a mu-receptor agonist/delta-receptor antagonist that neuromodulates colonic motility (Pacheco et al., 2019). Lubiprostone, a chloride channel regulator in the gut, can be prescribed for patients with IBS-C (Lacy et al., 2016).

Patients with all types of IBS complain of abdominal pain. This symptom may be mitigated by prescribing smooth muscle antispasmodic agents (e.g., dicyclomine). Antidepressants can assist in treating underlying anxiety and depression but also have secondary benefits. Antidepressants may affect serotonin levels, thus modulating intestinal transit time and improving abdominal comfort. Peppermint oil, a complementary medication, has proven effective in diminishing abdominal discomfort (Lacy et al., 2016). Other alternatives for IBS management include probiotics. Probiotics are bacteria that include *Lactobacillus* and *Bifidobacterium* that can be given to help decrease abdominal bloating and gas (Lacy et al., 2016).

Nursing Management

The nurse's role is to provide patient and family education and encourage self-care activities. The nurse may provide education on the appropriate use of a bowel habit diary, such as the Bristol Stool Form Scale (see Fig. 41-2A). The nurse emphasizes and reinforces good sleep habits and good dietary habits (e.g., avoidance of food triggers). A good way to identify problem foods is to keep a 1- to 2-week food diary and correlate symptoms with food intake. Patients are encouraged to eat at regular times and to avoid food triggers. They should understand that although adequate fluid intake is necessary, fluid should not be taken with meals because this results in abdominal distention. Alcohol use and cigarette smoking are discouraged. Stress management via relaxation techniques, cognitive-behavioral therapy, yoga, and exercise can be recommended.

DISORDERS OF MALABSORPTION

The inability of the digestive system to absorb one or more of the major vitamins (especially A and B$_{12}$), minerals (i.e., iron and calcium), and nutrients (i.e., carbohydrates, fats, and proteins) occurs in disorders of malabsorption. Interruptions in the complex digestive process may occur anywhere in the digestive system and cause decreased absorption (Norris, 2019). The conditions that cause malabsorption can be grouped into the following categories (Norris, 2019):

- Mucosal (transport) disorders causing generalized malabsorption (e.g., celiac disease, Crohn's disease, radiation enteritis)
- Luminal disorders causing malabsorption (e.g., bile acid deficiency, Zollinger-Ellison syndrome, pancreatic insufficiency, small bowel bacterial overgrowth, or chronic pancreatitis)
- Lymphatic obstruction, interfering with transport of fat by products of digestion into the systemic circulation (e.g., neoplasms, surgical trauma).

Chart 41-3

PATIENT EDUCATION

Managing Lactose Intolerance

The nurse instructs the patient to:

- Recognize that deficiency of lactase, a digestive enzyme essential for the digestion and absorption of lactose ("milk sugar") from the intestines, results in an intolerance to milk.
- Prevent symptoms by eliminating milk and milk substances.
- Eliminate processed foods that have fillers, such as dried milk, added to them; recognizing this can help determine which foods may need to be eliminated.
- Reduce symptoms by pretreating foods with lactase preparations (e.g., Lactaid drops) before ingestion or by ingesting lactase enzyme tablets with the first bite of food.
- Understand that most people can tolerate 1 to 2 cups of milk or milk products daily without major problems; they are best tolerated if ingested in small amounts during the day.
- Be aware that lactase activity of yogurt with "active cultures" helps the digestion of lactose within the intestine better than lactase preparations.
- Recognize that milk and milk products are rich sources of calcium and vitamin D; elimination of milk from the diet may result in calcium and vitamin D deficiencies; decreased intake without supplements can lead to osteoporosis.

Table 41-2 lists the clinical and pathologic aspects of select malabsorptive disorders. Chart 41-3 provides an education plan for a patient with lactose intolerance, a common malabsorptive disorder caused by a deficiency in lactase.

Celiac Disease

Celiac disease is a disorder of malabsorption caused by an autoimmune response to consumption of products that contain the protein gluten. Gluten is most commonly found in wheat, barley, rye, and other grains, malt, dextrin, and brewer's yeast. Celiac disease has become more common in the past decade, with an estimated prevalence of 1% in the United States. Women are afflicted twice as often as men. This disease is more common among Caucasians, although the rates of celiac disease are on the rise among non-Caucasians. Celiac disease also has a familial risk component, particularly among first-degree relatives. Others at heightened risk include those with type 1 diabetes, Down syndrome, and Turner syndrome. Celiac disease may manifest at any age in a person who is genetically predisposed (NIDDK, 2016a).

Pathophysiology

Nearly 30% of the population in the United States may be genetically predisposed to developing celiac disease. Individuals who are predisposed share a major histocompatibility complex (MHC) class II allele human leukocyte antigen (HLA), HLA-DQ2 or HLA-DQ8. Those who develop celiac disease exhibit an autoimmune response to gluten products that is both humoral and cell mediated. It is not known what trigger or triggers may incite this autoimmune response, although it cannot occur if gluten is not ingested. As a result of this response, the epithelial cells that line the small intestines become inflamed, particularly the proximal portion, where most absorption of nutrients occurs. Eventually, the mucosal villi of the small intestine become denuded and cannot function. This results

TABLE 41-2 Select Disorders of Malabsorption

Diseases/Disorders	Pathophysiology	Clinical Features
Gastric resection with gastrojejunostomy	Decreased pancreatic stimulation because of duodenal bypass; poor mixing of food, bile, pancreatic enzymes; decreased intrinsic factor	Weight loss, moderate steatorrhea, anemia (combination of iron deficiency, vitamin B_{12} malabsorption, folate deficiency)
Pancreatic insufficiency (chronic pancreatitis, pancreatic carcinoma, pancreatic resection, cystic fibrosis)	Reduced intraluminal pancreatic enzyme activity, with maldigestion of lipids and proteins	History of abdominal pain followed by weight loss; marked steatorrhea, azotorrhea (excess of nitrogenous matter in the feces or urine); also frequent glucose intolerance (70% in pancreatic insufficiency)
Ileal dysfunction (resection or disease)	Loss of ileal absorbing surface leads to reduced bile salt pool size and reduced vitamin B_{12} absorption; bile in colon inhibits fluid absorption	Diarrhea, weight loss with steatorrhea, especially when >100-cm resection, decreased vitamin B_{12} absorption
Stasis syndromes (surgical strictures, blind loops, enteric fistulas, multiple jejunal diverticula, scleroderma)	Overgrowth of intraluminal intestinal bacteria, especially anaerobic organisms, to >10^6/mL results in deconjugation of bile salts, leading to decreased effective bile salt pool size, also bacterial utilization of vitamin B_{12}	Weight loss, steatorrhea; low vitamin B_{12} absorption; may have low D-xylose absorption
Zollinger-Ellison syndrome	Hyperacidity in duodenum inactivates pancreatic enzymes	Ulcer diathesis, steatorrhea
Lactose intolerance	Deficiency of intestinal lactase results in high concentration of intraluminal lactose with osmotic diarrhea	Varied degrees of diarrhea and cramps after ingestion of lactose-containing foods; positive lactose intolerance test, decreased intestinal lactase
Celiac disease (gluten-sensitive enteropathy)	Toxic response to a gluten fraction gliadin by surface epithelium results in destruction of absorbing surface of intestine	Weight loss, diarrhea, bloating, anemia (low iron, folate), osteomalacia, steatorrhea, azotorrhea, low D-xylose absorption; folate and iron malabsorption
Tropical sprue	Unknown toxic factor results in mucosal inflammation, partial villous atrophy	Weight loss, diarrhea, anemia (low folate, vitamin B_{12}); steatorrhea; low D-xylose absorption, low vitamin B_{12} absorption
Whipple disease	Bacterial invasion of intestinal mucosa	Arthritis, hyperpigmentation, lymphadenopathy, serous effusions, fever, weight loss, steatorrhea, azotorrhea
Certain parasitic diseases (giardiasis, strongyloidiasis, coccidiosis, capillariasis)	Damage to or invasion of surface mucosa	Diarrhea, weight loss; steatorrhea; organism may be seen on jejunal biopsy or recovered in stool
Immunoglobulinopathy	Decreased local intestinal defenses, lymphoid hyperplasia, lymphopenia	Frequent association with *Giardia*: hypogammaglobulinemia or isolated immunoglobulin A deficiency

Adapted from Hammami, M. B. (2019). Malabsorption. *Medscape.* Retrieved on 2/29/2019 at: emedicine.medscape.com/article/180785-overview; Norris, T. L. (2019). *Porth's pathophysiology: Concepts of altered health states* (10th ed.). Philadelphia, PA: Wolters Kluwer.

in loss of ability to absorb both micronutrients and macronutrients, causing systemic nutritional deficits (Norris, 2019).

Clinical Manifestations

The most common GI clinical manifestations of celiac disease include diarrhea, steatorrhea, abdominal pain, abdominal distention, flatulence, and weight loss. However, these manifestations are more common among children than adults. Adults can present with non-GI signs and symptoms of celiac disease, which are highly variable and can include fatigue, general malaise, depression, hypothyroidism, migraine headaches, osteopenia, anemia, seizures, paresthesias in the hands and feet, and a red, shiny tongue. Some adults and children may evidence ridges in the enamel of their adult teeth, as well as discoloration or yellowing. Dermatitis herpetiformis is a rash that is frequently associated with celiac disease in adults; it manifests as clusters of erythematous macules that develop into itchy papules and vesicles on the forearms, elbows, knees, face, or buttocks (NIDDK, 2016a).

Assessment and Diagnostic Findings

A comprehensive assessment of the patient's presenting signs and symptoms, as well as a family history and risk factor assessment, may provide the first clues that the patient may have celiac disease. The definitive diagnosis is based upon a series of serologic tests and endoscopic biopsy. It is important that the patient continues to consume gluten products during testing, or there could be a false-negative serologic finding. The first serologic test is the immunoglobulin A (IgA) anti-tissue transglutaminase (tTG), which is 90% sensitive and 95% specific to celiac disease. Findings are confirmed with upper endoscopy with biopsies of the proximal small intestine (Goebel, 2019).

Medical Management

Celiac disease is a chronic, noncurable, lifelong disease. There are no drugs that induce remission; the treatment is to refrain from exposure to gluten in foods and other products (see later discussion). A consultation with a dietician may be advisable. The patient should be advised that it will likely take time before bothersome signs and symptoms resolve; it will take a full year before the integrity of the intestinal villi can be restored. The patient should be cautioned that despite adhering to a gluten-free diet, symptoms can still occur and can have an impact on quality of life (Roos, Liedberg, Hellström, et al., 2019). Other manifestations of celiac disease may require specific, targeted treatment. For instance, patients who present with anemia may require folate, cobalamin, or iron supplements (see Chapter 29). Patients with osteopenia may require treatment for osteoporosis (see Chapter 36).

Nursing Management

The nurse provides patient and family education regarding adherence to a gluten-free diet (see Chart 41-4), and how to avoid other gluten products. For instance, oats are not contraindicated in gluten-free diets; however, many oat products are produced in facilities that are cross-contaminated with wheat or other contraindicated grains. Likewise, gluten-free foods prepared in restaurants or dining areas that share preparatory space can become gluten-contaminated. For instance, gluten-free toast prepared in a toaster that is also used for wheat-based toast can become gluten-contaminated. Patients must become vigilant in asking restaurant and dining hall staff about how gluten-free foods are prepared.

Products that are not foods can also contain gluten. Many generic and over-the-counter drugs can be prepared with gluten gels. Toothpastes, communion wafers, and some cosmetics (e.g., lipsticks) and art supplies (e.g., modeling clay) can also contain gluten. Patients must understand how to carefully read labels on both foods and nonfood products to determine if they contain gluten. The U.S. Food and Drug Administration (FDA) regulates and monitors the appropriate application of gluten-free labels.

ACUTE ABDOMEN

An acute abdomen, sometimes called a *surgical abdomen* is characterized by an acute onset of abdominal pain that does not have a traumatic etiology and that most typically requires swift surgical intervention to prevent peritonitis, sepsis, and septic shock. Disorders of the lower GI tract that may cause similar initial presenting clinical manifestations, causing acute abdominal pain and an acute abdomen include appendicitis, severe diverticulitis, and intestinal obstruction, all of which may lead to peritonitis.

Peritonitis

Peritonitis is inflammation of the peritoneum, which is the serous membrane lining the abdominal cavity and covering the viscera. Usually, it is a result of bacterial infection but may occur secondary to a fungal or mycobacterial infection; the organisms come from diseases or disorders of the GI tract or, in women, from the internal reproductive organs (e.g., fallopian tube). The most common bacteria implicated are *Escherichia coli* and *Klebsiella*, *Proteus*, *Pseudomonas*, and *Streptococcus* species. Peritonitis can also result from external sources such as abdominal surgery or trauma (e.g., gunshot wound, stab wound) or an inflammation that extends from an organ outside the peritoneal area, such as the kidney, or from continuous ambulatory peritoneal dialysis (CAPD) (see Chapter 48). Peritonitis can be categorized as (Daley, 2019):

- Primary peritonitis, also called *spontaneous bacterial peritonitis (SBP)*, occurs as a spontaneous bacterial infection of ascitic fluid. This occurs most commonly in adult patients with liver failure (see Chapter 43).
- Secondary peritonitis occurs secondary to perforation of abdominal organs with spillage that infects the serous peritoneum. The most common causes include a perforated appendix (see later discussion), perforated peptic ulcer (see Chapter 40), perforated sigmoid colon caused by severe diverticulitis (see later discussion), volvulus of the colon (see later discussion), and strangulation of the small intestine (see later discussion). The major focus of this section is on secondary peritonitis.

Chart 41-4 **PATIENT EDUCATION**
How to Avoid Gluten

The nurse instructs the patient to choose foods that are naturally gluten-free such as:

- Fresh fruits and vegetables
- Meat and poultry
- Fish and seafood
- Dairy
- Beans, legumes, and nuts
- Corn, rice, soy, quinoa, and potato

The nurse instructs the patient to avoid foods that commonly contain gluten, including the following:

- Wheat (wheat-free does not mean gluten-free), barley, bran, durum, spelt, faro, rye, bulgur, graham, semolina, farina, emmer, and triticale; these are generally used in:
  - Cakes, pastries, cookies
  - Breads, pastas, rolls, pizza, crackers
- Brewer's yeast; this generally includes beer, ale, and porter
- Malt, malt extract, and malt flavoring
- Modified food starch made from wheat (commonly contained in sour cream)

The nurse instructs the patient to exercise caution and carefully read labels on foods,[a] particularly before consuming the following:

- Candies (gluten-free candy list is available on Celiac Disease Foundation site)
- Caramel-colored foods
- Cornflakes and puffed rice cereals (these often contain malt flavoring or extract, which contains gluten)
- Oat products not specifically labeled as produced in gluten-free facilities
- Processed lunch meats and "shaped" foods (e.g., cheese sticks)
- Salad dressings, condiments, soy sauce, seasonings
- Sauces (wheat is often used as thickening agent)
- Soft drinks

[a]The U.S. Food and Drug Administration (FDA) standard for "gluten-free" is that the product must contain less than 200 parts per million (ppm) of gluten.

Adapted from Celiac Disease Foundation. Gluten-Free Living. Retrieved on 2/29/2020 at: celiac.org/gluten-free-living/gluten-free-foods/

- Tertiary peritonitis occurs as a result of a superinfection in a patient who is immunocompromised. Tuberculous peritonitis in a patient with AIDS is an example of tertiary peritonitis; these are rare causes of peritonitis.

Pathophysiology

Secondary peritonitis is caused by leakage of contents from abdominal organs into the abdominal cavity, usually as a result of inflammation, infection, ischemia, trauma, or tumor perforation. Bacterial proliferation occurs. Edema of the tissues results, and exudation of fluid develops in a short time. Fluid in the peritoneal cavity becomes turbid with increasing amounts of protein, white blood cells, cellular debris, and blood. The immediate response of the intestinal tract is hypermotility, soon followed by paralytic ileus with an accumulation of air and fluid in the bowel (Daley, 2019; Norris, 2019).

Clinical Manifestations

Symptoms depend on the location and extent of the inflammation. The early clinical manifestations of peritonitis frequently are the signs and symptoms of the disorder causing the condition (e.g., manifestations of infection). At first, pain is diffuse but then becomes constant, localized, and more intense over the site of the pathologic process (site of maximal peritoneal irritation). Movement usually aggravates the pain. The affected area of the abdomen becomes extremely tender and distended, and the muscles become rigid. Rebound tenderness may be present. Usually, anorexia, nausea, and vomiting occur and peristalsis is diminished, followed by paralytic ileus. An initial temperature of 37.8° to 38.3°C (100° to 101°F) can be expected, along with an increased pulse rate. With progression of the condition, patients may become hypotensive and oliguric or anuric. Without swift and decisive intervention, clinical manifestations will mirror those of sepsis and septic shock (Daley, 2019) (see Chapter 11).

Assessment and Diagnostic Findings

The white blood cell count is elevated (> 11,000/mm^3) and may demonstrate a relative increase in the bands (i.e., immature neutrophils), consistent with bacterial infection (Daley, 2019). The hemoglobin and hematocrit levels may be low if blood loss has occurred. Serum electrolyte studies may reveal altered levels of potassium, sodium, and chloride. Blood chemistry panels and arterial blood gases may reveal dehydration and acidosis.

An abdominal x-ray may show free air and fluid as well as distended bowel loops. Abdominal ultrasound may reveal **abscesses** (localized collection of purulent material surrounded by inflamed tissues) and fluid collections, and ultrasound-guided aspiration may assist in easier placement of drains. A computed tomography (CT) scan of the abdomen may show abscess formation. Peritoneal aspiration and culture and sensitivity studies of the aspirated fluid may reveal infection and identify the causative organisms. Ultrasound-guided paracentesis may be indicated for the patient with ascites. MRI may be used for diagnosis of intra-abdominal abscesses (Daley, 2019).

Medical Management

Fluid, colloid, and electrolyte replacement is the major focus of medical management. The administration of several liters of an isotonic solution is prescribed. Hypovolemia occurs because massive amounts of fluid and electrolytes move from the intestinal lumen into the peritoneal cavity and deplete the fluid in the vascular space.

Analgesic medications are prescribed for pain. Antiemetic agents are given as prescribed for nausea and vomiting. Intestinal intubation and suction assist in relieving abdominal distention and in promoting intestinal function. Fluid in the abdominal cavity can cause pressure that restricts expansion of the lungs and causes respiratory distress. Oxygen therapy by nasal cannula or mask generally promotes adequate oxygenation, but airway intubation and ventilatory assistance occasionally are required.

Antibiotic therapy is initiated early in the treatment of peritonitis. Large doses of a broad-spectrum antibiotic are given IV until the specific organism causing the infection is identified and appropriate antibiotic therapy can be initiated.

The main focus of treatment in secondary peritonitis is to identify and control the source of infection, maintain organ function, and prevent complications (Daley, 2019). Treatment is multidisciplinary and involves hemodynamic support, fluid and electrolyte replacement, systemic broad-spectrum antibiotics, and nutritional support. Control of the source of infection can be treated surgically and nonsurgically depending on the patient's condition and underlying pathology. Nonsurgical treatment includes percutaneous drainage of abscesses and endoscopic stent placement. In select instances, ultrasound-guided and CT-guided peritoneal drainage of abdominal and extraperitoneal abscesses has allowed for avoidance or delay of surgical therapy until the acute septic process has subsided (Daley, 2019). Surgical treatment is directed toward excision (e.g., appendix), resection with or without anastomosis (e.g., intestine), repair (e.g., perforation), and drainage (e.g., abscess). With extensive sepsis, a fecal diversion may need to be created (see later discussions). Antibiotic therapy is continued postoperatively.

 Nursing Management

Intensive care is needed for the patient with septic shock (see Chapter 11). Signs indicating that peritonitis is subsiding include a decrease in temperature and pulse rate, softening of the abdomen, return of peristaltic sounds, passing of flatus, and bowel movements. The nurse increases fluid and food intake gradually and reduces parenteral fluids as prescribed. A worsening clinical condition may indicate a complication, and the nurse must prepare the patient for emergency surgery. The nursing management of a patient treated for secondary peritonitis is based upon the patient's primary diagnosis and treatment (see later discussions of Nursing Management of Patients with Appendicitis, Diverticular Disease, and Intestinal Obstruction).

Appendicitis

The appendix is a small, vermiform (i.e., wormlike) appendage about 8 to 10 cm (3 to 4 inches) long that is attached to the cecum just below the ileocecal valve. The appendix fills with byproducts of digestion and empties regularly into the cecum. Because it empties inefficiently and its lumen is small, the appendix is prone to obstruction and is particularly vulnerable to infection (i.e., appendicitis). Appendicitis, the most frequent cause of acute abdomen in the United States, is the most common reason for emergency abdominal surgery. Although it can occur at any age, it typically occurs between the ages of 10 and 30 years. Its incidence is slightly higher among males and there is a familial predisposition (Craig, 2018; NIDDK, 2014a).

Pathophysiology

The appendix becomes inflamed and edematous as a result of becoming kinked or occluded by a fecalith, lymphoid hyperplasia (secondary to inflammation or infection), or rarely, foreign bodies (e.g., fruit seeds) or tumors. The inflammatory process increases intraluminal pressure, causing edema and obstruction of the orifice. Once obstructed, the appendix becomes ischemic, bacterial overgrowth occurs, and eventually gangrene or perforation occurs (Craig, 2018).

Clinical Manifestations

Vague periumbilical pain (i.e., visceral pain that is dull and poorly localized) with anorexia progresses to right lower quadrant pain (i.e., parietal pain that is sharp, discrete, and well localized) and nausea in approximately 50% of patients with appendicitis (Craig, 2018). A low-grade fever may be present. Local tenderness may be elicited at McBurney's point when pressure is applied (see Fig. 41-3). Rebound tenderness (i.e., production or intensification of pain when pressure is released) may be present. Rovsing's sign may be elicited by palpating the left lower quadrant; this paradoxically causes pain to be felt in the right lower quadrant (see Fig. 41-3). If the appendix has ruptured, the pain becomes consistent with

peritonitis (see previous discussion); abdominal distention develops as a result of paralytic ileus, and the patient's condition worsens (Craig, 2018).

Constipation can also occur with appendicitis. Laxatives given in this instance may result in perforation of the inflamed appendix. In general, a laxative or cathartic should not be given when a person has fever, nausea, and abdominal pain.

Assessment and Diagnostic Findings

Diagnosis is based on the results of a complete history and physical examination, laboratory findings, and imaging studies. The white blood cell (WBC) count is useful when determining diagnosis; between 80% and 85% of adults with appendicitis will have a WBC count >10,500/mm^3; 78% of patients have neutrophilia, where neutrophils comprise >75% of the WBCs (Daley, 2019). C-reactive protein levels are typically elevated, especially within the first 12 hours of symptoms, but may return to normal in patients who are symptomatic longer than 24 hours (Daley, 2019). A CT scan or ultrasound is used to confirm the diagnosis. A pregnancy test may be ordered for women of childbearing age to rule out ectopic pregnancy and before radiologic studies are done. As an alternative, a transvaginal ultrasound may be used to confirm the diagnosis (Craig, 2018). A urinalysis is usually obtained to rule out urinary tract infection or renal calculi.

Complications

The major complications of appendicitis are gangrene or perforation of the appendix, which can lead to peritonitis, abscess formation, or portal pylephlebitis, which is septic thrombosis of the portal vein caused by vegetative emboli that arise from septic intestines. Perforation generally occurs within 6 to 24 hours after the onset of pain and leads to peritonitis (Craig, 2018; Spelman, 2019).

 ## Gerontologic Considerations

Acute appendicitis is uncommon in older adults. When appendicitis does occur, classic signs and symptoms are altered and may vary greatly. Pain may be absent or minimal. Symptoms may be vague, suggesting bowel obstruction or another process. Fever and leukocytosis may not be present. As a result, diagnosis and prompt treatment may be delayed, causing complications and mortality. The patient may have no symptoms until the appendix becomes gangrenous or perforates. The incidence of complications is higher in older adults because many of these patients do not seek health care as quickly as younger patients (Craig, 2018; Eliopoulos, 2018).

Medical Management

Immediate surgery is typically indicated if appendicitis is diagnosed (Craig, 2018). To correct or prevent fluid and electrolyte imbalance, dehydration, and sepsis, antibiotics, and IV fluids are given until surgery is performed. Appendectomy (i.e., surgical removal of the appendix) is performed as soon as possible to decrease the risk of perforation. Appendectomy has traditionally been performed under general anesthesia with an open technique via transverse incision in the right

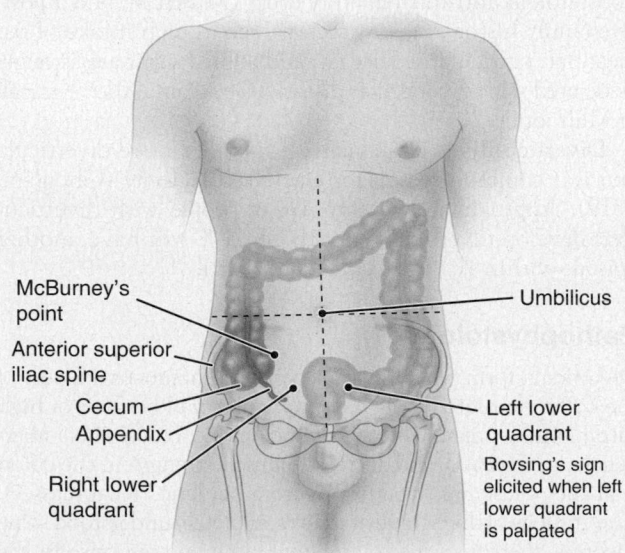

McBurney's point
Anterior superior iliac spine
Cecum
Appendix
Right lower quadrant
Umbilicus
Left lower quadrant
Rovsing's sign elicited when left lower quadrant is palpated

Figure 41-3 • When the appendix is inflamed, tenderness can be noted in the right lower quadrant at McBurney's point, which is between the umbilicus and the anterior superior iliac spine. Rovsing's sign is pain felt in the right lower quadrant after the left lower quadrant has been palpated.

lower quadrant (laparotomy). The laparoscopic approach is becoming the procedure of choice; it allows the patient an earlier return to normal activities (Santacroce, 2019). Both laparotomy and laparoscopy are safe and effective in the treatment of appendicitis with or without perforation. Antibiotic prophylaxis is recommended for less than 24 hours for nonperforated appendicitis and for <5 days for perforated appendicitis (Daley, 2019). Antibiotic selection should follow guidelines outlined by the CDC to prevent surgical site infections (CDC, 2017a).

Some patients may have abscess formation that involves the cecum or terminal ileum. In these select cases, appendectomy may be deferred until the mass is drained. Most commonly, these abscesses are drained percutaneously or surgically. The patient continues to receive treatment with antibiotics. After the abscess is drained and there is no further evidence of infection, an appendectomy is then performed (Craig, 2018).

Nursing Management

Goals include relieving pain, preventing fluid volume deficit, reducing anxiety, preventing or treating surgical site infection, preventing atelectasis, maintaining skin integrity, and attaining optimal nutrition.

The nurse prepares the patient for surgery, which includes an IV infusion to replace fluid loss and promote adequate renal function, antibiotic therapy to prevent infection, and administration of analgesic agents for pain. An enema is not given because it can lead to perforation.

After surgery, the nurse places the patient in a high Fowler position. This position reduces the tension on the incision and abdominal organs, helping to reduce pain. It also promotes thoracic expansion, diminishing the work of breathing, and decreasing the likelihood of atelectasis. The patient is educated on the use of an incentive spirometer and encouraged to use it at least every 2 hours while awake (see Chapter 19 for discussion on atelectasis and incentive spirometry). A parenteral opioid (e.g., morphine) is typically prescribed to relieve pain; this is switched to an oral agent when the patient is able to tolerate oral fluids and foods. Any patient who was dehydrated before surgery receives IV fluids. When tolerated, oral fluids are given. Food is provided as desired and tolerated on the day of surgery when bowel sounds are present. The nurse auscultates for the return of bowel sounds and queries the patient for passing of flatus. Urine output is monitored to ensure that the patient is not hampered by postoperative urinary retention and to ensure that hydration status is adequate. The patient is encouraged to ambulate the day of surgery to reduce risks of atelectasis and venous thromboembolism (VTE) formation.

The patient may be discharged on the day of surgery if the temperature is within normal limits, there is no undue discomfort in the operative area, and the appendectomy was performed laparoscopically. Discharge instruction for the patient and family is imperative. The nurse instructs the patient to make an appointment to have the surgeon remove any sutures and inspect the wound between 1 and 2 weeks after surgery. Incision care and activity guidelines are discussed; heavy lifting is to be avoided postoperatively, although normal activity can usually be resumed within 2 to 4 weeks.

Patients with a gangrenous or perforated appendix are at greater risk for infection and peritonitis; therefore, they may be kept in the hospital for several days. Secondary abscesses may form in the pelvis, under the diaphragm, or in the liver, causing elevation of the temperature, pulse rate, and white blood cell count. When the patient is ready for discharge, the patient and family are educated about how to care for the incision and perform dressing changes and irrigations as prescribed. A home health nurse may be needed to assist with this care and to monitor the patient for complications and wound healing.

Diverticular Disease

A **diverticulum** is a saclike herniation of the lining of the bowel that extends through a defect in the muscle layer. True diverticula are herniations of all layers of the GI wall (mucosa, muscularis propria, and adventitia), while pseudo-diverticula only involve the mucosa and submucosa (Ghoulam, 2019). Diverticula may occur anywhere in the GI tract, from the esophagus to the colon, but occur most commonly in the colon. In the colon there is only one complete muscle layer, in contrast to the small intestine and rectum which have two muscular layers. People with Asian ancestry are more likely to develop diverticula in the right colon, while people of European descent are more prone to diverticular disease in the sigmoid colon (Ghoulam, 2019).

Diverticulosis is defined by the presence of multiple diverticula without inflammation or symptoms. Diverticular disease of the colon is very common in developed countries, and its prevalence increases with increasing age; it is present in half of all adults over 65 years of age, and 70% of adults over 80 years of age (Krzyzak & Mulrooney, 2019). Diverticulosis is the most common pathologic incidental finding on colonoscopy. Approximately 80% of patients with diverticulosis never develop any complications or symptoms of disease. Risk factors include low intake of dietary fiber, slow colonic transit time, obesity, a history of cigarette smoking, regular use of nonsteroidal anti-inflammatory drugs (NSAIDs), and a positive family history. Dietary factors such as high intake of red meat, fat, particularly dairy fat, and refined sugar are strongly associated with diverticular disease (Ghoulam, 2019; Krzyzak & Mulrooney, 2019).

Diverticulitis is inflammation of one or more diverticula and is a common reason for elective colectomy (Ghoulam, 2019). Approximately 1% to 4% of people with diverticulosis develop diverticulitis; of those, 20% will have another episode within 10 years (Ghoulam, 2019).

Pathophysiology

Diverticula form when the mucosal and submucosal layers of the colon herniate through the muscular wall because of high intraluminal pressure, low volume in the colon (i.e., fiber-deficient contents), and decreased muscle strength in the colon wall (i.e., muscular hypertrophy from hardened fecal masses). The etiology of diverticulitis is not completely understood. One theory is the cause due to an altered immune response in the gut microbiome (Krzyzak & Mulrooney, 2019). Other explanations are feces or food particles become trapped in diverticula, resulting in bacterial overgrowth, distention, increased intraluminal pressure, muscle spasms, vascular compromise, and subsequent micro- or macroperforation. Complications include intra-abdominal abscesses, peritonitis, **fistula** (abnormal tract formation), and hemorrhage (Krzyzak & Mulrooney, 2019). Repeated bouts of diverticulitis can result in scar tissue formation, which may lead to narrowing of the colonic lumen and bowel obstruction.

Bowel contents can accumulate in a diverticulum and decompose, causing inflammation and infection. The diverticulum can also become obstructed and then inflamed if the obstruction continues. The inflammation of the weakened colonic wall of the diverticulum can cause it to perforate, giving rise to irritability and spasticity of the colon (i.e., diverticulitis). In addition, abscesses may develop and may eventually perforate, leading to peritonitis and erosion of the arterial blood vessels, resulting in bleeding. When a patient develops symptoms of diverticulitis, microperforation of the colon has occurred.

Clinical Manifestations

Chronic constipation sometimes precedes the development of diverticulosis by many years. Most commonly, no problematic symptoms occur with diverticulosis. Some patients may have mild signs and symptoms that include bowel irregularity with intervals of alternating constipation and diarrhea, with nausea, anorexia, and bloating or abdominal distention.

With diverticulitis, up to 70% of patients report an acute onset of mild to severe cramping pain in the left lower quadrant (Ghoulam, 2019). This may be accompanied by a change in bowel habits, most typically constipation or obstipation (i.e., severe constipation) and bloating, with nausea, fever, and leukocytosis. Acute complications of diverticulitis may include abscess formation, bleeding, and peritonitis. If an abscess develops, the associated findings are tenderness, a palpable mass, fever, and leukocytosis. Inflamed diverticula may erode areas adjacent to arterial branches, causing massive rectal bleeding. An inflamed diverticulum that perforates results in abdominal pain localized over the involved segment, usually the sigmoid; local abscess or peritonitis follows (see previous discussion).

Recurrent episodes of diverticulitis may cause chronic complications that include fistula formation, including colovesicular fistulas (i.e., between the colon and bladder) and, in women, colovaginal fistulas (i.e., between the colon and vagina). As a response to repeated inflammation, the colon may narrow with scar tissue and fibrotic strictures, leading to cramps, narrow stools, and increased constipation, or, at times, intestinal obstruction (see later discussion).

Assessment and Diagnostic Findings

Diverticulosis is typically diagnosed by colonoscopy, which permits visualization of the extent of diverticular disease. Laboratory tests that assist in diagnosis of diverticulitis include a CBC; if the patient has frank blood in the stool, the hemoglobin level should be analyzed. The WBC is frequently elevated; however, a normal WBC count does not rule out diverticulitis. Up to 40% of patients with diverticulitis have a normal WBC count (Ghoulam, 2019). Urinalysis and urine cultures should be analyzed in patients with suspected colovesicular fistulas.

An abdominal CT scan with contrast agent is the diagnostic test of choice to confirm diverticulitis; it can also reveal perforation and abscesses. Abdominal x-rays may demonstrate free air under the diaphragm if a perforation has occurred from the diverticulitis. Results from these radiologic tests confirm whether or not the patient has uncomplicated diverticulitis or complicated diverticulitis that could require surgical intervention. The Modified Hinchey Classification System is used as a guide to determine treatment (Hinchey, Schaal, & Richards, 1978; Krzyzak & Mulrooney, 2019) (see Table 41-3).

 Gerontologic Considerations

The incidence of diverticular disease increases with age because of degeneration and structural changes in the circular muscle layers of the colon and because of cellular hypertrophy. The symptoms are less pronounced in the older adult than in other adults. Older adults may not have abdominal pain until infection occurs. They may delay reporting symptoms because they fear surgery or are afraid that they may have cancer (Eliopoulos, 2018).

Medical Management

Medical management is guided by the severity of disease and the presence of comorbid diagnoses and complications. Treatment for patients with uncomplicated diverticulitis is on an outpatient basis with diet and medication. This is the typical treatment for most patients with diagnosed diverticulitis. Rest, oral fluids, and analgesic medications are recommended. Initially, a clear liquid diet is consumed until the inflammation subsides; then a high-fiber, low-fat diet is recommended. This type of diet helps increase stool volume, decrease colonic transit time, and reduce intraluminal pressure. The American Gastroenterology Association recommends selective use of

TABLE 41-3	Modified Hinchey Classification: Staging of Acute, Complicated Diverticulitis	
Modified Hinchey Classification Stage	**Description**	**Category**
0	Mild diverticulitis or diverticula with colonic thickening on CT	Uncomplicated
Ia	Colonic reaction with inflammatory reaction in the pericolic fate	Uncomplicated
Ib	Localized pericolic or mesenteric abscess	Complicated
II	Intra-abdominal, pelvic, or retroperitoneal abscess	Complicated
III	Perforated diverticulitis causing generalized purulent peritonitis	Complicated
IV	Rupture of diverticula into the peritoneal cavity with generalized fecal peritonitis	Complicated

Adapted from Ghoulam, E. M. (2019). Diverticulitis. *Medscape*. Retrieved on 2/29/2020 at: emedicine.medscape.com/article/173388-overview; Krzyzak, M., & Mulrooney, S. (2019). Diverticulitis: A review of diagnosis, treatment, and prevention. *Consultant*, 59(2), 35–37, 44.

antibiotics for patients with acute, uncomplicated diverticulitis (Ghoulam, 2019).

In acute cases of diverticulitis with significant symptoms, hospitalization is required. Hospitalization is often indicated for those who are older, immunocompromised, taking corticosteroids, or unable to tolerate oral fluids. Patients with complicated disease (see Table 41-3) can require hospitalization; those with higher stages require surgery and hospitalization (see later discussion). Withholding oral intake, administering IV fluids, and instituting nasogastric (NG) suctioning if vomiting or distention occurs are used to rest the bowel. Broad-spectrum antibiotics (e.g., ampicillin/sulbactam, ticarcillin/clavulanate) are prescribed. An opioid or other analgesic agent may be prescribed for pain relief. Oral intake is increased as symptoms subside. A low-fiber diet may be necessary until signs of infection decrease.

Surgical Management

Although acute diverticulitis usually subsides with medical management, immediate surgical intervention is necessary if complications (e.g., perforation, peritonitis, hemorrhage, obstruction) occur. In cases of abscess formation without peritonitis, hemorrhage, or obstruction, CT-guided percutaneous drainage may be performed to drain the abscess, and IV antibiotics are given. After the abscess is drained and the acute episode of inflammation has subsided (after approximately 6 weeks), surgery may be recommended to prevent repeated episodes. Two types of surgery are typically considered either to treat acute complications or prevent further episodes of inflammation:

- One-stage resection, in which the inflamed area is removed and a primary end-to-end anastomosis is completed
- Multiple-stage procedures for complications such as obstruction or perforation (see Fig. 41-4)

The type of surgery performed depends on the extent of complications found during the procedure. When possible, the area of diverticulitis is resected and the remaining bowel

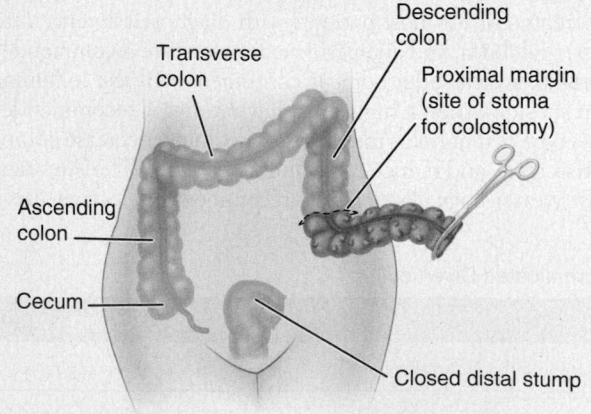

Figure 41-4 • Hartmann procedure for diverticulitis: primary resection for diverticulitis of the colon. The affected segment (*clamp attached*) has been divided at its distal end. In a primary anastomosis, the proximal margin (*dotted line*) is transected and the bowel attached end to end. In a two-stage procedure, a colostomy is constructed at the proximal margin with the distal stump oversewn (Hartmann procedure, as shown) and the stump is left in the pelvis. The distal stump may be brought to the surface as a mucous fistula if there is concern about blood supply. The second stage consists of colostomy takedown and anastomosis.

is joined end to end (i.e., primary resection and end-to-end anastomosis). This is performed using traditional surgical or laparoscopically assisted colectomy with lavage. A two-stage resection may be performed in patients with Hinchey Stage IV diverticulitis; the diseased colon is resected (as in a one-stage procedure) but no anastomosis is performed. In this procedure, one end of the bowel is brought out to the abdominal wall and the distal end is closed over and left in the abdomen (Hartmann procedure), or if the blood supply to the distal colon is questionable, both ends of the bowel are brought out to the abdominal wall (double-barrel). Both Hartmann procedures and double-barrel colostomies usually can be reanastomosed at a later time.

Nursing Management

The nurse recommends a fluid intake of 2 L/day (within limits of the patient's cardiac and renal reserve) and suggests foods that are soft but have increased fiber, such as prepared cereals or soft-cooked vegetables, to increase the bulk of the stool and facilitate peristalsis, thereby promoting defecation. An individualized exercise program is encouraged to improve abdominal muscle tone. It is important to review the patient's daily routine to establish a schedule for meals and a set time for defecation and to assist in identifying habits that may have suppressed the urge to defecate. The nurse encourages daily intake of bulk laxatives such as psyllium, which helps propel feces through the colon. Some people with diverticulosis may have food triggers such as nuts and popcorn that bring on a diverticulitis attack, whereas others may not report food triggers. If triggers are identified, patients should be urged to avoid them.

For the patient who has had a colostomy placed, refer to the later section on Nursing Management of the Patient Requiring an Ostomy.

Intestinal Obstruction

Intestinal obstruction exists when blockage prevents the normal flow of intestinal contents through the intestinal tract. Two types of processes can impede this flow (Norris, 2019; Ramnarine, 2017):

- *Mechanical obstruction:* *Extrinsic* lesions from outside the intestines or *intrinsic* lesions within the intestines can obstruct flow. Examples of extrinsic lesions include adhesions, hernias, and abscesses. Examples of intrinsic lesions include intestinal tumors (benign and cancerous), strictures (from prior surgery or radiation), or *intraluminal* lesions due to a defect in the bowel lumen (e.g., intussusception).
- *Functional or paralytic obstruction:* The intestinal musculature cannot propel the contents along the bowel either due to interruption of innervation or vascular supply to the bowel. Examples are amyloidosis, muscular dystrophy, endocrine disorders such as diabetes, or neurologic disorders such as Parkinson's disease. The blockage also can be temporary and the result of the manipulation of the bowel during surgery (i.e., ileus).

Obstruction can occur in the large or small intestine and can be partial or complete. Severity depends on the region of bowel affected, the degree to which the lumen is occluded, and especially the degree to which the vascular supply to

TABLE 41-4	Mechanical Causes of Intestinal Obstruction	
Cause	**Description**	**Result**
Adhesions	Loops of intestine become adherent to areas that heal slowly or scar after abdominal surgery; occurs most commonly in small intestine	After surgery, adhesions produce a kinking of an intestinal loop.
Intussusception (see Fig. 41-5A)	One part of the intestine slips into another part located below it (like a telescope shortening); occurs more commonly in infants than adults	The intestinal lumen becomes narrowed, and blood supply becomes strangulated.
Volvulus (see Fig. 41-5B)	Bowel twists and turns on itself and occludes the blood supply	Intestinal lumen becomes obstructed. Gas and fluid accumulate in the trapped bowel.
Hernia (see Fig. 41-5C)	Protrusion of intestine through a weakened area in the abdominal muscle wall	Intestinal flow may be completely obstructed. Blood flow to the area may be obstructed as well.
Tumor	A tumor that exists within the wall of the intestine extends into the intestinal lumen, or a tumor outside the intestine causes pressure on the wall of the intestine. Most common type is colorectal adenocarcinoma	Intestinal lumen becomes partially obstructed; if the tumor is not removed, complete obstruction results.

the bowel wall is disturbed. Most obstructions occur in the small intestine. Adhesions, hernia, and tumor account for 90% of obstructions in the small intestines (Bordeianou & Yeh, 2019). Other causes of small bowel obstruction include Crohn's disease, intussusception, volvulus, and paralytic ileus. Most obstructions in the large intestines occur in the sigmoid colon. The most common causes of large bowel obstruction are cancer (60%), diverticular disease (20%), and volvulus (5%). Other causes of large bowel obstruction include benign tumors, strictures, and obstipation or fecal impaction (Hopkins, 2017). Table 41-4 and Figure 41-5 list mechanical causes of obstruction and describe how they occur.

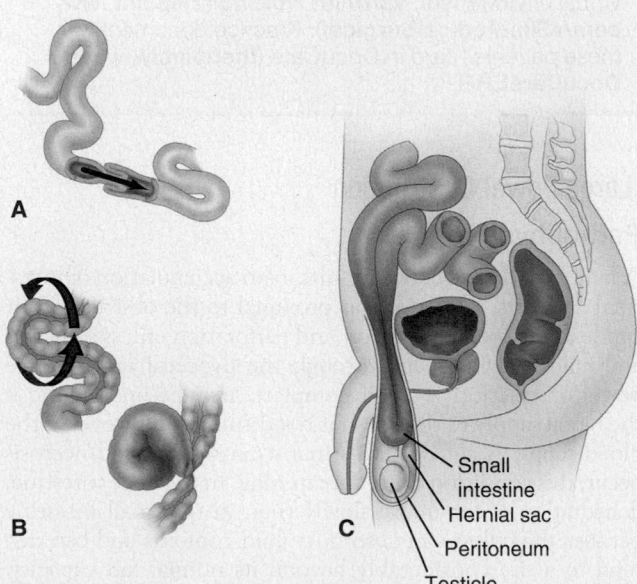

Figure 41-5 • Three causes of intestinal obstruction. **A.** Intussusception; invagination or shortening of the colon caused by the movement of one segment of bowel into another. **B.** Volvulus of the sigmoid colon; the twist is counterclockwise in most cases. Note the edematous bowel. **C.** Hernia (inguinal). The sac of the hernia is a continuation of the peritoneum of the abdomen. The hernial contents are intestine, omentum, or other abdominal contents that pass through the hernial opening into the hernial sac.

Small Bowel Obstruction

Pathophysiology

Intestinal contents, fluid, and gas accumulate proximal to the intestinal obstruction. The abdominal distention and retention of fluid reduce the absorption of fluids and stimulate more gastric secretion. With increasing distention, pressure within the intestinal lumen increases, causing a decrease in venous and arteriolar capillary pressure. Third-spacing of fluids, electrolytes, and proteins into the intestinal lumen occurs, resulting in decreased circulating fluid volume and dehydration. With continued intestinal distention and edema, perfusion to the affected intestinal segment can be compromised, leading to ischemia, necrosis, and eventual rupture or perforation of the intestinal wall, with resultant peritonitis (Bordeianou & Yeh, 2019; Ramnarine, 2017).

Clinical Manifestations

The initial symptom is usually crampy pain that is wavelike and colicky due to persistent peristalsis both above and below the blockage. The patient may pass blood and mucus but no fecal matter and no flatus. Vomiting occurs. If the obstruction is complete, the peristaltic waves initially become extremely vigorous and eventually assume a reverse direction, with the intestinal contents propelled toward the mouth instead of toward the rectum. The signs of dehydration become evident: intense thirst, drowsiness, oliguria, generalized malaise, aching, and a parched tongue and mucous membranes. The patient may continue to have flatus and stool early in the process due to distal peristalsis. The abdomen becomes distended. The lower the obstruction in the GI tract, the more marked the abdominal distention; this may cause reflux vomiting. Vomiting results in loss of hydrogen ions and potassium from the stomach, leading to reduction of chloride and potassium in the blood and to metabolic alkalosis. Dehydration and acidosis develop from loss of water and sodium. With acute fluid losses, hypovolemic shock may occur; septic shock may also occur (Bordeianou & Yeh, 2019; Ramnarine, 2017) (see Chapter 11).

Assessment and Diagnostic Findings

Diagnosis is based on the symptoms, physical assessment findings, and the results of imaging studies. Early in the process, bowel sounds are high-pitched and hyperactive in an attempt to pass the obstruction; later, bowel sounds will be hypoactive. Changes in the pattern (constant) or increased intensity of bowel sounds may also be indicative of strangulation or ischemic bowel (Bordeianou & Yeh, 2019; Ramnarine, 2017). Abdominal x-ray and CT scan findings include abnormal quantities of gas, fluid, or both in the intestines and sometimes collapsed distal bowel. Laboratory studies (i.e., electrolyte studies and a CBC) reveal a picture of dehydration, loss of plasma volume, and possible infection. The approach to small bowel obstruction focuses on confirming the diagnosis, identifying the etiology, and determining the likelihood of strangulation.

Medical Management

Decompression of the bowel through insertion of an NG tube is necessary for all patients with small bowel obstruction; this may be tried for up to 3 days for patients with partial obstructions, as resting the bowel in this manner can result in resolution of the obstruction (Ramnarine, 2017). For patients with adhesions, administration of hypertonic water-soluble GI contrast media (Gastrografin) may be of benefit in stimulating peristalsis and determining the probability of needing surgical intervention. The dye is administered via NG tube, the tube is clamped for 2 to 4 hours, then an abdominal x-ray is taken within 6 to 24 hours; evidence of the dye in the large intestine is predictive of resolution of obstruction without surgical intervention (Bordeianou & Yeh, 2019).

Surgical Management

Approximately 25% of patients with obstruction will need surgical intervention (Bordeianou & Yeh, 2019). When the bowel is completely obstructed, the possibility of strangulation and tissue necrosis warrants surgical intervention. Before surgery, IV fluids are necessary to replace the depleted water, sodium, chloride, and potassium.

The surgical treatment of intestinal obstruction depends on the cause of the obstruction. For the most common causes of obstruction, such as hernia and adhesions, the surgical procedure involves repairing the hernia or dividing the adhesion to which the intestine is attached. In some instances, the portion of affected bowel may be removed and an anastomosis performed. The complexity of the surgical procedure depends on the duration of the intestinal obstruction and the condition of the intestine. Open or laparoscopic technique can be used.

Nursing Management

Nursing management of the patient with a small bowel obstruction who does not require surgery includes maintaining the function of the NG tube, assessing and measuring the NG output, assessing for fluid and electrolyte imbalance, monitoring nutritional status, and assessing for manifestations consistent with resolution (e.g., return of normal bowel sounds, decreased abdominal distention, subjective improvement in abdominal pain and tenderness, passage of flatus or stool).

> ### ▶ Quality and Safety Nursing Alert
>
> *Maintaining fluid and electrolyte balance is a priority to monitor in the patient with a small bowel obstruction. The presence of the NG tube in conjunction with the patient's nothing-by-mouth (NPO) status places the patient at significant risk of fluid imbalance. Thus, measures to promote fluid balance are critically important.*

The nurse reports discrepancies in the patient's intake and output, worsening of pain or abdominal distention, and increased NG output. If the patient's condition does not improve, the nurse prepares them for surgery. This preparation includes preoperative education as the patient's condition indicates. Nursing care of the patient after surgical repair of a small bowel obstruction is similar to that for other abdominal surgeries (see Chapter 16).

Unfolding Patient Stories: Stan Checketts • Part 2

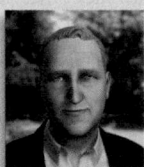

Recall from Chapter 9 **Stan Checketts,** who arrived in the emergency department with severe abdominal pain. He is diagnosed with a small bowel obstruction. He is NPO and has an NG tube placed to low intermittent suction. Describe the steps of a focused GI assessment performed by the nurse. How would the nurse explain the rationale for an NG tube and NPO status? What are specific assessments and nursing care responsibilities for an NG tube?

Care for Stan and other patients in a realistic virtual environment: *vSim for Nursing* (**thepoint.lww.com/vSimMedicalSurgical**). Practice documenting these patients' care in DocuCare (**thepoint.lww.com/DocuCareEHR**).

Large Bowel Obstruction

Pathophysiology

A large bowel obstruction results in an accumulation of intestinal contents, fluid, and gas proximal to the obstruction. It can lead to severe distention and perforation unless some gas and fluid can flow back through the ileocecal valve. Large bowel obstruction, even if complete, may be undramatic if the blood supply to the colon is not disturbed. However, if the blood supply is cut off, intestinal strangulation and necrosis occur; this condition is life threatening. In the large intestine, dehydration occurs more slowly than in the small intestine because the colon can absorb its fluid contents and can distend to a size considerably beyond its normal full capacity. Similar to small bowel obstruction, complications include perforation, peritonitis, and sepsis.

Clinical Manifestations

Large bowel obstruction differs clinically from small bowel obstruction in that the symptoms develop and progress relatively slowly. In patients with obstruction in the sigmoid colon or the rectum, constipation may be the only symptom for weeks. The shape of the stool is altered as it passes the obstruction that is gradually increasing in size. Blood loss in the stool may result in iron deficiency anemia. The patient may experience weakness, weight loss, and anorexia. Eventually, the abdomen becomes markedly distended, loops of large bowel become visibly outlined through the abdominal wall, and the patient has crampy lower abdominal pain (Hopkins, 2017).

Assessment and Diagnostic Findings

Diagnosis is based on symptoms, physical assessment findings, and on imaging studies. The abdomen may be distended, bowel sounds may be normal early in the obstruction, but later hypoactive to absent, and the abdomen hyperresonant (Hopkins, 2017).

Abdominal x-ray and abdominal CT or MRI findings reveal a distended colon and pinpoint the site of the obstruction (Hopkins, 2017).

Medical Management

Restoration of intravascular volume, correction of electrolyte abnormalities, and NG aspiration and decompression are instituted immediately. A colonoscopy may be performed to untwist and decompress the bowel. A rectal tube may be used to decompress an area that is lower in the bowel. As an alternative, a metal colonic stent may be used as either a palliative intervention or as a bridge to definitive surgery. The colonic stent is placed endoscopically with the assistance of an image intensifier, which creates a fluoroscopic image (Hopkins, 2017). The usual treatment is surgical resection to remove the obstructing lesion. A temporary or permanent colostomy may be necessary. An ileoanal anastomosis may be performed if removal of the entire large bowel is necessary (Hopkins, 2017).

Nursing Management

The nurse's role is to monitor the patient for symptoms indicating that the intestinal obstruction is worsening or resolving and to provide emotional support and comfort. The nurse administers IV fluids and electrolytes as prescribed. If the patient's condition does not respond to nonsurgical treatment, the nurse prepares the patient for surgery. This preparation includes preoperative education as the patient's condition indicates. After surgery, routine postoperative nursing care is provided, including abdominal wound care (see Chapter 16).

INFLAMMATORY BOWEL DISEASE

Inflammatory bowel disease (IBD) is a group of chronic disorders: Crohn's disease and ulcerative colitis that result in inflammation or ulceration (or both) of the bowel. Both disorders have striking similarities but also several differences. Approximately 10% to 15% of patients with IBD have characteristics of both disorders and cannot be definitively diagnosed with either disorder and are classified as having indeterminate colitis (Rowe, 2020). Table 41-5 compares Crohn's disease and ulcerative colitis.

The prevalence of IBD in the United States has increased in the past century; it is estimated that 1.3% of adults are diagnosed with IBD (CDC, 2019). Prevalence is highest in Europe (particularly in Germany and Norway), the United States, and Canada, although the incidence has been increasing in South America, Africa, and Asia (Piovani, Danese, Peyrin-Biroulet, et al., 2019).

Family history predisposes people to IBD, particularly if a first-degree relative has the disease (Rowe, 2020). Other risk factors for IBD include being Caucasian, of Ashkenazi Jewish descent, living in a northern climate, and living in an urban area (Rowe, 2020). Both diseases are commonly diagnosed in people 15 to 40 years of age, with a second peak incidence in adults 55 to 65 years of age (Rowe, 2020). Current smokers are at risk for Crohn's disease, but those who are ex-smokers or nonsmokers are at risk for ulcerative colitis (Piovani et al., 2019).

Despite extensive research, the cause of IBD is still unknown. Three underlying factors are genetic predisposition, altered immune response, and an altered response to gut microorganisms (Rowe, 2020). Researchers theorize that environmental triggers (e.g., exposure to air pollutants), food, tobacco, and viral illnesses in people genetically predisposed to developing an IBD can trigger the cell-mediated immune response that results in the inflammatory changes that characterize IBDs (Rowe, 2020). Inflammatory cytokines have been identified in the pathologic and clinical characteristics of both disorders (Rowe, 2020; Walfish, 2019). Both disorders have extra-intestinal manifestations; systemic symptoms common to both include fever, arthralgias, malaise, and episodes of diaphoresis (Rowe, 2020).

Crohn's Disease (Regional Enteritis)

Crohn's disease, also called regional enteritis, is characterized by a subacute and chronic inflammation of the GI tract wall that extends through all layers (i.e., transmural lesion). Although its characteristic histopathologic changes can occur anywhere in the GI tract, it most commonly occurs in the distal ileum and the ascending colon. Approximately 35% of patients have ileitis (only ileal involvement); 45% have ileocolitis (diseased ileum and colon); and 20% have granulomatous colitis (only colon involvement) (Rowe, 2020).

Pathophysiology

The inflammatory process in Crohn's disease begins with crypt inflammation and abscesses, which develop into small, focal ulcers. These initial lesions then deepen into longitudinal and transverse ulcers, separated by edematous patches, creating a characteristic *cobblestone* appearance in the affected bowel. Fistulas, fissures, and abscesses form as the inflammation extends into the peritoneum. Granulomas can occur in lymph nodes, the peritoneum, and through the layers of the bowel in about half of patients. Diseased bowel segments are sharply demarcated by adjoining areas of normal bowel tissue. These are called *skip* lesions, from which the label *regional enteritis* is derived. As the disease advances, the bowel wall thickens and becomes fibrotic, and the intestinal lumen narrows. Diseased bowel loops sometimes adhere to other loops surrounding them (Rowe, 2020).

TABLE 41-5	Comparison of Crohn's Disease and Ulcerative Colitis	
	Crohn's Disease	**Ulcerative Colitis**
Course	Prolonged, variable	Exacerbations, remissions
Pathology		
Early	Transmural thickening	Mucosal ulceration
Late	Deep, penetrating granulomas	Minute, mucosal ulcerations
Clinical Manifestations		
Location	Ileum, ascending colon (usually)	Rectum, descending colon
Bleeding	Usually not, but if it occurs, it tends to be mild	Common—severe
Perianal involvement	Common	Rare—mild
Fistulas	Common	Rare
Diarrhea	Less severe	Severe
Abdominal mass	Common	Rare
Diagnostic Study Findings		
Barium studies	Regional, discontinuous skip lesions	Diffuse involvement
	Narrowing of colon	No narrowing of colon
	Thickening of bowel wall	No mucosal edema
	Mucosal edema	Stenosis rare
	Stenosis, fistulas	Shortening of colon
Sigmoidoscopy	May be unremarkable unless accompanied by perianal fistulas	Abnormal inflamed mucosa
Colonoscopy	Distinct ulcerations separated by relatively normal mucosa in ascending colon	Friable mucosa with pseudopolyps or ulcers in descending colon
Therapeutic Management	Corticosteroids, aminosalicylates (sulfasalazine)	Corticosteroids, aminosalicylates (sulfasalazine) useful in preventing recurrence
	Immunomodulators (e.g., azathioprine) or monoclonal antibodies (e.g., infliximab, adalimumab) may be tried if refractory to corticosteroids and aminosalicylates	Immunomodulators (e.g., azathioprine) or monoclonal antibodies (e.g., infliximab, adalimumab) may be tried if refractory to corticosteroids and aminosalicylates
	Antibiotics	Bulk hydrophilic agents
	Parenteral nutrition	Antibiotics
	Partial or complete colectomy, with ileostomy or anastomosis	Proctocolectomy, with ileostomy
	Rectum can be preserved in some patients	Rectum can be preserved in only a few patients "cured" by colectomy
	Recurrence common	
Systemic Complications	Small bowel obstruction	Toxic megacolon
	Right-sided hydronephrosis	Perforation
	Nephrolithiasis	Hemorrhage
	Colon cancer	Colon cancer
	Cholelithiasis	Pyelonephritis
	Arthritis	Nephrolithiasis
	Uveitis	Cholangiocarcinoma
	Erythema nodosum	Arthritis
		Uveitis
		Erythema nodosum

Adapted from Walfish, A. E. (2019). Inflammatory bowel disease. *Merck Manual: Professional Version.* Retrieved on 3/1/2020 at: www.merckmanuals.com/professional/gastrointestinal-disorders/inflammatory-bowel-disease-ibd/overview-of-inflammatory-bowel-disease

Clinical Manifestations

The onset of symptoms is usually insidious in Crohn's disease, with diarrhea and prominent right lower quadrant abdominal pain unrelieved by defecation. Scar tissue and the formation of granulomas interfere with the ability of the intestine to transport products of upper intestinal digestion through the constricted lumen, resulting in crampy abdominal pain. There is abdominal tenderness and spasm. Because eating stimulates intestinal peristalsis, the crampy pains occur after meals. To avoid these bouts of crampy pain, the patient tends to limit food intake, reducing the amounts and types of food to such a degree that normal nutritional requirements are often not met. As a result, weight loss, malnutrition, and secondary anemia occur. Ulcers in the membranous lining of the intestine and other inflammatory changes result in a weeping, edematous intestine that continually empties an irritating discharge into the colon. Disrupted absorption causes chronic diarrhea and nutritional deficits, which can lead to significant weight loss and dehydration. In some patients, the inflamed intestine may perforate, leading to intra-abdominal and anal abscesses. Fever and leukocytosis occur. Chronic symptoms include diarrhea, abdominal pain, **steatorrhea** (i.e., excessive fat in the feces), anorexia, weight loss, and nutritional deficiencies.

Manifestations may extend beyond the GI tract and can include joint disorders (e.g., arthritis), skin lesions (e.g., erythema nodosum), ocular disorders (e.g., uveitis), and oral ulcers. The clinical course and symptoms can vary; in some patients, periods of remission and exacerbation occur, but in others, the disease follows a fulminating course. When intestinal symptoms worsen, some extraintestinal manifestations can worsen, whereas the clinical course of some extraintestinal manifestations seems independent of the clinical course of the Crohn's disease (Walfish, 2019).

Assessment and Diagnostic Findings

CT scan is indicated to find bowel wall thickening and mesenteric edema, as well as obstructions, abscesses, and fistulas, and may help specify abscess formation and location, guiding percutaneous access and drainage. MRI is both highly sensitive and specific in terms of identifying pelvic and perianal abscesses and fistulas (Rowe, 2020).

A CBC is performed to assess hematocrit and hemoglobin levels (which may be decreased) as well as the WBC count (may be elevated). The erythrocyte sedimentation rate (ESR) is usually elevated. Albumin and protein levels may be decreased, indicating malnutrition (Rowe, 2020).

Complications

Complications of Crohn's disease include intestinal obstruction or stricture formation, perianal disease, fluid and electrolyte imbalances, malnutrition from malabsorption, and fistula and abscess formation. The most common type of small bowel fistula caused by Crohn's disease is the enterocutaneous fistula (i.e., an abnormal opening between the small bowel and the skin). Abscesses can be the result of an internal fistula that results in fluid accumulation and infection. Patients with colonic Crohn's disease are also at increased risk of colon cancer (NIDDK, 2017d).

Ulcerative Colitis

Ulcerative colitis is a chronic ulcerative and inflammatory disease of the mucosal and submucosal layers of the colon and rectum that is characterized by unpredictable periods of remission and exacerbation with bouts of abdominal cramps and bloody or purulent diarrhea. The inflammatory changes typically begin in the rectum and progress proximally through the colon (Basson, 2019b).

Pathophysiology

Ulcerative colitis affects the superficial mucosa of the colon and is characterized by multiple ulcerations, diffuse inflammations, and desquamation or shedding of the colonic epithelium. Bleeding occurs as a result of the ulcerations. The mucosa becomes edematous and inflamed. The lesions are contiguous, occurring one after the other. Eventually, the bowel narrows, shortens, and thickens because of muscular hypertrophy and fat deposits. Because the inflammatory process is not transmural (i.e., it affects the inner lining only), abscesses, fistulas, obstruction, and fissures are uncommon in ulcerative colitis (Walfish, 2019).

Clinical Manifestations

The clinical course is usually one of remissions and exacerbations. The predominant symptoms of ulcerative colitis include diarrhea, with passage of mucus, pus, or blood; left lower quadrant abdominal pain; and intermittent tenesmus. The bleeding may be mild or severe, and pallor, anemia, and fatigue result. The patient may have anorexia, weight loss, fever, vomiting, and dehydration, as well as cramping, and the passage of six or more liquid stools each day. The disease is classified as mild, severe, or fulminant, depending on the severity of the symptoms. Hypoalbuminemia, electrolyte imbalances, and anemia frequently develop. Extraintestinal manifestations include skin lesions (e.g., erythema nodosum), eye lesions (e.g., uveitis), joint abnormalities (e.g., arthritis), and liver disease (Basson, 2019b).

Assessment and Diagnostic Findings

Abdominal x-ray studies are useful for determining the cause of symptoms. Free air in the peritoneum and bowel dilation or obstruction should be excluded as a source of the presenting symptoms. Colonoscopy is the definitive screening test that can distinguish ulcerative colitis from other diseases of the colon with similar symptoms. It may reveal friable, inflamed mucosa with exudate and ulcerations. Biopsies are typically taken to determine histologic characteristics of the colonic tissue and extent of disease. CT scanning, MRI, and ultrasound studies can identify abscesses and perirectal involvement (Basson, 2019b).

The stool is positive for blood, and laboratory test results reveal low hematocrit and hemoglobin levels in addition to an elevated WBC count, low albumin levels (indicating malabsorptive disorders), and an electrolyte imbalance. C-reactive protein levels are elevated. Elevated antineutrophil cytoplasmic antibody levels are common. Careful stool examination for parasites and other microbes is performed to rule out dysentery caused by common intestinal organisms, especially *Entamoeba histolytica*, *C. difficile* and *Campylobacter*, *Salmonella*, *Shigella*, and *Cryptospora* species (Basson, 2019b).

Complications

Complications of ulcerative colitis include toxic megacolon, perforation, and bleeding as a result of ulceration. In toxic megacolon, the inflammatory process extends into the muscularis, inhibiting its ability to contract and resulting in colonic distention. Symptoms include fever, abdominal pain and distention, vomiting, and fatigue. If the patient with toxic megacolon does not respond within 72 hours to medical management with NG suction, IV fluids with electrolytes, corticosteroids, and antibiotics, surgery is required. A subtotal colectomy may be performed if bowel perforation has not occurred. Otherwise, colectomy is indicated; it is ultimately needed in up to one third of patients with severe ulcerative colitis (Walfish, 2019). For many patients, surgery becomes necessary to relieve the effects of the disease and to treat these serious complications; an ileostomy usually is performed. The surgical procedures involved and the care of patients with this type of fecal diversion are discussed later in this chapter.

Patients with ulcerative colitis also have a significantly increased risk of osteoporotic fractures due to decreased bone mineral density. Corticosteroid therapy may also contribute to the diminished bone density. Patients with ulcerative colitis are also at increased risk for colon cancer. Approximately 20 years post diagnosis, an estimated 7% to 10% of patients with extensive ulcerative colitis (i.e., not contained to the rectum) will have colon cancer (Walfish, 2019).

Management of Inflammatory Bowel Disease

Most patients with either Crohn's disease or ulcerative colitis have long periods of well-being interspersed with short intervals of illness. Medical treatment for both of these types of IBD is aimed at inducing disease remission, using a management process called induction therapy, and preventing flare-ups of the disease process while maximizing quality of life, using a management process called maintenance therapy (Basson, 2019b; Rowe, 2020; Rubin, Ananthakrishnan, Siegel, et al., 2019; Walfish, 2019). Pharmacologic therapy is indicated to meet the goals of inducing and maintaining remission of IBD.

Medical Management

Pharmacologic Therapy

Aminosalicylates such as sulfasalazine are typically the first pharmacologic agents selected to induce and maintain remission of mild to moderate IBD (Rowe, 2020; Wilhelm & Love, 2017). Sulfa-free aminosalicylates (e.g., mesalamine, olsalazine, balsalazide) are indicated for patients with sulfa allergies; these drugs tend to be better tolerated by most patients, including those without sulfa allergies, and are effective in preventing and treating recurrence of inflammation. Aminosalicylates tend to be more effective agents in treating ulcerative colitis than Crohn's disease, although they are indicated as first-line agents for both types of IBDs (Wilhelm & Love, 2017). These drugs are administered orally or topically (by enema or rectal suppository) for patients with more distal disease involvement (Rowe, 2020). Common adverse effects of aminosalicylates include headaches, nausea, and diarrhea (Comerford & Durkin, 2020).

Some select patients with perianal fistulas or inflammatory abdominal masses that occur from flare-ups of Crohn's disease may be prescribed antibiotics as first line agents, rather than aminosalicylates. The most commonly prescribed antibiotics include a combination therapy of both metronidazole and ciprofloxacin, taken orally. These drugs are not prescribed longterm, however. Therefore, another medication regimen must be selected for maintenance therapy. These antibiotics are associated with adverse effects that include nausea and diarrhea, and increased risk of *Clostridium difficile* infection. Furthermore, metronidazole can cause peripheral neuropathy that, if present, can warrant its discontinuance (Rowe, 2020; Walfish, 2019).

Tapering dosages of corticosteroids may be prescribed for patients who are refractory to inducing remission with other drugs such as aminosalicylates, or who are experiencing an exacerbation of the disease process (i.e., a flare-up or acute episode). These medications have potent anti-inflammatory effects (Rowe, 2020). Corticosteroids can be given orally (e.g., prednisone) in outpatient treatment or parenterally (e.g., hydrocortisone) in patients who are hospitalized. Topical (i.e., rectal administration) corticosteroids (e.g., budesonide) are widely used in the treatment of proctitis and colon disease associated with IBD. Because corticosteroids can adversely affect intestinal wound healing, they are only indicated for shortterm use. Other adverse effects of corticosteroids are discussed in Chapter 45 and summarized in Table 45-3 (Walfish, 2019).

Immunomodulators (e.g., azathioprine, mercaptopurine, methotrexate, cyclosporine) alter the pathologic immune response present in IBD. The exact mechanism of action of these medications in treating IBD is unclear. These agents have demonstrated effectiveness in reducing inflammation and decreasing the need for corticosteroids, hospitalization, and surgery. Because it takes at least 2 months before they are effective, these agents tend to not be used to induce remission, but are useful as maintenance therapy, particularly for patients intolerant to aminosalicylates or in those who would otherwise require long-term use of corticosteroids to maintain remission (Rowe, 2020; Wilhelm & Love, 2017). These agents depress bone marrow function; therefore, the CBC must be periodically monitored for neutropenia (i.e., low WBC counts) and pancytopenia (i.e., generally low blood cells counts) that may warrant reducing the dosage or changing to a different agent (Rowe, 2020). Liver function should also be monitored periodically as these agents can be toxic to the liver (see Chapter 43, Table 43-1 for Common Laboratory Tests to Assess Liver Function). These agents can be immunosuppressive, placing patients at increased risk for pneumonia and cancers. Because of these risks, adults receiving these agents should be advised to receive pneumococcal vaccination with both PCV13 and PPSV23 (see Chapter 19 for further discussion of PCV13 and PPSV23); women should be screened for cervical cancer annually (i.e., Papanicolaou [Pap] Smear; see Chapter 50 for further discussion). Patients taking azathioprine or mercaptopurine should be screened annually for squamous cell carcinoma, particularly if they are over 50 years of age (Farraye, Melmed, Lichtenstein, et al., 2017).

Anti-tumor necrosis factor (TNF) medications incorporate monoclonal antibodies that inhibit the inflammatory effects of the cytokine TNF in the gut. These agents are indicated for use in patients with moderate to severe IBD that is refractory to treatment with immunomodulators (Wilhelm & Love, 2017). The first drug in this class that was approved for treatment of both types of IBD is infliximab. Infliximab has proven to be effective at inducing and maintaining remission of IBD, especially Crohn's disease. However, it must be administered by IV infusion. Infliximab is generally well tolerated by most patients, although it can rarely be associated with flulike symptoms. For those patients who experience these symptoms, premedication with diphenhydramine and acetaminophen seems to mitigate those unpleasant effects. Newer alternative anti-TNF medications include adalimumab (for both types of IBD), certolizumab (for Crohn's disease only), and golimubab (for ulcerative colitis only). Each of these agents may be administered by subcutaneous injections (Walfish, 2019). Since all of these anti-TNF agents can potentially reactivate latent viral infections, patients must be tested for tuberculosis and hepatitis B before treatment commences (Rowe, 2020; Wilhelm & Love, 2017). Furthermore, all age-appropriate immunizations should be up to date prior to commencing treatment with these medications (Farraye et al., 2017) (see Chapter 3, Table 3-3 for adult immunizations). Patients prescribed these medications over the long-term need to be educated that they are at higher risk for cancers, particularly lymphomas and melanomas (Farraye et al., 2017; Rowe, 2020; Wilhelm & Love, 2017).

Nutritional Therapy

During induction therapy, oral fluids and a low-residue, highprotein, high-calorie diet with supplemental vitamin therapy and iron replacement are prescribed to meet nutritional needs, reduce inflammation, and control pain and diarrhea

(Rowe, 2020). Patients prescribed corticosteroids may require supplemental calcium and vitamin D to prevent osteopenia (Rowe, 2020). Fluid and electrolyte imbalances from dehydration caused by diarrhea are corrected by IV therapy as necessary if the patient is hospitalized, or by oral fluids if the patient is managed at home. Any foods that cause or exacerbate bothersome symptoms, such as bloating or diarrhea, are avoided. Cold foods and smoking are avoided because both increase intestinal motility. Some patients may experience an improvement in symptoms if they follow the FODMAP diet that is commonly indicated for patients with IBS (see previous discussion), while others experience symptomatic improvement by restricting intake of milk and treating lactose intolerance (see Chart 41-3) (DeLegge, 2020).

Once remission is induced, patients with IBD are educated to avoid food triggers and maintain a diet that best meets their nutritional needs. Probiotic supplements (e.g., *Escherichia coli Nissle, Lactobacillus rhamnosus*) might be indicated to maintain remission in patient with ulcerative colitis, but have not been found to be similarly effective in patients with Crohn's disease (Bischoff, Escher, Hebuterne, et al., 2020). Most patients who achieve remission need not restrict fiber during maintenance therapy (DeLegge, 2020). A consultation with a dietician may be indicated (Bischoff et al., 2020).

Patients with IBD are at risk for becoming malnourished. Fewer patients with IBD are malnourished and require intensive nutritional therapy than was the case 30 years ago (DeLegge, 2020). In general, patients with IBD who have lost more than 10% of their lean body mass are considered malnourished, and are at risk for increased morbidity (e.g., infections, poor wound healing). These patients may require intensive nutritional therapy, which might include enteral nutrition (see Chapter 39) or parenteral nutrition (DeLegge, 2020). Oral nutrition or enteral nutrition is generally preferable to parenteral nutrition. However, parenteral nutrition may be indicated for patients intolerant of oral and enteral nutrition, or those with bowel obstruction or short bowel syndrome, or in patients with Crohn's disease and proximal fistula formation (see later discussion of parenteral nutrition) (Bischoff et al., 2020).

Surgical Management

When nonsurgical measures fail to relieve severe symptoms of IBD, surgery may be necessary. Nearly one third of patients with severe ulcerative colitis and between 60% and 70% of patients with Crohn's disease require surgery (Walfish, 2019). Common indications for surgery in patients with ulcerative colitis include the presence of colon cancer or colonic dysplasia/polyps (see later discussion); megacolon; severe, intractable bleeding; or perforation (Walfish, 2019). The most common indication for surgery in patients with Crohn's disease is small bowel obstruction, which occurs in 30% to 50% of patients; other indications for surgery include abscess, perforation, hemorrhage, or fistula formation (Ghazi, 2019; Walfish, 2019).

Patients with either ulcerative colitis or Crohn's disease may require surgery to relieve strictures. A common procedure performed for strictures of the small bowel is laparoscope-guided strictureplasty, in which blocked or narrowed sections of the intestines are widened, leaving the intestines intact. In some cases, a small bowel resection is performed; diseased segments of the small intestines are resected, and the remaining portions of the intestines are anastomosed. Surgical removal of up to 80% of the small bowel usually can be tolerated (Gilroy, 2018).

Some patients with severe Crohn's disease may benefit from an intestinal transplant. This technique is now available to children and to young and middle-aged adults who have lost intestinal function from disease. It may improve quality of life for some patients. The associated technical and immunologic problems remain formidable, and the costs and mortality rates continue to be high (Gilroy, 2018).

Proctocolectomy and Total Colectomy with Ileostomy

Proctocolectomy (i.e., surgical excision of the colon and rectum) with **ileostomy** (i.e., a surgical opening into the ileum by means of a stoma to allow drainage of bowel contents) is recommended in the patient with IBD with a severely diseased colon and rectum that is refractory to medical therapy. This surgery cures the disease in patients with ulcerative colitis; however surgical cure is not possible with Crohn's disease (Ghazi, 2019; Walfish, 2019).

An ileostomy is a type of fecal diversion that allows for drainage of fecal matter, called *effluent,* from the ileum to the outside of the body. The drainage is liquid to unformed and occurs at frequent intervals. Nursing management of the patient with an ileostomy is discussed later in this chapter.

An ileostomy is indicated after a proctocolectomy or a total colectomy (i.e., surgical excision of the entire colon) and is either temporary or permanent. For patients with severe ulcerative colitis, restorative proctocolectomy with ileal pouch anal anastomosis (IPAA) is the procedure of choice. This option is not generally recommended for patients with Crohn's disease, however, as the surgically formed ileal pouch frequently becomes diseased in these patients. A permanent ileostomy is typically indicated for the patient with Crohn's disease who must have a total colectomy.

Restorative Proctocolectomy with Ileal Pouch Anal Anastomosis

A restorative proctocolectomy with IPAA is the surgical procedure of choice in cases where the rectum can be preserved because it eliminates the need for a permanent ileostomy. It establishes an ileal reservoir that functions as a "new" rectum, and anal sphincter control of elimination is retained. The procedure involves connecting the ileum to the anal pouch (made from a small intestine segment), and the surgeon connects the pouch to the anus in conjunction with removing the colon and the rectal mucosa (i.e., total abdominal colectomy and mucosal proctectomy) (see Fig. 41-6). A temporary diverting loop ileostomy that promotes healing of the surgical anastomoses is constructed at the time of surgery and closed about 3 months later.

With IPAA or restorative proctocolectomy, the diseased colon and rectum are removed, voluntary defecation is maintained, and anal continence is preserved. The ileal reservoir decreases the number of bowel movements significantly. Nighttime elimination is gradually reduced to one bowel movement. Complications of ileoanal anastomosis include irritation of the perianal skin from leakage of fecal contents, stricture formation at the anastomosis site, pelvic abscess, fistula, small bowel obstruction, and *pouchitis* (i.e., inflammation of the ileoanal pouch) (Wu, Ke, Kiran, et al., 2020). This

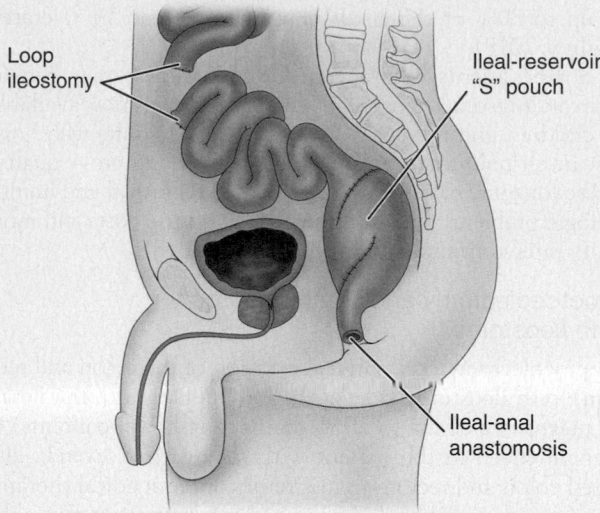

Loop
ileostomy

Ileal-reservoir
"S" pouch

Ileal-anal
anastomosis

Figure 41-6 • A mucosal proctectomy precedes anastomosis of the ileal reservoir. A temporary loop ileostomy diverts effluent for several months to allow healing.

procedure involves pelvic dissection; therefore, it is also associated with the risk of infertility in women. Women wanting to become pregnant may want to consider other treatment options (Rowe, 2020). Dietary intolerances may persist after the IPAA is formed. Increased stool output, flatulence, and perineal irritation are associated with consumption of nuts, corn, chocolate, spicy foods, onions, and citrus fruits. Consequently, some patients may need to alter their diet to avoid complications and perineal breakdown.

Continent Ileostomy

The procedure consists of a proctocolectomy, with 30 to 45 cm of the terminal ileum used to create a J- or S-shaped continent ileal reservoir (i.e., Kock pouch) by diverting a portion of the distal ileum to the abdominal wall and creating a stoma. This procedure eliminates the need for an external fecal collection bag. A nipple valve is created by pulling a portion of the terminal ileal loop back into the ileum. GI effluent can accumulate in the pouch for several hours and then be removed by means of a catheter inserted through the nipple valve. Possible indications for a total colectomy with Kock pouch placement (rather than a restorative proctocolectomy with IPAA) include a badly diseased rectum, lack of rectal sphincter tone, or inability to achieve fecal continence post IPAA (Wu et al., 2020). Variations on the Kock pouch include the Barnett continent intestinal reservoir and T-pouch (Wu et al., 2020).

The major challenge with the Kock pouch is malfunction of the nipple valve, which often requires additional corrective surgery. Other potential postoperative complications include fistulas, stoma-related problems (strictures, parastomal hernia, difficulty with catheterization), pouchitis, and short-bowel syndrome (i.e., nutritional deficits that occur from loss of part of the small intestines). Kock pouches are used less commonly because they have greater complication rates than does restorative proctocolectomy with IPAA (Wu et al., 2020). A major advantage of the procedure is potential improved body image and lack of external drainage appliance (Wu et al., 2020).

NURSING PROCESS

Management of the Patient with Inflammatory Bowel Disease

Assessment

The nurse obtains a health history to identify the onset, duration, and characteristics of abdominal pain; the presence of diarrhea, fecal urgency, or tenesmus; nausea, anorexia, or weight loss; and family history of IBD. It is important to discuss dietary patterns and smoking habits. The nurse asks about patterns of bowel elimination, including character, frequency, and presence of blood, pus, fat, or mucus. Allergies and food intolerance, especially milk (lactose) intolerance, must be noted. The patient may identify sleep disturbances if diarrhea or pain occurs at night.

Diagnosis

NURSING DIAGNOSES
Based on the assessment data, nursing diagnoses may include the following:
- Diarrhea associated with the inflammatory process
- Acute pain associated with increased peristalsis and GI inflammation
- Hypovolaemia associated with anorexia, nausea, and diarrhea
- Impaired nutritional status associated with dietary restrictions, nausea, and malabsorption
- Activity intolerance associated with generalized weakness
- Anxiety associated with impending surgery
- Difficulty coping associated with repeated episodes of diarrhea
- Risk for impaired skin integrity associated with malnutrition and diarrhea
- Lack of knowledge concerning the process and management of the disease

COLLABORATIVE PROBLEMS/POTENTIAL COMPLICATIONS
Potential complications may include the following:
- Electrolyte imbalance
- Cardiac arrhythmias related to electrolyte imbalances
- GI bleeding with fluid volume loss
- Perforation of the bowel

Planning and Goals

The major goals for the patient include attainment of normal bowel elimination patterns, relief of abdominal pain and cramping, prevention of fluid volume deficit, maintenance of optimal nutrition and weight, avoidance of fatigue, reduction of anxiety, promotion of effective coping, absence of skin breakdown, increased knowledge about the disease process and self-health management, and avoidance of complications.

Nursing Interventions

MAINTAINING NORMAL ELIMINATION PATTERNS
The nurse assists the patient in determining if there is a relationship between diarrhea and certain foods, activities, or emotional stressors. Identifying precipitating factors, the frequency of bowel movements, and the character, consistency, and amount of stool passed is important. The nurse provides ready access to a bathroom, commode, or bedpan

and keeps the environment clean and odor free. It is important to administer antidiarrheal medications as prescribed. Loperamide may be prescribed 30 minutes before meals (see previous discussion on interventions for diarrhea). The nurse should record the frequency and consistency of stools after therapy is initiated.

RELIEVING PAIN

The character of the pain is described as dull, burning, or crampy. It is important to ask about its onset. Does it occur before or after meals, during the night, or before elimination? Is the pattern constant or intermittent? Is it relieved with medications? The nurse administers analgesic agents as prescribed for pain. Position changes, local application of heat (as prescribed), diversional activities, and prevention of fatigue also are helpful for reducing pain.

MAINTAINING FLUID INTAKE

To detect fluid volume deficit, the nurse keeps an accurate record of intake and output. The nurse monitors daily weights for fluid gains or losses and assesses the patient for signs of fluid volume deficit (i.e., dry skin and mucous membranes, decreased skin turgor, oliguria, fatigue, decreased temperature, increased hematocrit, elevated urine specific gravity, and hypotension). It is important to encourage oral intake of fluids and to monitor the flow rate of any IV fluids. The nurse initiates measures to decrease diarrhea (e.g., dietary restrictions, stress reduction, antidiarrheal agents).

MAINTAINING OPTIMAL NUTRITION

Nursing interventions focus on optimizing the patient's nutritional status and include ensuring that the patient maintains adequate intake of fluids and nutrients and recognizes and avoids foods that exacerbate symptoms (DeLegge, 2020). The nurse assesses the patient's nutrition, including usual dietary habits, changes in appetite and body mass index (BMI) and trends in weight loss or gain (see Chapter 4 for further discussion of nutritional assessment). Laboratory studies to detect vitamin and mineral deficiencies may help identify the need for supplementation, especially vitamin D and B_{12} (Rowe, 2020). During the induction therapy, if oral foods are tolerated, small, frequent, low-residue feedings are given to avoid overdistending the stomach and stimulating peristalsis. For the patient with IBD who is malnourished and hospitalized, enteral nutrition or parenteral nutrition may be prescribed (see Chapter 39 for further discussion of enteral nutrition). Parenteral nutrition is indicated in patients who have short-bowel syndrome, bowel obstruction, or Crohn's disease with severe malnutrition and intolerance to enteral nutrition and who are expected to likely remain intolerant to enteral nutrition for more than 1 to 2 weeks (DeLegge, 2020) (see later discussion on parenteral nutrition in this chapter).

PROMOTING REST

The nurse recommends intermittent rest periods during the day and schedules or restricts activities to conserve energy and reduce the metabolic rate. It is important to encourage activity within the limits of the patient's capacity. The nurse suggests naps and periods of bed rest for a patient who is febrile, has frequent diarrheal stools, or is bleeding. However, the patient should perform active exercises to maintain muscle tone and prevent venous thromboembolic complications. If the patient cannot perform these active exercises, the nurse performs passive exercises and joint range of motion. Activity restrictions are modified as needed on a day-to-day basis.

REDUCING ANXIETY

Anxiety is nearly twice as prevalent in individuals with IBD than in the general population. The prevalence of anxiety in patients with IBD is not dependent upon whether or not the disease is active or in remission (Farraye et al., 2017). Therefore, the nurse must recognize that the patient with IBD may experience anxiety throughout the spectrum of disease; that is, during periods of remission as well as exacerbation. Rapport can be established by being attentive and displaying a calm, confident manner. The nurse allows time for the patient to ask questions and express feelings. Careful listening and sensitivity to nonverbal indicators of anxiety (e.g., restlessness, tense facial expressions) are helpful. The patient may be emotionally labile because of the consequences of the disease and the uncertainty of exacerbations with complications. The nurse tailors information about possible impending surgery to the patient's level of understanding and desire for detail. If surgery with placement of a stoma is planned, photographs, illustrations, websites, and blogs help explain the surgical procedure and help the patient visualize what a stoma looks like.

ENHANCING COPING MEASURES

Because the patient may feel isolated, helpless, and out of control, understanding and emotional support are essential. The patient may respond to stress in a variety of ways that may alienate others (e.g., anger, denial, social self-isolation).

The nurse needs to recognize that the patient's behavior may be affected by a number of factors. Any patient suffering the discomforts of frequent bowel movements and rectal soreness is anxious, discouraged, and unhappy. It is important to develop a relationship with the patient that supports their attempts to cope with these stressors. It is also important to communicate that the patient's feelings are understood by encouraging the patient to talk and express their feelings and to discuss any concerns. Stress reduction measures that may be used include relaxation techniques, visualization, breathing exercises, and biofeedback. Professional counseling may be needed to help the patient and family manage issues associated with chronic illness and resulting disability.

PREVENTING SKIN BREAKDOWN

The nurse examines the patient's skin frequently, especially the perianal skin. Perianal care, including the use of a skin barrier (e.g., petroleum ointment), is important after each bowel movement. The nurse gives immediate attention to reddened or irritated areas over bony prominences and uses pressure-relieving devices to prevent skin breakdown. Consultation with a wound-ostomy-continence (WOC) nurse (or WOCN; a nurse specially educated in the management of a variety of fecal and urinary diversions) is often helpful.

MONITORING AND MANAGING POTENTIAL COMPLICATIONS

Serum electrolyte levels are monitored daily, and electrolyte replacements are given as prescribed. Evidence of arrhythmias or changes in level of consciousness must be reported immediately.

The nurse closely monitors rectal bleeding and administers blood component therapy and volume expanders as prescribed to prevent hypovolemia. It is important to monitor the blood pressure for hypotension and to obtain coagulation profiles and hemoglobin and hematocrit levels frequently. Vitamin K may be prescribed to increase clotting factors.

The nurse closely monitors the patient for indications of perforation (i.e., acute increase in abdominal pain, rigid abdomen, vomiting, or hypotension) and obstruction and toxic megacolon (i.e., abdominal distention, decreased or absent bowel sounds, change in mental status, fever, tachycardia, hypotension, dehydration, and electrolyte imbalances).

PROMOTING HOME, COMMUNITY-BASED, AND TRANSITIONAL CARE

Educating Patients About Self-Care. The nurse assesses the patient's understanding of the disease process and their need for additional information about medical management (e.g., medications, diet) and surgical interventions. The nurse provides information about nutritional management and foods that might relieve symptoms and decrease diarrhea (e.g., FODMAP diet). It is important to explain the rationale for the use of corticosteroids and anti-inflammatory, antibacterial, and antidiarrheal medications. The nurse emphasizes the importance of taking medications as prescribed and not abruptly discontinuing them (especially corticosteroids) to avoid development of serious medical problems (see Chart 41-5). Patients over the age of 50 should be educated about the importance of receiving the herpes zoster vaccination; all patients should receive the influenza vaccination annually (Farraye et al., 2017). Patient education information can be obtained from the Crohn's and Colitis Foundation of America (CCFA) and from a patient skills education program developed by the American College of Surgeons (see Resources section).

Continuing and Transitional Care. For patients who have been hospitalized to treat IBD, readmission rates are as high as 18% at 30 days, and as high as 36% at 90 days (Nguyen, Koola, Dulai, et al., 2020). Overall, readmission rates were higher for patients with Crohn's disease than for those with ulcerative colitis. The most common reasons for rehospitalization were IBD flare-ups, infections, postoperative complications, pain management, or need for parenteral nutrition or surgery (Nguyen et al., 2020). Risk factors for readmission include history of chronic disease, psychiatric comorbidities, smoking, and opioid dependence (Cohen-Mekekburg, Rosenblatt, Wallace, et al., 2019; George, Martin, Gupta, et al., 2019; Micic, Gaetano, Rubin, et al., 2017; Nguyen et al., 2020). Patients treated at large centers with IBD specialty departments tend to have lower rates of readmission (George et al., 2019).

Patients with IBD are managed at home with follow-up care by their primary provider or through an outpatient clinic. Those whose nutritional status is compromised and who are receiving enteral or parenteral nutrition need the home health or transitional care nurse to consult and ensure that their nutritional requirements are being met and that they or their caregivers can follow through with the instructions for maintaining the nutrition plan. Patients who are undergoing medical treatment need to understand that their disease can be controlled and that they can lead a healthy life between exacerbations. Control implies management based on an understanding of the disease and its treatment. Patients in the home or transitional setting need information about their medications (i.e., name, dose, side effects, and frequency of administration) and need to take medications on schedule. Medication reminders such as containers that separate pills according to day and time or daily checklists are helpful.

During a flare-up, the nurse encourages the patient to rest as needed and to modify activities according to their energy level. Patients should limit tasks that impose strain on the lower abdominal muscles. They should sleep in a room close to the bathroom because of the frequent diarrhea; quick access to a toilet helps alleviate worry about having an "accident." Room deodorizers help control odors.

Dietary modifications can control but do not cure the disease; the nurse recommends a low-residue, high-protein, high-calorie diet, especially during an acute phase. It is important to encourage the patient to keep a record of the foods that irritate the bowel and to avoid them and to drink at least eight glasses of water each day.

The prolonged nature of the disease has an impact on the patient and often strains their family life and financial resources. Family support is vital; however, some family members may be resentful or feel guilty, tired, or unable to cope

---

Chart 41-5 **HOME CARE CHECKLIST**

The Patient with Inflammatory Bowel Disease

At the completion of education, the patient and/or caregiver will be able to:

- State the impact of inflammatory bowel disease on physiologic functioning, ADLs, IADLs, roles, relationships, and spirituality.
- Discuss nutritional management: high-protein, high-vitamin diet; identify foods to include and foods to be avoided.
- Explain the importance of and necessity for adherence with prescribed medication regimen.
- Demonstrate methods of keeping track of the medication regimen, storing the prescribed medications, and using reminders such as beepers and/or pillboxes.
- State the name, dose, side effects, frequency, and schedule for all medications.
- Identify measures to be used to treat exacerbation of symptoms, to include rest, dietary modifications, and medications.

- Identify measures to be used to promote fluid and electrolyte balance during acute exacerbations.
- Demonstrate management of enteral or parenteral nutrition therapy, if applicable; identify possible complications and interventions.
- State how to reach primary provider with questions or complications.
  - State time and date of follow-up appointments, testing.
- Verbalize ways to cope with stress successfully, plans for regular exercise, and rationale for obtaining adequate rest.
- Identify the need for health promotion (e.g., cessation of use of tobacco products), disease prevention and screening activities.

ADLs, activities of daily living; IADLs, instrumental activities of daily living.

with the emotional demands of the illness and the physical demands of providing care. Some patients with IBD do not socialize for fear of being embarrassed. Because they have lost control over elimination, they may fear losing control over other aspects of their lives. They need time to express their fears and frustrations. Individual and family counseling may be helpful.

Evaluation

Expected patient outcomes may include:

1. Reports a decrease in the frequency of diarrheal stools
   a. Adheres to dietary restrictions; maintains bed rest
   b. Takes medications as prescribed
2. Has reduced pain
3. Maintains fluid volume balance
   a. Drinks 1 to 2 L of oral fluids daily
   b. Has normal body temperature
   c. Displays adequate skin turgor and moist mucous membranes
4. Attains optimal nutrition; tolerates small, frequent feedings without diarrhea
5. Avoids fatigue
   a. Rests periodically during the day
   b. Adheres to activity restrictions
6. Is less anxious
   a. Seeks emotional support as appropriate
   b. Verbalizes fewer feelings of anxiety and concern
7. Copes successfully with diagnosis
   a. Verbalizes feelings freely
   b. Uses appropriate stress reduction behaviors
8. Maintains skin integrity
   a. Cleans perianal skin after defecation
   b. Uses appropriate skin barrier
9. Acquires an understanding of the disease process
   a. Modifies diet appropriately to decrease diarrhea
   b. Adheres to medication regimen as prescribed
   c. Recognizes signs and symptoms of complications
10. Recovers without complications
    a. Electrolytes within normal ranges
    b. Normal sinus or baseline cardiac rhythm
    c. Maintains fluid balance
    d. Experiences no perforation or rectal bleeding

DELIVERING NUTRITION PARENTERALLY

Parenteral nutrition is a method of providing nutrients to the body by an IV route. The nutrients are a complex admixture containing proteins, carbohydrates, fats, electrolytes, vitamins, trace minerals, and sterile water in a single container. The goals of parenteral nutrition are similar to the goals of enteral feedings (see Chapter 39); namely, to improve nutritional status, establish a positive nitrogen balance, maintain muscle mass, promote weight maintenance or gain, and enhance the healing process (Seres, 2020). Parenteral nutrition is indicated in adults who are malnourished or at risk for becoming malnourished and who cannot tolerate receiving nutrition orally or by the enteral route (Worthington, Balint, Bechtold, et al., 2017).

Nursing Management

Establishing Positive Nitrogen Balance

Most IV fluids do not provide sufficient calories or protein to meet the body's daily requirements. Parenteral nutrition solutions can provide enough calories and nitrogen to meet the patient's daily nutritional needs. The patient with fever, trauma, burns, major surgery, or hypermetabolic disease requires additional daily calories (Norris, 2019). When highly concentrated dextrose is given, caloric requirements are satisfied and the body uses amino acids for protein synthesis rather than for energy. Additionally, electrolytes such as calcium, phosphorus, magnesium, and sodium chloride are added to the solution to maintain proper electrolyte balance and to transport glucose and amino acids across cell membranes.

The volume of fluid necessary to provide these calories peripherally can surpass fluid tolerance. To provide the required calories in a smaller volume, it is necessary to increase the concentration of nutrients and use a route of administration that rapidly dilutes incoming nutrients to the proper levels of body tolerance. Typically, a large, high-flow vein such as the superior vena cava (at the right atriocaval junction) is the preferred site (Worthington et al., 2017).

Recognizing Clinical Indications

The indications for parenteral nutrition include an inability to ingest at least 50% of the daily required calories and nutrients within a 7-day timeframe for adults who are physiologically stable and well nourished, and within a 3- to 5-day time frame for adults who are malnourished. Enteral nutrition should be considered before parenteral support because it assists in maintaining gut mucosal integrity and improved immune function and is typically associated with fewer complications (Worthington et al., 2017). In both the home and hospital setting, parenteral nutrition is indicated in the situations listed in Table 41-6.

TABLE 41-6	Indications for Parenteral Nutrition
Condition or Need	**Examples**
Insufficient oral or enteral intake	Severe burns, malnutrition, short-bowel syndrome, acquired immune deficiency syndrome, sepsis, cancer
Impaired ability to ingest or absorb food orally or enterally	Paralytic ileus, Crohn's disease, short-bowel syndrome, postradiation enteritis, high-output enterocutaneous fistula
Patient unwilling or unable to ingest adequate nutrients orally or enterally	Major psychiatric illness (e.g., severe anorexia nervosa)
Prolonged preoperative and postoperative nutritional needs	Extensive bowel surgery, acute pancreatitis

Adapted from McClave, S. A., Taylor, B. E., Martindale, R. G., et al. (2016). Guidelines for the provision and assessment of nutrition support therapy in the adult critically ill patient: Society of Critical Care Medicine (SCCM) and American Society for Parenteral and Enteral Nutrition (ASPEN). *Journal of Parenteral and Enteral Nutrition*, 40(2), 159–211.

Administering Formulas

A total of 1 to 3 L of solution is given over a 24-hour period. The label of the solution is verified by at least two identifiers and compared with the prescription (Guenter, Worthington, Ayers, et al., 2018). When parenteral nutrition is delivered as a *2-in-1* admixture of dextrose and amino acids, they are typically supplemented with a **lipid injectable emulsion (ILE;** also called intravenous fat emulsions [IVFE] or lipid). The dextrose and amino acid solution should be administered using a 0.22-micron in-line filter, and the ILE should be administered using a 1.2-micron in-line filter. The ILE may be administered in the same IV line as the 2-in-1 solution; however, a Y-connector should be used for the ILE, and the connector should be placed closer to the patient so that it bypasses the 0.22-micron filter. The 2-in-1 solution is not to be piggybacked into the ILE. As an alternative, the ILE may be delivered via a separate IV line from the 2-in-1 solution (Guenter et al., 2018). Usually, 500 mL of a 10% ILE or 250 mL of 20% ILE is given over 6 to 12 hours, one to three times a week. ILEs can provide up to 30% of the total daily calorie intake.

> ### ◤ *Quality and Safety Nursing Alert*
>
> *Before a parenteral nutrition infusion is administered, the solution must be inspected for separation, oily appearance (also known as a "cracked solution"), or any precipitate (which appears as white crystals). If any of these are present, the solution is not used.*

ILEs can be mixed by the pharmacy staff with other components of parenteral nutrition to create a *3-in-1* admixture commonly called a **total nutrient admixture (TNA).** TNA is delivered using a 1.2-micron filter to prevent the administration of a precipitate (i.e., calcium, phosphorus, incompatibilities) that cannot be seen due to the opacity of the solution (Guenter et al., 2018). Advantages of TNA over parenteral nutrition are cost savings in preparation and equipment, decreased risk of catheter or nutrient contamination, decreased nursing time, and increased patient convenience and satisfaction (Gervasio, 2015). Ideally, the pharmacist, nutritionist, and primary provider should collaborate to determine the specific formula needed.

Initiating Therapy

Parenteral nutrition solutions are initiated slowly and advanced gradually each day to the desired rate as the patient's fluid and dextrose tolerance permits. The patient's laboratory test results and response to parenteral nutrition therapy are monitored on an ongoing basis by the primary provider. These parameters include the patient's weight, intake and output, blood glucose, CBC, and chemistry panel, including serum carbon dioxide, magnesium, phosphorus, and triglycerides. A 24-hour urine collection for nitrogen may be done to analyze nitrogen balance. In most hospitals, admixture solutions are prescribed on a daily standard parenteral nutrition form. The formulation of the parenteral nutrition solutions is calculated carefully each day to meet the complete nutritional needs of the individual patient.

Providing Parenteral Nutrition

Various vascular access devices are used to administer parenteral nutrition solutions in clinical practice. Parenteral nutrition may be given through either peripheral or central IV lines, depending on the patient's condition and the anticipated length of therapy.

Peripheral Method

To supplement oral intake, peripheral parenteral nutrition (PPN) may be prescribed. PPN is given through a peripheral vein; this is possible because the solution is less hypertonic than a full-calorie parenteral nutrition solution. PPN formulas are not nutritionally complete because of their low dextrose content. ILEs are given simultaneously to buffer the PPN and to protect the peripheral vein from irritation. The usual length of therapy using PPN is 5 to 7 days.

> ### ◤ *Quality and Safety Nursing Alert*
>
> *Formulations with dextrose concentrations of more than 10% should not be given through peripheral veins because they irritate the intima (innermost walls) of small veins, causing chemical phlebitis.*

Central Method

Because central parenteral nutrition solutions have at least five times the solute concentration of blood (and exert an osmotic pressure of about 2000 mOsm/L), they are given into the vascular system through a catheter inserted into a high-flow, large blood vessel, ideally at the superior vena cava/right atriocaval junction (Worthington et al., 2017). Concentrated solutions are then very rapidly diluted to isotonic levels by the blood in this vessel.

Several types of **central venous access devices (CVADs)** are available: percutaneous (or nontunneled), peripherally inserted central catheters (PICCs), surgically placed (or tunneled) catheters, and implanted vascular access ports.

Percutaneous (Nontunneled) Central Catheters

Percutaneous central catheters are used for short-term (less than 6 weeks) IV therapy in acute care settings. The subclavian vein is the most common vessel accessed because the subclavian area provides a stable insertion site to which the catheter can be anchored, is easily compressible (facilitating control of hemorrhage), allows the patient freedom of movement, and provides easy access to the dressing site. The subclavian access site should be avoided in patients with advanced kidney disease and those on hemodialysis to prevent subclavian vein stenosis. The second most common access sites include the basilic, brachial, or cephalic veins in the arm followed by the jugular vein. The femoral vein should be avoided for this purpose and should only be used as a last resort because of concerns about infection (Gorski, Hadaway, Hagle, et al., 2016). For a patient with limited IV access, a triple-lumen catheter can be used because it offers three ports for various uses (see Fig. 41-7). The use of a single-lumen catheter dedicated for the administration of parenteral nutrition is not typically feasible, because most patients require administration of medications and fluids in addition to parenteral nutrition, and the line used to administer parenteral nutrition cannot be used for other purposes (Gorski et al., 2016).

When a patient requires IV access for parenteral nutrition, the insertion procedure is first explained so that the patient is aware of what to expect. The patient is placed supine in the

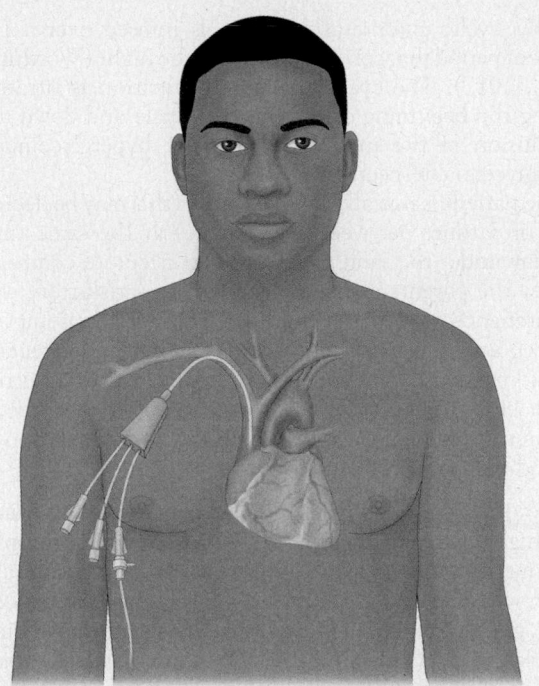

Figure 41-7 • Subclavian triple-lumen catheter used for parenteral nutrition and other adjunctive therapy. The catheter is threaded through the subclavian vein into the vena cava/right atriocaval junction. Each lumen is an avenue for solution administration. The lumens are secured with threaded needleless adapters or Luer lock–type caps when the device is not in use.

Trendelenburg position to produce dilation of neck and shoulder vessels, which makes insertion easier and decreases the risk of air embolus. The skin is cleansed with 2% chlorhexidine to remove surface oils. To afford maximal accuracy in the placement of the catheter, the patient is instructed to turn their head away from the site of venipuncture and to remain motionless while the catheter is inserted and the wound is dressed. The nurse maintains the sterile field and supports the patient throughout the procedure. Maximal barrier precautions mandate that full-body sterile drapes are applied and sterile gloves, cap, gown, and masks are donned to reduce risk of central line–associated bloodstream infection (CLABSI) (The Society for Healthcare Epidemiology of America [SHEA] Guideline Central, 2015) (see Chapter 11, Chart 11-2). Lidocaine is injected to anesthetize the skin and underlying issues. A large-bore needle on a syringe is inserted and moved parallel to and beneath the clavicle until it enters the vein. A radiopaque wire is inserted through the needle into the vein. The catheter is then advanced over the wire, the needle is withdrawn, and the hub of the catheter is attached to the IV tubing. Until the syringe is detached from the needle and the catheter is inserted, the patient may be asked to perform the Valsalva maneuver. The patient is instructed to take a deep breath, hold it, and bear down with the mouth closed to produce a positive phase in central venous pressure, thereby lessening the possibility of air being drawn into the circulatory system (air embolism). The catheter is sutured to the skin. A chlorhexidine-impregnated disc or gel with a semipermeable transparent dressing is applied using sterile technique (Gorski et al., 2016).

The position of the tip of the catheter is verified with x-ray or fluoroscopy to confirm its location in the superior vena cava at the junction of the right atrium and to rule out

a pneumothorax resulting from inadvertent puncture of the pleura. Once the catheter's position is confirmed, the prescribed central parenteral nutrition solution can be started. The initial rate of infusion is usually low, and the rate is gradually increased to the target rate.

An injection cap is attached to the end of each central catheter lumen, creating a closed system. IV infusion tubing is connected to the insertion cap of the central catheter with a threaded needleless adapter or Luer lock device. To ensure patency, all lumens are initially flushed according to institution policy with a 10-mL syringe. Smaller-volume syringes are not to be used because the pressure from smaller syringes is potentially harmful to the catheter. Lumens are flushed with normal saline or diluted heparin (10 U/mL) after each intermittent infusion and after blood drawing; this flushing is necessary daily when the catheter is not in use. Force is never used to flush the catheter (Gorski et al., 2016). If resistance is met, aspiration may restore lumen patency; if this is not effective, the primary provider is notified. Low-dose tissue plasminogen activator may be prescribed to dissolve a clot or fibrin sheath. If attempts to clear the lumen are ineffective, the catheter should be changed.

Peripherally Inserted Central Catheters

Peripherally inserted central catheters (PICCs) are used for intermediate-term (several days to months) IV therapy in the hospital, long-term care, or home setting. These catheters may be inserted at the bedside or in the outpatient setting by a primary provider or specially trained nurse. The basilic, brachial, or cephalic vein is accessed above the antecubital space, and the catheter is threaded to the superior vena cava/right atriocaval junction (see Chapter 12, Fig. 12-6). Taking of blood pressure and blood specimens from the extremity with the PICC is avoided.

Surgically Placed (Tunneled) Central Catheters

Surgically placed central catheters are for long-term use and may remain in place for many years. These catheters are cuffed and can have single or double lumens; examples are the Power line (Power injectable), Hickman, Groshong, and Permacath. These catheters are inserted surgically. They are threaded (or tunneled) under the skin (reducing the risk of ascending infection) to the subclavian vein and advanced into the superior vena cava.

Implanted Vascular Access Ports

Implanted vascular access ports are also used for long-term IV therapy; examples include the Power injectable Port-A-Cath, Mediport, Hickman Port, and P.A.S. Port. Instead of exiting from the skin, the end of the catheter is attached to a small chamber that is placed in a subcutaneous pocket, either on the anterior chest wall or on the forearm. The port requires minimal care and allows the patient complete freedom of activity. Implanted ports are more expensive than the external catheters, and access requires passing a special noncoring needle (Huber tipped) through the skin into the chamber to initiate IV therapy (see Chapter 12, Fig. 12-3).

Discontinuing Parenteral Nutrition

The parenteral nutrition solution is discontinued gradually to allow the patient to adjust to decreased levels of glucose.

If the parenteral nutrition solution is abruptly terminated, isotonic dextrose can be given at the same rate the parenteral nutrition solution was infusing for 1 to 2 hours to prevent rebound hypoglycemia. Symptoms of rebound hypoglycemia include weakness, faintness, sweating, shakiness, feeling cold, confusion, and increased heart rate. Once IV therapy is completed, the percutaneous central venous catheter or PICC is removed, pressure is held until hemostasis is achieved, and an occlusive dressing is applied to the exit site. Surgically placed central catheters and implanted vascular access ports are removed only by the primary provider.

NURSING PROCESS

The Patient Receiving Parenteral Nutrition

Assessment

The nurse assists in identifying patients unable to tolerate oral or enteral feedings who may be candidates for parenteral nutrition. Indicators include significant weight loss (10% or more of usual weight), a decrease in oral food intake for more than 1 week, muscle wasting, decreased tissue healing, abnormal urea nitrogen excretion, and persistent vomiting and diarrhea (McClave et al., 2016). The nurse carefully monitors the patient's hydration status, electrolyte levels, and calorie intake.

Diagnosis

NURSING DIAGNOSES

Based on the assessment data, major nursing diagnoses may include the following:
- Impaired nutritional intake associated with inadequate oral intake of nutrients
- Risk for infection associated with contamination of the central catheter site or infusion line
- Fluid imbalance associated with altered infusion rate
- Risk for activity intolerance associated with restrictions because of the presence of IV access device

COLLABORATIVE PROBLEMS/POTENTIAL COMPLICATIONS

The most common complications are pneumothorax, air embolism, a clotted or displaced catheter, sepsis, hyperglycemia, fluid overload, and rebound hypoglycemia. These problems and the associated collaborative interventions are described in Table 41-7.

Planning and Goals

The major goals for the patient receiving parenteral nutrition may include optimal level of nutrition, absence of infection, adequate fluid volume, optimal level of activity (within individual limitations), knowledge of and skill in self-care, and absence of complications.

Nursing Interventions

MAINTAINING OPTIMAL NUTRITION

A continuous, uniform infusion of parenteral nutrition solution over a 24-hour period is desired. However, in some cases (e.g., home care patients), cyclic parenteral nutrition may be appropriate. Cyclic parenteral nutrition is infused during a set period of time. The time periods for infusion are sufficient to meet the patient's nutritional and pharmacologic needs.

Ideally, cyclic parenteral nutrition is infused over a 10- to 14-hour period that continues through the night (Worthington et al., 2017). The cyclic parenteral nutrition is titrated up during the beginning of the infusion cycle and down at the conclusion of the infusion to prevent hyperglycemia and hypoglycemia, respectively.

The patient is initially weighed daily (this may be decreased to 2 or 3 times per week once stable) at the same time of the day under the same conditions for accurate comparison. Under the parenteral nutrition regimen, satisfactory weight maintenance or gain can usually be achieved. It is important to keep accurate intake and output records and calculations of fluid balance. A calorie count is kept of any oral nutrients. Trace elements (copper, zinc, chromium, manganese, and selenium) are included in parenteral nutrition solutions and are individualized for each patient.

PREVENTING INFECTION

The high dextrose and fat content of parenteral nutrition solutions makes them an ideal culture medium for bacterial and fungal growth, and CVADs provide a port of entry. Gram-positive cocci, gram-negative bacilli, and *Candida* species are frequently isolated as causes of CLABSI. Common organisms include *Staphylococcus aureus*, *Staphylococcus epidermidis*, *Pseudomonas aeruginosa*, *Acinetobacter* species, and *Klebsiella pneumoniae*.

 Quality and Safety Nursing Alert

Meticulous aseptic technique is essential to prevent infection any time the IV line setup is manipulated.

The skin and the catheter hub are the major sources for CLABSIs. The catheter site is covered with a chlorhexidine disc or gel and semipermeable transparent film dressing. The semipermeable transparent dressing allows frequent examination of the catheter site, adheres well to the skin, and is more comfortable for the patient. The transparent semipermeable membrane CVAD dressing is changed every 7 days unless the dressing is damp, bloody, loose, or soiled. Alternatively, an occlusive gauze dressing may be used and is changed every 48 hours or as needed (Gorski et al., 2016). During dressing changes, the nurse and patient wear masks to reduce the possibility of airborne contamination. Sterile technique is used (e.g., the nurse wears sterile gloves). The area is checked for leakage; bloody or purulent drainage; a kinked catheter; and skin reactions such as inflammation, redness, swelling, or tenderness. If chlorhexidine is used for skin asepsis, it is important to allow it to completely dry before applying the new dressing to avoid skin irritation.

The catheter is another major source of colonization and infection. The use of chlorhexidine/silver sulfadiazine- or minocycline/rifampin-impregnated catheters is recommended for a patient whose catheter is expected to remain in place for longer than 5 days if there is concern over a possibility of the patient acquiring a CLABSI (CDC, 2017b).

MAINTAINING FLUID BALANCE

The ubiquitous use of infusion pumps ensures that an accurate rate of parenteral nutrition administration can be achieved. A designated rate is set in milliliters per hour (i.e., mL/h), and the rate is routinely verified per institution policy, generally at least every 4 hours. The infusion rate should not be increased or decreased to compensate for fluids that have infused too

| TABLE 41-7 | Potential Complications of Parental Nutrition | | |

Complications	Causes	Select Nursing Interventions	
		Therapeutic	**Preventive**
Pneumothorax	Improper catheter placement and inadvertent puncture of the pleura	Place patient in Fowler position. Offer reassurance. Monitor vital signs. Prepare for thoracentesis or chest tube insertion.	Assist patient to remain still in Trendelenburg position during catheter insertion.
Air embolism	Disconnected tubing Cap missing from port Blocked segment of vascular system	Replace tubing immediately and notify primary provider. Replace cap and notify primary provider. Turn patient on left side and place in the head-low position. Notify primary provider.	Examine all tubing connection sites for their security.
Clotted catheter line	Inadequate/infrequent saline/ heparin flushes Disruption of infusion	At direction of primary provider, flush with thrombolytic medication as prescribed.	Flush lines per established protocols. Monitor infusion rate hourly and inspect integrity of the line.
Catheter displacement and contamination	Excessive movement, possibly with a nonsecured catheter Separation of tubing and contamination	Stop the infusion, and notify the primary provider.	Examine all tubing connection sites. Avoid interrupting the main line or piggybacking other lines.
Sepsis	Separation of dressings Contaminated solution Infection at insertion site of catheter	Reinforce or change dressing quickly using aseptic technique. Discard. Notify pharmacist. Notify primary provider. Monitor vital signs.	Maintain sterile technique when changing tubing, dressing, or parenteral nutrition bag. Scrub the hub for 15 s prior to accessing line for any reason; air-dry prior to use.
Hyperglycemia	Glucose intolerance	Notify primary provider; addition of insulin to parenteral nutrition solution may be prescribed.	Monitor glucose levels (blood and urine). Monitor urine output. Observe for stupor, confusion, or lethargy.
Fluid overload	Fluid infusing rapidly	Decrease infusion rate. Monitor vital signs. Notify primary provider. Treat respiratory distress by sitting patient upright and administering oxygen as needed, if prescribed.	Use infusion pump. Verify correct infusion rate ordered.
Rebound hypoglycemia	Feedings stopped too abruptly	Monitor for symptoms (weakness, tremors, diaphoresis, headache, hunger, and apprehension); notify primary provider.	Gradually wean patient from parenteral nutrition.

Adapted from McClave, S. A., Taylor, B. E., Martindale, R. G., et al. (2016). Guidelines for the provision and assessment of nutrition support therapy in the adult critically ill patient: Society of Critical Care Medicine (SCCM) and American Society for Parenteral and Enteral Nutrition (ASPEN). *Journal of Parenteral and Enteral Nutrition, 40*(2), 159–211.

quickly or too slowly. If the solution runs out, 10% dextrose and water is infused at the same rate to prevent hypoglycemia until the next parenteral nutrition solution is available for administration.

If the rate is too rapid, hyperosmolar diuresis can occur. Excess glucose is excreted by the renal tubules, pulling large volumes of water into the tubules via osmosis, resulting in higher-than-normal urine output and intravascular fluid volume deficit. If the flow rate is too slow, the patient does not receive the maximal benefit of calories and nitrogen. Intake and output is recorded on an ongoing basis so that fluid imbalance can be readily detected.

ENCOURAGING ACTIVITY

Activities and ambulation are encouraged when the patient is physically able. With a central catheter, the patient is free to move the extremities, and normal activity should be encouraged to maintain good muscle tone. If applicable, the education and exercise program initiated by occupational and physical therapists is reinforced.

PROMOTING HOME, COMMUNITY-BASED, AND TRANSITIONAL CARE

Educating Patients About Self-Care. Successful home parenteral nutrition requires educating the patient and family in specialized skills using an intensive training program and follow-up supervision in the home. This is best accomplished through a team effort. Initiation of a home program facilitates the patient's discharge from the hospital.

Ideal candidates for home parenteral nutrition are patients who have a reasonable life expectancy after return home, have a limited number of illnesses other than the one that has resulted in the need for parenteral nutrition, and are highly motivated and fairly self-sufficient. Ethical dilemmas occur when the patient and family, as well as the caregiver, do not thoroughly understand what is involved in home parenteral

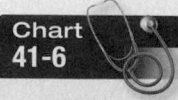

ASSESSMENT
Assessing for Home Nutrition Support

Be alert to the following assessment findings:

- *Water:* Water is necessary for hand hygiene and cleaning of work areas.
- *Electricity:* A reliable power source is needed to provide proper lighting and charging of pumps.
- *Refrigeration:* Refrigeration must be adequate for accommodation of several bags of parenteral nutrition solution.
- *Telephone:* A telephone is necessary for contacting home health personnel, arranging for prompt delivery of supplies, and for emergency purposes.
- *Environment:*
  - Should be free of rodents and insects
  - Should have storage that is not accessible to pets and small children
  - Should be assessed for stairs, carpets, and inaccessible areas, which can limit mobility with infusion pumps if the patient has a disability

Adapted from Worthington, P., Balint, J., Bechtold, M., et al. (2017). When is parenteral nutrition appropriate? *Journal of Parenteral and Enteral Nutrition, 41*(3), 324–377.

nutrition. In addition, the ability to learn, availability of family interest and support, adequate finances, and physical plan of the home are factors that must be assessed when the decision about home parenteral nutrition is made (Worthington et al., 2017) (see Chart 41-6).

Many home health care agencies have developed education brochures and videos for home parenteral nutrition treatment. Topics include catheter and dressing care, the use of an infusion pump, administration of lipid emulsions, and catheter maintenance. Education begins in the hospital and continues in the home or ambulatory infusion center.

Continuing and Transitional Care. The home, community-based, or transitional care nurse should be aware that the typical patient needs several instruction sessions for assessment of learning and reinforcement. More information about home patient education is presented in Chart 41-7.

Evaluation

Expected patient outcomes may include:

1. Attains or maintains nutritional balance
2. Is free of catheter-related infection
   a. Is afebrile
   b. Has no purulent drainage from the catheter insertion site
3. Is hydrated, as evidenced by good skin turgor
4. Achieves an optimal level of activity, within limitations
5. Demonstrates skill in managing parenteral nutrition regimen
6. Prevents complications
   a. Maintains proper catheter and equipment function
   b. Maintains metabolic balance within normal limits

MANAGEMENT OF THE PATIENT REQUIRING AN OSTOMY

Approximately 100,000 patients have surgery to create fecal diversions in the United States annually (Taneja, Netsch, Ralstad, et al., 2017). Common indications for these procedures include not only IBD and diverticulitis, but also advanced colorectal cancer (see later discussion) (Hendren, Hammond, Glasgow, et al., 2015). Fecal diversions may be either ileostomies or colostomies, both of which may be permanent or temporary. While an ileostomy surgically creates an opening into the small intestine, a **colostomy** surgically creates an opening into the colon; both divert fecal drainage to the abdominal wall by means of a stoma. The Plan of Nursing Care summarizes care for the patient requiring an ostomy (see Chart 41-8).

HOME CARE CHECKLIST
The Patient Receiving Parenteral Nutrition

At the completion of education, the patient and/or caregiver will be able to:

- State the goal and purpose of parenteral nutrition therapy and any impact on physiologic functioning, ADLs, IADLs, roles, relationships, and spirituality.
- State what types of changes are needed (if any) to support home parenteral nutrition therapy and maintain a clean home environment and prevent infection.
- State how to contact the primary provider, the team of home care professionals overseeing care, and parental nutrition supply vendor.
  - List emergency phone numbers
- State how to obtain medical supplies and carry out catheter and dressing care, and other prescribed regimens.
- Demonstrate how to perform catheter and dressing care.
- Discuss basic components of parenteral nutrition solution and intravenous fat emulsions.
- State the name, dose, side effects, frequency, and schedule for all medications.
- Demonstrate accurate and safe administration of medications.

- Demonstrate how to handle solutions and medications correctly.
- Demonstrate correct administration of parenteral nutrition
  - Operate infusion pump
  - Prime tubing and filter
  - Connect and disconnect parenteral nutrition infusion
  - Flush central line
  - Clean and maintain pump
  - Change tubing and filters as directed
- Discuss pump warning signals and how to address these signals.
- Identify possible parenteral nutrition complications and interventions.
- Identify a plan for refrigeration of parenteral nutrition solutions and operation of parental nutrition pump during a power outage or other emergency.
- State time and date of follow-up appointments and testing.
- Identify the need for health promotion, disease prevention, and screening activities.

ADLs, activities of daily living; IADLs, instrumental activities of daily living.

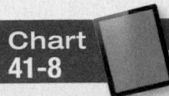

PLAN OF NURSING CARE
Chart 41-8
The Patient Undergoing Ostomy Surgery

NURSING DIAGNOSIS: Lack of knowledge about the surgical procedure and preoperative preparation
GOAL: Understands the surgical process and the necessary preoperative preparations

Nursing Interventions	Rationale	Expected Outcomes
Preoperative Care 1. Ascertain whether the patient has had a previous surgical experience, and ask for recollections of positive and negative impressions. 2. Determine what information the surgeon gave the patient and family and whether it was understood. Clarify and elaborate as necessary. Determine whether the stoma is permanent or temporary. Be aware of the patient's prognosis if carcinoma exists. 3. Use pictures, drawings, or websites to illustrate the location and appearance of the surgical wounds (abdominal, perineal) and the stoma if the patient is receptive. 4. Explain that oral/parenteral antimicrobial agents will be given to cleanse the bowel preoperatively. Mechanical cleansing may also be required. 5. Assist the patient during nasogastric/nasoenteric intubation, if indicated. Measure drainage from the tube.	1. Fear of a repeated negative experience increases anxiety. Talking about the experience with a nurse helps clarify misconceptions and helps the patient ventilate any repressed emotions. Positive experiences are reinforced. 2. Clarification prevents misunderstandings and alleviates anxiety. 3. Knowledge, for some, alleviates anxiety because fear of the unknown is decreased. Others choose not to know because it makes them more anxious. 4. Antimicrobial agents and mechanical cleansing (e.g., laxatives, enemas) reduce intestinal bacterial flora. 5. Nasoenteral intubation is used for decompression and drainage of GI contents before surgery.	• Expresses anxieties and fears about the surgical process • Projects a positive attitude toward the surgical procedure • Repeats in own words information given by the surgeon • Identifies normal anatomy and physiology of gastrointestinal (GI) tract and how it will be altered; can point to expected location of abdominal wound and stoma; describes stoma appearance and size • Adheres to "bowel prep" regimen of antimicrobial agents or mechanical cleansing • Tolerates the presence of nasogastric/nasoenteric tube, if present

NURSING DIAGNOSIS: Disturbed body image
GOAL: Attainment of a positive self-concept

Nursing Interventions	Rationale	Expected Outcomes
1. Encourage the patient to verbalize feelings about the stoma. Offer to be present when the stoma is first viewed and touched. 2. Suggest that the spouse or significant other view the stoma. 3. Offer counseling, if desired. 4. Arrange for a visit, phone call, or online chat with another patient with a stoma.	1. Free expression of feelings allows the patient the opportunity to verbalize and identify concerns. Expressed concerns can be therapeutically addressed by health care team members. 2. Helps patient to overcome fears about the response of significant other 3. Provides opportunity for additional support. 4. People with stomas can offer support and share mutual feelings and experiences.	• Freely expresses concerns and fears • Accepts support • Seeks help as needed • States is willing to talk with another patient with a stoma or participate in support groups or blog sites

NURSING DIAGNOSIS: Anxiety associated with the loss of bowel control
GOAL: Reduction of anxiety

Nursing Interventions	Rationale	Expected Outcomes

Postoperative Care
1. Provide information about expected bowel function:
  a. Characteristics of effluent
  b. Frequency of discharge
2. Explain how to prepare the appliance for an adequate fit.
  a. Choose the drainage appliance that will provide a secure fit around the stoma. Measure the stoma size with a measuring guide provided by the ostomy equipment manufacturer and compare with the opening on the pouch. The barrier opening should be sized to "hug" the stoma and cover the peristomal skin; wafer barriers can be pulled or molded to the size of the stoma.
	1. Emotional adjustment is facilitated if adequate information is provided at the level of the learner.
	
	2. Adequate fit is necessary for successful use of the appliance.
	  a. The appliance opening should be larger than the stoma for an adequate fit. Available brands come in different sizes to fit the stoma. Adjustments are made as necessary.
		• Expresses interest in learning about altered bowel function
		• Handles equipment correctly
		• Changes the appliance unassisted
		• Irrigates colostomy successfully, if indicated
		• Progresses toward a regular schedule of elimination

(continued on page 1320)

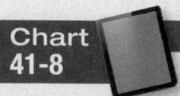

Chart 41-8 · PLAN OF NURSING CARE (continued)
The Patient Undergoing Ostomy Surgery

Nursing Interventions	Rationale	Expected Outcomes
b. Remove any plastic covering that protects the appliance adhesive. *Note:* The pouch is applied by pressing the adhesive for 30 seconds to the skin barrier.	**b.** The appliance is ready to apply directly to the skin or skin protector.	
3. Demonstrate how to change the appliance or empty the pouch before leakage occurs. Be aware that the older adult may have diminished vision and difficulty handling equipment.	**3.** Manipulation of the appliance is a learned motor skill that requires practice and positive reinforcement.	
4. If appropriate, demonstrate how to irrigate the colostomy (usually on the 4th or 5th day). Recommend that irrigation be performed at a consistent time, depending on the type of colostomy.	**4.** Colostomy irrigation is used to regulate the passage of fecal material; alternatively, the bowel can be allowed to evacuate naturally. Irrigation is not routinely indicated.	

NURSING DIAGNOSIS: Risk for impaired skin integrity associated with irritation of the peristomal skin by the effluent
GOAL: Maintenance of skin integrity

Nursing Interventions	Rationale	Expected Outcomes
1. Provide information about signs and symptoms of irritated or inflamed skin. Use pictures if possible.	**1.** Peristomal skin should be slightly pink without abrasions and similar to that of the entire abdomen.	• Describes appearance of healthy skin
2. Instruct patient how to cleanse the peristomal skin gently.	**2.** Mild friction with warm water and a gentle soap cleanses the skin and minimizes irritation and possible abrasions. After rinsing the soap, patting the skin dry prevents tissue trauma.	• Correctly cleanses the skin • Successfully applies a skin barrier • Gently removes the drainage appliance without skin damage • Demonstrates intact skin around the stoma
3. Demonstrate how to apply a skin barrier (e.g., wafer).	**3.** Skin barriers protect the peristomal skin from enzymes and bacteria.	
4. Demonstrate how to remove the pouch.	**4.** Gently separate adhesive from the skin to avoid irritation. Never pull!	

NURSING DIAGNOSIS: Impaired nutritional intake associated with avoidance of foods that may cause GI discomfort
GOAL: Achievement of an optimal nutritional intake

Nursing Interventions	Rationale	Expected Outcomes
1. Conduct a complete nutritional assessment to identify any foods that may increase peristalsis by irritating the bowel.	**1.** Patients react differently to certain foods because of individual sensitivity.	• Modifies diet to avoid offensive foods yet maintains adequate nutritional intake
2. Advise the patient to avoid food products with a cellulose or hemicellulose base (nuts, seeds).	**2.** Cellulose food products are the nondigestible residue of plant foods. They hold water, provide bulk, and stimulate elimination.	• Avoids cellulose-based foods, such as peanuts • Modifies intake of certain fruits
3. Recommend moderation in intake of certain irritating fruits such as prunes, grapes, and bananas.	**3.** These fruits tend to increase the quantity of effluent.	

NURSING DIAGNOSIS: Impaired sexual functioning associated with altered body image
GOAL: Attainment of satisfactory sexual performance

Nursing Interventions	Rationale	Expected Outcomes
1. Encourage the patient to verbalize concerns and fears. The sexual partner is welcomed to participate in the discussion.	**1.** Expressed needs help to develop a plan of care.	• Expresses fears and concerns • Discusses alternative sexual positions
2. Recommend alternative sexual positions.	**2.** Avoids patient embarrassment with the visual appearance of the stoma. Avoids peristomal skin irritation or stomal trauma secondary to friction.	• Accepts services of a professional counselor
3. Seek assistance from a sexual therapist or wound-ostomy-continence nurse.	**3.** Some patients may benefit from professional sexual counseling.	

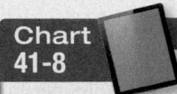

Chart 41-8 PLAN OF NURSING CARE (continued)
The Patient Undergoing Ostomy Surgery

NURSING DIAGNOSIS: Risk for hypovolaemia associated with anorexia and vomiting and increased loss of fluids and electrolytes from GI tract
GOAL: Attainment of fluid balance

Nursing Interventions	Rationale	Expected Outcomes
1. Estimate fluid intake and output: a. Record intake and output	1. Provides indication of fluid balance a. An early indicator of fluid imbalance is a daily, significant difference between intake and output. The average person ingests (food, fluids) and loses (from urine, feces, lungs) about 2 L of fluid every 24 hours.	• Maintains fluid balance • Maintains normal serum and urinary values for sodium and potassium • Normal skin turgor • Surface of tongue is pink, with a moist mucous membrane
b. Daily weights	b. A gain/loss of 1 L of fluid is reflected in a body weight change of 1 kg (2.2 lb).	
2. Assess serum and urinary values of sodium and potassium.	2. Sodium is the major electrolyte regulating water balance. Vomiting results in decreased urinary and serum sodium levels. Urinary sodium values, in contrast to serum values, reflect early, sensitive changes in sodium balance. Sodium works in conjunction with potassium, which is also decreased with vomiting. A significant deficiency in potassium is associated with a decrease in intracellular potassium bicarbonate, which leads to acidosis and compensatory hyperventilation.	
3. Observe and record skin turgor and the appearance of the tongue.	3. Adequate hydration is reflected by the skin's ability to return to its normal shape after being grasped between the fingers. *Note:* In the older person, it is normal for the return to be delayed. Changes in the mucous membrane covering the tongue are accurate and early indicators of hydration status.	

Preoperative Nursing Management

A period of preparation with replacement of fluid, blood, and protein is necessary prior to surgery. Antibiotics may be prescribed. If the patient has been taking corticosteroids (e.g., to treat IBD), they will be continued during the surgical phase to prevent steroid-induced adrenal insufficiency. Usually, the patient is given a low-residue diet, provided in frequent, small feedings. All other preoperative measures are similar to those for general abdominal surgery. The abdomen is marked for the proper placement of the stoma by the surgeon or the WOC nurse. Care is taken to ensure that the stoma is conveniently placed—for instance, ileostomy stomas are usually placed in the right lower quadrant about 5 cm (2 inches) below the waist, in an area away from previous scars, bony prominences, skin folds, or fistulas. The stoma site must be visible to the patient.

The patient must have a thorough understanding of the surgery to be performed and what to expect after surgery. Preoperative education ideally should be delivered by a WOC nurse and include information about the ostomy by means of written materials, models, websites, and discussion. Preoperative education should also include management of drainage from the stoma; the nature of drainage; an introduction to use of common stoma appliances; and the need for NG intubation, parenteral fluids, and possibly perineal packing (Francone, 2020).

Postoperative Nursing Management

General abdominal surgery care is required. As with other patients undergoing abdominal surgery, the nurse encourages those with an ostomy to engage in early ambulation. It is important to administer prescribed pain medications as required. The nurse observes the stoma for color and size. It should be pink to bright red and shiny. Typically, a temporary clear or transparent plastic bag (i.e., appliance or pouch) with an adhesive facing is placed over the ostomy in the operating room and firmly pressed onto the surrounding skin. The nurse monitors the ostomy for fecal drainage, which should begin about 24 to 48 hours after surgery for an ileostomy and within 3 to 6 days after surgery for a colostomy.

The drainage from an ileostomy is a continuous liquid from the small intestine because the stoma does not have a controlling sphincter. The contents drain into the pouch and are thus kept from coming into contact with the skin. They are collected, measured, and discarded when the pouch becomes full. If a continent ileal reservoir was created, as described for the Kock pouch, continuous drainage is provided by an indwelling reservoir catheter for 2 to 3 weeks after surgery.

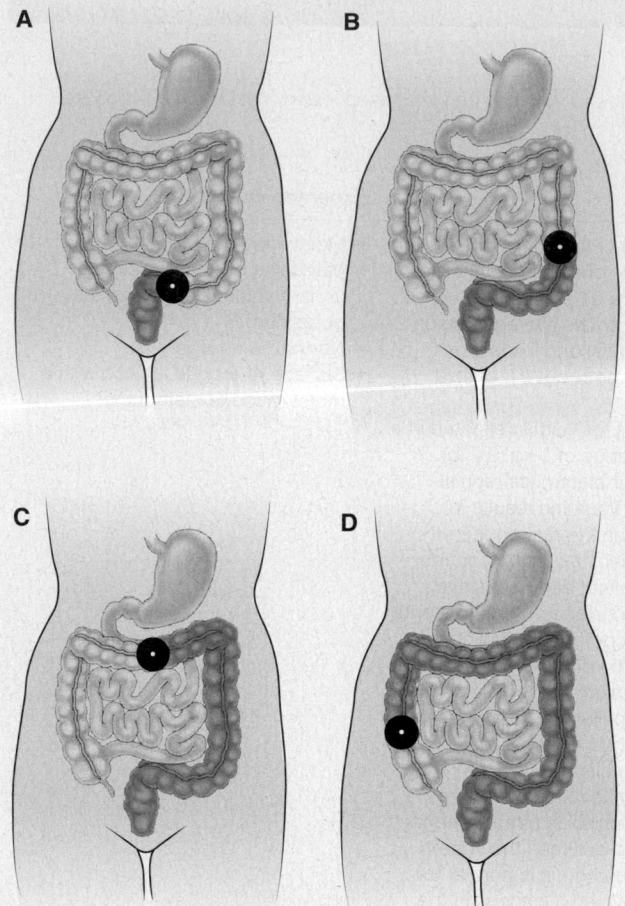

Figure 41-8 • Placement of permanent colostomies. The nature of the discharge varies with the site. *Shaded areas* show sections of bowel removed. **A.** With a sigmoid colostomy, the feces are formed. **B.** With a descending colostomy, the feces are semiformed. **C.** With a transverse colostomy, the feces are unformed. **D.** With an ascending colostomy, the feces are fluid.

This allows the suture lines to heal. Stool drainage from transverse colostomies may be soft and unformed; whereas, stool from descending and sigmoid colostomies is more solid (see Fig. 41-8).

Because patients lose large fluid volumes in the early postoperative period, an accurate record of fluid intake and output, including fecal discharge, is necessary to help gauge each patient's fluid needs. Between 600 and 1200 mL of daily output from an ileostomy and between 200 and 600 mL of daily output from a colostomy can be expected (Bridges, Nasser, & Parrish, 2019). With these losses, sodium and potassium are depleted. The nurse monitors laboratory values and administers electrolyte replacements as prescribed. Fluids may be given IV for 4 to 5 days to replace lost fluids.

NG suction may be a part of the immediate postoperative care, with the tube requiring frequent irrigation, as prescribed. The purpose of NG suction is to prevent a buildup of gastric contents while the intestines are not functioning. After the tube is removed, the nurse offers sips of clear liquids and gradually progresses the diet. Nausea and abdominal distention, which may indicate intestinal obstruction, must be reported immediately.

If rectal packing has been used, it is removed by the end of the first week. Because this procedure may be uncomfortable, the nurse may administer an analgesic agent an hour before the removal. After the packing is removed, the perineum is irrigated two or three times daily until full healing takes place.

Providing Emotional Support

The patient may think that everyone is aware of the ostomy and may view the stoma as a mutilation compared with other abdominal incisions that heal and are hidden. Because there is loss of a body part and a major change in anatomy and function, the patient often goes through the phases of grief—denial, anger, bargaining, depression, and acceptance. Nursing support through these phases is important, and understanding of the patient's emotional state should determine the approach taken. For example, education may be ineffective until the patient is ready to learn. Concern about body image may lead to questions related to family relationships, sexual function, and, for women of childbearing years, the ability to become pregnant and deliver a baby vaginally. Patients need to know that the nurse understands and cares about them; a calm, nonjudgmental attitude aids in gaining the patient's confidence. It is important to recognize that treatment of a possibly terminal illness (e.g., cancer) makes patients irritable, anxious, and unhappy. The nurse can coordinate patient care through meetings attended by consultants such as the primary provider, psychologist, psychiatrist, social worker, WOC nurse, and dietitian.

Conversely, a surgical procedure to create an ileostomy can produce dramatic positive changes in patients who have suffered from IBD for several years. After the discomfort of the disease has decreased and the patient learns how to take care of the ileostomy, they often develop a more positive outlook. Until the patient progresses to this phase, an empathetic and tolerant approach by the nurse plays an important part in recovery. The sooner the patient masters the physical care of the ostomy, the sooner they will psychologically accept it.

Support from other people with ostomies is also helpful. The United Ostomy Associations of America (UOAA) is dedicated to the rehabilitation of people with ostomies. This organization gives patients useful information about living with an ostomy through an educational program of literature, lectures, and exhibits (see Resources section at the end of this chapter). Local associations offer consultations by qualified members who provide hope and rehabilitation services to patients with new ostomies. Hospitals and other health care agencies may have a WOC nurse on staff who can serve as a valuable resource person for the patient with an ileostomy.

Managing Skin and Stoma Care

The patient with an ileostomy cannot establish regular bowel habits because the contents of the ileum are fluid and are discharged continuously. The patient must wear a pouch at all times. Stomal size and pouch size vary initially; the stoma should be rechecked 3 weeks after surgery, when the edema has subsided. The final size and type of appliance is selected in 3 months, after the patient's weight has stabilized and the stoma shrinks to a stable shape.

The incidence of complications related to a colostomy is usually less than that of an ileostomy. Postoperatively, the stoma is examined for swelling (slight edema from surgical manipulation is normal), color (a healthy stoma is pink or red), discharge (a small amount of oozing is normal), and bleeding (an abnormal sign if bright red or more than trace amounts).

Skin excoriation around the stoma can be a persistent problem, particularly for ileostomies. Peristomal skin integrity may be compromised by several factors, such as an allergic reaction to the ostomy appliance, skin barrier, or paste; chemical irritation from the effluent; mechanical injury from the removal of the appliance; and infection. If irritation and yeast growth occur, antifungal spray, water-based cream, or powder can be applied on the peristomal skin and a pouch with skin barrier is applied over the affected area (Stelton, 2019).

Changing an Appliance

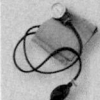

A regular schedule for changing the appliance before leakage occurs must be established for those with an ostomy. The patient should be educated to change the pouch.

> For the procedural guidelines for changing an ostomy appliance, go to **thepoint.lww.com/Brunner15e**.

The amount of time a person can keep the appliance sealed to the body surface depends on the location of the stoma and on body structure. The usual wearing time, which also depends on the type of skin barrier, is 5 to 10 days. The appliance is emptied every 4 to 6 hours, or at the same time the patient empties the bladder. An emptying spout at the bottom of the appliance is closed with a special clip or Velcro closure made for this purpose. If the patient wishes to bathe or shower before putting on a clean appliance, micropore tape applied to the sides of the pouch keeps it secure during bathing.

Most pouches are disposable and odor proof. Foods such as spinach and parsley act as deodorizers in the intestinal tract; foods that cause odors include asparagus, cabbage, onions, and fish. Bismuth subcarbonate tablets, which may be prescribed and taken orally three or four times each day, are effective in reducing odor. Oral diphenoxylate with atropine can be prescribed to diminish intestinal motility, thereby thickening the stool and assisting in odor control. Foods such as rice, mashed potatoes, and applesauce may also thicken stool.

Irrigating a Colostomy

The purpose of irrigating a colostomy is to empty the colon of gas, mucus, and feces so that the patient can go about social and business activities without fear of fecal drainage. A stoma does not have voluntary muscular control and may empty at irregular intervals. Regulating the passage of fecal material is achieved by irrigating the colostomy or allowing the bowel to evacuate naturally without irrigations. This choice depends on the person and the type of the colostomy (i.e., descending or sigmoid colostomies). By irrigating the stoma at a regular time, there is less gas and retention of the irrigant. The time for irrigating the colostomy should be consistent with the schedule that the person will follow after leaving the hospital.

Colostomy irrigation is not recommended for people with extensive pelvic irradiation because it carries a risk of perforation. Likewise, it is contraindicated in patients currently receiving chemotherapy, those with IBS, Crohn's disease, diverticulitis, and peristomal hernias (Bauer, Arnold-Long, & Kent, 2016).

As soon as the patient with a descending or sigmoid colostomy has established a routine for evacuation with irrigations, pouches may be dispensed with, and a closed ostomy appliance or a stoma cap is used to cover the stoma. Except for gas and a slight amount of mucus, nothing escapes from the colostomy opening between irrigations. New assistive devices and ostomy care algorithms are available to help nurses learn ostomy assessment and ostomy product selection (see Resources section at the end of this chapter).

Irrigating a Continent Ileostomy

In the first several days postoperatively after a continent ileostomy (i.e., Kock pouch) is created, a catheter extends from the stoma and is attached to a closed drainage suction system. To ensure patency of the catheter, the nurse instills 10 to 20 mL of normal saline gently into the pouch usually every 3 hours; return flow is not aspirated but is allowed to drain by gravity.

After approximately 2 weeks, when the healing process has progressed to the point at which the catheter is removed from the stoma, the patient is educated how to drain the pouch. A catheter is inserted into the reservoir to drain the fluid. The length of time between drainage periods is gradually increased until the reservoir needs to be drained only every 4 to 6 hours and irrigated once each day. A pouch is not necessary; instead, most patients wear a small dressing over the opening.

When the fecal discharge is thick, water can be injected through the catheter to loosen and soften it. The consistency of the effluent is affected by food intake. At first, drainage is only 60 to 80 mL, but as time goes on, the amount increases significantly. The internal Kock pouch stretches, eventually accommodating between 500 and 1000 mL. The patient learns to use the sensation of pressure in the pouch as a gauge to determine how often the pouch should be drained.

Managing Dietary and Fluid Needs

A low-residue diet is followed for the first 6 to 8 weeks. Strained fruits and vegetables are ingested. These foods are important sources of vitamins A and C. Later, there are few dietary restrictions, except for avoiding foods that are high in fiber or hard-to-digest kernels, such as celery, popcorn, corn, poppy seeds, caraway seeds, and coconut, which may result in a stomal obstruction (food blockage) for the person with an ileostomy. Foods are reintroduced one at a time.

Getting enough fluids during the summer may be a challenge, when fluid lost through perspiration adds to the fluid loss through the ileostomy. Fluids such as sports drinks (Gatorade) are helpful in maintaining electrolyte balance. If the fecal discharge is too watery, fibrous foods (e.g., whole-grain cereals, fresh fruit skins, beans, corn, nuts) are restricted. If the effluent is excessively dry, salt intake is increased. Increased intake of water or fluid does not increase the effluent, because excess water is excreted in the urine.

Gerontologic Considerations

Some older adults may require an ostomy but have difficulty managing care due to decreased vision, impaired hearing, and

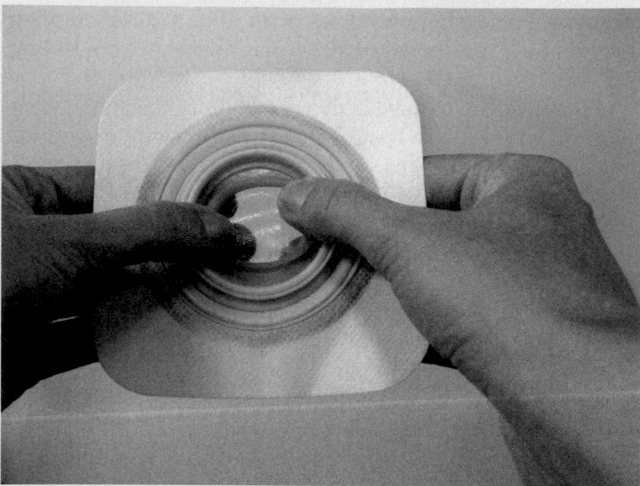

Figure 41-9 • Moldable stomal skin barrier. Reprinted with permission of ConvaTec, Inc.

difficulty with fine motor coordination. Skin care is a major concern in older patients with an ostomy because of the skin changes that occur with aging—the epithelial and subcutaneous fatty layers become thin, and the skin is irritated easily (Eliopoulos, 2018). To prevent skin breakdown, special attention is paid to skin cleansing and the proper fit of an appliance. Stoma skin barriers should be molded into shape around the stoma (e.g., ConvaTec; see Fig. 41-9). Arteriosclerosis may also be an issue; it causes decreased blood flow to the wound and stoma site, which may lead to delayed nutrient transport and prolonged healing time. Some patients have delayed elimination after irrigation because of decreased peristalsis and mucus production. Most patients require 6 months before they feel comfortable with their ostomy care.

Preventing Complications

Monitoring for complications is an ongoing activity for the patient with an ostomy. Peristomal skin irritation, which results from leakage of effluent, is the most common complication of an ileostomy. A drainable pouching system that does not fit well is often the cause. Components of the drainable pouching system include the pouch, a solid skin barrier, and adhesive. The WOC nurse typically recommends the appropriate drainable pouching system. The solid skin barrier is the component of this system that is most important in ensuring healthy peristomal skin. Solid skin barriers are typically shaped as rectangular or elliptical wafers and are composed of polymers and hydrocolloids. They protect the skin around the stoma from effluent from the stoma and provide a stable interface between the stoma and the pouch. It is critical that the barrier be sized appropriately to "hug" the stoma (up to the stoma but not touching) and not expose peristomal skin.

Other common complications include diarrhea, stomal stenosis, urinary calculi, and cholelithiasis. Even in the presence of a properly fitted drainable pouching system, diarrhea can be problematic. Diarrhea, manifested by very irritating effluent that rapidly fills the pouch (every hour or sooner), can quickly lead to dehydration and electrolyte losses. Supplemental water, sodium, and potassium are given to prevent hypovolemia and hypokalemia. Antidiarrheal agents are given. Stenosis is caused by circular scar tissue that forms

at the stoma site. The scar tissue must be surgically released. Urinary calculi may occur in patients with ileostomies and are at least partly attributed to dehydration from decreased fluid intake. Crohn's disease is a risk factor for cholelithiasis (i.e., gallstones) due to altered absorption of bile acids (see Chapter 44).

Promoting Home, Community-Based, and Transitional Care

 Educating Patients About Self-Care

Wound and ostomy care has been identified by family caregivers as one of the most challenging care responsibilities (Kirkland-Kyhn, Martin, Zaratkiewicz, et al., 2018). Ostomy care can be complex and may be viewed as unpleasant by caregivers, and some patients may have body image issues (Kirkland-Kyhn et al., 2018). Nurses can provide the patient and family with information and resources prior to discharge, so they are prepared when the patient arrives home. The family should be familiar with adjustments that will be necessary; for example, they need to know why it is necessary for the patient to occupy the bathroom for 10 minutes or more at certain times of the day and why certain equipment is needed. Their understanding is necessary to reduce tension; a relaxed patient tends to have fewer problems. Visits from a home health, WOC, or transitional care nurse may be arranged to ensure that the patient is progressing as expected and to provide additional guidance and education as needed.

Continuing and Transitional Care

The patient needs to know the commercial name of the drainable pouching system to be used so that they can obtain a ready supply; the patient should also know how to obtain other supplies. The names and contact information of a local WOC nurse and local self-help groups are often helpful. Any restrictions on driving or working also need to be reviewed. The nurse educates the patient about common postoperative complications and how to recognize and report them (see Chart 41-9).

COLORECTAL NEOPLASMS

The term *neoplasm* means new growth. Colorectal neoplasms encompass both cancerous and benign growths, including colorectal cancer and cancerous and benign colorectal polyps.

Colorectal Cancer

Tumors of the colon and rectum are relatively common; the colorectal area (the colon and rectum combined) is the third most common site of new cancer cases in the United States. In the United States, approximately 104,600 new cases and 53,200 deaths from colorectal cancer occur annually; these deaths include 3640 people under age 50 years (American Cancer Society [ACS], 2020). Colorectal cancer is the third leading cause of cancer death in men or women and the second leading cause of cancer death among all adults in the United States (ACS, 2020). The WHO estimates there were 1.8 million new cases and nearly 861,000 deaths worldwide in 2018 (Macrae & Bendell, 2020).

Chart 41-9

🏠 **HOME CARE CHECKLIST**

Managing Ostomy Care

At the completion of education, the patient and/or caregiver will be able to:

- Name the procedure that was performed and identify changes in anatomic structure or function as well as changes in ADLs, IADLs, roles, relationships, and spirituality.
  - Describe the frequency and character of effluent.
- Identify sources for obtaining ostomy care/appliance supplies.
- State the name, dose, side effects, frequency, and schedule for all medications.
- Demonstrate ostomy care, including wound cleansing, irrigation, and appliance changing.
- Describe the importance of assessing and maintaining peristomal skin integrity.
- Identify dietary restrictions (foods that can cause diarrhea and constipation), process for reintroduction of foods, as well as foods that may be encouraged.

- Identify measures to be used to promote fluid and electrolyte balance.
- Describe potential complications and necessary actions to be taken if complications occur.
- Relate how to reach primary provider with questions or complications.
  - Identify how to contact wound-ostomy-continence or home health nurse.
- State time and date of follow-up medical appointments, therapy, and testing.
- Identify sources of support (e.g., friends, relatives, faith community, ostomy support, caregiver support).
- Identify the need for health promotion, disease prevention, and screening activities.

ADLs, activities of daily living; IADLs, instrumental activities of daily living.

The most significant risk factor for colorectal cancer is older age. The median age at diagnosis is now 66 years of age compared to the median age 20 years ago of 72 years of age (ACS, 2020). The median age at diagnosis is younger for rectal cancer (62 years for men and 63 years for women) (ACS, 2020). The incidence of colorectal cancer in adults over 50 years of age has been declining by approximately 2% annually (Macrae & Bendell, 2020). This corresponds with an approximate 19% increase in colonoscopies being performed (Simonson, 2018). However, recent trends in epidemiologic data from the Surveillance, Epidemiology, and End Results registry (SEER) of the National Cancer Institute (NCI) revealed that nearly one in seven new diagnoses of colorectal cancer were among adults younger than 50 years of age; furthermore, these patients were more likely to have more advanced disease at the time of diagnosis. These cancers are largely left-sided cancers (i.e., more distal); rectal cancer is particularly prevalent among younger adults with colorectal cancer (Macrae & Bendell, 2020). Research findings suggest that sedentary behavior in adults younger than 50 years of age might be linked to colorectal cancer (Nguyen, Liu, Zheng, et al., 2018).

Approximately 30% of patients with colorectal cancer have a family history of the disease (ACS, 2020). The exact cause of colon and rectal cancer is still unknown, but risk factors have been identified (see Chart 41-10). A specific form of hereditary colorectal cancer is *Lynch syndrome*, or hereditary non-polyposis colorectal cancer (HNPCC). HNPCC-defining cancers include those of the colorectum, uterus, stomach, ovaries, urinary epithelium, and small bowel. HNPCC is characterized by early age of onset. Another disorder with high risk of colorectal cancer is familial adenomatous polyposis (FAP), in which patients develop hundreds of colonic polyps that can become malignant.

The stage at presentation affects the prognosis in colon cancer. If the disease is localized and treated before it spreads, the 5-year survival rate is 89%; with distant metastases, the survival rate drops to 15% (ACS, 2020). SEER estimates the overall 5-year survival rate for all stages at 67% (ACS, 2020). Many people are asymptomatic for long periods and seek health care only when they notice a change in bowel habits or rectal bleeding (ACS, 2020). Education, prevention, and early screening are key to detection and reduction of mortality rates.

Pathophysiology

Cancer of the colon and rectum is predominantly (95%) adenocarcinoma (i.e., arising from the epithelial lining of the intestine) (Dragovich, 2020). It may start as a mutation of the adenomatous polyposis gene (APC), leading to malignancy. The genetic mutations are associated with the transformation of a benign polyp to invasive adenocarcinoma, which can invade and destroy normal tissues and extend into

---

Chart 41-10

⚠️ **RISK FACTORS**

Colorectal Cancer

- Cigarette smoking
- Family history of colon cancer (especially if history of Lynch syndrome) or polyps (especially if history of familial adenomatous polyposis)
- High consumption of alcohol (i.e., >2 drinks daily in men, >1 drink daily in women)
- High-fat, high-protein (with high intake of beef), low-fiber diet
- History of genital cancer (e.g., endometrial cancer, ovarian cancer) or breast cancer (in women)
- History of inflammatory bowel disease
- History of radiation to the pelvis
- History of type 2 diabetes
- Increasing age
- Male gender
- Overweight or obesity
- Previous colon cancer or adenomatous polyps
- Racial/ethnic background: African American or Ashkenazi Jewish

Adapted from American Cancer Society (ACS). (2020). Colorectal cancer facts & figures 2020–2022, American Cancer Society, Inc., Surveillance Research; Colorectal (Colon) Cancer: What Are the Risk Factors for Colorectal Cancer? CDC. Retrieved on 3/09/2020 at: https://www.cdc.gov/cancer/colorectal/basic_info/risk_factors.htm

surrounding structures. Cancer cells may migrate away from the primary tumor and spread to other parts of the body, most often to the liver, peritoneum, and lungs.

Clinical Manifestations

The symptoms are determined by the location of the tumor, the stage of the disease, and the function of the affected intestinal segment. The most common presenting symptom is a change in bowel habits. The passage of blood in or on the stools is the second most common symptom. Symptoms may also include unexplained anemia, anorexia, weight loss, and fatigue (ACS, 2020). Patients younger than 50 years of age may report abdominal pain rather than the usual "alarm" symptoms associated with colorectal cancer, which include rectal bleeding, a change in bowel habits, the presence of an abdominal mass, or anemia (Dragovich, 2020).

The symptoms most commonly associated with right-sided lesions (i.e., more proximal tumors) are dull abdominal pain and melena (i.e., black, tarry stools). Patients with right-sided tumors tend to have poorer outcomes than those with left-sided tumors. The symptoms most commonly associated with left-sided lesions are a change in bowel habits or those associated with obstruction (i.e., abdominal pain and cramping, narrowing stools, constipation, distention), as well as hematochezia (i.e., bright red blood in the stool). Symptoms associated with rectal lesions are tenesmus, rectal pain, the feeling of incomplete evacuation after a bowel movement, alternating constipation and diarrhea, and bloody stool (Dragovich, 2020).

Assessment and Diagnostic Findings

Screening is an effective method to identify and prevent colorectal cancer. Screening colonoscopies can reduce mortality by decreasing the incidence of and increasing the survival rates for patients with colorectal cancer (ACS, 2020). Colorectal cancer develops slowly from polyps in the colon or rectum and if identified early, can be removed before undergoing malignant transformation (Simonson, 2018). Screening recommendations differ based on the organization publishing the guidelines; differences include the frequency and method of screening and age to begin and discontinue screening. The U.S. Preventive Services Task Force (USPSTF) recommends that all adults should begin periodic screening for colorectal cancer at the age of 50 years. Due to the increased incidence of colorectal cancer in people under age 50, the 2018 ACS guideline recommends screening begin at age 45 for people of average risk (ACS, 2020). Screening for high-risk people should begin earlier, based on their individual risk profile. The ACS offers information and guidelines for high-risk screening (see Resources). Whether or not to continue screening adults after the age of 75 years should be made based upon each patient's preference and overall health status. Adults older than 85 years of age should not continue to be screened (see Chapter 12, Table 12-3, for summary of colorectal cancer screening guidelines). Because colonoscopy is the only screening test that can also simultaneously remove precancerous polyps, thus preventing colorectal cancer, other experts recommend colonoscopies every 5 to 10 years beginning at the age of 50 years as the major screening test for colorectal cancer, including the American College of Gastroenterology

and the National Comprehensive Cancer Network (see Chapter 38 for discussion of colonoscopies) (Cabebe, 2020).

A patient who has a tumor found on screening colonoscopy should have the tumor biopsied and tattooed during the colonoscopy to facilitate further workup. For the patient whose tumor was found on a diagnostic test other than a colonoscopy (e.g., flexible sigmoidoscopy, FIT), a colonoscopy is indicated to biopsy and tattoo the tumor (Rex, 2018).

The patient is referred to a colorectal surgeon. The preoperative workup consists of a focused history, to determine if there are any symptoms suggestive of colorectal cancer (see previous discussion in Clinical Manifestations). A family history is done to screen for a genetic predisposition (e.g., Lynch syndrome, FAP). Laboratory studies are done, including a CBC (may or may not reveal anemia), chemistry panel (to determine baseline status), and liver function tests (to screen for possible liver metastasis). A baseline carcinoembryonic antigen (CEA) level is also obtained. CEA is a tumor marker that is recommended for assessing the presence of colorectal cancer, as well as its progression or recurrence, although it does yield both false positives and false negatives. However, at present there is no other readily available tumor marker test. Therefore, CEA is not used as the sole predictor of tumor status, including progression or recurrence. Other tests indicated include contrast CT scans of the abdomen, pelvis, and chest, to screen for extent of the tumor and any metastases (Macrae & Bendell, 2020).

Complications

Tumor growth may cause partial or complete bowel obstruction or perforation. Extension of the tumor and ulceration into the surrounding blood vessels can result in hemorrhage. Each of these complications can be treated surgically. Obstruction may be resected without anastomosis (e.g., Hartmann procedure) (see Fig. 41-4) or with anastomosis (e.g., colectomy or partial colectomy). Perforation typically carries a grim prognosis; it is typically treated with an ostomy. Acute hemorrhage is a rare complication; when it occurs, it is most effectively treated with surgical resection.

 Gerontologic Considerations

Carcinomas of the colon and rectum are common malignancies in advanced age. In men, only the incidence of prostate cancer and lung cancer exceeds that of colorectal cancer. In women, only the incidence of breast cancer and lung cancer exceeds that of colorectal cancer (ACS, 2020). Symptoms are often insidious. Patients with colorectal cancer may report fatigue, which can be caused by iron deficiency anemia. In early stages, minor changes in bowel patterns and occasional bleeding may occur. The later symptoms most commonly reported by the older adult are abdominal pain, obstruction, tenesmus, and rectal bleeding.

Colon cancer in the older adult has been closely associated with dietary carcinogens. Lack of fiber is a major causative factor because the passage of feces through the intestinal tract is prolonged, which extends exposure to possible carcinogens. Excess dietary fat, high alcohol consumption, and smoking all increase the incidence of colorectal tumors. Physical activity and NSAIDs and aspirin have protective effects (ACS, 2020).

Prevention

Several primary prevention strategies might thwart the onset of colorectal cancer. Use of tobacco products is implicated in one third of all cancers, including colorectal cancer (see Chapter 23 for discussion of smoking cessation programs). Physical activity, dietary modification, and weight reduction strategies mirror those for other cancers (see previous discussion of Life Style Factors in Chapter 12) (ACS, 2020). In addition to these strategies, the USPSTF recommends that adults between the ages of 50 and 59 who are also at risk for developing cardiovascular disease, and who have no contraindication to aspirin, take daily or alternate-day aspirin (dosage ≥ 75 mg) for 5 to 10 years, as an effective primary prevention strategy for both cardiovascular disease and colorectal cancer (Chubak, Kamineni, Buist, et al., 2015). To date, there is no expert consensus guideline that advocates routine prescription of aspirin postcolorectal cancer diagnosis.

Medical Management

Treatment for colorectal cancer depends on the stage of the disease (see Table 41-8) and consists of surgery to remove the tumor, supportive therapy, and adjuvant therapy. Definitive staging can only be done after surgical excision.

Surgical Management

Surgery is the mainstay of initial treatment for colorectal cancer. The goal is removal of the primary tumor with clean margins, including lymph nodes (Dragovich, 2020). It may be curative or palliative. Advances in surgical techniques can enable the patient with rectal cancer to have sphincter-sparing devices that restore continuity of the GI tract. The type of surgery recommended depends on the location and size of the tumor (Dragovich, 2020).

Patients who have Stage 0 tumors typically have endoscopic or laparoscopic excision of their tumors. Laparoscopic surgery for stage I, II, and III colorectal tumors achieves

TABLE 41-8	Staging of Colorectal Cancer: American Joint Committee on Cancer (AJCC) Stage Groupings	
Stage	**TNM**	**Description**
Stage 0	Tis, N0, M0	Tis: carcinoma *in situ*; intraepithelial or invasion of lamina propria N0: no regional lymph node spread M0: no distant metastasis
Stage I	T1–2, N0, M0	T1: Tumor invades submucosa T2: Tumor invades muscularis propria
Stage IIA	T3, N0, M0	T3: Tumor invades through the muscularis propria into pericolorectal tissues arriving at colorectal fat tissue
Stage IIB	T4, T4a, N0, M0	T4: Tumor directly invades other organs T4a: Tumor directly penetrates visceral peritoneum
Stage IIC	T4b, N0, M0 Nx	T4b: Tumor directly invades or is adherent to other organs or structures Nx: Regional lymph nodes cannot be assessed
Stage IIIA	T1–T2, N1–N1c, M0 T1, N2a, M0	N1: Metastases in 1–3 regional lymph nodes N1a: Spread to 1 regional lymph node N1b: Spread to 2–3 regional lymph nodes N1c: Tumor deposit(s) in the subserosa, mesentery, or nonperitonealized pericolic or perirectal tissues without regional nodal metastasis N2: Spread to ≥ 4 regional lymph nodes N2a: Spread to 4–6 regional lymph nodes
Stage IIIB	T3–T4a, N1–N1c, M0 T2–T3, N2a, M0 T1–T2, N2b, M0	N2b: Spread to ≥ 7 regional lymph nodes
Stage IIIC	T4a, N2a, M0 T3–T4a, N2b, M0 T4b, N1–N2, M0	
Stage IVA	Any T, Any N, M1a	M1a: Metastasis confined to 1 organ or site (e.g., liver, lung, ovary, nonregional node)
Stage IVB	Any T, Any N, M1b	M1b: Metastasis in >1 organ/site or the peritoneum
Stage IVC	Any T, Any N, M1c	M1c: Metastases to peritoneum with or without metastases to other organs

Note: This is based upon AJCC 8th Edition and National Cancer Institute (NCI) recommendations that at least 12 regional lymph nodes are examined in patients with colorectal cancer to confirm staging.

T, primary tumor; N, regional lymph nodes; M, distant metastasis. Not listed on table: Tx: tumor cannot be assessed, T0: No evidence of primary tumor

Adapted from Tong, G. J., Zhang, G. Y., Lui, J., et al. (2018). Comparison of the eighth version of the American Joint Committee on Cancer manual to the seventh version for colorectal cancer: A retrospective review of our data. *World Journal of Clinical Oncology, 9*(7), 148–161.

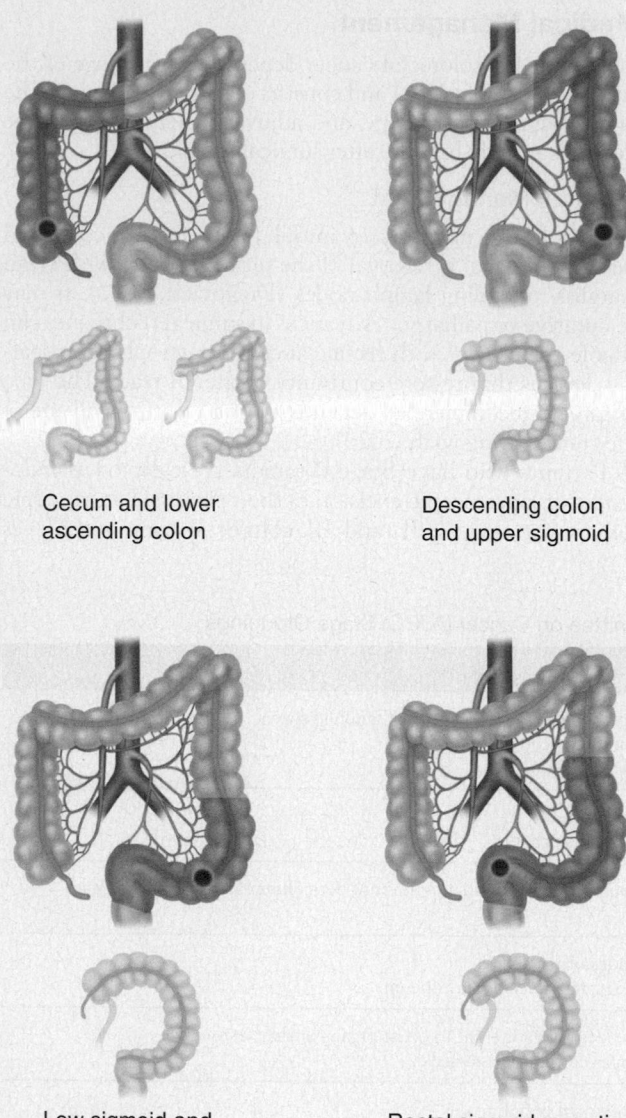

Cecum and lower
ascending colon

Descending colon
and upper sigmoid

Low sigmoid and
upper rectum

Rectal sigmoid resection

Figure 41-10 • Examples of areas where cancer can occur, the area that is removed, and how the anastomosis is performed (*small diagrams*).

equivalent oncologic outcomes to surgery done by traditional open laparotomy (Dragovich, 2020). In addition, laparoscopic surgery is associated with shorter hospital lengths of stay, fewer postoperative complications, improved pain control, and earlier progression to a normal diet. Possible surgical procedures include the following (note that only segmental resections with anastomoses may be done by laparoscope):

- Segmental resection with anastomosis (i.e., removal of the tumor and portions of the bowel on either side of the growth, as well as the blood vessels and lymphatic nodes) (see Fig. 41-10)
- Abdominoperineal resection with permanent sigmoid colostomy (i.e., removal of the tumor and a portion of the sigmoid and all of the rectum and anal sphincter, also called *Miles resection*) (see Fig. 41-11)
- Temporary colostomy followed by segmental resection and anastomosis and subsequent reanastomosis of the colostomy, allowing initial bowel decompression and bowel preparation before resection
- Permanent colostomy or ileostomy for palliation of unresectable obstructing lesions
- Construction of a coloanal reservoir called a *colonic J-pouch*, which is performed in two steps. A temporary loop ileostomy is constructed to divert intestinal flow, and the newly constructed J-pouch (made from 6 to 10 cm of colon) is reattached to the anal stump. About 3 months after the initial stage, the ileostomy is reversed and intestinal continuity is restored. The anal sphincter and therefore continence are preserved

The colostomy can be created as a temporary or permanent fecal diversion. It allows the drainage or evacuation of colon contents to the outside of the body. The consistency of the drainage is related to the placement of the colostomy, which is dictated by the location of the tumor and the extent of invasion into surrounding tissues (see Fig. 41-8).

Adjuvant Therapy and Ongoing Management

Patients diagnosed with colorectal cancer are referred to a medical oncologist for further management after they are discharged from the hospital after surgery. Patients at the lowest risk for recurrence (i.e., those with Stage 0 or I disease) do not require chemotherapy or radiation therapy. Those with Stage 0 disease do not require specific follow-up. Patients with stage I colorectal cancer should have follow-up colonoscopies 1-year postoperatively, then again in another 3 years, and then every 5 years.

Most patients with stage II disease do not require any adjuvant chemotherapy. However, some patients with stage II tumors have mutations in their DNA mismatch repair genes (MMR) that are classified as proficient (MMR-P). Patients in this subset have improved survival and less disease recurrence if they take the antimetabolite chemotherapeutic drug capecitabine for 6 months. In order to screen for the MMR-P gene, the tumor should be analyzed by a multigene assay (i.e., genetic test). Patients with stage II disease who may also benefit from capecitabine are those who had inadequately sampled lymph nodes, with T4-sized tumors, or with poorly differentiated tumors. Capecitabine is equivalent to the dual chemotherapeutic drugs 5-fluorouracil and leucovorin. It may be given either orally or intravenously. The most common adverse effects of capecitabine include anemia, neutropenia, fatigue, diarrhea, and palmar-plantar erythrodysesthesia (i.e., hand-foot syndrome), which manifests by reddening, pain, and swelling of the palms of the hands and soles of the feet (NCI, 2020).

Patients with stage III tumors are typically prescribed the combination chemotherapeutic drug of 5-fluorouracil, leucovorin, and oxaliplatin. This combination chemotherapeutic drug is usually given over 6 months, but there is some debate whether 3 months of treatment is as effective (Lee & Chu, 2018; Sougklakos, Boukovinas, Xynogalos,

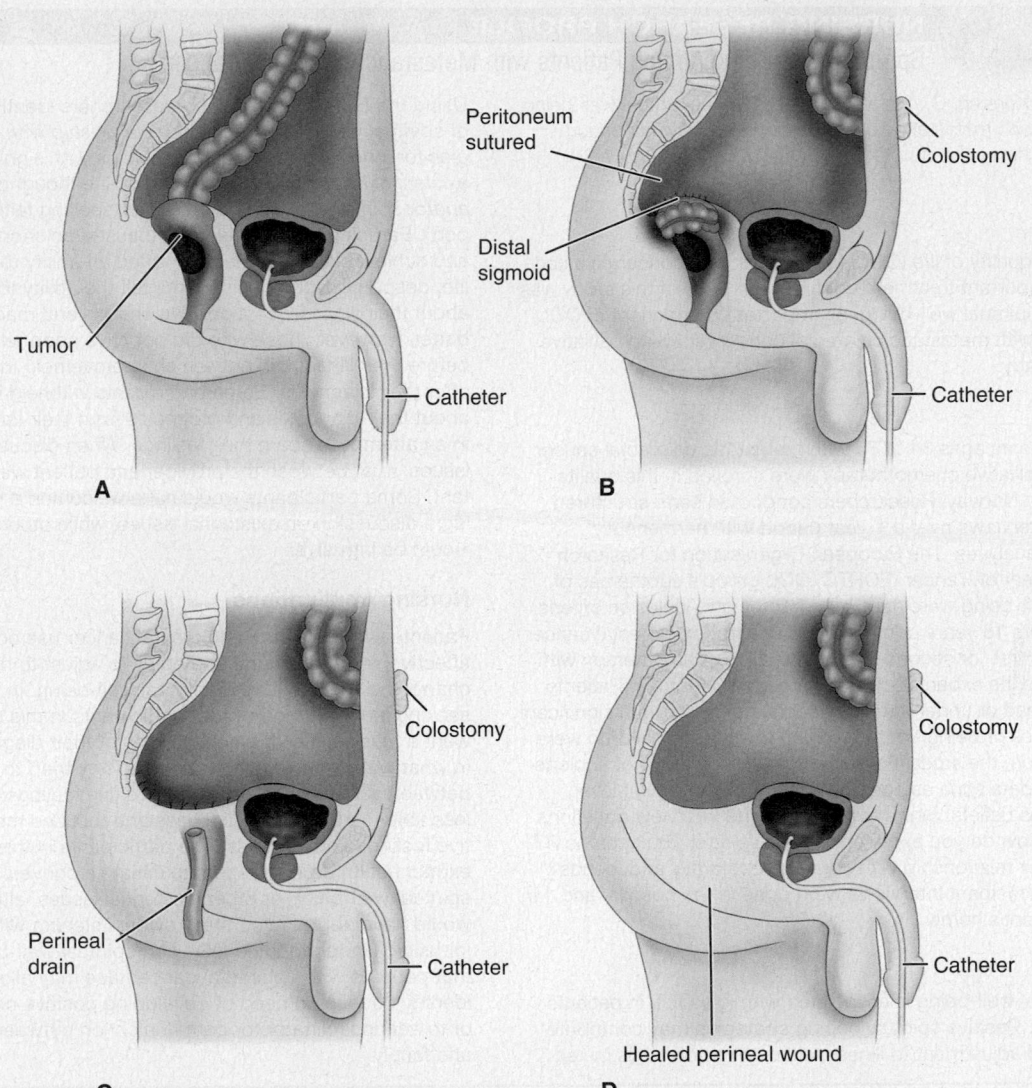

Figure 41-11 • Abdominoperineal resection for carcinoma of the rectum. **A.** Prior to surgery. Note tumor in rectum. **B.** During surgery, the sigmoid is removed and the colostomy is established. The distal bowel is dissected free to a point below the pelvic peritoneum, which is sutured over the closed end of the distal sigmoid and rectum. **C.** Perineal resection includes removal of the rectum and free portion of the sigmoid from below. A perineal drain is inserted. **D.** The final result after healing. Note the healed perineal wound and the permanent colostomy.

et al., 2019). The 3-month treatment regimen is associated with less neurotoxicity (Dragovich, 2020). The adverse effects mirror those of capecitabine, plus patients frequently experience cold sensitivity and paresthesias of their hands and feet, which typically cease after the chemotherapy is completed. An alternative treatment is now available, and consists of a combination drug of capecitabine and oxaliplatin for 3 or 6 months of therapy (Dragovich, 2020).

Patients with stage II or stage III tumors should have routine follow-ups and CEA testing every 3 to 6 months for 5 years. CT scans of the abdomen and chest should be done each year for 3 years. Colonoscopy should also be done 1-year postoperatively, and then every 5 years (NCI, 2020).

Patients with stage IV or recurrent colorectal tumors have metastases to distant organs. The treatment is highly variable

and individualized, based upon the extent of the tumor mass(es), and the health status and wishes of the patient. Treatment might consist of targeted therapy aimed at possible cure, or palliative care (see Chapter 13). Chemotherapeutic drugs that might be tried include those previously described for treating stage II or stage III disease, as well as other categories of agents, including monoclonal antibodies (e.g., cetuximab, panitumumab), and anti-vascular endothelial growth factor (anti-VEGF) agents (e.g., bevacizumab, aflibercept), to name a few. When metastasis occurs, the liver is implicated half the time. Therapy targeted to treat metastases to the liver can include surgical resection, radiofrequency ablation, and intra-arterial chemotherapy (Dragovich, 2020). Maintaining quality of life is an important goal for many patients with cancer, particularly those receiving palliative care (Rohde, Kersten, Vistad, et al., 2017) (see Chart 41-11: Nursing Research Profile).

Chart 41-11

NURSING RESEARCH PROFILE

Spiritual Well-Being Among Patients with Metastatic Colorectal Cancer

Rohde, G., Kersten, C., Vistad, I., et al. (2017). Spiritual well-being in patients with metastatic colorectal cancer receiving noncurative chemotherapy: A qualitative study. *Cancer Nursing, 40*(3), 209–216.

Purpose

Enhancing quality of life (QOL) for patients with noncurative cancer is an important treatment goal. The purpose of this study was to explore spiritual well-being, an important component of QOL, in patients with metastatic colorectal cancer receiving palliative chemotherapy.

Design

Twenty patients ages 34 to 75 with metastatic colorectal cancer receiving palliative chemotherapy were enrolled in this qualitative study in Norway. Researchers conducted semi-structured, in-depth interviews over a 1-year period with hermeneutic editing for analyses. The European Organisation for Research and Treatment of Cancer (EORTC) QOL group's subthemes of spiritual well-being were used as a framework. Inclusion criteria were patients 18 years or older with metastatic colorectal cancer referred for first- or second-line noncurative chemotherapy with an expected life expectancy that exceeded 6 months. Patients unable to read or understand Norwegian, or those with significant comorbidities or being treated with an investigational drug were excluded from the study. Participants varied in terms of sociodemographic data such as age, marital status, education level, and religious beliefs. Some examples of the interview questions included "How do you experience your life after you became ill?" "How is your relationship with your nearest family and friends?" Nineteen participant interviews were done in the hospital and 1 in the participant's home.

Findings

Low spiritual well-being is associated with low QOL in patients with cancer. Positive spiritual coping strategies may contribute to improved adjustment to illness, although evidence is mixed.

Using the EORTC's model, the researchers identified subthemes of spiritual well-being, including *relationship with others* (strategies for inner harmony, sharing feelings with significant others), *existential issues* (coping with end-of-life thoughts) and *religious and/or spiritual beliefs and practices* (seeking faith as inner support). Participants identified and focused on short-term, positive, and achievable goals. Many reported an ability to live a good life, despite the prognosis. Some felt the ability to speak openly about their illness was a positive change and made relationships better. However, those who did not have good relationships before their illness did not see an improvement in relationships after their diagnosis. Some participants withheld information about their diagnosis and prognosis from their families by choice in an attempt to spare their feelings. When discussing end-of-life issues, trust between the provider and patient was very important. Some participants would have welcomed a provider initiating a discussion on existential issues, while others thought it would be intrusive.

Nursing Implications

Patients with metastatic colorectal cancer use cognitive, affective, and behavioral strategies to adjust to health-related changes in their QOL and spiritual well-being. In the process of seeking inner harmony, most participants in this study underwent a response shift when learning of their diagnosis and shift in what was important in their lives. They tried to find a balance between sadness and grief and positive feelings; others were less able to adjust to their illness and focused more on negative feelings and sadness. The participants in this study did not expect health care providers to initiate a conversation about spiritual well-being or other existential issues, although many would have appreciated the provider listening without being intrusive. Understanding QOL and spiritual well-being issues that patients with colorectal cancer face may allow the nurse to identify patients in need of developing positive coping strategies or to act as facilitator for communication between the patient and family.

NURSING PROCESS

The Patient Having Surgery for Colorectal Cancer

Assessment

The nurse obtains a health history about the presence of fatigue, abdominal or rectal pain (e.g., location, frequency, duration, association with eating or defecation), past and present elimination patterns, and characteristics of stool (e.g., color, odor, consistency, presence of blood or mucus). Additional information includes a history of IBD or colorectal polyps, a family history of colorectal disease, Lynch syndrome, or FAP, and current medication therapy. The nurse assesses dietary patterns, including fat and fiber intake, as well as amounts of alcohol consumed and history of smoking. The nurse describes and documents a history of weight loss and feelings of weakness and fatigue.

Assessment includes auscultation of the abdomen for bowel sounds and palpation of the abdomen for areas of tenderness, distention, and solid masses. Stool specimens are inspected for character and presence of blood.

Diagnosis

NURSING DIAGNOSES

Based on the assessment data, major nursing diagnoses may include the following:

- Impaired nutritional intake associated with nausea and anorexia
- Risk for infection associated with surgery on bowel and disruption of colonic bacteria
- Risk for hypovolaemia associated with vomiting and dehydration
- Lack of knowledge concerning the diagnosis, the surgical procedure, and self-care after discharge
- Anxiety associated with impending surgery and the diagnosis of cancer
- Impaired skin integrity associated with the surgical incisions (abdominal or perianal)

COLLABORATIVE PROBLEMS/POTENTIAL COMPLICATIONS

Potential complications may include the following:

- Intraperitoneal infection
- Complete large bowel obstruction
- GI bleeding

- Bowel perforation
- Peritonitis, abscess, and sepsis

Planning and Goals

The major goals for the patient may include attainment of optimal level of nutrition; prevention of infection; maintenance of fluid balance; knowledge about the diagnosis, surgical procedure, and self-care after discharge; reduction of anxiety; maintenance of optimal tissue healing; and avoidance of complications.

Nursing Interventions

The patient awaiting surgery for colorectal cancer has many concerns, needs, and fears. They may be physically debilitated and emotionally distraught with concerns about lifestyle changes after surgery, prognosis, ability to perform in established roles, and finances. Priorities for nursing care include preparing the patient physically for surgery; providing information about postoperative care; and supporting the patient and family emotionally. An Enhanced Recovery After Surgery (ERAS) Society pathway, first developed in 2005 and last revised in 2018, provides a care path developed for patients undergoing elective colorectal surgery (i.e., colorectal surgery that is planned in advance, rather than done emergently) to reduce perioperative stress, reduce length of stay, and optimize patient outcomes (Gustafsson, Scott, Hubner, et al., 2018). Multidisciplinary strategies included in the pathway are evidence-based and are associated with a reduction in morbidity, comparable or reduced 30-day hospital readmission rates, faster recovery, earlier discharge, and decreased costs (Riccardi, MacKay, & Joshi, 2019). Despite advanced age, patients over 70 years managed with the ERAS pathway experienced similar benefits in terms of length of stay and postoperative outcomes as did younger patients who underwent colorectal surgery (Joris, Hans, Coimbra, et al., 2019). (See Chapter 15 for further discussion of ERAS pathways.)

PROVIDING PREOPERATIVE CARE

Maintaining Optimal Nutrition. Physical preparation for surgery involves building the patient's stamina in the days preceding surgery. If the patient's condition permits, the nurse recommends a diet high in calories, protein, and carbohydrates and low in residue for several days before surgery to provide adequate nutrition and minimize cramping by decreasing excessive peristalsis. If the patient is hospitalized in the days preceding surgery, parenteral nutrition may be required to replace depleted nutrients, vitamins, and minerals. In some instances, parenteral nutrition is given at home before surgery (Gustafsson et al., 2018).

Preventing Infection. Postoperative infection is a major cause of morbidity and mortality following colorectal surgery (Rollins, Javanmard-Emamghissi, & Lobo, 2018). Preoperative mechanical bowel preparations (e.g., enemas, oral laxatives) traditionally have been prescribed to reduce fecal bulk and colonic bacteria. It had been posited that these measures would prevent postoperative complications of infection. However, findings from a meta-analysis suggest that these interventions do not reduce the rates of postoperative infectious complications among patients having colorectal surgery (Rollins et al., 2018). Nonetheless, there is a lack of consensus regarding best practices that might reduce the rates of infections. The American Society of Colon and Rectal Surgeons supports the use of mechanical bowel preparations

for elective colorectal surgery only when accompanied by preoperative oral antibiotics (Migaly, Bafford, Francone, et al., 2019). Antibiotics typically prescribed may include kanamycin, ciprofloxacin, neomycin, metronidazole, and cephalexin to be administered orally the day before surgery. IV antibiotics such as cefazolin and metronidazole are usually given within 60 minutes of the surgical incision (Gustaffsson et al., 2018).

Maintaining Fluid Volume Balance. For the patient who is very ill and hospitalized, the nurse measures and records intake and output, including vomitus, to provide an accurate record of fluid balance. The patient's intake of oral food and fluids may be restricted to prevent vomiting. The nurse administers antiemetic agents as prescribed. Full or clear liquids may be tolerated, or the patient may be NPO. An NG tube may be inserted to drain accumulated fluids and prevent abdominal distention. The nurse monitors the abdomen for increasing distention, loss of bowel sounds, and pain or rigidity, which may indicate obstruction or perforation. It also is important to monitor IV fluids and electrolytes. Monitoring serum electrolyte levels can detect the hypokalemia and hyponatremia that occur with GI fluid loss. The nurse observes for signs of hypovolemia (e.g., tachycardia, hypotension, decreased pulse volume); assesses hydration status; and reports decreased skin turgor, dry mucous membranes, and concentrated urine.

Providing Preoperative Education. The nurse assesses the patient's knowledge about the diagnosis, prognosis, surgical procedure, and expected level of functioning after surgery. Education is provided about the preparations for surgery, the expected appearance and care of the wound, dietary restrictions, pain control, and medication management. All procedures are explained in language the patient understands. If the patient is going to have a colostomy, the nurse manages the plan of care as described previously (see Nursing Management of the Patient Requiring an Ostomy).

Providing Emotional Support. Patients anticipating bowel surgery for colorectal cancer may be very anxious. They may grieve about the diagnosis and the impending surgery. The nurse's role is to assess the patient's anxiety level and coping mechanisms and suggest methods for reducing anxiety, such as deep-breathing exercises and visualizing a successful recovery from surgery and cancer. The nurse can arrange a meeting with a spiritual advisor if the patient desires or with the primary provider if the patient wishes to discuss the treatment or prognosis. To promote patient comfort, the nurse projects a relaxed, professional, and empathetic attitude.

PROVIDING POSTOPERATIVE CARE

Postoperative nursing care for patients undergoing colon resection is similar to nursing care for any abdominal surgery patient (see Chapter 16), including pain management during the immediate postoperative period. The nurse also monitors the patient for complications. The nurse assesses the abdomen for returning peristalsis and assesses the initial stool characteristics. It is important to help patients out of bed on the first postoperative day to prevent atelectasis, VTE, and accelerate the return of peristalsis (Chan, LeRoux, Stutzman, et al., 2019; Kaff, Wehner, & Litkouhi, 2018).

Maintaining Optimal Nutrition. The nurse educates the patient having surgery for colorectal cancer about the health benefits to be derived from consuming a healthy diet. The diet is individualized as long as it is nutritionally sound and does not cause diarrhea or constipation. The return to normal diet is rapid.

Providing Wound Care. The nurse frequently examines the abdominal dressing during the first 24 hours after surgery to detect signs of hemorrhage or infection. It is important to help the patient splint the abdominal incision during coughing and deep breathing to lessen tension on the edges of the incision. The nurse monitors temperature, pulse, and respiratory rate for elevations that may indicate an infectious process.

If the malignancy has been removed using the perineal route, the perineal wound is observed for signs of hemorrhage. This wound may contain a drain or packing that is removed gradually. Bits of tissue may slough off for a week. This process is hastened by mechanical irrigation of the wound or with sitz baths performed two or three times each day initially. The condition of the perineal wound and any bleeding, infection, or necrosis is documented.

Monitoring and Managing Potential Complications. The patient is observed for signs and symptoms of complications. The nurse monitors vital signs for increased temperature, pulse, and respirations and for decreased blood pressure that may indicate an intra-abdominal infectious process. It is important to frequently assess the abdomen, including bowel sounds and abdominal girth, to detect bowel obstruction. Rectal bleeding must be reported immediately because it indicates hemorrhage. The nurse monitors hemoglobin and hematocrit levels and administers blood component therapy as prescribed. Any abrupt change in abdominal pain is reported promptly. Elevated white blood cell counts and temperature or symptoms of shock are reported because they may indicate sepsis. The nurse administers antibiotics as prescribed. Table 41-9 lists additional potential postoperative complications.

TABLE 41-9 Potential Complications and Nursing Interventions After Colorectal Surgery

Complication	Nursing Interventions
General Complications	
Paralytic ileus	Initiate or continue nasogastric intubation if prescribed (typically only indicated with vomiting or abdominal distention).
	Prepare patient for x-ray study or CT scan of abdomen.
	Ensure adequate fluid and electrolyte replacement; monitor serum electrolytes for abnormalities (e.g., hypokalemia, hyponatremia, hypomagnesemia).
	Prepare to institute or discontinue prescribed drugs or therapies that can increase motility (e.g., chewing gum increases motility, opioid analgesics can decrease motility).
Mechanical obstruction	Assess patient for intermittent colicky pain, nausea, and vomiting.
	Initiate or continue nasogastric intubation if prescribed.
	Prepare patient for x-ray study or CT scan of abdomen.
	Prepare patient for surgery.
Intra-abdominal Septic and Ischemic Conditions	
Peritonitis	Evaluate patient for nausea, hiccups, chills, spiking fever, tachycardia, rigid, boardlike abdomen.
	Administer antibiotics as prescribed.
	Prepare patient for drainage procedure.
	Administer parenteral fluid and electrolyte therapy as prescribed.
	Prepare patient for surgery if condition deteriorates.
Abscess formation	Administer antibiotics as prescribed.
	Apply warm compresses as prescribed.
	Prepare patient for surgical or percutaneous drainage.
Acute mesenteric ischemia	Assess patient for sudden onset of severe, colicky pain, abdominal distention, and sepsis.
	Prepare patient for x-ray study or CT scan of abdomen.
	Administer antibiotics as prescribed.
	Prepare patient for surgery.
Surgical Wound Complications	
Infection	Monitor temperature; report temperature elevation.
	Observe for redness, tenderness, induration (hardening), and pain around the surgical wound.
	Assist in establishing local drainage.
	Obtain specimen of drainage material for culture and sensitivity studies.
Wound dehiscence	Observe for sudden drainage of profuse serous fluid from wound.
	Cover wound area with sterile moist dressings.
Wound evisceration	Observe for wound dehiscence with protrusion of abdominal organs (e.g., intestines) through wound.
	Prepare patient immediately for surgery.
Abdominal wound infection	Monitor for evidence of constant or generalized abdominal pain, rapid pulse, and elevation of temperature.
	Prepare for tube decompression of bowel.
	Administer fluids and electrolytes by IV route as prescribed.
	Administer antibiotics as prescribed.
Anastomotic Complications	
Dehiscence of anastomosis	Prepare patient for surgery.
Fistulas	Prepare for tube decompression of bowel.
	Administer parenteral fluids as prescribed to correct fluid and electrolyte deficits.

Adapted from: Moyle, S. (2017). Postoperative complications: Clinical guidelines for nurses. *Ausmed*. Retrieved on 3/9/2020 at: www.ausmed.com/cpd/articles/postoperative-complications

Promoting Home, Community-Based, and Transitional Care

Educating Patients About Self-Care. Patient education and discharge planning require the combined efforts of the primary provider, nurse, social worker, and dietitian. Patients are given specific information about wound care and signs and symptoms of potential complications that is individualized to their needs. Dietary instructions are essential to help patients identify and eliminate irritating foods that can cause diarrhea or constipation. It is important to educate patients about their prescribed medications (i.e., action, purpose, and possible side and toxic effects).

Some patients who are older with multiple comorbid conditions may need referral to a home care agency and the telephone number of the local chapter of the ACS. The home health nurse provides further care and education and assesses the patient's and family's adjustment. The home environment is assessed for adequacy of resources that allow the patient to manage self-care activities. A family member may assume responsibility for purchasing the equipment and supplies needed at home.

Patients need very specific directions about when to call their primary provider. They need to know which complications require prompt attention (i.e., bleeding, abdominal distention and rigidity, diarrhea, fever, wound drainage, and disruption of suture line). If chemotherapy is planned, the possible side effects (e.g., diarrhea, fatigue, palmar-plantar erythrodysesthesia, neuropathies) are reviewed.

Continuing and Transitional Care. Ongoing care of the patient with cancer extends well beyond the initial hospital stay. Transitional care nurses who work in cancer care infusion centers manage follow-up care and coordinate adjuvant therapy and surveillance follow-ups. Some patients are interested in and can benefit from involvement in colorectal cancer support groups (see Resources section at the end of this chapter).

Evaluation

Expected patient outcomes may include:
1. Consumes a healthy diet
    a. Avoids foods and fluids that cause diarrhea, constipation, and obstruction
    b. Substitutes nonirritating foods and fluids for those that are restricted
2. Does not exhibit any signs or symptoms of infection
    a. Is afebrile
3. Maintains fluid balance
    a. Experiences no vomiting or diarrhea
    b. Experiences no signs or symptoms of dehydration
4. Acquires information about diagnosis, surgical procedure, preoperative preparation, and self-care after discharge
    a. Discusses the diagnosis, surgical procedure, and postoperative self-care
    b. Demonstrates techniques of ostomy care
5. Feels less anxious
    a. Expresses concerns and fears freely
    b. Uses coping measures to manage stress
6. Maintains clean wound(s)
7. Recovers without complications
    a. Regains normal bowel activity
    b. Exhibits no signs and symptoms of perforation or bleeding
    c. Identifies signs and symptoms that should be reported to the health care provider

Polyps of the Colon and Rectum

A polyp is a mass of tissue that protrudes into the lumen of the bowel. Polyps can occur anywhere in the intestinal tract and rectum. They can be classified as neoplastic (i.e., typically adenocarcinomas) or non-neoplastic (i.e., mucosal and hyperplastic). Non-neoplastic polyps, which are benign epithelial growths, are common in the Western world. They occur more commonly in the large intestine than in the small intestine. Because polyps might develop into malignant neoplasms, they should be removed when they are identified, typically during screening colonoscopy (Enders, 2020). Adenomatous polyps are more common in men. The proportion of these polyps arising in the proximal part of the colon increases with age. The prevalence among adults over 60 years of age is estimated to be 10% (Enders, 2020).

Clinical manifestations depend on the size of the polyp and the amount of pressure it exerts on intestinal tissue. Most commonly, there are no symptoms. When there are clinical manifestations, the most common is rectal bleeding. Lower abdominal pain may also occur. If the polyp is large enough, symptoms of obstruction occur. The diagnosis is based on history and digital rectal examination, double-contrast barium enema studies, sigmoidoscopy, or colonoscopy (NIDDK, 2017a).

After a polyp is identified, it should be removed. Several methods are used: colonoscopy with the use of special equipment (i.e., biopsy forceps and snares), laparoscopy, or colonoscopic excision with laparoscopic visualization. The latter technique enables immediate detection of potential problems and allows laparoscopic resection and repair of the major complications of perforation and bleeding that may occur with polypectomy. Microscopic examination of the polyp then identifies the type of polyp and indicates what further surgery is required, if any (NIDDK, 2017a).

DISORDERS OF THE ANORECTUM

Anorectal disorders are common. Patients with anorectal disorders seek medical care primarily because of pain, rectal bleeding, or change in bowel habits. Other common complaints are protrusion of hemorrhoids, anal discharge, perianal itching, swelling, anal tenderness, stenosis, and ulceration. Constipation results from delaying defecation because of anorectal pain.

Proctitis

Proctitis refers to inflammation of the mucosa of the rectum, which may be secondary to infection, IBD, celiac disease, rectal instrumentation, antibiotic treatment, or radiation. Infectious diseases are the most frequent cause of proctitis; these etiologies may be either from enteric organism (e.g., *Shigella*, *Salmonella*) or from sexually transmitted infections (STIs; also called *sexually transmitted diseases*, or STDs).

Proctitis secondary to an STI may occur in any gender but is more prevalent among gay men who practice anorectal intercourse. It is commonly associated with recent anal-receptive intercourse with an infected partner. Symptoms include mucopurulent discharge or bleeding, rectal pain, and diarrhea. The pathogens most frequently involved are *Neisseria gonorrhoeae*, *Chlamydia trachomatis*, syphilis, herpes simplex virus, and *Clostridium difficile*. These infections may progress into proctocolitis and enteritis. Proctocolitis involves the rectum and lowest portion of the descending colon. Symptoms are similar to proctitis but may also include watery or bloody diarrhea, cramps, pain, and bloating. Enteritis involves more of the descending colon, and symptoms include watery, bloody diarrhea; abdominal pain; and weight loss. The most common pathogens causing enteritis are *E. histolytica*, *Giardia lamblia, and Shigella*, and *Campylobacter* species (Irizarry, 2018).

Sigmoidoscopy is performed to identify portions of the anorectum involved. Samples are taken with rectal swabs, and cultures are obtained to identify the pathogens involved. Antibiotics (e.g., ceftriaxone, doxycycline) are the treatment of choice for gonorrheal proctitis. Acyclovir is given to patients with viral infections. Antiamebic therapy (i.e., metronidazole) is appropriate for infections with *E. histolytica* and *G. lamblia*. Metronidazole or oral vancomycin is recommended for patients with proctitis due to *C. difficile* infection (Irizarry, 2018).

Anorectal Abscess

An anorectal abscess is caused by obstruction of an anal gland with dried debris, resulting in retrograde infection. People with Crohn's disease or immunosuppressive conditions such as AIDS are particularly susceptible to these infections. Many of these abscesses result in fistulas (Hebra, 2018).

An abscess may occur in a variety of spaces in and around the rectum, usually in the path of least resistance, where anatomic structures are in close proximity without hard or thick structures to separate them. Most patients with anorectal abscesses will complain of dull perianal discomfort and itching, and increased pain with defecation. Approximately half will present with perianal edema; only one quarter will report any abnormal fecal discharge, such as pus, mucous, or blood. Only 21% report fever or chills (Hebra, 2018).

Prompt surgical treatment to incise and drain the abscess is the treatment of choice, to prevent complications such as fistula formation, fecal incontinence, and sepsis. This may be done in the emergency department or in an outpatient clinic office setting. The wound may be packed with an absorptive dressing (e.g., calcium alginate or hydrofiber) and allowed to heal by granulation (Hebra, 2018).

Anal Fistula

An anal fistula is a tiny, tubular, fibrous tract that extends into the anal canal from an opening located beside the anus in the perianal skin (see Fig. 41-12A). Fistulas usually result from an abscess. They may also develop from trauma, fissures, or Crohn's disease. Purulent drainage or stool may leak constantly from the cutaneous opening. Other symptoms may be the passage of flatus or feces from the vagina or bladder, depending on the location of the fistula tract. Untreated fistulas may cause systemic infection with related symptoms (Hebra, 2018).

Surgery is recommended because few fistulas heal spontaneously. A fistulectomy (i.e., excision of the fistulous tract) is the recommended surgical procedure. The lower bowel is evacuated thoroughly with several prescribed enemas. The fistula is dissected or laid open by an incision from its rectal opening to its outlet. The wound is packed with gauze. Postoperative medications include analgesics and antibiotics. Fistulas recur in up to half of patients (Hebra, 2018).

Anal Fissure

An anal fissure is a longitudinal tear or ulceration in the lining of the anal canal usually just distal to the dentate line (see Fig. 41-12B). Fissures are usually caused by the trauma of passing a large, firm stool or from persistent tightening of the anal canal because of stress and anxiety (leading to constipation). Other causes include childbirth, trauma, and or anal intercourse.

Painful defecation, burning, and bleeding characterize fissures. Bright red blood may be seen on the toilet tissue after

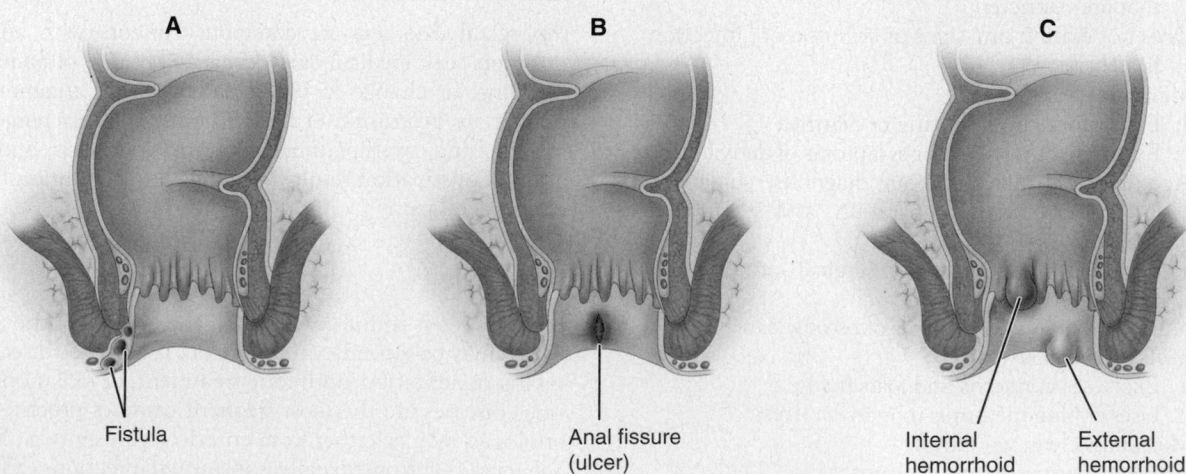

Fistula   Anal fissure (ulcer)   Internal hemorrhoid   External hemorrhoid

Figure 41-12 • Various types of anal lesions. A. Fistula. **B.** Fissure. **C.** External and internal hemorrhoids.

a bowel movement. Most of these fissures heal if treated by conservative measures that include dietary modification with addition of fiber supplements, stool softeners and bulk agents, an increase in water intake, and sitz baths (Poritz, 2018). Anal dilation under anesthesia may be required. Therapies such as perianal or intra-anal application of nitroglycerin ointment, calcium channel blockers, minoxidil, or botulinum toxin injections have increased the rate of healing and lowered pain levels in chronic anal fissures; these therapies should be tried before surgery. These agents work by increasing blood supply to the region and relaxing the anal sphincter (Poritz, 2018).

If fissures do not respond to conservative treatment, surgery is indicated. The procedure of choice is the lateral internal sphincterotomy with excision of the fissure.

Hemorrhoids

Hemorrhoids are dilated portions of veins in the anal canal. In the United States, approximately 10 million people have hemorrhoids; of these, nearly one third seek medical treatment for hemorrhoids annually (Perry, 2019). Shearing of the mucosa during defecation results in the sliding of the structures in the wall of the anal canal, including the hemorrhoidal and vascular tissues. Increased pressure in the hemorrhoidal tissue due to pregnancy may initiate hemorrhoids or aggravate existing ones. Hemorrhoids are classified into two types: those above the internal sphincter are called *internal hemorrhoids*, and those appearing outside the external sphincter are called *external hemorrhoids* (Perry, 2019) (see Fig. 41-12C). Internal hemorrhoids are classified by their degree of prolapse (Soweld, 2018):

- First degree—do not prolapse and protrude into anal canal
- Second degree—prolapse outside the anal canal during defecation but reduce spontaneously
- Third degree—prolapsed to the extent that they require manual reduction
- Fourth degree—prolapsed to the extent that they may not be reduced and are at risk for strangulation and thrombosis

Hemorrhoids cause itching and pain and are the most common cause of bright red bleeding with defecation. External hemorrhoids are associated with severe pain from the inflammation and edema caused by thrombosis (i.e., clotting of blood within the hemorrhoid). This may lead to ischemia of the area and eventual necrosis. Internal hemorrhoids are not usually painful until they bleed or prolapse when they become enlarged.

Hemorrhoid symptoms and discomfort can be relieved by good personal hygiene and by avoiding excessive straining during defecation. A high-residue diet that contains fruit and bran along with an increased fluid intake may be all the treatment that is necessary to promote the passage of soft, bulky stools to prevent straining. If this treatment is not successful, the addition of hydrophilic bulk-forming agents such as psyllium may help. Warm compresses, sitz baths, analgesic ointments and suppositories, and astringents (e.g., witch hazel) reduce engorgement (Perry, 2019).

There are several types of nonsurgical treatments for hemorrhoids. Infrared photocoagulation, bipolar diathermy, and laser therapy are used to affix the mucosa to the underlying muscle. Injection of sclerosing agents is also effective for small, bleeding hemorrhoids. Sclerotherapy involves injecting a sclerosing agent (5% phenol in saline) into the base of the hemorrhoid to cause blood vessel thrombosis. These procedures help prevent prolapse (Perry, 2019).

A conservative surgical treatment of internal hemorrhoids is the rubber band ligation procedure. The hemorrhoid is visualized through the anoscope, and its proximal portion above the mucocutaneous lines is grasped with an instrument. A small rubber band is then slipped over the hemorrhoid. Tissue distal to the rubber band becomes necrotic after several days and sloughs off. Fibrosis occurs; the result is that the lower anal mucosa is drawn up and adheres to the underlying muscle. Although this treatment has been satisfactory for some patients, it has proven painful for others and may cause secondary hemorrhage. It has also been known to cause perianal infection (Soweld, 2018).

Stapled hemorrhoidopexy uses surgical staples to treat prolapsing hemorrhoids and is associated with less postoperative pain and fewer complications. If it is not successful, hemorrhoidectomy, or surgical excision, may be performed to remove all of the redundant tissue involved in the process. During surgery, the rectal sphincter is usually dilated digitally, and the hemorrhoids are removed with a clamp and cautery or are ligated and then excised. After the surgical procedures are completed, a small tube may be inserted through the sphincter to permit the escape of flatus and blood; pieces of absorbable gelatin sponge (Gelfoam) or oxidized cellulose (Oxycel) gauze may be placed over the anal wounds (Perry, 2019).

Pilonidal Sinus or Cyst

A pilonidal sinus or cyst is found in the intergluteal cleft on the posterior surface of the lower sacrum (see Fig. 41-13). Current theories suggest that it results from local trauma, causing penetration of hairs into the epithelium and subcutaneous tissue. It may also be formed congenitally by an infolding of

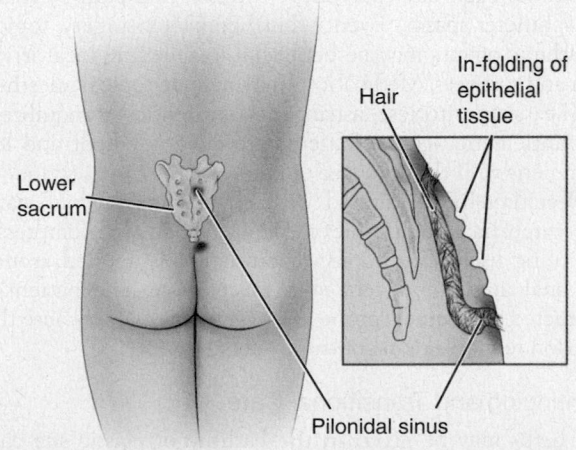

Figure 41-13 • (**Left**) Pilonidal sinus on lower sacrum about 5 cm (2 inches) above the anus in the intergluteal cleft. (**Right**) Hair particles emerge from the sinus tract, and localized indentations (pits) can appear on the skin near the sinus openings.

epithelial tissue beneath the skin, which may communicate with the skin surface through one or several small sinus openings. Hair frequently is seen protruding from these openings, and this gives the cyst its name, *pilonidal* (i.e., a nest of hair). The cysts rarely cause symptoms until adolescence or early adult life, when infection produces an irritating drainage or an abscess. Perspiration and friction easily irritate this area (Koyfman, 2019).

The abscess is incised and drained under local anesthesia. After the acute process resolves, further surgery might be indicated to excise the cyst and any secondary sinus tracts. The wound is allowed to heal by granulation. Absorptive dressings are placed in the wound to keep its edges separated while healing occurs (Koyfman, 2019).

Nursing Management of Patients with Anorectal Disorders

Most patients with anorectal disorders are not hospitalized. Those who undergo surgical procedures to correct the condition often are discharged directly from the outpatient surgical center. If they are hospitalized, it is for a short time, usually only 24 hours.

Promoting Home, Community-Based, and Transitional Care

 Educating Patients About Self-Care

Patient education is essential to facilitate recovery at home.

The nurse instructs the patient to keep the perianal area as clean as possible by gently cleansing with warm water and then drying with absorbent cotton wipes. The patient should avoid rubbing the area with toilet tissue. Instructions are provided about how to take a sitz bath and how to test the temperature of the water.

During the first 24 hours after rectal surgery, painful spasms of the sphincter and perineal muscles may occur. The nurse instructs the patient that ice and analgesic ointments may decrease the pain. Warm compresses may promote circulation and soothe irritated tissues. Sitz baths taken three to four times each day can relieve soreness and pain by relaxing sphincter spasm. Twenty-four hours after surgery, topical anesthetic agents may be beneficial in relieving local irritation and soreness. Medications may include topical anesthetics (i.e., suppositories), astringents, antiseptics, tranquilizers, and antiemetic agents. Patients are more adherent and less apprehensive if they are free of pain.

Wet dressings saturated with equal parts of cold water and witch hazel help relieve edema. When wet compresses are being used continuously, petrolatum is applied around the anal area to prevent skin maceration. The patient is instructed to assume a prone position at intervals because this position reduces edema of the tissue.

Continuing and Transitional Care

Sitz baths may be given in the bathtub or plastic sitz bath unit three to four times each day. Sitz baths should follow each bowel movement for 1 to 2 weeks after surgery. The nurse encourages intake of at least 2 L of water daily to provide adequate hydration and recommends high-fiber foods to promote bulk in the stool and to make it easier to pass fecal matter through the rectum. Bulk laxatives such as psyllium may be recommended, and stool softeners (e.g., docusate) may be prescribed. The patient is advised to set aside a time for bowel movements and to heed the urge to defecate as promptly as possible, in order to prevent constipation. The diet is modified to increase fluids and fiber. Moderate exercise is encouraged, and the patient is taught about the prescribed diet, the significance of proper eating habits and exercise, and the laxatives that can be taken safely.

CRITICAL THINKING EXERCISES

1 **ipc** You are a home health nurse making a first post-discharge visit for a 42-year-old female discharged home following a proctocolectomy with ileostomy. The patient has a 20-year history of Crohn's disease with multiple exacerbations, as well as a history of depression, anemia, malnutrition, and arthritis primarily affecting the metacarpal phalangeal (MCP) and proximal interphalangeal (PIP) joints of both hands. She is married and lives with her husband; an adult daughter lives out of state. The patient is a self-employed attorney. What interdisciplinary and community resources would you consider mobilizing that can facilitate the patient's recovery from surgery, help her to manage her ileostomy over the long-term, and improve her quality of life?

2 **pg** As a staff nurse on a hospital surgical unit, you are caring for a 68-year male admitted from the postanesthesia care unit (PACU) following emergent laparotomy for repair of an anastomotic leak of a segmental bowel resection done 10 days ago for stage II colon cancer. In addition to his history of colon cancer, the patient also has a history of hypertension, obstructive sleep apnea, and obesity (with a body mass index [BMI] of 36/m^2). The patient is drowsy, oriented to person, place, and time; he reports an abdominal pain score of "6" on a 0 to 10 numeric pain intensity scale. The patient's vital signs include: temperature 36.6°C (97.8°F), heart rate 82 bpm, respiratory rate 12/min, blood pressure 138/78, and SpO$_2$ of 99% on 2 L/min of O$_2$ by nasal cannula. The patient has a midline abdominal wound with staples with a small amount of serosanguinous drainage on the dressing and a Jackson-Pratt drain to bulb suction with scant bloody drainage, a Foley catheter to gravity drainage, and sequential compression devices in place bilaterally to his lower extremities. A peripheral IV line in his left forearm is infusing normal saline at 100 mL/h. What are your assessment priorities? Discuss the patient's risk for postoperative complications, and identify appropriate preventive interventions.

3 **ebp** You work in an outpatient gastroenterology clinic. The clinic manager asks you to develop an educational program for patients with inflammatory bowel disease. Describe your learning objectives for this program. What evidence-based health promotion strategies would you include? How might you monitor the effectiveness of your program?

REFERENCES

*Asterisk indicates nursing research.
**Double asterisk indicates classic reference.

Books

Chubak, J., Kamineni, A., Buist, D. S., et al. (2015). Aspirin use for the prevention of colorectal cancer: An updated systematic evidence review for the U.S. Preventive Services Task Force. *Evidence Synthesis No. 133.* AHRQ Publication No. 15–05228-EF-1. Rockville, MD: Agency for Healthcare Research and Quality.

Comerford, K. C., & Durkin, M. T. (Eds.). (2020). *Nursing2020 Drug Handbook.* Philadelphia, PA: Wolters Kluwer.

Eliopoulos, C. (2018). *Gerontological nursing* (9th ed.). Philadelphia, PA: Wolters Kluwer.

Mada, P. K., & Alam, M. U. (2019). Clostridium difficile. *StatPearls.* [Updated 2019 Jun 4]. In: StatPearls [Internet]. Treasure Island, FL: StatPearls Publishing. https://www.ncbi.nlm.nih.gov/books/NBK431054/

Norris, T. L. (2019). *Porth's pathophysiology: Concepts of altered health states* (10th ed.). Philadelphia, PA: Wolters Kluwer.

Taylor, C., Lynn, P., & Bartlette, J. L. (2019). *Fundamentals of Nursing: The art and science of person-centered care.* Philadelphia, PA: Wolters Kluwer.

Weber, J. R., & Kelley, J. H. (2018). *Health assessment in nursing* (6th ed.). Philadelphia, PA: Wolters Kluwer.

Journals and Electronic Documents

American Cancer Society (ACS). (2020). Key statistics for colorectal cancer. Retrieved on 3/9/2020 at: www.cancer.org/cancer/colon-rectal-cancer/about/key-statistics.html

Basson, M. D. (2019a). Constipation. *Medscape.* Retrieved on 2/29/2020 at: emedicine.medscape.com/article/184704-1

Basson, M. D. (2019b). *Ulcerative colitis. Medscape.* Retrieved on 3/1/2020 at: emedicine.medscape.com/article/183084-overview

Bauer, C., Arnold-Long, M., & Kent, D. J. (2016). Colostomy irrigation to maintain continence: An old method revived. *Nursing, 46*(8), 59–62.

Bischoff, S. C., Escher, J., Hebuterne, X., et al. (2020). ESPEN practical guideline: Clinical nutrition in inflammatory bowel disease. *Clinical Nutrition, 39*(2020), 632–653.

Bordeianou, L., & Yeh, D. D. (2019). Etiologies, clinical manifestations, and diagnosis of mechanical small bowel obstruction in adults. *UpToDate.* Retrieved on 3/1/20120 at: www.uptodate.com/contents/etiologies-clinical-manifestations-and-diagnosis-of-mechanical-small-bowel-obstruction-in-adults1

Bridges, M., Nasser, R., & Parrish, C. R. (2019). High-output ileostomies: The stakes are higher than the output. *Practical Gastroenterology, XLIII*(9), Retrieved on 3/1/2020 at: practicalgastro.com/2019/09/23/high-output-ileostomies-the-stakes-are-higher-than-the-output/

Cabebe, E. C. (2020). *Colorectal cancer guidelines. Medscape.* Retrieved on 3/9/2020 at: emedicine.medscape.com/article/2500006-overview

Celiac Disease Foundation. Gluten-free living. Retrieved on 2/29/2020 at: celiac.org/gluten-free-living/gluten-free-foods/

Centers for Disease Control and Prevention (CDC). (2017a). Surgical site infection. Guideline for prevention of surgical site infection. Retrieved on 2/29/2019 at: www.cdc.gov/infectioncontrol/guidelines/ssi/index.html

Centers for Disease Control and Prevention (CDC). (2017b). Guidelines for the prevention of intravascular catheter-related infections, 2011, with 2017 updates. Retrieved on 7/13/2020 at: www.cdc.gov/infectioncontrol/pdf/guidelines/bsi-guidelines-H.pdf

Centers for Disease Control and Prevention (CDC). (2019). *Inflammatory bowel disease (IBD) prevalence in the United States.* Retrieved on 3/01/2020 at: www.cdc.gov/ibd/data-statistics.htm

*Chan, L., LeRoux, S., Stutzman, S., et al. (2019). Gum chewing and prolonged postoperative ileus: An observational retrospective study examining the impact of an evidence based practice change. *MedSurg Nursing Journal, 28*(6), 387–392.

Cohen-Mekekburg, S., Rosenblatt, R., Wallace, B., et al. (2019). Inflammatory bowel disease readmissions are associated with utilization and comorbidity. *The American Journal of Managed Care, 25*(10), 474–481.

Craig, S. (2018). Appendicitis. *Medscape.* Retrieved on 3/1/2019 at: emedicine.medscape.com/article/773895-overview

Daley, B. J. (2019). Peritonitis and abdominal sepsis. *Medscape.* Retrieved on 2/29/2020 at: emedicine.medscape.com/article/180234-overview#a7

DeLegge, M. H. (2020). *Nutrition and dietary management for adults with inflammatory bowel disease. UpToDate.* Retrieved on 7/10/2020 at: www.uptodate.com/contents/nutrition-and-dietary-management-for-adults-with-inflammatory-bowel-disease/contributors

Dimidi, E., Cox, C., Grant, R., et al. (2019). Perceptions of constipation among the general public and people with constipation differ strikingly from those of general and specialist doctors and the Rome IV criteria. *The American Journal of Gastroenterology, 114*(7), 1116–1129.

Dragovich, T. (2020). *Colon cancer treatment & management. Medscape.* Retrieved on 3/9/2020 at: emedicine.medscape.com/article/277496-treatment

Emmanuel, A. (2019). *Neurogenic bowel dysfunction.* F1000Research, 8, F1000 Faculty Rev-1800. doi.org/10.12688/f1000research.20529.1

Enders, G. E. (2020). Colonic polyps. *Medscape.* Retrieved on 5/21/2020 at: emedicine.medscape.com/article/172674-overview#a2

Farraye, F. A., Melmed, G. Y., Lichtenstein, G. R., et al. (2017). ACG clinical practice guideline: Preventive care in inflammatory bowel disease. *The American Journal of Gastroenterology, 112*, 241–258.

Francone, T. D. (2020). *Overview of surgical ostomy for fecal diversion. UpToDate.* Retrieved on 7/14/2020 at: www.uptodate-com/contents/overview-of-surgical-ostomy-for-fecal-diversion

George, L. A., Martin, B., Gupta, N., et al. (2019). Predicting 30-day readmission rate in inflammatory bowel disease patients: Performance of LACE index. *Crohns & Colitis 360, 1*(1), otz007. doi.org/10.1093/crocol/otz007.

Gervasio, J. (2015). Total nutrient admixtures (3-in-1) pros vs cons for adults. *Nutrition in Clinical Practice, 30*(3), 331–335.

Ghazi, L. J. (2019). *Crohn disease treatment & management. Medscape.* Retrieved on 3/1/2020 at: emedicine.medscape.com/article/172940-treatment#d14

Ghoulam, E. M. (2019). Diverticulitis. *Medscape.* Retrieved on 2/29/2020 at: emedicine.medscape.com/article/173388-overview

Gilroy, R. K. (2018). *Intestinal and multivisceral transplantation. Medscape.* Retrieved on 3/2/2020 at: emedicine.medscape.com/article/430743-overview#a9

Goebel, S. U. (2019). *Celiac disease. Medscape.* Retrieved on 5/19/2020 at: emedicine.medscape.com/article/171805-clinical

Gorski, L., Hadaway, L., Hagle, M. E., et al. (2016). Infusion therapy standards of practice. *Journal of Infusion Nursing (Supplement), 39*(1 Suppl), S1–S159.

Guenter, P., Worthington, P., Ayers, P., et al. (2018). Standardized competencies for parenteral nutrition administration: The ASPEN Model. *Nutrition in Clinical Practice, 33*(2), 295–304.

Gump, K., & Schmelzer, M. (2016). Gaining control over fecal incontinence. *Medsurg Nursing, 25*(2), 97–103.

Gustafsson, U. O., Scott, M. J., Hubner, M., et al. (2018). Guidelines for perioperative care in elective colorectal surgery: Enhanced recovery after surgery (ERAS) society recommendations: 2018. *World Journal of Surgery, 43*, 659–695.

Hammami, M. B. (2019). Malabsorption. *Medscape.* Retrieved on 2/29/2019 at: emedicine.medscape.com/article/180785-overview

Hebra, A. (2018). Anorectal abscess. *Medscape.* Retrieved on 3/1/2020 at: emedicine.medscape.com/article/191975-overview#showall

Hendren, S., Hammond, K., Glasgow, S. C., et al. (2015). Clinical practice guidelines for ostomy surgery. *Diseases of the Colon & Rectum, 58*(4), 375–387.

**Hinchey, E. J., Schaal, P. G., & Richards, G. K. (1978). Treatment of perforated diverticular disease of the colon. *Advances in Surgery, 12*, 85–109.

Hopkins, C. (2017). *Large-bowel obstruction. Medscape.* Retrieved on 3/1/2020 at: emedicine.medscape.com/article/774045-overview#a6

Irizarry, L. (2018). *Acute proctitis. Medscape.* Retrieved on 3/2/2020 at: emedicine.medscape.com/article/775952-overview

Jones, L., & Cantor, R. M. (2019). In watery diarrhea cases, do probiotics affect outcome? ACEP Now. *American College of Emergency Physicians, 38*(1). Retrieved on 2/29/2020 at: www.acepnow.com/issue/acep-now-vol-38-no-01-january-2019/page/2/

Joris, J., Hans, G., Coimbra, C., et al. (2019). Elderly patients over 70 years benefit from enhanced recovery programme after colorectal surgery as much as younger patients. *Journal of Visceral Surgery, 157*(1), 23–31.

Kaff, J. C., Wehner, S., & Litkouhi, B. (2018). *Measures to prevent prolonged postoperative ileus. UpToDate.* Retrieved on 3/6/2020 at: www.uptodate.com/contents/measures-to-prevent-prolonged-postoperative-ileus#H547645413

Kirkland-Kyhn, H., Martin, S., Zaratkiewicz, S., et al. (2018). Ostomy care at home. *American Journal of Nursing, 118*(4), 63–68.

Koyfman, A. (2019). *Pilonidal cyst and sinus. Medscape.* Retrieved on 3/2/2020 at: emedicine.medscape.com/article/788127-overview

Krzyzak, M., & Mulrooney, S. (2019). Diverticulitis: A review of diagnosis, treatment, and prevention. *Consultant, 59*(2), 35–37, 44.

Lacy, B. E., Mearin, F., Chang, L., et al. (2016). Bowel disorders. *Gastroenterology, 150*(6), 1393–1407.

Lee, J. J., & Chu, E. (2018). The adjuvant treatment of stage III colon cancer; Might less be more? *Oncology Journal, 32*(9), 437–444.

Lehrer, J. K. (2019). *Irritable bowel syndrome (IBS). Medscape.* Retrieved on 2/29/2020 at: emedicine.medscape.com/article/180389-overview

Macrae, F. A., & Bendell, J. (2020). *Clinical presentation, diagnosis, and staging of colorectal cancer. UpToDate.* Retrieved on 3/9/2020 at: www.uptodate.com/contents/clinical-presentation-diagnosis-and-staging-of-colorectal-cancer

Mari, A., Mahamid, M., Amara, H., et al. (2020). Chronic constipation in the elderly patient: Updates in evaluation and management. *Korean Journal of Family Medicine, 41*(2). doi.org/10.4082/kjfm.18.0182.

McClave, S. A., Taylor, B. E., Martindale, R. G., et al. (2016). Guidelines for the provision and assessment of nutrition support therapy in the adult critically ill patient: Society of Critical Care Medicine (SCCM) and American Society for Parenteral and Enteral Nutrition (ASPEN). *Journal of Parenteral and Enteral Nutrition, 40*(2), 159–211.

Micic, D., Gaetano, J. N., Rubin, J. N., et al. (2017). Factors associated with readmission to the hospital within 30 days in patients with inflammatory bowel disease. *Plos One, 12*(8), e0182900.

Migaly, J., Bafford, A. C., Francone, T. D., et al. (2019). The American Society of Colon and Rectal Surgeons clinical practice guidelines for the use of bowel preparation in elective colon and rectal surgery. *Diseases of the Colon and Rectum, 62*(1), 3–8.

Moyle, S. (2017). *Postoperative complications: Clinical guidelines for nurses. Ausmed.* Retrieved on 3/9/2020 at: www.ausmed.com/cpd/articles/postoperative-complications

National Cancer Institute (NCI). (2020). PDQ colon cancer treatment, Bethesda, MD. Retrieved on 5/21/2020 at: www.cancer.gov/types/colorectal/hp/colon-treatment-pdq

National Institute of Diabetes and Digestive and Kidney Diseases (NIDDK). (2014a). Appendicitis. Retrieved on 4/8/2020 at: www.niddk.nih.gov/health-information/digestive-diseases/appendicitis

National Institute of Diabetes and Digestive and Kidney Diseases (NIDDK). (2014b). *Digestive diseases statistics for the United States.* Retrieved on 2/29/2020 at: www.niddk.nih.gov/health-information/health-statistics/Pages/digestive-diseases-statistics-for-the-united-states.aspx

National Institute of Diabetes and Digestive and Kidney Diseases (NIDDK). (2016a). *Celiac disease.* Retrieved on 4/8/2020 at: www.niddk.nih.gov/health-information/digestive-diseases/celiac-disease

National Institute of Diabetes and Digestive and Kidney Diseases (NIDDK). (2016b). *Diarrhea.* Retrieved on 2/29/2020 at: www.niddk.nih.gov/health-information/digestive-diseases/diarrhea

National Institute of Diabetes and Digestive and Kidney Diseases (NIDDK). (2017a). *Colon polyps.* Retrieved on 3/1/2020 at: www.niddk.nih.gov/health-information/digestive-diseases/colon-polyps/treatment

National Institute of Diabetes and Digestive and Kidney Diseases (NIDDK). (2017b). *Fecal incontinence.* Retrieved on 2/29/2020 at: www.niddk.nih.gov/health-information/digestive-diseases/bowel-control-problems-fecal-incontinence/symptoms-causes

National Institute of Diabetes and Digestive and Kidney Diseases (NIDDK). (2017c). *Irritable bowel syndrome.* Retrieved on 2/29/2020 at: www.niddk.nih.gov/health-information/digestive-diseases/irritable-bowel-syndrome

National Institute of Diabetes and Digestive and Kidney Diseases (NIDDK). (2017d). *Crohn's disease.* Retrieved on 3/1/2020 at: www.niddk.nih.gov/health-information/digestive-diseases/crohns-disease

National Institute of Diabetes and Digestive and Kidney Diseases (NIDDK). (2018). Constipation. Retrieved on 5/19/2020 at: www.niddk.nih.gov/health-information/digestive-diseases/constipation/definition-facts#whois

Nguyen, N. H., Koola, J., Dulai, P. S., et al. (2020). Rate of risk factors for and interventions to reduce hospital readmission in patients with inflammatory bowel diseases. *Clinical Gastroenterology and Hepatology, 18*(9), 1939–1948.

Nguyen, L. H., Liu, P. H., Zheng, X., et al. (2018). Sedentary behaviors, TV viewing time, and risk of young-onset colorectal cancer. *JNCI Cancer Spectrum, 2*(4), pky073.

Pacheco, R. L., Roizenblatt, A., Góis, A. F. T., et al. (2019). What do Cochrane systematic reviews say about the management of irritable bowel syndrome? *Sao Paulo Medical Journal, 137*(1), 82–91.

Perry, K. R. (2019). *Hemorrhoids treatment & management. Medscape.* Retrieved on 3/20/2020 at: emedicine.medscape.com/article/775407-treatment

Piovani, D., Danese, S., Peyrin-Biroulet, L., et al. (2019). Environmental risk factors for inflammatory bowel diseases: An umbrella review of meta-analyses. *Gastroenterology, 157*(3), 647–659.

Poritz, L. S. (2018). *Anal fissure treatment & management. Medscape.* Retrieved on 3/2/2020 at: emedicine.medscape.com/article/196297-treatment#d9

Ramnarine, M. (2017). *Small-bowel obstruction. Medscape.* Retrieved on 3/1/2020 at: emedicine.medscape.com/article/774140-overview#a5

Rao, S. S., & Patcharatrakul, T. (2016). Diagnosis and treatment of dyssenergic defecation, *Journal of Neurogastroenterology and Motility, 22*(3), 423–435. doi.org/10.5056/jnm16060.

Rao, S. S., Bharucha, A. E., Chiaroni, G., et al. (2016). Anorectal disorders. *Gastroenterology, 150*(6), 1430–1442.

Rao, S. S., Valestin, J. A., Xiang, X., et al. (2018). Home-based versus office-based biofeedback therapy for constipation with dyssynergic defecation: A randomised controlled trial. *The Lancet Gastroenterology & Hepatology, 3*(1), 768–777.

Rex, D. K. (2018). The appropriate use and techniques of tattooing in the colon. *Gastroenterology & Hepatology, 14*(5), 314–317.

Riccardi, R., MacKay, G., & Joshi, G. P. (2019). *Enhanced recovery after colorectal surgery. UpToDate.* Retrieved on 3/9/2020 at: www.uptodate.com/contents/enhanced-recovery-after-colorectal-surgery

*Rohde, G., Kersten, C., Vistad, I., et al. (2017). Spiritual well-being in patients with metastatic colorectal cancer receiving noncurative chemotherapy: A qualitative study. *Cancer Nursing, 40*(3), 209–216.

Rollins, K. E., Javanmard-Emamghissi, H., & Lobo, D. N. (2018). Impact of mechanical bowel preparation in elective colorectal surgery: A meta-analysis. *World Journal of Gastroenterology, 24*(4), 519–536.

*Roos, S., Liedberg, G. M., Hellström, I., et al. (2019). Persistent symptoms in people with celiac disease despite gluten-free diet: A concern? *Gastroenterology Nursing, 42*(6), 496–503.

Rowe, W. A. (2020). *Inflammatory bowel disease. Medscape.* Retrieved on 5/20/2020 at: emedicine.medscape.com/article/179037-overview#a4

Rubin, D. T., Ananthakrishnan, A. N., Siegel, C. A., et al. (2019). ACG Clinical guideline: Ulcerative colitis in adults. *American Journal of Gastroenterology, 114*(3), 384–413.

Santacroce, L. (2019). *Appendectomy technique. Medscape.* Retrieved on 2/29/2019 at: emedicine.medscape.com/article/195778-technique

Seres, D. (2020). *Nutrition support in critically ill patients: Parenteral nutrition. UpToDate.* Retrieved on 7/11/2020 at: www.uptodate.com/contents/nutrition-support-in-critically-ill-patients-parenteral-nutrition

Simonson, C. (2018). Colorectal cancer—An update for primary care nurse practitioners. *Journal for Nurse Practitioners, 14*(4), 344–350.

Simren, M., Palsson, O. S., & Whitehead, W. E. (2017). Update on Rome IV criteria for colorectal disorders: Implications for clinical practice. *Current Gastroenterology Reports, 19*(4), 15. doi: 10.1007/s11894-017-0554-0.

Sougklakos, I., Boukovinas, I., Xynogalos, S., et al. (2019). Three versus six months adjuvant FOLFOX or CAPOX for high risk stage II and stage III colon cancer patients: The efficacy results of Hellenic oncology research group (HORG) participation to the international duration evaluation of adjuvant chemotherapy (IDEA) project. *Journal of Clinical Oncology, 37*(15 Suppl), 3500–3500.

Soweld, A. M. (2018). *Internal hemorrhoid banding. Medscape.* Retrieved on 3/2/2020 at: emedicine.medscape.com/article/1829718-overview

Spelman, D. (2019). *Pylephlebitis. UpToDate.* Retrieved on 3/1/2020 at: www.uptodate.com/contents/pylephlebitis

Stelton, S. (2019). Stoma care: A clinical review. *Am J Nurs, 119*(6), 38–45.

Taneja, C., Netsch, D., Ralstad, B. S., et al. (2017). Clinical and economic burden of peristomal skin complications in patients with recent ostomies. *Journal of Wound, Ostomy, and Continence Nursing, 44*(4), 350–357.

The Society for Healthcare Epidemiology of America SHEA Guideline Central. (2015). *Central line-associated bloodstream infections.* Retrieved on 9/10/2019 at: www.cambridge.org/core/journals/infection-control-and-hospital-epidemiology/article/strategies-to-prevent-central-lineassociated-bloodstream-infections-in-acute-care-hospitals-2014-update/CB398EB001FEADE0D9B4FF1A096ECA52

Tong, G. J., Zhang, G. Y., Lui, J., et al. (2018). Comparison of the eighth version of the American Joint Committee on Cancer manual to the seventh version for colorectal cancer: A retrospective review of our data. *World Journal of Clinical Oncology, 9*(7), 148–161.

Walfish, A. E. (2019). *Inflammatory bowel disease.* Merck Manual: Professional Version. Retrieved on 3/1/2020 at: www.merckmanuals.com/professional/gastrointestinal-disorders/inflammatory-bowel-disease-ibd/overview-of-inflammatory-bowel-disease

Wilhelm, S. M., & Love, B. L. (2017). Management of patients with inflammatory bowel disease: Current and future treatments. *Clinical Pharmacist, 9*(3). doi: 10.1211/CP.2017.20202316.

Williams, B. A., Grant, L. J., Gidley, M. J., et al. (2017). Gut fermentation of dietary fibres: Physico-chemistry of plant cell walls and implications for health. *International Journal of Molecular Sciences, 18*(10), 2203. doi: 10.3390/ijms18102203.

Worthington, P., Balint, J., Bechtold, M., et al. (2017). When is parenteral nutrition appropriate? *Journal of Parenteral and Enteral Nutrition, 41*(3), 324–377.

Wu, X., Ke, H., Kiran, R. P., et al. (2020). Continent ileostomy as an alternative to end ileostomy. *Gastroenterology Research and Practice, 2020,* Article ID 9740980. doi.org/10.1155/2020/9740980.

Resources

American Cancer Society, www.cancer.org

American College of Surgeons, Ostomy Home Skills Program, www.facs.org/education/patient-education/skills-programs/ostomy-program

American Society for Parenteral and Enteral Nutrition (A.S.P.E.N.), www.nutritioncare.org

American Society of Colon and Rectal Surgeons (ASCRS), www.fascrs.org

Beyond Celiac Disease, www.beyondceliac.org

Celiac Disease Foundation, celiac.org

Colorectal Cancer Alliance, www.ccalliance.org

Crohn's and Colitis Foundation of America (CCFA), crohnscolitisfoundation.org

Gluten Free Drugs, www.glutenfreedrugs.com

International Foundation for Gastrointestinal Disorders (IFFGD), www.iffgd.org

J-Pouch Group (source for J-Pouch surgery support), www.j-pouch.org

Meet an OstoMate, www.meetanostomate.org

National Cancer Institute, National Institutes of Health, www.cancer.gov

National Celiac Association, nationalceliac.org

National Colorectal Cancer Roundtable, nccrt.org

National Comprehensive Cancer Network Guidelines for Patients with Colon Cancer, www.nccn.org/patients/guidelines/colon/index.html#114

National Institute of Diabetes and Digestive and Kidney Diseases (NIDDK), www.niddk.nih.gov

The Colon Club, colonclub.org

The Rome Foundation, theromefoundation.org

United Ostomy Associations of America (UOAA), www.ostomy.org

Wound Ostomy and Continence Nurses Society, www.wocn.org

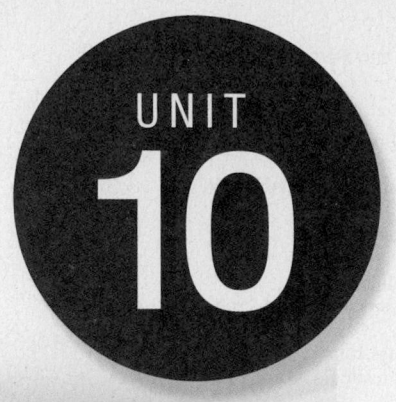

UNIT 10

Metabolic and Endocrine Function

APPLYING PATIENT-CENTERED CARE FOR THE PATIENT WITH DIABETES

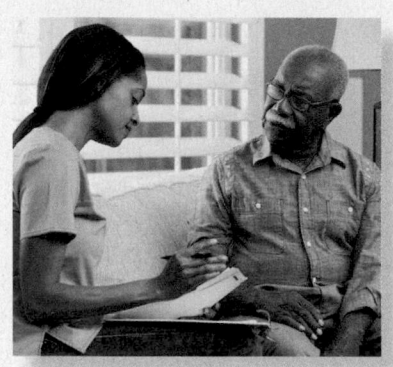

You are a certified diabetes care and education specialist in a community hospital. Today you are making a home visit to a 53-year-old Black man to follow up on the results of a 13% HgbA$_{1c}$ that was drawn a few weeks ago. He is 5′5″, weighs 180 lb, his finger stick glucose today is 310 mg/dL, and he lives with his adult daughter. While discussing the associations between an HgbA$_{1c}$ and poor blood glucose control, you review the pharmacologic and nonpharmacologic treatments. During the visit the patient and his daughter state they want to try cinnamon tea and other alternative and complementary therapies to help control his blood glucose naturally. You intend to collaborate with the family's preferences and educate them on the various ways he can maintain glucose control through diet, exercise, and medications.

QSEN Competency Focus: Patient-Centered Care

The complexities inherent in today's health care system challenge nurses to demonstrate integration of specific interdisciplinary core competencies. These competencies are aimed at ensuring the delivery of safe, quality patient care (Institute of Medicine, 2003). The Quality and Safety Education for Nurses project (Cronenwett, Sherwood, Barnsteiner, et al., 2007; QSEN, 2020) provides a framework for the knowledge, skills, and attitudes (KSAs) required for nurses to demonstrate competency in these key areas, which include *patient-centered care*, *interdisciplinary teamwork and collaboration*, *evidence-based practice*, *quality improvement*, *safety*, and *informatics.*

Patient-Centered Care Definition: Recognize the patient or designee as the source of control and full partner in providing compassionate and coordinated care based on respect for patient's preferences, values, and needs.

SELECT PRE-LICENSURE KSAs	APPLICATION AND REFLECTION
Knowledge	
Integrate understanding of multiple dimensions of patient centered care: • patient/family/community preferences, values • coordination and integration of care • information, communication, and education • physical comfort and emotional support • involvement of family and friends • transition and continuity Describe how diverse cultural, ethnic and social backgrounds function as sources of patient, family, and community values	Based on this patient's preferences, how can you provide education to this patient and his family regarding the management of his blood glucose? Identify how you can incorporate the patient's preferences for alternative and complementary therapies with diet and exercise management.
Skills	
Communicate patient values, preferences and expressed needs to other members of health care team	During the visit, you discuss with the patient and family ways they can adhere to a diet, exercise, and medication regimen. How can you communicate support of their choice to incorporate alternative and complementary therapies in managing the patient's blood glucose so that healthy glycemic control is achieved?
Attitudes	
Value seeing health care situations "through patients' eyes" Respect and encourage individual expression of patient values, preferences, and expressed needs	Reflect on the complex interrelationships between the patient's desire to manage his blood glucose with alternative therapies. Think about your own desire for this patient to adhere to a diet, exercise, and medications regimen. How might you demonstrate that you value the patient's preferences to utilize alternative and complementary therapies?

Cronenwett, L., Sherwood, G., Barnsteiner, J., et al. (2007). Quality and safety education for nurses. *Nursing Outlook*, *55*(3), 122–131; Institute of Medicine. (2003). *Health professions education: A bridge to quality*. Washington, DC: National Academies Press; QSEN Institute. (2020). *QSEN Competencies: Definitions and pre-licensure KSAs; Patient centered care*. Retrieved on 8/15/2020 at: qsen.org/competencies/pre-licensure-ksas/#patient-centered_care

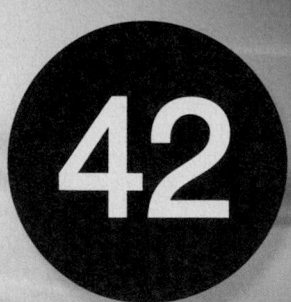

42

Assessment and Management of Patients with Obesity

Obesity in the United States and globally has reached pandemic proportions. Given the high prevalence of obesity, nurses will encounter adults with obesity in every inpatient and outpatient clinical setting. This chapter describes the etiology, risks, assessment, clinical manifestations, management, and related nursing care of the patient with obesity. The management of patients with obesity using both nonsurgical and surgical treatments is discussed.

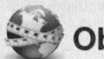 **Obesity**

Obesity is defined by the World Health Organization (WHO) as an "abnormal or excessive fat accumulation that may impair

health" (WHO, 2018, p. 1). As a response to endorsements by multiple health care organizations and societies, including the American College of Cardiology, the Endocrine Society, and the American College of Surgeons, to name a few, the American Medical Association (AMA) House of Delegates in 2013 officially resolved that obesity should be diagnosed and treated as a disease (AMA, 2013). This resolution was based on the scientific observation that obesity followed criteria commonly used for defining a disease; namely, it can be said that obesity impairs normal bodily function, possesses characteristic signs and symptoms, and causes morbidity (AMA, 2013).

Epidemiology of Obesity

Worldwide, over 650 million adults have obesity, and another 1.9 billion are overweight (WHO, 2018). Since 1975, the prevalence of obesity has more than tripled for men, and more than doubled for women. In particular, 3% of the world's men and 6% of the world's women had obesity in 1975, whereas 11% of the world's men and 15% of the world's women had obesity in 2016 (WHO, 2018). The burden of obesity is significant in both developed and developing nations. The WHO (2018) notes that many developing nations are now facing a "double-burden" effect from disorders linked to nutrition and metabolism; that is, these nations must simultaneously deal with the public health threats of both undernutrition and obesity. In developing nations, obesity has become particularly prevalent in urban settings (WHO, 2018).

Since 1980, the number of adults with obesity in the United States has continued to rise (Henry, 2018; Trust for America's Health [TFAH] & Robert Wood Johnson Foundation [RWJF], 2018). The prevalence of obesity in the United States is now the 12th highest among nations in the world, with Nauru, an island nation in Micronesia, being first, with an obesity prevalence of 61% (Hales, Carroll, Fryar, et al., 2020; Hales, Fryar, Carroll, et al., 2018). Among American adults, an estimated 42.4% have obesity (Hales et al., 2020); an estimated 70.9% have obesity or are overweight (Hales et al., 2018). The overall prevalence of overweight and obesity is slightly higher among American women than American men, and among African Americans and Hispanics than among Whites or Asian Americans (see Fig. 42-1). In general, those who are less educated and earn less income are more likely to have obesity, reflecting socioeconomic disparities in the disease burden of obesity (Hales et al., 2018; TFAH & RWJF, 2018). Being overweight or having obesity is the primary reason why young American adults are excluded from military service (Warren, Beck, & Rayburn, 2018) (see later discussion in Veterans Considerations section).

The economic burden of obesity to American society extends beyond limiting young adults with obesity from pursuing military service commitments. It is estimated that annual health care costs tied to obesity are approximately $190 billion (Warren et al., 2018), and that average annual health care expenditures for Americans with obesity are $3429 higher per person than for those Americans without obesity (Biener, Cawley, & Meyerhoefer, 2017).

Obesity Risks

The causes of obesity are complex and multifactorial, and include behavioral, environmental, physiologic, and genetic factors. While there are certain demographic groups who seem to be at risk for obesity (see Fig. 42-1) and while there are notable familial patterns of obesity, identification of risk factors that specify odds of being diagnosed with obesity is not as clearly elucidated as those for other diseases (Centers for Disease Control and Prevention [CDC], 2020), such as coronary artery disease (see Chapter 23) and cerebrovascular disease (see Chapter 62).

What is abundantly clear, however, is that obesity incurs a greater overall risk of mortality. Obesity alone does not decrease a person's lifespan (Kuk, Rotondi, Sui, et al., 2018). However, obesity is associated with a 2- to 6-year decrease in overall life expectancy when coupled with metabolic disease or another chronic illness (Khan, Ning, & Wilkins, 2018).

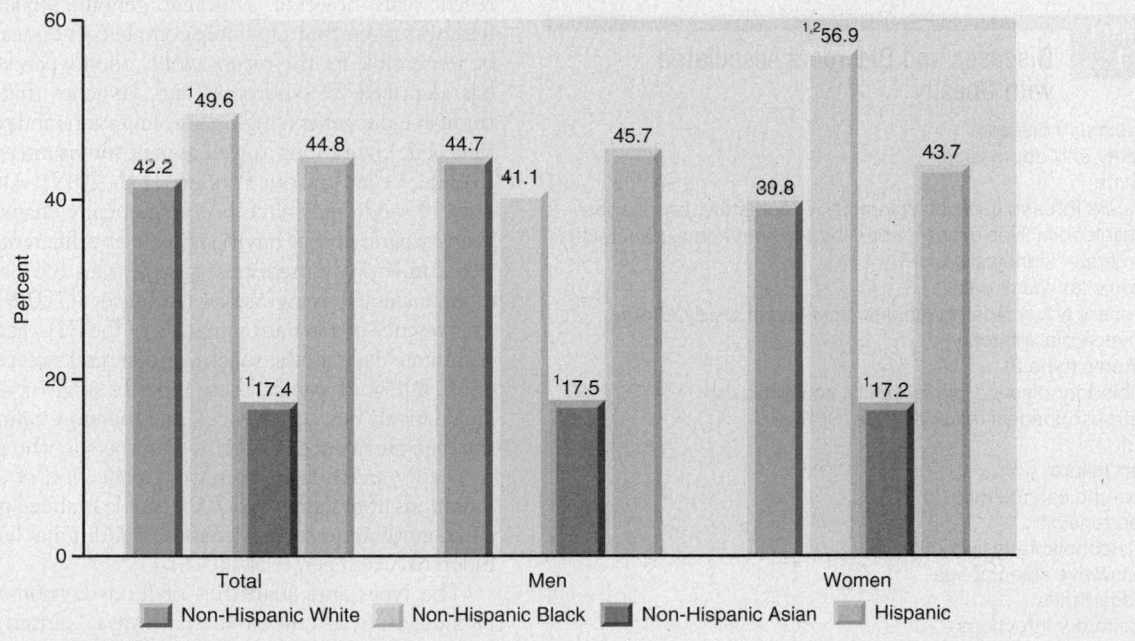

[1]Significantly different from all other race and Hispanic-origin groups.
[2]Significantly different from men for same race and Hispanic-origin group.
NOTES: Estimates were age adjusted by the direct method to the 2000 U.S. Census population using the age groups 20–39, 40–59, and 60 and over. Access data table for this figure at: https://www.cdc.gov/nchs/data/databriefs/db360_tables-508.pdf#2.
SOURCE: NCHS, National Health and Nutrition Examination Survey, 2017–2018.

Figure 42-1 • Prevalence of obesity among adults aged 20 and older, by gender and race/ethnicity in the United States (2017–2018). Reprinted from Hales, C. M., Carroll, M. D., Fryar, C. D., et al. (2020). Prevalence of obesity among adults and youth: United States, 2017–2018. Figure 2, page 2, National Center for Health Statistics. NCHS Data Brief, no. 360. Hyattsville, MD. Retrieved on 11/16/2020 at: www.cdc.gov/nchs/data/databriefs/db360-h.pdf

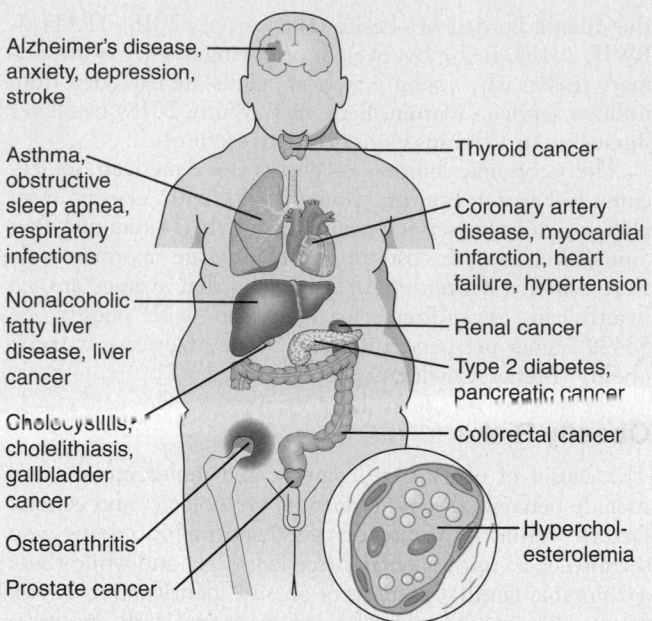

Alzheimer's disease, anxiety, depression, stroke

Asthma, obstructive sleep apnea, respiratory infections

Nonalcoholic fatty liver disease, liver cancer

Cholecystitis, cholelithiasis, gallbladder cancer

Osteoarthritis

Prostate cancer

Thyroid cancer

Coronary artery disease, myocardial infarction, heart failure, hypertension

Renal cancer

Type 2 diabetes, pancreatic cancer

Colorectal cancer

Hypercholesterolemia

Figure 42-2 • Morbid diseases and disorders associated with obesity.

Furthermore, obesity is associated with morbidity and mortality from numerous other diseases (see Fig. 42-2 and Chart 42-1). For instance, as body mass index (BMI) increases, so does the overall risk of cancer and risk for death from cancer; obesity is responsible for up to 90,000 deaths from cancer annually. Having obesity increases the likelihood of having type 2 diabetes by 10-fold and the likelihood of having either

asthma or hypertension by nearly fourfold (American Society for Metabolic and Bariatric Surgery [ASMBS], 2019b). Adults with obesity are twice as likely to eventually be diagnosed with Alzheimer's disease than those adults who maintain a normal weight (Biener et al., 2017).

Pathophysiology

Obesity is a chronic, relapsing disease characterized by an excessive accumulation of body fat and weight gain (ASMBS, 2019a). These increases in body fat cause **adiposopathy**, a dysfunction of adipose tissue, which promotes the development of metabolic, biomechanical, and psychosocial diseases and disorders (Fruh, 2017; Wu & Berry, 2010). Dysfunctional adipose tissue cells release biochemical mediators that cause chronic inflammatory changes, which can lead to a multitude of diseases, including heart disease, hypertension, and type 2 diabetes (ASMBS, 2018a).

At the most fundamental level, obesity results from a metabolic imbalance, characterized by an excess of caloric consumption relative to caloric expenditures. That is, too many foods are consumed and too little physical activity is conducted over the long term, resulting in weight gain (Norris, 2019). According to the "thrifty gene" hypothesis, the human **genome** (i.e., the total complement of genes in humans) was sequenced during times when finding and storing food sources expended more energy than during contemporary times. Hunting for scarce food sources during prehistoric times consumed a lot of energy, and food sources were not abundant. Storing fat to provide energy sources during times of food scarcity was a physiologic adaptive response to these environmental challenges (van Meijel, Blaak, & Goossens, 2018).

The "thrifty gene" hypothesis has come under scrutiny in recent years, however, as human genome sequencing research findings suggest that a far more complex genetic explanation may be responsible for the recent global obesity pandemic. Research has identified 79 syndromes and 31 genes that cause obesity through monogenic (single gene) mutations and polygenic (multiple gene) mutations as well as gene–environment interactions (Rohde, Keller, la Cour Poulsen, et al., 2019). Although to date only 19 syndromes have been genetically characterized, it has been recognized that having at least one different genetic mutation can strongly predispose people who have ready access to food sources to having obesity (Rohde et al., 2019). For instance, the presence of a variant mutation of the *FTO* gene is associated with more daily meals, snacks, and fat and sweet intake (Rohde et al., 2019). However, these types of single genetic mutations are relatively rare occurrences, and therefore cannot account for the high prevalence of obesity. Most people who are predisposed to obesity are thought to have a collection of several genetic mutations from more than 700 possible mutated genes that each can contribute to several pounds of additional body fat (Yengo, Sidorenko, Kemper, et al., 2018).

The types and quantities of foods consumed affect complex digestive and metabolic pathways. Certain processed and high caloric foods that contain fructose corn syrup, simple sugars, or trans fats, are hypothesized to be **obesogenic** (i.e., promote weight gain) because they are associated with food cravings consonant with other type of addictive cravings (Campana, Brasiel, de Aguiar, et al., 2019). Additionally, the portions of both entrees and desserts served in fast food restaurants have increased over the past 30 years, subtly affecting

---

Chart 42-1 Diseases and Disorders Associated with Obesity

Alzheimer's disease
Anxiety and depression
Asthma
Cancers (breast, cervical, colorectal, endometrial, esophageal, gallbladder, liver, ovarian, non-Hodgkin lymphoma, pancreatic, prostate, kidney, thyroid)
Chronic low back pain
Coronary artery disease (angina, acute coronary syndrome, myocardial infarction)
Diabetes (type 2)
Gallbladder disease (cholecystitis, cholelithiasis)
Gastroesophageal reflux disease (GERD)
Gout
Heart failure
Hypercholesterolemia
Hypertension
Nonalcoholic fatty liver disease
Obstructive sleep apnea
Osteoarthritis
Respiratory infections
Stroke

Adapted from American Society for Metabolic and Bariatric Surgery (ASMBS). (2019b). The impact of obesity on your body and health. Retrieved on 5/1/2020 at: www.asmbs.org/patients/impact-of-obesity; Centers for Disease Control and Prevention (CDC). (2020). Adult obesity causes & consequences. Retrieved on 5/1/2020 at: www.cdc.gov/obesity/adult/causes.html

consumers' feelings of **satiety** (i.e., feeling of having eaten sufficient amounts of food) (McCrory, Harbaugh, Appeadu, et al., 2019). Furthermore, there is a greater variety of entrees and desserts that may be selected on the menus of most fast food restaurants, providing the illusion of healthier meal options although there are actually less healthy food alternatives available for selection than 30 years ago (McCrory et al., 2019).

Multiple hormones that control food cravings and feelings of fullness could be affected by individual genes. In response to periods of fasting, the hormone ghrelin is secreted by the stomach and the hormone neuropeptide Y (NPY) is secreted by the small intestines. These hormones are **orexigenic**, meaning that they stimulate appetite through central nervous system (CNS) pathways that lead to the hypothalamus, signaling higher neural pathways that lead to eating behaviors. Once eating occurs, multiple hormones are released throughout the gastrointestinal (GI) tract that promote satiety, including somatostatin, cholecystokinin (CCK), and insulin, to name a few. CCK also slows gastric motility and emptying, stimulates gallbladder contraction and release of bile into the duodenum, and stimulates the release of pancreatic digestive enzymes, all of which serve to enhance the digestive process. Somatostatin also slows gastric emptying but has other effects that are in opposition to CCK, such as decreasing the secretion of bile, depending on foods consumed and metabolic needs (Gimeno, Briere, & Seeley, 2020).

Increases in fat stores, or adipose tissue, result in increases in the hormone leptin, which is secreted by fat cells. Leptin also has the effect of signaling satiety in the hypothalamus. Patients with obesity who lose weight are thought to also have drops in leptin levels that persist for the long term, creating persistent feelings of hunger, which may partially explain why many patients with obesity who lose weight tend to regain it (Campana et al., 2019).

By adulthood, the GI tract **microbiota**, which is the complement of microbes within the gut, has been found to contain up to 100 trillion microbes, or 10 times the cells present in the human body (McElroy, Chung, & Regan, 2017). The collective genome of the microbiota, or the gut **microbiome**, has more than 100 times more genes than in the human genome. It has long been known that gut microbes perform numerous digestive, metabolic, and immunologic functions. The composition and diversity of these microbes may very well be tied in with obesity (McElroy et al., 2017). For instance, patients with obesity tend to have less diverse microbiota than patients who are of normal weight. In turn, patients with obesity who have less diverse microbiota typically also have dyslipidemia, impaired glucose metabolism, and low-grade generalized inflammatory disorders. "Western-style diets," which are high in processed foods, fat, and sugars and low in fiber, are thought to not only negatively affect the diversity of the gut microbiota, but also to negatively affect the complement of *Bacteroidetes* species microbes, which are associated with a leaner type of microbiome (McElroy et al., 2017). Whether or not it is possible to regulate the composition of the gut microbiota and prevent or treat obesity is the focus of ongoing research.

Assessment of Obesity

Assessment of the patient with obesity includes a health history and physical examination that evaluates the effects of obesity on the health of the patient.

Health History

Nurses need to approach patients with obesity with the same respectful, courteous, and empathetic behavior that they extend to patients without obesity. Confronting their own attitudes and beliefs about patients with obesity may help to mitigate biases. For instance, using patient-first language for all patients with diagnosed diseases, including the disease of obesity, can be an effective way to dispel bias. By referencing *the patient with obesity*, the nurse is effectively noting that the patient, not the disease, is the central point of concern and that the disease is amenable to treatment. On the other hand, referencing *the obese patient* tends to define the person by having obesity, which can lead to subliminal impressions that the patient is somehow responsible for having obesity. Research studies report that many health care providers, including nurses, hold negative attitudes toward patients with obesity and believe that they are indulgent, lazy, and lack willpower (Robstad, Westergren, Siebler, et al., 2019; Smigelski-Theiss, Gampong, & Kurasaki, 2017).

Patients with obesity should be assessed to see if there have been any recent increases or decreases in body weight. If the patient has recently lost or gained weight, determining if that is intentional weight loss or gain may give clues to whether or not changes in weight might be secondary to another disease process. Other useful health history information to gather includes how long the patient has had obesity (e.g., since childhood, since a pregnancy) and whether or not there is a family history of obesity. Any patterns of weight loss over time, and prior successful or unsuccessful weight loss strategies should be analyzed. A history of exercise patterns and dietary patterns (see Chapter 4 for discussion of nutritional assessment) is also assessed. Some patients with obesity report sleep pattern disturbances (e.g., difficulty falling asleep, difficulty staying asleep); therefore, typical sleeping habits are evaluated. Some patients who quit smoking report significant weight gain after smoking cessation is achieved; consequently, the patient's smoking status is also determined (Perreault, 2020).

Some patients with obesity may develop secondary diseases or disorders (see Chart 42-1) and may be prescribed medications aimed at treating those secondary diseases or disorders that can exacerbate weight gain (see Chart 42-2). Other patients may not have had a previous history of obesity, but may gain weight after being prescribed specific medications associated with weight gain. A history of weight gain that parallels the time frame of commencing treatment with specific prescriptive medications may suggest that the medication has a key role in promoting weight gain. In some instances, prescription medication dosages may be adjusted or another medication may be prescribed. For instance, patients with type 2 diabetes and obesity may reap the dual benefits of achieving better glycemic control and weight loss by taking the prescription drug metformin (Apovian, Aronne, Bessesen, et al., 2015).

Physical Assessment

Patient's height and weight are measured to determine the **body mass index (BMI)**. The BMI is the definitive measure used to determine whether or not a patient has obesity; this is based on a ratio of body weight in kilograms and height in meters (see Chapter 4, Table 4-1). Patients identified as overweight or pre-obese have a BMI of 25 to 29.9 kg/m² and those with obesity have a BMI that exceeds 30 kg/m². Those with a BMI exceeding 40 kg/m² are considered to have severe

Chart 42-2 **PHARMACOLOGY**
Select Medications That Affect Body Weight

Many medications prescribed to treat a variety of chronic diseases and disorders have the untoward side effect of weight gain, whereas others are associated with weight loss. The following list contains some examples of each of these.

Medications Associated with Weight Gain

Anticonvulsant Medications:
- Carbamazepine
- Gabapentin
- Pregabalin
- Valproate
- Vigabatrin

Antidepressant Medications:
- Selective Serotonin Reuptake Inhibitors (SSRIs) (Note—these tend to be associated with early weight loss followed by gain within 6 months in some patients):
  - Citalopram
  - Escitalopram
  - Fluvoxamine
  - Paroxetine
  - Sertraline
- Tricyclic Antidepressants:
  - Amitriptyline
  - Clomipramine
  - Doxepin
  - Imipramine
  - Mirtazapine
  - Nortriptyline
  - Protriptyline
  - Trimipramine

Antihistamines:
- Azelastine
- Cetirizine
- Cyproheptadine
- Diphenhydramine
- Fexofenadine

Antihypertensive Medications:
- Alpha-Blocker:
  - Terazosin
- Beta-Blockers:
  - Atenolol
  - Metoprolol
  - Propranolol
- Dihydropyridine Calcium Channel Blockers:
  - Amlodipine
  - Felodipine
  - Nifedipine

Antipsychotic Medications:
- Asenapine
- Chlorpromazine
- Clozapine
- Haloperidol
- Iloperidone
- Olanzapine
- Paliperidone
- Quetiapine
- Risperidone

Diabetes Medications:
- Insulins:
  - Insulin aspart
  - Insulin glulisine
  - Insulin lispro
- Meglitinides:
  - Nateglinide
  - Repaglinide
- Sulfonylureas:
  - Chlorpropamide
  - Glimepiride
  - Glipizide
  - Glyburide
  - Tolbutamide
- Thiazolidinedione:
  - Pioglitazone

Hormones:
- Corticosteroids:
  - Prednisone
  - Budesonide
  - Methylprednisolone
- Hormonal Contraceptive:
  - Medroxyprogesterone

Mood Stabilizers:
- Lithium

Medications Associated with Weight Loss

Anticonvulsant Medications:
- Lamotrigine
- Topiramate
- Zonisamide

Antidepressant Medication:
- Bupropion
- Desvenlafaxine
- Venlafaxine

Diabetes Medication:
- Dulaglutide
- Exenatide
- Liraglutide
- Lixisenatide
- Metformin
- Semaglutide

Adapted from Comerford, K. C., & Durkin, M. T. (2020). *Nursing 2020 drug handbook*. Philadelphia, PA: Wolters Kluwer; VA/DoD Clinical Practice Guideline. (2020). Medications and their affects on weight. Retrieved on 3/7/2021 at: www.healthquality.va.gov/guidelines/CD/obesity/MedsEffectsWeightProviderToolFINAL50817Dec2020.pdf; Welcome, A. (2017). Medications that may increase weight. Retrieved on 5/1/2020 at: www.obesitymedicine.org/medications-that-cause-weight-gain

or extreme obesity (Nguyen, Brethauer, Morton, et al., 2020; WHO, 2017) (see Fig. 42-3 and Table 42-1).

Patients with obesity may also have their waist circumferences assessed. Women with waist circumferences more than 35 inches and men with waist circumferences more than 40 inches have greater risks for obesity-related morbidity (see Chart 42-1) than those with smaller waistlines (Meigs, 2019). The hip may also be measured and the waist-to-hip ratio assessed. Women with waist-to-hip ratios greater than 0.80 and men with waist-to-hip ratios greater than 0.90 are presumed to have proportionally more visceral (i.e., abdominal) fat stores. This morphologic appearance is called android obesity, and is sometimes referenced as an "apple-shaped" appearance. Patients with android obesity have greater risk for developing hypertension, coronary artery disease, stroke, and type 2 diabetes, than patients who have gynoid obesity, also called the "pear-shaped" body (Weber & Kelley, 2018) (see Fig. 42-4).

Body Mass Index Table

	Normal						Overweight					Obese										Extreme Obesity														
BMI	19	20	21	22	23	24	25	26	27	28	29	30	31	32	33	34	35	36	37	38	39	40	41	42	43	44	45	46	47	48	49	50	51	52	53	54
Height (inches)													Body Weight (pounds)																							
58	91	96	100	105	110	115	119	124	129	134	138	143	148	153	158	162	167	172	177	181	186	191	196	201	205	210	215	220	224	229	234	239	244	248	253	258
59	94	99	104	109	114	119	124	128	133	138	143	148	153	158	163	168	173	178	183	188	193	198	203	208	212	217	222	227	232	237	242	247	252	257	262	267
60	97	102	107	112	118	123	128	133	138	143	148	153	158	163	168	174	179	184	189	194	199	204	209	215	220	225	230	235	240	245	250	255	261	266	271	276
61	100	106	111	116	122	127	132	137	143	148	153	158	164	169	174	180	185	190	195	201	206	211	217	222	227	232	238	243	248	254	259	264	269	275	280	285
62	104	109	115	120	126	131	136	142	147	153	158	164	169	175	180	186	191	196	202	207	213	218	224	229	235	240	246	251	256	262	267	273	278	284	289	295
63	107	113	118	124	130	135	141	146	152	158	163	169	175	180	186	191	197	203	208	214	220	225	231	237	242	248	254	259	265	270	278	282	287	293	299	304
64	110	116	122	128	134	140	145	151	157	163	169	174	180	186	192	197	204	209	215	221	227	232	238	244	250	256	262	267	273	279	285	291	296	302	308	314
65	114	120	126	132	138	144	150	156	162	168	174	180	186	192	198	204	210	216	222	228	234	240	246	252	258	264	270	276	282	288	294	300	306	312	318	324
66	118	124	130	136	142	148	155	161	167	173	179	186	192	198	204	210	216	223	229	235	241	247	253	260	266	272	278	284	291	297	303	309	315	322	328	334
67	121	127	134	140	146	153	159	166	172	178	185	191	198	204	211	217	223	230	236	242	249	255	261	268	274	280	287	293	299	306	312	319	325	331	338	344
68	125	131	138	144	151	158	164	171	177	184	190	197	203	210	216	223	230	236	243	249	256	262	269	276	282	289	295	302	308	315	322	328	335	341	348	354
69	128	135	142	149	155	162	169	176	182	189	196	203	209	216	223	230	236	243	250	257	263	270	277	284	291	297	304	311	318	324	331	338	345	351	358	365
70	132	139	146	153	160	167	174	181	188	195	202	209	216	222	229	236	243	250	257	264	271	278	285	292	299	306	313	320	327	334	341	348	355	362	369	376
71	136	143	150	157	165	172	179	186	193	200	208	215	222	229	236	243	250	257	265	272	279	286	293	301	308	315	322	329	338	343	351	358	365	372	379	386
72	140	147	154	162	169	177	184	191	199	206	213	221	228	235	242	250	258	265	272	279	287	294	302	309	316	324	331	338	346	353	361	368	375	383	390	397
73	144	151	159	166	174	182	189	197	204	212	219	227	235	242	250	257	265	272	280	288	295	302	310	318	325	333	340	348	355	363	371	378	386	393	401	408
74	148	155	163	171	179	186	194	202	210	218	225	233	241	249	256	264	272	280	287	295	303	311	319	326	334	342	350	358	365	373	381	389	396	404	412	420
75	152	160	168	176	184	192	200	208	216	224	232	240	248	256	264	272	279	287	295	303	311	319	327	335	343	351	359	367	375	383	391	399	407	415	423	431
76	156	164	172	180	189	197	205	213	221	230	238	246	254	263	271	279	287	295	304	312	320	328	336	344	353	361	369	377	385	394	402	410	418	426	435	443

Adapted from *Clinical Guidelines on the Identification, Evaluation, and Treatment of Overweight and Obesity in Adults: The Evidence Report.*

Figure 42-3 • Body mass index table. Adapted from National Heart, Lung, and Blood Institute (NHLBI) of the National Institutes of Health (2020). Aim for a healthy weight: Body mass index table. Retrieved on 8/12/2020 at: www.nhlbi.nih.gov/health/educational/lose_wt/BMI/bmi_tbl.pdf

Diagnostic Evaluation

Patients with obesity may have other diagnostic laboratory studies done to screen for cardiovascular diseases, such as cholesterol and triglycerides (see Chapter 23), for type 2 diabetes, such as fasting blood glucose and glycosylated hemoglobin (hemoglobin A1c) (see Chapter 46), or for nonalcoholic fatty liver disease, such as aspartate aminotransferase (AST) and alanine aminotransferase (ALT) (Orringer, Harrison, Nichani, et al., 2020) (see Chapter 43). Obesity is the most important risk factor for obstructive sleep apnea (OSA), particularly among older men (Kline, 2020); therefore, the older male patient with obesity and sleep disturbances may undergo diagnostic sleep studies (see Chapter 18).

In some instances, obesity may be secondary to other diseases or disorders, such as hypothyroidism or Cushing's syndrome (see Chapter 45). In those particular cases, the diagnostic workup follows that prescribed for the primary disease or disorder, and, when the therapeutic regimen is implemented, the patient may lose weight and the obesity may even resolve (Orringer et al., 2020).

Medical Management

Treatment of obesity generally includes lifestyle modification, pharmacologic management, and nonsurgical or surgical interventions.

Lifestyle Modification

The first approach used to treat obesity consists of lifestyle modification aimed at weight loss and then weight maintenance. The U.S. Preventive Services Task Force (USPSTF) recommends that all adults with BMIs in excess of 30 kg/m² be advised to engage in multicomponent behavioral interventions that include (Curry, Krist, Owens, et al., 2018; LeBlanc, Patnode, Webber, et al., 2018):

- Setting weight loss goals,
- Improving lifestyle behaviors (e.g., diet habits, physical activity),
- Addressing barriers to change,

TABLE 42-1	Body Mass Index (BMI) Classification for Overweight and Obesity
Classification	**BMI Range (kg/m²)**
Overweight/pre-obese	25–29.9
Class I obesity	30–34.9
Class II obesity	35–39.9
Class III (also called "extreme" or "severe") obesity	≥40

Adapted from Centers for Disease Control and Prevention (CDC). (2017). Defining adult overweight and obesity. Retrieved on 8/3/2019 at: www.cdc.gov/obesity/adult/defining.html

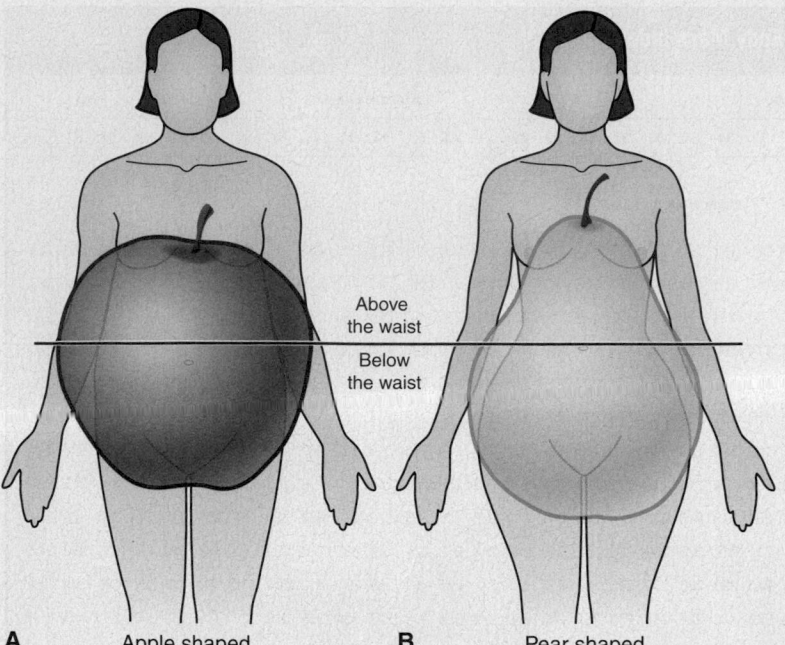

Above the waist

Below the waist

A Apple shaped   **B** Pear shaped

Figure 42-4 • **A.** Android obesity, with greater visceral/abdominal fat stores. **B.** Gynoid obesity. Reprinted with permission from Weber, J. R., & Kelley, J. H. (2018). *Health assessment in nursing* (6th ed.). Philadelphia, PA: Wolters Kluwer.

- Considering use of adjunctive pharmacotherapy agents, and
- Self-monitoring and strategizing ongoing lifestyle changes aimed at a healthy weight.

The most effective behavioral interventions are those considered high intensity; consisting of 12 to 24 sessions annually, which may include individual counseling sessions between the primary provider and patient, group nutrition education sessions, and physical activity sessions, to name a few (LeBlanc et al., 2018; Wadden, Tsai, & Tronieri, 2019). These interventions are called intensive behavioral therapy. The USPSTF notes that modest weight loss of 5% total body weight can be associated with significant clinical improvements and benefits to patients with obesity (LeBlanc et al., 2018).

A patient with obesity should be counseled to plan a caloric deficit of between 500 and 1000 calories daily from baseline, in order to achieve a 5% to 10% reduction in weight within about 6 months. This can be achieved through increasing physical activity and decreasing caloric dietary intake (Orringer et al., 2020).

Increasing physical activity through promotion of an exercise regimen is a key recommendation that can burn calories and result in weight loss. Physical activity recommendations for all adults (those with and without obesity) include at least 150 minutes of moderate-intensity aerobic exercise weekly or 75 minutes of vigorous-intensity aerobic exercise weekly. In addition, muscle-strengthening exercises that engage all major muscle groups should be done at least twice weekly (Orringer et al., 2020). Patients with obesity who were previously sedentary and deconditioned may not be able to achieve this at the start; however, encouragement to move more and sit less along with 10 to 20 minutes of daily physical activity can result in weight loss and improved exercise tolerance (Campbell & Rutherford, 2018; DiPietro & Stachenfeld, 2017; Orringer et al., 2020).

Patients with obesity should be counseled that reducing dietary caloric intake is a necessary component of weight loss

therapy. This must also include a change in dietary habits in order for weight loss to be sustained over the long term. It is important to identify current dietary patterns and typical daily caloric intake in order to recommend an appropriate diet plan. Assessing food records or 24-hour recalls or conducting dietary interviews are all effective methods to gather baseline dietary information from patients (see Chapter 4: Dietary Data). There are a plethora of commercial diets that patients may select (see Chart 42-3). Regardless of the diet plan chosen, successful weight loss occurs when patients consistently make healthier dietary choices (Thorn & Lean, 2017). To date, there have not been sufficiently rigorous longitudinal studies to determine which diet plans are superior to others in terms of achieving long-term weight loss, however (Yeh, Glick-Bauer, & Katz, 2017).

Patients need not purchase commercial diet plans in order to achieve weight loss and embrace healthy diet habits. Most nutritionists advocate that healthy diets include few processed foods, sugars, and trans fats, and are heavy in plant-based foods (Yeh et al., 2017). The Dietary Approaches to Stop Hypertension (DASH) diet is an example of a superior healthy noncommercial diet. Although initially promoted to manage hypertension, the DASH diet also provides a solid

---

Chart 42-3 **Select Popular Commercial Diets**

Atkins Diet, www.atkins.com
Jenny Craig, www.jennycraig.com
Ketogenic "keto" diet, www.dietdoctor.com/low-carb/keto
Medifast, www.medifast1.com/index.jsp
Nutrisystem, www.nutrisystem.com/jsps_hmr/home/index.jsp
Optifast, www.optifast.com
Ornish Diet, www.ornish.com/proven-program/nutrition
South Beach Diet, www.southbeachdiet.com/home/index.jsp
WW: Weight Watchers, www.weightwatchers.com/us
Zone Diet, www.zonediet.com

Chart 42-4 PATIENT EDUCATION
Healthy Eating Strategies

The nurse instructs the patient about the healthy eating strategies outlined below.

Limit or eliminate the following:
- Processed foods with limited nutritional value (e.g., packaged cakes, cookies, chips)
- High caloric beverages (sugar-sweetened, juices, cream-enhanced)
- Fast foods
- Vending machine foods
- Foods high in sugars (e.g., candies) and saturated fats (e.g., fried foods, hot dogs)

Track the following:
- Daily food intake (food journals, diaries, smartphone, and tablet applications)
- Nutritional value and caloric content on food labels

Encourage the following:
- Reduce portions; use smaller plates and measure foods
- Schedule and plan meals and snacks in advance for each day; prepack lunches and snacks when you are out of the home (e.g., for work)
- Eat at home more often than you would eat outside the home; when eating out or ordering take-out food, avoid fried foods and choose lean meats and vegetables and salads with condiments on the side
- Eat with your family members so that together you create a healthy eating environment
- Avoid screen time when eating
- Limit exposure to food and beverage marketing
- Eat breakfast
- Limit snacks
- Eat a variety of nutritious foods; monitoring quality of foods consumed is as important as the quantity of foods consumed
- Drink plenty of water
- Stay within your daily caloric intake plan; do not become discouraged if one day you do not adhere to your plan

Adapted from Orringer, K. A., Harrison, A. V., Nichani, S. S., et al. (2020). University of Michigan Health System Clinical Alignment and Performance Excellence Guideline: Obesity prevention and management. Retrieved on 5/1/2020 at: www.mcd.umich.edu/1info/FHP/practiceguides/obesity/obesity.pdf

foundation for achieving and maintaining weight loss due to its focus on low intake of fat and carbohydrates (Goldstein, Mayer, Graybill, et al., 2020; Thorn & Lean, 2017) (see Chapter 27, Table 27-3: The DASH Diet). Another healthy diet plan that may form a basis for weight loss, though not specifically designed for this purpose, is the Mediterranean Diet (see Chapter 23). Patient education tips for managing ongoing healthy eating strategies are noted in Chart 42-4.

In addition to promoting healthy exercise and diet habits, ensuring healthy sleep habits is an additional lifestyle strategy that is associated with weight loss and maintenance of a healthy weight. It is posited that sleep deprivation can cause changes in cortisol levels that promote weight gain (Orringer et al., 2020). Advising patients with sleep disturbances to plan to be in bed with lights out at least 7 hours prior to wake-up time, to create a dark, relaxing bedroom environment, to avoid activities that can cause arousal around bedtime (e.g., text messaging), and to avoid beverages with caffeine after lunchtime can all be helpful strategies aimed at ensuring a

restful night's sleep that is consonant with weight reduction (Orringer et al., 2020).

Pharmacologic Therapy

Patients who are not successful at meeting weight loss goals from lifestyle modification alone may be prescribed antiobesity medications. Some patients may exhibit initial success with lifestyle modifications, but be stymied with attempts to maintain a lower BMI over the long term. These patients may also benefit from antiobesity medications. Patients who are prescribed antiobesity medications should be counseled that these prescriptions are meant to supplement, not supplant diet modification and exercise (Coulter, Rebello, & Greenway, 2018; Saunders, Umashanker, Igel, et al., 2018). Indications for antiobesity medications include a BMI greater than 30 kg/m² or a BMI greater than 27 kg/m² with concomitant morbidity that is related to being overweight (e.g., type 2 diabetes, hypertension) (Saunders et al., 2018).

Antiobesity medications work by either inhibiting GI absorption of fats, or by altering central brain receptors to enhance satiety or reduce cravings (National Institute of Diabetes and Digestive and Kidney Diseases [NIDDK], 2016b). Each of these medications has distinct side effects and contraindications; therefore, selection of these agents is individualized (see Table 42-2). The patient is monitored while taking the selected medication; if the patient does not lose at least 5% body weight after 12 weeks, the prescription may need to be changed, or the patient may be referred for other weight-reduction therapy (e.g., bariatric surgery) (NIDDK, 2016b).

Quality and Safety Nursing Alert

Antiobesity medications are believed to be teratogenic. Women with obesity who are of childbearing years should be screened carefully and advised to avoid pregnancy if they seek a prescription for an antiobesity medication.

The class of antiobesity medications known as the sympathomimetic amines are only supposed to be prescribed for short-term use (i.e., no longer than 12 weeks). They have many side effects (see Table 42-2), and patients do tend to regain weight once they are no longer taking these medications (NIDDK, 2016b).

Nonsurgical Interventions

Adult patients with obesity that does not respond to lifestyle interventions or antiobesity medications and who have either Class III/severe/extreme obesity (i.e., BMI in excess of 40 kg/m²) or Class II obesity (BMI 35 to 39.9 kg/m²) with obesity-related diseases or disorders (e.g., OSA, type 2 diabetes) may be candidates for bariatric surgical interventions (see later discussion). As an alternative, some patients may elect to pursue minimally invasive interventions, which may include vagal blocking therapy, intragastric balloon therapy, or bariatric embolization.

Vagal blocking therapy, also known as gastric stimulation, involves placement of a pacemakerlike device (vBloc™) into the subcutaneous tissue in the lateral thoracic cavity with two leads that are laparoscopically implanted at the point where the vagus nerve truncates, at the gastroesophageal junction.

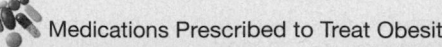

TABLE 42-2 Medications Prescribed to Treat Obesity

Medication	Adverse Effects	Nursing Considerations[a]
Gastrointestinal Lipase Inhibitor Mechanism of Action: Diminishes intestinal absorption and metabolism of fats, particularly triglycerides		
Orlistat Note: Also available in lower dosages over-the-counter	Diarrhea Flatus Oily stools Fecal incontinence	Patients may have associated problems with malabsorption of nutrients; advise them to take a concomitant daily multivitamin. Caution in patients with known history of renal insufficiency, liver disease, or gallbladder disease as concomitant use is associated with renal calculi, liver failure, and cholelithiasis. Do not administer with cyclosporine.
Selective Serotonin Receptor Agonist Mechanism of Action: Stimulates serotonin 5-HT2C receptors, causing excretion of the alpha-melanocortin–stimulating hormone (alpha-MSH) and elicits appetite suppression		
Lorcaserin	Fatigue Dizziness Nausea Headaches Cough Dry mouth Constipation	Encourage patient to stay well hydrated. Can be associated with deficits in attention or memory; administer with caution in patients who drive or work with hazardous equipment when first prescribed until effects are realized. Can cause hypoglycemia in patients with diabetes. Contraindicated for patients taking antidepressants or migraine medications due to synergistic effects. Discontinue in patients who express suicidal ideation. Rarely, serotonin syndrome may develop—be alert for high fevers, brisk reflexes, agitation, and diarrhea; notify primary provider immediately and hold medication if these occur.
GLP-1 Receptor Agonists Mechanism of Action: Mimics the effects of incretins, resulting in delayed gastric emptying, thus curbing appetite		
Liraglutide Note: Also available in lower dosages to treat type 2 diabetes	Nausea Diarrhea or constipation Headache Tachycardia	Must be given subcutaneously on a daily basis in the abdomen, thigh, or upper arm. Dosage increases weekly until week 5. Discontinue in patients who express suicide ideation. May be associated with pancreatitis; also associated with thyroid tumors in animal models.
Sympathomimetic Amines Mechanism of Action: Stimulate central noradrenergic receptors, causing appetite suppression		
Phentermine Benzphetamine Diethylpropion Phendimetrazine	Palpitations and tachycardia Tremors Hypertension Dizziness Insomnia Diarrhea or constipation Mouth dryness Restlessness Alterations in taste	These are only FDA approved for short-term use (i.e., no more than 12 weeks). Contraindications include heart disease, uncontrolled hypertension, hyperthyroidism, and glaucoma. Caution patients to not drink alcohol while taking one of these medications.
Dual Agents Mechanism of Action: Each of these medications combines two medications with known antiobesity effects; when taken together, the effects are synergistic		
Phentermine/topiramate-ER Mechanism of Action: combines the effectiveness of phentermine (see above) and topiramate, an anticonvulsant, which stimulates central GABA receptors and inhibits central glutamate receptors, suppressing appetite	Paresthesias Dizziness Insomnia Mouth dryness Alterations in taste Insomnia Constipation Tachycardia	Same contraindications apply as for phentermine (see above). May need to monitor electrolytes, as hypokalemia and metabolic acidosis are possible. Monitor creatinine and watch for manifestations of renal calculi.
Naltrexone/bupropion Mechanism of action: inhibits central opioid receptors and inhibits reuptake of dopamine and norepinephrine selectively, resulting in diminished appetite and cravings	Constipation or diarrhea Nausea Vomiting Insomnia Dizziness Mouth dryness Hypertension Tachycardia	Contraindications include uncontrolled hypertension, epilepsy, history of eating disorder such as anorexia nervosa or bulimia, and history of alcohol abuse or history of substance use disorder. Discontinue in patients who express suicidal ideation.

[a]All antiobesity medications may be teratogenic; pregnancy is a contraindication to all of these agents.
FDA, U.S. Food and Drug Administration.
Adapted from Coulter, A. A., Rebello, C. J., & Greenway, F. L. (2018). Centrally acting agents for obesity: Past, Present, and Future. *Drugs, 78*(11), 1113–1132; Munoz-Mantilla, D. (2018). Top weight loss medications. Retrieved on 12/15/2019 at: www.obesitymedicine.org/weight-loss-medications; National Institute of Diabetes and Digestive and Kidney Diseases (NIDDK). (2016b). Prescription medications to treat overweight and obesity. Retrieved on 2/18/2020 at: www.niddk.nih.gov/health-information/weight-management/prescription-medications-treat-overweight-obesity

A pre-programmed, pulsating signal is delivered for 12 hours daily. This signal causes intermittent "blocking" of the vagus nerve. Vagal blocking results in diminished gastric contraction and emptying, limited ghrelin secretion, and diminished pancreatic enzyme secretion; these cause increased satiety, decreased cravings, and diminished absorption of calories, all of which lead to weight loss (Papasavas, El Chaar, Kothari, et al., 2016). Results from a randomized controlled trial found greater initial and 2-year sustained weight loss with participants with obesity who received vagal blocking versus control sham device implantation (Vairavamurthy, Cheskin, Kraitchman, et al., 2017). There are few adverse effects noted with use of this device, which include GI symptoms (e.g., heartburn, belching). Patients must be educated to recharge the device twice weekly for about an hour with an external coil device.

Intragastric balloon therapy involves endoscopic placement of a gas-filled balloon (ORBERA™) or a saline-filled dual balloon (ReShape™) into the stomach. The mechanism by which these devices result in weight loss is poorly understood, but thought to be related to increased feelings of satiety and decreased gastric emptying (Kurian, Kroh, Chand, et al., 2018). Post insertion, the intragastric balloon(s) remain in place for 3 to 6 months, and are then deflated and removed. Studies suggest greater weight loss with these than with sham therapy or with lifestyle interventions alone (Ali, Moustarah, Kim, et al., 2015; Kurian et al., 2018). Early adverse effects include complaints of nausea and vomiting, which are generally transient and do not require balloon removal. Pancreatitis and gastric or esophageal perforation may also occur although these are rare adverse events (Moore & Rosenthal, 2018). Balloon rupture can occur over the long term, however, which may lead to intestinal obstruction. In order to monitor for this serious complication, it is recommended that the balloon be impregnated with methylene blue pre-insertion so that patients with silent ruptures can report the presence of green urine to their primary providers and receive timely interventions to remove the deflated balloons before they cause obstruction. Patients who seem unlikely to return for follow-up appointments should not be candidates for intragastric balloons. Balloons should be removed within 6 months of placement; longer placement periods are associated with increased likelihood of rupture and intestinal obstruction (Ali et al., 2015).

Endovascular bariatric embolization is in the process of undergoing clinical trials to validate its safety and effectiveness. During this procedure, the gastric fundus is embolized with microspheres (beads) via the left gastric artery. The gastric fundus secretes approximately 90% of the orexigenic hormone ghrelin that is secreted in the body; therefore, it is posited that embolizing the fundus should effectively result in diminished secretion of ghrelin (Hafezi-Nejad, Bailey, Gunn, et al., 2019; Kurian et al., 2018). Preliminary results from clinical trials report an estimated weight loss ranging from 8% to 18% that is sustained for at least 1 year, without reported adverse events (Vairavamurthy et al., 2017).

 Gerontologic Considerations

According to findings from the 2017–2018 United States National Health and Nutrition Examination Survey (NHANES), the prevalence of obesity for adults 60 years of age and older is 42.8%, slightly higher than the prevalence of obesity among all adults (Hales et al., 2020). Climbing rates of obesity among older adults mirrors the rate increases among all adults over the past few decades.

As adults age, lean skeletal mass decreases and adipose tissue increases. Adipose tissue does not burn calories as efficiently as lean skeletal mass; furthermore, basal metabolism drops by 2% for each additional decade of adult life. Therefore, older adults are more likely to gain weight unless they either increase activity levels or decrease their caloric intake (Eliopoulos, 2018).

Research suggests that older adults with obesity are at risk for complications that may negatively affect their quality of life. In particular, older adults with obesity may be at greater risk of falls and mobility impairments (Batsis & Zagaria, 2018; Messier, Resnik, Beavers, et al., 2018). Another study found that older adults with higher BMIs had more evidence of cognitive dysfunction compared to their normal weight counterparts (Rambod, Ghodsbin, & Moradi, 2020). More older adults with obesity are admitted to nursing homes than normal weight older adults (Zhou, Kozikowski, Pekmezaris, et al., 2017).

There is some evidence that older adults with an overweight body mass (i.e., between 25 and 29.9 kg/m^2) have reasonably good health outcomes; therefore, older adults who are overweight are not necessarily counseled to lose weight (Orringer et al., 2020). However, older adults with obesity (i.e., with BMIs in excess of 30 kg/m^2) should be encouraged to engage in lifestyle modifications, including diet and exercise, similar to younger adults (Orringer et al., 2020). Along with decreasing dietary caloric intake, older adult patients should be counseled that the quality of calories consumed should be the focus of the daily diet (see Chapter 8, Fig. 8-2). Fats should be limited to less than 30% of total calories, while proteins should comprise 10% to 20% of the daily diet. Intake of soluble fibers (e.g., oats, pectin) is particularly important since these can lower cholesterol levels and prevent cardiovascular diseases and cancers. Fewer than one third of older adults consume the recommended five servings of fruits and vegetables daily (Eliopoulos, 2018). Identifying barriers to consumption of these important sources of nutrients may help the older adult patient with obesity lose weight and adopt healthier eating habits. For instance, the older adult who has difficulty chewing raw fruits may enjoy fruit smoothies.

Whether or not older adult patients with obesity should be candidates for bariatric surgery (see later discussion) has been a point of ongoing debate. Research findings confirm that many older adults with obesity benefit from bariatric surgery, having outcomes and complications at rates comparable to their younger adult counterparts (Chouillard, Alsabah, Chahine, et al., 2018; Giordano & Victorzon, 2015). At present, there are no guidelines that identify the profile of which older adult patients with obesity can most benefit from bariatric surgery.

 Veterans Considerations

Recruits into any branch of the U.S. military must meet prescribed height and weight requirements. Although these requirements vary slightly between branches of service, their general aim is to restrict recruitment to only applicants of normal weight. Despite having to meet height and weight standards during the recruitment process and then demonstrate the ability to meet standards of physical fitness on at least an annual basis, the rates of service members who have obesity or are overweight has reportedly tripled in the past 20 years (McCarthy, Elshaw, Szekeley, et al., 2017). The U.S. Department of Defense (DoD, 2019) reported that the overall prevalence of obesity (i.e., BMI greater than or equal to 30 kg/m^2) among men and women of all ages who serve in the Army, Navy, Marine Corps, and Air Force was 17.4% in 2019, reflecting a steady annual increase since 2014. Obesity in service members can hamper their ability to functionally meet their job requirements; as such, obesity in large sectors of the military population may adversely affect overall military readiness (McCarthy et al., 2017; Shiozawa, Madsen, Banaag, et al., 2019). Furthermore, service members with obesity utilize more health service resources than those who are of normal weight and risk nonvoluntary separation from military service because they cannot meet physical fitness requirements (Shiozawa et al., 2019).

The prevalence of obesity and overweight among the nearly 21 million military veterans in the United States is estimated to be higher than that in the general civilian population, suggesting that weight gain is widespread after separation or retirement from military service (Tarlov, Zenk, Matthews, et al., 2017). Tarlov and colleagues (2017) found that 89% of all veterans (approximately 19 million veterans) lived in areas of the country where access to supermarkets, grocery stores, fitness facilities, and parks was limited, which could partially explain weight gain in veterans. Other researchers have noted that cessation of having to meet physical fitness standards, changes in daily routines, and stresses incurred during military service can also partially explain why veterans may be at greater risk of obesity (Bookwalter, Porter, Jacobson, et al., 2019). Bookwalter and colleagues (2019) prospectively studied over 28,000 veterans who separated or retired from military service and found that approximately 36% of normal weight veterans became overweight and 26% of overweight veterans had obesity within 6 years post separation. Factors that mitigated weight gains in these veterans included engaging in at least 150 minutes of moderate activity weekly, not engaging in more than 7 hours of sedentary lifestyle behaviors daily, eating fast foods less than once per week, sleeping between 7 and 9 hours nightly, not currently smoking, and drinking at least one but no more than 14 alcoholic beverages weekly for men and no more than seven alcoholic beverages weekly for women (Bookwalter et al., 2019). These findings are consonant with the tenets of the United States Veterans Administration (VA) MOVE program, whose aim is to improve the health status of veterans with obesity by encouraging physical activity, good dietary choices, and weight reduction strategies (McCarthy et al., 2017; Tarlov et al., 2017).

✹ COVID-19 Considerations

Several risks for both severe acute respiratory syndrome coronavirus 2 (SARS-CoV-2) infection and pathogenesis to coronavirus disease 2019 (COVID-19) have been posed (see Chapter 66). Early epidemiologic data from China did not identify obesity as a risk for becoming infected with SARS-CoV-2. However, with the spread of the pandemic to both Europe and North America, the two continents with the highest prevalence of obesity in the world, that risk became apparent (Moriconi, Masi, Rebelos, et al., 2020). In particular, obesity seems to be a significant risk factor for younger adults requiring hospitalization to manage COVID-19 (Kass, Duggal, & Cingolani, 2020). Obesity is also associated with prolonged hospitalization, admission to critical-care units, and overall poorer outcomes in patients with COVID-19 (Kalligeros, Shehadeh, Mylona, et al., 2020; Moriconi et al., 2020; Tamara & Tahapary, 2020).

Nursing Management

Patients with obesity report feeling socially marginalized, judged, and unsupported by society at large. Many times, patients with obesity report that they suffer stigmatization by their health care providers, including nurses (Eisenberg, Noria, Grover, et al., 2019). The bias that nurses may have against patients with obesity may not directly affect their nursing care; however, indirectly, the consequences of this stigmatization can lead to poor health outcomes. Patients with obesity who feel stigmatized by their health care providers report increased depression, low self-esteem, and avoidance of health care appointments and health maintenance activities (e.g., diet and exercise) (Smigelski-Theiss et al., 2017).

The patient with obesity who requires medical-surgical nursing care, whether it is because the patient is admitted to the hospital, needs home health care, or is admitted to a transitional care setting, merits special considerations. Obesity can adversely affect the mechanics of ventilation and circulation, pharmacokinetics and pharmacodynamics, skin integrity, and body mechanics and mobility. These adverse effects are more common with higher BMIs; thus, the patient with Class III obesity (BMI in excess of 40 kg/m^2) is particularly vulnerable.

Obesity can result in anatomic remodeling, including compression of the oropharynx and increased neck circumference and chest diameter. These changes can predispose the patient with obesity to OSA (see Chapter 18), respiratory failure, and obesity hypoventilation syndrome. Obesity hypoventilation syndrome is characterized by daytime hypoventilation with hypercapnea (i.e., PaCO$_2$ greater than 45 mm Hg) and hypoxemia (i.e., PaO$_2$ less than 80 mm Hg), and sleep-disordered breathing. Potential adverse effects of obesity hypoventilation syndrome can be mitigated by maintaining the patient in the low Fowler position, which maximizes diaphragmatic chest expansion. Continuous pulse oximetry monitoring may be advisable, as well as supplemental oxygen therapy (see Chapter 19) and frequent respiratory assessments (at least every shift). For the patient with a known diagnosis of OSA, ensuring that the patient utilizes prescribed therapy (e.g., oral appliance, continuous positive airway pressure [CPAP]) if newly hospitalized or in a different transitional care environment is important in order to ensure breathing effectiveness and avoid respiratory failure (Haesler, 2018; Holsworth & Gallagher, 2017; Petcu, 2017).

The patient with obesity may have central and peripheral circulatory compromise. Heart failure is more commonplace among patients with obesity (see Chapter 25). Hypertension is also more prevalent; the nurse must use appropriately sized blood pressure cuffs to obtain valid blood pressure readings (see Chapter 27). Peripheral blood flow can be compromised for the patient with obesity, resulting in stasis of blood flow, one of three components of the Virchow triad, which is the broad category of risk for venous thromboembolism (VTE) (see Chapter 26, Chart 26-8). Peripheral circulatory compromise not only can increase the risk for VTE formation (e.g., pulmonary embolism [PE] and deep vein thrombosis [DVT]), but it can also make finding venous access difficult when the patient with obesity requires intravenous (IV) therapy. Finding appropriate venous access can be exacerbated by the presence of increased adipose tissue in the extremities. Ultrasound guidance may be required in order to successfully gain IV access and place an IV cannula in the patient with obesity (Oliver, Oliver, Ohanyan, et al., 2019).

The patient with obesity may have differences in both pharmacokinetics (i.e., the movement of drug metabolites within the body) and pharmacodynamics (i.e., how drugs are metabolized and the effects of drugs) that can affect drug dosages, drug effectiveness, and patient safety. The effectiveness of many drugs is affected by the ratio of lean skeletal muscle mass to adipose tissue. The active metabolites of many drugs are protein bound in the plasma. In patients with greater adipose tissue, more of these active metabolites can be unbound in plasma, or free, and exert greater effects. Some drugs readily bind to adipose tissue, which may either inactivate them or prolong their effects. In addition, increased adiposity can have indirect effects on metabolic pathways within the liver, resulting in changes in drug metabolic pathways, which can result in either increased or decreased drug metabolism, depending on the drug and the affected metabolic pathway. In other words, some drugs have enhanced effects while others have diminished effects with patients with obesity compared to patients of normal weight. For instance, research studies have found that patients with obesity who are critically ill with sepsis require proportionally lower dosages of IV drip norepinephrine, which is typically given based on weight-based calculations, than patients with normal weight (Droege & Ernst, 2017; Radosevich, Patanwala, & Erstad, 2016). On the other hand, patients with obesity who require opioid agents to treat pain frequently require higher dosages of opioid agents to achieve pain relief, but are more likely to have serious adverse effects of sedation and respiratory depression (Meisenberg, Ness, Rao, et al., 2017). The nurse should be cognizant that weight-based calculations of drug dosages for patients with obesity may need to be altered, depending on the patient and the drug, and should consult with clinical pharmacologists and the patient's primary provider as needed to ensure optimal drug effectiveness and patient safety.

Patients with obesity are particularly vulnerable to developing pressure injuries (see Chart 42-5). Increased adipose tissue can diminish the supply of blood, oxygen, and nutrients

---

Chart 42-5 · ETHICAL DILEMMA
When Is Prescribed Care Beneficent and When Is It Paternalistic?

Case Scenario

T.N. is a 40-year-old woman admitted to the hospital 2 days ago for treatment of nonhealing and infected stage III pressure injuries. T.N. is 64 inches tall and weighs 275 pounds; thus, her BMI is 47.2 kg/m^2, consistent with Class III/severe obesity. T.N. has had obesity since childhood and reportedly has not been willing to listen to her family practice primary provider's repeated cautions to increased physical activity and decreased caloric dietary intake. The admitting primary provider has prescribed wound débridement, intravenous antibiotics, and a diet restricted to 1000 calories daily during her hospitalization. You are a staff nurse on the unit where T.N. has been admitted and are assigned to care for her. During oncoming shift report, you hear that staff members suspect T.N. is somehow having additional food brought into her room. During your initial assessment of T.N. she says to you "This hospital food is terrible. It tastes bad and I am not getting nearly enough to eat." The charge nurse suggests that T.N.'s visitors could be screened to discourage them from bringing T.N. outside food and to assist T.N. to adhere to the therapeutic regime to help facilitate healing.

Discussion

Patients with severe obesity are at risk for pressure injuries. Therefore, it seems reasonable to assume that T.N.'s overall health status will improve with weight reduction. Furthermore, it is common practice that patients are placed on dietary restrictions while hospitalized. For instance, patients with hypertension are typically prescribed low sodium diets. There are some bioethicists and clinicians who argue that patients should consent to such restrictions, and that placing patients on dietary restriction smacks of paternalism (i.e., "father knows best"). Others would argue that dietary restrictions are part of the holistic health care plan that benefits patients who are hospitalized.

Analysis

• Describe the ethical principles that are in conflict in this case (see Chapter 1, Chart 1-7). Does T.N. have the autonomous

right to not adhere to her prescribed diet? Is it reasonable to enforce a caloric restriction on her while she is being hospitalized? Should her visitors be subjected to requests that they not bring her food, or does that breach the confidentiality of her treatment plan?

• Does placing T.N. on a calorie restricted diet during her hospitalization benefit her? If she does lose weight while she is hospitalized, might that accelerate the healing of her pressure injuries? Or might she become malnourished? Do a risk analysis. Are there more potential risks or more potential benefits entailed with this prescribed diet?

• T.N. has reportedly been resistant to changing her habits. It is not known whether or not her motivation to lose weight has ever been assessed; yet, patients with severe obesity must be motivated to make changes in order to successfully manage their disease. Assume that her motivation is assessed and that she is motivated and ready to lose weight. What are the next steps? Admonishing her that she should adhere to the prescribed diet? Or are there other resources that might be mobilized to assist her to successfully manage her disease?

References

Anderson-Shaw, L. (2018). Forced calorie restrictions in the clinical setting. *The American Journal of Bioethics*, 18(7), 83–85.

Humbyrd, C. J. (2018). Complex obesity: Multifactorial etiologies and multifaceted responses. *The American Journal of Bioethics*, 18(7), 87–89.

Maginot, T. R., & Rhee, K. (2018). Challenges of obesity treatment: The question of decisional capacity. *The American Journal of Bioethics*, 18(7), 85–87.

Spike, J. P. (2018). Obesity, pressure ulcers, and family enablers. *The American Journal of Bioethics*, 18(7), 81–82.

Resources

See Chapter 1, Chart 1-10 for Steps of an Ethical Analysis and Ethics Resources.

to peripheral tissue. The presence of more folds in the skin is associated with more skin moisture and increased skin friction, which are pressure injury risks. Moreover, skin folds may be present in uncommon areas, including under the breasts, under the lower abdomen, within gluteal folds, and at the nape of the neck (Haesler, 2018; Williamson, 2020). In addition, patients with obesity frequently have more limitations in mobility than patients of normal weight. Immobility is another risk for pressure injury development (Williamson, 2020). Consultation with a wound-ostomy-continence (WOC) nurse may be advisable to ensure that pressure injury risks for the patient with obesity are minimized.

The nurse must ensure that appropriate specialty equipment is utilized as needed so that the patient with obesity who is immobilized is turned and mobilized as indicated to prevent pressure injuries. For many years, the traditional nursing protocol was that the patient who is immobilized and bedfast should be turned every 2 hours to prevent pressure injuries; that is now updated so that more frequent patient movements are encouraged, particularly in the patient with obesity (Haesler, 2018). Nurses should be familiar with and comfortable using specialized durable medical bariatric equipment (e.g., lifts, transport equipment, commodes) so that the patient with obesity receives necessary care. It is also important to enforce and implement safe patient handling protocols so that the nurse does not incur musculoskeletal injury.

The Patient Undergoing Bariatric Surgery

The term **bariatric** is derived from two Greek words meaning "weight" and "treatment." Thus, bariatric surgery is surgery indicated to treat obesity. Surgery is typically performed after other nonsurgical attempts at weight control have failed. Insurance coverage for bariatric surgery varies widely, but most insurance companies will consider surgery as a treatment if the patient has Class III obesity or Class II obesity with a related medical condition (e.g., type 2 diabetes, OSA) (see Table 42-1) (Obesity Action Coalition [OAC], 2019a).

According to estimates by the ASMBS (2018b), the number of bariatric surgeries performed in the United States grew by nearly 30% between 2011 and 2017. Bariatric surgical procedures work by restricting a patient's ability to eat (restrictive procedure), interfering with ingested nutrient absorption (malabsorptive procedures), or both. The different types of bariatric surgical procedures require unique lifestyle modifications. In order to optimize their success, patients should be well informed about the specific lifestyle changes, eating habits, and bowel habits that may result from each type of procedure.

Bariatric surgery typically results in a weight loss of 10% to 35% of total body weight within 2 years postoperatively, with the majority of weight loss occurring within the first year (OAC, 2019b; Shanti & Patel, 2019). Comorbid conditions such as type 2 diabetes, hypertension, and OSA may resolve; and dyslipidemia improves (Nguyen et al., 2020; Shanti & Patel, 2019). Bariatric surgery has been extended to carefully selected adolescents with severe obesity and comorbidity because of the positive results it has achieved in adults (Ruiz-Cota, Bacardí-Gascón, & Jiménez-Cruz, 2019). However, the long-term benefits for patients who undergo bariatric surgery during adolescence are debatable, as weight regain and risk reduction of comorbidities tend to resume within 5 years postoperatively (Ruiz-Cota et al., 2019).

Patient selection is critical, and the preliminary process may necessitate months of counseling, education, and evaluation by a multidisciplinary team, including social workers, dietitians, a nurse counselor, a psychologist or psychiatrist, and a bariatric surgeon. The selection criteria for patients has changed considerably since the advent of bariatric surgery, with patients with BMIs as low as 30 kg/m² now considered candidates for surgical intervention if they have comorbid conditions that may demonstrably improve post weight loss (e.g., type 2 diabetes) (Nguyen et al., 2020; NIDDK, 2016a) (see Chart 42-6).

Because bariatric surgery involves a drastic change in the functioning of the digestive system, patients need counseling before and after the surgery. Guidelines have been developed to assist in the care of patients having bariatric surgery (Mechanick, Apovian, Brethauer, et al., 2019).

Surgical Procedures

Sleeve gastrectomy, Roux-en-Y gastric bypass (RYGB), biliopancreatic diversion with duodenal switch, and gastric banding are the current bariatric procedures that might be performed. These procedures may be performed by laparoscopy or by an open surgical technique. Currently, the sleeve

---

Chart 42-6 Selection Criteria for Bariatric Surgery

Patients with the Following BMIs and Associated Factors

- BMI ≥40 kg/m² without excessive surgical risk
- BMI ≥35 kg/m² and one or more severe obesity-associated comorbid conditions (e.g., hyperlipidemia, obstructive sleep apnea, obesity hypoventilation syndrome, nonalcoholic fatty liver disease, hypertension, asthma, debilitating arthritis, or considerably impaired quality of life)
- BMI ≥30 kg/m² with type 2 diabetes with poor glycemic control despite optimal medical treatments and lifestyle changes

Inclusion Criteria

- Ability to perform activities of daily living and self-care
- Presence of a support network of family and friends
- Failure of previous nonsurgical attempts at weight loss, including nonprofessional programs
- Expectation that patient will adhere to postoperative care, follow-up visits, and recommended medical management, including the use of dietary supplements

Exclusion Criteria

Reversible endocrine or other disorders that can cause obesity
Current substance use disorder (SUD: e.g., drug or alcohol abuse)
Uncontrolled, severe psychiatric illness
Lack of comprehension of risks, benefits, expected outcomes, alternatives, and lifestyle changes required with bariatric surgery

Adapted from Mechanick, J. I., Apovian, C., Brethauer, S., et al. (2019). Clinical practice guidelines for the perioperative nutritional, metabolic, and nonsurgical support of the bariatric surgery patient—2019 update: Cosponsored by the American Association of Clinical Endocrinologists, The Obesity Society, and American Society for Metabolic & Bariatric Surgery. *Endocrine Practice, 25*(12), 1–75.

gastrectomy is the most commonly performed procedure, followed by the RYGB; postoperative outcomes are equally favorable between sleeve gastrectomy and RYGB, and generally better than outcomes with gastric banding (ASMBS, 2018b; Kizy, Jahansouz, Downey, et al., 2017; Mechanick et al., 2019). Gastric banding tends to be done less commonly, as there have been reports of problems with band failures and a need for more frequent patient postoperative monitoring (Tsai, Zehetner, Beel, et al., 2019). Biliopancreatic diversion with duodenal switch tends to result in the most postoperative weight loss, and is therefore more commonly indicated for patients with very high BMIs (Nguyen et al., 2020).

The RYGB is a combined restrictive and malabsorptive procedure. The gastric banding and sleeve gastrectomy are restrictive procedures, and the biliopancreatic diversion with duodenal switch combines gastric restriction with intestinal malabsorption. Figure 42-5A–D provides additional details about these procedures.

NURSING PROCESS

The Patient Undergoing Bariatric Surgery

Assessment

Preoperatively, the nurse assesses for contraindications to major abdominal surgery. Previous attempts at losing weight are also assessed, including strategies such as nutritional counseling, dieting, or exercise programs. The nurse ensures the patient has received education and counseling regarding the possible risks and benefits of bariatric surgery including the complications, postsurgical outcomes, dietary changes, and the need for lifelong follow-up. The nurse also confirms that the patient has been screened for behavioral disorders that may interfere with postsurgical outcomes. Dietary counseling is initiated preoperatively to prepare for postoperative dietary changes (Mechanick et al., 2019; OAC, 2019b).

The nurse ensures that preoperative screening tests are obtained and scrutinizes the results. Typical laboratory tests include a complete blood cell count (CBC), electrolytes, blood urea nitrogen (BUN), and creatinine. See Appendix A on thePoint for normal values for these laboratory tests. Patients with obesity may have OSA, gastroesophageal reflux disease (GERD), heart disease, nonalcoholic fatty liver disease, diabetes (or prediabetes), and vitamin and mineral deficiencies; thus, other screening tests that may be obtained include a sleep study, upper endoscopy, electrocardiogram (ECG), lipid panel, AST, ALT, glucose, and hemoglobin A1c, as well as iron, vitamin B_{12}, thiamine, folate, vitamin D, and calcium levels.

Postoperatively, the nurse assesses the patient to ensure that goals for recovery are met and that the patient exhibits absence of complications secondary to the surgical intervention. See Chapter 16 for general assessment of the postoperative patient.

Diagnosis

NURSING DIAGNOSES

Based on the assessment data, major nursing diagnoses may include the following:
- Lack of knowledge about the nature of the surgical procedure, dietary limitations, and activities

- Anxiety associated with impending surgery
- Acute pain associated with surgical procedure
- Risk for hypovolaemia associated with nausea, gastric irritation, and pain
- Risk for infection associated with anastomotic leak
- Impaired nutritional status associated with dietary restrictions
- Disturbed body image associated with body changes from bariatric surgery

COLLABORATIVE PROBLEMS/POTENTIAL COMPLICATIONS
Potential complications may include the following:
- Change in bowel habits, including diarrhea and/or constipation
- Hemorrhage
- Venous thromboembolism (VTE)
- Bile reflux
- Dumping syndrome
- Dysphagia
- Bowel or gastric outlet obstruction

Planning and Goals

Preoperative goals include that the patient will become knowledgeable about the preoperative and postoperative dietary routine/restrictions and will have decreased anxiety about the surgery. Postoperative goals include relief of pain, maintenance of homeostatic fluid balance, prevention of infection, adherence to detailed diet instructions to include progression of food intake as well as fluid intake (to prevent dehydration), knowledge about vitamin supplements and the need for lifelong follow-up, achievement of a positive body image, and maintenance of normal bowel habits (ASMBS, 2013; Mechanick et al., 2019).

Nursing Interventions

 FOSTERING PATIENT KNOWLEDGE

Although care of patients with obesity who are undergoing surgery is best achieved with a multidisciplinary care team, nurses have the opportunity to lead patient education initiatives. A systematic review noted that weight management centers within and outside of the United States have not extensively tested education practices for their effectiveness (Groller, 2017). Furthermore, patient education was not comparable across centers with much variance between educational content and delivery practices specific to teaching style and educator role (Groller, 2017).

Education for patients undergoing bariatric surgery should include information on the surgical procedure, nutrition requirements, activity, and psychosocial behaviors (Groller, 2017). Providing this education to patients in small group and individualized teaching sessions will enable patients to ask questions and have the nurse evaluate patient understanding to promote adherence to the treatment plan.

The nurse counsels the patient anticipating bariatric surgery to ingest nothing but clear liquids for a specified period of time preoperatively (typically about 24 to 48 hours before). Nutritional support for patients scheduled for bariatric surgery is tailored to meet each patient's individual need to ensure optimal consumption of micronutrients. Bariatric diets usually follow a slow progression from clear liquids only continuing

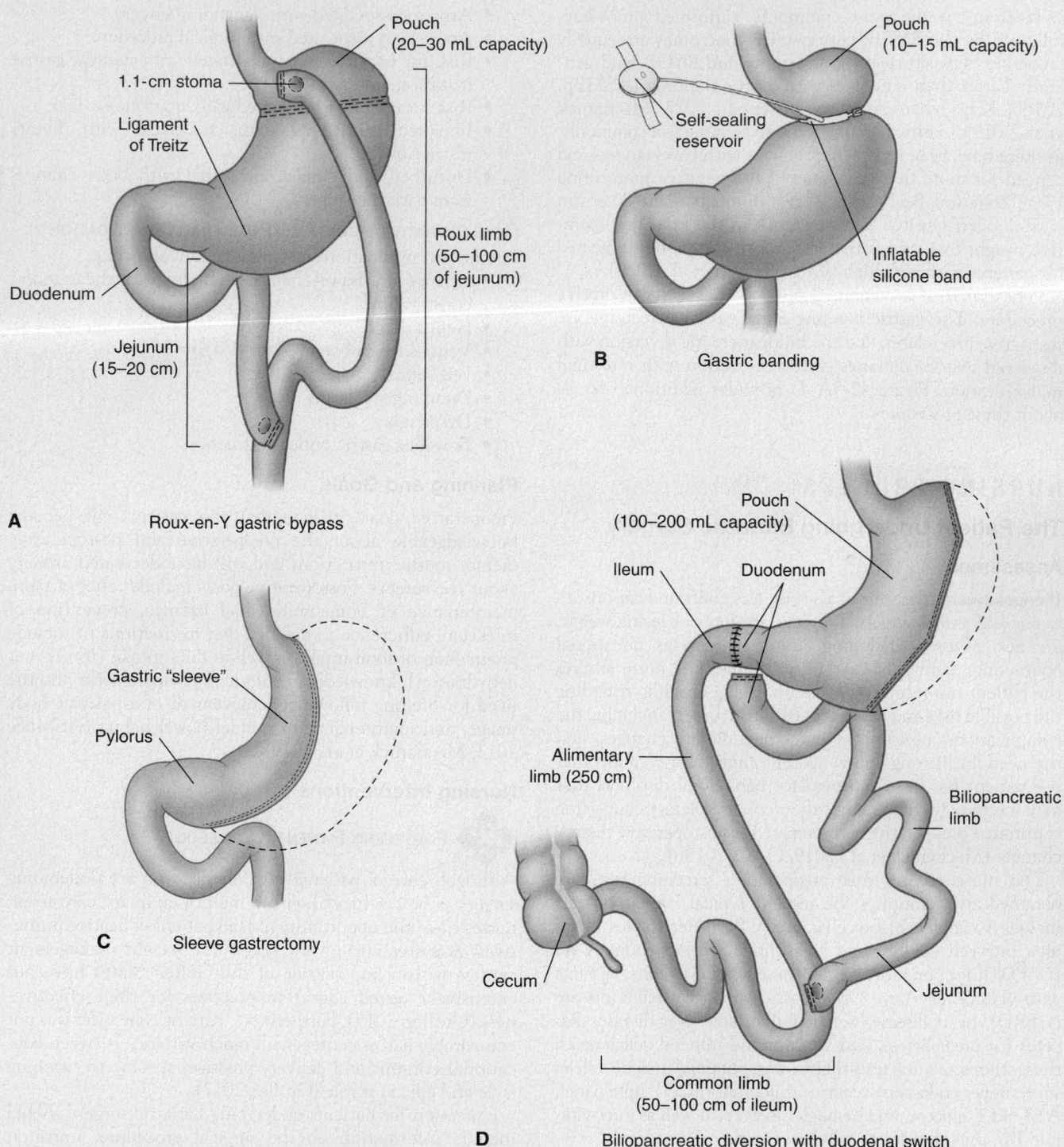

Figure 42-5 • Bariatric surgical procedures. **A.** Roux-en-Y gastric bypass. A horizontal row of staples across the fundus of the stomach creates a pouch with a capacity of 20 to 30 mL. The jejunum is divided distal to the ligament of Treitz, and the distal end is anastomosed to the new pouch. The proximal segment is anastomosed to the jejunum. **B.** Gastric banding. A prosthetic device is used to restrict oral intake by creating a small pouch of 10 to 15 mL that empties through the narrow outlet into the remainder of the stomach. **C.** Sleeve gastrectomy. The stomach is incised vertically and up to 85% of the stomach is surgically removed, leaving a "sleeve"-shaped tube that retains intact nervous innervation and does not obstruct or decrease the size of the gastric outlet. **D.** Biliopancreatic diversion with duodenal switch (also called *sleeve gastrectomy with duodenal switch*). Half of the stomach is removed, leaving a small area that holds about 60 mL. The entire jejunum is excluded from the rest of the gastrointestinal tract. The duodenum is disconnected and sealed off. The ileum is divided above the ileocecal junction, and the distal end of the jejunum is anastomosed to the first portion of the duodenum. The distal end of the biliopancreatic limb is anastomosed to the ileum.

for up to 48 hours postoperatively, to full liquids with sugar-free or low sugar options, to pureed diet, to soft solids and, eventually by approximately the 8-week postoperative time frame, to solid foods (Mechanick et al., 2019; Petcu, 2017). This slow progression is necessary to maximize weight loss, and to prevent complications such as nausea, vomiting, bile reflux, and diarrhea.

The patient's diet likely will be limited upon discharge from the hospital; because of this, patients scheduled for bariatric surgery are given guidelines prior to surgery on which foods and liquids they may consume postoperatively so that they may stock up on these items at home before they are admitted to the hospital. These typically include sugar-free drinks, gelatins and puddings, flavored electrolyte drinks, fat-free milk, protein drinks, sugar-free applesauce, and low-fat soups (Mechanick et al., 2019; Petcu, 2017).

REDUCING ANXIETY

The nurse provides the patient preparing for bariatric surgery anticipatory guidance as to what to expect during the surgery and postoperatively. In addition, the nurse may encourage the patient to join a bariatric surgery support group preoperatively, with the intent that the patient will continue to participate in this group postoperatively. Most bariatric surgery centers sponsor patient support groups that meet in person or online. These support groups provide a forum where patients contemplating bariatric surgery may talk with patients who have had the surgery and may provide them with guidance and tips that can help to lessen their anxiety (Mechanick et al., 2019).

RELIEVING PAIN

After surgery, analgesic agents may be given as prescribed to relieve pain and discomfort. In the past, patient-controlled analgesic pumps were used postoperatively; however, this is no longer recommended practice (Nguyen et al., 2020). The opioid crisis has stimulated research to question opioid prescription and use practices in this population (Heinberg, Pudalov, Alameddin, et al., 2019). New recommendations favor nonopioid agents and restriction to no more than 15 doses of oral opioids during any postoperative recovery (Friedman, Ghiassi, Hubbard, et al., 2019; Nguyen et al., 2020). Patients are usually prescribed oral immediate-release opioids (e.g., oxycodone) and other nonopioid agents, such as acetaminophen. The nurse should educate the patient about these medications and monitor their effectiveness. It is especially important to provide adequate pain relief so that the patient can perform pulmonary care activities (deep breathing and coughing) and leg exercises, turn from side to side, and ambulate. The nurse assesses the effectiveness of analgesic intervention and consults with other members of the health care team if pain is not adequately controlled (see Chapter 9). Positioning the patient in a low or high Fowler position promotes comfort and emptying of the stomach after any type of gastric surgery, including bariatric procedures.

ENSURING FLUID VOLUME BALANCE

Patients who have had bariatric surgery usually receive IV fluids for the first several hours postoperatively. Once they are awake and alert on the surgical unit, they are encouraged to begin intake of sugar-free oral fluids. Introducing small volumes of these liquids is believed to stimulate GI peristalsis and perfusion and thwart gastric reflux. Sugar-free fluids are preferred because they are not implicated in causing dumping syndrome (see later discussion). With a typical regimen, patients are encouraged to slowly sip 30 mL of these fluids every 15 minutes (Fencl, Walsh, & Vocke, 2015). Patients should stop ingesting fluids, however, if they feel nauseated or full. Antiemetic agents may be prescribed to relieve nausea and prevent vomiting, which could cause strain on the surgical site and cause either a hemorrhage or anastomotic leak (Mechanick et al., 2019).

PREVENTING INFECTION/ANASTOMOTIC LEAK

Disruption at the site of anastomosis (i.e., surgically resected site) may cause leakage of gastric contents into the peritoneal cavity, causing infection and possible sepsis. Patients at risk for this particular complication tend to be older, male, and with greater body mass. In addition, anastomotic leak is more commonly associated with open rather than laparoscopic procedures. Patients with anastomotic leaks typically exhibit nonspecific signs and symptoms that include fever, abdominal pain, tachycardia, and leukocytosis. This may progress to sepsis and possibly septic shock if not recognized and treated early (see Chapter 11). The nurse must be astute in recognizing these manifestations and alerting the patient's primary provider should they occur (Petcu, 2017).

A patient suspected of having an anastomotic leak may have an upper GI series that includes follow-up computed tomography (CT) scan with contrast dye, which may find leaking contrast dye, thus confirming the diagnosis. Treatment varies depending on the timing (early or late postoperatively) and severity of the leak. CT-guided drainage of the area may be appropriate for a less severe leak in the later postoperative phase of recovery, but an early or severe leak requires immediate open surgical intervention to repair the leak (Petcu, 2017).

ENSURING ADEQUATE NUTRITIONAL STATUS

After bowel sounds have returned and oral intake is resumed, six small feedings consisting of a total of 600 to 800 calories per day are provided, and consumption of fluids between meals is encouraged to prevent dehydration. The nurse instructs the patient to eat slowly and stop when feeling full. Eating too much or too fast or eating high-calorie liquids and soft foods can result in vomiting or painful esophageal distention. Gastric retention may be evidenced by abdominal distention, nausea, and vomiting. A nutritionist is typically consulted to assist with diet restrictions and diet progression (Mechanick et al., 2019; Nguyen et al., 2020) (see Chart 42-7).

Common dietary deficiencies in patients who have had bariatric surgery include malabsorption of organic iron, which may require supplementation with oral or parenteral iron, and a low serum level of vitamin B_{12}; the patient may be prescribed monthly vitamin B_{12} intramuscular injections to prevent pernicious anemia (Holsworth & Gallagher, 2017; Mechanick et al., 2019) (see Chapter 29 for further discussion of pernicious anemia).

SUPPORTING BODY IMAGE CHANGES

After bariatric surgery most patients report greatly improved perceptions of their body image, as well as improved quality of life. In particular, patients identified satisfaction with bariatric surgery when they achieved personal weight goals,

Chart 42-7 — PATIENT EDUCATION

Dietary Guidelines for the Patient Who Has Had Bariatric Surgery

The nurse instructs the patient to:

- Eat smaller but more frequent meals that contain protein and fiber; each meal size should not exceed 1 cup.
- Eat only foods high in nutrients (e.g., peanut butter, cheese, chicken, fish, beans).
- Consume fat as tolerated.
- Ensure a low carbohydrate intake; in particular, avoid concentrated sources of carbohydrates (e.g., candy).
- Eat two protein snacks daily; animal protein may be poorly tolerated after Roux-en-Y gastric bypass, however.
- Eat slowly and chew thoroughly or may feel food "sticking" in throat.
- Assume a low Fowler position during mealtime and then remain in that position for 20 to 30 minutes after mealtime—this delays stomach emptying and decreases the likelihood of dumping syndrome.
- Know that antispasmodic agents, as prescribed, also may aid in delaying the emptying of the stomach.
- Avoid drinking fluid with meals; instead, consume fluids up to 30 minutes before a meal and 60 minutes after mealtime.
- Do drink plenty of water; refrain from drinking liquid calories (e.g., alcoholic beverages, fruit drinks, nondiet sodas).
- Take prescribed dietary supplements of vitamins and medium-chain triglycerides.
- Follow up with primary provider for monthly injections of vitamin B_{12} and iron as prescribed.
- Walk for at least 30 minutes daily.

Adapted from Groller, K. D., Teel, C., Stegenga, K. H., et al. (2018). Patient perspectives about bariatric surgery unveil experiences, education, satisfaction, and recommendations for improvement. *Surgery for Obesity and Related Diseases, 14*(6), 785–796; Mechanick, J. I., Apovian, C., Brethauer S., et al. (2019). Clinical practice guidelines for the perioperative nutritional, metabolic, and nonsurgical support of the bariatric surgery patient—2019 update: Cosponsored by the American Association of Clinical Endocrinologists, The Obesity Society, and American Society for Metabolic & Bariatric Surgery. *Endocrine Practice, 25*(12), 1–75.

adhered to postoperative care rules, and saw physical health improvements (Groller, Teel, Stegenga, et al., 2018). However, some patients report lingering dissatisfaction with their body images. In particular, some patients may report dissatisfaction related to loose skin folds and may eventually seek elective body-contouring surgical options (e.g., breast reductions, breast lifts, abdominoplasty) (Groller et al., 2018). The nurse provides support to the patient who reports dissatisfaction with body image post weight loss by acknowledging the patient's feelings as real, sharing that these perceptions are not unusual, and providing links to live or online supports groups or counselors, as necessary (see the Nursing Research Profile in Chart 42-8).

MONITORING AND MANAGING POTENTIAL COMPLICATIONS

After surgery, the nurse assesses the patient for complications from the bariatric surgery, such as changes in bowel habits, hemorrhage, venous thromboembolism (VTE), bile reflux, dumping syndrome, dysphagia, and bowel or gastric outlet obstruction.

Change in Bowel Habits. Patients may complain of either diarrhea or constipation postoperatively. Diarrhea is more common an occurrence after bariatric surgery, particularly after malabsorptive procedures (Mechanick et al., 2019). Both may be prevented if the patient consumes a nutritious diet that is high in fiber. Steatorrhea also may occur as a result of rapid gastric emptying, which prevents adequate mixing with pancreatic and biliary secretions (Mechanick et al., 2019). In mild cases, reducing the intake of fat and administering an antimotility medication (e.g., loperamide) may control symptoms. Persistent diarrhea or steatorrhea may warrant further diagnostic testing, such as an upper endoscopy or colonoscopy with biopsies to rule out the presence of additional pathology, such as celiac disease or *Clostridium difficile* infection (Mechanick et al., 2019) (see Chapter 41).

Hemorrhage. Postoperative hemorrhage may be a complication following bariatric surgery. Intra-abdominal hemorrhage may be evident by frank, bright red oral or rectal bleeding, tarry melena, bloody output from the wound or drains, if present, as well as typical clinical manifestations of severe bleeding and hemorrhagic shock (e.g., tachycardia, hypotension, syncope) (see Chapter 11). Bleeding within the first 72 hours postoperatively is most likely caused by disruption in a staple or suture. Bleeding 72 hours to 30 days postoperatively is most likely from formation of a gastric or duodenal ulcer (Nguyen et al., 2020; Petcu, 2017) (see Chapter 40).

Venous Thromboembolism. Patients who have bariatric surgery are at moderate to high risk of VTE, including both PE and DVT. Patients who are older, have higher BMIs, and have a prior history of a VTE or coagulation defect are at higher risk (Holsworth & Gallagher, 2017; Nguyen et al., 2020). ASMBS guidelines for VTE prevention specify that in the immediate postoperative period, patients who have had bariatric surgery should be prescribed mechanical compression (e.g., intermittent pneumatic compression devices) and prophylactic anticoagulation with subcutaneous low-molecular-weight heparin (LMWH) agents (e.g., dalteparin, enoxaparin). The duration of time that mechanical compression and anticoagulation should continue postoperatively is not described, however, and is left to the discretion of the patient and primary provider. In addition to implementing this prescribed therapy, nurses caring for patients post bariatric surgery should encourage them to begin early ambulation to further deter the advent of VTE (Holsworth & Gallagher, 2017; Nguyen et al., 2020) (see Chapter 26).

Bile Reflux. Bile reflux may occur with procedures that manipulate or remove the pylorus, which acts as a barrier to the reflux of duodenal contents. Reflux of bile can cause gastritis or esophagitis (inflammation of the stomach or esophagus, respectively). Burning epigastric pain and vomiting of bilious material manifest this condition. Eating or vomiting does not relieve the symptoms. Bile reflux may be managed with proton pump inhibitors (e.g., omeprazole) (Nguyen et al., 2020).

Dumping Syndrome. **Dumping syndrome** is an unpleasant set of vasomotor and GI symptoms that commonly occur in patients who have had bariatric surgery. For many years, it had been theorized that the hypertonic gastric food boluses that quickly transit into the intestines drew extracellular fluid from the circulating blood volume into the small intestines to dilute the high concentration of electrolytes and sugars, resulting in symptoms. Now, it is thought that this rapid

Chart 42-8 — NURSING RESEARCH PROFILE
Patient Experiences with Education and Satisfaction in Weight Loss Surgery

Groller, K. D., Teel, C., Stegenga, K. H., et al. (2018). Patient perspectives about bariatric surgery unveil experiences, education, satisfaction, and recommendations for improvement. *Surgery for Obesity and Related Diseases*, 14(6), 785–796.

Purpose

Accreditation standards require weight management centers to provide programs before and after weight loss surgery (WLS) to educate and support patients throughout lifestyle transitions. The educational programs offered at weight management centers vary by curriculum, timing, and delivery approach and may not be evidence based or patient centered. Despite these educational efforts, up to 35% of patients who undergo WLS will experience some type of weight recidivism (gain) within the first 2 postoperative years. Patient risk of regaining 5% or more from maximum weight lost continues to increase each year postoperatively. First-line treatment for patients who regain previously lost weight after WLS is to enroll and participate in additional educational programs that reinforce previously learned concepts about lifestyle demands post surgery. This study sought to obtain patient perspectives about their WLS journey with emphasis on their experiences with education, satisfaction, and recommendations to enhance the experience for future patients.

Design

This qualitative descriptive study used a purposive sampling method to recruit adult patients from an accredited weight management center. Fifty percent of all WLS cases completed within the previous 6 months were randomly selected and were mailed an invitation letter to participate in the research study. English-speaking adult patients who responded to the invitation letter were interviewed. All 11 participants, 36% male, participated in an audio-recorded interview with one researcher using a semistructured interview guide. Interview recordings were transcribed verbatim and evaluated using Colaizzi's method for inductive content analysis. Interview responses were categorized and grouped into codes, subthemes, and main themes once data saturation was achieved. Member-checking occurred to confirm final themes and subthemes that emerged from the interview data.

Findings

The study sample was fairly homogenous and oversampled males to obtain perspectives from both genders. The concept of A New Me-Version 2.0 included three main themes that emerged from participant interviews. Programming and Tools (Theme 1) provided insight on how individuals undergoing WLS obtained support from the weight management center program. Updates and Upgrades (Theme 2) explained lifestyle challenges and routines before and after WLS and quality-of-life concerns. The last theme, Lessons Learned and Future Considerations (Theme 3), described satisfaction level through the lived experience and provided suggestions for improving the experience for future patients.

Nursing Implications

Results from this study provide insight into the lived WLS patient experience. Through emerged themes, WLS success was associated with meeting weight goals, adhering to new lifestyle routines, and seeing improved health. Participants emphasized education efforts should focus on explaining program objectives, incorporating technology to support monitoring of holistic transformations, and fostering a network of community members. This study also identified the need for future research to develop WLS education best practices and study the impact WLS education has on clinical outcomes.

---

transit of the food bolus from the stomach into the small intestines instead causes a rapid and exuberant release of metabolic peptides that are responsible for the symptoms of dumping syndrome (Mattar & Rogers, 2020).

Symptoms of dumping syndrome typically occur within a few minutes to 2 hours after eating and include tachycardia, dizziness, sweating, nausea, vomiting, bloating, abdominal cramping, and diarrhea (Mattar & Rogers, 2020). These symptoms typically resolve once the intestine has been evacuated (i.e., with defecation). Later, blood glucose rises rapidly, followed by increased insulin secretion. This results in a reactive hypoglycemia, which also is unpleasant for the patient. Vasomotor symptoms that occur 10 to 90 minutes after eating include pallor, perspiration, palpitations, headache, and feelings of warmth, dizziness, and even drowsiness. Anorexia may also result from dumping syndrome, because the patient may be reluctant to eat (Mattar & Rogers, 2020).

Dysphagia. **Dysphagia,** or difficulty swallowing, may occur in patients who have had any type of restrictive bariatric procedure. If it occurs, it tends to be most severe 4 to 6 weeks postoperatively and may persist for up to 6 months after surgery. Dysphagia may be prevented by educating patients to eat slowly, to chew food thoroughly, and to avoid eating tough foods such as steak or dry chicken or doughy bread. Patients with severe dysphagia who have had gastric banding may benefit from having their bands adjusted. Patients who have had other restrictive procedures may experience relief of symptoms after having stomal strictures relieved endoscopically (Mechanick et al., 2019).

Bowel and Gastric Outlet Obstruction. Bowel or gastric outlet obstruction may occur as a complication of bariatric surgery. The typical manifestations and treatments of gastric outlet obstruction are described in Chapter 40; however, there is a key difference in the treatment of a patient who has undergone bariatric surgery with a gastric outlet obstruction. It is contraindicated to insert a nasogastric (NG) tube in patients that have had bariatric surgery, even if they have a gastric outlet obstruction. Alternative treatment options may include endoscopic procedures aimed at relieving the obstruction, such as balloon dilation, or surgical revisions (King & Herron, 2020).

Quality and Safety Nursing Alert

Insertion of NG tubes is contraindicated in the patient post bariatric surgery. This procedure may disrupt the surgical suture line and cause anastomotic leak or hemorrhage.

PROMOTING HOME, COMMUNITY-BASED, AND TRANSITIONAL CARE

Patients are usually discharged from the hospital within 4 days postoperatively (this may be within 24 to 72 hours for patients who have had laparoscopic procedures) with detailed dietary instructions (see Chart 42-7) as well as instructions about how to either begin or resume an appropriate exercise regimen. Instructions on making follow-up appointments with the bariatric surgeon for routine postoperative visits or for complications are shared with the patient (Mechanick et al., 2019).

Educating Patients About Self-Care. The nurse provides education with the patient about nutrition, nutritional supplements, pain management, the importance of physical activity, and the symptoms of dumping syndrome and measures to prevent or minimize these symptoms. Patients who undergo laparoscopic or open RYGB procedures may have one or more Jackson–Pratt drains, which may remain in place after discharge. The nurse educates the patient or caregiver about how to empty, measure, and record the amount of drainage. Patients should be instructed to avoid taking nonsteroidal anti-inflammatory drugs (NSAIDs) (e.g., ibuprofen) post discharge, as they have been implicated in development of stomach ulcers (Mechanick et al., 2019; Peterson & Kempenich, 2020). The nurse must emphasize the continued need for follow-up (even after weight loss goals are met) and continued support group participation.

Continuing and Transitional Care. After bariatric surgery, all patients require lifelong monitoring of weight, comorbidities, metabolic and nutritional status, and dietary and activity behaviors because they are at risk for developing malnutrition or weight gain. Women of childbearing age who have bariatric surgery are advised to use contraceptives for at least 18 months after surgery to avoid pregnancy until their weight stabilizes. After weight loss, the patient may elect additional surgical interventions for body contouring. These may include breast reductions, lipoplasty to remove fat deposits, or a panniculectomy or abdominoplasty to remove excess abdominal skin folds (Mechanick et al., 2019; OAC, 2019b).

Evaluation

Expected patient outcomes may include the following:
1. Improved knowledge
   a. Reports appropriate expectations for surgical procedure
   b. Verbalizes understanding of diet and fluid restrictions post surgery
2. Diminished anxiety
   a. Exhibits calm demeanor
   b. Identifies support resources
3. Relief of pain
   a. Reports relief of pain
   b. Engages in early mobilization activities as prescribed
4. Maintenance of fluid balance
   a. Able to tolerate progressive fluid intake without complaints of nausea or gastric reflux
   b. Voids at least 400 mL in 24 hours and 0.5 mL/kg/h for any 6-hour time frame postoperatively
5. Maintenance of asepsis
   a. No evidence of infection (e.g., no fever, no leukocytosis, no complaints of abdominal pain)
6. Achievement of nutritional balance
   a. Able to consume small, frequent meals as prescribed
   b. Adheres to prescribed intake of vitamins and supplements
   c. Achieves and maintains weight reduction goals
7. Promotion of positive body image
   a. Verbalizes continued satisfaction with weight reduction plan and its effect on body image
8. Has no complications (e.g., no diarrhea, constipation, bleeding, VTE, bile reflux, dumping syndrome, dysphagia, or bowel or gastric outlet obstruction)

CRITICAL THINKING EXERCISES

1 ebp You work as a staff nurse in a women's health clinic. A 50-year-old female patient presents for her annual physical examination. You measure her height as 65 inches and weight as 196 pounds. As you record these into her electronic health record, you note that last year she weighed 180 pounds. What is her BMI? As you reconcile her medications and allergies, she discloses how unhappy she is with regard to her increase in body weight despite her daily physical activity regimen of brisk walking or strength training. She reports symptoms of menopause. She asks, "Can you recommend a diet that will help me lose the 16 pounds of weight I gained over this year? I just want to get back to the normal me." What other information will you need to elicit from this patient in order to provide her with guidance about a healthier lifestyle? What diet may you recommend for her? Describe the strength of the evidence you use to offer her the healthiest weight loss outcomes.

2 pg A 47-year-old male patient is 6 weeks postoperative from a sleeve gastrectomy procedure. He presents to the emergency department with vomiting and dehydration. His temperature is 99.9°F (37.7°C), BP is 130/76 mm Hg, heart rate is 118 bpm, and respiratory rate is 22 breaths/min with an SpO$_2$ of 97%. During triage, his wife shares that he has been unable to eat for the past 3 days as he vomits soon afterward. He has not been able "keep liquids down" for the past 12 hours. Explain what nursing assessments you will conduct. What nursing interventions would you implement and why?

3 ipc You are a nurse who works at a weight management center. A 25-year-old female patient is referred by her primary care provider to visit the weight management center for treatment as she has had repeated attempts of unsuccessful weight loss for the past 18 months. She is 5 feet tall with a current weight of 192 pounds. She reports being newly married with a history of polycystic ovary syndrome (PCOS). She wishes to become pregnant. Although her last menstrual period was 3 months ago, she is not currently pregnant. What members of the interdisciplinary team could be consulted to help this woman achieve her goals of both weight loss and pregnancy?

REFERENCES

*Asterisk indicates nursing research.

Books

Campbell, M. D., & Rutherford, Z. H. (2018). The role of physical activity and exercise in managing obesity and achieving weight loss. In J. R. Weaver (Ed.). *Practical guide to obesity medicine*. St. Louis, MO: Elsevier.

Comerford, K. C., & Durkin, M. T. (2020). *Nursing 2020 drug handbook*. Philadelphia, PA: Wolters Kluwer.

DiPietro, L., & Stachenfeld, N. S. (2017). Exercise treatment of obesity. In K. R. Feingold, B. Anawalt, & A. Boyce (Eds.). *Endotext [Internet]*. South Dartmouth, MA: MD Text.

Eliopoulos, C. (2018). *Gerontological nursing* (9th ed.). Philadelphia, PA: Lippincott Williams & Wilkins.

King, N. A., & Herron, D. M. (2020). Gastrointestinal obstruction after bariatric surgery. In N. T. Nguyen, S. A. Brethauer, J. M. Morton, et al. (Eds.). *The ASMBS textbook of bariatric surgery*. Switzerland, AG: Springer.

Mattar, S. G., & Rogers, A. M. (2020). Early and late dumping syndromes. In N. T. Nguyen, S. A. Brethauer, J. M. Morton, et al. (Eds.). *The ASMBS textbook of bariatric surgery*. Switzerland, AG: Springer.

Nguyen, N. T., Brethauer, S. A., Morton, J. M., et al. (2020). *The ASMBS textbook of bariatric surgery*. Switzerland, AG: Springer.

Norris, T. L. (2019). *Porth's pathophysiology: Concepts of altered health states* (10th ed.). Philadelphia, PA: Wolters Kluwer.

Peterson, R. M., & Kempenich, J. W. (2020). Management of marginal ulcers. In N. T. Nguyen, S. A. Brethauer, J. M. Morton, et al. (Eds.). *The ASMBS textbook of bariatric surgery*. Switzerland, AG: Springer.

van Meijel, R., Blaak, E. E., & Goossens, G. H. (2018). Adipose tissue metabolism and inflammation in obesity. In R. Johnston & B. Surat (Eds.). *Mechanisms and manifestations of obesity in lung disease*. (pp. 1–22). San Francisco, CA: Academic Press.

Weber, J. R., & Kelley, J. H. (2018). *Health assessment in nursing* (6th ed.). Philadelphia, PA: Lippincott Williams & Wilkins.

Yeh, M., Glick-Bauer, M., & Katz, D. L. (2017). Weight maintenance and weight loss: The adoption of diets based on predominantly plants. In F. Mariotti (Ed.). *Vegetarian and plant-based diets in health and disease prevention*. London, UK: Academic Press.

Journals and Electronic Documents

Ali, M. R., Moustarah, F., Kim, J. J., et al. (2015). ASMBS position statement on intragastric balloon therapy endorsed by SAGES. Retrieved on 12/15/2019 at: www.asmbs.org/resources/position-statement-on-intragastric-balloon-therapy-endorsed-by-sages

American Medical Association (AMA) House of Delegates. (2013). Recognition of obesity as a disease. Resolution: 420 (A-13); received 5/16/13. AMA: Author.

American Society for Metabolic and Bariatric Surgery (ASMBS). (2013). Medical and bariatric surgery: Medical outcomes of bariatric surgery. Retrieved on 8/3/2019 at: www.asmbs.org/resources/metabolic-and-bariatric-surgery

American Society for Metabolic and Bariatric Surgery (ASMBS). (2018a). Obesity in America: Fact sheet. Retrieved on 8/3/2019 at: www.asmbs.org/app/uploads/2018/11/Obesity-in-America-Fact-Sheet.pdf

American Society for Metabolic and Bariatric Surgery (ASMBS). (2018b). Estimate of bariatric surgery numbers, 2011–2017. Retrieved on 8/3/2019 at: www.asmbs.org/resources/estimate-of-bariatric-surgery-numbers

American Society for Metabolic and Bariatric Surgery (ASMBS). (2019a). Disease of obesity. Retrieved on 8/3/2019 at: www.asmbs.org/patients/disease-of-obesity

American Society for Metabolic and Bariatric Surgery (ASMBS). (2019b). The impact of obesity on your body and health. Retrieved on 5/1/2020 at: www.asmbs.org/patients/impact-of-obesity

Anderson-Shaw, L. (2018). Forced calorie restrictions in the clinical setting. *The American Journal of Bioethics*, 18(7), 83–85.

Apovian, C. M., Aronne, L. J., Bessesen, D. H., et al. (2015). Pharmacological management of obesity: An Endocrine Society Clinical Practice Guideline. *Journal of Clinical Endocrinology and Metabolism*, 100(2), 342–362.

Batsis, J. A., & Zagaria, A. B. (2018). Addressing obesity in aging patients. *Medical Clinics of North America*, 102(1), 65–85.

Biener, A., Cawley, J., & Meyerhoefer, C. (2017). The high and rising costs of obesity to the US health care system. *Journal of General Internal Medicine*, 32(Suppl 1), 6–8.

Bookwalter, D. B., Porter, B., Jacobson, I. G., et al. (2019). Healthy behaviors and incidence of overweight and obesity in military veterans. *Annals of Epidemiology*, 39, 26–32.e1.

Campana, B., Brasiel, P. G., de Aguiar, A. S., et al. (2019). Obesity and food addiction: Similarities to drug addiction. *Obesity Medicine*, 16, 1–5.

Centers for Disease Control and Prevention (CDC). (2017). Defining adult overweight and obesity. Retrieved on 8/3/2019 at: www.cdc.gov/obesity/adult/defining.html

Centers for Disease Control and Prevention (CDC). (2020). Adult obesity causes & consequences. Retrieved on 5/1/2020 at: www.cdc.gov/obesity/adult/causes.html

Chouillard, E., Alsabah, S., Chahine, E., et al. (2018). Changing the quality of life in old age bariatric patients. Cross-sectional study for 79 old age patients. *International Journal of Surgery*, 54(Pt A), 236–241.

Coulter, A. A., Rebello, C. J., & Greenway, F. L. (2018). Centrally acting agents for obesity: Past, present, and future. *Drugs*, 78(11), 1113–1132.

Curry, S. J., Krist, A. H., Owens, D. K., et al. (2018). Behavioral weight loss interventions to prevent obesity-related morbidity and mortality in adults: US Preventive Services Task Force recommendation statement. *JAMA: The Journal of the American Medical Association*, 320(11), 1163–1171.

Dreyer, J. L., & Liebl, A. L. (2018). Early colonization of the gut microbiome and its relationship with obesity. *Human Microbiome Journal*, 10(6), 1–5.

Droege, C. A., & Ernst, N. E. (2017). Impact of norepinephrine weight-based dosing compared with non-weight-based dosing in achieving time to goal mean arterial pressure in obese patients with septic shock. *Annals of Pharmacotherapy*, 51(7), 614–616.

Eisenberg, D., Noria, S., Grover, B., et al. (2019). ASMBS position statement on weight bias and stigma. *Surgery for Obesity and Related Diseases*, 15(6), 814–821.

Fencl, J. L., Walsh, A., & Vocke, D. (2015). The bariatric patient: An overview of perioperative care. *AORN Journal*, 102(2), 116–128.

Friedman, D., Ghiassi, S., Hubbard, M. O., et al. (2019). Postoperative opioid prescribing practices and evidence-based guidelines in bariatric surgery. *Obesity Surgery*, 29(7), 2030–2036.

*Fruh, S. M. (2017). Obesity: Risk factors, complications, and strategies for sustainable long-term weight management. *Journal of the American Association of Nurse Practitioners*, 29(S1), S3–S14.

Gimeno, R. E., Briere, D. A., & Seeley, R. J. (2020). Leveraging the gut to treat metabolic disease. *Cell Metabolism*, 31(4), 679–698.

Giordano, S., & Victorzon, M. (2015). Bariatric surgery in elderly patients: A systematic review. *Clinical Interventions in Aging*, 10, 1627–1635.

Goldstein, M., Mayer, S. B., Graybill, S., et al. (2020). *VA/DoD clinical practice guideline for the management of adult overweight and obesity*. Washington, DC: Department of Veterans Affairs. Retrieved on 3/7/2021 at: www.healthquality.va.gov/guidelines/CD/obesity

*Groller, K. D. (2017). Systematic review of patient education practices in weight loss surgery. *Surgery for Obesity and Related Diseases*, 13(6), 1072–1085.

*Groller, K. D., Teel, C., Stegenga, K. H., et al. (2018). Patient perspectives about bariatric surgery unveil experiences, education, satisfaction, and recommendations for improvement. *Surgery for Obesity and Related Diseases*, 14(6), 785–796.

*Haesler, E. (2018). Evidence Summary: Prevention of pressure injuries in individuals with overweight or obesity. *Wound Practice & Research*, 26(3), 158–161.

Hafezi-Nejad, N., Bailey, C. R., Gunn, A. J., et al. (2019). Weight loss after left gastric artery embolization: A systematic review and meta-analysis. *Journal of Vascular and Interventional Radiology*, 30(10), 1593–1603.e3.

Hales, C. M., Carroll, M. D., Fryar, C. D., et al. (2020). Prevalence of obesity among adults and youth: United States, 2017–2018. National Center for Health Statistics. NCHS Data Brief, no. 360. Hyattsville, MD. Retrieved on 5/1/2020 at: www.cdc.gov/nchs/data/databriefs/db360-h.pdf

Hales, C. M., Fryar, C. D., Carroll, M. D., et al. (2018). Differences in obesity prevalence by demographic characteristics and urbanization level among adults in the United States, 2013–2016. *JAMA: The Journal of the American Medical Association*, 319(23), 2419–2429.

Heinberg, L. J., Pudalov, L., Alameddin, H., et al. (2019). Opioids and bariatric surgery: A review and suggested recommendations for assessment and risk reduction. *Surgery for Obesity and Related Diseases, 15*(2), 314–321.

Henry, T. A. (2018). Adult obesity rates rise in 6 states, exceed 35% in 7. Retrieved on 12/20/2019 at: www.ama-assn.org/delivering-care/public-health/adult-obesity-rates-rise-6-states-exceed-35-7

Holsworth, C., & Gallagher, S. (2017). Managing care of critically ill bariatric patients. *AACN Advanced Critical Care, 28*(3), 275–283.

Humbyrd, C. J. (2018). Complex obesity: Multifactorial etiologies and multifaceted responses. *The American Journal of Bioethics, 18*(7), 87–89.

Kalligeros, M., Shehadeh, F., Mylona, E. K., et al. (2020). Association of obesity with disease severity among patients with coronavirus disease 2019. *Obesity, 28*(7), 1200–1204.

Kass, D. A., Duggal, P., & Cingolani, O. (2020). Obesity could shift severe COVID-19 disease to younger ages. *Lancet, 395*(10236), 1544–1545.

Khan, S. S., Ning, H., Wilkins, J. T., et al. (2018). Association of body mass index with lifetime risk of cardiovascular disease and compression of morbidity. *JAMA Cardiology, 3*(4), 280–287.

Kizy, S., Jahansouz, C., Downey, M. C., et al. (2017). National trends in bariatric surgery 2012–2015: Demographics, procedure selection, readmissions, and cost. *Obesity Surgery, 27*(11), 2933–2939.

Kline, L. R. (2020). Clinical presentation and diagnosis of obstructive sleep apnea in adults. *UpToDate.* Retrieved on 8/13/2020 at: www.uptodate.com/contents/search?search=clinical-presentation-and-diagnosis-of-obstructive-sleep-apnea-in-adults

Kuk, J., Rotondi, M., Sui, X., et al. (2018). Individuals with obesity but no other metabolic risk factors are not at significantly elevated all-cause mortality risk in men and women. *Clinical Obesity, 8*(5), 305–312.

Kurian, M., Kroh, M., Chand, B., et al. (2018). SAGES review of endoscopic and minimally invasive bariatric interventions: A review of endoscopic and non-surgical bariatric interventions. *Surgical Endoscopy, 32*(10), 4063–4067.

LeBlanc, E. S., Patnode, C. D., Webber, E. M., et al. (2018). Behavioral and pharmacotherapy weight loss interventions to prevent obesity-related morbidity and mortality in adults: Updated evidence report and systematic review for the US Preventive Services Task Force. *JAMA: The Journal of the American Medical Association, 320*(11), 1172–1191.

Maginot, T. R., & Rhee, K. (2018). Challenges of obesity treatment: The question of decisional capacity. *The American Journal of Bioethics, 18*(7), 85–87.

*McCarthy, M. S., Elshaw, E. B., Szekeley, B. M., et al. (2017). A randomized controlled trial of nurse coaching vs. herbal supplementation for weight reduction in soldiers. *Military Medicine, 182*(S1), 274–280.

McCrory, M. A., Harbaugh, A. G., Appeadu, S., et al. (2019). Fast-food offerings in the United States in 1986, 1991, and 2016 show large increases in food variety, portion size, dietary energy, and selected micronutrients. *Journal of the Academy of Nutrition and Dietetics, 119*(6), 923–933.

McElroy, K. G., Chung, S., & Regan, M. (2017). CE: Health and the human microbiome: A primer for nurses. *American Journal of Nursing, 117*(7), 24–30.

Mechanick, J. I., Apovian, C., Brethauer, S., et al. (2019). Clinical practice guidelines for the perioperative nutritional, metabolic, and nonsurgical support of the bariatric surgery patient—2019 update: Cosponsored by the American Association of Clinical Endocrinologists, The Obesity Society, and American Society for Metabolic & Bariatric Surgery. *Endocrine Practice, 25*(12), 1–75.

Meigs, J. B. (2019). The metabolic syndrome (insulin resistance syndrome or syndrome X). *UpToDate.* Retrieved on 8/13/2020 at: www.uptodate.com/contents/the-metabolic-syndrome-insulin-resistance-syndrome-or-syndrome-x

Meisenberg, B., Ness, J., Rao, S., et al. (2017). Implementation of solutions to reduce opioid-induced oversedation and respiratory depression. *American Journal of Health-System Pharmacy: AJHP: Official Journal of the American Society of Health-System Pharmacists, 74*(3), 162–169.

Messier, S. P., Resnik, A. E., Beavers, D. P., et al. (2018). Intentional weight loss in overweight and obese patients with knee osteoarthritis: Is more better? *Arthritis Care and Research: The Official Journal of the Arthritis Health Professions Association, 70*(11), 1569–1575.

Moore, R., & Rosenthal, R. (2018). Proposed addendum to position statement on intragastric balloon therapy. Retrieved on 12/15/2019 at: www.asmbs.org/app/uploads/2018/02/Balloon-Addemdum-Moore-Rosenthal.pdf

Moriconi, D., Masi, S., Rebelos, E., et al. (2020). Obesity prolongs the hospital stay in patients affected by COVID-19, and may impact on SARS-COV-2 shedding. *Obesity Research & Clinical Practice, 14*(3), 205–209.

Munoz-Mantilla, D. (2018). Top weight loss medications. Retrieved on 12/15/2019 at: www.obesitymedicine.org/weight-loss-medications

National Institute of Diabetes and Digestive and Kidney Diseases (NIDDK). (2016a). Potential candidates for bariatric surgery. Retrieved on 8/14/2020 at: www.niddk.nih.gov/health-information/weight-management/bariatric-surgery/potential-candidates

National Institute of Diabetes and Digestive and Kidney Diseases (NIDDK). (2016b). Prescription medications to treat overweight and obesity. Retrieved on 8/14/2020 at: www.niddk.nih.gov/health-information/weight-management/prescription-medications-treat-overweight-obesity

Obesity Action Coalition (OAC). (2019a). Access to care resources: Reviewing your insurance policy or employer sponsored medical benefits plan. Retrieved on 8/3/2019 at: www.obesityaction.org/action-through-advocacy/access-to-care/access-to-care-resources/reviewing-your-insurance-policy-or-employer-sponsored-medical-benefits-plan

Obesity Action Coalition (OAC). (2019b). What is obesity treatment? Bariatric surgery. Retrieved on 8/3/2019 at: www.obesityaction.org/obesity-treatments/what-is-obesity-treatment/bariatric-surgery

Oliver, L. A., Oliver, J. A., Ohanyan, S., et al. (2019). Ultrasound for peripheral and arterial access. *Best Practice & Research. Clinical Anaesthesiology, 33*(4), 523–537.

Orringer, K. A., Harrison, A. V., Nichani, S. S., et al. (2020). University of Michigan Health System Clinical Alignment and Performance Excellence Guideline: Obesity prevention and management. Retrieved on 5/1/2020 at: www.med.umich.edu/1info/FHP/practiceguides/obesity/obesity.pdf

Papasavas, P., El Chaar, M., Kothari, S. N., et al. (2016). American Society for Metabolic and Bariatric Surgery position statement on vagal blocking therapy for obesity. *Surgery for Obesity and Related Diseases, 12*(3), 460–461.

Perreault, L. (2020). Obesity in adults: Prevalence, screening, and evaluation. *UpToDate.* Retrieved on 8/12/2020 at: www.uptodate.com/contents/obesity-in-adults-prevalence-screening-and-evaluation

Petcu, A. (2017). Comprehensive care for bariatric surgery patients. *AACN Advanced Critical Care, 28*(3), 263–274.

Radosevich, J. J., Patanwala, A. E., & Erstad, B. L. (2016). Norepinephrine dosing in obese and nonobese patients with septic shock. *American Journal of Critical Care: An Official Publication, American Association of Critical-Care Nurses, 25*(1), 27–32.

*Rambod, M., Ghodsbin, F., & Moradi, A. (2020). The association between body mass index and comorbidity, quality of life, and cognitive function in the elderly population. *International Journal of Community Based Nursing and Midwifery (IJCBNM), 8*(1), 45–54.

*Robstad, N., Westergren, T., Siebler, F., et al. (2019). Intensive care nurses' implicit and explicit attitudes and their behavioural intentions towards obese intensive care patients. *Journal of Advanced Nursing, 75*(12), 3631–3642.

Rohde, K., Keller, M., la Cour Poulsen, L., et al. (2019). Genetics and epigenetics in obesity. *Metabolism: Clinical and Experimental, 92*, 37–50.

Ruiz-Cota, P., Bacardí-Gascón, M., & Jiménez-Cruz, A. (2019). Long-term outcomes of metabolic and bariatric surgery in adolescents with severe obesity with a follow-up of at least 5 years: A systematic review. *Surgery for Obesity and Related Diseases, 15*(1), 133–144.

Saunders, K. H., Umashanker, D., Igel, L. I., et al. (2018). Obesity pharmacotherapy. *Medical Clinics of North America, 102*(1), 135–148.

Shanti, H., & Patel, A. G. (2019). Surgery for obesity. *Medicine, 47*(3), 184–187.

Shiozawa, B., Madsen, C., Banaag, A., et al. (2019). Body mass index effect on health service utilization among active duty male United States Army soldiers. *Military Medicine, 184*(9–10), 447–453.

Smigelski-Theiss, R., Gampong, M., & Kurasaki, J. (2017). Weight bias and psychosocial implications for acute care of patients with obesity. *AACN Advanced Critical Care, 28*(3), 254–262.

Spike, J. P. (2018). Obesity, pressure ulcers, and family enablers. *The American Journal of Bioethics, 18*(7), 81–82.

Tamara, A., & Tahapary, D. L. (2020). Obesity as a predictor for a poor prognosis of COVID-19: A systematic review. *Diabetes & Metabolic Syndrome: Clinical Research & Reviews, 14*(4), 655–659.

*Tarlov, E., Zenk, S. N., Matthews, S. A., et al. (2017). Neighborhood resources to support healthy diets and physical activity among US military veterans. *Preventing Chronic Disease: Public Health Research, Practice, and Policy, 14*, E111.

Thorn, G., & Lean, M. (2017). Is there an optimal diet for weight management and metabolic health? *Gastroenterology, 152*(7), 1739–1751.

Trust for America's Health (TFAH) & Robert Wood Johnson Foundation (RWJF). (2018). The state of obesity 2018: Better policies for a healthier America. Retrieved on 12/17/2019 at: www.tfah.org/report-details/the-state-of-obesity-2018

Tsai, C., Zehetner, J., Beel, J., et al. (2019). Long-term outcomes and frequency of reoperative bariatric surgery beyond 15 years after gastric banding: A high band failure rate with safe revisions. *Surgery for Obesity and Related Diseases, 15*(6), 900–907.

U.S. Department of Defense (DoD). (2019). 2018 health of the DoD force: Obesity. *Medical Surveillance Monthly Report, 26*(8), 13–22.

VA/DoD Clinical Practice Guideline. (2020). Medications and their affects on weight. Retrieved on 3/7/2021 at: www.healthquality.va.gov/guidelines/CD/obesity/MedsEffectsWeightProviderTool-FINAL50817Dec2020.pdf

Vairavamurthy, J., Cheskin, L. J., Kraitchman, D. L., et al. (2017). Current and cutting-edge interventions for the treatment of obese patients. *European Journal of Radiology, 93*, 134–142.

Wadden, T. A., Tsai, A. G., & Tronieri, J. S. (2019). A protocol to deliver intensive behavioral therapy (IBT) for obesity in primary care settings: The MODEL-IBT program. *Obesity, 27*(10), 1562–1566.

Warren, M., Beck, S., & Rayburn, J. (2018). The state of obesity 2018: Better policies for a healthier America. Retrieved on 7/29/2019 at: www.tfah.org/report-details/the-state-of-obesity-2018

Welcome, A. (2017). Medications that may increase weight. Retrieved on 5/1/2020 at: www.obesitymedicine.org/medications-that-cause-weight-gain

Williamson, K. (2020). Nursing people with bariatric care needs: More questions than answers. *Wounds UK, 16*(1), 64–71.

World Health Organization (WHO). (2017). 10 facts on obesity. Retrieved on 12/15/2019 at: www.who.int/features/factfiles/obesity/en

World Health Organization (WHO). (2018). Obesity and overweight: Fact sheet. Retrieved on 7/29/2019 at: www.who.int/en/news-room/fact-sheets/detail/obesity-and-overweight

*Wu, Y. K., & Berry, D. C. (2018). Impact of weight stigma on physiological and psychological health outcomes for overweight and obese adults: A systematic review. *Journal of Advanced Nursing, 74*(5), 1030–1042.

Yengo, L., Sidorenko, J., Kemper, K. E., et al. (2018). Meta-analysis of genome-wide association studies for height and body mass index in ~700000 individuals of European ancestry. *Human Molecular Genetics, 27*(20), 3641–3649.

Zhou, W., Kozikowski, A., Pekmezaris, R. et al. (2017). Association between weight change, health outcomes, and mortality in older residents in long-term care. *Southern Medical Journal, 110*(7), 459–465.

Resources

American Society for Metabolic and Bariatric Surgery (ASMBS), www.asmbs.org

Centers for Disease Control and Prevention (CDC), www.cdc.gov/obesity

DASH Diet for Healthy Eating, www.dashdiet.org

National Heart, Lung, and Blood Institute of the National Institutes of Health, Aim for a Healthy Weight, www.nhlbi.nih.gov/health/educational/lose_wt/index.htm

National Institute of Diabetes and Digestive and Kidney Diseases, Weight Management, www.niddk.nih.gov/health-information/weight-management

Obesity Action Coalition, www.obesityaction.org

Obesity Medicine Association, www.obesitymedicine.org

The Obesity Society (TOS), www.obesity.org

Uconn Rudd Center for Food Policy and Obesity, www.uconnruddcenter.org

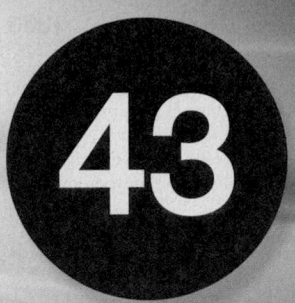

43

Assessment and Management of Patients with Hepatic Disorders

Liver function is complex, and hepatic dysfunction affects all body systems. For this reason, the nurse must understand how the liver functions and must have expert clinical assessment and management skills to care for patients undergoing diagnostic and treatment procedures. The nurse also must have an understanding of technologic advances in the management of hepatic disorders. Liver disorders are common and may result from a virus, obesity, insulin resistance, or exposure to toxic substances, such as alcohol, or tumors (Norris, 2019).

ASSESSMENT OF THE LIVER

Anatomic and Physiologic Overview

The liver, the largest gland of the body and a major organ, can be considered a chemical factory that manufactures, stores, alters, and excretes a large number of substances involved in metabolism (Hammer & McPhee, 2019; Sanyal, Boyer, Terrault, et al., 2018). The location of the liver is essential because it receives nutrient-rich blood directly from the gastrointestinal (GI) tract and then either stores or transforms these nutrients into chemicals that are used elsewhere in the body for metabolic needs. The liver is especially important in the regulation of glucose and protein metabolism. The liver manufactures and secretes bile, which has a major role in the digestion and absorption of fats in the GI tract. The liver removes waste products from the bloodstream and secretes them into the bile. The bile produced by the liver is stored temporarily in the gallbladder until it is needed for digestion, at which time the gallbladder empties and bile enters the intestine (see Fig. 43-1).

Anatomy of the Liver

The liver is a large, highly vascular organ located behind the ribs in the upper right portion of the abdominal cavity. It weighs between 1200 and 1500 g in the average adult and is divided into four lobes. A thin layer of connective tissue surrounds each lobe, extending into the lobe itself and dividing the liver mass into small, functional units called *lobules* (Barrett, Barman, Brooks, et al., 2019; Hammer & McPhee, 2019).

The circulation of the blood into and out of the liver is of major importance to liver function. The blood that perfuses the liver comes from two sources. Approximately 80% of the blood supply comes from the portal vein, which drains the GI tract and is rich in nutrients but lacks oxygen. The remainder of the blood supply enters by way of the hepatic artery and is rich in oxygen. Terminal branches of these two blood vessels join to form common capillary beds, which constitute the sinusoids of the liver (see Fig. 43-2). Thus, a mixture of venous and arterial blood bathes the hepatocytes (liver cells). The sinusoids empty into venules that occupy the center of each liver lobule and are called the *central veins*. The central veins join to form the hepatic vein, which constitutes the venous drainage from the liver and empties into the inferior vena cava, close to the diaphragm (Barrett et al., 2019; Hammer & McPhee, 2019; Sanyal et al., 2018).

In addition to hepatocytes, phagocytic cells belonging to the reticuloendothelial system are present in the liver. Other organs that contain reticuloendothelial cells are the spleen, bone marrow, lymph nodes, and lungs. In the liver, these cells are called *Kupffer cells* (Barrett et al., 2019; Hammer & McPhee, 2019). As the most common phagocyte in the human body, their main function is to engulf particulate matter (e.g., bacteria) that enters the liver through the portal blood.

The smallest bile ducts, called *canaliculi*, are located between the lobules of the liver. The canaliculi receive secretions from the hepatocytes and carry them to larger bile ducts, which eventually form the hepatic duct. The hepatic duct from the liver and the cystic duct from the gallbladder join to form the common bile duct, which empties into the small intestine. The sphincter of Oddi, located at the junction

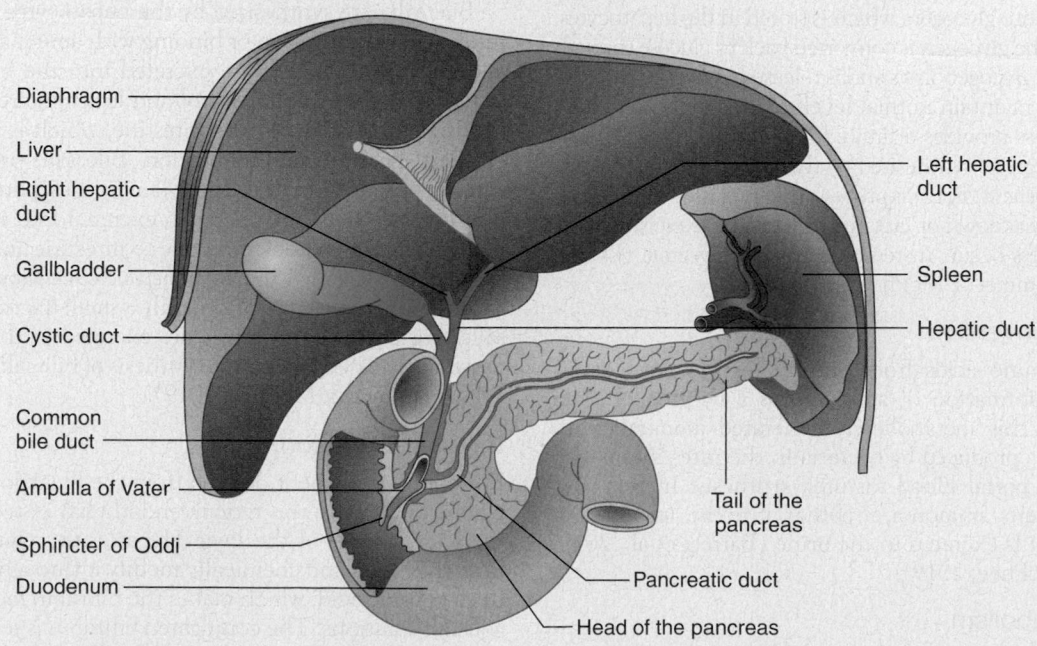

Diaphragm
Liver
Right hepatic duct
Gallbladder
Cystic duct
Common bile duct
Ampulla of Vater
Sphincter of Oddi
Duodenum

Left hepatic duct
Spleen
Hepatic duct
Tail of the pancreas
Pancreatic duct
Head of the pancreas

Figure 43-1 • The liver and biliary system, including the gallbladder and bile ducts. Reprinted with permission from Norris, T. L. (2019). *Porth's pathophysiology: Concepts of altered health states* (10th ed., Fig. 38.1). Philadelphia, PA: Wolters Kluwer.

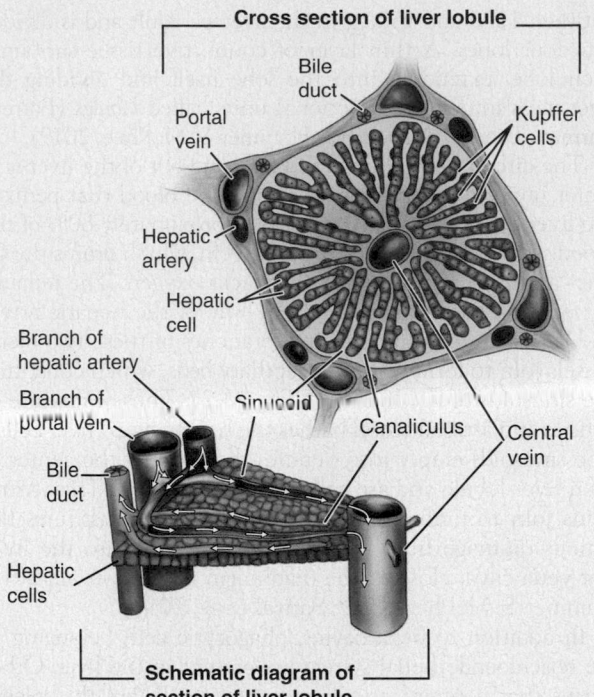

Cross section of liver lobule

Bile duct
Portal vein
Kupffer cells
Hepatic artery
Hepatic cell
Branch of hepatic artery
Branch of portal vein
Sinusoid
Canaliculus
Central vein
Bile duct
Hepatic cells

Schematic diagram of section of liver lobule

Figure 43-2 • A section of liver lobule showing the location of hepatic veins, hepatic cells, liver sinusoids, and branches of the portal vein and hepatic artery.

where the common bile duct enters the duodenum, controls the flow of bile into the intestine.

Functions of the Liver

Glucose Metabolism

The liver plays a major role in the metabolism of glucose and the regulation of blood glucose concentration. After a meal, glucose is taken up from the portal venous blood by the liver and converted into glycogen, which is stored in the hepatocytes. Subsequently, the glycogen is converted back to glucose through a process called glycogenolysis and is released as needed into the bloodstream to maintain normal levels of blood glucose. However, this process provides a limited amount of glucose. Additional glucose can be synthesized by the liver through a process called *gluconeogenesis*. For this process, the liver uses amino acids from protein breakdown or lactate produced by exercising muscles. This process occurs in response to hypoglycemia (Barrett et al., 2019; Hammer & McPhee, 2019).

Ammonia Conversion

The use of amino acids from protein for gluconeogenesis results in the formation of ammonia as a by-product. The liver converts this metabolically generated ammonia into urea. Ammonia produced by bacteria in the intestines is also removed from portal blood for urea synthesis. In this way, the liver converts ammonia, a potential toxin, into urea, a compound that is excreted in the urine (Barrett et al., 2019; Hammer & McPhee, 2019).

Protein Metabolism

The liver also plays an important role in protein metabolism. It synthesizes almost all of the plasma proteins (except gamma-globulin), including albumin, alpha-globulins and beta-globulins, blood clotting factors, specific transport proteins, and most of the plasma lipoproteins. Vitamin K is required by the liver for synthesis of prothrombin and some of the other clotting factors. Amino acids are used by the liver for protein synthesis (Barrett et al., 2019; Hammer & McPhee, 2019).

Fat Metabolism

The liver is also active in fat metabolism. Fatty acids can be broken down for the production of energy and ketone bodies (acetoacetic acid, beta-hydroxybutyric acid, and acetone). Ketone bodies are small compounds that can enter the bloodstream and provide a source of energy for muscles and other tissues. Breakdown of fatty acids into ketone bodies occurs primarily when the availability of glucose for metabolism is limited, as in starvation or in uncontrolled diabetes. Fatty acids and their metabolic products are also used for the synthesis of cholesterol, lecithin, lipoproteins, and other complex lipids (Hammer & McPhee, 2019; Sanyal et al., 2018).

Vitamin and Iron Storage

Vitamins A, B, and D and several of the B-complex vitamins are stored in large amounts in the liver. Certain substances, such as iron and copper, are also stored in the liver.

Bile Formation

Bile is continuously formed by the hepatocytes and collected in the canaliculi and bile ducts. It is composed mainly of water and electrolytes such as sodium, potassium, calcium, chloride, and bicarbonate, and it also contains significant amounts of lecithin, fatty acids, cholesterol, bilirubin, and bile salts. Bile is collected and stored in the gallbladder and is emptied into the intestine as needed for digestion. The functions of bile are excretory, as in the excretion of bilirubin; bile also serves as an aid to digestion through the emulsification of fats by bile salts.

Bile salts are synthesized by the hepatocytes from cholesterol. After conjugation or binding with amino acids (taurine and glycine), bile salts are excreted into the bile. The bile salts, together with cholesterol and lecithin, are required for emulsification of fats in the intestine, which is necessary for efficient digestion and absorption. Bile salts are then reabsorbed, primarily in the distal ileum, into portal blood for return to the liver and are again excreted into the bile. This pathway from hepatocytes to bile to intestine and back to the hepatocytes is called the *enterohepatic circulation*. Because of the enterohepatic circulation, only a small fraction of the bile salts that enter the intestine are excreted in the feces. This decreases the need for active synthesis of bile salts by the liver cells (Hammer & McPhee, 2019).

Bilirubin Excretion

Bilirubin is a pigment derived from the breakdown of hemoglobin by cells of the reticuloendothelial system, including the Kupffer cells of the liver. Hepatocytes remove bilirubin from the blood and chemically modify it through conjugation to glucuronic acid, which makes the bilirubin more soluble in aqueous solutions. The conjugated bilirubin is secreted by the hepatocytes into the adjacent bile canaliculi and is eventually carried in the bile into the duodenum.

In the small intestine, bilirubin is converted into urobilinogen, which is partially excreted in the feces and partially absorbed through the intestinal mucosa into the portal blood. Much of this reabsorbed urobilinogen is removed by the hepatocytes and secreted into the bile once again (enterohepatic circulation). Some of the urobilinogen enters the systemic circulation and is excreted by the kidneys in the urine. Elimination of bilirubin in the bile represents the major route of its excretion.

Drug Metabolism

The liver metabolizes many medications, such as barbiturates, opioids, sedatives, anesthetics, and amphetamines (Goldman & Schafer, 2019; Hammer & McPhee, 2019; Sanyal et al., 2018). Metabolism generally results in drug inactivation, although activation may also occur. One of the important pathways for medication metabolism involves conjugation (binding) of the medication with a variety of compounds, such as glucuronic acid or acetic acid, to form more soluble substances. These substances may be excreted in the feces or urine, similar to bilirubin excretion. Bioavailability is the fraction of the given medication that actually reaches the systemic circulation. The bioavailability of an oral medication (absorbed from the GI tract) can be decreased if the medication is metabolized to a great extent by the liver before it reaches the systemic circulation; this is known as first-pass effect. Some medications have such a large first-pass effect that their use is essentially limited to the parenteral route, or oral doses must be substantially larger than parenteral doses to achieve the same effect.

Gerontologic Considerations

Chart 43-1 summarizes age-related changes in the liver. In the older adult, the most common change in the liver is a decrease in size and weight, accompanied by a decrease in total hepatic blood flow. However, in general, these decreases are proportional to the decreases in body size and weight seen in normal aging. Results of liver function tests do not normally change with age; abnormal results in older patients indicate abnormal liver function and are not a result of the aging process itself.

Metabolism of medications by the liver decreases in the older adult, but such changes are usually accompanied by changes in intestinal absorption, renal excretion, and altered body distribution of some medications secondary to changes in fat deposition. These alterations necessitate careful medication administration and monitoring; if appropriate, reduced dosages may be needed to prevent medication toxicity.

Assessment

Health History

If liver function test results are abnormal, the patient is evaluated for liver disease. In such cases, the health history focuses on previous exposure of the patient to hepatotoxic substances or infectious agents. The patient's occupational, recreational, and travel history may assist in identifying exposure to hepatotoxins (e.g., industrial chemicals, other toxins). The patient's history of alcohol and drug use, including but not limited to the use of intravenous (IV) or injection drugs, provides additional information about exposure to toxins and infectious agents. Many medications (including acetaminophen, ketoconazole, and valproic acid) are responsible for hepatic dysfunction and disease (Friedman & Martin, 2018). A thorough medication history should address all current and past prescription medications, over-the-counter (OTC) medications, herbal remedies, illicit drugs, and dietary supplements.

Lifestyle behaviors that increase the risk of exposure to infectious agents are identified. IV or injection drug use, sexual practices, and foreign travel are all potential risk factors for liver disease. The amount and type of alcohol consumed are identified using screening tools (questionnaires) that have been developed for this purpose (see Chapter 4). The amount of alcohol required to produce chronic liver disease varies widely, but men who consume 60 to 80 g/day of alcohol (approximately four glasses of beer, wine, or mixed drinks) and women whose alcohol intake is 40 to 60 g/day are considered at high risk for cirrhosis. **Cirrhosis** is a chronic liver disorder characterized by fibrotic changes, the formation of dense connective tissue within the liver, subsequent degenerative changes, and loss of functional liver tissue (Barrett et al., 2019; Sanyal et al., 2018).

The history also includes an evaluation of the patient's past medical history to identify risk factors for the development of liver disease. Current and past medical conditions, including those of a psychological or psychiatric nature, are identified. The family history includes questions about familial liver disorders that may have their origin in alcohol abuse or gallstone disease, as well as other familial or genetic disorders (see Chart 43-2).

The history also addresses symptoms that suggest liver disease. Symptoms that may have their origin in liver disease but are not specific to hepatic dysfunction include jaundice, malaise, weakness, fatigue, pruritus, abdominal pain, fever, anorexia, weight gain, edema, increasing abdominal girth, hematemesis, melena, hematochezia (passage of bloody stools), easy bruising, changes in mental acuity, personality changes, sleep disturbances, and decreased libido in men and secondary amenorrhea in women.

Chart 43-1

Age-Related Changes of the Hepatobiliary System

- Atypical clinical presentation of biliary disease
- Decreases in the following:
  - Clearance of hepatitis B surface antigen
  - Drug metabolism and clearance capabilities
  - Intestinal and portal vein blood flow
  - Gallbladder contraction after a meal
  - Rate of replacement and or repair of liver cells after injury
  - Size and weight of the liver, particularly in women
- Increased prevalence of gallstones due to the increase in cholesterol secretion in bile
- More rapid progression of hepatitis C infection and lower response rate to therapy
- More severe complications of biliary tract disease

Adapted from Townsend, C. M., Beauchamp, R. D., Evers, B. M., et al. (2016). *Sabiston's textbook of surgery: The biological basis of modern surgical practice.* Philadelphia, PA: Elsevier.

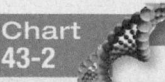

Chart 43-2 GENETICS IN NURSING PRACTICE
Hepatic Disorders

A number of hepatic disorders have an underlying genetic cause. However, other genetic disorders associated with metabolic, gastrointestinal, or bleeding disorders will also impact the function of the liver. Some examples of hepatic disorders caused by genetic abnormalities include:

Autosomal Dominant:
- Alagille syndrome
- Hereditary coproporphyria
- Polycystic liver disease

Autosomal Recessive:
- Crigler–Najjar syndrome
- Dublin–Johnson syndrome
- Hemochromatosis
- Progressive familial intrahepatic cholestasis
- Thalassemia
- Wilson disease

Inheritance Pattern is not distinct; however, there is a genetic predisposition for the disorder:
- Biliary atresia
- Gilbert syndrome

Other genetic disorders that impact the hepatic system:
- Alpha-1 antitrypsin deficiency
- Cystic fibrosis
- Glycogen storage disease
- Lysosomal storage disease
- Polycystic kidney disease
- Zellweger syndrome

Nursing Assessments

Refer to Chapter 4, Chart 4-2: Genetics in Nursing Practice: Genetic Aspects of Health Assessment

Family History Assessment Related to Hepatic Disorders

- Collect family history for three generations of maternal and paternal relatives in the patient's family
- Assess family history for relatives with early-onset hepatic disease

Patient Assessment Related to Genetic Hepatic Disorders

- Assess for physical signs or history of the following:
  - Abdominal bloating, and constipation
  - Changes to skin color or yellow hue to sclera
  - Enlarged liver, spleen, or abdomen
  - Episodes of nausea and vomiting
  - Hemorrhoids, esophageal varices, or gallstones
  - Intolerance to fatty foods or alcohol
  - Pale-colored stools
  - Presence and frequency of indigestion or reflux
  - Unexplained weight loss
- Assess for associated nervous system disorders such as depression and mood changes especially anger and irritability (Wilson disease).
- Assess for associated blood sugar problems such as hypoglycemia
- Inquire about and assess for abnormal bleeding or bruising
- Obtain and review laboratory values: Liver function tests, ammonia, bilirubin, fat soluble vitamins (e.g., vitamins A, D, E, K)

Genetics Resources

American Liver Foundation, www.liverfoundation.org
See Chapter 6, Chart 6-7 for components of genetic counseling.

Physical Assessment

The nurse assesses the patient for physical signs that may occur with liver dysfunction, including the pallor often seen with chronic illness and jaundice. The skin, mucosa, and sclerae are inspected for jaundice, and the extremities are assessed for muscle atrophy, edema, and skin excoriation secondary to scratching. The nurse observes the skin for petechiae or ecchymotic areas (bruises), spider angiomas (see Fig. 43-3), and palmar erythema. The male patient is assessed for unilateral or bilateral gynecomastia and testicular atrophy due to hormonal changes. The patient's cognitive status (recall, memory, abstract thinking) and neurologic status are assessed. The nurse observes for general tremor, **asterixis** (involuntary flapping movements of the hands), weakness, and slurred speech. These symptoms are discussed later.

In some conditions, lipids may accumulate in the hepatocytes, resulting in the abnormal condition called *fatty liver disease*. If unrelated to alcohol, this disease is referred to as nonalcoholic fatty liver disease (NAFLD). A condition known as nonalcoholic steatohepatitis (NASH) represents a more serious condition within the broad spectrum of NAFLDs and may result in damage, fibrotic changes in the liver, and cirrhosis (Hammer & McPhee, 2019).

NAFLD and NASH are two diseases within the spectrum of fatty liver disease to fibrosis and cirrhosis that are strongly associated with obesity (Barrett et al., 2019). Some studies suggest that being overweight and drinking too much alcohol can cause severe harm to the liver. People who are overweight and people with obesity who are heavy drinkers have a significantly increased risk of developing and dying of chronic liver disease (Bellentani, 2017; Friedman & Martin, 2018; Schiff, Maddrey, & Reddy, 2018). Studies have also identified that there is an increased risk of liver cancer in people with alcoholic cirrhosis who also have fatty liver

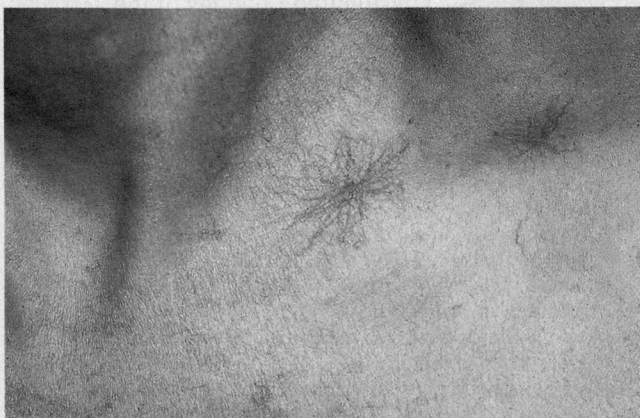

Figure 43-3 • Spider angioma. This vascular (arterial) spider appears on the skin. Beneath the elevated center and radiating branches, the blood vessels are looped and tortuous.

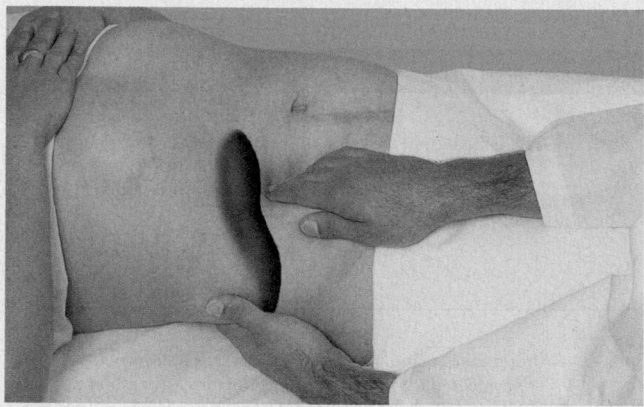

Figure 43-4 • Technique for palpating the liver. The examiner places one hand under the right lower rib cage and presses downward during inspiration with light pressure with the other hand. Reprinted with permission from Bickley, L. S. (2017). *Bates' guide to physical examination and history taking* (12th ed.). Philadelphia, PA: Lippincott Williams & Wilkins.

disease, type 2 diabetes, and are overweight or have obesity (Bellentani, 2017; Schiff et al., 2018). In patients who are overweight, have obesity, or have high alcohol intake, the nurse observes for signs of associated liver dysfunction.

The nurse assesses for the presence of an abdominal fluid wave (discussed later). The abdomen is palpated to assess liver size and to detect any tenderness over the liver. The liver may be palpable in the right upper quadrant. A palpable liver presents as a firm, sharp ridge with a smooth surface (see Fig. 43-4). The nurse estimates the size of the liver by percussing its upper and lower borders. If the liver is not palpable but tenderness is suspected, tapping the lower right thorax briskly may elicit tenderness. For comparison, the nurse then performs a similar maneuver on the left lower thorax.

If the liver is palpable, the nurse notes and records its size, its consistency, any tenderness, and whether its outline is regular or irregular. If the liver is enlarged, the degree to which it descends below the right costal margin is recorded to provide some indication of its size. The nurse determines whether the liver's edge is sharp and smooth or blunt and whether the enlarged liver is nodular or smooth. The liver of a patient with cirrhosis is small and hard in late-stage cirrhosis, whereas the liver of a patient with acute hepatitis is soft and the hand easily moves the edge.

Tenderness of the liver indicates recent acute enlargement with consequent stretching of the liver capsule. The absence of tenderness may imply that the enlargement is of longstanding duration. The liver of a patient with viral hepatitis is tender, whereas that of a patient with alcoholic hepatitis is not. Enlargement of the liver is an abnormal finding that requires evaluation (Hammer & McPhee, 2019).

Diagnostic Evaluation

A wide range of diagnostic studies may be performed in patients with hepatic disorders. The nurse should educate the patient about the purpose, what to expect, and any possible side effects related to these examinations prior to testing. The nurse should note trends in results because they provide information about disease progression as well as the patient's response to therapy.

Liver Function Tests

More than 70% of the parenchyma of the liver may be damaged before liver function test results become abnormal. Function is generally measured in terms of serum enzyme activity (i.e., serum aminotransferases, alkaline phosphatase, lactic dehydrogenase) and serum concentrations of proteins (albumin and globulins), bilirubin, ammonia, clotting factors, and lipids (Hammer & McPhee, 2019; Mansour & McPherson, 2018; Sanyal et al., 2018; Wendon, Cordoba, Dhawan, et al., 2017). Several of these tests may be helpful for assessing patients with liver disease. However, the nature and extent of hepatic dysfunction cannot be determined by these tests alone, because other disorders can affect test results.

Serum aminotransferases are sensitive indicators of injury to the liver cells and are useful in detecting acute liver disease such as hepatitis. Alanine aminotransferase (ALT), aspartate aminotransferase (AST), and gamma-glutamyl transferase (GGT) (also called gamma-glutamyl transpeptidase [GGTP]) are the most frequently used tests of liver damage (Friedman & Martin, 2018; Maher & Schreibman, 2018; Schiff et al., 2018). ALT levels increase primarily in liver disorders and may be used to monitor the course of hepatitis or cirrhosis or the effects of treatments that may be toxic to the liver. AST is present in tissues that have high metabolic activity; therefore, the level may be increased if there is damage to or death of tissues of organs such as the heart, liver, skeletal muscle, and kidney. Although not specific to liver disease, levels of AST may be increased in cirrhosis, hepatitis, and liver cancer. Increased GGT levels are associated with cholestasis but can also be due to alcoholic liver disease. Although the kidney has the highest level of the enzyme, the liver is considered the source of normal serum activity. The test determines liver cell dysfunction and is a sensitive indicator of cholestasis. Its main value in liver disease is confirming the hepatic origin of an elevated alkaline phosphatase level. Common liver function tests are summarized in Table 43-1, additional laboratory values can be found in Appendix A on thePoint.

Liver Biopsy

Liver biopsy is the removal of a small amount of liver tissue, usually through needle aspiration. It permits examination of liver cells. The most common indication is to evaluate diffuse disorders of the parenchyma and to diagnose space-occupying lesions. Liver biopsy is especially useful when clinical findings and laboratory tests are not diagnostic. Though rare due to the radiologic guidance now available, peritonitis caused by blood or bile after liver biopsy is the most common complication; therefore, coagulation studies are obtained, their values are noted, and abnormal results are treated before liver biopsy is performed (Schiff et al., 2018). Other techniques for liver biopsy are preferred if **ascites** (an accumulation of albumin-rich fluid in the peritoneal cavity) or coagulation abnormalities exist. A liver biopsy can be performed percutaneously with ultrasound guidance or transvenously through the right internal jugular vein to right hepatic vein under fluoroscopic control. Liver biopsy can also be performed laparoscopically.

TABLE 43-1	Common Laboratory Tests to Assess Liver Function	
Test	**Normal**	**Clinical Functions**
Pigment Studies		These studies measure the ability of the liver to conjugate and excrete bilirubin. Results are abnormal in liver and biliary tract disease and are associated with jaundice clinically.
Serum bilirubin, direct	0.1–0.4 mg/dL (1.7–3.7 mcmol/L)	
Serum bilirubin, total	0.3–1 mg/dL (5–17 mcmol/L)	
Urine bilirubin	<0.25 mg/24 h (<0.42 mcmol/L)	
Urine urobilinogen	(Urine urobilinogen) 0.05–2.5 mg/24 h (0.5–4 Ehrlich U/24 h)	
Fecal urobilinogen (infrequently used)	(Fecal urobilinogen) 50–300 mg/24 h (100–400 Ehrlich U/100 g)	
Protein Studies		Proteins are manufactured by the liver. Their levels may be affected in a variety of liver impairments: albumin is affected in cirrhosis, chronic hepatitis, edema; and ascites; globulins are affected in cirrhosis, liver disease, chronic obstructive jaundice, and viral hepatitis.
Total serum protein	7–7.5 g/dL (70–75 g/L)	
Serum albumin	3.5–5.2 g/dL (35–52 g/L)	
Serum globulin	2.3–3.5 g/dL (23–35 g/L)	
Serum protein electrophoresis		
Albumin	3.5–5.2 g/dL (35–52 g/L)	
α_1-Globulin	0.1–0.3 g/dL (1–3 g/L)	
α_2-Globulin	0.6–1 g/dL (6–10 g/L)	
β-Globulin	0.5–1 g/dL (5–10 g/L)	
γ-Globulin	0.6–1.3 g/dL (6–13 g/L)	
A/G ratio	A > G or 1.5:1–2.5:1	A/G ratio is reversed in chronic liver disease (decreased albumin and increased globulin).
Prothrombin Time/International Normalized Ratio (PT/INR)	100% or 11–13 s/the INR is a calculation based on results of the PT. INR levels <1.1 are considered normal	Prothrombin time and INR may be prolonged in liver disease. It is an indicator of synthetic hepatic function. It will not return to normal with vitamin K in severe liver cell damage.
Serum Alkaline Phosphatase	Varies with method: *Adults:* 52–142 U/L	Serum alkaline phosphatase is manufactured in bones, liver, kidneys, and intestine and excreted through biliary tract. In the absence of bone disease, it is a sensitive measure of biliary tract obstruction. Results may vary because this test is temperature and lab method dependent.
Serum Aminotransferase Studies		The studies are based on release of enzymes from damaged liver cells. These enzymes are elevated in liver cell damage. Normal values may differ in men and women.
AST	10–40 U/mL (0.34–0.68 U/L)	
ALT	8–40 U/mL (0.14–0.68 U/L)	
GGT, GGTP	0–30 U/L IU/L	Values are elevated in alcohol abuse and markers for biliary cholestasis.
LDH	100–200 units (100–225 U/L)	
Ammonia (plasma)	15–45 mcg/dL (11–32 mcmol/L)	Liver converts ammonia to urea. Ammonia level rises in liver failure.
Cholesterol		Cholesterol levels are elevated in biliary obstruction and decreased in parenchymal liver disease.
Ester	60–70% of total cholesterol, fraction of total cholesterol 0.60–0.70	
HDL	*Male:* 35–70 mg/dL; *Female:* 35–85 mg/dL	
LDL	<130 mcg/dL	

A/G, albumin/globulin; ALT, alanine aminotransferase; AST, aspartate aminotransferase; GGT, gamma-glutamyl transferase; GGTP, gamma-glutamyl transpeptidase; HDL, high-density lipoprotein; LDH, lactate dehydrogenase; LDL, low-density lipoprotein.
Adapted from Fischbach, F., & Fischbach, M. (2018). *A manual of laboratory and diagnostic tests* (10th ed.). Philadelphia, PA: Wolters Kluwer.

 For the procedural guidelines for assisting with percutaneous liver biopsy, go to **thepoint.lww.com/Brunner15e**.

Other Diagnostic Tests

Ultrasonography, computed tomography (CT) scans, and magnetic resonance imaging (MRI) are used to identify normal structures and abnormalities of the liver and biliary tree. A radioisotope liver scan may be performed to assess liver size, blood flow, and obstruction. Noninvasive liver stiffness measurements or elastography uses ultrasound-based vibration and scanning to identify liver fibrosis and determine its extent. Magnetic resonance elastography uses mechanical shear waves to identify stiff tissue (Schiff et al., 2018). Liver fibrosis and other liver diseases can be identified, evaluated and monitored with a variety of other noninvasive studies. These studies may reduce the need for liver biopsy (Friedman & Martin, 2018; Schiff et al., 2018).

Laparoscopy (insertion of a fiberoptic endoscope through a small abdominal incision) is used to examine the liver and other pelvic structures. It is also used to perform guided liver biopsy, to determine the cause of ascites, and to diagnose and stage tumors of the liver and other abdominal organs.

MANIFESTATIONS OF HEPATIC DYSFUNCTION

Hepatic dysfunction results from damage to the liver's parenchymal cells, directly from primary liver diseases, or indirectly from either obstruction of bile flow or derangements of hepatic circulation. Liver dysfunction may be acute or chronic; the latter is far more common.

Chronic liver disease, including cirrhosis, is the 12th leading cause of death in the United States among young and middle-aged adults (Schiff et al., 2018). At least 40% of those deaths are associated with alcohol use. The rate of chronic liver disease for men is twice that for women, and chronic liver disease is more common in Asian and African countries than it is in Europe and the United States. Compensated cirrhosis, in which the damaged liver is still able to perform normal functions, often goes undetected for extended periods, and as many as 1% of people may have subclinical or compensated cirrhosis (Bope & Kellerman, 2018; Schiff et al., 2018). Approximately 80% of patients diagnosed with cirrhosis compensate and remain asymptomatic for the next 10 years (Schiff et al., 2018).

Disease processes that lead to hepatocellular dysfunction may be caused by infectious agents such as bacteria and viruses and by anoxia, metabolic disorders, toxins and medications, nutritional deficiencies, and hypersensitivity states. The most common cause of parenchymal damage is malnutrition, especially that related to alcoholism (Moon, Singal, & Tapper, 2018). It is important to remember that even patients who are overweight or have obesity may suffer from not only malnutrition related to liver disease, but also from sarcopenia, the significant loss of muscle tissue. Sarcopenia is associated with increased morbidity and mortality in patients with end-stage liver disease (ESLD) (Aby & Saab, 2019).

The parenchymal cells respond to most noxious agents by replacing glycogen with lipids, producing fatty infiltration with or without cell death or necrosis. This is commonly associated with inflammatory cell infiltration and growth of fibrous tissue. Cell regeneration can occur if the disease process is not too toxic to the cells. The result of chronic parenchymal disease is the shrunken, fibrotic liver seen in cirrhosis.

The consequences of liver disease are numerous and varied. Their ultimate effects are often incapacitating or life-threatening, and their presence is ominous. Among the most common and significant manifestations of liver disease are jaundice, portal hypertension, ascites and varices, nutritional deficiencies (resulting from the inability of damaged liver cells to metabolize certain vitamins), and **hepatic encephalopathy** or coma.

Jaundice

The bilirubin concentration in the blood may be increased in the presence of liver disease, if the flow of bile is impeded (e.g., by gallstones in the bile ducts), or if there is excessive destruction of red blood cells. With bile duct obstruction, bilirubin does not enter the intestine; as a consequence, urobilinogen is absent from the urine and decreased in the stool (Hammer & McPhee, 2019).

When the bilirubin concentration in the blood is abnormally elevated, all of the body tissues, including the sclerae and the skin, become tinged yellow or greenish-yellow, a condition known as **jaundice**. Jaundice becomes clinically evident when the serum bilirubin level exceeds 2.0 mg/dL (34 mmol/L) (Hammer & McPhee, 2019). Increased serum bilirubin levels and jaundice may result from impairment of hepatic uptake, conjugation of bilirubin, or excretion of bilirubin into the biliary system. There are several types of jaundice: hemolytic, hepatocellular, and obstructive jaundice, and jaundice due to hereditary hyperbilirubinemia. Hepatocellular and obstructive jaundice are the two types commonly associated with liver disease.

Hemolytic Jaundice

Hemolytic jaundice is the result of an increased destruction of the red blood cells; the effect is that the plasma is rapidly flooded with bilirubin so that the liver, although functioning normally, cannot excrete the bilirubin as quickly as it is formed. This type of jaundice is encountered in patients with hemolytic transfusion reactions and other hemolytic disorders. In these patients, the bilirubin in the blood is predominantly unconjugated or free. Fecal and urine urobilinogen levels are increased, but the urine is free of bilirubin. Patients with this type of jaundice, unless their hyperbilirubinemia is extreme, do not experience symptoms or complications as a result of the jaundice per se. However, prolonged jaundice, even if mild, predisposes to the formation of pigment stones in the gallbladder, and extremely severe jaundice (levels of free bilirubin exceeding 20 to 25 mg/dL) poses a risk for central nervous system effects (Goldman & Schafer, 2019).

Hepatocellular Jaundice

Hepatocellular jaundice is caused by the inability of damaged liver cells to clear normal amounts of bilirubin from the blood. The cellular damage may be caused by hepatitis viruses, other viruses that affect the liver (e.g., yellow fever virus, Epstein–Barr virus), chemical toxins (e.g., carbon tetrachloride, phosphorus, arsenicals, certain medications), or alcohol. Cirrhosis of the liver is a form of hepatocellular disease that may produce jaundice. It is usually associated with excessive alcohol intake, but it may also be a late result of liver cell necrosis caused by viral infection. In prolonged obstructive jaundice, cell damage eventually develops, and both types of jaundice (i.e., obstructive and hepatocellular jaundice) appear together.

Patients with hepatocellular jaundice may be mildly or severely ill, with lack of appetite, nausea, malaise, fatigue, weakness, and possible weight loss. In some cases of hepatocellular disease, jaundice may not be obvious. The serum bilirubin concentration and the urine urobilinogen level may be elevated. In addition, AST and ALT levels may be increased, indicating cellular necrosis. The patient may report headache, chills, and fever if the cause is infectious. Depending on the cause and extent of the liver cell damage, hepatocellular jaundice may be completely reversible.

Obstructive Jaundice

Obstructive jaundice resulting from extrahepatic obstruction may be caused by occlusion of the bile duct from a gallstone, an inflammatory process, a tumor, or pressure from an enlarged organ (e.g., liver, gallbladder). The obstruction may also involve the small bile ducts within the liver (i.e., intrahepatic obstruction); this may be caused, for example, by pressure on these channels from inflammatory swelling of the liver or by an inflammatory exudate within the ducts themselves. Intrahepatic obstruction resulting from stasis and inspissation (thickening) of bile within the canaliculi may occur after the ingestion of certain medications, which are referred to as cholestatic agents. These include phenothiazines, antithyroid medications, sulfonylureas, tricyclic antidepressant agents, nitrofurantoin, androgens and estrogens, and some antibiotics.

Regardless of whether the obstruction is intra- or extrahepatic, and regardless of its cause, bile cannot flow normally into the intestine and becomes backed up into the liver. It is then reabsorbed into the blood and carried throughout the entire body, staining the skin, mucous membranes, and sclerae. It is excreted in the urine, which becomes deep orange and foamy. Because of the decreased amount of bile in the intestinal tract, the stools become light or clay colored. The skin may itch intensely, requiring repeated soothing baths. Dyspepsia and intolerance to fatty foods may develop because of impaired fat digestion in the absence of intestinal bile. In general, AST, ALT, and GGT levels rise only moderately, but bilirubin and alkaline phosphatase levels are elevated.

Hereditary Hyperbilirubinemia

Hyperbilirubinemia (increased serum bilirubin levels), resulting from any of several inherited disorders, can also produce jaundice. Gilbert syndrome is a familial disorder characterized by an increased level of unconjugated bilirubin that causes jaundice. Although serum bilirubin levels are increased, liver histology and liver function test results are normal, and there is no hemolysis. This syndrome affects 3% to 8% of the population, predominantly males (Bope & Kellerman, 2018).

Other conditions that are probably caused by inborn errors of biliary metabolism include Dubin–Johnson syndrome (chronic idiopathic jaundice, with pigment in the liver) and Rotor syndrome (chronic familial conjugated hyperbilirubinemia, without pigment in the liver); the "benign" cholestatic jaundice of pregnancy, with retention of conjugated bilirubin, probably secondary to unusual sensitivity to the hormones of pregnancy; and benign recurrent intrahepatic cholestasis.

Portal Hypertension

Portal hypertension is the increased pressure throughout the portal venous system that results from obstruction of blood flow into and through the damaged liver. Commonly associated with hepatic cirrhosis, it can also occur with noncirrhotic liver disease. Although splenomegaly (enlarged spleen) with possible hypersplenism is a common manifestation of portal hypertension, the two major consequences of portal hypertension are ascites and varices (Friedman & Martin, 2018).

Ascites

Pathophysiology

The mechanisms responsible for the development of ascites are not completely understood. Portal hypertension and the

resulting increase in capillary pressure and obstruction of venous blood flow through the damaged liver are contributing factors. The vasodilation that occurs in the splanchnic circulation (the arterial supply and venous drainage of the GI system from the distal esophagus to the midrectum, including the liver and spleen) is also a suspected causative factor. The failure of the liver to metabolize aldosterone increases sodium and water retention by the kidney. Sodium and water retention, increased intravascular fluid volume, increased lymphatic flow, and decreased synthesis of albumin by the damaged liver all contribute to the movement of fluid from the vascular system into the peritoneal space. The process becomes self-perpetuating; loss of fluid into the peritoneal space causes further sodium and water retention by the kidney in an effort to maintain the vascular fluid volume.

As a result of liver damage, large amounts of albumin-rich fluid, 20 L or more, may accumulate in the peritoneal cavity as ascites (Hammer & McPhee, 2019; Mansour & McPherson, 2018). Ascites may also occur with disorders such as cancer, kidney disease, and heart failure. With the movement of albumin from the serum to the peritoneal cavity, the osmotic pressure of the serum decreases. This, combined with increased portal pressure, results in movement of fluid into the peritoneal cavity (see Fig. 43-5).

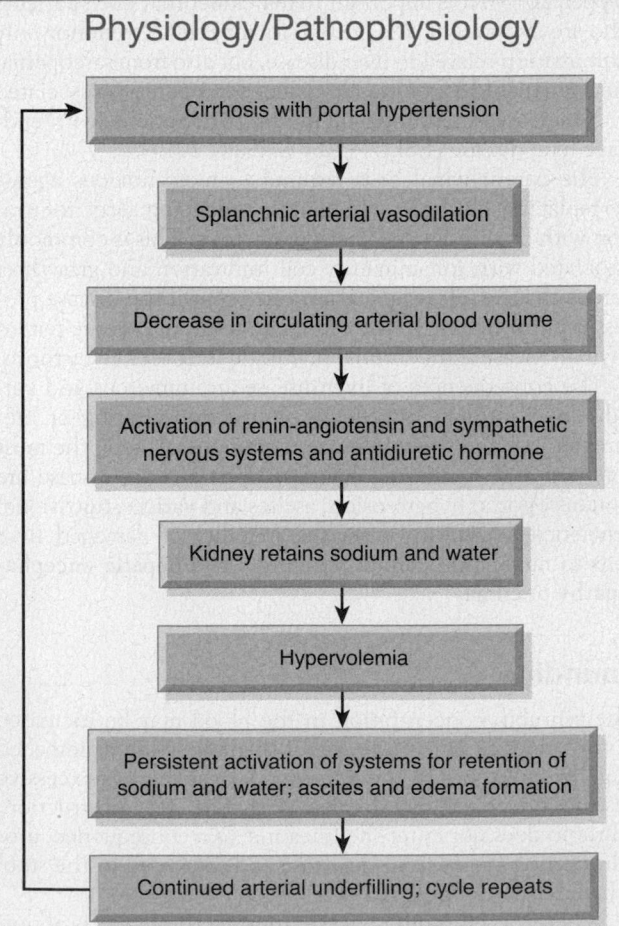

Physiology/Pathophysiology

Cirrhosis with portal hypertension

Splanchnic arterial vasodilation

Decrease in circulating arterial blood volume

Activation of renin-angiotensin and sympathetic nervous systems and antidiuretic hormone

Kidney retains sodium and water

Hypervolemia

Persistent activation of systems for retention of sodium and water; ascites and edema formation

Continued arterial underfilling; cycle repeats

Figure 43-5 • Pathogenesis of ascites (arterial vasodilation theory).

Clinical Manifestations

Increased abdominal girth and rapid weight gain are common presenting symptoms of ascites. The patient may be short of breath and uncomfortable from the enlarged abdomen; striae and distended veins may be visible over the abdominal wall. Umbilical hernias also occur frequently in those patients with cirrhosis. Fluid and electrolyte imbalances are common.

Assessment and Diagnostic Findings

The presence and extent of ascites are assessed by percussion of the abdomen. When fluid has accumulated in the peritoneal cavity, the flanks bulge when the patient assumes a supine position. The presence of fluid can be confirmed by percussing for shifting dullness or by detecting a fluid wave (see Fig. 43-6) (Weber & Kelley, 2018). A fluid wave is likely to be found only if a large amount of fluid is present (Hammer & McPhee, 2019). Daily measurement and recording of abdominal girth and body weight are essential to assess the progression of ascites and its response to treatment.

Medical Management

The medical management of the patient with ascites includes dietary modifications, pharmacologic therapy, bed rest, paracentesis, the use of shunts, and other therapies.

Nutritional Therapy

The goal of treatment for the patient with ascites is a negative sodium balance to reduce fluid retention. Table salt, salty foods, salted butter and margarine, and all canned and frozen foods that are not specifically prepared for low-sodium (2-g sodium) diets should be avoided (Hammer & McPhee, 2019; Simonetto, Liu, & Kamath, 2019). It may take 2 to

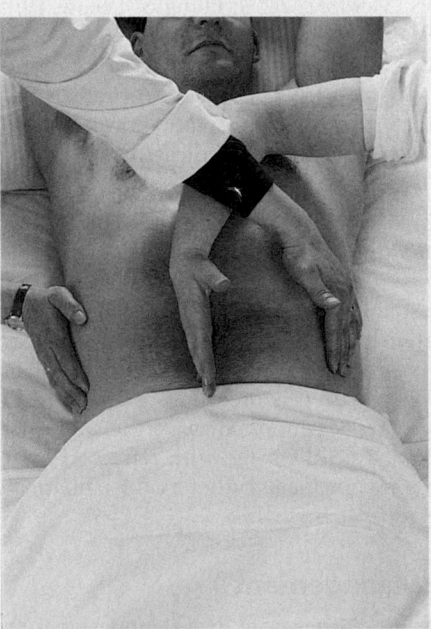

Figure 43-6 • Assessing for abdominal fluid wave. The examiner places the hands along the sides of the patient's flanks, then strikes one flank sharply, detecting any fluid wave with the other hand. An assistant's hand is placed (ulnar side down) along the patient's midline to prevent the fluid wave from being transmitted through the tissues of the abdominal wall.

3 months for the patient's taste buds to adjust to unsalted foods. In the meantime, the taste of unsalted foods can be improved by using salt substitutes such as lemon juice, oregano, and thyme. Commercial salt substitutes need to be approved by the patient's primary provider, because those that contain ammonia could precipitate hepatic encephalopathy and coma. Most salt substitutes contain potassium and should be avoided if the patient has impaired renal function. The patient should make liberal use of powdered, low-sodium milk and milk products. If fluid accumulation is not controlled with this regimen, the daily sodium allowance may be reduced further to 500 mg, and diuretic agents may be given. However, most patients will not accept such a severe sodium restriction as 500 mg, so clinicians often will not recommend it (Simonetto et al., 2019).

Dietary control of ascites via strict sodium restriction is difficult to achieve at home. The likelihood that the patient will follow a 2-g sodium diet increases if the patient and the person preparing meals understand the rationale for the diet and receive periodic guidance about selecting and preparing appropriate foods. Approximately 10% of patients with ascites respond to these measures alone. Patients who do not respond and those who find sodium restriction difficult require diuretic therapy (Hammer & McPhee, 2019; Simonetto et al., 2019).

Pharmacologic Therapy

The use of diuretic agents along with sodium restriction is successful in 90% of patients with ascites (Hammer & McPhee, 2019; Mansour & McPherson, 2018). Spironolactone, an aldosterone-blocking agent, is most often the first-line therapy in patients with ascites from cirrhosis. When used with other diuretic agents, spironolactone helps prevent potassium loss. Oral diuretic agents such as furosemide may be added but should be used cautiously, because long-term use may induce severe hyponatremia (sodium depletion). Ammonium chloride and acetazolamide are contraindicated because of the possibility of precipitating hepatic encephalopathy and coma. Daily weight loss should not exceed 1 kg (2.2 lb) in patients with ascites and peripheral edema or 0.5 to 0.75 kg (1.1 to 1.65 lb) in patients without edema (Bope & Kellerman, 2018; Hammer & McPhee, 2019; Simonetto et al., 2019). Fluid restriction is not attempted unless the serum sodium concentration is very low.

Possible complications of diuretic therapy include fluid and electrolyte disturbances (including hypovolemia, hypokalemia, hyponatremia, and hypochloremic alkalosis) (see Chapter 10) and encephalopathy. Encephalopathy may be precipitated by dehydration and hypovolemia. In addition, when potassium stores are depleted, the amount of ammonia in the systemic circulation increases, which may cause impaired cerebral functioning and encephalopathy.

Bed Rest

In patients with ascites, an upright posture is associated with activation of the renin–angiotensin–aldosterone system and sympathetic nervous system (Hammer & McPhee, 2019). This causes reduced renal glomerular filtration and sodium excretion and a decreased response to loop diuretics. Therefore, bed rest may be a useful therapy, especially for patients whose condition is refractory to diuretic agents.

Paracentesis

Paracentesis is the removal of fluid (ascites) from the peritoneal cavity through a puncture or a small surgical incision through the abdominal wall under sterile conditions (Hammer & McPhee, 2019; Simonetto et al., 2019). Ultrasound guidance may be indicated in some patients who are at high risk for bleeding because of an abnormal coagulation profile and in those who have had previous abdominal surgery and may have adhesions. Paracentesis was once considered a routine form of treatment for ascites. However, it is now performed primarily for diagnostic examination of ascitic fluid; in treatment for massive ascites that is resistant to nutritional and diuretic therapy and is causing severe problems to the patient; and as a prelude to diagnostic imaging studies, peritoneal dialysis, or surgery. A sample of the ascitic fluid may be sent to the laboratory for cell count, albumin and total protein levels, culture, and other tests.

Large-volume (5 to 6 L) paracentesis is a safe method for treating patients with severe ascites. The use of this therapeutic intervention should not be restricted to patients in whom diuretic therapy has failed but should be considered the treatment of choice for all patients with large-volume ascites (Hammer & McPhee, 2019; Mansour & McPherson, 2018; Simonetto et al., 2019). This technique, in combination with the IV infusion of salt-poor albumin or other colloid, has become a standard management strategy yielding an immediate effect. Refractive, massive ascites is unresponsive to multiple diuretic agents and sodium restriction for 2 weeks or more and can result in severe sequelae such as respiratory distress, which requires rapid intervention. Albumin infusions help to correct decreases in effective arterial blood volume that lead to sodium retention. The use of this colloid reduces the incidence of postparacentesis circulatory dysfunction with renal dysfunction, hyponatremia, and rapid reaccumulation of ascites associated with decreased effective arterial volume (Hammer & McPhee, 2019; Mansour & McPherson, 2018; Simonetto et al., 2019). The beneficial effects of albumin administration on hemodynamic stability and renal functional status may be related to an improvement in cardiac function as well as a decrease in the degree of arterial vasodilation. Although the patient with cirrhosis has a greatly increased extracellular blood volume, the kidney incorrectly senses that the intravascular volume has decreased. The renin–angiotensin–aldosterone axis is stimulated, and sodium is reabsorbed (Hammer & McPhee, 2019). In addition, antidiuretic hormone secretion increases, which leads to increased retention of free water and sometimes to the development of dilutional hyponatremia. Therapeutic paracentesis provides only temporary removal of fluid; ascites rapidly recurs, necessitating repeated fluid removal.

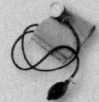 For the procedural guidelines for assisting with a paracentesis, go to **thepoint.lww.com/ Brunner15e.**

Transjugular Intrahepatic Portosystemic Shunt Assisting with Paracentesis

Transjugular intrahepatic portosystemic shunt (TIPS) is a method of treating ascites in which a cannula is threaded into

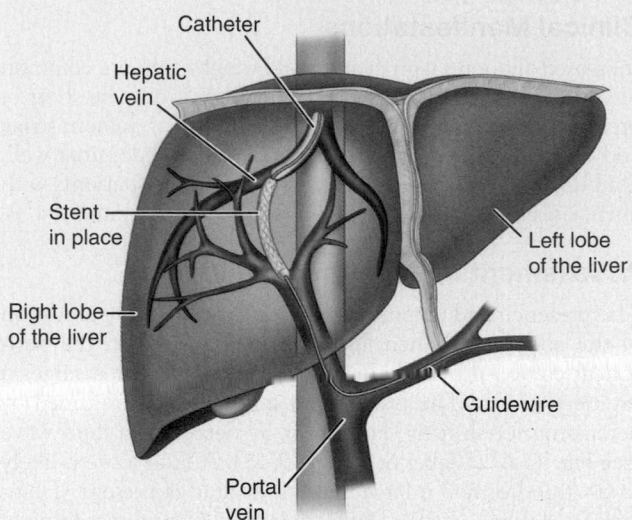

Figure 43-7 • Transjugular intrahepatic portosystemic shunt. A stent is inserted via catheter to the portal vein to divert blood flow and reduce portal hypertension.

the portal vein by the transjugular route (see Fig. 43-7). To reduce portal hypertension, an expandable stent is inserted to serve as an intrahepatic shunt between the portal circulation and the hepatic vein. This is extremely effective in decreasing sodium retention, improving the renal response to diuretic therapy, and preventing recurrence of fluid accumulation (Hammer & McPhee, 2019; Simonetto et al., 2019). TIPS is an effective management strategy for refractive ascites. However, due to a higher risk of encephalopathy and higher cost of TIPS compared with large-volume paracentesis plus albumin, many consider TIPS a second-line therapy for refractive ascites that continues to occur despite medical management (Hammer & McPhee, 2019; Hung & Lee, 2019; Simonetto et al., 2019).

Because the development of ascites in patients with cirrhosis is associated with a 50% mortality rate, patients considered candidates for liver transplantation may be referred for TIPS if paracentesis is contraindicated.

Other Methods of Treatment

Ascites can also be treated by the insertion of a peritoneovenous shunt to redirect ascitic fluid from the peritoneal cavity into the systemic circulation via an abdominal and a thoracic catheter that drain into the superior vena cava through a one-way valve (Hammer & McPhee, 2019; Simonetto et al., 2019). However, this procedure is rarely used due to the availability of newer, more effective therapies such as TIPS. In patients with ESLD, some with refractory ascites may be candidates for peritoneal catheters for palliation (Macken, Hashim, Mason, et al., 2019).

Nursing Management

If a patient with ascites from liver dysfunction is hospitalized, nursing measures include assessment and documentation of intake and output (I&O), abdominal girth, and daily weight to assess fluid status. The nurse also closely monitors the respiratory status because large volumes of ascites can compress the thoracic cavity and inhibit adequate lung expansion. The nurse monitors serum ammonia, creatinine, and electrolyte levels to assess electrolyte balance, response to therapy, and indications of hepatic encephalopathy.

Promoting Home, Community-Based, and Transitional Care

 Educating Patients About Self-Care

The patient treated for ascites is likely to be discharged with some ascites still present. Before hospital discharge, the nurse educates the patient and family about the treatment plan, including the need to avoid all alcohol intake, adhere to a low-sodium diet, take medications as prescribed, and check with the primary provider before taking any new medications, including OTC and herbal preparations. Additional home care education is summarized in Chart 43-3.

Continuing and Transitional Care

A referral for transitional, home, or community-based care may be warranted, especially if the patient lives alone or cannot provide self-care. The home visit enables the nurse to assess changes in the patient's condition and weight, abdominal girth, skin, and cognitive and emotional status. The nurse assesses the home environment and the availability of resources needed to adhere to the treatment plan (e.g., a scale to obtain daily weights, facilities to prepare and store appropriate foods, resources to purchase needed medications). The nurse also assesses the patient's adherence to the treatment plan and the ability to buy, prepare, and eat appropriate foods. The nurse reinforces previous education and emphasizes the need for regular follow-up and the importance of keeping scheduled health care appointments.

Esophageal Varices

Esophageal varices are present in 30% of patients with compensated cirrhosis and 60% of patients with decompensated cirrhosis at the time of diagnosis (Hammer & McPhee, 2019; Kovacs & Jensen, 2019; Simonetto et al., 2019) (see Clinical Manifestations in the Hepatic Cirrhosis section for further discussion). Varices are varicosities that develop from elevated pressure in the veins that drain into the portal system. They are prone to rupture and often are the source of massive hemorrhages from the upper GI tract and the rectum. In addition, abnormalities in blood clotting, often seen in patients with severe liver disease, increase the likelihood of bleeding with significant blood loss.

Once esophageal varices form, they increase in size over time and may eventually bleed (Hammer & McPhee, 2019; Kovacs & Jensen, 2019; Simonetto et al., 2019). In cirrhosis, varices are the most significant source of bleeding. The first bleeding episode has a mortality rate of 10% to 30% depending on the severity of the liver disease and is one of the major causes of death in patients with cirrhosis. Overall mortality associated with acute variceal bleeding ranges from 10% to 40%. The mortality rate is related to failure to control a bleeding episode and the occurrence of early rebleeding (Hammer & McPhee, 2019; Kovacs & Jensen, 2019; Simonetto et al., 2019). Patients surviving the first episode of variceal bleeding are at very high risk for recurrent bleeding (approximately 70%) and death (30% to 50%) (Hammer & McPhee, 2019; Kovacs & Jensen, 2019; Simonetto et al., 2019).

Pathophysiology

Esophageal varices are dilated, tortuous veins that are usually found in the submucosa of the lower esophagus but may

---

Chart 43-3 **HOME CARE CHECKLIST**

Management of Ascites

At the completion of education, the patient and/or caregiver will be able to:

- State the impact of ascites and treatment on physiologic functioning, ADLs, IADLs, roles, relationships, and spirituality.
- State the name, dose, side effects, frequency, and schedule for all medications.
- Describe effects, side effects, and monitoring parameters for diuretic therapy.
- Discuss importance of avoiding nonsteroidal anti-inflammatory agents, medications containing alcohol (e.g., cough mixtures), antibiotics, or antacids containing salt.
- Make appropriate dietary choices consistent with dietary prescription and recommendations.
  - Explain the use of salt substitutes must be approved by primary provider.
- State the importance of weighing self-daily and keeping a daily record of weight.
  - Maintain record of daily weight, and identify daily weight-loss goals.
  - List weight changes (loss or gain) that should be reported to the primary provider.
- Identify rationale for fluid restrictions (if needed), and for monitoring and keeping a daily record intake and output.
  - Maintain a record of daily intake and output.

- Identify changes in output that should be reported to primary provider (e.g., decreasing urine output).
- Identify need to stop all alcohol intake as critical to well-being.
- Explain how to contact Alcoholics Anonymous or alcohol counselors in related organizations if indicated.
- Demonstrate how to inspect and care for skin, alleviate pressure over bony prominences by turning when in bed or chair, and decrease edema by position changes.
- Identify early signs and symptoms of complications (encephalopathy, spontaneous bacterial peritonitis, dehydration, electrolyte abnormalities, azotemia).
- Relate how to reach primary provider with questions or complications.
- State time and date of follow-up medical appointments, therapy, and testing.
- Identify sources of support (e.g., friends, relatives, faith community).
- Identify the contact details for support services for patients and their caregivers/families.
- Identify the need for health promotion, disease prevention, and screening activities.

ADLs, activities of daily living; IADLs, instrumental activities of daily living.

Physiology/Pathophysiology

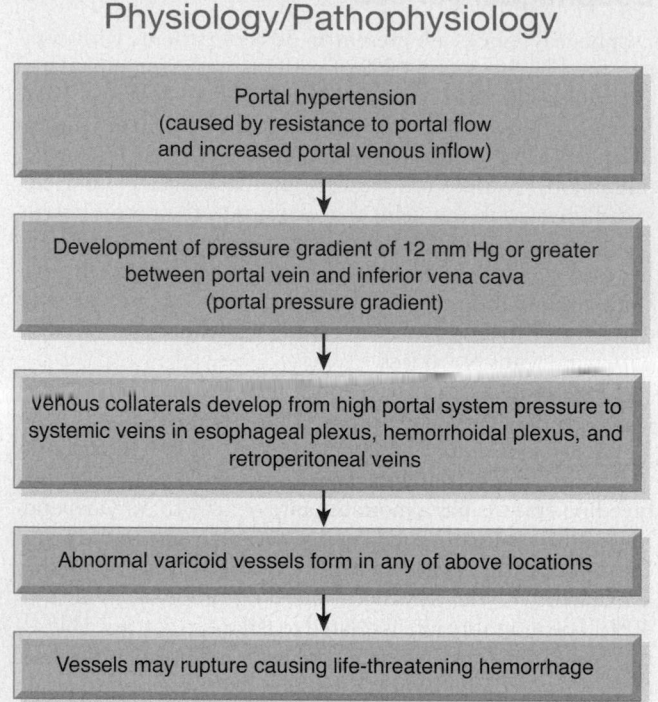

Figure 43-8 • Pathogenesis of bleeding esophageal varices.

develop higher in the esophagus or extend into the stomach. This condition is almost always caused by portal hypertension, which results from obstruction of the portal venous circulation within the damaged liver.

Because of increased obstruction of the portal vein, venous blood from the intestinal tract and spleen seeks an outlet through collateral circulation (new pathways for return of blood to the right atrium). The effect is increased pressure, particularly in the vessels in the submucosal layer of the lower esophagus and upper part of the stomach. These collateral vessels are not very elastic; rather, they are tortuous and fragile, and they bleed easily (see Fig. 43-8). Less common causes of varices are abnormalities of the circulation in the splenic vein or superior vena cava and hepatic venothrombosis.

Bleeding esophageal varices are life-threatening and can result in hemorrhagic shock that produces decreased cerebral, hepatic, and renal perfusion. In turn, there is an increased nitrogen load from bleeding into the GI tract and an increased serum ammonia level, increasing the risk of encephalopathy. Usually, the dilated veins cause no symptoms. However, if the portal pressure increases sharply and the mucosa or supporting structures become thin, massive hemorrhaging occurs.

Factors that contribute to hemorrhage are muscular exertion from lifting heavy objects; straining at stool; sneezing, coughing, or vomiting; esophagitis; irritation of vessels by poorly chewed foods or irritating fluids; and reflux of stomach contents (especially alcohol). Salicylates and any medication that erodes the esophageal mucosa or interferes with cell replication also may contribute to bleeding.

Clinical Manifestations

The patient with bleeding esophageal varices may present with hematemesis, melena, or general deterioration in mental or physical status and often has a history of alcohol abuse. Signs and symptoms of shock (cool clammy skin, hypotension, tachycardia) may be present (see Chapter 11).

Assessment and Diagnostic Findings

Endoscopy is used to identify the bleeding site, along with ultrasonography, CT scanning, and angiography. Another diagnostic tool, the endoscopic video capsule, can detect esophageal varices but does not substitute for endoscopy unless this test cannot be performed. Standard endoscopy is superior to video capsule for the diagnosis of esophageal varices (Hammer & McPhee, 2019; Kovacs & Jensen, 2019; Simonetto et al., 2019). Because varices are present in 50% of patients with cirrhosis, it is recommended that patients who have been diagnosed with cirrhosis undergo screening endoscopy. If no varices are detected on initial endoscopy, the test should be repeated in 2 to 3 years in an effort to identify and treat large varices, which are the ones most likely to bleed. If small varices are identified on initial endoscopy, the test should be repeated in 1 to 2 years (Hammer & McPhee, 2019; Kovacs & Jensen, 2019; Simonetto et al., 2019).

Endoscopy

Immediate endoscopy (see Chapter 38) is indicated to identify the cause and the site of bleeding; approximately 40% of patients with suspected bleeding from esophageal varices are actually bleeding from another source (gastritis, ulcer) (Hammer & McPhee, 2019; Kovacs & Jensen, 2019; Simonetto et al., 2019). Nursing support is essential during this often stressful experience. Careful monitoring can detect early signs of cardiac arrhythmias, perforation, and hemorrhage.

After the examination, fluids are not given until the patient's gag reflex returns. Lozenges and gargles may be used to relieve throat discomfort if the patient's physical condition and mental status permit. If the patient is actively bleeding, oral intake will not be permitted, and the patient will be prepared for further diagnostic and therapeutic procedures.

Portal Hypertension Measurements

Portal hypertension may be suspected if dilated abdominal veins and hemorrhoids are detected. Splenomegaly and ascites may also be present. Portal venous pressure can be measured directly or indirectly. Indirect measurement of the hepatic vein pressure gradient is the most common procedure. The measurement requires insertion of a catheter with a balloon into the antecubital or femoral vein. The catheter is advanced under fluoroscopy to a hepatic vein. Fluid is infused once the catheter is in position to inflate the balloon. A "wedged" pressure (similar to pulmonary artery wedge pressure) is obtained by occluding the blood flow in the blood vessel; pressure in the unoccluded vessel is also measured and the hepatic venous pressure gradient (HVPG) is obtained. An HVPG of over 10 mm Hg is indicative of clinically significant portal hypertension (Kovacs & Jensen, 2019). Although the values obtained may underestimate portal pressure, this measurement may be taken several times to evaluate the results of therapy (Kovacs & Jensen, 2019; Schiff et al., 2018).

Direct measurement of portal vein pressure can be obtained by several methods. One direct measurement requires insertion of a catheter into the portal vein or one of its branches (Kovacs & Jensen, 2019; Schiff et al., 2018). Endoscopic measurement of pressure within varices is used only in conjunction with endoscopic sclerotherapy (see later discussion).

Laboratory Tests

Laboratory studies may include various liver function tests, such as serum aminotransferases, bilirubin, alkaline phosphatase, and serum proteins. Splenoportography, which involves serial or segmental x-rays, is used to detect extensive collateral circulation in esophageal vessels, which would indicate varices. Other tests are hepatoportography and celiac angiography. These are usually performed in the operating room or x-ray department.

 ## Medical Management

Bleeding from esophageal varices is an emergency that can quickly lead to hemorrhagic shock. The patient is critically ill, requiring aggressive medical care and expert nursing care, and is usually transferred to the intensive care unit (ICU) for close monitoring and management. See Chapter 11 for a discussion of care of the patient in shock. The extent of bleeding is evaluated, and vital signs are monitored continuously if hematemesis and melena are present.

Because patients with bleeding esophageal varices have intravascular volume depletion and are subject to electrolyte imbalance, IV fluids, electrolytes, and volume expanders are provided to restore fluid volume and replace electrolytes. Transfusion of blood components also may be required.

Caution must be taken with volume resuscitation so that overhydration does not occur, because this would raise portal pressure and increase bleeding. An indwelling urinary catheter is usually inserted to permit frequent monitoring of urine output.

Although a variety of pharmacologic, endoscopic, and surgical approaches are used to treat bleeding esophageal varices, none is ideal, and most are associated with considerable risk to the patient. Nonsurgical treatment of bleeding esophageal varices is preferable because of the high mortality rate of emergency surgery to control bleeding esophageal varices and because of the poor physical condition that is typical of the patient with severe liver dysfunction.

Pharmacologic Therapy

In suspected variceal bleeding, vasoactive drugs such as octreotide or vasopressin need to be given as soon as possible and before endoscopy (Kovacs & Jensen, 2019; Simonetto et al., 2019). In a patient who is actively bleeding, medications are given initially because they can be obtained and given more quickly than other therapies. Octreotide, a synthetic analog of the hormone somatostatin, is effective in decreasing bleeding from esophageal varices, and lacks the vasoconstrictive effects of vasopressin. Because of this safety and efficacy profile, octreotide is considered the preferred treatment regimen for immediate control of variceal bleeding. These medications cause selective splanchnic vasoconstriction by inhibiting glucagon release and are used mainly in the management of active hemorrhage. Adverse effects are rare with octreotide but mild hypoglycemia and abdominal cramping can occur (Kovacs & Jensen, 2019; Simonetto et al., 2019).

Vasopressin may be the initial mode of therapy in urgent situations because it produces constriction of the splanchnic

arterial bed and decreases portal pressure. As described previously, splanchnic circulation comprises the arterial blood supply and venous drainage of the entire GI tract from the distal esophagus to the midrectum, including the liver and spleen. Vasopressin constricts distal esophageal and proximal gastric veins, thus reducing the inflow into the portal system and therefore the portal pressure. Vital signs and the presence or absence of blood in the gastric aspirate indicate the effectiveness of vasopressin. Monitoring of I&O and electrolyte levels is necessary because hyponatremia may develop, and vasopressin may have an antidiuretic effect.

Coronary artery disease is a contraindication to the use of vasopressin because coronary vasoconstriction is a side effect that may precipitate myocardial infarction. The combination of vasopressin with nitroglycerin (given by the IV, sublingual, or transdermal route) has been effective in reducing or preventing the side effects (constriction of coronary vessels and angina) caused by vasopressin alone. Side effects of vasopressin include myocardial and extremity ischemia as well as cardiac arrhythmias; therefore, vasopressin is used only in urgent situations or when other agents such as octreotide are not available. Vasopressin must be given with close monitoring (Kovacs & Jensen, 2019; Simonetto et al., 2019).

Beta-blocking agents such as propranolol, nadolol, or carvedilol that decrease portal pressure are the most common medications used both to prevent a first bleeding episode in patients with known varices and to prevent rebleeding (Bunchorntavakul & Reddy, 2019; Hammer & McPhee, 2019; Simonetto et al., 2019). Beta-blockers have been shown to effectively reduce the risk of variceal bleeding and its associated mortality. Beta-blockers should not be used in acute variceal hemorrhage, but they are effective prophylaxis against initial and recurrent bleeding episodes (Bunchorntavakul & Reddy, 2019; Hammer & McPhee, 2019; Simonetto et al., 2019). Nitrates such as isosorbide lower portal pressure by venodilation and decreased cardiac output and may be used in combination with beta-blockers to reduce the risk of recurrent variceal bleeding (Bunchorntavakul & Reddy, 2019; Kovacs & Jensen, 2019).

 ### Balloon Tamponade

Although used infrequently today, balloon tamponade therapy may be used to temporarily control hemorrhage and to stabilize a patient with massive bleeding prior to other definitive management (Kovacs & Jensen, 2019; Simonetto et al., 2019). This procedure involves the insertion of a tube from the nose into the stomach. This tube has two inflatable balloons, one esophageal and one gastric. When inflated from a port external to the patient, these balloons compress bleeding varices in the stomach or esophagus to inhibit bleeding.

When indicated, balloon tamponade can be successful; however, there are risks. Displacement of the tube and the inflated balloon into the oropharynx can cause life-threatening obstruction of the airway and asphyxiation. This may occur if the patient pulls on the tube because of confusion or discomfort. It may also result from rupture of the gastric balloon, which causes the esophageal balloon to move into the oropharynx. Sudden rupture of the balloon causes airway obstruction and aspiration of gastric contents into the lungs. Therefore, the tube must be tested before insertion to minimize this risk by ensuring that the balloons can attain and maintain inflation. Aspiration of blood and secretions into the lungs is frequently associated with balloon tamponade, especially in the stuporous or comatose patient. Endotracheal intubation before insertion of the tube protects the airway and minimizes the risk of aspiration. Ulceration and necrosis of the nose, the mucosa of the stomach, or the esophagus may occur if the tube is left in place too long, inflated too long, or inflated at too high a pressure. The therapy is used for as short a time as possible to control bleeding while emergency treatment is completed and definitive therapies are instituted (no longer than 12 hours, preferably less) (Kovacs & Jensen, 2019; Mansour & McPherson, 2018; Simonetto et al., 2019).

> ### ◢ Quality and Safety Nursing Alert
>
> *The patient being treated with balloon tamponade must remain under close observation in the ICU and must be monitored continuously because of the risk of serious complications such as aspiration, esophageal ulcer formation, and perforation. Precautions must be taken to ensure that the patient does not pull on or inadvertently displace the tube.*

Nursing measures include frequent mouth and nasal care. For secretions that accumulate in the mouth, tissues should be within easy reach of the patient. Oral suction may be necessary to remove secretions.

Although balloon tamponade stops the bleeding in 90% of patients, bleeding recurs in 60% to 70%, necessitating other treatment modalities, such as endoscopic therapies (see later discussion). Once the balloons are deflated or the tube is removed, the patient must be assessed frequently because of the high risk of recurrent bleeding (Kovacs & Jensen, 2019; Mansour & McPherson, 2018; Simonetto et al., 2019).

Endoscopic Sclerotherapy

In endoscopic **sclerotherapy** (see Fig. 43-9), also referred to as injection sclerotherapy, a sclerosing agent (i.e., sodium morrhuate, ethanolamine oleate, sodium tetradecyl sulfate, or ethanol) is injected through a fiberoptic endoscope into or adjacent to the bleeding esophageal varices to promote thrombosis and eventual sclerosis (Kovacs & Jensen, 2019; Mansour & McPherson, 2018). The process of sclerotherapy causes inflammation of the involved vein with eventual thrombosis and loss of the lumen of the vessel. The procedure has been used successfully to treat acute GI hemorrhage but

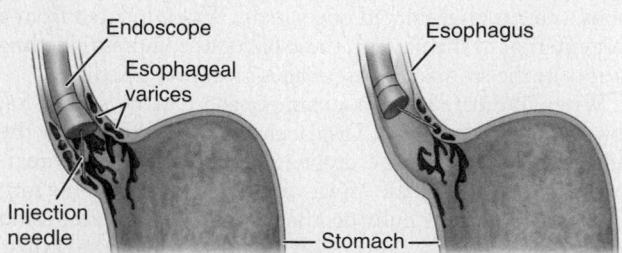

Figure 43-9 • Endoscopic or injection sclerotherapy. Injection of sclerosing agent into esophageal varices through an endoscope promotes thrombosis and eventual sclerosis, thereby obliterating the varices.

is not recommended for prevention of first and subsequent variceal bleeding episodes where **endoscopic variceal ligation (EVL)**, also known as esophageal banding therapy (discussed later), is the first-line treatment (Kovacs & Jensen, 2019; Mansour & McPherson, 2018).

After treatment for acute hemorrhage, the patient must be observed for bleeding, perforation of the esophagus, aspiration pneumonia, and esophageal stricture. Antacids, histamine-2 (H_2) antagonists such as cimetidine, or proton pump inhibitors such as pantoprazole may be given after the procedure to counteract the chemical effects of the sclerosing agent on the esophagus and the acid reflux associated with the therapy.

Endoscopic Variceal Ligation (Esophageal Banding Therapy)

In EVL (see Fig. 43-10), also referred to as variceal banding, a modified endoscope loaded with an elastic rubber band is passed through an overtube directly onto the varix (or varices) to be banded. After the bleeding varix is suctioned into the tip of the endoscope, the rubber band is slipped over the tissue, causing necrosis, ulceration, and eventual sloughing of the varix.

An EVL procedure is effective in controlling acute bleeding. Compared with sclerotherapy, EVL also significantly reduces the rebleeding rate, mortality, procedure-related complications, as well as number of sessions needed to eradicate varices and thus has replaced sclerotherapy as the treatment of choice in the management of esophageal varices (Kovacs & Jensen, 2019; Simonetto et al., 2019). Potential complications include superficial ulceration and dysphagia, transient chest discomfort, and, rarely, esophageal strictures. An EVL procedure in combination with pharmacologic therapy may

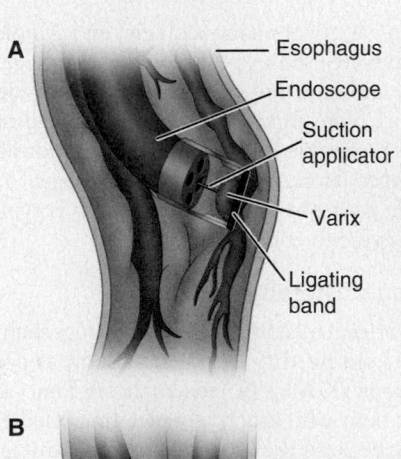

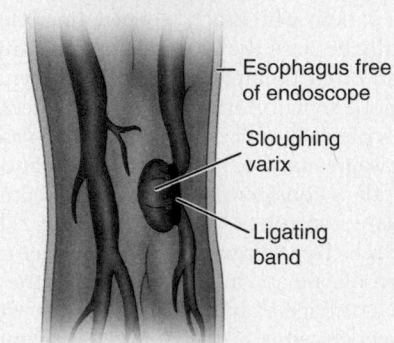

Figure 43-10 • Endoscopic variceal ligation. **A.** A rubber band–like ligature is slipped over an esophageal varix via an endoscope. **B.** Necrosis results, and the varix eventually sloughs off.

be more effective than monotherapy (i.e., a single mode of therapy) in the treatment of acute hemorrhage. EVL is also recommended for patients who have experienced variceal bleeding while receiving beta-blocker therapy and for those who cannot tolerate beta-blocking agents (Kovacs & Jensen, 2019; Simonetto et al., 2019).

Transjugular Intrahepatic Portosystemic Shunt

A TIPS procedure (see Fig. 43-9) is indicated for the treatment of an acute episode of uncontrolled variceal bleeding refractory to pharmacologic or endoscopic therapy. In 10% to 20% of patients for whom urgent band ligation or sclerotherapy and medications are not successful in eradicating bleeding, a TIPS procedure can effectively control acute variceal hemorrhage by rapidly lowering portal pressure. Polytetrafluoroethylene-covered TIPS placement should be considered in high-risk patients with cirrhosis and active bleeding at the time of endoscopy (Kovacs & Jensen, 2019; Simonetto et al., 2019). Potential complications of TIPS include bleeding, sepsis, heart failure, organ perforation, shunt thrombosis, and progressive liver failure.

Additional Therapies

The use of endoscopically placed tissue adhesives and fibrin glue has been successful in the treatment of gastric and esophageal varices. Coated expandable stents (placed via endoscope) have also been used effectively for the same purpose (Kovacs & Jensen, 2019; Simonetto et al., 2019). Portosystemic shunting into lower resistance vessels (those vessels not affected by the high pressure in the portal system) and the end-organ collateral variceal formation that results in bleeding may also be treated by a variety of embolization procedures, including balloon-occluded retrograde transvenous obliteration (BRTO) (Brunicardi, 2019; Philips, Rajesh, Augustine, et al., 2019).

Surgical Management

Several surgical procedures have been developed to treat esophageal varices and to minimize rebleeding, but these procedures have significant risk. Procedures that may be used for esophageal varices are direct surgical ligation of varices; splenorenal, mesocaval, and portacaval venous shunts to relieve portal pressure; and esophageal transection with devascularization. These procedures are rarely used and remain controversial, as studies regarding their effectiveness and outcomes continue. What is known is that these procedures are very effective in controlling variceal bleeding. They may be considered as second-line management (rescue therapy) in those patients for whom all other treatments have failed, those who are not candidates for liver transplantation, and those who require a bridge to transplantation. There is a high incidence of encephalopathy after the surgical shunting procedures, and morbidity and mortality statistics remain high (Kovacs & Jensen, 2019; Philips et al., 2019). The TIPS procedure has largely replaced the use of surgical decompression shunts and ligation procedures but these interventions may still be used in some cases to manage esophageal varices.

Surgical Bypass Procedures

Surgical decompression (shunt surgery) of the portal circulation may be used with the advent of a variceal bleeding episode. Although effective in eradicating bleeding, survival statistics

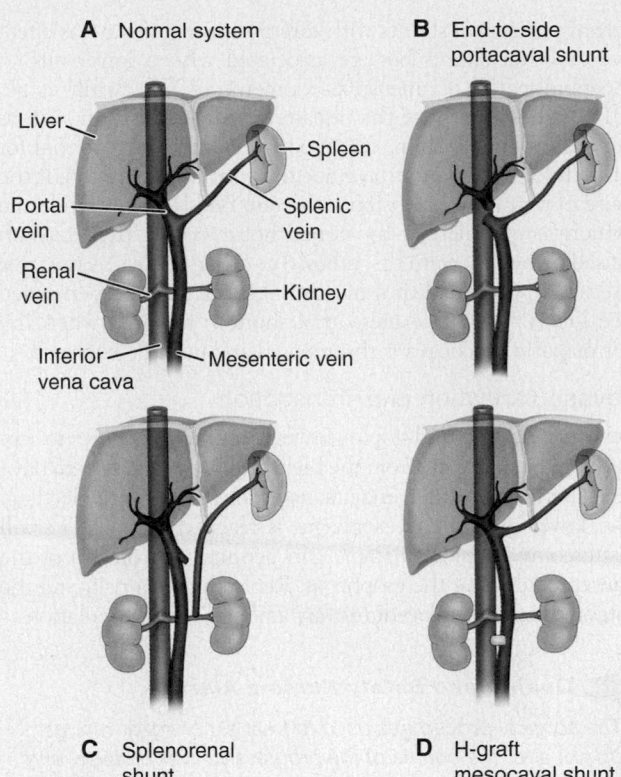

A Normal system **B** End-to-side portacaval shunt

Liver — Spleen
Portal vein — Splenic vein
Renal vein — Kidney
Inferior vena cava — Mesenteric vein

C Splenorenal shunt **D** H-graft mesocaval shunt

Figure 43-11 • Portosystemic shunts. **A.** Normal portal system. **B–D.** Examples of portal shunts to reduce portal pressure.

and encephalopathy are worse than other preventative measures such as a TIPS procedure when this method is employed for prophylaxis, and shunt surgery for this purpose has largely been abandoned worldwide (Brunicardi, 2019; Kovacs & Jensen, 2019). The current recommendation is that surgical shunts be considered only in patients who have Model for End-Stage Liver Disease (MELD) scores of <15, who are not candidates for hepatic transplantation, or who have limited access to TIPS therapy and needed follow-up. (See later discussion of MELD classification in Liver Transplantation section.)

An aim of a surgical shunt is to reduce portal venous pressure (Brunicardi, 2019). One surgical shunting procedure (see Fig. 43-11) is the distal splenorenal shunt, which is made between the splenic vein and the left renal vein after splenectomy. A mesocaval shunt is created by anastomosing the superior mesenteric vein to the proximal end of the vena cava or to the side of the vena cava using grafting material. The goal of distal splenorenal and mesocaval shunts is to decrease portal pressure by draining only a portion of venous blood from the portal bed; therefore, they are considered selective shunts. The liver continues to receive some portal flow, and the incidence of encephalopathy may be reduced. Portacaval shunts are considered nonselective shunts because they divert all portal flow to the vena cava via end-to-side or side-to-side approaches.

These procedures are extensive and are not always successful because of secondary thrombosis in the veins used for the shunt and because of complications (e.g., encephalopathy, accelerated liver failure). The effectiveness of these procedures has been studied extensively. All shunt procedures are equally effective in preventing recurrent variceal bleeding but may cause further impairment of liver function and encephalopathy.

Partial portacaval shunts with interposition grafts are as effective as other shunts but are associated with a lower rate of encephalopathy (Cameron & Cameron, 2020; Schiff et al., 2018). The severity of the disease (by a classification such as the Child–Pugh system, discussed later) and the potential for future liver transplantation guide the treatment decision. If the cause of portal hypertension is the rare Budd–Chiari syndrome (which is manifested by noncirrhotic portal hypertension caused by hepatic vein thrombosis) or other venous obstructive disease, a portacaval or a mesoatrial shunt may be performed (see Fig. 43-11). The mesoatrial shunt is required when the infrahepatic vena cava is thrombosed and must be bypassed.

Devascularization and Transection

Devascularization and staple-gun transection procedures to separate the bleeding site from the high-pressure portal system have been used in the emergency management of variceal bleeding. The lower end of the esophagus is reached through a small gastrostomy incision; a staple gun permits anastomosis of the transected ends of the esophagus. Rebleeding is a risk, and the outcomes of these procedures vary among patient populations.

Quality and Safety Nursing Alert

The surgical procedures used to treat esophageal varices do not alter the course of the progressive liver disease, and bleeding may recur as new collateral vessels develop. The risk of complications (hypovolemic or hemorrhagic shock, hepatic encephalopathy, electrolyte imbalance, metabolic and respiratory alkalosis, alcohol withdrawal syndrome, and seizures) is high.

Nursing Management

Nursing assessment includes monitoring the patient's physical condition and evaluating emotional responses and cognitive status. The nurse monitors and records vital signs and assesses the patient's nutritional and neurologic status. This assessment assists in identifying hepatic encephalopathy (see later discussion).

If complete rest of the esophagus is indicated because of bleeding, parenteral nutrition is initiated. Gastric suction usually is initiated to keep the stomach as empty as possible and to prevent straining and vomiting. The patient often complains of severe thirst, which may be relieved by frequent oral hygiene and moist sponges to the lips. The nurse closely monitors the blood pressure. Vitamin K therapy and multiple blood transfusions often are indicated because of blood loss. A quiet environment and calm reassurance may help to relieve the patient's anxiety and reduce agitation.

Bleeding anywhere in the body is anxiety provoking, resulting in a crisis for the patient and family. If the patient has been a heavy user of alcohol, delirium secondary to alcohol withdrawal can complicate the situation. The nurse provides support and explanations about medical and nursing interventions to prepare both the patient and the family, because these procedures can be difficult to undergo and observe. Close monitoring of the patient helps in detecting and managing complications. Management modalities and nursing care of the patient with bleeding esophageal varices are summarized in Table 43-2.

Hepatic Encephalopathy and Coma

Hepatic encephalopathy, or portosystemic encephalopathy, is a life-threatening complication of liver disease that occurs

TABLE 43-2	Select Modalities and Nursing Care for the Patient with Bleeding Esophageal Varices
Treatment Modality[a]	**Nursing Interventions**
Nonsurgical Modalities	
Pharmacologic agents	Observe response to therapy.
Propranolol	Monitor for side effects: *propranolol, carvedilol, nadolol*—decreased pulse pressure, impaired cardiovascular
Carvedilol	response to hemorrhage; *vasopressin*—angina (nitroglycerin may be prescribed to prevent or treat
Nadolol	angina).
Vasopressin	
Octreotide	Support patient during treatment.
Balloon tamponade	Explain procedure to patient briefly to obtain cooperation with insertion and maintenance of esophageal/gastric tamponade tube and reduce patient's fear of the procedure.
	Monitor closely to prevent inadvertent removal or displacement of tube, subsequent airway obstruction, and aspiration.
	Provide frequent oral hygiene.
Endoscopic sclerotherapy	Observe for aspiration, perforation of the esophagus, and recurrence of bleeding after treatment.
Endoscopic variceal ligation	Observe for recurrence of bleeding, esophageal perforation.
Transjugular intrahepatic portosystemic shunt (TIPS)	Observe for rebleeding and signs of infection.
Balloon-occluded retrograde transvenous obliteration (BRTO) procedure	Observe for rebleeding, signs of infection, or changes in mental status.
Surgical Modalities	
Portal-systemic shunt	Observe for development of portal-systemic encephalopathy (altered mental status, neurologic dysfunction), hepatic failure, and rebleeding.
	Requires intensive, expert nursing care for prolonged period.
Surgical ligation of varices	Observe for rebleeding.
Esophageal transection and devascularization	Observe for rebleeding.
	Provide postthoracotomy care.

[a]Several modalities may be used concurrently or in sequence.

Adapted from Brunicardi, F. C. (2019). *Schwartz's principles of surgery* (11th ed.). New York: McGraw-Hill Education; Feldman, M., Friedman, L. S., & Brandt, L. J. (2016). *Sleisinger & Fordtran's gastrointestinal & liver disease* (10th ed.). Philadelphia, PA: Saunders Elsevier.

with profound liver failure. Patients with this condition may have no overt signs of the illness but have abnormalities on neuropsychological testing (Hammer & McPhee, 2019; Simonetto et al., 2019; Yanny, Winters, Boutros, et al., 2019). Hepatic encephalopathy is the neuropsychiatric manifestation of hepatic failure associated with portal hypertension and the shunting of blood from the portal venous system into the systemic circulation (Mansour & McPherson, 2018; Yanny et al., 2019). This reversible metabolic form of encephalopathy can improve with recovery of liver function. The onset is often insidious and subtle, and initially the disease is termed *subclinical* or *minimal hepatic encephalopathy*.

Pathophysiology

Despite the frequency with which hepatic encephalopathy occurs, the precise pathophysiology is not fully understood (Yanny et al., 2019). Two major alterations underlie its development in acute and chronic liver disease. First, hepatic insufficiency may result in encephalopathy because of the inability of the liver to detoxify toxic by-products of metabolism. Second, portosystemic shunting, in which collateral vessels develop as a result of portal hypertension, allows elements of the portal blood (laden with potentially toxic substances usually extracted by the liver) to enter the systemic circulation (Yanny et al., 2019). Ammonia is considered the major etiologic factor in the development of encephalopathy. Ammonia enters the brain and excites peripheral benzodiazepine-type receptors on astrocyte cells, increasing neurosteroid synthesis, and stimulating gamma-aminobutyric acid (GABA) neurotransmission. GABA causes depression of the central nervous system that inhibits neurotransmission and synaptic regulation (Yanny et al., 2019), producing sleep and behavior patterns associated with hepatic encephalopathy.

Circumstances that increase serum ammonia levels tend to aggravate or precipitate hepatic encephalopathy. The largest source of ammonia is the enzymatic and bacterial digestion of dietary and blood proteins in the GI tract. Ammonia from these sources increases as a result of GI bleeding (i.e., bleeding esophageal varices, chronic GI bleeding), a high-protein diet, bacterial infection, or uremia. The ingestion of ammonium salts also increases the blood ammonia level. In the presence of alkalosis or hypokalemia, increased amounts of ammonia are absorbed from the GI tract and from the renal tubular fluid. Conversely, serum ammonia is decreased by elimination of protein from the diet and by the administration of antibiotics, such as neomycin sulfate, which reduce the number of intestinal bacteria capable of converting urea to ammonia (Hammer & McPhee, 2019; Yanny et al., 2019).

Other factors unrelated to increased serum ammonia levels that can cause hepatic encephalopathy in susceptible patients include excessive diuresis, dehydration, infections, surgery, fever, and some medications (sedatives, tranquilizers, analgesics, and diuretics that cause potassium loss). Additional causes include elevated levels of serum manganese (Schiff et al., 2018), as well as changes in the types of circulating amino acids, mercaptans, and levels of dopamine and other neurotransmitters in the central nervous system (Schiff et al., 2018). Mercaptans are toxic metabolites of sulfur-containing compounds that are excreted by the liver under normal conditions. Mercaptans and these other so-called "false" neurotransmitters may

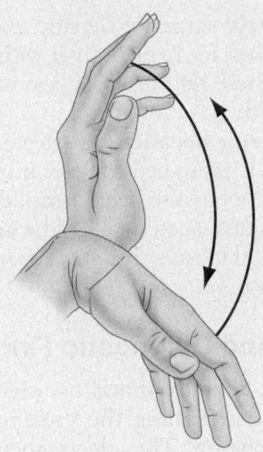

Figure 43-12 • Asterixis ("liver flap") may occur in hepatic encephalopathy. The patient is asked to hold the arm out with the handheld upward (dorsiflexed). Within a few seconds, the hand falls forward involuntarily and then quickly returns to the dorsiflexed position.

be generated from an intestinal source or from metabolism of protein by the liver and, with defective hepatic clearance, may precipitate encephalopathy.

Clinical Manifestations

The earliest symptoms of hepatic encephalopathy include mental status changes and motor disturbances. The patient appears confused and unkempt and has alterations in mood and sleep patterns. The patient tends to sleep during the day and has restlessness and insomnia at night. As hepatic encephalopathy progresses, the patient may become difficult to awaken and completely disoriented with respect to time and place. With further progression, the patient lapses into frank coma and may have seizures.

Asterixis, an involuntary flapping of the hands, may be seen in stage II encephalopathy (see Fig. 43-12). Simple tasks, such as handwriting, become difficult. A handwriting or drawing sample (e.g., star figure), taken daily, may provide graphic evidence of progression or reversal of hepatic encephalopathy. Inability to reproduce a simple figure in two or three dimensions (see Fig. 43-13) is referred to as **constructional**

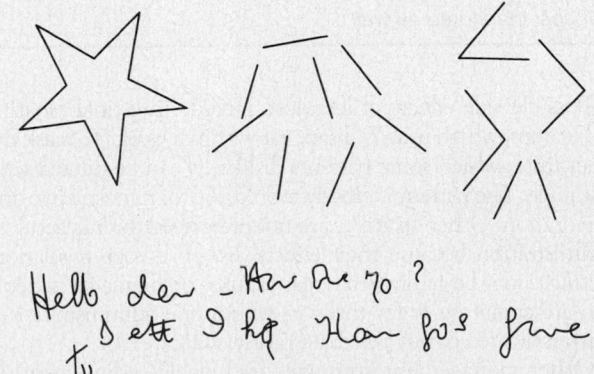

Figure 43-13 • Effects of constructional apraxia. Deterioration of handwriting and inability to draw a simple star figure occurs with progressive hepatic encephalopathy. Reprinted with permission from Morgan, M. (2018). Hepatic encephalopathy in patients with cirrhosis. In J. Dooley, A. S. Lok, G. Garcia-Tsao, & P. Massimo (Eds.). *Sherlock's diseases of the liver and biliary system* (13th ed.). Oxford, UK: John Wiley & Sons.

apraxia. In the early stages of hepatic encephalopathy, the deep tendon reflexes are hyperactive; with worsening of the encephalopathy, these reflexes disappear and the extremities may become flaccid.

Occasionally, **fetor hepaticus**, a sweet, slightly fecal odor to the breath that is presumed to be of intestinal origin, may be noticed. The odor has also been described as similar to that of freshly mowed grass, acetone, or old wine. Fetor hepaticus is prevalent with extensive collateral portal circulation in chronic liver disease.

Assessment and Diagnostic Findings

Several diagnostic algorithms and a variety of psychometric tests are used in determining the presence and severity of hepatic encephalopathy. The electroencephalogram shows generalized slowing, an increase in the amplitude of brain waves, and characteristic triphasic waves. The survival rate after a first episode of overt hepatic encephalopathy in patients with cirrhosis is approximately 40% at 1 year. Eligible patients should be referred for liver transplantation after this initial episode (Mansour & McPherson, 2018; Yanny et al., 2019).

Medical Management

Medical management focuses on identifying and eliminating the precipitating cause, if possible, initiating ammonia-lowering therapy, minimizing potential medical complications of cirrhosis and depressed consciousness, and reversing the underlying liver disease, if possible. Correction of the possible reasons for the deterioration such as bleeding, electrolyte abnormalities, sedation, or azotemia is essential. Lactulose is given to reduce serum ammonia levels. It acts by trapping and expelling the ammonia in the feces (Hammer & McPhee, 2019; Mansour & McPherson, 2018; Yanny et al., 2019). Two or three soft stools per day are desirable; this indicates that lactulose is performing as intended.

> ### ▶ Quality and Safety Nursing Alert
>
> *The patient receiving lactulose is monitored closely for the development of watery diarrhea stools, because they indicate a medication overdose. Serum ammonia levels are closely monitored as well.*

Possible side effects of lactulose include intestinal bloating and cramps, which usually disappear within a week. To mask the sweet taste, which some patients dislike, it can be diluted with fruit juice. The patient is closely monitored for hypokalemia and dehydration. Other laxatives are not prescribed during lactulose administration because their effects disturb dosage regulation. Lactulose may be given by nasogastric tube or enema for patients who are comatose or for those in whom oral administration is contraindicated or not possible (Yanny et al., 2019).

Other management strategies include IV administration of glucose to minimize protein breakdown, administration of vitamins to correct deficiencies, and correction of electrolyte imbalances (especially potassium). Antibiotics may also be added to the treatment regimen. Neomycin, metronidazole, and rifaximin have been used to reduce levels of ammonia-forming bacteria in the colon. However, no benefit has been shown for long-term treatment with these antibiotics (Mansour & McPherson, 2018; Yanny et al., 2019). Additional management strategies for hepatic encephalopathy include the following:

- Neurologic status is assessed frequently.
- Mental status is monitored by keeping a daily record of handwriting and arithmetic performance.
- I&O and body weight are recorded each day.
- Vital signs are measured and recorded every 4 hours.
- Potential sites of infection (peritoneum, lungs) are assessed frequently, and abnormal findings are reported promptly.
- Serum ammonia level is monitored daily.
- Dietary protein intake should not be restricted in hepatic encephalopathy as recommended in the past. Protein intake should be maintained at 1.2 to 1.5 g/kg/day (European Association for the Study of the Liver [EASL], 2019; Styskel, Natarajan, & Kanwal, 2019; Yanny et al., 2019; Yao, Fung, Chu, et al., 2018) (see Chart 43-4). The danger of protein malnutrition far outweighs the risk of worsening hepatic encephalopathy caused by increased protein intake (Styskel et al., 2019; Yanny et al., 2019; Yao et al., 2018).
- Enteral feeding is provided for patients whose encephalopathic state persists.
- Reduction in the absorption of ammonia from the GI tract is accomplished by the use of gastric suction, enemas, or oral antibiotics.
- Electrolyte status is monitored and corrected if abnormal.
- Sedatives, tranquilizers, and analgesic medications are discontinued.
- Benzodiazepine antagonists such as flumazenil may be administered IV to improve encephalopathy, whether or not the patient has previously taken benzodiazepines.

> ### Chart 43-4 Nutritional Management of Hepatic Encephalopathy
>
> - Minimize the formation and absorption of toxins, principally ammonia, from the intestine.
> - Keep daily protein intake between 1.2 and 1.5 g/kg body weight per day.
> - Avoid protein restriction if possible, even in those with encephalopathy.
> - For patients who are truly protein intolerant, provide additional nitrogen in the form of an amino acid supplement. The use of branched-chain amino acids should be a consideration in patients with cirrhosis. It has improved outcomes in varied populations with the disease.
> - Provide small, frequent meals and 3 small snacks per day in addition to a late-night snack before bed.
>
> Adapted from European Association for the Study of the Liver (EASL). (2019). EASL clinical practice guidelines on nutrition in chronic liver disease. *Journal of Hepatology, 70*(1), 172–193; Styskel, B., Natarajan, Y., & Kanwal, F. (2019). Nutrition in alcoholic liver disease: An update. *Clinics in Liver Disease, 23*(1), 99–114; Yanny, B., Winters, A., Boutros, S., et al. (2019). Hepatic encephalopathy challenges, burden, and diagnostic and therapeutic approach. *Clinics in Liver Disease, 23*(4), 607–623; Yao, C. K., Fung, J., Chu, N. H. S., et al. (2018). Dietary interventions in liver cirrhosis. *Journal of Clinical Gastroenterology, 52*(8), 663–673.

This action may have short-term efficacy because patients with hepatic encephalopathy have an increased concentration of benzodiazepine receptors (Friedman & Martin, 2018).

 Nursing Management

Table 43-3 presents the stages of hepatic encephalopathy, common signs and symptoms, and potential nursing diagnoses for each stage. The nurse is responsible for maintaining a safe environment to prevent injury, bleeding, and infection. The nurse administers the prescribed treatments and monitors the patient for the numerous potential complications. The potential for respiratory compromise is great given the patient's depressed neurologic status. The nurse encourages deep breathing and position changes to prevent the development of atelectasis, pneumonia, and other respiratory complications. Despite aggressive pulmonary care, patients may develop respiratory compromise. They may require intubation and mechanical ventilation to protect the airway, and they are frequently admitted to the ICU.

The nurse communicates with the patient's family to inform them about the patient's status and supports them by explaining the procedures and treatments that are part of the patient's care. If the patient recovers from hepatic encephalopathy and coma, rehabilitation is likely to be prolonged. Therefore, the patient and family will require assistance to understand the causes of this severe complication and to recognize that it may recur.

Promoting Home, Community-Based and Transitional Care

 Educating Patients About Self-Care

If the patient has recovered from hepatic encephalopathy and is to be discharged home, the nurse educates the family about subtle signs of recurrent encephalopathy. The goals for caloric intake and protein intake should be 35 to 40 kcal/kg body weight per day and 1.2 to 1.5 g/kg body weight per day (see Chart 43-4) (Styskel et al., 2019; Yanny et al., 2019; Yao et al., 2018). Protein intake should not be limited too severely, because doing so worsens nutritional status and increases mortality (Styskel et al., 2019; Yanny et al., 2019; Yao et al., 2018). Continued use of lactulose after discharge is not uncommon, and the patient and family should closely monitor its efficacy and side effects. They should also be cautioned that constipation can precipitate encephalopathy and may be prevented through the prescribed use of lactulose.

Continuing and Transitional Care

Referral for transitional, home, or community-based care is warranted for the patient who returns home after recovery from hepatic encephalopathy. The nurse assesses the patient's physical and mental status and collaborates closely with the primary provider. The home visit provides an opportunity for the nurse to assess the home environment and the ability of the patient and family to monitor signs and symptoms and follow the treatment regimen. The nurse must evaluate the patient's fluid volume status and be alert for changes indicative of hypovolemia due to decreased intake and for decreased urine output associated with hepatorenal syndrome (see later discussion). Monitoring of laboratory values continues to be important, and the nurse must obtain prescriptions to correct abnormalities, especially electrolyte imbalances, which also can worsen encephalopathy.

The safety of the home environment is assessed closely to identify areas of risk for falls and other injuries. Home or transitional care visits are especially important if the patient lives alone because encephalopathy may affect the patient's ability to remember or follow the treatment regimen. The nurse reinforces previous education and reminds the patient and family about the importance of dietary restrictions, close monitoring, and follow-up. In addition, the nurse must observe the patient for subtle behavior changes of worsening hepatic encephalopathy. Patients with all types and stages of hepatic encephalopathy should have periodic neurologic evaluations to determine their cognitive function so that they do not engage in potentially harmful activities. Even subtle

TABLE 43-3	Stages of Hepatic Encephalopathy and Applicable Nursing Diagnoses		
Stage	**Clinical Symptoms**	**Clinical Signs and EEG Changes**	**Select Potential Nursing Diagnoses[a]**
1	Normal level of consciousness with periods of lethargy and euphoria; reversal of day–night sleep patterns	Impaired writing and ability to draw line figures. Normal EEG.	Activity intolerance Impaired ability to manage regime Impaired sleep pattern
2	Increased drowsiness; disorientation; inappropriate behavior; mood swings; agitation	Asterixis; fetor hepaticus. Abnormal EEG with generalized slowing.	Impaired socialisation Impaired role performance Risk for injury Acute confusion
3	Stuporous; difficult to rouse; sleeps most of time; marked confusion; incoherent speech	Asterixis; increased deep tendon reflexes; rigidity of extremities. EEG markedly abnormal.	Impaired nutritional intake Impaired mobility Impaired verbal communication
4	Comatose; may not respond to painful stimuli	Absence of asterixis; absence of deep tendon reflexes; flaccidity of extremities. EEG markedly abnormal.	Risk for aspiration Impaired gas exchange Impaired tissue integrity

EEG, electroencephalogram.

[a]Nursing diagnoses are likely to progress; thus, most nursing diagnoses present at earlier stages will occur during later stages as well.

Adapted from information in Feldman, M., Friedman, L. S., & Brandt, L. J. (2016). *Sleisinger & Fordtran's gastrointestinal & liver disease* (10th ed.). Philadelphia, PA: Saunders Elsevier.

neuropsychiatric abnormalities may preclude patients from driving, operating machinery, or participating in other activities that require psychomotor coordination.

Patients and families may need additional support during those times that the patient exhibits mood disturbances and sleep disorders. Patients should be as active as possible during the day and develop a normal sleep–wake pattern. Sedating medications should be avoided because they may precipitate encephalopathy. Patients and families may require assistance in developing plans to cope with changes in mood and mental status changes. This plan should identify support persons to attend to the patient in the home if needed. Social workers and case managers may make appropriate referrals for assistance with physical and psychosocial support and care. Referrals to psychologists, psychiatric liaison nurses, case managers, social workers, or therapists may assist family members with coping. Spiritual advisors may also provide another outlet for communication and guidance. If alcohol played a role in the development of the liver disease and encephalopathy, referral to Alcoholics Anonymous or Al-Anon may provide needed support and education.

Other Manifestations of Hepatic Dysfunction

Edema and Bleeding

Many patients with liver dysfunction develop generalized edema caused by hypoalbuminemia due to decreased hepatic production of albumin. The production of blood clotting factors by the liver is also reduced, leading to an increased incidence of bruising, epistaxis, bleeding from wounds, and, as described previously, GI bleeding. Abnormalities in the number and effectiveness of platelets also contribute to the bleeding in liver dysfunction. Congestion of the spleen secondary to portal hypertension causes hypersplenism (increased pooling of platelets in the organ). The resultant thrombocytopenia generally correlates with spleen size. In patients who abuse alcohol, suppression of bone marrow by the acute toxic effects of alcohol or folate deficiency may contribute to the thrombocytopenia (Goldman & Schafer, 2019). These factors predispose patients to easy bruising, petechiae formation, and bleeding from a variety of sources such as the GI or genitourinary tract (Goldman & Shafer, 2019).

Vitamin Deficiency

Decreased production of several clotting factors may be partially due to deficient absorption of vitamin K from the GI tract. This probably is caused by the inability of liver cells to use vitamin K to make prothrombin (Barrett et al., 2019; Hammer & McPhee, 2019). Absorption of the other fat-soluble vitamins (vitamins A, D, and E) as well as dietary fats may also be impaired because of decreased secretion of bile salts into the intestine.

Another group of problems common to patients with severe chronic liver dysfunction results from inadequate intake of sufficient vitamins. These include the following:

- Vitamin A deficiency, resulting in night blindness and eye and skin changes
- Thiamine deficiency, leading to beriberi, polyneuritis, and Wernicke–Korsakoff psychosis
- Riboflavin deficiency, resulting in characteristic skin and mucous membrane lesions
- Pyridoxine deficiency, resulting in skin and mucous membrane lesions and neurologic changes
- Vitamin C deficiency, resulting in the hemorrhagic lesions of scurvy
- Vitamin K deficiency, resulting in hypoprothrombinemia, characterized by spontaneous bleeding and ecchymoses
- Folic acid deficiency, resulting in macrocytic anemia

Because of these potential vitamin deficiencies, the diet of every patient with chronic liver disease (especially if alcohol related) is supplemented with vitamins A, B complex, C, K, and folic acid (EASL, 2019; Styskel et al., 2019; Yao et al., 2018).

Metabolic Abnormalities

Abnormalities of glucose metabolism also occur; the blood glucose level may be abnormally high shortly after a meal (similar to that when diabetes is present), but hypoglycemia may occur during fasting because of decreased hepatic glycogen reserves and decreased gluconeogenesis. Medications must be used cautiously and in reduced dosages because the ability to metabolize medications is decreased in the patient with liver failure.

Many endocrine abnormalities also occur with liver dysfunction because the liver cannot properly metabolize hormones, including androgens and sex hormones. Failure of the damaged liver to inactivate estrogens normally can cause gynecomastia, amenorrhea, testicular atrophy, loss of pubic hair in the male, menstrual irregularities in the female, and other disturbances of sexual function and sex characteristics.

Pruritus and Other Skin Changes

Patients with liver dysfunction resulting from biliary obstruction commonly develop severe pruritus due to retention of bile salts. Patients may develop vascular (or arterial) spider angiomas on the skin (see Fig. 43-3), usually above the waistline. These are numerous small vessels resembling a spider's legs. They are most often associated with cirrhosis, especially in alcoholic liver disease. Patients may also develop palmar erythema ("liver palms" or reddened palms).

VIRAL HEPATITIS

Viral hepatitis is a systemic, viral infection in which necrosis and inflammation of liver cells produce a characteristic cluster of clinical, biochemical, and cellular changes. To date, five definitive types of viral hepatitis that cause liver disease have been identified: hepatitis A, B, C, D, and E. Hepatitis A and E are similar in mode of transmission (fecal–oral route), whereas hepatitis B, C, and D share many other characteristics.

Hepatitis is easily transmitted and causes high morbidity and prolonged loss of time from school or employment. Acute viral hepatitis affects 0.5% to 1% of people in the United States each year. Hepatitis A virus (HAV) was responsible for 3366 cases in the United States in 2017. Incidence rates decreased more than 95% from 1995 to 2011, then increased by 140% from 2011 to 2017. In 2017, large person-to-person outbreaks began occurring, among persons who use drugs and persons experiencing homelessness (Centers for Disease Control and Prevention [CDC], 2017). During the same year, the hepatitis B virus (HBV) was the offending agent in a total of 3407 cases of acute viral hepatitis nationwide. The occurrence rate of viral hepatitis C (HCV) in 2017 was 3186 cases, with an incidence of 1.0 cases per 100,000 population, which represents an increase since 2013. Rates have been influenced by the opioid crisis. An estimated 2.4 million people in the United States are living with HCV infection (CDC, 2017).

The number of reported acute hepatitis B cases has remained stable with a slight increase in 2017. The increase is most likely due to increasing injection drug use related to the opioid crisis, and improved surveillance (CDC, 2017). The overall decrease in HBV rates since 1990 is largely due to the use of hepatitis A and B vaccines, the introduction of universal precautions and blood supply safety measures as well as public health education regarding high-risk behaviors (Goldman & Schafer, 2019). Conversely, the incidence of HAV and HCV infections has been on the rise. It is estimated that 60% to 90% of viral hepatitis cases go unreported (CDC, 2017). The occurrence of subclinical cases, failure to recognize mild cases, and misdiagnosis are thought to contribute to the underreporting. Table 43-4 compares the major forms of viral hepatitis.

The clinical presentation of hepatitis varies with individual patients as well as with the specific causative virus. Four phases of infectious hepatitis describe the clinical presentation. Phase 1 is the viral replication phase in which patients are asymptomatic but laboratory studies will reveal markers of hepatitis. Phase 2 is the preicteric or prodromal phase when those affected may experience anorexia, nausea, vomiting, fatigue and pruritus. Phase 3 is the icteric phase which is characterized by jaundice and dark urine. Some patients experience abdominal pain from an enlarged liver. Phase 4 is the convalescent phase when signs and symptoms resolve and laboratory values return to normal. Not all patients will experience all phases, especially those with a mild form of the disease (Chi, Cleary, & Bocchini, 2018; Shin, 2018).

Hepatitis A Virus

The HAV accounts for 20% to 25% of cases of clinical hepatitis in the United States (CDC, 2017). Hepatitis A, formerly called *infectious hepatitis*, is caused by an RNA virus of the enterovirus family. In the United States, the disease is seen mainly in the adult population. HAV is transmitted primarily through the fecal–oral route, by the ingestion of food or liquids infected with the virus. It is more prevalent in countries with overcrowding and poor sanitation. The virus has been found in the stool of infected patients before the onset of symptoms and during the first few days of illness.

Typically, a child or a young adult acquires the infection at school through poor hygiene, hand-to-mouth contact, or other close contact. The virus is carried home, where haphazard sanitary habits spread it through the family. An infected food handler can spread the disease, and people can contract it by consuming water or shellfish from sewage-contaminated waters. Outbreaks have occurred in day care centers and institutions as a result of poor hygiene among people with

TABLE 43-4	Comparison of Major Forms of Viral Hepatitis				
	Hepatitis A	**Hepatitis B**	**Hepatitis C**	**Hepatitis D**	**Hepatitis E**
Previous Names	Infectious Hepatitis	Serum Hepatitis	Non-A, non-B Hepatitis		
Epidemiology					
Cause	Hepatitis A virus (HAV)	Hepatitis B virus (HBV)	Hepatitis C virus (HCV)	Hepatitis D virus (HDV)	Hepatitis E virus (HEV)
Immunity	*Average:* 30 days Homologous	*Average:* 70–80 days Homologous	*Average:* 50 days Second attack may indicate weak immunity or infection with another agent.	*Average:* 35 days Homologous	*Average:* 31 days Unknown
Nature of Illness					
Signs and symptoms	May occur with or without symptoms; flu-like illness *Preicteric phase:* Headache, malaise, fatigue, anorexia, fever *Icteric phase:* Dark urine, jaundice of sclera and skin, tender liver	May occur without symptoms May develop arthralgias, rash	Similar to HBV; less severe and anicteric	Similar to HBV	Similar to HAV; very severe in pregnant women
Outcome	Usually mild with recovery. No carrier state or increased risk of chronic hepatitis, cirrhosis, or hepatic cancer.	May be severe. Carrier state possible. Increased risk of chronic hepatitis, cirrhosis, and hepatic cancer.	Frequent occurrence of chronic carrier state and chronic liver disease, but effective therapies that provide a sustained virologic response (SVR) are available. SVR is indicative of a cure of HCV infection. Increased risk of hepatic cancer if disease is not treated.	Similar to HBV but greater likelihood of carrier state, chronic active hepatitis, and cirrhosis	Similar to HAV except very severe in pregnant women

Adapted from Goldman, L., & Schafer, A. I. (2019). *Goldman's Cecil medicine* (26th ed.). Philadelphia, PA: Saunders Elsevier.

developmental disability. Hepatitis A can be transmitted during sexual activity; this is more likely with oral–anal contact or anal intercourse and with multiple sex partners (Chi et al., 2018; Goldman & Schafer, 2019; Shin & Jeong, 2018). Hepatitis A is not transmitted by blood transfusions.

The incubation period is estimated to be between 2 and 6 weeks, with a mean of approximately 4 weeks (CDC, 2017; Chi et al., 2018; Shin & Jeong, 2018). The illness may be prolonged, lasting 4 to 8 weeks. It usually lasts longer and is more severe in those older than 40 years. Most patients recover from hepatitis A; it rarely progresses to acute liver necrosis or acute hepatic failure resulting in cirrhosis of the liver or death. The mortality rate of hepatitis A is approximately 0.5% for those younger than 40 years and 1% to 2% for older adults. In patients with underlying chronic liver disease, morbidity and mortality are increased in the presence of an acute hepatitis A infection. No carrier state exists, and no chronic hepatitis is associated with the HAV. The virus is present only briefly in the serum; by the time jaundice occurs, the patient is likely to be noninfectious. Although hepatitis A confers immunity against itself, the person may contract other forms of hepatitis.

Clinical Manifestations

Many patients are anicteric (without jaundice) and symptomless. When symptoms appear, they resemble those of a mild, flu-like upper respiratory tract infection, with low-grade fever. Anorexia, an early symptom, is often severe. It is thought to result from release of a toxin by the damaged liver or from failure of the damaged liver cells to detoxify an abnormal product. Later, jaundice and dark urine may become apparent. Indigestion is present in varying degrees, marked by vague epigastric distress, nausea, heartburn, and flatulence. The patient may also develop a strong aversion to the taste of cigarettes or the presence of cigarette smoke and other strong odors (Papadakis & McPhee, 2020; Shin & Jeong, 2018). These symptoms tend to clear as soon as the jaundice reaches its peak, perhaps 10 days after its initial appearance. Symptoms may be mild in children; in adults, they may be more severe and the course of the disease prolonged.

Assessment and Diagnostic Findings

The liver and spleen are often moderately enlarged for a few days after onset; other than jaundice, there are few other physical signs. An HAV antigen may be found in the stool 7 to 10 days before illness and for 2 to 3 weeks after symptoms appear. HAV antibodies are detectable in the serum, although usually not until symptoms appear. Analysis of subclasses of immunoglobulins can help determine whether the antibody represents acute or past infection.

Prevention

A number of strategies exist to prevent transmission of HAV. Patients and their families are encouraged to follow general precautions that can prevent transmission of the virus. Scrupulous hand hygiene, safe water supplies, and proper control of sewage disposal are just a few of these prevention strategies.

Effective (95% to 100% after two to three doses) and safe HAV vaccines are available (Link-Gelles, Hofmeister, & Nelson, 2018). It is recommended that the two-dose vaccine be given to adults 18 years of age or older, with the second dose given 6 to 12 months after the first. Protection against HAV develops within several weeks after the first dose of the vaccine. Children and adolescents 1 to 18 years of age receive three doses; the second dose is given 1 month after the first, and the third dose is given 6 to 12 months later. HAV routine immunization of young children has proved to be effective in reducing disease incidence and maintaining very low incidence levels among vaccine recipients and across all age groups in many settings (Chi et al., 2018; Goldman & Schafer, 2019). As a result of its effectiveness in decreasing HAV, the hepatitis A vaccination recommendations have been expanded to include all children at 1 year of age. Hepatitis A vaccine is also recommended for people traveling to locations where sanitation and hygiene are unsatisfactory. Vaccination is also recommended for those from high-risk groups, such as men who have sex with men, people who use IV or injection drugs, staff of day care centers, health care personnel and those who work with the virus in research or animal care settings (Chi et al., 2018). The vaccine has also been used to interrupt community-wide outbreaks. A combined HAV and HBV vaccine is available for vaccination of people 18 years of age and older with indications for both HAV and HBV vaccination. Vaccination consists of three doses, given on the same schedule as that used for single-antigen HBV vaccine.

For people who have not been previously vaccinated, HAV can be prevented by intramuscular administration of globulin during the incubation period, if given within 2 weeks of exposure. This bolsters the person's antibody production and provides 6 to 8 weeks of passive immunity. Immune globulin may suppress overt symptoms of the disease; the resulting subclinical case of HAV would produce immunity to subsequent episodes of the virus.

Immune globulin is also recommended for household members and sexual contacts of people with HAV. Susceptible people in the same household as the patient are usually also infected by the time the diagnosis is made and should receive immune globulin. Institutional contacts of patients with HAV should also receive post-exposure prophylaxis with immune globulin. Prophylaxis is not necessary for casual contacts of an infected person, such as classmates, coworkers, or hospital employees (Link-Gelles et al., 2018). Although rare, systemic reactions to immune globulin do occur. Caution is required when anyone who has previously had angioedema, hives, or other allergic reactions is treated with any human immune globulin. Epinephrine should be available in case of systemic, anaphylactic reaction.

Pre-exposure prophylaxis is recommended for those traveling to developing countries or settings with poor or uncertain sanitation conditions who do not have sufficient time to acquire protection by administration of hepatitis A vaccine (Chi et al., 2018). Prevention strategies for HAV are outlined in Chart 43-5.

Medical Management

Bed rest during the acute stage and a nutritious diet are important aspects of treatment. During the period of anorexia, the patient should receive frequent small feedings, supplemented if necessary by IV fluids with glucose. Because the patient

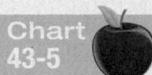

Chart 43-5 HEALTH PROMOTION
Prevention of Hepatitis

Hepatitis A

- Educate patients regarding safe practices for preparing and dispensing food.
- Encourage conscientious individual hygiene.
- Encourage proper community and home sanitation.
- Facilitate mandatory reporting of viral hepatitis to local health departments.
- Promote community health education programs.
- Promote vaccination to interrupt community-wide outbreaks.
- Recommend pre-exposure vaccination for all children 12–23 months of age. Continue existing immunization programs for children 1–18 years of age.
- Recommend vaccination for travelers to developing countries, illegal drug users (injection and noninjection drug users), men who have sex with men, people with chronic liver disease, people who work with HAV-infected animals or work with HAV in research facilities and recipients (e.g., hemophiliacs) of pooled plasma products for clotting factor disorders.
- Support effective health supervision of schools, dormitories, extended care facilities, barracks, and camps.

Hepatitis B

- Advise avoidance of high-risk behaviors.
- Avoid multidose vials in patient care settings.

- Monitor cleaning, disinfection, and sterilization of reusable devices in patient care settings.
- Recommend vaccination for international travelers to regions with high or intermediate levels of endemic hepatitis B virus infection and for persons with chronic liver disease or with human immune deficiency virus infection.
- Recommend vaccination for persons at risk for infection by sexual exposure, by percutaneous or mucosal exposure to blood.
- Recommend vaccination of all infants in the United States regardless of the mother's hepatitis B.
- Use barrier precautions in situations of contact with blood or body fluids.
- Use needleless IV and injection systems in health care.
- Use standard precautions in clinical care.

Hepatitis C

- Advise avoidance of high-risk behaviors such as IV drug use.
- Avoid multidose vials in patient care settings.
- Monitor cleaning, disinfection, and sterilization of reusable devices in patient care settings.
- Use barrier precautions in situations of contact with blood or body fluids.
- Use needleless IV and injection systems in health care.
- Use standard precautions in clinical care.

Adapted from Ferri, F. F. (Ed.). (2014). *Practical guide to the care of the medical patient* (9th ed.). Philadelphia, PA: Mosby Elsevier.

---

often has an aversion to food, gentle persistence, and creativity may be required to stimulate appetite. Optimal food and fluid levels are necessary to counteract weight loss and to speed recovery. Even before the icteric phase, however, many patients recover their appetites (see Chart 43-6).

The patient's sense of well-being and laboratory test results are generally appropriate guides to bed rest and restriction of physical activity. Gradual but progressive ambulation hastens recovery.

Chart 43-6 Dietary Management of Hepatitis

- Advise patient to avoid substances (medications, herbs, illicit drugs, and toxins) that may affect liver function, such as St. John's wort in patients taking hepatitis C virus protease inhibitors.
- Be aware that enteral feedings may be necessary if anorexia, nausea, and vomiting persist.
- Carefully monitor fluid balance.
- Instruct patient to abstain from alcohol during acute illness and for at least 6 months after recovery.
- Provide intake of 25–30 kcal/kg/day.
- Provide protein intake of 1.2–1.5 g/kg/day.
- Recommend small, frequent meals; minimize periods without food intake.

Adapted from European Association for the Study of the Liver (EASL). (2019). EASL clinical practice guidelines on nutrition in chronic liver disease. *Journal of Hepatology, 70*(1), 172–193; Styskel, B., Natarajan, Y., & Kanwal, F. (2019). Nutrition in alcoholic liver disease: An update. *Clinics in Liver Disease, 23*(1), 99–114.

Nursing Management

Management usually occurs in the home unless symptoms are severe. Therefore, the nurse assists the patient and family in coping with the temporary disability and fatigue that are common with HAV and educates them to seek additional health care if the symptoms persist or worsen. The patient and family also need specific guidelines about diet, rest, follow-up blood work, and the importance of avoiding alcohol, as well as sanitation and hygiene measures (particularly hand hygiene) to prevent spread of the disease to other family members.

Specific education for patients and families about reducing the risk of contracting HAV includes good personal hygiene, stressing careful hand hygiene (after bowel movements and before eating) and environmental sanitation (safe food and water supply, effective sewage disposal).

Hepatitis B Virus

Unlike HAV, the HBV is transmitted primarily through blood (percutaneous and permucosal routes). HBV can be found in blood, saliva, semen, and vaginal secretions and can be transmitted through mucous membranes and breaks in the skin. HBV is also transferred from carrier mothers to their infants, especially in areas with a high incidence (e.g., Southeast Asia). The infection usually is not transmitted via the umbilical vein but from the mother at the time of birth and during close contact afterward.

HBV has a long incubation period. It replicates in the liver and remains in the serum for relatively long periods, allowing transmission of the virus. Risk factors for HBV infection are summarized in Chart 43-7. Screening of blood donors has greatly reduced the occurrence of HBV after blood transfusion.

Most people (more than 90%) who contract HBV infection develop antibodies and recover spontaneously in 6 months. The mortality rate from acute HBV has been reported to be as high as 1%. Another 10% of patients who have HBV progress to a carrier state or develop chronic hepatitis with persistent HBV infection and hepatocellular injury and inflammation. It remains a major worldwide cause of cirrhosis and hepatocellular carcinoma (HCC) with higher mortality rates (Papadakis & McPhee, 2020; Sedhom, 2018; Schiff et al., 2018). In fact, approximately 15% of those who develop chronic hepatitis B during adulthood die of cirrhosis or liver cancer. Mortality rates are even higher (25%) for those whose chronic infection occurs during childhood (Chi et al., 2018). An estimated 730,000 adult residents of the United States are afflicted with chronic hepatitis B infection; however, there has been a small but significant decrease in the prevalence among U.S.-born adults who are 20 to 49 years of age (CDC, 2017; Sedhom, 2018).

Gerontologic Considerations

The immune system is altered in older adults. A less responsive immune system may be responsible for the increased incidence and severity of HBV among older adults and the increased incidence of liver abscesses secondary to decreased phagocytosis by the Kupffer cells. The older patient with HBV has a serious risk of severe liver cell necrosis or acute hepatic failure, particularly if other illnesses are present. With the advent of an HBV vaccine as the standard for prevention, the incidence of hepatic diseases may decrease in the future.

Clinical Manifestations

Clinically, HBV closely resembles HAV, but the incubation period is much longer (1 to 6 months). Signs and symptoms of HBV may be insidious and variable. Fever and respiratory symptoms are rare; some patients have arthralgias and rashes. The patient may have loss of appetite, dyspepsia, abdominal pain, generalized aching, malaise, and weakness. Jaundice may or may not be evident. If jaundice occurs, light-colored stools and dark urine accompany it. The liver may be tender and enlarged to 12 to 14 cm vertically. The spleen is enlarged and palpable in a few patients; the posterior cervical lymph nodes may also be enlarged. Subclinical episodes also occur frequently.

Assessment and Diagnostic Findings

HBV is a deoxyribonucleic acid (DNA) virus composed of the following antigenic particles:
- HBcAg—hepatitis B core antigen (antigenic material in an inner core)
- HBsAg—hepatitis B surface antigen (antigenic material on the viral surface, a marker of active replication and infection)
- HBeAg—an independent protein circulating in the blood
- HBxAg—gene product of X gene of HBV DNA

Each antigen elicits its specific antibody and is a marker for different stages of the disease process:
- anti-HBc—antibody to core antigen of HBV; persists during the acute phase of illness; may indicate continuing HBV in the liver
- anti-HBs—antibody to surface determinants on HBV; detected during late convalescence; usually indicates recovery and development of immunity
- anti-HBe—antibody to hepatitis B e-antigen; usually signifies reduced infectivity
- anti-HBxAg—antibody to the hepatitis B x-antigen; may indicate ongoing replication of HBV

HBsAg appears in the circulation in 80% to 90% of infected patients 1 to 10 weeks after exposure to HBV and 2 to 8 weeks before the onset of symptoms or an increase in transferase levels. Patients with HBsAg that persists for 6 months or longer after acute infection are considered to be HBsAg carriers (Chi et al., 2018; Sedhom, 2018). HBeAg is the next antigen of HBV to appear in the serum. It usually appears within 1 week of the appearance of HBsAg but before changes in aminotransferase levels; it disappears from the serum within 2 weeks. HBV DNA, detected by polymerase chain reaction testing, appears in the serum at about the same time as HBeAg. HBcAg is not always detected in the serum in HBV infection.

In the United States, the number of cases of chronic HBV is estimated to be 0.8 to 1.4 million persons. However, an accurate estimate is difficult to obtain because there is no national chronic-hepatitis surveillance program (CDC, 2017; Younossi, Stepanova, Younossi, et al., 2019). In 2013, males who died with HBV had a mortality rate that was nearly three times the mortality rate of females who died with HBV (0.8 deaths/100,000 population compared to 0.3 deaths/100,000 population). From 2009 to 2013, HBV-related mortality remained relatively stable for males and females (CDC, 2017). In 2015, hepatitis B resulted in an estimated 887,000 deaths worldwide, mostly from cirrhosis and HCC (World Health Organization [WHO], 2019).

Prevention

Prevention of hepatitis B transmission requires a multifaceted approach, including public health interventions and education as well as programs to foster immunization against this virulent virus in an effort to reduce the disease burden.

Preventing Transmission

Continued screening of blood donors for the presence of hepatitis B antigen (HBAg) further decreases the risk of transmission by blood transfusion. The use of disposable syringes, needles, and lancets and the introduction of needleless IV administration systems have reduced the risk of spreading this infection from one patient to another or to health care personnel during the collection of blood samples or the administration of parenteral therapy. In the clinical laboratory and the hemodialysis unit, work areas are disinfected daily. Gloves are worn when handling all blood and body fluids, as well as HBAg–positive specimens, or when there is potential exposure to blood (e.g., blood drawing) or to patients' secretions. Eating is prohibited in the laboratory and in other areas exposed to secretions, blood, or blood products. Patient education regarding the nature of the disease, its infectiousness, and prognosis is a critical factor in preventing transmission and protecting contacts (see Chart 43-5).

Active Immunization: HBV

Active immunization is recommended for people who are at high risk for HBV (e.g., health care personnel, patients undergoing hemodialysis). In addition, people with HCV and other chronic liver diseases should receive the vaccine. In 2018, the Advisory Committee on Immunization **Practices (ACIP)** recommended the use of a newly licensed hepatitis B vaccine, HEPLISAV-B, for people over the age of 18. This new vaccine is administered in two doses given 1 month apart. The decreased number of doses and abbreviated time period between doses may increase the rates of completion of the full vaccine series (Chi et al., 2018).

Prior to 2019, a yeast-recombinant hepatitis B vaccine was used to provide active immunity and has shown rates of protection greater than 90% in healthy people (Chan, Wong, Qin, et al., 2016; Terrault, Lok, McMahon, et al., 2018). Although antibody levels may become low or undetectable, immunologic memory may remain intact for at least 5 to 10 years. Measurable levels of antibodies may not be essential for protection. In general, in those with normal immune systems, booster doses are not required, and no data support the use of booster doses of hepatitis B vaccine among people who are immunocompetent and have responded to the vaccination series. However, booster doses are recommended for people who are immunocompromised (Chan et al., 2016; Terrault et al., 2018). A hepatitis B vaccine prepared from plasma of humans chronically infected with HBV is used only rarely in patients who are immunodeficient or allergic to recombinant yeast-derived vaccines.

Hepatitis B vaccines should be administered to adults in the deltoid muscle. Antibody response may be measured by anti-HBs levels 1 to 3 months after completion of the basic course of vaccine, but this testing is not routine and is not currently recommended. People who do not respond may benefit from additional doses (Terrault et al., 2018).

People at high risk, including nurses and other health care personnel exposed to blood or blood products, should receive active immunization. Health care workers who have had frequent contact with blood are screened for anti-HBs to determine whether immunity is already present from previous exposure. The vaccine produces active immunity to HBV in 90% to 95% of healthy people (Chi et al., 2018; Friedman & Martin, 2018; Terrault et al., 2018). It does not provide protection to those already exposed to HBV nor does it provide protection against other types of viral hepatitis.

Because HBV infection is frequently transmitted sexually, hepatitis B vaccination is recommended for all people who are unvaccinated and are being evaluated for a sexually transmitted infection (STI). It is also recommended for those with a history of an STI, people with multiple sex partners, people who have sex with people who use injection drugs, and men who are sexually active and have sex with other men (CDC, 2017; Chi et al., 2018; Terrault et al., 2018).

Universal childhood vaccination for hepatitis B prevention has been instituted in the United States, and universal vaccination of all infants is encouraged. Catch-up vaccination is recommended for all children and prepubertal adolescents up to the age of 19 years who have not been previously immunized (Feldman et al., 2016). Development of chronic carrier states has not been reported in adult responders to the vaccine.

Passive Immunity: Hepatitis B Immune Globulin

Hepatitis B immune globulin (HBIG) provides passive immunity to HBV and is indicated for people exposed to HBV who have never had hepatitis B and have never received hepatitis B vaccine. Specific indications for postexposure vaccine with HBIG include inadvertent exposure to HBAg-positive blood through percutaneous (needlestick) or transmucosal (splashes in contact with mucous membrane) routes, sexual contact with people positive for HBAg, and perinatal exposure (infants born to HBV-infected mothers should receive HBIG within 12 hours after delivery). HBIG is prepared from plasma selected for high titers of anti-HBs. Prompt immunization with HBIG (within hours to a few days after exposure to hepatitis B) increases the likelihood of protection. Both active and passive immunization are recommended for people who have been exposed to HBV through sexual contact or through the percutaneous or transmucosal routes. If HBIG and hepatitis B vaccines are given at the same time, separate sites and separate syringes should be used. HBIG is considered very safe, and there has been no evidence that infectious diseases have been transmitted due its administration (Chi et al., 2018; Terrault et al., 2018).

Medical Management

Goals are to minimize infectivity and liver inflammation and decrease symptoms. Of all the agents that have been used to treat chronic type B viral hepatitis, alpha-interferon is the single modality of therapy that offers the most promise. A regimen of 5 million U daily or 10 million U three times weekly for 16 to 24 weeks results in remission of disease in approximately one third of patients (Chan et al., 2016; Terrault et al., 2018). A prolonged course of treatment may also have additional benefits and is under study. Interferon must be given by injection and has significant side effects, including fever, chills, anorexia, nausea, myalgias, and fatigue. Delayed side effects are more serious and may necessitate dosage reduction or discontinuation. These include bone marrow suppression, thyroid dysfunction, alopecia, and bacterial infections. Several recombinant forms of alpha-interferon are also available, including the pegylated form (peginterferon alfa-2a), with once-weekly dosing. Pegylated interferon, also referred to as peginterferon, has largely replaced standard interferon due to its dosing schedule (Terrault et al., 2018). The American Association for the Study of Liver Diseases (AASLD) recommends pegylated interferon, entecavir or tenofovir, as preferred initial therapy for adults with chronic hepatitis B (AASLD, 2020; Terrault et al., 2018). These two antiviral agents, entecavir and tenofovir, are oral nucleoside analogs approved for use in chronic hepatitis B in the United States. They are the currently recommended agents for patients with HBV-related decompensated cirrhosis (AASLD, 2020, Terrault et al., 2018). Studies have revealed improved seroconversion rates and loss of detectable virus, improved liver function, and reduced progression to cirrhosis with entecavir and tenofovir. These agents can also be used for patients with decompensated cirrhosis who are awaiting liver transplantation (Chan et al., 2016; Terrault et al., 2018). Patients with decompensated cirrhosis have such severely damaged liver parenchyma that normal liver function severely deteriorates, resulting in life-threatening ascites, encephalopathy, or variceal hemorrhage (Chan et al., 2016; Schiff et al., 2018).

Bed rest may be recommended until the symptoms of hepatitis have subsided. Activities are restricted until the hepatic enlargement and levels of serum bilirubin and liver enzymes have decreased. Gradually, increased activity is then allowed.

Adequate nutrition should be maintained. Proteins are not restricted. Protein intake should be 1.2 to 1.5 g/kg/day (Schiff et al., 2018; Yao et al., 2018). Measures to control the dyspeptic symptoms and general malaise include the use of antacids and antiemetic agents, but all medications should be avoided if vomiting occurs. If vomiting persists, the patient may require hospitalization and fluid therapy. Because of the mode of transmission, the patient is evaluated for other bloodborne diseases (e.g., human immune deficiency virus infection).

Nursing Management

Convalescence may be prolonged, with complete symptomatic recovery sometimes requiring 3 to 4 months or longer (Papadakis & McPhee, 2020). During this stage, gradual resumption of physical activity is encouraged after the jaundice has resolved.

The nurse identifies psychosocial issues and concerns, particularly the effects of separation from family and friends if the patient is hospitalized during the acute and infective stages. Even if not hospitalized, the patient will be unable to work and must avoid sexual contact. Planning is required to minimize social isolation. Planning that includes the family helps to reduce their fears and anxieties about the spread of the disease.

Promoting Home, Community-Based and Transitional Care

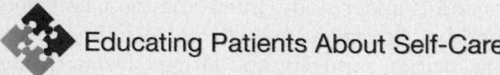

Educating Patients About Self-Care

Because of the prolonged period of convalescence, the patient and family must be prepared for care in the home. Provision

for adequate rest and nutrition must be ensured. The nurse educates family members and friends who have had intimate contact with the patient about the risks of contracting HBV and makes arrangements for them to receive hepatitis B vaccine or HBIG as prescribed. Those at risk must be made aware of the early signs of HBV and of ways to reduce risk by avoiding all modes of transmission. Patients with all forms of hepatitis should avoid drinking alcohol (Chan et al., 2016; Friedman & Martin, 2018; Schiff et al., 2018; Wang, Cheng, & Kao, 2020).

Continuing and Transitional Care

Follow-up visits by a transitional or home health nurse may be needed to assess the patient's progress and answer family members' questions about disease transmission. During a home visit, the nurse assesses the patient's physical and psychological status and confirms that the patient and family understand the importance of adequate rest and nutrition. The nurse also reinforces previous education. Because of the risk of transmission through sexual activity, strategies to prevent exchange of body fluids are recommended, such as abstinence or the use of condoms. The nurse emphasizes the importance of keeping follow-up appointments and participating in other health promotion activities and recommended health screenings.

Hepatitis C Virus

Blood transfusions and sexual contact once accounted for most cases of HCV in the United States, but other parenteral means, such as sharing of contaminated needles by those who use IV or injection drugs and unintentional needlesticks and other injuries in health care workers now account for a significant number of cases. In 2017, a total of 3186 cases of acute hepatitis C were reported to the CDC. After adjusting for under-ascertainment and under-reporting, an estimated 44,300 acute hepatitis C cases occurred in 2017. Approximately 2.5 million people in the United States are living with HCV, making it the most common chronic bloodborne infection nationally, though many of those infected are unaware of the disease (CDC, 2017). The highest prevalence of HCV is in adults 40 to 59 years of age; in this age group, its prevalence is highest among African Americans. In 2017, 17,253 U.S. death certificates had HCV recorded as an underlying or contributing cause of death but it has been suggested that deaths from this cause are underestimated (CDC, 2017; Houghton, 2019). HCV is the underlying cause of about one third of cases of HCC, and it is one of the most common reason for liver transplantation (CDC, 2017; Houghton, 2019).

People who are at particular risk for HCV include those who use IV or injection drugs, people who are sexually active with multiple partners, patients receiving frequent transfusions, those who require large volumes of blood, and health care personnel (see Chart 43-8). The incubation period is variable and may range from 15 to 160 days. The clinical course of acute HCV is similar to that of HBV; symptoms are usually mild or absent. However, a chronic carrier state occurs frequently, and there is an increased risk of chronic liver disease, including cirrhosis or liver cancer, after HCV. It is for this reason that those in high- and moderate-risk groups as well as those known to have high prevalence rates (e.g., those born in certain countries or regions) be screened for HCV as well as for HBV (CDC, 2017; Houghton, 2019; Schiff et al., 2018). Small amounts of alcohol taken regularly appear to cause progression of the disease. Therefore, alcohol and medications that may affect the liver should be avoided.

There is no benefit from rest, diet, or vitamin supplements. The treatment for HCV infection has evolved since the introduction of highly effective HCV protease inhibitor therapies in 2011. Currently available therapies can achieve sustained virologic response (SVR) defined as the absence of detectable virus 12 weeks after completion of treatment; an SVR is indicative of a cure of HCV infection. Over 90% of persons infected with HCV can be cured of HCV infection regardless of HCV genotype (there are over 67 identified subtypes but type 1 is most common), with 8 to 12 weeks of oral therapy (CDC, 2017). HCV direct-acting antivirals (DAA) including simeprevir plus sofosbuvir, ledipasvir-sofosbuvir, and ombitasvir-paritaprevir-ritonavir packaged with dasabuvir have fewer side effects, shorter treatment durations, and higher cure rates than previously recommended antiviral agents. A newer dual combination that includes another derivative of daclatasvir with sofosbuvir is equally effective against all HCV genotypes (Chan et al., 2016; Houghton, 2019). Prescribers must take into account the degree of cirrhosis in individual patients in order to determine the most appropriate protease inhibitor. The American Association for the Study of Liver Diseases (AASLD, 2020) recommends regimens of glecaprevir/pibrentasvir or sofusbuvir/velpatasvir for those patients who meet the criteria for simplified HCV treatment that includes treatment-naive adults without cirrhosis or those with compensated cirrhosis. The choice of medication is dependent on the genotype as well (AASLD, 2020).

There are HCV treatments in development that are expected to be more effective in curing the disease and better tolerated with fewer adverse effects and contraindications (Houghton, 2019). As a result of the rapidly changing landscape for treatment of viral infections, it is important to monitor related websites for the most up-to-date recommendations (CDC, 2017; Houghton, 2019). A key challenge remains how to deliver the currently expensive DAA drugs to all global carriers of HCV (Houghton, 2019).

Screening of blood has reduced the incidence of HCV associated with blood transfusion, and public health programs are helping to reduce the number of cases associated with shared needles in IV or injection drug use (see Chart 43-5).

Hepatitis D Virus

Hepatitis D virus (delta agent) infection occurs in some cases of hepatitis B. Because the virus requires HBsAg for its replication, only people with hepatitis B are at risk for hepatitis D. Anti-delta antibodies in the presence of HBAg on testing confirm the diagnosis. Hepatitis D is common among those who use IV or injection drugs, patients undergoing hemodialysis, and recipients of multiple blood transfusions. Sexual contact with those who have hepatitis B is considered to be an important mode of transmission of hepatitis B and D. The incubation period varies between 30 and 150 days (Schiff et al., 2018).

The symptoms of hepatitis D are similar to those of hepatitis B, except that patients are more likely to develop acute hepatic failure and to progress to chronic active hepatitis and cirrhosis. Treatment is similar to that of other forms of hepatitis. Currently, interferon alfa is the only licensed drug available in the treatment for HDV infection. The rate of recurrence is high, and the efficacy of interferon is related to the dose and duration of treatment. High-dose, long-duration therapy for at least a year is recommended (Friedman & Martin, 2018; Schiff et al., 2018; Sedhom, D'Souza, John, et al., 2018).

Hepatitis E Virus

It is believed that HEV is transmitted by the fecal–oral route, principally through contaminated water in areas with poor sanitation. The incubation period is variable, estimated to range between 15 and 65 days. In general, hepatitis E resembles hepatitis A. It has a self-limited course with an abrupt onset. Jaundice is almost always present. Chronic forms do not develop.

Avoiding contact with the virus through good hygiene, including handwashing, is the major method of prevention of hepatitis E. The effectiveness of immune globulin in protecting against HEV is uncertain.

Hepatitis G Virus and GB Virus-C

It has long been believed that there is another non-A–E agent causing hepatitis in humans. The incubation period for posttransfusion hepatitis is 14 to 145 days—too long for hepatitis B or C. In the United States, about 5% of chronic liver disease remains cryptogenic (i.e., does not appear to be autoimmune or viral in origin), and 50% of these patients have received blood transfusions before developing disease. Therefore, another form of hepatitis, referred to as hepatitis G virus (HGV) or GB virus-C (GBV-C), has been described; these are thought to be two different isolates of the same virus, which are percutaneously transmitted. Autoantibodies are absent.

The clinical significance of this virus remains uncertain. Risk factors are similar to those for hepatitis C. There is no clear relationship between HGV/GBV-C infection and progressive liver disease. Persistent infection does occur but does not affect the clinical course (Papadakis & McPhee, 2020; Sedhom et al., 2018).

NONVIRAL HEPATITIS

Certain chemicals have toxic effects on the liver and produce acute liver cell necrosis or toxic hepatitis when inhaled, injected parenterally, or taken by mouth. Some chemicals commonly implicated in this disease include carbon tetrachloride and phosphorus. These substances are true hepatotoxins. Many medications can induce hepatitis but are only sensitizing rather than toxic. Drug-induced hepatitis is similar to acute viral hepatitis, but parenchymal destruction tends to be more extensive. Medications that can lead to hepatitis include isoniazid, halothane, acetaminophen, methyldopa, and certain antibiotics, antimetabolites, and anesthetic agents.

Toxic Hepatitis

At the onset of disease, toxic hepatitis resembles viral hepatitis. Obtaining a history of exposure to hepatotoxic chemicals, medications, botanical agents, or other toxic agents assists in early treatment and removal of the causative agent. Anorexia, nausea, and vomiting are the usual symptoms; jaundice and hepatomegaly are noted on physical assessment. Symptoms are more intense for the more severely toxic patient.

Recovery from acute toxic hepatitis is rapid if the hepatotoxin is identified early and removed or if exposure to the agent has been limited. Recovery is unlikely if there is a prolonged period between exposure and onset of symptoms. There are no effective antidotes. The fever rises; the patient becomes toxic and prostrated. Vomiting may be persistent, with the emesis containing blood. Clotting abnormalities may be severe, and hemorrhages may appear under the skin. The severe GI symptoms may lead to vascular collapse. Delirium, coma, and seizures develop, and within a few days the patient may die of acute hepatic failure (discussed later) unless they receive a liver transplant.

Short of liver transplantation, few treatment options are available. Therapy is directed toward restoring and maintaining fluid and electrolyte balance, blood replacement, and comfort and supportive measures. A few patients recover from acute toxic hepatitis only to develop chronic liver disease. If the liver heals, there may be scarring, followed by postnecrotic cirrhosis.

Drug-Induced Hepatitis

Drug-induced liver disease is the most common cause of acute liver failure, accounting for more than 50% of all cases in the United States (Schiff et al., 2018; Stravitz & Lee, 2019; Thomas & Lewis, 2018). Manifestations of sensitivity to a medication may occur on the first day of its use or not until several months later. Usually, the onset is abrupt, with chills, fever, rash, pruritus, arthralgia, anorexia, and nausea. Later, there may be jaundice, dark urine, and an enlarged and tender liver. After the offending medication is withdrawn, symptoms may gradually subside. However, reactions can be severe, or even fatal, even if the medication is stopped. If fever, rash, or pruritus occurs from any medication, its use should be stopped immediately.

Although any medication can affect liver function, the use of acetaminophen (found in many OTC medications used to treat fever and pain) has been identified as the leading cause of acute liver failure (Schiff et al., 2018; Stravitz & Lee, 2019). Other causes commonly associated with liver injury include many anesthetic agents, medications used to

treat rheumatic and musculoskeletal disease, antidepressants, psychotropic medications, anticonvulsants, and antituberculosis agents (Schiff et al., 2018; Stravitz & Lee, 2019; Thomas & Lewis, 2018).

A short course of high-dose corticosteroids may be used in patients with severe hypersensitivity reactions, although its efficacy is uncertain. Liver transplantation is an option for drug-induced hepatitis, but outcomes may not be as successful as with other causes of liver failure.

ACUTE LIVER FAILURE

Acute hepatic failure or **acute liver failure** (ALF) is the clinical syndrome of sudden and severely impaired liver function in a person who was previously healthy. The definition of ALF includes neurologic dysfunction, an elevated prothrombin time and international normalized ratio (PT/INR) ≥1.5, no prior evidence of liver disease, and a disease course of ≤26 weeks (Friedman & Martin, 2018; Maher & Schreibman, 2018; Montrief, Koyfman, & Long, 2019; Schiff et al., 2018). The time from the onset of symptoms such as jaundice to the development of hepatic encephalopathy categorizes the different forms of acute liver failure: a very rapid injury (within hours) is referred to as hyperacute liver failure; and a slower, immune-based injury (days to weeks) is considered acute or subacute (Maher & Schreibman, 2018; Stravitz & Lee, 2019). In hyperacute liver failure, the duration of jaundice before the onset of encephalopathy is 0 to 7 days; in acute liver failure, it is 8 to 28 days; and in subacute liver failure, it is 28 to 72 days. The prognosis for acute hepatic failure is much worse than for chronic liver failure. However, in acute failure, the hepatic lesion is potentially reversible, and survival rates are approximately 20% to 50%, depending greatly on the cause. Those who do not survive die of massive hepatocellular injury and necrosis (Maher & Schreibman, 2018; Montrief et al., 2019; Stravitz & Lee, 2019).

Viral hepatitis is a common cause of ALF; other causes include toxic medications (e.g., acetaminophen) and chemicals (e.g., carbon tetrachloride), metabolic disturbances (e.g., Wilson disease, a hereditary syndrome with deposition of copper in the liver), and structural changes (e.g., Budd–Chiari syndrome, an obstruction to outflow in major hepatic veins) (Maher & Schreibman, 2018; Stravitz & Lee, 2019).

Jaundice and profound anorexia may be the initial reasons the patient seeks health care. ALF is often accompanied by coagulation defects, kidney disease and electrolyte disturbances, cardiovascular abnormalities, infection, hypoglycemia, encephalopathy, and cerebral edema (Maher & Schreibman, 2018; Montrief et al., 2019; Stravitz & Lee, 2019).

The key to optimized treatment is rapid recognition of ALF and intensive intervention. Supporting the patient in the ICU and assessing the indications for and feasibility of liver transplantation are hallmarks of management. The use of antidotes for certain conditions may be indicated, such as N-acetylcysteine for acetaminophen toxicity and penicillin for mushroom poisoning. Treatment modalities may include plasmapheresis to correct coagulopathy, to reduce serum ammonia levels, and to stabilize the patient awaiting liver transplantation, and prostaglandin therapy to enhance hepatic blood flow. Although these treatment modalities may be implemented, no evidence exists indicating any clinical improvement with their use (Maher & Schreibman, 2018; Montrief et al., 2019; Stravitz & Lee, 2019; Wendon et al., 2017). Hepatocytes within synthetic fiber columns have been tested as liver support systems (liver assist devices) to provide a bridge to transplantation.

Research into interventions for ALF has begun to focus on techniques that combine the efficacy of a whole liver with the convenience and biocompatibility of hemodialysis. The acronyms ELAD (*extracorporeal liver assist devices*) and BAL (*bioartificial liver*) have been used to describe these hybrid devices. These short-term devices, which remain experimental, may help patients survive until transplantation is possible (Villarreal & Sussman, 2019; Wendon et al., 2017). The BAL device exposes separated plasma to a cartridge containing porcine liver cells after the plasma has flowed through a charcoal column that removes substances toxic to hepatocytes. The ELAD exposes whole blood to cartridges containing human hepatoblastoma cells, resulting in removal of toxic substances. These approaches appear promising and have had success in animal studies. In human clinical application, the use of various BAL systems has resulted in improved neurologic and biochemical parameters. Adding albumin to extracorporeal dialysis in a process known as molecular adsorbent recirculating system (MARS), and therapeutic plasma exchanges (TPE) have been used to remove protein-bound toxins and is potentially useful in unstable patients with ALF or acute or chronic liver disease (Bañares et al., 2019; Larsen, 2019; Wendon et al., 2017).

In patients who have ALF with stage 4 encephalopathy (see Table 43-3), there is a high risk of cerebral edema, a life-threatening complication. The cause is not fully understood, although disruption of the blood–brain barrier and plasma leakage into the cerebrospinal fluid may be one cause. An increase in the intracellular osmolarity within cerebral astrocyte cells, possibly related to increased sodium and glutamine in these cells, may be another (Montrief et al., 2019; Stravitz & Lee, 2019). These patients require intracranial pressure monitoring. Measures to promote adequate cerebral perfusion include careful fluid balance and hemodynamic assessments, a quiet environment, and diuresis with mannitol, an osmotic diuretic.

The use of pharmacologic neuromuscular blockade (NMB) and sedation is indicated to prevent surges in intracranial pressure related to agitation. Other support measures include monitoring for and treating hypoglycemia, coagulopathies, and infection. Despite these treatment modalities, the mortality rate remains high. Consequently, liver transplantation (discussed later) is the treatment of choice for ALF.

HEPATIC CIRRHOSIS

Cirrhosis is a chronic disease characterized by replacement of normal liver tissue with diffuse fibrosis that disrupts the structure and function of the liver. There are three types of cirrhosis or scarring of the liver:

- Alcoholic cirrhosis, in which the scar tissue characteristically surrounds the portal areas. This is most frequently caused by chronic alcoholism and is the most common type of cirrhosis.

- Postnecrotic cirrhosis, in which there are broad bands of scar tissue. This is a late result of a previous bout of acute viral hepatitis.
- Biliary cirrhosis, in which scarring occurs in the liver around the bile ducts. This type of cirrhosis usually results from chronic biliary obstruction and cholangitis (bile duct infection); it is much less common.

The portion of the liver chiefly involved in cirrhosis consists of the portal and the periportal spaces, where the bile canaliculi of each lobule communicate to form the liver bile ducts. These areas become the sites of inflammation, and the bile ducts become occluded with inspissated (thickened) bile and pus. The liver attempts to form new bile channels; hence, there is an overgrowth of tissue made up largely of disconnected, newly formed bile ducts and surrounded by scar tissue.

Pathophysiology

Several factors have been implicated in the etiology of cirrhosis. Nutritional deficiency with reduced protein intake contributes to liver destruction in cirrhosis, but excessive alcohol intake is the major causative factor in fatty liver and its consequences. However, cirrhosis can occur in people who do not consume alcohol and in those who consume a normal diet and have a high alcohol intake.

Some people appear to be more susceptible than others to this disease, whether or not they have alcoholism or are malnourished. Other factors may play a role, including exposure to certain chemicals (carbon tetrachloride, chlorinated naphthalene, arsenic, or phosphorus) or infectious schistosomiasis. Twice as many men as women are affected, although, for unknown reasons, women are at greater risk for development of alcohol-induced liver disease. Most patients are between 40 and 60 years of age. Alcohol-associated cirrhosis contributes to up to 50% of the overall cirrhosis burden in the United States and worldwide (Lucey, 2019). From 1999 to 2016 in the United States, annual deaths from cirrhosis increased by 65% to approximately 35,000 (Baki, 2019; Tapper, 2018).

Alcoholic cirrhosis is characterized by episodes of necrosis involving the liver cells, which sometimes occur repeatedly throughout the course of the disease. The destroyed liver cells are gradually replaced by scar tissue. Eventually, the amount of scar tissue exceeds that of the functioning liver tissue. Islands of residual normal tissue and regenerating liver tissue may project from the constricted areas, giving the cirrhotic liver its characteristic hobnail appearance. The disease usually has an insidious onset and a protracted course, occasionally proceeding over a period of 30 or more years.

The prognoses for different forms of cirrhosis caused by various liver diseases have been investigated in several studies. Of the many prognostic indicators, the Child–Pugh classification seems most useful in predicting the outcome of patients with liver disease (see Table 43-5). It is also used in choosing management approaches.

Clinical Manifestations

Signs and symptoms of cirrhosis increase in severity as the disease progresses, and severity is used to categorize the disorder as compensated or decompensated cirrhosis (see Chart 43-9). Compensated cirrhosis, with its less severe, often vague symptoms, may be discovered secondarily at a routine

TABLE 43-5	Modified Child–Pugh Classification of the Severity of Liver Disease		
	Points Assigned		
Parameter	1	2	3
Ascites	Absent	Slight	Moderate
Bilirubin (mg/dL)	≤2	2–3	>3
Albumin (g/dL)	>3.5	2.8–3.5	<2.8
Prothrombin time (seconds over control)	1–3	4–6	>6
Encephalopathy	None	Grade 1–2	Grade 3–4

Total score of 5–6, grade A; 7–9, grade B; 10–15, grade C.
Adapted from Feldman, M., Friedman, L. S., & Brandt, L. J. (2016). *Sleisinger & Fordtran's gastrointestinal & liver disease* (10th ed.). Philadelphia, PA: Saunders Elsevier.

physical examination. The hallmarks of decompensated cirrhosis result from failure of the liver to synthesize proteins, clotting factors, and other substances and manifestations of portal hypertension (see earlier sections of this chapter for clinical manifestations and management of portal hypertension, ascites, varices, and hepatic encephalopathy).

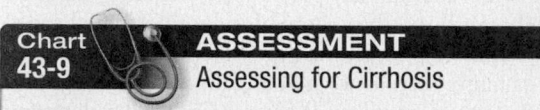

Chart 43-9 — ASSESSMENT
Assessing for Cirrhosis

Be alert to the following signs and symptoms:

Compensated

- Abdominal pain
- Ankle edema
- Firm, enlarged liver
- Flatulent dyspepsia
- Intermittent mild fever
- Palmar erythema (reddened palms)
- Splenomegaly
- Unexplained epistaxis
- Vague morning indigestion
- Vascular spiders

Decompensated

- Ascites
- Clubbing of fingers
- Continuous mild fever
- Epistaxis
- Gonadal atrophy
- Hypotension
- Jaundice
- Muscle wasting
- Purpura (due to decreased platelet count)
- Sparse body hair
- Spontaneous bruising
- Weakness
- Weight loss
- White nails

Adapted from Lee, S. S., & Moreau, R. (2015). *Cirrhosis: A practical guide to management* (1st ed.). Hoboken, NJ: John Wiley & Sons, Ltd.

Liver Enlargement

Early in the course of cirrhosis, the liver tends to be large, and the cells are loaded with fat. The liver is firm and has a sharp edge that is noticeable on palpation. Abdominal pain may be present because of recent, rapid enlargement of the liver, which produces tension on Glisson capsule (the fibrous covering of the liver). Later in the disease, the liver decreases in size as scar tissue contracts the liver tissue. The liver edge, if palpable, is nodular.

Portal Obstruction and Ascites

Portal obstruction and ascites—late manifestations of cirrhosis—are caused partly by chronic failure of liver function and partly by obstruction of the portal circulation. Almost all of the blood from the digestive organs is collected in the portal veins and carried to the liver. Because a cirrhotic liver does not allow free blood passage, blood backs up into the spleen and the GI tract, and these organs become the seat of chronic passive congestion—that is, they are stagnant with blood and therefore cannot function properly. Indigestion and altered bowel function result. Fluid rich in protein may accumulate in the peritoneal cavity, producing ascites. This can be detected through percussion for shifting dullness or a fluid wave (see Fig. 43-6).

Infection and Peritonitis

Bacterial peritonitis may develop in patients with cirrhosis and ascites in the absence of an intra-abdominal source of infection or an abscess. This condition is referred to as spontaneous bacterial peritonitis (SBP). Bacteremia due to translocation of intestinal flora is believed to be the most likely route of infection. Clinical signs may be absent, necessitating paracentesis for diagnosis. Antibiotic therapy is effective in the treatment and prevention of recurrent episodes of SBP. The development of SBP is a precipitating factor to the onset of hepatorenal syndrome, a form of acute kidney injury unresponsive to administration of fluid or diuretic agents (Adebayo, Neong, & Wong, 2019; Schiff et al., 2018). This type of kidney disease is characterized by a lack of pathologic changes in the kidney; there is no evidence of dehydration or obstruction of the urinary tract or any other renal disorder.

Gastrointestinal Varices

The obstruction to blood flow through the liver caused by fibrotic changes also results in the formation of collateral blood vessels in the GI system and shunting of blood from the portal vessels into blood vessels with lower pressures. As a result, the patient with cirrhosis often has prominent, distended abdominal blood vessels, called *caput medusae*, which are visible on abdominal inspection and distended blood vessels throughout the GI tract. The esophagus, stomach, and lower rectum are common sites of collateral blood vessels. These distended blood vessels form varices or hemorrhoids, depending on their location.

Because these vessels were not intended to carry the high pressure and volume of blood imposed by cirrhosis, they may rupture and bleed. Therefore, assessment must include observation for occult and frank bleeding from the GI tract.

Edema

Another late symptom of cirrhosis is edema, which is attributed to chronic liver failure. A reduced plasma albumin concentration predisposes the patient to the formation of edema. Although edema is generalized, it often affects the lower extremities, the upper extremities, and the presacral area. Facial edema is not typical. Overproduction of aldosterone occurs, causing sodium and water retention and potassium excretion.

Vitamin Deficiency and Anemia

Because of inadequate formation, use, and storage of certain vitamins (notably vitamins A, C, and K), signs of deficiency are common, particularly hemorrhagic phenomena associated with vitamin K deficiency. Chronic gastritis and impaired GI function, together with inadequate dietary intake and impaired liver function, account for the anemia that is often associated with cirrhosis. The patient's anemia, poor nutritional status, and poor state of health result in severe fatigue, which interferes with the ability to carry out routine activities of daily living.

Mental Deterioration

Additional clinical manifestations include deterioration of mental and cognitive function with impending hepatic encephalopathy and hepatic coma, as described previously. Serial neurologic assessment is indicated, including assessment of the patient's general behavior, cognitive abilities, orientation to time and place, and speech patterns.

Assessment and Diagnostic Findings

The extent of liver disease and the type of treatment are determined after review of the laboratory findings. The functions of the liver are complex, and many diagnostic tests provide information about liver function (see Table 43-1). The patient needs to know why these tests are being performed and how to cooperate.

In severe parenchymal liver dysfunction, the serum albumin level tends to decrease, and the serum globulin level rises. Enzyme tests indicate liver cell damage: serum alkaline phosphatase, AST, ALT, and GGT levels increase, and the serum cholinesterase level may decrease. Bilirubin tests are performed to measure bile excretion or retention; increased levels of bilirubin can occur with cirrhosis and other liver disorders. Prothrombin time is prolonged. Normal values for laboratory data are listed in Appendix A on thePoint.

Ultrasound scanning is used to measure the difference in density of parenchymal cells and scar tissue. CT, MRI, radioisotope liver scans, and elastography studies give information about liver size, hepatic blood flow and obstruction and the presence of liver fibrosis. Diagnosis is confirmed by liver biopsy. Arterial blood gas analysis may reveal a ventilation–perfusion imbalance and hypoxia.

Medical Management

Management of the patient with cirrhosis is usually based on the presenting symptoms. For example, antacids or H_2 antagonists are prescribed to decrease gastric distress and minimize the possibility of GI bleeding. Vitamins and nutritional supplements promote healing of damaged liver cells and improve the patient's general nutritional status. Potassium-sparing diuretic agents such as spironolactone or triamterene may be indicated to decrease ascites, if present; these diuretics

are preferred because they minimize the fluid and electrolyte changes commonly seen with other agents. An adequate diet and avoidance of alcohol are essential. Although the fibrosis of the cirrhotic liver cannot be reversed, its progression may be halted or slowed by such measures.

Many medications possess antifibrotic activity for the treatment of cirrhosis. Some of these medications include colchicine, angiotensin system inhibitors, statins, diuretics including spironolactone, immunosuppressants, and glitazones such as pioglitazone or rosiglitazone. Angiotensin receptor blocker (ARB) medications also have antifibrogenic properties and may also be prescribed (Schiff et al., 2018).

Many advances have been made in the treatment of liver fibrosis. Understanding of the pathogenic mechanisms of liver disease and fibrogenesis has led to the recent increase in the number of clinical trials, particularly for patients with NASH. Fibrosis is a key predictor of liver mortality in NASH, and many studies have focused on evaluating the potential of drugs to reduce liver fibrogenesis. Drugs that target different pathways in NASH are, therefore, being evaluated in isolation or as combination therapy. Some of the antifibrotic medications currently under study can reduce injury and inflammation and include vitamin E and chemokine receptor (CCR2/CCR5) inhibitors. Peroxisome proliferator-activated receptor (PPAR) agonists have been shown to cause cell death of hepatic stellate cells that potentiate fibrosis. Farnesoid X receptor agonists, such as obeticholic acid, have been reported to prevent chronic inflammation and liver fibrosis (Manka Zeller, & Syn, 2019; Schiff et al., 2018).

Many patients who have ESLD with cirrhosis use the herb milk thistle (*Silybum marianum*) to treat jaundice and other symptoms. This herb has been used for centuries because of its healing and regenerative properties for liver disease. Silymarin from milk thistle has anti-inflammatory and antioxidant properties that may have beneficial effects, especially in hepatitis, alcohol-induced liver injury and HCC (Weiskirchen, Weiskirchen, & Tacke, 2018). The natural compound SAM-e (S-adenosylmethionine) may improve outcomes in liver disease by improving liver function, possibly through enhancing antioxidant function. Primary biliary cirrhosis has been treated with ursodeoxycholic acid to improve liver function.

Nursing Management

Nursing management for the patient with cirrhosis of the liver is described in detail in Chart 43-10. Nursing interventions are directed toward promoting patient's rest, improving nutritional status, providing skin care, reducing risk of injury, and monitoring and managing potential complications.

Promoting Rest

The patient with cirrhosis requires rest and other supportive measures to permit the liver to reestablish its functional ability. If the patient is hospitalized, weight and I&O are measured and recorded daily. The nurse adjusts the patient's position in bed for maximal respiratory efficiency, which is especially important if ascites is marked, because it interferes with adequate thoracic excursion. Oxygen therapy may be required in liver failure to oxygenate the damaged cells and prevent further cell destruction.

(*text continued on page 1403*)

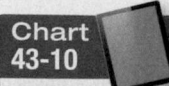

Chart 43-10

PLAN OF NURSING CARE
The Patient with Impaired Liver Function

NURSING DIAGNOSIS: Activity intolerance associated with fatigue, lethargy, and malaise
GOAL: Patient reports decrease in fatigue and reports increased ability to participate in activities

Nursing Interventions	Rationale	Expected Outcomes
1. Assess level of activity tolerance and degree of fatigue, lethargy, and malaise when performing routine activities of daily living. 2. Assist with activities and hygiene when fatigued. 3. Encourage rest when fatigued or when abdominal pain or discomfort occurs. 4. Assist with selection and pacing of desired activities and exercise. 5. Provide diet high in carbohydrates with protein intake of 1.2 to 1.5 g/kg/day. 6. Administer supplemental vitamins (A, B complex, C, and K).	1. Provides baseline for further assessment and criteria for assessment of effectiveness of interventions. 2. Promotes exercise and hygiene within patient's level of tolerance. 3. Conserves energy and protects the liver. 4. Stimulates patient's interest in selected activities. 5. Provides calories for energy and protein for healing. 6. Provides additional nutrients.	• Exhibits increased interest in activities and events • Participates in activities and gradually increases exercise within physical limits • Reports increased strength and well-being • Reports absence of abdominal pain and discomfort • Plans activities to allow ample periods of rest • Takes vitamins as prescribed

NURSING DIAGNOSIS: Impaired nutritional intake associated with abdominal distention, discomfort, and anorexia
GOAL: Positive nitrogen balance, no further loss of muscle mass; meets nutritional requirements

Nursing Interventions	Rationale	Expected Outcomes
1. Assess dietary intake and nutritional status through diet history and diary, daily weight measurements, and laboratory data. 2. Provide diet high in carbohydrates with protein intake of 1.2 to 1.5 g/kg/day. 3. Assist patient in identifying low-sodium foods. 4. Elevate the head of the bed during meals. 5. Provide oral hygiene before meals and pleasant environment for meals at mealtime. 6. Offer smaller, more frequent meals (6/day). 7. Encourage patient to eat meals and supplementary feedings. 8. Provide attractive meals and an aesthetically pleasing setting at mealtime. 9. Eliminate alcohol. 10. Administer medications prescribed for nausea, vomiting, diarrhea, or constipation. 11. Encourage increased fluid intake and exercise if the patient reports constipation.	1. Identifies deficits in nutritional intake and adequacy of nutritional state. 2. Provides calories for energy and protein for healing. 3. Reduces edema and ascites formation. 4. Reduces discomfort from abdominal distention and decreases sense of fullness produced by pressure of abdominal contents and ascites on the stomach. 5. Promotes positive environment and increased appetite; reduces unpleasant taste. 6. Decreases feeling of fullness, bloating. 7. Encouragement is essential for the patient with anorexia and gastrointestinal discomfort. 8. Promotes appetite and sense of well-being. 9. Eliminates "empty calories" and further damage from alcohol. 10. Reduces gastrointestinal symptoms and discomforts that decrease the appetite and interest in food. 11. Promotes normal bowel pattern and reduces abdominal discomfort and distention.	• Exhibits improved nutritional status by increased weight (without fluid retention) and improved laboratory data • States rationale for dietary modifications • Identifies foods high in carbohydrates and protein • Reports improved appetite • Participates in oral hygiene measures • Reports increased appetite; identifies rationale for smaller, frequent meals • Demonstrates intake of high-calorie diet; adheres to protein intake recommendations • Identifies foods and fluids that are nutritious and permitted on diet • Gains weight without increased edema or ascites formation • Reports increased appetite and well-being • Excludes alcohol from diet • Takes medications for gastrointestinal disorders as prescribed • Reports normal gastrointestinal function with regular bowel function

NURSING DIAGNOSIS: Impaired skin integrity associated with pruritus from jaundice and edema
GOAL: Decrease potential for pressure injury development; breaks in skin integrity

Nursing Interventions	Rationale	Expected Outcomes
1. Assess degree of discomfort related to pruritus and edema. 2. Note and record degree of jaundice and extent of edema.	1. Assists in determining appropriate interventions. 2. Provides baseline for detecting changes and evaluating effectiveness of interventions.	• Exhibits intact skin without redness, excoriation, or breakdown • Reports relief from pruritus • Exhibits no skin excoriation from scratching

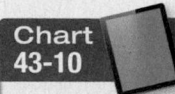

Chart 43-10

PLAN OF NURSING CARE (continued)

The Patient with Impaired Liver Function

Nursing Interventions	Rationale	Expected Outcomes
3. Keep patient's fingernails short and smooth.	3. Prevents skin excoriation and infection from scratching.	• Uses nondrying soaps and lotions; states rationale for the use of nondrying soaps and lotions
4. Provide frequent skin care; avoid the use of soaps and alcohol-based lotions.	4. Removes waste products from skin while preventing dryness of skin.	• Turns self periodically; exhibits reduced edema of dependent parts of the body
5. Massage every 2 hours with emollients; turn every 2 hours.	5. Promotes mobilization of edema.	• Exhibits no areas of skin breakdown
6. Initiate use of alternating-pressure mattress or low air loss bed.	6. Minimizes prolonged pressure on bony prominences susceptible to breakdown.	• Exhibits decreased edema; normal skin turgor
7. Recommend avoiding the use of harsh detergents.	7. May decrease skin irritation and need for scratching.	
8. Assess skin integrity every 4–8 hours. Instruct patient and family in this activity.	8. Edematous skin and tissue have compromised nutrient supply and are vulnerable to pressure and trauma.	
9. Restrict sodium as prescribed.	9. Minimizes edema formation.	
10. Perform range-of-motion exercises every 4 hours; elevate edematous extremities whenever possible.	10. Promotes mobilization of edema.	

NURSING DIAGNOSIS: Risk for injury associated with altered clotting mechanisms and altered level of consciousness
GOAL: Reduced risk of injury

Nursing Interventions	Rationale	Expected Outcomes
1. Assess level of consciousness and cognitive level.	1. Assists in determining patient's ability to protect self and comply with required self-protective actions; may detect deterioration of hepatic function.	• Is oriented to time, place, and person
2. Provide safe environment (pad side rails, remove obstacles in room, prevent falls).	2. Minimizes falls and injury if falls occur.	• Exhibits no hallucinations and demonstrates no efforts to get up unassisted or to leave hospital
3. Provide frequent surveillance to orient patient, and avoid the use of restraints.	3. Protects patient from harm while stimulating and orienting patient; the use of restraints may disturb patient further.	• Exhibits no ecchymoses (bruises), cuts, or hematoma
4. Replace sharp objects (razors) with safer items.	4. Avoids cuts and bleeding.	• Uses electric razor rather than sharp-edged razor
5. Observe each stool for color, consistency, and amount.	5. Permits detection of bleeding in gastrointestinal tract.	• Exhibits absence of frank bleeding from gastrointestinal tract
6. Be alert to symptoms of anxiety, epigastric fullness, weakness, and restlessness.	6. May indicate early signs of bleeding and shock.	• Exhibits absence of restlessness, epigastric fullness, and other indicators of hemorrhage and shock
7. Test each stool and emesis for occult blood.	7. Detects early evidence of bleeding.	• Exhibits negative results of test for occult gastrointestinal bleeding
8. Observe for hemorrhagic manifestations: ecchymosis, epistaxis, petechiae, and bleeding gums.	8. Indicates altered clotting mechanisms.	• Is free of ecchymotic areas or hematoma formation
9. Record vital signs at frequent intervals, depending on patient acuity (every 1–4 hours).	9. Provides baseline and evidence of hypovolemia and hemorrhagic shock.	• Exhibits normal vital signs
10. Keep patient quiet, and limit activity.	10. Minimizes risk of bleeding and straining.	• Maintains rest and remains quiet if active bleeding occurs
11. Assist provider in passage of tube for esophageal balloon tamponade, if its insertion is indicated.	11. Promotes nontraumatic insertion of tube in a patient who is anxious and combative for immediate treatment of bleeding.	• Identifies rationale for blood transfusions and measures to treat bleeding
12. Observe during blood transfusions.	12. Permits detection of transfusion reactions (risk increased with multiple blood transfusions needed for active bleeding from esophageal varices).	• Uses measures to prevent trauma (e.g., uses soft toothbrush, blows nose gently, avoids bumps, falls, straining during defecation)
13. Measure and record nature, time, and amount of vomitus.	13. Assists in evaluating extent of bleeding and blood loss.	• Experiences no side effects of medications
14. Maintain patient in fasting state, if indicated.	14. Reduces risk of aspiration of gastric contents and minimizes risk of further trauma to esophagus and stomach by preventing vomiting.	• Takes all medications as prescribed
		• Identifies rationale for precautions with the use of all medications
		• Adheres to prescribed treatment modalities

(continued on page 1398)

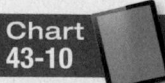

Chart 43-10

PLAN OF NURSING CARE (continued)
The Patient with Impaired Liver Function

Nursing Interventions	Rationale	Expected Outcomes
15. Administer vitamin K as prescribed.	15. Promotes clotting by providing fat-soluble vitamin necessary for clotting.	
16. Remain with patient during episodes of bleeding.	16. Reassures patient who is anxious and permits monitoring and detection of further needs of the patient.	
17. Offer cold liquids by mouth when bleeding stops (if prescribed).	17. Minimizes risk of further bleeding by promoting vasoconstriction of esophageal and gastric blood vessels.	
18. Institute measures to prevent trauma. a. Maintain safe environment.	18. Promotes safety of patient. a. Minimizes risk of trauma and bleeding by avoiding falls and cuts, etc.	
b. Encourage *gentle* blowing of nose.	b. Reduces risk of epistaxis (nosebleed) secondary to trauma and decreased clotting.	
c. Provide soft toothbrush, and avoid the use of toothpicks.	c. Prevents trauma to oral mucosa while promoting good oral hygiene.	
d. Encourage intake of foods with high content of vitamin C.	d. Promotes healing.	
e. Apply cold compresses where indicated.	e. Minimizes bleeding into tissues by promoting local vasoconstriction.	
f. Record location of bleeding sites.	f. Permits detection of new bleeding sites and monitoring of previous sites of bleeding.	
g. Use small-gauge needles for injections.	g. Minimizes oozing and blood loss from repeated injections.	
19. Administer medications carefully; monitor for side effects.	19. Reduces risk of side effects secondary to damaged liver's inability to detoxify (metabolize) medications normally.	

NURSING DIAGNOSIS: Disturbed body image associated with changes in appearance, sexual dysfunction, and role function
GOAL: Patient verbalizes feelings consistent with improvement of body image and self-esteem

Nursing Interventions	Rationale	Expected Outcomes
1. Assess changes in appearance and the meaning these changes have for patient and family.	1. Provides information for assessing impact of changes in appearance, sexual function, and role on the patient and family.	• Verbalizes concerns related to changes in appearance, life, and lifestyle • Shares concerns with significant others
2. Encourage patient to verbalize reactions and feelings about these changes.	2. Enables patient to identify and express concerns; encourages patient and significant others to share these concerns.	• Identifies past coping strategies that have been effective • Uses past effective coping strategies to deal with changes in appearance, life, and lifestyle
3. Assess patient's and family's previous coping strategies.	3. Permits encouragement of those coping strategies that are familiar to patient and have been effective in the past.	• Maintains good grooming and hygiene
4. Assist and encourage patient to maximize appearance (such as strategies to limit the appearance of jaundice and ascites through careful selection of colors and type of clothing) and explore alternatives to previous sexual and role functions.	4. Encourages patient to continue safe roles and functions while encouraging exploration of alternatives.	• Identifies short-term goals and strategies to achieve them • Takes an active role in decision making about self and care • Identifies resources that are not harmful
5. Assist patient in identifying short-term goals.	5. Accomplishing these goals serves as positive reinforcement and increases self-esteem.	• Verbalizes that some of previous lifestyle practices may have been harmful, if applicable • Uses healthy expressions of frustration, anger, anxiety
6. Encourage and assist patient in decision making about care.	6. Promotes patient's control of life and improves sense of well-being and self-esteem.	
7. Identify with patient resources to provide additional support (counselor, spiritual advisor).	7. Assists patient in identifying resources and accepting assistance from others when indicated.	
8. Assist patient in identifying previous practices that may have been harmful to self (substance use disorder). Involve patient in goal setting, and provide positive feedback for accomplishments.	8. Recognition and acknowledgment of the harmful effects of these practices are necessary for identifying a healthier lifestyle.	

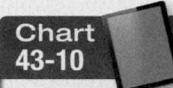

**Chart
43-10**

PLAN OF NURSING CARE (continued)
The Patient with Impaired Liver Function

NURSING DIAGNOSIS: Comfortable with respect to enlarged tender liver and ascites
GOAL: Increased level of comfort

Nursing Interventions	Rationale	Expected Outcomes
1. Maintain bed rest when patient experiences abdominal discomfort. 2. Administer antispasmodic and analgesic agents as prescribed. 3. Observe, record, and report presence and character of pain and discomfort. 4. Reduce sodium and fluid intake if prescribed. 5. Prepare patient and assist with procedures for management of ascites such as paracentesis or TIPS procedure, if indicated. 6. Encourage the use of distracting activities such as music, reading, or meditation.	1. Reduces metabolic demands and protects the liver. 2. Reduces irritability of the gastrointestinal tract and decreases abdominal pain and discomfort. 3. Provides baseline to detect further deterioration of status and to evaluate interventions. 4. Minimizes further formation of ascites. 5. Removal of ascites fluid may decrease abdominal discomfort. 6. Distraction may limit the perception of pain.	• Reports pain and discomfort if present • Maintains bed rest and decreases activity in presence of pain • Takes antispasmodic and analgesic agents as indicated and as prescribed • Reports decreased pain and abdominal discomfort • Reduces sodium and fluid intake to prescribed levels if indicated to treat ascites • Exhibits decreased abdominal girth and appropriate weight changes • Reports decreased discomfort after paracentesis or other procedure to manage ascites such as TIPS procedure

NURSING DIAGNOSIS: Hypervolemia associated with ascites and edema formation
GOAL: Restoration of normal fluid volume

Nursing Interventions	Rationale	Expected Outcomes
1. Restrict sodium and fluid intake if prescribed. 2. Administer diuretic agents, potassium, and protein supplements as prescribed. 3. Record intake and output every 1–8 hours depending on response to interventions and on patient acuity. 4. Measure and record abdominal girth and weight daily. 5. Explain rationale for sodium and fluid restriction. 6. Prepare patient and assist with paracentesis or TIPS procedure, if indicated.	1. Minimizes formation of ascites and edema. 2. Promotes excretion of fluid through the kidneys and maintenance of normal fluid and electrolyte balance. 3. Indicates effectiveness of treatment and adequacy of fluid intake. 4. Monitors changes in ascites formation and fluid accumulation. 5. Promotes patient's understanding of restriction and cooperation with it. 6. Paracentesis will temporarily decrease amount of ascites present and a TIPS procedure will lower portal pressure and thus limit the accumulation of ascitic fluid.	• Consumes diet low in sodium and within prescribed fluid restriction • Takes diuretic agents, potassium, and protein supplements as indicated without experiencing side effects • Exhibits increased urine output • Exhibits decreasing abdominal girth • Exhibits no rapid increase in weight • Identifies rationale for sodium and fluid restriction • Shows a decrease in ascites with decreased weight

NURSING DIAGNOSIS: Acute confusion associated with abnormal liver function and increased serum ammonia level
GOAL: Improved mental status; safety maintained; ability to cope with cognitive and behavioral changes

Nursing Interventions	Rationale	Expected Outcomes
1. Give frequent, small feedings of carbohydrates and protein. 2. Protect from infection. 3. Keep environment warm and draft free. 4. Pad the side rails of the bed. 5. Limit visitors.	1. Promotes consumption of adequate carbohydrates for energy requirements and protein for healing. 2. Minimizes risk of further increase in metabolic requirements. 3. Minimizes shivering, which would increase metabolic requirements. 4. Provides protection for the patient should hepatic coma and seizure activity occur. 5. Minimizes patient's activity and metabolic requirements.	• Demonstrates an interest in events and activities in environment • Demonstrates normal attention span • Follows and participates in conversation appropriately • Is oriented to person, place, and time • Remains in bed when indicated • Experiences no seizures • No neurologic or respiratory depression • Patient develops no cognitive impairments, but if they develop, they are quickly identified and treated, enhancing the potential of recovery

(continued on page 1400)

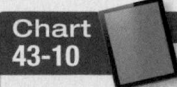

Chart 43-10

PLAN OF NURSING CARE (continued)
The Patient with Impaired Liver Function

Nursing Interventions	Rationale	Expected Outcomes
6. Provide careful nursing surveillance to ensure patient's safety.	6. Provides close monitoring of new symptoms and minimizes trauma to the patient who is confused.	• Patient and family describe adequate feelings of coping and lowered anxiety. They demonstrate ability to listen and to make decisions as able
7. Avoid opioids and barbiturates.	7. Prevents masking of symptoms of hepatic coma and prevents drug overdose secondary to reduced ability of the damaged liver to metabolize opioids and barbiturates; prevents respiratory depression.	• Patient and family communicate their feelings and their needs in a secure and caring environment
8. Awaken at intervals (every 2–4 hours during daytime hours for the patient who is stable) to assess cognitive status.	8. Provides stimulation to the patient and opportunity for observing patient's level of consciousness.	
9. Identify subtle changes in behavior or sleep–wake pattern (consistent staff caring for the patient enhances this assessment as they become familiar with patient's baseline).	9. These changes may herald worsening of encephalopathy, which requires rapid intervention, including medication.	
10. Assess handwriting or drawing skill daily as indication of cognitive ability.	10. These changes may herald worsening of encephalopathy, which requires rapid intervention, including medication.	
11. Encourage patient and family to participate in therapeutic strategies to enhance coping with episodes of mental deterioration.	11. Promoting activities such as listening to music, relaxation techniques, or preillness coping strategies can reduce anxiety.	
12. Encourage patient and family to discuss feeling of fear, powerlessness, or emotional distress related to patient's mental deterioration.	12. Actively listening demonstrates caring and concern.	

NURSING DIAGNOSIS: Risk for impaired thermoregulation: failure to maintain normal body temperature due to inflammatory process of cirrhosis or hepatitis

GOAL: Maintenance of normal body temperature, free from infection

Nursing Interventions	Rationale	Expected Outcomes
1. Record temperature regularly (every 4 hours).	1. Provides baseline to detect fever and to evaluate interventions.	• Exhibits normal temperature and reports absence of chills or sweating
2. Encourage fluid intake.	2. Corrects fluid loss from perspiration and fever and increases patient's level of comfort.	• Demonstrates adequate intake of fluids
3. Apply cool sponges or ice bag for elevated temperature.	3. Promotes reduction of fever and increases patient's comfort.	• Exhibits no evidence of local or systemic infection
4. Administer antibiotics as prescribed.	4. Ensures appropriate serum concentration of antibiotics to treat infection.	• Develops no health care–associated infections related to invasive procedures/ lines
5. Avoid exposure to infections by use of appropriate hand hygiene and limiting use of central lines and urinary catheters to the shortest period of time, only when they are necessary.	5. Minimizes risk of further infection and further increases in body temperature and metabolic rate.	
6. Keep patient at rest while temperature is elevated.	6. Reduces metabolic rate.	
7. Assess for abdominal pain, tenderness.	7. May occur with bacterial peritonitis.	
8. Use sterile technique for all invasive procedures.	8. Many evidence-based practice guidelines (e.g., central venous catheter care) recommend the use of sterile technique to prevent health care-associated infections.	

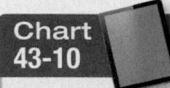

Chart 43-10 PLAN OF NURSING CARE (continued)
The Patient with Impaired Liver Function

NURSING DIAGNOSIS: Impaired breathing associated with restriction of thoracic excursion secondary to ascites, abdominal distention, and fluid in the thoracic cavity

GOAL: Improved respiratory status

Nursing Interventions	Rationale	Expected Outcomes
1. Elevate head of bed to at least 30 degrees.	1. Reduces abdominal pressure on the diaphragm and permits fuller thoracic excursion and lung expansion.	• Reports decreased shortness of breath • Reports increased strength and sense of well-being
2. Conserve patient's strength by providing rest periods and assisting with activities.	2. Reduces metabolic and oxygen requirements.	• Exhibits normal respiratory rate (12–18 breaths/min) with no adventitious sounds
3. Change position every 2 hours.	3. Promotes expansion and oxygenation of all areas of the lungs.	• Exhibits full thoracic excursion without shallow respirations
4. Assist with paracentesis, TIPS or thoracentesis, if indicated.	4. Paracentesis, TIPS, and thoracentesis (performed to remove fluid from the abdominal and thoracic cavities, respectively) may be frightening to the patient.	• Exhibits normal arterial blood gases • Exhibits adequate oxygen saturation by pulse oximetry • Absence of confusion or cyanosis • Reports improved comfort level • Exhibits no complications related to the indwelling catheter, as appropriate
a. Explain procedure and its purpose to patient.	a. Helps obtain patient's cooperation with procedures.	
b. Have patient void before paracentesis.	b. Prevents inadvertent bladder injury.	
c. Support and maintain position during procedure.	c. Prevents inadvertent organ or tissue injury.	
d. Record both the amount and the character of fluid aspirated.	d. Provides record of fluid removed and indication of severity of limitation of lung expansion by fluid.	
e. Observe for evidence of coughing, increasing dyspnea, or pulse rate.	e. Indicates irritation of the pleural space and evidence of pneumothorax or hemothorax.	
5. Provide education to patients who may be discharged with an indwelling peritoneal drainage catheter for palliation of refractory ascites.	5.	
a. Explain procedure and its purpose to patient.	a. Explaining the purpose of the catheter demonstrates respect for the patient's self-determination	
b. Explain care of the catheter and assessment of complications	b. Explanations promote patient adherence to the therapeutic regimen	

COLLABORATIVE PROBLEM: Gastrointestinal bleeding and hemorrhage

GOAL: Absence of episodes of gastrointestinal bleeding and hemorrhage

Nursing Interventions	Rationale	Expected Outcomes

1. Assess patient for evidence of gastrointestinal bleeding or hemorrhage. If bleeding does occur:
  a. Monitor vital signs (blood pressure, pulse, respiratory rate) every 4 hours or more frequently, depending on acuity.
  b. Assess skin temperature, level of consciousness every 4 hours or more frequently, depending on acuity.
  c. Monitor gastrointestinal secretions and output (emesis, stool for occult or obvious bleeding). Test emesis for blood once per shift and with any color change. Hematest each stool.
  d. Monitor hematocrit and hemoglobin for trends and changes.
	1. Allows early detection of signs and symptoms of bleeding and hemorrhage.	• Experiences no episodes of bleeding and hemorrhage
		• Vital signs are within acceptable range for patient
		• No evidence of bleeding from gastrointestinal tract
		• Hematocrit and hemoglobin levels within acceptable limits
		• Turns and moves without straining and increasing intra-abdominal pressure
		• No straining with bowel movements
		• No further bleeding episodes if aggressive treatment of bleeding and hemorrhage was needed
		• Patient and family state rationale for treatments

(continued on page 1402)

Chart 43-10

PLAN OF NURSING CARE (continued)

The Patient with Impaired Liver Function

2. Avoid activities that increase intra-abdominal pressure (straining, turning).
   a. Avoid coughing/sneezing.
   b. Assist patient to turn.
   c. Keep all needed items within easy reach.
   d. Use measures to prevent constipation such as adequate fluid intake, stool softeners.
   e. Ensure small meals.
3. Have equipment (balloon tamponade tube medications, IV fluids) available if indicated.

4. Assist with procedures and therapy needed to treat gastrointestinal bleeding and hemorrhage such as endoscopic variceal ligation (EVL) or sclerotherapy.

5. Monitor respiratory status every hour, and minimize risk of respiratory complications if balloon tamponade is needed.

6. Prepare patient physically and psychologically for other treatment modalities if needed.

7. Monitor patient for recurrence of bleeding and hemorrhage.

8. Keep family informed of patient's status.

9. Once recovered from bleeding episode, provide patient and family with information regarding signs and symptoms of gastrointestinal bleeding.

2. Minimizes increases in intra-abdominal pressure that could lead to rupture and bleeding of esophageal or gastric varices.

3. Equipment, medications, and supplies will be readily available if patient experiences bleeding from ruptured esophageal or gastric varices.

4. Gastrointestinal bleeding and hemorrhage require emergency measures (e.g., insertion of Sengstaken–Blakemore tube™, administration of fluids, medications).

5. The patient is at high risk for respiratory complications, including asphyxiation if gastric balloon of tamponade tube ruptures or migrates upward.

6. The patient who experiences hemorrhage is very anxious and fearful; minimizing anxiety assists in control of hemorrhage.

7. Risk of rebleeding is high with all treatment modalities used to halt gastrointestinal bleeding.

8. Family members are likely to be anxious about the patient's status; providing information will reduce their anxiety level and promote more effective coping.

9. Risk of rebleeding is high. Subtle signs may be more quickly identified.

- Patient and family identify supports available to them
- Patient and family describe signs and symptoms of a recurrent bleeding episode and identify needed action

---

COLLABORATIVE PROBLEM: Hepatic encephalopathy

GOAL: Absence of changes in cognitive status and of injury

Nursing Interventions	Rationale	Expected Outcomes

1. Assess cognitive status every 4–8 hours.
  a. Assess patient's orientation to person, place, and time.
  b. Monitor patient's level of activity, restlessness, and agitation. Assess for presence of asterixis (flapping hand tremors) (see Fig. 43-12).
  c. Obtain and record daily sample of patient's handwriting or ability to construct a simple figure (e.g., star) (see Fig. 43-13).
  d. Assess neurologic signs (deep tendon reflexes, ability to follow instructions).
	1. Data will provide baseline of patient's cognitive status and enable detection of changes.	• Remains awake, alert, and aware of surroundings
		• Is oriented to time, place, and person
		• Deep tendon reflexes remain within normal limits
		• Absence of asterixis
		• Exhibits no restlessness or agitation
		• Record of handwriting demonstrates no deterioration in cognitive function
		• States rationale for treatment used to prevent or treat hepatic encephalopathy
		• Demonstrates stable serum ammonia level within acceptable limits
		• Takes medications as prescribed
		• Breath sounds normal without adventitious sounds
		• Skin and tissue intact without evidence of pressure or breaks in integrity
		• Verbalizes understanding of need for treatments and procedures to promote recovery

2. Monitor medications to prevent administration of those that may precipitate hepatic encephalopathy (sedative, hypnotic, analgesic agents).	2. Medications are a common precipitating factor in development of hepatic encephalopathy in patients at risk.	
3. Monitor laboratory data, especially serum ammonia level.	3. Increases in serum ammonia level are associated with hepatic encephalopathy and coma.	

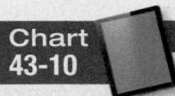

Chart 43-10

PLAN OF NURSING CARE (continued)
The Patient with Impaired Liver Function

Nursing Interventions	Rationale	Expected Outcomes
4. Notify primary provider of even subtle changes in patient's neurologic assessment, cognitive function, sleep pattern, or mood.	4. Allows early initiation of treatment of hepatic encephalopathy and prevention of hepatic coma.	
5. Administer medications prescribed to reduce serum ammonia level (e.g., lactulose, antibiotics, glucose, benzodiazepine antagonist [flumazenil] if indicated).	5. Reduces breakdown and conversion of protein to ammonia. Reduces serum ammonia level.	
6. Assess respiratory status, and initiate measures to prevent complications.	6. The patient who develops hepatic coma is at risk for respiratory complications (i.e., pneumonia, atelectasis, infection).	
7. Protect patient's skin and tissue from pressure and breakdown.	7. The patient in coma is at risk for skin breakdown and pressure injury formation.	
8. Provide support and active listening for patient and family as patient's mental status deteriorates.	8. The patient with hepatic encephalopathy can experience episodes of mental deterioration due to liver failure. This can produce feelings of fear and anxiety.	

Rest reduces the demands on the liver and increases the liver's blood supply. Because the patient is susceptible to the hazards of immobility, efforts to prevent respiratory, circulatory, and vascular disturbances are initiated. These measures may help prevent such problems as atelectasis, pneumonia, venous thromboemboli formation, and pressure injuries. After nutritional status improves and strength increases, the nurse encourages the patient to increase activity gradually. Activity and mild exercise, as well as rest, are planned.

Improving Nutritional Status

The patient with cirrhosis without ascites, edema, or signs of impending hepatic coma should receive a nutritious, high-protein diet, if tolerated, supplemented by vitamins of the B complex, as well as A, C, and K. The nurse encourages the patient to eat. If ascites is present, small, frequent meals may be better tolerated than three large meals because of the abdominal pressure exerted by ascites.

The use of probiotics for the management of hepatic encephalopathy is currently the topic of ongoing research. Imbalance of the intestinal flora is not uncommon. Some research suggests that the oral ingestion of 1 cup of probiotic yogurt three times a day reduces intestinal flora imbalance by decreasing *Escherichia coli* counts and promoting the growth of non–urease-producing bacteria. This strategy is thought to then reduce ammonia levels and improve mental status (Acharya & Bajaj, 2018).

Patients with steatorrhea (fatty stools) should receive water-soluble forms of fat-soluble vitamins A, D, and E. Folic acid and iron are prescribed to prevent anemia. Sodium restriction is also indicated to prevent ascites. Patients with prolonged or severe anorexia and those who are vomiting or eating poorly for any reason may receive nutrients by the enteral or parenteral route (see Chapter 39 for further details on enteral nutrition and Chapter 41 for further details on parenteral nutrition).

Providing Skin Care

Providing careful skin care is important because of subcutaneous edema, the patient's immobility, jaundice, and increased susceptibility to skin breakdown and infection. Frequent changes in position are necessary to prevent pressure injuries. Irritating soaps and the use of adhesive tape are avoided to prevent trauma to the skin. Lotion may be soothing to irritated skin; the nurse takes measures to minimize scratching by the patient.

Reducing Risk of Injury

The nurse protects the patient with cirrhosis from falls and other injuries. The side rails should be in place and pads used in case the patient becomes agitated or restless. To minimize agitation, the nurse orients the patient to time and place and explains all procedures. The nurse instructs the patient to ask for assistance to get out of bed. The nurse carefully evaluates any injury because of the possibility of internal bleeding.

Because of the risk for bleeding from abnormal clotting, the patient should use an electric razor rather than a safety razor. A soft-bristled toothbrush helps minimize bleeding gums, and pressure applied to all venipuncture sites helps minimize bleeding.

Monitoring and Managing Potential Complications

A major role of the nurse is monitoring of the patient with cirrhosis for complications.

Bleeding and Hemorrhage

The patient is at increased risk for bleeding and hemorrhage because of decreased production of prothrombin and decreased ability of the diseased liver to synthesize the necessary substances for blood coagulation (see the Esophageal Varices section).

 Hepatic Encephalopathy

Hepatic encephalopathy and coma, which are complications of cirrhosis, may manifest as deteriorating mental status (delirium) or as physical signs such as abnormal voluntary and involuntary movements. Hepatic encephalopathy was discussed earlier in the chapter in detail.

Monitoring is essential to identify early deterioration in mental status. The nurse monitors the patient's mental status closely and reports changes so that treatment for encephalopathy can be initiated promptly. An extensive baseline and ongoing neurologic evaluation is key to identify progression through the four stages of encephalopathy (see Table 43-3).

Each advancing stage demands more intensive nursing interventions aimed at providing for patient safety and prevention and early identification of life-threatening complications such as respiratory failure and cerebral edema, which would necessitate interventions in an ICU. Because electrolyte disturbances can contribute to encephalopathy, serum electrolyte levels are carefully monitored and corrected if abnormal. Oxygen is given if oxygen desaturation occurs. The nurse monitors for fever or abdominal pain, which may signal the onset of bacterial peritonitis or other infection (see earlier discussion of hepatic encephalopathy).

Fluid Volume Excess

Patients with advanced chronic liver disease develop cardiovascular abnormalities. These occur due to an increased cardiac output and decreased peripheral vascular resistance, possibly resulting from the release of vasodilators. A hyperdynamic circulatory state develops in patients with cirrhosis, and plasma volume increases. This increase in circulating plasma volume is probably multifactorial, but some studies have implicated excess production of nitrous oxide, such as that seen in sepsis, as one causative factor (Friedman & Martin, 2018). The greater the degree of hepatic decompensation, the more severe the hyperdynamic state. Close assessment of cardiovascular and respiratory status is of key importance for the care of patients with this disorder. Pulmonary compromise is always a potential complication of ESLD because of plasma volume excess; consequently, the nurse has an important role in preventing pulmonary complications. Administering diuretic agents, implementing fluid restrictions, and enhancing patient positioning can optimize pulmonary function. Fluid retention may be noted in the development of ascites, lower extremity swelling, and dyspnea. Monitoring of I&O, daily weight changes, changes in abdominal girth, and edema formation is part of nursing assessment in the hospital or in the home setting. Patients are also monitored for nocturia and, later, for oliguria, because these states indicate increasing severity of liver dysfunction (Mansour & McPherson, 2018; Schiff et al., 2018).

Promoting Home, Community-Based and Transitional Care

Educating Patients About Self-Care

During the hospital stay, the nurse and other health care providers prepare the patient with cirrhosis for discharge, focusing on dietary education. Of greatest importance is the exclusion of alcohol from the diet. The patient may benefit from referral to Alcoholics Anonymous, psychiatric care, or counseling or support from a spiritual advisor. The patient should avoid the consumption of raw shellfish.

Sodium restriction will continue for a considerable time, if not permanently. The patient will require written education, reinforcement, and support from the staff as well as family members.

Successful treatment depends on convincing the patient of the need to adhere completely to the therapeutic plan. This includes rest, lifestyle changes, adequate dietary intake, and the elimination of alcohol. The nurse also educates the patient and family about symptoms of impending encephalopathy, possible bleeding tendencies, and susceptibility to infection. Nurses should consider implementing the teach-back method when educating patients and families to insure that they are able to describe what they have been taught in their own words or perform a task as instructed (see Chapter 3 for further discussion of the teach-back method).

Recovery is neither rapid nor easy; there are frequent setbacks and apparent lack of improvement. Many patients find it difficult to refrain from using alcohol for comfort or escape. The nurse has a significant role in offering support and encouragement to the patient and in providing positive feedback when the patient experiences success.

Continuing and Transitional Care

Referral for transitional or home care may assist the patient in dealing with the transition from hospital to home. The use of alcohol may have been an important part of normal home and social life in the past. The nurse assesses the patient's progress at home and the manner in which the patient and family are coping with the elimination of alcohol and the dietary restrictions. The nurse also reinforces previous education and answers questions that may not have occurred to the patient or family until the patient is back home and trying to establish new patterns of eating, drinking, and lifestyle.

CANCER OF THE LIVER

Hepatic tumors may be malignant or benign. Benign liver tumors were uncommon until oral contraceptives were in widespread use in western countries. Now, benign liver tumors such as hepatic adenomas occur most frequently in women in their reproductive years who are taking oral contraceptives, though the incidence has decreased with the development of modern contraceptives which contain less estrogen. The risk of these tumors is increased in those who are overweight or have obesity. These lesions may be complicated by hemorrhage and conversion to a malignant state (Tsilimigras, Rahnemai-Azar, Ntanasis-Stathopoulos, et al., 2019).

Primary Liver Tumors

Few cancers originate in the liver. Primary liver tumors usually are associated with chronic liver disease, hepatitis B and C infections, and cirrhosis. HCC is the most common type of primary liver cancer, responsible for 75% of all liver cancers, with more than half a million cases diagnosed each year on a worldwide basis. HCC is the second leading cause of cancer-related mortality worldwide. It is rare in the United States and northern Europe, accounting for fewer than 6 cases per 100,000 inhabitants (Akinyemiju, Abera, Ahmed, et al., 2017; Schiff et al., 2018). Other types of primary liver cancer include fibrolamellar carcinoma, angiosarcoma, hepatoblastoma, cholangiocellular carcinoma, and combined hepatocellular and cholangiocellular carcinoma. HCC is usually nonresectable because of rapid growth and metastasis. If found early, resection of primary liver cancer may be possible; however, early detection is not common.

Cirrhosis, chronic infection with HBV and HCV, and exposure to certain chemical toxins (e.g., vinyl chloride, arsenic) have been implicated as causes of HCC. Cigarette smoking has also been identified as a risk factor, especially when combined with alcohol (Petrick, Campbell, Koshiol, et al., 2018). Some evidence suggests that aflatoxin, a metabolite of the fungus *Aspergillus flavus*, may be a risk factor for HCC. This is especially true in areas where HCC is endemic (i.e., Asia, Africa). Aflatoxin and other similar toxic molds can contaminate food such as ground nuts and grains and may act as co-carcinogens with hepatitis B (Friedman & Martin, 2018). The risk of contamination is greatest when these foods are stored unrefrigerated in tropical or subtropical climates.

Liver Metastases

Metastases from other primary sites, particularly the digestive system, breast, and lung, are found in the liver 2.5 times more frequently than tumors due to primary liver cancers (Friedman & Martin, 2018; Goldman & Schafer, 2019). Malignant tumors are likely to reach the liver eventually, by way of the portal system or lymphatic channels, or by direct extension from an abdominal tumor. Moreover, the liver apparently is an ideal place for these malignant cells to thrive. Often, the first evidence of cancer in an abdominal organ is the appearance of liver metastases; unless exploratory surgery or an autopsy is performed, the primary tumor may never be identified.

Clinical Manifestations

The early manifestations of malignancy of the liver include pain—a continuous dull ache in the right upper quadrant, epigastrium, or back. Weight loss, loss of strength, anorexia, and anemia may also occur. The liver may be enlarged and irregular on palpation. Jaundice is present only if the larger bile ducts are occluded by the pressure of malignant nodules in the hilum of the liver. Ascites develops if such nodules obstruct the portal veins or if tumor tissue is seeded in the peritoneal cavity.

Assessment and Diagnostic Findings

The diagnosis of liver cancer is based on clinical signs and symptoms, the history and physical examination, and the results of laboratory and x-ray studies. Increased serum levels of bilirubin, alkaline phosphatase, AST, GGT, and lactic dehydrogenase may occur. Leukocytosis (increased white blood cells), erythrocytosis (increased red blood cells), hypercalcemia, hypoglycemia, and hypocholesterolemia may also be seen on laboratory assessment.

The serum level of alpha-fetoprotein, which serves as a tumor marker, is elevated in 80% to 90% of patients with HCC, commonly to levels greater than 200 ng/mL (Friedman & Martin, 2018). Patients with small tumors (<5 cm in diameter) have normal or minimally elevated levels of alpha-fetoprotein. The level of carcinoembryonic antigen, a marker of advanced cancer of the digestive tract, may be elevated. These two markers together are useful to distinguish between metastatic liver disease and primary liver cancer.

Many patients have metastases from the primary liver tumor to other sites by the time the diagnosis is made; metastases occur primarily to the lung but may also occur to regional lymph nodes, adrenals, bone, kidneys, heart, pancreas, or stomach.

X-rays, liver scans, CT scans, ultrasound studies, MRI, arteriography, and laparoscopy may be part of the diagnostic workup and may be performed to determine the extent of the cancer. Positron emission tomography (PET) scans are used to evaluate a wide range of metastatic tumors of the liver.

Confirmation of a tumor's histology can be made by biopsy under imaging guidance (CT scan or ultrasound) or laparoscopically. Local or systemic dissemination of the tumor by needle biopsy or fine-needle biopsy can occur. Because of the small but real risks of tumor seeding (0.5% to 2%), hemorrhage, and false-negative results from biopsy, many transplant centers avoid biopsy, particularly in patients who may be candidates for liver resection or liver transplantation. Assessment of the imaging characteristics for the diagnosis of HCC is preferred in these instances, and a confirmed diagnosis of HCC is made by frozen section at the time of surgery (Goldman & Schafer, 2019).

Medical Management

Although surgical resection of the liver tumor is possible in some patients, the underlying cirrhosis is so prevalent in cancer of the liver that it increases the risks associated with surgery. Radiation therapy and chemotherapy have been used to treat cancer of the liver with varying degrees of success. Although these therapies may prolong survival and improve quality of life by reducing pain and discomfort, their major effect is palliative.

Radiation Therapy

The use of external-beam radiation for the treatment of liver tumors has been limited by the radiosensitivity of normal hepatocytes and the risk of destruction of normal liver parenchyma. More effective methods of delivering radiation to tumors of the liver include IV or transarterial injection of a lipiodol-ethanol (radiopaque agent) mixture (also known as transarterial chemoembolization [TACE]) that specifically attacks tumor-associated antigens, use of drug-eluding beads (DEB-TACE) and percutaneous placement of a high-intensity source for interstitial radiation therapy (delivery of radiation directly to the tumor cells). Internal radiotherapy can result in reduction in tumor size, but its effect on survival is yet to be determined (Friedman & Martin, 2018; Schiff et al., 2018).

Chemotherapy

Typically, studies of patients with advanced cases of liver cancer have shown that the use of systemic chemotherapeutic agents leads to poor outcomes. For patients with stable hepatic function (Child class A), a targeted molecular therapy, sorafenib, has been developed and approved for use and is the standard systemic treatment for patients with advanced HCC. Regorafenib may be used in patients who cease responding to sorafenib (Friedman & Martin, 2018). Systemic chemotherapy may be used to treat metastatic liver lesions. Embolization of tumor vessels with chemotherapy produces anoxic necrosis with high concentrations of trapped chemotherapeutic agents. This therapy has begun to show some promising results. An implantable pump has been used to deliver a high concentration of chemotherapy by constant infusion to the liver through the hepatic artery in cases of metastatic disease. This method has shown a moderate response rate (Friedman & Martin, 2018).

Percutaneous Biliary Drainage

Percutaneous biliary or transhepatic drainage is used to bypass biliary ducts obstructed by liver, pancreatic, or bile duct tumors in patients who have inoperable tumors or are considered poor surgical risks. Under fluoroscopy, a catheter is inserted through the abdominal wall and past the obstruction into the duodenum. Such procedures are used to reestablish biliary drainage, relieve pressure and pain from the buildup of bile behind the obstruction, and decrease pruritus and jaundice. As a result, the patient is made more comfortable, and quality of life and survival are improved.

For several days after its insertion, the catheter is opened to external drainage. The bile is observed closely for amount, color, and presence of blood and debris. Complications of percutaneous biliary drainage include sepsis, leakage of bile, hemorrhage, and reobstruction of the biliary system by debris in the catheter or by encroaching tumor. Therefore, the patient is observed for fever and chills, bile drainage around the catheter, changes in vital signs, and evidence of biliary obstruction, including increased pain or pressure, pruritus, and recurrence of jaundice.

Other Nonsurgical Treatments

Laser hyperthermia has been used to treat hepatic metastases. Heat has been directed to tumors through several methods to cause necrosis of the tumor cells while sparing normal tissue. In radiofrequency thermal ablation, a needle electrode is inserted into the liver tumor under imaging guidance. Radiofrequency energy passes through to the noninsulated needle tip, causing heat and tumor cell death from coagulation necrosis.

Immunotherapy is another treatment modality under investigation. In this therapy, lymphocytes with antitumor reactivity are given to the patient with hepatic cancer. Tumor regression has been demonstrated in patients with metastatic cancer for whom standard treatment has failed.

Transcatheter arterial embolization interrupts the arterial blood flow to small tumors by injecting small particulate embolic or chemotherapeutic agents (as described previously) into the artery supplying the tumor. As a result, ischemia and necrosis of the tumor occur.

For multiple small lesions, ultrasound-guided injection of alcohol promotes dehydration of tumor cells and tumor necrosis (Srinivasan & Friedman, 2018).

Surgical Management

Surgical resection is the treatment of choice when HCC is confined to one lobe of the liver and the function of the remaining liver is considered adequate for postoperative recovery. In the case of metastasis, hepatic resection can be performed if the primary site can be completely excised and the metastasis is limited. However, metastases to the liver are rarely limited or solitary. Capitalizing on the regenerative capacity of the liver cells, some surgeons have successfully removed 90% of the liver. However, the presence of cirrhosis limits the ability of the liver to regenerate. Laparoscopic liver resection for malignant tumors has also been described. Staging of liver tumors aids in predicting the likelihood of surgical cure (Cameron & Cameron, 2020; Friedman & Martin, 2018; Schiff et al., 2018).

In preparation for surgery, the patient's nutritional, fluid, and general physical status are assessed, and efforts are undertaken to ensure the best physical condition possible. Extensive diagnostic studies may be performed. Specific studies may include liver scan, liver biopsy, cholangiography, selective hepatic angiography, percutaneous needle biopsy, peritoneoscopy, laparoscopy, ultrasound, CT scan, PET scan, MRI, and blood tests, particularly determinations of serum alkaline phosphatase, AST, and GGT and its isoenzymes.

Lobectomy

Removal of a lobe of the liver is the most common surgical procedure for excising a liver tumor. If it is necessary to restrict blood flow from the hepatic artery and portal vein for longer than 15 minutes, it is likely that hypothermia will be used. For a right-liver lobectomy or an extended right lobectomy (including the medial left lobe), a thoracoabdominal incision is used. An extensive abdominal incision is made for a left lobectomy.

Local Ablation

In patients who are not candidates for resection or transplantation, ablation of HCC may be accomplished by chemicals such as ethanol or by physical means such as radiofrequency ablation (most frequently used local ablative therapy) or microwave coagulation. These techniques may be performed under ultrasound or CT guidance laparoscopically or percutaneously. Radiofrequency ablation is becoming a standard mode of treatment; a tumor up to 5 cm in size can be destroyed in one session. The most common complications following ablation are local pain or bleeding. Serious complications are rare (Friedman & Martin, 2018).

Immunotherapy with interferon may be used after surgical resection for HCC to prevent recurrence of the lesion in those patients who have developed the lesion related to hepatitis B or C.

Liver Transplantation

Liver transplantation offers good patient outcomes. Candidates with liver cancer meet stringent selection criteria, including having small, early-stage lesions (Friedman & Martin, 2018; Gerber, Baliga, & Karp, 2018; Yang, Larson, Watt, et al., 2017). The Milan criteria have been developed to limit transplantation to patients who are most likely to have better outcomes. The Milan criteria include that the patient must have a single tumor measuring less than 5 cm, or have three or fewer lesions with none over 3 cm in size (Friedman & Martin, 2018; Schiff et al., 2018). This treatment involves removing the liver and replacing it with a healthy donor organ. Studies report decreased recurrence rates of the primary liver malignancy after transplantation, with improvement in 4-year survival rates to approximately 85%, which is similar to survival rates seen in patients transplanted for nonmalignant disorders (Friedman & Martin, 2018; Schiff et al., 2018). Metastasis and recurrence may be enhanced by the immunosuppressive therapy that is needed to prevent rejection of the transplanted liver. In patients with small (less than 5 cm), single lesions, liver transplantation has been shown to be beneficial, but its use is limited by organ shortages. The increasing use of living donor transplantation may improve this situation and decrease the waiting time and tumor proliferation that is characteristic of patients with liver cancer (see later discussion).

Nursing Management

For patients with liver cancer anticipating surgery, support, education, and encouragement are provided to help them prepare psychologically for the surgery. After surgery, potential problems related to cardiopulmonary involvement may include vascular complications and respiratory and liver dysfunction. Metabolic abnormalities require careful attention. Because extensive blood loss may occur as well, the patient receives infusions of blood and IV fluids. The patient requires constant, close monitoring and care for the first 2 or 3 days, similar to postsurgical abdominal and thoracic nursing care.

If the patient is to receive chemotherapy or radiation therapy in an effort to relieve symptoms, they may be discharged home while still receiving one or both of these therapies. The patient may also go home with a biliary drainage system or hepatic artery catheter in place. In most cases, the hepatic artery catheter has been inserted surgically and has a prefilled infusion pump implanted subcutaneously that delivers a continuous chemotherapeutic dose until completed (Friedman & Martin, 2018; Schiff et al., 2018). A hepatic artery port may also be inserted to provide access for intermittent chemotherapy infusion. This port dwells under the skin, but because it provides direct arterial access, it is not used for continuous infusion therapy in the home environment; the access line is discontinued once the chemotherapeutic agent has infused. The patient and family require education about care of the biliary catheter and the effects and side effects of hepatic artery chemotherapy. This education is necessary because of participation of the patient and family in patient care in the home setting.

Promoting Home, Community-Based and Transitional Care

 Educating Patients About Self-Care

The nurse educates the patient to recognize and report the potential complications and side effects of the chemotherapy and the desirable and undesirable effects of the specific chemotherapy regimen. The nurse also emphasizes the importance of follow-up visits to assess the response to chemotherapy and radiation therapy. In addition, if the patient is receiving chemotherapy on an outpatient basis, the nurse explains the patient's and family's role in managing the chemotherapy infusion and in assessing the infusion or insertion site. The nurse encourages the patient to resume routine activities as soon as possible while cautioning about falls and activities that may damage the infusion pump or site.

Patients at home with a biliary drainage system in place typically fear that the catheter will become dislodged; this fear is often shared by the patient's family. Reassurance and education can help reduce their fear that the catheter will fall out easily. The patient and family also require education on catheter care, including instruction on how to keep the catheter site clean and dry and how to assess the catheter and its insertion site. Irrigation of the catheter with sterile normal saline solution or water may be prescribed to keep the catheter patent and free of debris. The patient and caregivers are taught proper technique to avoid introducing bacteria into the biliary system or catheter during irrigation. They are instructed not to aspirate or draw back on the syringe during irrigation in order to prevent entry of irritating duodenal contents into the biliary tree or catheter. The patient and caregivers are also educated about the signs of complications and are encouraged to notify the nurse or primary provider if problems or questions arise. The nurse should consider using the teach-back method when educating patients and family about these interventions (see Chapter 3 for further discussion of the teach-back method).

Patients with implantable ports are educated about the chemotherapy regimen, types of medications, effects and side effects that may occur, and appropriate management strategies if problems occur. If a hepatic artery port is inserted for intermittent chemotherapy, patients and their families are provided the same educational content. Such a port has an internal one-way valve; therefore, it is not aspirated for a blood return before the infusion is initiated. The patient is instructed to assess the port site between infusions and to note and report any sign of infection or inflammation.

Continuing and Transitional Care

In many cases, referral for transitional or home care enables the patient with liver cancer to be at home in a familiar environment with family and friends. Because of the poor prognosis associated with liver cancer, the nurse serves a vital role in assisting the patient and family to cope with the symptoms that may occur and the prognosis. The patient's physical and psychological statuses are assessed as well as adequacy of pain relief, nutritional status, and presence of symptoms indicating complications of treatment or progression of disease. During home visits, the nurse assesses the function of the chemotherapy pump, the infusion site, and the biliary drainage system, if indicated. The nurse collaborates with the other members of the health care team, the patient, and the family to ensure effective pain management and to manage potential problems, which include weakness, pruritus, inadequate dietary intake, jaundice, and symptoms associated with metastasis to other sites. The nurse also assists the patient and family in making decisions about hospice care and assists with initiation of referrals. The patient is encouraged to discuss preferences for end-of-life care with family members and health care providers (see Chapter 13).

LIVER TRANSPLANTATION

Liver transplantation is used to treat life-threatening ESLD for which no other form of treatment is available. The transplantation procedure involves total removal of the diseased liver and replacement with a healthy liver from a deceased donor or with the right lobe from a live donor in the same anatomic location, referred to as **orthotopic liver transplantation [OLT]**. Removal of the liver creates a space for the new liver and permits anatomic reconstruction of the hepatic vasculature and biliary tract as close to normal as possible.

The success of liver transplantation depends on successful immunosuppression. Immunosuppressant agents currently used include the calcineurin inhibitors cyclosporine and tacrolimus. Corticosteroids are commonly used for induction immunosuppression. Mycophenolate mofetil blocks lymphocyte proliferation and results in lower dose requirements of calcineurin inhibitors. Target of rapamycin inhibitors sirolimus (formerly known as rapamycin) and everolimus inhibit T- and B-cell proliferation. Antibody therapies such as antithymocyte globulin, basiliximab, and daclizumab deplete lymphocytes and inhibit T-cell proliferation (Friedman & Martin, 2018). There is no one, accepted, optimal immunosuppressive regimen. Most transplant centers have developed their own therapeutic practices, largely based on experience. Multiple immunosuppressive strategies can be used to prevent transplanted organ rejection. Most strategies involve the use of more than one agent, but current recommendations advise the minimization of immunosuppression in order to avoid toxicity (Friedman & Martin, 2018). Using multiple immunosuppressive agents has the effect of blocking multiple targets in the immune response cascade. This allows the use of lower doses of each drug, thus avoiding toxicity associated with high doses of these powerful drugs. Some patients are treated with "triple therapy" using corticosteroids, a calcineurin inhibitor, and either an antiproliferative agent (mycophenolate mofetil) or a target of rapamycin inhibitor (Friedman & Martin, 2018). Some transplant centers also prescribe steroid-free immunosuppressant regimens after liver transplantation. This regimen has been found to be a safe alternative. Still other transplant centers advocate monotherapy with a calcineurin inhibitor alone to provide long-term immunosuppression (Cameron & Cameron, 2020; Friedman & Martin, 2018). In order to prevent acute rejection in the early, high-risk months after liver transplantation, some centers employ induction therapy, which is the use of prophylactic, perioperative course of immunosuppressant drugs that suppress the body's response to the foreign, transplanted tissue and may improve graft survival by reducing the risk of acute cellular rejection (Friedman & Martin, 2018). Over time, withdrawal of all immunosuppressants is possible but rare; randomized, prospective studies are needed before this clinical practice is accepted.

Despite the success of immunosuppression in reducing the incidence of rejection of transplanted organs, liver transplantation is not routine and may be accompanied by complications related to the lengthy surgical procedure, immunosuppressive therapy, infection, and technical difficulties encountered in reconstructing the blood vessels and biliary tract. Long-standing systemic problems resulting from the primary liver disease may complicate the pre- and postoperative course. Previous surgery of the abdomen, including procedures to treat complications of advanced liver disease (i.e., shunt procedures used to treat portal hypertension, esophageal varices) increase the complexity of the transplantation procedure.

General indications for liver transplantation include irreversible advanced chronic liver disease, ALF, metabolic liver diseases, and some hepatic malignancies. Examples of disorders that are indications for liver transplantation include hepatocellular liver diseases (e.g., viral hepatitis, drug- or alcohol-induced liver disease, Wilson disease) and cholestatic diseases (primary biliary cirrhosis, sclerosing cholangitis, NASH, and biliary atresia).

The patient being considered for liver transplantation frequently has many systemic problems that influence pre- and postoperative care. Because transplantation is more difficult if the patient has developed severe GI bleeding and hepatic coma, efforts are made to perform the procedure before the disease progresses to this stage. The patient must undergo a thorough evaluation of hepatic reserve and general health. Part of this evaluation includes classification of the degree of medical need, an objective determination known as the MELD classification, which stratifies the level of illness of those awaiting a liver transplant. The MELD score is derived from a complex formula incorporating bilirubin levels, PT/INR, creatinine, and the cause of the liver disease (i.e., cholestatic, alcoholic, or other). The MELD score is an indicator of short-term mortality for those with ESLD. Organs are allocated using the MELD score in an effort to provide transplants to the most severely ill patients (Friedman & Martin, 2018; Schiff et al., 2018).

Liver transplantation is an established therapeutic modality, and the number of liver transplant centers is increasing. Patients requiring transplantation are often referred from distant hospitals to these centers. To prepare the patient and family for liver transplantation, nurses in all settings must understand the processes and procedures of liver transplantation.

Many ethical issues arise concerning liver transplantation, particularly concerning the allocation of organs. The way in which some persons contracted liver disease (e.g., alcohol use, hepatitis) leads others to question allocation of organs to them, and some believe that preference should be given to people who need liver transplants but do not have a history of socially unacceptable behavior. More issues arise when a patient requires a second transplant operation because of a return to alcohol or drug use or failure to follow immunosuppressive regimens. Transplant recipients must go through a rigorous selection and preparation process that includes counseling and education to aid them in making critical choices for their improved health. Nurses and other health care providers need to be aware of and confront their own biases and work toward improved understanding and acceptance.

Surgical Procedure

During the procedure, the donor liver is freed from other structures, the bile is flushed from the gallbladder to prevent damage to the walls of the biliary tract, and the liver is perfused with a preservative and cooled. Before the donor liver is placed in the recipient, it is flushed with cold lactated Ringer solution to remove potassium and air bubbles. The presence of portal hypertension increases the difficulty of the procedure.

Anastomoses (connections) of the blood vessels and bile duct are performed between the donor liver and the recipient liver. There are two types of biliary anastomoses. Biliary reconstruction is performed with an end-to-end anastomosis of the donor and recipient common bile ducts; a stented T-tube may be inserted for external drainage of bile. In patients with biliary disease such as primary sclerosing cholangitis or

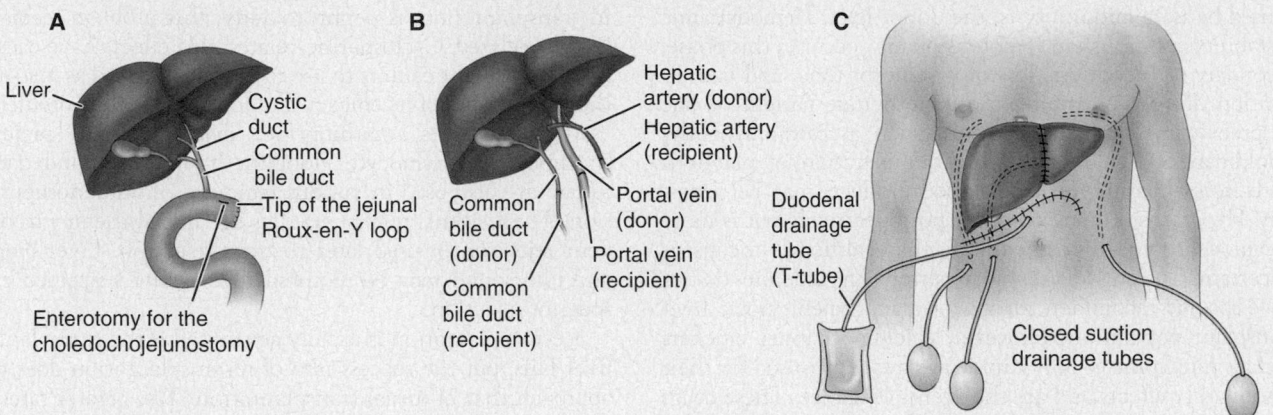

Figure 43-14 • **A.** Some transplant recipients have diseases or conditions that cause their bile ducts to be unusable for anastomosis to the donor liver bile duct. In this case, a loop of jejunum is used as a bridge from the donor liver bile duct to the recipient's small bowel for biliary continuity and drainage. This procedure is termed *Roux-en-Y hepaticojejunostomy*. **B.** Final appearance of implanted liver graft with an end-to-end biliary anastomosis. **C.** Final closure and drain placement after liver transplantation with an end-to-end biliary anastomosis and T-tube placement.

if the recipient's bile duct is not suitable for anastomosis for other reasons, a biliary-enteric end-to-side anastomosis with a 40- to 50-cm Roux-en-Y loop of jejunum is created for biliary drainage (known as a Roux-en-Y procedure) (see Fig. 43-14A); in this case, bile drainage is internal, and a T-tube is not inserted (Cameron & Cameron, 2020). Figure 43-14B,C illustrates the final appearance of the grafted liver and final closure and one method of drain placement. Some transplant centers may use fewer drains.

Several additional techniques have been developed to expand the donor pool for liver transplantation. In a split-liver transplant, a single organ is used to provide grafts for two individuals with ESLD, with the smaller patient receiving the smaller left lobe. This procedure has resulted in a higher complication rate and lower survival rate than traditional liver transplantation. Living donor transplantation is being increasingly performed from adult to adult using full right lobes, although it is controversial because it is a major surgical procedure for the donor, and some donor deaths have occurred.

Living donor liver transplantation (LDLT) is considered for patients who have a high potential for mortality while awaiting a deceased liver donor, such as those patients with HCC or those with severe complications of cirrhosis including GI bleeding or hepatic encephalopathy (Cameron & Cameron, 2020). The results thus far have indicated that this procedure is most successful when donor and recipient are appropriately selected using careful screening criteria (Cameron & Cameron, 2020). The option of LDLT decreases the waiting list mortality and produces positive recipient outcomes with a low risk of morbidity and mortality for the donor. The LDLT procedure involves transplantation of the right hepatic lobe from an adult donor to the recipient. Potential donors are evaluated by a donor advocate team. Donors must be completely healthy and have hepatic size and anatomy compatible with right lobe transplantation (Cameron & Cameron, 2020). There is an extensive informed consent process for live liver donors. The donor advocate ensures that the concern for donor safety is paramount, especially in the intra- and postoperative period when complications can occur. The

clear separation of donor and recipient teams ensures that the donor is treated without ulterior motives, which might occur if the same team cared for both the donor and recipient.

In the LDLT procedure, the surgeon performs a formal right hepatic lobectomy. The right lobe is then flushed with preservative solution and vascular reconstruction is completed to prepare for implantation. The recipient operation involves an inferior vena cava–sparing hepatectomy with anastomosis of the donor right-sided vascular and biliary structures to the corresponding recipient structures (Cameron & Cameron, 2020).

Liver transplantation is a long surgical procedure, partly because the patient with liver failure often has portal hypertension, requiring ligation of many venous collateral vessels. Blood loss during the surgical procedure may be extensive. If the patient has adhesions from previous abdominal surgery, lysis of adhesions is often necessary. If a shunt procedure was performed previously, it must be surgically reversed to permit adequate portal venous blood supply to the new liver. During the lengthy surgery, it is important to provide regular updates to the family about the progress of the operation and the patient's status.

Complications

The postoperative complication rate is high, primarily because of technical complications or infection. Immediate postoperative complications may include bleeding, infection, and rejection. Disruption, infection, obstruction of the biliary anastomosis, and impaired biliary drainage may occur. Vascular thrombosis and stenosis are other potential complications. These complications occur in patients receiving either a deceased donor or live donor organ. Despite the development of some complications, the 1-year patient survival rate approaches 90%, and the 5-year patient survival rate is approximately 80% (Cameron & Cameron, 2020; Friedman & Martin, 2018).

Bleeding

Bleeding is common in the postoperative period and may result from coagulopathy, portal hypertension, and fibrinolysis caused by ischemic injury to the donor liver. Hemodynamic instability and transient hypotension may occur in this phase, secondary to blood loss, loss of vasomotor tone, and vasodilatation due to rewarming the hypothermic patient or due to preexisting cardiac conditions such as cardiomyopathy (Goldman & Schafer, 2019). Administration of platelets, fresh-frozen plasma, or other blood products may be necessary. Hypertension may co-occur postoperatively but is more common later in the postoperative phase, although its cause is uncertain. Currently available hypertension guidelines do not have specific recommendations for management in the liver transplant population. However, calcium channel blockers such as nifedipine or amlodipine are frequently used for their vasodilatory effects and are the agents of choice. These drugs also are preferable due to their low interaction level with the cytochrome P450 enzyme system with resultant minimal risk of disruption of immunosuppressant levels. Angiotensin-converting enzyme (ACE) inhibitors and ARB medications are not first-line drugs for the treatment of hypertension during the first year after transplant due to low levels of renin during this time period. Thiazide diuretics are reserved for patients requiring more than one medication for blood pressure control (Friedman & Martin, 2018). Blood pressure elevation that is significant or sustained is also managed with lifestyle modifications, a low-sodium diet, and an exercise regimen.

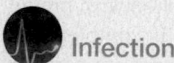 **Infection**

Infection is the leading cause of death after liver transplantation. Pulmonary and fungal infections are common; susceptibility to infection is increased by the immunosuppressive therapy that is needed to prevent rejection (Friedman & Martin, 2018). Therefore, precautions must be taken to prevent health care–associated infections. The nurse uses strict asepsis when manipulating central venous catheters, arterial lines, and urine, bile, and other drainage systems; obtaining specimens; and changing dressings. Meticulous hand hygiene is crucial. In the ICU, the nurse vigilantly monitors for early clinical manifestations of sepsis (see Chapter 11, Chart 11-6) and uses evidence-based practice guidelines (or bundles) developed by the Institute for Healthcare Improvement (IHI) in the care of the postoperative liver transplant patient. Some of these care guidelines include prevention of sepsis through prevention of central line–associated bloodstream infections and its rapid treatment (see Chapter 11, Chart 11-2) and prevention of ventilator-associated pneumonia (VAP) (see Chapter 19, Chart 19-6).

Rejection

Rejection is a major concern. A transplanted liver is perceived by the immune system as a foreign antigen. This triggers an immune response, leading to the activation of T lymphocytes that attack and destroy the transplanted liver. Immunosuppressive agents are used as long-term therapy to prevent this response and rejection of the transplanted liver. These agents inhibit the activation of immunocompetent T lymphocytes to prevent the production of effector T-cells.

Although the 1- and 5-year survival rates have increased dramatically with the use of new immunosuppressive therapies, these advances are not without major side effects. A major side effect of cyclosporine, which has been widely used

in transplantation, is nephrotoxicity; this problem seems to be dose related. Cyclosporine-related side effects have caused many transplant centers to use tacrolimus instead as first-line therapy because of its efficacy and lower side-effect profile.

Corticosteroids, azathioprine, mycophenolate mofetil, sirolimus, antithymocyte globulin, basiliximab, and daclizumab are also used in various regimens of immunosuppression. These agents may be used as the initial therapy to prevent rejection or used later to treat rejection. Liver biopsy and ultrasound may be required to evaluate suspected episodes of rejection.

Retransplantation is usually attempted if the transplanted liver fails, but the success rate of retransplantation does not approach that of initial transplantation. The greater rates of organ dysfunction and loss after a second or third liver transplant are related to technical intraoperative difficulties and higher bleeding risk (Cameron & Cameron, 2020; Friedman & Martin, 2018).

Complications of the LDLT Donor

Improved surgical techniques have made the LDLT procedure an increasingly safe one; however, complications do occur for donors as well. The most frequently occurring complications include pulmonary emboli, portal vein thrombosis, bile duct injury, and liver insufficiency secondary to a resection that is too extensive (Cameron & Cameron, 2020; Friedman & Martin, 2018).

Nursing Management

The patient considering transplantation, together with the family, must make difficult choices about treatment, the use of financial resources, and relocation to another area to be closer to the medical center. They must also be aware of the risks and benefits of the procedure and its consequences. In addition, they must also cope with the patient's long-standing health problems and any social and family problems associated with behaviors that may have caused the patient's liver failure. As a result, considerable emotional stress occurs while the patient and family consider liver transplantation and wait for an available liver. The nurse must be aware of these issues and attuned to the emotional and psychological status of the patient and family. Referral to a psychiatric liaison nurse, psychologist, psychiatrist, or spiritual advisor may help them cope with the stressors associated with ESLD and liver transplantation.

If the patient and family are considering undergoing an LDLT, they are subject to additional stressors. Both the patient and the potential donor must undergo a thorough and exhaustive physical and psychological workup to ensure that all involved parties are physically and emotionally prepared. Often, but not always, the donor is a close family member. Coercion must be excluded as influencing the decision to donate a portion of one's liver to another. The potential donor must be aware of the risks associated with the procedure.

If the patient and family believe that liver transplantation may be appropriate, the nurse, surgeon, hepatologist, and other health care team members provide the patient and family with full explanations about the procedure, the chances of success, and the risks (for the donor—bleeding and venous thromboembolism), including the side effects of long-term immunosuppression and postoperative complications in the recipient as well as bleeding and biliary abnormalities (Cameron & Cameron, 2020; Friedman & Martin, 2018). The need for close follow-up and lifelong adherence to the therapeutic regimen, including immunosuppression, is emphasized to the patient and family.

Preoperative Nursing Interventions

Once the patient has been accepted as a candidate, they are placed on a waiting list at the transplant center, and patient information is entered into the United Network for Organ Sharing (UNOS) computer system. The UNOS system uses the MELD score to determine organ allocation priorities so that the patient with the highest MELD score will receive the first available organ. Candidates may be matched with appropriate organs as they become available. MELD scores provide the necessary information regarding medical need.

Except in the case of LDLT, a liver becomes available for transplantation only with the death of another person, usually someone who had been healthy except for severe brain injury and brain death. Therefore, the patient and family undergo a stressful waiting period, and the nurse is often their major source of support. The patient must be accessible at all times in case an appropriate liver becomes available. During this time, liver function may deteriorate further, and the patient may experience complications from the progressing disease. Because of the shortage of donor organs, many patients die awaiting transplantation.

Malnutrition, massive ascites, and fluid and electrolyte disturbances are treated before surgery to increase the likelihood of a successful outcome. If the patient's liver dysfunction has a very rapid onset, as in ALF, there is little time or opportunity for the patient to consider and weigh options and their consequences; the patient may be in a coma and the decision to proceed with transplantation made by the family.

The nurse coordinator is an integral member of the transplant team and plays an important role in preparing the patient for liver transplantation. The nurse serves as an advocate for the patient and family and assumes the important role of liaison between the patient and the other members of the transplant team. The nurse also serves as a resource to other nurses and health care team members involved in evaluating and caring for the patient.

 Postoperative Nursing Interventions

The organ recipient is maintained in an environment as free from bacteria, viruses, and fungi as possible, because immunosuppressive medications reduce the body's natural defenses. In the immediate postoperative period, cardiovascular, pulmonary, renal, neurologic, and metabolic functions are monitored continuously. Mean arterial and pulmonary artery pressures are also monitored continuously. Cardiac output, central venous pressure, pulmonary artery wedge pressure, arterial and mixed venous blood gases, oxygen saturation, oxygen demand and delivery, urine output, heart rate, and blood pressure are used to evaluate the patient's hemodynamic status and intravascular fluid volume. Liver function tests, electrolyte levels, the coagulation profile, chest x-ray, electrocardiogram, and fluid output (including urine, bile from the T-tube, and drainage from Jackson–Pratt tubes)

are monitored closely. Because the liver is responsible for the storage of glycogen and the synthesis of protein and clotting factors, these substances need to be monitored and replaced in the immediate postoperative period.

There is a high risk of atelectasis and an altered ventilation–perfusion ratio caused by insult to the diaphragm during the surgical procedure, prolonged anesthesia, immobility, and postoperative pain. The patient may have an endotracheal tube in place and require mechanical ventilation during the initial postoperative period. Suctioning is performed as required, and sterile humidification is provided. Evidence-based practice guidelines are implemented to prevent the development of pneumonia in the postoperative liver transplant recipient (see Chapter 19, Chart 19-6).

As the patient's condition stabilizes, efforts are made to promote recovery from the trauma of this complex surgery. After removal of the endotracheal tube, the nurse encourages the patient to use an incentive spirometer to decrease the risk of atelectasis (see Chapter 19, Chart 19-1 for further details on incentive spirometry). Following extubation, the patient is assisted to get out of bed, to ambulate as tolerated, and to participate in self-care to prevent the complications associated with immobility (Pearson, Mangold, Kosiorek, et al., 2018). Close monitoring for signs and symptoms of liver dysfunction and rejection continue throughout the hospital stay. Plans are made for close follow-up after discharge as well. Education is initiated during the preoperative period and continues after surgery.

The live donor is frequently admitted to an ICU setting along with the recipient. The donor also requires close monitoring for cardiovascular, hemodynamic, and pulmonary stability. The nurse closely assesses the donor for signs of hemorrhage, biliary complication, respiratory decompensation, and infection. The donor is mobilized early in the postoperative phase to prevent the development of complications such as pulmonary embolism. Studies suggest that the donor may experience more pain than the recipient, possibly requiring more analgesia for pain control (Friedman & Martin, 2018). Patient education focuses on prevention and recognition of complications as well as activity progression and pain management.

Promoting Home, Community-Based and Transitional Care

 Educating Patients About Self-Care

Educating the patient, family, and caregivers about long-term measures to promote health is crucial for the success of transplantation and is an important role of the nurse. The patient and family must understand why they need to adhere closely to the therapeutic regimen, with special emphasis on the methods of administration, rationale, and side effects of the prescribed immunosuppressive agents. The nurse provides written and verbal education about how and when to take the medications. To avoid running out of medication or skipping a dose, the patient must make sure that an adequate supply of medication is available. Education is provided about the signs and symptoms that indicate problems necessitating consultation with the transplant team. The patient with a T-tube in place must be educated about how to manage the tube, drainage, and skin care.

Chart 43-11 NURSING RESEARCH PROFILE
Psychosocial Adjustments in Patients Undergoing Liver Transplantation

Yıldız, E., & Kılınç, G. (2018). The relationship between anxiety-depression status and psychosocial adjustments in the patients undergoing liver transplantation. *Perspectives in Psychiatric Care, 54*(2), 221–229.

Purpose

The purpose of this study was to determine the relationship between the anxiety-depression status and psychosocial adjustments in patients undergoing liver transplantation.

Design

This was a descriptive correlational study conducted with 90 participants who received a liver transplant in one transplant facility in Turkey. The participants included in the study were administered two questionnaires, the Hospital Anxiety and Depression Scale (HADS) and the Psychosocial Adjustment to Illness Self Report (PAIS).

Findings

The study found that as the anxiety risk of participants increased, their adjustments to their domestic and psychological environments were negatively affected.

In younger participants, the risk of experiencing anxiety increased and psychological adjustment to undergoing liver transplantation decreased. Women had a greater risk of anxiety. Most participants showed low psychosocial adjustment after liver transplantation, but this was most pronounced in those who were single, had a moderate socioeconomic level, and who were employed.

Nursing Implications

A psychiatric assessment is one element of the intensive preoperative evaluation of patients prior to undergoing liver transplantation. Psychiatric nurse practitioners may take part in such evaluations, and this information is important to have not only in the preoperative realm but after surgery should patients experience anxiety. It is important that patients are able to adjust socially and psychologically to their life changes after liver transplantation. Nurses are key participants in identifying methods to alleviate anxiety and improve coping strategies. Nurses provide encouragement for patients to participate in self-care activities that can promote effective psychosocial adjustment. Some of the patient education and support that is carried out preoperatively may facilitate this adjustment postoperatively.

Coordinating an effective plan with the interprofessional team, including psychiatric professionals, is part of the nursing role in caring for recipients of liver transplants and in helping these patients to achieve seamless transitions, less anxiety, and optimum levels of adjustment.

Following liver transplantation, the patient experiences a period of psychosocial adjustment (Ko, Muehrer, & Bratzke, 2018; Yıldız, & Kılınç, 2018). The nurse educates patients and caregivers to be alert for signs and symptoms of anxiety and depression and to report them to the transplant team so that appropriate referrals can be made for treatment as needed. See the Nursing Research Profile in Chart 43-11.

Continuing and Transitional Care

The nurse emphasizes the importance of follow-up laboratory tests and appointments with the transplant team. Trough blood levels of immunosuppressive agents are obtained, along with other blood tests that assess the function of the liver and kidneys. During the first months, the patient is likely to require blood tests two or three times a week. As the patient's condition stabilizes, laboratory studies and visits to the transplant team are less frequent. The importance of routine ophthalmologic examinations is emphasized because of the increased incidence of cataracts and glaucoma associated with the long-term corticosteroid therapy used with transplantation. Regular oral hygiene and follow-up dental care, with administration of prophylactic antibiotics before dental examinations and treatments, are recommended because of the immunosuppression.

The nurse reminds the patient that preventing rejection and infection is essential and increases the chances for survival and a more normal life than before transplantation. Many patients live successful and productive lives after receiving a liver transplant. Pregnancy may be considered after transplantation but it is not without risks. Despite advances in immunosuppressive therapy, increasing experience in the management of pregnancy after liver transplantation and some successful outcomes, these pregnancies are considered high risk for both mother and infant and referral should be made to a high-risk pregnancy center well before conception (Baskiran, Karakas, Ince, et al., 2017). Transplant recipients should be advised about birth control. The waiting period allows time to establish good health, stable liver function, and lower maintenance levels of immunosuppressive therapy (Baskiran et al., 2017).

LIVER ABSCESSES

Two categories of liver abscess have been identified: amebic and pyogenic. Amebic liver abscesses are most commonly caused by *Entamoeba histolytica*. Most amebic liver abscesses occur in the developing countries of the tropics and subtropics because of poor sanitation and hygiene. Pyogenic liver abscesses are much less common, but they are more common in developed countries than the amebic type (Friedman & Martin, 2018).

Pathophysiology

Whenever an infection develops anywhere along the biliary or GI tract, infecting organisms may reach the liver through the biliary system, portal venous system, or hepatic arterial or lymphatic system. Most bacteria are destroyed promptly, but occasionally some gain a foothold. The bacterial toxins destroy the neighboring liver cells, and the resulting necrotic tissue serves as a protective wall for the organisms.

Meanwhile, leukocytes migrate into the infected area. The result is an abscess cavity full of a liquid containing living and dead leukocytes, liquefied liver cells, and bacteria. Pyogenic abscesses of this type may be either single or multiple and small. Examples of causes of pyogenic liver abscess include cholangitis (usually related to benign or malignant obstruction of the biliary tree) and abdominal trauma.

Clinical Manifestations

The clinical picture is one of sepsis with few or no localizing signs. Fever with chills and diaphoresis, malaise, anorexia, nausea, vomiting, and weight loss may occur. The patient may complain of dull abdominal pain and tenderness in the right upper quadrant of the abdomen. Hepatomegaly, jaundice, anemia, and pleural effusion may develop. Sepsis and shock may be severe and life-threatening.

Appropriate diagnosis may be delayed and requires a high degree of clinical suspicion, especially in light of the lack of localizing signs in some patients. The diagnosis is made with the wide availability of various radiologic modalities including ultrasound, CT, and MRI (Goldman & Schaefer, 2019).

Assessment and Diagnostic Findings

Although blood cultures are obtained, the organism may not be identified with this test. Aspiration of the liver abscess, guided by ultrasound, CT, or MRI, may be performed to assist in diagnosis, obtain cultures and identify the organism. Percutaneous drainage of pyogenic abscesses is carried out to evacuate the abscess material and promote healing. A catheter may be left in place for continuous drainage; the patient must be educated about its management. Percutaneous drainage alone without catheter placement has received recent attention with patients followed with close clinical monitoring and serial ultrasounds. Results of this method are promising but controlled clinical trials are necessary to clarify effects and outcomes (Goldman & Schaefer, 2019).

Medical Management

Treatment includes IV antibiotic therapy; the specific antibiotic used in treatment depends on the organism identified. Continuous supportive care is indicated because of the serious condition of the patient. Open surgical drainage may be required if antibiotic therapy and percutaneous drainage are ineffective (Friedman & Martin, 2018; Schiff et al., 2018).

Nursing Management

Although the manifestations of liver abscess vary with the type of abscess, most patients appear acutely ill. Others appear to be chronically ill and debilitated. The nursing management depends on the patient's physical status and the medical management that is indicated. For patients who undergo evacuation and drainage of an abscess, monitoring the drainage and providing skin care are imperative. Strategies must be implemented to contain the drainage and to protect the patient from other sources of infection. Vital signs are monitored to detect changes in the patient's physical status. Deterioration in vital signs or the onset of new symptoms such as increasing pain, which may indicate rupture or extension of the abscess, is reported promptly. The nurse administers IV antibiotic therapy as prescribed. The white blood cell count and other laboratory test results are monitored closely for changes consistent with worsening infection. The nurse prepares the patient for discharge by providing education about symptom management, signs and symptoms that should be reported to the primary provider, management of drainage, and the importance of taking antibiotics as prescribed.

CRITICAL THINKING EXERCISES

1 pcs You are the nurse working with a 46-year-old woman who is at high risk for hepatitis B and C due to a history of IV drug abuse. What laboratory testing is likely to be done first for this patient? If laboratory testing is positive for either or both diseases, what invasive and noninvasive testing is warranted next? Describe the education you should provide about these tests. What are the priorities for the treatment plan if testing is positive for the diseases?

2 ipc A 58-year-old man underwent an orthotopic liver transplant for decompensated alcoholic cirrhosis. He is placed on an immunosuppressant regimen including corticosteroids, mycophenolate mofetil, and tacrolimus. On day 9 postoperatively, he develops a fever with an acute change in mental status and confusion. What nursing and interprofessional assessments are indicated for this patient? What interprofessional services should be engaged?

3 ebp A 44-year-old woman with obesity is diagnosed with NAFLD and is symptomatic with jaundice and fatigue. What are the best risk reduction tactics for this patient? How should you prepare and educate the patient to achieve specific evidence-based management goals and potentially control the disease? Should this patient be evaluated for malnutrition and sarcopenia even though she has obesity? If so, why would an evaluation for sarcopenia be important?

REFERENCES

*Asterisk indicates nursing research.

Books

Barrett, K. E., Barman, S. M., Brooks, H. L., & Yuan, J. (Eds.). (2019). *Ganong's review of medical physiology* (26th ed.). New York: McGraw-Hill Education.

Bickley, L. S. (2017). *Bates' guide to physical examination and history taking* (12th ed.). Philadelphia, PA: Lippincott Williams & Wilkins.

Bope, E. T., & Kellerman, R. D. (Eds.). (2018). *Conn's current therapy*. Philadelphia, PA: Saunders.

Brunicardi, F. C. (2019). *Schwartz's principles of surgery* (11th ed.). New York: McGraw-Hill Education.

Cameron, J. L., & Cameron, A. M. (2020). *Current surgical therapy* (13th ed.). Philadelphia, PA: Elsevier.

Feldman, M., Friedman, L. S., & Brandt, L. J. (2016). *Sleisinger & Fordtran's gastrointestinal & liver disease* (10th ed.). Philadelphia, PA: Saunders Elsevier.

Fischbach, F., & Fischbach, M. (2018). *A manual of laboratory and diagnostic tests* (10th ed.). Philadelphia, PA: Wolters Kluwer.

Friedman, L., & Martin, P. (2018). *Handbook of liver disease* (4th ed.). Philadelphia, PA: Elsevier.

Goldman, L., & Schafer, A. I. (2019). *Goldman's Cecil medicine* (26th ed.). Philadelphia, PA: Saunders Elsevier.

Hammer, G. D., & McPhee, S. J. (Eds.). (2019). *Pathophysiology of disease: An introduction to clinical medicine*. New York: McGraw-Hill.

Kumar, V., Abbas, A. K., Fausto, N., et al. (2014). *Robbins and Cotran pathologic basis of disease* (9th ed.). Philadelphia, PA: Saunders Elsevier.

Lee, S. S., & Moreau, R. (2015). *Cirrhosis: A practical guide to management* (1st ed.). Hoboken, NJ: John Wiley & Sons, Ltd.

Norris, T. L. (2019). *Porth's pathophysiology: Concepts of altered health states* (10th ed.). Philadelphia, PA: Wolters Kluwer.

Papadakis, M. A., & McPhee, S. J. (Eds.). (2020). *Current medical diagnosis and treatment* (59th ed.). New York: McGraw-Hill.

Sanyal, A., Boyer, T., & Terrault, N. (2018). *Zakim & Boyer's hepatology: A textbook of liver disease.* Philadelphia, PA: Elsevier.

Schiff, E. R., Maddrey, W. C., & Reddy, K. R. (2018). *Schiff's diseases of the liver* (12th ed.). Oxford, UK: John Wiley & Sons, Ltd.

Srinivasan, S., & Friedman, L. S. (2018). *Sitaraman & Friedman's essentials of gastroenterology* (2nd ed.). Hoboken, NJ: John Wiley & Sons, Ltd.

Weber, J., & Kelley, J. (2018). *Health assessment in nursing* (6th ed.). Philadelphia, PA: Wolters Kluwer.

Journals and Electronic Documents

AASLD-IDSA Hepatitis C Guidance Panel (2020). Hepatitis C Guidance 2019 Update: American Association for the Study of Liver Diseases—Infectious Diseases Society of America recommendations for testing, managing, and treating hepatitis C virus infection. *Hepatology, 71*(2), 686–721.

Aby, E. S., & Saab, S. (2019). Frailty, sarcopenia, and malnutrition in cirrhotic patients. *Clinics in Liver Disease, 23*(4), 589–605.

Acharya, C., & Bajaj, J. S. (2018). Current management of hepatic encephalopathy. *The American Journal of Gastroenterology, 113*(1), 1600–1612.

Adebayo, D., Neong, S. F., & Wong, F. (2019). Ascites and hepatorenal syndrome. *Clinics in Liver Disease, 23*(4), 659–682. doi:10.1016/j.cld.2019.06.002

Akinyemiju, T., Abera, S., Ahmed, M., et al. (2017). The burden of primary liver cancer and underlying etiologies from 1990 to 2015 at the global, regional, and national level: Results from the Global Burden of Disease Study 2015. *JAMA Oncology, 3*(12), 1683–1691.

Baki, J. A., & Tapper, E. B. (2019). Contemporary epidemiology of cirrhosis. *Current Treatment Options in Gastroenterology, 17*(2), 244–253.

Bañares, R., Ibáñez-Samaniego, L., Torner, J. M., et al. (2019). Meta-analysis of individual patient data of albumin dialysis in acute-on-chronic liver failure: Focus on treatment intensity. *Therapeutic Advances in Gastroenterology, 12*, 1–12.

Baskiran, A., Karakas, S., Ince, V., et al. (2017). Pregnancy after liver transplantation: Risks and outcomes. *Transplantation Proceedings, 49*(8), 1875–1878.

Bellentani, S. (2017). The epidemiology of non-alcoholic fatty liver disease. *Liver International, 37*(s1), 81–84.

Bunchorntavakul, C., & Reddy, K. R. (2019). Pharmacologic management of portal hypertension. *Clinics in Liver Disease, 23*(4), 713–736.

Centers for Disease Control and Prevention (CDC), Division of Viral Hepatitis. (2017). Viral hepatitis surveillance—United States, 2017. Retrieved on 12/10/2019 at: www.cdc.gov/hepatitis/Statistics/2010Surveillance/index.htm

Chan, S. L., Wong, V. W. S., Qin, S., et al. (2016). Infection and cancer: The case of hepatitis B. *Journal of Clinical Oncology, 34*(1), 83–91.

Chi, V., Cleary, S., & Bocchini, J. A. Jr. (2018). In pursuit of control and elimination: Update on hepatitis A and B epidemiology and prevention strategies. *Current Opinion in Pediatrics, 30*(5), 689–697.

European Association for the Study of the Liver (EASL). (2019). EASL clinical practice guidelines on nutrition in chronic liver disease. *Journal of Hepatology, 70*(1), 172–193.

Gerber, D. A., Baliga, P., & Karp, S. J. (2018). Allocation of donor livers for transplantation: A contemporary struggle. *JAMA Surgery, 153*(9), 787–788.

Houghton, M. (2019). Hepatitis C virus: 30 years after its discovery. *Cold Spring Harbor Perspectives in Medicine, 9*(12), 1–10. doi:10.1101/cshperspect.a037069

Hung, M. L., & Lee, E. W. (2019). Role of transjugular intrahepatic portosystemic shunt in the management of portal hypertension: Review and update of the literature. *Clinics in Liver Disease, 23*(4), 737–754.

*Ko, D., Muehrer, R. J., & Bratzke, L. C. (2018). Self-management in liver transplant recipients: A narrative review. *Progress in Transplantation, 28*(2), 100–115.

Kovacs, T. O., & Jensen, D. M. (2019). Varices: Esophageal, gastric, and rectal. *Clinics in Liver Disease, 23*(4), 625–642.

Larsen, F. S. (2019). Artificial liver support in acute and acute-on-chronic liver failure. *Current Opinion in Critical Care, 25*(2), 187–191.

Link-Gelles, R., Hofmeister, M. G., & Nelson, N. P. (2018). Use of hepatitis A vaccine for post-exposure prophylaxis in individuals over 40 years of age: A systematic review of published studies and recommendations for vaccine use. *Vaccine, 36*(20), 2745–2750.

Lucey, M. R. (2019). Alcohol-associated cirrhosis. *Clinics in Liver Disease, 23*(1), 115–126.

Macken, L., Hashim, A., Mason, L., et al. (2019). Permanent indwelling peritoneal catheters for palliation of refractory ascites in end-stage liver disease: A systematic review. *Liver International, 39*(9), 1594–1607.

Maher, S. Z., & Schreibman, I. R. (2018). The clinical spectrum and manifestations of acute liver failure. *Clinics in Liver Disease, 22*(2), 361–374.

Manka, P., Zeller, A., & Syn, W. K. (2019). Fibrosis in chronic liver disease: An update on diagnostic and treatment modalities. *Drugs, 79*(9), 903–927.

Mansour, D., & McPherson, S. (2018). Management of decompensated cirrhosis. *Clinical Medicine, 18*(Suppl 2), s60–s65.

Montrief, T., Koyfman, A., & Long, B. (2019). Acute liver failure: A review for emergency physicians. *The American Journal of Emergency Medicine, 37*(2), 329–337.

Moon, A. M., Singal, A. G., & Tapper, E. B. (2020). Contemporary epidemiology of chronic liver disease and cirrhosis. *Clinical Gastroenterology and Hepatology, 18*(12), 2650–2666. doi:10.1016/j.cgh.2019.07.060

*Pearson, J. A., Mangold, K., Kosiorek, H. E., et al. (2018). Registered nurse intent to promote physical activity for hospitalised liver transplant recipients. *Journal of Nursing Management, 26*(4), 442–448.

Petrick, J. L., Campbell, P. T., Koshiol, J., et al. (2018). Tobacco, alcohol use and risk of hepatocellular carcinoma and intrahepatic cholangiocarcinoma: The Liver Cancer Pooling Project. *British Journal of Cancer, 118*(7), 1005–1012.

Philips, C. A., Rajesh, S., Augustine, P., et al. (2019). Portosystemic shunts and refractory hepatic encephalopathy: Patient selection and current options. *Hepatic Medicine: Evidence and Research, 11*, 23–34.

Sedhom, D., D'Souza, M., John, E., et al. (2018). Viral hepatitis and acute liver failure: Still a problem. *Clinics in Liver Disease, 22*(2), 289–300.

Shin, E. C., & Jeong, S. H. (2018). Natural history, clinical manifestations, and pathogenesis of hepatitis A. *Cold Spring Harbor Perspectives in Medicine, 8*(9), 1–13. doi:10.1101/cshperspect.a031708.

Simonetto, D. A., Liu, M., & Kamath, P. S. (2019). Portal hypertension and related complications: Diagnosis and management. *Mayo Clinic Proceedings, 94*(4), 714–726.

Stravitz, R. T., & Lee, W. M. (2019). Acute liver failure. *The Lancet, 394*(10201), 869–881.

Styskel, B., Natarajan, Y., & Kanwal, F. (2019). Nutrition in alcoholic liver disease: An update. *Clinics in Liver Disease, 23*(1), 99–114.

Tapper, E. B., & Parikh, N. D. (2018). Mortality due to cirrhosis and liver cancer in the United States, 1999–2016: Observational study. *BMJ, 362*(k2817), 1–11.

Terrault, N. A., Lok, A. S., McMahon, B. J., et al. (2018). Update on prevention, diagnosis, and treatment of chronic hepatitis B: AASLD 2018 hepatitis B guidance. *Hepatology, 67*(4), 1560–1599.

Thomas, A. M., & Lewis, J. H. (2018). Nonacetaminophen drug-induced acute liver failure. *Clinics in Liver Disease, 22*(2), 301–324.

Tsilimigras, D. I., Rahnemai-Azar, A. A., Ntanasis-Stathopoulos, I., et al. (2019). Current approaches in the management of hepatic adenomas. *Journal of Gastrointestinal Surgery, 23*(1), 199–209.

Villarreal, J. A., & Sussman, N. L. (2019). Extracorporeal liver support in patients with acute liver failure. *Texas Heart Institute Journal, 46*(1), 67–68.

Wang, C. C., Cheng, P. N., & Kao, J. H. (2020). Systematic review: Chronic viral hepatitis and metabolic derangement. *Alimentary Pharmacology & Therapeutics, 51*(2), 216–230.

Weiskirchen, R., Weiskirchen, S., & Tacke, F. (2018). Recent advances in understanding liver fibrosis: Bridging basic science and individualized treatment concepts. *F1000Research. 7*, F1000 Faculty Rev-921, 1–46.

Wendon, J., Cordoba, J., Dhawan, A., et al. (2017). EASL clinical practical guidelines on the management of acute (fulminant) liver failure. *Journal of Hepatology, 66*(5), 1047–1081.

World Health Organization (WHO). (2019). Fact Sheet on Hepatitis B. Retrieved on 12/28/2019 at: www.who.int/news-room/fact-sheets/detail/hepatitis-b

Yang, J. D., Larson, J. J., Watt, K. D., et al. (2017). Hepatocellular carcinoma is the most common indication for liver transplantation and placement on the waitlist in the United States. *Clinical Gastroenterology and Hepatology, 15*(5), 767–775.

Yanny, B., Winters, A., Boutros, S., et al. (2019). Hepatic encephalopathy challenges, burden, and diagnostic and therapeutic approach. *Clinics in Liver Disease, 23*(4), 607–623.

Yao, C. K., Fung, J., Chu, N. H. S., et al. (2018). Dietary interventions in liver cirrhosis. *Journal of Clinical Gastroenterology, 52*(8), 663–673.

*Yıldız, E., & Kılınç, G. (2018). The relationship between anxiety-depression status and psychosocial adjustments in the patients undergoing liver transplantation. *Perspectives in Psychiatric Care, 54*(2), 221–229.

Younossi, Z. M., Stepanova, M., Younossi, I., et al. (2019). Long-term effects of treatment for chronic HBV infection on patient-reported outcomes. *Clinical Gastroenterology and Hepatology, 17*(8), 1641–1642.

Resources

Al-Anon Family Groups Headquarters, www.al-anon.alateen.org
Alcoholics Anonymous World Services (AAWS), www.aa.org
American Association for the Study of Liver Diseases (AASLD), www.aasld.org
American College of Gastroenterology (ACG), gi.org/
American Liver Foundation (ALF), www.liverfoundation.org
Hepatitis Foundation International (HFI), hepatitisfoundation.org
National Council on Alcoholism and Drug Dependence (NCADD), www.ncadd.org
National Digestive Diseases Information Clearinghouse (NDDIC), www.digestive.niddk.nih.gov
National Institute on Alcohol Abuse and Alcoholism (NIAAA), www.niaaa.nih.gov
United Network for Organ Sharing (UNOS), www.unos.org

44

Management of Patients with Biliary Disorders

LEARNING OUTCOMES

On completion of this chapter, the learner will be able to:

1. Identify the structure and function of the biliary tract and pancreas.
2. Describe the pathophysiology, clinical manifestations, and medical management of cholelithiasis.
3. Differentiate between acute and chronic pancreatitis.

4. Apply the nursing process as a framework for care of the patient with cholelithiasis, undergoing laparoscopic or open cholecystectomy, or with acute pancreatitis.
5. Explain the nutritional and metabolic effects of surgical treatment of tumors of the pancreas.

NURSING CONCEPTS

Comfort

Family

Infection

Inflammation

Metabolism

Nutrition

GLOSSARY

amylase: pancreatic enzyme; aids in the digestion of carbohydrates

cholecystectomy: removal of the gallbladder

cholecystitis: inflammation of the gallbladder which can be acute or chronic

cholecystojejunostomy: anastomosis of the jejunum to the gallbladder to divert bile flow

cholecystokinin (CCK): hormone; major stimulus for digestive enzyme secretion; stimulates contraction of the gallbladder

cholecystostomy: surgical opening and drainage of the gallbladder

choledocholithiasis: stones in the common bile duct

choledochostomy: opening into the common bile duct

cholelithiasis: calculi in the gallbladder

dissolution therapy: the use of medications to break up/dissolve gallstones

endocrine: secreting internally; hormonal secretion of a ductless gland

endoscopic retrograde cholangiopancreatography (ERCP): procedure using fiberoptic technology to visualize the biliary system

endoscopic ultrasound (EUS): invasive procedure using an ultrasound probe at the end of an endoscope to detect cholelithiasis and to decompress the gallbladder in the setting of acute cholecystitis

exocrine: secreting externally; hormonal secretion from excretory ducts

lipase: pancreatic enzyme; aids in the digestion of fats

lithotripsy: disintegration of gallstones by shock waves

pancreatitis: inflammation of the pancreas; may be acute or chronic

secretin: hormone responsible for stimulating bicarbonate secretion from the pancreas; also used as an aid in diagnosing pancreatic exocrine disease

steatorrhea: frothy, foul-smelling stools with a high fat content; results from impaired digestion of proteins and fats due to a lack of pancreatic juice in the intestine

trypsin: pancreatic enzyme; aids in the digestion of proteins

Zollinger-Ellison syndrome: hypersecretion of gastric acid that produces peptic ulcers as a result of a non–beta-cell tumor of the pancreatic islets

Disorders of the biliary tract and pancreas are common and include gallbladder stones and pancreatic dysfunction. An understanding of the structure and function of the biliary tract and pancreas is essential, along with an understanding of how biliary tract disorders are closely linked with liver disease. Patients with acute or chronic biliary tract or pancreatic disease require care from nurses who are knowledgeable about the diagnostic procedures and interventions that are used in the management of gallbladder and pancreatic disorders.

ANATOMIC AND PHYSIOLOGIC OVERVIEW

The Gallbladder

The gallbladder, a pear-shaped, hollow, saclike organ that is 7.5 to 10 cm (3 to 4 inches) long, lies in a shallow depression on the inferior surface of the liver, to which it is attached by loose connective tissue. The capacity of the gallbladder is 30 to 50 mL of bile. Its wall is composed largely of smooth muscle. The gallbladder is connected to the common bile duct (CBD) by the cystic duct (see Fig. 44-1).

The gallbladder functions as a storage depot for bile. Between meals, when the sphincter of Oddi is closed, bile produced by the hepatocytes enters the gallbladder. During storage, a large portion of the water in bile is absorbed through the walls of the gallbladder; thus, bile in the gallbladder is five to 10 times more concentrated than that originally secreted by the liver. When food enters the duodenum, the gallbladder contracts and the sphincter of Oddi (located at the junction of the CBD with the duodenum) relaxes. Relaxation of this sphincter allows the bile to enter the intestine. This response is mediated by secretion of the hormone **cholecystokinin (CCK)** from the intestinal wall (Norris, 2019). CCK is the major stimulus for digestive enzyme secretion and acts by stimulating the gallbladder to contract.

Bile is composed of water and electrolytes (sodium, potassium, calcium, chloride, and bicarbonate) along with significant amounts of lecithin, fatty acids, cholesterol, bilirubin, and bile salts. The bile salts, together with cholesterol, assist in emulsification of fats in the distal ileum. They are then reabsorbed into the portal blood for return to the liver, after which they are once again excreted into the bile. This pathway from hepatocytes to bile to intestine and back to the hepatocytes is called the *enterohepatic circulation*. Because of this circulation, only a small fraction of the bile salts that enter the intestine are excreted in the feces. This decreases the need for active synthesis of bile salts by the liver cells.

Approximately half of the bilirubin (a pigment derived from the breakdown of red blood cells) is a component of bile. It is converted by the intestinal flora into urobilinogen, which is a highly soluble substance. Urobilinogen is either excreted in the feces or returned to the portal circulation, where it is re-excreted into the bile. About 5% is normally absorbed into the general circulation and then excreted by the kidneys (Goldman & Schafer, 2019; Norris, 2019).

If the flow of bile is impeded (e.g., by gallstones in the bile ducts), bilirubin does not enter the intestine. As a result, blood levels of bilirubin increase. This causes increased renal excretion of urobilinogen, which results from conversion of bilirubin in the small intestine, and decreased excretion in the stool. These changes produce many of the signs and symptoms seen in gallbladder disorders.

The Pancreas

The pancreas is located in the upper abdomen (see Fig. 44-1). It has both **exocrine** (secreting externally; hormonal secretion from excretory ducts) and **endocrine** (secreting internally; hormonal secretion of a ductless gland) functions. The exocrine functions include secretion of pancreatic enzymes into the gastrointestinal (GI) tract through the pancreatic duct. The endocrine functions include secretion of insulin, glucagon, and somatostatin directly into the bloodstream.

The Exocrine Pancreas

The secretions of the exocrine portion of the pancreas are collected in the pancreatic duct, which joins the CBD and enters the duodenum at the ampulla of Vater. Surrounding the ampulla is the sphincter of Oddi, which partially controls the rate at which secretions from the pancreas and the gallbladder enter the duodenum.

The secretions of the exocrine pancreas are digestive enzymes high in protein content and an electrolyte-rich fluid. The secretions, which are very alkaline because of their high concentration of sodium bicarbonate, are capable of neutralizing the highly acidic gastric juice that enters the duodenum. Pancreatic enzymes include **amylase**, which aids in the digestion of carbohydrates; **trypsin**, which aids in the digestion of proteins; and **lipase**, which aids in the digestion of fats. Other enzymes that promote the breakdown of more complex foodstuffs are also secreted.

Hormones originating in the GI tract stimulate the secretion of these exocrine pancreatic juices. The hormone **secretin** is the major stimulus for increased bicarbonate secretion from the pancreas, and the major stimulus for digestive enzyme secretion is the hormone CCK. The vagus nerve also influences exocrine pancreatic secretion.

The Endocrine Pancreas

The islets of Langerhans, the endocrine part of the pancreas, are collections of cells embedded in the pancreatic tissue. They are composed of alpha, beta, and delta cells. The hormone produced by the beta cells is called *insulin*, the alpha cells secrete glucagon, and the delta cells secrete somatostatin.

Insulin

A major action of insulin is to lower blood glucose by permitting entry of glucose into the cells of the liver, muscle, and other tissues, where it is either stored as glycogen or used for energy. Insulin also promotes the storage of fat in adipose tissue and the synthesis of proteins in various body tissues.

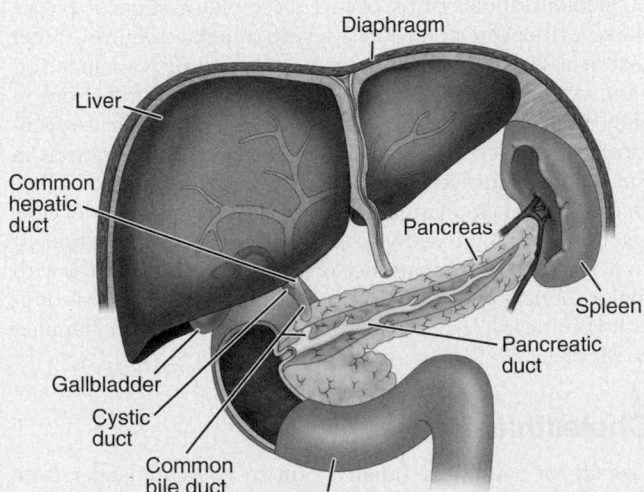

Figure 44-1 • The liver, biliary system, and pancreas.

In the absence of insulin, glucose cannot enter the cells and is excreted in the urine. This condition, called *diabetes*, can be diagnosed by high levels of glucose in the blood. In diabetes, stored fats and protein are used for energy instead of glucose, causing loss of body mass. Diabetes is discussed in detail in Chapter 46. The level of glucose in the blood normally regulates the rate of insulin secretion from the pancreas (Goldman & Schafer, 2019; Norris, 2019).

Glucagon

The effect of glucagon (opposite to that of insulin) is chiefly to raise the blood glucose by converting glycogen to glucose in the liver. Glucagon is secreted by the pancreas in response to a decrease in the level of blood glucose.

Somatostatin

Somatostatin exerts a hypoglycemic effect by interfering with release of growth hormone from the pituitary and glucagon from the pancreas, both of which tend to raise blood glucose levels.

Endocrine Control of Carbohydrate Metabolism

Glucose required for energy is derived by metabolism of ingested carbohydrates and also from proteins by the process of gluconeogenesis. Glucose can be stored temporarily in the form of glycogen in the liver, muscles, and other tissues. The endocrine system controls the level of blood glucose by regulating the rate at which glucose is synthesized, stored, and moved to and from the bloodstream. Through the action of hormones, blood glucose is normally maintained at less than 100 mg/dL (5.6 mmol/L) (Norris, 2019; Papadakis & McPhee, 2020). Insulin is the primary hormone that lowers the blood glucose level. Hormones that raise the blood glucose level are glucagon, epinephrine, adrenocorticosteroids, growth hormone, and thyroid hormone.

The endocrine and exocrine functions of the pancreas are interrelated. The major exocrine function is to facilitate digestion through secretion of enzymes into the proximal duodenum. Secretin and CCK are hormones from the GI tract that aid in the digestion of food substances by controlling the secretions of the pancreas. Neural factors also influence pancreatic enzyme secretion. Considerable dysfunction of the pancreas must occur before enzyme secretion decreases and protein and fat digestion becomes impaired. Pancreatic enzyme secretion is normally 1500 to 3000 mL/day (Norris, 2019; Papadakis & McPhee, 2020).

Gerontologic Considerations

There is little change in the size of the pancreas with age. However, there is an increase in fibrous material and some fatty deposition in the normal pancreas in people older than 70 years. Some localized arteriosclerotic changes occur with age. There is also a decreased rate of pancreatic enzyme secretion (i.e., amylase, lipase, and trypsin) and decreased bicarbonate output in older adults. Some impairment of normal fat absorption occurs with increasing age, possibly because of delayed gastric emptying and pancreatic insufficiency (Eliopoulos, 2018; Norris, 2019; Papadakis & McPhee, 2020). Decreased calcium absorption may also occur. These changes require care in interpreting diagnostic test results in the normal older patient and in providing dietary counseling.

DISORDERS OF THE GALLBLADDER

Several disorders affect the biliary system and interfere with normal drainage of bile into the duodenum. These disorders include inflammation of the biliary system and carcinoma that obstructs the biliary tree. Gallbladder disease with stones is the most common disorder of the biliary system. Not all occurrences of cholecystitis are related to stones (calculi) in the gallbladder (**cholelithiasis**) or stones in the CBD (**choledocholithiasis**). However, most of the 15 million Americans with gallstones have no pain and are unaware of the presence of stones (Cameron & Cameron, 2020; Kellerman & Rakel, 2018).

Cholecystitis

Cholecystitis (inflammation of the gallbladder which can be acute or chronic) causes pain, tenderness, and rigidity of the upper right abdomen that may radiate to the midsternal area or right shoulder and is associated with nausea, vomiting, and the usual signs of an acute inflammation. An empyema of the gallbladder develops if the gallbladder becomes filled with purulent fluid (pus).

Calculous cholecystitis is the cause of more than 90% of cases of acute cholecystitis (Brunicardi, 2019; Cameron & Cameron, 2020). In calculous cholecystitis, a gallbladder stone obstructs bile outflow. Bile remaining in the gallbladder initiates a chemical reaction; autolysis and edema occur; and the blood vessels in the gallbladder are compressed, compromising its vascular supply. Gangrene of the gallbladder with perforation may result. Bacteria play a minor role in acute cholecystitis; however, secondary infection of bile occurs in approximately 50% of cases. The organisms involved are generally enteric (normally live in the GI tract) and include *Escherichia coli*, *Klebsiella* species, and *Streptococcus*. Bacterial contamination is not believed to stimulate the actual onset of acute cholecystitis (Feldman, Friedman, & Brandt, 2016; Goldman & Schafer, 2019).

Acalculous cholecystitis describes acute gallbladder inflammation in the absence of obstruction by gallstones. Acalculous cholecystitis occurs after major surgical procedures, orthopedic procedures, severe trauma, or burns. Other factors associated with this type of cholecystitis include torsion, cystic duct obstruction, primary bacterial infections of the gallbladder, and multiple blood transfusions. It is speculated that acalculous cholecystitis is caused by alterations in fluids and electrolytes and alterations in regional blood flow in the visceral circulation. Bile stasis (lack of gallbladder contraction) and increased viscosity of the bile are also thought to play a role. The occurrence of acalculous cholecystitis with major surgical procedures or trauma makes its diagnosis difficult (Brunicardi, 2019; Cameron & Cameron, 2020; Hammer & McPhee, 2019).

Cholelithiasis

Calculi, or gallstones, usually form in the gallbladder from the solid constituents of bile; they vary greatly in size, shape, and composition (see Fig. 44-2). They are uncommon in

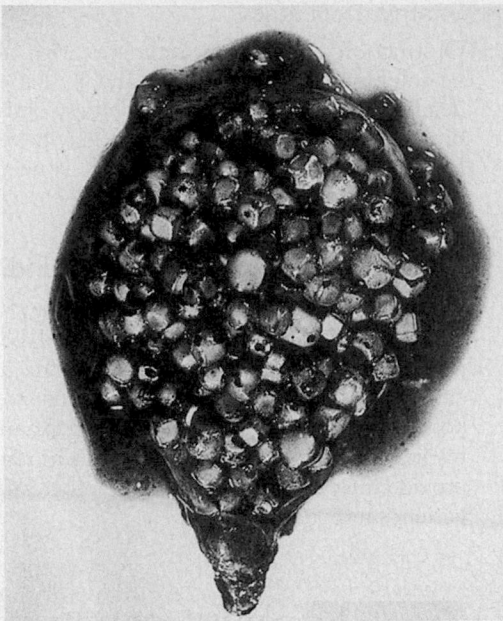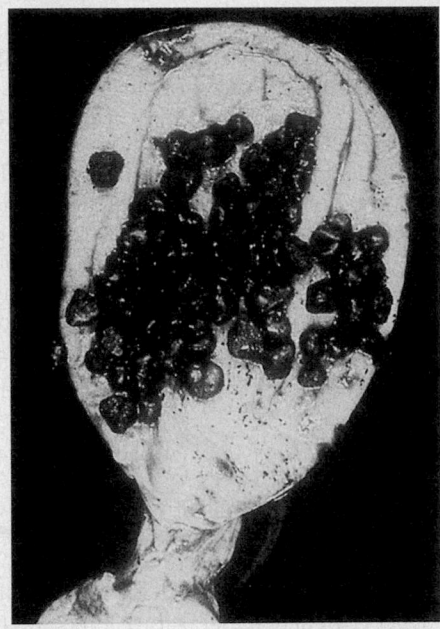

Figure 44-2 • Examples of cholesterol gallstones (**left**) made up of a coalescence of multiple small stones and pigment gallstones (**right**) composed of calcium bilirubinate. Reprinted with permission from Strayer, D. S., & Rubin, E. (2015). *Rubin's pathology: Clinicopathologic foundations of medicine* (7th ed.). Philadelphia, PA: Lippincott Williams & Wilkins.

children and young adults but become more prevalent with increasing age. It is estimated that the prevalence of gallstones ranges from 5% to 20% in women between the ages of 20 and 55 years and from 25% to 30% in women older than 50 years. Cholelithiasis affects approximately 50% of women by the age of 70 years (Littlefield & Lenahan, 2019).

Pathophysiology

The pathophysiology of gallstone development is multifactorial. There are two major types of gallstones: those composed predominantly of pigment and those composed primarily of cholesterol. Pigment stones probably form when unconjugated pigments in the bile precipitate to form stones; these stones account for about 10% to 25% of cases in the United States (Hammer & McPhee, 2019). The risk of developing such stones is increased in patients with cirrhosis, hemolysis, and infections of the biliary tract. Pigment stones cannot be dissolved and must be removed surgically.

Cholesterol stones account for most of the remaining 75% of cases of gallbladder disease in the United States. Cholesterol, which is a normal constituent of bile, is insoluble in water. Its solubility depends on bile acids and lecithin (phospholipids) in bile (Hammer & McPhee, 2019). In gallstone-prone patients, there is decreased bile acid synthesis and increased cholesterol synthesis in the liver, resulting in bile supersaturated with cholesterol, which precipitates out of the bile to form stones (Hammer & McPhee, 2019). The cholesterol-saturated bile predisposes to the formation of gallstones and acts as an irritant that produces inflammatory changes in the mucosa of the gallbladder (Hammer & McPhee, 2019).

Two to three times more women than men develop cholesterol stones and gallbladder disease; affected women are usually older than 40 years, multiparous, and have obesity (Feldman et al., 2016; Goldman & Schafer, 2019; Hammer & McPhee, 2019). Stone formation is more frequent in people who use oral contraceptives, estrogens, or clofibrate; these medications are known to increase biliary cholesterol saturation (Hammer & McPhee, 2019). The incidence of stone formation increases with age as a result of increased hepatic secretion of cholesterol and decreased bile acid synthesis (Hammer & McPhee, 2019). In addition, there is an increased risk because of malabsorption of bile salts in patients with GI disease or T-tube fistula and in those who have undergone ileal resection or bypass. The incidence is also greater in people with diabetes (see Chart 44-1). The role of diet in the causation of cholesterol stones has not been confirmed but is under study. Those at high risk may be encouraged to maintain an optimal body weight and consider reducing modifiable risk factors by avoiding consumption of sugar and sweet foods, low-fiber foods, and fast foods (Di Ciaula, Garruti, Frühbeck, et al., 2019).

> ### Chart 44-1 ⚠ RISK FACTORS
> #### Cholelithiasis
>
> - Cystic fibrosis
> - Diabetes
> - Frequent changes in weight
> - Ileal resection or disease
> - Low-dose estrogen therapy—carries a small increase in the risk of gallstones
> - Obesity
> - Rapid weight loss (leads to rapid development of gallstones and high risk of symptomatic disease)
> - Treatment with high-dose estrogen
> - Women, especially those who have had multiple pregnancies or who are of Native American or U.S. southwestern Hispanic ethnicity
>
> Adapted from Cox, M. R., Eslick, G. D., & Padbury, R. (2018). *The management of gallstone disease: A practical and evidence-based approach*. Cham, Switzerland: Springer Publishing.

Clinical Manifestations

Gallstones may be silent, producing no pain and only mild GI symptoms. Such stones may be detected incidentally during surgery or evaluation for unrelated problems (Hammer & McPhee, 2019; Srinivasan & Friedman, 2018).

The patient with gallbladder disease resulting from gallstones may develop two types of symptoms: those due to disease of the gallbladder itself and those due to obstruction of the bile passages by a gallstone. The symptoms may be acute or chronic. Epigastric distress, such as fullness, abdominal distention, and vague pain in the right upper quadrant of the abdomen, may occur. This distress may follow a meal rich in fried or fatty foods (Brunicardi, 2019; Cameron & Cameron, 2020; Hammer & McPhee, 2019).

Pain and Biliary Colic

If a gallstone obstructs the cystic duct, the gallbladder becomes distended, inflamed, and eventually infected (acute cholecystitis). The patient develops a fever and may have a palpable abdominal mass. The patient may have biliary colic with excruciating upper right abdominal pain that radiates to the back or right shoulder. Biliary colic is usually associated with nausea and vomiting, and it is noticeable several hours after a heavy meal. The patient moves about restlessly, unable to find a comfortable position. In some patients, the pain is constant rather than colicky (Brunicardi, 2019; Cameron & Cameron, 2020).

Such a bout of biliary colic is caused by contraction of the gallbladder, which cannot release bile because of obstruction by the stone. When distended, the fundus of the gallbladder comes in contact with the abdominal wall in the region of the right ninth and 10th costal cartilages. This produces marked tenderness in the right upper quadrant on deep inspiration and prevents full inspiratory excursion.

The pain of acute cholecystitis may be so severe that analgesic medications are required. The use of morphine has traditionally been avoided because of concern that it could cause spasm of the sphincter of Oddi. This is controversial, because morphine is the preferred analgesic agent for management of acute pain. Furthermore, all opioids stimulate the sphincter of Oddi to some degree (Littlefield & Lenahan, 2019; Papadakis & McPhee, 2020).

If the gallstone is dislodged and no longer obstructs the cystic duct, the gallbladder drains and the inflammatory process subsides after a relatively short time. If the gallstone continues to obstruct the duct, abscess, necrosis, and perforation with generalized peritonitis may result.

Jaundice

Jaundice occurs in a few patients with gallbladder disease, usually with obstruction of the common bile duct. The bile, which is no longer carried to the duodenum, is absorbed by the blood and gives the skin and mucous membranes a yellow color. This is frequently accompanied by marked pruritus (itching) of the skin.

Changes in Urine and Stool Color

The excretion of the bile pigments by the kidneys gives the urine a very dark color. The feces, no longer colored with bile pigments, are grayish (like putty) or clay colored.

Vitamin Deficiency

Obstruction of bile flow interferes with absorption of the fat-soluble vitamins A, D, E, and K. Patients may exhibit deficiencies of these vitamins if biliary obstruction has been prolonged. For example, a patient may have bleeding caused by vitamin K deficiency (vitamin K is necessary for normal blood clotting).

Assessment and Diagnostic Findings

A wide range of diagnostic studies may be performed in patients with biliary disorders. Table 44-1 identifies various procedures and their diagnostic uses. The nurse should educate the patient about the purpose, what to expect, and any possible side effects related to these examinations prior to testing. The nurse should note trends in results because they provide information about disease progression as well as the patient's response to therapy.

TABLE 44-1	Studies Used in the Diagnosis of Biliary Tract and Pancreatic Disease
Studies	**Diagnostic Uses**
Magnetic resonance cholangiopancreatography (MRCP)	Visualizes the biliary tree and capable of detecting biliary tract obstruction
Cholecystogram, cholangiogram	Visualize gallbladder and bile duct
Celiac axis arteriography	Visualizes liver and pancreas
Laparoscopy	Visualizes anterior surface of liver, gallbladder, and mesentery through a trocar
Ultrasonography	Shows size of abdominal organs and presence of masses
Helical computed tomography and magnetic resonance imaging	Detect neoplasms; diagnose cysts, pseudocysts, abscess, and hematomas; determine severity of pancreatitis based on the presence of necrosis or peripancreatic fluid collections
Endoscopic retrograde cholangiopancreatography	Visualizes biliary structures and pancreas via endoscopy
Endoscopic ultrasound (EUS)	Identifies small tumors and other abnormalities and facilitate fine-needle aspiration biopsy of tumors or lymph nodes for diagnosis
Serum alkaline phosphatase	In the absence of bone disease, to measure biliary tract obstruction
Gamma-glutamyl, gamma-glutamyl transpeptidase, lactate dehydrogenase	Markers for biliary stasis; also elevated in alcohol abuse
Cholesterol levels	Elevated in biliary obstruction; decreased in parenchymal liver disease

Adapted from Fischbach, F. T., & Fischbach, M. A. (2018). *Fischbach's manual of laboratory and diagnostic tests* (10th ed.). Philadelphia, PA: Wolters Kluwer.

Abdominal X-Ray

If the patient presents with symptoms of gallbladder disease, an abdominal x-ray may be obtained to exclude other causes of symptoms. However, only 10% to 15% of gallstones are calcified sufficiently to be visible on such x-ray studies (Brunicardi, 2019; Goldman & Shafer, 2019).

Ultrasonography

Ultrasonography is the diagnostic procedure of choice because it is rapid and accurate and can be used in patients with liver dysfunction and jaundice. It does not expose patients to ionizing radiation. The procedure is most accurate if the patient fasts overnight so that the gallbladder is distended. Ultrasonography can detect calculi in the gallbladder or a dilated CBD with 90% accuracy (Brunicardi, 2019; Goldman & Shafer, 2019; Littlefield & Lenahan, 2019; Mou, Tesfasilassie, Hirji, et al., 2019).

Radionuclide Imaging or Cholescintigraphy

Cholescintigraphy is used successfully in the diagnosis of acute cholecystitis or blockage of a bile duct (Brunicardi, 2019; Goldman & Schafer, 2019; Littlefield & Lenahan, 2019; Mou et al., 2019). During this procedure, a radioactive agent is administered intravenously (IV), which is taken up by the hepatocytes and excreted rapidly through the biliary tract. The biliary tract is then scanned, and images of the gallbladder and biliary tract are obtained. This test is more expensive than ultrasonography, takes longer to perform, and exposes the patient to radiation. It is often used when ultrasonography is not conclusive, such as in acalculous cholecystitis (Brunicardi, 2019; Goldman & Schafer, 2019; Littlefield & Lenahan, 2019; Mou et al., 2019).

Oral Cholecystography

Oral cholecystography is used if ultrasound equipment is not available or if the ultrasound results are inconclusive. This study may be performed to detect gallstones and to assess the ability of the gallbladder to fill, concentrate its contents, contract, and empty. If the patient is not allergic to iodine or seafood, an iodide-containing contrast agent that is excreted by the liver and concentrated in the gallbladder is given 10 to 12 hours before the x-ray study (Brunicardi, 2019; Goldman & Schafer, 2019; Littlefield & Lenahan, 2019; Mou et al., 2019). The normal gallbladder fills with this radiopaque substance. If gallstones are present, they appear as shadows on the x-ray image.

Oral cholecystography may be used as part of the evaluation of patients who have been treated with gallstone **dissolution therapy** (the use of medications to break up/dissolve gallstones) or **lithotripsy** (disintegration of gallstones by shock waves).

Endoscopic Retrograde Cholangiopancreatography

Endoscopic retrograde cholangiopancreatography (ERCP) permits direct visualization of structures that previously could be seen only during laparotomy. This procedure examines the hepatobiliary system via a side-viewing flexible fiberoptic endoscope inserted through the esophagus to the descending duodenum (see Fig. 44-3). Multiple position changes are

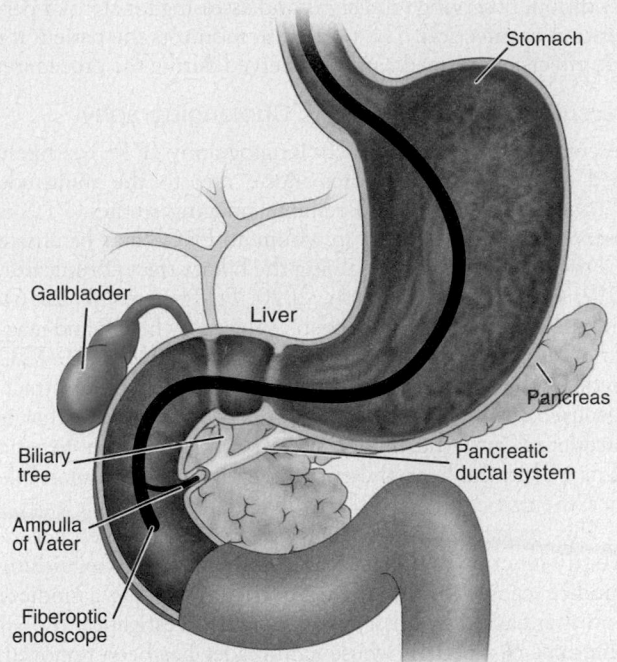

Figure 44-3 • Endoscopic retrograde cholangiopancreatography. A fiberoptic duodenoscope, with side-viewing apparatus, is inserted into the duodenum. The ampulla of Vater is catheterized, and the biliary tree is injected with contrast agent. The pancreatic ductal system is also assessed, if indicated. This procedure is of special value in visualizing neoplasms of the ampulla area and extracting a biopsy specimen.

required to pass the endoscope during the procedure, beginning in the left semiprone position.

Fluoroscopy and multiple x-rays are used during ERCP to evaluate the presence and location of ductal stones. Careful insertion of a catheter through the endoscope into the CBD is the most important step in sphincterotomy (division of the muscles of the biliary sphincter) for gallstone extraction via this technique (see later discussion). ERCP is not recommended for the evaluation of suspected CBD stones but can be used to treat confirmed choledocholithiasis before or during laparoscopic cholecystectomy (Brunicardi, 2019; Cameron & Cameron, 2020).

Nursing Implications

Before ERCP, the patient is educated about the procedure and their role in it. This preparation can allay anxiety and facilitate the insertion of the endoscope without damage to the GI tract structures, including the biliary tree. The patient takes nothing by mouth for several hours before the procedure. The procedure requires intravenous (IV) sedation and monitored anesthesia care. In some cases general anesthesia is required, and the sedated patient is monitored closely during and after the procedure (Brunicardi, 2019). It may be necessary to administer medications, such as glucagon or anticholinergic agents, to make cannulation easier by decreasing duodenal peristalsis. The nurse observes closely for signs of respiratory and CNS depression, hypotension, oversedation, and vomiting (if glucagon is given). During ERCP, the nurse monitors IV fluids, administers medications, and positions the patient. After the procedure, the nurse monitors the patient's condition, observing vital signs and assessing for signs of perforation or infection. The nurse also monitors the patient for side effects of any medications received during the procedure.

Percutaneous Transhepatic Cholangiography

Percutaneous transhepatic cholangiography (PTC) is rarely used for diagnostic purposes alone due to the multitude of other less invasive and reliable imaging studies. PTC is reserved for those patients in whom an ERCP may be unsafe due to previous surgery involving the biliary tract (Brunicardi, 2019; Cameron & Cameron, 2020; Feldman et al., 2016). The use of PTC has mainly been replaced by ERCP and magnetic resonance cholangiopancreatography (MRCP). PTC involves the injection of dye directly into the biliary tract. Because of the relatively large concentration of dye that is introduced into the biliary system, including the hepatic ducts within the liver, the entire length of the common bile duct, the cystic duct, and the gallbladder is outlined clearly.

This procedure can be carried out in the presence of liver dysfunction and jaundice. It is useful for distinguishing jaundice caused by liver disease (hepatocellular jaundice) from that caused by biliary obstruction, investigating the GI symptoms of a patient whose gallbladder has been removed, locating stones within the bile ducts, and diagnosing cancer involving the biliary system (Brunicardi, 2019; Cameron & Cameron, 2020; Feldman et al., 2016).

This sterile procedure is performed under moderate sedation on a patient who has been fasting; the patient also receives local anesthesia. Coagulation parameters and platelet count should be normal to minimize the risk of bleeding. Broad-spectrum antibiotics are given during the procedure because of the high prevalence of bacterial colonization from obstructed biliary systems (Feldman et al., 2016; Brunicardi, 2019; Cameron & Cameron, 2020). After infiltration with a local anesthetic agent has occurred, a flexible needle is inserted into the liver from the right side in the midclavicular line immediately beneath the right costal margin. Successful entry of a duct is noted when bile is aspirated or on injection of a contrast agent. Ultrasound can be used to guide puncture of the duct. Bile is aspirated, and samples are sent for bacteriology and cytology (Brunicardi, 2019; Feldman et al., 2016; Kellerman & Rakel, 2018). A water-soluble contrast agent is injected to fill the biliary system. The fluoroscopy table is tilted and the patient is repositioned to allow x-rays to be taken in multiple projections. Delayed x-ray views can identify abnormalities of more distant ducts and determine the length of a stricture or multiple strictures. Before the needle is removed, as much dye and bile as possible are aspirated to forestall subsequent leakage into the needle tract and eventually into the peritoneal cavity, thus minimizing the risk of bile peritonitis.

Nursing Implications

Although the complication rate after this procedure is low, the nurse must closely observe the patient for symptoms of bleeding, peritonitis, and sepsis. The nurse assesses the patient for pain and indications of these complications and reports them promptly to the primary provider, takes measures to reassure the patient, and ensures patient comfort. Antibiotic agents are often prescribed to minimize the risk of sepsis and septic shock.

Medical Management

The major objectives of medical therapy are to reduce the incidence of acute episodes of gallbladder pain and cholecystitis by supportive and dietary management and, if possible, to remove the cause of cholecystitis by pharmacologic therapy, endoscopic procedures, or surgical intervention. Although nonsurgical procedures eliminate risks associated with surgery, these approaches are associated with persistent symptoms or recurrent stone formation. Most of the nonsurgical approaches, including lithotripsy and dissolution of gallstones, provide only temporary solutions to gallstone problems and are infrequently used in the United States. In some instances, other treatment approaches may be indicated; these are described later.

Cholecystectomy (removal of the gallbladder) through traditional surgical approaches has largely been replaced by laparoscopic cholecystectomy (removal of the gallbladder through a small incision through the umbilicus) (see later discussion). As a result, surgical risks have decreased, along with the length of hospital stay and the long recovery period required after standard surgical cholecystectomy. In relatively rare instances, a standard surgical procedure may be necessary.

Nutritional and Supportive Therapy

Approximately 80% of the patients with acute gallbladder inflammation achieve remission with rest, IV fluids, nasogastric suction, analgesia, and antibiotic agents. Unless the patient's condition deteriorates, surgical intervention is delayed just until the acute symptoms subside (usually within a few days). At this time, the patient undergoes a laparoscopic cholecystectomy (Brunicardi, 2019; Cameron & Cameron, 2020; Goldman & Schafer, 2019).

The diet immediately after an episode is usually low-fat liquids. These can include powdered supplements high in protein and carbohydrate stirred into skim milk. Cooked fruits, rice or tapioca, lean meats, mashed potatoes, non–gas-forming vegetables, bread, coffee, or tea may be added as tolerated. The patient should avoid eggs, cream, pork, fried foods, cheese, rich dressings, gas-forming vegetables, and alcohol. It is important to remind the patient that fatty foods may induce an episode of cholecystitis. Dietary management may be the major mode of therapy in patients who have had only dietary intolerance to fatty foods and vague GI symptoms (Kellerman & Rakel, 2018).

Pharmacologic Therapy

Ursodeoxycholic acid (UDCA) and chenodeoxycholic acid (chenodiol or CDCA) have been used to dissolve small, radiolucent gallstones composed primarily of cholesterol (Goldman & Shafer, 2019). UDCA has fewer side effects than chenodiol and can be given in smaller doses to achieve the same effect. It acts by inhibiting the synthesis and secretion of cholesterol, thereby desaturating bile. Treatment with UDCA can reduce the size of existing stones, dissolve small stones, and prevent new stones from forming. Six to 12 months of therapy is required in many patients to dissolve stones, and monitoring of the patient for recurrence of symptoms or the occurrence of side effects (e.g., GI symptoms, pruritus, headache) is required during this time. The effective dose of medication depends on body weight. This method of

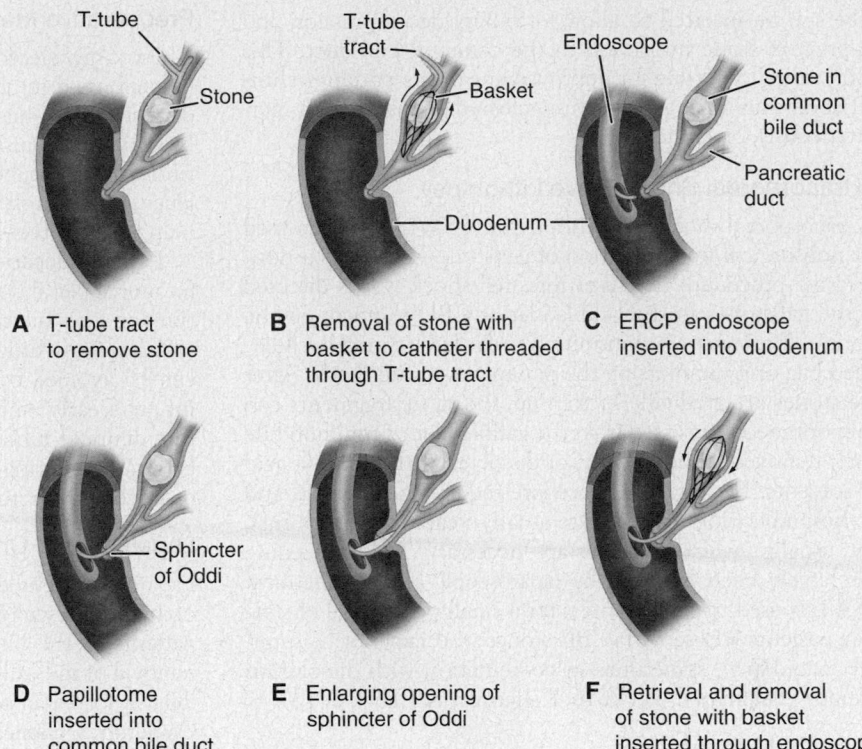

Figure 44-4 • A–F. Procedures for removing gallstones.

A T-tube tract to remove stone

B Removal of stone with basket to catheter threaded through T-tube tract

C ERCP endoscope inserted into duodenum

D Papillotome inserted into common bile duct

E Enlarging opening of sphincter of Oddi

F Retrieval and removal of stone with basket inserted through endoscope

treatment is generally indicated for patients who refuse surgery or for whom surgery is contraindicated. The success rate of this therapy is low as the recurrence following it is high (Goldman & Shafer, 2019).

Patients with frequent symptoms, cystic duct occlusion, or pigment stones are not candidates for pharmacologic therapy. Laparoscopic or open cholecystectomy is more appropriate for symptomatic patients with acceptable operative risk (Goldman & Shafer, 2019).

Nonsurgical Removal of Gallstones

Dissolving Gallstones

Several methods have been used to dissolve gallstones by infusion of a solvent (mono-octanoin or methyl tertiary butyl ether [MTBE]) into the gallbladder. The solvent can be infused through the following routes: through a tube or catheter inserted percutaneously directly into the gallbladder; through a tube or drain inserted through a T-tube tract to dissolve stones not removed at the time of surgery, endoscopically with ERCP; or via a transnasal biliary catheter, a rarely used procedure due to its lack of success, potential side effects, and recurrence rates of up to 50% (Goldman & Shafer, 2019; Townsend, Beauchamp, Evers, et al., 2016).

Laparoscopic cholecystectomy is the standard for management. Dissolution therapies are used for those patients who may not be candidates for the procedure due to safety concerns regarding general anesthesia (Goldman & Shafer, 2019; Townsend et al., 2016).

Stone Removal by Instrumentation

Several methods are used to remove stones that were not removed at the time of cholecystectomy or have become lodged in the CBD (see Fig. 44-4A,B). A catheter and instrument with a basket attached are threaded through the T-tube

tract or fistula formed at the time of T-tube insertion; the basket is used to retrieve and remove the stones lodged in the common bile duct.

A second procedure involves the use of the ERCP endoscope (see Fig. 44-4C). After the endoscope is inserted, a cutting instrument is passed through the endoscope into the ampulla of Vater of the common bile duct. It may be used to cut the submucosal fibers, or papilla, of the sphincter of Oddi, enlarging the opening, which may allow the lodged stones to pass spontaneously into the duodenum. Another instrument with a small basket or balloon at its tip may be inserted through the endoscope to retrieve the stones (see Fig. 44-4D–F). The patient is observed closely for bleeding, perforation, and the development of pancreatitis (see later discussion) or sepsis.

The ERCP procedure is particularly useful in diagnosis and treatment of patients who have symptoms after biliary tract surgery, patients with intact gallbladders, and patients for whom surgery is particularly hazardous.

Intracorporeal Lithotripsy

Stones in the gallbladder or CBD may be fragmented by means of laser pulse technology. A laser pulse is directed under fluoroscopic guidance with the use of devices that can distinguish between stones and tissue. The laser pulse produces rapid expansion and disintegration of plasma on the stone surface, resulting in a mechanical shock wave. Electrohydraulic lithotripsy uses a probe with two electrodes that deliver electric sparks in rapid pulses, creating expansion of the liquid environment surrounding the gallstones. This results in pressure waves that cause stones to fragment. This technique can be used percutaneously with a basket or balloon catheter system or by direct visualization through an endoscope. Repeated procedures may be necessary because of stone size, local anatomy, bleeding, or technical difficulty. A nasobiliary tube can be inserted to allow for biliary decompression and to prevent stone impaction in the common bile duct. This approach allows time for improvement in the patient's clinical condition until gallstones are cleared endoscopically, percutaneously, or surgically.

Extracorporeal Shock Wave Lithotripsy

Extracorporeal shock wave lithotripsy (ESWL) has been used for nonsurgical fragmentation of gallstones. ESWL is a noninvasive procedure that uses repeated shock waves directed at the gallstones in the gallbladder or CBD to fragment the stones. The waves are transmitted to the body through a fluid-filled bag or by immersing the patient in a water bath. After the stones are gradually broken up, the stone fragments can be spontaneously passed from the gallbladder or common bile duct, removed by endoscopy, or dissolved with oral bile acid or solvents. Because the procedure requires no incision and no hospitalization, patients are usually treated as outpatients, but usually several sessions are necessary. This procedure has largely been replaced by laparoscopic cholecystectomy. ESWL is used in some centers for a small percentage of suitable patients (those with CBD stones who may not be surgical candidates), sometimes in combination with dissolution therapy (Feldman et al., 2016; Kellerman & Rakel, 2018).

Surgical Management

Surgical treatment of gallbladder disease and gallstones is carried out to relieve persistent symptoms, to remove the cause of biliary colic, and to treat acute cholecystitis. Surgery may be delayed until the patient's symptoms have subsided, or it may be performed as an emergency procedure, if necessitated by the patient's condition.

Preoperative Measures

Chest x-ray, electrocardiogram, and liver function tests may be performed in addition to imaging studies of the gallbladder. Vitamin K may be given if the prothrombin level is low. Nutritional requirements are considered, and, if the nutritional status is suboptimal, it may be necessary to provide IV glucose with protein supplements to aid wound healing and help prevent liver damage.

Patient education for gallbladder surgery is similar to that for any upper abdominal laparotomy or laparoscopy. Instructions and explanations are given before surgery about turning and deep breathing. Postoperative pneumonia and atelectasis can be avoided by deep-breathing exercises, frequent turning, and early ambulation. The patient should be informed that drainage tubes and a nasogastric tube and suction might be required during the immediate postoperative period if an open cholecystectomy is performed.

Laparoscopic Cholecystectomy

Laparoscopic cholecystectomy (see Fig. 44-5) is the standard of therapy for symptomatic gallstones. Approximately 700,000 patients in the United States require surgery each year for removal of the gallbladder, and 80% to 90% of them are candidates for laparoscopic cholecystectomy (Brunicardi, 2019; Cameron & Cameron, 2020; Feldman et al., 2016; Goldman & Shafer, 2019). If the CBD is thought to be obstructed by a gallstone, an ERCP with sphincterotomy may be performed to explore the duct before laparoscopy (Brunicardi, 2019; Cameron & Cameron, 2020; Goldman & Shafer, 2019; Littlefield & Lenahan, 2019; Mou et al., 2019).

Before the procedure, the patient is educated that an open abdominal procedure may be necessary, and general

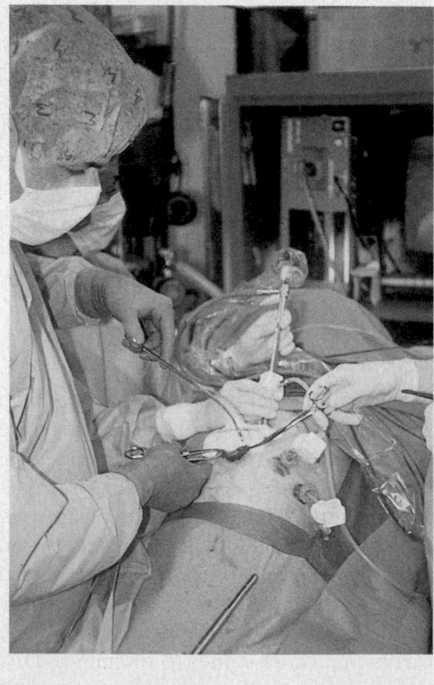
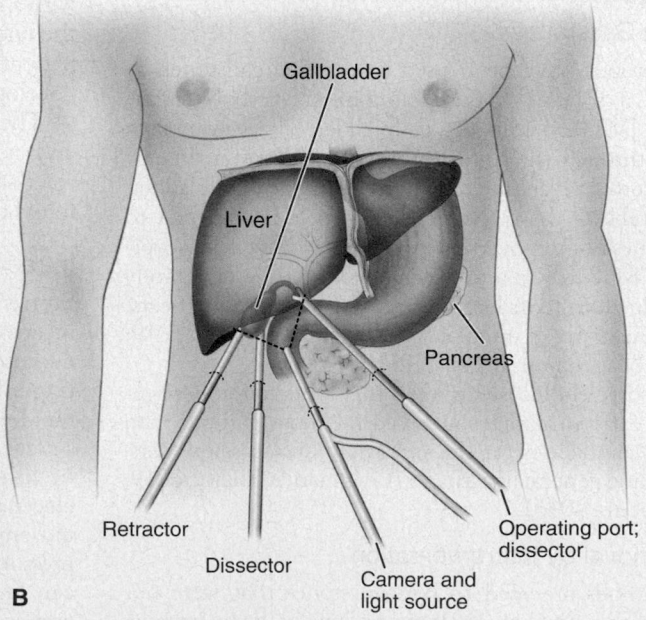

A   **B**

Figure 44-5 • In laparoscopic cholecystectomy (**A**), the surgeon makes four small incisions (less than one half inch each) in the abdomen and inserts a laparoscope with a miniature camera through the umbilical incision (**B**). The camera apparatus displays the gallbladder and adjacent tissues on a screen, allowing the surgeon to visualize the sections of the organ for removal.

Gallbladder

Liver

Pancreas

Retractor

Dissector

Camera and light source

Operating port; dissector

anesthesia is given. Laparoscopic cholecystectomy is performed through a small incision or puncture made through the abdominal wall at the umbilicus. The abdominal cavity is insufflated with carbon dioxide (pneumoperitoneum) to assist in inserting the laparoscope and to aid in visualizing the abdominal structures. The fiberoptic scope is inserted through the small umbilical incision. Several additional punctures or small incisions are made in the abdominal wall to introduce other surgical instruments into the operative field. A camera attached to the laparoscope permits the surgeon to view the intra-abdominal field and biliary system on a television monitor. After the cystic duct is dissected, the CBD can be visualized by ultrasound or cholangiography to evaluate the anatomy and identify stones. The cystic artery is dissected free and clipped. The gallbladder is separated from the hepatic bed and removed from the abdominal cavity after bile and small stones are aspirated. Stone forceps also can be used to remove or crush larger stones.

With the laparoscopic procedure, the patient does not experience the paralytic ileus that occurs with open abdominal surgery and has less postoperative abdominal pain. The patient is often discharged from the hospital on the same day of surgery or within 1 or 2 days and resumes full activity and employment within 1 week after the procedure.

Conversion to a traditional abdominal surgical procedure occurs in 2.2% of cases in the United States and 3.6% to 8.2% of cases internationally. Conversion to an open procedure occurs if there is inflammation in and around the gallbladder, making safe dissection of the porta hepatis difficult (Brunicardi, 2019; Feldman et al., 2016; Goldman & Shafer, 2019). The porta hepatis is the fissure of the liver where the portal vein and the hepatic artery enter and the hepatic ducts exit the liver.

The most serious complication after laparoscopic cholecystectomy is a bile duct injury, which may be identified and corrected at the time of the procedure. Patients with a postoperative bile leak may not develop symptoms until several days after the procedure, and some have an even more prolonged period before injury to the bile duct becomes apparent (Brunicardi, 2019; Cameron & Cameron, 2020). A bile leak may result in fluid collections, which can usually be managed by endoscopic stent placement. Bile peritonitis, a rare complication, may result in serious illness or death.

Because of the short length of hospital stay with uncomplicated laparoscopic cholecystectomies, it is important to provide patient education about managing postoperative pain and reporting signs and symptoms of intra-abdominal complications, including loss of appetite, vomiting, pain, distention of the abdomen, and temperature elevation. Although recovery from laparoscopic cholecystectomy is rapid, patients are drowsy afterward. The patient must have assistance at home during the first 24 to 48 hours. If pain occurs in the right shoulder or scapular area (from migration of the carbon dioxide used to insufflate the abdominal cavity during the procedure), the nurse may recommend a heating pad for 15 to 20 minutes hourly.

Cholecystectomy

In cholecystectomy, the gallbladder is removed through an abdominal incision (usually right subcostal) after the cystic duct and artery are ligated. The procedure is performed for acute and chronic cholecystitis. In some patients, a drain is placed close to the gallbladder bed and brought out through a puncture wound if there is a bile leak. The drain type is chosen based on the surgeon's preference. A small leak should close spontaneously in a few days, with the drain preventing accumulation of bile. Usually, only a small amount of serosanguineous fluid drains in the initial 24 hours after surgery; afterward, the drain is removed. The drain is typically maintained if there is excess oozing or bile leakage. Insertion of a T-tube (named for its shape) into the CBD during the open procedure is now uncommon; it is used only in the setting of a complication (i.e., retained CBD stone). A T-tube is inserted into the CBD at the time of surgical exploration. It allows external drainage of bile into a collection bag, allowing the surgical site to heal.

Bile duct injury is a serious complication of cholecystectomy, but it occurs less frequently than with the laparoscopic approach, which has largely replaced traditional surgical cholecystectomy.

Small-Incision Cholecystectomy

Small-incision cholecystectomy is a surgical procedure in which the gallbladder is removed through a small abdominal incision, as the name implies. If needed, the surgical incision is extended to remove larger gallbladder stones. Drains may or may not be used. The short length hospital stay has been identified as a major advantage of this type of procedure (Brunicardi, 2019; Cameron & Cameron, 2020; Goldman & Schafer, 2019). The procedure is controversial because it limits exposure to all involved biliary structures.

Choledochostomy

Choledochostomy is reserved for the patient with acute cholecystitis who may be too ill to undergo a surgical procedure. This procedure involves making an incision in the common duct, usually for removal of stones. After the stones have been evacuated, a tube is usually inserted into the duct for drainage of bile until edema subsides. This tube is connected to gravity drainage tubing; the patient is monitored closely, and a laparoscopic cholecystectomy is planned for a future date after acute inflammation has resolved.

Surgical Cholecystostomy

Cholecystostomy is performed when the patient's condition precludes more extensive surgery or when an acute inflammatory reaction is severe. The gallbladder is surgically opened, stones and the bile or the purulent drainage are removed, and a drainage tube is secured with a purse-string suture. The drainage tube is connected to a drainage system to prevent bile from leaking around the tube or escaping into the peritoneal cavity. After recovery from the acute episode, the patient may return for subsequent laparoscopic cholecystectomy. Despite its lower risk, surgical cholecystostomy has a high mortality rate (reported to be as high as 10% to 30%) because of the underlying infectious disease process (Brunicardi, 2019; Cameron & Cameron, 2020; Feldman et al., 2016; Goldman & Schafer, 2019).

Percutaneous Cholecystostomy

Percutaneous cholecystostomy has been used in the treatment and diagnosis of acute cholecystitis in patients who are poor risks for any surgical procedure or for general anesthesia. This at-risk population may include patients with sepsis or severe cardiac, renal, pulmonary, or liver failure (Goldman & Shafer, 2019; Roberts, Plotnik, Chick, et al., 2019). Under local anesthesia, a fine needle is inserted through the abdominal wall and liver edge into the gallbladder under the guidance of ultrasound or computed tomography (CT). Bile is aspirated to ensure adequate placement of the needle, and a catheter is inserted into the gallbladder to decompress the biliary tract. Almost immediate relief of pain and resolution of signs and symptoms of sepsis and cholecystitis have been reported with this procedure. Antibiotic agents are given before, during, and after the procedure.

Endoscopic Ultrasound

Endoscopic ultrasound (EUS) is a guided gallbladder drainage procedure that is an effective treatment option with success rates comparable to percutaneous drainage (Goldman & Shafer, 2019). EUS is described in more detail later in the chapter.

 Gerontologic Considerations

Surgical intervention for disease of the biliary tract is the most common operative procedure performed in the older adult. Cholesterol saturation of bile increases with age because of increased hepatic secretion of cholesterol and decreased bile acid synthesis.

Although the incidence of gallstones increases with age, the older patient may not exhibit the typical symptoms of fever, pain, chills, and jaundice. Symptoms of biliary tract disease in the older adult may be accompanied or preceded by those of septic shock, which include oliguria, hypotension, changes in mental status, tachycardia, and tachypnea.

Although surgery in the older adult presents a risk because of preexisting associated diseases, the mortality rate from serious complications of biliary tract disease itself is also high. The risk of death and complications is increased in the older patient who undergoes emergency surgery for life-threatening disease of the biliary tract. Despite the presence of chronic illness in many older patients, elective cholecystectomy is usually well tolerated and can be carried out with low risk if expert assessment and care are provided before, during, and after the surgical procedure (Rothrock, 2019).

The higher risk of complications and shorter length of hospital stay make it essential that older patients and their family members receive specific information about signs and symptoms of complications and measures to prevent them.

NURSING PROCESS

The Patient Undergoing Surgery for Gallbladder Disease

Assessment

The patient undergoing surgical treatment of gallbladder disease is often admitted to the hospital or same-day surgery unit on the morning of surgery. Preadmission testing is often completed a week or longer before admission. At that time, the nurse educates the patient about the need to avoid smoking, to enhance pulmonary recovery postoperatively, and to avoid

respiratory complications. The need to avoid aspirin, nonsteroidal antiinflammtory drugs, and other agents (over-the-counter medications and herbal remedies) that can alter coagulation and other biochemical processes is also emphasized.

Assessment should focus on the patient's respiratory status. If a traditional surgical approach is planned, the high abdominal incision required during surgery may interfere with full respiratory excursion. The nurse notes a history of smoking, previous respiratory problems, shallow respirations, a persistent or ineffective cough, and the presence of adventitious breath sounds. Nutritional status is evaluated through a dietary history and a general examination performed at the time of preadmission testing. The nurse also reviews previously obtained laboratory results to obtain information about the patient's nutritional status.

Diagnosis

NURSING DIAGNOSES

Based on the assessment data, major postoperative nursing diagnoses may include the following:

- Acute pain and discomfort associated with surgical incision
- Impaired gas exchange associated with the high abdominal surgical incision (if traditional surgical cholecystectomy was performed)
- Impaired skin integrity associated with altered biliary drainage after surgical intervention (if a T-tube was inserted because of retained stones in the common bile duct or another drainage device was employed)
- Impaired nutritional status associated with inadequate bile secretion
- Lack of knowledge about self-care activities associated with incision care, dietary modifications (if needed), medications, and reportable signs or symptoms (e.g., fever, bleeding, vomiting)

COLLABORATIVE PROBLEMS/POTENTIAL COMPLICATIONS

Potential complications may include the following:

- Bleeding
- GI symptoms (may be related to biliary leak or injury to the bowel)

Planning and Goals

The goals for the patient include relief of pain, adequate ventilation, intact skin and improved biliary drainage, optimal nutritional intake, absence of complications, and understanding of self-care routines.

Nursing Interventions

After recovery from anesthesia, the patient is placed in the low Fowler position. Fluids may be administered IV, and nasogastric suction (a nasogastric tube was probably inserted immediately before surgery for a nonlaparoscopic procedure) may be instituted to relieve abdominal distention. Water and other fluids are given within hours after laparoscopic procedures. A soft diet is started after bowel sounds return, which is usually the next day if the laparoscopic approach is used.

RELIEVING PAIN

The location of the subcostal incision in nonlaparoscopic gallbladder surgery often causes the patient to avoid turning and moving, to splint the affected site, and to take shallow breaths to prevent pain. Because full expansion of the lungs and gradually increased activity are necessary to prevent postoperative complications, the nurse administers analgesic agents as prescribed to relieve the pain and to help the patient turn, cough, breathe deeply, and ambulate as indicated. The use of a pillow or abdominal binder over the incision may reduce pain during these maneuvers.

IMPROVING RESPIRATORY STATUS

Patients undergoing biliary tract surgery are especially prone to pulmonary complications, as are all patients with upper abdominal incisions. Therefore, the nurse reminds the patient to take deep breaths and cough every hour to expand the lungs fully and prevent atelectasis. The early and consistent use of incentive spirometry also helps improve respiratory function. Early ambulation prevents pulmonary complications as well as other complications, such as venous thromboembolism (VTE) formation. Pulmonary complications are more likely to occur in patients who are older, those with obesity, and those with preexisting pulmonary disease.

MAINTAINING SKIN INTEGRITY AND PROMOTING BILIARY DRAINAGE

In patients who have undergone a cholecystostomy or choledochostomy, the drainage tube must be connected immediately to a drainage receptacle. The nurse should fasten the tubing to the dressings or to the patient's gown, with enough leeway for the patient to move without dislodging or kinking the tube. Because a drainage system remains attached when the patient is ambulating, the drainage bag may be placed in a bathrobe pocket or fastened so that it is below the waist or common duct level. If drains are used, the nurse changes the dressings as required.

After these surgical procedures, the patient is observed for indications of infection, leakage of bile into the peritoneal cavity, and obstruction of bile drainage. If bile is not draining properly, an obstruction is probably causing bile to be forced back into the liver and bloodstream. Because jaundice may result, the nurse should assess the color of the sclerae. The nurse should note and report right upper quadrant abdominal pain, nausea and vomiting, bile drainage around any drainage tube, clay-colored stools, and a change in vital signs.

Bile may continue to drain from the drainage tract in considerable quantities for some time, necessitating frequent changes of the outer dressings and protection of the skin from irritation (bile is corrosive to the skin).

To prevent total loss of bile, the surgeon may want the drainage tube (T-tube) or collection receptacle elevated above the level of the abdomen so that the bile drains externally only if pressure develops in the duct system. Every 24 hours, the nurse measures the bile collected and records the amount, color, and character of the drainage. After several days of drainage, the T-tube may be clamped for 1 hour before and after each meal to deliver bile to the duodenum to aid in digestion (Brunicardi, 2019; Cameron & Cameron, 2020; Townsend et al., 2016). Within 7 days to 3 weeks, the drainage tube is removed (Brunicardi, 2019; Cameron & Cameron, 2020; Townsend et al., 2016). The patient who goes home with a drainage tube in place requires instruction and reassurance about the function and care of the T-tube (Rothrock, 2019).

In all patients with biliary drainage, the nurse (or the patient, if at home) observes the color of stools daily. Urine and stool specimens may be sent to the laboratory for examination for bile pigments. In this way, it is possible to determine whether the bile pigment is disappearing from the blood and is draining again into the duodenum. Maintaining a careful record of fluid intake and output is important.

IMPROVING NUTRITIONAL STATUS

The nurse encourages the patient to eat a diet that is low in fats and high in carbohydrates and proteins immediately after surgery. At the time of hospital discharge, there are usually no special dietary instructions other than to maintain a healthy diet and avoid excessive fats. Fat restriction usually is lifted in 4 to 6 weeks, when the biliary ducts dilate to accommodate the volume of bile once held by the gallbladder and when the ampulla of Vater again functions effectively. After this time, when the patient eats fat, adequate bile will be released into the GI tract to emulsify the fats and allow their digestion. This is in contrast to the condition before surgery, when fats may not have been digested completely or adequately and flatulence may have occurred. One purpose of gallbladder surgery is to allow a normal diet.

MONITORING AND MANAGING POTENTIAL COMPLICATIONS

Bleeding may occur as a result of inadvertent puncture or injury to a major blood vessel. Postoperatively, the nurse closely monitors vital signs and inspects the surgical incisions and any drains for bleeding. The nurse also assesses the patient for increased tenderness and rigidity of the abdomen. If these signs and symptoms occur, they are reported to the surgeon. The patient and family are instructed to report any change in the color of stools, because this may indicate complications. GI symptoms, although not common, may occur with manipulation of the intestines during surgery.

After laparoscopic cholecystectomy, the nurse assesses the patient for anorexia, vomiting, pain, abdominal distension, and temperature elevation. These may indicate infection or disruption of the GI tract and should be reported to the surgeon promptly. Because the patient is discharged soon after laparoscopic surgery, the patient and family are instructed verbally and in writing about the importance of reporting these symptoms promptly. Nurses should consider implementing the teach-back method when educating patients and families to ensure that they are able to describe what they have been taught in their own words or perform a task as instructed (see Chapter 3 for discussion of the teach-back method).

PROMOTING HOME, COMMUNITY-BASED CARE, AND TRANSITIONAL CARE

Educating Patients About Self-Care. The nurse educates the patient about the medications that are prescribed (vitamins, anticholinergic and antispasmodic agents) and their actions. The nurse also informs the patient and family about symptoms that should be reported to the primary provider, including jaundice, dark urine, pale-colored stools, pruritus, and signs of inflammation and infection such as pain or fever.

Some patients report one to three bowel movements a day, which is a result of a continual trickle of bile through the

---

Chart 44-2

Managing Self-Care After Laparoscopic Cholecystectomy

The nurse instructs the patient about pain management, activity and exercise, wound care, nutrition, and follow-up care as described below.

Managing Pain

- You may experience pain or discomfort from the gas used to inflate your abdominal area during surgery. Sitting upright in bed or a chair, walking, or using a heating pad may ease the discomfort.
- Take analgesic medications as needed and as prescribed. Report to your surgeon if pain is unrelieved even with analgesic use.

Resuming Activity

- Begin light exercise (walking) immediately.
- Take a shower or bath after 1 or 2 days.
- Drive a car after 3 or 4 days.
- Avoid lifting objects exceeding 5 lb after surgery, usually for 1 week.
- Resume sexual activity when desired.

Caring for the Wound

- Check puncture site daily for signs of infection.
- Wash puncture site with mild soap and water.
- Allow special adhesive strips on the puncture site to fall off. Do not pull them off.

Resuming Eating

- Resume your normal diet.
- If you had fat intolerance before surgery, gradually add fat back into your diet in small increments.

Managing Follow-Up Care

- Make an appointment with your surgeon for 7 to 10 days after discharge.
- Call your surgeon if you experience any signs or symptoms of infection at or around the puncture site: redness, tenderness, swelling, heat, or drainage.
- Call your surgeon if you experience a fever of 37.7°C (100°F) or more for 2 consecutive days.
- Call your surgeon if you develop nausea, vomiting, or abdominal pain.

---

choledochoduodenal junction after cholecystectomy. Usually, such frequency diminishes over a period of a few weeks to several months.

If a patient is discharged from the hospital with a drainage tube still in place, the patient and family need education about its management. The nurse educates them in proper care of the drainage tube and the importance of reporting promptly any changes in the amount or characteristics of drainage. Assistance in securing the appropriate dressings reduces the patient's anxiety about going home with the drain or tube still in place. Chart 44-2 provides additional details about patient education for managing self-care after laparoscopic cholecystectomy.

Continuing and Transitional Care. With sufficient support at home, most patients recover quickly from a cholecystectomy. However, some patients may require a referral for transitional or home care. The hospital nurse can help ease the unpredictability of the postoperative and postdischarge experience for patients by providing relevant patient education, prompt pain relief, and an attentive approach to the nursing care (Rothrock, 2019). During home visits, the nurse assesses the patient's physical status, especially wound healing, and progress toward recovery. Assessing the patient for adequacy of pain relief and pulmonary exercises is also important. If the patient has a drainage system in place, the nurse assesses it for patency and appropriate management by the patient and family. Assessing for signs of infection and educating the patient about the signs and symptoms of infection are also important nursing interventions. The patient's understanding of the therapeutic regimen (medications, gradual return to normal activities) is assessed, and previous education is reinforced. The nurse emphasizes the importance of keeping follow-up appointments and reminds the patient and family of the importance of participating in health promotion activities and recommended health screening.

Evaluation

Expected patient outcomes may include:

1. Reports decrease in pain
   a. Splints abdominal incision to decrease pain
   b. Avoids foods that cause pain
   c. Uses postoperative analgesia as prescribed
2. Demonstrates appropriate respiratory function
   a. Achieves full respiratory excursion, with deep inspiration and expiration
   b. Coughs effectively, using pillow to splint abdominal incision
   c. Uses postoperative analgesia as prescribed
   d. Exercises as prescribed (e.g., turns, ambulates)
3. Exhibits normal skin integrity around biliary drainage site (if applicable)
   a. Is free of fever; abdominal pain; change in vital signs; and presence of bile, foul-smelling drainage, or pus around drainage tube
   b. Demonstrates correct management of drainage tube (if applicable)
   c. Identifies signs and symptoms of biliary obstruction to be noted and reported
   d. Has serum bilirubin level within normal range
4. Obtains relief from dietary intolerance
   a. Maintains adequate dietary intake and avoids foods that cause GI symptoms
   b. Reports decreased or absent nausea, vomiting, diarrhea, flatulence, and abdominal discomfort
5. Absence of complications
   a. Has normal vital signs (blood pressure, pulse, respiratory rate and pattern, and temperature)
   b. Reports absence of bleeding from GI tract and from biliary drainage tube or catheter (if present) and no evidence of bleeding in stool
   c. Reports return of appetite and no evidence of vomiting, abdominal distention, or pain
   d. Lists symptoms that should be reported to surgeon promptly and demonstrates an understanding of self-care, including wound care

DISORDERS OF THE PANCREAS

Pancreatitis (inflammation of the pancreas) is a serious disorder. The most basic classification system used to describe or categorize the various stages and forms of pancreatitis divides the disorder into acute and chronic forms. Acute pancreatitis can be a medical emergency associated with a high risk of life-threatening complications and mortality, whereas chronic pancreatitis often goes undetected because classic clinical and diagnostic findings are not always present in the early stages of the disease (Feldman et al., 2016; Papadakis & McPhee, 2020; Srinivasan & Friedman, 2018). By the time symptoms occur in chronic pancreatitis, approximately 90% of normal acinar cell function (exocrine function) has been lost (Feldman et al., 2016; Goldman & Shaffer, 2019; Papadakis & McPhee, 2020; Srinivasan & Friedman, 2018). Acute pancreatitis does not usually lead to chronic pancreatitis unless complications develop. However, chronic pancreatitis can be characterized by acute episodes.

Although the mechanisms causing pancreatic inflammation are unknown, pancreatitis is commonly described as autodigestion of the pancreas. It is believed that the pancreatic duct becomes temporarily obstructed, accompanied by hypersecretion of the exocrine enzymes of the pancreas. These enzymes enter the bile duct, where they are activated and, together with bile, back up (reflux) into the pancreatic duct, causing pancreatitis.

Acute Pancreatitis

Approximately 200,000 cases of acute pancreatitis occur in the United States each year, of which 80% are the result of cholelithiasis or sustained alcohol abuse (Faghih, Fan, & Singh, 2019; Olson, Perelman, & Birk, 2019). Acute pancreatitis ranges from a mild, self-limited disorder to a severe, rapidly fatal disease that does not respond to any treatment. These two main types of acute pancreatitis (mild and severe) are classified as interstitial edematous pancreatitis and necrotizing pancreatitis, respectively. Interstitial pancreatitis affects the majority of patients. It is characterized by a lack of pancreatic or peripancreatic parenchymal necrosis with diffuse enlargement of the gland due to inflammatory edema (Faghih et al., 2019; Olson et al., 2019). The edema and inflammation in interstitial pancreatitis is confined to the pancreas itself. Minimal organ dysfunction is present, and return to normal function usually occurs within 6 months. Although this is considered the milder form of pancreatitis, the patient is acutely ill and at risk for hypovolemic shock, fluid and electrolyte disturbances, and sepsis.

In the more severe form, necrotizing pancreatitis, there is tissue necrosis in either the pancreatic parenchyma or in the tissue surrounding the gland. This type can be sterile or infected; if the parenchyma is involved, this is a marker for more severe disease (Brunicardi, 2019; Faghih, et al., 2019; Olson et al., 2019). A more widespread and complete enzymatic digestion of the gland characterizes necrotizing pancreatitis. Enzymes damage the local blood vessels, and bleeding and thrombosis can occur. The tissue may become necrotic, with damage extending into the retroperitoneal tissues. Local complications include pancreatic cysts or abscesses and acute fluid collections in or near the pancreas. Patients who develop systemic complications with organ failure, such as pulmonary insufficiency with hypoxia, shock, kidney disease, and GI bleeding, are also characterized as having severe acute pancreatitis.

Gerontologic Considerations

Acute pancreatitis affects people of all ages, but the mortality rate associated with acute pancreatitis increases with age (Brunicardi, 2019; Faghih et al., 2019; Olson et al., 2019). In addition, the pattern of complications changes with age. Younger patients tend to develop local complications; the incidence of multiple organ dysfunction syndrome (MODS) increases with age, possibly as a result of progressive decreases in physiologic function of major organs with increasing age. Close monitoring of major organ function (i.e., lungs, kidneys) is essential, and aggressive treatment is necessary to reduce mortality from acute pancreatitis in the older adult patient.

Pathophysiology

Self-digestion of the pancreas by its own proteolytic enzymes, principally trypsin, causes acute pancreatitis. These patients usually have had undiagnosed chronic pancreatitis before their first episode of acute pancreatitis. Gallstones enter the CBD and lodge at the ampulla of Vater, obstructing the flow of pancreatic juice or causing a reflux of bile from the CBD into the pancreatic duct, thus activating the powerful enzymes within the pancreas. Normally, these remain in an inactive form until the pancreatic secretions reach the lumen of the duodenum (Brunicardi, 2019; Faghih et al., 2019; Norris, 2019; Olson et al., 2019). Activation of the enzymes can lead to vasodilation, increased vascular permeability, necrosis, erosion, and hemorrhage (Brunicardi, 2019; Faghih et al., 2019; Norris, 2019; Olson et al., 2019; Townsend et al., 2016).

Other less common causes of pancreatitis include bacterial or viral infection, with pancreatitis occasionally developing as a complication of mumps viral infection. Spasm and edema of the ampulla of Vater, caused by duodenitis, can probably produce pancreatitis. Blunt abdominal trauma, peptic ulcer disease, ischemic vascular disease, hyperlipidemia, hypercalcemia, and the use of corticosteroids, thiazide diuretics, oral contraceptives, and other medications have also been associated with an increased incidence of pancreatitis. Acute pancreatitis may develop after surgery on or near the pancreas or after instrumentation of the pancreatic duct. In addition to alcohol consumption, use of tobacco products is a risk factor for the development of acute and chronic pancreatitis (Aune, Yahya, Norat, et al., 2019). Acute idiopathic pancreatitis accounts for up to 10% of the cases of acute pancreatitis. Some postulate that these cases may be related to occult microlithiasis (small stones in the bile) (Goodchild, Chouhan, & Johnson, 2019; Olson et al., 2019; Townsend et al., 2016). In addition, there is a small incidence of hereditary pancreatitis.

The mortality rate of patients with acute pancreatitis is 2% to 10% because of shock, anoxia, hypotension, or fluid and electrolyte imbalances. This mortality rate may also be related to the 10% to 30% of patients with severe acute disease characterized by pancreatic and peripancreatic necrosis (Goodchild et al., 2019; Olson et al., 2019; Townsend et al.,

2016). Pancreatitis may result in complete recovery, may recur without permanent damage, or may progress to chronic pancreatitis. The patient who is admitted to the hospital with a diagnosis of pancreatitis is acutely ill and needs expert nursing and medical care.

Clinical Manifestations

Severe abdominal pain is the major symptom of pancreatitis that causes the patient to seek medical care. Abdominal pain and tenderness and back pain result from irritation and edema of the inflamed pancreas. Increased tension on the pancreatic capsule and obstruction of the pancreatic ducts also contribute to the pain. Typically, the pain occurs in the midepigastrium. Pain is frequently acute in onset, occurring 24 to 48 hours after a very heavy meal or alcohol ingestion, and it may be diffuse and difficult to localize. It is generally more severe after meals and is unrelieved by antacids. Pain may be accompanied by abdominal distention; a poorly defined, palpable abdominal mass; decreased peristalsis; and vomiting that fails to relieve the pain or nausea.

The patient appears acutely ill. Abdominal guarding is present. A rigid or boardlike abdomen may develop, usually indicating peritonitis (Goodchild et al., 2019; Olson et al., 2019). Ecchymosis (bruising) in the flank or around the umbilicus may indicate severe pancreatitis. Nausea and vomiting are common in acute pancreatitis. The emesis is usually gastric in origin but may also be bile stained. Fever, jaundice, mental confusion, and agitation may also occur.

Hypotension is typical and reflects hypovolemia and shock caused by the loss of large amounts of protein-rich fluid into the tissues and peritoneal cavity. In addition to hypotension, the patient may develop tachycardia; cyanosis; and cold, clammy skin. Acute kidney injury is common.

Respiratory distress and hypoxia are common, and the patient may develop diffuse pulmonary infiltrates, dyspnea, tachypnea, and abnormal blood gas values. Myocardial depression, hypocalcemia, hyperglycemia, and disseminated intravascular coagulation may also occur with acute pancreatitis.

Assessment and Diagnostic Findings

The diagnosis of acute pancreatitis is based on the fulfillment of two out of the three following criteria: a history of upper abdominal pain, biochemical changes with serum amylase or lipase levels greater than three times the upper limit of normal, or typical findings on imaging (CT, magnetic resonance imaging [MRI] or ultrasonography). The presence of known risk factors is also helpful for diagnostic purposes (Feldman et al., 2016; Goodchild et al., 2019; Olson et al., 2019; Żorniak, Beyer, & Mayerle, 2019). In most cases, serum amylase and lipase levels are elevated within 24 hours of the onset of the symptoms. Serum amylase usually returns to normal within 48 to 72 hours, but serum lipase levels may remain elevated for a longer period, often days longer than amylase. Urinary amylase levels also become elevated and remain elevated longer than serum amylase levels. The white blood cell count is usually elevated; hypocalcemia is present in many patients and correlates well with the severity of pancreatitis. Transient hyperglycemia and glucosuria and elevated serum bilirubin levels occur in some patients with acute pancreatitis.

X-ray studies of the abdomen and chest may be obtained to differentiate pancreatitis from other disorders that can cause similar symptoms and to detect pleural effusions. Ultrasound studies, contrast-enhanced CT scans, and MRI scans are used to identify an increase in the diameter of the pancreas and to detect pancreatic cysts, abscesses, or pseudocysts.

Hematocrit and hemoglobin levels are used to monitor the patient for bleeding. Peritoneal fluid, obtained through paracentesis or peritoneal lavage, may contain increased levels of pancreatic enzymes. ERCP is rarely used in the diagnostic evaluation of acute pancreatitis, because the patient is acutely ill; however, it may be valuable in the treatment of gallstone pancreatitis.

The severity of acute pancreatitis is difficult to predict early in the course of the disease, but mortality can be predicted based on clinical and laboratory data (see Chart 44-3). According to the revised Atlanta Classification, there are three degrees of severity: (1) mild with the absence of organ failure and no local or systemic complications, (2) moderately severe with the presence of transient organ failure or local or systemic complications, and (3) severe acute pancreatitis characterized by persistent organ failure (>48 hours) (Banks, Bollen, Dervenis, et al., 2013; Żorniak et al., 2019). Several risk stratification systems aim to predict persistent organ failure and complications. The Acute Physiology and Chronic Health Evaluation II (APACHE II), Ranson Criteria for Pancreatitis Mortality, and Bedside Index of Severity in Acute Pancreatitis (BISAP) are scoring systems that assess clinical and biochemical factors to determine the severity of acute pancreatitis. Laboratory values such as C-reactive protein, procalcitonin, and blood urea nitrogen (BUN) may also carry some predictive value (Żorniak et al., 2019). Early prediction of the severity of acute pancreatitis is important for guiding early treatment, choosing the optimal level of care, and identifying patients who might benefit from transfer to a center that specializes in the care of this disease (Żorniak et al., 2019).

Chart 44-3	**The Ranson Criteria for Pancreatic Mortality**

Criteria on Admission to Hospital

Age >55 years
White blood cells (WBCs) >16,000 mm^3
Serum glucose >200 mg/dL (>11.1 mmol/L)
Serum lactate dehydrogenase (LDH) >350 IU/L (>350 U/L)
Aspartate aminotransferase (AST) >250 IU/L

Criteria within 48 Hours of Hospital Admission

Fall in hematocrit >10% (>0.10)
Blood urea nitrogen (BUN) increase >5 mg/dL (>1.7 mmol/L)
Serum calcium <8 mg/dL (<2 mmol/L)
Base deficit >4 mEq/L (>4 mmol/L)
Fluid retention or sequestration >6 L
Partial pressure of oxygen (PO$_2$) <60 mm Hg
Two or fewer signs, 1% mortality; 3 or 4 signs, 15% mortality; 5 or 6 signs, 40% mortality; >6 signs, 100% mortality.

Note: The more risk factors a patient has, the greater the severity and likelihood of complications or death.
Adapted from Ranson, J. H., Rifkind, K. M., Roses, D. F., et al. (1974). Prognostic signs and the role of operative management in acute pancreatitis. *Surgery, Gynecology & Obstetrics, 139*(1), 69–81.

Medical Management

Management of acute pancreatitis is directed toward relieving symptoms and preventing or treating complications. All oral intake is withheld to inhibit stimulation of the pancreas and its secretion of enzymes. Ongoing research has shown positive outcomes with the use of enteral feedings. The current recommendation is that, whenever possible, the enteral route should be used to meet nutritional needs in patients with pancreatitis. This strategy also has been found to prevent infectious complications safely and cost-effectively (McClave, 2019; Mueller, 2017; Olson et al., 2019; Ramanathan & Aadam, 2019; Townsend et al., 2016). Enteral feedings should be started early in the course of acute pancreatitis (Goodchild et al., 2019; McClave, 2019; Mueller, 2017; Olson et al., 2019; Ramanathan & Aadam, 2019). Parenteral nutrition has a role in the nutritional support of patients with severe acute pancreatitis, particularly in those who are unable to tolerate enteral nutrition (Goodchild et al., 2019; Mueller, 2017; Olson et al., 2019). Nasogastric suction may be used to relieve nausea and vomiting and to decrease painful abdominal distention and paralytic ileus (Brunicardi, 2019). Research data do not support the routine use of nasogastric tubes to remove gastric secretions in an effort to limit pancreatic secretion. Though current literature discourages the use of acid-suppressive therapy, this practice is common for hospitalized patients. Histamine-2 (H_2) antagonists such as cimetidine may be prescribed to decrease pancreatic activity by inhibiting secretion of gastric acid. Proton pump inhibitors such as pantoprazole may be used for patients who do not tolerate H_2 antagonists or for whom this therapy is ineffective (Barbateskovic, Marker, Granholm, et al., 2019; Kavitt, Lipowska, Anyane-Yeboa, et al., 2019).

Pain Management

Adequate administration of analgesia is essential during the course of acute pancreatitis to provide sufficient pain relief and to minimize restlessness, which may stimulate pancreatic secretion further. Pain relief may require parenteral opioids such as morphine, fentanyl, or hydromorphone (Cameron & Cameron, 2020; Goodchild et al., 2019; Olson et al., 2019). The recommendation for pain management is the use of opioids, with assessment for their effectiveness, and altering therapy if pain is not controlled or is increased (Faghih et al., 2019; Goodchild et al., 2019; Olson et al., 2019). There is some evidence that implementing the World Health Organization (WHO) analgesia ladder provides a pragmatic approach to pain management in patients with pancreatitis (Żorniak et al., 2019). This stepwise escalation from low potency to higher potency of nonsteroidal anti-inflammatory drugs (NSAIDs) alone or in combination with opioids may provide an effective method of pain management and lower the potential for opioid dependency (Żorniak et al., 2019). NSAIDs must be avoided or used in caution in patients at risk for bleeding. GI paralysis and ileus are common problems in early acute pancreatitis that can be potentiated and aggravated with the use of high-dose opioids (Żorniak et al., 2019). More research is needed to identify the best option for pain management in the patient with acute pancreatitis (Faghih et al., 2019). Until evidence-based recommendations are developed, guidelines for acute pain management

in the perioperative setting should be followed (Rothrock, 2019). Antiemetic agents may be prescribed to prevent vomiting.

 Intensive Care

Correction of fluid and blood loss and low albumin levels is necessary to maintain fluid volume and prevent acute kidney injury. The patient is usually acutely ill and is monitored in the intensive care unit, where hemodynamic monitoring and arterial blood gas monitoring are initiated. Antibiotic agents may be prescribed if infection is present. Prophylactic antibiotics are not recommended for patients with acute pancreatitis (Faghih et al., 2019; Goodchild, 2019; Olson et al., 2019). Insulin may be required if hyperglycemia occurs. Intensive insulin therapy (continuous infusion) in the critically ill patient has undergone much study. The best practice recommendations, which have arisen from many investigations on this complex topic, include targeting a blood glucose level of 140 to 200 mg/dL if insulin therapy is required in critically ill medical and surgical patients. Additionally, clinicians are advised to avoid glucose targets <140 mg/dL because adverse effects are likely to increase with lower blood glucose targets (Horton, 2019).

Respiratory Care

Aggressive respiratory care is indicated because of the high risk of elevation of the diaphragm, pulmonary infiltrates and effusion, and atelectasis. Hypoxemia occurs in a significant number of patients with acute pancreatitis, even with normal x-ray findings. Respiratory care may range from close monitoring of arterial blood gases to the use of humidified oxygen to intubation and mechanical ventilation (see Chapter 19 for further discussion).

Biliary Drainage

Placement of biliary drains (for external drainage) and stents (indwelling tubes) in the pancreatic duct through endoscopy has been performed to reestablish drainage of the pancreas. This has resulted in decreased pain.

Surgical Intervention

Although the acutely ill patient is at high risk for surgical complications, surgery may be performed to assist in the diagnosis of pancreatitis (diagnostic laparotomy); to establish pancreatic drainage; or to resect or débride an infected, necrotic pancreas. The patient who undergoes pancreatic surgery may have multiple drains in place postoperatively, as well as a surgical incision that is left open for irrigation and repacking every 2 to 3 days to remove necrotic debris (see Fig. 44-6).

Postacute Management

Oral feedings that are low in fat and protein are initiated gradually. Caffeine and alcohol are eliminated from the diet. If the episode of pancreatitis occurred during treatment with thiazide diuretics, corticosteroids, or oral contraceptives, these medications are discontinued. Follow-up may include ultrasound, x-ray studies, or ERCP to determine whether the pancreatitis is resolving and to assess for abscesses and pseudocysts. ERCP may also be used to identify the cause of acute pancreatitis if it is in question and for endoscopic

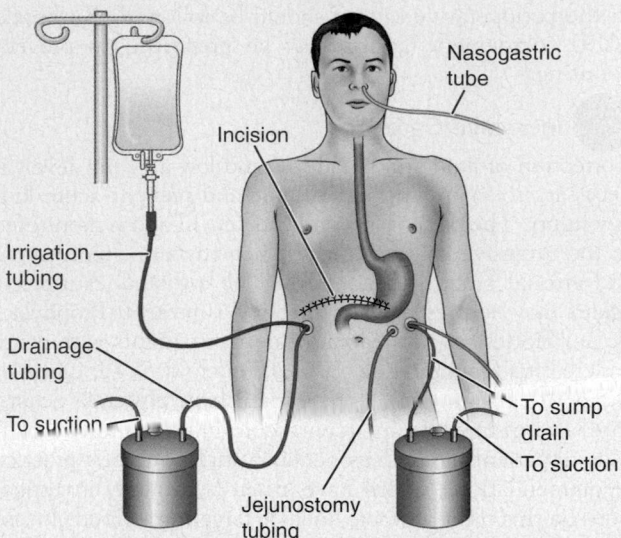

Figure 44-6 • Multiple sump tubes are used after pancreatic surgery. Triple-lumen tubes consist of ports that provide tubing for irrigation, air venting, and drainage.

sphincterotomy and removal of gallstones from the common bile duct.

Nursing Management

Relieving Pain and Discomfort

Because the pathologic process responsible for pain is autodigestion of the pancreas, the objectives of therapy are to relieve pain and decrease secretion of pancreatic enzymes. The pain of acute pancreatitis is often very severe, necessitating the liberal use of analgesic agents. The current recommendation for pain management in this population is parenteral opioids, including morphine, hydromorphone, or fentanyl via patient-controlled analgesia or bolus (Goodchild et al., 2019; Olson et al., 2019). In patients who are critically ill, a continuous infusion may be needed. Because most opioids stimulate spasm of the sphincter of Oddi to some degree, consensus has not been reached on the most effective agent. Ensuring patient comfort, regardless of the opioid prescribed, is the most essential aspect of care. The nurse frequently assesses the pain level and the effectiveness of the pharmacologic (and nonpharmacologic) interventions. Changes may be needed in the regimen for pain management based on the achievement of pain control. Pain assessment tools (see Chapter 9) are available for the nurse to ensure an accurate rating of pain. Nonpharmacologic interventions such as proper positioning, music, distraction, and imagery may be effective in reducing pain when used along with medications.

Oral feedings are withheld to decrease the secretion of secretin. Parenteral fluids and electrolytes are prescribed to restore and maintain fluid balance. Nasogastric suction may be used to relieve nausea and vomiting or to treat abdominal distention and paralytic ileus. The nurse provides frequent oral hygiene and care to decrease discomfort from the nasogastric tube and relieve dryness of the mouth.

The patient who is acutely ill is maintained on bed rest to decrease the metabolic rate and reduce the secretion of pancreatic and gastric enzymes. If the patient experiences increasing severity of pain, the nurse reports this to the primary provider because the patient may be experiencing hemorrhage of the pancreas or the dose of analgesic medication may be inadequate.

The patient with acute pancreatitis is often confused or delirious because of severe pain, fluid and electrolyte disturbances, and hypoxia. Therefore, the nurse provides frequent and repeated but simple explanations about the need for withholding fluids, maintenance of gastric suction, and bed rest.

Improving Breathing Pattern

The nurse maintains the patient in a semi-Fowler position to decrease pressure on the diaphragm by a distended abdomen and to increase respiratory expansion. Frequent changes of position are necessary to prevent atelectasis and pooling of respiratory secretions. Pulmonary assessment, including monitoring of pulse oximetry or arterial blood gases, is essential to detect changes in respiratory status so that early treatment can be initiated. The nurse instructs the patient in techniques of coughing and deep breathing and in the use of incentive spirometry to improve respiratory function and assists the patient to perform these activities every hour.

Improving Nutritional Status

The nurse assesses the patient's nutritional status and notes factors that alter the patient's nutritional requirements (e.g., temperature elevation, surgery, drainage). Laboratory test results and daily weights are useful to monitor the nutritional status.

Enteral or parenteral nutrition may be prescribed. In addition to administering enteral or parenteral nutrition, the nurse monitors serum glucose levels every 4 to 6 hours. As the acute symptoms subside, oral feedings are gradually reintroduced. Between acute attacks, the patient receives a diet that is high in protein and low in fat (Goodchild et al., 2019; Olson et al., 2019). The patient should avoid heavy meals and alcoholic beverages.

Maintaining Skin Integrity

The patient is at risk for skin breakdown because of poor nutritional status, enforced bed rest, and restlessness, which may result in pressure injuries and breaks in tissue integrity. In addition, the patient who has undergone surgery may have multiple drains or an open surgical incision and is at risk for skin breakdown and infection. The wound, drainage sites, and skin are carefully assessed for signs of infection, inflammation, and breakdown. The nurse carries out wound care as prescribed and takes precautions to protect intact skin from contact with drainage. Consultation with a wound-ostomy-continence (WOC) nurse, a nurse specially educated in appropriate skin, wound, ostomy, and continence care is often helpful in identifying appropriate skin care devices and protocols. The patient must be turned every 2 hours; the use of specialty beds may be indicated to prevent skin breakdown.

 Monitoring and Managing Potential Complications

Fluid and electrolyte disturbances are common complications because of nausea, vomiting, movement of fluid from the vascular compartment to the peritoneal cavity, diaphoresis, fever, and the use of gastric suction. The nurse assesses the patient's fluid and electrolyte status by noting skin turgor and moistness of mucous membranes. The nurse weighs the patient daily and carefully measures fluid intake and output, including urine output, nasogastric secretions, and diarrhea. In addition, it is important to assess for other factors that may affect fluid and electrolyte status, including increased body temperature and wound drainage. The patient is assessed for ascites, and abdominal girth is measured daily if ascites is suspected.

Fluids are administered IV and may be accompanied by infusion of blood or blood products to maintain the blood volume and to prevent or treat hypovolemic shock. Emergency medications must be readily available because of the risk of circulatory collapse and shock. The nurse promptly reports decreased blood pressure and reduced urine output, which indicate hypovolemia and shock or acute kidney injury. Low serum calcium and magnesium levels may occur and require prompt treatment.

Pancreatic necrosis is a major cause of morbidity and mortality in patients with acute pancreatitis because of resulting hemorrhage, septic shock, and MODS. The patient may undergo diagnostic procedures for confirmation of pancreatic necrosis. If the patient is found to have pancreatic necrosis with infection, this may require surgical, percutaneous or endoscopic débridement or insertion of multiple drains. Percutaneous or endoscopic catheter drainage is the first step of what is known as the "Step-Up Approach." Catheters are placed via the left or right retroperitoneal approach to drain the infection. Débridement, if required, may be performed through video-assisted retroperitoneal débridement. These interventions, coupled with appropriate, targeted antibiotic therapy, may be the only necessary treatment for some patients (Paulino, Ramos, & Veloso Gomes, 2019; Rashid, Hussain, Jehanzeb, et al., 2019; Sion & Davis, 2019; Wolbrink, Kolwijck, Ten Oever, et al., 2019). These procedures are considered first-line approaches, with surgery reserved for patients for whom these interventions do not work. Prophylactic antibiotics are not indicated (Paulino et al., 2019; Sion & Davis, 2019; Wolbrink et al., 2019). The patient with pancreatic necrosis with or without infection is usually critically ill and requires expert medical and nursing management, including hemodynamic monitoring in the intensive care unit.

In addition to carefully monitoring vital signs and other signs and symptoms, the nurse is responsible for administering prescribed fluids, medications, and blood products; assisting with supportive management, such as the use of a ventilator; preventing additional complications; and providing physical and psychological care.

Shock and MODS may occur with acute pancreatitis. Hypovolemic shock may occur as a result of hypovolemia and sequestering of fluid in the peritoneal cavity. Hemorrhagic shock may occur with hemorrhagic pancreatitis. Septic shock may occur with bacterial infection of the pancreas. Cardiac dysfunction may occur as a result of fluid and electrolyte disturbances, acid–base imbalances, and release of toxic substances into the circulation.

The nurse closely monitors the patient for early signs of neurologic, cardiovascular, renal, and respiratory dysfunction and must be prepared to respond quickly to rapid changes in the patient's status, treatments, and therapies. In addition, it is important to inform the family about the patient's status and progress and to allow them to spend time with the patient. Management of shock and MODS is discussed in detail in Chapter 11.

Promoting Home, Community-Based, and Transitional Care

 Educating Patients About Self-Care

After an episode of acute pancreatitis, the patient is often still weak and debilitated for weeks or months. A prolonged period may be needed to regain strength and return to the previous level of activity. Because of the severity of the acute illness, the patient may not recall education given during the acute phase. Patient education often needs to be repeated and reinforced. The nurse educates the patient about the factors implicated in the onset of acute pancreatitis and about the need to avoid high-fat foods, heavy meals, and alcohol. The patient and family should receive verbal and written instructions about signs and symptoms of acute pancreatitis and possible complications that should be reported promptly to the primary provider.

If acute pancreatitis is a result of biliary tract disease, such as gallstones and gallbladder disease, additional explanations are needed about required dietary modifications. If the pancreatitis is a result of alcohol abuse, the nurse reinforces the need to avoid all alcohol.

Continuing and Transitional Care

A referral for home, community-based or transitional care is often indicated. This enables the nurse to assess the patient's physical and psychological status and adherence to the therapeutic regimen. The nurse also assesses the home situation and reinforces instructions about fluid and nutrition intake and avoidance of alcohol. Nurses should consider implementing the teach-back method when educating patients and families about this vital information (see Chapter 3 for a discussion of the teach-back method). After the acute attack has subsided, some patients may be inclined to return to their previous drinking habits. The nurse provides specific information about resources and support groups that may be of assistance in avoiding alcohol in the future. Referral to Alcoholics Anonymous as appropriate or other support groups is essential. See the accompanying plan of nursing care in Chart 44-4 for care of the patient with acute pancreatitis.

Chronic Pancreatitis

Chronic pancreatitis is an inflammatory disorder characterized by progressive destruction of the pancreas. As cells are replaced by fibrous tissue with repeated attacks of pancreatitis, pressure within the pancreas increases. The result is obstruction of the pancreatic and common bile ducts and the duodenum. In addition, there is atrophy of the epithelium of the ducts, inflammation, and destruction of the secreting cells of the pancreas.

Alcohol consumption in Western societies and malnutrition worldwide are the major causes of chronic pancreatitis. Patients diagnosed with chronic pancreatitis due to alcohol

(text continued on page 1436)

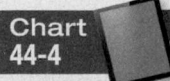

Chart 44-4

PLAN OF NURSING CARE
Care of the Patient with Acute Pancreatitis

NURSING DIAGNOSIS: Acute pain associated with edema, distention of the pancreas, peritoneal irritation, and excess stimulation of pancreatic secretions

GOAL: Relief of pain

Nursing Interventions	Rationale	Expected Outcomes
1. Using a pain scale, assess pain level at baseline, before and after administration of analgesic medications.	1. Baseline assessment and control of pain are important because restlessness increases the body's metabolism, which stimulates the secretion of pancreatic and gastric enzymes.	• Patient rates pain using pain scale • Reports relief of pain, discomfort, and abdominal cramping • Moves and turns without increasing pain and discomfort • Rests comfortably and sleeps for increasing periods • Reports increased feelings of well-being and security with the health care team
2. Administer morphine, fentanyl, or hydromorphone frequently, as prescribed, to achieve level of pain acceptable to patient. Depending on pain severity, non-steroidal anti-inflammatory drugs NSAIDs) may be considered alone or in combination with opioids.	2. Fentanyl and hydromorphone act by depressing the central nervous system and thereby increasing the patient's pain threshold.	
3. Maintain the patient NPO (nothing by mouth) as prescribed.	3. Pancreatic secretion is increased by food and fluid intake.	
4. Maintain the patient on bed rest.	4. Bed rest decreases body metabolism and thus reduces pancreatic and gastric secretions.	
5. Maintain continuous nasogastric drainage if paralytic ileus or nausea and vomiting, abdominal distention are present. a. Measure gastric secretions at specified intervals. b. Observe and record color and viscosity of gastric secretions. c. Ensure that the nasogastric tube is patent to permit free drainage.	5. Nasogastric suction relieves nausea, vomiting, and abdominal distention. Decompression of the intestines (if intestinal intubation is used) also assists in relieving respiratory distress.	
6. Report unrelieved pain or increasing intensity of pain.	6. Pain may increase pancreatic enzymes and may also indicate pancreatic hemorrhage.	
7. Assist patient to assume positions of comfort; turn and reposition every 2 hours.	7. Frequent turning relieves pressure and assists in preventing pulmonary and vascular complications.	
8. Use nonpharmacologic interventions for relieving pain (e.g., relaxation, focused breathing, diversion).	8. The use of nonpharmacologic methods will enhance the effects of analgesic medications.	
9. Listen to patient's expression of pain experience.	9. Demonstration of caring can help to decrease anxiety.	

NURSING DIAGNOSIS: Discomfort associated with nasogastric tube

GOAL: Relief of discomfort associated with nasogastric intubation used to treat ileus, vomiting, and distention

Nursing Interventions	Rationale	Expected Outcomes
1. Use water-soluble lubricant around external nares.	1. Prevents irritation of nares.	• Exhibits intact skin and tissue of nares at site of nasogastric tube insertion • Reports no pain or irritation of nares or oropharynx • Exhibits moist, clean mucous membranes of mouth and nasopharynx • States that thirst is relieved by oral hygiene • Identifies rationale for nasogastric tube and suction
2. Turn patient at intervals; avoid pressure or tension on nasogastric tube.	2. Relieves pressure of tube on esophageal and gastric mucosa.	
3. Provide oral hygiene and gargling solutions without alcohol.	3. Relieves dryness and irritation of oropharynx.	
4. Explain rationale for the use of nasogastric drainage.	4. Assists patient to cooperate with the drainage, nasogastric tube, and suction.	

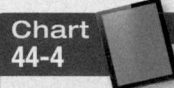

Chart 44-4

PLAN OF NURSING CARE (continued)
Care of the Patient with Acute Pancreatitis

NURSING DIAGNOSIS: Impaired nutritional status associated with inadequate dietary intake, impaired pancreatic secretions, increased nutritional needs secondary to acute illness, and increased body temperature

GOAL: Improvement in nutritional status

Nursing Interventions	Rationale	Expected Outcomes
1. Assess current nutritional status and increased metabolic requirements.	1. Alteration in pancreatic secretions interferes with normal digestive processes. Acute illness, infection, and fever increase metabolic needs.	• Maintains normal body weight • Demonstrates no additional weight loss • Maintains normal serum glucose levels • Reports decreasing episodes of vomiting and diarrhea
2. Monitor serum glucose levels and administer insulin as prescribed.	2. Impairment of endocrine function of the pancreas leads to increased serum glucose levels.	• Reports return of normal stool characteristics and bowel pattern • Consumes foods high in carbohydrates, low in fat and protein
3. Administer IV fluid and electrolytes, enteral or parenteral nutrition as prescribed.	3. Parenteral administration of fluids and electrolytes, and enteral or parenteral nutrients are essential to provide fluids, calories, electrolytes, and nutrients when oral intake is prohibited.	• Explains rationale for high-carbohydrate, low-fat, low-protein diet • Eliminates alcohol from diet
4. Provide high-carbohydrate, low-protein, and low-fat diet when tolerated.	4. These foods increase caloric intake without stimulating pancreatic secretions beyond the ability of the pancreas to respond.	• Explains rationale for limiting coffee intake and avoiding spicy foods • Participates in Alcoholics Anonymous as appropriate or other counseling approach
5. Instruct patient to eliminate alcohol, and refer to Alcoholics Anonymous, if indicated. 6. Counsel patient to avoid excessive use of coffee and spicy foods. 7. Monitor daily weights.	5. Alcohol intake produces further damage to pancreas and precipitates attacks of acute pancreatitis. 6. Coffee and spicy foods increase pancreatic and gastric secretions. 7. This provides a baseline and a means to measure weight gain or weight loss.	• Returns to and maintains desirable weight

NURSING DIAGNOSIS: Impaired breathing associated with splinting from severe pain, pulmonary infiltrates, pleural effusion, and atelectasis

GOAL: Improvement in respiratory function

Nursing Interventions	Rationale	Expected Outcomes
1. Assess respiratory status (rate, pattern, breath sounds), pulse oximetry, and arterial blood gases.	1. Acute pancreatitis produces retroperitoneal edema, elevation of the diaphragm, pleural effusion, and inadequate lung ventilation. Intra-abdominal infection and labored breathing increase the body's metabolic demands, which further decreases pulmonary reserve and leads to respiratory failure.	• Demonstrates normal respiratory rate and pattern and full lung expansion • Demonstrates normal breath sounds and absence of adventitious breath sounds • Demonstrates normal arterial blood gases and pulse oximetry • Maintains semi-Fowler position when in bed
2. Maintain semi-Fowler position.	2. Decreases pressure on diaphragm and allows greater lung expansion.	• Changes position in bed frequently • Coughs and takes deep breaths at least every hour
3. Instruct and encourage patient to take deep breaths and to cough every hour. 4. Assist patient to turn and change position every 2 hours.	3. Taking deep breaths and coughing will clear the airways and reduce atelectasis. 4. Changing position frequently assists aeration and drainage of all lobes of the lungs.	• Demonstrates normal body temperature • Exhibits no signs or symptoms of respiratory infection or impairment • Is alert and responsive to environment

5. Reduce the excessive metabolism of the body.
  a. Administer antibiotics as prescribed.
  b. Administer nasal oxygen as required for hypoxia.
  c. Use a hypothermia blanket if necessary.
	5. Pancreatitis produces a severe peritoneal and retroperitoneal reaction that causes fever, tachycardia, and accelerated respirations. Supporting the patient with oxygen therapy decreases the workload of the respiratory system and the tissue utilization of oxygen. Reduction of fever and pulse rate decreases the metabolic demands on the body.	

(continued on page 1436)

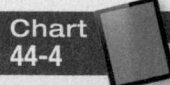

Chart 44-4 · PLAN OF NURSING CARE (continued)
Care of the Patient with Acute Pancreatitis

COLLABORATIVE PROBLEM: Fluid and electrolyte disturbances, hypovolemia, shock
GOAL: Improvement in fluid and electrolyte status, prevention of hypovolemia and shock

Nursing Interventions	Rationale	Expected Outcomes
1. Assess fluid and electrolyte status (skin turgor, mucous membranes, urine output, vital signs, hemodynamic parameters).	1. The amount and type of fluid and electrolyte replacement are determined by the status of the blood pressure, the laboratory evaluations of serum electrolyte and blood urea nitrogen levels, the urinary volume, and the assessment of the patient's condition	• Exhibits moist mucous membranes and normal skin turgor • Exhibits normal blood pressure without evidence of orthostatic hypotension • Excretes adequate urine volume • Exhibits normal, not excessive, thirst • Maintains normal pulse and respiratory rate
2. Assess sources of fluid and electrolyte loss (vomiting, diarrhea, nasogastric drainage, excessive diaphoresis).	2. Electrolyte losses occur from nasogastric suctioning, severe diaphoresis, and emesis, and as a result of the patient being in a fasting state.	• Remains alert and responsive • Exhibits normal arterial pressures and blood gases • Exhibits normal electrolyte levels

3. Combat shock if present.
  a. Administer corticosteroids as prescribed if patient does not respond to conventional treatment.
  b. Evaluate the amount of urinary output. Attempt to maintain this at ≥0.5 mL/kg/hr and ≥400 mL/day.
	3. Extensive acute pancreatitis may cause peripheral vascular collapse and shock. Blood and plasma may be lost into the abdominal cavity; therefore, there is a decreased blood and plasma volume. The toxins from the bacteria of a necrotic pancreas may cause shock.	• Exhibits no signs or symptoms of calcium deficit (e.g., tetany, carpopedal spasm)
		• Exhibits no additional losses of fluids and electrolytes through vomiting, diarrhea, or diaphoresis
		• Demonstrates no change in weight

4. Administer blood products, fluids, and electrolytes (sodium, potassium, chloride) as prescribed.	4. Patients with hemorrhagic pancreatitis lose large amounts of blood and plasma, which decreases effective circulation and blood volume.	• Demonstrates no increase in abdominal girth • Demonstrates no fluid wave on palpation of the abdomen
5. Administer plasma and blood products as prescribed.	5. Replacement with blood, plasma, or albumin assists in ensuring effective circulating blood volume.	• Demonstrates stable organ function without manifestations of failure
6. Keep a supply of IV calcium gluconate or calcium chloride readily available.	6. Calcium may be prescribed to prevent or treat tetany, which may result from calcium losses into retroperitoneal (peripancreatic) exudate.	

7. Assess abdomen for ascites formation.
  a. Measure abdominal girth daily.
  b. Weigh patient daily.
  c. Assess abdomen for ascites (see Chapter 43, Fig. 43-6).
	7. During acute pancreatitis, plasma may be lost into the abdominal cavity, which diminishes the blood volume.	

8. Monitor for manifestations of multiple organ dysfunction syndrome: neurologic, cardiovascular, renal, and respiratory dysfunction.	8. All body systems may fail if pancreatitis is severe and treatment is ineffective.	

typically present between the ages of 40 and 60 years (Singh, 2019). Frequently, at that age, patients already report a long history of alcohol abuse. Excessive and prolonged consumption of alcohol accounts for approximately 70% to 80% of all cases of chronic pancreatitis (Papadakis & McPhee, 2020; Srinivasan & Friedman, 2018; Townsend et al., 2016). The incidence of pancreatitis is 50 times greater in people with alcoholism than in those who do not abuse alcohol. Long-term alcohol consumption causes hypersecretion of protein in pancreatic secretions, resulting in protein plugs and calculi within the pancreatic ducts. Alcohol also has a direct toxic effect on the cells of the pancreas. Damage to these cells is more likely to occur and to be more severe in patients whose diets are poor in protein content and either very high or very low in fat.

Smoking is another factor in the development of chronic pancreatitis. Because smoking and alcohol are often associated, it is difficult to separate the effects of these two factors (Aune et al., 2019; Papadakis & McPhee, 2020; Singh, 2019).

Clinical Manifestations

Chronic pancreatitis is characterized by recurring attacks of severe upper abdominal and back pain, accompanied by vomiting. Attacks are often so painful that opioids, even in large doses, do not provide relief. The risk of opioid dependence is increased in pancreatitis because of the chronic nature and severity of the pain. As the disease progresses, recurring attacks of pain are more severe, more frequent, and of longer duration. Some patients experience continuous severe pain, and others have dull, nagging constant pain. Periods of well-being sometimes follow the episodes of pain (Singh, 2019). In some patients, chronic pancreatitis is painless. The natural history of abdominal pain (character, timing, severity) is variable, and many studies have documented a decrease in pain ("burnout") over time in a majority of patients (Singh, 2019).

Weight loss is a major problem in chronic pancreatitis. More than 80% of patients experience significant weight loss, which is usually caused by decreased dietary intake secondary to anorexia or fear that eating will precipitate another attack (Kellerman & Rakel, 2018; Singh, 2019). Malabsorption occurs late in the disease, when as little as 10% of pancreatic function remains (Kellerman & Rakel, 2018; Singh, 2019). As a result, digestion, especially of proteins and fats, is impaired. The stools become frequent, frothy, and foul smelling because of impaired fat digestion, which results in stools with a high fat content referred to as **steatorrhea**. As the disease progresses, calcification of the gland may occur, and calcium stones may form within the ducts.

Assessment and Diagnostic Findings

A CT scan is the initial diagnostic test that should be performed for patients in whom there is a suspicion of chronic pancreatitis. The presence of either calcifications, pancreatic ductal changes, or both of these findings can substantiate the diagnosis of chronic pancreatitis (Singh, 2019). MRCP is considered for further evaluation, should the CT findings be equivocal in patients with known risk factors. Transabdominal ultrasonography is frequently used as a screening method for patients with abdominal symptoms. EUS and laparoscopic ultrasound are capable of detecting very small abnormalities in the pancreas. EUS is frequently used early in the evaluation of patients with pancreatic disease, and MRCP is increasingly being used in select patients who are candidates for the most invasive imaging method, ERCP. EUS evaluates for parenchymal and ductal abnormalities that are useful for diagnosis and staging (Singh, 2019). The staging of disease is important in the care of patients, and a combination of imaging methods is usually used to confirm the stage (Brunicardi, 2019; Singh, 2019). ERCP provides details about the anatomy of the pancreas and the pancreatic and biliary ducts. It is also helpful in obtaining tissue for analysis and differentiating pancreatitis from other conditions, such as carcinoma (Singh, 2019).

A glucose tolerance test evaluates pancreatic islet cell function and provides necessary information for making decisions about surgical resection of the pancreas. An abnormal glucose tolerance test may indicate the presence of diabetes associated with pancreatitis. Acute exacerbations of chronic pancreatitis may result in increased serum amylase levels. Steatorrhea is best confirmed by laboratory analysis of fecal fat content (Kellerman & Rakel, 2018).

Medical Management

The management of chronic pancreatitis depends on its probable cause in each patient. Treatment is directed toward preventing and managing acute attacks, relieving pain and discomfort, and managing exocrine and endocrine insufficiency of pancreatitis (Singh, 2019; Papadakis & McPhee, 2020).

Nonsurgical Management

Nonsurgical approaches may be indicated for the patient who refuses surgery, is a poor surgical risk, or when the disease and symptoms do not warrant surgical intervention. Endoscopy to remove pancreatic duct stones, correct strictures with stenting, and drain cysts may be effective in select patients to manage pain and relieve obstruction via ERCP (Singh, 2019).

Management of abdominal pain and discomfort is similar to that of acute pancreatitis; however, the focus is usually on the use of nonopioid methods to manage pain and the implementation of the WHO's three-step ladder for the treatment of chronic pain. This involves initiating monotherapy and, if ineffective, instituting combination therapy with peripherally acting and centrally acting medications. Pain management in the early stages may respond to nonopioid analgesics, but if the pain becomes more constant or debilitating, introduction of opioid analgesics is appropriate. The abuse of opioids is possible in these patients, and may be more likely in patients with depression, higher pain intensity, and history of alcohol misuse or abuse (Singh, 2019). Adjunct means of pain modulation, such as use of antioxidants, antidepressants, and nonopioid agents as well as avoidance of smoking and alcohol, are recommended before starting opioids for pain control (Singh, 2019). Antioxidants assist in the relief of pain and in improving quality of life and are often given to patients with chronic pancreatitis (Jalal, Campbell, & Hopper, 2019; Singh, 2019). An EUS with guided placement of a celiac nerve block is a potential option for managing the chronic, unrelieved pain of this disease (Singh, 2019). Yoga and other mindfulness-based therapies may be effective nonpharmacologic methods for pain reduction and for relief of other coexisting symptoms of chronic pancreatitis (Jalal et al., 2019). Persistent, unrelieved pain is often the most difficult aspect of management (Jalal et al., 2019; Singh, 2019). The primary provider, nurse, and dietitian emphasize to the patient and family the importance of avoiding alcohol and foods that have produced abdominal pain and discomfort in the past. The health care team stresses to the patient that no other treatment is likely to relieve pain if the patient continues to consume alcohol.

Diabetes resulting from dysfunction of the pancreatic islet cells is treated with diet, insulin, or oral antidiabetic agents. The hazard of severe hypoglycemia with alcohol consumption is stressed to the patient and family. Pancreatic enzyme replacement is indicated for the patient with malabsorption and steatorrhea.

Surgical Management

Chronic pancreatitis is not often managed by surgery. However, surgery may be indicated to relieve persistent abdominal pain and discomfort, restore drainage of pancreatic secretions, and reduce the frequency of acute attacks of pancreatitis and hospitalization (Brunicardi, 2019; Jalal et al., 2019; Singh, 2019). The type of surgery performed depends on the anatomic and functional abnormalities of the pancreas, including the location of disease within the pancreas, the presence of diabetes, exocrine insufficiency, biliary stenosis, and pseudocysts of the pancreas. Other considerations for surgery selection include the patient's likelihood for continued use of alcohol and the likelihood that the patient will be able to manage the endocrine or exocrine changes that are expected after surgery.

Pancreaticojejunostomy (also referred to as Roux-en-Y), with a side-to-side anastomosis or joining of the pancreatic duct to the jejunum, allows drainage of the pancreatic secretions into the jejunum. Pain relief occurs within 6 months in more than 85% of the patients who undergo this procedure, but pain returns in a substantial number of patients as the disease progresses (Brunicardi, 2019; Cameron & Cameron, 2020; Yeo, 2019).

Other surgical procedures may be performed for different degrees and types of underlying disorders. These procedures include revision of the sphincter of the ampulla of Vater, internal drainage of a pancreatic cyst into the stomach (see later discussion), insertion of a stent, and wide resection or removal of the pancreas. A Whipple's resection (pancreaticoduodenectomy) can be carried out to relieve the pain of chronic pancreatitis (see later discussion under Tumors of the Head of the Pancreas). In an effort to provide permanent pain relief and avoid endocrine and exocrine insufficiency that ensue with major resections of the pancreas, some procedures combine limited resection of the head of the pancreas with a pancreaticojejunostomy. These procedures, known as the Beger or Frey operations, remove most of the head of the pancreas except for a shell of pancreatic tissue posteriorly (Brunicardi, 2019; Cameron & Cameron, 2020; Yeo, 2019).

When chronic pancreatitis develops as a result of gallbladder disease, surgery is performed to explore the common duct and remove the stones; usually, the gallbladder is removed at the same time. In addition, an attempt is made to improve the drainage of the CBD and the pancreatic duct by dividing the sphincter of Oddi, a muscle that is located at the ampulla of Vater (this surgical procedure is known as a sphincterotomy). A T-tube usually is placed in the common bile duct, requiring a drainage system to collect the bile postoperatively. Nursing care after such surgery is similar to that indicated after other biliary tract surgery.

Approximately two thirds of all patients with chronic pancreatitis can be managed with endoscopic or laparoscopic intervention (Jalal et al., 2019; Singh, 2019). Endoscopic and laparoscopic procedures such as distal pancreatectomy, longitudinal decompression of the pancreatic duct, nerve denervation, and stenting have been performed in patients with jaundice or recurrent inflammation and are being refined. Minimally invasive procedures to treat chronic pancreatitis may prove to be successful adjuncts in the management of this complex disorder (Jalal et al., 2019; Singh, 2019).

Patients who undergo surgery for chronic pancreatitis may experience weight gain and improved nutritional status; this may result from reduction in pain associated with eating rather than from correction of malabsorption. However, morbidity and mortality after these surgical procedures are high because of the poor physical condition of the patient before surgery and the frequent presence of cirrhosis. Even after undergoing these surgical procedures, the patient is likely to continue to have pain and impaired digestion secondary to pancreatitis.

Pancreatic Cysts

As a result of the local necrosis that occurs because of acute pancreatitis, collections of fluid may form close to the pancreas. These fluid collections become walled off by fibrous tissue and are called *pancreatic pseudocysts*. Pseudocysts are amylase-rich fluid collections contained within a wall of fibrous

granulation tissue and develop within 4 to 6 weeks after an episode of acute pancreatitis. They are a result of pancreatic necrosis, which produces a pancreatic ductal leak into pancreatic tissue weakened by extravasating enzymes (Feldman et al., 2016; Goldman & Schafer, 2019). Pseudocysts are distinguished from true cysts by the characteristics of the lining of the walls of these anomalies. The lining of pseudocysts consists of fibrous granulation tissue, whereas true cysts have epithelium-lined walls (Bansal, Gupta, Singh, et al., 2019; Feldman et al., 2016; Goldman & Schafer, 2019; Papadakis & McPhee, 2020). Pseudocysts are the most common type of pancreatic "cyst." Less common cysts occur as a result of congenital anomalies or secondary to chronic pancreatitis or trauma to the pancreas.

Diagnosis of pancreatic cysts and pseudocysts is made by ultrasound, CT scan, and ERCP. ERCP may be used to identify the anatomy of the pancreas and evaluate the patency of pancreatic drainage. Pancreatic pseudocysts may be of considerable size. When pancreatic pseudocysts enlarge, they impinge on and displace the adjacent stomach or the colon because of the location of pseudocysts behind the posterior peritoneum. Eventually, through pressure or secondary infection, they produce symptoms and require drainage.

Drainage into the GI tract or through the skin and abdominal wall may be established. In the latter instance, the drainage is likely to be profuse and destructive to tissue because of the enzyme contents. Hence, steps (including application of skin ointment) must be taken to protect the skin near the drainage site from excoriation. A suction apparatus may be used to continuously aspirate digestive secretions from the drainage tract so that skin contact with the digestive enzymes is avoided. Expert nursing attention is required to ensure that the suction tube does not become dislodged and suction is not interrupted. Consultation with a WOC nurse is indicated to identify appropriate strategies for maintaining drainage and protecting the skin.

Cancer of the Pancreas

Pancreatic cancer is the fourth leading cause of cancer death in men in the United States and the fifth leading cause of cancer death in women. It is very rare before the age of 45 years, and the majority of patients present in or beyond the sixth decade of life (Feldman et al., 2016; Papadakis & McPhee, 2020; Yeo, 2019). The incidence of pancreatic cancer increases with age, peaking in the seventh and eighth decades for both men and women (American Cancer Society [ACS], 2020). The frequency of pancreatic cancer has decreased slightly over the past 25 years among non-Caucasian men. There is a slight male preponderance; and in the United States, incidence is highest in African American males (ACS, 2020; Feldman et al., 2016). Exposure to industrial chemicals or toxins in the environment, and a diet high in fat, meat, or both are associated risk factors (ACS, 2020; Feldman et al., 2016; Papadakis & McPhee, 2020).

The risk of pancreatic cancer is greater in those with a history of increased pack years of cigarette smoking and in those with high alcohol intake. Diabetes, chronic pancreatitis, hereditary pancreatitis, and obesity are also associated with pancreatic cancer (Rawla, 2019; Yeo, 2019). The pancreas can also be the site of metastasis from other tumors.

Cancer may develop in the head, body, or tail of the pancreas; clinical manifestations vary depending on the site and whether functioning insulin-secreting pancreatic islet cells are involved. Approximately 70% of pancreatic cancers originate in the head of the pancreas and give rise to a distinctive clinical picture (Feldman et al., 2016; Rawla, 2019). Functioning islet cell tumors, whether benign (adenoma) or malignant (adenocarcinoma), are responsible for the syndrome of hyperinsulinism. The symptoms are typically nonspecific, and patients usually do not seek medical attention until late in the disease. Only about 7% of cases are diagnosed in early stages; 80% to 85% of patients have advanced, unresectable tumor when first detected. As a result, pancreatic carcinoma has only a 7% survival rate at 5 years regardless of the stage of disease at diagnosis or treatment (ACS, 2020; Rawla, 2019; Yeo, 2019).

Clinical Manifestations

Pain, jaundice, or both are present in more than 80% of patients and, along with weight loss, are considered classic signs of pancreatic carcinoma (Brunicardi, 2019; Feldman et al., 2016; Yeo, 2019). However, they often do not appear until the disease is far advanced. Other signs include rapid, profound, and progressive weight loss as well as vague upper or midabdominal pain or discomfort that is unrelated to any GI function and is often difficult to describe. Such discomfort radiates as a boring pain in the midback and is unrelated to posture or activity. It is often progressive and severe, requiring the use of opioids. It is often more severe at night and is accentuated when lying supine. Relief may be obtained by sitting up and leaning forward.

Malignant cells from pancreatic cancer are often shed into the peritoneal cavity, increasing the likelihood of metastasis. The formation of ascites is common. An important sign, if present, is the onset of symptoms of insulin deficiency: glucosuria, hyperglycemia, and abnormal glucose tolerance. Therefore, diabetes may be an early sign of carcinoma of the pancreas. Meals often aggravate epigastric pain, which usually occurs before the appearance of jaundice and pruritus.

Assessment and Diagnostic Findings

Spiral (helical) CT is more than 85% to 90% accurate in the diagnosis and staging of pancreatic cancer and currently is the most useful preoperative imaging technique. MRI/MRCP may also be used. EUS is useful in identifying small tumors and in performing fine-needle aspiration biopsy of the primary tumor or lymph nodes (Goldman & Schafer, 2019; Papadakis & McPhee, 2020). EUS can be superior to CT in localizing these small tumors, which can produce dramatic symptoms despite their size (<1 cm) (Brunicardi, 2019). ERCP may also be used in the diagnosis of pancreatic carcinoma.

Cells obtained during ERCP are sent to the laboratory for analysis. GI x-ray findings may demonstrate deformities in adjacent organs caused by the impinging pancreatic mass.

A histologic diagnosis is not usually required in patients who are candidates for surgery. The tissue diagnosis is made at the time of the surgical procedure. Percutaneous fine-needle aspiration biopsy of the pancreas, which is used to diagnose pancreatic tumors, is also used to confirm the diagnosis in patients whose tumors are not resectable so that a palliative plan of care can be determined. This may eliminate the stress and postoperative pain of ineffective surgery. In this procedure, a needle is inserted through the anterior abdominal wall into the pancreatic mass, guided by CT, ultrasound, ERCP, or other imaging techniques. The aspirated material is examined for malignant cells. Although percutaneous biopsy is a valuable diagnostic tool, it has some potential drawbacks: a false-negative result if small tumors are missed and the risk of seeding of cancer cells along the needle track. Low-dose radiation to the site may be used before the biopsy to reduce this risk.

PTC is another procedure that may be performed to identify obstructions of the biliary tract by a pancreatic tumor. Several tumor markers (e.g., cancer antigen 19-9, carcinoembryonic antigen, DU-PAN-2) may be used in the diagnostic workup, but they are nonspecific for pancreatic carcinoma. These tumor markers are useful as indicators of disease progression.

Angiography, CT scans, and laparoscopy may be performed to determine whether the tumor can be removed surgically. Intraoperative ultrasonography has been used to determine whether there is metastatic disease to other organs.

Medical Management

If the tumor is resectable and localized (typically tumors in the head of the pancreas), the surgical procedure to remove it is usually extensive (see later discussion). However, total excision of the lesion often is not possible for two reasons: (1) extensive growth of tumor before diagnosis, and (2) probable widespread metastases (especially to the liver, lungs, and bones). More often, treatment is limited to palliative measures.

Although pancreatic tumors may be resistant to standard radiation therapy, the patient may be treated with radiation and chemotherapy (5-fluorouracil, leucovorin, and gemcitabine). Currently, gemcitabine is the standard of care for patients with metastatic pancreatic cancer and has been found to lengthen survival (ACS, 2020; Feldman et al., 2016). The targeted anticancer drug erlotinib has demonstrated a slight improvement in advanced pancreatic cancer survival when used in combination with gemcitabine (ACS, 2020; Brunicardi, 2019). Agents such as S-1 (an oral fluoropyrimidine), or the use of nanoparticle albumin-bound paclitaxel with gemcitabine therapy, combined with radiation or surgery may also result in improved survival (ACS, 2020; Brunicardi, 2019; Kamisawa, Wood, Itoi, et al., 2016). Irinotecan, in combination with fluorouracil and leucovorin, was approved as treatment for metastatic pancreatic adenocarcinoma that has progressed following treatment with a gemcitabine-based therapy. 5-Fluorouracil or capecitabine, a similar but orally administered drug, are used as radiosensitizers during radiation therapy (Brunicardi, 2019). Single-agent gemcitabine may be used in patients who are not well enough to tolerate combination therapy (ACS, 2020; Brunicardi, 2019; O'Reilly, Fou, Hasler, et al., 2018).

If the patient undergoes surgery, intraoperative radiation therapy may be used to deliver a high dose of radiation to the tumor with minimal injury to other tissues; this may also be helpful in relief of pain. Interstitial implantation of radioactive sources has also been used, although the rate of complications is high. A large biliary stent inserted percutaneously or by endoscopy may be used to relieve jaundice (Brunicardi, 2019; O'Reilly et al., 2018).

Nursing Management

Pain management and attention to nutritional requirements are important nursing measures that improve the level of patient comfort. Skin care and nursing measures are directed toward relief of pain and discomfort associated with jaundice, anorexia, and profound weight loss. Specialty mattresses are beneficial and protect bony prominences from pressure. Pain associated with pancreatic cancer may be severe and may require liberal use of opioids; patient-controlled analgesia should be considered for the patient with severe, escalating pain.

There is growing evidence that symptoms frequently appear together in a phenomenon known as a symptom cluster. A symptom cluster is two (or more) symptoms occurring at the same time. The symptoms included in a cluster may have shared underlying mechanisms or outcomes, and pancreatic cancer is one of the diseases that appears to have associated symptom clusters. It may be beneficial to investigate these symptoms as a cluster, rather than individually (Miaskowski, Barsevick, Berger, et al., 2017).

Symptom clusters associated with pancreatic cancer have been identified in several studies and include affective, GI, gustatory, and discomfort-related symptoms (Burrell, Yeo, Smeltzer, et al., 2018a, 2018b). See the Nursing Research Profile in Chart 44-5.

Knowledge and awareness regarding symptom clusters is important to nursing care for patients with pancreatic cancer. Improving nursing assessments and interventions based upon this evidence may improve the quality of life and survival in patients with pancreatic cancer undergoing surgical resection for this disease (Burrell et al., 2018a, 2018b). Because of the poor prognosis and likelihood of short survival, end-of-life preferences are discussed and honored. If appropriate, the nurse refers the patient to hospice care. See Chapters 12 and 13 for care of the patient with cancer and end-of-life care, respectively.

Promoting Home, Community-Based, and Transitional Care

 Educating Patients About Self-Care

Specific education for the patient and family varies with the stage of disease and the treatment choices made by the patient. If the patient elects to receive chemotherapy, the nurse focuses on prevention of side effects and complications of the agents used. If surgery is performed to relieve obstruction and establish biliary drainage, education addresses management of the drainage system and monitoring for complications. The nurse educates the family about changes In the patient's status that should be reported to the primary provider.

Continuing and Transitional Care

A referral for home, community-based, or transitional care is indicated to help the patient and family deal with the physical problems and discomforts associated with pancreatic cancer and the psychological impact of the disease. The nurse assesses the patient's physical status, fluid and nutritional status, skin integrity, and the adequacy of pain management. The nurse educates the patient and family on strategies to prevent skin breakdown and relieve pain, pruritus, and anorexia. It is important to discuss and arrange palliative care (hospice services) as indicated in an effort to relieve patient discomfort, assist with care, and comply with the patient's end-of-life decisions and wishes.

Tumors of the Head of the Pancreas

Tumors of the head of the pancreas comprise 60% to 80% of all pancreatic tumors (Goldman & Schafer, 2019; Yeo, 2019). Tumors in this region of the pancreas obstruct the common bile duct where the duct passes through the head of the pancreas to join the pancreatic duct and empty at the ampulla of Vater into the duodenum. The tumors producing the obstruction may arise from the pancreas, the common bile duct, or the ampulla of Vater (Yeo, 2019).

Chart 44-5 **NURSING RESEARCH PROFILE**
Symptom Clusters in Patients with Pancreatic Cancer

Burrell, S. A., Yeo, T. P., Smeltzer, S. C., et al. (2018a). Symptom clusters in patients with pancreatic cancer undergoing surgical resection: Part I. *Oncology Nursing Forum, 45*(4), e36–e52.

Purpose

The purpose of this study was to describe patient-reported symptoms and symptom clusters in patients with pancreatic cancer undergoing surgical resection.

Design

The study recruited 143 patients with stage II pancreatic cancer undergoing surgical resection alone or with subsequent adjuvant chemoradiation or chemotherapy to participate in a nested, longitudinal, exploratory study through convenient sampling techniques. The Functional Assessment in Cancer Therapy–Hepatobiliary questionnaire was used to assess 17 pancreatic cancer symptoms preoperatively and at 3, 6, and 9 months

postoperatively. Exploratory and confirmatory factor analyses were used to identify symptom clusters.

Findings

Fatigue, trouble sleeping, poor appetite, trouble digesting food, and weight loss were consistently reported as the most prevalent and severe symptoms. Sixteen distinct symptom clusters were identified within 9 months of surgery. Four core symptom clusters persisted over time: affective, GI, gustatory, and discomfort.

Nursing Implications

The findings in this study may be used by nurses to provide anticipatory patient and family education and guidance as they begin and continue with their treatment.

Nurses and other health care providers will be knowledgeable about symptoms and symptom clusters in this population, which may guide assessments and interventions.

Clinical Manifestations

The obstructed flow of bile produces jaundice, clay-colored stools, and dark urine. Malabsorption of nutrients and fat-soluble vitamins may result if the tumor obstructs the entry of bile to the GI tract. Abdominal discomfort or pain and pruritus may be noted, along with anorexia, weight loss, and malaise. If these signs and symptoms are present, cancer of the head of the pancreas is suspected.

The jaundice of this disease must be differentiated from that due to a biliary obstruction caused by a gallstone in the common duct. Jaundice caused by a gallstone is usually intermittent and occurs more commonly in women and in people with obesity and who have had previous symptoms of gallbladder disease.

Assessment and Diagnostic Findings

Diagnostic studies may include duodenography, angiography by hepatic or celiac artery catheterization, pancreatic scanning, PTC, ERCP, and percutaneous needle biopsy of the pancreas. Results of a biopsy of the pancreas may aid in the diagnosis.

Medical Management

Before extensive surgery can be performed, a period of preparation is necessary because the patient's nutritional status and physical condition are often quite compromised. Various liver and pancreatic function studies are performed. A diet high in protein along with pancreatic enzymes, which aid digestion, is often prescribed. Preoperative preparation includes adequate hydration, correction of prothrombin deficiency with vitamin K, and treatment of anemia to minimize postoperative complications. Enteral or parenteral nutrition and blood component therapy are frequently required.

A biliary drainage procedure may be performed, usually with a catheter via percutaneous access, to relieve the jaundice and, perhaps, to provide time for a thorough diagnostic evaluation. Total pancreatectomy (removal of the pancreas) may be performed if there is no evidence of direct extension of the tumor to adjacent tissues or regional lymph nodes. A pancreaticoduodenectomy (Whipple's procedure or resection) is used for potentially resectable cancer of the head of the pancreas (see Fig. 44-7) (Brunicardi, 2019; Yeo, 2019). This procedure involves removal of the gallbladder, a portion of the stomach, duodenum, proximal jejunum, head of the pancreas, and distal common bile duct. Reconstruction involves anastomosis of the remaining pancreas and stomach to the jejunum (Cameron & Cameron, 2020; Townsend et al., 2016; Yeo, 2019). A pylorus-preserving pancreaticojejunostomy (PPPD) may also be performed for tumors of the head of the pancreas and may reduce postgastrectomy symptoms and improve overall GI function (Yeo, 2019). The result of these procedures is removal of the tumor, allowing flow of bile into the jejunum. If the tumor cannot be excised, the jaundice may be relieved by diverting the bile flow into the jejunum by anastomosing the jejunum to the gallbladder, a procedure known as **cholecystojejunostomy** (Brunicardi, 2019; Yeo, 2019).

The postoperative management of patients who have undergone a pancreatectomy or a pancreaticoduodenectomy is similar to the management of patients after extensive GI or biliary surgery. The patient's physical status is often suboptimal, increasing the risk of postoperative complications.

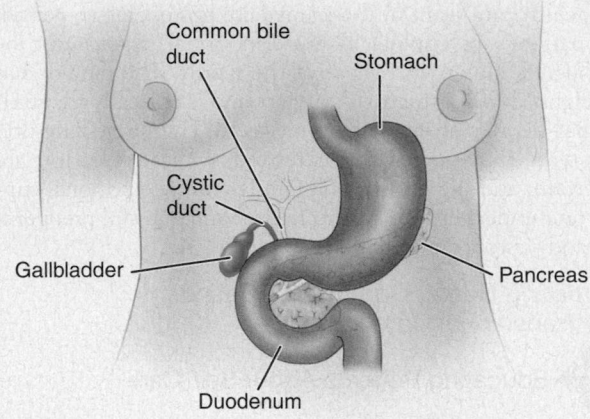

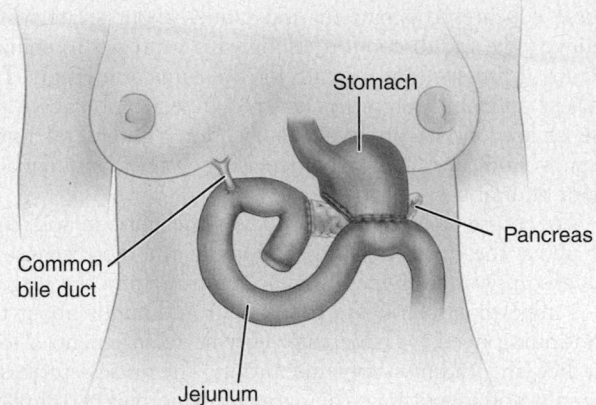

Figure 44-7 • Pancreatoduodenectomy (Whipple's procedure or resection). End result of resection of carcinoma of the head of the pancreas or the ampulla of Vater. The common duct is sutured to the side of the jejunum (choledochojejunostomy), and the remaining portion of the pancreas and the end of the stomach are sutured to the side of the jejunum.

Hemorrhage, vascular collapse, and hepatorenal failure remain the major postoperative complications. The mortality rate associated with these procedures has decreased because of advances in nutritional support and improved surgical techniques. A nasogastric tube with suction and parenteral nutrition allow the GI tract to rest while promoting adequate nutrition.

 ## Nursing Management

Preoperatively and postoperatively, nursing care is directed toward promoting patient comfort, preventing complications, and assisting the patient to return to and maintain as normal and comfortable a life as possible. The nurse closely monitors the patient in the intensive care unit after surgery; in the immediate postoperative period, multiple IV and arterial lines are used for fluid and blood replacement and hemodynamic monitoring, and a mechanical ventilator may be used. It is important to note and report changes in vital signs, arterial blood gases and pressures, pulse oximetry, laboratory values, and urine output. The nurse must also consider the patient's compromised nutritional status and risk of bleeding. Depending on the type of surgical procedure performed, malabsorption syndrome and diabetes are likely; the nurse must address these issues during acute and long-term patient care.

Although the patient's physiologic status is the focus of the health care team in the immediate postoperative period, the patient's psychological and emotional states must be considered, along with those of the family. The patient has undergone a major high-risk surgery and is critically ill; anxiety and depression may affect recovery. The immediate and long-term outcomes of this extensive surgical resection are uncertain, and the patient and family require emotional support and understanding in the critical and stressful preoperative and postoperative periods.

Promoting Home, Community-Based, and Transitional Care

 Educating Patients About Self-Care

The patient who has undergone this extensive surgery requires careful and thorough preparation for self-care at home. The nurse educates the patient and family about strategies to relieve pain and discomfort, along with strategies to manage drains, if present, and to care for the surgical incision. The patient and family members may require education about the use of appropriate analgesic medications, parenteral nutrition, wound care, skin care, increasing activity, and management of drainage.

The nurse may need to educate the patient and family about the need for modifications in the diet because of malabsorption and hyperglycemia resulting from the surgery. It is important to educate the patient and family about the continuing need for pancreatic enzyme replacement, a low-fat diet, and vitamin supplementation. The nurse describes—verbally and in writing—the signs and symptoms of complications and educates the patient and family about indicators of complications that should be reported promptly.

Discharge of the patient to a long-term care or rehabilitation facility may be warranted after surgery as extensive as pancreatectomy or pancreaticoduodenectomy, particularly if the patient's preoperative status is not optimal. Information about the education that has been provided is shared with the long-term care staff so that instructions can be clarified and reinforced. During the recovery or long-term phase of care, the patient and family receive further education about self-care in the home.

Continuing and Transitional Care

A referral for home, community-based, or transitional care may be indicated when the patient returns home. The nurse assesses the patient's physical and psychological status and the ability of the patient and family to manage needed care. The nurse provides needed physical care and monitors the adequacy of pain management. In addition, it is important to assess the patient's nutritional status and monitor the use of enteral or parenteral nutrition, if used. The nurse discusses the use of hospice services with the patient and family and makes a referral if indicated.

Pancreatic Islet Tumors

At least two types of tumors of the pancreatic islet cells are known: those that secrete insulin (insulinoma) and those in which insulin secretion is not increased (nonfunctioning islet cell cancer). All of these types of tumors combined are termed *neuroendocrine tumors* (NETs). Insulinomas produce hypersecretion of insulin and cause an excessive rate of glucose metabolism. The resulting hypoglycemia may produce symptoms of weakness, mental confusion, and seizures. These symptoms may be relieved almost immediately by oral or IV administration of glucose. The 5-hour glucose tolerance test is helpful to diagnose insulinoma and to distinguish a diagnosis of NET from other causes of hypoglycemia.

Surgical Management

If a tumor of the islet cells (a type of NET) has been diagnosed, surgical treatment with removal of the tumor is usually recommended (Brunicardi, 2019; Yeo, 2019). The tumors may be benign adenomas, or they may be malignant. Complete removal usually results in almost immediate relief of symptoms. In some patients, symptoms may be produced by simple hypertrophy of this tissue rather than a tumor of the islet cells. In such cases, a partial pancreatectomy (removal of the tail and part of the body of the pancreas) is performed.

Nursing Management

In preparing the patient for surgery, the nurse must be alert for symptoms of hypoglycemia and be ready to administer glucose as prescribed if symptoms occur. Postoperatively, the nursing management is the same as after other upper abdominal surgical procedures, with special emphasis on monitoring serum glucose levels. Patient education is determined by the extent of surgery and alterations in pancreatic function.

Hyperinsulinism

Hyperinsulinism is caused by overproduction of insulin by the pancreatic islets. Symptoms resemble those of excessive doses of insulin and are attributable to the same mechanism: an abnormal reduction in blood glucose levels. Clinically, it is characterized by episodes during which the patient experiences unusual hunger, nervousness, sweating, headache, and faintness; in severe cases, seizures and episodes of unconsciousness may occur. The findings at the time of surgery or at autopsy may indicate hyperplasia (overgrowth) of the islets of Langerhans or a benign or malignant tumor involving the islets that is capable of producing large amounts of insulin (see preceding discussion). Occasionally, tumors of nonpancreatic origin produce an insulinlike material that can cause severe hypoglycemia and may be responsible for seizures coinciding with blood glucose levels that are too low to sustain normal brain function (i.e., lower than 30 mg/dL [1.6 mmol/L]) (Goldman & Schafer, 2019; Kellerman & Rakel, 2018).

All of the symptoms that accompany spontaneous hypoglycemia are relieved by the oral or parenteral administration of glucose. Surgical removal of the hyperplastic or neoplastic tissue from the pancreas is the only successful method of treatment. About 15% of patients with spontaneous or functional hypoglycemia eventually develop diabetes.

Ulcerogenic Tumors

Some tumors of the islets of Langerhans are associated with hypersecretion of gastric acid that produces ulcers in the stomach, duodenum, and jejunum. This is referred to as

Zollinger-Ellison syndrome. The hypersecretion is so excessive that even after partial gastric resection, enough acid is produced to cause further ulceration. If a marked tendency to develop gastric and duodenal ulcers is noted, an ulcerogenic tumor of the islets of Langerhans is considered (Brunicardi, 2019; Yeo, 2019). The clinical manifestations include nausea, vomiting, diarrhea, and burning discomfort or pain in the upper abdomen. The diagnostic test for this disorder includes measuring a blood gastrin level. Imaging tests may include CT scan or MRI, EUS or upper endoscopy. Scintigraphy and positron emission tomography (PET)/CT are sensitive and specific tests for this disease (Brunicardi, 2019; Yeo, 2019).

These tumors, which may be benign or malignant, are treated by excision, if possible. Frequently, however, removal is not possible because of extension beyond the pancreas and because the tumors are often quite small and difficult to locate. Acid hypersecretion in patients with gastrinoma can be managed with proton pump inhibitors and this is often the first-line treatment intervention. Highly selective vagotomy may make management easier in some patients and should be considered in those with surgically untreatable or unresectable gastrinoma. Total gastrectomy for Zollinger-Ellison is not indicated (Brunicardi, 2019; Yeo, 2019). Embolization or radiofrequency ablation may also be used to control the tumor.

The many disorders of the biliary and pancreatic systems result in a host of clinical and biochemical abnormalities presented in detail in this chapter. The recognition and management of these illnesses pose a challenge to nurses. There is now much evidence about the prevention, diagnosis, and treatment of these disorders. However, there is still much to learn as the medical and nursing communities strive to provide optimum care to patients afflicted with biliary and pancreatic disorders.

CRITICAL THINKING EXERCISES

1 `pq` A 57-year-old man has been having symptoms over the past 2 months including burning discomfort or pain in his upper abdomen, nausea, and diarrhea. He thought that he had acid reflux with heartburn so he started an over-the-counter histamine antagonist. His appetite had decreased and he had lost several pounds. The patient's physician performed a complete physical examination and thinks that the patient may have Zollinger-Ellison syndrome. What laboratory testing might you anticipate? What diagnostic imaging will most likely be performed? What medication or medications may be prescribed? Since the patient continues to be symptomatic, surgery is recommended. What patient education can you provide to best prepare the patient for the surgical intervention and the postoperative care?

2 `ebp` A 58-year-old man presents to the emergency department with complaints of severe midepigastric pain. He is also nauseated and vomiting. His vital signs reveal hypotension and tachycardia and he is mildly febrile. His history is significant for alcohol abuse and hypertension. What laboratory and imaging studies do you expect to be performed? His CT scan revealed noninfected pancreatic necrosis. An evidence-based approach for managing pancreatic necrosis was implemented. Would surgery be included in this initial approach? What first-line intervention would you expect to be implemented in this case? What classification of pancreatitis is this patient experiencing? After 1 week in the hospital, the patient's fever is higher, he is having more abdominal pain and a repeat CT scan reveals multiple fluid collections and worsening edema consistent with infected pancreatic necrosis. What is the evidence for new therapies to effectively treat this patient?

3 `ipc` A 55-year-old woman has been experiencing upper abdominal pain for several weeks. She believes that she has gallbladder disease but is concerned because her mother died from pancreatic cancer. She visits her primary provider who prescribes diagnostic and laboratory studies. Which laboratory tests would you expect to be assessed? An MRI reveals a small mass at the head of the pancreas. What type of referrals might be appropriate for this patient? What members of the interprofessional health care team do you anticipate as being integral to the care of this patient?

REFERENCES

*Asterisk indicates nursing research.
**Double asterisk indicates classic reference.

Books

Brunicardi, F. C. (2019). *Schwartz's principles of surgery* (11th ed.). New York: McGraw-Hill Education.

Cameron, J. L., & Cameron, A. M. (2020). *Current surgical therapy* (13th ed.). Philadelphia, PA: Elsevier.

Cox, M. R., Eslick, G. D., & Padbury, R. (2018). *The management of gallstone disease: A practical and evidence-based approach.* Cham, Switzerland: Springer Publishing.

Eliopoulos, C. (2018). *Gerontological nursing* (9th ed.). Philadelphia, PA: Wolters Kluwer.

Feldman, M., Friedman, L. S., & Brandt, L. J. (2016). *Sleisenger and Fordtran's gastrointestinal and liver disease* (10th ed.). Philadelphia, PA: Saunders Elsevier.

Fischbach, F. T., & Fischbach, M. A. (2018). *Fischbach's a manual of laboratory and diagnostic tests* (10th ed.). Philadelphia, PA: Wolters Kluwer.

Goldman, L., & Schafer, A. I. (2019). *Goldman-Cecil medicine* (26th ed.). Philadelphia, PA: Saunders Elsevier.

Hammer, G. D., & McPhee, S. J. (Eds.). (2019). *Pathophysiology of disease: An introduction to clinical medicine.* New York: McGraw Hill.

Horton, W. B. (2019). *Inpatient Management of Diabetes and Hyperglycemia.* In Saldana, J. R. (Ed.). *The diabetes textbook.* Springer, Cham, Switzerland: Springer Publishing.

Kellerman, R. D., & Rakel, D. (Eds.). (2018). *Conn's current therapy.* Philadelphia, PA: Saunders.

Mueller, C. M. (2017). *The ASPEN adult nutrition support core curriculum* (3rd ed.). Silver Spring, MD: American Society for Parenteral and Enteral Nutrition.

Norris, T. L. (2019). *Porth's pathophysiology: Concepts of altered health states* (10th ed.). Philadelphia, PA: Wolters Kluwer.

Papadakis, M. A., & McPhee, S. J. (Eds.). (2020). *Current medical diagnosis and treatment* (59th ed.). New York: McGraw-Hill.

Rothrock, J. (2019). *Alexander's care of the patient in surgery* (16th ed.). St. Louis, MO: Elsevier.

Srinivasan, S., & Friedman, L. S. (2018). *Sitaraman and Friedman's essentials of gastroenterology* (2nd ed.). Hoboken, NJ: John Wiley & Sons, Ltd.

Townsend, C. M., Beauchamp, R. D., Evers, B. M., et al. (2016). *Sabiston textbook of surgery: The biological basis of modern surgical practice.* Philadelphia, PA: Elsevier.

Yeo, C. J. (Ed.) (2019). *Shackelford's surgery of the alimentary tract* (11th ed.). Philadelphia, PA: Elsevier.

Journals and Electronic Documents

American Cancer Society (ACS). (2020). Cancer facts & figures 2018. Retrieved on 12/12/2019 at: www.cancer.org/Research/CancerFactsFigures

Aune, D., Yahya, M. S., Norat, T., et al. (2019). Tobacco smoking and the risk of pancreatitis: A systematic review and meta-analysis of prospective studies. *Pancreatology, 19*(8), 1009–1022.

**Banks, P. A., Bollen, T. L., Dervenis, C., et al. (2013). Classification of acute pancreatitis—2012: Revision of the Atlanta classification and definitions by international consensus. *Gut, 62*(1), 102–111.

Bansal, A., Gupta, P., Singh, H., et al. (2019). Gastrointestinal complications in acute and chronic pancreatitis. *Journal of Gastroenterology & Hepatology Open, 3*(6), 450–455.

Barbateskovic, M., Marker, S., Granholm, A., et al. (2019). Stress ulcer prophylaxis with proton pump inhibitors or histamin-2 receptor antagonists in adult intensive care patients: A systematic review with meta-analysis and trial sequential analysis. *Intensive Care Medicine, 45*(2), 143–158.

*Burrell, S. A., Yeo, T. P., Smeltzer, S. C., et al. (2018a). Symptom clusters in patients with pancreatic cancer undergoing surgical resection: Part I. *Oncology Nursing Forum, 45*(4), e36–e52.

*Burrell, S. A., Yeo, T. P., Smeltzer, S. C., et al. (2018b). Symptom clusters in patients with pancreatic cancer undergoing surgical resection: Part II. *Oncology Nursing Forum, 45*(4), e53–e66.

Di Ciaula, A., Garruti, G., Frühbeck, G., et al. (2019). The role of diet in the pathogenesis of cholesterol gallstones. *Current Medicinal Chemistry, 26*(19), 3620–3638.

Faghih, M., Fan, C., & Singh, V. K. (2019). New advances in the treatment of acute pancreatitis. *Current Treatment Options in Gastroenterology, 17*(1), 146–160.

Goodchild, G., Chouhan, M., & Johnson, G. J. (2019). Practical guide to the management of acute pancreatitis. *Frontline Gastroenterology, 10*(3), 292–299.

Jalal, M., Campbell, J. A., & Hopper, A. D. (2019). Practical guide to the management of chronic pancreatitis. *Frontline Gastroenterology, 10*(3), 253–260.

Kamisawa, T., Wood, L. D., Itoi, T., et al. (2016). Pancreatic cancer. *The Lancet, 388*(10039), 73–85.

Kavitt, R. T., Lipowska, A. M., Anyane-Yeboa, A., et al. (2019). Diagnosis and treatment of peptic ulcer disease. *The American Journal of Medicine, 132*(4), 447–456.

Littlefield, A., & Lenahan, C. (2019). Cholelithiasis: Presentation and management. *Journal of Midwifery & Women's Health, 64*(3), 289–297.

McClave, S. A. (2019). Factors that worsen disease severity in acute pancreatitis: Implications for more innovative nutrition therapy. *Nutrition in Clinical Practice, 34*(Suppl 1), S43–S48.

Miaskowski, C., Barsevick, A., Berger, A., et al. (2017). Advancing symptom science through symptom cluster research: Expert panel proceedings and recommendations. *Journal of the National Cancer Institute, 109*(4), djw253.

Mou, D., Tesfasilassie, T., Hirji, S., et al. (2019). Advances in the management of acute cholecystitis. *Annals of Gastroenterological Surgery, 3*(3), 247–253.

Olson, E., Perelman, A., & Birk, J. W. (2019). Acute management of pancreatitis: The key to best outcomes. *Postgraduate Medical Journal, 95*(1124), 328–333.

O'Reilly, D., Fou, L., Hasler, E., et al. (2018). Diagnosis and management of pancreatic cancer in adults: A summary of guidelines from the UK National Institute for Health and Care Excellence. *Pancreatology, 18*(8), 962–970.

Paulino, J., Ramos, G., & Veloso Gomes, F. (2019). Together we stand, divided we fall: A multidisciplinary approach in complicated acute pancreatitis. *Journal of Clinical Medicine, 8*(10), 1607–1616.

Ramanathan, M., & Aadam, A. A. (2019). Nutrition management in acute pancreatitis. *Nutrition in Clinical Practice, 34*(Suppl 1), S7–S12.

**Ranson, J. H., Rifkind, K. M., Roses, D. F., et al. (1974). Prognostic signs and the role of operative management in acute pancreatitis. *Surgery, Gynecology & Obstetrics, 139*(1), 69–81.

Rashid, M. U., Hussain, I., Jehanzeb, S., et al. (2019). Pancreatic necrosis: Complications and changing trend of treatment. *World Journal of Gastrointestinal Surgery, 11*(4), 198–217.

Rawla, P., Sunkara, T., & Gaduputi, V. (2019). Epidemiology of pancreatic cancer: Global trends, etiology and risk factors. *World Journal of Oncology, 10*(1), 10–27.

Roberts, D. G., Plotnik, A. N., Chick, J. F., et al. (2019). Interventional radiology-operated percutaneous cholecystoscopy with ultrasonic lithotripsy and stone basket retrieval: A treatment for symptomatic cholelithiasis in non-operative candidates. *Journal of Medical Imaging and Radiation Oncology, 63*(3), 340–345.

Singh, V. K., Yadav, D., & Garg, P. K. (2019). Diagnosis and management of chronic pancreatitis: A review. *JAMA, 322*(24), 2422–2434.

Sion, M. K., & Davis, K. A. (2019). Step-up approach for the management of pancreatic necrosis: A review of the literature. *Trauma Surgery & Acute Care Open, 4*(1), e000308.

Wolbrink, D. R., Kolwijck, E., Ten Oever, J., et al. (2020). Management of infected pancreatic necrosis in the intensive care unit: A narrative review. *Clinical Microbiology and Infection, 26*(1), 18–25.

Żorniak, M., Beyer, G., & Mayerle, J. (2019). Risk stratification and early conservative treatment of acute pancreatitis. *Visceral Medicine, 35*(2), 82–89.

Resources

Al-Anon Family Groups Headquarters, www.al-anon.alateen.org
Alcoholics Anonymous World Services (AAWS), www.aa.org
American Gastroenterological Association (AGA), www.gastro.org
Endocrine Society, www.endo-society.org
National Pancreas Foundation (NPF), www.pancreasfoundation.org

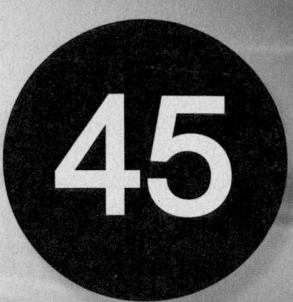

45

Assessment and Management of Patients with Endocrine Disorders

LEARNING OUTCOMES

On completion of this chapter, the learner will be able to:

1. Describe the functions of each of the endocrine glands and their hormones.
2. Differentiate diagnostic studies and clinical manifestations for endocrine disorders.
3. Demonstrate knowledge of management strategies for endocrine disorders.
4. Explain nursing interventions in the care of patients with endocrine disorders.
5. Use the nursing process as a framework for care of the patient with an endocrine disorder.

NURSING CONCEPTS

Cellular Regulation
Family
Infection

Inflammation
Metabolism
Mobility

Nutrition
Stress

GLOSSARY

acromegaly: progressive enlargement of peripheral body parts resulting from excessive secretion of growth hormone

Addison's disease: chronic adrenocortical insufficiency due to inadequate adrenal cortex function

Addisonian crisis: acute adrenocortical insufficiency; characterized by hypotension, cyanosis, fever, nausea/vomiting, and signs of shock

adrenalectomy: surgical removal of one or both adrenal glands

adrenocorticotropic hormone (ACTH): hormone secreted by the anterior pituitary, essential for growth and development

androgens: male sex hormones

basal metabolic rate: chemical reactions occurring when the body is at rest

calcitonin: hormone secreted by the thyroid gland; participates in calcium regulation

Chvostek sign: spasm of the facial muscles produced by sharply tapping over the facial nerve in front of the parotid gland and anterior to the ear; suggestive of latent tetany in patients with hypocalcemia

corticosteroids: hormones produced by the adrenal cortex or their synthetic equivalents

Cushing's syndrome: group of symptoms produced by an oversecretion of adrenocorticotropic hormone; characterized by truncal obesity, "moon face," acne, abdominal striae, and hypertension

diabetes insipidus: condition in which abnormally large volumes of dilute urine are excreted as a result of deficient production of vasopressin

euthyroid: state of normal thyroid hormone production

exophthalmos: abnormal protrusion of one or both eyeballs

glucocorticoids: steroid hormones secreted by the adrenal cortex in response to adrenocorticotropic hormone; produce a rise of liver glycogen and blood glucose

goiter: enlargement of the thyroid gland

Graves disease: a form of hyperthyroidism; characterized by a diffuse goiter and exophthalmos

hormones: chemical transmitter substances produced in one organ or part of the body and carried by the bloodstream to other cells or organs on which they have a specific regulatory effect

mineralocorticoids: steroid hormones secreted by the adrenal cortex

myxedema: severe hypothyroidism; can be with or without coma

negative feedback: regulating mechanism in which an increase or decrease in the level of a substance decreases or increases the function of the organ producing the substance

pheochromocytoma: adrenal medulla tumor

syndrome of inappropriate antidiuretic hormone (SIADH): excessive secretion of antidiuretic hormone from the pituitary gland despite low serum osmolality level

thyroidectomy: surgical removal of all or part of the thyroid gland

thyroiditis: inflammation of the thyroid gland; may lead to chronic hypothyroidism or may resolve spontaneously

thyroid-stimulating hormone (TSH): released from the pituitary gland; causes stimulation of the thyroid, resulting in release of T_3 and T_4

thyroid storm: life-threatening condition of the thyroid due to untreated hyperthyroidism

thyrotoxicosis: condition produced by excessive endogenous or exogenous thyroid hormone

thyroxine (T_4): thyroid hormone; active iodine compound formed and stored in the thyroid; deiodinated in peripheral tissues to form triiodothyronine; maintains body metabolism in a steady state

triiodothyronine (T_3): thyroid hormone; formed and stored in the thyroid; released in smaller quantities, biologically more active, and with faster onset of action than T_4; widespread effect on cellular metabolism

Trousseau sign: carpopedal spasm induced when blood flow to the arm is occluded using a blood pressure cuff or tourniquet, causing ischemia to the distal nerves; suggestive sign for latent tetany in hypocalcemia

vasopressin: antidiuretic hormone secreted by the posterior pituitary

The endocrine system plays a vital role in orchestrating transportation of chemicals across cell membranes, growth and development, metabolism, fluid and electrolyte balance, acid–base balance, adaptation, and reproduction (Norris, 2019). This interconnected network of glands is closely linked with the nervous and immune systems, regulating the functions of multiple body organs. The hypothalamus is responsible for this interrelationship. The pituitary gland, because of its status as the master gland, plays an important role in the regulation of endocrine hormones; its primary function is to secrete hormones into the bloodstream, which in turn affects endocrine glands such as the thyroid. Disorders of the endocrine system are common and are manifested as hyper- and hypofunction.

Nursing interventions are essential in the management of patients with endocrine disorders. This chapter focuses on the anatomy and physiology of the endocrine system; the most common endocrine disorders of the pituitary, thyroid, parathyroid, and adrenal glands; clinical manifestations; diagnostic studies; medical management; and nursing interventions. The unique endocrine and exocrine functions of the pancreas, pancreatic function, and associated pancreatic disorders are discussed in Chapter 44 and reproductive structures, including the ovaries and testes, are discussed in Chapters 50 and 53, respectively.

ASSESSMENT OF THE ENDOCRINE SYSTEM

Anatomic and Physiologic Overview

The endocrine system involves the release of chemical transmitter substances known as **hormones**. These substances regulate and integrate body functions by acting on local or distant target sites. Hormones are generally produced by the endocrine glands but may also be produced by specialized tissues such as those found in the gastrointestinal (GI) system, the kidney, and white blood cells. The GI mucosa produces hormones (e.g., gastrin, enterogastrone, secretin, cholecystokinin) that are important in the digestive process; the kidneys produce erythropoietin, a hormone that stimulates the bone marrow to produce red blood cells; and the white blood cells produce cytokines (hormonelike proteins) that actively participate in inflammatory and immune responses.

The endocrine system has a unique relationship with the immune and the nervous systems. Chemicals such as neurotransmitters (e.g., epinephrine) released by the nervous system can also function as hormones when needed. The immune system responds to the introduction of foreign agents by means of chemical messengers (cytokines), and is also subject to regulation by adrenal corticosteroid hormones (Norris, 2019).

Glands of the Endocrine System

The endocrine system is composed of the pituitary gland, thyroid gland, parathyroid glands, adrenal glands, pancreatic islets, ovaries, and testes. See Figure 45-1 for major hormonal secreting glands of the endocrine system. Most hormones secreted from endocrine glands are released directly into the bloodstream. However, exocrine glands, such as sweat glands, secrete their products through ducts onto epithelial surfaces or into the GI tract.

Function and Regulation of Hormones

Hormones help regulate organ function in concert with the nervous system. The rapid action by the nervous system is balanced by slower hormonal action. This dual regulatory system permits precise control of organ functions in response to changes within and outside the body.

The endocrine glands are composed of secretory cells arranged in minute clusters known as acini. A rich blood supply provides a vehicle for the hormones produced by the endocrine glands to enter the bloodstream rapidly. The amount of circulating hormones depends on their unique function and the body's needs. In the healthy physiologic state, hormone concentration in the bloodstream is maintained at a relatively constant level. To prevent accumulation, these hormones must be inactivated continuously by a **negative feedback** system so that when the hormone concentration increases, further production of that hormone is inhibited. Conversely, when the hormone concentration decreases, the rate of production of that hormone increases.

Classification and Action of Hormones

Hormones are classified into four categories according to their structure: (1) amines and amino acids (e.g., epinephrine, norepinephrine, and thyroid hormones); (2) peptides, polypeptides, proteins, and glycoproteins (e.g., thyrotropin-releasing hormone [TRH], follicle-stimulating hormone [FSH], and growth hormone [GH]); (3) steroids (e.g., **corticosteroids,**

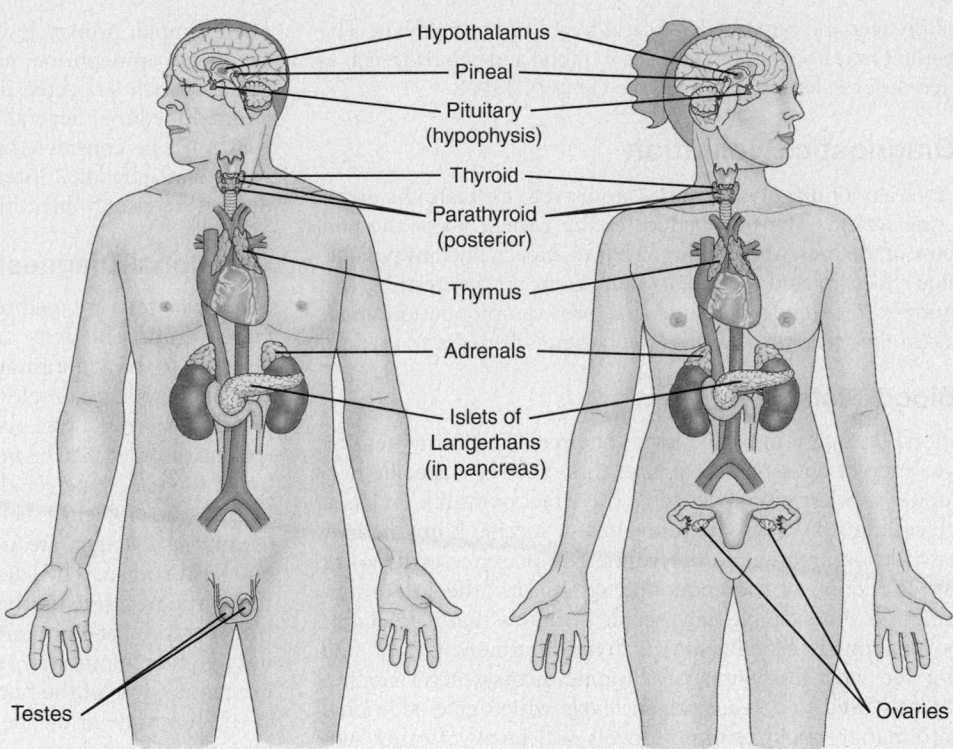

Hypothalamus
Pineal
Pituitary
(hypophysis)
Thyroid
Parathyroid
(posterior)
Thymus
Adrenals
Islets of
Langerhans
(in pancreas)
Testes
Ovaries

Figure 45-1 • Major hormone-secreting glands of the endocrine system.

which are hormones produced by the adrenal cortex or their synthetic equivalents); and (4) fatty acid derivatives (e.g., eicosanoid, retinoids) (Norris, 2019). Although most hormones released by endocrine glands can be transported to distant target sites for action, some hormones never enter the bloodstream because they act locally in the area where they are released; this is called *paracrine action* (e.g., the effect of sex hormones on the ovaries). Others may act on the actual cells from which they were released; this is called *autocrine action* (e.g., the effect of insulin from pancreatic beta cells on those cells) (Norris, 2019).

Hormones can alter the function of the target tissue by interacting with chemical receptors located either on the cell membrane or in the interior of the cell. For example, *peptide* and *protein hormones* interact with receptor sites on the cell surface, resulting in stimulation of the intracellular enzyme adenyl cyclase. This causes increased production of cyclic 3′,5′-adenosine monophosphate (AMP). The cyclic AMP inside the cell alters enzyme activity. Thus, cyclic AMP is the "second messenger" that links the peptide hormone at the cell surface to a change in the intracellular environment. Some protein and peptide hormones also act by changing membrane permeability and act within seconds or minutes. The mechanism of action for *amine hormones* is similar to that for peptide hormones (Norris, 2019).

Steroid hormones, because of their smaller size and higher lipid solubility, penetrate cell membranes and interact with intracellular receptors. The steroid–receptor complex modifies cell metabolism and the formation of messenger ribonucleic acid (mRNA) from deoxyribonucleic acid (DNA). The mRNA then stimulates protein synthesis within the cell. Steroid hormones require several hours to exert their effects, because they exert their action by the modification of protein synthesis.

Assessment

The nursing assessment of the patient with endocrine dysfunction includes a health history and physical examination that evaluates the effects of endocrine disorders on the patient.

Health History

Although specific endocrine disorders are often accompanied by specific clinical symptoms, more general manifestations may also occur. A thorough health history and review of systems are necessary for diagnosis and management of these disorders. Patients should be asked if they have experienced changes in the following areas: energy level, tolerance to heat or cold, weight, thirst, frequency of urination, bowel function, body proportions, muscle mass, fat and fluid distribution, secondary sexual characteristics (e.g., loss or growth of hair), menstrual cycle, memory, concentration, sleep patterns, mood, vision, joint pain, and sexual dysfunction. Documentation is important regarding the severity of these changes, the length of time the patient has experienced these changes, the way in which these changes have affected the patient's ability to carry out activities of daily living, the effect of the changes on the patient's self-perception, and family history.

Physical Assessment

The physical examination should include vital signs; head-to-toe inspection; and palpation of skin, hair, and thyroid. Findings should be compared with previous findings, if available. Physical, psychological, and behavioral changes should be noted. Examples of changes in physical characteristics on examination may include appearance of facial hair in women, "moon face," "buffalo hump," **exophthalmos** (abnormal protrusion of one or both eyeballs), vision changes, edema, thinning of the skin, obesity of the trunk, thinness of the extremities, increased size of the feet and hands, edema, and hypo- or hyperreflexia. The patient may also exhibit changes in mood and behavior such as nervousness, lethargy, and fatigue (Jensen, 2019).

Diagnostic Evaluation

A variety of diagnostic studies are used to evaluate the endocrine system. The nurse educates the patient about the purpose of the prescribed studies, what to expect, and any possible side effects related to these examinations prior to testing. The nurse notes trends in results that provide information about disease progression as well as the patient's response to therapy.

Blood Tests

Blood tests determine the levels of circulating hormones, the presence of autoantibodies, and the effect of a specific hormone on other substances (e.g., the effect of insulin on blood glucose levels). The serum levels of a specific hormone may provide information to determine the presence of hypo- or hyperfunction of the endocrine system and the site of dysfunction. An example of a specific hormone that is amenable to analyzing by blood testing is thyroid hormone (i.e., T_3 and T_4; see later discussion). Radioimmunoassay tests are frequently used to detect antigen levels which give additional information about hormone levels and levels of other substances (Fischbach & Fischbach, 2018).

Urine Tests

Urine tests are used to measure the amount of hormones or the end products of hormones excreted by the kidneys. One-time specimens or, in some disorders, 24-hour urine specimens are collected to measure hormones or their metabolites.

For example, urinary levels of free catecholamines (norepinephrine, epinephrine, and dopamine) may be measured in patients with suspected **pheochromocytoma,** a tumor of the adrenal medulla. Several disadvantages related to urine tests that must be considered are that patients may be unable to urinate at scheduled intervals and that some medications or disease states may affect the test results (Norris, 2019).

Additional Diagnostic Studies

Stimulation tests are used to confirm hypofunction of an endocrine organ. The tests determine how an endocrine gland responds to the administration of stimulating hormones that are normally produced or released by the hypothalamus or pituitary gland. If the endocrine gland responds to this stimulation, the specific disorder may be in the hypothalamus or pituitary. Failure of the endocrine gland to respond to this stimulation helps identify the problem as being in the endocrine gland itself.

Suppression tests are used to detect hyperfunction of an endocrine organ. They determine if the organ is not responding to the negative feedback mechanisms that normally control secretion of hormones from the hypothalamus or pituitary gland. Suppression tests measure the effect of a given exogenous dose of the hormone on the endogenous secretion of the hormone or on the secretion of stimulation hormones from the hypothalamus or pituitary gland.

Imaging studies include radioactive scanning, magnetic resonance imaging (MRI), computed tomography (CT), ultrasonography, positron emission tomography (PET), and dual-energy x-ray absorptiometry (DXA) (Norris, 2019).

Genetic screening is becoming more routine in the assessment of endocrine disorders (see Chart 45-1). DNA testing can be used for the identification of specific genes associated

---

Chart 45-1 **GENETICS IN NURSING PRACTICE**
Metabolic and Endocrine Disorders

Metabolic and endocrine disorders that are influenced by genetic factors are complex and typically impact multiple body systems. Some examples of genetic metabolic and endocrine disorders include:

- Diabetes
- Disorders in amino acids (e.g., phenylketonuria, homocystinuria, maple syrup urine disease)
- Disorders of carbohydrate metabolism (e.g., galactosemia)
- Disorders of fatty acid oxidation (e.g., medium-chain acyl-CoA dehydrogenase deficiency)
- Disorders of glycogen storage (e.g., Pompe disease, Von Gierke disease, Danon disease, Cori disease, Anderson disease, McArdle disease)
- Disorders of lysosomal storage disease (e.g., Tay Sachs, Gaucher, Niemann-Pick, Fabry disease)
- Disorders of mucopolysaccharides (e.g., Hurler syndrome, Hunter disease, Morquio syndrome)
- Disorders in urea cycle (e.g., ornithine transcarbamylase deficiency)
- Hemochromatosis
- McCune–Albright syndrome
- Multiple endocrine neoplasia type I and type II

Nursing Assessments

Refer to Chapter 4, Chart 4-2: Genetics in Nursing Practice: Genetic Aspects of Health Assessment

Family History Assessment

- Assess family history for relatives with early-onset hepatic, pancreatic, or endocrine disease.
- Inquire about family members with diabetes and their ages at onset.
- Assess family history of other related genetic conditions such as cystic fibrosis, alpha$_1$-antitrypsin deficiency, and hemochromatosis.

Patient Assessment

- Assess for physical symptoms such as mucosal neuromas, hypertrophied lips, skeletal abnormalities, and marfanoid appearance.
- Assess for signs of arthritis and hemochromatosis (bronze pigmentation of the skin).
- Assess for history of seizures, sweet smell to urine, jaundice, lethargy, vomiting, dehydration, acidosis, neutropenia, hepatomegaly, high ammonia levels

Genetics Resources

Association for Glycogen Storage Disease, www.agsdus.org
Society for Inherited Metabolic Disorders, www.simd.org
See Chapter 6, Chart 6-7, for components of genetic counseling.

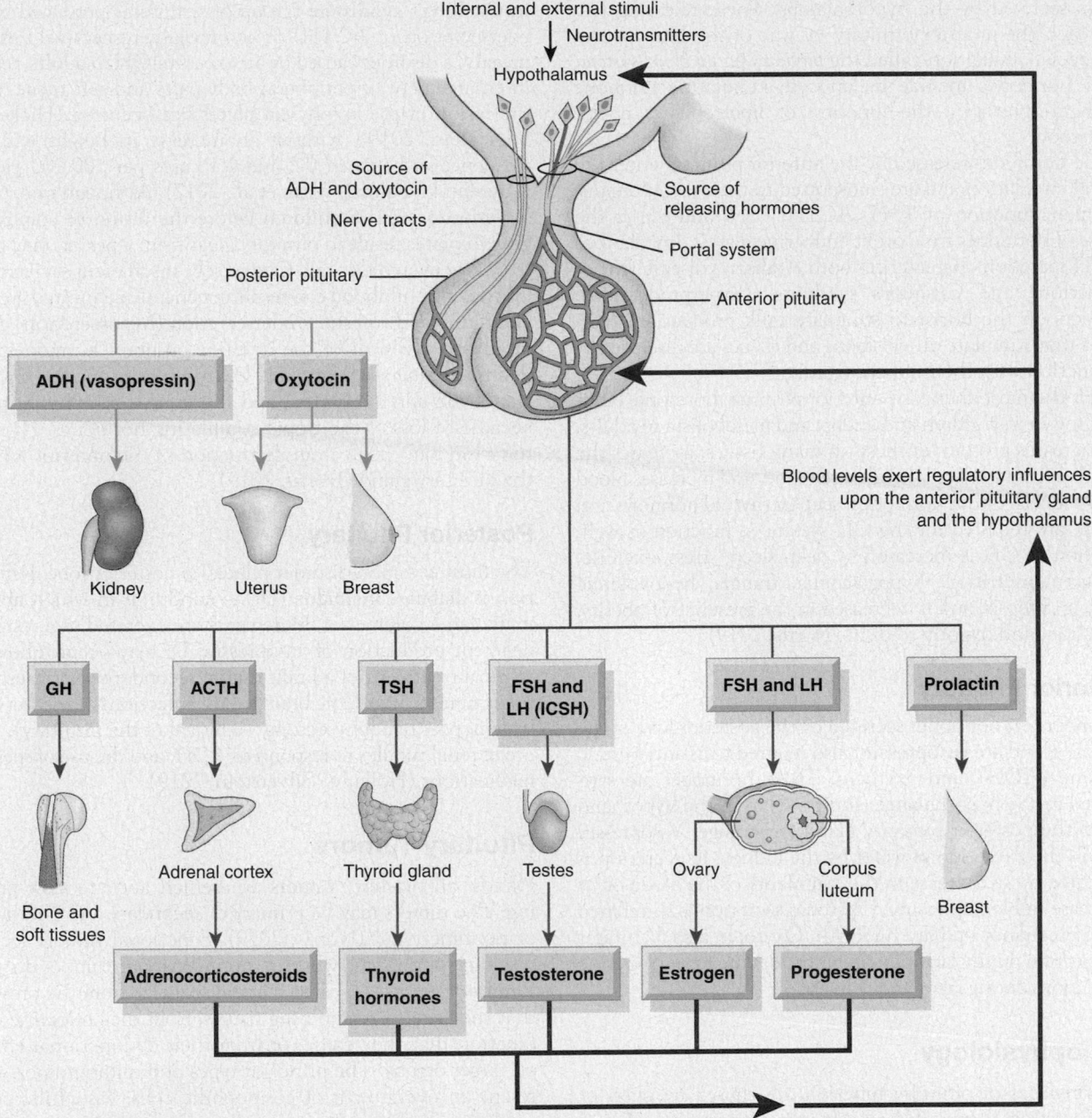

Figure 45-2 • The pituitary gland, the relationship of the brain to pituitary action, and the hormones secreted by the anterior and posterior pituitary lobes. ADH, antidiuretic hormone; GH, growth hormone; ACTH, adrenocorticotropic hormone; TSH, thyroid-stimulating hormone; FSH, follicle-stimulating hormone; LH, luteinizing hormone; ICSH, interstitial cell-stimulating hormone.

with endocrine disorders, selective targeting for drug development, and increased understanding of the function of the endocrine system. Genetic screening is used to determine the presence of a gene mutation that may predispose a person to a certain condition, the implications of which must be considered by the patient.

THE PITUITARY GLAND

Anatomic and Physiologic Overview

The pituitary gland, or hypophysis, is commonly referred to as the master gland because of the influence it has on secretion

of hormones by other endocrine glands (see Fig. 45-2). The round structure, about 1.27 cm (1/2 inch) in diameter, is located on the inferior aspect of the brain and is divided into anterior and posterior lobes. The gland is controlled by the hypothalamus, which is an adjacent area of the brain that is connected to the pituitary by the pituitary stalk.

Anterior Pituitary

The major hormones of the anterior pituitary gland are FSH, luteinizing hormone (LH), prolactin (PRL), **adrenocorticotropic hormone (ACTH)**, **thyroid-stimulating hormone (TSH)**, and GH (also referred to as somatotropin). The secretion of these major hormones is controlled by releasing factors secreted by the hypothalamus. These releasing factors reach the anterior pituitary by way of the bloodstream in a special circulation called the *pituitary portal blood system*. Other hormones include melanocyte-stimulating hormone and beta-lipotropin; the function of lipotropin is poorly understood.

The hormones released by the anterior pituitary enter the general circulation and are transported to their target organs. The main function of TSH, ACTH, FSH, and LH is the release of hormones from other endocrine glands. Imbalanced ACTH secretion characterizes both Addison's disease (hypoproduction) and Cushing's syndrome (hyperproduction). PRL acts on the breast to stimulate milk production. Hormones that stimulate other organs and tissues are discussed in conjunction with their target organs.

GH, the most abundant anterior pituitary hormone, regulates growth in children and energy and metabolism in adults. GH increases protein synthesis in many tissues, increases the breakdown of fatty acids in adipose tissue, and increases blood glucose levels. Other hormones, such as thyroid hormone and insulin, are required for the GH system to function as well. Secretion of GH is increased by deep sleep, stress, exercise, fasting, malnutrition, hypoglycemia, trauma, hypovolemic shock, and sepsis, and is decreased in the presence of obesity, depression, and hypothyroidism (Norris, 2019).

Posterior Pituitary

The important hormones secreted by the posterior lobe of the pituitary gland are **vasopressin**, also referred to as antidiuretic hormone (ADH), and oxytocin. These hormones are synthesized in the hypothalamus and travel from the hypothalamus to the posterior pituitary gland for storage. Vasopressin controls the excretion of water by the kidney; its secretion is stimulated by an increase in the osmolality of the blood or by a decrease in blood pressure. Oxytocin secretion is stimulated during pregnancy and at childbirth. Oxytocin also facilitates milk ejection during lactation and increases the force of uterine contractions during labor and delivery.

Pathophysiology

Abnormalities of pituitary function are caused by over- or undersecretion of any of the hormones produced or released by the gland. Abnormalities of the anterior and posterior portions of the gland may occur independently. Hypopituitarism, or hypofunction of the pituitary gland, can result from disease of the pituitary gland itself or disease of the hypothalamus; the outcome is essentially the same. Hypopituitarism can result from radiation therapy to the head and neck area. The total destruction of the pituitary gland by trauma, tumor, or vascular lesion removes all stimuli that are normally received by the thyroid, the gonads, and the adrenal glands. This leads to extreme weight loss, emaciation, atrophy of all endocrine glands and organs, hair loss, impotence, amenorrhea, hypometabolism, and hypoglycemia. Coma and death occur if the missing hormones are not replaced (Norris, 2019).

Anterior Pituitary

Oversecretion (hypersecretion) of the anterior pituitary gland most commonly involves ACTH or GH and results in **Cushing's syndrome** (group of symptoms produced by an oversecretion of ACTH) or acromegaly, respectively. **Acromegaly**, a disorder caused by an excess of GH in adults, results in enlargement of peripheral body parts and soft tissue, after the fusion of the epiphyseal plates has occurred (Hickey & Silverstein, 2019), without an increase in height with an incidence of between 0.2 and 1.1 cases per 100,000 people (Lavrentaki, Paluzzi, Wass, et al., 2017). Although rare, oversecretion of GH in children before the fusion of epiphyseal growth plates result in pituitary gigantism; a person may grow to be 7 or even 8 feet tall. Conversely, insufficient secretion of GH during childhood can result in generalized limited growth and pituitary dwarfism. Undersecretion (hyposecretion) commonly involves all of the anterior pituitary hormones and is termed *panhypopituitarism*. In this condition, the thyroid gland, the adrenal cortex, and the gonads atrophy (shrink) because of loss of the tropic-stimulating hormones. Hypopituitarism may result from destruction of the anterior lobe of the pituitary gland (Norris, 2019).

Posterior Pituitary

The most common disorder related to posterior lobe dysfunction is **diabetes insipidus** (DI), a condition in which abnormally large volumes of dilute urine are excreted as a result of deficient production of vasopressin. DI may occur following surgical treatment of a brain tumor, secondary to nonsurgical brain tumors, traumatic brain injury, infections of the nervous system, post hypophysectomy (removal of the pituitary), failure of renal tubules to respond to ADH, and the use of specific medications (Hollar & Silverstein, 2019).

Pituitary Tumors

Almost all pituitary tumors are benign and are slow growing. The tumors may be primary or secondary and functional or nonfunctional (Norris, 2019). Functional tumors secrete pituitary hormones, whereas nonfunctional tumors do not. Pituitary tumors can cause clinical sequelae from the pressure that they exert on adjoining tissues, from the endocrine dysfunction that they cause, or from their dysfunctional effects on target organs. The principal types of pituitary tumors represent an overgrowth of eosinophilic cells, basophilic cells, or chromophobic cells (i.e., cells with no affinity for either eosinophilic or basophilic stains).

Clinical Manifestations

Eosinophilic tumors that develop early in life result in gigantism. The affected person may be more than 7 feet tall and large in all proportions, yet so weak and lethargic that they can hardly stand. If the disorder begins during adult life, the excessive skeletal growth occurs only in the feet, the hands, the superciliary ridge, the molar eminences, the nose, and the chin, giving rise to the clinical picture called *acromegaly*. However, enlargement involves all tissues and organs of the body, and many of these patients suffer from severe headaches and visual disturbances because the tumors exert pressure on the optic nerves (Norris, 2019). Assessment of central vision and visual fields may reveal loss of color discrimination, diplopia (double vision), or blindness in a portion of a field of vision. Decalcification of the skeleton, muscular weakness, and endocrine disturbances, similar to those occurring in patients with hyperthyroidism, also are associated with this type of tumor.

Basophilic tumors give rise to Cushing's syndrome with features largely attributable to hyperadrenalism, including masculinization and amenorrhea in females, truncal obesity, hypertension, osteoporosis, and polycythemia.

Chromophobic tumors represent 90% of pituitary tumors. These tumors usually produce no hormones but destroy the rest of the pituitary gland, causing hypopituitarism. People with this disease often have obesity, are somnolent, and exhibit fine, scanty hair; dry, soft skin; a pasty complexion; and small bones. They also experience headaches, loss of libido, and visual defects progressing to blindness. Other signs and symptoms include polyuria, polyphagia, a lowering of the **basal metabolic rate** (chemical reactions occurring when the body is at rest), and a subnormal body temperature (Sadiq & Silverstein, 2019b).

Assessment and Diagnostic Findings

Diagnostic evaluation requires a careful history and physical examination, including assessment of visual acuity and visual fields. CT and MRI scans are used to diagnose the presence and extent of pituitary tumors. Serum levels of pituitary hormones may be obtained along with measurements of hormones of target organs (e.g., thyroid, adrenal) to assist in diagnosis.

Medical Management

Hypophysectomy, or surgical removal of the pituitary gland through a transsphenoidal approach, is the usual treatment. Stereotactic radiation therapy, which requires the use of a neurosurgery-type stereotactic frame, may be used to deliver external-beam radiation therapy precisely to the pituitary tumor with minimal effect on normal tissue (see Chapter 12). Other treatments include conventional radiation therapy, bromocriptine, and octreotide. These medications inhibit the production or release of GH and may bring about marked improvement of symptoms. Octreotide and lanreotide may also be used preoperatively to improve the patient's clinical condition and to shrink the tumor (American Association of Neurological Surgeons, 2019).

Surgical Management

Hypophysectomy is the treatment of choice in patients with Cushing's disease resulting from excessive production of ACTH by a pituitary tumor. Hypophysectomy may also be performed on occasion as a palliative measure to relieve bone pain secondary to metastasis of malignant lesions of the breast and prostate.

Several approaches are used to remove or destroy the pituitary gland, including surgical removal by transfrontal, subcranial, or oronasal–transsphenoidal approaches; irradiation; and cryosurgery. The transsphenoidal approach and the nursing management of a patient undergoing cranial surgery are discussed in Chapter 61. Features or symptoms of acromegaly are unaffected by surgical removal of the tumor.

The absence of the pituitary gland alters the function of many body systems. Menstruation ceases and infertility occurs after total or near-total ablation of the pituitary gland. Replacement therapy with corticosteroids and thyroid hormone is necessary.

Diabetes Insipidus

Diabetes insipidus (DI) is a rare disorder that occurs due to injury to the hypothalamus or pituitary gland with a deficiency of ADH (vasopressin) that results in excretion of large volumes of dilute urine and extreme thirst. DI is characterized as central, nephrogenic, or dipsogenic, as well as gestational (Hollar & Silverstein, 2019).

The primary etiology for central DI is head trauma but other causes include surgery, infection, inflammation, brain tumors, or cerebral vascular disease; it also may be idiopathic. Nephrogenic DI etiologic factors include kidney injury, medications such as lithium, hypokalemia, and hypercalcemia. Dipsogenic DI is caused by a defect in the hypothalamus and may be the result of damage to the pituitary gland from a head injury, surgery, infection, inflammatory process, or a tumor (National Institute of Diabetes and Digestive and Kidney Diseases, 2019). DI must be differentiated from diabetes, which may also cause polydipsia and excessive urination.

Clinical Manifestations

Without the action of ADH on the distal nephron of the kidney, an enormous daily output (greater than 250 mL per hour) of very dilute urine with a specific gravity of 1.001 to 1.005 occurs (Hollar & Silverstein, 2019). The urine contains no abnormal substances such as glucose or albumin. Because of the intense thirst, the patient tends to drink 2 to 20 L of fluid daily and craves cold water. In adults, the onset of DI may be insidious or abrupt.

The disease cannot be controlled by limiting fluid intake, because the high-volume loss of urine continues even without fluid replacement. Attempts to restrict fluids cause the patient to experience an insatiable craving for fluid and to develop hypernatremia and severe dehydration.

Assessment and Diagnostic Findings

The fluid deprivation test is carried out by withholding fluids for 8 to 12 hours or until 3% to 5% of the body weight is lost. The patient is weighed frequently during the test. Plasma and urine osmolality studies are performed at the beginning and end of the test. The inability to increase the specific gravity and osmolality of the urine is characteristic of DI. The patient continues to excrete large volumes of urine with low specific gravity and experiences weight loss, increasing serum osmolality, and elevated serum sodium levels. The patient's condition needs to be monitored frequently during the test, and the test is terminated if tachycardia, excessive weight loss, or hypotension develops.

Other diagnostic procedures include concurrent measurements of plasma levels of ADH and plasma and urine osmolality as well as a trial of desmopressin therapy and intravenous (IV) infusion of hypertonic saline solution. If the diagnosis is confirmed and the cause (e.g., head injury) is not obvious, the patient is carefully assessed for tumors that may be causing the disorder.

Medical Management

The objectives of therapy are to replace ADH (which is usually a long-term therapeutic program), ensure adequate fluid replacement, and identify and correct the underlying intracranial pathology. Nephrogenic causes require different management approaches (Hollar & Silverstein, 2019).

Pharmacologic Therapy

Desmopressin, a synthetic vasopressin without the vascular effects of natural ADH, is the drug of choice for central DI. The drug may be given orally or intranasally (Norris, 2019). Vasopressin causes vasoconstriction; therefore, it must be used cautiously in patients with coronary artery disease. Chlorpropamide and thiazide diuretics are also used in mild forms of the disease because they potentiate the action of vasopressin but are used with caution due to the risk for hypoglycemia (Norris, 2019).

If the DI is renal in origin, the previously described treatments are ineffective. Thiazide diuretics, mild salt depletion, and prostaglandin inhibitors (e.g., indomethacin and aspirin) are used to treat the nephrogenic form of DI.

Nursing Management

Ongoing physical assessment and patient education are the pillars of skilled nursing management of the patient with a diagnosis of DI. Initially, the nurse reviews the patient history and physical assessment and monitors for clinical manifestations of dehydration. Severe dehydration can lead to decreased cardiac output and, therefore, decreased perfusion of the vital organs, specifically the brain and kidneys. Ongoing monitoring of vital signs as well as intake and output (I&O) is essential. The nurse is responsible to educate the patient, family, and other caregivers about follow-up care, prevention of complications, and emergency measures. Specific verbal and written instructions should include the dose, actions, side effects, and administration of all medications and the signs and symptoms of hyponatremia. The nurse should demonstrate and observe a return demonstration of medication administration to ensure that the patient received the prescribed dosage. The patient should be advised to wear a medical identification bracelet and carry required medication and information about DI at all times.

Syndrome of Inappropriate Antidiuretic Hormone Secretion

The **syndrome of inappropriate antidiuretic hormone (SIADH)** results from a failure of the negative feedback system that regulates the release and inhibition of ADH (Norris, 2019). Patients with SIADH cannot excrete a dilute urine, retain fluids, and develop a sodium deficiency known as dilutional hyponatremia. SIADH is often of nonendocrine origin; for instance, the syndrome may occur in patients with bronchogenic carcinoma in which malignant lung cells synthesize and release ADH. SIADH has also occurred in patients with severe pneumonia, pneumothorax, and other disorders of the lungs, as well as malignant tumors that affect other organs (Norris, 2019).

Disorders of the central nervous system, such as head injury, brain surgery or tumor, and infection, are thought to produce SIADH by direct stimulation of the pituitary gland (Norris, 2019). Some medications (e.g., vincristine, phenothiazines, tricyclic antidepressants, thiazide diuretics) and nicotine have been implicated in SIADH; they either directly stimulate the pituitary gland or increase the sensitivity of renal tubules to circulating ADH.

Medical Management

SIADH is generally self-limiting and treatment is focused on eliminating the underlying cause, if possible, and restricting fluid intake (Parham & Silverstein, 2019). Because retained water is excreted slowly through the kidneys, the extracellular fluid volume contracts and the serum sodium concentration gradually increases toward normal. Diuretic agents such as furosemide may be used along with fluid restriction. In severe hyponatremia sometimes a hypertonic NaCl (3%) may be prescribed and administered IV (Norris, 2019).

Nursing Management

Close monitoring of fluid I&O, daily weight, urine and blood chemistries, and neurologic status is indicated for the patient at risk for SIADH. Supportive measures and explanations of procedures and treatments assist the patient in managing this disorder.

THE THYROID GLAND

The thyroid gland—the largest endocrine gland—is a butterfly-shaped organ located in the lower neck, anterior to the trachea (Fig. 45-3). It consists of two lateral lobes connected by an isthmus. The gland is about 5 cm long and 3 cm wide and weighs about 30 g. The blood flow to the thyroid is very high (about 5 mL/min per gram of thyroid tissue), approximately five times the blood flow to the liver. The thyroid gland produces three hormones: **thyroxine (T_4)**, **triiodothyronine (T_3)**, and **calcitonin**. Thyroxine and triiodothyronine are needed by all body cells for metabolism (Moore, 2018).

Anatomic and Physiologic Overview

Various hormones and chemicals are responsible for normal thyroid function. Key among them are thyroid hormone, calcitonin, and iodine.

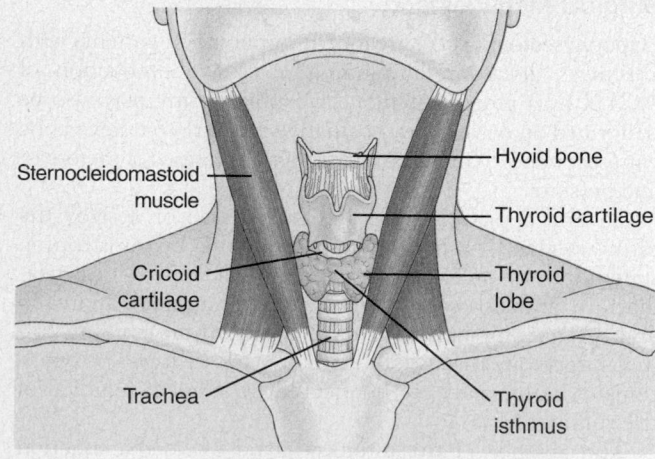

Figure 45-3 • The thyroid gland and surrounding structures.

Thyroid Hormone

Thyroid hormone is comprised of T_4 and T_3, two separate hormones produced by the thyroid gland. Both are amino acids that contain iodine molecules bound to the amino acid structure; T_4 contains four iodine atoms in each molecule, and T_3 contains three. These hormones are synthesized and stored bound to proteins in the cells of the thyroid gland until needed for release into the bloodstream. Three thyroid-binding hormones—thyroxine-binding globulin (TBG), transthyretin (formerly known as thyroid-binding prealbumin), and albumin—bind and transport T_3 and T_4 (Norris, 2019).

Synthesis of Thyroid Hormone

Iodine is essential to the thyroid gland for synthesis of its hormones. The major use of iodine in the body is by the thyroid, and the major derangement in iodine deficiency is alteration of thyroid function. Iodide is ingested in the diet and absorbed into the blood in the GI tract. The thyroid gland is extremely efficient at taking up iodide from the blood and concentrating it within the cells, where iodide ions are converted to iodine molecules, which react with tyrosine (an amino acid) to form the thyroid hormones (Norris, 2019).

Regulation of Thyroid Hormone

The secretion of T_3 and T_4 by the thyroid gland is controlled by TSH (also called *thyrotropin*) from the anterior pituitary gland. TSH controls the rate of thyroid hormone release through a negative feedback mechanism. In turn, the level of thyroid hormone in the blood determines the release of TSH. If the thyroid hormone concentration in the blood decreases, the release of TSH increases, which causes increased output of T_3 and T_4. The term **euthyroid** refers to thyroid hormone production that is normal.

TRH, secreted by the hypothalamus, exerts a modulating influence on the release of TSH from the pituitary. Environmental factors, such as a decrease in temperature, may lead to increased secretion of TRH, resulting in elevated secretion of thyroid hormones. Figure 45-4 shows the hypothalamic–pituitary–thyroid axis, which regulates thyroid hormone production.

Function of Thyroid Hormone

The main function of thyroid hormone is to control cellular metabolic activity. T_4, a relatively weak hormone, maintains body metabolism in a steady state. T_3 is about five times as potent as T_4 and has a more rapid metabolic action. These hormones accelerate metabolic processes by increasing the level of specific enzymes that contribute to oxygen consumption and altering the responsiveness of tissues to other hormones. The thyroid hormones influence cell replication, are important in brain development, and are necessary for normal growth. Thyroid hormones affect virtually every major organ system and tissue function, including the basal metabolic rate, tissue thermogenesis, serum cholesterol levels, and vascular resistance (Norris, 2019).

Calcitonin

Calcitonin, or thyrocalcitonin, is another important hormone secreted by the thyroid gland. The hormone is secreted in response to high plasma levels of calcium, and it reduces

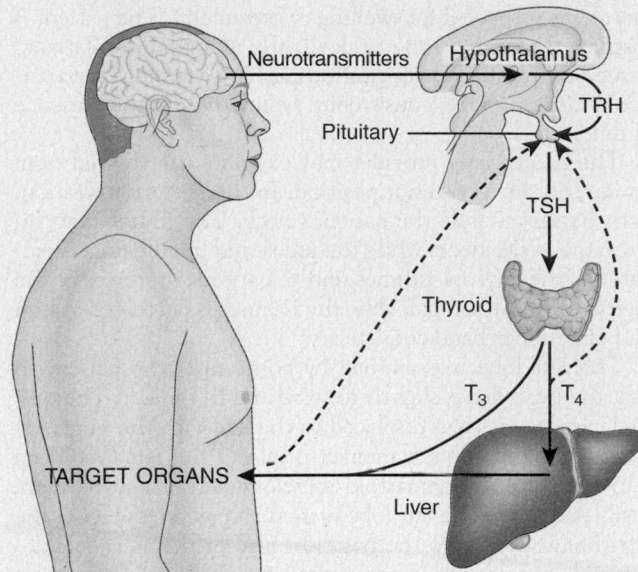

Figure 45-4 • The hypothalamic–pituitary–thyroid axis. Thyroid-releasing hormone (TRH) from the hypothalamus stimulates the pituitary gland to secrete thyroid-stimulating hormone (TSH). TSH stimulates the thyroid to produce thyroid hormone (triiodothyronine [T_3] and thyroxine [T_4]). High circulating levels of T_3 and T_4 inhibit further TSH secretion and thyroid hormone production through a negative feedback mechanism (*dashed lines*).

the plasma level of calcium by increasing its deposition in bone.

Pathophysiology

Congenital hypothyroidism, which occurs when there is inadequate secretion of thyroid hormone during fetal and neonatal development, results in intellectual disability and stunted physical growth because of general depression of metabolic activity (Norris, 2019). In adults, hypothyroidism manifests as lethargy, slow mentation, weight gain, constipation, cold intolerance, and generalized slowing of body functions (Singh & Clutter, 2019).

Hyperthyroidism (oversecretion of thyroid hormones) is manifested by a greatly increased metabolic rate. Many of the other characteristics of hyperthyroidism result from the increased response to circulating catecholamines (epinephrine and norepinephrine).

Oversecretion of thyroid hormones is usually associated with an enlarged thyroid gland known as a **goiter**. Goiter also commonly occurs with iodine deficiency. In this latter condition, lack of iodine results in low levels of circulating thyroid hormones, which causes increased release of TSH; the elevated TSH causes overproduction of thyroglobulin (a precursor of T_3 and T_4) and hypertrophy of the thyroid gland.

Assessment

Physical Examination

The thyroid gland is inspected and palpated routinely in all patients. Inspection begins with identification of landmarks. The lower neck region between the sternocleidomastoid muscles is inspected for swelling or asymmetry. The patient is instructed to extend the neck slightly and swallow. Thyroid tissue rises normally with swallowing. The thyroid is then palpated for size, shape, consistency, symmetry, and the presence of tenderness.

The health care provider may examine the thyroid from an anterior or a posterior position. In the posterior position, both hands encircle the patient's neck. The thumbs rest on the nape of the neck, while the index and middle fingers palpate for the thyroid isthmus and the anterior surfaces of the lateral lobes. When palpable, the isthmus is perceived as firm and of a rubber-band consistency.

The left lobe is examined by positioning the patient so that the neck flexes slightly forward and to the left. The thyroid cartilage is then displaced to the left with the fingers of the right hand. This maneuver displaces the left lobe deep into the sternocleidomastoid muscle, where it can be more easily palpated. The left lobe is then palpated by placing the left thumb deep into the posterior area of the sternocleidomastoid muscle, while the index and middle fingers exert opposite pressure in the anterior portion of the muscle. Having the patient swallow during the maneuver may assist the examiner to locate the thyroid as it ascends in the neck. The procedure is reversed to examine the right lobe. The isthmus is the only portion of the thyroid that is normally palpable. If a patient has a very thin neck, two thin, smooth, nontender lobes may also be palpable.

If palpation discloses an enlarged thyroid gland, both lobes are auscultated using the diaphragm of the stethoscope. Auscultation identifies the localized audible vibration of a bruit. This is indicative of increased blood flow through the thyroid gland associated with hyperthyroidism and necessitates referral to a primary provider. Other abnormal findings that require referral for further evaluation may include a soft texture (Graves disease), firmness (Hashimoto thyroiditis or malignancy), and tenderness (thyroiditis) (Jensen, 2019).

Diagnostic Evaluation

Assessment measures in addition to palpation and auscultation include thyroid function tests, such as laboratory measurement of thyroid hormones, thyroid scanning, biopsy, and ultrasonography. The most widely used tests are serum immunoassay for TSH and free T_4. Free T_4 levels correlate with metabolic status; they are elevated in hyperthyroidism and decreased in hypothyroidism (Fischbach & Fischbach, 2018). Ultrasound, CT, and MRI may be used to clarify or confirm the results of other diagnostic studies.

Thyroid Tests

Serum Thyroid-Stimulating Hormone

Measurement of the serum TSH concentration is the primary screening test of thyroid function. The ability to detect minute changes in serum TSH makes it possible to distinguish subclinical thyroid disease from euthyroid states in patients with low or high normal values. Measurement of TSH is also used for monitoring thyroid hormone replacement therapy and for differentiating between disorders of the thyroid gland itself and disorders of the pituitary or hypothalamus.

The American Thyroid Association recommends that pregnant women be screened for thyroid disease (Alexander, Pearce, Brent, et al., 2017); however, there is lack of consensus among professional organizations regarding routine screening of adults for thyroid disease. The US Preventive Services Task Force (USPSTF) does not recommend routine screening of adults (USPSTF, 2019).

Serum Free T_4

Serum free T_4 is a direct measurement of free (unbound) thyroxine, the only metabolically active fraction of T_4. The range of free T_4 in serum is normally 0.7 to 2.0 ng/dL (10 to 26 pmol/L) (Fischbach & Fischbach, 2018). When measured by the dialysis method, free T_4 is not affected by variations in protein binding and is the procedure of choice for monitoring the changes in T_4 secretion during treatment for hyperthyroidism.

Serum T_3 and T_4

Measurement of total T_3 or T_4 includes protein-bound and free hormone levels that occur in response to TSH secretion. T_4 is 70% bound to TBG; T_3 is bound less firmly. Only 0.03% of T_4 and 0.3% of T_3 are unbound. Serious systemic illnesses, medications (e.g., oral contraceptives, corticosteroids, carbamazepine, salicylates), and protein wasting as a result of nephrosis or the use of androgens may interfere with accurate test results. Normal range for T_4 is 5.4 to 11.5 µg/dL (57 to 148 nmol/L) (Fischbach & Fischbach, 2018). Although serum T_3 and T_4 levels generally increase or decrease together, the T_3 level appears to be a more accurate indicator of hyperthyroidism or severity of the disorder, as T_4 levels are often within normal range. The normal range for serum T_3 is 260 to 480 pg/dL (4.0 to 7.4 pmol/L) (Fischbach & Fischbach, 2018).

T_3 Resin Uptake Test

The T_3 resin uptake test is an indirect measure of unsaturated TBG. Its purpose is to determine the amount of thyroid hormone bound to TBG and the number of available binding sites. This provides an index of the amount of thyroid hormone already present in the circulation. Normally, TBG is not fully saturated with thyroid hormone, and additional binding sites are available to combine with radioiodine-labeled T_3 added to the blood specimen. The normal T_3 uptake value is 25% to 35% (relative uptake fraction, 0.25 to 0.35), which indicates that about one third of the available sites of TBG are occupied by thyroid hormone. If the number of free or unoccupied binding sites is low, as in hyperthyroidism, the T_3 uptake is greater than 35% (0.35). If the number of available sites is high, as occurs in hypothyroidism, the test result is less than 25% (0.25).

T_3 uptake is useful in evaluating thyroid hormone levels in patients who have received diagnostic or therapeutic doses of iodine. The test results may be altered by the use of estrogens, androgens, salicylates, phenytoin, anticoagulants, or corticosteroids (Fischbach & Fischbach, 2018).

Thyroid Antibodies

Autoimmune thyroid diseases include both hypo- and hyperthyroid conditions. Results of testing by immunoassay techniques for antithyroid antibodies are positive in chronic autoimmune thyroid disease (90%), Hashimoto thyroiditis

(100%), Graves disease (80%), and other organ-specific auto-immune diseases, such as systemic lupus erythematosus (SLE) and rheumatoid arthritis. Antithyroid antibody titers are normally present in 5% to 10% of the population and increase with age.

Radioactive Iodine Uptake

The radioactive iodine uptake test measures the rate of iodine uptake by the thyroid gland. The patient is given a tracer dose of iodine 123 (^{123}I) or another radionuclide, and a count is made over the thyroid gland with a scintillation counter, which detects and counts the gamma rays released from the breakdown of ^{123}I in the thyroid. The radioactive iodine uptake test is a simple test with reliable results. The test measures the proportion of the given dose that is present in the thyroid gland at a specific time after its administration. Since the test is affected by the patient's intake of iodide or thyroid hormone, a careful preliminary clinical history is essential in evaluating results. Normal values vary from one geographic region to another and with the intake of iodine. Patients with hyperthyroidism exhibit a high uptake of the ^{123}I (in some patients, as high as 90%), whereas patients with hypothyroidism exhibit a very low uptake.

Fine-Needle Aspiration Biopsy

The use of a small-gauge needle to sample the thyroid tissue for biopsy is a safe and accurate method of detecting malignancy and is often the initial test for evaluation of thyroid masses. Results are reported as benign, malignant, suspicious, or nondiagnostic/insufficient (Ross, Cooper, & Mulder, 2019). Within the malignancy category, masses are reported as a follicular neoplasm or a follicular lesion.

Thyroid Scan, Radioscan, or Scintiscan

In a thyroid scan, a scintillation detector or gamma camera moves back and forth across the area to be studied in a series of parallel tracks, and a visual image is made of the distribution of radioactivity in the area being scanned. The most commonly used isotopes of iodine are ^{123}I and ^{131}I (Fischbach & Fischbach, 2018).

Scans are helpful in determining the location, size, shape, and anatomic function of the thyroid gland, particularly when thyroid tissue is substernal or large (Fischbach & Fischbach, 2018). Identifying areas of increased function ("hot" areas) or decreased function ("cold" areas) can assist in diagnosis. Although most areas of decreased function do not represent malignancies, lack of function increases the likelihood of malignancy, particularly if only one nonfunctioning area is present. Scanning of the entire body, to obtain the total body profile, may be carried out in a search for a functioning thyroid metastasis (i.e., a lesion that produces thyroid hormones).

Serum Thyroglobulin

Thyroglobulin (Tg) can be measured reliably in the serum by radioimmunoassay. Clinically, it is used to detect persistence or recurrence of thyroid carcinoma.

Nursing Implications

Since thyroid tests involve the use of iodine, determining if the patient has any allergies to iodine or is taking medications that contain iodine is essential. The relationship

---

Chart 45-2 — PHARMACOLOGY
Select Medications That May Alter Thyroid Test Results

amiodarone
aspirin
cimetidine
diazepam
estrogens
furosemide
glucocorticoids
heparin
lithium
phenytoin and other anticonvulsants
propranolol

Adapted from Morton, P. G., & Fontaine, D. K. (2018). *Critical care nursing: A holistic approach* (10th ed.). Philadelphia, PA: Wolters Kluwer.

---

between having an allergy to shellfish and having an allergy to iodine is a long held belief; however, an allergy to shellfish is due to specific proteins in the shellfish and not iodine (American College of Allergy, Asthma and Immunology, 2019). Patients should be asked if they have had a reaction to iodine previously and to shellfish so that the radiologist can determine what precautions need to be taken, if any (American College of Allergy, Asthma and Immunology, 2019). Patients should be asked about obvious sources of iodine-containing medications such as contrast agents and those used to treat thyroid disorders such as radioactive iodine. They should also be asked whether they eat kelp or seaweed. Numerous medications may also affect test results because they affect the thyroid. Chart 45-2 gives a list of select medications that may interfere with accurate testing of thyroid gland function (Fischbach & Fischbach, 2018). This information should be documented in the patient's electronic health record (EHR) and communicated clearly to personnel conducting the test.

Hypothyroidism

Hypothyroidism results from suboptimal levels of thyroid hormone. Thyroid deficiency can affect all body functions and can range from mild, subclinical forms to **myxedema** (severe deficiency discussed later), an advanced life-threatening form. The most common cause of hypothyroidism in adults is autoimmune thyroiditis (Hashimoto disease), in which the immune system attacks the thyroid gland. Symptoms of hyperthyroidism may later be followed by those of hypothyroidism and myxedema. Hypothyroidism also commonly occurs in patients with previous hyperthyroidism that has been treated with radioiodine or antithyroid medications or **thyroidectomy** (surgical removal of all or part of the thyroid gland). Testing of thyroid function is recommended for all patients who receive radiation therapy to the neck. See Chart 45-3 for other causes of hypothyroidism.

More than 95% of patients with hypothyroidism have primary or thyroidal hypothyroidism, which refers to dysfunction of the thyroid gland itself. If the cause of the thyroid dysfunction is failure of the pituitary gland, the hypothalamus, or both, the hypothyroidism is known as central

Chart 45-3 Causes of Hypothyroidism

Autoimmune disease (Hashimoto thyroiditis, post-Graves disease)
Atrophy of thyroid gland with aging
Infiltrative diseases of the thyroid (amyloidosis, scleroderma, lymphoma)
Iodine deficiency, iodine excess, and iodine compounds
Medications (e.g., Lithium)
Radioactive iodine (^{131}I)
Therapy for hyperthyroidism
Thyroidectomy
Radiation to head and neck in treatment for head and neck cancers, lymphoma

hypothyroidism. If the cause is entirely a pituitary disorder, it may be referred to as pituitary or secondary hypothyroidism. If the cause is a disorder of the hypothalamus resulting in inadequate secretion of TSH due to decreased stimulation of TRH, it is referred to as hypothalamic or tertiary hypothyroidism. If thyroid deficiency is present at birth, it is referred to as neonatal hypothyroidism. In such instances, the mother may also have thyroid deficiency. The term *myxedema* refers to the accumulation of mucopolysaccharides in subcutaneous and other interstitial tissues. Although myxedema occurs in long-standing hypothyroidism, the term is used appropriately only to describe the extreme symptoms of severe hypothyroidism (Chaker, Bianco, Janklaas, et al., 2017).

Clinical Manifestations

Presenting clinical manifestations in adults frequently reflect the decrease in metabolism resulting from the decrease in thyroid function. Clinical manifestations include complaints of fatigue and lethargy that may interfere with activities of daily living, weight gain without an increased intake of calories, cold intolerance, dry skin, and, in some patients, a deepening of the voice. Other clinical manifestations are related to gender, age, and duration of the decrease in thyroid function (see Fig. 45-5). These include cardiovascular-related manifestations such as bradycardia and changes in electrical conduction of the heart which will be noted on the electrocardiogram (ECG). In women, changes in the menstrual cycle will be noted (Chaker et al., 2017).

Severe hypothyroidism results in a subnormal body temperature and pulse rate. The patient usually begins to gain weight even without an increase in food intake, although they may be cachectic. The skin becomes thickened because of an accumulation of mucopolysaccharides in the subcutaneous tissues. The hair thins and falls out, and the face becomes expressionless and masklike. The patient often complains of being cold even in a warm environment.

At first, the patient may be irritable and may complain of fatigue, but as the condition progresses, the emotional responses are subdued. The mental processes become dulled, and the patient appears apathetic. Speech is slow, the tongue enlarges, the hands and feet increase in size, and deafness may occur. The patient frequently reports constipation.

Advanced hypothyroidism may produce personality and cognitive changes characteristic of dementia. Inadequate

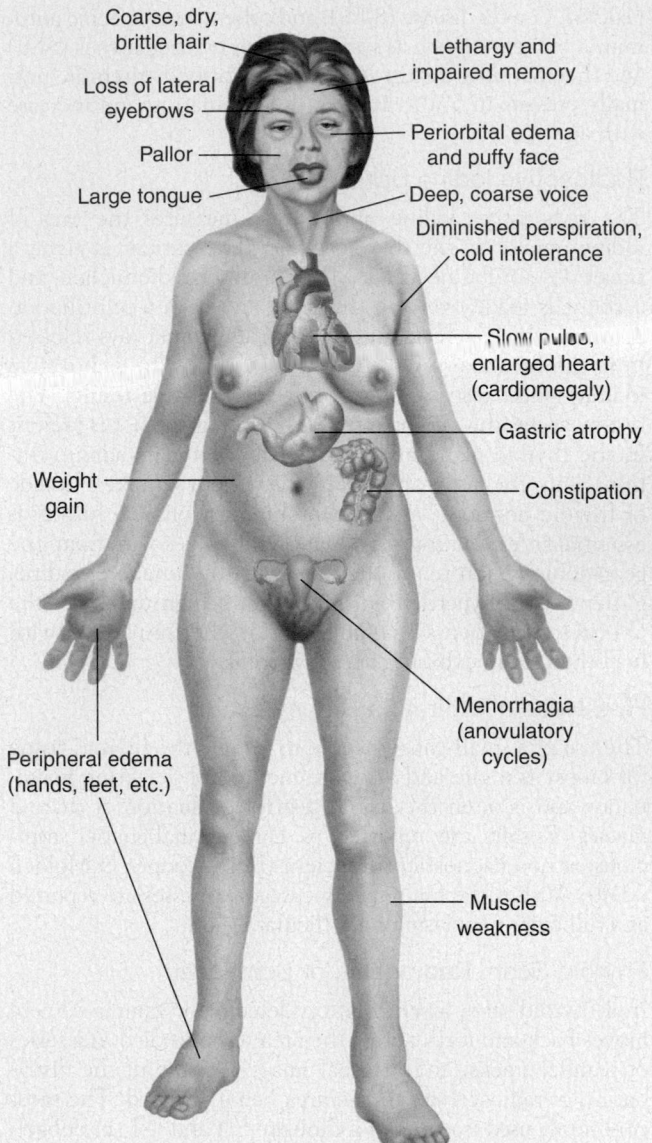

Figure 45-5 • Clinical manifestations of hypothyroidism. Reprinted with permission from Norris, T. L. (2019). *Porth's pathophysiology: Concepts of altered health states* (10th ed., Fig. 41.5). Philadelphia, PA: Wolters Kluwer.

ventilation and sleep apnea can occur with severe hypothyroidism. Pleural effusion, pericardial effusion, and respiratory muscle weakness may also occur (Chaker et al., 2017).

Severe hypothyroidism is associated with an elevated serum cholesterol level, atherosclerosis, coronary artery disease, and poor left ventricular function. The patient with advanced hypothyroidism is hypothermic and abnormally sensitive to sedative, opioid, and anesthetic agents, which must be given with extreme caution.

Patients with unrecognized hypothyroidism who are undergoing surgery are at increased risk for intraoperative hypotension, postoperative heart failure, and altered mental status.

Myxedema coma is a rare life-threatening condition and a decompensated state of severe hypothyroidism in which the patient is hypothermic and unconscious. This condition may develop with undiagnosed hypothyroidism and may be precipitated by infection or other systemic disease or by use of sedatives or opioid analgesic agents. Patients may also experience myxedema coma if they forget to take their thyroid replacement medication. The condition occurs most often among older women in the winter months and appears to be precipitated by cold. However, the disorder can affect any age group.

In myxedema coma, the patient may initially show signs of depression, diminished cognitive status, lethargy, and somnolence (Chaker et al., 2017).

Increasing lethargy may progress to stupor. The patient's respiratory drive is depressed, resulting in alveolar hypoventilation, progressive carbon dioxide retention, narcosis, and coma. In addition, patients with myxedema coma can also exhibit hyponatremia, hypoglycemia, hypoventilation, hypotension, bradycardia, and hypothermia. These symptoms, along with cardiovascular collapse and shock, require aggressive and intensive supportive and hemodynamic therapy if the patient is to survive. Although there has been a decline in mortality rates over the past two decades due to early intervention and improved therapies, the mortality rate remains at 40% despite treatment; proper diagnosis and prompt treatment is essential (Eledrisi, 2018).

Medical Management

The objectives in the management of hypothyroidism are to restore a normal metabolic state by replacing the missing hormone, as well as prevention of disease progression and complications.

Pharmacologic Therapy

Synthetic levothyroxine is the drug of choice for the treatment of hypothyroidism (Drake, 2018). The general range is 75 to 150 mcg per day and treatment is generally started at the lower dose and titrated slowly until desired levels of serum TSH concentration are achieved (Singh & Clutter, 2019). Older adult patients generally require a lower dose; normal TSH levels are often achieved with 50 mcg per day (Singh & Clutter, 2019). Some patients on thyroid hormone replacement may complain of continued clinical manifestations despite normal TSH levels (Chaker et al., 2017).

Prevention of Cardiac Dysfunction

Any patient who has had hypothyroidism for a long period usually has associated elevated serum cholesterol, atherosclerosis, and coronary artery disease. As long as metabolism is subnormal and the tissues (including the myocardium) require relatively little oxygen, a reduction in blood supply is tolerated without overt symptoms of coronary artery disease. When thyroid hormone is given, the oxygen demand increases, but oxygen delivery cannot be increased unless, or until, the atherosclerosis improves. This occurs very slowly, if at all. The occurrence of angina and acute coronary syndrome (see Chapter 23) is the signal that the oxygen needs of the myocardium exceed its blood supply. Angina or arrhythmias can occur when thyroid replacement is initiated because thyroid hormones enhance the cardiovascular effects of catecholamines.

Quality and Safety Nursing Alert

The nurse must monitor for signs and symptoms of cardiac dysfunction, which can occur in response to therapy in patients with severe, long-standing hypothyroidism or myxedema coma, especially during the early phase of treatment. Acute coronary syndrome must be aggressively treated to avoid morbid complications (e.g., myocardial infarction).

If angina or arrhythmias occur, thyroid hormone administration must be discontinued immediately. Later, when it can be resumed safely, it should be prescribed cautiously at a lower dosage and with close monitoring by the primary provider and the nurse.

Prevention of Medication Interactions

Oral thyroid hormones interact with many other medications. They increase the effect of warfarin and the cardiovascular effects of adrenergic agents (bronchodilators and vasopressors). In addition, the dosage of insulin and oral hypoglycemic medications used to treat diabetes may require adjustment. Caution is also needed in patients who are concomitantly taking estrogen, which may necessitate an increased dosage of the oral thyroid hormone. Absorption may be affected by any supplement or food that contains calcium, iron, magnesium or zinc (Vallerand & Sanoski, 2018).

Even in small IV doses, hypnotic and sedative agents may induce profound somnolence, lasting far longer than anticipated and leading to narcosis (stuporlike condition). Furthermore, they are likely to cause respiratory depression, which can easily be fatal because of decreased respiratory reserve and alveolar hypoventilation. The dose of these medications should be one half or one third of that typically prescribed for patients of similar age and weight with normal thyroid function.

Supportive Therapy

Severe hypothyroidism and myxedema coma require prompt, aggressive management to maintain vital functions. Arterial blood gases may be measured to determine carbon dioxide retention and to guide the use of assisted ventilation to combat hypoventilation. Oxygen saturation levels should be monitored using pulse oximetry. Fluids are given cautiously because of the danger of water intoxication. Passive rewarming with a blanket is recommended versus active rewarming such as application of external heat (e.g., heating pads). The latter should be avoided to prevent increased oxygen demands and hypotension.

Nursing Management

Nursing care of the patient with hypothyroidism and myxedema is summarized in the plan of nursing care in Chart 45-4. In patients with hypothyroidism, the effects of analgesic, sedative, and anesthetic agents are prolonged. The nurse should carefully monitor patients who are prescribed these agents for adverse effects. Older patients are at increased risk because of age-related changes in liver and renal function.

(text continued on page 1460)

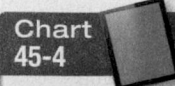

PLAN OF NURSING CARE
Care of the Patient with Hypothyroidism

Chart 45-4

NURSING DIAGNOSIS: Impaired breathing associated with depressed ventilation
GOAL: Improved respiratory status and maintenance of normal breathing pattern

Nursing Interventions	Rationale	Expected Outcomes
1. Assess respiratory rate, depth, pattern, pulse oximetry, and arterial blood gases.	1. Identifies patient's baseline to monitor further changes and evaluate effectiveness of interventions.	• Shows improved respiratory status and normal respiratory rate, depth, and pattern
2. Encourage deep breathing, coughing, and the use of incentive spirometry.	2. Prevents atelectasis and promotes adequate ventilation.	• Takes deep breaths, coughs and uses incentive spirometry
3. Verify with the provider orders to administer any hypnotic and sedative until euthyroid state achieved. If these medications are needed, monitor for adverse side effects.	3. Patients with hypothyroidism are susceptible to respiratory depression with the use of hypnotics and sedatives.	• Explains rationale for cautious use of medications • Maintains adequate oxygenation
4. Maintain patient airway through suction and ventilator support if needed (see Chapter 19 for care of patients requiring mechanical ventilation).	4. The use of artificial airway and ventilator support may be necessary.	

NURSING DIAGNOSIS: Risk for impaired cardiac function associated with altered metabolism
GOAL: Improved cardiac status and maintenance of adequate cardiac output

Nursing Interventions	Rationale	Expected Outcomes
1. Assess heart rate and rhythm and blood pressure	1. Identifies patient's baseline to monitor further changes and evaluate effectiveness of interventions	• Shows improved cardiac status and maintenance of normal cardiac pattern
2. Monitor serum cholesterol value and complaints of anginal pain.	2. The presence of atherosclerosis and cardiac disease prior to onset of hypothyroidism/myxedema may contribute to decreased perfusion	• Reports free of anginal pain • Maintains normal sinus rhythm
3. Monitor ECG for the presence of any arrhythmias, especially after thyroid hormone replacement therapy is initiated.	3. Initiation of thyroid therapy enhances the cardiovascular effects of catecholamines.	

NURSING DIAGNOSIS: Risk for impaired thermoregulation
GOAL: Maintenance of normal body temperature

Nursing Interventions	Rationale	Expected Outcomes
1. Provide extra layer of clothing or extra blanket.	1. Minimizes heat loss	• Experiences relief of discomfort and cold intolerance
2. Avoid and discourage the use of external heat source (e.g., heating pads, electric or warming blankets).	2. Reduces risk of peripheral vasodilation and vascular collapse	• Maintains baseline body temperature • Reports adequate feeling of warmth and lack of chilling
3. Monitor patient's body temperature and report decreases from patient's baseline value.	3. Detects decreased body temperature and onset of myxedema coma	• Uses extra layer of clothing or extra blanket
4. Protect from exposure to cold and drafts.	4. Increases patient's level of comfort and decreases further heat loss	• Explains rationale for avoiding external heat source

---

NURSING DIAGNOSIS: Acute confusion associated with altered cardiovascular and respiratory status and depression
GOAL: Improved thought process

Nursing Interventions	Rationale	Expected Outcomes
1. Orient patient to time, place, date, and events around them.	1. Provides reality orientation to patient	• Shows improved cognitive functioning • Identifies time, place, date, and events correctly
2. Provide stimulation through conversation and nonthreatening activities.	2. Provides stimulation within patient's level of tolerance for stress	• Responds appropriately when stimulated
3. Explain to patient and family that change in cognitive and mental functioning is a result of disease process.	3. Reassures patient and family about the cause of the cognitive changes and that a positive outcome is possible with appropriate treatment	• Responds spontaneously as treatment becomes effective • Interacts spontaneously with family and environment

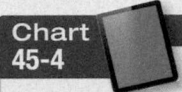

Chart 45-4

PLAN OF NURSING CARE (continued)

Care of the Patient with Hypothyroidism

Nursing Interventions	Rationale	Expected Outcomes
4. Monitor cognitive and mental processes and response of these to medication and other therapy.	4. Permits evaluation of the effectiveness of treatment	• Explains that change in mental and cognitive processes is a result of disease processes • Takes medications as prescribed to prevent decrease in cognitive processes

NURSING DIAGNOSIS: Activity intolerance associated with insufficient physiologic or psychological energy
GOAL: Increased participation in activities and increased independence

Nursing Interventions	Rationale	Expected Outcomes

1. Promote independence in self-care activities.
  a. Space activities to promote rest and exercise as tolerated.
  b. Assist with self-care activities when patient is fatigued.
  c. Provide stimulation through conversation and nonstressful activities.
  d. Monitor patient's response to increasing activities.
	1. Encouragement needed in patients with decreased energy
	  a. Encourages activities while allowing time for adequate rest
	  b. Permits patient to participate to the extent possible in self-care activities
	  c. Promotes interest without stressing the patient
	  d. Guards against over- and underexertion by the patient
		• Participates in self-care activities
		• Reports increased level of energy
		• Displays interest and awareness in environment
		• Participates in activities and events in environment
		• Participates in family events and activities
		• Reports free of chest pain, increased fatigue, or breathlessness with increased level of activity

NURSING DIAGNOSIS: Constipation associated with diminished gastrointestinal peristalsis
GOAL: Return of normal bowel function

Nursing Interventions	Rationale	Expected Outcomes
1. Encourage increased fluid intake within limits of fluid restriction. 2. Provide foods high in fiber. 3. Instruct patient about foods with high water content. 4. Monitor bowel function. 5. Encourage increased mobility within patient's exercise tolerance. 6. Encourage patient to use laxatives and enemas sparingly.	1. Promotes passage of soft stools 2. Increases bulk of stools and more frequent bowel movements 3. Provides rationale for patient to increase fluid intake 4. Permits detection of constipation and return to normal bowel pattern 5. Promotes evacuation of the bowel 6. Minimizes patient's dependence on laxatives and enemas and encourages normal pattern of bowel evacuation	• Reports normal bowel function • Identifies and consumes foods high in fiber • Drinks recommended amount of fluid each day • Participates in gradually increasing exercises • Uses laxatives as prescribed and avoids excessive dependence on laxatives and enemas

NURSING DIAGNOSIS: Lack of knowledge about the therapeutic regimen for lifelong thyroid replacement therapy
GOAL: Knowledge and acceptance of the prescribed therapeutic regimen

Nursing Interventions	Rationale	Expected Outcomes
1. Explain rationale for thyroid hormone replacement. 2. Describe desired effects of medication to patient. 3. Assist patient to develop schedule and checklist to ensure self-administration of thyroid replacement. 4. Describe signs and symptoms of over- and underdose of medication. 5. Explain the necessity for long-term follow-up to patient and family.	1. Provides rationale for patient to use thyroid hormone replacement as prescribed 2. Provides encouragement to patient by identifying improved physical status and well-being that will occur with thyroid hormone therapy and return to a euthyroid state 3. Increases chances that medication will be taken as prescribed 4. Serves as check for patient to determine if therapeutic goals are met 5. Increases likelihood that hypo- or hyperthyroidism will be detected and treated	• Describes therapeutic regimen correctly • Explains rationale for thyroid hormone replacement • Identifies positive outcomes of thyroid hormone replacement • Administers medication to self as prescribed • Identifies adverse side effects that should be reported promptly to primary provider: recurrence of symptoms of hypothyroidism and occurrence of symptoms of hyperthyroidism • Restates need for periodic/long-term follow-up visits to primary provider

(continued on page 1460)

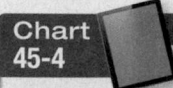

Chart 45-4

PLAN OF NURSING CARE (continued)

Care of the Patient with Hypothyroidism

COLLABORATIVE PROBLEM: Myxedema and myxedema coma
GOAL: Evidence of progression to pre-coma baseline without incurring additional complications

Nursing Interventions	Rationale	Expected Outcomes

1. Monitor patient for increasing severity of signs and symptoms of hypothyroidism:
  a. Decreased level of consciousness
  b. Decreased vital signs (blood pressure, respiratory rate, temperature, pulse rate)
  c. Increasing difficulty in awakening or arousing patient
	1. Extreme hypothyroidism may lead to myxedema, myxedema coma, and slowing of all body systems if untreated	• Exhibits reversal of myxedema and myxedema coma
		• Responds appropriately to questions and surroundings
		• Vital signs return to normal or near-normal ranges
		• Respiratory status improves with adequate spontaneous ventilatory effort
		• Reports free of angina or other indicators of cardiac insufficiency
		• Experiences minimal or no complications caused by immobility

2. Assist in ventilator support if respiratory depression and failure occur.	2. Ventilator support is necessary to maintain adequate oxygenation and maintenance of airway	
3. Administer prescribed medications (e.g., thyroxine) with extreme caution.	3. The slow metabolism and atherosclerosis of myxedema may result in angina with administration of thyroxine	
4. Turn and reposition patient at least every 2 hours.	4. Minimizes risks associated with immobility	
5. Avoid the use of hypnotic, sedative and analgesic agents.	5. Altered metabolism of these agents greatly increases the risks of their use in myxedema	

Quality and Safety Nursing Alert

Medications are given to the patient with hypothyroidism with extreme caution because of the potential for altered metabolism and excretion, as well as depressed metabolic rate and respiratory status.

Promoting Home, Community-Based, and Transitional Care

Educating Patients About Self-Care

The patient and family require education and support to manage this complex disorder at home. Oral and written instructions should be provided regarding the following:

• The importance of life-long therapy and the need to take thyroid medication everyday

• Desired actions and side effects of medications
• Correct medication administration ("Take first thing in the morning with a full glass of water on an empty stomach.")
• Importance of continuing to take the medications as prescribed even after symptoms improve
• When to seek medical attention
• Importance of nutrition and diet to promote weight loss and normal bowel patterns
• Importance of periodic follow-up testing

The patient and family should be educated that the symptoms observed during the course of the disorder will disappear with effective treatment (see Chart 45-5).

Continuing and Transitional Care

If indicated, a referral is made for home, community-based or transitional care. The nurse monitors the patient's recovery

Chart 45-5

HOME CARE CHECKLIST

The Patient with Hypothyroidism (Myxedema)

At the completion of education, the patient and/or caregiver will be able to:

• State the impact of hypothyroidism and treatment on physiologic functioning, ADLs, IADLs, roles, relationships, and spirituality.
• State the need to avoid extreme cold temperature until condition is stable.
• State precipitating factors and interventions for complications (hyperthyroidism, myxedema coma).
• State the continuing potential effects of hypothyroidism on the body.
• State the potential for menstrual irregularities and potential for pregnancy in women.

• State the importance of avoiding infection.
• Relate how to reach primary provider with questions or complications.
• State time and date of follow-up medical appointments, therapy, and testing.
• Identify sources of support (e.g., friends, relatives, faith community).
• Identify the contact details for support services for patients and their caregivers/families.
• Identify the need for health promotion, disease prevention, and screening activities.

ADLs, activities of daily living; IADLs, instrumental activities of daily living.

and ability to cope with changes, and assesses the patient's physical and cognitive status and the patient's and family's understanding of previous education. The nurse documents and reports to the patient's primary provider subtle signs and symptoms that may indicate either inadequate or excessive thyroid hormone.

Gerontologic Considerations

The prevalence of hypothyroidism increases with age, most often among women (Calsolaro, Niccolai, Pasqualetti, et al., 2019). The higher prevalence of hypothyroidism among older adults may be related to age-related alterations in immune function and complicated by multiple comorbidities.

Most patients with primary hypothyroidism present with long-standing mild to moderate hypothyroidism. Subclinical disease is common among older women and can be asymptomatic or mistaken for other medical conditions. Subtle symptoms of hypothyroidism, such as fatigue, muscle aches, and mental confusion, may be attributed to the normal aging process by patients, families, and health care providers; therefore, these symptoms require close attention (Calsolaro et al., 2019). In addition, signs and symptoms of hypothyroidism in older adults are often atypical, and manifestations of hypothyroidism and hyperthyroidism may blur. Patients may have few or no symptoms until dysfunction is severe. Depression, apathy, and decreased mobility or activity may be the major initial symptoms and may be accompanied by significant weight loss. Constipation affects one fourth of older patients.

In those with mild to moderate hypothyroidism, thyroid hormone replacement is individually tailored and must be started with low dosages and increased gradually to prevent serious cardiovascular side effects (Calsolaro et al., 2019). Angina, for example, may occur with rapid thyroid replacement in the presence of coronary artery disease secondary to the hypothyroid state. Heart failure and tachyarrhythmias may worsen during the transition from the hypothyroid state to the normal metabolic state. Dementia may become more apparent during early thyroid hormone replacement in older patients with concomitant dementia.

Older patients with severe hypothyroidism and atherosclerosis may become confused and agitated if their metabolic rate is increased too quickly. Marked clinical improvement follows the administration of hormone replacement; such medication must be continued for life, even though signs of hypothyroidism disappear within 3 to 12 weeks.

Older patients require periodic follow-up monitoring of serum TSH levels, because poor adherence with therapy may occur or the patient may take the medications erratically. A careful history can identify the need for further education about the importance of the medication.

Hyperthyroidism

Hyperthyroidism, a common endocrine disorder, is a form of **thyrotoxicosis** resulting from an excessive synthesis and secretion of endogenous or exogenous thyroid hormones by the thyroid (Norris, 2019). The most common causes are Graves disease, toxic multinodular goiter, and toxic adenoma. Other causes include **thyroiditis** (inflammation of the thyroid gland) and excessive ingestion of thyroid hormone.

Graves disease is an autoimmune disorder that results from an excessive output of thyroid hormones caused by abnormal stimulation of the thyroid gland by circulating immunoglobulins. This disease affects women eight times more frequently than men, with onset usually between the second and fourth decades. The disorder may appear after an emotional shock, stress, or an infection, but the exact significance of these relationships is not understood (Norris, 2019).

Clinical Manifestations

Patients with hyperthyroidism exhibit a characteristic group of signs and symptoms (see Fig. 45-6). Clinical manifestations are related to the increase in metabolic rate and increased oxygen consumption. The patient may appear anxious, seem restless and irritable, and exhibit fine tremors of the hands. The patient will be tachycardic and complain of palpitations.

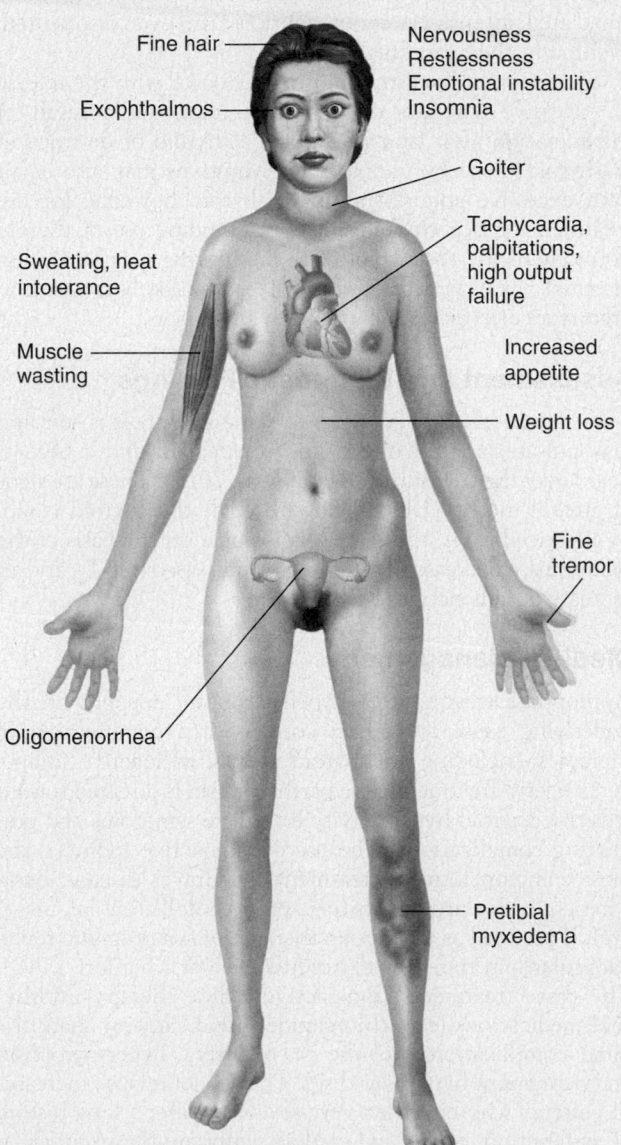

Fine hair

Exophthalmos

Nervousness
Restlessness
Emotional instability
Insomnia

Goiter

Tachycardia, palpitations, high output failure

Sweating, heat intolerance

Muscle wasting

Increased appetite

Weight loss

Fine tremor

Oligomenorrhea

Pretibial myxedema

Figure 45-6 • Clinical manifestations of hyperthyroidism. Reprinted with permission from Norris, T. L. (2019). *Porth's pathophysiology: Concepts of altered health states* (10th ed., Fig. 41.5). Philadelphia, PA: Wolters Kluwer.

Heat intolerance will be noted with increased perspiration. Additional clinical manifestations include an increase in appetite, diarrhea, weight loss, and thin skin. Patients with Graves disease may present with exophthalmos and may exhibit reduced blinking and lid retraction. Treatment may not reverse ocular manifestations (Medford, 2019). Women experience changes in menstruation including oligomenorrhea (Lee & Khardori, 2018).

Cardiac effects may include sinus tachycardia or arrhythmias, decreased cardiac output, increased pulse pressure, and palpitations; these changes may be related to increased sensitivity to catecholamines or to changes in neurotransmitter turnover. Myocardial hypertrophy and heart failure may occur if the hyperthyroidism is severe and untreated.

The course of the disease may be mild, characterized by remissions and exacerbations, and terminate with spontaneous recovery in a few months or years. Conversely, it may progress relentlessly, with the untreated person becoming emaciated, intensely nervous, delirious, and even disoriented; eventually, the heart fails.

Symptoms of hyperthyroidism may occur with the release of excessive amounts of thyroid hormone as a result of inflammation after irradiation of the thyroid or destruction of thyroid tissue by tumor. Such symptoms may also occur with excessive administration of thyroid hormone for the treatment of hypothyroidism. Long-standing use of thyroid hormone in the absence of close monitoring may be a cause of symptoms of hyperthyroidism. It is also likely to result in premature osteoporosis, particularly in women.

Assessment and Diagnostic Findings

The thyroid gland is enlarged to some extent. It is soft and may pulsate; a thrill often can be palpated, and a bruit is heard over the thyroid arteries (Norris, 2019). These are signs of greatly increased blood flow through the thyroid gland. In advanced cases, the diagnosis is made on the basis of the symptoms, a decrease in serum TSH, increased free T_4, and an increase in radioactive iodine uptake.

Medical Management

Appropriate treatment of hyperthyroidism depends on the underlying cause and often consists of a combination of therapies, including antithyroid agents, radioactive iodine, and surgery. Treatment of hyperthyroidism is directed toward reducing thyroid hyperactivity to relieve symptoms and preventing complications. The use of radioactive iodine is the most common form of treatment for Graves disease. Beta-adrenergic blocking agents (e.g., propranolol, atenolol, metoprolol) are used as adjunctive therapy for symptomatic relief, particularly in transient thyroiditis (Lee & Khardori, 2018). The three treatments (radioactive iodine therapy, antithyroid medications [e.g., thionamides], and surgery) share the same complications: relapse or recurrent hyperthyroidism and permanent hypothyroidism. The rate of relapse increases in patients who have had very severe disease, a long history of dysfunction, ocular and cardiac symptoms, large goiter, or relapse after previous treatment. Patients with Graves disease may sustain remission for up to 12 to 18 months but often experience recurrence within 12 months of treatment (Lee & Khardori, 2018).

Pharmacologic Therapy

Two forms of pharmacotherapy are available for treating hyperthyroidism and controlling excessive thyroid activity: (1) the use of irradiation by administration of the radioisotope ^{131}I for destructive effects on the thyroid gland and (2) antithyroid medications that interfere with the synthesis of thyroid hormones and other agents that control manifestations of hyperthyroidism.

Radioactive Iodine Therapy

Radioactive iodine has been used to treat toxic adenomas, toxic multinodular goiter, and most varieties of thyrotoxicosis and is considered the treatment of choice because a single dose is effective in treating 80% to 90% of cases (Bauerle & Clutter, 2019). Radioactive iodine is contraindicated during pregnancy because it crosses the placenta. Women of childbearing age should be given a pregnancy test 48 hours before administration of radioactive iodine. They should also be instructed to not conceive for at least 6 months following treatment. In addition, breast-feeding for up to 6 weeks prior to radioactive iodine treatment is contraindicated (Lee & Khardori, 2018).

The goal of radioactive iodine therapy (^{131}I) is to eliminate the hyperthyroid state with the administration of sufficient radiation in a single dose (Lee & Khardori, 2018). Almost all of the iodine that enters and is retained in the body becomes concentrated in the thyroid gland. Therefore, the radioactive isotope of iodine is concentrated in the thyroid gland, where it destroys thyroid cells without jeopardizing other radiosensitive tissues. Over a period of several weeks, thyroid cells exposed to the radioactive iodine are destroyed, resulting in reduction of the hyperthyroid state and inevitably hypothyroidism.

The use of an ablative dose of radioactive iodine initially causes an acute release of thyroid hormone from the thyroid gland and may cause increased symptoms. The patient is observed for signs of **thyroid storm** (see Chart 45-6), a life-threatening condition manifested by cardiac arrhythmias, fever, and neurologic impairment (Norris, 2019) which may lead to heart failure, circulatory collapse and dangerous elevation of body temperature, all related to the increase in metabolism. Beta-blockers are used to control these symptoms.

Thyroid hormone replacement is started 4 to 18 weeks after the antithyroid medications have been stopped based on the results of thyroid function tests. TSH measurements can be misleading in the early months following treatment with radioactive iodine. Therefore, serum free T_4 is the principal test measured at 3 to 6 weeks following administration of radioactive iodine and then every 1 to 2 months until normal thyroid function is established. If TSH and free T_4 are both persistently low, the total T_3 then must be measured to differentiate between persistent hyperthyroidism (T_3 elevated) or transient hypothyroidism (T_3 normal or low). Once a normal thyroid state has been established, TSH should be measured every 6 to 12 months for life (Fischbach & Fischbach, 2018).

A major advantage of treatment with radioactive iodine is that it avoids many of the side effects associated with antithyroid medications. However, some patients may elect to be treated with antithyroid medications rather than radioactive iodine for a variety of reasons, including fear of radiation.

Chart 45-6 Thyroid Storm (Thyrotoxic Crisis, Thyrotoxicosis)

Thyroid storm (thyrotoxic crisis) is a form of severe hyperthyroidism, usually of abrupt onset. Untreated, it is almost always fatal, but with proper treatment the mortality rate is reduced substantially. The patient with thyroid storm or crisis is critically ill and requires astute observation and aggressive and supportive nursing care during and after the acute stage of illness.

Clinical Manifestations

Thyroid storm is characterized by:

- Hyperpyrexia (high fever), >38.5°C (>101.3°F)
- Extreme tachycardia (>130 bpm)
- Exaggerated symptoms of hyperthyroidism with disturbances of a major system—for example, gastrointestinal (weight loss, diarrhea, abdominal pain) or cardiovascular (edema, chest pain, dyspnea, palpitations)
- Altered neurologic or mental state, which frequently appears as delirium psychosis, somnolence, or coma

Life-threatening thyroid storm is usually precipitated by stress, such as injury, infection, thyroid and nonthyroid surgery, tooth extraction, insulin reaction, diabetic ketoacidosis, pregnancy, digitalis intoxication, abrupt withdrawal of antithyroid medications, extreme emotional stress, or vigorous palpation of the thyroid. These factors can precipitate thyroid storm in the partially controlled or completely untreated patient with hyperthyroidism. Current methods of diagnosis and treatment for hyperthyroidism have greatly decreased the incidence of thyroid storm, making it uncommon today.

Management

Immediate objectives are reduction of body temperature and heart rate and prevention of vascular collapse. Measures to accomplish these objectives include:

- A hypothermia mattress or blanket, ice packs, a cool environment, hydrocortisone, and acetaminophen. Salicylates (e.g., aspirin) are not used because they displace thyroid hormone from binding proteins and worsen the hypermetabolism.
- Humidified oxygen is given to improve tissue oxygenation and meet the high metabolic demands. Arterial blood gas levels or pulse oximetry may be used to monitor respiratory status.
- IV fluids containing dextrose are given to replace liver glycogen stores that have been decreased in the patient who is hyperthyroid.
- Propylthiouracil or methimazole is given to impede formation of thyroid hormone and block conversion of T_4 to T_3, the more active form of thyroid hormone.
- Hydrocortisone is prescribed to treat shock or adrenal insufficiency.
- Iodine is given to decrease output of T_4 from the thyroid gland. For cardiac problems such as atrial fibrillation, arrhythmias, and heart failure, sympatholytic agents may be given. Propranolol, combined with digitalis, has been effective in reducing severe cardiac symptoms.

T_3, triiodothyronine; T_4, thyroxine.

Adapted from Morton, P. G., & Fontaine, D. K. (2018). *Critical care nursing: A holistic approach* (10th ed.). Philadelphia, PA: Wolters Kluwer; Comerford, K. C., & Durkin, M. T. (2020). *Nursing 2020 drug handbook*. Philadelphia, PA: Wolters Kluwer.

Patients who receive radioactive iodine should be informed that they can contaminate their household and other people through saliva, urine, or radiation emitting from their body. They should avoid sexual contact, sleeping in the same bed with other people, having close contact with children and pregnant women, and sharing utensils and cups. The patient should follow the instructions provided regarding the time restrictions for these cautions because they are dose related (Fischbach & Fischbach, 2018).

Antithyroid Medications

Antithyroid medications (thionamides) are summarized in Table 45-1. The objective of pharmacotherapy is to inhibit one or more stages in thyroid hormone synthesis or hormone release. Antithyroid agents block the utilization of iodine by interfering with the iodination of tyrosine and the coupling of iodotyrosines in the synthesis of thyroid hormones. This prevents the synthesis of thyroid hormone. The most commonly used antithyroid drugs in the United States are methimazole or propylthiouracil. The medications are used until the patient is euthyroid (i.e., neither hyperthyroid nor hypothyroid). These medications block extrathyroidal conversion of T_4 to T_3 (Bauerle & Clutter, 2019).

Prior to initiating therapy with these drugs, baseline blood tests are performed, including complete blood count (white blood cell [WBC] count with differential) and liver profile (transaminases and bilirubin) (Bauerle & Clutter, 2019). The therapeutic dose is determined on the basis of clinical criteria, including changes in pulse rate, pulse pressure, body weight, size of the goiter, and results of laboratory studies. The patient should be instructed to take the medication in the morning on an empty stomach 30 minutes before eating to avoid decrease in absorption associated with some foods such as walnuts, soybean flour, cottonseed meal, and dietary fiber. Because antithyroid medications do not interfere with release or activity of previously formed thyroid hormones, it may take several weeks until symptom relief occurs. At that time, the maintenance dose is established, and the medication is gradually tapered over several months.

Toxic complications of antithyroid medications are relatively uncommon; nevertheless, the importance of periodic follow-up is emphasized, because medication sensitization, fever, rash, urticaria, or even agranulocytosis and thrombocytopenia (decrease in granulocytes and platelets) may develop (Bauerle & Clutter, 2019). With any sign of infection, especially pharyngitis and fever or the occurrence of mouth ulcers, the patient is advised to stop the medication, notify the primary provider immediately, and undergo hematologic studies (Bauerle & Clutter, 2019). Propylthiouracil is recommended during the first trimester of pregnancy rather than methimazole due to the teratogenic effects of methimazole. Due to risk of hepatotoxicity, propylthiouracil should be discontinued after the first trimester and the patient should be switched to methimazole for the remainder of the pregnancy and when breast-feeding (Bauerle & Clutter, 2019).

TABLE 45-1 Pharmacologic Agents Used to Treat Hyperthyroidism		
Agent	**Action**	**Nursing Considerations**
Propylthiouracil	Blocks synthesis of hormones (conversion of T_4 to T_3)	Monitor cardiac parameters. Observe for conversion to hypothyroidism. Must be given by mouth. Watch for rash, nausea, vomiting, agranulocytosis, SLE.
Methimazole	Inhibits synthesis of thyroid hormone	More toxic than propylthiouracil. Watch for rash and other symptoms as for propylthiouracil.
Sodium iodide	Suppresses release of thyroid hormone	Given 1 h after propylthiouracil or methimazole. Watch for edema, hemorrhage, gastrointestinal upset.
Potassium iodide	Suppresses release of thyroid hormone	Discontinue for rash. Watch for signs of toxic iodinism.
Saturated solution of potassium iodide (SSKI)	Suppresses release of thyroid hormone	Mix with juice or milk. Given by straw to prevent staining of teeth.
Beta-blocker (e.g., propranolol)	Beta-adrenergic blocking agent	Monitor cardiac status. Hold for bradycardia or decreased cardiac output. Use with caution in patients with heart failure.

SLE, systemic lupus erythematosus; T_3, triiodothyronine; T_4, thyroxine.
Adapted from Bauerle, K. T., & Clutter, W. E. (2019). Hyperthyroidism. In T. J. Braranski, J. B. McGill, & J. M. Silverstein (Eds.). *The Washington manual endocrinology subspecialty consult* (4th ed.). Philadelphia, PA: Wolters Kluwer; Comerford, K. C., & Durkin, M. T. (2020). *Nursing 2020 drug handbook*. Philadelphia, PA: Wolters Kluwer.

Discontinuation of antithyroid medications before therapy is complete usually results in relapse within 6 months. It is important that the possibility of relapse be discussed so that a treatment strategy will be in place if relapse occurs.

Adjunctive Therapy

Additional medications may be necessary. Potassium iodide (SSKI) may be used in combination with antithyroid agents or beta-adrenergic blockers to prepare the patient with hyperthyroidism for surgery. The drugs reduce the effects of hyperthyroidism quickly and help to prevent the onset of thyroid storm. The usual dosage for SSKI is 5 drops every 6 hours. The usual dose of propylthiouracil is 200 mg every 6 hours and the usual dose of propranolol is 60 to 80 mg orally every 6 hours to prevent tachycardia. The patient will need to continue to take the propylthiouracil and any cardiac medication until the free T_4 and T_3 levels are near normal (Bauerle & Clutter, 2019).

Surgical Management

Surgery to remove thyroid tissue is reserved for special circumstances, for example, in pregnant women who are allergic to antithyroid medications, in patients with large goiters, or in patients who are unable to take antithyroid agents. Surgery for treatment of hyperthyroidism is performed soon after the thyroid function has returned to normal (4 to 6 weeks).

The surgical removal of about five sixths of the thyroid tissue (subtotal thyroidectomy) reliably results in a prolonged remission in most patients with exophthalmic goiter. Its use today is reserved for patients with obstructive symptoms, some pregnant women, and for patients with a need for rapid normalization of thyroid function. Before surgery, an antithyroid medication is given until signs of hyperthyroidism have disappeared. A beta-adrenergic blocking agent (e.g., propranolol) may be used to reduce the heart rate and other signs and symptoms of hyperthyroidism. Medications that may prolong clotting (e.g., aspirin) are stopped several weeks before surgery to reduce the risk of postoperative bleeding. Patients receiving iodine medication must be monitored for evidence of iodine toxicity, which requires immediate withdrawal of the medication. Symptoms of toxicity include mucosa membranes stained brown, burning pain in the mouth and esophagus, laryngeal edema, and shock (Fischbach & Fischbach, 2018).

Gerontologic Considerations

Although hyperthyroidism is much less common in older adults than hypothyroidism, patients 65 years and older need careful assessment to avoid missing subtle signs and symptoms. This age group may present with atypical vague and nonspecific signs and symptoms of thyroid disease such as anorexia and weight loss with absence of ocular signs, or isolated atrial fibrillation (Morton & Fontaine, 2018). New or worsening heart failure or angina is more likely to occur in older patients rather than in younger patients. Symptoms such as tachycardia, fatigue, mental confusion, weight loss, change in bowel habits, and depression can be attributed to age and other illnesses that are common in older adults (Eliopoulos, 2018). The older patient may complain of difficulty climbing stairs or rising from a chair because of muscle weakness. Evaluation for thyroid disease with a serum TSH measurement is indicated in older patients who have unexplained physical or mental deterioration (Samuels, 2018). Free T_4 and T_3 should be included in the initial screening when hyperthyroidism is highly suspected. Once thyrotoxicosis is confirmed, additional tests such as radioactive iodine uptake and thyroid scan are prescribed to differentiate between causes such as Graves disease, toxic nodular goiter, acute thyroiditis, and other disorders. Toxic nodular goiter is the most common cause of thyrotoxicosis in older patients. Patients have the option of treatment using antithyroid medications, radioactive iodine, and surgery. Radioactive iodine is generally recommended for treatment of thyrotoxicosis caused by toxic nodular goiter in older patients unless an enlarged thyroid gland is pressing on the airway. Long-term use of certain antithyroid medications such as propylthiouracil is not recommended for treatment of hyperthyroidism in older adults due to potential side effects (Samuels, 2018).

The use of beta-adrenergic blocking agents (e.g., propranolol and atenolol) may be indicated to decrease the cardiovascular and neurologic signs and symptoms of thyrotoxicosis. These agents must be used with extreme caution in older patients to minimize adverse effects on cardiac function that may produce heart failure. The dosage of other medications used to treat other chronic illnesses in older patients may also need to be modified because of the altered rate of metabolism associated with hyperthyroidism.

NURSING PROCESS

The Patient with Hyperthyroidism

Assessment

The health history and examination focus on symptoms related to accelerated or exaggerated metabolism. These include the patient's and family's reports of irritability and increased emotional reaction and the impact that these changes have had on the patient's interactions with family, friends, and coworkers. The history includes other stressors and the patient's ability to cope with stress.

The nurse initially and periodically assesses the patient's nutritional status and the presence of symptoms related to the hypermetabolic state. This hypermetabolic state may affect the cardiovascular system, causing changes in vital signs including heart rate and rhythm, blood pressure, heart sounds, and peripheral pulses. Other specific changes may include alteration in vision and appearance of the external eye. Because emotional changes are associated with hyperthyroidism, the patient's emotional state and psychological status are evaluated, as well as such symptoms as irritability, anxiety, sleep disturbances, apathy, and lethargy, all of which may occur with hyperthyroidism (Bauerle & Clutter, 2019). The family may also provide information about recent changes in the patient's emotional status.

Diagnosis

NURSING DIAGNOSES

Based on the assessment data, major priority nursing diagnoses may include the following:
- Risk for impaired cardiac function associated with alteration in heart rate and rhythm.
- Impaired nutritional status associated with exaggerated metabolic rate, excessive appetite, and increased GI activity
- Difficulty coping associated with irritability, hyperexcitability, apprehension, and emotional instability
- Situational low self-esteem associated with changes in appearance, excessive appetite, and weight loss
- Risk for impaired thermoregulation

COLLABORATIVE PROBLEMS/POTENTIAL COMPLICATIONS

Potential complications may include the following:
- Thyrotoxicosis or thyroid storm
- Hypothyroidism

Planning and Goals

The major goals for the patient may include maintenance of adequate cardiac function, maintenance of adequate nutritional status, improved coping ability, improved self-esteem, maintenance of normal body temperature, and absence of complications.

Nursing Interventions

MAINTAINING ADEQUATE CARDIAC OUTPUT

Due to the effects of hyperthyroidism on the cardiac system, it is important to critically assess vital signs, especially heart rate and rhythm and body temperature. Nurses need to be alert to complaints of palpitations which may be reported as "my heart is racing." The nurse monitors the patient for signs of heart failure (dyspnea, jugular vein distention, crackles, and peripheral edema; see Chapter 25).

In the presence of thyroid storm the patient should be placed on a cardiac monitor in order to adequately monitor for arrhythmias. Monitoring of electrolytes and strict I&O assessment is also essential. The nurse is prepared to administer beta-blockers as prescribed. Acetaminophen is the drug of choice to reduce elevated body temperature because medications containing salicylates may result in higher levels of unbound thyroid hormone. A cooling blanket as well as a cool environment may also be needed.

IMPROVING NUTRITIONAL STATUS

Hyperthyroidism affects all body systems, including the GI system. Rapid movement of food through the GI tract may result in nutritional imbalance and weight loss. In addition, the patient will report an increased appetite and should be encouraged to eat small frequent nutritious meals. If necessary, the patient is referred to a nutritionist or dietician to develop a meal plan to address dietary concerns.

Foods and fluids are selected to replace fluid lost through diarrhea and diaphoresis and to control the diarrhea that results from increased peristalsis. To reduce diarrhea, highly seasoned foods, coffee, tea, cola, and alcohol are discouraged while high-calorie, high-protein foods are encouraged. A quiet atmosphere during mealtime may aid digestion. The patient should be encouraged to record weight and dietary intake.

ENHANCING COPING MEASURES

The patient with hyperthyroidism needs reassurance that the emotional reactions being experienced are a result of the disorder and that with effective treatment those symptoms will be controlled. Because of the negative effect that these symptoms can have on family and friends, they too need reassurance that the symptoms are expected to disappear with treatment. A calm, unhurried approach is beneficial for the patient. Stressful experiences should be minimized and a quiet, uncluttered environment should be maintained. The patient should be instructed to balance periods of activity with rest.

If a thyroidectomy is planned, the patient needs to know that pharmacologic therapy is necessary to prepare the thyroid gland for surgical treatment. The nurse provides education and reminds the patient to take the medications as prescribed. Because of hyperexcitability and shortened attention span, the patient may require repetition of this education and written instructions.

IMPROVING SELF-ESTEEM

The patient with hyperthyroidism is likely to experience changes in appearance, appetite, and weight. These factors, along with the patient's inability to cope well with family and the illness, may result in loss of self-esteem. The nurse conveys an understanding of the patient's concern about these problems and promotes the use of effective coping strategies. The patient and family should be reassured that these changes are a result of the thyroid dysfunction and are, in fact, out of the patient's control. The nurse refers the patient to professional counseling as necessary.

If the patient experiences ocular changes secondary to hyperthyroidism, eye care and protection may be necessary. The nurse educates the patient about instillation of eye drops or ointment prescribed to soothe the eyes and protect the exposed corneas. Smoking should be highly discouraged, and smoking cessation strategies are recommended. The patient may be embarrassed by the need to eat large meals. The nurse explains the need for increased food consumption to caregivers and family members in order to address the possibility of their commenting on the patient's increased appetite.

MAINTAINING NORMAL BODY TEMPERATURE

The patient with hyperthyroidism frequently finds a normal room temperature too warm because of an exaggerated metabolic rate and increased heat production. If the patient is hospitalized, the environment should be maintained at a cool, comfortable temperature, and the bedding and clothing should be changed as needed. Cool baths and cool or cold fluids may also provide relief.

MONITORING AND MANAGING POTENTIAL COMPLICATIONS

The nurse closely monitors the patient with hyperthyroidism for signs and symptoms that may be indicative of thyroid storm. Cardiac and respiratory functions are assessed by measuring vital signs and cardiac output, electrocardiographic (ECG) monitoring, arterial blood gases, and pulse oximetry. Assessment continues after treatment is initiated because of the potential effects of treatment on cardiac function. Oxygen is given to prevent hypoxia, to improve tissue oxygenation, and to meet the high metabolic demands. IV fluids may be necessary to maintain blood glucose levels and to replace lost fluids. Antithyroid medications (methimazole or propylthiouracil) may be prescribed to reduce thyroid hormone levels. In addition, beta-blockers and digitalis may be prescribed to treat cardiac symptoms. If shock develops, treatment strategies must be implemented (see Chapter 11).

Hypothyroidism is likely to occur with any of the treatments used for hyperthyroidism. Therefore, the nurse periodically monitors the patient. Most patients report a greatly improved sense of well-being after treatment of hyperthyroidism, and some fail to continue to take prescribed thyroid replacement therapy. Therefore, part of patient and family education is instruction about the importance of continuing therapy indefinitely after discharge and a discussion of the consequences of failing to take medication.

PROMOTING HOME, COMMUNITY-BASED, AND TRANSITIONAL CARE

Educating Patients About Self-Care. The nurse educates the patient with hyperthyroidism about how and when to take prescribed medication and provides education about the essential role of the medication in the broader therapeutic plan. Because of the hyperexcitability and decreased attention span associated with hyperthyroidism, the nurse provides a written plan for the patient to take home and use. The type and amount of information given depend on the patient's stress and anxiety levels. The patient and family members receive verbal and written education about the actions and possible side effects of the medications as well as adverse effects that should be reported if they occur (see Chart 45-7).

Chart 45-7 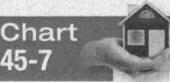 HOME CARE CHECKLIST
The Patient with Hyperthyroidism

At the completion of education, the patient and/or caregiver will be able to:

- State the impact of hyperthyroidism, treatment on physiologic functioning, ADLs, IADLs, roles, relationships, and spirituality.
- State that emotional lability is part of disease process.
- Identify the potential for menstrual irregularities and pregnancy, and increased risk of osteoporosis in women.
- State that long-term treatment and follow-up is necessary.
- Describe the potential benefits and risks of surgical intervention or radioactive iodine therapy.
- State the name, dose, side effects, frequency, and schedule for all medications.
- Explain the purpose, dose, route, schedule, side effects, and precautions of treatment of hyperthyroidism (antithyroid medications, radioactive iodine).
- State the need to contact primary provider before taking over-the-counter medications.
- State changes in lifestyle (e.g., diet, activity) necessary to maintain health.
- Identify the need for increased dietary intake until weight stabilizes.

- Identify foods to be avoided.
- Identify the need for planned rest periods and methods to improve sleep patterns.
- Identify areas of stress and management techniques.
- Identify rationale for smoking cessation and steps to stop use of any tobacco product.
- State precipitating factors and interventions for complications (hypothyroidism, thyroid storm).
- Relate how to reach primary provider with questions or complications.
- State time and date of follow-up medical appointments, therapy, and testing.
  - Identify sources of support (e.g., friends, relatives, faith community).
  - Identify the contact details for support services for patients and their caregivers/families.
- Identify the need for health promotion, disease prevention, and screening activities.

ADLs, activities of daily living; IADLs, instrumental activities of daily living.

If a total or subtotal thyroidectomy is anticipated, the patient needs to be educated about what to expect. Information is repeated as the time of surgery approaches. The nurse also advises the patient to avoid stressful situations that may precipitate thyroid storm.

Continuing and Transitional Care. Referral for home, community-based or transitional care, if indicated, allows the nurse to assess the home and family environment, as well as the patient's and family's understanding of the importance of adhering to the therapeutic regimen and the recommended follow-up monitoring. The nurse reinforces to the patient and family the importance of long-term follow-up because of the risk of hypothyroidism after thyroidectomy or treatment with antithyroid medications or radioactive iodine. The patient is assessed for changes indicating return to normal thyroid function and signs and symptoms of hyperthyroidism and hypothyroidism. Furthermore, the patient and family are reminded about the importance of health promotion activities and recommended health screening.

Evaluation

Expected patient outcomes may include:
1. Improved cardiac status
   a. Vital signs within normal limits
   b. Absence of dyspnea, crackles, and peripheral edema
   c. Reports absence of palpitations
2. Improved nutritional status
   a. Reports adequate dietary intake and decreased hunger
   b. Identifies high-calorie, high-protein foods; identifies foods to be avoided
   c. Avoids the use of alcohol and stimulants
   d. Stops smoking
   e. Reports decreased episodes of diarrhea
3. Demonstrates effective coping methods in dealing with family, friends, and coworkers
   a. Explains reasons for irritability and emotional instability
   b. Avoids stressful situations, events, and people
   c. Participates in relaxing, nonstressful activities
4. Achieves increased self-esteem
   a. Verbalizes feelings about self and illness
   b. Describes feelings of frustration and loss of control
   c. Describes reasons for increased appetite
5. Maintains normal body temperature
6. Absence of complications
   a. Serum thyroid hormone and TSH levels within normal limits
   b. Identifies signs and symptoms of thyroid storm and hypothyroidism
   c. Vital signs and results of ECG, arterial blood gases, and pulse oximetry within normal limits
   d. States importance of regular follow-up and lifelong maintenance of prescribed therapy

Thyroid Tumors

Tumors of the thyroid gland are classified on the basis of being benign or malignant, the presence or absence of associated thyrotoxicosis, and the diffuse or irregular quality of the glandular enlargement. If the enlargement is sufficient to cause a visible swelling in the neck, the tumor is referred to as a goiter.

All grades of goiter are encountered, from those that are barely visible to those producing disfigurement. Some are symmetric and diffuse; others are nodular. Some are accompanied by hyperthyroidism, in which case they are described as toxic; others are associated with a euthyroid state and are referred to as nontoxic goiters.

Endemic (Iodine-Deficient) Goiter

The most common type of goiter that occurs when iodine intake is deficient is the simple or colloid goiter. In addition to being caused by an iodine deficiency, simple goiter may be caused by an intake of large quantities of goitrogenic substances in patients with unusually susceptible glands. These substances include excessive amounts of iodine. Lithium prescribed for the treatment of bipolar disorder has also been found to also have antithyroid actions (Singh & Clutter, 2019).

Simple goiter is a compensatory hypertrophy of the thyroid gland, caused by stimulation by the pituitary gland. The pituitary gland produces thyrotropin or TSH, a hormone that controls the release of thyroid hormone from the thyroid gland. Its production increases if there is subnormal thyroid activity, as when insufficient iodine is available for production of the thyroid hormone. Such goiters usually cause no symptoms, except for the swelling in the neck, which may result in tracheal compression when excessive swelling is present.

Many goiters of this type recede after the iodine imbalance is corrected. Supplementary iodine, such as SSKI, is prescribed to suppress the pituitary's thyroid-stimulating activity. When surgery is indicated, the risk of postoperative complications is minimized by ensuring a preoperative euthyroid state through treatment with antithyroid medications and iodide to reduce the size and vascularity of the goiter. The introduction of iodized salt has been the single most effective means of preventing goiter in at-risk populations.

Nodular Goiter

Some thyroid glands are nodular because of areas of hyperplasia (overgrowth). No symptoms may arise as a result of this condition, but not uncommonly these nodules slowly increase in size, with some descending into the thorax, where they cause local pressure symptoms. Some nodules become malignant, and some are associated with a hyperthyroid state. Therefore, the patient with many thyroid nodules may eventually require surgery.

Thyroid Cancer

Cancer of the thyroid is less prevalent than other forms of cancer; however, the incidence has tripled in the last 30 years (American Cancer Society [ACS], 2019) and accounts for 90% of endocrine malignancies. Although it has the fastest-growing cancer rate among both men and women, women are three times more likely to develop this cancer than men. In addition, thyroid cancer is more likely to develop in patients that are younger than 50 years (ACS, 2019; Yoo, Yu, & Choi, 2018).

Chart 45-8

NURSING RESEARCH PROFILE

Lifestyle Factors and the Risk of Thyroid Cancer

Yoo, Y. G., Yu, B. J., & Choi, E. (2018) A comparison study: The risk factors in the lifestyles of thyroid cancer patients and healthy adults of South Korea. *Cancer Nursing, 41*(1), E48–E56.

Purpose

In South Korea and in the United States, rates of thyroid cancer have increased significantly. This study investigated which risk factors might be influencing the rates of thyroid cancer in South Korea.

Design

This retrospective comparison study compared a group of patients with thyroid cancer to a group of healthy adults. The Health Belief Model framework guided the study. The Lifestyle Measurement Scale was used to assess the 6 domains of dietary habits, alcohol consumption, smoking habits, rest and physical activity, stress management, and annual physical and health screenings. Participants self-completed the surveys.

Findings

There were 217 usable surveys completed. In the patient group ($n = 102$), mean age was 50 years; in the healthy adult group ($n = 115$), 52 years. In both the patient group and the healthy adult group, females made up the majority (85% and 76%, respectively) and most of the participants were married (94% and 93%, respectively). A history of previous smoking, lower physical activity levels, higher stress, and unhealthy eating habits (consumption of more instant food products and fewer vegetables) were all identified as risk factors for developing thyroid cancer.

Nursing Implications

All health care professionals can be instrumental in helping prevent thyroid cancer. Nurses should encourage higher physical activity levels, effective stress management, avoidance of direct and indirect exposure to smoking, and a healthy diet that includes consumption of fewer instant food products and more vegetables to help in prevention efforts.

External radiation of the head, neck, or chest in infancy and childhood increases the risk of thyroid carcinoma. The incidence of thyroid cancer appears to increase 5 to 40 years after irradiation. Consequently, people who underwent radiation treatment or were otherwise exposed to radiation as children should consult their primary provider, request an isotope thyroid scan as part of the evaluation, follow recommended treatment of abnormalities of the gland, and continue with annual checkups.

Additional risk factors that have been identified include smoking, low physical activity, unhealthy eating habits and high stress levels (Yoo et al., 2018). See the Nursing Research Profile in Chart 45-8 for more information on lifestyle risk factors.

Assessment and Diagnostic Findings

Lesions that are single, hard, and fixed on palpation or associated with cervical lymphadenopathy suggest malignancy. Thyroid function tests may be helpful in evaluating thyroid nodules and masses; however, results are rarely conclusive. An ultrasound-guided fine needle biopsy of the thyroid gland is the standard diagnostic procedure for evaluating thyroid nodules. It is performed as an outpatient procedure to make a diagnosis of thyroid cancer, to differentiate cancerous thyroid nodules from noncancerous nodules, and to stage the cancer if detected (Amdur & Dagan, 2019). The procedure is safe and usually requires only a local anesthetic agent. Additional diagnostic studies include ultrasound, MRI, CT, thyroid scans, radioactive iodine uptake studies, and thyroid suppression tests.

Medical Management

The medical management depends on the classification of cell type found on biopsy. The three common groups include well-differentiated thyroid cancer (DTC), papillary thyroid carcinoma (PTC), and follicular thyroid carcinoma (FTC) (Amdur & Dagan, 2019).

The treatment of choice for localized thyroid carcinoma is surgical removal (Amdur & Dagan, 2019). Total or near-total thyroidectomy is performed if possible (ACS, 2019). Modified neck dissection or more extensive radical neck dissection is performed if there is lymph node involvement.

Efforts are made to spare parathyroid tissue to reduce the risk of postoperative hypocalcemia and tetany. After surgery, ablation procedures are carried out with radioactive iodine to eradicate residual microscopic disease (ACS, 2019). Radioactive iodine is also used for thyroid cancers with metastasis (ACS, 2019).

After surgery, thyroid hormone is given to lower the levels of TSH to a euthyroid state (Bauerle & Riek, 2019). If the remaining thyroid tissue is inadequate to produce sufficient thyroid hormone, thyroxine is required permanently.

Several routes are available for administering radiation to the thyroid or tissues of the neck, including oral administration of radioactive iodine (Bauerle & Riek, 2019) and external administration of radiation therapy. Administration of radioactive iodine for DTC is the most successful targeted therapy in oncology (Amdur & Dagan, 2019). Short-term side effects of radioactive iodine treatment may include neck soreness, nausea, and upset stomach; tender and swollen salivary glands; dry mouth; changes in taste; and, rarely, pain (Bauerle & Riek, 2019). The patient who receives external sources of radiation therapy is at risk for mucositis, dryness of the mouth, dysphagia, redness of the skin, anorexia, and fatigue (see Chapter 12). Chemotherapy is infrequently used to treat thyroid cancer.

Patients whose thyroid cancer is detected early, who are younger than 50 years, and who are appropriately treated have a good prognosis (Amdur & Dagan, 2019). Patients who have had papillary cancer—the most common and least aggressive tumor—have the best prognosis of all thyroid cancers (ACS, 2019). Long-term survival is also common in follicular cancer, which is a more aggressive form of thyroid cancer (Bauerle & Riek, 2019). However, continued thyroid hormone therapy and periodic follow-up and diagnostic testing are important to ensure the patient's well-being.

Later follow-up includes clinical assessment for recurrence of nodules or masses in the neck and signs of hoarseness, dysphagia, or dyspnea. The recommendations for long-term follow-up of patients with differentiated thyroid cancer are based on the stage of cancer and results of the follow-up examination 1 year following the initial treatment. The first year evaluation includes clinical examination, TSH and free thyroxine, and measurement of serum thyroglobulin within 6 months following the initial treatment, and a routine neck ultrasound with the first 6 to 12 months following initial treatment. Tests used to confirm sites of metastasis if there is clinical evidence of recurrence include radioiodine imaging, CT, MRI, skeletal x-rays, and skeletal radionucleotide imaging.

Fluorodeoxyglucose (FDG) PET is useful to establish prognosis if there is evidence of distant metastases (ACS, 2019). Free T_4, TSH, and serum calcium and phosphorus levels are monitored to determine whether the thyroid hormone supplementation is adequate and to note whether calcium balance is maintained.

Patient education emphasizes the importance of taking prescribed medications and following recommendations for follow-up monitoring. The patient who is undergoing radiation therapy is also instructed in how to assess and manage side effects of treatment (see Chapter 12).

Nursing Management

Important preoperative goals are to prepare the patient for surgery and reduce anxiety. Often, the patient's home life has become tense because of their restlessness, irritability, and nervousness secondary to hyperthyroidism. Efforts are necessary to protect the patient from tension and stress to avoid precipitating thyroid storm. Suggestions are made to limit stressful situations. Quiet and relaxing activities are encouraged.

Providing Preoperative Care

The nurse educates the patient about the importance of eating a diet high in carbohydrates and proteins. A high daily caloric intake is necessary because of the increased metabolic activity and rapid depletion of glycogen reserves. Supplementary vitamins, particularly thiamine and ascorbic acid, may be prescribed. The patient is reminded to avoid tea, coffee, cola, and other stimulants.

The nurse also informs the patient about the purpose of preoperative tests, if they are to be performed, and explains what preoperative preparations to expect. This information should help to reduce the patient's anxiety about the surgery. In addition, special efforts are made to ensure a good night's rest before surgery.

Preoperative education includes demonstrating to the patient how to support the neck with the hands after surgery to prevent stress on the incision. This involves raising the elbows and placing the hands behind the neck to provide support and reduce strain and tension on the neck muscles and the surgical incision.

Providing Postoperative Care

In the postoperative period, the priorities are to observe for any difficulty in breathing due to edema of the glottis, hematoma formation, or injury to the recurrent laryngeal nerve which requires the insertion of an airway, and to monitor the pulse and blood pressure for any indication of internal bleeding. The nurse must be alert for complaints of a sensation of pressure or fullness at the incision site which may indicate subcutaneous hemorrhage and hematoma formation and should be reported. In addition, the nurse periodically assesses the surgical dressings and reinforces as necessary. When the patient is in a recumbent position, the nurse observes the sides and the back of the neck as well as the anterior dressing for bleeding. A tracheostomy set is kept at the bedside at all times, and the surgeon is summoned at the first indication of respiratory distress. If the respiratory distress is caused by hematoma, surgical evacuation is required.

The intensity of pain is assessed, and analgesic agents are given as prescribed for pain. The nurse should anticipate apprehension in the patient and should inform the patient that oxygen will assist breathing. When moving and turning the patient, the nurse carefully supports the patient's head and avoids tension on the sutures. The most comfortable position is the semi-Fowler position, with the head elevated and supported by pillows.

IV fluids are given during the immediate postoperative period. Water may be given by mouth as soon as nausea subsides and bowel sounds are present. Usually, there is a little difficulty in swallowing; initially, cold fluids and ice may be taken better than other fluids. Often, patients prefer a soft diet to a liquid diet in the immediate postoperative period.

The patient is advised to talk as little as possible to reduce edema to the vocal cords; however, when the patient does speak, any voice changes are noted, indicating possible injury to the recurrent laryngeal nerve, which lies just behind the thyroid next to the trachea. An overbed table is provided for access to frequently used items so that the patient avoids turning their head. The table can also be used to support a humidifier when vapor-mist inhalations are prescribed for the relief of excessive mucous accumulation.

> ### ▶ Quality and Safety Nursing Alert
>
> *An essential assessment following a thyroidectomy is of voice changes. Difficulty in speaking (the act of moving air to vibrate vocal cords) may indicate increasing edema, damage to laryngeal nerve, or hemorrhage and should be reported immediately.*

The patient is encouraged to be out of bed as soon as possible and to eat foods that are easily swallowed. A high-calorie diet may be prescribed to promote weight gain. The incision may be closed using absorbable sutures, nonabsorbable sutures, and adhesive strips. Absorbable sutures dissolve within the body. If nonabsorbable sutures are used, the timeline for removal may vary; however, these types of sutures are usually removed 5 to 7 days following surgery. Adhesives will peel off spontaneously. The patient is usually discharged from the hospital on the day of surgery or soon afterward if the postoperative course is uncomplicated.

Monitoring and Managing Potential Complications

Hemorrhage, hematoma formation, edema of the glottis, and injury to the laryngeal nerve are complications reviewed previously in this chapter. Occasionally in thyroid surgery, the parathyroid glands are injured or removed, producing a disturbance in calcium metabolism. As the blood calcium level falls, hyperirritability of the nerves occurs, with spasms of the hands and feet and muscle twitching (see Chapter 10). This group of symptoms is termed *tetany*, and the nurse must immediately report its appearance because laryngospasm, although rare, may occur and obstruct the airway. Tetany of this type is usually treated with IV calcium gluconate. This calcium abnormality is usually temporary after thyroidectomy unless all parathyroid tissues were removed.

> ▶ **Quality and Safety Nursing Alert**
>
> *Following thyroid surgery, the patient should be monitored closely for signs of tetany, including hyperirritability of the nerves, with spasms of the hands and feet and muscle twitching. Laryngospasm, although rare, may occur and obstruct the airway.*

Promoting Home, Community-Based, and Transitional Care

Predischarge education is essential because these patients have short hospital stays. The patient, family, and caregivers need to be knowledgeable about the signs and symptoms that should be reported. Discharge education includes strategies for managing postoperative pain at home and for increasing humidification. The nurse explains to the patient and family the need for rest, relaxation, and adequate nutrition and to avoid putting strain on the incision and sutures. The patient is permitted to resume their former activities and responsibilities completely once recovered from surgery.

Family responsibilities and factors relating to the home environment that produce emotional tension have often been implicated as precipitating causes of thyrotoxicosis. A home visit provides an opportunity to evaluate these factors and to suggest ways to improve the home and family environment. If indicated, a referral to home, community-based or transitional care is made. The nurse reviews the history; performs a physical assessment; assesses the surgical incision; develops a plan of care with the patient and family; and educates the patient, family, and caregivers about wound care, signs and symptoms to report, stress reduction, and the importance of keeping appointments with the primary provider.

THE PARATHYROID GLANDS

Anatomic and Physiologic Overview

The parathyroid glands (normally four) are situated in the neck and embedded in the posterior aspect of the thyroid gland (see Fig. 45-7). Parathormone (parathyroid hormone)—the protein hormone produced by the parathyroid glands—regulates calcium and phosphorus metabolism. Increased secretion of parathormone results in increased calcium absorption from the kidney, intestine, and bones, which raises the serum calcium level (Norris, 2019). Some actions of this hormone are increased by the presence of vitamin D. Parathormone also tends to lower the blood phosphorus level. The serum level of ionized calcium regulates the output of

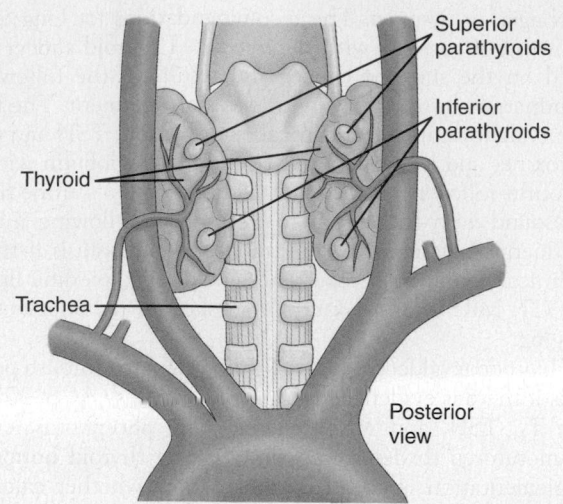

Figure 45-7 • The parathyroid glands are located behind the thyroid gland. The parathyroids may be embedded in the thyroid tissue.

parathormone. Increased serum calcium results in decreased parathormone secretion, creating a negative feedback system.

Pathophysiology

Excess parathormone can result in markedly increased levels of serum calcium, which is a potentially life-threatening situation. When the product of serum calcium and serum phosphorus (calcium × phosphorus) rises, calcium phosphate may precipitate in various organs of the body (e.g., the kidneys) and cause tissue calcification.

Hyperparathyroidism

Hyperparathyroidism is caused by overproduction of parathormone by the parathyroid glands and is characterized by bone decalcification and the development of renal calculi (kidney stones) containing calcium.

Primary hyperparathyroidism occurs two to four times more often in women than in men and is most common in people between 60 and 70 years of age. Its incidence is approximately 25 cases per 100,000 people. The disorder is rare in children younger than 15 years, but its incidence increases 10-fold between the ages of 15 and 65 years. Half of the people diagnosed with hyperparathyroidism do not have symptoms (Yalla & Hickey, 2019). Secondary hyperparathyroidism, with manifestations similar to those of primary hyperparathyroidism, occurs in patients who have chronic kidney failure and the so-called renal rickets as a result of phosphorus retention, increased stimulation of the parathyroid glands, and increased parathormone secretion.

Clinical Manifestations

The patient may have no symptoms or may experience signs and symptoms resulting from involvement of several body systems. Apathy, fatigue, muscle weakness, nausea, vomiting, constipation, hypertension, and cardiac arrhythmias may occur. All of these signs and symptoms are attributable to the increased concentration of calcium in the blood. Psychological effects may vary from irritability and neurosis to psychoses caused by the direct action of calcium on the brain and nervous system. An increase in calcium produces a decrease in the excitation potential of nerve and muscle tissue.

Nephrolithiasis (formation of stones in one or both kidneys), related to the increased urinary excretion of calcium and phosphorus, is one of the major complications of hyperparathyroidism. Although the incidence is on the decline in the United States, nephrolithiasis occurs in 15% to 20% of newly diagnosed patients (Yalla & Hickey, 2019). Kidney damage can result from the precipitation of calcium phosphate in the renal pelvis and parenchyma, which causes renal calculi, obstruction, pyelonephritis, and kidney injury.

Musculoskeletal symptoms accompanying hyperparathyroidism may be caused by demineralization of the bones or by bone tumors composed of benign giant cells resulting from overgrowth of osteoclasts. The patient may develop skeletal pain and tenderness, especially of the back and joints; pain on weight bearing; pathologic fractures; deformities; and shortening of body stature. Bone loss attributable to hyperparathyroidism increases the risk of fracture.

The incidence of peptic ulcer and pancreatitis is increased with hyperparathyroidism and may be responsible for many of the GI symptoms that occur.

Assessment and Diagnostic Findings

Primary hyperparathyroidism is diagnosed by persistent elevation of serum calcium levels and an elevated concentration of parathormone. Radioimmunoassays for parathormone are sensitive and differentiate primary hyperparathyroidism from other causes of hypercalcemia in more than 80% of patients with elevated serum calcium levels (Silverberg & Fuleihan, 2019). An elevated serum calcium level alone is a nonspecific finding, because serum levels may be altered by diet, medications, and kidney and bone changes. Bone changes may be detected on x-ray or bone scans in advanced disease. The double-antibody parathyroid hormone test is used to distinguish between primary hyperparathyroidism and malignancy as a cause of hypercalcemia. Ultrasound, MRI, thallium scan, and fine-needle biopsy have been used to evaluate the function of the parathyroid glands and to localize parathyroid cysts, adenomas, or hyperplasia.

Medical Management

Surgical Management

The recommended treatment for primary hyperparathyroidism is parathyroidectomy, the surgical removal of abnormal parathyroid tissue (Silverberg & Fuleihan, 2019). In the past, the standard parathyroidectomy involved a bilateral neck exploration under general anesthesia. Today, minimally invasive parathyroidectomy techniques allow for unilateral neck exploration using local anesthesia; these are performed on an outpatient basis. In some cases, only the removal of a single diseased gland is necessary, reducing morbidity rates associated with surgery. For asymptomatic patients who have only mildly elevated serum calcium concentrations and normal kidney function, surgery may be delayed and the patient monitored closely for worsening of hypercalcemia, bone deterioration, renal impairment, or the development of kidney stones.

Surgery is recommended for patients who are asymptomatic and who meet one or more of the following criteria: younger than 50 years; unable or unlikely to participate in follow-up care; serum calcium level more than 1 mg/dL (0.25 mmol/L) above normal reference range; GFR less than 60 mL/min; urinary calcium level greater than 400 mg per day (10 mmol per day); bone density at hip, lumbar spine, or distal radius with T score less than −2.5 or previous fracture at any site; or nephrolithiasis or nephrocalcinosis (Yalla & Hickey, 2019).

Hydration Therapy

Patients with hyperparathyroidism are at risk for renal calculi. Therefore, a daily fluid intake of 2000 mL or more is encouraged to help prevent calculus formation. The patient is instructed to report other manifestations of renal calculi, such as abdominal pain and hematuria. Thiazide diuretics are avoided, because they decrease the renal excretion of calcium and further elevate serum calcium levels. Because of the risk of hypercalcemic crisis (see later discussion), the patient is instructed to avoid dehydration and to seek immediate health care if conditions that commonly produce dehydration (e.g., vomiting, diarrhea) occur.

Mobility

The nurse encourages the patient to be mobile. The patient with limited mobility is encouraged to walk. Bones subjected to the normal stress of walking give up less calcium. Bed rest increases calcium excretion and the risk of renal calculi. Oral phosphates lower the serum calcium level in some patients; long-term use is not recommended because of the risk of ectopic calcium phosphate deposition in soft tissues.

Diet and Medications

Nutritional needs are met, but the patient is advised to avoid a diet with restricted or excess calcium. If the patient has a coexisting peptic ulcer, prescribed antacids and protein feedings are necessary. Because anorexia is common, efforts are made to improve the appetite. Prune juice, stool softeners, and physical activity, along with increased fluid intake, help offset constipation, which is common postoperatively.

Nursing Management

The insidious onset and chronic nature of hyperparathyroidism along with its diverse and commonly vague symptoms may result in depression and frustration. The family may have considered the patient's illness to be psychosomatic. An awareness of the course of the disorder and an understanding approach by the nurse may help the patient and family deal with their reactions and feelings.

The nursing management of the patient undergoing parathyroidectomy is essentially the same as that of a patient undergoing thyroidectomy. However, the previously described precautions about airway patency, dehydration, immobility, and diet are particularly important in the patient who is awaiting or recovering from parathyroidectomy. Although not all parathyroid tissue is removed during surgery in an effort to control the calcium–phosphorus balance, the nurse closely monitors the patient to detect symptoms of tetany (which may be an early postoperative complication). Most patients quickly regain function of the remaining parathyroid tissue

Chart 45-9 — HOME CARE CHECKLIST
The Patient with Hyperparathyroidism

At the completion of education, the patient and/or caregiver will be able to:

- State the impact of hyperparathyroidism and treatment on physiologic functioning, ADLs, IADLs, roles, relationships, and spirituality.
- Describe potential benefits and risks of parathyroidectomy.
- State the name, dose, side effects, frequency, and schedule for all medications.
- Explain the purpose, dose, route, schedule, side effects, and precautions of pharmacologic treatment (loop diuretics, phosphates, and calcitonin) of hyperparathyroidism.
- State the need to contact primary provider before taking over-the-counter medication containing calcium.
- State changes in lifestyle (e.g., diet, activity) necessary to maintain health, including:
- Recommended intake of dietary calcium.
- Maintenance of regular bowel habits and management of constipation (e.g., prune juice, stool softeners, increased physical activity and fluids).

- Monitoring of fluid intake as indicated, generally 2000 mL daily.
- Managing pain (medication and nonpharmacologic interventions).
- Increasing mobility as indicated.
- Relate how to reach primary provider with questions or complications.
- State time and date of follow-up medical appointments, therapy, and testing.
- Identify sources of support (e.g., friends, relatives, faith community).
- Identify the contact details for support services for patients and their caregivers/families.
- Identify the need for health promotion, disease prevention, and screening activities.

ADLs, activities of daily living; IADLs, instrumental activities of daily living.

---

and experience only mild, transient postoperative hypocalcemia. In patients with significant bone disease or bone changes, a more prolonged period of hypocalcemia should be anticipated. The nurse educates the patient and family about the importance of follow-up laboratory testing to ensure return of serum calcium levels to normal (see Chart 45-9).

 ## Complications: Hypercalcemic Crisis

Acute hypercalcemic crisis can occur with extreme elevation of serum calcium levels. Serum calcium levels greater than 13 mg/dL (3.25 mmol/L) result in neurologic, cardiovascular, and kidney symptoms that can be life-threatening (Fischbach & Fischbach, 2018). Rapid rehydration with large volumes of IV isotonic saline fluids to maintain urine output of 100 to 150 mL per hour is combined with administration of calcitonin (Shane & Berenson, 2019). Calcitonin promotes renal excretion of excess calcium and reduces bone resorption. The saline infusion should be stopped and a loop diuretic may be needed if the patient develops edema. Dosage and rates of infusion depend on the patient profile. The patient should be monitored carefully for fluid overload. Loop diuretics are not recommended as initial therapy in the absence of heart failure and kidney insufficiency. Bisphosphonates are added to promote a sustained decrease in serum calcium levels by promoting calcium deposition in bone and reducing the GI absorption of calcium. Cytotoxic agents (e.g., mithramycin), calcitonin, and dialysis may be used in emergency situations to decrease serum calcium levels quickly.

> ### ▶ Quality and Safety Nursing Alert
>
> *The patient in acute hypercalcemic crisis requires close monitoring for life-threatening complications (e.g., airway obstruction) and prompt treatment to reduce serum calcium levels.*

A combination of calcitonin and corticosteroids is given in emergencies to reduce the serum calcium level by increasing calcium deposition in bone. Other agents that may be given to decrease serum calcium levels include bisphosphonates (e.g., etidronate, pamidronate) (Shane & Berenson, 2019).

Expert assessment and care are required to minimize complications and reverse the life-threatening hypercalcemia. Medications are given with care, and attention is given to fluid balance to promote return of normal fluid and electrolyte balance. Supportive measures are necessary for the patient and family. See Chapter 12, Table 12-13, for further discussion of hypercalcemic crisis.

Hypoparathyroidism

Hypoparathyroidism is caused by abnormal parathyroid development, destruction of the parathyroid glands (surgical removal or autoimmune response), and vitamin D deficiency. The most common cause is the near-total removal of the thyroid gland. The result is inadequate secretion of parathormone (Goltzman, 2019).

Deficiency of parathormone results in hyperphosphatemia (increased blood phosphate levels) and hypocalcemia (decreased blood calcium levels). In the absence of parathormone, there is decreased intestinal absorption of dietary calcium and decreased resorption of calcium from bone and through the renal tubules. Decreased renal excretion of phosphate causes hypophosphaturia, and low serum calcium levels result in hypocalciuria.

Clinical Manifestations

Hypocalcemia causes irritability of the neuromuscular system and contributes to the chief symptom of hypoparathyroidism—tetany. Tetany is general muscle hypertonia, with tremor and spasmodic or uncoordinated contractions occurring with or without efforts to make voluntary movements. Symptoms of latent tetany are numbness, tingling, and cramps in the extremities, and the patient complains of stiffness in the hands and feet. In overt tetany, the signs include bronchospasm, laryngeal spasm, carpopedal spasm (flexion of the elbows and wrists and extension of the carpophalangeal joints and dorsiflexion of the feet), dysphagia, photophobia, cardiac arrhythmias, and seizures. Other symptoms include anxiety, irritability, depression, and even delirium. ECG changes and hypotension also may occur.

Assessment and Diagnostic Findings

A positive Chvostek sign or a positive Trousseau sign suggests latent tetany. **Chvostek sign** is positive when a sharp tapping over the facial nerve just in front of the parotid gland and anterior to the ear causes spasm or twitching of the mouth, nose, and eye (see Fig. 10-8A). **Trousseau sign** is positive when carpopedal spasm is induced by occluding the blood flow to the arm for 3 minutes with a blood pressure cuff (see Fig. 10-8B). The diagnosis of hypoparathyroidism often is difficult because of the vague symptoms, such as aches and pains. Therefore, laboratory studies are especially helpful. Tetany develops at very low serum calcium levels. Serum phosphate levels are increased, and x-rays of bone show increased density. Calcification is detected on x-rays of the subcutaneous or paraspinal basal ganglia of the brain.

Medical Management

The goal of therapy is to increase the serum calcium level to 9 to 10 mg/dL (2.2 to 2.5 mmol/L) and to eliminate the symptoms of hypoparathyroidism and hypocalcemia. Management is determined by the underlying cause and patient profile. Treatment may include combinations of calcium, magnesium, and ergocalciferol or calcitriol, the latter being preferred. A thiazide diuretic (e.g., hydrochlorothiazide) may be given to help decrease urinary calcium excretion (Goltzman, 2019). Recombinant parathyroid hormone has been approved for the treatment of osteoporosis but not for hypoparathyroidism at this time (Goltzman, 2019).

When hypocalcemia and tetany occur after a thyroidectomy, the immediate treatment is administration of IV calcium gluconate. If this does not decrease neuromuscular irritability and seizure activity immediately, sedative agents such as pentobarbital may be given.

Because of neuromuscular irritability, the patient with hypocalcemia and tetany requires an environment that is free of noise, drafts, bright lights, or sudden movement. If the patient develops respiratory distress, a tracheostomy or mechanical ventilation may become necessary, along with medications that cause bronchodilation in order to provide respiratory support.

Therapy for chronic hypoparathyroidism is determined after serum calcium levels are obtained. A diet high in calcium and low in phosphorus is prescribed. Although milk, milk products, and egg yolk are high in calcium, they are restricted because they also contain high levels of phosphorus. Spinach also is avoided because it contains oxalate, which would form insoluble calcium substances. Oral tablets of calcium salts, such as calcium gluconate, may be used to supplement the diet. Aluminum hydroxide gel or aluminum carbonate also is given after meals to bind phosphate and promote its excretion through the GI tract.

Nursing Management

Nursing management of the patient with possible acute hypoparathyroidism includes the following:

- Care of postoperative patients who have undergone thyroidectomy, parathyroidectomy, or radical neck dissection is directed toward detecting early signs of hypocalcemia and anticipating signs of tetany, seizures, and respiratory difficulties.
- Calcium gluconate should be available for emergency IV administration. If the patient requiring administration of calcium gluconate has a cardiac disorder, is subject to arrhythmias, or is receiving digitalis, the calcium gluconate is given slowly and cautiously.
- Calcium and digitalis increase systolic contraction and also potentiate each other; this can produce potentially fatal arrhythmias. Consequently, the cardiac patient requires continuous cardiac monitoring and careful assessment.

An important aspect of nursing care is patient education about medications and diet therapy. The patient needs to know the reason for high calcium and low phosphate intake and the symptoms of hypocalcemia and hypercalcemia; they should know to contact the primary provider immediately if these symptoms occur (see Chart 45-10).

Chart 45-10   🏠 **HOME CARE CHECKLIST**
The Patient with Hypoparathyroidism

At the completion of education, the patient and/or caregiver will be able to:

- State the impact of hypoparathyroidism and treatment on physiologic functioning, ADLs, IADLs, roles, relationships, and spirituality.
- State purpose, dose, route, schedule, side effects, and precautions of prescribed medications (calcium, phosphate binders).
- State changes in lifestyle (e.g., diet, activity) necessary to maintain health, including:
- Ensuring a diet high in calcium and vitamin D, low in phosphorous.
- Alternating activity and rest periods.
- State precipitating factors and interventions for complications (seizure, cardiac arrhythmias, cardiac arrest).

- State necessary actions for seizure activity.
- Relate how to reach primary provider with questions or complications.
- State time and date of follow-up medical appointments, therapy, and testing.
- Identify sources of support (e.g., friends, relatives, faith community).
- Identify the contact details for support services for patients and their caregivers/families.
- Identify the need for health promotion, disease prevention, and screening activities.

ADLs, activities of daily living; IADLs, instrumental activities of daily living.

THE ADRENAL GLANDS

Anatomic and Physiologic Overview

Each person has two adrenal glands, one attached to the upper portion of each kidney. Each adrenal gland is, in reality, two endocrine glands with separate, independent functions. The adrenal medulla at the center of the gland secretes catecholamines, and the outer portion of the gland, the adrenal cortex, secretes steroid hormones (Norris, 2019). The secretion of hormones from the adrenal cortex is regulated by the hypothalamic–pituitary–adrenal axis. The hypothalamus secretes corticotropin-releasing hormone (CRH), which stimulates the pituitary gland to secrete ACTH, which in turn stimulates the adrenal cortex to secrete glucocorticoid hormone (cortisol). Increased levels of the adrenal hormone then inhibit the production or secretion of CRH and ACTH. This system is an example of a negative feedback mechanism.

Adrenal Medulla

The adrenal medulla functions as part of the autonomic nervous system. Stimulation of preganglionic sympathetic nerve fibers, which travel directly to the cells of the adrenal medulla, causes release of the catecholamine hormones epinephrine and norepinephrine. About 90% of the secretion of the human adrenal medulla is epinephrine (also called *adrenaline*). Catecholamines regulate metabolic pathways to promote catabolism of stored fuels to meet caloric needs from endogenous sources. The major effects of epinephrine release are to prepare to meet a challenge (fight-or-flight response). Secretion of epinephrine causes decreased blood flow to tissues that are not needed in emergency situations, such as the GI tract, and increased blood flow to tissues that are important for effective fight or flight, such as cardiac and skeletal muscle. Catecholamines also induce the release of free fatty acids, increase the basal metabolic rate, and elevate the blood glucose level.

Adrenal Cortex

A functioning adrenal cortex is necessary for life; adrenocortical secretions make it possible for the body to adapt to stress of all kinds. The three types of steroid hormones produced by the adrenal cortex are glucocorticoids, mainly cortisol; mineralocorticoids, mainly aldosterone; and sex hormones, mainly androgens (Norris, 2019). Without the adrenal cortex, severe stress would cause peripheral circulatory failure, circulatory shock, and prostration. Survival in the absence of a functioning adrenal cortex is possible only with nutritional, electrolyte, and fluid replacement and appropriate replacement with exogenous adrenocortical hormones.

Glucocorticoids

The **glucocorticoids** are so named because they have an important influence on glucose metabolism: Increased cortisol secretion results in elevated blood glucose levels. However, the glucocorticoids have major effects on the metabolism of almost all organs of the body. Glucocorticoids are secreted from the adrenal cortex in response to the release of ACTH from the anterior lobe of the pituitary gland. This system represents an example of negative feedback. The presence of glucocorticoids in the blood inhibits the release of CRH from the hypothalamus and also inhibits ACTH secretion from the pituitary. The resultant decrease in ACTH secretion causes diminished release of glucocorticoids from the adrenal cortex.

Corticosteroids are the classification of drugs that include glucocorticoids. These drugs are given to inhibit the inflammatory response to tissue injury and to suppress allergic manifestations. Their side effects include the development of diabetes, osteoporosis, and peptic ulcer; increased protein breakdown resulting in muscle wasting and poor wound healing; and redistribution of body fat. When large doses of exogenous glucocorticoids are given, the release of ACTH and endogenous glucocorticoids are inhibited. This can cause the adrenal cortex to atrophy. If exogenous glucocorticoid administration is discontinued suddenly, adrenal insufficiency results because of the inability of the atrophied cortex to respond adequately.

Mineralocorticoids

Mineralocorticoids exert their major effects on electrolyte metabolism. They act principally on the renal tubular and GI epithelium to cause increased sodium ion absorption in exchange for excretion of potassium or hydrogen ions. ACTH only minimally influences aldosterone secretion. It is primarily secreted in response to the presence of angiotensin II in the bloodstream. Angiotensin II is a substance that elevates the blood pressure by constricting arterioles. Its concentration is increased when renin is released from the kidney in response to decreased perfusion pressure. The resultant increased aldosterone levels promote sodium reabsorption by the kidney and the GI tract, which tends to restore blood pressure to normal. The release of aldosterone is also increased by hyperkalemia. Aldosterone is the main hormone for the long-term regulation of sodium balance.

Adrenal Sex Hormones (Androgens)

Androgens, the third major type of steroid hormones produced by the adrenal cortex, exert effects similar to those of male sex hormones. The adrenal gland may also secrete small amounts of some estrogens, or female sex hormones. ACTH controls the secretion of adrenal androgens. When secreted in normal amounts, the adrenal androgens have little effect, but when secreted in excess, they produce masculinization in women, feminization in men, or premature sexual development in children. This is called the adrenogenital syndrome.

Pheochromocytoma

Pheochromocytoma is a rare tumor that is usually benign and originates from the chromaffin cells of the adrenal medulla. This tumor is the cause of high blood pressure in 0.1% of patients with hypertension and is usually fatal if undetected and untreated; however, it is usually cured by surgery. In 90% of patients the tumor arises in the medulla; in the remaining patients, it occurs in the extra-adrenal chromaffin tissue located in or near the aorta, ovaries, spleen, or other organs. Pheochromocytoma may occur at any age, but its peak incidence is between 40 and 50 years of age and affects men and women equally (U.S. National Library of Medicine, 2019). Ten percent of the tumors are bilateral, and 10% are malignant. Because of the high incidence of pheochromocytoma in family members of affected people, the patient's family members should be alerted and screened for this tumor. Pheochromocytoma may occur in the familial form as part of multiple endocrine neoplasia type 2; therefore, it should be considered a possibility in patients who have medullary thyroid carcinoma and parathyroid hyperplasia or tumor.

Clinical Manifestations

The nature and severity of symptoms of functioning tumors of the adrenal medulla depend on the relative proportions of epinephrine and norepinephrine secretion. The typical triad of symptoms is headache, diaphoresis, and palpitations in the patient with hypertension. Hypertension and other cardiovascular disturbances are common. The hypertension may be intermittent or persistent. If the hypertension is sustained, it may be difficult to distinguish from other causes of hypertension. Other symptoms may include tremor, headache, flushing, and anxiety. Hyperglycemia may result from conversion of liver and muscle glycogen to glucose due to epinephrine secretion; insulin may be required to maintain normal blood glucose levels.

The clinical picture in the paroxysmal form of pheochromocytoma is usually characterized by acute, unpredictable attacks lasting seconds or several hours. Symptoms usually begin abruptly and subside slowly. During these attacks, the patient is extremely anxious, tremulous, and weak. The patient may experience headache, vertigo, blurring of vision, tinnitus, air hunger, and dyspnea. Other symptoms include polyuria, nausea, vomiting, diarrhea, abdominal pain, and a feeling of impending doom. Palpitations and tachycardia are common (Singh & Herrick, 2019). Blood pressures exceeding 250/150 mm Hg have been recorded. Such blood pressure elevations are life-threatening and can cause severe complications, such as cardiac arrhythmias, dissecting aneurysm, stroke, and acute kidney failure. Orthostatic hypotension (decrease in systolic blood pressure, lightheadedness, dizziness on standing) occurs in 70% of patients with untreated pheochromocytoma.

Assessment and Diagnostic Findings

Pheochromocytoma is suspected if signs of sympathetic nervous system overactivity occur in association with marked elevation of blood pressure. These signs can be associated with the "five Hs": *h*ypertension, *h*eadache, *h*yperhidrosis (excessive sweating), *h*ypermetabolism, and *h*yperglycemia. The presence of these signs is highly predictive of pheochromocytoma. Paroxysmal symptoms of pheochromocytoma commonly develop in the fifth decade of life.

Measurements of urine and plasma levels of catecholamines and metanephrine (MN), a catecholamine metabolite, are the most direct and conclusive tests for overactivity of the adrenal medulla. A test for detecting pheochromocytoma measures free MN in plasma by high-pressure liquid chromatography and electrochemical detection. A negative test result virtually excludes pheochromocytoma. Measurements of catecholamine metabolites (MN and vanillylmandelic acid [VMA]) or free catecholamines have been extensively used in the clinical setting. In most cases, pheochromocytoma can be diagnosed or confirmed based on a properly collected 24-hour urine sample. Levels can be as high as two times the normal limit. A 24-hour urine specimen is collected to detect free catecholamines, MN, and VMA; the use of combined tests increases the diagnostic accuracy of testing. A number of medications and foods, such as coffee and tea (including decaffeinated varieties), bananas, chocolate, vanilla, and aspirin, may alter the results of these tests; therefore, careful instructions to avoid restricted items must be given to the patient. Urine collected over a 2- or 3-hour period after an attack of hypertension can be assayed for catecholamine content (Singh & Herrick, 2019).

The total plasma catecholamine (epinephrine and norepinephrine) concentration is measured with the patient supine and at rest for 30 minutes. To prevent elevation of catecholamine levels resulting from the stress of venipuncture, a butterfly needle, scalp vein needle, or venous catheter may be inserted 30 minutes before the blood specimen is obtained.

Factors that may elevate catecholamine concentrations must be controlled to obtain valid results; these factors include consumption of coffee or tea (including decaffeinated varieties), the use of tobacco, emotional and physical stress, and the use of many prescription and over-the-counter medications (e.g., amphetamines, nose drops or sprays, decongestant agents, bronchodilators).

Normal plasma values of epinephrine are 100 pg/mL (590 pmol/L); normal values of norepinephrine are generally less than 100 to 550 pg/mL (590 to 3240 pmol/L). Values of epinephrine greater than 400 pg/mL (2180 pmol/L) or norepinephrine values greater than 2000 pg/mL (11,800 pmol/L) are considered diagnostic of pheochromocytoma. Values that fall between normal levels and those diagnostic of pheochromocytoma indicate the need for further testing.

A clonidine suppression test may be performed if the results of plasma and urine tests of catecholamines are inconclusive. Clonidine is a centrally acting antiadrenergic medication that suppresses the release of neurogenically mediated catecholamines. The suppression test is based on the principle that catecholamine levels are normally increased through the activity of the sympathetic nervous system. In pheochromocytoma, increased catecholamine levels result from the diffusion of excess catecholamines into the circulation, bypassing normal storage and release mechanisms. Therefore, in patients with pheochromocytoma, clonidine does not suppress the release of catecholamines (Singh & Herrick, 2019).

Imaging studies, such as CT, MRI, and ultrasonography, may also be carried out to localize the pheochromocytoma and to determine whether more than one tumor is present. The use of ^{131}I-metaiodobenzylguanidine (MIBG) scintigraphy may be required to determine the location of the pheochromocytoma and to detect metastatic sites outside the adrenal gland. MIBG is a specific isotope for catecholamine-producing tissue. It has been helpful in identifying tumors not detected by other tests or procedures. MIBG scintigraphy is a noninvasive, safe procedure that has increased the accuracy of diagnosis of adrenal tumors (Fischbach & Fischbach, 2018).

Other diagnostic studies may focus on evaluating the function of other endocrine glands because of the association of pheochromocytoma in some patients with other endocrine tumors.

Medical Management

During an episode or attack of hypertension, tachycardia, anxiety, and the other symptoms of pheochromocytoma, bed rest with the head of the bed elevated is prescribed to promote an orthostatic decrease in blood pressure.

Pharmacologic Therapy

The patient may be treated preoperatively on an inpatient or outpatient basis. Regardless of the setting, monitoring of blood pressure and cardiac function is essential. The goals are to control hypertension before and during surgery and volume expansion, and to prevent a catecholamine storm as a result of surgery (Singh & Herrick, 2019).

Preoperatively, the patient may begin treatment with a low dose of an alpha-adrenergic blocker, either phenoxybenzamine or doxazosin, 10 to 14 days or longer prior to surgery (Singh & Herrick, 2019). The patient should be informed about the potential for adverse effects of these medications, which include orthostasis, nasal stuffiness, increased fatigue, and retrograde ejaculation in men. The medication dosages are started at a low dose and increased every 2 to 3 days as needed to control blood pressure. Patients may be required to consume a high-sodium diet or take salt supplements.

After administration of the alpha-blockers, the blood pressure should be monitored closely. In an outpatient setting, the blood pressure should be taken twice daily in a sitting and standing position. The targets are less than 130/80 mm Hg (seated) with a standing systolic pressure greater than 90 mm Hg and target heart rate of 60 to 70 beats per minute sitting and 70 to 80 beats per minute standing (Singh & Herrick, 2019). Age and comorbid disease should be taken into consideration when establishing and evaluating targets. Propranolol and metoprolol may be administered with caution to achieve the target heart rate (Singh & Herrick, 2019).

Calcium channel blockers such as nifedipine are sometimes used as an alternative or supplement to preoperative alpha- and beta-blockers, when blood pressure control is inadequate or the patient is unable to tolerate the side effects. Nifedipine and nicardipine may be used safely without causing undue hypotension. For episodes of severe hypertension, nifedipine is a fast and effective treatment, because the capsules can be pierced and chewed. The patient needs to be well hydrated before, during, and after surgery to prevent hypotension. Additional medications that may be used preoperatively include catecholamine synthesis inhibitors, such as alpha-methyl-*p*-tyrosine (metyrosine). These are occasionally used if adrenergic blocking agents (i.e., alpha- and beta-blockers) are not effective. Long-term use of metyrosine may result in many adverse effects, including sedation, depression, diarrhea, anxiety, nightmares, dysuria, impotence, elevated aspartate aminotransferase, anemia, thrombocytopenia, crystalluria, galactorrhea (breast discharge), and extrapyramidal signs (e.g., drooling, speech impairment, tremors).

Surgical Management

The definitive treatment of pheochromocytoma is surgical removal of the tumor, usually with **adrenalectomy** (removal of one or both adrenal glands); surgical treatment is considered high risk in this patient population. Surgery may be performed using a laparoscopic approach or an open operation. The laparoscopic approach is the preferred method for patients with pheochromocytomas including large tumors because of the decreased blood loss, decreased hospitalization time, and decreased morbidity. Bilateral adrenalectomy may be necessary if tumors are present in both adrenal glands. Patient preparation includes control of blood pressure and blood volumes; usually, this is carried out over 10 to 14 days, as described previously. A calcium channel blocker (nicardipine) can be given intraoperatively exclusively or in combination with the alpha- and beta-blockers to control blood pressure.

A hypertensive crisis, however, can still arise as a result of manipulation of the tumor during surgical excision, causing a release of stored epinephrine and norepinephrine, with marked increases in blood pressure and changes in heart rate. Exploration of other possible tumor sites is frequently undertaken to ensure removal of all tumor tissue. As a result, the patient is subject to the stress and effects of a long surgical procedure, which may increase the risk of hypertension postoperatively.

Corticosteroid replacement is required if bilateral adrenalectomy has been necessary. Corticosteroids may also be required for the first few days or weeks after removal of a single adrenal gland. IV administration of corticosteroids (methylprednisolone) may begin on the evening before surgery and continue during the early postoperative period to prevent adrenal insufficiency. Oral preparations of corticosteroids (prednisone) are prescribed after the acute stress of surgery diminishes.

Hypotension and hypoglycemia may occur in the postoperative period because of the sudden withdrawal of excessive amounts of catecholamines. Therefore, careful attention is directed toward monitoring and treating these changes. Hypertension may continue if not all pheochromocytoma tissue was removed, if pheochromocytoma recurs, or if the blood vessels were damaged by severe and prolonged hypertension. Several days after surgery, urine and plasma levels of catecholamines and their metabolites are measured to determine whether the surgery was successful.

Nursing Management

The patient who has undergone surgery to treat pheochromocytoma has experienced a stressful preoperative and postoperative course and may remain fearful of repeated attacks. Although it is usually expected that all pheochromocytoma tissue has been removed, there is a possibility that other sites were undetected and that attacks may recur. The patient is monitored until stable with special attention given to ECG changes, arterial pressures, fluid and electrolyte balance, and blood glucose levels. IV access will be required for administration of fluids and medications.

Promoting Home, Community-Based, and Transitional Care

 Educating Patients About Self-Care

During the pre- and postoperative phases of care, the nurse educates the patient about the importance of follow-up monitoring to ensure that pheochromocytoma does not recur undetected. After adrenalectomy, the use of corticosteroids may be needed. Therefore, the nurse educates the patient about their purpose, the medication schedule, and the risks of skipping doses or stopping their administration abruptly.

The patient and family are educated about how to measure the patient's blood pressure and when to notify the primary provider about changes in blood pressure. In addition, the nurse provides verbal and written instructions about the procedure for collecting 24-hour urine specimens to monitor urine catecholamine levels.

Continuing and Transitional Care

A follow-up visit from a home, community-based or transitional care nurse may be indicated to assess the patient's postoperative recovery, surgical incision, knowledge regarding medication, and adherence to the medication schedule. This may help reinforce previous education about management and monitoring. The nurse also obtains blood pressure measurements and assists the patient in preventing or dealing with problems that may result from long-term use of corticosteroids.

Because of the risk of recurrence of hypertension, periodic checkups are required, especially in young patients and in those whose families have a history of pheochromocytoma. The patient is scheduled for periodic follow-up appointments to observe for return of normal blood pressure and plasma and urine levels of catecholamines.

Adrenocortical Insufficiency (Addison's Disease)

Primary adrenal insufficiency, also called **Addison's disease**, is the result of dysfunction of the hypothalamus–pituitary gland–adrenal gland feedback loop which results in insufficient production of steroids by the adrenal glands (Norris, 2019). Addison's disease is considered rare. In 70% to 90% of cases, the cause is an autoimmune disorder but tuberculosis and histoplasmosis are also associated with destruction of adrenal tissue; therefore, both should be considered in the diagnostic workup. Other causes include surgical removal of both adrenal glands; medications such as rifampin, barbiturates, ketoconazole, and tyrosine kinase inhibitors; and metastatic cancers such as lung, breast, colon, and melanoma (Zhang & Carmichael, 2019). Secondary adrenal insufficiency may result from the sudden cessation of exogenous adrenocortical hormonal therapy, which suppresses the body's normal response to stress and interferes with normal feedback mechanisms. Treatment with daily administration of corticosteroids for 2 to 4 weeks may suppress function of the adrenal cortex; therefore, adrenal insufficiency should be considered in any patient who has been treated with corticosteroids (Zhang & Carmichael, 2019).

Clinical Manifestations

The loss of mineralocorticoids leads to increased excretion of sodium, chloride, and water with increased retention of potassium. This may lead to a deficiency in extracellular fluid causing decreased cardiac output. The loss of glucocorticoids results in hypoglycemia with complaints of muscle weakness, lethargy, and GI symptoms including anorexia, weight loss, nausea and vomiting. In addition, the increase in levels of ACTH results in hyperpigmentation of the skin and mucous membranes, especially of the knuckles, knees, and skin folds (Norris, 2019).

Patients with Addison's disease are at risk to develop an **Addisonian crisis**, a life-threatening complication in which severe hypotension, cyanosis, fever, nausea, vomiting, and signs of shock develop. In addition, the patient may have pallor; complain of headache, abdominal pain, and diarrhea; and may show signs of confusion and restlessness. Even slight overexertion, exposure to cold, acute infection, or a decrease in salt intake may lead to circulatory collapse, shock, and death, if untreated. The stress of surgery or dehydration resulting from preparation for diagnostic tests or surgery may precipitate an Addisonian or hypotensive crisis because of the inhibited feedback loop.

Assessment and Diagnostic Findings

Although the clinical manifestations presented appear specific, the onset of Addison's disease usually occurs with nonspecific symptoms. The diagnosis is confirmed by laboratory test results. Combined measurements of early-morning serum cortisol and plasma ACTH are performed to differentiate primary adrenal insufficiency from secondary adrenal insufficiency and from normal adrenal function. Patients with primary insufficiency have a greatly increased plasma ACTH level and a serum cortisol concentration lower than the normal range or in the low-normal range (Zhang & Carmichael, 2019). Other laboratory findings include hypoglycemia (decreased levels of blood glucose), hyponatremia (decreased levels of sodium), hyperkalemia (increased serum potassium concentration), and leukocytosis (increased white blood cell count).

Medical Management

Immediate treatment is directed toward combating circulatory shock: restoring blood circulation, administering fluids and corticosteroids, monitoring vital signs, and placing the patient in a recumbent position with the legs elevated. Hydrocortisone is administered by IV, followed by 3 to 4 L of normal saline or 5% dextrose solution. Vasopressors may be required if hypotension persists.

Antibiotics may be given if infection has precipitated adrenal crisis in a patient with chronic adrenal insufficiency. In addition, the patient is assessed closely to identify other factors, stressors, or illnesses that led to the acute episode.

Oral intake may be initiated as soon as tolerated. IV fluids are gradually decreased after oral fluid intake is adequate to prevent hypovolemia. If the adrenal gland does not regain function, the patient needs lifelong replacement of corticosteroids and mineralocorticoids to prevent recurrence of adrenal insufficiency. Patients who are undergoing stressful procedures, surgery, significant illnesses, or are in the third trimester of pregnancy require additional supplementary therapy with corticosteroid medications to prevent Addisonian crisis. In addition, dietary intake may need to be supplemented with additional salt to manage GI losses of fluids through vomiting and diarrhea (Zhang & Carmichael, 2019).

Nursing Management

Assessing the Patient

The health history and examination focus on the presence of symptoms of fluid imbalance and the patient's level of stress. The nurse should monitor the blood pressure and pulse rate as the patient moves from a lying, sitting, and standing position to assess for inadequate fluid volume. A decrease in systolic pressure (20 mm Hg or more) may indicate depletion of fluid volume, especially if accompanied by symptoms. The skin should be assessed for changes in color and turgor, which could indicate chronic adrenal insufficiency and hypovolemia. The patient is assessed for change in weight, muscle weakness, fatigue, and any illness or stress that may have precipitated the acute crisis.

Monitoring and Managing Addisonian Crisis

The patient at risk is monitored for signs and symptoms indicative of Addisonian crisis, which can include shock; hypotension; rapid, weak pulse; rapid respiratory rate; pallor, and extreme weakness (see Chapter 11). Physical and psychological stressors such as cold exposure, overexertion, infection, and emotional distress should be avoided.

The patient with Addisonian crisis requires immediate treatment with IV administration of fluid, glucose, and electrolytes, especially sodium; replacement of missing steroid hormones; and vasopressors. The nurse anticipates and meets the patient's needs to promote return to a precrisis state.

Restoring Fluid Balance

The nurse encourages the patient to consume foods and fluids that assist in restoring and maintaining fluid and electrolyte balance which in turn maintains adequate cardiac output. Along with the dietitian, the nurse helps the patient select foods high in sodium during GI disturbances and in very hot weather.

The nurse educates the patient and family to administer hormone replacement as prescribed and to modify the dosage during illness and other stressful situations. Written and verbal instructions are provided about the administration of exogenous glucocorticoids (i.e., corticosteroid medications such as hydrocortisone, cortisone, and prednisone) and mineralocorticoids (fludrocortisone) as prescribed. The patient should be instructed to take prescribed corticosteroids with antacids or meals. The patient should be informed that the steroid therapy usually corrects the mood swings and mental status changes which adrenal insufficiency frequently causes (Quintanar, 2019).

Improving Activity Tolerance

Until the patient's condition is stabilized, the nurse takes precautions to avoid unnecessary activity and stress that could precipitate another hypotensive episode. Efforts are made to detect signs of infection or the presence of other stressors. Explaining the rationale for minimizing stress during the acute crisis assists the patient to increase activity gradually.

Promoting Home, Community-Based, and Transitional Care

 Educating Patients About Self-Care

Because of the need for lifelong replacement of adrenal cortex hormones to prevent Addisonian crises, the patient and family members receive explicit education about the rationale for replacement therapy and proper dosage. In addition, the patient, family, and caregivers are educated about the signs of excessive or insufficient hormone replacement. Stress can precipitate an Addisonian crisis, and in times of stress the usual dose may need to be adjusted. The patient should have an emergency kit available with syringe and either hydrocortisone or dexamethasone as prescribed by the primary provider (Zhang & Carmichael, 2019). Specific verbal and written instructions about how and when to use the injection are also provided to the patient and family or caregivers. Chart 45-11 summarizes education for patients with Addison's disease and their caregivers.

Continuing and Transitional Care

Although most patients can return to their job and family responsibilities soon after hospital discharge, others cannot do so because of concurrent illnesses or incomplete recovery

---

Chart 45-11

HOME CARE CHECKLIST

The Patient with Adrenal Insufficiency (Addison's Disease)

At the completion of education, the patient and/or caregiver will be able to:

- State the impact of adrenal insufficiency and treatment on physiologic functioning, ADLs, IADLs, roles, relationships, and spirituality.
- State the purpose, dose, route, schedule, side effects, and precautions of prescribed medications (corticosteroid replacement).
- State that compliance with medical regimen is lifelong.
- Recognize the need for dosage adjustment during times of stress.
- State changes in lifestyle (e.g., diet, activity) necessary to maintain health, including:
- Wearing medical alert identification, and carrying medical information card.
- Avoiding strenuous activity in hot, humid weather.
- Identifying strategies for dealing with stress and avoiding adrenal crisis.
- Notifying primary providers about disease before treatment or procedure.

- Increasing fluid intake and salt with excessive perspiration.
- Ensuring high-carbohydrate, high-protein diet with adequate sodium intake.
- State warning signs of adrenal crisis and the need for emergency care.
- Explain components of an emergency kit and indications for their use; demonstrate how to use them.
- Relate how to reach primary provider with questions or complications.
- State time and date of follow-up medical appointments, therapy, and testing.
- Identify sources of support (e.g., friends, relatives, faith community).
- Identify the contact details for support services for patients and their caregivers/families.
- Identify the need for health promotion, disease prevention, and screening activities.

ADLs, activities of daily living; IADLs, instrumental activities of daily living.

from the episode of adrenal insufficiency. In these circumstances, a referral for home, community-based or transitional care enables the nurse to assess the patient's recovery, monitor hormone replacement, and evaluate stress in the home. The nurse assesses the patient's and family's knowledge about medication therapy and dietary modifications and provides education as needed. The home health nurse educates the patient and family on the importance of keeping follow-up visits with the primary provider and participating in health promotion activities and health screening.

Cushing's Syndrome

The most common cause of Cushing's syndrome (also known as Cushing's disease) is the use of corticosteroid medications, but the syndrome can also be due to excessive glucocorticoid production secondary to hyperplasia of the adrenal cortex (Sadiq & Silverstein, 2019a). However, overproduction of endogenous glucocorticoids may be caused by several mechanisms, including a tumor of the pituitary gland that produces ACTH and stimulates the adrenal cortex to increase its hormone secretion despite production of adequate amounts. Primary hyperplasia of the adrenal glands in the absence of a pituitary tumor is less common. Another less common cause of Cushing's syndrome is the ectopic production of ACTH by malignancies; bronchogenic carcinoma is the most common type. Regardless of the cause, the normal feedback mechanisms that control the function of the adrenal cortex become ineffective, and the usual diurnal pattern of cortisol is lost. The signs and symptoms of Cushing's syndrome are primarily a result of oversecretion of glucocorticoids and androgens, although mineralocorticoid secretion may be affected as well (Norris, 2019).

Clinical Manifestations

When overproduction of the adrenocortical hormone occurs, arrest of growth, obesity, and musculoskeletal changes occur along with glucose intolerance. The classic picture of Cushing's syndrome in the adult is that of central-type obesity, with a fatty "buffalo hump" in the neck and supraclavicular areas, a heavy trunk, and relatively thin extremities. The skin is thin, fragile, and easily traumatized; ecchymoses (bruises) and striae develop. The patient complains of weakness and lassitude. Sleep is disturbed because of altered diurnal secretion of cortisol.

Excessive protein catabolism occurs, producing muscle wasting and osteoporosis. Kyphosis, backache, and compression fractures of the vertebrae may result. Retention of sodium and water occurs as a result of increased mineralocorticoid activity, producing hypertension and heart failure.

The patient develops a "moon-faced" appearance and may experience increased oiliness of the skin and acne. Hyperglycemia or overt diabetes may develop. The patient may also report weight gain, slow healing of minor cuts, and bruises.

Women between the ages of 20 and 40 years are five times more likely than men to develop Cushing's syndrome. In females of all ages, virilization may occur as a result of excess androgens. Virilization is characterized by the appearance of masculine traits and the recession of feminine traits. Hirsutism (excessive growth of hair on the face) occurs, the breasts atrophy, menses cease, the clitoris enlarges, and the voice deepens. Libido is lost in men and women. Distress and

Chart 45-12 Clinical Manifestations of Cushing's Syndrome

Cardiovascular

Heart failure
Hypertension

Dermatologic

Acne
Ecchymoses
Petechiae
Striae
Thinning of skin

Endocrine/Metabolic

Adrenal suppression
Altered calcium metabolism
Buffalo hump
Hyperglycemia
Hypokalemia
Impotence
Menstrual irregularities
Metabolic alkalosis
Moon face
Negative nitrogen balance
Sodium retention
Truncal obesity

Gastrointestinal

Pancreatitis
Peptic ulcer

Immune Function

Decreased inflammatory
responses
Impaired wound healing
Increased susceptibility to
infections

Muscular

Muscle weakness
Myopathy

Ophthalmic

Cataracts
Glaucoma

Psychiatric

Mood alterations
Psychoses

Skeletal

Aseptic necrosis of femur
Osteoporosis
Spontaneous fractures
Vertebral compression
fractures

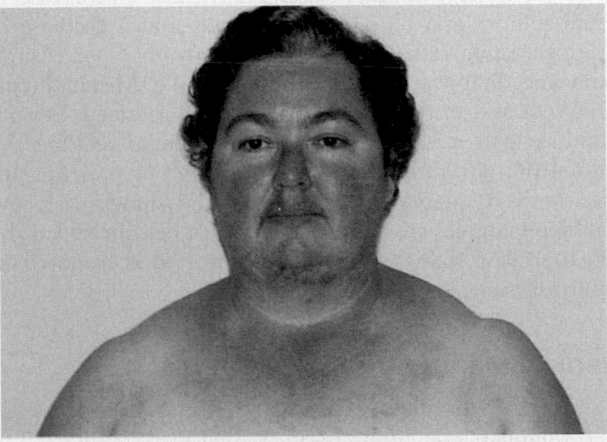

This woman with Cushing syndrome has several classic signs, including facial hair, buffalo hump, and moon face. Reprinted with permission from Rubin, R., Strayer, D. S., & Rubin, E. (2012). *Rubin's pathology* (6th ed.). Philadelphia, PA: Lippincott Williams & Wilkins.

depression are common and are increased by the severity of the physical changes that occur with this syndrome. If Cushing's disease is a consequence of pituitary tumor, visual disturbances may occur because of pressure of the growing tumor on the optic chiasm. Chart 45-12 summarizes the clinical manifestations of Cushing's syndrome.

Assessment and Diagnostic Findings

The three tests used to diagnose Cushing's syndrome are serum cortisol, urinary cortisol, and low-dose dexamethasone suppression tests. Two of these three tests need to be unequivocally abnormal to diagnose Cushing's syndrome. If the results of all three tests are normal, the patient likely does not have Cushing's syndrome (but may have a mild case, or the manifestations may be cyclic). For these patients, further testing is not recommended unless symptoms progress. If test results are either slightly abnormal or discordant, further testing is recommended.

Serum cortisol levels are usually higher in the early morning (6 to 8 AM) and lower in the evening (4 to 6 PM). This variation is lost in patients with Cushing's syndrome (Fischbach & Fischbach, 2018).

A urinary cortisol test requires a 24-hour urine collection. The nurse instructs the patient how to collect and store the specimen. If the results of the urinary cortisol test are three times the upper limit of the normal range and one other test is abnormal, Cushing's syndrome can be assumed.

An overnight dexamethasone suppression test is used to diagnosis pituitary and adrenal causes of Cushing's syndrome. It can be performed on an outpatient basis. Dexamethasone (1 or 8 mg) is given orally late in the evening or at bedtime, and a plasma cortisol level is obtained at 8 AM the next morning. Suppression of cortisol to less than 5 mg/dL indicates that the hypothalamic–pituitary–adrenal axis is functioning properly (Fischbach & Fischbach, 2018). Stress, obesity, depression, and medications such as anticonvulsant agents, estrogen (during pregnancy or as oral medications), and rifampin can falsely elevate cortisol levels.

Indicators of Cushing's syndrome include an increase in serum sodium and blood glucose levels and a decrease in serum potassium, a reduction in the number of blood eosinophils, and disappearance of lymphoid tissue. Measurements of plasma and urinary cortisol levels are obtained. Several blood samples may be collected to determine whether the normal diurnal variation in plasma levels is present; this variation is frequently absent in adrenal dysfunction. If several blood samples are required, they must be collected at the times specified, and the time of collection must be noted on the requisition slip.

Medical Management

If Cushing's syndrome is caused by pituitary tumors rather than tumors of the adrenal cortex, treatment is directed at the pituitary gland. Surgical removal of the tumor by transsphenoidal hypophysectomy (see Chapter 61) is the treatment of choice. Radiation of the pituitary gland has also been successful, although it may take several months for control of symptoms. Adrenalectomy is the treatment of choice in patients with unilateral primary adrenal hypertrophy. Medical management is recommended for bilateral adrenal dysplasia.

Postoperatively, symptoms of adrenal insufficiency may begin to appear 12 to 48 hours after surgery because of reduction of the high levels of circulating adrenal hormones. Temporary replacement therapy with hydrocortisone may be necessary for several months, until the adrenal glands begin to respond normally to the body's needs.

Adrenal enzyme inhibitors (e.g., metyrapone, aminoglutethimide, mitotane, and ketoconazole) may be used to reduce hyperadrenalism if the syndrome is caused by ectopic ACTH secretion by a tumor that cannot be eradicated. Close monitoring is necessary, because symptoms of inadequate adrenal function may result, and side effects of the medications may occur.

If Cushing's syndrome is a result of the administration of corticosteroids, an attempt is made to reduce or taper the medication to the minimum dosage needed to treat the underlying disease process (e.g., autoimmune or allergic disease, rejection of a transplanted organ). Frequently, alternate-day therapy decreases the symptoms of Cushing's syndrome and allows recovery of the adrenal glands' responsiveness to ACTH.

Diabetes and peptic ulcer are common in patients with Cushing's syndrome. Therefore, insulin therapy and medication to prevent or treat peptic ulcer are initiated if needed. Before, during, and after surgery, blood glucose monitoring and assessment of stools for blood are carried out to monitor for these complications. If the patient has other symptoms of Cushing's syndrome, these are considered in the preoperative preparation. For example, if the patient has experienced weight gain, special instruction is given about postoperative breathing exercises.

NURSING PROCESS

The Patient with Cushing's Syndrome

Assessment

The health history and examination focus on the effects on the body of high concentrations of adrenal cortex hormones and on the inability of the adrenal cortex to respond to changes in cortisol and aldosterone levels. The history includes information about the patient's level of activity and ability to carry out routine and self-care activities. The skin is observed and assessed for trauma, infection, breakdown, bruising, and edema. Changes in physical appearance are noted, and the patient's responses to these changes are elicited. The nurse assesses the patient's mental function, including mood, responses to questions, awareness of environment, and level of depression. The family is often a good source of information about gradual changes in the patient's physical appearance as well as emotional status.

Diagnosis

NURSING DIAGNOSES

Based on the assessment data, major priority nursing diagnoses include the following:

- Risk for impaired cardiac function associated with changes in cardiac function
- Risk for injury associated with weakness
- Risk for infection associated with altered immune system function
- Impaired skin integrity associated with edema, impaired healing, and thin and fragile skin
- Disturbed body image associated with altered physical appearance, impaired sexual functioning, and decreased activity level
- Difficulty coping associated with mood swings, irritability, and depression

COLLABORATIVE PROBLEMS/POTENTIAL COMPLICATIONS

Potential complications may include the following:
- Addisonian crisis
- Adverse effects of adrenocortical activity

Planning and Goals

The major goals for the patient include maintenance of adequate cardiac function, decreased risk of injury, decreased risk of infection, improved skin integrity, improved body image, improved mental function, and absence of complications.

Nursing Interventions

MAINTAINING ADEQUATE CARDIAC FUNCTION

The patient who is taking corticosteroid medications should be monitored for the presence of hypertension and hypokalemia. The nurse assesses fluid and electrolyte status by monitoring laboratory values and daily weights. The patient should be educated about foods low in sodium to decrease fluid retention and foods high in potassium; referral to a dietitian may be useful. The patient should also be instructed to report and pedal edema or changes in activity tolerance.

DECREASING RISK OF INJURY

Establishing a protective environment helps prevent falls, fractures, and other injuries to bones and soft tissues. The patient who is very weak may require assistance from the nurse in ambulating to avoid falling or bumping into sharp corners of furniture. Foods high in protein, calcium, and vitamin D are recommended to minimize muscle wasting and osteoporosis. Referral to a dietitian may assist the patient in selecting appropriate foods that are also low in sodium and calories.

DECREASING RISK OF INFECTION

The patient should avoid unnecessary exposure to others with infections. The nurse frequently assesses the patient for subtle signs of infection, because the anti-inflammatory effects of corticosteroids may mask the common signs of inflammation and infection.

PROMOTING SKIN INTEGRITY

Meticulous skin care is necessary to avoid traumatizing the patient's fragile skin. The use of adhesive tape is avoided, because it can irritate the skin and tear the fragile tissue when the tape is removed. The nurse frequently assesses the skin and bony prominences and encourages and assists the patient to change positions frequently to prevent skin breakdown.

IMPROVING BODY IMAGE

The patient may benefit from discussion of the effect the changes have had on their self-concept and relationships with others. Weight gain and edema may be modified by a low-carbohydrate, low-sodium diet, and a high-protein intake may reduce some of the other bothersome symptoms. The patient may also benefit from discussion of the changes being temporary if the treatment with corticosteroids is temporary.

IMPROVING COPING

Explanations to the patient and family members about the cause of emotional instability are important in helping them cope with the mood swings, irritability, and depression that may occur. Psychotic behavior may occur in a few patients and should be reported. The nurse encourages the patient and family members to verbalize their feelings and concerns.

MONITORING AND MANAGING POTENTIAL COMPLICATIONS

Addisonian Crisis. The patient with Cushing's syndrome whose symptoms are treated by withdrawal of corticosteroids, by adrenalectomy, or by removal of a pituitary tumor is at risk for adrenal hypofunction and Addisonian crisis. If high levels of circulating adrenal hormones have suppressed the function of the adrenal cortex, atrophy of the adrenal cortex is likely. If the circulating hormone level is decreased rapidly because of surgery or abrupt cessation of corticosteroid agents, manifestations of adrenal hypofunction and Addisonian crisis may develop. Therefore, the patient with Cushing's syndrome should be assessed for signs and symptoms of Addisonian crisis as discussed previously. If Addisonian crisis occurs, the patient is treated for circulatory collapse and shock (see Chapter 11).

Adverse Effects of Adrenocortical Activity. The nurse assesses fluid and electrolyte status by monitoring laboratory values and daily weights. Because of the increased risk of glucose intolerance and hyperglycemia, blood glucose monitoring is initiated. The nurse reports elevated blood glucose levels to the primary provider so that treatment can be prescribed if needed. If indicated, the patient may need to be educated in self-monitoring of blood glucose and insulin injections.

PROMOTING HOME, COMMUNITY-BASED, AND TRANSITIONAL CARE

Educating Patients About Self-Care. The patient, family, and caregivers should be educated that acute adrenal insufficiency and underlying symptoms will recur if medication is stopped abruptly without medical supervision. The nurse stresses the need for dietary modifications to ensure adequate calcium intake without increasing the risks for hypertension, hyperglycemia, and weight gain. The nurse educates the patient and family about how to monitor blood pressure, blood glucose levels, and weight. Patients should be advised to wear a medical alert bracelet and to notify other health care providers (e.g., dentist) about their condition (see Chart 45-13).

Continuing and Transitional Care. The need for follow-up depends on the origin and duration of the disease and its management. The patient who has been treated by adrenalectomy or removal of a pituitary tumor requires close monitoring to ensure that adrenal function has returned to normal and adequacy of circulating adrenal hormones. Home care referral may be indicated to ensure a safe environment that minimizes stress and risk of falls and other side effects. The home health nurse assesses the patient's physical and psychological status and reports changes to the primary provider. The nurse also assesses the patient's understanding of and ability to manage the medication regimen and reinforces previous education about the medications and the importance of taking them as prescribed. The nurse emphasizes the importance of regular medical follow-up, the side effects and toxic effects of medications, and the need to wear medical identification with Addison's and Cushing's diseases. In addition, the patient and family are reminded about the importance of health promotion activities and recommended health screening, including bone mineral density testing.

Chart 45-13 — HOME CARE CHECKLIST
The Patient with Cushing's Syndrome

At the completion of education, the patient and/or caregiver will be able to:

- State the impact of Cushing's syndrome and treatment on physiologic functioning, ADLs, IADLs, roles, relationships, and spirituality.
- State the relationship between adrenal hormones, emotional state, and stress.
- State the purpose, dose, route, schedule, side effects, and precautions for prescribed medications (adrenocortical inhibitors).
- State importance of compliance with medical regimen.
- State the need to contact primary provider before taking over-the-counter medications.
- State changes in lifestyle (e.g., diet, activity) necessary to maintain health, including:
- Wearing medical alert identification, and carrying medical information card.
- Identifying methods for managing labile emotions.
- Describing protective skin care measures and the use of protective devices and practices to decrease injury/fracture.

- Identifying foods high in potassium and low in sodium, calories, and carbohydrates.
- Describing measures to decrease risk of infection.
- Balancing rest and activity.
- Monitoring blood pressure, blood glucose levels, and weight.
- Identify signs and symptoms of excessive and insufficient adrenal hormone.
- Relate how to reach primary provider with questions or complications.
- State time and date of follow-up medical appointments, therapy, and testing.
- Identify sources of support (e.g., friends, relatives, faith community).
- Identify the contact details for support services for patients and their caregivers/families.
- Identify the need for health promotion, disease prevention, and screening activities.

ADLs, activities of daily living; IADLs, instrumental activities of daily living.

Evaluation

Expected patient outcomes may include:

1. Maintains adequate cardiac function
   a. Blood pressure is maintained within acceptable ranges
   b. Potassium levels are within normal ranges
   c. Absence of pedal edema
2. Decreases risk of injury
   a. Is free of fractures or soft tissue injuries
   b. Is free of ecchymotic areas
3. Decreases risk of infection
   a. Experiences no temperature elevation, redness, pain, or other signs of infection or inflammation
   b. Avoids contact with others who have infections
4. Attains/maintains skin integrity
   a. Has intact skin, without evidence of breakdown or infection
   b. Exhibits decreased edema in extremities and trunk
   c. Changes position frequently and inspects bony prominences daily
5. Achieves improved body image
   a. Verbalizes feelings about changes in appearance, sexual function, and activity level
   b. States that physical changes are a result of excessive glucocorticoids
6. Exhibits improved thought processes
7. Exhibits absence of complications
   a. Exhibits normal vital signs and weight and is free of symptoms of Addisonian crisis
   b. Identifies signs and symptoms of adrenocortical hypofunction that should be reported and measures to take in case of severe illness and stress
   c. Identifies strategies to minimize complications of Cushing's syndrome
   d. Adheres to recommendations for follow-up appointments and health screening

Primary Aldosteronism

The principal action of aldosterone is to conserve body sodium. Under the influence of this hormone, the kidneys excrete less sodium and more potassium and hydrogen. Primary aldosteronism is also known as Conn syndrome. Etiologic factors for primary aldosteronism include tumors of the adrenal gland, ovarian tumors that secrete aldosterone, and a family history. The true incidence of primary aldosteronism is unknown (Ma & Baranski, 2019) but studies have indicated that it is underestimated (Monticone, Burrello, Tizzani, et al., 2017). Excessive production of aldosterone causes a distinctive pattern of biochemical changes and a corresponding set of clinical manifestations that are diagnostic of this condition.

Clinical Manifestations

Hypertension is the most prominent and almost universal sign of primary aldosteronism. Patients with uncomplicated, complicated, and treatment-resistant hypertension and hypertension with hypokalemia should be considered at risk for this disorder. However, hypokalemia should no longer be considered a requisite for this diagnosis. It is now recognized that hypokalemia occurs in less than half of the patients (Ma & Baranski, 2019). If hypokalemia is present, it may be responsible for the variable muscle weakness or paralysis, cramping, and fatigue in patients with aldosteronism, as well as the kidneys' inability to acidify or concentrate the urine. Accordingly, the urine volume is excessive, leading to polyuria. Serum, by contrast, becomes abnormally concentrated, contributing to polydipsia (excessive thirst) and arterial hypertension. A secondary increase in blood volume and possible direct effects of aldosterone on nerve receptors, such as the carotid sinus, are other factors that result in hypertension.

Hypokalemic alkalosis may decrease the ionized serum calcium level and predispose the patient to tetany and paresthesias. Chvostek and Trousseau signs may be used to assess neuromuscular irritability before overt paresthesia and tetany occur. Glucose intolerance may occur, because hypokalemia interferes with insulin secretion from the pancreas.

Assessment and Diagnostic Findings

Withholding antihypertensive medication before laboratory testing is not required. If the patient is taking an antihypertensive agent, this information should be considered when interpreting the results of the PAC/PRA (plasma aldosterone concentration/plasma renin activity) study as well as the ARR (aldosterone-renin ratio) (Ma & Baranski, 2019).

Medical Management

The recommended treatment of unilateral primary aldosteronism is total surgical removal of the adrenal tumor through laparoscopic adrenalectomy rather than open surgery. Laparoscopic surgery is associated with shorter hospital stays and generally fewer complications following surgery (Ma & Baranski, 2019). During the preoperative period, blood pressure and potassium levels are closely monitored. During the immediate postoperative period, the patient is susceptible to fluctuations in adrenocortical hormones and requires administration of corticosteroids, fluids, and other agents to maintain blood pressure and prevent acute complications. If the adrenalectomy is bilateral, replacement of corticosteroids will be lifelong. A normal serum glucose level is maintained with insulin, appropriate IV fluids, and dietary modifications. Hypokalemia typically resolves for all patients after surgery and hypertension is resolved in 35% to 60%. Postoperatively, spironolactone and potassium supplements should be discontinued and antihypertensives should be decreased. Potassium levels should be checked once a week for 4 weeks postoperatively (Ma & Baranski, 2019). Medical treatment rather than surgery is recommended for patients with bilateral adrenal involvement due to poor blood pressure control and other risks.

Pharmacologic Therapy

Pharmacologic management is required for patients with bilateral adrenal hyperplasia or unilateral aldosterone hypersecretion who do not undergo surgery. Spironolactone is recommended as the first-line drug to control hypertension. Eplerenone, a more expensive drug, is recommended as a second-line drug if the patient cannot tolerate side effects of spironolactone (Ma & Baranski, 2019). Serum potassium and creatinine should be monitored frequently during the first 4 to 6 weeks of taking spironolactone. Ongoing monitoring will be determined by the clinical course. The half-life of digoxin may be increased when taken with spironolactone, and its dosage may need to be adjusted.

Nursing Management

Nursing management in the postoperative period includes frequent assessment of vital signs to detect early signs and symptoms of adrenal insufficiency and crisis or hemorrhage. Explaining all treatments and procedures, providing comfort measures, and providing rest periods can reduce the patient's stress and anxiety level.

TABLE 45-2 Commonly Used Corticosteroid Preparations	
Generic Names	Select Trade Names
beclomethasone	Beconase AQ, Qnasl
betamethasone	Beta-Val, Dermabet, Luxiq, Valnac
dexamethasone	Dexamethasone Intensol
hydrocortisone	Colocort, Cortef, Cortenema, Solu-Cortef
methylprednisolone	Depo-Medrol, Solu-Medrol
prednisone	Prednisone Intensol, Rayos
prednisolone	Prelone
triamcinolone	Kenalog, Triderm

Adapted from Comerford, K. C., & Durkin, M. T. (2020). *Nursing 2020 drug handbook.* Philadelphia, PA: Wolters Kluwer.

Corticosteroid Therapy

Corticosteroids are used extensively for adrenal insufficiency and are also widely used in suppressing inflammation and autoimmune reactions, controlling allergic reactions, and reducing the rejection process in transplantation. Commonly used corticosteroid preparations are listed in Table 45-2. Their anti-inflammatory and antiallergy actions make corticosteroids effective in treating rheumatic or connective tissue diseases, such as rheumatoid arthritis and SLE. They are also frequently used in the treatment of asthma, multiple sclerosis, and other autoimmune disorders.

High doses appear to allow patients to tolerate high degrees of stress. Such antistress action may be caused by the ability of corticosteroids to aid circulating vasopressor substances in keeping the blood pressure elevated; other effects, such as maintenance of the serum glucose level, also may keep blood pressure elevated.

Side Effects

Although the synthetic corticosteroids are safer for some patients because of relative freedom from mineralocorticoid activity, most natural and synthetic corticosteroids produce similar kinds of side effects. The dose required for anti-inflammatory and antiallergy effects also produces metabolic effects, pituitary and adrenal gland suppression, and changes in the function of the central nervous system. Therefore, although corticosteroids are highly effective therapeutically, they may also be very dangerous. Dosages of these medications are frequently altered to allow high concentrations when necessary and then tapered in an attempt to avoid undesirable effects. This requires that patients be observed closely for side effects and that the dose be reduced when high doses are no longer required. Suppression of the adrenal cortex may persist up to 1 year after a course of corticosteroids.

Therapeutic Uses of Corticosteroids

The dosage of corticosteroids is determined by the nature and chronicity of the illness as well as the patient's other medical conditions. Rheumatoid arthritis, bronchial asthma, and multiple sclerosis are chronic disorders that corticosteroids do not cure; however, these medications may be useful when other measures do not provide adequate control of symptoms. In addition, corticosteroids may be used to treat acute exacerbations of these disorders.

In such situations, the adverse effects of corticosteroids are weighed against the patient's current condition. These medications may be used for a period but then are gradually reduced or tapered as the symptoms subside. The nurse plays an important role in providing encouragement and understanding during times when the patient is experiencing (or is apprehensive about experiencing) recurrence of symptoms while taking smaller doses.

Treatment of Acute Conditions

Acute flare-ups and crises are treated with large doses of corticosteroids. Examples include emergency treatment for bronchial obstruction in status asthmaticus and for septic shock from septicemia caused by gram-negative bacteria. Other measures, such as anti-infective agents or medications, are also used with corticosteroids to treat shock and other major symptoms. At times, corticosteroids are continued past the acute flare-up stage to prevent serious complications.

Ophthalmologic Treatment

Outer eye infections can be treated by topical application of corticosteroid eye drops, because the agents do not cause systemic toxicity. However, long-term application can cause an increase in intraocular pressure, which leads to glaucoma in some patients. In addition, prolonged use of corticosteroids can sometimes lead to cataract formation.

Dermatologic Disorders

Topical administration of corticosteroids in the form of creams, ointments, lotions, and aerosols is especially effective in many dermatologic disorders. It may be more effective in some conditions to use occlusive dressings around the affected part to achieve maximum absorption of the medication. Penetration and absorption are also increased if the medication is applied when the skin is hydrated or moist (e.g., immediately after bathing).

Absorption of topical agents varies with body location. For example, absorption is greater through the layers of skin on the scalp, face, and genital area than on the forearm; as a result, the use of topical agents on these sites increases the risk of side effects. The availability of over-the-counter topical corticosteroids increases the risk of side effects in patients who are unaware of their potential risks. Excessive use of these agents, especially on large surface areas of inflamed skin, can lead to decreased therapeutic effects and increased side effects.

Dosage

Attempts have been made to determine the best time to administer pharmacologic doses of steroids. If symptoms have been controlled on a 6- or 8-hour program, a once-daily or every-other-day schedule may be implemented. In keeping with the natural secretion of cortisol, the best time of day for the total corticosteroid dose is in the early morning, between 7 and 8 AM. Large-dose therapy at 8 AM, when the adrenal gland is most active, produces maximal suppression of the gland. A large 8 AM dose is more physiologic because it allows the body to escape effects of the steroids from 4 PM to 6 AM, when serum levels are normally low, hence minimizing cushingoid effects. If symptoms of the disorder being treated are suppressed, alternate-day therapy is helpful in reducing pituitary–adrenal suppression in patients requiring prolonged therapy. Some patients report discomfort associated with symptoms of their primary illness on the second day; therefore, the nurse must explain to patients that this regimen is necessary to minimize side effects and suppression of adrenal function.

Tapering

Corticosteroid dosages are tapered (reduced gradually) to allow normal adrenal function to return and to prevent steroid-induced adrenal insufficiency. Up to 1 year or longer after the use of corticosteroids, the patient is still at risk for adrenal insufficiency in times of stress. For example, if surgery for any reason is necessary, the patient is likely to require IV corticosteroids during and after surgery to reduce the risk of acute adrenal crisis.

Nursing Management

Nursing management of corticosteroid therapy includes many important interventions. Table 45-3 provides an overview of the effects of corticosteroid therapy and the nursing implications.

Promoting Home, Community-Based, and Transitional Care

 Educating Patients About Self-Care

The nurse educates the patient, family, and caregivers that acute adrenal insufficiency and underlying symptoms will recur if corticosteroid therapy is stopped abruptly without medical supervision. The patient should be instructed to always have an adequate supply of the corticosteroid medication to avoid running out.

Continuing and Transitional Care

The patient who requires continued corticosteroid therapy is monitored to ensure understanding of the medications and the need for a dosage that treats the underlying disorder while minimizing the side effects. Home care referral may be indicated to ensure a safe environment that minimizes stress, risk of falls, and other side effects. The nurse assesses the patient's physical and psychological status and reports changes to the primary provider. The nurse also assesses the patient's understanding of and ability to manage the medication regimen and reinforces previous education about the medications and the importance of taking them as prescribed. The nurse emphasizes the importance of regular medical follow-up, the side effects of the medications, and the effects of abruptly discontinuing corticosteroids. In addition, the patient and family are reminded about the importance of health promotion activities and recommended health screening, including bone mineral density testing.

TABLE 45-3	Corticosteroid Therapy and Implications for Nursing Practice	
Side Effects	**Nursing Interventions**
Cardiovascular Effects	
Hypertension	Monitor for elevated blood pressure.
Thrombophlebitis	Assess for signs and symptoms of deep venous thrombosis: redness, warmth, tenderness, and edema of an extremity.
Thromboembolism	Remind patient to avoid positions and situations that restrict blood flow (e.g., crossing legs, prolonged sitting in same position).
Accelerated atherosclerosis	Encourage foot and leg exercises when recumbent.
	Encourage low-sodium diet.
	Encourage limited intake of fat.
Immunologic Effects	
Increased risk of infection and masking of signs of infection	Assess for subtle signs of infection and inflammation.
	Encourage patient to avoid exposure to others with upper respiratory infection.
	Monitor patient for fungal infections.
	Encourage good hand hygiene.
Ophthalmologic Changes	
Glaucoma	Encourage yearly eye examinations.
Corneal lesions	Refer patient to ophthalmologist if changes in visual acuity are detected.
Musculoskeletal Effects	
Muscle wasting	Encourage high-protein intake.
Poor wound healing	Encourage high-protein intake and vitamin C supplementation.
Osteoporosis with vertebral compression fractures, pathologic fractures of long bones, aseptic necrosis of head of the femur	Encourage diet high in calcium and vitamin D or calcium and vitamin D supplementation if indicated.
	Take measures to avoid falls and other trauma.
	Use caution in moving and turning patient.
	Encourage postmenopausal women on corticosteroids to consider bone mineral density testing and treatment, if indicated.
	Instruct patient to rise slowly from bed or chair to avoid falling due to orthostatic hypotension.
Metabolic Effects	
Alterations in glucose metabolism	Monitor blood glucose levels at periodic intervals.
Steroid withdrawal syndrome	Instruct patient about medications, diet, and exercise prescribed to control blood glucose level.
	Report signs of adrenal insufficiency.
	Administer corticosteroids and mineralocorticoids as prescribed.
	Instruct patient about importance of taking corticosteroids as prescribed without abruptly stopping therapy.
	Encourage patient to obtain and wear a medical identification bracelet.
	Advise patient to notify all health care providers (e.g., dentist) about the need for corticosteroid therapy.
Changes in Appearance	
Moon face	Encourage low-calorie, low-sodium diet.
Weight gain	Assure patient that most changes in appearance are temporary and will disappear if and when corticosteroid therapy is no longer necessary.
Acne	
Fluid and Electrolyte Imbalances	Monitor I&O and electrolytes.
	Administer fluids and electrolytes as prescribed.

I&O, intake and output.

CRITICAL THINKING EXERCISES

1 ebp A 62-year-old man has been recently diagnosed with hypothyroidismn and requires education to manage his condition. What evidence-based practices will you include when educating this patient? Identify at least three essential pieces of information you would include.

2 pq You are caring for a patient who requires long-term administration of prednisone. Identify three priority nursing diagnoses for this patient related to the use of the prednisone. State the expected outcomes and at least three priority interventions with scientific rationales for each nursing diagnosis.

3 ipc A patient with a 6-month history of Addison's disease is hospitalized for Addisonian crisis and is transferred to a medical unit after a 2-day stay in the intensive care unit. During interprofessional collaborative rounds, the team discusses this patient. What information will the primary provider, the nurse, the physical therapist, and the discharge planner contribute to the discussion? What patient-centered goals will each discipline set for the patient?

4 pq Identify the priorities, approach, and techniques you would use to perform a comprehensive assessment on a 60-year-old patient newly diagnosed with Cushing's syndrome. How will your priorities, approach, and techniques differ if the patient has a visual impairment or is hard of hearing? If the patient is from a culture with very different values from your own?

REFERENCES

*Asterisk indicates nursing research.

Books

Amdur, R. J., & Dagan, R. (2019). Thyroid cancer. In Halperin, E. C., Wazer, D. E., Perez, C.A., & Brady, L. W. (Eds.). *Perez & Brady's principles and practice of radiation oncology* (7th ed.). Philadelphia, PA: Wolters Kluwer.

Bauerle, K. T., & Clutter, W. E. (2019). Hyperthyroidism. In T. J. Braranski, J. B. McGill, & J. M. Silverstein (Eds.). *The Washington manual endocrinology subspecialty consult* (4th ed.). Philadelphia, PA: Wolters Kluwer.

Bauerle, K. T., & Riek, A. E. (2019). Thyroid cancer. In T. J. Braranski, J. B. McGill, & J. M. Silverstein (Eds.). *The Washington manual endocrinology subspecialty consult* (4th ed.). Philadelphia, PA: Wolters-Kluwer.

Comerford, K. C., & Durkin, M. T. (2020). *Nursing 2020 drug handbook*. Philadelphia, PA: Wolters Kluwer.

Eliopoulos, C. (2018). *Gerontological nursing* (9th ed.). Philadelphia, PA: Wolters-Kluwer.

Fischbach, F. T., & Fischbach, M. A. (2018). *Fischbach's manual of laboratory and diagnostic tests* (10th ed.). Philadelphia, PA: Wolters Kluwer.

Hickey, K., & Silverstein, J. M. (2019). Acromegaly. In T. J. Braranski, J. B. McGill, & J. M. Silverstein (Eds.). *The Washington manual endocrinology subspecialty consult* (4th ed.). Philadelphia, PA: Wolters Kluwer.

Hollar, L. N., & Silverstein, J. M. (2019). Diabetes insipidus. In T. J. Braranski, J. B. McGill, & J. M. Silverstein (Eds.). *The Washington manual endocrinology subspecialty consult* (4th ed.). Philadelphia, PA: Wolters Kluwer Health.

Jensen, S. (2019). *Nursing health assessment: A best practice approach* (3rd ed.). Philadelphia, PA: Wolters Kluwer.

Ma, N., & Baranski, T. J. (2019). Hyperaldosteronism. In T. J. Braranski, J. B. McGill, & J. M. Silverstein (Eds.). *The Washington manual endocrinology subspecialty consult* (4th ed.). Philadelphia, PA: Wolters Kluwer.

Medford, L. C. (2019). Disorders of endocrine control of growth and metabolism. In T. J. Braranski, J. B. McGill, & J. M. Silverstein (Eds.). *The Washington manual endocrinology subspecialty consult* (4th ed.). Philadelphia, PA: Wolters Kluwer.

Morton, P. G., & Fontaine, D. K. (2018). *Critical care nursing: A holistic approach* (10th ed.). Philadelphia, PA: Wolters Kluwer.

Norris, T. L. (2019). *Porth's pathophysiology: Concepts of altered health status* (10th ed.). Philadelphia, PA: Wolters Kluwer.

Parham, J. S., & Silverstein, J. M. (2019). Syndrome of inappropriate diuretic hormone. In T. J. Braranski, J. B. McGill, & J. M. Silverstein (Eds.). *The Washington manual endocrinology subspecialty consult* (4th ed.). Philadelphia, PA: Wolters Kluwer Health.

Quintanar, A. (2019). Endocrine care. In D. Kantor (Ed.). *Lippincott visual nursing: A guide to clinical diseases, skills, and treatments* (3rd ed.). Philadelphia, PA: Wolters Kluwer.

Sadiq, S., & Silverstein, J. M. (2019a). Cushing syndrome. In T. J. Braranski, J. B. McGill, & J. M. Silverstein (Eds.). *The Washington manual endocrinology subspecialty consult* (4th ed.). Philadelphia, PA: Wolters Kluwer.

Sadiq, S., & Silverstein, J. M. (2019b). Sellar and suprasellar masses. In T. J. Braranski, J. B. McGill, & J. M. Silverstein (Eds.). *The Washington manual endocrinology subspecialty consult* (4th ed.). Philadelphia, PA: Wolters Kluwer.

Samuels, M. H. (2018). Hyperthyroidism in the elderly. In K. Feingold, B. Anawalt, A. Boyce, et al. (Eds.). *Endotex*. South Darthmouth, MA: MDText.com, Inc.

Singh, S., & Clutter, W. E. (2019). Hypothyroidism. In T. J. Braranski, J. B. McGill, & J. M. Silverstein (Eds.). *The Washington manual endocrinology subspecialty consult* (4th ed.). Philadelphia, PA: Wolters Kluwer.

Singh, S., & Herrick, C. J. (2019). Pheochromocytoma and paraganglioma. In T. J. Braranski, J. B. McGill, & J. M. Silverstein (Eds.). *The Washington manual endocrinology subspecialty consult* (4th ed.). Philadelphia, PA: Wolters Kluwer.

Vallerand, A. H., & Sanoski, C. A. (2018). *Davis's drug guide for nurses* (16th ed.). Philadelphia, PA: F.A. Davis.

Yalla, N., & Hickey, K. (2019). Hypercalcemia and hyperparathyroidism. In T. J. Braranski, J. B. McGill, & J. M. Silverstein (Eds.). *The Washington manual endocrinology subspecialty consult* (4th ed.). Philadelphia, PA: Wolters Kluwer.

Zhang, R. M., & Carmichael, K. (2019). Adrenal insufficiency. In T. J. Braranski, J. B. McGill, & J. M. Silverstein (Eds.). *The Washington manual endocrinology subspecialty consult* (4th ed.). Philadelphia, PA: Wolters Kluwer.

Journals and Electronic Documents

Alexander, E., Pearce, E., Brent, G., et al. (2017). 2017 Guidelines of the American Thyroid Association for the diagnosis and management of thyroid disease during pregnancy and the postpartum. *Thyroid, 27*(3), 315–389.

American Association of Neurological Surgeons. (2019). Pituitary gland and pituitary tumors. Retrieved on 4/14/2019 at: www.aans.org/Patients/Neurosurgical-Conditions-and-Treatments/Pituitary-Gland-and-Pituitary-Tumors

American Cancer Society (ACS). (2019). About thyroid cancer. Retrieved on 6/11/2019 at: www.cancer.org/cancer/thyroid-cancer/about.html

American College of Allergy, Asthma and Immunology. (2019). Is shellfish allergy related to iodine? Retrieved on 5/11/2019 at: acaai.org/resources/connect/ask-allergist/shellfish-allergy-related-iodine

Calsolaro, V., Niccolai, F., Pasqualetti, F., et al. (2019). Hypothyroidism in the elderly: Who should be treated and how? *Journal of the Endocrine Society, 3*(1), 146–158.

Chaker, L., Bianco, A. C., Janklaas, J., et al. (2017). Hypothyroidism. *The Lancet, 390*(10101), 1550–1562.

Drake, M. (2018). Hypothyroidism in clinical practice. *Mayo Clinic Proceedings*. Retrieved on 6/11/2019 at: doi.org/10.1016/j.mayocp.2018.07.015

Eledrisi, M. S. (2018). Myxedema coma or crisis. *Medscape*. Retrieved on 5/10/2019 at: emedicine.medscape.com/article/123577-overview#a1

Goltzman, D. (2019). Hypoparathyroidism. *UpToDate*. Retrieved on 6/11/2019 at: www.uptodate.com/contents/hypoparathyroidism

Lavrentaki, A., Paluzzi, A., Wass, J. A., et al. (2017). Epidemiology of acromegaly: Review of population studies. *Pituitary, 20*(1), 4–9.

Lee, S. L., & Khardori, R. (2018). Hyperthyroidism and thyrotoxicosis. *Medscape*. Retrieved on 5/15/2019 at: emedicine.medscape.com/article/121865-overview

Monticone, S., Burrello, J., Tizzani, D., et al. (2017). Prevalence and clinical manifestations of primary aldosteronism encountered in primary care practice. *Journal of the American College of Cardiology, 69*(14), 1811–1820.

Moore, D. (2018). Hypothyroidism and nursing care. *American Nurse Today, 13*(2), 45–46.

Naranjo, J., & Dodd, S. M. (2017). Perioperative management of pheochromocytoma. *Journal of Cardiothoracic Vascular Anesthesia, 31*(4), 1427–1439.

National Institute of Diabetes and Digestive and Kidney Diseases. (2019). Diabetes insipidus. Retrieved on 4/14/2019 at: www.niddk.nih.gov/health-information/kidney-disease/diabetes-insipidus

Ross, D. S., Cooper, D. S., & Mulder, J. E. (2019). Patient education: Thyroid nodules beyond the basics. *UpToDate*. Retrieved on 7/11/2019 at: www.uptodate.com/contents/thyroid-nodules-beyond-the-basics

Shane, E., & Berenson, J. R. (2019). Treatment of hypercalcemia. *UpToDate*. Retrieved on 6/11/2019 at: www.uptodate.com/contents/treatment-of-hypercalcemia

Silverberg, S. J., & Fuleihan, G.-E. H. (2019). Primary hyperparathyroidism: Management. *UpToDate*. Retrieved on 6/11/2019 at: www.uptodate.com/contents/primary-hyperparathyroidism-management

US National Library of Medicine. (2019). Pheochromocytoma. Retrieved on 4/1/2019 at: medlineplus.gov/ency/article/000340.htm

US Preventive Services Task Force. (2019). Final recommendation statement: Screening for thyroid dysfunction. Retrieved on 7/11/2019 at: www.uspreventiveservicestaskforce.org/Announcements/News/Item/final-recommendation-statement-screening-for-thyroid-dysfunction

*Yoo, Y. G., Yu, B. J., & Choi, E. (2018). A comparison study: The risk factors in the lifestyles of thyroid cancer patients and healthy adults of South Korea. *Cancer Nursing, 41*(1), E48–E56.

Resources

American Association of Clinical Endocrinologists (AACE), www.aace.com

American Cancer Society, www.cancer.org

American Thyroid Association, www.thyroid.org

Cushing's Support and Research Foundation (CSRF), www.csrf.net

Endocrine Society, www.endocrine.org

Hormone Health Network, www.hormone.org

National Adrenal Diseases Foundation (NADF), www.nadf.us

National Cancer Institute, Cancer Net for Health Professionals, www.cancer.gov

National Institute of Diabetes and Digestive and Kidney Disease, www.niddk.nih.gov

46 Management of Patients with Diabetes

LEARNING OUTCOMES

On completion of this chapter, the learner will be able to:

1. Differentiate between the types of diabetes, associated etiologic factors, and pathophysiologic alterations.
2. Identify the diagnostic and clinical significance of blood glucose test results.
3. Describe the relationships among diet and dietary modifications, exercise, and medication (i.e., insulin or oral antidiabetic agents) for people with diabetes.
4. Use the nursing process as a framework for care of the patient who has hyperglycemia with diabetic ketoacidosis or hyperglycemic hyperosmolar syndrome.
5. Describe management strategies for a person with diabetes to use during "sick days."
6. Outline the major complications of diabetes and the self-care behaviors that are important in their prevention.

NURSING CONCEPTS

Acid–Base Balance	Fluids and Electrolytes	Metabolism
Family	Infection	Patient Education

GLOSSARY

diabetes: a group of metabolic diseases characterized by hyperglycemia resulting from defects in insulin secretion, insulin action, or both

diabetic ketoacidosis (DKA): a metabolic derangement, most commonly occurring in type 1 diabetes, that results from a deficiency of insulin; highly acidic ketone bodies are formed, resulting in acidosis

fasting plasma glucose (FPG): blood glucose determination obtained in the laboratory after fasting for at least 8 hours

gestational diabetes: any degree of glucose intolerance with its onset during pregnancy

glycated hemoglobin: a measure of glucose control that is a result of glucose molecule attaching to hemoglobin for the life of the red blood cell (120 days) (*synonyms:* glycosylated hemoglobin, HgbA$_{1C}$, or A1C)

glycemic index: the amount a given food increases the blood glucose level compared with an equivalent amount of glucose

hyperglycemia: elevated blood glucose level

hyperglycemic hyperosmolar syndrome (HHS): a metabolic disorder, most commonly of type 2 diabetes resulting from a relative insulin deficiency initiated by an illness that raises the demand for insulin

hypoglycemia: low blood glucose level

impaired fasting glucose (IFG) or impaired glucose tolerance (IGT): a metabolic stage intermediate between normal glucose homeostasis and diabetes; referred to as prediabetes

insulin: a hormone secreted by the beta cells of the islets of Langerhans of the pancreas that is necessary for the metabolism of carbohydrates, proteins, and fats; a deficiency of insulin results in diabetes

ketone: a highly acidic substance formed when the liver breaks down free fatty acids in the absence of insulin

latent autoimmune diabetes of adults (LADA): a subtype of diabetes

medical nutrition therapy (MNT): nutritional therapy prescribed for management of diabetes that usually is given by a registered dietitian

nephropathy: a long-term complication of diabetes in which the kidney cells are damaged; characterized by microalbuminuria in early stages and progressing to end-stage kidney disease

neuropathy: a long-term complication of diabetes resulting from damage to the nerve cell

prediabetes: impaired glucose metabolism in which blood glucose concentrations fall between normal levels and those considered diagnostic for diabetes; includes impaired fasting glucose and impaired glucose tolerance, not clinical entities in their own right but risk factors for future diabetes and cardiovascular disease

retinopathy: a condition that occurs when the small blood vessels that nourish the retina in the eye are damaged

self-monitoring of blood glucose (SMBG): a method of capillary blood glucose testing

type 1 diabetes: a metabolic disorder characterized by an absence of insulin production and secretion from autoimmune destruction of the beta cells of the islets of Langerhans in the pancreas (*formerly*: insulin-dependent diabetes, or juvenile diabetes)

type 2 diabetes: a metabolic disorder characterized by the relative deficiency of insulin production and a decreased insulin action and increased insulin resistance (*formerly*: non–insulin-dependent diabetes, or adult-onset diabetes)

Diabetes is a group of metabolic diseases characterized by **hyperglycemia** (an elevated level of glucose in the blood) resulting from defects in insulin secretion, insulin action, or both (Centers for Disease Control and Prevention [CDC], 2020). Care of the patient with diabetes, formerly known as diabetes mellitus but now more commonly referred to as diabetes, requires an understanding of the epidemiology, pathophysiology, diagnostic testing, medical and nursing care, and rehabilitation of patients with diabetes. The field of diabetes is dynamic with constant advances in technology, research, and medications that can improve the life and well-being of people with diabetes. Nurses care for patients with diabetes in all settings. This chapter focuses on the nursing management of patients with diabetes.

DIABETES

Epidemiology

It is estimated that more than 34.1 million adults in the United States have diabetes, although almost one third of these cases are undiagnosed (CDC, 2020). The number of people older than 20 years newly diagnosed with diabetes increases by 1.7 million per year. If this trend continues, one in every three adults in the United States could have diabetes by 2050. In 2018, the percentage of adults with diabetes increased with age, reaching 28.3% of those age 65 years or older (CDC, 2020).

The rate of prediabetes is also steadily increasing. It is estimated that 35.5% of U.S. adults aged 18 years or older (88 million people) had prediabetes in 2018, based on laboratory findings. Nearly half (48.3%) of adults aged 65 years or older had prediabetes (CDC, 2020). Over $237 billion a year is spent in medical costs and $90 billion a year is lost in productivity related to diabetes (CDC, 2020).

Ethnic and racial minority populations are disproportionately affected by diabetes. The age-adjusted prevalence of diabetes is increasing among all gender and racial groups, but compared with Caucasians, African Americans, and members of other racial and ethnic groups (Native Americans and persons of Hispanic origin) are more likely to develop diabetes, are at greater risk for many of the complications, and have higher death rates due to diabetes (CDC, 2020). Chart 46-1 summarizes risk factors for diabetes.

Diabetes can have far-reaching and devastating physical, social, and economic consequences, including the following (CDC, 2020; Virani, Alonso, Benjamin, et al., 2020):

- In the United States, diabetes is the leading cause of nontraumatic amputations and end-stage kidney disease (ESKD).

- Diabetes is the seventh leading cause of death in the United States and the leading cause of new blindness in adults aged 18 to 64 years.
- Emergency department visits and hospitalization rates for adults and children with diabetes are greater than for the general population.

The economic cost of diabetes continues to increase because of increasing health care costs and an aging population.

Classification

The major classifications of diabetes are type 1 diabetes, type 2 diabetes, gestational diabetes, latent autoimmune diabetes of adults (LADA), and diabetes associated with other conditions or syndromes (American Diabetes Association [ADA], 2020). The different types of diabetes vary in cause, clinical course, and treatment (see Table 46-1). The classification system is dynamic in two ways. First, research findings suggest many differences among individuals within each category. Second, except for people with type 1 diabetes, patients may move from one category to another. For example, a woman with gestational diabetes may, after delivery, move into type 2 diabetes. **Prediabetes** is classified as **impaired glucose tolerance (IGT) or impaired fasting glucose (IFG)** and refers to a condition in which blood glucose concentrations fall between normal levels and those considered diagnostic for diabetes (ADA, 2020; CDC, 2020).

Chart 46-1 ⚠ **RISK FACTORS**
Diabetes

- Age >30 years for type 2 and <30 years for type 1
- High-density lipoprotein (HDL) cholesterol level ≤35 mg/dL (0.90 mmol/L) and/or triglyceride level ≥250 mg/dL (2.8 mmol/L)
- History of gestational diabetes or delivery of a baby over 9 lb
- Hypertension
- Family history of diabetes (e.g., parents or siblings with diabetes)
- Obesity (i.e., ≥20% over desired body weight or body mass index ≥30 kg/m^2)
- Previously identified impaired fasting glucose or impaired glucose tolerance
- Race/ethnicity (e.g., African Americans, Hispanic Americans, Native Americans, Asian Americans, Pacific Islanders)

Adapted from American Diabetes Association (ADA). (2020). Standards of medical care in diabetes—2020. *Diabetes Care, 43*(Suppl 1), S1–S212.

TABLE 46-1	Common Types of Diabetes and Related Glucose Intolerances
Classification	**Clinical Characteristics and Implications**
Type 1 (5–10% of all patients with diabetes; formerly juvenile diabetes, or insulin-dependent diabetes)	Onset any age, but usually young (<30 yrs) Usually thin at diagnosis; recent weight loss Etiology includes genetic, immunologic, and environmental factors (e.g., virus) Often have islet cell antibodies Often have antibodies to insulin even before insulin treatment Little or no endogenous insulin Need exogenous insulin to preserve life Ketosis prone when insulin absent Acute complication of hyperglycemia: diabetic ketoacidosis
Type 2 (90–95% of all diabetes: patients with obesity—80% of type 2, patients without obesity—20% of type 2; formerly adult-onset diabetes, or non–insulin-dependent diabetes)	Onset any age, usually ≥30 yrs Usually obesity is present at diagnosis Causes include obesity, heredity, and environmental factors No islet cell antibodies Decrease in endogenous insulin, or increased with insulin resistance Most patients can control blood glucose through weight loss if they have obesity Oral antidiabetic agents may improve blood glucose levels if dietary modification and exercise are unsuccessful May need insulin on a short- or long-term basis to prevent hyperglycemia Ketosis uncommon, except in stress or infection Acute complication: hyperglycemic hyperosmolar syndrome
Diabetes associated with other conditions or syndromes (previously classified as secondary diabetes)	Accompanied by conditions known or suspected to cause the disease: pancreatic diseases, hormonal abnormalities, medications such as corticosteroids and estrogen-containing preparations Depending on the ability of the pancreas to produce insulin, the patient may require treatment with oral antidiabetic agents or insulin.
Gestational diabetes	Onset during pregnancy, usually in the second or third trimester Because of hormones secreted by the placenta, which inhibit the action of insulin Above-normal risk for perinatal complications, especially macrosomia (abnormally large babies) Treated with diet and, if needed, insulin to strictly maintain normal blood glucose levels Occurs in about 18% of pregnancies Glucose intolerance transitory but may recur: • In subsequent pregnancies • 35–60% will develop diabetes (usually type 2) within 10–20 yrs, especially if they have obesity Risk factors include obesity, age >30 yrs, family history of diabetes, previous large babies (>9 lb) Screening tests (glucose challenge test) should be performed on all pregnant women between 24 and 28 wks of gestation Should be screened for diabetes every 3 yrs
Prediabetes (previously classified as abnormality of glucose tolerance)	Previous history of hyperglycemia (e.g., during pregnancy or illness) Current normal glucose metabolism Impaired glucose tolerance or impaired fasting glucose screening after age 40 yrs if there is a family history of diabetes or if symptomatic Encourage ideal body weight, because loss of 10–15 lb may improve glycemic control

Adapted from American Diabetes Association (ADA). (2020). Standards of medical care in diabetes—2020. *Diabetes Care, 43*(Suppl 1), S1–S212; Virani, S. S., Alonso, A., Benjamin, E. J., et al. (2020). Heart disease and stroke statistics—2020 update: A report from the American Heart Association. *Circulation, 141*(9), e139–e596.

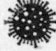 ## COVID-19 Considerations

The coronavirus disease 2019 (COVID-19) pandemic began in Wuhan, China, in late 2019. Since that time, several risks for both severe acute respiratory syndrome coronavirus 2 (SARS-CoV-2) infection and pathogenesis to COVID-19 have been posed (see Chapter 66). Epidemiologic data from China suggest that having any type of diabetes could be an important risk factor for becoming infected with SARS-CoV-2 as well as for being hospitalized to manage COVID-19 (Sommerstein, Kochen, Messerli, et al., 2020). Patients with diabetes who are hospitalized with COVID-19 have higher rates of intubation and mortality. Researchers who looked at 486 patients hospitalized with COVID-19 reported those who were older than 60 years of age, male, and had a history of diabetes were at greater risk of requiring intubation (Hur, Price,

Gray, et al., 2020). Another study reported that increased mortality in patients with diabetes was associated with older age, having a positive C-reactive protein laboratory finding, and being on insulin (Chen, Yang, Chen, et al., 2020).

Pathophysiology

Insulin is a hormone secreted by beta cells, which are one of four types of cells in the islets of Langerhans in the pancreas (Norris, 2019). Insulin is an anabolic, or storage, hormone. When a person eats a meal, insulin secretion increases and moves glucose from the blood into muscle, liver, and fat cells. In those cells, insulin has the following actions:

- Transports and metabolizes glucose for energy
- Stimulates storage of glucose in the liver and muscle (in the form of glycogen)

- Signals the liver to stop the release of glucose
- Enhances storage of dietary fat in adipose tissue
- Accelerates transport of amino acids (derived from dietary protein) into cells
- Inhibits the breakdown of stored glucose, protein, and fat

During fasting periods (between meals and overnight), the pancreas continuously releases a small amount of insulin (basal insulin); another pancreatic hormone called *glucagon* (secreted by the alpha cells of the islets of Langerhans) is released when blood glucose levels decrease, which stimulates the liver to release stored glucose. The insulin and the glucagon together maintain a constant level of glucose in the blood by stimulating the release of glucose from the liver.

Initially, the liver produces glucose through glycogenolysis (the breakdown of glycogen). After 8 to 12 hours without food, the liver forms glucose from the breakdown of noncarbohydrate substances, including amino acids, through the process of gluconeogenesis.

Type 1 Diabetes

Type 1 diabetes is characterized by the destruction of the pancreatic beta cells (Norris, 2019). Combined genetic, immunologic, and possibly environmental (e.g., viral) factors are thought to contribute to beta-cell destruction. Although the events that lead to beta-cell destruction are not fully understood, it is generally accepted that a genetic susceptibility is a common underlying factor in the development of type 1 diabetes. People do not inherit type 1 diabetes itself but rather a genetic predisposition, or tendency, toward the development of type 1 diabetes. This genetic tendency has been found in people with certain human leukocyte antigen types. There is also evidence of an autoimmune response in type 1 diabetes. This is an abnormal response in which antibodies are directed against normal tissues of the body, responding to these tissues as if they were foreign. Autoantibodies against islet cells and against endogenous (internal) insulin have been detected in people at the time of diagnosis and even several years before the development of clinical signs of type 1 diabetes. In addition to genetic and immunologic components, environmental factors such as viruses or toxins that may initiate destruction of the beta cell continue to be investigated.

Regardless of the specific cause, the destruction of the beta cells results in decreased insulin production, increased glucose production by the liver, and fasting hyperglycemia. In addition, glucose derived from food cannot be stored in the liver but instead remains in the bloodstream and contributes to postprandial (after meals) hyperglycemia. If the concentration of glucose in the blood exceeds the renal threshold for glucose, usually 180 to 200 mg/dL (9.9 to 11.1 mmol/L), the kidneys may not reabsorb all of the filtered glucose; glycosuria then occurs (i.e., the glucose then appears in the urine). When excess glucose is excreted in the urine, it is accompanied by excessive loss of fluids and electrolytes. This is called *osmotic diuresis*.

Because insulin normally inhibits glycogenolysis and gluconeogenesis, these processes occur in an unrestrained fashion in people with insulin deficiency and contribute further to hyperglycemia. In addition, fat breakdown occurs, resulting in an increased production of **ketone** bodies, a highly acidic substance formed when the liver breaks down free fatty acids in the absence of insulin.

Diabetic ketoacidosis (DKA) is a metabolic derangement that occurs most commonly in persons with type 1 diabetes and results from a deficiency of insulin; highly acidic ketone bodies are formed, and metabolic acidosis occurs. The three major metabolic derangements are hyperglycemia, ketosis, and metabolic acidosis (Norris, 2019). DKA is commonly preceded by a day or more of polyuria, polydipsia, nausea, vomiting, and fatigue with eventual stupor and coma if not treated. The breath has a characteristic fruity odor due to the presence of ketoacids.

 ### Type 2 Diabetes

Type 2 diabetes occurs more commonly among people who are older than 30 years and who have obesity, although its incidence is rapidly increasing in younger people because of the growing epidemic of obesity in children, adolescents, and young adults (CDC, 2020).

The two main problems related to insulin in type 2 diabetes are insulin resistance and impaired insulin secretion. Insulin resistance refers to a decreased tissue sensitivity to insulin. Normally, insulin binds to special receptors on cell surfaces and initiates a series of reactions involved in glucose metabolism. In type 2 diabetes, these intracellular reactions are diminished, making insulin less effective at stimulating glucose uptake by the tissues and at regulating glucose release by the liver (see Fig. 46-1). The exact mechanisms that lead to insulin resistance and impaired insulin secretion in type 2 diabetes are unknown, although genetic factors are thought to play a role.

To overcome insulin resistance and to prevent the buildup of glucose in the blood, increased amounts of insulin must be secreted to maintain the glucose level at a normal or slightly elevated level. If the beta cells cannot keep up with the increased demand for insulin, the glucose level rises and type 2 diabetes develops. Insulin resistance may also lead to metabolic syndrome, which is a constellation of symptoms, including hypertension, hypercholesterolemia, abdominal obesity, and other abnormities (Norris, 2019).

Despite the impaired insulin secretion that is characteristic of type 2 diabetes, there is enough insulin present to prevent the breakdown of fat and the accompanying production of ketone bodies. Therefore, DKA does not typically occur in

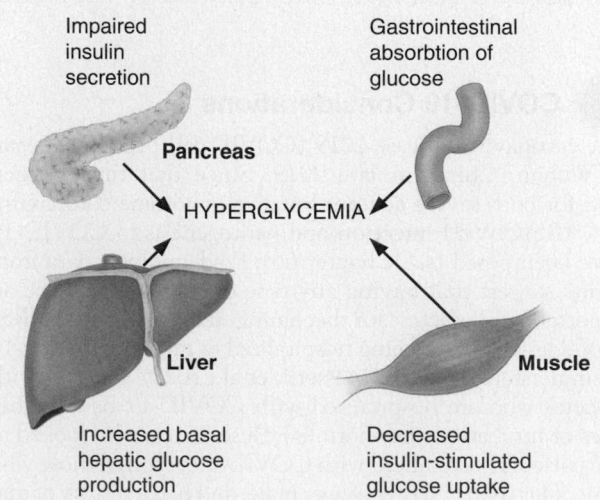

Physiology/Pathophysiology

Impaired insulin secretion

Gastrointestinal absorbtion of glucose

Pancreas

HYPERGLYCEMIA

Liver

Muscle

Increased basal hepatic glucose production

Decreased insulin-stimulated glucose uptake

Figure 46-1 • Pathogenesis of type 2 diabetes.

type 2 diabetes. However, uncontrolled type 2 diabetes may lead to another acute problem—**hyperglycemic hyperosmolar syndrome (HHS)** (see discussion later in chapter).

Because type 2 diabetes is associated with a slow, progressive glucose intolerance, its onset may go undetected for many years. If the patient experiences symptoms, they are frequently mild and may include fatigue, irritability, polyuria, polydipsia, poorly healing skin wounds, vaginal infections, or blurred vision (if glucose levels are very high).

For most patients (approximately 75%), type 2 diabetes is detected incidentally (e.g., when routine laboratory tests or ophthalmoscopic examinations are performed). One consequence of undetected diabetes is that long-term diabetes complications (e.g., eye disease, peripheral neuropathy, peripheral vascular disease) may have developed before the actual diagnosis of diabetes is made (ADA, 2020), signifying that the blood glucose has been elevated for a time before diagnosis.

Gestational Diabetes

Gestational diabetes is any degree of glucose intolerance with its onset during pregnancy (Norris, 2019). Hyperglycemia develops during pregnancy, particularly in the second and third trimesters, because of the secretion of placental hormones that cause insulin resistance.

Women who are considered to be at high risk for gestational diabetes and should be screened by blood glucose testing at their first prenatal visit are those with marked obesity, a personal history of gestational diabetes, glycosuria, or a strong family history of diabetes. High-risk ethnic groups include Hispanic Americans, Native Americans, Asian Americans, African Americans, and Pacific Islanders. If these high-risk women do not have gestational diabetes at initial screening, they should be retested between 24 and 28 weeks of gestation. All women of average risk should be tested at 24 to 28 weeks of gestation. Testing is not specifically recommended for women identified as being at low risk. Low-risk women are those who meet all of the following criteria: age younger than 25 years, normal weight before pregnancy, member of an ethnic group with low prevalence of gestational diabetes, no history of abnormal glucose tolerance, no known history of diabetes in first-degree relatives, and no history of poor obstetric outcomes (ADA, 2020). Women considered to be at high or average risk should have either an oral glucose tolerance test or a glucose challenge test followed by an oral glucose tolerance test in women who exceed the glucose threshold value of 140 mg/dL (7.8 mmol/L) (ADA, 2020).

Initial management includes dietary modification and blood glucose monitoring. Between 70% and 85% of women with gestational diabetes can control blood glucose levels with lifestyle modifications alone. Dietary recommendations include a daily minimum of 175 g of carbohydrates, 71-g protein, 28-g fiber, and low saturated fats (ADA, 2020). If hyperglycemia persists, insulin is prescribed. Target ranges for blood glucose levels during pregnancy are 140 to 180 mg/dL (7.8 to 10 mmol/L) (ADA, 2020).

After delivery, blood glucose levels in women with gestational diabetes usually return to normal. However, many women who have had gestational diabetes develop type 2 diabetes later in life. Women with a history of gestational diabetes should be screened for the development of diabetes or prediabetes every 3 years (ADA, 2020).

Latent Autoimmune Diabetes of Adults (LADA)

In adults, **LADA** is a subtype of diabetes in which the progression of autoimmune beta cell destruction in the pancreas is slower than in types 1 and 2 diabetes. Patients with LADA are at high risk of becoming insulin dependent. Most patients with LADA have at least two of the following: age of onset less than 50 years, body mass index (BMI) less than 25 kg/m^2, history of autoimmune disease, acute symptoms prior to diagnosis, or positive family history of autoimmune disease (Fischbach & Fischbach, 2018).

Prevention

The Diabetes Prevention Program Research Group (2002) reported that type 2 diabetes can be prevented with appropriate changes in lifestyle. Participants at high risk for type 2 diabetes (BMI greater than 24 kg/m^2, fasting and postprandial plasma glucose levels elevated but not to levels diagnostic of diabetes) received standard lifestyle recommendations plus metformin, an oral antidiabetic agent; standard lifestyle recommendations plus placebo; or an intensive program of lifestyle modifications. The 16-lesson curriculum of the intensive program of lifestyle modifications focused on weight reduction of greater than 7% of initial body weight and physical activity of moderate intensity. It also included behavior modification strategies designed to help patients achieve the goals of weight reduction and participation in exercise. Compared to the placebo group, the lifestyle intervention group had a 58% lower incidence of diabetes and the metformin group had a 31% lower incidence of diabetes. These findings were found in both genders and all racial and ethnic groups. This research demonstrates that type 2 diabetes can be prevented or delayed in persons at high risk for the disease (Diabetes Prevention Program Research Group, 2002). The Diabetes Prevention Program Outcomes Study followed participants for 15 years and demonstrated that those who enrolled in the program continued to develop type 2 diabetes at a lower rate compared to controls (Diabetes Prevention Program Research Group, 2015).

Researchers have also reported in a study of more than 7000 participants followed for 8 years that those who took glucosamine, a supplement that decreases osteoarthritis and joint pain, had a lower risk of developing type 2 diabetes compared to those not taking the supplement (Ma, Li, Zhou, et al., 2020).

Clinical Manifestations

Clinical manifestations depend on the patient's level of hyperglycemia. Classic clinical manifestations of diabetes include the "three Ps": *p*olyuria, *p*olydipsia, and *p*olyphagia. Polyuria (increased urination) and polydipsia (increased thirst) occur as a result of the excess loss of fluid associated with osmotic diuresis. Patients also experience polyphagia (increased appetite) that results from the catabolic state induced by insulin deficiency and the breakdown of proteins and fats (Norris, 2019). Other symptoms include fatigue and weakness, sudden vision changes, tingling or numbness in hands or feet, dry skin, skin lesions or wounds that are slow to heal, and recurrent infections. The onset of type 1 diabetes may also be associated with sudden weight loss or nausea, vomiting, or abdominal pains, if DKA has developed.

> **Chart 46-2** Criteria for the Diagnosis of Diabetes
>
> - Symptoms of diabetes plus casual plasma glucose concentration equal to or greater than 200 mg/dL (11.1 mmol/L). Casual is defined as any time of day without regard to time since last meal. The classic symptoms of diabetes include polyuria, polydipsia, and unexplained weight loss.
>
>   **Or**
>
> - Fasting plasma glucose greater than or equal to 126 mg/dL (7.0 mmol/L). Fasting is defined as no caloric intake for at least 8 hours.
>
>   **Or**
>
> - Two-hour postload glucose equal to or greater than 200 mg/dL (11.1 mmol/L) during an oral glucose tolerance test. The test should use a glucose load containing the equivalent of 75-g anhydrous glucose dissolved in water.
>
>   **Or**
>
> - Hemoglobin A1C ≥6.5% (48 mmol/mol).
>
> In the absence of unequivocal hyperglycemia with acute metabolic decompensation, these criteria should be confirmed by repeat testing on a different day. The third measure is not recommended for routine clinical use.
>
> A1C, glycosylated hemoglobin
> Adapted from American Diabetes Association (ADA). (2020). Standards of medical care in diabetes—2020. *Diabetes Care, 43*(Suppl 1), S1–S212.

Assessment and Diagnostic Findings

An abnormally high blood glucose level is the basic criterion for the diagnosis of diabetes. **Fasting plasma glucose (FPG)** (blood glucose determination obtained in the laboratory after fasting for at least 8 hours), random plasma glucose, and glucose level 2 hours after receiving glucose (2-hour postprandial load) may be used (Fischbach & Fischbach, 2018). See Chart 46-2 for the ADA's diagnostic criteria for diabetes (ADA, 2020).

In addition to the assessment and diagnostic evaluation performed to diagnose diabetes, ongoing specialized assessment of patients with known diabetes and evaluation for complications in patients with newly diagnosed diabetes are important components of care. Parameters that should be regularly assessed are discussed in Chart 46-3.

 ## Gerontologic Considerations

Diabetes is particularly prevalent in older adults. In fact, type 2 diabetes is the seventh leading cause of death and affects approximately 20% of older adults (Eliopoulos, 2018). There is a high prevalence among African Americans and those who are 65 to 74 years of age (Eliopoulos, 2018).

Early detection is important but may be challenging because symptoms may be absent or nonspecific. A glucose tolerance test is more effective in diagnosis than urine testing for glucose in older patients due to the higher renal threshold for glucose (Eliopoulos, 2018).

Medical Management

The main goal of diabetes treatment is to normalize insulin activity and blood glucose levels to reduce the development of complications. The Diabetes Control and Complications

> **Chart 46-3** 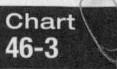 **ASSESSMENT**
> Assessing the Patient with Diabetes
>
> **History**
>
> - Symptoms related to the diagnosis of diabetes:
>   Symptoms of hyperglycemia
>   Symptoms of hypoglycemia
>   Frequency, timing, severity, and resolution
> - Results of blood glucose monitoring
> - Status, symptoms, and management of chronic complications of diabetes:
>   Eye; kidney; nerve; genitourinary and sexual, bladder, and gastrointestinal
>   Cardiac; peripheral vascular; foot complications associated with diabetes
> - Adherence to/ability to follow prescribed dietary management plan
> - Adherence to prescribed exercise regimen
> - Adherence to/ability to follow prescribed pharmacologic treatment (insulin or oral antidiabetic agents)
> - Use of tobacco, alcohol, and prescribed and over-the-counter medications/drugs
> - Lifestyle, cultural, psychosocial, and economic factors that may affect diabetes treatment
> - Effects of diabetes or its complications on functional status (e.g., mobility, vision)
>
> **Physical Examination**
>
> - Blood pressure (sitting and standing to detect orthostatic changes)
> - Body mass index (height and weight)
> - Funduscopic examination and visual acuity
> - Foot examination (lesions, signs of infection, pulses)
> - Skin examination (lesions and insulin injection sites)
> - Neurologic examination
>   Vibratory and sensory examination using monofilament
>   Deep tendon reflexes
> - Oral examination
>
> **Laboratory Examination**
>
> - HgbA1C (A1C)
> - Fasting lipid profile
> - Test for microalbuminuria
> - Serum creatinine level
> - Urinalysis
> - Electrocardiogram
>
> **Need for Referrals**
>
> - Ophthalmologist
> - Podiatrist
> - Dietitian
> - Diabetes educator
> - Others if indicated
>
> A1C, glycosylated hemoglobin
> Adapted from American Diabetes Association (ADA). (2020). Standards of medical care in diabetes—2020. *Diabetes Care, 43*(Suppl 1), S1–S212.

Trial Research Group (DCCT), a 10-year prospective clinical trial conducted from 1983 to 1993, demonstrated the importance of achieving blood glucose control in the normal, nondiabetic range. This landmark trial demonstrated that intensive glucose control dramatically reduced the development and progression of complications such as **retinopathy** (damage to small blood vessels that nourish the retina), **nephropathy** (damage to kidney cells), and **neuropathy** (damage to nerve cells). Intensive treatment is defined as 3 or 4 insulin injections per day or an insulin pump (i.e., a continuous subcutaneous insulin infusion) plus frequent blood glucose monitoring and weekly contacts with diabetes educators (DCCT, 1993). The ADA recommends that all patients with diabetes strive for glucose control (HgbA$_{1C}$ less than 7%) to reduce their risk of complications (ADA, 2020a).

Intensive therapy must be initiated with caution and must be accompanied by thorough education of the patient and family and by responsible behavior of the patient. Careful screening of patients for capability and responsibility is a key step in initiating intensive therapy.

The therapeutic goal for diabetes management is to achieve euglycemia (normal blood glucose levels) without **hypoglycemia** while maintaining a high quality of life. Diabetes management has five components: nutritional therapy, exercise, monitoring, pharmacologic therapy, and education. Diabetes management involves constant assessment and modification of the treatment plan by health professionals and daily adjustments in therapy by the patient. Although the health care team directs the treatment, it is the individual patient who must manage the complex therapeutic regimen. For this reason, patient and family education is an essential component of diabetes treatment and is as important as all other components of the regimen.

Nutritional Therapy

Nutrition, meal planning, weight control, and increased activity are the foundation of diabetes management (ADA, 2020; Evert, Dennison, Gardner, et al., 2019; Franz, MacLeod, Evert, et al., 2017). The most important objectives in the dietary and nutritional management of diabetes are control of total caloric intake to attain or maintain a reasonable body weight, control of blood glucose levels, and normalization of lipids and blood pressure to prevent heart disease. Success in this area alone is often associated with reversal of hyperglycemia in type 2 diabetes. However, achieving these goals is not easy. Because **medical nutrition therapy (MNT)**— nutritional therapy prescribed for management of diabetes usually given by a registered dietitian—is complex, a registered dietitian who understands the therapy has the major responsibility for designing and educating about this aspect of the therapeutic plan. Nurses and all other members of the health care team must be knowledgeable about nutritional therapy and supportive of patients who need to implement nutritional and lifestyle changes. Nutritional management of diabetes includes the following goals:

1. To achieve and maintain:
   a. Blood glucose levels in the normal range or as close to normal as is safely possible
   b. A lipid and lipoprotein profile that reduces the risk for vascular disease
   c. Blood pressure levels in the normal range or as close to normal as is safely possible
2. To prevent, or at least slow, the rate of development of the chronic complications of diabetes by modifying nutrient intake and lifestyle
3. To address individual nutrition needs, taking into account personal and cultural preferences and willingness to change

4. To maintain the pleasure of eating by only limiting food choices when indicated by scientific evidence

For patients who have obesity and diabetes (especially those with type 2 diabetes), weight loss is the key to treatment. (It is also a major factor in preventing diabetes.) In general, overweight is considered to be a BMI of 25 kg/m^2 to 29 kg/m^2; obesity is defined as 20% above ideal body weight or a BMI equal to or greater than 30 kg/m^2 (ADA, 2020; WHO, 2018). Calculation of BMI is discussed in Chapter 4, and obesity is discussed further in Chapter 42. Patients who have obesity, type 2 diabetes, and require insulin or oral agents to control blood glucose levels may be able to reduce or eliminate the need for medication through weight loss. A weight loss of 5% to 10% of total weight may significantly improve blood glucose levels. For patients who have obesity and diabetes but do not take insulin or an oral antidiabetic medication, consistent meal content or timing is important but not as critical. Rather, decreasing the overall caloric intake is of greater importance. Meals should not be skipped. Pacing food intake throughout the day decreases demands on the pancreas.

The actions of several oral antidiabetic medications include weight loss. For example, the glucagonlike peptide-1 (GLP-1) agonists are associated with delayed gastric emptying and weight loss. The dipeptidyl peptidase-4 (DPP4) and sodium-glucose cotransporter-2 (SGLT2) inhibitors improve glucose control assisting with weight loss (Keresztes & Peacock-Johnson, 2019). See discussion later in the chapter about oral antidiabetic medications.

Consistently following a meal plan is one of the most challenging aspects of diabetes management. It may be more realistic to restrict calories only moderately. For patients who have lost weight incorporating new dietary habits into their lifestyles, diet education, behavioral therapy, group support, and ongoing nutrition counseling are encouraged to maintain weight loss.

Meal Planning and Related Education

The meal plan must consider the patient's food preferences, lifestyle, usual eating times, and ethnic and cultural background. For patients who require insulin to help control blood glucose levels, maintaining as much consistency as possible in the amount of calories and carbohydrates ingested at each meal is essential. In addition, consistency in the approximate time intervals between meals, with the addition of snacks if necessary, helps prevent hypoglycemic reactions and maintain overall blood glucose control. For patients who can master the insulin-to-carbohydrate calculations, lifestyle can be more flexible and diabetes control more predictable. For those using intensive insulin therapy, there may be greater flexibility in the timing and content of meals by allowing adjustments in insulin dosage for changes in eating and exercise habits. Newer insulin analogues, insulin algorithms, and insulin pumps permit greater flexibility of schedules than was previously possible. This contrasts with the concept of maintaining a constant dose of insulin, requiring strict scheduling of meals to match the onset and duration of the insulin.

The first step in preparing a meal plan is a thorough review of the patient's diet history to identify eating habits and lifestyle and cultural eating patterns (ADA, 2020; Evert et al., 2019; Franz et al., 2017). This includes a thorough assessment of the patient's need for weight loss, gain, or maintenance. In most instances, people with type 2 diabetes require weight reduction.

In educating about meal planning, clinical dietitians use various tools, materials, and approaches. Initial education addresses the importance of consistent eating habits, the relationship of food and insulin, and the provision of an individualized meal plan. In-depth follow-up education then focuses on management skills, such as eating at restaurants; reading food labels; and adjusting the meal plan for exercise, illness, and special occasions. The nurse plays an important role in communicating pertinent information to the dietitian and reinforcing the patient's understanding. Communication between the team is important.

Certain aspects of meal planning, such as the food exchange system, may be difficult to learn. This may be related to limitations in the patient's intellectual level or to emotional issues, such as difficulty accepting the diagnosis of diabetes or feelings of deprivation and undue restriction in eating. In any case, it helps to emphasize that using the exchange system (or any food classification system) provides a new way of thinking about food rather than a new way of eating. It is also important to simplify information as much as possible and to provide opportunities for the patient to practice and repeat activities and information.

Caloric Requirements

Calorie-controlled diets are planned by first calculating a person's energy needs and caloric requirements based on age, gender, height, and weight. An activity element is then factored in to provide the actual number of calories required for weight maintenance. To promote a 1- to 2-lb weight loss per week, 500 to 1000 calories are subtracted from the daily total. The calories are distributed into carbohydrates, proteins, and fats, and a meal plan is then developed, taking into account the patient's lifestyle and food preferences.

Patients may be underweight at the onset of type 1 diabetes because of rapid weight loss from severe hyperglycemia. The goal initially may be to provide a higher-calorie diet to regain lost weight and blood glucose control.

Caloric Distribution

A meal plan for diabetes focuses on the percentages of calories that come from carbohydrates, proteins, and fats (Evert et al., 2019; Franz et al., 2017).

Carbohydrates. The caloric distribution currently recommended is higher in carbohydrates than in fat and protein. In general, carbohydrate foods have the greatest effect on blood glucose levels because they are more quickly digested than other foods and are converted into glucose rapidly. However, research into the appropriateness of a higher-carbohydrate diet in patients with decreased glucose tolerance is ongoing, and recommendations may change accordingly. Currently, the ADA and the Academy of Nutrition and Dietetics (formerly the American Dietetic Association) recommend that for all levels of caloric intake, 50% to 60% of calories should be derived from carbohydrates, 20% to 30% from fat, and the remaining 10% to 20% from protein (Evert et al., 2019). The majority of the selections for carbohydrates should come from whole grains. These recommendations are also consistent with those of the American Heart Association and American Cancer Society.

Carbohydrates consist of sugars (e.g., sucrose) and starches (e.g., rice, pasta, bread). Low glycemic index diets (described later) may reduce postprandial glucose levels. Therefore, the nutrition guidelines recommend that all carbohydrates should be eaten in moderation to avoid high postprandial blood glucose levels (Evert et al., 2019; Franz et al., 2017).

Foods high in carbohydrates, such as sucrose (concentrated sweets), are not totally eliminated from the diet but should be eaten in moderation (up to 10% of total calories), because they are typically high in fat and lack vitamins, minerals, and fiber.

Fats. The recommendations regarding fat content of the diabetic diet include both reducing the total percentage of calories from fat sources to less than 30% of total calories and limiting the amount of saturated fats to 10% of total calories. Additional recommendations include limiting the total intake of dietary cholesterol to less than 300 mg/day. This approach may help reduce risk factors such as increased serum cholesterol levels, which are associated with the development of coronary artery disease—the leading cause of death and disability among people with diabetes (ADA, 2020; Evert et al., 2019).

Protein. The meal plan may include the use of some nonanimal sources of protein (e.g., legumes, whole grains) to help reduce saturated fat and cholesterol intake. In addition, the amount of protein intake may be reduced in patients with early signs of kidney disease.

Fiber. Increased fiber in the diet may improve blood glucose levels, decrease the need for exogenous insulin, and lower total cholesterol and low-density lipoprotein levels in the blood (Evert et al., 2019).

There are two types of dietary fibers: soluble and insoluble. Soluble fiber—in foods such as legumes, oats, and some fruits—plays more of a role in lowering blood glucose and lipid levels than does insoluble fiber, although the clinical significance of this effect is probably small (Evert et al., 2019). Soluble fiber slows stomach emptying and the movement of food through the upper digestive tract. The potential glucose-lowering effect of fiber may be caused by the slower rate of glucose absorption from foods that contain soluble fiber. Insoluble fiber is found in whole-grain breads and cereals and in some vegetables. This type of fiber along with soluble fiber increases satiety, which is helpful for weight loss. At least 28 g of fiber should be ingested daily (ADA, 2020).

One risk involved in suddenly increasing fiber intake is that it may require adjusting the dosage of insulin or oral agents to prevent hypoglycemia. Other problems may include abdominal fullness, nausea, diarrhea, increased flatulence, and constipation if fluid intake is inadequate. If fiber is added to or increased in the meal plan, it should be done gradually and in consultation with a dietitian. Exchange lists (ADA, 2020) serve as an excellent guide for increasing fiber intake. Fiber-rich food choices within the vegetable, fruit, and starch/bread exchanges are highlighted in the lists.

Food Classification Systems

To educate about diet principles and help in meal planning, several systems have been developed in which foods are organized into groups with common characteristics, such as number of calories, composition of foods (i.e., amount of protein, fat, carbohydrate in the food), or effect on blood glucose levels. Several of these are listed next.

TABLE 46-2	Select Sample Menus from Exchange Lists		
Exchanges	Sample Lunch #1	Sample Lunch #2	Sample Lunch #3
2 starch	2 slices bread	Hamburger bun	1 cup cooked pasta
3 meat	2-oz sliced turkey and 1-oz low-fat cheese	3-oz lean beef patty	3-oz boiled shrimp
1 vegetable	Lettuce, tomato, onion	Green salad	½ cup plum tomatoes
1 fat	1-tsp mayonnaise	1-tbsp salad dressing	1-tsp olive oil
1 fruit	1 medium apple	1¼ cup watermelon	1¼ cup fresh strawberries
"Free" items (optional)	Unsweetened iced tea Mustard, pickle, hot pepper	Diet soda 1 tbsp catsup, pickle, onions	Ice water with lemon Garlic, basil

Exchange Lists. A commonly used tool for nutritional management is the exchange lists for meal planning (ADA, 2020). There are six main exchange lists: bread/starch, vegetable, milk, meat, fruit, and fat. Foods within one group (in the portion amounts specified) contain equal numbers of calories and are approximately equal in grams of protein, fat, and carbohydrate. Meal plans can be based on a recommended number of choices from each exchange list. Foods on one list may be interchanged with one another, allowing for variety while maintaining as much consistency as possible in the nutrient content of foods eaten. Table 46-2 presents three sample lunch menus that are interchangeable in terms of carbohydrate, protein, and fat content.

Exchange list information on combination foods such as pizza, chili, and casseroles, as well as convenience foods, desserts, snack foods, and fast foods, is available from the ADA (see the Resources section). Some food manufacturers and restaurants publish exchange lists that describe their products.

Nutrition Labels. Food manufacturers are required to have the nutrition content of foods listed on their packaging, and reading food labels is an important skill for patients to learn and use when food shopping. The label includes information about how many grams of carbohydrate are in a serving of food. This information can be used to determine how much medication is needed. For example, a patient who takes premeal insulin may use the algorithm of 1 unit of insulin for 15 g of carbohydrate. Patients can also be educated to have a "carbohydrate budget" per meal (e.g., 45 to 60 g).

Carbohydrate counting is a nutritional tool used for blood glucose management because carbohydrates are the main nutrients in food that influence blood glucose levels. This method provides flexibility in food choices, can be less complicated to understand than the diabetic food exchange list, and allows more accurate management with multiple daily injections (insulin before each meal). However, if carbohydrate counting is not used with other meal-planning techniques, weight gain can result. A variety of methods are used to count carbohydrates. When developing a diabetic meal plan using carbohydrate counting, all food sources should be considered.

Once digested, 100% of carbohydrates are converted to glucose. Approximately 50% of protein foods (meat, fish, and poultry) are also converted to glucose, and this has minimal effect on blood glucose levels.

While carbohydrate counting is commonly used for blood glucose management with type 1 and type 2 diabetes, it is not

a perfect system. All carbohydrates affect the blood glucose level to different degrees, regardless of equivalent serving size (i.e., the glycemic index—see later discussion). When carbohydrate counting is used, reading labels on food items is the key to success. Knowing what the "carbohydrate budget" for the meal is and knowing how many grams of carbohydrate are in a serving of a food, the patient can calculate the amount in one serving.

Healthy Food Choices. An alternative to counting grams of carbohydrate is measuring servings or choices. This method is used more often by people with type 2 diabetes. It is similar to the food exchange list and emphasizes portion control of total servings of carbohydrate at meals and snacks. One carbohydrate serving is equivalent to 15 g of carbohydrate. Examples of one serving are an apple 2 inches in diameter and one slice of bread. Vegetables and meat are counted as one third of a carbohydrate serving. This system works well for those who have difficulty with more complicated systems.

MyPlate Food Guide. The Food Guide (i.e., MyPlate) is another tool used to develop meal plans. It is commonly used for patients with type 2 diabetes who have a difficult time following a calorie-controlled diet. Foods are categorized into five major groups (grains, vegetables, fruits, dairy, and protein), plus fats and oils (see Chapter 4, Fig. 4-5). Foods (grains, fruits, and vegetables) that are lowest in calories and fat and highest in fiber should make up the basis of the diet. For those with diabetes, as well as for the general population, 50% to 60% of the daily caloric intake should be from these three groups. Foods higher in fat (particularly saturated fat) should account for a smaller percentage of the daily caloric intake. Fats, oils, and sweets should be used sparingly to obtain weight and blood glucose control and to reduce the risk for cardiovascular disease. Reliance on MyPlate may result in fluctuations in blood glucose levels, however, because high-carbohydrate foods may be grouped with low-carbohydrate foods. The guide is appropriately used only as a first-step educational tool for patients who are learning how to control food portions and how to identify which foods contain carbohydrate, protein, and fat.

Glycemic Index. One of the main goals of diet therapy in diabetes is to avoid sharp, rapid increases in blood glucose levels after food is eaten. The term **glycemic index** is used to describe how much a given food increases the blood glucose level compared with an equivalent amount of glucose. The effects of the use of the glycemic index on blood glucose levels and on long-term patient outcomes are unclear, but it may be beneficial (ADA, 2020; Evert et al., 2019). Although more research is necessary, the following guidelines may be helpful when making dietary recommendations:

- Combining starchy foods with protein- and fat-containing foods tends to slow their absorption and lower the glycemic index.
- In general, eating foods that are raw and whole results in a lower glycemic index than eating chopped, puréed, or cooked foods (except meat).
- Eating whole fruit instead of drinking juice decreases the glycemic index, because fiber in the fruit slows absorption.
- Adding foods with sugars to the diet may result in a lower glycemic index if these foods are eaten with foods that are more slowly absorbed.

Patients can create their own glycemic index by monitoring their blood glucose level after ingestion of a particular food. This can help improve blood glucose control through individualized manipulation of the diet. Many patients who use frequent monitoring of blood glucose levels can use this information to adjust their insulin doses in accordance with variations in food intake.

Other Dietary Concerns

Alcohol Consumption

Patients with diabetes do not need to give up alcoholic beverages entirely, but patients and primary providers must be aware of the potential adverse effects of alcohol specific to diabetes. Alcohol is absorbed before other nutrients and does not require insulin for absorption. Large amounts can be converted to fats, increasing the risk for DKA. In general, the same precautions regarding the use of alcohol by people without diabetes should be applied to patients with diabetes. Moderation is recommended. A major danger of alcohol consumption by the patient with diabetes is hypoglycemia, especially for patients who take insulin or insulin secretagogues (medications that increase the secretion of insulin by the pancreas). Alcohol may decrease the normal physiologic reactions in the body that produce glucose (gluconeogenesis). Therefore, if a patient with diabetes consumes alcohol on an empty stomach, there is an increased likelihood of hypoglycemia. In addition, excessive alcohol intake may impair the patient's ability to recognize and treat hypoglycemia or to follow a prescribed meal plan to prevent hypoglycemia. To reduce the risk of hypoglycemia, the patient should be cautioned to consume food along with the alcohol; however, carbohydrate consumed with alcohol may raise blood glucose.

Alcohol consumption may lead to excessive weight gain (from the high caloric content of alcohol), hyperlipidemia, and elevated glucose levels (especially with mixed drinks and liqueurs). Patient education regarding alcohol intake must emphasize moderation in the amount of alcohol consumed. Moderate intake is considered to be one alcoholic beverage per day for women and two per day for men. Lower-calorie or less-sweet drinks (e.g., light beer, wine) and food intake along with alcohol consumption are advised (ADA, 2020; Evert et al., 2019). Patients with type 2 diabetes who wish to control their weight should incorporate the calories from alcohol into the overall meal plan.

Sweeteners

The use of artificial sweeteners is acceptable, especially if it assists in overall dietary adherence. Moderation in the amount of sweetener used is encouraged to avoid potential adverse effects. There are two main types of sweeteners: nutritive and nonnutritive. The nutritive sweeteners contain calories, and the nonnutritive sweeteners have few or no calories in the amounts normally used.

Nutritive sweeteners include fructose (fruit sugar), sorbitol, and xylitol, all of which provide calories in amounts similar to those in sucrose (table sugar). They cause less elevation in blood sugar levels than sucrose does and are often used in sugar-free foods. Sweeteners containing sorbitol may have a laxative effect.

Nonnutritive sweeteners have minimal or no calories. They are used in food products and are also available for table use. They produce minimal or no elevation in blood glucose levels, and the U.S. Food and Drug Administration (FDA) lists them as safe for people with diabetes.

Misleading Food Labels

Foods labeled "sugarless" or "sugar-free" may still provide calories equal to those of the equivalent sugar-containing products if they are made with nutritive sweeteners. Therefore, these foods should not be considered "free" foods to be eaten in unlimited quantity, because they can elevate blood glucose levels. Foods labeled "dietetic" are not necessarily reduced-calorie foods. Patients are advised that foods labeled dietetic may still contain significant amounts of sugar or fat.

Patients must read the labels of "health foods"—especially snacks—because they often contain carbohydrates (e.g., honey, brown sugar, corn syrup, flour) and saturated vegetable fats (e.g., coconut or palm oil), hydrogenated vegetable fats, or animal fats, which may be contraindicated in people with elevated blood lipid levels.

Exercise

Exercise is extremely important in diabetes management because of its effects on lowering blood glucose and reducing cardiovascular risk factors (ADA, 2020). Exercise lowers blood glucose levels by increasing the uptake of glucose by body muscles and by improving insulin utilization. It also improves circulation and muscle tone. Resistance (strength) training, such as weight lifting, can increase lean muscle mass, thereby increasing the resting metabolic rate. These effects are useful in diabetes in relation to losing weight, easing stress, and maintaining a feeling of well-being. Exercise also alters blood lipid concentrations, increasing levels of high-density lipoproteins and decreasing total cholesterol and triglyceride levels. This is especially important for people with diabetes because of their increased risk of cardiovascular disease.

Exercise Recommendations

Ideally, a person with diabetes should engage in regular exercise. General considerations for exercise in patients with diabetes are presented in Chart 46-4. Exercise recommendations must be altered as necessary for patients with diabetic complications, such as retinopathy, autonomic neuropathy, sensorimotor neuropathy, and cardiovascular disease (ADA, 2020). Increased blood pressure associated with exercise may aggravate diabetic retinopathy and increase the risk of a hemorrhage into the vitreous or retina.

In general, a slow, gradual increase in the exercise period is encouraged. For many patients, walking is a safe and beneficial form of exercise that requires no special equipment (except for proper shoes) and can be performed anywhere. People with diabetes should discuss an exercise program with their primary provider and undergo a careful medical evaluation with appropriate diagnostic studies before beginning a program (ADA, 2020).

For patients who are older than 30 years and who have two or more risk factors for heart disease, an exercise stress test is recommended prior to starting an exercise program (ADA, 2020). Risk factors for heart disease include hypertension, obesity, high cholesterol levels, abnormal resting electrocardiogram (ECG), sedentary lifestyle, smoking, male gender, and a family history of heart disease. An abnormal stress test may indicate cardiac ischemia. Typically, an abnormal stress test is followed by a cardiac catheterization and, in some cases, with an intervention such as angioplasty, stent placement, or cardiac surgery.

Exercise Precautions

Patients who have blood glucose levels exceeding 250 mg/dL (14 mmol/L) and who have ketones in their urine should not begin exercising until the urine test results are negative for ketones and the blood glucose level is closer to normal. Exercising with elevated blood glucose levels increases the secretion of glucagon, growth hormone, and catecholamines. The liver then releases more glucose, and the result is an increase in the blood glucose level (ADA, 2020).

The physiologic decrease in circulating insulin that normally occurs with exercise cannot occur in patients treated with insulin. Initially, patients who require insulin should be taught to eat a 15-g carbohydrate snack (a fruit exchange) or a snack of complex carbohydrates with a protein before engaging in moderate exercise to prevent unexpected

hypoglycemia. The exact amount of food needed varies from person to person and should be determined by blood glucose monitoring.

Another concern for patients who take insulin is hypoglycemia that occurs many hours after exercise. To avoid post-exercise hypoglycemia, especially after strenuous or prolonged exercise, the patient may need to eat a snack at the end of the exercise session and at bedtime and monitor the blood glucose level more frequently. Patients who are capable, knowledgeable, and responsible can learn to adjust their own insulin doses by working closely with a diabetes educator. Others need specific instructions on what to do when they exercise.

Patients taking insulin and participating in extended periods of exercise should test their blood glucose levels before, during, and after the exercise period, and they should snack on carbohydrates as needed to maintain blood glucose levels. Other participants or observers should be aware that the person exercising has diabetes, and they should know what assistance to give if severe hypoglycemia occurs.

In people with type 2 diabetes who are overweight or have obesity, exercise in addition to dietary management both improves glucose metabolism and enhances loss of body fat. Exercise coupled with weight loss improves insulin sensitivity and may decrease the need for insulin or oral antidiabetic agents (ADA, 2020). Eventually, the patient's glucose tolerance may return to normal. Patients with type 2 diabetes who are not taking insulin or an oral agent may not need extra food before exercise.

 ### Gerontologic Considerations

Physical activity that is consistent and realistic is beneficial to older adults with diabetes. Physical fitness in the older adult population with diabetes may lead to improved glycemic control, decreased risk for chronic vascular disease, and an improved quality of life (Eliopoulos, 2018). Advantages of exercise in this population include a decrease in hyperglycemia, a general sense of well-being, and better use of ingested calories, resulting in weight reduction. Because there is an increased incidence of cardiovascular problems in older adults, a physical examination and exercise stress test may be warranted before an exercise program is initiated. A pattern of gradual, consistent exercise, including a combination of stretching, aerobic exercise, and resistance training, should be planned that does not exceed the patient's physical capacity. Physical impairment because of other chronic diseases must also be considered. In some cases, a physical therapy evaluation may be indicated, with the goal of determining exercises specific to the patient's needs and abilities. Tools such as the Go4Life senior fitness booklet may be helpful (see Resources section at the end of chapter).

Monitoring Glucose Levels and Ketones

Blood glucose monitoring is a cornerstone of diabetes management, and **self-monitoring of blood glucose (SMBG)** levels have dramatically altered diabetes care. SMBG is a method of capillary blood glucose testing in which the patient pricks their finger and applies a drop of blood to a test strip that is read by a meter. It is recommended that SMBG occurs when circumstances call for it (e.g., before meals, snacks, exercise) for many patients taking insulin (ADA, 2020).

Self-Monitoring of Blood Glucose

Using SMBG and learning how to respond to the results enable people with diabetes to individualize their treatment regimen to obtain optimal blood glucose control. This allows for detection and prevention of hypoglycemia and hyperglycemia and plays a crucial role in normalizing blood glucose levels, which in turn may reduce the risk of long-term diabetic complications.

Various methods for SMBG are available. Most involve obtaining a drop of blood from the fingertip, applying the blood to a special reagent strip, and allowing the blood to stay on the strip for the amount of time specified by the manufacturer (usually 5 to 30 seconds). The meter gives a digital readout of the blood glucose value. The meters available for SMBG offer various features and benefits such as monthly averages, tracking of events such as exercise and food consumption, and downloading capacity. Most meters are biosensors that can use blood obtained from alternative test sites, such as the forearm. There is a special lancing device that is useful for patients who have painful fingertips or experience pain with fingersticks.

Because laboratory methods measure plasma glucose, most blood glucose monitors approved for patient use in the home and some test strips calibrate blood glucose readings to plasma values. Plasma glucose values are 10% to 15% higher than whole blood glucose values, and it is crucial for patients with diabetes to know whether their monitor and strips provide whole blood or plasma results.

Methods for SMBG must match the skill level and physical capabilities of patients. Factors affecting SMBG performance include visual acuity, fine motor coordination, cognitive ability, comfort with technology and willingness to use it, and cost (Eliopoulos, 2018). Some meters can be used by patients with visual impairments; these meters have audio components to assist in performing the test and obtaining the result. In addition, meters are available to check both blood glucose and blood ketone levels by those who are particularly susceptible to DKA. Most insurance companies, and programs such as Medicare and Medicaid, cover some or all of the costs of meters and strips.

All methods of SMBG carry the risk that patients may obtain and report erroneous blood glucose values as a result of incorrect techniques. Some common sources of error include improper application of blood (e.g., drop too small), damage to the reagent strips caused by heat or humidity, the use of outdated strips, and improper meter cleaning and maintenance.

Nurses play an important role in providing initial education about SMBG techniques. Equally important is evaluating the techniques of patients who are experienced in self-monitoring. Every 6 to 12 months, patients should conduct a comparison of their meter result with a simultaneous laboratory-measured blood glucose level in their provider's office and have their technique observed. The accuracy of the meter and strips can also be assessed with control solutions specific to that meter whenever a new vial of strips is used and whenever the validity of the reading is in doubt.

Candidates for Self-Monitoring of Blood Glucose

SMBG is a useful tool for managing self-care for everyone with diabetes. It is a key component of treatment for any intensive insulin therapy regimen (i.e., 2 to 4 injections per day or the use of an insulin pump) and for diabetes management during pregnancy. It is also recommended for patients with the following conditions:

- Unstable diabetes (severe swings from very high to very low blood glucose levels within a 24-hour day)
- A tendency to develop severe ketosis or hypoglycemia
- Hypoglycemia without warning symptoms

For patients not taking insulin, SMBG is helpful for monitoring the effectiveness of exercise, diet, and oral antidiabetic agents. For patients with type 2 diabetes, SMBG is recommended during periods of suspected hyperglycemia (e.g., illness) or hypoglycemia (e.g., unusual increased activity levels) and when the medication or dosage of medication is modified (ADA, 2020).

Frequency of Self-Monitoring of Blood Glucose

For most patients who require insulin, SMBG is recommended two to four times daily (usually before meals and at bedtime). For patients who take insulin before each meal, SMBG is required at least three times daily before meals to determine each dose (ADA, 2020). Those not receiving insulin may be instructed to assess their blood glucose levels at least two or three times per week, including a 2-hour postprandial test. For all patients, testing is recommended whenever hypoglycemia or hyperglycemia is suspected; with changes in medications, activity, or diet; and with stress or illness.

Responding to Self-Monitoring of Blood Glucose Results

Patients are asked to keep a record or logbook of blood glucose levels so that they can detect patterns. Testing is done at the peak action time of the medication to evaluate the need for dosage adjustments. To evaluate basal insulin and determine bolus insulin doses, testing is performed before meals. To determine the need for bolus doses of regular or rapid-acting insulin (lispro, aspart, or glulisine), testing is done 2 hours after meals. Patients with type 2 diabetes are encouraged to test daily before and 2 hours after the largest meal of the day until individualized blood glucose levels are reached. Thereafter, testing should be done periodically before and after meals. Patients who take insulin at bedtime or who use an insulin infusion pump should also test at 3 AM once a week to document that the blood glucose level is not decreasing during the night. If the patient is unwilling or cannot afford to test frequently, then once or twice a day may be sufficient if the time of testing is varied (e.g., before breakfast one day, before lunch the next day).

Patients are more likely to discontinue SMBG if they are not instructed how to use the results to alter the treatment regimen, if they receive no positive reinforcement, and if testing costs increase. At the very least, the patient should be given parameters for contacting the primary provider. Patients using intensive insulin therapy regimens may be instructed in the use of algorithms (rules or decision trees) for changing the insulin doses based on patterns of values greater or less than the target range and the amount of carbohydrate to be consumed. Baseline patterns should be established by SMBG for 1 to 2 weeks.

Using a Continuous Glucose Monitoring System

A continuous glucose monitoring (CGM) system is an advanced way that people living with diabetes can use to

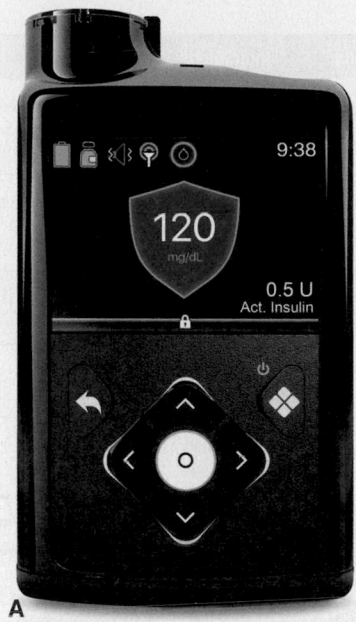

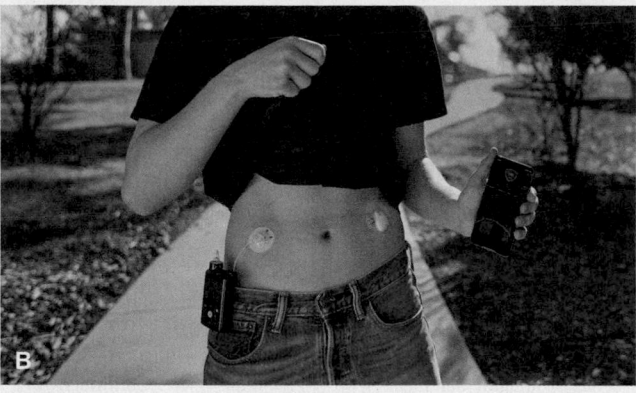

Figure 46-2 • A. The MiniMed™ 770G Hybrid Closed Loop System offers SmartGuard™, a feature using continuous glucose monitoring to automatically adjust insulin delivery. **B.** Patient using this insulin pump for self-management of blood glucose and insulin doses. Parts A and B: Manufactured by the diabetes division of Medtronic, Inc. Used with permission.

monitor blood glucose levels. A CGM can be used with or without an insulin pump (see Fig. 46-2A). A sensor attached to a transmitter is inserted subcutaneously in the abdomen or back of the arm and connected to a wireless monitoring device, where the glucose levels are displayed in real time (see Fig. 46-2B). Sensors are replaced every 7 to 14 days. The data from the CGM device are downloaded, and blood glucose readings are analyzed. The newest CGM is implantable and can be worn for 90 days (Kropff, Choudhary, Neupane, et al., 2017). Although the CGM cannot be used for making decisions about specific insulin doses, it can be used to determine whether treatment is adequate over a 24-hour period. This device is most useful in patients with type 1 diabetes (ADA, 2020).

Testing for Glycated Hemoglobin

Glycated hemoglobin (also referred to as glycosylated hemoglobin, HgbA$_{1C}$, or A1C) is a measure of glucose control for the past 3 months (ADA, 2020). When blood glucose levels are elevated, glucose molecules attach to hemoglobin in red blood cells. The longer the amount of glucose in the blood remains above normal, the more glucose binds to hemoglobin and the higher the glycated hemoglobin level becomes. This complex (hemoglobin attached to the glucose) is permanent and lasts for the life of an individual red blood cell, approximately 120 days. If near-normal blood glucose levels are maintained, with only occasional increases, the overall value will not be greatly elevated. However, if the blood glucose values are consistently high, then the test result is also elevated. If the patient reports mostly normal SMBG results but the glycated hemoglobin is high, there may be errors in the methods used for glucose monitoring, errors in recording results, or frequent elevations in glucose levels at times during the day when the patient is not usually monitoring blood sugar levels. Normal values typically range from 4% to 6% and indicate consistently near-normal blood glucose concentrations. The target range for people with diabetes is less than 7% (53 mmol/mol) (ADA, 2020).

Testing for Ketones

Ketones (or ketone bodies) are by-products of fat breakdown, and they accumulate in the blood and urine. Ketones in the urine signal that there is a deficiency of insulin and control of type 1 diabetes is deteriorating. When there is almost no effective insulin available, the body starts to break down stored fat for energy.

The patient may use a urine dipstick (Ketostix or Chemstrip uK) to detect ketonuria. The reagent pad on the strip turns purple when ketones are present. (One of the ketone bodies is called *acetone*, and this term is frequently used interchangeably with the term *ketones*.) Other strips are available for measuring both urine glucose and ketones (Keto-Diastix or Chemstrip uGK). Large amounts of ketones may depress the color response of the glucose test area, meters that text the blood for ketones are available.

Urine ketone testing should be performed whenever patients with type 1 diabetes have glycosuria or persistently elevated blood glucose levels (more than 240 mg/dL or 13.2 mmol/L for two testing periods in a row) and during illness, in pregnancy with preexisting diabetes, and in gestational diabetes (ADA, 2020).

Pharmacologic Therapy

Insulin is secreted by the beta cells of the islets of Langerhans and lowers the blood glucose level after meals by facilitating the uptake and utilization of glucose by muscle, fat, and liver cells. In the absence of adequate insulin, pharmacologic therapy is essential.

Insulin Therapy

In type 1 diabetes, exogenous insulin must be given for life because the body loses the ability to produce insulin. In type 2 diabetes, insulin may be necessary on a long-term basis to control glucose levels if meal planning and oral agents are ineffective or when insulin deficiency occurs. In addition, some patients in whom type 2 diabetes is usually controlled by meal planning alone or by meal planning and an oral

TABLE 46-3	Select Categories of Insulin				
Time Course	Agent	Onset	Peak	Duration	Indications
Rapid acting	lispro aspart glulisine	15–30 min 15 min 5–15 min	30–90 min 1–3 h 1 h	≤5 h 3–4 h 5 h	Used for rapid reduction of glucose level, to treat postprandial hyperglycemia, or to prevent nocturnal hypoglycemia
Short acting	regular	30–60 min	2–3 h	4–6 h	Usually given 15 min before a meal; may be taken alone or in combination with longer-acting insulin
Intermediate acting	NPH (neutral protamine Hagedorn)	1–1.5 h	4–12 h	Up to 24 h	Food should be taken around the time of onset and peak
Long acting	glargine detemir	3–6 h unknown	Continuous (no peak)	24 h 24 h	Used for basal dose
Rapid-acting inhalation powder	Afrezza	<15 min	~50 min	2–3 h	Administer at the beginning of a meal

Adapted from Comerford, K. C., & Durkin, M. T. (2020). *Nursing 2020 drug handbook*. Philadelphia, PA: Wolters Kluwer; Keresztes, P., & Peacock-Johnson, A. (2019). Type 2 diabetes: A pharmacological update. *American Journal of Nursing, 119*(2), 32–40.

antidiabetic agent may require insulin temporarily during illness, infection, pregnancy, surgery, or some other stressful event. In many cases, insulin injections are given two or more times daily to control the blood glucose level. Because the insulin dose required by the individual patient is determined by the level of glucose in the blood, accurate monitoring of blood glucose levels is essential; thus, SMBG is a cornerstone of insulin therapy.

Preparations

A number of insulin preparations are available. They vary according to three main characteristics: time course of action, species (source), and manufacturer (Comerford & Durkin, 2020). Human insulins are produced by recombinant deoxyribonucleic acid (DNA) technology and are the only type of insulin available in the United States.

Time Course of Action. Insulins may be grouped into several categories based on the onset, peak, and duration of action (see Table 46-3).

Rapid-acting insulins produce a more rapid effect that is of shorter duration than regular insulin. Because of their rapid onset, the patient should be instructed to eat no more than 5 to 15 minutes after injection. Because of the short duration of action of these insulin analogues, patients with type 1 diabetes and some patients with type 2 or gestational diabetes also require a long-acting insulin (basal insulin) to maintain glucose control. Basal insulin is necessary to maintain blood glucose levels irrespective of meals. A constant level of insulin is required at all times. Intermediate-acting insulins function as basal insulins but may have to be split into 2 injections to achieve 24-hour coverage.

Short-acting insulins are called *regular insulin* (marked R on the bottle). Regular insulin is a clear solution and is usually given 15 minutes before a meal, either alone or in combination with a longer-acting insulin. Regular insulin can be administered IV (Comerford & Durkin, 2020).

Intermediate-acting insulins are called *NPH insulin* (neutral protamine Hagedorn), which are similar in their time course of action, appear uniformly milky and cloudy. If an NPH insulin is taken alone, it is not crucial that it be taken

before a meal but patients should eat some food around the time of the onset and peak of these insulins.

"Peakless" basal or long-acting insulins are used as a basal insulin—that is, the insulin is absorbed very slowly over 24 hours and can be given once a day (Comerford & Durkin, 2020). Because the insulin is in a suspension with a pH of 4, it cannot be mixed with other insulins because this would cause precipitation. It is administered once a day at any time of the day but must be given at the same time each day to prevent overlap of action. Many patients fall asleep, forgetting to take their bedtime insulin, or may be wary of taking insulin before going to sleep. Having these patients take their insulin in the morning ensures that the dose is taken.

> ### ▶ Quality and Safety Nursing Alert
>
> *When administering insulin, it is very important to read the label carefully and to be sure that the correct type and dose of insulin is given.*

The nurse should emphasize which meals—and snacks—are being "covered" by which insulin doses. In general, the rapid- and short-acting insulins are expected to cover the increase in glucose levels after meals, immediately after the injection; the intermediate-acting insulins are expected to cover subsequent meals; and the long-acting insulins provide a relatively constant level of insulin and act as a basal insulin.

Insulin Regimens

Insulin regimens vary from 1 to 4 injections per day. Usually, there is a combination of a short-acting insulin and a longer-acting insulin. The normally functioning pancreas continuously secretes small amounts of insulin during the day and night. In addition, whenever blood glucose increases after ingestion of food, there is a rapid burst of insulin secretion in proportion to the glucose-raising effect of the food. The goal of all but the simplest, 1-injection insulin regimens is to mimic this normal pattern of insulin secretion in response to food intake and activity patterns. Table 46-4 describes several insulin regimens and the advantages and disadvantages of each.

TABLE 46-4 Insulin Regimens

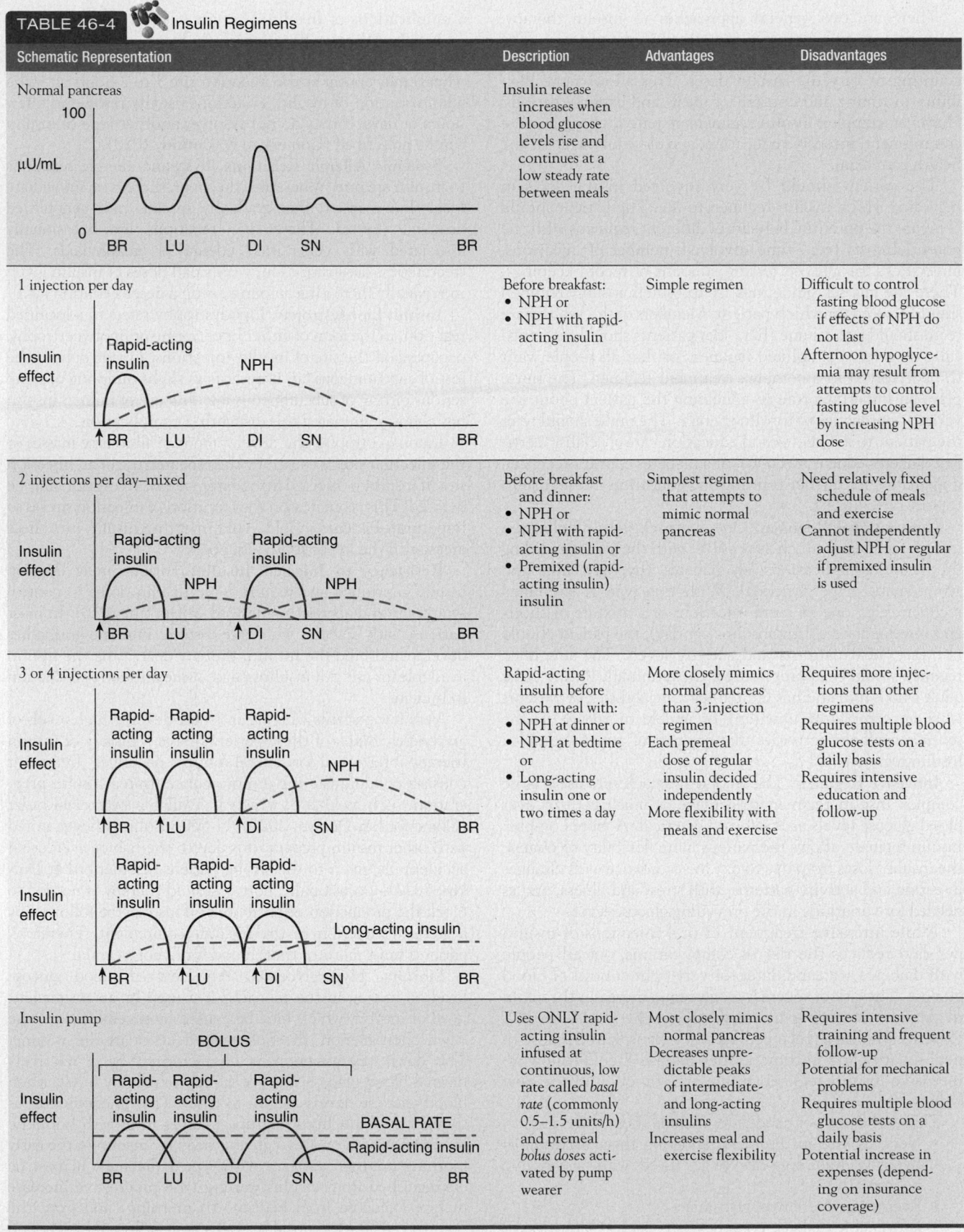

Schematic Representation	Description	Advantages	Disadvantages
Normal pancreas	Insulin release increases when blood glucose levels rise and continues at a low steady rate between meals		
1 injection per day	Before breakfast: • NPH or • NPH with rapid-acting insulin	Simple regimen	Difficult to control fasting blood glucose if effects of NPH do not last Afternoon hypoglycemia may result from attempts to control fasting glucose level by increasing NPH dose
2 injections per day–mixed	Before breakfast and dinner: • NPH or • NPH with rapid-acting insulin or • Premixed (rapid-acting insulin) insulin	Simplest regimen that attempts to mimic normal pancreas	Need relatively fixed schedule of meals and exercise Cannot independently adjust NPH or regular if premixed insulin is used
3 or 4 injections per day	Rapid-acting insulin before each meal with: • NPH at dinner or • NPH at bedtime or • Long-acting insulin one or two times a day	More closely mimics normal pancreas than 3-injection regimen Each premeal dose of regular insulin decided independently More flexibility with meals and exercise	Requires more injections than other regimens Requires multiple blood glucose tests on a daily basis Requires intensive education and follow-up
Insulin pump	Uses ONLY rapid-acting insulin infused at continuous, low rate called *basal rate* (commonly 0.5–1.5 units/h) and premeal *bolus doses* activated by pump wearer	Most closely mimics normal pancreas Decreases unpredictable peaks of intermediate- and long-acting insulins Increases meal and exercise flexibility	Requires intensive training and frequent follow-up Potential for mechanical problems Requires multiple blood glucose tests on a daily basis Potential increase in expenses (depending on insurance coverage)

Note: Rapid-acting insulin—lispro, aspart, or glulisine.
BR, breakfast; DI, dinner; ↑, insulin injections; LU, lunch; NPH, neutral protamine Hagedorn; regular; SN, snack.
Adapted from Comerford, K. C., & Durkin, M. T. (2020). *Nursing 2020 drug handbook.* Philadelphia, PA: Wolters Kluwer.

There are two general approaches to insulin therapy: conventional and intensive (described in detail later). The patient can learn to use SMBG results and carbohydrate counting to vary the insulin doses. This allows more flexibility in timing and content of meals and exercise periods. However, complex insulin regimens require a strong level of commitment, intensive education, and close follow-up by the health care team.

The patient should be very involved in the decision regarding which insulin regimen to use. The patient should compare the potential benefits of different regimens with the potential costs (e.g., time involved, number of injections, fingersticks for glucose testing, amount of record keeping). There are no set guidelines as to which insulin regimen should be used for which patient. Members of the health care team should not assume that older patients should automatically be given a simplified regimen, or that all people want to be involved in a complex treatment regimen. The nurse plays an important role in educating the patient about the various approaches to insulin therapy. The nurse should refer the patient to a diabetes and education care specialist, certified diabetes educator (CDE), or a diabetes education center, if available, for further training and education in the insulin treatment regimens.

Conventional Regimen. One approach is to simplify the insulin regimen as much as possible, with the aim of avoiding the acute complications of diabetes (hypoglycemia and symptomatic hyperglycemia). With this type of simplified regimen (e.g., one or more injections of a mixture of short- and intermediate-acting insulins per day), the patient should not vary meal patterns and activity levels. The simplified regimen would be appropriate for the terminally ill, the older adult who is frail and has limited self-care abilities, or patients who are completely unwilling or unable to engage in the self-management activities that are part of a more complex insulin regimen.

Intensive Regimen. The second approach is to use a more complex insulin regimen to achieve as much control over blood glucose levels as is safe and practical. A more complex insulin regimen allows the patient more flexibility to change the insulin doses from day to day in accordance with changes in eating and activity patterns, with stress and illness, and as needed for variations in the prevailing glucose level.

While intensive treatment (3 or 4 injections of insulin per day) reduces the risk of complications, not all people with diabetes are candidates for very tight control of blood glucose. The risk of severe hypoglycemia increases threefold in patients receiving intensive treatment (ADA, 2020). Patients who have received a kidney transplant because of nephropathy and chronic kidney disease should follow an intensive insulin regimen to preserve function of the new kidney.

Those who are not candidates include those with:
- Nervous system disorders rendering them unaware of hypoglycemic episodes (e.g., those with autonomic neuropathy)
- Recurring severe hypoglycemia
- Irreversible diabetic complications, such as blindness or ESKD
- Severe cerebrovascular or cardiovascular disease
- Ineffective self-care skills

Complications of Insulin Therapy

Local Allergic Reactions. A local allergic reaction (redness, swelling, tenderness, and induration or a 2- to 4-cm wheal) may appear at the injection site 1 to 2 hours after the administration of insulin. Reactions usually resolve in a few hours or days. If they do not resolve, another type of insulin can be prescribed (Comerford & Durkin, 2020).

Systemic Allergic Reactions. Systemic allergic reactions to insulin are rare. When they do occur, there is an immediate local skin reaction that gradually spreads into generalized urticaria (hives). These rare reactions are occasionally associated with generalized edema or anaphylaxis. The treatment is desensitization, with small doses of insulin given in gradually increasing amounts using a desensitization kit.

Insulin Lipodystrophy. Lipodystrophy refers to a localized reaction, in the form of either lipoatrophy or lipohypertrophy, occurring at the site of insulin injections. Lipoatrophy is the loss of subcutaneous fat; it appears as slight dimpling or more serious pitting of subcutaneous fat. The use of human insulin has almost eliminated this disfiguring complication.

Lipohypertrophy, the development of fibrofatty masses at the injection site, is caused by the repeated use of an injection site. If insulin is injected into scarred areas, absorption may be delayed. This is one reason that rotation of injection sites is so important. Patients should avoid injecting insulin into these areas until the hypertrophy disappears.

Resistance to Injected Insulin. Patients may develop insulin resistance and require large insulin doses to control symptoms of diabetes (Comerford & Durkin, 2020). In most patients with diabetes who take insulin, immune antibodies develop and bind the insulin, thereby decreasing the insulin available for use. All insulins cause some antibody production in humans.

Very few patients who are resistant develop high levels of antibodies. Many of these patients have a history of insulin therapy interrupted for several months or longer. Treatment consists of administering a more concentrated insulin preparation, such as U-500, which is available by special order (Comerford & Durkin, 2020). U-500 insulin is never stored with other insulin preparations due to the risk of overdose if accidentally given to the wrong patient (Comerford & Durkin, 2020). Occasionally, corticosteroid therapy is needed to block the production of antibodies. This may be followed by a gradual reduction in the insulin requirement. Therefore, patients must monitor their blood for hypoglycemia.

Morning Hyperglycemia. An elevated blood glucose level on arising in the morning is caused by an insufficient level of insulin, which may be caused by several factors: the dawn phenomenon, the Somogyi effect, or insulin waning. The dawn phenomenon is characterized by a relatively normal blood glucose level until approximately 3 AM, when blood glucose levels begin to rise. The phenomenon is thought to result from nocturnal surges in growth hormone secretion, which creates a greater need for insulin in the early morning hours in patients with type 1 diabetes. It must be distinguished from insulin waning (the progressive increase in blood glucose from bedtime to morning) and from the Somogyi effect (nocturnal hypoglycemia followed by rebound hyperglycemia). Insulin waning is frequently seen if the evening NPH dose is given before dinner; it is prevented by moving the evening dose of NPH insulin to bedtime.

Characteristics and Treatment of Morning Hyperglycemia

Insulin Waning

Progressive rise in blood glucose from bedtime to morning.
Treated by increasing evening (predinner or bedtime) dose of
  intermediate- or long-acting insulin, or instituting a dose of
  insulin before the evening meal if one is not already part
  of the treatment regimen.

Dawn Phenomenon

Relatively normal blood glucose until early morning hours when
  levels begin to rise.
Treated by changing time of injection of evening intermediate-
  acting insulin from dinnertime to bedtime.

Somogyi Effect

Normal or elevated blood glucose at bedtime, early morning
  hypoglycemia, and a subsequent increased blood glucose
  caused by the production of counter-regulatory hormones.
Treated by decreasing evening (predinner or bedtime) dose of
  intermediate-acting insulin, or increasing bedtime snack.

Adapted from Norris, T. L. (2019). *Porth's pathophysiology:
  Concepts of altered health state* (10th ed.). Philadelphia, PA:
  Wolters Kluwer.

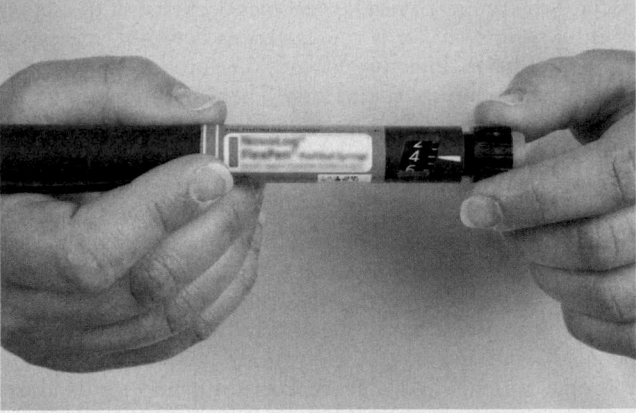

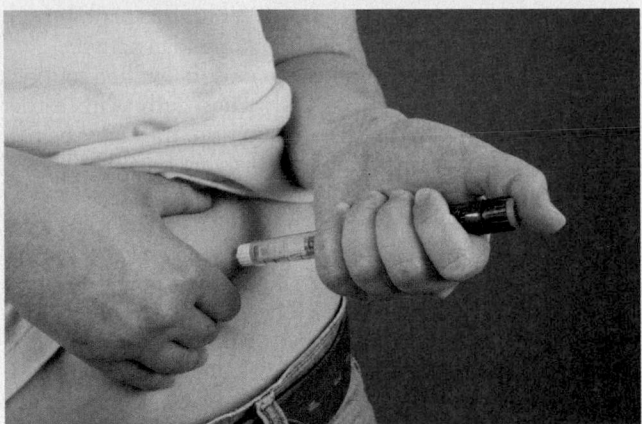

Figure 46-3 • Prefilled insulin syringe.

It may be difficult to tell from a patient's history what the cause is for morning hyperglycemia. To determine the cause, the patient must be awakened once or twice during the night to test blood glucose levels. Testing at bedtime, at 3 AM, and on awakening provides information that can be used to make adjustments in insulin to avoid morning hyperglycemia.

Chart 46-5 summarizes the differences among insulin waning, the dawn phenomenon, and the Somogyi effect.

Methods of Insulin Delivery

Methods of insulin delivery include traditional subcutaneous injections, insulin pens, jet injectors, and insulin pumps. (See later Nursing Management discussion of traditional subcutaneous injections.)

Insulin Pens. Insulin pens use small (150- to 300-unit) prefilled insulin cartridges that are loaded into a penlike holder. A disposable needle is attached to the device for insulin injection. Insulin is delivered by dialing in a dose or pushing a button for every 1- or 2-unit increment given. People using these devices still need to insert the needle for each injection (see Fig. 46-3); however, they do not need to carry insulin bottles or draw up insulin before each injection. These devices are most useful for patients who need to inject only one type of insulin at a time (e.g., premeal rapid-acting insulin three times a day, bedtime NPH insulin) or who can use the premixed insulins. These pens are convenient for those who administer insulin before dinner if eating out or traveling. They are also useful for patients with impaired manual dexterity, vision, or cognitive function, which makes the use of traditional syringes difficult.

Jet Injectors. As an alternative to needle injections, jet injection devices deliver insulin through the skin under pressure in an extremely fine stream. These devices are more expensive and require thorough training and supervision when first used. In addition, patients should be cautioned that absorption rates, peak insulin activity, and insulin levels may be different when changing to a jet injector. (Insulin given by jet injector is usually absorbed faster.) The use of jet injectors has been associated with bruising in some patients.

Insulin Pumps. Continuous subcutaneous insulin infusion involves the use of small, externally worn devices called insulin pumps (ADA, 2020). This technology mimics the functions of a healthy pancreas by providing automated systems that can adjust insulin delivery based on basal (background) insulin every 5 minutes. Insulin pumps contain a 3-mL syringe attached to a long (24- to 42-inch), thin, narrow-lumen tube with a needle or Teflon catheter attached to the end. The patient inserts the needle or catheter into subcutaneous tissue (usually on the abdomen) and secures it with tape or a transparent dressing. The needle or catheter is changed at least every 3 days. The pump is then worn either on the patient's clothing or in a pocket. Some women keep the pump tucked into the front or side of the bra. Additional accessories, such as belt, clip or pouch can be used to carry an insulin pump.

When an insulin pump is used, insulin is delivered by subcutaneous infusion at a basal rate that ranges from 0.25 to 2 units per hour depending on the device. When a meal is consumed, the patient calculates a dose of insulin to metabolize the meal by counting the total amount of carbohydrate for the meal using a predetermined insulin-to-carbohydrate ratio; for example, a ratio of 1 unit of insulin for every 15 g of carbohydrate would require 3 units for a meal with 45 g of carbohydrate. This allows flexibility of meal timing and content.

Possible disadvantages of insulin pumps are unexpected disruptions in the flow of insulin from the pump that may occur if the tubing or needle becomes occluded, if the supply of insulin runs out, or if the battery is depleted, increasing the risk of DKA. Effective education to produce knowledgeable patients minimizes this risk. There is the potential for infection at needle insertion sites. Hypoglycemia may occur with insulin pump therapy; however, this is usually related to the lowered blood glucose levels that many patients achieve rather than to a specific problem with the pump itself. The tight diabetes control associated with the use of an insulin pump may increase the incidence of hypoglycemia unawareness because of the very gradual decline in serum glucose level, from more than 70 mg/dL (3.9 mmol/L) to less than 60 mg/dL (3.3 mmol/L).

Some patients find that wearing the pump for 24 hours each day is inconvenient. However, the pump can easily be disconnected, per patient preference, for limited periods, such as for showering, exercise, swimming, or sexual activity.

Candidates for the insulin pump must be willing to assess their blood glucose level several times daily with either SMBG or CGM (ADA, 2020). In addition, they must be psychologically stable and comfortable about having diabetes, because the insulin pump is often a visible sign to others and a constant reminder to patients that they have diabetes. Most important, patients using insulin pumps must have extensive education in the use of the pump and in self-management of blood glucose and insulin doses. They must work closely with a team of health care professionals who are experienced in insulin pump therapy—specifically, a diabetologist/endocrinologist, a dietitian, and a diabetes and education specialist or CDE.

The most common risk of insulin pump therapy is DKA which can occur if there is an occlusion in the infusion set or tubing. Because only rapid-acting insulin is used in the pump, any interruption in the flow of insulin may rapidly cause the patient to be without insulin. The patient should be taught to administer insulin by manual injection if an insulin interruption is suspected (e.g., no response in blood glucose level after a meal bolus).

Many insurance companies cover the cost of pump therapy. If not, the extra expense of the pump and associated supplies may be a deterrent for some patients. Medicare covers insulin pump therapy for patients with type 1 diabetes.

Insulin pumps have been used in patients with type 2 diabetes whose beta-cell function has diminished and who require insulin. Patients with a hectic lifestyle often do well with an insulin pump. There is no risk of DKA when there is an interruption of the flow of insulin in people with type 2 diabetes wearing an insulin pump.

Transplantation of Pancreatic Cells. Transplantation of the whole pancreas or a segment of the pancreas is being performed on a limited population (mostly patients with diabetes who are receiving a kidney transplantation simultaneously) (Aref, Zayan, Pararajasingam, et al., 2019). Patients must weigh the risks of antirejection medications against the advantages of pancreas transplantation. Implantation of insulin-producing pancreatic islet cells is another approach. This latter approach involves a less extensive surgical procedure and a potentially lower incidence of immunogenic problems. However, thus far, independence from exogenous insulin has been limited to 2 years after transplantation of islet cells. Results of studies of patients younger than 50 years of age with islet cell transplants

using less toxic antirejection drugs have shown some promise (Aref et al., 2019). These procedures are not widely available due to a shortage of organs for transplantation.

Oral Antidiabetic Agents

Oral antidiabetic agents may be effective for patients who have type 2 diabetes that cannot be treated effectively with MNT and exercise alone. In the United States, oral antidiabetic agents include second-generation sulfonylureas, biguanides, alpha-glucosidase inhibitors, non-sulfonylurea insulin secretogogues (meglitinides, phenylalanine derivatives), thiazolidinediones (glitazones), dipeptide peptidase-4 (DPP-4) inhibitors, glucagonlike peptide-1 receptor agonists (GLP-1), and sodium-glucose cotransporter 2 (SGL-2) inhibitors (see Table 46-5). The thiazolidinediones are a class of oral antidiabetic medications that reduce insulin resistance in target tissues, enhancing insulin action without directly stimulating insulin secretion. Second-generation sulfonylureas and meglitinides are insulin secretagogues (Keresztes & Peacock-Johnson, 2019). Patients must understand that oral agents are prescribed as an addition to (not a substitute for) other treatment modalities, such as MNT and exercise. The use of oral antidiabetic medications may need to be halted temporarily and insulin prescribed if hyperglycemia develops that is attributable to infection, trauma, or surgery. See later section on glycemic control in the patient who is hospitalized.

Because mechanisms of action vary (see Fig. 46-4), effects may be enhanced with the use of a multidose, or more than one medication (ADA, 2020). A combination of oral agents with insulin, usually glargine at bedtime, has also been used as a treatment for some patients with type 2 diabetes. Insulin therapy may be used from the onset for newly diagnosed patients with type 2 diabetes who are symptomatic and have high blood glucose and A1C levels (ADA, 2020).

Other Pharmacologic Therapy

Additional medications are available for use in the pharmacologic management of diabetes. These injectables are adjunct therapies, not a substitute for insulin if insulin is required to control diabetes.

Pramlintide, a synthetic analogue of human amylin, a hormone that is secreted by the beta cells of the pancreas, is approved for treatment of both type 1 and type 2 diabetes (Comerford & Durkin, 2020). It is used to control hyperglycemia in adults who have not achieved acceptable levels of glucose control despite the use of insulin at mealtimes. It is used with insulin, not in place of insulin. It acts to slow the rate at which food leaves the stomach and reduces appetite (Comerford & Durkin, 2020). The goal of therapy is to minimize fluctuations in daily glucose levels and provide better glucose control. Pramlintide must be injected subcutaneously 2 in from an insulin injection site (Comerford & Durkin, 2020). Patients are instructed to monitor their blood glucose levels closely during the initial period of use of pramlintide.

Nursing Management

Nursing management of patients with diabetes can involve treatment of a wide variety of physiologic disorders, depending on the patient's health status and whether the patient is newly diagnosed or seeking care for an unrelated health problem.

TABLE 46-5 Select Oral Antidiabetic Medications

Generic Name	Action/Indications	Side Effects	Nursing Implications
Alpha-Glucosidase Inhibitors acarbose miglitol	Delay absorption of complex carbohydrates in the intestine and slow entry of glucose into systemic circulation Does not increase insulin secretion Can be used alone or in combination with sulfonylureas, metformin, or insulin to improve glucose control	Hypoglycemia (risk increased if used with insulin or other antidiabetic agents) GI side effects (abdominal discomfort or distention, diarrhea, flatulence) Drug–drug interactions	Must be taken with first bite of food to be effective Monitor for GI side effects (diarrhea, abdominal distention). Monitor for blood glucose levels to assess effectiveness of therapy. Monitor liver function studies every 3 mo for 1 yr, then periodically. Contraindicated in patients with GI or kidney dysfunction, or cirrhosis. *Alert:* Hypoglycemia must be treated with glucose, not sucrose.
Biguanides metformin metformin with glyburide	Inhibit production of glucose by the liver Increase body tissue sensitivity to insulin Decrease hepatic synthesis of cholesterol	Lactic acidosis Hypoglycemia if metformin is used in combination with insulin or other antidiabetic agents Drug–drug interaction GI disturbances Contraindicated in patients with impaired kidney or liver function, respiratory insufficiency, severe infection, or alcohol abuse	Monitor for lactic acidosis and hypoglycemia. Monitor kidney function. Patients taking metformin are at increased risk for acute kidney injury and lactic acidosis with the use of iodinated contrast material for diagnostic studies; metformin should be stopped 48 h prior to and for 48 h after the use of contrast agent or until kidney function is evaluated and normal. Check for interactions with other medications.
Dipeptidyl Peptidase-4 (DPP-4) Inhibitors alogliptin linagliptin saxagliptin sitagliptin vildagliptin	Increase and prolong the action of incretin, a hormone that increases insulin release and decreases glucagon levels, with the result of improved glucose control	Upper respiratory infection Stuffy or runny nose and sore throat Headache Stomach discomfort and diarrhea Hypoglycemia, if used with sulfonylurea	Usually given once a day. Used alone or with other oral antidiabetic agents. Instruct patient about signs and symptoms of hypoglycemia and other adverse effects to report. Monitor kidney function.
Glucagonlike peptide-1 agonist (GLP-1) dulaglutide liraglutide	Enhances glucose-dependent insulin secretion and exhibit other antihyperglycemic actions following their release into the circulation from the gastrointestinal tract.	Pancreatitis, weight loss, diarrhea, nausea, vomiting, reaction at injection site, cough	Given once a day by subcutaneous injection.
Non-Sulfonylurea Insulin Secretagogues nateglinide categorized as a D-phenylalanine derivative repaglinide categorized as a meglitinide	Stimulate pancreas to secrete insulin Can be used alone or in combination with metformin or thiazolidinediones to improve glucose control	Hypoglycemia/weight gain less likely than sulfonylureas Drug–drug interactions (with ketoconazole, fluconazole, erythromycin, rifampin, isoniazid)	Monitor blood glucose levels to assess effectiveness of therapy. Has rapid action and short half-life Should be taken only if able to eat a meal immediately. Educate patients about symptoms of hypoglycemia. Monitor patients with impaired liver function and renal impairment. Has no effect on plasma lipids. Is taken before each meal. Check for interactions with other medications.
Second-Generation Sulfonylureas glimepiride glipizide glyburide	Stimulate beta cells of the pancreas to secrete insulin; may improve binding between insulin and insulin receptors or increase the number of insulin receptors Have more potent effects than first-generation sulfonylureas May be used in combination with metformin or insulin to improve glucose control	Hypoglycemia Mild GI symptoms Weight gain Drug–drug interactions (NSAIDs, warfarin, sulfonamides)	Monitor patient for hypoglycemia. Monitor blood glucose and urine ketone levels to assess effectiveness of therapy. Patients at high risk for hypoglycemia: advanced age, renal insufficiency. When taken with beta-adrenergic blocking agents, may mask usual warning signs and symptoms of hypoglycemia. Instruct patients to avoid the use of alcohol. Contraindicated with sulfa allergy.

(continued on page 1506)

TABLE 46-5	Select Oral Antidiabetic Medications (continued)		
Generic Name	**Action/Indications**	**Side Effects**	**Nursing Implications**
Sodium-glucose co-transporter 2 (SGL-2) Inhibitors			
anagliflozin dapagliflozin empagliflozin	Prevents the kidneys from reabsorbing glucose back into the blood, therefore lowering glucose by releasing glucose into the urine	Urinary tract infections 　Hypoglycemia May increase LDL and HDL cholesterol	Should be taken once daily before first meal in the morning. Monitor for genital or urinary tract infections.
Thiazolidinediones (or Glitazones)			
pioglitazone rosiglitazone	Sensitize body tissue to insulin; stimulate insulin receptor sites to lower blood glucose and improve action of insulin May be used alone or in combination with sulfonylurea, metformin, or insulin	Hypoglycemia (risk increased with the use of insulin or other antidiabetic agents) Anemia Weight gain, edema Decrease effectiveness of oral contraceptives Possible liver dysfunction Drug–drug interactions Hyperlipidemia (has variable effect on lipids; pioglitazone may be preferred choice in patients with lipid abnormalities) Impaired platelet function	Monitor blood glucose levels to assess effectiveness of therapy. Monitor liver function tests. Arrange dietary education to establish weight control program Instruct patient taking oral contraceptives about increased risk of pregnancy.

GI, gastrointestinal; NSAIDs, nonsteroidal anti-inflammatory drugs.
Adapted from Comerford, K. C., & Durkin, M. T. (2020). *Nursing 2020 drug handbook*. Philadelphia, PA: Wolters Kluwer.

Glucose control in patients diagnosed with diabetes as well as those who have not been diagnosed is an important consideration in the hospital setting. Nursing management of patients with DKA and HHS and of those with diabetes as a secondary diagnosis is discussed in subsequent sections of this chapter.

Because all patients with diabetes must master the concepts and skills necessary for long-term management and avoidance of potential complications of diabetes, a solid educational foundation is necessary for competent self-care and is an ongoing focus of nursing care.

Managing Glucose Control in the Hospital Setting

Hyperglycemia can prolong lengths of stay and increase infection rates and mortality; thus, nurses need to address glucose management in all hospital patients. Hyperglycemia occurs most often in patients with known diabetes (i.e., type 1, type 2,

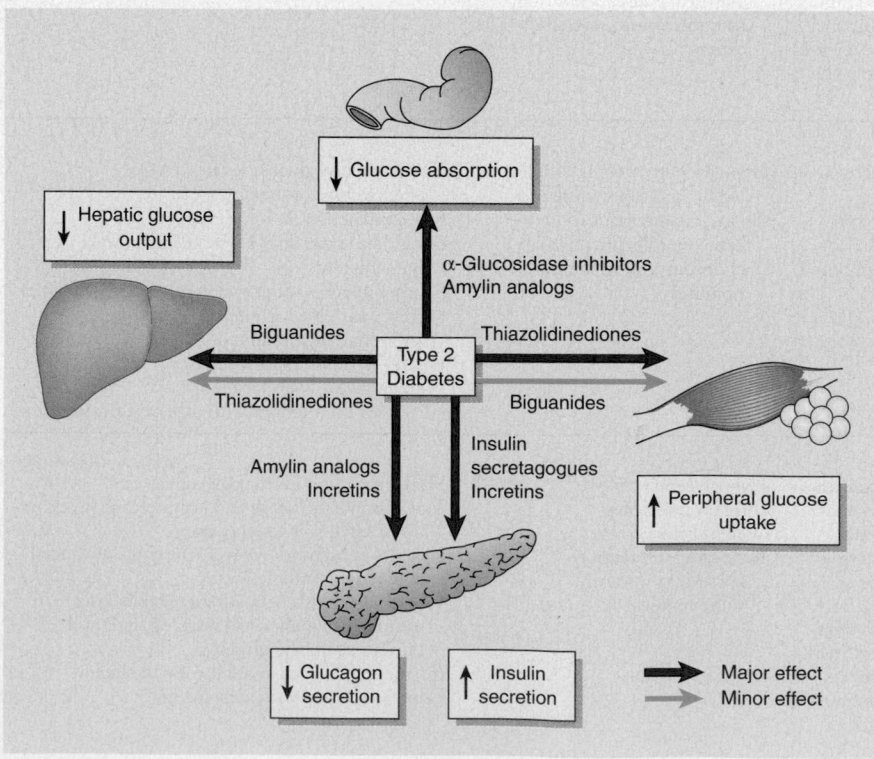

Figure 46-4 • Action sites of hypoglycemic agents and mechanisms of lowering blood glucose in type 2 diabetes. The incretins are the dipeptidyl peptidase-4 inhibitors and glucagonlike peptide-1 agonists.

gestational) and in those newly diagnosed with diabetes or stress hyperglycemia. Nursing management of hyperglycemia in the hospital uses the following principles (ADA, 2020):

- Blood glucose targets are 140 to 180 mg/dL.
- Insulin (subcutaneous or IV) is preferred to oral antidiabetic agents to manage hyperglycemia.
- Hospital insulin protocols or order sets should minimize complexity, ensure adequate staff training, include standardized hypoglycemic treatment, and make guidelines available for glycemic goals and insulin dosing.
- Appropriate timing of blood glucose checks, meal consumption, and insulin dose are all crucial for glucose control and to avoid hypoglycemia.

Providing Patient Education

Diabetes is a chronic illness that requires a lifetime of special self-management behaviors (ADA, 2020). Because MNT, physical activity, medication, and physical and emotional stress affect diabetic control, patients must learn to balance a multitude of factors.

Developing a Diabetes Education Plan

Patients with new-onset type 1 diabetes are hospitalized for short periods or may be managed completely on an outpatient basis. Patients with new-onset type 2 diabetes are rarely hospitalized for initial care. Outpatient diabetes education and training programs have proliferated with the availability of third-party reimbursement. All encounters with patients with diabetes are opportunities for reinforcement of self-management skills, regardless of the setting.

Many health systems employ nurses and registered dietitians who specialize in diabetes education and management and who are certified by the National Certification Board for Diabetes Educators as CDEs. However, because of the large number of patients with diabetes all nurses play a vital role in identifying patients with diabetes, assessing self-care skills, providing basic education, reinforcing the education provided by the specialist, and referring patients for follow-up care. Diabetes patient education programs that have been peer-reviewed by the ADA as meeting National Standards for Diabetes Self-Management Education can be reimbursed for education (Davidson, Ross, & Castor, 2018).

Unfolding Patient Stories: Skyler Hansen • Part 2

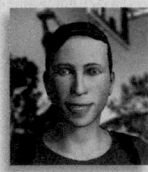

Recall from Chapter 5 **Skyler Hansen,** a high school student recently diagnosed with type 1 diabetes. Outline a diabetes education plan for Skyler and his parents. What are important patient education topics, resources, and methods for the nurse to consider? How would the nurse evaluate whether the patient and his family understand the education provided?

Care for Skyler and other patients in a realistic virtual environment: **v*Sim*** *for Nursing* (**thepoint.lww. com/vSimMedicalSurgical**). Practice documenting these patients' care in DocuCare (**thepoint.lww.com/ DocuCareEHR**).

Organizing Information

There are various strategies for organizing and prioritizing the vast amount of information that must be taught to patients with diabetes. In addition, many hospitals and outpatient diabetes centers have devised written guidelines, care plans, and documentation forms (often based on ADA guidelines) that may be used to document and evaluate education (Davidson et al., 2018).

A general approach is to organize information and skills into two main categories: basic or initial, and in-depth (advanced) or continuing education.

Educating Patients About Basic Skills. Basic skills must be learned by all patients with newly diagnosed type 1 or type 2 diabetes and all patients receiving insulin for the first time. Basic information that patients must know is included in Chart 46-6.

For patients with newly diagnosed type 2 diabetes, emphasis is initially placed on meal planning, exercise, and weight loss if applicable. Those who are starting to take oral antidiabetic agents need to know about detecting, preventing, and treating hypoglycemia. If diabetes has gone undetected for many years, the patient may already be experiencing some chronic complications from diabetes. Therefore, for some patients with newly diagnosed type 2 diabetes, basic diabetes education must include information on preventive skills, such as foot care (Davidson et al., 2018) and eye care (e.g., planning yearly or more frequent complete [dilated eye] examinations by an ophthalmologist, understanding that retinopathy is largely asymptomatic until advanced stages).

Patients also need to realize that once they master the basic skills and information, diabetes education is a life-long process. Acquiring in-depth and advanced diabetes knowledge occurs both formally through programs of continuing

---

Chart 46-6 **PATIENT EDUCATION**
Basic Skills for People with Diabetes

The nurse includes the following basic information in education:

1. Pathophysiology
   a. Basic definition of diabetes (having a high blood glucose level)
   b. Normal blood glucose ranges and target blood glucose levels
   c. Effect of insulin and exercise (decrease glucose)
   d. Effect of food and stress, including illness and infections (increase glucose)
   e. Basic treatment approaches
2. Treatment modalities
   a. Administration of insulin and oral antidiabetic medications
   b. Meal planning (food groups, timing of meals)
   c. Monitoring of blood glucose and urine ketones
3. Recognition, treatment, and prevention of acute complications
   a. Hypoglycemia
   b. Hyperglycemia
4. Pragmatic information
   a. Where to buy and store insulin, syringes, and glucose monitoring supplies
   b. When and how to contact the primary provider

Adapted from American Diabetes Association (ADA). (2020). Standards of medical care in diabetes—2020. *Diabetes Care,* 43(Suppl 1), S1–S212.

education and informally through experience and sharing of information with other people with diabetes.

Planning In-Depth and Continuing Education. This education involves more details related to basic skills (e.g., learning to vary food choices [carbohydrate counting], type of insulin, preparing for travel) as well as learning preventive measures for avoiding long-term complications from diabetes. Preventive measures include foot care, eye care, general hygiene (e.g., skin care, oral hygiene), and risk factor management (e.g., control of blood pressure, blood glucose, cholesterol, weight) (ADA, 2020; Davidson et al., 2018).

More advanced continuing education may include alternative methods for insulin delivery, such as the insulin pump, CGM, and algorithms or rules for evaluating and adjusting insulin doses. The degree of advanced diabetes education to be provided depends on the patient's interest and ability. However, learning preventive measures (especially foot and eye care) is mandatory for early detection and treatment to reduce the occurrence of amputations and blindness in patients with diabetes.

Assessing Readiness to Learn

Before initiating diabetes education, the nurse assesses the patient's (and family's) readiness to learn. When patients are first diagnosed with diabetes (or first told of their need for insulin), they often go through stages of the grieving process. These stages may include shock and denial, anger, depression, negotiation, and acceptance. The amount of time it takes for the patient and family members to work through the grieving process varies from patient to patient. They may experience helplessness, guilt, altered body image, loss of self-esteem, and concern about the future. The nurse must assess the patient's coping strategies and reassure the patient and family that feelings of depression and shock are normal.

Asking the patient and family about their major concerns or fears is an important way to learn about any misinformation that may be contributing to anxiety. Simple, direct information should be provided to dispel misconceptions. Once the patient masters basic skills, more information is provided.

Patients who are in the hospital rarely have the luxury of waiting until they feel ready to learn; short lengths of hospital stay necessitate initiation of basic skill education as early as possible. This gives the patient the opportunity to practice skills with supervision by the nurse before discharge. Follow-up in the home is often necessary for reinforcement of skills.

The nurse evaluates the patient's social situation for factors that may influence the diabetes treatment and education plan, such as:

- Low literacy level (may be evaluated while assessing for visual deficits by having the patient read from educational materials)
- Limited financial resources or lack of health insurance
- Presence or absence of family support
- Typical daily schedule (the patient is asked about the timing and number of usual daily meals, work and exercise schedule, plans for travel)
- Cognitive deficits or other disabling conditions, obtained from the patient's health history and physical assessment (the patient is assessed for aphasia or decreased ability to follow simple commands)

Cultural beliefs may also impact adherence to a regimen.

Educating Experienced Patients

Nurses need to annually assess the skills and self-care behaviors of patients who have had diabetes for many years (Davidson et al., 2018). Assessment of these patients must include direct observation of skills, not just the patient's self-report of self-care behaviors. In addition, these patients must be fully aware of preventive measures related to foot care, eye care, and risk factor management. Those experiencing long-term complications from diabetes for the first time may go through the grieving process again. Some patients may have a renewed interest in diabetes self-care in the hope of delaying further complications. Others may have guilt and depression. The patient is encouraged to discuss feelings and fears related to complications. Meanwhile, the nurse provides appropriate information regarding complications from diabetes.

Determining Education Methods

Maintaining flexibility with regard to education approaches is important. Providing education on skills and information in a logical sequence is not always the most helpful method for patients. For example, many patients fear self-injection. Before they learn how to prepare, purchase, store, and mix insulins, they should be taught to insert the needle and inject insulin (or practice with saline solution).

Various tools can be used to complement education. Many of the companies that manufacture products for diabetes self-care also provide booklets, videotapes, DVDs, or on-line materials to assist in patient education. Educational materials are also available from many sources (see the Resources section). It is important to use a variety of written handouts that match the patient's learning needs (including different languages, low-literacy information, and large print) and reading level and to ensure that these materials are technically accurate. Patients can continue learning about diabetes care by participating in community-based educational programs and other sources such as Web-based programs (Davidson et al., 2018).

Educating Patients to Self-Administer Insulin

Insulin injections are self-administered into the subcutaneous tissue with the use of special insulin syringes. Basic information includes explanations of the equipment, insulins, and syringes and how to mix insulin, if necessary.

Storing Insulin

Whether insulin is the short- or the long-acting preparation, vials not in use, including spare vials or pens, should be refrigerated. Extremes of temperature should be avoided; insulin should not be allowed to freeze and should not be kept in direct sunlight or in a hot car. The insulin vial in use should be kept at room temperature to reduce local irritation at the injection site, which may occur if cold insulin is injected. If a vial of insulin will be used up within 1 month, it may be kept at room temperature. The patient should be instructed to always have a spare vial of the type or types of insulin used (ADA, 2020). Cloudy insulins should be thoroughly mixed by gently inverting the vial or rolling it between the hands before drawing the solution into a syringe or a pen (Comerford & Durkin, 2020). The patient needs to be educated to pay attention to the expiration date on any type of insulin.

Bottles of intermediate-acting insulin should also be inspected for flocculation, which is a frosted, whitish coating inside the bottle. This occurs most commonly with insulins that are exposed to extremes of temperature. If a frosted, adherent coating is present, some of the insulin is bound, inactive, and should not be used.

Selecting Syringes

Syringes must be matched with the insulin concentration (e.g., U-100). Currently, three sizes of U-100 insulin syringes are available:

- 1-mL syringe, 100-unit capacity
- 0.5-mL syringe, 50-unit capacity
- 0.3-mL syringe, 30-unit capacity

The concentration of insulin used in the United States is U-100; that is, there are 100 units per milliliter (or cubic centimeter). Small syringes allow patients who require small amounts of insulin to measure and draw up the amount of insulin accurately. There is a U-500 (500 units/mL) concentration of insulin available by special order for patients who have severe insulin resistance and require massive doses of insulin.

Most insulin syringes have a disposable 27- to 29-gauge needle that is approximately 0.5 in long. The smaller syringes are marked in 1-unit increments and may be easier to use for patients with visual deficits and those taking very small doses of insulin. The 1-mL syringes are marked in 1- and 2-unit increments. A small disposable insulin needle (31 gauge, 8 mm long) is available for very thin patients and children.

Mixing Insulins

When rapid- or short-acting insulins are to be given simultaneously with longer-acting insulins, they are usually mixed together in the same syringe; the longer-acting insulins must be mixed thoroughly before drawing into the syringe. It is important that patients prepare their insulin injections consistently from day to day.

There are varying opinions regarding which type of insulin (short- or longer-acting) should be drawn up into the syringe first when they are going to be mixed, but the ADA recommends that the regular insulin be drawn up first. The most important issues are that patients are consistent in technique, so as not to draw up the wrong dose in error or the wrong type of insulin, and that patients not inject one type of insulin into the bottle containing a different type of insulin. Injecting cloudy insulin into a vial of clear insulin contaminates the entire vial of clear insulin and alters its action.

For patients who have difficulty mixing insulins, several options are available. They may use a premixed insulin, they may have prefilled syringes prepared (see Fig. 46-3), or they may take 2 injections. Premixed insulins are available in many different ratios of NPH insulin to regular insulin (Comerford & Durkin, 2020). The ratio of 70/30 (70% NPH and 30% regular insulin in one bottle) is most common. Combinations with a ratio of 75% NPL (neutral protamine lispro) and 25% insulin lispro are also available. The appropriate initial dosage of premixed insulin must be calculated so that the ratio of NPH to regular insulin most closely approximates the separate doses needed.

For patients who can inject insulin but who have difficulty drawing up a single or mixed dose, syringes may be prefilled with the help of home health nurses or family and friends. A 3-week supply of insulin syringes may be prepared and kept in the refrigerator but warmed to room temperature before administration. The prefilled syringes should be stored with the needle in an upright position to avoid clogging of the needle; they should be mixed thoroughly by inverting syringe several times before the insulin is injected.

Withdrawing Insulin

Most (if not all) of the printed materials available on insulin dose preparation instruct patients to inject air into the bottle of insulin equivalent to the number of units of insulin to be withdrawn. The rationale for this is to prevent the formation of a vacuum inside the bottle, which would make it difficult to withdraw the proper amount of insulin.

Selecting and Rotating the Injection Site

The four main areas for injection are the abdomen, upper arms (posterior surface), thighs (anterior surface), and hips (see Fig. 46-5). Insulin is absorbed faster in some areas of the body than others. The speed of absorption is greatest in the abdomen and decreases progressively in the arm, thigh, and hip, respectively.

Systematic rotation of injection sites within an anatomic area is recommended to prevent lipodystrophy (localized changes in fatty tissue). In addition, to promote consistency in insulin absorption, the patient should be encouraged to use all available injection sites within one area rather than randomly rotating sites from area to area. For example, some patients almost exclusively use the abdominal area, administering each injection 0.5 to 1 inch away from the previous injection. Another approach to rotation is always to use the same area at the same time of day. For example, patients may inject morning doses into the abdomen and evening doses into the arms or legs.

A few general principles apply to all rotation patterns. First, the patient should try not to use the exact same site more than once in 2 to 3 weeks. In addition, if the patient is planning to exercise, insulin should not be injected into the limb that will be exercised because this will cause the drug to be absorbed faster, which may result in hypoglycemia.

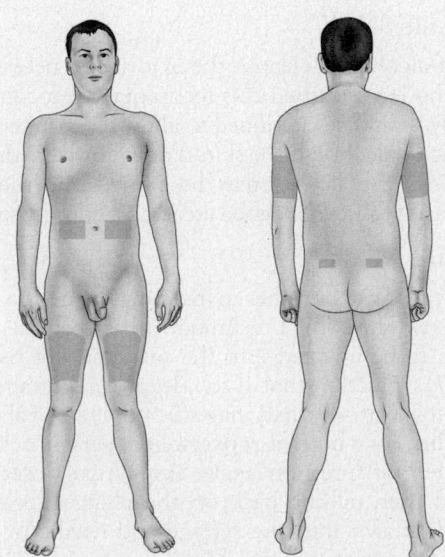

Figure 46-5 • Suggested areas for insulin injection.

Chart 46-7

Self-Injection of Insulin

The nurse instructs the patient to:

1. With one hand, stabilize the skin by spreading it or pinching up a large area.

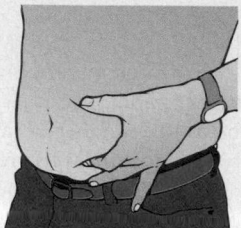

Pinching the skin

2. Pick up syringe with the other hand, and hold it as you would a pencil. Insert needle straight into the skin.[a]

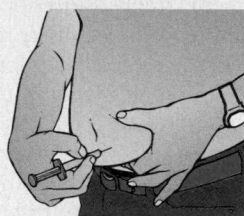

Inserting the needle into the skin

3. To inject the insulin, push the plunger all the way in.

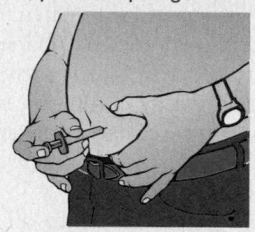

Injecting the insulin

4. Pull needle straight out of skin. Press cotton ball over injection site for several seconds.

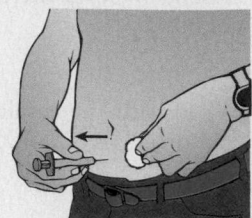

Removing the needle and holding cotton ball over site

5. Use disposable syringe only once and discard into hard plastic container (with a tight-fitting top) such as an empty bleach or detergent container.[b] Follow state regulations for disposal of syringes and needles.

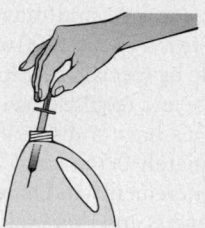

Disposing of syringe

[a]Some patients may be taught to insert the needle at a 45-degree angle.
[b]Although some studies suggest that reusing disposable syringes may be safe, it is recommended that this be done only in the absence of poor personal hygiene, an acute concurrent illness, open wounds on the hands, or decreased resistance to infection.

Preparing the Skin

The use of alcohol to cleanse the skin is not necessary, but patients who have learned this technique often continue to use it. They should be cautioned to allow the skin to dry after cleansing with alcohol. If the skin is not allowed to dry before the injection, the alcohol may be carried into the tissues, resulting in a localized reddened area and a burning sensation.

Inserting the Needle

There are varying approaches to inserting the needle for insulin injections. The correct technique is based on the need for the insulin to be injected into the subcutaneous tissue (see Chart 46-7). Injection that is too deep (e.g., intramuscular) or too shallow (intradermal) may affect the rate of absorption of the insulin. For a normal or overweight person, a 90-degree angle is the best insertion angle. Aspiration (inserting the needle and then pulling back on the plunger to assess for blood being drawn into the syringe and needle in vein) is not necessary. Many patients who have been using insulin for an extended period have eliminated this step from their

insulin injection routine with no apparent adverse effects. Chart 46-8 details how to evaluate the effectiveness of self-injection of insulin education.

Disposing of Syringes and Needles

Insulin syringes and pens, needles, and lancets should be disposed of according to local regulations. If community disposal programs are unavailable, used sharps should be placed in a puncture-resistant container. The patient should contact local trash authorities for instructions about proper disposal of filled containers, which should not be mixed with containers to be recycled.

Promoting Home, Community-Based, and Transitional Care

 Educating the Patient About Self-Care

If poor glucose control or preventable complications occur, the nurse needs to assess the reasons for the patient's ineffective management of the treatment regimen. It should not be

Chart 46-8 Criteria for Determining Effectiveness of Self-Injection of Insulin Education

Equipment

Insulin

1. Identifies information on label of insulin bottle:
   - Type (e.g., NPH, regular, 70/30)
   - Manufacturer
   - Concentration (e.g., U-100)
   - Expiration date
2. Checks appearance of insulin:
   - Clear or milky white
   - Checks for flocculation (clumping, frosted appearance)
   - Identifies where to purchase and store insulin:
   - Indicates approximately how long bottle will last (1000 units per bottle U-100 insulin)
   - Indicates how long opened bottles can be used

Syringes

1. Identifies concentration (U-100) marking on syringe
2. Identifies size of syringe (e.g., 100 units, 50 units, 30 units)
3. Describes appropriate disposal of used syringe

Preparation and Administration of Insulin Injection

1. Draws up correct amount and type of insulin
2. Properly mixes 2 insulins if necessary
3. Inserts needle and injects insulin
4. Describes site rotation:
   - Demonstrates injection with all anatomic areas to be used
   - Describes pattern for rotation, such as using abdomen only or using certain areas at the same time of day
   - Describes system for remembering site locations, such as horizontal pattern across the abdomen as if drawing a dotted line

Knowledge of Insulin Action

1. Lists prescription:
   - Type and dosage of insulin
   - Timing of insulin injections
2. Describes approximate time course of insulin action:
   - Identifies long- and short-acting insulins by name
   - States approximate time delay until the onset of insulin action
   - Identifies need to delay food until 5 to 15 minutes after injection of rapid-acting insulin (lispro, aspart, glulisine)
   - Knows that longer time delays are safe when blood glucose level is high and that time delays may need to be shortened when blood glucose level is low

Incorporation of Insulin Injections into Daily Schedule

1. Recites proper order of premeal diabetes activities:
   - May use mnemonic device such as the word "tie," which helps the patient remember the order of activities ("t" = test [blood glucose], "i" = insulin injection, "e" = eat)
   - Describes daily schedule, such as test, insulin, eat before breakfast and dinner; test and eat, before lunch and bedtime
2. Describes information regarding hypoglycemia:
   - Symptoms: shakiness, sweating, nervousness, hunger, weakness
   - Causes: too much insulin, too much exercise, not enough food
   - Treatment: 15-g concentrated carbohydrate, such as 2 or 3 glucose tablets, 1 tube glucose gel, 0.5 cup juice
   - After initial treatment, follow with snack including starch and protein, such as cheese and crackers, milk and crackers, half sandwich.
3. Describes information regarding prevention of hypoglycemia:
   - Avoids delays in meal timing
   - Eats a meal or snack approximately every 4 to 5 hours (while awake)
   - Does not skip meals
   - Increases food intake before exercise if blood glucose level is less than 100 mg/dL
   - Checks blood glucose regularly
   - Identifies safe modification of insulin doses consistent with management plan
   - Carries a form of fast-acting sugar at all times
   - Wears a medical identification bracelet
   - Educates family, friends, and coworkers about signs and treatment of hypoglycemia
   - Has family, roommates, and traveling companions learn to use injectable glucagon for severe hypoglycemic reactions
4. Maintains regular follow-up for evaluation of diabetes control:
   - Keeps written record of blood glucose, insulin doses, hypoglycemic reactions, variations in diet
   - Keeps all appointments with health professionals
   - Sees primary provider regularly (usually two to four times per year)
   - States how to contact primary provider in case of emergency
   - States when to call primary provider to report variations in blood glucose levels

assumed that problems with diabetes management are related to the patient's decision to ignore self-management. The patient may have forgotten or may have never learned certain information, or there may be cultural or religious beliefs that interfere with adherence. The problem may be correctable simply through providing complete information and ensuring that the patient understands the information. The focus of diabetes education should be patient empowerment. Patient education must address behavior change, self-efficacy, and health beliefs.

If knowledge deficit is not the issue, physical or emotional factors may be impairing the patient's ability to perform self-care skills. For example, decreased visual acuity may impair the patient's ability to administer insulin accurately, measure the blood glucose level, or inspect the skin and feet. In addition, decreased joint mobility (especially in older adults) or preexisting disability may impair the patient's ability to inspect the bottom of the feet. Denial of the diagnosis or depression may impair the patient's ability to carry out multiple daily self-care measures. The patient whose family, personal, or work problems may be of higher priority may benefit from assistance in establishing priorities. The nurse must also assess the patient for infection or emotional stress, which may lead to elevated blood glucose levels despite adherence to the treatment regimen.

The following approaches are helpful for promoting self-care management skills:

- Address any underlying factors (e.g., knowledge deficit, self-care deficit, illness) that may affect control of diabetes.

- Simplify the treatment regimen if it is too difficult for the patient to follow.
- Adjust the treatment regimen to meet patient requests (e.g., adjust diet or insulin schedule to allow increased flexibility in meal content or timing).
- Establish a specific plan or contract with each patient with simple, measurable goals.
- Provide positive reinforcement of self-care behaviors performed instead of focusing on behaviors that were neglected (e.g., positively reinforce blood glucose tests that were performed instead of focusing on the number of missed tests).
- Help the patient identify personal motivating factors rather than focusing on wanting to please primary providers.
- Encourage the patient to pursue life goals and interests, and discourage an undue focus on diabetes.

Continuing and Transitional Care

The degree to which patients interact with primary providers to obtain ongoing care depends on many factors. Age, socioeconomic level, existing complications, type of diabetes, and comorbid conditions may dictate the frequency of follow-up visits. Many patients with diabetes are seen by home health, community-based, or transitional care nurses for diabetes education, wound care, insulin preparation, or assistance with glucose monitoring. Even patients who achieve excellent glucose control and have no complications can expect to see their primary provider at least twice a year for ongoing evaluation and should receive routine nutrition updates. In addition, the nurse should remind the patient to participate in recommended health promotion activities (e.g., annual flu vaccines) and age-appropriate health screenings (e.g., pelvic examinations, mammograms).

Participation in support groups (in person or online) is encouraged for patients who have had diabetes for many years as well as for those who are newly diagnosed. Such participation may help the patient and family cope with changes in lifestyle that occur with the onset of diabetes and its complications. People who participate in support groups often share valuable information and experiences and learn from others. Support groups provide an opportunity for discussion of strategies to deal with diabetes and its management and to clarify and verify information with nurses or other health care professionals leading to healthier behaviors.

ACUTE COMPLICATIONS OF DIABETES

There are three major acute complications of diabetes related to short-term imbalances in blood glucose levels: hypoglycemia, DKA, and HHS (Fayfman, Pasquel, & Umpeirrez, 2017).

Hypoglycemia (Insulin Reactions)

Hypoglycemia means low (hypo) sugar in the blood (glycemia) and occurs when the blood glucose falls to less than 70 mg/dL (3.9 mmol/L) (ADA, 2020). It can occur when there is too much insulin or oral hypoglycemic agents, too little food, or excessive physical activity. Hypoglycemia may

occur at any time of the day or night. It often occurs before meals, especially if meals are delayed or snacks are omitted. For example, midmorning hypoglycemia may occur when the morning insulin is peaking, whereas hypoglycemia that occurs in the late afternoon coincides with the peak of the morning NPH insulin. Middle-of-the-night hypoglycemia may occur because of peaking evening or predinner NPH insulins, especially in patients who have not eaten a bedtime snack.

 Gerontologic Considerations

In older patients with diabetes, hypoglycemia is a particular concern for many reasons:

- Older adults frequently live alone and may not recognize the symptoms of hypoglycemia.
- With decreasing kidney function, it takes longer for oral hypoglycemic agents to be excreted by the kidneys.
- Skipping meals may occur because of decreased appetite or financial limitations.
- Decreased visual acuity may lead to errors in insulin administration.

Clinical Manifestations

The clinical manifestations of hypoglycemia may be grouped into two categories: adrenergic symptoms and central nervous system (CNS) symptoms.

In mild hypoglycemia, as the blood glucose level falls, the sympathetic nervous system is stimulated, resulting in a surge of epinephrine and norepinephrine. This causes symptoms such as sweating, tremor, tachycardia, palpitation, nervousness, and hunger.

In moderate hypoglycemia, the drop in blood glucose level deprives the brain cells of needed fuel for functioning. Signs of impaired function of the CNS may include inability to concentrate, headache, lightheadedness, confusion, memory lapses, numbness of the lips and tongue, slurred speech, impaired coordination, emotional changes, irrational or combative behavior, double vision, and drowsiness. Any combination of these symptoms (in addition to adrenergic symptoms) may occur with moderate hypoglycemia.

In severe hypoglycemia, CNS function is so impaired that the patient needs the assistance of another person for treatment of hypoglycemia. Symptoms may include disoriented behavior, seizures, difficulty arousing from sleep, or loss of consciousness.

 Concept Mastery Alert

It is important to check the patient's blood glucose level and correlate it with the patient's symptoms. If the blood glucose level is low but the patient is not exhibiting any symptoms, the nurse should double-check the glucose level to ensure that it is correct.

Assessment and Diagnostic Findings

Symptoms of hypoglycemia may occur suddenly and vary considerably from person to person. Decreased hormonal (adrenergic) response to hypoglycemia may contribute to lack of symptoms of hypoglycemia. This occurs in some patients who have had diabetes for many years. It may be related to autonomic neuropathy, which is a chronic diabetic complication (see later discussion). As the blood glucose level falls, the normal surge in adrenalin does not occur, and the usual adrenergic symptoms, such as sweating and shakiness, do not take place. The hypoglycemia may not be detected until moderate or severe CNS impairment occurs. Affected patients must perform SMBG on a frequent regular basis, especially before driving or engaging in other potentially dangerous activities.

Management

Treating with Carbohydrates

Immediate treatment must be given when hypoglycemia occurs (ADA, 2020). The usual recommendation is for 15 to 20 g of a fast-acting concentrated source of carbohydrate. It is not necessary to add sugar to juice, even if it is labeled as unsweetened juice, because the fruit sugar in juice contains enough carbohydrate to raise the blood glucose level. Adding table sugar to juice may cause a sharp increase in the blood glucose level, and patients may experience hyperglycemia for hours after treatment.

Initiating Emergency Measures

In adults whose glucose level is less than 54 mg/dL (3.0 mmol/L) or who are unconscious and cannot swallow, an injection of glucagon 1 mg can be given either subcutaneously or intramuscularly (ADA, 2020). Glucagon is a hormone produced by the alpha cells of the pancreas that stimulates the liver to breakdown glycogen, the stored glucose. Injectable glucagon is packaged as a powder in 1-mg vials and must be mixed with a diluent immediately before being injected. After injection of glucagon, the patient may take as long as 20 minutes to regain consciousness. A concentrated source of carbohydrate followed by a snack should be given to the patient on awakening to prevent recurrence of hypoglycemia (because the duration of the action of 1 mg of glucagon is brief—its onset is 8 to 10 minutes, and its action lasts 12 to 27 minutes) and to replenish liver stores of glucose. Some patients experience nausea after the administration of glucagon. If this occurs, the patient should be turned to the side to prevent aspiration in case the patient vomits.

Glucagon is sold by prescription only and should be part of the emergency supplies available to patients with diabetes who require insulin. Family members, caregivers, and coworkers should be instructed in the use of glucagon, especially for patients who have little or no warning of hypoglycemic episodes (ADA, 2020). Patients should be instructed to notify their primary provider after severe hypoglycemia has occurred and been treated. Close monitoring for 24 hours following a hypoglycemic episode is indicated because the patient is at increased risk of another episode (ADA, 2020).

In hospitals and emergency departments, for patients who are unconscious or cannot swallow, 25 to 50 mL of dextrose 50% in water ($D_{50}W$) may be administered IV. The effect is usually seen within minutes. The patient may complain of a headache and of pain at the injection site. Ensuring patency of the IV line used for injection of 50% dextrose is essential because hypertonic solutions such as 50% dextrose are very irritating to veins.

 Providing Patient Education

Hypoglycemia is prevented by a consistent pattern of eating, administering insulin, and exercising. Between-meal and bedtime snacks may be needed to counteract the maximum insulin effect. In general, the patient should cover the time of peak activity of insulin by eating a snack and by taking additional food when physical activity is increased. Routine blood glucose tests are performed so that changing insulin requirements may be anticipated and the dosage adjusted. Because unexpected hypoglycemia can occur, all patients treated with insulin should wear an identification bracelet or tag stating that they have diabetes.

Patients, family members, and coworkers must be instructed to recognize the symptoms of hypoglycemia. Family members in particular must be made aware that any subtle (but unusual) change in behavior may be an indication of hypoglycemia. They should be taught to encourage and even insist that the person with diabetes assess blood glucose levels if hypoglycemia is suspected. Some patients become very resistant to testing or eating and become angry with family members who are trying to treat the hypoglycemia. Family members must be taught to persevere and to understand that the hypoglycemia can cause irrational behavior, due to low supply of glucose to the brain.

Autonomic neuropathy or beta-blockers such as propranolol to treat hypertension or cardiac arrhythmias may mask the typical symptoms of hypoglycemia. It is very important that patients taking these medications perform blood glucose tests on a frequent and regular basis. Patients who have type 2 diabetes and who take oral sulfonylurea agents may also develop hypoglycemia, which can be prolonged and severe; this is a particular risk for older adult patients.

It is important that patients with diabetes, especially those receiving insulin, learn to carry some form of simple sugar with them at all times (ADA, 2020; Davidson et al., 2018). There are commercially prepared glucose tablets and gels that the patient may find convenient to carry. If the patient has a hypoglycemic reaction and does not have any of the recommended emergency foods available, any available food (preferably a carbohydrate food) should be eaten.

Patients are advised to refrain from eating high-calorie, high-fat dessert foods (e.g., cookies, cakes, doughnuts, ice cream) to treat hypoglycemia because their high-fat content may slow the absorption of the glucose and resolution of the hypoglycemic symptoms. The patient may subsequently eat more of the foods when symptoms do not resolve rapidly, which may cause very high blood glucose levels for several hours and may contribute to weight gain.

Patients who feel unduly restricted by their meal plan may view hypoglycemic episodes as a time to reward themselves with desserts. Instructing these patients to incorporate occasional desserts into the meal plan may be more effective, because this may make it easier for them to limit their treatment of hypoglycemic episodes to simple (low-calorie) carbohydrates such as juice or glucose tablets. Patients should be instructed to report all severe hypoglycemic episodes in addition to any increase in the incidence, frequency, and severity to the primary provider.

 ## Diabetic Ketoacidosis

DKA is caused by an absence or markedly inadequate amount of insulin. This deficit in available insulin results in disorders in the metabolism of carbohydrate, protein, and fat. The three main clinical features of DKA are as follows:

- Hyperglycemia
- Dehydration and electrolyte loss
- Acidosis

Pathophysiology

Without insulin, the amount of glucose entering the cells is reduced, and gluconeogenesis (the production and release of glucose by the liver) is increased, leading to hyperglycemia (see Fig. 46-6). In an attempt to rid the body of the excess glucose, the kidneys excrete the glucose along with water and electrolytes (e.g., sodium, potassium). This osmotic diuresis, which is characterized by polyuria, leads to dehydration and marked electrolyte loss (Norris, 2019). Patients with severe DKA may lose up to 6.5 L of water and up to 400 to 500 mEq each of sodium, potassium, and chloride over a 24-hour period.

Another effect of insulin deficiency or deficit is lipolysis, the breakdown of fat into free fatty acids and glycerol. The free fatty acids are converted into ketone bodies by the liver. Ketone bodies are acids; their accumulation in the circulation due to lack of insulin leads to metabolic acidosis.

Three main causes of DKA are decreased or missed dose of insulin, illness or infection, and undiagnosed and untreated diabetes (DKA may be the initial manifestation of type 1 diabetes). An insulin deficiency may result from an insufficient dosage of insulin prescribed or from insufficient insulin being given by the patient. Errors in insulin dosage may be made by patients who are ill and who assume that if they are eating less or if they are vomiting, they must decrease their insulin doses. (Because illness, especially infections, can cause increased blood glucose levels, the patient does not need to decrease the insulin dose to compensate for decreased food intake when ill and may even need to increase the insulin dose.)

Other potential causes of decreased insulin include patient error in drawing up or injecting insulin (especially in patients with visual impairments), intentional skipping of insulin doses (especially in adolescents with diabetes who are having difficulty coping with diabetes or other aspects of their lives), or equipment problems (e.g., occlusion of insulin pump tubing). Illness and infections are associated with insulin resistance. In response to physical (and emotional) stressors, there is an increase in the level of "stress" hormones—glucagon, epinephrine, norepinephrine, cortisol, and growth hormone. These hormones promote glucose production by the liver and interfere with glucose utilization by muscle and fat tissue, counteracting the effect of insulin. If insulin levels are not increased during times of illness and infection, hyperglycemia may progress to DKA (ADA, 2020).

Prevention

For prevention of DKA related to illness, "sick day rules" for managing diabetes when ill (see Chart 46-9) should be reviewed with patients. The most important concept in this is to never eliminate insulin doses when nausea and vomiting occur. Instead, the patient should take the usual insulin dose (or previously prescribed special sick day doses) and then attempt to consume frequent small portions of carbohydrates (including foods usually avoided, such as juices, regular sodas, and gelatin). Drinking fluids every hour is important to prevent dehydration. Blood glucose and urine ketones must be assessed every 3 to 4 hours.

Physiology/Pathophysiology

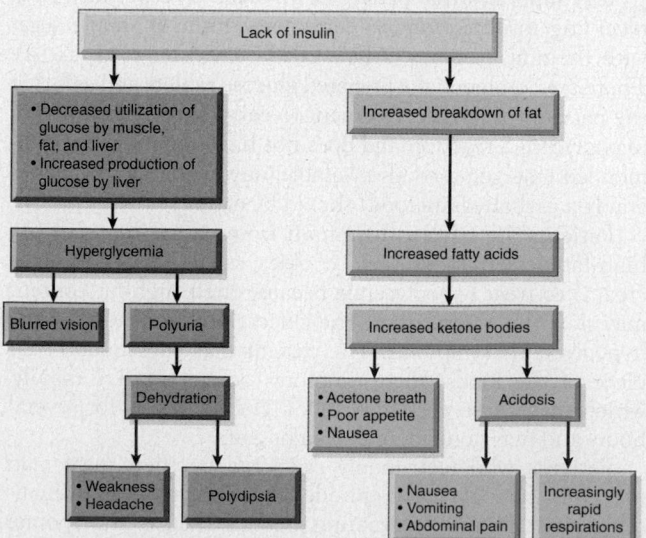

Figure 46-6 • Abnormal metabolism causes signs and symptoms of diabetic ketoacidosis. Redrawn from Pearce, M. A., Rosenberg, C. S., & Davidson, M. D. (2003). Patient education. In Davidson, M. B. (Ed.). *Diabetes mellitus: Diagnosis and treatment.* New York: Churchill Livingstone.

Chart 46-9 — **PATIENT EDUCATION**

Guidelines to Follow During Periods of Illness ("Sick Day Rules")

The nurse instructs the patient to:

- Take insulin or oral antidiabetic agents as usual.
- Test blood glucose and urine ketones every 3 to 4 hours.
- Report elevated glucose levels as specified or urine ketones to your primary provider.
- Take supplemental doses of regular insulin every 3 to 4 hours, if needed, if you take insulin.
- Substitute soft foods (e.g., 1/3 cup regular gelatin, 1 cup cream soup, ½ cup custard, 3 squares graham crackers) six to eight times a day if you cannot follow your usual meal plan.
- Take liquids (e.g., ½ cup regular cola or orange juice, ½ cup broth, 1 cup sports drink [Gatorade]) every ½ to 1 hour to prevent dehydration and to provide calories, if vomiting, diarrhea, or fever persists.
- Report nausea, vomiting, and diarrhea to your primary provider, because extreme fluid loss may be dangerous.
- Be aware that if you are unable to retain oral fluids, you may require hospitalization to avoid diabetic ketoacidosis and possibly coma.

If the patient cannot take fluids without vomiting, or if elevated glucose or ketone levels persist, the provider must be contacted. Patients are taught to have foods available for use on sick days (Down, 2018). In addition, a supply of urine test strips (for ketone testing) and blood glucose test strips should be available. The patient must know how to contact their primary provider 24 hours a day. These materials should be assembled in a "sick day" kit.

After the acute phase of DKA has resolved, the nurse should assess for underlying causes. If there are psychological reasons for the patient missing insulin doses, the patient and family may be referred for evaluation and counseling or therapy.

Clinical Manifestations

The hyperglycemia of DKA leads to polyuria, polydipsia, and marked fatigue. In addition, the patient may experience blurred vision, weakness, and headache. Patients with marked intravascular volume depletion may have orthostatic hypotension (drop in systolic blood pressure of 20 mm Hg or more on changing from a reclining to a standing position). Volume depletion may also lead to frank hypotension with a weak, rapid pulse.

The ketosis and acidosis of DKA lead to gastrointestinal symptoms, such as anorexia, nausea, vomiting, and abdominal pain. The patient may have acetone breath (a fruity odor), which occurs with elevated ketone levels. In addition, hyperventilation (with very deep, but not labored, respirations) may occur. These Kussmaul respirations represent the body's attempt to decrease the acidosis, counteracting the effect of the ketone buildup (Norris, 2019). In addition, mental status in DKA varies widely. The patient may be alert, lethargic, or comatose.

Assessment and Diagnostic Findings

Blood glucose levels may vary between 250 and 800 mg/dL (16.6 and 44.4 mmol/L). Some patients have lower glucose values, and others have values of 1000 mg/dL (55.5 mmol/L) or higher (usually depending on the degree of dehydration). The severity of DKA is not necessarily related to the blood glucose level. Evidence of ketoacidosis is reflected in low serum bicarbonate (0 to 15 mEq/L) and low pH (6.8 to 7.3) values. A low partial pressure of carbon dioxide ($PaCO_2$ 10 to 30 mm Hg) reflects respiratory compensation (Kussmaul respirations) for the metabolic acidosis. Accumulation of ketone bodies (which precipitates the acidosis) is reflected in blood and urine ketone measurements (Down, 2018).

Sodium and potassium concentrations may be low, normal, or high, depending on the amount of dehydration present. Despite the plasma concentration, there has been a marked total body depletion of these (and other) electrolytes, and they will need to be replaced. Increased levels of creatinine, blood urea nitrogen (BUN), and hematocrit may also be seen with dehydration. After rehydration, continued elevation in the serum creatinine and BUN levels suggests underlying renal insufficiency.

Management

In addition to treating hyperglycemia, management of DKA is aimed at correcting dehydration, electrolyte loss, and acidosis before correcting the hyperglycemia with insulin (Fayfman et al., 2017; Joyner Blair, Hamilton, & Spurlock, 2018).

Rehydration

In dehydrated patients, rehydration is important for maintaining tissue perfusion. In addition, fluid replacement enhances the excretion of excessive glucose by the kidneys. The patient may need as much as 6 to 10 L of IV fluid to replace fluid losses caused by polyuria, hyperventilation, diarrhea, and vomiting.

Initially, 0.9% sodium chloride (normal saline [NS]) solution is given at a rapid rate, usually 0.5 to 1 L per hour for the first 2 to 4 hours (Fayfman et al., 2017). Half-strength NS (0.45%) solution (also known as hypotonic saline solution) may be used for patients with hypertension or hypernatremia and those at risk for heart failure. After the first few hours, half-strength NS solution is the fluid of choice for continued rehydration, provided the blood pressure is stable and the sodium level is not low. Moderate to high rates of infusion (200 to 500 mL per hour) may be needed for several more hours. When the blood glucose level reaches 300 mg/dL (16.6 mmol/L) or less, the IV solution may be changed to dextrose 5% in water (D_5W) to prevent a precipitous decline in the blood glucose level (Fayfman et al., 2017).

Monitoring of fluid volume status involves frequent measurements of vital signs (including monitoring for orthostatic changes in blood pressure and heart rate), lung assessment, and monitoring of intake and output. Initial urine output lags behind IV fluid intake as dehydration is corrected. Plasma expanders may be necessary to correct severe hypotension that does not respond to IV fluid treatment. Monitoring for signs of fluid overload is especially important for patients who are older, have renal impairment, or are at risk for heart failure.

Restoring Electrolytes

The major electrolyte of concern during treatment of DKA is potassium. The initial plasma concentration of potassium may be low, normal, or high, but more often than not, tends to be high (hyperkalemia) from disruption of the cellular sodium-potassium pump (in the face of acidosis). Therefore, the serum potassium level must be monitored frequently. Some of the factors related to treating DKA that affect potassium concentration include rehydration, which leads to increased plasma volume and subsequent decreases in the concentration of serum potassium. Rehydration also leads to increased urinary excretion of potassium. Insulin administration enhances the movement of potassium from the extracellular fluid into the cells.

Cautious but timely potassium replacement is vital to avoid arrhythmias that may occur with hypokalemia. As much as 40 mEq/h may be needed for several hours. Because extracellular potassium levels decrease during DKA treatment, potassium must be infused even if the plasma potassium level is normal.

Frequent (every 2 to 4 hours initially) ECGs and laboratory measurements of potassium are necessary during the first 8 hours of treatment. Potassium replacement is withheld only if hyperkalemia is present or if the patient is not urinating.

> ◤ *Quality and Safety Nursing Alert*
>
> *Because a patient's serum potassium level may drop quickly as a result of rehydration and insulin treatment, potassium replacement must begin once potassium levels drop to normal in the patient with DKA.*

Reversing Acidosis

Ketone bodies (acids) accumulate as a result of fat breakdown. The acidosis that occurs in DKA is reversed with insulin, which inhibits fat breakdown, thereby ending ketone production and acid buildup. Insulin is usually infused IV at a slow, continuous rate (e.g., 5 units per hour). Hourly blood glucose values must be measured. IV fluid solutions with higher concentrations of glucose, such as NS solution (e.g., D_5NS, D_5 0.45% NS), are given when blood glucose levels reach 250 to 300 mg/dL (13.9 to 16.6 mmol/L) to avoid too rapid a drop in the blood glucose level (i.e., hypoglycemia) during treatment.

Regular insulin, the only type of insulin approved for IV use, may be added to IV solutions. The nurse must convert hourly rates of insulin infusion (frequently prescribed as units per hour) to IV drip rates. For example, if 100 units of regular insulin are mixed into 500 mL of 0.9% NS, then 1 unit of insulin equals 5 mL; therefore, an initial insulin infusion rate of 5 units per hour would equal 25 mL per hour. The insulin is often infused separately from the rehydration solutions to allow frequent changes in the rate and content of the latter (Fayfman et al., 2017).

Insulin must be infused continuously until subcutaneous administration of insulin can be resumed. Any interruption in administration may result in the reaccumulation of ketone bodies and worsening acidosis. Even if blood glucose levels are decreasing and returning to normal, the insulin drip must not be stopped until subcutaneous insulin therapy has been started. Rather, the rate or concentration of the dextrose infusion may be increased to prevent hypoglycemia. Blood glucose levels are usually corrected before the acidosis is corrected. Therefore, IV insulin may be continued for 12 to 24 hours, until the serum bicarbonate level increases (to at least 15 to 18 mEq/L) and until the patient can eat. In general, bicarbonate infusion to correct severe acidosis is avoided during treatment of DKA because it precipitates further,

sudden (and potentially fatal) decreases in serum potassium levels. Continuous insulin infusion is usually sufficient for reversal of DKA (Down, 2018; Fayfman et al., 2017).

 Quality and Safety Nursing Alert

When hanging the insulin drip, the nurse must flush the insulin solution through the entire IV infusion set and discard the first 50 mL of fluid. Insulin molecules adhere to the inner surface of plastic IV infusion sets; therefore, the initial fluid may contain a decreased concentration of insulin.

 ## Hyperglycemic Hyperosmolar Syndrome

HHS is a metabolic disorder most often of type 2 diabetes resulting from a relative insulin deficiency initiated by an illness that raises the demand for insulin. This is a serious condition in which hyperosmolality and hyperglycemia predominate, with alterations of the sensorium (sense of awareness). At the same time, ketosis is usually minimal or absent. The basic biochemical defect is the lack of effective insulin (i.e., insulin resistance). Persistent hyperglycemia causes osmotic diuresis, which results in losses of water and electrolytes. To maintain osmotic equilibrium, water shifts from the intracellular fluid space to the extracellular fluid space. With glycosuria and dehydration, hypernatremia and increased osmolarity occur. Table 46-6 compares DKA and HHS.

HHS occurs most often in older adults (50 to 70 years of age) who have no known history of diabetes or who have type 2 diabetes (Fayfman et al., 2017). HHS often can be traced to an infection or a precipitating event such as an acute illness (e.g., stroke), medications that exacerbate hyperglycemia (e.g., thiazides), or treatments such as dialysis. The

TABLE 46-6	Comparison of Diabetic Ketoacidosis and Hyperglycemic Hyperosmolar Syndrome	
Characteristics	**DKA**	**HHS**
Patients most commonly affected	Can occur in type 1 or type 2 diabetes; more common in type 1 diabetes	Can occur in type 1 or type 2 diabetes; more common in type 2 diabetes, especially older adults with type 2 diabetes
Precipitating event	Omission of insulin; physiologic stress (infection, surgery, stroke, MI, untreated type 1 diabetes)	Physiologic stress (infection, surgery, stroke, MI), medications (e.g., thiazides), treatments (e.g., dialysis)
Onset	Rapid (<24 h)	Slower (over several days)
Blood glucose levels	Usually >250 mg/dL (>13.9 mmol/L)	Usually >600 mg/dL (>33.3 mmol/L)
Arterial pH level	<7.3	Normal
Serum and urine ketones	Present	Absent
Serum osmolality	275–320 mOsm/L	>320 mOsm/L
Plasma bicarbonate level	<15 mEq/L	Normal
BUN and creatinine levels	Elevated	Elevated
Mortality rate	<1%	5–16%

BUN, blood urea nitrogen; DKA, diabetic ketoacidosis; HHS, hyperglycemic hyperosmolar syndrome; MI, myocardial infarction.
Adapted from Fayfman, M., Pasquel, F. J., & Umpeirrez, G. E. (2017). Management of hyperglycemic crises: Diabetic ketoacidosis and hyperglycemic hyperosmolar state. *Medical Clinics of North America, 101*(3), 587–606.

history includes days to weeks of polyuria with adequate fluid intake. What distinguishes HHS from DKA is that ketosis and acidosis generally do not occur in HHS, partly because of differences in insulin levels. In DKA, no insulin is present, and this promotes the breakdown of stored glucose, protein, and fat, which leads to the production of ketone bodies and ketoacidosis. In HHS, the insulin level is too low to prevent hyperglycemia (and subsequent osmotic diuresis), but it is high enough to prevent fat breakdown. Patients with HHS do not have the ketosis-related gastrointestinal symptoms that lead them to seek medical attention. Instead, they may tolerate polyuria and polydipsia until neurologic changes or an underlying illness (or family members or others) prompts them to seek treatment.

Clinical Manifestations

The clinical picture of HHS is one of hypotension, profound dehydration (dry mucous membranes, poor skin turgor), tachycardia, and variable neurologic signs (e.g., alteration of consciousness, seizures, hemiparesis) (Down, 2018; Fayfman et al., 2017) (see Table 46-6).

Assessment and Diagnostic Findings

Diagnostic assessment includes a range of laboratory tests, including blood glucose, electrolytes, BUN, complete blood count, serum osmolality, and arterial blood gas analysis. The blood glucose level is greater than 600 mg/dL, the osmolality exceeds 320 mOsm/kg, and ketoacidosis is absent (Fayfman et al., 2017). Electrolyte and BUN levels are consistent with the clinical picture of severe dehydration (see Chapter 10). Mental status changes, focal neurologic deficits, and hallucinations are common secondary to the cerebral dehydration that results from extreme hyperosmolality. Orthostatic hypotension accompanies the dehydration (Fayfman et al., 2017).

Management

The overall approach to the treatment of HHS is similar to that of DKA: fluid replacement, correction of electrolyte imbalances, and insulin administration. Because patients with HHS are typically older, close monitoring of volume and electrolyte status is important for prevention of fluid overload, heart failure, and cardiac arrhythmias. Fluid treatment is started with 0.9% or 0.45% NS, depending on the patient's sodium level and the severity of volume depletion. Central venous or hemodynamic pressure monitoring guides fluid replacement. Potassium is added to IV fluids when urinary output is adequate and is guided by continuous ECG monitoring and frequent laboratory determinations of potassium (Fayfman et al., 2017).

Extremely elevated blood glucose concentrations decrease as the patient is rehydrated. Insulin plays a less important role in the treatment of HHS because it is not needed for reversal of acidosis, as in DKA. Nevertheless, insulin is usually given at a continuous low rate to treat hyperglycemia, and replacement IV fluids with dextrose are given (as in DKA) after the glucose level has decreased to the range of 250 to 300 mg/dL (13.8 to 16.6 mmol/L) (Fayfman et al., 2017).

Other therapeutic modalities are determined by the underlying illness and the results of continuing clinical and laboratory evaluation. It may take 3 to 5 days for neurologic symptoms to clear, and treatment of HHS usually continues well after metabolic abnormalities have resolved. After recovery from HHS, many patients can control their diabetes with MNT alone or with MNT and oral antidiabetic medications. Insulin may not be needed once the acute hyperglycemic complication is resolved. Frequent SBGM is important in prevention of recurrence of HHS (Fayfman et al., 2017).

NURSING PROCESS

The Patient with Diabetic Ketoacidosis or Hyperglycemic Hyperosmolar Syndrome

Assessment

For the patient with DKA, the nurse monitors the ECG for arrhythmias indicating abnormal potassium levels. Vital signs (especially blood pressure and pulse), arterial blood gases, breath sounds, and mental status are assessed every hour and recorded on a flow sheet. Neurologic status checks are included as part of the hourly assessment because cerebral edema can be a severe and sometimes fatal outcome. Blood glucose levels are checked every hour (Fayfman et al., 2017).

For the patient with HHS, the nurse assesses vital signs, fluid status, and laboratory values. Fluid status and urine output are closely monitored because of the high risk of kidney failure secondary to severe dehydration. Because HHS tends to occur in older patients, the physiologic changes that occur with aging should be considered. Careful assessment of cardiovascular, pulmonary, and kidney function throughout the acute and recovery phases of HHS is important (Fayfman et al., 2017).

Diagnosis

NURSING DIAGNOSES

Based on the assessment data, major nursing diagnoses may include the following:

- Risk for hypovolemia associated with polyuria and dehydration
- Fluid imbalance associated with fluid loss or shifts
- Lack of knowledge about diabetes self-care skills or information
- Anxiety associated with loss of control, fear of inability to manage diabetes, misinformation associated with diabetes, fear of diabetes complications

COLLABORATIVE PROBLEMS/POTENTIAL COMPLICATIONS

Potential complications may include the following:

- Fluid overload, pulmonary edema, and heart failure
- Hypokalemia
- Hyperglycemia and ketoacidosis
- Hypoglycemia
- Cerebral edema

Planning and Goals

The major goals for the patient may include maintenance of fluid and electrolyte balance, increased knowledge about diabetes basic skills and self-care, decreased anxiety, and absence of complications.

Nursing Interventions

MAINTAINING FLUID AND ELECTROLYTE BALANCE

Intake and output are measured. IV fluids and electrolytes are given as prescribed, and oral fluid intake is encouraged when it is permitted. Laboratory values of serum electrolytes (especially sodium and potassium) are monitored. Vital signs are monitored hourly for signs of dehydration (tachycardia, orthostatic hypotension) along with assessment of breath sounds, level of consciousness, presence of edema, and cardiac status (ECG rhythm strips).

INCREASING KNOWLEDGE ABOUT DIABETES MANAGEMENT

The development of DKA or HHS suggests the need for the nurse to carefully assess the patient's understanding of and adherence to the diabetes management plan. Furthermore, factors that may have led to the development of DKA or HHS are explored with the patient and family. If the patient's blood glucose monitoring, dietary intake, use of antidiabetic medications (insulin or oral agents), and exercise patterns differ from those identified in the diabetes management plan, their relationship to the development of DKA or HHS is discussed, along with early manifestations of DKA or HHS. If other factors, such as trauma, illness, surgery, or stress, are implicated, appropriate strategies to respond to these and similar situations in the future are described so that the patient can respond in the future without developing life-threatening complications. The nurse may need to provide education about basic skills again to patients who may not be able to recall the instructions. If the patient has omitted insulin or oral antidiabetic agents that have been prescribed, the nurse explores the reasons for doing so and addresses those issues to prevent future recurrence and readmissions for treatment of these complications.

If the patient has not previously been diagnosed with diabetes, the opportunity is used to educate the patient about the need for maintaining blood glucose at a normal level and learning about diabetes management and basic skills.

DECREASING ANXIETY

Educating the patient about cognitive strategies may be useful for relieving tension, overcoming anxiety, decreasing fear, and achieving relaxation (see Chapter 3). Examples include:

- *Imagery:* The patient concentrates on a pleasant experience or restful scene.
- *Distraction:* The patient thinks of an enjoyable story or recites a favorite poem or song.
- *Optimistic self-recitation:* The patient recites optimistic thoughts ("I know all will go well").
- *Music:* The patient listens to soothing music (an easy-to-administer, inexpensive, noninvasive intervention).

MONITORING AND MANAGING POTENTIAL COMPLICATIONS

Fluid Overload. Fluid overload can occur because of the administration of a large volume of fluid at a rapid rate, which is often required to treat patients with DKA or HHS. This risk is increased in older patients and in those with preexisting cardiac or kidney disease. To avoid fluid overload and resulting heart failure and pulmonary edema, the nurse monitors the patient closely during treatment by measuring vital signs and intake and output at frequent intervals. Central venous pressure monitoring and hemodynamic monitoring may be initiated to provide additional measures of fluid status.

Physical examination focuses on assessment of cardiac rate and rhythm, breath sounds, venous distention, skin turgor, and urine output. The nurse monitors fluid intake and keeps careful records of IV and other fluid intake, along with urine output measurements.

Hypokalemia. Hypokalemia is a potential complication during the treatment of DKA. Low serum potassium levels may result from rehydration, increased urinary excretion of potassium, movement of potassium from the extracellular fluid into the cells with insulin administration, and restoration of the cellular sodium–potassium pump. Prevention of hypokalemia includes cautious replacement of potassium; however, before its administration, it is important to ensure that a patient's kidneys are functioning. Because of the adverse effects of hypokalemia on cardiac function, monitoring of the cardiac rate, cardiac rhythm, ECG, and serum potassium levels is essential.

Cerebral Edema. Although the exact cause of cerebral edema is unknown, rapid correction of hyperglycemia, resulting in fluid shifts, is thought to be the cause. Cerebral edema, which occurs more often in children than in adults, can be prevented by a gradual reduction in the blood glucose level. An hourly flow sheet is used to enable close monitoring of the blood glucose level, serum electrolyte levels, fluid intake, urine output, mental status, and neurologic signs. Precautions are taken to minimize activities that could increase intracranial pressure.

 EDUCATING PATIENTS ABOUT SELF-CARE

The patient is educated about basic skills, including treatment modalities (diet, insulin administration, monitoring of blood glucose, and, for type 1 diabetes, monitoring of urine ketones); the patient is also educated about recognition, treatment, and prevention of DKA and HHS (Down, 2018; Fayfman et al., 2017). Education addresses those factors leading to DKA or HHS. Follow-up education is arranged with a home health nurse and dietitian or an outpatient diabetes education center. This is particularly important for patients who have experienced DKA or HHS because of the need to address factors that led to its occurrence (e.g., dehydration). For patients who have had HHS, avoiding dehydration and paying attention to increased urination or thirst are even more important than insulin administration. The importance of self-monitoring and of monitoring and follow-up by primary providers is reinforced, and the patient is reminded about the importance of keeping follow-up appointments.

Evaluation

Expected patient outcomes may include:

1. Achieves fluid and electrolyte balance
   a. Demonstrates intake and output balance
   b. Exhibits electrolyte values within normal limits
   c. Exhibits vital signs that remain stable, with resolution of orthostatic hypotension and tachycardia
2. Demonstrates knowledge about DKA and HHS
   a. Identifies factors leading to DKA and HHS
   b. Describes signs and symptoms of DKA and HHS
   c. Describes short- and long-term consequences of DKA and HHS

d. Identifies strategies to prevent the development of DKA and HHS

e. States when contact with primary provider is needed to treat early signs of DKA and HHS

3. Decreased anxiety

a. Identifies strategies to decrease anxiety and fear

4. Absence of complications

a. Exhibits normal cardiac rate and rhythm and normal breath sounds

b. Exhibits no jugular venous distention

c. Exhibits blood glucose and urine ketone levels within target range

d. Exhibits no manifestations of hypoglycemia or hyperglycemia

e. Shows improved mental status without signs of cerebral edema

LONG-TERM COMPLICATIONS OF DIABETES

The number of deaths attributable to ketoacidosis and infection in patients with diabetes has steadily declined, but diabetes related complications have increased. Long-term complications are becoming more common as more people live longer with diabetes; these complications can affect almost every organ system of the body and are a major cause of disability. The general categories of long-term diabetic complications are macrovascular disease, microvascular disease, and neuropathy.

The causes and pathogenesis of each type of complication are still being investigated. However, it appears that increased levels of blood glucose play a role in neuropathic disease, microvascular complications, and risk factors contributing to macrovascular complications. Hypertension may also be a major contributing factor, especially in macrovascular and microvascular diseases (ADA, 2020).

Long-term complications are seen in both type 1 and type 2 diabetes but usually do not occur within the first 5 to 10 years after diagnosis. However, evidence of these complications may be present at the time of diagnosis of type 2 diabetes, because patients may have had undiagnosed diabetes for many years. Kidney (microvascular) disease is more prevalent in patients with type 1 diabetes, and cardiovascular (macrovascular) complications are more prevalent in older patients with type 2 diabetes.

Macrovascular Complications

Diabetic macrovascular complications result from changes in the medium to large blood vessels. Blood vessel walls thicken, sclerose, and become occluded by plaque that adheres to the vessel walls. Eventually, blood flow is blocked. These atherosclerotic changes tend to occur more often and at an earlier age in patients with diabetes. Coronary artery disease, cerebrovascular disease, and peripheral vascular disease are the three main types of macrovascular complications that occur frequently in patients with diabetes.

Myocardial infarction (MI) is twice as common in men with diabetes and three times as common in women with diabetes, compared with people without diabetes. There

is also an increased risk of complications resulting from MI and an increased likelihood of a second MI. Coronary artery disease accounts for an increased incidence of death among patients with diabetes. The typical ischemic symptoms may be absent in patients with diabetes. Therefore, the patient may not experience the early warning signs of decreased coronary blood flow and may have "silent" MIs, which may be discovered only as changes on the ECG. In some cases, ECG changes may not be apparent. This lack of ischemic symptoms may be secondary to autonomic neuropathy (see later discussion). See Chapter 23 for a detailed discussion of coronary vascular disorders.

Cerebral blood vessels are similarly affected by accelerated atherosclerosis. Occlusive changes or the formation of an embolus elsewhere in the vasculature that lodges in a cerebral blood vessel can lead to transient ischemic attacks and strokes. People with diabetes have twice the risk of developing cerebrovascular disease and an increased risk of death from stroke (Virani et al., 2020). In addition, recovery from a stroke may be impaired in patients who have elevated blood glucose levels at the time of and immediately after a stroke. Because symptoms of a stroke may be similar to symptoms of acute diabetic complications (HHS or hypoglycemia), it is very important to assess the blood glucose level (and treat abnormal levels) rapidly in patients with these symptoms so that testing and treatment of a stroke can be initiated promptly if indicated.

Atherosclerotic changes in the large blood vessels of the lower extremities are responsible for the increased incidence (two to three times higher than in people without diabetes) of occlusive peripheral arterial disease in patients with diabetes (ADA, 2020). Signs and symptoms of peripheral vascular disease include diminished peripheral pulses and intermittent claudication (pain in the buttock, thigh, or calf during walking). The severe form of arterial occlusive disease in the lower extremities is largely responsible for the increased incidence of gangrene and subsequent amputation in patients with diabetes. Neuropathy and impairments in wound healing also play a role in diabetic foot disease (see later discussion).

Role of Diabetes in Macrovascular Diseases

Researchers continue to investigate the relationship between diabetes and macrovascular diseases. The main feature unique to diabetes is elevated blood glucose; however, a direct link has not been found between hyperglycemia and atherosclerosis. Although it may be tempting to attribute the increased prevalence of macrovascular diseases to the increased prevalence of certain risk factors (e.g., obesity, increased triglyceride levels, hypertension) in patients with diabetes, there is a higher-than-expected rate of macrovascular diseases among patients with diabetes compared with patients without diabetes who have the same risk factors (ADA, 2020). Therefore, diabetes itself is seen as an independent risk factor for accelerated atherosclerosis. Other potential factors that may play a role in diabetes-related atherosclerosis include platelet and clotting factor abnormalities, decreased flexibility of red blood cells, decreased oxygen release, changes in the arterial wall related to hyperglycemia, and possibly hyperinsulinemia.

Management

The focus of management is an aggressive modification and reduction of risk factors. This involves prevention and treatment of the commonly accepted risk factors for atherosclerosis. MNT and exercise are important in managing obesity, hypertension, and hyperlipidemia. In addition, the use of medications to control hypertension and hyperlipidemia is indicated. Smoking cessation is essential. Control of blood glucose levels may reduce triglyceride concentrations and can significantly reduce the incidence of complications (ADA, 2020; Evert et al., 2019).

Microvascular Complications

Diabetic microvascular disease (or microangiopathy) is characterized by capillary basement membrane thickening. The basement membrane surrounds the endothelial cells of the capillary. Researchers believe that increased blood glucose levels react through a series of biochemical responses to thicken the basement membrane to several times its normal thickness. Two areas affected by these changes are the retina and the kidneys (Norris, 2019).

Diabetic Retinopathy

Diabetic retinopathy is the leading cause of blindness among people between 20 and 74 years of age in the United States; it occurs in both type 1 and type 2 diabetes (ADA, 2020).

People with diabetes are subject to many visual complications (see Table 46-7). The pathology referred to as diabetic retinopathy is caused by changes in the small blood vessels in the retina, which is the area of the eye that receives images and sends information about the images to the brain (see Fig. 46-7). The retina is richly supplied with blood vessels of all kinds: small arteries and veins, arterioles, venules, and capillaries. Retinopathy has three main stages: nonproliferative (background), preproliferative, and proliferative.

Almost all patients with type 1 diabetes and the majority of patients with type 2 diabetes have some degree of retinopathy after 20 years (ADA, 2020). Changes in the microvasculature include microaneurysms, intraretinal hemorrhage, hard exudates, and focal capillary closure. Although most patients do not develop visual impairment, it can be devastating if it occurs. A complication of nonproliferative retinopathy—macular edema—occurs in approximately 10% of people with

TABLE 46-7	Ocular Complications of Diabetes
Eye Disorder	**Characteristics**
Retinopathy	Damage to the small blood vessels that nourish the retina.
Background	Early-stage, asymptomatic retinopathy. Blood vessels within the retina develop microaneurysms that leak fluid, causing swelling and forming exudates (deposits). In some cases, macular edema causes distorted vision.
Preproliferative	Represents increased destruction of retinal blood vessels.
Proliferative	Abnormal growth of new blood vessels on the retina. New vessels rupture, bleeding into the vitreous and blocking light. Ruptured blood vessels in the vitreous form scar tissue, which can pull on and detach the retina.
Cataracts	Opacity of the lens of the eye; cataracts occur at an earlier age in patients with diabetes.
Lens Changes	The lens of the eye can swell when blood glucose levels are elevated. For some patients, visual changes related to lens swelling may be the first symptoms of diabetes. It may take up to 2 mo of improved blood glucose control before hyperglycemic swelling subsides and vision stabilizes. Therefore, patients are advised not to change eyeglass prescriptions during the 2 mo after discovery of hyperglycemia.
Extraocular Muscle Palsy	This may occur as a result of diabetic neuropathy. The involvement of various cranial nerves responsible for ocular movements may lead to double vision. This usually resolves spontaneously.
Glaucoma	Results from occlusion of the outflow channels by new blood vessels. Glaucoma may occur with slightly higher frequency among patients with diabetes.

Adapted from Norris, T. L. (2019). *Porth's pathophysiology: Concepts of altered health state* (10th ed.). Philadelphia, PA: Wolters Kluwer.

type 1 or type 2 diabetes and may lead to visual distortion and loss of central vision (ADA, 2020).

An advanced form of background retinopathy—preproliferative retinopathy—is considered to be a precursor to the more serious proliferative retinopathy. In preproliferative retinopathy, there are more widespread vascular changes

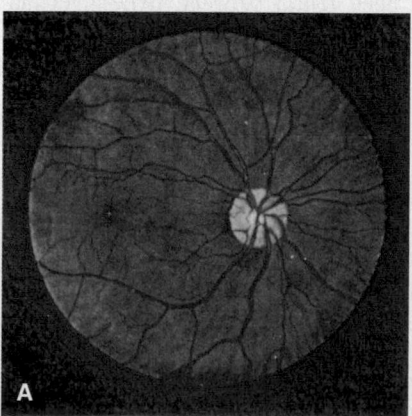
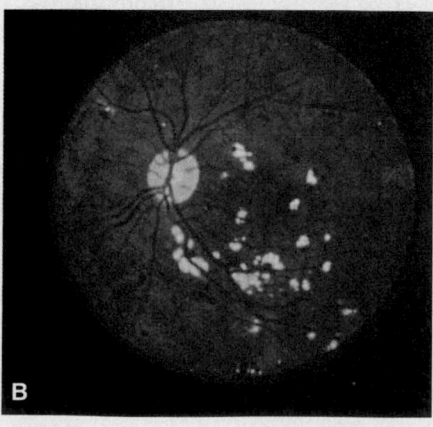

Figure 46-7 • Diabetic retinopathy. **A.** In the fundus photograph of a normal eye, the light circular area over which a number of blood vessels converge is the optic disc, where the optic nerve meets the back of the eye. **B.** The fundus photograph of a patient with diabetic retinopathy shows characteristic waxy-looking retinal lesions, microaneurysms of the vessels, and hemorrhages. Courtesy of American Optometric Association.

and loss of nerve fibers. Epidemiologic evidence suggests that 10% to 50% of patients with preproliferative retinopathy will develop proliferative retinopathy within a short time (possibly as little as 1 year). As with background retinopathy, if visual changes occur during the preproliferative stage, they are usually caused by macular edema.

Proliferative retinopathy represents the greatest threat to vision and is characterized by the proliferation of new blood vessels growing from the retina into the vitreous. These new vessels are prone to bleeding. The visual loss associated with proliferative retinopathy is caused by this vitreous hemorrhage, retinal detachment, or both. The vitreous is normally clear, allowing light to be transmitted to the retina. When there is a hemorrhage, the vitreous becomes clouded and cannot transmit light, resulting in loss of vision. Another consequence of vitreous hemorrhage is that resorption of the blood in the vitreous leads to the formation of fibrous scar tissue. This scar tissue may place traction on the retina, resulting in retinal detachment and subsequent visual loss.

Clinical Manifestations

Retinopathy is a painless process. In non- and preproliferative retinopathy, blurry vision secondary to macular edema occurs in some patients, although many patients are asymptomatic. Even patients with a significant degree of proliferative retinopathy and some hemorrhaging may not experience major visual changes. However, symptoms indicative of hemorrhaging include floaters or cobwebs in the visual field, sudden visual changes including spotty or hazy vision, or complete loss of vision.

Assessment and Diagnostic Findings

Diagnosis is by direct visualization of the retina through dilated pupils with an ophthalmoscope or with a technique known as fluorescein angiography. Fluorescein angiography can document the type and activity of the retinopathy. Dye is injected into an arm vein and is carried to various parts of the body through the blood, but especially through the vessels of the retina of the eye. This technique allows an ophthalmologist, using special instruments, to see the retinal vessels in bright detail and gives useful information that cannot be obtained with just an ophthalmoscope.

Side effects of this diagnostic procedure may include nausea during the dye injection; yellowish, fluorescent discoloration of the skin and urine lasting 12 to 24 hours; and occasionally allergic reactions, usually manifested by hives or itching. However, the diagnostic procedure is generally safe.

Medical Management

The first focus of management of retinopathy is on primary and secondary prevention. The DCCT study (1993) demonstrated that in patients without preexisting retinopathy, maintenance of blood glucose to a normal or near-normal level in type 1 diabetes through intensive insulin therapy and patient education decreased the risk of retinopathy by 76%, compared with conventional therapy. The progression of retinopathy was decreased by 54% in patients with very mild to moderate nonproliferative retinopathy at the time of initiation of treatment. Additional research demonstrated similar results in patients with type 2 diabetes (Action to Control Cardiovascular Risk in Diabetes Follow-On [ACCORDIAN] Eye Study Group, 2016). Thus, control of blood glucose levels in patients with both types of diabetes reduces the risk of retinopathy as well (ADA, 2020).

Other strategies that may slow the progression of diabetic retinopathy include control of hypertension, control of blood glucose, and cessation of smoking.

For advanced cases of diabetic retinopathy, the main treatment is argon laser photocoagulation. The laser treatment destroys leaking blood vessels and areas of neovascularization. For patients who are at increased risk for hemorrhage, panretinal photocoagulation may significantly reduce the rate of progression to blindness. Panretinal photocoagulation involves the systematic application of multiple (more than 1000) laser burns throughout the retina (except in the macular region). This stops the widespread growth of new vessels and hemorrhaging of damaged vessels. The role of "mild" panretinal photocoagulation (with only one third to one half as many laser burns) in the early stages of proliferative retinopathy or in patients with preproliferative changes is being investigated. For patients with macular edema, focal photocoagulation is used to apply smaller laser burns to specific areas of microaneurysms in the macular region. This may reduce the rate of visual loss from macular edema (ADA, 2020).

Photocoagulation treatments are usually performed on an outpatient basis, and most patients can return to their usual activities by the next day. Limitations may be placed on activities involving weight bearing or bearing down. In most cases, the treatment does not cause intense pain, although patients may report varying degrees of discomfort such as a headache. Usually, an anesthetic eye drop is all that is needed during the treatment. A few patients may experience slight visual loss, loss of peripheral vision, or impairments in adaptation to the dark. However, the risk of slight visual changes from the laser treatment itself is much less than the potential for loss of vision from progression of retinopathy.

A major hemorrhage into the vitreous may occur, with the vitreous fluid becoming mixed with blood, preventing light from passing through the eye; this can cause blindness. A vitrectomy is a surgical procedure in which vitreous humor filled with blood or fibrous tissue is removed with a special drill-like instrument and replaced with saline or another liquid. A vitrectomy is performed for patients who already have visual loss and in whom the vitreous hemorrhage has not cleared on its own after 6 months. The purpose is to restore useful vision; recovery to near-normal vision is not usually expected.

Nursing Management

Nursing management of patients with diabetic retinopathy or other eye disorders involves implementing the individual plan of care and providing patient education. Education focuses on prevention through regular ophthalmologic examinations, blood glucose control, and self-management of eye care regimens. The effectiveness of early diagnosis and prompt treatment is emphasized in educating the patient and family.

If vision loss occurs, nursing care must also address the patient's adjustment to impaired vision and the use of adaptive devices for diabetes self-care as well as activities of daily living. See Chapter 58 for discussion of nursing care for patients with low vision and blindness.

Promoting Home, Community-Based, and Transitional Care

 Educating Patients About Self-Care

Because the course of the retinopathy may be long and stressful, patient education is essential. In educating and counseling patients, it is important to stress the following:

- Retinopathy may appear after many years of diabetes, and its appearance does not necessarily mean that the diabetes is on a downhill course.
- The odds for maintaining vision are in the patient's favor, especially with adequate control of glucose levels and blood pressure.
- Frequent eye examinations allow for the detection and prompt treatment of retinopathy.

A patient's response to vision loss depends on personality, self-concept, and coping mechanisms. Acceptance of blindness occurs in stages; some patients may learn to accept blindness in a rather short period, and others may never do so. An important issue in educating patients is that several complications of diabetes may occur simultaneously. For example, a patient who is blind due to diabetic retinopathy may also have peripheral neuropathy and may experience impairment of manual dexterity and tactile sensation, or kidney failure. This can be devastating to the patient and family. Psychological counseling may be warranted. To prevent further losses, glycemic control remains a priority.

Continuing and Transitional Care

The importance of careful diabetes management is emphasized as one means of slowing the progression of visual changes. The patient is reminded of the need to see an ophthalmologist regularly. If eye changes are progressive and unrelenting, the patient should be prepared for inevitable blindness. Therefore, consideration is given to making referrals for educating the patient in Braille and for training the patient with guide (i.e., service) dogs. Referral to state agencies should be made to ensure that the patient receives services for the blind. Family members are also taught how to assist the patient to remain as independent as possible despite decreasing visual acuity.

Referral for home care may be indicated for some patients, particularly those who live alone, those who are not coping well, and those who have other health problems or complications of diabetes that may interfere with their ability to perform self-care. During home visits, the nurse can assess the patient's home environment and their ability to manage diabetes despite visual impairments. See Chapter 58 for a detailed discussion of medical management and nursing care for patients with visual disturbances.

Nephropathy

Nephropathy, or kidney disease secondary to diabetic microvascular changes in the kidney, is a common complication of diabetes (ADA, 2020). In the United States each year, people with diabetes account for almost 50% of new cases of ESKD, and about 25% of those require dialysis or transplantation. About 20% to 30% of people with type 1 or types 2 diabetes develop nephropathy, but fewer of those with type 2 diabetes progress to ESKD. Native American, Latino, African American, Asian American, and Pacific Island people with type 2 diabetes are at greater risk for ESKD than non-Latino Whites (ADA, 2020).

Patients with type 1 diabetes frequently show initial signs of kidney disease after 10 to 15 years, while patients with type 2 diabetes tend to develop kidney disease within 10 years after the diagnosis of diabetes. Many patients with type 2 diabetes have had diabetes for many years before the diabetes is diagnosed and treated. Therefore, they may have evidence of nephropathy at the time of diagnosis (ADA, 2020). If blood glucose levels are elevated consistently for a significant period of time, the kidney's filtration mechanism is stressed, allowing blood proteins to leak into the urine. As a result, the pressure in the blood vessels of the kidney increases. It is thought that this elevated pressure serves as the stimulus for the development of nephropathy. Various medications and diets are being tested to prevent these complications.

The DCCT (1993) results showed that intensive treatment for type 1 diabetes with a goal of achieving a glycolated hemoglobin level as close to the nondiabetic range as possible reduced the occurrence of early signs of nephropathy. Similarly, the United Kingdom Prospective Diabetes Study Group (UKPDS, 1998) demonstrated a reduced incidence of overt nephropathy in patients with type 2 diabetes who controlled their blood glucose levels.

Clinical Manifestations

Most of the signs and symptoms of kidney dysfunction in patients with diabetes are similar to those seen in patients without diabetes (see Chapter 48). In addition, as kidney failure progresses, the catabolism (breakdown) of both exogenous and endogenous insulin decreases, and frequent hypoglycemic episodes may result. Insulin needs change as a result of changes in the catabolism of insulin, changes in diet related to the treatment of nephropathy, and changes in insulin clearance that occur with decreased kidney function.

Assessment and Diagnostic Findings

Albumin is one of the most important blood proteins that leak into the urine. Although small amounts may leak undetected for years, its leakage into the urine is among the earliest signs that can be detected. Clinical nephropathy eventually develops in more than 85% of people with microalbuminuria but in fewer than 5% of people without microalbuminuria. The urine should be checked annually for the presence of microalbumin. If the microalbuminuria exceeds 30 mg/24 hours on two consecutive random urine tests, a 24-hour urine sample should be obtained and tested. If results are positive, treatment is indicated (see later discussion).

In addition, tests for serum creatinine and BUN levels should be conducted annually. Diagnostic testing for cardiac or other systemic disorders may also be required with progression of other complications, and caution is indicated if contrast agents are used with these tests. Contrast agents and dyes used for some diagnostic tests may not be easily cleared by the damaged kidney, and the potential benefits of these diagnostic tests must be weighed against their potential risks.

Hypertension often develops in patients (with and without diabetes) who are in the early stages of kidney disease. However, hypertension is the most common complication in all people with diabetes (ADA, 2020). Therefore, this symptom may or may not be due to kidney disease; other diagnostic criteria must also be present.

Management

In addition to achieving and maintaining near-normal blood glucose levels, management for all patients with diabetes should include careful attention to the following:

- Control of hypertension (the use of angiotensin-converting enzyme [ACE] inhibitors, such as captopril), because control of hypertension may also decrease or delay the onset of early proteinuria
- Prevention or vigorous treatment of urinary tract infections
- Avoidance of nephrotoxic medications and contrast dye
- Adjustment of medications as kidney function changes
- Low-sodium diet
- Low-protein diet

If the patient has already developed microalbuminuria with levels that exceed 30 mg/24 hours on two consecutive tests, an ACE inhibitor should be prescribed. ACE inhibitors lower blood pressure and reduce microalbuminuria, thereby protecting the kidney. Alternatively, angiotensin receptor–blocking agents may be prescribed. This preventive strategy should be part of the standard of care for all people with diabetes (ADA, 2020). Carefully designed low-protein diets also appear to reverse early leakage of small amounts of protein from the kidney.

In chronic or ESKD, two types of treatment are available: dialysis (hemodialysis or peritoneal dialysis) and transplantation from a relative or a deceased donor. Hemodialysis for patients with diabetes is similar to that for patients without the disease (see Chapter 48). Because hemodialysis creates additional stress on patients with cardiovascular disease, it may not be appropriate for some patients.

Continuous ambulatory peritoneal dialysis is being used by patients with diabetes, mainly because of the independence it allows. In addition, insulin can be mixed into the dialysate, which may result in better blood glucose control and end the need for insulin injections. Some patients may require higher doses of insulin because the dialysate contains glucose. Major risks of peritoneal dialysis are infection and peritonitis. The mortality rate for patients with diabetes undergoing dialysis is higher than that for patients without diabetes undergoing dialysis and is closely related to the severity of cardiovascular problems.

Kidney disease is frequently accompanied by advancing retinopathy that may require laser treatments and surgery. Severe hypertension also worsens eye disease because of the additional stress it places on the blood vessels. Patients being treated with hemodialysis who require eye surgery may be changed to peritoneal dialysis and have their hypertension aggressively controlled for several weeks before surgery to prevent bleeding and damage to the retina. The rationale for this change is that hemodialysis requires anticoagulant agents that can increase the risk of bleeding after the surgery, and peritoneal dialysis minimizes pressure changes in the eyes.

In medical centers performing large numbers of transplantations, the chances are 75% to 80% that the transplanted kidney will continue to function in patients with diabetes for at least 5 years. Like the original kidneys, transplanted kidneys can eventually be damaged if blood glucose levels are consistently high after the transplantation. Therefore, monitoring blood glucose levels frequently and adjusting insulin levels in patients with diabetes are essential for long-term success of kidney transplantation. Optimal treatment is a simultaneous kidney and pancreatic transplantation (Aref et al., 2019).

Diabetic Neuropathies

Diabetic neuropathy refers to a group of diseases that affect all types of nerves, including peripheral (sensorimotor), autonomic, and spinal nerves. The disorders appear to be clinically diverse and depend on the location of the affected nerve cells. The prevalence increases with the age of the patient and the duration of the disease (National Institute of Diabetes and Digestive and Kidney Diseases [NIDDK], 2018).

The etiology of neuropathy may involve elevated blood glucose levels over a period of years. Control of blood glucose levels to normal or near-normal levels decreases the incidence of neuropathy. The pathogenesis of neuropathy may be attributed to either a vascular or metabolic mechanism or both. Capillary basement membrane thickening and capillary closure may be present. In addition, there may be demyelinization of the nerves, which is thought to be related to hyperglycemia. Nerve conduction is disrupted when there are aberrations of the myelin sheaths.

The two most common types of diabetic neuropathy are sensorimotor polyneuropathy and autonomic neuropathy. Sensorimotor polyneuropathy is also called *peripheral neuropathy*. Cranial mononeuropathies—those affecting the oculomotor nerve—also occur in diabetes, especially in older adults.

Peripheral Neuropathy

Peripheral neuropathy most commonly affects the distal portions of the nerves, especially the nerves of the lower extremities; it affects both sides of the body symmetrically and may spread in a proximal direction.

Clinical Manifestations

Although approximately half of patients with diabetic neuropathy do not have symptoms, initial symptoms may include paresthesias (prickling, tingling, or heightened sensation) and burning sensations (especially at night). As the neuropathy progresses, the feet become numb. In addition, a decrease in proprioception (awareness of posture and movement of the body and of position and weight of objects in relation to the body) and a decreased sensation of light touch may lead to an unsteady gait. Decreased sensations of pain and temperature place patients with neuropathy at increased risk for injury due to falls and undetected foot infections (Hickey & Strayer, 2020). Deformities of the foot may also occur; neuropathy-related joint changes are sometimes referred to as Charcot joints. These joint deformities result from the abnormal weight distribution on joints resulting from lack of proprioception.

On physical examination, a decrease in deep tendon reflexes and vibratory sensation is found. For patients with fewer or no symptoms of neuropathy, these physical findings may be the only indication of neuropathic changes. For patients with signs or symptoms of neuropathy, it is important to rule out other possible causes, including alcohol-induced and vitamin-deficiency neuropathies.

Management

Intensive insulin therapy and control of blood glucose levels delay the onset and slow the progression of neuropathy. Pain, particularly of the lower extremities, is a disturbing symptom in some people with neuropathy secondary to diabetes. In some cases, neuropathic pain spontaneously resolves within 6 months; for others, pain persists for many years. Various approaches to pain management can be tried. These include analgesic agents (preferably nonopioid); tricyclic antidepressants and other antidepressant medications (duloxetine); anticonvulsant medications (pregabalin or gabapentin); mexiletine, an antiarrhythmic agent; and transcutaneous electrical nerve stimulation (Hickey & Strayer, 2020).

Autonomic Neuropathies

Neuropathy of the autonomic nervous system results in a broad range of dysfunctions affecting almost every organ system of the body (NIDDK, 2018).

Clinical Manifestations

Three manifestations of autonomic neuropathy are related to the cardiac, gastrointestinal, and renal systems. Cardiovascular symptoms range from a fixed, slightly tachycardic heart rate and orthostatic hypotension to silent, or painless, myocardial ischemia and infarction. Research suggests that cardiovascular health may also be impacted by diabetes distress and depressive symptoms (McCarthy, Whittemore, Gholson, et al., 2019). See the Nursing Research Profile in Chart 46-10.

Delayed gastric emptying may occur with the typical gastrointestinal symptoms of early satiety, bloating, nausea, and vomiting. "Diabetic" constipation or diarrhea (especially nocturnal diarrhea) may occur as a result. In addition, there may be unexplained wide swings in blood glucose levels related to inconsistent absorption of the glucose from ingested foods secondary to the inconsistent gastric emptying.

Urinary retention, a decreased sensation of bladder fullness, and other urinary symptoms of neurogenic bladder result from autonomic neuropathy. The patient with a neurogenic bladder is predisposed to development of urinary tract infections because of the inability to empty the bladder completely. This is especially true of patients with poorly controlled diabetes because hyperglycemia impairs resistance to infection.

Hypoglycemic Unawareness

Autonomic neuropathy affecting the adrenal medulla is responsible for diminished or absent adrenergic symptoms of hypoglycemia. Patients may report that they no longer feel the typical shakiness, sweating, nervousness, and palpitations associated with hypoglycemia. Frequent blood glucose monitoring is recommended for these patients. The inability to detect and treat these warning signs of hypoglycemia puts patients at risk for development of dangerously low blood glucose levels. Therefore, goals for blood glucose levels may need to be adjusted to reduce the risk for hypoglycemia. Patients and families need to be taught to recognize subtle and atypical symptoms of hypoglycemia, such as numbness around the mouth and impaired ability to concentrate.

Sudomotor Neuropathy

The neuropathic condition called *sudomotor neuropathy* refers to a decrease or absence of anhidrosis (sweating) of the extremities, with a compensatory increase in upper body anhidrosis. Dryness of the feet increases the risk for the development of foot ulcerations.

Sexual Dysfunction

Sexual dysfunction, especially erectile dysfunction in men, is a complication of diabetes. The effects of autonomic neuropathy on female sexual functioning are not well documented. Reduced vaginal lubrication has been mentioned as a possible neuropathic effect. Other possible changes in sexual function in women with diabetes include decreased libido and lack of

---

Chart 46-10

NURSING RESEARCH PROFILE

Health Factors in Adults with Type 1 Diabetes

McCarthy, M. M., Whittemore, R., Gholson, G., et al. (2019). Diabetes distress, depressive symptoms, and cardiovascular health in adults with type 1 diabetes. *Nursing Research, 68*(6), 445–452.

Purpose

The prevalence of type 1 diabetes in adults is increasing. The purpose of this study was to describe the relationships among the psychological factors of depressive symptoms and diabetes distress and six cardiovascular risk factors.

Design

This was a cross-sectional survey of a sample of 83 adults with type 1 diabetes. Data were collected about sociodemographic information, depressive symptoms, diabetes distress, and cardiovascular health factors (body mass index [BMI], blood pressure, cholesterol, smoking, hemoglobin A1C, and physical activity).

Findings

The mean age of participants was 45 years, with a mean duration of 20 years with type 1 diabetes. The majority had low

scores on the Diabetes Distress Scale while 18% had moderate, and another 18% had high scores. Twenty-two percent of participants had an increased level of depressive symptoms. Significant correlations were found between diabetes distress and fear of hypoglycemia ($r = .65$, $p < .0001$), depressive symptoms ($r = .55$, $p < .0001$), hemoglobin A1C ($r = .41$, $p < .001$), and total cholesterol ($r = .26$, $p < .05$). There were significant correlations between depressive symptom scores and fear of hypoglycemia ($r = .35$, $p < .01$), as well as hemoglobin A1C ($r = .25$, $p < .05$). There were small to medium nonsignificant correlations between depressive symptoms scores and weekly step counts and BMI.

Nursing Implications

Nurses working with patients with type 1 diabetes need to be aware that elevated diabetes distress and depressive symptoms may further affect these patients' already high risk of cardiovascular disease. Interventions are needed that affect both physical and psychological factors that have the potential to adversely affect cardiovascular health.

orgasm. Vaginal infection, which increases in the incidence in women with diabetes, may be associated with decreased lubrication and vaginal pruritus (itching) and tenderness. Urinary tract infections and vaginitis may also affect sexual function.

Erectile dysfunction occurs with greater frequency in men with diabetes than in other men of the same age. Some men with autonomic neuropathy have normal erectile function and can experience orgasm but do not ejaculate normally. Retrograde ejaculation occurs; seminal fluid is propelled backward through the posterior urethra and into the urinary bladder. Examination of the urine confirms the diagnosis because of the large number of active sperm present. Fertility counseling may be necessary for couples attempting conception.

Diabetic neuropathy is not the only cause of erectile dysfunction in men with diabetes. Medications such as antihypertensive agents, psychological factors, and other medical conditions (e.g., vascular insufficiency) that may affect other men also play a role in erectile dysfunction in men with diabetes (see Chapter 53).

Management

Management strategies for autonomic neuropathy focus on alleviating symptoms and on modification and management of risk factors. Detection of painless cardiac ischemia is important so that education about avoiding strenuous exercise can be provided. Orthostatic hypotension may respond to a diet high in sodium, discontinuation of medications that impede autonomic nervous system responses, the use of sympathomimetic and other agents (e.g., caffeine) that stimulate an autonomic response, mineralocorticoid therapy, and the use of lower-body elastic garments that maximize venous return and prevent pooling of blood in the extremities.

Treatment of delayed gastric emptying includes a low-fat diet, frequent small meals, frequent blood glucose monitoring, and the use of agents that increase gastric motility (e.g., metoclopramide, bethanechol). Treatment of diabetic diarrhea may include bulk-forming laxatives or antidiarrheal agents. Constipation is treated with a high-fiber diet and adequate hydration; medications, laxatives, and enemas may be necessary if constipation is severe. Management of sexual dysfunction in women and men is discussed in Chapters 51 and 53, respectively. Intermittent straight catheterization may be necessary to prevent urinary tract infections in patients with neurogenic bladders.

Treatment of sudomotor dysfunction focuses on education about skin care and heat intolerance.

Foot and Leg Problems

Lower limb amputations in adults with diabetes increased by 50% between 2009 and 2015 compared to prior years (Virani et al., 2020). Amputations are preventable, provided patients are taught appropriate foot care measures and practice them on a daily basis (ADA, 2020). Complications of diabetes that contribute to the increased risk of foot problems and infections include the following:

- *Neuropathy:* Sensory neuropathy leads to loss of pain and pressure sensation, and autonomic neuropathy leads to increased dryness and fissuring of the skin (secondary to decreased sweating). Motor neuropathy results in muscular atrophy, which may lead to changes in the shape of the foot.

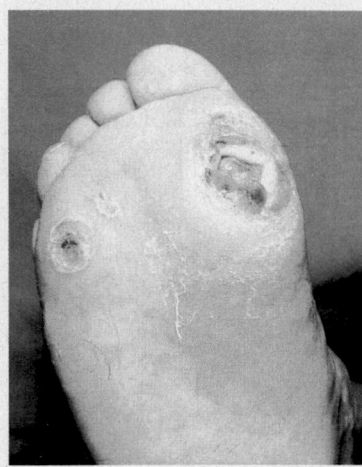

Figure 46-8 • Neuropathic ulceration occurs on pressure points in areas with diminished sensation in diabetic polyneuropathy. Because pain is absent, the ulceration may go unnoticed.

- *Peripheral vascular disease:* Poor circulation of the lower extremities contributes to poor wound healing and the development of gangrene.
- *Immunocompromise:* Hyperglycemia impairs the ability of specialized leukocytes to destroy bacteria. Therefore, in poorly controlled diabetes, there is a lowered resistance to certain infections.

The typical sequence of events in the development of a diabetic foot ulceration begins with a soft tissue injury of the foot, formation of a fissure between the toes or in an area of dry skin, or formation of a callus (see Fig. 46-8). Patients with an insensitive foot do not feel injuries, which may be thermal (e.g., from using heating pads, walking barefoot on hot concrete, testing bathwater with the foot), chemical (e.g., burning the foot while using caustic agents on calluses, corns, or bunions), or traumatic (e.g., injuring skin while cutting nails, walking with an undetected foreign object in the shoe, or wearing ill-fitting shoes and socks).

If the patient is not in the habit of thoroughly inspecting both feet on a daily basis, the injury or fissure may go unnoticed until a serious infection has developed. Drainage, swelling, redness of the leg (from cellulitis), or gangrene may be the first sign of foot problems that the patient notices. Treatment of foot ulcerations involves keeping the patient off their feet, antibiotics, and débridement. In addition, controlling glucose levels, which tend to increase when infections occur, is important for promoting wound healing. When peripheral vascular disease is present, foot ulcerations may not heal because of the decreased ability of oxygen, nutrients, and antibiotics to reach the injured tissue. Amputation (see Chapter 37) may be necessary to prevent the spread of infection, particularly if it involves the bone (osteomyelitis) (see Chapter 36).

Foot assessment and foot care instructions are most important when caring for patients who are at high risk for foot infections (Johnson, Osbourne, Rispoli, et al., 2018). Some of the high-risk characteristics include:

- Duration of diabetes more than 5 years
- Age greater than 40 years
- Current smoker and history of smoking
- Decreased peripheral pulses
- Decreased sensation

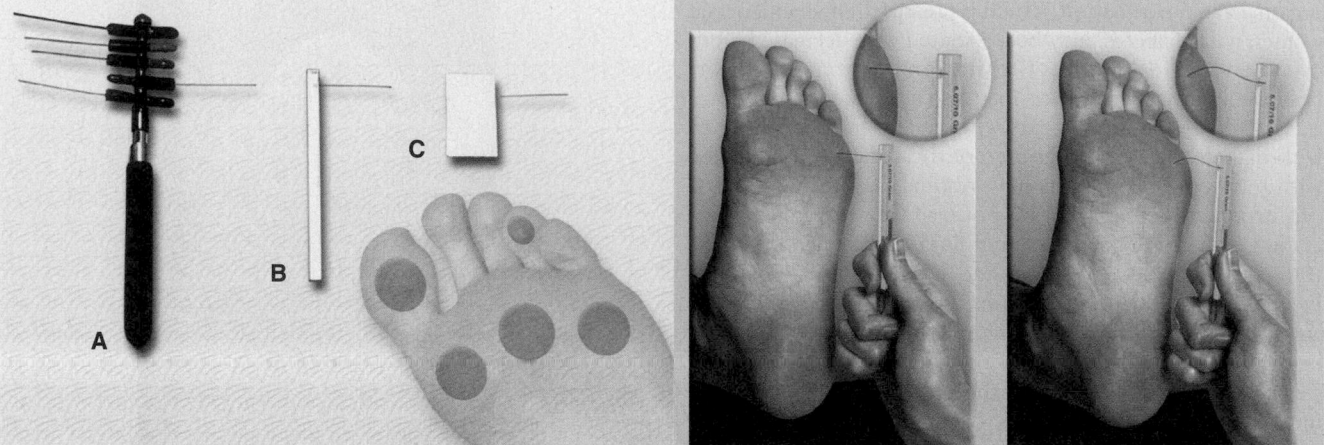

Figure 46-9 • The monofilament test is used to assess the sensory threshold in patients with diabetes. The test instrument—a monofilament—is gently applied to about five pressure points on the foot (as shown in image on *left*). **A.** Example of a monofilament used for advanced quantitative assessment. **B.** Semmes-Weinstein monofilament used by clinicians. **C.** Disposable monofilament used by patients. The examiner applies the monofilament to the test area to determine whether the patient feels the device. Adapted with permission from Cameron, B. L. (2002). Making diabetes management routine. *American Journal of Nursing, 102*(2), 26–32.

- Anatomic deformities or pressure areas (e.g., bunions, calluses, hammer toes)
- History of previous foot ulcerations or amputation

Medical Management

The feet of a patient with diabetes should be examined during every health care visit or at least once per year (more often if there is an increase in risk) by a podiatrist, physician, or nurse (ADA, 2020; Johnson et al., 2018). All patients should be assessed for neuropathy and undergo evaluation of neurologic status by an experienced examiner using a monofilament device (ADA, 2020; Johnson et al., 2018) (see Fig. 46-9). Pressure areas, such as calluses, or thick toenails should be treated by a podiatrist in addition to routine trimming of nails. Blood glucose control is essential for avoiding decreased resistance to infections and for preventing diabetic neuropathy.

Nursing Management

The nurse facilitates or conducts a foot assessment at each visit to a health care provider (Johnson et al., 2018). Educating patients about proper foot care is an essential nursing intervention that can prevent costly and painful complications that result in disability (see Chart 46-11).

SPECIAL ISSUES IN DIABETES CARE

Patients with Diabetes Who Are Undergoing Surgery

During periods of physiologic stress, such as surgery, blood glucose levels tend to increase, because levels of stress hormones (epinephrine, norepinephrine, glucagon, cortisol, and growth hormone) increase. If hyperglycemia is not controlled during surgery, the resulting osmotic diuresis may lead to excessive loss of fluids and electrolytes. Patients with type 1 diabetes also risk developing DKA during periods of stress.

Hypoglycemia is also a concern in patients with diabetes who are undergoing surgery. This is a special concern during the preoperative period if surgery is delayed beyond the morning in a patient who received a morning injection of intermediate-acting insulin.

There are various approaches to managing glucose control during the perioperative period. Frequent blood glucose monitoring is essential throughout the pre- and postoperative periods, regardless of the method used for glucose control. Examples of these approaches are described in Chart 46-12. The use of IV insulin and dextrose has become widespread with the increased availability of intraoperative glucose monitoring.

During the postoperative period, patients with diabetes must also be closely monitored for cardiovascular complications because of the increased prevalence of atherosclerosis, wound infections, and skin breakdown (especially in patients with decreased sensation in the extremities due to neuropathy). Maintaining adequate nutrition and blood glucose control promote wound healing.

Management of Patients with Diabetes Who Are Hospitalized

At any one time, as many as 25% of hospitalized general medical-surgical patients have diabetes (ADA, 2020). Often, diabetes is not the primary medical diagnosis, yet problems with control of diabetes frequently result from changes in the patient's normal routine or from surgery or illness. Patients who are hospitalized and have a diagnosis of diabetes should have this clearly indicated on their electronic health record (EHR), and glucose monitoring needs to be prescribed (ADA, 2020). During the course of treatment, blood glucose control may worsen. Control of blood glucose levels is important because hyperglycemia in patients who are hospitalized can increase the length of hospital stay, the risk of infection, and mortality (ADA, 2020).

In addition, this is an opportunity for patients with diabetes to update their knowledge about diabetes self-care and prevention of complications. Nurses caring for patients with diabetes should focus attention on the diabetes as well as the primary health issue.

Chart 46-11 PATIENT EDUCATION
Foot Care Tips

The nurse instructs the patient to:

Take care of your diabetes.

- Work with your health care team to keep your blood glucose level within a normal range.

Inspect your feet every day.

- Look at your bare feet every day for cuts, blisters, red spots, and swelling.
- Use a mirror to check the bottoms of your feet, or ask a family member for help if you have trouble seeing.
- Check for changes in temperature.

Wash your feet every day.

- Wash your feet in warm, not hot, water.
- Dry your feet well. Be sure to dry between the toes.
- Do not soak your feet.
- Do not check water temperature with your feet; use a thermometer or elbow.

Keep the skin soft and smooth.

- Rub a thin coat of skin lotion over the tops and bottoms of your feet, but not between your toes.

Smooth corns and calluses gently.

- Use a pumice stone to smooth corns and calluses.
- Do not shave calluses.
- See a podiatrist as needed.

Trim your toenails each week or when needed.

- Trim your toenails straight across, and file the edges with an emery board or nail file.

Wear shoes and socks at all times.

- Never walk barefoot.
- Wear comfortable shoes that fit well and protect your feet.
- Feel inside your shoes before putting them on each time to make sure that the lining is smooth and there are no objects inside.
- Be aware that a podiatrist can provide inserts (orthotics) to remove pressure from pressure points on the foot.
- Break in new shoes slowly (i.e., wear for 1 to 2 hours initially, with gradual increases in the length of time worn) to avoid blister formation.
- If you have bony deformities, custom-made shoes with extra width or depth may be needed.

Protect your feet from hot and cold.

- Wear shoes at the beach or on hot pavement.
- Wear socks at night if your feet get cold.

Keep the blood flowing to your feet.

- Put your feet up when sitting.
- Wiggle your toes and move your ankles up and down for 5 minutes, two or three times a day.
- Do not cross your legs for long periods of time.
- Do not smoke.

Check with your primary provider.

- Have your primary provider check your bare feet and find out whether you are likely to have serious foot problems. Remember that you may not feel the pain of an injury.
- Call your primary provider right away if a cut, sore, blister, or bruise on your foot does not begin to heal after 1 day.
- Follow your primary provider's advice about foot care.
- Do not self-medicate or use home remedies or over-the-counter agents to treat foot problems.

Adapted from Johnson, R., Osbourne, A., Rispoli, J., et al. (2018). The diabetic foot assessment. *Orthopaedic Nursing, 37*(1) 13–21.

Chart 46-12 Approaches to Management of Glucose Control During the Perioperative Period for Those with a Diagnosis of Diabetes

- Monitor blood glucose levels frequently (every 1 to 2 hours).
- For patients taking insulin:
  1. The morning of surgery, all subcutaneous insulin doses are withheld, unless the blood glucose level is elevated (e.g., >200 mg/dL [11.1 mmol/L]), in which case a small dose of subcutaneous regular insulin may be prescribed. The blood glucose level is controlled during surgery with the IV infusion of regular insulin, which is balanced by an infusion of dextrose. The insulin and dextrose infusion rates are adjusted according to frequent (hourly) capillary glucose determinations. After surgery, the insulin infusion may be continued until the patient can eat. If IV insulin is discontinued, subcutaneous regular insulin may be given at set intervals (every 4 to 6 hours), or intermediate-acting insulin may be given every 12 hours with supplemental regular insulin as necessary until the patient is eating and the usual pattern of insulin dosing is resumed.
     - Carefully monitor the insulin infusion rate and blood glucose levels in a patient with diabetes who is receiving IV insulin. IV insulin has a much shorter duration of action than subcutaneous insulin. If the infusion is interrupted or discontinued, hyperglycemia will develop rapidly (within 1 hour in type 1 diabetes and within a few hours in type 2 diabetes).
     - Ensure that subcutaneous insulin is given 30 minutes before the IV insulin infusion is discontinued.
  2. One half to two thirds of the patient's usual morning dose of insulin (either intermediate-acting insulin alone or both short- and intermediate-acting insulins) is given subcutaneously in the morning before surgery. The remainder is then given after surgery.
  3. The patient's usual daily dose of subcutaneous insulin is divided into 4 equal doses of regular insulin. These are then given at 6-hour intervals. The last 2 approaches do not provide the control achieved by IV administration of insulin and dextrose.
     - Patients with type 2 diabetes who do not usually take insulin may require insulin during the perioperative period to control blood glucose elevations. Patients who are taking metformin may be instructed to discontinue the oral agent 24 to 48 hours before surgery, if possible. Some of these patients may resume their usual regimen of diet and oral agent during the recovery period. Other patients (whose diabetes is probably not well controlled with diet and an oral antidiabetic agent before surgery) need to continue with insulin injections after discharge.
     - For patients with type 2 diabetes who are undergoing minor surgery but who do not normally take insulin, glucose levels may remain stable provided no dextrose is infused during the surgery. After surgery, these patients may require small doses of regular insulin until the usual diet and oral agent are resumed.

Adapted from Comerford, K. C., & Durkin M. T. (2020). *Nursing 2020 drug handbook*. Philadelphia, PA: Wolters Kluwer.

Self-Care Issues

For patients who are actively involved in diabetes self-management (especially insulin dose adjustment), relinquishing control over meal timing, insulin timing, and insulin dosage can be particularly difficult and anxiety provoking. The patient may fear hypoglycemia and express much concern over possible delays in receiving attention from the nurse if hypoglycemic symptoms occur or may disagree with a planned dose of insulin.

The nurse acknowledges the patient's concerns and involves the patient in the plan of care as much as possible. If the patient disagrees with certain aspects of the care related to diabetes, the nurse must communicate this to other members of the health care team. Nurses and other health care providers must pay particular attention to patients who are successful in managing self-care; they should assess these patients' self-care management skills and encourage them to continue if their performance is correct and effective.

Hospitalization of a patient with diabetes should be considered an opportunity to evaluate the patient's self-care skills and to reinforce or deliver education that might be needed. The nurse observes the patient preparing and injecting the insulin, monitoring blood glucose, and performing foot care. Simply questioning the patient about these skills without actually observing performance of the skills is not sufficient. The patient's knowledge about diet can be assessed with the help of a dietitian through direct questioning and review of the patient's menu choices. The patient's understanding about signs and symptoms, treatment, and prevention of hypoglycemia and hyperglycemia is assessed, along with knowledge of risk factors for macrovascular disease, including hypertension, increased lipids, and smoking. In addition, the patient is asked the date of their last eye examination (including dilation of the pupils). Education about these issues is critical.

Hyperglycemia During Hospitalization

Hyperglycemia may occur in patients who are hospitalized as a result of the original illness that led to the need for hospitalization. A number of other factors may contribute to hyperglycemia; examples include:

- Changes in the usual treatment regimen (e.g., increased food, decreased insulin, decreased activity)
- Medications (e.g., corticosteroids such as prednisone, which are used in the treatment of a variety of inflammatory disorders)
- IV dextrose, which may be part of the maintenance fluids or may be used for the administration of antibiotics and other medications, without adequate insulin therapy
- Overly vigorous treatment of hypoglycemia
- Inappropriate withholding of insulin or inappropriate use of "sliding scales"
- Mismatched timing of meals and insulin (e.g., postmeal hyperglycemia may occur if short-acting insulin is given immediately before or even after a meal)

Nursing actions to correct some of these factors are important for avoiding hyperglycemia. Assessment of the patient's usual home routine is important. The nurse should try to approximate as much as possible the home schedule of insulin, meals, and activities. Monitoring blood glucose levels has been identified by the ADA as an additional "vital sign" essential in assessment of patients (ADA, 2020). The results of blood glucose monitoring provide information needed to obtain orders for extra doses of insulin (at times when insulin is usually taken), which is an important nursing function. Insulin doses must not be withheld when blood glucose levels are normal. It is very important to test blood glucose before a meal and administer insulin at that time, not on a rigid set time schedule as other medications are given. Insulin should be given when the meal is served to prevent hypoglycemia and elicit a physiologic response.

Short-acting insulin is usually needed to avoid postprandial hyperglycemia (even in patients with normal premeal glucose levels), and NPH insulin does not peak until many hours after the dose is given. IV antibiotics should be mixed in NS (if possible) to avoid excess infusion of dextrose (especially in patients who are eating). It is important to avoid overly vigorous treatment of hypoglycemia, which may lead to hyperglycemia.

Hypoglycemia During Hospitalization

Hypoglycemia in patients who are hospitalized is usually the result of too much insulin or delays in eating. Specific examples include:

- Overuse of sliding-scale regular insulin, particularly as a supplement to regularly scheduled, twice-daily short- and intermediate-acting insulins
- Lack of change in insulin dosage when dietary intake is changed (e.g., in the patient taking nothing by mouth [NPO])
- Overly vigorous treatment of hyperglycemia (e.g., giving too-frequent successive doses of regular insulin before the time of peak insulin activity is reached), resulting in a cumulative effect
- Delayed meal after administration of lispro, aspart, or glulisine insulin (patient should eat within 5 to 15 minutes after insulin administration)

Treatment of hypoglycemia should be based on the established hospital protocol (ADA, 2020). If the initial treatment does not increase the glucose level adequately, the same treatment may be repeated after 15 minutes. The nurse must assess the pattern of glucose values and avoid giving doses of insulin that repeatedly lead to hypoglycemia. Successive doses of subcutaneous regular insulin should be given no more frequently than every 3 to 4 hours. For patients receiving intermediate insulin before breakfast and dinner, the nurse must use caution in administering supplemental doses of regular insulin at lunch and bedtime. Hypoglycemia may occur when two insulins peak at similar times (e.g., morning NPH peaks with lunchtime regular insulin and may lead to late-afternoon hypoglycemia; dinnertime NPH peaks with bedtime regular insulin and may lead to nocturnal hypoglycemia). To avoid hypoglycemic reactions caused by delayed food intake, the nurse should arrange for snacks to be given to the patient if meals are going to be delayed because of procedures, physical therapy, or other activities.

Common Alterations in Diet

Dietary modifications commonly prescribed during hospitalization require special consideration for patients who have diabetes (ADA, 2020).

Nothing by Mouth

For patients who must be NPO in preparation for diagnostic or surgical procedures, the nurse must ensure that the usual insulin dosage has been changed. These changes may include eliminating the rapid-acting insulin and giving a decreased amount (e.g., half the usual dose) of intermediate-acting insulin. Another approach is to use frequent (every 3 to 4 hours) dosing of rapid-acting insulin only. IV dextrose may be given to provide calories and to avoid hypoglycemia.

Even without food, glucose levels may increase as a result of hepatic glucose production, especially in patients with type 1 diabetes and lean patients with type 2 diabetes. Furthermore, in type 1 diabetes, elimination of the insulin dose may lead to the development of DKA. Administration of basal insulin to patients with type 1 diabetes who are NPO is an important nursing action.

For patients with type 2 diabetes who are taking insulin, DKA does not usually develop when insulin doses are eliminated because the patient's pancreas produces some insulin. Therefore, skipping the insulin dose altogether (when the patient is receiving IV dextrose) may be safe; however, close monitoring of blood glucose levels is essential.

For patients who are NPO for extended periods (24 hours), glucose testing and insulin administration should be performed at regular intervals, usually four times per day. Insulin regimens for the patient who is NPO for an extended period may include NPH insulin every 12 hours, rapid-acting insulin only every 4 to 6 hours, or an IV insulin drip. These patients should receive dextrose infusions to provide some calories and limit ketosis.

To prevent the problems that result from the need to withhold food, diagnostic tests and procedures and surgery should be scheduled early in the morning when possible.

Clear Liquid Diet

When the diet is advanced to include clear liquids, patients with diabetes receive more simple carbohydrate foods, such as juice and gelatin desserts, than are usually included in the diabetic diet. Because patients who are hospitalized should maintain their nutritional status as much as possible to promote healing, the use of reduced-calorie substitutes such as diet soda or diet gelatin desserts would not be appropriate when the only source of calories is clear liquids. Simple carbohydrates, if eaten alone, cause a rapid rise in blood glucose levels; therefore, it is important to try to match peak times of insulin effect with peaks in the blood glucose concentration. If the patient receives insulin at regular intervals while NPO, the scheduled times for glucose tests and insulin injections should match mealtimes.

Enteral Tube Feedings

Tube feeding formulas contain more simple carbohydrates and less protein and fat than the typical meal plan for diabetes (see Chapter 39). This results in increased levels of glucose in patients with diabetes who are receiving tube feedings. Insulin doses must be given at regular intervals (e.g., NPH every 12 hours or regular insulin every 4 to 6 hours) when continuous tube feedings are given. If insulin is administered at routine (prebreakfast and predinner) times, hypoglycemia during the day may result (because the patient receives more insulin without more calories); hyperglycemia may occur during the night if feedings continue but insulin action decreases.

A common cause of hypoglycemia in patients receiving both continuous tube feedings and insulin is inadvertent or purposeful discontinuation of the feeding. The nurse must discuss with the medical team any plans for temporarily discontinuing the

tube feeding (e.g., when the patient is away from the unit). Planning ahead may allow for alterations to be made in the insulin dose or for administration of IV dextrose. In addition, if problems with the tube feeding develop unexpectedly (e.g., the patient pulls out the tube, the tube clogs, the feeding is discontinued when residual gastric contents are found), the nurse must notify the primary provider, assess blood glucose levels more frequently, and administer IV dextrose if indicated.

Parenteral Nutrition

Patients receiving parenteral nutrition may receive both IV insulin (added to the parenteral nutrition IV bag) and subcutaneous intermediate- or short-acting insulins. If the patient is receiving continuous parenteral nutrition, the blood glucose level should be monitored and insulin given at regular intervals. If the parenteral nutrition is infused over a limited number of hours, subcutaneous insulin should be given so that peak times of insulin action coincide with times of parenteral nutrition infusion (see Chapter 41 for discussion of parenteral nutrition).

Hygiene

Nurses caring for hospitalized patients with diabetes must focus attention on oral hygiene and skin care. Because these patients are at increased risk for periodontal disease, the nurse assists with at least daily dental care. The patient may also require assistance in keeping the skin clean and dry, especially in areas of contact between two skin surfaces (e.g., groin, axilla, under the breasts), where chafing and fungal infections tend to occur.

Careful assessments of the oral cavity and the skin are important. The skin is assessed for dryness, cracks, breakdown, and redness, especially at pressure points and on the lower extremities. The patient is asked about symptoms of neuropathy, such as tingling and pain or numbness of the feet. Deep tendon reflexes are assessed.

As with any patient confined to bed, nursing care must emphasize the prevention of skin breakdown at pressure points. The heels are particularly susceptible to breakdown because of loss of sensation of pain and pressure associated with sensory neuropathy.

Feet should be cleaned, dried, lubricated with lotion (but not between the toes), and inspected frequently. If the patient is in the supine position, pressure on the heels can be alleviated by elevating the lower legs on a pillow, with the heels positioned over the edge of the pillow. When the patient is seated in a chair, the feet should be positioned so that pressure is not placed on the heels. If the patient has an ulceration on one foot, the nurse provides preventive care to the unaffected foot as well as special care of the affected foot.

As always, every opportunity should be taken to educate the patient about diabetes self-management, including daily oral, skin, and foot care. Female patients should also be instructed about measures for the avoidance of vaginal infections, which occur more frequently when blood glucose levels are elevated. Patients often take their cues from nurses and realize the importance of daily personal hygiene if this is emphasized during their hospitalization.

Stress

Physiologic stress, such as infections and surgery, contributes to hyperglycemia and may precipitate DKA or HHS.

Emotional stress related to hospitalization for any reason can also have a negative impact on diabetic control. An increase in stress hormones leads to an increase in glucose levels, especially if intake of food and insulin remains unchanged. In addition, during periods of emotional stress, people with diabetes may alter their usual pattern of meals, exercise, and medication. This can contribute to hyperglycemia or even hypoglycemia (e.g., in the patient taking insulin or oral antidiabetic agents who stops eating in response to stress).

People with diabetes must be made aware of the potential deterioration in diabetic control that can accompany emotional stress. They must be encouraged to follow the diabetes treatment plan as much as possible during times of stress. In addition, learning strategies for minimizing stress and coping with stress when it does occur are important aspects of diabetes education.

 ### Gerontologic Considerations

Because people with diabetes are living longer, both type 1 and type 2 diabetes are being seen more frequently in older patients hospitalized for various reasons. Regardless of the type or duration of diabetes, the goals of diabetes treatment may need to be altered when caring for older adults who are hospitalized. The focus is on quality-of-life issues, such as maintaining independent functioning and promoting general well-being.

Some of the barriers to learning and self-care during hospital stays and in preparing patients for discharge include decreased vision, hearing loss, memory deficits, decreased mobility and fine motor coordination, increased tremors, depression and isolation, decreased financial resources, and limitations related to disability and other medical disorders. Assessing these barriers is important in planning diabetes treatment and educational activities. Presenting brief, simplified instructions with ample opportunity for practice of skills is important. The use of special devices such as a magnifier for the insulin syringe, an insulin pen, or a mirror for foot inspection is helpful. Frequent evaluation of self-care skills (insulin administration, blood glucose monitoring, foot care, diet planning) is essential, especially in patients with deteriorating vision and memory. Providing written instructions with handouts to take home also assists with management in the home setting.

If appropriate, family members may be called on to assist with diabetes basic skills, and referral to community resources may be made. It is preferable to educate the patient or family members to test blood glucose at home; the choice of meter should be tailored to the patient's visual and cognitive status and dexterity.

> **Quality and Safety Nursing Alert**
>
> *Careful monitoring for complications of diabetes in older adults is vital. Hypoglycemia is especially dangerous, because it may go undetected and result in falls. Dehydration is a concern in patients who have chronically elevated blood glucose levels. Assessment for long-term complications, especially eye and foot problems, is important. Avoiding blindness and amputation through early detection and treatment of retinopathy and foot ulcerations may mean the difference between placement in a long-term care facility and continued independent living for the older adult with diabetes.*

Nursing Management

Monitoring and Managing Potential Complications

Assessment for hypo- and hyperglycemia involves frequent blood glucose monitoring (usually prescribed before meals and at bedtime) and monitoring for signs and symptoms of hypoglycemia or prolonged hyperglycemia (including DKA or HHS), as described previously. Inadequate control of blood glucose levels may hinder recovery from the primary health problem. Blood glucose levels are monitored, and insulin is given as prescribed. The nurse must ensure that prescribed insulin dosage is modified as needed to compensate for changes in the patient's schedule or eating pattern. Treatment is given for hypoglycemia (with oral glucose) or hyperglycemia (with supplemental regular insulin no more often than every 3 to 4 hours). Blood glucose records are assessed for patterns of hypo- and hyperglycemia at the same time of day, and findings are reported to the primary provider for modification in insulin orders. In the patient with prolonged elevations in blood glucose, laboratory values and the patient's physical condition are monitored for signs and symptoms of DKA or HHS.

Promoting Home, Community-Based, and Transitional Care

 #### Educating Patients About Self-Care

Even if patients have had diabetes for many years, their knowledge and adherence to the plan of care must be assessed. A new plan of care may need to be devised using updated evidence. The nurse also reminds the patient and family about the importance of health promotion activities and recommended health screening.

Continuing and Transitional Care

A patient who is hospitalized may require referral for home, community-based or transitional care. The nurse can use this opportunity to assess the patient's knowledge about diabetes management and the patient's and family's ability to carry out that management. The nurse reinforces the education provided in the hospital, clinic, office, or diabetes education center and assesses the home care environment to determine its adequacy for self-care and safety.

CRITICAL THINKING EXERCISES

1 **ipc** An 18-year-old woman is newly diagnosed with type 1 diabetes in the clinic where you work. How will you educate this patient about this new diagnosis? Which referrals are appropriate to help this patient manage her type 1 diabetes? What steps will the interdisciplinary team take to address the patient's health care needs?

2 **ebp** A 45-year-old patient has had type 2 diabetes for 6 years. During his annual examination at the clinic where you work, a small ulceration is identified on the bottom of his foot. What is the evidence for management of a foot ulceration in this patient? What criteria would you use to assess the strength of the evidence? What is the evidence for the timing of future foot assessments?

3 [pq] A 65-year-old patient is admitted to the emergency department with possible HHS. Identify the pathophysiology and signs and symptoms of HHS. What are your priorities for the assessment, medical management, and nursing care for this patient with HHS? What are your priorities for discharge planning to prevent another episode?

REFERENCES

*Asterisk indicates nursing research.
**Double asterisk indicates classic reference.

Books

Centers for Disease Control and Prevention (CDC). (2020). *National Diabetes Statistics Report, 2020*. Atlanta, GA: Centers for Disease Control and Prevention, US Department of Health and Human Services.

Comerford, K. C., & Durkin, M. T. (2020). *Nursing 2020 drug handbook*. Philadelphia, PA: Wolters Kluwer.

Eliopoulos, C. (2018). *Gerontological nursing* (9th ed.). Philadelphia, PA: Wolters Kluwer.

Fischbach, F., & Fischbach, M. A. (2018). *A manual of laboratory and diagnostic tests* (10th ed.). Philadelphia, PA: Wolters Kluwer.

Hickey, J. V., & Strayer, A. L. (2020). *The clinical practice of neurological and neurosurgical nursing* (8th ed.). Philadelphia, PA: Wolters Kluwer.

Norris, T. L. (2019). *Porth's pathophysiology: Concepts of altered health state* (10th ed.). Philadelphia, PA: Wolters Kluwer.

Journals and Electronic Documents

Action to Control Cardiovascular Risk in Diabetes Follow-On (ACCORDION) Eye Study Group and the Action to Control Cardiovascular Risk in Diabetes Follow-On (ACCORDION) Study Group. (2016). Persistent effects of intensive glycemic control on retinopathy in type 2 diabetes in the action to Control Cardiovascular Risk in Diabetes (ACCORD) follow-on study. *Diabetes Care, 39*(7), 1089–1100.

American Diabetes Association (ADA). (2020). Standards of medical care in diabetes—2020. *Diabetes Care, 43*(Suppl 1), S1–S212.

Aref, A., Zayan, T., Pararajasingam, R., et al. (2019). Pancreatic transplantation: Brief review of the current evidence. *World Journal of Transplantation, 9*(4), 81–93.

Chen, Y., Yang, D., Chen, B., et al. (2020). Clinical characteristics and outcomes of patients with diabetes and COVID-19 in association with glucose-lowering medication. *Diabetes Care, 43*(7), 1399–1407. doi: 10.2337/dc20-0660

Davidson, P., Ross, T., & Castor, C. (2018). Academy of nutrition and dietetics: Revised 2017 standards of practice and standards of professional performance for registered dietitian nutritionists (competent, proficient, and expert) in diabetes care. *Journal of the Academy of Nutrition and Dietetics, 118*(5), 932–946.e48.

**Diabetes Control and Complications Trial Research Group (DCCT), Nathan, D. M., Genuth, S., et al. (1993). The effect of intensive treatment of diabetes on the development and progression of long-term complications in insulin-dependent diabetes mellitus. *New England Journal of Medicine, 329*(14), 977–986.

**Diabetes Prevention Program Research Group. (2002). Reduction in the incidence of type 2 diabetes with lifestyle intervention or metformin. *New England Journal of Medicine, 346*(6), 393–403.

Diabetes Prevention Program Research Group. (2015). Long-term effects of lifestyle intervention or metformin on diabetes development and microvascular complications over 15-year follow-up: The Diabetes Prevention Program Outcomes Study. *Lancet, Diabetes and Endocrinology, 3*(11), 866–875.

Down, S. (2018). How to advise on sick day rules. *Diabetes and Primary Care, 20*(1), 15–16.

Evert, A. B., Dennison, M., Gardner, C. D., et al. (2019). Nutrition therapy for adults with diabetes or prediabetes: A consensus report. *Diabetes Care, 42*(5), 731–754.

Fayfman, M., Pasquel, F. J., & Umpeirrez, G. E. (2017). Management of hyperglycemic crises: Diabetic ketoacidosis and hyperglycemic hyperosmolar state. *Medical Clinics of North America, 101*(3), 587–606.

Franz, M. J., MacLeod, J., Evert, A., et al. (2017). Academy of Nutrition and Dietetics Nutrition Practice Guideline for Type 1 and Type 2 diabetes in adults: Systematic review of evidence for medical nutrition therapy effectiveness and recommendations for integration into the nutrition care process. *Journal of the Academy of Nutrition and Dietetics, 117*(10), 1659–1679.

Hur, K., Price, C. P. E., Gray, E. L., et al. (2020). Factors associated with intubation and prolonged intubation in hospitalized patients with COVID-19. *Otolaryncology-Head and Neck Surgery,* 1–9. doi: 10.1177/0194599820929640

Johnson, R., Osbourne, A., Rispoli, J., et al. (2018). The diabetic foot assessment. *Orthopaedic Nursing, 37*(1) 13–21.

Joyner Blair, A. M., Hamilton, B. K., & Spurlock, A. (2018). Evaluating an order set for improvement of quality outcomes in diabetic ketoacidosis. *Advanced Emergency Nursing Journal, 40*(1), 59–72.

Keresztes, P., & Peacock-Johnson, A. (2019). Type 2 diabetes: A pharmacological update. *American Journal of Nursing, 119*(2), 32–40.

Kropff, J., Choudhary, P., Neupane, S., et al. (2017). Accuracy and longevity of an implantable continuous glucose sensor in the PRECISE Study: A 180-day, prospective, multicenter, pivotal trial. *Diabetes Care, 40*(1), 63–68.

Ma, H., Li, Z., Zhou, T., et al. (2020). Glucosamine use, inflammation, and genetic susceptibility, and incidence of type 2 diabetes: A prospective study in UK biobank. *Diabetes Care, 43*(4), 719–725.

*McCarthy, M. M., Whittemore, R., Gholson, G., et al. (2019). Diabetes distress, depressive symptoms, and cardiovascular health in adults with type 1 diabetes. *Nursing Research, 68*(6), 445–452.

National Institute of Diabetes and Digestive and Kidney Diseases (NIDDK). (2018). Diabetic neuropathies: The nerve damage of diabetes. Retrieved on 1/2/2020 at: www.niddk.nih.gov/health-information/diabetes/overview/preventing-problems/nerve-damage-diabetic-neuropathies?dkrd=hispt0026

Sommerstein, R., Kochen, M. M., Messerli, F. H., et al. (2020). Coronavirus disease 2019 (COVID-19): Do angiotensin-converting enzyme inhibitors/angiotensin receptor blockers have a biphasic effect? *Journal of the American Heart Association, 9*(7), e016509. doi: 10.1161/JAHA.120.016509.

**United Kingdom Prospective Diabetes Study Group. (1998). Intensive blood glucose control with sulfonylureas or insulin compared with conventional treatment and risk of complications with type 2 diabetes. *Lancet, 352*(9131), 837–853.

Virani, S. S., Alonso, A., Benjamin, E. J., et al. (2020). Heart disease and stroke statistics—2020 update: A report from the American Heart Association. *Circulation, 141*(9), e139–e596.

World Health Organization (WHO). (2018). Diabetes. Retrieved on 1/2/2020 at: www.who.int/news-room/fact-sheets/detail/diabetes

Resources

Academy of Nutrition and Dietetics (formerly the American Dietetic Association), www.eatright.org
American Association of Diabetes Educators (AADE), www.diabeteseducator.org
American Diabetes Association, www.diabetes.org
American Foundation for the Blind (AFB), www.afb.org
Go4Life, www.healthinaging.org/tools-and-tips/go4life-national-institute-aging
JDRF (formerly the Juvenile Diabetes Research Foundation), www.jdrf.org
MedicAlert Foundation, www.medicalert.org
National Diabetes Information Clearinghouse, www.niddk.nih.gov
National Library Services for the Blind and Physically Handicapped (NLS), www.loc.gov/nls/

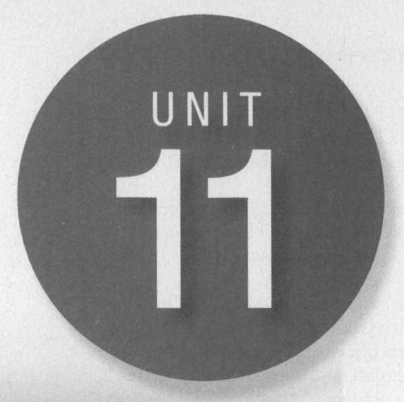

UNIT 11

Kidney and Urinary Tract Function

Case Study AVOIDING FALLS FOR THE PATIENT AT RISK

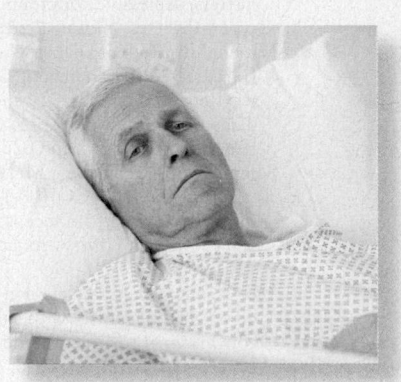

Y ou are a nurse working in an intermediate medical unit caring for a 78-year-old man who was admitted from the emergency department (ED) with a change in level of consciousness and falling at home. His diagnostic and laboratory findings show that he has a lower urinary tract infection (UTI). Your initial assessment reveals the patient is still not oriented to person, place, or time. In addition, he is trying to get up to the bathroom due to urinary urgency caused by the UTI. Because of his change in level of consciousness and urgency, you determine that safety is a priority. You implement falls precautions.

QSEN Competency Focus: Safety

The complexities inherent in today's health care system challenge nurses to demonstrate integration of specific interdisciplinary core competencies. These competencies are aimed at ensuring the delivery of safe, quality patient care (Institute of Medicine, 2003). The Quality and Safety Education for Nurses project (Cronenwett, Sherwood, Barnsteiner, et al., 2007; QSEN, 2020) provides a framework for the knowledge, skills, and attitudes (KSAs) required for nurses to demonstrate competency in these key areas, which include **patient-centered care**, **interdisciplinary teamwork and collaboration**, **evidence-based practice**, **quality improvement**, **safety**, and **informatics.**

Safety Definition: Minimizes risk of harm to patients and providers through both system effectiveness and individual performance.

SELECT PRE-LICENSURE KSAs	APPLICATION AND REFLECTION
Knowledge	
Examine human factors and other basic safety design principles as well as commonly used unsafe practices (such as, work-arounds and dangerous abbreviations)	Describe how you will prioritize care for this patient. How does safety impact priority decisions for this patient? Based on the assessment findings, why was the patient placed on falls precautions?
Skills	
Demonstrate effective use of technology and standardized practices that support safety and quality	Identify the technology and standardized practices you will use to implement falls precautions for this patient. How will you determine when the falls precautions can be discontinued?
Attitudes	
Value vigilance and monitoring (even of own performance of care activities) by patients, families, and other members of the health care team	Reflect on what you learned from this case study. The nurse's role in patient safety is essential. How can the nurse educate the patient and family to value safety in the home environment to prevent falls? Which additional health care team members could be consulted to assist the patient and family in a home assessment for safety?

Cronenwett, L., Sherwood, G., Barnsteiner, J., et al. (2007). Quality and safety education for nurses. *Nursing Outlook, 55*(3), 122–131; Institute of Medicine. (2003). *Health professions education: A bridge to quality.* Washington, DC: National Academies Press; QSEN Institute. (2020). *QSEN competencies: Definitions and pre-licensure KSAs; Safety.* Retrieved on 8/15/2020 at: qsen.org/competencies/pre-licensure-ksas/#safety

LEARNING OUTCOMES

On completion of this chapter, the learner will be able to:

1. Describe the structure and function of the renal and urinary systems.
2. Explain the role of the kidneys in regulating fluid and electrolyte balance, acid–base balance, and blood pressure.
3. Identify the diagnostic studies used to determine upper and lower urinary tract function and related nursing implications.
4. Discriminate between normal and abnormal assessment findings of upper and lower urinary tract function.
5. Initiate education and preparation for patients undergoing assessment of the urinary system.

NURSING CONCEPTS

Acid–Base Balance
Acid–Base Balance Assessment
Comfort

Elimination
Fluids and Electrolytes
Infection

Patient Education

GLOSSARY

aldosterone: hormone synthesized and released by the adrenal cortex; causes the kidneys to reabsorb sodium

antidiuretic hormone (ADH): hormone secreted by the posterior pituitary gland; causes the kidneys to reabsorb more water (*synonym:* vasopressin)

anuria: decreased urine output of less than 50 mL in 24 hours

bacteriuria: bacteria in the urine

creatinine: endogenous waste product of muscle energy metabolism

diuresis: increased urine volume

dysuria: painful or difficult urination

erythropoietin: glycoprotein produced by kidney; stimulates bone marrow to produce red blood cells

glomerular filtration rate (GFR): amount of plasma filtered through the glomeruli per unit of time

glomerulus: tuft of capillaries forming part of the nephron through which filtration occurs

glycosuria: excretion of glucose in the urine

hematuria: red blood cells in the urine

micturition: urination or voiding

nephrons: structural and functional units of the kidney responsible for urine formation

nocturia: awakening at night to urinate

oliguria: urine output less than 400 mL in 24 hours or less than 0.5 mL/kg/h over 6 hours

proteinuria: protein in the urine

pyuria: white blood cells in the urine

renal clearance: ability of the kidneys to clear solutes from the plasma

specific gravity: expression of the degree of concentration of the urine

urea nitrogen: end product of protein metabolism (*synonym:* blood urea nitrogen [BUN])

urinary frequency: voiding more frequently than every 3 hours

Function of the renal and urinary systems is essential to life. The primary purpose of the renal and urinary systems is to maintain the body's state of homeostasis by carefully regulating fluid and electrolytes, removing wastes, and providing other functions (see Chart 47-1). Dysfunction of the kidneys and lower urinary tract is common and may occur at any age and with varying degrees of severity. Assessment of upper and lower urinary tract function is part of every health examination and requires the nurse to understand the anatomy and physiology of the urinary system as well as the effects of changes in the system on other physiologic functions.

<table>
<tr><td colspan="2">

Chart 47-1 Functions of the Kidney

</td></tr>
</table>

Control of blood pressure
Control of water balance
Excretion of waste products
Regulation of electrolytes
Regulation of acid–base balance
Regulation of red blood cell production
Renal clearance
Secretion of prostaglandins
Synthesis of vitamin D to active form
Urine formation

Adapted from Norris, T. L. (2019). *Porth's pathophysiology: Concepts of altered health states* (10th ed.). Philadelphia, PA: Wolters Kluwer.

Anatomic and Physiologic Overview

A focused assessment of kidney and urinary tract function requires an understanding of the anatomy and physiology of these systems.

Anatomy of the Kidney and Urinary Systems

The kidney and urinary systems include the kidneys, ureters, bladder, and urethra. Urine is formed by the kidney and flows through the other structures to be eliminated from the body.

Kidneys

The kidneys are a pair of bean-shaped, brownish-red structures located retroperitoneally (behind and outside the peritoneal cavity) on the posterior wall of the abdomen—from the 12th thoracic vertebra to the 3rd lumbar vertebra in the adult (see Fig. 47-1A). The rounded outer convex surface of each kidney is called the hilum. Each hilum is penetrated with blood vessels, nerves, and the ureter. The average adult kidney weighs approximately 113 to 170 g (about 4.5 oz) and is 10 to 12 cm long, 6 cm wide, and 2.5 cm thick (Norris, 2019; Russell, 2017). The right kidney is slightly lower than the left due to the location of the liver.

Externally, the kidneys are well protected by the ribs and by the muscles of the abdomen and back. Internally, fat deposits surround each kidney, providing protection against jarring. The kidneys and surrounding fat are suspended from the abdominal wall by renal fascia made of connective tissue which holds the kidney in place (Norris, 2019). The fibrous connective tissue, blood vessels, and lymphatics surrounding each kidney are known as the renal capsule. An adrenal gland lies on top of each kidney. The kidneys and adrenals are independent in function, blood supply, and innervation.

The renal parenchyma is divided into two parts: the cortex and the medulla (see Fig. 47-1B). The medulla, which is approximately 5 cm wide, is the inner portion of the kidney. It contains the loops of Henle, the vasa recta, and the collecting ducts of the juxtamedullary nephrons. The collecting ducts from both the juxtamedullary and the cortical nephrons connect to the renal pyramids, which are triangular and are situated with the base facing the concave surface of the kidney and the point (papilla) facing the hilum, or pelvis. Each kidney contains approximately 8 to 18 pyramids. The pyramids drain into minor calyces, which drain into major calyces that open directly into the renal pelvis. The tip of each pyramid is called a papilla and projects into the minor calyx. The renal pelvis is the beginning of the collecting system and is composed of structures that are designed to collect and transport urine. Once the urine leaves the renal pelvis, the composition or amount of urine does not change.

The cortex, which is approximately 1 cm wide, is located farthest from the center of the kidney and around the outermost edges (Norris, 2019). It contains the **nephrons** (the structural and functional units of the kidney responsible for urine formation), which are discussed later.

Blood Supply to the Kidneys

The hilum is the concave portion of the kidney through which the renal artery enters and the ureters and renal vein exit. The kidneys receive 20% to 25% of the total cardiac output, which means that all of the body's blood circulates through the kidneys approximately 12 times per hour (Norris, 2019). The renal artery (arising from the abdominal aorta) divides into smaller and smaller vessels, eventually forming the afferent arterioles. Each afferent arteriole branches to form a **glomerulus**, which is the tuft of capillaries forming

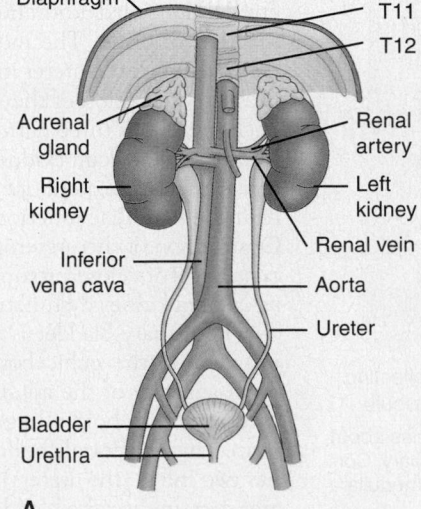

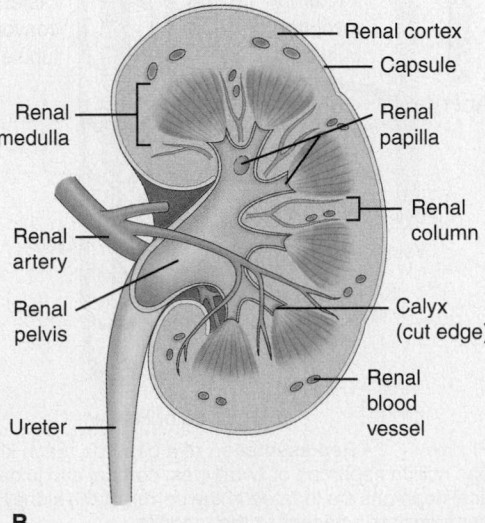

Figure 47-1 • A. Kidneys, ureters, and bladder. **B.** Internal structure of the kidney. Redrawn with permission from Porth, C. M., & Matfin, G. (2009). *Pathophysiology: Concepts of altered health states* (8th ed.). Philadelphia, PA: Lippincott Williams & Wilkins.

A

Diaphragm — T11 — T12
Adrenal gland
Right kidney
Renal artery
Left kidney
Renal vein
Inferior vena cava
Aorta
Ureter
Bladder
Urethra

B

Renal cortex
Capsule
Renal medulla
Renal papilla
Renal artery
Renal column
Renal pelvis
Calyx (cut edge)
Ureter
Renal blood vessel

part of the nephron through which filtration occurs. Blood leaves the glomerulus through the efferent arteriole and flows back to the inferior vena cava through a network of capillaries and veins.

Nephrons

Each kidney has one million nephrons that are located within the renal parenchyma and are responsible for the formation of filtrate that will become urine (Norris, 2019). The large number of nephrons allows for adequate renal function even if the opposite kidney is damaged or becomes nonfunctional. If the total number of functioning nephrons is less than 20% of normal, kidney replacement therapy needs to be considered.

There are two types of nephrons. The cortical nephrons (80% to 85%) are located in the outermost part of the cortex, and the juxtamedullary nephrons (15% to 20%) are located deeper in the cortex (Norris, 2019). The juxtamedullary nephrons are distinguished by long loops of Henle and are surrounded by long capillary loops called vasa recta that dip into the medulla of the kidney. The length of the tubular component of the nephron is directly related to its ability to concentrate urine.

Nephrons are made up of two basic components: a filtering element composed of an enclosed capillary network (the glomerulus) and the attached tubule (see Fig. 47-2). The glomerulus is a unique network of capillaries suspended between the afferent and efferent blood vessels, which are

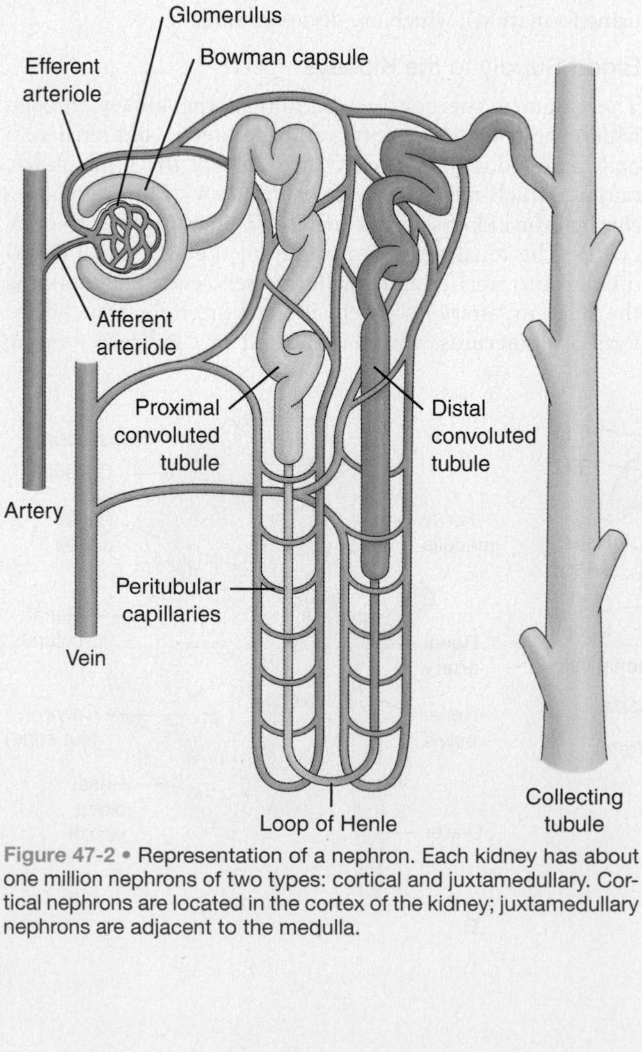

enclosed in an epithelial structure called the Bowman capsule. The glomerular membrane is composed of three filtering layers: the capillary endothelium, the basement membrane, and the epithelium. This membrane normally allows filtration of fluid and small molecules yet limits passage of larger molecules, such as blood cells and albumin. Pressure changes and the permeability of the glomerular membrane of the Bowman capsule facilitate the passage of fluids and various substances from the blood vessels, filling the space within the Bowman capsule with this filtered solution.

The tubular component of the nephron begins in the Bowman capsule. The filtrate created in the Bowman capsule travels first into the proximal tubule, which is made up of epithelial cells resting on the basement membrane, then the loop of Henle, the distal tubule, and either the cortical or medullary collecting ducts. The structural arrangement of the tubule allows the distal tubule to lie in close proximity to where the afferent and efferent arterioles, respectively, enter and leave the glomerulus. The distal tubular cells located in this area, known as the macula densa, function with the adjacent afferent arteriole and create what is known as the juxtaglomerular apparatus. This is the site of renin production. Renin is a hormone directly involved in the control of arterial blood pressure; it is essential for proper functioning of the glomerulus (see later discussion).

The tubular component consists of the Bowman capsule, the proximal tubule, the descending and ascending limbs of the loop of Henle, and the cortical and medullary collecting ducts. This portion of the nephron is responsible for making adjustments in the filtrate based on the body's needs. Changes are continually made as the filtrate travels through the tubules until it enters the collecting system and is expelled from the body (see Fig. 47-2).

Ureters, Bladder, and Urethra

The urine formed in the nephrons flows through the renal calyces and then into the ureters, which are long fibromuscular tubes that connect each kidney to the bladder (Verlander & Clapp, 2019). These narrow tubes, each 24 to 30 cm long, originate at the lower portion of the renal pelvis and terminate in the trigone (tissue between the opening of the ureters and urethra) of the bladder wall.

The lining of the ureters is made up of transitional cell epithelium called urothelium. The urothelium prevents reabsorption of urine. The movement of urine from each renal pelvis through the ureter into the bladder is facilitated by peristaltic contraction of the smooth muscles in the ureter wall. Each ureter has three narrow areas that are prone to obstruction by renal calculi (kidney stones) or stricture. These three areas include the ureteropelvic junction, the ureteral segment near the sacroiliac junction, and the ureterovesical junction. Obstruction of the ureteropelvic junction is the most serious because of its close proximity to the kidney and the risk of associated kidney dysfunction.

The urinary bladder is a distensible muscular sac located just behind the pubic bone (Weber & Kelley, 2018). The usual capacity of the adult bladder is 400 to 500 mL, but it can distend to hold a larger volume. The bladder is characterized by its central, hollow area, called the vesicle, which has two inlets (the ureters) and one outlet (the urethra). The area surrounding the bladder neck is called the ureterovesical

Figure 47-2 • Representation of a nephron. Each kidney has about one million nephrons of two types: cortical and juxtamedullary. Cortical nephrons are located in the cortex of the kidney; juxtamedullary nephrons are adjacent to the medulla.

junction. The angling of the ureterovesical junction is the primary means of providing antegrade, or downward, movement of urine, also referred to as efflux of urine. This angling prevents vesicoureteral reflux (retrograde, or backward, movement of urine) from the bladder, up the ureter, toward the kidney.

The wall of the bladder contains four layers. The outermost layer is the adventitia, which is made up of connective tissue. Immediately beneath the adventitia is a smooth muscle layer known as the detrusor. Beneath the detrusor is a submucosal layer of loose connective tissue that serves as an interface between the detrusor and the innermost layer, a mucosal lining. The inner layer contains specialized transitional cell epithelium, a membrane that is impermeable to water and prevents reabsorption of urine stored in the bladder. The bladder neck contains bundles of involuntary smooth muscle that form a portion of the urethral sphincter known as the internal sphincter. An important portion of the sphincter mechanism that helps maintain continence is the external urinary sphincter at the anterior urethra, which is the segment most distal from the bladder (Norris, 2019). During **micturition** (voiding or urination), increased intravesical pressure keeps the ureterovesical junction closed and urine within the ureters. As soon as micturition is completed, intravesical pressure returns to its normal low baseline value, allowing efflux of urine to resume. Therefore, the only time that the bladder is completely empty is in the last seconds of micturition, before efflux of urine resumes.

The urethra arises from the base of the bladder: In the male, it passes through the penis; in the female, it opens just anterior to the vagina. In the male, the prostate gland, which lies just below the bladder neck, surrounds the urethra posteriorly and laterally.

Physiology of the Kidney and Urinary Systems

Understanding the physiology of the kidney and urinary systems includes comprehending urine formation, antidiuretic hormone, osmolarity and osmolality; the regulation of water excretion, electrolyte excretion, and acid–base balance; autoregulation of blood pressure, renal clearance, regulation of red blood cell (RBC) production, vitamin D synthesis, secretion of prostaglandins and other substances, excretion of waste products, urine storage as well as bladder emptying.

Urine Formation

The healthy human body is composed of approximately 60% water. Water balance is regulated by the kidneys and results in the formation of urine. Urine is formed in the nephrons through a complex three-step process: glomerular filtration, tubular reabsorption, and tubular secretion (see Fig. 47-3). Each nephron functions independently from other nephrons because each has its own blood supply (Norris, 2019). The various substances normally filtered by the glomerulus, reabsorbed by the tubules, and excreted in the urine include sodium, chloride, bicarbonate, potassium, glucose, urea, creatinine, and uric acid. Within the tubule, some of these substances are selectively reabsorbed into the blood. Others are secreted from the blood into the filtrate as it travels down the tubule.

Physiology/Pathophysiology

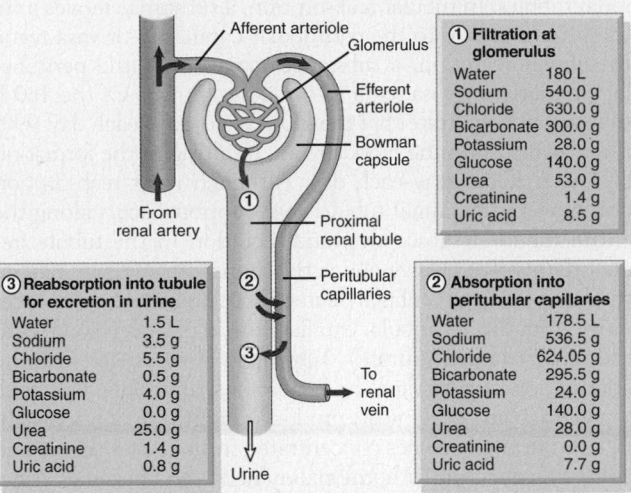

Figure 47-3 • Urine is formed in the nephrons in a three-step process: filtration, reabsorption, and secretion. Water, electrolytes, and other substances, such as glucose and creatinine, are filtered by the glomerulus; varying amounts of these substances are reabsorbed in the renal tubule or excreted in the urine. Approximate normal volumes of these substances during the steps of urine formation are shown at the top. Wide variations may occur in these values depending on diet.

Amino acids and glucose are usually filtered at the level of the glomerulus and reabsorbed so that neither is excreted in the urine. Normally, glucose does not appear in the urine. However, **glycosuria** (excretion of glucose in the urine) occurs if the amount of glucose in the blood and glomerular filtrate exceeds the amount that the tubules are able to reabsorb. Renal glycosuria can occur on its own as a benign condition. It also occurs in poorly controlled diabetes—the most common condition that causes the blood glucose level to exceed the kidney's reabsorption capacity.

Protein molecules also are not usually found in the urine; however, low-molecular-weight proteins (globulins and albumin) may periodically be excreted in small amounts. Protein in the urine is referred to as **proteinuria** (Fischbach & Fischbach, 2018).

Glomerular Filtration

The normal blood flow through the kidneys is between 1000 and 1300 mL/min (Norris, 2019). As blood flows into the glomerulus from an afferent arteriole, filtration occurs. The filtered fluid, also known as filtrate or ultrafiltrate, then enters the renal tubules. Under normal conditions, about 20% of the blood passing through the glomeruli is filtered into the nephron, amounting to about 180 L/day of filtrate (Norris, 2019). The filtrate normally consists of water, electrolytes, and other small molecules, because water and small molecules are allowed to pass, whereas larger molecules stay in the bloodstream. As blood enters the glomerulus from the afferent arteriole, filtration depends on adequate blood flow that maintains a consistent pressure through the glomerulus called hydrostatic pressure. Many factors can alter this blood flow and pressure, including hypotension, decreased oncotic pressure in the blood, and increased pressure in the renal tubules from an obstruction (Norris, 2019).

Tubular Reabsorption and Tubular Secretion

The second and third steps of urine formation occur in the renal tubules. In tubular reabsorption, a substance moves from the filtrate back into the peritubular capillaries or vasa recta. In tubular secretion, a substance moves from the peritubular capillaries or vasa recta into tubular filtrate. Of the 180 L (45 gallons) of filtrate that the kidneys produce each day, 99% is reabsorbed into the bloodstream, resulting in the formation of 1 to 2 L of urine each day. Although most reabsorption occurs in the proximal tubule, reabsorption occurs along the entire tubule. Reabsorption and secretion in the tubule frequently involve passive and active transport and may require the use of energy. Tubular secretion occurs when substances move from the peritubular capillary blood plasma (blood) into the tubular lumen (filtrate). Tubular secretion helps with the elimination of potassium, hydrogen ions, ammonia, uric acid, some drugs, and other waste products (Fischbach & Fischbach, 2018). Filtrate becomes concentrated in the distal tubule and collecting ducts under hormonal influence and becomes urine, which then enters the renal pelvis. In the absence of tubular reabsorption, volume depletion would rapidly occur.

Antidiuretic Hormone

Antidiuretic hormone (ADH), also known as vasopressin, is a hormone that is secreted by the posterior portion of the pituitary gland in response to changes in osmolality of the blood. With decreased water intake, blood osmolality tends to increase, stimulating ADH release. ADH then acts on the kidney, increasing reabsorption of water and thereby returning the osmolality of the blood to normal. With excess water intake, the secretion of ADH by the pituitary is suppressed; therefore, less water is reabsorbed by the kidney tubule, leading to **diuresis** (increased urine volume).

A dilute urine with a fixed **specific gravity** (about 1.010) or fixed osmolality (about 300 mOsm/L) indicates an inability to concentrate and dilute the urine, which is a common early sign of kidney disease (Fischbach & Fischbach, 2018).

Osmolarity and Osmolality

Osmolarity refers to the ratio of solute to water. The regulation of salt and water is paramount for control of the extracellular volume and both serum and urine osmolarity. Controlling either the amount of water or the amount of solute can change osmolarity. Osmolarity and ionic composition are maintained by the body within very narrow limits. As little as a 1% to 2% change in the serum osmolarity can cause a conscious desire to drink and conservation of water by the kidneys (Emmett & Palmer, 2018).

The degree of dilution or concentration of the urine is also measured in terms of osmolality (the number of osmoles [the standard unit of osmotic pressure] dissolved per kilogram of solution). The filtrate in the glomerular capillary normally has the same osmolality as the blood—280 to 300 mOsm/kg. Serum and urine osmolality and osmolarity are discussed in more detail in Chapter 10.

Regulation of Water Excretion

Regulation of the amount of water excreted is an important function of the kidney. With high fluid intake, a large volume of dilute urine is excreted. Conversely, with a low fluid intake, a small volume of concentrated urine is excreted. A person normally ingests about 1300 mL of oral liquids and 1000 mL of water in food per day. Of the fluid ingested, approximately 800 mL is lost through the skin and lungs and 200 mL through feces (called insensible loss). It is important to consider all fluid gained and lost when evaluating total fluid status. Daily weight measurements are a reliable means of determining overall fluid status. One pound (1 lb) equals approximately 500 mL, so a weight change of as little as 1 lb could suggest an overall fluid gain or loss of 500 mL (Norris, 2019).

Regulation of Electrolyte Excretion

When the kidneys are functioning normally, the volume of electrolytes excreted per day is equal to the amount ingested. For example, the average American daily diet contains 6 to 15 g each of sodium chloride (salt) and 8 g potassium chloride, and approximately the same amounts are excreted in the urine.

The regulation of sodium volume excreted depends on **aldosterone,** a hormone synthesized and released by the adrenal cortex. With increased aldosterone in the blood, less sodium is excreted in the urine, because aldosterone fosters renal reabsorption of sodium. Release of aldosterone from the adrenal cortex is largely under the control of angiotensin II. Angiotensin II levels are in turn controlled by renin, an enzyme that is released from specialized cells in the kidneys (see Fig. 47-4). This complex system is activated when pressure in the renal arterioles falls below normal levels, as occurs with shock, dehydration, or decreased sodium chloride delivery to the tubules. Activation of this system increases the retention of water and expansion of the intravascular fluid volume, thereby maintaining enough pressure within the glomerulus to ensure adequate filtration.

The regulation of serum sodium and potassium is discussed in detail in Chapter 10.

Physiology/Pathophysiology

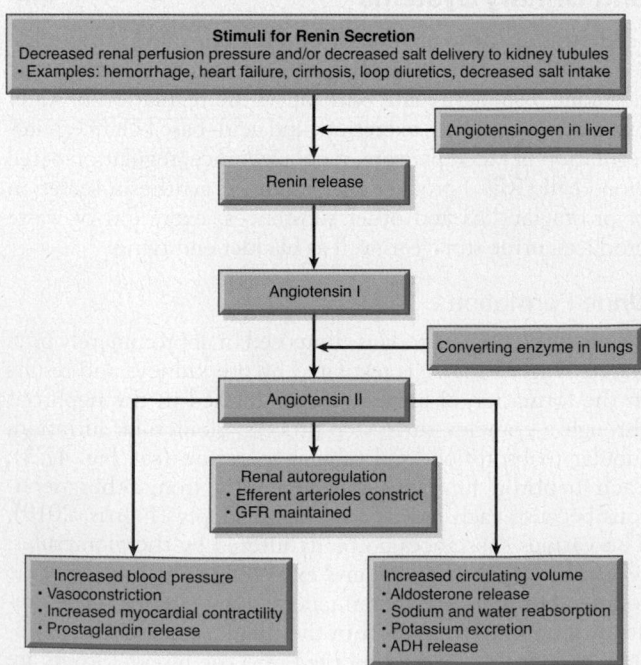

Figure 47-4 • The renin–angiotensin system. ADH, antidiuretic hormone; GFR, glomerular filtration rate.

Regulation of Acid–Base Balance

The normal serum pH is about 7.35 to 7.45 and must be maintained within this narrow range for optimal physiologic function (Norris, 2019). The kidney performs major functions to assist in this balance. One function is to reabsorb and return to the body's circulation any bicarbonate from the urinary filtrate; other functions are to excrete or reabsorb acid, synthesize ammonia, and excrete ammonium chloride (Fischbach & Fischbach, 2018). Because bicarbonate is a small ion, it is freely filtered at the glomerulus. The renal tubules actively reabsorb most of the bicarbonate in the urinary filtrate. To replace any lost bicarbonate, the renal tubular cells generate new bicarbonate through a variety of chemical reactions. This newly generated bicarbonate is then reabsorbed by the tubules and returned to the body.

The body's acid production is the result of catabolism, or breakdown, of proteins, which produces acid compounds, particularly phosphoric and sulfuric acids. The normal daily diet also includes a certain amount of acid materials. Unlike carbon dioxide (CO_2), phosphoric and sulfuric acids cannot be eliminated by the lungs. Because accumulation of these acids in the blood lowers pH (making the blood more acidic) and inhibits cell function, they must be excreted in the urine. However, if the hydrogen ions are low, they will be reabsorbed. A person with normal kidney function excretes about 70 mEq of acid each day. The kidney is able to excrete some of this acid directly into the urine until the urine pH reaches 4.5, which is 1000 times more acidic than blood (Norris, 2019).

However, more acid usually needs to be eliminated from the body than can be secreted directly as free acid in the urine. These excess acids are bound to chemical buffers so that they can be excreted in the urine. Two important chemical buffers are phosphate ions and ammonia (NH_3). When buffered with acid, ammonia becomes ammonium (NH_4). Phosphate is present in the glomerular filtrate, and ammonia is produced by the cells of the renal tubules and secreted into the tubular fluid. Through the buffering process, the kidney is able to excrete large quantities of acid in a bound form without further lowering the pH of the urine.

Autoregulation of Blood Pressure

Regulation of blood pressure is an important function of the kidney. Specialized vessels of the kidney, called the vasa recta, constantly monitor blood pressure as blood begins its passage into the kidney. When the vasa recta detect a decrease in blood pressure, specialized juxtaglomerular cells near the afferent arteriole, distal tubule, and efferent arteriole secrete the hormone renin. Renin converts angiotensinogen to angiotensin I, which is then converted to angiotensin II—the most powerful vasoconstrictor known; angiotensin II causes the blood pressure to increase (Norris, 2019). The adrenal cortex secretes aldosterone in response to stimulation by the pituitary gland, which occurs in response to poor perfusion or increasing serum osmolality. The result is an increase in blood pressure. When the vasa recta recognize the increase in blood pressure, renin secretion stops. Failure of this feedback mechanism is one of the primary causes of hypertension (see Fig. 47-4).

Renal Clearance

Renal clearance refers to the ability of the kidneys to clear solutes from the plasma. A 24-hour collection of urine is the primary test of renal clearance used to evaluate how well the kidney performs this important excretory function. Renal clearance depends on several factors: how quickly the substance is filtered across the glomerulus, how much of the substance is reabsorbed along the tubules, and how much of the substance is secreted into the tubules. It is possible to measure the renal clearance of any substance, but the one measure that is particularly useful is the creatinine clearance.

Creatinine is an endogenous waste product of skeletal muscle that is filtered at the glomerulus, passed through the tubules with minimal change, and excreted in the urine. Hence, creatinine clearance is a good measure of the **glomerular filtration rate (GFR),** the amount of plasma filtered through the glomeruli per unit of time. To calculate creatinine clearance, a 24-hour urine specimen is collected. Midway through the collection, the serum creatinine level is measured. The following formula is then used to calculate the creatinine clearance:

$$\frac{(\text{Volume of urine [mL/min]} \times \text{Urine creatinine [mL/dL]})}{\text{Serum creatinine (mg/dL)}}$$

The adult glomerular filtration rate (GFR) can vary from a normal of approximately 125 mL/min (1.67 to 2 mL/s) to a high of 200 mL/min (Norris, 2019). Creatinine clearance is the best approximation of renal function. As renal function declines, both creatinine clearance and renal clearance (the ability to excrete solutes) decrease.

Regulation of Red Blood Cell Production

When the kidneys detect a decrease in the oxygen tension in renal blood flow, because of anemia, arterial hypoxia, or inadequate blood flow, they release erythropoietin. **Erythropoietin** is a glycoprotein from the kidney that stimulates the bone marrow to produce RBCs, which carry oxygen throughout the body (Norris, 2019).

Vitamin D Synthesis

The kidneys are also responsible for the final conversion of inactive vitamin D to its active form, 1,25-dihydroxycholecalciferol. Vitamin D is necessary for maintaining normal calcium balance in the body.

Secretion of Prostaglandins and Other Substances

The kidneys also produce prostaglandin E and prostacyclin, thromboxanes, and leukotrienes, which have vasoactive effects. These substances help the afferent and efferent arterioles maintain renal blood flow by causing selective vasodilation or vasoconstriction (Norris, 2019).

Excretion of Waste Products

The kidneys eliminate the body's metabolic waste products. The major waste product of protein metabolism is urea, of which about 25 to 30 g are produced and excreted daily (Norris, 2019). All of this urea must be excreted in the urine; otherwise, it accumulates in body tissues. Other waste products of metabolism that must be excreted are creatinine, phosphates, and sulfates. Uric acid, formed as a waste product of purine metabolism, is also eliminated in the urine. The kidneys serve as the primary mechanism for excreting drug metabolites.

Urine Storage

The bladder is the reservoir for urine. Both filling and emptying of the bladder are mediated by coordinated sympathetic and parasympathetic nervous system control mechanisms involving the detrusor muscle and the bladder outlet. Conscious awareness of bladder filling occurs as a result of sympathetic neuronal pathways that travel via the spinal cord to the level of T10 through T12, where peripheral, hypogastric nerve innervation allows for continued bladder filling. As bladder filling continues, stretch receptors in the bladder wall are activated, coupled with the desire to void. This information from the detrusor muscle is relayed back to the cerebral cortex via the parasympathetic pelvic nerves at the levels of S1 through S4 (Norris, 2019). Overall bladder pressure remains low due to the bladder's compliance (ability to expand or collapse) as urine volume changes.

Bladder compliance is due in part to the smooth muscle lining of the bladder and collagen deposits within the wall of the bladder, as well as to neuronal mechanisms that inhibit the detrusor muscle from contracting (specifically, adrenergic receptors that mediate relaxation). To maintain adequate kidney filtration rates, bladder pressure during filling must remain lower than 40 cm water (H_2O). This low pressure allows the urine to freely leave the renal pelvis and enter the ureters. The sensation of bladder fullness is transmitted to the central nervous system when the bladder has reached about 150 to 200 mL in adults, and an initial desire to void occurs (Weber & Kelley, 2018). A marked sense of fullness and discomfort with a strong desire to void usually occurs when the bladder reaches its functional capacity of 400 to 500 mL of urine. Neurologic changes to the bladder at the level of the supraspinal nerves, the spinal nerves, or the bladder wall itself can cause abnormally high volumes (up to 2000 mL) of urine to be stored due to a decreased or absent urge to void.

Under normal circumstances with average fluid intake of approximately 1 to 2 L/day, the bladder should be able to store urine for periods of 2 to 4 hours at a time during the day (Norris, 2019). At night, the release of vasopressin in response to decreased fluid intake causes a decrease in the production of urine and makes it more concentrated. This phenomenon usually allows the bladder to continue filling for periods of 6 to 8 hours in adolescents and adults, making them able to sleep for longer periods before needing to void. In older adults, decreasing bladder compliance and decreased vasopressin levels often cause **nocturia** (awakening during the night to urinate).

Bladder Emptying

Micturition normally occurs approximately eight times in a 24-hour period. It is activated via the micturition reflex arc within the sympathetic and parasympathetic nervous systems, which causes a coordinated sequence of events. Initiation of voiding occurs when the efferent pelvic nerve, which originates in the S1 to S4 area, stimulates the bladder to contract, resulting in complete relaxation of the striated urethral sphincter. This is followed by a decrease in urethral pressure, contraction of the detrusor muscle, opening of the vesical neck and proximal urethra, and flow of urine. This coordinated effort by the parasympathetic system is mediated by muscarinic and, to a lesser extent, cholinergic receptors within the detrusor muscle. The pressure generated

in the bladder during micturition is about 20 to 40 cm H_2O in females. It is somewhat higher and more variable in males 45 years and older due to the normal hyperplasia of the cells of the middle lobes of the prostate gland, which surround the proximal urethra. Any obstruction of the bladder outlet, such as in advanced benign prostatic hyperplasia (BPH), results in a high voiding pressure. High voiding pressures make it more difficult to start urine flow and maintain it.

If the spinal pathways from the brain to the urinary system are destroyed (e.g., after a spinal cord injury), reflex contraction of the bladder is maintained, but voluntary control over the process is lost. In both situations, the detrusor muscle can contract and expel urine, but the contractions are generally insufficient to empty the bladder completely, so residual urine (urine left in the bladder after voiding) remains. Normally, residual urine amounts to no more than 50 mL in the middle-age adult and less than 50 to 100 mL in the older adult (Weber & Kelley, 2018).

 ### Gerontologic Considerations

Upper and lower urinary tract function changes with age. The GFR decreases, starting between 35 and 40 years of age, and a yearly decline of about 1 mL/min continues thereafter. Older adults are more susceptible to acute kidney injury and chronic kidney disease due to the structural and functional changes in the kidney. Examples include sclerosis of the glomerulus and renal vasculature, decreased blood flow, decreased GFR, altered tubular function, and acid–base imbalance. Although renal function usually remains adequate, renal reserve is decreased and may reduce the kidneys' ability to respond effectively to drastic or sudden physiologic changes. This steady decrease in glomerular filtration, combined with the use of multiple medications in which metabolites are cleared by the kidneys, puts the older person at higher risk for adverse drug effects and drug–drug interactions (Eliopoulos, 2018).

Older adults are more prone to develop hypernatremia and fluid volume deficit, because increasing age is also associated with diminished osmotic stimulation of thirst. Thirst is defined as one's awareness of the desire to drink. The sense of thirst is so protective that hypernatremia almost never occurs in adults younger than 60 years.

Structural or functional abnormalities that occur with aging may also prevent complete emptying of the bladder. This may be due to decreased bladder wall contractility; secondary to myogenic or neurogenic factors; or related to bladder outlet obstruction, such as in BPH or after prostatectomy. Vaginal and urethral tissues atrophy (become thinner) in aging women due to decreased estrogen levels. This causes decreased blood supply to the urogenital tissues, resulting in urethral and vaginal irritation and urinary incontinence.

Urinary incontinence is present in 15% to 30% of community-dwelling older adults, 50% of older adults who are institutionalized, and 30% of older adults who are hospitalized (Eliopoulos, 2018). Many older adults and their families are unaware that urinary incontinence stems from many causes. The nurse needs to inform the patient and family that with appropriate evaluation, urinary incontinence can often be managed at home, and in many cases it can be eliminated. Many treatments are available for urinary incontinence in older adults, including noninvasive, behavioral interventions that the patient or caregiver can carry out. Treatment modalities for urinary incontinence are described in further detail in Chapter 49.

Preparation of the older adult patient for diagnostic tests must be managed carefully to prevent dehydration, which might precipitate kidney disease in a patient with marginal renal function. Limitations in mobility may affect an older patient's ability to void adequately or to consume an adequate volume of fluids. The patient may limit fluid intake to minimize the frequency of voiding or the risk of incontinence.

 Concept Mastery Alert

Providing education about the dangers of an inadequate fluid intake is an important role of the nurse caring for the older patient. The nurse emphasizes the need to drink throughout the day even if the patient does not feel thirsty, because the thirst stimulation is decreased.

Older adults often have incomplete emptying of the bladder and urinary stasis, which may result in urinary tract infection (UTI) or increasing bladder pressure, leading to overflow incontinence, hydronephrosis, pyelonephritis, or chronic kidney disease (Eliopoulos, 2018). Urologic symptoms can mimic disorders such as appendicitis, peptic ulcer disease, and cholecystitis, which can make diagnosis difficult in older adults due to decreased neurologic innervation (Eliopoulos, 2018).

Assessment of the Kidney and Urinary Systems

An assessment of the kidney and urinary systems involves conducting a health history and physical assessment.

Health History

Obtaining a urologic health history requires excellent communication skills, because many patients are embarrassed or uncomfortable discussing genitourinary function or symptoms (Ball, Dains, Flynn, et al., 2019; Weber & Kelley, 2018). It is important to use language the patient can understand and to avoid medical jargon. It is also important to review risk factors, particularly for those patients who are at high risk. For example, the nurse needs to be aware that multiparous women delivering their children vaginally have a high risk for stress urinary incontinence, which, if severe enough, can also lead to urge incontinence. People with neurologic disorders such as diabetic neuropathy, multiple sclerosis, or Parkinson's disease often have incomplete emptying of the bladder and urinary stasis, which may result in UTI or increasing bladder pressure, leading to overflow incontinence, hydronephrosis, pyelonephritis, or chronic kidney disease (Eliopoulos, 2018). Risk factors for specific disorders and kidney and lower urinary tract dysfunction are summarized in Table 47-1 and discussed in Chapters 48 and 49.

TABLE 47-1 ⚠ Risk Factors for Select Kidney or Urologic Disorders

Risk Factor	Possible Kidney or Urologic Disorder
Advanced age	Incomplete emptying of bladder, leading to urinary tract infection and urosepsis
Benign prostatic hyperplasia	Obstruction to urine flow, leading to frequency, oliguria, anuria
Diabetes	Chronic kidney disease, neurogenic bladder
Gout, hyperparathyroidism, Crohn's disease, ileostomy	Kidney stone formation
Hypertension	Renal insufficiency, chronic kidney disease
Instrumentation of urinary tract, cystoscopy, catheterization	Urinary tract infection, incontinence
Immobilization	Kidney stone formation
Multiple sclerosis	Incontinence, neurogenic bladder, and other complications
Occupational, recreational, or environmental exposure to chemicals (plastics, pitch, tar, rubber)	Acute kidney injury
Obstetric injury, tumors	Incontinence
Parkinson's disease	Incontinence and other complications
Pregnancy	Proteinuria, urinary frequency
Radiation therapy to pelvis	Cystitis, fibrosis of ureter, or fistula in urinary tract
Recent pelvic surgery	Inadvertent trauma to ureters or bladder
Sickle cell disease, multiple myeloma	Chronic kidney disease
Spinal cord injury	Neurogenic bladder, urinary tract infection, incontinence
Strep throat, impetigo, nephrotic syndrome	Chronic kidney disease
Systemic lupus erythematosus	Nephritis, chronic kidney disease

Adapted from Norris, T. L. (2019). *Porth's pathophysiology: Concepts of altered health states* (10th ed.). Philadelphia, PA: Wolters Kluwer.

TABLE 47-2 Identifying Characteristics of Genitourinary Pain

Type	Location	Characteristics	Associated Signs and Symptoms	Possible Etiology
Kidney	Costovertebral angle; may extend to umbilicus	Dull constant ache; if sudden distention of capsule, pain is severe, sharp, stabbing, and colicky in nature	Nausea and vomiting, diaphoresis, pallor, signs of shock	Acute obstruction, kidney stone, blood clot, acute pyelonephritis, trauma
Bladder	Suprapubic area	Dull, continuous pain that may be intense with voiding; may be severe if bladder full	Urgency, pain at end of voiding, painful straining	Overdistended bladder, infection, interstitial cystitis; tumor
Ureteral	Costovertebral angle, flank, lower abdominal area, testis, or labium	Severe, sharp, stabbing pain, colicky in nature	Nausea and vomiting, paralytic ileus	Ureteral stone, edema or stricture, blood clot
Prostatic	Perineum and rectum	Vague discomfort, feeling of fullness in perineum, vague back pain	Suprapubic tenderness, obstruction to urine flow; frequency, urgency, dysuria, nocturia	Prostatic cancer, acute or chronic prostatitis
Urethral	*Male:* Along penis to meatus *Female:* Urethra to meatus	Pain variable, most severe during and immediately after voiding	Frequency, urgency, dysuria, nocturia, urethral discharge	Irritation of bladder neck, infection of urethra, trauma, foreign body in lower urinary tract

Adapted from Norris, T. L. (2019). *Porth's pathophysiology: Concepts of altered health states* (10th ed.). Philadelphia, PA: Wolters Kluwer; Weber, J. R., & Kelley, J. H. (2018). *Health assessment in nursing* (6th ed.). Philadelphia, PA: Wolters Kluwer.

When obtaining the health history, the nurse should inquire about the following:

- The patient's chief concern or reason for seeking health care, the onset of the problem, and its effect on the patient's quality of life
- The location, character, and duration of **dysuria** (painful or difficult urination), if present, and its relationship to voiding; factors that precipitate dysuria, and those that relieve it
- History of UTIs, including past treatment or hospitalization for UTI
- Fever or chills
- Previous renal or urinary diagnostic tests, surgeries or procedures; or the use of indwelling urinary catheters
- Hesitancy, straining to urinate, or frequency of urination
- Urinary incontinence (stress incontinence, urge incontinence, overflow incontinence, or functional incontinence)
- **Hematuria** (RBCs in the urine) or change in color or volume of urine
- Nocturia and its date of onset
- Renal calculi (kidney stones), passage of stones or gravel in urine
- In female patients, the number and type (vaginal or cesarean) of deliveries; the use of forceps; vaginal infection, discharge, or irritation; contraceptive practices
- History of **anuria** (decreased urine production of less than 50 mL in 24 hours) or other kidney problem
- Presence or history of genital lesions or sexually transmitted infections
- The use of tobacco, alcohol, or recreational drugs
- Any prescription and over-the-counter medications (including those prescribed for renal or urinary problems)

Common Symptoms

Dysfunction of the kidney can produce a complex array of symptoms throughout the body. Pain, changes in voiding, and gastrointestinal symptoms are particularly suggestive of urinary tract disease.

Pain

Genitourinary pain is usually caused by distention of some portion of the urinary tract as a result of obstructed urine flow or inflammation and swelling of tissues. Severity of pain is related to the sudden onset, rather than the extent of distention.

Table 47-2 lists the various types of genitourinary pain, characteristics of the pain, associated signs and symptoms, and possible causes. However, kidney disease does not always involve pain. It tends to be diagnosed because of other symptoms that cause a patient to seek health care, such as pedal edema, shortness of breath, and changes in urine elimination (Weber & Kelley, 2018).

Changes in Voiding

Micturition is normally a painless function that occurs approximately eight times in a 24-hour period. The average person voids 1 to 2 L of urine in 24 hours, although this amount varies depending on fluid intake, sweating, environmental temperature, vomiting, or diarrhea. Common problems associated with voiding include **urinary frequency** (voiding more frequently than every 3 hours), urgency, dysuria, hesitancy, incontinence, enuresis, polyuria, **oliguria** (urine output less than 400 mL in 24 hours or less than 0.5 mL/kg/h over 6 hours), and hematuria. These problems and others are described in Table 47-3. Increased urinary urgency and frequency, coupled with decreasing urine volumes strongly suggest urine retention. Depending on the acuity of the onset of these symptoms, immediate bladder emptying via catheterization and evaluation may be necessary to prevent kidney dysfunction.

Gastrointestinal Symptoms

Gastrointestinal signs and symptoms are often associated with urologic conditions because of shared autonomic and sensory

TABLE 47-3	Problems Associated with Changes in Voiding	
Problem	**Definition**	**Possible Etiology**
Anuria	Urine output <50 mL/day	Acute kidney injury or chronic kidney disease (see Chapter 48), complete obstruction
Bacteriuria	Bacterial count >100,000 colonies/mL in the urine	Infection
Dysuria	Painful or difficult voiding	Lower urinary tract infection, inflammation of bladder or urethra, acute prostatitis, stones, foreign bodies, tumors in bladder
Enuresis	Involuntary voiding during sleep	Delay in functional maturation of central nervous system (bladder control usually achieved by 5 yrs of age), obstructive disease of lower urinary tract, genetic factors, failure to concentrate urine, urinary tract infection, psychological stress
Frequency	Frequent voiding—more than every 3 h	Infection, obstruction of lower urinary tract leading to residual urine and overflow, anxiety, diuretic agents, benign prostatic hyperplasia, urethral stricture, diabetic neuropathy
Hematuria	Red blood cells in the urine	Cancer of genitourinary tract, acute glomerulonephritis, renal stones, renal tuberculosis, blood dyscrasia, trauma, extreme exercise, rheumatic fever, hemophilia, leukemia, sickle cell trait or disease
Hesitancy	Delay, difficulty in initiating voiding	Benign prostatic hyperplasia, compression of urethra, outlet obstruction, neurogenic bladder
Incontinence	Involuntary loss of urine	External urinary sphincter injury, obstetric injury, lesions of bladder neck, detrusor dysfunction, infection, neurogenic bladder, medications, neurologic abnormalities
Nocturia	Awakening during the night to urinate	Decreased renal concentrating ability, heart failure, diabetes, incomplete bladder emptying, excessive fluid intake at bedtime, nephrotic syndrome, cirrhosis with ascites
Oliguria	Urine output <400 mL in 24 h or <0.5 mL/kg/h over 6 h	Acute kidney injury or chronic kidney disease, inadequate fluid intake
Polyuria	Increased volume of urine voided	Diabetes, diabetes insipidus, the use of diuretics, excess fluid intake, lithium toxicity, some forms of kidney disease (hypercalcemic and hypokalemic nephropathy)
Proteinuria	Protein in the urine	Acute kidney injury or chronic kidney disease, nephrotic syndrome, vigorous exercise, heatstroke, severe heart failure, diabetic nephropathy, multiple myeloma
Urgency	Strong desire to void	Infection, chronic prostatitis, urethritis, obstruction of lower urinary tract leading to residual urine and overflow, anxiety, diuretic agents, benign prostatic hyperplasia, urethral stricture, diabetic neuropathy

innervation and renointestinal reflexes (see Table 47-3). The proximity of the right kidney to the colon, duodenum, head of the pancreas, common bile duct, liver, and gallbladder may cause gastrointestinal disturbances. The proximity of the left kidney to the colon (splenic flexure), stomach, pancreas, and spleen may also result in intestinal symptoms. The most common signs and symptoms are nausea, vomiting, diarrhea, abdominal discomfort, and abdominal distention.

Unexplained Anemia

Gradual kidney dysfunction can be insidious in its presentation, although fatigue is a common symptom. Fatigue, shortness of breath, and exercise intolerance all result from the condition known as anemia of inflammation formerly known as anemia of chronic disease. See Chapter 29 for more information on anemia of inflammation.

Past Health, Family, and Social History

Data collection about previous health problems or diseases provides the health care team with useful information for evaluating the patient's current urinary status. People with diabetes who have hypertension are at risk for renal dysfunction. Older men are at risk for prostatic enlargement, which causes urethral obstruction and can result in UTIs and kidney disease. People with a family history of urinary tract problems are at increased risk for renal disorders. Genetics may also influence renal conditions (see Chart 47-2).

It is also important to assess the patient's psychosocial status, level of anxiety, perceived threats to body image, available support systems, and sociocultural patterns.

Physical Assessment

Several body systems can affect upper and lower urinary tract dysfunction, and conversely that dysfunction can affect several end organs; therefore, a head-to-toe assessment is indicated. Areas of emphasis include the abdomen, suprapubic region, genitalia, lower back, and lower extremities.

The kidneys are not usually palpable. However, palpation of the kidneys may detect an enlargement that could prove to be very important (Weber & Kelley, 2018). The correct technique for palpation is illustrated in Figure 47-5. It may be possible to palpate the smooth, rounded lower pole of the kidney between the hands. The right kidney is easier to detect, because it is somewhat lower than the left one. In patients with obesity, palpation of the kidneys is more difficult.

Chart 47-2 · GENETICS IN NURSING PRACTICE
Kidney and Urinary Disorders

Various conditions that affect the renal system and urinary tract function are influenced by genetic factors. Some examples of these genetic disorders are:

Autosomal Dominant:

- Familial Wilms tumor
- Polycystic kidney disease
- Renal cystic disease in tuberous sclerosis complex

X-Linked Recessive:

- Alport syndrome (primarily X-linked but autosomal dominant and recessive forms exist)

Congenital Kidney Disorders:

- Congenital absence of the vas deferens (caused by *CFTR* gene mutation for cystic fibrosis)
- Horseshoe kidney
- Multicystic dysplastic kidneys

Other Genetic Disorders that Impact the Renal System:

- Alpha$_1$-antitrypsin deficiency
- Anderson–Fabry disease
- Diabetes
- Coronary artery disease
- Pulmonary hypertension
- von Hippel–Lindau syndrome

Nursing Assessments

Refer to Chapter 4, Chart 4-2: Genetics in Nursing Practice: Genetic Aspects of Health Assessment

Family History Specific to Kidney and Urinary Disorders

- Inquire about other family members with a history of renal and/or urinary tract malformations, kidney disease, or end-stage kidney disease and age of onset.

- Determine if other family members have diabetic kidney disease (clustering of this within the family could indicate genetic susceptibility).
- Identify family history of male infertility and cystic fibrosis (congenital absence of vas deferens).
- Be alert to family members with history of early-onset renal (Wilms tumor) or other cancers.

Physical Assessment Specific to Genetic Kidney and Urinary Disorders

- Be alert to signs and symptoms of kidney disease at an early age.
- Ascertain for presence and frequency of kidney stones or urinary tract infections.
- Assess for the presence and frequency of:
  - Abdominal pain or presence of an abdominal mass
  - Hematuria
  - Hypertension
  - Peripheral or orbital edema
  - Proteinuria
- Assess for clinical findings suggesting that kidney disease is a component of a genetic syndrome (e.g., seizures, intellectual disability, skin involvement).
- Assess for bleeding tendencies, abnormal clotting, or history of anemia.

Genetics Resources

Alport Syndrome Foundation, www.alportsyndrome.org
American Kidney Fund, www.kidneyfund.org
See Chapter 6, Chart 6-7 for components of genetic counseling resources.

Renal dysfunction may produce tenderness over the costovertebral angle, which is the angle formed by the lower border of the 12th, or bottom, rib and the spine (see Fig. 47-6). The abdomen (just slightly to the right and left of the midline in both upper quadrants) is auscultated to assess for bruits (low-pitched murmurs that indicate renal artery stenosis or an aortic aneurysm). The abdomen is also assessed for the presence of ascites (accumulation of fluid in the peritoneal

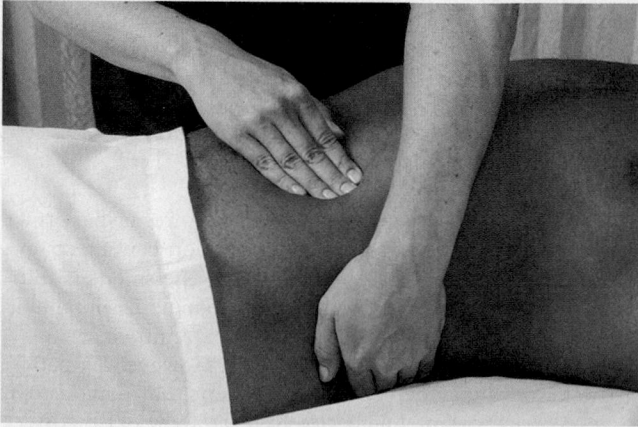

Figure 47-5 • The left kidney is palpated by reaching over to the patient's left side and placing the right hand beneath the patient's lower left rib. Push the hand on top forward as the patient inhales deeply. Reprinted with permission from Weber, J. R., & Kelley, J. H. (2018). *Health assessment in nursing* (6th ed., Fig. 23-27). Philadelphia, PA: Wolters Kluwer.

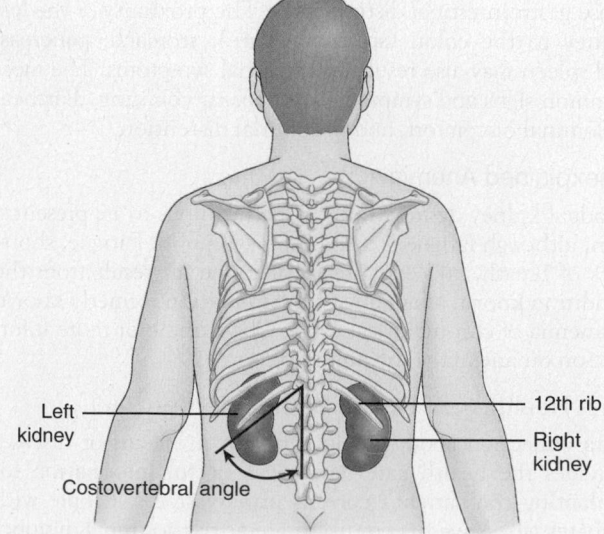

Left kidney — 12th rib — Right kidney — Costovertebral angle

Figure 47-6 • Location of the costovertebral angle.

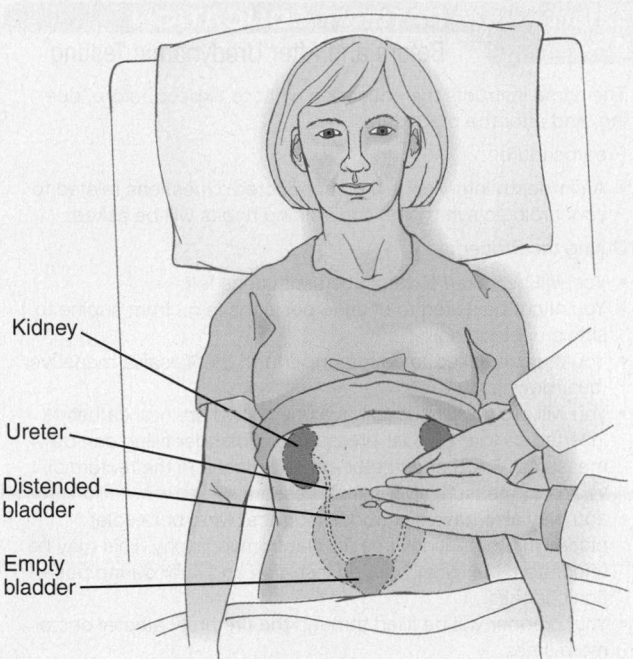

Kidney

Ureter

Distended bladder

Empty bladder

Figure 47-7 • Palpating distended bladder (larger *dotted line* is area of distention). Reprinted with permission from Weber, J. R., & Kelley, J. H. (2018). *Health assessment in nursing* (6th ed., Fig. 23-28). Philadelphia, PA: Wolters Kluwer.

cavity), which may occur with kidney as well as liver dysfunction (see Chapter 43 for further discussion of ascites and liver disorders).

To check for residual urine, the bladder can be percussed after the patient voids. Percussion of the bladder begins at the midline just above the umbilicus and proceeds downward. The sound changes from tympanic to dull when percussing over the bladder. The bladder, which can be palpated only if it is moderately distended, feels like a smooth, firm, round mass rising out of the abdomen, usually at midline (see Fig. 47-7). Dullness to percussion of the bladder after

voiding indicates incomplete bladder emptying (Weber & Kelley, 2018).

Portable bladder ultrasound is another method of detecting urinary retention. These devices provide a three-dimensional image of the bladder and should be used after voiding to detect urine retention. Researchers have reported that the use of a portable bladder ultrasound reduces the rate of UTIs and shortens the length of stay for patients who have had an ischemic stroke (Chen, Chen, Chen, et al., 2018). See the Nursing Research Profile in Chart 47-3 and the later discussion in the bladder ultrasonography section.

In older men, BPH or prostatitis can cause difficulty with urination. Because the signs and symptoms of prostate cancer can mimic those of BPH, the prostate gland is palpated by digital rectal examination (DRE) as part of the yearly physical examination in men 40 years and older (see Chapter 53). In addition, a blood specimen is obtained to test the prostate-specific antigen (PSA) level annually; the results of the DRE and PSA are then correlated. Blood is drawn for PSA before the DRE, because manipulation of the prostate can cause the PSA level to increase temporarily. The inguinal area is examined for enlarged nodes, an inguinal or femoral hernia, and varicocele (varicose veins of the spermatic cord).

In women, the vulva, urethral meatus, and vagina are examined (Weber & Kelley, 2018). The urethra is palpated for diverticula, and the vagina is assessed for adequate estrogen effect and any of five types of herniation: urethrocele, cystocele, pelvic prolapse, enterocele, and rectocele. Urethrocele is the bulging of the anterior vaginal wall into the urethra. Cystocele is the herniation of the bladder wall into the vaginal vault. Pelvic prolapse is bulging of the cervix into the vaginal vault. Enterocele is herniation of the bowel into the posterior vaginal wall. Rectocele is herniation of the rectum into the vaginal wall. These prolapses are graded depending on the degree of herniation. See Chapter 51 for more information.

The woman is asked to cough and perform a Valsalva maneuver to assess the urethra's system of muscular and ligament support. If urine leakage occurs, the index and

---

Chart 47-3

NURSING RESEARCH PROFILE

Positive Outcomes with the Use of a Portable Bladder Ultrasound

Chen, S., Chen, P., Chen, G., et al. (2018). Portable bladder ultrasound reduces incidence of urinary tract infection and shortens hospital length of stay in patients with acute ischemic stroke. *Journal of Cardiovascular Nursing, 31*(6), 551–558.

Purpose

Certain patient populations, such as those who have had a stroke, have high rates of urinary tract infections (UTIs). The purpose of this study was to investigate whether there was a change in patient outcomes, such as UTI rates, following implementation of the use of portable bladder ultrasound to measure postvoid urine residuals on a unit that provided care for patients following an acute ischemic stroke.

Design

The medical records of all patients admitted to one unit for a 3-year period prior to the implementation of the use of portable bladder ultrasound were retrospectively reviewed and outcomes

compared to all patients admitted for a 3-year period after the implementation of the use of portable bladder ultrasound.

Findings

Those patients admitted during the period after the implementation of the portable bladder ultrasound had a lower incidence of UTI (4% vs. 6.9%) and a shorter hospital length of stay (11.9 days vs. 13.6 days). Multivariate analysis revealed that patients at higher risk of UTI were patients 75 years of age or older, women, and those with a more severe stroke.

Nursing Implications

Nurses can make a difference in patient outcomes by using portable bladder ultrasound to measure postvoid urine residuals in patients at risk for UTI when this technology is available. This study reported that UTI rates and hospital length of stay were lower following implementation of this technology. This study needs to be replicated in other patient populations at high risk for UTI.

middle fingers of the examiner's gloved hand are used to support either side of the urethra as the woman is asked to repeat the Valsalva maneuver; this is called the *Marshall–Bonney maneuver*. If this produces urinary leakage, referral is suggested.

The patient is assessed for edema and changes in body weight. Edema may be observed, particularly in the face and dependent parts of the body, such as the ankles and sacral areas, and suggests fluid retention. An increase in body weight commonly accompanies edema. A 1 kg weight gain equals approximately 1000 mL of fluid (1 lb is approximately 500 mL) (Weber & Kelley, 2018).

The deep tendon reflexes of the knee are examined for quality and symmetry. This is an important part of testing for neurologic causes of bladder dysfunction, because the sacral area, which innervates the lower extremities, is the same peripheral nerve area responsible for urinary continence. The gait pattern of the person with bladder dysfunction is also noted, as well as the patient's ability to walk toe to heel. These tests evaluate possible supraspinal causes for urinary incontinence.

Unfolding Patient Stories: Lloyd Bennett • Part 2

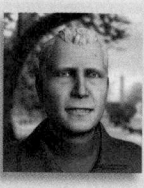

Recall from Chapter 28 **Lloyd Bennett**, who presented to the emergency department with a hip fracture. What effect can significant blood loss from surgery to repair the fracture have on renal function? What clinical findings would indicate to the nurse that kidney function is impaired? What clinical assessment findings would alert the nurse of potential trauma to the urinary tract resulting from the hip fracture? What diagnostic tests may be used to identify a urinary tract complication that the nurse would consider for preparatory patient education?

Care for Lloyd and other patients in a realistic virtual environment: *vSim for Nursing* (thepoint.lww.com/.vSimMedicalSurgical). Practice documenting these patients' care in DocuCare (thepoint.lww.com/DocuCareEHR).

Diagnostic Evaluation

A wide range of diagnostic studies may be performed in patients with urinary conditions. A comprehensive health history is used to determine the appropriate laboratory and diagnostic tests. The following sections review some of the specific tests that might be used.

The nurse educates the patient about the purpose, what to expect, and any possible side effects related to these examinations prior to testing. The nurse should also note trends in results, because they provide information about disease progression as well as the patient's response to therapy.

Most patients undergoing urologic testing or imaging studies are apprehensive, even those who have had these tests in the past. Patients frequently feel discomfort and embarrassment about such a private and personal function as voiding. Voiding in the presence of others can frequently cause

---

Chart 47-4 **PATIENT EDUCATION**
Before and After Urodynamic Testing

The nurse instructs the patient on what to expect before, during, and after the procedure:

Preprocedure
- An in-depth interview will be conducted. Questions related to your urologic symptoms and voiding habits will be asked.

During the Procedure
- You will be asked to describe sensations felt.
- You might be asked to change positions (e.g., from supine to sitting or standing).
- You may be asked to cough or perform the Valsalva maneuver (bear down).
- You will probably need to have one or two urethral catheters inserted so that bladder pressure and bladder filling can be measured. Another catheter may be placed in the rectum or vagina to measure abdominal pressure.
- You may also have electrodes (surface, wire, or needle) placed in the perianal area for electromyography. This may be uncomfortable initially during insertion and later during position changes.
- Your bladder will be filled through the urethral catheter one or more times.

After the Procedure
- You may experience urinary frequency, urgency, or dysuria from the urethral catheters. Avoid caffeinated, carbonated, and alcoholic beverages because they can further irritate the bladder. These symptoms usually decrease or subside by the day after the procedure.
- You might notice slight hematuria (blood-tinged urine) right after the procedure (especially in men with benign prostatic hyperplasia). Drinking fluids will help to clear the hematuria.
- If the urinary meatus is irritated, a warm sitz bath may be helpful.
- Be alert to signs of a urinary tract infection. Contact your primary provider if you experience fever, chills, lower back pain, or continued dysuria and hematuria.
- If you receive an antibiotic medication before the procedure, you should continue taking the complete course of medication after the procedure. This is a measure to prevent infection.

---

guarding, a natural reflex that inhibits voiding due to situational anxiety. Because the outcomes of these studies determine the plan of care, the nurse must help the patient relax by providing as much privacy and explanation about the procedure as possible (see Chart 47-4). In addition, Chart 47-5 provides a plan of nursing care for the patient undergoing diagnostic testing.

Urinalysis and Urine Culture

The urinalysis provides important clinical information about kidney function and helps diagnose other diseases, such as diabetes. The urine culture determines whether bacteria are present in the urine, as well as their strains and concentration. Urine culture and sensitivity also identify the antimicrobial therapy that is best suited for the particular strains identified, taking into consideration the antibiotic agents that have the best rate of resolution in that particular geographic region. Appropriate evaluation of any abnormality can assist in detecting serious underlying diseases.

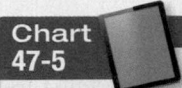

Chart 47-5

PLAN OF NURSING CARE
Care of the Patient Undergoing Diagnostic Testing of the Renal–Urologic System

NURSING DIAGNOSIS: Lack of knowledge about procedures and diagnostic tests
GOAL: Patient demonstrates increased understanding of the procedure and tests and expected behaviors

Nursing Interventions	Rationale	Expected Outcomes
1. Assess patient's level of understanding of planned diagnostic tests 2. Provide a description of tests in language the patient can understand 3. Assess patient's understanding of test results after their completion 4. Reinforce information provided to patient about test results and implications for follow-up care	1. Provides basis for education and gives indication of patient's perception of tests 2. Understanding what is expected enhances patient adherence and cooperation 3. Apprehension may interfere with patient's ability to understand information and results provided by health care team 4. Provides opportunity for patient to clarify information and anticipate follow-up care	• States rationale for planned diagnostic tests and what tasks and behaviors are expected during the procedure • Adheres to prescribed urine collection, fluid modifications, or other procedures required for diagnostic evaluation • Restates in own words results of diagnostic tests • Asks for clarification of terms and procedures • Explains rationale for follow-up care • Participates in follow-up care

NURSING DIAGNOSIS: Acute pain associated with infection, edema, obstruction, or bleeding along urinary tract or associated with invasive diagnostic tests
GOAL: Patient reports decrease in pain and absence of discomfort

Nursing Interventions	Rationale	Expected Outcomes
1. Assess level of pain: dysuria, burning on urination, abdominal or flank pain, bladder spasm 2. Encourage fluid intake (unless contraindicated) 3. Encourage warm sitz baths 4. Report increased pain to primary provider 5. Administer analgesic and antispasmodic agents for pain and spasm as prescribed 6. Assess voiding patterns and hygiene practices and provide instructions about recommended voiding patterns and hygienic practices	1. Provides baseline for evaluation of pain-relief strategies and progression of dysfunction 2. Promotes dilute urine and flushing of the lower urinary tract 3. Relieves local discomfort and promotes relaxation 4. May indicate progression or recurrence of dysfunction, or untoward signs (e.g., bleeding, calculi) 5. Prescribed to relieve pain or spasm 6. Delayed emptying of the bladder and poor hygiene may contribute to pain secondary to renal or urinary tract dysfunction	• Reports decreasing levels of pain • Reports absence of local symptoms • States ability to start and stop urinary stream without discomfort • Increases fluid intake, if indicated • Uses sitz bath as indicated • Identifies signs and symptoms to be reported to the primary provider • Takes medications as prescribed • Does not delay in emptying bladder • Uses appropriate hygienic measures, avoids bubble baths, uses appropriate hygiene after bowel movements

NURSING DIAGNOSIS: Fear associated with potential alteration in renal function and embarrassment secondary to discussion of urinary function and invasion of genitalia
GOAL: Patient appears relaxed and reports decreased fear and anxiety

Nursing Interventions	Rationale	Expected Outcomes
1. Assess patient's level of fear and apprehension 2. Explain all procedures and tests to patient 3. Provide privacy and respect patient's modesty by closing doors and keeping patient covered. Keep urinal and bedpan covered and out of sight 4. Use correct terminology in a factual manner when questioning patient about urinary tract dysfunction 5. Assess patient's fears about perceived changes associated with tests and other procedures 6. Instruct patient in relaxation techniques	1. A high level of fear or apprehension can interfere with learning and cooperation 2. Knowledge about what is expected helps reduce fear and apprehension 3. Communicates that you are aware of and accept patient's need for privacy and modesty 4. Conveys that you are comfortable discussing patient's urinary dysfunction and symptoms with patient 5. May uncover fears and misconceptions of the patient that can be alleviated by correct understanding 6. Promotes relaxation and assists patient in coping with uncertainty about outcomes	• Appears relaxed with a low level of fear or apprehension • States rationale for tests and procedures in a calm, relaxed manner • Maintains usual privacy and modesty • Discusses own urinary tract dysfunction using correct terminology without overt indications of embarrassment or discomfort • Relates fears and concerns • Demonstrates correct understanding of procedures and possible outcomes • Appears relaxed with low level of fear and apprehension

TABLE 47-4	Changes in Urine Color and Possible Causes
Urine Color	**Possible Cause**
Colorless to pale yellow	Dilute urine due to diuretic agents, alcohol consumption, diabetes insipidus, glycosuria, excess fluid intake, chronic kidney disease
Yellow to milky white	Pyuria, infection, vaginal cream
Bright yellow	Multiple vitamin preparations
Pink to red	Hemoglobin breakdown, red blood cells, gross blood, menses, bladder or prostate surgery, beets, blackberries, medications (phenytoin, rifampin, thioridazine, cascara sagrada, senna products)
Blue, blue green	Dyes, methylene blue, *Pseudomonas* species organisms, medications (amitriptyline HCl, triamterene)
Orange to amber	Concentrated urine due to dehydration, fever, bile, excess bilirubin or carotene, medications (phenazopyridine hydrochloride, nitrofurantoin)
Brown to black	Old red blood cells, urobilinogen, bilirubin, melanin, porphyrin, extremely concentrated urine due to dehydration, medications (cascara sagrada, metronidazole, iron preparations, quinine sulfate, senna products, methyldopa, nitrofurantoin)

Adapted from Comerford, K. C., & Durkin, M. T. (Eds.). (2020). *Nursing 2020 drug handbook*. Philadelphia, PA: Wolters Kluwer.

Components

Urine examination includes the following:

- Urine color (see Table 47-4)
- Urine clarity and odor
- Urine pH and specific gravity
- Tests to detect protein, glucose, and ketone bodies in the urine (proteinuria, renal glycosuria, and ketonuria, respectively)
- Microscopic examination of the urine sediment after centrifugation to detect hematuria, **pyuria** (white blood cells), casts (cylindruria), crystals (crystalluria), and **bacteriuria** (bacteria) (see Table 47-3)

Significance of Findings

Several abnormalities, such as hematuria and proteinuria, produce no symptoms but may be detected during a routine urinalysis using a dipstick. Normally, about one million RBCs pass into the urine daily, which is equivalent to one to three RBCs per high-power field. Hematuria (more than three RBCs per high-power field) can develop from an abnormality anywhere along the genitourinary tract and is more common in women than in men. Common causes include acute infection (cystitis, urethritis, or prostatitis), renal calculi, and neoplasm. Other causes include systemic disorders, such as bleeding disorders; malignant lesions; and medications, such as warfarin and heparin. Although hematuria may initially be detected using a dipstick test, further evaluation is necessary and more accurate with a 24-hour collection (Fischbach & Fischbach, 2018).

Proteinuria may be a benign finding, or it may signify serious disease. Occasional loss of up to 150 mg/day of protein in the urine, primarily albumin and Tamm–Horsfall protein (also known as uromodulin), is considered normal and usually does not require further evaluation. A dipstick examination, which can detect from 30 to 1000 mg/dL of protein, should be used as a screening test only, because urine concentration, pH, hematuria, and radiocontrast materials all affect the results. Because dipstick analysis does not detect protein concentrations of less than 30 mg/dL, the test cannot be used for early detection of diabetic nephropathy. Microalbuminuria (excretion of 20 to 200 mg/dL of protein in the urine) is an early sign of diabetic nephropathy. Common benign causes of transient proteinuria are fever, strenuous exercise, and prolonged standing.

Causes of persistent proteinuria include glomerular diseases, malignancies, collagen diseases, diabetes, preeclampsia, hypothyroidism, heart failure, exposure to heavy metals, and the use of medications, such as nonsteroidal anti-inflammatory drugs and angiotensin-converting enzyme inhibitors (Comerford & Durkin, 2020).

Specific Gravity

Specific gravity is an expression of the degree of concentration of the urine that measures the density of a solution compared to the density of distilled water, which is 1.000. Specific gravity is altered by the presence of blood, protein, and casts in the urine. The normal range of urine specific gravity is 1.005 to 1.025 (Fischbach & Fischbach, 2018; Norris, 2019).

Methods for determination of specific gravity include the following:

- Multiple-test dipstick (most common method), with a specific reagent area for specific gravity
- Urinometer (least accurate method), in which urine is placed in a small cylinder and the urinometer is floated in the urine; a specific gravity reading is obtained at the meniscus level of the urine
- Refractometer, an instrument used in a laboratory setting, which measures differences in the speed of light passing through air and the urine sample; this is the most accurate test

Urine specific gravity depends largely on hydration status. When fluid intake decreases, specific gravity normally increases. With high fluid intake, specific gravity decreases. In patients with kidney disease, urine specific gravity does not vary with fluid intake, and the patient's urine is said to have a fixed specific gravity. Disorders or conditions that cause decreased urine specific gravity include diabetes insipidus, glomerulonephritis, and severe renal damage. Those that can cause increased specific gravity include diabetes, nephritis, and fluid deficit.

Osmolality

Osmolality is the most accurate measurement of the kidney's ability to dilute and concentrate urine. It measures the number of solute particles in a kilogram of water. Serum and urine osmolality are measured simultaneously to assess the body's fluid status. In healthy adults, serum osmolality is 275 to 290 mOsm/kg, and normal urine osmolality is 200 to 800 mOsm/kg. For a 24-hour urine sample, the normal value is 300 to 900 mOsm/kg (Fischbach & Fischbach, 2018).

TABLE 47-5	Renal Function Tests	
Test	**Purpose**	**Normal Values**
Renal Concentration Specific gravity Urine osmolality	A measure of the degree of concentration of the urine. Concentrating ability is lost early in kidney disease; hence, these test findings may disclose early defects in renal function.	1.005–1.025 300–900 mOsm/kg/24 h, 50–1200 mOsm/kg random sample
24-h Urine Creatinine clearance	Detects and evaluates progression of kidney disease. Test measures volume of blood cleared of endogenous creatinine in 1 min, which provides an approximation of the glomerular filtration rate. Sensitive indicator of kidney disease used to follow progression of kidney disease.	Measured in mL/min/1.73 m^2

Age (Years)	Male	Female
<30	88–146	81–134
30–40	82–140	75–128
40–50	75–133	69–122
50–60	68–126	64–116
60–70	61–120	58–110
70–80	55–113	52–105

Serum Creatinine level	Measures effectiveness of renal function. Creatinine is the end product of muscle energy metabolism. In normal function, the level of creatinine, which is regulated and excreted by the kidneys, remains fairly constant in the body.	Males: 0.6–1.2 mg/dL (71–106 mmol/L) Females: 0.4–1.0 mg/dL (36–90 mmol/L)
BUN	Serves as index of renal function. Urea is the nitrogenous end product of protein metabolism. Test values are affected by protein intake, tissue breakdown, and fluid volume changes.	8–20 mg/dL; patients >60 yrs: 8–23 mg/dL
BUN to creatinine ratio	Evaluates hydration status. An elevated ratio is seen in hypovolemia; a normal ratio with an elevated BUN and creatinine is seen with intrinsic kidney disease.	About 10:1

BUN, blood urea nitrogen.
Adapted from Fischbach, F. T., & Fischbach, M. A. (2018). *A manual of laboratory and diagnostic tests* (10th ed.). Philadelphia, PA: Wolters Kluwer.

Renal Function Tests

Renal function tests are used to evaluate the severity of kidney disease and to assess the status of the patient's kidney function. These tests also provide information about the effectiveness of the kidney in carrying out its excretory function. Renal function test results may be within normal limits until the GFR is reduced to less than 50% of normal. Renal function can be assessed most accurately if several tests are performed and their results are analyzed together. Common tests of renal function include renal concentration tests, creatinine clearance, and serum creatinine and blood **urea nitrogen** (end product of protein metabolism) levels (see Table 47-5).

Other tests for evaluating renal function that may be helpful include serum electrolyte levels as well as urinary biomarkers to detect acute kidney injury (Fischbach & Fischbach, 2018) (see Chapter 10).

Diagnostic Imaging

There are a wide range of diagnostic studies used for the assessment of kidney and urinary function.

Kidney, Ureter, and Bladder Studies

An x-ray study of the abdomen or kidneys, ureters, and bladder (KUB) may be performed to delineate the size, shape, and position of the kidneys and to reveal urinary system abnormalities (Fischbach & Fischbach, 2018).

General Ultrasonography

Ultrasonography is a noninvasive procedure that uses sound waves passed into the body through a transducer to detect abnormalities of internal tissues and organs. Abnormalities such as fluid accumulation, masses, congenital malformations, changes in organ size, and obstructions can be identified. During the test, the lower abdomen and genitalia may need to be exposed. Ultrasonography requires a full bladder; therefore, fluid intake is encouraged before the procedure.

Bladder Ultrasonography

Bladder ultrasonography is a noninvasive method of measuring urine volume in the bladder. It may be indicated for urinary frequency, inability to void after removal of an indwelling urinary catheter, measurement of postvoiding residual urine volume, inability to void postoperatively, or assessment of the need for catheterization during the initial stages of an intermittent catheterization training program. Portable, battery-operated devices are available for bedside use. The scan head is placed on the patient's abdomen and directed toward the bladder (see Fig. 47-8). These devices automatically calculate and display an estimated urine volume (Taylor, Lynn, & Bartlett, 2019).

Computed Tomography and Magnetic Resonance Imaging

Computed tomography (CT) and magnetic resonance imaging (MRI) are noninvasive techniques that provide excellent cross-sectional views of the anatomy of the kidney and urinary tract. They are used to evaluate genitourinary masses, nephrolithiasis, chronic renal infections, renal or urinary tract trauma, metastatic disease, and soft tissue abnormalities. Occasionally, an oral or intravenous (IV) radiopaque contrast agent is used in CT scanning to enhance visualization.

Nursing Interventions

Preparation includes educating the patient about relaxation techniques and explaining that they will be able to

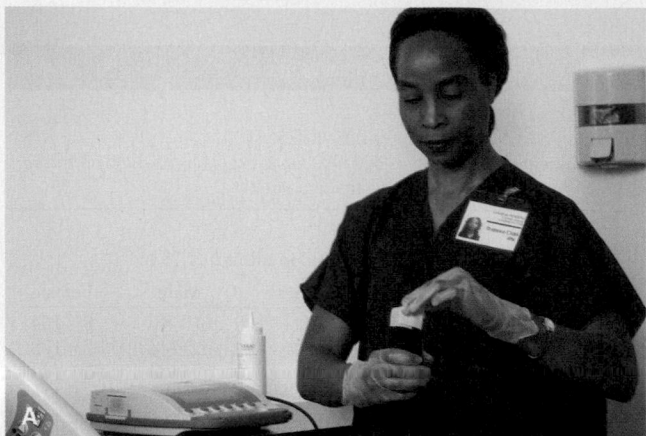
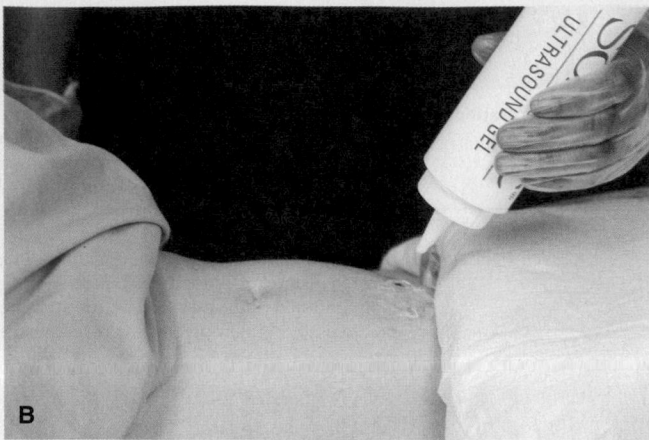

Figure 47-8 • Portable bladder ultrasound. **A.** The nurse puts on gloves and cleans the rounded end of the scan head with an alcohol pad. **B.** The nurse places ultrasound gel 2.5 cm (1 inch) superior to the symphysis pubis. (Photos by B. Proud.) Reprinted with permission from Taylor, C., Lynn, P., & Bartlett, J. L. (2019). *Fundamentals of nursing: The art and science of person-centered care* (9th ed.). Philadelphia, PA: Wolters Kluwer.

communicate with the staff by means of a microphone located inside the scanner. Many MRI suites provide headphones so that patients can listen to the music of their choice during the procedure. Nursing care guidelines for patient preparation and precautions for any imaging procedure that requires a contrast agent (contrast medium) are explained in Chart 47-6.

Before the patient enters the room where the MRI is to be performed, all metal objects and credit cards (the magnetic field can erase them) are removed. This includes medication patches (e.g., nicotine and nitroglycerin) that have a metal backing, which can cause burns if they are not removed. No metal objects (e.g., oxygen tanks, ventilators, stethoscopes) may be brought into the MRI room. The magnetic field is so strong that any metal-containing items will be pulled toward the magnet, causing severe injury and possible death. Patients with any type of cardiac implantable electronic device need to be screened to see if it is safe for the patient to undergo MRI (Indik, Gimbel, Abe, et al., 2017). A patient history is obtained to determine the presence of any internal objects containing metal such as aneurysm clips, orthopedic hardware, artificial heart valves, or intrauterine devices. These objects could malfunction, be dislodged, or heat up as they absorb energy. Cochlear implants are inactivated by MRI; therefore, other imaging procedures are considered. A sedative agent may be prescribed, because claustrophobia is a problem for some patients.

Prior to MRI of the urinary system, the patient needs to be informed to avoid alcohol, caffeine-containing beverages, and smoking for at least 2 hours and food for at least 1 hour prior to the scan. Patients should continue taking their usual medication, except for iron supplements, which can interfere with the imaging (Fischbach & Fischbach, 2018).

Nuclear Scans

Nuclear scans require injection of a radioisotope (a technetium 99m–labeled compound or iodine 123 [^{123}I] hippurate) into the circulatory system; the isotope is then monitored as it moves through the blood vessels of the kidneys. A scintillation camera is placed behind the kidney with the patient in a supine, prone, or seated position. Hypersensitivity to the

---

Chart 47-6

Patient Care During Urologic Testing with Contrast Agents

For some patients, contrast agents are nephrotoxic and allergenic. Emergency equipment and medications should be available in case of an anaphylactic reaction to the contrast agent. Emergency supplies include epinephrine, corticosteroids, vasopressors, oxygen, and airway and suction equipment.

The following guidelines can help the nurse respond quickly in the event of a problem.

Nursing Actions for Patient Preparation

- Obtain the patient's allergy history with emphasis on allergy to iodine, shellfish, and other seafood, because many contrast agents contain iodine.
- Notify primary provider and radiologist if the patient is allergic or suspected to be allergic to iodine.
- Obtain health history. Contrast agents should be used with great caution in older patients and in patients who have multiple myeloma, renal impairment, or volume depletion.
- Obtain medication history. Nephrotoxic medications such as vancomycin, amphotericin B, metformin, and nonsteroidal anti-inflammatory drugs should be discontinued before contrast media administration.
- The use of both nonionic low osmolar contrast media (LOCM, e.g., iohexol) and ionic high osmolar contrast media (HOCM, e.g., diatrizoate), is indicated in patients with renal impairment and other risk factors to prevent contrast-induced nephropathy.
- Check kidney function in patients who are at risk. Patients should receive IV hydration prior to the procedure.
- Inform the patient that they may experience a temporary feeling of warmth, flushing of the face, and an unusual flavor (similar to that of seafood) in the mouth when the contrast agent is infused.

Nursing Actions During and Post Procedure

- Monitor patient closely for allergic reaction, and monitor urine output.
- Maintain hydration status.

Adapted from Andreucci, M., Solomon, R., & Tasanarong, A. (2014). Side effects of radiographic contrast media: Pathogenesis, risk factors, and prevention. Retrieved on 3/17/2020 at: www.hindawi.com/journals/bmri/2014/741018

radioisotope is rare. The technetium scan provides information about kidney perfusion. The ^{123}I-hippurate renal scan provides information about kidney function, such as GFR.

Nuclear scans are used to evaluate acute and chronic kidney injury, renal masses, and blood flow before and after kidney transplantation. The radioisotope is injected at a specified time to achieve the proper concentration in the kidneys. After the procedure is completed, the patient is encouraged to drink fluids to promote excretion of the radioisotope by the kidneys.

Intravenous Urography

IV urography includes various tests such as excretory urography, intravenous pyelography (IVP), and infusion drip pyelography. A radiopaque contrast agent is given IV. An IVP shows the kidneys, ureter, and bladder via x-ray imaging as the dye moves through the upper and then the lower urinary system. A nephrotomogram may be carried out as part of the study to visualize different layers of the kidney and the diffuse structures within each layer and to differentiate solid masses or lesions from cysts in the kidneys or urinary tract.

IV urography may be used as the initial assessment of many suspected urologic conditions, especially lesions in the kidneys and ureters. It also provides an approximate estimate of renal function. After the contrast agent (sodium diatrizoate or meglumine diatrizoate) is given IV, multiple x-rays are obtained to visualize drainage structures in the upper and lower urinary systems.

Infusion drip pyelography requires IV infusion of a large volume of a dilute contrast agent to opacify the renal parenchyma and fill the urinary tract. This examination method is useful when prolonged opacification of the drainage structures is desired so that tomograms (body-section radiography) can be made. Images are obtained at specified intervals after the start of the infusion. These images show the filled and distended collecting system. The patient preparation is the same as for excretory urography, except fluids are not restricted.

Retrograde Pyelography

In retrograde pyelography, catheters are advanced through the ureters into the renal pelvis by means of cystoscopy. A contrast agent is then injected. Retrograde pyelography is usually performed if IV urography provides inadequate visualization of the collecting systems. It may also be used before extracorporeal shock wave lithotripsy and in patients with urologic cancer who need follow-up and have an allergy to IV contrast agents. Possible complications include infection, hematuria, and perforation of the ureter. Retrograde pyelography is used infrequently because of improved techniques in excretory urography.

Cystography

Cystography aids in evaluating vesicoureteral reflux (backflow of urine from the bladder into one or both ureters) and in assessing for bladder injury. A catheter is inserted into the bladder, and a contrast agent is instilled to outline the bladder wall. The contrast agent may leak through a small bladder perforation stemming from bladder injury, but such leakage is usually harmless. Cystography can also be performed with simultaneous pressure recordings inside the bladder.

Voiding Cystourethrography

Voiding cystourethrography uses fluoroscopy to visualize the lower urinary tract and assess urine storage in the bladder. It is commonly used as a diagnostic tool to identify vesicoureteral reflux. A urethral catheter is inserted, and a contrast agent is instilled into the bladder. When the bladder is full and the patient feels the urge to void, the catheter is removed, and the patient voids.

Renal Angiography

A renal angiogram, or renal arteriogram, provides an image of the renal arteries. The femoral (or axillary) artery is pierced with a needle, and a catheter is threaded up through the femoral and iliac arteries into the aorta or renal artery. A contrast agent is injected to opacify the renal arterial supply. Angiography is used to evaluate renal blood flow in suspected renal trauma, to differentiate renal cysts from tumors, and to evaluate hypertension. It is used preoperatively for renal transplantation.

Nursing Interventions

Before the procedure, a laxative may be prescribed to evacuate the colon so that unobstructed x-rays can be obtained. Injection sites (groin for femoral approach or axilla for axillary approach) may be shaved. The peripheral pulse sites (radial, femoral, and dorsalis pedis) are marked for easy access during postprocedural assessment. See Chart 47-6 for considerations for the patient receiving a contrast agent.

After the procedure, vital signs are monitored until stable. If the axillary artery was the injection site, blood pressure measurements are taken on the opposite arm. The injection site is examined for swelling and hematoma. Peripheral pulses are palpated, and the color and temperature of the involved extremity are noted and compared with those of the uninvolved extremity. Cold compresses may be applied to the injection site to decrease edema and pain. Possible complications include hematoma formation, arterial thrombosis or dissection, false aneurysm formation, and altered renal function.

MAG3 Renogram

This scan is used to further evaluate kidney function in some centers by permitting visualization of renal clearance (Fischbach & Fischbach, 2018). The patient is given an injection containing a small amount of radioactive material, which will show how the kidneys are functioning. The patient needs to lie still for about 35 minutes while special cameras take images (Fischbach & Fischbach, 2018).

Urologic Endoscopic Procedures

Endourology, or urologic endoscopic procedures, can be performed in one of two ways: using a cystoscope inserted into the urethra, or percutaneously, through a small incision.

The cystoscopic examination is used to directly visualize the urethra and bladder. The cystoscope, which is inserted through the urethra into the bladder, has an optical lens system that provides a magnified, illuminated view of the bladder (see Fig. 47-9). The use of high-intensity light and interchangeable lenses allows excellent visualization and permits still and motion pictures to be taken. The cystoscope is manipulated to allow complete visualization of the urethra and bladder

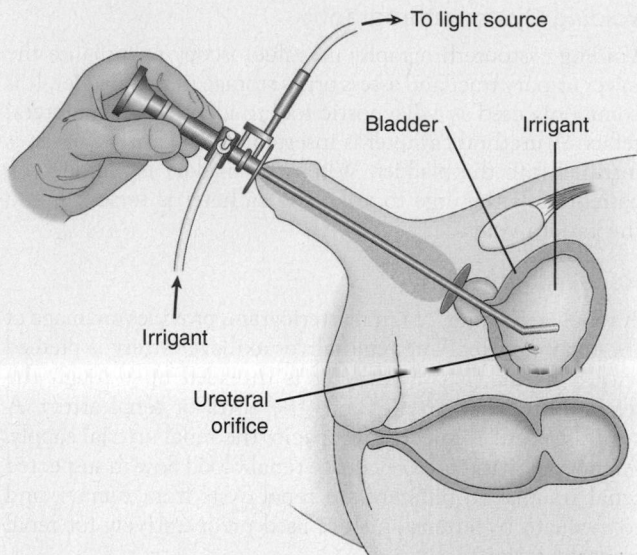

Figure 47-9 • Cystoscopic examination. A rigid or semirigid cystoscope is introduced into the bladder. The upper cord is an electric line for the light at the distal end of the cystoscope. The lower tubing leads from a reservoir of sterile irrigant that is used to inflate the bladder.

as well as the ureteral orifices and prostatic urethra. Small ureteral catheters can be passed through the cystoscope for assessment of the ureters and the pelvis of each kidney.

The cystoscope also allows the urologist to obtain a urine specimen from each kidney to evaluate its function. Cup forceps can be inserted through the cystoscope for biopsy. Calculi may be removed from the urethra, bladder, and ureter using cystoscopy. If a lower tract cystoscopy is performed, the patient is usually conscious, and the procedure is usually no more uncomfortable than a catheterization. To minimize posttest urethral discomfort, viscous lidocaine is given several minutes before the study. If the cystoscopy includes examination of the upper tracts, a sedative agent may be given before the procedure. General anesthesia is usually given to ensure that there are no involuntary muscle spasms when the scope is being passed through the ureters or kidneys.

Nursing Interventions

The nurse describes the procedure to the patient and family to prepare them and to allay their fears. If an upper cystoscopy is to be performed, the patient is usually restricted to nothing by mouth (NPO) for several hours beforehand.

Postprocedural management is directed at relieving any discomfort resulting from the examination. Some burning on voiding, blood-tinged urine, and urinary frequency from trauma to the mucous membranes can be expected. Moist heat to the lower abdomen and warm sitz baths are helpful in relieving pain and relaxing the muscles.

After a cystoscopic examination, the patient with obstructive pathology may experience urine retention if the instruments used during the examination caused edema. The nurse carefully monitors the patient with prostatic hyperplasia for urine retention. Warm sitz baths and antispasmodic medication, such as flavoxate, may be prescribed to relieve temporary urine retention caused by poor relaxation of the urinary sphincter; however, intermittent catheterization may be necessary for a few hours after the examination. The nurse

monitors the patient for signs and symptoms of UTI. Because edema of the urethra secondary to local trauma may obstruct urine flow, the patient is also monitored for signs and symptoms of obstruction.

Biopsy

Renal and Ureteral Brush Biopsy

Brush biopsy techniques provide specific information when abnormal x-ray findings of the ureter or renal pelvis raise questions about whether a defect is a tumor, a stone, a blood clot, or an artifact. First, a cystoscopic examination is conducted. Then, a ureteral catheter is introduced, followed by a biopsy brush that is passed through the catheter. The suspected lesion is brushed back and forth to obtain cells and surface tissue fragments for histologic analysis.

Kidney Biopsy

Biopsy of the kidney is used to help diagnose and evaluate the extent of kidney disease. Indications for biopsy include unexplained acute kidney injury, persistent proteinuria or hematuria, transplant rejection, and glomerulopathies. A small section of renal cortex is obtained either percutaneously (needle biopsy) or by open biopsy through a small flank incision. Before the biopsy is carried out, coagulation studies are conducted to identify any risk of postbiopsy bleeding. Contraindications to kidney biopsy include bleeding tendencies, uncontrolled hypertension, sepsis, a solitary kidney, large polycystic kidneys, kidney neoplasm, UTI, and morbid obesity.

The patient may be prescribed a fasting regimen 6 to 8 hours before the test. An IV line is established. A urine specimen is obtained and saved for comparison with the postbiopsy specimen.

If a needle biopsy is to be performed, the patient is instructed to breathe in and hold that breath (to prevent the kidney from moving) while the needle is being inserted. The sedated patient is placed in a prone position with a sandbag under the abdomen. The skin at the biopsy site is infiltrated with a local anesthetic agent. The biopsy needle is introduced just inside the renal capsule of the outer quadrant of the kidney. The location of the needle may be confirmed by fluoroscopy or by ultrasound, in which case a special probe is used.

With open biopsy, a small incision is made over the kidney, allowing direct visualization. Preparation for an open biopsy is similar to that for any major abdominal surgery.

Nursing Interventions

After a biopsy procedure, nursing care includes monitoring vital signs to detect signs and symptoms of bleeding or infection (Fischbach & Fischbach, 2018). The nurse should assess for other signs and symptoms of internal bleeding such as pallor, dizziness, and flank or back pain. IV fluids may be given to help clear the kidneys and prevent clot formation. Urine may contain blood (usually clearing in 24 to 48 hours) from oozing at the site. Bed rest should be maintained and pressure dressings applied for prescribed periods of time to control bleeding. Puncture sites should be examined for signs and symptoms of infection. Analgesic agents should be given as prescribed and needed for pain.

CRITICAL THINKING EXERCISES

1 pq A 53-year-old female is scheduled for urodynamic testing. Describe your priorities for educating this patient about aspects of care during and after this procedure.

2 ebp You make a home visit to a 72-year-old male who had a cystoscopic examination the day before your visit. He complains of difficulty urinating since his return home. Identify assessments and possible interventions that you would use to evaluate and manage the patient's symptoms. Identify the evidence for the assessments and nursing interventions you chose and the strength of that evidence.

REFERENCES

*Asterisk indicates nursing research.

Books

Ball, J. W., Dains, J. E., Flynn, J. A., et al. (2019). *Seidel's guide to physical examination* (9th ed.). St. Louis, MO: Elsevier.

Comerford, K. C., & Durkin, M. T. (Eds.). (2020). *Nursing 2020 drug handbook*. Philadelphia, PA: Wolters Kluwer.

Eliopoulos, C. (2018). *Gerontological nursing* (9th ed.). Philadelphia, PA: Wolters Kluwer.

Fischbach, F. T., & Fischbach, M. A. (2018). *A manual of laboratory and diagnostic tests* (10th ed.). Philadelphia, PA: Wolters Kluwer.

Norris, T. L. (2019). *Porth's pathophysiology: Concepts of altered health states* (10th ed.). Philadelphia, PA: Wolters Kluwer.

Russell, S. S. (2017). Physiology of the kidney. In S. M. Bodin (Ed.). *Contemporary nephrology nursing* (3rd ed.). Pitman, NJ: American Nephrology Nurses Association.

Taylor, C., Lynn, P., & Bartlett, J. L. (2019). *Fundamentals of nursing: The art and science of person-centered care* (9th ed.). Philadelphia, PA: Wolters Kluwer.

Verlander, J. W., & Clapp, W. L. (2019). Anatomy of the kidney. In A. S. L. Yu, G. M. Certow, V. Luyckx, et al. (Eds.). *Brenner and Rector's the kidney* (11th ed.). Philadelphia, PA: Elsevier.

Weber, J. R., & Kelley, J. H. (2018). *Health assessment in nursing* (6th ed.). Philadelphia, PA: Wolters Kluwer.

Journals and Electronic Documents

Andreucci, M., Solomon, R., & Tasanarong, A. (2014). Side effects of radiographic contrast media: Pathogenesis, risk factors, and prevention. *BioMed Research International*. Retrieved on 3/17/2020 at: www.hindawi.com/journals/bmri/2014/741018

*Chen, S., Chen, P., Chen, G., et al. (2018). Portable bladder ultrasound reduces incidence of urinary tract infection and shortens hospital length of stay in patients with acute ischemic stroke. *Journal of Cardiovascular Nursing, 31*(6), 551–558.

Emmett, M., & Palmer, B. F. (2018). Serum osmol gap. *UpToDate*. Retrieved on 6/14/2019 at: www.uptodate.com/contents/serum-osmol-gap

Indik, J. H., Gimbel, J. R., Abe, H., et al. (2017). 2017 HRS expert consensus statement on magnetic resonance imaging and radiation exposure in patients with cardiovascular implantable electronic devices. *Heart Rhythm, 14*(7), e97–e153.

Resources

American Association of Kidney Patients (AAKP), www.aakp.org

National Institute of Diabetes and Digestive and Kidney Diseases, National Institutes of Health, www.niddk.nih.gov

National Kidney Foundation, www.kidney.org

48

Management of Patients with Kidney Disorders

exchange: denotes a complete cycle including fill, dwell, and drain phases of peritoneal dialysis

glomerular filtration rate (GFR): amount of plasma filtered through the glomeruli per unit of time

glomerulonephritis: inflammation of the glomerular capillaries

hemodialysis (HD): procedure during which a patient's blood is circulated through a dialyzer to remove waste products and excess fluid

interstitial nephritis: inflammation within the renal tissue

nephrosclerosis: hardening of the renal arteries

nephrotic syndrome: type of kidney disease with increased glomerular permeability and massive proteinuria

nephrotoxic: any substance, medication, or action that is toxic to kidney tissue

oliguria: urine output less than 400 mL in 24 hours or less than 0.5 mL/kg/h over 6 hours

osmosis: movement of water through a semipermeable membrane from an area of lower solute concentration to an area of higher solute concentration

peritoneal dialysis (PD): procedure that uses the lining of the patient's peritoneal cavity, the peritoneal membrane, as the semipermeable membrane for exchange of fluid and solutes

peritonitis: inflammation of the peritoneal membrane

polyuria: excessive urine production

ultrafiltration: process whereby water is removed from the blood by means of a pressure gradient between the patient's blood and the dialysate

uremia: an excess of urea and other nitrogenous wastes in the blood

urinary casts: proteins secreted by damaged kidney tubules

The kidneys and urinary system help regulate the body's internal environment and are essential for the maintenance of life. Nurses working in all clinical settings will encounter patients with various kidney injuries and diseases and need to be knowledgeable about these disorders. This chapter provides an overview of electrolyte imbalances and systemic manifestations that are common in patients with kidney disorders. The main causes are discussed, together with management strategies to prevent damage and preserve renal function. Chronic kidney disease (CKD) and acute kidney injury (AKI) are discussed, as is the care of patients with other renal conditions requiring dialysis, continuous renal replacement therapy (CRRT), transplantation, and kidney surgery.

FLUID AND ELECTROLYTE IMBALANCES IN KIDNEY DISORDERS

Patients with kidney disorders commonly experience fluid and electrolyte imbalances and require careful assessment and close monitoring for signs of potential problems. The patient whose fluid intake exceeds the ability of the kidneys to excrete fluid is said to have fluid overload. If fluid intake is inadequate, the patient is said to be volume depleted and may show signs and symptoms of fluid volume deficit. The intake and output (I&O) record, a key monitoring tool, is used to document important fluid parameters, including the amount of fluid taken in (orally or parenterally), the volume of urine excreted, and other fluid losses (diarrhea, vomiting, diaphoresis). Patient weight is considered a more accurate indication of volume status than I&O, due to the challenges and multiple variables involved in accurately monitoring I&O. Documenting trends in weight is a key assessment strategy essential for determining the daily fluid allowance and indicating signs of fluid volume excess or deficit.

> ### Quality and Safety Nursing Alert
>
> *The most accurate indicator of fluid loss or gain in patients who are acutely ill is weight. An accurate daily weight must be obtained and recorded. A 1-kg weight gain is equal to 1 L (1000 mL) of retained fluid.*

Clinical Manifestations

The signs and symptoms of common fluid and electrolyte disturbances that can occur in patients with kidney disorders and general management strategies are listed in Table 48-1. The nurse continually assesses, monitors, and informs appropriate members of the health care team if the patient exhibits any of these signs. Management strategies for fluid and electrolyte disturbances in kidney disease are discussed in greater depth later in this chapter (see Chapter 10 for more discussion of fluid and electrolyte disturbances).

 ### Gerontologic Considerations

With aging, the kidney is less able to respond to acute fluid and electrolyte changes. Older adult patients may develop atypical and nonspecific signs and symptoms of altered renal function and fluid and electrolyte imbalances. A fluid balance deficit in older adults can lead to falls, medication toxicity, constipation, urinary tract and respiratory tract infections, delirium, seizures, electrolyte imbalances, hyperthermia, and delayed wound healing. Recognition of acute changes in fluid and electrolytes is further hampered by their association with preexisting disorders and the misconception that they are normal changes of aging (Hain, 2017).

KIDNEY DISORDERS

Chronic Kidney Disease

Chronic kidney disease (CKD) is an umbrella term that describes kidney damage or a decrease in the glomerular filtration rate (GFR) lasting for 3 or more months. CKD is associated with decreased quality of life, increased health care expenditures, and premature death. Untreated CKD can result in **end-stage kidney disease (ESKD**, formerly known as end-stage renal disease [ESRD]), which is the final stage of CKD. ESKD results in retention of uremic waste products and the need for renal replacement therapy (RRT), such as dialysis or kidney transplantation (Chicca, 2020). Risk factors include cardiovascular disease, diabetes, hypertension, and obesity.

TABLE 48-1   Common Fluid and Electrolyte Disturbances in Kidney Disorders

Disturbance	Manifestations	General Management Strategies
Fluid volume deficit	Acute weight loss ≥5%, decreased skin turgor, dry mucous membranes, oliguria or anuria, increased hematocrit, BUN level increased out of proportion to creatinine level, hypothermia	Fluid challenge, fluid replacement orally or parenterally
Fluid volume excess	Acute weight gain ≥5%, edema, crackles, shortness of breath, decreased BUN, decreased hematocrit, distended neck veins	Fluid and sodium restriction, diuretic agents, dialysis
Hyponatremia (sodium deficit)	Nausea, malaise, lethargy, headache, abdominal cramps, apprehension, seizures	Diet, normal saline or hypertonic saline solutions
Hypernatremia (sodium excess)	Dry, sticky mucous membranes, thirst, rough dry tongue, fever, restlessness, weakness, disorientation	Fluids, diuretic agents, dietary restriction
Hypokalemia (potassium deficit)	Anorexia, abdominal distention, paralytic ileus, muscle weakness, ECG changes, arrhythmias	Diet, oral or parenteral potassium replacement therapy
Hyperkalemia (potassium excess)	Diarrhea, colic, nausea, irritability, muscle weakness, ECG changes	Dietary restriction, diuretics, IV glucose, insulin and sodium bicarbonate, cation-exchange resin, calcium gluconate, dialysis
Hypocalcemia (calcium deficit)	Abdominal and muscle cramps, stridor, carpopedal spasm, hyperactive reflexes, tetany, positive Chvostek or Trousseau sign, tingling of fingers and around mouth, ECG changes	Diet, oral or parenteral calcium salt replacement
Hypercalcemia (calcium excess)	Deep bone pain, flank pain, muscle weakness, depressed deep tendon reflexes, constipation, nausea and vomiting, confusion, impaired memory, polyuria, polydipsia, ECG changes	Fluid replacement, etidronate, pamidronate, mithramycin, calcitonin, corticosteroids, phosphate salts
Metabolic acidosis (bicarbonate deficit)	Headache, confusion, drowsiness, increased respiratory rate and depth, nausea and vomiting, warm flushed skin	Bicarbonate replacement, dialysis
Metabolic alkalosis (bicarbonate excess)	Depressed respirations, muscle hypertonicity, dizziness, tingling of fingers and toes	Fluid replacement if volume depleted; ensure adequate chloride
Hypoalbuminemia (protein deficit)	Chronic weight loss, emotional depression, pallor, fatigue, soft flabby muscles	Diet, dietary supplements, hyperalimentation, albumin
Hypomagnesemia (magnesium deficit)	Dysphagia, muscle cramps, hyperactive reflexes, tetany, positive Chvostek or Trousseau sign, tingling of fingers, arrhythmias, vertigo	Diet, oral or parenteral magnesium replacement therapy
Hypermagnesemia (magnesium excess)	Facial flushing, nausea and vomiting, sensation of warmth, drowsiness, depressed deep tendon reflexes, muscle weakness, respiratory depression, cardiac arrest	Calcium gluconate, mechanical ventilation, dialysis
Hypophosphatemia (phosphorus deficit)	Deep bone pain, flank pain, muscle weakness and pain, paresthesia, apprehension, confusion, seizures	Diet, oral or parenteral phosphorus supplementation therapy

BUN, blood urea nitrogen; ECG, electrocardiographic; IV, intravenous.
Adapted from Fischbach, F., & Fischbach, M. (2018). *A manual of laboratory and diagnostic tests* (10th ed.). Philadelphia, PA: Wolters Kluwer.

Recent research reported that 15% of the adult U.S. population, 37 million people or 1 in 7 individuals, have CKD and 9 of 10 affected individuals are unaware of their disease (Centers for Disease Control and Prevention [CDC], 2019). On December 31, 2017, there were more than 746,000 Americans diagnosed with ESKD (United States Renal Data System [USRDS], 2019). The majority of people with CKD will die of a cardiovascular event (heart attack or stroke) prior to reaching ESKD (Subbiah, Chhabra, & Mahajan, 2016).

Diabetes and hypertension cause approximately 70% of cases of CKD (Chicca, 2020). About one in three adults with diabetes may have CKD (CDC, 2019). Diabetes is the leading cause of kidney disease in patients starting RRT. About one in five adults with hypertension may have CKD (CDC, 2019). Other causes include glomerulonephritis,

pyelonephritis; polycystic, hereditary, or congenital disorders; and renal cancers.

Pathophysiology

In the early stages of CKD, there can be significant damage to the kidneys without signs or symptoms. The pathophysiology of CKD is not yet clearly understood, but the damage to the kidneys is thought to be caused by prolonged acute inflammation that is not organ specific and thus has subtle systemic manifestations.

Stages of Chronic Kidney Disease

CKD has been classified into five stages by the National Kidney Foundation (NKF) (see Chart 48-1). Stage 5 results

Chart 48-1 Stages of Chronic Kidney Disease

Stages are based on the GFR. The normal GFR is 125 mL/min/1.73 m².

Stage 1

GFR ≥90 mL/min/1.73 m²
Kidney damage with normal or increased GFR

Stage 2

GFR = 60–89 mL/min/1.73 m²
Mild decrease in GFR

Stage 3

GFR = 30–59 mL/min/1.73 m²
Moderate decrease in GFR

Stage 4

GFR = 15–29 mL/min/1.73 m²
Severe decrease in GFR

Stage 5

GFR <15 mL/min/1.73 m²
End-stage kidney disease or chronic kidney disease

Adapted from Norris, T. L. (2019). *Porth's pathophysiology: Concepts of altered health states* (10th ed.). Philadelphia, PA: Wolters Kluwer.
GFR, glomerular filtration rate.

when the kidneys cannot remove the body's metabolic wastes or perform their regulatory functions; thus, RRT is required to sustain life. Screening and early intervention are important, because not all patients progress to stage 5 CKD. Patients with CKD are at increased risk for cardiovascular disease, which is the leading cause of morbidity and mortality (Carey & Whelton, 2018). Treatment of hypertension, anemia, and hyperglycemia and detection of proteinuria all help to slow disease progression and improve patient outcomes (Brooks, 2017).

Clinical Manifestations

Elevated serum creatinine levels indicate underlying kidney disease; as the creatinine level increases, symptoms of CKD begin. Those with CKD are one of the most symptomatic groups among patients with chronic diseases (Kalfoss, Schick-Makaroff, & Molzahn, 2019). Anemia, due to decreased erythropoietin production by the kidney, metabolic acidosis, and abnormalities in calcium and phosphorus balance herald the development of CKD (Brooks, 2017). Fluid retention, evidenced by both edema and congestive heart failure, develops. As the disease progresses, abnormalities in electrolytes occur, heart failure worsens, and hypertension becomes more difficult to control, often due to fluid volume excess (Ku, Lee, Wei, et al., 2019).

Assessment and Diagnostic Findings

The **glomerular filtration rate (GFR)** is the amount of plasma filtered through the glomeruli per unit of time. Creatinine clearance is a measure of the amount of creatinine the kidneys are able to clear in a 24-hour period. Normal values

differ in men and women. Calculation of GFR, an important assessment parameter in CKD, is discussed in Chapter 47.

Medical Management

The management of patients with CKD includes treatment of the underlying causes. Regular clinical and laboratory assessment is important to keep the blood pressure below 125 to 130/80 mm Hg (Ku et al., 2019). Controlling cardiovascular risk factors, treating hyperglycemia, managing anemia, encouraging smoking cessation, weight loss, and exercise programs as well as reducing salt and alcohol intake and minimizing nephrotoxins all slow progression toward ESKD. Medical management also includes early referral for initiation of RRT as indicated by the patient's renal status. Patient engagement and education are essential as many of these factors are under the patient's control.

 Gerontologic Considerations

Changes in kidney function with normal aging increase the susceptibility of older patients to kidney dysfunction and kidney disease (Hain, 2017). With aging, the number of nephrons decline. In addition, the incidence of systemic diseases, such as atherosclerosis, hypertension, heart failure, diabetes, and cancer, increases with advancing age, predisposing older adults to kidney disease associated with these disorders. Therefore, acute problems need to be prevented if possible or recognized and treated quickly to avoid kidney damage. Nurses in all settings need to be alert to signs and symptoms of kidney dysfunction in older patients.

Older patients frequently take multiple prescription and over-the-counter medications. Because alterations in renal blood flow, glomerular filtration, and renal clearance increase the risk of medication-associated changes in renal function, precautions are indicated with all medications. When older patients undergo extensive diagnostic tests or when new medications (e.g., diuretic agents) are added, precautions must be taken to prevent dehydration, which can compromise marginal renal function and exacerbate preexisting kidney dysfunction (Hain, 2017).

Nephrosclerosis

Nephrosclerosis (hardening of the renal arteries) is most often due to prolonged hypertension, diabetes, the aging process, and other factors. Individuals with nephrosclerosis generally experience slowly elevating blood urea nitrogen (BUN) and creatinine, and mild proteinuria (spilling of protein in the urine). Nephrosclerosis is a major cause of CKD and ESKD secondary to many disorders. Groups at increased risk include African Americans, those with uncontrolled hypertension, and individuals with underlying CKD, especially those with diabetic nephropathy. African American patients have an approximate eightfold elevation in the risk of hypertension-induced ESKD (Mann & Hilgers, 2019).

Pathophysiology

There are two forms of nephrosclerosis: acute hypertensive and benign. Acute hypertensive nephrosclerosis is often associated with significant and prolonged hypertension.

Damage is caused by decreased blood flow to the kidney resulting in patchy necrosis of the renal parenchyma. Over time, fibrosis occurs and glomeruli are destroyed. Untreated, the disease process can progress rapidly. Benign nephrosclerosis can be found in older adults, associated with atherosclerosis, hypertension, and diabetes (Parikh, Haddad, & Hebert, 2019).

Assessment and Diagnostic Findings

Symptoms are rare early in the disease, even though the urine usually contains protein and occasional casts. CKD and associated signs and symptoms occur late in the disease.

Medical Management

Treatment of nephrosclerosis is antihypertensive therapy. An angiotensin-converting enzyme (ACE) inhibitor, alone or in combination with other antihypertensive medications, significantly reduces its incidence. See Chapter 27 for additional information on hypertension.

Primary Glomerular Diseases

Diseases that destroy the glomerulus of the kidney are the third most common cause of stage 5 CKD (USRDS, 2019). The glomeruli (a Greek word meaning "filter") are the multiple small blood vessels within the nephron that remove urea from the blood. There are two major categories of glomerular diseases: glomerulonephritis and glomerulosclerosis. Primary glomerular diseases are within the kidney itself, while secondary glomerular kidney disease is a result of systemic disease, such as diabetes or lupus nephritis. Primary glomerulonephritis means that the kidney is inflamed, often due to an autoimmune disorder (Norris, 2019).

Antigen–antibody complexes form in the blood and become trapped in the glomerular capillaries (the filtering portion of the kidney), inducing an inflammatory response. Immunoglobulin G (IgG)—the major immunoglobulin (antibody) found in the blood—can be detected in the glomerular capillary walls. The major clinical manifestations of glomerular injury include proteinuria, hematuria, decreased GFR, decreased excretion of sodium, edema, and hypertension (Mahaffey, 2017) (see Chart 48-2).

Chart 48-2

Terms Typically Used When Describing Glomerular Disease

Primary: Disease is mainly in glomeruli
Secondary: Glomerular diseases that are the consequence of systemic disease
Idiopathic: Cause is unknown
Acute: Occurs over days or weeks
Chronic: Occurs over months or years
Rapidly progressing: Constant, rapid loss of renal function with better chance of recovery with early diagnosis
Diffuse: Involves all glomeruli
Focal: Involves some glomeruli
Segmental: Involves portions of individual glomeruli
Membranous: Evidence of thickened glomerular capillary walls
Proliferative: Number of glomerular cells involved is increasing

---

Acute Nephritic Syndrome

Glomerulonephritis is an inflammation of the glomerular capillaries that can occur in acute and chronic forms. **Acute nephritic syndrome** is a type of acute glomerulonephritis. In acute nephritic syndrome, hematuria due to glomerular bleeding is seen as well as pus and cellular and granular casts in the urine. Variable proteinuria is noted. A decreased glomerular filtration rate is seen in severe cases of nephritic glomerular injury (Mahaffey, 2017; Norris, 2019).

Pathophysiology

Primary glomerular diseases include postinfectious glomerulonephritis, rapidly progressive glomerulonephritis, membrane proliferative glomerulonephritis, and membranous glomerulonephritis. Postinfectious causes are group A beta-hemolytic streptococcal infection of the throat that precedes the onset of glomerulonephritis by 2 to 3 weeks (see Fig. 48-1). Postinfectious glomerulonephritis may also follow impetigo (infection of the skin) and acute viral infections (upper respiratory tract infections, mumps, varicella zoster virus, Epstein–Barr virus, hepatitis B, and human immune deficiency virus [HIV] infection). In some patients, antigens outside the body (e.g., medications, foreign serum) initiate the process, resulting in antigen–antibody complexes being deposited in the glomeruli. In other patients, the kidney tissue itself serves as the inciting antigen (autoimmune phenomenon). With early

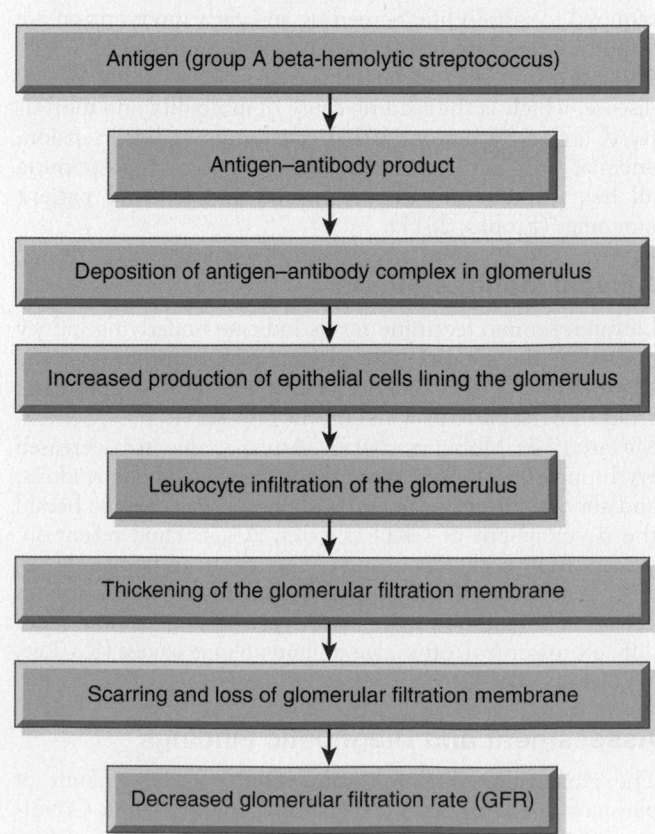

Physiology/Pathophysiology

Antigen (group A beta-hemolytic streptococcus)

↓

Antigen–antibody product

↓

Deposition of antigen–antibody complex in glomerulus

↓

Increased production of epithelial cells lining the glomerulus

↓

Leukocyte infiltration of the glomerulus

↓

Thickening of the glomerular filtration membrane

↓

Scarring and loss of glomerular filtration membrane

↓

Decreased glomerular filtration rate (GFR)

Figure 48-1 • Sequence of events in acute nephritic syndrome.

diagnosis and treatment, the kidney damage is generally reversible (Mahaffey, 2017).

Clinical Manifestations

The primary presenting features of an acute glomerular inflammation are hematuria, edema, **azotemia** (an abnormal concentration of nitrogenous wastes in the blood), and **proteinuria** (excess protein in the urine) (Mahaffey, 2017; Norris, 2019). The hematuria may be microscopic (identifiable only through microscopic examination) or macroscopic (visible to the eye). The urine may appear cola-colored because of red blood cells (RBCs) and protein plugs or casts; RBC casts indicate glomerular injury. Glomerulonephritis may be mild and the hematuria discovered incidentally through a routine urinalysis, or the disease may be severe, with AKI and oliguria.

Some degree of edema and hypertension is present in most patients. Marked proteinuria due to the increased permeability of the glomerular membrane may also occur, with associated pitting edema, hypoalbuminemia, hyperlipidemia, and fatty casts in the urine. BUN and serum creatinine levels may increase as urine output decreases. In addition, anemia may be present.

In the more severe form of the disease, patients also complain of headache, malaise, and flank pain. Older patients may experience circulatory overload with dyspnea, engorged neck veins, cardiomegaly, and pulmonary edema. Atypical symptoms include confusion, somnolence, and seizures, which are often confused with the symptoms of a primary neurologic disorder.

Assessment and Diagnostic Findings

In acute nephritic syndrome, the kidneys become large, edematous, and congested. All renal tissues, including the glomeruli, tubules, and blood vessels, are affected to varying degrees. Patients with an immunoglobulin A (IgA) nephropathy have an elevated serum IgA and low to normal complement levels. Electron microscopy and immunofluorescent analysis help identify the nature of the lesion; however, a kidney biopsy may be needed for definitive diagnosis. See Chapter 47 for discussion of kidney biopsy.

If the patient improves, the amount of urine will increase and the urinary protein and sediment will diminish. Some patients develop severe **uremia** (an excess of urea and other nitrogenous wastes in the blood) within weeks and require dialysis for survival. Others, after a period of apparent recovery, insidiously develop chronic glomerulonephritis.

Complications

Complications of acute glomerulonephritis include hypertensive encephalopathy, heart failure, and pulmonary edema. Hypertensive encephalopathy is a medical emergency, and therapy is directed toward reducing the blood pressure without impairing renal function. This can occur in acute nephritic syndrome or preeclampsia with chronic hypertension of greater than 130/80 mm Hg.

Rapidly progressive glomerulonephritis is characterized by a rapid decline in renal function. Without treatment, ESKD develops in a matter of weeks or months. Signs and symptoms are similar to those of acute glomerulonephritis (hematuria and proteinuria), but the course of the disease is more severe

and rapid. Crescent-shaped cells accumulate in Bowman space, disrupting the filtering surface. Therapeutic plasma exchange and treatment with high-dose corticosteroids, cytotoxic agents or monoclonal antibodies have been used to reduce the inflammatory response.

Dialysis is initiated in acute glomerulonephritis if signs and symptoms of uremia are severe. However, the prognosis for patients with acute nephritic syndrome is excellent and it rarely causes CKD (Mahaffey, 2017).

Medical Management

Management consists primarily of treating symptoms, attempting to preserve kidney function, and treating complications promptly. Treatment may include prescribing corticosteroids, managing hypertension, and controlling proteinuria. Pharmacologic therapy depends on the cause of acute glomerulonephritis. If residual streptococcal infection is suspected, penicillin is the agent of choice. However, other antibiotic agents may be prescribed. Dietary protein may be restricted when renal insufficiency and nitrogen retention (elevated BUN) develop. Sodium is restricted when the patient has hypertension, edema, and heart failure.

Nursing Management

Although most patients with acute uncomplicated glomerulonephritis are cared for as outpatients, nursing care is important in every setting.

Providing Care in the Hospital

In a hospital setting, carbohydrates are given liberally to provide energy and reduce the catabolism of protein. I&O is carefully measured and recorded. Fluids are prescribed based on the patient's fluid losses and daily body weight. Insensible fluid loss through the lungs (300 mL) and skin (500 mL) is considered when estimating fluid loss (see Chapter 10, Table 10-2) (Norris, 2019). If treatment is effective, diuresis will begin, resulting in decreased edema and blood pressure. Proteinuria and microscopic hematuria may persist for many months. Other nursing interventions focus on patient education about the disease process, explanations of laboratory and other diagnostic tests, and preparation for safe and effective self-care at home.

Promoting Home, Community-Based, and Transitional Care

 Educating Patients About Self-Care

Patient education is directed toward managing symptoms and monitoring for complications. Fluid and diet restrictions must be reviewed with the patient to avoid worsening of edema and hypertension. The patient is instructed verbally and in writing to notify the primary provider if symptoms of kidney disease occur (e.g., fatigue, nausea, vomiting, loss of appetite, diminishing urine output) or at the first sign of any infection.

Continuing and Transitional Care

The importance of follow-up evaluations of blood pressure, laboratory blood studies for BUN and creatinine levels, and urinalysis for protein, to determine if the disease has progressed, is stressed to the patient. A referral for transitional, home, or community-based care may be indicated. A home visit from a nurse provides an opportunity for careful assessment of the patient's progress and detection of early signs and symptoms of renal insufficiency. If corticosteroids, immunosuppressant agents, or antibiotic medications are prescribed, the nurse uses the opportunity to review the dosages, desired actions, and adverse effects of medications and the precautions to be taken.

Chronic Glomerulonephritis

Chronic glomerulonephritis may be due to repeated episodes of acute nephritic syndrome, hypertensive nephrosclerosis, hyperlipidemia, chronic tubulointerstitial injury, or hemodynamically mediated glomerular sclerosis. Secondary glomerular diseases that can have systemic effects include systemic lupus erythematosus, Goodpasture syndrome (caused by antibodies to the glomerular basement membrane), and diabetic glomerulosclerosis (Mahaffey, 2017).

Pathophysiology

The kidneys are reduced to as little as one fifth their normal size (consisting largely of fibrous tissue). The cortex layer shrinks to 1 to 2 mm in thickness or less. Bands of scar tissue distort the remaining cortex, making the surface of the kidney rough and irregular. Numerous glomeruli and their tubules become scarred, and the branches of the renal artery are thickened. The resulting severe glomerular damage can progress to stage 5 CKD and require RRT. Patients who initially have impaired kidney function or notable proteinuria tend to have increased progression of kidney disease (Parikh et al., 2019).

Clinical Manifestations

The symptoms of chronic glomerulonephritis vary. Some patients with severe disease have no symptoms at all for many years. The condition may be discovered when hypertension or elevated BUN and serum creatinine levels or proteinuria are detected. Most patients report general symptoms, such as loss of weight and strength, increasing irritability, and nocturia (an increased need to urinate at night). Headaches, dizziness, and digestive disturbances are also common. Early diagnosis and treatment are key to preventing CKD and ESKD and the development of late complications.

As chronic glomerulonephritis progresses, signs and symptoms of CKD may develop. With undiagnosed or untreated disease, the patient appears poorly nourished, with a yellow-gray pigmentation of the skin and periorbital and peripheral (dependent) edema. Blood pressure may be normal or severely elevated. Retinal findings include hemorrhage, exudate, narrowed tortuous arterioles, and papilledema. Anemia causes pale mucous membranes. Cardiomegaly, a gallop rhythm, distended neck veins, and other signs and symptoms of heart failure may be present. Crackles can be heard in the bases of the lungs.

Peripheral neuropathy with diminished deep tendon reflexes and neurosensory changes occur late in the disease. The patient becomes confused and demonstrates a limited attention span. Additional late findings include evidence of pericarditis with a pericardial friction rub and pulsus paradoxus (difference in blood pressure during inspiration and expiration of greater than 10 mm Hg). Pleural effusions may be seen on chest x-ray.

Assessment and Diagnostic Findings

A number of laboratory abnormalities occur. Urinalysis reveals a fixed specific gravity of about 1.010, variable proteinuria, and **urinary casts** (proteins secreted by damaged kidney tubules). As kidney disease progresses and the GFR falls below 50 mL/min, the following changes occur:

- Anemia secondary to decreased erythropoiesis (production of RBCs)
- Decreased serum calcium level (calcium binds to phosphorus to compensate for elevated serum phosphorus levels)
- Hyperkalemia due to decreased urinary potassium excretion, acidosis, catabolism, and potassium intake from food and medications
- Hypoalbuminemia with edema secondary to protein loss through the damaged glomerular membrane
- Increased serum phosphorus level due to decreased renal excretion of phosphorus
- Impaired nerve conduction due to electrolyte abnormalities and uremia resulting in peripheral neuropathy
- Mental status changes
- Metabolic acidosis from decreased acid secretion by the kidney and inability to regenerate bicarbonate

Chest x-rays may show cardiac enlargement and pulmonary edema due to volume overload. The electrocardiogram (ECG) may be normal or may indicate left ventricular hypertrophy associated with hypertension and signs of electrolyte disturbances, such as tall, tented (or peaked) T waves associated with hyperkalemia. Renal ultrasound shows decreased renal mass in both kidneys (Norris, 2019).

Medical Management

Management of symptoms guides the treatment. If the patient has hypertension, efforts are made to reduce the blood pressure with sodium and water restriction, antihypertensive agents, or both. Weight is monitored daily, and diuretic medications are prescribed to treat fluid overload. Proteins of high-biologic value (eggs, meats, fish) are provided to promote good nutritional status. Adequate calories are provided to spare protein for tissue growth and repair. Urinary tract infections (UTIs) must be treated promptly to prevent further kidney damage. Nonsteroidal anti-inflammatory drugs (NSAIDs) are avoided as well as other nephrotoxic medications and diagnostic studies which necessitate the administration of intravenous (IV) contrast dye (Nahar, 2017).

Dialysis is initiated early in the course of the disease to keep the patient in optimal physical condition, prevent fluid and electrolyte imbalances, and minimize the risk of complications of kidney disease. The course of dialysis is smoother if treatment begins before the patient develops complications.

Nursing Management

Whether the patient is hospitalized or cared for in the home, the nurse observes the patient for common fluid and electrolyte disturbances in kidney disease (see Table 48-1). Changes in fluid and electrolyte status and in cardiac and neurologic status are promptly reported to the primary provider. Throughout the course of the disease and treatment, the nurse gives emotional support by providing opportunities for the patient and family to verbalize their concerns, have their questions answered, and explore their options (Mahaffey, 2017).

Promoting Home, Community-Based, and Transitional Care

 #### Educating Patients About Self-Care

The nurse has a major role in educating the patient and family about the prescribed treatment plan and the risks associated with nonadherence. Instructions to the patient include explanations and scheduling for follow-up evaluations: blood pressure, urinalysis for protein and casts, and laboratory studies of BUN and serum creatinine levels. If long-term dialysis is needed, the nurse educates the patient and family about the procedure, how to care for the access site, dietary and fluid restrictions, and other necessary lifestyle modifications. These topics are discussed later in this chapter.

Periodic hospitalization, visits to the outpatient clinic or office, and home care referrals provide the nurse in each setting with the opportunity for careful assessment of the patient's progress and continued education about changes to report to the primary provider (worsening signs and symptoms of kidney disease, such as nausea, vomiting, loss of appetite, and diminished urine output). Specific education may include explanations of recommended diet and fluid modifications; medications (purpose, desired effects, adverse effects, dosage, and administration schedule); and encouragement to achieve and maintain a healthy weight (Chicca, 2020). The nurse consults with the renal dietitian for detailed dietary education.

Continuing and Transitional Care

Periodic laboratory evaluations of creatinine clearance and BUN and serum creatinine levels are carried out to assess residual renal function and the need for dialysis or transplantation. If dialysis is initiated, the patient and family require considerable assistance and support in dealing with therapy and its long-term implications. The patient and family are reminded of the importance of participation in health promotion activities, including health screening. The patient is instructed to inform all health care providers about the diagnosis of glomerulonephritis so that all medical management, including pharmacologic therapy, is based on altered renal function.

Nephrotic Syndrome

Nephrotic syndrome is a type of kidney disease characterized by increased glomerular permeability and is manifested by massive proteinuria (Mahaffey, 2017). Clinical findings include proteinuria (a marked increase in protein [particularly albumin] in the urine), hypoalbuminemia (a decrease in albumin in the blood), diffuse edema, high serum cholesterol, and hyperlipidemia (elevated low-density lipoproteins). A hypercoagulable state is often present and the patient has an increased risk of deep venous thrombosis, renal vein thrombosis, and pulmonary embolism (Kelepouris & Rovin, 2019).

Physiology/Pathophysiology

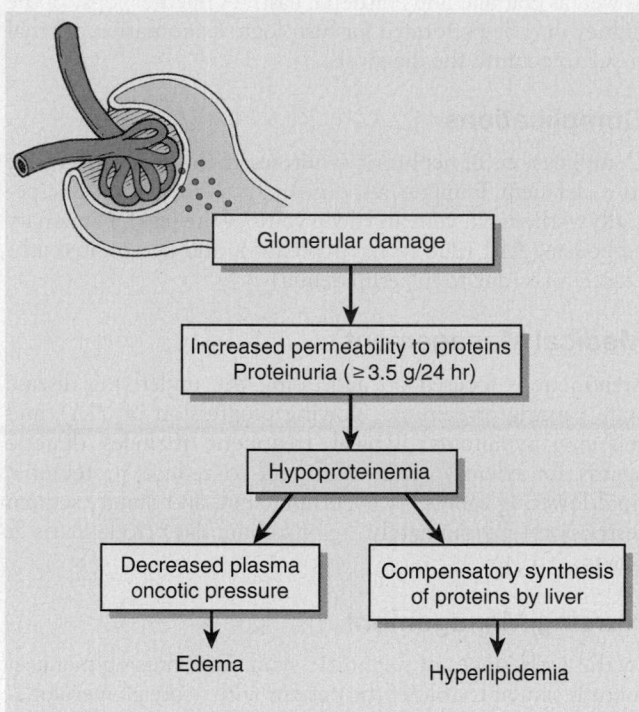

Figure 48-2 • Pathophysiology of the nephrotic syndrome. Reprinted with permission from Norris, T. L. (2019). *Porth's pathophysiology: Concepts of altered health state* (10th ed., Fig. 33-14). Philadelphia, PA: Wolters Kluwer.

The syndrome is apparent in any condition that seriously damages the glomerular capillary membrane and results in increased glomerular permeability to plasma proteins. Although the liver is capable of increasing the production of albumin, it cannot keep up with the daily loss of albumin through the kidneys. Thus, hypoalbuminemia results (see Fig. 48-2).

Pathophysiology

Nephrotic syndrome occurs with many intrinsic kidney diseases and systemic diseases that cause glomerular damage. It is not a specific glomerular disease but a constellation of clinical findings that result from the glomerular damage.

Clinical Manifestations

The major manifestation of nephrotic syndrome is edema. It is usually soft and pitting and commonly occurs around the eyes (periorbital), in dependent areas (sacrum, ankles, and hands), and in the abdomen (ascites). Patients may also exhibit irritability, headache, and malaise.

Assessment and Diagnostic Findings

Proteinuria (predominately albumin) exceeding 3.5 g/day is the hallmark of the diagnosis of nephrotic syndrome. Protein excretion can be measured on a 24-hour urine collection; the normal value is less than 150 mg/day (Kelepouris & Rovin, 2019). Urine protein electrophoresis and immunofixation may be performed to categorize the type of proteinuria. The urine may also contain increased white blood cells (WBCs) as well as granular and epithelial casts. A needle biopsy of the kidney may be performed for histologic examination of renal tissue to confirm the diagnosis.

Complications

Complications of nephrotic syndrome include infection (due to a deficient immune response), thromboembolism (especially of the renal vein and deep veins of the legs), pulmonary embolism, AKI (due to hypovolemia), and accelerated atherosclerosis (due to hyperlipidemia).

Medical Management

Treatment is focused on addressing the underlying disease state causing proteinuria, slowing progression of CKD, and relieving symptoms. Typical treatment includes diuretic agents for edema, ACE inhibitors to reduce proteinuria, lipid-lowering agents for hyperlipidemia, and dietary sodium restriction (approximately 2 g of sodium/day) (Kelepouris & Rovin, 2019).

Nursing Management

In the early stages of nephrotic syndrome, nursing management is similar to that of the patient with acute glomerulonephritis, but as the condition worsens, management is similar to that of the patient with ESKD (see the following section).

Patients with nephrotic syndrome need adequate education about the importance of following all medication and dietary regimens so that their condition can remain stable for as long as possible. Patients must be educated about the importance of promptly communicating any health-related change to their primary providers so that appropriate medication and dietary changes can be made before further changes occur within the glomeruli.

Polycystic Kidney Disease

Polycystic kidney disease (PKD) is a genetic disorder characterized by the growth of numerous fluid-filled cysts in the kidneys, which destroy the nephrons. PKD cysts can profoundly enlarge the kidneys while replacing much of the normal structure, resulting in reduced kidney function and leading to kidney failure (Mahaffey, 2017).

Pathophysiology

Patients with PKD can also have cysts in the liver and pancreas, aneurysms in blood vessels in the brain, and cardiovascular abnormalities. The number of cysts and the resulting complications distinguish PKD from the usually harmless cysts that can form in the kidneys in later years of life.

PKD is the most common inherited genetic cause of kidney failure (Bolignano, Palmer, Ruospo, et al., 2015). Two major inherited forms of PKD exist: autosomal dominant PKD and autosomal recessive PKD.

- Autosomal dominant PKD is the most common inherited form (90%). There are two subtypes. PKD1 has a mutation on chromosome 16 and is the most prevalent form with 78% of patients having this mutation. The second subtype is PKD2 with a mutation on chromosome 4. PKD2 progresses more slowly than PKD1. The average age for patients to progress to ESKD is 54.3 years among patients with PKD1 versus 74.0 years among patients with PKD2 (Torres & Bennett, 2019).
- Autosomal recessive PKD is a rare inherited form (10%) of PKD. Symptoms of autosomal recessive PKD begin in the earliest months of life or in utero. Since the gene is recessive, both parents are carriers but neither parent is affected (Mahaffey, 2017).

Clinical Manifestations

Signs and symptoms of PKD result from loss of renal function and the increasing size of the kidneys as the cysts grow. Kidney damage can result in hematuria, hypertension, and development of renal calculi with associated UTIs and proteinuria. As the cysts grow in size and number, the patient reports increasing abdominal fullness and flank pain (back and lower sides).

Assessment and Diagnostic Findings

PKD is a genetic disease; therefore, a careful evaluation of family history is necessary. Palpation of the abdomen will often reveal enlarged cystic kidneys. Ultrasound imaging of the kidneys is the preferred technique for diagnosis. Genetic testing is performed if imaging results are uncertain (Torres & Bennett, 2019).

Medical Management

PKD has no cure, but tolvaptan slows the decrease in kidney function in patients with PKD. The most common side effects are **polyuria** (excessive urine production) and rare, but potentially serious liver injury, which is most often reversible when the drug is stopped (Comerford & Durkin, 2020). Other treatments are largely supportive and include blood pressure control, pain management, and antibiotic agents to resolve infections. Once the kidneys fail, RRT is indicated (see later discussion in chapter). Genetic studies and counseling may be indicated, particularly when screening family members for potential kidney donation (Torres & Bennett, 2019).

RENAL CANCER

Renal cancer is relatively rare in the United States and accounts for about 4.2% of all cancers. However, an increased incidence of renal cancer at all stages has been noted in the past two decades (National Cancer Institute, 2019). This increase may be due to improved detection as a result of incidental findings during other diagnostic tests. The incidence of renal cell carcinoma is higher in men and in individuals with an increased body mass index. Tobacco use continues to be a significant risk factor (see Chart 48-3). In addition, African Americans have higher rates of renal cancer than Caucasians (Conde & Workman, 2017).

Ninety percent of renal cancers derive from the renal parenchyma and are known as renal cell carcinomas or renal adenocarcinomas. Between 70% and 80% of all renal cell carcinomas are clear cell carcinoma (also known as conventional or nonpapillary) and arise from the proximal renal tubule.

The next most prevalent form (10%) is papillary renal cell carcinomas (American Cancer Society [ACS], 2020). These tumors may metastasize to the lungs, abdominal and mediastinal lymph nodes, brain, bone, and liver; metastatic disease is seen in 30% of patients at diagnosis (ACS, 2020).

Staging is based on tumor size, lymph node involvement, and distant metastasis. The 5-year survival rate based on the stage of renal cancer at diagnosis is 92% with only local involvement, 65% with regional spread, and 12% with distant metastases (Conde & Workman, 2017). Although enhanced imaging techniques account for improved detection of early-stage kidney cancer, it is unknown why the rate of late-stage, metastatic renal cancers is high. Over 50% of renal cancers are found incidentally on radiologic studies in individuals who have no symptoms (Conde & Workman, 2017).

Clinical Manifestations

Many renal tumors produce no symptoms and are discovered on a routine physical examination as a palpable abdominal or flank mass. Signs and symptoms, which occur in only 10% of patients, include hematuria, pain, and a mass in the flank. The usual sign that first calls attention to the tumor is painless hematuria, which may be either intermittent and microscopic, or continuous and overt (gross hematuria) (Conde & Workman, 2017). There may be a dull pain in the back from the pressure produced by compression of the ureter, extension of the tumor into the perirenal area, or hemorrhage into the kidney tissue. Colicky pains occur if a clot or mass of tumor cells passes down the ureter. Symptoms from metastasis may be the first manifestations of a renal tumor and may include unexplained weight loss, fatigue, and anemia.

Assessment and Diagnostic Findings

The diagnosis of a renal tumor may require IV urography, cystoscopic examination, renal angiograms, ultrasonography, or a CT or MRI scan (see Chapter 47). These tests may be exhausting for patients already debilitated by the systemic effects of a tumor as well as for older patients and those who are anxious about the diagnosis and outcome. The nurse assists the patient to prepare physically and psychologically for these procedures and monitors carefully for signs and symptoms of dehydration and impaired coping.

Medical Management

The goal of medical management is to detect the tumor early and to eradicate tumors before metastasis occurs. Treatment most often includes a combination of surgery and pharmacologic management. Radiation therapy may be used for palliation in patients who are not candidates for surgery or other treatments or in those with metastatic disease (ACS, 2020).

Surgical Management

Nephrectomy

Open, laparoscopic, or robotic surgical procedures are utilized for radical and partial nephrectomies (ACS, 2020). A radical nephrectomy is the primary treatment if the tumor can be removed and if the tumor has spread to the inferior vena cava (Conde & Workman, 2017). This includes removal of the kidney (and tumor), adrenal gland, surrounding perinephric fat and Gerota fascia, and lymph nodes. Laparoscopic nephrectomy can be performed for removal of the kidney with a small tumor. This procedure incurs less morbidity and a shorter recovery time. Radiation therapy, hormonal therapy, or immunotherapy may be used along with surgery. Nephron-sparing surgery, or partial nephrectomy, is increasingly being used to treat patients with bilateral tumors, cancer of a functional single kidney, and for small local tumors with a normal contralateral kidney. This is the preferred surgery for local disease as well as for those individuals with risk factors for CKD. The success rate of partial nephrectomies is excellent with operative morbidity and mortality both low (Richie, Atkins, & Chen, 2019).

Renal Artery Embolization

In patients with metastatic renal carcinoma, the renal artery may be occluded to impede the blood supply to the tumor and thus kill the tumor cells. After angiographic studies are completed, a catheter is advanced into the renal artery, and embolizing materials (e.g., Gelfoam, autologous blood clot, steel coils) are injected into the artery and carried with the arterial blood flow to occlude the tumor vessels mechanically. This decreases the local blood supply, making nephrectomy easier. After renal artery embolization and tumor infarction, a characteristic symptom complex called postinfarction syndrome occurs, lasting 2 to 3 days. The patient has pain localized to the flank and abdomen, elevated temperature, and gastrointestinal (GI) symptoms. Pain is treated with parenteral analgesic agents, and acetaminophen is given to control fever. Antiemetic medications, restriction of oral intake, and IV fluids are used to treat the GI symptoms.

Minimally Invasive Technologies

Radiofrequency ablation, cryoablation, or microwave ablation are minimally invasive technologies performed by urologists or interventional radiologists. They are used instead of surgery in select patients for many types of tumors, including renal cell carcinomas. In renal cell carcinomas these nephron-sparing procedures can be used for either small, localized renal tumors, if patients are poor surgical candidates and/or to preserve renal function. In these procedures, temperature extremes are used to kill tumor cells (Hines & Goldberg, 2018).

Pharmacologic Therapy

Depending on the stage of the tumor, partial or radical nephrectomy may be followed by treatment with immunotherapy.

Standard chemotherapy has not improved survival rates and is only used for those patients in whom immunotherapy has not been successful (ACS, 2020). For stage IV clear cell renal cell carcinomas, treatment with biologic response modifiers such as interleukin 2 (IL-2) and interferon has largely been replaced by targeted therapies, antiangiogenic therapy, and checkpoint inhibitors (George & Jonasch, 2019).

Experimental approaches to stimulate the host immune recognition of tumor through autologous tumor cell immunotherapy are being actively pursued in patients with stage IV renal cell carcinomas (George & Jonasch, 2019).

Nursing Management

The patient with a renal tumor usually undergoes extensive diagnostic and therapeutic procedures. Treatments may include surgery, radiation therapy, and immunotherapy. After surgery, the patient usually has catheters and drains in place to maintain a patent urinary tract, to remove drainage, and to permit accurate measurement of urine output. Because of the location of the surgical incision, the patient's position during surgery, and the nature of the surgical procedure, pain and muscle soreness are common. Pharmacologic management may include immunotherapy agents. Therefore, patients are monitored for infection.

The patient requires frequent analgesia during the postoperative period and assistance with turning, coughing, the use of incentive spirometry, and deep breathing to prevent atelectasis and other pulmonary complications (see Chapter 19). The patient and family require assistance and support to cope with the diagnosis and uncertain prognosis. See discussion later in this chapter of postoperative care of the patient undergoing kidney surgery and Chapter 12 for discussion of care of the patient with cancer.

Promoting Home, Community-Based, and Transitional Care

 Educating Patients About Self-Care

The nurse educates the patient and family about how to inspect and care for the incision and to perform other general postoperative care including activity, lifting and driving restrictions, and pain management. Instructions are provided about when to notify the primary provider about problems (e.g., fever, respiratory difficulty, wound drainage, blood in the urine, pain or swelling of the legs).

The nurse encourages the patient to eat a healthy diet and to drink adequate liquids to avoid constipation and to maintain an adequate urine volume. Stool softeners, mild stimulants (e.g., senna), and polyethylene glycol may also be prescribed to avoid constipation. Education and emotional support are provided related to the diagnosis, treatment, and continuing care because many patients are concerned about the loss of the other kidney, the possible need for dialysis, or the recurrence of cancer.

Continuing and Transitional Care

Follow-up care is essential to detect any signs of metastases and to reassure the patient and family about the patient's status and well-being. The patient who has had surgery for renal carcinoma should have a yearly physical examination and chest x-ray, because late metastases are not uncommon

(George & Jonasch, 2019). All subsequent symptoms should be evaluated with possible metastases in mind.

If follow-up immunotherapy is necessary, the patient and family are informed about the treatment plan or immunotherapy protocol, what to expect with each visit, and when to notify the primary provider. Evaluation of remaining renal function (creatinine clearance, BUN, and serum creatinine levels) may also be carried out periodically. A home health nurse may monitor the patient's physical status and psychological well-being and coordinate other indicated services and resources.

KIDNEY DISEASE

Kidney disease results when the kidneys cannot remove the body's metabolic wastes or perform their regulatory functions. The substances normally eliminated in the urine accumulate in the body fluids as a result of impaired renal excretion, affecting endocrine and metabolic functions as well as resulting in fluid, electrolyte, and acid–base disturbances. Kidney disease is a systemic disease and a final common pathway of many different kidney and urinary tract diseases. The impact of kidney failure in the United States continues to increase due to the aging of the U.S. population and the increasing incidence of obesity and diabetes (USRDS, 2019).

Acute Kidney Injury

Acute kidney injury (AKI) is a rapid loss of renal function due to damage to the kidneys. Depending on the duration and severity of AKI, a wide range of potentially life-threatening metabolic complications can occur, including metabolic acidosis as well as fluid and electrolyte imbalances. Treatment is aimed at replacing renal function temporarily to minimize potentially lethal complications and reduce potential causes of increased kidney injury with the goal of minimizing long-term loss of renal function.

AKI is a problem seen in patients who are hospitalized and those in outpatient settings. A widely accepted criterion for AKI is a 50% or greater increase in serum creatinine above baseline (normal creatinine is less than 1 mg/dL) (The Acute Dialysis Quality Initiative, 2004). Urine volume may be normal, or changes may occur including nonoliguria (greater than 800 mL/day), **oliguria** (less than 400 mL/day or 0.5 mL/kg/h over 6 hours), or **anuria** (less than 50 mL/day) (Odom, 2017).

COVID-19 Considerations

The coronavirus disease 2019 (COVID-19) pandemic began in Wuhan, China, in late 2019. Since that time, several risks for both severe acute respiratory syndrome coronavirus 2 (SARS-CoV-2) infection and pathogenesis to COVID-19 have been identified (see Chapter 66, Chart 66-8). Findings from a retrospective, single-center study of 1392 patients hospitalized with COVID-19 in Wuhan, China, reported that 7% developed AKI during hospitalization (Cheng, Luo, Wang, et al., 2020). Factors associated with high risk of developing AKI included more severe disease, a high serum creatinine at baseline, lymphopenia, and elevated D-dimer level (Cheng et al., 2020). Patients who developed AKI were more likely to be admitted to an intensive care unit and had a higher mortality rate compared to patients who did not develop AKI. Of those patients who survived to be discharged from the hospital, 68% recovered from AKI (Cheng et al., 2020).

Pathophysiology

Although the pathogenesis of AKI and oliguria is not always known, many times there is a specific underlying cause. Some of the factors may be reversible if identified and treated promptly, before kidney function is impaired. This is true of the following conditions that reduce blood flow to the kidney and impair kidney function: hypovolemia; hypotension; reduced cardiac output and heart failure; obstruction of the kidney or lower urinary tract by tumor, blood clot, or kidney stone; and bilateral obstruction of the renal arteries or veins. If these conditions are treated and corrected before the kidneys are permanently damaged, the increased BUN and creatinine levels, oliguria, and other signs may be reversed.

Although renal stones are not a common cause of AKI, some recurrent types may increase the risk of AKI. Some hereditary stone diseases (see Chapter 49), primary struvite stones, and infection-related urolithiasis associated with anatomic and functional urinary tract anomalies and spinal cord injury may cause repeated bouts of obstruction as well as crystal-specific damage to tubular epithelial cells and interstitial renal cells (Odom, 2017).

Classifications of Acute Kidney Injury

The term acute kidney injury has replaced the term acute renal failure because it better describes this syndrome, in both those who require RRT and also in those patients who experience minor changes in renal function. Classification criteria for AKI include assessment of three grades of severity and two outcome-level classifications. This 5-point system is known as the RIFLE classification system. RIFLE stands for *risk, injury, failure, loss, and ESKD* (Bellomo et al., 2004). Risk, injury, and failure are considered grades of AKI severity, whereas loss and ESKD are considered outcomes of loss that require some form of RRT, at least temporarily (Bellomo et al., 2004). Table 48-2 lists the classification criteria for the RIFLE system for AKI (Bellomo et al., 2004). This classification system is used by health care professionals to identify kidney injury and improve patient outcomes. A diagnosis of AKI results in significantly longer hospital stays, has an increased mortality rate, and is a major risk factor for the development of CKD (Medel-Herrero, Mitchell, & Moyce, 2019).

Categories of Acute Kidney Injury

The major categories of AKI are prerenal (hypoperfusion of kidney), intrarenal (actual damage to kidney tissue), and postrenal (obstruction to urine flow). Prerenal AKI, which occurs in 60% to 70% of cases, is the result of impaired blood flow that leads to hypoperfusion of the kidney commonly caused by volume depletion (burns, hemorrhage, GI losses), hypotension (sepsis, shock), and obstruction of renal vessels, ultimately leading to a decrease in the GFR (Odom, 2017). Intrarenal or intrinsic AKI is the result of actual parenchymal damage to the glomeruli or kidney tubules. **Acute tubular necrosis (ATN)**, or AKI in which there is damage to the kidney tubules, is the most common type of intrinsic AKI. Characteristics of ATN are intratubular obstruction, tubular back leak (abnormal reabsorption of filtrate and decreased urine

TABLE 48-2	The RIFLE Classification for Acute Kidney Injury	
Class	**GFR Criteria**	**Urinary Output Criteria**
R (Risk)	Increased serum creatinine 1.5 × baseline OR GFR decreased ≥25%	0.5 mL/kg/h for 6 hrs
I (Injury)	Increased serum creatinine 2 × baseline OR GFR decreased ≥50%	0.5 mL/kg/h for 12 hrs
F (Failure)	Increased serum creatinine 3 × baseline OR GFR decreased ≥75% OR Serum creatinine ≥354 mmol/L with an acute rise of at least 44 mmol/L	<0.3 mL/kg/h for 24 hrs OR Anuria for 12 hrs
L (Loss)	Persistent acute kidney injury = complete loss of kidney function >4 wks	
E (ESKD)	ESKD >3 mo	

ESKD, end-stage kidney disease; GFR, glomerular filtration rate.
Adapted from Bellomo, R., Ronco, C., Kellum, J. A., et al. (2004). Acute renal failure-definition, outcome measures, animal models, fluid therapy and information technology needs: the Second International Consensus Conference of the Acute Dialysis Quality Initiative (ADQI) Group. *Critical Care, 8*, B204.

flow through the tubule), vasoconstriction, and changes in glomerular permeability. These processes result in a decrease of GFR, progressive azotemia, and fluid and electrolyte imbalances. CKD, diabetes, heart failure, hypertension, and cirrhosis can contribute to ATN. Postrenal AKI usually results from obstruction distal to the kidney by conditions such as renal calculi, strictures, blood clots, benign prostatic hyperplasia, malignancies, and pregnancy. Pressure rises in the kidney tubules, and eventually the GFR decreases. Common causes of each type of AKI are further summarized in Chart 48-4.

Phases of Acute Kidney Injury

There are four phases of AKI: initiation, oliguria, diuresis, and recovery.

- The initiation period begins with the initial insult and ends when oliguria develops.
- The oliguria period is accompanied by an increase in the serum concentration of substances usually excreted by the kidneys (urea, creatinine, uric acid, organic acids, phosphorus, and the intracellular cations [potassium and magnesium]). The minimum amount of urine needed to rid the body of normal metabolic waste products is approximately 400 mL in 24 hours or 0.5 mL/kg/h over 6 hours. In this phase, uremic symptoms first appear and life-threatening conditions such as hyperkalemia develop.
- The diuresis period is marked by a gradual increase in urine output, which signals that glomerular filtration has started to recover. Laboratory values stabilize and eventually decrease. Although the volume of urinary output may

---

Chart 48-4 — Causes of Acute Kidney Injury

Prerenal Failure

- Volume depletion resulting from:
  - Gastrointestinal losses (vomiting, diarrhea, nasogastric suction)
  - Hemorrhage
  - Renal losses (diuretic agents, osmotic diuresis)
- Impaired cardiac efficiency resulting from:
  - Arrhythmias
  - Cardiogenic shock
  - Heart failure
  - Myocardial infarction
- Vasodilation resulting from:
  - Anaphylaxis
  - Antihypertensive medications or other medications that cause vasodilation
  - Sepsis

Intrarenal Failure

- Prolonged renal ischemia resulting from:
  - Hemoglobinuria (transfusion reaction, hemolytic anemia)
  - Pigment nephropathy (associated with the breakdown of blood cells containing pigments that in turn occlude kidney structures)

- Rhabdomyolysis/myoglobinuria (trauma, crush injuries, burns)
- Nephrotoxic agents such as:
  - Aminoglycoside antibiotics (gentamicin, tobramycin)
  - Angiotensin-converting enzyme inhibitors
  - Heavy metals (lead, mercury)
  - Nonsteroidal anti-inflammatory drugs
  - Radiopaque contrast agents
  - Solvents and chemicals (ethylene glycol, carbon tetrachloride, arsenic)
- Infectious processes such as:
  - Acute glomerulonephritis
  - Acute pyelonephritis

Postrenal Failure

- Urinary tract obstruction, including:
  - Benign prostatic hyperplasia
  - Blood clots
  - Calculi (stones)
  - Strictures
  - Tumors

Adapted from Norris, T. L. (2019). *Porth's pathophysiology: Concepts of altered health states* (10th ed.). Philadelphia, PA: Wolters Kluwer.

---

reach normal or elevated levels, renal function may still be markedly abnormal, since the filtration of urea and creatinine has not yet commenced. Because uremic symptoms may still be present, the need for expert medical and nursing management continues. The patient must be observed closely for dehydration during this phase; if dehydration occurs, the uremic symptoms are likely to increase and an elevated serum BUN and creatinine will be noted.

- The recovery period signals the improvement of renal function and may take 3 to 12 months. Laboratory values return to the patient's normal level. Although a permanent 1% to 3% reduction in the GFR may occur, it is not clinically significant. However, in those patients with preexisting CKD, an episode of AKI may necessitate beginning CRRT.

Some patients have decreased renal function with increasing nitrogen retention but actually excrete normal amounts of urine (1 to 2 L/day). This is the nonoliguric form of kidney injury and occurs predominantly after exposure of the patient to **nephrotoxic** agents (any substance or medication that damages kidney tissue), burns and traumatic injury.

Clinical Manifestations

Almost every system of the body is affected with failure of the normal renal regulatory mechanisms. The patient may appear critically ill and lethargic. Central nervous system signs and symptoms include drowsiness, headache, muscle twitching, and seizures. Table 48-3 summarizes common clinical characteristics in all three categories of AKI.

TABLE 48-3 — Comparing Clinical Characteristics of Acute Kidney Injury

Characteristics	Categories		
	Prerenal	Intrarenal	Postrenal
Etiology	Hypoperfusion due to shock, hypovolemia	Parenchymal damage	Obstruction
Blood urea nitrogen value	↑ (out of normal 20:1 proportion to creatinine)	↑	↑
Creatinine	↑	↑	↑
Urine output	↓	Varies, often ↓	Varies, may be ↓, or sudden anuria
Urine sodium	↓ to <20 mEq/L	↑ to >40 mEq/L	Varies, often ↓ to ≤20 mEq/L
Urinary sediment	Normal, few hyaline casts	Abnormal casts and debris	Usually normal
Urine osmolality	↑ to 500 mOsm	~350 mOsm, similar to serum	Varies, ↑ or equal to serum
Urine specific gravity	↑	Low normal	Varies

↑, increased; ↓, decreased.

Assessment and Diagnostic Findings

Assessment of the patient with AKI includes evaluation for changes in the urine, diagnostic tests that evaluate the kidney contour, and a variety of laboratory values. See Chapter 47 for information about the normal characteristics of urine, diagnostic findings, and laboratory values in the renal system.

In AKI, urine output varies from scanty to a normal volume, hematuria may be present, and the urine has a low specific gravity (compared with a normal value of 1.010 to 1.025). One of the earliest manifestations of tubular damage is the inability to concentrate the urine (Odom, 2017). Patients with prerenal azotemia have a decreased amount of sodium in the urine (less than 20 mEq/L) and normal urinary sediment. Patients with intrarenal azotemia usually have increased urinary sodium levels greater than 40 mEq/L with **urinary casts** and other cellular debris.

Ultrasonography is a critical component of the evaluation of patients with kidney disease. A renal sonogram or a non-contrast CT scan may show evidence of anatomic changes.

The BUN level increases steadily at a rate that depends on the degree of catabolism (breakdown of protein), renal perfusion, and protein intake. Serum creatinine levels are useful in monitoring kidney function and disease progression and increase with glomerular damage.

With a decline in the GFR, oliguria, and anuria, patients are at high risk for hyperkalemia. Protein catabolism results in the release of cellular potassium into the body fluids, causing severe hyperkalemia (high serum potassium levels). Hyperkalemia may lead to cardiac arrhythmias, such as ventricular tachycardia and cardiac arrest. Sources of potassium include normal tissue catabolism, dietary intake, blood in the GI tract, or blood transfusion and other sources (e.g., IV infusions, potassium penicillin, and extracellular shift in response to metabolic acidosis).

Progressive metabolic acidosis occurs in kidney disease because patients cannot eliminate the daily metabolic load of acid-type substances produced by the normal metabolic processes. In addition, normal renal buffering mechanisms fail. This is reflected by decreased serum carbon dioxide (CO_2) and pH levels.

Blood phosphorus concentrations may increase; calcium levels may be low due to decreased absorption of calcium from the intestine and as a compensatory mechanism for the elevated blood phosphate levels. Anemia is another common laboratory finding in AKI, as a result of reduced erythropoietin production, uremic GI lesions, reduced RBC lifespan, and blood loss from the GI tract.

Prevention

AKI has a high mortality rate that ranges from 10% to 80%. Factors that influence mortality include severity of kidney injury, level and availability of medical care, requirements for RRT, increased age, increased number of comorbid conditions, and preexisting kidney and vascular diseases and respiratory failure (Odom, 2017). Therefore, prevention of AKI is essential (see Chart 48-5).

A careful history is obtained to identify exposure to nephrotoxic agents or environmental toxins. The kidneys are susceptible to the adverse effects of medications because the metabolic by-products of most medications are excreted by

---

Chart 48-5 | **Preventing Acute Kidney Injury**

- Continually assess renal function (urine output, laboratory values) when appropriate.
- Monitor central venous and arterial pressures and hourly urine output of patients who are critically ill to detect the onset of kidney dysfunction as early as possible.
- Pay special attention to wounds, burns, and other precursors of sepsis.
- Prevent and treat infections promptly. Infections can produce progressive kidney damage.
- Prevent and treat hypotensive shock promptly with blood and fluid replacement.
- Provide adequate hydration to patients at risk for dehydration, including:
  - Before, during, and after surgery
  - Patients undergoing intensive diagnostic studies requiring fluid restriction and contrast agents (e.g., barium enema, IV pyelograms), especially older patients who may have marginal renal reserve or CKD
  - Patients with neoplastic disorders or disorders of metabolism (e.g., gout) and those receiving chemotherapy with potential tumor lysis syndrome
  - Patients with skeletal muscle injuries (e.g., crush injuries, compartment syndrome)
  - Patients with heat-induced illnesses (e.g., heat stroke, heat exhaustion)
- To prevent infections from ascending in the urinary tract, give meticulous care to patients with indwelling catheters. Remove catheters as soon as possible.
- To prevent toxic drug effects, closely monitor dosage, duration of use, and blood levels of all medications metabolized or excreted by the kidneys.

---

the kidneys. Patients taking nephrotoxic medications (e.g., aminoglycosides, such as gentamicin and tobramycin, polymyxin B, amphotericin B, vancomycin, amikacin, cyclosporine, tacrolimus) should have drug levels monitored closely, since high serum levels will cause changes in renal function. Kidney function needs to be monitored prior to initiation of these medications and during therapy (Schira, 2017).

Chronic use of analgesic agents, particularly NSAIDs, may cause **interstitial nephritis** (inflammation within the renal tissue) and papillary necrosis. Patients with heart failure or cirrhosis with ascites are at particular risk for NSAID-induced kidney disease. Increased age, preexisting kidney disease, diabetes, and the simultaneous administration of several nephrotoxic agents increase the risk of kidney damage (Schira, 2017; Schonder, 2017).

Contrast-induced acute kidney injury is a major cause of hospital-acquired AKI. However, this is potentially preventable in many, but not all, cases. Patients at high risk for the development of contrast-induced AKI are those with CKD and/or elevated creatinine due to dehydration. Those who need to undergo a coronary interventional procedure, which requires larger amounts of contrast media to be given, are at the greatest risk. Limiting the patient's exposure to contrast agents and nephrotoxic medications will reduce the risk of contrasted-induced AKI. Prehydration with IV normal saline is considered the most effective method to prevent contrast-induced AKI. N-acetylcysteine administration is no longer recommended as a preventative measure (Nahar, 2017).

Gerontologic Considerations

About half of all patients who develop AKI during hospitalization are older than 60 years and 40% have diabetes (Pavkov, Harding, & Burrows, 2018). The etiology of AKI in older adults includes prerenal causes such as dehydration, intrarenal causes such as nephrotoxic agents (e.g., medications, contrast agents), and complications of major surgery (Hain, 2017). Suppression of thirst, enforced bed rest, lack of access to drinking water, and confusion all contribute to the older patient's failure to consume adequate fluids and may lead to dehydration, further compromising already decreased renal function.

AKI in older adults is also often seen in the community setting. Nurses in the ambulatory setting need to be aware of the risk to patients taking medications that could result in damage to the kidney either through reduced circulation or nephrotoxicity. Outpatient procedures that require fasting or a bowel preparation may cause dehydration and, therefore, patients undergoing such procedures need careful monitoring.

Medical Management

The kidneys have a remarkable ability to recover from insult. The objectives of treatment for AKI are to restore normal chemical balance and prevent complications until repair of renal tissue and restoration of renal function can occur. Management includes eliminating the underlying cause; maintaining fluid balance; avoiding fluid excesses; and, when indicated, providing RRT. Prerenal azotemia is treated by optimizing renal perfusion, whereas postrenal failure is treated by relieving the obstruction. Intrarenal or intrinsic azotemia is treated with supportive therapy, with removal of causative agents, aggressive management of pre- and postrenal failure, and avoidance of associated risk factors. Shock and infection, if present, are treated promptly (see Chapter 11). The patient who has had a crush injury, compartment syndrome, or heat-induced illness with subsequent myoglobinuria (myoglobin in the urine) is treated for rhabdomyolysis (Odom, 2017) (see Chapter 67).

Maintenance of fluid balance is based on daily body weight, serial measurements of central venous pressure, serum and urine concentrations, fluid intake and output, blood pressure, and the clinical status of the patient. The parenteral and oral intake and the output of urine, gastric drainage, stools, wound drainage, and perspiration are calculated and are used as the basis for fluid replacement. The insensible fluid produced through the normal metabolic processes and lost through the skin and lungs is also considered in fluid management.

Fluid excesses can be detected by the clinical findings of dyspnea, tachycardia, and distended neck veins. The patient's lungs are auscultated for moist crackles. Because pulmonary edema may be caused by excessive administration of parenteral fluids, extreme caution must be used to prevent fluid overload. The development of generalized edema is assessed by examining the presacral and pretibial areas several times daily. Furosemide or bumetanide, both loop diuretics, may be prescribed to initiate diuresis, although there is no consensus regarding the use of loop diuretics in AKI (Odom, 2017).

Adequate renal blood flow in patients with prerenal causes of AKI may be restored by IV fluids or transfusions of blood products. If AKI is caused by hypovolemia secondary to hypoproteinemia, an infusion of albumin may be prescribed. Dialysis may be initiated to prevent complications of AKI, such as hyperkalemia, metabolic acidosis, pericarditis, and pulmonary edema. Dialysis corrects many biochemical abnormalities; allows for liberalization of fluid, protein, and sodium intake; diminishes bleeding tendencies; and promotes wound healing. **Hemodialysis (HD)** (a procedure that circulates the patient's blood through an artificial kidney [dialyzer] to remove waste products and excess fluid), **peritoneal dialysis (PD)**; a procedure that uses the patient's peritoneal membrane (the lining of the peritoneal cavity) as the semipermeable membrane to exchange fluid and solutes, or a variety of **continuous renal replacement therapy (CRRT)** (methods used to replace normal kidney function by circulating the patient's blood through a hemofilter) may be performed (Odom, 2017). These and other treatment modalities for patients with renal dysfunction are discussed later in this chapter.

Pharmacologic Therapy

Hyperkalemia is the most life-threatening of the fluid and electrolyte changes that occur in patients with kidney disorders. Therefore, the patient is monitored for hyperkalemia through serial serum electrolyte levels (potassium value greater than 5.0 mEq/L [5 mmol/L]), ECG changes (tall, tented, or peaked T waves), and changes in clinical status (see Chapter 10). Other symptoms of hyperkalemia include irritability, abdominal cramping, diarrhea, paresthesia, and generalized muscle weakness. Muscle weakness may present as slurred speech, difficulty breathing, paresthesia, and paralysis. As the potassium level increases, both cardiac and other muscular function declines, making this a medical emergency.

The elevated potassium levels may be reduced by administering cation-exchange resins such as sodium polystyrene sulfonate orally or by retention enema that works by exchanging sodium ions for potassium ions in the intestinal tract. The slow onset of action of more than 6 hours limits its use to those patients without emergent hyperkalemia causing ECG changes. Sorbitol may be given in combination with sodium polystyrene sulfonate to induce a diarrhea-type effect (by inducing water loss in the GI tract). If a sodium polystyrene sulfonate retention enema is given (the colon is the major site of potassium exchange), a rectal catheter with a balloon may be used to facilitate retention if necessary (Schonder, 2017). Afterward, a cleansing enema may be prescribed to remove remaining medication as a precaution against fecal impaction.

If the patient is experiencing ECG changes, IV dextrose 50%, insulin, and calcium replacement may be given to shift potassium back into the cells. Since the medications are administered IV, they take effect quickly. The shift of potassium into the intracellular space is temporary, so arrangements for dialysis need to be made on an emergent basis. The capillary glucose level is monitored for hypoglycemia with insulin administration (Ross, Nissenson, & Daugirdas, 2015).

Many medications are eliminated through the kidneys; therefore, dosages must be reduced when a patient has AKI. Examples of commonly used agents that require adjustment are antibiotic medications (especially aminoglycosides), digoxin, phenytoin, ACE inhibitors, and magnesium-containing agents.

In patients with severe acidosis, the arterial blood gases and serum bicarbonate levels must be monitored because the patient may require sodium bicarbonate therapy or dialysis. If respiratory problems develop, appropriate ventilatory measures must be instituted. The elevated serum phosphorus level may be controlled with phosphate-binding agents (e.g., calcium or lanthanum carbonate) that help prevent a continuing rise in serum phosphorus levels by binding with the phosphate from food in the intestinal tract and eliminating it in the stool, thus preventing absorption (Schonder, 2017).

Nutritional Therapy

AKI causes severe nutritional imbalances (because nausea and vomiting contribute to inadequate dietary intake), impaired glucose use and protein synthesis, and increased tissue catabolism. The patient is weighed daily and loses 0.2 to 0.5 kg (0.5 to 1 lb) daily if the nitrogen balance is negative (i.e., caloric intake falls below caloric requirements). If the patient gains or does not lose weight or develops hypertension, fluid retention should be suspected.

Nutritional support is based on the underlying cause of AKI, the catabolic response, the type and frequency of RRT, comorbidities, and nutritional status. Replacement of dietary proteins is individualized to provide the maximum benefit and minimize uremic symptoms. Caloric requirements are met with high-carbohydrate meals, because carbohydrates have a protein-sparing effect (i.e., in a high-carbohydrate diet, protein is not used for meeting energy requirements but is "spared" for growth and tissue healing). Foods and fluids containing sodium, potassium, or phosphorus (e.g., bananas, citrus fruits and juices, dairy foods) are restricted.

The oliguric phase of AKI may last 10 to 14 days and is followed by the diuretic phase, at which time urine output begins to increase, signaling the patient is in the recovery phase (Odom, 2017). Results of blood chemistry tests are used to determine the amounts of sodium, potassium, and water needed for replacement, along with assessment for over- or under hydration (daily weights). Following the diuretic phase, the patient is placed on a high-protein, high-calorie diet and is encouraged to resume activities gradually.

Nursing Management

The nurse has an important role in caring for the patient with AKI. The nurse monitors for complications, participates in emergency treatment of fluid and electrolyte imbalances, assesses the patient's progress and response to treatment, and provides physical and emotional support. In addition, the nurse keeps family members informed about the patient's condition, helps them understand the treatments, and provides psychological support. Although the development of AKI may be the most serious problem, the nurse continues to provide nursing care indicated for the primary disorder (e.g., burns, shock, trauma, obstruction of the urinary tract).

Monitoring Fluid and Electrolyte Balance

Because of the serious fluid and electrolyte imbalances that can occur with AKI, the nurse monitors the patient's serum electrolyte levels and physical indicators of these complications during all phases of the disorder. IV solutions must be carefully selected based on the patient's fluid and electrolyte status. The patient's cardiac function and musculoskeletal status are monitored closely for signs of hyperkalemia.

Quality and Safety Nursing Alert

Hyperkalemia is the most immediate life-threatening imbalance seen in AKI. Parenteral fluids, all oral intake, and all medications are screened carefully to ensure that sources of potassium are not inadvertently given or consumed.

The nurse monitors fluid status by paying careful attention to fluid intake (IV medications should be given in the smallest volume possible), urine output, apparent edema, distention of the jugular veins, alterations in heart sounds and breath sounds, and increasing difficulty in breathing. Accurate daily weights, as well as I&O records, are essential. Indicators of deteriorating fluid and electrolyte status are reported immediately to the primary provider, and preparation is made for emergency treatment. Severe fluid and electrolyte disturbances may be treated with HD, PD, or CRRT.

Reducing Metabolic Rate

The nurse takes steps to reduce the patient's metabolic rate. Fever and infection, both of which increase the metabolic rate and catabolism, are prevented and treated promptly; blood, urine and wound cultures are ordered as indicated.

Promoting Pulmonary Function

Attention is given to pulmonary function, and the patient is assisted to turn, cough, and take deep breaths frequently to prevent atelectasis and respiratory tract infection. Drowsiness and lethargy may prevent the patient from moving and turning without encouragement and assistance.

Preventing Infection

Asepsis is essential with invasive lines and catheters to minimize the risk of infection and increased metabolism. An indwelling urinary catheter is avoided whenever possible due to the high risk of UTI associated with its use, but may be required to provide ongoing data required to accurately monitor fluid I&O.

Providing Skin Care

The skin may be dry or susceptible to breakdown as a result of edema; therefore, meticulous skin care is important. In addition, excoriation and itching of the skin may result from the deposit of irritating toxins in the patient's tissues. Bathing the patient with cool water, frequent turning, and keeping the skin clean and well moisturized and the fingernails trimmed to avoid scratching are often comforting and prevent skin breakdown.

Providing Psychosocial Support

The patient with AKI may require treatment with HD, PD, or CRRT. The length of time that these treatments are necessary varies with the cause and extent of damage to the kidneys. The patient and family need assistance, explanation, and support during this period. The purpose of the treatment is explained to the patient and family by the primary provider. However, high levels of anxiety and fear may necessitate repeated explanation and clarification by the nurse. The family members may initially be afraid to touch and talk to the patient during these procedures but should be encouraged and assisted to do so.

In an intensive care setting, many of the nurse's functions are devoted to the technical aspects of patient care; however, it is essential that the psychological needs and other concerns of the patient and family be addressed. Continued assessment of the patient for complications of AKI and precipitating causes is essential (Odom, 2017).

End-Stage Kidney Disease or Chronic Kidney Disease

When a patient has sustained enough kidney damage to require RRT on a permanent basis, the patient has moved into the fifth or final stage of CKD, also referred to as ESKD. In 2017, 86.9% of patients newly diagnosed with ESKD began RRT with HD, 10.1% started with PD, and 2.9% received a preemptive kidney transplant. A preemptive transplant is when a patient undergoes kidney transplantation from a living donor before dialysis is initiated. Of great concern is that 33% of patients diagnosed with ESKD had received little or no pre-ESKD nephrology care and 19.2% received no nephrology care prior to requiring RRT. As of December 31, 2017, 62.7% of all patients previously diagnosed with ESKD were receiving HD therapy, 7.1% were being treated with PD, and 29.9% had a functioning kidney transplant. Among patients being treated with HD, 98.0% used in-center HD (USRDS, 2019).

In July 2019, the President, the U.S. Department of Health and Human Services (HHS) Secretary, and the Administrator of the Centers for Medicare and Medicaid Services (CMS) issued an Executive Order, with the goal of improving the lives of Americans with ESKD by expanding treatment options and reducing health care costs. As part of this Executive Order, a mandatory payment model promotes moving patients from in-center to home dialysis (both PD and home HD) and increasing the number of patients receiving kidney transplants. There is much work and policy development that will need to be done to reach this goal by the projected date of 2025 (Kear, Bednarski, Smith, et al., 2019).

Pathophysiology

As renal function declines, the end products of protein metabolism (normally excreted in urine) accumulate in the blood. Uremia develops and adversely affects every system in the body. The greater the buildup of waste products, the more pronounced the symptoms.

The rate of decline in renal function and progression of ESKD is related to the underlying disorder, the urinary excretion of protein, and the presence of hypertension. The disease tends to progress more rapidly in patients who excrete significant amounts of protein or have elevated blood pressure than in those without these conditions (Mahaffey, 2017).

Clinical Manifestations

Because virtually every body system is affected in ESKD, patients exhibit a number of signs and symptoms. The severity of these signs and symptoms depends in part on the degree of renal impairment, other underlying conditions, and the patient's age. Cardiovascular disease is the predominant cause of death in patients with ESKD (Subbiah et al., 2016). Peripheral neuropathy, a disorder of the peripheral nervous system, is present in some patients, especially those with diabetes. Patients complain of severe pain and discomfort. Restless leg syndrome and burning feet can occur in the early

stage of uremic peripheral neuropathy. The precise mechanisms for many of these systemic signs and symptoms have not been identified. However, it is generally thought that the accumulation of uremic waste products is the probable cause. Chart 48-6 summarizes the systemic signs and symptoms.

Assessment and Diagnostic Findings

Glomerular Filtration Rate

As the GFR decreases (due to nonfunctioning glomeruli), the creatinine clearance decreases, whereas the serum creatinine and BUN levels increase. Serum creatinine is a more sensitive indicator of renal function than BUN. The BUN is affected not only by kidney disease but also by protein intake in the diet, catabolism (tissue and RBC breakdown), parenteral nutrition, and medications such as corticosteroids.

Sodium and Water Retention

The kidney cannot concentrate or dilute the urine normally in ESKD. Appropriate responses by the kidney to changes in the daily intake of water and electrolytes, therefore, do not occur. Some patients retain sodium and water, increasing the risk for edema, heart failure, and hypertension. Hypertension may also result from activation of the renin–angiotensin–aldosterone axis and the concomitant increased aldosterone secretion. Other patients have a tendency to lose sodium and run the risk of developing hypotension and hypovolemia. Vomiting and diarrhea may cause water depletion, which may worsen the uremic state.

Acidosis

Metabolic acidosis occurs in ESKD because the kidneys are unable to excrete increased loads of acid. Decreased acid secretion results from the inability of the kidney tubules to excrete ammonia (NH_3^-) and to reabsorb sodium bicarbonate (HCO_3^-). There is also decreased excretion of phosphorus and other organic acids.

Anemia

Anemia develops as a result of inadequate erythropoietin production, the shortened lifespan of RBCs, nutritional deficiencies, and the patient's tendency to bleed, particularly from the GI tract. Erythropoietin, a substance normally produced by the kidneys, stimulates bone marrow to produce RBCs. In ESKD, erythropoietin production decreases and profound anemia results, producing fatigue, angina, and shortness of breath (Evans, 2017).

Calcium and Phosphorus Imbalance

Another abnormality seen in ESKD is a disorder in calcium and phosphorus metabolism. Serum calcium and phosphate levels have a reciprocal relationship in the body: As one increases, the other decreases. With a decrease in filtration through the glomerulus of the kidney, there is an increase in the serum phosphorus level and a reciprocal or corresponding decrease in the serum calcium level. The decreased serum calcium level causes increased secretion of parathormone from the parathyroid glands. However, in kidney disease, the body cannot respond normally to the increased secretion of parathormone. As a result, calcium leaves the bone, often producing bone changes and bone disease as well as calcification of major blood vessels in the body. In addition, the active

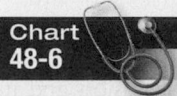

Chart 48-6

ASSESSMENT
Assessing for End-Stage Kidney Disease

Be alert to the following signs and symptoms:

Neurologic

- Asterixis
- Behavior changes
- Burning of soles of feet
- Confusion
- Disorientation
- Inability to concentrate
- Restlessness of legs
- Seizures
- Tremors
- Weakness and fatigue

Integumentary

- Coarse, thinning hair
- Dry, flaky skin
- Ecchymosis
- Gray-bronze skin color
- Pruritus
- Purpura
- Thin, brittle nails

Cardiovascular

- Engorged neck veins
- Hyperkalemia
- Hyperlipidemia
- Hypertension
- Pericardial effusion
- Pericardial friction rub
- Pericardial tamponade
- Pericarditis
- Periorbital edema
- Pitting edema (feet, hands, sacrum)

Pulmonary

- Crackles
- Depressed cough reflex
- Kussmaul-type respirations
- Pleuritic pain
- Shortness of breath
- Tachypnea
- Thick, tenacious sputum
- Uremic pneumonitis

Gastrointestinal

- Ammonia odor to breath ("uremic fetor")
- Anorexia, nausea, and vomiting
- Bleeding from gastrointestinal tract
- Constipation or diarrhea
- Hiccups
- Metallic taste
- Mouth ulcerations and bleeding

Hematologic

- Anemia
- Thrombocytopenia

Reproductive

- Amenorrhea
- Decreased libido
- Infertility
- Testicular atrophy

Musculoskeletal

- Bone fractures
- Bone pain
- Foot drop
- Loss of muscle strength
- Muscle cramps
- Renal osteodystrophy

Adapted from Weber, J. R., & Kelley, J. H. (2018). *Health assessment in nursing* (6th ed.). Philadelphia, PA: Wolters Kluwer.

---

metabolite of vitamin D (1,25-dihydroxycholecalciferol) normally manufactured by the kidney decreases as kidney disease progresses (Brooks, 2017). Uremic bone disease, often called renal osteodystrophy, develops from the complex changes in calcium, phosphate, and parathormone balance. There is also evidence of calcification of blood vessels.

Complications

There are a number of potential complications of ESKD that necessitate a collaborative approach to care. These include the following:

- Anemia due to decreased erythropoietin production, decreased RBC lifespan, bleeding in the GI tract from irritating toxins and ulcer formation, and blood loss in the dialysis circuit and dialyzer after HD has been completed
- Bone disease and metastatic and vascular calcifications due to retention of phosphorus, low serum calcium levels, and abnormal vitamin D metabolism
- Hyperkalemia due to decreased excretion, metabolic acidosis, catabolism, and excessive potassium intake from diet, medications, or IV solutions

- Hypertension due to sodium and water retention and malfunction of the renin–angiotensin–aldosterone system
- Pericarditis, pericardial effusion, and pericardial tamponade due to retention of uremic waste products and inadequate dialysis

Medical Management

The goal of management is to maintain kidney function and homeostasis for as long as possible. All factors that contribute to ESKD and all factors that are reversible (e.g., obstruction) are identified and treated. Management is accomplished primarily with medications and diet therapy, although dialysis may also be needed to decrease the level of uremic waste products in the blood and to control electrolyte balance. The close collaboration of a renal dietitian is essential in dietary therapy.

Pharmacologic Therapy

Complications can be prevented or delayed with the appropriate medication. Phosphate-binding agents, calcium and vitamin D supplements, antihypertensive and cardiac medications, as well as recombinant human erythropoietin are frequently prescribed (Parikh et al., 2019).

Calcium and Phosphorus Binders

Hyperphosphatemia and hypocalcemia are treated with medications that bind dietary phosphorus in the GI tract. Binders such as calcium carbonate or calcium acetate are prescribed, but there is a risk of hypercalcemia. If calcium is high or the calcium–phosphorus product exceeds 55 mg/dL, a polymeric phosphate binder such as sevelamer carbonate may be prescribed (Schonder, 2017). This medication binds dietary phosphorus in the intestinal tract; one to four tablets are given with the first bite of food to be effective.

Antihypertensive and Cardiovascular Agents

Hypertension is managed by intravascular volume control and a variety of antihypertensive agents (Schonder, 2017). Heart failure and pulmonary edema may also require treatment with fluid restriction, low-sodium diets, diuretic agents, inotropic agents, and dialysis. The metabolic acidosis of ESKD usually produces no symptoms and requires no treatment. However, sodium bicarbonate supplements or dialysis may be needed to correct the acidosis if it causes symptoms.

Erythropoietin

Anemia associated with ESKD is treated with erythrocyte-stimulating agents (recombinant human erythropoietin). Patients with anemia present with nonspecific symptoms, such as malaise, general fatigability, and decreased activity tolerance. Erythrocyte stimulation therapy is initiated to achieve a target hemoglobin of 10 to 11 g/dL, which generally alleviates many of the symptoms of anemia without causing an increased risk of death and cardiovascular complications (Evans, 2017; Schonder, 2017).

Recombinant human erythropoietin may be administered IV or subcutaneously once or three times a week in ESKD. It will take 2 to 6 weeks for the hemoglobin to increase. Therefore, the medication is not indicated for patients who need immediate correction of severe anemia. Adverse effects seen with erythropoietin therapy include hypertension (especially during early stages of treatment), increased clotting of vascular access sites, seizures, cardiovascular events, and depletion of body iron stores (Evans, 2017; Schonder, 2017).

Management involves adjustment of heparin to prevent clotting of the lines during HD treatments and monitoring of hemoglobin and hematocrit, serum iron and transferrin levels. Prior to beginning therapy, iron studies are indicated and if iron deficiency is noted, a course of IV iron is prescribed since adequate stores of iron are needed for an adequate response. In addition, vitamin deficiencies are ruled out including folate or vitamin B_{12}. Common iron supplements include iron sucrose and ferric gluconate (Evans, 2017).

In addition, the patient's blood pressure and serum potassium level are monitored to detect hypertension and increasing serum potassium levels, which may occur with therapy and the increasing RBC mass. Recombinant erythropoietin therapy should be used cautiously in patients with uncontrolled hypertension (Schonder, 2017). The occurrence of hypertension requires initiation or adjustment of the patient's antihypertensive therapy.

Patients who have received erythropoietin therapy have reported decreased levels of fatigue, increased feelings of well-being, better tolerance of dialysis, higher-energy levels, and improved exercise tolerance (Evans, 2017). In addition, this therapy has decreased the need for transfusion and its associated risks, including bloodborne infectious disease, antibody formation, and iron overload (Evans, 2017).

Nutritional Therapy

A referral to a renal dietitian is essential. Dietary intervention is necessary with deterioration of renal function and includes careful regulation of protein intake, fluid intake to balance fluid losses, and restriction of potassium and sodium. At the same time, adequate caloric intake and vitamin supplementation must be ensured. Patients on dialysis need a higher intake of protein than healthy adults and current protein recommendations for stable patients on HD is 1.2 g/kg/day and PD is 1.2 to 1.3 g/kg/day (National Kidney Foundation Kidney Disease Outcomes Quality Initiative [NKF KDOQI], 2000). The allowed protein must be of high-biologic value (eggs, meats, fish). High–biologic-value proteins are those that are complete proteins and supply the essential amino acids necessary for growth and cell repair.

Usually, the fluid allowance per day for patients who receive in-center HD who are anuric is about 1000 mL daily. For those who produce urine, recommendations are individualized based on the patient's 24-hour urinary volume. This is done in order to limit interdialytic weight gains to less than 4% of estimated dry weight (Gonyea, 2017). Adequate calories are supplied by carbohydrates, protein, and fat to prevent wasting. In addition, the patient on dialysis loses water-soluble vitamins during the dialysis treatment, so an oral vitamin B and C supplement is prescribed to be taken after dialysis.

Hyperkalemia is usually prevented by ensuring adequate dialysis treatments with potassium removal and careful restriction of diet, medications, and fluids for their potassium content.

Dialysis

The patient with increasing symptoms of kidney disease is referred to a dialysis and transplantation center early in the course of progressive kidney disease. Dialysis is usually initiated when the patient cannot maintain a reasonable quality of life with conservative treatment.

Nursing Management

The patient with ESKD requires astute nursing care to avoid the complications of reduced renal function and the stresses and anxieties of dealing with a life-threatening illness.

Nursing care is directed toward assessing fluid status and identifying potential sources of imbalance, working with a renal dietitian to implement a dietary program to ensure proper nutritional intake within the limits of the treatment regimen, and engaging the patient by encouraging increased self-care and greater independence. It is extremely important to provide explanations and information to the patient and family concerning ESKD, treatment options, and potential complications. A great deal of emotional support is needed by the patient and family because of the numerous changes experienced. A social worker is also a vital part of the interprofessional care at the dialysis center. Specific interventions, along with rationale and evaluation criteria, are presented in more detail in the plan of nursing care for the patient with ESKD (see Chart 48-7).

(text continued on page 1576)

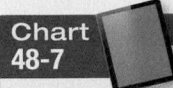

Chart 48-7 PLAN OF NURSING CARE
The Patient with End-Stage Kidney Disease

NURSING DIAGNOSIS: Hypervolaemia associated with decreased urine output, dietary excesses, and retention of sodium and water
GOAL: Maintenance of ideal body weight without excess fluid

Nursing Interventions	Rationale	Expected Outcomes

1. Assess fluid status:
  a. Daily weight
  b. Intake and output balance
  c. Skin turgor and presence of edema
  d. Distention of neck veins
  e. Blood pressure, pulse rate, and rhythm
  f. Respiratory rate and effort
2. Limit fluid intake to prescribed volume.
 	
3. Identify potential sources of fluid:
  a. Medications and fluids used to take or administer medications: oral and IV
  b. Foods
4. Explain to patient and family the rationale for fluid restriction.
5. Assist patient to cope with the discomforts resulting from fluid restriction.
6. Provide or encourage frequent oral hygiene.
	1. Assessment provides baseline and ongoing database for monitoring changes and evaluating interventions.
	
	2. Fluid restriction will be determined on basis of weight, urine output, and response to therapy.
	3. Unrecognized sources of excess fluids may be identified.
	
	4. Understanding promotes patient and family cooperation with fluid restriction.
	5. Increasing patient comfort promotes adherence to dietary restrictions.
	6. Oral hygiene minimizes dryness of oral mucous membranes.
		• Demonstrates no rapid weight changes
		• Maintains dietary and fluid restrictions
		• Exhibits normal skin turgor without edema
		• Exhibits normal vital signs
		• Exhibits no neck vein distention
		• Reports no difficulty breathing or shortness of breath
		• Performs oral hygiene frequently
		• Reports decreased thirst
		• Reports decreased dryness of oral mucous membranes

NURSING DIAGNOSIS: Impaired nutritional intake associated with anorexia, nausea, vomiting, dietary restrictions, and altered oral mucous membranes
GOAL: Maintenance of adequate nutritional intake

Nursing Interventions	Rationale	Expected Outcomes

1. Consult with renal dietitian for recommendations regarding appropriate diet: potassium, phosphorus, sodium restrictions, and protein requirements
2. Assess nutritional status:
  a. Weight changes
  b. Laboratory values (serum electrolyte, blood urea nitrogen [BUN], creatinine, protein, transferrin, and iron levels) (see Appendix A on thePoint)
3. Assess patient's nutritional dietary patterns:
  a. Diet history
  b. Food preferences
  c. Calorie counts
4. Assess for factors contributing to altered nutritional intake:
  a. Anorexia, nausea, or vomiting
  b. Diet unpalatable to patient
  c. Depression
  d. Lack of understanding of dietary restrictions
  e. Stomatitis
5. Provide patient's food preferences within dietary restrictions.
6. Promote intake of high–biologic-value protein foods: eggs, fish, meats.
 	
7. Encourage high-calorie, low-phosphorus, low-sodium, and low-potassium snacks between meals.
 	
8. Alter schedule of medications so that they are not given immediately before meals (except for phosphate binders which are given with the first bite of food).
	1. Involve multidisciplinary team in patient management.
	
	2. Baseline data allow for monitoring of changes and evaluating effectiveness of interventions.
	
	3. Past and present dietary patterns are considered in planning meals.
	
	4. Information about other factors that may be altered or eliminated to promote adequate dietary intake is provided.
	
	5. Increased dietary intake is encouraged.
	6. Complete proteins are provided for positive nitrogen balance needed for growth and healing.
	7. Reduces source of restricted foods and proteins and provides calories for energy, sparing protein for tissue growth and healing.
	8. Ingestion of medications just before meals may produce anorexia and feeling of fullness.
		• Consumes protein of high-biologic value
		• Chooses foods within dietary restrictions that are appealing
		• Consumes high-calorie foods within dietary restrictions
		• Explains in own words rationale for dietary restrictions and relationship to urea and creatinine levels
		• Takes medications on schedule that does not produce anorexia or feeling of fullness
		• Consults written lists of acceptable foods
		• Reports increased appetite at meals
		• Exhibits no rapid increases or decreases in weight
		• Demonstrates normal skin turgor without edema; wound healing and acceptable plasma albumin levels

(continued on page 1574)

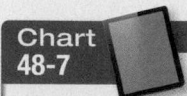

Chart 48-7

PLAN OF NURSING CARE (continued)

The Patient with End-Stage Kidney Disease

Nursing Interventions	Rationale	Expected Outcomes
9. Explain rationale for dietary restrictions and relationship to kidney disease and increased urea and serum creatinine levels.	9. Promotes patient understanding of relationships between diet and urea and creatinine levels to kidney disease.	
10. Provide written lists of foods allowed and suggestions for improving their taste without the use of sodium or potassium.	10. Lists provide a positive approach to dietary restrictions and a reference for patient and family to use when at home.	
11. Provide pleasant surroundings at mealtimes.	11. Unpleasant factors that contribute to patient's anorexia are eliminated.	
12. Weigh patient daily.	12. Allows monitoring of fluid and nutritional status.	

13. Assess for evidence of inadequate protein intake:
  a. Edema formation
  b. Delayed wound healing
  c. Decreased serum albumin levels
	13. Inadequate protein intake can lead to decreased albumin and other proteins, edema formation, and delay in wound healing.	

NURSING DIAGNOSIS: Lack of knowledge regarding condition and treatment
GOAL: Increased knowledge about condition and related treatment

Nursing Interventions	Rationale	Expected Outcomes

1. Assess understanding of cause of kidney disease, consequences of kidney disease, and its treatment:
  a. Cause of patient's kidney disease
  b. Meaning of kidney disease
  c. Understanding of renal function
  d. Relationship of fluid and dietary restrictions to kidney disease
  e. Rationale for treatment (HD, PD, transplantation)
	1. Provides baseline for further explanations and education.	• Verbalizes relationship of cause of kidney disease to consequences
		• Explains fluid and dietary restrictions as they relate to failure of kidney's regulatory functions
		• States in own words relationship of kidney disease and need for treatment
		• Asks questions about treatment options, indicating readiness to learn
		• Verbalizes plans to continue as normal a life as possible
		• Uses written information and instructions to clarify questions and seek additional information

2. Provide explanation of renal function and consequences of kidney disease at patient's level of understanding and guided by patient's readiness to learn.	2. Patient can learn about kidney disease and treatment as they become ready to understand and accept the diagnosis and consequences.	
3. Assist patient to identify ways to incorporate changes related to illness and its treatment into lifestyle.	3. Patient can see that their life does not have to revolve around the disease.	

4. Provide oral and written information as appropriate about:
  a. Renal function and failure
  b. Fluid and dietary restrictions
  c. Medications
  d. Reportable problems, signs, and symptoms
  e. Follow-up schedule
  f. Community resources
  g. Treatment options
	4. Provides patient with information that can be used for further clarification at home.	

NURSING DIAGNOSIS: Activity intolerance associated with fatigue, anemia, retention of waste products, and dialysis procedure
GOAL: Participation in activity within tolerance

Nursing Interventions	Rationale	Expected Outcomes

1. Assess factors contributing to activity intolerance:
  a. Fatigue
  b. Anemia
  c. Fluid and electrolyte imbalances
  d. Retention of waste products
  e. Depression
	1. Indicates factors contributing to severity of fatigue.	• Participates in increasing levels of activity and exercise
		• Reports increased sense of well-being
		• Alternates rest and activity
		• Participates in selected self-care activities

2. Promote independence in self-care activities as tolerated; assist if fatigued.	2. Promotes improved self-esteem.	
3. Encourage alternating activity with rest.	3. Promotes activity and exercise within limits and adequate rest.	
4. Encourage patient to rest after dialysis treatments.	4. Adequate rest is encouraged after dialysis treatments, which are exhausting to many patients.	

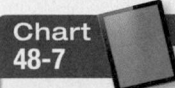

Chart 48-7

PLAN OF NURSING CARE (continued)
The Patient with End-Stage Kidney Disease

NURSING DIAGNOSIS: Risk for situational low self-esteem associated with dependency, role changes, change in body image, and change in sexual function

GOAL: Improved self-esteem

Nursing Interventions	Rationale	Expected Outcomes
1. Assess patient's and family's responses and reactions to illness and treatment.	1. Provides data about problems encountered by patient and family in coping with changes in life.	• Identifies previously used coping styles that have been effective and those no longer possible due to disease and treatment (alcohol or drug use; extreme physical exertion)
2. Assess relationship of patient and significant family members.	2. Identifies strengths and supports of patient and family.	
3. Assess usual coping patterns of patient and family members.	3. Coping patterns that may have been effective in past may be harmful in view of restrictions imposed by disease and treatment.	• Patient and family identify and verbalize feelings and reactions to disease and necessary changes in their lives
4. Encourage open discussion of concerns about changes produced by disease and treatment: a. Role changes b. Changes in lifestyle c. Changes in occupation d. Sexual changes e. Dependence on health care team	4. Encourages patient to identify concerns and steps necessary to deal with them.	• Seeks professional counseling, if necessary, to cope with changes resulting from kidney disease
5. Explore alternative ways of sexual expression other than penile-vaginal intercourse.	5. Alternative forms of sexual expression may be acceptable.	• Reports satisfaction with method of sexual expression
6. Discuss role of giving and receiving love, warmth, and affection.	6. Sexuality means different things to different people, depending on stage of maturity.	
7. Consult with medical social worker (MSW), psychiatry for unresolved problems	7. Collaborate with interprofessional team for unresolved patient care issues.	

COLLABORATIVE PROBLEMS: Hyperkalemia; pericarditis, pericardial effusion, and pericardial tamponade; hypertension; anemia; bone disease and metastatic calcifications

GOAL: Absence of complications

Nursing Interventions	Rationale	Expected Outcomes
Hyperkalemia		
1. Monitor serum potassium levels. Notify primary provider if level is at or approaching >5.5 mEq/L, and prepare to treat hyperkalemia.	1. Hyperkalemia causes potentially life-threatening changes in the body.	• Has normal potassium level • Experiences no muscle weakness or diarrhea
2. Assess patient for muscle weakness, diarrhea, electrocardiographic (ECG) changes (tall-tented T waves and widened QRS).	2. Cardiovascular signs and symptoms are characteristic of hyperkalemia.	• Exhibits normal ECG pattern • Vital signs are within normal limits
Pericarditis, Pericardial Effusion, and Pericardial Tamponade		
1. Assess patient for fever, chest pain, and a pericardial friction rub (signs of pericarditis); if present, notify primary provider.	1. Patients with chronic kidney disease may develop pericarditis due to uremia; fever, chest pain, and a pericardial friction rub are classic signs.	• Has strong and equal peripheral pulses • Absence of a paradoxical pulse
2. If patient has pericarditis, assess for the following every 4 hours: a. Paradoxical pulse, >10 mm Hg b. Extreme hypotension c. Weak or absent peripheral pulses d. Altered level of consciousness e. Jugular venous distention	2. Pericardial effusion is a common sequela of pericarditis. Signs of an effusion include a paradoxical pulse (>10 mm Hg drop in blood pressure during inspiration) and signs of shock due to compression of the heart by a large effusion. Cardiac tamponade, which may be fatal, exists when the patient is severely compromised hemodynamically.	• Absence of pericardial effusion or tamponade on cardiac ultrasound • Has normal heart sounds
3. Prepare patient for echocardiogram to aid in diagnosis of pericardial effusion and cardiac tamponade.	3. Echocardiogram is useful in visualizing pericardial effusions and cardiac tamponade.	
4. If cardiac tamponade develops, prepare patient for emergency pericardiocentesis.	4. Cardiac tamponade is a life-threatening condition, with a high mortality rate. Immediate drainage of fluid from the pericardial space via a pericardial window procedure is essential.	

(continued on page 1576)

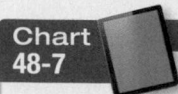

Chart 48-7

PLAN OF NURSING CARE (continued)
The Patient with End-Stage Kidney Disease

Nursing Interventions	Rationale	Expected Outcomes
Hypertension		
1. Monitor and record blood pressure as indicated.	1. Provides objective data for monitoring. Elevated levels may indicate nonadherence to the treatment regimen.	• Blood pressure and weight within normal limits
2. Administer antihypertensive medications as prescribed.	2. Antihypertensive medications play a key role in treatment of hypertension associated with chronic kidney disease.	• Reports no headaches, visual problems, or seizures
3. Encourage adherence to dietary and fluid restriction therapy.	3. Adherence to diet and fluid restrictions and dialysis schedule prevents excess fluid and sodium accumulation.	• Edema is absent • Demonstrates adherence to dietary and fluid restrictions
4. Instruct patient to report signs of fluid overload, vision changes, headaches, edema, or seizures.	4. These are indications of inadequate control of hypertension and the need to alter therapy.	
Anemia		
1. Monitor red blood cell (RBC) count and hemoglobin and hematocrit levels as indicated.	1. Provides assessment of degree of anemia.	• Patient has a normal skin color without pallor
2. Administer medications as prescribed, including iron and folic acid supplements, an erythrocyte-stimulating agent, and multivitamins.	2. RBCs need iron, folic acid, and vitamins to be produced. An erythrocyte-stimulating agent stimulates the bone marrow to produce RBCs.	• Exhibits hemoglobin levels within acceptable limits • Experiences no bleeding from any site
3. Avoid drawing unnecessary blood specimens.	3. Anemia is worsened by drawing numerous specimens.	
4. Educate patient to prevent bleeding: Avoid vigorous nose blowing and contact sports, and use a soft toothbrush.	4. Bleeding from anywhere in the body worsens anemia.	
5. Administer blood component therapy as indicated.	5. Blood component therapy may be needed if the patient has symptoms.	
Bone Disease and Metastatic Calcifications		
1. Administer the following medications as prescribed: phosphate binders, calcium supplements, vitamin D supplements, calcimimetics.	1. Chronic kidney disease causes numerous physiologic changes affecting calcium, phosphorus, and vitamin D metabolism.	• Takes phosphate binders with the first bite of food.
2. Monitor serum laboratory values as indicated (calcium, phosphorus, ionized parathyroid [iPTH] hormone), and report abnormal findings to primary provider.	2. Hyperphosphatemia, hypocalcemia, and hyperparathyroidism are common in chronic kidney disease.	• Exhibits serum calcium, phosphorus, and iPTH levels within acceptable ranges • Exhibits no symptoms of hypocalcemia
3. Assist patient with an exercise program.	3. Bone demineralization increases with immobility, hyperphosphatemia, hyperparathyroidism.	• Has no bone demineralization on bone scan • Discusses importance of maintaining activity level and exercise program
4. Consult with renal dietitian	4. Involve interprofessional team in patient management.	

Promoting Home, Community-Based, and Transitional Care

 ### Educating Patients About Self-Care

The nurse plays an important role in educating the patient with ESKD. Because of the extensive education needed, the home health nurse, dialysis nurse, and nurses in the hospital and outpatient settings, as well as a renal dietitian, all provide ongoing education and reinforcement while monitoring the patient's progress and adherence to the treatment regimen. The patient is instructed to check the vascular access for patency and to use appropriate precautions, such as avoiding venipuncture and blood pressure measurements on the arm with the access device. In addition, the patient and family need to know what problems to report to the primary provider. These include the following:

- Worsening signs and symptoms of kidney disease (nausea, vomiting, change in usual urine output, metallic taste in the mouth, ammonia odor on breath)
- Signs and symptoms of hyperkalemia (muscle weakness, diarrhea, abdominal cramps)
- Signs and symptoms of access problems (clotted fistula or graft, infection)

Signs and symptoms of decreasing renal function, in addition to increasing BUN and serum creatinine levels, may indicate a need to alter the dialysis prescription. The dialysis nurses also provide ongoing education and support at each treatment visit.

Continuing and Transitional Care

The importance of follow-up examinations and treatment is stressed with the patient and family because of changing physical status, renal function, and dialysis requirements. Referral for home care provides the home health nurse with the opportunity to assess the patient's environment, emotional status, and the coping strategies used by the patient and family to deal with the changes in family roles often associated with chronic illness.

The home health nurse also assesses the patient for further deterioration of renal function and signs and symptoms of complications resulting from the primary kidney disorder, the resulting kidney disease, and effects of treatment strategies (e.g., dialysis, medications, dietary restrictions). Patients need education and reinforcement of the dietary restrictions required, including fluid, sodium, potassium, and phosphorus restriction. Reminders about the need for health promotion activities and health screening are an important part of nursing care for the patient with kidney disease.

 ## Gerontologic Considerations

Diabetes, hypertension, chronic glomerulonephritis, interstitial nephritis, and urinary tract obstruction are among the causes for ESKD in older adults. The fastest growing group of patients with CKD is older adults who also have more comorbidities (Brooks, 2017). The signs and symptoms of kidney disease in older adults are often nonspecific. The occurrence of symptoms of other disorders (heart failure, dementia) can mask the symptoms of kidney disease and delay or prevent diagnosis and treatment (Hain, 2017).

HD and PD are used effectively in treating older patients with ESKD. Initiation of dialysis among older adults has increased in the past decade as baby boomers have come of age. Implementation of palliative care has also increased among patients who choose not to start dialysis or who decide to stop dialysis. Although there is no specific age limitation for kidney transplantation, concomitant disorders (e.g., coronary artery disease, peripheral vascular disease) have made it a less common treatment for older adults. However, in the United States, when adults age 60 and older who have significant comorbidities are ruled out (i.e., not considered to be suitable) as transplant candidates, those who do receive a kidney transplant survive longer than patients on dialysis and those who remain on the transplant waiting list (Bunnapradist, Abdalla, & Reddy, 2017).

Some older patients elect not to undergo dialysis or transplantation. Conservative management and palliative care, also known as supportive care, including nutritional therapy, fluid control, and medications such as phosphate binders, may be considered in patients who are not suitable for or elect not to have dialysis or transplantation (Molzahn & Schick-Makaroff, 2017). Palliative care for the patient with ESKD focuses on relieving suffering, promoting health-related quality of life, and facilitating dignity at the end-of-life (see Chapter 13).

RENAL REPLACEMENT THERAPY (RRT)

The use of RRT becomes necessary when the kidneys can no longer remove wastes, maintain electrolytes, and regulate fluid balance. This can occur rapidly or over a long period of time, and the need for replacement therapy can be acute (short term) or chronic (long term). RRT includes the various types of dialysis and kidney transplantation.

Dialysis

Types of dialysis include HD, CRRT, and PD. Acute or urgent dialysis is indicated when there is a high and increasing level of serum potassium, fluid overload, or impending pulmonary edema, increasing acidosis, pericarditis, and advanced uremia. It may also be used to remove medications or toxins (poisoning or medication overdose) from the blood or for edema or hypertension that does not respond to other treatment, and hyperkalemia.

Chronic or maintenance dialysis is indicated in advanced CKD and ESKD in the following instances: the presence of uremic signs and symptoms affecting all body systems (nausea and vomiting, severe anorexia, increasing lethargy, mental confusion), hyperkalemia, fluid overload not responsive to diuretics and fluid restriction, and a general lack of well-being. An urgent indication for dialysis in patients with kidney disease is pericardial friction rub, which is indicative of uremic pericarditis.

The decision to initiate dialysis should be reached only after thoughtful discussion among the patient, family, primary provider, and other health care team members. The nurse can assist the patient and family by answering their questions, clarifying the information provided, and supporting their decision.

Successful kidney transplantation eliminates the need for dialysis. Not only is the quality of life much improved in patients with ESKD who undergo transplantation, but physiologic function is improved as well. Patients who undergo kidney transplantation from living donors before dialysis is initiated (preemptive transplant) generally have longer survival of the transplanted kidney than patients who receive transplantation after dialysis treatment is initiated (Bunnapradist, Abdalla, & Reddy, 2017).

Hemodialysis (HD)

HD is used for patients who are acutely ill and require short-term dialysis for days to weeks until kidney function resumes, as in patients with AKI, and for patients with advanced CKD and ESKD who require long-term or permanent RRT. HD prevents death but does not cure kidney disease and does not compensate for the loss of endocrine or metabolic activities of the kidneys. Approximately 62.7% of patients requiring long-term RRT are on chronic HD (USRDS, 2019). Most patients receive intermittent HD that involves treatments three times a week with an average treatment duration of 3 to 4 hours in an outpatient setting. HD can also be performed at home by the patient and a caregiver. See later discussion on home HD.

The objectives of HD are to extract toxic nitrogenous substances from the blood and to remove excess fluid. A **dialyzer** (also referred to as an artificial kidney) is a synthetic semipermeable membrane through which blood is filtered to remove uremic toxins and a desired amount of fluid. In HD, the blood, laden with toxins and nitrogenous wastes, is diverted from the patient to a machine via the use of a blood pump to the dialyzer, where toxins are filtered from the blood and the cleansed blood is returned to the patient.

Diffusion, osmosis, and **ultrafiltration** are the principles on which HD is based (see Chapter 10). The toxins and wastes in the blood are removed by **diffusion**—that is, they move from an area of higher concentration in the blood to an area of lower concentration in the dialysate. The **dialysate** is a solution that circulates through the dialyzer, made up of all the electrolytes in their ideal extracellular concentrations. The electrolyte level in the patient's blood can be brought under control by properly adjusting the electrolytes in the dialysate solution. The semipermeable membrane impedes the diffusion of large molecules, such as RBCs and proteins.

Excess fluid is removed from the blood by **osmosis**, in which water moves from an area of low concentration potential (the blood) to an area of high concentration potential (the dialysate bath). In **ultrafiltration**, fluid moves under high pressure to an area of lower pressure. This process is much more efficient than osmosis for fluid removal and is accomplished by applying negative pressure (a suctioning-type force) to the dialysis membrane. Because patients with ESKD requiring dialysis usually cannot excrete enough water, this force is necessary to remove fluid to achieve fluid balance.

The body's buffer system is maintained using a dialysate bath made up of bicarbonate (most common) or acetate, which is metabolized to form bicarbonate. The anticoagulant heparin is given to keep blood from clotting in the extracorporeal dialysis circuit. Cleansed blood is returned to the body with the goal of removing fluid, balancing electrolytes, and managing acidosis (Hellebrand, Allen, & Hoffman, 2017).

Dialyzers

Dialyzers are hollow-fiber devices containing thousands of tiny capillary tubes that carry the blood through the artificial kidney. The tubes are porous and act as a semipermeable membrane, allowing toxins, fluid, and electrolytes to pass across the membrane. The constant flow of the solution maintains the concentration gradient to facilitate the exchange of wastes from the blood across the semipermeable membrane into the dialysate solution, where they are removed and discarded (see Fig. 48-3).

Dialyzers have undergone many technologic changes in performance and biocompatibility. High-flux dialysis uses highly permeable membranes to increase the clearance of low- and mid–molecular-weight molecules. These special membranes are used with higher than traditional rates of flow for the blood entering and exiting the dialyzer (500 to 550 mL/min). High-flux dialysis increases the efficiency of treatments while shortening their duration and reducing the need for heparin.

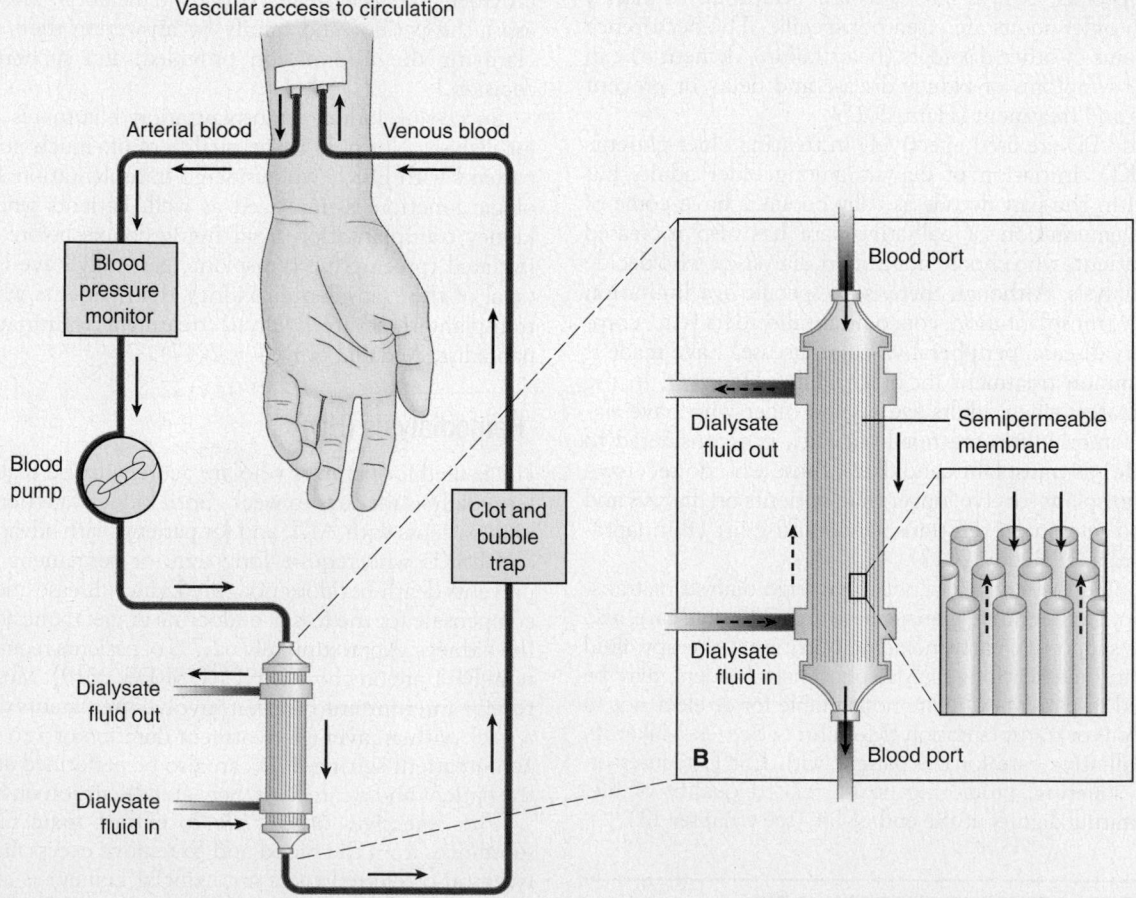

Figure 48-3 • HD system. Blood from the arteriovenous fistula or graft is pumped (**A**) into a dialyzer, where it flows through the synthetic capillary tubes (**B**), which act as the semipermeable membrane (*inset*). The dialysate, which has a particular chemical composition, flows into the dialyzer around the capillary tubes that the blood flows through. The waste products in the blood diffuse across the semipermeable membrane into the dialysate solution and flows out to the drain.

Vascular Access

Access to the patient's vascular system must be established to allow blood to be removed, cleansed, and returned to the patient's vascular system at the rapid rates of 300 and 500 mL/min. Several types of access can be surgically created or placed during procedures performed in interventional radiology suites or at the bedside.

Vascular Access Devices

Immediate access to the patient's circulation for acute HD is achieved by inserting a double-lumen, noncuffed, large-bore catheter into the right or left internal jugular or femoral vein of either leg by the physician, nurse practitioner, or physician assistant (see Fig. 48-4). The subclavian vein is rarely used as there is an increased risk for central stenosis (Pryor & Brouwer-Maier, 2017). This method of vascular access involves some risk (e.g., hematoma, bleeding, pneumothorax, infection, thrombosis of the vein, inadequate flow). The catheter is removed when no longer needed (e.g., because the patient's condition has improved or another type of permanent access has been established). Double-lumen, cuffed catheters may also be inserted, usually by either a surgeon or interventional radiologist, into the internal jugular vein of the patient. Because these catheters have cuffs under the skin, the insertion site heals, sealing the wound and reducing the risk for ascending infection. This feature makes these catheters safe for longer-term use. However, infection rates remain high, and sepsis continues to be a common cause for hospital admission (Pryor & Brouwer-Maier, 2017).

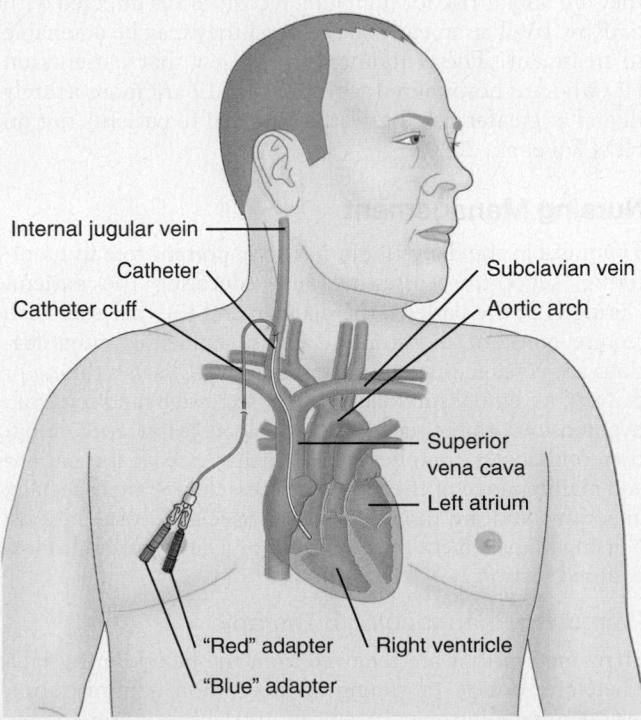

Figure 48-4 • Double-lumen, cuffed HD catheter used in acute HD. The red catheter lumen is attached to a blood line through which blood is pumped from the patient to the dialyzer. After the blood passes through the dialyzer (artificial kidney), it returns to the patient through the other lumen of the catheter.

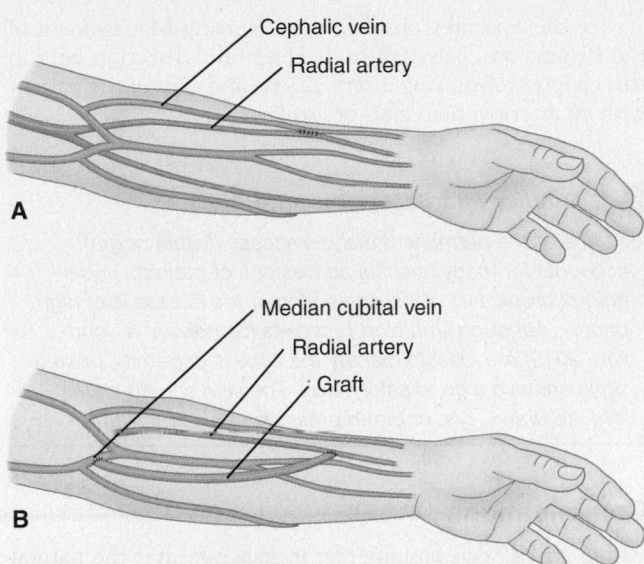

Figure 48-5 • **A.** Arteriovenous fistulas are created by anastomosing a patient's vein to an artery. This illustrates a side-to-side anastomosis. **B.** Arteriovenous grafts are established by connecting the artery and vein using synthetic tubing.

Arteriovenous Fistula

The preferred method of permanent vascular access for dialysis is an **arteriovenous fistula** (AVF) that is created surgically (usually in the forearm) by anastomosing (joining) an artery to a vein, either side to side or end to side (see Fig. 48-5A). Needles are inserted into the vessel to obtain blood flow which is adequate to pass through the dialyzer. The arterial segment of the fistula is used for outflow to the dialyzer and the venous segment for reinfusion of the dialyzed blood. This access will need time (at least 3 months) to "mature" before it can be used. As the AVF matures, the venous segment dilates due to the increased blood flow coming directly from the artery. Once sufficiently dilated, it will then accommodate two large-bore (14-, 15-, or 16-gauge) needles that are inserted for each dialysis treatment. The patient is encouraged to perform hand exercises (e.g., squeezing a rubber ball) to increase the size of these vessels to accommodate the large-bore needles. Once established, this access has the longest useful life and thus is considered the best option for vascular access for the patient requiring ongoing HD (Inglese, 2017).

Arteriovenous Graft

An **arteriovenous graft** can be created by subcutaneously interposing a biologic, semibiologic, or synthetic graft material between an artery and vein (see Fig. 48-5B). Usually, a graft is created when the patient's vessels are not suitable for creation of an AVF. Patients with compromised vascular systems (e.g., from diabetes) often require a graft because their native vessels may not be suitable for creation of an AVF. Grafts are usually placed in the arm but may be placed in the thigh or chest wall. Stenosis, infection, and thrombosis are the most common complications of this access. It is not at all uncommon to see a dialysis patient with numerous "old" or "nonfunctioning" accesses present on their arms. The patient is asked to identify the current access in use, and it is assessed carefully and regularly for the presence of a bruit and thrill.

See the Special Considerations: Nursing Management of the Patient on Dialysis Who Is Hospitalized section later in this chapter for nursing interventions and care of the patient with an arteriovenous graft or fistula.

> ▶ **Quality and Safety Nursing Alert**
>
> *Failure of the permanent dialysis access (fistula or graft) accounts for many hospital admissions of patients undergoing chronic HD. Thus, protection of the access is of high priority. Although limb alert bracelets (Sturdivant & Johnson, 2019) are ideal to identify the access extremity, posted signs are also a good safety alert. The sign should state, "No lab draws, IVs, or blood pressures on access arm."*

Complications

Although HD can prolong life, it does not alter the natural course of the underlying CKD, nor does it completely replace kidney function. The CKD complications previously discussed will continue to worsen and require treatment. With the initiation of dialysis, disturbances of lipid metabolism are accelerated and contribute to cardiovascular complications. Heart failure, coronary artery disease, angina, stroke, and peripheral vascular disease may occur and can incapacitate the patient. Cardiovascular disease remains the leading cause of death in patients receiving dialysis as well as for patients with CKD.

Many complications result from both the underlying ESKD and the HD treatments. The anemia of ESKD is compounded by blood loss during HD. Gastric ulcers may result from the physiologic stress of chronic illness, medication, and preexisting medical conditions (e.g., diabetes). Patients with uremia often report a metallic taste and nausea. Vomiting may occur during the HD treatment when rapid fluid shifts and hypotension occur. These contribute to the malnutrition seen in patients on dialysis. Disordered calcium metabolism and renal osteodystrophy can result in bone pain and fractures, interfering with mobility. As time on dialysis continues, calcification of major blood vessels has been reported and linked to hypertension and other vascular complications. Phosphorus deposits in the skin can occur and cause itching.

Many people undergoing HD experience major sleep problems that further complicate their overall health status. Early-morning or late-afternoon dialysis may be a risk factor for developing sleep disturbances.

Other complications of dialysis may include the following:
- Episodes of shortness of breath often occur as fluid accumulates between dialysis treatments.
- Hypotension may occur during the treatment as fluid is removed. Nausea and vomiting, diaphoresis, tachycardia, and dizziness are common signs of hypotension.
- Painful muscle cramping may occur, usually late in dialysis as fluid and electrolytes rapidly leave the extracellular space.
- Exsanguination may occur if blood lines separate or dialysis needles become dislodged.
- Arrhythmias may result from electrolyte and pH changes or from removal of antiarrhythmic medications during dialysis.

- Air embolism is very rare since the advent of venous air detectors, but can occur if air enters the vascular system.
- Chest pain may occur in patients with anemia or arteriosclerotic heart disease.
- Dialysis disequilibrium results from cerebral fluid shifts. Signs and symptoms include headache, nausea and vomiting, restlessness, decreased level of consciousness, and seizures. It is rare and more likely to occur in AKI or when BUN levels are very high (exceeding 150 mg/dL) and the patient is dialyzed with high blood and dialysate flows. Therefore, short treatments with low blood and dialysate flow rates are prescribed (Hellebrand et al., 2017).

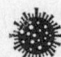 **COVID-19 Considerations**

Patients undergoing outpatient HD are at high risk of contracting the SARS-CoV-2 virus due to comorbidities (e.g., hypertension), their relatively suppressed immune status, and more frequent hospitalizations (Wu, Li, Zhu, et al., 2020). Travel to an outpatient dialysis center three times a week also increases their risk of contracting the virus (Ajaimy & Melamed, 2020). Findings from a retrospective, single-center study of 49 patients on HD compared to 52 patients without kidney disease all hospitalized with COVID-19 pneumonia in Wuhan, China, reported that the main symptoms of fever and cough were less prevalent in patients who were undergoing HD (Wu et al., 2020). Patients on HD were also more likely to be admitted to intensive care, need ventilator support, and had a higher mortality rate compared to controls (Wu et al., 2020). These early findings suggest that patients receiving HD are not only at greater risk for COVID-19, they are also at risk for not being recognized as infected with SARS-CoV-2 at an early stage, when they may be amenable to treatment. These findings also suggest that patients on HD who are hospitalized with COVID-19 are more acutely ill and at greater risk for death compared to patients not on HD (Wu et al., 2020).

Nursing Management

The nurse in the dialysis unit has an important role in monitoring, supporting, assessing, and educating the patient. During HD, the patient, the dialyzer, and the dialysate bath require constant monitoring because numerous complications are possible, including clotting of the dialysis tubing or dialyzer, air embolism, inadequate or excessive fluid removal, hypotension, cramping, vomiting, blood leaks, contamination, and access complications. Nursing care of the patient and maintenance of the vascular access device are especially important and are discussed in the Special Considerations: Nursing Management of the Patient on Dialysis Who Is Hospitalized section.

Promoting Pharmacologic Therapy

Many medications are removed from the blood during HD. Therefore, dosage or timing of medication administration may require adjustment. Medications that are water soluble are readily removed during HD treatment, and those that are fat soluble or adhere to other substances (like albumin) are not dialyzed out very well. This is the reason some drug overdoses are treated with emergency HD and others are not.

Patients undergoing HD who require medications (e.g., cardiac glycosides, antibiotic agents, antiarrhythmic medications, antihypertensive agents) are monitored closely to ensure that blood and tissue levels of these medications are maintained without toxic accumulation. Antihypertensive therapy, often part of the regimen of patients on dialysis, is one example when communication, education, and evaluation can make a difference in patient outcomes. The patient must know when—and when not—to take the medication. For example, if an antihypertensive agent is taken on a dialysis day, hypotension may occur during dialysis, causing dangerously low blood pressure. Many medications that are taken once daily should be administered after the dialysis treatment.

Promoting Nutritional and Fluid Therapy

Diet is important for patients on HD. Goals of nutritional therapy are to minimize uremic symptoms and fluid and electrolyte imbalances; to maintain good nutritional status through adequate protein, calorie, vitamin, and mineral intake; and to enable the patient to eat a palatable and enjoyable diet. Restriction of fluid is also part of the dietary prescription because fluid accumulation may occur, leading to fluid volume excess, heart failure, and pulmonary edema.

With the initiation of HD, the patient usually requires some restriction of dietary sodium, potassium, phosphorus, and fluid intake. Close collaboration with a renal dietitian is essential in helping the patient make good food choices. Protein intake is restricted to about 1.2 g/kg ideal body weight per day; therefore, protein must be of high-biologic quality. Sodium is usually restricted to 2 g/day; the fluid prescription is individualized based on residual urine output (generally 1000 to 1500 mL/day). The goal for patients on HD is to keep their interdialytic (between dialysis treatments) weight gain less than 4% of their estimated dry weight (Gonyea, 2017). Potassium restriction depends on the amount of residual renal function and the frequency of dialysis.

Dietary restriction is an unwelcome change in lifestyle for many patients with ESKD. Patients can feel stigmatized in social situations because there may be few food choices available for their diet. If the restrictions are ignored, life-threatening complications, such as hyperkalemia and pulmonary edema, may result. Thus, the patient may feel punished for responding to basic human drives to eat and drink. The nurse and renal dietitian who care for a patient with symptoms or complications resulting from dietary indiscretion must avoid harsh, judgmental, or punitive tones when communicating with them. Regular education with reinforcement is needed to achieve these difficult changes in lifestyle.

Meeting Psychosocial Needs

Patients requiring long-term HD, as they engage in psychosocial adaptation, tend to feel mired in a cyclical routine (Lin, Han, & Pan, 2015). They often have financial problems, difficulty holding a job, waning sexual desire and impotence, clinical depression, and fear of dying. Younger patients worry about marriage, having children, and the burden that they bring to their families. The regimented lifestyle that frequent dialysis treatments and restrictions in food and fluid intake impose can be demoralizing to the patient and family. Researchers have studied how patients on HD perceive and cope with the treatment by developing resilience (Kim, Lee, & Chang, 2019). (See the Nursing Research Profile in Chart 48-8.)

Dialysis alters the lifestyle of the patient and family. The amount of time required for dialysis and primary provider visits and being chronically ill can create conflict, frustration, guilt, and depression. It may be difficult for the patient, spouse, and family to express anger and negative feelings.

The nurse needs to give the patient and family the opportunity to express feelings of anger and concern about the limitations that the disease and treatment impose, possible financial problems, and job insecurity. If anger is not expressed, it

---

Chart 48-8 · NURSING RESEARCH PROFILE

Resilience in Patients Receiving Dialysis

Kim, E., Lee, Y., & Chang, S. (2019). How do patients on hemodialysis perceive and overcome hemodialysis?: Concept development of the resilience of patients on hemodialysis. *Nephrology Nursing Journal, 46*(5), 521–530.

Purpose

This qualitative study was designed to identify and conceptualize the concept of resilience in patients receiving HD.

Design

This study was conducted in three phases. In the first phase, called the theoretical phase, a literature review was undertaken and a definition of the resilience of patients on HD was constructed. In the fieldwork phase, interviews were held with 10 patients. Qualitative data from the 10 interviews were analyzed for patterns to identify attributes of resilience for patients on HD. The last phase compared the theoretical definition with the data collected in the fieldwork phase.

Findings

The purposive patient sample included 10 participants from one HD center at a university hospital in Korea who were chosen by nurses with expertise in HD who assessed the patients to have characteristics of resilience. The length of time participants had been on HD ranged between 1 and 10 years, and 60% were female. Through in-depth interviews, the concept of the resilience of patients on HD was found to have three dimensions: a willingness to actively solve problems, building daily routine strategies continuing roles as a family member and asserting the will to grow through overcoming HD; an acceptance of the HD situation, maintaining the homeostasis of the body and deliberating on death; and a positive self-perception and positively reinterpreting human relationships.

Nursing Implications

The nurse should assess and reinforce positive coping strategies that patients are using to cope with the issues encountered with the HD routine and change in lifestyle. By identifying the concept of resilience, nurses can encourage patients to use their positive coping skills to manage the financial, psychosocial, and medical challenges they may experience. The findings of this study could be used as a foundation for intervention strategies that incorporate the inventory of patients' strengths.

Chart 48-9

ETHICAL DILEMMA

How Can Patient Rights Be Discerned during a Pandemic?

Case Scenario

B.J. is a 74-year-old widow with chronic kidney disease (CKD) managed with HD three times weekly in an outpatient dialysis center. She is admitted to the medical unit where you work as a staff nurse with fluid retention and dyspnea. It is reported that B.J. had been a "no show" at the dialysis center for at least the past week. As part of her therapeutic plan, she is supposed to be dialyzed while in the hospital. As you enter her room to prepare her for transport to the hospital's dialysis center, you find B.J. humming to herself, clapping her hands, and smiling. When you explain to her that she is going to be transported to the dialysis center, she says "Honey, I am not going anywhere. I want to see Jesus. It is my time and I am ready to see the Lord." You have heard from the medical social worker that this is not B.J.'s first admission to the hospital for poor adherence to her outpatient dialysis treatment. During past hospitalizations, her three adult daughters would visit her together and effectively cajole her into receiving dialysis treatments. Reportedly, the daughters have a loving and supportive relationship with each other and their mother. However, there is an outbreak of coronavirus disease 2019 (COVID-19) within your community and the hospital has responded with a no-visitor policy throughout the facility, so B.J.'s daughters may not visit her.

Discussion

The principle of autonomy is considered sacrosanct. Patients have the right to refuse treatments, even if those treatments are life-saving. However, in this particular instance, B.J. could be delirious as a manifestation of her poorly managed CKD. If she is delirious, it may be determined that she lacks the capacity to

make her own decisions. Her daughters might be her surrogates and legally responsible to make health care decisions for her. However, her daughters' prohibition to visit her while she is hospitalized hampers their ability to discuss her options with her and gain her assent for treatment.

Analysis

- Describe the ethical principles that are in conflict in this case (see Chapter 1, Chart 1-7). Can the principle of beneficence and wishing to "do good" for B.J. trump her autonomous right to refuse treatment? Can she be forced to undergo dialysis?
- What if it is determined that B.J. lacks the capacity to make informed decisions? On the contrary, what if it is determined that B.J. is not delirious and has the capacity to refuse to be dialyzed? Describe methods that you might employ to engage B.J.'s daughters so that they might be able to communicate with her and with each other as a family unit.
- What resources might be mobilized to be of assistance to B.J., her daughters, and the health care team so that a treatment plan that preserves B.J.'s dignity during this pandemic might be devised?

References

Hulkower, A. (2020). Learning from COVID. *Hastings Center Report*, 50(3), 16–17.

Resources

See Chapter 1, Chart 1-10 for Steps of an Ethical Analysis and Ethics Resources.

---

may be directed inward and lead to depression, despair, and attempts at suicide; however, if anger is projected outward to other people, it may damage family relationships.

Although these feelings are normal in this situation, they are often profound. Counseling and psychotherapy may be useful. All patients receiving dialysis should be screened for depression using a standard screening tool such as the Patient Health Questionnaire 9 (PHQ-9) or the Beck Depression Inventory (BDI) (Shirazian, Grant, Aina, et al., 2017). Depression may require treatment. Referring the patient and family to a mental health provider with expertise in the care of patients receiving dialysis may also be helpful. Clinical nurse specialists, psychologists, and social workers may be helpful in assisting the patient and family to cope with the changes brought about by kidney disease and its treatment by encouraging the development of resilience (Kim et al., 2019; Lieser, 2017).

The sense of loss that the patient experiences cannot be underestimated because every aspect of a "normal life" is disrupted. Some patients use denial to deal with the array of medical problems (e.g., infections, hypertension, anemia, neuropathy). Staff who are tempted to label the patient as nonadherent must consider the impact of kidney disease and its treatment on the patient and family and the coping strategies that they may use.

Palliative care principles that focus on symptom control are becoming increasingly important as greater attention is focused on quality-of-life issues. Patients and their families are encouraged to discuss end-of-life options and to develop

advanced directives or living wills (Molzahn & Schick-Makaroff, 2017) (see Chart 48-9).

Promoting Home, Community-Based, and Transitional Care

Educating Patients About Self-Care

Preparing a patient for HD is essential. Assessment helps identify the learning needs of the patient and family members. In many cases, the patient is discharged home before learning needs and readiness to learn can be thoroughly evaluated; therefore, hospital-based nurses, dialysis staff, and home health nurses must work together to provide appropriate education that meets the patient's and family's changing needs and readiness to learn (see Chart 48-10).

The diagnosis of ESKD and the need for dialysis is a big adjustment for the patient and family. In addition, many patients with ESKD have clinical depression, and chronic uremia contributes to a shortened attention span, a decreased level of concentration, and altered perception. Therefore, education must occur in brief, 10- to 15-minute sessions, with time added for clarification, repetition, reinforcement, and questions from the patient and family. The nurse needs to convey a nonjudgmental attitude to enable the patient and family to discuss options and their feelings about those options. Team conferences are helpful for sharing information and providing every team member the opportunity to discuss the needs of the patient and family.

Chart 48-10 — HOME CARE CHECKLIST
The Patient Undergoing HD

At the completion of education, the patient and/or caregiver will be able to:

- Discuss kidney disease and its effects on the body.
- State the goal and purpose of HD and its impact on physiologic functioning, ADLs, IADLs, roles, relationships, and spirituality.
- Discuss common problems that may occur during HD and their prevention and management.
- State the name, dose, side effects, frequency, and schedule for all medications on dialysis and nondialysis days.
- Describe commonly measured laboratory values, results, and implications.
- State changes in lifestyle (e.g., diet, activity) necessary to maintain health.
  - Acknowledge dietary and fluid restrictions, rationale, and consequences of nonadherence.
  - State dietary restrictions and changes required to provide adequate protein, calorie, vitamin, and mineral intake.
- List guidelines for prevention and detection of fluid overload, meaning of "dry" weight, and how to weigh self.

- Demonstrate vascular access care, how to check patency, signs and symptoms of infection, and prevention of complications.
- Develop strategies to manage or reduce anxiety and maintain independence.
- Discuss strategies for detection, management, and relief of pruritus, neuropathy, and other potential complications of kidney disease.
- Relate how to reach primary provider with questions or complications.
- State time and date of follow-up medical appointments, therapy, and testing.
- Coordinate financial arrangements for HD and strategies to identify and obtain resources.
- Identify sources of support (e.g., friends, relatives, faith community).
- Identify the contact details for support services for patients and their caregivers/families.
- Identify the need for health promotion, disease prevention, and screening activities.

ADLs, activities of daily living; IADLs, instrumental activities of daily living.

Home Hemodialysis

Most patients who undergo HD do so in an outpatient setting, but home HD is an option for some. Prior to the COVID-19 pandemic, approximately 2% of patients receiving RRT were on home HD (USRDS, 2019). Home HD requires a highly motivated patient who is willing to take responsibility for the procedure and is able to adjust each treatment to meet the body's changing needs. It also requires the commitment and cooperation of a caregiver to assist the patient. However, many patients are not comfortable imposing on others and do not wish to subject family members to the feeling that their home is being turned into a clinic. The health care team never forces a patient to use home HD, because this treatment requires changes in the home and family. Home HD must be the patient's and family's decision (Harwood & Dominski, 2017). However, more patients needing RRT are being encouraged to reassess the home dialysis option as this modality allows the patient to self-isolate and to avoid having to enter an HD center thrice weekly, thus lowering the risk of contracting the SARS-CoV-2 virus (Ajaimy & Melamed, 2020).

The patient undergoing home HD and the caregiver assisting that patient must be trained to prepare, operate, and disassemble the dialysis machine; maintain and clean the equipment; administer medications (e.g., heparin) into the machine lines; and handle emergency problems (HD dialyzer rupture, electrical or mechanical problems, hypotension, shock, and seizures) (Harwood & Dominski, 2017). Because home HD places primary responsibility for the treatment on the patient and the family member, they must understand and be capable of performing all aspects of the HD procedure.

Before home HD is initiated, the home environment, household and community resources, and ability and willingness of the patient and family to carry out this treatment are assessed. The home is surveyed to see if electrical outlets, plumbing facilities, and storage space are adequate.

Modifications may be needed to enable the patient and caregiver to perform dialysis safely and to deal with emergencies.

Once home HD is initiated, the home health nurse must visit periodically to evaluate adherence with the recommended techniques, to assess the patient for complications, to reinforce previous education, and to provide feedback and reassurance.

Continuing and Transitional Care

The health care team's goal in treating patients with CKD is to maximize their vocational potential, functional status, and quality of life (Browne & Johnstone, 2017). To facilitate renal rehabilitation, appropriate follow-up and monitoring by members of the health care team (physicians, dialysis nurses, renal dietitian, social worker, psychologist, home health nurses, and others as appropriate) are essential to early identification and resolution of problems. Many patients with CKD can resume relatively normal lives, doing the things that are important to them: traveling, exercising, working, or actively participating in family activities. If appropriate interventions are available early in the course of dialysis, the potential for better health improves, and the patient can remain active in family and community life. Outcome goals for renal rehabilitation include employment for those able to work, improved physical functioning of all patients, improved understanding about adaptation and options for living well, increased control over the effects of kidney disease and dialysis, and resumption of activities enjoyed before dialysis.

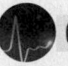 **Continuous Renal Replacement Therapy**

CRRT may be indicated for patients with acute or chronic kidney disease who are too clinically unstable for traditional HD, for patients with fluid overload secondary to oliguric (low urine output) kidney disease, and for patients whose kidneys cannot handle their acutely high metabolic

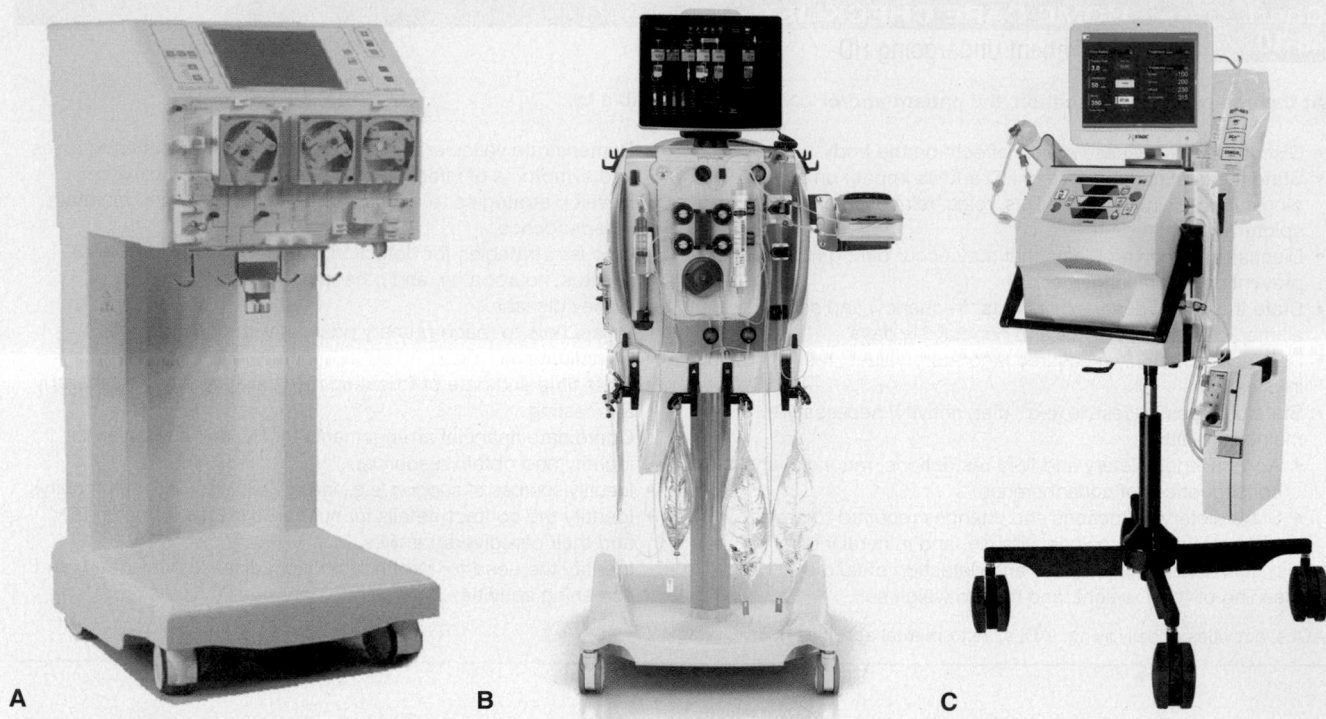

Figure 48-6 • Devices for administering continuous renal replacement therapy (CRRT) offer an integrated fluid warmer for the heating of infusion and dialysate fluids, a weighing or volumetric measuring system to reduce the possibility of error in assessing fluid balance, and a battery backup that allows treatments to continue when the patient is moved. **A.** Diapact CRRT System, B-Braun Medical, Inc., Bethlehem, PA. **B.** PrisMax, Baxter International, Inc., Chicago, Il. **C.** System One with NxView, NxStage Medical Inc. Photo courtesy of Fresenius Medical Care.

or nutritional needs. Some forms of CRRT may not require dialysis machines or dialysis personnel to carry out the procedures and can be initiated quickly in the critical-care unit. Several types of CRRT are available and widely used in critical-care units (see Fig. 48-6). The methods are similar, as they require access to the circulation and blood to pass through an artificial filter. A hemofilter (an extremely porous blood filter containing a semipermeable membrane) is used in all types.

 Continuous Venovenous Hemofiltration

Continuous venovenous hemofiltration (CVVH) is often used to manage AKI. Blood from a double-lumen venous catheter is pumped (using a small blood pump) through a hemofilter and then returned to the patient through a different lumen of the same catheter (Odom, 2017). CVVH provides **ultrafiltration** (continuous slow fluid removal); therefore, hemodynamic effects are mild and better tolerated by patients with unstable conditions. CVVH requires a dual-lumen venous catheter, a specialized machine, and critical-care nurses trained in management of the therapy who can set up, initiate, maintain, and terminate the system. Many hospitals have developed a collaborative approach to managing the CVVH therapy between the critical-care and nephrology nursing staff (Odom, 2017).

 Continuous Venovenous Hemodialysis

Continuous venovenous hemodialysis (CVVHD) is similar to CVVH. Blood is pumped from a double-lumen venous catheter through a hemofilter and returned to the patient through a different lumen of the same catheter. In addition to the benefits of ultrafiltration, CVVHD uses a concentration gradient to facilitate the removal of uremic toxins and fluid by adding a dialysate solution into the jacket of the dialyzer, surrounding the blood in the fibers. Hemodynamic effects are usually mild and critical-care nurses can set up, initiate, maintain, and terminate the system with the support of the nephrology nursing staff (Odom, 2017).

Peritoneal Dialysis (PD)

The goals of PD are to remove toxic substances and metabolic wastes and to reestablish normal fluid and electrolyte balance. PD may be the treatment of choice for patients with kidney disease who are unable or unwilling to undergo HD or kidney transplantation. Patients who are susceptible to the rapid fluid, electrolyte, and metabolic changes that occur during HD experience fewer of these problems with the slower rate of PD. Therefore, patients with diabetes or cardiovascular disease, many older patients, and those who may be at risk for adverse effects of systemic heparin are likely candidates for PD. In addition, severe hypertension, heart failure, and pulmonary edema not responsive to usual treatment regimens have been successfully treated with PD. Fewer than 8% of patients with ESKD receive PD as their treatment modality (USRDS, 2019). Chart 48-11 discusses suitability for PD.

In PD, the peritoneal membrane that covers the abdominal organs and lines the abdominal wall serves as the semipermeable membrane. Sterile dialysate fluid, containing dextrose and electrolytes, is introduced into the peritoneal cavity

Chart 48-11 Considerations for Peritoneal Dialysis

Although peritoneal dialysis (PD) is not suitable for all patients with end-stage kidney disease (ESKD), it is a viable therapy for those who can perform self-care and fluid exchanges and fit therapy into their own routines. Often, patients report having more energy and feeling healthier once they begin PD. Nurses can be instrumental in helping patients with ESKD find the dialysis therapy that best suits their lifestyle. Those considering PD need to understand the advantages and disadvantages along with the indications and contraindications for this form of therapy.

Advantages

- Freedom from a hemodialysis (HD) machine
- More control over daily activities
- Opportunities to eat a more liberal diet than allowed with HD; usually increased fluid allowance; improved serum hematocrit values; improved blood pressure control; avoidance of venipuncture; and improved sense of well-being.

Disadvantages

- Need for dialysis 7 days a week
- Dietary alterations related to protein and potassium losses. Patients may be encouraged to increase the intake of protein and potassium in the diet due to these losses with PD fluid exchanges

Indications

- Patient's willingness, motivation, and ability to perform dialysis at home
- Strong family or community support system (essential for success), particularly if the patient is an older adult
- Special problems with long-term HD, such as dysfunctional or failing vascular access devices, excessive thirst, severe hypertension, post-dialysis headaches, and severe anemia requiring frequent transfusion
- Interim therapy while awaiting kidney transplantation
- ESKD secondary to diabetes because hypertension, uremia, and hyperglycemia are easier to manage with PD than with HD

Contraindications

- Adhesions from previous surgery (adhesions reduce clearance of solutes) or systemic inflammatory disease
- Chronic backache and preexisting disc disease, which could be aggravated by the continuous pressure of dialysis fluid in the abdomen
- Severe arthritis or poor hand strength necessitating assistance in performing the exchange. However, patients who are blind or partially blind and those with other physical limitations can learn to perform PD

---

through an abdominal catheter at established intervals. Once the sterile solution is in the peritoneal cavity, uremic toxins such as urea and creatinine begin to be cleared from the blood. Diffusion of these solutes occurs as waste products move from an area of higher concentration (the bloodstream) to an area of lesser concentration (the dialysate fluid) through a semipermeable membrane (the peritoneum). This movement of solute from the blood into the dialysate fluid is called clearance. Because substances cross the peritoneal membrane at different rates, adjustments in solution dwell time and volume are made to facilitate the process of clearance. Ultrafiltration occurs in PD through an osmotic gradient created by using a dialysate fluid with a higher glucose concentration than the blood.

Procedure

As with other forms of treatment, the decision to begin PD is made by the patient and family in consultation with the nephrologist. With PD, the patient generally has ESKD and will need to receive ongoing treatments.

Preparing the Patient

The nurse's preparation of the patient and family for PD depends upon the assessment of the patient's physical and psychological status, mental status, previous experience with dialysis, and understanding of and familiarity with the procedure.

The nurse and surgeon or interventional radiologist or nephrologist explain the procedure to the patient. The nurse assists the provider in obtaining signed consent for insertion of the catheter. Baseline vital signs, weight, and serum electrolyte levels are recorded. Evaluation of the abdomen for placement of the catheter exit site is done to facilitate self-care. Typically, the catheter is placed on the nondominant side to allow the patient easier access to the catheter connection site when exchanges are done. The patient is instructed to empty the bladder and bowel to reduce the risk of puncture of internal organs during the insertion procedure. A prophylactic antibiotic agent will be given to prevent infection. The peritoneal catheter can be inserted in interventional radiology, in the operating room, or, rarely, at the bedside. Depending on the situation, this will need to be explained to the patient and family.

Preparing the Equipment

In addition to assembling the equipment to administer PD, the nurse consults with the physician to determine the concentration of dialysate to be used and the medications to be added. Heparin may be added to prevent fibrin formation and resultant occlusion of the peritoneal catheter. Potassium chloride may be prescribed to prevent hypokalemia. Antibiotic agents may be added to treat **peritonitis** (inflammation of the peritoneal membrane) caused by infection. Insulin is rarely added to PD fluid due to widespread use of subcutaneous insulin pumps and sliding scales (Kelman & Watson, 2017). Aseptic technique is imperative whenever medications are added to the PD solution. In a hospital setting, to prevent contamination, a pharmacist generally adds all medications to the dialysate bags in the pharmacy under a laminar flow hood. In the home setting, the nurse instructs the patient or family on how to aseptically add medications to PD fluid.

The dialysate is warmed to body temperature to prevent patient discomfort and abdominal pain and to dilate the vessels of the peritoneum to increase urea clearance. Solutions that are too cold cause pain, cramping, and vasoconstriction and reduce clearance. Dry heating (heating cabinet, incubator, or heating pad) is recommended. Methods that are never recommended include soaking the bags of solution in warm water (introduces bacteria to the exterior of the bags of solution and increases the chance of peritonitis) and using a microwave oven to heat the fluid (increases the danger of burning the peritoneum) (Kelman & Watson, 2017).

Immediately before initiating dialysis, using aseptic technique, the nurse assembles the dialysate with attached tubing and drainage bag. All PD dialysate fluid, tubing, and drainage bags are manufactured as closed systems and no spiking of solution is needed. The tubing is primed with the prepared dialysate to prevent air from entering the catheter and peritoneal cavity, which would cause abdominal discomfort and interfere with instillation and drainage of the fluid.

Inserting the Catheter

In most cases, the peritoneal catheter is inserted in the operating room or radiology suite to maintain surgical asepsis and minimize the risk of contamination. Catheters for long-term use are usually soft and flexible and made of silicone with a radiopaque strip to permit visualization on x-ray. These catheters have three sections: an intraperitoneal section, with numerous openings and an open tip to allow dialysate to flow freely; a subcutaneous section that passes from the peritoneal membrane and tunnels through muscle and subcutaneous fat to the skin; and an external section for connection to the manufacturer specific transfer set which then connects to the dialysate tubing with attached dialysate. Most adult catheters have 2 cuffs made of Dacron polyester. The cuffs stabilize the catheter, limit movement, prevent leaks, and provide a barrier against microorganisms. One cuff is placed just distal to the peritoneum, and the other cuff is placed subcutaneously. The subcutaneous tunnel (5 to 10 cm long) further protects against bacterial infection (see Fig. 48-7).

Performing the Exchange

All types of PD involve a series of exchanges or cycles. An **exchange** is the entire cycle including drainage of the **effluent** (fluid), instillation of the dialysate, and dwell. This cycle is repeated throughout the course of the dialysis.

At the end of the dwell time, the drainage portion of the exchange begins. The dialysate is infused by gravity into the peritoneal cavity. A period of about 10 minutes is usually required to infuse 2 to 3 L of fluid. A sterile cap is applied to the transfer set and the patient can perform ADLs. The prescribed dwell, or equilibration time, allows diffusion and osmosis to occur. At the end of the prescribed dwell, the patient performs hand hygiene, dons a mask, removes the sterile cap, unclamps the transfer set, and the solution drains from the peritoneal cavity by gravity through a closed system. Drainage is usually completed in 20 to 30 minutes. The drainage fluid is normally colorless or straw-colored and should not be cloudy. Bloody or pink-colored drainage may be seen in the first few exchanges after insertion of a new catheter, but should not occur after that time (Kelman & Watson, 2017).

The number of cycles or exchanges and their frequency are prescribed based on monthly laboratory values and the presence of uremic symptoms. The exchanges can be performed manually during the waking hours by the patient (continuous ambulatory peritoneal dialysis [CAPD]) or via the use of a PD machine (cycler) that automatically performs exchanges, usually while the patient is sleeping at night (continuous cycling peritoneal dialysis [CCPD]).

The removal of excess water during PD occurs because dialysate has a high dextrose concentration, making it hypertonic. An osmotic gradient is created between the blood and the dialysate solution. Dextrose solutions of 1.5%, 2.5%, and

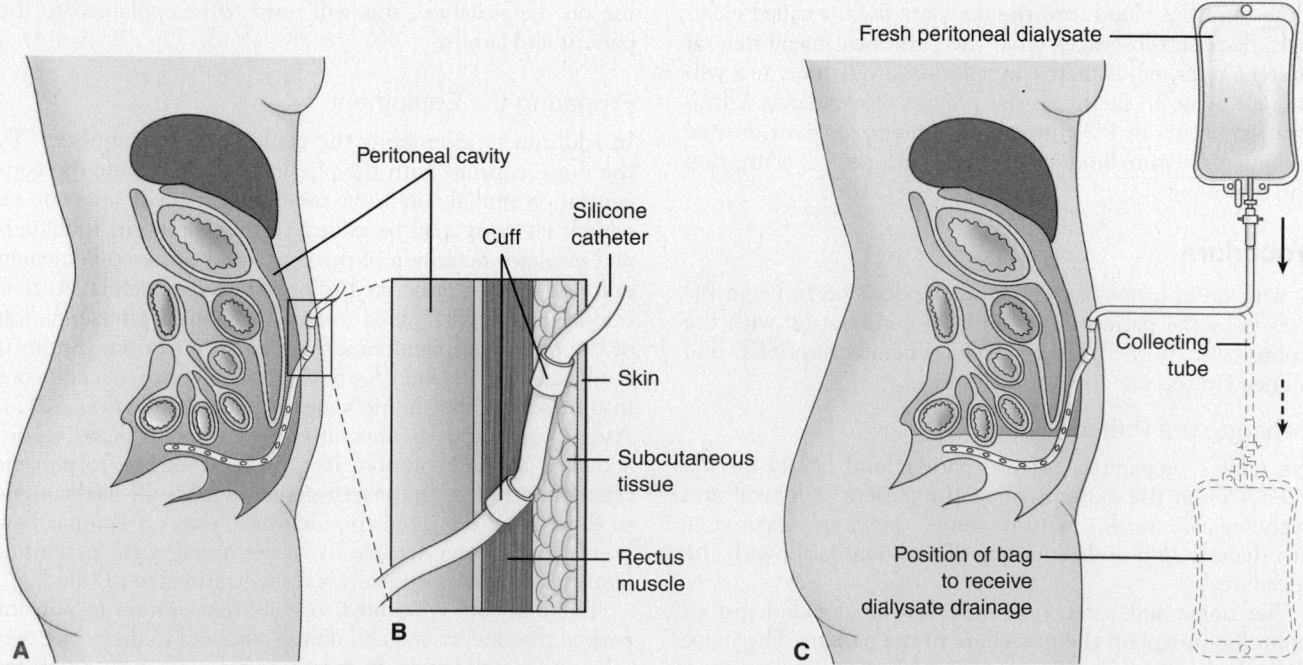

Figure 48-7 • Peritoneal dialysis. **A.** The peritoneal catheter is implanted through the abdominal wall. **B.** Dacron cuffs and a subcutaneous tunnel provide protection against bacterial infection. **C.** Continuous Ambulatory Peritoneal Dialysis (CAPD): Dialysate flows by gravity through the peritoneal catheter into the peritoneal cavity. After a prescribed period of time, the fluid is drained by gravity and discarded. New solution is then infused into the peritoneal cavity until the next drainage period. Dialysis thus continues on a 24-hour-a-day basis, during which the patient is free to move around and engage in their usual activities.

4.25% are available in several volumes, from 1000 to 3000 mL. The higher the dextrose concentration, the greater the osmotic gradient and the more water will be removed. Selection of the appropriate solution is based on the patient's fluid status (Kelman & Watson, 2017).

Complications

Most complications of PD are often minor; however, several, if unattended, can have serious consequences.

Acute Complications

Peritonitis

Peritonitis is the most common and serious complication of PD. The first sign of peritonitis is cloudy dialysate effluent (Kelman & Watson, 2017). Diffuse abdominal pain and rebound tenderness often occur later. Hypotension and other signs of shock may also occur with advancing infection. The patient with peritonitis may be treated as an inpatient or outpatient (most common), depending on the severity of the infection and the patient's clinical status. Effluent is examined for WBC count. Gram stain and culture are used to identify the organism and guide treatment. If the effluent WBC count is greater than 100 μL (after a dwell time of at least 2 hours) with over 50% polymorphonuclear cells, then broad-spectrum antibiotic agents (aminoglycosides or cephalosporins) are usually added to subsequent exchanges until Gram stain or culture results are available for specific antibiotic sensitivity. Intraperitoneal administration of antibiotic agents is as effective as IV administration and, therefore, most often used. Antibiotic therapy continues for 14 to 21 days (Kelman & Watson, 2017). Careful selection and calculation of the antibiotic dosages are needed to prevent nephrotoxicity and further compromise of residual renal function.

During an episode of peritonitis, the patient loses large amounts of protein through the peritoneal membrane due to inflammation and increased permeability. Acute malnutrition and delayed healing and recovery from the peritonitis may result. Therefore, attention must be given to educating the patient to detect and promptly seek treatment for peritonitis.

Leakage

In general, use of the PD catheter is delayed for at least 2 weeks post insertion to allow healing to occur and to prevent leakage through the tunnel and exit site. It also allows the exit site time to heal. However, leakage of dialysate through the catheter site may occur even after a healing period. Usually, the leak stops spontaneously when dialysis is withheld for several days, giving the tissue the opportunity to heal around the catheter cuffs and to seal the insertion tunnel. During this time, it is important to reduce factors that might delay healing, such as undue abdominal muscle activity (bending, lifting over 5 lb) and straining during bowel movements. In many cases, leakage can be avoided by using small volumes (500 mL) of dialysate, gradually increasing the volume up to 2000 to 3000 mL (Payton & Kennedy, 2017).

Bleeding

Bloody effluent may be observed occasionally, especially in young, menstruating women. (The hypertonic fluid pulls blood from the uterus, through the opening in the fallopian tubes, and into the peritoneal cavity.) Bleeding is also common during the first few exchanges after a new catheter insertion because some blood enters the abdominal cavity following insertion. The bleeding most often clears up after several exchanges. In many cases, no cause can be found for the bleeding, although catheter displacement from the pelvis has occasionally been associated with bleeding. Some patients have had bloody effluent after an enema or from minor trauma. Most often, bleeding stops in 1 to 2 days and requires no specific intervention. More frequent exchanges and the addition of heparin to the dialysate during this time may be necessary to prevent blood clots from obstructing the catheter (Kelman & Watson, 2017).

Long-Term Complications

Hypertriglyceridemia, likely due to the use of glucose containing dialysate, is common in patients on long-term PD, suggesting that the therapy may contribute to atherogenesis. Cardiovascular disease is the leading cause of morbidity and mortality in patients with both CKD and ESKD, and many patients have suboptimal blood pressure control which contributes to cardiovascular disease. Beta-blockers and ACE inhibitors are often used to control hypertension, decrease proteinuria, and protect the heart, and the use of aspirin and statins should be considered (Schonder, 2017).

Other complications that may occur with long-term PD include abdominal hernias (incisional, inguinal, diaphragmatic, and umbilical), likely resulting from continuously increased intra-abdominal pressure. The persistently elevated intra-abdominal pressure also aggravates symptoms of hiatal hernia and hemorrhoids. Low back pain and anorexia from fluid in the abdomen and a constant sweet taste related to glucose absorption may also be experienced by the patient.

Mechanical problems occasionally occur and may interfere with instillation or drainage of the dialysate. Formation of clots and fibrin in the peritoneal catheter and constipation are factors that may contribute to these problems.

Approaches

PD can be performed using several different approaches: acute intermittent peritoneal dialysis, CAPD, and CCPD.

Acute Intermittent Peritoneal Dialysis

Indications for acute intermittent PD, a variation of PD, include uremic signs and symptoms (nausea, vomiting, fatigue, altered mental status), fluid overload, acidosis, and hyperkalemia. Although PD is not as efficient as HD in removing solute and fluid, it permits a more gradual change in the patient's fluid volume status and in waste product removal. Therefore, it may be the treatment of choice for the patient who is hemodynamically unstable. It can be carried out manually (the nurse warms and hangs each container of dialysate) or by a cycler machine. Exchange times range from 30 minutes to 2 hours. One example of a routine is hourly exchanges consisting of a 10-minute infusion, a 30-minute dwell time, and a 20-minute drain time. Acute intermittent PD is not indicated for long-term patient management, but for specific situations such as patients who are referred late in the course of CKD (CKD stage 5) and require immediate dialysis (Kelman & Watson, 2017).

Maintaining the PD cycle is a nursing responsibility. Aseptic technique is maintained when changing solution bags and emptying effluent bags. Vital signs, weight, I&O, laboratory values, and patient status are frequently monitored. The nurse uses a flow sheet on paper or within the electronic health record to document each exchange and records vital signs, dialysate concentration, medications added, exchange volume, dwell time, dialysate fluid balance for each exchange (fluid lost or gained), and cumulative fluid balance. The nurse also carefully assesses skin turgor and mucous membranes to evaluate fluid status and monitor the patient for edema. Daily weight is the most accurate indicator of fluid volume status. Patients receiving CAPD are generally weighed with a dwell, while those on CCPD may not carry a daytime dwell and may be weighed without a dwell. The presence of absence of a dwell during the daily weight should be documented.

> ### ◣ *Quality and Safety Nursing Alert*
>
> *If the peritoneal fluid does not drain properly, the nurse can facilitate drainage by turning the patient from side to side, having the patient sit or stand, or raising the head of the bed. The peritoneal catheter should never be manipulated.*

Other measures to promote drainage include checking the patency of the catheter by inspecting for kinks, closed clamps, or an air lock. The nurse monitors for complications, including peritonitis, bleeding, respiratory difficulty, and leakage of peritoneal fluid around the catheter. In addition, the nurse must ensure that the PD catheter remains secure and that the dressing remains dry and is changed on a routine basis. The patient and family are educated about the procedure and are kept informed about progress (fluid loss, weight loss, laboratory values). Emotional support and encouragement are given to the patient and family during this stressful and uncertain time.

Continuous Ambulatory Peritoneal Dialysis (CAPD)

Continuous ambulatory peritoneal dialysis (CAPD) works on the same principles as other forms of PD: diffusion and osmosis. Less extreme fluctuations in the patient's laboratory values occur with CAPD than with intermittent PD or HD because the dialysis is constantly in progress. The serum electrolyte levels often remain in the normal range.

Procedure

The patient performs exchanges four or five times a day, 24 hours a day, 7 days a week, at intervals scheduled throughout the day. Different manufacturers supply slightly different equipment. A closed Y-shaped system is most commonly used, in which a bag containing dialysate solution comes connected to one branch of the "Y" and a sterile empty bag is connected to the second branch. This leaves the third part of the "Y" open and available for connection to the transfer set on the PD catheter. To perform an exchange, the patient (or person doing the exchange) washes their hands, dons a mask, and then removes the cap from the transfer set while maintaining sterility. The open end of the "Y" set is connected to the end of the transfer set and the dialysate is drained into the attached empty sterile bag (effluent) (over about 20 to 30 minutes). Then the attached dialysate is infused, the patient clamps off the transfer set and the tubing set, disconnects the tubing set, and applies a new sterile cap to the transfer set, making it a closed system.

For some patients, depending on the characteristic of the peritoneal membrane, the longer the dwell time, the better the clearance of uremic toxins. If dwell time is excessive (e.g., overnight dwells), the patient will absorb some of the effluent back into the body simply because the osmotic gradient is lost. Once equilibrium is reached, the movement of fluid and toxins stops (Kelman & Watson, 2017).

Complications

To reduce the risk of peritonitis, the patient (and all caregivers) must use meticulous aseptic care to avoid contaminating the catheter, fluid, or tubing and to avoid accidentally disconnecting the catheter from the tubing. Whenever a connection or disconnection is made, hand hygiene must be performed and a mask worn by anyone within 6 ft of the area to avoid contamination with airborne bacteria. Excess manipulation should be avoided, and meticulous care of the catheter exit site is provided using a standardized protocol. At home, a patient is taught to use clean technique for exit site care (Payton & Kennedy, 2017). In the hospital, due to the increased risk of infection, sterile technique is employed by the nurse and patient.

Continuous Cyclic Peritoneal Dialysis

Continuous cyclic peritoneal dialysis (CCPD) uses a machine called a cycler to provide the fluid exchanges. It is programmed to deliver an established amount of PD solution that will dwell in the peritoneal cavity for a programmed period of time before it drains from the peritoneal cavity via gravity. The cycler is also set to deliver a specific number of fluid changes in a designated period of time. Because it is programmed, it also keeps track of the total amounts removed and will sound an alarm if limits are not met. It requires that a person set up and break down the system for use, which typically takes about 30 minutes.

CCPD may combine overnight intermittent PD with a prolonged dwell time during the day. However, some patients are drained completely after completing the nighttime exchanges and do not carry a dwell during the day. This avoids reabsorption of fluid during the long daytime dwell. Every evening, the patient connects the peritoneal catheter to tubing on the cycler machine, usually just before the patient goes to sleep for the night. Because the machine is very quiet, the patient can sleep, and the extra-long tubing allows the patient to move and turn normally. In the morning, the patient disconnects from the cycler. This process is done every day to achieve the effects of dialysis required.

CCPD has a lower infection rate than other forms of PD because there are fewer opportunities for contamination with bag changes and tubing disconnections. It also allows the patient to be free from exchanges throughout the day, making it possible to engage in work and activities of daily living more freely (Kelman & Watson, 2017).

Nursing Management

Meeting Psychosocial Needs

In addition to the complications of PD described previously, patients who elect to do PD may experience altered body image because of the presence of the abdominal catheter, bag, tubing, and cycler. Waist size increases from 1 to 2 inches (or more) with fluid in the abdomen. This affects clothing selection and may make the patient feel distended or fat. The nurse may arrange for the patient to talk with other patients who have adapted well to PD. Although some patients have no psychological problems with the catheter—they think of it as their lifeline and as a life-sustaining device—other patients feel they are doing exchanges all day long and have no free time, particularly in the beginning. They may experience depression because they feel overwhelmed with the responsibility of self-care.

Patients undergoing PD may also experience altered sexuality patterns and sexual dysfunction. The patient and partner may be reluctant to engage in sexual activities, partly because of the catheter being psychologically "in the way" of sexual performance. In patients on CCPD, the presence of the dialysis cycler in the bedroom and the continual connection during the sleeping hours can also cause interference with intimacy. Although these problems may resolve with time, some problems may warrant special counseling. Questions by the nurse about concerns related to sexuality and sexual function often provide the patient with a welcome opportunity to discuss these issues and a first step toward assisting in their resolution.

Promoting Home, Community-Based, and Transitional Care

 Educating Patients About Self-Care

Patients are educated as inpatients or outpatients to perform PD once their condition is medically stable. Education generally takes 5 days to 2 weeks. Patients are taught according to their own learning ability and knowledge level and only as much at one time as they can handle without feeling uncomfortable or becoming saturated. Education topics for the patient and family who will be performing PD at home are described in Chart 48-12. The use of an adult learning theory–based curriculum may decrease peritonitis and exit site infection rates (Kelman & Watson, 2017).

Because of protein loss with PD, the patient is instructed to eat a high-protein (1.2 to 1.3g/kg/day), low phosphorus, nutritious diet (NKF KDOQI, 2000). The patient is also encouraged to increase their daily fiber intake to help prevent constipation, which can impede the flow of dialysate into or out of the peritoneal cavity. Patients may gain 3 to 5 lb within a month of initiating PD, so they may be asked to limit their carbohydrate intake to avoid weight gain. Potassium and fluid restrictions are not usually necessary. Patients commonly lose at least 1 to 2 L of fluid over and above the volume of dialysate infused into the abdomen during a 24-hour period, permitting a moderate fluid intake.

Continuing and Transitional Care

Follow-up care through phone calls, visits to the dialysis clinic, outpatient department, and continuing home care assists patients in the transition to home and promotes their active participation in their own health care. Patients often check with the nurse to see if they are making the correct choices about dialysate or control of blood pressure, or simply to discuss a problem.

Patients may be seen by the PD team as outpatients once a month or more often if needed. The exchange procedure is

---

Chart 48-12 — HOME CARE CHECKLIST
Peritoneal Dialysis, Continuous Ambulatory Peritoneal Dialysis, or Continuous Cycling Peritoneal Dialysis

At the completion of education, the patient and/or caregiver will be able to:

- Discuss kidney disease and its effects on the body.
- State the goal and purpose of dialysis and its impact on physiologic functioning, ADLs, IADLs, roles, relationships, and spirituality.
- Describe the basic principles of peritoneal dialysis (PD) and exchange options such as continuous ambulatory peritoneal dialysis (CAPD), or continuous cycling peritoneal dialysis (CCPD).
- State what types of changes are needed (if any) to support home PD therapy and maintain a clean home environment and prevent infection.
- State how to contact the primary provider, the team of home care professionals overseeing care, and supply vendor.
  - Discuss ordering, storage, and inventory of dialysis supplies.
  - List emergency phone numbers.
- State the name, dose, side effects, frequency, and schedule for all medications.
  - Demonstrate procedure for adding medications to the dialysis solution.
- Demonstrate catheter and exit site care.
- Demonstrate measurement of vital signs and weight measurement.
- Discuss monitoring and management of fluid balance.
- Discuss basic principles of aseptic technique.
- Demonstrate the CAPD or CCPD exchange procedure using aseptic technique (patients receiving CCPD should also

- demonstrate exchange procedure in case of failure or unavailability of cycling machine) and discuss cycling machine warning signals and how to address these signals.
- Demonstrate maintenance of home dialysis records.
- Demonstrate procedure for obtaining sterile PD fluid samples.
- Discuss routine laboratory tests needed and implications of results.
- Discuss high protein diet and diet to avoid constipation, any other dietary restrictions as indicated.
- Discuss complications of PD; prevention, recognition, and management of complications.
- Describe actions in case of emergency.
- Relate how to reach primary provider with questions or complications.
- State time and date of follow-up medical appointments, therapy, and testing.
- Collaborate with renal/dialysis social worker to coordinate financial arrangements for PD and strategies to identify and obtain resources.
- Identify sources of support (e.g., friends, relatives, faith community).
- Identify the contact details for support services for patients and their caregivers/families.
- Identify the need for health promotion, disease prevention, and screening activities.

ADLs, activities of daily living; IADLs, instrumental activities of daily living.

evaluated at that time to reassess that strict aseptic technique is followed. Blood chemistry and effluent values are followed closely to make certain the therapy is adequate for the patient.

If a referral is made for home care, the home health nurse assesses the home environment and suggests modifications to accommodate the equipment and facilities needed to carry out PD. In addition, the nurse assesses the patient's and family's understanding of PD and evaluates their technique in performing PD. Assessments include checking for changes related to kidney disease; any complications such as peritonitis; medication management; and treatment-related problems such as heart failure, inadequate drainage, and weight gain or loss. The nurse continues to reinforce and clarify education about PD and ESKD and assesses the patient's and family's progress in coping with the procedure. This is also an opportunity to remind patients about the need to participate in appropriate health promotion activities and health screening (e.g., gynecologic examinations, colonoscopy).

Special Considerations: Nursing Management of the Patient on Dialysis Who Is Hospitalized

Whether undergoing HD or PD, the patient may be hospitalized for treatment of complications related to the dialysis treatment, the underlying kidney disorder, or health problems not related to renal dysfunction or its treatment.

Protecting Vascular Access

When the patient undergoing HD is hospitalized for any reason, care must be taken to protect the vascular access. The nurse assesses the vascular access for patency and takes precautions to ensure that the extremity with the vascular access is not used for measuring blood pressure or for obtaining blood specimens. Constricting dressings, restraints, or jewelry over the vascular access must be avoided as well (Inglese, 2017).

The bruit, or "thrill," over the venous access site must be evaluated at least every 8 to 12 hours. Absence of a palpable thrill or audible bruit may indicate blockage or clotting in the vascular access. Clotting can occur if the patient has an infection anywhere in the body (serum viscosity increases) or if the blood pressure has dropped. When blood flow is reduced through the access for any reason (hypotension, application of blood pressure cuff or tourniquet), the access can clot. When a patient has an HD catheter, the nurse must observe for signs and symptoms of infection such as redness, swelling, drainage from the exit site, fever, and chills. The nurse must assess the integrity of the dressing and change it as needed. Patients with kidney disease are more prone to infection; therefore, appropriate infection control measures must be used for all procedures. The patient's vascular access should not be used for any purpose other than dialysis, unless it is an emergency situation and no other access is available. In this situation, a dialysis nurse or physician should cannulate the vascular access. If accessing an HD catheter in an emergency, the catheter dwell volume should be withdrawn prior to medication or fluid administration.

Taking Precautions during Intravenous Therapy

When the patient needs IV therapy, the rate of administration must be as slow as possible to avoid volume overload in the patient with renal disease or ESKD. Accurate I&O records are essential.

 Quality and Safety Nursing Alert

Because patients on dialysis cannot excrete water, rapid administration of IV fluid can result in pulmonary edema.

Monitoring Symptoms of Uremia

As metabolic end products accumulate, symptoms of uremia worsen. Patients whose metabolic rate accelerates (those receiving corticosteroid medications or parenteral nutrition, those with infections or bleeding disorders, those undergoing surgery) accumulate waste products more quickly and may require daily dialysis. These same patients are more likely than other patients receiving dialysis to experience complications.

Detecting Cardiac and Respiratory Complications

Cardiac and respiratory assessment must be conducted frequently. As fluid builds up, fluid overload, heart failure, and pulmonary edema develop. Crackles in the bases of the lungs, moist cough and frothy, blood-tinged sputum may indicate pulmonary edema.

Pericarditis may result from the accumulation of uremic toxins. If not detected and treated promptly, this serious complication may progress to pericardial effusion and cardiac tamponade. Pericarditis is detected by the patient's report of substernal chest pain, low-grade fever, and pericardial friction rub. A pulsus paradoxus (a decrease in blood pressure of more than 10 mm Hg during inspiration) is often present. When pericarditis progresses to effusion, the friction rub disappears, heart sounds become distant and muffled, ECG waves show very low voltage, and the pulsus paradoxus worsens (see Chapter 24 for further discussion of pericarditis).

The effusion may progress to life-threatening cardiac tamponade, noted by narrowing of the pulse pressure in addition to muffled or inaudible heart sounds, crushing chest pain, dyspnea, and hypotension. An emergent pericardial window procedure is performed and a chest tube is inserted to drain the pericardial effusion. The effusion fluid is sent for laboratory and cytology analysis.

 Quality and Safety Nursing Alert

Although pericarditis, pericardial effusion, and cardiac tamponade can be detected by chest x-ray, they should also be detected through astute nursing assessment. Because of their clinical significance, assessment of the patient for these complications is a priority.

Controlling Electrolyte Levels and Diet

Electrolyte alterations are common, and potassium changes can be life-threatening. All IV solutions and medications to be given are evaluated for their electrolyte content. Serum laboratory values are assessed daily. If blood transfusions are required, they may be given during HD, if possible, so that excess potassium and fluid can be removed and hypervolemia is avoided. Dietary intake must also be monitored. The patient's frustrations related to dietary restrictions typically increase if the food is unappetizing. The nurse needs to recognize that this may lead to dietary indiscretion with resultant hyperkalemia.

Hypoalbuminemia is an indicator of malnutrition in patients undergoing long-term or maintenance dialysis. Although some patients can be treated with adequate nutrition alone, some patients remain hypoalbuminemic for reasons that are poorly understood.

Managing Discomfort and Pain

Complications such as pruritus and pain secondary to neuropathy must be managed. Antihistamine agents, such as diphenhydramine, are commonly used, and analgesic medications may be prescribed. However, because elimination of the metabolites of medications occurs through dialysis rather than through renal excretion, medication dosages often need to be adjusted. Keeping the skin clean and well moisturized using bath oils, superfatted soap, and creams or lotions helps promote comfort and reduce itching. Instructing the patient to keep the nails trimmed to avoid scratching and excoriation also promotes comfort.

Monitoring Blood Pressure

Hypertension in kidney disease is common. It is usually the result of fluid overload and, in part, oversecretion of renin. Many patients undergoing dialysis receive some form of antihypertensive therapy. Patients require detailed education and reinforcement of information regarding their antihypertensive regimen, because it is not uncommon for patients to need more than one antihypertensive agent. Rapid fluid fluctuations in patients receiving dialysis also create challenges to maintaining blood pressure control. Antihypertensive agents are often withheld before dialysis and administered after dialysis to avoid hypotension due to the combined effect of fluid removal with the dialysis treatment and the medication (Campoy, 2017). Typically, these patients require multiple antihypertensive agents to achieve normal blood pressure, thus adding to the total number of medications needed on an ongoing basis (Campoy, 2017).

Preventing Infection

Patients with ESKD commonly have decreased phagocytic ability with low WBC counts, low RBC counts (anemia), impaired platelet function, and are often prescribed anticoagulants to prevent heart attacks and strokes. Together, these pose a high risk of infection and potential for bleeding after even minor trauma. Preventing and controlling infection are essential because the incidence of infection is high. Infection of the vascular access site and pneumonia are common (Inglese, 2017).

Caring for the Catheter Site

Patients receiving CAPD usually know how to care for the catheter exit site. However, the hospital stay is an opportunity to assess catheter care technique and correct misperceptions or deviations from recommended technique. Recommended daily or 3 or 4 times weekly routine catheter site care is typically performed during showering or bathing (Payton & Kennedy, 2017). The exit site should not be submerged in bathwater. The most common cleaning method is soap and water; liquid soap is recommended. During care, the nurse and patient need to make sure that the catheter remains secure to avoid tension and trauma. The patient may wear a gauze dressing over the exit site.

Administering Medications

All medications and the dosage prescribed for any patient on dialysis must be closely monitored to avoid those that are toxic to the kidneys and may threaten residual renal function. Medications are also scrutinized for potassium and magnesium content; those medications that contain them are avoided. Care must be taken to evaluate all problems and symptoms that the patient reports without automatically attributing them to kidney disease or to dialysis therapy.

Providing Psychological Support

Over time, patients undergoing chronic dialysis may begin to reevaluate their status, the treatment modality, their satisfaction with life, and the impact of these factors on their families and support systems. Nurses must provide opportunities for these patients to express their feelings and reactions and to explore options. The decision to begin dialysis does not require that dialysis be continued indefinitely, and it is not uncommon for patients to consider discontinuing treatment. These feelings and reactions must be taken seriously, and the patient should have the opportunity to discuss them with the dialysis team as well as with a psychologist, psychiatrist, psychiatric nurse, trusted friend, or spiritual advisor. After a psychiatric evaluation has ruled out depression, the patient's informed decision about discontinuing treatment should be respected. If the patient is thought to be depressed, treatment for depression should be initiated and the patient stabilized prior to participating in decisions on advanced directives (Molzahn & Schick-Makaroff, 2017).

KIDNEY SURGERY

A patient may undergo surgery or procedures in the interventional radiology department to remove obstructions that affect the kidney (tumors or calculi), to insert a tube for draining the kidney (nephrostomy, ureterostomy), or to remove the kidney involved in unilateral kidney disease, renal carcinoma, or kidney transplantation.

Management of Patients Undergoing Kidney Surgery

Preoperative Considerations

Surgery is performed only after a thorough evaluation of renal function. Patient preparation to ensure that optimal renal function is maintained is essential. Fluids are encouraged to promote increased excretion of waste products before surgery unless contraindicated because of preexisting renal or cardiac dysfunction. If kidney infection is present preoperatively, broad-spectrum antimicrobial agents may be prescribed to prevent bacteremia. Antibiotic agents must be given with extreme care because many are toxic to the kidneys. Coagulation studies (prothrombin time, partial thromboplastin time, platelet count) may be indicated if the patient has a history of bruising and bleeding. The preoperative preparation is similar to that described in Chapter 14.

Because many patients facing kidney surgery are apprehensive, the nurse encourages the patient to recognize and verbalize concerns. Confidence is reinforced by establishing

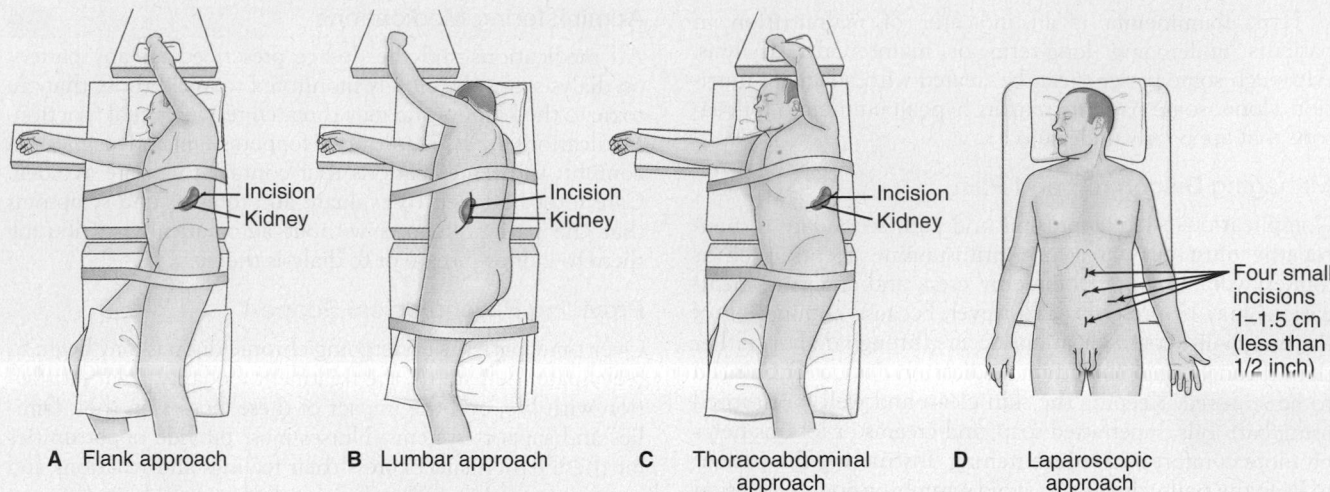

| **A** Flank approach | **B** Lumbar approach | **C** Thoracoabdominal approach | **D** Laparoscopic approach |

Figure 48-8 • Patient positioning and incisional approaches for nephrectomy—flank (**A**), lumbar (**B**), thoracoabdominal (**C**)—for kidney surgery are associated with significant postoperative discomfort. (**D**) Laparoscopic nephrectomy is associated with less discomfort and faster recovery times.

a relationship of trust and by providing expert care. Patients faced with the prospect of losing a kidney may think that they will have to depend on dialysis for the rest of their lives. The nurse reassures the patient and family that normal renal function can be maintained by a single healthy kidney.

Perioperative Concerns

Kidney surgery requires various patient positions to expose the surgical site adequately. Three surgical approaches are common: flank, lumbar, and thoracoabdominal (see Fig. 48-8A–C). Laparoscopic urologic surgery is often performed as a less invasive option than open surgery (see Fig. 48-8D). During surgery, plans are carried out for managing altered urinary drainage. These may include inserting a nephrostomy or other drainage tube.

Postoperative Management

Because the kidney is a highly vascular organ, hemorrhage and shock are the chief potential complications of kidney surgery. Fluid and blood component replacement is frequently necessary in the immediate postoperative period to treat intraoperative blood loss.

Abdominal distention and paralytic ileus may occur after renal and ureteral surgery and are thought to be due to a reflex paralysis of intestinal peristalsis and manipulation of the colon or duodenum during surgery. Abdominal distention is relieved by decompression through a nasogastric tube. See Chapter 41 for treatment of paralytic ileus. Oral fluids are permitted when the passage of flatus is noted.

If infection occurs, antibiotics are prescribed after a culture reveals the causative organism. The toxic effects that antibiotic agents have on the kidneys (nephrotoxicity) must be kept in mind when assessing the patient. Low-dose heparin therapy may be initiated postoperatively to prevent thromboembolism in patients who have had any type of urologic surgery.

Nursing Management

In addition to those interventions listed in this section, Chart 48-13 provides a plan of nursing care for the patient undergoing kidney surgery.

Providing Immediate Postoperative Care

Immediate postoperative care of the patient who has undergone kidney surgery includes assessment of all body systems. Respiratory and circulatory status, pain level, fluid and electrolyte status, and patency and adequacy of urinary drainage systems are assessed.

Respiratory Status

As with any surgery, the use of anesthesia increases the risk of respiratory complications. Noting the location of the surgical incision assists the nurse in anticipating respiratory problems and pain. Respiratory status is assessed by monitoring the rate, depth, and pattern of respirations. The location of the incision frequently causes pain on inspiration and coughing; therefore, the patient tends to splint the chest wall and take shallow respirations. Auscultation is performed to assess normal and adventitious breath sounds.

Circulatory Status and Blood Loss

The patient's vital signs and arterial or central venous pressure are monitored. Skin color and temperature and urine output provide information about circulatory status. The surgical incision and drainage tubes are observed frequently to help detect unexpected blood loss and hemorrhage.

Pain

Postoperative pain is a major problem for the patient because of the location of the surgical incision and patient's position on the operating table to permit access to the kidney. The location and severity of pain are assessed before and after analgesic medications are given. Abdominal distention, which increases discomfort, is also noted.

Urinary Drainage

Urine output and drainage from tubes inserted during surgery are monitored for amount, color, and type or characteristics. Decreased or absent drainage is promptly reported to the primary provider because it may indicate obstruction that could cause pain, infection, and disruption of the suture lines.

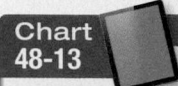

Chart 48-13

LAN OF NURSING CARE

Care of the Patient Undergoing Kidney Surgery

NURSING DIAGNOSIS: Impaired airway clearance associated with pain of high abdominal or flank incision, abdominal discomfort, and immobility; impaired breathing pattern associated with high abdominal incision
GOAL: Improved airway clearance

Nursing Interventions	Rationale	Expected Outcomes
1. Assess respiratory status: a. Rate b. Breath sounds 2. Administer analgesic agent as prescribed. 3. Splint incision with hands or pillow to assist patient in coughing. 4. Assist patient to change positions frequently. 5. Encourage the use of incentive spirometer as indicated or prescribed. 6. Assist with and encourage early ambulation.	1. Baseline data allow for monitoring of changes and evaluating effectiveness of interventions. 2. Adequate pain relief enables patient to take deep breaths and cough. 3. Splints incision and promotes adequate cough and prevention of atelectasis. 4. Promotes drainage and inflation of all lobes of the lungs. 5. Encourages adequate deep breaths. 6. Mobilizes pulmonary secretions.	• Exhibits respiratory rate of 12 to 18 breaths/min and normal breath sounds without adventitious sounds • Takes deep breaths and coughs adequately when encouraged and assisted • Exhibits full thoracic excursion without shallow respirations • Uses incentive spirometer with encouragement • Splints incision while taking deep breaths and coughing • Reports progressively less pain and discomfort with coughing and deep breaths

NURSING DIAGNOSIS: Acute pain and discomfort associated with surgical incision, positioning, and stretching of muscles during kidney surgery
GOAL: Relief of pain and discomfort

Nursing Interventions	Rationale	Expected Outcomes
1. Assess level of pain based on measureable scale rating. 2. Administer analgesic agents as prescribed. 3. Splint incision with hands or pillow during movement or deep breathing and coughing exercises. 4. Assist and encourage early ambulation. 5. Offer and educate patient how to use appropriate nonpharmacologic interventions. 6. Evaluate the effectiveness of pain relief using a scale rating.	1. Provides baseline for later evaluation of pain relief strategies. 2. Promotes pain relief. 3. Minimizes sensation of pulling or tension on incision and provides sense of support to the patient. 4. Promotes resumption of muscle activity exercise. 5. Many nonpharmacologic interventions, such as music, relaxation exercises, and imagery assist patients to decrease their pain. 6. A scale provides an objective measure of the efficacy of pain relief strategies.	• Reports decreased pain on pain scale to a level that is acceptable to the patient. • Takes analgesia as prescribed • Exercises aching muscles within recommendations • Uses music, relaxation exercises, and imagery to relieve pain • Exhibits no behavioral manifestations of pain and discomfort (e.g., restlessness, perspiration, verbal expressions of pain) • Participates in deep-breathing and coughing exercises • Gradually increases physical activity and exercise

NURSING DIAGNOSIS: Fear and anxiety associated with diagnosis, outcome of surgery, and alteration in urinary function
GOAL: Reduction of fear and anxiety

Nursing Interventions	Rationale	Expected Outcomes
1. Assess patient's anxiety and fear before surgery if possible. 2. Assess patient's knowledge about procedure and expected surgical outcome preoperatively. 3. Evaluate the meaning of alterations resulting from surgical procedure for the patient and family or partner. 4. Encourage patient to verbalize reactions, feelings, and fears. 5. Encourage patient to share feelings with spouse or partner. 6. Offer and arrange for visit from member of support group (e.g., ostomy group, transplant group, if indicated).	1. Provides a baseline for postoperative assessment. 2. Provides a basis for further education. 3. Enables understanding of patient's reactions and responses to expected and unexpected results of surgery. 4. Affirms patient's understanding of and ultimate resolution of feelings and fears. 5. Enables patient and partner to receive mutual support and reduces sense of isolation from each other. 6. Provides support from another person who has encountered the same or a similar surgical procedure and an example of how others have coped with the alteration.	• Verbalizes reactions and feelings to staff • Shares reactions and feelings with family or partner • Grieves appropriately for self and for changes in role and function • Identifies information needed to promote own adaptation and coping • Participates in activities and events in immediate environment • Accepts visit from support group if indicated • Identifies support person or support group

(continued on page 1594)

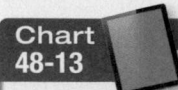

LAN OF NURSING CARE (continued)

Chart 48-13
Care of the Patient Undergoing Kidney Surgery

NURSING DIAGNOSIS: Impaired urination associated with urinary drainage; risk for urinary infection associated with altered urinary drainage

GOAL: Maintenance of urinary elimination; infection-free urinary tract

Nursing Interventions	Rationale	Expected Outcomes
1. Assess urinary drainage system immediately.	1. Provides basis for further assessment and action.	• Exhibits adequate urinary output and patent drainage system
2. Assess adequacy of urinary output and patency of drainage system.	2. Provides baseline.	• Exhibits urinary output consistent with fluid intake
3. Assess pertinent laboratory values (see Chapter 47, Table 47-5).	3. Provides basis for further assessment and action.	• Demonstrates normal laboratory values: blood urea nitrogen, serum creatinine levels, urine specific gravity, and osmolality
4. Use asepsis and hand hygiene when providing care and manipulating drainage system.	4. Prevents or reduces risk of contamination of urinary drainage system.	• Exhibits sterile urine on urine culture
5. Maintain closed urinary drainage system.	5. Reduces risk of bacterial contamination and infection.	• Exhibits clear, dilute urine without debris or encrustation in the drainage system
6. If irrigation of the drainage system is necessary, use sterile gloves and sterile irrigating solution and a closed drainage and irrigation system.	6. Permits irrigation when necessary while maintaining closed drainage system, minimizing risk of infection.	• States rationale for avoiding manipulation of catheter, drainage, or irrigation system
7. If irrigation is necessary and prescribed, perform it gently with sterile saline and the prescribed amount of irrigating fluid.	7. Maintains patency of the catheter or drainage system and prevents sudden increases in pressure in the urinary tract that may cause trauma, pressure on sutures or urinary tract structures, and pain.	• Exhibits normal placement of urinary stent or ureteral catheters until removed by physician
8. Assist patient in turning and moving in bed and when ambulating to prevent displacement or inadvertent removal of urinary stent or ureteral catheters if in place.	8. Prevents trauma from accidental displacement of urinary stent or ureteral catheter necessitating repeated instrumentation of the urinary tract (e.g., cystoscopy) to replace them.	• Maintains closed urinary drainage system
9. Observe urine color, volume, odor, and components.	9. Provides information about adequacy of urine output, condition and patency of drainage system, and debris in urine.	• Exhibits normal body temperature without signs or symptoms of urinary tract infection
10. Minimize trauma and manipulation of catheter, drainage system, and urethra.	10. Reduces risk of contamination of drainage system and eliminates site of bacterial invasion.	• Cleans catheter twice daily with soap and water or antibacterial meatal cleansing cloths
11. Clean catheter gently with soap during bathing, avoiding any to-and-fro movement of catheter.	11. Removes debris and encrustations without causing trauma to or contamination of urethra.	• Consumes adequate fluid intake (6 to 8 glasses of water or more per day, unless contraindicated)
12. Anchor drainage tube with hospital-approved device (e.g., Stat-Lock).	12. Prevents movement or slipping of drainage tube, minimizing trauma to and contamination of urethra or catheter.	• Urinary drainage system remains in place until physician orders discontinuation.
13. Maintain adequate fluid intake.	13. Promotes adequate urine output and prevents urinary stasis.	• Maintains urinary drainage system without infection or obstruction
14. Assist with and encourage early ambulation while ensuring placement of urinary drainage system.	14. Minimizes cardiovascular and pulmonary complications while preventing loss, dislodging, or disruption of drainage system.	• Maintains urinary diversion as instructed
15. If patient is to be discharged with urinary drainage system (catheter) in place or a urinary diversion, instruct patient and family member in care.	15. Knowledge and understanding of the drainage system or urinary diversion are essential to prevent infection and other complications.	• Maintains self-care so that environment is odor free

NURSING DIAGNOSIS: Risk for fluid imbalance associated with surgical fluid loss, altered urinary output, parenteral fluid administration

GOAL: Normal fluid balance will be maintained

Nursing Interventions	Rationale	Expected Outcomes
1. Weigh patient daily.	1. Daily weight is the most sensitive indicator of fluid loss or gain.	• Patient's weight will be within 2 to 3 lb of patient's baseline.
2. Document accurate intake and output.	2. Assists in detection of fluid retention due to poor cardiac or renal output.	• Intake that exceeds output will be detected early.
3. Place all parenteral therapy on an infusion pump.	3. Ensures that the patient does not receive excess or insufficient IV fluids.	• The exact amount of solution is infused with no adverse effects resulting from over- or underinfusion.
4. Monitor amount and characteristics of urine.	4. Assists in early detection of possible complications of surgery or tube insertion.	• Urine is clear and absent of blood, pus, or any foreign substances.
5. Monitor vital signs: temperature, pulse, respirations, and blood pressure.	5. When fluid volume or cardiac output is altered, vital signs are affected.	• Temperature, pulse, respiration, and blood pressure are within defined limits.
6. Auscultate heart and lungs sounds every shift.	6. When fluid volume is increased because of poor cardiac or renal output, fluid accumulates in the lungs. In addition, heart sounds change as heart failure develops; frequent auscultation ensures early detection.	• Normal heart and lung sounds are present.

Monitoring and Managing Potential Complications

Bleeding is a major complication of kidney surgery. If undetected and untreated, it can result in hypovolemia and hemorrhagic shock. The nurse's role is to observe for these complications, to report their signs and symptoms, and to administer prescribed parenteral fluids and blood and blood components. Monitoring of vital signs, skin condition, the urinary drainage system, the surgical incision, and the level of consciousness is necessary to detect evidence of bleeding, decreased circulating blood, and fluid volume and cardiac output. Frequent monitoring of vital signs (initially monitored at least at hourly intervals) and urinary output is necessary for early detection of these complications.

If bleeding goes undetected or is not detected promptly, the patient may lose significant amounts of blood and may experience hypoxemia. In addition to hypovolemic shock due to hemorrhage, this type of blood loss may precipitate a myocardial infarction or transient ischemic attack. Bleeding may be suspected when the patient experiences fatigue and shortness of breath and when urine output is less than 400 mL within 24 hours. As bleeding persists, late signs of hypovolemia occur, such as cool skin, flat neck veins, and change in level of consciousness or responsiveness. Transfusions of blood components are indicated, along with surgical repair of the bleeding vessel.

Pneumonia may be prevented through the use of an incentive spirometer, adequate pain control, and early ambulation. Early signs of pneumonia include fever, increased heart and respiratory rates, and adventitious breath sounds.

Preventing infection involves using asepsis when changing dressings and handling and preparing catheters, other drainage tubes, central venous catheters, and IV catheters for administration of fluids. Insertion sites are monitored closely for signs and symptoms of inflammation: redness, drainage, heat, and pain. Special care must be taken to prevent UTI, which is associated with the use of indwelling urinary catheters. Catheters and other invasive tubes are removed as soon as they are no longer needed.

Antibiotics are commonly given postoperatively to prevent infection. If antibiotic agents are prescribed, serum creatinine and BUN values must be monitored closely because many antibiotic agents are toxic to the kidney or can accumulate to toxic levels if renal function is compromised.

Preventing fluid imbalance is critical when caring for a patient undergoing kidney surgery, because both fluid loss and fluid excess are possible adverse effects of the surgery. Fluid loss may occur during surgery as a result of excessive urinary drainage when the obstruction is removed, or it may occur if diuretic agents are used. Such loss may also occur with GI losses, with diarrhea resulting from antibiotic use, or with nasogastric drainage. When postoperative IV therapy is inadequate to match the output or fluids lost, a fluid deficit results. Fluid excess, or overload, may result from cardiac effects of anesthesia, administration of excessive amounts of fluids, or the patient's inability to excrete fluid because of changes in renal function. Decreased urine output may be an indication of fluid excess.

Astute assessment skills are needed to detect early signs of fluid excess (such as weight gain, pedal edema, urine output below 400 mL/day, and slightly elevated pulmonary artery wedge pressure if available) before they become severe (appearance of adventitious breath sounds, shortness of breath).

Fluid excess may be treated with fluid restriction and administration of furosemide or other diuretic agents. If renal insufficiency is present, these medications may prove ineffective; therefore, dialysis may be necessary to prevent heart failure and pulmonary edema.

Deep vein thrombosis (DVT) may occur postoperatively because of surgical manipulation of the iliac vessels during surgery or prolonged immobility. Anti-embolism stockings are applied, and the patient is monitored closely for signs and symptoms of thrombosis and encouraged to exercise the legs. Heparin or other anticoagulants may be given postoperatively to reduce the risk of thrombosis.

Promoting Home, Community-Based, and Transitional Care

 Educating Patients About Self-Care

If the patient has a drainage system in place, measures are taken to ensure that both the patient and family understand the importance of maintaining the system correctly at home and preventing infection. Verbal and written instructions and guidelines are provided to the patient and family at the time of hospital discharge. The patient may be asked to demonstrate or "teach back" management of the drainage system to validate understanding (see Chapter 3 for further discussion of the teach-back technique). Strategies to prevent postoperative complications (urinary tract obstruction and infection, DVT, atelectasis, and pneumonia) are stressed to the patient and family. With both the patient and family, the nurse reviews the signs, symptoms, problems, and questions that should be referred to the physician or other primary provider.

Continuing and Transitional Care

The need for postoperative assessment and care after kidney surgery continues regardless of the setting: the home, subacute care unit, outpatient clinic or office, or rehabilitation facility. Referral for home care is indicated for the patient who is going home with a urinary drainage system in place. During the home visit, the home health nurse reviews the instructions and guidelines given to the patient at hospital discharge. The nurse assesses the patient's ability to carry out the instructions in the home and answers questions that the patient or family has about management of the drainage system and the surgical incision.

In addition, the home health nurse obtains vital signs and assesses the patient for signs and symptoms of urinary tract obstruction and infection. The nurse also ensures that pain is adequately controlled and that the patient is adhering to recommendations. The home health nurse encourages adequate fluid intake and increased levels of activity. Together, the nurse, patient, and family review the signs, symptoms, problems, and questions that should be referred to the primary provider. If the patient has a drainage tube in place, the nurse assesses the site and the patency of the system and monitors the patient for complications, such as DVT, bleeding, or pneumonia.

Because it is easy for the patient, family, and health care team to focus on the patient's immediate disorder to the exclusion of other health issues, the nurse reminds the patient and family about the importance of participating in health promotion activities, including appropriate health screenings.

Kidney Transplantation

Kidney transplantation is the treatment of choice for select and appropriately screened patients with ESKD. It is not considered a cure for ESKD since, in general, the transplant will not continue to function for the entire lifespan of most recipients (Danovitch, 2017). Patients choose kidney transplantation for various reasons, such as the desire to avoid dialysis or to improve their sense of well-being and the wish to lead a more normal life. Kidney transplantation is an elective procedure, not an emergency lifesaving procedure. Therefore, patients should be in the best possible physical condition prior to transplantation.

In the United States and globally, there are many more patients on the waiting list for kidney transplantation than there are organ donors. More than 103,356 Americans are on the waiting list to receive a kidney (Organ Procurement and Transplantation Network [OPTN], 2019). In the United States, the cost of a kidney transplant annually per person is estimated at $34,084 versus about $88,750 annually per person for in center HD (Saran, Robinson, Abbott, et al., 2018). Kidney transplantation involves transplanting a kidney from a living or deceased donor to a recipient who no longer has renal function. A living donor may or may not be related to the recipient. A deceased donor transplant comes from someone who has died and donated their organs. The term "cadaveric donor" is no longer used and the appropriate terminology is "deceased donor." Transplantation from well-matched living donors (those with compatible ABO and human leukocyte antigens) is more successful than from deceased donors, especially long term (Woodard & Arnold, 2017).

The NKF provides written information describing the organ donation program and a card specifying the organs to be donated in the event of death. The organ donation card is signed by the donor and two witnesses and should be carried by the donor at all times. In many states in the United States, drivers can indicate their desire to be organ donors on their driver's license application or renewal. However, the donor should discuss this decision with family members because the organ procurement agency will approach the family to explore this option.

Contemporary developments in kidney transplantation are paired exchanges and chains. In paired donor exchanges and chains, recipients swap compatibly matched kidneys with willing donors, who are unrelated or unknown to the recipient. Although medically eligible to donate a kidney, a willing donor may be incompatible with the intended recipient due to blood type or antigens. The donor then agrees to donate the kidney to a compatible and unknown recipient, with the intention that the donor's originally intended organ recipient will be part of the donation chain and be the recipient of a donated kidney through organized donor and recipient matches. Several national registry programs have organized systems to find a matching pair on the national level (Woodard & Arnold, 2017). See Resources at the end of the chapter.

Prior to either receiving or donating an organ, an extensive medical evaluation is performed; first on the potential recipient and then, if the recipient is deemed suitable for a transplant, the living donor is evaluated. Not everyone is suitable for kidney transplantation. Contraindications include recent malignancy, active or chronic infection (e.g., HIV, hepatitis B and C), severe irreversible extrarenal disease (e.g., inoperable cardiac disease, chronic lung disease, severe peripheral vascular disease), Class II obesity (body mass index greater than 35 kg/m^2), current substance use disorder (SUD), inability to give informed consent, active psychiatric disease, and history of nonadherence to treatment regimens (Bunnapradist et al., 2017; Woodard & Arnold, 2017).

Donors may be rejected for the same reasons or any condition that is determined to have an impact on the remaining kidney. Examples include hypertension and diabetes because both are known causes of kidney disease. It is imperative when donors are evaluated that serious consideration be given to the overall long-term health of the donor. Every precaution must be taken to ensure that the remaining kidney in the donor will remain healthy. When these conditions are met, the donor should remain healthy after donation and have a normal lifespan. Because one kidney can easily handle the body's needs, no long-term adjustments will need to be made. Routine health maintenance visits are stressed for blood pressure monitoring and preventative care.

The recipient's native kidneys are not usually removed, except for enlarged polycystic kidneys with cysts that may rupture or become infected (Bunnapradist et al., 2017). In some centers, for the patient with polycystic kidneys, the surgeon may perform a bilateral nephrectomy simultaneously with the renal transplant, while in others, the native nephrectomy precedes or is scheduled after the transplant procedure.

The transplanted kidney is placed in the patient's iliac fossa anterior to the iliac crest because it allows for easier access to the blood supply needed to perfuse the kidney. The ureter of the newly transplanted kidney is transplanted into the bladder or anastomosed to the ureter of the recipient (see Fig. 48-9). Once the blood supply has been reestablished to the transplanted kidney in the operating room, urine should begin to flow. For deceased donor kidneys, the production of urine at this stage is an important indicator of the overall success of the procedure and ultimate long-term outcome (Longton, 2017).

Preoperative Management

Preoperative management goals include bringing the patient's metabolic state to a level as close to normal as possible through diet, possibly dialysis and medical management, ensuring that the patient is free of infection, and educating the patient for surgery and the postoperative course.

Medical Management

A complete physical examination is performed on the living donor and the recipient to detect and treat any conditions that could cause complications after the living donor nephrectomy and recipient transplantation procedure. Tissue typing, blood typing, and antibody screening are performed to determine compatibility of the tissues and cells of the donor and recipient. Other diagnostic tests must be completed for both potential donor and recipient to identify conditions requiring treatment before the transplant procedure.

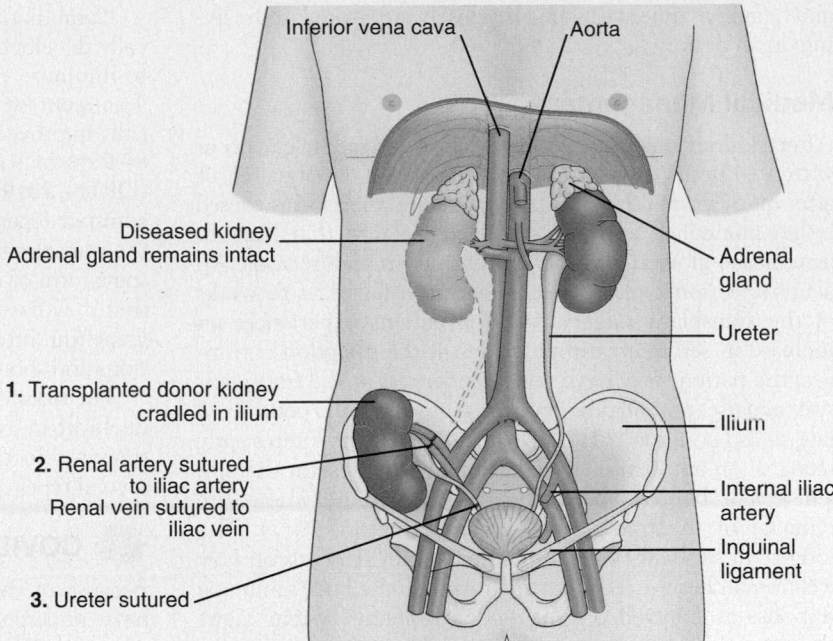

Figure 48-9 • Kidney transplantation. **1.** The transplanted kidney is placed in the iliac fossa. **2.** The renal vein of the donated kidney is sutured to the iliac vein, and the renal artery is sutured to the iliac artery. **3.** The ureter of the donated kidney is sutured to the bladder or to the patient's ureter.

Both patients must be free of infection at the time of kidney transplantation. After surgery, medications to prevent transplant rejection will be prescribed for the transplant recipient. These medications suppress the immune response, leaving the patient at risk for infection. Therefore, both the donor and recipient are evaluated and treated for any infections, including gingival (gum) disease and dental caries.

A psychosocial evaluation is conducted to assess the organ recipient's ability to adjust to the transplant, coping styles, social history, social support available, and financial resources. Psychiatric conditions are often aggravated by the corticosteroids and other medications needed for immunosuppression after transplantation, so a history of psychiatric illness is important to obtain (Shenoy & Danovitch, 2017). A psychosocial evaluation is also conducted to assess the motive of the donor for giving the organ. The donor should not be coerced to donate this organ; it should be an altruistic act (Rastogi, Hersh-Rifkin, Gritsch, et al., 2017).

Nursing Management

The nursing aspects of preoperative care for the patient undergoing kidney transplant and donation are similar to those for patients undergoing other types of kidney or elective abdominal surgery. Preoperative education can be conducted in a variety of settings, including the outpatient preadmission area, the hospital, or the transplantation clinic during the preliminary work up phase. Patient education for the kidney transplant donor and recipient addresses postoperative pulmonary hygiene, pain management options, dietary restrictions, IV lines, tubes (indwelling catheter), and early ambulation. Most patients have been on dialysis for months or years before transplantation, eagerly awaiting a kidney transplant, and are anxious about the surgery, possible rejection, and the need to return to dialysis. Helping the patient to deal with these concerns is part of the nurse's role in preoperative management, as is educating the patient about what to expect after surgery. HD may be performed before the kidney

transplantation procedure. When the patient is receiving peritoneal dialysis, the patient will continue to dialyze until the surgery. The dwell will be drained prior to going to the operating room.

The patient who receives a kidney from a living related donor is often concerned about the donor and how the donor will tolerate the surgical procedure. If the patient is receiving a deceased donor transplant, the recipient may express sadness and grief over the loss of the donor's life. The nurse must maintain open communication with the recipient of the organ and allow the patient to express these concerns.

The nurse working in an intensive care setting may provide care to the organ donor who is declared brain dead prior to organ removal. In the absence of brain death, deceased donation may also occur after the heart has stopped beating (donation after cardiac death or non–heart-beating donor). The overall goal is to preserve the function of the organs through maintaining hemodynamic stability, decreasing the risk for infection, and monitoring laboratory values while providing dignified care to the donor and family members (Woodard & Arnold, 2017). Continuing care for the donor can be complex and last for more than several hours. Care is often provided in collaboration with the organ procurement and transplant coordinators.

Postoperative Management

The goal of postoperative care is to maintain homeostasis until the transplanted kidney is functioning well. The patient whose kidney functions immediately has a more favorable prognosis than the patient whose kidney does not (Longton, 2017).

Often, the living organ donor will be on the same unit as the transplant recipient. The donor will require the same level of care provided to the recipient, including follow-up at prescribed intervals after the procedure and long-term. The organ donor often experiences more pain than the recipient, requiring more analgesia for pain control. Fluid, electrolyte, and hemodynamic status are also closely monitored in the living organ donor.

Medical Management

After a kidney transplantation, rejection and failure can occur within 24 hours (hyperacute), within 3 to 14 days (acute), or after many years (chronic). A hyperacute rejection is caused by an immediate antibody-mediated reaction that leads to generalized glomerular capillary thrombosis and necrosis. An acute rejection typically occurs within a few days to weeks of the transplant surgery, and the patient experiences an increase in serum creatinine values. If the rejection continues, the patient may have fever, tenderness at the transplant site, malaise, and oliguria, but these are generally considered late signs (Longton, 2017). An acute rejection requires early recognition and treatment with immunosuppressant therapy, whereas a hyperacute reaction would require immediate removal of the transplanted organ (Longton, 2017). The long-term survival of a transplanted kidney depends on how well it matches the recipient and how well the body's immune response is controlled. The body's immune system views the transplanted kidney as "foreign." Therefore, it continually works to reject it. To overcome or minimize the body's defense mechanisms, immunosuppressive agents are given. Optimally, medications modify the immune system enough to prevent rejection, although not enough to allow infections or malignancies to develop (see Table 48-4).

Combinations of corticosteroids and medications specifically developed to affect the action of lymphocytes are used to minimize the body's reaction to the transplanted organ. Treatment with combinations of new agents has dramatically improved patient and graft survival rates, and now 90% to 95% of transplanted kidneys still function after 1 year (OPTN, 2019). Doses of immunosuppressive agents are often adjusted depending on the patient's immunologic response to the transplant. However, the patient will be required to take some form of immunosuppressive therapy for the entire time that they have the transplanted kidney. Grapefruit juice and grapefruit interact with many immunosuppressant medications and should be avoided (Comerford & Durkin, 2020).

The risks associated with taking these medications include nephrotoxicity, hypertension, hyperlipidemia, hirsutism, tremors, blood dyscrasias, cataracts, gingival hyperplasia, and several types of cancer (Sievers, Lum, & Danovitch, 2017).

COVID-19 Considerations

Because of the need for immunosuppression, patients who have undergone kidney transplantation are at higher risk of contracting SARS-CoV-2 (Ajaimy & Melamed, 2020). One study reported outcomes of 41 patients who had a transplanted kidney, 22 of whom had confirmed COVID-19 and 19 of whom had suspected COVID-19 (Husain, Dube, Morris, et al., 2020). Among the 41 patients, 13 needed to be hospitalized while the rest were managed on an outpatient

TABLE 48-4	Immunosuppressant Agents Used Following Organ Transplant	
Agent	**Action**	**Nursing Implications**
tacrolimus	Calcineurin inhibitor: inhibits helper T lymphocytes	Monitor for nephrotoxicity, hyperkalemia, neurotoxicity (tremors). Assess for hypertension. Monitor tacrolimus levels
cyclosporine	Calcineurin inhibitor: selective and reversible inhibition of first phase of T-cell activation with T lymphocytes	Monitor for nephrotoxicity, hirsutism, gingival hyperplasia. Give medication with food to reduce gastrointestinal upset. Administer medication at the same time each day and ensure consistent food intake. Monitor cyclosporine levels.
sirolimus	mTOR inhibitor: inhibits the response of helper T and B lymphocytes	Instruct patient to swallow tablets whole and to avoid chewing or crushing tablets. Instruct patient to avoid grapefruit juice and grapefruit. Instruct the patient to limit exposure to sunlight. Administer 4 hours after oral cyclosporine.
mycophenolate mofetil mycophenolic acid	Antiproliferative: inhibition of T- and B-lymphocyte responses, thus inhibiting antibody formation and generation of cytotoxic T cells	Causes GI upset, diarrhea. Administer with food. Do not crush or open capsules and avoid contact with powder in capsules; wash hands thoroughly with soap and water if contact occurs. Obtain baseline complete blood count with differential prior to initiating therapy. Instruct the patient to avoid over-the-counter antacids.
belatacept	Costimulation blocker: inhibits T-lymphocyte proliferation and cytokine production	Contraindicated in patients with EBV seronegativity or unknown EBV serostatus, liver transplantation, breast-feeding. Monitor for symptoms of infection, anemia, GI symptoms, and, rarely, progressive multifocal leukoencephalopathy. Administer IV.
everolimus	mTOR inhibitor-proliferation signal inhibitors	Monitor for hypersensitivity reaction. Watch for changes in pulmonary status and cough. Avoid administration of live vaccines. Administer at the same time each day with food; do not crush or allow patient to chew tablet.

EBV, Epstein–Barr virus; GI, gastrointestinal; IV, intravenous; mTOR, mammalian target of rapamycin.
Adapted from Alquadan, K., Womer, K., & Casey, M. (2019). Immunosuppressive medications in kidney transplantation. In J. Feehally, J. Floege, M. Tonelli, et al. (Eds.), *Comprehensive clinical nephrology* (6th ed.). Philadelphia, PA: Elsevier.

basis being closely monitored with telehealth. The majority (80%) of patients reported fever but those requiring hospitalization were more likely to report dyspnea compared to those not requiring hospitalization. Patients requiring hospitalization also had higher serum creatinine levels upon admission, suggesting compromise of the function of their transplanted kidneys. More than half of the patients (63%), whether hospitalized or not, had a reduction in the immunosuppressive regimen but there was no reported mortality (Husain et al., 2020). These findings suggest that it may be safe to lower the immunosuppressive regimen of patients who have undergone kidney transplantation to augment the ability of their immune system to fight COVID-19.

Nursing Management

Assessing the Patient for Transplant Rejection

After kidney transplantation, the nurse assesses the patient for signs and symptoms of transplant rejection: oliguria, edema, fever, increasing blood pressure, weight gain, and swelling or tenderness over the transplanted kidney or graft. Patients receiving cyclosporine may not exhibit the usual signs and symptoms of acute rejection. In these patients, the only sign may be an asymptomatic rise in the serum creatinine level (Longton, 2017).

Preventing Infection

The results of blood chemistry tests and leukocyte and platelet counts are monitored closely because immunosuppression depresses the formation of leukocytes and platelets. The patient is closely monitored for infection because of susceptibility to impaired healing and infections related to immunosuppressive therapy and complications of kidney disease. Clinical manifestations of infection include shaking chills, fever, tachycardia (rapid heartbeat), tachypnea (rapid respirations), as well as either leukocytosis (increase in WBCs) or leukopenia (decrease in WBCs).

Infection may be introduced through many sources. Urine cultures are performed frequently because of the high incidence of bacteriuria during early and late stages of transplantation. Any type of wound drainage should be viewed as a potential source of infection because drainage is an excellent culture medium for bacteria. Catheter and drain tips may be cultured when removed by cutting off the tip of the catheter or drain (using aseptic technique) and placing the tip in a sterile container to be sent to the laboratory for culture (see Chart 48-14).

The nurse ensures that the patient is protected from exposure to infection by hospital staff and in the environment (e.g., fresh flowers are not permitted in the transplant unit), visitors, and other patients with active infections. Attention to hand hygiene by all who come in contact with the patient is imperative.

Monitoring Urinary Function

A kidney from a living donor who is related to the patient usually begins to function immediately after surgery and may produce large quantities of dilute urine. A kidney from a deceased donor may undergo ATN and therefore may not function for 2 or 3 weeks, during which time anuria, oliguria, or polyuria may be present. During this stage, the patient may experience significant changes in fluid and electrolyte

---

Chart 48-14 | **Kidney Transplant Rejection and Infection**

Renal graft rejection and failure may occur within 24 hours (hyperacute), within 3 to 14 days (acute), or after many years (chronic). It is not uncommon for a treatable rejection episode to occur during the first year after transplantation.

Detecting Rejection

Ultrasonography may be used to detect hydronephrosis (enlargement of the kidney) due to obstruction of urine flow; percutaneous renal biopsy (most reliable) and nuclear medicine studies are used to evaluate transplant rejection. If the body rejects the transplanted kidney, the patient needs to commence dialysis. The rejected kidney may or may not be removed, depending on when the rejection occurs (acute vs. chronic) and the risk for infection if the kidney is left in place.

Potential Infection

Infection continues to be a major cause of morbidity and mortality in kidney transplant recipients, both due to the surgical procedure, the high doses of induction immunosuppression given in the postoperative period, and the continuing need for maintenance immunosuppression. The majority of infections happen in the first month after transplantation and are generally due to the complications of the surgery or invasive medical devices (IV, central line, and urinary catheters and ureteral stents) and mostly involve the genitourinary tract (since this is the focus of the surgery). The most common infections include genitourinary infections, pneumonia, wound and abdominal fluid collection infections, device-related infections, and, later in the transplant course, viral diseases. After 6 months, patients who have stable kidney function, have not required treatment for rejection or a need for reoperation are considered as having a successful outcome with stable maintenance immunosuppression and, thus, decreased infectious risks. When recipients have poor renal function, have had rejection treatments which have necessitated increased immunosuppression, and have ongoing issues with genitourinary dysfunction, opportunistic infections are more likely to present, such as cytomegalovirus (CMV) and other human herpesviruses (HHV) and polyoma virus. Despite the continuing menace of infection in renal transplant recipients, the 1-year patient survival rates are close to 100% and graft survival exceeds 90%.

Adapted from Schaenman, J., & Kubak, B. (2017). Infections in kidney transplantation. In G. Danovitch (Ed.), *Handbook of kidney transplantation* (6th ed.). Philadelphia, PA: Wolters Kluwer.

---

status. Therefore, careful monitoring is indicated. The output from the urinary catheter is measured every hour. IV fluids are given on the basis of urine volume and serum electrolyte levels, as prescribed by the primary provider. HD may be necessary postoperatively to maintain homeostasis until the transplanted kidney is functioning well. It also may be required if fluid overload and hyperkalemia occur. The vascular access for HD is assessed to ensure patency and to evaluate for evidence of infection.

Addressing Psychological Concerns

The rejection of a transplanted kidney is of great and ongoing concern to the patient, the family, and the health care team. The fear of kidney rejection and the complications of immunosuppressive therapy (Cushing's syndrome, diabetes, capillary fragility, osteoporosis, glaucoma, cataracts, acne, nephrotoxicity) place tremendous psychological stress on the patient. If the organ donor was a family member there may be added emotional responses that need to be addressed. Anxiety and uncertainty about the future and difficult post transplantation adjustment are often sources of stress for the patient and family.

An important nursing function is the assessment of the patient's stress and coping. Psychosocial issues are common in individuals and families with chronic diseases, and ESKD is a chronic disease (Shenoy & Danovitch, 2017). The nurse uses each visit with the patient to determine if the patient and family are coping effectively and the patient is adhering to the prescribed medication regimen. If indicated or requested, the nurse refers the patient for counseling (Longton, 2017).

Monitoring and Managing Potential Complications

The patient undergoing kidney transplantation is at risk for the postoperative complications that are associated with any surgical procedure. In addition, the patient's physical condition may be compromised because of the effects of long-standing kidney disease and its treatment. Therefore, careful assessment of the complications related to kidney disease and often, diabetes and hypertension, and those associated with a major surgery are important aspects of nursing care. Breathing exercises, early ambulation, and care of the surgical incision are priorities of postoperative care.

GI ulceration and corticosteroid-induced bleeding may occur. Therefore, preventative medications such as H_2-blockers (e.g., famotidine) or proton pump inhibitors (PPIs) (e.g., omeprazole) are prescribed. Fungal colonization of the GI tract (especially the mouth) and urinary bladder may occur secondary to immunosuppressive and antibiotic therapy; thus, prophylactic oral antifungal mouth rinses are prescribed. Closely assessing the patient and notifying the primary provider about the occurrence of these complications are important nursing interventions. In addition, the patient is monitored for any signs and symptoms of adrenal insufficiency if the immunosuppressive regimen has included the use of long-term corticosteroids.

Promoting Home, Community-Based, and Transitional Care

 Educating Patients About Self-Care

The nurse works closely with the patient and family to be sure that they understand the need for continuing immunosuppressive therapy as prescribed. In addition, the patient and family are educated on how to assess for and report signs and symptoms of transplant rejection, infection, or significant adverse effects of the immunosuppressive regimen. The patient and family are educated about the need to report decreased urine output; weight gain; malaise; fever; respiratory distress; tenderness over the transplanted kidney; anxiety; depression; changes in eating, drinking, or other habits; and changes in blood pressure. The patient is instructed to inform all health care providers (e.g., dentist) about the kidney transplant and the use of immunosuppressive agents.

Continuing and Transitional Care

The patient needs to know that follow-up care after transplantation is a lifelong necessity. Individual written instructions with verbal explanations are provided concerning diet, medication,

fluids, daily weight, daily measurement of urinary output, management of oral intake, prevention of infection and rejection, resumption of activity, and avoidance of contact sports in which the transplanted kidney may be injured. Because of the risk of other potential complications, the patient is followed closely by a health care team that includes the nephrologist, transplant surgeon, transplant coordinator or nurse, social worker, transplant pharmacist, and dietitian. Medications are often obtained at one pharmacy or through the pharmacy at the hospital where the transplant surgery was performed for the purpose of accurate medication reconciliation. Follow-up with providers from the transplant team will initially occur once or twice a week upon discharge from the hospital and taper over time. Laboratory studies will also be obtained and followed on an ongoing basis to monitor the function of the kidney.

Cardiovascular disease is the major cause of morbidity and mortality after transplantation, due in part to the increasing age of patients with transplants. An additional problem is possible malignancy; patients receiving long-term immunosuppressive therapy are at higher risk for cancers than the general population (Huang & Kasiske, 2017). The nurse reminds the patient of the importance of health promotion and health screening and provides information on local transplantation support groups at the transplant hospital or through the procurement organization.

The American Association of Kidney Patients (AAKP) and the NKF (listed in the Resources section of this chapter) are nonprofit organizations that serve the needs of those with kidney disease. These groups can provide many helpful suggestions for patients and family members learning to cope with the journey of dialysis and transplantation.

RENAL TRAUMA

The kidneys are protected by the rib cage and musculature of the back posteriorly and by a cushion of abdominal wall and viscera anteriorly. They are highly mobile and are fixed only at the renal pedicle (stem of renal blood vessels and the ureter). With traumatic injury, the kidneys can be thrust against the lower ribs, resulting in contusion and rupture. Rib fractures or fractures of the transverse process of the upper lumbar vertebrae may be associated with renal contusion or laceration.

Motor vehicle crashes, falls from heights, and assaults cause the majority of blunt renal trauma (Santucci & Chen, 2016). Failure to wear seat belts contributes to the incidence of renal trauma in motor vehicle crashes. Injuries may be blunt (deceleration forces in motor vehicle crashes, falls, athletic injuries, assaults) or penetrating (gunshot wounds, stabbings). Gunshot wounds are responsible for 86% of penetrating trauma, while stab wounds account for about 14% (Santucci & Chen, 2016).

Blunt renal trauma is classified into one of four groups, as follows:

- Contusion: Bruises or hemorrhages under the renal capsule; capsule and collecting system intact
- Minor laceration: Superficial disruption of the cortex; renal medulla and collecting system are not involved
- Major laceration: Parenchymal disruption extending into cortex and medulla, possibly involving the collecting system
- Vascular injury: Tears of renal artery or vein

Physiology/Pathophysiology

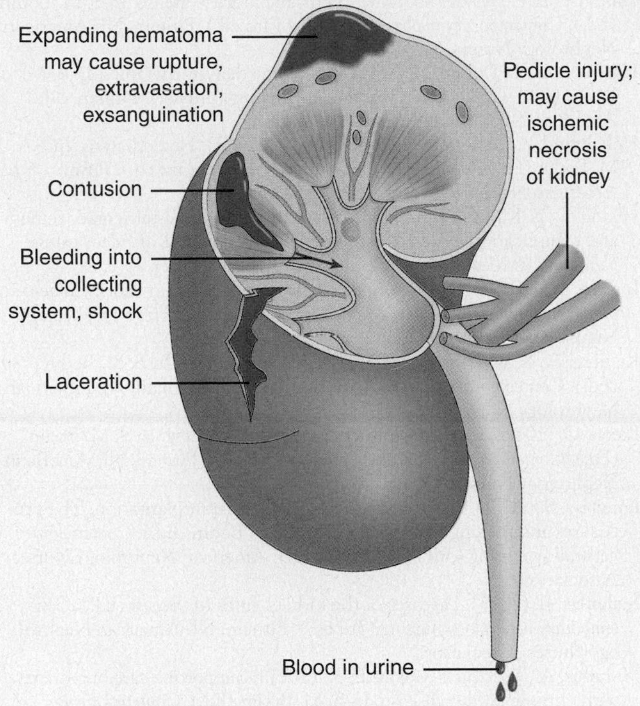

Expanding hematoma may cause rupture, extravasation, exsanguination

Pedicle injury; may cause ischemic necrosis of kidney

Contusion

Bleeding into collecting system, shock

Laceration

Blood in urine

Figure 48-10 • Types and pathophysiologic effects of kidney injuries: contusions, lacerations, rupture, and pedicle injury.

The most common renal injuries are contusions, lacerations, ruptures, and renal pedicle injuries or small internal lacerations of the kidney (see Fig. 48-10). The kidneys receive half of the blood flow from the abdominal aorta; therefore, even a fairly small renal laceration can produce massive bleeding. The majority of patients are in shock when admitted to the hospitals. In some cases, there is an isolated renal artery thrombosis.

The best indicators of urinary system injury are gross and microscopic hematuria (on urinalysis or dipstick), especially in association with a history of injury or trauma (Santucci & Chen, 2016). Other clinical manifestations include pain, renal colic (due to blood clots or fragments obstructing the collecting system), mass or swelling in the flank, ecchymoses, and lacerations or wounds of the lateral abdomen and flank. There is no relationship between the degree of hematuria and the degree of injury. Signs and symptoms of hypovolemia and shock (see Chapter 11) are likely with significant hemorrhage.

Medical Management

The goals of management in patients with renal trauma are to control hemorrhage, pain, and infection as well as to preserve and restore renal function. All urine is saved and sent to the laboratory for analysis to detect RBCs and to evaluate the course of bleeding. Serial hematocrit and hemoglobin levels are monitored closely; decreasing values indicate hemorrhage.

The patient is monitored for oliguria and signs of hemorrhagic shock, because a pedicle injury or shattered kidney can lead to rapid exsanguination (lethal blood loss). An expanding hematoma may cause rupture of the kidney capsule. To detect hematoma, the area around the lower ribs, upper lumbar

vertebrae, flank, and abdomen is palpated for tenderness. A palpable flank or abdominal mass with local tenderness, swelling, and ecchymosis suggests renal hemorrhage. The area of the original mass can be outlined with a surgical marking pen so that the examiner can evaluate the area for change.

Renal trauma is often associated with other injuries to the abdominal organs (liver, colon, small intestines); therefore, the patient is assessed for skin abrasions, lacerations, and entry and exit wounds of the upper abdomen and lower thorax, because these may be associated with kidney injury. A contrast-enhanced computed tomography (CT) scan is the standard for genitourinary imaging in renal trauma when the patient is stable and not suspected of acute hemorrhage (Santucci & Chen, 2016).

With a contusion of the kidney, healing may take place with conservative measures. If the patient has microscopic hematuria and a normal CT scan, outpatient management is possible. If gross hematuria or a minor laceration is present, the patient is hospitalized and kept on bed rest until the hematuria clears. Antimicrobial medications may be prescribed to prevent infection from perirenal hematoma or urinoma (a cyst containing urine). Patients with retroperitoneal hematomas may develop low-grade fever as absorption of the clot takes place.

Surgical Management

Depending on the patient's condition and the nature of the injury, major lacerations may be treated through surgical intervention or interventional radiology treatment (angioembolization) or conservatively (bed rest, no surgery). The majority of blunt and penetrating injuries to the kidneys no longer require open surgical intervention (Santucci & Chen, 2016). However, any sudden change in the patient's condition suggests hemorrhage and requires rapid surgical intervention. Vascular injuries require immediate exploratory surgery because of the high incidence of involvement of other organ systems and the serious complications that may result if these injuries are untreated. The patient is often in shock and requires aggressive fluid resuscitation. Nephrectomy, or surgery to remove the damaged kidney, may be required.

Early postoperative complications (within 6 months) include rebleeding, perinephric abscess formation, sepsis, urine extravasation, and fistula formation. Other complications include stone formation, infection, cysts, vascular aneurysms, and loss of renal function. Hypertension can be a complication of any surgery but usually is a late complication of kidney injury.

Nursing Management

The patient with renal trauma must be assessed frequently during the first few days after injury to detect flank and abdominal pain, muscle spasm, and swelling over the flank. During this time, the patient who has undergone surgery is educated about care of the incision and the importance of an adequate fluid intake. In addition, instructions are provided about changes that should be reported to the physician, such as fever, hematuria, flank pain, or any signs and symptoms of decreasing kidney function. Guidelines for gradually increasing activity, lifting, and driving are also explained in accordance with the physician's prescription.

Follow-up nursing care includes monitoring the blood pressure to detect hypertension and advising the patient to restrict activities for about 1 month after trauma to minimize the incidence of delayed or secondary bleeding. The patient should be advised to schedule periodic follow-up assessments of renal function (creatinine clearance, BUN, and serum creatinine analyses). If a nephrectomy was necessary, the patient is advised to wear medical identification.

CRITICAL THINKING EXERCISES

1 **pq** You are a staff nurse in an outpatient dialysis facility. A 28-year-old woman with ESKD is seen in the clinic for the first time and states that she wants to begin PD. The patient lives alone and is employed full-time. What are your priorities for educating this patient about the options for dialysis and what is involved with each method? How should the priorities change if the patient decides on home HD?

2 **ipc** A 62-year-old man who normally has HD 3 times a week has been admitted to the medical unit where you work. What nursing and interprofessional assessments are indicated during your initial interactions with him? What other interprofessional services might you try to engage?

3 **ebp** You are caring for a 45-year-old patient who is postoperative following a kidney transplant. What is the evidence base for treatment options for immunosuppression? Identify the criteria used to evaluate the strength of the evidence.

REFERENCES

*Asterisk indicates nursing research.
**Double asterisk indicates classic reference.

Books

Alquadan, K., Womer, K., & Casey, M. (2019). Immunosuppressive medications in kidney transplantation. In J. Feehally, J. Floege, M. Tonelli, et al. (Eds.). *Comprehensive clinical nephrology* (6th ed.). Philadelphia, PA: Elsevier.

Brooks, D. (2017). Chronic kidney disease: Diagnosis, classification, and management. In S. M. Bodin (Ed.). *Contemporary nephrology nursing* (3rd ed.). Pitman, NJ: American Nephrology Nurses Association.

Browne, T., & Johnstone, S. (2017). Psychosocial issues in nephrology nursing. In S. M. Bodin (Ed.). *Contemporary nephrology nursing* (3rd ed.). Pitman, NJ: American Nephrology Nurses Association.

Bunnapradist, S., Abdalla, B., & Reddy, U. (2017). Evaluation of adult kidney transplant candidates. In G. Danovitch (Ed.). *Handbook of kidney transplantation* (6th ed.). Philadelphia, PA: Wolters Kluwer.

Campoy, S. (2017). Hypertension. In S. M. Bodin (Ed.). *Contemporary nephrology nursing* (3rd ed.). Pitman, NJ: American Nephrology Nurses Association.

Comerford, K. C., & Durkin, M. T. (2020). *Nursing 2020 drug handbook.* Philadelphia, PA: Wolters Kluwer.

Conde, F., & Workman, T. (2017). Genitourinary cancers. In S. Newton, M. Hickey, & J. Brant (Eds.). *Oncology nursing advisor: A comprehensive guide to clinical practice* (2nd ed.). St. Louis, MO: Elsevier.

Danovitch, G. (Ed.). (2017). *Handbook of kidney transplantation* (6th ed.). Philadelphia, PA: Wolters Kluwer.

Evans, E. (2017). Anemia. In S. M. Bodin (Ed.). *Contemporary nephrology nursing* (3rd ed.). Pitman, NJ: American Nephrology Nurses Association.

Fischbach, F., & Fischbach, M. (2018). *A manual of laboratory and diagnostic tests* (10th ed.). Philadelphia, PA: Wolters Kluwer.

Gonyea, J. (2017). Nutrition and chronic kidney disease. In S. M. Bodin (Ed.). *Contemporary nephrology nursing* (3rd ed.). Pitman, NJ: American Nephrology Nurses Association.

Hain, D. (2017). Older adults with chronic kidney disease. In S. M. Bodin (Ed.). *Contemporary nephrology nursing* (3rd ed.). Pitman, NJ: American Nephrology Nurses Association.

Harwood, L., & Dominski, C. (2017). Home dialysis therapies. In S. M. Bodin (Ed.). *Contemporary nephrology nursing* (3rd ed.). Pitman, NJ: American Nephrology Nurses Association.

Hellebrand, A., Allen, D., & Hoffman, M. (2017). Hemodialysis. In S. M. Bodin (Ed.). *Contemporary nephrology nursing* (3rd ed.). Pitman, NJ: American Nephrology Nurses Association.

Huang, E., & Kasiske, B. (2017). Post-transplant: Long-term management and complications. In G. Danovitch (Ed.). *Handbook of kidney transplantation* (6th ed.). Philadelphia, PA: Wolters Kluwer.

Inglese, M. (2017). Arteriovenous fistula. In S. M. Bodin (Ed.). *Contemporary nephrology nursing* (3rd ed.). Pitman, NJ: American Nephrology Nurses Association.

Kelman, E., & Watson, D. (2017). Peritoneal dialysis. In S. M. Bodin (Ed.). *Contemporary nephrology nursing* (3rd ed.). Pitman, NJ: American Nephrology Nurses Association.

Lieser, C. (2017). Depression in chronic kidney disease. In S. M. Bodin (Ed.). *Contemporary nephrology nursing* (3rd ed.). Pitman, NJ: American Nephrology Nurses Association.

Longton, S. (2017). Kidney, pancreas, and liver transplantation: The procedures and nursing management. In S. M. Bodin (Ed.). *Contemporary nephrology nursing* (3rd ed.). Pitman, NJ: American Nephrology Nurses Association.

Mahaffey, L. (2017). Diseases of the kidney. In S. M. Bodin (Ed.). *Contemporary nephrology nursing* (3rd ed.). Pitman, NJ: American Nephrology Nurses Association.

Molzahn, A., & Schick-Makaroff, K. (2017). Supportive care of patients with chronic kidney disease. In S. M. Bodin (Ed.). *Contemporary nephrology nursing* (3rd ed.). Pitman, NJ: American Nephrology Nurses Association.

Norris, T. L. (2019). *Porth's pathophysiology: Concepts of altered health states* (10th ed.). Philadelphia, PA: Wolters Kluwer.

Odom, B. (2017). Acute kidney injury. In S. M. Bodin (Ed.). *Contemporary nephrology nursing* (3rd ed.). Pitman, NJ: American Nephrology Nurses Association.

Parikh, S., Haddad, N., & Hebert, L. (2019). Retarding progression of kidney disease. In R. Johnson, J. Feehally, J. Floege, et al. (Eds.). *Comprehensive clinical nephrology* (6th ed.). China: Elsevier.

Payton, J., & Kennedy, S. (2017). Peritoneal dialysis access. In S. M. Bodin (Ed.). *Contemporary nephrology nursing* (3rd ed.). Pitman, NJ: American Nephrology Nurses Association.

Pryor, L., & Brouwer-Maier, D. (2017). Central venous catheter. In S. M. Bodin (Ed.). *Contemporary nephrology nursing* (3rd ed.). Pitman, NJ: American Nephrology Nurses Association.

Rastogi, A., Hersh-Rifkin, M., Gritsch, H. A., et al. (2017). Living donor kidney transplantation. In G. M. Danovitch (Ed.). *Handbook of kidney transplantation* (6th ed.). Philadelphia, PA: Wolters Kluwer.

Ross, E., Nissenson, A., & Daugirdas, J. (2015). Acute hemodialysis prescription. In J. Daugirdas, P. Blake, & T. Ing, (Eds.). *Handbook of dialysis* (5th ed.). Philadelphia, PA: Wolters Kluwer.

Santucci, R., & Chen, M. (2016). *Upper urinary tract trauma.* In A. Wein, L. Kavoussi, A. Partin, et al. (Eds.). *Campbell-Walsh urology* (11th ed.). Philadelphia, PA: Elsevier.

Schaenman, J., & Kubak, B. (2017). Infections in kidney transplantation. In G. Danovitch (Ed.). *Handbook of kidney transplantation* (6th ed.). Philadelphia, PA: Wolters Kluwer.

Schira, M. (2017). Medication-related nephrotoxicity. In S. M. Bodin (Ed.). *Contemporary nephrology nursing* (3rd ed.). Pitman, NJ: American Nephrology Nurses Association.

Schonder, K. (2017). Pharmacology of kidney disease. In S. M. Bodin (Ed.). *Contemporary nephrology nursing* (3rd ed.). Pitman, NJ: American Nephrology Nurses Association.

Shenoy, A., & Danovitch, I. (2017). Psychiatric aspects of kidney transplantation. In G. M. Danovitch (Ed.). *Handbook of kidney transplantation* (6th ed.). Philadelphia, PA: Wolters Kluwer.

Sievers, T., Lum, E., & Danovitch, G. (2017). Immunosuppressive medications and protocols for kidney transplantation. In G. M. Danovitch (Ed.). *Handbook of kidney transplantation* (6th ed.). Philadelphia, PA: Wolters Kluwer.

Weber, J. R., & Kelley, J. H. (2018). *Health assessment in nursing* (6th ed.). Philadelphia, PA: Wolters Kluwer.

Woodard, A., & Arnold, E. (2017). Kidney transplantation: Organ donation. In S. M. Bodin (Ed.). *Contemporary nephrology nursing* (3rd ed.). Pitman, NJ: American Nephrology Nurses Association.

Journals and Electronic Documents

Ajaimy, M., & Melamed, M. (2020). COVID-19 in patient with kidney disease. *Clinical Journal of the American Society of Nephrology, 15*(8), 1087–1089.

American Cancer Society. (2020). Kidney cancer. Retrieved on 1/1/2020 at: www.cancer.org/cancer/kidney-cancer/causes-risks-prevention/what-causes.html

**Bellomo, R., Ronco, C., Kellum, J. A., et al. (2004). Acute renal failure-definition, outcome measures, animal models, fluid therapy and information technology needs: The Second International Consensus Conference of the Acute Dialysis Quality Initiative (ADQI) Group. *Critical Care, 8*(4), B204.

Bolignano, D., Palmer, S. C., Ruospo, M., et al. (2015). Interventions for preventing the progression of autosomal dominant polycystic kidney disease. *Cochrane Database of Systematic Reviews, 7*, CD010294.

Carey, R., & Whelton, P. (2018). Prevention, detection, evaluation, and management of high blood pressure in adults: Synopsis of the 2017 American College of Cardiology/American Heart Association Hypertension Guideline. *Annals of Internal Medicine, 168*(5), 351–358.

Centers for Disease Control and Prevention (CDC). (2019). Chronic kidney disease in the United States, 2019. Retrieved on 1/13/2020 at: www.cdc.gov/kidneydisease/publications-resources/2019-national-facts.html

Cheng, Y., Luo, R., Wang, X., et al. (2020). The incidence, risk factors, and prognosis of acute kidney injury in adult patients with coronavirus 2019. *Clinical Journal of the American Society of Nephrology, 15*(10), 1394–1402.

Chicca, J. (2020). Adults with chronic kidney disease: Overview and nursing care goals. *American Nurse Journal, 15*(3), 16–22.

George, D., & Jonasch, E. (2019). Systemic therapy of advanced clear cell renal carcinoma. *UpToDate.* Retrieved on 1/4/2020 at: www.uptodate.com/contents/systemic-therapy-of-advanced-clear-cell-renal-carcinoma

Hines, A., & Goldberg, S. (2018). Radiofrequency ablation and cryoablation for renal cell carcinoma. *UpToDate.* Retrieved on 1/13/2020 at: www.uptodate.com/contents/radiofrequency-ablation-and-cryoablation-for-renal-cell-carcinoma

Hulkower, A. (2020). Learning from COVID. *Hastings Center Report, 50*(3), 16–17.

Husain, S. A., Dube, G., Morris, H., et al. (2020). Early outcomes of outpatient management of kidney transplant recipients with coronavirus 2019. *Clinical Journal of the American Society of Nephrology, 15*(8), 1174–1178.

Kalfoss, M., Schick-Makaroff, K., & Molzahn, A. (2019). Living with chronic kidney disease: Illness perceptions, symptoms, coping, and quality of life. *Nephrology Nursing Journal, 46*(3), 277–290.

Kear, T., Bednarski, D., Smith, L., et al. (2019). Letter from the ANNA Board of Directors to the Centers for Medicare and Medicaid Services Regarding the Advancing American Kidney Health Initiative. *Nephrology Nursing Journal, 46*(5), 477–481.

Kelepouris, E., & Rovin, B. (2019). Overview of heavy proteinuria and the nephrotic syndrome. *UpToDate.* Retrieved on 1/13/2020 at:www.uptodate.com/contents/overview-of-heavy-proteinuria-and-the-nephrotic-syndrome

*Kim, E., Lee, Y., Chang, S. (2019). How do patients on hemodialysis perceive and overcome hemodialysis? Concept development of the resilience of patients on hemodialysis. *Nephrology Nursing Journal, 46*(5), 521–530.

Ku, E., Lee, B. J., Wei, J., et al. (2019). Hypertension in CKD: Core curriculum 2019. *American Journal of Kidney Disease, 74*(1), 120–131.

*Lin, C. C., Han, C., & Pan, I. J. (2015). A qualitative approach of psychosocial adaptation process in patients undergoing long-term hemodialysis. *Asian Nursing Research, 9*(1), 35–41.

Mann, J., & Hilgers, K. (2019). Clinical features, diagnosis, and treatment of hypertensive nephrosclerosis. *UpToDate.* Retrieved on 1/12/2019 at: www.uptodate.com/contents/clinical-features-diagnosis-and-treatment-of-hypertensive-nephrosclerosis

Medel-Herrero, A., Mitchell, D., & Moyce, S. (2019). The expanding burden of acute kidney injury in California: Impact of the epidemic of diabetes on kidney injury hospital admissions. *Nephrology Nursing Journal, 46*(6), 629–640.

Nahar, D. (2017). Prophylactic management of contrast-induced acute kidney injury in high-risk patients. *Nephrology Nursing Journal, 44*(3), 244–249.

National Cancer Institute. (2019). Kidney cancer. Retrieved on 12/8/2019 at: seer.cancer.gov/statistics/preliminary-estimates/preliminary.html

**National Kidney Foundation Kidney Disease Outcomes Quality Initiative (NKF KDOQI). (2000). Clinical practice guidelines for nutrition in chronic renal failure. *American Journal of Kidney Diseases, 35*(6 Suppl 2), S1–S140.

Organ Procurement and Transplantation Network (OPTN). (2019). Waiting list candidates as of today. Retrieved on 12/11/2019 at: optn.transplant.hrsa.gov/data

Pavkov, M. E., Harding, J. L., & Burrows, N. R. (2018). Trends in hospitalizations for acute kidney injury—United States, 2000–2014. *MMWR, 67*(10), 289–293.

Richie, J., Atkins, M., & Chen, W. (2019). Definitive surgical management of renal cell carcinoma. *UpToDate.* Retrieved on 4/14/2020 at: www.uptodate.com/contents/definitive-surgical-management-of-renal-cell-carcinoma?search=Definitive%20surgical%20management%20of%20renal%20cell%20carcinoma

Saran, R., Robinson, B., Abbott, K. C., et al. (2018). 2017 USRDS annual data report: Epidemiology of kidney disease in the United States. *American Journal of Kidney Diseases, 71*(3 Suppl 1), A7.

Shirazian, S., Grant, C. D., Aina, O., et al. (2017). Depression in chronic kidney disease and end-stage renal disease: Similarities and differences in diagnosis, epidemiology, and management. *Kidney International Reports, 2*(1), 94–107.

Sturdivant, T., & Johnson, P. (2019). Protecting restricted extremities: The implementation of a pink wristband. *Nephrology Nursing Journal 46*(4), 423–452.

Subbiah, A., Chhabra, Y., & Mahajan, S. (2016). Cardiovascular disease in patients with chronic kidney disease: A neglected subgroup. *Heart Asia, 8*(2), 56–61.

Torres, V., & Bennett, W. (2019). Autosomal dominant polycystic kidney disease (ADPKD) in adults: Epidemiology, clinical presentation, and diagnosis. *UpToDate.* Retrieved on 4/15/2020 at: www.uptodate.com/contents/autosomal-dominant-polycystic-kidney-disease-adpkd-in-adults-epidemiology-clinical-presentation-and-diagnosis

United States Renal Data System (USRDS). (2019). 2019 USRDS annual data report: Epidemiology of kidney disease in the United States. National Institutes of Health, National Institute of Diabetes and Digestive and Kidney Diseases. Bethesda, MD. Retrieved on 1/14/2020 at: www.usrds.rg/2019/view/Default.aspx

Wu, J., Li, J., Zhu, G., et al. (2020). Clinical features of maintenance hemodialysis patients with novel coronavirus pneumonia in Wuhan, China. *Clinical Journal of the American Society of Nephrology, 15*(8), 1139–1145.

Resources

Alliance for Paired Donation (APD), paireddonation.org
American Association of Kidney Patients (AAKP), www.aakp.org
American Kidney Fund, www.kidneyfund.org
American Nephrology Nurses' Association (ANNA), www.annanurse.org
American Urological Association (AUA), www.auanet.org
Arteriovenous Fistula First, www.fistulafirst.org
National Institute of Diabetes and Digestive and Kidney Diseases (NIDDK), www.niddk.nih.gov
National Kidney Registry (NKR), www.kidneyregistry.org
National Kidney and Urologic Diseases Information Clearinghouse (NKUDIC), digestive.niddk.nih.gov
National Kidney Foundation (NKF), www.kidney.org
United Network for Organ Sharing (UNOS), www.unos.org
United States Renal Data System (USRDS), www.usrds.org

49

Management of Patients with Urinary Disorders

LEARNING OUTCOMES

On completion of this chapter, the learner will be able to:

1. Explain the factors contributing to upper and lower urinary tract infections.
2. Use the nursing process as a framework for care of the patient with a lower urinary tract infection.
3. Differentiate between the various adult dysfunctional voiding patterns and develop an education plan for a patient who has urinary incontinence.
4. Identify potential causes of an obstruction of the urinary tract along with the medical, surgical, and nursing management of the patient with this condition.
5. Describe the pathophysiology, clinical manifestations, medical management, and nursing management for patients with genitourinary trauma and urinary tract cancers.
6. Use the nursing process as a framework for care of the patient with renal calculi and for care of the patient undergoing urinary diversion surgery.

NURSING CONCEPTS

Cellular Regulation

Comfort

Elimination

Family

Inflammation

Patient Education

GLOSSARY

bacteriuria: bacteria in the urine

catheter-associated urinary tract infection (CAUTI): a urinary tract infection (UTI) associated with indwelling urinary catheters

cystectomy: surgical removal of the urinary bladder

cystitis: inflammation of the urinary bladder

functional incontinence: involuntary loss of urine due to physical or cognitive impairment

iatrogenic incontinence: involuntary loss of urine due to extrinsic medical factors

ileal conduit: transplantation of the ureters to an isolated section of the terminal ileum, with one end of the ureters brought to the abdominal wall (*synonym:* ileal loop)

interstitial cystitis: inflammation of the bladder wall that eventually causes disintegration of the lining and loss of bladder elasticity

micturition: voiding or urination

mixed incontinence: involuntary urinary leakage associated with urgency and also with exertion, effort, sneezing, or coughing

neurogenic bladder: bladder dysfunction that results from a disorder or dysfunction of the nervous system and leads to urinary incontinence

nocturia: awakening at night to urinate

overflow incontinence: involuntary urine loss associated with overdistention of the bladder

prostatitis: inflammation of the prostate gland

pyelonephritis: inflammation of the renal pelvis

pyuria: white blood cells in the urine

residual urine: urine that remains in the bladder after voiding

stress incontinence: involuntary loss of urine through an intact urethra as a result of exertion, sneezing, coughing, or changing position

suprapubic catheter: a urinary catheter that is inserted through a suprapubic incision into the bladder

ureterovesical or vesicoureteral reflux: backward flow of urine from the bladder into one or both ureters

urethritis: inflammation of the urethra

urethrovesical reflux: an obstruction to free-flowing urine leading to the reflux of urine from the urethra into the bladder

urge incontinence: involuntary loss of urine associated with a strong urge to void that cannot be suppressed

urinary frequency: voiding more often than every 3 hours

urinary incontinence: unplanned, involuntary, or uncontrolled loss of urine from the bladder

urosepsis: spread of infection from the urinary tract to the bloodstream that results in a systemic infection

The urinary system is responsible for providing the route for drainage of urine formed by the kidneys. Care of the patient with disorders of the urinary tract requires an understanding of the anatomy, physiology, diagnostic testing, medical, and nursing care, as well as rehabilitation of patients with the multiple processes that affect the urinary system. Nurses care for patients with urologic disorders in all settings. This chapter focuses on the nursing management of patients with common urinary dysfunctions, including infections, dysfunctional voiding patterns, urolithiasis, genitourinary trauma, cancer of the urinary tract, and urinary diversions.

INFECTIONS OF THE URINARY TRACT

Urinary tract infections (UTIs) are caused by pathogenic microorganisms in the urinary tract (the normal urinary tract is sterile above the urethra). UTIs are generally classified by location as infections of the lower urinary tract, involving the bladder and structures below the bladder, or upper urinary tract, involving the kidneys and ureters.

A UTI is the second most common infection in the body. UTIs account for nearly 25% of all infections and are commonly diagnosed in women visiting emergency departments in the United States. Approximately 8.1 million women are diagnosed with UTIs in the United States annually (Freeman, Martin, & Uithoven, 2017). In addition, UTIs are the cause of more than 100,000 hospital admissions annually (Freeman et al., 2017).

Fifty percent of all hospital-acquired infections are UTIs, and in the majority of cases these are **catheter-associated urinary tract infections (CAUTI)** (Freeman et al., 2017). A CAUTI is a UTI associated with indwelling urinary catheters. The definition used for ongoing monitoring is a UTI that occurs while the patient had an indwelling urinary catheter in place for more than 2 calendar days on the day that the infection was detected.

Lower Urinary Tract Infections

The sterility of the bladder is maintained by several mechanisms, especially important since the urethra is considered a clean, not a sterile space. The physical barrier of the urethra assists in keeping bacteria away from the bladder, while urine flow helps to carry any bacteria away from the bladder. In addition, ureterovesical junction competence, various antibacterial enzymes and antibodies, and antiadherent effects mediated by the mucosal cells of the bladder all play a major part in protecting the sterility of the bladder. Abnormalities or dysfunctions of any of these mechanisms are contributing risk factors for lower UTIs (see Chart 49-1).

Lower UTIs include bacterial **cystitis** (inflammation of the urinary bladder), bacterial **prostatitis** (inflammation of the prostate gland), and bacterial **urethritis** (inflammation of the urethra).

Pathophysiology

For infection to occur, bacteria must gain access to the bladder, attach to and colonize the epithelium of the urinary tract to avoid being washed out with voiding, evade host defense mechanisms, and initiate inflammation. Many UTIs result

---

> **Chart 49-1** ⚠️ **RISK FACTORS**
> **Urinary Tract Infection**
>
> - Contributing conditions such as:
>   - Female gender
>   - Diabetes
>   - Pregnancy
>   - Neurologic disorders
>   - Gout
>   - Altered states caused by incomplete emptying of the bladder and urinary stasis
> - Decreased natural host defenses or immunosuppression
> - Inability or failure to empty the bladder completely
> - Inflammation or abrasion of the urethral mucosa
> - Instrumentation of the urinary tract (e.g., catheterization, cystoscopic procedures)
> - Obstructed urinary flow caused by:
>   - Congenital abnormalities
>   - Urethral strictures
>   - Contracture of the bladder neck
>   - Bladder tumors
>   - Calculi (stones) in the ureters or kidneys
>   - Compression of the ureters
>
> Adapted from Eliopoulos, C. (2018). *Gerontological nursing* (9th ed.). Philadelphia, PA: Wolters Kluwer; Norris, T. L. (2019). *Porth's pathophysiology: Concepts of altered health state* (10th ed.). Philadelphia, PA: Wolters Kluwer.

---

from fecal organisms ascending from the perineum to the urethra and the bladder and then adhering to the mucosal surfaces.

Bacterial Invasion of the Urinary Tract

By increasing the normal slow shedding of bladder epithelial cells (resulting in bacteria removal), the bladder can clear large numbers of bacteria. Glycosaminoglycan (GAG), a hydrophilic protein, normally exerts a nonadherent protective effect against various bacteria. The GAG molecule attracts water molecules, forming a water barrier that serves as a defensive layer between the bladder and the urine. GAG may be impaired by certain agents (cyclamate, saccharin, aspartame, and tryptophan metabolites). The normal bacterial flora of the vagina and urethral area also interfere with adherence of *Escherichia coli*. Urinary immunoglobulin A (IgA) in the urethra may also provide a barrier to bacteria.

Reflux

An obstruction to free-flowing urine is a condition known as **urethrovesical reflux**, which is the reflux (backward flow) of urine from the urethra into the bladder (see Fig. 49-1). With coughing, sneezing, or straining, the bladder pressure increases, which may force urine from the bladder into the urethra. When the pressure returns to normal, the urine flows back into the bladder, bringing into the bladder bacteria from the anterior portions of the urethra. Urethrovesical reflux is also caused by dysfunction of the bladder neck or urethra. The urethrovesical angle and urethral closure pressure may be altered with menopause, increasing the incidence of infection in postmenopausal women.

Ureterovesical or vesicoureteral reflux refers to the backward flow of urine from the bladder into one or both ureters (see Fig. 49-1). Normally, the ureterovesical junction

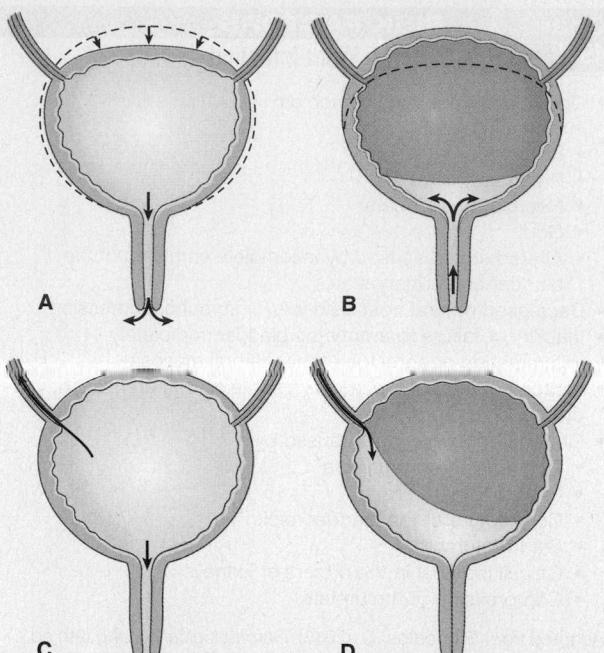

Figure 49-1 • Mechanisms of urethrovesical and ureterovesical reflux may cause urinary tract infection. *Urethrovesical reflux:* With coughing and straining, bladder pressure rises, which may force urine from the bladder into the urethra. **A.** When bladder pressure returns to normal, the urine flows back to the bladder (**B**), which introduces bacteria from the urethra to the bladder. *Ureterovesical reflux:* With failure of the ureterovesical valve, urine moves up the ureters during voiding (**C**) and flows into the bladder when voiding stops (**D**). This prevents complete emptying of the bladder. It also leads to urinary stasis and contamination of the ureters with bacteria-laden urine.

prevents urine from traveling back into the ureter. The ureters tunnel into the bladder wall so that the bladder musculature compresses a small portion of the ureter during normal voiding. When the ureterovesical valve is impaired by congenital causes or ureteral abnormalities, the bacteria may reach the kidneys and eventually destroy them.

Uropathogenic Bacteria

Bacteriuria is the term used to describe the presence of bacteria in the urine. Because urine samples (especially in women) can be easily contaminated by the bacteria normally present in the urethral area, a clean-catch midstream urine specimen is the measure used to establish bacteriuria. In men, contamination of the collected urine sample occurs less frequently.

Routes of Infection

Bacteria enter the urinary tract in three ways: by the transurethral route (ascending infection), through the bloodstream (hematogenous spread), or by means of a fistula from the intestine (direct extension).

The most common route of infection is transurethral, in which bacteria (often from fecal contamination) colonize the periurethral area and subsequently enter the bladder by means of the urethra (Freeman et al., 2017; Norris, 2019). In women, the short urethra offers little resistance to the movement of uropathogenic bacteria. Penile-vaginal intercourse forces the bacteria from the urethra into the bladder. This accounts for the increased incidence of UTIs in women who

engage in penile-vaginal intercourse. Bacteria may also enter the urinary tract by means of the blood from a distant site of infection or through direct extension by way of a fistula from the intestinal tract.

Clinical Manifestations

Signs and symptoms of UTI depend on whether the infection involves the lower (bladder) or upper (kidney) urinary tract and whether the infection is acute or chronic. Signs and symptoms of an uncomplicated lower UTI include burning on urination, **urinary frequency** (voiding more than every 3 hours), urgency, **nocturia** (awakening at night to urinate), incontinence, and suprapubic or pelvic pain. Hematuria and back pain may also be present (Martin, Wingo, & Holland, 2019). In older adults, these symptoms are less common (see Gerontologic Considerations section).

In patients with complicated UTIs, manifestations can range from asymptomatic bacteriuria to gram-negative sepsis with shock. Complicated UTIs often are caused by a broader spectrum of organisms, have a lower response rate to treatment, and tend to recur. Many patients with CAUTIs are asymptomatic; however, any patient with a catheter who suddenly develops signs and symptoms of septic shock should be evaluated for **urosepsis** (the spread of infection from the urinary tract to the bloodstream that results in a systemic infection).

 ## Gerontologic Considerations

The incidence of bacteriuria in older adults differs from that in younger adults. Bacteriuria increases with age and disability, and women are affected more frequently than men. UTI is the most common infection of older adults and increases in prevalence with age. UTIs occur more frequently in women than in men at younger ages but the gap between the sexes narrows in later life, which is due to reduced penile-vaginal intercourse in women and a higher incidence of bladder outlet obstruction secondary to benign prostatic hyperplasia in men (Eliopoulos, 2018).

In older adults, structural abnormalities secondary to decreased bladder tone, **neurogenic bladder** (dysfunctional bladder) secondary to stroke, or autonomic neuropathy of diabetes may prevent complete emptying of the bladder and increase the risk of UTI (Eliopoulos, 2018). When indwelling catheters are used, the risk of CAUTI increases dramatically. Older women often have incomplete emptying of the bladder and urinary stasis. In the absence of estrogen, postmenopausal women are susceptible to colonization and increased adherence of bacteria to the vagina and urethra. Oral or topical estrogen has been used to restore the glycogen content of vaginal epithelial cells and an acidic pH for some postmenopausal women with recurrent cystitis.

The antibacterial activity of prostatic secretions that protect men from bacterial colonization of the urethra and bladder decreases with aging. The use of catheterization or cystoscopy in evaluation or treatment for prostatic hyperplasia or carcinoma, strictures of the urethra, and neuropathic bladder may contribute to the higher incidence of UTIs in men. The incidence of bacteriuria also increases in men with confusion, dementia, or bowel or bladder incontinence. The most common cause of recurrent UTIs in older males is chronic bacterial prostatitis. Resection of the prostate gland may help reduce its incidence (see Chapter 53).

<table>
<tr><td>

Chart 49-2

Factors That Contribute to Urinary Tract Infection in Older Adults

- Cognitive impairment
- Frequent use of antimicrobial agents
- High incidence of multiple chronic medical conditions
- Immune compromised
- Immobility and incomplete emptying of bladder
- Low fluid intake and excessive fluid loss
- Obstructed flow of urine (e.g., urethral strictures, neoplasms, clogged indwelling catheter)
- Poor hygiene practices

Adapted from Eliopoulos, C. (2018). *Gerontological nursing* (9th ed.). Philadelphia, PA: Wolters Kluwer.

</td></tr>
</table>

Chart 49-2 lists other factors that may contribute to UTI in older patients. Diligent hand hygiene, careful perineal care, and frequent toileting may decrease the incidence of UTIs.

The organisms responsible for UTIs in older adults residing in institutions may differ from those found in patients residing in the community; this is thought to result in part from the frequent use of antibiotic agents by patients in long-term care facilities. *Escherichia coli* is the most common organism seen in older patients in the community or hospital. However, patients with indwelling catheters are more likely to be infected with organisms such as *Proteus, Klebsiella, Pseudomonas,* or *Staphylococcus*. Patients who have been previously treated with antibiotics may be infected with *Enterococcus* species. Frequent reinfections are common in older adults.

Early symptoms of UTI in postmenopausal women and older adults include malaise, nocturia, urinary incontinence, or a complaint of foul-smelling urine. Additional early symptoms include burning, urgency, and fever (Eliopoulos, 2018; Freeman et al., 2017). Some patients develop incontinence and delirium with the onset of a UTI.

Antibiotics are prescribed when bacteriuria is present (Eliopoulos, 2018). Treatment regimens are generally the same as those for younger adults, although age-related changes in the intestinal absorption of medications and decreased kidney function and hepatic flow may necessitate alterations in the antimicrobial regimen. Kidney function must be monitored, and medication dosages should be altered accordingly. The nurse carefully monitors fluid intake and output. Increasing fluid intake is advisable, provided that the patient's cardiac status does not contraindicate this action (Eliopoulos, 2018).

Assessment and Diagnostic Findings

Results of various tests, such as bacterial colony counts, cellular studies, and urine cultures, help confirm the diagnosis of UTI. In an uncomplicated UTI, the strain of bacteria determines the antibiotic of choice (Norris, 2019).

Urine Cultures

Urine cultures are useful for documenting a UTI and identifying the specific organism present. UTI is diagnosed by bacteria in the urine culture. A colony count greater than 100,000 CFU/mL of urine on a clean-catch midstream or catheterized specimen indicates infection (Fischbach & Fischbach, 2018). However, symptoms of UTI and subsequent sepsis have occurred with lower bacterial colony counts. The presence of any bacteria in specimens obtained by suprapubic needle aspiration of the urinary bladder, straight catheterization (insertion of a tube into the urinary bladder), or during surgery or cystoscopy is considered clinically significant (Fischbach & Fischbach, 2018).

The following groups of patients should have urine cultures obtained when bacteriuria is present (Fischbach & Fischbach, 2018; Norris, 2019):

- All children
- All men (because of the likelihood of structural or functional abnormalities)
- Patients who have been recently hospitalized or who live in long-term care facilities
- Patients who have undergone recent instrumentation (including catheterization) of the urinary tract
- Patients with diabetes
- Patients with prolonged or persistent symptoms
- Patients with three or more UTIs in the previous year
- Women who are postmenopausal
- Women who are pregnant
- Women who are sexually active
- Women who have new sexual partners
- Women with a history of compromised immune function or renal problems

Cellular Studies

Microscopic hematuria is present in about half of patients with an acute UTI (see Chapter 47). **Pyuria** (white blood cells [WBCs] in the urine) occurs in all patients with UTI; however, it is not specific for bacterial infection. Pyuria can also be seen with renal calculi, interstitial nephritis, and renal tuberculosis.

Other Studies

A multiple-test dipstick often includes testing for WBCs, known as the leukocyte esterase test, and nitrite testing (Norris, 2019). Tests for sexually transmitted infections may be performed because acute urethritis caused by sexually transmitted organisms (i.e., *Chlamydia trachomatis, Neisseria gonorrhoeae,* herpes simplex) or acute vaginitis infections (caused by *Trichomonas* or *Candida* species) may be responsible for symptoms similar to those of UTIs.

X-ray images, computed tomography (CT) scan, ultrasonography, and kidney scans are useful diagnostic tools. A CT scan may detect pyelonephritis or abscesses. Ultrasonography and kidney scans are extremely sensitive for detecting obstruction, abscesses, tumors, and cysts (Norris, 2019).

Medical Management

Management of UTIs typically involves pharmacologic therapy and patient education. Various prescribed medication regimens are used to treat UTI. The American Urological Association (AUA) guidelines for treatment of UTIs, particularly for recurrent uncomplicated UTIs in women, guide medical management (AUA, 2019a, 2019b).

Acute Pharmacologic Therapy

The ideal medication for treatment of UTI in women is an antibacterial agent that eradicates bacteria from the urinary tract with minimal effects on fecal and vaginal flora, thereby minimizing the incidence of vaginal yeast infections. The

TABLE 49 -1	Select Medications Used to Treat Urinary Tract Infections and Pyelonephritis	
Drug Classes	**Generic Name**	**Major Indications**
Anti-infective, urinary tract Bactericidal	Nitrofurantoin	UTI
	Cephalexin	Genitourinary infection
Cephalosporin	Cefadroxil	UTI
Fluoroquinolone	Ciprofloxacin Ofloxacin Norfloxacin Gatifloxacin	UTI Pyelonephritis
Fluoroquinolone	levofloxacin	Uncomplicated UTI
Penicillin	ampicillin amoxicillin	UTI—not commonly used alone due to *Escherichia coli* resistance Pyelonephritis UTI—not commonly used alone due to *E. coli* resistance
Trimethoprim–sulfamethoxazole combination	Co-trimoxazole	UTI Pyelonephritis
Urinary analgesic agent	Phenazopyridine	For relief of burning, pain, and other symptoms associated with UTI

UTI, urinary tract infection.
Adapted from Comerford, K. C., & Durkin, M. A. (2020). *Nursing 2020 drug handbook* (40th ed.). Philadelphia, PA: Wolters Kluwer.

antibacterial agent should be affordable and should have few adverse effects and low resistance. Because the organism in initial, uncomplicated UTIs in women is most likely *E. coli* or other fecal flora, the agent should be effective against these organisms. Various treatment regimens have been successful in treating uncomplicated lower UTIs in women: single-dose administration, short-course (3-day) regimens, or 7-day regimens (Freeman et al., 2017). The trend is toward a shortened course of antibiotic therapy for uncomplicated UTIs, because most cases are cured after 3 days of treatment. Medications commonly used to treat UTIs are listed in Table 49-1. Regardless of the regimen prescribed, the patient is instructed to take all doses prescribed, even if relief of symptoms occurs promptly. Longer medication courses are indicated for men, pregnant women, and women with pyelonephritis and other types of complicated UTIs. Men with UTIs should be evaluated for possible prostatitis (Eliopoulos, 2018). Hospitalization and intravenous (IV) antibiotics are occasionally necessary (Freeman et al., 2017).

Long-Term Pharmacologic Therapy

Although pharmacologic treatment of UTIs for 3 days is usually adequate in women, infection recurs in about 20% of women treated for uncomplicated UTIs. Infections that recur within 2 weeks of therapy do so because organisms of the original offending strain remain. Relapses suggest that the source of bacteriuria may be the upper urinary tract or that initial treatment was inadequate or given for too short a time. Recurrent infections in men are usually caused by persistence

of the same organism; further evaluation and treatment are indicated (Eliopoulos, 2018).

If infection recurs after completing antimicrobial therapy, another short course (3 to 4 days) of full-dose antimicrobial therapy followed by a regular bedtime dose of an antimicrobial agent may be prescribed.

A meta-analysis of nine studies reported the daily intake of cranberry, especially in the form of capsules, significantly reduced the rate of recurrent UTI compared to placebo with minor adverse effects such as rash and gastrointestinal symptoms (Tambunan & Rahardjo, 2019). The same meta-analysis reported that antibiotics were more effective for the treatment of recurrent UTI compared to cranberry capsules but had more severe adverse effects including gastrointestinal symptoms and Stevens–Johnson syndrome (Tambunan & Rahardjo, 2019).

NURSING PROCESS

The Patient with a Lower Urinary Tract Infection

Nursing care of the patient with a lower UTI focuses on treating the underlying infection and preventing a recurrence.

Assessment

A history of pertinent signs and symptoms is obtained from the patient with a suspected UTI. The presence of pain, frequency, urgency, hesitancy, and changes in urine are assessed, documented, and reported. The patient's usual pattern of voiding is assessed to detect factors that may predispose them to UTI. Infrequent emptying of the bladder, the association of symptoms of UTI with penile-vaginal intercourse, contraceptive practices, and personal hygiene are assessed. The patient's knowledge about prescribed antimicrobial medications and preventive health care measures is also assessed. In addition, the urine is assessed for volume, color, concentration, cloudiness, and odor—all of which are altered by bacteria in the urinary tract. Patients need to be asked specifically about the use of complementary and alternative medicine (CAM) therapies. Women with **interstitial cystitis** (inflammation of the bladder wall) use both complementary and conventional therapies. CAM therapies reported include behavioral therapy, physical therapy, stress reduction, and dietary manipulation (Oh-oka, 2017). Clinical efficacy was reported in a year-long clinical trial of intensive dietary manipulation (Oh-oka, 2017).

Diagnosis

NURSING DIAGNOSES

Based on the assessment data, nursing diagnoses may include the following:

- Acute pain associated with infection within the urinary tract
- Lack of knowledge about factors predisposing the patient to infection and recurrence, detection and prevention of recurrence, and pharmacologic therapy

COLLABORATIVE PROBLEMS/POTENTIAL COMPLICATIONS

Potential complications may include the following:

- Sepsis (urosepsis)
- The long term result of either extensive infective or inflammatory processes have the potential to result in either acute kidney injury or chronic kidney disease.

Planning and Goals

Major goals for the patient may include relief of pain and discomfort, increased knowledge of preventive measures and treatment modalities, and absence of complications.

Nursing Interventions

RELIEVING PAIN

The pain associated with a UTI is quickly relieved once effective antimicrobial therapy is initiated. Antispasmodic agents may also be useful in relieving bladder irritability and pain. Analgesic agents and the application of heat to the perineum help relieve pain and spasm. The patient is encouraged to drink liberal amounts of fluids (water and cranberry juice are the best choices) to promote renal blood flow and to flush the bacteria from the urinary tract. Urinary tract irritants (e.g., coffee, tea, citrus, spices, colas, alcohol) should be avoided. Frequent voiding (every 2 to 3 hours) is encouraged to empty the bladder completely, because doing so can lower urine bacterial counts, reduce urinary stasis, and prevent reinfection (Wu, Grealish, Moyle, et al., 2020).

MONITORING AND MANAGING POTENTIAL COMPLICATIONS

Early recognition of UTI and prompt treatment are essential to prevent recurrent infection and the possibility of complications, such as kidney disease, sepsis (urosepsis), strictures, and obstructions. The goal of treatment is to prevent infection from progressing and causing permanent kidney damage and injury. Thus, the patient must be educated to recognize early signs and symptoms, to test for bacteriuria, and to initiate treatment as prescribed. Appropriate antimicrobial therapy, liberal fluid intake, frequent voiding, and hygienic measures are commonly prescribed for managing UTIs. The patient is instructed to notify the primary provider if fatigue, nausea, vomiting, fever, or pruritus occurs. Periodic monitoring of renal function and evaluation for strictures, obstructions, or stones may be indicated for patients with recurrent UTIs.

Patients with UTIs are at increased risk for gram-negative sepsis. For each day a urinary catheter is in place, the risk of developing CAUTI increases by 3% to 7% per day of catheterization (Gould, Umscheid, Agarwal, et al., 2019). The Centers for Medicare and Medicaid Services has classified a CAUTI as a "never event" which means no reimbursement to pay for the cost of treatment will be covered by CMS or other insurers if the CAUTI is incurred within an acute care or rehabilitation hospital (Gould et al., 2019). Urosepsis mortality rates following catheterization are reported to be 25% to 60% (Newman, 2017).

Careful assessment of vital signs and level of consciousness may alert the nurse to kidney involvement or impending sepsis. Positive blood cultures and elevated WBC counts must be reported immediately. At the same time, appropriate antibiotic therapy and increased fluid intake are prescribed (IV antibiotic therapy and fluids may be required). Aggressive early treatment is the key to reducing the mortality rate associated with CAUTI especially in older patients, those with anemia, and those with elevated blood glucose levels (McCoy, Paredes, Allen, et al., 2017; Taylor, 2018).

PROMOTING HOME, COMMUNITY-BASED, AND TRANSITIONAL CARE

 Educating Patients About Self-Care. In helping patients learn about and prevent or manage a recurrent UTI, the nurse implements education that meets the patient's needs. Health-related behaviors that help prevent recurrent UTIs include practicing careful personal hygiene, increasing fluid intake to promote voiding and dilution of urine, urinating regularly and more frequently, and adhering to the therapeutic regimen (Martin et al., 2019). For a detailed discussion of patient education, see Chart 49-3.

Chart 49-3

PATIENT EDUCATION

Preventing Recurrent Urinary Tract Infections

The nurse instructs the patient on the following basic information:

Hygiene

- Shower rather than bathe in the tub because bacteria in the bathwater may enter the urethra.
- Clean the perineum and urethral meatus from front to back after each bowel movement. This will help reduce concentrations of pathogens at the urethral opening and, in women, the vaginal opening.

Fluid Intake

- Drink liberal amounts of fluids daily to flush out bacteria. It may be helpful to include at least one glass of cranberry juice per day.
- Avoid coffee, tea, colas, alcohol, and other fluids that are urinary tract irritants.

Voiding Habits

Void every 2 to 3 hours during the day, and completely empty the bladder. This prevents overdistention of the bladder and compromised blood supply to the bladder wall. Both predispose the patient to urinary tract infection. Precautions expressly for women include voiding immediately after penile-vaginal intercourse.

Interventions

- Take medication *exactly* as prescribed. Special timing of administration may be required.
- Keep in mind that if bacteria continue to appear in the urine, long-term antimicrobial therapy may be required to prevent colonization of the periurethral area and recurrence of infection.
- For recurrent infection, consider daily consumption of cranberry juice or capsules.
- If prescribed, test urine for presence of bacteria following manufacturer's and health care provider's instructions.
- Notify the primary provider if fever occurs or if signs and symptoms persist.
- Consult the primary provider regularly for follow-up.

Adapted from Tambunan, M. P., & Rahardjo, H. E. (2019). Cranberries for women with recurrent urinary tract infection: A meta-analysis. *Medical Journal of Indonesia*, 28(3), 268–275.

Evaluation

Expected patient outcomes may include:

1. Experiences relief of pain
   a. Reports absence of pain, urgency, frequency, nocturia, or hesitancy on voiding
   b. Takes analgesic, antispasmodic, and antibiotic agents as prescribed
2. Explains UTIs and their treatment
   a. Demonstrates knowledge of preventive measures and prescribed treatments
   b. Drinks 8 to 10 glasses of fluids daily
   c. Voids every 2 to 3 hours
   d. Produces urine that is clear and odorless
3. Experiences no complications
   a. Reports no symptoms of infection (fever, frequency)
   b. Has normal kidney function, negative urine and blood cultures
   c. Exhibits normal vital signs and temperature; no signs or symptoms of sepsis (urosepsis)
   d. Maintains adequate urine output more than 400 mL/day

Upper Urinary Tract Infections

Upper UTIs are much less common than those in the lower urinary tract. Acute pyelonephritis and chronic pyelonephritis are thought to be the most likely type, with interstitial nephritis (inflammation of the kidney) and kidney abscesses also a potential cause. Upper UTIs are a common cause of urosepsis (Freeman et al., 2017).

Pyelonephritis is a bacterial infection of the renal pelvis, tubules, and interstitial tissue of one or both kidneys. Causes involve either the upward spread of bacteria from the bladder or spread from systemic sources reaching the kidney via the bloodstream. Bacteria from a bladder infection can ascend into the kidney, resulting in pyelonephritis. An incompetent ureterovesical valve or obstruction occurring in the urinary tract increases the susceptibility of the kidneys to infection (see Fig. 49-1), because static urine provides a good medium for bacterial growth. Bladder or prostate tumors, strictures, benign prostatic hyperplasia, and urinary stones are some potential causes of obstruction that can lead to infections. Systemic infections (such as tuberculosis) can spread to the kidneys and result in abscesses. Pyelonephritis may be acute or chronic.

Acute Pyelonephritis

Acute pyelonephritis is the cause of more than 25,000 hospital admissions annually and usually leads to enlargement of the kidneys with interstitial infiltrations of inflammatory cells (Freeman et al., 2017; Norris, 2019). Abscesses may be noted on or within the renal capsule and at the corticomedullary junction. Eventually, atrophy and destruction of tubules and the glomeruli may result.

Clinical Manifestations

The patient with acute pyelonephritis has chills, fever, leukocytosis, bacteriuria, and pyuria. Low back pain, flank pain, nausea and vomiting, headache, malaise, and painful urination are common findings. Physical examination reveals pain and tenderness in the area of the costovertebral angle (see Chapter 47, Fig. 47-6). In addition, symptoms of lower urinary tract involvement, such as urgency and frequency, are common.

Assessment and Diagnostic Findings

An ultrasound study or a CT scan may be performed to locate an obstruction in the urinary tract. Relief of obstruction is essential to prevent complications and eventual kidney damage. An IV pyelogram may be indicated if functional and structural renal abnormalities are suspected (Fischbach & Fischbach, 2018). Radionuclide imaging with gallium citrate and indium-111 (^{111}In)–labeled WBCs may be useful to identify sites of infection that may not be visualized on CT scan or ultrasound. Urine culture and sensitivity tests are performed to determine the causative organism so that appropriate antimicrobial agents can be prescribed (Fischbach & Fischbach, 2018).

Medical Management

Patients with acute uncomplicated pyelonephritis are most often treated on an outpatient basis if they are not exhibiting acute symptoms of sepsis, dehydration, nausea, or vomiting. Patients treated on an outpatient basis must be willing and able to take their medications as prescribed. For outpatients, a 2-week course of antibiotic agents is recommended because renal parenchymal disease is more difficult to eradicate than mucosal bladder infections. Commonly prescribed agents include many of the same medications prescribed for the treatment of UTIs (see Table 49-1).

Following acute pyelonephritis treatment, the patient may develop a chronic or recurring symptomless infection persisting for months or years. After the initial antibiotic regimen, the patient may need antibiotic therapy for up to 6 weeks if a relapse occurs. A follow-up urine culture is obtained 2 weeks after completion of antibiotic therapy to document clearing of the infection.

Hydration with oral or parenteral fluids is essential in all patients with UTIs when there is adequate kidney function. Hydration helps facilitate "flushing" of the urinary tract and reduces pain and discomfort.

Chronic Pyelonephritis

Repeated bouts of acute pyelonephritis may lead to chronic pyelonephritis. When pyelonephritis becomes chronic, the kidneys become scarred, contracted, and nonfunctioning. Chronic pyelonephritis is a cause of chronic kidney disease that can result in the need for renal replacement therapy (RRT) such as transplantation or dialysis (see Chapter 48 for discussion of RRT).

Clinical Manifestations

The patient with chronic pyelonephritis usually has no symptoms of infection unless an acute exacerbation occurs. Noticeable signs and symptoms may include fatigue, headache, poor appetite, polyuria, excessive thirst, and weight loss. Persistent and recurring infection may produce progressive scarring of the kidney, resulting in chronic kidney disease (see Chapter 48).

Assessment and Diagnostic Findings

The extent of the disease is assessed by an IV urogram and measurements of creatinine clearance, blood urea nitrogen, and creatinine levels (Fischbach & Fischbach, 2018).

Complications

Complications of chronic pyelonephritis include end-stage kidney disease (from progressive loss of nephrons secondary to chronic inflammation and scarring), hypertension, and formation of renal calculi (from chronic infection with urea-splitting organisms).

Medical Management

Bacteria, if detected in the urine, are eradicated if possible. Long-term use of prophylactic antimicrobial therapy may help limit recurrence of infections and kidney scarring. Impaired kidney function alters the excretion of antimicrobial agents and necessitates careful monitoring of kidney function, especially if the medications are potentially toxic to the kidneys.

Nursing Management

The patient may require hospitalization or may be treated as an outpatient. When the patient requires hospitalization, fluid intake and output are carefully measured and recorded. Unless contraindicated, 3 to 4 L of fluids per day is encouraged to dilute the urine, decrease burning on urination, and prevent dehydration. The nurse assesses the patient's temperature every 4 hours and administers antipyretic and antibiotic agents as prescribed.

Patient education focuses on prevention of further infection by consuming adequate fluids, emptying the bladder regularly, and performing recommended perineal hygiene. The importance of taking antimicrobial medications exactly as prescribed is stressed, as is the need for keeping follow-up appointments.

ADULT VOIDING DYSFUNCTION

The **micturition** (voiding or urination) process involves several highly coordinated neurologic responses that mediate bladder function. A functional urinary system allows for appropriate bladder filling and complete bladder emptying (see Chapter 47). If voiding dysfunction goes undetected and untreated, the upper urinary system may be compromised. Both neurogenic and nonneurogenic disorders can cause adult voiding dysfunction (see Table 49-2). Chronic incomplete bladder emptying from poor detrusor pressure results in recurrent bladder infection. Incomplete bladder emptying due to bladder outlet obstruction (such as benign prostatic hyperplasia), causing high-pressure detrusor contractions, can result in hydronephrosis from the high detrusor pressure that radiates up the ureters to the renal pelvis.

Urinary Incontinence

More than 25 million adults in the United States are estimated to have **urinary incontinence** (unplanned, involuntary, or uncontrolled loss of urine from the bladder); however, it is difficult to determine exact numbers as there are many

TABLE 49-2	Conditions Causing Adult Voiding Disorders	
Disorder	**Voiding Dysfunction**	**Treatment**
Neurogenic Disorders		
Cerebellar ataxia	Incontinence or dyssynergia	Timed voiding; anticholinergic agents
Stroke	Retention or incontinence	Anticholinergic agents; bladder retraining
Dementia	Incontinence	Prompted voiding; anticholinergic agents
Diabetes	Incontinence and/or incomplete bladder emptying	Timed voiding; EMG/biofeedback; pelvic floor nerve stimulation; anticholinergic/antispasmodic agents; well-controlled blood glucose levels
Multiple sclerosis	Incontinence or incomplete bladder emptying	Timed voiding; EMG/biofeedback to learn pelvic muscle exercises and urge inhibition; pelvic floor nerve stimulation; antispasmodic agents
Parkinson's disease	Incontinence	Anticholinergic/antispasmodic agents
Spinal Cord Dysfunction		
Acute injury	Urinary retention	Indwelling catheter
Degenerative disease	Incontinence and/or incomplete bladder emptying	EMG/biofeedback; pelvic floor nerve stimulation; anticholinergic agents
Nonneurogenic Disorder		
"Bashful bladder"	Inability to initiate voiding in public bathrooms	Relaxation therapy; EMG/biofeedback
Overactive bladder	Urgency, frequency, and/or urge incontinence	EMG/biofeedback; pelvic floor nerve stimulation; bladder drill (see Chart 49-6); anticholinergic agents
Post general surgery	Acute urine retention	Catheterization
Postprostatectomy	Incontinence	*Mild:* Biofeedback; bladder drill (see Chart 49-6); pelvic floor nerve stimulation *Moderate/severe:* Surgery—artificial sphincter
Stress incontinence	Incontinence with cough, laugh, sneeze, position change	*Mild:* Biofeedback; bladder drill (see Chart 49-6); periurethral bulking with collagen *Moderate/severe:* Surgery

EMG, electromyogram.
Adapted from Hickey, J. V., & Strayer, A. L. (2020). *The clinical practice of neurological and neurosurgical nursing* (8th ed.). Philadelphia, PA: Wolters Kluwer.

types of urinary incontinence. The prevalence is thought to be 9% to 12% of all adults in the United States, but women are affected twice as often as men (Norris, 2019). Urinary incontinence is more common in older adults, with rates of between 50% and 90% reported in older adults residing in institutions (Eliopoulos, 2018).

Despite widespread media coverage, urinary incontinence remains underdiagnosed, underreported, and undertreated. Patients may be too embarrassed to seek help, causing them to ignore or conceal symptoms. Many patients use absorbent pads or other devices without having their condition properly diagnosed and appropriately treated. Health care providers must be alert to subtle cues of urinary incontinence and stay informed about current management strategies.

The costs of care for patients with urinary incontinence include the expenses of absorbent products, medications, and surgical or nonsurgical treatment modalities, as well as psychosocial costs (i.e., embarrassment, loss of self-esteem, and social isolation) (Norris, 2019).

Although urinary incontinence is commonly regarded as a condition that occurs in older multiparous women, it can occur in young nulliparous women, especially during vigorous high-impact activity. Age, gender, and number of vaginal deliveries are established risk factors that explain, in part, the increased incidence in women (see Chart 49-4). Men can have urinary incontinence, especially those with certain comorbid conditions. Researchers have reported that 40% of men with Parkinson's disease reported urinary incontinence (McDonald, Winge, & Burn, 2017). Urinary incontinence may be a symptom of other disorders, such as UTI or fecal impaction.

Types of Urinary Incontinence

There are many types of urinary incontinence, including the following:

Stress incontinence is the involuntary loss of urine through an intact urethra as a result of exertion, sneezing, coughing, or changing position (Wooldridge, 2017). It predominantly affects women who have had vaginal deliveries and is thought to be the result of decreasing ligament and pelvic floor support of the urethra and decreasing or absent estrogen levels within the urethral walls and bladder base. In men, stress incontinence is often experienced after a radical prostatectomy for prostate cancer because of the loss of urethral compression that the prostate had supplied before the surgery, and possibly bladder wall irritability.

Urge incontinence is the involuntary loss of urine associated with a strong urge to void that cannot be suppressed (Wooldridge, 2017). The patient is aware of the need to void but is unable to reach a toilet in time. An uninhibited detrusor contraction is the precipitating factor. This can occur in a patient with neurologic dysfunction that impairs inhibition of bladder contraction or in a patient without overt neurologic dysfunction.

Functional incontinence is the involuntary loss of urine due to physical or cognitive impairment. This occurs when the lower urinary tract function is intact but other factors, such as severe cognitive impairment (e.g., Alzheimer's dementia), make it difficult for the patient to identify the need to void or physical impairments make it difficult or impossible for the patient to reach the toilet in time for voiding (Miller, 2019; Wooldridge, 2017).

Iatrogenic incontinence is the involuntary loss of urine due to extrinsic medical factors, predominantly medications. One such example is the use of alpha-adrenergic agents to decrease blood pressure. In some people with an intact urinary system, these agents adversely affect the alpha receptors responsible for bladder neck closing pressure; the bladder neck relaxes to the point of incontinence with a minimal increase in intra-abdominal pressure, thus mimicking stress incontinence. As soon as the medication is discontinued, the apparent incontinence resolves.

Mixed incontinence, which encompasses several types of urinary incontinence, is involuntary leakage associated with urgency and also with exertion, effort, sneezing, or coughing (Miller, 2019; Wooldridge, 2017).

Overflow incontinence occurs when there is continual leakage of urine from an overdistended bladder (Norris, 2019). This can occur because of detrusor muscle underactivity or an outlet obstruction caused by benign prostatic hyperplasia, pelvic organ prolapse, or tumors, among other things.

Only with appropriate recognition of the problem, assessment, and referral for diagnostic evaluation and treatment can the outcome of incontinence be determined. All people with incontinence should be considered for evaluation and treatment.

 ## Gerontologic Considerations

Although urinary incontinence is not a normal consequence of aging, age-related changes in the urinary tract do predispose the older person to incontinence. However, if nurses and other health care providers accept incontinence as an inevitable part of illness or aging or consider it irreversible and untreatable, it cannot be treated successfully. Collaborative, interdisciplinary efforts are essential in assessing and effectively treating urinary incontinence. Urinary incontinence can decrease an older person's ability to maintain an independent lifestyle, which increases dependence on caregivers and may lead to institutionalization. Between 35% and 41% of older women have urinary incontinence (Wooldridge, 2017).

Many older adults experience transient episodes of incontinence that tend to be abrupt in onset. When this occurs, the nurse should question the patient, as well as the family if possible, about the onset of symptoms and any signs or symptoms of a change in other organ systems. Acute UTI, infection elsewhere in the body, constipation, decreased fluid intake, and a change in a chronic disease pattern, such as elevated blood glucose levels in patients with diabetes or decreased estrogen levels in menopausal women, can provoke the onset of urinary incontinence. If the cause is identified and modified or eliminated early at the onset of incontinence, the incontinence itself may be eliminated. Although the bladder of the older person is more vulnerable to altered detrusor activity, age alone is not a risk factor for urinary incontinence (Miller, 2019; Wooldridge, 2017).

Decreased bladder muscle tone is a normal age-related change found in older adults. This leads to decreased bladder capacity, increased **residual urine** (urine remaining in the bladder after voiding), and an increase in urgency.

Many medications affect urinary continence in addition to causing other unwanted or unexpected effects (Miller, 2019; Wooldridge, 2017). All medications need to be assessed for potential interactions.

Assessment and Diagnostic Findings

Once incontinence is recognized, a thorough history is necessary. This includes a detailed description of the problem and a history of medication use. The patient's voiding history, a diary of fluid intake and output, and bedside tests (e.g., residual urine, stress maneuvers) may be used to help determine the type of urinary incontinence involved. Urodynamic tests may be performed (see Chapter 47). Urinalysis and urine culture are performed to identify infection.

Urinary incontinence may be transient or reversible if the underlying cause is successfully treated and the voiding pattern reverts to normal. Chart 49-5 provides causes of transient incontinence.

Medical Management

Management depends on the type of urinary incontinence and its causes. Management of urinary incontinence may be behavioral, pharmacologic, or surgical.

Behavioral Therapy

Behavioral therapies, also known as nonpharmacologic, or conservative treatments, are the first choice to decrease or eliminate urinary incontinence (see Chart 49-6). These are recommended as first-line treatment for nonneurologic causes of incontinence in adults (AUA, 2019b). In using these techniques, health care professionals help patients avoid potential adverse effects of pharmacologic or surgical interventions. Pelvic floor muscle exercises (sometimes referred to as Kegel exercises) represent the cornerstone of behavioral intervention for addressing symptoms of stress, urge, and mixed incontinence (Miller, 2019; Wooldridge, 2017). Other behavioral treatments include the use of a voiding diary, biofeedback, verbal instruction (prompted voiding), and physical therapy (AUA, 2019b; Wooldridge, 2017).

Pharmacologic Therapy

Pharmacologic therapy works best when used as an adjunct to behavioral interventions. The particular antibiotic used will be dependent on the type of incontinence diagnosed (AUA, 2019a). Anticholinergic agents inhibit bladder contraction and are considered first-line medications for urge incontinence (AUA, 2019a; Wooldridge, 2017). Mirabegron, a beta-3 adrenergic agonist, may be used for urge incontinence and overactive bladder but should be used with caution in patients with hypertension as it can cause increased blood pressure (Wooldridge, 2017). A tricyclic antidepressant medication (e.g., amitriptyline) can also decrease bladder contractions as well as increase bladder neck resistance (Wooldridge, 2017). Pseudoephedrine sulfate, which acts on alpha-adrenergic receptors, causing urinary retention, may be used to treat stress incontinence; it needs to be used with caution in men with prostatic hyperplasia and in patients with hypertension.

Surgical Management

Surgical correction may be indicated in patients who have not achieved continence using behavioral and pharmacologic therapy. Surgical options vary according to the underlying anatomy and the physiologic problem. Most procedures involve lifting and stabilizing the bladder or urethra to restore the normal urethrovesical angle or to lengthen the urethra.

Women with stress incontinence may undergo an anterior vaginal repair, retropubic suspension, or needle suspension to reposition the urethra. Procedures to compress the urethra and increase resistance to urine flow include sling procedures and placement of periurethral bulking agents such as artificial collagen.

Periurethral bulking is a minimally invasive procedure in which small amounts of artificial collagen are placed within the walls of the urethra to enhance the closing pressure of the urethra (Norris, 2019). This procedure takes only 10 to 20 minutes and may be performed under local anesthesia or moderate sedation. A cystoscope is inserted into the urethra. An instrument is inserted through the cystoscope to deliver a small amount of collagen into the urethral wall at locations selected by the urologist. The patient is usually discharged home after voiding. There are no restrictions following the procedure, although multiple sessions may be necessary for a cure (Norris, 2019). Collagen placement anywhere in the body is considered semipermanent because its durability averages between 12 and 24 months, until the body absorbs the material. Periurethral bulking with collagen is a relatively safe alternative to surgery. It is also an option for people who

---

Chart 49-5	**Causes of Transient Incontinence**

- Atrophic vaginitis, urethritis, prostatitis
- Delirium or confusion
- Excessive urine production (increased intake, diabetes, diabetic ketoacidosis)
- Limited or restricted activity
- Pharmacologic agents (anticholinergic agents, sedatives, alcohol, analgesic agents, diuretics, muscle relaxants, adrenergic agents)
- Psychological factors (depression, regression)
- Stool impaction or constipation
- Urinary tract infections (UTI)

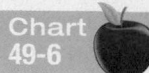

Chart 49-6

HEALTH PROMOTION
Interventions for Urinary Incontinence

Behavioral strategies are largely carried out, coordinated, and monitored by the nurse. These interventions may or may not be augmented by the use of medications.

Fluid Management

An adequate daily fluid intake of approximately 1500 to 1600 mL, taken as small increments between breakfast and the evening meal, helps to reduce urinary urgency related to concentrated urine production, decreases the risk of urinary tract infection, and maintains bowel functioning. (Constipation, resulting from inadequate daily fluid intake, can increase urinary urgency and urine retention.) The best fluid is water, although some suggest it may be helpful to include at least one glass of cranberry juice per day. Fluids containing caffeine, carbonation, alcohol, or artificial sweetener should be avoided because they irritate the bladder wall, thus resulting in urinary urgency. Some patients who have heart failure or end-stage kidney disease need to discuss their daily fluid limit with their primary provider.

Standardized Voiding Frequency

After establishing a patient's natural voiding and urinary incontinence tendencies, voiding on a schedule can be very effective in those with and without cognitive impairment, although patients with cognitive impairment may require assistance with this technique from nursing personnel or family members. The object is to purposely empty the bladder before the bladder reaches the critical volume that would cause an urge or stress incontinence episode. This approach involves the following:

- **Timed voiding** involves establishing a set voiding frequency (such as every 2 hours if incontinent episodes tend to occur 2 or more hours after voiding). The individual chooses to "void by the clock" at the given interval while awake rather than wait until a voiding urge occurs.
- **Prompted voiding** is timed voiding that is carried out by staff or family members when the individual has cognitive difficulties that make it difficult to remember to void at set intervals. The caregiver checks the patient to assess if they have remained dry and, if so, assists the patient to use the bathroom while providing positive reinforcement for remaining dry.
- **Habit retraining** is timed voiding at an interval that is more frequent than the individual would usually choose. This technique helps to restore the sensation of the need to void in individuals who are experiencing diminished sensation of bladder filling due to various medical conditions such as a stroke.
- **Bladder retraining**, also known as "bladder drill," incorporates a timed voiding schedule and urinary urge inhibition exercises to inhibit voiding, or leaking urine, in an attempt to remain dry for a set time. When the first timing interval is easily reached on a consistent basis without urinary urgency or incontinence, a new voiding interval, usually 10 to 15 minutes beyond the last,

is established. Again, the individual practices urge inhibition exercises to delay voiding or avoid incontinence until the next preset interval arrives. When an acceptable voiding interval is reached, the patient continues that timed voiding sequence throughout the day.

Pelvic Muscle Exercise

Also known as Kegel exercises, pelvic muscle exercise (PME) aims to strengthen the voluntary muscles that assist in bladder and bowel continence in both men and women. Written or verbal instruction alone is usually inadequate to educate an individual about how to identify and strengthen the pelvic floor for sufficient bladder and bowel control. Biofeedback-assisted PME uses either electromyography or manometry to help the individual identify the pelvic muscles as they attempt to learn which muscle group is involved when performing PME. The biofeedback method also allows assessment of the strength of this muscle area.

PME involves gently tightening the same muscles used to stop flatus or the stream of urine for 5- to 10-second increments, followed by 10-second resting phases. To be effective, these exercises need to be performed two or three times a day for at least 6 weeks. Depending on the strength of the pelvic musculature when initially evaluated, anywhere from 10 to 30 repetitions of PME are prescribed at each session. Older patients may need to exercise for an even longer time to strengthen the pelvic floor muscles. Pelvic muscle exercises are helpful for women with stress, urge, or mixed incontinence and for men who have undergone prostate surgery.

Vaginal Cone Retention Exercises

Vaginal cone retention exercises are an adjunct to the Kegel exercises. Vaginal cones of varying weight are inserted intravaginally twice a day. The patient tries to retain the cone for 15 minutes by contracting the pelvic muscles.

Transvaginal or Transrectal Electrical Stimulation

Commonly used to treat urinary incontinence, electrical stimulation is known to elicit a passive contraction of the pelvic floor musculature, thus re-educating these muscles to provide enhanced levels of continence. This modality is often used with biofeedback-assisted pelvic muscle exercise training and voiding schedules. At high frequencies, it is effective for stress incontinence. At low frequencies, electrical stimulation can also relieve symptoms of urinary urgency, frequency, and urge incontinence. Intermediate ranges are used for mixed incontinence.

Neuromodulation

Neuromodulation via transvaginal or transrectal nerve stimulation of the pelvic floor inhibits detrusor overactivity and hypersensory bladder signals and strengthens weak sphincter muscles.

Adapted from Hickey, J. V., & Strayer, A. L. (2020). *The clinical practice of neurological and neurosurgical nursing* (8th ed.). Philadelphia, PA: Wolters Kluwer.

---

are seeking help with stress incontinence who prefer to avoid surgery and who do not have access to behavioral therapies.

An artificial urinary sphincter can be used to close the urethra and promote continence. Two types of artificial sphincters are a periurethral cuff and a cuff inflation pump.

Men with overflow and stress incontinence may undergo a transurethral resection to relieve symptoms of prostatic enlargement. An artificial sphincter can be used after prostatic surgery for sphincter incompetence (see Fig. 49-2). After

surgery, periurethral bulking agents can be injected into the periurethral area to increase compression of the urethra.

Nursing Management

The nurse may encounter the patient with incontinence either in the hospital or as an outpatient. Nursing management of the patient with urinary incontinence in any setting is based on the premise that incontinence is not inevitable with illness

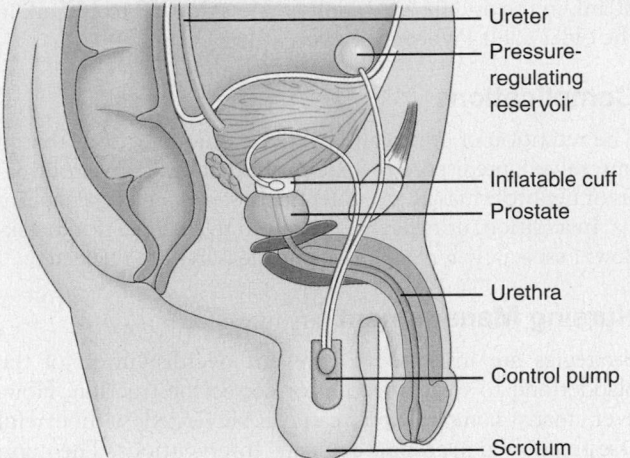

Ureter

Pressure-
regulating
reservoir

Inflatable cuff

Prostate

Urethra

Control pump

Scrotum

Figure 49-2 • Male artificial urinary sphincter. An inflatable cuff is inserted surgically around the urethra or neck of the bladder. To empty the bladder, the cuff is deflated by squeezing the control pump located in the scrotum.

Chart 49-8

PATIENT EDUCATION

Strategies for Promoting Urinary Continence

The nurse instructs the patient to:

- Avoid bladder irritants, such as caffeine, alcohol, and artificial sweeteners such as aspartame (NutraSweet).
- Avoid taking diuretic agents after 4 PM.
- Increase awareness of the amount and timing of all fluid intake.
- Perform all pelvic floor muscle exercises as prescribed, every day.
- Stop smoking (smokers usually cough frequently, which increases incontinence).
- Take steps to avoid constipation: Drink adequate fluids, eat a well-balanced diet high in fiber, exercise regularly, and take stool softeners if recommended.
- Void regularly, five to eight times a day (about every 2 to 3 hours):
  - First thing in the morning
  - Before each meal
  - Before retiring to bed
  - Once during the night if necessary

---

or aging and that it is often reversible and treatable. Patients who are incontinent and hospitalized need routine skin assessment to distinguish between incontinence-associated dermatitis (IAD) and pressure injury (Francis, 2019; Qiang, Xian, Bin, et al., 2020). When either IAD or pressure injury are identified, appropriate management techniques must be implemented to avoid complications (Francis, 2019; Qiang et al., 2020). See the Nursing Research Profile in Chart 49-7.

The nursing interventions in the outpatient setting are determined in part by the type of treatment that is undertaken. For behavioral therapy to be effective, the nurse must provide support and encouragement, because it is easy for the patient to become discouraged if therapy does not quickly improve the level of continence. Patient education is important and should be provided verbally and in writing (see

Chart 49-8). The patient should be educated to develop and use a log or diary to record timing of pelvic floor muscle exercises, frequency of voiding, any changes in bladder function, and any episodes of incontinence (Miller, 2019).

If pharmacologic treatment is used, the patient and family are educated about its purpose. Patients with mixed incontinence must be informed that anticholinergic and antispasmodic agents can help decrease urinary urgency and frequency and urge incontinence but do not decrease the urinary incontinence related to stress incontinence. If surgical correction is undertaken, the procedure and its desired outcomes are described to the patient and family. Follow-up contact with the patient enables the nurse to answer

---

Chart 49-7

NURSING RESEARCH PROFILE

Understanding Incontinence-Associated Dermatitis

Qiang, L., Xian, L. W., Bin, P. Y., et al. (2020). Investigating ICU nurses' understanding of incontinence-associated dermatitis: An analysis of influencing factors. *World Council of Enterostomal Therapists Journal*, *40*(1), 32–38.

Purpose

Patients with urinary and bowel incontinence are at high risk for incontinence-associated dermatitis (IAD) in the hospital setting. The purpose of this study was to investigate the knowledge, attitude, and preventive behavior of ICU nurses related to IAD.

Design

This was a prospective study that used a questionnaire designed by the researchers. A convenience sample of 508 nurses who had been working in an ICU in China with at least 1 year of experience were asked to fill out an online version of the questionnaire which resulted in 500 useable surveys.

Findings

The mean score on the knowledge of IAD was 7 out of a possible 11, indicating the need to educate nurses on their

knowledge of IAD. The mean score on the attitude toward prevention of IAD was 23 out of a possible 28. The lowest scores on this portion of the questionnaire were in the section about conducting quality control and monitoring of IAD that indicated the need to have a quality improvement program that recorded and followed rates of IAD. The mean score on prevention behaviors was 43 out of a possible 59, indicating the need for more education about daily behaviors such as assessment. Experience was the main influence on knowledge, attitude, and preventive behaviors, as nurses with the most years of experience scored highest.

Nursing Implications

This study provided information about the knowledge, attitude, and preventive behaviors associated with IAD. Nurses have a positive attitude but lack the knowledge and protocols needed to help prevent IAD. This study provides evidence for the need for educational programs and the implementation of standardized quality control and monitoring protocols.

the patient's questions and to provide reinforcement and encouragement.

Urinary Retention

Urinary retention is the inability to empty the bladder completely during attempts to void. Chronic urine retention often leads to overflow incontinence (described previously). In a healthy adult younger than 60 years, complete bladder emptying should occur with each voiding, with no residual. In adults older than 60 years, 50 to 100 mL of residual urine may remain after each voiding because of the decreased contractility of the detrusor muscle.

Urinary retention can occur postoperatively in any patient, particularly if the surgery affected the perineal or anal regions and resulted in reflex spasm of the sphincters. General anesthesia reduces bladder muscle innervation and suppresses the urge to void, impeding bladder emptying.

Pathophysiology

Urinary retention may result from diabetes, prostatic enlargement, urethral pathology (infection, tumor, calculus), trauma (pelvic injuries), pregnancy, or neurologic disorders (e.g., stroke, spinal cord injury, multiple sclerosis, Parkinson's disease). Some medications cause urinary retention either by inhibiting bladder contractility or by increasing bladder outlet resistance (AUA, 2019b; Wooldridge, 2017).

Assessment and Diagnostic Findings

The assessment of a patient for urinary retention is multifaceted because the signs and symptoms are challenging to detect. The following questions serve as a guide in assessment:

- What was the time of the last voiding, and how much urine was voided?
- Is the patient voiding small amounts of urine frequently?
- Is the patient dribbling urine?
- Does the patient complain of pain or discomfort in the lower abdomen? (Discomfort may be relatively mild if the bladder distends slowly.)
- Is the pelvic area rounded and swollen (could indicate urine retention and a distended bladder)?
- Does percussion of the suprapubic region elicit dullness (possibly indicating urine retention and a distended bladder)?
- Are other indicators of urinary retention present, such as restlessness and agitation?
- Does a postvoid bladder ultrasound test reveal residual urine?

The patient may verbalize an awareness of bladder fullness and a sensation of incomplete bladder emptying. Signs and symptoms of UTI (hematuria, urgency, frequency, and nocturia) may be present. A series of urodynamic studies (described in Chapter 47) may be performed to identify the type of bladder dysfunction and to aid in determining appropriate treatment. A voiding diary can be used to provide a written record of the amount of urine voided and the frequency of voiding. Postvoid residual urine may be assessed by using either straight catheterization or an ultrasound bladder scanner (see Chapter 47, Fig. 47-8) and is considered diagnostic of urinary retention. Normally, residual urine amounts to no more than 50 mL in the middle-aged adult and less than 50 to 100 mL in the older adult (Weber & Kelley, 2018).

Complications

The retention of urine can lead to chronic infections that, if unresolved, predispose the patient to renal calculi (urolithiasis or nephrolithiasis), pyelonephritis, sepsis, or hydronephrosis. In addition, urine leakage can lead to perineal skin breakdown, especially if regular hygiene measures are neglected.

Nursing Management

Strategies are instituted to prevent overdistention of the bladder and to treat infection or correct obstruction. However, many complications can be prevented with careful assessment and appropriate nursing interventions. The nurse explains to the patient why normal voiding is not occurring and monitors urine output closely. The nurse also provides reassurance about the temporary nature of retention and successful management strategies.

Promoting Urinary Elimination

Nursing measures to encourage normal voiding patterns include providing privacy, ensuring an environment and body position conducive to voiding, and assisting the patient with the use of the bathroom or bedside commode, rather than a bedpan, to provide a more natural setting for voiding. If his condition allows, the male patient may stand beside the bed to use the urinal; most men find this position more comfortable and natural.

Additional measures include applying warmth to relax the sphincters (e.g., sitz baths, warm compresses to the perineum, showers), giving the patient hot caffeine-free beverage and offering encouragement and reassurance. Simple trigger techniques, such as turning on the water faucet while the patient is trying to void, may also be used. Other examples of trigger techniques are stroking the abdomen or inner thighs, tapping above the pubic area, and dipping the patient's hands in warm water. After surgery or childbirth, prescribed analgesic agents should be given because pain in the perineal area can make voiding difficult. A combination of techniques may be necessary to initiate voiding.

When the patient cannot void, bladder scanning is used to assess for distention, then straight catheterization (as prescribed) is used to prevent overdistention of the bladder (see later discussion of neurogenic bladder and catheterization). In the case of prostatic obstruction, attempts at catheterization (by the urologist) may not be successful, requiring insertion of a **suprapubic catheter** (catheter inserted through a small abdominal incision into the bladder) (see Fig. 49-4, below). After urinary drainage is restored, bladder retraining is initiated for the patient who cannot void spontaneously.

Promoting Home, Community-Based, and Transitional Care

In addition to the strategies listed for promoting urinary continence found in Chart 49-8, modifications to the home environment can provide simple and effective ways to assist in treating urinary incontinence and retention. For example, the patient may need to remove obstacles, such as throw rugs or other objects, to provide easy, safe access to the bathroom.

Other modifications that the nurse may recommend include installing support bars in the bathroom; placing a bedside commode, bedpan, or urinal within easy reach; leaving lights on in the bedroom and bathroom; and wearing clothing that is easy to remove quickly.

Neurogenic Bladder

Neurogenic bladder is a dysfunction that results from a disorder or dysfunction of the nervous system and leads to urinary incontinence. It may be caused by spinal cord injury, spinal tumor, herniated vertebral disc, multiple sclerosis, congenital disorders (spina bifida or myelomeningocele), infection, or complications of diabetes (Alley, 2017) (see Chapters 63 and 64).

Pathophysiology

The two types of neurogenic bladder are spastic (or reflex) bladder and flaccid bladder. Spastic bladder is the more common type and is caused by any spinal cord lesion above the voiding reflex arc (upper motor neuron lesion) (Hickey & Strayer, 2020). The result is a loss of conscious sensation and cerebral motor control. A spastic bladder empties on reflex, with minimal or no controlling influence to regulate its activity.

Flaccid bladder is caused by a lower motor neuron lesion, commonly resulting from trauma. This form of neurogenic bladder is also increasingly being recognized in patients with diabetes. The bladder continues to fill and becomes greatly distended, and overflow incontinence occurs. The bladder muscle does not contract forcefully at any time. Because sensory loss may accompany a flaccid bladder, the patient feels no discomfort.

Assessment and Diagnostic Findings

Evaluation for neurogenic bladder involves measurement of fluid intake, urine output, and residual urine volume; urinalysis; and assessment of sensory awareness of bladder fullness and degree of motor control. Comprehensive urodynamic studies are also performed.

Complications

The most common complication of neurogenic bladder is infection resulting from urinary stasis and catheterization. Other complications include renal calculi, impaired skin integrity, and urinary incontinence or retention.

Medical Management

The problems resulting from neurogenic bladder disorders vary considerably from patient to patient and are a major challenge to the health care team. Several long-term objectives appropriate for all types of neurogenic bladders include preventing overdistention of the bladder, emptying the bladder regularly and completely, maintaining urine sterility with no stone formation, and maintaining adequate bladder capacity with no reflux.

Specific interventions include continuous, intermittent, or self-catheterization (discussed later in this chapter); the use of an external condom-type catheter; a diet low in calcium (to prevent calculi); and encouragement of mobility and ambulation. A liberal fluid intake is encouraged to reduce the urinary bacterial count, reduce stasis, decrease the concentration of calcium in the urine, and minimize the precipitation of urinary crystals and subsequent stone formation.

A bladder retraining program may be effective in treating a spastic bladder or urine retention. The use of a timed, or habit, voiding schedule may be established. To further enhance emptying of a flaccid bladder, the patient may be taught to "double void." After each voiding, the patient is instructed to remain on the toilet, relax for 1 to 2 minutes, and then attempt to void again in an effort to further empty the bladder.

Pharmacologic Therapy

Parasympathomimetic medications, such as bethanechol, may help to increase the contraction of the detrusor muscle.

Surgical Management

Surgery may be carried out to correct bladder neck contractures or vesicoureteral reflux, or to perform a urinary diversion procedure.

Urinary Catheters

In patients with a urologic disorder or with marginal kidney function, care must be taken to ensure that urinary drainage is adequate and that kidney function is preserved. When urine cannot be eliminated naturally and must be drained artificially, catheters may be inserted directly into the bladder, the ureter, or the renal pelvis.

Catheterization is performed to achieve the following (Gould et al., 2019; Taylor, 2018):
- Assist with postoperative drainage in urologic and other surgeries
- Provide a means to monitor accurate urine output in patients who are critically ill
- Promote urinary drainage in patients with neurogenic bladder dysfunction, urine retention, or at end-of-life care
- Prevent urinary leakage in patients with stage III to IV pressure injuries (see Chapter 56)
- Relieve urinary tract obstruction

An indwelling urinary catheter should be placed only if necessary because catheterization commonly leads to CAUTI. Figure 49-3 summarizes the pathophysiology of CAUTI.

Indwelling Catheters

If an indwelling catheter is necessary, the following specific nursing interventions are initiated to prevent CAUTI (McCoy et al., 2017; Taylor, 2018):
- Use strict aseptic technique during insertion of the smallest catheter possible
- Secure the catheter to prevent movement
- Frequently inspect urine color, odor, and consistency
- Perform daily perineal care with soap and water
- Maintain a closed system
- Follow the manufacturer's instructions when using the catheter port to obtain urine specimens
- Discontinue use as soon as feasible

Physiology/Pathophysiology

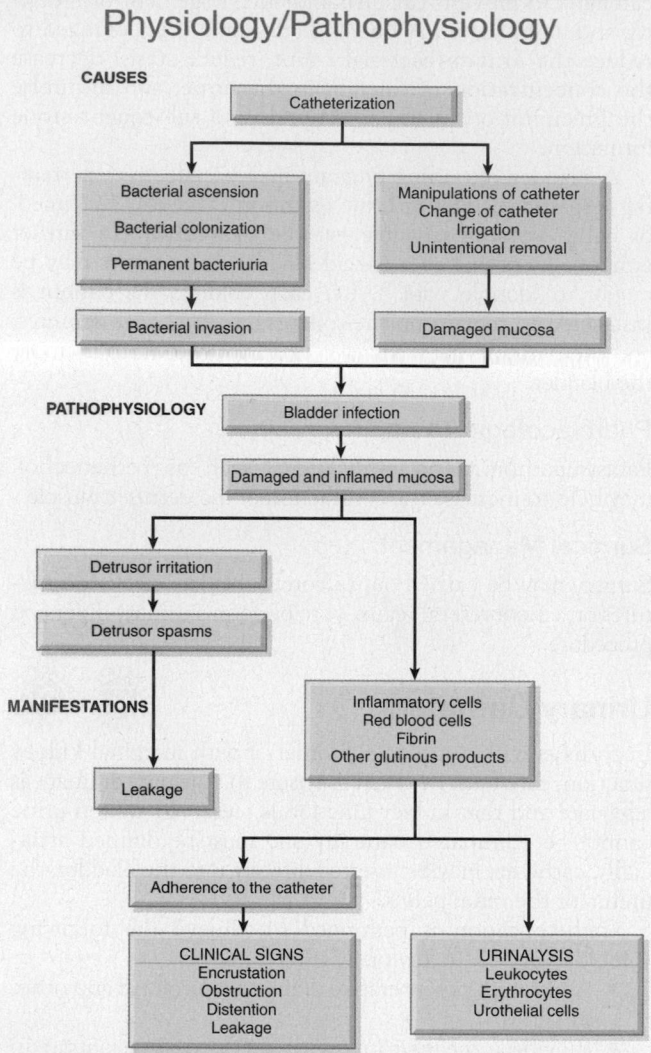

Figure 49-3 • Pathophysiology of CAUTI.

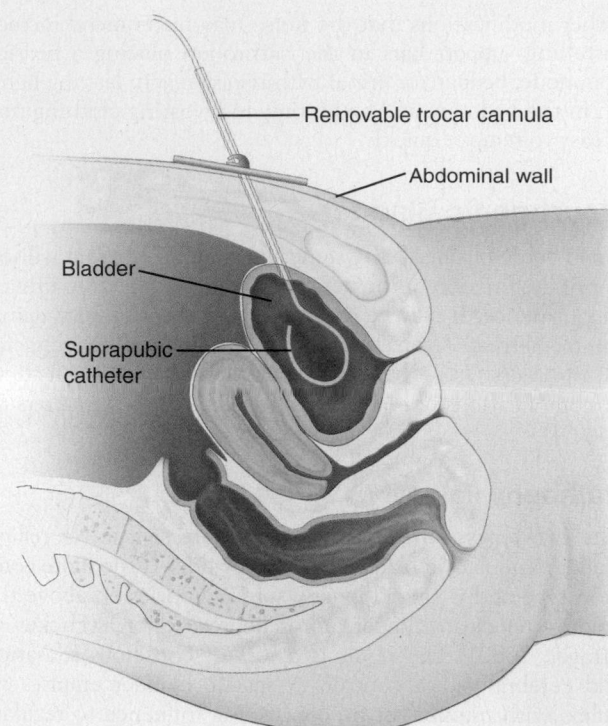

Figure 49-4 • Suprapubic bladder drainage. A trocar cannula is used to puncture the abdominal and bladder walls. The catheter is threaded through the trocar cannula, which is then removed, leaving the catheter in place. The catheter is secured by tape or sutures to prevent unintentional removal.

Suprapubic Catheters

Suprapubic catheterization allows bladder drainage by inserting a catheter or tube into the bladder through a suprapubic (above the pubis) incision or puncture (see Fig. 49-4). The catheter or suprapubic drainage tube is then threaded into the bladder and secured with sutures or tape, and the area around the catheter is covered with a sterile dressing. The catheter is connected to a sterile closed drainage system, and the tubing is secured to prevent tension on the catheter. This may be a temporary measure to divert the flow of urine from the urethra when the urethral route is impassable (because of injuries, strictures, prostatic obstruction), after gynecologic or other abdominal surgery when bladder dysfunction is likely to occur, and occasionally after pelvic fractures. A permanent indwelling suprapubic catheter may be needed in the patient who is incontinent following a spinal cord injury (Hickey & Strayer, 2020).

Suprapubic bladder drainage may be maintained continuously for several weeks. When the patient's ability to void is to be tested, the catheter is clamped for 4 hours, during which time the patient attempts to void. After the patient voids, the catheter is unclamped, and the residual urine is measured.

If the amount of residual urine is less than 100 mL on two separate occasions (morning and evening), the catheter is usually removed. However, if the patient complains of pain or discomfort, the suprapubic catheter is usually left in place until the patient can void successfully.

Suprapubic drainage offers certain advantages. Patients can usually void sooner after surgery than those with urethral catheters, and they may be more comfortable. The catheter allows greater mobility, permits measurement of residual urine without urethral instrumentation, and presents less risk of bladder infection. The suprapubic catheter is removed when it is no longer required, and a sterile dressing is placed over the site.

The patient requires liberal amounts of fluid to prevent encrustation around the catheter. Other potential problems include the formation of bladder stones, acute and chronic infections, and problems collecting urine. A wound-ostomy-continence (WOC) nurse may be consulted to assist the patient and family in selecting the most suitable urine collection system and to educate them about its use and care.

Nursing Management

Assessing the Patient and the System

Patients at high risk for CAUTI need to be identified and monitored carefully. These include women; older adults; and patients who are debilitated, malnourished, chronically ill, immunosuppressed, or have diabetes (Newman, 2017). They are observed for signs and symptoms of CAUTI: cloudy malodorous urine, hematuria, fever, chills, anorexia, and malaise. Any drainage and excoriation in the area around the urethral orifice is noted. Urine cultures provide the most accurate means of assessing a patient for infection.

Preventing Infection

Certain principles of care are essential to prevent infection in patients with a closed urinary drainage system (see Chart 49-9). The catheter is an object foreign to the body and produces a reaction in the urethral mucosa with some urethral discharge. Cleansing should be done on a daily basis

---

Chart 49-9

Preventing Infection in the Patient with an Indwelling Urinary Catheter

- Avoid contamination of the drainage spout. A receptacle in which to empty the bag is provided for each patient.
- Avoid routine catheter changes. The catheter is changed only to correct problems such as leakage, blockage, or encrustations.
- Avoid unnecessary handling or manipulation of the catheter by the patient or staff.
- Carry out hand hygiene before and after handling the catheter, tubing, or drainage bag.
- Ensure a free flow of urine to prevent infection. Improper drainage occurs when the tubing is kinked or twisted, allowing pools of urine to collect in the tubing loops.
- Evaluate the benefit of placing an indwelling urinary catheter versus the risk of the patient developing a catheter-associated urinary tract infection (CAUTI).
- If the collection bag *must* be raised above the level of the patient's bladder, clamp the drainage tube. This prevents backflow of contaminated urine into the patient's bladder from the bag.
- Monitor the patient's voiding when the catheter is removed. The patient must void within 8 hours; if unable to void, the patient may require catheterization with a straight catheter.
- Never disconnect the tubing to obtain urine samples, to irrigate the catheter, or to ambulate or transport the patient.
- Never irrigate the catheter routinely. If the patient is prone to obstruction from clots or large amounts of sediment, use a three-way system with continuous irrigation.
- Never leave the catheter in place longer than is necessary to decrease the risk of CAUTI.
- Obtain a urine specimen for culture at the first sign of infection.
- To prevent contamination of the closed system, *never* disconnect the tubing. The drainage bag must *never* touch the floor. The bag and collecting tubing are changed if contamination occurs, if urine flow becomes obstructed, or if tubing junctions start to leak at the connections.
- To reduce the risk of bacterial proliferation, empty the collection bag at least every 8 hours through the drainage spout—more frequently if there is a large volume of urine.
- Use scrupulous aseptic technique during insertion of the catheter. Use a preassembled, sterile, closed urinary drainage system of the smallest catheter size possible to minimize trauma.
- Wash the perineal area with soap and water at least twice a day; avoid a to-and-fro motion of the catheter. Dry the area well, but avoid applying powder because it may irritate the perineum.

Adapted from McCoy, C., Paredes, M., Allen, S., et al. (2017). Catheter-associated urinary tract infections. *Clinical Journal of Oncology Nursing, 21*(4), 460–465; Gould, C. V., Umscheid, C. A., Agarwal, R. K., et al. (2019). Guideline for prevention of catheter-associated urinary tract infections 2009. Retrieved on 5/13/2020 at: www.cdc.gov/infectioncontrol/guidelines/cauti/

---

and after bowel movements/contamination. A clean washcloth or wipe is used, cleansing from the catheter along its length from the meatus away from the patient. Disinfectants or antibacterial lubricants have not been found to decrease infections. Water in the wash basin used for daily cleansing is avoided as it may harbor microbes. Using disposable wipes that contain purified water, aloe, and vitamin E has been shown to decrease the incidence of CAUTIs (Newman, 2017). Vigorous cleansing of the meatus while the catheter is in place is discouraged because the cleansing action can move the catheter back and forth, increasing the risk of infection. The catheter is anchored as securely as possible to prevent it from moving in the urethra (Gould et al., 2019). Special care should be taken to ensure that any patient who is confused does not remove the catheter with the retention balloon still inflated, because this could cause bleeding and considerable injury to the urethra.

A liberal fluid intake, within the limits of the patient's cardiac and renal reserve, and an increased urine output must be ensured to flush the catheter and to dilute urinary substances that might form encrustations (Newman, 2017).

Urine cultures are obtained as prescribed or indicated when monitoring the patient for infection; many catheters have an aspiration (puncture) port from which a specimen can be obtained.

Bacteriuria is considered inevitable in patients with indwelling catheters; therefore, controversy remains about the usefulness of taking cultures and treating asymptomatic bacteriuria, because overtreatment may lead to resistant strains of bacteria. Continual observation for fever, chills, and other signs and symptoms of systemic infection is necessary. Infections are treated aggressively.

Retraining the Bladder

When an indwelling urinary catheter is in place, the detrusor muscle does not actively contract the bladder wall to stimulate emptying because urine is continuously draining from the bladder. As a result, the detrusor may not immediately respond to bladder filling when the catheter is removed, resulting in either urine retention or urinary incontinence. This condition, known as postcatheterization detrusor instability, can be managed with bladder retraining (see Chart 49-10).

Immediately after the indwelling catheter is removed, the patient is placed on a timed voiding schedule, usually every 2 to 3 hours. At the given time interval, the patient is instructed to void. The bladder is then scanned using a portable ultrasonic bladder scanner, and if the bladder has not emptied completely, straight catheterization may be performed (Newman, 2017). After a few days, as the nerve endings in the bladder wall become resensitized to the bladder filling and emptying, bladder function usually returns to normal. If the patient has had an indwelling catheter in place for an extended period (e.g., greater than 1 month), bladder retraining will take longer; in some cases, function may never return to normal, and long-term intermittent catheterization may become necessary.

Assisting with Intermittent Self-Catheterization

Intermittent self-catheterization provides periodic drainage of urine from the bladder. By promoting drainage and eliminating excessive residual urine, intermittent catheterization

Chart 49-10

Bladder Retraining After Indwelling Catheterization

- Instruct the patient to drink a measured amount of fluid from 8 AM to 10 PM to avoid bladder overdistention. Offer no fluids (except sips) after 10 PM.
- At specific times, ask the patient to void by applying pressure over the bladder, tapping the abdomen, or running water to trigger the bladder.
- Immediately after the voiding attempt, perform a bladder scan to determine the amount of residual urine (see Chapter 47, Fig. 47-8).
- Measure the volumes of urine voided.
- Palpate the bladder at repeated intervals to assess for distention.
- Instruct the patient who has no voiding sensation to be alert to any signs that indicate a full bladder, such as perspiration, cold hands or feet, or feelings of anxiety.
- Perform straight catheterization, as prescribed, usually for residual urine of >300 mL.
- Lengthen the intervals between catheterizations as the volume of residual urine decreases. Catheterization is usually discontinued when the volume of residual urine is <100 mL.

Adapted from Newman, D. (2017). Catheters, devices, products, and catheter-associated urinary tract infections. In D. K. Newman, J. F. Wyman, & V. W. Welch (Eds.). *Core curriculum for urologic nursing*. Pitman, NJ: Society of Urologic Nurses and Associates.

protects the kidneys, reduces the incidence of UTIs, and improves continence. It is the treatment of choice in some patients with spinal cord injury and other neurologic disorders, such as multiple sclerosis, when the ability to empty the bladder is impaired. Self-catheterization promotes independence, results in few complications, and enhances self-esteem and quality of life.

When educating the patient about how to perform self-catheterization, the nurse often teaches the patient to use a "clean technique" (nonsterile) at home (Hickey & Strayer, 2020). Antibacterial liquid soap is recommended for cleaning urinary catheters at home. The catheter is thoroughly rinsed with warm tap water and must be dried before reuse. It should be kept in its own container, such as a plastic food storage bag.

In educating the patient, the nurse emphasizes the importance of frequent catheterization and emptying the bladder at the prescribed time. The average daytime clean intermittent catheterization schedule is every 4 to 6 hours and just before bedtime. If the patient is awakened at night with an urge to void, catheterization may be performed after an attempt is made to void normally.

The female patient assumes a Fowler position and uses a mirror to help locate the urinary meatus. She lubricates the catheter and inserts it 7.5 cm (3 inches) into the urethra, in a downward and backward direction. The male patient assumes a Fowler or sitting position, lubricates the catheter, and retracts the foreskin of the penis with one hand while grasping the penis and holding it at a right angle to the body. (This maneuver straightens the urethra and makes it easier to insert the catheter.) He inserts the catheter 15 to 25 cm (6 to 10 inches) until urine begins to flow. After removal, the catheter is cleaned, rinsed, dried, and placed in a plastic bag or case. Patients who follow an intermittent catheterization

routine should consult a primary provider at regular intervals to assess urinary function and to detect complications. If the patient cannot perform intermittent self-catheterization, a family member or caregiver may be taught to carry out the procedure at regular intervals during the day.

An alternative to self-catheterization is creation of the Mitrofanoff umbilical appendicovesicostomy, which provides easy access to the bladder but requires an extensive surgical procedure (King, 2017). In this procedure, the bladder neck is closed and the appendix is used to create access to the bladder from the skin surface through a submucosal tunnel created with the appendix. One end of the appendix is brought to the skin surface and used as a stoma, and the other end is tunneled into the bladder. The appendix serves as an artificial urinary sphincter when an alternative is necessary to empty the bladder. A surgically prepared continent urine reservoir with a sphincter mechanism is required in cases of bladder cancer and severe interstitial cystitis. Various types of urinary diversions may be used when a radical **cystectomy** (surgical removal of the bladder) is necessary (see discussion later in chapter).

UROLITHIASIS AND NEPHROLITHIASIS

Urolithiasis and nephrolithiasis refer to stones (calculi) in the urinary tract and kidney, respectively. Urinary stones predominantly occur in the third to fifth decades of life and affect men twice as often as women (Norris, 2019). The prevalence of renal calculi is 10.6% for males and 7.1% for females; however, recent studies show that rates are increasing among women with estimates that the ratio of affected males-to-females is 1.3 to 1 (Flagg & Joiner, 2017). Stones may develop in one or both kidneys (Norris, 2019).

Pathophysiology

Stones are formed in the urinary tract when urinary concentrations of substances such as calcium oxalate, calcium phosphate, and uric acid increase. Referred to as supersaturation, this depends on the amount of the substance, ionic strength, and pH of the urine. Stones may be found anywhere from the kidney to the bladder and may vary in size from minute granular deposits, called *sand* or *gravel*, to bladder stones as large as an orange. The different sites of calculi formation in the urinary tract are shown in Figure 49-5.

Certain factors favor the formation of stones, including infection, urinary stasis, and periods of immobility, all of which slow kidney drainage and alter calcium metabolism (Norris, 2019). In addition, increased calcium concentrations in the blood and urine promote precipitation of calcium and formation of stones (the most common are calcium based) (Norris, 2019). Causes of hypercalcemia (high serum calcium) and hypercalciuria (high urine calcium) may include the following (Norris, 2019):

- Hyperparathyroidism
- Renal tubular acidosis
- Cancers (e.g., leukemia, multiple myeloma)
- Dehydration
- Granulomatous diseases (e.g., sarcoidosis, tuberculosis), which may cause increased vitamin D production by the granulomatous tissue

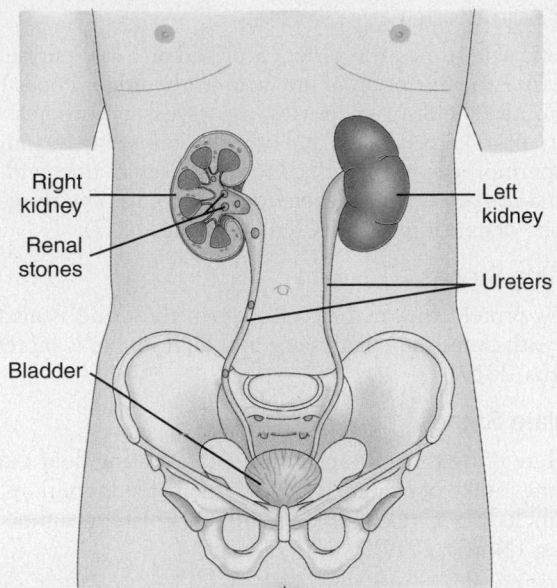

Figure 49-5 • Examples of potential sites of calculi formation in the urinary tract (urolithiasis) and kidney (nephrolithiasis).

- Excessive intake of vitamin D
- Excessive intake of milk and alkali
- Myeloproliferative diseases such as polycythemia vera, which produce an unusual proliferation of blood cells from the bone marrow
- Intestinal bypass surgery

For patients with stones containing uric acid, struvite, or cystine, a thorough physical examination and metabolic workup are indicated because of associated disturbances contributing to the stone formation. Uric acid stones account for 72% of stones in men (Flagg & Joiner, 2017). These may be seen in patients with gout or myeloproliferative disorders. Seventy-two percent of stones diagnosed in women are struvite stones (Flagg & Joiner, 2017) which form in persistently alkaline, ammonia-rich urine caused by the presence of bacteria such as *Proteus, Pseudomonas, Klebsiella, Staphylococcus,* or *Mycoplasma.* Predisposing factors for struvite stones include neurogenic bladder, foreign bodies, and recurrent UTIs (Norris, 2019).

Several conditions, as well as certain metabolic risk factors, predispose patients to stone formation. These include anatomic derangements such as polycystic kidney disease, horseshoe kidneys, chronic strictures, and medullary sponge disease. Urinary stone formation can occur in patients with inflammatory bowel disease and in those with an ileostomy or bowel resection because these patients absorb more oxalate. Medications known to cause stones in some patients include antacids, acetazolamide, vitamin D, laxatives, and high doses of aspirin (Comerford & Durkin, 2020). However, in many patients, no cause may be found.

Clinical Manifestations

Signs and symptoms of stones in the urinary system depend on the presence of obstruction, infection, and edema. When stones block the flow of urine, obstruction develops, producing an increase in hydrostatic pressure and distending the renal pelvis and proximal ureter (Norris, 2019). Infection (pyelonephritis and UTI with chills, fever, and frequency) can be a contributing factor with struvite stones. Some stones cause few, if any, symptoms while slowly destroying the functional units (nephrons) of the kidney; others cause excruciating pain and discomfort (Flagg & Joiner, 2017). Stones in the renal pelvis may be associated with an intense, deep ache in the costovertebral region. Hematuria is often present; pyuria may also be noted. Pain originating in the renal area radiates anteriorly and downward toward the bladder in the female and toward the testes in the male. If the pain suddenly becomes acute, with tenderness over the costovertebral area, and nausea and vomiting occur, the patient is having an episode of renal colic. Diarrhea and abdominal discomfort are due to renointestinal reflexes and the anatomic proximity of the kidneys to the stomach, pancreas, and large intestine.

Stones lodged in the ureter (ureteral obstruction) cause acute, excruciating, colicky, wavelike pain that radiates down the thigh and to the genitalia. Often, the patient has a desire to void, but little urine is passed, and it usually contains blood because of the abrasive action of the stone. This group of symptoms is called *ureteral colic.* Colic is mediated by prostaglandin E, a substance that increases ureteral contractility and renal blood flow and that leads to increased intraureteral pressure and pain. In general, the patient is able to pass stones 0.5 cm in diameter (Norris, 2019). Stones larger than 1 cm in diameter usually must be removed or fragmented (broken up by lithotripsy) so that they can be removed or passed spontaneously.

Stones lodged in the bladder usually produce symptoms of irritation and may be associated with UTI and hematuria. If the stone obstructs the bladder neck, urinary retention occurs. If infection is associated with a stone, the condition is far more serious, with the potential for urosepsis developing.

Assessment and Diagnostic Findings

The diagnosis is confirmed by a noncontrast CT scan (Flagg & Joiner, 2017). Blood chemistries and a 24-hour urine test for measurement of calcium, uric acid, creatinine, sodium, pH, and total volume may be part of the diagnostic workup. Dietary and medication histories and family history of renal calculi are obtained to identify factors predisposing the patient to the formation of stones.

When stones are recovered (whether freely passed by the patient or removed through special procedures), chemical analysis is carried out to determine their composition. Stone analysis can provide a clear indication of the underlying disorder. For example, calcium oxalate or calcium phosphate stones usually indicate disorders of oxalate or calcium metabolism, whereas urate stones suggest a disturbance in uric acid metabolism (Flagg & Joiner, 2017).

Medical Management

The goals of management are to eradicate the stone, determine the stone type, prevent nephron destruction, control infection, and relieve any obstruction that may be present. The immediate objective of treatment of renal or ureteral colic is to relieve the pain until its cause can be eliminated. Opioid analgesic agents are given to prevent shock and syncope that may result from the excruciating pain. Nonsteroidal anti-inflammatory drugs (NSAIDs) are effective in treating renal calculus pain because they provide specific pain relief. They also inhibit the synthesis of prostaglandin E, reducing swelling and facilitating passage of the stone. Generally, once the stone has passed, the pain is relieved. Unless the patient is vomiting or has heart failure or any other condition requiring fluid restriction, fluids are encouraged. This increases the hydrostatic pressure behind the stone, assisting it in its downward passage. A high, around-the-clock fluid intake reduces the concentration of urinary crystalloids, dilutes the urine, and ensures a high urine output.

Nutritional Therapy

Nutritional therapy plays an important role in preventing renal calculi (Flagg & Joiner, 2017) (see Chart 49-11). Fluid intake is the mainstay of most medical therapy for renal calculi. Unless fluids are contraindicated, patients with renal calculi should drink eight to ten 8-oz glasses of water daily or have IV fluids prescribed to keep the urine dilute. A urine output exceeding 2 L/day is advisable.

Calcium Stones

Historically, patients with calcium-based renal calculi were advised to restrict calcium in their diet. However, evidence has questioned this practice, except for patients with type 2 absorptive hypercalciuria (half of all patients with calcium stones), as stones in these patients are clearly the result of excess dietary calcium. Liberal fluid intake is encouraged. Medications such as ammonium chloride may be used, and if increased parathormone production (resulting in increased serum calcium levels in blood and urine) is a factor in the formation of stones, therapy with thiazide diuretics may be beneficial in reducing the calcium loss in the urine and lowering the elevated parathormone levels (Cahill & Haras, 2017).

Uric Acid Stones

For uric acid stones, the patient is placed on a low-purine diet to reduce the excretion of uric acid in the urine. Foods high in purine (shellfish, anchovies, asparagus, mushrooms, and organ meats) are avoided, and other proteins may be limited. Allopurinol may be prescribed to reduce serum uric acid levels and urinary uric acid excretion, and to dissolve or reduce the size of existing stones (Cahill & Haras, 2017).

Cystine Stones

A low-protein diet may be prescribed, the urine is alkalinized with potassium alkali salts, and fluid intake is increased (Norris, 2019).

Oxalate Stones

A dilute urine is maintained through increasing fluid intake, and the intake of oxalate is limited. Many foods contain oxalate including spinach, Swiss chard, chocolate, peanuts, and pecans (Norris, 2019).

Interventional Procedures

If the stone does not pass spontaneously or if complications occur, common interventions include endoscopic or other procedures. For example, ureteroscopy, extracorporeal shock wave lithotripsy (ESWL), or endourologic (percutaneous) stone removal may be necessary (Norris, 2019).

Ureteroscopy (see Fig. 49-6A) involves first visualizing the stone and then destroying it. Access to the stone is accomplished by inserting a ureteroscope into the ureter and then inserting a laser, electrohydraulic lithotripter, or ultrasound device through the ureteroscope to fragment and remove the stones. A stent may be inserted and left in place for 48 hours or more after the procedure to keep the ureter patent. Length of hospital stay is generally brief, and some patients can be treated as outpatients.

ESWL, commonly referred to as lithotripsy, is a noninvasive procedure used to break up stones in the calyx of the kidney (see Fig. 49-6B). After the stones are fragmented to the size of grains of sand, the remnants of the stones are spontaneously voided. In ESWL, a high-energy amplitude of pressure, or shock wave, is generated by the abrupt release of energy and transmitted through water and soft tissues. When the shock wave encounters a substance of different intensity (a renal calculus), a compression wave causes the surface of the stone to fragment. Repeated shock waves focused on the stone eventually reduce it to many small pieces that are excreted in the urine.

Discomfort from the multiple shocks may occur, although the shock waves usually do not cause damage to other tissue. The patient is observed for obstruction and infection resulting from blockage of the urinary tract by stone fragments. All urine is strained after the procedure; voided gravel or sand is sent to the laboratory for chemical analysis. Several treatments may be necessary to ensure disintegration of stones.

Endourologic methods of stone removal (see Fig. 49-6C) may be used to extract kidney calculi that cannot be removed by other procedures. A percutaneous nephrostomy or a percutaneous nephrolithotomy (which are similar procedures) may be performed. A nephroscope is introduced through a percutaneous route into the renal parenchyma. Depending on its size, the stone may be extracted with forceps or by a

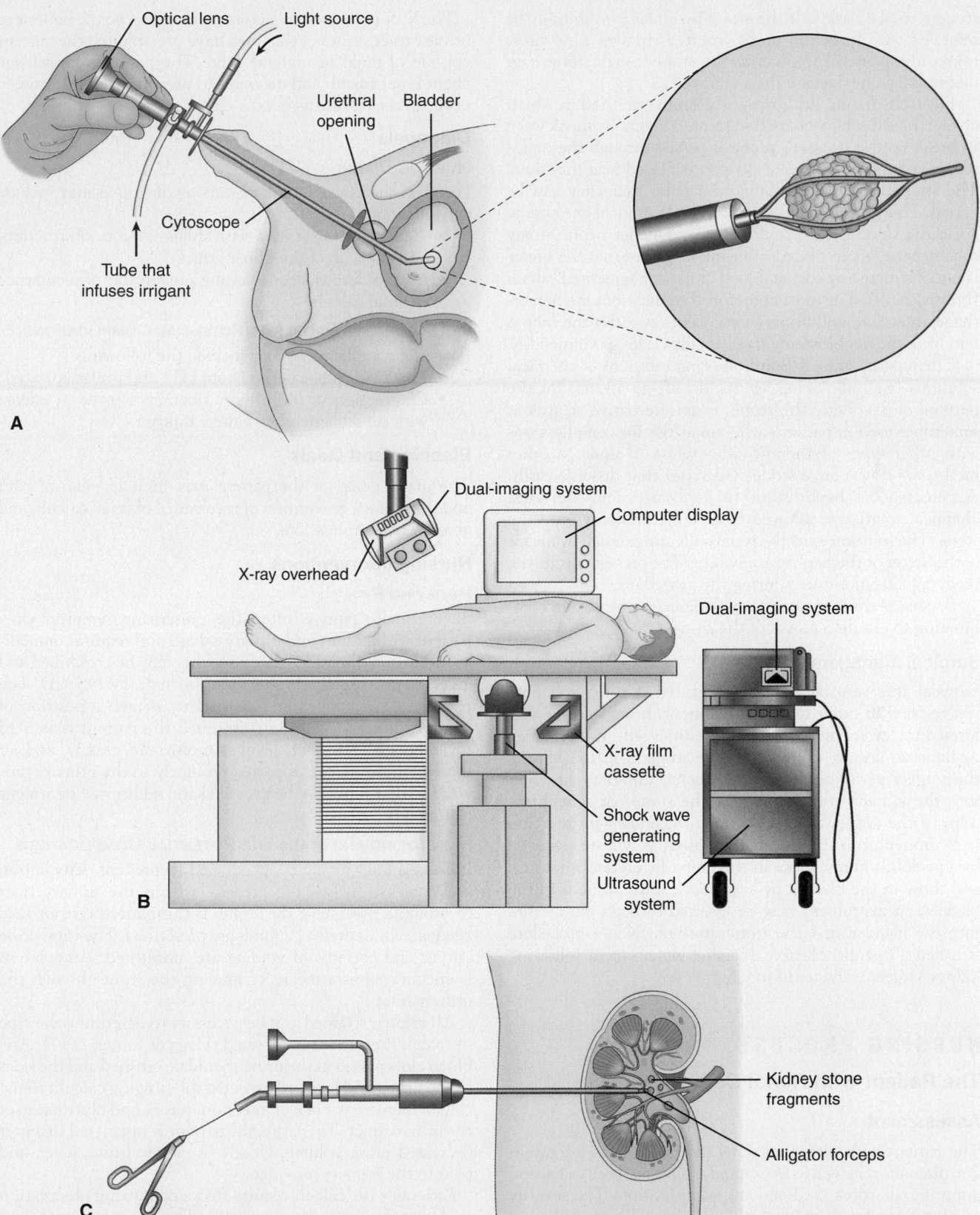

Figure 49-6 • Methods of treating renal calculi. **A.** During ureteroscopy, which is used for removing small stones located in the ureter close to the bladder, a ureteroscope is inserted into the ureter to visualize the stone. The stone is then fragmented or captured and removed. **B.** Extracorporeal shock water lithotripsy is used for most symptomatic, nonpassable upper urinary stones. Electromagnetically generated shock waves are focused over the area of the renal calculus. The high-energy dry shock waves pass through the skin and fragment the stone. **C.** Percutaneous nephrolithotomy is used to treat larger stones. A percutaneous tract is formed, and a nephroscope is inserted through it. Then, the stone is extracted or pulverized.

stone retrieval basket. If the stone is too large to initially be removed, an ultrasound probe inserted through a nephrostomy tube is used to pulverize the stone. Small stone fragments and stone dust are then removed.

Electrohydraulic lithotripsy is a similar method in which an electrical discharge is used to create a hydraulic shock wave to break up the stone. A probe is passed through the cystoscope, and the tip of the lithotripter is placed near the stone. The strength of the discharge and pulse frequency can be varied. This procedure is performed under topical anesthesia. After the stone is extracted, the percutaneous nephrostomy tube may be left in place for a time to ensure that the ureter is not obstructed by edema, blood clots, or fragmented calculi (Norris, 2019). The most common complications are hemorrhage, infection, and urinary extravasation. After the tube is removed, the nephrostomy tract usually closes spontaneously.

Chemolysis, stone dissolution using infusions of chemical solutions (e.g., alkylating agents, acidifying agents) for the purpose of dissolving the stone, is an alternative treatment sometimes used in patients who are at risk for complications with other types of therapy, who refuse to undergo other methods, or who have stones (struvite) that dissolve easily. A percutaneous nephrostomy is performed, and the warm chemical solution is allowed to flow continuously onto the stone. The solution exits the renal collecting system by means of the ureter or the nephrostomy tube. The pressure inside the renal pelvis is monitored during the procedure.

Several of these treatment modalities may be used in combination to ensure removal of the stones.

Surgical Management

Surgical intervention may be indicated if the stone does not respond to other forms of treatment. It may also be performed to correct anatomic abnormalities within the kidney to improve urinary drainage. If the stone is in the kidney, the surgery performed may be a nephrolithotomy (incision into the kidney with removal of the stone) or a nephrectomy, if the kidney is nonfunctional secondary to infection or hydronephrosis. Stones in the kidney pelvis are removed by a pyelolithotomy, those in the ureter by ureterolithotomy, and those in the bladder by cystotomy. If the stone is in the bladder, an instrument may be inserted through the urethra into the bladder, and the stone crushed. Such a procedure is called a cystolitholapaxy. Nursing management following kidney surgery is discussed in Chapter 48.

NURSING PROCESS

The Patient with Renal Calculi

Assessment

The patient with suspected renal calculi is assessed for pain and discomfort as well as associated symptoms, such as nausea, vomiting, diarrhea, and abdominal distention. The severity and location of pain are determined, along with any radiation of the pain. Nursing assessment also includes observing for signs and symptoms of UTI (chills, fever, frequency, and hesitancy) and obstruction (frequent urination of small amounts, oliguria, or anuria). The urine is inspected for blood and is strained for stones or gravel.

The history focuses on factors that predispose the patient to urinary tract stones or that may have precipitated the current episode of renal or ureteral colic. The patient's knowledge about renal calculi and measures to prevent their occurrence or recurrence is also assessed.

Diagnosis

NURSING DIAGNOSES

Based on the assessment data, nursing diagnoses may include the following:

- Acute pain associated with inflammation, obstruction, and abrasion of the urinary tract
- Lack of knowledge regarding prevention of recurrence of renal calculi

COLLABORATIVE PROBLEMS/POTENTIAL COMPLICATIONS

Potential complications may include the following:

- Infection and urosepsis (from UTI and pyelonephritis)
- Obstruction of the urinary tract by a stone or edema with subsequent acute kidney injury

Planning and Goals

The major goals for the patient may include relief of pain and discomfort, prevention of recurrence of renal calculi, and absence of complications.

Nursing Interventions

RELIEVING PAIN

Severe acute pain is often the presenting symptom of a patient with kidney and urinary calculi and requires immediate attention. Opioid analgesic agents may be prescribed and given to provide rapid relief along with an IV NSAID. The patient is encouraged and assisted to assume a position of comfort. If activity brings pain relief, the patient is assisted to ambulate. The pain level is monitored closely, and an increase in severity is reported promptly to the primary provider so that relief can be provided and additional treatment initiated.

MONITORING AND MANAGING POTENTIAL COMPLICATIONS

Increased fluid intake is encouraged to prevent dehydration and increase hydrostatic pressure within the urinary tract to promote passage of the stone. If the patient cannot take adequate fluids orally, IV fluids are prescribed. The total urine output and patterns of voiding are monitored. Ambulation is encouraged as a means of moving the stone through the urinary tract.

All urine is strained as it be necessary to determine the type of calculi the patient has formed (Flagg & Joiner, 2017). Any blood clots passed in the urine should be crushed and the sides of the urinal and bedpan inspected for clinging calculi. Renal calculi increase the risk of infection, sepsis, and obstruction of the urinary tract. Therefore, the patient is instructed to report decreased urine volume, bloody or cloudy urine, fever, and pain to the primary provider.

Patients with calculi require frequent nursing observation to detect the spontaneous passage. The patient is instructed to immediately report any sudden increases in pain intensity because of the possibility of a stone fragment obstructing a ureter. Vital signs, including temperature, are monitored closely to detect early signs of infection. UTIs may be associated with renal calculi due to an obstruction from the stone or from the stone itself. All infections should be treated with the appropriate antibiotic agent before efforts are made to dissolve the stone.

PROMOTING HOME, COMMUNITY-BASED, AND TRANSITIONAL CARE

Educating Patients About Self-Care. Because the risk of recurring renal calculi is high, the nurse provides education about the causes of renal calculi and recommendations to prevent their recurrence (see Chart 49-11).

The patient is encouraged to follow a regimen to avoid further stone formation, including maintaining a high fluid intake because stones form more readily in concentrated urine. A patient who has shown a tendency to form stones should drink enough fluid to excrete greater than 2000 mL (preferably 3000 to 4000 mL) of urine every 24 hours (Flagg & Joiner, 2017).

Urine cultures may be performed every 1 to 2 months in the first year and periodically thereafter. Recurrent UTI is treated promptly. Because prolonged immobilization slows renal drainage and alters calcium metabolism, increased mobility is encouraged whenever possible. In addition, excessive ingestion of vitamins (especially vitamin D) and minerals is discouraged.

If lithotripsy, percutaneous stone removal, ureteroscopy, or other surgical procedures for stone removal have been performed, the nurse educates the patient about the signs and symptoms of complications (e.g., urinary retention, infection) that need to be reported to the primary provider. The importance of follow-up is to assess kidney function and to ensure the eradication or removal of all renal calculi is emphasized to the patient and family.

If ESWL has been performed, the nurse must provide instructions for home care and necessary follow-up. The patient is encouraged to increase fluid intake to assist in the passage of stone fragments, which may occur for 6 weeks to several months after the procedure. The patient and family are educated about signs and symptoms of complications. It is also important to inform the patient to expect hematuria (it is anticipated in all patients), but it should disappear within 4 to 5 days. If the patient has a stent in the ureter, hematuria may be expected until the stent is removed. The patient is instructed to check their temperature daily and notify the primary provider if the temperature is greater than 38°C (about 101°F) or the pain is unrelieved by the prescribed medication. The patient is also informed that a bruise may be observed on the treated side of the back.

Continuing and Transitional Care. Close monitoring of the patient in follow-up care is essential to ensure that treatment has been effective and that no complications develop. The nurse has the opportunity to assess the patient's understanding of ESWL and possible complications. In addition, the nurse has the opportunity to assess the patient's understanding of factors that increase the risk of recurrence of renal calculi and strategies to reduce those risks.

The nurse must assess the patient's ability to monitor urinary pH and interpret the results during follow-up visits. Because of the high risk of recurrence, the patient with renal calculi needs to understand the signs and symptoms of stone formation, obstruction, and infection and the

importance of reporting these signs promptly. If medications are prescribed for the prevention of stone formation, the nurse explains their actions, importance, and side effects to the patient.

Evaluation

Expected patient outcomes may include:
1. Reports relief of pain
2. States increased knowledge of health-seeking behaviors to prevent recurrence
    a. Consumes increased fluid intake (at least eight 8-oz glasses of fluid per day)
    b. Participates in appropriate activity
    c. Consumes diet prescribed to reduce dietary factors predisposing to stone formation
    d. Recognizes symptoms (fever, chills, flank pain, hematuria) to be reported to primary provider
    e. Monitors urinary pH as directed
    f. Takes prescribed medication as directed to reduce stone formation
3. Experiences no complications
    a. Reports no signs or symptoms of infection or urosepsis
    b. Voids 200 to 400 mL per voiding of clear urine without evidence of bleeding
    c. Experiences absence of urgency, frequency, and hesitancy
    d. Maintains normal body temperature

GENITOURINARY TRAUMA

Various types of injuries to the flank, back, or upper abdomen may result in trauma to the ureters, bladder, or urethra. Blunt trauma is responsible for approximately 85% of all genitourinary trauma and another 15% is from penetrating trauma (Blair, 2017). Kidney trauma is discussed in Chapter 48.

Specific Injuries

Ureteral Trauma

The main causes of ureteral trauma are motor vehicle crashes, sports injuries, falls, and assaults. Penetrating trauma, such as gunshot wounds, is the most frequent etiology, accounting for 90% of ureteral injuries (Blair, 2017). Injuries range from contusions to complete transection. Unintentional injury to the ureter may occur during gynecologic or urologic surgery. There are no specific signs or symptoms of ureteral injury; many traumatic injuries are discovered during exploratory surgery. Surgical repair with placement of stents (to divert urine away from an anastomosis) is usually necessary. If the ureteral trauma is not detected and urine leakage continues, fistulas can develop (Norris, 2019).

Bladder Trauma

Injury to the bladder may occur with pelvic fractures, multiple trauma, or from a blow to the lower abdomen when the bladder is full. Blunt trauma may result in contusion evident as an ecchymosis—a large bruise resulting from escape of blood into the tissues and involving a segment of the bladder wall—or in rupture of the bladder extraperitoneally, intraperitoneally, or both. Because of the bladder's protected location within the bony pelvis, bladder trauma is relatively uncommon (Blair, 2017). Complications from these injuries include hemorrhage, shock, sepsis, and extravasation of blood into the tissues, which must be treated promptly.

Urethral Trauma

Urethral injuries usually occur with blunt trauma to the lower abdomen or pelvic region. Many patients with urethral injuries also have associated pelvic fractures. The classic triad of symptoms include blood at the urinary meatus, inability to void, and a distended bladder. Complete rupture is seen more often in children because their urethras are less elastic and tear more easily than the adult urethra. Men have five times the risk of urethral injury than women because of the exposed nature of the male urethra (Blair, 2017).

Medical Management

The goals of management in patients with genitourinary trauma are to control hemorrhage, pain, and infection and to maintain urinary drainage. Genitourinary trauma is frequently associated with kidney trauma (see Chapter 48). Hematocrit and hemoglobin levels are monitored closely; decreasing values can indicate hemorrhage within the genitourinary system. The patient is also monitored for oliguria, signs of hemorrhagic shock, and signs and symptoms of acute peritonitis.

Surgical Management

In urethral trauma, a patient whose condition is unstable and who needs monitoring of urine output may need a suprapubic catheter inserted. The patient is catheterized after urethrography has been performed to minimize the risk of urethral disruption and extensive, long-term complications, such as stricture, incontinence, and impotence. Surgical repair may be performed using either open or laparoscopic approaches (Blair, 2017). After surgery, an indwelling urinary catheter may remain in place for 1 to 2 months to allow the system to heal.

Nursing Management

The patient with genitourinary trauma should be assessed frequently during the first few days after injury to detect flank and abdominal pain, muscle spasm, and swelling over the flank.

During this time, patients are educated about care of the incision and the importance of adequate fluid intake. In addition, instructions about changes that should be reported to the primary provider, such as fever, hematuria, flank pain, or any signs and symptoms of decreasing kidney function, are provided (Blair, 2017). The patient with a ruptured bladder may have gross bleeding for several days after repair. Guidelines for increasing activity gradually, lifting, and driving are also provided.

Follow-up nursing care includes monitoring the blood pressure to detect hypertension and advising the patient to restrict activities for about 1 month after trauma to minimize the incidence of delayed or secondary bleeding.

URINARY TRACT CANCERS

Urinary tract cancers include those of the urinary bladder; kidney and renal pelvis; ureters; and other urinary structures, such as the prostate. Kidney cancer is discussed in Chapter 48, and prostate cancer is discussed in Chapter 53.

Cancer of the Bladder

Twenty-five percent of cancers of the urinary bladder occur in adults older than 65 years (Caruso, Tyler, & Wolkowicz, 2017). It is the sixth most common cancer with a much higher incidence in men than women for reasons that are still not well understood (National Cancer Institute [NCI], 2020). Bladder cancer is a leading cause of death, accounting for more than 15,000 deaths in the United States annually (NCI, 2020). Cancers arising from the prostate, colon, and rectum in males and from the lower gynecologic tract in females may metastasize to the bladder.

Tobacco use, especially cigarettes, continues to be a leading risk factor for all urinary tract cancers (NCI, 2020) (see Chart 49-12).

Clinical Manifestations

Bladder tumors usually arise at the base of the bladder and involve the ureteral orifices and bladder neck. Visible, painless hematuria is the most common symptom of bladder cancer. Infection of the urinary tract is a common complication, producing frequency and urgency. However, any alteration in voiding or change in the urine may indicate cancer of the bladder. Pelvic or back pain may occur with metastasis.

Assessment and Diagnostic Findings

The diagnostic evaluation includes cystography, excretory urography, CT and MRI scans, ultrasonography, and bimanual examination with the patient anesthetized. Noninvasive detection using molecular markers is currently under investigation (Caruso et al., 2017). Biopsies of the tumor and adjacent mucosa are the definitive diagnostic procedures (NCI,

---

Chart 49-12 | ⚠ **SELECT RISK FACTORS**
Bladder Cancer

- Certain genetic mutations including:
  - *HRAS* mutation (Costello syndrome, Facio-cutaneous-skeletal syndrome).
  - *Rb1* mutation.
  - *PTEN/MMAC1* mutation (Cowden syndrome).
  - *NAT2* slow acetylator phenotype.
  - *GSTM1* null phenotype.
- Exposure to arsenic
- Occupational exposure to chemicals in processed paint, dye, metal, and petroleum products
- Positive family history of bladder cancer
- Pelvic radiation therapy or treatment for other cancers
- Tobacco use, cigarette smoking in particular

Adapted from National Cancer Institute (NCI). (2020). Bladder cancer treatment (PDQ®)—Health professional version. Retrieved on 01/11/2020 at: www.cancer.gov/types/bladder/hp/bladder-treatment-pdq#section/all

2020; Norris, 2019). Transitional cell carcinomas and carcinomas in situ shed recognizable cancer cells. Cytologic examination of fresh urine and saline bladder washings provides information about the prognosis and staging, especially for patients at high risk for recurrence of primary bladder tumors. See Chapter 12 for more information on cancer grading and staging.

Medical Management

Treatment of bladder cancer depends on the grade of the tumor (the degree of cellular differentiation) and the stage of tumor growth (the degree of local invasion and the presence or absence of metastasis) (NCI, 2020). The patient's age and physical, mental, and emotional status are considered when determining treatment modalities.

Surgical Management

Transurethral resection or fulguration (cauterization) may be performed for simple papillomas (benign epithelial tumors) (Caruso et al., 2017). These procedures eradicate the tumors through surgical incision or electrical current with the use of instruments inserted through the urethra. After this bladder-sparing surgery, intravesical administration of bacille Calmette–Guérin (BCG) is the treatment of choice. BCG Live is an attenuated live strain of *Mycobacterium bovis*, the causative agent in tuberculosis; treatment is recommended for a minimum of 1 year (NCI, 2020). The exact action of BCG is unknown, but it is thought to produce a local inflammatory and a systemic immunologic response.

Management of superficial bladder cancers presents a challenge because there are usually widespread abnormalities in the bladder mucosa. The entire lining of the urinary tract, or urothelium, is at risk because carcinomatous changes can occur in the mucosa of the bladder, kidney pelvis, ureter, and urethra.

A simple cystectomy or a radical cystectomy is performed for invasive or multifocal bladder cancer. Radical cystectomy in men involves removal of the bladder, prostate, and seminal vesicles and immediate adjacent perivesical tissues. In women, radical cystectomy involves removal of the bladder, lower ureter, uterus, fallopian tubes, ovaries, anterior vagina, and urethra. It may include removal of pelvic lymph nodes. Removal of the bladder requires a urinary diversion procedure, which is described later in this chapter.

Although radical cystectomy remains the standard of care for invasive bladder cancer in the United States, clinical trials continue to explore other options in an effort to spare patients the need for radical cystectomy (NCI, 2020). Other options for managing transitional cell bladder cancer mandate lifelong surveillance with periodic cystoscopy. Although most patients respond completely and their bladders remain free from invasive relapse, one fourth develop a relapse of noninvasive disease. This may be managed with transurethral resection of the bladder tumor and intravesical therapies but carries an additional risk that a late cystectomy may be required.

Pharmacologic Therapy

Chemotherapy with a combination of methotrexate, 5-fluorouracil, vinblastine, doxorubicin, and cisplatin has been effective in producing partial remission of transitional cell carcinoma of the bladder in some patients. IV chemotherapy may be accompanied by radiation therapy (NCI, 2020). Topical chemotherapy (intravesical chemotherapy or instillation of antineoplastic agents into the bladder, resulting in contact of the agent with the bladder wall) is considered when there is a high risk of recurrence, when cancer in situ is present, or when tumor resection has been incomplete. Topical chemotherapy delivers a high concentration of medication (thiotepa, doxorubicin, mitomycin, and BCG Live) to the tumor to promote tumor destruction. Bladder cancer may also be treated by direct infusion of the cytotoxic agent through the bladder's arterial blood supply to achieve a higher concentration of the chemotherapeutic agent with fewer systemic toxic effects (Blair, 2017; NCI, 2020).

BCG Live is now considered the most predominant and conservative intravesical agent for recurrent bladder cancer, especially superficial transitional cell carcinoma, because it is an immunotherapeutic agent that enhances the body's immune response to cancer. BCG Live has a 43% advantage in preventing tumor recurrence, a significantly better rate than the 16% to 21% advantage of intravesical chemotherapy. In addition, BCG Live is particularly effective in the treatment of carcinoma in situ, eradicating it in more than 80% of cases. In contrast to intravesical chemotherapy, BCG Live has also been shown to decrease the risk of tumor progression. Although BCG Live treatment is the current standard of care, this treatment is most effective when some form of maintenance therapy is utilized (Caruso, et al., 2017; NCI, 2020).

The optimal course of BCG Live appears to be a 6-week course of weekly instillations, followed by a 3-week course at 3 months for tumors that do not respond. In high-risk cancers, maintenance BCG Live given in a 3-week course at 6, 12, 18, and 24 months may limit recurrence and prevent progression. However, the adverse effects associated with this prolonged therapy may limit its widespread applicability.

The patient is allowed to eat and drink before the instillation procedure. Once the bladder is full, the patient must retain the intravesical solution for 2 hours before voiding. At the end of the procedure, the patient is encouraged to void and to drink liberal amounts of fluid to flush the medication from the bladder.

Radiation Therapy

Radiation of the tumor may be performed preoperatively to reduce microextension of the neoplasm and viability of tumor cells, thus decreasing the chances that the cancer may recur in the immediate area or spread through the circulatory or lymphatic systems. Radiation therapy is also used in combination with surgery or to control the disease in patients with inoperable tumors.

For more advanced bladder cancer or for patients with intractable hematuria (especially after radiation therapy), a large, water-filled balloon placed in the bladder produces tumor necrosis by reducing the blood supply of the bladder wall (hydrostatic therapy). The instillation of formalin, phenol, or silver nitrate relieves hematuria and strangury (slow and painful discharge of urine) in some patients.

URINARY DIVERSIONS

Urinary diversion procedures are performed to divert urine from the bladder to a new exit site, usually through a surgically created opening (stoma) in the skin. These procedures are primarily performed when a bladder tumor necessitates cystectomy (NCI, 2020) and are most commonly associated with a high-grade or muscle-invasive bladder cancer (Caruso et al., 2017). Urinary diversion has also been used in managing pelvic malignancy, birth defects, strictures, trauma to the ureters and urethra, neurogenic bladder, chronic infection causing severe ureteral and kidney damage, and intractable interstitial cystitis. It may also be used as a last resort in managing incontinence.

Controversy exists about the best method of establishing permanent diversion of the urinary tract. New techniques are frequently introduced in an effort to improve patient outcomes and quality of life (Shi, Yu, Bellmont, et al., 2018). The age of the patient, condition of the bladder, body build, presence of obesity, degree of ureteral dilation, status of kidney function, and the patient's learning ability, and willingness to participate in postoperative care are all taken into consideration when determining the appropriate surgical procedure.

The types of urinary diversions are an ileal conduit, an orthotopic neobladder reconstruction, or various other continent urinary diversions (Chang & Lawrentschuk, 2015; Yang, Bai, Wang, et al., 2019). The choice of a urinary diversion surgical procedure depends on the patient's and surgeon's preferences, the extent of comorbidity, and the quality of life goal in the postoperative period (Chang & Lawrentschuk, 2015). Variations in urinary diversion surgical procedures are devised frequently in an effort to identify and perfect procedures that will improve patient outcomes and reduce the incidence of postoperative problems (Yang et al., 2019).

Ileal Conduit

The **ileal conduit** (ileal loop) is the oldest and most common of the urinary diversion procedures in use because of the low number of complications and the simplicity of the procedure (Chang & Lawrentschuk, 2015; Shi et al., 2018) (Fig 49-7). Additional advantages include that it is well known to health care professionals, there is no need for bladder retraining, and no nocturnal incontinence (Chang & Lawrentschuk, 2015).

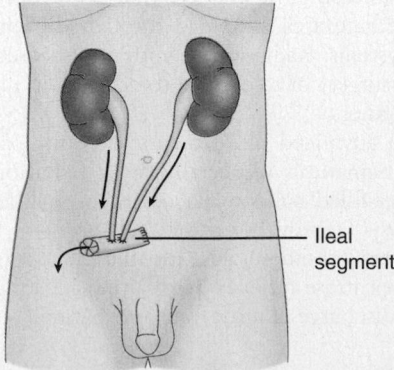

Figure 49-7 • Conventional ileal conduit. The surgeon transplants the ureters to an isolated section of the terminal ileum (ileal conduit), bringing one end to the abdominal wall. The ureter may also be transplanted into the transverse sigmoid colon (colon conduit) or proximal jejunum (jejuna conduit).

When an ileal conduit surgical procedure is performed, the urine is diverted by implanting the ureter into a 12-cm loop of ileum that is led out through the abdominal wall. This loop of ileum is a simple conduit (passageway) for urine from the ureters to the surface. A loop of the sigmoid colon may also be used. An ileostomy bag is used to collect the urine. The resected (cut) ends of the remaining intestine are anastomosed (connected) to provide an intact bowel (Wound Ostomy Continence Nurses [WOCN] Society, 2018).

Stents, usually made of thin, pliable tubing, are placed in the ureters to prevent occlusion secondary to postsurgical edema (Yang et al., 2019). The bilateral ureteral stents allow urine to drain from the kidney to the stoma and provide a method for accurate measurement of urine output. They may be left in place 10 to 21 days postoperatively. Jackson–Pratt drains or other types of drains are inserted to prevent the accumulation of fluid in the space created by removal of the bladder.

The outcome for a patient with an ileal conduit depends to a large degree on the location or position of the stoma, whether the drainage device (bag) establishes a watertight seal to the skin, and the patient's ability to manage the appliance.

After surgery, a skin barrier and a transparent, disposable urinary drainage bag are applied around the conduit and connected to drainage. A custom-cut appliance is used until the edema subsides and the stoma shrinks to normal size. The clear bag allows the stoma to be inspected and the patency of the stent and the urine output to be monitored. The ileal bag drains urine (not feces) continuously. The appliance (bag) usually remains in place as long as it is watertight; it is changed when necessary to prevent leakage of urine.

Complications

Complications that may follow placement of an ileal conduit include wound infection or wound dehiscence, urinary leakage, ureteral obstruction, hyperchloremic acidosis, small bowel obstruction, ileus, and gangrene of the stoma. Delayed complications include ureteral obstruction, contraction or stenosis (narrowing) of the stoma, kidney deterioration due to chronic reflux, peristomal hernia, retraction, pyelonephritis, renal calculi, and cancer recurrence (WOCN Society, 2018).

Nursing Management

During the preoperative period, the nurse helps facilitate the marking of the stoma on the abdominal wall as this is associated with decreased complications postoperatively, fewer problems with the fitting of the appliance, and increased quality of life and independence postoperatively (WOCN Society, 2018). Preoperative education is initiated about basic self-care skills for managing the ileal conduit (WOCN Society, 2018). Because the patient requires specialized care, a consultation is initiated with a WOC nurse.

In the immediate postoperative period, urine volumes are monitored hourly. Throughout the patient's hospitalization, the nurse monitors closely for complications, reports signs and symptoms of them promptly, and intervenes quickly to prevent their progression.

A urine output below 0.5 mL/kg/h may indicate dehydration or an obstruction in the ileal conduit, with possible backflow or leakage from the ureteroileal anastomosis. A catheter may be inserted through the urinary conduit to monitor the patient for possible stasis or residual urine from a constricted stoma. Urine may drain through the bilateral ureteral stents as well as around the stents. If the ureteral stents are not draining, the nurse may be instructed to carefully irrigate with 5 to 10 mL sterile normal saline solution, being careful not to exert tension that could dislodge the stent. Hematuria may be noted in the first 48 hours after surgery but usually resolves spontaneously.

Providing Stoma and Skin Care

The stoma is inspected frequently for color and viability. A healthy stoma is pink or red. A change from this normal color to purple, brown, or black suggests that the vascular supply may be compromised. If cyanosis and a compromised blood supply persist, surgical intervention may be necessary. The stoma is not sensitive to touch, but the skin around the stoma becomes sensitive if urine or the appliance causes irritation. The skin is inspected for signs of irritation and bleeding of the stoma mucosa, encrustation and skin irritation around the stoma (from alkaline urine coming in contact with exposed skin), rashes, redness, pruritus, or other signs of impairment and wound infections (WOCN Society, 2018).

Caring for the Ostomy

Moisture in bed linens or clothing or the odor of urine around the patient should alert the nurse to the possibility of leakage from the appliance, potential infection, or a problem in hygienic management. A properly fitted appliance is essential to prevent exposure of the skin around the stoma to urine (WOCN Society, 2018). If the urine smells foul, the stoma is catheterized, if prescribed, to obtain a urine specimen for culture and sensitivity testing.

Encouraging Fluids and Relieving Anxiety

Because mucous membrane is used in forming the conduit, the patient may excrete a large amount of mucus mixed with urine. This causes anxiety in many patients. To help relieve this anxiety, the nurse reassures the patient that this is a normal occurrence after an ileal conduit procedure. The nurse encourages adequate fluid intake to flush the ileal conduit and decrease the accumulation of mucus.

Selecting the Ostomy Appliance

The nurse is instrumental (often with consultation with a WOC nurse) in selecting an appropriate ostomy appliance. The urinary appliance may consist of one or two pieces and may be disposable (usually used once and discarded) or reusable. The choice of appliance is determined by the location of the stoma and by the patient's normal activity, manual dexterity, visual function, body build, economic resources, and preference.

Promoting Home, Community-Based, and Transitional Care

 Educating Patients About Self-Care

Patient education begins in the hospital but continues in the home setting because patients are usually discharged within days of surgery. The nurse educates the patient how to assess and manage the urinary diversion as well as how to deal with changes in body image. A WOC nurse is invaluable in consulting with the nurse on various aspects of care and patient education (WOCN Society, 2018).

Changing the Appliance

The patient and family are educated about how to apply and change the appliance so that they are comfortable carrying out the procedure and can do so proficiently. Ideally, the appliance system is changed before the system leaks and at a time that is convenient for the patient. Many patients find that early morning is most convenient because the urine output is reduced. A variety of appliances are available (WOCN Society, 2018).

Regardless of the type of appliance used, a skin barrier is essential to protect the skin from irritation and excoriation (WOCN Society, 2018). To maintain skin integrity, a skin barrier or leaking pouch is never patched with tape to prevent accumulation of urine under the skin barrier or faceplate. The patient is instructed to avoid moisturizing soaps and body washes when cleaning the area because they interfere with the adhesion of the pouch. The degree to which the stoma protrudes is not the same in all patients; thus, there are various accessories and custom-made appliances to solve individual problems. Patient guidelines for applying reusable and disposable systems are presented in Chart 49-13.

Controlling Odor

The patient is instructed to avoid foods that give the urine a strong odor (e.g., asparagus, cheese, eggs). Most appliances contain odor barriers, but, if needed, a few drops of liquid deodorizer or diluted white vinegar may be introduced through the drain spout into the bottom of the pouch with a syringe or eyedropper to reduce odors. The patient is reminded that odor will develop if the pouch is worn longer than recommended and not cared for properly (WOCN Society, 2018).

Managing the Ostomy Appliance

The patient is instructed to empty the pouch by means of a drain valve when it is one third full because the weight of more urine will cause the pouch to separate from the skin. Some patients prefer wearing a leg bag attached with an adapter to the drainage apparatus. To promote uninterrupted sleep, a collecting bottle and tubing (one unit) are snapped onto an adapter that connects to the ileal appliance. A small amount of urine is left in the bag when the adapter is attached to prevent the bag from collapsing against itself. The tubing may be threaded down the pajama or pants leg to prevent kinking. The collecting bottle and tubing are rinsed daily with cool water and once a week with a 3:1 solution of water and white vinegar.

Cleaning and Deodorizing the Appliance

Usually, the reusable appliance is rinsed in warm water and soaked in a 3:1 solution of water and white vinegar or a commercial deodorizing solution for 30 minutes. It is rinsed with tepid water and air-dried away from direct sunlight as hot water and exposure to direct sunlight dry the pouch and increase the incidence of cracking. After drying, the appliance

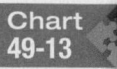

Chart 49-13   **PATIENT EDUCATION**

Using Urinary Diversion Collection Appliances

Applying a Reusable Pouch System

The nurse instructs the patient to:

1. Gather all necessary supplies. Perform hand hygiene.
2. Prepare new appliance according to the manufacturer's directions:
   - Apply double-faced adhesive disc that has been properly sized to fit the reusable pouch faceplate.
   - Remove paper backing and set pouch aside, or apply thin layer of contact cement to one side of the reusable pouch faceplate.
   - Set pouch aside.
3. Remove soiled pouch gently. Lay aside to clean later.
4. Clean peristomal skin (skin around stoma) with small amount of soap and water. Rinse thoroughly and dry. If a film of soap remains on the skin and the site does not dry, the appliance will not adhere adequately.
5. Use a wick (rolled gauze pad or tampon) over the stoma to absorb urine and keep the skin dry throughout the appliance change.
6. Inspect peristomal skin for irritation.
7. Note that a skin protector wipe or barrier ring may be applied before centering the faceplate opening directly over the stoma.
8. Position appliance over stoma, and press gently into place.
9. If desired, use a pouch cover or apply cornstarch under the pouch to prevent perspiration and skin irritation.
10. Clean soiled pouch, and prepare for reuse.

Applying a Disposable Pouch System

The nurse instructs the patient to:

1. Gather all necessary supplies. Perform hand hygiene.
2. Measure stoma, and prepare an opening in the skin barrier about 1/8-inch larger than the stoma and the same shape as the stoma.
3. Remove paper backing from skin barrier, and set aside.
4. Gently remove old appliance, and set aside.
5. Clean peristomal skin with warm water, and dry thoroughly.
6. Inspect peristomal skin (skin around stoma) for irritation.
7. Use a wick (rolled gauze pad or tampon) over the stoma to absorb urine, and keep the skin dry during the appliance change.
8. Center opening of skin barrier over stoma, and apply with firm, gentle pressure to attain a watertight seal.
9. If using a two-piece system, snap pouch onto the flanged wafer that adheres to skin.
10. Close drainage tap or spout at bottom of pouch.
11. Note that a pouch cover can be used or cornstarch applied under pouch to prevent perspiration and skin irritation.
12. Apply hypoallergenic tape around the skin barrier in a picture-frame manner.
13. Dispose of soiled appliance.

Adapted from Wound Ostomy Continence Nurses (WOCN) Society. (2018). WOCN Society Clinical Guideline: Management of the adult patient with a fecal or urinary ostomy—An executive summary. *Journal of Wound Ostomy Continence Nursing, 45*(1), 50–58.

may be powdered with cornstarch and stored. Two appliances are necessary—one to be worn while the other is air-drying.

Continuing and Transitional Care

Follow-up care is essential to determine how the patient has adapted to the altered body image and lifestyle changes.

Referral for home health is indicated to determine how well the patient and family are coping with the urinary drainage diversion. The nurse assesses the patient's physical status and emotional response. In addition, the nurse assesses the ability of the patient and family to manage the urinary diversion and appliance, reinforces previous education, and provides additional information (e.g., community resources, sources of ostomy supplies, insurance coverage for supplies).

As the postoperative edema subsides, the nurse assists in determining the appropriate changes needed in the ostomy appliance. The size of the stoma is measured every 3 to 6 weeks for the first few months postoperatively. The correct appliance size is determined by measuring the widest part of the stoma with a ruler. The permanent appliance should be no more than 1.6 mm (1/8 inch) larger than the diameter of the stoma and the same shape as the stoma to prevent contact of the skin with drainage.

The nurse educates the patient and family about resources (see the Resources section at the end of this chapter). Local chapters of the American Cancer Society (ACS) can provide medical equipment and supplies and other resources for the patient who has undergone ostomy surgery for cancer.

The home health nurse assesses the patient for potential long-term complications such as ureteral obstruction, strictures, hernias, or deterioration of kidney function (Yang et al., 2019). The nurse also reinforces previous education about potential complications and self-care management (WOCN Society, 2018).

Orthotopic Neobladder

An orthotopic neobladder reconstruction is performed in approximately 38% of patients who have undergone cystectomy for invasive bladder cancer (Shi et al., 2018). During this surgery, a new bladder is constructed from segments of the intestine (Chang & Lawrentschuk, 2015) (see Fig. 49-8). There are several advantages of this type of urinary diversion compared to the more common ileal conduit including that the newly reconstructed bladder is attached to the urethra, achieving functional and anatomical restoration (Shi et al., 2018). The new voiding system is similar to the natural preoperative state, and researchers have reported a higher quality of life in patients who undergo this procedure compared to

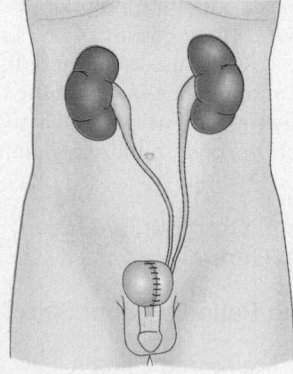

Figure 49-8 • Orthotopic neobladder. The surgeon constructs a new bladder from segments of intestine.

patients with an ileal conduit (Chang & Lawrentschuk, 2015; Shi et al., 2018; Yang et al., 2019).

There are several disadvantages to orthotopic neobladder reconstruction as well. Not all patients are suitable for the surgery (see later discussion). Other disadvantages include the need for bladder retraining and the potential for incontinence postoperatively (Chang & Lawrentschuk, 2015). The intestine used to create the neobladder does not have the stimulation to contract that the natural bladder had, leading to the need for bladder retraining. Even with bladder retraining, only 80% of patients achieve full continence (Shi et al., 2018).

Surgical Management

In the preoperative period, the patient undergoes careful evaluation as not all patients are suitable for this surgery. Major contraindications include renal and liver impairment, intestinal disease, and cancer in specific parts of the bladder (Chang & Lawrentschuk, 2015). See Chart 49-14 for a list of patient characteristics that contraindicate performing an orthotopic neobladder reconstruction. However, this surgery is a viable alternative to an ileal conduit in the patient who is free of these contraindications, does not want a stoma, and is willing to adhere to the neobladder training (Chang & Lawrentschuk, 2015).

When the surgery is performed, the surgeon constructs a sphere-shaped neobladder, also referred to as a pouch, from intestinal segments to replace the bladder that has been removed. The most common intestinal segments used are the ileum, colon, and sigmoid portions of the intestine (Chang & Lawrentschuk, 2015).

Complications

This is a more complex surgery than the creation of an ileal conduit; therefore, there is a higher risk of several complications including fluid and electrolyte imbalances, postoperative ileus, and incontinence. The patient is at risk for metabolic acidosis as the wall of the neobladder is now made of intestinal mucosa that is more permeable to urinary electrolytes compared to the original bladder wall (Chang & Lawrentschuk, 2015). The shift in electrolytes also leads to the urine being more concentrated, which can lead to dehydration (Chang & Lawrentschuk, 2015). Patients are at higher risk of postoperative ileus at the fifth postoperative day and later compared to those undergoing an ileal conduit procedure (Chang & Lawrentschuk, 2015).

Nursing Management

In the preoperative period, the nurse assists in the assessment of the suitability of the patient to undergo an orthotopic neobladder reconstruction. In conjunction with the surgeon the nurse assesses for potential patient contraindications to the surgery (see Chart 49-14). It is important to begin education about what the patient can expect in the postoperative period, especially the time and effort that will be needed for bladder retraining. The patient needs to clearly understand the risk for incontinence both in the short term postoperatively and possibly on a long-term basis.

Postoperative nursing care of the patient with an orthotopic neobladder reconstruction is similar to nursing care of the patient with an ileal conduit. In addition to the usual postoperative care (see Chapter 16), the patient will have an indwelling and subrapubic catheter (Chang & Lawrentschuk, 2015). Procedures may vary between surgical centers that perform this procedure, but commonly an irrigation of 100 mL normal saline every 6 to 8 hours is prescribed to prevent catheter blockage due to an increase in the amount of mucous discharged from the intestine compared to a regular bladder wall (Chang & Lawrentschuk, 2015).

Monitoring Fluid and Electrolytes

Fluid and electrolyte balance is maintained in the immediate postoperative period by closely monitoring the serum electrolyte levels and administering appropriate IV fluids. The patient is monitored for signs and symptoms of metabolic acidosis and dehydration. Electrolyte replacement may be required to return values to within normal limits.

Encouraging Adequate Nutrition

The patient has additional carbohydrate and protein needs in order to heal from the complex surgery (Chang & Lawrentschuk, 2015). Dietary instructions include increasing the fiber content in the diet to decrease the risk of postoperative ileus, particularly on the fifth postoperative day and following discharge. Increased dietary fiber and other measures are needed to prevent constipation as the intestine is now shorter.

Promoting Home, Community-Based, and Transitional Care

Patient education begins in the hospital but continues in the home setting because patients are usually discharged within days of surgery. The neobladder needs 2 to 3 weeks to heal and therefore the patient is discharged home with an indwelling and subrapubic catheter (Chang & Lawrentschuk, 2015). The nurse instructs the patient how to assess and manage the indwelling catheters and irrigate as needed. Once it is determined that the neobladder is watertight, neobladder retraining begins.

> ## Chart 49-14 Contraindications to Orthotopic Neobladder Reconstruction Surgery
>
> - Acute kidney injury with a serum creatinine of >150 umol/L
> - Lack of motivation or intellectual ability to follow a strict postoperative voiding regimen
> - Impaired liver function
> - Inability to accept incontinence postoperatively (mainly nocturnal) in the short term and possibly long term
> - Intestinal disease due to radiation or inflammatory bowel disease
> - Histologically confirmed cancer at the prostatic apex (males) or bladder neck (females)
> - Physical limitations preventing the performance of self-catheterization
> - Presence of metastatic cancer
>
> Adapted from Chang, D. T. S., & Lawrentschuk, N. (2015). Orthotopic neobladder reconstruction. *Urology Annals*, 7(1), 1–7.

PATIENT EDUCATION

Neoblation Training

The nurse instructs the patient to:

- Void in a sitting position using the Valsalva maneuver to empty the neobladder
- Perform all pelvic floor muscle exercises as prescribed, every day.
- Take steps to avoid constipation: Drink adequate fluids, eat a well-balanced diet high in fiber, exercise regularly, and take stool softeners if recommended.
- Void regularly, five to eight times a day (about every 2 to 3 hours):
  - First thing in the morning
  - Before each meal
  - Before retiring to bed
  - Once during the night if necessary

Adapted from Chang, D. T. S., & Lawrentschuk, N. (2015). Orthotopic neobladder reconstruction. *Urology Annals*, 7(1), 1–7.

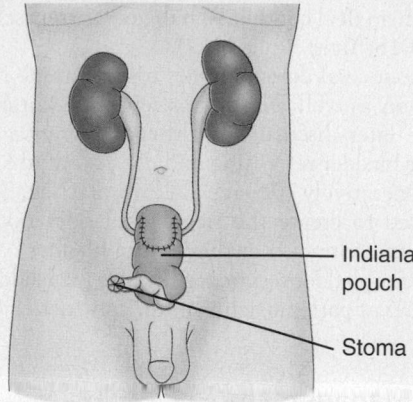

Figure 49-9 • Indiana pouch. The surgeon introduces the ureters into a segment of ileum and cecum. Urine is drained periodically by inserting a catheter into the stoma.

Educating Patients About Self-Care

Patient education is important and should be provided verbally and in writing (see Chart 49-15). The patient should be educated to develop and use a log or diary to record timing of pelvic floor muscle exercises, frequency of voiding and intermittent catheterization, any changes in bowel function, and any episodes of incontinence.

Continuing and Transitional Care

Follow-up care is essential to determine how the patient has adapted to the changes needed to manage the neobladder. Referral for home health is indicated to continue the neobladder training and determine how well the patient and family are coping with the urinary drainage diversion. The nurse assesses the patient's physical status and emotional response. In addition, the nurse assesses the ability of the patient and family to manage the urinary diversion, reinforces previous education, and provides additional information (e.g., community resources, insurance coverage for supplies).

Other Continent Urinary Diversion Procedures

Another type of continent urinary diversion is the Indiana pouch, created for the patient whose bladder is removed (Chang & Lawrentschuk, 2015). The Indiana pouch uses a segment of the ileum and cecum to form the reservoir for urine (see Fig. 49-9). The ureters are tunneled through the muscular bands of the intestinal pouch and anastomosed. The reservoir is made continent by narrowing the efferent portion of the ileum and sewing the terminal ileum to the subcutaneous tissue, forming a continent stoma flush with the skin. The pouch is sewn to the anterior abdominal wall around a cecostomy tube. Urine collects in the pouch until a catheter is inserted and the urine is drained.

The pouch must be drained at regular intervals by a catheter to prevent absorption of metabolic waste products from the urine, reflux of urine to the ureters, and UTI. Postoperative

nursing care of the patient with a continent ileal urinary pouch is similar to nursing care of the patient with an ileal conduit. However, these patients usually have additional drainage tubes (cecostomy catheter from the pouch, stoma catheter exiting from the stoma, ureteral stents, and Penrose drain, as well as a urethral catheter). All drainage tubes must be carefully monitored for patency and amount and type of drainage. In the immediate postoperative period, the cecostomy tube is irrigated two or three times daily to remove mucus and prevent blockage.

Other variations of continent urinary reservoirs are used occasionally (Chang & Lawrentschuk, 2015). With these methods, the pouch must be drained at regular intervals by inserting a catheter.

NURSING PROCESS

The Patient Undergoing Urinary Diversion Surgery

Preoperative Assessment

The following are key preoperative nursing assessment concerns:

- Cardiopulmonary function assessments are performed because patients undergoing cystectomy are often older adults who may be at greater risk for cardiac and respiratory complications.
- A nutritional status assessment is important because of possible poor nutritional intake related to underlying health problems.
- Learning needs are assessed in consultation with a WOC nurse to evaluate the patient's and the family's understanding of the procedure as well as the changes in physical structure and function that result from the surgery. The patient's self-concept and self-esteem are assessed in addition to methods for coping with stress and loss. The patient's mental status, manual dexterity and coordination, vision, and preferred method of learning are noted because they affect postoperative self-care.

Preoperative Diagnosis

NURSING DIAGNOSES

Based on the assessment data, preoperative nursing diagnoses may include the following:

- Anxiety associated with anticipated losses associated with the surgical procedure
- Impaired nutritional intake associated with inadequate nutritional ingestion
- Lack of knowledge about the surgical procedure and postoperative care

Preoperative Planning and Goals

The major goals for the patient may include relief of anxiety; improved preoperative nutritional status; and increased knowledge about the surgical procedure, expected outcomes, and postoperative care.

Preoperative Nursing Interventions

RELIEVING ANXIETY

The threat of cancer and removal of the bladder create anxiety related to changes in body image. Patients may face problems adapting to an external appliance, a stoma, a surgical incision, and altered toileting habits. Men must also adapt to sexual impotency; a penile implant is considered if the patient is a candidate for the procedure. Women also have anxiety related to altered appearance, body image, and self-esteem. A supportive approach, both physical and psychosocial, is needed and includes assessing the patient's self-concept and manner of coping with stress and loss; helping the patient to identify ways to maintain their lifestyle and independence with as few changes as possible; and encouraging the patient to express fears and anxieties about the ramifications of the upcoming surgery. Support services are available through ostomy societies and agencies, and can provide emotional support and make adaptation easier both before and after surgery (see Resources section at the end of this chapter).

ENSURING ADEQUATE NUTRITION

A low-residue diet is prescribed to cleanse the bowel to minimize fecal stasis, decompress the bowel, and minimize postoperative ileus. In addition, antibiotic medications are given to reduce pathogenic flora in the bowel and to reduce the risk of infection. Because the patient undergoing a urinary diversion procedure for cancer may be severely malnourished due to the tumor, previous treatments, and anorexia, enteral or parenteral nutrition may be prescribed to promote healing. Adequate preoperative hydration is imperative to ensure urine flow during surgery and to prevent hypovolemia during the prolonged surgical procedure.

EXPLAINING SURGERY AND ITS EFFECTS

Participation of a WOC nurse in patient education and care is invaluable for informed preoperative education and postoperative planning. Explanations of the surgical procedure, the appearance of the stoma, the rationale for preoperative bowel preparation, the reasons for wearing a collection device, and the anticipated effects of the surgery on sexual functioning are part of patient education. The placement of the stoma site is planned preoperatively with the patient standing, sitting, and lying down to locate the stoma away from bony prominences, skin creases, and folds. The stoma should also be placed away from old scars, the umbilicus, and the belt line.

For ease of self-care, the patient must be able to see and reach the site comfortably. The site is marked with indelible ink so that it can be located easily during surgery. The patient is assessed for allergies or sensitivity to tape or adhesives. Patch testing of certain appliances may be necessary before the ostomy equipment is selected. This is particularly important if the patient is or may be allergic to latex (see Chapter 14, Fig. 14-2).

Preoperative Evaluation

To measure the effectiveness of care, the nurse evaluates the patient's preoperative anxiety level and nutritional status as well as preexisting knowledge and expectations of surgery.

Expected patient outcomes may include:

1. Exhibits reduced anxiety about surgery and expected losses
   a. Verbalizes fears with health care team and family
   b. Expresses positive attitude about outcome of surgery
2. Exhibits adequate nutritional status
   a. Maintains adequate intake before surgery
   b. Maintains body weight
   c. States rationale for enteral or parenteral nutrition if needed
   d. Exhibits normal skin turgor, moist mucous membranes, adequate urine output, and absence of excessive thirst
3. Demonstrates knowledge about the surgical procedure and postoperative course
   a. Identifies limitations expected after surgery
   b. Discusses expected immediate postoperative environment (tubes, equipment, nursing surveillance)
   c. Practices deep-breathing, coughing, and foot exercises

Postoperative Assessment

The role of the nurse in the immediate postoperative period is to prevent complications and to assess the patient carefully for any signs and symptoms of complications. The catheters and any drainage devices are monitored closely. Urine volume, patency of the drainage system, and color of the drainage are assessed. A sudden decrease in urine volume or increase in drainage is reported promptly to the primary provider, because these may indicate obstruction of the urinary tract, inadequate blood volume, or bleeding. In addition, the patient's need for pain control is assessed regularly, as with all postoperative patients.

Postoperative Diagnosis

NURSING DIAGNOSES

Based on the assessment data, major postoperative nursing diagnoses may include the following:

- Risk for impaired skin integrity associated with problems in managing the urine collection appliance
- Acute pain associated with surgical incision
- Disturbed body image associated with urinary diversion
- Impaired sexual functioning associated with structural and physiologic alterations
- Lack of knowledge about management of urinary function

COLLABORATIVE PROBLEMS/POTENTIAL COMPLICATIONS

Potential complications may include the following:

- Peritonitis due to disruption of anastomosis
- Stoma ischemia and necrosis due to compromised blood supply to stoma
- Stoma retraction and separation of mucocutaneous border due to tension or trauma

Postoperative Planning and Goals

The major goals for the patient may include maintaining skin integrity, relieving pain, increasing self-esteem, developing appropriate coping mechanisms to accept and deal with altered urinary function and sexuality, increasing knowledge about management of urinary function, and preventing potential complications.

Postoperative Nursing Interventions

Postoperative management focuses on monitoring urinary function, preventing postoperative complications (infection and sepsis, respiratory complications, fluid and electrolyte imbalances, fistula formation, and urine leakage), and promoting patient comfort. Catheters or drainage systems are monitored, and urine output is monitored carefully. A nasogastric tube is inserted during surgery to decompress the GI tract and to relieve pressure on the intestinal anastomosis. It is usually kept in place for several days after surgery. As soon as bowel function resumes—as indicated by bowel sounds, the passage of flatus, and a soft abdomen—oral fluids are permitted. Until that time, IV fluids and electrolytes are given. The patient is assisted to ambulate as soon as possible to prevent complications of immobility.

MAINTAINING SKIN INTEGRITY

Strategies to promote skin integrity begin with reducing and controlling those factors that increase the patient's risk of poor nutrition and poor healing. Meticulous skin care and management of the drainage system are provided by the nurse until the patient can manage them and is comfortable doing so. Care is taken to keep the system intact to protect the skin from exposure to drainage. Supplies must be readily available to manage the drainage in the immediate postoperative period. Consistency in implementing the skin care program throughout the postoperative period results in maintenance of skin integrity and patient comfort. In addition, maintenance of skin integrity around the stoma enables the patient and family to adjust more easily to the alterations in urinary function and helps them learn skin care techniques.

RELIEVING PAIN

Analgesic medications are administered liberally postoperatively to relieve pain and promote comfort, thereby allowing the patient to turn, cough, and perform deep-breathing exercises. Patient-controlled analgesia and regular administration of analgesic agents around the clock are two options that may be used to ensure adequate pain relief. A pain intensity scale is used to evaluate the adequacy of the medication and the approach to pain management. See Chapter 9 for further discussion of pain management.

IMPROVING BODY IMAGE

The patient's ability to cope with the changes associated with the surgery depends to some degree on their body image and self-esteem before the surgery and the support and reaction of others. Allowing the patient to express concerns and anxious feelings can help, especially in adjusting to the changes in toileting habits. The nurse can also help improve the patient's self-concept by educating about skills needed to be independent in managing the urinary drainage devices. Education about ostomy care is conducted in a private setting to encourage the patient to ask questions without fear of embarrassment. Explaining why the nurse must wear gloves when performing ostomy care can prevent the patient from misinterpreting the use of gloves as a sign of aversion to the stoma.

EXPLORING SEXUALITY ISSUES

Patients who experience altered sexual function as a result of the surgical procedure may mourn this loss. Encouraging the patient and partner to share their feelings about this loss with each other and acknowledging the importance of sexual function and expression may encourage the patient and partner to seek sexual counseling and to explore alternative ways of expressing sexuality. Using the support and expertise from another patient with an ostomy who is functioning fully in society and family life may also assist the patient and family in recognizing that full recovery is possible.

MONITORING AND MANAGING POTENTIAL COMPLICATIONS

Complications are not unusual because of the complexity of the surgery, the underlying reason (cancer, trauma) for the urinary diversion procedure, and the patient's frequently less-than-optimal nutritional status. Complications may include respiratory disorders (e.g., atelectasis, pneumonia), fluid and electrolyte imbalances, breakdown of any anastomosis, sepsis, fistula formation, fecal or urine leakage, and skin irritation. If these occur, the patient will remain hospitalized for an extended length of time and will probably require parenteral nutrition, GI decompression by means of nasogastric suction, and further surgery. The goals of management are to establish drainage, provide adequate nutrition for healing to occur, and prevent sepsis.

Peritonitis. Peritonitis can occur postoperatively if urine leaks at the anastomosis. Signs and symptoms include abdominal pain and distention, muscle rigidity with guarding, nausea and vomiting, paralytic ileus (absence of bowel sounds), fever, and leukocytosis.

Urine output must be monitored closely, because a sudden decrease in output with a corresponding increase in drainage from the incision or drains may indicate urine leakage. In addition, the urine drainage device is observed for leakage. The pouch is changed if a leak is observed. Small leaks in the anastomosis may seal themselves, but surgery may be needed for larger leaks.

Vital signs (blood pressure, pulse and respiratory rates, temperature) are monitored. Changes in vital signs, as well as increasing pain, nausea and vomiting, and abdominal distention, are reported and may indicate peritonitis.

Stoma Ischemia and Necrosis. The stoma is monitored because ischemia and necrosis of the stoma can result from tension on the mesentery blood vessels, twisting of the bowel segment (conduit) during surgery, or arterial insufficiency. The new stoma must be inspected at least every 4 hours to assess the adequacy of its blood supply. The stoma should be red or pink. If the blood supply to the stoma is compromised, the color changes to purple, brown, or black. These changes are reported immediately. The surgeon or WOC nurse may insert a small, lubricated tube into the stoma and shine a flashlight into the lumen of the tube to assess for superficial ischemia or necrosis. A necrotic stoma requires surgical intervention. If the ischemia is superficial, the dusky stoma is observed and may slough its outer layer in several days.

Stoma Retraction and Separation. Stoma retraction and separation of the mucocutaneous border can occur as a result of trauma or tension on the internal bowel segment used for creation of the stoma. In addition, mucocutaneous separation can occur if the stoma does not heal as a result of accumulation of urine on the stoma and mucocutaneous border. Using a collection drainage pouch with an antireflux valve is helpful because the valve prevents urine from pooling on the stoma and mucocutaneous border. Meticulous skin care to keep the area around the stoma clean and dry promotes healing. If a separation of the mucocutaneous border occurs, surgery is not usually needed. The separated area is protected by applying karaya powder, stoma adhesive paste, and a properly fitted skin barrier and pouch. By protecting the separation, healing is promoted. If the stoma retracts into the peritoneum, surgical intervention is mandatory.

If surgery is needed to manage these complications, the nurse provides explanations to the patient and family. The need for additional surgery is usually perceived as a setback by the patient and family. Emotional support of the patient and family is provided along with physical preparation of the patient for surgery.

PROMOTING HOME, COMMUNITY-BASED, AND TRANSITIONAL CARE

Educating Patients About Self-Care. A major postoperative objective is to assist the patient to achieve the highest level of independence and self-care possible. The nurse and WOC nurse work closely with the patient and family to educate and assist them in all phases of managing the ostomy. Adequate supplies and complete instruction are necessary to enable the patient and a family member to develop competence and confidence in their skills. Written and verbal instructions are provided, and the patient is encouraged to contact the nurse or primary provider with follow-up questions. Follow-up telephone calls from the nurse to the patient and family after discharge may provide added support and provide another opportunity to answer their questions. Follow-up visits and reinforcement of correct skin care and appliance management techniques also promote skin integrity. Specific techniques for managing the appliance are described in Chart 49-13.

The patient is encouraged to participate in decisions regarding the type of collecting appliance and the time of day to change the appliance. The patient is assisted and encouraged to look at and touch the stoma early to overcome any fears. The patient and family need to know the characteristics of a normal stoma:

- Pink or red and moist, like the inside of the mouth
- Insensitive to pain because it has no nerve endings
- Vascular, which means it may bleed when cleaned

In addition, if a segment of the GI tract was used to create the urinary diversion, mucus may be visible in the urine. By learning what is normal, the patient and family become familiar with what signs and symptoms they should report and what problems they can handle themselves.

Information provided to the patient and the extent of involvement in self-care are determined by the patient's physical recovery and ability to accept and acquire the knowledge and skill needed for independence. Verbal and written instructions are provided, and the patient is given the opportunity to practice and demonstrate the knowledge and skills needed to manage urinary drainage.

Continuing and Transitional Care. Follow-up care is essential to determine how the patient has adapted to the changes in body image and lifestyle adjustments. Visits from a nurse are important to assess the patient's adaptation to the home setting and management of the ostomy. Education and reinforcement may assist the patient and family to cope with altered urinary function. It is important to assess for long-term complications that may occur, such as pouch leakage or rupture, stone formation, stenosis of the stoma, deterioration in kidney function, or incontinence.

Long-term monitoring for anemia is performed to identify vitamin B_{12} deficiency, which may occur when a significant portion of the terminal ileum is removed. This may take several years to develop and can be treated with vitamin B_{12} injections. The patient and family are informed about the United Ostomy Associations of America (UOAA) and any local ostomy support groups to provide ongoing support, assistance, and education (see Resources section at the end of this chapter).

Postoperative Evaluation

Expected patient outcomes may include:
1. Maintains skin integrity
   a. Maintains intact skin and demonstrates skill in managing drainage system and appliance
   b. States actions to take if skin excoriation occurs
2. Reports relief of pain
3. Exhibits improved body image as evidenced by the following:
   a. Voices acceptance of urinary diversion, stoma, and appliance
   b. Demonstrates increasingly independent self-care, including hygiene and grooming
   c. States acceptance of support and assistance from family members, health care providers, and another patient with an ostomy
4. Copes with sexuality issues
   a. Verbalizes concern about possible alterations in sexuality and sexual function
   b. Reports discussion of sexual concerns with partner and appropriate counselor
5. Demonstrates knowledge needed for self-care
   a. Performs self-care and proficient management of urinary diversion and appliance
   b. Asks questions relevant to self-management and prevention of complications
   c. Identifies signs and symptoms needing care from primary provider, nurse, or other health care providers

6. Absence of complications as evidenced by the following:
   a. Reports absence of pain or tenderness in abdomen
   b. Has temperature within normal range
   c. Reports no urine leakage from incision or drains
   d. Has urine output within desired volume limits
   e. Maintains stoma that is red or pink, moist, and appropriate in size without edema
   f. Has intact and healed border of the stoma

CRITICAL THINKING EXERCISES

1 **ipc** You are caring for a 53-year-old woman in the outpatient clinic where you work; she is newly diagnosed with urinary incontinence. What type of referrals might be appropriate for this patient? What members of the interprofessional health care team do you anticipate as being integral to the care of this patient?

2 **ebp** You notice an increase in the number of CAUTIs among patients on the medical-surgical unit where you work. What are the evidence-based management techniques used in CAUTI prevention? Identify the criteria used to evaluate the strength of the evidence for these practices. How will you individualize these techniques for your unit?

3 **pq** A 65-year-old man is admitted to the medical-surgical nursing unit where you work with bladder cancer. He is scheduled for a radical cystectomy with an orthotopic neobladder reconstruction. Identify the priorities, approach, and techniques you would use to provide care for this patient in the preoperative phase of care. How will your priorities, approach, and techniques differ in the postoperative phase of care?

REFERENCES

*Asterisk indicates nursing research.

Books

Alley, M. (2017). Congenital anomalies and malformations of the lower urinary tract. In D. K. Newman, J. F. Wyman, & V. W. Welch (Eds.). *Core curriculum for urologic nursing.* Pitman, NJ: Society of Urologic Nurses and Associates.

Blair, M. (2017). Genitourinary trauma. In D. K. Newman, J. F. Wyman, & V. W. Welch (Eds.). *Core curriculum for urologic nursing.* Pitman, NJ: Society of Urologic Nurses and Associates.

Cahill, M., & Haras, M. (2017). Disorders of calcium and phosphorus metabolism. In S. Bodin (Ed.). *Contemporary nephrology nursing.* Pitman, NJ: American Nephrology Nurses Association.

Caruso, A. M., Tyler, A., & Wolkowicz, S. B. (2017). Bladder cancer. In D. K. Newman, J. F. Wyman, & V. W. Welch (Eds.). *Core curriculum for urologic nursing.* Pitman, NJ: Society of Urologic Nurses and Associates.

Comerford, K. C., & Durkin, M. A. (2020). *Nursing 2020 drug handbook* (40th ed.). Philadelphia, PA: Wolters Kluwer.

Eliopoulos, C. (2018). *Gerontological nursing* (9th ed.). Philadelphia, PA: Wolters Kluwer.

Fischbach, F. T., & Fischbach, M. A. (2018). *A manual of laboratory and diagnostic tests* (10th ed.). Philadelphia, PA: Wolters Kluwer.

Flagg, L., & Joiner, C. J. (2017). Urinary stone disease. In D. K. Newman, J. F. Wyman, & V. W. Welch (Eds.). *Core curriculum for urologic nursing.* Pitman, NJ: Society of Urologic Nurses and Associates.

Freeman, J., Martin, K., & Uithoven, R. (2017). Urinary tract infections. In D. K. Newman, J. F. Wyman, & V. W. Welch (Eds.). *Core curriculum for urologic nursing.* Pitman, NJ: Society of Urologic Nurses and Associates.

Hickey, J. V., & Strayer, A. L. (2020). *The clinical practice of neurological and neurosurgical nursing* (8th ed.). Philadelphia, PA: Wolters Kluwer.

King, S. J. (2017). Reconstructive surgery for incontinence. In D. K. Newman, J. F. Wyman, & V. W. Welch (Eds.). *Core curriculum for urologic nursing.* Pitman, NJ: Society of Urologic Nurses and Associates.

Miller, C. A. (2019). *Nursing for wellness in older adults* (8th ed.). Philadelphia, PA: Wolters Kluwer.

Newman, D. K. (2017). Catheters, devices, products, and catheter-associated urinary tract infections. In D. K. Newman, J. F. Wyman, & V. W. Welch (Eds.). *Core curriculum for urologic nursing.* Pitman, NJ: Society of Urologic Nurses and Associates.

Norris, T. L. (2019). *Porth's pathophysiology: Concepts of altered health state* (10th ed.). Philadelphia, PA: Wolters Kluwer.

Weber, J., & Kelley, J. (2018). *Health assessment in nursing* (6th ed.). Philadelphia, PA: Wolters Kluwer.

Wooldridge, L. S. (2017). Urinary incontinence. In D. K. Newman, J. F. Wyman, & V. W. Welch (Eds.). *Core curriculum for urologic nursing.* Pitman, NJ: Society of Urologic Nurses and Associates.

Journals and Electronic Documents

American Urological Association (AUA). (2019a). Diagnosis and treatment of non-neurogenic overactive bladder in adults: An AUA/SUFU Guideline (2019). Retrieved on 5/13/2020 at: www.auanet.org/guidelines

American Urological Association (AUA). (2019b). Recurrent uncomplicated urinary tract infections in women: AUA/CUA/SUFU Guideline (2019). Retrieved on 5/13/2020 at: www.auanet.org/Guidelines

Chang, D. T. S., & Lawrentschuk, N. (2015). Orthotopic neobladder reconstruction. *Urology Annals, 7*(1), 1–7.

Francis, K. (2019). Damage control: Differentiating incontinence-associated dermatitis from pressure injury. *Nursing 2019 Critical Care, 14*(6), 28–35.

Gould, C. V., Umscheid, C. A., Agarwal, R. K., et al. (2019). Guideline for prevention of catheter-associated urinary tract infections 2009. Retrieved on 5/13/2020 at: www.cdc.gov/infectioncontrol/guidelines/cauti/

Martin, C. D., Wingo, N., & Holland, A. C. (2019). Evaluating suppressive therapies to prevent recurrent urinary tract infections: A literature review. *Women's Healthcare, 7*(1), 28–32, 43.

McCoy, C., Paredes, M., Allen, S., et al. (2017). Catheter-associated urinary tract infections. *Clinical Journal of Oncology Nursing, 21*(4), 460–465.

McDonald, C., Winge, K., & Burn, D. J. (2017). Lower urinary tract symptoms in Parkinson's disease: Prevalence, etiology, and management. *Parkinsonism and Related Disorders, 35,* 8–16.

National Cancer Institute (NCI). (2020). Bladder cancer treatment (PDQ®)—Health professional version. Retrieved on 01/11/2020 at: www.cancer.gov/types/bladder/hp/bladder-treatment-pdq#section/all

Oh-oka, H. (2017). Clinical efficacy of 1-year intensive systematic dietary manipulation as complementary and alternative medicine therapies on female patients with interstitial cystitis/bladder pain syndrome. *Urology, 106,* 50–54.

*Qiang, L., Xian, L. W., Bin, P. Y., et al. (2020). Investigating ICU nurses' understanding of incontinence-associated dermatitis: An analysis of influencing factors. *World Council of Enterostomal Therapists Journal, 40*(1), 32–38.

Shi, H., Yu, H., Bellmont, J., et al. (2018). Comparison of health-related quality of life (HRQoL) between ileal conduit diversion and orthotopic neobladder based on validated questionnaires: A systematic review and meta-analysis. *Quality Of Life Research, 27*(11), 2759–2775.

Tambunan, M. P., & Rahardjo, H. E. (2019). Cranberries for women with recurrent urinary tract infection: A meta-analysis. *Medical Journal of Indonesia, 28,* 268–275.

*Taylor, J. (2018). Reducing the incidence of inappropriate indwelling catheterisation. *Journal of Community Nursing, 32*(3), 50–56.

Wound Ostomy Continence Nurses (WOCN) Society. (2018). WOCN Society Clinical Guideline: Management of the adult patient with a fecal or urinary ostomy—An executive summary. *Journal of Wound Ostomy Continence Nursing, 45*(1), 50–58.

*Wu, M., Grealish, L., Moyle, W., et al. (2020). The effectiveness of nurse-led interventions for preventing urinary tract infections in older adults in residential age care facilities: A systematic review. *Journal of Clinical Nursing, 29*(9-10), 1432–1444.

Yang, Y., Bai, Y., Wang, X., et al. (2019). Internal double-J stent was associated with a lower incidence of ureteroileal anastomosis stricture than external ureteral catheter for patient undergoing radical cystectomy and orthotopic neobladder: A systematic review and meta-analysis. *International Journal of Surgery, 72*(2019), 80–84.

Resources

American Urological Association, www.auanet.org

National Association for Continence (NAFC), www.nafc.org

National Institute of Diabetes and Digestive and Kidney Diseases (NIDDK), National Institutes of Health, www.niddk.nih.gov

National Kidney and Urologic Diseases Information Clearinghouse (NKUDIC), kidney.niddk.nih.gov/

National Kidney Foundation, www.kidney.org

United Ostomy Associations of America, www.ostomy.org

Wound Ostomy and Continence Nurses Society, www.wocn.org

Reproductive Function

IMPLEMENTING ALTERNATIVE, COMPLEMENTARY, AND SPIRITUAL PRACTICES

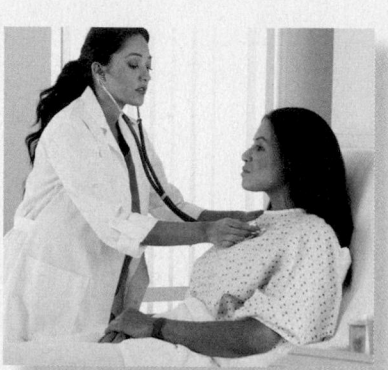

You work on an oncology unit and are caring for a 37-year-old woman from Brazil who reported a growing lump on her right breast after it became painful to touch. She is positive for metastatic breast cancer and is admitted for bilateral mastectomy. She is married with two children, ages 6 and 10. The oncologist, radiologist, surgical oncologist, and oncology nurse meet with her to discuss the plan of care. She will need radiation and chemotherapy following the mastectomy. The patient states that she wants "everything done," including the use of alternative and complementary therapies her family is sending from her home country. She also states that maintaining her spiritual practices is imperative as part of her healing process. The team discusses how to implement these requests into the plan of care.

QSEN Competency Focus: Patient-Centered Care

The complexities inherent in today's health care system challenge nurses to demonstrate integration of specific interdisciplinary core competencies. These competencies are aimed at ensuring the delivery of safe, quality patient care (Institute of Medicine, 2003). The Quality and Safety Education for Nurses project (Cronenwett, Sherwood, Barnsteiner, et al., 2007; QSEN, 2020) provides a framework for the knowledge, skills, and attitudes (KSAs) required for nurses to demonstrate competency in these key areas, which include *patient-centered care*, *interdisciplinary teamwork and collaboration*, *evidence-based practice*, *quality improvement*, *safety*, and *informatics*.

Patient-Centered Care Definition: Recognize the patient or designee as the source of control and full partner in providing compassionate and coordinated care based on respect for patient's preferences, values, and needs.

SELECT PRE-LICENSURE KSAs	APPLICATION AND REFLECTION
Knowledge	
Integrate understanding of multiple dimensions of patient-centered care: • patient/family/community preferences, values • coordination and integration of care • information, communication, and education • physical comfort and emotional support • involvement of family and friends • transition and continuity Describe how diverse cultural, ethnic and social backgrounds function as sources of patient, family, and community values	Describe how you can integrate the patient's preferences and values into her treatment regimen for metastatic breast cancer. How does the involvement of the patient's family impact the plan of care? What are the cultural implications for a patient from Brazil in terms of traditional medicine, spirituality, and care?
Skills	
Elicit patient values, preferences and expressed needs as part of clinical interview, implementation of care plan and evaluation of care	Identify the skills needed by members of the health care team to incorporate patient-centered care and consideration for this patient. How can you be more culturally aware and sensitive to the patient's requests for alternative and complementary therapy?
Attitudes	
Respect and encourage individual expression of patient values, preferences, and expressed needs	Reflect on your attitudes toward use of alternative and complementary therapy by patients who have cancer. Do you feel that these alternative treatment methods are beneficial or harmful? How might your attitude encourage or discourage trust between you and your patients who are managing a serious disease process?

Cronenwett, L., Sherwood, G., Barnsteiner, J., et al. (2007). Quality and safety education for nurses. *Nursing Outlook*, *55*(3), 122–131; Institute of Medicine. (2003). *Health professions education: A bridge to quality*. Washington, DC: National Academies Press; QSEN Institute. (2020). *QSEN Competencies: Definitions and pre-licensure KSAs; Patient centered care*. Retrieved on 8/15/2020 at: qsen.org/competencies/pre-licensure-ksas/#patient-centered_care

50 Assessment and Management of Patients with Female Physiologic Processes

GLOSSARY

adnexa: the fallopian tubes and ovaries
amenorrhea: absence of menstrual flow
cervix: bottom (inferior) part of the uterus that is located in the vagina
corpus luteum: site within a follicle that changes after ovulation
cystocele: a bulge caused by the bladder protruding into the vagina
dysmenorrhea: painful menstruation
dyspareunia: difficult or painful penile-vaginal intercourse
endometrial ablation: procedure performed through a hysteroscope in which the lining of the uterus is burned away or ablated to treat abnormal uterine bleeding
endometrium: mucous membrane lining of the uterus
estrogens: several hormones produced in the ovaries that develop and maintain the female reproductive system
follicle-stimulating hormone (FSH): hormone released by the pituitary gland to stimulate estrogen production and ovulation
fornix: upper part of the vagina
fundus: the rounded upper portion of the uterus
graafian follicle: cystic structure that develops on the ovary as ovulation begins
hymen: tissue that covers the vaginal opening partially or completely before vaginal penetration
hysteroscopy: an endoscopic procedure performed using a long telescope like instrument inserted through the cervix to diagnose uterine problems

introitus: perineal opening to the vagina
luteal phase: stage in the menstrual cycle in which the endometrium becomes thicker and more vascular
luteinizing hormone (LH): hormone released by the pituitary gland that stimulates progesterone production
menarche: beginning of menstrual function
menopause: permanent cessation of menstruation resulting from the loss of ovarian follicular activity
menstruation: sloughing and discharge of the lining of the uterus if conception does not take place
ovaries: almond-shaped reproductive organs that produce eggs at ovulation and play a major role in hormone production
ovulation: discharge of a mature ovum from the ovary
perimenopause: the period around menopause
progesterone: hormone produced by the corpus luteum that prepares the uterus for receiving the fertilized ovum
proliferative phase: stage in the menstrual cycle before ovulation when the endometrium increases
rectocele: bulging of the rectum into the vagina
secretory phase: stage of the menstrual cycle in which the endometrium becomes thickened, becomes more vascular, and ovulation occurs
uterine prolapse: the cervix and uterus descend into the lower vagina

Nurses who work with women need an understanding of the physical, developmental, psychological, and sociocultural influences on women's health, as well as health practices. It is necessary to consider how medications and diseases specifically affect women. In addition, women's sexuality is complex and often affected by many factors, and related issues need careful evaluation and treatment.

CHALLENGES IN WOMEN'S HEALTH

Women face unique challenges in their roles, lifestyles, and family patterns. Furthermore, they encounter increasing environmental hazards and stress, prompting greater attention to health and health-promoting practices. As a result, many women are taking a greater interest in and responsibility for their own health and health care. Nurses encounter women with health care needs in all settings and they need a solid understanding of the unique issues related to women's health to provide optimal care. The Affordable Care Act (ACA) had made major changes to the health insurance market, and millions of women have gained coverage since its implementation (Kaiser Family Foundation, 2018).

The ACA expands coverage to the uninsured through a combination of Medicaid expansions, private insurance reforms, and tax credits (Kaiser Family Foundation, 2018). The affordability of health coverage and care is a problem that affects both sexes; however, women consistently are more likely than men to report cost-related barriers to care (Lee, Monuteaux, & Galbraith, 2019). Among the 97.4 million American women ages 19 to 64, most had some form of insurance coverage in 2017. However, gaps in private sector and publicly funded programs still leave almost one in ten women uninsured. Women with low incomes, women of color, and those who are immigrants are still at greater risk of being uninsured. Single mothers are much more likely to be uninsured (13%) than women in two-parent households (10%) (Kaiser Family Foundation, 2018).

The ACA set new standards for the scope of benefits offered in private plans. In addition to the broad categories of essential health benefits (EHBs) offered by the state-based marketplace plans, the law also requires that new private plans cover preventive services without copayments or other cost sharing. This includes Pap tests, mammograms, bone density tests, as well as the human papilloma virus (HPV) vaccine. New plans are required to cover additional preventive services for women, including prescribed contraceptives, breast-feeding supplies, and resources such as breast pumps, screening for intimate partner violence, well woman visits, and several counseling and screening services (Kaiser Family Foundation, 2018; Lee et al., 2019).

ASSESSMENT OF THE FEMALE REPRODUCTIVE SYSTEM

Anatomic and Physiologic Overview

The female reproductive system is complex because it involves many external and internal structures that are under hormonal control.

Anatomy of the Female Reproductive System

The female reproductive system consists of external and internal pelvic structures. Other anatomic structures that affect the female reproductive system include the hypothalamus and pituitary gland of the endocrine system. The female breast is covered in Chapter 52.

External Genitalia

The female external genitalia are composed of a variety of tissue types starting with the mons pubis, which is a thick pad of adipose tissue that covers the symphysis pubis and cushions it during penile-vaginal intercourse (see Fig. 50-1). Moving downward are two thick folds of connective tissue covered with pubic hair known as the labia majora, which extend from the mons pubis to the perineum. The labia majora cover the oval-shaped area known as the vestibule, where the labia minora originate. The labia minora are two narrow folds of hairless skin, beginning at the clitoris and extending to the fourchette. This area is highly vascular and rich in nerve supply and glands that lubricate the vulva, the collective name for the external genitalia. The labia minora join at the top to form the prepuce, a hoodlike structure that partially covers the clitoris. The clitoris, an erectile organ located beneath the pubic arch, consists of a shaft and glans. It secretes smegma, a pheromone (olfactory erotic stimulant), and is sensitive to touch and temperature. Below the clitoris is the urinary meatus, the external opening of the female urethra that has a slit appearance. Below the meatus is the **introitus** (vaginal opening). On each side of the introitus are Bartholin glands, which secrete mucus through tiny ducts that lie within the labia minora and are external to the **hymen** (membrane that encircles the introitus). The vestibule is bounded by the clitoris, fourchette, and labia minora and contains the urethral meatus. Skene glands, located within the urethral meatus, produce mucus for lubrication (Ball, Dains, Flynn, et al., 2019). The Bartholin glands on either side of the entrance to the vagina also produce mucus for lubrication (Ball et al., 2019).

The hymen opening varies widely among women, and the size of the opening is an unreliable indicator of sexual experience (Ball et al., 2019). The fourchette is located in the midline below the vaginal opening where the labia majora and

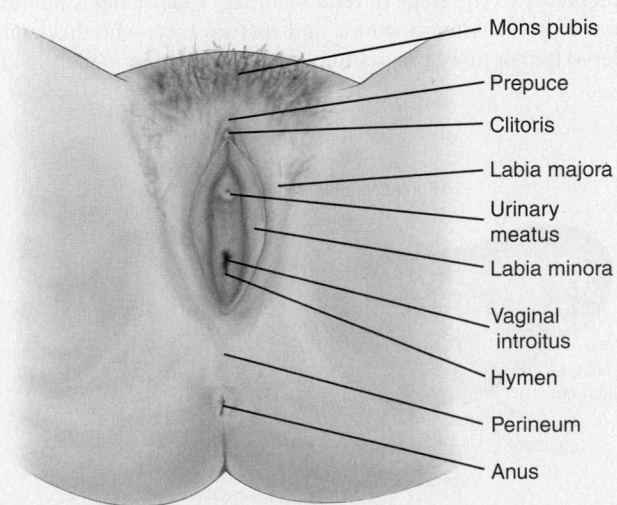

Figure 50-1 • External female genitalia.

- Mons pubis
- Prepuce
- Clitoris
- Labia majora
- Urinary meatus
- Labia minora
- Vaginal introitus
- Hymen
- Perineum
- Anus

labia minora merge. The perineum is the area between the vagina and the rectum or anus; it is a skin-covered muscular tissue (Ball et al., 2019).

A number of muscles support the external genitalia. Support for the pelvic organs is from the deep muscle layer known as the levator ani. This muscle, which forms most of the pelvic diaphragm, is composed of the iliococcygeus, pubococcygeus, and the puborectalis muscles. It supports the organs of reproduction and provides elasticity of the pelvic floor. When viewed from above, it looks like joined cupped hands. Its main function is to provide support to the organs of the pelvis when increased pressure from coughing and sneezing occurs. When this muscle group is contracted, the pelvic floor is lifted upward, supporting continence (Eickmeyer, 2017). Muscles that contribute to the strength of the pelvic floor may be damaged during childbirth (Eickmeyer, 2017). The bulbocavernosus, ischiocavernosus, and transverse perineal muscles encircle and support the vagina and urethra as well as the anal sphincter.

Internal Reproductive Structures

The internal structures consist of the vagina, uterus, ovaries, and fallopian or uterine tubes (see Fig. 50-2).

Vagina

The vagina, a tubular-shaped canal lined with glandular mucous membrane, is 7.5 to 10 cm (3 to 4 inches) long and extends upward and backward from the vulva to the cervix. It is thin walled and can be distended during birth. It is highly vascular and has little sensation. Anterior to it are the bladder and the urethra, and posterior to it lies the rectum. The anterior and posterior walls of the vagina normally touch each other. The **fornix** (the upper part of the vagina) surrounds the **cervix** (the inferior part of the uterus) (Ball et al., 2019).

Uterus

The uterus, a pear-shaped, muscular organ, is about 7.5 cm (3 inches) long and 5 cm (2 inches) wide at its upper part. Its walls are about 1.25 cm (0.5 inch) thick. The size of the uterus varies, depending on parity (number of pregnancies), size of the infants, and uterine abnormalities (e.g., fibroids, which are a type of tumor that may distort the uterus). A woman who is nulliparous (one who has not completed a pregnancy to the stage of fetal viability) usually has a smaller uterus than a woman who is multiparous (one who has completed two or more pregnancies to the stage of fetal viability).

The uterus lies posterior to the bladder and is held in position by several ligaments. The round ligaments extend anteriorly and laterally to the internal inguinal ring and down the inguinal canal, where they blend with the tissues of the labia majora. The broad ligaments are folds of peritoneum extending from the lateral pelvic walls and enveloping the fallopian tubes. The uterosacral ligaments extend posterior to the sacrum (Eickmeyer, 2017).

The uterus has four parts: the cervix, fundus, corpus, and isthmus. The cervix is the opening to the uterus and projects into the vagina. A larger upper part, the **fundus**, is the rounded portion above the insertion of the fallopian tubes. The corpus or body is the main portion of the uterus located between the fundus and the isthmus. The isthmus is referred to as the lower uterine segment during pregnancy and joins the corpus to the cervix.

The cervix is divided into two portions. The portion above the site of attachment of the cervix to the vaginal vault is known as the supravaginal portion; the portion below the attachment site that protrudes into the vagina is known as the vaginal portion. The cervix is composed of fibrous connective tissue. The diameter varies from 2 to 5 cm depending on the childbearing history. The length is usually 2.5 to 3 cm in the woman who is not pregnant. The vaginal portion is smooth, firm, and doughnut shaped with a visible central opening referred to as the external os. The external os is round before the first birth and is often slitlike in shape after childbirth. The internal os is the opening in the cervix to the uterine cavity. In response to cyclic hormones, the cervix produces mucus, which is an important factor in fertility awareness. The vaginal surface of the cervix is covered with squamous epithelium, a rapid cellular growth site of cervical cancer and precancerous changes.

The uterine wall has three layers. The **endometrium**, the innermost layer, is highly vascular and responds to hormone stimulation to prepare to receive the developing ovum. It sloughs if pregnancy does not occur, resulting in menstruation; if pregnancy occurs, it sloughs after delivery. The myometrium, the middle layer, is made up of several smooth muscle layers. The outer layer of the myometrium is composed of longitudinal fibers, chiefly in the fundus, which provide the power to expel the fetus. The middle layer of the myometrium is composed of fibers interlaced with blood vessels in a figure-eight pattern called a *living ligature* because it contracts after childbirth to help control blood loss (Eickmeyer, 2017). The inner layer of the myometrium is composed of circular fibers that are concentrated around the internal cervical os to help keep the cervix closed during pregnancy. The outer layer of the uterus is composed of parietal peritoneum, which covers most of the uterus. From here, the oviducts or fallopian (or uterine) tubes extend outward, and their lumina are internally continuous with the uterine cavity (Ball et al., 2019). The fallopian tubes or oviducts are the passageway for eggs from the ovary to the uterus. They curve around each ovary and are attached to the uterine fundus. Fallopian tubes are about 10 cm in length and are comprised of four parts. The infundibulum, the most distal portion, is covered in fimbriae, whose wavelike motion helps to pull the egg into the tube. The ampulla is usually the site of fertilization of the egg or ovum. The fallopian tube then narrows from its 0.6 cm diameter in the isthmus, ending in the narrowest part of the interstitial portion, which opens into the uterine cavity. The fallopian tube also secretes nutrients for

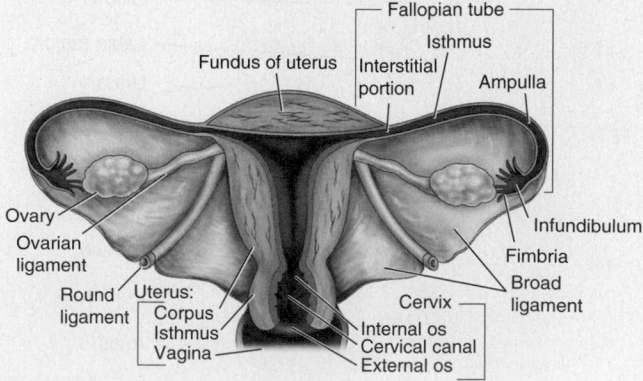

Figure 50-2 • Internal female reproductive structures.

growth and development of the ovum after fertilization while it passes down the tube to the uterus.

Ovaries

The **ovaries** lie behind the broad ligaments and behind and below the fallopian tubes. They are almond-shaped bodies about 3 cm (1.2 inches) long. At birth, they contain thousands of tiny egg cells, or ova. The ovaries and the fallopian tubes together are referred to as the **adnexa**.

Function of the Female Reproductive System

Ovulation

At puberty (usually between 11 and 13 years of age), the ova begin to mature and menstrual cycles begin. In the follicular phase, an ovum enlarges into a cystic structure called a **graafian follicle** until it reaches the surface of the ovary, where transport occurs. The ovum (or oocyte) is discharged into the peritoneal cavity. This periodic discharge of matured ovum is referred to as **ovulation**. The ovum usually finds its way into the fallopian tube, where it is carried to the uterus. If it is penetrated by a spermatozoon, the male reproductive cell, a union occurs, and conception takes place. After the discharge of the ovum, the cells of the graafian follicle undergo a rapid change. Gradually, they become yellow and produce **progesterone**, a hormone that prepares the uterus for receiving the fertilized ovum. Ovulation usually occurs 2 weeks prior to the next menstrual period (Casanova, Chuang, Goepfert, et al., 2019).

Menstrual Cycle

The menstrual cycle is a complex process involving the reproductive and endocrine systems. The ovaries produce steroid hormones, predominantly estrogens and progesterone. Several different estrogens are produced by the ovarian follicle, which consists of the developing ovum and its surrounding cells. The most potent of the ovarian estrogens is estradiol. **Estrogens** are responsible for developing and maintaining the female reproductive organs and the secondary sex characteristics associated with the adult female. Estrogens play an important role in breast development and in monthly cyclic changes in the uterus (Casanova et al., 2019).

Progesterone is also important in regulating the changes that occur in the uterus during the menstrual cycle. It is secreted by the **corpus luteum** (site within a follicle that changes after ovulation) or the ovarian follicle after the ovum has been released. Progesterone is the most important hormone for conditioning the endometrium (the mucous membrane lining of the uterus) in preparation for implantation of a fertilized ovum. If pregnancy occurs, the progesterone secretion becomes largely a function of the placenta and is essential for maintaining a normal pregnancy. In addition, progesterone, working with estrogen, prepares the breast for producing and secreting milk. Androgens are hormones produced by the ovaries and adrenal glands in small amounts. These hormones affect many aspects of female health, including follicle development, libido, oiliness of hair and skin, and hair growth (Casanova et al., 2019).

Two gonadotropic hormones are released by the pituitary gland: **follicle-stimulating hormone (FSH)** and **luteinizing hormone (LH)**. FSH is primarily responsible for stimulating

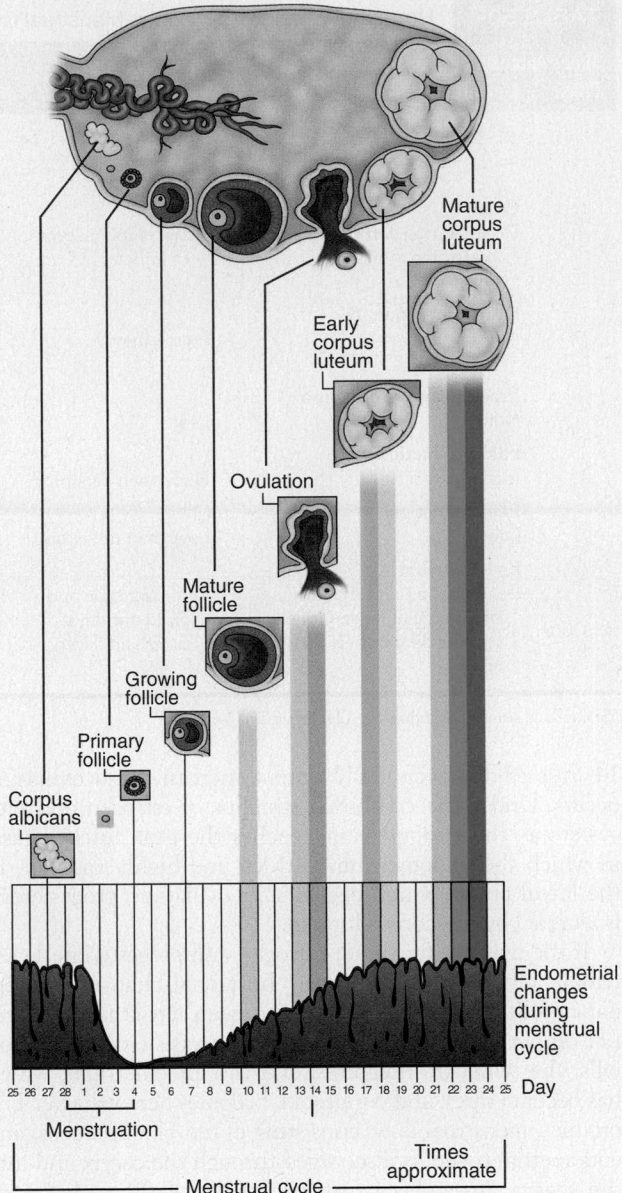

Figure 50-3 • The menstrual cycle and corresponding changes in the endometrium.

the ovaries to secrete estrogen. LH is primarily responsible for stimulating progesterone production. Feedback mechanisms, in part, regulate FSH and LH secretion. For example, elevated estrogen levels in the blood inhibit FSH secretion but promote LH secretion, whereas elevated progesterone levels inhibit LH secretion. In addition, gonadotropin-releasing hormone (GnRH) from the hypothalamus affects the rate of FSH and LH release (Casanova et al., 2019).

The secretion of ovarian hormones follows a cyclic pattern that results in changes in the uterine endometrium and in menstruation (see Fig. 50-3 and Table 50-1). This cycle is typically 28 days in length, but there are many normal variations (from 21 to 42 days). In the **proliferative phase** at the beginning of the cycle (just after menstruation), FSH output increases, and estrogen secretion is stimulated. This causes the endometrium to thicken and become more vascular. In the **secretory phase** near the middle portion of the cycle (day

TABLE 50-1 Hormonal Changes during the Menstrual Cycle

Times Approximate Phase	Menstrual	Follicular	Ovulation	Luteal	Premenstrual
Days	1 2 3 4 5 6 7 8 9	10 11 12 13 14	15 16 17 18 19	20 21 22 23 24	25 26 27 28 1 2
Ovary	Degenerating corpus luteum; beginning follicular development	Growth and maturation of follicle	Ovulation	Active corpus luteum	Degenerating corpus luteum
Estrogen production	Low	Increasing	High	Declining, then a secondary rise	Decreasing
Progesterone production	None	Low	Low	Increasing	Decreasing
FSH production	Increasing	High, then declining	Low	Low	Increasing
LH production	Low	Low, then increasing	High	High	Decreasing
Endometrium	Degeneration and shedding of superficial layer. Coiled arteries dilate, then constrict again.	Reorganization and proliferation of superficial layer	Continued growth	Active secretion and glandular dilation; highly vascular; edematous	Vasoconstriction of coiled arteries; beginning degeneration

FSH, follicle-stimulating hormone; LH, luteinizing hormone.

14 in a 28-day cycle), LH output increases, and ovulation occurs. Under the combined stimulus of estrogen and progesterone, the endometrium reaches the peak **luteal phase**, in which the endometrium is thick and highly vascular. In the luteal phase, which begins after ovulation, progesterone is secreted by the corpus luteum.

If the ovum is fertilized, estrogen and progesterone levels remain high, and the complex hormonal changes of pregnancy follow. If the ovum has not been fertilized, FSH and LH output diminishes; estrogen and progesterone secretion falls; the ovum disintegrates; and the endometrium, which has become thick and congested, becomes hemorrhagic. The product, menstrual flow, consisting of old blood, mucus, and endometrial tissue, is discharged through the cervix and into the vagina. After the menstrual flow stops, the cycle begins again; the endometrium proliferates and thickens from estrogenic stimulation, and ovulation recurs (Ball et al., 2019).

Menopausal Period

The menopausal period marks the end of a woman's reproductive capacity. It usually occurs between 41 and 59 years of age (Ball et al., 2019). Perimenopause precedes this and can begin as early as 35 years of age. Physical, emotional, and menstrual changes may occur, and this transition offers another opportunity for health promotion and disease prevention education and counseling. Menopause is a normal part of aging and maturation. Menstruation ceases, and because the ovaries are no longer active, the reproductive organs become smaller. No more ova mature; therefore, no ovarian hormones are produced. (An earlier menopause may occur if the ovaries are surgically removed or are destroyed by radiation or chemotherapy or because of an unknown etiology.) Multifaceted changes also occur throughout the woman's body. These changes are neuroendocrine, biochemical, and metabolic and are related to normal maturation or aging (see Table 50-2).

TABLE 50-2 Age-Related Changes in the Female Reproductive System

The age-related changes described below pertain to women ages 41 yrs and older.

Changes	Physiologic Effects	Signs and Symptoms
Cessation of ovarian function and decreased estrogen production	Decreased ovulation	Decreased/loss of ability to conceive; increased infertility
	Onset of menopause	Irregular menses with eventual cessation of menses
	Vasomotor instability and hormonal fluctuations	Hot flashes or flushing; night sweats, sleep disturbances; mood swings; fatigue
	Decreased bone formation	Bone loss and increased risk for osteoporosis and osteoporotic fractures; loss of height
	Decreased vaginal lubrication	Dyspareunia, resulting in lack of interest in sex
	Thinning of urinary and genital tracts	Increased risk for urinary tract infection
	Increased pH of vagina	Increased incidence of inflammation (atrophic vaginitis) with discharge, itching, and vulvar burning
	Thinning of pubic hair and shrinking of labia	
Relaxation of pelvic musculature	Prolapse of uterus, cystocele, rectocele	Dyspareunia, incontinence, feelings of perineal pressure

Adapted from Casanova, R., Chuang, A., Goepfert, A. R., et al. (2019). *Beckman and Ling's obstetrics and gynecology* (8th ed.). Philadelphia. PA: Wolters Kluwer.

Chart 50-1 Select Health Screening and Counseling Issues for Women

Ages 19–39 Years

Sexuality and Reproductive Issues

Annual pelvic examination to begin at 21 years of age
Annual clinical breast examination
Contraceptive options
High-risk sexual behaviors

Health and Risk Behaviors

Hygiene
Injury prevention
Nutrition
Exercise patterns
Risk for abuse, maltreatment, and neglect
Use of tobacco, drugs, and alcohol
Life stresses
Immunizations

Diagnostic Testing[a]

Cervical cytology (Pap smear) alone every 3 years from ages 21 to 29. From ages 30 to 64: cervical cytology alone every 3 years; or cytology and HPV testing every 5 years.
Sexually transmitted infection screening as indicated

Ages 40–64 Years

Sexuality and Reproductive Issues

Annual pelvic examination
Annual clinical breast examination
Contraceptive options
High-risk sexual behaviors
Menopausal concerns

Health and Risk Behaviors

Hygiene
Bone loss and injury prevention
Nutrition
Exercise patterns
Risk for abuse, maltreatment, and neglect
Use of tobacco, drugs, and alcohol
Life stresses
Immunizations

Diagnostic Testing[a]

Cervical cytology (Pap smear) every 3 years; or cytology and HPV testing every 5 years.
Annual mammography for women ages 45 to 54 years, women ages 40 to 44 years have the option to begin yearly screening.
- Women 55 and older may continue yearly screening or transition to every 2 years.
- Screening should continue as long as a woman is in good health and is expected to live 10 more years or longer.

Cholesterol and lipid profile
Colorectal cancer screening beginning at age 50 years
Bone mineral density testing
Thyroid-stimulating hormone testing
Hearing and eye examinations

Age 65 Years and Older

Sexuality and Reproductive Issues

Annual pelvic examination
Annual clinical breast examination
High-risk sexual behaviors

Health and Risk Behaviors

Hygiene
Injury prevention, falls
Nutrition
Exercise patterns
Risk for abuse, maltreatment, and neglect
Use of tobacco, drugs, and alcohol
Life stresses
Immunizations

Diagnostic Testing[a]

No cervical cytology (Pap smear) following adequate negative prior screenings
Mammography
Cholesterol and lipid profile
Colorectal cancer screening
Bone mineral density testing
Thyroid-stimulating hormone testing
Hearing and eye examinations

HPV, human papilloma virus.
[a]Each person's risks (family history, personal history) influence the need for specific assessments and their frequency.
Adapted from American Cancer Society (ACS). (2019). Breast cancer facts & figures 2019–2020. Retrieved on 9/9/2019 at: www.cancer.org/content/dam/cancer-org/research/cancer-facts-and-statistics/breast-cancer-facts-and-figures/breast-cancer-facts-and-figures-2019-2020.pdf; Eliopoulos, C. (2018). *Gerontological nursing* (9th ed.). Philadelphia, PA: Lippincott Williams & Wilkins.

Assessment

A nurse who is obtaining information from a woman for the health history and performing physical assessment is in an ideal position to discuss the woman's general health issues, health promotion, and health-related concerns. Relevant topics include fitness, nutrition, cardiovascular risks, health screening, sexuality, menopause, abuse, health risk behaviors, emotional well-being, and immunizations. Select health screening and counseling issues are summarized in Chart 50-1.

Health History

In addition to the general health history, the nurse asks about past illnesses and experiences specific to a woman's health. Data should be collected about the following:

- Menstrual history (including onset, length of cycles, duration and amount of flow, presence of cramps or pain, bleeding between periods or after penile-vaginal intercourse, bleeding after menopause)
- Pregnancies (number of pregnancies, outcomes of pregnancies)
- Exposure to medications (diethylstilbestrol, immunosuppressive agents, others)
- **Dysmenorrhea** (pain with menses), **dyspareunia** (pain with penile-vaginal intercourse), pelvic pain
- Symptoms of vaginitis (i.e., odor or itching)
- Problems with urinary function, including frequency, urgency, and incontinence
- Bowel problems
- Sexual history

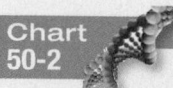

Chart 50-2 · GENETICS IN NURSING PRACTICE
Female Reproductive Processes

Various female reproductive disorders are influenced by genetic factors. Some examples include:

- Hereditary breast or ovarian cancer syndromes
- Hereditary nonpolyposis colon cancer syndrome (risk for uterine cancer)
- Kallmann syndrome
- Müllerian aplasia
- 21-Hydroxylase deficiency (female masculinization)
- Turner syndrome (45, XO)

Nursing Assessments

Refer to Chapter 4, Chart 4-2: Genetics in Nursing Practice: Genetic Aspects of Health Assessment

Family History Assessment Specific to Female Reproductive Processes

- Assess family history for other family members with similar reproductive problems/abnormalities. If the female is a carrier of fragile X, she may be at risk for premature ovarian failure.
- Ask about age at the start and completion of puberty. Failure to complete puberty can lead to infertility.
- The absence of the sense of smell is noted with Kallmann syndrome which, if untreated, can lead to infertility.
- Inquire about ethnic background (e.g., Ashkenazi Jewish populations and hereditary breast/ovarian cancer mutations).

- Inquire about relatives with other cancers, including early-onset ovarian, uterine, renal, prostate cancers.
- Obtain family history that includes a thorough review of reproductive history which addresses spontaneous abortions (miscarriages), infant deaths, or difficulties during pregnancy.
- If possible, obtain ages of the parents during pregnancy.

Patient Assessment Specific to Female Reproductive Processes

- In females with delayed puberty or primary amenorrhea, assess for clinical features of Turner syndrome (short stature, webbing of the neck, widely spaced nipples).
- Assess for other congenital anomalies in females with Müllerian defect, including renal and vertebral anomalies.
- Assess for exposure to toxic chemicals, radiation, or medications during pregnancy.
- Obtain prior reproductive history.
- Inquire about use and frequency of alcohol or tobacco during pregnancy.

Genetics Resources

American Cancer Society, www.cancer.org
Association for X and Y Chromosome Variations, www.genetic.org
March of Dimes Birth Defects Foundation, www.marchofdimes.org
Turner Syndrome Society, www.turnersyndrome.org
See Chapter 6, Chart 6-7 for components of genetic counseling.

- Sexually transmitted infections (STIs) and methods of treatment
- Current or previous sexual abuse or physical abuse
- Past surgery or other procedures on reproductive tract structures (including female genital mutilation [FGM] or female circumcision)
- Chronic illness or disability that may affect health status, reproductive health, need for health screening, or access to health care
- Presence or family history of a genetic disorder. Chart 50-2 presents information about genetic reproductive disorders.

In collecting data related to reproductive health, the nurse can educate the patient about normal physiologic processes, such as menstruation and menopause, and assess possible abnormalities. Many problems experienced by young or middle-aged women can be corrected easily. However, if they are not treated, they may result in anxiety and health problems. Issues related to sexuality and sexual function are typically more often brought to the attention of the gynecologic or women's health care provider than other health care providers; however, nurses caring for all women should consider these issues part of routine health assessment.

Sexual History

A sexual assessment includes both subjective and objective data and should be included in care of people from adolescence through advanced age. Health and sexual histories, physical examination findings, and laboratory results are all part of the database. The purpose of a sexual history is to obtain information that provides a picture of a woman's sexuality and sexual practices and to promote sexual health. It may lead to discussion about sexually transmitted illnesses,

unintended pregnancies, and ways of reducing high-risk sexual behaviors (Herbert, 2018). The sexual history may enable a patient to discuss sexual matters openly and to discuss sexual concerns with an informed health professional. Due to the sensitive nature of the subject matter, excellent communication skills are essential when taking a sexual history (Herbert, 2018). This information can be obtained after the gynecologic–obstetric or genitourinary history is completed. By incorporating the sexual history into the general health history, the nurse can move from areas of lesser sensitivity to areas of greater sensitivity after establishing initial rapport.

Taking the sexual history becomes a dynamic process reflecting an exchange of information between the patient and the nurse and provides the opportunity to clarify myths and explore areas of concern that the patient may not have felt comfortable discussing in the past. In obtaining a sexual history, the nurse must not assume the patient's sexual orientation until clarified. When asking about sexual health, the nurse also cannot assume that the patient is married or unmarried. Asking a patient to label herself as single, married, widowed, or divorced may be considered by some women as inappropriate. Asking about a partner or about current meaningful relationships may be a less offensive way to initiate a sexual history.

The PLISSIT (permission, limited information, specific suggestions, intensive therapy) model of sexual assessment and intervention may be used to provide a framework for nursing interventions (Annon, 1976). The assessment begins by introducing the topic and asking the woman for permission to discuss issues related to sexuality with her. See Chapter 53 for further discussion of sexual history.

The nurse can begin by explaining the purpose of obtaining a sexual history (e.g., "I ask all my patients about their sexual health. May I ask you some questions about this?"). History taking continues by inquiring about gender identity and sexual orientation (see Chapter 54, Chart 54-1 for further discussion about how to assess for personal information), followed by inquiring about sexual activity (e.g., "Are you currently having sex? With a man, woman, both, or a gender questioning or nonconforming person?"). Inquiries about possible sexual dysfunction may include, "Are you having any problems related to your current sexual performance?" Such problems may be related to medication, life changes, disability, or the onset of physical or emotional illness. A patient can be asked about her thoughts on what is causing the current problem (Weber & Kelley, 2018).

Information about sexual function can be introduced during the health history (see Chapter 4). By initiating an assessment about sexual concerns, the nurse communicates to the patient that issues about changes or problems in sexual functioning are valid health issues, which provides a safe environment for discussing these sensitive topics. Young women may be apprehensive about having irregular periods, may be concerned about STIs, or may need contraception. They may want information about using tampons, emergency contraception, or issues related to pregnancy. Women who are perimenopausal may have concerns about irregular menses. Women who are menopausal may be concerned about vaginal dryness and discomfort with penile-vaginal intercourse. Women of any age may have concerns about relationships, sexual satisfaction, orgasm, or masturbation.

Risk of STIs can be assessed by asking about the number of sexual partners in the past year or in the patient's lifetime. An open-ended question related to the patient's need for further information should be included (e.g., "Do you have any questions or concerns about your sexual health?"). Women can be advised that sexual activity should never be painful; pain should be investigated by a care provider. They should also be encouraged to talk openly about their sexual feelings with their partner; in an intimate relationship, feelings are facts.

Female Genital Mutilation or Cutting

Female genital mutilation (FGM) comprises all procedures that involve partial or total removal of the external female genitalia, or other injuries to the female genital organs for nonmedical reasons. FGM is recognized internationally as a violation of the human rights of girls and women. It reflects deep-rooted inequality between the sexes and constitutes an extreme form of discrimination against women. It is nearly always carried out on minors and is a violation of the rights of children. The practice also violates a person's rights to health, security and physical integrity, the right to be free from torture and cruel, inhuman or degrading treatment, and the right to life when the procedure results in death (World Health Organization [WHO], 2018).

Complications for patients who have undergone FGM can include infertility, childbirth complications, impaired bladder function, and urinary complications. The practice is most common in the western, eastern, and north-eastern regions of Africa, in some countries in Asia and the Middle East, and among migrants from these areas (WHO, 2018).

Nurses caring for patients who have undergone FGM need to be sensitive, empathetic, knowledgeable, culturally competent, and nonjudgmental. Respect for others' health beliefs, practices, and behaviors, as well as recognition of the complexity of issues involved, is crucial. The nurse should use terminology with which the woman is familiar; *cutting* is usually a more acceptable term than *mutilation*. Speculums are not used in some developing countries; the function of this instrument should be explained, and an appropriately sized speculum used to examine women who have experienced FGM.

Intimate Partner Violence

Intimate partner violence (IPV) is a preventable public health problem affecting more than 32 million Americans (Weil, 2019). IPV involves four main types of violence: physical violence, sexual violence, stalking, and psychological aggression (Centers for Disease Control and Prevention [CDC], 2019a).

Approximately one in four women in the United States has experienced one or more of the four forms of IPV, with lifetime costs of more than $6.3 trillion (CDC, 2019a). Violence is rarely a one-time occurrence in a relationship; it usually continues and escalates in severity. This is an important point to emphasize when a woman states that her partner has hurt her but has promised to change. Perpetrators can change their behavior, although not without extensive counseling and motivation. Sixteen percent of homicide victims are killed by an intimate partner (CDC, 2019a). If a woman states that she is being hurt, sensitive care is required (see Chart 50-3).

By knowing about this major public health problem, being alert to abuse-related problems, and learning how to elicit information from women about abuse, maltreatment, and neglect in their lives, nurses can intervene to assist the patient in addressing a problem that might otherwise go undetected and thus save lives by making women safer through education and support. As part of a comprehensive assessment, the nurse should ensure a safe environment (i.e., a private room with the door closed) and ask each woman about violence in her life. More information on family violence, abuse, and neglect, including sexual assault and rape, can be found in Chapter 67.

No specific signs or symptoms are diagnostic of abuse; however, nurses may see an injury that does not fit the account of how it happened (e.g., a bruise on the side of the upper arm after "I walked into a door"). Manifestations of abuse, maltreatment, and neglect may involve suicide attempts, drug and alcohol abuse, frequent emergency department visits, vague pelvic pain, somatic complaints, and depression. However, there may be no obvious signs or symptoms. Women in abusive situations have higher levels of depression (CDC, 2019a) and often report that they "do not feel well," possibly due to the stress or fear and anticipation of impending abuse.

Incest and Childhood Sexual Abuse

Nurses may encounter women who have been sexually traumatized. Female survivors of sexual abuse are reported to have more mental and physical health problems than women who were not victims of abuse (Hailes, Yu, Danese, et al., 2019). Victims of childhood sexual abuse are reported to experience more depression (Hailes et al., 2019), posttraumatic stress disorder, morbid obesity, marital instability, gastrointestinal problems, and headaches, as well as use health care services more frequently than people who were not victims. In women, chronic pelvic pain is often associated with physical violence,

Chart 50-3 Strategies for Providing Sensitive Care Following Intimate Partner Violence, Maltreatment, and Neglect

Strategy	Rationale
Reassure the woman that she is not alone	Women often believe that they are alone in experiencing abuse, maltreatment, and neglect at the hands of their partners.
Express your belief that no one should be hurt, that abuse is the fault of the batterer and is against the law.	Doing so lets the woman know that no one deserves to be abused and that she has not caused the abuse.
Assure the woman that her information is confidential, although it does become part of her medical record. *If children are suspected of being abused or are being abused, the law requires that this be reported to the authorities.* Some states require reporting of spousal or partner abuse. Domestic violence agencies and medical and nursing groups disagree with this policy and are trying to have it changed. Serious opposition is based on the fact that reporting does not and cannot currently guarantee a woman's safety and may place her in more danger. It may also interfere with a patient's willingness to discuss her personal life and concerns with health care providers. This places a serious barrier in the way of comprehensive nursing care. If nurses are in doubt about laws on reporting abuse, they need to check with their local or state domestic violence agency.	Women are often afraid that their information will be reported to the police or protective services and their children may be taken away.
Document the woman's statement of abuse and take photographs of any visible injuries if written formal consent has been obtained. (Emergency departments usually have a camera available if one is not on the nursing unit.)	Doing so provides documentation of injuries that may be needed for later legal or criminal proceedings.
Provide education that includes the following: • Inform the woman that shelters are available to ensure safety for her and her children. (Lengths of stay in shelters vary by state but are often up to 2 months. Staff often assists with housing, jobs, and the emotional distress that accompanies the breakup of the family.) Provide list of shelters. • Inform the woman that violence gets worse, not better. • If the woman chooses to go to a shelter, let her make the call. • If the woman chooses to return to the abuser, remain nonjudgmental and provide information that will make her safer than she was before disclosing her situation. • Make sure that the woman has a 24-hour hotline telephone number that provides information and support (Spanish translation and a device for the deaf are also available), police number, and 911. • Assist her to set up a safety plan in case she decides to return home. (A safety plan is an organized plan for departure with packed bags and important papers hidden in a safe spot.)	Options may be lifesaving for the woman and her children.

Adapted from Centers for Disease Control and Prevention (CDC). (2019a). Understanding intimate partner violence fact sheet. Retrieved on 11/9/2019 at: www.cdc.gov/violenceprevention/intimatepartnerviolence/fastfact.html

emotional neglect, and sexual abuse in childhood (Harris, Wieser, Vitonis, et al., 2018). Women who have experienced rape or sexual abuse may be very anxious about pelvic examinations, labor, pelvic or breast irradiation, or any treatment or examination that involves hands-on treatment or requires removal of clothing. Nurses should be prepared to offer support and referral to psychologists, community resources, and self-help groups.

Health Issues in Women with Disability

Approximately 20% of women have disability and encounter physical, architectural, and attitudinal barriers that may limit their full participation in society (Okoro, Hollis, Cyrus, et al., 2018). Women with disability may experience stereotyping and increased risk of abuse, maltreatment, and neglect. They have reported that others, including health care providers, often equate them with their disability. Studies have reported that women with disability receive less primary health care and preventive health screening than other women, often because of access problems and health care providers who focus on the causes of disability rather than on health issues that are of concern to all women (Horner-Johnson, 2019; Okoro et al., 2018). To address these issues, the health history must include questions about barriers to health care encountered by women with disability and the effect of their disability on their health status and health care.

The CDC and the Association of Maternal Child Health Programs partnered to develop a central resource tool made of existing resources for nurses, physicians, physician assistants, and nurse practitioners who work with women with disability.

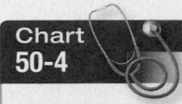

Chart 50-4 ASSESSMENT
Assessing a Woman with a Disability

Health History

Address questions directly to the woman herself rather than to people accompanying her. Ask about:

- Self-care limitations resulting from her disability (ability to feed and dress self, the use of assistive devices, transportation requirements, other assistance needed)
- Sensory limitations (lack of sensation, low vision, deaf or hard of hearing)
- Accessibility issues (ability to get to health care provider, transfer to examination table, accessibility of office/clinic of health care provider, previous experiences with health care providers, health screening practices, her understanding of physical examination)
- Cognitive or developmental changes that affect understanding
- Limitations secondary to disability that affect general health issues and reproductive health and health care
- Sexual function and concerns (those of all women and those that may be affected by the presence of a disabling condition)
- Menstrual history and menstrual hygiene practices
- Physical, sexual, or psychological abuse (including abuse by care providers; abuse by neglect, withholding or withdrawing assistive devices or personal or health care) (see Chart 50-3)
- Presence of secondary disability (i.e., those resulting from the patient's primary disability: pressure injuries, spasticity, osteoporosis, etc.)
- Health concerns related to aging with a disability

Physical Assessment

Provide instructions directly to the woman herself rather than to people accompanying her; provide written or audiotaped instructions.

Ask the woman what assistance she needs for the physical examination and provide assistance if needed:

- Undressing and dressing
- Providing a urine specimen
- Standing on scale to be weighed (provide alternative means of obtaining weight if she is unable to stand on scale)
- Moving on and off the examination table
- Assuming, changing, and maintaining positions

Consider the fatigue experienced by the woman during a lengthy examination and allow rest.

Provide assistive devices and other aids/methods needed to allow adequate communication with the patient (interpreters, signers, large-print written materials).

Complete examination that would be indicated for any other woman; having a disability is *never* justification for omitting parts of the physical examination, including the pelvic examination.

Adapted from Konig-Bachman, M., Zenzmaier, C., & Schildberger, B. (2019). Health professionals' views on maternity care for women with physical disabilities: A qualitative study. *BMC Health Services Research, 19*(1), 551.

People Who Identify as Lesbian, Gay, Bisexual, Transgender, or Queer (LGBTQ)

As the nature of family changes in our society, so must the health care providers' understanding of the people who make up the family unit (Gregg, 2018). Many health assessments presume a heterosexual orientation. Many health care providers are insufficiently prepared to meet the health needs of patients who identify as lesbian, gay, bisexual, transgender, or queer (LGBTQ) (see Chapter 54) (Wingo, Ingraham, & Roberts, 2018).

Those who identify themselves as LGBTQ may have concerns about disclosure and confidentiality, discriminatory attitudes, and treatment (Gregg, 2018; Wingo et al., 2018) (see Chart 50-5). Some research has reported that transgender people abuse alcohol and drugs to a greater degree than their nontransgender counterparts because their social venues may contribute to alcohol and drug use.

Youth who identify as LGBTQ are at higher risk of human immune deficiency virus (HIV) and STIs (Wingo et al., 2018). In addition, youth who self-identify as lesbian, gay, or

Chart 50-5 Health Care for Those Who Identify as LGBTQ

Nurses working with those who identify as LGBTQ should consider that these people:

- Are found in every ethnic group and socioeconomic class.
- Are seen in all age groups, including teens and seniors.
- Can be single, celibate, or divorced.
- Have often encountered insensitivity in health care encounters.
- Are typically offered contraception when asked if they are sexually active and respond affirmatively, as health care providers may assume incorrectly that they practice heterosexual intercourse.
- Have lower health screening rates than other women.
- Often feel invisible and underuse health care, similar to many other marginalized groups of women.

Nurses need to:

- Use gender-neutral questions and terms that are nonjudgmental and accepting.
- Recognize that lesbian teens are at risk for suicide and screen for those at risk.
- Recognize that many lesbians do participate in heterosexual activity but consider themselves at low risk for STIs. Because human papilloma virus, herpes infections, and other organisms implicated in STIs are transmitted by secretions and contact, lesbians may need information on STIs and contraception. If sex toys are used and not cleaned, pelvic infections can occur.

Women who identify as LGBTQ are at high risk for cancer, heart disease, depression, and alcohol abuse. They may have a higher body mass index, may bear fewer or no children, and often have fewer health preventive screenings than women who are heterosexual. These factors may increase the risk of colon, endometrial, ovarian, and breast cancer, as well as cardiovascular disease and diabetes. Adolescents are at risk for smoking and suicide/depression.

Adapted from Gregg, I. (2018). The health care experiences of lesbian women becoming mothers. *Nursing for Women's Health, 22*(1), 40–50; Wingo, E., Ingraham, N., & Roberts, S. (2018). Reproductive health care priorities and barriers to effective care for LGBTQ people assigned female at birth: A qualitative study. *Women's Health Issues, 28*(4), 350–357.

The Toolbox provides links to existing tools to help facilitate preventive services (such as routine physical examinations, teeth cleanings, hepatitis B vaccinations, cervical cancer and breast cancer screenings, and family planning services) to women with disability (CDC, 2019b). Other issues to be addressed regarding the care of women with disability are identified in Chart 50-4.

bisexual or who lack support from parents and families may experience increased physical and mental health issues (e.g., depression, obesity) as well as isolation (Lapinski, Covas, Perkins, et al., 2018). Nurses need to understand the unique needs of this population and provide appropriate and sensitive care.

 ### Gerontologic Considerations

Older women function at various levels across the health spectrum; some function at a high level in their jobs or families, whereas others may be very ill. Nurses need to be prepared to care for older women who may be bright, energetic, and ambitious or who are coping with multiple family crises, including their own health issues, as well as for those who are experiencing a life-altering or life-threatening health problem. Older women are at risk for several conditions, including diabetes, dyslipidemia, hypertension, and thyroid disease, all of which have symptoms that may be dismissed as typical aging. Nurses can help prevent morbidity and mortality from these conditions by encouraging women to obtain regular health screenings (Eliopoulos, 2018). Knowledge about heart disease prevention, pharmacology, diet, signs of dementia or cognitive decline, fall prevention, osteoporosis prevention, gynecologic and breast cancers, and sexuality are important for providing high-level nursing care. Health disparities, cultural competency, and end-of-life issues also need to be considered.

Physical Assessment

Periodic examinations and routine cancer screening are important for all women (Bibbins-Domingo, 2017). Patients need understanding and support due to the emotional and physical considerations associated with gynecologic examinations. Women may be embarrassed by the usual questions asked by a gynecologist or women's health care provider. Because gynecologic conditions are of a personal and private nature to most women, such information is shared only with those directly involved in patient care.

The approach to the gynecologic examination needs to be systematic and thorough (Weber & Kelley, 2018). The nurse can alleviate feelings of anxiety with explanations and education (see Chart 50-6). It may be helpful to emphasize that a pelvic examination should not usually be uncomfortable. Before the examination begins, the patient is asked to empty her bladder and to provide a urine specimen if urine tests are part of the assessment. Voiding ensures patient comfort and eases the examination because a full bladder can make palpation of pelvic organs uncomfortable for the patient and difficult for the examiner.

Positioning

The supine lithotomy position is used most commonly (Weber & Kelley, 2018). If the patient chooses, alternative positions are sometimes used (Ball et al., 2019). The lithotomy position offers several advantages:

- It is more comfortable for some women.
- It allows better eye contact between patient and examiner.
- It may provide an easier means for the examiner to carry out the bimanual examination.

Chart 50-6

PATIENT EDUCATION
The Pelvic Examination

A pelvic examination includes assessment of the appearance of the vulva, vagina, and cervix and the size and shape of the uterus and ovaries to ensure reproductive health and absence of illness. Providing education for the patient should make the examination proceed more smoothly.

The nurse instructs the patient to:

- Expect to have a feeling of fullness or pressure during the examination, but you should not feel pain. It is important to relax, because if you are very tense, you may feel discomfort.
- Recognize that it is normal to feel uncomfortable and apprehensive.
- Be aware that a narrow, warmed speculum will be inserted to visualize the cervix and a Papanicolaou (Pap) smear will be obtained, if indicated, and should not be uncomfortable.
- Note that you may watch the examination with a mirror if you choose; the examination usually takes no longer than 5 minutes.
- Understand that draping will be used to minimize exposure and reduce embarrassment.

Adapted from Weber, J., & Kelley, J. (2018). *Health assessment in nursing* (6th ed.). Philadelphia, PA: Lippincott Williams & Wilkins.

- It enables the woman to use a mirror to see her anatomy (if she chooses) to visualize any conditions that require treatment or to learn about using certain contraceptive methods.

Inspection

After the patient is prepared, the examiner inspects the external genitalia by looking at the labia majora and minora, noting the epidermal tissue of the labia majora; the skin fades to the pink mucous membrane of the vaginal introitus. Lesions of any type (e.g., genital warts, pigmented lesions [melanoma]) are evaluated. In the woman who is nulliparous, the labia minora come together at the opening of the vagina. In a woman who has delivered children vaginally, the labia minora may gape and vaginal tissue may protrude.

Trauma to the anterior vaginal wall during childbirth may have resulted in incompetency of the musculature, and **cystocele** (a bulge caused by the bladder protruding into the submucosa of the anterior vaginal wall) may be seen. Childbirth trauma may also have affected the posterior vaginal wall, producing a **rectocele** (a bulge caused by rectal cavity protrusion). **Uterine prolapse**, in which the cervix and uterus descend under pressure through the vaginal canal and may be seen at the introitus, may also occur. To identify such protrusions, the examiner asks the patient to "bear down."

The introitus should be free of superficial mucosal lesions. The labia minora may be separated by the fingers of the gloved hand and the lower part of the vagina palpated. In women who have not had penile-vaginal intercourse, a hymen of variable thickness may be felt circumferentially within the vaginal opening. The hymenal ring usually permits the insertion of one finger. Rarely, the hymen totally occludes the vaginal entrance (imperforate hymen).

Examination

Examination techniques include the speculum examination and several palpation methods.

Speculum Examination

The bivalve speculum, either metal or plastic, is available in many sizes (Ball et al., 2019). Metal specula are cleaned and sterilized between patients; plastic specula are for one-time use. Water-soluble lubricant or warm water is used to lubricate the speculum (Ball et al., 2019).

The speculum is gently inserted into the posterior portion of the introitus and slowly advanced to the top of the vagina; this should not be painful or uncomfortable for the woman. The speculum is then slowly opened. In the metal types, a setscrew of the thumb rest is tightened; in the plastic types, a clip is locked to hold the blades in place (Ball et al., 2019).

Inspecting the Cervix

The cervix is inspected for color, position, size, surface characteristics, discharge, and size and shape of the cervical os (Ball et al., 2019). In women who are nulliparous, the cervix usually is 2 to 3 cm wide and smooth. In women who have borne children, the cervix may have a laceration, usually transverse, giving the cervical os a "fishmouth" appearance. Epithelium from the endocervical canal may have grown onto the surface of the cervix, appearing as beefy-red surface epithelium circumferentially around the os. Occasionally, the cervix of a woman whose mother took diethylstilbestrol during pregnancy has a hooded appearance (a peaked aspect superiorly or a ridge of tissue surrounding it); this is evaluated by colposcopy when identified.

Malignant changes may not be obviously differentiated from the rest of the cervical mucosa. Small, benign cysts may appear on the cervical surface. Called *nabothian (retention) cysts*, these are usually bluish or white and are a normal finding after childbirth (Ball et al., 2019). A polyp of endocervical mucosa may protrude through the os and usually is dark red. Polyps can cause irregular bleeding; they are rarely malignant and usually are removed easily in an office or clinic setting. A carcinoma may appear as a cauliflowerlike growth (Ball et al., 2019). Bluish coloration of the cervix is a sign of early pregnancy (Chadwick sign).

Obtaining Pap Smears and Other Samples

A Papanicolaou (Pap) smear is a screening test for abnormal cells of the cervix. Usually, a Pap test is obtained using liquid-based cytology. A cytobrush collection device is rotated in the cervical os. The nurse or provider should be sure to follow the manufacturer's instructions to collect and preserve the specimen appropriately. The liquid sample is also used to test for the presence of HPV (Ball et al., 2019). Immediately after the Pap smear, DNA testing for organisms or a wet mount and potassium hydroxide procedures can be completed before the speculum is removed (Ball et al., 2019).

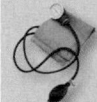 For the procedural guidelines for obtaining an optimal Pap smear, go to **thepoint.lww.com/ Brunner15e**.

A specimen of any purulent material appearing at the cervical os is obtained for culture. A sterile applicator is used to obtain the specimen, which is immediately placed in an appropriate medium for transfer to a laboratory. In a patient who has a high risk for infection, routine cultures for gonococcal and chlamydial organisms are recommended because of the high incidence of both diseases and the complications of pelvic infection, fallopian tube damage, and subsequent infertility (Ball et al., 2019).

Vaginal discharge, which may be normal or may result from vaginitis, may be present. Table 50-3 summarizes the characteristics of vaginal discharge found in different conditions.

Inspecting the Vagina

The vagina is inspected as the examiner withdraws the speculum. It is smooth in young girls and thickens after puberty, with many rugae (folds) and redundancy in the epithelium. In women who are menopausal, the vagina thins and has fewer rugae because of decreased estrogen.

Bimanual Palpation

To complete the pelvic examination, the examiner performs a bimanual examination. The examiner should inform the woman that she will be examined internally with the examiners' fingers. The gloved fingers are then advanced vertically along the vaginal canal, and the vaginal wall is palpated. Any firm part of the vaginal wall may represent old scar tissue from childbirth trauma but may also require further evaluation (Ball et al., 2019).

Cervical Palpation

The cervix is palpated and assessed for its consistency, mobility, size, and position. The normal cervix is uniformly firm but not hard. Softening of the cervix is a finding in early pregnancy. Hardness and immobility of the cervix may reflect invasion by a neoplasm. Pain on gentle movement of the cervix is called a *positive chandelier sign* (positive cervical motion tenderness; recorded as + CMT) and usually indicates a pelvic infection.

TABLE 50-3	Characteristics of Vaginal Discharge		
Cause of Discharge	**Symptoms**	**Odor**	**Consistency/Color**
Physiologic	None	None	Mucus/white
Candida species infection	Itching, irritation	Yeast odor or none	Thin to thick, curdlike/white
Bacterial vaginosis	Odor	Fishy, often noticed after penile-vaginal intercourse	Thin/grayish or yellow
Trichomonas species infection	Irritation, odor	Malodorous	Copious, often frothy/yellow-green
Atrophic	Vulvar or vaginal dryness	Occasional mild malodor	Usually scant and mucoid/may be blood tinged

Uterine Palpation

To palpate the uterus, the examiner places the opposite hand on the abdominal wall halfway between the umbilicus and the pubis and presses firmly toward the vagina. Movement of the abdominal wall causes the body of the uterus to descend, and the organ becomes freely movable between the hand used to examine the abdomen and the fingers of the hand used to examine the pelvis. Uterine size, mobility, and contour can be estimated through palpation. Fixation of the uterus in the pelvis may be a sign of endometriosis or malignancy.

The body of the uterus is normally twice the diameter and twice the length of the cervix, curving anteriorly toward the abdominal wall. Some women have a retroverted or retroflexed uterus, which tips posteriorly toward the sacrum, whereas others have a uterus that is neither anterior nor posterior and is described as midline.

Adnexal Palpation

The right and left adnexal areas are palpated to evaluate the fallopian tubes and ovaries. The fingers of the hand examining the pelvis are moved first to one side, then to the other, while the hand palpating the abdominal area is moved correspondingly to either side of the abdomen and downward. The adnexa (ovaries and fallopian tubes) are trapped between the two hands and palpated for an obvious mass, tenderness, and mobility. Commonly, the ovaries are slightly tender, and the patient is informed that slight discomfort on palpation is normal.

Vaginal and Rectal Palpation

Bimanual palpation of the vagina and cul-de-sac is accomplished by placing the index finger in the vagina and the middle finger in the rectum. To prevent cross-contamination between the vaginal and rectal orifices, the examiner puts on new gloves. A gentle movement of these fingers toward each other compresses the posterior vaginal wall and the anterior rectal wall and assists the examiner in identifying the integrity of these structures. During this procedure, the patient may sense an urge to defecate. The nurse assures the patient that this is unlikely to occur. Ongoing explanations are provided to reassure and educate the patient about the procedure.

 Gerontologic Considerations

Yearly examinations aid early identification of reproductive system disorders in aging women (Eliopoulos, 2018). Nurses play an important role in encouraging all women to have an annual gynecologic examination. Women older than 65 years may stop cervical cancer screening if they have had a hysterectomy or have had three normal cytology tests and no abnormal test in the past 10 years (U.S. Preventive Services Task Force [USPSTF], 2018).

Perineal pruritus is abnormal in older women and should be evaluated because it may indicate a disease process (diabetes or malignancy). Vulvar dystrophy (a thickened or whitish discoloration of tissue) may be visible, and biopsy is needed to rule out abnormal cells. Topical cortisone and hormone creams may be prescribed for symptomatic relief.

With relaxing pelvic musculature, uterine prolapse and relaxation of the vaginal walls can occur (Eliopoulos, 2018). Appropriate evaluation and surgical repair can relieve the discomfort and pressure of the prolapse if the patient is a candidate for surgery. The patient should be informed that tissue repair and healing after surgery may require more time with aging. A pessary (rubber or plastic device that provides support) is often used before surgery to see if surgery can be avoided. It is fitted by a gynecologic health care provider and may reduce the patient's discomfort and pressure. Pessaries also are used if surgery is contraindicated. The use of a pessary requires the patient to have routine gynecologic examinations to monitor for irritation or infection. The patient must be assessed for allergy prior to insertion of a latex pessary. See Chapter 51, Figure 51-4, for details about pessaries.

Diagnostic Evaluation

A wide range of diagnostic studies may be performed in the management of female physiologic processes. The nurse should educate the patient about the purpose, what to expect, and any possible side effects related to these examinations prior to testing. The nurse should be aware of contraindications, potential complications, and trends in results. Trends provide information about disease progression as well as the patient's response to therapy.

Cytologic Test for Cancer (Pap Smear)

The Pap smear is used to detect cervical cancer. Cervical secretions are gently removed from the cervical os and may be transferred to a glass slide and fixed immediately by spraying with a fixative or immersed in solution. If the Pap smear reveals atypical cells, the liquid method allows for HPV testing. See Chapter 51 for further discussion of HPV.

Terminology used to describe findings includes the following categories:

- No abnormal or atypical cells
- Atypical squamous cells of undetermined significance
- Inflammatory reactions and microbes identified
- Positive deoxyribonucleic acid (DNA) test for HPV
- Precancerous and cancerous lesions of the cervix identified

The patient may incorrectly assume that an abnormal Pap smear signifies cancer. If the Pap smear (liquid immersion method) shows atypical cells and no high-risk HPV types, the next Pap smear is performed in 1 year. If a specific infection is causing inflammation, it is treated appropriately, and the Pap smear is repeated. If the repeat Pap smear reveals atypical squamous cells with high-risk HPV types, colposcopy may be indicated. Pap smears that indicate precancerous lesions should be repeated in 4 to 6 months and colposcopy performed if the lesion has not resolved. Patients with Pap smears that indicate cancerous lesions require prompt colposcopy (Casanova et al., 2019).

If the Pap smear results are abnormal, prompt notification, evaluation, and treatment are crucial. Notification of patients is often the responsibility of nurses in a women's health care practice or clinic. Pap smear follow-up is essential because it can provide early detection of cervical cancer. Interventions are tailored to meet the needs and health beliefs of the particular patient. Intensive telephone counseling, tracking systems, brochures, videos, and financial incentives have all been used to encourage follow-up. The nurse provides clear explanations and emotional support along with a carefully designed setting-specific follow-up protocol designed to meet the needs of the patient.

Colposcopy and Cervical Biopsy

If the cervical cytology screening result requires evaluation, a colposcopy is performed. The colposcope is an instrument with a magnifying lens that allows the examiner to visualize the cervix and obtain a sample of abnormal tissue for analysis (Casanova et al., 2019). Nurse practitioners and gynecologists require special training in this diagnostic technique.

After inserting a speculum and visualizing the cervix and vaginal walls, the examiner applies acetic acid to the cervix. Subsequent abnormal findings that indicate the need for biopsy include leukoplakia (white plaque visible before applying acetic acid), acetowhite tissue (white epithelium after applying acetic acid), punctation (dilated capillaries occurring in a dotted or stippled pattern), mosaicism (a tile-like pattern), and atypical vascular patterns. If biopsy specimens show precancerous cells, the patient usually requires cryotherapy, laser therapy, or a cone biopsy (excision of an inverted tissue cone from the cervix).

Cryotherapy and Laser Therapy

Cryotherapy (freezing cervical tissue with nitrous oxide) and laser treatment are used in the outpatient setting. Cryotherapy may result in cramping and occasional feelings of faintness (vasovagal response). A watery discharge is normal for a few weeks after the procedure as the cervix heals; however, excessive bleeding, pain, or fever should be reported to the primary provider (Casanova et al., 2019).

Cone Biopsy and Loop Electrosurgical Excision Procedure

If endocervical curettage findings indicate abnormal changes or if the lesion extends into the canal, the patient may undergo a cone biopsy. This can be performed surgically or with a procedure called *loop electrosurgical excision procedure* (LEEP), which uses a laser beam (Casanova et al., 2019).

Usually performed in the outpatient setting, LEEP is associated with a high success rate in removal of abnormal cervical tissue. The gynecologist excises a small amount of cervical tissue, and the pathologist examines the borders of the specimen to determine if disease is present. A patient who has received anesthesia for a surgical cone biopsy is advised to rest for 24 hours after the procedure and to leave any vaginal packing in place until it is removed (usually the next day). The patient is instructed to report any excessive bleeding.

The nurse or primary provider provides guidelines regarding postoperative sexual activity, bathing, and other activities. Because open tissue may be potentially exposed to HIV and other pathogens, the patient is cautioned to avoid penile-vaginal intercourse until healing is complete and verified at follow-up.

Endometrial (Aspiration) Biopsy

Endometrial biopsy, a method of obtaining endometrial tissue, is performed as an outpatient procedure. This procedure is usually indicated in cases of midlife irregular bleeding,

postmenopausal bleeding, and irregular bleeding while taking hormone therapy or tamoxifen. A tissue sample obtained through biopsy permits diagnosis of cellular changes in the endometrium. The only absolute contraindication to an endometrial biopsy is the presence of a viable and desired pregnancy (Del Priore, 2019).

Women who undergo endometrial biopsy may experience slight discomfort. The examiner may apply a tenaculum (a clamplike instrument that stabilizes the uterus) after the pelvic examination and then inserts a thin, hollow, flexible suction tube (Pipelle or sampler) through the cervix into the uterus.

Findings on aspiration may include normal endometrial tissue, hyperplasia, or endometrial cancer. Simple hyperplasia is an overgrowth of the uterine lining and is usually treated with progesterone. Complex hyperplasia, which refers to overgrowth of cells with abnormal features, is a risk factor for uterine cancer and is treated with progesterone and careful follow-up. Women who are overweight, who are older than 45 years, who have a history of nulliparity and infertility, or who have a family history of colon cancer seem to be at higher risk for hyperplasia. See Chapter 51 for discussion of endometrial cancer.

Dilation and Curettage

Dilation and curettage (D&C) may be diagnostic (identifies the cause of irregular bleeding) or therapeutic (often temporarily stops irregular bleeding). The cervical canal is widened with a dilator, and the uterine endometrium is scraped with a curette. The purpose of the procedure is to secure endometrial or endocervical tissue for cytologic examination, to control abnormal uterine bleeding, and as a therapeutic measure for incomplete abortion.

Because D&C is usually carried out under anesthesia and requires surgical asepsis, it is usually performed in the operating room (Casanova et al., 2019). However, it may take place in the outpatient setting with the patient receiving a local anesthetic supplemented with diazepam or midazolam.

The nurse explains the procedure, preparation, and expectations regarding postoperative discomfort and bleeding. The patient is instructed to void before the procedure. The patient is placed in the lithotomy position, the cervix is dilated with a dilating instrument, and endometrial scrapings are obtained by a curette. A perineal pad is placed over the perineum after the procedure, and excessive bleeding is reported. No restrictions are placed on dietary intake. If pelvic discomfort or low back pain occurs, mild analgesic medications usually provide relief. The primary provider indicates when sexual activity may be safely resumed. To reduce the risk of infection and bleeding, most gynecologists advise no vaginal penetration or use of tampons for 2 weeks.

Endoscopic Examinations

Laparoscopy (Pelvic Peritoneoscopy)

A laparoscopy, minimally invasive surgery, involves inserting a laparoscope (a tube about 10 mm wide and similar to a small periscope) into the peritoneal cavity through a 2-cm (0.75-inch) incision below the umbilicus to allow visualization of the pelvic structures (see Fig. 50-4). Laparoscopy may be used for diagnostic purposes (e.g., in cases of pelvic

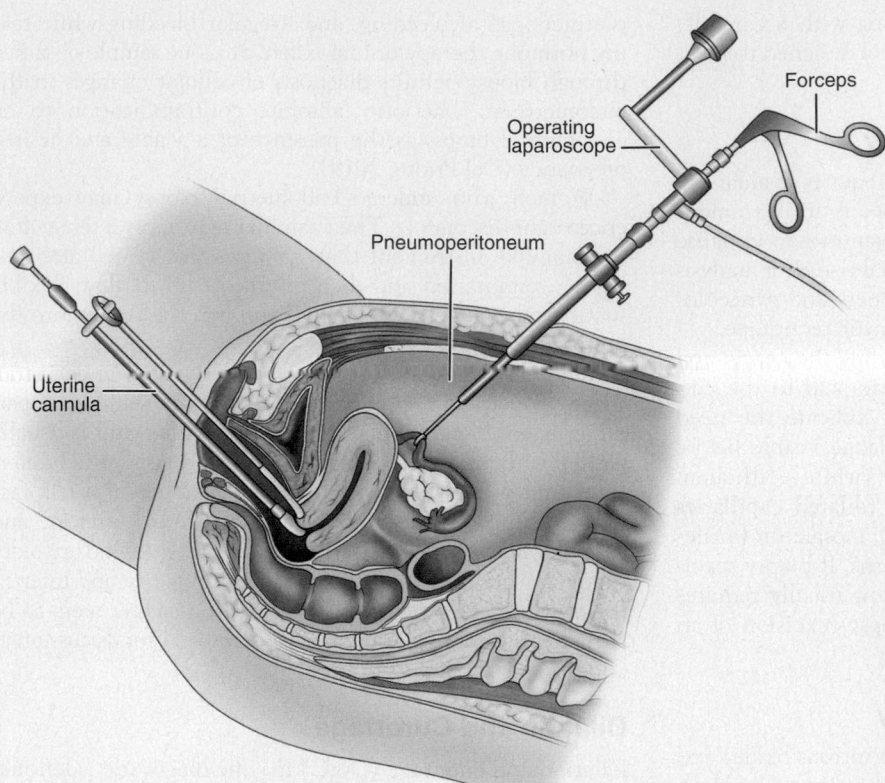

Forceps

Operating
laparoscope

Pneumoperitoneum

Uterine
cannula

Figure 50-4 • Laparoscopy. The laparoscope (*right*) is inserted through a small incision in the abdomen. A forceps is inserted through the scope to grasp the fallopian tube. To improve the view, a uterine cannula (*left*) is inserted into the vagina to push the uterus upward. Insufflation of gas creates an air pocket (pneumoperitoneum), and the pelvis is elevated (note the angle), which forces the intestines higher in the abdomen.

pain when no cause can be found) or treatment. Laparoscopy facilitates many surgical procedures, such as tubal ligation, ovarian biopsy, myomectomy, hysterectomy, and lysis of adhesions (scar tissue that can cause pelvic discomfort) (Sharp, 2019). A surgical instrument (intrauterine sound or cannula) may be positioned inside the uterus to permit manipulation or movement during laparoscopy, affording better visualization. The pelvic organs can be visualized after the injection of carbon dioxide intraperitoneally into the cavity. Called *insufflation,* this technique separates the intestines from the pelvic organs (Sharp, 2019). If a patient is undergoing sterilization, the fallopian or uterine tubes may be electrocoagulated, sutured, or ligated and a segment removed for histologic verification (clips are an alternative device for occluding the tubes).

After the laparoscopy is completed, the laparoscope is withdrawn, carbon dioxide is allowed to escape through the outer cannula, the small skin incision is closed with sutures or a clip, and the incision is covered with an adhesive bandage. The patient is carefully monitored for several hours to detect any untoward signs indicating bleeding (most commonly from vascular injury to the hypogastric vessels), bowel or bladder injury, or burns from the coagulator. These complications are rare, making laparoscopy a cost-effective and safe short-stay procedure. The patient may experience abdominal or shoulder pain related to the use of carbon dioxide gas (Casanova et al., 2019).

Hysteroscopy

Hysteroscopy (transcervical intrauterine endoscopy) allows direct visualization of all parts of the uterine cavity by means of a lighted optical instrument. The procedure is best performed about 5 days after menstruation ceases, in the estrogenic phase of the menstrual cycle. The vagina and vulva are cleansed, and a paracervical anesthetic block is performed or lidocaine spray is used. The instrument used for the procedure, a hysteroscope, is passed into the cervical canal and advanced 1 or 2 cm under direct vision. Uterine-distending fluid (normal saline solution or dextrose 5% in water) is infused through the instrument to dilate the uterine cavity and enhance visibility. Hysteroscopy, which has few complications, is useful for evaluating endometrial pathology or for evaluating and treating retained products of conception (Bradley, 2018).

Hysteroscopy may be indicated as an adjunct to a D&C and laparoscopy in cases of infertility, unexplained bleeding, retained intrauterine device (IUD), and recurrent early pregnancy loss (Bradley, 2018). Treatment for some conditions (e.g., fibroid tumors) can be accomplished during this procedure, and sterilization may also be performed. Hysteroscopy is contraindicated in patients with cervical or endometrial carcinoma or acute pelvic inflammation.

An **endometrial ablation** (destruction of the uterine lining) procedure is performed with a hysteroscope and resector (cutting loop), roller ball (a barrel-shaped electrode), or laser beam in cases of severe bleeding not responsive to other therapies. Completed in an outpatient setting under general, regional, or local anesthesia, this rapid procedure is an alternative to hysterectomy for some patients. Following uterine distention with fluid infusion, the lining of the uterus is destroyed. Hemorrhage, perforation, and burns can occur.

Other Diagnostic Procedures

Additional diagnostic procedures may be helpful in evaluating pelvic conditions; these include x-rays, barium enemas, gastrointestinal x-ray series, intravenous (IV) urography, and cystography studies. In addition, because the uterus, ovaries, and fallopian tubes are near the structures of the urinary tract, urologic diagnostic studies, such as x-ray study of the kidney, ureters, and bladder (KUB) and pyelography are used, as are angiography and radioisotope scanning, if needed. Other diagnostic procedures include hysterosalpingography (HSG) and computed tomography (CT) scanning.

Hysterosalpingography or Uterotubography

HSG is an x-ray study of the uterus and the fallopian tubes after injection of a contrast agent. The diagnostic procedure is performed to evaluate infertility or tubal patency and to detect any abnormal condition in the uterine cavity. Sometimes, the procedure is therapeutic because the flowing contrast agent flushes debris or loosens adhesions.

Prior to HSG, laxatives and an enema may be given to evacuate the intestinal tract so that gas shadows do not distort the x-ray findings. A mild sedative or an analgesic agent, such as ibuprofen, may be prescribed. The patient is placed in the lithotomy position and the cervix is exposed with a bivalve speculum. A cannula is inserted into the cervix, and the contrast agent is injected into the uterine cavity and the fallopian tubes. X-rays are taken to show the path and the distribution of the contrast agent.

Some patients experience nausea, vomiting, cramps, and faintness. After the test, the patient is advised to wear a perineal pad for several hours, because the radiopaque contrast agent may stain clothing.

Computed Tomography

CT scans have several advantages over ultrasonography, but they involve radiation exposure and are more costly. They are more effective than ultrasonography for patients with obesity or for patients with a distended bowel. CT scans can also demonstrate a tumor and any extension into the retroperitoneal lymph nodes and skeletal tissue, although they have limited value in diagnosing other gynecologic abnormalities (Casanova et al., 2019).

Ultrasonography

Ultrasonography (or ultrasound) is a useful adjunct to the physical examination, particularly in patients receiving obstetric care or in patients with abnormal pelvic examination findings. It is a simple procedure based on sound wave transmission that uses pulsed ultrasonic waves at frequencies exceeding 20,000 Hz (formerly cycles per second) by way of a transducer placed in contact with the abdomen (abdominal scan) or a vaginal probe (vaginal ultrasound). Mechanical energy is converted into electrical impulses, which in turn are amplified and recorded on an oscilloscope screen while a photograph or video recording of the patterns is taken. The entire procedure takes 15 to 30 minutes and involves no ionizing radiation and no discomfort other than a full bladder, which is necessary for good visualization during an abdominal scan. A vaginal ultrasound or sonogram does not require a full bladder; however, the vaginal probe may cause mild discomfort in some women (Casanova et al., 2019).

Magnetic Resonance Imaging

Magnetic resonance imaging (MRI) produces patterns that are finer and more definitive than other imaging procedures, and it does not expose patients to radiation. However, MRI is more costly.

> ### ▶ Quality and Safety Nursing Alert
>
> *All metal devices, including medication skin patches with foil backing, must be removed before MRI is performed to avoid burns.*

MANAGEMENT OF FEMALE PHYSIOLOGIC PROCESSES

Many health concerns of women are related to normal changes or abnormalities of the menstrual cycle and may result from women's lack of understanding of the menstrual cycle, developmental changes, and factors that may affect the pattern of the menstrual cycle. Educating women about the menstrual cycle and changes over time is an important aspect of the nurse's role in providing quality care to women. Education should begin early so that menstruation and the lifelong changes in the menstrual cycle can be anticipated and accepted as a normal part of life.

Menstruation

Menstruation, the sloughing and discharge of the lining of the uterus that takes place if conception does not occur, happens about every 28 days during the reproductive years, although normal cycles can vary from 25 to 35 days (Welt, 2019) (see Fig. 50-3). The flow usually lasts 4 to 5 days, during which time 50 to 60 mL of blood is lost.

A perineal pad or tampon is generally used to absorb menstrual discharge. Tampons are used extensively. There is no significant evidence of untoward effects from their use, provided that there is no difficulty in inserting them. However, a tampon should not be used for more than 4 to 8 hours, and the lowest absorbency should be used to prevent toxic shock syndrome (Mayo Clinic, 2017). If a tampon is difficult to remove or shreds when removed, less absorbent tampons should be used. If the string breaks or retracts, the woman should squat in a comfortable position, insert one finger into the vagina, try to locate the tampon, and remove it. If she feels uncomfortable attempting this maneuver or cannot remove the tampon, she should consult a gynecologic health care provider promptly.

Psychosocial Considerations

Girls who are approaching **menarche** (the onset of menstruation) should be educated about the normal process of the menstrual cycle before it occurs. Psychologically, it is much healthier and appropriate to refer to this event as a "period" rather than as "being sick." With adequate nutrition, rest, and exercise, most women feel little discomfort, although some report breast tenderness and a feeling of fullness 1 or 2 days before menstruation begins. Others report fatigue and some discomfort in the lower back, legs, and pelvis on the first day and temperament or mood changes. Slight deviations from a usual pattern of daily living are considered normal, but excessive deviation may require evaluation. Regular exercise and a healthy diet have been found to decrease discomfort for some women. Heating pads or nonsteroidal anti-inflammatory drugs (NSAIDs) may be very effective for cramps. For women with excessive cramping or dysmenorrhea, referral to a women's health care provider is appropriate; following evaluation, providers may prescribe oral contraceptive agents.

Cultural Considerations

Cultural views and beliefs about menstruation differ. Some women believe that it is detrimental to change a pad or tampon too frequently; they think that allowing the discharge to accumulate increases the flow, which is considered desirable. Some women believe they are vulnerable to illness during menstruation. Others believe it is harmful to swim, shower, have their hair permed, have their teeth filled, or eat certain foods during menstruation. They may also avoid using contraception during menstruation.

In such situations, nurses are in a position to provide women with facts in an accepting and culturally sensitive manner. The objective is to be mindful of these unexpressed, deep-rooted beliefs and to provide the facts with care. Aspects of gynecologic problems cannot always be expressed easily. The nurse needs to convey confidence and openness and to offer facts to facilitate communication. Suggestions to improve care include overcoming language barriers, providing appropriate materials in the patient's language, asking about traditional beliefs and dietary practices, and asking about fears regarding care. Patience, sensitivity, and a desire to learn about other cultures and groups will enhance the nursing care of all women.

Menstrual Disorders

Menstrual disorders may include premenstrual syndrome (PMS); dysmenorrhea; amenorrhea; and excessive bleeding, irregular bleeding, or bleeding between cycles or unrelated to cycles. These disorders need to be discussed with a health care provider and managed individually.

Premenstrual Syndrome

PMS is a cluster of physical, emotional, and behavioral symptoms that are usually related to the luteal phase of the menstrual cycle. PMS is very common, affecting many women at some time in their lives (Gnanasambanthan & Datta, 2019) (see Chart 50-7).

Clinical Manifestations

Major symptoms of PMS include physical symptoms such as headache, fatigue, low back pain, painful breasts, and a feeling of abdominal fullness. Behavioral and emotional symptoms may include general irritability, mood swings, fear of losing control, binge eating, and crying spells. Symptoms vary widely from one woman to another and from one cycle to the next in the same woman. Great variability is found in the degree of symptoms. Many women are affected to some degree, but

---

Chart 50-7 **Causes, Manifestations, and Treatment of Premenstrual Syndrome**

Cause

- Unknown; may be related to hormonal changes combined with other factors (diet, stress, and lack of exercise)
- Many women have some symptoms related to menses, but premenstrual syndrome affects 75% to 95% of women at some point and is a complex of symptoms that result in dysfunction.

Physical Symptoms

- Fluid retention (e.g., bloating, breast tenderness)
- Headache
- Low back pain

Affective Symptoms

- Depression
- Anger
- Irritability
- Anxiety
- Confusion
- Withdrawal
- Symptoms begin in the 5 days preceding menses, and relief occurs within 4 days of onset of menses. Dysfunction usually occurs in relationships, parenting, work, or school.

Treatment

- The use of social support and family resources
- Nutritious diet consisting of whole grains, fruits, and vegetables; increased water intake may help.
- Selective serotonin reuptake inhibitors
- Alprazolam has been effective, but risk of physical and psychological dependence is high
- Spironolactone, a diuretic agent, may be effective in treating fluid retention
- Initiation/maintenance of exercise program
- Stress reduction techniques

Adapted from Casper, R. F., & Yonkers, K. A. (2019). Treatment of premenstrual syndrome and premenstrual dysphoric disorder. *UpToDate.* Retrieved on 11/17/2019 at: www.uptodate.com/contents/treatment-of-premenstrual-syndrome-and-premenstrual-dysphoric-disorder; Gnanasambanthan, S., & Datta, S. (2019). Premenstrual syndrome. *Obstetrics, Gynaecology and Reproductive Medicine, 29*(10), 281–285.

---

some are severely affected. Premenstrual dysphoric disorder (PMDD) is a severe form of PMS with significant severity of symptoms (Casper & Yonkers, 2019; Gnanasambanthan & Datta, 2019).

Medical Management

Because there is no single treatment or known cure for PMS, it is helpful for women to keep a record of their symptoms so they can anticipate and therefore cope with them. Regular exercise may be helpful. Although women have been advised to avoid caffeine, high-fat foods, and refined sugars, little research demonstrates the efficacy of dietary changes. Alternative therapies that have been used include vitamins B_6 (pyridoxine) and E, calcium, magnesium, and oil of primrose capsules (Casper & Yonkers, 2019; Gnanasambanthan & Datta, 2019).

Pharmacologic treatments include selective serotonin reuptake inhibitors (e.g., fluoxetine), prostaglandin inhibitors (e.g., ibuprofen and naproxen), diuretic agents, antianxiety agents, and calcium supplements. Oral contraceptives containing drospirenone (a synthetic progestin) and extended regimens also may be effective (Gnanasambanthan & Datta, 2019).

Nursing Management

The nurse obtains a health history, noting the time when symptoms began and their nature and intensity. The nurse then determines whether symptoms occur before or shortly after the menstrual flow begins. In addition, the nurse can show the patient how to record the timing and intensity of symptoms. A nutritional history is also elicited to determine if the diet is high in salt, caffeine, or alcohol or low in essential nutrients.

The patient's goals may include reduction of anxiety, mood swings, crying, binge eating, fear of losing control, improved coping with day-to-day stressors, improved relationships with family and coworkers, and increased knowledge about PMS. Positive coping measures are promoted. This may involve encouraging the woman's partner to offer support and assistance with childcare. The patient can try to plan her working time to accommodate the days she is less productive because of PMS. The nurse encourages the patient to use exercise, meditation, imagery, and creative activities to reduce stress. The nurse also encourages the patient to take medications as prescribed and provides instructions about the desired effects of the medications. Contact details for PMS support services should also be provided.

If the patient has severe symptoms of PMS or PMDD, the nurse assesses her for suicidal, uncontrollable, and violent behavior. An immediate psychiatric evaluation is necessary for women with any suggestions of suicidal tendencies. In rare cases, uncontrollable behavior may lead to violence toward family members. If abuse, maltreatment, and neglect of any member of a patient's family are suspected, it is important to implement and follow reporting protocols.

Dysmenorrhea

Primary dysmenorrhea is painful menstruation, with no identifiable pelvic pathology. It occurs at the time of menarche or shortly thereafter. It is characterized by crampy pain that begins before or shortly after the onset of menstrual flow and continues for 48 to 72 hours. Pelvic examination findings are normal. Dysmenorrhea is thought to result from excessive production of prostaglandins, which causes painful contraction of the uterus. In secondary dysmenorrhea, pelvic pathology such as endometriosis, tumors such as leiomyomata or malignancies, polyps, or pelvic inflammatory disease (PID) contributes to symptoms. Patients frequently have pain that occurs several days before menses, with ovulation, and occasionally with penile-vaginal intercourse. It may be accompanied by nausea, diarrhea, dizziness, and backache (Kulkarni & Deb, 2019).

Assessment and Diagnostic Findings

A pelvic examination is performed to rule out possible disorders, such as endometriosis, PID, adenomyosis, and uterine fibroids. A laparoscopy may be performed to identify organic causes (see Fig. 50-4).

Management

In primary dysmenorrhea, the reason for the discomfort is explained, and the patient is assured that menstruation is a normal function of the reproductive system. If the patient is young and accompanied by her mother, the mother may also need reassurance. Many young women expect to have painful periods if their mothers did. The discomfort of cramps can be treated once anxiety and concern about its cause are dispelled by adequate explanation. Symptoms usually subside with appropriate medication. Useful medications include prostaglandin antagonists such as NSAIDs (e.g., ibuprofen, naproxen, and mefenamic acid, or aspirin). If one medication does not provide relief, another may be recommended. Usually, these medications are well tolerated, but some women experience gastrointestinal side effects. Contraindications include allergy, peptic ulcer history, sensitivity to aspirin-containing medications, asthma, and pregnancy. Low-dose oral contraceptives may be prescribed for women with dysmenorrhea who are sexually active but do not desire pregnancy (Kulkarni & Deb, 2019).

Continuous low-level local heat, such as a heating pad, may be effective in relieving primary dysmenorrhea. Heat therapy and medication have been found to work well in combination. The patient is encouraged to continue her usual activities and to increase physical exercise if possible because this relieves discomfort for some women. Taking analgesic agents before cramps start, in anticipation of discomfort, is advised.

Management of secondary dysmenorrhea is directed at diagnosis of and treatment for the underlying cause (e.g., endometriosis, PID) (see Chapter 51).

Amenorrhea

Amenorrhea, or the absence of menstrual flow, is a symptom of a variety of disorders and dysfunctions. Primary amenorrhea (delayed menarche) refers to the situation in which a young woman who by age 15 years has not begun developing secondary sex characteristics or who by age 16 years or older has developed secondary sex characteristics but has not started menstruation (Welt & Barbieri, 2018). There are many reasons for primary amenorrhea, including genetic and anatomical disorders, Turner syndrome, anorexia, and polycystic ovarian syndrome (Welt & Barbieri, 2018).

The nurse encourages the patient to express her concerns and anxiety about this problem because the patient may feel that she is different from her peers. A complete physical examination, careful health history, and laboratory tests help rule out possible causes, such as metabolic or endocrine disorders and systemic diseases. Treatment is directed toward correcting any abnormalities.

Secondary amenorrhea (an absence of menses for three cycles or 6 months after a normal menarche) may be caused by functional hypothalamic amenorrhea, pituitary disease, primary ovarian failure, pregnancy, breast-feeding, menopause, too little body fat (about 22% required for menses), eating disorder, thyroid disease, or polycystic ovary syndrome (Welt & Barbieri, 2018). In adolescents, secondary amenorrhea can be caused by minor emotional upset related to being away from home, attending college, tension due to schoolwork, or interpersonal problems.

Secondary nutritional disturbances may also be factors. Obesity can result in anovulation and subsequent amenorrhea. Eating disorders, such as anorexia and bulimia, often result in lack of menses because the decrease in body fat and caloric intake affects hormonal function. Intense exercise can induce menstrual disturbances. Females who are competitive athletes often experience amenorrhea. Oligomenorrhea (infrequent periods) may be related to thyroid disorders, polycystic ovarian syndrome, or premature ovarian failure. Women who are HIV positive are apt to miss menstrual periods and need to be evaluated for pregnancy, thyroid disorders, hyperprolactinemia, and menopause.

Abnormal Uterine Bleeding

Dysfunctional uterine bleeding is defined as irregular, painless bleeding of endometrial origin that may be excessive, prolonged, or without pattern. Dysfunctional uterine bleeding can occur at any age but is most common at opposite ends of the reproductive lifespan. It is usually secondary to anovulation (lack of ovulation) and is common in adolescents and women approaching menopause.

Adolescents account for many cases of abnormal uterine bleeding; they often do not ovulate regularly as the pituitary–ovarian axis matures. Women who are perimenopausal also experience this condition because of irregular ovulation secondary to decreasing ovarian hormone production. Other causes may include fibroids, obesity, and hypothalamic dysfunction.

Abnormal or unusual vaginal bleeding that is atypical in time or amount must be evaluated because it could possibly be a manifestation of a major disorder. A physical examination is performed, and the patient is evaluated for conditions such as pregnancy, neoplasm, infection, anatomic abnormalities, endocrine disorders, trauma, blood dyscrasias, platelet dysfunction, and hypothalamic disorders.

Menorrhagia

Menorrhagia is prolonged or excessive bleeding at the time of the regular menstrual flow. In young women, the cause is usually related to endocrine disturbance; in later life, it usually results from inflammatory disturbances, tumors of the uterus, or hormonal imbalance.

Women with menorrhagia are urged to see a primary provider and to describe the amount of bleeding by pad count and saturation (i.e., absorbency of perineal pad or tampon and number saturated hourly). Persistent heavy bleeding can result in anemia. It can also be a sign of a bleeding disorder or a result of anticoagulant therapy. Treatment may involve endometrial ablation or hysterectomy.

Metrorrhagia

Metrorrhagia (vaginal bleeding between regular menstrual periods) is probably the most significant form of menstrual dysfunction because it may signal cancer, benign tumors of the uterus, or other gynecologic problems. This condition warrants prompt evaluation and treatment. Although bleeding between menstrual periods by women taking oral contraceptive agents is usually not serious, irregular bleeding by women taking hormone therapy should be evaluated (Goodman, 2020).

Menometrorrhagia is heavy vaginal bleeding between and during periods. It, too, requires evaluation.

Dyspareunia

Dyspareunia (difficult or painful penile-vaginal intercourse) can be superficial, deep, primary, or secondary and may occur at the beginning of, during, or after penile-vaginal intercourse. Dyspareunia may be related to many factors, including injury during childbirth; lack of vaginal lubrication; a history of incest, sexual abuse, or assault; endometriosis; pelvic or vaginal infection; vaginal dryness due to breast-feeding or menopause; gastrointestinal disorders; fibroids; urinary tract infection; STIs; or vulvodynia (vulvar pain that affects women of all ages without any discernible physical cause). Depending on the cause of dyspareunia, counseling, extra lubrication, or antidepressant medications may be prescribed (Mayo Clinic, 2018). Women's health issues related to sexuality may be affected by many factors. Thus, these issues need to be taken seriously, carefully assessed, and treated.

Contraception

Approximately 61 million women in the United States are in their childbearing years (i.e., between the ages of 15 and 44 years). Those who are sexually active and do not want to become pregnant but could become pregnant if they and their partners fail to use a contraceptive method, are at risk of unintended pregnancy. Thus, approximately 43 million women of childbearing age are at risk for unintended pregnancy (Alan Guttmacher Institute, 2018). Approximately 45% of the pregnancies each year in the United States are unintended and can result in negative health consequences and are an enormous financial burden to the health care system (American College of Obstetricians and Gynecologists [ACOG], 2019). Family planning benefits mothers, newborns, families, and communities.

Nurses who are involved in helping patients make contraceptive choices need to listen, take time to answer questions, and educate and assist patients in choosing the contraceptive method they prefer (see Chart 50-8). It is important for women to receive unbiased and nonjudgmental information, understand the benefits and risks of each contraceptive method, learn about alternatives and how to use them, and receive positive reinforcement and acceptance of their choice. Nurses also have the opportunity to dispel myths and misinformation surrounding contraception. Figure 50-5 provides an overview of the effectiveness of family planning methods.

Contraindications

Coexisting medical disorders may make contraception a complex issue. Contraception needs to be addressed individually in women with preexisting conditions. With the aid of a thorough history, nurses are well positioned to aid patients in choosing the safest, most effective method of contraception to meet their individual needs.

Chart 50-8 • PATIENT EDUCATION

Using Contraceptives

The nurse provides education to enhance the chosen method of contraception.

The nurse instructs patients who have chosen male or female sterilization to:

- Use another contraceptive method for the first 3 months.
- Use condoms to protect against sexually transmitted infections.

The nurse instructs women who have chosen an injectable method to:

- Use condoms to protect against sexually transmitted infections.
- Obtain repeat injections on time.

The nurse instructs women who have chosen pills to:

- Use condoms to protect against sexually transmitted infections.
- Take the pill at exactly the same time every day.

The nurse instructs women who have chosen the patch to:

- Use condoms to protect against sexually transmitted infections.
- Change the patch once a week.

The nurse instructs women who have chosen a ring to:

- Use condoms to protect against sexually transmitted infections.
- Remove the vaginal ring after 3 weeks.

The nurse instructs women who have chosen a diaphragm to:

- Use correctly each time you have sex.

The nurse instructs women who have chosen condoms, a sponge, withdrawal, or spermicides to:

- Use correctly each time you have sex.

Adapted from Holland, A. C., Strachan, A. T., Pair, L., et al. (2018). Highlights from the U.S. selected practice recommendations for contraception use. *Nursing for Women's Health*, 22(2), 181–190.

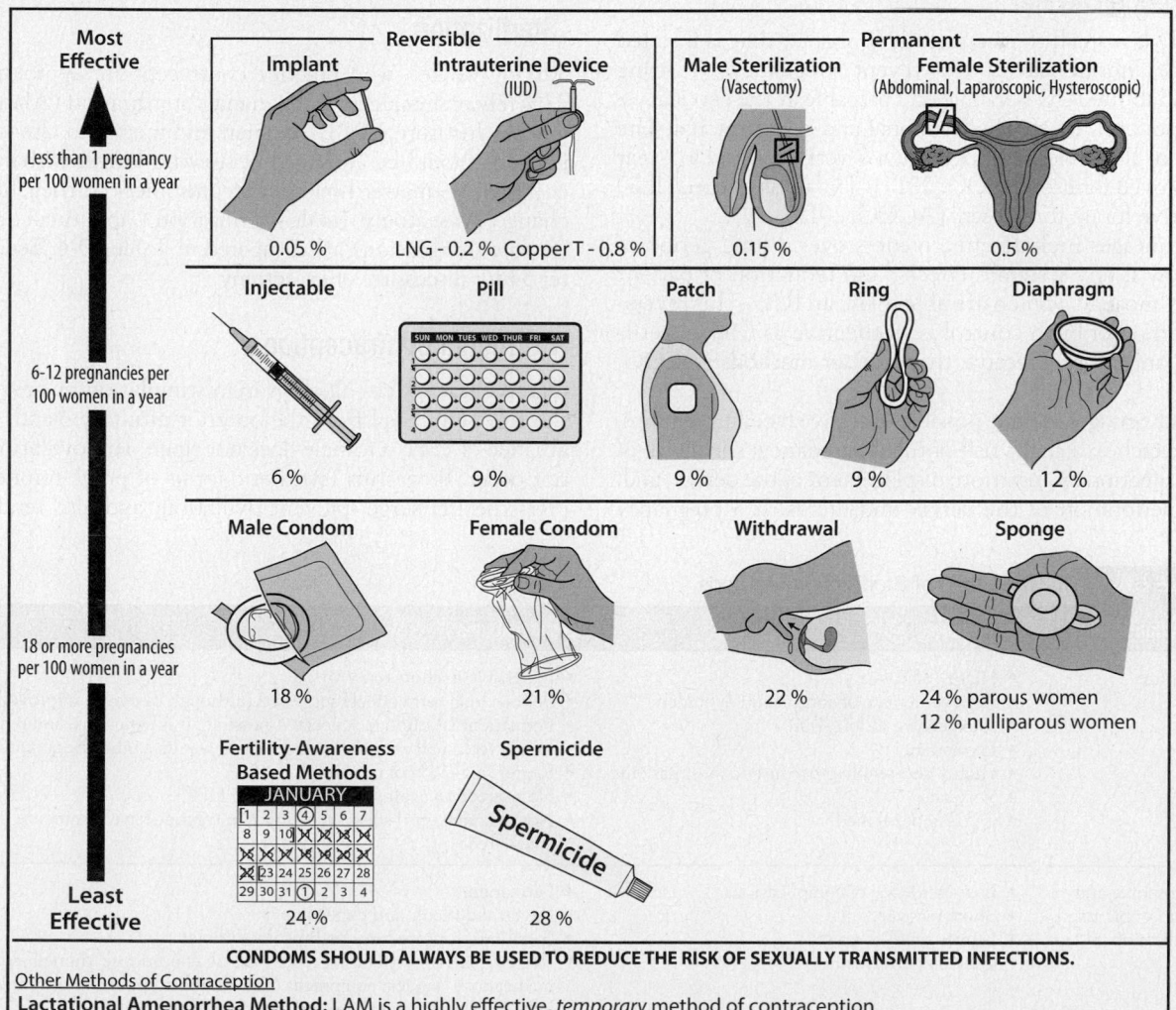

Figure 50-5 • Overview of the effectiveness of select family planning methods. Adapted from Centers for Disease Control and Prevention (CDC). (2016). U.S. selected practice recommendations for contraceptive use, 2016. *Morbidity and Mortality Weekly Report*, 65(4), 1–72.

Abstinence

Abstinence, or celibacy, is the only completely effective means of preventing pregnancy. Abstinence may not be a desired or available option for many women because of cultural expectations and their own and their partner's values and sexual needs.

Long-Acting Reversible Contraceptive (LARC) Methods

Long-acting reversible contraception (LARC) methods are the most effective reversible methods for pregnancy prevention with a failure rate of less than 1% (Moore, Edie, Johnson, et al., 2019). Encouraging the use of LARC methods for appropriate candidates may help lower unintended pregnancy rates in the United States. With few contraindications, the LARC methods should be offered as first-tier contraception to most women (ACOG, 2015 reaffirmed 2018; Moore et al., 2019). LARC methods include the IUD and the single-rod implant (ACOG, 2017).

Intrauterine Device

An IUD is a small device, usually T shaped that is inserted into the uterine cavity to prevent pregnancy. A string attached to the IUD is visible and palpable at the cervical os. Two types of IUDs are the hormonal and nonhormonal. The hormonal IUD releases progestin; a 3-year type and a 5-year are approved for use (ACOG, 2017). The nonhormonal IUD is effective for up to 10 years (ACOG, 2017).

Advantages include effectiveness over a long period of time, few if any systemic effects, and reduction of patient error. Almost all women are able to use an IUD. This reversible method of birth control is as effective as female sterilization and more effective than barrier methods (ACOG, 2017).

Disadvantages include possible excessive bleeding, cramps, and backaches; a slight risk of tubal pregnancy; slight risk of pelvic infection on insertion; displacement of the device; and, rarely, perforation of the cervix and uterus. If a pregnancy occurs with an IUD in place, the device is removed immediately to avoid infection. Spontaneous abortion (miscarriage) may occur on removal (ACOG, 2017).

Implants

One type of single-rod subdermal implant, effective for 3 years, is approved for use in the United States and is usually placed inside the upper arm using a small incision (ACOG, 2017). After implant insertion, changes in menstrual bleeding are common and include amenorrhea or frequent, infrequent, or prolonged bleeding (ACOG, 2017). Women should be warned about possible discomforts that can be treated with NSAIDs. Heavy or prolonged bleeding should be evaluated for an underlying gynecologic problem, such as interactions with other medications, an STI, pregnancy, or new pathologic uterine conditions (e.g., polyps, fibroids) (ACOG, 2017).

Almost all women are able to use the implant, even those who are lactating. The implant is very convenient as once it is in place the patient does not have to do anything else to prevent pregnancy.

Sterilization

Among women who practice contraception, approximately 22% rely on female and 7% on male sterilization (Alan Guttmacher Institute, 2018). Women and men who choose sterilization should be certain that they no longer wish to have children, no matter how the circumstances in their life may change. Vasectomy (male sterilization) and tubal ligation (female sterilization) are compared in Table 50-4. See Chapter 53 for discussion of vasectomy.

Hormonal Contraception

Oral contraceptives block ovarian stimulation by preventing the release of FSH from the anterior pituitary gland. In the absence of FSH, a follicle does not ripen, and ovulation does not occur. Progestins (synthetic forms of progesterone) suppress the LH surge, prevent ovulation, and also render the

TABLE 50-4	Comparison of Sterilization Methods	
Sterilization Method	**Advantages**	**Disadvantages**
Vasectomy	• Highly effective • Relieves female of contraceptive burden • Inexpensive in long run • Permanent • Highly acceptable procedure to most patients • Very safe • Quickly performed	• Expensive in short term • Serious long-term effects suggested (although currently unproved) • Permanent (Although reversal is possible, it is expensive and requires highly technical and major surgery, and results cannot be guaranteed.) • Regret in 5–10% of patients • No protection against STIs, including HIV • Not effective until sperm remaining in reproductive system are ejaculated
Hysteroscopic and laparoscopic tubal sterilization	• Low incidence of complications • Short recovery • Leaves small or no scar • Quickly performed	• Permanent • Reversal difficult and expensive • Sterilization procedures technically difficult • Requires surgeon, operating room (aseptic conditions), trained assistants, medications, surgical equipment. (Essure [insertion of coil or spring in fallopian tubes] requires hysteroscopy rather than surgery.) • Expensive at the time performed • If failure, high probability of ectopic pregnancy • No protection against STIs, including HIV

HIV, human immune deficiency virus; STIs, sexually transmitted infections.

Chart 50-9 PHARMACOLOGY
Benefits and Risks of Hormonal Contraceptives

Benefits

- Highly effective at preventing unintended pregnancy
- Decreased cramps and bleeding
- Decreased incidence of anemia
- Decreased incidence of ectopic pregnancy
- Decreased incidence of pelvic infection
- Protection from benign breast disease
- Protection from uterine and ovarian cancer
- Regular bleeding cycle

Risks

- Bothersome side effects (e.g., breakthrough bleeding, breast tenderness)
- Nausea, weight gain, mood changes
- No protection from sexually transmitted infections (possible increased risk with unsafe sex)
- Possible increased incidence of benign liver tumors and gallbladder disorders
- Small increased risk of developing blood clots, stroke, or heart attack, related more to smoking than to oral contraceptive use alone
- Rare in women who are healthy

Adapted from Casanova, R., Chuang, A., Goepfert, A. R., et al. (Eds.). (2019). *Beckman and Ling's obstetrics and gynecology* (8th ed.). Philadelphia, PA: Wolters Kluwer.

cervical mucus impenetrable to sperm. Hormonal contraceptive agents may be intrauterine, implantable, injectable, oral, transdermal, or intravaginal. (See previous discussion of LARC methods.) These methods contain either a combination of estrogen and progestin or progestin-only. The combined methods include combination oral contraceptives, the transdermal patch, and the intravaginal ring. The progestin-only methods include the intrauterine system, the implant, the injectable, and the "mini-" pill. Hormonal contraception methods work by inhibiting ovulation (with the exception of the mini-pill and the intrauterine system).

Chart 50-9 describes the benefits and risks of hormonal contraceptive use.

Methods of Hormonal Contraception

A wide variety of hormonal methods of birth control are available. Combination methods include the combination of oral contraceptive pills, vaginal ring, and transdermal patch. Progestin-only methods include the progestin-only pills or "mini-pills," once-every-3-month injection, levonorgestrel-releasing intrauterine system, and single-rod subdermal implant (Casanova et al., 2019).

Quality and Safety Nursing Alert

Patients need to be aware that hormonal contraceptives protect them from pregnancy but not from STIs or HIV infection. In addition, sex with multiple partners or sex without a condom may also result in chlamydial and other infections, including HIV infection.

Oral Contraceptives

Many women use oral contraceptive preparations of synthetic estrogens and progestins. A variety of formulations are available. Extended regimens of oral hormonal contraceptive agents are an option for women who have heavy or uncomfortable menstrual bleeding or who wish to have fewer periods. With the use of these regimens, women may have an increased occurrence of breakthrough bleeding; the blood may be dark brown rather than red. It may be more difficult to tell if a pregnancy occurs with this method, although pregnancy is unlikely if pills are taken as prescribed (Casanova et al., 2019).

Transdermal Contraceptives

Transdermal contraception is done through a thin, beige, matchbook-size skin patch that releases an estrogen and a progestin continuously. It is changed every week for 3 weeks, and no patch is used during the fourth week, resulting in withdrawal bleeding. The effectiveness of transdermal contraception is comparable to that of oral contraceptives. Its risks are similar to those of oral contraceptives and include an increased risk of venous thromboemboli formation. The patch may be applied to the torso, chest, arms, or thighs; it should not be applied to the breasts. The patch is convenient and more easily remembered than a daily pill but is not as effective for women who weigh more than 90 kg (198 lb). One additional side effect with the patch includes possible skin reaction such as irritation, redness, pigment changes, or rash at the site of the patch (Casanova et al., 2019).

Vaginal Contraceptives

An etonogestrel/ethinyl estradiol vaginal ring is a combination hormonal contraceptive that releases estrogen and progestin. It is as effective as oral contraceptive agents and results in lower hormone blood levels than oral contraceptives. The ring is flexible, does not require sizing or fitting, and is effective when placed anywhere in the vagina. Patients are occasionally reluctant to consider vaginal methods of contraception unless discussed openly and as a convenient alternative to other routes of administration. Some women are uncomfortable with this method and may fear that the ring may migrate or be uncomfortable or be noticed by a partner. The ring is usually more expensive than oral contraceptives as well.

Injectable Contraceptives

An intramuscular injection of a long-acting progestin every 13 weeks inhibits ovulation and provides a reliable, private, and convenient contraceptive method (Casanova et al., 2019). A subcutaneous formulation is also available. It can be used by women who are lactating and those with hypertension, liver disease, migraine headaches, heart disease, and hemoglobinopathies. With continued use, women must be prepared for irregular bleeding episodes and spotting decrease, or amenorrhea.

Advantages of long-acting progestin include reduction of menorrhagia, dysmenorrhea, and anemia due to heavy menstrual bleeding. It may reduce the risk of pelvic infection, has been associated with improvement in hematologic status in women with sickle cell disease, and does not interfere with the efficacy of seizure agents. It decreases the risk of endometrial cancer, PID, endometriosis, and uterine fibroids (Casanova et al., 2019).

Possible side effects of long-acting progestin include irregular menstrual bleeding, bloating, headaches, hair loss, decreased sex drive, bone loss, and weight loss or weight gain. The contraceptive does not protect against STIs. Although bone loss may occur while using the injections, when the injections are stopped, sometimes all of the bone loss is regained. Use of this method should be limited to 2 years of use because of loss of bone mineral density (Casanova et al., 2019).

Long-acting progestin is contraindicated in women who are pregnant and those who have abnormal vaginal bleeding of unknown cause, breast or pelvic cancer, or sensitivity to synthetic progestin.

Mechanical Barriers

Diaphragm

The diaphragm is an effective contraceptive device that consists of a round, flexible spring (50 to 90 mm wide) covered with a domelike latex rubber cup. A spermicidal (contraceptive) jelly or cream is used to coat the concave side of the diaphragm before it is inserted deep into the vagina, covering the cervix completely. The spermicide inhibits spermatozoa from entering the cervical canal. The diaphragm is not felt by the user or her partner when properly fitted and inserted. Because women vary in size, the diaphragm must be sized and fitted by an experienced clinician. The woman is instructed in using and caring for the device. A return demonstration ensures that the woman can insert the diaphragm correctly and that it covers the cervix.

Each time the woman uses the diaphragm, she should examine it carefully. By holding it up to a bright light, she should ensure that it has no pinpoint holes, cracks, or tears; if any are present, the diaphragm should not be used. She then applies spermicidal jelly or cream and inserts the diaphragm. The diaphragm should remain in place at least 6 hours after coitus (no more than 12 hours). Additional spermicide is necessary if more than 6 hours have passed before penile-vaginal intercourse occurs and before each act of repeated penile-vaginal intercourse. On removal, the diaphragm should be cleansed thoroughly with mild soap and water, rinsed, and dried before being stored in its original container.

Disadvantages include allergic reactions in those who are sensitive to latex and an increased incidence of urinary tract infections. Toxic shock syndrome has been reported in some diaphragm users but is rare.

> ### ▶ *Quality and Safety Nursing Alert*
>
> *The nurse must assess the woman for possible latex allergy because the use of latex barrier methods (e.g., diaphragm, cervical cap, male condoms) may cause severe allergic reactions, including anaphylaxis, in patients with latex allergy.*

Cervical Cap

The cervical cap is much smaller (22 to 35 mm) than the diaphragm and covers only the cervix. If a woman can feel her cervix, she can usually learn to use a cervical cap. The chief advantage is that the cap may be left in place for 2 days after coitus. Although convenient to use, the cervical cap may cause cervical irritation; therefore, before fitting a cap, most primary providers obtain a Pap smear and repeat the smear after 3 months. The cap is used with a spermicide and does not require additional spermicide for repeated penile-vaginal intercourse.

Female Condom

The female condom was developed to give control of barrier protection to women—to provide them with protection from STIs and HIV as well as pregnancy. The female condom consists of a cylinder of polyurethane enclosed at one end by a closed ring that covers the cervix and at the other end by an open ring that covers the perineum (see Fig. 50-6). Advantages include some degree of protection from STIs (i.e., HPV, herpes simplex virus, and HIV) (Casanova et al., 2019). Disadvantages are that female condoms are more costly than male condoms and the inability to use the female condom with some positions (i.e., standing).

Spermicides

Spermicides are made from nonoxynol-9 or octoxynol and are available over the counter as foams, gels, films, suppositories, and sponges and also on condoms. Spermicides do not protect women from HIV or other STIs (Casanova et al., 2019). Advantages of spermicides include they are nonhormonal, are user controlled, do not cause systemic side effects, and are immediately effective (Casanova et al., 2019).

Male Condom

The male condom is an impermeable, snug-fitting cover applied to the erect penis before it enters the vaginal canal. The tip of the condom is pinched while being applied to leave space for ejaculate. If no space is left, ejaculation may cause a tear or hole in the condom and reduce its effectiveness. The penis, with the condom held in place, is removed from the vagina while still erect to prevent the ejaculate from leaking. Condoms are available in large and small sizes.

The latex condom also creates a barrier against transmission of STIs (gonorrhea, chlamydial infection, and HIV) by body fluids and may reduce the risk of herpes virus transmission. However, natural condoms (those made from animal tissue) do not protect against HIV infection. Nurses need to reassure women that they have a right to insist that their male partners use condoms and a right to refuse sex without condoms, although women in abusive relationships may increase their risk of abuse, maltreatment, and neglect by doing so. Some women carry condoms with them to be certain that one is available. Nurses should be familiar and comfortable with instructions about using condoms because many women need to know about this way of protecting themselves from HIV and other STIs. Condoms do not provide complete protection from STIs, however, because HPV may be transmitted by skin-to-skin contact. Other STIs may be transmitted if any abraded skin is exposed to body fluids. This information should be included in patient education.

The nurse needs to consider the possibility of latex allergy. Swelling and itching can also occur. Possible warning signs of latex allergy include oral itching after blowing up a balloon or eating kiwis, bananas, pineapples, passion fruit, avocados,

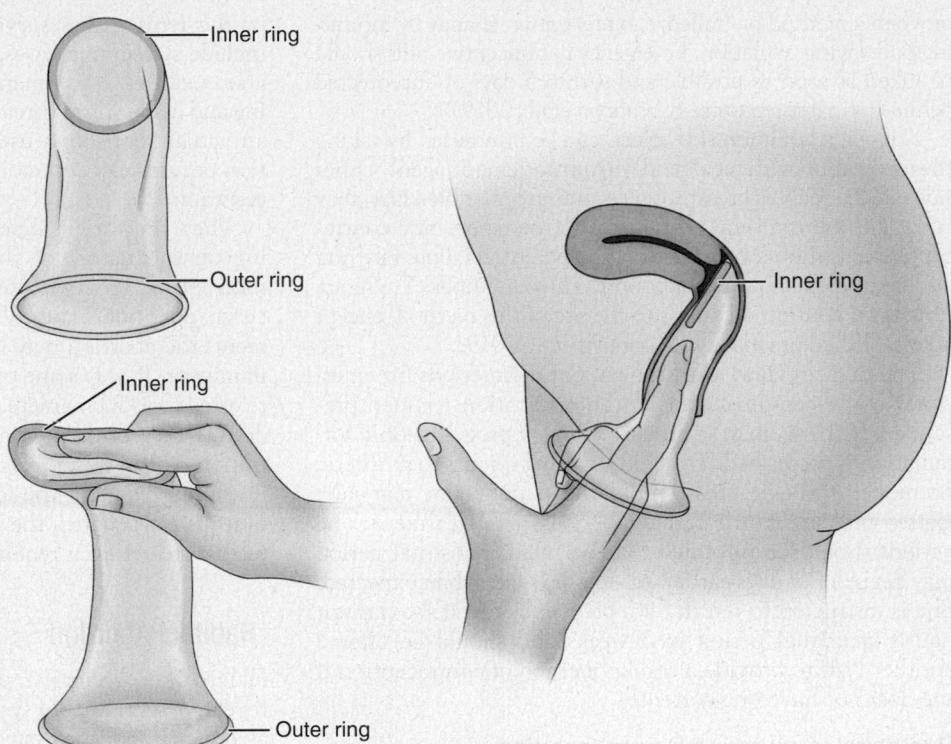

Figure 50-6 • Female condom. To insert the female condom, hold the inner ring between the thumb and middle finger. Put the index finger on the pouch between the thumb and other fingers and squeeze the ring. Slide the condom into the vagina as far as it will go. The inner ring keeps the condom in place.

or chestnuts. Because many contraceptives are made of latex, patients who experience burning or itching while using latex contraceptives are instructed to see their primary provider. Alternatives to latex condoms include the female condom (Reality) and the male condom (Avanti), made of polyurethane.

Coitus Interruptus or Withdrawal

Coitus interruptus (removing the penis from the vagina before ejaculation) requires careful control by the male partner. Although it is a frequently used method of preventing pregnancy and better than no method, it is considered an unreliable method of contraception.

Fertility Awareness–Based Methods

Fertility awareness is knowing and recognizing when the fertile time occurs in the menstrual cycle. If a couple is practicing fertility awareness as a birth control method to prevent pregnancy, the couple needs to avoid having penile-vaginal intercourse or use a barrier method during the fertile period. If the woman would like to get pregnant, the couple should have penile-vaginal intercourse during the women's fertile days. When used to prevent pregnancy, during the first year of typical use, up to 24 women out of 100 will become pregnant (Alan Guttmacher Institute, 2018).

The most common fertility awareness–based method is the Standard Days method. With this method, users must avoid unprotected penile-vaginal intercourse on days 8 to 19 of the menstrual cycle. The Standard Days method requires the woman to determine the fertile days of her cycle. This method works best if the woman has a regular menstrual cycle.

The advantages of using fertility awareness–based methods to prevent pregnancy are that they are safe, inexpensive, and approved by some religions that do not approve of other methods of contraception. The disadvantage is that they require discipline by the couple, who must monitor the menstrual cycle and abstain from penile-vaginal intercourse during the fertile phase.

Ovulation detection methods are available in most pharmacies. The presence of the enzyme guaiacol peroxidase in cervical mucus signals ovulation 6 days beforehand and also affects mucosal viscosity. Over-the-counter test kits are easy to use and reliable but can be expensive. Ovulation prediction kits are more effective for planning conception than for avoiding it.

Emergency Contraception

Emergency contraception are methods that can be used by women after unprotected penile-vaginal intercourse to prevent pregnancy (Casanova et al., 2019). Nurses need to be aware of emergency contraception as an option for women and the indications for its use. It is clearly not suitable for long-term avoidance of pregnancy because it is not as effective as oral contraceptives or other reliable methods used regularly. However, it is valuable following penile-vaginal intercourse when a pregnancy is not intended and in emergency situations such as rape, a defective or torn condom or diaphragm, or other situations that may result in unintended conception.

Methods of Emergency Contraception
Emergency Contraceptive Pills

Three kinds of emergency contraceptive pills are available in the United States. A properly timed, adequate dose of medication after penile-vaginal intercourse without effective contraception, or when a method has failed, can prevent pregnancy by inhibiting or delaying ovulation. Emergency contraceptive pills should be taken as soon as possible and within 5 days of unprotected penile-vaginal intercourse (Casanova et al., 2019).

Nausea, a common side effect, can be minimized by taking the medication with meals and with an antiemetic agent. Other side effects, such as breast soreness and irregular bleeding, may occur but are transient. Patients who use emergency contraceptive pills should be advised of the potential failure rate and also counseled about other contraceptive methods. There are no known contraindications to the use of this method, except an established pregnancy (Casanova et al, 2019).

The nurse reviews with the patient instructions for emergency contraception based on the medication regimen prescribed. If the woman is breast-feeding, a progestin-only formulation is prescribed. To avoid exposing infants to synthetic hormones through breast milk, the patient can manually express milk and bottle-feed for 24 hours after treatment. The patient should be informed that her next menstrual period may begin a few days earlier or a few days later than expected. She is instructed to return for a pregnancy test if she has not had a menstrual period in 3 weeks and should be offered another visit to provide a regular method of contraception if she does not have one currently.

Postcoital Intrauterine Device Insertion

Postcoital IUD insertion, another form of emergency contraception, involves insertion of a copper-bearing IUD within 5 days of coitus (Casanova et al., 2019). The copper-bearing IUD prevents fertilization by causing a chemical change in sperm and egg before they can meet. The patient may experience discomfort on insertion and may have heavier menstrual periods and increased cramping. Contraindications include a confirmed or suspected pregnancy or any contraindication to regular IUD use. The patient must be informed that there is a risk that insertion of an IUD may disrupt a pregnancy that is already present.

Nursing Management

Patients who use emergency contraception may be anxious, embarrassed, and lacking information about birth control. The nurse must be supportive and nonjudgmental and provide facts and appropriate patient education. If the patient repeatedly uses this method of birth control, she should be informed that the failure rate with this method is higher than with a regularly used method. Nurses can educate and inform women about emergency contraception options to reduce unintended pregnancies and abortions. See the Resources section at the end of this chapter for more information.

Abortion

Interruption of pregnancy or expulsion of the product of conception before the fetus is viable is called *abortion*. The fetus is generally considered to be viable any time after the fifth to sixth month of gestation.

Spontaneous Abortion

It is estimated that 1 of every 5 to 10 conceptions ends in spontaneous abortion. Most of these occur because an abnormality in the fetus makes survival impossible. Other causes may include systemic diseases, hormonal imbalance, or anatomic abnormalities. If a woman who is pregnant experiences bleeding and cramping, a threatened abortion is diagnosed because an actual abortion is usually imminent. Spontaneous abortion occurs most commonly in the second or third month of gestation.

There are various types of spontaneous abortion, depending on the nature of the process (threatened, inevitable, incomplete, or complete). In a threatened abortion, the cervix does not dilate. With bed rest and conservative treatment, the abortion may be prevented. If not, an abortion is imminent. If only some of the tissue is passed, the abortion is referred to as incomplete. An emptying or evacuation procedure (D&C, or dilation and evacuation [D&E]) or administration of oral misoprostol is usually required to remove the remaining tissue. If the fetus and all related tissue are spontaneously evacuated, the abortion is termed *complete*, and no further treatment is required.

Habitual Abortion

Habitual or recurrent abortion is defined as successive, repeated, spontaneous abortions of unknown cause. As many as 60% of abortions may result from chromosomal anomalies (Casanova et al., 2019). After two consecutive abortions, the patient is referred for genetic counseling and testing, and other possible causes are explored.

If bleeding occurs in a woman who is pregnant with a past history of habitual abortion, conservative measures, such as bed rest and administration of progesterone to support the endometrium, are attempted to save the pregnancy. Supportive counseling is crucial in this stressful condition. Bed rest, sexual abstinence, a light diet, and no straining on defecation may be recommended in an effort to prevent spontaneous abortion. If infection is suspected, antibiotic agents may be prescribed.

In the condition known as incompetent or dysfunctional cervix, the cervix dilates painlessly in the second trimester of pregnancy, often resulting in a spontaneous abortion. In such cases, a surgical procedure called *cervical cerclage* may be used to prevent the cervix from dilating prematurely. It involves placing a purse-string suture around the cervix at the level of the internal os (Casanova et al., 2019). Bed rest is usually advised to keep the weight of the uterus off the cervix. About 2 to 3 weeks before term or at the onset of labor, the suture is cut. Delivery is usually by cesarean section.

Medical Management

After a spontaneous abortion, all tissue passed vaginally is saved for examination, if possible. The patient and all personnel who care for her are alerted to save any discharged material. In the rare case of heavy bleeding, the patient may require blood component transfusions and fluid replacement. An estimate of the bleeding volume can be determined by recording the number of perineal pads and the degree of saturation over 24 hours. When an incomplete abortion occurs, oxytocin may be prescribed to cause uterine contractions before D&E or uterine suctioning.

Nursing Management

Because patients experience loss and anxiety, emotional support and understanding are important aspects of nursing care. Women may be grieving or relieved, depending on their feelings about the pregnancy. Providing opportunities for the patient to talk and express her emotions is helpful and also provides clues for the nurse in planning more specific care.

Induced Abortion

A voluntary induced termination of pregnancy is performed by skilled health care providers. Decisions about abortion reside with a woman and her primary provider in the first trimester. During the second trimester, the state may regulate practice in the interest of a woman's health and during the final weeks of pregnancy may choose to protect the life of the fetus, except when necessary to preserve the life or health of the woman.

In the United States, 42% of all unintended pregnancies were terminated by abortion (Allan Guttmacher Institute, 2018). These numbers indicate the need for effective contraceptive education, information about emergency contraception, and counseling.

Medical Management

Before the abortion procedure is performed (see Chart 50-10), a nurse or counselor trained in pregnancy counseling should talk with the patient and explore her fears, feelings, and options. The nurse then identifies the patient's choice (i.e., continuing pregnancy and parenthood, continuing pregnancy followed by adoption, or terminating pregnancy by abortion). If abortion is chosen, the patient has a pelvic examination to determine uterine size. A pelvic ultrasound may also be performed. Laboratory studies before an abortion must include a pregnancy test to confirm the pregnancy, hematocrit to rule out anemia, and Rh determination. Patients with anemia will require an iron supplement, and patients who are Rh negative may require Rho(D) immune globulin (RhoGAM) to prevent isoimmunization. Before the procedure, all patients should be screened for STIs to prevent introducing pathogens upward through the cervix during the procedure.

Chart 50-10 Types of Induced Abortions

Vacuum Aspiration

- The cervix is dilated manually with instrumentation or by laminaria (small suppositories made of seaweed that swells as it absorbs water).
- A uterine aspirator is introduced.
- Suction is applied, and tissue is removed from the uterus.

This is the most common type of termination procedure and is used early in pregnancy, up to 14 weeks. Laminaria may be used to soften and dilate the cervix prior to the procedure.

Dilation and Evacuation

Cervical dilation with laminaria followed by vacuum aspiration

Labor Induction

These procedures account for fewer than 1% of all terminations and generally take place in an inpatient setting.

1. Installation of normal saline or urea results in uterine contractions.
   - Although rare, serious complications can occur, including cardiovascular collapse, cerebral edema, pulmonary edema, kidney disease, and disseminated intravascular coagulopathy.
2. Prostaglandins
   - Prostaglandins are introduced into the amniotic fluid or by vaginal suppository or intramuscular injection in later pregnancy.
   - Strong uterine contractions begin within 4 hours and usually result in abortion.
   - Gastrointestinal side effects (e.g., nausea, vomiting, diarrhea, and abdominal cramping) and fever can occur.
3. IV oxytocin
   - Used for later abortions for genetic indications. Requires patient to go through labor.

Medical Abortion

Mifepristone

- Mifepristone is a progesterone antagonist that prevents implantation of the ovum.
- Given orally within 10 days of an expected menstrual period, mifepristone produces a medical abortion in most patients.
- Combined with a prostaglandin suppository, mifepristone causes abortion in up to 95% of patients.
- Prolonged bleeding may occur. Other side effects may include abdominal pain, nausea, vomiting, and diarrhea. This method may not be used in women with adrenal failure, asthma, long-term corticosteroid therapy, an intrauterine device in place, porphyria, or a history of allergy to mifepristone or other prostaglandins. It is less effective when used in pregnancies more than 49 days from the beginning of the last menstrual period.

Methotrexate

- Methotrexate has also been used to terminate pregnancy because it is lethal to the fetus. It has been found to have minimal risk and few side effects in the woman. Its low cost may provide an alternative for some women.

Misoprostol

- Misoprostol is a synthetic prostaglandin analog that produces cervical effacement and uterine contractions.
- Inserted vaginally, misoprostol is effective in terminating a pregnancy in about 75% of cases.
- When combined with methotrexate or mifepristone, misoprostol's effectiveness rate is high.

Adapted from Bartz, D. A., & Blumenthal, P. D. (2019). First-trimester pregnancy termination: Medical abortion. *UpToDate*. Retrieved on 12/8/2019 at: www.uptodate.com/contents/first-trimester-pregnancy-termination-medication-abortion; Hammond, C. (2019). Second-trimester pregnancy termination: Induction (medication) termination. *UpToDate*. Retrieved on 5/12/2020 at: www.uptodate.com/contents/second-trimester-pregnancy-termination-induction-medication-termination; Shih, G., & Wallace, R. (2020). First-trimester pregnancy termination: Uterine aspiration. *UpToDate*. Retrieved on 5/12/2020 at: www.uptodate.com/contents/first-trimester-pregnancy-termination-uterine-aspiration

> ### ◄ Quality and Safety Nursing Alert
>
> *Women who have resorted to unskilled attempts to end a pregnancy may become critically ill because of infection, hemorrhage, or uterine rupture. If a woman has undergone such efforts to end a pregnancy, prompt medical attention, broad-spectrum antibiotics, and replacement of fluids and blood components may be required before careful attempts are made to evacuate the uterus.*

Surgical terminations include D&C or vacuum aspiration of uterine contents. Medications can also be used. Mifepristone is used only in early pregnancy (up to 49 days from the last menstrual period). It works by blocking progesterone. Cramping and bleeding similar to a heavy menstrual period occur. After counseling and consent and often a sonogram to confirm the pregnancy, mifepristone is given. This is followed by a dose of misoprostol orally or vaginally. If the pregnancy persists, a suction aspiration is performed. Contraindications include ectopic pregnancy, adrenal failure, allergy to the medications, bleeding disorder, irritable bowel syndrome, or uncontrolled seizure disorders. Several deaths from sepsis have occurred following medical abortion; researchers and the FDA are closely monitoring the morbidity and mortality associated with medical abortion. Medical and surgical abortions used in the first trimester are both highly effective with low complication rates (Bartz & Blumenthal, 2019).

Nursing Management

Patient education is an important aspect of care for women who elect to terminate a pregnancy. A patient undergoing induced abortion is informed about what the procedure entails and the expected course after the procedure. The patient is scheduled for a follow-up appointment 2 weeks after the procedure and is instructed about signs and symptoms (i.e., fever, heavy bleeding, or pain) that should be reported.

Available contraceptive methods are reviewed with the patient. Effectiveness depends on the method used and the extent to which the woman and her partner follow the instructions for use. A woman who has used any method of birth control should be assessed for her understanding of the method and its potential side effects as well as her satisfaction with the method. If the woman has not been using contraception, the nurse explains all methods and their benefits and risks and helps the patient make a contraceptive choice for use after abortion. Related education issues, such as the need to use barrier contraceptive devices (i.e., condoms) for protection against transmission of STIs and HIV infection and the availability of emergency contraception, are also important.

Psychological support is another important aspect of nursing care. The nurse needs to be aware that women terminate pregnancies for many reasons. Some women terminate pregnancies because of severe genetic defects. Women who have been raped or impregnated in incestuous relationships or by an abusive partner may elect to terminate their pregnancies. The care of a woman undergoing termination of pregnancy is stressful, and assistance needs to be provided in a safe and nonjudgmental way. Nurses have the right to refuse to participate in a procedure that is against their religious beliefs but are professionally obligated not to impose their beliefs or judgments on their patients.

Infertility

In the United States, infertility affects approximately 1 in 8 couples between ages 15 and 44 (over 7 million women) and is defined as a couple's inability to achieve pregnancy after 1 year of unprotected penile-vaginal intercourse (Lee, 2019). Primary infertility refers to a couple who has never had a child. Secondary infertility means that at least one conception has occurred, but currently the couple cannot achieve a pregnancy. It is often a complex physical problem and causes are related to endometriosis, uterine factors, anovulation, tubal obstruction, and male factors.

Diagnostic Findings

Ovarian and Ovulation Factors

Diagnostic studies performed to determine if ovulation is regular and whether the progestational endometrium is adequate for implantation may include a serum progesterone level and an ovulation index. The ovulation index involves a urine dipstick test to determine whether the surge in LH that precedes follicular rupture has occurred.

Tubal and Uterine Factors

HSG is used to rule out uterine or tubal abnormalities. A contrast agent injected into the uterus through the cervix produces an outline of the shape of the uterine cavity and the patency of the tubes. This process sometimes removes mucus or tissue that is lodged in the tubes. Laparoscopy permits direct visualization of the tubes and other pelvic structures and can assist in identifying conditions that may interfere with fertility (e.g., endometriosis).

Fibroids, polyps, and congenital malformations are possible causative factors affecting the uterus. Their presence may be determined by pelvic examination, hysteroscopy, saline sonogram (a variation of a sonogram), and HSG. Endometriosis, even if mild, is associated with reduced fertility (Schenken, 2019).

Male Factors

An analysis of semen provides information about the number of sperm (density), percentage of moving forms, quality of forward movement (forward progression), and morphology (shape and form). From 2 to 6 mL of watery alkaline semen is normal. A normal count has 60 to 100 million sperm/mL. However, the incidence of impregnation is lessened only when the count decreases to fewer than 15 million sperm/mL (Anawat & Page, 2019).

Men may also be affected by varicoceles (varicose veins around the testicle), which decrease semen quality by increasing testicular temperature. Retrograde ejaculation or ejaculation into the bladder is assessed by urinalysis after ejaculation. Blood tests for male partners may include measuring testosterone, FSH, and LH (both of which are involved in maintaining testicular function), and prolactin levels (Anawat & Page, 2019).

Medical Management

The treatment of infertility is complex and often requires advanced technology. The specific type of treatment depends on the cause of the problem, if it can be identified. Many couples with infertility have normal test results for ovulation, sperm production, and fallopian tube patency.

Ovulatory dysfunction is complex, but many women with ovulation disorders have polycystic ovary syndrome (see Chapter 51) and may be treated with 5 days of clomiphene to induce ovulation (Comerford & Durkin, 2020). Insulin sensitizing agents are sometimes used, and once insulin levels are normalized, ovulation often occurs. Some women have high prolactin levels, which inhibit ovulation, and they are treated with dopaminergic drugs after a pituitary adenoma is ruled out by MRI. If a woman has premature ovarian failure, oocyte donation may be considered.

Pharmacologic Therapy

Pharmacologically induced ovulation is undertaken when women do not ovulate on their own or ovulate irregularly. These couples are often treated with clomiphene to stimulate ovulation. Gonadotropin treatment may also be used if conception does not occur. Various other medications are used, depending on the main cause of infertility (see Chart 50-11).

Blood tests and ultrasounds are used to monitor ovulation. Multiple pregnancies (i.e., twins, triplets, or more) may occur with the use of these medications. Ovarian hyperstimulation syndrome (OHSS) may also occur. This condition is characterized by enlarged multicystic ovaries and is complicated by a shift of fluid from the intravascular space into the abdominal cavity. The fluid shift can result in ascites, pleural effusion, and edema; hypovolemia may also occur. Risk factors include younger age, history of polycystic ovarian syndrome, high serum estradiol levels, a larger number of follicles, and pregnancy.

Artificial Insemination

Artificial insemination is the deposit of semen into the female genital tract by artificial means. If the sperm cannot penetrate the cervical canal normally, artificial insemination using a partner's or husband's semen or that of a donor may be considered. When the sperm of the woman's partner is defective or absent (azoospermia) or when there is a risk of transmitting a genetic disease, donor sperm may be used. Safeguards are put in place to address legal, ethical, emotional, and religious issues. Written consent is obtained to protect all parties involved, including the woman, the donor, and the resulting child. The donor's semen is frozen, and the donor is evaluated to ensure that he is free of genetic disorders and STIs, including HIV infection (Ginsburg & Srouji, 2019).

Conditions must be optimal for conception before semen is transferred to the vagina or uterus. The woman must have no abnormalities of the genital system, the fallopian tubes must be patent, and ova must be available. In the male, sperm need to be normal in shape, amount, motility, and endurance. The time of ovulation should be determined as accurately as possible so that the 2 or 3 days during which fertilization is possible each month can be targeted for the treatment.

Ultrasonography and blood studies of varying hormone levels are used to pinpoint the best time for insemination and to monitor for OHSS. Fertilization seldom occurs from

Chart 50-11	PHARMACOLOGY

Medications That Induce Ovulation

- Clomiphene citrate is an estrogen antagonist that increases gonadotropin release, resulting in follicular rupture or ovulation. Clomiphene is used when the hypothalamus is not stimulating the pituitary gland to release follicle-stimulating hormone (FSH) and luteinizing hormone (LH). This medication stimulates follicles in the ovary. It is usually taken for 5 days beginning on the 5th day of the menstrual cycle. Ovulation should occur 4 to 8 days after the last dose. Patients receive instructions about timing penile-vaginal intercourse to facilitate fertilization.
- Menotropins, a combination of FSH and LH, may be used to stimulate the ovaries to produce eggs. These agents are used for women with deficiencies in FSH and LH. When followed by administration of human chorionic gonadotropin, menotropins stimulates the ovaries, so monitoring by ultrasound and hormone levels is essential because overstimulation may occur.
- Follitropin alfa, follitropin beta, and urofollitropin may be used to treat ovulation disorders or to stimulate a follicle and egg production for intrauterine insemination or in vitro fertilization or other assisted reproductive technologies.
- Gonadotropin-releasing hormone agonists (leuprolide, nafarelin acetate) suppress FSH, prevent premature egg release, and shrink fibroids.
- Bromocriptine may be used in treatment for infertility due to elevated prolactin levels.
- Progesterone vaginal suppositories help improve the uterine lining after ovulation.
- Urofollitropin, which contains FSH with a small amount of LH, is used in some disorders (e.g., polycystic ovarian syndrome) to stimulate follicle growth. Clomiphene is then used to stimulate ovulation.
- Chorionic gonadotropin, which mimics LH, releases an egg after hyperstimulation and supports the corpus luteum.
- Metformin may be used in polycystic ovarian syndrome to induce regular ovulation.
- Aspirin and heparin may be used to prevent recurrent pregnancy loss in patients with elevated antiphospholipid antibodies.

Adapted from Comerford, K. C., & Durkin, M. T. (2020). *Nursing 2020 drug handbook*. Philadelphia, PA: Wolters Kluwer.

a single insemination. Usually, insemination is attempted between days 10 and 17 of the cycle; three different attempts may be made during one cycle. The woman may have received clomiphene or other medications to stimulate ovulation before insemination. The recipient is placed in the lithotomy position on the examination table, a speculum is inserted, and the vagina and cervix are swabbed with a cotton-tipped applicator to remove any excess secretions. The sperm are washed before insertion to remove biochemicals and to select the most active sperm. Semen is drawn into a sterile syringe, and a cannula is attached. The semen is then directed to the external os. In intrauterine insemination, semen is placed into the uterine cavity.

Assisted Reproductive Technologies

Assisted reproductive technologies include in vitro fertilization (IVF) and its modifications. Currently, between 1% and 3% of all live births each year in the United States are achieved through assisted technology (Paulson, 2019).

IVF refers to a set of procedures that, if successful, results in a pregnancy. These procedures involve ovarian stimulation, egg retrieval, fertilization, and embryo transfer. The ovaries are stimulated to produce multiple eggs or ova, usually with medications, because success rates are greater with more than one embryo. Many different protocols exist for inducing ovulation with one or more agents (Paulson, 2019). Patients are carefully selected and evaluated, and cycles are carefully monitored using ultrasound and monitoring hormone levels. At the appropriate time, the ova are recovered by transvaginal ultrasound retrieval. Sperm and eggs are coincubated for up to 36 hours, and the embryos are transferred about 48 hours after retrieval. Implantation should occur in 3 to 5 days.

Gamete intrafallopian transfer (GIFT), a variation of IVF, is the treatment of choice for patients with ovarian failure. GIFT is considered in unexplained infertility and when there is religion-based discomfort with IVF. The most common indications for IVF and GIFT are irreparable tubal damage, endometriosis (see Chapter 51), unexplained infertility, inadequate sperm, and exposure to diethylstilbestrol. Success rates for GIFT are similar to those for IVF (Paulson, 2019).

Additional Assisted Reproductive Technologies

In intracytoplasmic sperm injection (ICSI), an ovum is retrieved, and a single sperm is injected through the zona pellucida, through the egg membrane, into the cytoplasm of the oocyte. The fertilized egg is then transferred back to the donor. ICSI is the treatment of choice in severe male factor infertility.

Women who cannot produce their own eggs (i.e., premature ovarian failure) have the option of using the eggs of a donor after stimulation of the donor's ovaries. The recipient also receives hormones in preparation for these procedures. Couples may also choose this modality if the female partner has a genetic disorder that may be passed on to children.

Tubal embryo transfer (TET) involves the placement of fertilized eggs or embryos into the fallopian tube. A laparoscopic procedure is needed to place the embryos in the fallopian tubes. Some women choose TET after IVF failure (Paulson, 2019).

Nursing Management

Nursing interventions when working with couples during infertility evaluations include assisting in reducing stress in the relationship, encouraging cooperation, protecting privacy, fostering understanding, and referring the couple to appropriate resources when necessary. Because infertility evaluations and treatments are expensive, time-consuming, invasive, stressful, and not always successful, couples need support in working together to deal with this process (Stevenson, Cebert, & Silva, 2019) (see the Nursing research Profile in Chart 50-12).

Smoking cessation is encouraged because smoking, smokeless tobacco, electronic nicotine delivery systems (ENDS) including e-cigarettes, e-pens, e-pipes, e-hookah, and e-cigars, have an adverse effect on the success of assisted reproduction (Rodriguez, 2020). Diet, exercise, stress reduction techniques, folic acid supplementation, health maintenance, and disease prevention are emphasized in many infertility programs. Couples may also consider adoption, child-free living, and gestational carriers (the use of a surrogate to carry the fetus for the couple with infertility). Nurses can be helpful listeners and information resources in these deliberations.

Preconception/Periconception Health Care

Nurses can be instrumental in encouraging all women of childbearing age, including those with chronic illness or disabilities, to consider issues that may affect health during pregnancy (Lammers, Hulme, Wey, et al., 2017). Preconception health care is a concept that expands on the definition of prenatal care to include the time before conception

---

Chart 50-12 · NURSING RESEARCH PROFILE

Stress and Anxiety in Couples Who Conceive via In Vitro Fertilization

Stevenson, E. L., Cebert, M., & Silva, S. (2019). Stress and anxiety in couples who conceive via In Vitro fertilization compared with those who conceive spontaneously. *Journal of Obstetric, Gynecologic and Neonatal Nursing, 48*(6), 635–644.

Purpose

Infertility, which impacts roughly 15% of couples worldwide, is a stressful event for couples. Few studies have examined the continued stress and anxiety experienced after successful in vitro fertilization (IVF). Even less investigated is the partners' experience during infertility and IVF. The aim of this pilot study was to examine the levels of stress and anxiety of women and their partners who conceived via IVF compared with each other, as well as compared to couples who conceived spontaneously.

Design

The longitudinal, descriptive pilot study enrolled 48 women and their partners (*n* = 96). The 22 couples (*n* = 44) who conceived by IVF and 26 (*n* = 52) couples who conceived spontaneously were recruited from 2 fertility clinics and a well women clinic throughout the northeast and southeast United States. Participants were

asked to complete three instruments during each trimester of pregnancy to measure the perceptual and emotional response components of stress and anxiety.

Results

The analysis of the instruments across the 3 trimesters showed significant differences between women and their male partners. All women showed greater levels of stress and anxiety during each trimester compared to their male partners. Anxiety was not consistent throughout the pregnancy, showing a gradual decline as the pregnancy progressed. The study also reported no significant difference in the levels of stress and anxiety between couples who conceived by IVF and those who conceived spontaneously.

Nursing Implications

It is imperative that nurses and other professionals recognize the impact infertility can have on a couple's level of stress and anxiety. In addition to care of the couple, nurses need to care for the individual, taking into full account the differences in experiences of the woman and her partner during the pregnancy.

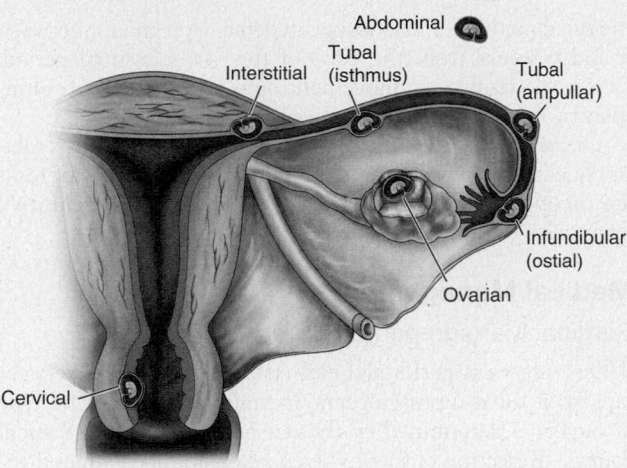

Figure 50-7 • Sites of ectopic pregnancy.

(Lammers et al., 2017). Women who plan their pregnancies and are healthy and well informed tend to have better outcomes. There are currently nine consensus recommendations for advancing preconception health (see Chart 50-13).

Nurses can make a difference in preconception health through education and counseling. Women who use tobacco products, by smoking or ENDS, should be encouraged to stop their use; it may help to offer cessation classes. Women should take folic acid supplements to prevent neural tube defects. Women with diabetes should have good glycemic control prior to conception. It is necessary to assess rubella immunity and other immunizations as well as a family history of genetic defects; genetic counseling may be appropriate. Women taking teratogenic medications and women concerned about genetic disorders should be encouraged to discuss effective contraception and childbearing plans with their primary provider (see Chart 50-2).

Ectopic Pregnancy

The incidence of ectopic pregnancy and the risk of death due to ectopic pregnancy are decreasing. However, ectopic pregnancy remains the leading cause of pregnancy-related death in the first trimester (ACOG, 2018). Ectopic pregnancy occurs when a fertilized ovum (a blastocyst) becomes implanted on any tissue other than the uterine lining, most commonly along the fallopian tube (ACOG, 2018) (see Fig. 50-7).

Possible causes of ectopic pregnancy include salpingitis, peritubal adhesions (after pelvic infection, endometriosis, appendicitis), structural abnormalities of the fallopian tube, previous ectopic pregnancy, previous tubal surgery, multiple previous induced abortions, and tumors that distort the tube (ACOG, 2018). Additional risk factors include use of tobacco products, IUD use, history of PID, and use of fertility drugs to induce ovulation (ACOG, 2018).

Risk factors are important, but all women need to be educated about early treatment and have a high index of suspicion in the case of a period that does not seem normal, the presence of pain, or pain with a suspected pregnancy. Women may have fatal hemorrhage with ruptured ectopic pregnancies if they delay seeking attention or if their primary providers are not alert to the possibility of this diagnosis.

Clinical Manifestations

Signs and symptoms vary depending on whether tubal rupture has occurred. Delay in menstruation from 1 to 2 weeks followed by slight bleeding (spotting) or a report of a slightly abnormal period suggests the possibility of an ectopic pregnancy. Symptoms may begin late, with vague soreness on the affected side (probably due to uterine contractions and distention of the tube), and may proceed to sharp, colicky pain. Most patients experience some pelvic or abdominal pain and some spotting or bleeding. Gastrointestinal symptoms, dizziness, or lightheadedness may occur. Patients may think the abnormal bleeding is a menstrual period, especially if a recent period occurred and was normal.

If implantation occurs in the fallopian tube, the tube becomes more and more distended and can rupture if the ectopic pregnancy remains undetected for 4 to 6 weeks or longer after conception. When the tube ruptures, the ovum is discharged into the abdominal cavity, and the woman experiences agonizing pain, dizziness, faintness, and nausea and vomiting due to the peritoneal reaction to blood escaping from the tube. Dyspnea and symptoms of shock may occur, and the signs of hemorrhage—rapid and thready pulse, decreased blood pressure, subnormal temperature, restlessness, pallor, and sweating—are evident. Later, the pain becomes generalized in the abdomen and radiates to the shoulder and neck because of accumulating intraperitoneal blood that irritates the diaphragm.

Assessment and Diagnostic Findings

Ectopic pregnancies must be diagnosed promptly to prevent life-threatening hemorrhage, which is the major complication of rupture. During vaginal examination, a large mass of clotted blood that has collected in the pelvis behind the uterus or a tender adnexal mass may be palpable, although there are often no abnormal findings. If an ectopic pregnancy is suspected, the patient is evaluated by sonography and human chorionic gonadotropin (hCG) levels. Serial hCG tests may be needed (Tulandi, 2019). The levels of hCG (the diagnostic hormone of pregnancy) double in early normal pregnancies every 3 days but are reduced in abnormal or ectopic pregnancies. A less-than-normal increase is cause for suspicion. Transvaginal ultrasound, the usual method of diagnosis, can detect a pregnancy between 5 and 6 weeks from the time of the last menstrual period. Detectable fetal heart movement outside the uterus on ultrasound is firm evidence of an ectopic pregnancy.

Occasionally, the clinical picture makes the diagnosis relatively easy. However, when the clinical signs and symptoms are inconclusive, laparoscopy may be required for definitive diagnosis (Tulandi, 2019).

Medical Management

Surgical Management

When surgery is performed early, almost all patients recover rapidly; if tubal rupture occurs, mortality increases. The type of surgery is determined by the size and extent of local tubal damage. Resection of the involved fallopian tube with end-to-end anastomosis may be effective. Some surgeons attempt to salvage the tube with a salpingotomy, which involves opening and evacuating the tube and controlling bleeding. More extensive surgery includes salpingectomy (removing the tube alone) or salpingo-oophorectomy (removing the tube and ovary).

Pharmacologic Therapy

Another option is the use of methotrexate without surgery (ACOG, 2018). Because methotrexate stops the pregnancy from progressing by interfering with DNA synthesis and the multiplication of cells, it interrupts early, small, unruptured ectopic pregnancies. The patient must be hemodynamically stable; have no active renal or hepatic disease; have no evidence of thrombocytopenia or leukopenia; and have a very small, unruptured ectopic pregnancy on ultrasound. Other indications may include no fetal cardiac activity and no active abdominal bleeding. Methotrexate is occasionally used to eliminate residual ectopic pregnancy tissue following a laparoscopy (ACOG, 2018).

NURSING PROCESS

The Patient with an Ectopic Pregnancy

Assessment

The health history includes the menstrual pattern and any (even slight) bleeding since the last menstrual period. The nurse elicits the patient's description of pain and its location. The nurse asks the patient whether any sharp, colicky pains have occurred and whether pain radiates to the shoulder and neck (possibly caused by rupture and pressure on the diaphragm).

In addition, the nurse monitors vital signs, level of consciousness, and the nature and amount of vaginal bleeding. If possible, the nurse assesses how the patient is coping with the abnormal pregnancy and likely loss.

Diagnosis

NURSING DIAGNOSES

Based on the assessment data, major nursing diagnoses may include the following:

- Acute pain associated with the progression of the ectopic pregnancy
- Grief associated with the loss of pregnancy and anticipatory effect on future pregnancies

- Lack of knowledge associated with the treatment and effect on future pregnancies

COLLABORATIVE PROBLEMS/POTENTIAL COMPLICATIONS

Potential complications may include:
- Hemorrhage
- Hemorrhagic shock

Planning and Goals

The major goals may include relief of pain; acceptance and resolution of grief and pregnancy loss; increased knowledge about ectopic pregnancy, its treatment, and its outcome; and absence of complications.

Nursing Interventions

RELIEVING PAIN

The abdominal pain associated with ectopic pregnancy may be described as cramping or severe continuous pain. If the patient is to have surgery, preanesthetic medications may provide pain relief. Postoperatively, analgesic agents are given liberally; this promotes early ambulation and enables the patient to cough and take deep breaths.

SUPPORTING THE GRIEVING PROCESS

Patients experience varying levels of distress. If the pregnancy was desired, loss may or may not be expressed verbally by the patient and her partner. The impact may not be fully realized until much later. The nurse should be available to listen and provide support. The patient's partner, if appropriate, should participate in this process. Even if the pregnancy was unintended, a loss has been experienced, and a grief reaction may occur.

MONITORING AND MANAGING POTENTIAL COMPLICATIONS

Potential complications of ectopic pregnancy are hemorrhage and shock. Careful assessment is essential to detect the development of these complications. Continuous monitoring of vital signs, level of consciousness, amount of bleeding, and intake and output provide information about the possibility of hemorrhage and the need to prepare for IV therapy. Bed rest is indicated. Hematocrit, hemoglobin, and blood gases are monitored to assess hematologic status and adequacy of tissue perfusion. Significant deviations in these laboratory values are reported immediately, and the patient is prepared for possible surgery. Blood component therapy may be required if blood loss has been rapid and extensive. If hypovolemic shock occurs, the treatment is directed toward reestablishing tissue perfusion and adequate blood volume. See Chapter 11 for a discussion of the IV fluids and medications used in treating shock.

The nurse has an important role in prevention by being alert to patients with abnormal bleeding who may be at risk for an ectopic pregnancy and referring them immediately for care. It is necessary to keep a high index of suspicion in daily practice when a woman of childbearing age, particularly one who is not using an effective method of contraception consistently, reports abdominal discomfort or abnormal bleeding.

PROMOTING HOME, COMMUNITY-BASED, AND TRANSITIONAL CARE

 Educating Patients About Self-Care. If the patient has experienced life-threatening hemorrhage and shock, these complications are addressed and treated before education can begin. At this time, the patient's and the nurse's attention is focused on the crisis, not on learning.

Once hemodynamically stable, the patient begins to ask questions about what happened and why certain procedures were performed. Procedures are explained in terms that are understandable to a patient who is distressed and apprehensive. The patient's partner is included in education when possible. After the patient recovers from postoperative discomfort, it may be more appropriate to address any questions and concerns that she and her partner have, including the effect of this pregnancy or its treatment on future pregnancies. The patient should be advised that ectopic pregnancies may recur. The patient is educated about possible complications and instructed to report early signs and symptoms. It is important to review signs and symptoms with the patient and instruct her to report an abnormal menstrual period promptly.

Continuing and Transitional Care. Because of the risk of subsequent ectopic pregnancies, the patient is advised to seek preconception counseling before considering future pregnancies and to seek early prenatal care. Follow-up contact allows the nurse to answer questions and clarify information for the patient and her partner.

Evaluation

Expected patient outcomes may include:
1. Experiences relief of pain
   a. Reports a decrease in pain and discomfort
   b. Ambulates as prescribed; performs coughing and deep breathing
2. Begins to accept loss of pregnancy and expresses grief by verbalizing feelings and reactions to loss
3. Verbalizes an understanding of the causes of ectopic pregnancy
4. Experiences no complications
   a. Exhibits no signs of bleeding, hemorrhage, or shock
   b. Has decreased amounts of discharge (on perineal pad)
   c. Has normal skin color and turgor
   d. Exhibits stable vital signs and adequate urine output
   e. Levels of beta-hCG return to normal

Perimenopause

Perimenopause is the menstrual transition period before menopause that begins on average 4 years before the last menstrual period (Casper, 2019). Perimenopause is characterized by marked hormonal fluctuations and irregular menstrual cycles (Casper, 2019). Women often have varied beliefs about aging, and these must be considered when caring for or educating patients who are perimenopausal.

Nursing Management

Women who are perimenopausal often benefit from information about the subtle physiologic changes they are experiencing. Perimenopause has been described as an opportune time for educating women about health promotion and disease prevention strategies. When discussing health-related concerns with women who are in midlife, nurses should consider the following issues:

- Sexuality, fertility, contraception, and STIs
- Unintended pregnancy (if contraception is not used correctly and consistently)
- Oral contraceptive use. Oral contraceptives provide women with protection against uterine cancer, ovarian cancer, anemia, pregnancy, and fibrocystic breast changes as well as relief from perimenopausal symptoms (Casanova et al., 2019). This option should be discussed with women who are perimenopausal. Women who smoke and are 35 years or older should not take oral contraceptive agents because of an increased risk of cerebrovascular disease. Contraception is discussed in detail earlier in this chapter.
- Breast health. About 16% of cases of breast cancer occur in women who are perimenopausal, so breast self-examination, routine physical examinations, and mammograms are essential.

Menopause

Menopause is the permanent physiologic cessation of menses associated with declining ovarian function evidenced by 12 consecutive months with no menstrual bleeding (Casanova et al., 2019). Most women stop menstruating between 41 and 59 years of age. Postmenopause is the period beginning from about 1 year after menses cease. Due to a decrease in estrogen levels, menopause may be associated with some atrophy of breast tissue and genital organs, loss in bone density, and vascular changes.

Menopause starts gradually and is usually signaled by changes in menstruation. The monthly flow may increase or decrease, become irregular, and finally cease. Often, the interval between periods is longer; a lapse of several months between periods is not uncommon. Ovulation occurs less frequently, estrogen levels fluctuate, and FSH levels increase in an attempt to stimulate estrogen production (Casanova et al., 2019).

Postmenopausal Bleeding

Bleeding 1 year after menses cease at menopause must be investigated, and a malignant condition must be considered until proven otherwise. A transvaginal ultrasound can be used to measure the thickness of the endometrial lining (Goodman, 2020). The uterine lining in women who are postmenopausal should be thin because of low estrogen levels. A thicker lining warrants further evaluation by endometrial biopsy or a D&C.

Clinical Manifestations

Menopause has systemic effects that include an increase in body fat and intra-abdominal deposition of body fat. Also, levels of total and LDL cholesterol increase. Hot flashes occur in many women going through menopause due to alterations in thermoregulation. Because of these hormonal changes, some women notice irregular menses, breast tenderness, and mood changes long before menopause occurs (Casanova et al., 2019). The hot or warm flashes and night sweats reported by some women are thought to be caused by hormonal changes and denote vasomotor instability. They may vary in intensity from a barely perceptible warm feeling to a sensation of extreme warmth accompanied by profuse sweating, causing discomfort, sleep disturbances, and subsequent fatigue. Other physical changes may include increased bone loss (see Chapter 36).

- An annual physical examination can help screen for problems and promote general health.
- Changes in lifestyle (e.g., diet, activity) to promote health and wellness.
  - A nutritious diet (decrease fat and calories, increase fiber and whole grains) and weight control will enhance physical and emotional well-being.
  - Exercise for at least 30 minutes 3 or 4 times a week to maintain good health.
  - Involvement in outside activities is beneficial in reducing anxiety and tension.
- Recognize the following about sexual activity:
  - Sexual functioning may be enhanced at midlife.
  - Frequent sexual activity helps to maintain the elasticity of the vagina.
  - Contraception is advised until 1 year passes without menses.
  - Safer sex is important at any age.
- Strategies and methods to prevent or manage potential problems:
  - *Hot flashes:* See primary provider to discuss hormone replacement therapy indications (lowest dose for shortest period of time) and alternative therapy (e.g., vitamin therapy, black cohosh, and other herbal preparations). Fatigue and stress may worsen hot flashes.
  - *Itching or burning of vulvar areas:* See primary provider to rule out dermatologic abnormalities and, if appropriate,

to obtain a prescription for a lubricating or hormonal cream.
  - *Dyspareunia due to vaginal dryness:* Use a water-soluble lubricant, hormone cream, or contraceptive foam.
  - *Decreased perineal muscle tone and bladder control:* Practice Kegel exercises daily (contract the perineal muscles as though stopping urination; hold for 5 to 10 seconds and release; repeat frequently during the day).
  - *Dry skin:* Use mild emollient skin cream and lotions to prevent dry skin.
  - *Weight control:* Join a weight reduction support group such as Weight Watchers or a similar group if appropriate or consult a registered dietitian for guidance about the tendency to gain weight, particularly around the hips, thighs, and abdomen.
  - *Osteoporosis:* Observe recommended calcium and vitamin D intake, including calcium supplements, if indicated, to slow the process of osteoporosis; avoid smoking, alcohol, and excessive caffeine, all of which increase bone loss. Perform weight-bearing exercises. Undergo bone density testing when appropriate.
  - *Risk for urinary tract infection (UTI):* Drink 6 to 8 glasses of water daily as a possible way to reduce the incidence of UTI related to atrophic changes of the urethra.
  - *Vaginal bleeding:* Report any bleeding after 1 year of no menses to the primary provider *immediately, no matter how minimal.*

The entire genitourinary system is affected by the reduced estrogen level. Changes in the vulvovaginal area may include a gradual thinning of pubic hair and a gradual shrinkage of the labia. Vaginal secretions decrease, and women may report dyspareunia. The vaginal pH increases during menopause, predisposing women to bacterial infections and atrophic vaginitis. Discharge, itching, and vulvar burning may result.

Some women report fatigue, forgetfulness, weight gain, irritability, trouble sleeping, feeling "blue," and feelings of panic. Menopausal complaints need to be evaluated carefully because they may indicate other disorders. Most women have few problems and are relieved to be free from menstrual periods. Nurses should provide women with education and health promotion strategies appropriate for those approaching menopause (see Chart 50-14).

Psychological Considerations

Women's reactions and feelings related to loss of reproductive capacity may vary. Some women may experience role confusion, whereas others experience a sense of sexual and personal freedom. Women may be relieved that the childbearing phase of their lives is over. Each woman's personal views about menopause and circumstances affect her response and must be considered on an individual basis. Nurses need to be sensitive to all possibilities and take their cues from the patient.

Medical Management

Women approaching menopause often have many concerns about their health. Some have concerns based on a family history of heart disease, osteoporosis, or cancer. Each woman needs to be as knowledgeable as possible about her health

options and should be encouraged to discuss her concerns with her primary provider so that she can make an informed decision about managing menopausal symptoms and maintaining her health.

Hormone Therapy

HT or menopausal hormonal therapy (previously referred to as hormone replacement therapy [HRT]) is medication that contains estrogen or estrogen and progestin together, to replace the ones the body is no longer making. HT is controversial but it is prescribed to treat moderate to severe menopause-related vasomotor symptoms (hot flashes and night sweats) in women without contraindications to estrogen and progesterone whose quality of life is being affected (Martin & Barbieri, 2019). The current recommendation for treatment of hot flashes with HT is to use the lowest dose possible for the shortest time possible (Martin & Barbieri, 2019).

Methods of Administration

Both estrogen and progestin are prescribed for women who have not had a hysterectomy; progestin prevents proliferation of the uterine lining and hyperplasia. Women who no longer have a uterus because of hysterectomy can take estrogen without progestin (i.e., unopposed estrogen) because there is no longer a risk of estrogen-induced hyperplasia of the uterine lining. Although there is a slight increase of risk of stroke in women taking estrogen alone following hysterectomy, the risk of breast cancer is unchanged (Martin & Barbieri, 2019).

Some women take both estrogen and progestin daily; others take estrogen for 25 consecutive days each month, with progestin taken in cycles (e.g., 10 to 14 days of the month).

Women who take HT for 25 days often experience bleeding after completing the progestin. Other women take estrogen and progestin every day and usually experience no bleeding. They occasionally have irregular spotting, which should be evaluated by their primary provider. Progestin administration may be oral, transdermal, vaginal, or intrauterine.

Estrogen patches, which are replaced once or twice weekly, are another option but require a progestin along with them if the woman still has a uterus. Another type of patch provides estrogen and progestin treatment (Comerford & Durkin, 2020). Skin should be dry at the area of application and cleansing the site with alcohol may improve adhesiveness. Vaginal treatment with an estrogen cream, suppository, or a vaginal ring may be used for vasomotor symptoms, vaginal dryness, or atrophy (Comerford & Durkin, 2020).

Risks and Benefits

HT is contraindicated in women with a history of breast cancer, vascular thrombosis, impaired liver function, uterine cancer, and undiagnosed abnormal vaginal bleeding. The risk of venous thromboembolism is increased with HT (Martin & Barbieri, 2019). Women who elect to take HT should be educated about the signs and symptoms of deep vein thrombosis (DVT) and pulmonary embolism (PE) and instructed to report these signs and symptoms (i.e., leg redness, tenderness, chest pain, shortness of breath) immediately. Women who take HT need to be informed about the importance of regular follow-up care, including a yearly physical examination and mammograms as needed and age appropriate. An endometrial biopsy is indicated for any irregular bleeding. Because the risk of complications increases the longer HT is used, HT should be used for the shortest time possible (Martin & Barbieri, 2019). Estrogen alone or in combination with a progestin does not reduce the risk of dementia or cognitive impairment.

Alternative Therapy for Hot Flashes

Because women often seek information about alternatives to the use of HT, nurses must be knowledgeable about other approaches that women can use to promote their health in the peri- and postmenopausal periods. Problematic hot flashes have been treated with low-dose venlafaxine, psychoeducational approaches, and diet and lifestyle changes (Santen, Loprinzi, & Casper, 2019). Similarly, vitamin B_6 and vitamin E may be effective. Some women have expressed interest in other alternative treatments (e.g., natural estrogens and progestins, black cohosh, ginseng, dong quai, soy products, and several other herbal preparations); however, scant data exist about their safety or effectiveness. A few studies have shown some improvement in vasomotor symptoms (hot flashes and night sweats) with the use of complementary therapies. These include reflexology, aromatherapy, yoga, hypnotherapy, breathing exercises, and meditation (Santen et al., 2019). When taking a medical history of a patient who is perimenopausal or menopausal, the nurse should always address their use of complementary and alternative therapies and supplements.

Maintaining Bone Health

Acceleration of bone loss resulting in osteoporosis and microarchitectural deterioration of bone tissue occurs at menopause and leads to increased bone fragility and risk of fracture (see Chapter 36).

Maintaining Cardiovascular Health

A variety of strategies can help to lower the risk of heart disease in women, including lifestyle changes and behavioral strategies (see Chapter 21).

Behavioral Strategies

As stated previously, regular physical exercise is beneficial. It may also reduce stress, enhance well-being, and improve self-image. In addition, weight-bearing exercise may prevent loss of muscle tissue and bone tissue.

Women are also encouraged to participate in other health-promoting activities. These include regular health screening recommended for women at the time of menopause: gynecologic examinations, mammograms, colonoscopy, fecal occult blood testing, and bone mineral density testing if at risk for osteoporosis.

Nutritional Therapy

Women are encouraged to decrease their fat and caloric intake and increase their intake of whole grains, fibers, fruits, and vegetables.

Nursing Management

Nurses can encourage women to view menopause as a natural change resulting in freedom from symptoms related to menses. No relationship exists between menopause and mental health problems; however, social circumstances (e.g., adolescent children, ill partners, and dependent or ill parents) that may coincide with menopause can be stressful.

Measures should be taken to promote general health. The nurse explains to the patient that cessation of menses is a normal occurrence that is rarely accompanied by nervous symptoms or illness. The current expected lifespan after menopause for the average woman is 30 to 35 years, which may encompass as many years as the childbearing phase of her life. Normal sexual urges continue, and women retain their usual response to sex long after menopause. Many women enjoy better health after menopause than before, especially those who have experienced dysmenorrhea. The individual woman's evaluation of herself and her worth, now and in the future, is likely to affect her emotional reaction to menopause. Patient education and counseling regarding healthy lifestyles, health promotion, and health screening are of paramount importance (Santen et al., 2019).

CRITICAL THINKING EXERCISES

1 **ebp** During an outpatient visit, your 33-year-old female patient and her spouse mention they are interested in infertility evaluation. What information will you need to determine if infertility treatment is an option? What is the evidence base for infertility methods for this couple? Specify the criteria used to evaluate the strength of the evidence for the practices that you identify.

2 ipc A 40-year-old woman was admitted to your unit for complications from a recent induced abortion. You notice bruising in various stages of healing and suspect she may be a victim of intimate partner violence. What type of referrals might be appropriate for this patient? What members of the interprofessional health care team do you anticipate as being integral to the care of this patient?

3 pq During her annual physical examination, a 21-year-old woman is anxious about her first pelvic examination. What are the immediate nursing priorities in providing care to this patient? How will your priorities and approach differ if the patient were older adult or from a different culture than your own?

REFERENCES

*Asterisk indicates nursing research.
**Double asterisk indicates classic reference.

Books

**Annon, J. S. (1976). *The behavioral treatment of sexual problems.* Honolulu, HI: Enabling Systems.
Ball, J., Dains, J., Flynn, J., et al. (2019). *Seidel's guide to physical examination* (9th ed.). St. Louis, MO: Elsevier Mosby.
Casanova, R., Chuang, A., Goepfert, A. R., et al. (Eds.). (2019). *Beckman and Ling's obstetrics and gynecology* (8th ed.). Philadelphia, PA: Wolters Kluwer.
Comerford, K. C., & Durkin, M. T. (2020). *Nursing 2020 drug handbook.* Philadelphia, PA: Wolters Kluwer.
Eliopoulos, C. (2018). *Gerontological nursing* (9th ed.). Philadelphia, PA: Lippincott Williams & Wilkins.
Weber, J., & Kelley, J. (2018). *Health assessment in nursing* (6th ed.). Philadelphia, PA: Lippincott Williams & Wilkins.

Journals and Electronic Documents

Alan Guttmacher Institute. (2018). Contraceptive use in the United States. Retrieved on 11/23/2019 at: www.guttmacher.org/fact-sheet/contraceptive-use-united-states
American Cancer Society (ACS). (2019). Breast cancer facts & figures 2019-2020. Retrieved on 9/9/2019 at: www.cancer.org/content/dam/cancer-org/research/cancer-facts-and-statistics/breast-cancer-facts-and-figures/breast-cancer-facts-and-figures-2019-2020.pdf
American College of Obstetricians and Gynecologists (ACOG). (2015, reaffirmed 2018). Committee Opinion Number 642. Increasing access to contraceptive implants and intrauterine devices to reduce unintended pregnancy. Retrieved on 12/8/2019 at: www.acog.org/Clinical-Guidance-and-Publications/Committee-Opinions/Committee-on-Gynecologic-Practice/Increasing-Access-to-Contraceptive-Implants-and-Intrauterine-Devices-to-Reduce-Unintended-Pregnancy
American College of Obstetricians and Gynecologists (ACOG). (2017). Practice Bulletin # 186. Long-acting reversible contraception: Implants and intrauterine devices. Retrieved on 12/8/2019 at: www.acog.org/Clinical-Guidance-and-Publications/Practice-Bulletins/Committee-on-Practice-Bulletins-Gynecology/Long-Acting-Reversible-Contraception-Implants-and-Intrauterine-Devices
American College of Obstetricians and Gynecologists (ACOG). (2018). Practice Bulletin # 193. Tubal ectopic pregnancy. Retrieved on 12/8/2019 at: www.acog.org/Clinical-Guidance-and-Publications/Practice-Bulletins/Committee-on-Practice-Bulletins-Gynecology/Tubal-Ectopic-Pregnancy
American College of Obstetricians and Gynecologists (ACOG). (2019). Committee Opinion Number 762. Prepregnancy counseling. Retrieved on 11/23/2019 at: www.acog.org/clinical/clinical-guidance/committee-opinion/articles/2019/01/prepregnancy-counseling

Anawat, B. D., & Page, S. T. (2019). Approach to the male with infertility. *UpToDate.* Retrieved on 5/9/2020 at: www.uptodate.com/contents/approach-to-the-male-withinfertility
Bartz, D. A., & Blumenthal, P. D. (2019). First-trimester pregnancy termination: Medical abortion. *UpToDate.* Retrieved on 12/8/2019 at: www.uptodate.com/contents/first-trimester-pregnancy-termination-medication-abortion?search=surgical%20abortion&topicRef=3287&source=see_link
Bibbins-Domingo, K. (2017). Screening for gynecologic conditions with pelvic exam US Preventive Services Task Force recommendation statement. *Journal of the American Medical Association, 317*(9), 947–953.
Bradley, L. D. (2018). Overview of hysteroscopy. *UpToDate.* Retrieved on 12/17/19 at: www.uptodate.com/contents/overview-of-hysteroscopy
Casper, R. F. (2019). Clinical manifestations and diagnosis of menopause. *UpToDate.* Retrieved on 12/15/19 at: www.uptodate.com/contents/clinical-manifestations-and-diagnosis-of-menopause?search=perimenopause&source=search_result&selectedTitle=1~91&usage_type=default&display_rank=1
Casper, R. F., & Yonkers, K. A. (2019). Treatment of premenstrual syndrome and premenstrual dysphoric disorder. *UpToDate.* Retrieved on 11/17/2019 at: www.uptodate.com/contents/treatment-of-premenstrual-syndrome-and-premenstrual-dysphoric-disorder
Centers for Disease Control and Prevention (CDC). (2019a). Understanding intimate partner violence fact sheet. Retrieved on 11/9/2019 at: www.cdc.gov/violenceprevention/intimatepartnerviolence/fastfact.html
Centers for Disease Control and Prevention (CDC). (2019b). Tools for improving clinical preventative services receipt among women with disabilities of childbearing ages and beyond. Retrieved on 11/16/2019 at: www.amchp.org/programsandtopics/womens-health/Focus%20Areas/WomensHealthDisability/Pages/CliniciansandWomenInteractions.aspx
Del Priore, G. (2019). Endometrial sampling procedure. *UpToDate.* Retrieved on 11/17/2019 at: www.uptodate.com/contents/endometrial-sampling-procedures
Eickmeyer, S. (2017). Anatomy and physiology of the pelvic floor. *Physical Medicine and Rehabilitation Clinics of North America, 28*(3), 455–460.
Ginsburg, E. S., & Srouji, S. S. (2019). Donor insemination. *UpToDate.* Retrieved on 12/8/2019 at: www.uptodate.com/contents/donor-insemination?search=artificial%20insemination&source=search_result&selectedTitle=1~15&usage_type=default&display_rank=1
Gnanasambanthan, S., & Datta, S. (2019). Premenstrual syndrome. *Obstetrics, Gynaecology and Reproductive Medicine, 29*(10), 281–285.
Goodman, A. (2020). Postmenopausal uterine bleeding. *UpToDate.* Retrieved on 5/9/2020 at: www.uptodate.com/contents/postmenopausal-uterine-bleeding
Gregg, I. (2018). The health care experiences of lesbian women becoming mothers. *Nursing for Women's Health, 22*(1), 40–50.
Hailes, H. P., Yu, R., Danese, A., et al. (2019). Long term outcomes of childhood sexual abuse: An umbrella review. *The Lancet Psychiatry, 6*(10), 803–839.
Hammond, C. (2019). Second-trimester pregnancy termination: Induction (medication) termination. *UpToDate.* Retrieved on 5/12/2020 at: https://www.uptodate.com/contents/second-trimester-pregnancy-termination-induction-medicationtermination
Harris, H. R., Wieser, F., Vitonis, A. F., et al. (2018). Early life abuse and risk of endometriosis. *Human Reproduction, 33*(9), 1657–1668.
Herbert, S. (2018). Sexual history and examination in men and women. *Medicine, 46*(5), 272–276.
Holland, A. C., Strachan, A. T., Pair, L., et al. (2018). Highlights from the U.S. selected practice recommendations for contraception use. *Nursing for Women's Health, 22*(2), 181–190.
Horner-Johnson, W. (2019). Shining a light on reproductive health care needs of women with disabilities. *Journal of Women's Health, 28*(7), 888–889.
Kaiser Family Foundation. (2018). Women's health insurance coverage: Fact sheet. Retrieved on 11/9/2019 at: www.kff.org/womens-health-policy/fact-sheet/womens-health-insurance-coverage/
Konig-Bachman, M., Zenzmaier, C., & Schildberger, B. (2019). Health professionals' views on maternity care for women with physical disabilities: A qualitative study. *BMC Health Services Research, 19*(1), 551.
Kulkarni, A., & Deb, S. (2019). Dysmenorrhea. *Obstetrics, Gynaecology and Reproductive Medicine, 29*(10), 286–291.

Lammers, C. R., Hulme, P. A., Wey, H., et al. (2017). Understanding women's awareness and access to preconception health care in rural population: A cross-sectional study. *Journal of Community Health, 42*(3), 489–499.

Lapinski, J., Covas, T., Perkins, J., et al. (2018). Best practices in transgender health: A clinician's guide. *Primary Care. Clinics in Office Practices, 45*(4), 687–703.

Lee, L. K., Monuteaux, M. C., & Galbraith, A. A. (2019). Women's affordability, access, and preventative care after the affordable care act. *American Journal of Preventative Medicine, 56*(5), 631–638.

*Lee, M. (2019). I wish I had known sooner: Stratified reproduction as a consequence of disparities in infertility awareness, diagnosis, and management. *Women & Health, 59*(10), 1185–1198.

Martin, K. A., & Barbieri, R. L. (2019). Treatment of menopausal symptoms with hormone therapy. *UpToDate*. Retrieved on 12/15/2019 at: www.uptodate.com/contents/treatment-of-menopausal-symptoms-with-hormone-therapy?search=hormone%20replacement%20therapy&topicRef=7427&source=see_link

Mayo Clinic. (2017). Toxic shock syndrome. Retrieved on 11/17/2019 at: www.mayoclinic.org/diseases-conditions/toxic-shock-syndrome/symptoms-causes/syc-20355384

Mayo Clinic. (2018). Painful intercourse (dyspareunia). Retrieved on 11/23/2019 at: www.mayoclinic.org/diseases-conditions/painful-intercourse/diagnosis-treatment/drc-20375973

Moore, C. L., Edie, A. L., Johnson, J. L., et al. (2019). Long-acting reversible contraception: Assessment of knowledge and interest among college females. *Journal of American College Health, 67*(7), 615–619.

Okoro, C. A., Hollis, N. D., Cyrus, A. C., et al. (2018). Prevalence of disabilities and health care access by disability status and type among adults—United States, 2016. *MMWR Morbidity and Mortality Weekly Report, 67*(32), 882–887.

Paulson, R. (2019). In vitro fertilization. *UpToDate*. Retrieved on 12/8/2019 at: www.uptodate.com/contents/in-vitro-fertilization

Rodriguez, D. (2020). Cigarette and tobacco products in pregnancy: Impact on pregnancy and the neonate. *UpToDate*. Retrieved on 5/9/2020 at: www.uptodate.com/contents/cigarette-and-tobacco-products-in-pregnancy-impact-on-pregnancy-and-theneonate

Santen, R. J., Loprinzi, C. L., & Casper, R. F. (2019). Menopausal hot flashes. *UpToDate*. Retrieved on 12/15/2019 at: www.uptodate.com/contents/menopausal-hot-flashes

Schenken, R. S. (2019). Endometriosis: Pathogenesis, clinical features and diagnosis. *UpToDate*. Retrieved on 12/8/2019 at: www.uptodate.com/contents/endometriosis-pathogenesis-clinical-features-and-diagnosis

Sharp, H. T. (2019). Overview of gynecologic laparoscopic surgery and non-umbilical entry sites. *UpToDate*. Retrieved on 11/17/2019 at: www.uptodate.com/contents/overview-of-gynecologic-laparoscopic-surgery-and-non-umbilical-entry-sites

Shih, G., & Wallace, R. (2020). First-trimester pregnancy termination: Uterine aspiration. *UpToDate*. Retrieved on 5/12/2020 at: www.uptodate.com/contents/first-trimester-pregnancy-termination-uterine-aspiration

*Stevenson, E. L., Cebert, M., & Silva, S. (2019). Stress and anxiety in couples who conceive via In Vitro fertilization compared with those who conceive spontaneously. *Journal of Obstetric, Gynecologic and Neonatal Nursing, 48*(6), 635–644.

Tulandi, T. (2019). Ectopic pregnancy: Clinical manifestations and diagnosis. *UpToDate*. Retrieved on 12/8/2019 at: www.uptodate.com/contents/ectopic-pregnancy-clinical-manifestations-and-diagnosis

U.S. Preventive Services Task Force (USPSTF). (2018). Cervical cancer screening recommendations of the U.S. Preventive Services Task Force. Retrieved on 11/16/2019 at: www.uspreventiveservicestaskforce.org/Page/Name/uspstf-a-and-b-recommendations/

Weil, W. (2019). Intimate partner violence: Epidemiology and health consequences. *UpToDate*. Retrieved on 11/9/2019 at: www.uptodate.com/contents/intimate-partner-violence-epidemiology-and-health-consequences

Welt, C. K. (2019). Physiology of the normal menstrual cycle. *UpToDate*. Retrieved on 11/17/2019 at: www.uptodate.com/contents/physiology-of-the-normal-menstrual-cycle

Welt, C. K., & Barbieri, R. L. (2018). Evaluation and management of primary amenorrhea. *UpToDate*. Retrieved on 11/23/2019 at: www.uptodate.com/contents/evaluation-and-management-of-primary-amenorrhea

Wingo, E., Ingraham, N., & Roberts, S. (2018). Reproductive health care priorities and barriers to effective care for LGBTQ people assigned female at birth: A qualitative study. *Women's Health Issues, 28*(4), 350–357.

World Health Organization (WHO). (2018). Female genital mutilation fact sheet. Retrieved on 11/9/2019 at: www.who.int/news-room/fact-sheets/detail/female-genital-mutilation

Resources

American Congress of Obstetricians and Gynecologists (ACOG), www.acog.org

American Society for Reproductive Medicine (ASRM), www.asrm.org

Association of Women's Health, Obstetric and Neonatal Nurses (AWHONN), www.awhonn.org

DES Action USA, www.desaction.org

Emergency Contraception, ec.princeton.edu

Female Genital Cutting Education and Networking Project (provides fact sheets, state policies, periodicals), www.fgmnetwork.org

Futures Without Violence, www.futureswithoutviolence.org

Health Promotion for Women With Disabilities, Villanova University College of Nursing, www1.villanova.edu/villanova/nursing/community/womendisabilities.html

National Coalition Against Domestic Violence (NCADV), www.ncadv.org

North American Menopause Society (NAMS), www.menopause.org

Nurse Practitioners in Women's Health (NPWH), www.npwh.org

Planned Parenthood Federation of America, www.plannedparenthood.org

LEARNING OUTCOMES

On completion of this chapter, the learner will be able to:

1. Compare the various types of vaginal infections and the signs, symptoms, and treatments of each.
2. Discuss the signs and symptoms, management, and nursing care of patients with inflammatory processes, structural disorders, and benign and malignant conditions of the female reproductive tract.

3. Use the nursing process as a framework for care of the patient with a vulvovaginal infection or with genital herpes, or who is undergoing a hysterectomy.
4. Describe the nursing management of the patient undergoing radiation therapy for cancer of the female reproductive tract.

NURSING CONCEPTS

Comfort
Family

Infection
Reproduction

Sexuality

GLOSSARY

abscess: a collection of purulent material

Bartholin cyst: a cyst in a paired Bartholin or vestibular gland in the vulva

brachytherapy: delivery of radiation therapy through internal implants to a localized area of tissue

candidiasis: infection caused by *Candida* species or yeast; also referred to as monilial vaginitis or yeast infection

condylomata: warty growths indicative of the human papillomavirus

cryotherapy: destruction of tissue by freezing (e.g., with liquid nitrogen)

cystocele: displacement of the bladder downward into the vagina

douche: rinsing the vaginal canal with fluid

dysplasia: term related to abnormal cell changes; may be found on Pap smear and cervical biopsy reports

endocervicitis: inflammation of the mucosa and the glands of the cervix

endometriosis: endometrial tissue in abnormal locations; causes pain with menstruation, scarring, and possible infertility

enterocele: a protrusion of the intestinal wall into the vagina

fibroid tumor: usually benign tumor arising from the muscle tissue of the uterus

fistula: abnormal opening between two organs or sites (e.g., vesicovaginal, between bladder and vagina; rectovaginal, between rectum and vagina)

hyphae: long, branching filamentous structures characteristic of fungi such as *Candida* seen under microscopic examination

hysterectomy: surgical removal of the uterus

loop electrocautery excision procedure (LEEP): procedure in which a laser is used to remove a thin layer of cervical tissue after abnormal biopsy findings

myomectomy: surgical removal of uterine fibroids

oophorectomy: surgical removal of an ovary

pelvic exenteration: major surgical procedure in which the pelvic organs are removed

pelvic inflammatory disease (PID): inflammatory condition of the pelvic cavity, usually from a sexually transmitted infection

polycystic ovary syndrome (PCOS): complex endocrine condition resulting in chronic anovulation, androgen excess, and multiple ovarian cysts

rectocele: bulging of the rectum into the vagina

salpingitis: inflammation of the fallopian tube

salpingo-oophorectomy: removal of the ovary and its fallopian tube (removal of the fallopian tube alone is a salpingectomy)

vaginitis: inflammation of the vagina, usually secondary to infection

vulvar dystrophy: thickening or lesions of the vulva; usually causes itching and may require biopsy to exclude malignancy

vulvectomy: removal of the tissue of the vulva

vulvitis: inflammation of the vulva, usually secondary to infection or irritation

vulvodynia: painful condition that affects the vulva

Disorders of the female reproductive system can be minor or serious but are often anxiety producing and distressing. Some disorders are self-limited and cause only minor inconvenience; others are life-threatening and require immediate attention and long-term therapy. Many disorders are managed by the patient at home, whereas others require hospitalization and surgical intervention. Nurses not only need to be knowledgeable about these disorders but need to be sensitive to patient concerns and possible discomfort in discussing and managing these disorders.

VULVOVAGINAL INFECTIONS

Vulvovaginal infections are common, and nurses have an important role in providing information that may prevent their occurrence. To help prevent these infections, women need to understand their anatomy and normal vulvovaginal health.

The Bartholin glands on either side of the entrance to the vagina can become blocked (cyst formation) or infected (abscess formation) (Ball, Dains, Flynn, et al., 2019). Treatment is different for both cyst and abscess formation, but pain is common with both. Pain can interfere with sitting and walking.

The vagina is protected against infection by its normally low pH (3.5 to 4.5), which is maintained in part by the actions of *Lactobacillus acidophilus*, the dominant bacteria in a healthy vaginal ecosystem. These bacteria suppress the growth of anaerobes and produce lactic acid, which maintains normal pH. They also produce hydrogen peroxide, which is toxic to anaerobes (Paavonen & Brunham, 2018). The risk of infection increases if a woman's resistance is reduced by stress or illness, if the pH is altered, or if a pathogen is introduced (see Chart 51-1). Continued research into causes and treatments is needed, along with better ways to encourage growth of lactobacilli.

Chart 51-1   ⚠️ **RISK FACTORS**
Vulvovaginal Infections

- Allergies
- Diabetes
- Frequent douching
- HIV infection
- Long-term or repeated use of broad-spectrum antibiotics
- Low estrogen levels
- Oral–genital contact (yeast can inhabit the mouth and intestinal tract)
- Perimenopause/Menopause
- Poor personal hygiene
- Pregnancy
- Premenarche
- Sex with infected partner
- Synthetic clothing
- Tight undergarments
- Use of oral contraceptives

HIV, human immune deficiency virus.
Adapted from Singh, J., Kalia, N., & Kaur, M. (2018). Recurrent vulvovaginal infections: Etiology, diagnosis, treatment and management. In P. Sing (Ed.). *Infectious diseases and your health*. Singapore: Springer; Zapata, M. R. (2017). Diagnosis and treatment of vulvovaginitis. In D. Shoupe (Ed.). *Handbook of gynecology*. Switzerland: Springer.

The epithelium of the vagina is highly responsive to estrogen, which induces glycogen formation. The subsequent breakdown of glycogen into lactic acid assists in producing a low vaginal pH. When estrogen decreases during lactation and menopause, glycogen also decreases. With reduced glycogen formation, infections may occur. In addition, as estrogen production ceases during the peri- and postmenopausal periods, the vagina and labia may atrophy (thin), making the vaginal area more susceptible to infection. When patients are treated with antibiotic agents, the normal vaginal flora is reduced. This results in altered pH and growth of fungal organisms. Other factors that may initiate or predispose to infections include contact with an infected partner and wearing tight, nonabsorbent, and heat- and moisture-retaining clothing.

Vaginitis (inflammation of the vagina) is a group of conditions that cause vulvovaginal symptoms such as itching, irritation, burning, and abnormal discharge. Bacterial vaginitis is the most common cause, followed by trichomoniasis and vulvovaginal candidiasis (Paladine & Desai, 2018) (see Table 51-1). Other types include desquamative vaginitis, atrophic vaginitis, various vulvar dermatologic conditions, and vulvodynia. Normal vaginal discharge, which may occur in slight amounts during ovulation or just before the onset of menstruation, is clear to white, odorless, and viscous. It becomes more profuse when vaginitis occurs. Urethritis may accompany vaginitis because of the proximity of the urethra to the vagina. Discharge that occurs with vaginitis may produce itching, odor, redness, burning, or edema, which may be aggravated by voiding and defecation. After the causative organism has been identified, appropriate treatment (discussed later) is prescribed. This may include an oral medication or a local medication that is inserted into the vagina using an applicator.

Candidiasis

Vulvovaginal **candidiasis** is a fungal or yeast infection caused by strains of *Candida* (see Table 51-1). It is the second most common type of vaginal infection and accounts for an estimated 1.4 million outpatient visits annually in the United States (Centers for Disease Control and Prevention [CDC], 2019a). An estimated 75% of women will experience at least one yeast infection, and 40% to 45% will experience two or more in their lifetime (CDC, 2019a). *Candida albicans* accounts for approximately 90% of the cases, but other strains, such as *Candida glabrata*, may also be implicated (Casanova, Chuang, Goepfert, et al., 2019). Many women with a healthy vaginal ecosystem harbor *Candida* but are asymptomatic. Certain conditions favor the change from an asymptomatic state to colonization with symptoms. For example, the use of antibiotic agents decreases bacteria, thereby altering the natural protective organisms usually present in the vagina. Although infections can occur at any time, they occur more commonly in pregnancy or with a systemic condition such as diabetes or human immune deficiency virus (HIV) infection, or when patients are taking medications such as corticosteroids or oral contraceptive agents (Casanova et al., 2019).

Clinical Manifestations

Clinical manifestations include a vaginal discharge that causes pruritus (itching) and subsequent irritation. The discharge may be watery or thick but usually has a white, cottage

TABLE 51-1	Vaginal Infections and Vaginitis		
Infection	**Cause**	**Clinical Manifestations**	**Management Strategies**
Candidiasis	*Candida albicans,* *C. glabrata,* or *C. tropicalis*	Inflammation of vaginal epithelium, producing itching, reddish irritation White, cheeselike discharge clinging to epithelium	Eradicate the fungus by administering an antifungal agent. Some more frequently used vaginal creams and suppositories are miconazole and clotrimazole. Review other causative factors (e.g., antibiotic therapy, nylon underwear, tight clothing, pregnancy, oral contraceptive agents). Assess for diabetes and HIV infection in patients with recurrent monilia.
Gardnerella-associated bacterial vaginosis	*Gardnerella vaginalis* and vaginal anaerobes	Usually no edema or erythema of vulva or vagina Gray-white to yellow-white discharge clinging to external vulva and vaginal walls	Administer metronidazole, with instructions about avoiding alcohol while taking this medication. If infection is recurrent, may treat partner.
Trichomonas vaginalis vaginitis	*Trichomonas vaginalis*	Inflammation of vaginal epithelium, producing burning and itching Frothy yellow-white or yellow-green vaginal discharge	Relieve inflammation, restore acidity, and reestablish normal bacterial flora; provide oral metronidazole for patient and partner.
Bartholinitis (infection of the greater vestibular gland)	*Escherichia coli* *T. vaginalis* Staphylococcus Streptococcus Gonococcus	Erythema around vestibular gland Swelling and edema Abscessed vestibular gland	Drain the abscess; provide antibiotic therapy; excise gland of patients with chronic bartholinitis.
Cervicitis—acute and chronic	Chlamydia Gonococcus Streptococcus Many pathogenic bacteria	Profuse purulent discharge Backache Urinary frequency and urgency	Determine the cause—perform cytologic examination of cervical smear and appropriate cultures. Eradicate the gonococcal organism, if present: penicillin (as directed) or spectinomycin or tetracycline, if patient is allergic to penicillin. Tetracycline, doxycycline to eradicate chlamydia. Eradicate other causes.
Atrophic vaginitis	Lack of estrogen; glycogen deficiency	Discharge and irritation from alkaline pH of vaginal secretions	Provide topical vaginal estrogen therapy; improve nutrition if necessary; relieve dryness through the use of moisturizing medications.

HIV, human immune deficiency virus.
Adapted from Paladine, H. L., & Desai, U. A. (2018). Vaginitis: Diagnosis and treatment. *American Family Physician, 97*(5), 321–329.

cheese–like appearance. Symptoms are usually more severe just before menstruation and may be less responsive to treatment during pregnancy. Diagnosis is made by microscopic identification of spores and **hyphae** (long, branching filamentous structures) on a glass slide prepared from a discharge specimen mixed with potassium hydroxide. With candidiasis, the pH of the discharge is 4 to 5 (Casanova et al., 2019). Manifestations may be uncomplicated, occurring sporadically in women who are healthy, or recurrent and complicated in women who have diabetes, are pregnant, have a compromised immune system, or have obesity.

Medical Management

The goal of management is to eliminate symptoms. Treatments include antifungal agents such as miconazole, nystatin, clotrimazole, and terconazole cream. These agents are inserted into the vagina with an applicator at bedtime. There are 1-, 3-, and 7-night treatment courses available (Paladine & Desai, 2018). Oral medication (fluconazole) is also available in a one-pill dose. Relief should be noted within 3 days.

Some vaginal creams are available without a prescription; however, patients are cautioned to use these creams only if they are certain that they have a yeast or monilial infection. Patients often use these remedies for problems other than yeast infections. If a woman is uncertain about the cause of her symptoms or if relief has not been obtained after using these creams, she should be instructed to seek health care promptly. Yeast infections can become recurrent or complicated. Women may have more than four infections in a year and severe symptoms due to preexisting conditions such as diabetes or immunosuppression. Cell-mediated immunity may be a factor. Women with recurrent yeast infections benefit from a comprehensive gynecologic assessment.

Bacterial Vaginosis

Bacterial vaginosis is caused by an overgrowth of anaerobic bacteria and *Gardnerella vaginalis* normally found in the vagina and an absence of lactobacilli (see Table 51-1). Risk factors include douching after menses, smoking, multiple sex partners, and other sexually transmitted infections (STIs) (also referred to as sexually transmitted diseases [STDs]). Bacterial vaginosis is not considered an STI but is associated with sexual activity, and incidence is increased in female same-sex partners (Paavonen & Brunham, 2018).

Clinical Manifestations

Bacterial vaginosis can occur throughout the menstrual cycle and does not produce local discomfort or pain. More than half of patients with bacterial vaginosis do not notice any symptoms. Discharge, if noticed, is heavier than normal and gray to yellowish white in color. It is characterized by a fishlike odor that is particularly noticeable after penile–vaginal intercourse or during menstruation as a result of an increase in vaginal pH. The pH of the discharge is usually greater than 4.7 because of the amines that result from enzymes from anaerobes. The fishlike odor can be detected readily by adding a drop of potassium hydroxide to a glass slide with a sample of vaginal discharge, which releases amines; this is referred to as a positive "whiff" test. Under the microscope, vaginal cells are coated with bacteria and are described as "clue cells." Lactobacilli, which serve as a natural host defense, are usually absent. Bacterial vaginosis is not usually considered a serious condition, although it can be associated with premature labor, premature rupture of membranes, endometritis, and pelvic infection (Casanova et al., 2019; Paavonen & Brunham, 2018).

Medical Management

Metronidazole, given orally twice a day for 1 week, is effective; a vaginal gel is also available. Clindamycin vaginal cream or ovules (oval suppositories) are also effective. Treatment of patients' partners does not seem to be effective, but the use of condoms may be helpful. Bacterial vaginosis is highly persistent and tends to recur after treatment; therefore, women are encouraged to seek follow-up care if symptoms recur (CDC, 2015; Paladine & Desai, 2018).

Trichomoniasis

Trichomonas vaginalis is a flagellated protozoan that causes a common STI often called *trich*. About 3.7 million cases occur each year in the United States; however, only about 30% of those will exhibit symptoms of the disease (CDC, 2017a). Trichomoniasis may be transmitted by an asymptomatic carrier who harbors the organism in the urogenital tract (see Table 51-1). It may increase the risk of contracting HIV from an infected partner and may play a role in development of cervical neoplasia, postoperative infections, adverse pregnancy outcomes, pelvic inflammatory disease (PID), and infertility.

Clinical Manifestations

Clinical manifestations include a vaginal discharge that is thin (sometimes frothy), yellow to yellow-green, malodorous, and very irritating. An accompanying vulvitis may result, with vulvovaginal burning and itching. Diagnosis is made most often by microscopic detection of the motile causative organisms or less frequently by culture. Inspection with a speculum often reveals vaginal and cervical erythema (redness) with multiple small petechiae ("strawberry spots") (Casanova et al., 2019). Testing of a trichomonal discharge demonstrates a pH greater than 4.5.

Medical Management

The most effective treatment for trichomoniasis is metronidazole or tinidazole. All partners receive a one-time loading dose or a smaller dose twice a day for 7 days (CDC, 2015). The one-time dose is more convenient; consequently, adherence tends to be greater. The week-long treatment has occasionally been noted to be more effective. Some patients complain of an unpleasant but transient metallic taste when taking metronidazole. Nausea and vomiting, as well as a hot, flushed feeling can occur when this medication is taken with an alcoholic beverage. Patients are strongly advised to abstain from alcohol during treatment and for 24 hours after taking metronidazole or 72 hours after completion of a course of tinidazole (CDC, 2015). About 1 in 5 people will be reinfected with trichomoniasis within 3 months of treatment. All sexual partners should be treated, and patients are encouraged to abstain from sexual activity for 7 to 10 days after treatment (CDC, 2017a).

 ## Gerontologic Considerations

After menopause, the vaginal mucosa becomes thinner and may atrophy. While vulvovaginal atrophy can occur at any time in a woman's life, it is most common in women who are postmenopausal, with an incidence of nearly 50% (Naumova & Castelo-Branco, 2018). This condition can be complicated by infection from phylogenic bacteria, resulting in atrophic vaginitis (see Table 51-1). Leukorrhea (vaginal discharge) may cause itching and burning. Management is similar to bacterial vaginosis. Estrogenic hormones, either taken orally or inserted into the vagina in a cream form, can also be effective in restoring the epithelium.

Desquamative inflammatory vaginitis is an uncommon but severe purulent form of vaginal infection that occurs mostly in Caucasian women who are perimenopausal. It results in vaginal inflammation, burning, discharge, and dyspareunia (pain with penile–vaginal intercourse). Topical anti-inflammatory and antibiotic treatment is usually effective (Mills, 2017).

NURSING PROCESS

The Patient with a Vulvovaginal Infection

Assessment

The woman with vulvovaginal symptoms should be examined as soon as possible after the onset of symptoms. She should be instructed not to **douche** (rinse the vaginal canal), because doing so removes the discharge needed to make the diagnosis. The area is observed for erythema, edema, excoriation, and discharge. Each of the infection-producing organisms produces its own characteristic discharge and effect (see Table 51-1). The patient is asked to describe any discharge and other symptoms, such as odor, itching, or burning. Dysuria often occurs as a result of local irritation of the urinary meatus. A urinary tract infection may need to be ruled out by obtaining a urine specimen for culture and sensitivity testing.

The patient is asked about the occurrence of factors that may contribute to vulvovaginal infection:

- Physical and chemical factors, such as constant moisture from tight or synthetic clothing, perfumes and powders, soaps, bubble bath, poor hygiene, and the use of feminine hygiene products

- Psychogenic factors (e.g., stress, fear of STIs, intimate partner violence [IPV])
- Medical conditions or endocrine factors, such as a predisposition to Monilia in a patient who has diabetes
- The use of medications such as antibiotics, which may alter the vaginal flora and allow an overgrowth of monilial organisms
- New sex partner, multiple sex partners, previous vaginal infection

The patient is also asked about factors that could contribute to infection, including hygiene practices (douching) and the use or nonuse of condoms.

The nurse may prepare a vaginal smear (wet mount) to assist in diagnosing the infection. A common method for preparing the smear is to collect vaginal secretions with an applicator and place the secretions on two separate glass slides. A drop of saline solution is added to one slide and a drop of 10% potassium hydroxide is added to another slide for examination under a microscope. If bacterial vaginosis is present, the slide with normal saline solution added shows epithelial cells dotted with bacteria (clue cells). If *Trichomonas* species is present, small motile cells are seen. In the presence of yeast, the potassium hydroxide slide reveals branching hyphae (Casanova et al., 2019). Discharge associated with bacterial vaginosis produces a strong odor when mixed with potassium hydroxide. Testing the pH of the discharge with Nitrazine paper assists in proper diagnosis (Casanova et al., 2019).

Diagnosis

NURSING DIAGNOSES

Based on the assessment data, major nursing diagnoses may include the following:

- Discomfort associated with distressing symptoms and feelings of discomfort from the infectious process
- Anxiety associated with worry about symptoms
- Risk for infection or spread of infection
- Lack of knowledge about proper hygiene and preventive measures

Planning and Goals

Major goals may include increased comfort, reduction of anxiety related to symptoms, prevention of reinfection or infection of sexual partner, and acquisition of knowledge about methods for preventing vulvovaginal infections and managing self-care.

Nursing Interventions

RELIEVING IMPAIRED COMFORT

Treatment with the appropriate medication usually relieves discomfort. Sitz baths may be occasionally recommended and may provide temporary relief of symptoms.

REDUCING ANXIETY

Vulvovaginal infections are upsetting and require treatment. The patient who experiences such an infection may be very anxious about the significance of the symptoms and possible causes. Explaining the cause of symptoms may reduce anxiety related to fear of a more serious illness. Discussing ways to help prevent vulvovaginal infections may help patients adopt specific strategies to decrease infection and the related symptoms.

PREVENTING REINFECTION OR SPREAD OF INFECTION

Patient education should include the fact that vulvovaginal candidiasis is not an STI and incidence can be decreased by completing treatment, avoiding unnecessary antibiotic agents, wearing cotton underwear, and not douching.

The patient needs to be informed about the importance of adequate treatment for herself and her partner, if indicated. Other strategies to prevent persistence or spread of infection include abstaining from penile–vaginal intercourse when infected, treatment for sexual partners, and minimizing irritation of the affected area. When medications such as antibiotic agents are prescribed for any infection, the nurse instructs the patient about the usual precautions related to using these agents. If vaginal itching occurs several days after use, the patient can be reassured that this is usually not an allergic reaction but may be a yeast or monilial infection resulting from altered vaginal bacteria. Treatment for monilial infection is prescribed if indicated.

Another goal of treatment is to reduce tissue irritation caused by scratching or wearing tight clothing. The area needs to be kept clean by daily bathing and adequate hygiene after voiding and defecation. The use of a hair dryer on a cool setting will dry the area, and application of topical corticosteroids may decrease irritation.

When educating the patient about medications such as suppositories and devices such as applicators to dispense cream or ointment, the nurse may demonstrate the procedure by using a plastic model of the pelvis and vagina. The nurse should also stress the importance of hand hygiene before and after each administration of medication. To prevent the medication from escaping from the vagina, the patient should recline for 30 minutes after it is inserted, if possible. The patient is informed that seepage of medication may occur, and the use of a perineal pad may be helpful.

PROMOTING HOME, COMMUNITY-BASED, AND TRANSITIONAL CARE

Educating Patients About Self-Care. Vulvovaginal conditions are treated on an outpatient basis unless a patient has other medical problems. Patient education, tact, and reassurance are important aspects of nursing care. Women may express embarrassment, guilt, or anger and may be concerned that the infection could be serious or that it may have been acquired from a sex partner. In some instances, treatment plans include the partner.

The nurse assesses the patient's learning needs about the immediate problem. The patient needs to know the characteristics of normal as opposed to abnormal discharge. Questions often arise about douching. Normally, douching and the use of feminine hygiene sprays are unnecessary because daily baths or showers and proper hygiene after voiding and defecating keep the perineal area clean. Douching tends to eliminate normal flora, reducing the body's ability to ward off infection. In addition, repeated douching may result in vaginal epithelial breakdown and chemical irritation and has been associated with other pelvic disorders. In the case of recurrent yeast infections, the perineum should be kept as dry as possible. Loose-fitting cotton instead of tight-fitting synthetic, nonabsorbent, heat-retaining underwear is recommended.

Vulvar self-examination is a good health practice for all women. Becoming familiar with one's own anatomy and reporting anything that seems new or different may result in early detection and treatment of any new disorders. Nurses can also play a role in educating women about the risks of unprotected penile–vaginal intercourse, particularly with partners who have had sex with others.

Evaluation

Expected patient outcomes may include:

1. Experiences increased comfort
   a. Cleans the perineum as instructed
   b. Reports that itching is relieved
   c. Maintains urine output within normal limits and without dysuria
2. Experiences relief of anxiety
3. Remains free from infection
   a. Has no signs of inflammation, pruritus, odor, or dysuria
   b. Notes that vaginal discharge appears normal (thin, clear, not frothy)
4. Participates in self-care
   a. Takes medication as prescribed
   b. Wears absorbent underwear
   c. Avoids unprotected penile–vaginal intercourse
   d. Douches only as prescribed
   e. Performs vulvar self-examination regularly and reports any new findings to primary provider

Human Papillomavirus

Human papillomavirus (HPV) is the most common STI in the United States, affecting 79 million Americans and about 14 million newly acquired infections each year. Most adults who are sexually active will be infected with at least one type of HPV during their lifetime (CDC, 2019b). Most infections are self-limiting and without symptoms, and others can cause cervical and anogenital cancers. Infections can be latent (asymptomatic and detected only by deoxyribonucleic acid [DNA] hybridization tests for HPV), subclinical (visualized only after application of acetic acid followed by inspection under magnification), or clinical (visible condylomata acuminata).

Pathophysiology

HPV can be found in lesions of the skin, cervix, vagina, anus, penis, and oral cavity. Of the more than 100 genotypes of HPV that exist, about 40 genotypes affect the anogenital tract (Casanova et al., 2019). Some are low risk in that they are unlikely to cause cancerous changes. These include types 6, 11, 42, 43, 44, 54, 61, 70, and 72. The most common strains of HPV, 6 and 11, usually cause **condylomata** (warty growths) that can appear on the vulva, vagina, cervix, and anus. These are often visible or may be palpable by patients. Condylomata are rarely premalignant but are an outward manifestation of the virus (Casanova et al., 2019). High-risk oncogenic types, including 16, 18, 31, 33, 45, and 52 affect the cervix, causing abnormal cell changes or **dysplasia** (found on a Papanicolaou [Pap] smear). HPV types 16 and 18 account for 66% of cervical cancer cases, while types 31, 33, 45, and 52 account for another 15% (American College of Obstetricians and Gynecologists [ACOG], 2017a). The incidence of HPV in young women who are sexually active is high. The infection often disappears as the result of an effective immune system response. It is thought that two proteins produced by high-risk types of HPV interfere with tumor suppression by normal cells. Risk factors include being young, being sexually active, having multiple sex partners, and having sex with a partner who has or has had multiple partners. It can be transmitted by other means, however, as it has been found in young girls who have not been sexually active.

Medical Management

Options for the treatment of external genital warts by a primary provider include topical application of trichloroacetic acid, podophyllin, cryotherapy, as well as surgical removal. Topical agents that can be applied by patients to external lesions include podofilox and imiquimod. Because the safety of podophyllin, imiquimod, and podofilox during pregnancy has not been determined, these agents should not be used during pregnancy. Electrocautery and laser therapy are alternative therapies that may be indicated for patients with a large number or area of genital warts.

Treatment usually eradicates perineal warts or condylomata. However, they may resolve spontaneously without treatment and may also recur even with treatment. Genital warts are more resistant to treatment in patients with diabetes, those who are pregnant, who smoke, or are immunocompromised (Casanova et al., 2019).

If the treatment includes application of a topical agent by the patient, she needs to be carefully instructed in the use of the agent prescribed and must be able to identify the warts and be able to apply the medication to them. The patient is instructed to anticipate mild pain or local irritation with the use of these agents.

Women with HPV should have annual Pap smears because of the potential of HPV to cause dysplasia.

 For the procedural guidelines for obtaining an optimal Pap smear, go to **thepoint.lww.com/Brunner15e**.

Much remains unknown about subclinical and latent HPV disease. Women are often exposed to HPV by partners who are unknowing carriers. The use of condoms can reduce the likelihood of transmission, but transmission can also occur during skin-to-skin contact in areas not covered by condoms.

In many cases, patients are angry about having warts or HPV and do not know who infected them because the incubation period can be long, and partners may have no symptoms. Acknowledging the emotional distress that occurs when an STI is diagnosed and providing support and facts are important nursing actions.

Prevention

The best strategy is prevention of HPV. The Advisory Committee on Immunization Practices (ACIP) of the CDC recommends routine vaccination of boys and girls 11 to 12 years of age, before they become sexually active. Vaccination is also recommended for females aged 13 through 26 years and males aged 13 through 21 years for those who were not previously vaccinated (Meites, Szilagyi, Chesson, et al., 2019). The ACIP recommends the 9-valent human papillomavirus (9vHPV) vaccine for routine vaccinations. In addition to the four noninfectious virus–like particles (VLPs) HPV 6, 11, 16, and 18 found in 4vHPV, 9vHPV also contains HPV 31, 33, 45, 52, and 58 VLPs (Meites et al., 2019). The vaccination is given in two intramuscular doses, with the initial dose followed by a second dose 6 to 12 months after the first dose. Completion of both doses of the vaccine is important for immunity to develop. If the doses are less than 5 months apart a third dose is required. The vaccination is contraindicated for use in women who are pregnant (National Cancer Institute [NCI], 2018).

Although this vaccine is considered an important medical breakthrough with the potential to decrease the impact of HPV-related disease in men and women, it does not replace other strategies important in prevention of HPV. Women still need cervical cancer screening (CDC, 2019b).

Herpes Virus Type 2 Infection (Herpes Genitalis, Herpes Simplex Virus)

Herpes simplex virus 2 (HSV-2) is a recurrent, lifelong viral infection that causes herpetic lesions (blisters) on the external genitalia and occasionally the vagina and cervix. It is an STI but possibly may also be transmitted asexually from wet surfaces or by self-transmission (i.e., touching a cold sore and then touching the genital area). The initial infection is usually very painful, and blisters may take 2 to 4 weeks to heal, but it can also be asymptomatic. Over 87% of infected individuals are unaware of their infection; most HSV transmission occurs from asymptomatic viral shedding (CDC, 2017b). Recurrences are less painful, self-limited, and usually produce less severe symptoms. Some patients have few or no recurrences, whereas others have frequent bouts (CDC, 2017b). Recurrences can be associated with stress, sunburn, dental work, or inadequate rest or poor nutrition, or any situations that tax the immune system.

There are more than 400 million people affected by HSV-2 worldwide (Cohen, 2017). The prevalence of other STIs has decreased slightly, possibly because of increased condom use, but herpes can be transmitted by contact with skin that is not covered by a condom. Transmission is possible even when a carrier does not have symptoms (subclinical shedding). Lesions increase vulnerability to HIV infection and other STIs.

Pathophysiology

Herpes simplex virus (HSV) is a double-stranded DNA virus that is differentiated into two types of HSV infection (Casanova et al., 2019). These include herpes simplex type 1 (HSV-1), usually associated with cold sores of the lips (herpes labialis) and gingivostomatitis as well as herpes simplex type 2 (HSV-2), usually associated with genital herpes.

Close human contact by the mouth, oropharynx, mucosal surface, vagina, or cervix appears necessary to acquire the infection. Other susceptible sites are skin lacerations and conjunctivae. Usually, the virus is killed at room temperature by drying. When viral replication diminishes, the virus ascends the peripheral sensory nerves and remains inactive in the nerve ganglia. Another outbreak may occur when the host is subjected to stress. In women who are pregnant and have active herpes, infants delivered vaginally may become infected with the virus. There is a risk of fetal morbidity and mortality if this occurs; therefore, a cesarean delivery may be performed if the virus recurs near the time of delivery.

Clinical Manifestations

Itching and pain occur as the infected area becomes red and edematous. Infection may begin with macules and papules and progress to vesicles and ulcers. The vesicular state often appears as a blister, which later coalesces, ulcerates, and encrusts. In women, the labia are the usual primary site, although the cervix, vagina, and perianal skin may be affected. In men, the glans penis, foreskin, or penile shaft is typically affected. Influenzalike symptoms may occur 3 or 4 days after the lesions appear. Inguinal lymphadenopathy (enlarged lymph nodes in the groin), minor temperature elevation, malaise, headache, myalgia (aching muscles), and dysuria (pain on urination) are often noted. Pain is evident during the first week and then decreases. The lesions last 2 to 12 days before crusting over (CDC, 2017b).

Rarely, complications may arise from extragenital spread, such as to the buttocks, upper thighs, or even the eyes, as a result of touching lesions and then touching other areas. Patients should be advised to wash their hands after contact with lesions. Other potential problems are aseptic meningitis, neonatal transmission, and severe emotional stress related to the diagnosis.

Medical Management

Currently, there is no cure for genital herpes infection, but treatment is aimed at relieving the symptoms. Management goals include preventing the spread of infection, making patients comfortable, decreasing potential health risks, and initiating a counseling and education program. Three oral antiviral agents—acyclovir, valacyclovir, and famciclovir—can suppress symptoms and shorten the course of the infection (King, 2017). These agents are effective at reducing the duration of lesions and preventing recurrences. Antispasmodic agents and a saline compress can provide additional relief of symptoms. Resistance and long-term side effects do not appear to be major problems. Recurrent episodes are often milder than the initial episode. Prophylactic vaccine and topical gel development for genital herpes continues to be investigated in clinical trials (King, 2017).

NURSING PROCESS

The Patient with a Genital Herpes Infection

Assessment

The health history and a physical and pelvic examination are important in establishing the nature of the infectious condition. In addition, patients are assessed for risk of STIs. The perineum is inspected for painful lesions. Inguinal nodes are assessed and are often enlarged and tender during an occurrence of genital herpes.

Diagnosis

NURSING DIAGNOSES

Based on the assessment data, major nursing diagnoses may include the following:

- Acute pain associated with the genital lesions
- Risk for infection or spread of infection
- Anxiety associated with worry about the diagnosis
- Lack of knowledge about the disease and its management

Planning and Goals

Major goals may include relief of pain and discomfort, control of infection and its spread, relief of anxiety, knowledge of and adherence to the treatment regimen and self-care, and knowledge about implications for the future.

Nursing Interventions

RELIEVING PAIN

The lesions should be kept clean, and proper hygiene practices are advocated. Sitz baths may ease discomfort. Additional strategies for relieving pain during a herpes outbreak can be found in Chart 51-2.

Chart 51-2 **HEALTH PROMOTION**

Strategies for the Patient with Genital Herpes

Herpes is transmitted mainly by direct contact. Sexual activity during a herpes outbreak not only increases the risk of transmission but also increases the likelihood of contracting HIV and other STIs. The patient therefore takes the following measures:

- Abstains from sexual activity during treatment for active disease (other options such as hand-holding and kissing are acceptable).
- Avoids exposure to the sun, which can cause recurrences (and skin cancer).
- Avoids self-infection by not touching lesions during an outbreak.
- Uses barrier methods when engaging in sexual activity to provide protection against viral transmission.
- Informs sexual partners of herpes diagnosis as transmission is possible even in the absence of active lesions.
- Informs obstetric care provider about the history of genital herpes. In cases of recurrence at time of delivery, cesarean section may be considered.
- Utilizes available support services (see Resources section).
- Keeps follow-up appointments with health care provider, and reports repeated recurrences (may not be as severe as the initial episode).
- Takes medication prescribed for outbreaks and avoids occlusive ointments, strong perfumed soaps, or bubble bath.
- Takes aspirin and other analgesic agents to control pain during outbreaks.
- Uses the appropriate hygiene practices including hand hygiene, perineal cleanliness, gentle washing of lesions with mild soap and running water and lightly drying lesions (i.e., lesions can become infected from germs on the hand, and the virus from the lesion can be transmitted from the hand to another area of the body or another person).
- Wears loose, comfortable clothing; eats a balanced diet; ingests adequate fluids gets adequate rest during outbreaks.

HIV, human immune deficiency virus; STIs, sexually transmitted infections.

The patient is encouraged to increase fluid intake, to be alert for possible bladder distention, and to contact her primary provider immediately if she cannot void because of discomfort. Painful voiding may occur if urine comes in contact with the herpes lesions. Discomfort with urination can be reduced by pouring warm water over the vulva during voiding. When oral antiviral agents are prescribed, the patient is instructed about when to take the medication and what side effects to note, such as rash and headache.

PREVENTING INFECTION AND ITS SPREAD

The risk of reinfection and spread of infection to others or to other structures of the body can be reduced by proper hand hygiene, the use of barrier methods with sexual contact, and adherence to prescribed medication regimens. Avoidance of contact when obvious lesions are present does not eliminate the risk because the virus can be shed in the absence of symptoms, and lesions may not be visible.

RELIEVING ANXIETY

Concern about the presence of herpes infection, future occurrences of lesions, and the impact of the infection on future relationships and childbearing may cause considerable patient anxiety. Nurses serve as important sources of support by listening to patients' concerns and providing information and education. The patient may be angry with her partner if the partner is the probable source of the infection. The patient may need assistance in discussing the infection and its implications with her current sexual partners and in future sexual relationships. The nurse can provide the patient with contact details for support services to assist in coping with the diagnosis (see the Resources section).

INCREASING KNOWLEDGE ABOUT THE DISEASE AND ITS TREATMENT

Patient education is an essential part of nursing care of the patient with a genital herpes infection. This includes an adequate explanation about the infection and how it is transmitted, management and treatment strategies, strategies to minimize spread of infection, the importance of adherence to the treatment regimen, and self-care strategies. Because of the increased risk of HIV and other STIs in the presence of skin lesions, an important part of education involves informing the patient of strategies to protect herself from exposure to HIV and other STIs.

PROMOTING HOME, COMMUNITY-BASED, AND TRANSITIONAL CARE

 Educating Patients About Self-Care. Health promotion strategies and self-care measures for the patient with genital herpes are described in Chart 51-2.

Evaluation

Expected patient outcomes may include:

1. Experiences a reduction in pain and discomfort
2. Keeps infection under control
   a. Demonstrates proper hygiene techniques
   b. Takes medication as prescribed
   c. Consumes adequate fluids
   d. Assesses own current lifestyle (diet, adequate fluid intake, safer sex practices, stress management)

3. Uses strategies to reduce anxiety
   a. Verbalizes issues and concerns related to genital herpes infection
   b. Discusses strategies to deal with issues and concerns with current and future sexual partners
   c. Utilizes available support services if indicated
4. Demonstrates knowledge about genital herpes and strategies to control and minimize recurrences
   a. Identifies methods of transmission of herpes infection and strategies to prevent transmission to others
   b. Discusses strategies to reduce recurrence of lesions
   c. Takes medications as prescribed
   d. Reports no recurrence of lesions

Endocervicitis and Cervicitis

Endocervicitis is an inflammation of the mucosa and the glands of the cervix that may occur when organisms gain access to the cervical glands after penile–vaginal intercourse and, less often, after procedures such as abortion, intrauterine manipulation, or vaginal delivery. If untreated, the infection may extend into the uterus, fallopian tubes, and pelvic cavity. Inflammation can irritate the cervical tissue, resulting in spotting or bleeding and mucopurulent cervicitis (inflammation of the cervix with exudate).

Chlamydia and Gonorrhea

Chlamydia and gonorrhea are the most common causes of endocervicitis, although *Mycoplasma* may also be involved. Chlamydia causes about 2.86 million infections every year in the United States; it is most commonly found in young people who are sexually active with more than one partner and is transmitted through sexual contact (CDC, 2016). Untreated chlamydia infections can spread to the fallopian tubes and uterus leading to serious complications including PID, an increased risk of ectopic pregnancy, and infertility (CDC, 2016). Chlamydial infections of the cervix often produce no symptoms, but cervical discharge, dyspareunia, dysuria, and bleeding may occur. Other complications include conjunctivitis and perihepatitis (Fitz-Hugh–Curtis syndrome) (CDC, 2016). Gonorrhea is the second most commonly reported STI, with over a million new infections each year (CDC, 2019). The inflamed cervix that results from infection may leave a woman more vulnerable to HIV transmission from an infected partner. Gonorrhea is often asymptomatic and a major cause of PID, tubal infertility, ectopic pregnancy, and chronic pelvic pain (CDC, 2019). Diagnosis can be confirmed by urine culture or other methods such as using a swab to obtain a sample of cervical or penile discharge from the patient's partner (CDC, 2019).

Medical Management

The CDC recommends treating chlamydia with doxycycline for 1 week or with a single dose of azithromycin (CDC, 2016). Antimicrobial resistance to fluoroquinolones in the treatment of gonorrhea has left cephalosporins as the remaining recommended treatment (ACOG, 2018a; CDC, 2019). Dual therapy with azithromycin and ceftriaxone given simultaneously on the same day is the recommended first-line treatment for gonorrhea infection (ACOG, 2018a; CDC, 2019). Partners must also be treated. Women who are pregnant are cautioned not to take tetracycline because of potential adverse effects on the fetus. In these cases, erythromycin may be prescribed. Results are usually good if treatment begins early. Possible complications from delayed or no treatment are tubal disease, ectopic pregnancy, PID, and infertility.

Cultures for chlamydia and other STIs should be obtained from all patients who have been sexually assaulted when they first seek medical attention; patients are treated prophylactically. Cultures should then be repeated in 2 weeks. Annual screening for chlamydia is recommended for all young women who are sexually active and older women with new sex partners or multiple partners (CDC, 2016).

Nursing Management

All women who are sexually active may be at risk for chlamydia, gonorrhea, and other STIs, including HIV. Nurses can assist patients in assessing their own risk. Recognition of risk is a first step before changes in behavior occur. Patients should be discouraged from assuming that a partner is "safe" without open, honest discussion. Nonjudgmental attitudes, educational counseling, and role-playing may be helpful.

Because chlamydia, gonorrhea, and other STIs may have a serious effect on future health and fertility, and because many of these disorders can be prevented by the use of condoms and spermicides and careful choice of partners, nurses can play a major role in counseling patients about safer sex practices. Exploring options with patients, addressing knowledge deficits, and correcting misinformation may reduce morbidity and mortality.

Patients should be advised to refer partners for evaluation and treatment. All women aged 25 and younger who are sexually active should be screened annually. Those older than 25 years should be screened if risk factors are present. Repeat testing should occur 3 months after treatment (CDC, 2016).

Promoting Home, Community-Based, and Transitional Care

 Educating Patients About Self-Care

Nurses can educate women and help them improve communication skills and initiate discussions about sex with their partners. Communicating with partners about sex, risk, postponing penile–vaginal intercourse, and using safer sex behaviors, including the use of condoms, may be lifesaving. Some young women report having sex but not being comfortable enough to discuss sexual risk issues. Nurses can help women to advocate for their own health by discussing safety with partners prior to sexual activity.

Reinforcing the need for annual screening for chlamydia and other STIs is an important part of patient education. Instructions also include the need for the patient to abstain from penile–vaginal intercourse until all her sex partners are treated (CDC, 2016).

Pelvic Inflammatory Disease

Pelvic inflammatory disease (PID) is an inflammatory condition of the pelvic cavity that may begin with cervicitis and involve the uterus (endometritis), fallopian tubes (salpingitis), ovaries (oophoritis), pelvic peritoneum, or pelvic vascular system. Infection, which may be acute, subacute, recurrent, or chronic and localized or widespread, is usually caused by bacteria but may be attributed to a virus, fungus, or parasite. Gonorrheal and chlamydial organisms are common causes, but most cases of PID are polymicrobial. While incidence has been declining over the past decades, data from a recent survey indicates the rate of PID in sexually experienced women of reproductive age (18 to 44 years of age) is 4.4% or 2.5 million women (CDC, 2017c; Curry, Williams, & Penny, 2019).

Short- and long-term consequences can occur. The fallopian tubes become narrow and scarred, which increases the risk of ectopic pregnancy (fertilized eggs trapped in the tube), infertility, recurrent pelvic pain, tubo-ovarian **abscess** (a collection of purulent material), and recurrent disease (Curry et al., 2019).

Pathophysiology

The exact pathogenesis of PID has not been determined, but it is presumed that organisms usually enter the body through the vagina, pass through the cervical canal, colonize the endocervix, and move upward into the uterus. Under various conditions, the organisms may proceed to one or both fallopian tubes and ovaries and into the pelvis. In bacterial infections that occur after childbirth or abortion, pathogens are disseminated directly through the tissues that support the uterus by way of the lymphatics and blood vessels (see Fig. 51-1A). In pregnancy, the increased blood supply required by the placenta provides a wider pathway for infection. These postpartum and postabortion infections tend to be unilateral. Infections can cause perihepatic inflammation when the organism invades the peritoneum.

In gonorrheal infections, the gonococci pass through the cervical canal and into the uterus, where the environment, especially during menstruation, allows them to multiply rapidly and spread to the fallopian tubes and into the pelvis (see Fig. 51-1B). The infection is usually bilateral.

In rare instances, organisms (e.g., tuberculosis) gain access to the reproductive organs by way of the bloodstream from the lungs (see Fig. 51-1C). One of the most common causes of **salpingitis** (inflammation of the fallopian tube) is chlamydia, possibly accompanied by gonorrhea.

Pelvic infection is most often sexually transmitted but can also occur with invasive procedures such as endometrial biopsy, abortion, hysteroscopy, or insertion of an intrauterine device. Bacterial vaginosis (a vaginal infection) may predispose women to pelvic infection. Risk factors include early age at first sexual experience multiple sexual partners, frequent penile–vaginal intercourse, penile–vaginal intercourse without condoms, sex with a partner with an STI, and a history of STIs or previous pelvic infection.

Clinical Manifestations

Symptoms of pelvic infection usually begin with vaginal discharge, dyspareunia, dysuria, pelvic or lower abdominal pain, tenderness that occurs after menses, and postcoital bleeding. Other symptoms include fever, general malaise, anorexia, nausea, headache, and possibly vomiting (Norris, 2019). On pelvic examination, intense tenderness may be noted on palpation of the uterus or movement of the cervix (cervical motion tenderness). Symptoms may be acute and severe or low grade and subtle (CDC, 2017c; Curry et al., 2019).

Complications

Pelvic or generalized peritonitis, abscesses, strictures, and fallopian tube obstruction may develop. Obstruction may cause an ectopic pregnancy in the future if a fertilized egg cannot pass a tubal stricture, or scar tissue may occlude the tubes, resulting in sterility. Adhesions are common and often result in chronic pelvic pain; they eventually may require removal of the uterus, fallopian tubes, and ovaries.

Medical Management

Broad-spectrum antibiotic therapy is prescribed, usually a combination of ceftriaxone, doxycycline, and metronidazole. Women are most often treated as outpatients and monitored carefully. Indications for hospitalization include surgical emergencies, pregnancy, no clinical response to outpatient oral antimicrobial therapy, inability to follow or tolerate an outpatient oral regimen, severe illness (i.e., nausea, vomiting, or high fever), and tubo-ovarian abscess (Curry et al., 2019; Norris, 2019). Treatment of sexual partners is necessary to prevent reinfection.

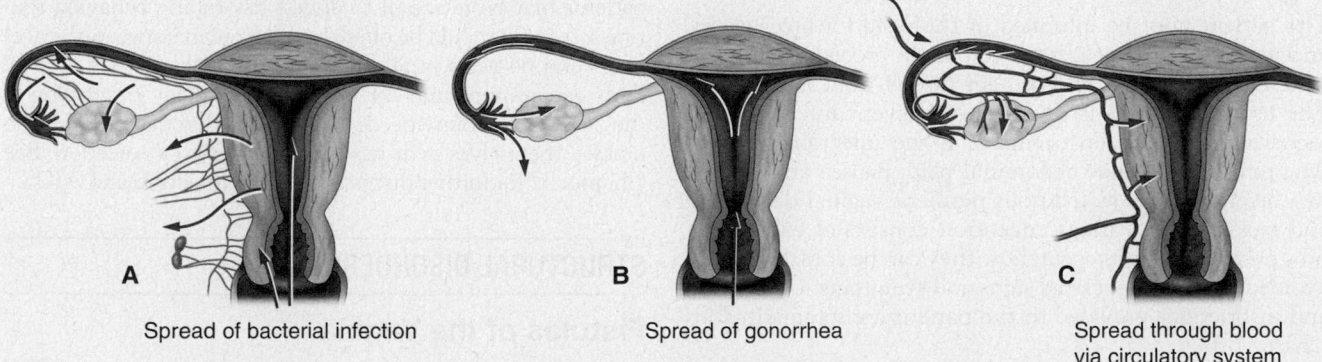

A	B	C
Spread of bacterial infection	Spread of gonorrhea	Spread through blood via circulatory system

Figure 51-1 • Pathway by which microorganisms spread in pelvic infections. **A.** Bacterial infection spreads up the vagina into the uterus and through the lymphatics. **B.** Gonorrhea spreads up the vagina into the uterus and then to the tubes and ovaries. **C.** Bacterial infection can reach the reproductive organs through the bloodstream (hematogenous spread).

Nursing Management

The nurse assesses for both the physical and emotional effects of PID. The patient may feel well one day and experience vague symptoms and discomfort the next. She may also suffer from constipation and menstrual difficulties.

If the patient is hospitalized, the nurse prepares the patient for further diagnostic evaluation and surgical intervention as prescribed. Accurate recording of vital signs, intake and output, and the characteristics and amount of vaginal discharge is necessary as a guide to therapy.

The nurse administers analgesic agents as prescribed for pain relief. Adequate rest and a healthy diet are encouraged. In addition, the nurse minimizes the transmission of infection by adhering to appropriate infection control practices and performing meticulous hand hygiene.

Promoting Home, Community-Based, and Transitional Care

Educating Patients About Self-Care

The patient must be informed of the need for precautions and must be encouraged to take part in procedures to prevent infecting others and protect herself from reinfection. The use of condoms is essential to prevent infection and sequelae. If reinfection occurs or if the infection spreads, symptoms may include abdominal pain, nausea and vomiting, fever, malaise, malodorous purulent vaginal discharge, and leukocytosis. Patient education consists of explaining how pelvic infections occur, how they can be controlled and avoided, and the associated signs and symptoms. Guidelines and instructions provided to the patient are summarized in Chart 51-3.

All patients who have had PID need to be informed of the signs and symptoms of ectopic pregnancy (pain, abnormal bleeding, delayed menses, faintness, dizziness, and shoulder pain), because they are prone to this complication. See Chapter 50 for a discussion of ectopic pregnancy.

Human Immune Deficiency Virus Infection and Acquired Immune Deficiency Syndrome

Any discussion of vulvovaginal infections and STIs must include the topic of HIV and acquired immune deficiency syndrome (AIDS). Although the incidence of HIV diagnosis among women has declined in recent years, more than 7000 (19%) of all new HIV diagnoses are adolescent and adult women (CDC, 2019c). Because HIV infection may be detected during prenatal testing and screening for STIs, nurses and other women's health care clinicians may be the first professionals to provide care for a woman with HIV infection. Thus, clinicians need to be knowledgeable about this disorder and sensitive to women's issues and concerns.

After informed consent is obtained, women who are at risk for HIV are offered testing by a nurse or counselor. Because patients may be reluctant to discuss risk-taking behavior, routine screening should be offered to all women between the ages of 13 and 64 years in all health care settings (CDC, 2019d). Early detection permits early treatment to delay progression of the disease. The nurse needs to remember that many women do not see themselves as at risk for acquiring HIV infection. See Chapter 32 for further discussion of HIV infection and AIDS.

STRUCTURAL DISORDERS

Fistulas of the Vagina

A **fistula** is an abnormal opening between two internal hollow organs or between an internal hollow organ and the exterior of the body. The name of the fistula indicates the two areas

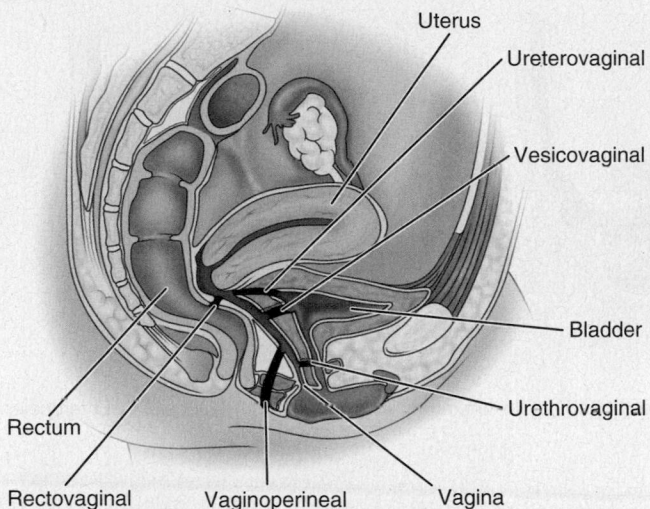

Figure 51-2 • Common sites for vaginal fistulas. *Vesicovaginal*—bladder and vagina. *Urethrovaginal*—urethra and vagina. *Vaginoperineal*—vagina and perineal area. *Ureterovaginal*—ureter and vagina. *Rectovaginal*—rectum and vagina.

that are connected abnormally—for example, a vesicovaginal fistula is an opening between the bladder and the vagina, and a rectovaginal fistula is an opening between the rectum and the vagina (see Fig. 51-2). Fistulas may be congenital in origin but are most common in developing countries due to obstructed labor complications. In developed countries, they occur most often as a result of injury during pelvic surgery, vaginal delivery, radiation therapy, complications from surgical insertion of vaginal mesh, or disease processes such as carcinoma (El-Azab, Abolella, & Farouk, 2019).

Clinical Manifestations

Symptoms depend on the specific defect. For example, in a patient with a vesicovaginal fistula, urine escapes continuously into the vagina. With a rectovaginal fistula, there is fecal incontinence, and flatus is discharged through the vagina. The combination of fecal discharge with leukorrhea results in malodor that is difficult to control.

Assessment and Diagnostic Findings

A history of the symptoms experienced by the patient is important to identify the structural alterations and to assess the impact of the symptoms on the patient's quality of life. Although there is no reported specificity for its use, methylene blue dye is commonly used to help delineate the course of the fistula (El-Azab et al., 2019). In a vesicovaginal fistula, the dye is instilled into the bladder along with placement of vaginal packing known as the "tampon test"; stained vaginal packing can be indicative of a fistula (El-Azab et al., 2019). Cystourethroscopy is useful in identifying fistula while cystoscopy or IV pyelography may then be used to determine the exact location.

Medical Management

The goal is to eliminate the fistula and to treat infection and excoriation. A fistula may heal without surgical intervention, but surgery is often required. If the primary provider determines that a fistula will heal without surgical intervention, care is

planned to relieve discomfort, prevent infection, and improve the patient's self-concept and self-care abilities. Measures to promote healing include proper nutrition, cleansing douches and enemas, rest, and administration of prescribed intestinal antibiotic agents. A rectovaginal fistula heals faster when the patient eats a low-residue diet and when the affected tissue drains properly. Warm perineal irrigations promote healing.

Sometimes, a fistula does not heal and cannot be surgically repaired. In this situation, care must be planned and implemented on an individual basis. Cleanliness, frequent sitz baths, and deodorizing douches are required, as are perineal pads and protective undergarments. Meticulous skin care is necessary to prevent excoriation. Applying bland creams or lightly dusting with cornstarch may be soothing. In addition, attending to the patient's social and psychological needs is an essential aspect of care.

If the patient is to have a fistula repaired surgically, preoperative treatment of any existing vaginitis is important to ensure success. Usually, the vaginal approach is used to repair vesicovaginal and urethrovaginal fistulas; the abdominal approach is used to repair fistulas that are large or complex. Fistulas that are difficult to repair or very large may require surgical repair with a urinary or fecal diversion. Tissue transfer techniques (skin or tissue grafting) may be used (El-Azab et al., 2019).

Because fistulas usually are related to obstetric, surgical, or radiation trauma, occurrence in a patient without previous vaginal delivery or a history of surgery must be evaluated carefully. Crohn's disease and lymphogranuloma venereum are other possible causes.

Despite the best surgical intervention, fistulas may recur. After surgery, medical follow-up continues for at least 2 years to monitor for a possible recurrence.

Pelvic Organ Prolapse: Cystocele, Rectocele, Enterocele

Age and parity can put strain on the ligaments and structures that make up the female pelvis and pelvic floor. Childbirth can result in tears of the levator sling musculature, resulting in structural weakness. Hormone deficiency also may play a role. Some degree of prolapse (weakening of the vaginal walls allowing the pelvic organs to descend and protrude into the vaginal canal) may be found in older women. Risk factors include age, parity (particularly vaginal delivery), menopause, previous pelvic surgery, and possibly a genetic predisposition (ACOG, 2017b; Casanova et al., 2019).

Cystocele is a downward displacement of the bladder toward the vaginal orifice (see Fig. 51-3) from damage to the anterior vaginal support structures. It usually results from injury and strain during childbirth. The condition usually appears years later when genital atrophy associated with aging occurs, but younger women who are multiparous and premenopausal may also be affected.

Rectocele is an upward pouching of the rectum that pushes the posterior wall of the vagina forward. Both rectoceles and perineal lacerations, which occur because of muscle tears below the vagina, may affect the muscles and tissues of the pelvic floor and may occur during childbirth. Sometimes, the lacerations may completely sever the fibers of the anal sphincter (complete tear). An **enterocele** is a protrusion of the intestinal wall into the vagina. Prolapse results from a

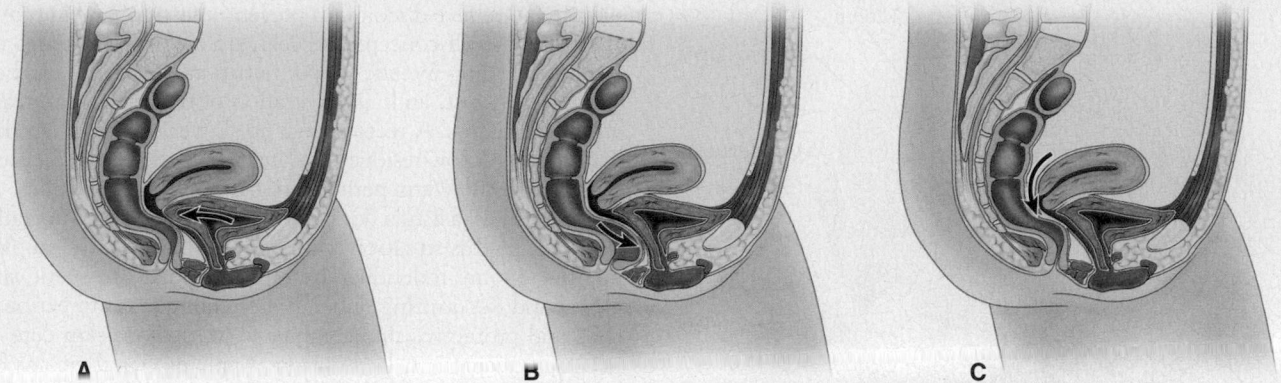

Figure 51-3 • Diagrammatic representation of the three most common types of pelvic floor relaxation. **A.** Cystocele. **B.** Rectocele. **C.** Enterocele. *Arrows* depict sites of maximum protrusion.

weakening of the support structures of the uterus itself; the cervix drops and may protrude from the vagina. If complete prolapse occurs (cervix descending beyond vulva), it may also be referred to as procidentia.

Clinical Manifestations

Because a cystocele causes the anterior vaginal wall to bulge downward, the patient may report a sense of pelvic pressure and urinary problems such as incontinence, frequency, and urgency. Back pain and pelvic pain may occur as well. The symptoms of rectocele resemble those of cystocele, with one exception: Instead of urinary symptoms, patients may experience rectal pressure. Constipation, uncontrollable gas, and fecal incontinence may occur in patients with complete tears. Prolapse can result in feelings of pressure and ulcerations and bleeding. Dyspareunia may occur with these disorders.

Medical Management

Kegel exercises, which involve contracting or tightening the vaginal muscles, are prescribed to help strengthen these weakened muscles (Good & Solomon, 2019). The exercises are more effective in the early stages of a cystocele. Kegel exercises are easy to perform and are recommended for all women, including those with strong pelvic floor muscles (see Chart 51-4). Pelvic floor PT is another treatment option for

early-stage pelvic organ prolapse. It often requires multiple visits and use of manometers and internal examinations, which can be distressing to some (Good & Solomon, 2019).

A pessary can be used alone or in conjunction with other treatments to avoid surgery (ACOG, 2017b; Good & Solomon, 2019). This device is inserted into the vagina and positioned to keep an organ, such as the bladder, uterus, or intestine, properly aligned when a cystocele, rectocele, or prolapse has occurred. Pessaries are usually ring- or doughnut shaped and are made of various materials, such as rubber or plastic (see Fig. 51-4). Rubber pessaries must be avoided in women with latex allergy. The size and type of pessary are selected and fitted by a gynecologic health care provider. The patient should have the pessary removed, examined, and cleaned by her health care provider at prescribed intervals. At these checkups, vaginal walls should be examined for pressure points or signs of irritation. Normally, the patient experiences no pain, discomfort, or discharge with a pessary, but if chronic irritation, excessive discharge, or bleeding occur, alternative measures may be needed (ACOG, 2017b; Good & Solomon, 2019).

A Colpexin Sphere is another nonsurgical device used to treat pelvic organ prolapse. This intravaginal device is similar to a pessary, but it supports the pelvic floor muscles and facilitates exercise of these muscles. It is removed daily for cleaning.

Surgical Management

In many cases, surgery helps correct structural abnormalities. The procedure to repair the anterior vaginal wall is called anterior colporrhaphy, repair of a rectocele is referred to as a posterior colporrhaphy, and repair of perineal lacerations is called a perineorrhaphy. These repairs are frequently performed laparoscopically, resulting in short hospital lengths of stay and good outcomes. A laparoscope is inserted through a small abdominal incision, the pelvis is visualized, and surgical repairs are performed. Transvaginal surgical mesh as a treatment option has been associated with the complications of vaginal erosion, pain and infection leading to the U.S. Food and Drug Administration (FDA) ordering manufacturers of surgical mesh to stop selling and distributing these products (FDA, 2019).

Uterine Prolapse

Usually, the uterus and the cervix lie at right angles to the long axis of the vagina with the body of the uterus inclined

---

Chart 51-4

PATIENT EDUCATION

Performing Kegel (Pelvic Muscle) Exercises

Purposes: To strengthen and maintain the tone of the pubococcygeal muscle, which supports the pelvic organs; reduce or prevent stress incontinence and uterine prolapse; enhance sensation during penile–vaginal intercourse; and hasten postpartum healing.

The nurse instructs the patient to:

1. Become aware of pelvic muscle function by "drawing in" the perivaginal muscles and anal sphincter as if to control urine or defecation, but not contracting the abdominal, buttock, or inner thigh muscles.
2. Sustain contraction of the muscles for up to 10 seconds, followed by at least 10 seconds of relaxation.
3. Perform these exercises 30–80 times a day.

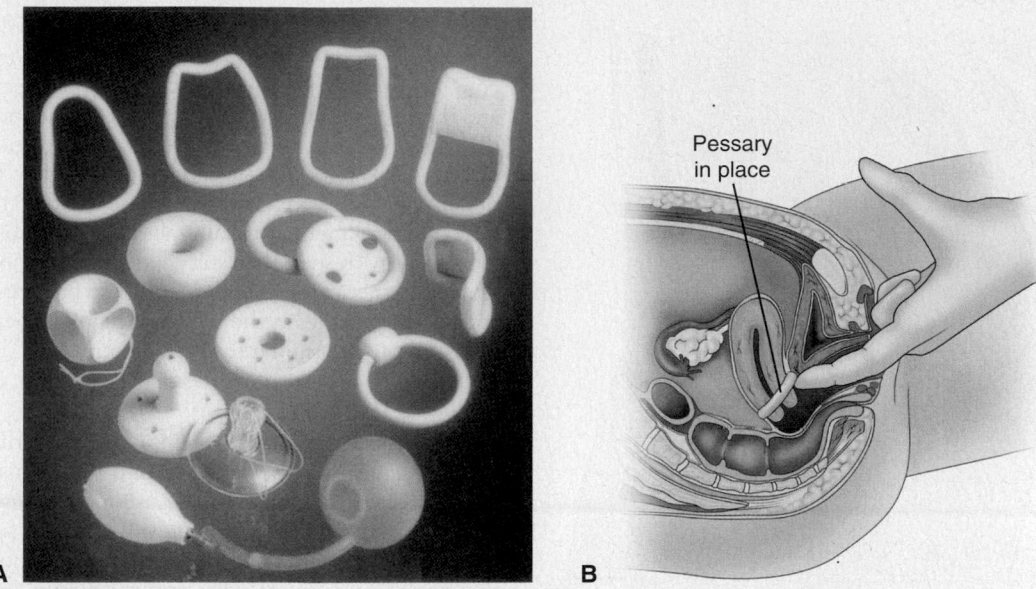

Figure 51-4 • Examples of pessaries. **A.** Various shapes and sizes of pessaries available. **B.** Insertion of one type of pessary.

slightly forward. The uterus is normally freely movable on examination. Individual variations may result in an anterior, middle, or posterior uterine position. A backward positioning of the uterus, known as retroversion and retroflexion, is not uncommon (see Fig. 51-5).

If the structures that support the uterus weaken (typically from childbirth), the uterus may prolapse, or move down the vaginal canal; in severe prolapse, called procidentia, the uterus may appear outside the vaginal orifice (see Fig. 51-6). As the uterus descends, it may pull the vaginal walls and even

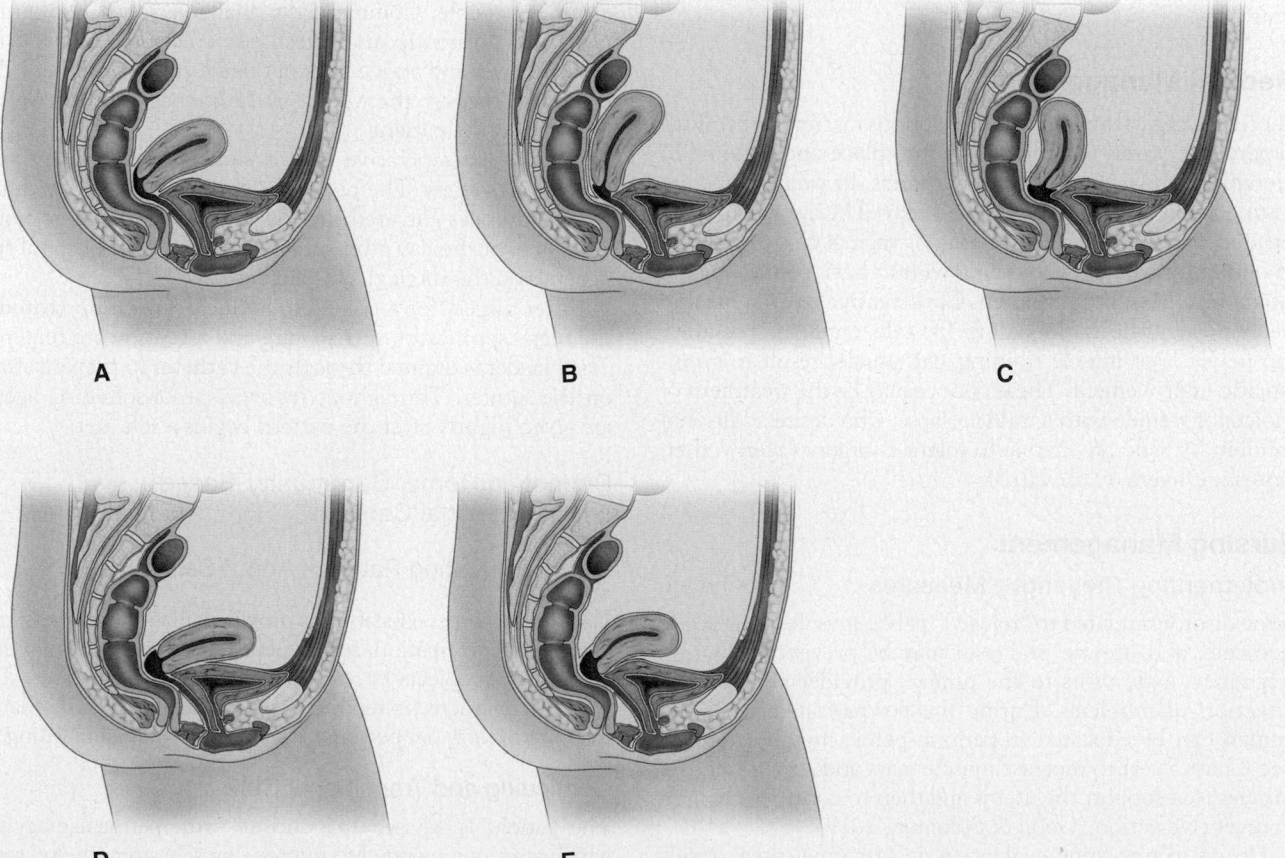

Figure 51-5 • Positions of the uterus. **A.** The most common position of the uterus detected on palpation. **B.** In *retroversion,* the uterus turns posteriorly as a whole unit. **C.** In *retroflexion,* the fundus bends posteriorly. **D.** In *anteversion,* the uterus tilts forward as a whole unit. **E.** In *anteflexion,* the uterus bends anteriorly.

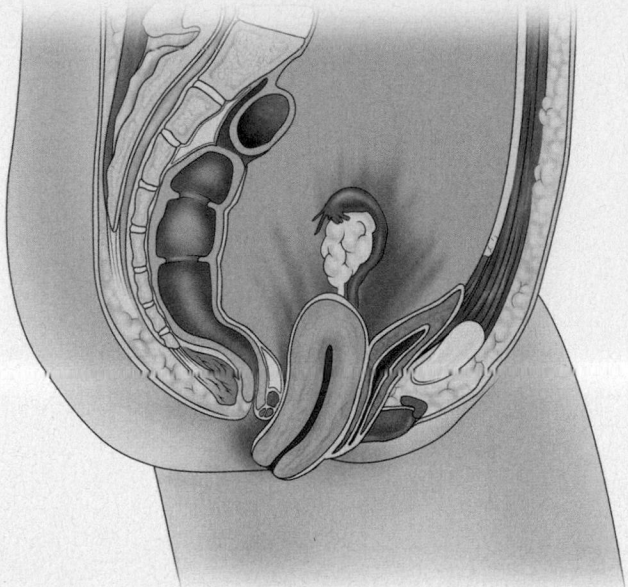

Figure 51-6 • Complete prolapse of the uterus through the introitus.

the bladder and rectum with it. Symptoms include pressure and urinary problems (incontinence or retention) from displacement of the bladder. The symptoms are aggravated when a woman coughs, lifts a heavy object, or stands for a long time. Normal activities, even walking up stairs, may aggravate the symptoms.

Medical Management

There are surgical and nonsurgical options for treatment. With surgery, the uterus is sutured back into place and repaired to strengthen and tighten the muscle bands. In women who are postmenopausal, the uterus may be removed by hysterectomy or repaired by colpopexy. Colpocleisis, or vaginal closure, may be an option for women who do not wish to have penile–vaginal intercourse or to bear children. Conservative treatments and mechanical options, including lifestyle changes, pessaries, and pelvic floor muscle training, can usually result in symptomatic improvement. These options may be the treatment of choice for women with a mild prolapse, who desire additional children, or who are unable to tolerate surgery (Meriwether, Antosh, Olivera, et al., 2018).

Nursing Management

Implementing Preventive Measures

Some disorders related to "relaxed" pelvic muscles (cystocele, rectocele, and uterine prolapse) may be prevented. During pregnancy, early visits to the primary provider permit early detection of problems. During the postpartum period, the woman can be educated to perform pelvic muscle exercises (see Chart 51-4) to increase muscle mass and strengthen the muscles that support the uterus and then to continue them as a preventive action (Good & Solomon, 2019).

Delays in obtaining evaluation and treatment may result in complications such as infection, cervical ulceration, cystitis, and hemorrhoids. The nurse encourages the patient to obtain prompt treatment for these structural disorders.

Implementing Preoperative Nursing Care

Before surgery, the patient needs to know the extent of the proposed surgery, the expectations for the postoperative period, and the effect of surgery on future sexual function. In addition, the patient having a rectocele repair needs to know that before surgery, a laxative and a cleansing enema may be prescribed. She may be asked to administer these at home the day before surgery. The patient is usually placed in a lithotomy position for surgery, with special attention given to moving both legs in and out of the stirrups simultaneously to prevent muscle strain and excess pressure on the legs and thighs. Other preoperative interventions are similar to those described in Chapter 14.

Initiating Postoperative Nursing Care

Immediate postoperative goals include preventing infection and pressure on any existing suture line. This may require perineal care and may preclude using dressings. The patient is encouraged to void within a few hours after surgery for cystocele and complete tear. If the patient does not void within this period and reports discomfort or pain in the bladder region after 6 hours, catheterization is needed. An indwelling catheter may be indicated for 2 to 4 days, so some women may return home with a catheter in place. Various other bladder care methods are described in Chapter 49. After each voiding or bowel movement, the perineum may be cleaned with warm, sterile saline solution and dried with sterile absorbent material if a perineal incision has been made.

After an external perineal repair, the perineum is kept as clean as possible. Commercially available sprays containing combined antiseptic and anesthetic solutions are soothing and effective, and an ice pack applied locally may relieve discomfort. However, the weight of the ice bag must rest on the bed, not on the patient.

Routine postoperative care is similar to that given after abdominal surgery. The patient is positioned in bed with the head and knees elevated slightly. The patient may go home the day of or the day after surgery; the length of hospital stay depends on the surgical approach used.

After surgery for a complete perineal laceration (through the rectal sphincter), special care and attention are required. The bladder is drained through the catheter to prevent strain on the sutures. Throughout recovery, stool-softening agents are given nightly after the patient begins a soft diet.

Promoting Home, Community-Based, and Transitional Care

 Educating Patients About Self-Care

Prior to discharge, education is provided about cleanliness, prevention of constipation, recommended exercises, and avoiding lifting heavy objects or standing for prolonged periods. The patient is instructed to report any pelvic pain, unusual discharge, inability to carry out personal hygiene, and vaginal bleeding.

Continuing and Transitional Care

The patient is advised to continue with perineal exercises, which are recommended to improve muscle strength and tone. She is reminded to return to the gynecologist for a follow-up visit and to consult with the primary provider about when it is safe to resume sexual activity.

BENIGN DISORDERS

Vulvitis and Vulvodynia

Vulvitis (an inflammation of the vulva) may occur with other disorders, such as diabetes, dermatologic problems, or poor hygiene, or it may be secondary to irritation from a vaginal discharge related to a specific vaginitis.

Vulvodynia is a chronic vulvar pain syndrome. Symptoms may include burning, stinging, irritation, or stabbing pain. The syndrome has been described as primary, with onset at first tampon insertion or sexual experience, or secondary, beginning months or years after first tampon insertion or sexual experience. Women affected by this are usually between 18 and 25 years of age. The cause of vulvodynia is not well understood; many believe it is multifactorial. Future research is critical to understanding the pathophysiology and cause of vulvodynia. It can be chronic or unremitting, intermittent or episodic, or may occur only in response to contact (Stenson, 2017). The pathophysiology is unknown. Vestibulodynia is the most frequent type of vulvodynia, producing sharp pain on pressure on the vestibule or posterior aspect of the vaginal opening.

Medical Management

Treatment methods for vulvodynia vary and depend on cause. Topical treatments, self-management care (strict vulvar care/hygiene), surgery, as well as biofeedback and dietary changes, have been used. Some cases seem to be similar to peripheral neuralgia and may respond to treatment with tricyclic antidepressant agents. Patients with dyspareunia may benefit from referral to a behavioral or mental health professional. Psychotherapy is a validated noninvasive treatment option (Stenson, 2017).

Vulvar Cysts

Bartholin cyst results from the obstruction of a duct in one of the paired Bartholin or vestibular mucous-secreting glands located in the posterior third of the vulva, near the vestibule. This cyst is the most common vulvar disorder. A simple cyst may be asymptomatic, but an infected cyst or abscess may cause discomfort. Infection may be due to a gonococcal organism, *Escherichia coli*, or *Staphylococcus aureus* and can cause an abscess with or without involving the inguinal lymph nodes. Skene duct cysts may result in pressure, dyspareunia, altered urinary stream, and pain, especially if infection is present. Vestibular cysts, located inferior to the hymen, may also occur. Cysts can be treated by resection or with laser, ablation with silver nitrate, and puncture. Asymptomatic cysts do not require treatment. Malignancy can occur, usually in women older than 40 years, so drainage and biopsy may be considered (Mahonski & Hu, 2019).

Medical Management

The usual treatment for a symptomatic Bartholin cyst or abscess is drainage. If a cyst is asymptomatic, treatment is unnecessary. Moist heat or sitz baths may promote drainage and resolution.

If drainage is necessary, several techniques are available. The simplest technique is incision and drainage. Using a Word catheter provides another method. This catheter, which is a short latex stem with an inflatable bulb at the distal end, creates a tract that preserves the gland and allows for drainage. A nonopioid analgesic agent may be given before this outpatient procedure. A local anesthetic agent is injected, and the cyst is incised or lanced and irrigated with normal saline; the catheter is inserted and inflated with 2 to 3 mL of water. The catheter stem is then tucked into the vagina to allow freedom of movement. The catheter is left in place for 4 to 6 weeks (Mahonski & Hu, 2019). The patient is informed that discharge should be expected because the catheter allows drainage of the cyst. She is instructed to contact her primary provider if pain occurs, in which case the bulb may be too large for the cavity and fluid may need to be removed. Routine hygiene is encouraged. Marsupialization (creation of small pouch) and gland removal are additional treatment options (Mahonski & Hu, 2019).

Vulvar Dystrophy

Vulvar dystrophy is a condition found in older women that causes dry, thickened skin on the vulva or slightly raised, whitish papules, fissures, or macules. Symptoms usually consist of varying degrees of itching, but some patients have no symptoms. A few patients with vulvar cancer have associated dystrophy (vulvar cancer is discussed later in this chapter). Biopsy with careful follow-up is the standard intervention. Benign dystrophies include lichen planus, lichen simplex chronicus, lichen sclerosus (benign disorder of the vulva), squamous cell hyperplasia, vulvar **vestibulitis** (inflammation of the vulvar vestibule), and other dermatoses (Chibnall, 2017).

Medical Management

Topical corticosteroids (i.e., hydrocortisone creams) are the usual treatment. Petrolatum jelly may relieve pruritus. Use is decreased as symptoms resolve. Topical corticosteroids are effective in treating squamous cell hyperplasia. Treatment is often complete in 2 to 3 weeks, but ongoing assessment for vulvar atrophy should occur at least annually (Chibnall, 2017).

If malignant cells are detected on biopsy, local excision, laser therapy, local chemotherapy, and immunologic treatment are used. Vulvectomy is avoided, if possible, to spare the patient from the stress of disfigurement and possible sexual dysfunction.

Nursing Management

Key nursing responsibilities for patients with vulvar dystrophies focus on education. Important topics include hygiene and self-monitoring for signs and symptoms of complications.

Promoting Home, Community-Based, and Transitional Care

 Educating Patients About Self-Care

Education for patients with benign vulvar dystrophies includes the importance of maintaining good personal hygiene and keeping the vulva dry. Lanolin or hydrogenated vegetable oil is recommended for relief of dryness. Sitz baths may help but should not be overused because dryness may result or increase. The patient is instructed to notify the primary provider about any change or ulceration because biopsy may be necessary to rule out squamous cell carcinoma.

By encouraging all patients to perform genital self-examinations regularly and have any itching, lesions, or unusual symptoms assessed by a primary provider, nurses can help prevent complications and progression of vulvar lesions. Ongoing assessment should occur at least annually.

Ovarian Cysts

The ovary is a common site for cysts, which may be simple enlargements of normal ovarian constituents, the graafian follicle, or the corpus luteum, or they may arise from abnormal growth of the ovarian epithelium. Ovarian cysts are often detected on routine pelvic examination. Although these cysts are typically benign, they nevertheless should be evaluated to exclude ovarian cancer, particularly in women who are postmenopausal (Casanova et al., 2019).

The patient may or may not report acute or chronic abdominal pain. Symptoms of a ruptured cyst mimic various acute abdominal emergencies, such as appendicitis or ectopic pregnancy. Larger cysts may produce abdominal swelling and exert pressure on adjacent abdominal organs.

Postoperative nursing care after surgery to remove an ovarian cyst is similar to that after abdominal surgery, with one exception. The marked decrease in intra-abdominal pressure resulting from removal of a very large cyst usually leads to considerable abdominal distention. This may be prevented to some extent by applying a snug-fitting abdominal binder.

Some surgeons discuss the option of a hysterectomy when a woman is undergoing bilateral ovary removal because of a suspicious mass; it may increase life expectancy and avoid a later second surgery. Patient preference is a priority in determining its appropriateness.

Polycystic ovary syndrome (PCOS) is a type of hormonal imbalance or cystic disorder that affects the ovaries. This complex endocrine condition involves a disorder in the hypothalamic-pituitary and ovarian network or axis, resulting in chronic anovulation and hyperandrogenism, often along with multiple small ovarian cysts. It is common and occurs in approximately 6% to 20% of women of childbearing age (Pfieffer, 2019). Features can include obesity, insulin resistance, glucose intolerance, dyslipidemia, sleep apnea, and infertility. Symptoms are related to androgen excess. Irregular menstrual periods, resulting from lack of regular ovulation, infertility, obesity, and hirsutism, may be a presenting complaint. Cysts form in the ovaries because the hormonal milieu cannot cause ovulation on a regular basis.

Diagnosis is based on clinical criteria, including hyperandrogenism, chronic anovulation, and polycystic ovaries on ultrasound examination. Two out of three of these criteria must be present to make the diagnosis (ACOG, 2018b; Pfieffer, 2019). Women with PCOS are at increased risk for diabetes, increased blood lipids, cardiovascular disease, nonalcoholic fatty liver disease as well as anxiety and depression (Pfieffer, 2019).

Medical Management

The treatment of polycystic ovary syndrome consists of lifestyle changes including weight loss and pharmacotherapy. Oral contraceptive agents are often prescribed to treat PCOS (ACOG, 2018b; Pfieffer, 2019). When pregnancy is desired, medications to stimulate ovulation (clomiphene citrate) are often effective. Lifestyle modification is critical, and weight management is part of the treatment plan.

Weight loss as little as 5% to 10% of total body weight can help with hormone imbalance and infertility. Metformin often regulates periods and can help with weight loss (ACOG, 2018b; Pfieffer, 2019). Women with this diagnosis are at increased risk for endometrial cancer due to anovulation.

Benign Tumors of the Uterus: Fibroids (Leiomyomas, Myomas)

Most women will develop myomatous or **fibroid tumors** of the uterus at some point in their life. It is estimated that by the age of 50, up to 70% of White women and 80% of African American women will experience uterine fibroids (National Institutes of Health [NIH], 2018). It is thought that women are genetically predisposed to develop this condition, which is almost always benign. Fibroids arise from the muscle tissue of the uterus and can be solitary or multiple, intracavitary (in the lining of the uterus), intramural (in the muscle wall), and serosal (in the outside surface). They usually develop slowly in women between 25 and 40 years of age and may become quite large. A growth spurt with enlargement of the fibroid tumor may occur in the decade before menopause, possibly related to anovulatory cycles and high levels of unopposed estrogen. Fibroids are a common reason for hysterectomy because they often result in menorrhagia, which can be difficult to control.

Clinical Manifestations

Fibroids may cause no symptoms, or they may produce abnormal vaginal bleeding. Other symptoms result from pressure on the surrounding organs and include pain, backache, pressure, bloating, constipation, and urinary problems. Menorrhagia (excessive bleeding) and metrorrhagia (irregular bleeding) may occur because fibroids may distort the uterine lining (see Fig. 51-7). Fibroids may interfere with fertility.

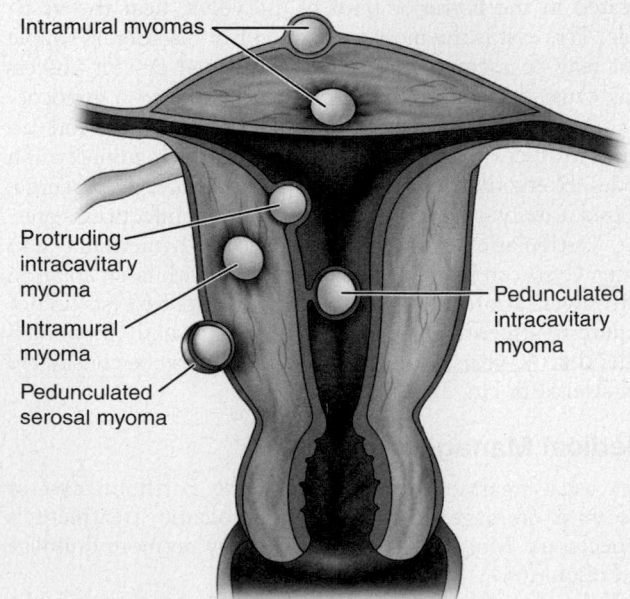

Intramural myomas

Protruding intracavitary myoma

Intramural myoma

Pedunculated serosal myoma

Pedunculated intracavitary myoma

Figure 51-7 • Myomas (fibroids). Those that impinge on the uterine cavity are called *intracavitary myomas.*

Medical Management

Treatment of uterine fibroids may include medical or surgical intervention and depends to a large extent on the size, symptoms, and location, as well as the woman's age and her reproductive plans. Fibroids usually shrink and disappear during menopause, when estrogen is no longer produced. Simple observation and follow-up may be all the management that is necessary. The patient with minor symptoms is closely monitored. If she plans to have children, treatment is as conservative as possible. As a rule, **myomectomy** (surgical removal of uterine fibroids) is performed for large tumors that produce pressure symptoms. A hysterectomy may be performed if symptoms are severe and childbearing is completed (see later discussion of nursing care for a patient having a hysterectomy).

Several alternatives to hysterectomy have been developed for the treatment of excessive bleeding due to fibroids (Fortin, Flyckt, & Falcone, 2017). These include the following:

- *Hysteroscopic resection of myomas:* A laser is used through a hysteroscope passed through the cervix; no incision or overnight stay is needed.
- *Laparoscopic myomectomy:* Removal of a fibroid through a laparoscope inserted through a small abdominal incision.
- *Laparoscopic myolysis:* The use of a laser or electrical needles to cauterize and shrink the fibroid.
- *Laparoscopic cryomyolysis:* Electric current is used to coagulate the fibroid.
- *Uterine artery embolization (UAE):* Polyvinyl alcohol or gelatin particles are injected into the blood vessels that supply the fibroid via the femoral artery, resulting in infarction and resultant shrinkage. This percutaneous image-guided therapy offers an alternative to hormone therapy or surgery. UAE may result in infrequent but serious complications such as pain, infection, amenorrhea, necrosis, and bleeding. Although rare, deaths and ovarian failure may occur. Women need to weigh the risks and benefits carefully, especially if they have not completed childbearing.
- *Magnetic resonance–guided focused ultrasound surgery (MRgFUS):* Ultrasonic energy is passed through the abdominal wall to target and destroy the fibroid. This noninvasive procedure is approved by the FDA for women who are premenopausal with bothersome symptoms due to fibroids and who do not want more children. It is an outpatient treatment.

Medications (e.g., leuprolide) or other gonadotropin-releasing hormone (GnRH) analogues, which induce a temporary menopause like environment, may be prescribed to shrink the fibroids. This treatment consists of monthly injections, which may cause hot flashes and vaginal dryness. Treatment is usually short term (i.e., before surgery) to shrink the fibroids, allowing easier surgery, and to alleviate anemia, which may occur as a result of heavy menstrual flow. This treatment is used on a temporary basis because it leads to vasomotor symptoms and loss of bone density.

Antifibrotic agents are under investigation for long-term treatment of fibroids. Mifepristone, a progesterone antagonist, is also utilized.

Endometriosis

Endometriosis is a chronic disease affecting between 7% and 10% of women of reproductive age, occurring more frequently in women who have never had children (Casanova et al., 2019). **Endometriosis** consists of a benign lesion or lesions that contain endometrial tissue (similar to that lining the uterus) found in the pelvic cavity outside the uterus. Extensive endometriosis may cause few symptoms, or an isolated lesion may produce severe symptoms. It is a major cause of chronic pelvic pain and infertility.

Endometriosis has been diagnosed more frequently as a result of the increased use of laparoscopy. There is a high incidence among patients who bear children late and among those who have fewer children. In countries where tradition favors early marriage and early childbearing, endometriosis is rare. There also appears to be a familial predisposition to endometriosis; it is more common in women whose close female relatives are affected. Other factors that may suggest increased risk include a shorter menstrual cycle (less than every 27 days), flow longer than 7 days, outflow obstruction, and younger age at menarche.

Pathophysiology

Misplaced endometrial tissue responds to and depends on ovarian hormonal stimulation. During menstruation, this ectopic tissue bleeds, mostly into areas having no outlet, which causes pain and adhesions. The lesions are typically small and puckered, with a blue/brown/gray powder-burn appearance and brown or blue-black appearance, indicating concealed bleeding.

Endometrial tissue contained within an ovarian cyst has no outlet for the bleeding; this formation is referred to as a pseudocyst or chocolate cyst. Adhesions, cysts, and scar tissue may result, causing pain and infertility (Casanova et al., 2019). Endometriosis may increase the risk of ovarian cancer.

Currently, the best-accepted theory regarding the origin of endometrial lesions is the transplantation theory, which suggests that a backflow of menses (retrograde menstruation) transports endometrial tissue to ectopic sites through the fallopian tubes. Why some women with retrograde menstruation develop endometriosis and others do not is unknown. Endometrial tissue can also be spread by lymphatic or venous channels.

Clinical Manifestations

Symptoms vary but include dysmenorrhea (menstrual pain), dyspareunia, and pelvic discomfort or pain. Dyschezia (pain with bowel movements) and radiation of pain to the back or leg may occur. Depression, loss of work due to pain, and relationship difficulties may result. Infertility may occur because of fibrosis and adhesions or because of a variety of substances (prostaglandins, cytokines, other factors) produced by the implants of endometriosis and scar tissue on anatomic sites.

Assessment and Diagnostic Findings

A health history, including an account of the menstrual pattern, is necessary to elicit specific symptoms. On bimanual pelvic examination, fixed tender nodules are sometimes palpated, and uterine mobility may be limited, indicating adhesions. Laparoscopic examination confirms the diagnosis and helps stage the disease. In stage 1, patients have superficial or minimal lesions; stage 2, mild involvement; stage 3, moderate involvement; and stage 4, extensive involvement and dense adhesions, with obliteration of the cul-de-sac. Ultrasonography, magnetic resonance imaging (MRI), and CT scans may also be useful to visualize endometriosis (Casanova et al., 2019).

Medical Management

Treatment depends on the symptoms, the patient's desire for pregnancy, and the extent of the disease. If the woman does not have symptoms, routine examination may be all that is required. Other therapy for varying degrees of symptoms may be NSAIDs, oral contraceptive agents, GnRH agonists, or surgery. Pregnancy often alleviates symptoms, because neither ovulation nor menstruation occurs.

Pharmacologic Therapy

Palliative measures include the use of medications, such as analgesic agents and prostaglandin inhibitors, for pain. Hormonal therapy is effective in suppressing endometriosis and relieving dysmenorrhea. Oral contraceptive agents provide effective pain relief and may prevent disease progression (Casanova et al., 2019). Infrequently, side effects may occur with oral contraceptives, such as fluid retention, weight gain, and nausea. These can usually be managed by changing brands or formulations.

Several types of hormonal therapy are also available in addition to oral contraceptive agents. A synthetic androgen, danazol, causes atrophy of the endometrium and subsequent amenorrhea. The medication inhibits the release of gonadotropin with minimal overt sex hormone stimulation. The drawbacks of this medication are that it is expensive and may cause troublesome side effects such as fatigue, depression, weight gain, oily skin, decreased breast size, mild acne, hot flashes, and vaginal atrophy (Casanova et al., 2019; Comerford & Durkin, 2020). GnRH agonists decrease estrogen production and cause subsequent amenorrhea. Side effects are related to low estrogen levels (e.g., hot flashes and vaginal dryness). Loss of bone density is often offset by concurrent use of estrogen. If side effects from GnRH develop, treatment is needed long term or repeated treatments are necessary, additional therapy should be considered. Norethindrone acetate (low-dose hormone) given along with GnRH agonist will mitigate the bone density side effects as well as not affect the drug's control of pelvic pain. Aromatase inhibitor therapy is emerging as an alternative therapy (Casanova et al., 2019). Most women continue treatment despite side effects, and symptoms diminish for 80% to 90% of women with mild to moderate endometriosis. Hormonal medications are not used in patients with a history of abnormal vaginal bleeding or liver, heart, or kidney disease. Bone density is followed carefully because of the risk of bone loss; hormone therapy is usually short term.

Surgical Management

If conservative measures are not helpful, surgery may be necessary to relieve pain and improve the possibility of pregnancy. Surgery may be combined with the use of medical therapy. The procedure selected depends on the patient. Laparoscopy may be used to fulgurate (cut with high-frequency current) endometrial implants and to release adhesions. Laser surgery is another option made possible by laparoscopy. Laser therapy vaporizes or coagulates the endometrial implants, thereby destroying this tissue. Other surgical options include endocoagulation and electrocoagulation, laparotomy, abdominal hysterectomy, **oophorectomy** (removal of the ovary), bilateral **salpingo-oophorectomy** (removal of the ovary and its fallopian tube), and appendectomy. Many women need further intervention following conservative surgeries; therefore, total hysterectomy is the definitive procedure (Casanova et al., 2019).

Nursing Management

The health history and physical examination focus on specific symptoms (e.g., pelvic pain), the effect of prescribed medications, and the woman's reproductive plans. This information helps in determining the treatment plan. Explaining the various diagnostic procedures may help to alleviate the patient's anxiety. Patient goals include relief of pain, dysmenorrhea, dyspareunia, and avoidance of infertility.

As the treatment progresses, the woman with endometriosis and her partner may find that pregnancy is not easily possible, and the psychosocial impact of this realization must be recognized and addressed. Alternatives, such as assisted reproductive technologies or adoption, may be discussed at an appropriate time and referrals offered.

The nurse's role in patient education is to dispel myths and encourage the patient to seek care if dysmenorrhea or dyspareunia occur. The Endometriosis Association (see the Resources section) is a helpful resource for patients seeking further information and support for this condition, which can cause disabling pain and severe emotional distress.

Chronic Pelvic Pain

Chronic pelvic pain is a common disorder of women that may be related to several of the previously discussed gynecologic disorders. Chronic pelvic pain is defined as noncyclic pain concentrated in the pelvis, anterior abdominal wall, and buttock or lumbosacral region for a period greater than 6 months (Andrew & Pickett, 2019). Causes may be of reproductive, genitourinary, or gastrointestinal origin. A history of sexual abuse, IPV, PID, endometriosis, interstitial cystitis, musculoskeletal disorders, irritable bowel syndrome, and previous surgery resulting in abdominal adhesions may be associated with chronic pelvic pain. Dysmenorrhea, dyspareunia, and lower abdominal pain may also be associated with sexual abuse and IPV.

Chronic pelvic pain is often difficult to treat. Treatment depends on physical and diagnostic test results and may include antidepressant, analgesic, anxiolytic, and oral contraceptive agents; GnRH agonists; exercise; diet modification; and various surgical procedures (Andrew & Pickett, 2019).

Adenomyosis

In adenomyosis, the tissue that lines the endometrium invades the uterine wall. Symptoms include hypermenorrhea (excessive and prolonged bleeding), dysmenorrhea, polymenorrhea (abnormally frequent bleeding), and pelvic pain. Physical examination findings on palpation include a symmetrically enlarged, tender, and boggy uterus (Casanova et al., 2019). Treatment depends on the severity of bleeding and pain. Hysterectomy may be the best option in providing relief of symptoms.

Endometrial Hyperplasia

Endometrial hyperplasia (a buildup of endometrial tissue) is the most common precursor to endometrial cancer and often results from unopposed estrogen from any source. Estrogen therapy alone without progesterone in a woman with a uterus can cause this condition. Women with anovulatory cycles, PCOS, or obesity may have high circulating levels of estrogen. Tamoxifen may also be a causative factor. Diagnosis is by biopsy or ultrasound findings of thickness of the endometrium. Hyperplasia with atypia on a pathology or biopsy report indicates risk of progression. Progestin treatment may be effective, but hysterectomy may be advised if pathology from an endometrial biopsy shows atypia. Abnormal bleeding is the most common symptom.

MALIGNANT CONDITIONS

Gynecologic cancer is any cancer that starts in a woman's reproductive organs (CDC, 2019e). According to the American Cancer Society (ACS, 2019a), the projected incidence for female reproductive cancers in the United States includes about 61,880 new cases of uterine cancer; 22,530 new cases of ovarian cancer; 13,170 new cases of cervical cancer; 6070 new cases of vulvar cancer; and 5350 new cases of vaginal cancer per year. Ovarian cancer is responsible for 5% of all cancer deaths in women and is the leading cause of death in female reproductive cancers.

Although some cancers are difficult to detect or prevent, annual pelvic examination with a Pap smear is a painless and relatively inexpensive method of early detection (CDC, 2019e). Primary providers can encourage women to follow this health practice by providing examinations that are educational and supportive and offer women an opportunity to ask questions and clarify misinformation.

Women diagnosed with gynecologic malignancies experience anxiety related to their prognosis. The occurrence of physical symptoms may cause more psychological distress. Intervention directed toward physical and psychological symptoms requires a multidisciplinary approach.

Nurses should be aware of ongoing clinical trials to identify options for many conditions. They are often able to answer questions about clinical trials and to encourage patients to consider participation if appropriate. Women's participation in cancer research may not occur in part because women are unaware of ongoing relevant research (see ClinicalTrials.gov in the Resources section).

Cancer of the Cervix

Death from cervical cancer is less common due to early detection of cell changes by Pap smear (ACS, 2019b). However, it is still the third most common female reproductive cancer in the United States (ACS, 2019b). Risk factors are presented in Chart 51-5.

Preventive measures include regular pelvic examinations and Pap tests for all women, especially older women past childbearing age. Preventive counseling should encourage delaying first penile–vaginal intercourse, avoiding HPV infection, engaging only in safer sex, ceasing smoking, and receiving HPV immunization.

Chart 51-5 ⚠ **RISK FACTORS**
Cervical Cancer

Chronic cervical infection

- Early childbearing
- Exposure to diethylstilbestrol in utero
- Exposure to human papillomavirus, types 16 and 18
- Family history of cervical cancer
- HIV infection and other causes of immune deficiency
- Low socioeconomic status (may be related to early marriage and early childbearing)
- Nutritional deficiencies (folate, beta-carotene, and vitamin C levels are lower in women with cervical cancer than in women without it)
- Overweight status
- Prolonged use of oral contraceptives
- Sexual activity:
  - Multiple sex partners
  - Early age (<20 years) at first coitus (exposes the vulnerable young cervix to potential viruses from a partner)
- Sexual contact with men whose partners have had cervical cancer
- Sex with uncircumcised men
- Smoking and exposure to secondhand smoke

HIV, human immune deficiency virus.
Adapted from American Cancer Society. (2019b). *Cervical cancer.* Retrieved on 10/28/2019 at: www.cancer.org/cancer/cervical-cancer/about/key-statistics.html; Casanova, R., Chuang, A., Goepfert, A. R., et al. (Eds.). (2019). *Beckman and Ling's obstetrics and gynecology* (8th ed.). Philadelphia, PA: Wolters Kluwer.

There are several different types of cervical cancer. Most of these cancers are squamous cell carcinomas, and the rest are adenocarcinomas or mixed adenosquamous carcinomas. Adenocarcinomas begin in mucous-producing glands and are often due to HPV infection. Most cervical cancers, if not detected and treated, spread to regional pelvic lymph nodes, and local recurrence is not uncommon (ACS, 2019b).

Clinical Manifestations

Early cervical cancer rarely produces symptoms. If symptoms are present, they may go unnoticed as a thin, watery vaginal discharge often noticed after penile–vaginal intercourse or douching. When symptoms such as discharge, irregular bleeding, or pain or bleeding after penile–vaginal intercourse occur, the disease may be advanced. Advanced disease should not occur if all women have access to gynecologic care and avail themselves to it. The nurse's role in access to care and its utilization is crucial.

In advanced cervical cancer, the vaginal discharge gradually increases and becomes watery and, finally, dark and foul smelling from necrosis and infection. The bleeding, which occurs at irregular intervals between periods (metrorrhagia) or after menopause, may be slight (just enough to spot the undergarments) and occurs usually after mild trauma or pressure (e.g., penile–vaginal intercourse, douching, or bearing down during defecation). As the disease continues, the bleeding may persist and increase. Leg pain, dysuria, rectal bleeding, and edema of the extremities signal advanced disease.

As the cancer advances, it may invade the tissues outside the cervix, including the lymph glands anterior to the sacrum. In one third of patients with invasive cervical cancer, the disease involves the fundus. The nerves in this region may be affected, producing excruciating pain in the back and the legs that is relieved only by large doses of opioid analgesic agents. If the disease progresses, it often produces extreme emaciation and anemia that usually is accompanied by fever (due to secondary infection and abscesses in the ulcerating mass) and by fistula formation. Because the survival rate for in situ cancer is 100% and the rate for women with more advanced stages of cervical cancer decreases dramatically, early detection is essential.

Assessment and Diagnostic Findings

Diagnosis may be made on the basis of abnormal Pap smear results, followed by biopsy results identifying severe dysplasia (cervical intraepithelial neoplasia type III [CIN III], high-grade squamous intraepithelial lesions [HGSILs, also referred to as HSILs], or carcinoma in situ). HPV infections are usually implicated in these conditions. Carcinoma in situ is technically classified as severe dysplasia and is defined as cancer that has extended through the full thickness of the epithelium of the cervix, but not beyond. This is often referred to as preinvasive cancer.

In its very early stages, cervical cancer is found microscopically by Pap smear. In later stages, pelvic examination may reveal a large, reddish growth or a deep, ulcerating lesion. The patient may report spotting or bloody discharge.

When the patient has been diagnosed with invasive cervical cancer, clinical staging estimates the extent of the disease so that treatment can be planned more specifically, and prognosis reasonably predicted. Staging is based on the International Federation of Gynecology and Obstetrics (FIGO) Staging Classification (Casanova et al., 2019):

- Stage I, the carcinoma is strictly confined to the cervix.
- Stage II, the carcinoma invades beyond the uterus but not the pelvic wall or vagina.
- Stage III, the tumor spreads to the pelvic wall and/or the vagina, and/or causes hydronephrosis of the kidneys.
- Stage IV, the tumor has extended beyond the pelvis and involves the bladder or rectum.

Signs and symptoms are evaluated, and x-rays, laboratory tests, and special examinations, such as biopsy and colposcopy, are performed (Casanova et al., 2019). Depending on the stage of the cancer, other tests and procedures may be performed to determine the extent of disease and appropriate treatment. These tests may include dilation and curettage (D&C), CT scan, MRI scan, IV urography, cystography, positron emission tomography (PET) scan, and barium x-ray studies. Treatment depends on the stage of the disease.

Medical Management

Precursor or Preinvasive Lesions

When precursor lesions, such as low-grade squamous intraepithelial lesions (LGSILs, also referred to as LSILs; CIN I and II or mild to moderate dysplasia), are found by colposcopy and biopsy, careful monitoring by frequent Pap smears or conservative treatment is possible. Conservative treatment may consist of monitoring, **cryotherapy** (freezing with liquid nitrogen), or laser therapy. A **loop electrocautery excision procedure (LEEP)** may also be used to remove abnormal cells. In this procedure, a thin wire loop with laser is used to cut away a thin layer of cervical tissue. LEEP is an outpatient procedure that usually is performed in a gynecologist's office; it takes only a few minutes. Analgesia is given before the procedure, and a local anesthetic agent is injected into the area. This procedure allows the pathologist to examine the removed tissue sample to determine if the borders of the tissue are disease free. Another procedure referred to as a cone biopsy or conization (removing a cone-shaped portion of the cervix) is performed when biopsy findings demonstrate CIN III or HGSIL (equivalent to severe dysplasia) and carcinoma in situ.

If preinvasive cervical cancer (carcinoma in situ) occurs when a woman has completed childbearing, a simple hysterectomy (removal of the uterus only) is usually recommended (Casanova et al., 2019). If a woman is pregnant or wishes to have children and invasion is less than 1 mm, conization may be sufficient. Frequent follow-up examinations are necessary to monitor for recurrence (Casanova et al., 2019).

Patients who have precursor or premalignant lesions need reassurance that they do not have invasive cancer. However, the importance of close follow-up is emphasized because the condition, if untreated for a long time, may progress to cancer. Patients with cervical cancer in situ also need to know that this is usually a slow-growing and nonaggressive type of cancer that is not expected to recur after appropriate treatment.

Invasive Cancer

Treatment of invasive cervical cancer depends on the stage of the lesion, the patient's age and general health. Surgery and radiation treatment (intracavitary and external) are most often used. Surgical procedures that may be used to treat cervical cancer are summarized in Chart 51-6. Robot-assisted technology for the treatment of cervical cancer is a rapidly growing alternative to more invasive surgical options with decreased length of stay, recovery time, decreased blood loss, and increase in total number of retrievable lymph nodes (ACOG, 2017c).

Chart 51-6 Surgical Procedures for Cervical Cancer

- Total hysterectomy—removal of the uterus, cervix, and ovaries
- Radical hysterectomy—removal of the uterus, ovaries, fallopian tubes, proximal vagina, and bilateral lymph nodes through an abdominal incision (*Note:* "Radical" indicates that an extensive area of the paravaginal, paracervical, parametrial, and uterosacral tissues is removed with the uterus.)
- Radical vaginal hysterectomy—vaginal removal of the uterus, ovaries, fallopian tubes, and proximal vagina
- Bilateral pelvic lymphadenectomy—removal of the common iliac, external iliac, hypogastric, and obturator lymphatic vessels and nodes
- Pelvic exenteration—removal of the pelvic organs, including the bladder or rectum and pelvic lymph nodes, and construction of diversional conduit, colostomy, and vagina
- Radical trachelectomy—removal of the cervix and selected nodes to preserve childbearing capacity in a woman of reproductive age with cervical cancer

Adapted from American Cancer Society. (2019b). *Cervical cancer*. Retrieved on 10/28/2019 at: www.cancer.org/cancer/cervical-cancer/about/key-statistics.html; Casanova, R., Chuang, A., Goepfert, A. R., et al. (Eds.). (2019). *Beckman and Ling's obstetrics and gynecology* (8th ed.). Philadelphia PA: Wolters Kluwer.

Frequent follow-up after surgery is imperative because the risk of recurrence is high and usually occurs within the first 2 years. Recurrences are often in the upper quarter of the vagina, and ureteral obstruction may be a sign. Weight loss, leg edema, and pelvic pain may be signs of lymphatic obstruction and metastasis.

Radiation, which is often part of treatment to reduce recurrent disease, may be delivered by an external beam or by **brachytherapy** (method by which the radiation source is placed near the tumor in a sealed source) or both. The field to be irradiated as well as the dose and method of radiation are determined by stage, volume of tumor, and lymph node involvement (Casanova et al., 2019).

A variety of chemotherapeutic approaches are used to treat advanced cervical cancer. They are often used in combination with surgery and radiation. Vaginal stenosis is a frequent side effect of radiation. Preventive therapy (i.e., vaginal dilator) can be used to avoid severe permanent vaginal stenosis.

Some patients with recurrences of cervical cancer are considered for **pelvic exenteration**, in which several pelvic organs are removed. This is a complex, extensive surgical procedure that is reserved for women with a high likelihood of cure. Unilateral leg edema, sciatica, and ureteral obstruction indicate likely disease progression. Patients with these symptoms have advanced disease and are not considered candidates for this major surgical procedure. Surgery is complex because it is performed close to the bowel, bladder, ureters, and great vessels. Possible complications include pulmonary embolism (PE), pulmonary edema, myocardial infarction, cerebrovascular disease, hemorrhage, sepsis, small bowel obstruction, fistula formation, obstruction of the ileal conduit, bladder dysfunction, and pyelonephritis, most often in the first 18 months postoperatively. Vein constriction must be avoided postoperatively. Patients with varicose veins or a history of thromboembolic disease may be treated prophylactically with heparin. Anti-embolism stockings are prescribed to reduce the risk of deep vein thrombosis (DVT). Nursing care of these patients is complex and requires coordination and care by experienced health care professionals. Pelvic exenteration is discussed in further detail later in this chapter.

Cancer of the Uterus (Endometrium)

Over the last decade there has been an increase in both the incidence and death rates of cancer of the uterine endometrium (fundus or corpus), possibly because of increased lifespan and coexisting comorbidities. This cancer is the most frequently occurring gynecologic cancer in the United States. After breast, lung, and colorectal cancer, endometrial cancer is the fourth most common cancer in women. Most women are diagnosed after menopause, with only 15% diagnosed before age 50 (ACOG, 2019). Many women with endometrial cancer have obesity, which increases the risk of morbidity and mortality from this disease. Cumulative exposure to estrogen is considered the major risk factor (see Chart 51-7). This exposure occurs with the use of estrogen therapy without the use of progestin, early menarche, late menopause, nulliparity, and anovulation. Other risk factors include infertility, diabetes, and the use of tamoxifen. Tamoxifen, which is taken for treatment or prevention of breast cancer, may cause proliferation of the uterine lining (ACOG, 2019). Women who

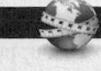

Chart 51-7 | **RISK FACTORS**
Uterine Cancer

- Age—usually >50 years; average age, 63 years
- Obesity that results in increased estrone levels (related to excess weight) resulting from conversion of androstenedione to estrone in body fat, which exposes the uterus to unopposed estrogen
- Unopposed estrogen therapy (estrogen used without progesterone, which offsets the risk of unopposed estrogen)
- Other—nulliparity, truncal obesity, early menarche, late menopause (after 52 years of age) and the use of tamoxifen

Adapted from American College of Obstetricians and Gynecologists. (2015, reaffirmed 2019). Practice Bulletin No. 149: Endometrial cancer. *Obstetrics and Gynecology, 125*(4), 1006–1026.

take tamoxifen should be monitored by their oncologists and/or gynecologic health care providers.

Pathophysiology

Most uterine cancers are endometrioid (i.e., originating in the lining of the uterus). There are two types. Type 1, which accounts for about 90% of cases, is estrogen dependent. It is usually low grade with a favorable prognosis. Type 2, which occurs in about 10% of cases, is high grade and usually serous cell or clear cell. Type 2 is considered to be estrogen independent. Older and African American women are at higher risk for type 2 (ACOG, 2019; Casanova et al., 2019).

Assessment and Diagnostic Findings

All women should be encouraged to have annual checkups, including a gynecologic examination. Any woman who is experiencing irregular bleeding should be evaluated promptly. If a menopausal woman experiences bleeding, an endometrial aspiration or biopsy is performed to rule out hyperplasia, which is a possible precursor of endometrial cancer. The procedure is quick and usually not painful. Transvaginal ultrasound can also be used to measure the thickness of the endometrium (ACOG, 2019). (Women who are postmenopausal should have a very thin endometrium due to low levels of estrogen; a thicker lining warrants further investigation.) A biopsy or aspiration for tissue pathology is diagnostic.

Medical Management

Treatment for endometrial cancer consists of surgical staging, total or radical hysterectomy (discussed later in this chapter), and bilateral salpingo-oophorectomy and lymph node sampling. Laparoscopy or a robot-assisted laparoscopic surgery is less invasive than abdominal surgery (ACOG, 2019). Lymph node sampling and visualization of the peritoneum can be accomplished in many women in this manner. Cancer antigen 125 (CA-125) levels must be monitored, because elevated levels are a significant predictor of extrauterine disease or metastasis. Depending on the stage, the therapeutic approach is individualized and is based on stage, type, differentiation, degree of invasion, and node involvement. Radiation may be used in the form of external-beam radiation or vaginal brachytherapy (ACOG, 2019). Whole pelvis radiotherapy may be used if there is any spread beyond the uterus.

Recurrent cancer usually occurs inside the vaginal vault or in the upper vagina, and metastasis usually occurs in lymph nodes or the ovary. Recurrent lesions in the vagina are treated with surgery and radiation. Recurrent lesions beyond the vagina are treated with hormonal therapy or chemotherapy. Progestin therapy is used frequently. Patients should be prepared for such side effects as nausea, depression, rash, or mild fluid retention with progestin therapy.

Cancer of the Vulva

Primary cancer of the vulva is rare, representing less than 1% of all cancers (Weinberg & Gomez-Martinez, 2019). It is most common in women who are postmenopausal, although its incidence in younger women is increasing. Possible risk factors include smoking, HPV infection, HIV infection, and immunosuppression. Squamous cell carcinoma accounts for most primary vulvar tumors. Less common are Bartholin gland cancer, vulvar sarcoma, and malignant melanoma. Little is known about what causes this disease; however, increased risk may be related to chronic vulvar irritation. In younger women, HPV infection may be implicated, especially types 16, 18, and 31. Prevention includes delaying onset of sexual activity to avoid early exposure to HPV, administration of the HPV vaccine, and avoidance of smoking. Regular pelvic examinations, Pap smears, and vulvar self-examination are helpful in early detection. Women with persistent irritation or itching should be encouraged to seek evaluation.

Clinical Manifestations

Vulvar cancers are rarely asymptomatic (Weinberg & Gomez-Martinez, 2019). Long-standing pruritus and soreness are the most common symptoms of vulvar cancer. Itching occurs in half of all patients with vulvar malignancy. Bleeding, dysuria, foul-smelling discharge, and pain may also be present and are usually signs of advanced disease. Cancerous lesions of the vulva are visible and accessible and grow relatively slowly. Early lesions appear as a chronic dermatitis; later, patients may note a lump that continues to grow and becomes a hard, ulcerated, cauliflowerlike growth. Biopsy should be performed on any vulvar lesion that persists, ulcerates, or fails to heal quickly with proper therapy. Vulvar malignancies may appear as a lump or mass, redness, or a lesion that fails to heal.

Medical Management

Vulvar intraepithelial lesions are preinvasive and are also called *vulvar carcinoma in situ*. They may be treated by local excision, laser ablation, application of chemotherapeutic creams, or cryosurgery.

When invasive vulvar carcinoma exists, treatment may include wide excision of the vulva and **vulvectomy** (removal of the vulva). An effort is made to individualize treatment, depending on the extent of the disease. A wide excision is performed only if lymph nodes are normal. More pervasive lesions require vulvectomy with deep pelvic node dissection. Vulvectomy is very effective at prolonging life but is frequently followed by complications (i.e., scarring, wound breakdown, leg swelling, vaginal stenosis, or rectocele). To reduce complications, only necessary tissue is removed. External-beam radiation may be used, resulting in sunburnlike irritation that usually resolves in 6 to 12 months. Laser therapy and chemotherapy are other possible treatment options.

If a widespread area is involved or the disease is advanced, a radical vulvectomy with bilateral groin dissection may be performed. Antibiotic and heparin prophylaxis may be prescribed preoperatively and continued postoperatively to prevent infection, DVT, and PE. Sequential compression devices (SCDs) are applied to reduce the risk of venous thromboembolism (VTE).

Although the role of systemic chemotherapy in the treatment of vulvar cancer remains to be determined, chemotherapy may be helpful when used in combination with radiation therapy in treatment for advanced disease. The combination of radiation and chemotherapy may reduce the size of the cancer, resulting in less extensive subsequent surgery (Weinberg & Gomez-Martinez, 2019).

Clinical trials to determine the most effective treatment are difficult to conduct because there are few patients with this condition. Morbidity with recurrence of the disease is high, and patterns of recurrence vary. Reconstruction after vulvectomy is performed by plastic surgeons when appropriate and desired.

Nursing Management

Obtaining the Health History

The health history is a valuable tool for establishing rapport with the patient. The reason the patient is seeking health care is apparent. What the nurse can tactfully elicit is the reason a delay, if any, occurred in seeking health care—for example, because of modesty, economics, denial, neglect, or fear (partners who are abusive sometimes prevent women from seeking health care). Factors involved in any delay in seeking health care and treatment may also affect recovery. The patient's health habits and lifestyle are assessed, and her receptivity to education is evaluated. Psychosocial factors are also assessed. Preoperative preparation and psychological support begin at this time.

Providing Preoperative Care

Relieving Anxiety

Prior to surgery, the patient must be allowed time to talk and ask questions. Fear often decreases when a woman who is to undergo wide excision of the vulva or vulvectomy learns that the possibility for subsequent sexual relations is good. The nurse reinforces the information the surgeon has given to the patient and addresses the patient's questions and concerns.

Preparing Skin for Surgery

Skin preparation may include cleansing the lower abdomen, inguinal areas, upper thighs, and vulva with chlorhexidine for several days before the surgical procedure. The patient may be instructed to do this at home.

Providing Postoperative Care

Relieving Pain

Because of the wide excision, the patient may experience severe pain and discomfort even with minimal movement. Therefore, analgesic agents are given preventively (i.e., around the clock at designated times) to relieve pain, increase the patient's comfort level, and allow mobility. Patient-controlled analgesia (see Chapter 9) may be used to relieve pain and promote patient comfort. Careful positioning using pillows usually increases comfort, as do soothing backrubs. A low Fowler position or, occasionally, a pillow placed under the knees reduces pain by relieving tension on the incision; however, efforts must be made to avoid pressure behind the knees, which increases the risk of DVT. Positioning the patient on her side, with pillows between her legs and against the lumbar region, provides comfort and reduces tension on the surgical wound.

Improving Skin Integrity

A pressure-reducing mattress may be used to prevent pressure injuries. Moving from one position to another requires time and effort; the use of an overbed trapeze bar may help the patient move herself more easily. The extent of the surgical incision and the type of dressing are considered when choosing strategies to promote skin integrity. Intact skin needs to be protected from drainage and moisture. Dressings are changed as needed to ensure patient comfort, to perform wound care and irrigation (if prescribed), and to permit observation of the surgical site.

The wound is usually cleansed daily with warm, normal saline irrigations or other antiseptic solutions as prescribed, or a transparent dressing may be in place over the wound to minimize exposure to the air and subsequent pain. The appearance of the surgical site and the characteristics of drainage are assessed and documented. After the dressings are removed, a bed cradle may be used to keep the bed linens away from the surgical site.

Supporting Positive Sexuality and Sexual Function

The patient who undergoes vulvar surgery usually experiences concerns about body image, sexual attractiveness, and functioning. Establishing a trusting nurse–patient relationship is important for the patient to feel comfortable with expressing her concerns and fears. The patient is encouraged to discuss her concerns with her sexual partner as well.

Because alterations in sexual sensation and functioning depend on the extent of surgery, the nurse needs to know about any structural and functional changes resulting from the surgery. Referral of the patient and her partner to a sex counselor may help them address these changes and resume satisfying sexual activity.

Monitoring and Managing Potential Complications

Location, extent, and exposure of the surgical site and incision put the patient at risk for contamination of the site, infection, and sepsis. The patient is monitored closely for local and systemic signs and symptoms of infection: purulent drainage, redness, increased pain, fever, and increased white blood cell count. The nurse assists in obtaining specimens for culture if infection is suspected and administers antibiotic agents as prescribed. Hand hygiene—always a crucial infection-preventing measure—is of particular importance along with wearing masks whenever there is an extensive area of exposed tissue. Catheters, drains, and dressings are handled carefully with gloves on to avoid cross-contamination. A low-residue diet prevents straining on defecation and wound contamination.

The patient is at risk for complications of VTE, which include DVT and PE, because of the positioning required during surgery, postoperative edema, and the immobility needed to promote healing. SCDs are applied, and other prophylactic measures may be prescribed for patients at high risk. The patient is encouraged and reminded to perform ankle exercises to minimize venous pooling, which leads to VTE. The patient is encouraged and assisted in changing positions by using the overbed trapeze bar. Pressure behind the knees is avoided when positioning the patient, because this may increase venous pooling. The patient is assessed for signs and symptoms of DVT (leg pain, redness, warmth, edema) and PE (chest pain, tachycardia, dyspnea). Fluid intake is encouraged to prevent dehydration, which also increases the risk of DVT.

The extent of the surgical incision and possibly wide excision of tissue increase the risk of postoperative bleeding and hemorrhage. Pressure dressings are applied after surgery to minimize this risk.

> ### ▶ *Quality and Safety Nursing Alert*
>
> The patient must be monitored closely for signs of hemorrhage and resulting hypovolemic shock. These signs may include decreased blood pressure; increased pulse rate; decreased urine output; decreased mental status; and cold, clammy skin.

If hemorrhage and shock occur, interventions include fluid replacement, blood component therapy, and vasopressor medications. Laboratory results (e.g., hematocrit and hemoglobin levels) and hemodynamic monitoring are used to assess the patient's response to treatment. Depending on the specific cause of hemorrhage, the patient may be returned to the operating room. See Chapter 11 for a detailed discussion of shock.

Promoting Home, Community-Based, and Transitional Care

 Educating Patients About Self-Care

Preparing the patient for hospital discharge begins before hospital admission. The patient and family are informed about what to expect during the immediate postoperative and recovery periods. Depending on the changes resulting from the surgery, the patient and her family may need education about wound care, urinary catheterization, and possible complications. The patient is encouraged to share her concerns and to assume increasing responsibility for her own care. She is encouraged and assisted in learning to care for the surgical site. A referral for transitional, home, or community-based care is made as indicated.

Nurses are in an ideal position to educate women about performing regular vulvar self-examinations. Using a mirror, patients can see what constitutes normal female anatomy and learn about changes that should be reported (e.g., lesions, ulcers, masses, persistent itching). Nurses must urge women to seek health care if they notice anything abnormal, because vulvar cancer is one of the most curable of all malignant conditions.

Continuing and Transitional Care

Patients may be discharged early in their postoperative recovery to home or a subacute facility. During this phase, the patient's physical status and psychological responses to the surgery are assessed. In addition, the patient is assessed for complications and healing of the surgical site. During home visits, the nurse assesses the home to determine if modifications are needed to facilitate care. The home visit is used to reinforce previous education and to assess the patient's and the family's understanding of and adherence to the prescribed treatment strategies. Follow-up phone calls by the nurse to the patient between home visits are usually reassuring to the patient and family, who may be responsible for performing complex care procedures. Attention to the patient's psychological responses is important because the patient may become discouraged and depressed because of alterations in body image and a slow recovery. Communication between the nurse involved in the patient's immediate postoperative care and the home health nurse is essential to ensure continuity of care.

Cancer of the Vagina

Cancer of the vagina is uncommon, representing 1% to 3% of gynecologic cancers; it is usually squamous in origin (Casanova et al., 2019). Malignant melanoma and sarcomas can occur. Most vaginal cancers are secondary and invasive at the time of diagnosis. Risk factors include previous cervical cancer, in utero exposure to diethylstilbestrol, previous vaginal or vulvar cancer, previous radiation therapy, history of HPV, or pessary use. Any patient with previous cervical cancer should be examined regularly for vaginal lesions.

Vaginal pessaries, which are used to support prolapsed tissues, can be a source of chronic irritation. As such, they have been associated with vaginal cancer, but only when the devices were not cared for properly (i.e., the device was not cleaned regularly or the patient did not return to the primary provider regularly for vaginal examinations).

Patients often do not have symptoms but may report slight bleeding after penile–vaginal intercourse, spontaneous bleeding, vaginal discharge, pain, and urinary or rectal symptoms (or both). Diagnosis is often by Pap smear. Encouraging close follow-up is the focus of nursing interventions with women who were exposed to diethylstilbestrol in utero. Emotional support for mothers who received diethylstilbestrol before its risks were discovered and their daughters who were exposed to diethylstilbestrol in utero is essential.

Medical Management

Treatment of early lesions may include local excision, topical chemotherapy, or laser. Laser therapy is a common treatment option in early vaginal and vulvar cancer. Surgery for more advanced lesions depends on the size and the stage of the cancer. If radical vaginectomy is required, a vagina can be reconstructed with tissue from the intestine, muscle, or skin grafts. After vaginal reconstructive surgery and radiation, regular penile–vaginal intercourse may be helpful in preventing vaginal stenosis. Water-soluble lubricants are helpful in reducing dyspareunia.

Following surgery, radiation therapy may be given by a variety of methods, including external-beam radiation, which is usually an outpatient procedure, or brachytherapy, which is internal radiation therapy. Internal radiation may be given with intracavitary radioactive material contained in a seed, wire, needle, or tube, which is placed into a cavity such as the uterus or vagina. Interstitial radiation is another type of internal radiation treatment in which the radioactive material is placed in or near the cancer but not into a body cavity and is used in cervical and ovarian malignancies. These treatments may be high dose for a short period or low dose, which may take longer. Treatment during hospitalization or during outpatient therapy depends on several factors, including the status of the patient and the mode of delivery.

Cancer of the Fallopian Tubes

Malignancies of the fallopian tube are the least common type of genital cancer (ACS, 2019a). Although this type of cancer can occur at any age, it is most common in women who are postmenopausal. Symptoms are often minimal, causing diagnosis to be made at an advanced stage (Casanova et al., 2019). Symptoms include abdominal pain, abnormal bleeding, and vaginal discharge. An enlarged fallopian tube may be found on sonogram if dilated and fluid filled, or it may appear or be palpated as a mass. Surgery followed by radiation therapy is the usual treatment.

Cancer of the Ovary

Ovarian cancer is the leading cause of gynecologic cancer deaths in the United States, and the fifth deadliest cancer for women following lung, breast, colorectal, and pancreatic (Casanova et al., 2019; Stewart, Ralyea, & Lockwood, 2019). Despite careful physical examination, ovarian tumors are often difficult to detect because they are usually deep in the pelvis. Often called the "Silent Killer," about 70% of ovarian cancers are not diagnosed until stage III or IV. Tumor-associated antigens are helpful in determining follow-up care after diagnosis and treatment and to evaluate for recurrent disease but are not useful in early general screening (Casanova et al., 2019).

Epidemiology

One in 70 women will develop ovarian cancer in her lifetime. The incidence of this type of cancer increases with age until 70 years, with most cases diagnosed by age 60 (Stewart et al., 2019). The frequency of ovarian cancer is highest in industrialized countries and affects women of all races and ethnic backgrounds.

Family history is the most significant risk factor. Most cases are random, but 8% to 13% of ovarian cancers are familial (Casanova et al., 2019). In most cases, the mutations are in the *BRCA1* gene and sometimes in the *BRCA2* gene. A family history in a first-degree relative (mother, daughter, or sister), older age, early menarche, late menopause, and obesity may increase the risk of ovarian cancer. However, most women who develop ovarian cancer have no known risk factors, and no definitive causative factors have been determined.

Patients with concerns about their family history should be referred to a cancer genetics center to obtain information and testing, if indicated (see Chapter 6). Women with inherited types of ovarian cancer tend to be younger when the diagnosis is made than the average age at the time of diagnosis. Hereditary non-polyposis colorectal cancer (HNPCC, also known as Lynch syndrome) increases the risk of ovarian cancer by 5% to 10% (Casanova et al., 2019). Lifetime risk of developing ovarian cancer has been shown to be decreased by 40% to 50% with long-term suppression (greater than 5 years) of ovulation through use of oral contraceptives (Stewart et al., 2019).

Pathophysiology

Types of tumors include germ cell tumors, which arise from the cells that produce eggs and are the most common cause of ovarian cancer in women younger than 20 years (Casanova et al., 2019); stromal cell tumors, which arise in connective tissue cells that produce hormones; and epithelial tumors, which originate from the outer surface of the ovary. Most ovarian cancers are epithelial in origin. Of the many different cell types in ovarian cancer, epithelial tumors constitute 90%. Germ cell and stromal tumors make up the other 10% (Casanova et al., 2019).

Primary peritoneal carcinoma is closely related to ovarian cancer. Extraovarian primary peritoneal carcinoma (EOPPC) resembles ovarian cancer histologically and can occur in women with and without ovaries. Symptoms and treatment are similar. Because of the possibility of EOPPC, oophorectomy lessens the chance but does not guarantee that the patient will not develop carcinoma.

Clinical Manifestations

Symptoms of ovarian cancer are nonspecific and may include increased abdominal girth, pelvic pressure, bloating, back pain, constipation, abdominal pain, urinary urgency, indigestion, flatulence, increased waist size, leg pain, and pelvic pain. Symptoms are often vague, so many women tend to ignore them. Ovarian cancer is often silent, but enlargement of the abdomen from an accumulation of fluid is a common sign. All women with gastrointestinal symptoms without a known cause must be evaluated for potential ovarian cancer. Vague, undiagnosed, persistent gastrointestinal symptoms should alert the nurse to the possibility of an early ovarian malignancy. A palpable ovary in a woman who has gone through menopause is investigated immediately, because ovaries normally become smaller and less palpable after menopause.

Assessment and Diagnostic Findings

Any enlarged ovary must be investigated. Pelvic examination often does not detect early ovarian cancer, and pelvic imaging techniques are not always definitive. Ovarian tumors are classified as benign if there is no proliferation or invasion, borderline if there is proliferation but no invasion, and malignant if there is invasion. Of all new cases of ovarian tumors, 20% are classified as borderline and have low malignancy potential. However, by the time of diagnosis, most ovarian cancers are advanced (Casanova et al., 2019; Stewart et al., 2019).

Diagnostic test may include an MRI scan, transvaginal and pelvic ultrasound, chest x-rays, and a blood test for CA-125. An abdominal CT scan with and without contrast may be used to rule out metastasis (Casanova et al., 2019).

Medical Management

Surgical Management

Surgical staging, exploration, and reduction of tumor mass are the basics of treatment. Surgical removal is the treatment

---

Chart 51-8 — Main Stages of Ovarian Cancer

I. Cancer is contained within the ovary (or ovaries).

II. Cancer is in one or both ovaries and has involved other organs (i.e., uterus, fallopian tubes, bladder, the sigmoid colon, or the rectum) within the pelvis.

III. Cancer involves one or both ovaries, and one or both of the following are present: (1) cancer has spread beyond the pelvis to the lining of the abdomen; (2) cancer has spread to lymph nodes.

IV. The most advanced stage of ovarian cancer. Cancer is in one or both ovaries. There is distant metastasis to the liver, lungs, or other organs outside the peritoneal cavity; ovarian cancer cells in the pleural cavity are evidence of stage IV disease.

Adapted from Casanova, R., Chuang, A., Goepfert, A. R., et al. (Eds.). (2019). *Beckman and Ling's obstetrics and gynecology* (8th ed.). Philadelphia, PA: Wolters Kluwer.

---

of choice. Staging the tumor by the FIGO staging system is performed to guide treatment (see Chart 51-8). Likely treatment involves a total abdominal hysterectomy with removal of the fallopian tubes and ovaries and possibly the omentum (bilateral salpingo-oophorectomy and omentectomy), tumor debulking, para-aortic and pelvic lymph node sampling, diaphragmatic biopsies, random peritoneal biopsies, and cytologic washings. Postoperative management may include taxanes or platinum-based chemotherapy (discussed in the next section).

Borderline tumors resemble ovarian cancer but have much more favorable outcomes. Women diagnosed with this type of cancer tend to be younger (early 40s). A conservative surgical approach is used. The affected ovary is removed, but the uterus and the contralateral ovary may remain in place. Adjuvant therapy may not be warranted.

Pharmacologic Therapy

Chemotherapy is usually administered IV on an outpatient basis using a combination of platinum and taxane agents. Paclitaxel plus carboplatin are most often used because of their excellent clinical benefits and manageable toxicity. Leukopenia, neurotoxicity, and fever may occur.

Because paclitaxel often causes leukopenia, patients may need to take granulocyte colony-stimulating factor as well. Paclitaxel is contraindicated in patients with hypersensitivity to medications formulated in polyoxyethylated castor oil and in patients with baseline neutropenia. Because of possible adverse cardiac effects, paclitaxel is not used in patients with cardiac disorders. Hypotension, dyspnea, angioedema, and urticaria indicate severe reactions that usually occur soon after the first and second doses are given. Nurses who administer chemotherapy are prepared to assist in treating anaphylaxis. Patients should be prepared for inevitable hair loss.

Carboplatin may be used in the initial treatment and in patients with recurrence. It is used with caution in patients with renal impairment. Usually, six cycles are given. A positive clinical response is normalization of the tumor marker CA-125, negative CT results, and a normal physical and gynecologic examination.

Liposomal therapy, delivery of chemotherapy in a liposome, allows the highest possible dose of chemotherapy to the tumor target with a reduction in adverse effects. Liposomes are used as drug carriers because they are nontoxic, biodegradable, easily available, and relatively inexpensive. This encapsulated chemotherapy allows increased duration of action and better targeting. The encapsulation of doxorubicin lessens the incidence of nausea, vomiting, and alopecia. Patients must be monitored for bone marrow suppression and gastrointestinal and cardiac effects.

Combination IV and intraperitoneal chemotherapy is an option for some patients. However, this treatment is more toxic and side effects are more severe than regular chemotherapy (ACS, 2018). Intraperitoneal chemotherapy is reserved for women with good kidney function (ACS, 2018).

Genetic engineering and identification of cancer genes may make gene therapy a future possibility; gene therapy is under investigation. Emerging proteomic technologies (tissue-based protein analysis) look promising; they may allow earlier diagnosis and treatment decision making. New biomarkers need further validation, but protein signature patterns are now being tested. These technologies may result in individualized treatment strategies for epithelial ovarian cancer (ACS, 2018).

Recurrence of ovarian cancer is common, and many patients may require treatment with multiple agents. Treatment is directed toward control of the cancer, maintenance of quality of life, and palliation. Liposomal preparations, intraperitoneal drug administration, anticancer vaccines, monoclonal antibodies directed against cancer antigens, gene therapy, and antiangiogenic treatments (to prevent formation of new blood vessels in an effort to halt growth of ovarian cancer) may be used in the treatment for recurrence.

Nursing Management

Nursing measures involve those related to the patient's treatment plan, which may include surgery, chemotherapy, palliative care, or a combination of these. Nursing interventions after pelvic surgery to remove the tumor are similar to those after other abdominal surgeries. If ovarian cancer occurs in a young woman and the tumor is unilateral, it is removed. Childbearing, if desired, is encouraged in the near future. After childbirth, surgical re-exploration may be performed, and the remaining ovary may be removed. If both ovaries are involved, bilateral oophorectomy is performed and chemotherapy follows.

Patients with advanced ovarian cancer may develop ascites and pleural effusion. Nursing care may include administering IV fluids prescribed to alleviate fluid and electrolyte imbalances, administering parenteral nutrition to provide adequate nutrition, providing postoperative care after intestinal bypass to alleviate any obstruction, controlling pain, and managing drainage tubes. Comfort measures for women with ascites may include providing small frequent meals, decreasing fluid intake, administering diuretic agents, and providing rest. Patients with pleural effusion may experience shortness of breath, hypoxia, pleuritic chest pain, and cough. Thoracentesis is usually performed to relieve these symptoms. The patient with ovarian cancer often has complex needs and benefits from the assistance and support of an oncology clinical nurse specialist.

Hysterectomy

Hysterectomy is the surgical removal of the uterus to treat cancer, dysfunctional uterine bleeding, endometriosis, nonmalignant growths, persistent pain, pelvic relaxation and prolapse, and previous injury to the uterus. Hysterectomies have been steadily declining over the last decade as the number of other therapeutic options (i.e., laser therapy, endometrial ablation, UAE, medications to shrink fibroid tumors) has increased (Morgan, Kamdar, Swenson, et al., 2017). Despite the decline in hysterectomies, it is still the second most common gynecologic procedure; 90% of all hysterectomies are for benign causes (ACOG, 2017d).

A total hysterectomy involves removal of the uterus and the cervix. Hysterectomy can be supracervical or subtotal, in which the uterus is removed but the cervix is spared. Radical hysterectomy involves removal of the uterus as well as the surrounding tissue, including the upper third of the vagina and pelvic lymph nodes. The procedure can be performed through the vagina, through an abdominal incision, or laparoscopically (in which the uterus is removed in sections through small incisions using a laparoscope). Malignant conditions usually require a total abdominal hysterectomy and bilateral salpingo-oophorectomy.

A laparoscopically assisted approach can also be used for vaginal hysterectomy. This procedure is performed as a short-stay procedure or ambulatory surgery in patients who are carefully selected. Robot-assisted hysterectomies are performed in more than 20% of cases, with similar outcomes compared to laparoscopic and vaginal methods at a higher cost (ACOG, 2017d).

Preoperative Management

Patients are advised to discontinue anticoagulant medications, NSAIDs such as aspirin, and vitamin E prior to surgery to reduce the risk of bleeding. Pregnancy is ruled out on the day of surgery. Prophylactic antibiotic agents may be given prior to surgery and discontinued the next day. Prevention of thromboembolic events is critical, and methods depend on the risk profile of the patient.

Postoperative Management

The principles of general postoperative care for abdominal surgery apply. Major risks are infection and hemorrhage. In addition, because the surgical site is close to the bladder, voiding problems may occur, particularly after a vaginal hysterectomy. Edema or nerve trauma may cause temporary bladder atony (loss of bladder tone), and an indwelling catheter may be inserted.

NURSING PROCESS

The Patient Undergoing a Hysterectomy

Assessment

The health history and the physical and pelvic examination are completed, and laboratory tests are performed. Additional assessment data include the patient's psychosocial responses, because the need for a hysterectomy may elicit strong emotional reactions. If the hysterectomy is performed to remove a malignant tumor, anxiety related to fear of cancer and its consequences adds to the stress of the patient and her family. Women who have had a hysterectomy may be at risk for psychological and physical symptoms. Alternatively, women may note improved physical and mental health after hysterectomy as troublesome symptoms may be alleviated.

Diagnosis

NURSING DIAGNOSES

Based on the assessment data, major nursing diagnoses may include the following:

- Anxiety associated with the diagnosis of cancer, fear of pain, possible perception of loss of femininity or childbearing potential
- Disturbed body image associated with altered body function
- Acute pain associated with surgery and other adjuvant therapy
- Lack of knowledge of the perioperative aspects of hysterectomy and postoperative self-care

COLLABORATIVE PROBLEMS/POTENTIAL COMPLICATIONS

Potential complications may include the following:

- Hemorrhage
- VTE
- Bladder dysfunction
- Infection

Planning and Goals

The major goals may include relief of anxiety, acceptance of loss of the uterus, absence of pain or discomfort, increased knowledge of self-care requirements, and absence of complications.

Nursing Interventions

RELIEVING ANXIETY

Anxiety stems from several factors: unfamiliar environment; the effects of surgery on body image and reproductive ability; fear of pain and other discomfort; and, possibly, feelings of embarrassment about exposure in the perioperative period. The nurse determines what the experience means to the patient and encourages her to verbalize her concerns. Throughout the preoperative, postoperative, and recovery periods, explanations are given about physical preparations and procedures that are performed.

IMPROVING BODY IMAGE

The patient may have strong emotional reactions to having a hysterectomy and personal feelings related to the diagnosis, views of significant others who may be involved (family, partner), religious beliefs, and fears about prognosis. Concerns such as the inability to have children and the effect on femininity may surface, as may questions about the effects of surgery on sexual relationships, function, and satisfaction. The patient needs reassurance that she will still have a vagina and that she can experience sexual activity after temporary postoperative abstinence while tissues heal. Information that sexual satisfaction and orgasm arise from clitoral stimulation rather than from the uterus reassures many women. Most women note some change in sexual feelings after hysterectomy, but they vary in intensity. In some cases, the vagina is shortened by surgery, and this may affect sensitivity or comfort.

When hormonal balance is upset, as often occurs with reproductive system disorders, the patient may experience depressed mood and heightened emotional sensitivity to people and situations. The nurse needs to approach and evaluate each patient individually in light of these factors. A nurse who exhibits interest, concern, and willingness to listen to the patient's fears will help the patient progress through the surgical experience.

RELIEVING PAIN

Postoperative pain and discomfort are common. Therefore, the nurse assesses the intensity of the patient's pain and assists the patient with analgesia as prescribed. If the patient has abdominal distention or flatus, a rectal tube and application of heat to the abdomen may be prescribed. When abdominal auscultation reveals return of bowel sounds and peristalsis, additional fluids and a soft diet are permitted. Early ambulation facilitates the return of normal peristalsis.

ADDRESSING LEARNING NEEDS

Patient education should address learning needs specific to the surgical procedure being performed. Research indicates that women undergoing robotic or laparoscopic surgeries have different learning needs (Kurt, Loerzel, Hines, et al., 2018). See the Nursing Research Profile in Chart 51-9.

Chart 51-9 | **NURSING RESEARCH PROFILE**
Gynecologic Surgery Learning Needs

Kurt, G., Loerzel, V. W., Hines, R. B., et al. (2018). Learning needs of women who undergo robotic versus open gynecologic surgery. *Journal of Obstetric, Gynecologic, and Neonatal Nursing: JOGNN, 47*(4), 490–497.

Purpose

The purpose of this study was to determine and compare the specific learning needs of women who undergo open gynecologic surgery via laparotomy or robotic surgery.

Design

The study used a descriptive exploratory design. The sample consisted of 226 women who underwent laparotomy ($n = 71$) or robotic surgery ($n = 155$) in one hospital. Participants were 18 years of age or older, able to speak, understand and read English or Spanish and scheduled for a laparotomy or robotic surgical procedure. Learning needs were measured using a 50-item patient learning needs scale (PLNS).

Findings

Study findings reported that at the time of discharge, participants in the robotic surgery group had significantly more learning needs overall on the PLNS, with means of 179.67 in the group that had robotic surgery compared to 159.66 in the group that had laparotomy ($p < 0.001$). Specifically, learning needs were greater in the topics of medications, activities of daily living, feelings related to condition, treatment and complications, skin care, and enhancing quality of life.

Nursing Implications

Nurses need to be proactive in educating women about postoperative care following robotic surgery for gynecologic conditions. Nurses caring for these women should consider providing education earlier in the surgical process, ideally prior to surgery. A learning needs assessment done prior to surgery will help the nurse develop an individualized education plan.

Patient education also addresses the outcomes of surgery, possible feelings of loss, and options for management of any symptoms that occur. Women vary in their preferences for information and participation in decision making, including choice of treatment options, accurate and useful information at the appropriate time, support from their health care providers, and access to professional and lay support systems.

Monitoring and Managing Potential Complications

HEMORRHAGE

Vaginal bleeding and hemorrhage may occur after hysterectomy. To detect these complications early, the nurse counts the perineal pads used or checks the incision site, assesses the extent of saturation with blood, and monitors vital signs. Abdominal dressings are monitored for drainage if an abdominal surgical approach has been used. In preparation for hospital discharge, the nurse gives prescribed guidelines for activity restrictions to promote healing and to prevent postoperative bleeding. Because many women may go home the day of surgery or within a day or two, they are instructed to contact the nurse or surgeon if bleeding is beyond what is expected, which should be minimal.

VENOUS THROMBOEMBOLISM

Because of positioning during surgery, postoperative edema, and decreased activity postoperatively, the patient is at risk for DVT and PE. To minimize the risk, anti-embolism stockings are applied. In addition, the patient is encouraged and assisted to change positions frequently, although pressure under the knees is avoided, and to exercise her legs and feet while in bed. The nurse helps the patient ambulate early in the postoperative period. The nurse also assesses for DVT (leg pain, redness, warmth, edema) and PE (chest pain, tachycardia, dyspnea). If the patient is being discharged home soon after surgery, she is instructed to avoid prolonged sitting in a chair with pressure at the knees, sitting with crossed legs, and inactivity. Furthermore, she is instructed to contact her primary provider if symptoms of DVT or PE occur.

BLADDER DYSFUNCTION

Because of possible difficulty in voiding postoperatively, occasionally an indwelling catheter may be inserted before or during surgery and is left in place in the immediate postoperative period. If a catheter is in place, it is usually removed shortly after the patient begins to ambulate. After the catheter is removed, urinary output is monitored; additionally, the abdomen is assessed for distention. If the patient does not void within a prescribed time, measures are initiated to encourage voiding (e.g., assisting the patient to the bathroom, pouring warm water over the perineum). If the patient cannot void, catheterization may be necessary. On rare occasions, the patient may be discharged home with the catheter in place and is instructed in its management.

PROMOTING HOME, COMMUNITY-BASED, AND TRANSITIONAL CARE

Educating Patients About Self-Care. The information provided to the patient is tailored to her needs. She must know what limitations or restrictions, if any, to expect. She is instructed to check the surgical incision daily and to contact her primary provider if redness or purulent drainage or discharge occurs. She is reminded that

her periods are now over but that she may have a slightly bloody discharge for a few days; if bleeding recurs after this time, it should be reported immediately. The patient is educated about the importance of an adequate oral intake and of maintaining bowel and urinary tract function. The patient is informed that she is likely to recover quickly but that postoperative fatigue is not unusual.

The patient should resume activities gradually. This does not mean sitting for long periods, because doing so may cause blood to pool in the pelvis, increasing the risk of VTE. The nurse explains that showers are preferable to tub baths to reduce the possibility of infection and to avoid the dangers of injury that may occur when getting in and out of the bathtub. The patient is instructed to avoid straining, lifting, having penile–vaginal intercourse, or driving until permitted. Vaginal discharge, foul odor, excessive bleeding, any leg redness or pain, or an elevated temperature should be reported, and the nurse reinforces education regarding activities and restrictions.

Continuing and Transitional Care. Follow-up telephone contact provides the nurse with the opportunity to determine whether the patient is recovering without problems and to answer any questions that may have arisen. The patient is reminded about postoperative follow-up appointments. If the patient's ovaries were removed and she finds vasomotor symptoms troublesome, hormone therapy may be considered at a low dose for a short amount of time. The patient is reminded to discuss risks and benefits of hormone therapy and alternative therapies with her primary provider and gynecologic care provider. Decisions about use of hormone therapy need to be made individually in consultation with these providers.

Evaluation

Expected patient outcomes may include:
1. Experiences decreased anxiety
   a. Has improved body image
   b. Discusses changes resulting from surgery with her partner
   c. Verbalizes understanding of her disorder and the treatment plan
2. Displays minimal depression or anxiety
3. Experiences minimal pain and discomfort
   a. Reports relief of abdominal pain and discomfort
   b. Ambulates without pain
4. Verbalizes knowledge and understanding of self-care
   a. Practices deep-breathing, turning, and leg exercises as instructed
   b. Increases activity and ambulation daily
   c. Reports adequate fluid intake and adequate urinary output
   d. Identifies reportable symptoms
   e. Schedules and keeps follow-up appointments
5. Absence of complications
   a. Has minimal vaginal bleeding and exhibits normal vital signs
   b. Ambulates early
   c. Notes no chest or calf pain and no redness, tenderness, or swelling in the extremities
   d. Reports no urinary problems or abdominal distention

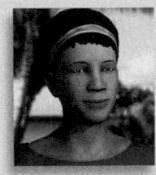
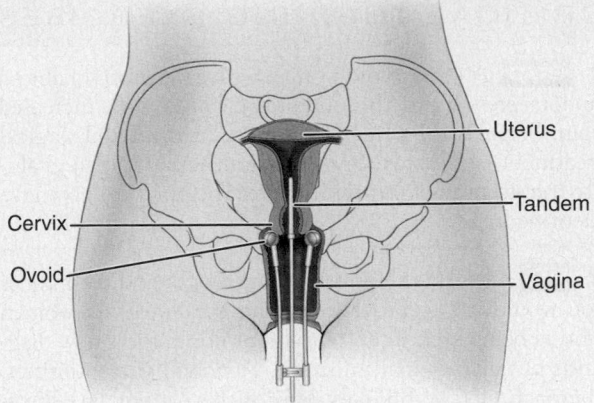

Figure 51-8 • Placement of tandem and ovoids for internal radiation therapy.

Radiation Therapy

Radiation may be used in the treatment of cervical, uterine, and less frequently in ovarian cancers either alone or in combination with surgery and chemotherapy. Several approaches are used to deliver radiation to the female reproductive system: external radiation, intraoperative radiation therapy (IORT), and internal (intracavitary) irradiation or brachytherapy (Smith & Jhingran, 2017). The cervix and uterus can serve as a receptacle for radioactive sources for internal radiation therapy.

Methods of Radiation Therapy

External Radiation Therapy

This method of delivering radiation destroys cancerous cells at the skin surface or deeper in the body. Other methods of delivering radiation therapy are more commonly used to treat cancer of the female reproductive system than this method.

Intraoperative Radiation Therapy

IORT allows radiation to be applied directly to the affected area during surgery. An electron beam is directed at the disease site. This direct-view irradiation may be used when para-aortic nodes are involved or for unresectable (inoperable) or partially resectable neoplasms. Benefits include accurate beam direction (which precisely limits the radiation to the tumor) and the ability during treatment to block sensitive organs from radiation. IORT is usually combined with external-beam irradiation pre- or postoperatively.

Internal (Intracavitary) Irradiation

After the patient receives an anesthetic agent and an examination, specially prepared applicators are inserted into the endometrial cavity and vagina. These devices are not loaded with radioactive material until the patient returns to her room. X-rays are obtained to verify the precise relationship of the applicator to the normal pelvic anatomy and to the tumor. When this step is completed, the radiation oncologist loads the applicators with predetermined amounts of radioactive material. This procedure, called *afterloading*, allows for precise control of the radiation exposure received by the patient, with minimal exposure of physicians, nurses, and other health care personnel. A patient undergoing internal radiation treatment remains isolated in a private room until the application is completed. Adjacent rooms may need to be evacuated and a lead shield placed at the doorway to the patient's room.

Of the various applicators developed for intracavitary treatment, some are inserted into the endometrial cavity and endocervical canal as multiple small irradiators (e.g., Heyman capsules). Others consist of a central tube (a tandem or intrauterine "stem") placed through the dilated endocervical canal into the uterine cavity, which remains in a fixed relationship with the irradiators placed in the upper vagina on each side of the cervix (vaginal ovoids) (see Fig. 51-8).

When the applicator is inserted, an indwelling urinary catheter is also inserted. Vaginal packing is inserted to keep the applicator in place and to keep other organs, such as the bladder and rectum, as far from the radioactive source as possible. The objective of the internal treatment is to maintain the distribution of internal radiation at a fixed dosage throughout the application, which may last 24 to 72 hours, depending on dose calculations made by the radiation physicist.

Automated high-dose rate intracavitary brachytherapy systems have been developed that allow outpatient radiation therapy. Treatment time is shorter, thereby decreasing patient discomfort. Staff exposure to radiation is also avoided. Isotopes of radium and cesium are used for intracavitary irradiation.

Nursing Considerations for Radiation Safety

Special precautions for the safety of the patient and the nurse are important considerations when the patient is receiving radiation therapy. The radiation safety department will identify specific safety precautions to those people who will be in contact with the patient, including health care providers and family. Nursing concerns include providing the patient with emotional support and physical comfort. Further details about nursing management are provided in Chapter 12.

CRITICAL THINKING EXERCISES

1 **ebp** A 48-year-old woman with a diagnosis of fibroid tumors presents to the outpatient clinic with increased pain. What is the evidence base for medical and surgical treatment of fibroids? Specify the criteria used to evaluate the strength of the evidence for the practices you have identified.

2 **pq** Identify the priorities, approach, and techniques you would use to provide care for a 20-year-old woman who is being seen in an outpatient clinic for a new diagnosis of vulvovaginal infection. How will your priorities, approach, and techniques differ if the patient says she is not in a monogamous relationship? If the patient is from a culture with very different values from your own? Describe your priorities, approach, and techniques to prevent reinfection or spread of the infection.

3 **ipc** A 32-year-old woman has been admitted to your unit for a radical vulvectomy after a new diagnosis of vulvar cancer. Describe the preoperative education for her and the postoperative care that can be anticipated. What modifications in postoperative education and discharge planning may be necessary if the patient tells you she is a newlywed and is anxious about future sexual experiences? Describe how you will collaborate with her physician during her recovery process. What other professionals might you wish to include as part of her interdisciplinary care team?

REFERENCES

*Asterisk indicates nursing research.

Books

American Cancer Society (ACS). (2019a). *Cancer facts and figures 2019*. Atlanta, GA: Author.

Ball, J., Dains, J., Flynn, J., et al. (2019). *Seidel's guide to physical examination* (9th ed.). St. Louis, MO: Elsevier Mosby.

Casanova, R., Chuang, A., Goepfert, A. R., et al. (Eds.). (2019). *Beckman and Ling's obstetrics and gynecology* (8th ed.). Philadelphia, PA: Wolters Kluwer.

Comerford, K. C., & Durkin, M. T. (2020). *Nursing 2020 drug handbook*. Philadelphia, PA: Wolters Kluwer.

Norris, T. L. (2019). *Porth's pathophysiology: Concepts of altered health state* (10th ed.). Philadelphia, PA: Wolters Kluwer.

Singh, J., Kalia, N., & Kaur, M. (2018). Recurrent vulvovaginal infections: Etiology, diagnosis, treatment and management. In P. Sing (Ed.). *Infectious diseases and your health*. Singapore: Springer.

Smith, J. A., & Jhingran, A. (2017). Principles of radiation therapy and chemotherapy in gynecologic cancer: Basic principles, uses and complications. In R. A. Lobo, D. M. Gershenson, G. M. Lentz, et al. (Eds.). *Comprehensive gynecology* (7th ed., pp. 635–654). Philadelphia, PA: Elsevier.

Zapata, M. R. (2017). Diagnosis and treatment of vulvovaginitis. In D. Shoupe (Ed.). *Handbook of gynecology*. Switzerland: Springer International, Inc.

Journals and Electronic Documents

American Cancer Society (ACS). (2018). Ovarian cancer. Retrieved on 11/02/2019 at: www.cancer.org/cancer/ovarian-cancer/treating/chemotherapy.html

American Cancer Society (ACS). (2019b). Cervical cancer. Retrieved on 10/28/2019 at: www.cancer.org/cancer/cervical-cancer/about/key-statistics.html

American College of Obstetricians and Gynecologists (ACOG). (2017a). Human papillomavirus vaccination. *Committee Opinion No. 704*. Retrieved on 8/3/2019 at: www.acog.org/-/media/Committee-Opinions/Committee-on-Adolescent-Health-Care/co704.pdf?dmc=1&ts=20190803T1615020443

American College of Obstetricians and Gynecologists (ACOG). (2017b). Pelvic organ prolapse. *Practice Bulletin No. 185*. Retrieved on 10/19/2019 at: www.acog.org/Clinical-Guidance-and-Publications/Practice-Bulletins/Committee-on-Practice-Bulletins-Gynecology/Pelvic-Organ-Prolapse

American College of Obstetricians and Gynecologists (ACOG). (2015, reaffirmed 2017c). Robotic surgery in gynecology. *Committee Opinion No. 628*. Retrieved on 10/28/2019 at: www.acog.org/Clinical-Guidance-and-Publications/Committee-Opinions/Committee-on-Gynecologic-Practice/Robotic-Surgery-in-Gynecology

American College of Obstetricians and Gynecologists (ACOG). (2017d). Choosing the route of hysterectomy for benign disease. *Committee Opinion No. 701*. Retrieved on 11/2/2019 at: www.acog.org/-/media/Committee-Opinions/Committee-on-Gynecologic-Practice/co701.pdf?dmc=1&ts=20191102T1844228661

American College of Obstetricians and Gynecologists (ACOG). (2015, reaffirmed 2019). Practice Bulletin No. 149: Endometrial cancer. *Obstetrics and Gynecology, 125*(4), 1006–1026.

American College of Obstetricians and Gynecologists (ACOG). (2018a). Dual therapy for gonococcal infections. *Committee Opinion No. 645*. Retrieved on 10/17/2019 at: www.acog.org/Clinical-Guidance-and-Publications/Committee-Opinions/Committee-on-Gynecologic-Practice/Dual-Therapy-for-Gonococcal-Infections

American College of Obstetricians and Gynecologists (ACOG). (2018b). Practice Bulletin No. 194: Polycystic ovary syndrome. *Obstetrics and Gynecology, 131*(6), 157–171.

Andrew, N., & Pickett, C. (2019). Making chronic pelvic pain a little less painful. *Contemporary OB/GYN, 64*(7), 12–28.

Centers for Disease Control and Prevention (CDC). (2015). 2015 Sexually transmitted disease treatment guidelines. Retrieved on 9/01/2019 at: www.cdc.gov/std/tg2015/default.htm

Centers for Disease Control and Prevention (CDC). (2016). Chlamydia—CDC fact sheet. Retrieved on 10/17/2019 at: www.cdc.gov/std/chlamydia/stdfact-chlamydia-detailed.htm

Centers for Disease Control and Prevention (CDC). (2017a). Trichomoniasis—CDC fact sheet. Retrieved on 9/1/2019 at: www.cdc.gov/std/trichomonas/stdfact-trichomoniasis.htm

Centers for Disease Control and Prevention (CDC). (2017b). Genital herpes—CDC fact sheet (detailed). Retrieved on 10/6/2019 at: www.cdc.gov/std/herpes/stdfact-herpes-detailed.htm

Centers for Disease Control and Prevention (CDC). (2017c). Pelvic inflammatory disease (PID)—CDC fact sheet. Retrieved on 10/17/2019 at: www.cdc.gov/std/pid/stdfact-pid-detailed.htm

Centers for Disease Control and Prevention (CDC). (2019). Gonorrhea—CDC fact sheet. Retrieved on 9/1/2020 at: www.cdc.gov/std/gonorrhea/stdfact-gonorrhea-detailed.htm

Centers for Disease Control and Prevention (CDC). (2019a). Vaginal candidiasis. Retrieved on 8/10/2019 at: www.cdc.gov/fungal/diseases/candidiasis/genital

Centers for Disease Control and Prevention (CDC). (2019b). Genital HPV infection—CDC fact sheet. Retrieved on 10/6/2019 at: www.cdc.gov/std/hpv/stdfact-hpv.htm

Centers for Disease Control and Prevention (CDC). (2019c). HIV among women. Retrieved on 10/17/2019 at: www.cdc.gov/hiv/group/gender/women/index.html

Centers for Disease Control and Prevention (CDC). (2019d). HIV basics. Retrieved on 10/1/2019 at: www.cdc.gov/hiv/basics/testing.html

Centers for Disease Control and Prevention (CDC). (2019e). Basic information about gynecologic cancers. Retrieved on 10/26/2019 at: www.cdc.gov/cancer/gynecologic/basic_info/what-is-gynecologic-cancer.htm

Chibnall, R. (2017). Vulvar pruritus and lichen simplex chronicus. *Obstetrics and Gynecology Clinics of North America, 44*(3), 379–388.

Cohen, J. I. (2017). Vaccination to reduce reactivation of herpes simplex virus type 2. *The Journal of Infectious Diseases, 215*(6), 844–846.

Curry, A., Williams, T., & Penny, M. L. (2019). Pelvic inflammatory disease: Diagnosis, management, and prevention. *American Family Physician, 100*(6), 357–364.

El-Azab, A. S., Abolella, H. A., & Farouk, M. (2019). Update on vesicovaginal fistula: A systematic review. *Arab Journal of Urology, 17*(1), 61–68.

Fortin, C., Flyckt, R., & Falcone, T. (2017). Alternatives to hysterectomy: The burden of fibroids and the quality of life. *Best Practice & Research: Clinical Obstetrics & Gynaecology, 46,* 31–42.

Good, M. M., & Solomon, E. R. (2019). Pelvic floor disorders. *Obstetrics and Gynecology Clinics of North America, 46*(3), 527–540.

King, M. (2017). Prophylaxis and treatment of herpetic infections. *The Journal of Clinical and Aesthetic Dermatology, 10*(1), E5–E7.

*Kurt, G., Loerzel, V. W., Hines, R. B., et al. (2018). Learning needs of women who undergo robotic versus open gynecologic surgery. *Journal of Obstetric, Gynecologic, and Neonatal Nursing: JOGNN, 47*(4), 490–497.

Mahonski, S., & Hu, K. M. (2019). Female nonobstetric genitourinary emergencies. *Emergency Medicine Clinics of North America, 37*(4), 771–784.

Meites, E., Szilagyi, P. G., Chesson, H. W., et al. (2019). Human papillomavirus vaccination for adults: Updated recommendations of the Advisory Committee on Immunization Practices. *MMWR. Morbidity and Mortality Weekly Report, 68*(32), 698–702.

Meriwether, K. V., Antosh, D. D., Olivera, C. K, et al. (2018). Uterine preservation vs hysterectomy in pelvic organ prolapse surgery: A systematic review with meta-analysis and clinical practice guidelines. *American Journal of Obstetrics and Gynecology, 219*(2), 129–146.e2.

Mills, B. B. (2017). Vaginitis: Beyond the basics. *Obstetrics and Gynecology Clinics of North America, 44*(2), 159–177.

Morgan, D. M., Kamdar, N. S., Swenson, C. W., et al. (2017). Nationwide trends in the utilization of and payments for hysterectomy in the United States among commercially insured women. *American Journal of Obstetrics and Gynecology, 218*(4), 425.e1–425.e18.

National Cancer Institute (NCI). (2018). Human papillomavirus (HPV) vaccines. Retrieved on 10/6/2019 at: www.cancer.gov/about-cancer/causes-prevention/risk/infectious-agents/hpv-vaccine-fact-sheet

National Institutes of Health (NIH). (2018). Uterine fibroids—NIH fact sheet. Retrieved on 10/26/2019 at: www.nichd.nih.gov/health/topics/factsheets/uterine

Naumova, I., & Castelo-Branco, C. (2018). Current treatment options for postmenopausal vaginal atrophy. *International Journal of Women's Health, 10,* 387–395.

Paavonen, J., & Brunham, R. C. (2018). Bacterial vaginosis and desquamative inflammatory vaginitis. *The New England Journal of Medicine, 379*(23), 2246–2254.

Paladine, H. L., & Desai, U. A. (2018). Vaginitis: Diagnosis and treatment. *American Family Physician, 97*(5), 321–329.

Pfieffer, M. L. (2019). Polycystic ovary syndrome: An update. *Nursing, 49*(8), 34–40.

Stenson, A. L. (2017). Vulvodynia: Diagnosis and management. *Obstetrics and Gynecology Clinics of North America, 44*(3), 493–508.

Stewart, C., Ralyea, C., & Lockwood, S. (2019). Ovarian cancer: An integrated review. *Seminars in Oncology Nursing, 35*(2), 151–156.

U.S. Food and Drug Administration (FDA). (2019). Medical devices: Urogynecologic surgical mesh implants. Retrieved on 10/19/2019 at: www.fda.gov/medical-devices/implants-and-prosthetics/urogynecologic-surgical-mesh-implants

Weinberg, D., & Gomez-Martinez, R. A. (2019). Vulvar cancer. *Obstetrics and Gynecology Clinics of North America, 46*(1), 125–135.

Resources

American Cancer Society, www.cancer.org

American Sexual Health Association, www.ashasexualhealth.org

Association of Women's Health, Obstetric and Neonatal Nurses (AWHONN), www.awhonn.org

Centers for Disease Control and Prevention (CDC), Office of Women's Health, www.cdc.gov/women

ClinicalTrials.gov, National Institutes of Health, www.clinicaltrials.gov

Endometriosis Association, www.endometriosisassn.org

Foundation for Women's Cancer (formerly the Gynecologic Cancer Foundation), www.foundationforwomenscancer.org

Gay and Lesbian Medical Association (GLMA), www.glma.org

Herpes Hotline, 1-919-361-8488

National Ovarian Cancer Coalition (NOCC), www.ovarian.org

National STD Hotline, 1-800-232-4636

Office on Women's Health, www.womenshealth.gov/patient-materials/health-topic/reproductive-health

Oncology Nursing Society (ONS), www.ons.org

Ovarian Cancer Research Alliance, www.ocrahope.org

Planned Parenthood Federation of America, Inc. www.plannedparenthood.org

RESOLVE: The National Infertility Association, www.resolve.org

The American College of Obstetricians and Gynecologists (ACOG), www.acog.org

52

Assessment and Management of Patients with Breast Disorders

GLOSSARY

adjuvant chemotherapy: the use of anticancer medications in addition to other treatments to delay or prevent a recurrence of the disease

adjuvant hormonal therapy: the use of synthetic hormones or other medications given after primary treatment to increase the chances of a cure by stopping or slowing the growth of certain cancers that are affected by hormone stimulation, also called endocrine or antiestrogen therapy

aromatase inhibitors: medications that block the production of estrogens by the adrenal glands

atypical hyperplasia: abnormal increase in the number of cells in a specific area within the ductal or lobular areas of the breast; this abnormal proliferation increases the risk for cancer

benign proliferative breast disease: various types of atypical, yet noncancerous, breast tissue that increase the risk of breast cancer

brachytherapy: delivery of radiation therapy through internal implants placed inside or adjacent to a tumor

BRCA1 and *BRCA2*: genes on chromosome 17 that, when damaged or mutated, increase a person's risk for breast or ovarian cancer compared with people without the mutation

breast conservation treatment: surgery to remove a breast tumor and a margin of tissue around the tumor without removing any other part of the breast; may or may not include lymph node removal and radiation therapy

dose-dense chemotherapy: administration of chemotherapeutic agents at standard doses with shorter time intervals between each cycle of treatment

ductal carcinoma in situ (DCIS): cancer cells starting in the ductal system of the breast but not penetrating surrounding tissue

fibrocystic breast changes: term used to describe certain benign changes in the breast, typically palpable nodularity, lumpiness, swelling, or pain

fine-needle aspiration (FNA): removal of fluid for diagnostic analysis from a cyst or cells from a mass using a needle and syringe

gynecomastia: firm, overdeveloped breast tissue typically seen in adolescent boys

HER-2/neu: a protein that, when found in larger amounts, indicates an aggressive tumor

lobular carcinoma in situ (LCIS): atypical change and pro-liferation of the lobular cells of the breast

lymphedema: chronic swelling of an extremity due to inter-rupted lymphatic circulation, typically from an axillary lymph node dissection

mammoplasty: surgery to reconstruct or change the size or shape of the breast; can be performed for reduction or augmentation

mastalgia: breast pain, usually related to hormonal fluctua-tions or irritation of a nerve

mastectomy: removal of the breast tissue and nipple–areola complex

mastitis: inflammation or infection of the breast

modified radical mastectomy: removal of the breast tis-sue, nipple–areola complex, and a portion of the axillary lymph nodes

Paget disease: form of breast cancer that begins in the ductal system and involves scaly changes in the nipple, areola, and surrounding skin

sentinel lymph node: first lymph node(s) in the lymphatic basin that receives drainage from the primary tumor in the breast; identified by a radioisotope or blue dye

stereotactic core biopsy: computer-guided method of core needle biopsy that is useful when masses or calcifi-cations in the breast cannot be felt but can be visualized using mammography

surgical biopsy: surgical removal of all or a portion of a mass for microscopic examination by a pathologist

transverse rectus abdominal myocutaneous (TRAM) flap: method of breast reconstruction in which a flap of skin, fat, and muscle from the lower abdomen, with its attached blood supply, is rotated to the mastectomy site

Nurses care for patients with breast disorders in many set-tings. To care for these patients effectively, nurses require an understanding of the assessment, diagnostic testing, nurs-ing management, and rehabilitation needs of patients with multiple processes that affect the breasts. A breast disorder, whether benign or malignant, can cause great anxiety and fear of potential disfigurement, loss of sexual attractiveness, and even death. Nurses, therefore, must have expertise in the assessment and management of not only the physical symp-toms but also the psychosocial symptoms associated with various breast disorders.

BREAST ASSESSMENT

Anatomic and Physiologic Overview

Male and female breasts mature comparably until puberty, when estrogen and other hormones initiate breast develop-ment in females. This development usually occurs from 10 to 16 years of age, although the range can vary from 9 to 18 years. Stages of breast development are described as Tanner stages 1 through 5:

- Stage 1 describes a prepuberty breast.
- Stage 2 is breast budding, the first sign of puberty in a female.
- Stage 3 involves further enlargement of breast tissue and the areola (a darker tissue ring around the nipple).
- Stage 4 occurs when the nipple and areola form a sec-ondary mound on top of the breast tissue.
- Stage 5 is the continued development of a larger breast with a single contour.

The breasts are located between the second and sixth ribs over the pectoralis muscle from the sternum to the midaxil-lary line. An area of breast tissue, called the *tail of Spence*, extends into the axilla (Bland, Copeland, & Klimberg, 2018). Fascial bands, called *Cooper ligaments*, support the breast on the chest wall. The inframammary fold (or crease) is a ridge of fat at the bottom of the breast.

Each breast contains 12 to 20 cone-shaped lobes, which are made up of glandular elements (lobules and ducts) and sepa-rated by fat and fibrous tissue that binds the lobes together.

Milk is produced in the lobules and then carried through the ducts to the nipple. Figure 52-1 shows the anatomy of the fully developed breast.

Assessment

Breast assessment includes a targeted health history and physical examination.

Health History

When a patient presents with a breast problem, the nurse con-ducts a general health assessment, including history of medical disorders and previous surgery; family history of diseases, partic-ularly cancer; gynecologic and obstetric history; present medi-cations (including prescriptions, vitamins, and herbals); past and present use of hormonal contraceptives, hormone therapy (HT) (formerly referred to as hormone replacement therapy [HRT]), or fertility treatments; and social habits (e.g., smoking, drinking alcohol, illicit drug use). Psychosocial information, such as the patient's marital status, occupation, and availability of resources and support people, is obtained. Any recent x-rays or other diagnostic tests are noted. Focused questions pertain-ing to the breast disorder are asked concerning the onset of the disorder and the length of time it has been present. In addition, the patient is asked if any masses are palpable and if there is any associated pain, swelling, redness, nipple discharge, or change in the skin. Knowledge and comfort related to breast self-awareness, which can include breast self-examination (BSE), should also be ascertained from the patient.

Physical Assessment: Female Breast

A female breast examination can be conducted during any general physical or gynecologic examination or whenever the patient reports an abnormality. While the American Cancer Society (ACS) no longer recommends regular clini-cal breast examinations for average-risk women, this doesn't mean that the examination should never be performed. Pro-viders may still examine women's breasts, offer education about breast awareness to all women, and women should get screening imaging based upon their risks (see later discussion) (American Cancer Society [ACS], 2019).

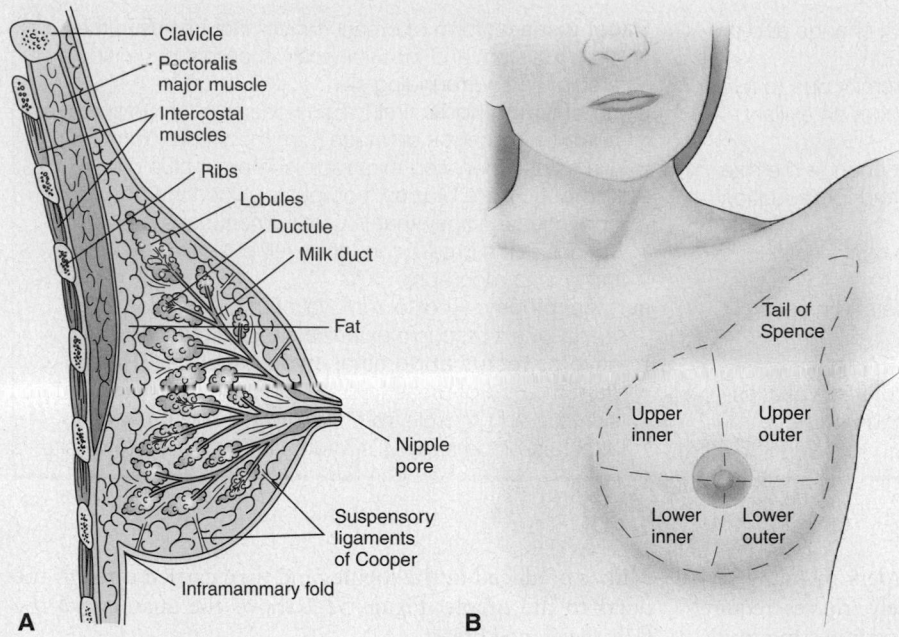

Figure 52-1 • **A.** Anatomy of the breast. **B.** Areas of breast, including the tail of Spence.

Inspection

Examination begins with inspection. The patient is asked to disrobe to the waist and sit in a comfortable position facing the examiner. The breasts are inspected for size and symmetry. A slight variation in the size of each breast is common and generally normal. The skin is inspected for color, venous pattern, thickening, or edema. Erythema (redness) may indicate benign local inflammation or superficial lymphatic invasion by a neoplasm. A prominent venous pattern can signal increased blood supply required by a tumor. Edema and pitting of the skin may result from a neoplasm blocking lymphatic drainage, giving the skin an orange peel appearance; this is called peau d'orange—a classic sign of advanced breast cancer. Nipple inversion of one or both breasts is not uncommon and is significant only when of recent origin. Ulceration, rashes, or spontaneous nipple discharge requires evaluation. Examples of abnormal breast findings on inspection can be found in Chart 52-1.

To elicit skin dimpling or retraction that may otherwise go undetected, the examiner instructs the patient to raise both arms overhead. This maneuver normally elevates both breasts equally. The patient is then instructed to place her hands on her waist and push in. These movements, which cause contraction of the pectoral muscles, do not normally alter the breast contour or nipple direction. Any dimpling or retraction during these position changes suggests an underlying mass. The clavicular and axillary regions are inspected for swelling, discoloration, lesions, or enlarged lymph nodes (Mallory & Golshan, 2018).

Palpation

The breasts are palpated with the patient upright (sitting up) and supine (lying down). In the supine position, the patient's shoulder is first elevated with a small pillow to help balance the breast on the chest wall. Failure to do this allows the breast tissue to slip laterally and a breast mass may be missed. The entire surface of the breast and the axillary tail is systematically palpated using the flat part (pads) of the second,

third, and fourth fingertips, held together, making dime-size circles. The examiner may choose to proceed in a clockwise direction, following imaginary concentric circles from the outer limits of the breast toward the nipple. Other acceptable methods are to palpate from each number on the face of the clock toward the nipple in a clockwise fashion or along imaginary vertical lines on the breast (see Fig. 52-2).

Palpation of the axillary and clavicular areas is easily performed with the patient seated (see Fig. 52-3). To examine the axillary lymph nodes, the examiner gently abducts the patient's arm from the thorax. With the left hand, the patient's right forearm is grasped and supported. The right hand is then free to palpate the axilla. Any lymph nodes that may be lying against the thoracic wall are noted. Normally, these lymph nodes are not palpable, but if they are enlarged, their location, size, mobility, and consistency are noted. During palpation, the examiner notes any patient-reported tenderness or masses. If a mass is detected, it is described by its location (e.g., right breast, 2 cm from the nipple at 2 o'clock position). Size, shape, consistency, border delineation, and mobility are included in the description (Mallory & Golshan, 2018). The examiner then modifies these steps to use the right hand to grasp the patient's left forearm, and then uses the left hand to palpate the axilla of the left breast.

The breast tissue of the adolescent is usually firm and lobular, whereas that of the postmenopausal woman is more likely to feel thinner and fattier. During pregnancy and lactation, the breasts are firmer and larger with lobules that are more distinct. Hormonal changes cause the areola to darken.

Obesity may have a proinflammatory effect on the breast that can contribute to increased rates of atypia. Atypia in breast ductal lavage and C-reactive protein levels in the nipple are significantly correlated with body mass index (BMI). Excessive body weight, as reflected by a BMI of 25 kg/m^2 or higher, is associated with postmenopausal breast cancer and increases the risk of dying of this disease; conversely, being overweight or having obesity seems to provide protection to women aged 40 to 49 (ACS, 2019).

Chart 52-1 · ASSESSMENT

Abnormal Assessment Findings during Inspection of the Breasts

Retraction Signs

- Signs include skin dimpling, creasing, or changes in the contour of the breast or nipple
- They may be secondary to contraction of fibrotic tissue that can occur with underlying malignancy
- They may be secondary to scar tissue formation after breast surgery
- Retraction signs may appear only with position changes

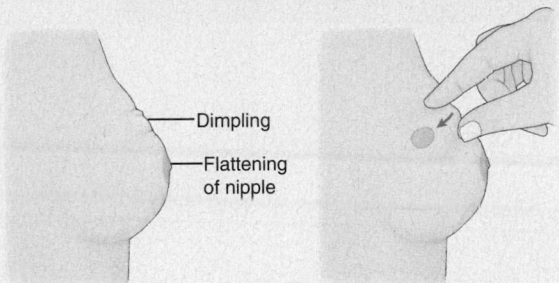

Retraction signs   Retraction with compression

Increased Venous Prominence

- Unilateral localized increase in venous pattern associated with malignant tumors
- Normal with bilateral and symmetrical breast enlargement associated with pregnancy and lactation

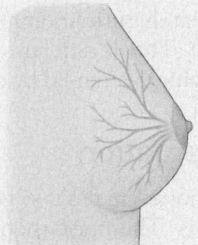

Increased venous prominence

Peau d'Orange (Edema)

- Associated with inflammatory breast cancer
- Caused by interference with lymphatic drainage
- Breast skin has orange peel appearance
- Skin pores enlarge
- May be noted on the areola
- Skin becomes thick, hard, and immobile

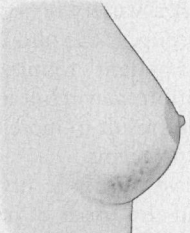

Peau d'orange

Nipple Inversion

- Considered normal if long-standing
- Associated with fibrosis and malignancy if recent development

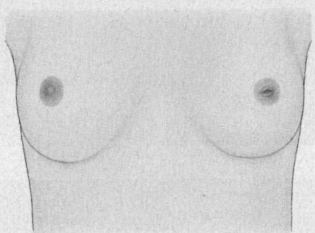

Nipple inversion

Acute Mastitis (Inflammation of the Breasts)

- Associated with lactation but may occur at any age
- Nipple cracks or abrasions noted
- Breast skin reddened and warm to touch
- Tenderness
- Systemic signs include fever and increased pulse

Paget Disease (Malignancy of Mammary Ducts)

- Early signs—erythema of nipple and areola
- Late signs—thickening, scaling, and erosion of the nipple and areola

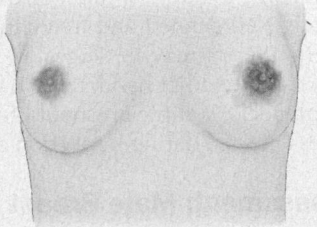

Paget's disease

Adapted from Stanford Medicine 25. (2020). Breast exam. Retrieved on 5/13/2020 at: www.stanfordmedicine25.stanford.edu/the25/Breast-Exam.html and Newton, E., & Grethlein, S. (2018). Breast examination. Retrieved on 5/13/2020 at: https://emedicine.medscape.com/article/1909276-overview.

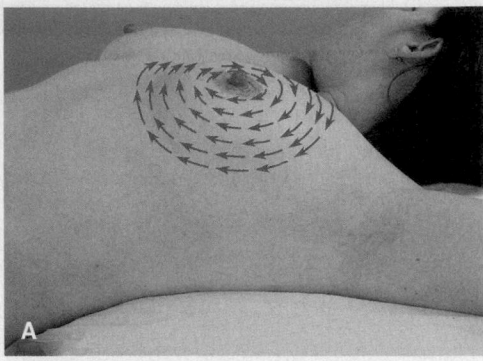

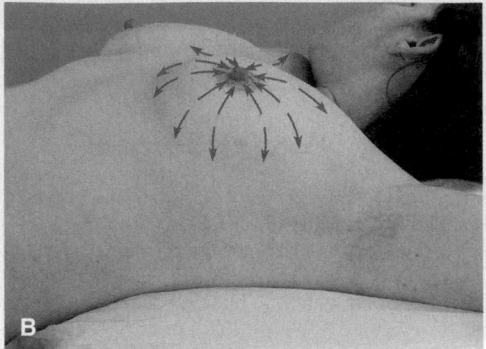

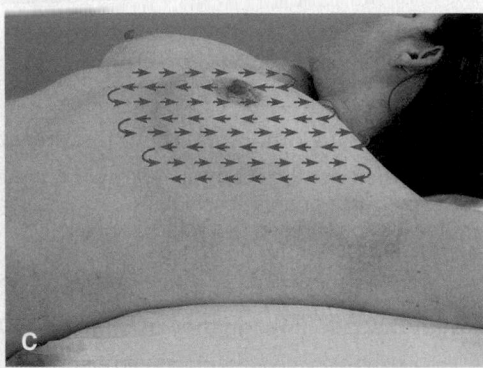

Figure 52-2 • Breast examination with the woman in a supine position. The entire surface of the breast is palpated from the outer edge of the breast to the nipple; palpation patterns are circular or clockwise (**A**), wedge (**B**), and vertical strip (**C**).

Cysts are commonly found in women who are menstruating and are usually well defined and freely movable. In the premenstrual period, cysts may be larger and more tender. Malignant tumors, on the other hand, tend to be hard, poorly defined, and nontender. A clinician should further evaluate any abnormalities detected during inspection and palpation.

Physical Assessment: Male Breast

Breast cancer can occur in men. Assessment of the male breast and axilla is brief but important and should be included in a physical examination. The nipple and areola are inspected for swelling, nodules, ulcerations, and nipple discharge. The flat disc of undeveloped breast tissue under the nipple is palpated. The same procedure for palpating the female breast is used to assess the male breast (Canadian Cancer Society, 2020).

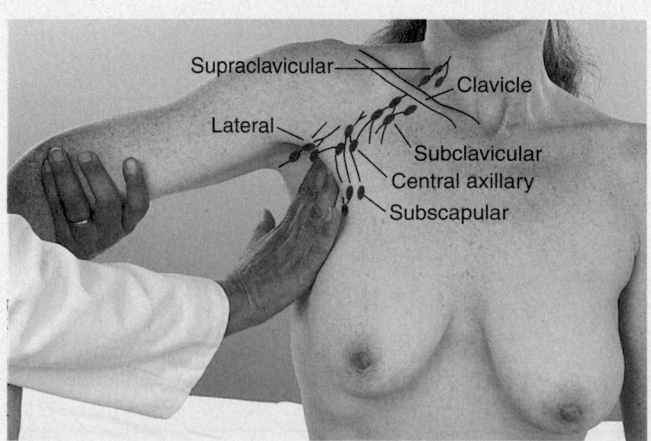

Figure 52-3 • Palpating axillary nodes in breast examination.

Gynecomastia is the firm enlargement of glandular tissue beneath and immediately surrounding the areola of the male (see later discussion). This is different from the enlargement of soft, fatty tissue, which is caused by obesity.

Diagnostic Evaluation

A wide range of diagnostic studies may be performed in patients with breast conditions. The nurse should educate the patient about the purpose, what to expect, and any possible side effects related to these examinations prior to testing. The nurse should note trends in the patient's test results, because they often provide information about disease progression as well as the patient's response to therapy.

Breast Self-Examination

The nurse plays a critical role in breast awareness education—a modality used for the early detection of breast cancer. BSE can be taught in a variety of settings, either on a one-to-one basis or in a group. It can also be initiated by a health care provider during a patient's routine physical examination. Regular self-examinations may result in early identification of problems and may also result in more diagnostic workups for benign or malignant problems.

Variations in breast tissue occur during the menstrual cycle, pregnancy, and the onset of menopause. Women on HT can also experience fluctuations. Normal changes must be distinguished from those that may signal disease. Most women notice increased tenderness and lumpiness before their menstrual periods; therefore, BSE is best performed after menses (day 5 to day 7, counting the first day of menses as day 1). In addition, many women have grainy-textured breast tissue, but such areas are usually less nodular after menses.

Younger women may find BSE particularly difficult because of the density of their breast tissue. As women age, their breasts become fattier and may be easier to examine.

Current practice is shifting from educating about BSE to promoting breast self-awareness, which is a woman's attentiveness to the normal appearance and feel of her breasts. However, self-examination still may be appropriate for some women who are at high risk and for those who prefer it. Breast self-awareness can include self-examination. For every woman, knowing how her breasts normally feel helps detect any changes or signs of a problem. BSE may play an important role in screening, especially for women who develop cancer in the interval after a negative result on mammography or clinical breast examination or who have a false-negative imaging or clinical examination result. It can also promote detection in women who have not been screened. The goal, with or without BSE, is to report any breast changes to a primary provider.

Family history can increase the risk of breast cancer in men, particularly if other men in the family have had breast cancer. The risk is also higher if there is a breast cancer gene abnormality in the family. *BRCA2* mutations are much more common than *BRCA1* mutations in males (Jain & Gradishar, 2018). Instructions about BSE should be provided to men if they have a family history of breast cancer.

Patients who elect to perform BSE should receive proper instruction on technique (see Chart 52-2). They should be informed that routine, monthly BSE will help them become familiar with their "normal abnormalities." If a change is detected, they should seek medical attention.

Patients should be instructed about optimal timing for BSE (5 to 7 days after menses begin for women who are premenopausal and once monthly for women who are postmenopausal or not menstruating). When demonstrating examination techniques, the feel of normal breast tissue should be reviewed and ways to identify breast changes discussed. Patients should then perform a BSE demonstration on themselves or on a breast model. Patients who have had breast cancer surgery should be instructed to examine their breast or chest wall for any new changes or nodules that may indicate a recurrence of the disease.

Mammography

The ACS has changed the mammography recommendations to state that healthy women should have mammography every year beginning at age 45; women aged 40 to 44 have the option to begin yearly screening early (ACS, 2019). Women 55 and older may continue yearly screening or transition to every 2 years. This change was based on calculations that starting annual screening mammography later and getting it less often would cause less harm and be as safe as starting it earlier and getting it more often. Screening every other year may, however, result in a missed diagnosis and a small increase in the probability of being diagnosed with later-stage cancer.

Mammography is a breast imaging technique using a low-dose x-ray system to visualize the anatomy of the breasts; this aids in the early detection and diagnosis of malignant or benign disease (American College of Radiology [ACR], 2019). The procedure takes about 30 minutes and can be performed in a hospital radiology department or independent imaging center. Two views are taken of each breast. The breast is mechanically compressed from top to bottom (craniocaudal view) (see Fig. 52-4) and side to side (mediolateral oblique view). Women may experience some discomfort because maximum compression is necessary for proper visualization. The new mammogram is compared with previous mammograms, and any changes may indicate a need for further investigation. Mammography may detect a breast tumor before it is clinically palpable. Younger women, or those taking HTs, may have dense breast tissue, making it more difficult to detect lesions with mammography.

Patients scheduled for a mammogram may voice concern about exposure to radiation. The radiation exposure is equivalent to about 7 weeks of natural background radiation exposure (ACR, 2019), so patients would have to have many mammograms in a year to increase their cancer risk. To ensure that a mammogram is reliable, it is important that a woman find a reputable facility. Mammographic facilities are certified by the U.S. Food and Drug Administration (FDA), and the machines are accredited by either the American College of Radiology or the States of Arkansas, Iowa or Texas (U.S. Food and Drug Administration [FDA], 2018).

Additional techniques for breast screening include digital mammography and 3D mammography. Digital mammography records x-ray images on a computer instead of on film, thus allowing radiologists to adjust the contrast and focus on an image without having to take additional x-rays. Although the accuracy of both film and digital screening mammography is similar for most women, digital mammography has been shown to be better at detecting estrogen receptor–negative tumors and cancer in extremely dense breasts. Both of these subgroups are more common in younger women, who may therefore choose digital mammography if they wish to have screening mammography. The 3D mammography obtains multiple projections of the compressed breast and results in lower false-positive interpretation rates and improved cancer detection rates (Bassett & Lee-Felker, 2018). Computer-aided detection (CAD) is an option for radiologists and can be helpful in finding abnormal areas that should be checked more closely for early cancers. Refinements and improvements have been made to CAD software with a focus on increasing sensitivity for masses and reducing false-positive rates.

Contrast Mammography

A contrast mammography (i.e., ductogram, galactogram) is a diagnostic procedure that involves injection of less than 1 mL of radiopaque material through a cannula inserted into a ductal opening on the areola, which is followed by a mammogram (Bassett & Lee-Felker, 2018). It is performed to evaluate an abnormality within the duct when the patient has bloody nipple discharge on expression, spontaneous nipple discharge, or a solitary dilated duct noted on mammography.

Ultrasonography

Ultrasonography (ultrasound) is used as a diagnostic adjunct to mammography to help distinguish fluid-filled cysts from other lesions. A thin coating of lubricating jelly is spread over the area to be imaged. A transducer is then placed on the breast. The transducer transmits high-frequency sound waves

Chart 52-2

Breast Self-Examination

The nurse instructs the patient to perform the following steps:

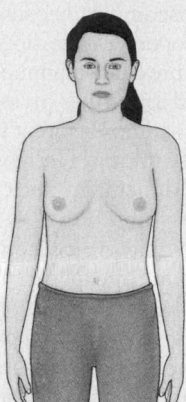

Step 1

1. Stand in front of a mirror.
2. Check both breasts for anything unusual.
3. Look for discharge from the nipple, puckering, dimpling, or scaling of the skin.

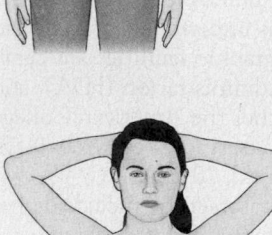

Step 2

Steps 2 and 3 are done to check for any changes in the contour of your breasts. As you do them, you should be able to feel your muscles tighten.

1. Watch closely in the mirror as you clasp your hands behind your head and press your hands forward.
2. Note any change in the contour of your breasts.

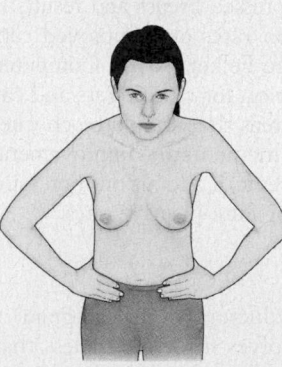

Step 3

1. Next, press your hands firmly on your hips and bow slightly toward the mirror as you pull your shoulders and elbows forward.
2. Note any change in the contour of your breasts.

Step 4

Some women do step 4 of the examination in the shower. Your fingers will glide easily over soapy skin, so you can concentrate on feeling for changes inside the breast.

1. Raise your left arm.
2. Use three or four fingers of your right hand to feel your left breast firmly, carefully, and thoroughly.
3. Beginning at the outer edge, press the flat part of your fingers in small circles, moving the circles slowly around the breast.
4. Gradually work toward the nipple.
5. Be sure to cover the whole breast.
6. Pay special attention to the area between the breast and the underarm, including the underarm itself.
7. Feel for any unusual lumps or masses under the skin.
8. If you have any spontaneous discharge during the month—whether or not it is during your breast self-examination—see your primary provider.
9. Repeat the examination on your right breast.

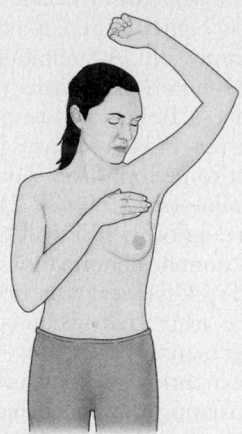

Step 5

Step 4 should be repeated lying down.

1. Lie flat on your back with your left arm over your head and a pillow or folded towel under your left shoulder. (This position flattens your breast and makes it easier to check.)
2. Use the same circular motion described earlier.
3. Repeat on your right breast.

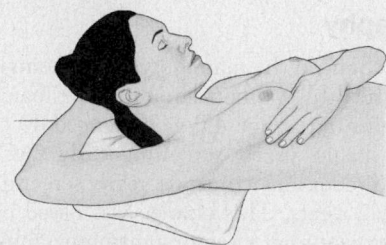

Adapted from Boraas, M., & Gupta, S. (2019). Breast self-exam. Retrieved on 5/14/2020 at: www.breastcancer.org/symptoms/testing/types/self_exam

through the skin toward the area of concern. The sound waves are reflected back from a two-dimensional image, which is then displayed on a computer screen. No radiation is emitted during the procedure. Ultrasound is also used as an adjunct to mammography in women with dense breast tissue. Ultrasound may be used as an aid for interventional procedures.

Ultrasonography has advantages and disadvantages. Although it can diagnose cysts with great accuracy, it cannot definitively rule out malignant lesions. Microcalcifications, which are detectable on mammography, cannot be identified on ultrasonography. Finally, examination techniques and interpretation criteria are not standardized.

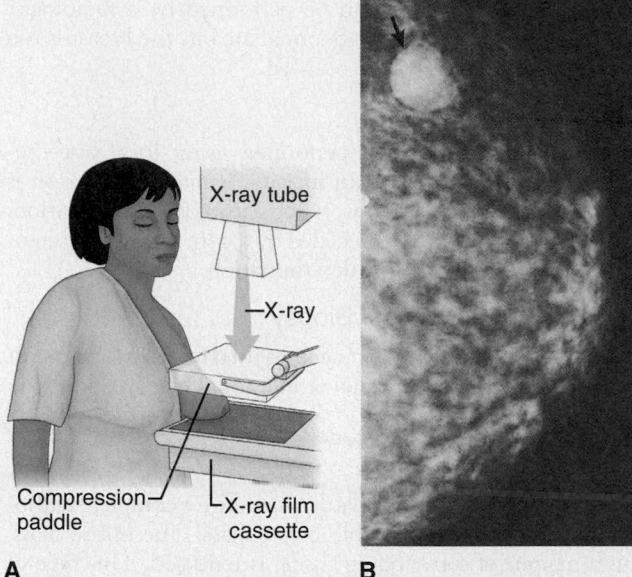

A   **B**

Figure 52-4 • The mammography procedure **(A)** relies on x-ray imaging to produce the mammogram **(B)**, which in this case reveals a breast lump (see *arrow*).

Magnetic Resonance Imaging

Magnetic resonance imaging (MRI) of the breast is a highly sensitive test that has become a useful diagnostic adjunct to mammography. A magnet is linked to a computer that creates detailed images of the breast without exposure to radiation. An intravenous (IV) injection of gadolinium, a contrast dye, is given to improve visibility. The patient lies face down, and the breast is placed through a depression in the table. A coil is placed around the breast, and the patient is placed inside the MRI machine. The entire procedure takes about 30 to 40 minutes.

Breast MRI is useful for evaluation of contralateral disease, invasive lobular carcinoma, and assessment of chemotherapeutic response. Additionally, screening guidelines provided by the National Comprehensive Cancer Network (NCCN)

recommend an annual MRI scan in addition to mammography in women at high risk for breast cancer (i.e., those with greater than 20% lifetime risk). Candidates include women who have a *BRCA1* or *BRCA2* mutation, a first-degree relative with either of these mutations, certain rare genetic syndromes, or radiation to the chest between 10 and 30 years of age (National Comprehensive Cancer Network [NCCN], 2019). MRI should be used in addition to mammography, not instead of it.

Some disadvantages of MRI include high cost, variations in technique and interpretation, and the potential for patient claustrophobia. The procedure cannot always accurately distinguish between malignant and benign breast conditions, so false-positive results may occur. MRI is contraindicated in patients with implantable metal devices (e.g., aneurysm clips, ports of tissue expanders). Patients with any type of cardiac implantable electronic device need to be screened to see if it is safe for them to undergo an MRI (Indik, Gimbel, Abe, et al., 2017). Foil-backed medication patches (e.g., nicotine, nitroglycerin, fentanyl) must be removed prior to MRI to avoid burns to the skin.

Procedures for Tissue Analysis

Percutaneous Biopsy

Percutaneous biopsy is performed on an outpatient basis to sample palpable and nonpalpable lesions. Less invasive than a surgical biopsy, percutaneous biopsy is a needle or core biopsy that obtains tissue by making a small puncture in the skin. Table 52-1 outlines the different types of biopsies that can be performed to obtain a tissue diagnosis.

 *Concept Mastery Alert*

It is important to understand the differences between common procedures used for patients with breast disorders. Mammography is used to detect breast abnormalities, whereas biopsy is performed to confirm a diagnosis of breast cancer.

TABLE 52-1	Types of Breast Biopsies		
Procedure	**Palpable Mass**	**Health Professional Who Performs Procedure**	**Nature of Breast Tissue Removed**
Fine-needle aspiration	Yes	Surgeon	Cellular material
Core needle biopsy	Yes	Surgeon	Tissue core
Stereotactic core biopsy	No	Radiologist	Tissue core
Ultrasound-guided core biopsy	No	Radiologist	Tissue core
Magnetic resonance imaging (MRI)-guided core biopsy	No	Radiologist	Tissue core
Excisional biopsy	Yes	Surgeon	Entire mass
Incisional biopsy	Yes	Surgeon	Tissue core
Wire needle localization biopsy; may be guided by mammogram, ultrasound, or MRI	No	Radiologist inserts wire; surgeon performs biopsy	Entire mass

Fine-Needle Aspiration

Fine-needle aspiration (FNA) is a biopsy technique that is generally well tolerated by most women. A local anesthetic may or may not be used. A small-gauge needle (20- to 27-gauge) attached to a syringe is inserted into the mass or area of nodularity. Suction is applied to the syringe, and multiple passes are made through the mass. A simple cyst often disappears on aspiration, and the fluid is usually discarded if it is nonbloody. If the material is bloody, however, it most likely indicates malignancy and should be sent for cytology; this is performed either directly as a smear or after the fluid is centrifuged (Obeng-Gyasi, Grimm, Hwang, et al., 2018). For nonpalpable masses, the same procedure can be performed by a radiologist using ultrasound guidance (ultrasound-guided FNA).

FNA is less expensive than other diagnostic methods, and results are usually available quickly. However, false-negative or false-positive results are possible, and appropriate follow-up depends on the clinical judgment of the treating physician.

Core Needle Biopsy

Core needle biopsy is similar to FNA, except that a larger-gauge needle is used (usually 11- to 18-gauge). A local anesthetic is applied, and tissue cores are removed via a spring-loaded device. This procedure allows for a more definitive diagnosis than FNA, because actual tissue, not just cells, is removed. It is often performed for relatively large tumors that are close to the skin surface, but is also utilized for smaller, deeper lesions that are visible on ultrasound.

Stereotactic Core Biopsy

Stereotactic core biopsy is performed on nonpalpable lesions detected by mammography. The patient lies prone on the stereotactic table. The breast is suspended through an opening in the table and compressed between two x-ray plates. Images are then obtained using digital mammography. The exact coordinates of the lesion to be sampled are located with the aid of a computer. Next, a local anesthetic is injected into the entry site on the breast. A small nick is made in the skin, a core needle is inserted, and samples of the tissue are taken for pathologic examination. Often, several passes are taken to ensure that the lesion is well sampled. Postbiopsy images are then taken to check that sampling has been adequate. A small titanium clip is almost always placed at the biopsy site so that the site can easily be located if further treatment is indicated (Obeng-Gyasi et al., 2018). Stereotactic biopsy is quite accurate and often allows the patient to avoid a surgical biopsy. However, there is a small false-negative rate. Appropriate follow-up depends on the final pathologic diagnosis and the clinical judgment of the primary provider. The use of a titanium clip does not preclude subsequent MRIs.

Ultrasound-Guided Core Biopsy

The principles for ultrasound-guided core biopsy are similar to those of stereotactic core biopsy, but by using ultrasound guidance, computer coordination and mammographic compression are not necessary. An ultrasound-guided core biopsy does not use radiation and is also usually faster and less expensive than stereotactic core biopsy.

Magnetic Resonance Imaging–Guided Core Biopsy

MRI-guided core biopsy can be performed by a radiologist and technologist when the abnormal area in the breast is too small to be felt but is visible on MRI.

Surgical Biopsy

Surgical biopsy is usually performed using local anesthesia and IV sedation. After an incision is made, the lesion is excised and sent to a laboratory for pathologic examination. Surgical biopsy is usually preceded by a core biopsy or stereotactic biopsy for pathologic determination.

Types of Surgical Breast Biopsy

There are several types of procedures used for a surgical breast biopsy including an excisional or incisional biopsy, and a wire needle localization.

Excisional Biopsy

Excisional biopsy is the standard procedure for complete pathologic assessment of a palpable breast mass. The entire mass, plus a margin of surrounding tissue, is removed. This type of biopsy may also be referred to as a lumpectomy. Depending on the clinical situation, a frozen-section analysis of the specimen may be performed at the time of the biopsy by the pathologist, who does an immediate reading intraoperatively and provides a provisional diagnosis. This can help confirm a diagnosis in a patient who has had no previous tissue analysis performed.

Incisional Biopsy

Incisional biopsy surgically removes a portion of a mass. This is performed to confirm a diagnosis and to conduct special studies (e.g., ER/PR, HER-2/neu [also referred to as ERBB2]; see later discussion for explanation of these terms) that will aid in determining treatment, which is discussed later in this chapter. Complete excision of the area may not be possible or immediately beneficial to the patient, depending on the clinical situation. This procedure is often performed on women with locally advanced breast cancer or on women with suspected cancer recurrence, whose treatment may depend on the results of these special studies. However, pathologic information may be easily obtained from core needle biopsy, and incisional biopsy is becoming less common.

Wire Needle Localization

Wire needle localization is a technique used to locate nonpalpable masses or suspicious calcium deposits detected on a mammogram, ultrasound, or MRI that require an excisional biopsy. The radiologist inserts a long, thin wire through a needle, which is then inserted into the area of abnormality using x-ray or ultrasound guidance (whichever imaging technique originally identified the abnormality). The wire remains in place after the needle is withdrawn to ensure the precise location. The patient is then taken to the operating room, where the surgeon follows the wire to the tip and excises the area.

Nursing Implications

During the preoperative or preprocedure visit, the nurse assesses the patient for any specific educational, physical, or psychosocial needs. This can be accomplished by reviewing the medical and psychosocial history and encouraging the patient to verbalize fears, concerns, and questions. Patients are often worried not only about the procedure but also about the potential implications of the pathology results. Providing a thorough explanation about what to expect in a supportive manner can help alleviate anxiety. Patients often have difficulty absorbing all the information given to them; therefore, written materials to take home are often provided to reinforce and clarify education.

The nurse instructs the patient to discontinue any agents that can increase the risk of bleeding, including products containing aspirin, nonsteroidal anti-inflammatory drugs, vitamin E supplements, herbal substances (such as ginkgo biloba and garlic supplements). Patients on prescription anticoagulants need to check with the prescriber prior to temporary cessation for the procedure, as biopsies done without cessation of these drugs can result in prolonged bleeding and hematomas. The patient may be instructed not to eat or drink for several hours prior to the procedure or after midnight the night before the procedure, depending on the type of biopsy and anesthesia planned. Most breast biopsy procedures are performed with the use of the combination of sedation and local anesthesia.

Immediate assessment after the procedure includes monitoring the effects of the anesthesia and inspecting the surgical dressing for any signs of bleeding. Once the sedation has worn off, the nurse reviews the care of the biopsy site, pain management, and activity restrictions with the patient. Prior to discharge from the ambulatory surgical center or the office, the patient must be able to tolerate fluids, ambulate, and void. The patient must be accompanied home by an adult. The dressing covering the incision is usually removed after 48 hours, but the Steri-Strips, which are applied directly over the incision, should remain in place for approximately 7 to 10 days or until they fall off. The use of a supportive bra following surgery is encouraged to limit movement of the breast and reduce discomfort. A follow-up telephone call from the nurse 24 to 48 hours after the procedure can provide the patient with the opportunity to ask any questions and can be a source of great comfort and reassurance.

Most women return to their usual activities the day after the procedure but are encouraged to avoid jarring or high-impact activities for 1 week to promote healing of the biopsy site. Discomfort is usually minimal, and most women find acetaminophen sufficient for pain relief, although a mild opioid analgesic agent may be prescribed if needed.

Follow-up after the biopsy includes a return visit to the surgeon for discussion of the final pathology report and assessment of the healing of the biopsy site. Depending on the results of the biopsy, the nurse's role varies. If the pathology report is benign, the nurse reviews incision care and explains what the patient should expect as the biopsy site heals (i.e., changes in sensation may occur weeks or months after the biopsy due to nerve injury within the breast tissue). If a diagnosis of cancer is made, the nurse's role changes dramatically. This is discussed in depth later in this chapter.

CONDITIONS AFFECTING THE NIPPLE

Nipple Discharge

Nipple discharge in a woman who is not lactating may be related to many causes, such as carcinoma, papilloma, pituitary adenoma, cystic breasts, and various medications. Oral contraceptives, pregnancy, HT, chlorpromazine, and frequent breast stimulation may be contributing factors. In some women, nipple discharge may occur during running or aerobic exercises. Nipple discharge should be evaluated by a health care provider, but it is not often a cause for alarm. One in three women has clear discharge on expression, which is usually normal. A green discharge could indicate an infection. Any discharge that is spontaneous, persistent, or unilateral is of concern. Although bloody discharge can indicate a malignancy, it is often caused by a benign wartlike growth on the lining of the duct called an *intraductal papilloma*.

Nipple discharge should be evaluated for the presence of occult (hidden) blood by performing a guaiac test. A negative test can be reassuring as it indicates that there is no blood, but it does not prove there is no malignancy. A galactogram can also be performed to detect abnormalities within the duct that may be causing the discharge. If there is a high level of suspicion, an excisional biopsy may be indicated. (See procedures for tissue analysis earlier in this chapter.)

Fissure

A fissure is a longitudinal ulcer that may develop in women who are breast-feeding. If the nipple becomes irritated, a painful, raw area may form and become a site of infection. Daily washing with water, massage with breast milk or lanolin, and exposure to air are helpful. Breast-feeding can continue with the use of a nipple shield. However, if the fissure is severe or extremely painful, the woman may be advised to stop breast-feeding. A breast pump can be used until breast-feeding can be resumed. Persistent ulceration requires further diagnosis and therapy. Guidance from a nurse or lactation consultant may be helpful, because nipple irritation can result from improper positioning or poor latching on (i.e., the infant has not grasped the areola fully) during breast-feeding.

BREAST INFECTIONS

Mastitis

Mastitis, an inflammation or infection of breast tissue, occurs most commonly in women who are breast-feeding, although it may also occur in women who are nonlactating. The infection may result from a transfer of microorganisms to the breast by the patient's hands or from a breast-fed infant with an oral, eye, or skin infection. Mastitis may also be caused by bloodborne organisms. As inflammation progresses, the breast texture becomes tough or doughy, and the patient complains of dull to severe pain in the infected region. A nipple that is discharging purulent material, serum, or blood should be investigated promptly.

Treatment consists of antibiotics and local application of cold compresses to relieve discomfort. A broad-spectrum antibiotic agent may be prescribed for 7 to 10 days. The patient should wear a snug bra and perform personal hygiene carefully. Adequate rest and hydration are important aspects of management.

Lactational Abscess

A breast abscess may develop as a consequence of acute mastitis. The area affected becomes tender and red. Purulent matter can usually be aspirated with a needle, but incision and drainage may be required. Specimens of the aspirated material are obtained for culture so that an organism-specific antibiotic agent can be prescribed.

BENIGN CONDITIONS OF THE BREAST

Breast Pain

Mastalgia (breast pain) may be cyclical or noncyclical. Cyclical pain is usually related to hormonal fluctuations, usually during the menstrual cycle, and accounts for the majority of complaints. Noncyclical pain is far less common and does not vary with the menstrual cycle. Women who experience injury or trauma to the breast or those who have had a breast biopsy may experience noncyclical pain. Patients should be reassured that breast pain is rarely indicative of cancer. However, if the pain persists after menses begin, the patient should see her primary provider.

Nursing Management

The nurse may recommend that the patient wear a supportive bra both day and night for a week, avoiding the use of underwire bras, decrease her salt and caffeine intake, and take ibuprofen as needed for its anti-inflammatory actions. Vitamin E supplements may also be helpful.

Cysts

Cysts are fluid-filled sacs that develop as breast ducts dilate. Cysts occur most commonly in women 30 to 55 years of age and may be exacerbated during perimenopause. Although their cause is unknown, cysts usually disappear after menopause, suggesting that estrogen is a factor. Cystic areas often fluctuate in size and are usually larger premenstrually. They may be painless or may become very tender premenstrually. Occasionally, a patient may report an intermittent shooting sensation or a dull ache. Various breast masses are compared in Table 52-2. Cysts that are confirmed on an ultrasound and are not bothersome can often be left alone. To confirm a diagnosis or to relieve pain, FNA can be performed. Cysts are rarely malignant (Sasaki, Geletzke, Kass, et al., 2018).

Fibrocystic breast changes, often incorrectly called *fibrocystic breast disease*, is a nonspecific term used to describe an array of benign findings including palpable nodularity, lumpiness, swelling, or pain. The changes do not necessarily indicate a cystic or disease process.

TABLE 52-2 Comparison of Various Breast Masses

The most common breast masses are due to cysts, fibroadenomas, or malignancy. Biopsy is usually needed for confirmation, but the following characteristics are diagnostic clues:

Characteristics	Cysts	Fibroadenomas	Malignancy
Age	30–55 yrs, regress after menopause except with use of estrogen therapy	Puberty to menopause	30–90 yrs; most common, 40–80 yrs
Number	Single or multiple	Usually single	Usually single
Shape	Round	Round, disc, or lobular	Irregular or stellate
Consistency	Soft to firm, usually elastic	Usually firm	Firm or hard
Mobility	Mobile	Mobile	May be fixed to skin or underlying tissues
Tenderness	Usually tender	Usually nontender	Usually nontender
Retraction signs	Absent	Absent	May be present

Adapted from Bland, K., Copeland, E., Klimberg, V., et al. (Eds.). *The breast: Comprehensive management of benign and malignant diseases* (5th ed.). Philadelphia, PA: Elsevier.

Fibroadenomas

Fibroadenomas are firm, round, movable, benign tumors. They can occur from puberty to menopause with a peak incidence at 30 years of age. These masses are nontender and are sometimes biopsied or removed for definitive diagnosis.

Benign Proliferative Breast Disease

The two most common types of **benign proliferative breast disease** (atypical, yet noncancerous, breast tissue) found on biopsy are atypical hyperplasia and lobular carcinoma in situ (LCIS). These diagnoses increase a woman's risk of breast cancer.

Atypical Hyperplasia

Atypical hyperplasia can be ductal or lobular and is a premalignant lesion of the breast. It is recognized as a precursor lesion to both noninvasive and invasive breast cancer. Imbalance in the normal regulation of cell proliferation is a defining feature. Women with atypical hyperplasia have a fourfold increased risk of breast cancer compared to women in the general population (Sasaki et al., 2018).

Lobular Carcinoma In Situ

Lobular carcinoma in situ (LCIS) is an incidental microscopic finding of abnormal tissue growth in the lobules of the breast. Many types of LCIS have been identified; some types are associated with a 4- to 10-fold increased risk of invasive breast cancer (Klimberg & Bland, 2018). Affected women should undergo rigorous breast cancer surveillance that consists of annual mammography and clinical breast examination every 6 months (NCCN, 2019). Patients should be offered information about chemoprevention with selective estrogen receptor modulators (SERMs), such as tamoxifen. See the discussion of chemoprevention later in this chapter.

Other Benign Conditions

Cystosarcoma phyllodes is a rare fibroepithelial tumor that tends to grow rapidly. It is rarely malignant and is treated with surgical excision. If it is malignant, mastectomy may follow. Lymph node removal is usually not performed, because metastasis is rare.

Fat necrosis is a condition of the breast that is often associated with a history of trauma. Surgical procedures such as a breast biopsy, lumpectomy, or mastectomy can cause fat necrosis. It may be indistinguishable from carcinoma, and the entire mass may be excised or biopsied. If excision is not indicated, it is followed with regular breast imaging.

Intraductal papilloma is a wartlike growth that often involves the large milk ducts near the nipple, causing bloody nipple discharge. Surgery usually involves removal of the papilloma and a segment of the duct where the papilloma is found.

Superficial thrombophlebitis of the breast (Mondor disease) is an uncommon condition that is usually associated with pregnancy, trauma, or breast surgery. Pain and redness occur as a result of a superficial thrombophlebitis in the vein that drains the outer part of the breast. The mass is usually linear, tender, and erythematous. Treatment consists of analgesic agents and heat.

MALIGNANT CONDITIONS OF THE BREAST

Breast cancer is a major health problem in the United States. Current statistics indicate that over a lifetime (birth to death), a woman's risk of developing breast cancer is about 12%, or one in eight. Currently, about 268,600 new cases of invasive breast cancer are diagnosed in women each year. Risk of developing breast cancer increases with increasing age. About two of three invasive breast cancers are found in women 55 years or older. About 5% to 10% of breast cancer cases are thought to be hereditary, resulting directly from gene defects (cell mutations) inherited from a biologic parent (ACS, 2019). Female breast cancer incidence rates vary substantially by race and ethnicity. Non-Hispanic African American women have higher incidence of breast cancer than non-Hispanic Caucasian women before the age of 40 and are more likely to die from breast cancer at every age. Higher death rates in African Americans have been attributed to later stage at diagnosis and poorer stage-specific survival (ACS, 2019).

Types of Breast Cancer

Ductal Carcinoma In Situ

Ductal carcinoma in situ (DCIS) is characterized by the proliferation of malignant cells inside the milk ducts without invasion into the surrounding tissue. Unlike invasive breast cancer, DCIS does not metastasize and a woman generally does not die of DCIS unless it develops into invasive breast cancer. DCIS can develop into invasive breast cancer if left untreated. The best estimates are that 14% to 53% of untreated DCIS progresses to invasive breast cancer over a period of 10 years or more. However, the natural history of DCIS is not well understood, and it is currently not possible to accurately predict which women with DCIS will go on to develop invasive breast cancer (ACS, 2019). DCIS is frequently manifested on a mammogram with the appearance of calcifications and is considered breast cancer stage 0.

Medical Management

Current management takes into account the assurance of an accurate diagnosis, assessment of DCIS size and grade, and careful margin evaluation. The pathologist analyzes the piece of breast tissue removed to determine the type and grade of the DCIS or how abnormal the cells look when compared with normal breast cells and how fast they are growing. Grade III (high-grade DCIS) cells tend to grow more quickly than grade I (low-grade) and grade II (moderate-grade) cells and look very different from normal breast cells. Accurate grading of DCIS is critical, because high nuclear grade and the presence of necrosis (the premature death of cells in living tissue) are highly predictive of the inability to achieve adequate margins or borders of healthy tissue around the cancer, of local recurrence, and of the probability of missed areas of invasion. The pros and cons of irradiating patients with DCIS who are treated conservatively should be carefully weighed on a case-by-case basis, considering recent trials have shown that radiation has a beneficial effect on distant recurrence, breast cancer–specific mortality, and overall survival. Breast conservation (treatment of a breast cancer without the loss of the breast) can be curative for well-defined subsets of women with DCIS, especially if the area of concern is very small (ACS, 2019).

Invasive Cancer

Invasive breast cancer includes several types of carcinoma and Paget disease.

Infiltrating Ductal Carcinoma

Infiltrating ductal carcinoma—the most common histologic type of breast cancer—accounts for 70% to 80% of all cases (Komen, 2019b). The tumors arise from the duct system and invade the surrounding tissues. They often form a solid irregular mass in the breast (Komen, 2019b).

Micropapillary invasive ductal carcinoma is a rare type of aggressive ductal cancer characterized by a high rate of axillary node metastasis and skin involvement (Komen, 2019b).

Infiltrating Lobular Carcinoma

Infiltrating lobular carcinoma accounts for 10% to 15% of breast cancers (Komen, 2019b). The tumors arise from the lobular epithelium and typically occur as an area of ill-defined thickening in the breast. They are often multicentric and can be bilateral (Komen, 2019b).

Medullary Carcinoma

Medullary carcinoma accounts for less than 1% of breast cancers (Komen, 2019b), and it tends to be diagnosed more often in women younger than 50 years. The tumors grow in a capsule inside a duct. They can become large and may be mistaken for a fibroadenoma. The prognosis is often favorable (Komen, 2019b).

Mucinous Carcinoma

Mucinous carcinoma accounts for about 2% of breast cancers and often presents in women who are postmenopausal and are 75 years and older (Komen, 2019b). A mucin producer, the tumor is also slow growing; thus, the prognosis is more favorable than in many other types (Komen, 2019b).

Tubular Carcinoma

Tubular carcinoma accounts for 1% to 5% of breast cancers (Komen, 2019b). Because axillary metastases are uncommon with this histology, prognosis is usually excellent.

Inflammatory Carcinoma

Inflammatory carcinoma is a rare (1% to 5%) (ACS, 2019; Komen, 2019b) and aggressive type of breast cancer that has unique symptoms. The cancer is characterized by diffuse edema and erythema of the skin, often referred to as peau d'orange. This is caused by malignant cells blocking the lymph channels in the skin. An associated mass may or may not be present; if there is a mass, it is often a large area of indiscrete thickening. Inflammatory carcinoma can be confused with an infection because of its presentation (Komen, 2019b). The disease can spread to other parts of the body rapidly. Chemotherapy often plays an initial role in controlling disease progression, but radiation and surgery may also follow (Komen, 2019b).

Paget Disease

Paget disease of the breast accounts for 1% to 4% of diagnosed cases of breast cancer; it is more common in men than in women (Komen, 2019b). Symptoms typically include a scaly, erythematous, pruritic lesion of the nipple. Paget disease often represents DCIS of the nipple but may have an invasive component. If no lump can be felt in the breast tissue and the biopsy shows DCIS without invasion, the prognosis is very favorable (Komen, 2019b).

Risk Factors

There is no single, specific cause of breast cancer. A combination of genetic, hormonal, and possibly environmental factors may increase the risk of its development (see Table 52-3). More than 80% of all cases of breast cancer are sporadic, meaning that patients have no known family history of the disease. The remaining cases are either familial (there is a family history of breast cancer, but it is not passed on genetically) or genetically acquired. Research suggests that obesity, alcohol use, and smoking (especially when started before the first pregnancy) may increase risk (ACS, 2019). There is some evidence that late-in-life weight gain, a sedentary lifestyle, and night shift work may increase the risk for breast cancer (ACS, 2019). There is no evidence that silicone breast implants, the use of antiperspirants, underwire bras, or abortion (induced or spontaneous) increases the risk of the disease (ACS, 2019).

As stated previously, breast cancer can be genetically inherited, resulting in significant risk. Approximately 5% to 10% of breast cancer cases have been linked to specific genetic mutations. Factors that may indicate a genetic link include multiple first-degree relatives with early-onset breast cancer, breast and ovarian cancer in the same family, male breast cancer, and Ashkenazi Jewish background. **BRCA1 and BRCA2** are tumor suppressor genes that normally function to identify damaged deoxyribonucleic acid (DNA) and thereby restrain abnormal cell growth (O'Donnell, Axilbund, & Euhus, 2018). Mutations in these genes on chromosome 17 are responsible for the majority of hereditary breast cancer in the United States. *BRCA* mutations in women have been associated with an overall risk of breast cancer up to 70% (ACS, 2019). Currently, women who are *BRCA* positive are counseled to start screening, typically using mammography, once a year and then MRI 6 months after the yearly mammography by 25 years of age, or 5 to 10 years earlier than their youngest affected family member. Mutations in the *PALB2* gene confer similar risk. Males who carry the *BRCA2* mutation may have a lifetime risk of 6% to 7% of developing breast cancer (Jain & Gradishar, 2018).

Protective Factors

Certain factors may be protective against the development of breast cancer. Breast-feeding for at least 1 year, regular or moderate physical activity, and maintaining a healthy body weight are cited as protective (ACS, 2019). Some research suggests that the use of extra virgin olive oil, as is found in a

TABLE 52-3 ⚠ Risk Factors for Breast Cancer	
Risk Factor	**Comments**
Female gender	99% of cases occur in women.
Increasing age	Increasing age is associated with an increased risk.
Personal history of breast cancer	Once treated for breast cancer, the risk of developing breast cancer in same or opposite breast is significantly increased.
Family history of breast cancer	Having first-degree relative with breast cancer (mother, sister, daughter) increases the risk twofold; having two first-degree relatives increases the risk fivefold. The risk is higher if the relative was premenopausal at the time of diagnosis. The risk is increased if a father or brother had breast cancer (exact risk is unknown).
Genetic mutation	*BRCA1* and *BRCA2* mutations account for majority of inherited cases of breast cancer (see additional information in text).
Hormonal Factors • Early menarche • Late menopause • Nulliparity • Late age at first full-term pregnancy • Hormone therapy (formerly referred to as hormone replacement therapy)	 Before 12 yrs of age After 55 yrs of age No full-term pregnancies After 30 yrs of age Current or recent use of combined postmenopausal hormone therapy (estrogen and progesterone) Long-term use (several years or more)
Exposure to ionizing radiation during adolescence and early adulthood	The risk is highest if breast tissue was exposed while still developing (during adolescence), such as women who received mantle radiation (to the chest area) for treatment of Hodgkin lymphoma in their younger years.
History of benign proliferative breast disease	Having had atypical ductal or lobular hyperplasia or lobular carcinoma in situ increases the risk.
Obesity	Obesity and weight gain during adulthood increases the risk of postmenopausal breast cancer. During menopause, estrogen is primarily produced in fat tissue. More fat tissue can increase estrogen levels, thereby increasing breast cancer risk.
High-fat diet	More research is needed.
Alcohol intake (beer, wine, or liquor)	Two to five drinks daily increases the risk about one and a half times.

Adapted from National Comprehensive Cancer Network (NCCN). (2019). Clinical practice guidelines: Breast. Retrieved on 9/9/2019 at: www.nccn.org/professionals/physician_gls/pdf/breast_risk.pdf

Mediterranean diet, might be preventive, but recent research is inconclusive (Mayo Clinic, 2018).

Breast Cancer Prevention Strategies in the Patient Who Is at High Risk

Patients often over- or underestimate their risk of developing breast cancer. A consultation with a breast specialist is of paramount importance prior to embarking on any of the prevention strategies that follow. Once patients have an accurate assessment of their risk, along with the knowledge of the pros and cons of each prevention strategy, they can make a decision that is most appropriate for their situation.

Long-Term Surveillance

Long-term surveillance focuses on early detection. As recommended by the NCCN (2019), women at high risk for breast cancer benefit from additional screening using MRI along with a yearly mammogram. Clinical breast examinations may be performed twice a year starting as early as 25 years of age. Mammograms may also be performed as early as 25 years of age. Data concerning the effectiveness of BSE are limited. In addition to yearly mammography and MRI, other screening tests, including ultrasonography, may be useful.

Chemoprevention

Chemoprevention is the main modality that aims to prevent the disease. Several national, randomized clinical trials have led to FDA approval of tamoxifen and raloxifene as effective chemopreventive agents for use in women who are at high risk (Mayo Clinic, 2019a). Tamoxifen has been shown to reduce risk by up to 50% even in women in whom up to three first-degree relatives are also affected (O'Donnell et al., 2018). Because tamoxifen is associated with an increased risk for endometrial cancer and thromboembolic events, especially in postmenopausal women, it is more frequently recommended for premenopausal women. In women previously diagnosed with LCIS, who are at risk for developing invasive cancer, tamoxifen has been approved for use premenopausally, while raloxifene is recommended postmenopausally (Calhoun & Anderson, 2018). Postmenopausally, anastrozole and exemestane are also now used for chemoprevention (Mayo Clinic, 2019a). Nurses can help women who are considering chemoprevention by providing them with information about the benefits, risks, and possible side effects of these medications.

Prophylactic Mastectomy

Prophylactic mastectomy is another primary prevention modality that can reduce the risk of breast cancer by 90% to 95% (Mayo Clinic, 2019b) and is sometimes referred to as a "risk-reducing" mastectomy. The procedure consists of a total **mastectomy** (removal of breast tissue) and is usually accompanied by immediate breast reconstruction. Possible candidates include women with a strong family history of breast cancer, a diagnosis of LCIS or atypical hyperplasia, a mutation in a *BRCA* gene, and previous cancer in one breast. Because of physical and psychological ramifications including anxiety, depression, and altered body image, this procedure should be undertaken only after extensive counseling related to its risks and benefits. The procedure does not confer 100% protection against the development of breast cancer (Mayo Clinic, 2019b).

A multidisciplinary approach is used to help the patient arrive at a decision that is best for her. Consultation with a genetic counselor, plastic surgeon, medical oncologist, and psychiatrist can be invaluable. The patient needs to understand that this surgery is elective and not emergent. The nurse can play a valuable role in providing the patient with information, clarification, and support during the decision-making process.

Clinical Manifestations

Breast cancers can occur anywhere in the breast but are usually found in the upper outer quadrant, where the most breast tissue is located. In general, the lesions are nontender, fixed rather than mobile, and hard with irregular borders. Complaints of diffuse breast pain and tenderness with menstruation are usually associated with benign breast disease.

Because of mammography, more women are seeking treatment at earlier stages of the disease. These women often have no signs or symptoms other than a mammographic abnormality. Some women with advanced disease seek initial treatment after ignoring symptoms. Advanced signs may include skin dimpling, nipple retraction, or skin ulceration.

Assessment and Diagnostic Findings

Techniques to determine the diagnosis of breast cancer include various types of biopsy, which have been described previously. Tumor staging and analysis of additional prognostic factors are used to determine the prognosis and optimal treatment regimen (see below).

Staging

Staging involves classifying the cancer by the extent of the disease in the body. It is based on whether the cancer is invasive or noninvasive, the size of the tumor, how many lymph nodes are involved, and if it has spread to other parts of the body. The stage of a cancer is one of the most important factors in determining prognosis and treatment options. The most common system used to describe the stages of breast cancer is the American Joint Committee on Cancer (AJCC) TNM (tumor, nodes, metastasis) system (see Chapter 12, Chart 12-3). Other factors considered in staging include hormone receptors and genetic mutations.

Other diagnostic tests may be performed before or after surgery to help in the staging of the disease. The extent of testing often depends on the clinical presentation of the disease and may include chest x-rays, computed tomography (CT) scan, MRI scan, positron emission tomography (PET) scan, bone scans, and blood work (complete blood count, comprehensive metabolic panel, and tumor markers [i.e., carcinoembryonic antigen, cancer antigen 15-3]).

Prognosis

Several different factors must be taken into consideration when determining the prognosis of a patient with breast cancer. Two of the most important factors are tumor size and whether the tumor has spread to the axillary (underarm) lymph nodes.

In general, the smaller the tumor appears, the better the prognosis. A tumor starts with a genetic alteration in a single cell and takes time to divide and double in size. A carcinoma may double in size 30 times to become 1 cm or larger, at which point it becomes clinically apparent. Doubling time varies, but breast tumors are often present for several years before they become palpable. Nurses can reassure patients that once breast cancer is diagnosed, they have a safe period of several weeks to make decisions regarding treatment; however, a lengthy delay is not advisable.

Prognosis also depends on the extent of spread of the breast cancer. The 5-year survival rate is approximately 88% for a stage I breast cancer and 15% for a stage IV breast cancer (ACS, 2019). The most common route of regional spread is to the axillary lymph nodes. Other sites of lymphatic spread include the internal mammary and supraclavicular nodes (see Fig. 52-5). Distant metastasis can affect any organ, but the most common sites are bone, lung, liver, and brain (Breastcancer.org, 2018).

In addition to the type of breast cancer and the stage, other factors may help determine prognosis (see Chart 52-3). Amplification (excessive number of copies of certain genes) or overexpression (excessive amounts of their protein product) may represent a poorer prognosis. The HER-2/neu

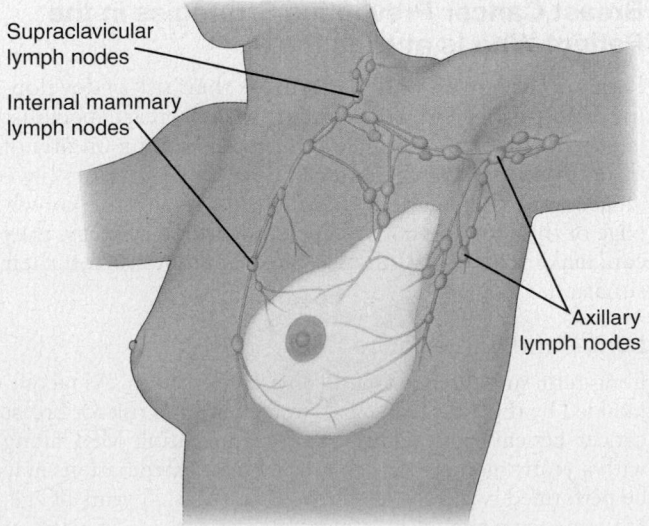

Supraclavicular lymph nodes

Internal mammary lymph nodes

Axillary lymph nodes

Figure 52-5 • Lymphatic drainage of the breast.

Chart 52-3	Factors Associated with Favorable Prognosis for Breast Cancer

- Noninvasive tumors or invasive tumors <1 cm
- Negative axillary lymph nodes
- Estrogen receptor (ER) and progesterone receptor (PR) proteins
- Well-differentiated tumors
- Low expression of HER-2/neu oncogene (also known as *ERBB2*)
- No vascular or lymphatic invasion
- Diploid tumors with low S-phase fraction

Adapted from Chalasani, P. (2020). Breast cancer. Retrieved on 5/14/2020 at: www.emedicine.medscape.com/article/1947145-overview#a8

(also known as *ERBB2*) oncogene is the classic example; approximately 20% of invasive breast cancers, which typically involve the more aggressive tumors, have amplification or overexpression of this gene (Mayo Clinic, 2020). The proliferative rate or rapidity in growth rate (S-phase fraction) and DNA content (ploidy) of a tumor are factors that are also associated with overall survival rate.

Surgical Management

The main goal of surgery is to gain local control of the disease. With breast cancer being diagnosed today at earlier stages, options for less invasive, breast conserving surgical procedures are available. Surgical treatment options for noninvasive and invasive breast cancer are summarized in Table 52-4.

Modified Radical Mastectomy

Modified radical mastectomy is performed to treat invasive breast cancer. The procedure involves removal of breast tissue, including the nipple–areola complex. In addition, a portion of the axillary lymph nodes are also removed in axillary lymph node dissection (ALND). If immediate breast reconstruction is desired, the patient is referred to a plastic surgeon prior to the mastectomy so that the patient has the opportunity to explore all available options (see Chart 52-4). In modified radical mastectomy, the pectoralis major and pectoralis minor muscles are left intact, unlike in radical mastectomy, in which the muscles are removed.

TABLE 52-4	Surgical Treatment Options for Noninvasive and Invasive Breast Cancer

Noninvasive Breast Cancer	Invasive Breast Cancer
Breast conservation[a] alone	Breast conservation[a] with one of the following: Sentinel lymph node biopsy Axillary lymph node dissection
Total mastectomy alone	Total mastectomy with sentinel lymph node biopsy *or* Modified radical mastectomy

[a]Breast conservation treatment includes lumpectomy, wide excision, partial or segmental mastectomy, and quadrantectomy. These are relatively synonymous terms that describe removal of varying amounts of breast tissue.

Total Mastectomy

Like modified radical mastectomy, total mastectomy (i.e., simple mastectomy) also involves removal of the breast and nipple–areola complex but does not include ALND. Total mastectomy may be performed in patients with noninvasive breast cancer (e.g., DCIS), which does not have a tendency to spread to the lymph nodes. It may also be performed prophylactically in patients who are at high risk for breast cancer (e.g., LCIS, *BRCA* mutation). A total mastectomy may also be performed in conjunction with sentinel lymph node biopsy (SLNB) for patients with invasive breast cancer.

Breast Conservation Treatment

The goal of **breast conservation treatment** (i.e., lumpectomy, wide excision, partial or segmental mastectomy, quadrantectomy) is to excise the tumor in the breast completely and obtain clear margins while achieving an acceptable cosmetic result. If the procedure is being performed to treat a noninvasive breast cancer, lymph node removal is not necessary. For an invasive breast cancer, lymph node removal (SLNB or ALND) is indicated. The lymph nodes are removed through a separate semicircular incision in the axilla.

Sentinel Lymph Node Biopsy

The status of the lymph nodes is the most important prognostic factor in breast cancer. The SLNB is a less invasive alternative to ALND and is considered a standard of care for the treatment of early-stage breast cancer. ALND is associated with potential morbidity, including lymphedema, cellulitis, decreased arm mobility, and sensory changes. Studies suggest that SLNB is highly accurate and is associated with a low axillary recurrence rate (Prati, Chang, & Chung, 2018). Table 52-5 compares SLNB and ALND.

The **sentinel lymph node**, which is the first node (or nodes) in the lymphatic basin that receives drainage from the primary tumor in the breast, is identified by injecting a radioisotope or blue dye into the breast; the radioisotope or dye then travels via the lymphatic pathways to the node. In SLNB, the surgeon uses a handheld probe to locate the sentinel lymph node, excises it, and sends it for pathologic analysis, which is often performed immediately during the surgery using frozen-section analysis. If the sentinel lymph node is positive, the surgeon can proceed with an immediate ALND, thus sparing the patient a return trip to the operating room and additional anesthesia. (The patient could also return for additional surgery at a later time.) If the sentinel lymph node is negative, a standard ALND is not needed, thus sparing the patient the possible complications of the procedure. After the procedure is complete, all specimens are sent to pathology for more thorough analysis.

Nursing Management

Patients who undergo SLNB in conjunction with breast conservation treatments are generally discharged the same day. Patients who undergo SLNB with total mastectomy usually stay in the hospital overnight, possibly longer if breast reconstruction is being performed. The patient must be informed that although frozen-section analysis is highly accurate, false-negative results can occur. A negative sentinel lymph node on frozen-section analysis may show metastatic disease on subsequent analysis, indicating that ALND is still necessary. The patient should also be reassured that

Chart 52-4 ETHICAL DILEMMA
What Is Acceptable Treatment for a Patient with Breast Cancer during a Pandemic?

Case Scenario

You work as a staff nurse on an oncology surgery unit. K.M. is a 37-year-old woman who is one day postoperative for a mastectomy for an invasive ductal carcinoma of her left breast. There is an outbreak of coronavirus disease 2019 (COVID-19) within your community. K.M. does not have COVID-19 and the surgical unit where you work has been designated to manage patients without COVID-19; nonetheless, a no visitor policy is enforced throughout your hospital and K.M. may not receive any visitors. When you enter K.M.'s room to perform your baseline assessment, you find her crying. She says to you, "This is terrible. When my sister had a mastectomy 3 years ago, she was able to have breast reconstruction done at the same time. I did not have that choice because only the mastectomy was considered essential—the reconstruction was considered elective! I have to wait before I can have that done and go through surgery all over again! It is so unfair! And it is so unfair that my husband had to drop me off at the curb and cannot be with me! He is worried sick!" K.M. is not the only patient you have cared for during this pandemic who has faced obstacles receiving what had previously been considered standard care. Additionally, many of your patients have voiced anger, frustration, anxiety, and fear because their loved ones are barred from being able to visit them postoperatively.

Discussion

Access to health care resources can drastically change during a pandemic. Resources may be scarce not only for patients who are directly infected by the pathogen responsible for the pandemic, but for all patients. For instance, access to the services rendered by health care personnel (e.g., surgeons), facilities (e.g., surgical centers, operating rooms), pharmacologic agents, medical devices, to name a few, may all be disrupted or delayed because of societal needs to divert maximum resources to mitigate the effects of the pandemic. Diversion of these resources can result in a scarcity of resources considered as standard

therapy during other times. The COVID-19 pandemic has caused disruptions to and delays in access to care for many patients with breast cancer, as well as patients with other cancers.

Analysis

- Describe the ethical principles that are in conflict in this case (see Chapter 1, Chart 1-7). K.M. feels that she should have been eligible to have reconstruction done at the same time as her mastectomy. Her availability of choices and her personhood were arguably threatened by not being able to select her preferred surgical procedure. She might have elected to wait to have her mastectomy until such time as the breast reconstruction could have also been done; however, her risk of an adverse outcome related to her cancer would have been greater. Is it just to enforce these types of resource delays during a pandemic?
- K.M. expresses frustration at not being able to see her husband postoperatively. Are visitor prohibitions during a pandemic so much a threat to beneficence that they should not be enforced? Or are these types of universal prohibitions justifiable?
- What resources might be mobilized to assist you in caring for K.M. and other patients on your unit? How can you assure that your professional need to deliver quality care to your patients is not threatened? How can you preserve your own sense of self-worth?

References

Papautsky, E. L., & Hamlish, T. (2020). Patient-reported treatment delays in breast cancer care during the COVID-19 pandemic. *Breast Cancer Research and Treatment*, 184(1), 249–254.

Veronesi, P., & Corso, G. (2020). Impact of COVID-19 pandemic on clinical and surgical breast cancer management. *EClinicalMedicine*, 26, 100523.

Resources

See Chapter 1, Chart 1-10 for Steps of an Ethical Analysis and Ethics Resources.

---

the radioisotope and blue dye are generally safe. The nurse informs patients that they may notice a blue-green discoloration in the urine or stool for the first 24 hours as the blue dye is excreted. The incidence of lymphedema, decreased arm mobility, and seroma formation (collection of serous fluid) in the axilla is generally low, but the patient should be prepared for these possibilities. Women

who have SLNB alone have neuropathic sensations similar to those who undergo ALND, although the prevalence and severity of these sensations and the resulting distress are lower with SLNB.

The nurse must not overlook the psychosocial needs of the patient who has undergone SLNB. Although SLNB is a less invasive procedure than ALND and results in a shorter recovery

TABLE 52-5	Comparison of Sentinel Lymph Node Biopsy and Axillary Lymph Node Dissection
Sentinel Lymph Node Biopsy	**Axillary Lymph Node Dissection**
Shorter operating room time (~15–30 mins)	Longer operating room time (~60–90 mins)
No surgical drain	Surgical drain
Local anesthesia with IV moderate sedation as outpatient surgery (unless being performed in conjunction with total mastectomy)	General anesthesia; usually overnight admission (sometimes done as outpatient surgery)
Lymphedema risk minimal	Lymphedema risk higher
Presence of neuropathic sensations postoperatively (prevalence lower than after axillary lymph node dissection)	Presence of neuropathic sensations postoperatively
Decreased range of motion in affected arm unlikely postoperatively but may occur	Decreased range of motion likely postoperatively
Seroma (collection of serous fluid in the axilla) may occur postoperatively, but less likely	Seroma may occur postoperatively

Adapted from Breastcancer.org. (2019). Lymph node removal. Retrieved on 5/13/2020 at: https://www.breastcancer.org/treatment/surgery/lymph_node_removal

period, a patient who has undergone SLNB also has many difficult issues surrounding her breast cancer diagnosis and treatment. The nurse must listen, provide emotional support, and refer the patient to appropriate specialists when indicated.

NURSING PROCESS

The Patient Undergoing Surgery for Breast Cancer

Assessment

The health history is a valuable tool to assess the patient's reaction to the diagnosis and her ability to cope with it. Pertinent questions include the following:

- How is the patient responding to the diagnosis?
- What coping mechanisms does she find most helpful?
- What psychological or emotional supports does she have and use?
- Is there a partner, family member, or friend available to assist her in making treatment choices?
- What are her educational needs?
- Is she experiencing any discomfort?

Diagnosis

PREOPERATIVE NURSING DIAGNOSES

Based on the assessment data, major preoperative nursing diagnoses may include the following:

- Lack of knowledge about the planned surgical treatments
- Anxiety associated with the diagnosis of cancer
- Fear associated with specific treatments and body image changes
- Risk for difficulty with coping associated with the diagnosis of breast cancer and related treatment options
- Decisional conflict associated with treatment options

POSTOPERATIVE NURSING DIAGNOSES

Based on the assessment data, major postoperative nursing diagnoses may include the following:

- Acute pain and discomfort associated with surgical procedure
- Risk for impaired peripheral neurovascular function associated with nerve irritation in affected arm, breast, or chest wall
- Disturbed body image associated with loss or alteration of the breast
- Risk for difficulty with coping associated with the diagnosis of cancer and surgical treatment
- Impaired ability to perform hygiene, impaired ability to dress, impaired self feeding, and impaired self toileting associated with partial immobility of upper extremity on operative side
- Lack of knowledge: drain management after breast surgery, arm exercises to regain mobility of affected extremity, hand and arm care after ALND

COLLABORATIVE PROBLEMS/POTENTIAL COMPLICATIONS

Potential complications may include the following:

- Lymphedema
- Hematoma/Seroma formation
- Infection
- Changes in sexual function

Planning and Goals

The major goals may include increased knowledge about the disease and its treatment; reduction of preoperative and postoperative fear, anxiety, and emotional stress; improvement of decision-making ability; pain management; neurovascular function management; maintenance of a positive body image; improvement in coping abilities; increased self-care abilities; improvement in sexual function; and the absence of complications.

Preoperative Nursing Interventions

PROVIDING EDUCATION AND PREPARATION ABOUT SURGICAL TREATMENTS

Many cancer centers have coordinators to help patients navigate appointments, decision-making, and care-paths. Nurses can encourage patients and their support persons to establish and maintain contact with these coordinators and utilize available resources as needed along their journeys. The nurse will reinforce a coordinator's support, if available; if no coordinator is available, nurses assume much of this responsibility.

Patients with newly diagnosed breast cancer are expected to absorb an abundance of new information during a very emotionally difficult time, and this may lead to difficulty in making treatment decisions. The nurse plays a key role in reviewing treatment options by reinforcing information provided to the patient and answering any questions. The nurse fully prepares the patient for what to expect before, during, and after surgery. Patients undergoing breast conservation with ALND, or a total or modified radical mastectomy, generally remain in the hospital overnight (or longer if they have immediate reconstruction). Surgical drains will be inserted in the mastectomy incision and in the axilla if the patient undergoes ALND. A surgical drain is generally not needed after SLNB. The patient should be informed that she will go home with the drain(s) and that complete instructions about drain care will be provided prior to discharge. In addition, the patient should be informed that she will often have decreased arm and shoulder mobility after ALND and that she will be shown range-of-motion exercises prior to discharge. The patient should also be reassured that appropriate analgesia and comfort measures will be provided to alleviate any postoperative discomfort.

REDUCING FEAR AND ANXIETY AND IMPROVING COPING ABILITY

The nurse helps the patient cope with the physical and emotional effects of surgery. Many fears may emerge during the preoperative phase. These can include fear of pain, mutilation (after mastectomy), and loss of sexual attractiveness; concern about inability to care for oneself and one's family; concern about taking time off from work; and coping with an uncertain future. Providing the patient with realistic expectations about the healing process and expected recovery can help alleviate fears. Maintaining open communication and assuring the patient that she can contact the nurse at any time with questions or concerns can be a source of comfort. The patient should also be made aware of available resources at the treatment facility as well as in the breast cancer community such as social workers, psychiatrists, and support groups. Some women find it helpful and reassuring to talk to a survivor of breast cancer who has undergone similar treatments.

PROMOTING DECISION-MAKING ABILITY

The patient may be eligible for more than one therapeutic approach; she may be presented with treatment options and then asked to make a choice. This can be very frightening for some patients, and they may prefer to have someone else make the decision for them (e.g., surgeon, family member). The nurse can be instrumental in ensuring that the patient and family members truly understand their options. The nurse can then help the patient weigh the risks and benefits of each option. The patient may be presented with the option of having breast conservation treatment followed by radiation or a mastectomy. The nurse can explore the issues with the patient by asking questions such as the following:

- How do you think you might feel about losing your breast?
- Are you considering breast reconstruction?
- If you choose to retain your breast, would you consider undergoing radiation treatments 5 days a week for 5 to 6 weeks?

Questions such as these can help the patient focus. Once the patient's decision is made, it is very important to support it.

Postoperative Nursing Interventions

RELIEVING PAIN AND DISCOMFORT

Many patients tolerate breast surgery well and have minimal pain during the postoperative period. This is particularly true of less invasive procedures such as breast conservation treatment with SLNB. However, all patients must be carefully assessed, because individual patients can have varying degrees of pain. Patients who have had more invasive procedures, such as a modified radical mastectomy with immediate reconstruction, may have considerably more pain. All patients are discharged home with analgesic medication (e.g., oxycodone and acetaminophen) and are encouraged to take it if needed. An over-the-counter analgesic agent such as acetaminophen may provide sufficient relief. Patients sometimes complain of a slight increase in pain after the first few days of surgery; this may occur as patients regain sensation around the surgical site and become more active. However, patients who report more than moderate pain must be evaluated to rule out any potential complications such as infection or hematoma. Postoperative pain may be more common in patients who have had axillary dissection: the amount of discomfort may increase with each additional node removed. (Komen, 2019a). Alternative methods of pain management, such as taking warm showers (if permitted by the surgeon) and using distraction methods (e.g., guided imagery), may also be helpful. See Chapter 9 for further discussion of methods that relieve pain.

MANAGING POSTOPERATIVE SENSATIONS

Because nerves in the skin and axilla are often ligated or injured during breast surgery, patients experience a variety of sensations. Common sensations include tenderness, soreness, numbness, tightness, pulling, and twinges. These sensations may occur along the chest wall, in the axilla, and along the inside aspect of the upper arm. After mastectomy, some patients experience phantom sensations and report a feeling that the breast or nipple is still present. Overall, patients do not find these sensations severe or distressing. Sensations usually persist for several months and then begin to diminish, although some may persist for as long as 5 years and possibly longer. Patients should be reassured that this is a normal part of healing and that these sensations are not indicative of a problem.

PROMOTING POSITIVE BODY IMAGE

Patients who have undergone mastectomy may find it difficult to view the surgical site for the first time. No matter how prepared the patient may think she is, the appearance of an absent breast can be very emotionally distressing. Ideally, the patient sees the incision for the first time when she is with the nurse or another health care provider who is available for support.

The nurse first assesses the patient's readiness and provides gentle encouragement. It is important to maintain the patient's privacy while assisting her as she views the incision; this allows her to express feelings safely to the nurse. Asking the patient what she perceives, acknowledging her feelings, and allowing her to express her emotions are important nursing actions. Reassuring the patient that her feelings are a normal response to breast cancer surgery may be comforting. If the patient has not had immediate reconstruction, providing her with a temporary breast form or soft padding to place in her bra on discharge can help alleviate feelings of embarrassment or self-consciousness.

PROMOTING POSITIVE ADJUSTMENT AND COPING

Providing ongoing assessment of how the patient is coping with her diagnosis of breast cancer and her surgical treatment is important in determining her overall adjustment. Assisting the patient in identifying and mobilizing her support systems can be beneficial to her well-being. The patient's spouse or partner may also need guidance, support, and education. The patient and partner may benefit from a wide network of available community resources, including the Reach to Recovery program of the ACS, advocacy groups, social worker, or a spiritual advisor. Encouraging the patient to discuss issues and concerns with other patients who have had breast cancer may help her to understand that her feelings are normal and that other women who have had breast cancer can provide invaluable support and understanding.

The patient may also have considerable anxiety about the treatments that will follow surgery (i.e., chemotherapy and radiation) and their implications. Providing her with information about the plan of care and referring her to the appropriate members of the health care team also promote coping during recovery. Some women require additional support to adjust to their diagnosis and the changes that it brings. If a woman displays difficulty coping, consultation with a mental health provider may be indicated. Nurse navigators can help those undergoing breast biopsy to cope.

MONITORING AND MANAGING POTENTIAL COMPLICATIONS

Lymphedema. **Lymphedema** is a complication characterized by a chronic swelling of an extremity due to interrupted lymphatic circulation. The swelling is due to the accumulation of protein-rich fluid in the interstitial space and is a somewhat common postoperative complication after ALND. It often affects both the breast and ipsilateral limb. It is associated with a painful swelling of the arm as well as weakness, shoulder pain, and tingling sensations in the arm and shoulder. After ALND, the risk of developing lymphedema may be as low as 11% or as high as 57% (Rivere & Klimberg, 2018). Because sentinel lymph node dissection (SLND) involves more focused surgery and less disruption of the axilla, the risk is only up to 7% within 5 years (Rivere & Klimberg, 2018). Risk factors for lymphedema in mixed-age groups include ALND, concomitant radiation therapy, increased age, presence of a concomitant infection, preexisting cardiovascular conditions, and obesity (Rivere & Klimberg, 2018).

Lymphedema results if functioning lymphatic channels are inadequate to ensure a return flow of lymph fluid to the general circulation. After axillary lymph nodes are removed, collateral circulation must assume this function. Transient edema in the postoperative period occurs until collateral circulation has completely taken over this function, which generally occurs within a month. Performing prescribed exercises, elevating the arm above the heart several times a day, and gentle muscle pumping (making a fist and releasing) can help reduce the transient edema. The patient needs reassurance that this transient swelling is not lymphedema.

Once lymphedema develops, it tends to be chronic, so preventive strategies are vital. After ALND, the patient is taught hand and arm care to prevent injury or trauma to the affected extremity, thus decreasing the likelihood for development of lymphedema (see Chart 52-5). The patient is instructed to follow these guidelines for the rest of her life. She is also instructed to contact her primary provider immediately if she suspects that she has lymphedema, because early intervention provides the best chance for control. If allowed to progress without treatment, the swelling can become more difficult to manage. Treatment may consist of a course of antibiotic agents if an infection is present. A referral to a rehabilitation specialist (e.g., occupational or physical therapist) may be necessary for a compression sleeve or glove, exercises, manual lymph drainage, and a discussion of ways to modify daily activities to avoid worsening lymphedema. Ongoing research is seeking to identify which lymph nodes drain the arm before surgery so that they can be preserved when possible, helping to prevent the development of lymphedema. The practice of yoga may result in improved shoulder range of motion and upper extremity strength in women with postoperative

lymphedema (Mazor, Lee, Peled, et al., 2018). See the Nursing Research Profile in Chart 52-6.

Hematoma or Seroma Formation. Hematoma formation (collection of blood inside a cavity) may occur after either mastectomy or breast conservation and usually develops within the first 12 hours after surgery. The nurse assesses for signs and symptoms of hematoma at the surgical site, which may include swelling, tightness, pain, and bruising of the skin. The surgeon should be notified immediately if there is gross swelling or increased bloody output from the drain. Depending on the surgeon's assessment, a compression wrap may be applied to the incision for approximately 12 hours, or the patient may be returned to the operating room so that the incision may be reopened to identify the source of bleeding. Some hematomas are small, and the body absorbs the blood

---

Chart 52-5 PATIENT EDUCATION
Hand and Arm Care After Axillary Lymph Node Dissection

The nurse instructs the patient to:

- Avoid blood pressures, injections, and blood draws in affected extremity.
- Use sunscreen (higher than 15 SPF) for extended exposure to sun.
- Apply insect repellent to avoid insect bites.
- Wear gloves for gardening.
- Use cooking mitt for removing objects from oven.
- Avoid cutting cuticles; push them back during manicures.
- Use electric razor for shaving armpit.
- Avoid lifting objects heavier than 5 to 10 lb.
- If a trauma or break in the skin occurs, wash the area with soap and water, and apply an over-the-counter antibacterial ointment. Observe the area and extremity for 24 hours; if redness, swelling, or a fever occurs, call the surgeon or nurse.

Chart 52-6 NURSING RESEARCH PROFILE
Effect of Yoga on Lymphedema

Mazor, M., Lee, J. Q., Peled, A., et al. (2018). The effect of yoga on arm volume, strength, and range of motion in women at risk for breast cancer-related lymphedema. *Journal of Alternative and Complementary Medicine, 24*(2), 154–160.

Purpose

Breast cancer-related lymphedema (BCRL) is a complication of breast cancer that causes considerable morbidity. The intent of this study was to assess the feasibility, safety, and initial estimates of efficacy of a yoga program in the postoperative care of women at increased risk for BCRL.

Design

Twenty-one women were recruited at a breast care center in California. All participants were over 18 years of age, had undergone surgical intervention for breast cancer, and were at high risk for lymphedema. Women participated in an 8-week regimen of Ashtanga yoga, taking one instructor-led class weekly and also completing one self-led session weekly. Poses focused on upper-body strength and flexibility, while also avoiding placing the affected arm in a dependent position. Measurements of upper extremity volume, range of motion, and strength were assessed.

Findings

Twenty of the 21 participants finished the 8-week intervention and 17 completed the final assessment. The mean age was 52 years and body mass index was 24.8 kg/m^2. Postintervention mean upper extremity volumes were slightly decreased in the at-risk arm ($p = 0.397$). Range of motion in both shoulder flexion ($p < 0.01$) and external rotation ($p < 0.05$) improved significantly. After the intervention, strength also improved on the affected side for shoulder abduction, grip strength, and bilaterally for elbow flexion ($p < 0.05$ for all).

Nursing Implications

Nurses should know that yoga is feasible and safe to recommend for women at risk for BCRL and may result in small improvements in shoulder range of motion and upper extremity strength. Many women may have already been exposed to yoga or similar exercises prior to their cancer diagnosis and nurses can encourage these women to facilitate integration of this intervention into their postoperative care. The added benefits of yoga in providing stress reduction, mindfulness, breathing practices, and meditation may also contribute to a woman's sense of well-being and self-care.

naturally. The patient may take warm showers (if permitted by the surgeon) or apply warm compresses to help increase the absorption. A hematoma usually resolves in 4 to 5 weeks.

A seroma, a collection of serous fluid, may accumulate under the breast incision after mastectomy or breast conservation or in the axilla. Signs and symptoms may include swelling, heaviness, discomfort, and a sloshing of fluid. Seromas may develop temporarily after the drain is removed or if the drain is in place and becomes obstructed. Seromas rarely pose a threat and may be treated by unclogging the drain or manually aspirating the fluid with a needle and syringe. Large, long-standing seromas that have not been aspirated may lead to infection. Small seromas that are not bothersome to the patient usually resolve on their own.

Infection. Although infection is rare, it is a risk after any surgical procedure. This risk may be higher in patients with conditions such as diabetes, immune disorders, and advanced age, as well as in those with poor hygiene. Patients are taught to monitor for signs and symptoms of infection (redness, warmth around incision, tenderness, foul-smelling drainage, temperature greater than 38°C [100.4°F], chills) and to contact the surgeon or nurse for evaluation. Treatment consists of oral or IV antibiotics (for more severe infections) for 1 or 2 weeks. Cultures are taken of any foul-smelling discharge.

Changes in Sexual Function. Once discharged from the hospital and feeling well, most patients are physically allowed to engage in sexual activity, if interested. However, any change in the patient's body image, self-esteem, or the response of her partner may increase her anxiety level and affect sexual function. Some partners may have difficulty looking at the incision, whereas others may be completely unaffected. Encouraging the patient to openly discuss how she feels about herself and about possible reasons for a decrease in libido (e.g., fatigue, anxiety, self-consciousness) may help clarify issues for her. Helpful suggestions for the patient may include varying the time of day for sexual activity (when the patient is less tired), assuming positions that are more comfortable, and expressing affection using alternative measures (e.g., hugging, kissing, manual stimulation).

Most patients and their partners adjust with minimal difficulty if they openly discuss their concerns. However, if issues cannot be resolved, a referral for counseling (e.g., psychologist, psychiatrist, psychiatric clinical nurse specialist, social worker, sex therapist) may be helpful. The ambulatory care nurse in the outpatient clinic or hospital should inquire whether the patient who was sexually active prior to surgery has resumed activities, because many patients are reluctant or embarrassed to bring this topic up themselves.

PROMOTING HOME, COMMUNITY-BASED, AND TRANSITIONAL CARE

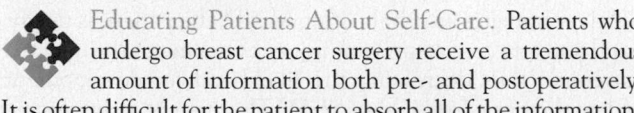

Educating Patients About Self-Care. Patients who undergo breast cancer surgery receive a tremendous amount of information both pre- and postoperatively. It is often difficult for the patient to absorb all of the information, partly because of the emotional distress that often accompanies the diagnosis and treatment. Prior to discharge, the nurse must assess the patient's readiness to assume self-care responsibilities and identify any gaps in knowledge. A review of education provided in written and oral forms, with reinforcement, may be required to ensure that the patient and family are prepared to manage the necessary care at home. The nurse reiterates symptoms that the patient should report, such as infection, seroma, hematoma, or arm swelling. All instruction should be reinforced during office visits and by telephone.

Most patients are discharged 1 or 2 days after ALND or mastectomy (possibly later if they have had immediate reconstruction) with surgical drains in place. Initially, the drainage fluid appears bloody, but it gradually changes to a serosanguineous and then a serous fluid over the next several days. The patient is given instructions about drainage management at home (see Chart 52-7). If the patient lives alone and drainage management

---

Chart 52-7 — HOME CARE CHECKLIST

Patient with a Drainage Device Following Breast Surgery

At the completion of education, the patient and/or caregiver will be able to:

- Name the procedure that was performed and identify changes in anatomic structure or function as well as changes in ADLs, IADLs, roles, relationships, and spirituality.
- Identify interventions and strategies (e.g., prosthesis) used in adapting to any permanent changes in structure or function.
- Describe ongoing postoperative therapeutic regimen, including diet and activities to perform (e.g., when to shower, arm exercises) and to limit or avoid (e.g., lifting weights, driving a car, contact sports).
- State the name, dose, side effects, frequency, and schedule for all medications.
  - Describe approaches to controlling pain (e.g., take analgesics as prescribed; use nonpharmacologic interventions).
- State how to obtain medical supplies and carry out dressing changes, wound care, and other prescribed regimens.
  - Care for the drain site and incision as per surgeon's recommendation.
  - Demonstrate how to empty and measure fluid from the drainage device.

- Demonstrate how to milk clots through the tubing of the drainage device.
- Identify when the drain is ready for removal (usually when draining <30 mL for 24 to 48 hours).
- Describe signs and symptoms of complications.
  - State observations that require contacting the primary provider or nurse (e.g., sudden change in color of drainage, sudden cessation of drainage, signs or symptoms of an infection).
- Relate how to reach primary provider with questions or complications.
- State time and date of follow-up appointments, therapy, and testing.
- Identify sources of support (e.g., friends, relatives, faith community).
- Identify the contact details for support services (for patients and their caregivers/families).
- Identify the need for health promotion, disease prevention, and screening activities (e.g., gynecologic examination, mammogram).

ADL, activities of daily living; IADL, instrumental activities of daily living.

is difficult, a referral for a home health nurse should be made. The drains are usually removed when the output is less than 30 mL in two consecutive 24-hour periods (approximately 7 to 10 days) (Grobmyer & Bland, 2018). The home health nurse also reviews pain management and incision care.

In general, the patient may shower on the second postoperative day and wash the incision and drain site with soap and water to prevent infection. Some surgeons do not permit showers until 48 hours after drains are removed. If immediate reconstruction has been performed, showering may be contraindicated until the drain is removed. A dry dressing may be applied to the incision each day for 7 days. The patient should realize that sensation may be decreased in the operative area because the nerves were disrupted during surgery, and she should be informed that gentle care is needed to avoid injury. After the incision has completely healed (usually after 4 to 6 weeks), lotions or creams may be applied to the area to increase skin elasticity. The patient can begin to use deodorant on the affected side, although many women note that they no longer perspire as much as before the surgery.

After ALND, patients are taught arm exercises on the affected side to restore range of motion (see Chart 52-8).

Chart 52-8

PATIENT EDUCATION

Exercise After Breast Surgery

The nurse instructs the patient to perform the following exercises:

1. *Wall hand climbing.* Stand facing the wall with feet apart and toes as close to the wall as possible. With elbows slightly bent, place the palms of the hand on the wall at shoulder level. By flexing the fingers, work the hands up the wall until arms are fully extended. Then reverse the process, working the hands down to the starting point.

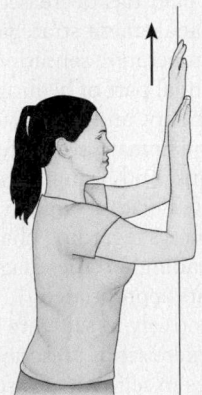

2. *Rope turning.* Tie a light rope to a doorknob. Stand facing the door. Take the free end of the rope in the hand on the side of surgery. Place the other hand on the hip. With the rope-holding arm extended and held away from the body (nearly parallel with the floor), turn the rope, making as wide swings as possible. Begin slowly at first; speed up later.

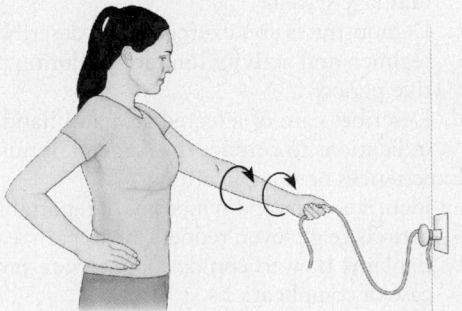

3. *Rod or broomstick lifting.* Grasp a rod with both hands, held about 2 feet apart. Keeping the arms straight, raise the rod over the head. Bend elbows to lower the rod behind the head. Reverse maneuver, raising the rod above the head, then return to the starting position.

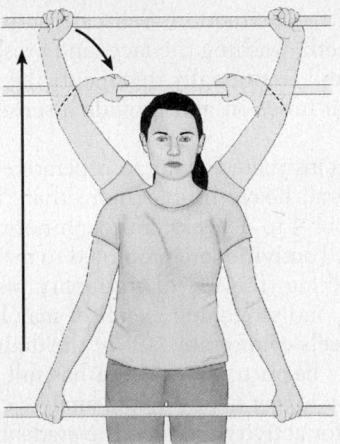

4. *Pulley tugging.* Toss a light rope over a shower curtain rod or doorway curtain rod. Stand as close to the rope as possible. Grasp an end in each hand. Extend the arms straight and away from the body. Pull the left arm up by tugging down with the right arm, then the right arm up and the left down in a see-sawing motion.

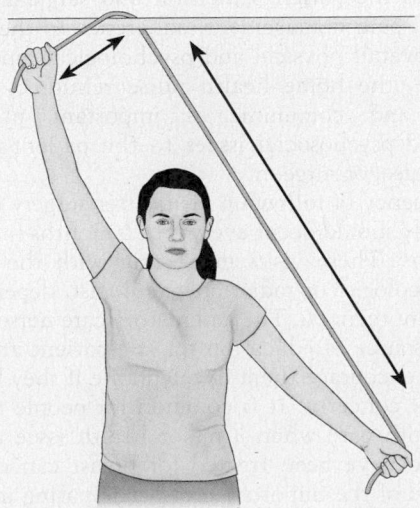

After SLNB, patients may also benefit from these exercises, although they are less likely to have decreased range of motion than those who have undergone ALND. Range-of-motion exercises are initiated on the second postoperative day; however, instruction often occurs on the first postoperative day. The goals of the exercise regimen are to increase circulation and muscle strength, prevent joint stiffness and contractures, and restore full range of motion. The patient is instructed to perform range-of-motion exercises at home three times a day for 20 minutes at a time until full range of motion is restored (generally 4 to 6 weeks). Most patients find that after the drain is removed, range of motion returns quickly if they have adhered to their exercise program.

If the patient is having any discomfort, taking an analgesic agent 30 minutes before beginning the exercises can be helpful. Taking a warm shower before exercising can also loosen stiff muscles and provide comfort. When exercising, the patient is encouraged to use the muscles in both arms and to maintain proper posture. Specific exercises may need to be prescribed and introduced gradually if the patient has had skin grafts; has a tense, tight surgical incision; or has had immediate reconstruction. Self-care activities, such as brushing the teeth, washing the face, and brushing the hair, are physically and emotionally therapeutic because they aid in restoring arm function and provide a sense of normalcy for the patient.

The patient is instructed about postoperative activity limitation. In general, heavy lifting (more than 5 to 10 lb) is avoided for about 4 to 6 weeks, although normal household and work-related activities are promoted to maintain muscle tone. Brisk walking, the use of stationary bikes and stepping machines, and stretching exercises may begin as soon as the patient feels comfortable. Once the drain is removed, the patient may begin to drive if she has full arm range of motion and is no longer taking opioid analgesic agents. General guidelines for activity focus on the gradual introduction of previous activities (e.g., bowling, weight training) once fully healed.

Continuing and Transitional Care. Patients who have difficulty managing their postoperative care at home may benefit from a referral for home health, transitional, or community-based care. The nurse making a home visit assesses the patient's incision and surgical drain(s), adequacy of pain management, adherence to the exercise plan, and overall physical and psychological functioning. In addition, the home health nurse reinforces previous education and communicates important physiologic findings and psychosocial issues to the patient's primary provider, nurse, or surgeon.

The frequency of follow-up visits after surgery may vary but generally should occur every 3 to 6 months for the first several years. These visits may occur with the surgeon, medical oncologist or radiation oncologist, depending on the treatment regimen. The ambulatory care nurse can also be a great source of education for the patient and family and should encourage them to telephone if they have any questions or concerns. It is common for people to ignore routine health care when a major health issue arises, so women who have been treated for breast cancer should be reminded of the importance of participating in routine health screening.

Evaluation

Expected preoperative patient outcomes may include:
1. Exhibits knowledge about diagnosis and surgical treatment options
   a. Asks relevant questions about diagnosis and available surgical treatments
   b. States rationale for surgery
   c. Describes advantages and disadvantages of treatment options
2. Verbalizes willingness to deal with anxiety and fears related to the diagnosis and the effects of surgery on self-image and sexual functioning
3. Demonstrates ability to cope with diagnosis and treatment
   a. Verbalizes feelings appropriately and recognizes normalcy of mood lability
   b. Proceeds with treatment in timely fashion
   c. Discusses impact of diagnosis and treatment on family and work
4. Makes decisions regarding treatment options in timely fashion

Expected postoperative patient outcomes may include:
1. Reports that pain has decreased and states pain and discomfort management strategies are effective
2. Identifies postoperative sensations and recognizes that they are a normal part of healing
3. Exhibits clean, dry, and intact surgical incisions without signs of inflammation or infection
4. Lists the signs and symptoms of infection to be reported to the nurse or surgeon
5. Verbalizes feelings regarding change in body image
6. Discusses meaning of the diagnosis, surgical treatment, and fears appropriately
7. Participates actively in self-care measures
   a. Performs exercises as prescribed
   b. Participates in self-care measures as prescribed
8. Discusses issues of sexuality and resumption of sexual relations
9. Demonstrates knowledge of post discharge recommendations and restrictions
   a. Describes follow-up care and activities
   b. Demonstrates appropriate care of incisions and drainage system
   c. Demonstrates arm exercises, and describes exercise regimen and activity limitations during postoperative period
   d. Describes care of affected arm and hand, and lists indications to contact the surgeon or nurse
10. Experiences no complications
    a. Identifies signs and symptoms of reportable complications (e.g., fever, redness, heat, pain, edema)
    b. Explains how to contact appropriate providers in case of complications

Radiation Therapy

Radiation therapy is used to decrease the chance of a local recurrence in the breast by eradicating residual microscopic cancer cells. Breast conservation treatment followed by radiation therapy for stages I and II breast cancer results in

| **Chart 52-9** | Contraindications to Breast Conservation Treatment |

Note: Breast-conservation treatment includes both surgery and radiation.

Absolute Contraindications

- First or second trimester of pregnancy
- Prior radiation to the breast or chest region
- Patient preference for mastectomy

Relative Contraindications

- History of collagen vascular disease
- Large tumor-to-breast ratio
- High probability of recurrence
- High probability of problems with radiation therapy
- Two or more tumors in different quadrants of the breast

Adapted from Rivere, A., & Klimberg, V. (2018). Lymphedema in the postmastectomy patient. Pathophysiology, prevention, and management. In K. Bland, E. Copeland, V. Klimberg, et al. (Eds.). *The breast: comprehensive management of benign and malignant diseases* (5th ed.). Philadelphia, PA: Elsevier.

a survival rate equal to that of a mastectomy (Freedman, 2018a). If radiation therapy, which is part of breast conservation treatment (see Chart 52-9), is contraindicated, a mastectomy would then be indicated.

External-beam radiation (the most common type) typically begins about 6 weeks after breast conservation to allow the surgical site to heal. If systemic chemotherapy is indicated, radiation therapy usually begins after its completion. Before radiation begins, the patient undergoes a planning session called a *simulation*, in which the anatomic areas to be treated are mapped out and then identified with small permanent ink markings (National Cancer Institute, 2018b). External-beam radiation, which delivers high-energy photons from a linear accelerator, is given to the entire breast region (whole breast radiation). Each treatment lasts only a few minutes and is generally given 5 days a week for 5 to 6 weeks. After completion of radiation to the entire breast, many patients receive a "boost"—a dose of radiation to the lumpectomy site where the cancer cells were located. The boost consists of the same dose of radiation but is less penetrating and directed to a smaller area. The treatments are not painful.

Because most breast cancer recurrences appear at or near the lumpectomy site, the need for whole breast radiation has been questioned. Partial breast radiation (radiation to the lumpectomy site alone) continues be evaluated at some institutions in patients who have been carefully selected. One approach is **brachytherapy**, in which radiation is delivered by an internal device that is placed inside or adjacent to the tumor within the breast. This technique can lead to an improved quality of life because the treatments are given over 4 to 5 days instead of 5 to 6 weeks. After mastectomy, postoperative radiation may be indicated for women at high risk for cancer recurrence (i.e., chest wall involvement, four or more positive lymph nodes, tumors larger than 5 cm, positive surgical margins).

Side Effects

In general, radiation therapy is well tolerated. Acute side effects consist of mild to moderate erythema, breast edema,

and fatigue. Occasionally, skin breakdown may occur in the inframammary fold or near the axilla toward the end of treatment; breakdown may be managed by application of topical medications between treatments (Freedman, 2018b). Fatigue can be depressing, as can the frequent trips to the radiation oncology unit for treatment. The patient needs to be reassured that the fatigue is normal and not a sign of recurrence. Side effects usually resolve within a few weeks to a few months after treatment is completed. Some long-term effects of radiation therapy include lung disease, dental disease, osteoporosis, and heart and vascular disease (Pedersen & Klemp, 2018).

Nursing Management

Nurses play a significant role in supporting patients throughout their treatment with radiation therapy. During brachytherapy, the radiation source will give off radiation. Patients must be educated about safety measures, including any restrictions to visitors, especially young children and pregnant women (National Cancer Institute, 2018a). See Chapter 12 for discussion of radiation therapy.

Self-care instructions for patients receiving radiation are provided to assist in the maintenance of skin integrity during the treatments and for several weeks after completion. They pertain only to the area being treated and not to the rest of the body. Instructions from the National Cancer Institute (2018c) include:

- Use mild soap with minimal rubbing.
- Avoid perfumed soaps or deodorants.
- Use hydrophilic lotions for dryness.
- Use a nondrying, antipruritic soap if pruritus occurs.
- Avoid tight clothes, underwire bras, excessive temperatures, and ultraviolet light.

Follow-up care includes educating the patient to minimize sun exposure to the treated area (i.e., using sunblock with sun protection factor [SPF] of 15 or higher) and reassuring the patient that short-term minor twinges and pain in the breast are normal after radiation treatment.

Systemic Treatments

Chemotherapy

Adjuvant chemotherapy involves the use of anticancer agents in addition to other treatments (i.e., surgery, radiation) to delay or prevent a recurrence of breast cancer. It is generally recommended for patients who have positive lymph nodes or who have invasive tumors greater than 1 cm in size, regardless of nodal status. It is considered in patients with smaller tumors; involvement of lymph nodes affects the decision-making process (NCCN, 2019). Table 52-6 outlines general indications for adjuvant chemotherapy. A survival benefit has been shown in both women who are pre- and postmenopausal and who have received chemotherapy, although data are limited in women older than 70 years. Chemotherapy is most commonly initiated after breast surgery and before radiation. Preoperative therapy may be considered in order to shrink tumor size to support breast conservation (Telli, 2018). Patients with triple-negative breast cancer (cancer that tests negative for estrogen receptors, progesterone receptors, and excess HER2 protein) who delay initiation of chemotherapy beyond 30 days postsurgery have an increased risk

TABLE 52-6	General Indications for Adjuvant Chemotherapy for Breast Cancer
Nodal Status, Tumor Size	**Adjuvant Chemotherapy**
Node negative, ≤0.5 cm	None
Node negative 0.6–1 cm (well differentiated)	None
Node negative, 0.6–1 cm (moderately or poorly differentiated and unfavorable features)	Consider chemotherapy
Node negative, >1 cm	Chemotherapy
Node positive, any tumor size	Chemotherapy

- In addition to chemotherapy, patients with HER-2/neu-positive tumors will receive trastuzumab if they have node-positive disease; or node-negative disease with a tumor >1 cm. Trastuzumab is a monoclonal antibody that targets and inactivates the HER-2/neu protein. HER-2/neu is overproduced in 25–30% of tumors and is associated with rapid growth and poor prognosis.
- Following chemotherapy, patients with hormone receptor positive (ER+/PR+) tumors will receive hormonal therapy (tamoxifen or aromatase inhibitor) if they have either node-positive disease; node-negative disease with a tumor >1 cm; or node-negative disease with a tumor 0.6–1 cm and moderately or poorly differentiated and unfavorable features.

Note: These are only general guidelines. Recommendations may vary depending on factors such as prognostic variables, patient age, and comorbid conditions.
Adapted from National Comprehensive Cancer Network (NCCN). (2019). Clinical practice guidelines: Breast. Retrieved on 9/9/2019 at: www.nccn.org/professionals/physician_gls/pdf/breast_risk.pdf

of recurrence (DePolo, 2018). Nurses encourage and assist in facilitating timely treatment to optimize outcomes.

Chemotherapy regimens for breast cancer combine several agents (polychemotherapy), generally given over a period of 3 to 6 months. Decisions regarding the optimal regimen are based on a variety of factors, including tumor characteristics (i.e., tumor size, lymph node status, hormone receptor status, HER-2/neu status) and the patient's age, physical status, and existing comorbid conditions. A regimen that includes cyclophosphamide, methotrexate, and fluorouracil (collectively referred to as CMF) has been the most widely used adjuvant therapy. It is usually well tolerated and may be considered for patients with a low risk of recurrence. CMF also may be considered for use in patients who have a high risk of cardiac toxicity or who have other limiting comorbidities. Anthracycline-based regimens (e.g., doxorubicin, epirubicin) have shown longer survival in patients. However, the benefit relative to CMF is modest and is accompanied by increased toxicity, especially to the bone marrow (Santa-Maria & Gradishar, 2018). Selection of patients most likely to benefit from anthracycline therapy would allow better use of current cytotoxic agents and reduce the risk of patients receiving toxicity with little or no effect. Cyclophosphamide, doxorubicin (trade name Adriamycin), and fluorouracil (CAF) and doxorubicin and cyclophosphamide (AC) are examples of the trade names of combination regimens often given to patients who are at high risk. Identifying biomarkers that can accurately predict benefit from specific chemotherapeutic agents will also highlight key resistance/susceptibility pathways that can then be exploited clinically to further increase

efficacy and ensure timely treatment (Korourian, Kumarapeli, & Klimberg, 2018).

The taxanes (paclitaxel, docetaxel) are generally incorporated into treatment regimens for patients with larger, node-negative cancers and for those with positive axillary lymph nodes. The addition of four cycles of paclitaxel after a standard course of AC has been found to increase the disease-free period and improve overall survival in patients with operable breast cancer and positive lymph nodes (NCCN, 2019).

Much attention has been focused on **dose-dense chemotherapy**, which is the administration of chemotherapeutic agents at standard doses with shorter time intervals between each cycle of treatment. Cells are more sensitive to chemotherapy during rapid growth phase, so more frequent doses kill more cancer cells than increased doses (Santa-Maria & Gradishar, 2018). Dose density is standard of care with some breast cancers, but is still controversial with estrogen-receptor positive disease.

Side Effects

Many of the side effects of adjuvant chemotherapy can be managed well, allowing patients to maintain their daily routines and work schedules. In large part, this is the result of the meticulous educational and psychological preparation provided to patients and their families by oncology nurses, oncologists, social workers, and other members of the health care team. In addition, strides have been made in the effectiveness of antiemetic agents used to alleviate nausea and vomiting and the use of hematopoietic growth factors to treat neutropenia and anemia.

Common physical side effects of chemotherapy for breast cancer may include nausea, vomiting, bone marrow suppression, taste changes, alopecia (hair loss), mucositis, neuropathy, skin changes, and fatigue. A weight gain of more than 10 lb occurs in about half of all patients; the cause is unknown. Women who are premenopausal may also experience temporary or permanent amenorrhea.

Specific side effects vary with the type of chemotherapeutic agent used. In general, CMF and the taxanes are better tolerated than the anthracyclines. However, the taxanes can cause peripheral neuropathy, arthralgias, and myalgias, particularly at high doses. During taxane administration, hypersensitivity reactions may occur; therefore, the patient must be premedicated with corticosteroids and antihistamines. Alopecia is also common. The side effects of the anthracyclines may be severe and include cardiotoxicity in addition to nausea and vomiting, bone marrow suppression, and alopecia. Their vesicant properties can lead to tissue necrosis if infiltration of the medication infusion occurs.

Nursing Management

Nurses play an important role in helping patients manage the physical and psychosocial sequelae of chemotherapy. (Chapter 12 provides an in-depth discussion of side effect management.) Educating the patient about the use of antiemetic agents and reviewing the optimal dosage schedule can help minimize nausea and vomiting. The different classes of antiemetic agents include serotonin (5-HT$_3$) receptor antagonists (palonosetron, granisetron, ondansetron); neurokinin-1 receptor antagonists (aprepitant); dopamine receptor antagonists (prochlorperazine, metoclopramide); benzodiazepines (lorazepam); and corticosteroids (dexamethasone). Measures to ease the symptoms of mucositis may include rinsing with normal saline or sodium bicarbonate solution, avoiding hot and spicy foods, and using a soft toothbrush.

Some patients may require hematopoietic growth factors to minimize the effects of chemotherapy-induced neutropenia and anemia. Granulocyte colony-stimulating factors boost the white blood cell count, helping to reduce the incidence of neutropenic fever and infection. The short-acting form, filgrastim, is injected subcutaneously or IV for 7 to 10 days after chemotherapy administration. The long-acting form, pegfilgrastim, is injected once, no earlier than 24 hours after chemotherapy (Vallerand & Sanoski, 2018). Erythropoietin growth factor increases the production of red blood cells, thus decreasing the symptoms of anemia. The short-acting form, epoetin alfa is usually given weekly. The long-acting form, darbepoetin alfa, can be given every 2 to 3 weeks. The nurse instructs the patient and family on proper injection technique of hematopoietic growth factors and about symptoms that require follow-up with a primary provider (see Chart 52-10).

To prevent some of the emotional trauma associated with alopecia, it often helps to have a patient obtain a wig before hair loss begins to occur. The nurse may provide a list of wig suppliers in the patient's geographic region. Familiarity with creative ways to use scarves and turbans may also help minimize the patient's distress. The patient needs reassurance that new hair will grow back when treatment is completed, although the color and texture may be different. The ACS offers the Look Good Feel Better program, which provides useful tips for applying cosmetics during the period a patient is receiving chemotherapy (see Resources section).

Chemotherapy may negatively affect the patient's self-esteem, sexuality, and sense of well-being. This, combined with the stress of a potentially life-threatening disease, can be acute. Providing support and promoting open communication are important aspects of nursing care. Referring the patient to the dietitian, social worker, psychiatrist, or spiritual advisor can provide additional support. Numerous community support and advocacy groups are available for patients and their families. Complementary therapies, such as guided imagery, meditation, and relaxation exercises, can also be used in conjunction with conventional treatments.

Hormonal Therapy

The use of **adjuvant hormonal therapy**, with or without the addition of chemotherapy, is considered in women who have hormone receptor–positive tumors. Its use can be determined by the results of an estrogen and progesterone receptor assay (a test to determine whether the breast tumor is nourished by hormones). About two thirds of breast cancers depend on estrogen for growth and express a nuclear receptor that binds to the estrogen; thus, they are estrogen receptor positive (ER+). Similarly, tumors that express the progesterone receptor are progesterone receptor positive (PR+). Hormonal therapy involves the use of synthetic hormones or other medications that compete with estrogen by binding to the receptor sites (SERMs), or the use of **aromatase inhibitors**, which block estrogen production by the adrenal glands. In general, tumors that are ER+/PR+ have the greatest likelihood of responding to hormonal therapy and have a more favorable prognosis than those that are ER−/PR−. Women who are pre- and perimenopausal are more likely to have non–hormone-dependent lesions, whereas women who are postmenopausal are more likely to have hormone-dependent lesions.

Traditionally, the SERM tamoxifen has been the main hormonal agent used in treatment of pre- and postmenopausal breast cancer and remains the mainstay in women who are premenopausal. As an SERM, tamoxifen has estrogen antagonistic (estrogen-blocking) and agonistic (estrogen-like) effects on certain tissues. Its antagonistic effects in the breast prevent estrogen from binding to the receptor sites, thus preventing tumor growth. Tamoxifen has positive agonistic effects on blood lipid profiles and bone mineral density in women who are postmenopausal. It also has agonistic effects on endometrial tissue and blood coagulation processes, leading to an increased incidence of endometrial cancer and thromboembolic events (e.g., deep vein thrombosis [DVT], superficial phlebitis, pulmonary embolism). Nevertheless, the benefits in most women with breast cancer outweigh the risks.

The aromatase inhibitors anastrozole, letrozole, and exemestane are important components in the hormonal management of women who are postmenopausal. Most of the circulating estrogens in women who are postmenopausal are derived from the conversion of the adrenal androgen androstenedione to estrone and the conversion of testosterone to estradiol. Aromatase inhibitors work by blocking the enzyme aromatase from performing the conversion, thereby decreasing the level of circulating estrogen in peripheral tissues. Clinical trials have demonstrated that the aromatase inhibitors are superior to tamoxifen in terms of overall response rate and clinical benefit and that inhibitors appear to be effective and feasible compared with tamoxifen as first-line hormonal therapy in women who are postmenopausal with advanced breast cancer (Santa-Maria & Gradishar, 2018). These data ensure that aromatase inhibitors will play an increasingly central role in the long-term management of breast cancer. Trials are ongoing to determine the optimal treatment regimen and the timing of the treatment; possible eligibility for a clinical trial should be discussed between the patient and the care team. Table 52-7 outlines the adverse effects of adjuvant hormonal therapy. Chart 52-11 outlines appropriate patient education to manage the adverse effects.

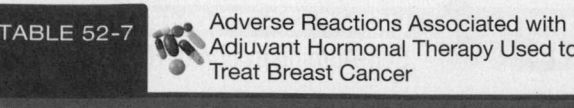

TABLE 52-7 Adverse Reactions Associated with Adjuvant Hormonal Therapy Used to Treat Breast Cancer

Therapeutic Agent	Adverse Reactions/Side Effects
Selective Estrogen Receptor Modulator	
tamoxifen	Hot flashes, vaginal dryness/discharge/bleeding, irregular menses, nausea, mood disturbances, rashes; increased risk for endometrial cancer; increased risk for thromboembolic events (deep vein thrombosis, pulmonary embolism, superficial phlebitis)
Aromatase Inhibitors	
anastrozole letrozole exemestane	Musculoskeletal symptoms (arthritis, arthralgia, myalgia), increased risk of osteoporosis/fractures, nausea/vomiting, hot flashes, fatigue, mood disturbances, rashes

Adapted from Vallerand, A., & Sanoski, C. (2018). *Davis's drug guide for nurses* (15th ed.). Philadelphia, PA: Davis.

Targeted Therapy

An exciting area of research in the systemic treatment of breast cancer involves the use of targeted therapies. Trastuzumab is a monoclonal antibody that binds specifically to the **HER-2/neu** protein. This protein, which regulates cell growth, is present in small amounts on the surface of normal breast cells and in most breast cancers. Approximately 20% of tumors overexpress (overproduce) the HER-2/neu protein and are associated with rapid growth and poor prognosis (Mayo Clinic, 2020). Trastuzumab targets and inactivates the HER-2/neu protein, thus slowing tumor growth.

Unlike chemotherapy, trastuzumab spares the normal cells and has limited adverse reactions, which may include fever, chills, nausea, vomiting, diarrhea, and headache. However, when trastuzumab is given to patients who have previously been treated with an anthracycline, the risk of cardiac toxicity is increased. The medication has been shown to improve

---

Chart 52-11 **PATIENT EDUCATION**
Managing Side Effects of Adjuvant Hormonal Therapy in Breast Cancer

The nurse instructs the patient in strategies to manage the following side effects:

Hot Flashes

- Wear breathable, layered clothing.
- Avoid caffeine and spicy foods.
- Perform breathing exercises (paced respirations).
- Consider medications (vitamin E, antidepressants) or acupuncture.

Vaginal Dryness

- Use vaginal moisturizers for everyday dryness (e.g., Replens, vitamin E suppository).
- Apply vaginal lubrication during penile–vaginal intercourse (e.g., Astroglide, K-Y Jelly).

Nausea and Vomiting

- Consume a bland diet.
- Try to take medication in the evening.

Musculoskeletal Symptoms

- Take nonsteroidal analgesic agents as recommended.
- Take warm baths.

Risk of Endometrial Cancer

- Report any irregular bleeding to a gynecologist for evaluation.

Risk for Thromboembolic Events

- Report any redness, swelling, or tenderness in the lower extremities, or any unexplained shortness of breath.

Risk for Osteoporosis or Fractures

- Undergo a baseline bone density scan.
- Perform regular weight-bearing exercises.
- Take calcium supplements with vitamin D.
- Take bisphosphonates (e.g., alendronate) or calcitonin as prescribed.

survival rates in women with HER-2/neu–positive metastatic breast cancer and is now regarded as standard therapy. Recently, three other HER2-targeting agents have entered routine clinical practice. These include a small molecule receptor tyrosine kinase inhibitor (lapatinib) and two novel HER2-targeting monoclonal antibodies (pertuzumab and ado-trastuzumab emtansine). Assessing the benefits and risks of these medications is complex, and medical oncologists often use a variety of aids in their decision making (Sledge, 2018).

Treatment of Recurrent and Metastatic Breast Cancer

Despite the advances made in the treatment of breast cancer, it may recur locally (on the chest wall or in the conserved breast), regionally (in the remaining lymph nodes), or systemically (in distant organs). In metastatic disease, the bone, usually the hips, spine, ribs, skull, or pelvis, is the most common site of spread. Other sites of metastasis include the lungs, liver, pleura, and brain.

The overall prognosis and optimal treatment are determined by a variety of factors such as the site and extent of recurrence, the time to recurrence from the original diagnosis, history of prior treatments, the patient's performance status, and any existing comorbid conditions. Patients with bone metastases generally have a longer overall survival compared with metastases in visceral organs.

Local recurrence in the absence of systemic disease is treated aggressively with surgery, radiation, and hormonal therapy. Chemotherapy may also be used for tumors that are not hormonally sensitive. Identifying a local recurrence may be an indicator of occult systemic disease (Wapnir, Tsai, & Aebi, 2018).

Metastatic breast cancer involves control of the disease rather than cure, individualized to location of the metastasis (NCCN, 2019). Treatment includes hormonal therapy, chemotherapy, and targeted therapy. Surgery or radiation may be indicated in select situations. Women who are premenopausal and who have hormonally dependent tumors may eliminate the production of estrogen by the ovaries through oophorectomy (removal of the ovaries) or suppression of estrogen production by medications such as leuprolide or goserelin.

Patients with advanced breast cancer are monitored closely for signs of disease progression. Baseline studies are obtained at the time of recurrence. These may include complete blood count; comprehensive metabolic panel; tumor markers (i.e., carcinoembryonic antigen, cancer antigen 15-3); bone scan; CT of the chest, abdomen, and pelvis; and MRI of symptomatic areas. Additional x-rays may be performed to evaluate areas of pain or abnormal areas seen on bone scan (e.g., long bones, pelvis). These studies are repeated at regular intervals to assess for effectiveness of treatment and to monitor progression of disease.

Nursing Management

Nurses play an important role in not only educating patients and managing their symptoms but also in providing emotional support. Many patients find that recurrence of the disease is more distressing than the initial cancer diagnosis. They not only have to contend with another round of treatments but

are also faced with a greater uncertainty about their future and long-term survival. The nurse can help the patient identify coping strategies and set priorities to optimize quality of life. Family members and significant others should be included in the treatment plan and follow-up care. Referrals to support groups, as well as psychiatry or psychiatric clinical nurse specialist, social work, and complementary medicine programs (e.g., guided imagery, meditation, yoga), should be made as indicated.

Nurses can also be instrumental in providing palliative care, if indicated. The highest priorities include alleviating pain and providing comfort measures. A frank discussion with the patient and family regarding their preferences for end-of-life care should occur before the need arises to ensure a smooth transition without disruption of care. Referrals to hospice and home health care should be initiated as necessary (see Chapters 12 and 13).

Reconstructive Procedures After Mastectomy

Breast reconstruction can provide a significant psychological benefit for women who are already struggling with the emotional distress of losing a breast. A consultation with a plastic surgeon can help the patient understand procedures for which she is a candidate and the pros and cons of each. Factors to consider include body size and shape, comorbid conditions (e.g., hypertension, diabetes, obesity), personal habits such as smoking, and patient preference. The patient must be informed that although breast reconstruction can provide a good cosmetic result, it will never precisely duplicate the natural breast. Realistic preparation can help the patient avoid unrealistic expectations. Once reconstruction is complete, the opposite breast may require augmentation, reduction, or mastopexy to achieve symmetry on both sides. The patient must also be informed that breast reconstruction will not affect the risk of cancer recurrence. Reconstruction is considered an integral component in the surgical treatment of breast cancer and is usually covered by insurance companies.

Many women elect immediate reconstruction at the time of the mastectomy operation. This can be beneficial in that it saves the woman from undergoing general anesthesia a second time and saves the cost and stress of future hospitalizations. However, it does increase the length of the surgical procedure. Delayed reconstruction is preferable in women who are having a difficult time deciding on the type of reconstruction that they desire. It may also be preferable in patients with advanced disease such as inflammatory breast cancer, where the breast cancer treatments should begin without delay; delayed reconstruction may also be beneficial if radiation is planned, as radiation therapy is technically less complicated on an unreconstructed chest wall (Fayanju, Garvey, Karuturi, et al., 2018). Any delays in healing after immediate reconstruction may interfere with the initiation of treatment.

Tissue Expander Followed by Permanent Implant

Breast reconstruction using a tissue expander followed by a permanent implant is the simplest and most common method

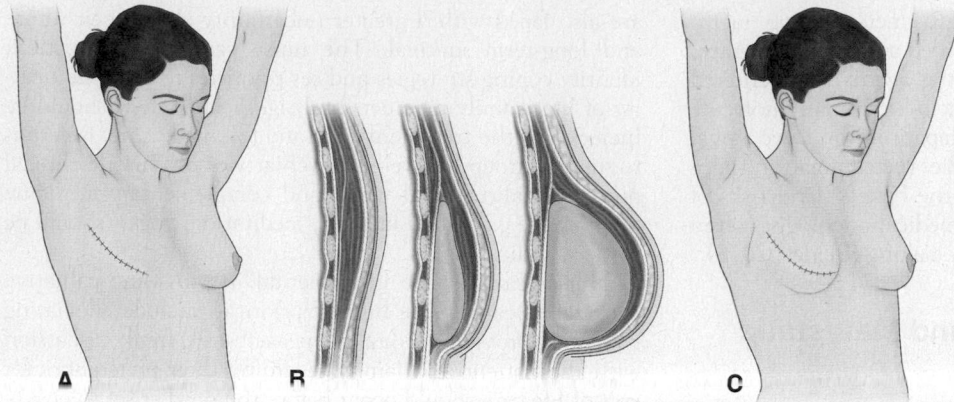

Figure 52-6 • Breast reconstruction with tissue expander. **A.** Mastectomy incision line prior to tissue expansion. **B.** The expander is placed under the pectoralis muscle and is gradually filled with saline solution through a port to stretch the skin enough to accept a permanent implant. **C.** The breast mound is restored. Although permanent, scars will fade with time. The nipple and areola are reconstructed later. Adapted from American Society of Plastic Surgeons.

in use (see Fig. 52-6). To accommodate an implant, the skin remaining after a mastectomy and the underlying muscle must gradually be stretched by a process called *tissue expansion.* The surgeon places a tissue expander (a balloonlike device) through the mastectomy incision underneath the pectoralis muscle. A small amount of saline is injected through a metal port intraoperatively to partially inflate the expander. Then, for about 6 to 8 weeks, at weekly intervals, the patient receives additional saline injections through the port until the expander is fully inflated. It remains fully expanded for about 6 weeks to allow the skin to loosen. The expander is then exchanged for a permanent implant. This is usually performed as an outpatient surgical procedure.

Advantages of the expansion procedure are a shorter operating time and a shorter recuperation period than for autologous reconstruction (see the Tissue Transfer Procedures section). A disadvantage is a tendency for the implant to feel firm and round, with little natural ptosis (sag). Women with a small to medium opposite breast with little ptosis are good candidates for this procedure. Women who have had radiation or who have connective tissue disease are not good candidates because of the decreased elasticity of the skin.

> ◣ **Quality and Safety Nursing Alert**
>
> *The patient must be cautioned not to have an MRI while the tissue expander is in place because the port contains metal. This is not an issue once the permanent implant is in place because it does not contain any metal.*

The patient should be informed that for the rest of her life she should not engage in any exercises that will develop the pectoralis muscle, because this can result in distortion of the reconstructed breast.

Tissue Transfer Procedures

Autologous reconstruction is the use of the patient's own tissue to create a breast mound. A flap of skin, fat, and muscle with its attached blood supply is rotated to the mastectomy site to create a mound that simulates the breast. Donor sites may include the **transverse rectus abdominal myocutaneous (TRAM) flap** (abdominal muscle) (see Fig. 52-7), gluteal flap (buttock muscle), or the latissimus dorsi flap (back muscle) (see Fig. 52-8). The results more closely resemble a real breast

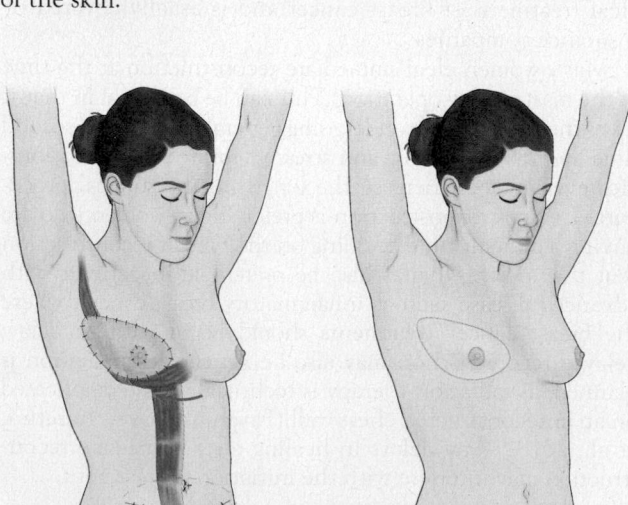

Figure 52-7 • Breast reconstruction: transverse rectus abdominal myocutaneous flap. **A.** A breast mound is created by tunneling abdominal skin, fat, and muscle to the mastectomy site. **B.** Final location of scars. Adapted from American Society of Plastic Surgeons.

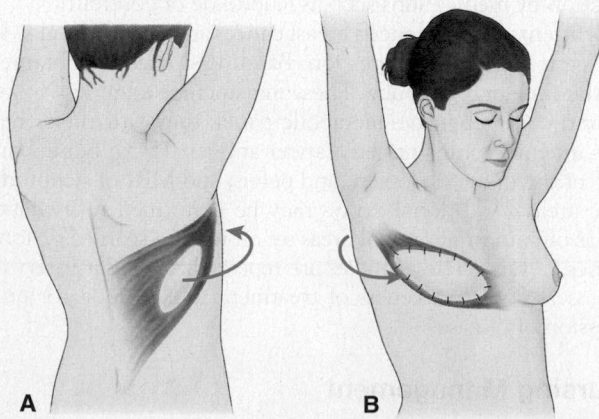

Figure 52-8 • Breast reconstruction: latissimus dorsi flap. **A.** The latissimus muscle with an ellipse of skin is rotated from the back to the mastectomy site. **B.** Because the flap is usually not bulky enough to provide an adequate breast mound, an implant is often also required. Adapted from American Society of Plastic Surgeons.

because the skin and fat from the donor sites are similar in consistency to a natural breast. These procedures avoid the use of synthetic material. However, they involve longer recuperation than a tissue expander procedure. The risk of potential complications (e.g., infection, bleeding, flap necrosis) is also greater. Therefore, patients must be in relatively good health, and those with medical conditions (e.g., atherosclerosis, pulmonary disease, heart failure) that affect circulation or compromise oxygen delivery are not good candidates. Other candidates who are poor risks include those with poorly controlled diabetes or morbid obesity and those who smoke.

The TRAM flap is the most commonly performed tissue transfer procedure. A free TRAM procedure may also be performed; in this case, the skin, fat, muscle, and blood supply are completely detached from the body and then transplanted to the mastectomy site using microvascular surgery (the use of a microscope to reconnect the vessels). Postoperatively, patients who have undergone TRAM procedures often face a lengthy recovery (often 6 to 8 weeks) and have incisions both at the mastectomy site and at the donor site in the abdomen. Other free flap procedures include deep inferior epigastric perforator (DIEP) flap and superficial inferior epigastric artery (SIEA) flap depending on whether the superior gluteal artery perforator or the inferior one is utilized. Free flaps involve microsurgery for blood vessel transfer.

Deep breathing and leg exercises are essential because the patient is more limited in her activity and is at greater risk for respiratory complications and DVT. Measures to help the patient reduce tension on the abdominal incision during the first postoperative week include elevating the head of the bed 45 degrees and flexing the patient's knees.

Once the patient is able to ambulate, she can protect the surgical incision by splinting it and will gradually achieve a more upright position. The patient is instructed to avoid high-impact activities and lifting (more than 5 to 10 lb for 6 to 8 weeks after surgery) to prevent stress on the incision.

Nipple–Areola Reconstruction

After the breast mound has been created and the site has healed, some women choose to have nipple–areola reconstruction. This is a minor surgical procedure carried out either in the physician's office or at an outpatient surgical facility. The most common method of creating a nipple is with the use of local flaps (skin and fat from the center of the new breast mound), which are wrapped around each other to create a projecting nipple. The areola is created using a skin graft. The most common donor site is the upper inner thigh, because this skin has darker pigmentation than the skin on the reconstructed breast. After the nipple graft has healed, micropigmentation (tattooing) can be performed to achieve a more natural color. The surgeon can usually match the reconstructed nipple–areola complex with that of the contralateral breast for an acceptable cosmetic result.

Prosthetics

Not all patients desire or are candidates for reconstructive surgery. A breast prosthesis—an external form that simulates the breast—is another option. Prostheses are available in different shapes, sizes, colors, and materials, although they are most often made of silicone. They can be placed inside a pocket in a bra or can adhere directly to the chest wall. The nurse can provide the patient with the names of shops where she can be fitted for a prosthesis, or the patient can call the Reach to Recovery program of the ACS for appropriate referrals. The patient should be encouraged to find a shop with a comfortable, supportive atmosphere that employs a certified prosthetics consultant. In general, medical supply shops are not recommended because often they do not have the appropriate resources to ensure the proper fitting of a prosthesis.

Prior to discharge from the hospital, the nurse usually provides the patient with a temporary, lightweight, cotton-filled form that can be worn until the surgical incision is well healed (4 to 6 weeks). After that, the patient can be fitted for a prosthesis. Insurance companies generally cover the cost of the prosthesis and the special bras that hold it in place. A breast prosthesis can provide a psychological benefit and assist the woman in resuming proper posture because it helps balance the weight of the remaining breast.

Special Issues in Breast Cancer Management

Implications of Genetic Testing

The rapid advancement in genetics not only has brought new knowledge about inherited breast cancer, but it has also raised potential ethical and psychosocial issues. Although the actual testing for the *BRCA1* and *BRCA2* and several other genes that increase risk involves a simple blood or saliva test, ethical and psychosocial issues must first be addressed. Before undergoing genetic testing, a person should meet either with a clinician who has expertise in this area or with a certified genetic counselor to discuss risk factors as well as the benefits, sequelae, and limitations of testing.

How people react when they receive their actual test results is not always easy to predict. A negative test in a person who comes from a family with a known mutation may lead to enormous relief. However, a negative test in a family with no known mutation may be a source of undue reassurance; the possibility of existing genes that cannot yet be detected remains. A negative test may also lead to feelings of guilt in a person whose family members did not receive favorable test results; this is known as survivor's guilt. A positive test could act as a motivator in a person to pursue appropriate screening or treatment, or it could cause tremendous anxiety, depression, and worry.

In addition, test results may be ambiguous, leading to feelings of confusion and uncertainty. People must be informed that not all gene carriers develop breast cancer (incomplete penetrance) and that not all noncarriers are protected or immune.

People must be well informed of all issues and potential implications prior to undergoing genetic testing (see Chapter 6). Nurses play a role in educating and counseling patients and their family members about the implications of genetic testing. Nurses provide support and clarification and make referrals to appropriate specialists when indicated.

Pregnancy and Breast Cancer

Breast cancer during pregnancy is defined as breast cancer diagnosed during gestation or within 1 year of childbirth.

According to the NCCN, in a California registry study, 1.3 breast cancers are diagnosed in 10,000 live births (NCCN, 2019). Because of increased levels of hormones produced during pregnancy and subsequent lactation, the breast tissue becomes tender and swollen, making it more difficult to detect a mass. If a mass is found during pregnancy, ultrasound is the preferred diagnostic method because it involves no exposure to radiation. If indicated, mammography with appropriate shielding, FNA, and biopsy can be performed. Modified radical mastectomy remains the most common form of surgical treatment. SLNB is typically not offered under 30-week gestation because of the unknown effects of the radioisotope and the blue dye on the fetus (NCCN, 2019). Breast conservation treatment may be considered if the breast cancer is diagnosed during the third trimester. Radiation can then be delayed until after delivery because it is contraindicated during pregnancy. If a woman is close to term, a cesarean section may be performed as soon as maturation of the fetus allows and then treatment is initiated. If aggressive disease is detected early in pregnancy and chemotherapy is advised, termination of the pregnancy may be considered. If a mass is found while a woman is breast-feeding, she is urged to stop to allow the breast to involute (return to its baseline state) before any type of surgery is performed. Endocrine therapy is also contraindicated during pregnancy and should be postponed until the postpartum period.

Fertility issues and the future desire for children are major concerns of young women who are survivors of breast cancer. Most cancer therapies have a substantial morbidity on reproductive function, not only because they increase the risk of early menopause but also because they are associated with a decreased ovarian reserve and a loss of fertility. It is estimated that physiologic age of the ovaries in a survivor of cancer may be 10 years older than the actual chronologic age.

Chemotherapy causes a progressive dose-related depletion of ovarian follicles and granulosa cells that translates into oligomenorrhea and subsequent premature ovarian failure, ultimately leading to what is known as chemotherapy-induced amenorrhea (CIA). Regardless of the beneficial effects that hormonal changes can have as part of the adjuvant endocrine strategy, CIA is an adverse event to consider when selecting the best adjuvant treatment. Patients with cancer need to be informed about their reproductive future and options to preserve fertility before treatment (Petersen, Moravek, Woodruff, et al., 2018). SaveMyFertility, a national nonprofit organization, can also provide updated information on reproduction (see the Resources section).

Quality of Life and Survivorship

With increased early detection and improved treatment modalities, women with breast cancer have become the largest group of cancer survivors. Ninety-nine percent of women diagnosed with early-stage cancer localized to the breast will survive beyond 5 years (Mehra, Berkowitz, & Sanft, 2018). However, the treatment or simply the diagnosis of breast cancer may have long-term effects that negatively affect the patient and her family. The patient should be prepared early on for the potential long-term effects of the disease so that she has realistic expectations and can make informed decisions.

Survivors of breast cancer may experience a variety of issues as a result of their diagnosis and treatment. Estrogen withdrawal from chemotherapy-induced menopause and hormonal treatments can lead to a variety of symptoms, including hot flashes, vaginal dryness, urinary tract infections, weight gain, decreased sex drive, and increased risk of osteoporosis. HT to alleviate symptoms is contraindicated in women with breast cancer. Certain chemotherapeutic agents can cause long-term cardiac effects and neuropathy. In addition, patients may experience impaired cognitive functioning, such as difficulty concentrating (often referred to as "chemo brain"). Studies have shown some correlation between levels of post-chemotherapy cognitive dysfunction and chemotherapy dosing; higher doses increase dysfunction (Shahpar, Mhatre, & Oza, 2018). Rare long-term effects of radiation can include pneumonitis, rib fractures, heart disease, and breast fibrosis or necrosis (Pederson & Klemp, 2018). Long-term sequelae after breast surgery may include lymphedema (mainly after ALND), pain, and sensory disturbances. Once lymphedema develops, it tends to be a chronic problem, so prevention strategies (discussed earlier) are vital. Weight gain and infections are risk factors for lymphedema (Makhoul, Banderudrappagari, & Pennisi, 2018). Nurses need to encourage patients to maintain an active lifestyle and avoid weight gain.

Long-term psychosocial sequelae may include fears of recurrence; mood changes (e.g., worry, sadness, anger, frustration); an increased sense of vulnerability, uncertainty, feelings of loss (e.g., fertility); concerns about body image, self-concept, and sexuality; emotional distress related to role adjustments and family response; and concerns about finances and employment. Depression and anxiety have been documented in 20% to 30% of women with breast cancer. Interventions should be targeted to meet informational needs, manage uncertainty, control symptoms, address cultural differences, and enhance social and emotional support (Makhoul et al., 2018).

 ## Gerontologic Considerations

Breast cancer reconstruction in older women with breast cancer is a feasible option that should be offered to patients. Most women tolerate the procedure well and have good cosmetic outcomes. Patients can be offered both implant-based reconstruction and autologous tissue transfer with minimal complications as long as appropriate preoperative selection criteria are used. The safety of reconstruction, together with increase in perceived quality of life, life expectancy, and healthier lifestyles, makes breast reconstruction after mastectomy desirable at any age (van Ee, Smits, Honkoop, et al., 2019).

A thorough assessment must be performed before any treatment is initiated, and careful monitoring must occur throughout the course of treatment to avoid complications. The physical and psychosocial assessment of the older woman should include general health, currently existing comorbidities, performance status, cognitive status, current medications, available resources, and support systems.

Breast Health of Women with Disability

Disparities in obtaining a mammogram at recommended screening intervals persist for many women, including those with disability. Prevalence of self-reported use of mammography is lower for women with a disability. Thirty-six million women in the United States are disabled (Centers for Disease Control and Prevention [CDC], 2019a). Efforts to reduce disparities in breast cancer screening might be more effective if all segments of the population are targeted. Possible barriers to the use of mammography in women with disability include physical inaccessibility of office space and medical equipment; limited transportation and parking options; and time and assistance constraints associated with undressing, transferring, and positioning for medical examinations. People who are lesbian, gay, bisexual, transgender, and those questioning their gender may also be uncomfortable with the health care system and avoid screening (Kates, Ranji, Beamesderfer, et al., 2018). To promote health and wellness, health agencies, providers, and health care plans must promote cancer prevention and educational programs that are inclusive and responsive to the special needs of women with disability (CDC, 2019b).

An essential role of the nurse is to assist all women, including those with disability, to identify accessible health screening and to advocate for greater accessibility of imaging centers and other health care facilities. Reminding women of the need for recommended clinical breast examinations and mammograms is an important part of nursing care.

RECONSTRUCTIVE BREAST SURGERY

Breast reconstruction surgery, called **mammoplasty**, is an elective procedure that can enhance a woman's self-image and sense of well-being. Women desire reconstruction for a variety of physical and psychological reasons. Therefore, it is important for the health care team to conduct a thorough assessment prior to reconstructive surgery to evaluate the woman's underlying desire, motivation, and expectations. Preparing a woman realistically could help her to avoid potential disappointment. A variety of reconstructive options are available today for women who desire a correction in the size or the shape of the breast, including reduction mammoplasty (breast reduction), augmentation mammoplasty (breast enlargement), and mastopexy (breast lift). Several options are also available to reconstruct the breast after a mastectomy.

Reduction Mammoplasty

Reduction mammoplasty is usually performed on women who have breast hypertrophy (excessively large breasts). The weight of the enlarged breasts can cause discomfort, fatigue, embarrassment, and poor posture.

Reduction mammoplasty is an outpatient procedure that is performed under general anesthesia. Most commonly, an anchor-shaped incision that circles the areola is made, extending downward and following the natural curve of the inframammary fold. Depending on the size of the breast, the nipple may be moved up to a higher position while still attached to the breast tissue, or it may be separated and transplanted to a new location. Drains are placed in the incision and remain for 2 to 5 days.

During the preoperative consultation, the patient should be informed that there is a possibility that sensory changes of the nipple (such as numbness) may occur. These sensations are normal and usually resolve after several months but can sometimes persist. The procedure may also make breastfeeding impossible, although some women have breast-fed successfully. The patient must also be aware that if she gains weight (usually more than 10 lb), her breasts may also enlarge.

After reduction mammoplasty, many women verbalize feelings of extreme satisfaction, possibly because of the relief they experience. The patient is instructed to wear a supportive bra 24 hours a day for 2 weeks to prevent tension on the swollen breast and incision line. Vigorous exercise (e.g., jumping, jogging) should be avoided for about 6 weeks after surgery.

Augmentation Mammoplasty

Augmentation mammoplasty is requested by women who desire larger or fuller breasts. The procedure is performed by placing a breast implant either under the pectoralis muscle (subpectoral) or under the breast tissue (subglandular). The subpectoral approach is preferred because it interferes less with clinical breast examinations and mammograms. The incision line can be placed in the inframammary fold, in the axilla, or around the areola. The procedure is performed as an outpatient procedure under general anesthesia. A drain is not necessary. Postoperative instructions are the same as for reduction mammoplasty.

Saline implants are typically used for augmentation mammoplasty. The FDA has approved the use of silicone gel–filled implants manufactured by three companies. FDA approval for use of these implants applies to women of all ages for breast reconstruction, and women 22 years and older for breast augmentation (FDA, 2019). Women with breast implants should be aware that mammograms may be more difficult to read, so they should seek experienced breast radiologists.

Mastopexy

Mastopexy is performed when the patient is happy with the size of her breasts but wishes to have the shape improved and a lift performed. This is also an outpatient surgical procedure, and postoperative instructions are the same as for reduction mammoplasty.

DISEASES OF THE MALE BREAST

Gynecomastia

Gynecomastia is the most common breast condition in the male. Adolescent boys can be affected because of hormones secreted by the testes. This type of gynecomastia is virtually always benign and resolves spontaneously in 1 to 2 years. Gynecomastia can also occur in older men and usually presents as a firm, tender mass underneath the areola. In these patients, gynecomastia may be diffuse and related to the use of certain medication (e.g., digitalis). It may also be associated with certain conditions, including feminizing testicular tumors, infection in the testes, and liver disease resulting from factors such as alcohol abuse or a parasitic infection.

Patients in their late teens to late 40s presenting with idiopathic (unknown cause) gynecomastia should have a testicular examination and possibly a testicular ultrasound. Treatment of the enlarged breast tissue is based on patient preference and is usually reserved for those men who cannot tolerate the cosmetic appearance of the breast or who have severe pain associated with the condition. Mammography and ultrasound are utilized if there is a concern about malignancy. Observation is acceptable in most cases because gynecomastia may resolve on its own. Surgical removal of the tissue through a small incision around the areola is the best treatment option. Liposuction performed by a plastic surgeon is another possibility, although this does not allow for pathologic examination of the tissue.

Male Breast Cancer

The lifetime risk of breast cancer in men is about 1 in 1000. The number of breast cancer cases in men relative to the population has been fairly stable over the past 30 years. Nearly 2670 new cases of invasive breast cancer were expected to be diagnosed in men in 2019 (ACS, 2019). The ratio of women to men diagnosed with breast cancer worldwide is 122:1 (Jain & Gradishar, 2018). Although breast carcinoma in both genders share certain characteristics, notable differences have emerged. Familial cases in men usually have *BRCA2* rather than *BRCA1* mutations. Klinefelter syndrome, a chromosomal condition reflecting decreased testosterone levels, is the strongest risk factor for developing male breast carcinoma. Presentation is usually a painless lump, but is often late, with more than 40% of individuals having stage III or IV disease. When survival is adjusted for age at diagnosis and stage of disease, outcomes for male and female patients with breast cancer is similar (Jain & Gradishar, 2018).

Early detection is uncommon in male breast cancer because of the rare nature of the disease. Often, neither patient nor provider suspects male breast cancer early in its development. There is no role for screening mammogram in males, but biopsies may be performed to determine hormone receptor status (Jain & Gradishar, 2018). Treatment generally consists of a total mastectomy with either SLNB or ALND. As in women with breast cancer, prognosis depends on the stage of disease at presentation. Involvement of the axillary lymph nodes is the most important prognostic indicator. Male breast cancers are very likely to be ER+, and tamoxifen, although it has several side effects, is a mainstay of treatment.

Because breast cancer is primarily a disease of women, men may feel that a certain stigma is attached to their diagnosis. This may cause poor adherence to treatment plans, especially long-term medication management. Health care professionals must be sensitive to their needs and provide information and support to improve survivorship.

CRITICAL THINKING EXERCISES

1 **ebp** A 34-year-old woman calls the breast clinic where you work in a panic. She explains that her mom was recently diagnosed with breast cancer. She is convinced that she also has cancer, because she woke up this morning with unilateral breast inflammation. After further questioning, you learn that she is breast-feeding her 10-day-old infant. What evidence-based recommendation would you make for genetic testing for this patient?

2 **pcq** A 45-year-old woman arrives to the medical-surgical unit where you work after having a mastectomy this morning. She plans a delayed implant and has a tissue expander in place. How do you prioritize her physical care and her education?

3 **ipc** A 70-year-old woman who had a mastectomy without reconstruction 7 years ago comes to the clinic where you work. She intermittently wears her compression garment and is faithful about her follow-up care. What members of the health care team should be included in the care of this patient?

REFERENCES

*Asterisk indicates nursing research.
**Double asterisk indicates classic reference.

Books

Bassett, L., & Lee-Felker, S. (2018). Breast imaging screening and diagnosis. In K. Bland, E. Copeland, V. Klimberg, et al. (Eds.). *The breast: Comprehensive management of benign and malignant diseases* (5th ed.). Philadelphia, PA: Elsevier.

Bland, K., Copeland, E., & Klimberg, V. (2018). Anatomy of the breast, axilla, chest wall and related metastatic sites. In K. Bland, E. Copeland, V. Klimberg, et al. (Eds.). *The breast: Comprehensive management of benign and malignant diseases* (5th ed.). Philadelphia, PA: Elsevier.

Calhoun, K., & Anderson, B. (2018). Lobular carcinoma in situ of the breast. In K. Bland, E. Copeland, V. Klimberg, et al. (Eds.). *The breast: Comprehensive management of benign and malignant diseases* (5th ed.). Philadelphia, PA: Elsevier.

Fayanju, O., Garvey, P., Karuturi, M., et al. (2018). Surgical procedures for advanced local and regional malignancies of the breast. In K. Bland, E. Copeland, V. Klimberg, et al. (Eds.). *The breast: Comprehensive management of benign and malignant diseases* (5th ed.). Philadelphia, PA: Elsevier.

Freedman, G. (2018a). Breast conserving therapy for invasive breast cancers. In K. Bland, E. Copeland, V. Klimberg, et al. (Eds.). *The breast: Comprehensive management of benign and malignant diseases* (5th ed.). Philadelphia, PA: Elsevier.

Freedman, G. (2018b). Radiation complications and their management. In K. Bland, E. Copeland, V. Klimberg, et al. (Eds.). *The breast: Comprehensive management of benign and malignant diseases* (5th ed.). Philadelphia, PA: Elsevier.

Grobmyer, S., & Bland, K. (2018). Wound care and complications of mastectomy. In K. Bland, E. Copeland, V. Klimberg, et al. (Eds.). *The breast: Comprehensive management of benign and malignant diseases* (5th ed.). Philadelphia, PA: Elsevier.

Jain, S., & Gradishar, W. (2018). Male breast cancer. In K. Bland, E. Copeland, V. Klimberg, et al. (Eds.). *The breast: Comprehensive management of benign and malignant diseases* (5th ed.). Philadelphia, PA: Elsevier.

Klimberg, V., & Bland, K. (2018). In situ carcinomas of the breast: Ductal carcinoma in situ and lobular carcinoma in situ. In K. Bland, E. Copeland, V. Klimberg, et al. (Eds.). *The breast: Comprehensive management of benign and malignant diseases* (5th ed.). Philadelphia, PA: Elsevier.

Korourian, S., Kumarapeli, A., & Klimberg, V. (2018). Breast biomarker immunocytochemistry. In K. Bland, E. Copeland, V. Klimberg, et al. (Eds.). *The breast: Comprehensive management of benign and malignant diseases* (5th ed.). Philadelphia, PA: Elsevier.

Makhoul, I., Banderudrappagari, R., & Pennisi, A. (2018). General considerations for follow-up. In K. Bland, E. Copeland, V. Klimberg, et al. (Eds.). *The breast: Comprehensive management of benign and malignant diseases* (5th ed.). Philadelphia, PA: Elsevier.

Mallory, M., & Golshan, M. (2018). Examination techniques: Roles of the physician and patient in evaluating breast disease. In K. Bland, E. Copeland, V. Klimberg, et al. (Eds.). *The breast: Comprehensive management of benign and malignant diseases* (5th ed.). Philadelphia, PA: Elsevier.

Mehra, K., Berkowitz, A., & Sanft, T. (2018). Psychosocial consequences and lifestyle interventions. In K. Bland, E. Copeland, V. Klimberg, et al. (Eds.). *The breast: Comprehensive management of benign and malignant diseases* (5th ed.). Philadelphia, PA: Elsevier.

O'Donnell, M., Axilbund, J., & Euhus, D. (2018). Breast cancer genetics: Syndromes, genes, pathology, counseling, testing, and treatment. In K. Bland, E. Copeland, V. Klimberg, et al. (Eds.). *The breast: Comprehensive management of benign and malignant diseases* (5th ed.). Philadelphia, PA: Elsevier.

Obeng-Gyasi, S., Grimm, L., Hwang, E., et al. (2018). Indications and techniques for biopsy. In K. Bland, E. Copeland, V. Klimberg, et al. (Eds.). *The breast: Comprehensive management of benign and malignant diseases* (5th ed.). Philadelphia, PA: Elsevier.

Pederson, H., & Klemp, J. (2018). Breast cancer survivorship. In K. Bland, E. Copeland, V. Klimberg, et al. (Eds.). *The breast: Comprehensive management of benign and malignant diseases* (5th ed.). Philadelphia, PA: Elsevier.

Petersen, L., Moravek, M., Woodruff, T., et al. (2018). Oncofertility options for young women with breast cancer. In K. Bland, E. Copeland, V. Klimberg, et al. (Eds.). *The breast: Comprehensive management of benign and malignant diseases* (5th ed.). Philadelphia, PA: Elsevier.

Prati, R., Chang, H., & Chung, M. (2018). Therapeutic value of axillary node dissection and selective management of the axilla in small breast cancers. In K. Bland, E. Copeland, V. Klimberg, et al. (Eds.). *The breast: Comprehensive management of benign and malignant diseases* (5th ed.). Philadelphia, PA: Elsevier.

Rivere, A., & Klimberg, V. (2018). Lymphedema in the postmastectomy patient: Pathophysiology, prevention, and management. In K. Bland, E. Copeland, V. Klimberg, et al. (Eds.). *The breast: Comprehensive management of benign and malignant diseases* (5th ed.). Philadelphia, PA: Elsevier.

Santa-Maria, C., & Gradishar, W. (2018). Adjuvant and neoadjuvant systemic therapies for early-stage breast cancer. In K. Bland, E. Copeland, V. Klimberg, et al. (Eds.). *The breast: Comprehensive management of benign and malignant diseases* (5th ed.). Philadelphia, PA: Elsevier.

Sasaki, J., Geletzke, A., Kass, R., et al. (2018). Etiology and management of benign breast disease. In K. Bland, E. Copeland, V. Klimberg, et al. (Eds.). *The breast: Comprehensive management of benign and malignant diseases* (5th ed.). Philadelphia, PA: Elsevier.

Shahpar, S., Mhatre, P., & Oza, S. (2018). Rehabilitation. In K. Bland, E. Copeland, V. Klimberg, et al. (Eds.). *The breast: Comprehensive management of benign and malignant diseases* (5th ed.). Philadelphia, PA: Elsevier.

Sledge, G. (2018). HER2-positive breast cancer. In K. Bland, E. Copeland, V. Klimberg, et al. (Eds.). *The breast: Comprehensive management of benign and malignant diseases* (5th ed.). Philadelphia, PA: Elsevier.

Telli, M. (2018). Principles of preoperative therapy for operable breast cancer. In K. Bland, E. Copeland, V. Klimberg, et al. (Eds.). *The breast: Comprehensive management of benign and malignant diseases* (5th ed.). Philadelphia, PA: Elsevier.

Vallerand, A., & Sanoski, C. (2018). *Davis's drug guide for nurses* (16th ed.). Philadelphia, PA: Davis.

Wapnir, I., Tsai, J., & Aebi, S. (2018). Locoregional recurrence after mastectomy. In K. Bland, E. Copeland, V. Klimberg, et al. (Eds.). *The breast: Comprehensive management of benign and malignant diseases* (5th ed.). Philadelphia, PA: Elsevier.

Journals and Electronic Documents

American Cancer Society (ACS). (2019). Breast cancer facts & figures 2019-2020. Retrieved on 9/9/2019 at: www.cancer.org/content/dam/cancer-org/research/cancer-facts-and-statistics/breast-cancer-facts-and-figures/breast-cancer-facts-and-figures-2019-2020.pdf

American College of Radiology (ACR). (2019). Radiation dose in x-ray and CT exams. Retrieved on 10/11/2019 at: www.radiologyinfo.org/en/info.cfm?pg=safety-xray

Boraas, M., & Gupta, S. (2019). Breast self-exam. Retrieved on 5/14/2020 at: www.breastcancer.org/symptoms/testing/types/self_exam

Breastcancer.org. (2018). Metastatic breast cancer symptoms and diagnosis. Retrieved on 11/7/2019 at: www.breastcancer.org/symptoms/types/recur_metast/mctastic

Breastcancer.org. (2019). Lymph node removal. Retrieved on 5/13/2020 at: www.breastcancer.org/treatment/surgery/lymph_node_removal

Canadian Cancer Society. (2020). Breast cancer in men. Retrieved on 1/12/2020 at: www.cancer.ca/en/cancer-information/cancer-type/breast/breast-cancer/breast-cancer-in-men/?region=on

Centers for Disease Control and Prevention (CDC). (2019a). Disability and health information for women with disabilities. Retrieved on 1/10/2020 at: www.CDC.gov/ncbddd/disabilityandhealth/women.html

Centers for Disease Control and Prevention (CDC). (2019b). Women with disabilities and breast cancer screening. Retrieved on 5/13/2020 at: www.cdc.gov/ncbddd/disabilityandhealth/breast-cancer-screening.html

DePolo, J. (2018). Delaying chemotherapy more than 30 days linked to worse outcomes for triple-negative breast cancer. Retrieved on 1/14/2020 at: www.breastcancer.org/research-news/chemo-delay-30-days-plus-worse-for-trip-neg

Indik, J. H., Gimbel, J. R., Abe, H., et al. (2017). 2017 HRS expert consensus statement on magnetic resonance imaging and radiation exposure in patients with cardiovascular implantable electronic devices. *Heart Rhythm*, 14(7), e97–e153.

Kates, J., Ranji, U., Beamesderfer, A., et al. (2018). Health and access to care and coverage for lesbian, gay, bisexual, and transgender (LGBT) individuals in the U.S. Retrieved on 5/12/2020 at: www.kff.org/disparities-policy/issue-brief/health-and-access-to-care-and-coverage-for-lesbian-gay-bisexual-and-transgender-individuals-in-the-u-s/view/print/

Komen, S. G. (2019a). Managing pain related to treatment for early breast cancer. Retrieved on 5/12/2020 at: ww5.komen.org/BreastCancer/ManagingPainRelatedtoTreatment.html

Komen, S. G. (2019b). Types of tumors. Retrieved on 12/17/2019 at: ww5.komen.org/AboutBreastCancer/DiagnosingBreastCancer/UnderstandingaDiagnosis/TumorTypesSizesGrades.html

Mayo Clinic. (2018). Breast cancer prevention: How to reduce your risk. Retrieved on 1/13/2020 at: www.mayoclinic.org/healthy-lifestyle/womens-health/in-depth/breast-cancer-prevention/art-20044676

Mayo Clinic. (2019a). Breast cancer chemoprevention: Medicines that reduce breast cancer risk. Retrieved on 12/31/2019 at: www.mayoclinic.org/diseases-conditions/breast-cancer/in-depth/breast-cancer/art-20045353

Mayo Clinic. (2019b). Preventive (prophylactic) mastectomy: Surgery to reduce breast cancer risk. Retrieved on 12/17/2019 at: www.mayoclinic.org/tests-procedures/mastectomy/in-depth/prophylactic-mastectomy/art-20047221

Mayo Clinic. (2020). HER-2 positive breast cancer: What is it? Retrieved on 5/8/2020 at: www.mayoclinic.org/breast-cancer/expert-answers/faq-20058066

*Mazor, M., Lee, J. Q., Peled, A., et al. (2018). The effect of yoga on arm volume, strength, and range of motion in women at risk for breast cancer-related lymphedema. *Journal of Alternative and Complementary Medicine*, 24(2), 154–160.

National Cancer Institute. (2018a). Brachytherapy to treat cancer. Retrieved on 1/3/2020 at: www.cancer.gov/about-cancer/treatment/types/radiation-therapy/brachytherapy

National Cancer Institute. (2018b). External beam radiation therapy for cancer. Retrieved on 1/3/2020 at: www.cancer.gov/about-cancer/treatment/types/radiation-therapy/external-beam

National Cancer Institute. (2018c). Skin and nail changes during cancer treatment. Retrieved on 1/3/2020 at: www.cancer.gov/about-cancer/treatment/side-effects/skin-nail-changes

National Comprehensive Cancer Network. (2019). NCCN clinical practice guidelines in oncology. Retrieved on 9/9/2019 at: www.nccn.org/professionals/physician_gls/pdf/breast.pdf

Newton, E., & Grethlein, S. (2018). Breast examination. Retrieved on 5/13/2020 at: https://emedicine.medscape.com/article/1909276-overview

Papautsky, E. L., & Hamlish, T. (2020). Patient-reported treatment delays in breast cancer care during the COVID-19 pandemic. *Breast Cancer Research and Treatment*, 184(1), 249–254.

Stanford Medicine 25. (2020). Breast exam. Retrieved on 5/13/2020 at: www.stanfordmedicine25.stanford.edu/the25/BreastExam.html

U.S. Food and Drug Administration (FDA). (2018). Frequently asked questions about MQSA. Retrieved on 10/11/2019 at: www.fda.gov/radiation-emitting-products/consumer-information-mqsa/frequently-asked-questions-about-mqsa#certs

U.S. Food and Drug Administration (FDA). (2019). Types of breast implants. Retrieved on 1/6/2020 at: www.fda.gov/medical-devices/breast-implants/types-breast-implants

*van Ee, B., Smits, C., Honkoop, A., et al. (2019). Open wounds and healed scars: A qualitative study of elderly women's experiences with breast cancer. *Cancer Nursing, 42*(3), 190–197.

Veronesi, P., & Corso, G. (2020). Impact of COVID-19 pandemic on clinical and surgical breast cancer management. *EClinicalMedicine, 26,* 100523.

Resources

ABCD: After Breast Cancer Diagnosis, www.abcdbreastcancersupport.org
American Cancer Society, www.cancer.org

American Society of Plastic Surgeons (ASPS), www.plasticsurgery.org
Cancer Care, www.cancercare.org
National Cancer Institute (NCI), www.cancer.gov/cancertopics/types/breast
National Comprehensive Cancer Network (NCCN), www.nccn.org
National Lymphedema Network (NLN), www.lymphnet.org
Oncology Nursing Society (ONS), www.ons.org
Reach To Recovery, cancer.org/treatment/support-programs-and-services/reach-to-recovery.html
Save My Fertility, www.savemyfertility.org
Susan G. Komen for the Cure, ww5.komen.org

53

Assessment and Management of Patients with Male Reproductive Disorders

LEARNING OUTCOMES

On completion of this chapter, the learner will be able to:

1. Describe structures and function of the male reproductive system.
2. Discuss nursing assessment of the male reproductive system, identifying diagnostic tests used and their related nursing implications.
3. Explain the causes and management of male sexual dysfunction.
4. Compare the types of prostatectomy with regard to advantages and disadvantages.
5. Use the nursing process as a framework for care of the patient with male reproductive disorders and conditions, including prostate, testicular, and penis disorders.

NURSING CONCEPTS

Assessment	Inflammation	Sexuality
Family	Mobility	Stress
Infection	Reproduction	

GLOSSARY

androgen deprivation therapy: surgical (orchiectomy) or medical castration (e.g., with luteinizing hormone–releasing hormone agonists)

benign prostatic hyperplasia (BPH): noncancerous enlargement or hypertrophy of the prostate; the most common pathologic condition in older men

brachytherapy: delivery of radiation therapy through internal implants placed inside or adjacent to a tumor

circumcision: excision of the foreskin, or prepuce, of the glans penis

cystostomy: surgical creation of an opening into the urinary bladder

epididymitis: infection of the epididymis that usually descends from an infected prostate or urinary tract; also may develop as a complication of gonorrhea, chlamydia, or *Escherichia coli*

erectile dysfunction: the inability to either achieve or maintain an erection sufficient to accomplish sexual intercourse (*synonym*: impotence)

hydrocele: a collection of fluid, generally in the tunica vaginalis of the testis, although it also may collect within the spermatic cord

orchiectomy: surgical removal of one or both testes

orchitis: acute inflammation of the testes (testicular congestion) caused by pyogenic, viral, spirochetal, parasitic, traumatic, chemical, or unknown factors

phimosis: condition in which the foreskin is constricted so that it cannot be retracted over the glans; can occur congenitally or from inflammation and edema

priapism: an uncontrolled, persistent erection of the penis from either neural or vascular causes, including medications, sickle cell thrombosis, leukemic cell infiltration, spinal cord tumors, and tumor invasion of the penis or its vessels

prostatectomy: surgical removal of the entire prostate, the prostate urethra, and the attached seminal vesicles plus the ampulla of the vas deferens

prostate-specific antigen (PSA): substance that is produced by the prostate gland; is used in combination with digital rectal examination to screen for prostate cancer

prostatitis: inflammation of the prostate gland caused by infectious agents (bacteria, fungi, mycoplasma) or various other problems (e.g., urethral stricture, prostatic hyperplasia)

retrograde ejaculation: during ejaculation, semen travels to the urinary bladder instead of exiting through the penis

spermatogenesis: production of sperm in the testes

testosterone: male sex hormone secreted by the testes; induces and preserves the male sex characteristics

transurethral resection of the prostate (TURP): resection of the prostate through endoscopy; the surgical and optical instrument is introduced directly through the urethra to the prostate, and the gland is then removed in small chips with an electrical cutting loop

varicocele: an abnormal dilation of the veins of the pampiniform venous plexus in the scrotum (the network of veins from the testis and the epididymis, which constitute part of the spermatic cord)

vasectomy: ligation and transection of part of the vas deferens, with or without removal of a segment of the vas, to prevent the passage of the sperm from the testes (*synonym:* male sterilization)

Disorders of the male reproductive system include a wide variety of conditions that usually affect both urinary and reproductive systems. Because these disorders involve the genitalia and often affect sexuality, the patient may experience anxiety and embarrassment. The nurse must be aware of the patient's need for privacy as well as the need for education and support. This requires an openness to discuss critical and sensitive issues with the patient, including a partner when appropriate, as well as effective assessment, management, and communication. Nurses must be comfortable when examining male genitalia and must recognize their own attitudes and perceptions about male reproductive disorders. Education of the patient and partner about treatment and self-care strategies is essential (Tabloski, 2019).

ASSESSMENT OF THE MALE REPRODUCTIVE SYSTEM

Anatomic and Physiologic Overview

In the male, several organs serve as parts of both the urinary tract and the reproductive system. Disorders in the male reproductive organs may interfere with the functions of one or both of these systems. As a result, diseases of the male reproductive system are usually treated by a urologist. The structures in the male reproductive system include the (1) external male genitalia, consisting of the testes, epididymis, scrotum, and penis, and the (2) internal male genitalia, consisting of the vas deferens (ductus deferens), ejaculatory duct, and prostatic and membranous sections of the urethra, seminal vesicles, and certain accessory glands, such as the prostate gland and Cowper glands (bulbourethral glands) (see Fig. 53-1).

The testes have a dual function: **spermatogenesis** (production of sperm) and secretion of the male sex hormone **testosterone**, which induces and preserves the male sex characteristics. The testes are formed in the embryo, within the abdominal cavity near the kidney. During the last month of fetal life, they descend posterior to the peritoneum and pierce the abdominal wall in the groin. Later, they progress along the inguinal canal into the scrotal sac. In this descent, they are accompanied by blood vessels, lymphatics, nerves, and ducts, which support the tissue and make up the spermatic cord. This cord extends from the internal inguinal ring through the abdominal wall and the inguinal canal to the scrotum. As the testes descend into the scrotum in the final 2 to 3 months of gestation, a tubular extension of peritoneum accompanies them (Rhoades & Bell, 2017). Normally, this tissue is obliterated during fetal development; only the tunica vaginalis, which covers the testes, remains. If the peritoneal process remains open into the abdominal cavity, a potential sac remains into which abdominal contents may enter to form an indirect inguinal hernia.

The testes, or ovoid sex glands, are encased in the scrotum, which keeps them at a slightly lower temperature than the rest of the body to facilitate spermatogenesis (Rhoades & Bell, 2017). The testes consist of numerous seminiferous tubules in which the spermatozoa form. Collecting tubules transmit the spermatozoa into the epididymis, a hoodlike structure lying on the testes and containing winding ducts that lead into the vas deferens. This firm, tubular structure passes upward through the inguinal canal to enter the abdominal cavity behind the peritoneum. It then extends downward toward the base of the bladder. An outpouching from this structure is the seminal vesicle, which acts as a reservoir for testicular secretions. The tract is continued as the ejaculatory

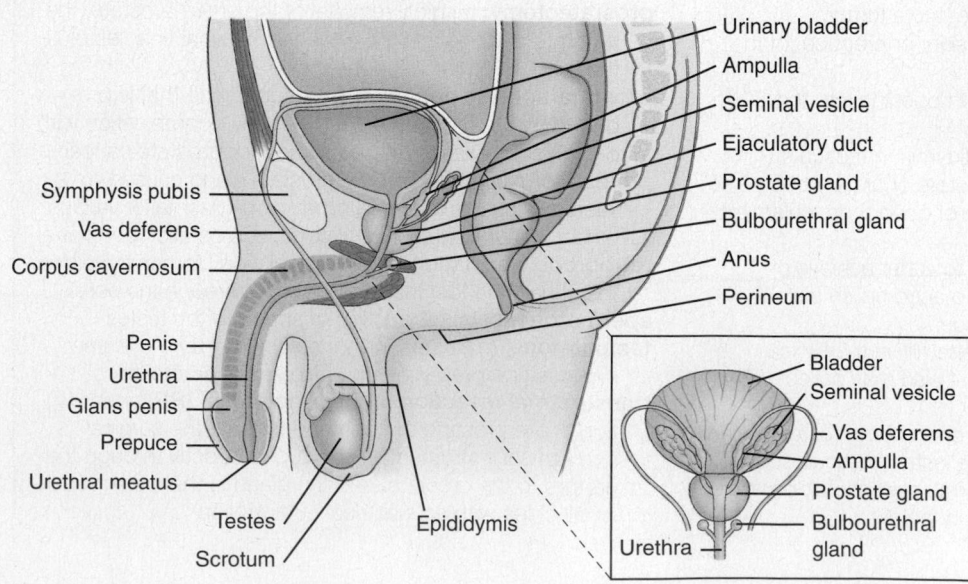

Figure 53-1 • Structures of the male reproductive system.

duct, which passes through the prostate gland to enter the urethra. Testicular secretions take this pathway when they exit the penis during ejaculation.

The penis is the organ for both copulation and urination. It consists of the glans penis, the body, and the root. The glans penis is the soft, rounded portion at the distal end of the penis. The urethra (the tube that carries urine) opens at the tip of the glans. The glans is naturally covered by elongated penile skin—the foreskin—which may be retracted to expose the glans. However, many men as newborns have undergone circumcision, which is a procedure to remove the foreskin. The body of the penis is composed of erectile tissues containing numerous blood vessels that become dilated, leading to an erection during sexual excitement. The urethra, which passes through the penis, extends from the bladder through the prostate to the distal end of the penis.

The prostate gland, lying just below the neck of the bladder, is composed of four zones and four lobes. It surrounds the urethra and is traversed by the ejaculatory duct, a continuation of the vas deferens. This gland produces a secretion that is chemically and physiologically suitable to the needs of the spermatozoa in their passage from the testes. Cowper glands lie below the prostate, within the posterior aspect of the urethra. This gland empties its secretions into the urethra during ejaculation, providing lubrication.

 ### Gerontologic Considerations

As men age, the prostate gland enlarges; prostate secretion decreases; the scrotum hangs lower; the testes decrease in weight, atrophy, and become softer; and pubic hair becomes sparser and stiffer. Changes in gonadal function include a decline in plasma testosterone levels and reduced production of progesterone (see Table 53-1). Libido and potency often decrease in as many as two thirds of men older than 70 years (Tabloski, 2019). Vascular problems cause about half of the cases of erectile dysfunction in men older than 50 years.

However, male reproductive capability is maintained with advancing age. Although degenerative changes occur in the seminiferous tubules and sperm production decreases, spermatogenesis continues, allowing men to produce viable sperm throughout their lives (McCance, Huether, Braskers, et al., 2018).

Male hypogonadism (decreased function of the testes) starts gradually at approximately 50 years of age, resulting in decreased testosterone production. The older man notices that the sexual response slows, erection takes longer, full erections may not be attained, ejaculation takes longer to occur, and control or resolution may occur without orgasm. Sexual function can be affected by psychological problems, illnesses, and medications (Sikka & Hellstrom, 2017). In general, the entire sexual act takes longer. Sexual activity is closely correlated with the man's sexual activity in his earlier years; if he was more active than average as a young man, he will most likely continue to be more active than average in his later years.

Men older than 50 years are at increased risk for genitourinary tract cancers, including those of the kidney, bladder, prostate, and penis. The digital rectal examination (DRE), prostate-specific antigen (PSA) test, and urinalysis, which screens for hematuria, may uncover a higher percentage of malignancies at earlier stages and lead to lower treatment-associated morbidity as well as a lower mortality.

Urinary incontinence occurs in one fifth of community-dwelling older men and rises to nearly 50% in men in long-term care settings (Tabloski, 2019). Older adults admitted to acute care settings should be screened for this problem. Urinary incontinence may have many causes, including medications, neurologic disease, or benign prostatic hyperplasia (BPH). Incontinence may also be linked to erectile dysfunction when there is damage to the neural pathways that initiate an erection (Rantell, Apostolidis, Anding, et al., 2017). Diagnostic tests are performed to exclude reversible causes. New-onset urinary incontinence is a nursing priority that requires evaluation.

Assessment

Assessing the male reproductive system includes a targeted health history and physical examination.

Health History

Male sexuality is a complex phenomenon that is strongly influenced by personal, cultural, religious, and social factors. Sexuality and male reproductive function become concerns in the presence of illness and disability (Kaufman, Lapauw, Mahmoud, et al., 2019). Throughout the assessment process, the nurse must recognize the significance of sexuality to the patient. Assessment of male reproductive function begins with an evaluation of urinary function and symptoms. The patient is asked about his usual state of health and any recent change in general physical and sexual activity. Any symptoms or

TABLE 53-1 Age-Related Changes in the Male Reproductive System

Age-Related Changes	Physiologic Changes	Manifestations
Decrease in sex hormone secretion, especially testosterone	Decreased muscle strength and sexual energy	Changes in sexual response—prolonged time to reach full erection, rapid penile detumescence, and prolonged refractory period
	Decrease in number of viable sperm	
	Shrinkage and loss of firmness of testes; thickening of seminiferous tubules	Smaller testes
	Fibrotic changes of corpora cavernosa	Erectile dysfunction
	Enlargement of prostate gland	Weakening of prostatic contractions
		Hyperplasia of prostate gland
		Signs and symptoms of obstruction of lower urinary tract (urgency, frequency, nocturia)

Adapted from Tabloski, P. A. (2019). *Gerontological nursing: The essential guide to clinical practice* (4th ed.). New York: Pearson.

changes in function are explored fully and described in detail. Symptoms related to bladder function and urination, collectively referred to as prostatism, are explored further. Symptoms may occur with an obstruction caused by an enlarged prostate gland and may include increased urinary frequency, decreased force of urine stream, and "double" or "triple" voiding (the patient needs to urinate two or three times over a period of several minutes to completely empty his bladder). The patient is also assessed for dysuria (painful urination), hematuria (blood in the urine), nocturia (urination during the night), and hematospermia (blood in the ejaculate).

Assessment also involves addressing sexual function, including manifestations of sexual dysfunction. The extent of the history depends on the patient's presenting symptoms and the presence of factors that may affect sexual function such as chronic illnesses or disability (e.g., diabetes, multiple sclerosis, stroke, cardiac disease), the use of medications that affect sexual function (e.g., antihypertensive and anticholesterolemic medications, psychotropic agents), stress, the use of alcohol, and the patient's willingness to discuss sexual issues.

By initiating an assessment about sexual concerns, the nurse conveys the message that changes in sexual functioning are valid topics and provides a safe environment for discussing these sensitive topics. Several models are available to assist in assessing patient's problems and concerns. The PLIS-SIT (permission, limited information, specific suggestions, intensive therapy) model of sexual assessment and intervention may be used to provide a framework for nursing interventions (Annon, 1976; Messelis, Kazer, & Gelmetti, 2019). It provides a graded counseling approach that allows health care professionals to deal with sexual issues with a level of comfort and expertise. The model begins by asking the patient's permission (P) to discuss sexual functioning. Limited information (LI) about sexual function may then be provided to the patient. As the discussion progresses, the nurse may offer specific suggestions (SS) for interventions. A professional who specializes in sex therapy may provide more intensive therapy (IT) as needed. The BETTER (bringing up the topic, explaining, telling, timing, educate about treatment-related sexual side effects, recording) model was developed more recently to assist health care professionals to include sexuality in the assessment of patients with cancer (Campbell, 2020).

Patients may find it difficult to express their feelings and concerns regarding their sexuality, especially after a body image change (e.g., after major surgery such as amputation). Discussing sexuality with patients who have an illness or disability can be uncomfortable for nurses and other health care providers; this, in turn, makes discussion of these issues more difficult and uncomfortable for patients. Some health care professionals may unconsciously have stereotypes about the sexuality of people who are ill or have a disability (e.g., the belief that people with disability are asexual or should be sexually inactive). In addition, patients are often embarrassed to initiate a discussion about sexual issues with their health care providers (Campbell, 2020; Katz, Cherven, Ballard, et al., 2019).

Physical Assessment

In addition to the usual aspects of the physical examination, two essential components address disorders of the male

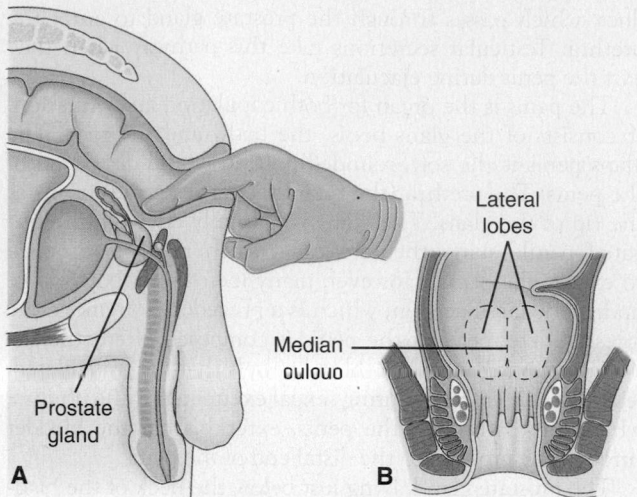

Figure 53-2 • **A.** Palpation of the prostate gland during digital rectal examination enables the examiner to assess the size, shape, and texture of the gland. **B.** The prostate is round, with a palpable median sulcus or groove separating the lateral lobes. It should feel rubbery and free of nodules and masses.

genital or reproductive system: the DRE and the testicular examination.

Digital Rectal Examination

The DRE is used to screen for prostate cancer and is recommended annually for every man older than 50 years (45 years for men at high risk [African American men and men with a family history of prostate cancer in first-degree relatives]) (American Cancer Society [ACS], 2020). The DRE enables the skilled examiner, using a lubricated, gloved finger placed in the rectum, to assess the size, symmetry, shape, and consistency of the posterior surface of the prostate gland (see Fig. 53-2). The clinician assesses for tenderness of the prostate gland on palpation and for the presence and consistency of any nodules. The DRE may be performed with the patient leaning over an examination table or positioning the man in a side-lying position with legs flexed toward the abdomen or supine with legs resting in stirrups. To minimize discomfort and relax the anal sphincter during the rectal examination, the patient is instructed to take a deep breath and exhale slowly as the practitioner inserts a finger. If possible, he should turn his feet inward, so that his toes are touching. Although this examination may be uncomfortable and embarrassing for the patient, it is an important screening tool.

Testicular Examination

The male genitalia are inspected for abnormalities and palpated for masses. The scrotum is palpated carefully for nodules, masses, or inflammation. Examination of the scrotum can reveal such disorders as hydrocele, inguinal hernia, testicular torsion, orchitis, epididymitis, or a tumor of the testis. The penis is inspected and palpated for ulcerations, nodules, inflammation, discharge, and curvature. If the patient is uncircumcised, the foreskin should be retracted for visualization of the glans penis. The testicular examination provides an excellent opportunity to educate the patient on how to perform a testicular self-examination (TSE) and its importance in early detection of testicular cancer. TSE should begin during adolescence. For more details on TSE, see later discussion in the chapter.

Diagnostic Evaluation

A wide range of diagnostic studies may be performed in men with reproductive disorders. The nurse should educate the patient about the purpose, what to expect, and any possible side effects related to these tests and examinations prior to testing. The nurse should note trends in results because they provide information about disease progression as well as the patient's response to therapy.

Prostate-Specific Antigen Test

The cells within the prostate gland produce a protein that can be measured in the blood called the **prostate-specific antigen (PSA)**. It is a sensitive but not specific test for prostate cancer. In the absence of prostate cancer, serum PSA levels vary with age, race, and prostate volume. Increased levels may indicate prostate cancer. However, a number of other conditions such as BPH, acute urinary retention, and acute prostatitis may cause high PSA levels. Values of PSA may also increase after ejaculation. PSA levels are measured in nanograms per milliliter (ng/mL). In most laboratories, values less than 4 ng/mL are generally considered normal, and values greater than 4 ng/mL are considered elevated in men 60 years of age or younger (Law, Nguyen, Barkin, et al., 2020; Pagana & Pagana, 2018). The use of age-specific reference ranges is encouraged to help minimize unnecessary biopsies (see Appendix A on the**Point**).

A serum PSA level and a DRE, which are recommended by the ACS (2020), are used to screen for prostate cancer for men with at least a 10-year life expectancy and for men at high risk, including those with a strong family history of prostate cancer and of African American ethnicity. The perceptions of some African American men and women reflect the belief that PSA screening saves lives and needs to be done despite recommendations against screening due to false positives potentially resulting in unnecessary treatment (Arace, Flores, Monaghan, et al., 2020; Kearns, Adeyemi, Anderson, et al., 2020). The PSA test is also used to monitor patients for recurrence after treatment for cancer of the prostate, based on evidence-based guidelines (National Comprehensive Cancer Network [NCCN], 2020b). Neither the DRE nor PSA is 100% accurate, but when used together, their accuracy increases.

Ultrasonography

Transrectal ultrasound (TRUS) may be performed in patients with abnormalities detected by DRE and in those with elevated PSA levels. After DRE has been completed, a lubricated, condom-covered, rectal probe transducer is inserted into the rectum (Lim, Jun, Chang, et al., 2019). Water may be introduced into the condom to help transmit sound waves to the prostate. TRUS may be used in detecting nonpalpable prostate cancers and in staging localized prostate cancer. Needle biopsies of the prostate are commonly guided by TRUS.

Prostate Fluid or Tissue Analysis

Specimens of prostate fluid or tissue may be obtained for culture if disease or inflammation of the prostate gland is suspected. A biopsy of the prostate gland may be necessary to obtain tissue for histologic examination. This may be performed at the time of prostatectomy or by means of a perineal or transrectal needle biopsy. Six to 12 biopsies from all four prostate zones may be obtained during a TRUS-guided biopsy.

Tests of Male Sexual Function

If the patient cannot engage in sexual activity to his satisfaction, a detailed history is obtained. Nocturnal erections occur in healthy males of all ages. Nocturnal penile tumescence tests may be conducted in a sleep laboratory to monitor changes in penile circumference during sleep using various methods to determine number, duration, rigidity, and circumference of penile erections; the results help identify whether the erectile dysfunction is caused by physiologic or psychological factors. Additional tests, including psychological evaluations, are also part of the diagnostic workup and are usually conducted by a specialized team of health care providers.

DISORDERS OF MALE SEXUAL FUNCTION

Erectile Dysfunction

Erectile dysfunction, also called *impotence*, is the inability to achieve or maintain an erect penis (Norris, 2019). The man may report decreased frequency of erections, inability to achieve a firm erection, or rapid detumescence (subsiding of erection). In the United States, 30 million men experience erectile dysfunction; more than half of men 40 to 70 years of age are unable to attain or maintain an erection sufficient for satisfactory sexual performance (Smith, Howards, Preminger, et al., 2019). The physiology of erection and ejaculation is complex and involves parasympathetic and sympathetic components. Erection involves the release of nitric oxide into the corpus cavernosum during sexual stimulation. Its release activates cyclic guanosine monophosphate (cGMP), causing smooth muscle relaxation. This allows flow of blood into the corpus cavernosum, resulting in erection (Cheng, MacLennan, & Bostwick, 2019; Norris, 2019).

Erectile dysfunction has both psychogenic and organic causes. Psychogenic causes include anxiety, fatigue, depression, pressure to perform sexually, negative body image, absence of desire, and privacy, as well as trust and relationship issues. Organic causes include cardiovascular disease, endocrine disease (diabetes, pituitary tumors, testosterone deficiency, hyperthyroidism, and hypothyroidism), cirrhosis, chronic kidney injury, genitourinary conditions (radical pelvic surgery), hematologic conditions (Hodgkin lymphoma, leukemia), neurologic disorders (neuropathies, parkinsonism, spinal cord injury [SCI], multiple sclerosis), trauma to the pelvic or genital area, smoking, medications (see Chart 53-1), and substance use disorder.

Assessment and Diagnostic Findings

The diagnosis of erectile dysfunction requires a sexual and medical history; an analysis of presenting symptoms; a physical examination, including a neurologic examination; a detailed assessment of all medications, alcohol, and drugs used; and various laboratory studies. Nocturnal penile tumescence tests are conducted to monitor changes in penile circumference. This test can help to determine if erectile dysfunction has an organic or a psychological cause. In healthy men, nocturnal penile erections closely parallel rapid eye movement (REM) sleep in occurrence and duration. Organically, men with erectile dysfunction show inadequate sleep-related erections that correspond to their waking performance. Arterial blood flow to the penis is measured using a Doppler probe. In addition, nerve conduction tests and extensive psychological evaluations may be carried out. Figure 53-3 describes the evaluation and treatment of erectile dysfunction.

Medical Management

Treatment can be medical, surgical, or both, depending on the cause. Treatment of erectile dysfunction includes therapy for associated disorders (e.g., alcoholism, diabetes) or adjustment of medications (McMahon, 2019). Endocrine therapy instituted to treat erectile dysfunction secondary to hypothalamic–pituitary–gonadal dysfunction may reverse the condition. Insufficient penile blood flow may be treated with vascular surgery. Patients with erectile dysfunction from psychogenic causes are referred to a health care provider or therapist who specializes in sexual dysfunction. Patients with erectile dysfunction secondary to organic causes may be candidates for penile implants.

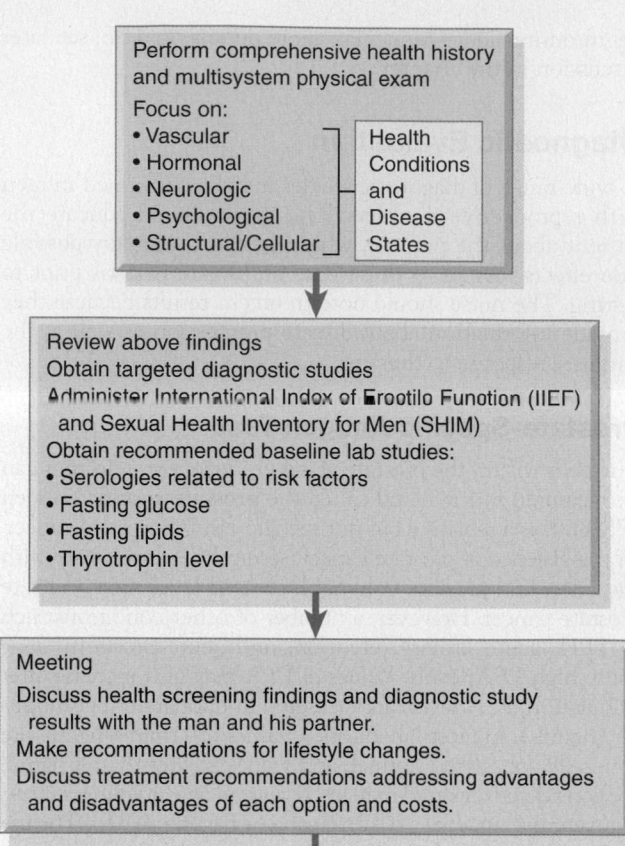

Figure 53-3 • Evaluation and treatment of erectile dysfunction.

Currently available therapies for the treatment of erectile dysfunction include pharmacologic therapy (including urethral suppositories), penile implants, and vacuum constriction devices (see Table 53-2). These options should be considered in a stepwise fashion, with increasing invasiveness and risk

TABLE 53-2	Treatments for Erectile Dysfunction			
Method	**Description**	**Advantages and Disadvantages**	**Duration**	
Pharmacologic Therapy Oral medications (sildenafil, vardenafil, tadalafil) Oral medication	Smooth muscle relaxant causing blood to flow into penis	Can cause headache, flushing, dyspepsia, diarrhea, nasal congestion, and lightheadedness See contraindications in Table 53-3	Taken orally before sexual activity. Stimulation is required to achieve erection. Erection can last up to 1 h.	
Injection (alprostadil, papaverine, phentolamine) Penile injection	Smooth muscle relaxant causing blood to flow into penis	Firm erections are achievable in >50% of cases Pain at injection site; plaque formation, risk of priapism	Injection 20 min before sexual activity. Erection can last up to 1 h.	
Urethral suppository (alprostadil) Penile suppository	Smooth muscle relaxant causing blood to flow into penis	May be used twice a day Urethral and genital pain; risk of hypertension and syncope Not recommended with pregnant partners	Inserted 10 min before sexual activity. Erection can last up to 1 h.	
Penile Implants • Semirigid rod • Inflatable • Soft silicone Penile implant	Surgically implanted into corpus cavernosum	Reliable Requires surgery Healing takes up to 3 wks Subsequent cystoscopic surgery is difficult Semirigid rod results in permanent semierection	Indefinite Inflatable prosthesis—saline returns from penile receptacle to reservoir.	
Negative-Pressure (Vacuum) Devices Penile vacuum pump	Induction of erection with vacuum; maintained with constriction band around base of penis	Few side effects Cumbersome to use before sexual activity Vasocongestion of penis can cause pain or numbness	To prevent penile injury, constriction band must not be left in place >1 h.	

balanced against the likelihood of efficacy. The patient and, if possible, his partner, should be informed of the relevant treatment options and their associated risks and benefits. The choice of treatment is made jointly by the primary provider, patient, and partner, taking into consideration patient preferences and expectations.

Pharmacologic Therapy

Phosphodiesterase type 5 (PDE-5) inhibitors (oral medications that are used to treat erectile dysfunction) are first-line therapy (Allen, 2019). Currently available PDE-5 inhibitors include sildenafil, vardenafil, and tadalafil. Each of these agents has a similar mechanism of action but a different pharmacologic action and clinical use. Erection involves the release of nitric oxide in the vasculature of the corpus cavernosum as a result of sexual stimulation. This subsequently leads to smooth muscle relaxation in blood vessels supplying the corpus cavernosum, resulting in increased blood flow and an erection. During sexual stimulation, PDE-5 inhibitors increase blood flow to the penis (Norris, 2019).

When PDE-5 inhibitors are taken about 1 hour before sexual activity, they are effective in producing an erection with sexual stimulation; the erection can last about 1 to 2 hours. The most common side effects of these medications include headache, flushing, dyspepsia, diarrhea, nasal congestion, and lightheadedness. These agents are contraindicated in men who take organic nitrates (e.g., isosorbide, nitroglycerin), because taken together, these medications can cause side effects such as severe hypotension (Cheng et al., 2019; Norris, 2019). In addition, PDE-5 inhibitors must be used with caution in patients with retinopathy, especially in those with diabetic retinopathy. Patient education about the use of these medications and their side effects is summarized in Table 53-3.

For patients in whom PDE-5 inhibitors are contraindicated or ineffective, other pharmacologic measures to induce erections include injecting vasoactive agents, such as alprostadil, papaverine, and phentolamine, directly into the penis. Complications include **priapism** (a persistent abnormal erection) and development of fibrotic plaques at the injection sites. Alprostadil is also formulated in a gel pellet that can be inserted into the tip of the urethra with an applicator to create an erection.

Penile Implants

Two general types of penile implants are available: the malleable, noninflatable, nonhydraulic prosthesis (also called the *semirigid rod*) and the inflatable, hydraulic prostheses (Lindsey, Lue, & Shindel, 2020). The semirigid rod (e.g., the

TABLE 53-3	Pharmacologic Treatment of Erectile Dysfunction		
	Sildenafil	**Vardenafil**	**Tadalafil**
When to take	Take the medication 30 min to 4 h before penile-vaginal intercourse. *There must be sexual stimulation to produce an erection.*	Take the medication 1 h before penile-vaginal intercourse. The peak action occurs in 30–120 min. *There must be sexual stimulation to produce an erection.*	Take the medication before sexual activity. Effect peaks at 30 min to 6 h; effect may last up to 36 h. *There must be sexual stimulation to produce an erection.*
Frequency of use	If you take this medication more than once a day, it will not have an increased effect. You may take it 7 days per week if you wish, but only once in 24 h. It does not build up in your bloodstream. Remember to take it only when you want to have penile-vaginal intercourse.	The recommended frequency for this medication is 10 mg in 24 h.	The effects of this medication may last up to 36 h. This allows for increased spontaneity in the sexual experience.
Side effects	Side effects include headache, flushing, indigestion, nasal congestion, abnormal vision, diarrhea, dizziness, and rash. You may also have low blood sugar and abnormal liver function tests; your primary provider can determine this.	Side effects include headache, flushing, runny nose, indigestion, sinusitis, flulike syndrome, dizziness, nausea, back pain, and joint pain. Tell your primary provider if you experience any of these effects. You may also have abnormally elevated liver enzymes; your primary provider can determine this.	Side effects are similar to those of sildenafil and vardenafil. Tadalafil may also cause back pain and muscle aches. Tell your primary provider if you experience any of these side effects.
Contraindications	Do not take if you are taking nitrate medications such as nitroglycerin or isosorbide mononitrate. Do not take if you have high uncontrolled blood pressure, coronary artery disease, or have had a heart attack within the past 6 mo. Do not take if you have been diagnosed with a cardiac arrhythmia or kidney or liver dysfunction.		
Drug interactions	This medication can react with other medications that you may be taking. Provide your primary provider and pharmacist with a complete list of all prescribed and over-the-counter medications that you are using.		
Use of PDE-5 inhibitors with penile injections or urethral suppositories	The use of PDE-5 inhibitors with other forms of therapy for erectile dysfunction has not been tested and should be avoided.		

PDE-5, phosphodiesterase type 5.
Adapted from McMahon, C. G. (2019). Current diagnosis and management of erectile dysfunction. *Medical Journal of Australia, 2*(10), 469–476.

Small–Carrion prosthesis) results in a permanent semierection but can be bent into an unnoticeable position when appropriate. The inflatable prosthesis simulates natural erections and natural flaccidity. Complications after implantation include infection, erosion of the prosthesis through the skin (more common with the semirigid rod than with the inflatable prosthesis), and persistent pain, which may require removal of the implant. Subsequent cystoscopic surgery is more difficult with a semirigid rod than with the inflatable prosthesis.

Factors to consider in choosing a penile prosthesis are the patient's activities of daily living, social activities, and the expectations of the patient and his partner. Ongoing counseling for the patient and his partner is usually necessary to help them adapt to the prosthesis.

Penis Transplants

In the United States, a few medical centers have protocols for penis transplants. Candidates for transplantation include military veterans and other men who have suffered traumatic penile injuries. It is believed that men undergoing this surgery will have their ability to urinate and their sexual functioning restored (Ngaage, Elegbede, Sugarman, et al., 2020). For more details on organ transplantation, see discussion in Chapter 48.

Negative-Pressure Devices

Negative-pressure (vacuum) devices may also be used to induce an erection. A plastic cylinder is placed over the flaccid penis, and negative pressure is applied. When an erection is attained, a constriction band is placed around the base of the penis to maintain the erection. To avoid penile injury, the patient is instructed not to leave the constricting band in place for longer than 1 hour. Only devices with a vacuum limiter are recommended for use (Sikka & Hellstrom, 2017). Although many men find this method satisfactory, others experience premature loss of penile rigidity or pain when applying suction or during sexual activity.

Nursing Management

Personal satisfaction and the ability to sexually satisfy a partner are common concerns of patients. Men with illnesses and disability may need the assistance of a sex therapist to identify, implement, and integrate their sexual beliefs and behaviors into a healthy and satisfying lifestyle. The nurse can inform patients about support groups for men with erectile dysfunction and their partners.

Disorders of Ejaculation

Premature ejaculation is defined as the occurrence of ejaculation sooner than desired, either before or shortly after penetration, causing distress to either one or both partners. It is one of the most common complaints of men or couples, affecting 20% to 30% of men (Cheng et al., 2019; Smith et al., 2019). The spectrum of responses ranges from occasional ejaculation with penile-vaginal intercourse or self-stimulation to complete inability to ejaculate under any circumstances. Various forms have been identified including lifelong premature ejaculation caused by neurobiologic or genetic conditions, acquired (medical or psychological), natural variable (normal variation), and premature like ejaculatory dysfunction (psychological). In young men aged 18 to 25 years, factors associated with premature ejaculation and erectile dysfunction include smoking, use of illegal drugs or medications without prescriptions, poor physical and mental health, lack of physical activity, and lack of sexual experience (Barbonetti, D'Andrea, Cavallo, et al., 2019). Other ejaculatory problems may include inhibited (delayed or retarded) ejaculation, which is the involuntary inhibition of the ejaculatory reflex (see Chart 53-2). **Retrograde ejaculation** occurs when semen travels toward the bladder instead of exiting through the penis, resulting in infertility. This form of premature ejaculation may occur after prior prostate or urethral surgery, with diabetes, or with the use of medications such as antihypertensive agents.

Chart 53-2 GENETICS IN NURSING PRACTICE
Male Reproductive Disorders

Various male reproductive disorders are influenced by genetic factors. Some examples are:

- 21-Hydroxylase deficiency
- Congenital absence of the vas deferens, prostate gland, or seminal vesicles
- Kallmann syndrome
- Klinefelter syndrome (47, XXY)
- Prostate cancer
- Y chromosome deletions

Nursing Assessments

Refer to Chapter 4, Chart 4-2: Genetics in Nursing Practice: Genetic Aspects of Health Assessment

Family History Assessment Specific to Male Reproductive Disorders

- Collect a three-generation family history on both maternal and paternal sides of the family.
- Assess family history for other family members with similar reproductive problems/abnormalities.

Patient Assessment Specific to Male Reproductive Disorders

- In males with delayed puberty or infertility, assess for clinical features of Klinefelter syndrome (tall stature, gynecomastia, learning disability).
- Assess males with delayed or absent puberty for clinical features of Kallmann syndrome (cleft lip with or without cleft palate, abnormal eye movements, hearing loss, and abnormalities of tooth development).
- Assess males for history of early growth spurt, which is a symptom of 21-hydroxylase deficiency.
- Inquire about history of prostate inflammation, genital infections, medication use (steroids), or prior history of mumps.
- Assess for physical abnormalities of the genitalia.

Genetics Resources

Association for X and Y Chromosome Variations, www.genetic.org
Klinefelter Syndrome Support Group, www.klinefeltersyndrome.org
See Chapter 6, Chart 6-7 for components of genetic counseling.

Evaluation of premature ejaculation involves a thorough sexual history focusing on the duration of symptoms, time to ejaculation, degree of voluntary control over ejaculation, frequency of occurrence, and course of the problem since the first sexual encounter (Cheng et al., 2019; Smith et al., 2019). Treatment, which depends on the nature, severity, and perceived distress that it causes, includes behavioral and psychological approaches, as well as pharmacologic therapy that attempts to alter the sensory input or retard the ejaculatory response. Behavioral therapy (e.g., counseling, sex therapy, psychoeducation, and couples therapy) often involves both the man and his sexual partner. The couple is encouraged to identify their sexual needs and to communicate those needs to each other. Pharmacologic management involves selective serotonin reuptake inhibitors, dapoxetine, alpha$_1$ adrenoceptor antagonists, the tricyclic antidepressant clomipramine, and topical anesthetic agents. In some cases, a combination of pharmacologic and behavioral therapy may be effective.

Inhibited ejaculation is most often caused by psychological factors, neurologic disorders (e.g., SCI, multiple sclerosis, neuropathy secondary to diabetes), surgery (prostatectomy), and medications. Chemical, vibratory, and electrical methods of stimulation have been used with some success. Treatment usually addresses the physical and psychological factors involved in inhibited ejaculation (Bartlik, Espinosa, & Mindes, 2019). Although outpatient therapy may involve numerous sessions (12 to 18), it often results in a success rate of 70% to 80%. The outcome depends on a previous satisfying sexual experience history, a short duration of the ejaculatory problem, communication about feelings of sexual desire and attraction to one's sexual partner, motivation for treatment, and absence of serious psychological problems.

For men with retrograde ejaculation, the urine may be collected shortly after ejaculation, revealing a large amount of sperm in the urine. This urine may also be collected to obtain adequate viable sperm for use in artificial insemination. In men with SCI, techniques that may be used to obtain sperm for artificial insemination include self-stimulation, vibratory stimulation, or electroejaculation. Electroejaculation involves the use of a specially designed probe that is inserted into the rectum next to the prostate. The probe delivers a current that stimulates the nerves and produces contraction of the pelvic muscles and ejaculation. However, spontaneous or stimulated ejaculation may cause autonomic dysreflexia (overstimulation of the autonomic nervous system) in patients with SCI at T6 or higher, creating a life-threatening situation (see Chapter 63). If this disorder is not treated promptly, it may lead to seizures, stroke, and even death.

INFECTIONS OF THE MALE GENITOURINARY TRACT

Acute uncomplicated cystitis in adult men is uncommon but occasionally occurs. Asymptomatic bacteriuria may also result from genitourinary manipulation, catheterization, or instrumentation. Urinary tract infections (UTIs) are discussed in Chapter 49.

According to the Centers for Disease Control and Prevention (CDC, 2019), more than 20 million people develop sexually transmitted infections (STIs) annually in the United States; almost half of all STIs occur in people 15 to 24 years of age. The CDC (2019) also reported that the incidence of STIs has increased over the past several years from 2013 through 2017, except in specific populations, such as men who have sex with men. Routine human papillomavirus (HPV) vaccination for all males has become the standard of preventative care since 2011, as recommended by the Advisory Committee on Immunization Practices (ACIP) (Meites, Szilagyi, Chesson, et al., 2019).

STIs affect people from all walks of life—from all social, educational, economic, and racial backgrounds. The single greatest risk factor for contracting an STI is the number of sexual partners. As the number of partners increases, so does the risk of exposure to a person infected with an STI. For men who have sex with men, the CDC recommends annual testing for human immune deficiency virus (HIV), syphilis, *Chlamydia*, gonorrhea, hepatitis B viral infection, and herpes simplex virus type 2, along with counseling (An, Bernstein, & Balaji, 2020; CDC, 2019). Additionally, it is now encouraged that primary providers screen for STI at extragenital sites such as the oropharyngeal and anal areas (Keenan, Thomas, & Cotler, 2020).

There are many causes of urethritis (gonococcal and nongonococcal), genital ulcers (genital herpes infections, primary syphilis, chancroid, granuloma inguinale, and lymphogranuloma venereum), genital warts (HPV), scabies, pediculosis pubis, molluscum contagiosum, hepatitis and enteric infections, proctitis, and acquired immune deficiency syndrome (AIDS). Trichomoniasis and STIs characterized by genital ulcers are thought to increase susceptibility to HIV infection. Trichomoniasis is associated with nonchlamydial, nongonococcal urethritis.

Current treatment guidelines for STIs are available from the CDC (2019; Kuehn, 2019). Treatment must target the patient as well as his sexual partners and sometimes an unborn child. A thorough history, including a sexual history, is crucial to identify patients at risk and to direct care and education. It is essential for patient education to focus on partner safety as people can misjudge partner safety with known acquaintances, thus causing individuals to be at greater risk of STI/HIV transmission (Dennin & Sinn, 2020).

Partners of men with STIs must also be examined, treated, and counseled to prevent reinfection and complications in both partners and to limit the spread of the disease. Sexual abstinence during treatment and recovery is advised to prevent the transmission of STIs. The use of synthetic condoms for at least 6 months after completion of treatment is recommended to decrease transmission of HPV infection as well as other STIs. It is important to assess and test for other STIs because patients who have one STI may also have another. The use of spermicides with nonoxynol-9 (known as N-9) is discouraged; these agents do not protect against HIV infection and may increase the risk of transmission of the virus. See Chapters 32 and 66 for more detailed discussions of HIV infection, AIDS, and other STIs.

PROSTATIC DISORDERS

Prostatitis

Prostatitis is an inflammation of the prostate gland that is often associated with lower urinary tract symptoms and symptoms of sexual discomfort and dysfunction. The condition affects 5% to 10% of men. It is the most common urologic diagnosis in men younger than 50 years and the third most common such diagnosis in men older than 50 years (Cheng et al., 2019). Prostatitis may be caused by infectious agents (bacteria, fungi, mycoplasma) or other conditions (e.g., urethral stricture, BPH). *Escherichia coli* is the most commonly isolated organism, although *Klebsiella* and *Proteus* species are also found (Wu, Jiang, Tan, et al., 2020). The microorganisms colonize the urinary tract and ascend to the prostate, ultimately causing infection. The causal pathogen is usually the same in recurrent infections.

There are four types of prostatitis: acute bacterial prostatitis (type I), chronic bacterial prostatitis (type II), chronic prostatitis/chronic pelvic pain syndrome (CP/CPPS) (type III), and asymptomatic inflammatory prostatitis (type IV). Type III, which occurs in more than 90% of cases, is further classified as type IIIA or type IIIB, depending on the presence (type IIIA) or absence (type IIIB) of white blood cells in semen after prostate massage (Rhoades & Bell, 2017).

Clinical Manifestations

Acute prostatitis is characterized by the sudden onset of fever, dysuria, perineal prostatic pain, and severe lower urinary tract symptoms including dysuria, frequency, urgency, hesitancy, and nocturia. Approximately 5% of cases of type I prostatitis (acute bacterial prostatitis) progress to type II prostatitis (chronic bacterial prostatitis) (Cheng et al., 2019). Patients with type II disease are typically asymptomatic between episodes. Patients with type III prostatitis often have no bacteria in the urine in the presence of genitourinary pain. Patients with type IV prostatitis are usually diagnosed incidentally during a workup for infertility, an elevated PSA test, or other disorders.

Medical Management

The goal of treatment is to eradicate the causal organisms. Hospital admission may be necessary for patients with unstable vital signs, sepsis, or intractable pelvic pain; those who are frail or immunosuppressed; or those who have diabetes or renal insufficiency. Specific treatment is based on the type of prostatitis and on the results of culture and sensitivity testing of the urine (Farmer, Johnston, Milica, et al., 2019). If bacteria are cultured from the urine, antibiotic agents, including trimethoprim-sulfamethoxazole or a fluoroquinolone (e.g., ciprofloxacin), may be prescribed, and continuous therapy with low-dose antibiotic agents may be used. If the patient is afebrile and has a normal urinalysis, anti-inflammatory agents may be used. Alpha-adrenergic blocker therapy (e.g., tamsulosin) may be prescribed to promote bladder and prostate relaxation.

Factors contributing to prostatitis, including stress, neuromuscular factors, and myofascial pain, are also addressed. Supportive, nonpharmacologic therapies may be prescribed. These include biofeedback, pelvic floor training, physical therapy, reduction of prostatic fluid retention by ejaculation through penile-vaginal intercourse or masturbation, sitz baths, stool softeners, and evaluation of sexual partners to reduce the possibility of cross-infection.

Nursing Management

If the patient experiences symptoms of acute prostatitis (fever, severe pain and discomfort, inability to urinate, malaise), he may be hospitalized for intravenous (IV) antibiotic therapy. Nursing management includes administration of prescribed antibiotic agents and provision of comfort measures, including prescribed analgesic agents and sitz baths.

The patient with chronic prostatitis is usually treated on an outpatient basis and needs to be educated about the importance of continuing antibiotic therapy and recognizing recurrent signs and symptoms of prostatitis.

Promoting Home, Community-Based, and Transitional Care

 Educating Patients About Self-Care

The nurse educates the patient about the importance of completing the prescribed course of antibiotic therapy. If IV antibiotic agents are to be given at home, the nurse educates the patient and family about correct and safe administration. Arrangements for a home health nurse to oversee administration may be needed. Warm sitz baths (10 to 20 minutes) may be taken several times daily. Fluids are encouraged to satisfy thirst but are not "forced," because an effective medication level must be maintained in the urine. Foods and liquids with diuretic action or that increase prostatic secretions, such as alcohol, coffee, tea, chocolate, cola, and spices, should be avoided. A suprapubic catheter may be necessary for severe urinary retention. During periods of acute inflammation, any sexual activity should be avoided. To minimize discomfort, the patient should avoid sitting for long periods. Medical follow-up is necessary for at least 6 months to 1 year, because prostatitis caused by the same or different organisms can recur. The patient is advised that the UTI may recur and is educated to recognize its symptoms.

Benign Prostatic Hyperplasia (Enlarged Prostate)

Benign prostatic hyperplasia (BPH), a noncancerous enlargement or hypertrophy of the prostate, is one of the most common diseases in aging men. It can cause bothersome lower urinary tract symptoms that affect quality of life by interfering with normal daily activities and sleep patterns (Cheng et al., 2019). BPH typically occurs in men older than 40 years. By the time they reach 60 years, 50% of men will have BPH. It affects as many as 90% of men by 85 years of age. BPH is the second most common cause of surgical intervention in men older than 60 years.

Pathophysiology

The cause of BPH is not well understood, but testicular androgens have been implicated. Dihydrotestosterone (DHT), a metabolite of testosterone, is a critical mediator of prostatic growth. Estrogens may also play a role in the cause of BPH; BPH generally occurs when men have elevated estrogen levels and when prostate tissue becomes more sensitive to estrogens and less responsive to DHT. Smoking, heavy alcohol consumption, obesity, reduced activity level, hypertension, heart disease, diabetes, and a Western diet (high in animal fat and protein and refined carbohydrates, low in fiber) are risk factors for BPH (Cheng et al., 2019; El Jalby, Thomas, Elterman, et al., 2019).

BPH develops over a prolonged period; changes in the urinary tract are slow and insidious. BPH is a result of complex interactions involving resistance in the prostatic urethra to mechanical and spastic effects, bladder pressure during voiding, detrusor muscle strength, neurologic functioning, and general physical health (McCance et al., 2018). The hypertrophied lobes of the prostate may obstruct the bladder neck or urethra, causing incomplete emptying of the bladder and urinary retention. As a result, hydroureter (dilation of the ureters) and hydronephrosis (dilation of the kidneys) can gradually occur. Urinary retention may result in UTIs because urine that remains in the urinary tract serves as a medium for infective organisms.

Clinical Manifestations

BPH may or may not lead to lower urinary tract symptoms; if symptoms occur, they may range from mild to severe. Severity of symptoms increases with age, and half of men with BPH report having moderate to severe symptoms. Obstructive and irritative symptoms may include urinary frequency, urgency, nocturia, hesitancy in starting urination, decreased and intermittent force of stream and the sensation of incomplete bladder emptying, abdominal straining with urination, a decrease in the volume and force of the urinary stream, dribbling (urine dribbles out after urination), and complications of acute urinary retention and recurrent UTIs. Normally, residual urine amounts to no more than 50 mL in the middle-aged adult and less than 50 to 100 mL in the older adult (Weber & Kelley, 2018). Ultimately, chronic urinary retention and large residual volumes can lead to azotemia (accumulation of nitrogenous waste products) and kidney failure.

Generalized symptoms may also be noted, including fatigue, anorexia, nausea, vomiting, and pelvic discomfort. Other disorders that produce similar symptoms include urethral stricture, prostate cancer, neurogenic bladder, and urinary bladder stones.

Assessment and Diagnostic Findings

The health history focuses on the urinary tract, previous surgical procedures, general health issues, family history of prostate disease, and fitness for possible surgery (DeNunzio, Lombardo, Cicione, et al., 2020). A voiding diary is used by the patient to record voiding frequency and urine volume. A DRE often reveals a large, rubbery, and nontender prostate gland. A urinalysis to screen for hematuria and UTI is recommended. A PSA level is obtained if the patient is without a terminal disease and for whom knowledge of the presence of prostate cancer would change management. The American Urological Association (AUA) Symptom Index or International Prostate Symptom Score (IPSS) can be used to assess the severity of symptoms (Smith et al., 2019).

Other diagnostic tests may include recording urinary flow rate and the measurement of postvoid residual urine. If invasive therapy is considered, urodynamic studies, urethrocystoscopy, and ultrasound may be performed. Complete blood studies are performed. Cardiac status and respiratory function are assessed because a high percentage of patients with BPH have cardiac or respiratory disorders due to their age.

Medical Management

The goals of medical management of BPH are to improve quality of life, improve urine flow, relieve obstruction, prevent disease progression, and minimize complications. Treatment depends on the severity of symptoms, the cause of disease, the severity of the obstruction, and the patient's condition.

If a patient is admitted on an emergency basis because he is unable to void, he is immediately catheterized. The ordinary catheter may be too soft and pliable to advance through the urethra into the bladder. In such cases, a stylet (thin wire) is introduced (by a urologist) into the catheter to prevent the catheter from collapsing when it encounters resistance. A metal catheter with a pronounced prostatic curve may be used if obstruction is severe. A **cystostomy** (incision into the bladder) may be needed to provide urinary drainage.

Discussion of all treatment options by the primary provider enables the patient to make an informed decision based on symptom severity, the effect of BPH on his quality of life, and preference. Patients with mild symptoms and those with moderate or severe symptoms, who are not bothered by them and have not developed complications, may be managed with "watchful waiting." With this approach, the patient is monitored and reexamined annually but receives no active intervention (DeNunzio et al., 2020). Other therapeutic choices include pharmacologic treatment, minimally invasive procedures, and surgery.

Pharmacologic Therapy

Pharmacologic treatment for BPH includes the use of alpha-adrenergic blockers and 5-alpha-reductase inhibitors (Cheng et al., 2019). Alpha-adrenergic blockers, which include alfuzosin, terazosin, doxazosin, and tamsulosin, relax the smooth muscle of the bladder neck and prostate. This improves urine flow and relieves symptoms of BPH. Side effects include dizziness, headache, asthenia/fatigue, orthostatic hypotension, rhinitis, and sexual dysfunction (Chapple, Steers, & Evans, 2020; Cheng et al., 2019).

Another method of treatment involves hormonal manipulation with antiandrogen agents. The 5-alpha-reductase inhibitors, finasteride and dutasteride, are used to prevent the conversion of testosterone to DHT and decrease prostate size. Side effects include decreased libido, ejaculatory dysfunction, erectile dysfunction, gynecomastia (breast enlargement), and flushing. Combination therapy (doxazosin and finasteride) has decreased symptoms and reduced clinical progression of BPH (Chapple et al., 2020; Cheng et al., 2019).

The use of alternative and complementary phytotherapeutic agents and other dietary supplements (*Serenoa repens* [saw palmetto berry] and *Pygeum africanum* [African plum]) are not recommended by the medical community, although they are commonly used (Rowland, McNabney, & Donarski, 2019). They may function by interfering with the conversion of testosterone to DHT. In addition, *S. repens* may directly block the ability of DHT to stimulate prostate cell growth. These agents should not be used with finasteride, dutasteride, or estrogen-containing medications (Rowland et al., 2019).

Surgical Management

Other treatment options include minimally invasive procedures and resection of the prostate gland.

Minimally Invasive Therapy

Several forms of minimally invasive therapy may be used to treat BPH. Transurethral microwave thermotherapy involves the application of heat to prostatic tissue. High-energy devices (CoreTherm, Prostatron, Targis) and low-energy devices (TherMatrx) are available (Cheng et al., 2019). A transurethral probe is inserted into the urethra, and microwaves are directed to the prostate tissue. The targeted tissue becomes necrotic and sloughs. To minimize damage to the urethra and decrease the discomfort from the procedure, some systems have a water-cooling apparatus.

Other minimally invasive treatment options include transurethral needle ablation by radiofrequency energy and insertion of a stent. Transurethral needle ablation uses low-level radiofrequencies delivered by thin needles placed in the prostate gland to produce localized heat that destroys prostate tissue while sparing other tissues. The body then reabsorbs the dead tissue. Prostatic stents are associated with significant complications (e.g., encrustation, infection, chronic pain); therefore, they are used only for patients with urinary retention and in patients who are at poor surgical risks (Cheng et al., 2019).

Surgical Resection

Surgical resection of the prostate gland is another option for patients with moderate to severe lower urinary tract symptoms of BPH and for those with acute urinary retention or other complications. The specific surgical approach (open or endoscopic) and the energy source (electrocautery vs. laser) are based on the surgeon's experience, the size of the prostate gland, the presence of other medical disorders, and the patient's preference. If surgery is to be performed, all clotting defects must be corrected and medications for anticoagulation withheld because bleeding is a potential complication of prostate surgery.

Transurethral resection of the prostate (TURP) remains the benchmark for surgical treatment for BPH. It involves the surgical removal of the inner portion of the prostate through an endoscope inserted through the urethra; no external skin incision is made. It can be performed with ultrasound guidance. The treated tissue either vaporizes or becomes necrotic and sloughs. The procedure is performed in the outpatient setting and usually results in less postoperative bleeding than a traditional surgical prostatectomy.

Other surgical options for BPH include transurethral incision of the prostate (TUIP), transurethral electrovaporization, laser therapy, and open prostatectomy (Chapple et al., 2020; Smith et al., 2019). TUIP is an outpatient procedure used to treat smaller prostates. One or two cuts are made in the prostate and prostate capsule to reduce constriction of the urethra and decrease resistance to flow of urine out of the bladder; no tissue is removed. Open **prostatectomy** involves the surgical removal of the inner portion of the prostate via a suprapubic, retropubic, or perineal (rare) approach for large prostate glands. Prostatectomy may also be performed laparoscopically or by robotic-assisted laparoscopy.

Nursing management of patients undergoing these procedures is described later in this chapter.

Cancer of the Prostate

Prostate cancer is the most common cancer in men other than nonmelanoma skin cancer. It is the second most common cause of cancer death in American men, exceeded only by lung cancer, and is responsible for 10% of cancer-related deaths in men. Among men diagnosed with prostate cancer, 98% survive at least 5 years, 84% survive at least 10 years, and 56% survive 15 years (ACS, 2020).

Prostate cancer is common in the United States and northwestern Europe but is rare in Africa, Central America, South America, China, and other parts of Asia. African American men have a high risk of prostate cancer; furthermore, they are more than twice as likely to die of prostate cancer as men of other racial or ethnic groups. Health care providers need to offer education about prostate cancer and appropriate screening in African American men, who are at higher risk compared to all other ethnic communities (Riviere, Luterstein, Kumar, et al., 2020). Health care providers should also ensure the delivery of culturally sensitive education programs and counseling about prostate cancer screening not only to the African American patient at risk for prostate cancer, but also to his friends and family (Kelly, Morgan, Connelly, et al., 2019; Owens, Kim, & Tavakoli, 2019).

Other risk factors for prostate cancer include increasing age; the incidence of prostate cancer increases rapidly after the age of 50 years. More than 70% of cases occur in men older than 65 years. A familial predisposition may occur in men who have a father or brother previously diagnosed with prostate cancer, especially if their relatives were diagnosed at a young age. Genes that may be associated with increased risk of prostate cancer include hereditary prostate cancer 1 (*HPC1*) and *BRCA1* and *BRCA2* mutations (Cheng et al., 2019). The risk of prostate cancer is also greater in men whose diet contains excessive amounts of red meat or dairy products that are high in fat (ACS, 2020). Endogenous hormones, such as androgens and estrogens, also may be associated with the development of prostate cancer.

Clinical Manifestations

Cancer of the prostate in its early stages rarely produces symptoms. Usually, symptoms that develop from urinary obstruction occur in advanced disease. Prostate cancer tends to vary in its course. If the cancer is large enough to encroach on the bladder neck, signs and symptoms of urinary obstruction occur (difficulty and frequency of urination, urinary retention, and decreased size and force of the urinary stream). Other symptoms may include blood in the urine or semen and painful ejaculation. Hematuria may occur if the cancer invades the urethra or bladder. Sexual dysfunction is common before the diagnosis is made.

Prostate cancer can spread to lymph nodes and bones. Symptoms of metastases include backache, hip pain, perineal and rectal discomfort, anemia, weight loss, weakness, nausea, oliguria (decreased urine output), and spontaneous pathologic fractures. These symptoms may be the first indications of prostate cancer.

Assessment and Diagnostic Findings

If prostate cancer is detected early, the likelihood of cure is high (Brant, 2019). It can be diagnosed through an abnormal finding with the DRE, serum PSA, and TRUS with biopsy. Detection is more likely with the use of combined diagnostic procedures. Routine repeated DRE (preferably by the same examiner) is important because early cancer may be detected as a nodule within the gland or as an extensive hardening in the posterior lobe. The more advanced lesion is "stony hard" and fixed. DRE also provides useful clinical information about the rectum, anal sphincter, and quality of stool.

The diagnosis of prostate cancer is confirmed by a histologic examination of tissue removed surgically by TURP, open prostatectomy, or ultrasound-guided transrectal needle biopsy. Fine-needle aspiration is a quick, painless method of obtaining prostate cells for cytologic examination and determining the stage of disease.

Most prostate cancers are detected when a man seeks medical attention for symptoms of urinary obstruction or are found by routine DRE and PSA testing. Cancer detected incidentally when TURP is performed for clinically benign disease and lower urinary tract symptoms occurs in about 1 of 10 cases.

 Concept Mastery Alert

DRE and PSA testing are important screening procedures because abnormal DRE and elevated levels of PSA may raise suspicion of prostate cancer. However, a diagnosis of cancer requires confirmation with a prostate biopsy.

TRUS helps detect nonpalpable prostate cancers and assists with staging of localized prostate cancer. Needle biopsies of the prostate are commonly guided by TRUS. The biopsies are examined by a pathologist to both determine if cancer is present and to grade the tumor. The most commonly used tumor grading system is the Gleason score. This system assigns a grade of 1 to 5 for the most predominant architectural pattern of the glands of the prostate and a secondary grade of 1 to 5 to the second most predominant pattern. The Gleason score is then reported as, for example, 2 + 4; the combined value can range from 2 to 10. With each increase in Gleason score, there is an increase in tumor aggressiveness. Lower Gleason scores indicate well-differentiated and less aggressive tumor cells; higher Gleason scores indicate undifferentiated cells and more aggressive cancer. A total score of 8 to 10 indicates a high-grade cancer (Smith et al., 2019; Zhou, Salles, Samarska, et al., 2019).

Categorization of low-, intermediate-, and high-risk prostate cancer is determined by the extent of cancer in the prostate gland, whether or not the cancer is localized to the prostate, the aggressiveness of the cells, and the spread to the lymph nodes and beyond. Level of risk, in turn, is used to determine treatment options.

Bone scans, skeletal x-rays, and magnetic resonance imaging (MRI) may be used to identify metastatic bone disease. Pelvic computed tomography (CT) scans may be performed to determine if the cancer has spread to the lymph nodes. The radiolabeled monoclonal antibody capromab pendetide with indium 111 is an antibody that can be used to detect either recurrent prostate cancer at low PSA levels or metastatic disease (NCCN, 2020b).

Medical Management

Treatment is based on the patient's life expectancy, symptoms, risk of recurrence after definitive treatment, size of the tumor, Gleason score, PSA level, likelihood of complications, and patient preference. Therapy is often guided by the use of a nomogram or risk stratification scheme suggested by the NCCN (2020b) clinical practice guidelines. A multidisciplinary team approach is essential for the development of appropriate treatment. Management may be nonsurgical and involve watchful waiting or be surgical and entail prostatectomy. Nursing care of the patient with cancer of the prostate is summarized in Chart 53-3.

For patients with prostate cancer who choose nonsurgical watchful waiting, this approach involves actively monitoring the course of disease and intervening only if the cancer progresses or if symptoms warrant other intervention. It is an option for patients with life expectancy of less than 5 years and low-risk cancers. Advantages include absence of side effects of more aggressive treatment, improved quality of life, avoidance of unnecessary treatment, and decreased initial costs. Disadvantages include missed chance at cure, risk of metastasis, subsequent need for more aggressive treatment, anxiety about living with untreated cancer, and need for frequent monitoring (NCCN, 2020b).

Therapeutic vaccines kill existing cancer cells and provide long-lasting immunity against further cancer development. Sipuleucel-T is the first therapeutic cancer vaccine approved by the U.S. Food and Drug Administration (FDA) for use in men with metastatic prostate cancer that is no longer responding to hormone therapy. This is an immunotherapy treatment that stimulates the patient's own immune system to identify and target prostate cancer cells, and it has minimal side effects (Caram, Ross, Lin, et al., 2019).

In addition, two other medications, abiraterone acetate and cabazitaxel, are treatment options for patients requiring care for the management of metastatic castration–resistant prostate cancer, which does not respond to sipuleucel-T or the usual treatment options (Nuhn, De Bono, Fizazi, et al., 2019).

Surgical Management

Radical prostatectomy is considered first-line treatment for prostate cancer and is used with patients whose tumor is confined to the prostate (Smith et al., 2019). It is the complete surgical removal of the prostate, seminal vesicles, tips of the vas deferens, and often the surrounding fat, nerves, and blood vessels. Laparoscopic radical prostatectomy and robotic-assisted laparoscopic radical prostatectomy have become the standard surgical approaches for localized cancer of the prostate. Although erectile dysfunction is a common side effect, these laparoscopic radical prostatectomy approaches result in low morbidity and more favorable postoperative outcomes, including improved quality of life and less sexual dysfunction if the nerves are spared. Surgical approaches are discussed in detail later in this chapter.

Radiation Therapy

Two major forms of radiation therapy are used to treat cancer of the prostate: teletherapy (external) and **brachytherapy** (internal). Teletherapy (external-beam radiation therapy [EBRT]) is prescribed by the radiation oncologist for a total dose over a certain time frame—for example, 28 treatments over 5½ weeks (Cheng et al., 2019). It is a treatment option for patients with low-risk prostate cancer; progression-free

(text continued on page 1760)

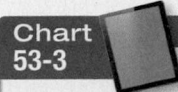

Chart 53-3

PLAN OF NURSING CARE
The Patient with Prostate Cancer

NURSING DIAGNOSIS: Anxiety associated with concern and lack of knowledge about the diagnosis, treatment plan, and prognosis
GOAL: Reduced stress and improved ability to cope

Nursing Interventions	Rationale	Expected Outcomes
1. Obtain health history to determine the following: a. Patient's concerns b. His level of understanding of his health problem c. His past experience with cancer d. Whether he knows his diagnosis of malignancy and its prognosis e. His support systems and coping methods 2. Provide education about diagnosis and treatment plan. a. Explain in simple terms what diagnostic tests to expect, how long they will take, and what will be experienced during each test. b. Review treatment plan and encourage patient to ask questions. 3. Assess his psychological reaction to his diagnosis/prognosis and how he has coped with past stresses. 4. Provide information about institutional and community resources for coping with prostate cancer: social services, support services, community agencies.	1. Nurse clarifies information and facilitates patient's understanding and coping. 2. Helping the patient to understand the diagnostic tests and treatment plan will help decrease his anxiety and promote cooperation. 3. This information provides clues in determining appropriate measures to facilitate coping. 4. Institutional and community resources can help the patient and family cope with the illness and treatment on an ongoing basis.	• Appears relaxed • States that anxiety has been reduced or relieved • Demonstrates understanding of illness, diagnostic tests, and treatment when questioned • Verbalizes adequate coping ability • Engages in open communication with others

NURSING DIAGNOSIS: Urinary retention associated with inability to empty bladder completely
GOAL: Improved pattern of urinary elimination

Nursing Interventions	Rationale	Expected Outcomes
1. Determine patient's usual pattern of urinary function. 2. Assess for signs and symptoms of urinary retention: amount and frequency of urination, suprapubic distention, complaints of urgency and discomfort. 3. Initiate measures to treat retention. a. Encourage assuming normal position for voiding. b. Recommend using Valsalva maneuver preoperatively, if not contraindicated. c. Administer prescribed medication. d. Monitor effects of medication. 4. Consult with primary provider regarding intermittent or indwelling catheterization; assist with procedure as required. 5. Monitor catheter function; maintain sterility of closed system; irrigate as required. 6. Prepare patient for surgery if indicated.	1. Provides a baseline for comparison and goal to work toward. 2. Voiding 20 to 30 mL frequently and output less than intake suggest retention. 3. Promotes voiding: a. Usual position provides relaxed conditions conducive to voiding. b. Valsalva maneuver exerts pressure to force urine out of bladder. c. Stimulates bladder contraction. d. If unsuccessful, another measure may be required. 4. Catheterization will relieve urinary retention until the specific cause is determined; it may be an obstruction that can be corrected only surgically. 5. Adequate functioning of catheter is to be ensured to empty bladder and to prevent infection. 6. Surgical removal of obstruction may be necessary.	• Voids at normal intervals • Reports absence of frequency, urgency, or bladder fullness • Displays no palpable suprapubic distention after voiding • Maintains balanced intake and output

(continued on page 1758)

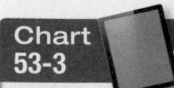

Chart 53-3 PLAN OF NURSING CARE (continued)
The Patient with Prostate Cancer

NURSING DIAGNOSIS: Lack of knowledge associated with the diagnosis of cancer, urinary difficulties, and treatment modalities

GOAL: Understanding of the diagnosis and ability to care for self

Nursing Interventions	Rationale	Expected Outcomes
1. Encourage communication with the patient.	1. This is designed to establish rapport and trust.	• Discusses his concerns and problems freely
2. Review the anatomy of the involved area.	2. Orientation to one's anatomy is basic to understanding its function.	• Asks questions and shows interest in his disorder
3. Be specific in selecting information that is relevant to the patient's particular treatment plan.	3. This is based on the treatment plan because it varies with each patient, individualization is desirable.	• Describes activities that help or hinder recovery
4. Identify ways to reduce pressure on the operative area after prostatectomy.	4. This is to prevent bleeding; such precautions are in order for 6 to 8 weeks postoperatively.	• Identifies ways of attaining/maintaining bladder control
a. Instruct patient to avoid prolonged sitting (in a chair, long automobile rides), standing, walking.		• Demonstrates satisfactory technique and understanding of catheter care
b. Instruct patient to avoid straining, such as during exercises, bowel movement, lifting, and sexual activity.		• Lists signs and symptoms that must be reported should they occur (e.g., abnormal bleeding, infection)
5. Familiarize patient with ways of attaining/maintaining bladder control.	5. These measures will help control frequency and dribbling and aid in preventing retention.	
a. Encourage urination every 2 to 3 hours; discourage voiding when supine.	a. By sitting or standing, patient is more likely to empty his bladder.	
b. Instruct patient to avoid drinking cola and caffeine beverages; urge a cutoff time in the evening for drinking fluids to minimize frequent voiding during the night.	b. Spacing the kind and amount of liquid intake will help to prevent frequency.	
c. Describe perineal exercises to be performed every hour.	c. Exercises will assist him in starting and stopping the urinary stream.	
d. Develop a schedule with patient that will fit into his routine.	d. A schedule will assist in developing a workable pattern of normal activities.	
6. Demonstrate catheter care; encourage his questions; stress the importance of position of urinary receptacle.	6. By requiring a return demonstration of care, collection, and emptying of the device, he will become more independent and also can prevent backflow of urine, which can lead to infection.	

NURSING DIAGNOSIS: Impaired nutritional intake associated with decreased oral intake because of anorexia, nausea, and vomiting caused by cancer or its treatment

GOAL: Maintain optimal nutritional status

Nursing Interventions	Rationale	Expected Outcomes
1. Assess the amount of food eaten.	1. This assessment will help determine nutrient intake.	• Responds positively to his favorite foods
2. Routinely weigh patient.	2. Weighing the patient on the same scale under similar conditions can help monitor changes in weight.	• Assumes responsibility for his oral hygiene
3. Elicit patient's explanation of why he is unable to eat more.	3. His explanation may present easily corrected practices.	• Reports absence of nausea and vomiting
4. Cater to his individual food preferences (e.g., avoiding foods that are too spicy or too cold).	4. He will be more likely to consume larger servings if food is palatable and appealing.	• Notes increase in weight after improved appetite
5. Recognize effect of medication or radiation therapy on appetite.	5. Many chemotherapeutic agents and radiation therapy promote anorexia.	
6. Inform patient that alterations in taste can occur.	6. Aging and the disease process can reduce taste sensitivity. In addition, smell and taste can be altered as a result of the body's absorption of by-products of cellular destruction (brought on by malignancy and its treatment).	

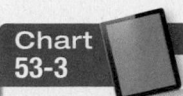

Chart 53-3

PLAN OF NURSING CARE (continued)
The Patient with Prostate Cancer

Nursing Interventions	Rationale	Expected Outcomes
7. Educate patient about appropriate oral hygiene interventions.	7. Food will be more palatable and appealing following good oral hygiene.	
8. Use measures to control nausea and vomiting. a. Administer prescribed antiemetic agents, around the clock if necessary. b. Provide oral hygiene after vomiting episodes. c. Provide rest periods after meals.	8. Prevention of nausea and vomiting can stimulate appetite.	
9. Provide frequent small meals and a comfortable and pleasant environment.	9. Smaller portions of food are more tolerable for the patient.	
10. Assess patient's ability to obtain and prepare foods.	10. Disability or lack of social support can hinder the patient's ability to obtain and prepare foods.	

NURSING DIAGNOSIS: Impaired sexual functioning associated with effects of therapy: chemotherapy, hormonal therapy, radiation therapy, surgery
GOAL: Ability to resume/enjoy modified sexual functioning

Nursing Interventions	Rationale	Expected Outcomes
1. Determine from nursing history what effect patient's medical condition is having on his sexual functioning.	1. Usually, decreased libido and, later, erectile dysfunction may be experienced.	• Describes the reasons for changes in sexual functioning • Discusses with appropriate health care personnel alternative approaches and methods of sexual expression • Includes partner in discussions related to changes in sexual function
2. Inform patient of the effects of prostate surgery, orchiectomy (when applicable), chemotherapy, irradiation, and hormonal therapy on sexual function.	2. Treatment modalities may alter sexual function, but each is evaluated separately regarding its effect on a particular patient.	
3. Include his partner in developing understanding and in discovering alternative, satisfying close relations with each other.	3. The bond between a couple may be strengthened with new appreciation and support that had not been evident before the current illness.	

NURSING DIAGNOSIS: Acute pain associated with progression of disease and treatment modalities
GOAL: Relief of pain

Nursing Interventions	Rationale	Expected Outcomes
1. Evaluate nature of patient's pain, its location, and intensity using pain rating scale.	1. Determining nature and causes of pain and its intensity help to select proper pain relief modality and provide baseline for later comparison.	• Reports relief of pain • Expects exacerbations, reports their quality and intensity, and obtains relief • Uses pain relief strategies appropriately and effectively • Identifies strategies to avoid complications of analgesic use (e.g., constipation)
2. Avoid activities that aggravate or worsen pain.	2. Bumping the bed is an example of an action that can intensify the patient's pain.	
3. Because pain is usually related to bone metastasis, ensure that patient's bed has a bed board or a firm mattress. In addition, protect the patient from falls/injuries.	3. This will provide added support and is more comfortable. Protecting the patient from injury protects him from additional pain.	
4. Provide support for affected extremities.	4. More support, coupled with reduced movement of the part, helps in pain control.	
5. Prepare patient for radiation therapy if prescribed.	5. Radiation therapy may be effective in controlling pain.	
6. Administer analgesic or opioid agents at regularly scheduled intervals as prescribed.	6. Analgesic agents alter perception of pain and provide comfort. Regularly scheduled analgesics around the clock rather than PRN (as needed) provide more consistent pain relief.	
7. Initiate bowel program to prevent constipation.	7. Opioid analgesic agents and inactivity contribute to constipation.	

(continued on page 1760)

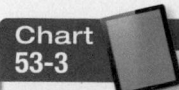

Chart 53-3

PLAN OF NURSING CARE (continued)
The Patient with Prostate Cancer

NURSING DIAGNOSIS: Impaired mobility associated with limitations in independent, purposeful movement of the body or one or more extremities
GOAL: Improved physical mobility

Nursing Interventions	Rationale	Expected Outcomes
1. Assess for factors causing limited mobility (e.g., pain, hypercalcemia, limited exercise tolerance). 2. Provide pain relief by administering prescribed medications. 0. Encourage the use of assistive devices: cane, walker. 4. Involve significant others in helping patient with range-of-motion exercises, positioning, and walking. 5. Provide positive reinforcement for achievement of small gains. 6. Assess nutritional status.	1. This information offers clues to the cause; if possible, cause is treated. 2. Analgesic/opioid agents allow the patient to increase his activity more comfortably. 3. Support may offer the security needed to become mobile. 4. Assistance from partner or others encourages patient to repeat activities and achieve goals. 5. Encouragement stimulates improvement of performance. 6. See Nursing Diagnosis: Impaired nutritional intake	• Achieves improved physical mobility • Relates that short-term goals are encouraging him because they are attainable

COLLABORATIVE PROBLEMS: Hemorrhage, infection, bladder neck obstruction
GOAL: Absence of complications

Nursing Interventions	Rationale	Expected Outcomes

1. Alert the patient to changes that may occur (after discharge) and that need to be reported:
  a. Continued bloody urine; passing blood clots
  b. Pain; burning around the catheter
 	
  c. Frequency of urination
 	
  d. Diminished urinary output
 	
  e. Increasing loss of bladder control
	1. Certain changes signal beginning complications, which call for nursing and medical interventions.
	  a. Hematuria with or without blood clot formation may occur postoperatively.
	  b. Indwelling urinary catheters may be a source of pain or infection.
	  c. Urinary frequency may be caused by urinary tract infections or by bladder neck obstruction, resulting in incomplete voiding.
	  d. Bladder neck obstruction decreases the amount of urine that is voided.
	  e. Urinary incontinence may be a result of urinary retention.
		• Experiences no bleeding or passage of blood clots
		• Reports no infection or pain around the catheter
		• Experiences normal frequency or urination
		• Reports normal urinary output
		• Maintains bladder control

survival is similar to that of low-risk patients treated with radical prostatectomy. Patients with intermediate- and high-risk cancers receive higher doses of EBRT. They may also be candidates for both pelvic lymph node irradiation and **androgen deprivation therapy** that entails surgical (orchiectomy) or medical castration (e.g., with luteinizing hormone–releasing hormone agonists) (NCCN, 2020b). Intensity-modulated radiation therapy is one method of delivery of EBRT. Intensity-modulated radiation therapy sets a dose for the target volume and restricts the dose to surrounding tissue. Another approach to delivery of radiation uses a computer-controlled robotic arm to deliver a course of radiotherapy (i.e., stereotactic radiosurgery) to localized prostate cancer. This method, referred to as the CyberKnife, is considered a safe and reliable method of delivering radiation to treat prostate cancer (Pollom, Wang, Gibbs, et al., 2019).

Brachytherapy involves the implantation of interstitial radioactive seeds under anesthesia. It has become a commonly used monotherapy treatment option for early, clinically organ-confined prostate cancer. The surgeon uses ultrasound guidance to place 80 to 100 seeds (depending on the prostate volume), and the patient returns home after the procedure. Exposure of others to radiation is minimal, but the patient should avoid close contact with pregnant women and infants for up to 2 months. Radiation safety guidelines include straining urine for seeds and using a condom during penile-vaginal intercourse for 2 weeks after implantation to catch any seeds that pass through the urethra. This approach can be completed in 1 day, with little lost time from normal activities. Brachytherapy may be combined with EBRT with or without neoadjuvant androgen deprivation therapy for patients considered at intermediate risk. High-risk patients are considered poor candidates for permanent brachytherapy (Brant, 2019).

Although cure rates with radiation are comparable to those of radical prostatectomy, radiation therapy possesses its own unique set of side effects, which differ depending on the method of radiation administration. Patients receiving EBRT or brachytherapy may experience inflammation of the rectum, bowel, and bladder (proctitis, enteritis, and cystitis) because of the proximity of these structures to the prostate and the radiation doses. Inflammation and mucosal loss at the bladder neck, prostate, and urethra can cause acute urinary dysfunction. Both irritative and obstructive urinary symptoms can cause pain with urination and ejaculation until the irritation subsides. Rectal urgency, diarrhea, and tenesmus may occur as a result of radiation of the anterior rectal wall. Late side effects include rectal proctitis, bleeding, and rectal fistula; painless hematuria; chronic interstitial cystitis; urethral stricture erectile dysfunction; and, rarely, secondary cancers of the rectum and bladder (Brant, 2019).

Hormonal Strategies

The number of survivors of prostate cancer in the United States is estimated at 2 million; approximately one third of these men currently receive androgen deprivation therapy (Jeong, Cowan, Broering, et al., 2019). Androgen deprivation therapy is commonly used to suppress androgenic stimuli to the prostate by decreasing the level of circulating plasma testosterone or interrupting the conversion to or binding of DHT. As a result, the prostatic epithelium atrophies (decreases in size). This effect is accomplished either by surgical castration through bilateral **orchiectomy** (removal of one or both testes), which has traditionally been the mainstay of hormonal treatment, or by medical castration with the administration of medications, such as luteinizing hormone–releasing hormone (LHRH) agonists. Bilateral orchiectomy decreases plasma testosterone levels significantly because approximately 93% of circulating testosterone is of testicular origin (7% is from the adrenal glands). Thus, the testicular stimulus required for continued prostatic growth is removed, resulting in prostatic atrophy.

However, orchiectomy often results in significant morbidity. Although the procedure does not cause the side effects associated with other hormonal therapies (described later), it is associated with considerable emotional impact. Because patients who have prostate cancer are living longer with the disease, health care providers are focusing on effective therapeutic modalities that promote an acceptable quality of life. Patients may be given the option for testicular prostheses to be placed during surgery.

LHRH agonists include leuprolide and goserelin. Additional hormonal manipulation with antiandrogens may be prescribed for patients who do not show adequate serum testosterone suppression (less than 50 ng/mL) with medical or surgical castration. Antiandrogen receptor antagonists include flutamide, bicalutamide, and nilutamide. LHRH agonists suppress testicular androgen, whereas antiandrogen receptor antagonists cause adrenal androgen suppression. When LHRH agonists are initiated, a testosterone flare may occur, causing pain in bony metastatic disease. Antiandrogens given for the first 7 days may reduce this uncomfortable symptom. The most common uses of LHRH agonists are in the adjuvant and neoadjuvant setting in combination with radiation therapy, after radical prostatectomy, and in the treatment of recurrence indicated by an elevation in the PSA but without clinical or x-ray evidence. Medical and surgical castration causes hot flushing because these treatment modalities increase hypothalamic activity, which stimulates the thermoregulatory centers of the body (Kunath, Goebell, Wullich, et al., 2020; Shore, Guerrero, Sanahuja, et al., 2019).

The management of hormone-refractory prostate cancer remains somewhat controversial. Another category of medication used as a second-line hormonal intervention is the adrenal ablating drugs. Ketoconazole is used to inhibit cytochrome P450 enzymes, which are required for the synthesis of androgens and other steroids. High-dose ketoconazole lowers testosterone by decreasing both testicular and endocrine production of androgen. Administration of this medication requires steroid supplementation to prevent adrenal insufficiency.

Hypogonadism is responsible for the adverse effects of androgen deprivation therapy, which include vasomotor flushing, loss of libido, decreased bone density (resulting in osteoporosis and fractures), anemia, fatigue, increased fat mass, lipid alterations, decreased muscle mass, gynecomastia (increased breast tissue), and mastodynia (breast/nipple tenderness). Hypogonadism is associated with an increased risk of diabetes, resulting from insulin resistance, metabolic syndrome, and cardiovascular disease (Cheng et al., 2019).

Chemotherapy

Recent studies have shown clear benefits in terms of survival with chemotherapy treatment that includes a docetaxel-based regimen for non–androgen-dependent prostate cancer (NCCN, 2020b). Other studies are under way to determine the importance of the vascular endothelial growth factor system. Tumor angiogenesis is essential for tumor growth, including growth of prostate carcinomas and other high-grade cancers. Therefore, antiangiogenic treatment in combination with conventional therapies may play a future role in treatment. Gene-based therapy in prostate cancer is an emerging and promising adjuvant to conventional treatment strategies.

Possible complications related to chemotherapy are specific to the type of chemotherapy given (see Chapter 12, Chart 12-4).

Other Therapies

Cryosurgery of the prostate is used to ablate prostate cancer in patients who cannot tolerate surgery and in those with recurrent prostate cancer. Transperineal probes are inserted into the prostate under ultrasound guidance to freeze the tissue directly.

Keeping the urethral passage patent may require repeated TURPs. If this is impractical, catheter drainage is instituted by way of the suprapubic or transurethral route. For men with advanced prostate cancer, palliative measures are indicated. Although cure is unlikely with advanced prostate cancer, many men survive for long periods, free of debilitating symptoms.

Bone lesions that result from metastasis of prostate cancer can be very painful and result in pathologic fractures. Opioid and nonopioid medications are used to control bone pain. EBRT can be delivered to skeletal lesions to relieve pain. Radiopharmaceuticals, such as strontium or samarium, can be injected IV to treat multiple sites of bone metastasis. Antiandrogen therapies are used in an effort to reduce the circulating androgens. If antiandrogen therapies are not effective, medications such as prednisone have been effective in reducing pain and improving quality of life (Dong, Zieren, Xue, et al., 2019; Sargon, Lamb, & Patel, 2019). Bisphosphonate therapy with pamidronate can be given to reduce the risk of pathologic fracture. In advanced prostate cancer, blood transfusions are given to maintain adequate hemoglobin levels when bone marrow is replaced by tumor.

More than one third of men with a diagnosis of prostate cancer elect to use some form of complementary and integrative health. Because research on many forms of complementary, alternative, and integrative health is lacking, patients often rely on anecdotal information to make decisions about which modalities to use. Nurses and other health care professionals play a vital role in assisting patients to locate and evaluate available information about these practices to ensure that harmful forms are avoided (Brant, 2019). The National Center for Complementary and Integrative Health (NCCIH) website can assist nurses in providing patients with evidence-based information (see the Resources section at the end of the chapter).

The Patient Undergoing Prostate Surgery

Prostate surgery may be indicated for the patient with BPH or prostate cancer. The objectives before prostate surgery are to assess the patient's general health status and to establish optimal kidney function. Prostate surgery should be performed before acute urinary retention develops and damages the upper urinary tract and collecting system or, in the case of prostate cancer, before cancer progresses.

Surgical Procedures

Several approaches can be used to remove the hypertrophied portion of the prostate gland: TURP, suprapubic prostatectomy, perineal prostatectomy, retropubic prostatectomy, TUIP, and laparoscopic radical prostatectomy and robotic-assisted laparoscopic radical prostatectomy (see Table 53-4). With these approaches, all cancerous or hyperplastic tissue is removed, leaving behind only the capsule of the prostate.

Transurethral Resection of the Prostate

TURP, which is the most common procedure used, can be carried out through endoscopy. The prostate gland is removed in small chips with an electrical cutting loop (see Fig. 53-4A). This procedure decreases the risk of transurethral resection syndrome (hyponatremia, hypervolemia). Transurethral resection syndrome is a potential but rare complication of TURP that occurs in approximately 2% of men who undergo the procedure (Hahn, 2019) (see Chart 53-4).

Urethral strictures are more frequent than with nontransurethral procedures, and repeated procedures may be necessary because the residual prostatic tissue grows back. TURP rarely causes erectile dysfunction but may trigger retrograde ejaculation, because removal of prostatic tissue at the bladder neck can cause the seminal fluid to flow backward into the bladder rather than forward through the urethra during ejaculation.

Suprapubic Prostatectomy

A suprapubic prostatectomy is an open surgical procedure (see Fig. 53-4B). Disadvantages include blood loss, the need for an abdominal incision, and the risks associated with any major abdominal surgical procedure.

Perineal Prostatectomy

A perineal prostatectomy (see Fig. 53-4C) is practical when other approaches are not possible and is useful for an open biopsy. However, incontinence, sexual dysfunction, and rectal injury are more likely to occur with this approach.

Retropubic Prostatectomy

Retropubic prostatectomy is used more commonly than the suprapubic approach (see Fig. 53-4D). This procedure is suitable for large glands located high in the pelvis. Although blood loss can be better controlled and the surgical site is easier to visualize, infections can readily start in the retropubic space.

Transurethral Incision of the Prostate

TUIP is indicated when the prostate gland is small (30 g or less), and it is an effective treatment for many cases of BPH (see Fig. 53-4E). TUIP can be performed as an outpatient procedure and has a lower complication rate than other more invasive prostate procedures.

Laparoscopic Radical Prostatectomy

A laparoscopic radical prostatectomy has fewer risks compared with open radical prostatectomy (Smith et al., 2019).

Robotic-Assisted Laparoscopic Radical Prostatectomy

Robotic-assisted laparoscopic radical prostatectomy is a minimally invasive approach that uses a computer console and a robot to move instruments, replicating the movements of the surgeon's hands (Peard, Goodwin, Hensley, et al., 2019; Smith et al., 2019).

Pelvic Lymph Node Dissection

Pelvic lymph node dissection (PLND) is not always performed. It may be used in some patients to provide information for staging the tumor and to remove an area of microscopic metastasis. The planned treatment may influence the surgeon's decision to perform PLND and the extent (limited vs. extended) of the dissection. Dissection of nodes anterior and lateral to the external iliac vessels is associated with an increased risk of lymphedema (NCCN, 2020a).

Complications

Postoperative complications depend on the type of prostatectomy performed and may include hemorrhage, clot formation, catheter obstruction, and sexual dysfunction. All prostatectomies carry a risk of erectile dysfunction because of potential damage to the pudendal nerves. In most instances, sexual activity may be resumed in 6 to 8 weeks, which is the time required for the prostatic fossa to heal. The anatomic changes in the posterior urethra can lead to retrograde ejaculation. During ejaculation, the seminal fluid goes into the bladder and is excreted with the urine. A vasectomy may be performed during surgery to prevent infection from spreading from the prostatic urethra through the vas and into the epididymis.

After total prostatectomy (usually for cancer), the risk of erectile dysfunction is high. If this is unacceptable to the patient, options are available to produce erections sufficient for sexual activity: prosthetic penile implants, negative-pressure (vacuum) devices, and pharmacologic interventions (see earlier discussion and Table 53-2).

TABLE 53-4	Surgical Approaches for Treatment of Prostate Disorders		

The surgical approach of choice depends on the size of the gland, the severity of the obstruction, the age of the patient, the condition of the patient, and the presence of associated diseases.

Surgical Approach	Advantages	Disadvantages	Nursing Implications
Transurethral Resection of the Prostate (TURP) Removal of prostatic tissue by optical instrument introduced through urethra; used for glands of varying size. Ideal for patients who are at poor surgical risks (see Fig. 53-4A).	Avoids abdominal incision Safer for surgical-risk patient Shorter length of hospital stay and recovery periods Lower morbidity rate Causes less pain Can be used as a palliative approach with history of radiation therapy	Recurrent obstruction, urethral trauma, and stricture may develop Delayed bleeding may occur	Monitor for hemorrhage. Observe for symptoms of urethral stricture (dysuria, straining, weak urinary stream).
Open Surgical Removal *Suprapubic approach* Removal of prostatic tissue through abdominal incision; can be used for gland of any size (see Fig. 53-4B).	Technically simple Offers wide area of exploration Permits exploration for cancerous lymph nodes Allows more complete removal of obstructing gland Permits treatment of associated bladder lesions	Requires surgical approach through the bladder Control of hemorrhage is difficult Urine may leak around the suprapubic tube Recovery may be prolonged and uncomfortable	Monitor for indications of hemorrhage and shock. Provide meticulous aseptic care to the area around suprapubic tube.
Perineal approach Removal of gland through an incision in the perineum; preferred approach for patients with obesity (see Fig. 53-4C).	Offers direct anatomic approach Permits gravity drainage Particularly effective for radical cancer therapy Allows hemostasis under direct vision Low mortality rate Low incidence of shock Ideal for patients with large prostate who are very old, frail, and at poor surgical risks	Higher postoperative incidence of erectile dysfunction and urinary incontinence Possible damage to rectum and external sphincter Restricted operative field Greater potential for contamination and infection of incision	Avoid using rectal tubes or thermometers and enemas after perineal surgery. Use drainage pads to absorb excess urinary drainage. Provide foam rubber ring for patient comfort in sitting. Anticipate urinary leakage around the wound for several days after the catheter is removed.
Retropubic approach Low abdominal incision; bladder is not entered (see Fig. 53-4D).	Avoids incision into the bladder Permits surgeon to see and control bleeding Shorter recovery period Less bladder sphincter damage Suitable for removal of large glands	Cannot treat associated bladder disease Increased incidence of hemorrhage from prostatic venous plexus; osteitis pubis	Monitor for hemorrhage. Anticipate posturinary leakage for several days after removing the catheter.
Transurethral Incision of the Prostate (TUIP) Urethral approach; 1–2 cuts are made in the prostate and prostate capsule to reduce pressure on the urethra and to reduce urethral constriction (see Fig. 53-4E).	Results comparable to TURP Low incidence of erectile dysfunction and retrograde ejaculation No bladder neck contracture	Recurrent obstruction and urethral trauma Delayed bleeding	Monitor for hemorrhage.
Laparoscopic Radical Prostatectomy In this approach, 4–6 small (1 cm [0.5 inch]) incisions are made in the abdomen; laparoscopic instruments inserted through the incisions are used to dissect the prostate.	Minimally invasive technique Improved patient satisfaction and quality of life Shorter length of hospital stay Short convalescence More rapid return to normal activity Short indwelling catheter duration Decreased blood loss to 400 mL Reduced infection risk Less scarring Better visualization of surgical field than other approaches	Lack of tactile sensation available with open prostatectomy Inability to palpably assess for induration and palpable nodules Inability to delineate the proximity of involvement of the neurovascular bundles due to lack of palpation Long surgical time (4–5 h)	Observe for symptoms of urethral stricture (dysuria), straining, and weak urinary stream. Monitor for hemorrhage and shock. Provide meticulous aseptic care to area around suprapubic tube. Monitor for changes in bowel function. Avoid using rectal tubes or thermometers and enemas after perineal surgery. Use drainage pads to absorb excess urinary drainage. Provide foam rubber ring for patient comfort in sitting. Anticipate urinary leakage around the wound for several days after the catheter is removed.

(continued on page 1764)

TABLE 53-4 Surgical Approaches for Treatment of Prostate Disorders (continued)

Surgical Approach	Advantages	Disadvantages	Nursing Implications
Robotic-Assisted Laparoscopic Radical Prostatectomy Involves using computer console and da Vinci (see Chapter 14, Fig. 14-1). In this approach, 6 small (1 cm [0.5 inch]) incisions are made in the abdomen; laparoscopic instruments inserted through the incisions are used to dissect the prostate.	Minimally invasive technique Improved patient satisfaction and quality of life Shorter length of hospital stay Short convalescence More rapid return to normal activity Short indwelling catheter duration Decreased blood loss to 150 mL Improved magnification of operative field, using a three-dimensional view (includes, magnification, high resolution, and depth perception) Less postoperative pain Reduced risk of infection Less scarring Laparoscopic instruments have 6 degrees of movement with joints, allowing extensive range of motion and precision Nerve sparing with less incontinence and sexual dysfunction	Lack of tactile sensation available with open prostatectomy Inability to palpably assess for induration and palpable nodules Inability to delineate the proximity of involvement of the neurovascular bundles due to lack of palpation	Observe for symptoms of urethral stricture (dysuria), straining, and weak urinary stream. Monitor for hemorrhage and shock. Provide meticulous aseptic care to the area around suprapubic tube. Monitor for changes in bowel function. Avoid using rectal tubes or thermometers and enemas after perineal surgery. Use drainage pads to absorb excess urinary drainage. Provide foam rubber ring for patient comfort in sitting. Anticipate urinary leakage around the wound for several days after the catheter is removed.

Adapted from Cheng, L., MacLennan, G. T., & Bostwick, D. G. (2019). *Urologic surgical pathology* (4th ed.). Philadelphia, PA: Elsevier; Smith, J. A., Howards, S. S., Preminger, G. M., et al. (2019). *Hinman's atlas of urologic surgery* (4th ed.). Philadelphia, PA: Wolters Kluwer.

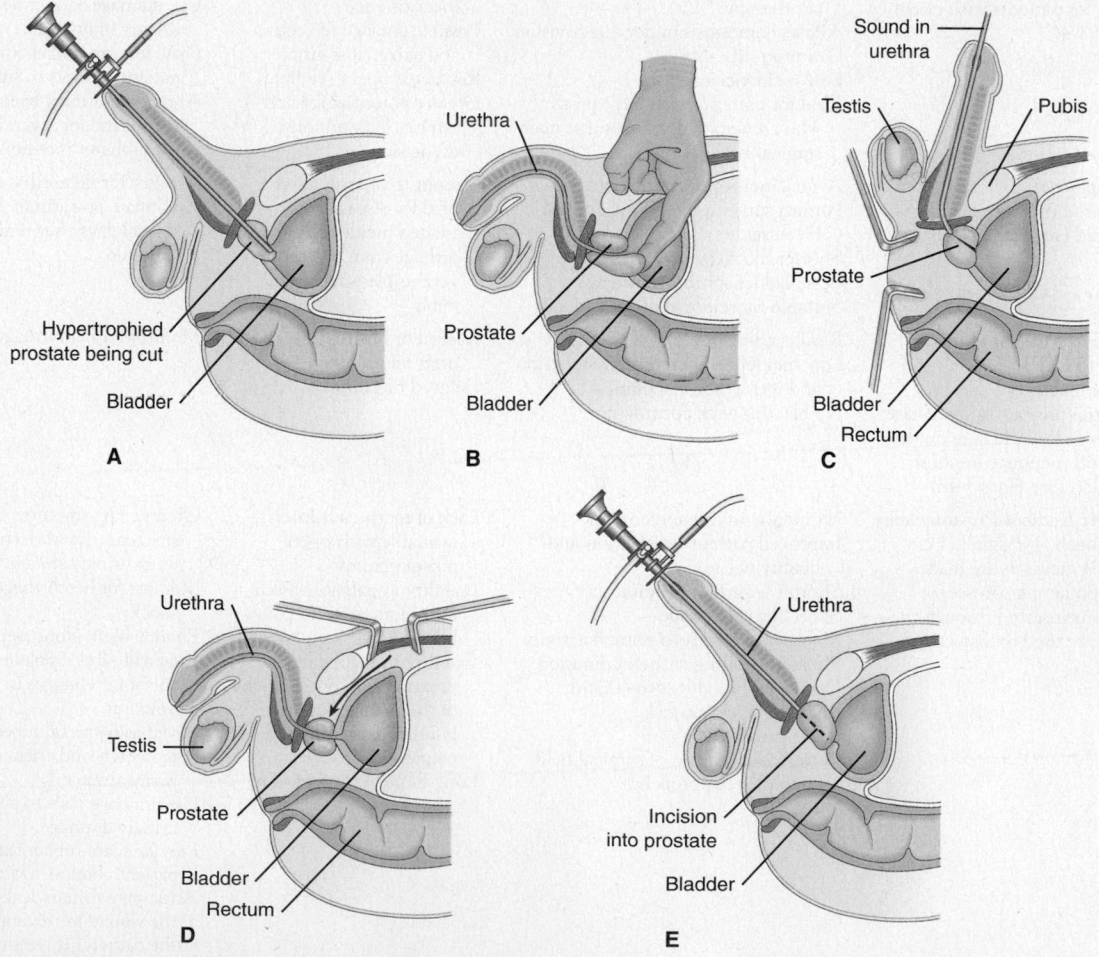

Figure 53-4 • Prostate surgery procedures. **A.** Transurethral resection of the prostate. A loop of wire connected with a cutting current is rotated in the cystoscope to remove shavings of prostate at the bladder orifice. **B.** Suprapubic prostatectomy. With an abdominal approach, the prostate is shelled out of its bed. **C.** Perineal prostatectomy. Two retractors on the left spread the perineal incision to provide a view of the prostate. **D.** Retropubic prostatectomy is performed through a low abdominal incision. Note two abdominal retractors and *arrow* pointing to the prostate gland. **E.** Transurethral incision of the prostate involves one or two incisions into the prostate to reduce pressure on the urethra.

Chart 53-4	Transurethral Resection Syndrome

Transurethral resection syndrome is a rare but potentially serious complication of transurethral resection of the prostate (TURP). Signs and symptoms are caused by neurologic, cardiovascular, and electrolyte imbalances associated with absorption of the solution used to irrigate the surgical site during the surgical procedure. Hyponatremia, hypervolemia, and occasionally hyperammonemia may occur.

Signs and Symptoms

- Collapse
- Headache
- Hypotension
- Lethargy and confusion
- Muscle spasms
- Nausea and vomiting
- Seizures
- Tachycardia

Interventions

- Discontinue irrigation.
- Administer diuretic agents as prescribed.
- Replace bladder irrigation with normal saline.
- Monitor intake and output.
- Monitor the patient's vital signs and level of consciousness.
- Differentiate lethargy and confusion of TURP syndrome from postoperative disorientation and hyponatremia.
- Maintain patient safety during times of confusion.
- Assess lung and heart sounds for indications of pulmonary edema, heart failure, or both as fluid moves back into the intravascular space.

Adapted from Hahn, R. G. (2019). What the intensive care physician should know about the transurethral resection syndrome. In J. L. Vincent (Ed). *Annual update in intensive care and emergency medicine 2019*. New York: Springer.

NURSING PROCESS

Patient Undergoing Prostatectomy

Assessment

The nurse assesses how the underlying disorder (BPH or prostate cancer) has affected the patient's lifestyle. Questions to ask during assessment include the following: Has the patient's activity level or activity tolerance changed? What is his presenting urinary problem (described in the patient's own words)? Has he experienced decreased force of urinary flow, decreased ability to initiate voiding, urgency, frequency, nocturia, dysuria, urinary retention, or hematuria? Does the patient report back pain, flank pain, and lower abdominal or suprapubic discomfort? Possible causes of such discomfort include infection, retention, and renal colic. Has the patient experienced erectile dysfunction or changes in frequency or enjoyment of sexual activity?

The nurse obtains further information about the patient's family history of cancer and heart or kidney disease, including hypertension. Has he lost weight? Does he appear pale? Can he raise himself out of bed and return to bed without assistance? Can he perform usual activities of daily living? A comprehensive functional assessment helps determine how soon the patient will be able to return to normal activities after prostatectomy.

Diagnosis

PREOPERATIVE NURSING DIAGNOSES

Based on the assessment data, major preoperative nursing diagnoses may include the following:

- Anxiety about surgery and its outcome
- Acute pain associated with bladder distention
- Lack of knowledge about factors associated with the disorder and the treatment protocol

POSTOPERATIVE NURSING DIAGNOSES

Based on the assessment data, major postoperative nursing diagnoses may include the following:

- Risk for hypovolaemia
- Acute pain associated with the surgical incision, catheter placement, and bladder spasms
- Lack of knowledge about postoperative care

COLLABORATIVE PROBLEMS/POTENTIAL COMPLICATIONS

Potential complications may include the following:

- Hemorrhage and shock
- Infection
- Venous thromboembolism (VTE)
- Catheter obstruction
- Complications with catheter removal
- Urinary incontinence
- Sexual dysfunction

Planning and Goals

The major preoperative goals for the patient may include reduced anxiety and learning about his prostate disorder and the perioperative experience. The major postoperative goals may include maintenance of fluid volume balance, relief of pain and discomfort, ability to perform self-care activities, and absence of complications.

Preoperative Nursing Interventions

REDUCING ANXIETY

The patient is usually admitted to the hospital or surgical center on the morning of surgery. Because contact with the patient may be limited before surgery, the nurse must establish communication with the patient to assess his understanding of the diagnosis and of the planned surgical procedure. The nature of the surgery and expected postoperative outcomes are clarified. In addition, the nurse familiarizes the patient with the pre- and postoperative routines and initiates measures to reduce anxiety. Because the patient may be sensitive and embarrassed discussing problems related to the genitalia and sexuality, the nurse provides privacy and establishes a trusting and professional relationship. The patient is encouraged to verbalize his feelings and concerns.

RELIEVING DISCOMFORT

If the patient experiences discomfort before surgery, bed rest may be prescribed, analgesic agents are given, and measures are initiated to relieve anxiety. If he is hospitalized, the nurse monitors his voiding patterns, watches for bladder distention, and assists with catheterization if indicated. An indwelling catheter is inserted if the patient has continuing urinary retention or if close monitoring is needed because of laboratory test results that indicate azotemia. The catheter can help decompress the bladder gradually over several days, especially if the patient is an older adult and hypertensive and has diminished kidney function or urinary retention that has existed for many weeks. For a few days after the bladder begins draining, the blood pressure may fluctuate, and kidney function may decline. If the patient cannot tolerate a urinary catheter, he is prepared for a cystostomy and insertion of a suprapubic catheter.

PROVIDING EDUCATION

Before surgery, the nurse reviews with the patient the anatomy of the affected structures and their function in relation to the urinary and reproductive systems, using diagrams and other educational aids as indicated. Web-based prostate cancer education both before and after surgery, along with phone and internet communication, promotes self-care management and support for patients, their partners, and families (Meyer, 2020; Remacle, 2019). This education can occur during the preadmission testing visit, with the nurse in prescribed settings, or in the urologist's office. The nurse explains what will take place while the patient is prepared for diagnostic tests and then for surgery (depending on the type of prostatectomy planned). The nurse also reinforces information given by the surgeon about the type of incision, which varies with the surgical approach (see Table 53-4), and describes the likely type of urinary drainage system (urethral or suprapubic) and the recovery room procedure. The amount of information given is based on the patient's needs and questions. The nurse explains procedures expected to occur during the immediate perioperative period; answers questions the patient, family, or significant other may have; and provides emotional support. In addition, the patient is given information about postoperative care and pain management.

PREPARING THE PATIENT

If the patient is scheduled for a prostatectomy, the preoperative preparation described in Chapter 14 is provided. Antiembolism stockings are applied before surgery and are particularly important to prevent VTE if the patient is placed in a lithotomy position during surgery. An enema is usually given at home on the evening before surgery or on the morning of surgery to prevent postoperative straining, which can induce bleeding.

Postoperative Nursing Interventions

MAINTAINING FLUID BALANCE

During the postoperative period, the patient is at risk for deficient fluid volume because of the irrigation of the surgical site during and after surgery. With irrigation of the urinary catheter to prevent its obstruction by blood clots, fluid may be absorbed through the open surgical site and retained, increasing the risk of excessive fluid retention, fluid imbalance, and water intoxication. The urine output and the amount of fluid used for irrigation must be closely monitored to determine whether irrigation fluid is being retained and to ensure an adequate urine output. An intake and output record, including the amount of fluid used for irrigation, must be maintained. The patient is also monitored for electrolyte imbalances (e.g., hyponatremia), increasing blood pressure, confusion, and respiratory distress. These signs and symptoms are documented and reported to the surgeon. The risk of fluid and electrolyte imbalance is greater in older patients with preexisting cardiovascular or respiratory disease.

RELIEVING PAIN

After a prostatectomy, the patient is assisted to sit and dangle his legs over the side of the bed on the day of surgery. The next morning, he is assisted to ambulate. If pain is present, the cause and location are determined, and the severity of pain and discomfort is assessed (Brant, 2019). The pain may be related to the incision or may be the result of excoriation of the skin at the catheter site. It may be in the flank area, indicating a kidney problem, or it may be caused by bladder spasms. Bladder irritability can initiate bleeding and result in clot formation, leading to urinary retention.

Patients experiencing bladder spasms may report urgency to void, a feeling of pressure or fullness in the bladder, and bleeding from the urethra around the catheter. Medications that relax the smooth muscles can help ease the spasms, which can be intermittent and severe; these medications include flavoxate and oxybutynin. Warm compresses to the pubis or sitz baths may also relieve the spasms.

The nurse monitors the drainage tubing and irrigates the system as prescribed to relieve any obstruction that may cause discomfort. Usually, the catheter is irrigated with 50 mL of irrigating fluid at a time. It is important to make sure that the same amount is recovered in the drainage receptacle. Securing the catheter drainage tubing to the leg or abdomen can help decrease tension on the catheter and prevent bladder irritation. Discomfort may be caused by dressings that are too snug, saturated with drainage, or improperly placed. Analgesic agents are given as prescribed. The nurse notifies the primary provider if the analgesic medications do not relieve the patient's pain and obtains a prescription for new doses or different medications.

After the patient is ambulatory, he is encouraged to walk but not to sit for prolonged periods, because this increases intra-abdominal pressure and the possibility of discomfort and bleeding. Prune juice and stool softeners are provided to ease bowel movements and to prevent excessive straining. An enema, if prescribed, is given with caution to avoid rectal perforation.

MONITORING AND MANAGING POTENTIAL COMPLICATIONS

After prostatectomy, the patient is monitored for major complications such as hemorrhage, infection, VTE, catheter problems, and sexual dysfunction.

Hemorrhage. Although patients are advised to discontinue all aspirin, nonsteroidal anti-inflammatory drugs, and platelet inhibitors 10 to 14 days before the surgery to prevent excessive bleeding, bleeding and hemorrhagic shock remain risks. The risk is increased with BPH because a hyperplastic prostate gland is very vascular. Bleeding may occur from the prostatic bed. Bleeding may also result in the formation of clots, which then obstruct urine flow. The drainage normally begins as reddish-pink and then clears to a light pink within 24 hours after surgery. Bright-red bleeding with increased viscosity and numerous clots usually indicates arterial bleeding. Venous blood appears darker and less viscous. Arterial hemorrhage usually requires surgical intervention (e.g., suturing or transurethral coagulation of bleeding vessels), whereas venous bleeding may be controlled by applying prescribed traction to the catheter so that the balloon holding the catheter in place applies pressure to the prostatic fossa. The surgeon applies traction by securely taping the catheter to the patient's thigh if hemorrhage occurs. Less blood loss (150 mL) is expected with robotic-assisted laparoscopic radical prostatectomy, compared to the 500 to 900 mL loss that may occur with open prostatectomy.

Nursing management includes assistance in implementing strategies to stop the bleeding and to prevent or reverse hemorrhagic shock. If blood loss is extensive, fluids and blood component therapy may be given. If hemorrhagic shock occurs, treatments described in Chapter 11 are initiated.

Nursing interventions include closely monitoring vital signs; administering medications, IV fluids, and blood component therapy as prescribed; maintaining an accurate record of intake and output; and carefully monitoring drainage to ensure adequate urine flow and patency of the drainage system. The patient who experiences hemorrhage and his family are often anxious and benefit from explanations and reassurance about the event and the procedures that are performed.

Infection. After perineal prostatectomy, the surgeon usually changes the dressing on the first postoperative day. Further dressing changes may become the responsibility of the nurse in the inpatient setting or the home health nurse upon discharge. Careful aseptic technique is used because the potential for infection is great. Dressings can be held in place by a double-tailed, T-binder bandage or a padded athletic supporter.

Rectal thermometers, rectal tubes, and enemas are avoided because of the risk of injury and bleeding in the prostatic fossa. After the perineal sutures are removed, the perineum is cleansed as indicated. Sitz baths are also used to promote comfort and healing.

UTIs and epididymitis are possible complications after prostatectomy. The patient is assessed for their occurrence; if they occur, the nurse administers antibiotic agents as prescribed. Because the risk of infection continues after discharge from the hospital, the patient and family need to be educated to monitor for signs and symptoms of infection (fever, chills, sweating, myalgia, dysuria, urinary frequency, and urgency). The patient and family are instructed to contact the urologist if these symptoms occur.

Venous Thromboembolism. Patients undergoing prostatectomy are at risk for VTE, including deep vein thrombosis and pulmonary embolism; therefore, the nurse assesses the patient frequently after surgery for manifestations of VTE. Early postoperative ambulation is essential to reduce the risk of VTE. Medical and nursing management of VTE is described in Chapter 26. In addition, if the patient is at high risk for clot formation, additional antithrombotic interventions may be prescribed (Klaassen, Wallis, Lavallée, et al., 2020).

Potential Catheter Problems. After TURP, the catheter must drain well; an obstructed catheter produces distention of the prostatic capsule and resultant hemorrhage. Furosemide may be prescribed to promote urination and initiate postoperative diuresis, thereby helping to keep the catheter patent.

The nurse observes the lower abdomen to ensure that the catheter has not become blocked. A distinct, rounded swelling above the pubis is a manifestation of an overdistended bladder. If the nurse ascertains that the client's bladder is distended, a portable bladder scanner may be used to determine if urine retention is a problem (see Chapter 47).

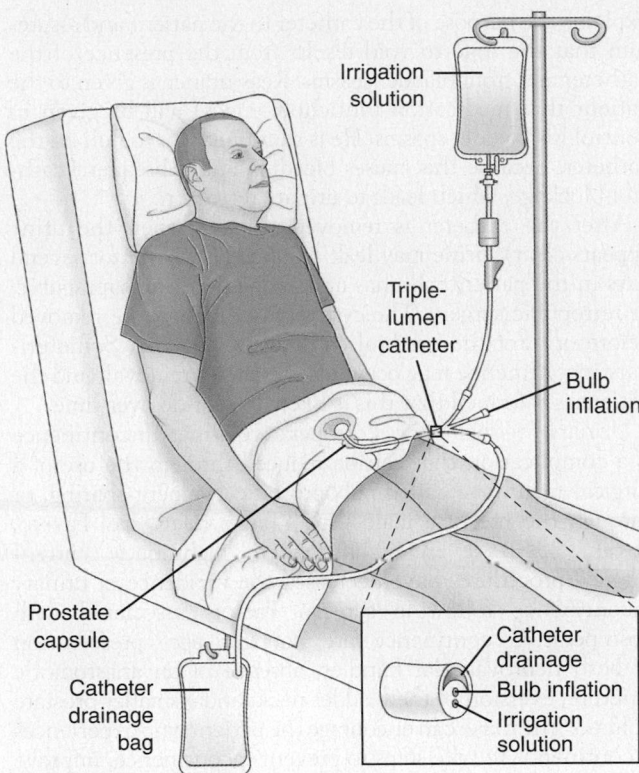

Figure 53-5 • A three-way system for bladder irrigation.

The drainage bag is monitored for bloody urine, and the dressings and surgical incision are examined for bleeding. The color of the urine is carefully noted and documented; a change in color from pink to amber indicates reduced bleeding. Blood pressure, pulse, and respirations are monitored and compared with baseline preoperative vital signs to detect hypotension. The nurse also observes the patient for restlessness, diaphoresis, pallor, any drop in blood pressure, and an increasing pulse rate.

Drainage of the bladder may be accomplished by gravity through a closed sterile drainage system. A three-way drainage system is useful in irrigating the bladder and preventing clot formation (see Fig. 53-5). Continuous irrigation may be used with TURP. Some urologists leave an indwelling catheter attached to a dependent drainage system. Gentle irrigation of the catheter may be prescribed to remove any obstructing clots.

If the patient complains of pain, the tubing is examined. The drainage system is irrigated with irrigating fluid (usually 50 mL), if indicated and prescribed, to clear any obstruction.

> ### ▶ *Quality and Safety Nursing Alert*
>
> *The amount of fluid recovered in the drainage bag must equal the amount of fluid instilled. Overdistention of the bladder should be avoided because it can induce secondary hemorrhage by stretching the coagulated blood vessels in the prostatic capsule.*

To prevent traction on the bladder, the drainage tube (not the catheter) is secured to the inner thigh. If a cystostomy catheter is in place, it is secured to the abdomen. The nurse explains the purpose of the catheter to the patient and assures him that the urge to void results from the presence of the catheter and from bladder spasms. Reassurance is given to the patient that medication (anticholinergics) will be given to control his bladder spasms. He is cautioned not to pull on the catheter, because this causes bleeding and subsequent catheter blockage, which leads to urinary retention.

After the catheter is removed (usually when the urine appears clear), urine may leak around the wound for several days in the patient who has undergone perineal, suprapubic, or retropubic surgery. The cystostomy tube may be removed before or after the urethral catheter is removed. Some urinary incontinence may occur after catheter removal, and the patient is informed that this is likely to subside over time.

Urinary Incontinence. Postoperative urinary incontinence is a complication that can be reduced through the use of a surgical technique called puboprostatic ligament-sparing, or through the use of a male sling (Tasso, Beels, Del Favero, et al., 2020). Even without these techniques, current surgical procedures have decreased the incidence of urinary incontinence following surgery. Factors associated with postoperative continence are younger age, preservation of both neurovascular bundles, absence of an anastomotic stricture, eversion of the bladder neck, and a smaller prostate volume. The nurse can encourage the patient who experiences incontinence to take steps to prevent incontinence, improve continence, anticipate leakage, and cope with lack of complete control (Remacle, 2019). Preventing incontinence involves increasing voiding frequency, avoiding positions that encourage the urge to void, and decreasing fluid intake prior to activities. Promoting continence involves pelvic floor exercises (see the Educating Patients About Self-Care section that follows), biofeedback, and electrical stimulation. Anticipating leakage may entail lifestyle modifications such as using absorbent pads and carrying extra clothes to prevent urinary incontinence; this can improve confidence when bathroom access is limited. It also helps to know the location of public bathrooms. Coping long term with complete lack of control may involve collagen injections, artificial sphincter implants, medications, and leg bags (Cheng et al., 2019; Remacle, 2019).

Sexual Dysfunction. Depending on the type of surgery, the patient may experience sexual dysfunction related to erectile dysfunction, decreased libido, and fatigue. These issues may become a concern to the patient soon after surgery or in the weeks to months of rehabilitation. With nerve-sparing radical prostatectomy, the likelihood of recovering the ability to have erections is better for men who are younger and men in whom both neurovascular bundles are spared. A decrease in libido is usually related to the impact of the surgery on the body. Reassurance that the usual level of libido will return after recuperation from surgery is often helpful to the patient and his partner. The patient should be aware that he may experience fatigue during rehabilitation from surgery. This fatigue may also decrease his libido and alter his enjoyment of usual activities.

Several options to restore erectile function are discussed with the patient by the surgeon or urologist. These options may include medications, surgically placed implants, or negative-pressure devices. PDE-5 inhibitors (see Table 53-3) may be effective for treatment of erectile dysfunction in men after radical prostatectomy, especially if the neurovascular bundles have been preserved. They may also improve erectile function in men with partial or moderate erectile dysfunction after radiation therapy for localized prostate cancer.

Nursing interventions include assessing for sexual dysfunction after surgery. Providing a private and confidential environment to discuss issues of sexuality is important. The emotional challenges of prostate surgery and its consequences need to be carefully explored with the patient and his partner. Providing the opportunity to discuss these issues can be very beneficial to the patient. For patients who have significant difficulty adjusting to sexual dysfunction, a referral to a sex therapist may be indicated.

PROMOTING HOME, COMMUNITY-BASED, AND TRANSITIONAL CARE

Educating Patients About Self-Care. The length of the hospital stay for the patient undergoing prostatectomy depends on the surgical approach used and ranges from 1 to 2 days for robotic-assisted laparoscopic prostatectomy to 3 to 5 days for open prostatectomy. The patient and family require education about how to manage the drainage system, how to assess for complications, and how to promote recovery. The nurse provides verbal and written education about the need to maintain the drainage system and to monitor urinary output; about wound care; and about strategies to prevent complications, such as infection, bleeding, and thrombosis. In addition, the patient and family need to know about signs and symptoms that should be reported to the primary provider (e.g., blood in urine, decreased urine output, fever, change in wound drainage, calf tenderness).

As the patient recovers and drainage tubes are removed, he may become discouraged and depressed because he cannot regain bladder control immediately. Furthermore, urinary frequency and burning may occur after the catheter is removed. Educating the patient about the following exercises may help him regain urinary control:

- Tense the perineal muscles by pressing the buttocks together, hold this position, and then relax. This exercise can be performed 10 to 20 times each hour while sitting or standing (Brant, 2019).
- Try to interrupt the urinary stream after starting to void; wait a few seconds and then continue to void.

Perineal exercises should continue until the patient gains full urinary control. The patient is educated to urinate as soon as he feels the first urge to do so. It is important to let the patient know that regaining urinary control is a gradual process; he may continue to "dribble" after being discharged from the hospital, but this should gradually diminish (usually within 1 year). The urine may be cloudy for several weeks after surgery but should clear as the prostate area heals.

While the prostatic fossa heals (6 to 8 weeks), the patient should avoid activities that produce Valsalva effects (straining, heavy lifting) because they may increase venous pressure and produce hematuria. He should avoid long motor trips and strenuous exercise, which increase the tendency to bleed. He should also know that spicy foods, alcohol, and coffee may cause bladder discomfort. The patient should be cautioned to drink enough fluids to avoid dehydration, which increases the tendency for a blood clot to form and obstruct the flow of urine. Signs of complications, such as bleeding, passage of

---

Chart 53-5

HOME CARE CHECKLIST

Postprostatectomy Care

At the completion of education, the patient and/or caregiver will be able to:

- Name the procedure that was performed and identify any permanent changes in anatomic structure or function as well as changes in ADLs, IADLs, roles, relationships, and spirituality.
- Locate list of names and telephone numbers of resource personnel involved in care (e.g., health care professionals, home health nurse, urinary catheter/dressing supply vendor).
- Identify the equipment necessary and how to obtain medical supplies to carry out dressing changes, wound care, and other prescribed regimens.
- Describe ongoing postoperative therapeutic regimen, including diet and activities to perform (e.g., increased activity and ambulation, perineal exercises) and to limit or avoid (e.g., lifting weights, driving a car, contact sports).
  - Describe measures to relieve postoperative pain and discomfort (e.g., take analgesics as prescribed; use nonpharmacologic interventions).
  - Demonstrate appropriate care of urinary catheter and collection receptacle.
  - Demonstrate appropriate dressing change/wound care.

- When appropriate, demonstrate performance of perineal muscle exercises to facilitate bladder control.
- State the name, dose, side effects, frequency, and schedule for all medications.
- Identify signs and symptoms of complications that should be reported to surgeon (e.g., decreased output, blood or clots in urine or urine drainage system, change in wound drainage, fever or symptoms of urinary tract infections, calf tenderness).
- Explain treatment plan and importance of follow-up care to all health care providers.
- State time and date of follow-up appointments, therapy, and testing.
- Identify community resources for peer and caregiver/family support:
  - Identify sources of support (e.g., friends, relatives, faith community).
  - Identify the contact details for support services for people with cancer and their caregivers/families.
- Identify the need for health promotion, disease prevention, and screening activities.

ADL, activities of daily living; IADL, instrumental activities of daily living.

---

blood clots, a decrease in the urinary stream, urinary retention, or symptoms of UTIs, should be reported to the primary provider (see Chart 53-5). Patients who have undergone robotic-assisted prostatectomy are often able to return to their usual activities in approximately 7 to 10 days (Cheng et al., 2019).

Continuing and Transitional Care. Referral for home, community-based, or transitional care may be indicated if the patient is an older adult or has other health problems, if the patient and family cannot provide care in the home, or if the patient lives alone without available supports. The nurse making a home visit assesses the patient's physical status (cardiovascular and respiratory status, fluid and nutritional status, patency of the urinary drainage system, wound and nutritional status) and provides catheter and wound care, if indicated. The nurse reinforces previous education, assesses the ability of the patient and family to manage required care, and encourages the patient to ambulate and to carry out perineal exercises as prescribed. The patient may need to be reminded that return of bladder control may take time.

The patient is reminded about the importance of routine health screening and other health promotion activities. If the prostatectomy was performed to treat prostate cancer, the patient and family are also instructed about the importance of follow-up and monitoring with the primary provider.

Evaluation

Expected preoperative patient outcomes may include:
1. Demonstrates reduced anxiety
2. States that pain and discomfort are decreased
3. Relates understanding of the surgical procedure and postoperative course and practices perineal muscle exercises and other techniques useful in facilitating bladder control

Expected postoperative patient outcomes may include the following:
1. Reports relief of discomfort
2. Exhibits fluid and electrolyte balance
   a. Irrigation fluid and urinary output are within parameters determined by surgeon
   b. Experiences no signs or symptoms of fluid retention
3. Participates in self-care measures
   a. Increases activity and ambulation daily
   b. Produces urine output within normal ranges and consistent with intake
   c. Performs perineal exercises and interrupts urinary stream to promote bladder control
   d. Avoids straining and lifting heavy objects
4. Is free of complications
   a. Maintains vital signs within normal limits
   b. Exhibits wound healing, without signs of inflammation or hemorrhage
   c. Maintains acceptable level of urinary elimination
   d. Maintains optimal drainage of catheter and other drainage tubes
   e. Reports understanding of changes in sexual function

DISORDERS AFFECTING THE TESTES AND ADJACENT STRUCTURES

Orchitis

Orchitis is an acute inflammation of one or both testes as a complication of systemic infection or as an extension of an associated epididymitis caused by bacterial, viral, spirochetal, or parasitic organisms. Microorganisms may reach the testes through the blood, lymphatic system, or, more commonly, by traveling through the urethra, vas deferens, and epididymis; bacteria usually spread from an associated epididymitis in sexually active men. The majority of cases are caused by viral mumps but other causative organisms include *Neisseria gonorrhoeae*, *Chlamydia trachomatis*, *E. coli*, *Klebsiella*, *Pseudomonas aeruginosa*, *Staphylococcus* species, and *Streptococcus* species (Norris, 2019).

Signs and symptoms of orchitis include fever; pain, which may range from mild to severe; tenderness in one or both testicles; bilateral or unilateral testicular swelling; penile discharge; blood in the semen; and leukocytosis.

Treatment of orchitis is based on whether the causative organism is bacterial or viral. Bacterial orchitis is treated with antibiotic agents and supportive comfort measures. If the cause of the orchitis is an STI, the partner should be treated as well. Viral orchitis is treated using supportive treatments of rest, elevation of the scrotum, ice packs to reduce scrotal edema, analgesic agents, and anti-inflammatory medications. Bilateral orchitis can cause sterility in some men. Mumps vaccination is recommended for men who have not had mumps or received inadequate immunization in childhood. Orchitis develops in approximately 30% of males who are post puberty with mumps 4 to 6 days after parotitis starts, and one third of men have irreversible loss of spermatogenesis (Norris, 2019).

Epididymitis

Epididymitis is an infection of the epididymis, which usually spreads from an infected urethra, bladder, or prostate. The incidence is less than 1 in 1000 males per year. Prevalence is greatest in men 19 to 35 years of age. Acute epididymitis occurs bilaterally in 5% to 10% of affected patients (Cheng et al., 2019). Risk factors for epididymitis include recent surgery or a procedure involving the urinary tract, participation in high-risk sexual practices, personal history of an STI, past prostate infections or UTIs, lack of circumcision, history of an enlarged prostate, and the presence of a chronic indwelling urinary catheter.

Pathophysiology

A causative organism can be identified in 80% of patients. In prepubertal males, older men, and gay men, the predominate causal organism is *E. coli*; although in older men, the condition may also be a result of urinary obstruction. In sexually active men 35 years and younger, the pathogens usually are related to bacteria associated with STIs (e.g., *C. trachomatis*, *N. gonorrhoeae*). The infection moves in an upward direction, through the urethra and the ejaculatory duct, and then along the vas deferens to the epididymis (Teelin, Babu, & Urban, 2019).

Clinical Manifestations

Epididymitis often slowly develops over 1 to 2 days, beginning with a low-grade fever, chills, and heaviness in the affected testicle. The testicle becomes increasingly tender to pressure and traction. The patient may report unilateral pain, soreness in the inguinal canal along the course of the vas deferens, and pain and swelling in the scrotum and the groin. The epididymis becomes increasingly swollen, with extreme pain in the lower abdomen and pelvis. Occasionally, there may be

discharge from the urethra, blood in the semen, pyuria and bacteriuria (pus and bacteria in the urine), and pain during sexual activity and ejaculation. The patient may report urinary frequency, urgency, or dysuria, and testicular pain aggravated by bowel movement.

Assessment and Diagnostic Findings

Laboratory assessment includes urinalysis, complete blood cell count, Gram stain of urethral drainage, urethral culture or deoxyribonucleic acid (DNA) probe, and referral for syphilis and HIV testing in sexually active patients. Acute testicular pain should never be ignored, and it should be distinguished from testicular torsion, which is a surgical emergency.

Medical Management

The selection of an antibiotic depends on the causative organism; if epididymitis is associated with an STI, the patient's partner should also receive antimicrobial therapy. The spermatic cord may be infiltrated with a local anesthetic agent to relieve pain if the patient is seen within the first 24 hours after onset of pain. Supportive interventions also include reduction in physical activity, scrotal support and elevation, ice packs, anti-inflammatory agents, analgesics (including nerve blocks), and sitz baths. Urethral instrumentation (e.g., catheter insertion) is avoided. The patient is observed for scrotal abscess formation as well.

In chronic epididymitis, a 4- to 6-week course of antibiotic therapy for bacterial pathogens is prescribed. An epididymectomy (excision of the epididymis from the testis) may be performed for patients who have recurrent, refractory, and incapacitating episodes of this infection. With long-term epididymitis, the passage of sperm may be obstructed. If the obstruction is bilateral, infertility may result.

Nursing Management

Bed rest is prescribed, and the scrotum is elevated with a scrotal bridge or folded towel to prevent traction on the spermatic cord, to promote venous drainage, and to relieve pain. Antimicrobial agents are given as prescribed until the acute inflammation subsides. Intermittent cold compresses to the scrotum may help ease the pain. Later, local heat or sitz baths may help resolve the inflammation. Analgesic medications are given for pain relief as prescribed.

The nurse instructs the patient to avoid straining, lifting, and sexual stimulation until the infection is under control. He should continue taking analgesic agents and antibiotics as prescribed and using ice packs if necessary, to relieve discomfort. He needs to know that it may take 4 weeks or longer for the inflammation to resolve.

Testicular Torsion

Testicular torsion is a surgical emergency requiring immediate diagnosis to avoid loss of the testicle. Torsion of the testis is rotation of the testis, which twists the blood vessels in the spermatic cord and therefore impedes the arterial and venous supply to the testicle and surrounding structures in the scrotum. The patient presents with sudden pain in the testicle, developing over 1 to 2 hours, with or without a predisposing event. Nausea, lightheadedness, and swelling of the scrotum may develop. On physical examination, testicular tenderness, an elevated testis, a thickened spermatic cord, and a swollen, painful scrotum may be present. If the torsion cannot be reduced manually, surgery to untwist the spermatic cord and anchor both testes in their correct position to prevent recurrence should occur within 6 hours of the onset of symptoms in order to save the testis (Norris, 2019). After 6 hours of impaired blood supply, the risk of loss of the testicle increases.

Testicular Cancer

Although only accounting for about 1% of all cancers in men, testicular cancer is the most common cancer diagnosed in men between 15 and 35 years of age; approximately 9610 new cases and 440 deaths occur in the United States annually (ACS, 2020). It is the second most common malignancy in those 35 to 39 years of age. For unknown reasons, worldwide incidence of testicular tumors has more than doubled in the past 40 years. Because of advances in cancer therapy, testicular cancer is a highly treatable and usually curable form of cancer. The 5-year relative survival rate for all testicular cancers is more than 95% and approaches 99% if the cancer has not spread outside of the testes (ACS, 2020). After treatment, most patients with testicular cancer have a near-normal life expectancy.

Classification of Testicular Tumors

The testicles contain several types of cells, each of which may develop into one or more types of cancer. The type of cancer cell determines the appropriate treatment and affects the prognosis. Testicular cancer is classified as germinal or nongerminal (stromal). Secondary testicular cancers may also occur.

Germinal Tumors

Germinal tumors make up approximately 90% of all cancers of the testis; germinal tumors are further classified as seminomas or nonseminomas. These cancers grow from the germ cells that produce sperm, thus the name *germinal tumors*. Seminomas are slow-growing forms of testicular cancer that are usually found in men in their 30s and 40s (ACS, 2020; NCCN, 2020c). Although seminomas can spread to the lymph nodes, the cancer is usually localized in the testes. Nonseminomas are more common and tend to grow more quickly than seminomas. Nonseminomas are often made up of different cell types and are identified according to the cells in which they start to grow. Nonseminoma testicular cancers include choriocarcinomas (rare), embryonal carcinomas, teratomas, and yolk sac tumors. It is crucial to distinguish between seminomas and nonseminomas because the differences affect prognosis and treatment.

Nongerminal Tumors

Nongerminal tumors account for less than 10% of testicular cancers. These cancers may develop in the supportive and hormone-producing tissues, or stroma, of the testicles. The two main types of stromal tumors are Leydig cell tumors and Sertoli cell tumors. Although these tumors infrequently spread beyond the testicle, a small number metastasize and tend to be resistant to chemotherapy and radiation therapy.

Secondary Testicular Tumors

Secondary testicular tumors are those that have metastasized to the testicle from other organs. Lymphoma is the most common cause of secondary testicular cancer. Cancers may also spread to the testicles from the prostate gland, lung, skin (melanoma), kidney, and other organs. The prognosis with these cancers is usually poor because they typically also spread to other organs. Treatment depends on the specific type of cancer (ACS, 2020).

Risk Factors

Risk factors for testicular cancer include cryptorchidism (undescended testicles), family history of testicular cancer, and personal history of testicular cancer (ACS, 2020). Other risk factors include race and ethnicity: Caucasian American men have a five times greater risk than African American men and more than two to three times greater risk than Asian, Native American, and Hispanic American men. The risk of developing testicular cancer is higher in HIV-positive men (ACS, 2020). Occupational hazards, including exposure to chemicals encountered in mining, oil and gas production, and leather processing, have been suggested as possible risk factors. No evidence has linked testicular cancer to prenatal exposure to diethylstilbestrol or to vasectomy (ACS, 2020).

Clinical Manifestations

The symptoms appear gradually, with a mass or lump on the testicle and usually painless enlargement of the testis. The patient may report heaviness in the scrotum, inguinal area, or lower abdomen. Backache (from retroperitoneal node extension), abdominal pain, weight loss, and general weakness may result from metastasis. Enlargement of the testis without pain is a significant diagnostic finding. Some testicular tumors tend to metastasize early, spreading from the testis to the lymph nodes in the retroperitoneum and to the lungs.

Assessment and Diagnostic Findings

Educating young men about testicular cancer and the need for urgent evaluation of any mass or enlargement or unexplained testicular pain is key to early detection (Li, Lu, Wang, et al., 2020). Education about TSE, starting in adolescence, alerts men to the importance of seeking medical attention if a testicle becomes indurated, enlarged, atrophied, nodular, or painful (see Chart 53-6). TSE should be performed monthly. Testicular cancers generally grow rapidly and are easily detected against a typically smooth and homogeneous texture. Annual testicular examination by a clinician can reveal signs and lead to early diagnosis and treatment of testicular cancer. Promoting awareness of this disease is an important health promotion intervention; men should seek medical evaluation for signs or symptoms of testicular cancer without delay (Li et al., 2020; Ustundag, 2019). See the Nursing Research Profile in Chart 53-7. Any suspicious testicular mass warrants prompt evaluation with a thorough history and physical examination, focusing on palpation of the affected testicle.

The tumor markers, alpha-fetoprotein (AFP) and beta-human chorionic gonadotropin (beta-hCG), may be elevated in patients with testicular cancer. Tumor marker levels in the blood are used for diagnosis, staging, and monitoring the

PATIENT EDUCATION

Chart 53-6

Testicular Self-Examination

Testicular self-examination is to be performed once a month. The test is neither difficult nor time-consuming. A convenient time is usually after a warm bath or shower when the scrotum is more relaxed.

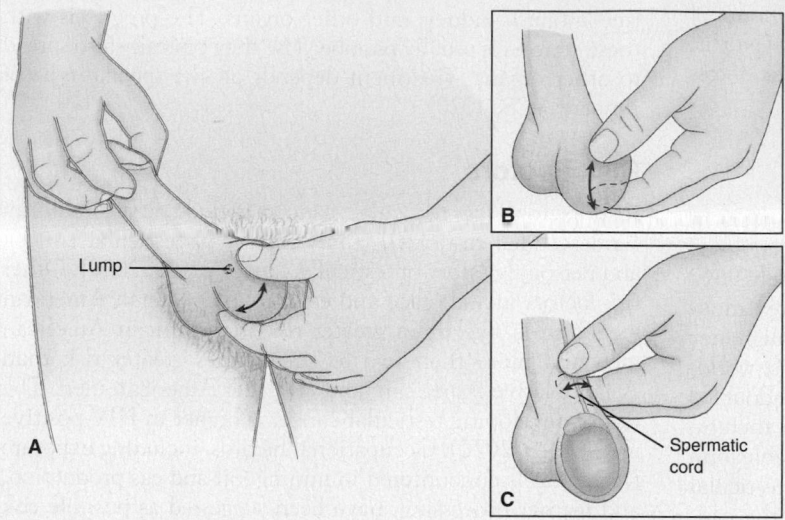

Lump
A
B
Spermatic cord
C

The nurse instructs the patient to:

1. Use both hands to palpate the testis. The normal testicle is smooth and uniform in consistency.
2. Place the index and middle fingers under the testis and the thumb on top; roll the testis gently in a horizontal plane between the thumb and fingers (**A**).
3. Feel for any evidence of a small lump or abnormality.
4. Follow the same procedure and palpate upward along the testis (**B**).
5. Locate and palpate the epididymis (**C**), a cordlike structure on the top and back of the testicle that stores and transports sperm. In addition, locate and palpate the spermatic cord.
6. Repeat the examination for the other testis, epididymis, and spermatic cord. It is normal to find that one testis is larger than the other.
7. If you find any evidence of a small, pea-sized lump or if the testis is swollen (possibly from an infection or tumor), consult your primary provider.

Adapted from Weber, J. R., & Kelley, J. H. (2018). *Health assessment in nursing* (6th ed.). Philadelphia, PA: Lippincott Williams & Wilkins.

NURSING RESEARCH PROFILE

Chart 53-7

Testicular Self-Examination Knowledge

Ustundag, H. (2019). Assessment of the testicular self-examination knowledge and Health Belief Model of health sciences students. *International Journal of Caring Sciences, 12*(2), 972–978.

Purpose

Early detection of testicular cancer is possible if men perform monthly testicular self-examinations. However, many men are not aware of the benefits of doing a testicular self-examination. The purpose of this study was to describe young male health sciences students' knowledge of testicular cancer and practice of testicular self-examination, along with their personal health beliefs.

Design

This descriptive survey research study was conducted in a state university in Turkey. There were 372 male students who were given the opportunity to participate, and 262 students (70%) completed the demographic data form and the Turkish version of the Champion Health Belief Model Scale. This scale contains five subscales: (1) Sensitiveness, an individual's perception of personal risks or sensitivities to a disease or health problem; (2) Caring/Seriousness, an individual's view of the seriousness of the disease outcomes; (3) Benefits, an individual's belief in the benefit of protective behavior to prevent the disease from occurring or decrease the severity of symptoms if it occurs; (4) Perceived barriers to instituting new behaviors and adapting to new situations; and (5) Self-efficacy/Confidence, an individual's belief in the ability to take on the new initiative. Each subscale has its own minimum and maximum scores, and a separate score is determined for each of the five subscales. There is no total calculated score. The statistical analysis was performed using basic descriptive statistics such as frequency, percentage, mean scores, and the nonparametric tests, the Kruskal–Wallis test and Mann–Whitney U test.

Findings

The study participants were 18 to 27 years of age, with approximately 60% of participants in the 18- to 21-year-old age range. Most of the participants (40%, $n = 104$) were in their second year of education at the university. All the participants indicated that they had knowledge about testicular cancer, with 42% ($n = 109$) revealing that their knowledge was obtained from the internet or from social media. There were 7% of the sample ($n = 18$) who acknowledged that they had had a testicular health problem. In their family histories, 93% ($n = 244$) of the participants stated that there was no history of testicular health problems. There were 225 of the participants (86%) who had no experience doing a self-examination. The most common reason for not performing a testicular self-examination was that 74% ($n = 195$) did not take the reason for doing the self-examination seriously. The Champion Health Beliefs Model Scale identified that the caring/seriousness subscale had the highest score and that the perceived benefits of performing a testicular self-examination had the lowest score.

Nursing Implications

The study confirmed that young males lack knowledge about testicular cancer and lack experience performing a testicular self-examination. It is important for nurses and other health care providers to address the patient's need for knowledge and practical education on the performance of testicular self-examination. Emphasis must be placed on the fact that testicular self-examination is a significant risk reduction strategy for testicular cancer. The screening for testicular cancer is a topic that not only must be addressed by health care providers, but also included in the curriculum of health science and other educational programs. Frequent discussion and materials about testicular screening must be made available to all males.

response to treatment. Blood chemistry, including lactate dehydrogenase, is also necessary.

A chest x-ray to assess for metastasis in the lungs and a transscrotal testicular ultrasound will be performed. Microscopic analysis of tissue is the only definitive way to determine if cancer is present, but it is usually performed at the time of surgery rather than as a part of the diagnostic workup to reduce the risk of promoting spread of the cancer (ACS, 2020). Inguinal orchiectomy is the standard way to establish the diagnosis of testicular cancer. Other staging tests to determine the extent of the disease in the retroperitoneum, pelvis, and chest include an abdominal/pelvic CT scan and chest CT scan (if the abdominal CT or chest x-ray is abnormal). A brain MRI and bone scan may be obtained if indicated (NCCN, 2020c). Discussion of the option to bank sperm should take place prior to orchiectomy and treatment.

Medical Management

Testicular cancer—one of the most curable solid tumors—is highly responsive to treatment. Early-stage disease is curable more than 95% of the time; thus, prompt diagnosis and treatment are essential. The NCCN practice consensus guidelines for testicular cancer are used to guide diagnostic workup, primary treatment, follow-up, and salvage therapy (treatment given when the cancer does not respond to standard treatment) for both seminomas and nonseminomas (NCCN, 2020c). The goals of management are to eradicate the disease and achieve a cure. Therapy is based on the cell type, the stage of the disease, and risk classification tables (determined as good, intermediate, and poor risk). Primary treatment includes removal of the affected testis by orchiectomy through an inguinal incision with a high ligation of the spermatic cord. The patient is offered the option of implantation of a testicular prosthesis during the orchiectomy. Although most patients experience no impairment of endocrine function after unilateral orchiectomy for testicular cancer, some patients have decreased hormonal levels, suggesting that the unaffected testis is not functioning normally. Retroperitoneal lymph node dissection may be performed after orchiectomy to diagnose and prevent lymphatic spread of the cancer. Alternatives to the more invasive open retroperitoneal lymph node dissection for early-stage germ cell testicular cancer include nerve-sparing and laparoscopic retroperitoneal lymph node dissection, which improve sexual function and promote rapid recovery (Mano, Di Natale, & Sheinfeld, 2019). Although libido and orgasm are usually unimpaired after a retroperitoneal lymph node dissection, ejaculatory dysfunction with resultant infertility may develop. Two thirds of men who are newly diagnosed with testicular cancer may be considering future fatherhood, and sperm quality is reduced in men with testicular cancer; therefore, sperm banking before treatment may be considered (Mano et al., 2019). Half of patients will not recover fertility as a result of radiation therapy, cytotoxic therapy, unilateral excision of a testis, and retroperitoneal lymph node dissection. Counseling about fertility issues may help the patient make the appropriate choices (Halpern, Brannigan, & Schlegel, 2019).

Radiation therapy is more effective with seminomas than with nonseminomas. Postoperatively, radiation may be used in early-stage seminomas. It is delivered only to the affected side; the other testis is shielded from radiation to preserve fertility. Radiation is also used in patients whose disease does not respond to chemotherapy and in those for whom lymph node surgery is not recommended.

Chemotherapy may be used for seminomas, nonseminomas, and advanced metastatic disease. Cisplatin can be used in combination with other chemotherapeutic agents, such as etoposide, bleomycin, paclitaxel, ifosfamide, and vinblastine, and results in a high percentage of complete remissions. With nonseminomas, aggressive surgical resection of all residual masses following chemotherapy is standard therapy. Good results may also be obtained by combining different types of treatment, including surgery, radiation therapy, and chemotherapy. Even with metastatic testicular cancer, the prognosis is favorable because of advances in treatment. However, for patients who do not respond to high-dose salvage chemotherapy, the cancer is nearly always incurable.

A patient with a history of one testicular tumor has a greater chance of developing subsequent tumors. Late relapse of testicular cancer is currently defined as tumor recurrence more than 2 years after complete remission following primary treatment that included chemotherapy. The most common site of recurrence is the retroperitoneum. Follow-up studies include chest x-rays, excretory urography, radioimmunoassay of beta-hCG and AFP levels, and examination of lymph nodes.

Long-term side effects associated with treatment for testicular cancer include renal insufficiency from kidney damage, hearing problems, gonadal damage, peripheral neuropathy, and, rarely, secondary cancers. Management of a patient with testicular carcinoma is therapy aimed at cure followed by close monitoring to detect and promptly treat any recurrences (NCCN, 2020c). Investigations of new medications, combinations of chemotherapeutic agents, and stem cell transplantation are ongoing.

Nursing Management

Nursing management includes assessment of the patient's physical and psychological status and monitoring of the patient for response to and possible effects of surgery, chemotherapy, and radiation therapy (see Chapter 12). Pre- and postoperative care is described in Chapters 14 and 16, respectively. In addition, because the patient may have difficulty coping with his condition, issues related to body image and sexuality should be addressed.

Patients may be required to endure a long course of therapy and will need encouragement to maintain a positive attitude. After completing treatment, patients enter a follow-up surveillance period. Nurses educate these cancer survivors about the importance of adhering to follow-up appointments for early detection of cancer recurrence (most often occurring within 2 years posttreatment) and evaluation of late effects of treatment (including secondary cancers). Additional concerns include infertility, cardiotoxicity, neurotoxicity, nephrotoxicity, pulmonary toxicity, and metabolic syndrome; and alterations in quality of life (Brant, 2019). The nurse carefully assesses cultural aspects of care related to testicular cancer and its treatment. The nurse reminds the patient about the importance of performing TSE in the treated or remaining testis. The patient is encouraged to participate in healthy behaviors, including smoking cessation, healthy diet, minimization of alcohol intake, and cancer screening activities. Most experts agree that couples should use birth control for 18 to 24 months after the last cycle of chemotherapy as this is the usual period of time after treatment for sperm to return to normal (Brant, 2019).

Hydrocele

A **hydrocele** is a collection of fluid most commonly located between the visceral and parietal layers of the tunica vaginalis of the testis, although it may also collect within the spermatic cord. This condition is the most common cause of scrotal swelling. At birth, 1 in 10 infants has a hydrocele, which usually resolves without treatment within the first year of life. Acute hydroceles primarily develop in adults older than 40 years; they may occur in association with inflammation (e.g., radiation therapy), infection, epididymitis, local injury, or systemic infectious disease (e.g., mumps). Chronic hydroceles may occur related to the imbalance between fluid secretion and reabsorption in the tunica vaginalis. On physical examination, an easily transilluminated, painless, extratesticular mass is found. Hydrocele can be differentiated from a hernia by transillumination; a hydrocele transmits light, whereas a hernia does not. Ultrasonography is recommended for large hydroceles to differentiate them from testicular tumors (Chapple et al., 2020).

Treatment is usually not required unless the hydrocele is large, bulky, tense, or uncomfortable; compromises testicular circulation; or causes an undesirable appearance. Treatment may involve surgical excision or needle aspiration. Hydrocelectomy (surgical excision) may be performed in an outpatient setting under general or spinal anesthesia with the goal of prevention of recurrence by excising the tunica vaginalis or sclerosing the visceral and parietal layers. Surgical excision involves resection or suturing together the two layers. A drainage tube may be required, and the patient is advised to wear a bulky dressing over the incisional site for a few days after the procedure. To reduce swelling, ice packs are applied to the scrotal area during the first 24 hours. A scrotal athletic supporter may be worn for a period of time postoperatively for comfort and support. Surgical risks include hematoma in the loose scrotal tissues, infection, or injury to the scrotum.

Needle aspiration is another option used to remove the fluid in the scrotum. Because it is common for fluid to reaccumulate, this treatment may be followed by the injection of a sclerosing agent to prevent this recurrence. This option may be used for men who are at poor surgical risks. Potential risks include infection and scrotal pain.

Varicocele

A **varicocele** is an abnormal dilation of the pampiniform venous plexus and the internal spermatic vein in the scrotum (the network of veins from the testis and the epididymis, which constitute part of the spermatic cord). Varicoceles occur in approximately 15% to 20% of healthy adult men and 40% of men with infertility; the large majority (95%) are in the left testicle because incompetent valves are more common in the left internal spermatic veins (Norris, 2019). Although men may report scrotal pain, tenderness, heaviness in the inguinal area, and infertility, varicoceles are often asymptomatic.

If the varicocele is mild and fertility is not an issue, no treatment is required, and a scrotal support is usually sufficient to relieve symptoms of heaviness. If the condition results in ongoing distressing symptoms or fertility is an issue, the varicocele can be corrected surgically. Postprocedural education and care include an ice pack applied to the scrotum for the first few hours after surgery to relieve edema, dressing removal after 48 hours, nonstrenuous exercise for the first 2 days, scrotal support, pain control, and reporting complications such as infection and hematoma.

Vasectomy

Vasectomy, or male sterilization, involves the surgical interruption of both vas deferens—the tubes that carry the sperm from the testicles and epididymis to the seminal vesicles—to prevent fertilization of an egg after ejaculation. During the outpatient procedure, the surgeon exposes the vas deferens through a small surgical opening or puncture in the scrotum using a sharp, curved hemostat (see Fig. 53-6). The vas is then ligated (cut) or cauterized (burned), with the severed ends occluded by ties or clips to seal the lumens and then placed back into the scrotum. A section of the vas deferens may or may not be removed. The spermatozoa, which are manufactured in the testes, cannot travel up the vas deferens after this surgery (Cheng et al., 2019).

Because seminal fluid is manufactured predominantly in the seminal vesicles and prostate gland, which are unaffected by vasectomy, no noticeable decrease in the amount of ejaculate occurs (volume decreases approximately 3%), even though it contains no spermatozoa. Because the sperm cells have no exit, they are resorbed into the body. A vasectomy usually has no effect on sexual potency, erection, ejaculation, or production of male hormones and provides no protection against STIs.

Couples who were once worried about pregnancy resulting from contraceptive failure often report a decrease in concern and an increase in spontaneous sexual arousal after vasectomy. Concise and factual preoperative explanations may minimize or relieve the patient's concerns related to pain and reduced masculinity. The patient is advised that he will be

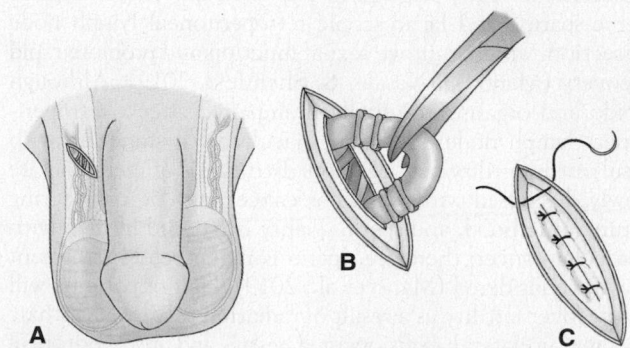

Figure 53-6 • A vasectomy is a resection of the vas deferens to prevent passage of sperm from the testes to the urethra during ejaculation. **A.** An incision or small puncture is made to expose the vas deferens. **B.** The vas deferens is isolated and severed. **C.** The severed ends are occluded with ligatures or clips, or the lumen of each vas is sealed by electrocautery and the incision is sutured closed. (Suturing may not be required if a puncture approach has been used.)

sterile, but that potency will not be altered after a bilateral vasectomy. On rare occasions, a spontaneous reanastomosis of the vas deferens occurs, making it possible to impregnate a partner.

Complications of vasectomy include scrotal ecchymoses and swelling, superficial wound infection, vasitis (inflammation of the vas deferens), epididymitis or epididymo-orchitis, hematomas, chronic pain, and spermatic granuloma. A spermatic granuloma is an inflammatory response to the collection of sperm leaking from the severed end of the proximal vas deferens into the scrotal tissue. A painless small lump is formed, which usually does not require surgical intervention.

Nursing Management

Nursing education focuses on self-management of swelling and discomfort post vasectomy. Applying ice bags intermittently to the scrotum for several hours after surgery can reduce swelling and relieve discomfort. The nurse advises the patient to wear snug cotton underwear or a scrotal support for added comfort and support. Explanation of expected discoloration of the scrotal skin and superficial swelling may alleviate anxiety and concerns. These conditions may be relieved by sitz baths.

Sexual activity may be resumed as desired, usually after 1 week. Fertility remains for a varying time after vasectomy until the spermatozoa stored distally in the seminal vesicles have been evacuated. Sterility is often achieved after 10 to 20 ejaculations following the vasectomy procedure but may take longer. A reliable method of contraception should be used until infertility is confirmed by examination of an ejaculate specimen in the urologist's office at a follow-up appointment, usually 4 to 8 weeks after the vasectomy.

Vasovasostomy (Sterilization Reversal)

Men choosing to undergo vasectomy should not consider the surgical procedure as reversible. However, microsurgical techniques can be used sometimes to reverse a vasectomy and restore patency to the vas deferens in a procedure called vasovasostomy. Many men have sperm in their ejaculate after a reversal, and 50% to 70% can impregnate a partner. The success of the procedure depends on the vasectomy method performed and the amount of time since the vasectomy. The procedure can be very costly, is not covered by insurance, is not permanent with occlusion of the vas recurring 2 or more years after vasovasostomy, and results in sperm counts at lower than prevasectomy levels (Sun & Premal, 2020).

Semen Cryopreservation (Sperm Banking)

Storing fertile semen in a sperm bank before a vasectomy is an option for men who experience a major life change and may want to father a child at a later time. In addition, if a man has just sustained an injury to the spinal cord or is about to undergo a procedure or treatment (e.g., radiation therapy to the pelvis, chemotherapy, orchiectomy) that may affect his fertility, sperm banking may be considered (Halpern, Hill, & Brannigan, 2020). This procedure usually requires several visits to the facility where the sperm is stored under hypothermic conditions. The semen is obtained by masturbation and collected in a sterile container for storage. Insurance carriers rarely cover the cost of semen collection and banking. The costs of semen cryopreservation vary according to facility, method of sperm retrieval, number of specimens, and length of time in storage, making the process cost-prohibitive for some men.

DISORDERS AFFECTING THE PENIS

Phimosis

Phimosis is a condition in which the prepuce (foreskin) cannot be retracted over the glans in uncircumcised males. With the decrease in routine circumcision of newborns, early education should be given to parents about cleansing the foreskin and the need for retraction to cleanse the glans. If the glans is not cleaned, secretions accumulate, causing balanitis (inflammation of the glans penis), which can later lead to adhesions and fibrosis. Phimosis often develops in adults as a result of inflammation, edema, and constriction because of poor hygiene or underlying medical conditions such as diabetes. The thickened secretions, called smegma, can become encrusted with urinary salts and calcify, forming calculi in the prepuce and increasing the risk of penile carcinoma. Treatment for phimosis secondary to inflammation is the application of steroidal cream to the foreskin to soften and correct the narrowness, resulting in decreased constriction. Although phimosis is the most common indication for adult circumcision, it is rarely necessary to surgically correct the condition by loosening or removing the foreskin.

Paraphimosis is a condition in which the foreskin, once retracted over the glans, cannot be returned to its usual position. Chronic inflammation under the foreskin leads to formation of a tight ring of skin when the foreskin is retracted behind the glans, causing venous congestion, edema, and enlargement of the glans, which makes the condition worse. As the condition progresses, arterial occlusion and necrosis of the glans may occur. Paraphimosis usually can be treated by firmly compressing the glans for 5 minutes to reduce the tissue edema and size and then pushing the glans back while simultaneously moving the foreskin forward (manual reduction). The constricting skin ring may require incision under local anesthesia. Circumcision is usually indicated after the inflammation and edema subside (Chapple et al., 2020).

Cancer of the Penis

Penile cancer accounts for less than 1% of cancers among men in the United States. An estimated 1290 new cancer cases and 300 expected deaths occur each year (ACS, 2020). The 5-year survival rates for cancer localized to the penis approaches 80%, but this statistic drops to 52% if the lymph nodes are involved and to 18% if the cancer has spread beyond the inguinal lymph nodes (Chapple et al., 2020). Penile cancer is much more common in some parts of Africa and South America, where it accounts for up to 10% of cancers in men. Because the penis contains different cell types, penile cancer can arise in each type of cell, which determines the prognosis. Types of penile cancer include squamous cell carcinoma (most common; 95% of cases), epidermoid penile cancer, verrucous carcinoma, adenocarcinoma, in situ carcinomas (erythroplasia of Queyrat and Bowen disease), basal cell penile cancer, melanoma, and sarcomas (Cheng et al., 2019). Several risk factors for penile cancer have been identified, including lack of circumcision, poor genital hygiene, phimosis, HPV, smoking, ultraviolet light treatment of psoriasis on the penis, increasing age (two thirds of cases occur in men older than 65 years), penile metastasis secondary to bladder cancer, lichen sclerosus, and balanitis xerotica obliterans (Chapple et al., 2020). However, the exact cause remains unclear. Because penile cancer is rare, there has been little improvement in diagnostic and staging tests, understanding of risk factors, and development of treatment modalities.

Clinical Manifestations

The penile lesion usually alerts the patient to the presence of penile cancer; however, men may delay seeking treatment for more than a year because of embarrassment, fear, or lack of understanding. Common clinical presentations are a painless lump, ulcer, or wartlike growth on the skin of the penis; a change in skin color such as a red rash, bluish growths, or whitish patches; and malodorous and persistent discharge in late stages.

Assessment and Diagnostic Findings

Penile cancer involves the glans most frequently (48%), followed by lesions of the foreskin (21%), the coronal sulcus (6%), the penile shaft (less than 2%), the urethra, and regional or distant lymph nodes (Chapple et al., 2020). A thorough physical examination is necessary, including assessment and palpation of the penis and the inguinal lymph nodes. The size, location, borders, consistency, fixation, and character and time of onset of the penile lesions should be noted. Incisional or excisional biopsy is performed to determine the cell types of the penile cancer. Further staging tests using ultrasonography, MRI, or CT scan may be obtained to determine the extent of local lesions, if metastatic disease is present, and treatment options.

Prevention

The best way to reduce the risk of penile cancer is to avoid known risk factors whenever possible (ACS, 2020). Avoidance of sexual practices that are likely to result in HPV infection may reduce the risk of penile cancer. Gardasil, a vaccine that protects against infection with HPV, the cause of 90% of genital warts, is recommended for males 9 through 26 years old (ACS, 2020). Although men who are uncircumcised have a greater incidence of penile cancer than men who are circumcised, the more important factor in preventing penile cancer is good genital hygiene. Circumcision is not recommended as a prevention strategy (ACS, 2020).

Medical Management

Treatment varies depending on the type and stage of penile cancer, location of the lesion, overall physical health, and personal preferences about treatments and side effects. Treatment emphasis is on minimizing the cancer's invasiveness and preserving organ function (Goonewardene, Pietrzak, & Albala, 2019). The goal of treatment in invasive penile cancer is complete excision with adequate margins. Surgery

is the most common treatment method used in all forms of the disease. Depending on the stage and invasiveness of the cancer, therapeutic options may include simple excision, electrodesiccation and curettage, cryosurgery, Mohs surgery (microscopically controlled surgery), yttrium aluminum garnet (YAG) laser surgery, wide local excision, circumcision, and penectomy (surgical removal of part of the penis or the entire penis). Organ-sparing surgical approaches are preferable. Partial penectomy is preferred to total penectomy because patients can then participate in sexual activity, stand for urination, and maintain cosmesis. Modern reconstructive surgical techniques are providing more options for patients. The shaft of the penis can still respond to sexual arousal with an erection and has the sensory capacity for orgasm and ejaculation. Total penectomy is indicated if the tumor is not amenable to conservative treatment. After a total penectomy, the patient may still experience orgasm with stimulation of the perineum and scrotal area.

Topical chemotherapy with 5-fluorouracil cream or biologic therapy may also be effective. Radiation therapy is used to treat small squamous cell carcinomas of the penis and for palliation in advanced tumors or cases of lymph node metastasis.

Penile cancer spreads primarily to the inguinal lymph nodes; thus, appropriate lymph node management plays a significant role in survival. Because enlarged inguinal lymph nodes are caused by inflammation in 50% of cases, patients who present with enlarged lymph nodes should undergo treatment of the primary lesion followed by a 4- to 6-week course of oral broad-spectrum antibiotic agents. Persistent enlarged lymph nodes after antibiotic therapy should be considered to be metastatic disease and treated with either a sentinel lymph node biopsy (to determine presence of cancer) or with pelvic and bilateral inguinal lymph node dissection. If extensive pelvic lymph node involvement is present, the patient should receive adjuvant or neoadjuvant chemotherapy and postoperative radiation therapy (Goonewardene et al., 2019).

Priapism

Priapism, a relatively uncommon disorder, is defined as a persistent penile erection that may or may not be related to sexual stimulation. The penis becomes large, hard, and painful. Priapism results from either neural or vascular causes, including sickle cell disease, leukemic cell infiltration, polycythemia, spinal cord tumors or injury, and tumor invasion of the penis or its vessels. It may also occur with use of vasoactive agents that affect the central nervous system, antihypertensive agents, antipsychotic and antidepressant medications, substances injected into the penis to treat erectile dysfunction, alcohol, and cocaine. There are three forms of priapism: ischemic (venoocclusive; low flow), nonischemic (high flow), and stuttering (intermittent).

The ischemic form, which is described as nonsexual, persistent erection with little or no cavernous blood flow, must be treated promptly to prevent permanent damage to the penis. The goal of therapy is to improve venous drainage of the corpora cavernosa to prevent ischemia, fibrosis, and erectile dysfunction. The initial treatment is directed at relieving the erection, preventing penile damage, and simultaneously treating the underlying disease. Recommended treatment is aspiration of the corpora cavernosa (with or without irrigation) or injection of sympathomimetic agents (e.g., phenylephrine). Repeated injections may be needed to resolve priapism. Surgical shunts are used to reestablish penile circulation if repeated injections of the sympathomimetic are ineffective (Goonewardene et al., 2019).

Nonischemic priapism and stuttering are generally not considered emergencies and often resolve without treatment. Conservative treatment (e.g., application of ice and site-specific compression to the injury) may be used. If repeated episodes occur, surgical shunting is considered. Patients with the intermittent form of priapism may be instructed in intra-cavernosal self-injection of phenylephrine.

Peyronie Disease

Peyronie disease is an acquired, benign condition that involves the buildup of fibrous plaques in the sheath of the corpus cavernosum. These plaques are not visible when the penis is relaxed. However, when the penis is erect, curvature occurs that can be painful and can make penile-vaginal intercourse difficult or impossible. Peyronie disease typically begins between 45 and 65 years of age. Medical management in the first year of active disease includes systemic, topical, intralesional, or extracorporeal techniques, with 50% of men experiencing spontaneous resolution. Surgical removal of mature plaques is used to treat severe disease. Patients should be fully informed of available treatment options and their likely outcomes (Martins, Kulkarni, & Kohler, 2020).

Urethral Stricture

Urethral stricture is a condition in which a section of the urethra is narrowed. It can occur congenitally or from a scar along the urethra. Traumatic injury to the urethra (e.g., from instrumentation or infections) can result in strictures that restrict urine flow and decrease the urinary stream, leading to spraying or double stream, postvoiding dribbling, and dilation of the proximal urethra and prostatic ducts. Prostatitis is a common complication. Treatment involves dilation of the urethra or, in severe cases, urethrotomy (surgical removal of the stricture). Antimicrobial agents are necessary for resolution of UTIs, followed by long-term prophylactic therapy until the stricture is corrected. Treatment should not be considered successful until at least 1 year has passed, because strictures may recur anytime during that period (Spilotros, Venn, Anderson, et al., 2019).

Circumcision

Circumcision is the surgical excision of the prepuce (foreskin) of the glans penis. Approximately 80% of men are circumcised in the United States, and circumcision is one of the oldest surgical procedures performed worldwide (CDC, 2019). There is controversy about the guidelines to determine the validity of male circumcision as a prevention of disease transmission (Osinibi, Smith, & Henderson, 2020). In adults, circumcision may be indicated as part of treatment for phimosis, paraphimosis, and recurrent infections of the glans and foreskin. It also may be performed at the patient's request.

The primary method of circumcision in adults is surgical excision. Postoperatively, a petrolatum gauze dressing is applied and changed as indicated. The patient is observed for bleeding. Because considerable pain may occur after circumcision, analgesic agents are given as needed.

CRITICAL THINKING EXERCISES

1 **pq** Address the priorities and the approach you would use to care for and to educate a 46-year-old male patient and his wife from the Middle East about self-care management priorities after undergoing surgery for prostate cancer. How will your priorities and approach to care and patient education integrate cultural considerations into essential information required for effective self-care management for discharge?

2 **ebp** A 78-year-old male patient who has a history of myocardial infarction with quadruple bypass surgery, hypertension, and type II diabetes is diagnosed with cancer of the penis. What evidence-based information would you provide to the patient and his spouse to assist in preventing postoperative complications during the recovery period? Identify the evidence for and the criteria used to evaluate the strength of the evidence for the nursing care identified.

3 **ipc** Your patient is a 28-year-old man diagnosed with testicular cancer. You are providing education for the patient and his spouse about the treatment and management of his pre- and postoperative care. The patient asks you about infertility and requests information on sperm banking. Which members of the interdisciplinary health team would you consult to provide this patient with the requested information on sperm banking?

REFERENCES

*Asterisk indicates nursing research.
**Double asterisk indicates classic reference.

Books

American Cancer Society (ACS). (2020). *Cancer facts and figures.* Atlanta, GA: Author.
**Annon, J. S. (1976). *The behavioral treatment of sexual problems.* Honolulu, HI: Enabling Systems.
Bartlik, B., Espinosa, G., & Mindes, J. (2019). *Integrative sexual health.* New York: Oxford University Press.
Brant, J. M. (2019). *Core curriculum for oncology nursing.* Philadelphia, PA: Elsevier Health Sciences.
Campbell, C. (2020). *Contemporary sex therapy: Skills in managing sexual problems.* New York: Routledge.
Centers for Disease Control and Prevention (CDC). (2019). *CDC work preventing HIV, viral hepatitis, STIs, and TB prevention in the United States.* Atlanta, GA: Author.
Chapple, C. R., Steers, W. D., & Evans, C. P. (Eds.). (2020). *Urologic principles and practices* (2nd ed.). New York: Springer.
Cheng, L., MacLennan, G. T., & Bostwick, D. G. (2019). *Urologic surgical pathology* (4th ed.). Philadelphia, PA: Elsevier.
DeNunzio, C., Lombardo, R., Cicione, A. M., et al. (2020). Benign prostatic hyperplasia. In C. R. Chapple, W. D. Steers, & C. P. Evans (Eds.). *Urologic principles and practice* (2nd ed.). New York: Springer.

Goonewardene, S. S., Pietrzak, P., & Albala, D. (2019). *Basic urological management*. New York: Springer.

Hahn, R. G. (2019). What the intensive care physician should know about the transurethral resection syndrome. In J. L. Vincent (Ed). *Annual update in intensive care and emergency medicine 2019*. New York: Springer.

Karch, A. M. (2020). *2020 Lippincott pocket drug guide for nurses* (8th ed.). Philadelphia, PA: Wolters Kluwer.

Katz, A., Cherven, B., Ballard, L., et al. (2019). Male sexuality. In T. Woodruff, D. K. Shah, & W. S. Vitek (Eds.). *Textbook of onco-fertility research and practice: A multidisciplinary approach*. New York: Springer.

Martins, F. E., Kulkarni, S. B., & Köhler, T. S. (2020). *Textbook of male genitourethral reconstruction*. New York: Springer.

McCance, K. L., Huether, S. E., Braskers, V. L., et al. (Eds.). (2018). *Pathophysiology: The biologic basis for disease in adults and children* (8th ed.). St. Louis, MO: Mosby Elsevier.

Messelis, E., Kazer, M. W., & Gelmetti, J. A. (2019). Sexuality, intimacy, and healthy aging. In P. P. Colls (Ed.). *Healthy aging*. New York: Springer.

Norris, T. L. (2019). *Porth's pathophysiology: Concepts of altered health states* (10th ed.). Philadelphia, PA: Wolters Kluwer.

Pagana, K. D., & Pagana, T. J. (2018). *Mosby's diagnostic and laboratory test reference* (13th ed.). St. Louis, MO: Mosby Elsevier.

Pollom, E., Wang, L., Gibbs, I. C., et al. (2019). CyberKnife robotic stereotactic radiosurgery. In D. M. Trifiletti, S. T. Chao, A. Sahgal, et al. (Eds.). *Stereotactic radiosurgery and stereotactic body radiation therapy*. New York: Springer.

Remacle, C. (2019). The patient journey in prostate cancer: Key points for nurses. In F. Charnay-Sonnek & A. E. Murphy (Eds.). *Principle of nursing in oncology*. New York: Springer.

Rhoades, R. A., & Bell, D. R. (2017). *Medical physiology: Principles for clinical medicine*. Philadelphia, PA: Wolters Kluwer.

Sikka, S., & Hellstrom, W. (2017). *Bioenvironmental issues affecting men's reproductive and sexual health*. Philadelphia, PA: Elsevier.

Smith, J. A., Howards, S. S., Preminger, G. M., et al. (2019). *Hinman's atlas of urologic surgery* (4th ed.). Philadelphia, PA: Wolters Kluwer.

Tabloski, P. A. (2019). *Gerontological nursing: The essential guide to clinical practice* (4th ed.). New York: Pearson.

Teelin, K. L., Babu, T. M., & Urban, M. A. (2019). Prostatitis, epididymitis, and orchitis. In J. Domachowske (Ed.). *Introduction to clinical infectious diseases*. New York: Springer.

Weber, J. R., & Kelley, J. H. (2018). *Health assessment in nursing* (6th ed.). Philadelphia, PA: Wolters Kluwer.

Journals and Electronic Documents

Allen, M. S. (2019). Physical activity as an adjunct treatment for erectile dysfunction. *Nature Reviews. Urology, 16*(9), 553–562.

An, Q., Bernstein, K. T., Balaji, A. B., et al. (2020). Sexually transmitted infection screening and diagnosis among adolescent men who have sex with men, three US cities, 2015. *International Journal of STD & AIDS, 31*(1), 53–61.

Arace, J., Flores, V., Monaghan, T., et al. (2020). Rates of clinically significant prostate cancer in African Americans increased significantly following the 2012 US Preventative Services Task Force recommendation against prostate specific antigen screening: A single institution retrospective study. *The International Journal of Clinical Practice, 74*(2), e13447.

Barbonetti, A., D'Andrea, S., Cavallo, F., et al. (2019). Erectile dysfunction and premature ejaculation in homosexual and heterosexual men: A systemic review and meta-analysis of comparative studies. *The Journal of Sexual Medicine, 16*(5), 624–632.

Caram, M. E. V., Ross, R., Lin, P., et al. (2019). Factors associated with use of Sipuleucel-T to treat patients with advanced prostate cancer. *Journal of the American Medical Association Network Open, 2*(4), e192589.

Dennin, R. H., & Sinn, A. (2020). HIV prevention concepts—Counter movements challenging societies. *World Journal of AIDS, 10*, 46–68.

Dong, L., Zieren, R. C., Xue, W., et al. (2019). Metastatic prostate cancer remains incurable, why? *Asian Journal of Urology, 6*(1), 26–41.

El Jalby, M., Thomas, D., Elterman, D., et al. (2019). The effect of diet on BPH, LUTS and ED. *World Journal of Urology, 37*(1), 1001–1005.

Farmer, T., Johnston, M., Milica, A., et al. (2019). Chronic prostatitis/chronic pelvic pain syndrome: A literature review of NIH III Prostatitis. *Current Bladder Dysfunction Reports, 14*, 83–89.

Halpern, J. A., Brannigan, R. E., & Schlegel, P. N. (2019). Fertility-enhancing male reproductive surgery: Glimpses into the past and thoughts for the future. *Fertility & Sterility, 112*(3), 426–437.

Halpern, J. A., Hill, R., & Brannigan, R. E. (2020). Guideline based approach to male fertility preservation. *Urologic Oncology, 38*(1), 31–35.

Jeong, C. W., Cowan, J. E., Broering, J. M., et al. (2019). Robust health utility assessment among long-term survivors of prostate cancer: Results from the Cancer of the Prostate Strategic Urologic Research Endeavor Registry. *European Urology, 76*(6), 743–751.

Kaufman, J., Lapauw, B., Mahmoud, A., et al. (2019). Aging and the male reproductive system. *Endocrine Reviews, 40*(4), 906–972.

*Kearns, J. T., Adeyemi, O., Anderson, W. E., et al. (2020). Contemporary racial disparities in PSA screening in a large, integrated health care system. *Journal of Clinical Oncology, 38*(6 Suppl), 308–318.

Keenan, M., Thomas, P., & Cotler, K. (2020). Increasing sexually transmitted infection detection through screening at extragenital sites. *The Journal for Nurse Practitioners, 16*(2), e27–e30.

Kelly, E., Morgan, K., Connelly, Z., et al. (2019). PSA density performs better in Caucasian men than in African American men in predicting prostate cancer and significant cancer on prostate biopsy. *The Urology Journal, 201*(Suppl 4), e654.

Klaassen, Z., Wallis, C. J. D., Lavallée, L. T., et al. (2020). Perioperative venous thromboembolism prophylaxis in prostate cancer surgery. *World Journal of Urology, 38*(3), 593–600.

Kuehn, B. M. (2019). A proactive approach needed to combat rising STIs. *JAMA, 321*(4), 330–332.

Kunath, F., Goebell, P. J., Wullich, B., et al. (2020). Timing of androgen deprivation monotherapy and combined treatments in castration-sensitive and castration-resistant prostate cancer: A narrative review. *World Journal of Urology, 38*(3), 601–611.

Law, K. W., Nguyen, D. D., Barkin, J., et al. (2020). Diagnosis of prostate cancer: The implications and proper utilization of PSA and its variants; indications of use of MRI and biomarkers. *Canadian Journal of Urology, 27*(Suppl 1), 3–10.

Li, Y., Lu, Q., Wang, Y., et al. (2020). Racial differences in testicular cancer in the United States: Descriptive epidemiology. *BMC Cancer, 20*(1), 1–10.

Lim, S., Jun, C., Chang, D., et al. (2019). Robotic transrectal ultrasound guided prostate biopsy. *IEEE Transactions on Biomedical Engineering, 66*(9), 2527–2537.

Lindsey, J. P., Lue, T. F., & Shindel, A. W. (2020). The future of penile prostheses for the treatment of erectile dysfunction. *Translational Andrology and Urology, 9*(Suppl 2), 244–251.

Mano, R., Di Natale, R., & Sheinfeld, J. (2019). Current controversies on the role of retroperitoneal lymphadenectomy for testicular cancer. *Urologic Oncology, 37*(3), 209–218.

McMahon, C. G. (2019). Current diagnosis and management of erectile dysfunction. *Medical Journal of Australia, 2*(10), 469–476.

Meites, E., Szilagyi, P. G., Chesson, H. W., et al. (2019). Human papillomavirus vaccination for adults: Updated recommendations of the Advisory Committee on Immunization Practices. *Morbidity and Mortality Weekly Report, 68*(32), 698–702.

Meyer, C. J. (2020). Sexual dysfunction after prostate cancer treatment: Patient education of optimal treatment choices for risk reduction. *Lynchburg Journal of Medical Science, 2*(2), 1–10.

National Comprehensive Cancer Network (NCCN). (2020a). Cancer guidelines. Retrieved on 4/10/2020 at: www.nccn.org/patients/guidelines/cancers.aspx

National Comprehensive Cancer Network (NCCN). (2020b). Clinical practice guidelines in oncology: Prostate cancer. Retrieved on 4/10/2020 at: www.nccn.org/professionals/default.aspx

National Comprehensive Cancer Network (NCCN). (2020c). Clinical practice guidelines in oncology: Testicular cancer. Retrieved on 4/10/2020 at: www.nccn.org/professionals/default.aspx

Ngaage, L. M., Elegbede, A., Sugarman, J., et al. (2020). The Baltimore Criteria for an ethical approach to penile transplantation: A clinical guideline. *Transplant International, 33*, 471–482.

Nuhn, P., De Bono, J. S., Fizazi, K., et al. (2019). Update on systemic prostate cancer therapies: Management of metastatic castration-resistant prostate cancer in the era of precision oncology. *European Urology, 75*(1), 88–99.

Osinibi, E., Smith, T., & Henderson, A. (2020). A primary care update to circumcision. *InnovAiT: Education and Inspiration for General Practice, 13*(3), 173–178.

*Owens, O. L., Kim, S., & Tavakoli, A. S. (2019). Are decision aids leading to shared prostate cancer screening decisions among African American men?: iDecide. *Cancer Causes & Control, 30*(7), 713–719.

*Peard, L., Goodwin, J., Hensley, P., et al. (2019). Examining and understanding value: The impact of preoperative characteristics, intraoperative variables, and postoperative complications on cost of robot-assisted laparoscopic radical prostatectomy. *Journal of Endourology, 33*(7), 541–548.

Rantell, A., Apostolidis, A., Anding, R., et al. (2017). How does lower urinary tract dysfunction affect sexual function in men and women? *Neurourology and Urodynamics, 36*, 949–952.

Riviere, P., Luterstein, E., Kumar, A., et al. (2020). Survival of African American and non-Hispanic white men with prostate cancer in an equal-access health care system. *Cancer, 126*(8), 1683–1690.

Rowland, D. L., McNabney, S. M., & Donarski, A. M. (2019). Plant-derived supplements for sexual health and problems: Part 1—Trends over the past decade. *Current Sexual Health Reports, 11*, 132–143.

Sargon, J., Lamb, J. V., & Patel, M. I. (2019). Preventing osteoporosis in men taking androgen deprivation therapy for prostate cancer: A systematic review and meta-analysis. *European Urology Oncology, 2*(5), 551–561.

Shore, N. D., Guerrero, S., Sanahuja, R. M., et al. (2019). A new sustained-release, 3-month leuprolide acetate formulation achieves and maintains castrate concentrations of testosterone in patients with prostate cancer. *Clinical Therapeutics, 41*(3), 412–425.

Spilotros, M., Venn, S., Anderson, P., et al. (2019). Penile urethral stricture disease. *Journal of Clinical Urology, 12*(2), 145–157.

Sun, R., & Premal, P. (2020). Predicting patency after vasovasostomy and heterogeneity in defining success. *Fertility & Sterility, 113*(4), 755–755.

*Tasso, G., Beels, E., Del Favero, L., et al. (2020). Non-obstructive slings (nos) for stress urinary incontinence after prostate surgery. Analysis of outcomes in different subgroups of patients. *Journal of Urology, 203*(Suppl 4), e593.

*Ustundag, H. (2019). Assessment of the testicular self-examination knowledge and Health Belief Model of health sciences students. *International Journal of Caring Sciences, 12*(2), 972–978.

Wu, Y., Jiang, H., Tan, M., et al. (2020). Screening for chronic prostatitis pathogens using high-throughput next-generation sequencing. *The Prostate, 80*(7), 577–587.

Zhou, A. G., Salles, D. C., Samarska, I. V., et al. (2019). How are Gleason Scores categorized in the current literature: An analysis and comparison of articles published in 2016–2017. *European Urology, 75*(1), 25–31.

Resources

American Cancer Society, www.cancer.org/cancer/prostate-cancer.html
American Urological Association, www.auanet.org
CancerCare, www.cancercare.org
Centers for Disease Control and Prevention (CDC), www.cdc.gov/cancer
National Cancer Institute (NCI), www.cancer.gov
National Comprehensive Cancer Network (NCCN), www.nccn.org
National Institutes of Health, National Center for Complementary and Integrative Health (NCCIH), www.nccih.nih.gov
Prostate Cancer Foundation, www.pcf.org
Testicular Cancer Society (TCS), www.testicularcancersociety.org
Urology Care Foundation, www.urologyhealth.org
Us TOO International Prostate Cancer Education and Support Network, www.ustoo.org

54 Assessment and Management of Patients Who Are LGBTQ

NURSING CONCEPTS

Assessment	Family	Sexuality
Communication	Identity	
Development/Human Development	Professionalism/Professional Behaviors	

GLOSSARY

bisexual: people who are romantically, emotionally, or sexually attracted to both male and female genders

cisgender: people who identify with the gender that matches the sex assigned to them at birth

gay: people who are romantically, emotionally, or sexually attracted to the same gender, such as men attracted to men

gender: set of socially constructed norms and behaviors that are taught to women and men

gender dysphoria: distress a person feels due to a mismatch between their gender identity and sex assigned at birth

gender identity: the internal self-conception of one's gender

intersex: a term used for a person who is born with biological traits that do not fit into those that traditionally characterize either male or female

lesbian: a term that gay women, or those women who are romantically, emotionally, or sexually attracted to other women, may prefer to use

LGBTQ: acronym that stands for lesbian, gay, bisexual, transgender, and queer

queer: people who are romantically, emotionally, or sexually attracted to numerous genders (male, female, transgender, intersex, etc.) or people who identify as nonheterosexual but do not want to use labels, such as gay, lesbian, or bisexual

questioning: a person who is unsure or is still exploring their sexual orientation or is concerned about applying a social label to themselves

sex: refers to the physical or biological characteristics that distinguish women and men, such as chromosomes, genitals, and hormones

sexual orientation: umbrella term that refers to romantic, emotional, or sexual attraction to persons of the opposite gender, the same gender, or to both or more than one gender

third-person pronouns: a way of referencing a person other than the self that may or may not use gender-specific labels (e.g., he/him, she/her, they/them)

transgender: umbrella term used to describe the full range of people whose gender identity does not match with the sex assigned to them at birth

transgender man: refers to a person who was assigned a female sex at birth but identifies with a male or masculine gender

transgender woman: refers to a person who was assigned a male sex at birth but identifies with a female or feminine gender

transition: process of aligning a person's gender expression with their self-identified gender identity, which can include social, medical, surgical, and legal changes

People who are **LGBTQ** (lesbian, gay, bisexual, transgender, and queer) have unique health care needs. They also experience particular health risks and disparities based on sexuality and gender identity. Increasingly, nursing and medical professionals are recognizing these risks and disparities; furthermore, these professionals are acknowledging the importance of providing culturally appropriate care to people who identify as LGBTQ. Nurses will encounter people who are LGBTQ and their families in every practice setting. As they would for other diverse populations, nurses should be prepared to provide quality and culturally appropriate care. This chapter focuses on the terminology around sexuality and gender identity, culturally appropriate assessment and communication, and assessment and management of patients who identify as LGBTQ, and, in particular, the unique health care needs of those patients seeking gender reassignment. The management of patients seeking gender reassignment using both nonsurgical and surgical treatments is discussed.

Sexuality and Gender Identity

Understanding the meaning and significance of the concepts and terminology for sexuality and gender identity is important to caring for patients who are LGBTQ.

Sexuality

Human sexuality is the way people experience and express themselves sexually. This involves biological, physical, emotional, or social feelings. Sexual orientation, which is a component of sexuality, is different than gender (see discussion below). **Sexual orientation** is an umbrella term that refers to romantic, emotional, or sexual attraction to persons of the opposite gender, the same gender, or to more than one gender. There are many terms that people use to describe their sexual orientation; however, the most commonly used terms are *heterosexual* or *straight*, *gay* or *lesbian*, *bisexual*, and *queer*.

People who are attracted to a different gender, such as women who are attracted to men, typically identify as heterosexual or straight. People who are attracted to the same gender, such as men attracted to men, often identify as **gay**. Gay women may prefer the term **lesbian**. People who are attracted to both male and female genders usually identify as **bisexual**.

Although the term *queer* was historically used as a word of insult, many people now choose to use it to identify their sexual orientation. People who are **queer** typically experience attractions to numerous genders (male, female, transgender, intersex, etc.). A person who does not want to use labels, such as gay, lesbian, or bisexual, may also use the term queer to identify as a nonheterosexual.

People who are exploring or are unsure of their sexual orientation may refer to themselves as **questioning**. Questioning one's own sexuality can be difficult and confusing and can take years to understand. This term can also apply to people who are concerned about applying a social label (e.g., gay, lesbian, bisexual, queer) to themselves and may prefer to use this term.

Gender Identity

To fully understand the term *gender identity*, the concepts of *sex* and *gender* must be discussed first. **Sex** in the context of gender identity refers to the physical or biological characteristics that distinguish women and men, such as chromosomes, genitals, and hormones (Eliason & Chinn, 2018). For example, women have XX chromosomes, a uterus and ovaries, and the primary sex hormone is estrogen; whereas, men have XY chromosomes, a penis and testicles, and the primary sex hormone is testosterone. In most societies, people are assigned either the male or female sex at birth. However, some persons do not clearly have these defined binary sets of sex chromosomes or may not have clearly distinguishable genitalia. **Intersex** is a term used for a person who is born with biological traits that do not fit into those that traditionally characterize either male or female.

Gender is a set of socially constructed characteristics of women and men (World Health Organization, 2019). Although a person is either assigned as male or female at birth based on sex characteristics, they are taught norms and behaviors that are appropriate for their gender. Gender is usually the first thing we notice about a person based on cues, such as voice, communication style, hairstyle, clothing, and mannerisms. Gender norms, behaviors, and cues vary from society to society and can be changed.

Gender identity refers to how a person feels about themselves or their self-concept as female or male, feminine or masculine, or as something on the continuum between the two extremes (Eliason & Chinn, 2018). **Cisgender** is a term that often refers to people who identify with the gender that matches the sex assigned to them at birth (e.g., a person with a female sex that identifies as a woman). **Transgender** is an umbrella term used to describe the full range of people whose gender identity does not match with the sex assigned to them at birth. Although there is a diversity of terms that transgender people may use to identify their gender (e.g., trans, gender nonconforming, agender, and genderqueer), this chapter will use two main terms: transgender woman and transgender man. **Transgender woman**, or male to female, refers to a person who was assigned a male sex at birth but identifies with a female or feminine gender. **Transgender man**, or female to male, refers to a person who was assigned a female sex at birth but identifies with a male or masculine gender.

It is important to remember that gender identity and sexual orientation are two different self-concepts. Sexual orientation refers to a person's attraction, and gender identity refers to how a person feels about their gender. For example, a transgender man who is attracted only to men has a male gender identity and a gay sexual orientation. Health care professionals should never assume a person's sexual orientation or gender identity based on physical characteristics, mannerisms, communication style, voice, clothing, or hairstyle.

Statistics on LGBTQ Populations

There are many challenges to estimating the LGBTQ population in the United States. The biggest challenge is the lack of federal-level data. Historically, the U.S. government has not collected sexual orientation and gender identity data on surveys such as the census count. Consequently, researchers have had to use statistical modeling to estimate LGBTQ population sizes.

The Williams Institute (2018), a prominent LGBTQ public policy organization, estimates that approximately 4.5%

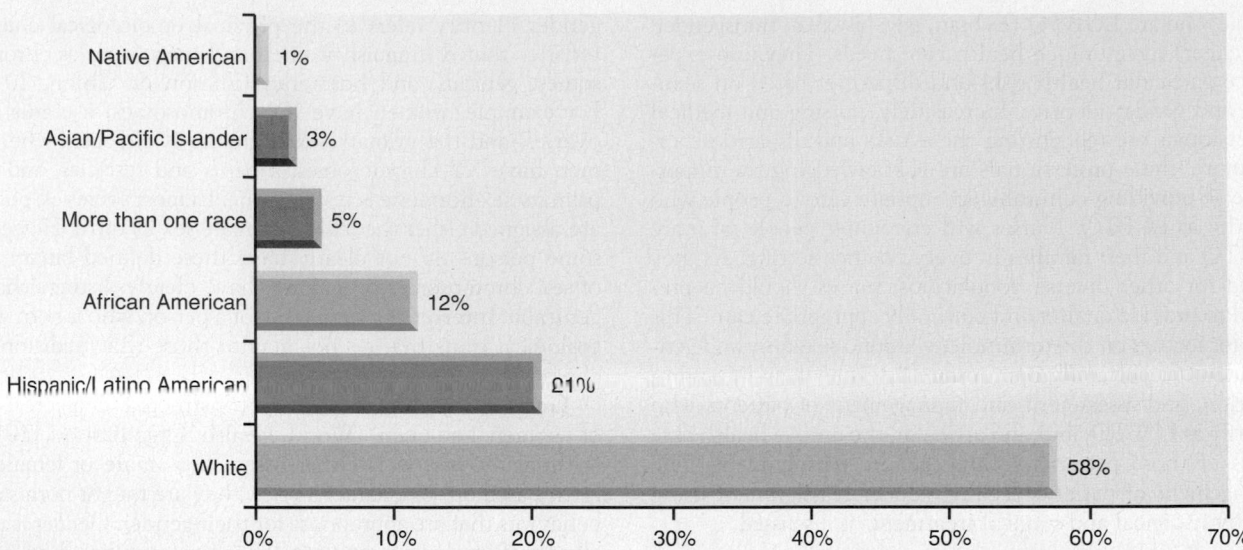

Figure 54-1 • Distribution of race among people in the United States who are LGBTQ. Adapted from The Williams Institute. (2019). LGBT demographic data interactive. Retrieved on 2/17/2020 at: williamsinstitute.law.ucla.edu/visualization/lgbt-stats/?topic=LGBT

of the U.S. population is LGBTQ. That percentage translates into nearly 15 million people. Although that number encompasses sexual orientation and gender identity, at least 1 million people in the United States identify as transgender (Meerwijk & Sevelius, 2017). Of the 15 million people who are LGBTQ, 58% identify as female and 42% as male; it is important to note that these survey data did not include nonbinary or gender-fluid gender identity options. The distribution of race and age among the LGBTQ population is shown in Figures 54-1 and 54-2, respectively (The Williams Institute, 2019).

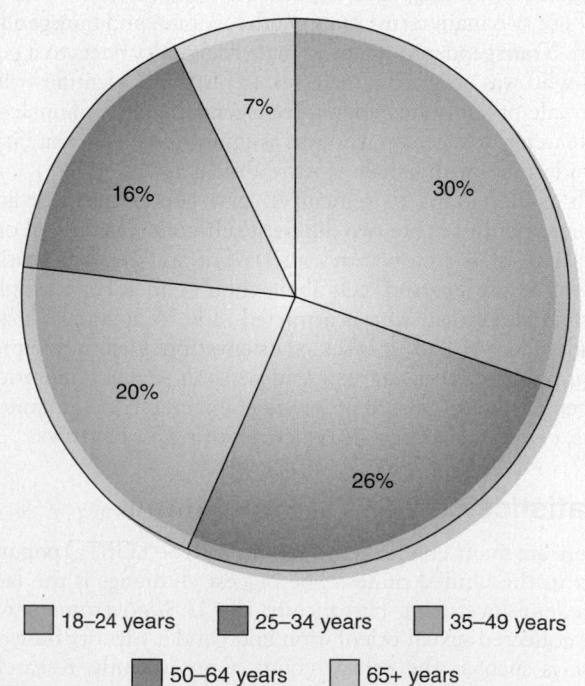

Figure 54-2 • Distribution of age among people in the United States who are LGBTQ. Adapted from The Williams Institute. (2019). LGBT demographic data interactive. Retrieved on 2/17/2020 at: williamsinstitute.law.ucla.edu/visualization/lgbt-stats/?topic=LGBT

Like parents who are heterosexual, parents who are LGBTQ are married, unmarried and cohabiting, separated or divorced, and single. There are intact families and blended families, and children who live between households. There are at least 1.1 million people who are LGBTQ in a legal same-sex marriage, over 1.2 million people who are LGBTQ who are in an unmarried same-sex relationship, and upwards of 3.7 million children under the age of 18 with at least one parent who is LGBTQ (Family Equality Council, 2017). Given the numerous limitations to accurately counting the number of families headed by people who are LGBTQ, these numbers are likely much higher. Also, it is important to note that on June 26, 2015, the U.S. Supreme Court ruled in *Obergefell v. Hodges* (576 U.S.) that the Constitution guarantees same-sex couples the right to marry and have their marriages recognized by the states. In the United States, there are over 1000 statutory provisions classified in the U.S. Code that provide benefits, rights, and privileges to legally married couples. This ruling was important to protecting couples who are LGBTQ and their children, especially in the health care setting. For example, marriage allows people to make medical, legal, and financial decisions on behalf of an incapacitated spouse even when the spouse does not designate a durable power of attorney. Without legal marriage, people can be barred from visiting their partner in the hospital. Without marriage, people could not easily cover the health care needs of their entire family with health insurance.

Health Risks

The root cause of health risks or disparities among people who are LGBTQ is stigma (i.e., negative and unfair beliefs). For reasons beyond the scope of this chapter, people learn to stigmatize some human differences such as skin color and sexual orientation, whereas other differences are not stigmatized, such as eye color or left-handedness (Eliason & Chinn, 2018). People who are LGBTQ have historically been viewed as different or deviant, which is known as stigmatization. The stigma of people who are LGBTQ has led to many social effects, such as lack of recognition of relationships and family, the right to adopt, hate crimes and violence, discrimination in employment and education, and discrimination in housing (Eliason & Chinn, 2018). A person who is LGBTQ does not experience health risks simply because they identify as gay, lesbian, bisexual, or transgender; the stigma associated with their LGBTQ identity is what puts them at risk for certain health disparities.

As compared to people who are heterosexual and cisgender, people who are LGBTQ are at greater risk for certain physical and mental health issues. In terms of mental health disorders, people who are LGBTQ have a higher rate of depression and anxiety (Bostwick, Hughes, Steffen, et al., 2019; Ross, Salway, Tarasoff, et al., 2018; Witcomb, Bouman, Claes, et al., 2018) and experience more suicidality (Lyons, Walters, Jack, et al., 2019; McNeil, Ellis, & Eccles, 2017). Nearly 50% of people who are transgender have reported suicide attempts. Moreover, people who are LGBTQ tend to experience more victimization, such as physical or verbal harassment, which is associated with higher rates of depression and suicidality (Burks, Cramer, Henderson, et al., 2018).

Women who are lesbian, bisexual, or queer tend to be at greater risk for obesity and cardiovascular disease as compared to heterosexual women (Simoni, Smith, Oost, et al., 2017). Obesity in women who are lesbian, bisexual, or queer is linked to dysregulated eating, such as emotional- or binge-eating. The causes of dysregulated eating are complex and include biological, psychological, and social factors. In women who are lesbian, bisexual, or queer, stigma is one of the root causes of obesity. Stigmatizing experiences, such as discrimination or victimization, leads to emotional distress, which in turn is associated with dysregulated eating as a coping strategy (Mason, Smith, & Lavender, 2019) (see Chapter 42 for further discussion on obesity).

Men who are gay or bisexual and transgender women have higher rates of infection with the human immune deficiency virus (HIV) as compared to the general population. Men who are gay or bisexual is the population most affected by HIV in the United States (Centers for Disease Control and Prevention [CDC], 2019a). People who are transgender receive an HIV diagnosis at three times the rate of the national average (CDC, 2019b). Among these populations, rates of HIV are even higher among certain subgroups, especially people who are African American and young adult (see Chapter 32 for further discussion on HIV).

Assessment

Nurses should strive to create a welcoming, inclusive, and therapeutic relationship with every patient. To better achieve this type of relationship with people who are LGBTQ, nurses should use inclusive terms and language. This will increase the likelihood of eliciting accurate information from anyone whose experience is different from cultural norms (Eliason & Chinn, 2018). Using inclusive language conveys to the person who is LGBTQ that the interviewer is open to hearing about their sexuality, gender identity, and relationships. If a nurse does not yet know a patient's sexual orientation and gender identity, they should always use neutral language to ensure the patient is comfortable during the assessment (see the Resources section at the end of the chapter for educational

TABLE 54-1	Sample Questions and Statements Using Gender-Neutral Language	
Question/Statement	Question/Statement with Neutral Language
Good morning, sir.	Good morning.
How may I help you, ma'am?	How may I help you?
She is scheduled for an x-ray.	They are scheduled for an x-ray.
Do you have a husband?	Are you in a relationship?
What are the names of your mom and dad?	What are the names of your parents or guardians?

materials that promote developing welcoming and inclusive patient–provider relationships).

In the United States, people tend to communicate using a binary gender system (female or male) and based on the assumption that people are heterosexual. This type of communication practice can be harmful to people who are LGBTQ, especially in the health care setting. Nurses should strive to use language terms that avoid assumptions about a patient's gender identity and sexual orientation. For example, nurses should avoid using singular **third-person pronouns** (a way of referencing a person other than the self that may use gender-specific labels) and salutations that use gender-specific labels (e.g., sir/miss/madam, Mr./Mrs./Ms.) until confirming the patient's preferences. They should also avoid using terms that assume sexual orientation of the patient and their family (e.g., wife/husband, boyfriend/girlfriend, mother/father). Table 54-1 provides specific examples of neutral questions and statements.

Nurses should routinely assess each patient's sexual orientation and gender identity (SO/GI), including preferred pronouns. In fact, national and federal recommendations for routine collection of SO/GI in health care settings have spanned nearly 20 years (Maragh-Bass, Torain, Adler, et al., 2017). Assessing for SO/GI in the health care setting facilitates the provision of enhanced, holistic, person-centered care. For example, people who are LGBTQ may have unique health risks that need attention or may have a diverse family structure. People who are LGBTQ typically want to disclose their SO/GI to health care professionals. However, most health care professionals do not ask about SO/GI and instead make assumptions about a patient's gender identity and presume every patient is heterosexual. These assumptions put the burden on the patient to disclose ("come out" about their SO/GI), putting them in a vulnerable position (Eliason & Chinn, 2018). Thus, nurses should be skilled at properly assessing for SO/GI and preferred pronouns (Chart 54-1).

Assessing for family structure and other important relationships should be routine for every patient. People who are LGBTQ may have diverse or nontraditional family structures and may include people who are not biologically related. Nurses should assess for family and family of choice. Family of choice is a commonly used term among people who are LGBTQ. Some people who are LGBTQ have been rejected by their family of origin and thus create their own family network of people who support and care for them (Eliason

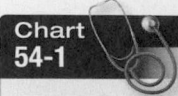

Chart 54-1 · ASSESSMENT
Personal Information

The nurse introduces these assessment questions by stating:

- "I am going to ask you a few questions about your sexual orientation and gender identity so we can provide personalized and affirmative care to you. These are questions I ask every patient. If you do not feel comfortable answering these questions, we can skip them."

The nurse assesses for gender identity using a two-step question:

- "What sex was listed on your birth certificate?"
- "What is your current gender identity?" or "How do you describe your gender identity?"

Assessing for pronouns:

- "What pronouns do you prefer we use?"
- If the patient is unsure of what this means, you can ask, "Do you use the pronouns he/him, she/her, or something else?"

Assessing sexual orientation:

- "What is your sexual orientation?" or "How do you describe your sexual orientation?"

Assessing for preferred name:

- "What name do you preferred to be called?" or "What is the name that you would like us to use?"

Adapted from Centers for Disease Control and Prevention (CDC). (2020). Collecting sexual orientation and gender identity information. Retrieved on 4/20/2020 at: www.cdc.gov/hiv/clinicians/transforming-health/health-care-providers/collecting-sexual-orientation.html; The Fenway Institute. (2017). Collecting sexual orientation and gender identity (SO/GI) data in electronic health records. Retrieved on 4/20/2020 at: www.lgbthealtheducation.org/wp-content/uploads/2017/05/SOGI-Office-Hours-Update-Final.pdf; The Fenway Institute. (2018). Ready, set go! Guidelines and tips for collecting patient data on sexual orientation and gender identity. Retrieved on 4/21/2020 at: www.lgbthealtheducation.org/wp-content/uploads/2018/03/Ready-Set-Go-publication-Updated-April-2018.pdf

& Chinn, 2018). Moreover, some people who are LGBTQ fear discrimination and exclusion of not only themselves but also their family. This is especially true of people who live in states that sanction narrow definitions of legal relationships (Eliason & Chinn, 2018).

Nurses should use neutral terms and be sensitive when interviewing all people about their family structure. Since some people who are LGBTQ have nontraditional family structures and families of choice, it is best to start the interview with an open-ended question, such as "Tell me about your family and social support system." As the nurse asks follow-up questions, neutral terms should be used when inquiring about partners/significant others and parents/guardians (examples are listed in Table 54-1). Also, the nurse should not assume a person who is LGBTQ does not have children. Many people who are LGBTQ have children through adoption, surrogacy, and previous relationships. If the patient has children, the nurse should avoid making assumptions about the family structure. Finally, the nurse should mirror the language and terms used by the patient and their family. For example, if a male-identifying patient refers to his significant other as "husband," the nurse should not choose to use a different term, such as "partner."

In terms of health assessment, people who are LGBTQ typically do not require specific assessments or diagnostic tests. They should receive nursing and medical person-centered care like any other patient. Depending on the health care setting, the nurse may want to focus parts of their assessment on those health risks mentioned earlier in the chapter. Time could be spent asking the person who is LGBTQ about anxiety, depression, suicidality, and discrimination and victimization. Since gay and bisexual men and transgender women have higher rates of HIV, sexual activity, safe sex practices, and HIV status should be assessed. People who identify as transgender should be asked about hormone treatment and surgical procedures only if it is relevant to the care being provided.

Gerontologic Considerations

In understanding older adults who are LGBTQ, it is important to recognize their social, historical, and cultural experiences. The lived experience of older adults who are LGBTQ is vastly different than younger people who are LGBTQ. Older adults who are LGBTQ lived their younger years in stigmatizing and dangerous environments (Ducheny, Hardacker, Claybren, et al., 2019). They frequently experienced discrimination and abuse in multiple areas, including physical, mental, and verbal abuse (Witten & Eyler, 2016). For many decades, it was dangerous for people who were LGBTQ to "come out" (disclose their sexual orientation or gender identity) and extremely difficult to find affirming health care services. Before the 1960s, people who identified as transgender were often committed to psychiatric institutions or forced to live in seclusion. From 1960 through 1990, people who identified as transgender could access rigid and isolating treatment and were made to adhere to narrow requirements (Ducheny et al., 2019). Until 1973, homosexuality was a diagnosed psychiatric mental illness. Moreover, older people who are LGBTQ faced significant discrimination that was sanctioned by state and federal governments. This history has profoundly affected the way in which older adults who are LGBTQ view and access all facets of health care, including clinics, hospitals, and assisted living/nursing homes (Witten & Eyler, 2016). To care for and promote the health of older adults who are LGBTQ, nurses should be mindful and understanding of this background. Moreover, this amplifies the importance of nurses needing to always provide a safe and welcoming space for all patients that promotes human dignity. Older adults who have hidden their sexual orientation or gender identity for many years due to fears of discrimination will be more likely to disclose this information if the nurse uses language and questions that signals to the patient that they are accepting and safe.

Assessment and Management of Patients Seeking Gender Reassignment

People who are transgender may experience **gender dysphoria**, which is the distress caused by the dissonance between the person's gender identity and that person's sex assigned at birth. To assist people with this distress and find a gender role that is comfortable for them, treatment is available and may include medical and surgical interventions. Treatment is individualized, meaning that interventions that effectively alleviate gender dysphoria in one patient may not work for a different patient.

Health care teams who provide psychological, medical, and surgical treatments to people who are transgender often follow the Standards of Care published by the World Professional Association for Transgender Health (WPATH, 2012). Even though the latest version of the Standards of Care was released in 2012, at the time of this book print, it is still the leading resource for the care of people who are transgender. Other important resources include the Guidelines for the Primary and Gender-Affirming Care of Transgender and Gender Nonbinary People from the University of California, San Francisco (Deutsch, 2016) and the Principles of Transgender Medicine and Surgery (Ettner, Monstrey, & Coleman, 2016) (see References and Resources sections at the end of the chapter).

Providing treatment to people who are seeking gender reassignment almost always starts with confirming a diagnosis of gender dysphoria. Many health insurance companies require a gender dysphoria or related diagnosis before covering the costs of gender reassignment treatments. Gender dysphoria is a diagnosis in the *Diagnostic and Statistical Manual of Mental Disorders* (DSM-5). Chart 54-2 lists the criteria used to diagnose a person with gender dysphoria. In short, to be diagnosed with gender dysphoria, a person must exhibit specific thoughts and feelings about the incongruence of their gender identity and their secondary sex characteristics for a period of at least 6 months (American Psychiatric Association, 2013).

An experienced mental health care professional, such as a psychiatric mental health nurse practitioner, clinical social worker, psychologist, or psychiatrist, can assess, diagnose, and provide psychological treatment for gender dysphoria. Before a health care provider prescribes medical or surgical treatments (e.g., hormones, gender reassignment surgery), they usually require that the person has consulted with a mental health care provider and received a diagnosis of gender dysphoria.

When a person wants to address the distress or other negative emotions associated with having a gender that does not align with their sex assigned at birth (gender dysphoria), they will usually work with an interdisciplinary health care team. This team typically includes a mental health care professional, a health care provider experienced in endocrinology, and a surgeon. The mental health care professional will provide psychological support to the person during their gender identity journey; the endocrinology health care provider will prescribe hormones and monitor outcomes; the surgeon will handle gender reassignment surgeries. Depending on the treatment settings, nurses are involved in various capacities along the treatment continuum.

Medical Management

Hormone Therapy

In addition to alleviating gender dysphoria, the goal of hormone gender-affirming therapy is the acquisition of the secondary sex characteristics of the other gender, to the fullest extent possible (Gooren, 2016). To achieve the secondary sex characteristics of the opposite gender, sex steroids/hormones are needed. There is no known difference in sensitivity to the action of sex hormones on the basis of genetics or gonadal/sex status (Gooren, 2016), meaning that a person can develop secondary sex characteristics of the opposite gender by taking sex hormones. However, certain effects of sex hormones cannot be reversed. For example, in people who are transgender women (male to female), the previous effects of androgens on the skeleton (average greater height; size and shape of hands, feet, and jaw; and pelvic structure) cannot be reversed by hormones (Gooren, 2016) (Table 54-2).

For patients who are transgender women, estrogen is prescribed to produce the desired physical changes. The prescribed dose of estrogen is individualized and depends on many different factors, such as the patient's goals, risk/benefit ratio, presence of other medical conditions, presence or absence of gonads, and social and economic issues (WPATH, 2012). Estrogen treatment should produce changes in body hair, breast development, skin, body fat composition, muscle mass, testes, and prostate. In addition to estrogen, androgen-reducing medications to reduce testosterone levels are also often prescribed, which diminish masculine characteristics and minimize the dosage of estrogen needed to suppress testosterone. Common androgen-reducing medications include spironolactone, cyproterone acetate, GnRH agonists (e.g., goserelin, buserelin, triptorelin), and 5-alpha reductase inhibitors (e.g., finasteride, dutasteride) (WPATH, 2012). Progestogen does not add to the feminization process and is typically not recommended due to the higher incidence of breast cancer and cardiovascular disease (Gooren, 2016). See Table 54-3 for commonly prescribed medications.

Chart 54-2 DSM-5[a] Diagnostic Criteria for Gender Dysphoria in Adolescents and Adults

A. A marked incongruence between one's experienced/expressed gender and assigned gender, of at least 6 months duration, as manifested by at least two of the following:
  1. Marked incongruence between one's experienced/expressed gender and primary and/or secondary sex characteristics (or in young adolescents, the anticipated secondary sex characteristics).
  2. A strong desire to be rid of one's primary and/or secondary sex characteristics because of a marked incongruence with one's experienced/expressed gender (or in young adolescents, a desire to prevent the development of the anticipated secondary sex characteristics).
  3. A strong desire for the primary and/or secondary sex characteristics of the other gender.
  4. A strong desire to be of the other gender (or some alternative gender different from one's assigned gender).
  5. A strong desire to be treated as the other gender (or some alternative gender different from one's assigned gender).
  6. A strong conviction that one has the typical feelings and reactions of the other gender (or some alternative gender different from one's assigned gender).

B. The condition is associated with clinically significant distress or impairment in social, occupational, or other important areas of functioning.

[a]DSM-5, *Diagnostic and Statistical Manual of Mental Disorders* (5th edition).

Reprinted with permission from American Psychiatric Association. (2013). *Diagnostic and statistical manual of mental disorders* (5th ed.). Arlington, VA: Author.

TABLE 54-2	Physical Effects of Hormone Treatment for Gender Reassignment
Feminizing Hormones (Male to Female)	**Masculinizing Hormones (Female to Male)**
Reduction in growth and thinning of body hair	Growth of facial and body hair; scalp hair loss
Breast formation	Decrease in glandular activity of breasts
Softening of skin and decreased oiliness	Skin oiliness and acne
Increase in body fat and decrease in muscle mass	Decrease in subcutaneous fat, increase in abdominal fat, and increase in muscle mass
Testicular and prostate volume atrophy	Clitoral enlargement and vaginal atrophy
Decreased sperm production	Cessation of menses
Male sexual dysfunction	Deepening of voice

Adapted from World Professional Association for Transgender Health (WPATH). (2012). Standards of care for the health of transsexual, transgender, and gender-nonconforming people (version 7). Retrieved on 2/17/2020 at: www.wpath.org/publications/soc

In people who are transgender men (female to male), testosterone is prescribed to produce the desired physical changes. Like estrogen, the prescribed dose of testosterone is individualized and depends on many different factors. Testosterone treatment should produce changes in scalp hair, skin oiliness, facial and body hair, voice, body fat composition, muscle mass, menses, clitoris, and vagina (see Tables 54-2 and 54-3).

As with any medical treatment, hormones carry risks to the person. The likelihood of a serious adverse event is dependent on numerous factors, such as dose, route of administration (e.g., oral vs. transdermal vs. intramuscular), and the patient's characteristics (e.g., age, comorbidities, health behaviors). People who take estrogen are at increased risk of venous thromboembolism (VTE), gallstones, elevated liver enzymes, weight gain, and hypertriglyceridemia. People

TABLE 54-3	Medications Prescribed to Facilitate Gender Transition	
Feminizing Hormone Medications for Male to Female		
Medication	**Adverse Effects[a]**	**Nursing Considerations**
Androgen-Reducing Medications (Antiandrogen)		
Spironolactone (off-label use) Mechanism of action: diuretic that also directly inhibits testosterone secretion and androgen binding to the androgen receptor	Electrolyte imbalances, especially hyperkalemia Decreased blood pressure	This medication is a diuretic and patients must be advised of frequent urination and need to increase water intake. Caution in patients with adrenal insufficiency, diabetes, hyperkalemia, and chronic kidney disease.
Cyproterone acetate Mechanism of action: antiandrogenic and progestogenic/ antigonadotropic properties, resulting in blocked binding of the active metabolite of testosterone and decreased production of testicular testosterone	Thromboembolism Hyperlipidemia Hepatotoxicity Glucose intolerance Mood changes Prostatic hyperplasia	Assess for signs and symptoms of thromboembolism. Monitor mood changes (anxiety, depression, insomnia), especially during the first 4–6 wks. Monitor liver function tests prior to and during therapy for symptoms of hepatotoxicity.
Dutasteride Finasteride Mechanism of action: inhibits the enzyme 5-alpha reductase, which is responsible for converting testosterone to its potent metabolite		Assess for urinary hesitancy, feeling of incomplete bladder emptying, interruption of urinary stream, and dysuria.
Estrogen		
Ethinyl estradiol Mechanism of action: semisynthetic estrogen that binds to estrogen receptors, increasing estrogen levels and decreasing testosterone levels	Thromboembolism Edema Hypertension Pancreatitis	Assess for signs and symptoms of thromboembolism. Assess blood pressure before and during therapy. Monitor hepatic function during therapy.
Masculinizing Hormone Medication for Female to Male		
Medication	**Adverse Effects**	**Nursing Considerations**
Androgen		
Testosterone undecanoate Mechanism of action: synthetic testosterone that binds to androgen receptors throughout body	Glucose intolerance Hypertension	Assess blood pressure before and during therapy. Monitor for hypoglycemia, especially in people taking diabetes medications.

[a]Erectile dysfunction and gynecomastia are side effects of these medications. However, people who are male-to-female transgender are expecting these side effects.
Adapted from Comerford, K. C., & Durkin, M. T. (Eds.). (2020). *Nursing2020 drug handbook*. Philadelphia, PA: Wolters Kluwer.

who take testosterone are at increased risk for polycythemia, weight gain, acne, androgenic alopecia (male-patterned balding), and sleep apnea. In addition, both estrogen and testosterone can increase the risk of the person developing type 2 diabetes when they have additional risk factors, such as older age (WPATH, 2012).

Hair Removal

Hormone treatment does not typically fully eliminate unwanted hair, and thus people who are transgender may seek additional gender-affirming medical procedures. Transgender women typically seek hair removal on the face, neck, and in the genital area as preoperative preparation for vaginoplasty. Transgender men typically seek hair removal on the forearm and thigh when needing graft sites for phalloplasty. Like hormone treatment, hair removal is associated with both decreased dysphoria and increased well-being among people who are transgender (Bradford, 2019). Although numerous treatments exist to help manage unwanted hair, there are two primary medical procedures used for long-term treatment: laser hair removal and electrolysis (Reeves, Deutsch, & Stark, 2016).

Laser hair removal is the leading therapy option for long-term results and works on the principle of selective photothermolysis, whereby photons destroy the hair follicle while sparing the surrounding tissue (Thomas & Houreld, 2019). The main risks of this procedure are overheating resulting in redness, blisters, and burns. Treatments should be avoided when photosensitizing medications are being used, such as acne medications (e.g., isotretinoin, minocycline, doxycycline), antibiotics (e.g., tetracyclines, sulfonamides, quinolones), and spironolactone. Nurses should review a patient's medication list and identify those that are photosensitive. Electrolysis involves the use of an electric current that destroys the root of individual hair follicles. This treatment is more time consuming and more painful than laser hair removal. The main risks of electrolysis are redness and pigment changes. To help manage the pain during laser hair removal and electrolysis, topical anesthetics (lidocaine-containing products) and acetaminophen are used (Reeves et al., 2016).

Acne Treatment

In transgender men, testosterone is the mainstay of masculinizing hormonal therapy. Although the exact mechanism in the pathogenesis of acne is not yet fully understood, testosterone increases the production of sebum (oily secretion) in sebaceous glands, leading to acne. Facial acne in transgender men who use testosterone peaks within the first 4 months of treatment; over 80% of testosterone-treated transgender men experience facial acne in the first year (Motosko, Zakhem, Pomeranz, et al., 2018). General guidelines for acne treatment can be followed for transgender men (Thiboutot, Dréno, Abanmi, et al., 2018); however, there are some specific considerations and risks. First, combining testosterone with some acne medications, especially minocycline, may lead to hepatotoxicity; thus, frequent monitoring of liver function tests is warranted. Second, some acne medications are teratogenic, such as minocycline, doxycycline, and isotretinoin. For transgender men who are still at risk of pregnancy (intact uterus and ovaries), careful sexual history and counseling should be performed before the initiation of any acne treatment. Third, some acne medications, especially isotretinoin, may delay

wound healing and lead to keloid formation after surgery; thus, a discussion about surgical plans is needed before starting acne treatment (Motosko et al., 2018).

Fertility and Reproductive Health

Many people who are transgender will want to have biological children, but because hormone treatment limits fertility, patients should be educated about their options before starting hormone treatment or undergoing surgery to remove or alter their reproductive organs. Although the long-term effects of gender-affirming hormone therapy using testosterone or estrogen on fertility are not known, limited research suggests that testosterone and estrogen can affect the reproductive abilities of ovaries and testes, respectively (Cheng, Pastuszak, Myers, et al., 2019). There are cases of transgender women and men stopping hormone treatment and still having fertile oocytes or sperm; however, there are many cases to the contrary and thus patients who are transgender should be fully informed of the possible implications that hormones have on fertility and preservation options.

In the postpuberty age group, transgender men should be educated about oocyte cryopreservation, embryo cryopreservation, and uterus preservation. Transgender women should be educated about sperm cryopreservation. In the prepuberty age group, trials are ongoing to determine the effectiveness of ovarian tissue cryopreservation and testicular tissue cryopreservation in transgender men and transgender women, respectively (Cheng et al., 2019).

 Gerontologic Considerations

The synthesis and secretion of many endogenous hormones change and the expression of cell receptors in tissues changes in numbers and signaling capacity as the human body ages (Houlberg, 2019). Although there is very little research on the effect of exogenous cross-sex hormones in older adults who are transgender, there are important considerations given the endocrine changes in aging bodies. The major consideration for nurses is the effects of sex steroids on the metabolism of medication. With aging, the metabolism and excretion of many drugs decrease (Ruscin & Linnebar, 2018). Sex hormones also influence the absorption, metabolism, pharmacodynamics, and adverse effects of medications (Gooren & T'Sjoen, 2018). Nurses may need to take additional precautions to monitor for adverse effects and toxicity of certain medications when working with people who are transgender and taking exogenous sex hormones. The other two considerations are cardiovascular disease and bone health. In transgender women, estrogen increases the risk of cardiovascular morbidity and mortality. Additional preventive screening is warranted in these patients and lowering the dose of estrogen in transgender women over the age of 55 should be considered. Lastly, cross-sex hormone treatment can decrease bone health in both transgender women and men (Gooren & T'Sjoen, 2018). Findings from a pilot study suggest that despite having an increased risk for osteoporosis, transgender individuals' knowledge of their risks for osteoporosis can be poor (Sedlak, Roller, van Dulmen, et al., 2017) (see the Nursing Research Profile in Chart 54-3). To help reduce the risk of reduced bone mineral density, nurses should educate about osteoporosis risks and promote physical exercise and intake

Chart 54-3

NURSING RESEARCH PROFILE
Osteoporosis Prevention Among Transgender Persons

Sedlak, C. A., Roller, C. G., van Dulmen, M., et al. (2017). Transgender individuals and osteoporosis prevention. *Orthopaedic Nursing, 36*(4), 259–268.

Purpose

Many people who are transgender take sex hormones in order to achieve desirable characteristics of the gender that they feel is consonant with their personal identity. An adverse effect of these medications is that bone mineral density can become prematurely depleted, leading to early osteoporosis. The purpose of this mixed methods pilot study was to identify osteoporosis knowledge, beliefs, and prevention behaviors among transgender adults.

Design

Participants were recruited by advertising flyers at LGBTQ community centers and by advertising via LGBTQ support groups on the Internet. In order to be included in the study, participants had to be at least 30 years of age, the age when bone mineral density is considered maximal. Eligible participants could identify with male or female gender, and had to be able to read and speak English. Thirty-one participants were recruited and consented to complete a survey, which included a series of scales such as the *Osteoporosis Knowledge Test,* the *Osteoporosis Health Belief Scale,* the *Osteoporosis Self-Efficacy Scale,* the *Dietary Calcium Rapid Assessment Tool,* and the *Yale Physical Activity Survey.* Fifteen of these participants were randomly selected to participate in online qualitative interviews that focused on their views of bone health and osteoporosis.

Findings

The majority of participants (90.3%) took sex hormones. Most participants had poor knowledge of their osteoporosis risks, with 81% receiving failing scores on the *Osteoporosis Knowledge Test.* Participants selected to partake in the interviews confirmed that their knowledge of osteoporosis and their knowledge of their osteoporosis risks were poor. Several expressed frustration that health care providers had not disclosed these risks to them previously. The mean daily dietary calcium intake for the sample was less than recommended standards as was the minutes of average daily exercise. Most participants were not taking vitamin D supplements. Of those participants who were taking vitamin D supplements, more than half were taking less than recommended dosages.

Nursing Implications

Sex hormones are commonly taken by persons who are transgender; yet, findings from this study suggest that few people who are transgender and take sex hormones have knowledge of their associated higher risk for osteoporosis. Nurses should educate people who are transgender regarding the risk for osteoporosis that is associated with sex hormones. In addition, nurses should encourage persons who are transgender and taking sex hormones to engage in strategies that can mitigate the effects of sex hormones on their bone mineral density, including increasing their dietary calcium and physical activities, and taking appropriate dosages of vitamin D supplements.

---

of vitamin D and calcium to people who are transgender and taking sex hormones (see Chapter 36 for further discussion of osteoporosis). Given these considerations, the risks of hormone treatment can be managed and rarely pose an absolute contraindication (Houlberg, 2019).

Surgical Management

People who are transgender have many different gender reassignment surgeries available to them as they **transition** from their sex assigned at birth to their gender identity (Table 54-4). Just like hormone treatment, gender reassignment surgeries help reduce gender dysphoria and improve quality of life. The WPATH (2012) recommends that people who are seeking gender reassignment surgeries meet certain criteria. They recommend that the person seeking surgery have (a) persistent, well-documented gender dysphoria; (b) capacity to make a fully informed decision and to give consent for treatment; (c) age of majority in a given country; and (d) any significant medical or mental health concerns be well controlled. For certain surgeries, including hysterectomy, phalloplasty, and vaginoplasty, WPATH (2012) also recommends that the person has had 12 continuous months of hormone therapy and has had 12 continuous months of living in a gender role that is congruent with their gender identity. This is based on clinical consensus, not empirical evidence, that living 12 months in a gender role that is congruent with their gender identity gives them ample opportunity to experience and socially adjust before undergoing irreversible surgery (Colebunders, Verhaeghe, Bonte, et al., 2016).

Male-to-Female Gender Reassignment Surgeries

There are numerous different gender reassignment surgeries for transgender women (see Table 54-4). Over the years, researchers have identified common differences between male and female faces. Typically, the female face is oval and heart-shaped with smooth lines, pointed chin, less pronounced mandibular angles, less nasal prominence, and less

TABLE 54-4 Select Gender Reassignment Surgeries

Male to Female	Female to Male
Facial feminization • Angle of mandible • Cheeks • Chin • Forehead • Nose • Upper lip	Facial masculinization • Angle of mandible • Cheekbones • Chin • Forehead
Hair transplantation	Subcutaneous mastectomy
Chondrolaryngoplasty (tracheal shave)	Hysterectomy and salpingo-oophorectomy
Voice feminization	Phalloplasty
Breast augmentation	
Orchiectomy	
Vaginoplasty	

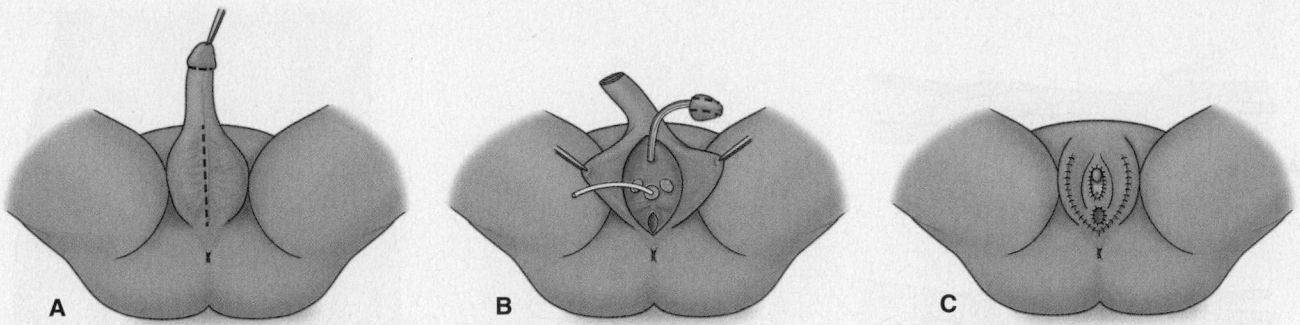

Figure 54-3 • Vaginoplasty in transgender woman (male to female). **A.** Surgically created penile skin flap and dorsal scrotal flap. **B.** Resection of penile and scrotal tissue. **C.** End surgical result is clitoroplasty.

angular nasal tip (Colebunders, Verhaeghe, et al., 2016). For people who desire a more feminine face, surgeries are available to modify most structures in the face. Chondrolaryngoplasty, reducing the prominent thyroid cartilage, commonly referred to as the Adam's apple, and feminizing the voice are commonly desired changes in people who are male-to-female transgender; both surgeries can be performed during the same procedure. Feminizing the voice involves shortening the vocal cord length or increasing the vocal cord tension (Colebunders, Verhaeghe, et al., 2016).

For most transgender women, breast augmentation greatly increases subjective feelings of femininity. Surgeons typically recommend the person take estrogen for at least 12 months prior to the surgery to maximize breast growth and obtain better aesthetic results. Mammogenesis in transgender women receiving estrogen follows a pattern like the Tanner stages of breast development (see Breast Assessment in Chapter 52 for discussion of Tanner stages). Although there are some sexual differences in chest wall and mammary anatomy, the implantation of breast prostheses is not very different from breast augmentation in a female natal patient. The incision is typically made axillary, inframammary, or periareolar. The implant is created behind the glandular tissue or behind the pectoralis muscle (Colebunders, Verhaeghe, et al., 2016).

Some transgender women choose to have genital reassignment surgery. The goal of genital reassignment surgery in transgender women is to create a perineogenital complex as feminine in appearance and function as possible and free of poorly healed areas, scars, and neuromas. To achieve this goal, two procedures are required, including an orchiectomy (removal of the testicles) and vaginoplasty. The major steps of a vaginoplasty (Fig. 54-3) include amputation of the penis, creation of the neovaginal cavity and the lining, reconstruction of a urethral meatus, and construction of the labia and clitoris (Colebunders, Verhaeghe, et al., 2016). Lining the neovaginal cavity requires either a skin flap or skin graft. The penile–scrotal skin flap, or penile inversion vaginoplasty, is the technique of choice and involves inverting the penile and scrotal skin (Ferrando, 2018). If the skin graft technique is used by the surgeon, skin tissue can be harvested from numerous different areas on the body, such as the penile or scrotal area, abdomen, intestines, or buccal mucosa.

The goals of postoperative care of the patient undergoing male-to-female genital reassignment surgery are to prevent complications and infection and to ensure patency of the neovaginal cavity. After surgery, the patient typically remains in bed for five days with a vaginal dilator in place while receiving subcutaneous low-molecular-weight heparin (LMWH) (e.g., enoxaparin; see Chapter 26 for further discussion on anticoagulation medications). After the fifth day, the dilator is periodically removed and daily cleansing of the neovaginal cavity begins. The patient will typically remain in the hospital for 8 days. After discharge, the patient is educated on how to dilate and cleanse their vaginal cavity for 3 to 6 months. Once fully healed, the patient can begin having penetrative vaginal intercourse and stop using the vaginal dilator. If the patient does not engage in regular intercourse, they will need to continue using the vaginal dilator (Colebunders, Verhaeghe, et al., 2016).

Female-to-Male Gender Reassignment Surgeries

There are also numerous different gender reassignment surgeries for transgender men (see Table 54-4). Male-sexed faces tend to have larger facial skeletons, be squarer with sharper angles and stronger jaws. Although facial masculinization procedures are far less common than facial feminization, surgeries are available to modify the forehead, angle of the mandible, chin, and cheekbones. Although the vocal cords can be surgically modified to reduce tension resulting in a more masculine voice, most people who are transgender male achieve their desired voice through testosterone treatment and behavioral therapies (Irwig, 2017; Schneider & Courey, 2016).

Testosterone treatment has little effect on reducing breast size, thus transgender men who desire a flat chest require a subcutaneous mastectomy (Fig. 54-4). From an anatomical standpoint, subcutaneous mastectomy in transgender males is nearly identical to mastectomies for breast disease. The main difference is the removal of breast tissue and excess skin and

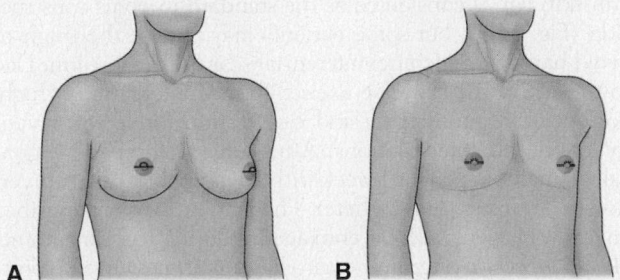

Figure 54-4 • Subcutaneous mastectomy in transgender man (female to male). **A.** Breast tissue with transareolar incision. **B.** Appearance postmastectomy.

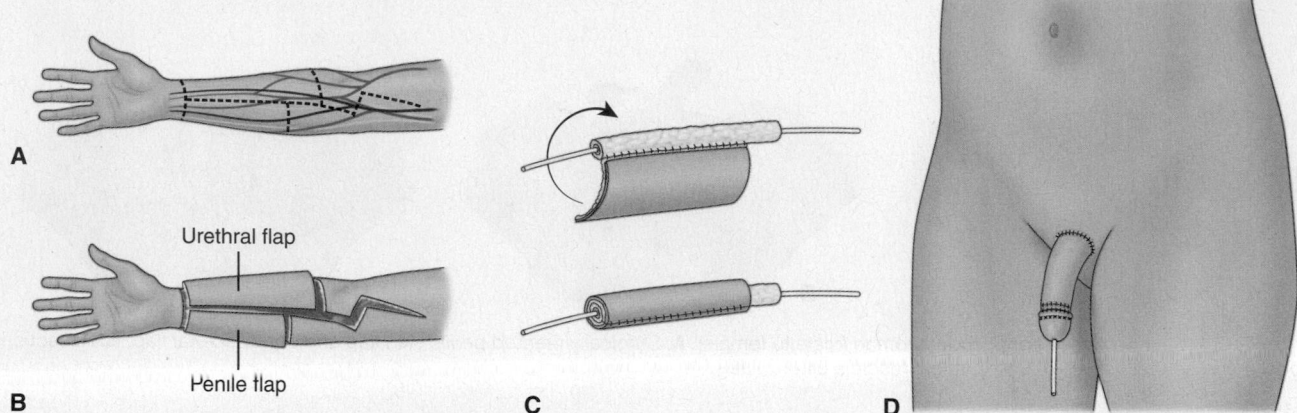

Figure 54-5 • Phalloplasty in transgender man (female to male). **A.** Selection of radial flap on forearm. **B.** The urethral (longer) and penile parts are dissected. **C.** Creation of a urethral tube within a penile tube. **D.** Postoperative results of phalloplasty.

reduction and repositioning of the nipple and areola to create an aesthetically pleasing male chest (Colebunders, D'Arpa, Weijers, et al., 2016). The complication rate of subcutaneous mastectomy is very low and carries similar risk to mastectomies for breast disease (Cuccolo, Kang, Boskey, et al., 2019) (see Chapter 52 for further discussion on mastectomy).

Some transgender men choose to have phalloplasty, which is the construction of a penis. The goals of phalloplasty include (Colebunders, D'Arpa, et al., 2016):

- having an aesthetic appearing penis,
- achieving tactile and erogenous sensation,
- having the ability to urinate while standing, and
- having the ability to have an erection and engage in penetrative intercourse.

Phalloplasty is a complicated surgery that involves numerous subprocedures. Although the selection of subprocedures will depend on the patient's goals, they typically include phallic shaft creation, penile urethroplasty, urethral lengthening, perineoplasty (reconstructing the perineum), scrotoplasty, vaginectomy, hysterectomy and oophorectomy, glansplasty (constructing the head of penis), testicular implants, and erectile device implant (Heston, Esmonde, Dugi, et al., 2019). To help retain erogenous sensation and the ability to achieve orgasm, surgeons try to maintain clitoral nerves. Patients can also elect to have clitoral transposition where the clitoris is placed in a superficial location just below the surface of the neophallus.

Constructing the penis requires a flap of skin to be excised from either the radial forearm or anterolateral thigh. The forearm skin flap is considered as the standard in penis construction (Fig. 54-5), but some patients may choose the thigh to avoid having a wide circumferential scar on the forearm. Due to the size of the skin flap excised from the forearm or thigh, postoperative monitoring and care is imperative to prevent infection and complications. After surgery, the patient typically remains in bed for 1 week with a suprapubic urinary diversion and transurethral catheter. The patient may be prescribed an LMWH agent, such as enoxaparin, during this time frame. However, pelvic or groin hematomas sometimes develop postphalloplasty, which must then be managed by either drains or surgical drainage, and thus the individual risks versus the benefits of prescribing an LMWH agent are carefully considered

(Crane, 2016). After the 1-week mark, the transurethral catheter is removed, and the suprapubic catheter is clamped so the patient can begin voiding. The patient will typically remain hospitalized for 2 to 3 weeks after a phalloplasty for close monitoring. To increase the aesthetic aspect of the phalloplasty, the patient may choose to tattoo the glans (head) of the penis after it has healed. Tattooing the glans allows for more natural coloring (Colebunders, D'Arpa, et al., 2016).

There are numerous challenges to achieving the last two goals of phalloplasty; namely, to urinate while standing and to achieve an erection. There have been many reported complications in patients who had urethral lengthening through construction of a neourethra, especially postoperative urethra fistulas and strictures/stenoses. Further, the long-term effects of urethral lengthening on bladder function is unknown. Lifelong follow-up with a urologist is usually required. Achieving rigidity (erection) after a phalloplasty remains a real challenge. There are numerous surgical approaches to creating rigidity, each with unique limitations and complications. One of the more common approaches is implanting an erectile device. Although infections can be a problem with penile implants, the latest erectile devices show promise in being durable and allowing the person to achieve an erection and sexual pleasure (Colebunders, D'Arpa, et al., 2016) (for further discussion of penile implants, see Chapter 53, Table 53-2).

An alternative technique to phalloplasty is metoidioplasty, which uses the clitoris to construct a microphallus. In metoidioplasty, the clitoris is detached from the pubic bone, allowing it to extend out further. This approach usually requires at least 12 months of testosterone treatment, which results in a hormonally hypertrophied clitoris. Metoidioplasty is the only procedure that enables creation of male genitalia with completely preserved protective and erogenous sensitivity. This means that the sexual sensation of the clitoris is preserved and intact, which differs from a phalloplasty that often requires reconstruction or transposition of the clitoris. The scrotum is usually created from labia majora flaps allowing for testicular implants. Compared to phalloplasty, metoidioplasty has a shorter hospital stay and minimal donor site complications. However, metoidioplasty does not allow the person to void while standing nor engage in penetrative sex (Djinovic, 2018).

NURSING PROCESS

The Patient Undergoing Gender Reassignment Surgery

Assessment

Preoperatively, the nurse should first gather details about the patient's gender identity, preferred name, preferred pronouns, and surgery. A person who is undergoing gender reassignment surgery will likely feel vulnerable and emotional. Gender reassignment surgery is a monumental moment for a person who is transgender. The nurse needs to ensure the patient and their family feel welcomed and safe. Using gender-neutral language (see Table 54-1) and properly assessing for gender identity and pronouns (see Chart 54-1) is imperative to creating a welcoming environment.

Preoperatively, the nurse ensures the patient has received education and counseling about their gender reassignment surgery, the possible risks and benefits, including complications, postsurgical outcomes, and need for possible long-term follow-up appointments. The nurse needs to assess the last time the patient took their hormone treatment (e.g., estrogen or testosterone) because certain procedures require the patient to stop hormones 2 to 3 weeks in advance of surgery. The nurse should ensure the patient completed their bowel preparation, especially in genital reassignment surgery. For patients undergoing phalloplasty, the nurse needs to assess smoking status because most surgeons require the patient to be free of tobacco products or inhaling nicotine and marijuana. This includes electronic nicotine delivery systems (ENDS) including e-cigarettes, e-pens, e-pipes, e-hookah, and e-cigars (Colebunders, D'Arpa, et al., 2016). Laboratory results, including complete blood count (CBC), electrolytes, blood urea nitrogen (BUN), and creatinine, should be assessed; however, the nurse should be aware that people who receive hormones may have alterations in their laboratory values (Tollinche, Walters, Radix, et al., 2018). For patients who are transitioning, regardless of whether the transition is female to male or male to female, the upper limit for creatinine, hemoglobin and hematocrit, and alkaline phosphatase should be based on male values. For patients who are transitioning from female to male, the lower limit of hemoglobin and hematocrit should be based on male values. For patients who are transitioning from male to female, the lower limit of hemoglobin and hematocrit should be based on female values (WPATH, 2012).

Postoperatively, the nurse assesses the patient to ensure the goals for recovery are met and that the patient exhibits absence of complications secondary to the surgical procedure(s). Gender reassignment surgeries often require very specific assessments to ensure proper healing and prevent complications. It is imperative that the nurse follow the surgeon's prescribed postoperative care guidelines and educate the patient to prevent both complications and revisional surgeries (Colebunders, Verhaeghe, et al., 2016).

Diagnosis

NURSING DIAGNOSES

Based on the assessment data, major nursing diagnoses may include the following:

- Risk for compromised dignity associated with stigmatization

- Anxiety associated with impending surgery
- Acute pain associated with surgical procedure
- Risk for infection associated with surgical procedure
- Hope associated with gender reassignment surgery

COLLABORATIVE PROBLEMS/POTENTIAL COMPLICATIONS

Potential complications may include the following:

- Hemorrhage
- Venous thromboembolism (VTE)
- Tissue necrosis

Planning and Goals

The major goals for the patient include enhanced sense of dignity and respect, reduction of anxiety about the surgery and postoperative care, relief of pain, absence of infection, enhancement of hope related to life after surgery, effective peripheral tissue perfusion, and absence of postoperative complications.

Nursing Interventions

ENSURING HUMAN DIGNITY

The nurse needs to promote a welcoming and safe environment for the patient undergoing gender reassignment surgery. In addition, the nurse needs to promote the use of gender-neutral language, preferred third-person pronouns, and utmost respect for the patient and their family (Johnson, Wakefield, & Garthe, 2020). The patient should be able to safely disclose their gender identity and sexual orientation. In addition, nurses and other health care providers should avoid having discussions about the patient that can be overheard by neighboring patients and staff who are not involved in care. While this principle should be applied to all patients, it is of the utmost importance to the care of people who are transgender because of concerns over discriminatory health care treatment (Tollinche et al., 2018).

People who are transgender should be roomed in accordance with their gender identity. Careful communication between the nurse and individuals responsible for room assignments (e.g., charge nurse) is necessary. If a private room is available, it should be offered as an option because it will provide increased privacy and comfort to the patient. However, the patient should not be forced into a private room because it may make the patient feel isolated (Tollinche et al., 2018).

REDUCING ANXIETY

The nurse provides the patient preparing for gender reassignment surgery anticipatory guidance as to what to expect during the surgery and postoperatively. The patient's preferred family should be included when possible to help reduce anxiety. Additionally, some surgery centers promote the use of relaxation techniques, such as aromatherapy, nature sounds, and relaxation exercises; the nurse should use these if available (Ertug, Olusoylu, Bal, et al., 2017). People who are transgender are often connected to larger networks, but the nurse can promote local and online support groups. Often, online support groups can become the main support resource after gender reassignment surgery (Cipolletta, Votadoro, & Faccio, 2017) (see Resources section).

Additionally, to help ease the patient's anxiety about postoperative care, the nurse can assist in coordinating services. People who are transgender have higher rates of anxiety and depression than cisgender people. These issues may be exacerbated during a prolonged hospital stay. Thus, the nurse should advocate for the involvement of mental health, social work, and spiritual care as needed to address all of the patient's needs (Tollinche et al., 2018).

RELIEVING PAIN

Evidence shows that patients experiencing postoperative pain should be offered multimodal analgesia, which is the pharmacologic method of combining various groups of medications for pain relief (Manworren, Gordon, & Montgomery, 2018) (see Chapter 9 for further discussion). After surgery, patients are usually prescribed opioid (morphine, hydromorphone) and nonopioid (acetaminophen or NSAIDs) agents. The nurse can administer these agents as prescribed to relieve pain and discomfort. Inadequately controlled postoperative pain can impede functional recovery and reduce quality of life (Manworren et al., 2018), thus nurses need to be vigilant about controlling the patient's pain. Patients undergoing genital reassignment surgery typically need to stay in bed for numerous days; thus, the nurse should help the patient reposition themselves to promote comfort.

PREVENTING AND MONITORING FOR INFECTION

Unless the patient undergoing gender reassignment surgery has risk factors (e.g., older adult, weak immune system, smoker, poor nutrition, overweight), they are not at greater risk for developing a postsurgical infection. The nurse should follow usual procedures to prevent and monitor for infection. Preventing infection after surgery requires proper and frequent hand hygiene, maintenance of the surgical site, and administration of prescribed prophylactic antibiotics. Early signs of infection should be reported to the surgeon immediately, including increased skin redness, pain, or swelling, cloudy or discolored discharge from the surgical site, and fever.

PROMOTING HOPE

People who are transgender often experience greater levels of depression and decreased quality of life as compared with cisgender people. However, people who undergo gender reassignment surgery often experience improved quality of life (Cai, Hughto, Reisner, et al., 2019; Passos, Teixeira, & Almeida-Santos, 2019). The nurse should promote open communication about the patient's feelings, hopes, and goals after their gender reassignment surgery and show a positive regard and sense of hope for the patient. Additionally, the nurse may want to explore unresolved emotions or anxieties.

MONITORING AND MANAGING POTENTIAL COMPLICATIONS

After surgery, the nurse assesses the patient for complications from the procedure, such as hemorrhage, VTE, and tissue necrosis.

Hemorrhage. Postoperative hemorrhage is a possible complication after gender reassignment surgery, especially following vaginectomy, which is one of the procedures during a phalloplasty (Colebunders, D'Arpa, et al., 2016). Signs and symptoms of possible hemorrhage include increased pain, frank red blood from the surgical site or rectum, increase in bloody output from any drain that might be in place (e.g., for mastectomy), and typical clinical manifestations (e.g., tachycardia, hypotension, lightheadedness, syncope).

Venous Thromboembolism. People who undergo gender reassignment surgery, especially those undergoing genital surgery and those who are transgender women, are at risk of VTE, including both pulmonary embolism (PE) and deep vein thrombosis (DVT) (Shatzel, Connelly, & DeLoughery, 2017). People who undergo genital reassignment surgery often need to stay in bed for up to 7 days, putting them especially at risk. Additionally, the estrogen hormone treatment among transgender women increases the risk. The patient is typically prescribed mechanical compression (e.g., intermittent pneumatic compression devices) and prophylactic anticoagulation with subcutaneous LMWH agents (e.g., enoxaparin) during hospitalization. Even with these prophylactic measures, some patients still develop DVT and PE, and thus the nurse should monitor for clinical signs (Colebunders, Verhaeghe, et al., 2016; Shatzel et al., 2017) (see Chapter 26 for further discussion on VTE).

Tissue Necrosis. Tissue necrosis from vascular compromise is a complication with certain gender reassignment surgeries, including subcutaneous mastectomy and phalloplasty. After the subcutaneous mastectomy, vascular compromise may occur around the reconstructed nipple and areola (Colebunders, Verhaeghe, et al., 2016). After the phalloplasty, vascular compromise may occur in the reconstructed shaft, penis glans, or scrotum (Colebunders, D'Arpa, et al., 2016). Signs of tissue necrosis from vascular compromise include skin/tissue discoloration (blue or black), feeling cool to the touch, increased pain or decreased sensation, and poor wound healing. Tissue necrosis is a medical emergency that needs to be addressed immediately.

PROMOTING HOME, COMMUNITY-BASED, AND TRANSITIONAL CARE

Educating Patients About Self-Care. People who undergo gender reassignment surgery are typically discharged to home from the hospital within seven days after surgery. General postoperative discharge education includes promptly notifying the surgeon for a temperature greater than 38°C (100.4°F) or for the presence of unusual or bloody drainage from the wound(s). The patient is encouraged to advance the diet as tolerated at home to promote wound healing and to abstain from all tobacco products at least until the surgical wound(s) has healed. Additional education provided is dependent upon the nature of the surgery. For instance, the patient who has had a vaginoplasty or phalloplasty will receive very specific education (Charts 54-4 and 54-5). If the patient has had a mastectomy and has a drain in place, then the patient needs to be educated on managing the drain at home (see Chapter 52, Chart 52-7: Home Care Checklist: Patient with a Drainage Device Following Breast Surgery).

The patient is discharged with specific instructions about follow-up appointments, including visits with their surgical, medical, and psychosocial providers to address their complex needs. Nurses should advocate that these follow-up appointments be made prior to hospital discharge. Additionally, the discharge process should assist the patient in coordinating any type of necessary equipment pickup, transportation to follow-up appointments, and filling medication prescriptions, as needed.

Continuing and Transitional Care. Gender reassignment surgery is very complex, involves numerous different procedures, and can be different from surgeon to surgeon. For these reasons, it is impossible to describe every postsurgical

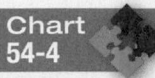

Chart 54-4 · PATIENT EDUCATION
Postoperative Education for Patients Who Have Had a Vaginoplasty

The nurse instructs the patient about activity, bathing, swelling, hygiene, and vaginal intercourse as described below.

Activity

- Avoid strenuous activity for 6 weeks
- Avoid swimming or bike riding for 3 months
- May be uncomfortable to sit for the first month; may use donut ring to relieve pressure

Bathing

- Resume showering following first postoperative visit
- Do not submerge groin area in water for 8 weeks

Swelling

- Labial swelling is normal and will resolve in 6 to 8 weeks
- Apply ice to perineum for 20 minutes every hour while awake for 1 week postoperatively
- Increased swelling with pain should be reported to surgeon

Hygiene

- Wash hands before and after contact with genital area
- Wipe genital area from front to back to avoid contamination by bacteria from anal region

Vaginal Intercourse

- May engage in vaginal intercourse 3 months after surgery

Adapted from Meltzer, T. (2016). Vaginoplasty procedures, complications and aftercare. Retrieved on 7/10/2020 at: transcare.ucsf.edu/guidelines/vaginoplasty; University of Utah.

Chart 54-5 · PATIENT EDUCATION
Postoperative Education for Patients Who Have Had a Phalloplasty

The nurse instructs the patient about activity, bathing, swelling, hygiene, and sexual activity as described below.

Activity

- Avoid strenuous activity for 6 weeks
- Do not flex at waist more than 90 degrees
- Do not lift anything heavier than 5 lb with arm with skin graft donor site

Bathing

- Lightly sponge bathe for 1 week postoperatively and then begin gently washing penis with warm soapy water
- Keep skin graft donor site dry; may use plastic bag to protect from water

Swelling

- Minor swelling is expected; however, report increased swelling in groin or change in girth of penis to surgeon

Hygiene

- Wash hands before and after contact with genital area

Sexual Activity

- Do not use penis for any sexual activities until approved by surgeon (including oral, vaginal, or anal insertion)

Adapted from Phalloplasty guide: How to prepare & what to expect during your recovery. Retrieved on 7/10/2020 at: healthcare.utah.edu/transgender-health/gender-affirmation-surgery/phalloplasty-recovery.php

---

self-care activity. The nurse needs to carefully review the discharge instructions provided by the surgical team. Genital reassignment surgery often has very specific self-care requirements of the patient. The nurse's role is to ensure the patient fully understands the self-care instructions and knows how to monitor for complications.

The patient will usually continue to see their surgeon for follow-up appointments for many months. Some procedures, such as a phalloplasty, may require follow-up appointments for up to a year after surgery. The patient will typically need lifelong hormonal treatment and should continue to follow-up with their endocrinology health care provider. Additionally, many people who undergo gender reassignment surgery continue to visit a mental health care provider for counseling.

Evaluation

Expected patient outcomes may include the following:

1. Enhanced human dignity
   a. Verbalizes feelings of satisfaction related to the level of respect given to them
2. Minimal anxiety
   a. Has facial expressions, gestures, and activity levels that reflect decreased distress
   b. Demonstrates ability to reassure self
3. Relief of pain
   a. Reports relief of pain
   b. Engages in early mobilization activities as prescribed

4. Maintenance of asepsis
   a. No evidence of infection (e.g., no fever, no leukocytosis, no increased redness or swelling of surgical sites)
5. Enhanced hope
   a. Verbalizes feelings about their quality of life after having had gender reassignment surgery
   b. Identifies future-oriented goals and hopes
6. Has no complications (no hemorrhage, VTE, or tissue necrosis)

CRITICAL THINKING EXERCISES

1 A 38-year-old patient is admitted to your hospital unit for a sickle cell crisis. During report from the emergency room nurse, you learn that this patient identifies as transgender. As you prepare to go and greet the patient and conduct the initial history and assessment, you recognize how important it is to provide an inclusive and welcoming environment for this patient. Describe how you should initially greet the patient. Prepare a list of questions to collect information about their preferred name, gender identity, and gender pronouns.

2 `ebp` An adult patient confides in you that they have been struggling with their gender identity since adolescence. They were assigned male sex at birth but have a strong desire to be a woman. The patient has been seeing a therapist who diagnosed them with gender dysphoria, but they have not yet started medical treatment. The patient plans to see a health care provider to start hormone treatment but says to you, "I would really like some information about hormones before I see my provider." Describe the types of feminizing hormones and the physical effects. Identify evidence-based information you can provide to the patient to inform them about hormone treatment.

3 `ipc` You are a nurse working in an emergency department when a 60-year-old person who identifies as a transgender woman is admitted. You overhear a resident physician and nurse talk about the patient using derogatory terms. Describe how you can educate the resident physician and nurse to be more culturally sensitive to this patient. Discuss ways to advocate for the unit to be more welcoming, inclusive, and safe for people who identify as LGBTQ. Identify resources that can be shared with fellow staff members.

4 `pg` A 55-year-old patient who identifies as a transgender woman is admitted to the medical-surgical unit for fever and shortness of breath two weeks after having a vaginoplasty. The patient is taking daily oral estrogen. The patient's BP is 128/95 mm Hg, HR 110 bpm, RR 28 breaths/min, T 38.40 °C (101.1 °F) and SpO$_2$ of 90%. Describe your priority nursing assessments for this patient. What nursing interventions would you implement first? Discuss the potential causes of this patient's abnormal vital signs.

REFERENCES

*Asterisk indicates nursing research.

Books

American Psychiatric Association. (2013). *Diagnostic and statistical manual of mental disorders* (5th ed.). Arlington, VA: Author.

Colebunders, B., D'Arpa, S., Weijers, S., et al. (2016). Female-to-male gender reassignment surgery. In R. Ettner, S. Monstrey, & E. Coleman (Eds.). *Principles of transgender medicine and surgery* (2nd ed., pp. 279–317). New York: Routledge.

Colebunders, B., Verhaeghe, W., Bonte, K., et al. (2016). Male-to-female gender reassignment surgery. In R. Ettner, S. Monstrey, & E. Coleman (Eds.). *Principles of transgender medicine and surgery* (2nd ed., pp. 250–278). New York: Routledge.

Comerford, K. C., & Durkin, M. T. (Eds.). (2020). *Nursing2020 Drug Handbook*. Philadelphia, PA: Wolters Kluwer.

Ducheny, K., Hardacker, C. T., Claybren, T., et al. (2019). The essentials: Foundational knowledge to support affirmative care for transgender and gender nonconforming (TGNC) older adults. In C. Hardacker, K. Ducheny, & M. Houlberg (Eds.). *Transgender and gender nonconforming health and aging* (pp. 1–20). Switzerland: Springer International Publishing.

Eliason, M. J., & Chinn, P. L. (2018). *LGBTQ cultures: What health care professionals need to know about sexual and gender diversity* (3rd ed.). Philadelphia, PA: Wolters Kluwer.

Ettner, R., Monstrey, S., & Coleman, E. (2016). *Principles of transgender medicine and surgery* (2nd ed.). New York: Routledge.

Gooren, L. J. (2016). Hormone treatment of adult transgender people. In R. Ettner, S. Monstrey, & E. Coleman (Eds.). *Principles of transgender medicine and surgery* (2nd ed., pp. 167–179). New York: Routledge.

Houlberg, M. (2019). Endocrinology, hormone replacement therapy (HRT), and aging. In C. Hardacker, K. Ducheny, & M. Houlberg (Eds.). *Transgender and gender nonconforming health and aging* (pp. 21–35). Switzerland: Springer International Publishing.

Ruscin, J. M., & Linnebar, S. A. (2018). Pharmacokinetics in older adults. *Merck manual*. Retrieved on 2/17/2020 at: merckmanuals.com/professional/geriatrics/drug-therapy-in-older-adults/pharmacokinetics-in-older-adults

Schneider, S., & Courey, M. (2016). Transgender voice and communication—vocal health and considerations. In M. B. Deutsch (Ed.). *Guidelines for the primary and gender-affirming care of transgender and gender nonbinary people*. Retrieved on 2/17/2020 at: transcare.ucsf.edu/guidelines/vocal-health

Witten, T. M., & Eyler, A. E. (2016). Care of aging transgender and gender non-conforming patients. In R. Ettner, S. Monstrey, & E. Coleman (Eds.). *Principles of transgender medicine and surgery* (2nd ed., pp. 344–378). New York: Routledge.

Journals and Electronic Documents

Bostwick, W. B., Hughes, T. L., Steffen, A., et al. (2019). Depression and victimization in a community sample of bisexual and lesbian women: An intersectional approach. *Archives of Sexual Behavior*, 48(1), 131–141.

Bradford, N. J., Rider, G. N., & Spencer, K. G. (2019). Hair removal and psychological well-being in transfeminine adults: Associations with gender dysphoria and gender euphoria. *Journal of Dermatological Treatment*, 22, 1–8.

Burks, A. C., Cramer, R. J., Henderson, C. E., et al. (2018). Frequency, nature, and correlates of hate crime victimization experiences in an urban sample of lesbian, gay, and bisexual community members. *Journal of Interpersonal Violence*, 33(3), 402–420.

Cai, X., Hughto, J. M. W., Reisner, S. L., et al. (2019). Benefit of gender-affirming medical treatment for transgender elders: Later-life alignment of mind and body. *LGBT Health*, 6(1), 34–39.

Centers for Disease Control and Prevention (CDC). (2019a). HIV and gay and bisexual men. Retrieved on 2/17/2020 at: www.cdc.gov/hiv/group/msm/index.html

Centers for Disease Control and Prevention (CDC). (2019b). HIV and transgender people. Retrieved on 2/17/2020 at: www.cdc.gov/hiv/group/gender/transgender/index.html

Centers for Disease Control and Prevention (CDC). (2020). Collecting sexual orientation and gender identity information. Retrieved on 4/20/2020 at: www.cdc.gov/hiv/clinicians/transforming-health/health-care-providers/collecting-sexual-orientation.html

Cheng, P. J., Pastuszak, A. W., Myers, J. B., et al. (2019). Fertility concerns of the transgender patient. *Translational Andrology and Urology*, 8(3), 209–218.

Cipolletta, S., Votadoro, R., & Faccio, E. (2017). Online support for transgender people: An analysis of forums and social networks. *Health and Social Care in the Community*, 25(5), 1542–1551.

Crane, C. (2016). Phalloplasty and metoidioplasty—overview and postoperative considerations. Retrieved on 7/8/2020 at: transcare.ucsf.edu/guidelines/phalloplasty

Cuccolo, N. G., Kang, C. O., Boskey, E. R., et al. (2019). Mastectomy in transgender and cisgender patients: A comparative analysis of epidemiology and postoperative outcomes. *Plastic and Reconstructive Surgery. Global Open*, 7(6), e2316.

Deutsch, M. B. (2016). Guidelines for the primary and gender-affirming care of transgender and gender nonbinary people. Retrieved on 2/17/2020 at: transcare.ucsf.edu/guidelines

Djinovic, R. P. (2018). Metoidioplasty. *Clinics in Plastic Surgery*, 45(3), 381–386.

*Ertug, N., Olusoylu, O., Bal, A., et al. (2017). Comparison of the effectiveness of two different interventions to reduce preoperative anxiety: A randomized controlled trial. *Nursing & Health Sciences*, 19(2), 250–256.

Family Equality Council. (2017). LGBTQ family fact sheet. Retrieved on 2/17/2020 at: www2.census.gov/cac/nac/meetings/2017-11/LGBTQ-families-factsheet.pdf

Ferrando, C. A. (2018). Vaginoplasty complications. *Clinics in Plastic Surgery*, 45(3), 361–368.

Gooren, L. J., & T'Sjoen, G. (2018). Endocrine treatment of aging transgender people. *Reviews in Endocrine and Metabolic Disorders, 19*(3), 253–262.

Heston, A. L., Esmonde, N. O., Dugi, D. D., et al. (2019). Phalloplasty: Techniques and outcomes. *Translational Andrology and Urology, 8*(3), 254–265.

Irwig, M. S. (2017). Testosterone therapy for transgender men. *The Lancet Diabetes & Endocrinology, 5*(4), 301–311.

*Johnson, M., Wakefield, C., & Garthe, K. (2020). Qualitative socioecological factors of cervical cancer screening use among transgender men. *Preventive Medicine Reports, 17*, 101052.

Lyons, B. H., Walters, M. L., Jack, S. P. D., et al. (2019). Suicides among lesbian and gay male individuals: Findings from the national violent death reporting system. *American Journal of Preventive Medicine, 56*(4), 512–521.

*Manworren, R. C. B., Gordon, D. B., & Montgomery, R. (2018). Managing postoperative pain. *American Journal of Nursing, 118*(1), 36–43.

Maragh-Bass, A. C., Torain, M., Adler, R., et al. (2017). Risks, benefits, and importance of collecting sexual orientation and gender identity data in healthcare settings: A multi-method analysis of patient and provider perspectives. *LGBT Health, 4*(2), 141–152.

Mason, T. B., Smith, K. E., & Lavender, J. M. (2019). Stigma control model of dysregulated eating: A momentary maintenance model of dysregulated eating among marginalized/stigmatized individuals. *Appetite, 132*(1), 67–72.

McNeil, J., Ellis, S. J., & Eccles, F. J. R. (2017). Suicide in trans populations: A systematic review of prevalence and correlates. *Psychology of Sexual Orientation and Gender Diversity, 4*(3), 341–353.

*Meerwijk, E. L., & Sevelius, J. M. (2017). Transgender population size in the United States: A meta-regression of population-based probability samples. *American Journal of Public Health, 107*(2), e1–e8.

Meltzer, T. (2016). Vaginoplasty procedures, complications and aftercare. Retrieved on 7/10/2020 at: transcare.ucsf.edu/guidelines/vaginoplasty

Motosko, C. C., Zakhem, G. A., Pomeranz, M. K., et al. (2018). Acne: A side-effect of masculinizing hormonal therapy in transgender patients. *British Journal of Dermatology, 180*(1), 26–30.

Passos, T. S., Teixeira, M. S., & Almeida-Santos, M. A. (2019). Quality of life after gender affirmation surgery: A systematic review and network meta-analysis. *Sexuality Research and Social Policy, 17*(2), 252–262.

Reeves, C., Deutsch, M. B., & Stark, J. W. (2016). Hair removal. In M. B. Deutsch (Ed.). *Guidelines for the primary and gender-affirming care of transgender and gender nonbinary people.* Retrieved on 2/17/2020 at: transcare.ucsf.edu/guidelines/hair-removal

Ross, L. E., Salway, T., Tarasoff, L. A., et al. (2018). Prevalence of depression and anxiety among bisexual people compared to gay, lesbian, and heterosexual individuals: A systematic review and meta-analysis. *Journal of Sex Research, 55*(4-5), 435–456.

*Sedlak, C. A., Roller, C. G., van Dulmen, M., et al. (2017). Transgender individuals and osteoporosis prevention. *Orthopaedic Nursing, 36*(4), 259–268.

Shatzel, J. J., Connelly, K. J., & DeLoughery, T. G. (2017). Thrombotic issues in transgender medicine: A review. *American Journal of Hematology, 92*(2), 204–208.

Simoni, J. M., Smith, L., Oost, K. M., et al. (2017). Disparities in physical health conditions among lesbian and bisexual women: A systematic review of population-based studies. *Journal of Homosexuality, 64*(1), 32–44.

The Fenway Institute. (2017). Collecting sexual orientation and gender identity (SO/GI) data in electronic health records. Retrieved

on 4/20/2020 at: www.lgbthealtheducation.org/wp-content/uploads/2017/05/SOGI-Office-Hours-Update-Final.pdf

The Fenway Institute. (2018). Ready, set go! Guidelines and tips for collecting patient data on sexual orientation and gender identity. Retrieved on 4/21/2020 at: www.lgbthealtheducation.org/wp-content/uploads/2018/03/Ready-Set-Go-publication-Updated-April-2018.pdf

The Williams Institute. (2018). LGBT stats. Retrieved on 2/17/2020 at: williamsinstitute.law.ucla.edu/impact/data-in-review-2018/

The Williams Institute. (2019). LGBT demographic data interactive. Retrieved on 2/17/2020 at: williamsinstitute.law.ucla.edu/visualization/lgbt-stats/?topic=LGBT

Thiboutot, D. M., Dréno, B., Abanmi, A., et al. (2018). Practical management of acne for clinicians: An international consensus from the Global Alliance to Improve Outcomes in Acne. *Journal of the American Academy of Dermatology, 78*(2), S1–S23.

Thomas, M. M., & Houreld, N. N. (2019). The "in's and outs" of laser hair removal: A mini review. *Journal of Cosmetic and Laser Therapy, 21*(6), 316–322.

Tollinche, L. E., Walters, C. B., Radix, A., et al. (2018). The perioperative care of the transgender patient. *Anesthesia and Analgesia, 127*(2), 359–366.

University of Utah. (2020). Phalloplasty guide: How to prepare & what to expect during your recovery. Retrieved on 7/10/2020 at: healthcare.utah.edu/transgender-health/gender-affirmation-surgery/phalloplasty-recovery.php

Witcomb, G. L., Bouman, W. P., Claes, L., et al. (2018). Levels of depression in transgender people and its predictors: Results of a large matched control study with transgender people accessing clinical services. *Journal of Affective Disorders, 235*(1), 308–315.

World Health Organization (WHO). (2019). Gender, equity and human rights. Retrieved on 2/17/2020 at: www.who.int/gender-equity-rights/knowledge/glossary/en/

World Professional Association for Transgender Health (WPATH). (2012). Standards of care for the health of transsexual, transgender, and gender-nonconforming people. Retrieved on 2/17/2020 at: www.wpath.org/publications/soc

Resources

Centers for Disease Control and Prevention (CDC) Lesbian, Gay, Bisexual, and Transgender Health, www.cdc.gov/lgbthealth/index.htm

Family Equality Council, www.familyequality.org

Gay and Lesbian Medical Association, www.glma.org

Human Rights Campaign Healthcare Equality Index, www.hrc.org/hei

Lavender Health LGBTQ Resource Center, www.lavenderhealth.org

National LGBT Cancer Network, LGBT Cultural Competence Toolkit, www.lgbtcultcomp.org

National LGBT Cancer Network, *Vanessa Goes to the Doctor* training video on YouTube, produced on 3/15/2015; retrieved on 6/29/2020 at: www.youtube.com/watch?v=S3eDKf3PFRo

National LGBT Health Education Center, www.lgbthealtheducation.org/

Nurses Advancing LGBTQ Health Equality, glmanursing.org/

The Fenway Health Institute, www.fenwayhealth.org

The Williams Institute on Sexual Orientation and Gender Identity Law and Public Policy, williamsinstitute.law.ucla.edu/

World Professional Association for Transgender Health (WPATH), www.wpath.org

Integumentary Function

Case Study MANAGING AND PREVENTING SKIN CANCER

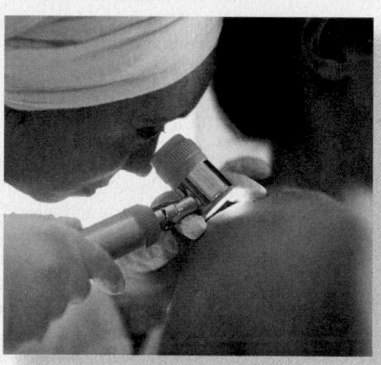

You are a nurse working in an outpatient dermatology clinic. A 22-year-old White woman with a family history of melanoma presents to the clinic with three moles that look atypical. She undergoes excision and biopsy of the moles. One week later she returns to the clinic for her results. Two of the moles are within normal limits; however, one mole on her right shoulder is positive for melanoma *in situ*. The dermatologist recommends a total excision of the area with 2.5 cm (1 in) margins. As the patient is leaving the clinic, she asks you if this is the best treatment option and what she can do to prevent further skin cancers. What is the evidence base for managing melanoma *in situ*? What evidence-based recommendations will you make to help her prevent further skin cancers?

QSEN Competency Focus: Evidence-Based Practice (EBP)

The complexities inherent in today's health care system challenge nurses to demonstrate integration of specific interdisciplinary core competencies. These competencies are aimed at ensuring the delivery of safe, quality patient care (Institute of Medicine, 2003). The Quality and Safety Education for Nurses project (Cronenwett, Sherwood, Barnsteiner, et al., 2007; QSEN, 2020) provides a framework for the knowledge, skills, and attitudes (KSAs) required for nurses to demonstrate competency in these key areas, which include *patient-centered care*, *interdisciplinary teamwork and collaboration*, *evidence-based practice*, *quality improvement*, *safety*, and *informatics.*

Evidence-Based Practice Definition: Integrate best current evidence with clinical expertise and patient/family preferences and values for delivery of optimal health care.

SELECT PRE-LICENSURE KSAs	APPLICATION AND REFLECTION
Knowledge	
Differentiate clinical opinion from research and evidence summaries Describe reliable sources for locating evidence reports and clinical practice guidelines	Identify the sources you would use for evidence-based reports and clinical guidelines for managing abnormal dermatologic skin findings in this patient as well as in others who have similar risk factors. Identify the evidence base for skin cancer prevention recommendations.
Skills	
Read original research and evidence reports related to area of practice Locate evidence reports related to clinical practice topics and guidelines	What is the strength of the evidence for management of melanoma *in situ* and for melanoma prevention in those with a family history? What criteria will you use to judge the strength of the evidence you have identified?
Attitudes	
Appreciate the importance of regularly reading relevant professional journals	Reflect upon what you learned by reviewing current evidence-based practice. Think about how patients rely on the best evidence to determine the most effective treatment. If a patient with a melanoma *in situ* were being treated in 10 years' time, do you think the same evidence-based guidelines or reports will be in use?

Cronenwett, L., Sherwood, G., Barnsteiner, J., et al. (2007). Quality and safety education for nurses. *Nursing Outlook, 55*(3), 122–131; Institute of Medicine. (2003). *Health professions education: A bridge to quality*. Washington, DC: National Academies Press; QSEN Institute. (2020). *QSEN Competencies: Definitions and pre-licensure KSAs; Evidence based practice*. Retrieved on 8/15/2020 at: qsen.org/competencies/pre-licensure-ksas/#evidence-based_practice

55 Assessment of Integumentary Function

In the United States, as many as one in three people will have a skin disorder or disease at any given time. Skin disorders are commonly observed in inpatient and outpatient nursing practice settings. The assessment of the skin can provide important information about the general health of the patient or clues to systemic conditions that manifest in the skin.

Any medical treatment can suddenly induce an episode of skin symptoms such as itching, skin discomfort, or rash. The psychological stress of illness or various personal and family problems may be exhibited outwardly as dermatologic disorders. In certain systemic conditions, such as hepatitis and some cancers, dermatologic manifestations may be the first sign of the disorder and the main reason a patient seeks health care.

Anatomic and Physiologic Overview

The skin is the largest organ system of the body and is essential for human life. It participates in many vital body functions; it forms a barrier between the internal and external environment protecting the body from pathogens, helps regulate temperature and water loss, and provides sensory input.

Anatomy of the Skin, Hair, Nails, and Glands of the Skin

Skin

The skin is composed of three layers: epidermis, dermis, and subcutaneous tissue (Fig. 55-1). The epidermis is an outermost layer of stratified epithelial cells, composed predominantly of keratinocytes. It ranges in thickness from about 0.05 mm on the eyelids to about 1.5 mm on the palms of the hands and soles of the feet. Four distinct layers compose the epidermis; from innermost to outermost, they are the stratum germinativum, stratum granulosum, stratum lucidum, and stratum corneum. Each layer becomes more differentiated (i.e., mature and with more specific functions) as it rises from the basal stratum germinativum layer to the outermost stratum corneum layer.

Epidermis

The epidermis, which is contiguous with the mucous membranes and the lining of the ear canals, consists of live, continuously dividing cells called **keratinocytes,** which differentiate and randomly migrate upward. These cells synthesize keratin; eventually they become metabolically inactive and form a thick and protective outer layer. This external layer, called the stratum corneum, is almost completely replaced every 3 to 4 weeks. The dead cells contain large amounts of

keratin, an insoluble, fibrous protein that forms the outer barrier of the skin and has the capacity to repel pathogens and prevent excessive fluid loss from the body. Keratin is the principal hardening ingredient of the hair and nails.

Melanocytes are the special cells of the epidermis that are primarily involved in producing the pigment **melanin,** which colors the skin and hair. A person's normal skin color is determined by the amount of melanin produced. Most of the skin of people who are dark skinned and the darker areas of the skin on people who are light skinned (e.g., the nipple) contain larger amounts of melanin and are not related to numbers of melanocytes. Normal skin color depends on race and varies from pale, almost ivory, to deep brown, almost pure black. Systemic disease can affect skin color. For example, insufficient oxygenation of the blood will induce cyanosis (a bluish hue in the skin of individuals who are light skinned), significant liver disease manifests as jaundice or icterus (a yellow green skin tone), and **erythema** (a pink or red skin shade caused by dilation of the capillaries) is seen when there is inflammation or fever.

Production of melanin is influenced by several factors including a hormone secreted from the hypothalamus of the brain called *melanocyte-stimulating hormone*. It is believed that melanin production responds in a protective manner with increased ultraviolet light in sunlight.

Two other types of cells are common to the epidermis: Merkel and Langerhans cells. **Merkel cells** are not fully understood but may have a role as receptors that transmit stimuli to the axon (long projection of a nerve cell) through a chemical synapse. **Langerhans cells** are believed to play a significant role in cutaneous immune system reactions. These accessory cells of the afferent immune system process invading antigens and transport the antigens to the lymph system to activate the T lymphocytes.

The characteristics of the epidermis vary in different areas of the body. It is thickest over the palms of the hands and

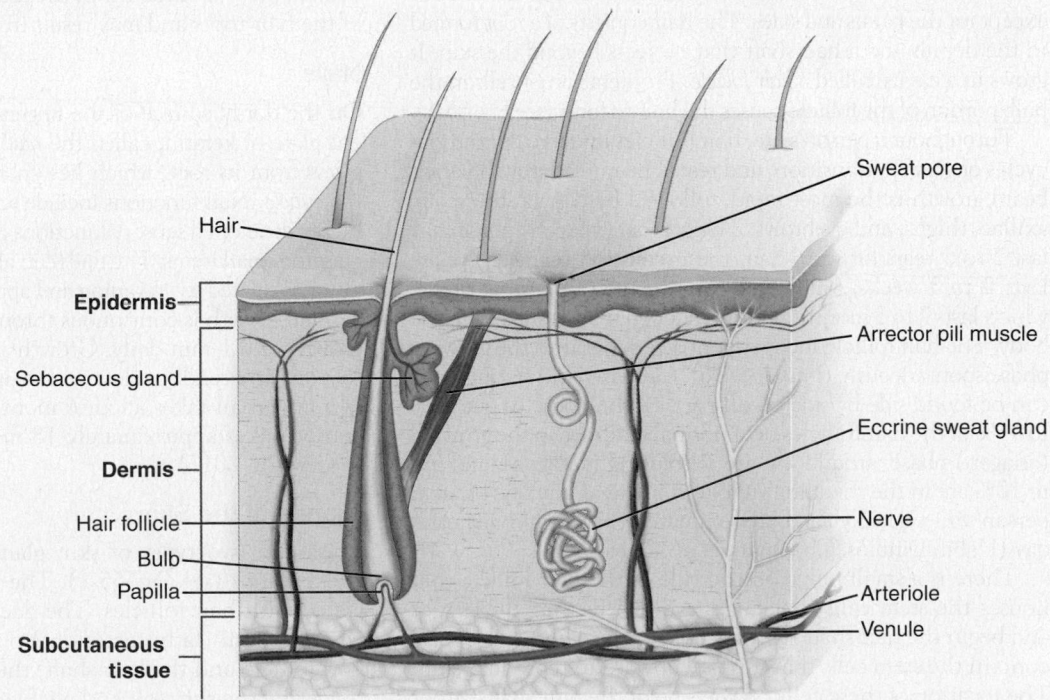

Figure 55-1 • Anatomic structures of the skin.

Hair

Epidermis

Sebaceous gland

Dermis

Hair follicle

Bulb

Papilla

Subcutaneous tissue

Sweat pore

Arrector pili muscle

Eccrine sweat gland

Nerve

Arteriole

Venule

soles of the feet and contains increased amounts of keratin. The thickness of the epidermis can increase with friction and pressure and can result in calluses forming on the hands or corns forming on the feet.

The junction of the epidermis and dermis is an area of undulations and furrows called **rete ridges** on the epidermal side and dermal papillae on the dermal side. Anchors found in this junction hold together the epidermis and dermis, permitting the free exchange of essential nutrients between the two layers. This interlocking between the dermis and epidermis produces ripples on the surface of the skin. On the fingertips, these ripples are called *fingerprints*. They are a person's most individual physical characteristic, and they rarely change over time (Wilhelmi & Molnar, 2018).

Dermis

The dermis makes up the largest portion of the skin, the connective tissue between the epidermis and subcutaneous tissue. It provides strength and structure in the form of collagen and elastic fibers. It is composed of two layers: papillary and reticular. Collagen fibers are loosely organized in the papillary dermis and are more tightly packed in the reticular dermis. The dermis also contains blood and lymph vessels, nerves, sweat and sebaceous glands, and hair roots.

Subcutaneous Tissue

The subcutaneous tissue, or hypodermis, is the innermost layer of the skin. It is primarily adipose and connective tissue, which provides a cushion between the skin layers and the muscles and bones. This layer also protects the nerve and vascular structures that transect the layers. It promotes skin mobility, molds body contours, and insulates the body. The subcutaneous tissues and the amount of fat deposited are important factors in body temperature regulation.

Hair

An outgrowth of the skin, hair is present over the entire body except for the palms and soles. The hair consists of a root formed in the dermis and a hair shaft that projects beyond the skin. It grows in a cavity called a *hair follicle*. Proliferation of cells in the bulb portion of the follicle causes the hair to form (see Fig. 55-1).

Throughout a person's life, hair follicles undergo continuous cycles of growth, transition, and rest. The rate of growth varies; beard growth is the most rapid, followed by hair on the scalp, axillae, thighs, and eyebrows. The growth (anagen) phase may last 2 to 6 years for scalp hair, the involution (catagen) phase lasts 2 to 3 weeks, followed by the telogen or resting phase, which lasts 2 to 3 months. During telogen, hair is shed from the body. The hair follicle independently recycles into the growing phase spontaneously (Nicol, 2016). Growing and resting hairs can be found side by side on all parts of the body. About 90% to 95% of the hair follicles on a normal scalp are in the growing (anagen) phase, around 1% are involuting (catagen), and 5% to 10% are in the shedding (telogen) phase at any one time. A person will typically shed approximately 100 scalp hairs each day (Habif, Dinulos, Chapman, et al., 2018).

There is a small bulge on the side of the hair follicle that houses the stem cells that migrate down to the follicle root and begin the hair shaft reproduction cycle. These bulges also contain the stem cells that migrate upward to reproduce skin. The location of these cells on the side of the hair shaft, rather than at the base, is a factor in hair loss. In conditions in which inflammation causes damage to the root of the hair, regrowth is possible. However, if inflammation causes damage to the side of the hair follicle, stem cells are destroyed, and the hair will not grow.

In certain locations on the body, hair growth is controlled by sex hormones. The most obvious example is the growth of hair on the face (i.e., beard, mustache), chest, and back, which is controlled by the male hormones known as androgens. Both men and women produce and need androgens, but in differing amounts. Women with higher levels of the androgen testosterone have hair in the areas generally thought of as masculine, such as the face, chest, and lower abdomen. This is often a normal genetic variation, but if it appears along with irregular menses and weight changes, it may indicate a hormonal imbalance (Habif et al., 2018).

Hair in different parts of the body serves different functions. The hairs of the eyes (i.e., eyebrows, lashes), nose, and ears filter out dust, bugs, and airborne debris. The hair of the skin provides thermal insulation in mammals with hair or fur. This function is enhanced during cold or fright by piloerection (i.e., hairs standing on end), caused by contraction of the tiny erector muscles attached to the hair follicle. The piloerector response that occurs in humans is probably vestigial (i.e., rudimentary), no longer serving its original purpose.

Hair color is supplied by varying amounts of melanin within the hair shaft. Gray or white hair reflects the loss of pigment. Hair quantity and distribution can be affected by endocrine conditions. For example, Cushing's syndrome causes **hirsutism** (i.e., excessive hair growth), especially in women, and hypothyroidism (i.e., underactive thyroid) causes changes in hair texture. Various factors can cause localized or generalized loss of hair, or **alopecia.** Chemotherapy and radiation therapy cause reversible hair thinning or weakening of the hair shaft. Several autoimmune disorders, including systemic lupus erythematosus and alopecia areata, cause hair loss in smaller defined areas. Folliculitis of the scalp will cause inflammation of the hair roots and may result in scarring hair loss.

Nails

On the dorsal surface of the fingers and toes, a hard, transparent plate of keratin, called the *nail*, overlies the skin. The nail grows from its root, which lies under a thin fold of skin called the *cuticle.* Nail functions include scratching and protecting the highly developed sensory functions of fingers and toes to assist in grasping small items. The nails can also be of psychosocial importance as related to grooming and appearance (Nicol, 2016).

Nail growth is continuous throughout life, with an average growth of 0.1 mm daily. Growth is faster in fingernails than toenails and tends to slow with aging. Complete regeneration of a fingernail takes about 6 months, whereas toenail regeneration takes approximately 18 months (Bolognia, Schaffer, & Cerroni, 2017).

Glands of the Skin

There are two types of skin glands: **sebaceous glands** and sweat glands (see Fig. 55-1). The sebaceous glands are associated with hair follicles. The ducts of the sebaceous glands empty **sebum** (fatty secretions) onto the space between the hair follicle and the hair shaft, thus lubricating the hair and rendering the skin soft and pliable.

Sweat glands are found in the skin over most of the body surface, but they are most heavily concentrated in the palms of the hands and soles of the feet. Only the glans penis, clitoris, labia minora, the margins of the lips, the external ear, and the nail bed are devoid of sweat glands. Sweat glands are subclassified into two categories: eccrine and apocrine.

The eccrine sweat glands are found in all areas of the skin. Their ducts open directly onto the skin surface. The thin, watery secretion called *sweat* is produced in the basal coiled portion of the eccrine gland and is released into its narrow duct. Sweat is composed predominantly of water and contains about half of the salt content of blood plasma. Sweat is released from eccrine glands in response to elevated ambient temperature and elevated body temperature. The rate of sweat secretion is under the control of the sympathetic nervous system. Excessive sweating of the palms and soles, axillae, forehead, and other areas may occur in response to pain and stress.

The apocrine sweat glands are larger than eccrine sweat glands and are located in the axillae, periumbilical area, nipple, anal region, scrotum, and labia majora. Their ducts generally open onto hair follicles. The apocrine glands become active at puberty. In women, they enlarge and recede with each menstrual cycle. Apocrine glands produce an oily sweat that is sometimes broken down by bacteria, such as *Corynebacterium* species, to produce the characteristic underarm odor. Specialized apocrine glands called *ceruminous glands* are found in the external ear, where they produce cerumen (i.e., wax).

Functions of the Skin

Protection

The skin covering most of the body is no more than 1 mm thick, but intact skin provides highly effective protection against invasion by bacteria and other foreign matter. The thickened skin of the palms and soles protects against the effects of the constant trauma that occurs in these areas.

The stratum corneum—the outer layer of the epidermis—provides the most effective barrier to epidermal water loss and penetration of environmental factors such as ultraviolet radiation, chemicals, microbes, and insect bites.

Various lipids are synthesized in the stratum corneum and are the basis for the barrier function of this layer. These are long-chain lipids that are suited for water-resistant ceramides, cholesterol, and free fatty acids (Bolognia et al., 2017). The presence of these lipids in the stratum corneum creates a relatively impermeable barrier for water loss and for the entry of toxins, microbes, and other substances that contact the surface of the skin.

Some substances do penetrate the skin but meet resistance in trying to move through the channels between the cell layers of the stratum corneum. Microbes and fungi, which are part of the body's normal flora, cannot penetrate unless there is a break in the skin barrier.

The basal layer, at the junction of the epidermis and dermis, is composed of collagen, anchoring fibers, and macromolecules. The basal layer serves four functions. It acts as a support structure for tissue organization and a template for regeneration; it provides selective permeability for migration of cells and proteins; it is a physical barrier between different types of cells; and it binds the epithelium to underlying cell layers (Bolognia et al., 2017).

Sensation

The receptor endings of nerves in the skin allow the body to constantly monitor the conditions of the immediate environment. The main functions of the receptors in the skin are to sense temperature, pain, light touch, and pressure (or heavy touch). Different nerve endings respond to each of the different stimuli. Although the nerve endings are distributed over the entire body, they are more concentrated in the head and distal extremities.

Fluid Balance

The stratum corneum—the outermost layer of the epidermis—has the capacity to absorb water, thereby preventing an excessive loss of water and electrolytes from the internal body and retaining moisture in the subcutaneous tissues. When skin is damaged, as occurs with a severe burn, large quantities of fluids and electrolytes may be lost rapidly, possibly leading to circulatory collapse, shock, and death (see Chapter 57).

The skin is not completely impermeable to water. Small amounts of water continuously evaporate from the skin surface. This evaporation, called *insensible perspiration*, amounts to approximately 500 mL daily in an average-sized adult (Norris, 2019). Insensible water loss varies with temperature, both body and ambient. In a person with a fever, the loss can increase in a predictable fashion, approximately 12% for every 1°C (1.8°F) increase in body temperature (Norris, 2019).

Temperature Regulation

The body, in the process of creating energy, continuously produces heat as a result of the metabolism of food. This heat is dissipated primarily through the skin. Three major physical processes are involved in loss of heat from the body to the environment. The first process—radiation—is the transfer of heat to another object of lower temperature situated at a distance. The second process—conduction—is the transfer of heat from the body to a cooler object in contact with it. The third process—convection, which consists of movement of warm air molecules away from the body—is the transfer of heat by conduction to the air surrounding the body.

Evaporation from the skin aids heat loss by conduction. Heat is conducted through the skin into water molecules on its surface, causing the water to evaporate. The water on the skin surface may be from insensible perspiration, sweat, or the environment.

Normally, all these heat loss mechanisms are used. When the ambient temperature is extremely high, evaporation becomes the only effective means to disperse generated body heat.

Under normal conditions, metabolic heat production is balanced by heat loss, and the internal temperature of the body is maintained constant at approximately 37°C (98.6°F). The rate of heat loss depends primarily on the surface temperature of the skin, which is a function of the skin blood flow. Under normal conditions, the total blood circulated through the skin is approximately 450 mL/min, or 10 to 20 times the amount of blood required to provide necessary metabolites and oxygen. Blood flow through these skin vessels is controlled primarily by the sympathetic nervous system. Increased blood flow to the skin results in more heat delivered to the skin and a greater rate of heat loss from the body. In contrast, decreased skin blood flow reduces the skin temperature and helps conserve heat for the body. When the temperature of the body begins to fall, as occurs on a cold day, the blood vessels of the skin constrict, thereby reducing heat loss from the body (Bolognia et al., 2017).

Sweating is another process by which the body can regulate the rate of heat loss. Sweating does not occur until the core body temperature exceeds 37°C (98.6°F), regardless of skin temperature. In extremely hot environments, the rate of sweat production may be as high as 1 L/h. Under some circumstances (e.g., emotional stress), sweating may occur as a reflex and may be unrelated to the need to lose heat from the body (Bolognia et al., 2017).

Vitamin Production

Skin exposed to ultraviolet light can synthesize vitamin D (cholecalciferol). Vitamin D is essential for preventing osteoporosis and rickets, a condition that causes bone deformities and results from a deficiency of vitamin D, calcium, and phosphorus. Estimations vary on the amount of sunlight necessary for this synthesis to occur since numerous individual and environmental variables make a uniform recommendation difficult. In some projections, most people would need 5 to 30 minutes of sun exposure twice a week. No studies to date have determined if vitamin D synthesis in the skin can occur without increasing skin cancer risk (Office of Dietary Supplements, National Institutes of Health, 2019). Adequate amounts of Vitamin D should be obtained from a healthy diet and supplementation rather than intentional sun exposure (U.S. Department of Health and Human Services and U.S. Department of Agriculture, 2015).

Immune Response Function

The skin functions not only as a barrier defense against environmental hazards, but also produces immune responses. The skin has the capacity to generate innate and adaptive immune responses (Bolognia et al., 2017). Innate immune functions of the skin include the closely packed layers of the stratum corneum, the nonspecific inflammatory response of pattern recognition receptors, and a chemical environment that inhibits microbial colonization (Norris, 2019). The Langerhans cells of the skin are part of adaptive immunity. They function as antigen-presenting cells, with the ability to transport foreign substances to nearby lymph nodes for cell-mediated immune reaction (Norris, 2019).

 Gerontologic Considerations

The skin undergoes many physiologic changes associated with normal aging that affect functioning; these changes include decreased dermal thickness, degeneration of collagen, decreased sebum production, and increased vascular fragility (Norris, 2019). Other factors such as lifetime of excessive sun exposure, systemic diseases, and poor nutrition can increase the range of skin conditions and the rapidity with which they appear. In addition, certain medications (e.g., antihistamine, antibiotic, and diuretic agents) are photosensitizing and increase the damage that results from sun exposure.

The visible changes in the skin of older adults include dryness, wrinkling, uneven pigmentation, and various proliferative lesions. Cellular changes associated with aging include a thinning at the junction of the dermis and epidermis. The result of this thinning is fewer anchoring sites between the two skin layers, which means that even minor injury or stress

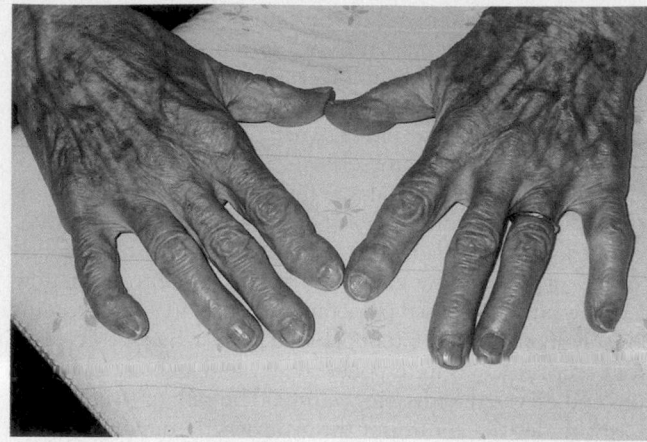

Figure 55-2 • Hands with skin atrophy common to aging skin.

to the epidermis can cause it to shear away from the dermis. This phenomenon may account for the increased vulnerability of aged skin to trauma. With increasing age, the epidermis and dermis thin and flatten, causing wrinkles, sags, and overlapping skin folds (Fig. 55-2).

Loss of the subcutaneous tissue substances of elastin, collagen, and fat diminishes the protection and cushioning of underlying tissues and organs, decreases muscle tone, and results in the loss of the insulating properties of fat.

Cellular replacement slows as a result of aging. As the dermal layers thin, the skin becomes fragile and transparent. The blood supply to the skin also changes with age. Vessels, especially the capillary loops, decrease in number and size. These vascular changes contribute to the delayed wound healing commonly seen in the older adult patient. The dry scaly skin common in aging is likely the consequence of decreased water retention by an impaired stratum corneum and the decreased number and functional ability of sweat and sebaceous glands (Bolognia et al., 2017). Reduced androgen levels are thought to contribute to declining sebaceous gland function.

Hair growth gradually diminishes, especially over the lower legs and dorsum of the feet. Thinning is common in the scalp, axillae, and pubic areas. Other functions affected by normal aging include the barrier function of skin, sensory perception, and thermoregulation.

Damage from excessive sun exposure, called photoaging, has detrimental effects on the normal aging of skin. A lifetime of outdoor work or outdoor activities (e.g., construction work, lifeguarding, sunbathing) without prudent use of covering clothing and sunscreens can lead to profound wrinkling, increased loss of elasticity, mottled, pigmented areas, cutaneous atrophy, and benign or malignant lesions.

Many skin lesions are part of normal aging. Recognizing and differentiating these lesions enables the examiner to assist the patient to feel less anxious about changes in skin. Chart 55-1 summarizes some skin lesions that are expected to appear as the skin ages. These are normal and require no special attention unless the skin becomes infected or irritated.

Assessment

When caring for patients with dermatologic disorders, the nurse obtains important information through the health

Chart 55-1

Benign Changes in the Skin of the Older Adult

- Cherry angiomas (bright red "moles")
- Diminished hair, especially on scalp and pubic area
- Dyschromias (color variations)
  - Solar lentigo (liver spot)
  - Melasma (dark discoloration of the skin)
  - Lentigines (freckles)
- Neurodermatitis (itchy spots)
- Seborrheic keratoses (crusty brown "stuck-on" patches)
- Spider angiomas (see Chapter 43, Fig. 43-3)
- Telangiectasias (red marks on skin caused by stretching of the superficial blood vessels)
- Wrinkles
- Xerosis (dryness)
- Xanthelasma (yellowish waxy deposits on upper and lower eyelids)

Unfolding Patient Stories: Vincent Brody • Part 2

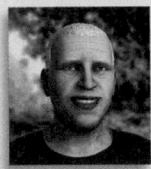

Recall from Chapter 3 **Vincent Brody**, with chronic obstructive pulmonary disease (COPD), who spends most of the day in a recliner chair smoking and has a poor nutritional intake due to shortness of breath. He is admitted to the hospital with COPD exacerbation. What are factors related to his diagnosis? What background information can influence skin breakdown? Describe the skin assessment performed by the nurse.

Care for Vincent and other patients in a realistic virtual environment: **vSim** *for Nursing* (**thepoint.lww.com/vSimMedicalSurgical**). Practice documenting these patients' care in DocuCare (**thepoint.lww.com/DocuCareEHR**).

history and direct observations. The nurse's skill in physical assessment and an understanding of the anatomy and function of the skin can ensure that deviations from normal are recognized, reported, and documented.

Health History

During the health history interview, the nurse asks about use of hair and skin products, as well as any family and personal history of skin allergies; allergic reactions to food, medications, and chemicals; previous skin conditions; and skin cancer (Weber & Kelley, 2018). The health history addresses the onset, signs and symptoms, location, and duration of any pain, itching, rash, or other discomfort experienced by the patient. The names of cosmetics, soaps, shampoos, and other personal hygiene products are obtained if there have been any recent skin conditions noticed with the use of these products. The patient is questioned about nonprescription or herbal preparations that are being used. Chart 55-2 lists selected questions useful in obtaining appropriate information, and Chart 55-3 provides genetic factors influencing skin conditions.

Physical Assessment

Assessment of the skin involves the entire skin area, including the mucous membranes, scalp, hair, and nails. The skin reflects a person's overall health, and alterations commonly correspond to disease in other organ systems. Inspection and palpation are techniques commonly used in examining the skin. The room must be well lighted and warm. A penlight may be used to highlight lesions. The patient completely disrobes and is adequately draped. Gloves are worn during skin examination.

The general appearance of the skin is assessed by observing color, temperature, moisture or dryness, skin texture (rough or smooth), lesions, vascularity, mobility, and the condition of the hair and nails. Skin turgor, possible edema, and elasticity are assessed by palpation.

Assessing Skin Color

The color gradations that occur in people with dark skin are largely determined by genetics; they may be described as light, medium, or dark. In people with dark skin, melanin is

Chart 55-2

ASSESSMENT

Assessing for Skin Disorders

Patient history relevant to skin disorders may be obtained by asking the following questions:

- When did you first notice this skin problem? (In addition, investigate duration and intensity.)
- Has it occurred previously?
- Are there any other symptoms?
- What site was first affected?
- What did the rash or lesion look like when it first appeared?
- Where and how fast did it spread?
- Do you have any itching, burning, tingling, or crawling sensations?
- Is there any loss of sensation?
- Is the problem worse at a particular time or season?
- How do you think it started?
- Do you have a history of hay fever, asthma, hives, eczema, or allergies?
- Who in your family has skin problems or rashes?
- Did the eruptions appear after certain foods were eaten? Which foods?
- When the problem occurred, had you recently consumed alcohol?
- What relation do you think there may be between a specific event and the outbreak of the rash or lesion?
- What medications are you taking?
- What topical medication (ointment, cream, salve) have you put on the lesion (including over-the-counter medications)?
- What skin products or cosmetics do you use?
- What is your occupation?
- What in your immediate environment (plants, animals, chemicals, infections) might be precipitating this disorder? Is there anything new, or are there any changes in the environment?
- Does anything touching your skin cause a rash?
- How has this affected you (or your life)?
- Is there anything else you wish to talk about in regard to this disorder?

Chart 55-3 GENETICS IN NURSING PRACTICE
Integumentary Conditions

Integumentary conditions influenced by genetic factors include the following:

Autosomal Dominant:

- Ehlers–Danlos
- Legius syndrome
- Loeys–Dietz syndrome
- Neurofibromatosis type 1
- Tuberous sclerosis

Autosomal Recessive:

- Albinism
- Congenital ichthyosis

X-Linked Dominant:

- Incontinentia pigmenti

X-Linked Recessive:

- Hypohidrotic ectodermal dysplasia
- Pseudoxanthoma elasticum

Inheritance pattern is not distinct; however, there is a genetic predisposition for the disease:

- Ectodermal dysplasias
- Eczema
- Port-wine stain
- Psoriasis

Nursing Assessments

Refer to Chapter 4, Chart 4-2: Genetics in Nursing Practice: Genetic Aspects of Health Assessment

Family History Assessment Specific to Skin Disorders

- Assess for family members in the past three generations with integumentary impairment or abnormalities.
- Inquire about the nature and type of skin lesions and age at onset (e.g., skin involvement with incontinentia pigmenti

occurs in the first few weeks of life with blistering of the skin, whereas lesions of neurofibromatosis type 1 may appear in early childhood through adulthood).

- Note gender of affected individuals (e.g., mostly females with incontinentia pigmenti, mostly males with hypohidrotic ectodermal dysplasia).
- Inquire about the presence of other clinical features, such as unusual hair, teeth, or nails; thrombocytopenia; recurrent infections.

Patient Assessment

- Assess for related clinical features, such as sparse eyebrows and eyelashes, abnormally shaped teeth, alopecia, nail abnormalities (e.g., hypohidrotic ectodermal dysplasia).
- Assess for related alterations in vision, such as nystagmus or strabismus; albinism; retinal abnormalities (e.g., pseudoxanthoma elasticum); Lisch nodules and/or optic glioma (neurofibromatosis type 1).
- Perform a thorough skin assessment.
- Inquire about sensitivity to the sun.
- Obtain history of wounds and delayed healing time.
- Assess for receding gum line (as seen with Ehlers–Danlos).
- Assess, record location and size of all skin lesions (e.g., *café-au-lait* spots, port-wine stains, bruises).
- Assess for abdominal pulsations or distention (abdominal aneurysm common in Loeys–Dietz syndrome).
- Inspect skin for presence and location of freckles (axillary freckles are associated with genetic disorders). Inquire if freckles were present upon birth and if the amount or location of freckles has grown.

Genetics Resources

The Ehlers–Danlos Society, www.ehlers-danlos.com
Neurofibromatosis Network, www.nfnetwork.org
See Chapter 6, Chart 6-7 for components of genetic counseling.

---

produced at a faster rate and in larger quantities than in people with light skin. Healthy dark skin has a reddish base or undertone. The buccal mucosa, tongue, lips, and nails normally are pink. The skin of exposed portions of the body, especially in sunny, warm climates, tends to be more pigmented than the rest of the body. Almost every process that occurs on the skin causes some color change. For example, **hypopigmentation** (i.e., loss of pigmentation) may be caused by a fungal infection, eczema, or **vitiligo** (i.e., white patches); **hyperpigmentation** (i.e., increase in pigmentation) can occur after sun injury or as a result of aging. Dark pigment responds with discoloration after injury or inflammation, and patients with dark skin more often experience postinflammatory hyperpigmentation than those with lighter skin. The hyperpigmentation eventually fades but may require months to do so.

Changes in skin color in people with dark skin are more noticeable and may cause more concern because the discoloration is more readily visible. Because of the increased activity of melanocytes in darker skin, pigment changes can become obvious and cause great psychological discomfort. Some variation in skin pigment levels is considered normal. Examples include the pigmented crease across the bridge of the nose, some pigmented streaks in the nails, and pigmented spots on the sclera of the eye. Women often develop a dark line along

the midline of the lower abdomen during pregnancy (Weber & Kelley, 2018).

Table 55-1 provides an overview of select color changes in people who are light and dark skinned.

Cyanosis

Cyanosis is the bluish discoloration that results from a lack of oxygen in the blood (Fig. 55-3). It appears with shock or with respiratory or circulatory compromise. In people with light skin, cyanosis manifests as a bluish hue to the lips, fingertips, and nail beds. Other indications of decreased tissue perfusion include cold, clammy skin; a rapid, thready pulse; and rapid, shallow respirations. The conjunctivae of the eyelids are examined for pallor and **petechiae** (i.e., pinpoint red spots that result from blood leakage into skin) (see Chapter 29, Fig. 29-4).

In a person with dark skin, the skin usually assumes a grayish cast. To detect cyanosis, the areas around the mouth and lips and over the cheekbones and earlobes should be observed.

Ecchymosis

Ecchymosis results from blood leaking into the skin and appears as varied discoloration (e.g., purple, black) which

TABLE 55-1	Select Color Changes in Light and Dark Skin	
Etiology	**Light Skin**	**Dark Skin**
Pallor Anemia—decreased hematocrit Shock—decreased perfusion, vasoconstriction	Generalized pallor	Brown skin appears yellow-brown, dull; black skin appears ashen gray, dull. (Observe areas with least pigmentation: conjunctivae, mucous membranes.)
Local arterial insufficiency	Marked localized pallor (lower extremities, especially when elevated)	Ashen gray, dull; cool to palpation
Albinism—total absence of pigment melanin	Whitish pink	Tan, cream, white
Vitiligo—a condition characterized by destruction of the melanocytes in circumscribed areas of the skin (may be localized or widespread)	Patchy, milky white spots, often symmetric bilaterally	Same
Cyanosis Increased amount of unoxygenated hemoglobin:	Dusky blue	Dark but dull, lifeless; only severe cyanosis is apparent in skin, and may appear grayish. (Observe conjunctivae, oral mucosa, nail beds.)
Central—chronic heart and lung diseases cause arterial desaturation Peripheral—exposure to cold, anxiety	Nail beds dusky	
Erythema Hyperemia—increased blood flow through engorged arterial vessels, as in inflammation, fever, alcohol intake, blushing	Red, bright pink	Purplish-gray tinge, but difficult to see. (Palpate for increased warmth with inflammation, taut skin, and hardening of deep tissues.)
Polycythemia—increased red blood cells, capillary stasis	Ruddy blue in face, oral mucosa, conjunctivae, hands and feet	Well concealed by pigment. (Observe for redness in lips.)
Carbon monoxide poisoning	Bright, cherry red in face and upper torso	Cherry red nail beds, lips, and oral mucosa
Venous stasis—decreased blood flow from area, engorged venules	Dusky rubor of dependent extremities (a prelude to necrosis with pressure injury)	Easily masked. (Use palpation to identify warmth or edema.)
Jaundice Increased serum bilirubin concentration (>2 mg/dL) due to liver dysfunction or hemolysis, as after severe burns or some infections	Yellow first in sclerae, hard palate, and mucous membranes; then over skin	Check sclerae for yellow near limbus; do not mistake normal yellowish fatty deposits in the periphery under eyelids for jaundice. (Jaundice is best noted at junction of hard and soft palate, on palms.)
Carotenemia—increased level of serum carotene from ingestion of large amounts of carotene-rich foods	Yellow-orange tinge in forehead, palms and soles, and nasolabial folds, but no yellowing in sclerae or mucous membranes	Yellow-orange tinge in palms and soles
Uremia—kidney injury causes retained urochrome pigments in the blood	Orange-green or gray overlying pallor of anemia; may also have ecchymoses and purpura	Easily masked. (Rely on laboratory and clinical findings.)
Brown-Tan Addison disease—cortisol deficiency stimulates increased melanin production	Bronzed appearance, an "external tan"; most apparent around nipples, perineum, genitalia, and pressure points (inner thighs, buttocks, elbows, axillae)	Easily masked. (Rely on laboratory and clinical findings.)
Café-au-lait spots—caused by increased melanin pigment in basal cell layer	Tan to light brown, irregularly shaped, oval patch with well-defined borders	Often not visible in the person who is very dark skinned

Adapted from Taylor, S. C., Kelly, A. P., Lim, H., et al. (2016). *Dermatology for skin of color* (2nd ed.). New York: McGraw-Hill Medical; Weber, J. W., & Kelley, J. H. (2018). *Health assessment in nursing* (6th ed.). Philadelphia, PA: Wolters Kluwer.

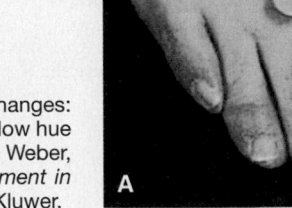
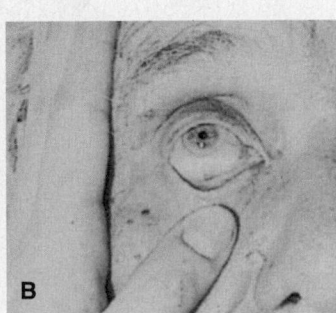

Figure 55-3 • Examples of skin color changes: (**A**) the bluish tint of cyanosis and (**B**) the yellow hue of jaundice. Reprinted with permission from Weber, J. W., & Kelley, J. H. (2018). *Health assessment in nursing* (6th ed.). Philadelphia, PA: Wolters Kluwer.

fades to green, yellow, or brown hues over time. It is most often seen following trauma (e.g., skin being struck with a solid object, fall) (Bickley & Szilagyi, 2017; Weber & Kelley, 2018). It is easier to observe in patients who have lighter skin color and may be seen more frequently in older adults due to increased skin fragility associated with collagen loss, decreased elasticity, and ultraviolet damage. The nurse should assess for unusual patterns or changes in ecchymoses that may indicate health disorders or abuse (Bickley & Szilagyi, 2017).

Erythema

Erythema is redness of the skin caused by the dilation of capillaries. In people who are light skinned, it is easily observable. To determine possible inflammation, the skin is palpated for increased warmth and for smoothness (i.e., edema) or hardness (i.e., intracellular infiltration). Because dark skin tends to assume a purple-gray cast when an inflammatory process is present, it may be difficult to detect erythema.

Jaundice

Jaundice, a yellowing of the skin, is directly related to elevations in serum bilirubin and is often first observed in the sclerae and mucous membranes (see Fig. 55-3).

Assessing Rash

In instances of pruritus (i.e., itching), the patient is asked to indicate which areas of the body are involved. The skin is then stretched gently to decrease the reddish tone and make the rash more visible. Pointing a penlight laterally across the skin may highlight the rash, making it easier to observe. The differences in skin texture are then assessed by running the tips of the fingers lightly over the skin. The borders of the rash may be palpable. The patient's mouth and ears are included in the examination (rubeola, or measles, causes a red cast to appear on the ears, and skin cancers are quite common on the top of the ears). The patient's temperature is assessed, and the lymph nodes are palpated especially in the axillae, inguinal fold, and popliteal area (behind the knees).

Assessing Skin Lesions

Skin lesions are the most prominent characteristics of dermatologic conditions. They vary in size, shape, and cause and are classified according to their appearance and origin. Skin lesions can be described as primary or secondary. Primary lesions are the initial lesions and are characteristic of the disease itself. Secondary lesions result from changes in primary lesions resulting from external causes, such as scratching, trauma, infections, or changes caused by wound healing. Depending on the stage of development, skin lesions are further categorized by type and appearance (Table 55-2).

A preliminary assessment of the eruption or lesion helps identify the type of dermatosis (i.e., abnormal skin condition) and indicates whether the lesion is primary or secondary. At the same time, the anatomic distribution of the eruption or

TABLE 55-2	Primary and Secondary Skin Lesions	
Lesion	**Description**	**Examples**
Primary Lesions		
MACULE, PATCH Macule Patch	Flat, nonpalpable skin color change (color may be brown, white, tan, purple, red) • *Macule:* <1 cm; circumscribed border • *Patch:* >1 cm; may have irregular border	Freckles, flat moles, petechia, rubella, vitiligo, port-wine stains, ecchymosis
PAPULE, PLAQUE Papule Plaque	Elevated, palpable, solid mass with a circumscribed border Plaque may be coalesced papules with flat top • *Papule:* <0.5 cm • *Plaque:* >0.5 cm	*Papules:* Elevated nevi, warts, lichen planus *Plaques:* Psoriasis, actinic keratosis
NODULE, TUMOR Tumor	Elevated, palpable, solid mass that extends deeper into the dermis than a papule • *Nodule:* 0.5–2 cm; circumscribed • *Tumor:* >1–2 cm; tumors do not always have sharp borders	*Nodules:* Lipoma, squamous cell carcinoma, poorly absorbed injection, dermatofibroma *Tumors:* Larger lipoma, carcinoma

TABLE 55-2	Primary and Secondary Skin Lesions (continued)	
Lesion	**Description**	**Examples**
VESICLE, BULLA Bulla Vesicle	Circumscribed, elevated, palpable mass containing serous fluid • *Vesicle:* <0.5 cm • *Bulla:* >0.5 cm	*Vesicles:* Herpes simplex/zoster, varicella, poison ivy, second-degree burn (blister) *Bulla:* Pemphigus, contact dermatitis, large burn blisters, poison ivy, bullous impetigo
WHEAL	Elevated mass with transient borders; often irregular; size and color vary Caused by movement of serous fluid into the dermis; does not contain free fluid in a cavity (e.g., as a vesicle does)	Urticaria (hives), insect bites
PUSTULE	Pus-filled vesicle or bulla	Acne, impetigo, furuncles, carbuncles
CYST	Encapsulated fluid-filled or semisolid mass in the subcutaneous tissue or dermis	Sebaceous cyst, epidermoid cysts

Secondary Lesions

Lesion	Description	Examples
EROSION	Loss of superficial epidermis that does not extend to dermis; depressed, moist area	Ruptured vesicles, scratch marks
ULCER	Skin loss extending past epidermis; necrotic tissue loss; bleeding and scarring possible	Stasis ulcer of venous insufficiency, pressure injury
FISSURE	Linear crack in the skin that may extend to dermis	Chapped lips or hands, tinea pedis
SCALES	Flakes secondary to desquamated, dead epithelium that may adhere to skin surface; color varies (silvery, white); texture varies (thick, fine)	Dandruff, psoriasis, dry skin, pityriasis rosea

(continued on page 1808)

TABLE 55-2	Primary and Secondary Skin Lesions (continued)	
Lesion	**Description**	**Examples**
CRUST	Dried residue of serum, blood, or pus on skin surface Large, adherent crust is a scab	Residue left after vesicle rupture: impetigo, herpes, eczema
SCAR (CICATRIX)	Skin mark left after healing of a wound or lesion; represents replacement by connective tissue of the injured tissue • *Young scars:* Red or purple • *Mature scars:* White or glistening	Healed wound or surgical incision
KELOID	Hypertrophied scar tissue secondary to excessive collagen formation during healing; elevated, irregular, red Greater incidence among African Americans	Keloid of ear piercing or surgical incision
ATROPHY	Thin, dry, transparent appearance of epidermis; loss of surface markings; secondary to loss of collagen and elastin; underlying vessels may be visible	Aged skin, arterial insufficiency
LICHENIFICATION	Thickening and roughening of the skin or accentuated skin markings that may be secondary to repeated rubbing, irritation, scratching	Contact dermatitis

Adapted from Bickley, L. S., & Szilagyi, P. G. (2017). *Bates' guide to physical examination and history taking* (12th ed.). Philadelphia, PA: Wolters Kluwer; Weber, J. W., & Kelley, J. H. (2018). *Health assessment in nursing* (6th ed.). Philadelphia, PA: Wolters Kluwer.

lesion should be observed because certain diseases more regularly affect certain sites of the body and are distributed in characteristic patterns and shapes (Figs. 55-4 and 55-5). To determine the extent of the regional distribution, the left and right sides of the body should be compared while the color and shape of the lesions are assessed. The degree of pigmentation of the patient's skin may affect the appearance of a lesion. Lesions may be black, purple, or gray on dark skin and tan or red in patients with light skin. A metric ruler is used to measure the size of the lesions so that any further extension can be compared with this baseline measurement. After observation, the nurse palpates the lesions with gloves on to determine their texture, shape, and border and to see if they are soft and filled with fluid or hard and fixed to the surrounding tissue.

Skin lesions are described clearly and in detail on the patient's health record, using precise terminology:

• Color of the lesion
• Any redness, heat, pain, or swelling
• Size and location of the involved area
• Pattern of eruption (e.g., macular, papular, scaling, oozing, discrete, confluent)
• Distribution of the lesion (e.g., bilateral, symmetric, linear, circular)

If acute open wounds or lesions are found on inspection of the skin, a comprehensive assessment should be made and documented. This assessment should address the following issues:

• *Wound bed:* Inspect for necrotic and granulation tissue, epithelium, exudate, color, and odor.
• *Wound edges and margins:* Observe for undermining (i.e., extension of the wound under the surface skin), and evaluate for condition of skin (i.e., necrotic).
• *Wound size:* Measure in centimeters, as appropriate, to determine diameter and depth of the wound and surrounding erythema.
• *Surrounding skin:* Assess for color, suppleness and moisture, irritation, and scaling.

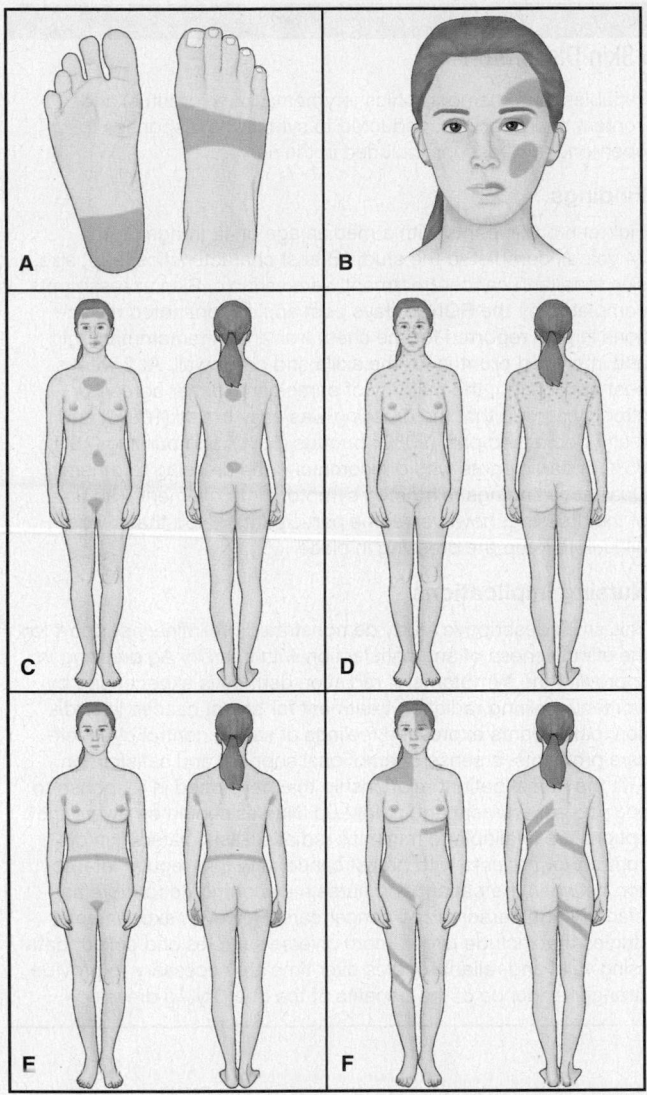

Figure 55-4 • Anatomic distribution of common skin disorders. **A.** Contact dermatitis (shoes). **B.** Contact dermatitis (cosmetics, perfumes, earrings). **C.** Seborrheic dermatitis. **D.** Acne. **E.** Scabies. **F.** Herpes zoster (shingles).

It is also important for the nurse to assess for other signs and symptoms associated with new skin lesions, such as pain, burning, or pruritus (see the Nursing Research Profile in Chart 55-4).

Assessing Vascularity and Hydration

After the color of the skin has been evaluated and lesions have been inspected, an assessment of vascular changes in the skin is performed. A description of vascular changes includes location, distribution, color, size, and the presence of pulsations. Common vascular changes include petechiae, ecchymoses, **telangiectasias** (vascular structures), and angiomas (Table 55-3).

Skin moisture, temperature, and texture are assessed primarily by palpation. The turgor (i.e., elasticity) of the skin, which decreases in normal aging, may be a factor in assessing the hydration status of a patient. To assess skin turgor, the skin should be gently pinched between the thumb and forefinger. The skin is observed to see how long it takes to return to

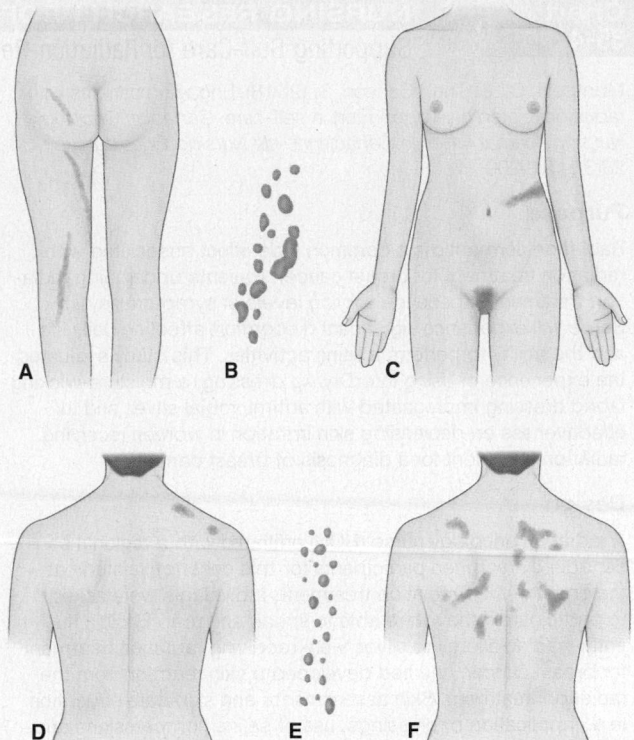

Figure 55-5 • Skin lesion configurations. **A.** Linear (in a line). **B.** Annular and arciform (circular or arcing). **C.** Zosteriform (linear along a nerve route). **D.** Grouped (clustered). **E.** Discrete (separate and distinct). **F.** Confluent (merged).

baseline. People who are dehydrated or those with dry skin will display decreased skin turgor, where the skin remains tented after being pinched rather than returning to normal almost immediately. Edema is indicated when the skin appears tense and shiny, when a finger gently pressed into the skin leaves an indentation or "pit" (see Chapter 25, Fig. 25-2). Assessing the depth of the pit and length of time to resolution indicates the extent of edema (Bickley & Szilagyi, 2017).

Assessing the Nails

A brief inspection of the nails includes observation of configuration, color, and consistency. Many alterations in the nail or nail bed reflect local or systemic abnormalities in progress or resulting from past events (Fig. 55-6). Beau lines, a transverse depression in the nails, may reflect retarded growth of the nail matrix because of severe illness or, more commonly, local trauma. Ridging, hypertrophy, and other changes may also be visible because of local trauma. Paronychia, an inflammation of the skin around the nail, is usually accompanied by tenderness and erythema. Pitted surface of the nails is a definite indication of psoriasis. Spoon-shaped nails can indicate severe iron-deficiency anemia. The angle between the normal nail and its base is 160 degrees. When palpated, the nail base is usually firm. Clubbing of the nails is manifested by a straightening of the normal angle (180 degrees or greater) and softening of the nail base. The softened area feels spongelike when palpated (Bickley & Szilagyi, 2017). Clubbing can be a normal variant, but it is most often associated with pulmonary disease and can be a sign of chronic hypoxia (Norris, 2019).

Chart 55-4

NURSING RESEARCH PROFILE

Supporting Self-Care for Radiation-Related Skin Discomfort

Montpetit, C., & Singh-Carlson, S. (2018). Engaging patients with radiation related skin discomfort in self-care. *Canadian Oncology Nursing Journal = Revue Canadienne de Nursing Oncologique, 28*(3), 191–200.

Purpose

Radiation dermatitis is a common side effect associated with radiation treatment for breast cancer. Patients undergoing radiation treatment experience varying levels of symptom severity. Some will experience significant discomfort affecting daily life and the ability to perform routine activities. This study evaluated the experience of using InterDry Ag dressing, a moisture-wicking fabric dressing impregnated with antimicrobial silver, and its effectiveness on decreasing skin irritation in women receiving radiation treatment for a diagnosis of breast cancer.

Design

A radiation oncology nurse (RON) affiliated with a regional cancer agency recruited participants for this descriptive study at the onset of their radiation treatment. Individuals were asked to participate if they were able to speak and read English fluently, had no allergy to silver, were receiving radiation treatment for breast cancer, and had developed a skin reaction from the radiation treatment. Skin assessments and skin care education (e.g., application of dressings, use of saline compressions and moisturizers) were provided to all participants receiving radiation. The InterDry Ag dressing was utilized in participants with moderate erythema, pruritus, or burning and evaluated during therapy using the National Cancer Institute: Common Terminology Criteria for Adverse Events (NCI CTCAE) (version 4.03) radiation dermatitis tool. In addition, a questionnaire to assess participants' discomfort and ease of dressing use was administered 5 days after dressing application. Follow-up was also conducted both 1-week (via telephone) and 2-week (in-person) post radiation by the RON. Descriptive statistics were generated to assess study variables (e.g., demographics, erythema, pain, pruritus) and content analysis was conducted to synthesize responses to open-ended questions included in the survey.

Findings

Eighteen participants with a median age of 42 (range 36 to 74 years), completed the study. Breast characteristics (e.g., size, skin tone) and cancer treatment were variable. Skin assessments completed by the RON (5 days post application) noted reductions in pain reported for the chest wall and inframammary fold and improved pruritus for the axilla and chest wall. At 2 weeks post application, the majority of participants either agreed or strongly agreed that the dressing was easy to use (100%) and that it decreased pain (90%), pruritus (88%), and burning (78%); 95% of participants would recommend the dressing to others. Qualitative findings reinforced symptom improvement with use of the dressing; however, some participants noted that it was difficult to keep the dressing in place.

Nursing Implications

This small descriptive study demonstrated preliminary support for the effectiveness of and satisfaction with InterDry Ag dressing in improving the symptoms of radiation dermatitis experienced by women receiving radiation treatment for breast cancer. In addition, participants expressed feelings of safety, control over self-care problems, a sense of emotional support, and satisfaction with the nurse–patient relationship that developed in response to ongoing assessment and follow-up. Nurses should be aware that options are available to minimize radiation-associated skin discomfort for patients with breast cancer and that regular interaction between the patient and nurse may contribute to more satisfactory and personalized cancer care. However, experimental studies that include larger, more diverse samples and collect data using valid and reliable scales over time are necessary to provide stronger evidence of the benefits of the InterDry Ag dressing.

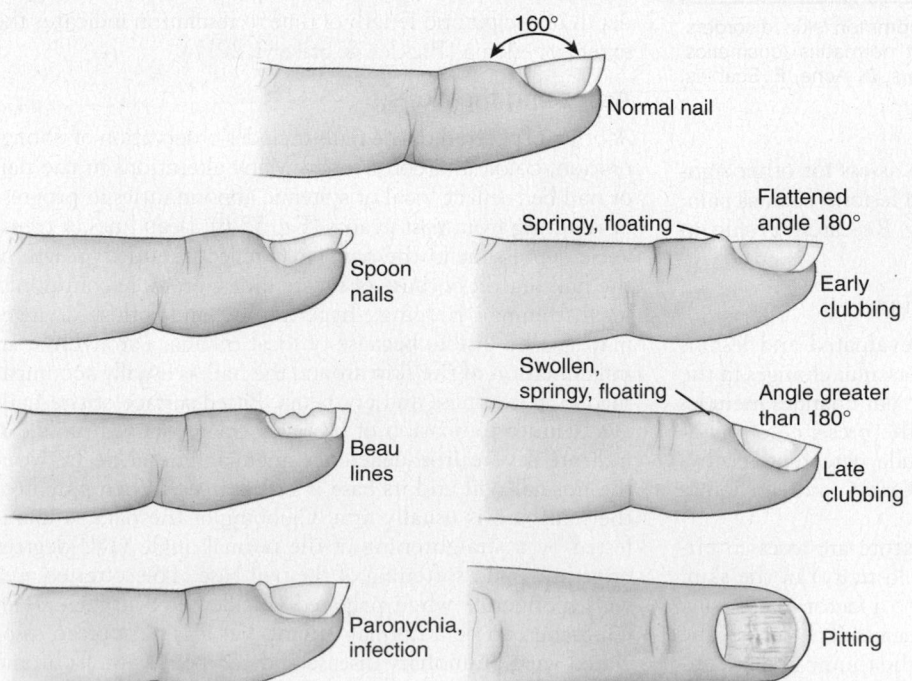

Figure 55-6 • Common nail disorders.

TABLE 55-3	Vascular Lesions
PETECHIA (PL. PETECHIAE) 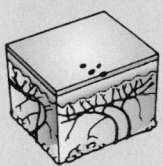	Round red or purple macule Small (1–2 mm) Secondary to blood extravasation Associated with bleeding tendencies or emboli to skin
ECCHYMOSIS (PL. ECCHYMOSES) 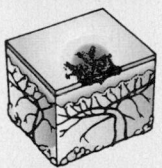	Round or irregular macular lesion Larger than petechia Color varies and changes—purple, black, yellow, and green hues Secondary to blood extravasation Associated with trauma, bleeding tendencies
CHERRY ANGIOMA 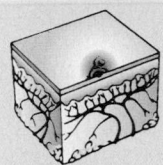	Papular and round Red or purple Noted on trunk, extremities May blanch with pressure Normal age-related skin alteration Usually not clinically significant
SPIDER ANGIOMA 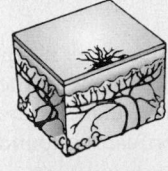	Red, arteriole lesion Central body with radiating branches Noted on face, neck, arms, trunk Rare below the waist May blanch with pressure Associated with liver disease, pregnancy, vitamin B deficiency
TELANGIECTASIA (VASCULAR STRUCTURE) 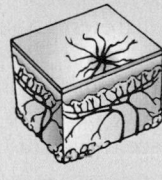	Shape varies—spiderlike or linear Color bluish or red Does not blanch when pressure is applied Noted on legs, anterior chest Secondary to superficial dilation of venous vessels and capillaries Associated with increased venous pressure states (varicosities)

Adapted from Bickley, L. S., & Szilagyi, P. G. (2017). *Bates' guide to physical examination and history taking* (12th ed.). Philadelphia, PA: Wolters Kluwer; Weber, J. W., & Kelley, J. H. (2018). *Health assessment in nursing* (6th ed.). Philadelphia, PA: Wolters Kluwer.

Assessing the Hair

The hair assessment is carried out by inspection and palpation. Gloves are worn by the examiner, and the examination room should be well lighted. The hair is separated so that the condition of the skin underneath can be easily seen. The examiner notes the color, texture, and distribution of hair shafts. The wooden end of a cotton swab can be used to make small parts in the hair so that the scalp can be inspected. Any abnormal lesions, evidence of itching, inflammation, scaling, or signs of infestation (i.e., lice or mites) are documented.

Color and Texture

Natural hair color ranges from white to black. Hair begins to turn gray or white with age, when loss of melanin in the hair

shaft becomes apparent. Loss of melanin in hair can occur at a younger age and may be due to heredity or genetic traits. The person with albinism (i.e., partial or complete absence of pigmentation) has a genetic predisposition to white hair from birth. The natural state of the hair can be altered by using hair dyes, bleaches, and curling or relaxing products. The use of these products has varying impact on hair, depending on its natural characteristics. For example, the use of straightening chemicals on the hair of most people can cause extensive breakage and hair loss (Bobonich & Nolen, 2014; Richardson, Agidi, Eaddy, et al., 2017).

The texture of scalp hair ranges from fine to coarse, silky to brittle, oily to dry, and shiny to dull, and hair can be straight, curly, or kinky. Dry, brittle hair may result from the overuse of hair dyes, hair dryers, and curling irons or from endocrine disorders, such as thyroid dysfunction. Oily hair is usually caused by increased secretion from the sebaceous glands close to the scalp. If the patient reports a recent change in hair texture, the underlying reason is pursued; the alteration may arise simply from the overuse of commercial hair products or from changing to a new shampoo.

Distribution

Body hair distribution varies with location. Hair over most of the body is fine, except in the axillae and pubic areas, where it is coarse. Pubic hair, which develops at puberty, forms a diamond shape extending up to the umbilicus in cisgender boys and men. Cisgender female pubic hair resembles an inverted triangle. If the pattern found is more characteristic of the opposite gender, it may indicate an endocrine disorder and further investigation is in order. Racial differences in hair are expected, such as straight hair in people of Asian descent and curly, coarse hair in people of African descent.

Men tend to have more body and facial hair than women. Alopecia can occur over the entire body or be localized to a specific area. Scalp hair loss may be patchy or may range from generalized thinning to total baldness. When assessing scalp hair loss, it is important to investigate the underlying cause with the patient. Patchy hair loss may be from habitual hair pulling or twisting; excessive traction on the hair (e.g., braiding too tightly); excessive use of dyes, straighteners, and oils; chemotherapeutic agents (e.g., doxorubicin, cyclophosphamide); bacterial or fungal infection; or moles or lesions on the scalp. Well-defined patches of localized hair loss generally indicate the condition called *alopecia areata*. The precise mechanism is unknown but may be triggered by an interaction between genetic and environmental factors. Regrowth in most cases is spontaneous and occurs in 1 to 3 months, though in some rarer patterns, the hair loss is recurrent or even permanent (Habif et al., 2018).

Hair Loss

The most common cause of male pattern hair loss or baldness is androgenic alopecia, which affects more than half of the male population and is believed to be related to heredity, aging, and androgen (male hormone) levels. Androgen is necessary for male pattern hair loss to develop. The pattern of hair loss begins with receding of the hairline in the frontal temporal area and may progress to gradual thinning and complete loss of hair over the top of the scalp and crown. The typical pattern of male hair loss is illustrated in Figure 55-7A.

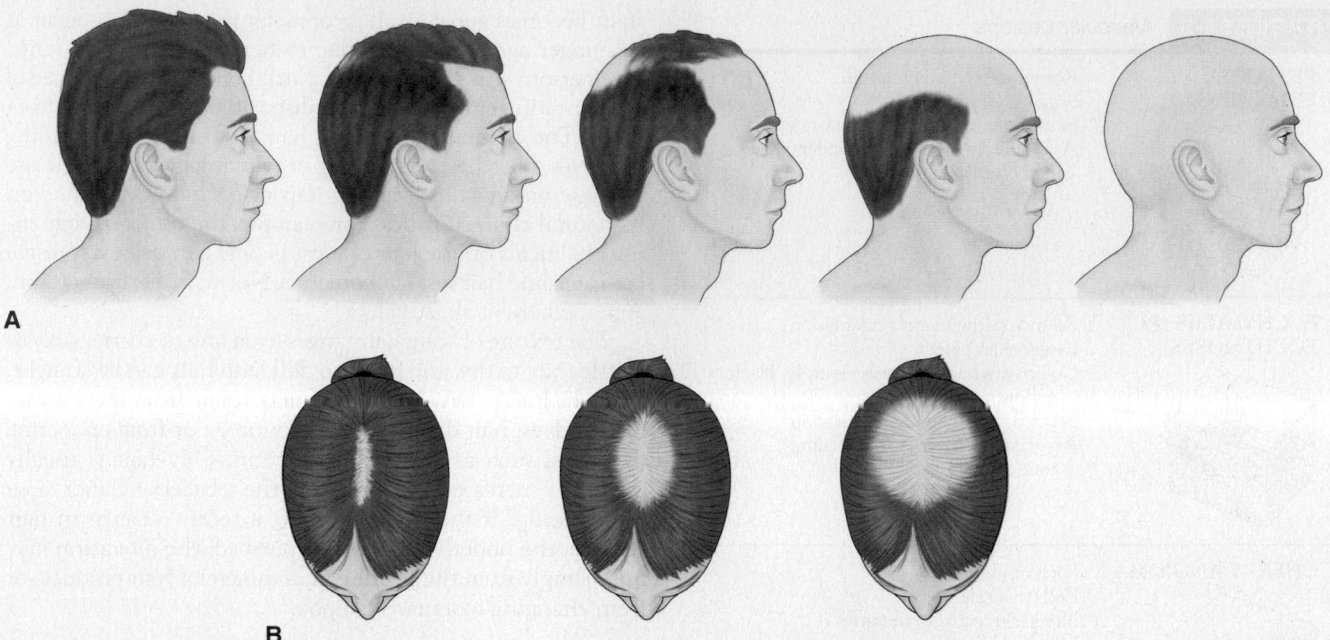

Figure 55-7 • Hair loss. **A.** Progression of male pattern hair loss. **B.** Progression of female pattern hair loss.

Although androgenic alopecia is considered a male disorder, millions of women experience female pattern hair loss, which is typically not seen with other signs of hyperandrogenism. For women complete baldness is rare; the typical pattern of hair loss is seen on the vertex scalp, sparing the frontal area (Nicol, 2016) (Fig. 55-7B).

Other Changes

Male pattern hair distribution may be seen in some women at the time of menopause, when the hormone estrogen is no longer produced by the ovaries. In women with hirsutism, excessive hair may grow on the face, chest, shoulders, and pubic area. If menopause is ruled out as the underlying cause, other hormonal changes related to pituitary or adrenal dysfunction must be investigated.

Because patients with skin conditions may be viewed negatively by others, these patients may experience psychological distress and avoid interactions and intimacy. Skin conditions can lead to isolation, job loss, and economic hardship as well as poor self-esteem.

Some conditions may lead to feelings of depression, frustration, self-consciousness, poor self-image, and rejection. Itching and skin irritation (features of many skin diseases) may be constant sources of physical distress. These discomforts may result in loss of sleep, anxiety, and depressive symptoms, all of which reinforce the general distress and fatigue that frequently accompany skin disorders.

For patients experiencing physical and psychological discomforts, the nurse needs to provide understanding, explanations of the problem, appropriate education related to treatment, nursing support, and encouragement. It is imperative to overcome any aversion that may be felt when caring for patients with unattractive skin disorders. The nurse should show no sign of hesitancy when approaching patients with skin disorders. Such hesitancy only reinforces the psychological trauma of the disorder.

Skin Consequences of Select Systemic Diseases

Diabetes

Because diabetes causes changes in circulation and cell nutrition, it can have a great impact on skin status. Some of the more common skin conditions encountered in diabetes are discussed in this section. Further information can be found in Chapter 46.

Diabetic Dermopathy

Diabetic dermopathy (shin spots or pigmented pretibial papules) is a frequent occurrence in people with diabetes. These lesions are found most often on the lower anterior legs. They are thought to be caused by diabetes-associated changes in the small vessels that supply the skin and trauma. Each cluster starts as dull red papules that slowly coalesce to brownish atrophic patches (Nicol, 2016).

Stasis Dermatitis

Stasis dermatitis is an eczematous eruption that occurs on the lower legs of patients with venous insufficiency. It is very common in patients with diabetes. Large vessels are damaged, compromising circulation to the lower arms and legs. The skin suffers from lack of nutrients, becoming very dry and fragile. Minor injuries heal slowly, and ulcers form easily. It initially presents with variable erythema and scale and pruritus. When chronic, it leads to permanent changes in skin color, hyper- or hypopigmentation, and either fragile or thicker skin texture (fibrosis).

Skin Infections

Bacterial infections may appear as small pimples around hair follicles (i.e., folliculitis). The most frequently affected sites include the lower legs, lower abdomen, and buttocks. Sometimes, these lesions enlarge to become furuncles or carbuncles.

Furuncles begin in a hair follicle, progressively enlarging and invading deeper into tissue to form an abscess. Carbuncles are formed by multiple contiguous lesions (Habif et al., 2018). The skin of patients with diabetes is prone to bacterial and fungal infections. If the blood glucose level is not well controlled, these infections may be very slow to heal.

Fungal infections are quite common in areas that remain moist (under breasts, upper thighs, in axillae). *Candida* (i.e., yeast) infections appear beefy red and often have small pustules around the border of the area, with the skin appearing moist and raw.

Dermatophyte infections are dry and only minimally red, with more scale. Common sites are the toenails and feet.

Nurses must be alert to the signs of these common infections. If necessary, they should bring them to the attention of the patient's primary provider and help the patient or family learn basic skin maintenance techniques.

Leg and Foot Ulcers

Because of changes in peripheral nerves, patients with diabetes do not always sense minor injuries to the lower legs and feet. Infections begin and, if untreated, may lead to ulcerations. Ulcerations are often not noticed and become quite large before being treated. Ulcerations unresponsive to treatment are a leading cause of diabetic foot and leg amputations (Johnson, Osburne, Rispoli, et al., 2018).

Human Immune Deficiency Virus Disease

Cutaneous signs may be the first manifestation of human immune deficiency virus (HIV), appearing in more than 90% of people who are HIV infected as immune function deteriorates. These skin signs correlate with low CD4$^+$ counts. Some disorders such as Kaposi sarcoma, oral hairy leukoplakia, facial molluscum contagiosum, and oral candidiasis may suggest that CD4$^+$ counts are less than 200 to 300 cells/mcL. Skin infections, both bacterial and viral, are common and will appear more severe than expected. Acute flare of chronic conditions such as seborrhea or acne may indicate a new infection. Being sensitive to these changes can alert the nurse so that early interventions can be initiated (Schwartz, 2019).

Diagnostic Evaluation

A wide range of diagnostic studies may be performed in patients with altered integumentary function. The nurse educates the patient about the purpose, what to expect, and any possible side effects related to these examinations prior to testing. The nurse also notes trends in results because they provide information about whether lesions are primary or secondary, disease progression, and the patient's response to therapy.

Skin Biopsy

Performed to obtain tissue for microscopic examination, a skin biopsy may be obtained by shave, excision, or by a skin punch instrument that removes a small core of tissue. Biopsies are performed on skin nodules, plaques, blisters, and other lesions to rule out malignancy, to aid in diagnosis, and to perform additional testing such as Gram stain for bacteria or periodic acid–Schiff (PAS) for fungal elements.

Patch Testing

Performed to identify substances to which the patient has developed an allergy, patch testing involves applying the suspected allergens, such as nickel or fragrances, to normal skin under occlusive patches. Patients wear these occluded strips on their backs for 48 hours, and the area is assessed after 72 hours. The development of redness, fine elevations, or itching is considered a weak positive reaction; fine blisters, papules, and severe itching indicate a moderately positive reaction; and blisters, pain, and ulceration indicate a strong positive reaction. The nurse educates the patient on means to avoid the reactive allergens, which is often quite difficult, due to the prevalence of many of these substances in the patient's environment.

Skin Scrapings

Tissue samples are scraped from suspected fungal lesions with a scalpel blade that has been moistened with oil so that the scraped skin adheres to the blade. The scraped material is transferred to a glass slide, covered with a coverslip, and examined microscopically. The spores and hyphae of dermatophyte infections, as well as infestations such as scabies, can be visualized.

Tzanck Smear

The Tzanck smear is a test used to examine cells from blistering skin conditions, such as herpes zoster, varicella, herpes simplex, and all forms of pemphigus. The secretions from a suspected lesion are applied to a glass slide, stained, and examined.

Wood Light Examination

Wood light is a special lamp that produces long-wave ultraviolet rays, which result in a characteristic blue to dark purple fluorescence. The color of the fluorescent light is best seen in a darkened room, where it is possible to differentiate epidermal from dermal lesions and hypo- and hyperpigmented lesions from normal skin. The patient is reassured that the light is not harmful to skin or eyes. Lesions that still contain melanin almost disappear under ultraviolet light, whereas lesions that are devoid of melanin increase in whiteness with ultraviolet light.

Clinical Photographs

Photographs are taken to document the nature and extent of the skin condition and are used to determine progress or improvement resulting from treatment. They are sometimes used to track the status of moles to document if the characteristics of the mole are changing.

Nursing Implications

The nurse may be responsible to ensure that consent forms are completed for surgical procedures and for clinical photography, that all specimens collected are managed according to protocol, that a log is maintained tracking specimens to and from the laboratory, and that results are received in a timely manner. The nurse educates the patient regarding appropriate care of surgical sites and implication of test results.

CRITICAL THINKING EXERCISES

1 `ebp` As a recent graduate nurse, you are aware that the U.S. Preventive Service Task Force (USPSTF) has given a grade B recommendation for providing sun protection education for individuals who are fair skinned, parents of young children, adolescents, and young adults. You share this recommendation with a patient, and the patient asks you to explain what a grade B recommendation means. How would you respond? Discuss sun protection behaviors you will include when providing this education. What other factors found when performing a skin examination or in the patient's history may make sun protection counseling advisable outside of this recommendation?

2 `pq` A 28-year-old woman who has rheumatoid arthritis was recently diagnosed with vitiligo and is expressing concerns about living with this condition. She has questions about how to protect her skin and how to cope with feelings of embarrassment. She also wants to know if her children are at risk for developing this condition. In providing patient education, which question will you address first? What education and resources will you provide and how will you counsel the patient to prioritize her physical, psychological, and emotional health?

REFERENCES

*Asterisk indicates nursing research.

Books

Bickley, L. S., & Szilagyi, P. G. (2017). *Bates' guide to physical examination and history taking* (12th ed.). Philadelphia, PA: Lippincott Williams & Wilkins.

Bobonich, M. A., & Nolen, M. E. (2014). *Dermatology for advanced practice clinicians*. Philadelphia, PA: Wolters Kluwer.

Bolognia, J., Schaffer, J., & Cerroni, L. (2017). *Dermatology* (4th ed.). Philadelphia, PA: Elsevier Saunders.

Habif, T., Dinulos, J., Chapman, M., et al. (2018). *Skin disease* (4th ed.). Philadelphia, PA: Elsevier.

Nicol, N. (2016). *Dermatologic nursing essentials: A core curriculum* (3rd ed.). Philadelphia, PA: Wolters Kluwer.

Norris, T. L. (2019). *Porth's pathophysiology: Concepts of altered health states* (10th ed.). Philadelphia, PA: Wolters Kluwer. Kindle edition.

Taylor, S. C., Kelly, A. P., Lim, H., et al. (2016). *Dermatology for skin of color* (2nd ed.). New York: McGraw-Hill Medical.

Weber, J. W., & Kelley, J. H. (2018). *Health assessment in nursing* (6th ed.). Philadelphia, PA: Wolters Kluwer.

Journals and Electronic Documents

Johnson, R., Osburne, A., Rispoli, J., et al. (2018). The diabetic foot assessment. *Orthopedic Nursing, 37*(1), 13–21.

*Montpetit, C., & Singh-Carlson, S. (2018). Engaging patients with radiation related skin discomfort in self-care. *Canadian Oncology Nursing Journal = Revue Canadienne de Nursing Oncologique, 28*(3), 191–200.

Office of Dietary Supplements, National Institutes of Health. (2019). Vitamin D: Fact sheet for health professionals. Retrieved on 2/6/2020 at: www.ods.od.nih.gov/factsheets/VitaminD-HealthProfessional

Richardson, V., Agidi, A. T., Eaddy, E. R., et al. (2017). Ten pearls every dermatologist should know about the appropriate use of relaxers. *Journal of Cosmetic Dermatology, 16*(1), 9–11.

Schwartz, R. A. (2019). Cutaneous manifestations of HIV. *Medscape.* Retrieved on 2/6/2020 at: www.emedicine.medscape.com/article/1133746-overview

U.S. Department of Health and Human Services and U.S. Department of Agriculture. (2015). *2015–2020 Dietary guidelines for Americans* (8th ed.). Retrieved on 7/6/2020 at: www.health.gov/dietaryguidelines/2015/guidelines

Wilhelmi, B. J., & Molnar, J. A. (2018). Finger nail and tip injuries. *Medscape.* Retrieved on 2/6/2020 at: www.emedicine.medscape.com/article/1285680-overview

Resources

American Academy of Dermatology Association (AAD), www.aad.org/public

Centers for Disease Control and Prevention, Skin Cancer, www.cdc.gov/cancer/skin/index.htm

Dermatology Atlas (DermIS), a cooperation between the Department of Clinical Social Medicine (University of Heidelberg) and the Department of Dermatology (University of Erlangen), www.dermis.net/dermisroot/en/home/index.htm

National Institutes of Health, National Institute on Aging, Skin Care and Aging, www.nia.nih.gov/health/skin-care-and-aging

New Zealand Dermatology Society (DermNet NZ), www.dermnetnz.org

Skin Cancer Foundation (lists approved sunscreens and other sun protection products), www.skincancer.org

56 Management of Patients with Dermatologic Disorders

LEARNING OUTCOMES

On completion of this chapter, the learner will be able to:

1. Describe the medical and nursing management of the patient with a wound, pruritus, dermatologic secretory disorder, infections of the skin, parasitic skin diseases, or noninfectious inflammatory dermatoses.
2. Use the nursing process as a framework for care of the patient with a pressure injury, or with a blistering disorder including toxic epidermal necrolysis and Stevens–Johnson syndrome.
3. Discuss the medical and nursing management of the patient with skin tumors (benign, malignant, and metastatic).
4. Identify the medical and nursing management of the patient undergoing plastic or cosmetic procedures.

NURSING CONCEPTS

Functional Ability   Mobility   Tissue Integrity

GLOSSARY

acantholysis: separation of epidermal cells from each other due to damage or abnormality of the intracellular substance

bullae: large, fluid-filled blisters

carbuncle: localized skin infection involving several hair follicles

cheilitis: inflammation of the lips

comedones: the primary lesions of acne, caused by sebum blockage in the hair follicle

cytotoxic: destructive of cells

débridement: removal of necrotic or dead tissue by mechanical, surgical, chemical, or autolytic means

dermatitis: any inflammation of the skin

dermatosis: any abnormal skin lesion

epidermopoiesis: development of epidermal cells

furuncle: localized skin infection of a single or a few hair follicles (*synonym*: boil)

hydrophilic: a material that absorbs moisture

hydrophobic: a material that repels moisture

hygroscopic: a material that absorbs moisture from the air

lichenification: thickening of the horny layer of the skin (*synonym*: scaling)

liniments: lotions with added oil for increased softening of the skin

pressure injury: localized area of skin breakdown and/or underlying soft tissue damage due to prolonged pressure and insufficient blood supply; formerly known as *pressure ulcer*

pruritus: itching

pyodermas: pus-forming bacterial skin infections

sinus tract: course or path of tissue destruction occurring in any direction from the surface or edge of a wound (*synonym*: tunneling)

slough: soft, moist avascular (devitalized) tissue; may be white, yellow, tan, gray, or green; may be loose or firmly adherent

striae: bandlike streaks on the skin, distinguished by color, texture, depression, or elevation from the tissue in which they are found; usually purplish or white

suspensions: liquid preparations in which powder is suspended, requiring shaking before use

tinea: a common superficial fungal infection on the skin or scalp (*synonym*: ringworm)

undermining: area of destroyed tissue that extends extensively under intact skin along the periphery of a wound

xerosis: overly dry, rough skin

Dermatologic disorders are encountered frequently by nurses across many practice settings. Nursing management of patients with dermatologic disorders can range from simple interventions such as administering topical and systemic medications for prevention to treating complex pressure injuries.

The nurse can also be instrumental in educating patients how to care for their skin and provide self-care for wounds. The objectives of nursing interventions are to prevent additional skin and tissue damage, prevent secondary infection, reverse the inflammatory process, and relieve the symptoms.

SKIN CARE

Some skin problems are markedly aggravated by soap and water; therefore, bathing routines are modified according to the condition. Denuded skin, whether the area of desquamation is large or small, is excessively prone to damage by chemicals, trauma, and even bathing. Friction occurs when skin rubs against another surface, which may happen when the skin is vigorously dried with a towel, resulting in damage to the epidermal and upper dermal skin layers (Bryant & Nix, 2016).

Protecting the Skin

The goal of routine skin care should be to maintain the acidic pH of the skin; therefore, alkaline soaps should be avoided. No-rinse, pH-balanced soap is the best. Moisturizing products, such as emollients and humectants, can be applied to help maintain skin moisture. Emollients moisturize and soften the skin; conversely, humectants attract water to moisturize skin with **xerosis** (very dry, rough skin) (Doughty & McNichol, 2016).

Basic skin care in bathing a patient with a skin disorder is as follows:

- A mild, lipid-free soap or soap substitute is used (e.g., Dove sensitive skin™, Cetaphil™, CeraVe™, VANICREAM™).
- The area is rinsed completely and blotted dry with a soft cloth.
- Deodorant soaps are avoided.
- Laundry detergents and fabric softener free of fragrance are used.

Special care is necessary when changing dressings. Sterile saline, or another prescribed solution, helps loosen crusts, remove exudates, or free an adherent dry dressing.

Preventing Secondary Infection

Skin lesions should be regarded as potentially infectious, and proper safety precautions should be observed until the diagnosis is established. Most lesions with purulent drainage contain infectious material. The nurse and primary provider must adhere to standard precautions and wear gloves when inspecting the skin or changing a dressing. The use of standard personal protective equipment (PPE) and proper disposal of any contaminated dressing is carried out according to the Occupational Safety and Health Administration (OSHA) regulations (OSHA, 2011).

Wound Dressing Care

Dressings can be categorized in several ways. An overview of select types of dressings and their indications is provided; however, this is not an exhaustive list of dressing types.

Passive dressings have only a protective function and maintain a moist environment for natural healing. They include those that just cover the area (e.g., DuoDERM™, Tegaderm™) and may remain in place for several days. *Interactive dressings* are capable of absorbing wound exudate while maintaining a moist environment in the area of the wound and allowing the surrounding skin to remain dry. They include hydrocolloids, alginates, and hydrogels. It is thought that interactive dressings are able to modify the physiology of the wound environment by modulating and stimulating cellular activity and by releasing growth factors (Dabiri, Damstetter, & Phillips, 2016). *Active dressings* improve the healing process and decrease the healing time. They include skin grafts and biologic skin substitutes. Both interactive and active dressings create a moist environment at the interface of the wound with the dressing.

Wicker dressings are ropelike dressings used to manage sinus tracts or wounds that have undermining (see later discussion of sinus tracts and undermining in Pressure Injuries). These are effective at absorbing drainage. Wicker dressings can be plain or antimicrobial. *Filler dressings* are best for deeper wounds; these fill the contour of the wound, allowing the wound to heal by secondary intention. *Cover dressings* are appropriate for surface wounds and also can be used as a secondary dressing over filler dressings. These dressings can be absorptive or hydrating, plain or antimicrobial (Doughty & McNichol, 2016).

Because so many wound care products are available, it is often difficult to select the most appropriate product for a specific wound. Selection of products should be made carefully because of their expense. Both clinical efficacy and health-related outcomes (e.g., decreased pain, increased mobility) should be used to measure the success of a wound care product. Even with the availability of a large variety of dressings, an appropriate selection can be made if certain principles are maintained. These principles are referred to as the five rules of wound care (Dabiri et al., 2016).

1. *Rule 1: Categorization.* The nurse learns about dressings by generic category and compares new products with those that already make up the category. The nurse becomes familiar with indications, contraindications, and side effects. The best dressing may be created by combining products in different categories to achieve several goals at the same time. These categories are discussed in subsequent sections.
2. *Rule 2: Selection.* The nurse selects the safest and most effective, easy-to-use, and cost-effective dressing possible. Nurses follow the primary provider's prescriptions for dressings. They must be prepared to give the primary provider feedback about the dressing's effect on the wound, ease of use for the patient, and other considerations when applicable.
3. *Rule 3: Change.* The nurse changes dressings based on patient, wound, and dressing assessments, not on standardized routines.
4. *Rule 4: Evolution.* As the wound progresses through the phases of wound healing, the dressing protocol is altered to optimize healing. It is rare, especially in cases of chronic wounds, that the same dressing material is appropriate throughout the healing process. The nurse educates the patient or family caregiver about wound care and ensures that the family has access to appropriate dressing choices.
5. *Rule 5: Practice.* Practice with dressing material is required for the nurse to learn the performance parameters of the particular dressing. Refining the skills of applying appropriate dressings correctly and learning about new dressing products are essential nursing responsibilities. Dressing changes should not be delegated to unlicensed personnel; these techniques require the knowledge base and assessment skills of professional nurses.

TABLE 56-1	Functions and Actions of Wound Dressings	
Function	**Action**	**Example**
Absorption	Absorbs exudates	Alginates, composite dressings, foams, gauze, hydrocolloids, hydrogels
Antimicrobial	Alters wound bed bioburden	Alginates, foams, collagens, composites, contact layers, hydrogels, transparent films, impregnated dressings, wound fillers
Cleansing	Removes purulent drainage, foreign debris, and devitalized tissue	Acetic acid, saline, sodium hypochlorite (Dakin's solution), Vashe Wound Solution™
Débridement	*Autolytic*—covers a wound and allows enzymes to self-digest sloughed skin	Absorption beads, pastes, powders; alginates; composite dressings; foams; gelling fiber; hydrate gauze; hydrogels; hydrocolloids; transparent films; wound care systems
	Chemical or enzymatic—applied topically to break down devitalized tissue	Enzymatic débridement agents
	Mechanical—removes devitalized tissue with mechanical force	Wound cleansers, gauze (wet to dry), whirlpool
Diathermy	Produces electrical current to promote warmth and new tissue growth	
Hydration	Adds moisture to a wound	Gauze (saturated with saline solution), hydrogels, wound care systems
Maintain moist environment	Manages moisture levels in a wound and maintains a moist environment	Composites, contact layers, foams, gauze (impregnated or saturated), hydrogels, hydrocolloids, transparent films, wound care systems
Manage high-output wounds	Manages excessive quantities of exudates	Pouching systems
Pack or fill dead space	Prevents premature wound closure or fills shallow areas and provides absorption	Absorbent beads, powders, pastes; alginates; composites, foams; gauze (impregnated and nonimpregnated)
Protect and cover wound	Provides protection from the external environment	Composites, compression bandages/wraps, foams, gauze dressings, hydrogels, hydrocolloids, transparent film dressings
Protect periwound skin	Prevents moisture and mechanical trauma from damaging delicate tissue around wound	Composites, foams, hydrocolloids, pouching systems, skin sealants, transparent film dressings
Provide therapeutic compression	Provides appropriate levels of support to the lower extremities in venous stasis disease	Compression bandages, wraps, graduated compression stockings

Adapted from Miline, C. (Ed.). (2019). *Wound source 2019*. Atlantic Beach, FL: Kestrel Health Information, Inc.

Autolytic Débridement

Autolytic **débridement** is a process that uses the body's own digestive enzymes to break down necrotic tissue. The wound is kept moist with occlusive dressings. Eschar and necrotic debris are softened, liquefied, and separated from the bed of the wound.

Several commercially available products mirror the enzymes that the body produces naturally and are referred to as enzymatic débriding agents; an example is collagenase. Application of these products speeds the rate at which necrotic tissue is removed. This method, although slower than surgical débridement, is more discriminating for tissue removal and does not damage healthy tissue surrounding the wound. When enzymatic débridement is being used under an occlusive dressing, a foul odor and exudate is produced by the breakdown of cellular debris. This odor does not indicate that the wound is infected. The nurse should expect this reaction and help the patient and family understand the reason for the odor. Silver and iodine inactivate collagenase and therefore should not be used with it. Application of collagenase should be nickel thick and changed daily to be effective (Bryant & Nix, 2016).

Categories of Dressings

Table 56-1 provides a guide to the functions and actions of wound dressings.

Occlusive Dressings

Occlusive dressings may be commercially produced or made inexpensively from sterile or nonsterile gauze squares or wrap. Occlusive dressings cover topical medication that is applied to a skin lesion. The area is kept airtight by using plastic film (e.g., plastic wrap). Plastic film is thin and readily adapts to all sizes, body shapes, and skin surfaces. In general, plastic wrap should be used no more than 12 hours each day. Plastic surgical tape containing a corticosteroid in the adhesive layer can be cut to size and applied to individual lesions. Occlusive dressings are often used to cover surgical incisions for the first 48 hours postoperatively (Doughty & McNichol, 2016).

Moisture-Retentive Dressings

Commercially produced moisture-retentive dressings are efficient at removing exudate because of their higher moisture–vapor transmission rate; some have reservoirs that can hold excessive exudate. A number of moisture-retentive dressings are already impregnated with saline solution, petrolatum, zinc-saline solution, hydrogel, or antimicrobial agents, thereby eliminating the need to coat the skin to avoid maceration. The main advantages of moisture-retentive dressings are improved fibrinolysis, accelerated epidermal resurfacing, reduced pain, fewer infections, less scar tissue, gentle autolytic débridement, and decreased frequency of dressing changes. Depending on the product used and the type of dermatologic conditions encountered, most moisture-retentive dressings may remain in place from 12 to 24 hours; some can remain in place as long as 3 days (Bryant & Nix, 2016; Doughty & McNichol, 2016).

Hydrogels

Hydrogels are polymers with 90% to 95% water content. They are available in impregnated sheets or as gels. Hydrogels provide moisture to maintain a moist wound bed to promote healing. Their high moisture content makes them ideal for autolytic débridement of wounds. They are semitransparent, allowing for wound inspection without dressing removal. They are comfortable and soothing for the painful wound. They require a secondary dressing to keep them in place. Hydrogels are appropriate for partial- and full-thickness, dry to light exudative wounds such as necrotic wounds, minor burns, and radiation burns (Bryant & Nix, 2016; Miline, 2019).

Hydrocolloids

Hydrocolloids are composed of a water-impermeable, polyurethane outer covering separated from the wound by a hydrocolloid material. They are adherent and nonpermeable to water vapor and oxygen. As water evaporates over the wound, it is absorbed into the dressing, which softens and discolors with the increased water content. Hydrocolloids promote autolysis, reduce the risk for infection and pain, protect the wound, and promote healing (Bryant & Nix, 2016). The dressing can be removed without causing damage to the wound. As the dressing absorbs water, it produces a foul-smelling, yellowish covering over the wound. This is a normal chemical interaction between the dressing and wound exudate and should not be confused with purulent drainage from the wound. Unfortunately, most of the hydrocolloid dressings are opaque, preventing inspection of the wound without removal of the dressing.

Available in sheets and in gels, hydrocolloids are a good choice for both partial- and full-thickness wounds, with light to moderate exudate. They are not recommended for infected wounds and are used cautiously in patients with diabetes (Bryant & Nix, 2016; Miline, 2019). Easy-to-use and comfortable hydrocolloid dressings promote débridement and formation of granulation tissue. Most are changed every 3 to 5 days and most can be submerged in water for bathing or showering.

Foam Dressings

Foam dressings consist of microporous polyurethane with an absorptive **hydrophilic** (water-absorbing) surface that covers the wound and a **hydrophobic** (water-resistant) backing to block leakage of exudate. They are nonadherent; most are designed so that they require a secondary dressing to keep them in place. Adhesive borders are available on some foam dressings, negating the need for a second dressing.

Moisture is absorbed into the foam layer, decreasing maceration of the surrounding tissue. A moist environment is maintained, and removal of the dressing does not damage the wound. The foams are opaque and must be removed for wound inspection. Foams are a good choice for partial- and full-thickness, moderate to heavy exudative wounds. They are especially helpful over bony prominences because they provide contoured cushioning (Bryant & Nix, 2016; Miline, 2019).

Calcium Alginates

Calcium alginates are derived from algae or kelp polysaccharides and consist of very absorbent calcium alginate fibers (Dabiri et al., 2016). They are hemostatic and bioabsorbable and can be used as sheets or mats of absorbent material. As the exudate is absorbed, the fibers turn into a viscous hydrogel. They are useful in areas where the tissue is more irritated or macerated. The alginate dressing forms a moist pocket over the wound while the surrounding skin stays dry. The dressing also reacts with wound fluid, which forms a foul-smelling coating. Alginates work well when packed into a deep cavity, wound, or sinus tract with heavy drainage. They are nonadherent and require a secondary dressing. Alginates are used for moderate to highly exudative full-thickness wounds, such as pressure injuries, infected wounds, and venous insufficiency ulcers (Bryant & Nix, 2016; Miline, 2019). Wound experts suggest that alginates are superior to other modern dressings for débriding necrotic wounds (Bryant & Nix, 2016).

Antimicrobials

Antimicrobial dressings contain antiseptics, cadexomer iodine, honey, hydrofera blue, mupirocin, or silver to reduce the risk of infection. They are available in many different types of dressings, such as gauze, foams, films, or absorptive or nonadherent materials. Antimicrobial dressings are indicated for partial- or full-thickness wounds that have a risk for infection, such as surgical wounds (Bryant & Nix, 2016; Miline, 2019).

Collagens

Collagen dressings are protein based and derived from animal sources (bovine, equine, porcine, or avian) that promote wound healing. Collagens are used for partial- or full-thickness noninfected wounds with light to moderate drainage, such as pressure injuries, vascular ulcers, skin donor sites, surgical wounds, diabetic ulcerations, and traumatic wounds (Miline, 2019).

Composites

Composite dressings combine components from several dressing types into a single dressing that is absorptive and that provide protection from bacteria and fluids (Bryant & Nix, 2016; Miline, 2019).

Contact Layers

Contact layers are thin, nonadherent, conforming dressings that are directly applied to wounds for protection. They are porous, thus allowing exudate to drain through to a secondary dressing. Contact layers are appropriate for partial- and full-thickness wounds, infected wounds, skin donor sites, and split-thickness skin grafts (Bryant & Nix, 2016; Miline, 2019).

TABLE 56-2	Select Topical Preparations and Medications	
Preparation	**Indications**	**Product Name**
Moisture barriers	Prevent excess moisture on skin to avoid maceration; protect skin	Calmoseptine™, Cavilon™, Proshield™
Moisturizer creams	Soothe, soften, moisturize, and protect skin	Acid Mantle Cream™, Curél Cream™, Dermasil™, Eucerin™, Lubriderm™, Noxzema Skin Cream™, Remedy™, Resta™
Moisturizer ointments	Soothe, soften, moisturize, and protect skin	Aquaphor Ointment™, Eutra Swiss Skin Cream™, Vaseline Ointment™
Topical anesthetic agents	Relieve pain	Lidocaine of various strengths in the form of spray, ointment, gel; lidocaine 2.5% and prilocaine 2.5%
Topical antibiotic agents	Second-line therapy when infection present; antibiotics are not first choice for treating wounds as they are associated with hypersensitivity reactions and development of antibiotic resistant organisms	Bacitracin™, bacitracin and polymyxin B, mupirocin 2%, erythromycin 2%, clindamycin phosphate 1%, gentamicin sulfate 1%, 1% silver sulfadiazine cream
Topical antimicrobials	Antimicrobial (bactericidal or bacteriostatic)	Acetic acid 0.25%, cadexomer iodine, chlorhexidine 0.02%, honey (medical grade), hydrofera blue, hydrogen peroxide, mupirocin 2%, povidone iodine, silver, sodium hypochlorite, 1% silver sulfadiazine cream

Adapted from Doughty, D., & McNichol, L. (2016). *WOCN Society core curriculum: Wound management.* Philadelphia, PA: Wolters Kluwer; Miline, C. (Ed.). (2019). *Wound source 2019.* Atlantic Beach, FL: Kestrel Health Information, Inc.

Transparent Film Dressings

Transparent film dressings are polymer membranes, permeable to moisture vapors and oxygen, but impermeable to water, liquids, and bacteria. Transparency allows for direct visualization of the wound. The purposes of films are to protect, provide a moist wound bed environment, promote autolysis, and lessen friction. Transparent films are used for partial or closed wounds with little to no exudate, such as intravenous access sites, skin donor sites, lacerations, and abrasions (Bryant & Nix, 2016; Miline, 2019).

Medical Management

Medical management of skin disorders includes a host of prescribed and over-the-counter (OTC) pharmacologic therapies.

Pharmacologic Therapy

Medicated lotions, creams, ointments, gels, and powders are frequently used to treat skin disorders. In general, moisture-retentive dressings, with or without medication, are used in the acute stage; lotions and creams are reserved for the subacute stage; and ointments are used when inflammation has become chronic and the skin is dry with scaling or **lichenification** (thickening of the horny layer of the skin).

High concentrations of some medications can be applied directly to the affected site with little systemic absorption and with few systemic side effects. However, some medications are readily absorbed through the skin and can produce systemic effects. Because topical preparations may induce allergic contact **dermatitis** (skin inflammation) in patients who are sensitive, any untoward response should be reported immediately and the medication discontinued.

With all types of topical medication, the patient is educated to apply the medication gently but thoroughly and, when necessary, to cover the medication with a dressing to protect clothing. Table 56-2 lists select topical preparations and medications.

Lotions

Lotions are frequently used to replenish lost skin oils or to relieve pruritus. They must be applied every 3 or 4 hours for sustained therapeutic effect. They are usually applied directly to the skin, but a dressing soaked in the lotion can be placed on the affected area. However, if left in place for a longer period, it may crust and cake on the skin.

Lotions are of two types: suspensions and liniments. **Suspensions** consist of either a powder in water that requires shaking before application, or clear solutions, which contain completely dissolved active ingredients. A suspension such as calamine lotion provides a rapid cooling and drying effect as it evaporates, leaving a thin, medicinal layer of powder on the affected skin. **Liniments** are lotions with oil added to prevent crusting. Because lotions are easy to use, therapeutic adherence is generally good.

Powders

Powders usually have a talc, zinc oxide, bentonite, or cornstarch base and are dusted on the skin with a shaker or with cotton sponges. Although their therapeutic action is brief, powders act as **hygroscopic** agents that absorb and retain moisture from the air and reduce friction between skin surfaces and clothing or bedding.

Creams

Creams may be suspensions of oil in water or emulsions of water in oil, with additional ingredients to prevent bacterial and fungal growth. Both may cause an allergic reaction such as contact dermatitis. Oil-in-water creams are easily applied and usually are the most cosmetically acceptable to the patient. Although they can be used on the face, they tend to have a drying effect. Water-in-oil emulsions are greasier and are preferred for drying and flaking dermatoses. Creams usually are rubbed into the skin by hand. They are used for their moisturizing and emollient effects.

Gels

Gels are semisolid emulsions that become liquid when applied to the skin or scalp. They are cosmetically acceptable to the patient because they are not visible after application, and they are greaseless and nonstaining. Water-based gels penetrate the skin more effectively and cause less stinging on application. They are especially useful for acute dermatitis in which there is weeping exudate (e.g., poison ivy) and are applied the same way as creams.

Pastes

Pastes are mixtures of powders and ointments and are used in inflammatory blistering conditions. They adhere to the skin and may be difficult to remove without using an oil (e.g., olive oil, mineral oil). Pastes are applied with a wooden tongue depressor or gloved hand.

Ointments

Ointments retard water loss and lubricate and protect the skin. They are the preferred vehicle for delivering medication to chronic or localized dry skin conditions, such as eczema or psoriasis. Ointments are applied with a wooden tongue depressor or gloved hand.

Sprays and Aerosols

Spray and aerosol preparations may be used on any widespread dermatologic condition. They evaporate on contact and are used infrequently.

Topical Corticosteroids

Corticosteroids are widely used in treating dermatologic conditions to provide anti-inflammatory, antipruritic, and vasoconstrictive effects. The patient is educated to apply this medication according to strict guidelines, using it sparingly but rubbing it into the prescribed area thoroughly. Absorption of topical corticosteroids is enhanced when the skin is hydrated or the affected area is covered by an occlusive or moisture-retentive dressing (Comerford & Durkin, 2020). Inappropriate use of topical corticosteroids can result in local and systemic side effects, especially when the medication is absorbed through inflamed and excoriated skin; it is used under occlusive dressings, or is used for longer time periods on sensitive areas. Local side effects may include skin atrophy and thinning, **striae** (bandlike streaks), and telangiectasias (dilated blood vessels). Thinning of the skin results from the ability of corticosteroids to inhibit skin collagen synthesis. The thinning process can be reversed by discontinuing the medication, but striae and telangiectasia are permanent. Systemic side effects may include hyperglycemia and symptoms of Cushing syndrome (see Chapter 45). Caution is required when applying corticosteroids around the eyes because long-term use may cause glaucoma or cataracts, and the anti-inflammatory effect of corticosteroids may mask existing viral or fungal infections.

Concentrated (fluorinated) corticosteroids should never be applied on the face or intertriginous areas (i.e., axillae and groin) because these areas have a thinner stratum corneum and therefore absorption is enhanced. Persistent use of concentrated topical corticosteroids in any location may produce acnelike dermatitis, known as steroid-induced acne, and hypertrichosis (excessive hair growth). Because some topical corticosteroid preparations are available without prescription, patients should be cautioned about prolonged and inappropriate use. Table 56-3 lists select topical corticosteroid preparations according to potency.

Intralesional Therapy

Intralesional therapy consists of injecting a sterile suspension of medication (usually a corticosteroid) into or just below a

---

TABLE 56-3 Potency: Select Topical Corticosteroids

Potency	Topical Corticosteroid	Preparations
OTC	0.5–1% hydrocortisone	Cream, lotion, ointment
Lowest	Dexamethasone 0.1% Alclometasone 0.05% Hydrocortisone 2.5%	Cream, ointment, aerosol, gel Cream, ointment Cream, lotion, ointment
Low–medium	Desonide 0.05% Fluocinolone acetonide 0.025% Hydrocortisone valerate 0.2% Betamethasone valerate 0.1% Fluticasone propionate 0.05%	Cream, lotion, ointment Cream, solution Cream, solution Cream, ointment Cream, ointment
Medium–high	Triamcinolone acetonide 0.1–0.5% Fluocinonide 0.05% Desoximetasone 0.05–0.25% Fluocinolone 0.2% Diflorasone diacetate 0.05%	Cream, ointment, lotion Cream, ointment, gel Cream, ointment, gel Cream, ointment Cream, ointment
Very high	Clobetasol propionate 0.05% Betamethasone dipropionate 0.05% Halobetasol propionate 0.05%	Cream, ointment, gel Cream, ointment, gel Cream, ointment

OTC, over the counter.
Adapted from Comerford, K. C., & Durkin, M. T. (2020). *Nursing 2020 drug handbook.* Philadelphia, PA: Wolters Kluwer.

lesion. Although this treatment may have an anti-inflammatory effect, local atrophy and discoloration may result if the medication is injected into subcutaneous fat. Skin lesions treated with intralesional therapy include psoriasis, keloids, and cystic acne. Occasionally, immunotherapeutic and antifungal agents are given as intralesional therapy.

Systemic Medications

Systemic medications are also prescribed for skin conditions. These include corticosteroids for short-term therapy of contact dermatitis or for long-term treatment of a chronic **dermatosis** (skin lesion), such as pemphigus vulgaris. Other frequently used systemic medications include antibiotic, antifungal, antihistamine, sedative, analgesic, tranquilizing, **cytotoxic** (destructive of cells), and immunosuppressive agents.

Nursing Management

Nursing management of the patient prescribed pharmacologic therapy to treat a skin disorder begins with a focused dermatologic health history, direct observation, and a complete physical examination (see Chapter 55). Because of its visibility, a skin condition is usually difficult to ignore or conceal from others and may therefore cause the patient emotional distress. The major goals for the patient may include maintenance of skin integrity, relief of discomfort, promotion of restful sleep, self-acceptance, knowledge about skin care, and avoidance of complications.

Nursing management for patients who must perform self-care for skin problems, such as applying medications and dressings, focuses on educating the patient about how to cleanse the affected area and pat it dry; apply medication to the lesion while the skin is moist; cover the area with plastic (e.g., Telfa™ pads, plastic wrap, vinyl gloves, plastic bag) if recommended; and cover it with an elastic bandage, dressing, or paper tape to seal the edges. Dressings that contain or cover a topical corticosteroid should be removed for 12 of every 24 hours to prevent adverse events.

Other forms of dressings, such as those used to cover topical medications, include soft cotton cloth and stretchable cotton dressings (e.g., Surgitube™, Tubegauz™) that can be used for fingers, toes, hands, and feet. The hands can be covered with disposable polyethylene or vinyl gloves sealed at the wrists; the feet can be wrapped in plastic bags covered by cotton socks. Gloves and socks that are already impregnated with emollients, making application to the hands and feet more convenient, are also available. When large areas of the body must be covered, cotton cloth topped by an expandable stockinette can be used. Disposable diapers or cloths folded in diaper fashion are useful for dressing the groin and the perineal areas. Axillary dressings can be made of cotton cloth, or a commercially prepared dressing may be used and taped in place or held by dress shields. A turban or plastic shower cap is useful for holding dressings on the scalp. A face mask, made from gauze with holes cut out for the eyes, nose, and mouth, may be held in place with gauze ties looped through holes cut in the four corners of the mask.

Pressure Injury

Pressure injury, formerly called pressure ulcer, is a localized area of necrotic soft tissue that occurs when pressure applied to the skin is greater than the normal capillary closure pressure (approximately 32 mm Hg) over a period of time sufficient to cause tissue injury. Patients who are critically ill have a lower capillary closure pressure and a greater risk of pressure injuries, as are patients who are exposed to prolonged pressure due to immobility, have motor or sensory dysfunction, or have muscular atrophy that reduces padding between the overlying skin and the underlying bone.

A landmark 10-year pressure injury prevalence survey conducted among 918,621 inpatients in the United States from 2006 through 2015 showed an overall decrease in prevalence of pressure injury from 13.5% in 2006 to 9.3% in 2015 (Van-Gilder, Lachenbruch, Algrim-Boyle, et al., 2017). Despite declining prevalence, pressure injuries nonetheless result in significant pain and suffering, increased morbidity and mortality, higher medical costs and resource use, and lower odds of discharge to the community (VanGilder et al., 2017).

The American Nurses Association tracks hospital-acquired pressure injuries (HAPI) quarterly as part of the National Database of Nursing Quality Indicators® (NDNQI®). In the United States, an estimate of 2.5 million patients in acute care facilities develop HAPIs annually, with approximately 60,000 patient deaths associated with complications from HAPIs. The cost of treatment for a single, full-thickness pressure injury may be as high as $70,000 with an estimated annual total cost of $11 billion for pressure injury treatment in the United States (Agency for Healthcare Research & Quality [AHRQ], 2014). All possible efforts to prevent skin breakdown must be made because the treatment of pressure injuries is costly in terms of health care dollars and quality of life for patients at risk.

The initial sign of pressure is erythema (redness of the skin) caused by reactive hyperemia, which normally resolves in less than 1 hour. Unrelieved pressure results in tissue ischemia or anoxia. The cutaneous tissues become broken or destroyed, leading to progressive destruction and necrosis of underlying soft tissue, and the resulting pressure injury is painful and slow to heal.

NURSING PROCESS

The Patient with Pressure Injury

Assessment

Nursing assessment involves identifying and evaluating risk for development of pressure injuries as well as assessment of the skin.

ASSESSMENT OF RISK FACTORS

Immobility, impaired sensory perception or cognition, decreased tissue perfusion, decreased nutritional status, friction and shear forces, increased moisture, and age-related skin changes and comorbidities all contribute to the development of pressure injuries (Doughty & McNichol, 2016). Chart 56-1 lists risk factors for pressure injuries. Scales such as the Braden scale (Table 56-4) or Norton scale (Norton, McLaren, & Exton-Smith, 1962) may be used to facilitate systematic assessment and quantification of a patient's risk for pressure injury, although the nurse should recognize that the reliability of these scales is not well established for all patient populations.

Chart 56-1

RISK FACTORS ⚠
Pressure Injuries

- Advanced age
- Comorbidities, such as diabetes, peripheral vascular disease, cancer, stroke, obesity, cognitive impairment
- Excessive moisture, including incontinence of urine or feces
- Excessive skin dryness
- Friction, shearing forces, trauma
- High-acuity patients, such as those in intensive care units
- History of having recurrent pressure injuries
- Immobility, compromised mobility
- Loss of protective reflexes, sensory deficit/loss
- Malnutrition, hypoproteinemia, anemia, vitamin deficiency
- Medical devices, such as casts, traction, restraints
- Medications, such as analgesics or sedatives
- Poor skin perfusion, edema
- Preexisting skin problems on admission
- Prolonged hospitalization
- Prolonged pressure on tissue
- Smoking
- Surgical procedures >3 hours

Adapted from Doughty, D., & McNichol, L. (2016). *Wound, Ostomy and Continence Nurses Society core curriculum: Wound management*. Philadelphia, PA: Wolters Kluwer.

Specific nursing actions related to assessing risk include:
- Evaluate level of mobility.
- Note safety and assistive devices (e.g., restraints, splints).
- Assess neurovascular status.
- Evaluate circulatory status (e.g., peripheral pulses, edema).
- Note present health problems.
- Evaluate nutritional and hydration status.
- Review the results of the patient's laboratory studies, including hematocrit, hemoglobin, electrolytes, albumin, prealbumin, transferrin, and creatinine.
- Determine presence of incontinence.
- Review current medications.

> ▶ *Quality and Safety Nursing Alert*
>
> *Pressure injuries are associated with increased costs of treatment and length of hospital stay as well as diminished quality of life for patients. It is imperative that nurses perform a skin assessment on every patient admitted to a hospital, inpatient rehabilitation facility, or skilled nursing facility.*

Immobility. When a person is immobile and inactive, pressure is exerted on the skin and subcutaneous tissue by objects on which the person rests, such as a mattress, chair seat, or cast. The development of pressure injuries is directly related to the duration of immobility. If pressure continues long enough, small-vessel thrombosis and tissue necrosis occur and a pressure injury is the result. Weight-bearing bony prominences are most susceptible to pressure injury development because they are covered only by skin and small amounts of subcutaneous tissue. Susceptible areas include the sacrum and coccygeal areas, ischial tuberosities (especially in people who sit for prolonged periods), greater trochanter, heel, knee, malleolus, medial condyle of the tibia, fibular

head, scapula, and elbow, with the sacrum and heels the most common sites (Doughty & McNichol, 2016) (Fig. 56-1).

Impaired Sensory Perception or Cognition. Patients with sensory loss, impaired level of consciousness, or paralysis may not be aware of the discomfort associated with prolonged pressure on the skin and therefore may not change their positions to relieve the pressure. This prolonged pressure impedes blood flow, reducing nourishment of the skin and underlying tissues. A pressure injury may develop in a short period of time, sometimes within minutes.

Decreased Tissue Perfusion. Any condition that reduces the circulation and nourishment of the skin and subcutaneous tissue (altered peripheral tissue perfusion) increases the risk of pressure injury development. Patients with diabetes have compromised microcirculation. Similarly, patients with edema have impaired circulation and poor nourishment of the skin tissue. Patients with obesity have large amounts of poorly vascularized adipose tissue, which is susceptible to breakdown.

Nutritional Status. Nutritional deficiencies, anemias, and metabolic disorders also contribute to the development of pressure injuries. Anemia, regardless of its cause, decreases the blood's oxygen-carrying ability and predisposes the patient to pressure injuries. Maintaining good nutrition and preventing malnutrition are essential to prevent pressure injuries and promote wound healing (Doughty & McNichol, 2016). Serum albumin and prealbumin levels are sensitive indicators of protein deficiency. Serum albumin levels of less than 3 g/dL are associated with hypoalbuminemic tissue edema and increased risk of pressure injuries. Prealbumin levels are more sensitive indicators of protein status than the albumin levels, but they are costlier to assess. The nurse should assess the patient's prealbumin and albumin values and electrolyte panel (Bryant & Nix, 2016).

Friction and Shear. Mechanical forces also contribute to the development of pressure injuries. Friction is the force of rubbing two surfaces against each another and is often caused by pulling a patient over a bed sheet or from a poorly fitted prosthetic device. Shear is the result of exerting a parallel force on the patient's body, such as the resistance between the patient and the chair or bed when the patient slides down (Edsberg, Black, Goldberg, et al., 2016). When shear occurs, tissue layers slide over one another, blood vessels stretch and twist, and the microcirculation of the skin and subcutaneous tissue is disrupted. Evidence of deep tissue damage may be slow to develop and may present through the development of a **sinus tract** (also called tunneling), which is an area of destroyed tissue that extends from the edge of a wound; this results in dead space that is susceptible to abscess formation. The sacrum and heels are most susceptible to the effects of shear. Pressure injuries from friction and shear occur when the patient slides down in bed (Fig. 56-2) or when the patient is positioned or moved improperly (e.g., dragged up in bed). Spastic muscles and paralysis increase the patient's vulnerability to pressure injuries related to friction and shear.

Increased Moisture. Prolonged contact with moisture from perspiration, urine, feces, or drainage produces maceration (softening) of the skin. The skin reacts to caustic substances in the excreta or drainage and becomes irritated. Moist, irritated skin is more vulnerable to pressure breakdown. Once the skin breaks, the area is invaded by microorganisms (e.g., streptococci, staphylococci, *Pseudomonas aeruginosa*, *Escherichia coli*), and infection occurs. Foul-smelling infectious

| TABLE 56-4 | Braden Scale for Predicting Pressure Injury Risk |

Patient's Name _____   Evaluator's Name _____

Date of Assessment

Sensory Perception Ability to respond meaningfully to pressure-related discomfort	**1. Completely Limited** Unresponsive (does not moan, flinch, or grasp) to painful stimuli, due to diminished level of consciousness or sedation OR limited ability to feel pain over most of body.	**2. Very Limited** Responds only to painful stimuli. Cannot communicate discomfort except by moaning or restlessness OR has a sensory impairment that limits the ability to feel pain or discomfort over half of body.	**3. Slightly Limited** Responds to verbal commands, but cannot always communicate discomfort or the need to be turned. OR has some sensory impairment that limits ability to feel pain or discomfort in one or two extremities.	**4. No Impairment** Responds to verbal commands. Has no sensory deficit that would limit ability to feel or voice pain or discomfort.			
Moisture Degree to which skin is exposed to moisture	**1. Constantly Moist** Skin is kept moist almost constantly by perspiration, urine, etc. Dampness is detected every time patient is moved or turned.	**2. Very Moist** Skin is often, but not always, moist. Linen must be changed at least once a shift.	**3. Occasionally Moist** Skin is occasionally moist, requiring an extra linen change approximately once a day.	**4. Rarely Moist** Skin is usually dry, linen only requires changing at routine intervals.			
Activity Degree of physical activity	**1. Bedfast** Confined to bed.	**2. Chairfast** Ability to walk severely limited or nonexistent. Cannot bear own weight and/or must be assisted into chair or wheelchair.	**3. Walks Occasionally** Walks occasionally during day, but for very short distances, with or without assistance. Spends majority of each shift in bed or chair.	**4. Walks Frequently** Walks outside room at least twice a day and inside room at least once every 2 hrs during waking hours.			
Mobility Ability to change and control body position	**1. Completely Immobile** Does not make even slight changes in body or extremity position without assistance.	**2. Very Limited** Makes occasional slight changes in body or extremity position but unable to make frequent or significant changes independently.	**3. Slightly Limited** Makes frequent though slight changes in body or extremity position independently.	**4. No Limitation** Makes major and frequent changes in position without assistance.			
Nutrition Usual food intake pattern	**1. Very Poor** Never eats a complete meal. Rarely eats more than a 1/3 of any food offered. Eats 2 servings or less of protein (meat or dairy products) per day. Takes fluids poorly. Does not take a liquid dietary supplement OR is NPO and/or maintained on clear liquids or IVs for more than 5 days.	**2. Probably Inadequate** Rarely eats a complete meal and generally eats only about 1/2 of any food offered. Protein intake includes only 3 servings of meat or dairy products per day. Occasionally will take a dietary supplement OR receives less than optimum amount of liquid diet or tube feeding.	**3. Adequate** Eats half of most meals. Eats a total of 4 servings of protein (meat, dairy products) per day. Occasionally will refuse a meal, but will usually take a supplement when offered OR is on a tube feeding or TPN regimen, which probably meets most of nutritional needs.	**4. Excellent** Eats most of every meal. Never refuses a meal. Usually eats a total of 4 or more servings of meat and dairy products. Occasionally eats between meals. Does not require supplementation.			
Friction and Shear	**1. Problem** Requires moderate to maximum assistance in moving. Complete lifting without sliding against sheets is impossible. Frequently slides down in bed or chair, requiring frequent repositioning with maximum assistance. Spasticity, contractures, or agitation leads to almost constant friction.	**2. Potential Problem** Moves feebly or requires minimum assistance. During a move, skin probably slides to some extent against sheets, chair, restraints, or other devices. Maintains relatively good position in chair or bed most of the time but occasionally slides down.	**3. No Apparent Problem** Moves in bed and in chair independently and has sufficient muscle strength to lift up completely during move. Maintains good position in bed or chair.				
			Total Score				

NPO, nothing by mouth; TPN, total parenteral nutrition.

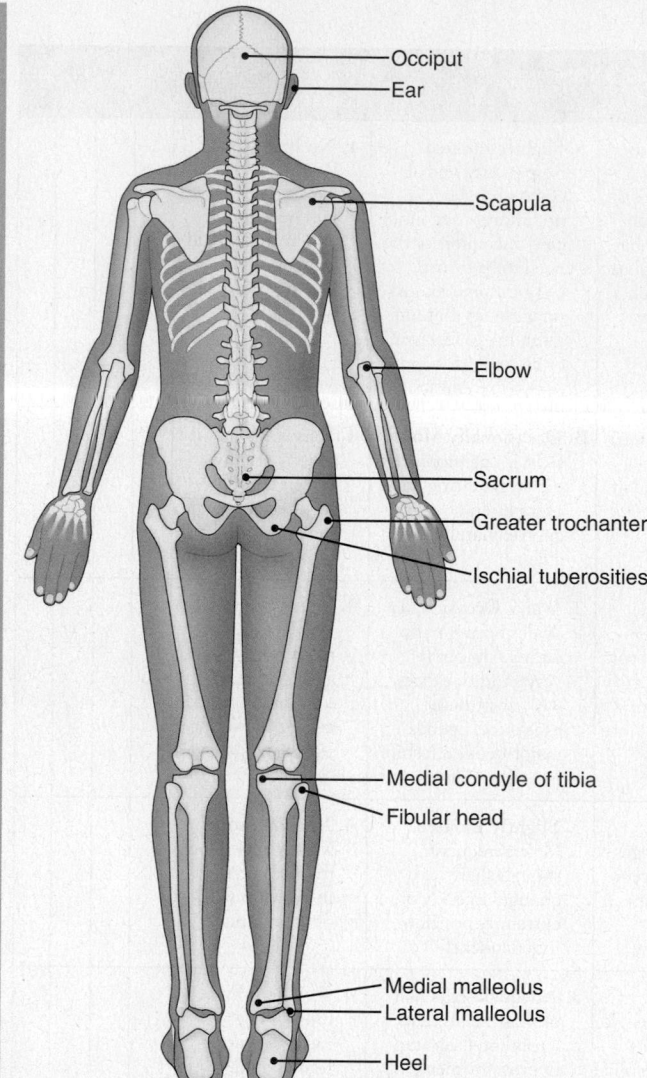

Figure 56-1 • Areas susceptible to pressure injuries.

drainage is present. The lesion may enlarge and allow a continuous loss of serum, which may further deplete the body of essential protein needed for tissue repair and maintenance. The lesion may continue to enlarge and extend deep into the

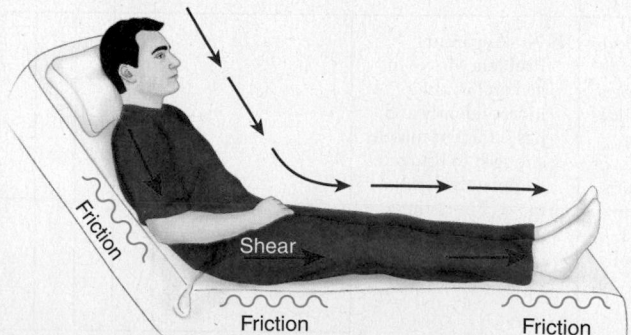

Figure 56-2 • Mechanical forces contribute to pressure injury development. As the person slides down or is improperly pulled up in bed, *friction* resists this movement. *Shear* occurs when one layer of tissue slides over another, disrupting microcirculation of skin and subcutaneous tissue.

fascia, muscle, and bone, with multiple sinus tracts radiating from the pressure injury. With extensive pressure injuries, life-threatening infections and sepsis may develop, frequently from gram-negative organisms.

Gerontologic Considerations. In older adults, the normal aging process leads to diminished epidermal thickness, dermal collagen, and tissue elasticity. The skin is drier as a result of diminished sebaceous and sweat gland activities. Cardiovascular changes result in decreased tissue perfusion. Muscles atrophy and bone structures become prominent. Diminished sensory perception and reduced ability to reposition oneself contribute to prolonged pressure on the skin. Therefore, older adults are more susceptible to pressure injuries, which cause pain, suffering, and reduced quality of life (Eliopoulos, 2018).

Obesity Considerations. In 2019, an international collaborative comprising members from the European Pressure Ulcer Advisory Panel (EPUAP), the U.S. National Pressure Injury Advisory Panel (NPIAP), and the Pan-Pacific Pressure Injury Alliance (PPPIA) released the third edition of the *Prevention and Treatment of Pressure Ulcers: Clinical Practice Guideline* (EPUAP, NPIAP, & PPPIA, 2019) to aid clinicians in leveraging the best evidence-based practices to prevent and treat pressure injuries. These updated guidelines include recommendations for adults who have obesity, with specific organization-level considerations, as well as recommendations for bed and equipment selection and repositioning. Please see the NPIAP Web site link at the end of this chapter to review the electronic version of the quick reference guideline.

ASSESSMENT OF SKIN AND EXISTING PRESSURE INJURIES

In addition to assessing risk, nursing actions to assess skin for pressure injuries include:

- Assess total skin condition at least twice a day.
- Inspect each pressure site for erythema.
- Assess areas of erythema for blanching response.
- Palpate the skin for increased warmth.
- Inspect for dry skin, moist skin, and breaks in skin.
- Note amount of drainage (scant to heavy); drainage characteristic (bloody, serosanguinous, serous, purulent); and odor.

If a pressure injury is seen, the nurse documents its size and location and uses a grading system to describe its severity and provides a description of the site (Chart 56-2). The appearance of purulent drainage or foul odor suggests an infection. With an extensive pressure injury, deep pockets of infection are often present. Drying and crusting of exudate may be present. Infection of a pressure injury may advance to osteomyelitis, pyarthrosis (pus formation within a joint cavity), sepsis, and septic shock.

Diagnosis

NURSING DIAGNOSES

Based on the assessment data, nursing diagnoses may include the following:

- Risk for impaired skin integrity
- Impaired skin integrity associated with immobility, decreased sensory perception, decreased tissue perfusion, decreased nutritional status, friction and shear forces, excessive moisture, or advanced age

Chart 56-2 Stages in the Development of Pressure Injuries

Deep Tissue Pressure Injury: Persistent Non-Blanchable Deep Red, Maroon or Purple Discoloration

Intact or non-intact skin with localized area of persistent non-blanchable deep red, maroon, purple discoloration or epidermal separation revealing a dark wound bed or blood filled blister. Pain and temperature change often precede skin color changes. Discoloration may appear differently in darkly pigmented skin. This injury results from intense and/or prolonged pressure and shear forces at the bone-muscle interface. The wound may evolve rapidly to reveal the actual extent of tissue injury, or may resolve without tissue loss. If necrotic tissue, subcutaneous tissue, granulation tissue, fascia, muscle or other underlying structures are visible, this indicates a full thickness pressure injury (Unstageable, Stage 3 or Stage 4). Do not use DTPI to describe vascular, traumatic, neuropathic, or dermatologic conditions.

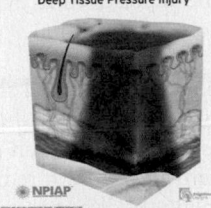

Deep Tissue Pressure Injury

Stage 1 Pressure Injury: Non-Blanchable Erythema of Intact Skin

Intact skin with a localized area of non-blanchable erythema, which may appear differently in darkly pigmented skin. Presence of blanchable erythema or changes in sensation, temperature, or firmness may precede visual changes. Color changes do not include purple or maroon discoloration; these may indicate deep tissue pressure injury.

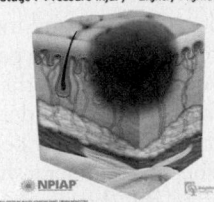

Stage 1 Pressure Injury – Lightly Pigmented

Stage 2 Pressure Injury: Partial-Thickness Skin Loss with Exposed Dermis

Partial-thickness loss of skin with exposed dermis. The wound bed is viable, pink or red, moist, and may also present as an intact or ruptured serum-filled blister. Adipose (fat) is not visible and deeper tissues are not visible. Granulation tissue, slough and eschar are not present. These injuries commonly result from adverse microclimate and shear in the skin over the pelvis and shear in the heel. This stage should not be used to describe moisture associated skin damage (MASD) including incontinence associated dermatitis (IAD), intertriginous dermatitis (ITD), medical adhesive related skin injury (MARSI), or traumatic wounds (skin tears, burns, abrasions).

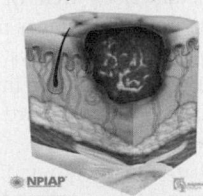

Stage 2 Pressure Injury

Stage 3 Pressure Injury: Full-Thickness Skin Loss

Full-thickness loss of skin, in which adipose (fat) is visible in the ulcer and granulation tissue and epibole (rolled wound edges) are often present. Slough and/or eschar may be visible. The depth of tissue damage varies by anatomical location; areas of significant adiposity can develop deep wounds. Undermining and tunneling may occur. Fascia, muscle, tendon, ligament, cartilage and/or bone are not exposed. If slough or eschar obscures the extent of tissue loss this is an Unstageable Pressure Injury.

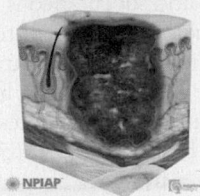

Stage 3 Pressure Injury

Stage 4 Pressure Injury: Full-Thickness Skin and Tissue Loss

Full-thickness skin and tissue loss with exposed or directly palpable fascia, muscle, tendon, ligament, cartilage or bone in the ulcer. Slough and/or eschar may be visible. Epibole (rolled edges), undermining and/or tunneling often occur. Depth varies by anatomical location. If slough or eschar obscures the extent of tissue loss this is an Unstageable Pressure Injury.

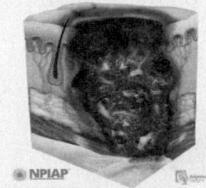

Stage 4 Pressure Injury

Unstageable Pressure Injury: Obscured Full-Thickness Skin and Tissue Loss

Full-thickness skin and tissue loss in which the extent of tissue damage within the ulcer cannot be confirmed because it is obscured by slough or eschar. If slough or eschar is removed, a Stage 3 or Stage 4 pressure injury will be revealed. Stable eschar (i.e. dry, adherent, intact without erythema or fluctuance) on the heel or ischemic limb should not be softened or removed.

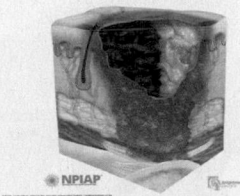

Planning and Goals

The major goals may include relief of pressure, improved mobility, maintenance of skin integrity, improved sensory perception, improved tissue perfusion, improved nutritional status, minimized friction and shear forces, dry surfaces in contact with skin, and healing of pressure injury, if present.

Nursing Interventions

RELIEVING PRESSURE

Frequent changes of position are needed to relieve and redistribute the pressure on the patient's skin and to promote blood flow to the skin and subcutaneous tissues. This can be accomplished by instructing the patient to change position or by turning and repositioning the patient. The patient's family members should be educated about how to position and turn the patient at home to prevent pressure injuries. Shifting weight allows the blood to flow into the ischemic areas and helps tissues recover from the effects of pressure. Elevating the head of bed no more than 30 degrees will prevent the patient from sliding down in bed and avoid the effects of shearing (Bryant & Nix, 2016).

For patients who spend long periods in a wheelchair, pressure can be relieved by:

- *Push-ups:* The patient pushes down on armrests and raises buttocks off the seat of the chair (Fig. 56-3).
- *One half push-up:* The patient repeats the push-up on the right side and then the left, pushing up on one side by pushing down on the armrest.

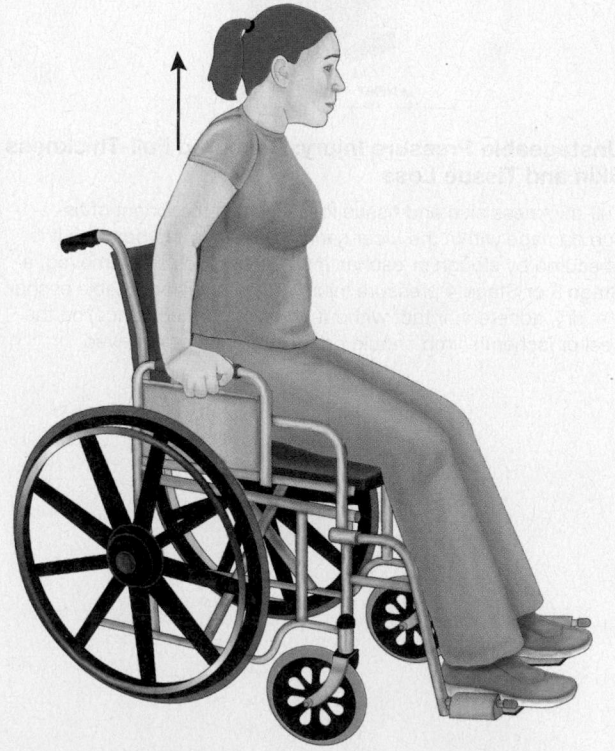

Figure 56-3 • Wheelchair push-up to prevent ischial pressure injuries. These push-ups should become an automatic routine (every 15 minutes) for the person with paraplegia. The person should stay up and out of contact with the seat for several seconds. The wheels are kept in the locked position during the exercise.

- *Moving side to side:* The patient moves from one side to the other while sitting in the chair.
- *Shifting:* The patient bends forward with the head down between the knees (if able) and constantly shifts in the chair.

POSITIONING THE PATIENT

The degree of ability to move independently—the comfort, fatigue, loss of sensation, overall physical and mental status, and specific disorder—influences plans for changing position. Patients should be positioned laterally, prone, and dorsally in sequence unless a position is not tolerated or is contraindicated. Generally, those who experience discomfort after 30 to 60 minutes of lying prone need to be repositioned. Patients able to shift their weight every 15 to 20 minutes and move independently may change total position every 2 to 4 hours. Indications for routine repositioning every 2 hours or more frequently include loss of sensation, paralysis, coma, and edema.

In addition to regular turning, small shifts of body weight, such as repositioning of an ankle, elbow, or shoulder, are necessary. The skin is inspected at each position change and assessed for temperature elevation. If redness or heat is noted or if the patient complains of discomfort, pressure on the area must be relieved.

Another way to relieve pressure over bony prominences is the bridging technique, accomplished through the correct positioning of pillows. Just as a bridge is supported on pillars to allow traffic to move underneath, the body can be supported by pillows to allow for space between bony prominences and the mattress. A pillow or commercial heel protector may be used to support the heels off the bed when the patient is supine. Placing pillows superior and inferior to the sacrum relieves sacral pressure. Supporting the patient in a 30-degree side-lying position avoids pressure on the trochanter; wedges can be used to accomplish this. In older adult patients, frequent small shifts of body weight may be effective. Placing a small rolled towel or sheepskin under a shoulder or hip allows a return of blood flow to the skin in the area on which the patient is sitting or lying. The towel or sheepskin is moved around the patient's pressure points in a clockwise fashion. A turning schedule can help the family keep track of the patient's turns.

USING PRESSURE-RELIEVING DEVICES

At times, specialty beds or alternative bed surfaces may be indicated to help relieve the pressure on the skin (EPUAP, NPIAP, & PPPIA, 2019). These are referred to as pressure redistribution surfaces because they aim to redistribute pressure. Ideally, they should also control moisture and temperature and minimize friction. These devices are designed to provide support for specific body areas or to distribute pressure evenly. Pressure redistribution surfaces may include specialty mattresses as well as mattress overlays. The use of pressure redistribution surfaces is particularly important for patients who cannot get out of bed and who are at high risk for pressure injury development.

A patient who sits in a wheelchair for prolonged periods should have wheelchair cushions fitted and adjusted on an individualized basis, using pressure measurement techniques as a guide to selection and fitting. The aim is to redistribute pressure away from areas at risk for injuries; however, no cushion can eliminate excessive pressure completely. The patient should be reminded to shift weight frequently and to rise for a few seconds every 15 minutes while sitting in a chair.

Static support devices (e.g., high-density foam, air, or liquid mattress overlays) distribute pressure evenly by bringing more of the patient's body surface into contact with the supporting surface. Gel-type flotation pads and air-fluidized beds reduce pressure. The weight of a body floating on a fluid system is evenly distributed over the entire supporting surface. Therefore, as the body sinks into the fluid, additional surface becomes available for weight bearing, body weight per unit area is decreased, and there is less pressure on the body parts.

Soft, moisture-absorbing padding is also useful because the softness and resilience of padding provide for more even distribution of pressure and the dissipation and absorption of moisture, along with freedom from wrinkles and friction. Bony prominences may be protected by gel pads, sheepskin padding, or soft foam rubber beneath the sacrum, the trochanters, heels, elbows, scapulae, and back of the head when there is pressure on these sites. Applying a gentle adhesive foam dressing to the sacral area is an effective pressure injury preventive measure (Doughty & McNichol, 2016).

Specialized beds are designed to prevent pressure on the skin. Air-fluidized beds allow the patient to float. Dynamic support surfaces, such as low–air-loss pockets, alternatively inflate and deflate sections to change support pressure for patients at high risk for pressure injuries and who are critically ill and cannot be repositioned to relieve pressure. Oscillating or kinetic beds change pressure by means of rocking movements of the bed that redistribute the patient's weight and stimulate circulation. These beds may be used with patients who have injuries attributed to multiple trauma. The specific needs of each individual patient are considered when choosing an appropriate pressure redistribution surface (Bryant & Nix, 2016).

IMPROVING MOBILITY

The patient is encouraged to remain active and is ambulated whenever possible. When sitting, the patient is reminded to change positions frequently to redistribute weight. Active and passive exercises increase muscular, skin, and vascular tone. For patients at risk for pressure injuries, turning and exercise schedules are essential, and repositioning must occur around the clock.

IMPROVING SENSORY PERCEPTION

The nurse helps the patient recognize and compensate for altered sensory perception. Depending on the origin of the alteration (e.g., decreased level of consciousness, spinal cord lesion), specific interventions are selected. Strategies to improve cognition and sensory perception may include stimulating the patient to increase awareness of self in the environment, encouraging the patient to participate in self-care, or supporting the patient's efforts toward active compensation for loss of sensation (e.g., a patient with paraplegia lifting up from the sitting position every 15 minutes). A patient with tetraplegia should be weight shifted every 30 minutes while sitting in a wheelchair. When decreased sensory perception exists, the patient and caregivers are taught to inspect potential pressure areas visually every morning and evening, using a mirror if necessary, for evidence of pressure injury development.

IMPROVING TISSUE PERFUSION

Activity, exercise, and repositioning improve tissue perfusion. Massage of erythematous areas is avoided because damage to the capillaries and deep tissue may occur (EPUAP, NPIAP, & PPPIA, 2019).

In patients who have evidence of compromised peripheral circulation (e.g., edema), positioning and elevation of the edematous body part to promote venous return and diminish congestion improve tissue perfusion. In addition, the nurse or family must be alert to environmental factors (e.g., wrinkles in sheets, pressure of tubes) that may contribute to pressure on the skin and diminished circulation and remove the source of pressure.

IMPROVING NUTRITIONAL STATUS

The patient's nutritional status must be adequate, and a positive nitrogen balance must be maintained because pressure injuries develop more quickly and are more resistant to treatment in patients with nutritional disorders. The nurse should assess the patient's nutritional status (see Chapter 4). To assess the patient's nutritional status in response to therapeutic strategies, the nurse monitors the patient's hemoglobin, prealbumin level, and body weight weekly.

Carbohydrates, proteins, fats, vitamins, and minerals are essential for wound healing (Bryant & Nix, 2016). Iron preparations may be necessary to raise the hemoglobin concentration so that tissue oxygen levels can be maintained within acceptable limits. Ascorbic acid (vitamin C) is necessary for tissue healing. Other nutrients associated with healthy skin include vitamins A, B, D, E, and K, copper, and zinc. With adequate nutrition and hydration, the skin can remain healthy, and damaged tissues can be repaired (Norris, 2019).

REDUCING FRICTION AND SHEAR

Raising the head of the bed by even a few centimeters increases the shearing force over the sacral area; therefore, the semireclining position is avoided in patients at risk. Proper positioning with adequate support is also important when the patient is sitting in a chair.

 Quality and Safety Nursing Alert

To avoid shearing forces when repositioning patients, the nurse must lift and avoid dragging patients across a surface. Lift devices should be used to prevent occupational injuries.

MINIMIZING IRRITATING MOISTURE

Continuous moisture on the skin must be prevented by meticulous hygiene measures. It is important to pay special attention to skin folds, including areas under the breasts, arms, and groin, and between the toes. Perspiration, urine, stool, and drainage must be removed from the skin promptly. The soiled skin should be washed immediately with mild soap and water and blotted dry with a soft towel. The skin may be lubricated with a bland lotion to keep it soft and pliable. Drying agents and powders are avoided. Topical barrier ointments (e.g., petroleum jelly) may be helpful in protecting the skin of patients who are incontinent.

Absorbent pads that wick moisture away from the body should be used to absorb drainage. Patients who are incontinent need to be checked regularly and have their wet incontinence pads and linens changed promptly. Their skin needs to be cleansed and dried promptly.

PROMOTING PRESSURE INJURY HEALING

Regardless of the stage of the pressure injury, the pressure on the area must be eliminated because the injured tissue will not heal until all pressure is removed. The patient must not lie or sit on the pressure injury, even for a few minutes. Individualized positioning and turning schedules must be written in the plan of nursing care and followed meticulously.

In addition, inadequate nutritional status as well as fluid and electrolyte abnormalities must be corrected to promote healing. Wounds from which body fluids and protein drain place the patient in a catabolic state and predispose to hypoproteinemia and serious secondary infections. Protein deficiency must be corrected to promote the healing of the pressure injury. Carbohydrates are necessary to "spare" the protein and to provide an energy source. Vitamin C and trace elements, especially zinc, are necessary for collagen formation and wound healing. (Refer to Chart 56-2 for descriptions of stages of pressure injuries.)

Deep Tissue Pressure Injury. These tissue injuries may evolve rapidly, and immediate pressure relief to the affected area is indicated. Therefore, the nurse must be vigilant in assessing for these types of injuries (EPUAP, NPIAP, & PPPIA, 2019).

Stage 1 Pressure Injury. To permit healing of stage 1 pressure injuries, the pressure is removed to allow increased tissue perfusion, nutritional and fluid and electrolyte balance is maintained, friction and shear are reduced, and moisture to the skin is avoided (EPUAP, NPIAP, & PPPIA, 2019).

Stage 2 Pressure Injury. In addition to measures listed for stage 1 pressure injuries, a moist environment, in which migration of epidermal cells over the injury surface occurs more rapidly, should be provided to aid wound healing in stage 2 pressure injury. The injured area is gently cleansed with sterile saline solution. The use of a heat lamp to dry the open wound is avoided, as is the use of antiseptic solutions that damage healthy tissues and delay wound healing. Semipermeable occlusive dressings, hydrocolloid wafers, or wet saline dressings are helpful in providing a moist environment for healing and in minimizing the loss of fluids and proteins from the body (EPUAP, NPIAP, & PPPIA, 2019).

Stage 3 Pressure Injury. Stage 3 pressure injuries are characterized by extensive tissue damage, including **slough** (i.e., soft, moist avascular tissue, which may be white, yellow, tan, gray, or green and may be loose or firmly adherent), formation of a sinus tract, and undermining (commonly seen in sheer injuries), to name a few. **Undermining** results in extensive tunneling under the edges of the wound; it is distinguished from a sinus tract in that there is a significant portion of the wound edge involved, whereas sinus tract involves only a small portion of the wound edge. Given the extensive damage to tissue and necrosis that characterize stage 3 pressure injuries, they must be débrided (cleaned) to create an area that will heal, in addition to the measures listed for stage 1 pressure injuries. Necrotic, devitalized tissue favors bacterial growth, delays granulation, and inhibits healing. Wound cleaning and dressing are uncomfortable; therefore, the nurse must prepare the patient for the procedure by explaining what will occur and administering prescribed analgesia (EPUAP, NPIAP, & PPPIA, 2019).

Stage 4 Pressure Injury. Surgical interventions are required for these extensive pressure injuries (EPUAP, NPIAP, & PPPIA, 2019). (See the following Other Treatment Methods section.)

OTHER TREATMENT METHODS

Débridement may be accomplished by wet-to-damp dressing changes, mechanical flushing of necrotic and infective exudate, application of prescribed enzyme preparations that dissolve necrotic tissue, or surgical dissection. If eschar (dry scab) covers the pressure injury, it is removed surgically to ensure the wound is clean and vitalized. Exudate may be absorbed by dressings or special hydrophilic powders, beads, or gels. Cultures of infected pressure injuries are obtained to guide the selection of antibiotic therapy.

After the pressure injury is clean, a topical treatment is prescribed to promote granulation. New granulation tissue must be protected from reinfection, drying, and damage, and care should be taken to prevent pressure and further trauma to the area. Dressings, solutions, and ointments should not disrupt the healing process. For chronic, noninfected injuries that are healing by secondary intention (healing of an open wound from the base upward by laying down new tissue), vacuum-assisted closure (VAC) or hyperbaric oxygen treatment may be used. VAC involves the use of a negative-pressure sponge dressing in the wound to increase blood flow, increasing formation of granulation tissue and nutrient uptake and decreasing bacterial load. Hyperbaric oxygen therapy involves either applying topical oxygen at increased pressure directly to the wound or placing the patient into a hyperbaric oxygen chamber. Both methods of hyperbaric oxygen therapy promote wound healing by stimulating new vascular growth and aiding in the preservation of damaged tissue. In a randomized control study comparing standard wound care with standard wound care and hyperbaric oxygen therapy for patients with diabetic foot ulcerations, Chen, Wu, Hsu, and colleagues (2017) reported improved wound healing and decreased risk of amputation among study participants who received hyperbaric oxygen therapy.

Multiple agents and protocols are used to treat pressure injuries; however, consistency is an important key to success. Objective evaluation of the pressure injury (e.g., measurement of the size and depth of the pressure injury, inspection for granulation tissue) for response to the treatment protocol must be made every 4 to 6 days. Taking photographs at weekly intervals is a reliable strategy for monitoring the healing process, which may take weeks to months.

Surgical intervention is necessary when the injury is extensive, when complications (e.g., fistula) exist, and when the pressure injury does not respond to treatment. Surgical procedures include débridement, incision and drainage, bone resection, and skin grafting. Osteomyelitis is a common complication of wounds of stage 4 depth. (See Chapter 36 for more information on osteomyelitis.)

PREVENTING RECURRENCE

It may take more than a year for healing tissue to regain the strength of preinjury skin; thus, care must be taken to prevent recurrence of pressure injuries. However, recurrence of pressure injuries should be anticipated; therefore, active, preventive intervention and frequent continuing assessments are essential. Patients with spinal cord injuries are particularly susceptible to pressure injuries and recurrence of pressure injuries; results from one meta-analysis suggest that globally, 23% of patients with spinal cord injuries will have a pressure injury during their lifetime (Chen, Cai, Du, et al., 2020).

The patient's tolerance for sitting or lying on the healed pressure area is increased gradually by increasing the time that pressure is allowed on the area in 5- to 15-minute increments. The patient is instructed to increase mobility and to follow a regimen of turning, weight shifting, and repositioning. The patient education plan includes strategies to reduce the risk for pressure injuries and methods to detect, inspect, and minimize pressure areas. Early recognition and intervention are keys to long-term management of potential impaired skin integrity.

Evaluation

Expected patient outcomes may include:

1. Maintains intact skin
   a. Exhibits no areas of nonblanchable erythema at bony prominences
   b. Avoids massage of bony prominences
   c. Exhibits no breaks in skin
2. Limits pressure on bony prominences
   a. Changes position every 1 to 2 hours
   b. Uses bridging techniques to reduce pressure
   c. Uses special equipment as appropriate
   d. Raises self from the seat of wheelchair every 15 minutes
3. Increases mobility
   a. Performs range-of-motion exercises
   b. Adheres to turning schedule
   c. Advances sitting time as tolerated
4. Has improved sensory and cognitive ability
   a. Demonstrates improved level of consciousness
   b. Remembers to inspect potential pressure injury areas every morning and evening
5. Demonstrates improved tissue perfusion
   a. Exercises to increase circulation
   b. Elevates body parts susceptible to edema
6. Attains and maintains adequate nutritional status
   a. Verbalizes the importance of protein and vitamin C in diet
   b. Eats diet high in protein and vitamin C
   c. Exhibits acceptable levels of hemoglobin, electrolyte, prealbumin, transferrin, and creatinine
7. Avoids friction and shear
   Avoids semireclining position
   Uses heel protectors when appropriate
   Lifts body instead of sliding across surfaces
8. Maintains clean, dry skin
   a. Avoids prolonged contact with wet or soiled surfaces
   b. Keeps skin clean and dry
   c. Uses lotion to keep skin lubricated

PRURITUS

Pruritus (itching) is the most common symptom of patients with dermatologic disorders (Song, Xian, Yang, et al., 2018). Pruritus may be general (over all body skin surfaces) or confined to specific regions.

Chart 56-3

Systemic Disorders Associated with Generalized Pruritus

- Chronic kidney disease
- Endocrine disease (thyrotoxicosis, hypothyroidism, diabetes)
- Folliculitis (bacterial, candidiasis, dermatophyte)
- Hematologic disorders (iron deficiency anemia)
- Infestations (scabies, lice, other insects)
- Malignancies (polycythemia vera, Hodgkin lymphoma, lymphoma, leukemia, multiple myeloma, mycosis fungoides, and cancers of the lung, breast, central nervous system, and gastrointestinal tract)
- Neurologic disorders (multiple sclerosis, brain abscess, brain tumor)
- Obstructive biliary disease (primary biliary cirrhosis, extrahepatic biliary obstruction, drug-induced cholestasis)
- Pruritus of pregnancy (pruritic urticarial papules of pregnancy, cholestasis of pregnancy, pemphigoid of pregnancy)
- Psychiatric disorders (emotional stress, anxiety, neurosis, phobias)
- Skin conditions (seborrheic dermatitis, folliculitis, atopic dermatitis)

Adapted from Song, J., Xian, D., Yang, L., et al. (2018). Pruritus: Progress toward pathogenesis and treatment. *BioMed Research International*, *2018*, 9625936.

General Pruritus

Itch receptors are unmyelinated, penicillate (brushlike) nerve endings that are found exclusively in the skin, mucous membranes, and cornea. Although pruritus is usually caused by primary skin disease with resultant rash or lesions, it may occur without a rash or lesion. This is referred to as essential pruritus, which generally has a rapid onset, may be severe, and interferes with normal daily activities.

Pruritus may be the first indication of a systemic internal disease such as diabetes, blood disorders, or cancer (occult malignancy of the breast or colon, lymphoma). It may also accompany kidney, hepatic, and thyroid diseases (Chart 56-3). Some common oral medications such as aspirin, antibiotics, hormones (e.g., estrogens, testosterone, or oral contraceptives), and opioids (e.g., morphine) may cause pruritus directly or by increasing sensitivity to ultraviolet (UV) light. Certain soaps and chemicals, radiation therapy, miliaria (prickly heat), and contact with woolen garments are associated with pruritus as well. Pruritus may also be caused by psychological factors, such as excessive stress in family or work situations, and is called *psychogenic pruritus* (Song et al., 2018).

Gerontologic Considerations

Pruritus occurs frequently in older adults as a result of dry skin. Older adults are also more likely to have a systemic illness that triggers pruritus, are at higher risk for occult malignancy, and are more likely to be taking multiple medications than younger people. All of these factors increase the incidence of pruritus in older adults (Eliopoulos, 2018).

Pathophysiology

Scratching the pruritic area causes the inflamed cells and nerve endings to release histamine, which produces more pruritus, generating a vicious itch–scratch cycle. If the patient responds to an itch by scratching, the integrity of the skin may be altered, and excoriation, redness, wheals (raised areas), infection, or changes in pigmentation may result. Pruritus usually is more severe at night and is less frequently reported during waking hours, probably because the person is distracted by daily activities. At night, when there are fewer distractions, the slightest pruritus cannot be easily ignored. Severe itching can be debilitating (Bolier, Elferink, & Beuers, 2016).

Medical Management

A thorough history and physical examination usually provide clues to the underlying cause of the pruritus, such as hay fever, allergy, recent administration of a new medication, or a change of cosmetics or soaps. After the cause has been identified, treatment of the condition should relieve the pruritus. Signs of infection and environmental clues, such as warm, dry air or irritating bed linens, should be identified. In general, washing with soap and hot water is avoided. Bath oils containing a surfactant that allows the oil to mix with bathwater (e.g., Lubath™, Alpha Keri™) may be sufficient for cleaning. However, an older adult patient or a patient with unsteady balance should avoid adding oil because it increases the danger of slipping in the bathtub. A warm bath with a mild soap followed by application of a bland emollient to moist skin can control xerosis. Tepid baths, or applying cool compresses or cool agents that contain menthol and camphor (which constrict blood vessels) may also help relieve pruritus (Cornish, 2019).

Pharmacologic Therapy

Topical antipruritic agents (e.g., lidocaine, prilocaine) or capsaicin cream may be useful in providing relief from localized pruritus. Topical corticosteroids are effective when used to diminish pruritus that occurs secondary to inflammatory conditions because of their anti-inflammatory effects. Oral antihistamines are frequently prescribed and may be effective when the pruritus is nocturnal, particularly agents such as diphenhydramine or hydroxyzine, which also cause somnolence, resulting in a restful and comfortable sleep. Other nonsedating antihistamines are not beneficial in relieving pruritus. Selective serotonin reuptake inhibitors (e.g., fluoxetine, sertraline) may be effective, particularly in patients with pruritus that is secondary to cholestasis or the uremia of chronic kidney disease (Bolier et al., 2016; Song et al., 2018).

Nursing Management

The nurse reinforces the reasons for the prescribed therapeutic regimen and educates the patient about specific points of care. The effectiveness of therapy may be gauged by asking the patient to rate the extent of itching pre- and post-therapy (Bolier et al., 2016). If baths have been prescribed, the patient is reminded to use tepid (not hot) water and to shake off the excess water and blot between intertriginous areas (body folds) with a towel. Rubbing vigorously with the towel is avoided because this overstimulates the skin and causes more itching. It also removes water from the stratum corneum. Immediately after bathing, the skin should be lubricated with an emollient to trap moisture.

The patient is instructed to avoid situations that cause vasodilation. Examples include exposure to an overly warm environment and ingestion of alcohol or hot foods and liquids, all of which can induce or intensify pruritus. Using a humidifier is helpful if environmental air is dry. Activities that result in perspiration should be limited because perspiration may irritate and promote pruritus. If itching interferes with sleep, the nurse can advise the patient to wear cotton clothing next to the skin rather than synthetic materials. The room should be kept cool and humidified. Vigorous scratching should be avoided and nails kept trimmed to prevent skin damage and infection. When the underlying cause of pruritus is unknown and further testing is required, the nurse explains each test and its expected outcome.

Perineal and Perianal Pruritus

Pruritus of the genital and anal regions may be caused by small particles of fecal material lodged in the perianal crevices or attached to anal hairs. Alternatively, it may result from perianal skin damage caused by scratching, moisture, and decreased skin resistance as a result of corticosteroid or antibiotic therapy. Other possible causes of perianal itching include local lesions such as hemorrhoids, fungal or yeast infections, and pinworm infestation. Conditions reviewed in Chart 56-3 may also result in pruritus. Occasionally, no cause can be identified.

Management

The patient is instructed to follow proper hygiene measures and to discontinue home and OTC remedies. The perineal or anal area should be rinsed with lukewarm water and blotted dry with cotton balls. Premoistened tissues may be used after defecation (Breen & Bleday, 2020).

As part of health education, the nurse instructs the patient to avoid bathing in water that is too hot and to avoid using bubble baths, sodium bicarbonate, and detergent soaps, all of which aggravate dryness. To keep the perineal or perianal skin as dry as possible, patients should avoid wearing underwear made of synthetic fabrics. The patient should also avoid vasodilating agents (e.g., alcohol), stimulants (e.g., caffeine), and mechanical irritants (e.g., rough or woolen clothing). A diet that includes adequate fiber may help maintain soft stools and prevent minor trauma to the anal mucosa (Breen & Bleday, 2020).

SECRETORY DISORDERS

The main secretory function of the skin is performed by the sweat glands, which help regulate body temperature. These glands excrete perspiration that evaporates, thereby cooling the body. The sweat glands are located in various parts of the body and respond to different stimuli. Those on the trunk generally respond to thermal stimulation; those on the palms and soles respond to nervous stimulation; and those in the axillae and on the forehead respond to both kinds of stimulation. Normal perspiration has no odor. Body odor is produced by the increase in bacteria on the skin and the interaction of bacterial waste products with the chemicals of perspiration (Norris, 2019). As a rule, moist skin is warm, and dry skin is cool, but this is not always true. It is not unusual to observe warm, dry skin in patients who are dehydrated and very hot, dry skin in patients with some febrile states.

Normally, sweat can be controlled with the use of antiperspirants and deodorants. Most antiperspirants are aluminum salts that block the opening to the sweat duct. Pure deodorants inhibit bacterial growth and block the metabolism of sweat; they have no antiperspirant effect. Fragrance-free deodorants are available for those with sensitive skin.

Hidradenitis Suppurativa

Hidradenitis suppurativa is a chronic suppurative folliculitis of the perianal, axillary, and genital areas or under the breasts. It can produce abscesses or sinuses with scarring. It develops after puberty and diminishes in incidence after 50 years of age. Black Americans are at greater risk for hidradenitis suppurativa, as are patients who smoke and who have obesity. In addition, men are at greater risk for anogenital hidradenitis suppurativa, whereas women are at greater risk for axillary hidradenitis suppurativa. The cause is unknown, but it appears to have a genetic basis (Tchero, Herlin, Bekara, et al., 2019).

Pathophysiology

It had been assumed for many years that hidradenitis suppurativa was caused by the blockage and infection of the sweat glands. However, recent evidence suggests that it is a primary disorder of follicular occlusion, often resulting in infection, that causes eventual hypertrophic formation of scar tissue in the area of the sweat glands (Doughty & McNichol, 2016).

Clinical Manifestations

Hidradenitis suppurativa occurs more frequently in the axillae but also appears in inguinal folds, on the mons pubis, around the buttocks, areolae of the breasts, submammary fold, nape of the neck, and shoulders. The patient may present with a firm, pea-sized nodule that causes discomfort, or with a history of this type of nodule that then ruptures and discharges purulent drainage. The nodule then propagates, and multiple similar nodules will form adjacent to the initial nodule. The nodules become deep seated and, as they rupture, form scars. The nodules may coalesce or form "bridges," become infected, and result in abscesses. As they coalesce, the patient will present with complaints of persistent pain (Doughty & McNichol, 2016).

Management

The patient is educated to use warm compresses and wear loose-fitting clothes over the nodules or lesions. Oral antibiotic agents such as erythromycin, tetracycline, minocycline, and doxycycline are frequently prescribed. Nonsteroidal anti-inflammatory drugs (NSAIDs) may be indicated to relieve the pain. Silver-impregnated alginate dressings may be useful with some lesions. Incision and drainage of large suppurating areas with gauze packs inserted to facilitate drainage are often necessary. Rarely, the entire area is excised, removing the scar tissue and any infection. This surgery is drastic in that it may require the use of skin grafts (see Chapter 57) and is performed only as a last resort. Carbon dioxide laser surgery (see later discussion) may be more effective than this type of excisional surgery (Tchero et al., 2019).

Seborrheic Dermatitis

Seborrhea is excessive production of sebum (secretion of sebaceous glands), which typically occurs in areas where sebaceous glands are normally found in large numbers, such as the face, scalp, eyebrows, eyelids, sides of the nose and upper lip, malar regions (cheeks), ears, axillae, under the breasts, groin, and gluteal crease of the buttocks. *Dermatosis* refers to a skin disorder; thus, the seborrheic dermatoses are skin disorders caused by an excessive production of sebum. *Dermatitis* refers to an inflammatory skin disorder. Seborrheic dermatitis is a chronic inflammatory disease of the skin with a predilection for areas that are well supplied with sebaceous glands or lie between skin folds, where the bacterial count is high (Doughty & McNichol, 2016).

Clinical Manifestations

Two forms of seborrheic dermatitis can occur: an oily form and a dry form. Either form may start in childhood and continue throughout life. The oily form appears moist or greasy. There may be patches of sallow, greasy skin, with or without scaling, and slight erythema, predominantly on the forehead, nasolabial fold, beard area, scalp, and between adjacent skin surfaces in the regions of the axillae, groin, and breasts. Small pustules or papulopustules resembling acne may appear on the trunk. The dry form, consisting of flaky desquamation of the scalp with a profuse amount of fine, powdery scales, is commonly called *dandruff*. The mild forms of the disease are asymptomatic. When scaling occurs, it is often accompanied by pruritus, which may lead to scratching and secondary infections and excoriation.

Seborrheic dermatitis has a genetic predisposition. Hormones, nutritional status, infection, and emotional stress influence its course. The remissions and exacerbations of this condition should be explained to the patient. If a person has not previously been diagnosed with this condition and suddenly appears with a severe outbreak, a complete history and physical examination should be conducted. Infrequently, it may be a manifestation of a serious disorder, such as Parkinson's disease or human immune deficiency virus (HIV) infection (Sasseville, 2020).

Medical Management

Because there is no known cure for seborrhea, the objectives of therapy are to control the disorder and allow the skin to repair itself. Seborrheic dermatitis of the body and face may respond to a topically applied corticosteroid cream, which allays the secondary inflammatory response. However, this medication should be used with caution near the eyelids because it can lead to glaucoma and cataracts. As an alternative treatment, patients can wash the eyelids using baby shampoo and cotton swabs (Handler, 2019).

Patients with seborrheic dermatitis may develop a secondary candidal (yeast) infection in body creases or folds. To avoid this, patients should be advised to ensure maximum aeration of the skin and to clean carefully areas where there are creases or folds in the skin (Doughty & McNichol, 2016). Patients with persistent candidiasis should be evaluated for diabetes.

The mainstay of dandruff treatment is proper, frequent shampooing (at least three times weekly) with medicated shampoos. Two or three different types of shampoo should be used in rotation to prevent the seborrhea from becoming resistant to a particular shampoo. The shampoo is left on at least 5 to 10 minutes. As the condition of the scalp improves, the treatment can be less frequent. Antiseborrheic shampoos include those containing selenium sulfide suspension, zinc pyrithione, salicylic acid, or sulfur compounds, and tar shampoo that contains sulfur or salicylic acid (Handler, 2019; Sasseville, 2020).

Nursing Management

The patient is educated that seborrheic dermatitis is a chronic condition that tends to reappear. The goal is to keep it under control through adherence to the treatment program (Handler, 2019; Sasseville, 2020). The patient is advised to avoid external irritants, excessive heat, and perspiration; rubbing and scratching prolong the disorder. To avoid secondary infection, the patient should air the skin and keep skin folds clean and dry.

Instructions for using medicated shampoos are reinforced for people with dandruff who require treatment. Frequent shampooing is contrary to some cultural practices; the nurse should be sensitive to these differences when educating the patient.

Acne Vulgaris

Acne vulgaris is a common disorder affecting susceptible pilosebaceous units (hair follicles and sebaceous glands), most commonly on the face, neck, torso, and upper arms (Dlugasch & Story, 2021; Thiboutot & Zaenglein, 2019). It is a chronic dermatosis characterized by **comedones** (primary acne lesions), both closed (whiteheads) and open (blackheads), and by papules, pustules, nodules, and cysts (Zaenglein, Pathy, Schlosser, et al., 2016) (see Chapter 55, Table 55-2).

Acne is the most commonly encountered skin condition that affects up to 80% of Americans at some time during their lives. Acne is most prevalent during adolescence among males but is more prevalent in adulthood among females. Acne is traditionally considered a skin disorder of adolescence; however, by age 45 years, up to 5% of adults report having acne (Rao & Chen, 2020). Acne appears to stem from an interplay of genetic, hormonal, and bacterial factors (Dlugasch & Story, 2021; Thiboutot & Zaenglein, 2019).

Pathophysiology

During puberty, androgens stimulate the sebaceous glands, causing them to enlarge and secrete sebum (a naturally occurring endogenous oil) that rises to the top of the hair follicle and flows out onto the skin surface. In adolescents who develop acne, androgenic stimulation produces a heightened response in the sebaceous glands, with increased sebum production and hyperkeratinization, causing sebum plug formation within the pilosebaceous ducts. Sebaceous plugging then causes a localized inflammatory response (Dlugasch & Story, 2021; Thiboutot & Zaenglein, 2019).

Clinical Manifestations

The main lesions of acne are comedones. Closed comedones form from impacted lipids or oils and keratin that plug the dilated follicle. Closed comedones may evolve into open comedones, in which the contents of the ducts are in open communication with the external environment. The color of open comedones results from an accumulation of lipid, bacterial, and epithelial debris. Some closed comedones may rupture, resulting in an inflammatory reaction caused by leakage of follicular contents (e.g., sebum, keratin, bacteria) into the dermis. The resultant inflammation is seen clinically as erythematous papules, inflammatory pustules, and inflammatory cysts. Mild papules and cysts drain and heal without treatment. Deeper papules and cysts cause scarring of the skin (Thiboutot & Zaenglein, 2019).

Assessment and Diagnostic Findings

The diagnosis of acne is based on the history and physical examination, evidence of lesions characteristic of acne, and age. Women may report a history of flare-ups a few days before menses. The presence of the typical comedones along with oily skin is characteristic (Rao & Chen, 2020). Oiliness is more prominent in the midfacial area; other parts of the face may appear dry.

Acne vulgaris can be classified as mild, moderate, or severe based upon the number and type of acne lesions, severity location and scarring. However, currently there is no consensus on the exact number of lesions that constitute mild, moderate, and severe acne (Zaenglein et al., 2016). Generally speaking, mild acne is characterized by the presence of comedones and a few papulopustules; moderate acne is characterized by a greater number of papulopustules and comedones along with the presence of inflammatory pustules; and, severe acne is characterized by the presence of cysts (also called nodules or nodulocysts) that are greater than 5 mm in diameter (Rao & Chen, 2020).

Medical Management

The goals of management are to reduce bacterial colonies, decrease sebaceous gland activity, prevent the follicles from becoming plugged, reduce inflammation, combat secondary infection, minimize scarring, and eliminate factors that predispose the person to acne. The therapeutic regimen depends on the type of lesion (e.g., comedones, papule, pustule, cyst). The duration of treatment depends on the extent and severity of the acne. In severe cases, treatment may extend over years.

Nutrition and Hygiene Therapy

The association between diet and acne is not established. In particular, the association between acne and milk products, chocolate, and fried foods is not well defined. However, there does appear to be a correlation between foods high in refined sugars and acne; therefore, these foods should be avoided (Zaenglein et al., 2016). In general, maintenance of good nutrition equips the immune system for effective action against bacteria and infection.

For mild cases of acne, washing twice a day with a cleansing soap and use of OTC products that contain benzoyl peroxide or salicylic acid (see later discussion) may be all that is required (Dlugasch & Story, 2021; Zaenglein et al., 2016). Oil-free cosmetics and creams should be chosen. These products are usually designated as useful for acne-prone skin.

TABLE 56-5	Medications Indicated for Treatment of Acne Vulgaris
Classification	**Recommended Medications**
Mild acne	Benzoyl peroxide -or- Topical retinoid -or- Combination[a] topical antibiotic and benzoyl peroxide -or- Combination[a] topical retinoid and benzoyl peroxide -or- Combination[a] topical retinoid and benzoyl peroxide and topical antibiotic
Moderate acne	Combination[a] topical antibiotic and benzoyl peroxide -or- Combination[a] topical retinoid and benzoyl peroxide -or- Combination[a] topical retinoid and benzoyl peroxide and topical antibiotic -or- Oral antibiotic and combination[a] topical retinoid and benzoyl peroxide -or- Oral antibiotic and combination[a] topical retinoid and benzoyl peroxide and topical antibiotic
Severe acne	Oral antibiotic and combination[a] topical retinoid and benzoyl peroxide -or- Oral antibiotic and combination[a] topical antibiotic and benzoyl peroxide -or- Oral antibiotic and combination[a] topical retinoid and benzoyl peroxide and topical antibiotic -or- Oral antibiotic and oral isotretinoin

[a]May be prescribed as combination products or as singular products.
Adapted from Zaenglein, A. L., Pathy, A. L., Schlosser, B. J., et al. (2016). Guidelines of care for the management of acne vulgaris. *Journal of the American Academy of Dermatology, 74*(5), 945–973.

Pharmacologic Therapy

Pharmacologic treatments for acne are based upon the severity of the acne (Zaenglein et al., 2016). Table 56-5 summarizes medications recommended to manage acne vulgaris based upon severity.

Topical Therapy

Recommended OTC acne medications contain benzoyl peroxide, which is very effective at removing the sebaceous follicular plugs. Benzoyl peroxide preparations produce a rapid and sustained reduction of inflammatory lesions. They depress sebum production and promote breakdown of comedo plugs and have an antibacterial effect (Zaenglein et al., 2016). Initially, benzoyl peroxide causes redness and scaling, but the skin usually adjusts quickly to its use. However, the skin of some people can be overly sensitive to these products, which can cause irritation or excessive dryness, especially when used with some prescribed topical medications. The patient should be instructed to discontinue use of the product if severe irritation occurs. Typically, the patient applies a gel of benzoyl peroxide once daily. In many instances, this is the only treatment needed (Comerford & Durkin, 2020).

OTC salicylic acid preparations are also available for use by patients with mild acne. The effects of these agents are similar to those of benzoyl peroxide products. Although salicylic acid products have long been used by patients with acne, their efficacy has not been demonstrated in clinical trials (Zaenglein et al., 2016). Prescription topical agents used for years that have also not demonstrated efficacy in clinical trials include zinc, sulfur, and resorcinol; and are therefore not recommended for treatment (Zaenglein et al., 2016).

Synthetic vitamin A acids, also called retinoids (e.g., tretinoin, adapalene, tazarotene), are applied topically to clear the keratin plugs from the pilosebaceous ducts. The patient should be informed that symptoms may worsen during early weeks of therapy because inflammation, erythema, and peeling may occur. The patient is cautioned against sun exposure while using this topical medication because it may cause sunburn. Package insert directions should be followed carefully. Improvement may take 8 to 12 weeks. Some patients may benefit from being treated with both a retinoid and benzoyl peroxide and may be prescribed a combination topical gel (e.g., adapalene–benzoyl peroxide) (Zaenglein et al., 2016).

Topical antibiotic treatment for acne is common. Topical antibiotic agents suppress bacterial growth; reduce superficial free fatty acid levels; decrease comedones, papules, and pustules; and produce no systemic side effects (Comerford & Durkin, 2020). Commonly prescribed agents include clindamycin and erythromycin. Topical combination gels that include both benzoyl peroxide and an antibiotic (e.g., benzoyl erythromycin) are commonly prescribed and can be very effective treatment (Zaenglein et al., 2016).

Other less commonly prescribed topical agents that may be effective in treating acne vulgaris include azelaic acid and dapsone gel. Azelaic acid has comedolytic, antibacterial, and anti-inflammatory effects. It may also have a lightening effect on skin that can be hyperpigmented as a consequence of acne (Zaenglein et al., 2016). Dapsone reduces inflammatory lesions and for reasons poorly understood, seems to work better in female adult patients than in adolescent or male patients (Zaenglein et al., 2016).

Systemic Therapy

Oral antibiotic agents given in small doses over a long period are very effective in treating moderate and severe acne, especially when the acne is inflammatory and results in pustules, abscesses, and scarring. Therapy may continue for months to years. Antibiotics most commonly selected are of the tetracycline class (e.g., tetracycline, doxycycline, minocycline) (Zaenglein et al., 2016). The tetracycline family of antibiotics is contraindicated in pregnant women. Side effects of tetracyclines include photosensitivity (sensitivity to the sun), nausea, diarrhea, cutaneous infection, and vaginitis in women (Comerford & Durkin, 2020). Alternative antibiotics that may be selected include erythromycin, azithromycin, and trimethoprim–sulfamethoxazole (Zaenglein et al., 2016).

Oral retinoids (e.g., isotretinoin) are used with dramatic results in patients with nodular cystic acne unresponsive to conventional therapy. This may prevent scarring that can result from cyst formation. Retinoids reduce sebaceous gland size and inhibit sebum production. They also cause epidermal desquamation (shedding of the epidermis), thereby unseating and expelling existing comedones. The most common side effect is **cheilitis** (inflammation of the lips). Dry and chafed skin and mucous membranes are also frequent side effects. These changes are reversible with the withdrawal of the medication. Retinoids are teratogenic, meaning that they may cause fetal defects. Effective contraceptive measures for women of childbearing age are mandatory during treatment and for about 4 to 8 weeks thereafter (Dlugasch & Story, 2021). To avoid additive toxic effects, patients are cautioned not to take vitamin A supplements while taking retinoids (Comerford & Durkin, 2020).

Estrogen therapy (including progesterone–estrogen preparations) suppresses sebum production and reduces skin oiliness. It is usually reserved for young women when the acne begins somewhat later than usual and tends to flare up at certain times in the menstrual cycle. Estrogen-dominant oral contraceptive compounds may be given on a prescribed cyclic regimen (Rao & Chen, 2020). Estrogen is not given to male patients because of the undesirable side effects such as enlargement of the breasts and decrease in body hair.

Phototherapy

The use of antibiotic therapy runs the risk of developing antibiotic resistance; therefore, phototherapy has been proposed as a potentially viable alternative treatment. The use of light-emitting diode (LED) phototherapy using blue light (i.e., directing wavelengths of 407 to 420 nm to targeted skin) has shown preliminary promise for the treatment of mild to moderate acne. The blue light is believed to cause photoactivation of naturally occurring porphyrins, resulting in free radical formation, which causes cell membrane destruction of *Propionibacterium acne*, the common culprit in inciting comedo formation (Ablon, 2018; Scott, Stehlik, Clark, et al., 2019). To date, there have been no reported adverse effects associated with blue light phototherapy. Patients must commit time to these treatments, which may be self-administered at home twice daily for 30 to 60 minutes for 5 weeks (Scott et al., 2019). At present, the efficacy of phototherapy remains under investigation.

Surgical Management

Treatment includes comedo extraction; injections of corticosteroids into the inflamed lesions; and incision and drainage of large, fluctuant (moving in palpable waves), nodular cystic lesions. Patients with deep scars may be treated with dermabrasion (deep abrasive therapy), in which the epidermis and some superficial dermis are removed down to the level of the scars (Rao & Chen, 2020).

Comedones may be removed with a comedo extractor. The site is first cleaned with alcohol. The opening of the extractor is then placed over the lesion, and direct pressure is applied to cause extrusion of the plug through the extractor. Removal of comedones leads to erythema, which may take several weeks to subside. Recurrence of comedones after extraction is common (Rao & Chen, 2020).

Nursing Management

Nursing care of patients with acne includes monitoring and managing potential complications of skin treatments. Major nursing activities include providing patient education, particularly in proper skin care techniques, and managing potential

problems related to the skin disorder or therapy. Providing positive reassurance, listening attentively, and being sensitive to the feelings of the patient with acne are essential to the patient's psychological well-being and understanding of the disease and treatment plan. Having acne, particularly if it persists into adulthood, can lead to anxiety and depression (Zaenglein et al., 2016).

Preventing Scarring

Prevention of scarring is the ultimate goal of therapy. The chance of scarring increases with the severity of the grade of acne. Severe acne usually requires longer-term therapy with systemic antibiotic agents and other treatments that may include combination topical agents or isotretinoin (see Table 56-5). Patients should be warned that discontinuing these medications may lead to more flare-ups and increase the chance of deep scarring. Furthermore, manipulation of the comedones, papules, and pustules increases the potential for scarring.

When acne surgery is prescribed to extract deep-seated comedones or inflamed lesions or to incise and drain cystic lesions, the intervention itself may result in further scarring. Dermabrasion, which levels existing scar tissue, can also increase scar formation. Hyper- or hypopigmentation also may affect the tissue involved. The patient should be informed of these potential outcomes before choosing surgical intervention for acne.

Promoting Home, Community-Based, and Transitional Care

 Educating Patients About Self-Care

In addition to providing instructions for taking prescribed medications, the nurse advises patients to wash the face and other affected areas with mild soap and water twice a day to remove surface oils and prevent obstruction of the oil glands. Mild abrasive soaps and drying agents are prescribed to eliminate the oily feeling that troubles many patients. At the same time, patients are cautioned to avoid excessive abrasion, because it makes acne worse.

All forms of friction and trauma are avoided, including propping the hands against the face, rubbing the face, and wearing tight collars, helmets, and face masks. Patients are instructed to avoid manipulation of pimples or blackheads. Squeezing merely worsens the problem, because a portion of the blackhead is pushed down into the skin, which may cause the follicle to rupture. Because cosmetics, shaving creams, and lotions can aggravate acne, these should be avoided.

INFECTIOUS DERMATOSES

Various dermatoses can be caused by bacterial, viral, fungal, or parasitic infections.

Bacterial Skin Infections

Also called **pyodermas**, pus-forming bacterial infections of the skin may be primary or secondary. Primary skin infections originate in previously normal-appearing skin and are usually caused by a single organism. Secondary skin infections arise from a preexisting skin disorder or from disruption of the skin integrity from injury or surgery. In either case, several microorganisms may be implicated (e.g., *Staphylococcus aureus*, group A streptococci). Common primary bacterial skin infections are impetigo and folliculitis. Folliculitis may lead to furuncles or carbuncles.

Impetigo

Impetigo is a superficial infection of the skin caused by staphylococci, streptococci, or multiple bacteria. Bullous impetigo, a more deep-seated infection of the skin caused by *S. aureus*, is characterized by the formation of **bullae** (i.e., large, fluid-filled blisters) from original vesicles. The bullae rupture, leaving raw, red areas. Nonbullous impetigo accounts for approximately 70% of the cases. This type of impetigo tends to affect skin that has already been disrupted by cuts, abrasions, bites, or other types of trauma. *S. aureus* is also commonly implicated, including methicillin-resistant *S. aureus* (MRSA) and gentamycin-resistant *S. aureus*, as well as *Streptococcus pyogenes* (Lewis, 2019).

The exposed areas of the body, face, hands, neck, and extremities are most frequently involved. Impetigo is contagious and may spread to other parts of the patient's skin or to other members of the family who touch the patient or use towels or combs that are soiled with the exudate of the lesions (Lewis, 2019).

Impetigo is seen in people of all races and ages. It is particularly common in children living in poor hygienic conditions. Chronic health problems, poor hygiene, and malnutrition may predispose an adult to impetigo. It is more prevalent in warm, humid climates and is therefore more commonly seen in the southeastern United States than in northern climates (Lewis, 2019).

Clinical Manifestations

The lesions of impetigo are most commonly seen on the face or extremities. They begin as small, red macules, which quickly become discrete, thin-walled vesicles that rupture and become covered with a loosely adherent honey-yellow crust (Fig. 56-4). These crusts are easily removed to reveal smooth, red, moist surfaces on which new crusts soon develop (Lewis, 2019).

Medical Management

Topical antibacterial therapy (e.g., mupirocin, retapamulin) is typically prescribed when the disease is limited to a small area. The medication must be applied to the lesions several times daily for 5 to 7 days. Lesions are first soaked or washed with soap solution to remove the central site of bacterial growth, giving the topical antibiotic an opportunity to reach the infected site. After the crusts are removed, the prescribed topical antibiotic cream is applied. Gloves are worn when providing patient care (Lewis, 2019).

Systemic antibiotic agents may be prescribed to treat infections that are widespread or in cases where there are systemic manifestations (e.g., fever is present). These antibiotics are effective in reducing contagious spread, treating deep infections, and preventing acute glomerulonephritis (kidney infection), which may occur as a consequence of streptococcal skin diseases. Amoxicillin–clavulanate, cloxacillin, or dicloxacillin may be prescribed. In cases where MRSA is present, antibiotics prescribed may include clindamycin, trimethoprim–sulfamethoxazole, levofloxacin, or ciprofloxacin (Lewis, 2019).

Nursing Management

The nurse educates the patient and family members to bathe at least once daily with bactericidal soap. Cleanliness and good hygiene practices help to prevent the spread of the lesions from one skin area to another and from one person to another. In particular, patients and family members must be educated to practice hand hygiene every time after a lesion is touched. Each person should have a separate towel and washcloth. Because impetigo is a contagious disorder, people who are infected should avoid contact with other people until the lesions heal (Lewis, 2019).

Folliculitis, Furuncles, and Carbuncles

Infectious folliculitis is an inflammatory condition of the cells within the wall and ostia of the hair follicles that may be caused by a bacterial, viral, fungal, or parasitic infection. Lesions may be superficial or deep. Single or multiple papules or pustules appear close to the hair follicles. Folliculitis can affect any hairy part of the body, most commonly the beard area of men who shave, as well as women's legs, if they shave. Other commonly affected areas include the axillae, trunk, and buttocks (Bryant & Nix, 2016).

Pseudofolliculitis barbae (shaving bumps) occur predominantly on the faces of Black men as a result of shaving. The sharp ingrowing hairs have a curved root that grows at a more acute angle and pierces the skin, provoking an irritative reaction. The only entirely effective treatment is to avoid shaving. Other treatments include using special lotions or antibiotics or using a hand brush to dislodge the hairs mechanically. If the patient must remove facial hair, a depilatory cream or electric razor may be used.

A **furuncle** (boil) is an acute inflammation arising deep in one or more hair follicles and spreading into the surrounding dermis (Fig. 56-5). This inflammation is a deep form of folliculitis. Furunculosis refers to multiple or recurrent lesions. Furuncles may occur anywhere on the body but are more prevalent in areas subjected to irritation, pressure, friction, and excessive perspiration, such as the back of the neck, the axillae, and the buttocks.

A furuncle may start as a small, red, raised, painful pimple. Frequently, the infection progresses and involves the skin

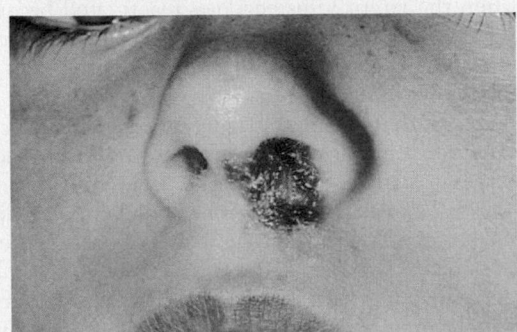

Figure 56-4 • Impetigo of the nostril.

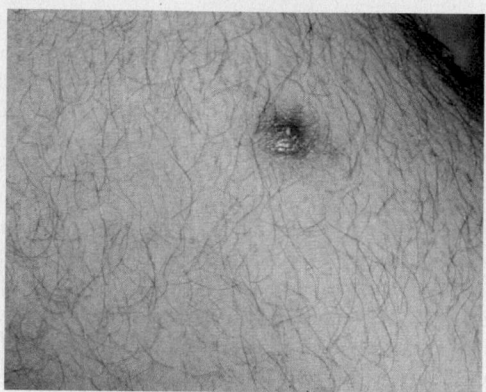

Figure 60-5 • Painful furuncle on the thigh. Reprinted with permission from Goodheart, H. P. (2003). *Goodheart's photoguide of common skin disorders* (2nd ed.). Philadelphia, PA: Lippincott Williams & Wilkins.

and subcutaneous fatty tissue, causing tenderness, pain, and cellulitis. The area of redness and induration represents an effort of the body to keep the infection localized. The bacteria (usually staphylococci) produce necrosis of the invaded tissue (Motswaledi, 2018). The characteristic pointing of a boil follows in a few days. When this occurs, the center becomes yellow or black, and the boil is said to have "come to a head."

A **carbuncle** is an abscess of the skin and subcutaneous tissue that represents an extension of a furuncle that has invaded several follicles and is large and deep seated. It is usually caused by a staphylococcal infection. Carbuncles appear most commonly in areas where the skin is thick and inelastic; the back of the neck and the back are common sites (Ahmad & Siddiqui, 2017). The extensive inflammation frequently prevents a complete walling off of the infection; purulent material may be absorbed, resulting in high fever, pain, leukocytosis, and sepsis.

Furuncles and carbuncles are more likely to occur in older adult patients with underlying systemic diseases, such as diabetes or hematologic malignancies, and in those receiving immunosuppressive therapy for other diseases. Both are more prevalent in hot climates, especially on skin beneath occlusive clothing (Ahmad & Siddiqui, 2017).

Medical Management

In treating staphylococcal infections, it is important not to rupture or destroy the protective wall of induration that localizes the infection. The boil or pimple should never be squeezed. Systemic antibiotic therapy, selected by culture and sensitivity study, is generally indicated. Oral dicloxacillin and cephalosporins are first-line medications. If MRSA is suspected, antibiotic agents selected may include clindamycin, trimethoprim–sulfamethoxazole, doxycycline, or minocycline (Harris, 2019).

When the pus has localized and is fluctuant, a small incision with a scalpel can speed resolution by relieving the tension and ensuring direct evacuation of the pus and debris. The patient is instructed to keep the draining lesion covered with a dressing.

Nursing Management

Intravenous (IV) fluids, fever reduction, and other supportive treatments are indicated for patients who are acutely ill

from infection. Warm, moist compresses hasten resolution of the furuncle or carbuncle. The surrounding skin may be cleansed gently with antibacterial soap, and an antibacterial ointment may be applied. Soiled dressings are handled according to standard precautions. Nursing personnel should carefully follow standard precautions to avoid becoming carriers of staphylococci.

> **Quality and Safety Nursing Alert**
>
> *Nurses must take special precautions in caring for boils on the patient's face because the skin area drains directly into the cranial venous sinuses. Sinus thrombosis can develop after manipulating a boil in this location. The infection can travel through the sinus tract and penetrate the brain cavity, causing a brain abscess.*

Promoting Home, Community-Based, and Transitional Care

 Educating Patients About Self-Care

To prevent and control staphylococcal skin infections such as boils and carbuncles, the staphylococcal pathogen must be eliminated from the skin and environment. Efforts must be made to provide a hygienic environment. If lesions are actively draining, the mattress and pillow should be covered with plastic material and wiped with disinfectant daily; the bed linens, towels, and clothing should be laundered after each use; and the patient should use an antibacterial soap and shampoo for an indefinite period, often several months.

Viral Skin Infections

Cutaneous manifestations may ensue because of viral infections. Viruses implicated in causing dermatologic disorders include the varicella-zoster virus (VZV), the herpes simplex viruses, and the severe acute respiratory syndrome coronavirus 2 (SARS-CoV-2).

Herpes Zoster

Herpes zoster, also called *shingles*, is an infection caused by VZV. The disease is characterized by painful vesicular eruptions along the areas of distribution of dermatomes (sensory nerves) from one or more posterior ganglia. After a case of primary varicella (chickenpox) runs its course, the VZV lies dormant inside nerve cells near the brain and spinal cord. Later, when the latent virus becomes reactivated because of declining cellular immunity, it travels by way of the peripheral nerves to the skin, where it replicates and create a red rash of small, fluid-filled blisters.

It is thought that during the aging process, natural immunity to the varicella virus wanes, facilitating viral reactivation. Herpes zoster develops naturally over the lifetime of about 10% to 20% of all adults who had chickenpox earlier in life, usually after 50 years of age. The rates of occurrence tend to be the same in both men and women but are slightly lower in Black adults than White adults. There is an increased frequency of herpes zoster infections in patients with weakened immune systems, including those with HIV infection and in those with cancer. In these patients, the infection can become widespread and cause significant complications (Janniger, Eastern, Hospenthal, et al., 2020).

Clinical Manifestations

Manifestations typically occur in three phases, including the preeruptive, acute eruptive, and postherpetic neuralgia phases. During the preeruptive phase, the previously dormant VZV becomes reactivated within the dorsal root ganglia of the spinal cord. Manifestations that follow, therefore, tend to follow the dermatomes that correspond with the ganglia that are affected. The patient will typically complain of pain, or sometimes pruritus or paresthesias, over the sensory region that follows affected dermatomes. This phase lasts from 1 to 10 days, with 48 hours being typical (Janniger et al., 2020).

The acute eruptive phase is heralded by the appearance of unilateral patchy erythematous areas in the dermatomal area that is affected. Vesicles develop that appear initially clear, then become cloudy, and eventually rupture and crust (Fig. 56-6). The pain that accompanies this stage is typically described as severe and unrelenting. This phase typically lasts between 10 and 15 days (Janniger et al., 2020).

The last phase—postherpetic neuralgia—is variable in terms of both duration and manifestations. The pain is typically localized to the dermatomal area that was affected. Approximately 50% of adults older than 60 years with herpes zoster experience postherpetic neuralgia pain for longer than 60 days (Janniger et al., 2020).

Herpes zoster ophthalmicus is a rare subtype of herpes zoster that causes severe consequences. Typically in herpes zoster ophthalmicus, a branch of the trigeminal nerve is affected that innervates the ocular and periocular structures. This may cause significant pain and morbid ocular complications, including blindness (Janniger et al., 2020).

Medical Management

The effects of herpes zoster can be diminished if oral antiviral agents such as acyclovir, valacyclovir, or famciclovir

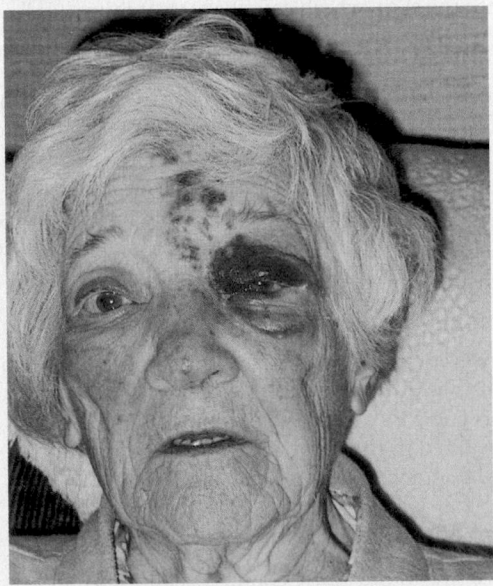

Figure 56-6 • Herpes zoster (shingles).

are given within 72 hours of the onset of symptoms; the prescribed antiviral agent then must continue to be taken for 7 to 10 days in patients who are immune competent. IV acyclovir may be indicated in patients who are immune compromised; length of therapy may continue for up to 21 days (Janniger et al., 2020).

The goals of herpes zoster management are to relieve the pain and to reduce or avoid complications, which include infection, scarring, and postherpetic neuralgia and eye complications. Pain is controlled with analgesic agents because adequate pain control during the acute phase helps prevent persistent pain patterns. Analgesic agents may include NSAIDs or acetaminophen for mild pain, or opioids such as oxycodone for moderate to severe pain (Beuscher, Reeves, & Harrell, 2017). Systemic corticosteroids have traditionally been prescribed; however, their routine use is currently controversial as benefits have not been seen in research studies (Janniger et al., 2020). Patients with postherpetic neuralgia may be prescribed pregabalin or gabapentin to mitigate its unpleasant effects. Alternative agents that might be prescribed to treat postherpetic neuralgia include tricyclic antidepressants (e.g., amitriptyline, nortriptyline) (Beuscher et al., 2017). Patients with herpes zoster ophthalmicus require emergent treatment by an ophthalmologist (Janniger et al., 2020).

Since 1995, the widespread vaccination of children with the VZV vaccine has led to a marked reduction in the incidence of primary varicella, which presumably will result in marked decrease in rates of herpes zoster in the future. A zoster vaccine live (ZVL) was introduced to boost VZV cellular immunity in adults 60 years of age and older in 2006. Since that time, consensus guidelines have lowered the age for vaccination to 50 years, and include those with a history of herpes zoster, because it may recur (Janniger et al., 2020). A nonlive, recombinant zoster vaccine (RZV) was approved by the U.S. Food and Drug Administration (FDA) in 2017. In response, the Centers for Disease Control and Prevention (CDC) revised its herpes zoster vaccination guidelines to recommend that adults 50 years of age and older should receive 2 doses of RZV 2 to 6 months apart, regardless of whether or not they have previously received the ZVL vaccine. For those adults who have received the ZVL vaccine, they should not receive a first dose of the RZV vaccine until at least 2 months have elapsed from receipt of the ZVL vaccine (Dooling, Guo, Patel, et al., 2018).

Nursing Management

The patient and family members are instructed about the importance of taking antiviral agents as prescribed and in keeping follow-up appointments with the primary provider. The nurse assesses the patient's discomfort and response to medication and collaborates with the primary provider to make necessary adjustments to the treatment regimen. Vesicles and rashes may be soothed by applying OTC calamine lotion or 5% aluminum acetate (Burow's solution) wet dressings for 30 to 60 minutes four to six times daily (Janniger et al., 2020). The patient is educated about how to follow proper hand hygiene techniques to avoid spreading the virus.

Diversionary activities and relaxation techniques are encouraged to ensure restful sleep and to alleviate discomfort. A caregiver may be required to assist with dressings, particularly if the patient is an older adult and unable to apply them. Food preparation for patients who cannot care for themselves or prepare nourishing meals must be arranged.

Herpes Simplex

Herpes simplex is a common skin infection. There are two types of the causative virus, which are identified by viral typing. In general, herpes simplex type 1 occurs on the skin of the lips, mouth, gums, or tongue (or on the skin around the mouth) and type 2 occurs in the genital area, but both viral types can be found in both locations. See Chapters 18 and 51 for discussion of herpes simplex type 1 and type 2, respectively.

COVID-19 Considerations

SARS-CoV-2, the virion implicated in causing the global pandemic of coronavirus disease 2019 (COVID-19), primarily manifests with respiratory ailments in patients who are infected (e.g., pneumonia, acute respiratory distress syndrome, acute respiratory failure), as its name implies. However, there have been notable dermatologic manifestations of COVID-19; these have been tracked by an international registry of patients with cutaneous manifestations of COVID-19, sponsored by the American Academy of Dermatology (AAD) and the International League of Dermatologic Societies (ILDS). At the time of this writing, the registry has reported dermatologic manifestations of COVID-19 among 716 patients from 31 countries (Freeman, McMahon, Lipoff, et al., 2020b). Although many diverse cutaneous manifestations of COVID-19 have been reported, one that is of particular note involves perniolike acral (fingers, toes) skin lesions (Freeman, McMahon, Lipoff, et al., 2020a; Freeman et al., 2020b).

Pernio (chilblains) is a dermatologic inflammatory manifestation of the superficial vasculature that occurs in response to cold. It exhibits as edema and erythema, sometimes with plaque formation, of affected fingers or toes; ulcerations are sometimes present. The unique perniolike acral manifestations of COVID-19, sometimes called *COVID toes*, are not related to cold/ambient temperature and are not believed to be caused by a vascular response. At the present time, researchers posit that its underlying cause may be idiopathic (unknown), or related to a simple inflammatory response, or related to a prothrombotic coagulopathy incited by the infection (Freeman et al., 2020a). Irrespective of the pathophysiologic mechanisms responsible for this phenomenon, the perniolike acral skin lesions apparently have a predilection for children and young adults rather than middle-aged or older adults with COVID-19. It more commonly affects the toes than the fingers, and in some instances, is the sole manifestation of SARS-CoV-2 infection (Freeman et al., 2020a; Freeman et al., 2020b). Furthermore, the infection tends to be mild and generally may be managed on an outpatient basis (see Chapter 19 for discussion of management of mild COVID-19). Based upon these observations, it is recommended that patients who are otherwise apparently healthy but who present with perniolike acral skin lesions should be tested for COVID-19, regardless of their history of COVID-19 exposure or the presence or absence of other symptoms suggestive of COVID-19 (Feldman & Freeman, 2020).

Fungal (Mycotic) Skin Infections

Fungi are eukaryotic microorganisms that belong to neither the plant nor the animal kingdoms. They are culprits in causing various common skin infections. In some cases, they affect only the skin and its appendages (hair and nails). In other cases, internal organs are involved, and the diseases may be life-threatening. However, superficial infections rarely cause even temporary disability and respond readily to treatment. Secondary infection with bacteria, *Candida*, or both organisms may occur.

The most common fungal skin infection is **tinea**, which is also called *ringworm* because of its characteristic appearance of a ring or rounded tunnel under the skin. Tinea infections affect the head, body, groin, feet, and nails (Sahoo & Mahajan, 2016). Table 56-6 summarizes the tinea infections and treatments.

To obtain a specimen for diagnosis, the lesion is cleaned and a scalpel or glass slide is used to remove scales from the margin of the lesion. The scales are dropped onto a slide to which potassium hydroxide has been added. The diagnosis is made by examination of the infected scales microscopically for spores and hyphae or by isolating the organism in culture. Under Wood's light, a specimen of infected hair appears fluorescent; this may be helpful in diagnosing some cases of tinea capitis (Sahoo & Mahajan, 2016).

Parasitic Skin Infestations

Parasitic skin infestations include those of the skin by lice (pediculosis) and the itch mite (scabies).

Pediculosis: Lice Infestation

Lice infestation affects people of all ages. Three varieties of lice infest humans: *Pediculus humanus capitis* (head louse), *Pediculus humanus corporis* (body louse), and *Pthiriasis pubis* (pubic louse or "crab"). Lice are called *ectoparasites* because they live on the outside of the host's body. They depend on the host for their nourishment, feeding on human blood several times a day. They inject their digestive juices and excrement into the skin, which causes severe itching (CDC, 2017).

Pediculosis Capitis

Pediculosis capitis is an infestation of the scalp by the head louse. The female louse lays her eggs (nits) close to the scalp. The nits become firmly attached to the hair shafts with a tenacious substance. The young lice hatch in about 6 to 9 days and reach maturity in 7 days. Head lice may be transmitted directly by physical contact or indirectly by infested combs, brushes, wigs, hats, helmets, and bedding (CDC, 2017).

Pediculosis Corporis and Pthiriasis Pubis

Pediculosis corporis is an infestation of the body by the body louse. This is a disease of those who live in close quarters. Pthiriasis pubis is extremely common. The infestation is generally localized in the genital region and is transmitted chiefly by sexual contact (Guenther & Maguiness, 2020).

Clinical Manifestations

Head lice are found most commonly along the back of the head and behind the ears. To the naked eye, the eggs look like

TABLE 56-6	Tinea (Ringworm) Infections	
Type and Location	**Clinical Manifestations**	**Treatment**
Tinea barbae (fungal infection of beard or moustache of men)	• Red, inflamed abscesslike lesions, pustules, or crusting • May develop secondary infection	• Griseofulvin for 4–6 wks or terbinafine for 2–4 wks • Shampoo beard or moustache twice weekly with selenium sulfide shampoo for 2 wks
Tinea capitis (scalp or eyebrows; contagious fungal infection of the hair shaft)	• Oval, scaling, erythematous patches • Small papules or pustules on the scalp or eyebrows • Brittle hair that breaks easily; patchy alopecia	• Griseofulvin for 4–6 wks or terbinafine for 2–4 wks • Shampoo hair or eyebrows twice weekly with selenium sulfide shampoo for 2 wks
Tinea corporis (body)	• Begins with red macule, which spreads to a ring of papules or vesicles with central clearing • Lesions found in clusters; many spread to the hair, scalp, or nails • Pruritis is a common complaint	• Local infections—topical antifungal creams once or twice daily (e.g., clotrimazole, econazole, ketoconazole) • Extensive infections or concomitant tinea capitis or immunosuppressive conditions (e.g., active neoplasms)—oral antifungal medications (e.g., fluconazole for 2–4 wks, itraconazole for 1 wk, terbinafine for 2 wks)
Tinea cruris (groin area; "jock itch")	• Begins with small, red scaling patches, which spread to form circular elevated plaques • Very pruritic • Clusters of pustules may be seen around borders	• Local infections—see treatment for tinea corporis • Extensive infections or concomitant tinea pedis or immunosuppressive conditions (e.g., active neoplasms)—see treatment for tinea corporis • Educate patients to avoid wearing clothing that is tight over the groin; patients should pat dry skin folds thoroughly (avoid rubbing) after bathing and use separate towels for groin and other body parts
Tinea pedis (foot; "athlete's foot")	• Soles of one or both feet have scaling and mild redness with maceration in the toe webs • More acute infections may have clusters of clear vesicles on dusky base	• Local infections—see treatment for tinea corporis • Extensive infections or concomitant tinea pedis or immunosuppressive conditions (e.g., active neoplasms)—see treatment for tinea corporis • Educate patients: • to put on socks before underwear to avoid cross-contamination to groin • to either dispose of old shoes or treat them with antifungal powder to prevent reinfection • to wear protective footwear at communal pools and tubs
Tinea unguium (toenails; onychomycosis)	• Nails thicken, crumble easily, and lack luster • Whole nail may be destroyed • If untreated, can result in pain, loss of balance, and candida infection	• Oral antifungal medications for 12 wks (e.g., itraconazole, terbinafine) with or without concomitant topical ciclopirox olamine nail lacquer • Nail avulsion may be indicated, either surgically or chemically using a 40–50% urea compound

Adapted from Handler, M. Z., Stephany, M. P., & Schwartz, R. A. (2020). Tinea capitis. *Medscape.* Retrieved on 10/12/2020 at: emedicine.medscape.com/article/1091351-overview; Robbins, C. M., & Elewski, B. E. (2020). Tinea pedis. *Medscape.* Retrieved on 10/12/2020 at: emedicine.medscape.com/article/1091684-overview; Schwartz, R. A., & Szepietowski, J. C. (2020). Tinea barbae. *Medscape.* Retrieved on 10/12/2020 at: emedicine.medscape.com/article/1091252-overview; Shukla, S., & Khachemoune, A. (2020). Tinea corporis. *Medscape.* Retrieved on 10/12/2020 at: emedicine.medscape.com/article/1091473-overview; Tosti, A. (2020). Onychomycosis. *Medscape.* Retrieved on 10/12/2020 at: emedicine.medscape.com/article/1105828-overview; Weiderkehr, M., & Schwartz, R. A. (2020). Tinea cruris. *Medscape.* Retrieved on 10/12/2020 at: emedicine.medscape.com/article/1091806-overview.

silvery, glistening oval bodies. The bite of the insect causes intense pruritus, and the resultant scratching often leads to secondary bacterial infection, such as impetigo or furunculosis. The infestation is more common in children and people with long hair (CDC, 2017).

With body lice, the areas of the skin that come in closest contact with the underclothing (i.e., neck, trunk, and thighs) are chiefly involved. The body louse lives primarily in the seams of underwear and clothing, to which it clings as it pierces the skin with its proboscis. Its bites cause characteristic minute hemorrhagic points. Widespread excoriation may appear as a result of intense pruritus and scratching, especially on the trunk and neck. Among the secondary lesions produced are parallel linear scratches and a slight degree of eczema. In long-standing cases, the skin may become thick, dry, and scaly, with dark pigmented areas (Dlugasch & Story, 2021).

Pruritus, particularly at night, is the most common symptom of lice infestation. Reddish-brown dust (i.e., excretions of the insects) may be found in the patient's underclothing. The pubic area should be examined with a magnifying glass for lice crawling down a hair shaft or nits cemented to the hair or at the junction with the skin. Infestation by pubic lice may coexist with sexually transmitted infections (STIs) such as gonorrhea, herpes, or syphilis. There may also be infestation of the hairs of the chest, axillae, beard, and eyelashes. Gray-blue macules may sometimes be seen on the trunk, thighs, and axillae as a result of either the reaction of the insects' saliva with bilirubin (converting it to biliverdin) or an excretion produced by the salivary glands of the louse (Guenther & Maguiness, 2020).

Medical Management

Treatment of head and pubic lice involves washing the hair with a shampoo containing pyrethrin compounds with piperonyl butoxide or rinsing with permethrin (CDC, 2019). The patient is instructed to shampoo the scalp and hair according to the product directions. After the hair is rinsed thoroughly, it is combed with a fine-toothed comb dipped in vinegar to remove any remaining nits or nit shells freed from the hair shafts. They are extremely difficult to remove and may have to be picked off one by one (CDC, 2019).

The patient with body lice is instructed to bathe with soap and water. Typically, no medications are indicated because the lice live on the patient's clothing. Topical medications used to treat head and pubic lice may be applied to the clothing, however, particularly in the seams of garments (see following discussion about general hygiene measures). If the eyelashes are involved, petrolatum may be thickly applied twice daily for 8 days, followed by mechanical removal of any remaining nits (CDC, 2019).

All articles of clothing, towels, and bedding that may have lice or nits should be washed in hot water—at least 54°C (130°F)—or dry-cleaned to prevent reinfestation. Upholstered furniture, rugs, and floors should be vacuumed frequently. Combs, brushes, and helmets are disinfected or discarded. All family members and close contacts are treated (CDC, 2019).

Complications, such as severe pruritus, pyoderma, and dermatitis, are treated with antipruritics, systemic antibiotics, and topical corticosteroids. Body lice can transmit epidemic rickettsial disease (e.g., epidemic typhus, relapsing fever, and trench fever) to humans. The causative organism may be in the gastrointestinal tract of the insect and may be excreted on the skin surface of the infested person (CDC, 2019).

Nursing Management

The nurse informs the patient that head lice may infest anyone and are not a sign of uncleanliness. Because the condition spreads rapidly, treatment must be started immediately. Epidemics among those living in close quarters (e.g., dormitories, military barracks, camps) may be managed by having everyone shampoo their hair on the same night. Cohabitants and family members should be warned not to share combs, brushes, and hats; they should be inspected for head lice daily for at least 2 weeks.

Treatment is necessary for all family members and sexual contacts of patients with body or pubic lice. The nurse educates them about personal hygiene and methods to prevent or control infestation. The patient and partner must also be scheduled for a diagnostic workup for coexisting STIs.

Scabies

Scabies is an infestation of the skin by the itch mite *Sarcoptes scabiei*. The disease is most commonly found in people living in substandard hygienic conditions and in people who are sexually active. People at increased risk include children, older adults, and those who are immune compromised. The mites frequently involve the fingers, and hand contact may produce infection (Cheng, Mzahim, Koenig, et al., 2020).

Clinical Manifestations

It takes approximately 4 weeks from the time of contact for the patient's symptoms to appear. The patient complains of severe itching caused by a delayed type of immunologic reaction to the mite or its fecal pellets. During examination, the patient is asked where the pruritus is most severe. A magnifying glass and a penlight are held at an oblique angle to the skin while a search is made for the small, raised burrows created by the mites. The burrows may be multiple, straight or wavy, brown or black, threadlike lesions, most commonly observed between the fingers and on the wrists. Other sites are the extensor surfaces of the elbows, the knees, the edges of the feet, the points of the elbows, around the nipples, in the axillary folds, under pendulous breasts, and in or near the groin or gluteal fold, penis, or scrotum. Red, pruritic eruptions usually appear between adjacent skin areas. However, the burrow is not always visible (Cheng et al., 2020).

One classic sign of scabies is the increased itching that occurs during the evening hours, perhaps because the increased warmth of the skin has a stimulating effect on the parasite. Hypersensitivity to the organism and its products of excretion also may contribute to the pruritus. If the infection has spread, other members of the family and close friends also complain of pruritus about 1 month later (Cheng et al., 2020).

Secondary lesions are quite common and include vesicles, papules, excoriations, and crusts. Bacterial superinfection may result from persistent excoriation of the burrows and papules (Cheng et al., 2020).

 Gerontologic Considerations

Older adult patients living in long-term care facilities are susceptible to outbreaks of scabies because of close living quarters, poor hygiene due to limited physical ability, and the potential for incidental spread of the organisms by staff members. The vivid inflammatory reaction seen in younger people seldom occurs; rather, the older adult may have peripheral sensory deficits and be less prone to scratch or may be physically unable to scratch. Scratching is an effective mechanism that partially eradicates mite infestation; thus, this results in a more severe subtype. The lesions crust over (causing "crusted scabies") and, in time, may become hyperkeratotic (Cheng et al., 2020).

Health care personnel in extended-care facilities should wear gloves when providing hands-on care to a patient suspected of having scabies until the diagnosis is confirmed and treatment is completed. It is advisable to treat all residents, staff, and families of patients at the same time to prevent reinfection. The scales that are present with crusted scabies must be removed so that the antiscabicidal medication may be effective. Crusts may be removed with warm water soaks followed by application of 5% salicylic acid in petrolatum cream (Cheng et al., 2020).

Assessment and Diagnostic Findings

The diagnosis is confirmed by recovering *S. scabiei* or the mites' byproducts from the skin. A sample of superficial epidermis is scraped from the top of the burrows or papules with a small scalpel blade. The scrapings are placed on a microscope slide and examined through a microscope at low power to demonstrate evidence of the mite (Cheng et al., 2020).

Medical Management

The patient is instructed to take a warm, soapy bath or shower to remove the scaling debris from the crusts and then to pat the skin dry thoroughly and allow it to cool. A prescription scabicide, 5% permethrin, is considered the medication of choice. It is applied thinly to the entire skin from the neck down, sparing only the face and scalp (which are not affected in scabies). The medication is left on for 12 to 24 hours, after which the patient is instructed to wash thoroughly. One application may be curative, but it is advisable to repeat the treatment for 1 week (Cheng et al., 2020).

Nursing Management

The patient should wear clean clothing and sleep between freshly laundered bed linens. All bedding and clothing should be washed in hot water and dried on the hot dryer cycle. If bed linens or clothing cannot be washed in hot water, dry cleaning is advised.

After treatment is completed, the patient may apply an ointment, such as a topical corticosteroid, to skin lesions because the scabicide may irritate the skin. The patient's hypersensitivity does not cease on destruction of the mites. Pruritus may continue for several weeks as a manifestation of hypersensitivity, particularly in people who are atopic (allergic). This is not a sign that the treatment has failed. The patient is instructed not to apply more scabicide, because it will cause more irritation and increased itching, and not to take frequent hot showers, because they can dry the skin and produce pruritus. Oral antihistamines such as diphenhydramine or hydroxyzine can help control the pruritus. If a secondary infection is present, treatment with oral antibiotic agents may be indicated (Cheng et al., 2020).

All family members and close contacts should be treated simultaneously to eliminate the mites. Some scabicides are approved for use in infants and pregnant women. If scabies is sexually transmitted, the patient may require treatment for coexisting STI. Scabies may also coexist with pediculosis.

NONINFECTIOUS INFLAMMATORY DERMATOSES

Noninfectious inflammatory dermatoses include dermatologic disorders such as irritant contact dermatitis, psoriasis, and generalized exfoliative dermatitis (also called *erythroderma*).

Irritant Contact Dermatitis

Contact dermatitis (also called *eczema*) is an inflammatory reaction of the skin to physical, chemical, or biologic agents. The epidermis is damaged by repeated physical and chemical irritations. Contact dermatitis may be of the primary irritant type, in which a nonallergic reaction results from exposure to an irritating substance, or it may be an allergic reaction resulting from exposure of sensitized people to contact allergens (see Chapter 33).

Common causes of irritant contact dermatitis are soaps, detergents, scouring compounds, and industrial chemicals. Predisposing factors include extremes of heat and cold, frequent contact with soap and water, and a preexisting skin disease. Persons at risk include those whose occupations require repeated handwashing (e.g., nurses) or repeated exposure to food or other irritants (e.g., food preparation workers, cleaners, hairdressers). Women tend to be affected more commonly than men (Goldner & Fransway, 2018).

Clinical Manifestations

The eruptions begin when the causative agent contacts the skin. The first reactions include pruritus, burning, and erythema, followed closely by edema, papules, vesicles, and oozing or weeping. In the subacute phase, these vesicular changes are less marked, and they occur alternatively with crusting, drying, fissuring, and peeling. If repeated reactions occur or if the patient continually scratches the skin, lichenification and pigmentation occur. Secondary bacterial invasion may follow (Goldner & Fransway, 2018).

Management

The objectives of management are to soothe and heal the involved skin and protect it from further damage. The distribution pattern of the reaction is identified to differentiate between allergic and irritant contact dermatitis. A detailed history is obtained. If possible, the offending irritant is removed. Local irritation should be avoided, and soap is not generally used until healing occurs.

Many preparations are advocated for relieving dermatitis. In general, a barrier cream that contains ceramide or dimethicone is used for small patches of erythema. A thin layer of cream or ointment containing a corticosteroid is commonly used, although the efficacy of corticosteroids has not been demonstrated in research (Goldner & Fransway, 2018). The patient is educated about how to treat and prevent future bouts of irritant contact dermatitis (Chart 56-4).

COVID-19 Considerations

The first known outbreak of COVID-19 began in Wuhan, China, in late 2019 and quickly spread through the province

---

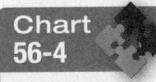

Chart 56-4

PATIENT EDUCATION

Strategies for Avoiding Irritant Contact Dermatitis

The precautions listed below may help prevent repeated cases of irritant contact dermatitis and should be followed for at least 4 months after skin appears to be completely healed.

The nurse instructs the patient to:

- Study the pattern and location of your dermatitis and think about which things have touched your skin and which things may have caused the problem; try to avoid contact with these materials.
- Avoid heat, soap, and rubbing, all of which are external irritants.
- Choose bath soaps, laundry detergents, and cosmetics that do not contain fragrance.
- Avoid using a fabric softener dryer sheet. Fabric softeners that are added to the washer may be used.
- Avoid topical medications, lotions, or ointments, except those specifically prescribed for your condition.
- Wash your skin thoroughly immediately after exposure to possible irritants.
- Ensure that when wearing gloves (such as for washing dishes or general cleaning), they are cotton lined. Do not wear them more than 15 or 20 minutes at a time.

Adapted from Goldner, R., & Fransway, A. F. (2018). Irritant contact dermatitis in adults. *UpToDate*. Retrieved on 10/12/2020 at: www.uptodate.com/contents/irritant-contact-dermatitis-in-adults

of Hubei. Working for long hours caring for patients with COVID-19, Hubei health care workers (HCWs), including nurses and physicians, wore PPE, such as N95 respirators, goggles, face shields, double gloves, and gowns, for extended hours (see Chapter 66 for discussion on PPE). In addition, HCWs spent more time than typical engaging in hand hygiene protocols. As a consequence of these practices that were aimed at protecting themselves and others from SARS-CoV-2 infection, many HCWs on the frontlines of the pandemic in Hubei reported high rates of irritant contact dermatitis. One study of 700 frontline HCWs reported an overall prevalence of irritant contact dermatitis of 97%, with 83.1% of HCWs reporting nasal bridge irritation, presumably from prolonged usage of N95 respirators and goggles (Lan, Song, Miao, et al., 2020). Another group of researchers found that among 61 frontline HCWs, 68.9% reported nasal bridge scarring. These same researchers reported that the incidence of adverse skin reactions to N95 respirators was 95.1%, to gloves 88.5%, and to other PPE 60.7% (Hu, Fan, Li, et al., 2020). In response to these reports, the AAD promulgated a white paper of guidelines that HCWs could adopt to avoid occupationally induced skin disorders during the COVID-19 pandemic. Key recommendations include the following (AAD, 2020):

- HCWs should use a moisturizer after engaging in hand hygiene. Continued hand moisturization when off work is also recommended in order to better protect the skin. Moisturizers that contain at least 5% petrolatum are most effective.
- If an HCW uses an N95 respirator that is irritating, the HCW should notify their respective safety officer and request an alternative N95 respirator that might be less irritating. If that is not possible, then a liquid skin sealant/protectant should be applied to the irritated area and dried before the mask is donned. Petrolatum should *not* be used as a protectant, however, as it can interfere with the seal of the mask.
- All HCWs who utilize PPE should keep their skin clean, dry, and well-moisturized. In particular, the face should be well-moisturized when off work. Cosmetics that include foundations and concealers should not be used. If skin moisturizers are applied, they should be applied at least one hour prior to donning PPE. Irritated areas, particularly the forehead, cheeks, and bridge of the nose, may be treated with petrolatum when off work.
- If masks must be reused, they should be thoroughly dry before they are donned a second time.

Psoriasis

Psoriasis is a chronic inflammatory multisystem disorder of the skin that affects approximately 3.2% of Americans (Nicpon, 2017). Although the primary manifestation of this noncommunicable disease tends to involve the skin, psoriasis may involve the oral cavity, eyes (including the lids, conjunctivae, and corneas), and joints. Psoriasis is typically characterized by the appearance of silvery plaques that most commonly appear on the skin over the elbows, knees, scalp, lower back, and buttocks (Habashy & Robles, 2019). Onset may occur at any age, with a median onset at 28 years. It is more prevalent among women and White Americans. It is thought that most patients with psoriasis have a genetic

predisposition to develop the disease. Psoriasis is characterized by periods of remission and exacerbation throughout life (Habashy & Robles, 2019).

Pathophysiology

Current evidence supports an autoimmune basis for psoriasis. Periods of emotional stress and anxiety aggravate the condition, and trauma, infections, and seasonal and hormonal changes may also serve as triggers (Habashy & Robles, 2019).

In this disease, the epidermis becomes infiltrated by activated T cells and cytokines, resulting in both vascular engorgement and proliferation of keratinocytes. Epidermal hyperplasia results. These epidermal cells tend to improperly retain their nuclei, crippling their ability to release lipids that encourage cellular adhesion. This results in rapid turnover of poorly matured cells that do not adhere well to each other, resulting in the classic presentation of plaquelike lesions that have a silvery, scaly, and flaky appearance (Habashy & Robles, 2019).

Clinical Manifestations

Psoriasis may range in severity from a cosmetic source of annoyance to a physically disabling and disfiguring disorder. Lesions appear as red, raised patches of skin covered with silvery scales. The scaly patches are formed by the buildup of living and dead skin (Fig. 56-7). If the scales are scraped away, the dark red base of the lesion is exposed, producing multiple bleeding points. The patches are not moist and may be pruritic. In many cases, the nails are also involved, with pitting, discoloration, crumbling beneath the free edges, and separation of the nail plate (Habashy & Robles, 2019). Psoriasis is classified as mild if the plaques involve less than 5% body surface area (BSA), moderate if they involve between 5% and 10% of BSA, and severe if more than 10% BSA is affected by plaque formation (Nicpon, 2017).

Complications

Asymmetric rheumatoid factor—negative arthritis of multiple joints occurs in up to 42% of people with psoriasis, most typically after the skin lesions appear (Nicpon, 2017). The

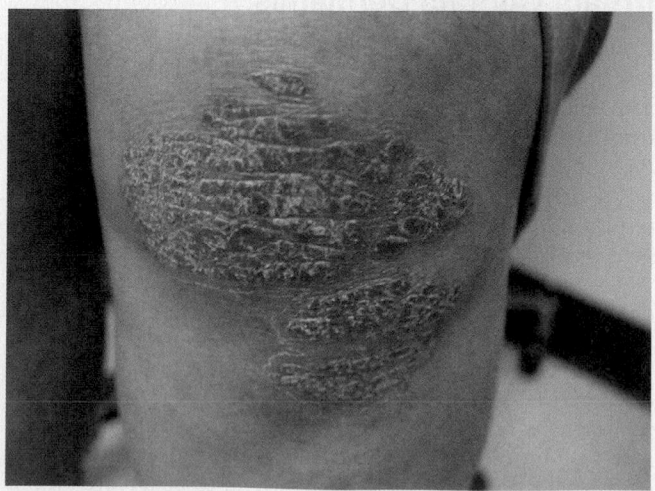

Figure 56-7 • Psoriasis.

most typical joints affected include those in the hands or feet, although sometimes larger joints such as the elbows, knees, or hips may be affected (Habashy & Robles, 2019). A rheumatologist should be consulted to assist in the diagnosis and long-term treatment of this disorder. See Chapter 34 for further discussion of spondyloarthropathies, including psoriatic arthritis. Generalized exfoliative dermatitis may also result from psoriasis (see discussion later in this chapter).

Assessment and Diagnostic Findings

The presence of the classic plaque-type lesions generally confirms the diagnosis of psoriasis. If in doubt, the health care provider should assess for signs of nail and scalp involvement and for a positive family history. Biopsy of the skin is of little diagnostic value. The presence and extent of plaque should be assessed carefully, to calculate BSA involvement.

Medical Management

The goals of management are to slow the rapid turnover of epidermis, to promote resolution of the psoriatic lesions, and to control the natural cycles of the disease. There is no known cure.

The therapeutic approach should be one that the patient understands; it should be cosmetically acceptable and minimally disruptive of lifestyle. Treatment involves the commitment of time and effort by the patient and possibly the family. Any precipitating or aggravating factors are addressed. An assessment is made of lifestyle because psoriasis is significantly affected by stress. Management of emotional factors should be addressed as part of the overall treatment of psoriasis. The patient is informed that treatment of severe psoriasis can be time-consuming, expensive, and aesthetically unappealing at times. Many patients report difficulty adhering to treatment plans, either for time reasons or lack of response to the treatment (Feldman, 2020).

Gentle removal of scales is an important principle of psoriasis treatment. This can be accomplished by taking baths with added oils (e.g., olive oil, mineral oil), colloidal oatmeal preparations, or coal tar preparations. A soft brush may be used to gently scrub the psoriatic plaques. After bathing, the application of emollient creams containing alpha-hydroxy acids or salicylic acid can soften thick scales. The patient and family should be encouraged to establish a regular skin care routine that can be maintained even when the psoriasis is not in an acute stage (Feldman, 2020).

Pharmacologic Therapy

Three types of therapy are commonly indicated: topical, phototherapy, and systemic. Topical agents, possibly in tandem with phototherapy, are recommended for mild disease. Patients with moderate or severe disease should receive topical agents, phototherapy, and systemic treatment (Nicpon, 2017).

Topical Agents

Topically applied agents are used to slow the overactive epidermis. Topical corticosteroids may be applied for their anti-inflammatory effects (see Table 56-3). Choosing the correct strength of corticosteroid for the involved site and choosing the most effective vehicle base are important aspects of topical treatment. In general, high-potency topical corticosteroids

should not be used on the face and intertriginous areas, and their use on other areas should be limited to a 4-week course of twice-daily applications. A 4-week break should be taken before repeating treatment with the high-potency corticosteroids. For long-term therapy, moderate-potency corticosteroids are used. On the face and intertriginous areas, only low-potency corticosteroids are appropriate for long-term use (Doughty & McNichol, 2016).

Occlusive dressings may be applied to increase the effectiveness of the corticosteroid. Large plastic bags may be used—one for the upper body with openings cut for the head and arms and one for the lower body with openings for the legs. Large rolls of tubular plastic can be used to cover the arms and legs. Another option is a vinyl jogging suit. The medication is applied, and the suit is put on over it. The hands can be wrapped in gloves, the feet in plastic bags, and the head in a shower cap. Occlusive dressings should not remain in place longer than 8 hours. The skin should be inspected carefully for the appearance of atrophy, hypopigmentation, striae, and telangiectasias—all of which are side effects of corticosteroids.

When psoriasis involves large areas of the body, topical corticosteroid treatment can be expensive and involve some systemic risk. The more potent corticosteroids, when applied to large areas of the body, have the potential to cause adrenal suppression through percutaneous absorption of the medication. In this event, other treatment modalities (e.g., nonsteroidal topical medications, UV light) may be used instead or in combination to decrease the need for corticosteroids (Doughty & McNichol, 2016).

Treatment with topical nonsteroidal agents, such as calcipotriene and tazarotene, can suppress **epidermopoiesis** (i.e., development of epidermal cells) and cause sloughing of the rapidly growing epidermal cells. Calcipotriene 0.05% is a derivative of vitamin D_2. It works by decreasing the mitotic turnover of the psoriatic plaques. Its most common side effect is local irritation. The intertriginous areas and face should be avoided when using this medication. The patient should be monitored for symptoms of hypercalcemia. Calcipotriene is available as a cream for use on the body and a solution for the scalp. It is not recommended for use by older adult patients because of their more fragile skin or by pregnant or lactating women (Feldman, 2020).

Tazarotene, a retinoid, causes sloughing of the scales covering psoriatic plaques. As with other retinoids, it causes increased sensitivity to sunlight by loss of the outermost layer of skin, so the patient should be cautioned to use an effective sunscreen and avoid other photosensitizers (e.g., tetracycline, antihistamines). Tazarotene is teratogenic, and the risk of use in pregnant women clearly outweighs any possible benefits. A negative result on a pregnancy test should be obtained before initiating this medication in women of childbearing age, and an effective contraceptive should be continued during treatment. Side effects include burning, erythema, or irritation at the site of application, and worsening of psoriasis (Feldman, 2020).

Intralesional injections of the corticosteroid triamcinolone can be given directly into highly visible or isolated patches of psoriasis that are resistant to other forms of therapy. Care must be taken to ensure that the medication is not injected into normal skin (Habashy & Robles, 2019).

Phototherapy

For patients who do not respond well to topical treatments, phototherapy using narrow-band ultraviolet-B (UVB) therapy may be effective as a single-therapy modality. However, phototherapy is generally more effective when it is given as ultraviolet-A (UVA) in conjunction with a photosensitizing oral medication (a combination referred to as PUVA). Here, the patient takes a photosensitizing medication (i.e., psoralen) in a standard dose and is subsequently exposed to long-wave UV light as the medication plasma levels peak. It is thought that when psoralen-treated skin is exposed to UVA light, the psoralen binds with DNA and decreases epidermal cellular proliferation. PUVA has been associated with long-term risks of skin cancer, cataracts, and premature aging of the skin (Habashy & Robles, 2019).

The patient is usually treated two or three times each week until the psoriasis clears. An interim period of 48 hours between treatments is necessary to allow any burns resulting from PUVA therapy to become evident. After the psoriasis clears, the patient begins a maintenance program. Once little or no disease is active, less potent therapies are used to keep minor flare-ups under control (Habashy & Robles, 2019).

Systemic Agents

Although systemic corticosteroids may cause rapid improvement of psoriasis, the usual risks and the possibility of triggering a severe flare-up on withdrawal limit their use; therefore, they are not indicated for treatment of psoriasis.

Methotrexate, a systemic cytotoxic agent, is the first-line drug for treating moderate to severe psoriasis (Nicpon, 2017). Methotrexate appears to inhibit DNA synthesis in epidermal cells, thereby reducing the turnover time of the psoriatic epidermis. However, the medication can be toxic, especially to the liver, kidneys, and bone marrow. Laboratory studies must be monitored to ensure that the hepatic, hematopoietic, and renal systems are functioning adequately. The patient should avoid drinking alcohol while taking methotrexate because alcohol ingestion increases the possibility of liver damage. The medication is teratogenic and thus should not be given to pregnant women.

Cyclosporine, a cyclic peptide immunosuppressive agent, may be considered in treatment of severe, therapy-resistant cases of psoriasis. However, its use is limited by side effects such as hypertension and nephrotoxicity and is only indicated for short-term use, generally no longer than 3 to 6 months (Habashy & Robles, 2019).

Another line of treatments for psoriasis includes a group called *biologic agents* because of their derivation from immunomodulators and bioengineered proteins (such as antibodies or recombinant cytokines) and their targeted action directly on the T cells. These agents act by inhibiting activation and migration, eliminating the T cells completely, slowing postsecretory cytokines or inducing immune deviation.

Infliximab is a monoclonal antibody that binds to tumor necrosis factor-alpha (TNF-α) and can only be given by IV infusion. Ustekinumab is also a monoclonal antibody that specifically interferes with the effect of interleukins (ILs), particularly IL-12 and IL-23. Etanercept is a fusion protein that binds with soluble TNF-α and blocks its interaction with the cell surface receptors. Alefacept is a fusion protein that inhibits T-cell proliferation. Adalimumab is a recombinant human immunoglobulin G1 (IgG1) monoclonal antibody against TNF-α. Secukinumab is a human IgG1 monoclonal antibody and ixekizumab is a humanized monoclonal IgG4 antibody; both of these agents neutralize the effects of the proinflammatory cytokine IL-17A and are administered subcutaneously. All of these biologic agents have significant side effects, making close monitoring essential (Habashy & Robles, 2019).

Nursing Management

Psoriasis may cause despair and frustration for the patient; observers may stare, comment, ask embarrassing questions, or even avoid the person. The disease can eventually exhaust the patient's resources, interfere with their job, and negatively affect many aspects of life.

The nurse assesses the impact of the disease on the patient and the coping strategies used for conducting normal activities and interactions with family and friends. Many patients need reassurance that the condition is not infectious, not a reflection of poor personal hygiene, and not skin cancer. The nurse can create an environment in which the patient feels comfortable discussing important quality of life issues related to their psychosocial and physical response to this chronic illness.

The nurse explains with sensitivity that although there is no cure for psoriasis and lifetime management is necessary, the condition can usually be controlled. The pathophysiology of psoriasis is reviewed, as are the factors that provoke it—irritation or injury to the skin (e.g., cut, abrasion, sunburn), current illness (e.g., pharyngeal streptococcal infection), and emotional stress. It is emphasized that repeated trauma to the skin and an unfavorable environment (e.g., cold) may exacerbate psoriasis. The patient is cautioned about taking any nonprescription medications because some may aggravate mild psoriasis. As well, the patient is advised to seek treatment from the same primary provider for any acute illnesses or chronic conditions to minimize chances of receiving prescriptions that may interfere with each other (Nicpon, 2017).

Reviewing and explaining the treatment regimen are essential to ensure adherence to the therapeutic regimen. For example, if the patient has a mild condition confined to localized areas, such as the elbows or knees, application of an emollient to maintain softness and minimize scaling may be all that is required. Most patients need a comprehensive plan of care that ranges from using topical medications and shampoos to more complex and lengthy treatment with systemic medications and photochemotherapy, such as PUVA therapy. Patient education materials that include a description of the therapy and specific guidelines are helpful but cannot replace face-to-face discussions (either in-person or online) of the treatment plan.

To avoid injuring the skin, the patient is advised not to pick at or scratch the affected areas. Measures to prevent dry skin are encouraged because dry skin worsens psoriasis. Too-frequent washing produces more soreness and scaling. Water should be warm, not hot, and the skin should be dried by patting with a towel rather than by rubbing. Emollients have a moisturizing effect, providing an occlusive film on the skin surface so that normal water loss through the skin is halted and allowing the trapped water to hydrate the stratum corneum. A bath oil or emollient cleansing agent can comfort sore and scaling skin. Softening the skin can prevent fissures.

A therapeutic relationship between health care professionals and the patient with psoriasis includes education and support. Introducing the patient to successful coping strategies used by others with psoriasis and making suggestions for reducing or coping with stressful situations at home, school, and work can facilitate a more positive outlook and acceptance of the chronicity of the disease.

Promoting Home, Community-Based, and Transitional Care

Educating Patients About Self-Care

Printed patient education materials may be provided to reinforce face-to-face discussions about treatment guidelines and other considerations. Patients using topical corticosteroid preparations repeatedly on the face and around the eyes should be aware that cataract development is possible. Strict guidelines for applying these medications should be emphasized, because overuse can result in skin atrophy, striae, and medication resistance.

PUVA, which is reserved for moderate to severe psoriasis, produces photosensitization. If exposure to the sun is unavoidable, the skin must be protected with sunscreen and clothing. Gray- or green-tinted wraparound sunglasses should be worn to protect the eyes during and after treatment, and ophthalmologic examinations should be performed on a regular basis (Nicpon, 2017).

If indicated, referral may be made to a mental health professional who can help to ease emotional strain and give support. Belonging to a support group may also help patients recognize that they are not alone in experiencing life adjustments in response to a visible, chronic disease. The National Psoriasis Foundation publishes periodic bulletins and reports about new and relevant developments in this condition (see Resources section).

Generalized Exfoliative Dermatitis

Generalized exfoliative dermatitis, also called *erythroderma*, is characterized by a scaling erythematous dermatitis that may involve more than 90% of the skin (César, Cruz, Mota, et al., 2016). Generalized exfoliative dermatitis has a variety of causes. It may occur as a result of a reactive process (e.g., drug allergy) or may be secondary to an underlying skin disease (e.g., psoriasis, contact dermatitis, atopic dermatitis) or a systemic disease (e.g., lymphoma, leukemia). The cause is idiopathic (i.e., unknown) in approximately 16% of cases (Kellen & Berlin, 2016; Umar & Kelly, 2019). Although generalized exfoliative dermatitis may occur at any age, it more commonly appears in those between the ages of 41 and 61 years. It occurs two to four times more commonly in men than in women (Kellen & Berlin, 2016).

Clinical Manifestations

This condition starts as a patchy or generalized erythematous eruption accompanied by fever, malaise, and chills. The skin color changes from pink to dark red. Afterward, the characteristic exfoliation (i.e., scaling) begins, usually in the form of thin flakes that leave the underlying skin smooth and red, with new scales forming as the older ones come off. It may be associated with chills, fever, prostration, and severe pruritus. There is a profound loss of stratum corneum (i.e., outermost layer of the skin), which causes capillary leakage, hypoalbuminemia, and negative nitrogen balance. Because of widespread dilation of cutaneous vessels, large amounts of body heat can be lost. Hair loss may accompany this disorder. The progression of these clinical manifestations varies, depending on the underlying cause. For instance, the progression from fever and scaling may be acute and progress over hours or a couple of days when generalized exfoliative dermatitis results from a drug reaction, or may be insidious and progress over weeks when it is secondary to a skin disease, such as psoriasis (Umar & Kelly, 2019).

Assessment and Diagnostic Findings

The presence of scaling erythematous dermatitis, particularly when it occurs in tandem with a known skin disease or a new prescription medication, increases the suspicion that generalized exfoliative dermatitis may be diagnosed. The patient frequently also presents with hypoalbuminemia and a negative nitrogen balance, as described previously, as well as an increased erythrocyte sedimentation rate that is consistent with an underlying acute inflammatory process. A skin biopsy is indicated, because it may confirm the underlying cause and diagnosis (Umar & Kelly, 2019).

Medical Management

The objectives of management are to discern and treat any underlying disorder, to maintain fluid and electrolyte balance, and to prevent infection. The treatment is individualized and supportive and should be initiated as soon as the condition is diagnosed.

The patient may be hospitalized. All medications that may be implicated are discontinued. A comfortable room temperature should be maintained because the patient does not have normal thermoregulatory control as a result of temperature fluctuations caused by vasodilation and evaporative water loss. Fluid and electrolyte balance must be maintained because there is considerable water and protein loss from the skin surface. Patients in a negative nitrogen balance may be prescribed enteral or parenteral therapy (Umar & Kelly, 2019) (see Chapters 39 and 41).

Nursing Management

Continual nursing assessment is carried out to prevent sepsis. The disrupted, erythematous, moist skin is susceptible to infection and becomes colonized with pathogenic organisms, which produce more inflammation. Antibiotic agents, which are prescribed if infection is present, are selected on the basis of culture and sensitivity.

Hypothermia may occur because of the increased blood flow in the skin, coupled with increased water loss through the skin, leads to heat loss by radiation, conduction, and evaporation. Changes in vital signs are closely monitored and reported. Intake and output are also closely monitored and reported if there is variance.

Topical therapy is used to provide symptomatic relief. Soothing baths, compresses, and lubrication with emollients are used to treat the extensive dermatitis. Topical corticosteroids are the mainstay of treatment (see Table 56-3). The patient is likely to be extremely irritable because of the severe pruritus; sedating antihistamines (e.g., hydroxyzine) administered before bedtime may be prescribed to relieve the itching and promote sleep (Umar & Kelly, 2019).

The use of oral or parenteral corticosteroids may be prescribed; however, their use is controversial. They are contraindicated when the cause of the condition is either not known or is suspected to be secondary to an underlying skin disease, such as psoriasis. When generalized exfoliative dermatitis occurs as a complication of psoriasis, systemic corticosteroids can exacerbate the condition (Umar & Kelly, 2019). When a specific cause is known, more specific therapy may be used. The patient is advised to avoid all irritants in the future, particularly medications that are known to cause the condition (Kellen & Berlin, 2016).

BLISTERING DISEASES

Blisters of the skin have many origins, including bacterial, fungal, or viral infections; allergic contact reactions; burns; metabolic disorders; and immunologically mediated (i.e., autoimmune) reactions. Some of these have been discussed previously (e.g., herpes simplex and zoster infections, contact dermatitis).

Immunoglobulin-mediated blistering skin diseases are referred to as *pemphigus* disorders. Of these, there are five subtypes. Three of these are immunoglobulin G (IgG)-mediated disorders, including pemphigus vulgaris, pemphigus foliaceus, and paraneoplastic pemphigus; the remaining two are immunoglobulin A (IgA)-mediated, and include subcorneal pustular dermatosis and intraepidermal neutrophilic dermatosis. Of these five pemphigus disorders, pemphigus vulgaris is the most common; the other four are relatively rare (Estupiñan & Sandhu, 2017; Hertl & Sitaru, 2020). Bullous pemphigoid, another type of IgG-mediated blistering disorder, has distinct characteristics that make this disease different from the pemphigus disorders. Dermatitis herpetiform is another nonpemphigus IgA-mediated blistering skin disorder that occurs as a consequence of gluten sensitivity. The diagnosis for all of these types of blistering skin disorders is made by immunofluorescent and histologic examination of a biopsy specimen (Hertl & Sitaru, 2020).

Pemphigus Vulgaris

Pemphigus vulgaris is characterized by the appearance of bullae of various sizes on apparently normal skin and mucous membranes. Pemphigus vulgaris is an autoimmune disease in which the IgG antibody is directed against a specific cell surface antigen in epidermal cells causing separation between the epidermis and dermis with subsequent blister formation (Doughty & McNichol, 2016). The blisters form from the antigen–antibody reaction. The level of serum antibody is predictive of disease severity. Genetic factors may also have a role in its development, with the highest incidence in people of Jewish or Mediterranean descent. This disorder usually occurs in men and women in middle and late adulthood (Hertl & Sitaru, 2020).

Assessment and Diagnostic Findings

Most patients present with oral lesions appearing as irregularly shaped erosions that are painful, bleed easily, and heal slowly. The skin bullae enlarge, rupture, and leave large, painful eroded areas that are accompanied by crusting and oozing. A characteristic odor emanates from the bullae and the exuding serum. There is blistering or sloughing of uninvolved skin when minimal pressure is applied (Nikolsky sign). The eroded skin heals slowly, and large areas of the body eventually are involved.

Specimens from the blister and surrounding skin demonstrate **acantholysis** (separation of epidermal cells from each other because of damage to or an abnormality of the intracellular substance), and immunofluorescent studies show intraepidermal presence of IgG (Doughty & McNichol, 2016).

The most common complications arise when the disease process is widespread. Skin bacteria have relatively easy access to the bullae as they ooze, rupture, and leave denuded areas exposed to the environment. Fluid and electrolyte imbalance results from fluid and protein loss as the bullae rupture.

Management

The goals of therapy are to bring the disease under control as rapidly as possible, to prevent loss of serum and the development of secondary infection, and to promote reepithelization (i.e., renewal of epithelial tissue).

Corticosteroids are given to control the disease and keep the skin free of blisters. The dosage level is maintained until remission is apparent. Immunosuppressive agents (e.g., azathioprine, mycophenolate mofetil) are prescribed early in the course of the disease to help control the disease and reduce the corticosteroid dose. The monoclonal antibody rituximab may be chosen as an alternative agent, as well as intravenous immunoglobulin (IVIG). The immunosuppressant agent cyclophosphamide may be tried when other medications fail to induce remission (Hertl & Geller, 2020; Kridin, 2018).

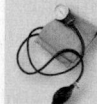

For the procedural guidelines for managing immunoglobulin therapy, go to **thepoint.lww. com/Brunner15e**.

Bullous Pemphigoid

Bullous pemphigoid is a chronic disease that is characterized by periodic flare-up and remission. If untreated, it may be fatal. It is most commonly seen in older adults, with a peak incidence at about 65 years of age. There is no gender or racial predilection, and the disease can be found throughout the world (Chan, 2018).

Assessment and Diagnostic Findings

Bullous pemphigoid is characterized most commonly by the general appearance of tense bullae that have a particular tendency to appear on the flexor surfaces of the arms. When the blisters break, the skin has shallow erosions that heal fairly quickly. Pruritus can be intense, even before the appearance of the blisters (Chan, 2018).

Immunofluorescent studies of skin biopsy specimens from patients with bullous pemphigoid reveal depositions of IgG and complement C3 at the junction of the dermis and epidermis (Chan, 2018).

Management

Medical treatment includes topical corticosteroids for localized eruptions and systemic anti-inflammatory or immunosuppressant medications for widespread involvement. Systemic corticosteroids (e.g., prednisone) may be continued for months, in alternative-day doses. The patient needs to understand the implications of long-term corticosteroid therapy (see Chapter 45). Tetracycline may be prescribed, although not for its antimicrobial effectiveness but because its anti-inflammatory properties are believed to be particularly efficacious in treating this disorder. Alternative medications may include immunosuppressive agents (e.g., azathioprine) or monoclonal antibodies (e.g., rituximab). Most patients will achieve remission, although this may require from 6 to 60 months of treatment (Chan, 2018).

Dermatitis Herpetiformis

Dermatitis herpetiformis is an intensely pruritic, chronic disease that manifests with small, tense blisters that are distributed over the extensor surfaces of the elbows and knees, as well as the buttocks and back. It most commonly occurs between 20 and 40 years of age but can appear at any age. It is more common in people of northern European heritage and is slightly more common in men. Patients with dermatitis herpetiformis have a defect in gluten metabolism; many have a concomitant diagnosis of celiac disease (Miller & Zaman, 2020).

Assessment and Diagnostic Findings

Patients typically present with erythematous papules with small, clustered (i.e., herpetiform) vesicles that tend to have a symmetrical distribution on affected extensor surfaces of the skin. Erosions and crusts may also be present, which may result from excoriation and scratching as a reaction to the intense pruritus (Miller & Zaman, 2020).

Immunofluorescent studies of skin biopsy specimens from patients with dermatitis herpetiformis reveal granular patterns of IgA deposits in the papillary dermis (Miller & Zaman, 2020).

Management

Most patients respond to dapsone and to a gluten-free diet. All patients should be screened for glucose-6-phosphate dehydrogenase deficiency because dapsone can induce severe hemolysis in those with this deficiency. Patients benefit from dietary counseling because the dietary restrictions are lifelong, and a gluten-free diet is often difficult to follow (see Chapter 41 for further discussion of gluten-free diets) (Miller & Zaman, 2020). Patients need emotional support as they deal with the process of learning new habits and accepting major changes in their lives.

NURSING PROCESS

Care of the Patient with a Blistering Disease

Assessment

Patients with blistering disorders may experience significant disability. There is constant itching and possible pain in the denuded areas of skin. There may be drainage from the denuded areas, which may be malodorous. Effective assessment and nursing management become a challenge.

Disease activity is monitored clinically by examining the skin for the appearance of new blisters. Particular attention is given to assessing for signs and symptoms of infection. Hyperpigmentation may be seen in areas of resolving blisters.

Diagnosis

NURSING DIAGNOSES

Based on the assessment data, major nursing diagnoses may include the following:

- Acute pain of skin and oral cavity associated with blistering and erosions
- Impaired skin integrity associated with ruptured bullae and denuded areas of the skin
- Disturbed body image associated with the appearance of the skin
- Risk for infection associated with loss of protective barrier of skin and mucous membranes
- Hypovolemia associated with loss of tissue fluids

Planning and Goals

The major goals for the patient may include relief of discomfort from lesions, skin healing, improved body image, absence of infection, and achievement of fluid and electrolyte balance.

Nursing Interventions

RELIEVING ORAL DISCOMFORT

Depending on the skin disorder, the patient's entire oral cavity may be affected with erosions and denuded surfaces. Necrotic tissue may develop over these areas, adding to the patient's discomfort and interfering with eating. Weight loss and hypoproteinemia may result. Meticulous oral hygiene is important to keep the oral mucosa clean and allow the epithelium to regenerate. Frequent rinsing of the mouth with chlorhexidine solution is prescribed to rid the mouth of debris and to soothe ulcerated areas. Commercial mouthwashes are avoided. The lips are kept moist with petrolatum. Cool mist therapy helps humidify environmental air.

ENHANCING SKIN INTEGRITY AND RELIEVING DISCOMFORT

The patient with painful and extensive lesions should be premedicated with analgesic agents before skin care is initiated. Patients with large areas of blistering have a characteristic odor that decreases when secondary infection is controlled. After the patient's skin is bathed, it is dried carefully. Tape should never be used because it may produce more blisters. Hypothermia is common, and measures to keep the patient warm and comfortable are priority nursing activities. The nursing management of patients with bullous skin conditions can be similar to that for patients with extensive burns (see Chapter 57).

PROMOTING A POSITIVE BODY IMAGE

Attention to the psychological needs of the patient requires listening to the patient, being available, providing expert nursing care, and educating the patient and the family. The patient is encouraged to express anxieties, discomfort, and feelings of hopelessness. Arranging for a family member or a close friend to spend more time with the patient, either live or via distance technology, can be supportive. When patients receive information about the disease and its treatment, uncertainty and anxiety often decrease, and the patient's capacity to act on their own behalf is enhanced. Psychological counseling may assist the patient in dealing with fears, anxiety, and promote positive self-esteem.

PREVENTING INFECTION

The patient is susceptible to infection because the barrier function of the skin is compromised. Bullae are also susceptible to infection, and sepsis may follow (see Chapter 11). The skin is cleaned to remove debris and dead skin and to prevent infection.

Secondary infection may be accompanied by an unpleasant odor from skin or oral lesions. *Candida albicans* of the mouth (i.e., thrush) commonly affects patients receiving corticosteroid therapy. The oral cavity is inspected daily, and any changes are reported. Oral lesions are slow to heal.

> ### ▶ Quality and Safety Nursing Alert
>
> *Because infection is the leading cause of death in patients with blistering diseases, meticulous assessment for signs and symptoms of local and systemic infection is required. Seemingly trivial complaints or minimal changes are investigated because corticosteroids can mask or alter typical signs and symptoms of infection.*

The patient's vital signs are monitored, and temperature fluctuations are documented. The patient is observed for chills, and all secretions and excretions are monitored for changes suggesting infection. Results of culture and sensitivity tests are monitored. Antimicrobial agents are given as prescribed, and response to treatment is assessed. Health care personnel must perform effective hand hygiene and wear gloves.

In patients who are hospitalized, environmental contamination is reduced as much as possible. Isolation measures, standard precautions, and the use of appropriate PPE are warranted. See Chapter 32, Chart 32-5 for a description of standard precautions.

PROMOTING FLUID BALANCE

Extensive denudation of the skin leads to fluid and electrolyte imbalance because of significant loss of fluids and sodium chloride from the skin. This sodium chloride loss is responsible for many of the systemic symptoms associated with the disease and is treated by IV administration of saline solution.

A large amount of protein and blood is also lost from the denuded skin areas. Blood component therapy may be prescribed to maintain the blood volume, hemoglobin level, and plasma protein concentration. Serum albumin, protein, hemoglobin, and hematocrit values are monitored.

The patient is encouraged to maintain adequate oral fluid intake. Cool, nonirritating fluids are encouraged to maintain hydration. Small, frequent meals or snacks of high-protein, high-calorie foods (e.g., oral nutritional supplements, eggnog, milk shakes) help maintain nutritional status. Parenteral nutrition is considered if the patient cannot eat an adequate diet.

Evaluation

Expected patient outcomes may include:
1. Reports relief from pain of oral lesions
   a. Identifies therapies that reduce pain
   b. Uses mouthwashes and anesthetic or antiseptic aerosol mouth spray
   c. Drinks chilled fluids at 2-hour intervals
2. Achieves skin healing
   a. States purpose of therapeutic regimen
   b. Adheres to soaks and bath regimen
3. Reports body image has improved
   a. Verbalizes concerns about condition, self, and relationships with others
   b. Participates in self-care
4. Remains free of infections and sepsis
   a. Has cultures from bullae, skin, and orifices that are negative for pathogenic organisms
   b. Has no purulent drainage
   c. Shows signs that skin is clearing
   d. Has normal body temperature
5. Maintains fluid and electrolyte balance
   a. Keeps intake record to ensure adequate fluid intake and normal fluid and electrolyte balance
   b. Verbalizes the rationale for IV infusion therapy
   c. Has urine output that is greater than 400 mL daily
   d. Has serum chemistry and hemoglobin and hematocrit values within normal limits

Toxic Epidermal Necrolysis and Stevens–Johnson Syndrome

Toxic epidermal necrolysis and Stevens–Johnson syndrome are potentially fatal acute skin disorders characterized by widespread erythema and macule formation with blistering, resulting in epidermal detachment or sloughing and erosion formation. These diseases are believed to be one and the same but manifest along a spectrum of reactions, with toxic epidermal necrolysis being the most severe. The mortality rate from toxic epidermal necrolysis is estimated to be 25% to 35% and from Stevens–Johnson syndrome is 1% to 5% (Kellen & Berlin, 2016). Up to 75% of cases of toxic epidermal necrolysis and Stevens–Johnson syndrome are triggered by a reaction to medications, with antibiotics (especially sulfonamides), anticonvulsants, NSAIDs, allopurinol, and oxicam NSAIDs (e.g., meloxicam) frequently implicated (Kellen & Berlin, 2016).

Toxic epidermal necrolysis and Stevens–Johnson syndrome occur in all ages and have a slight predilection for women. The mean age for patients with toxic epidermal necrolysis and Stevens–Johnson syndrome is reported to be between 46 and 63 years. However, older adults who take multiple medications may be at greater risk. There appears to be a genetic component to developing toxic epidermal necrolysis and Stevens–Johnson syndrome. The mechanism leading to toxic epidermal necrolysis and Stevens–Johnson syndrome seems to be a cell-mediated cytotoxic reaction (Cohen, Jellinek, & Schwartz, 2018).

Clinical Manifestations

Toxic epidermal necrolysis and Stevens–Johnson syndrome are characterized initially by conjunctival burning or itching, cutaneous tenderness, fever, cough, sore throat, headache, extreme malaise, and myalgias (i.e., aches and pains). These signs are followed by a rapid onset of erythema involving much of the skin surface and mucous membranes, including the oral mucosa, conjunctiva, and genitalia. In severe cases of mucosal involvement, there may be danger of damage to the larynx, bronchi, and esophagus from ulcerations. Large, flaccid bullae develop in some areas; in other areas, large sheets of epidermis are shed, exposing the underlying dermis. Fingernails, toenails, eyebrows, and eyelashes may be shed along with the surrounding epidermis. The skin is excruciatingly tender, and the loss of skin leaves a weeping surface similar to that of a total-body, partial-thickness burn (Cohen et al., 2018; Kellen & Berlin, 2016).

Complications

Keratoconjunctivitis, sepsis, and multiple organ dysfunction syndrome (MODS) are potential complications of toxic epidermal necrolysis and Stevens–Johnson syndrome. Keratoconjunctivitis can impair vision and result in conjunctival retraction, scarring, and corneal lesions. Sepsis and MODS can be life-threatening (Cohen et al., 2018; Kellen & Berlin, 2016) (see Chapter 11).

Assessment and Diagnostic Findings

Histologic studies of frozen skin cells from a fresh lesion and cytodiagnosis of collections of cellular material from a freshly denuded area are conducted. A history of the use of medications known to precipitate toxic epidermal necrolysis or Stevens–Johnson syndrome may confirm medication reaction as the underlying cause, especially if the medications were prescribed within 4 weeks prior to the onset of illness (Cohen et al., 2018).

Results from a complete blood count (CBC) may show leukopenia and a normochromic normocytic anemia. Skin biopsy results confirm the diagnosis, showing necrotic keratinocytes with full-thickness epithelial necrosis and detachment (Cohen et al., 2018).

Medical Management

The goals of treatment include control of fluid and electrolyte balance, prevention of sepsis, and prevention of ophthalmic complications. Supportive care is the mainstay of treatment.

Any medications that may be implicated as precipitating toxic epidermal necrolysis or Stevens–Johnson syndrome are discontinued immediately. The patient is treated in a regional burn center because aggressive treatment similar to that for severe burns is required. Tissue samples from the nasopharynx, eyes, ears, blood, urine, skin, and unruptured blisters are obtained for culture to identify pathogenic organisms. IV crystalloid fluids are prescribed to maintain fluid and electrolyte balance, using parameters similar to those used to guide care of patients with burns. Similarly, thermoregulation, wound care,

and pain management guidelines used to treat patients with burns are also implemented (Cohen et al., 2018) (see Chapter 57). Patients frequently require nutritional and metabolic support with total parenteral nutrition (see Chapter 41).

Initial treatment with systemic corticosteroids (e.g., methylprednisolone), although frequently tried, remains controversial. In many cases, the risk of infection, fluid and electrolyte imbalance, delayed healing, and difficulty in initiating oral corticosteroids early in the course of the disease outweigh its benefits. Administration of IVIG may provide rapid improvement and skin healing at dosages of 1 g/kg/day for 4 days. Other medications that may be effective include the immunosuppressive agents cyclosporine or cyclophosphamide (Cohen et al., 2018; Kellen & Berlin, 2016).

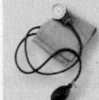

For the procedural guidelines for managing immunoglobulin therapy, go to **thepoint.lww.com/Brunner15e**.

Protecting the skin with topical agents is crucial. Various topical antibacterial and anesthetic agents are used to prevent wound sepsis and to assist with pain management. Temporary biologic dressings (e.g., pigskin, amniotic membrane) or plastic semipermeable dressings (e.g., Vigilon™) may be used to reduce pain, decrease evaporation, and prevent secondary infection until the epithelium regenerates. Meticulous oropharyngeal and eye care is essential when there is involvement of the mucous membranes and the eyes.

NURSING PROCESS

Care of the Patient with Toxic Epidermal Necrolysis or Stevens–Johnson Syndrome

Assessment

A careful inspection of the skin is made, including its appearance and the extent of involvement. The normal skin is closely observed to determine if new areas of blisters are developing. Drainage from blisters is monitored for amount, color, and odor. The oral cavity is inspected daily for blistering and erosive lesions; the patient is assessed daily for itching, burning, and dryness of the eyes. The patient's ability to swallow and drink fluids, as well as speak normally, is determined.

The patient's vital signs are monitored, and special attention is given to the presence and character of fever and the respiratory rate, depth, rhythm, and cough. The characteristics and amount of respiratory secretions are observed. Assessment for high fever, tachycardia, and extreme weakness and fatigue is essential because these factors indicate the process of epidermal necrosis, increased metabolic needs, and possible gastrointestinal and respiratory mucosal sloughing. Urine volume, specific gravity, and color are monitored. The insertion sites of IV lines are inspected for signs of local infection. Body weight is recorded daily.

The patient is asked to describe fatigue and pain levels. An attempt is made to evaluate the patient's level of anxiety. The patient's basic coping mechanisms are assessed, and effective coping strategies are identified.

Diagnosis

NURSING DIAGNOSES

Based on the assessment data, major nursing diagnoses may include the following:

- Impaired tissue integrity (i.e., oral, eye, and skin) associated with epidermal shedding
- Hypovolemia associated with loss of fluids from denuded skin
- Risk for hypothermia associated with heat loss secondary to skin loss
- Acute pain associated with denuded skin and oral lesions
- Anxiety associated with the physical appearance of the skin and prognosis

COLLABORATIVE PROBLEMS/POTENTIAL COMPLICATIONS

Potential complications may include the following:

- Sepsis
- Conjunctival retraction, scars, and corneal lesions

Planning and Goals

The major goals for the patient may include skin and oral tissue healing, fluid balance, prevention of heat loss, relief of pain, reduced anxiety, and absence of complications.

Nursing Interventions

MAINTAINING SKIN AND MUCOUS MEMBRANE INTEGRITY

The local care of the skin is an important area of nursing management. The skin denudes easily, especially when the patient is lifted and turned. The nursing staff must take special care to avoid friction involving the skin when moving the patient in bed. The skin should be checked after each position change to ensure that no new denuded areas have appeared. The nurse applies the prescribed topical agents to reduce the bacterial population of the wound surface. Warm compresses, if prescribed, should be applied gently to denuded areas. The topical antibacterial agent may be used in conjunction with hydrotherapy in a tank, bathtub, or shower. The nurse monitors the patient's condition during the treatment and encourages the patient to exercise the extremities during hydrotherapy.

The painful oral lesions make oral hygiene difficult. Careful oral hygiene is performed to keep the oral mucosa clean. Prescribed chlorhexidine mouthwashes, anesthetics, or coating agents are used frequently to rid the mouth of debris, soothe ulcerative areas, and control foul mouth odor. The oral cavity is inspected several times each day, and any changes are documented and reported. Petrolatum or a prescribed ointment is applied to the lips.

ATTAINING FLUID BALANCE

The patient's vital signs, urine output, and mental status are assessed for indications of hypovolemia. Mental changes from fluid and electrolyte imbalance, sensory overload, or sensory deprivation may occur. Laboratory test results are evaluated, and abnormal results are reported. The patient is weighed daily.

Oral lesions may result in dysphagia, making tube feeding or parenteral nutrition necessary until oral ingestion can be tolerated. A daily calorie count and accurate recording of all intake and output are essential.

PREVENTING HYPOTHERMIA

The patient with toxic epidermal necrolysis is prone to chilling. Dehydration may be made worse by exposing the denuded skin to a continuous current of warm air. The patient is usually sensitive to changes in room temperature. Measures similar to those implemented for a patient with burns, such as cotton blankets, ceiling-mounted heat lamps, and heat shields, are useful in maintaining body temperature. To minimize shivering and heat loss, the nurse should work rapidly and efficiently when large wounds are exposed for wound care. The patient's temperature is monitored frequently.

RELIEVING PAIN

The nurse assesses the patient's pain, its characteristics, factors that influence the pain, and the patient's behavioral responses. Prescribed analgesic agents are given on a regular schedule, and the nurse documents pain relief and any side effects. Analgesics are given before painful treatments are performed. Providing thorough explanations and speaking calmly to the patient during treatments can allay the anxiety that may intensify pain. Offering emotional support and reassurance and implementing measures that promote rest and sleep are basic in achieving pain control. As the pain diminishes and the patient has more physical and emotional energy, the nurse may educate the patient in self-management techniques for pain relief, such as progressive muscle relaxation and imagery (see Chapter 9).

REDUCING ANXIETY

Because the lifestyle of the patient with toxic epidermal necrolysis or Stevens–Johnson syndrome has been abruptly changed to one of complete dependence, an assessment of their emotional state may reveal anxiety, depression, and fear of dying. The patient can be reassured that these reactions are normal. The patient also needs nursing support, honest communication, and hope that the situation can improve. The patient is encouraged to express their feelings. Listening to the patient's concerns and being readily available with skillful and compassionate care are important anxiety-relieving interventions. Emotional support by a psychiatric nurse, spiritual advisor, psychologist, or psychiatrist may be helpful to promote coping during the long recovery period.

MONITORING AND MANAGING POTENTIAL COMPLICATIONS

Sepsis. The major cause of death from toxic epidermal necrolysis is from sepsis. Monitoring vital signs closely and noticing changes in respiratory, kidney, and gastrointestinal function may quickly detect the beginning of an infection. Strict asepsis is always maintained during routine skin care measures. Hand hygiene and wearing sterile gloves when carrying out procedures are essential. Visitors should wear protective garments and wash their hands before and after coming into contact with the patient. People with any infections or infectious disease should not visit the patient until they are no longer a danger to the patient. The nurse is critical in identifying early signs and symptoms of infection and notifying the primary provider. Antibiotic agents are not generally begun until there are signs and symptoms of an infection (Cohen et al., 2018).

Conjunctival Retraction, Scars, and Corneal Lesions. The eyes are inspected daily for signs of pruritus, burning, and dryness, which may indicate progression to keratoconjunctivitis—the principal eye complication. Applying a cool, damp cloth over the eyes may relieve burning sensations. The eyes are kept clean and observed for signs of discharge or discomfort, and the progression of symptoms is documented and reported. Administering an eye lubricant, when prescribed, may alleviate dryness and prevent corneal abrasion. Using eye patches or reminding the patient to blink periodically may also counteract dryness. The patient is instructed to avoid rubbing the eyes or putting any medication into the eyes that has not been prescribed or recommended by the primary provider.

PROMOTING HOME, COMMUNITY-BASED, AND TRANSITIONAL CARE

Educating Patients About Self-Care. Patients with toxic epidermal necrolysis or Stevens–Johnson syndrome with involvement of large areas of the skin require care that is similar to that of patients with thermal burns. As the patient completes the acute inpatient stage of illness, the focus is directed toward rehabilitation and outpatient care or care in a rehabilitation center. The patient and family members are involved throughout this care and are instructed in the procedures, such as wound care and dressing changes, that will continue at home. The patient and family members are assisted in acquiring dressing supplies that will be needed at home.

The patient and family members are also provided with education about pain management; nutrition; measures to increase mobility; and prevention of complications, including prevention of infection. They are educated about the signs and symptoms of complications and instructed when to notify the health care provider. Written instructions are provided to the patient and family so that they can refer to this information when necessary (Trommel, Hofland, van Komen, et al., 2019).

Continuing and Transitional Care. Interdisciplinary follow-up care is imperative to ensure that the patient's progress continues. Some patients will require care in a rehabilitation center before returning home. Others will require outpatient physical and occupational therapy for an extended period. When the patient returns home, the home health nurse coordinates the care provided by the various members of the health care team (e.g., physician, physical therapist, occupational therapist, dietician). The nurse also monitors the patient's progress, provides ongoing assessment to identify complications, and monitors the patient's adherence to the plan of care. The patient's adaptation to the home care environment and the patient's and family's needs for support and assistance are also assessed. Referrals to community agencies are made as appropriate (Trommel et al., 2019).

Evaluation

Expected patient outcomes may include:
1. Achieves increasing skin and oral tissue healing
   a. Demonstrates areas of healing skin
   b. Swallows fluids and speaks clearly
2. Attains fluid balance
   a. Demonstrates laboratory values within normal ranges
   b. Maintains urine volume and specific gravity within acceptable range
   c. Shows stable vital signs
   d. Increases intake of oral fluids without discomfort
   e. Maintains weight or gains weight, if appropriate

3. Attains thermoregulation
   a. Registers body temperature within normal range
   b. Reports no chills
4. Achieves pain relief
   a. Uses analgesic agents as prescribed
   b. Applies self-management techniques for relief of pain
5. Reports less anxiety
   a. Discusses concerns freely
   b. Sleeps for progressively longer periods
6. Absence of complications, such as sepsis and impaired vision
   a. Has body temperature within normal range
   b. Demonstrates laboratory values within normal ranges
   c. Has no abnormal discharges or signs of infection
   d. Continues to see objects at baseline acuity level
   e. Shows no signs of keratoconjunctivitis

SKIN TUMORS

Tumors of the skin are common and occur along a spectrum from those that are benign to those that are highly malignant.

Benign Skin Tumors

Cysts

Cysts of the skin are epithelium-lined cavities that contain fluid or solid material. Epidermal cysts (epidermoid cysts) occur frequently and may be described as slow-growing, firm, elevated tumors found most frequently on the face, neck, upper chest, and back. Surgical removal with biopsy of the cyst is typically performed (Docik, Johnson, & Rizk, 2019).

Trichilemmal or pilar cysts are most frequently found on the scalp. They originate from the middle portion of the hair follicle and from the cells of the outer hair root sheath. Treatment is surgical removal (Al Aboud, Yarrarapu, & Patel, 2020).

Seborrheic and Actinic Keratoses

Seborrheic keratoses are benign, wartlike lesions of various sizes and colors, ranging from light tan to black. They are usually located on the face, shoulders, chest, and back and are the most common skin tumors seen in middle-aged and older adults. Although these lesions are benign, they should be assessed periodically for changes in appearance that may suggest malignant transformation (see later discussion) (Norris, 2019). They may be cosmetically unacceptable to the patient. Treatment is removal of the tumor tissue by excision, electrodesiccation (destruction of the skin lesions by monopolar high-frequency electric current) and curettage, or application of carbon dioxide or liquid nitrogen.

Actinic keratoses are premalignant skin lesions that develop in chronically sun-exposed areas of the body. They appear as rough, scaly patches with underlying erythema. These lesions may gradually transform into squamous cell carcinoma (see later discussion); they are usually removed by cryotherapy, electrodesiccation, or lasers, or they may be treated with topical chemotherapeutic creams (e.g., 5-fluoro-uracil cream) (Doughty & McNichol, 2016).

Verrucae: Warts

Warts are common, benign skin tumors caused by infection with the human papillomavirus, which belongs to the DNA virus group. People of all ages may be affected, but the warts occur most frequently between the ages of 12 and 16 years. There are many types of warts.

As a rule, warts are asymptomatic, except when they occur on weight-bearing areas, such as the soles of the feet. They may be treated with locally applied laser therapy, liquid nitrogen, salicylic acid plasters, or electrodesiccation (Dlugasch & Story, 2021).

Warts occurring on the genitalia and perianal areas are known as condylomata acuminata. They may be transmitted sexually and are treated with liquid nitrogen, cryosurgery, electrosurgery, topically applied trichloroacetic acid, and curettage. Condylomata that affect the uterine cervix predispose the patient to cervical cancer (see Chapter 51).

Angiomas

Angiomas are benign vascular tumors that involve the skin and the subcutaneous tissues. They are present at birth and may occur as flat, violet-red patches (port-wine angiomas) or as raised, bright red, nodular lesions (i.e., hemangiomas of infancy, formerly known as strawberry angiomas). The latter tend to involute spontaneously within the first few years of life, but port-wine angiomas usually persist indefinitely. Most patients use masking cosmetics to camouflage the lesions. Cherry angiomas are small, smooth deep red papules found on the trunk of most adults older than 30 years of age that are benign and generally not considered cosmetically problematic (Norris, 2019).

Pigmented Nevi: Moles

Moles are common skin tumors of various sizes and shades, ranging from yellowish brown to black. They may be flat, macular lesions or elevated papules or nodules that occasionally contain hair. Most pigmented nevi are harmless lesions. However, in rare cases, malignant changes occur, and a melanoma develops at the site of the nevus. Nevi that show a change in color or size, become symptomatic (e.g., itch), or develop irregular borders should be removed to determine if malignant changes have occurred. Moles that occur in unusual places should be examined carefully for any irregularity and for notching of the border and variation in color. Nevi larger than 6 mm should be examined carefully. Excised nevi should be examined histologically (Hunt, Schaffer, & Bolognia, 2020).

Keloids

Keloids are benign overgrowths of fibrous tissue at the site of a scar or trauma. They are more common among people with dark skin. Keloids are asymptomatic but may cause disfigurement and cosmetic concerns. Treatment may consist of surgical excision, intralesional corticosteroid therapy or chemotherapy, laser therapy, or radiation (Doughty & McNichol, 2016).

Dermatofibroma

A dermatofibroma is a common, benign tumor of connective tissue that occurs predominantly on the lower extremities. It is a firm, dome-shaped nodule that may be of the same color as the patient's skin, or may present in a variety of colors, most commonly pink or brown. Treatment is not typically indicated, unless the patient finds it cosmetically unappealing. The tumor may be removed surgically, although scarring can occur. If the tumor is prominently raised, liquid nitrogen application may be a better option for treatment (Goldstein & Goldstein, 2020).

Neurofibromatosis: Von Recklinghausen Disease

Neurofibromatosis is an autosomal dominant genetic disorder manifested by *café-au-lait* macules (pigmented patches), axillary and inguinal freckling, cutaneous neurofibromas (soft, fleshy, benign skin tumors), and peripheral neurofibromas (benign peripheral nerve sheath tumors) that vary in size. Patients with neurofibromatosis are at risk for developing other benign and malignant tumors (e.g., sarcomas, astrocytomas) (Korf, Lobbous, & Metrock, 2020).

Malignant Skin Tumors

Skin cancer is the most common cancer in the United States. Each year, more people are diagnosed with skin cancer than all other cancers combined. It is estimated that at least one in five Americans will have skin cancer by age 70. The cost of treating Americans with skin cancers is estimated at $8.1 billion annually (Skin Cancer Foundation, 2020a). Because the skin is easily inspected, skin cancer is readily seen and detected and is therefore believed to be amenable to early intervention.

Exposure to UV radiation, including the sun and artificial UV rays (e.g., tanning booths) is the leading preventable cause of skin cancer; incidence is related to the total amount of exposure to UV radiation. Damage is cumulative, and harmful effects may be severe by 18 years of age (Skin Cancer Foundation, 2020a). Skin cancers in adults tend to manifest after a 20- to 50-year latency period post-UV radiation exposure (Bader, 2020) (Chart 56-5). Over 99% of all skin cancers include melanoma and the two most common types of nonmelanoma skin cancers, basal cell carcinoma and squamous cell carcinoma (American Cancer Society [ACS], 2020a).

Basal Cell Carcinoma and Squamous Cell Carcinoma

Basal cell carcinoma is the most prevalent skin cancer in the United States, responsible for 80% of all skin cancers in both men and women. It is rarely associated with any morbidity and rarely causes death. It is twice as common in men than women (Bader, 2020). Although less common than basal cell carcinoma, squamous cell carcinoma is the second most prevalent skin cancer in the United States. It is two to three times more common in men than women (Najjar, 2020). Although less aggressive than melanoma, squamous cell carcinoma is believed to be responsible for at least 15,000 deaths annually (Skin Cancer Foundation, 2020a).

Clinical Manifestations

Basal cell carcinoma generally appears on sun-exposed areas of the body, such as the face, neck, hands, and scalp. Basal cell carcinoma usually begins as a small, waxy nodule with rolled, translucent, pearly borders; telangiectatic vessels may be present. As it grows, it undergoes central ulceration and sometimes crusting (Fig. 56-8A). The tumors appear most frequently on the face. Basal cell carcinoma is characterized by invasion and erosion of contiguous (adjoining) tissues. It rarely metastasizes, but recurrence is common. However, a neglected lesion can result in the loss of a nose, an ear, or a lip. Other variants of basal cell carcinoma may appear as shiny, flat, gray, or yellowish plaques (Bader, 2020).

Squamous cell carcinoma is a malignant proliferation arising from the epidermis. Its precursor is typically actinic keratosis (see previous discussion). Although it usually appears on sun-damaged skin, it may arise from normal skin or from preexisting skin lesions. It is of greater concern than basal cell carcinoma because it is an invasive carcinoma, metastasizing in 4% to 8% of cases by the blood or lymphatic system (Najjar, 2020).

Squamous cell carcinoma appears as a rough, thickened, scaly tumor that may be asymptomatic or may bleed (Fig. 56-8B). The border of a squamous cell carcinoma lesion may be wider, more infiltrated, and more inflammatory than that of a basal cell carcinoma lesion. Secondary infection can occur. Exposed areas, especially of the upper extremities and of the face, lower lip, ears, nose, and forehead, are common sites (Najjar, 2020). The prognosis for squamous cell carcinoma depends on the incidence of metastases, which is related to the histologic type and the level or depth of invasion. Regional lymph nodes should be evaluated for metastases (Najjar, 2020).

Medical Management

The goal of treatment is to eradicate the tumor. The treatment method depends on the tumor location; the cell type, location, and depth; the cosmetic desires of the patient; the history of previous treatment; whether the tumor is invasive; and whether metastatic nodes are present. Management of basal cell carcinoma and squamous cell carcinoma includes surgical excision, which may include Mohs micrographic surgery, electrosurgery, or cryosurgery. In patients who are not surgical candidates, alternatives such as radiation therapy, photodynamic therapy, or topical chemotherapeutic creams may be viable options (Bader, 2020).

Surgical Management

The main goal is to remove the tumor entirely. The best way to maintain cosmetic appearance is to place the incision properly along natural skin tension lines and natural anatomic body lines. In this way, scars are less noticeable. The size of the incision depends on the tumor size and location but usually involves a length-to-width ratio of 3:1.

The adequacy of the surgical excision is verified by microscopic evaluation of sections of the specimen. When the

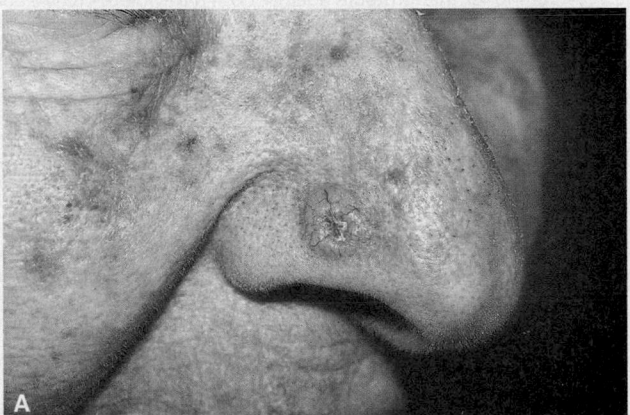
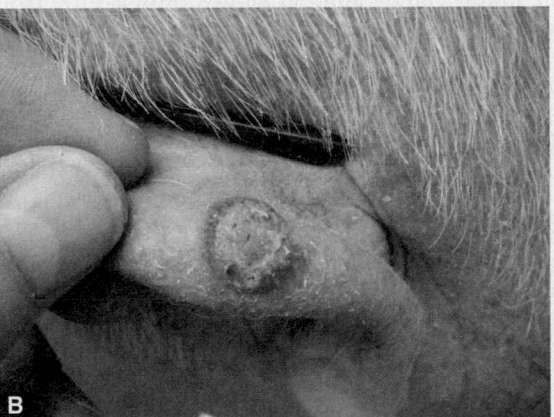

Figure 56-8 • Basal cell carcinoma (**A**) and squamous cell carcinoma (**B**). Reprinted with permission from Goodheart, H. P. (2011). *Goodheart's same-site differential diagnosis: A rapid method of diagnosing and treating common skin disorders*. Philadelphia, PA: Lippincott Williams & Wilkins.

tumor is large, reconstructive surgery with the use of a skin flap or skin grafting may be required. The incision is closed in layers to enhance cosmetic effect. A pressure dressing applied over the wound provides support. Infection after a simple excision is uncommon if proper surgical asepsis is maintained.

Mohs Micrographic Surgery

This technique is the most accurate surgical technique and best conserves normal tissue. The procedure removes the tumor layer by layer. The first layer excised includes all evident tumor and a small margin of normal-appearing tissue. The specimen is frozen and analyzed by section to determine if all of the tumor has been removed. If not, additional layers of tissue are shaved and examined until all tissue margins are tumor free. In this manner, only the tumor and a safe, normal tissue margin are removed. Mohs surgery is the recommended tissue-sparing procedure, with extremely high cure rates for basal cell carcinoma and squamous cell carcinoma. It is the treatment of choice and the most effective for tumors around the eyes, nose, upper lip, and auricular and periauricular areas (Najjar, 2020).

Electrosurgery

Electrosurgery is the destruction or removal of tissue by electrical energy. The current is converted to heat, which then passes to the tissue from a cold electrode. Electrosurgery may be preceded by curettage (excising the skin tumor by scraping its surface with a curette). Electrodesiccation is then implemented to achieve hemostasis and to destroy any viable malignant cells at the base of the wound or along its edges. Electrodesiccation and curettage is useful for lesions smaller than 1 to 2 cm (0.4 to 0.8 inch) in diameter.

This method takes advantage of the fact that the tumor is softer than the surrounding skin and therefore can be outlined by a curette, which "feels" the extent of the tumor. The tumor is removed and the base cauterized. The process is repeated twice. Usually, healing occurs within 1 month (Bader, 2020).

Cryosurgery

Cryosurgery destroys the tumor by deep-freezing the tissue. A thermocouple needle apparatus is inserted into the skin, and liquid nitrogen is directed to the center of the tumor until the tumor base is $-40°$ to $-60°C$ ($-40°$ to $-76°F$). Liquid nitrogen has the lowest boiling point of all cryogens, is inexpensive, and is easy to obtain. The tumor tissue is frozen, allowed to thaw, and then refrozen. The site thaws naturally and then becomes gelatinous and heals spontaneously. Swelling and edema follow the freezing. The appearance of the lesion varies. Normal healing, which may take 4 to 6 weeks, occurs faster in areas with a good blood supply (Bader, 2020).

Nonsurgical Alternative Therapies

Some older adult patients may defer surgical treatment options. Furthermore, in some cases, lesions may be extensive or are located on sites where wide surgical excision is not practical to achieve (e.g., cancer of the eyelid, tip of the nose). In these cases, local radiation therapy (see Chapter 12) or photodynamic therapy may prove reasonable alternatives. Photodynamic therapy involves application of 5-aminolevulinic acid to the lesion, which is then followed by photoactivation with directed blue light for approximately 1 hour. This has the effect of locally destroying the neoplastic cells, with good cosmetic results. Topical application of 5-fluorouracil cream (a chemotherapeutic agent) may be tried as another alternative to managing superficial basal cell carcinoma (Bader, 2020).

The patient should be informed that the skin may become red and blistered after any of these therapies. A bland skin ointment prescribed by the primary provider may be applied to relieve discomfort. The patient should also be cautioned to avoid exposure to the sun.

Nursing Management

Because many skin cancers are removed by excision, patients are usually treated in outpatient surgical units. The role of the nurse is to educate the patient about prevention of skin cancer (Chart 56-6) and self-care after treatment.

Promoting Home, Community-Based, and Transitional Care

 Educating Patients About Self-Care

The wound is usually covered with a dressing to protect the site from physical trauma, external irritants, and contaminants. The patient is advised when to report for a dressing change or is given written and verbal information on how to change dressings, including the type of dressing to purchase, how to remove dressings and apply fresh ones, and the importance of hand hygiene before and after the procedure.

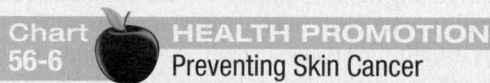

Chart 56-6 · **HEALTH PROMOTION**
Preventing Skin Cancer

Minimize sun exposure:

- To the extent possible, avoid sun between the hours of 10 AM and 4 PM.
- Wear protective clothing (e.g., long-sleeved clothing, broad-brimmed hats).
- Seek shady areas when outdoors.
- Wear sunglasses when outdoors to protect the sensitive skin around the eyes.
- Use caution around snow and water because of reflective sun rays.

Use sunscreen:

- Use a sunscreen with a sun protection factor (SPF) of 15 or higher that protects against both ultraviolet-A (UVA) and ultraviolet-B (UVB) rays.
- Apply generously 20 minutes prior to sun exposure (e.g., going outdoors).
- Reapply every 2 hours, or immediately after swimming.
- Use lip balm with SPF of 15 or higher.

Do not use artificial ultraviolet sources (e.g., tanning beds and booths).

Check your skin regularly:

- Perform self-examination monthly.
- Schedule an examination by primary provider yearly, if over the age of 50 years.

Strengthen your immune system:

- Do not smoke/quit smoking.

Adapted from American Cancer Society (ACS). (2019a). Can basal and squamous cell skin cancers be prevented? Retrieved on 4/5/2020 at: www.cancer.org/cancer/basal-and-squamous-cell-skin-cancer/causes-risks-prevention/prevention.html

The patient is advised to watch for excessive bleeding and tight dressings that compromise circulation. If the lesion is in the perioral area, the patient is instructed to drink liquids through a straw and limit talking and facial movement. Dental work should be avoided until the area is completely healed.

After the sutures are removed, an emollient cream may be used to help reduce dryness. Applying a sunscreen over the wound is advised to prevent postoperative hyperpigmentation if the patient spends time outdoors.

Follow-up examinations should be at regular intervals, usually every 3 months for a year, and should include palpation of the adjacent lymph nodes. The patient should also be instructed to seek treatment for any moles that are subject to repeated friction and irritation and to watch for indications of potential malignancy in moles as described previously. The importance of lifelong follow-up evaluations is emphasized.

Melanoma

A melanoma is a cancerous neoplasm characterized by neoplastic melanocytes present in the epidermis and the dermis (and sometimes the subcutaneous cells). Although melanoma only accounts for 1% of all skin cancers, it is responsible for approximately 6,850 deaths annually (Siegel, Miller, & Jemal, 2020). White Americans are 20 times more at risk for melanoma than Black Americans. It may strike adults of any age; however, the average age at diagnosis is 65 years. It is more prevalent among women than men younger than 50 years of age; by 65 years of age, it is twice as common among men than women and, by 80 years of age, is three times as common among men than women (Tan, 2020). Risk factors for melanoma are noted in Chart 56-5.

Clinical Manifestations

Melanoma may manifest as a change in a nevus or a new growth on the skin, arising from cutaneous epidermal melanocytes. A malignant melanoma is typically dark, red or blue colored, or a mix of any of these, and irregular in shape. It may be associated with itching, rapid growth, ulceration, or bleeding. This type of malignancy is found more frequently in the lower extremities in women, and in the trunk, neck, or head in men (National Cancer Institute [NCI], 2020). Rarely, melanomas may develop in the uveal tract of the eye or the mucosal lining of the gastrointestinal or genitourinary tract (Tan, 2020).

Melanoma can occur in one of the several forms: superficial spreading, lentigo maligna, nodular, acral lentiginous, mucosal lentiginous, desmoplastic, and verrucous melanoma (the last three are rarely seen) (Fig. 56-9). Each of these types have specific histologic features; however, the histologic features do not dictate treatment options and are not associated with differential prognoses (NCI, 2020).

Melanomas spread in two growth phases: radial and vertical. During the first growth phase—the radial phase—the tumor tends to spread radially within the epidermis. It is during this earlier phase of radial growth that the tumor is most amenable to treatment. The second growth phase—the vertical phase—is characterized by vertical tumor growth into

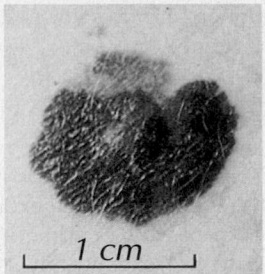 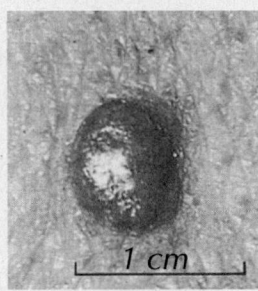

Figure 56-9 • Two forms of melanoma: superficial spreading (**left**) and nodular (**right**).

the dermal layer and eventual metastasis. Melanomas that progress more rapidly from the radial to the vertical growth phase are considered more aggressive types and have a poorer prognosis (Tan, 2020).

Assessment and Diagnostic Findings

Biopsy results confirm the diagnosis of melanoma. An excisional biopsy specimen provides information on the type, level of invasion, and thickness of the lesion. A specimen that includes a 1- to 2-cm margin of normal tissue and a portion of underlying subcutaneous fatty tissue is sufficient for staging a melanoma in situ or an early, noninvasive melanoma. Incisional biopsy should be performed when the suspicious lesion is too large to be removed safely without extensive scarring. Biopsy specimens obtained by shaving, curettage, or needle aspiration are not considered reliable histologic proof of disease (Tan, 2020).

A thorough history and physical examination should include a meticulous skin examination and palpation of regional lymph nodes that may drain the area surrounding the tumor. Because melanoma occurs in families, a positive family history of melanoma is investigated so that first-degree relatives, who may be at high risk for melanoma, can be evaluated for atypical lesions. After the diagnosis of melanoma has been confirmed, a chest x-ray, CBC, complete chemistry panel with creatinine, liver function tests, and lactate dehydrogenase (LDH) are usually performed. The LDH may be elevated in the presence of metastatic disease. Depending on the results of these tests, magnetic resonance imaging of the brain, computed tomography scans of the chest, abdomen, or pelvis, and positron emission tomography scans of the lymphatics may be indicated to further stage the extent of disease (Tan, 2020).

Staging of the tumor follows the TNM (tumor, nodes, metastasis) classification system (see Chapter 12) and is used to determine appropriate treatment (NCI, 2020):

- Stage 0: tumor in situ with only epidermal lesion
- Stage 1: tumor 2 mm thick or less without lymph node involvement or distant metastasis
- State 2: tumor more than 2 mm thick without lymph node involvement or distant metastasis
- Stage 3: tumor of any thickness with involvement of at least one lymph node but no distant metastasis
- Stage 4: tumor of any thickness, with or without lymph node involvement, and with distant metastasis

Patients with either stage 0 or stage 1 disease have a better than 99% likelihood of survival 5 years post diagnosis (ACS,

2019c). Early detection and treatment are thus key to ensuring good outcomes over the long term.

Medical Management

Treatment depends on the stage of the tumor and the tumor type. Surgical excision is the treatment of choice for small, superficial lesions. Deeper lesions require wide local excision, after which skin grafting may be necessary. Sentinel lymph node biopsy is commonly performed to examine the nodes nearest the tumor and to spare the patient the long-term sequelae of extensive removal of lymph nodes if the sampled nodes are negative. If these are positive, lymph node dissection may be indicated (Tan, 2020).

Patients with tumor cells present in multiple lymph nodes may benefit from radiation therapy to that chain of lymph nodes post dissection. It is thought that radiation therapy not only thwarts the recurrence of tumor cells within the lymphatics, but also improves the overall efficacy of checkpoint inhibitor therapy, a clear benefit for patients for whom that treatment is indicated (i.e., patients who are *BRAF* negative) (see following discussion) (NCI, 2020).

Patients with stage 2 tumors considered at risk for relapse were traditionally prescribed interferon alfa-2 therapy; however, long-term data did not support its therapeutic benefit. These patients tend to be managed with surgical excision only and then close ongoing monitoring for recurrence or metastasis (ACS, 2019c; NCI, 2020; Tan, 2020).

Patients with stage 3 and stage 4 tumors may be managed with intravenous checkpoint inhibitors, such as pembrolizumab, nivolumab, or ipilimumab. Checkpoint inhibitors enhance the action of T cells by inhibiting a specific "off" switch on their cellular surfaces, making them more effective in targeting and attacking cancer cells (ACS, 2019c; NCI, 2020; Tan, 2020). At least half of all patients with melanoma have a *BRAF* genetic mutation (NIC, 2020; Tan, 2020). These patients may be prescribed a *BRAF* inhibitor, to turn off the function of the *BRAF* mutation responsible for tumor growth. This therapy is typically prescribed along with an *MEK* inhibitor, as the *MEK* gene works in tandem with the *BRAF* mutation. This type of therapeutic regimen, called *targeted therapy*, may be prescribed in lieu of checkpoint inhibitors. Both *BRAF* inhibitors (dabrafenib, encorafenib, and vemurafenib) and *MEK* inhibitors (trametinib, cobemetinib, and binimetinib) may be administered orally. *BRAF* inhibitors are associated with an increased incidence of squamous cell carcinomas of the skin, however (NCI, 2020).

Patients who are diagnosed with melanoma are at high risk for a second melanoma or a recurrence of their primary tumor. Intralesional injection of an immunotherapeutic vaccine, talimogene laherparepvec, may be indicated in patients with recurrence of tumor that is considered nonresectable. Talimogene laherparepvec is a genetically modified oncolytic agent that is derived from herpes simplex-1 virus. Its use is associated with decreased tumor mass, although there is not an overall improvement in long-term survival (NCI, 2020).

Nursing Management

The best hope for decreasing the incidence of advanced melanoma lies in educating patients to recognize its early signs, when it is amenable to treatment and cure. The nurse educates patients at risk to examine their skin and scalp monthly in a systematic manner and to seek prompt medical attention if changes are detected. This is especially true for patients with a prior history of melanoma, as the likelihood of a second melanoma is higher than in patients without a personal history of having had melanoma (Tan, 2020). The AAD provides multimedia resources on performing skin self-examination (see the Resources section at the end of this chapter).

An important risk factor in the development of melanoma is exposure to UV radiation (e.g., sunlight). Irrespective of the presence or absence of other risks, all patients should be educated about the risks of UV radiation exposure and methods to mitigate that risk (e.g., sunscreen, shade). A group particularly at risk is young adult athletes, especially women (McGuffin, Jordan, Langford, et al., 2019; Orsimarsi, 2019). See the Nursing Research Profile in Chart 56-7.

The presence of nevi, particularly multiple nevi, is another risk factor for melanoma that should be addressed. The nurse educates patients with nevi how to self-assess for signs that may suggest malignant transformation, referred to as the *ABCDEs of Moles* (Chart 56-8). Evidence of these types of changes should be promptly reported to the patient's primary provider for further evaluation. Patients should also be on the alert for formation of the proverbial *Ugly Duckling* nevus, which may appear different from other nevi. In addition, reportable symptoms that may be consistent with a melanotic malignancy include pruritus, tenderness, and pain at the site of a nevus (Skin Care Foundation, 2020b).

The patient with a new diagnosis of advanced melanoma must be prepared for wide surgical excision. A melanoma may present on any skin surface, although they tend to appear on surfaces exposed to sun (e.g., extremities, head). Surgical removal of melanoma in different locations presents different challenges, taking into consideration the removal of the primary melanoma, and whether or not multiple sentinel lymph nodes evidence cancerous spread, necessitating lymph node dissection. A split- or full-thickness skin graft may be necessary when large defects are created by surgical removal of a melanoma (see Chapter 57 for further discussion of skin grafts). Nursing interventions after surgery for melanoma center on promoting comfort, including anticipating the need for and administration of appropriate analgesic medications (see Chapter 9).

Psychological support is essential when surgery that might be disfiguring is performed (Chart 56-9). Support includes encouraging the patient to express anxieties and feelings about the seriousness of the neoplasm and conveying understanding of these feelings. During the diagnostic workup and staging of the depth, type, and extent of the tumor, the nurse answers questions, provides information, and helps clarify misconceptions. Learning that they have a melanoma can cause the patient considerable fear and anguish. Pointing out the patient's resources, past effective coping mechanisms, and social support systems helps the patient cope with the diagnosis and need for treatment and continuing follow-up. Family members should be included in all discussions to enable them to clarify information, ask questions that the patient might be reluctant to ask, and provide emotional support to the patient.

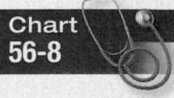

Chart 56-7 NURSING RESEARCH PROFILE
Sun Safety in Female College Athletes

McGuffin, K. S., Jordan, K., Langford, D., et al. (2019). Assessing knowledge, attitudes, and behaviors regarding sun safety in female collegiate athletes. *Journal of the Dermatology Nurses' Association*, *11*(1), 20–33.

Purpose

Melanoma is a common type of cancer among young adults, and its incidence has been rising for the past 30 years. Young adult athletes who compete in outdoor sports are at high risk for melanoma because they spend long hours exposed to ultraviolet (UV) radiation (i.e., sunlight) during games, matches, and practices. Young women are at greater risk for melanoma than young men, and frequently develop melanotic lesions in their extremities. Thus, women college athletes who compete in outdoor sports are especially at risk for melanoma, since their extremities are subjected to long–UV-radiation exposure. The purpose of this research study was to find if an education intervention would improve knowledge, attitudes, and behaviors on sun protection practices among female college athletes.

Design

The setting for this study was a public university in North Carolina. All varsity women athletes who competed in track, soccer, softball, tennis, and cross country were eligible and invited to participate, and all consented (N = 81). The researchers designed a brief 15-minute education intervention with PowerPoint™ images on sun safety practices, and delivered the intervention in a classroom setting in the university athletic offices. Participants took a pretest immediately prior to the intervention, which was a modified version of the Melanoma Risk Behavior Survey. The same survey was taken as the posttest immediately after the intervention was completed, and again 3 months after the intervention was completed. A paired *t*-test was done between the pretest and the posttests to determine whether or not there were improvements in knowledge, attitudes, and behaviors on sun safety practices among participants.

Findings

Participants' knowledge of sun safety significantly improved from pretest to the first posttest ($t = 15.232$, $p \leq 0.001$). This improvement was sustained from pretest to the second posttest 3 months post intervention ($t = 14.366$, $p \leq 0.001$). Moreover, 3 months postintervention, 79.1% of participants self-reported that they applied sunscreen more often than they had preintervention and experienced fewer sunburns post intervention; 91.6% affirmed that they would continue to engage in sun safety in the future.

Nursing Implications

On an anecdotal level, the researchers noted that many participants were surprised to learn of their melanoma risks. In particular, women athletes with dark skin did not see the need to use sunscreen and practice sun safety. While individuals with darker skin are at lesser risk of skin cancer than those with lighter skin, anyone afflicted with a sunburn has a higher risk of melanoma. This education intervention was concise and yet focused and ultimately, effective in its aim. It can be readily replicated in other college and high school settings. Future interventions could be delivered not only to the athletes, but also to their trainers and coaches, who could continue to encourage sun safety among young adult athletes.

Promoting Home, Community-Based, and Transitional Care

The patient with advanced melanoma will be prescribed either targeted therapy or a checkpoint inhibitor, depending upon the patient's *BRAF* status (see previous discussion). Because the agents that comprise targeted therapy for the patient who is *BRAF* positive may be administered orally, the patient can self-administer them at home, a key advantage. These agents

Chart 56-8 ASSESSMENT
Assessing the ABCDEs of Moles

Melanomas may be distinguished from benign nevi, using the following characteristics:

A for Asymmetry

- The lesion does not appear balanced on both sides. If an imaginary line was drawn down the middle, the two halves would not look alike.
- The lesion has an irregular surface with irregular topography (uneven elevations) either palpable or visible. A change in the surface may be noted from smooth to scaly.

B for Irregular Border

- Angular indentations or multiple notches appear in the border.
- The border is fuzzy or indistinct, as if rubbed with an eraser.

C for Variegated Color

- Benign moles are usually a uniform light to medium brown. Darker coloration indicates that the melanocytes have penetrated to a deeper layer of the dermis.

- Colors that may indicate malignancy if found together within a single lesion are shades of red, white, and blue; shades of blue are ominous.
- White areas within a pigmented lesion are suspicious.
- Some melanomas, however, are not variegated but are uniformly colored (bluish-black, bluish-gray, bluish-red).

D for Diameter

- A diameter >6 mm (about the size of a pencil eraser) is considered more suspicious, although this finding without other signs is not significant. Many benign skin growths are larger than 6 mm, whereas some early melanomas may be smaller.

E for Evolving

- Benign moles appear the same over time; when a mole starts to change in appearance, in size, shape, color, or elevation, it may suggest malignancy.

Adapted from Skin Cancer Foundation. (2020b). Warning signs: The ABCDEs of melanoma. Retrieved on 10/23/2020 at: www.skincancer.org/skin-cancer-information/melanoma/melanoma-warning-signs-and-images/#abcde

---

Chart 56-9 ETHICAL DILEMMA
Should Crowdfunding for Nonevidence–Based Therapies Be Permitted?

Case Scenario

You work as a nurse navigator in a surgical oncology clinic. O.G. is a 29-year-old woman who was referred to the clinic by her dermatologist for evaluation of a melanoma on her right upper arm. The surgical oncologist that examined O.G. wishes to perform a wide excision of her tumor with graft placement. You have an appointment set up with O.G. to coordinate her care between the surgical oncologist, a plastic surgeon (for the anticipated skin graft that will be performed after the tumor is excised), and a medical oncologist (for coordination of postoperative treatments). During your visit, O.G. states that she is reluctant to have the surgery since she believes it will be disfiguring. She tells you that her older sister was diagnosed with a melanoma 2 years ago that was successfully treated using black salve prescribed by a homeopathic physician in Mumbai, India. Although O.G. cannot afford to travel to India to pursue these treatments, her sister has offered to manage a GoFundMe™ site for her so that she might be able to pursue this option, which she finds more palatable than the treatment plan proposed by the surgical oncologist.

Discussion

Using social media to engage in crowdfunding, or online solicitation for donations, has become very popular over the past several years. Crowdfunding to solicit donations for medical procedures, therapies, or travel and other expenses related to pursuing medical treatment, is particularly commonplace. Bioethicists have criticized the use of medical crowdfunding for several reasons. Arguably, donors to crowdfunding platforms tend to favor people who seem more appealing or relatable, which can result in further widening of disparities in access to health care resources (causing a *distributive justice* dilemma). For instance, few people seeking donor support for obesity-related medical services are successful in raising funds on these sites, as persons with obesity may seem less appealing to some donors. Likewise, fewer people from ethnic minority groups tend to be successful in fundraising efforts than people who appear to be White and middle-class. Furthermore, not all people for whom funds are ostensibly raised may fully understand or consent to the setup of their fundraising platforms. These individuals may be coerced to do so by others, or lack the ability to fully comprehend what is being done on their behalf, or may be deceived by their fundraisers and not receive the funds raised for their relief.

Many patients with cancer use complementary and alternative medicine to assist them in managing the myriad of symptoms associated with cancer. Most patients use complementary and alternative therapies to complement mainstream medical treatments (i.e., allopathic medicine). However, some patients may elect to singularly pursue complementary and alternative therapy in lieu of evidence-based allopathic medical treatment. Crowdfunding can be used to try to finance these treatments, which are not covered by health insurance policies. Crowdfunding platforms have been criticized for not blocking the setup of these types of solicitations from their sites.

Analysis

- Describe the ethical principles that are in conflict in this case (see Chapter 1, Chart 1-7). Do you believe that O.G. has the right to determine what treatment options are best for her, even when the treatment option she chooses is not evidence-based? How would you assure your role to do what is in O.G.'s best interests without threatening her right to self-determination and without taking on a paternalistic tone (i.e., *I know what is best for you*)?

- How might family dynamics be affecting O.G.'s decision to pursue treatment options? It is not uncommon for patients with melanoma to have first-degree relatives who also have melanoma. How might O.G.'s relationship with her older sister, and her sister's previous treatment for melanoma, affect O.G.'s decision making now?

- What resources might you use to help you advocate for O.G. and assure that resources targeted to treat her melanoma are used in a just manner? How might O.G.'s medical crowdfunding platform affect the well-being of other patients with melanoma?

References

Kubheka, B. Z. (2020). Bioethics and the use of social media for medical crowdfunding. *BMC Medical Ethics*, 21(96), 1–5.

Moore, B. (2019). Medical crowdfunding and the virtuous donor. *Bioethics*, 33(2), 238–244.

Snyder, J., & Caulfield, T. (2019). Patients' crowdfunding campaigns for alternative cancer treatments. *The Lancet Oncology*, 20(1), 28–29.

Snyder, J., & Cohen, I. G. (2019). Medical crowdfunding for unproven medical treatments: Should Gofundme become a gatekeeper? *Hastings Center Report*, 49(6), 32–38.

Resources

See Chapter 1, Chart 1-10 for Steps of an Ethical Analysis and Ethics Resources.

---

have few side effects, most of which tend to be cutaneous (e.g., rashes, photosensitivity). In addition, patients taking these agents are at greater risk for developing squamous cell carcinomas (ACS, 2019d). Patients on these regimens should be educated to self-assess their skin and promptly report any signs to their primary provider for definitive follow-up. The importance of engaging in sun safety protocols including seeking shade whenever feasible when outdoors, and applying sunscreen, cannot be overemphasized.

The patient who is *BRAF* negative likely will be prescribed a checkpoint inhibitor. These agents must be administered IV; therefore, the patient must anticipate receiving treatments in an infusion center. Treatments are typically administered every 2 to 3 weeks for up to a year. However, the checkpoint inhibitors may be administered via a peripheral vein, and so the patient need not have an IV port placed. Furthermore, these agents tend to be tolerated better than most chemotherapeutic agents. The most commonly noted side effects include fatigue, rash, and diarrhea or constipation (ACS, 2020b). Patients receiving these agents should be educated to monitor for and promptly report side effects and to engage in sun safety protocols.

 ### Educating Patients About Self-Care

Until a few years ago, patients with metastatic disease had a grim prognosis. With the advent of targeted therapy and checkpoint inhibitors within the past decade, hope for remission and even cure is possible. Patients with metastatic disease and their family members should be given this positive news when they seek treatment. However, there are still instances where remission or cure is not possible. There is some evidence that patients with metastatic disease who are at end-of-life are not linked into palliative care services appropriately when they are near death, as it is becoming difficult to clearly identify when treatments aimed at remission have failed (Fox, Rosenberg, Ekberg, et al., 2020). The nurse caring for a patient with metastatic melanoma who is nearing end-of-life must advocate for the patient and family so that they receive appropriate and timely palliative care services (see Chapter 13).

Metastatic Skin Tumors

The skin is an important yet uncommon site of metastatic cancer. All types of cancer may metastasize to the skin. Cancers with a predilection to metastasize to the skin include melanomas and cancers of the breast, nasal sinuses, larynx, and oral cavity. Of these, skin metastases from carcinoma of the breast are most frequently seen, accounting for 30% of all cases. The clinical appearance of metastatic skin lesions is not distinctive, except perhaps in some cases of breast cancer in which diffuse, brawny hardening of the skin of the involved breast is seen. In most instances, metastatic lesions occur as multiple cutaneous or subcutaneous nodules of various sizes that may be skin colored or different shades of red (American Osteopathic College of Dermatology, 2020).

Kaposi Sarcoma

Kaposi sarcoma is a malignancy of endothelial cells that line the small blood vessels. Kaposi sarcoma is manifested clinically by lesions of the skin, oral cavity, gastrointestinal tract, and lungs. The skin lesions consist of reddish-purple to dark blue macules, plaques, or nodules. Kaposi sarcoma is subdivided into four categories (ACS, 2018):

- *Classic Kaposi sarcoma* occurs predominantly in older adult men of Mediterranean or Jewish ancestry. Most patients have nodules or plaques on the lower extremities that rarely metastasize beyond this area. Classic Kaposi sarcoma is chronic, relatively benign, and rarely fatal.
- *Endemic (African) Kaposi sarcoma* affects people predominantly in the eastern half of Africa near the equator. Men are affected more often than women, and children can be affected as well. The disease may resemble classic Kaposi sarcoma, or it may infiltrate and progress to lymphadenopathic forms.
- *Iatrogenic/organ transplant–associated Kaposi sarcoma* occurs in transplant recipients and in patients receiving long-term immunosuppressants, such as azathioprine, cyclosporine, or corticosteroids, such as prednisone.
- *AIDS-related or epidemic Kaposi sarcoma* occurs in people with AIDS. This form of Kaposi sarcoma is characterized by local skin lesions and disseminated visceral and mucocutaneous diseases. This is a more aggressive tumor type than other forms of Kaposi sarcoma. More information on AIDS-related Kaposi sarcoma can be found in Chapter 32.

PLASTIC, RECONSTRUCTIVE, AND COSMETIC PROCEDURES

The word *plastic* comes from a Greek word meaning "to form." Plastic or reconstructive procedures are performed to reconstruct or alter congenital or acquired defects to restore or improve the body's form and function. Often the terms *plastic* and *reconstructive* are used interchangeably. This type of surgery includes closure of wounds, removal of skin tumors, repair of soft tissue injuries or burns, correction of deformities, and repair of cosmetic defects. Plastic surgery can be used to repair many parts of the body and numerous structures, such as bone, cartilage, fat, fascia, mucous membrane, muscle, nerve, and cutaneous structures. Bone inlays and transplants for deformities and nonunion can be performed, muscle can be transferred, nerves can be reconstructed and spliced, and cartilage can be replaced. As important as any of these measures is the reconstruction of the cutaneous tissues around the neck and the face; this is usually referred to as aesthetic or cosmetic surgery.

Cosmetic procedures are generally considered to be ones that correct defects that are not life-threatening or caused by diseases. An example would be removal of a benign mole or sebaceous cyst from the face. Most health insurance plans do not cover procedures deemed to be cosmetic, and these procedures can be expensive. Procedures that are performed to correct a surgical defect, such as removal of a skin cancer or correction of a significant congenital defect such as a cleft lip are generally covered by insurance.

Wound Coverage: Grafts and Flaps

Various surgical techniques, including skin grafts and flaps, are used to cover skin wounds.

Skin Grafts

Skin grafting is a technique in which a section of skin is detached from its own blood supply and transferred as free tissue to a distant (recipient) site. Skin grafting can be used to repair almost any type of wound and is the most common form of reconstructive surgery.

Skin grafts are commonly used to repair surgical defects such as those that result from excision of skin tumors, to cover areas denuded of skin (e.g., burns), and to cover wounds in which insufficient skin is available to permit wound closure. They are also used when primary closure of the wound increases the risk of complications or when primary wound closure would interfere with function. Skin grafts may be classified as autografts, homografts, or xenografts (see Chapter 57 for further discussion of skin grafts).

Flaps

Another form of wound coverage is provided by flaps. A flap is a segment of tissue that remains attached at one end (i.e., a base or pedicle) while the other end is moved to a recipient area. Its survival depends on functioning arterial and venous blood supplies and lymphatic drainage in its pedicle or base (del Rosario & Barkley, 2017). A flap differs from a graft in that a portion of the tissue is attached to its original site and retains its blood supply. An exception is the free flap, which is described later.

Flaps may consist of skin, mucosa, muscle, adipose tissue, omentum, and bone. They are used for wound coverage and provide bulk, especially when bone, tendon, blood vessels, or nerve tissue is exposed. Flaps are used to repair defects caused by congenital deformity, trauma, or tumor ablation (removal, usually by excision) in an adjacent part of the body (del Rosario & Barkley, 2017).

Flaps offer an aesthetic solution because a flap retains the color and texture of the donor area; is more likely to survive than a graft; and can be used to cover nerves, tendons, and blood vessels. However, several surgical procedures are usually required to advance a flap. The major complication is necrosis of the pedicle or base as a result of failure of the blood supply.

A free flap or free tissue transfer is completely severed from the body and transferred to another site. A free flap receives early vascular supply from microvascular anastomosis with vessels at the recipient site. The procedure usually is completed in one step, eliminating the need for a series of surgical procedures to move the flap. Microvascular surgery allows surgeons to use a variety of donor sites for tissue reconstruction (Hsieh & Bhatt, 2020).

Cosmetic Procedures

A variety of cosmetic procedures may be performed, including chemical face peels, dermabrasion, facial reconstructive surgery, and rhytidectomy (i.e., face-lift).

Chemical Face Peeling

Chemical face peeling involves application of a chemical mixture to the face for superficial destruction of the epidermis and the upper layers of the dermis to treat fine wrinkles, keratoses, and pigment problems. It is especially useful for wrinkles at the upper and lower lip, forehead, and periorbital areas. The type of chemical used depends on the planned depth of the peel. The patient who is conscious feels a burning sensation that continues for 12 to 24 hours. Frequent small doses of analgesic and tranquilizing agents are prescribed to keep the patient comfortable. The most common complications include discoloration of the skin, infection of the burned area, persistent sensory changes or itching, and occasionally permanent scarring of the skin (Fabbrocini, 2017).

Dermabrasion

Dermabrasion is a form of skin abrasion used to treat acne scarring, aging, and sun-damaged skin. A special instrument (e.g., motor-driven wire brush, diamond-impregnated disc) is used. The epidermis and some superficial dermis are removed by a sanding-type action, and enough of the dermis is preserved to allow reepithelization of the treated areas. Results are best in the face because it is rich in intradermal epithelial elements (Bharti, Kirman, Molnar, et al., 2018).

Patients with a history of herpes simplex viral infection are typically prescribed with prophylactic antiviral medications (e.g., valacyclovir) preprocedurally so that the physiologic stress of the procedure is less likely to cause a cutaneous herpes eruption. Tretinoin cream may be prescribed with instructions to apply it 2 to 3 weeks preoperatively; this is associated with accelerating reepithelialization post dermabrasion. Patients must be educated preprocedurally about the postprocedural dressing regimen and when to return to the primary provider to have dressing changes performed (Wong, Arnold, & Boeckmann, 2016).

Facial Reconstructive Surgery

Reconstructive procedures on the face are individualized to the patient's needs and desired outcomes. They are performed to repair deformities or restore normal function. They may vary from closure of small defects to complicated procedures involving implantation of prosthetic devices to conceal a large defect or reconstruct a lost part of the face (e.g., nose, ear, jaw). Each surgical procedure is customized and involves a variety of incisions, flaps, and grafts. Multiple surgical procedures may be required.

The process of facial reconstruction is often slow and tedious. Because a person's facial appearance affects self-esteem so greatly, this type of reconstruction is often a very emotional experience for the patient.

Rhytidectomy

Rhytidectomy (i.e., face-lift) is a surgical procedure that removes soft tissue folds and minimizes cutaneous wrinkles on the face. It is performed to create a more youthful appearance. Psychological preparation requires that the patient recognize the limitations of surgery and the fact that miraculous rejuvenation will not occur. The patient is informed that the face may appear bruised and swollen after the dressings are removed and that several weeks may pass before the edema subsides. Corticosteroids (e.g., methylprednisolone) and vitamin C are prescribed postoperatively to minimize edema. Prophylactic antibiotic agents such as cephalexin may also be prescribed postoperatively (Neligan, Warren, & Van Beek, 2017).

Laser Treatment of Cutaneous Lesions

Lasers are devices that amplify or generate highly specialized light energy. They can mobilize immense heat and power when focused at close range and are valuable tools in providing dermatologic abrasion therapy. The laser modalities used for this purpose today include scanned carbon dioxide laser, pulsed carbon dioxide laser, pulsed erbium/yttrium-aluminum-garnet (Er:YAG) laser, fractional Er:YAG laser resurfacing, combination of carbon dioxide and Er:YAG lasers, and fractionated photothermolysis (Husain & Alster, 2016).

Each of these lasers is a precise surgical instrument that vaporizes and excises water-containing tissues with minimal damage. Because the beams used can seal blood and lymphatic vessels, they create a dry surgical field that makes many procedures easier and quicker. Therefore, these lasers are generally safe to use on patients with bleeding disorders or those receiving anticoagulant therapy. They are primarily used to improve the appearance of facial wrinkles, although they are also useful in removing epidermal nevi, tattoos, certain warts, skin cancer, ingrown toenails, and keloids. Incisions made with

TABLE 56-7	Select Nursing Considerations in Cosmetic Procedures
Nursing Consideration	**Interventions and Patient Education**
Maintaining airway and pulmonary function	Cosmetic surgeries involving the face and neck can cause considerable swelling; bandages can restrict breathing or eating. Check dressings frequently, and ensure that no constriction occurs as swelling develops.
Relieving pain and achieving comfort	Procedures that involve a large surface area will cause considerable pain. Cool compresses or ice packs will relieve the burning of dermabrasion or chemical peels. Oral analgesic agents should be administered regularly to control pain.
Maintaining adequate nutrition	When the face is involved, the patient may be unable to fully open the mouth, and chewing may be painful. Provide soft or liquid diet that is rich in protein to assist with healing.
Enhancing communication	Depending on the type of cosmetic procedure, a nonverbal method of communication might be necessary until pain and swelling have subsided.
Improving self-concept	Recovery time from cosmetic procedures is slow. Expected results will take weeks to become apparent. Patients with darker skin will experience increased pigmentation long after the initial wounds have healed. Helping patients to understand postoperative expectations will allow them to feel more comfortable with the healing process.
Promoting family coping	Most cosmetic procedures are performed in an outpatient facility; therefore, family members are integral to postoperative care. They should understand what to expect as the patient emerges from the procedure room: the type of dressings that will be in place, the skin care plan that is prescribed, and how to help the patient cope with pain.
Monitoring and managing potential complications	Infection is the most common complication, but excessive pain, nerve damage, and emotional distress about appearance are also common. If opioid analgesic agents are used, there may be gastrointestinal upset, mental status changes, or allergic reaction to the medication. Alert the caregiver to signs of these complications and how and when to report changes in status.

the laser beam heal and scar much like those made by a scalpel. Patients with a history of herpes simplex viral infection typically receive preprocedural antiviral prophylaxis (Husain & Alster, 2016).

Nursing Management

The majority of dermatologic and reconstructive procedures are performed in the physician's office or in an outpatient surgical department; therefore, most care takes place in the home. Most procedures, except very extensive reconstruction, are performed under local anesthesia or moderate sedation, therefore requiring a very short recovery time. Unless there are complications, the patient does not need hospitalization. The nurse must prepare both the patient and the family for what to expect during the postoperative recovery time. Table 56-7 lists select nursing considerations that must be reviewed in educating the patient and family.

CRITICAL THINKING EXERCISES

1 **pg** You work as a staff nurse in an emergency department (ED). A 46-year-old woman presents to the ED with complaints of fever, sore throat, and muscle aches for the past 48 hours. Today she began to feel markedly worse and had the sudden onset of widespread erythema, with blistering in her perineum. She has a history of epilepsy and is currently taking prescribed anticonvulsants. The ED physician tells you that the provisional diagnosis might be toxic epidermal necrolysis. What risks might the patient have for toxic epidermal necrolysis? What are your assessment priorities?

2 **ipc** A 25-year-old man is admitted to the medical-surgical unit where you work to manage his stage 3 sacral pressure injury. The patient had a spinal cord injury 2 years ago that resulted in paraplegia. He had extensive inpatient rehabilitation for the first several months post injury; however, for the past several months he has been living in his own apartment and able to maintain an at-home job as a data analyst. He has not had pressure injuries prior to this and is uncertain how the injuries happened and how to prevent recurrence. What resources might be available to help him effectively manage his own care so that he avoids recurrent pressure injury?

3 **ebp** You work in a college health office. A 21-year-old woman presents to the health office with a fever and sore throat. During your assessment, you note that she has tenderness of her shoulders and arms, with some mild erythema that is consistent with a sunburn. She plays on the varsity tennis team. You take the opportunity to talk to her about her risks for melanoma and the advisability of using sunscreen during meets and practices. She tells you that she is Latina, and does not need to worry about skin cancer. What is the strength of the evidence that this young woman is at risk for melanoma? How important is it that she engage in sun safety?

REFERENCES

*Asterisk indicates nursing research.
**Double asterisk indicates classic reference.

Books

Al Aboud, D. M., Yarrarapu, S. N., & Patel, B. C. (2020). *Pilar cyst*. StatPearls. Treasure Island, FL: StatPearls Publishing.

Bryant, R., & Nix, D. (2016). *Acute & chronic wounds: Current management concepts* (5th ed.). Philadelphia, PA: Elsevier.

Comerford, K. C., & Durkin, M. T. (2020). *Nursing2020 drug handbook.* Philadelphia, PA: Wolters Kluwer.

Dlugasch, L., & Story, L. (2021). *Applied pathophysiology for the advanced practice nurse.* Burlington, MA: Jones & Bartlett Learning.

Doughty, D. B., & McNichol, L. L. (2016). *WOCN Society core curriculum: Wound management.* Philadelphia, PA: Wolters Kluwer.

Eliopoulos, C. (2018). *Gerontological nursing* (9th ed.). Philadelphia, PA: Lippincott Williams & Wilkins.

Miline, C. (Ed.). (2019). *Wound source 2019.* Atlantic Beach, FL: Kestrel Health Information, Inc.

Neligan, P. C., Warren, R. J., & Van Beek, A. (2017). *Plastic surgery* (4th ed.). London, UK: Elsevier.

Norris, T. L. (2019). *Porth's pathophysiology: Concepts of altered health states* (10th ed.). Philadelphia, PA: Wolters Kluwer.

**Norton, D., McLaren, R., & Exton Smith, A. N. (1962). *An investigation of geriatric nursing problems in hospital.* Edinburgh: Churchill Livingstone.

Wong, B. J.-F, Arnold, M. G., & Boeckmann, J. O. (2016). *Facial plastic and reconstructive surgery.* New York: Springer.

Journals and Electronic Documents

Ablon, G. (2018). Phototherapy with light emitting diodes: Treating a broad range of medical and aesthetic conditions in dermatology. *Journal of Aesthetic Dermatology, 11*(2), 21–27.

Agency for Healthcare Research & Quality (AHRQ). (2014). Preventing pressure ulcers in hospitals: A toolkit for improving quality of care. Retrieved on 4/15/2020 at: www.ahrq.gov/patient-safety/settings/hospital/resource/pressureulcer/tool/index.html

Ahmad, H., & Siddiqui, S. S. (2017). An unusually large carbuncle of the temporofacial regions demonstrating remarkable post-debridement wound healing process: A case report. *Wounds: A Compendium of Clinical Research & Practice, 29*(4), 92–95.

American Academy of Dermatology (AAD). (2020). Preventing and treating occupationally induced dermatologic conditions during COVID-19. Retrieved on 10/16/2020 at: www.assets.ctfassets.net/1ny4yoiyrqia/1evNAmDqSmw6w9dhozuJGZ/303efdeff53db6e0347df52c65baf4bc/OCC_Derm_Conditions_V11_30Apr2020.pdf

American Cancer Society (ACS). (2018). About Kaposi sarcoma. Retrieved on 10/17/2020 at: www.cancer.org/content/dam/CRC/PDF/Public/8654.00.pdf

American Cancer Society (ACS). (2019a). Can basal and squamous cell skin cancers be prevented? Retrieved on 4/5/2020 at: www.cancer.org/cancer/basal-and-squamous-cell-skin-cancer/causes-risks-prevention/prevention.html

American Cancer Society (ACS). (2019b). Melanoma skin cancer causes, risk factors, and prevention. Retrieved on 10/19/2020 at: www.cancer.org/content/dam/CRC/PDF/Public/8824.00.pdf

American Cancer Society (ACS). (2019c). Survival rates for melanoma skin cancer. Retrieved on 10/22/2020 at: www.cancer.org/cancer/melanoma-skin-cancer/detection-diagnosis-staging/survival-rates-for-melanoma-skin-cancer-by-stage.html

American Cancer Society (ACS). (2019d). Targeted therapy drugs for melanoma skin cancer. Retrieved on 10/25/2020 at: www.cancer.org/cancer/melanoma-skin-cancer/treating/targeted-therapy.html

American Cancer Society (ACS). (2020a). About basal and squamous cell skin cancer. Retrieved on 10/19/2020 at: www.cancer.org/content/dam/CRC/PDF/Public/8818.00.pdf

American Cancer Society (ACS). (2020b). Immunotherapy for melanoma skin cancer. Retrieved on 10/25/2020 at: www.cancer.org/cancer/melanoma-skin-cancer/treating/immunotherapy.html

American Osteopathic College of Dermatology. (2020). Metastatic skin cancer. Retrieved on 5/16/2020 at: www.aocd.org/page/MetastaticSkinCancer

Bader, R. S. (2020). Basal cell carcinoma. *Medscape.* Retrieved on 10/19/2020 at: emedicine.medscape.com/article/276624-overview

Beuscher, L., Reeves, G., & Harrell, D. (2017). Managing herpes zoster in older adults: Prescribing considerations. *The Nurse Practitioner, 42*(6), 24–29.

Bharti, G., Kirman, C. N., Molnar, J. A., et al. (2018). Dermabrasion. *Medscape.* Retrieved on 10/17/2020 at: emedicine.medscape.com/article/1297069-overview#a3

Bolier, R., Elferink, R. P., & Beuers, U. (2016). Advances in pathogenesis and treatment of pruritus. *Clinics in Liver Disease, 17*(2), 319–329.

Breen, E., & Bleday, R. (2020). Approach to the patient with anal pruritus. *UpToDate.* Retrieved on 10/6/2020 at: www.uptodate.com/contents/approach-to-the-patient-with-anal-pruritus

Centers for Disease Control and Prevention (CDC). (2017). Parasites—lice. Retrieved on 10/12/2020 at: www.cdc.gov/parasites/lice/

Centers for Disease Control and Prevention (CDC). (2019). DPDx—pediculosis. Retrieved on 10/12/2020 at: www.cdc.gov/dpdx/pediculosis/

Centers for Disease Control and Prevention (CDC). (2020). What are the risk factors for skin cancer? Retrieved on 10/19/2020 at: www.cdc.gov/cancer/skin/basic_info/risk_factors.htm

César, A., Cruz, M., Mota, A., et al. (2016). Erythroderma. A clinical and etiological study of 103 patients. *Journal of Dermatological Case Reports, 10*(1), 1–9.

Chan, L. S. (2018). Bullous pemphigoid. *Medscape.* Retrieved on 10/13/2020 at: emedicine.medscape.com/article/1062391-overview

*Chen, C. Y., Wu, R. W., Hsu, M. C., et al. (2017). Adjunctive hyperbaric oxygen therapy for healing of chronic diabetic foot ulcers: A randomized controlled trial. *Journal of Wound Ostomy & Continence Nursing, 44*(6), 536–545.

Chen, H. L, Cai, J. Y., Du, L., et al. (2020). Incidence of pressure injury in individuals with spinal cord injury. *Journal of Wound, Ostomy, & Continence Nursing, 47*(3), 215–223.

Cheng, T. A., Mzahim, B., & Koenig, K. L. (2020). Scabies: Application of the identify-isolate-inform tool for detection and management. *Western Journal of Emergency Medicine, 21*(2), 191–198.

Cohen, V., Jellinek, S. P., & Schwartz, R. A. (2018). Toxic epidermal necrolysis. *Medscape.* Retrieved on 10/13/2020 at: emedicine.medscape.com/article/229698-overview

Cornish, L. (2019). Holistic management of malignant wounds in palliative patients. *British Journal of Community Nursing, 24*(Suppl 9), S19–S23.

Dabiri, G., Damstetter, E., & Phillips, T. (2016). Choosing a wound dressing based on common wound characteristics. *Advances in Wound Care, 5*(1), 32–41.

del Rosario, C., & Barkley, T. W. (2017). Postoperative graft and flap care: What clinical nurses need to know. *MedSurg Nursing, 26*(3), 180–192.

Docik, Y., Johnson, E., & Rizk, C. (2019). Small, asymptomatic nodules. *Clinical Advisor, 22*(2), 35–38.

Dooling, K. L., Guo, A., Patel, M., et al. (2018). Recommendations of the advisory committee for immunization practices for use of herpes zoster vaccinations. *Morbidity and Mortality Weekly Report (MMWR), 67*(3), 103–108.

Edsberg, L. E, Black, J. M., Goldberg, M., et al. (2016). Revised National Pressure Ulcer Advisory Panel Pressure Injury Staging System. *Journal of Wound, Ostomy, and Continence Nursing, 43*(6), 585–597.

Estupiñan, B. A., & Sandhu, N. (2017). IgA pemphigus. *Medscape.* Retrieved on 10/13/2020 at: emedicine.medscape.com/article/1063776-overview

European Pressure Ulcer Advisory Panel, National Pressure Injury Advisory Panel and Pan Pacific Pressure Injury Alliance (EPUAP, NPIAP, & PPPIA). (2019). *Prevention of pressure ulcers/injuries: Clinical practice guideline* (3rd ed.). Retrieved on 4/15/2020 at: www.internationalguideline.com/guideline

Fabbrocini, G. (2017). Chemical peels. *Medscape.* Retrieved on 10/17/2020 at: emedicine.medscape.com/article/1829120-overview

Feldman, S. R. (2020). Treatment of psoriasis in adults. *UpToDate.* Retrieved on 10/12/2020 at: www.uptodate.com/contents/treatment-of-psoriasis-in-adults

Feldman, S. R., & Freeman, E. E. (2020). Coronavirus disease 2019 (COVID-19): Cutaneous manifestations and issues related to dermatologic care. *UpToDate.* Retrieved on 10/16/2020 at: www.uptodate.com/contents/coronavirus-disease-2019-covid-19-cutaneous-manifestations-and-issues-related-to-dermatologic-care

*Fox, J. A., Rosenberg, J., Ekberg, S., et al. (2020). Palliative care in the context of immune and targeted therapies: A qualitative study of carers' experiences in metastatic melanoma. *Palliative Medicine, 34*(10), 1351–1360.

Freeman, E. E., McMahon, D. E., Lipoff, J. B., et al. (2020a). Pernio-like skin lesions associated with COVID-19: A case series of 318 patients from 8 countries. *Journal of the American Academy of Dermatology, 83*(2), 486–492.

Freeman, E. E., McMahon, D. E., Lipoff, J. B., et al. (2020b). The spectrum of COVID-19-associated dermatologic manifestations: An international registry of 716 patients from 31 countries. *Journal of the American Academy of Dermatology, 83*(4), 1118–1129.

Goldner, R., & Fransway, A. F. (2018). Irritant contact dermatitis in adults. *UpToDate*. Retrieved on 10/12/2020 at: www.uptodate.com/contents/irritant-contact-dermatitis-in-adults

Goldstein, B. G., & Goldstein, A. O. (2020). Overview of benign lesions of the skin. *UpToDate*. Retrieved on 10/19/2020 at: www.uptodate.com/contents/overview-of-benign-lesions-of-the-skin

Guenther, L. C. C., & Maguiness, S. (2020). Pediculosis and pthiriasis (lice infestation). *Medscape*. Retrieved on 10/12/2020 at: emedicine.medscape.com/article/225013-overview

Habashy, J., & Robles, D. T. (2019). Psoriasis. *Medscape*. Retrieved on 10/12/2020 at: emedicine.medscape.com/article/1943419-overview

Handler, M. Z. (2019). Seborrheic dermatitis treatment and management. *Medscape*. Retrieved on 10/6/2020 at: emedicine.medscape.com/article/1108312-treatment

Handler, M. Z., Stephany, M. P., & Schwartz, R. A. (2020). Tinea capitis. *Medscape*. Retrieved on 10/12/2020 at: emedicine.medscape.com/article/1091351-overview

Harris, A. (2019). Patient education: Methicillin-resistant staphylococcus aureus (MRSA) (Beyond the basics). *UpToDate*. Retrieved on 10/9/2020 at: www.uptodate.com/contents/methicillin-resistant-staphylococcus-aureus-mrsa-beyond-the-basics

Hertl, M., & Geller, S. (2020). Initial management of pemphigus vulgaris and pemphigus foliaceus. *UpToDate*. Retrieved on 10/13/2020 at: www.uptodate.com/contents/initial-management-of-pemphigus-vulgaris-and-pemphigus-foliaceus

Hertl, M., & Sitaru, C. (2020). Pathogenesis, clinical manifestations, and diagnosis of pemphigus. *UpToDate*. Retrieved on 10/13/2020 at: www.uptodate.com/contents/pathogenesis-clinical-manifestations-and-diagnosis-of-pemphigus

Hsieh, S. T., & Bhatt, R. A. (2020). Free tissue transfer flaps. *Medscape*. Retrieved on 10/17/2020 at: emedicine.medscape.com/article/1284841-overview#a2

Hu, K., Fan, J., Li, X., et al. (2020). The adverse skin reactions of health care workers using personal protective equipment for COVID-19. *Medicine, 99*(24), e20603.

Hunt, R., Schaffer, J. V., & Bolognia, J. L. (2020). Acquired melanocytic nevi (moles). *UpToDate*. Retrieved on 10/19/2020 at: www.uptodate.com/contents/acquired-melanocytic-nevi-moles

Husain, Z., & Alster, T. S. (2016). The role of lasers and intense pulsed light technology in dermatology. *Clinical, Cosmetic and Investigational Dermatology, 9,* 29–40.

Janniger, C. K., Eastern, J. S., Hospenthal, D. R., et al. (2020). Herpes zoster. *Medscape*. Retrieved on 10/12/2020 at: emedicine.medscape.com/article/1132465-overview

Kellen, R., & Berlin, J. M. (2016). Dermatology emergencies. *Journal of the Dermatology Nurses' Association, 8*(3), 193–202.

Korf, B. R., Lobbous, M., & Metrock, L. K. (2020). Neurofibromatosis type 1 (NF1): Pathogenesis, clinical features, and diagnosis. *UpToDate*. Retrieved on 10/19/2020 at: www.uptodate.com/contents/neurofibromatosis-type-1-nf1-pathogenesis-clinical-features-and-diagnosis

Kridin, K. (2018). Emerging treatment options for the management of pemphigus vulgaris. *Therapeutics and Clinical Risk Management, 14,* 757–778.

Kubheka, B. Z. (2020). Bioethics and the use of social media for medical crowdfunding. *BMC Medical Ethics, 21*(96), 1–5.

Lan, J., Song, Z., Miao, X., et al. (2020). Skin damage among health care workers managing coronavirus disease-2019. *Journal of the American Academy of Dermatology, 82*(5), 1215–1216.

Lewis, L. S. (2019). Impetigo. *Medscape*. Retrieved on 10/8/2020 at: emedicine.medscape.com/article/965254-overview

*McGuffin, K. S., Jordan, K., Langford, D., et al. (2019). Assessing knowledge, attitudes, and behaviors regarding sun safety in female collegiate athletes. *Journal of the Dermatology Nurses' Association, 11*(1), 20–33.

Miller, J. L., & Zaman, S. A. K. (2020). Dermatitis herpetiformis. *Medscape*. Retrieved on 10/13/2020 at: emedicine.medscape.com/article/1062640-overview

Moore, B. (2019). Medical crowdfunding and the virtuous donor. *Bioethics, 33*(2), 238–244.

Motswaledi, M. H. (2018). Superficial skin infections and the use of topical and systemic antibiotics in general practice. *Professional Nursing Today, 22*(4), 15–20.

Najjar, T. (2020). Cutaneous squamous cell carcinoma. *Medscape*. Retrieved on 10/19/2020 at: emedicine.medscape.com/article/1965430-overview

National Cancer Institute (NCI). (2020). Melanoma treatment—Health professional version. Retrieved on 10/22/2020 at: www.cancer.gov/types/skin/hp/melanoma-treatment-pdq

Nicpon, J. (2017). Psoriasis management: Quality, cost, and coordination. *Journal of the Dermatology Nurses' Association, 9*(1), 21–25.

Occupational Safety and Health Administration (OSHA). (2011). Bloodborne pathogens and needlestick prevention: Evaluating and controlling exposure. Retrieved on 10/5/2020 at: www.osha.gov/bloodborne-pathogens/evaluating-controlling-exposure

*Orsimarsi, G. (2019). Skin cancer knowledge and prevention practices among young adult athletes. *Journal of the Dermatology Nurses' Association, 11*(3), 113–128.

Rao, J., & Chen, J. (2020). Acne vulgaris. *Medscape*. Retrieved on 10/8/2020 at: emedicine.medscape.com/article/1069804-overview

Robbins, C. M., & Elewski, B. E. (2020). Tinea pedis. *Medscape*. Retrieved on 10/12/2020 at: emedicine.medscape.com/article/1091684-overview

Sahoo, A. K., & Mahajan, R. (2016). Management of tinea corporis, tinea cruris, and tinea pedis: A comprehensive review. *Indian Dermatology Online Journal, 7*(2), 77–86.

Sasseville, D. (2020). Seborrheic dermatitis in adolescents and adults. *UpToDate*. Retrieved on 10/6/2020 at: www.uptodate.com/contents/seborrheic-dermatitis-in-adolescents-and-adults

Schwartz, R. A., & Szepietowski, J. C. (2020). Tinea barbae. *Medscape*. Retrieved on 10/12/2020 at: emedicine.medscape.com/article/1091252-overview

Scott, A. M., Stehlik, P., Clark, J., et al. (2019). Blue-light therapy for acne vulgaris: A systematic review and meta-analysis. *Annals of Family Medicine, 17*(6), 545–552.

Shukla, S., & Khachemoune, A. (2020). Tinea corporis. *Medscape*. Retrieved on 10/12/2020 at: emedicine.medscape.com/article/1091473-overview

Siegel, R. L., Miller, K. D., & Jemal, A. (2020). Cancer statistics, 2020. *CA: A Cancer Journal for Clinicians, 70*(1), 7–30.

Skin Cancer Foundation. (2020a). Skin cancer facts and statistics: What you need to know. Retrieved on 10/19/2020 at: www.skincancer.org/skin-cancer-information/skin-cancer-facts/

Skin Cancer Foundation. (2020b). Warning signs: The ABCDEs of melanoma. Retrieved on 10/23/2020 at: www.skincancer.org/skin-cancer-information/melanoma/melanoma-warning-signs-and-images/#abcde

Snyder, J., & Caulfield, T. (2019). Digital oncology: Patients' crowdfunding campaigns for alternative cancer treatments. *The Lancet Oncology, 20,* 28–29.

Snyder, J., & Cohen, I. G. (2019). Medical crowdfunding for unproven medical treatments: Should Gofundme become a gatekeeper? *Hastings Center Report, 49*(6), 32–38.

Song, J., Xian, D., Yang, L., et al. (2018). Pruritus: Progress toward pathogenesis and treatment. *BioMed Research International, 2018,* Article ID 9625936, 12 pages.

Tan, W. W. (2020). Malignant melanoma. *Medscape*. Retrieved on 10/22/2020 at: emedicine.medscape.com/article/280245-overview

Tchero, H., Herlin, C., Bekara, F., et al. (2019). Hidradenitis suppurativa: A systematic review and meta-analysis of therapeutic interventions. *Indian Journal of Dermatology Venereology and Leprology, 85*(3), 248–257.

Thiboutot, D., & Zaenglein, A. (2019). Pathogenesis, clinical manifestations, and diagnosis of acne vulgaris. *UpToDate*. Retrieved on 10/8/2020 at: www.uptodate.com/contents/pathogenesis-clinical-manifestations-and-diagnosis-of-acne-vulgaris

Tosti, A. (2020). Onychomycosis. *Medscape*. Retrieved on 10/12/2020 at: emedicine.medscape.com/article/1105828-overview

*Trommel, N., Hofland, H. W., van Komen, R. S., et al. (2019). Nursing problems in patients with toxic epidermal necrolysis and Stevens-Johnson syndrome in a Dutch burn centre: A 30-year retrospective study. *Burns: Journal of the International Society for Burn Injuries, 45*(7), 1625–1633.

Umar, S. H., & Kelly, A. P. (2019). Erythroderma (generalized exfoliative dermatitis). *Medscape*. Retrieved on 10/13/2020 at: emedicine.medscape.com/article/1106906-overview

VanGilder, C., Lachenbruch, C., Algrim-Boyle, C., et al. (2017). The International Pressure Ulcer Prevalence Survey: 2006–2015: A 10-year pressure injury prevalence and demographic trend analysis by care setting. *Journal of Wound, Ostomy, and Continence Nursing, 44*(1), 20–28.

Weiderkehr, M., & Schwartz, R. A. (2020). Tinea cruris. *Medscape*. Retrieved on 10/12/2020 at: emedicine.medscape.com/article/1091806-overview

Zaenglein, A. L., Pathy, A. L., Schlosser, B. J., et al. (2016). Guidelines of care for the management of acne vulgaris. *Journal of the American Academy of Dermatology, 74*(5), 945–973.

Resources

American Academy of Dermatology (AAD), www.aad.org

American Cancer Society, www.cancer.org

American Melanoma Foundation (AMF), www.melanomafoundation.org

Dermatology Information System (DermIS), a cooperation between the Department of Clinical Social Medicine (University of Heidelberg) and the Department of Dermatology (University of Erlangen), www.dermis.net

National Eczema Association, www.nationaleczema.org

National Pressure Injury Advisory Panel (NPIAP), 2019 Clinical Practice Guideline, www.npiap.com/page/2019Guideline

National Psoriasis Foundation, www.psoriasis.org

New Zealand Dermatology Society (DermNET NZ), www.dermnetnz.org

Skin Cancer Foundation, www.skincancer.org

Wound, Ostomy, and Continence Nurses Society, www.wocn.org

LEARNING OUTCOMES

On completion of this chapter, the learner will be able to:

1. Identify the incidence and factors that affect severity of burn injury in the United States.
2. Describe the local and systemic effects of a major burn injury.
3. Use the nursing process as a framework for care of the patient in the emergent/resuscitative, acute/intermediate, and rehabilitative phases of a burn injury.
4. Compare priorities of care, including fluid replacement, wound management and psychosocial support, and potential complications for each phase of burn recovery.

NURSING CONCEPTS

Fluids and Electrolytes

Medical Emergencies

Metabolism

Tissue Integrity

GLOSSARY

autograft: a graft derived from one part of a patient's body and used on another part of that same patient's body

carboxyhemoglobin: a compound of carbon monoxide (CO) and hemoglobin formed in the blood with exposure to CO

collagen: a protein present in skin, tendon, bone, cartilage, and connective tissue

contracture: shrinkage of burn scar through collagen maturation

débridement: removal of foreign material and devitalized tissue until surrounding healthy tissue is exposed

donor site: the area from which skin is taken to provide a skin graft for another part of the body

eschar: devitalized tissue resulting from a burn or wound

escharotomy: a linear excision made through eschar to release constriction of underlying tissue

excision: surgical removal of tissue

fasciotomy: an incision made through the fascia to release constriction of underlying muscle

homograft: a graft transferred from one human (living or cadaveric) to another human (*synonym:* allograft)

xenograft: a graft obtained from an animal of a species other than that of the recipient (e.g., pigskin) (*synonym:* heterograft)

Burn injuries can be painful, costly, and disfiguring; they may require intensive and extensive rehabilitation therapy and are often associated with long-term disability. An extensive burn injury is associated with a complex, multisystem pathophysiology that continues to challenge health systems, despite advances that have resulted in significantly reduced comorbidities and length of stay (LOS). These advances in treatment of patients with severe burns include critical-care management, fluid resuscitation, nutrition, surgical débridement, wound coverage, and antimicrobial therapies (Jones, Williams, Cairns, et al., 2017; Weissman, Wagman, Givon, et al., 2017). The role of the nurse in the interdisciplinary treatment team includes provision of holistic evidence-based care during all phases of burn injury recovery to optimize patient outcomes.

Overview of Burn Injury

Burn injuries, which result from damage to the skin or other tissues from heat, chemicals, electricity, or radiation, most commonly occur in the home or work setting. Globally, they account for approximately 180,000 deaths and significant morbidity each year; however, many are preventable (World Health Organization [WHO], 2018).

Incidence

A burn injury can affect people of all ages, ethnicities, and socioeconomic groups. In the United States, an estimated 486,000 people are treated for burns and approximately 40,000 are hospitalized annually (American Burn Association [ABA], 2016). The largest proportion of burns, 41%, was reported as flame related, 35% were scalds, 10% were from direct source contact, 3% were electrical, 3% were chemical contact, 3% were inhalation only, and the remaining 5% were from unspecified or miscellaneous categories. Of those admitted to burn centers, the incidence of burn injuries for men was generally more than twice that for women; for both men and women, adults between 20 and 30 years of age had the highest prevalence of burn injuries. Of the reported injuries, 73% occurred in the home, 8% were industry related, 5% were recreationally related, and the remaining 14% of injuries were from other sources (American Burn Association National Burn Repository [ABA NBR], 2018).

Patients with burn injuries have particularly prolonged hospital LOS. Many require multiple surgical interventions, extensive pain control interventions, prolonged periods of immobilization and rehabilitation, and protracted intravenous (IV) medication regimens, particularly opioids and antibiotics. Historically, LOS projection was one hospital day per percent total body burn surface area (TBSA) burn. This underestimates LOS and resource utilization, most particularly in those over 40 years of age or those with an inhalation injury (Taylor, Sen, Greenhalgh, et al., 2017).

 ### Gerontologic Considerations

Age-related changes such as diminished mobility, postural stability, strength, coordination, sensation, visual acuity, and declining memory predispose older adults to burn injury. The population of older adults continues to grow, as does the number of burn injuries among older adults. Burn Injury Registry data over a 10-year period from 212,820 hospitalized patients with burns suggest that 15% of burn injuries requiring hospitalization occurred in patients 60 years of age and older, with fire/flame sources accounting for 56% of reported injuries (ABA NBR, 2018). Mortality associated with burns is greater in older adult patients than in younger adult patients when comparing injuries with similar severity. The overall mortality from burns in the adult over 59 years of age is approximately 13%; compared to a 2.9% overall mortality rate for all ages (ABA NBR, 2018). The lethal dose 50 describes the percentage of TBSA burn that results in 50% mortality for a population; for older adults, this remains 30% to 35% TBSA despite advances in treatment (Jeschke & Peck, 2017).

Complications associated with burn injuries are also highest in patients 60 years and older. Of all reported complications, pneumonia was the most common, followed closely by urinary tract infections. Other reported complications include respiratory failure, septicemia, cellulitis, wound infection, kidney injury, arrhythmias, and other hospital-acquired infections such as central line bloodstream infections (ABA NBR, 2018). There is evidence that frailty and high comorbidities can cause critical decompensation in even small TBSA burns for those 50 years of age and older (Maxwell, Rhee, Drake, et al., 2018; Romanowski, Curtis, Palmieri, et al., 2018). Therefore, premorbid physiology should be considered when planning care for the older adult patient with a burn injury.

The skin of the older adult is thinner and less elastic, which affects the depth of injury and its ability to heal. Pulmonary function becomes impaired with age affecting airway exchange, lung elasticity, and ventilation; these effects can be exacerbated by a history of smoking. Decreased cardiac output, presence of coronary artery disease, and decreased cardiovascular compensatory response increase the risk of complications in older adult patients with burn injuries. There may be a very fine line between adequate fluid resuscitation and fluid overload in this population. Decreased kidney and hepatic function can affect medication dosing due to altered medication clearance. Malnutrition may affect morbidity and mortality in older adults, especially those who are institutionalized. Additionally, older adult patients may have varying degrees of mental capacity on admission or throughout the course of care, rendering assessment of pain, anxiety, and delirium a challenge for the burn team.

Comorbidities are common among older adults and, when combined with treatments, result in polypharmacy (i.e., multiple medication prescriptions), which contribute to in-hospital complications and increase the need for discharge to a facility other than the patient's home after acute recovery. Nurses need to assess the older adult patient's ability to safely perform activities of daily living (ADLs), assist older adult patients and families to modify their environment to ensure safety, and make referrals as needed. In addition, an assessment of instrumental activities of daily living (IADLs) is warranted (see Chapter 2 for further discussion of IADLs). This is an assessment of the ability to carry out more complex tasks such as meal preparation, traveling to appointments, etc., and is particularly important for those returning home without a caregiver (American Psychological Association, 2020).

Prevention

Almost all burns are preventable. An important goal of nurses in community and home settings is to provide education regarding prevention of burn injuries (see Chart 57-1). The

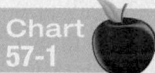

Chart 57-1 **HEALTH PROMOTION**
Burn Prevention

- Advise that matches and lighters be kept out of the reach of children.
- Emphasize the importance of never leaving children unattended around fire or in bathroom/bathtub.
- Educate about the installation and maintenance of smoke and CO detectors on every level of the home and changing batteries annually on birthday.
- Recommend the development and practice of a home exit fire drill with all members of the household.
- Advocate setting the water heater temperature no higher than 48.9°C (120°F).
- Educate about the perils of smoking in bed, smoking while using home oxygen, or falling asleep while smoking.
- Caution against using flammable liquids to start fires and/or throwing flammable liquids onto an already burning fire.
- Warn of the danger of removing the radiator cap from a hot car engine.
- Recommend avoidance of overhead electrical wires and underground wires when working outside.
- Advise that hot irons and curling irons be kept out of the reach of children.
- Discourage running electric cords under carpets or rugs.
- Recommend storage of flammable liquids well away from a fire source, such as a pilot light.
- Educate about the importance of being aware of loose clothing when cooking over a stovetop or flame.
- Recommend having a working fire extinguisher in the home and knowing how to use it.

WHO recommends heightened awareness of the burden of burn injury and its risk factors as imperatives to the development of an effective burn prevention program (WHO, 2018).

Outlook for Survival and Recovery

The WHO (2018) estimated 265,000 annual deaths worldwide are caused by burns, the majority occurring in middle- to low-income populations, while nonfatal burns are a leading cause of morbidity including disfigurement, disability, and social stigma. The overall mortality rate for all TBSA burns in the United States reported to the National Burn Repository is 3% (ABA NBR, 2018). The strongest predictors for mortality in burn injuries include increased percent of TBSA burned, presence of inhalation injury, and increased age. Provision of evidenced-based, multidisciplinary, holistic care is crucial to improving both survival and recovery culminating in reintegration of the survivor into society.

Great strides in research on burn wound treatments and critical care have improved the survival rate of patients with burn injuries. Evaluation of long-term outcomes is possible because patients with very large burns are surviving their injuries. Continued research and advances in the areas of critical care, rehabilitation, and psychosocial and scar management are essential for continued progress in burn care (Bielson, Duethman, Howard, et al., 2017).

Severity

Multiple factors determine the severity of each burn injury. These factors include age of the patient; depth of the burn; amount of surface area of the body burned; the presence of inhalation injury; presence of other injuries; location of the injury in areas such as the face, the perineum, hands, or feet; and the presence of comorbid conditions. Careful assessment enables the burn team to estimate the likelihood of survival and develop an individualized plan of care for each patient (ABA, 2018).

Age

Young children and older adults have increased morbidity and mortality when compared to other age groups with similar injuries and present a challenge for the burn team. Thinner skin at both ends of the age spectrum leads to deeper burns with more complications. This is an important factor when determining the severity of injury and potential outcomes for the patient.

Burn Depth

Burns are classified according to the depth of tissue destruction as depicted in Table 57-1. First-degree burns are superficial injuries that involve only the outermost layer of skin. These burns are painful and erythematous, but the epidermis is intact; if rubbed, the burned tissue does not separate from the underlying dermis. This is known as a negative Nikolsky's sign. A typical first-degree burn is a sunburn or superficial scald burn.

Second-degree (partial-thickness) burns involve the entire epidermis and varying portions of the dermis. They are painful and typically associated with blister formation. Healing time depends on the depth of dermal injury, typically ranging

TABLE 57-1	Characteristics of Burns According to Depth			
Causes	**Skin Involvement**	**Clinical Manifestations**	**Wound Appearance**	**Recuperative Course and Treatment**
First Degree (Superficial) Sunburn Low-intensity flash Superficial scald	Epidermis	Tingling Hyperesthesia (hypersensitivity) Pain that is soothed by cooling Peeling Itching	Reddened; blanches with pressure; dry Minimal or no edema Possible blisters	Complete recovery within a few days Oral pain medications, cool compresses, skin lubricants (e.g., ointments, emollients); topical antimicrobial agents not indicated
Second Degree (Partial Thickness) Scalds Flash flame Contact	Epidermis, portion of dermis	Pain Hyperesthesia Sensitive to air currents	Blistered, mottled red base; disrupted epidermis; weeping surface Edema	Recovery in 2–3 wks Some scarring and depigmentation possible; may require grafting
Third Degree (Full Thickness) Flame Prolonged exposure to hot liquids Electric current Chemical Contact	Epidermis, dermis, and sometimes subcutaneous tissue; may involve connective tissue and muscle	Insensate Shock Myoglobinuria (red pigment in urine) and possible hemolysis (blood cell destruction) Possible contact points (entrance or exit wounds in electrical burns)	Dry; pale white, red brown, leathery, or charred Coagulated vessels may be visible. Edema	Eschar may slough Grafting necessary Scarring and loss of contour and function
Fourth Degree (Full Thickness That Includes Fat, Fascia, Muscle, and/or Bone) Prolonged exposure or high-voltage electrical injury	Deep tissue, muscle and bone	Shock Myoglobinuria (red pigment in urine) and possible hemolysis (blood cell destruction)	Charred	Amputations likely Grafting of no benefit given depth and severity of wound(s)

Adapted from American Burn Association. (2018). *Advanced burn life support (ABLS) course provider manual 2018.* Chicago, IL.

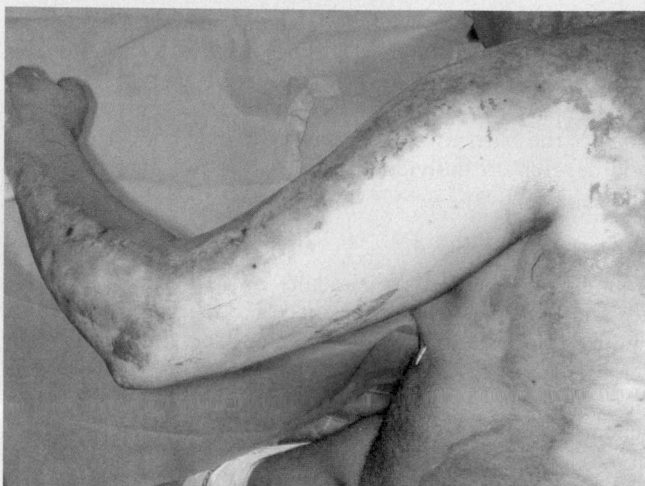

Figure 57-1 • Third-degree (full-thickness) burn to arm and upper back with surrounding second-degree (partial-thickness) burn. Used with permission from University of Texas Medical Branch, Galveston, TX.

from 2 to 3 weeks. Hair follicles and skin appendages remain intact. The wound bed is moist due to serous leakage from the peripheral microcirculation.

Third-degree (full-thickness) burns involve total destruction of the epidermis, dermis, and, in some cases, damage of underlying tissue. Wound color ranges widely from pale white to red, brown, or charred. The deeply burned area lacks sensation because the nerve fibers are damaged. The wound appears leathery and dry due to the destruction of the microcirculation. Skin organelles such as hair follicles and sweat glands may be affected. The severity of this burn is often deceiving to patients because they have no pain in the injury area (see Fig. 57-1).

Fourth-degree burns (deep burn necrosis) are those injuries that extend into deep tissue, muscle, or bone (see Fig. 57-2) (ABA, 2018; Strauss & Gillespie, 2018).

Burn depth determines whether spontaneous reepithelialization will occur. Determining burn depth can be difficult

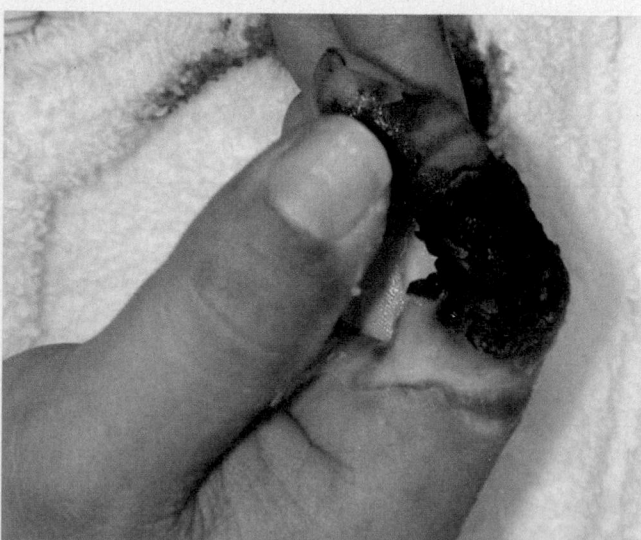

Figure 57-2 • Fourth-degree burn to second digit. Used with permission from University of Texas Medical Branch, Galveston, TX.

even for the experienced burn care provider. The following factors are considered in determining the depth of a burn: how the injury occurred, causative agent (such as flame or scalding liquid), temperature and duration of contact with the causative agent, and thickness of the skin at the injury site.

Extent of Body Surface Area Injured

Various methods are utilized to estimate the TBSA affected by burns; among them are the rule of nines, the Lund and Browder method, and the palmer method. These tools assist the treatment team in making decisions about the plan of care, which may include transfer of the patient to a burn center. Burn centers are hospital based and are specially equipped with the resources and personnel to treat patients with burns from the time of injury through their rehabilitation. Burn center designation is conferred jointly by the ABA and the American College of Surgeons (ABA, 2019). Chart 57-2 provides the ABA criteria for referral to a burn center.

Rule of Nines

The most common method of estimating the extent of burns in adults is the rule of nines (see Fig. 57-3). This system is based on anatomic regions, each representing approximately 9% of the TBSA, allowing clinicians to rapidly estimate percent of body burned. If the burn affects only a portion of an anatomic area, the TBSA is calculated accordingly—for example, if approximately half of one arm were burned, the TBSA burned would be 4.5%.

Lund and Browder Method

A more precise method of estimating the extent of a burn is the Lund and Browder method, which recognizes the percentage of surface area of various anatomic parts, especially the head and legs, as it relates to the age of the patient. By dividing the body into very small areas and providing an estimate of the proportion of TBSA accounted for by each body part, clinicians can obtain a reliable estimate of TBSA burned. The initial evaluation made on arrival of the patient to the

Chart 57-2

American Burn Association Criteria for Referral to a Burn Center

- Partial-thickness burns covering 10% of total body surface area or greater
- Burns involving the face, hands, feet, genitalia, perineum, or major joints
- Third-degree burns
- Electrical burns, including lightning injury
- Chemical burns
- Inhalation injury
- Burn injury in patients with preexisting medical disorders
- Any patients with burns and concomitant trauma
- Children with burn injuries in facilities that do not specialize in pediatric care
- Patients who will require special social, emotional, or long-term rehabilitation

Adapted from American Burn Association. (2018). *Advanced burn life support (ABLS) course provider manual 2018.* Chicago, IL: Author.

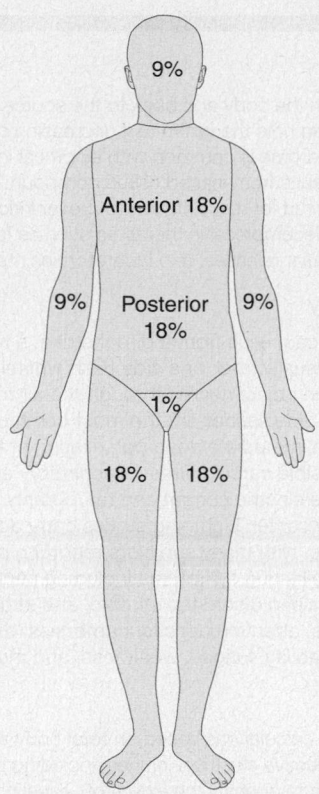

Figure 57-3 • The rule of nines. Estimated percentage of total body surface area (TBSA) in the adult is calculated by sectioning the body surface into areas with a numerical value related to nine. (*Note:* The anterior and posterior head total 9% of TBSA.)

hospital should be revised within the first 72 hours, because demarcation of the wound and its depth present themselves more clearly by this time. The Lund and Browder chart is readily available in both printed and electronic formats (ABA, 2018).

Palmer Method

In patients with scattered burns, or very large burns with minimal sparing, the palmer method is an expeditious method to determine extent of injury. The size of the patient's hand, including the fingers, is approximately 1% of that patient's TBSA (ABA, 2018).

Pathophysiology

Burns are exceptionally traumatic injuries as the initial injury evolves and worsens over time. Burn injury is the result of a chemical exposure or heat transfer from one site to another, causing tissue destruction through coagulation, protein denaturation, or ionization of cellular contents. The burn wound is not homogenous; rather, tissue necrosis generally occurs at the center of the injury with regions of tissue viability toward the periphery. The central area of the wound is termed the *zone of coagulation* due to the characteristic coagulation necrosis of cells that occurs (see Fig. 57-4). The surrounding zone, the *zone of stasis*, describes an area of injured cells that may remain viable but, with persistent ischemia, will undergo necrosis within 24 to 48 hours. The outermost zone, the *zone of hyperemia*, sustains minimal injury and may fully recover spontaneously over time.

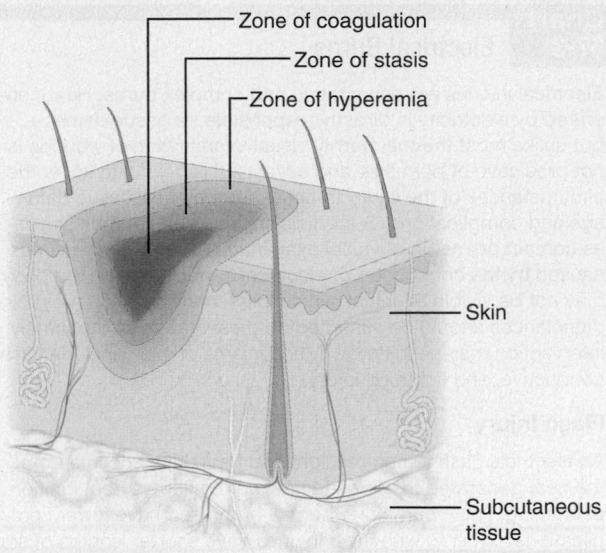

Figure 57-4 • Zones of burn injury. Each burned area has three zones of injury. The zone of coagulation (the innermost area, where cellular death occurs) sustains the most damage. The zone of stasis (the middle area) has a compromised blood supply, inflammation, and tissue injury. The zone of hyperemia (the outermost area) sustains the least damage.

The skin and the mucosa of the upper airways are the most common sites of tissue destruction, although deep tissues, including the viscera, can be damaged by electrical burns (see Chart 57-3) or prolonged contact with a heat or chemical source. The release of local mediators, changes in blood flow, tissue edema, and infection can cause progression in severity of the burn injury.

Another potential mechanism of burn injury is radiation exposure. This has received increased attention because of threats of terrorism and recent world events. Radiation injuries produce two detrimental effects. The first is a thermal effect, which results in cutaneous burn injuries. The second effect is damage to the cellular deoxyribonucleic acid (DNA), which may be localized or affect the whole body. Morbidity and mortality are dose dependent (see Chapter 68). Treatment for the cutaneous injury is the same as other burns discussed in this chapter.

The depth of a burn injury depends on the temperature of the burning agent and the duration of contact with the agent. In adults, exposure to temperatures of 54°C (130°F) for 30 seconds will result in burn injury. At 60°C (140°F), tissue destruction occurs in 5 seconds (this is a common setting for home water heaters; see Chart 57-1 for discussion of appropriate water heater setting). At 71°C (160°F) or higher, a full-thickness burn occurs instantaneously (ABA, 2018).

It is important to recognize injuries that affect more than approximately 20% TBSA as severe injuries, as they produce both local and systemic effects. The systemic inflammatory response to a severe burn injury signals the release of proinflammatory and anti-inflammatory cytokines, prompting hypermetabolism effects that produce organ dysfunction, a pronounced catabolic response, systemic compromise and, potentially, mortality (Rehou, Shahrokhi, Natanson, et al., 2018).

Chart 57-3 Electrical Burns

Electrical injuries are devastating and complex burns. Heat generated by electricity is directly responsible for tissue damage, but unlike most thermal burns, visual examination of wounds is not predictive of burn size and severity. It is helpful to know the circumstances of the injury to anticipate potential tissue damage and complications. Superficial injuries present themselves as contact points on physical examination. Deep tissue injuries caused by the conduction of electrical current through the body may not be visible on initial clinical presentation, but in most circumstances should be assumed on presentation so that timely intervention may be initiated. Mechanisms of injury include flash, conductive, and lightning injury.

Flash Injury

An electrical flash generates light and heat. Injury occurs from the heat generated to exposed areas or by flames from ignition of clothing. Flash burns are thermal burns and have fewer complications; patients with flash injuries have shorter lengths of stay than those with conductive injuries.

Conductive Injury

Conductive electrical injuries occur when the current overcomes the skin's resistance and travels through the body. The amount and severity of tissue damage is directly proportional to the strength of the current (voltage), duration of contact with the source, which organs lay along the pathway of current, and whether the current is direct or alternating. Conduction of electricity through the nerves and vessels and along the outside of bones generates heat, causing damage to adjacent tissues and direct injury to the peripheral nerves. Deep muscle injury may be present without injury to superficial muscles, masking the true extent of the injury. In addition, electrical current immediately contracts muscles as it travels through the body causing possible skeletal and joint injuries in high-voltage contact. Although the majority of reported electrical injuries are high-voltage (>1000 volts) injuries, significant physical and psychological morbidity also occur with low-voltage (<1000 volts) injuries as well.

Entrance and exit wounds or contact points can help identify the probable current path and therefore anticipated tissue and organ involvement. Direct current (DC) travels in one direction, is associated with an explosion and likely concomitant trauma from the blast. Alternating current (AC) passes back and forth from the point of contact, through the body and back to the source many times per second and can hold the victim to it, increasing contact time. Compartment syndrome is common with electrical injuries due to the edema that results from injured tissue compounded by the large fluid volumes required for resuscitation to prevent kidney failure. As a result, invasive decompressive therapies such as fasciotomies, nerve releases, ocular releases, and laparotomies may be required.

Lightning Injury

Lightning injuries can result from a direct strike, a high-voltage DC injury that is usually fatal, or a side flash wherein the current discharges from an object nearby through the air to an adjacent object or person. Side flashes are the most common cause of injury and result in immediate deep polarization of the entire myocardium with possible cardiac arrest. Respiratory arrest is also expected because electric current can temporarily inactivate the brain's respiratory center. Lightning strikes carry approximately 10% mortality rate, with many survivors reporting permanent morbidity and debilitating symptoms including neurologic disabilities, depression, sleep disorders, chronic, and at times, intense pain, memory loss, attention deficits, numbness, dizziness, stiffness in joints, irritability, fatigue, weakness, and muscle spasms.

Management

Resuscitation fluid calculations based on total body surface area are inaccurate in conductive electrical injuries, including some lightning injuries. It is difficult to quantify the extent of tissue injury without surgical exploration because the damage may not be visible on physical examination. Serum creatinine kinase levels are useful in determining the degree of muscle injury in the early phases of care. Myoglobinuria, common with muscle damage, may cause kidney failure if not treated. Intravenous (IV) fluid administration titrated to a higher target of urine output per hour than usual may be indicated until the urine is no longer red. It is common practice to add 50 mEq of sodium bicarbonate per liter of IV fluid in an effort to assist in alkalinizing the urine. Serum myoglobin and urine myoglobin levels may be monitored as indicators of the need for continued resuscitation.

Finally, the surgical treatment of an electrical injury is as complex as the injury itself. Vasculature is commonly affected; thus, progressive tissue necrosis occurs over time. Sequential surgical débridement may be necessary, using caution to preserve viable tissue.

Adapted from American Burn Association. (2018). *Advanced burn life support (ABLS) course provider manual 2018*. Chicago, IL; Culnan, D. M., Farner, K., Bitz, G. H., et al. (2018). Volume resuscitation in patients with high-voltage electrical injuries. *Annals of Plastic Surgery, 80*(3 Suppl 2), S113–S118; National Weather Service. (n.d.). *Lightning safety tips and resources*. Retrieved on 11/30/2019 at: www.weather.gov/safety/lightning; Walker, A., & Salerno, A. (2019). Shocking injuries: Knowing the risks and management for electrical injuries. *Trauma Reports, 20*(4), 1–25.

Severe injuries ultimately encompass changes in pathophysiology of all body systems as presented in Table 57-2. These pathologic responses occur in trauma injuries, but the magnitude, duration, and severity are significantly higher with burn injuries.

Cardiovascular Alterations

When a burn injury occurs, there is an immediate decrease in cardiac output that precedes the loss of plasma volume. The systemic inflammation causes the release of free oxygen radicals that increase capillary permeability, causing increased plasma loss and subsequent peripheral edema as water migrates to the interstitium. As a compensatory response to intravascular fluid loss, the sympathetic nervous system releases catecholamines, resulting in an increase in peripheral resistance (vasoconstriction) and an increase in pulse rate that further decreases tissue perfusion. Due to vasoconstrictive compensatory responses secondary to plasma volume loss through capillary leak, the workload of the heart and oxygen demand increase (Gillenwater & Garner, 2017; Wurzer, Culnan, Cancio, et al., 2018).

Hypovolemia is the immediate consequence of ensuing plasma volume loss and results in decreased perfusion and oxygen delivery to organs and tissues. As capillary leakage continues, vascular volume, cardiac output, and blood pressure decrease. This is the onset of early burn shock. Burn shock is initially a type of hypovolemic shock secondary to intravascular volume loss (see Chapter 11).

Unlike traumatic injuries, often characterized by blood loss, only plasma is lost in the burn injury. Prompt, appropriate

TABLE 57-2	Pathophysiologic Changes with Severe Burns
Body System	**Physiologic Changes**
Cardiovascular	Cardiac depression, edema, hypovolemia
Pulmonary	Vasoconstriction, edema
Gastrointestinal	Impaired motility and absorption, vasoconstriction, loss of mucosal barrier function with bacterial translocation, increased pH
Kidney	Vasoconstriction
Other	Altered thermoregulation, immunodepression, hypermetabolism

Adapted from Bielson, C. B., Duethman, N. C., Howard, J. M., et al. (2017). Burns: Pathophysiology of systemic complications and current management. *Journal of Burn Care & Research, 38*(1), e469–e481.

enteral or parenteral fluid resuscitation maintains the blood pressure in the low to normal range and improves cardiac output (see later discussion). However, even with adequate fluid resuscitation, cardiac filling pressures (central venous pressure, pulmonary artery pressure, and pulmonary artery wedge pressure) remain low during the initial burn shock period. Unless sufficient IV fluids are administered to maintain vascular volume, distributive shock occurs (see Chapter 11).

Generally, the greatest volume of intravascular fluid leak occurs in the first 24 to 36 hours after the burn injury, peaking at approximately 6 to 8 hours after the initial burn injury. As the capillaries begin to regain their integrity, burn shock resolves and fluid shifts back into the vascular compartment. Intrinsic diuresis will begin and continue for several days to 2 weeks in the previously healthy adult.

Fluid and Electrolyte Alterations

Edema forms rapidly after a burn injury. A superficial burn will cause localized edema to form within 4 hours, whereas a deeper burn will continue to form edema up to 18 hours post injury. The increased perfusion to the injured area in the presence of increased capillary permeability reflects the amount of microvascular and lymphatic damage to the tissue. In burns greater than 20% TBSA, inflammatory mediators stimulate local and systemic reactions resulting in extensive shift of intravascular fluid, electrolytes, and proteins into the surrounding interstitium (Gillenwater & Garner, 2017).

 *Concept Mastery Alert*

For patients in the emergent/resuscitative phase, nurses should do a primary survey and closely monitor circulation. As the taut, burned tissue becomes unyielding to the edema beneath its surface, it begins to act like a tourniquet, especially if the burn is circumferential. As edema increases, pressure on small blood vessels in the distal extremities obstructs blood flow resulting in consequent tissue ischemia and potentially acute compartment syndrome. See Chapter 37 for discussion of acute compartment syndrome. Patients in the acute/intermediate phase must be closely monitored for the development of venous thromboembolism (VTE).

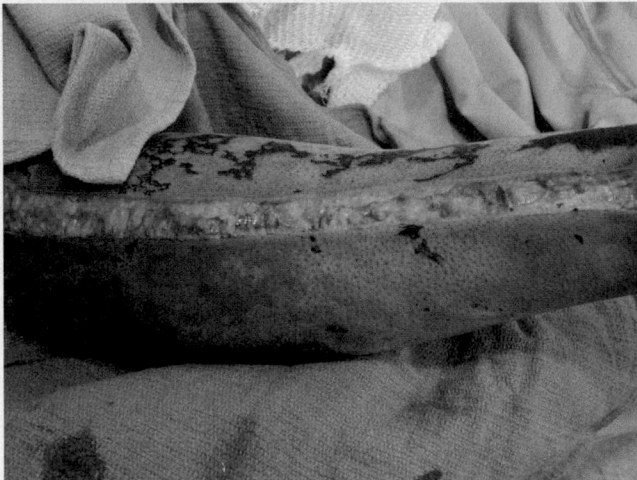

Figure 57-5 • Escharotomy of forearm. Used with permission from University of Texas Medical Branch, Galveston, TX.

Treatments for edema may include elevation of the extremity or, in severe cases, cutting of the **eschar** (i.e., devitalized tissue) via **escharotomy** (i.e., surgical incision through eschar), or decompression of edema formation via **fasciotomy** (i.e., surgical incision through fascia to relieve constricted muscle) to restore tissue perfusion (see Figs. 57-5 and 57-6).

Reabsorption of edema begins about 4 hours post injury and is complete approximately 4 days postburn injury. However, the rate of reabsorption depends on the depth of injury to the tissue. Although adequate fluid resuscitation is paramount to maintaining tissue perfusion, excessive fluid administration increases edema formation in both burned and unburned tissue causing ischemia and necrosis.

Immediately after burn injury, hyperkalemia (excessive potassium) may result from massive cell destruction. Hypokalemia (potassium depletion) may occur later with fluid shifts and inadequate potassium replacement. Serum sodium levels vary in response to fluid resuscitation. Hyponatremia (serum sodium depletion) may be present from plasma loss or may occur during the first week of the acute phase, as water

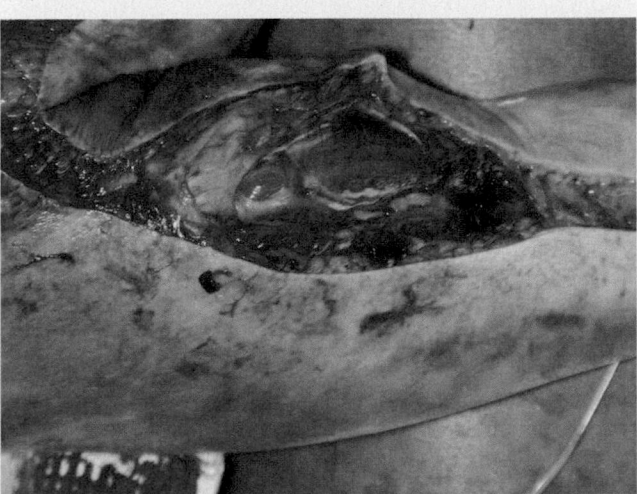

Figure 57-6 • Fasciotomy of upper arm. Used with permission from University of Texas Medical Branch, Galveston, TX.

shifts from the interstitial space and returns to the vascular space.

At the time of burn injury, some red blood cells may be destroyed, and others damaged. Despite this, the early hematocrit may be elevated due to plasma loss (hemoconcentration). Abnormalities in coagulation, including a decrease in platelets (thrombocytopenia) and prolonged clotting and prothrombin times also occur.

Pulmonary Alterations

Inhalation injuries, caused by inhalation of thermal and/or chemical irritants, are categorized as upper airway injury (above the glottis) or lower airway injury (below the glottis). Injuries above the vocal cords can be thermal or chemical, whereas injuries below the vocal cords are usually chemical (ABA, 2018). Approximately 2% to 14% of patients admitted to burn centers have an inhalation injury (ABA, 2018). The presence of inhalation injury is important to recognize, as it is one of the highest causes of mortality, along with age of the patient and burn size. History of the injury, such as a flame injury occurring in an enclosed space, and clinical signs such as singed facial hair or carbonaceous sputum (i.e., sputum with carbon particles which appears black; soot), are indicators for the potential presence of a smoke inhalation injury. Bronchoscopy is considered the standard test for definitive diagnosis as initial chest x-rays appear normal. The extent of pulmonary damage is directly related to the temperature and the concentration of toxic gases.

Upper Airway Injury

Upper airway injury is obstructive; it is caused by severe upper airway edema from direct thermal injury or secondary edema from face or neck burns in the early postburn period. Protective intubation is often warranted to maintain patency of the airway (ABA, 2018; Jones et al., 2017). Because of the cooling effect of rapid vaporization in the oropharynx, direct heat injury does not normally occur below the level of the glottis. However, with steam exposure or in blast injuries, thermal injury to the lower airways is possible because the upper airway cannot effectively protect the lower airway in these cases (Jones et al., 2017).

Lower Airway Injury

Inhalation injury below the glottis results from inhaling the products of incomplete combustion or noxious gases and is often the source of death at the scene of a fire. Smoke inhalation causes loss of ciliary action, triggers an inflammatory response causing hypersecretion, producing severe mucosal edema and potential bronchospasm. A reduction in alveolar surfactant production produces atelectasis (collapse of alveoli) in the parenchyma. Expectoration of carbon particles in the sputum is the cardinal sign of a lower airway inhalation injury. Aggressive pulmonary toilet is critical to maintain airway patency and clear resulting viscous sputum. Outcomes are improved in lower airway injuries when patients can expectorate carbonaceous sputum naturally (i.e., among patients who are not endotracheally intubated and mechanically ventilated) (Jones et al., 2017).

Noxious gases, such as carbon monoxide (CO) and hydrogen cyanide, contribute to lower airway injuries. CO poisoning is a factor in most fatalities at the scene of a fire as it combines with hemoglobin and displaces oxygen to form **carboxyhemoglobin.** The affinity of hemoglobin for CO is 200 times greater than that for oxygen, and if significant quantities of CO are present, then tissue hypoxia will occur. Treatment is administration of 100% oxygen to displace the CO molecules bound to hemoglobin, bringing the half-life of CO down to 45 minutes (ABA, 2018).

Hydrogen cyanide is a rapid systemic toxin also associated with mortality. Signs and symptoms are similar to CO poisoning and can include shortness of breath, headache, vertigo, confusion, and mucous membrane irritation. The cardiopulmonary effects initially cause a hyperdynamic response followed by bradycardia and hypotension leading to death. Hydrogen cyanide poisoning may be suspected in a patient with persistent lactic acidosis after resuscitation (ABA, 2018). Gaseous cyanide is a result from incomplete combustion of many items found in homes today.

Bronchoconstriction (caused by release of histamine, serotonin, and thromboxane [a powerful vasoconstrictor]) and chest constriction secondary to circumferential torso burns can contribute to deterioration. Even without pulmonary injury, hypoxia may be present. Early in the postburn period, catecholamine release in response to the stress of the burn injury alters peripheral blood flow, thereby reducing oxygen delivery to the periphery. Later, hypermetabolism and continued catecholamine release lead to increased tissue oxygen consumption, which can also lead to hypoxia. Administration of supplemental oxygen will ensure that adequate oxygen is available to the tissues. Restrictive pulmonary excursion may occur with full-thickness burns encircling the thorax resulting in decreased tidal volume. In such situations, an escharotomy may be necessary to restore adequate chest excursion (ABA, 2018).

Kidney Alterations

Kidney function may be altered as a result of decreased blood volume postburn injury due to the compensatory response to intravascular volume loss. Adequate fluid volume replacement can restore renal blood flow, increasing the glomerular filtration rate and urine volume. Additionally, destruction of red blood cells at the injury site may result in free hemoglobin in the urine. If muscle damage occurs (e.g., from electrical burns), myoglobin is released from the muscle cells and excreted by the kidneys causing the urine to be red. If there is inadequate blood flow through the kidneys caused by the hemoglobin and myoglobin occluding the renal tubules, acute tubular necrosis and acute kidney injury will occur (see Chapter 48). Increased abdominal pressure from the injury can also cause kidney ischemia.

Immunologic Alterations

The immunologic defenses of the body are significantly altered by a burn injury. Skin, the largest barrier to infection, when compromised continually exposes the patient to the environment. The burn injury itself produces systemic release of cytokines and other substances that cause leukocyte and endothelial cell dysfunction. Burn centers must provide an infection-controlled environment to protect the patient and minimize exposure to potentially harmful organisms (Palmieri, 2019).

Thermoregulatory Alterations

Integumentary loss also causes an inability to regulate body temperature resulting in various complications. Patients with burn injuries often exhibit low body temperatures in the early hours after injury not necessarily due to initial first aid, which may include cooling of the wounds, but more likely from the amount of TBSA involved, the IV resuscitation fluids administered, and exposure resulting in increased evaporative heat loss (Ehrl, Heidekrueger, Rubenbauger, et al., 2018). Burn centers often have additional heating sources to help maintain the patient's body temperature through environmental warming.

Gastrointestinal Alterations

Patients who are critically ill, especially those with burns, are predisposed to altered gastrointestinal (GI) motility. Impaired enteric nerve and smooth muscle function, inflammation, surgery, medications such as vasopressors, and inadequate tissue perfusion are some causes of GI dysfunction. Indicators of GI organ ischemia include increased bladder pressure, increasing serum lactate, and feeding intolerance. Three of the most common GI alterations in patients with burns are paralytic ileus (absence of intestinal peristalsis), Curling's ulcer, and translocation of bacteria. Decreased peristalsis and bowel sounds are manifestations of paralytic ileus. Gastric distention and nausea may lead to vomiting; therefore, gastric decompression is advised. Gastric bleeding secondary to massive physiologic stress may be signaled by occult blood in the stool, regurgitation of "coffee-ground" material from the stomach, or bloody vomitus. These signs suggest gastric or duodenal erosion (Curling's ulcer). Probiotics may be useful in maintaining intestinal barrier function through avoidance of colonization of pathogenic microorganisms (Culnan, Capek, & Sheridan, 2018).

Thermal injury damages the liver through induction of hepatic edema, apoptosis, insulin resistance associated with metabolic derangements, and development of a fatty liver. In addition, with severe burn injury, acute pancreatitis is common and may result in a threefold increase in amylase or lipase, feeding intolerance, or abdominal pain (Culnan et al., 2018).

Patients with large TBSA burns are also at risk for life-threatening abdominal compartment syndrome (ACS) due to large volumes of fluid required for resuscitation, fluid shifts to the interstitium causing edema formation, and decreased abdominal wall compliance due to eschar formation. Increased pressure in the abdominal cavity contributes to GI tract and abdominal organ ischemia (see Chapter 11). Ramirez, Palmieri, Greenhalgh, and colleagues (2018) reviewed 10 years of cases of ACS in patients with burns and found support for early laparotomy as definitive treatment of ACS.

Management of Burn Injury

Burn recovery generally occurs in three phases: emergent/resuscitative, acute/intermediate, and rehabilitation. Although priorities exist for each of the phases, assessment and management of problems and complications will overlap. Table 57-3 summarizes the priorities of care for each phase.

Emergent/Resuscitative Phase

On-the-Scene Care

The first step in management is to remove the patient from the source of injury and stop the burning process while preventing injury to the rescuer. Rescue workers' priorities include establishing an airway, supplying oxygen (100% oxygen if CO poisoning is suspected), inserting at least one large-bore IV catheter for fluid administration, and covering the wound with a clean, dry cloth or gauze. Continuous irrigation of chemical injury must begin immediately. Chart 57-4 describes the procedures and care required at the burn scene. The outward physical appearance of the person burned is often distracting, but the internal systemic effects pose the greater threat to life.

An immediate primary survey of the patient is performed assessing the ABCDEs: *a*irway (A) with consideration given to protecting the cervical spine, gas exchange or *b*reathing (B), *c*irculatory and *c*ardiac status (C), *d*isability (D) including neurologic deficit, and *e*xpose and *e*xamine (E) while maintaining a warm environment (ABA, 2018).

TABLE 57-3	Phases of Burn Care	
Phase	**Duration**	**Priorities**
Emergent/resuscitative	From onset of injury to completion of fluid resuscitation	• Primary survey: A, B, C, D, E • Prevention of shock • Prevention of respiratory distress • Detection and treatment of concomitant injuries • Wound assessment and initial care
Acute/intermediate	From beginning of diuresis to near completion of wound closure	• Wound care and closure • Prevention or treatment of complications, including infection • Nutritional support
Rehabilitation	From major wound closure to return to individual's optimal level of physical and psychosocial adjustment	• Prevention and treatment of scars and contractures • Physical, occupational, and vocational rehabilitation • Functional and cosmetic reconstruction • Psychosocial counseling

Adapted from American Burn Association. (2018). *Advanced burn life support (ABLS) course provider manual 2018.* Chicago, IL: Author; Serghiou, M. A., Ott, S., Cowan, A., et al. (2018). Burn rehabilitation along the continuum of care. In D. Herndon (Ed.). *Total burn care* (5th ed.). Edinburgh: Saunders Elsevier.

| Chart 57-4 | Emergency Procedures at the Burn Scene |

- **Extinguish the flames or remove from source.** A fire requires oxygen and fuel once ignited. When clothing catches fire, the flames can be extinguished if the person drops to the floor or ground and rolls ("stop, drop, and roll") or uses anything available, such as a blanket, rug, or coat, to smother the flames. The older adult, or others with impaired mobility, could be instructed to "stop, sit, and pat" to prevent concomitant musculoskeletal injuries. Standing still forces the person to breathe flames and smoke, while running fans the flames. If the burn source is electrical, the electrical source must be disconnected safely before approaching the patient.
- **Cool the burn.** After the flames are extinguished, the burned area and adherent clothing are soaked with *cool* water to cool the wound and halt the burning process. However, *never* apply ice directly to the burn, *never* wrap the person in ice, and *never* use cold soaks or dressings for longer than 20 or so minutes; such procedures may worsen tissue damage and lead to hypothermia in people with larger burns.
- **Remove restrictive objects.** If possible, remove affected, nonadherent clothing immediately. Adherent clothing may be left in place once cooled. Other clothing and all jewelry, including all piercings, should be removed to allow for assessment and to prevent constriction secondary to rapidly developing edema.
- **Cover the wound.** The burn should be covered as quickly as possible to minimize bacterial contamination, maintain body temperature by decreasing evaporative heat loss, and decrease pain by preventing air currents from coming in contact with the exposed nerves in the injured surface. Any clean, dry cloth can be used as an emergency dressing. Ointments and salves should *not* be used. Other than the dressing, no medication or material should be applied to the burn wound at the scene.
- **Irrigate chemical burns.** Chemical burns resulting from contact with a corrosive material are irrigated immediately and continuously with copious amounts of water. Most chemical laboratories have a shower for these types of emergencies. If a chemical contact occurs at home, brush off the chemical agent if dry, remove contaminated and all potentially contaminated clothes immediately, and rinse all areas of the body that have come in contact with the chemical. Rinsing can occur in the shower or any other source of continuous running water. If a chemical gets in or near the eyes, the eyes should be flushed with cool, clean water immediately and copiously. Outcomes for the patient with chemical burns are significantly improved by rapid, sustained flushing of the injury with water at the scene.

Adapted from American Burn Association. (2018). *Advanced burn life support (ABLS) course provider manual 2018.* Chicago, IL.

> **Quality and Safety Nursing Alert**

Airway patency and breathing must be assessed during the initial minutes of emergency care. Immediate therapy is directed toward establishing a patent airway and giving humidified 100% oxygen. If qualified personnel and equipment are available and the patient with burns has severe respiratory distress and/or airway edema, the rescuers must insert an endotracheal tube and initiate mechanical ventilation. No food or fluid is given by mouth, and the patient is placed in a position that will prevent aspiration of vomitus, because nausea and vomiting may occur, and protection of the airway is always a priority.

The secondary survey focuses on obtaining a history, the completion of the total body systems assessment, initial fluid resuscitation, and provision of psychosocial support of the conscious patient (see Chapter 67) (ABA, 2018).

Medical Management

Long-term outcomes are impacted by the quality of care received in the first few hours after injury (ABA, 2018). Initially, the patient is transported to the nearest emergency department (ED) so that lifesaving measures can be initiated. Early referral to a burn center is then made if indicated.

Initial priorities in the ED remain airway, breathing, and circulation. For mild pulmonary injury, 100% humidified oxygen is given, and the patient is encouraged to cough so that secretions can be expectorated or removed by suctioning. For more severe situations, it may be necessary to remove secretions by bronchial suctioning and administer bronchodilators and mucolytic agents. Continuous monitoring of airway patency is critical; a previously stable airway may rapidly deteriorate as edema increases and toxic effects of smoke inhalation become apparent.

Once urgent respiratory needs are appropriately addressed, fluid resuscitation is initiated. Fluid resuscitation in patients with burns greater than 20% TBSA addresses the intravascular volume deficit to improve tissue and organ perfusion caused by plasma loss, with the least amount of fluid possible. Daily weights and trends in laboratory test results require close monitoring in the immediate postburn (resuscitation) period to monitor fluid status. Both underresuscitation and overresuscitation with IV fluids are associated with poor outcomes. Shock, ischemic complications, and multiple organ dysfunction syndrome (MODS) occur with underresuscitation (see Chapter 11), and heart failure and pulmonary edema occur with overresuscitation (see Chapter 25).

In order to facilitate fluid administration, peripheral IV access may be obtained initially; however, in larger burns, central venous access is recommended due to the large volumes required. Once the TBSA is calculated, fluid resuscitation with lactated Ringer (LR) should be initiated using ABA resuscitation formulas. LR is the crystalloid of choice because its pH and osmolality most closely resemble human plasma.

The ABA (2018) fluid resuscitation formula for adults within 24 hours post thermal or chemical burn is as follows:

$$2 \text{ mL LR} \times \text{patient's weight in kilograms} \times \%\text{TBSA second-, third-, and fourth-degree burns}$$

For adults with electrical burns:

$$4 \text{ mL LR} \times \text{patient's weight in kilograms} \times \%\text{TBSA second-, third-, and fourth-degree burns}$$

Timing is one of the most important considerations in calculating fluid needs in the first 24 hours post burn. The starting point is the time of injury—not the time of arrival to the treating facility (ABA, 2018). The infusion is regulated so that half of the total calculated volume is given in the first 8 hours postburn injury. The second half of the calculated volume is infused over the next 16 hours.

These formulas are only guidelines. It is imperative that the rate of infusion be titrated hourly as indicated by physiologic monitoring of the patient's response. Each patient has a unique injury and optimum results require individualized treatments based on patient response (Gillenwater & Garner, 2017). Urinary output continues to be the standard for assessing patient response to fluid resuscitation. A urine output of 0.5 to 1 mL/kg/h in adults indicates appropriate resuscitation in thermal and chemical injuries, whereas in electrical injuries a urine output of 75 to 100 mL/h is desired (ABA, 2018). Other indicators such as blood pressure or heart rate are not useful in assessing adequate intravascular volume in patients with major burns due to the marked inflammatory response.

After adequate respiratory function and circulatory status have been established, the patient is assessed for cervical spine and/or head injuries if involved in a traumatic or electrical injury. All clothing and jewelry are removed because they may contain chemicals, retain heat, or become constrictive as edema rapidly develops. For chemical burns, flushing of the exposed areas with copious amounts of clean water is continued. The patient is checked for contact lenses. These are removed immediately if chemicals have come in contact with the eyes or if facial burns have occurred. In addition, the eyes are examined promptly for injury to the corneas. An ophthalmologist may be consulted for complete assessment via fluorescent staining to assess for corneal damage.

The patient's temperature must be monitored because hypothermia may develop rapidly, and manipulation of the environment may be necessary. A temperature less than 35°C (95°F) causes vasoconstriction, which may increase tissue ischemia and necrosis.

It is important to validate an account of the burn scenario provided by the patient, witnesses at the scene, and first responders. Information should include the time and the source of the burn injury, the scene of injury (particularly if the patient was in an enclosed space), length of exposure, prior treatment, and any history of concomitant traumatic injury. A history of preexisting medical conditions, allergies, medications, and the use of drugs, alcohol, and tobacco is obtained to assist with the treatment plan.

An indwelling urinary catheter is inserted to permit accurate monitoring of urine output and fluid needs and as a measure of kidney function for patients with moderate to severe burns. If the burn exceeds 20% to 25% TBSA, a nasogastric tube is inserted and connected to low intermittent suction. All patients who are intubated should have a nasogastric tube inserted to decompress the stomach, and to prevent vomiting and aspiration. Often, patients with large burns become nauseated as a result of the GI effects of the burn injury, such as paralytic ileus, and the effects of medications such as opioids.

Clean sheets are placed under and over the patient to protect the burn wound from contamination, maintain body temperature, and reduce pain caused by air currents passing over exposed nerve endings. Baseline height, weight, arterial blood gases, hematocrit, serum electrolytes, blood alcohol level, drug panel, urinalysis, and chest x-rays may be obtained. Because poor tissue perfusion accompanies burn injuries, only IV analgesia is given in small repeated doses, which is crucial for pain reduction in the emergent phase. If the patient has an electrical burn, a baseline electrocardiogram is also obtained and continuous cardiac monitoring is initiated. Because burns are contaminated wounds, tetanus prophylaxis is given if the patient's immunization status is not current or is unknown.

> ### ◣ Quality and Safety Nursing Alert
>
> *If necessary, a blood pressure cuff may be placed around a patient's burned extremity. The cuff must be of the correct size with accommodations made for edema.*

Although the major focus of care during the emergent phase is physiologic stabilization, the nurse must also attend to the patient's and the family's psychological needs. Anxiety accompanies burn injuries and must be addressed on an ongoing basis. A burn injury is a crisis—one that causes varying emotional responses that may result in conflicts that may precipitate ethical dilemmas. The patient's and family's coping abilities and available supports are assessed. The nurse must consider special circumstances surrounding the burn injury when providing care. Examples include cases of abuse, neglect, suicide attempts, and injury/death of other family members or friends from the same event.

Nursing Management

Nursing assessment in the emergent phase of burn injury focuses on the major priorities for any trauma patient; the burn wound is a secondary consideration to stabilization of airway, breathing, and circulation. The nurse monitors respiratory status closely, and pulses are evaluated, particularly in areas of circumferential burn injury to an extremity. Initially, cardiac monitoring is indicated if the patient has a history of cardiac disease, electrical injury, or altered respiratory conditions. The nurse should monitor vital signs with knowledge of expected abnormalities consistent with burn injury such as tachycardia, tachypnea.

If all extremities are burned, determining blood pressure may be difficult. A clean dressing applied under the blood pressure cuff protects the wound from contamination. Because increasing edema makes blood pressure difficult to auscultate, a Doppler (ultrasound) device or a noninvasive electronic blood pressure device may be helpful. In patients with severe burns, an arterial catheter is preferred for blood pressure measurement and is helpful for collecting blood specimens. Peripheral pulses in burned extremities are checked frequently either by palpation or the use of a Doppler. Elevation of burned extremities above the level of the heart is indicated for edema reduction. Large-bore IV catheters (e.g., 16 to 18 gauge) and an indwelling urinary catheter are inserted, if not already in situ, and the nurse's documentation must include hourly assessment of fluid intake and urine output.

Red-colored urine suggests the presence of hemochromogens from damage to red blood cells and myoglobin, the by-product of muscle damage (ABA, 2018). This anomaly is associated with deep burns caused by electrical injury or prolonged contact with heat or flame. Glycosuria, a common finding in the early postburn hours, results from the release of liver glycogen stores in response to stress.

The nurse assists with calculating the patient's expected fluid requirements and monitoring the patient's response to fluid resuscitation. Nurse-driven resuscitation protocols have been shown to decrease the amount of fluid given and improve patient outcomes in the emergent/resuscitative phase (Stewart, Ladd, Kovler, et al., 2019). Nursing responsibilities consist of appropriate fluid administration, strict monitoring of intake and output, monitoring the patient's response, and notifying the treatment team of significant assessment findings and any abnormal laboratory values.

To help guide treatment, the following are essential: documentation of body temperature, body weight, and pre-burn weight; history of allergies, tetanus immunization, past medical and surgical history, and current illnesses; and a list of current medications. The nurse performs a head-to-toe assessment, focusing on signs and symptoms of concomitant illness, associated trauma, or developing complications. Assessing the extent of the burn wound using the rule of nines or facilitated with anatomic diagrams (described previously) is performed. Additionally, the nurse works with the primary provider to clinically assess and document the initial areas of full- and partial-thickness injury. Psychosocial considerations of the patient and family and communication with the treatment team are imperative early in the course of care.

Nursing care of the patient in the emergent/resuscitative phase of burn injury is detailed in Chart 57-5.

 ## Acute/Intermediate Phase

The acute/intermediate phase of burn care follows the emergent/resuscitative phase and begins 48 to 72 hours after the burn injury. During this phase, attention is directed toward continued assessment and maintenance of respiratory and circulatory status, fluid and electrolyte balance, and GI and kidney function. Infection prevention and control, burn wound care (e.g., wound cleaning and débridement, topical antibacterial/antimicrobial therapy, application of dressings, wound grafting), pain management, modulation of the hypermetabolic response, and early positioning/mobility are priorities in the acute/intermediate stage of recovery.

Medical Management

Pulmonary complications are common in burn injury. Airway obstruction caused by upper airway edema can take as long as 48 hours to develop. Changes detected by x-ray and arterial blood gas analysis may occur as the effects of resuscitative fluid and the chemical reactions of smoke ingredients with lung tissues become evident. Diagnosis is largely based on history and clinical presentation, monitoring of arterial blood gases with carboxyhemoglobin levels, and direct observation of the airway by fiberoptic bronchoscopy (ABA, 2018). To lessen the effects of upper airway edema, elevation of the patient's head of the bed may be helpful. Stridor and dyspnea are ominous because they are late signs of impending airway obstruction. Early protective intubation to maintain airway patency should be considered as obstruction may occur very rapidly. However, intubation and mechanical ventilation are significant contributors to pulmonary infections. Ideally, the best practice is to remove the endotracheal tube as soon as possible so that a route for pathogens is not accessible to the lungs (ABA, 2018).

Late pulmonary complications secondary to inhalation injuries include mucosal sloughing of the airway and cast formation from cellular debris, which can lead to obstruction, increased secretions, inflammation, atelectasis, airway ulceration, pulmonary edema, and tissue hypoxia. Although research results are mixed, nebulized heparin therapy may be administered because it is thought to have some effect on the inflammatory cascade and formation of fibrin casts in the airways (Suresh & Dries, 2018). Pneumonia, acute lung injury (ALI), and acute respiratory distress syndrome (ARDS) may also occur.

Ventilator-associated pneumonia (VAP) is a common complication of any patient who is hospitalized and mechanically ventilated and is particularly exacerbated in the patient with an inhalation injury. It affects as many as 10% to 20% of patients on mechanical ventilation longer than 48 hours. See Chapter 19, Chart 19-6, for discussion of "bundled" strategies to prevent VAP and Chapter 19 for discussion of respiratory failure and ARDS.

As capillaries regain their integrity, 48 or more hours after the burn, fluid shifts from the interstitial to the intravascular compartment and intrinsic diuresis begins. If cardiac or kidney function is inadequate, fluid overload may occur, and symptoms of heart failure may emerge (see Chapter 25). Administration of fluids and electrolytes continues cautiously during this phase of burn care due to fluid shifts, evaporative fluid loss from large burn wounds, and the patient's physiologic responses to the burn injury. Blood components are given as needed to treat surgical blood loss and anemia.

Hyperthermia is common in patients after burn shock resolves. A resetting of the core body temperature in patients who are severely burned results in a body temperature a few degrees higher than normal for several weeks after the burn. This can be compounded by body temperature increases from sepsis.

Central venous, arterial, or specialty catheters (e.g., hemodialysis catheters, Zoll® catheters) may be required for monitoring hemodynamics. Commonly, patients with major burns need multiple invasive line sites due to the amount and frequency of fluid and medications required. Whenever possible, burned areas of the body are avoided as insertion sites for invasive lines.

One of the most important medical interventions for patients with burns that have positively affected mortality is early **excision** (surgical removal of tissue). The presence of the open wounds or invasive organisms triggers the response to a large burn injury, a systemic cascade of events (Culnan, Sherman, Chung, et al., 2018). Excising the necrotic tissue can ameliorate this response and preserve underlying viable tissue.

Infection Prevention and Control

There are multifactorial reasons why patients with burns incur some of the highest risks for health care–associated infections (HAIs). The systemic response to a burn injury results in dysregulation of the immune system, predisposing the patient to invasion by environmental pathogens (Lachiewicz, Hauck, Weber, et al., 2017). The wound provides a perfect medium for bacterial proliferation, as well as a conduit to the bloodstream (Ramos, Cornistein, Cerino, et al., 2017). Because of the loss of the epidermal barrier, presence of transmittable bacteria, and the ubiquity of mold species in the environment, it is critical that the nurse prioritizes infection prevention in the plan of care (Sood, Vaidya, Dam, et al., 2018). In addition, to support vital organs and bodily functions, invasive procedures are required which may undermine the body's natural defenses (Ramos et al., 2017).

(text continued on page 1879)

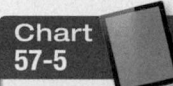

Chart 57-5

PLAN OF NURSING CARE
Care of the Patient during the Emergent/Resuscitative Phase of Burn Injury

NURSING DIAGNOSIS: Impaired gas exchange associated with carbon monoxide (CO) poisoning, smoke inhalation, and upper airway obstruction
GOAL: Maintenance of adequate tissue oxygenation

Nursing Interventions	Rationale	Expected Outcomes
1. Provide 100% humidified oxygen.	1. Humidification provides moisture to injured tissues; supplemental oxygen increases alveolar oxygenation.	• Absence of dyspnea • Arterial oxygen saturation >95% by pulse oximetry (in the absence of CO poisoning)
2. Assess breath sounds, and respiratory rate, rhythm, depth and symmetry of chest excursion. Monitor patient for signs of hypoxia. Report abnormalities to primary provider.	2. These factors provide baseline data of assessment and evidence of increasing respiratory compromise.	• Arterial blood gas levels within normal limits • Respiratory rate, pattern, and breath sounds normal

3. Observe for the following:
  a. Erythema or blistering of lips or buccal mucosa
  b. Singed nasal hairs
  c. Burns of face, neck, or chest
  d. Increasing hoarseness
  e. Soot in sputum or tracheal tissue in respiratory secretions
	3. These signs indicate possible inhalation injury and risk of respiratory dysfunction.	

4. Monitor arterial blood gas values, pulse oximetry readings, and carboxyhemoglobin levels.	4. Increasing $PaCO_2$ and decreasing PaO_2 and O_2 saturation may indicate need for mechanical ventilation.	
5. Prepare to assist with intubation and escharotomies of chest.	5. Intubation allows airway protection and mechanical ventilation. Escharotomy enables adequate chest excursion in circumferential chest burns.	

NURSING DIAGNOSIS: Impaired airway clearance associated with exposure to smoke
GOAL: Maintain patent airway and adequate airway clearance

Nursing Interventions	Rationale	Expected Outcomes
1. Maintain patent airway through proper patient positioning, removal of secretions, and artificial airway if needed.	1. A patent airway is crucial to respiration.	• Patent airway • Respiratory secretions are minimal, colorless, and thin.
2. Provide humidified oxygen as prescribed.	2. Humidification liquefies secretions and facilitates expectoration.	
3. Encourage patient to turn, cough, and deep breathe. Encourage patient to use incentive spirometry. Perform endotracheal suction as needed.	3. These activities promote mobilization and removal of secretions.	

NURSING DIAGNOSIS: Hypovolaemia associated with increased capillary permeability and evaporative losses from the burn wound
GOAL: Restoration of optimal fluid and electrolyte balance and perfusion of vital organs

Nursing Interventions	Rationale	Expected Outcomes
1. Monitor vital signs, hemodynamics, and urine output, as well as record strict intake and output and daily weights.	1. Hypovolemia is a major risk immediately following a burn injury. Overresuscitation with IV fluids might cause fluid overload.	• Urine output between 0.5 and 1.0 mL/kg/h (30–50 mL/h; 75–100 mL/h if electrical burn injury)
2. Maintain IV lines and regulate fluids at prescribed and appropriate rates following urine output.	2. Adequate fluids are necessary for perfusion of vital organs and maintenance of fluid and electrolyte balance.	• Mean arterial pressure ≥60 mm Hg • Voids clear yellow urine with specific gravity within normal limits
3. Observe for symptoms of deficiency or excess of serum sodium, potassium, calcium, phosphorus, and bicarbonate.	3. Rapid shifts in fluid and electrolyte status are possible in the postburn period.	• Serum electrolytes within normal limits
4. Elevate head of patient's bed and burned extremities, if not contraindicated.	4. Elevation promotes venous return.	
5. Notify primary provider immediately of decreased urine output and hemodynamic changes.	5. Rapid fluid shifts must be detected early to prevent complications.	

(continued on page 1878)

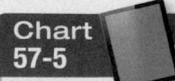

Chart 57-5   **PLAN OF NURSING CARE** (continued)
Care of the Patient during the Emergent/Resuscitative Phase of Burn Injury

NURSING DIAGNOSIS: Hypothermia associated with loss of skin microcirculation and open wounds
GOAL: Maintenance of adequate body temperature

Nursing Interventions	Rationale	Expected Outcomes
1. Assess core body temperature frequently.	1. Frequent temperature assessments help detect hypothermia.	• Body temperature remains >37°C (98.6°F)
2. Provide a warm environment by increasing room temperature or adjunct therapies as needed (overbed warmers, blankets, heat lamps, etc.).	2. Minimizes resting energy expenditure.	• Absence of chills or shivering
3. Work quickly when wounds must be exposed.	3. Limiting exposure minimizes evaporative heat loss from wound(s).	

NURSING DIAGNOSIS: Acute pain associated with chemical or physical injury
GOAL: Control of pain

Nursing Interventions	Rationale	Expected Outcomes
1. Use pain intensity scale to assess pain level. Differentiate restlessness due to pain from restlessness due to hypoxia.	1. Pain scales provide baselines for evaluating effectiveness of pain relief measures. Hypoxia can cause similar signs and must be ruled out before analgesic medication is given.	• States pain level is decreased and is acceptable to patient's pain goal
2. Administer IV antispasmodic agents as prescribed and assess for effectiveness.	2. IV administration is necessary because of altered tissue perfusion from burn injury.	• Absence of nonverbal cues of pain
3. Provide emotional support and reassurance.	3. Fear and anxiety increase the perception of pain.	

NURSING DIAGNOSIS: Anxiety associated with fear and the emotional impact of burn injury
GOAL: Minimization of patient's and family's anxiety

Nursing Interventions	Rationale	Expected Outcomes
1. Assess patient's and family's understanding of burn injury, coping skills, and family dynamics.	1. Previous successful coping strategies can be fostered for use in the present crisis. Assessment allows planning of individualized interventions.	• Patient and family verbalize understanding and acceptance of emergent burn care
2. Explain all procedures to the patient and the family in clear, simple terms.	2. Increased understanding alleviates fear of the unknown. High levels of anxiety may interfere with understanding of complex explanations.	• Patient and family's anxiety levels will be minimized
3. Administer prescribed antianxiety medications if the patient remains extremely anxious despite nonpharmacologic interventions.	3. Anxiety levels during the emergent phase may exceed the patient's coping abilities.	

COLLABORATIVE PROBLEMS: Acute respiratory failure, distributive shock, acute kidney injury, compartment syndrome, paralytic ileus, Curling's ulcer
GOAL: Absence of complications

Nursing Interventions	Rationale	Expected Outcomes
Acute Respiratory Failure		
1. Assess for increasing dyspnea, stridor, changes in respiratory patterns.	1. Such signs reflect deteriorating respiratory status.	• Breathes spontaneously with adequate tidal volume
2. Monitor pulse oximetry, arterial blood gas values.	2. Abnormal findings may indicate respiratory failure.	• Arterial blood gas values within acceptable limits
3. Monitor chest x-ray results.	3. X-ray may disclose pulmonary injury or infection.	• Chest x-ray findings normal
4. Assess for restlessness, confusion, difficulty attending to questions, or decreasing level of consciousness.	4. Such manifestations may indicate cerebral hypoxia.	• Absence of cerebral signs of hypoxia
5. Report deteriorating respiratory status immediately to primary provider.	5. Acute respiratory failure is life-threatening, and immediate intervention is required.	
6. Prepare to assist with intubation or escharotomies as indicated.	6. Intubation allows mechanical ventilation. Escharotomies allow adequate chest excursion with respirations.	

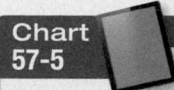

Chart 57-5   PLAN OF NURSING CARE (continued)
Care of the Patient during the Emergent/Resuscitative Phase of Burn Injury

Nursing Interventions	Rationale	Expected Outcomes
Distributive Shock		
1. Assess for decreasing urine output and alterations in vital signs and hemodynamics. 2. Assess for progressive edema as fluid shifts occur. 3. Adjust fluid resuscitation in collaboration with the primary provider in response to physiologic findings.	1. Such signs and symptoms may indicate distributive shock and inadequate intravascular volume. 2. As fluid shifts into the interstitial spaces in burn shock, edema occurs and may compromise tissue perfusion. 3. Optimal fluid resuscitation prevents distributive shock and improves patient outcomes.	• Urine output between 0.5 and 1.0 mL/kg/h (30–50 mL/h; 75–100 mL/h if electrical burn injury) • Blood pressure within patient's normal range • Hemodynamics remain within normal limits • No signs or symptoms of impaired perfusion
Acute Kidney Injury		
1. Monitor urine output, blood urea nitrogen (BUN), and serum creatinine levels. 2. Report decreased urine output or increased BUN and creatinine values to primary provider. 3. Assess urine for hemoglobin or myoglobin. Administer increased fluids as prescribed.	1. These values reflect renal function. 2. These laboratory values indicate possible kidney failure. 3. Hemoglobin or myoglobin in the urine predisposes patient to increased risk of kidney failure. Fluids help to flush hemoglobin and myoglobin from renal tubules.	• Adequate urine output • BUN and serum creatinine values remain normal
Compartment Syndrome		
1. Assess peripheral pulses frequently (with Doppler ultrasound device if needed). 2. Assess warmth, capillary refill, sensation, and movement of extremity frequently. Compare affected with unaffected extremity if possible. 3. Remove blood pressure cuff after each reading. 4. Elevate burned extremities if not contraindicated. 5. Report loss of pulse or sensation or presence of pain to primary provider immediately. 6. Prepare to assist with escharotomies.	1. Pulse assessments are crucial to assess for adequate perfusion. 2. These assessments may signal worsening peripheral perfusion. 3. Cuff may act as a tourniquet as extremities swell. 4. Elevation reduces edema formation. 5. These signs and symptoms may indicate impaired tissue perfusion. 6. Escharotomies relieve the constriction caused by edema.	• Peripheral pulses detectable • Signs of adequate peripheral perfusion
Paralytic Ileus		
1. Auscultate for bowel sounds, abdominal distention. 2. Maintain nasogastric tube on low intermittent suction until bowel sounds resume.	1. Presence of bowel sounds indicates normal peristalsis. Abdominal distention reflects inadequate decompression. 2. This measure relieves gastric and abdominal distention.	• Normal bowel sounds • Absence of abdominal distention
Curling's Ulcer		
1. Assess gastric aspirate and stools for blood. 2. Administer histamine-2 blockers and/or antacids as prescribed.	1. Blood indicates possible gastric or duodenal ulcer bleeding. 2. Such medications reduce gastric acidity and risk of ulceration.	• Gastric aspirate and stools do not contain blood

Causative agents of burn infections include bacteria, fungi, or viruses. Hydrotherapy equipment, direct or indirect contamination from healthcare workers' hands, environmental surfaces, and translocation of microorganisms from other body systems—most notably, the GI tract—are all common sources of potential contamination in the burn unit that require hypervigilance. Whether the burn wound is healing through spontaneous reepithelialization or is being prepared for skin grafting, protection from pathogens is crucial. Infection impedes burn wound healing by promoting excessive inflammation and damaging tissue. Clinical signs of infection include progressive erythema, warmth, tenderness, and malodorous exudate.

A multiple-strategy approach is crucial in prevention and control of burn wound infections. Such strategies include:

- The use of barrier techniques (e.g., gowns, gloves, eye protection, and masks if needed)

- Environmental cleaning with periodic cultures of patient care equipment (with special attention to hydrotherapy equipment)
- Application of appropriate topical antimicrobial agents
- Appropriate use of systemic antibiotic and antifungal agents (careful use and close monitoring of culture sensitivities are needed due to increasing challenges of antibiotic resistance in healthcare environments)
- Early excision and closure of the burn wound
- Control of hyperglycemia (with insulin as indicated, even in a patient without a prior diagnosis of diabetes)
- Management of the hypermetabolic response (see Chapter 11)

There are varying practices in the burn community regarding obtaining cultures for surveillance. In some burn centers, patients may be cultured on admission to screen for the presence of regionally known pathogens. Wounds are generally cultured on admission, prior to cleaning, with each surgical case, and for clinical suspicion of infection. Antimicrobial therapy is tailored to culture results. The broad use of prophylactic antibiotics is not supported by current research (Ramos et al., 2017).

Wound Cleaning

Proper management of burn wounds prevents wound deterioration. The goal of wound care is removal of nonviable tissue and wound exudate, and elimination of previously applied topical agents. Gentle cleaning with mild soap, water, and a washcloth can prevent infection by decreasing the bacteria and debris on the wound surface. Hair in and around the burn area, except the eyebrows, should be clipped short or shaved.

Various processes may facilitate cleaning burn wounds. Patients who are hemodynamically unstable may have their wounds washed at the bedside, whereas patients who are ambulatory may shower themselves or with assistance. Patients who are nonambulatory can be bathed and receive wound care using shower carts—mobile stretchers made with removable sides, drainage holes, and positioning capabilities. Retractable water hoses suspended from walls and ceilings provide the nurse with easy access to a clean water source for washing the wounds. Whatever method employed, the goal is to protect the wound from acute proliferation of pathogenic organisms on the surface through mechanical washing to prevent invasion of deeper tissues until the wounds are closed through spontaneous healing or skin grafting. Strategies for the prevention of cross-contamination include the use of plastic liners on the shower carts and chairs, water filtration systems or point-of-care filters, and thorough decontamination of equipment after each use.

Patient comfort and ability to participate in the prescribed treatment are important considerations. During bathing, patient participation is encouraged to promote exercise and range of motion of the extremities. During wound cleaning, the nurse inspects all skin for any signs of redness, breakdown, or local infection. This also provides the nurse an opportunity for targeted patient education.

During treatment, the patient is continuously assessed for signs of hypothermia. The temperature of the water is maintained at 37.8°C (100°F), and the temperature of the room should be maintained between 26.6° and 29.4°C (80° and 85°F) to prevent hypothermia. Other assessment considerations include patient fatigue, changes in hemodynamic status, and pain unrelieved by analgesic medications or relaxation techniques.

Topical Antibacterial Therapy

Variations in topical wound care for nonsurgical burn wounds exist among burn centers across the country. Selections are based on the individualized needs of each patient. The goal of topical therapy is to provide a dressing with the following characteristics:

- Effective against gram-positive and gram-negative organisms and fungi
- Penetrates the eschar but is not systemically toxic
- Is cost-effective, available, and acceptable to the patient
- Is easy to apply and remove, decreases the frequency of dressing changes, decreases pain, and minimizes nursing time

No single topical medication is universally effective, and the use of different agents at different times in the postburn period is best practice.

 Quality and Safety Nursing Alert

Prudent use and alternation of antimicrobial agents can result in reduction of resistant strains of bacteria, greater effectiveness of the agents, and a decreased risk of sepsis. Table 57-4 describes select topical antimicrobial agents.

Wound Dressing

After the prescribed topical agents are applied, the wound is covered with several layers of dry dressings with lighter dressing over joints to allow for mobility. Dressings may also require modification to accommodate splints or other positioning devices. Circumferential dressings should always be applied distally to proximally to promote return of excess fluid into the central circulation. In the case of hand or foot burns, the fingers and toes should be wrapped individually to promote mobility and function while healing.

Burns to the face may be left open to air once cleaned and the topical agent has been applied to maintain a moist environment. Careful attention ensures the topical agent does not come in contact with the eyes or mouth. A light, nonrestrictive dressing may be applied to the face to absorb excess exudate if needed.

Occlusive dressings, bulky gauze, and a topical antimicrobial agent may be used over areas with new skin grafts to protect the new graft and promote an optimal condition for its adherence to the recipient site. Ideally, these surgical dressings remain in place for 3 to 5 days, to allow growth of the microcirculation into the new graft before removal for inspection of the graft. When occlusive dressings are applied, precautions are taken to prevent two body surfaces from touching one another, such as fingers or toes, ear and scalp, the areas under the breasts, any point of flexion, or between the genital folds. Functional body alignment positions are maintained by using splints or by regular repositioning of the patient.

 Quality and Safety Nursing Alert

Dressings can impede circulation if they are wrapped too tightly. The peripheral pulses must be checked frequently and burned extremities elevated. If the patient's pulse is diminished, this is a critical situation and must be addressed immediately.

TABLE 57-4 Overview of Select Topical Antimicrobial Agents Used for Burn Wounds

Agent	Indication/Comment	Application	Nursing Implications
General			
Antimicrobial ointment	Antibacterial coverage and promotion of a moist wound environment	Apply 1/16-inch layer of ointment with a clean glove daily.	Ensure removal of residual ointment at the time of wound cleaning prior to applying a new layer. Monitor closely for signs and symptoms of local infection.
Specific Agents			
Silver sulfadiazine 1% water-soluble cream	Bactericidal agent for many gram-positive and gram-negative organisms, as well as yeast and *Candida albicans* Minimal penetration of eschar	Apply 1/16-inch layer of cream with a clean glove 1–3 times daily.	Anticipate formation of pseudoeschar (proteinaceous gel), which can be removed.
Mafenide acetate 5% hydrophilic-based solution or cream	Antimicrobial agent for gram-positive and gram-negative organisms Diffuses through eschar and avascular tissue (e.g., cartilage)	Apply twice a day with a clean glove.	Is a strong carbonic anhydrase inhibitor and may cause metabolic acidosis. Application may cause considerable pain initially.
Silver nitrate 0.5% aqueous solution	Effective against most strains of *Staphylococcus* and *Pseudomonas* and many gram-negative organisms. Does not penetrate eschar	Apply solution to gauze dressing and place over wound. Keep the dressing wet but covered with dry gauze and dry blankets to decrease vaporization.	Monitor serum sodium (Na^+) and potassium (K^+) levels and replace as prescribed. Silver nitrate solution is hypotonic and acts as a wick for sodium and potassium. Protect bed linens and clothing from contact with silver nitrate, which stains everything it touches.
Silver-impregnated dressings (sheets or mesh)	Broad antimicrobial effects (product specific) Delivers a uniform, antimicrobial concentration of silver ions to the burn wound.	Apply directly to wound. Cover with absorbent secondary dressing if needed.	May produce a pseudoeschar from silver after application. Can be left in place for several days (product specific).

Adapted from IBM Micromedix®. (2020). *Formulary advisor, New York Presbyterian Weill Cornell Medicine*. New York. Available pass-protected. Retrieved on 4/14/2020 at: www.micromedexsolutions.com/micromedex2/librarian/ssl/true

Dressings that adhere to the wound bed may be removed more comfortably and with less damage to healing tissue by moistening the dressing with water or saline. The patient may participate in removing the dressings, providing some degree of control over this painful procedure. The wounds are then cleaned and débrided to remove any remaining topical agent, exudate, and nonviable tissue. Sterile scissors and forceps may be used to trim loose eschar and encourage separation of devitalized tissue. During this procedure, the wound and surrounding skin are carefully inspected. Documentation should include color, odor, size, exudate, signs of reepithelialization, any changes from the previous dressing change, and other key characteristics.

Wound Débridement

The goals of **débridement** (removal of *devitalized* tissue) are:
- Removal of devitalized tissue or burn eschar in preparation for grafting and wound healing
- Removal of tissue contaminated by bacteria and foreign bodies, thereby protecting the patient from invasion of bacteria

There are four types of débridement—natural, mechanical, chemical, and surgical.

Natural Débridement

With natural débridement, the devitalized tissue separates from the underlying viable tissue spontaneously. Bacteria present at the interface of the burned tissue and healthy viable tissue gradually liquefy the fibrils of **collagen,** a protein present in skin, tendon, bone, cartilage, and connective tissue, that hold the eschar in place. Proteolytic and other natural enzymes cause this phenomenon. The process may take weeks to months to occur.

Mechanical Débridement

Mechanical débridement involves the use of surgical tools to separate and remove the eschar. This technique, performed by primary providers, specially trained nurses, or physical therapists, is usually performed with routine dressing changes. If bleeding occurs, hemostatic agents or pressure may be applied to achieve hemostasis. Dressing changes and wound cleaning aid the removal of wound debris. Wet-to-dry dressings are not advised for burn care because of the possibility of removing viable epithelial cells along with necrotic tissue. Wet-to-wet or wet-to-moist dressings may be used instead.

Chemical Débridement

Topical enzymatic agents are available to promote débridement of burn wounds. Because such agents usually do not have antimicrobial properties, they may be combined with topical antibacterial therapy to protect the patient from bacterial invasion. Heavy metals such as silver can deactivate débriding agents; therefore, caution is necessary to ensure that the topical antimicrobial agent does not interfere with the chemical débridement. Alternating topical medications may also be effective in achieving débridement without infection.

Surgical Débridement

Early surgical excision to remove devitalized tissue along with early burn wound closure has long been recognized as one of the most important factors contributing to survival in a patient with a major burn injury. Surgical débridement occurs before the natural separation of eschar transpires from bacterial lysis of collagen fibers at the dermal–eschar junction. This may be performed as soon as possible after the burn, once the patient is hemodynamically stable and edema has decreased. Ideally, the wound is covered immediately with a skin graft (if necessary) and a dressing. If the wound bed is not ready for a skin graft at the time of excision, a temporary biologic or synthetic dressing may be applied until an autograft can be successfully applied during a subsequent surgery.

The use of surgical excision carries with it risks and complications, especially with large burns. The procedure creates a high risk of extensive blood loss with lengthy operating and anesthesia times. Blood losses sustained during surgical procedures, wound care, and ongoing hemolysis exacerbate anemia. Blood transfusions may be required periodically to maintain adequate hemoglobin levels for oxygen delivery to the myocardium. See Chapter 28 for discussion of blood component therapy.

When conducted in a timely and efficient manner, surgical excision results in shorter lengths of stay and decreased risk of complications from invasive burn wound sepsis. Once débrided, granulation tissue fills the void created by the wound, creates a barrier to bacteria, and serves as a bed for epithelial cell growth. A wound covering is applied to keep the wound bed moist and promote the granulation process.

Wound Grafting

The patient with deep partial- or full-thickness burns may be a candidate for skin grafting to decrease the risk of infection; prevent further loss of protein, fluid, and electrolytes through the wound; minimize evaporative heat loss; and reduce scarring. Special attention is warranted when grafting the face (for cosmetic, functional, and psychological reasons); functional areas, such as the hands and feet; and areas over joints. Grafting permits earlier function and reduces scar **contractures** (shrinkage of burn scar through collagen maturation). When burns are very extensive, the order in which areas are grafted is chosen based on the ability to achieve wound closure as soon as possible; therefore, the chest and abdomen or back may be grafted first to reduce the overall open wound size.

Autografts

Autografting remains the preferred autologous method for definitive burn wound closure after excision. **Autografts** are the ideal means of covering burn wounds because the grafts are the patient's own skin and therefore are not rejected by the patient's immune system. They can be split-thickness, full-thickness, or epithelial grafts. Because the **donor site** (the area from which skin is taken to provide the autograft) for a full-thickness graft includes both the epidermis and dermis, its use must be cautiously considered because the donor site cannot heal spontaneously.

Split-thickness autografts are most commonly used and can be applied in sheets (see Fig. 57-7), or they can be expanded by meshing so that they cover more than a given donor site area (see Fig. 57-8). Skin meshers enable the surgeon to cut

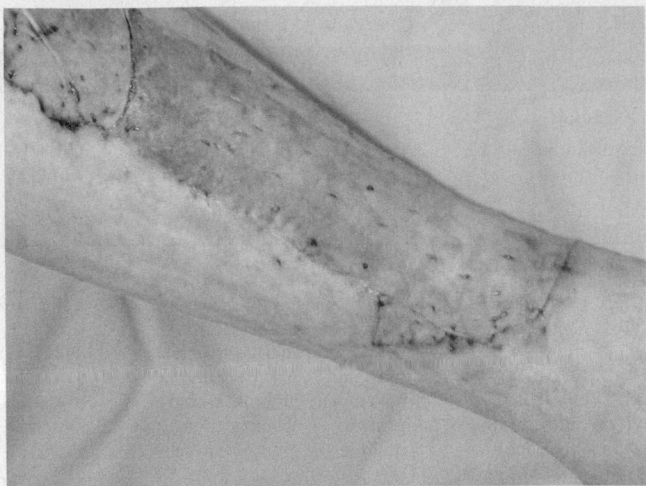

Figure 57-7 • Split-thickness sheet graft. Used with permission from University of Texas Medical Branch, Galveston, TX.

tiny slits into a sheet of donor skin, making it possible to expand, covering larger areas with smaller amounts of donor skin. Expanded grafts adhere to the recipient site more easily than sheet grafts and prevent the accumulation of blood, serum, air, or purulent material under the graft that would prevent revascularization and adherence. However, any kind of graft other than a sheet graft contributes to scar formation as it heals. The use of widely meshed (largely expanded) grafts may be necessary in large wounds but should be viewed as a compromise in terms of cosmesis.

If blood, serum, air, fat, or necrotic tissue is present between the recipient site and the graft, there may be partial or total loss of the graft. Infection, mishandling of the graft, sheer injury with mobilization or trauma during dressing changes account for most other instances of graft loss. The use of split-thickness grafts allows the remaining donor site to retain sweat glands and hair follicles, minimizing healing time.

Cultured epithelial autograft (CEA) has emerged as an important procedure in the management of massive burns. In burns that cover more than 90% TBSA, CEA may be the

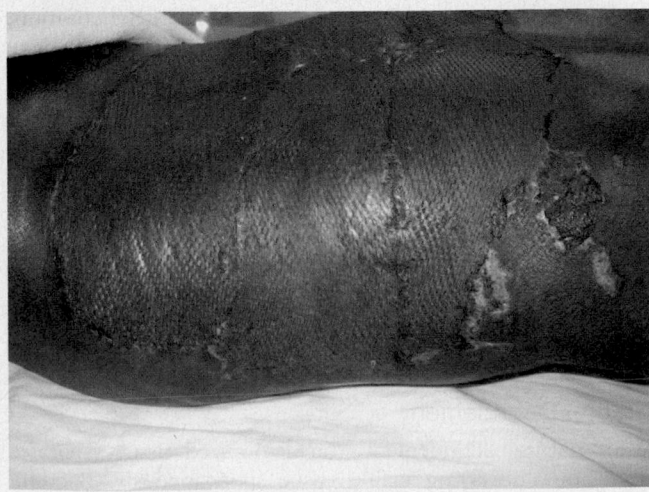

Figure 57-8 • Split-thickness meshed graft. Used with permission from University of Texas Medical Branch, Galveston, TX.

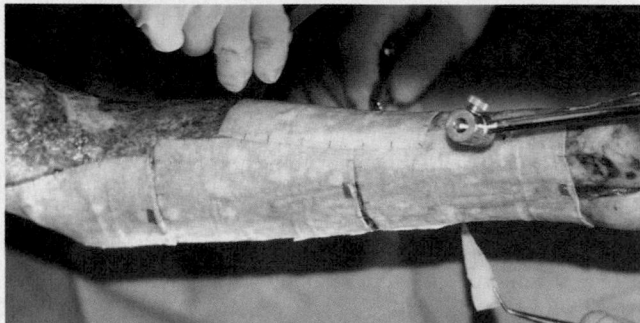

Figure 57-9 • Application of cultured epithelial autologous grafts. Used with permission from University of Texas Medical Branch, Galveston, TX.

only option because the availability of nonburned skin as donor sites will not be sufficient for grafting. CEA involves obtaining full-thickness biopsies of the patient's unburned skin that are cultured to promote growth of keratinocytes. The final product is available approximately 3 weeks later for grafting (see Fig. 57-9). Meticulous attention is required to apply CEA to body surfaces because it is extremely fragile and prone to graft loss. Use of CEA can be cost prohibitive; besides its direct costs, it also requires inordinately extended LOS for the patient.

Care of the graft site

Protection and immobility are key in caring for skin grafts postoperatively. Occlusive dressings encased in bulky gauze wraps are commonly used initially after grafting to immobilize the graft and support the humid environment required for optimal healing. Occupational or physical therapists may construct splints to immobilize joints affecting newly grafted areas. Homograft, xenograft, or synthetic dressings (discussed later) may also be used to protect fragile grafts or widely expanded meshed grafts.

The first dressing change is usually performed 3 to 5 days after surgery, or earlier if clinical signs of infection or bleeding are present. Infection, bleeding beneath the graft, and shearing forces are the most common reasons for graft loss in the early postoperative period. Patients must be positioned and turned carefully to avoid disturbing the graft or applying pressure on the graft site. If an extremity has been grafted, it is elevated to reduce edema. The patient may begin actively exercising the grafted area 5 to 7 days after surgery. This may vary with individual burn center's protocols.

Care of the donor site

The donor site is a clean, usually superficial wound created in a surgical environment that the surgeon uses to obtain a piece of skin for grafting of the wound bed. After the skin is excised, a hemostatic agent such as thrombin or epinephrine may be applied directly to the donor site to promote hemostasis. A myriad of dressings are available to cover donor sites once hemostasis is obtained. Because a donor site is usually a partial-thickness wound, it is very painful, an additional potential site of infection, and very susceptible to pressure injury. With proper care, the donor site should heal spontaneously within 7 to 14 days in an adult who was previously healthy and nonsmoking (Foster, Richey, Osborn, et al., 2020).

Homografts and Xenografts

Homografts (or allografts) and **xenografts** (or heterografts) are also referred to as biologic dressings and are intended as temporary wound coverage. Homografts are pieces of skin obtained from recently deceased or living humans other than the patient. Xenografts consist of skin taken from animals (usually pigs). Therefore, the body's immune response will eventually reject either of them as a foreign substance.

In extensive burns, biologic dressings provide temporary wound coverage and protection of granulation tissue until autografting is possible. As a temporary dressing, they also decrease the wound's evaporative water and protein loss, provide an effective barrier against entry of bacteria, and decrease pain by protecting nerve endings. Biologic dressings can be left open to air or covered with a dressing. They stay in place for varying lengths of time, but are removed in instances of bacterial colonization, infection, or rejection of the dressing by the body. They may also be used as a test graft in preparation for autografting to determine if the wound bed will accept the graft. Once the biologic dressing appears to be "taking," or adhering to the granulating surface with minimal underlying exudation, the patient is ready for an autologous skin graft. Another advantage of biologic dressings is that fewer dressing changes may be required.

Homografts tend to be the most expensive biologic dressings. They are available from skin banks in fresh and cryopreserved (frozen) forms. Homografts are thought to provide the best infection control of all biologic or biosynthetic dressings available. Revascularization occurs within 48 hours, and the graft may be left in place for several weeks.

Pigskin, an effective xenograft, is available from commercial suppliers. It is available fresh, frozen, or lyophilized (freeze-dried) for longer shelf life. Pigskin is used for temporary covering of clean wounds such as superficial partial-thickness wounds and donor sites. Although pigskin does not vascularize, it adheres to clean superficial wounds, providing pain control and reducing evaporative fluid loss allowing the underlying wound to reepithelialize (Aly, Dannoun, Jimenez, et al., 2018).

When grafting is not possible, surgically applied skin substitutes have been created that replace the epidermis or the dermis either temporarily or permanently. Each provides advantages and disadvantages that are important to consider in product selection.

Biosynthetic and Synthetic Dressings

Problems with availability, sterility, and cost have prompted the search for biosynthetic and synthetic dressings, which may eventually replace biologic dressings as temporary wound coverings. There are currently many products on the market, but they tend to be cost prohibitive for most patients and in most healthcare settings.

Pain Management

A burn injury is considered one of the most painful types of trauma that a person can experience. The nature of the injury may expose nerve endings to the atmosphere; and the patient may require multiple procedures, débridements, surgeries, and treatments. Moving, changing position, and receiving occupational and physical therapy cause additional discomfort. Adequate pain management must address background, breakthrough, and procedural pain.

Background pain is a continuous level of discomfort experienced even when the patient is inactive or not undergoing any procedures. The goal of treatment is to provide a long-acting analgesic agent that will provide uniform coverage for this long-term discomfort. It is helpful to use small escalating doses when initiating analgesia to reach the level of pain control that is acceptable to the patient and facilitates their participation in recovery. The use of patient-controlled analgesia gives control to the patient and often achieves this goal.

Breakthrough pain is described as acute, intense, and episodic. It is generally related to an activity or movement of the affected area. Short-acting agents are used for breakthrough pain to achieve pain control if needed. Procedural pain is discomfort that occurs with procedures such as daily wound treatments, invasive line insertions, and physical and occupational therapy. The goal is to plan proper analgesia to facilitate comfort for the patient throughout the procedure.

Most severe burns are a combination of partial- and full-thickness burns that influence the amount of pain the patient experiences. Superficial and partial-thickness burns are very painful because the nerve endings are not protected, resulting in excruciating pain with exposure to temperature, pressure, air currents, and movement. In a full-thickness burn, the nerve endings are destroyed, and there is numbness and decreased sensation to that area. Thus, the patient often underestimates severe injuries. Memories of the pain patients experience may persist for a long time. Educating patients and their families about burn pain and its relationship to the depth of injury as well as the pain management plan is an important priority for the nurse.

Pharmacologic treatment for the management of burn pain includes the use of opioids, nonsteroidal anti-inflammatory drugs, anxiolytics, and anesthetic agents. These and other pain management strategies are discussed in Chapter 9. For treatment of anxiety, benzodiazepines may be used in conjunction with opioids. The use of anesthetics in a nonoperative setting (i.e., moderate sedation) requires administration and monitoring by qualified personnel. Recent advances include the use of agents with rapid onset and short duration, which have been very effective in pain control during a planned procedure. In the provision of holistic patient care, the use of nonpharmacologic pain and anxiety interventions must not be overlooked. Nonpharmacologic therapies include relaxation techniques, distraction, guided imagery, hypnosis, therapeutic touch, humor, music therapy, and virtual reality techniques.

Modulation of Hypermetabolism

Burn injuries produce profound metabolic abnormalities fueled by the exaggerated stress response to the injury. The body's response has been classified as hyperdynamic, hypermetabolic, and hypercatabolic. Hypermetabolism can affect morbidity and mortality by increasing the risk of infection and slowing the healing rate.

Nutrition should be provided as soon as possible upon arrival to the burn center and may require placement of a nasogastric tube for adequate calorie delivery. Patients who are critically ill may even have their feedings continued intraoperatively if the airway is protected. Several formulas exist for estimating the daily metabolic expenditure and caloric requirements of patients with burn injuries. Carbohydrates are the most important energy source for patients who are severely burned (Culnan et al., 2018). Fat, although a required nutrient, should be provided in more limited quantities. When the oral route is used, high-protein, high-calorie meals and supplements are given. Dietary consultations are useful in helping patients meet their nutritional needs. Daily calorie counts aid in assessing the adequacy of nutritional intake.

Early excision and grafting of the burn wound is one of the most important factors in ameliorating hypermetabolism by removing eschar, thereby lessening the effects of inflammatory mediators. Appropriate manipulation of environmental temperatures decreases energy expenditure by the patient (Rizzo, Rowan, Driscoll, et al., 2017). Insulin therapy in patients with burns is required to treat the hyperglycemia that occurs from accelerated gluconeogenesis and is beneficial in muscle protein synthesis. Oxandrolone, an anabolic steroid, is commonly given to patients with burns because it improves protein synthesis and metabolism. Administration of propranolol (a beta-blocker) decreases heart rate and blocks harmful catecholamine effects.

Nursing Management

Nursing management of the patient in the acute/intermediate phase is focused on the following priorities: restoring fluid balance, preventing infection, modulating hypermetabolism, promoting skin integrity, relieving pain and discomfort, promoting mobility, strengthening coping strategies, supporting patient and family processes, and monitoring and managing complications.

Restoring Normal Fluid Balance

To reduce the risk of fluid overload and consequent heart failure and pulmonary edema, daily weights and careful calculation of intake and output measurement are utilized to guide therapy. Thirst, a normal body response to hypovolemia, may cause the patient to drink excessive amounts of water, driving the serum sodium to dangerously low levels. Serum sodium levels should be trended as fluid shifts may lead to metabolic derangements. Changes in physical assessment and hemodynamic indicators are also useful in evaluating the patient's response to treatment.

Preventing Infection

The patient with burns is at risk for infection from multiple sources, which may include open wounds, lung injury, GI ischemia, and indwelling catheters. Increased temperature, tachycardia, tachypnea, and leukocytosis are inherently present in the patient with burns, masking clinical signs of infection. Therapeutic interventions are complex due to the patient's altered physiology.

A major part of the nurse's role during the acute phase of burn care is detection and prevention of infection. The nurse is responsible for providing a clean environment, including the promotion of protective isolation interventions. The nurse protects the patient from sources of contamination, including other patients, staff members, visitors, and equipment. Patients can inadvertently promote migration of microorganisms from one burned area to another by touching their wounds or dressings. Bed linens can also spread infection through either colonization with wound microorganisms or fecal contamination. Regular bathing of unburned areas and changing of linens can help prevent infection. Fresh flowers, plants, and fresh fruit baskets are not permitted in the patient's room because of the risk of microorganism growth. Changing invasive lines and tubing routinely in accordance with Centers for Disease Control and Prevention (CDC) recommendations and institutional policy, and then promptly removing them when no longer indicated, will prevent many HAIs.

Modulating Hypermetabolism

The nurse collaborates with the dietitian or nutrition support team to develop a plan that meets the needs of the patient. Family members may be encouraged to bring nutritious and favorite foods to the hospital. High-calorie nutritional supplements may be necessary. Nutritional intake must be accurately documented. Vitamin and mineral supplements may be prescribed.

If caloric goals cannot be met by oral feeding, a feeding tube is inserted and used for continuous or bolus feedings of specific formulas. The volume of residual gastric secretions should be checked periodically to ensure absorption. The patient should be weighed each day and the results tracked to properly assess appropriate weight parameters and to attenuate catabolism of lean muscle mass.

Promoting Skin Integrity

Wound care is usually the single most time-consuming element of burn care after the emergent phase. The primary provider prescribes the desired topical antibacterial agents and specific biologic, biosynthetic, or synthetic wound coverings and plans for surgical excision and grafting. The nurse needs to make astute assessments of wound status, use creative approaches to dressing of wounds, and support the patient during the emotionally distressing and significantly painful experience of wound care.

Assessment of the burn wound requires an experienced eye, hand, and sense of smell. Important wound assessment features include size, color, odor, presence of eschar and exudate, epithelial buds (small pearl-like clusters of cells on the wound surface), bleeding, granulation tissue, the status of graft take, healing of the donor site, and the condition of the surrounding skin. Any significant changes in the wound are reported to the primary provider because they may indicate burn wound infection and require immediate intervention.

The nurse also assists the patient and family by providing education, support, and encouragement to take an active part in dressing changes and wound care when appropriate. Discharge planning needs for wound care must be anticipated early in the course of burn management, and the strengths of the patient and family are assessed and used in preparing for the patient's eventual discharge and home care needs. Family presence during dressing changes promotes feelings of readiness for discharge.

Relieving Pain and Discomfort

Pain management continues to be a priority during the acute phase of burn recovery. Frequent assessment of pain is required, and analgesic and anxiolytic medications are administered as prescribed. To increase its effectiveness, analgesic medication is provided before the pain becomes severe. Nonpharmacologic interventions can be used to alter the patient's perceptions of and responses to pain. Frequent reassessment of responses to interventions, whether pharmacologic or nonpharmacologic, is essential.

Postburn pruritus (itching) affects almost all patients with burns and is one of the most distressing symptoms in the postburn period. Oral antipruritic agents, environmental conditions, frequent lubrication of the skin with water or silica-based lotion, and diversion activities all help to promote comfort in this phase. The instructions "pat, don't scratch" must be reinforced with patients in order to prevent further discomfort and infectious complications

Lack of sleep and rest interfere with healing, comfort, and restoration of energy. If necessary, sleep aids may be prescribed on a regular basis in addition to analgesic and anxiolytic agents.

Promoting Physical Mobility

An early priority is prevention of the complications of immobility. Deep breathing, turning, and proper positioning are essential nursing practices that prevent atelectasis and pneumonia, control edema, and prevent pressure injuries and contractures. Specialty beds may be useful, and early mobility is strongly encouraged. If the lower extremities are burned, elastic pressure bandages should be applied before the patient is placed in an upright position to promote venous return and minimize edema formation.

The burn wound is in a dynamic state for at least 1 year after wound closure. During this time, aggressive efforts must be made to prevent contracture and hypertrophic scarring. Both passive and active range-of-motion exercises are initiated from the day of admission and are continued after grafting within prescribed limitations. Splints or functional devices applied to the extremities may lessen contractures through compression and stretch. The nurse monitors the splinted areas for signs of vascular insufficiency, nerve compression, and skin breakdown. Occupational and physical therapists are consulted to develop a patient-specific plan of care throughout hospitalization and recovery.

Strengthening Coping Strategies

Much of the patient's energy goes into maintaining vital physical functions and wound healing in the early postburn weeks, leaving little emotional energy for coping. In the acute phase of burn care, the patient is facing the reality of the burn injury. Grief, depression, anger, regression, and manipulative behavior are common responses of patients who have burn injuries. Withdrawal from participation in required treatments and regression must be viewed with an understanding that such behavior may help the patient cope with an enormously stressful event.

The patient may experience feelings of anger. At times, the anger may be directed inward because of a sense of guilt, perhaps for causing the fire or even for surviving when others perished. The anger may also be directed outward toward those who escaped unharmed or those who are now providing care. One way to help the patient handle these emotions is to enlist someone to whom the patient can express feelings without fear of retaliation. A nurse, social worker, psychiatric liaison nurse, peer supporter, spiritual advisor, or counselor who is not involved in direct care activities may fill this role successfully.

Patients with burn injuries are very dependent on health-care team members during the long period of treatment and recovery. However, even when physically unable to contribute much to self-care, they should be included in decisions regarding care and encouraged to assert their individuality in terms of preferences and recognition of their unique identities. As the patient improves in mobility and strength, the nurse works with the patient to set realistic expectations for self-care and planning for the future. Many patients respond positively to the use of contractual agreements and other strategies that recognize their independence, set expectations for behavior, and encourage positive communication.

Supporting Patient and Family Processes

The life-altering burn injury has tremendous psychological, economic, and social impact on the patient and family. The nurse is instrumental in providing support to the patient and family as they adapt to the burn injury. Referrals for social services or psychological counseling should be made as appropriate. This support continues into the rehabilitation phase. Some burn centers offer structured support programs which provide evidenced-based communication training to patients who have survived a burn injury with the goal of helping them to become more effective peer supporters. The peer supporter will visit the hospitalized patient to provide psychosocial support. Many patients appreciate the opportunity to be able to share their experience with another person who has had a burn injury.

With only 70 verified burn centers in the United States (ABA, 2019), patients who experience major burns are commonly sent to burn centers far from home. Because burn injuries are sudden and unexpected, family roles are disrupted. If the primary caregiver or wage earner in the family is injured, roles may change, which adds more stress to the family. Therefore, both the patient and the family need thorough information regarding the patient's burn care and expected course of treatment. Barriers to learning and preferred learning styles are assessed and considered. This information is used to tailor education activities. Patient and family education is a priority and is best provided with a multimedia approach.

Monitoring and Managing Potential Complications

Acute Respiratory Failure and Acute Respiratory Distress Syndrome

The patient's respiratory status is monitored closely for increased difficulty in breathing, change in respiratory pattern, or onset of adventitious (abnormal) breath sounds. Typically, at this stage, signs and symptoms of injury to the respiratory tract become apparent. As described previously, signs of hypoxia, diminished breath sounds, wheezing, tachypnea, stridor, and sputum tinged with soot (or in some cases containing sloughed tracheal tissue) are among the many possible findings. Medical management of the patient with acute respiratory failure requires intubation and mechanical ventilation (if not already in use). If ARDS has developed, higher oxygen levels, positive end-expiratory pressure, and pressure support are used with mechanical ventilation to promote gas exchange across the alveolar–capillary membrane (see Chapter 19).

Heart Failure and Pulmonary Edema

If the cardiac and renal systems cannot compensate for the excess vascular volume as fluid shifts back to the intravascular space, heart failure and pulmonary edema may result. The patient is assessed for signs of heart failure, including decreased cardiac output, oliguria, jugular vein distention, persistent edema, and the onset of an S_3 or S_4 heart sound. If invasive hemodynamic monitoring is used, increasing central venous, pulmonary artery, and pulmonary artery wedge pressures indicate increased fluid volume.

Crackles in the lungs and increased difficulty with breathing may indicate pulmonary edema, which should be reported promptly to the primary provider. In the meantime, the patient is positioned comfortably, with the head of the bed raised (if not contraindicated by other treatments or injuries) to promote lung expansion and gas exchange. Management of this complication includes providing supplemental oxygen, administering IV diuretic agents, carefully assessing the patient's response, and providing vasoactive medications, if indicated (see Chapter 25).

Sepsis

Sepsis is a leading cause of morbidity and mortality in patients with burn injuries. The signs of early sepsis are subtle, requiring a high index of suspicion and very close monitoring of changes in the patient's status. One of the challenges in recognizing sepsis is that burns are a noninfectious condition that triggers the systemic inflammatory response syndrome (SIRS), making it difficult to predict and diagnosis sepsis (Hill, Percy, Velamuri, et al., 2018). Because patients with burns are hypermetabolic, they display tachycardia, tachypnea, and elevated body temperature. These physiologic norms in patients with burns make the diagnosis of sepsis more challenging. See Chapter 11 for treatment recommendations for sepsis.

Delirium

Delirium, a transient and often reversible state of acute brain dysfunction which manifests as alterations in consciousness or cognitive function compared to the patient's baseline, may occur in patients secondary to the trauma sustained. Symptoms include restlessness, disorientation, sleep disorders, or anxiety; some patients experience hallucinations, delusions, or even become combative or suicidal. In patients with burns, a higher incidence of delirium has been found in those with a history of psychiatric issues or substance abuse, or in those with larger burns (Low, Meyer, Willebrand, et al., 2018).

There is ample literature to support the negative impact that pain, anxiety, and agitation have on both clinical and functional outcomes for patients with critical illnesses, yet this is not so for patients with burns who are in critical-care units. Depetris, Raineri, Pantet, and colleagues (2018) sought to assess current analgesia, sedation, and delirium monitoring and treatments in critical burn care to evaluate practice variations and adherence to current evidence-based practices. Although they found increasing awareness of patient delirium among burn care providers, delirium prevention practices vary widely, and they recommend further studies to establish burn-specific guidelines for prevention and treatment of this critical complication of severe burns (see Nursing Research Profile in Chart 57-6).

Powell, T. L., Nolan, M., Yang, G., et al. (2019). Nursing understanding and perceptions of delirium: Assessing current knowledge, attitudes, and beliefs in a burn ICU. *Journal of Burn Care and Research, 40*(4), 471–477.

Chart 57-6 NURSING RESEARCH PROFILE

Nursing Knowledge, Attitudes, and Beliefs About Delirium in a Burn ICU

Purpose

Patients with burns are at high risk for the development of delirium due to analgesia and sedation needs, prolonged mechanical ventilation, multiple operative procedures, and extended intensive care unit (ICU) stays. Delirium has grave negative effects on morbidity, mortality, and cognitive function and is common in this population. As the caregiver who spends the most time with the patient, the nurse must be attuned to early signs of delirium and initiate treatment. The purpose of this study was to evaluate and improve nurses' perceptions, attitudes, and knowledge about delirium while increasing compliance with administration of the Confusion Assessment Method for the ICU (CAM-ICU) tool and preventive interventions.

Design

The setting for this study was an 18-bed multispecialty burn ICU for both adults and children. Participants completed a survey that assessed attitudes regarding delirium, use of the CAM-ICU, and general knowledge of delirium before and after an educational intervention designed to improve recognition, prevention, and management of delirium The researchers conducted a review of the literature and sought expert consultation to inform the development of the survey, which included select items used in the American Nurses Association (2015), study on delirium. In addition, post intervention, participants were asked to evaluate the effectiveness of the educational activities. The educational intervention, which occurred over 7 months, consisted of training

a group of delirium nurse champions to serve as expert resources for the staff, creating an education board that addressed common questions and myths regarding delirium, and coordinating a week dedicated to delirium educational activities, including short videos and question and answer sessions.

Findings

Twenty-seven (38%) of the 71 burn ICU nurses participated in the project. Staff compliance with administration of the CAM-ICU assessment increased to 90% during the review time, and positive scores on the CAM-ICU decreased from 21% to 14%. Survey results indicated that nurses recognized the importance of assessing delirium and providing interventions. However, 26% of the nurses did not endorse the need for the CAM-ICU as a screening tool. Qualitative themes described existing knowledge of delirium and knowledge gaps, barriers to implementation of the CAM-ICU, and views on nonpharmacologic and pharmacologic nursing interventions.

Nursing Implications

The results from this study support that targeted education increased awareness and general knowledge of delirium, as well as appropriate nursing interventions. However, the authors found that participants perceived challenges to using the CAM-ICU, including the time it takes to conduct the assessment and the complexity of using it with patients who are non-English speaking, sedated, or intubated, which limited behavioral change or consistent use of the tool. In general, staff perceived the project as empowering, specifically as the project helped to reinforce the role that nurses play in delirium prevention and management and the positive difference that their interventions make in this patient population.

Rehabilitation Phase

Rehabilitation begins immediately after the burn has occurred and often extends for years after the initial injury. For nurses who care for patients with burns, this can be one of the more physically demanding and challenging phases. One important focus of the burn team is to evaluate the patient carefully for late complications related to burn injuries as described in Table 57-5.

Burn rehabilitation is comprehensive, complex, and requires a multidisciplinary approach to optimize the patient's physical and psychosocial recovery related to the injury. As patients begin to recover, they become more aware of the injuries and challenges they face. Individualized plans of care that are specific to the severity and location of injury are developed and reevaluated frequently. The increased survival of patients with significant burn injuries has translated into the need for additional and comprehensive burn rehabilitation programs worldwide. The ultimate goal is to return patients to the highest level of function possible within the context of their injuries. Specially trained occupational and physical therapists are essential for optimal patient outcomes.

Psychological Support

A patient's outlook, motivation, and support system are important to their overall well-being and ability to progress

through the rehabilitation phase. Psychiatric disorders may have contributed to the cause of the burn injury itself. Examples include self-inflicted burns, suicide attempts, or intentional infliction on one person by another in cases of abuse. These are a few examples that illustrate the critical need for psychosocial resources in burn recovery. Although psychiatric disorders are not contributory to all burn injuries, the life-altering nature of burn injuries almost always causes temporary or permanent impairment of psychosocial adaptation.

In the acute phase of the injury, acute shock, terror, disbelief, confusion, and anxiety are common. Patients may be at risk for delirium and may experience temporary psychoses. Patients may be confused from medications they are taking, but they have an underlying sense of fear, anxiety, and pain. Early consultation with mental health professionals will assist in best meeting individual needs, which may include pharmacologic interventions with concurrent counseling. The rehabilitation phase may present a new set of challenges. While the patient is physically recovering, the reality and impact of the injury begin to set in as patients recognize that survival is expected. Patients may experience devastating grief and loss. The sense of loss may originate from physical injury, loss of control from the forced dependency on others for care, or loss of family members/friends who may have died from burn injuries. In residential fires, survivors may have lost their homes and all of their possessions.

TABLE 57-5	Complications in Rehabilitation Phase of Burn Care	
Complications	**Contributing Factors**	**Interventions**
Neuropathies and nerve entrapment	Electrical injury, large deep burns, improper positioning, edema, scar tissue	Assess peripheral pulses and sensation (neurovascular checks). Prevent edema and pressure by elevation, positioning, and prevention of constricting dressings. Assess splints for proper fit and application. Consult OT and PT departments for positioning.
Wound breakdown and/or pressure injury formation	Shearing, pressure, inadequate nutrition	Protect wound from pressure and shearing forces. Educate patient about importance of good nutrition.
Hypertrophic scarring	Partial- and full-thickness burns	Keep skin pliable and soft by using emollients. Apply pressure garments as prescribed. Massage.
Contractures	Partial- and full-thickness burns	Maintain position of joints in alignment. Perform gentle range-of-motion exercises. Consult OT and PT departments for exercises and positioning recommendations.
Joint instability	Burn wound, burn scar, and contractures	Maintain appropriate joint positioning through appropriate application of splints. Monitor joint pinning if indicated.
Complex pain	Trauma and burns	Provide adequate pain management. Consult OT and PT departments for exercises and desensitization. Promote gentle motion of affected extremities.

OT, occupational therapy; PT, physical therapy.
Adapted from Serghiou, M. A., Ott, S., Cowan, A., et al. (2018). Burn rehabilitation along the continuum of care. In D. Herndon (Ed.). *Total burn care* (5th ed.). Edinburgh: Saunders Elsevier; Thananopavarn, P., & Hill J. J. (2017). Rehabilitation of the complex burn patient with multiple injuries or comorbidities. *Clinics in Plastic Surgery*, *44*(4), 695–701.

Posttraumatic stress disorder (PTSD) is a common psychiatric disorder in patients with burns. Patients with PTSD re-experience the injury event, exhibit an intensified perception of threat, and employ avoidance behaviors that sustain the symptoms (Low et al., 2018). Other psychological disorders that may be experienced by patients with burns include anxiety, depression, and sleep disturbances. The symptoms and psychological responses to stress are discussed further in Chapter 5.

As recovery progresses, discharge planning must include strategies to assist the patient in reintegrating into their home, community, workplace, and school. For many patients, issues regarding quality of life may become very real at this point in recovery. This is an emotional time as the patient and family begin to live with new physical limitations and challenges in relationships. In addition to preparing the patient's support system, the patient and family must also prepare for the reactions from strangers.

Organizations such as the Phoenix Society for Burn Survivors, an international support group for patients with burns, offer a myriad of resources, education, opportunities for peer support, and strategies for reintegration. Alan Breslau, a survivor of burn injuries, who recognized the importance of peer support in psychosocial recovery (see the Resources section), founded the Phoenix Society in 1977. Peer support provides opportunities for reflection and personal growth and gives new meaning for the patient with burns through sharing experiences with others with similar burn injuries. Each year, the Phoenix Society hosts the World Burn Congress, which is a conference for survivors, their families, caregivers, burn care professionals, and firefighters. This forum offers education as well as an opportunity for patients with burns and their families to connect with others who have experienced similar

life-changing events. Such interaction allows the patient and family to see that adaptation to a burn injury is possible.

Organizations that provide support for reintegration are able to offer education and training geared specifically to patients with burn injuries. Workshops on how to apply makeup to reduce the appearance of scars can benefit those with obvious facial scarring. This is one example of a strategy available to assist patients with burns who have body image disturbances. Cultural influences play a strong factor in this process, because some cultures are particularly sensitive to physical appearance, a focus of importance which may also be reinforced by current media practices. The role of the nurse is to encourage patients to voice their concerns, provide empathy, and provide them with assistive resources.

Abnormal Wound Healing

Partial-thickness wounds involving the epidermis and superficial dermis tend to heal without scarring. Deeper wounds will likely develop scarring of variable degrees. As with other disorders, risk factors may be stratified as modifiable or nonmodifiable. For example, a nonmodifiable risk factor for scarring is heredity, because some patients are simply more prone to hypertrophic scar formation. The focus of patient education for nurses must be on how to best change or adapt the *modifiable* risk factors. Patients should be strongly encouraged to follow occupational therapist recommendations for scar prevention and management.

Normal scarring occurs in a superficial tissue injury and begins forming within 7 to 10 days post injury and progresses over the next 6 to 12 months. Abnormal scarring occurs after a longer period of wound healing and may form either hypertrophic or keloid scars.

Hypertrophic and Keloid Scars

Hypertrophic scars form within the boundaries of the initial wound and push outward on the perimeter of the wound. They are common in areas over joints and in the younger population. The scar becomes red (due to its hypervascularity), raised, and hard.

Keloid scars are irregularly formed and extend beyond the margins of the original wound. They are large, nodular, and ropelike, often causing itching and tenderness. They are more common in dark-pigmented skin, uncommon in children and older adults, and have familial tendencies.

Prevention and Treatment of Scars

Preventive treatment modalities aimed at scar contractures and excess hypertrophic tissue are routinely employed. Compression is introduced early in burn wound treatment. Elastic bandage wraps used initially help promote adequate circulation, but they can also be used as the first form of compression for scar management, followed by elasticized tubular bandages until the patient can be measured for a customized garment. Application of elastic pressure garments loosens collagen bundles and encourages parallel orientation of the collagen to the skin surface. As pressure continues over time, collagen restructures and vascularity decreases. Although this therapy is somewhat controversial, pressure has shown to be beneficial in controlling scar formation over time (DeBruler, Baumann, Blackstone, et al., 2019). Recommended garment wear time is 23 hours per day; removing for bathing or wound care only.

Many areas of the body are difficult to compress due to the contours or location of the injury. Inserts, such as silicone sheets, are helpful for these small troublesome areas and are placed beneath the garment or compression dressing to enhance scar compression. Gentle superficial scar massage can be performed with a moisturizer several times a day.

Burn reconstruction is a treatment option after scars have matured and is discussed within the first few years after injury. This decision requires individualized planning, realistic expectations, and patience. The treatment team and the patient will ultimately decide on the best approach for long-term functionality and cosmesis.

NURSING PROCESS

Care of the Patient during the Rehabilitation Phase

Assessment

The nurse obtains information about the patient's education level, occupation, leisure activities, cultural background, religion, and family interactions. The patient's self-concept, mental status, emotional response to the injury and subsequent hospitalization, level of intellectual functioning, previous hospitalizations, response to pain and pain relief measures, and sleep pattern are also essential components of a comprehensive assessment. Information about the patient's general self-concept, self-esteem, and coping strategies in the past are valuable in assessing emotional needs.

Ongoing physical assessments related to rehabilitation goals include range of motion of affected joints, functional abilities in ADLs, early signs of skin breakdown, evidence of neuropathies (nerve damage), activity tolerance, and quality or condition of healing skin. The patient's participation in care and ability to demonstrate self-care in such areas as ambulation, eating, wound cleaning, toileting, and applying pressure wraps are documented on a regular basis.

Diagnosis

NURSING DIAGNOSES

Based on the assessment data, nursing diagnoses may include the following:

- Activity intolerance associated with pain with exercise, limited joint mobility, muscle wasting, and limited endurance
- Disturbed body image associated with altered physical appearance and self-concept
- Impaired mobility due to contractures or hypertrophic scarring
- Lack of knowledge about postdischarge home care and recovery needs

COLLABORATIVE PROBLEMS/POTENTIAL COMPLICATION

Potential complications may include the following:

- Inadequate psychological adaptation to burn injury

Planning and Goals

The major goals for the patient include increased mobility and participation in ADLs; adaptation and adjustment to alterations in body image, self-concept, and lifestyle; increased understanding and knowledge of the injury, treatment, and planned follow-up care; and absence of complications.

Nursing Interventions

PROMOTING ACTIVITY TOLERANCE

The extensive physical rehabilitation can be painful and challenging for the patient. Strategies to maintain motivation and participation may be beneficial during this critical phase. The nurse incorporates physical and occupational therapy exercises in the patient's care to prevent muscle atrophy and to maintain the mobility required for daily activities. The patient's activity tolerance, strength, and endurance gradually increase if activity occurs over increasingly longer periods. Monitoring of fatigue and pain tolerance will assist with determining the amount of activity to be encouraged on a daily basis. Activities such as family visits and recreational therapy (e.g., video games, radio, television) can provide diversion, improve the patient's outlook, and increase tolerance for physical activity. In older adult patients and those with chronic illness and disability, rehabilitation must take into account preexisting functional abilities and limitations.

The nurse must schedule care in such a way that the patient has periods of rest and uninterrupted sleep. A good time for planned patient rest is after the stress of dressing changes and exercise, while pain interventions and sedatives are still effective. This plan must be clearly communicated to family members and other care providers. The patient may have insomnia related to frequent nightmares about the burn injury or other fears and anxieties about the outcome of the injury. The nurse reassures the patient and administers agents, as prescribed, to promote sleep. Reducing metabolic stress by relieving pain, preventing chilling or fever, and promoting the physical integrity of all body systems helps the patient conserve energy for therapeutic activities and wound healing.

IMPROVING BODY IMAGE AND SELF-CONCEPT

Patients who have survived burn injuries may lack the benefit of anticipatory grief often seen in a patient who is approaching surgery or dealing with the terminal illness of a loved one. As care progresses, the patient who is recovering from burns becomes aware of daily improvement and begins to express basic concerns: Will I be disfigured or be disabled? How long will I be in the hospital? What about my job and family? Will I ever be independent again? How will this injury affect my sexual relationships? How can I pay for my care? Was my burn the result of my carelessness? Where will I live now?

When caring for a patient with a burn injury, the nurse needs to be aware that there are prejudices and misunderstandings in society about those viewed as different. Opportunities and accommodations available to others are often denied to those disfigured by scarring associated with a burn injury. These include social participation, employment, prestige, various roles, and status. The healthcare team must actively promote a healthy body image and self-concept in patients with burn injuries so that they can accept or challenge others' perceptions of those who are disfigured or disabled. Survivors themselves must show others who they are, how they function, and how they want to be treated.

PROMOTING PHYSICAL MOBILITY THROUGH PREVENTING CONTRACTURES OR HYPERTROPHIC SCAR FORMATION

With early and aggressive physical and occupational therapy, contractures or hypertrophic scars are rarely a long-term complication. However, surgical intervention is indicated if full range of motion in the patient with burns is not achieved.

MONITORING AND MANAGING POTENTIAL COMPLICATIONS

Impaired Psychological Adaptation to the Burn Injury. Some patients, particularly those with limited coping skills or psychological function, or a history of psychiatric problems before the burn injury, may not achieve adequate psychological adaptation to the burn injury. Psychological counseling or psychiatric referral may be made to assess the patient's emotional status, to help the patient develop coping skills, and to intervene if major psychological issues or ineffective coping is identified.

PROMOTING HOME, COMMUNITY-BASED, AND TRANSITIONAL CARE

Educating the Patient About Self-Care. The focus of rehabilitative interventions is directed toward outpatient care, home care, or care in a rehabilitation center. This includes wound care, dressing changes, pain management, nutrition, prevention of complications, and other care needs. Information and written instructions are provided about specific exercises and the use of pressure garments and splints. The patient and family are provided education to assist them in their continued care needs after discharge (see Chart 57-7).

Continuing and Transitional Care. After discharge, care by a multidisciplinary treatment team is necessary. Some patients may require the services of an inpatient rehabilitation center before returning home. Patients should receive follow-up from a burn center when possible for periodic evaluation by the burn team, modification of outpatient treatment plan, and evaluation for reconstructive surgery. Many patients require outpatient physical or occupational therapy several times a week. The nurse coordinates all aspects of care and ensures that the patient's needs are met. Such coordination is an important aspect of assisting the patient to achieve independence.

Some patients may require referral for transitional care after discharge. The nurse assesses the patient's physical and psychological status as well as the adequacy of the home setting for safe and adequate care. The nurse monitors the patient's progress; assesses adherence to the plan of care; and assists the patient and family with wound care, exercises, and other physical needs. Patients experiencing difficulties with psychosocial adjustments are identified and appropriate referrals are made (see Chapter 2, Chart 2-6, for further discussion about assisting the patient's preparation for home care).

Evaluation

Expected patient outcomes may include:
1. Demonstrates adequate activity tolerance
   a. Has energy available to perform daily activities
   b. Shows gradual increased tolerance and endurance in physical activities
   c. Obtains adequate sleep and rest daily
2. Adapts to altered body image
   a. Verbalizes accurate description of alterations in body image and accepts physical appearance
   b. Demonstrates interest in resources that may improve function and perception of body appearance (e.g., cosmetics, wigs, and prostheses as appropriate)
   c. Socializes with significant others, peers, and usual social group
   d. Seeks and achieves return to role in family, school, and community as a contributing member
3. Demonstrates physical mobility adequate to perform ADLs
   a. Demonstrates range of motion appropriate for injury
   b. Absence of complications from wound healing
4. Demonstrates knowledge of required self-care and follow-up care
   a. Verbalizes detailed plan for follow-up care
   b. Demonstrates ability to perform or direct wound care and prescribed exercises
   c. Returns for follow-up appointments as scheduled
   d. Identifies resource people and agencies to contact for specific problems
5. Exhibits no complications
   a. Exhibits psychosocial adaptation to burn injury
   b. Verbalizes understanding of diagnosis and treatment plan

Outpatient Burn Care

The increased availability of outpatient surgery and access to expert burn care in outpatient settings make this option possible for the treatment of minor burns as well as follow-up for the patient with more severe burns once discharged. The goals for treatment in an outpatient setting may include burn wound management, pain management, scar and reconstructive care, psychosocial care, and rehabilitation. However, a

Chart 57-7	**HOME CARE CHECKLIST**
	The Patient with a Burn Injury

At the completion of education, the patient and/or caregiver will be able to:

- State the impact of the burn injury and treatment on physiologic functioning, performance of ADLs and IADLs, roles, relationships, and spirituality.
- State how to contact all members of the treatment team (e.g., interdisciplinary burn team, healthcare providers, home care professionals, and durable medical equipment and supply vendors).
- State the name, dose, side effects, frequency, and schedule for all medications.
- Demonstrate psychosocial adaptation and social integration through verbalizing understanding of the following:
  - Changes in lifestyle and emotional adjustment to injury take time. It is not uncommon for patients to report nightmares or "flashbacks" of the injury. If this becomes disruptive, it should be discussed with the treatment team.
  - Resume previous interests and activities gradually.
  - Consider community and other resources such as burn support groups. Many books, videos, and Web sites are also available and may be invaluable in assisting with burn recovery.
  - Programs are available to assist with school reintegration and return to work. The treatment team should be consulted as needed.
  - Burn care (dressings, medications, therapy) can be very expensive. A social worker or care manager may find funding assistance programs if needed.
- Demonstrate adaptation of the home environment, assisted as needed by team members (e.g., social worker, care manager).
- State burn skin precautions:
  - Apply sunblock with the highest sun protection factor (SPF) possible to protect exposed burned skin from the sun. Light-colored clothing, long pants, and long-sleeved shirts may also be necessary to protect from the sun.
  - Use wide-brimmed hats if face or ears have been burned to protect the area from the sun.
  - Avoid further trauma to burned skin; leave blisters that may form intact.
  - Lubricate healed burned skin with lotion (as prescribed); avoid scratching.
  - Use only mild soaps and lotions (i.e., products without perfume or deodorants) on burned areas. Keeping skin clean overall is important to support good hygiene and prevent infection.
  - Avoid tight clothing over burned areas so as not to restrict movement or irritate newly healed areas.
  - Select white cotton, loose-fitting clothing so that dyes in colored clothes do not irritate healing skin.
  - Wear clothing and gloves to protect healing skin from unnecessary bruises, bumps, and scratches.
  - Be aware that tolerance to extremes in temperatures may be affected.
  - Itching is a normal, uncomfortable part of healing and burn recovery; do not scratch, pat areas; apply mild moisturizers

to decrease itching from dryness. Medications for itching can be discussed with the treatment team.
- Demonstrate wound care technique:
  - Take prescribed pain medications if needed 30 minutes prior to wound care to achieve maximum effectiveness.
  - Use mild soap, water, and a clean washcloth to clean wounds.
  - Apply prescribed topical medications and dressings as instructed.
  - Inspect wounds carefully with each dressing change for signs of infection, including increased redness, swelling, drainage, or foul odor.
- State aspects of ADLs and exercise:
  - Perform as much of own care as possible.
  - Adhere to the exercise regimen given by the therapists. Although physical rehabilitation is tiring, daily participation is essential.
  - Plan for adequate rest and sleep.
  - When at rest, swollen limbs should be elevated.
  - Describe approaches to controlling pain (e.g., take antispasmodic agents as prescribed; use nonpharmacologic interventions).
  - State changes in diet necessary to promote health (e.g., nutrient-rich foods, rather than empty calories).
  - State changes in fluid intake needed to prevent constipation associated with the use of analgesic medications.
- Discuss management of burn scar:
  - Massage with mild lotion or cream to stretch skin to maintain/increase its elasticity.
  - Wear compression garments 23 hours a day if instructed.
  - Discoloration of the skin for many months is an expected normal part of healing.
- Discuss resumption of intimacy:
  - Resumption of sexual relationships is the rule rather than the exception and should occur when comfortable for all.
  - Expect sensitivity of and around the genital area for several months if these areas were burned.
- State correct use of medical devices:
  - Follow occupational therapist's instructions for splint use and cleaning.
  - Use crutches, walkers, or other assistive devices as instructed.
  - If devices such as shower chairs or grab bars are needed in the home, this should be arranged prior to discharge.
- State time and date of follow-up appointments, therapy, and testing:
  - Keep a list of questions to ask team members.
  - Bring medications, or a list of current medications, to each visit for the team to review.
- Identify the need for health promotion, disease prevention, and screening activities.
- Identify the contact details for support services for patients and their caregivers/families.

ADLs, activities of daily living; IADLs, instrumental activities of daily living.

number of factors must be considered when determining if outpatient care is appropriate for the patient: age, past medical history, extent and depth of the burn, location of the burn wounds, availability of family support systems and community resources, the patient's ability and willingness to adhere to a therapeutic regimen, distance from home to the outpatient setting, and availability of transportation to and from home and the outpatient setting.

The frequency of follow-up visits is individualized. The initial outpatient visit for a discharged patient with burn injuries is usually scheduled within 3 to 5 days after hospital discharge. A survivor's follow-up appointment schedule will vary and decrease in frequency over time, based on patient's needs. Patient and family education is paramount and should include verbal and written instructions as well as return demonstration of the wound or scar care required. The importance of notifying the outpatient setting about changes in symptoms and of keeping follow-up appointments is emphasized to the patient and family. Physical therapy and occupational therapy are often provided in the outpatient burn setting. The rehabilitation goals are to increase range of motion, strengthen muscles, and build the patient's activity tolerance through a specific, individualized plan of care that includes routine visits for up to 2 years or more following the injury.

The patient's adaptation to lifestyle changes and emotional status should be assessed during the outpatient visits and proper referrals made for counseling services. These assessments may be difficult to recognize due to the infrequent nature of the visits; therefore, it is helpful to incorporate family response and interactions into the assessment. The healthcare team must also be alert to issues of substance abuse, safety concerns, suicidal thoughts, depression, and PTSD.

CRITICAL THINKING EXERCISES

1 **ebp** A 55-year-old man is hospitalized for a smoke inhalation injury with a 15% TBSA burn to his upper torso and extremities. He has been placed on 100% oxygen per non-rebreather mask and started on a morphine drip for pain control. He awakens when verbally stimulated, but he does not consistently follow directions. Which evidence-based tools should you use to assess the patient's neurologic and pulmonary status, and his response to pain management? What evidence-based nursing interventions should be integrated into the plan of care to support his pulmonary status and to manage the distress associated with his burn and high oxygen requirement?

2 **pq** A 65-year-old man was admitted overnight to the burn unit with an 18% partial-thickness scald burn. The day after admission, in the early afternoon, you note that the patient's heart rate has increased to 160 bpm, temperature is 38.7°C (101.7°F), and his capillary refill time has increased to greater than 2 seconds. After alerting the charge nurse, what interventions do you anticipate? What are your priority interventions?

3 **ipc** An 85-year-old woman is admitted to the burn center with a 65% TBSA full-thickness burn. She is a widow, with no living children, but has a neighbor who is her identified surrogate decision maker. Her body mass index (BMI) on admission is 16.7 kg/m² and she reports weight loss over the last year and a poor appetite. She takes no medications and has not seen a medical provider for many years. She reports a strong religious background and states that she believes that God has always watched over her and is doing so now. She consents to a workup for a mass that was observed in a routine chest x-ray. A biopsy of the lesion obtained after consent shows a poorly differentiated adenocarcinoma. She continues to agree to daily wound care but refuses surgery. The oncology consulting service states that she may benefit from chemotherapy. The surgery team believes that she would benefit from supplemental feeding via a feeding tube. Her pain is well controlled. What interprofessional consultation service could help to best facilitate patient-centered outcomes for this patient? Describe how the various members of this team could support this patient.

REFERENCES

*Asterisk indicates nursing research.

Books

Aly, M. E. I., Dannoun, M., Jimenez, C. J., et al. (2018). Operative wound management. In D. Herndon (Ed.). *Total burn care* (5th ed.). Edinburgh: Saunders Elsevier.

American Burn Association (ABA). (2018). *Advanced burn life support (ABLS) course provider manual 2018*. Chicago, IL: Author.

American Nurses Association. (2015). *Code of ethics for nurses with interpretive statements*. Washington, DC: American Nurses Publishing, American Nurses Foundation/American Nurses Association.

Culnan, D. M., Capek, K. D., & Sheridan, R. L. (2018). Etiology and prevention of multisystem organ failure. In D. Herndon (Ed.). *Total burn care* (5th ed.). Edinburgh: Saunders Elsevier.

Culnan, D. M., Sherman, W. C., Chung, K. K., et al. (2018). Critical care in the severely burned: Organ support and management of complications. In D. Herndon (Ed.). *Total burn care* (5th ed.). Edinburgh: Saunders Elsevier.

Low, J. F. A., Meyer, W. J., Willebrand, M., et al. (2018). Psychiatric disorders associated with burn injury. In D. Herndon (Ed.). *Total burn care* (5th ed.). Edinburgh: Saunders Elsevier.

Serghiou, M. A., Ott, S., Cowan, A., et al. (2018). Comprehensive rehabilitation of the burn patient. In D. Herndon (Ed.). *Total burn care* (5th ed.). Edinburgh: Saunders Elsevier.

Wurzer, P., Culnan, D., Cancio, L. C., et al. (2018). Pathophysiology of burn shock and burn edema. In D. Herndon (Ed.). *Total burn care* (5th ed.). Edinburgh: Saunders Elsevier.

Journals and Electronic Documents

American Burn Association (ABA). (2016). Burn incidence and treatment in the United States: 2016 fact sheet. Retrieved on 9/3/2019 at: www.ameriburn.org/resources_factsheet.php

American Burn Association (ABA). (2019). Burn center verification. Retrieved on 9/13/2019 at: www.ameriburn.org/verification_verified-centers.php

American Burn Association (ABA). (2019). Verified burn centers. Retrieved on 1/12/2020 at: www.ameriburn.org/public-resources/find-a-burn-center

American Burn Association National Burn Repository (ABA NBR). (2018). National Burn Repository 2017 update: Report of data from 2008–2017. Retrieved on 9/3/2019 at: www.ameriburn.org/2017NBRAnnualReport.pdf

American Psychological Association. (2020). *Instrumental activities of daily living scale*. Washington, DC. Retrieved on 1/2/2020 at: www.apa.org/pi/about/publications/caregivers/practice-settings/assessment/tools/daily-activities

Bielson, C. B., Duethman, N. C., Howard, J. M., et al. (2017). Burns: Pathophysiology of systemic complications and current management. *Journal of Burn Care & Research*, 38(1), e469–e481.

Culnan, D. M., Farner, K., Bitz, G. H., et al. (2018). Volume resuscitation in patients with high-voltage electrical injuries. *Annals of Plastic Surgery*, 80(3 Suppl 2), S113–S118.

DeBruler, D. M., Baumann, M. E., Blackstone, B. N., et al. (2019). Role of early application of pressure garments following burn injury and autografting. *Plastic and Reconstructive Surgery*, 143(2), 310e–321e.

Depetris, N., Raineri, S., Pantet, O., et al. (2018). Management of pain, anxiety, agitation and delirium in burn patients: A survey of clinical practice and a review of the current literature. *Annals of Burns and Fire Disasters, 31*(2), 97–108.

Ehrl, D., Heidekrueger, P. I., Rubenbauger, J., et al. (2018). Impact of prehospital hypothermia on the outcomes of severely burned patients. *Journal of Burn Care and Research, 39*(5), 739–743.

Foster, K. N., Richey, K. J., Osborn, S. C., et al. (2020). Healing of donor sites with an autologous skin cell suspension for large TBSA burn injuries: A prospective evaluation. *Journal of Burn Care & Research, 41*(1), S225–S226.

Gillenwater, J., & Garner, W. (2017). Acute fluid management of large burns: Pathophysiology, monitoring, and resuscitation. *Clinics in Plastic Surgery, 44*(3), 495–503.

Hill, D. M., Percy, M. D., Velamuri, S. R., et al. (2018). Predictors for identifying burn sepsis and performance vs existing criteria. *Journal of Burn Care and Research, 39*(6), 982–988.

IBM Micromedix®. (2020). Formulary advisor, New York Presbyterian Weill Cornell Medicine, New York. Available pass-protected. Retrieved on 2/14/2020 at: www.micromedexsolutions.com/micromedex2/librarian/ssl/true

Jeschke, M. G., & Peck, M. D. (2017). Burn care of the elderly. *Journal of Burn Care and Research, 38*(3), e625–e628.

Jones, S. W., Williams, F. N., Cairns, B. A., et al. (2017). Inhalation injury: Pathophysiology, diagnosis, and treatment. *Clinics in Plastic Surgery, 44*(3), 505–511.

Lachiewicz, A. M., Hauck, C. G., Weber, D. J., et al. (2017). Bacterial infections after burn injuries: Impact of multidrug resistance. *Clinical Infectious Diseases, 65*(12), 2130–2136.

Maxwell, D., Rhee, P., Drake, M., et al. (2018). Development of the burn frailty index: A prognostication index for elderly patients sustaining burn injuries. *The American Journal of Surgery, 218*(1), 87–94. Retrieved on 8/1/2019 at: www.doi.org/10.1016/j.amjsurg.2018.11.012

National Weather Service. (n.d.). Lightning safety for you and your family. Retrieved on 11/30/2019 at: www.weather.gov/media/safety/Lightning-Brochure18.pdf

Palmieri, T. L. (2019). Infection prevention: Unique aspects of burn units. *Surgical Infections, 20*(2), 111–114.

*Powell, T. L., Nolan, M., Yang, G., et al. (2019). Nursing understanding and perceptions of delirium: Assessing current knowledge, attitudes, and beliefs in a burn ICU. *Journal of Burn Care and Research, 40*(4), 471–477.

Ramirez, J. I., Sen, S., Palmieri, T. L., et al. (2018). Timing of laparotomy and closure in burn patients with abdominal compartment syndrome: Effects on survival. *Journal of the American College of Surgeons, 226*(6), 1175–1180.

Ramos, G., Cornistein, W., Cerino, G. T., et al. (2017). Systemic antimicrobial prophylaxis in burn patients: Systematic review. *Journal of Hospital Infection, 97*(2), 105–114.

Rehou, S., Shahrokhi, S., Natanson, R., et al. (2018). Antioxidant and trace element supplementation reduce the inflammatory response in critically ill burn patients. *Journal of Burn Care and Research, 39*(1), 1–9.

Rizzo, J. A., Rowan, M. P., Driscoll, I. R., et al. (2017). Perioperative temperature management during burn care. *Journal of Burn Care and Research, 38*(1), e277–e283.

Romanowski, K. S., Curtis, E., Palmieri, T. L., et al. (2018). Frailty is associated with mortality in patients aged 50 years and older. *Journal of Burn Care and Research, 39*(5), 703–707.

Sood, G., Vaidya, D., Dam, L., et al. (2018). A polymicrobial fungal outbreak in a regional burn center after Hurricane Sandy. *American Journal of Infection Control, 46*(9), 1047–1050.

Stewart, D., Ladd, M., Kovler, M., et al. (2019). Implementation of a nurse-driven fluid resuscitation protocol reduces total fluid given for resuscitation in large pediatric burns. *Journal of Burn Care and Research, 40*, Issue Supplement 1, S8–S9.

Strauss, S., & Gillespie, G. L. (2018). Initial assessment and management of burn patients. *American Nurse Today, 13*(6), 15–19.

Suresh, M. R., & Dries, D. J. (2018). Burn care: Resuscitation and respiratory care. *Air Medical Journal, 37*(1), 12–15.

Taylor, S. L., Sen, S., Greenhalgh, D. G., et al. (2017). Not all patients meet the 1 day per percent burn rule: A simple method for predicting hospital length of stay in patients with burn. *Burns, 43*(2), 282–289.

Thananopavarn, P., & Hill, J. J., 3rd. (2017). Rehabilitation of the complex burn patient with multiple injuries or comorbidities. *Clinics in Plastic Surgery, 44*(4), 695–701.

Walker, A., & Salerno, A. (2019). Shocking injuries: Knowing the risks and management for electrical injuries. *Trauma Reports, 20*(4), 1–25.

Weissman, O., Wagman, Y., Givon, A., et al. (2017). Examination of the life expectancy of patient burns over 20% of their total body surface area in comparison to the rest of the population. *Journal of Burn Care and Research, 38*(6), e906–e912.

World Health Organization (WHO). (2018). Burns. Retrieved on 9/3/2019 at: www.who.int/en/news-room/fact-sheets/detail/burns

Resources

Alisa Ann Ruch Burn Foundation, www.aarbf.org
American Burn Association (ABA), www.ameriburn.org
American Red Cross, www.redcross.org
Burn Foundation, www.burnfoundation.org
Burn Institute, www.burninstitute.org
Burn Prevention Network, www.burnprevention.org
Firefighters Burn Institute, www.ffburn.org
International Association of Fire Fighters, www.iaff.org
International Society for Burn Injuries (ISBI), https://www.worldburn.org/Home/First.cfm?CFID=10612098&CFTOKEN=c69aae52dd45 b2f3-8019C1B9-D023-BB0D-6B70CDBF44D65DE1
Lund-Browder Classification, medical-dictionary.thefreedictionary.com/Lund-Browder+classification
National Fire Protection Association (NFPA), www.nfpa.org
Phoenix Society for Burn Survivors, www.phoenix-society.org
U.S. Fire Administration, www.usfa.fema.gov

Sensory Function

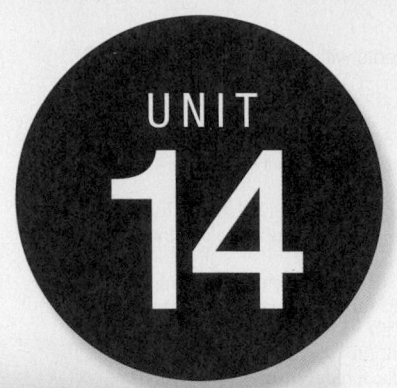

Case Study   MAKING A RAPID CHANGE TO TELEHEALTH

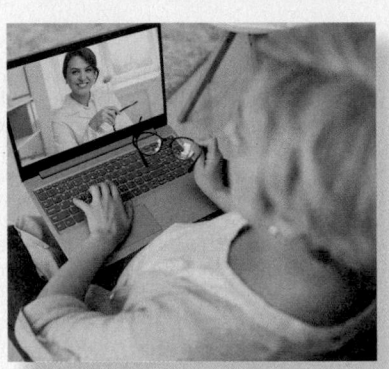

A 72-year-old female is due for a follow-up appointment at the outpatient ophthalmology clinic where you work. She has a history of type 2 diabetes, hypertension, and elevated cholesterol. During her previous visit, she reported her vision was blurred when watching television and that she stopped driving after dark as she could not see properly; she was subsequently diagnosed with diabetic retinopathy. However, there is an outbreak of coronavirus disease 2019 (COVID-19) within your community; the health network system that manages the ophthalmology clinic has responded by mandating that telehealth be used through video conference service to manage all patients for clinic visits. How will you assist the clinic staff as well as the patients, particularly this patient with poor vision, to make a rapid transition to telehealth visits while also assuring continued quality outcomes?

QSEN Competency Focus: Informatics

The complexities inherent in today's health care system challenge nurses to demonstrate integration of specific interdisciplinary core competencies. These competencies are aimed at ensuring the delivery of safe, quality patient care (Institute of Medicine, 2003). The Quality and Safety Education for Nurses project (Cronenwett, Sherwood, Barnsteiner, et al., 2007; QSEN, 2020) provides a framework for the knowledge, skills, and attitudes (KSAs) required for nurses to demonstrate competency in these key areas, which include *patient-centered care*, *interdisciplinary teamwork and collaboration*, *evidence-based practice*, *quality improvement*, *safety*, and *informatics.*

Informatics Definition: Use information and technology to communicate, manage knowledge, mitigate error, and support decision-making.

SELECT PRE-LICENSURE KSAs	APPLICATION AND REFLECTION
Knowledge	
Identify essential information that must be available in a common database to support patient care	Transitioning to telehealth in a short period of time can be challenging. How can you help communicate essential information and streamline the process of change?
Contrast benefits and limitations of different communication technologies and their impact on safety and quality	What are the benefits and limitations of using telehealth, especially with patients with low vision?
Describe examples of how technology and information management are related to the quality and safety of patient care	Describe how the implementation of telehealth in an outpatient clinic will increase the quality and safety for the patients who receive care there during a pandemic.
Recognize the time, effort, and skill required for computers, databases, and other technologies to become reliable and effective tools for patient care	How does the use of telehealth help the team in the ophthalmology clinic improve outcomes for patients?
Skills	
Seek education about how information is managed in care settings before providing care	How can you influence the safe and effective implementation of telehealth?
Apply technology and information management tools to support safe processes of care	How can you support safe processes of care utilizing this new technology?
Navigate the electronic health record	How will the telehealth system be integrated with the existing electronic health record and used to monitor outcomes of care processes?
Document and plan patient care in an electronic health record	Patients must now navigate the video conference system through the existing patient portal for follow-up visits. How will you communicate these changes to the ophthalmology clinic's mostly older adult patients, many of whom have poor vision and may feel challenged utilizing these types of technologic platforms?
Employ communication technologies to coordinate care for patients	
Respond appropriately to clinical decision-making supports and alerts	
Use information management tools to monitor outcomes of care processes	
Attitudes	
Value technologies that support clinical decision-making, error prevention, and care coordination	Reflect upon how rapid change is implemented within an organization during times of a pandemic. How can you find value in the use of telehealth for clinical decision-making, prevention of errors, and coordination of care?

Cronenwett, L., Sherwood, G., Barnsteiner, J., et al. (2007). Quality and safety education for nurses. *Nursing Outlook, 55*(3), 122–131; Institute of Medicine. (2003). *Health professions education: A bridge to quality*. Washington, DC: National Academies Press; QSEN Institute. (2020). *QSEN competencies: Definitions and pre-licensure KSAs; Informatics*. Retrieved on 8/15/2020 at: qsen.org/competencies/pre-licensure-ksas/#informatics

58

Assessment and Management of Patients with Eye and Vision Disorders

LEARNING OUTCOMES

On completion of this chapter, the learner will be able to:

1. Identify the major internal and external structures and functions of the eye.
2. Specify assessment and diagnostic findings used in the evaluation of ocular disorders.
3. Describe assessment and management strategies for patients with low vision and blindness.
4. List the pharmacologic actions and nursing management of common ophthalmic medications.
5. Recognize the clinical features, assessment and diagnostic findings, as well as the medical or surgical management, and nursing management of the patient with glaucoma, cataracts, and other ocular disorders.

NURSING CONCEPTS

Assessment	Infection	Patient Education
Comfort	Inflammation	Sensory Perception

GLOSSARY

anterior chamber: aqueous-containing space in the eye between the posterior (endothelial) cornea and the anterior iris and pupil

aqueous humor: transparent, nutrient-containing fluid that fills the anterior and posterior chambers of the eye

astigmatism: refractive error due to an irregularity in the curvature of the cornea

binocular vision: normal ability of both eyes to focus on one object and fuse the two images into one

blindness: inability to see, defined as corrected visual acuity of 20/400 or less, or a visual field of no more than 20 degrees in the better eye

cataract: progressive opacity of the lens of the eye

chemosis: edema of the conjunctiva

diplopia: seeing one object as two (*synonym:* double vision)

ectropion: turning out of the lower eyelid

emmetropia: normal refractive condition resulting in clear focus on retina; no optical defects

endophthalmitis: intraocular infection

entropion: turning in of the lower eyelid

enucleation: removal of the eyeball and part of the optic nerve

evisceration: removal of the intraocular contents through a corneal or scleral incision; the optic nerve, sclera, extraocular muscles, and sometimes the cornea are left intact

exenteration: surgical removal of the entire contents of the orbit, surrounding soft tissue, and most or all of the eyelids

exophthalmos: abnormal protrusion of the eyeball (*synonym:* proptosis)

glaucoma: group of conditions characterized by increased intraocular pressure

hyperemia: red eyes resulting from dilation of the vasculature of the conjunctiva

hyperopia: farsightedness; light rays focus behind the retina

hyphema: blood in the anterior chamber

hypopyon: collection of inflammatory cells in the anterior chamber of the eye

injection: congestion of blood vessels

keratoconus: cone-shaped deformity of the cornea

myopia: nearsightedness; light rays focus in front of the retina

neovascularization: growth of abnormal new blood vessels

nystagmus: involuntary oscillation of the eyeball

papilledema: swelling of the optic disc usually due to increased intracranial pressure

photophobia: ocular pain on exposure to light

presbyopia: the loss of accommodative power in the lens due to age

ptosis: drooping eyelid
refraction: determination of the refractive errors of the eye for the purpose of vision correction
scotomas: blind or partially blind areas in the visual field
sympathetic ophthalmia: an inflammatory condition created in the fellow eye by the affected eye

trachoma: an infectious disease caused by the bacterium *Chlamydia trachomatis*—the leading cause of preventable blindness in the world
trichiasis: turning in of the eyelashes
vitreous humor: transparent, colorless gelatinous material that fills the vitreous chamber behind the lens

The eye is a sensitive, highly specialized sense organ subject to various disorders, many of which can lead to impaired vision. Impaired vision may affect individuals in many ways, including their independence in self-care, sense of self-esteem, safety, and overall quality of life. Many of the leading causes of visual impairment are associated with aging (e.g., cataracts, glaucoma, macular degeneration). Younger people are also at risk for eye disorders, particularly traumatic injuries.

Assessment and management of patients with eye and vision disorders occur in various health care settings. In addition to understanding the prevention, treatment, and consequences of eye disorders, nurses in all settings assess visual acuity in patients at risk (e.g., older adults, those with hypertension, diabetes, acquired immune deficiency syndrome [AIDS]), refer patients to eye care specialists as appropriate, implement measures to prevent further visual loss, and help patients adapt to impaired vision.

ASSESSMENT OF THE EYE

Anatomic and Physiologic Overview

Unlike most organs of the body, the eye is available for external examination, and its anatomy is more easily assessed than other body parts (see Fig. 58-1). The eyeball, or globe, is situated in the bony protective orbit (Shaw & Lee, 2017). Lined

with muscle and connective and adipose tissues, the orbit is shaped like a four-sided pyramid, surrounded on three sides by the sinuses: ethmoid (medially), frontal (superiorly), and maxillary (inferiorly). The optic nerve and the ophthalmic artery enter the orbit at its apex through the optic foramen. The eyeball is moved through all fields of gaze by the extraocular muscles. The four rectus muscles and two oblique muscles (see Fig. 58-2) are innervated by cranial nerves (CNs) III, IV, and VI. Normally, the movements of the two eyes are coordinated and the brain perceives a single image.

The eyelids are composed of thin, elastic skin that covers striated and smooth muscles and protect the anterior portion of the eye. The eyelids contain multiple glands (sebaceous, sweat, and lacrimal). The upper lid normally covers the uppermost portion of the iris and is innervated by the oculomotor nerve (CN III). The lid margins contain meibomian glands, the inferior and superior puncta, and the eyelashes. The triangular spaces formed by the junction of the eyelids are known as the inner or medial canthus and the outer or lateral canthus. With every blink, the eyelids wash the cornea and conjunctiva with tears.

Tears are vital to eye health. Formed by the lacrimal gland and the accessory lacrimal glands, tears are secreted in response to reflex or emotional stimuli. A healthy tear is composed of three layers: lipoid, aqueous, and mucoid. These layers nourish the cornea and create a smooth optical surface of the cornea and conjunctival epithelium. If there is a defect in the composition of any of these layers, the integrity of the cornea may be compromised.

The conjunctiva, a thin transparent mucous membrane, provides a barrier to the external environment extending under the eyelids (palpebral conjunctiva) and over the sclera

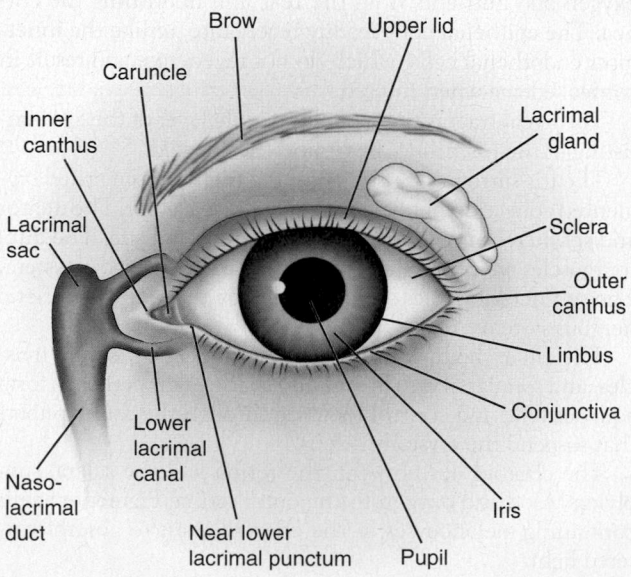

Figure 58-1 • External structures of the eye and position of the lacrimal structures.

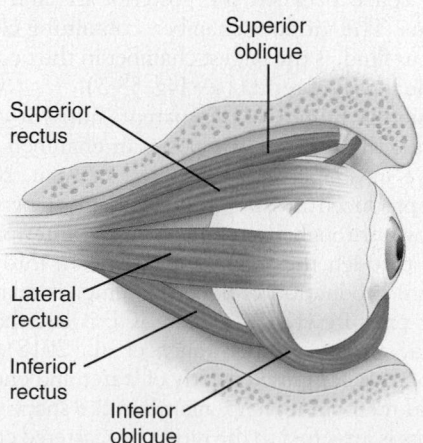

Figure 58-2 • The extraocular muscles responsible for eye movement. The medial rectus muscle (not shown) is responsible for opposing the movement of the lateral rectus muscle.

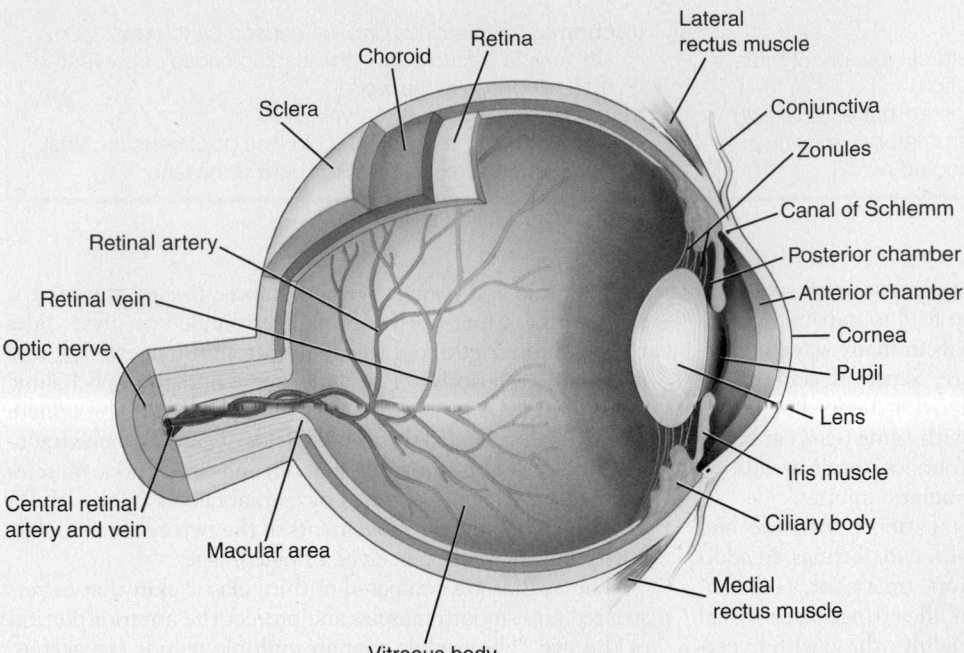

Figure 58-3 • Three-dimensional cross-section of the eye.

(bulbar conjunctiva). The junction of the two portions is known as the fornix. The conjunctiva meets the cornea at the limbus on the outermost edge of the iris.

The eyeball is composed of the following three layers:

- The outer dense fibrous layer, including the sclera and transparent cornea
- The middle vascular layer, containing the iris, ciliary body, and choroid
- The inner neural layer, including the retina, optic nerve, and visual pathway

The eyeball is divided anatomically into two segments. The anterior segment is between the anterior cornea and posterior iris, including the anterior and posterior chambers. The posterior segment is between the posterior lens and the retina, including the vitreous chamber. The eyeball also has three fluid-containing chambers. The aqueous-filled **anterior chamber** lies between the posterior cornea and the anterior iris and pupil. The posterior chamber is a small aqueous-containing space between the posterior iris and pupil and anterior lens. The vitreous chamber, containing clear gelatinous vitreous fluid, is the largest chamber in the ocular fundus between the lens and retina (see Fig. 58-3).

The **aqueous humor** is transparent, nutrient-containing fluid that fills the anterior and posterior chambers and helps give the eye its shape (Moore, Dalley, & Agur, 2018). The aqueous is produced in the posterior chamber by the ciliary body; it flows through the pupil into the anterior chamber and drains through the trabecular meshwork into the canal of Schlemm. Production of aqueous humor is related to the intraocular pressure (IOP). Normal IOP is less than 21 mm Hg (Sihota, Angmo, Ramaswamy, et al., 2018). **Vitreous humor,** which is composed mostly of water and encapsulated by a hyaloid membrane, helps maintain the shape of the eye. The vitreous is attached to the retina by scattered collagenous filaments. The vitreous shrinks and shifts with age. Through this degenerative process, the gel-like characteristics liquefy, causing stringy debris known as floaters.

The sclera is the white avascular dense fibrous structure that helps maintain the shape of the eyeball and protects the intraocular contents. Scleral thinning and changes of the scleral collagen fibers can cause the underlying uveal pigment to be seen, resulting in a blue or gray sclera. The episclera is a vascularized loose elastic tissue that overlies the sclera supplying nutritional support and reacting to inflammation.

The cornea, a vulnerable transparent avascular dome-like structure, forms the most anterior portion of the eyeball and is the main refracting surface of the eye. It is composed of five layers: the epithelium, Bowman's membrane, stroma, Descemet's membrane, and endothelium. It contains high concentrations of nerve fibers and is extremely sensitive to pain. The epithelium, the outermost protective layer, absorbs oxygen and nutrients from the tear film nourishing the cornea. The epithelial cells readily regenerate, unlike the innermost endothelial cells, which do not regenerate and result in corneal edema when injured.

The uveal tract is the vascular middle layer of the eye consisting of the iris, ciliary body, and the choroid.

The iris surrounding the pupil is a highly vascularized pigmented collection of fibers that give the eye color. The dilator and sphincter muscles of the iris control pupil size. The dilator muscles are controlled by the sympathetic nervous system. The sphincter muscles are controlled by the parasympathetic nervous system.

The ciliary body consists of ciliary processes, ciliary muscles, and zonular fibers (ligaments) that work together to form aqueous fluid and control focusing through the zonular fibers that suspend the crystalline lens.

The choroid lies between the retina and the sclera, supplying blood and oxygen to the outer retina. Pigmented cells containing melanocytes in the choroid assist to absorb scattered light.

Directly behind the pupil and iris lies the lens, an avascular and almost completely transparent biconvex structure held in position by zonular fibers in the ciliary body. The lens enables focusing for near and distance vision through accommodation, the process by which the lens of the eye adjusts the focal length to focus a clear image on the retina. With aging and certain conditions (e.g., diabetes or trauma), the lens loses its transparency and ability to focus due to formation of a cataract (see later discussion).

The retina—the innermost surface of the fundus composed of neural tissue—is an extension of the optic nerve. Viewed through the pupil, the landmarks of the retina are the optic disc, the retinal vessels, and the macula. The point of entrance of the optic nerve into the retina is the optic disc. The optic disc is pink, either oval or circular in shape, and has sharp margins. In the disc, a physiologic depression or cup is present centrally, with the retinal blood vessels emerging from it. The retinal tissues arise from the optic disc and line the inner surface of the vitreous chamber. The retinal vessels enter the eye through the optic disc, branching out through the retina and forming superior and inferior branches. The macula is the area of the retina responsible for central vision. The rest of the retina is responsible for peripheral vision. In the center of the macula is the most sensitive area—the fovea—which is avascular and surrounded by the superior and inferior vascular arcades. Two important layers of the retina are the retinal pigment epithelium and the sensory retina. A single layer of cells constitutes the retinal pigment epithelium. These cells have numerous functions, including the absorption of light. The sensory retina contains the photoreceptor cells: rods and cones. The rods are responsible for night or low light vision. The cones are retinal photoreceptor cells essential for visual acuity, color discrimination, and fine detail. Cones are distributed throughout the retina, with their greatest concentration in the fovea. Rods are absent in the fovea.

Visual acuity depends on a healthy functioning eye and an intact visual pathway. This pathway is made up of the retina, optic nerve, optic chiasm, optic tracks, lateral geniculate bodies, optic radiations, and the visual cortex area of the brain. The visual pathway is part of the central nervous system (see Fig. 58-4).

The optic nerve (CN II) transmits impulses from the retina to the occipital lobe of the brain. The optic nerve head, or optic disc, is the physiologic blind spot in each eye. The optic nerve leaves the eye and then meets the optic nerve from the other eye at the optic chiasm. The chiasm is the anatomic point at which the nasal fibers from the nasal retina of each eye cross to the opposite side of the brain. The nerve fibers from the temporal retina of each eye remain uncrossed. Fibers from the right half of each eye, which would be the left visual field, carry impulses to the right occipital lobe. Fibers from the left half of each eye, or the right visual field, carry impulses to the left occipital lobe. Beyond the chiasm, these fibers are known as the optic tract. The optic tract continues on to the lateral geniculate body. The lateral geniculate body is connected by the optic radiations to the cortex of the occipital lobe of the brain.

Assessment

Ocular History

The nurse, through careful questioning, elicits the necessary information that can assist in diagnosis of an ophthalmic condition. Pertinent questions to ask when taking an ocular

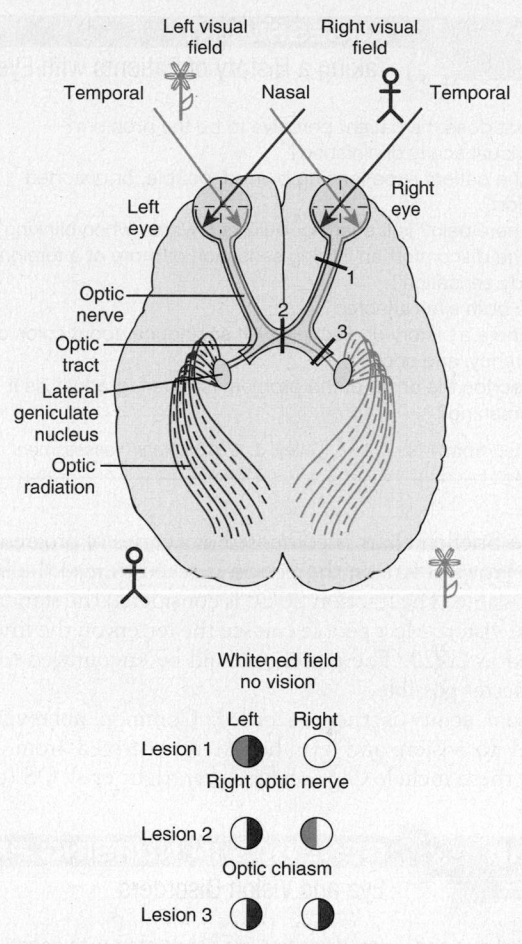

Figure 58-4 • Diagram of optic pathways. The *red* lines indicate the right visual field and the *blue* lines the left visual field. Note the crossing of the fibers from the medial half of each retina at the optic chiasm. Lesion 1 (right optic nerve) produces unilateral blindness. Lesion 2 (optic chiasm) may involve only those fibers that originate in the nasal half of each retina and cross to the opposite side in each field (bitemporal hemianopia). Lesion 3 (right optic tract) interrupts fibers (and vision) originating on the same side of both eyes (homonymous) with loss of vision from half of each field (hemianopia). Reprinted with permission from Norris, T. L. (2019). *Porth's pathophysiology: Concepts of altered health states* (10th ed., Fig. 19.23). Philadelphia, PA: Wolters Kluwer.

history are presented in Chart 58-1. Genetics may play a role in the causation and progression of eye and vision disorders (Singh & Tyagi, 2018) (see Chart 58-2).

Visual Acuity

Following the health history, the patient's visual acuity is assessed. This is an essential part of the eye examination and a measure against which all therapeutic outcomes are based.

Visual acuity is tested for both near (14 inches away) and distance (20 feet away) vision and is performed on each eye separately with a standardized Snellen chart for distance and a Rosenbaum pocket screener for near vision. A tumbling "E," "illiterate E," number, or picture chart is used if the person is illiterate or unable to read the English alphabet (Weber & Kelley, 2018).

Chart 58-1

ASSESSMENT

Taking a History of Patients with Eye and Vision Disorders

- What does the patient perceive to be the problem?
- Is visual acuity diminished?
- Is the patient experiencing blurred, double, or distorted vision?
- Is there pain? Is it sharp or dull? Is it worse when blinking?
- Is the discomfort an itching sensation or more of a foreign-body sensation?
- Are both eyes affected?
- Is there a history of discharge? If so, inquire about color, consistency, and odor.
- Describe the onset of the problem (sudden, gradual). Is it worsening?

- What is the duration of the problem?
- Is this a recurrence of a previous condition?
- How has the patient self-treated?
- What makes the symptoms improve or worsen?
- Has the condition affected performance of activities of daily living?
- Are there any systemic diseases? What medications are used in their treatment?
- What other eye conditions does the patient have?
- Is there a history of eye surgery?
- Have other family members had the same symptoms or condition?

Adapted from Weber, J., & Kelley, J. (2018). *Health assessment in nursing* (6th ed.). Philadelphia, PA: Wolters Kluwer.

The Snellen chart is composed of a series of progressively smaller rows of letters; the person is asked to read the lowest line possible. The fraction 20/20 is considered the standard of normal vision. Most people can see the letters on the line designated as 20/20. The patient should be encouraged to read every letter possible.

Visual acuity is then recorded. Common abbreviations related to vision and eye health are derived from Latin terms; these include OD (*oculus dexter*, right eye), OS (*oculus* sinister, left eye), and OU (*oculus uterque*, both eyes). The following would be an example of visual acuity documentation: A patient reads all five letters from the 20/20 line on the Snellen chart with the right eye (OD) and three of the five letters on the 20/30 line with the left eye (OS); the visual acuity is documented as OD: 20/20 and OS: 20/30 (Weber & Kelley, 2018).

If the patient cannot see the big "E" at the top of the Snellen chart, the examiner should determine next if the

---

Chart 58-2

GENETICS IN NURSING PRACTICE

Eye and Vision Disorders

Several eye and vision disorders are associated with genetic abnormalities. Some examples include:

Autosomal dominant:

- Aniridia
- Vitelliform macular dystrophy

Autosomal recessive:

- Achromatopsia
- Homocystinuria
- Leber congenital amaurosis

X linked:

- Choroideremia
- Color blindness

Mitochondrial inheritance:

- Leber hereditary optic neuropathy

Multiple inheritance patterns identified:

- Glaucoma
- Macular degeneration
- Retinitis pigmentosa

Other genetic illnesses that will impact vision:

- Albinism
- Isolated familial congenital cataracts
- Marfan syndrome
- Stickler syndrome
- Tay-Sachs disease
- Usher syndrome

Nursing Assessments

Refer to Chapter 4, Chart 4-2: Genetics in Nursing Practice: Genetic Aspects of Health Assessment

Family History Assessment Specific to Vision

- Assess history of family members in the past three generations with glaucoma, cataracts, night blindness (retinitis pigmentosa), color blindness, or other vision impairment.
- Inquire about the age of onset of symptoms (the onset of Leber congenital amaurosis is in childhood, whereas the onset of Leber hereditary optic neuropathy is in young adulthood).
- Inquire about family members with other disorders that may include visual impairment, such as cutaneous, metabolic, or connective tissue disorders and hearing loss.

Patient Assessment Specific to Vision

- Assess for other systemic and/or clinical features such as cutaneous or skeletal conditions, or hearing loss.
- Look for color and clarity of iris.
- Assess for presence of strabismus (cross-eyes), amblyopia (lazy eye), nystagmus, astigmatism, and near- or farsightedness.
- Assess for changes in visual acuity.
- Assess field of vision.
- Inquire about photophobia, night blindness, or double vision.

Genetics Resources

National Ophthalmic Disease Genotyping Network, eyegene.nih. gov/

See Chapter 6, Chart 6-7 for additional components of genetic counseling.

patient can count fingers ("CF" in documentation). Initially, the examiner stands 5 feet from the person, holds up a random number of fingers, and then asks the patient to count the number of fingers seen. If the patient is unable to count fingers at 5 feet, the examiner keeps moving a foot closer until either 1 foot away or the person can correctly count fingers. If the patient correctly counts the number of fingers at 3 feet, for example, the examiner would record vision as CF/3 feet.

If the patient cannot count fingers, the examiner raises one hand up and down or moves it side to side and asks in which direction the hand is moving. This level of vision is known as hand motion. A patient who can perceive only light is described as having light perception. The vision of a patient who cannot perceive light is described as no light perception.

External Eye Examination

The nurse uses a systematic approach to perform an external eye examination by first assessing for symmetry and placement of eyelids, pupils, and muscles. CNs III, IV, and VI control movement and pupil size. The eyelids should rest just above and below the corneal limbus without exposure of the sclera. The nurse observes for **ptosis** (drooping of the eyelid), **ectropion** (turning out of the lower eyelid), or **entropion** (turning in of the lower eyelid). Entropion may involve **trichiasis** (turning in of the eyelashes). Eyelids and lashes should be free of drainage or scaling.

The room should be darkened so that the pupils can be examined. The pupillary response is checked with a penlight to determine if the pupils are equally reactive and regular. A normal pupil is black. An irregular pupil may result from trauma, previous surgery, or a disease process.

The patient's eyes are observed in primary or direct gaze, and any head tilt is noted. A head tilt may indicate CN palsy. The patient is asked to stare at a target; each eye is covered and uncovered quickly while the examiner looks for any shift in gaze. The examiner observes for **nystagmus** (involuntary oscillating movement of the eyeball). The extraocular movements of the eyes are tested by having the patient follow the examiner's finger, pencil, or a hand light through the six cardinal directions of gaze (i.e., up, down, right, left, and both diagonals).

Diagnostic Evaluation

A wide range of diagnostic studies may be performed in patients with eye disorders. The nurse should educate the patient about the purpose, what to expect, and any possible side effects related to these examinations prior to testing. The nurse should be aware of contraindications, potential complications, and trends in results. Trends provide information about disease progression as well as the patient's response to therapy.

Direct Ophthalmoscopy

A direct ophthalmoscope is a handheld instrument with various plus and minus lenses (Weber & Kelley, 2018). The lenses can be rotated into place, enabling the examiner to bring the cornea, lens, and retina into focus sequentially. The examiner holds the ophthalmoscope in the right hand and uses the right eye to examine the patient's right eye. The examiner switches to the left hand and left eye when examining the patient's left eye. During this examination, the room should be darkened, and the patient's eye should be on the same level as the examiner's eye. The patient and the examiner should be comfortable, and both should breathe normally. The patient is given a target to gaze at and is encouraged to keep both eyes open and steady.

When the fundus is examined, the vasculature comes into focus first. The veins are larger in diameter than the arteries. The examiner focuses on a large vessel and then follows it toward the midline of the body, which leads to the optic nerve. The central depression in the disc is known as the cup. The normal cup is about one third the size of the diameter of the disc. The size of the physiologic optic cup should be estimated, and the disc margins described as sharp or blurred. A silvery or coppery appearance, which indicates arteriolosclerosis, should be noted. The periphery of the retina is examined by having the patient shift their gaze. The last area of the fundus to be examined is the macula, because this area is the most sensitive to light. The retina of a young person often has a glistening effect, sometimes referred to as a cellophane reflex.

The healthy fundus should be free of any lesions. The examiner looks for intraretinal hemorrhages, which may appear as red smudges, and, if the patient has hypertension, they may be somewhat flame shaped. Lipid with a yellowish appearance may be present in the retina of patients with hypercholesterolemia or diabetes. Soft exudates that have a fuzzy, white appearance (cotton-wool spots) should be noted. The examiner looks for microaneurysms, which look like little red dots, and nevi. Drusen (small, hyaline, globular deposits), commonly found in macular degeneration, appear as yellowish areas with indistinct edges. Small drusen have a more distinct edge. The examiner should sketch the fundus and document any abnormalities.

Indirect Ophthalmoscopy

The indirect ophthalmoscope is an instrument commonly used by the ophthalmologist to see larger areas of the retina, although in an unmagnified state. It produces a bright and intense light. The light source is affixed with a pair of binocular lenses mounted on the examiner's head. The ophthalmoscope is used with a handheld, 20-diopter lens.

Slit-Lamp Examination

The slit lamp is a binocular microscope mounted on a table. This instrument enables the user to examine the eye with magnification of 10 to 40 times the real image. The illumination can be varied from a broad to a narrow beam of light for different parts of the eye. For example, by varying the width and intensity of the light, the anterior chamber can be examined for signs of inflammation. Cataracts may be evaluated by changing the angle of the light. When a handheld contact lens, such as a three-mirror lens, is used with the slit lamp, the angle of the anterior chamber may be examined, as may the ocular fundus.

Tonometry

Tonometry is a common procedure to measure IOP. The device used for measuring IOP is an accurately calibrated applanation tonometer, which measures the pressure needed to flatten the cornea. This procedure is most commonly used to screen for and monitor IOP in glaucoma.

Nursing Interventions

Providing patient education prior to tonometry helps avoid possible errors in IOP measurement. Patients are cautioned to avoid squeezing the eyelids, holding their breath, or performing a Valsalva maneuver, because these may result in abnormally increased IOP.

Color Vision Testing

The ability to differentiate colors has a dramatic effect on the activities of daily living (ADLs). For example, the inability to differentiate between red and green can compromise traffic safety. Some careers (e.g., commercial artist, [color] photographer, airline pilot, electrician) may be closed to people with significant color deficiencies. The photoreceptor cells responsible for color vision are the cones, and the greatest area of color sensitivity is in the macula—the area of densest cone concentration.

A screening test, such as the polychromatic plates discussed in the next paragraph, can be used to establish whether a person's color vision is within normal range. Color vision deficits can be inherited. For example, red–green color deficiencies are inherited in an X-linked manner, affecting approximately 8% of men and 0.5% of women (Colour Blind Awareness, 2019). Acquired color vision losses may be caused by medications (e.g., digitalis) or pathology (e.g., cataracts). A simple test, such as asking a patient if the red top on a bottle of eye drops appears redder to one eye than the other, can be an effective tool. A difference in the perception of the intensity of the color red between the two eyes can be a symptom of a neurologic problem and may provide information about the location of the lesion.

Because alteration in color vision sometimes indicates conditions of the optic nerve, color vision testing is often performed in a neuro-ophthalmologic workup. The most common color vision test is performed using Ishihara polychromatic plates. These plates are bound together in a booklet. On each plate of this booklet are dots of primary colors that are integrated into a background of secondary colors. The dots are arranged in simple patterns, such as numbers or geometric shapes. Patients with diminished color vision may be unable to identify the hidden shapes. Patients with central vision conditions (e.g., macular degeneration) have more difficulty identifying colors than those with peripheral vision conditions (e.g., glaucoma) because central vision identifies color.

Amsler Grid

The Amsler grid is a test often used for patients with macular problems, such as macular degeneration. It consists of a geometric grid of identical squares with a central fixation point. The grid should be viewed by the patient wearing normal reading glasses. Each eye is tested separately. The patient is instructed to stare at the central fixation spot on the grid and report any distortion in the squares of the grid itself. For patients with macular disorders, some of the squares may look faded, or the lines may be wavy. Patients with age-related macular degeneration (AMD) are commonly given these Amsler grids to take home. The patient is encouraged to check the grids frequently, as often as daily, to monitor macular function for early detection of changes requiring immediate attention (Gerstenblith & Rabinowitz, 2017; Weber & Kelley, 2018).

Ultrasonography

Lesions in the globe or the orbit may not be directly visible and are evaluated by ultrasonography. Ultrasonography is a valuable diagnostic technique, especially when the view of the retina is obscured by opaque media such as cataract or hemorrhage. An ultrasonography B-scan identifies pathology such as orbital tumors, retinal detachment, and vitreous hemorrhage. Ultrasonography A-scans are used to measure the axial length for implants prior to cataract surgery (Gerstenblith & Rabinowitz, 2017).

Optical Coherence Tomography

Optical coherence tomography is a technology that involves low-coherence interferometry (Gerstenblith & Rabinowitz, 2017). Light is used to evaluate retinal and macular diseases as well as anterior segment conditions. This method is noninvasive and involves no physical contact with the eye.

Fundus Photography

Fundus photography is used to detect and document retinal lesions. The patient's pupils are usually widely dilated before the procedure. The resulting fundus photographs can be viewed stereoscopically so that elevations such as macular edema can be identified.

Laser Scanning

Various scanning techniques use laser light in the diagnostic evaluation of eye disorders. Confocal laser scanning ophthalmoscopy provides a three-dimensional image of the optic nerve topography and is used alone or in conjunction with fundus photography to provide comparative data for suspected optic nerve disease such as glaucoma and **papilledema** (swelling of the optic disc due to increased intracranial pressure) (Gerstenblith & Rabinowitz, 2017). Laser scanning polarimetry is used to measure nerve fiber layer thickness and is an important indicator of glaucoma progression.

Angiography

Angiography is done using fluorescein or indocyanine green as contrast agents. Fluorescein angiography is used to evaluate clinically significant macular edema, document macular capillary nonperfusion, and identify retinal and choroidal **neovascularization** (growth of abnormal new blood vessels) in AMD. It is an invasive procedure in which fluorescein dye is injected, usually into an antecubital vein. Within 10 to 15 seconds, this dye can be seen coursing through the retinal vessels. Over a 10-minute period, serial black-and-white photographs are taken of the retinal vasculature (Fischbach & Fischbach, 2018).

Indocyanine green angiography is used to evaluate abnormalities in the choroidal vasculature, which often are seen in macular degeneration. Indocyanine green dye is injected intravenously (IV), and multiple images are captured using digital video angiography. The dye is quickly removed from circulation by the liver, mostly clearing within 10 to 20 minutes (Norat, Soldozy, Elsarrag, et al., 2019).

Nursing Interventions

Prior to the angiography, the patient's blood urea nitrogen and creatinine should be checked to ensure that the kidneys will excrete the contrast agent (Fischbach & Fischbach, 2018). The patient should be well hydrated, and clear liquids are usually permitted up to the time of the test. The patient is instructed to remain immobile during the angiogram process and is told to expect a brief feeling of warmth in the face, behind the eyes, or in the jaw, teeth, tongue, and lips, and a metallic taste when the contrast agent is injected.

Nursing care after angiography includes observation of the injection site (usually the antecubital vein) for bleeding or hematoma formation (a localized collection of blood). Fluorescein may impart a gold tone to the skin in some patients, and urine may turn deep yellow or orange. This discoloration usually disappears in 24 hours. Indocyanine green dye is generally well tolerated, but some patients experience nausea and vomiting. Allergic reactions are rare; however, indocyanine green angiography is contraindicated in patients with a history of iodide reactions. Fluids are encouraged following the procedure to facilitate excretion of the contrast agent (Fischbach & Fischbach, 2018).

Perimetry Testing

Perimetry testing evaluates the field of vision. Visual field testing (i.e., perimetry) helps identify which parts of the patient's central and peripheral visual fields have useful vision. It is most helpful in detecting central **scotomas** (blind or partially blind areas in the visual field) in macular degeneration and the peripheral field defects in glaucoma and retinitis pigmentosa. Visual field evaluation and optic nerve assessment are major components of monitoring and detecting glaucoma progression.

IMPAIRED VISION

Refractive Errors

In refractive errors, vision is impaired because a shortened or elongated eyeball prevents light rays from focusing sharply on the retina. Blurred vision from refractive error can be corrected with eyeglasses or contact lenses. Ophthalmic **refraction** is the determination of the refractive errors of the eye for the purpose of vision correction and consists of placing various types of lenses in front of the patient's eyes to determine which lens best improves the patient's vision.

The depth of the eyeball is important in determining refractive error (see Fig. 58-5). Patients for whom the visual image focuses precisely on the macula and who do not need eyeglasses or contact lenses are said to have **emmetropia,** a normal refractive condition resulting in clear focus on retina with no optical defects (normal vision). Some people have deeper eyeballs, in which case the distant visual image focuses in front of, or short of, the retina; those with **myopia** are said to be nearsighted and have blurred distance vision. Other people have shallower eyeballs, in which case the visual image focuses beyond the retina; those with **hyperopia** are said to be farsighted and have excellent distance vision but blurry near vision (Weber & Kelley, 2018).

Wavefront technology to measure unique refractive imperfections of the cornea or higher aberrations (i.e., myopia, hyperopia, astigmatism) can be used to customize laser-assisted in situ keratomileusis (LASIK) procedures. These procedures are described later in this chapter.

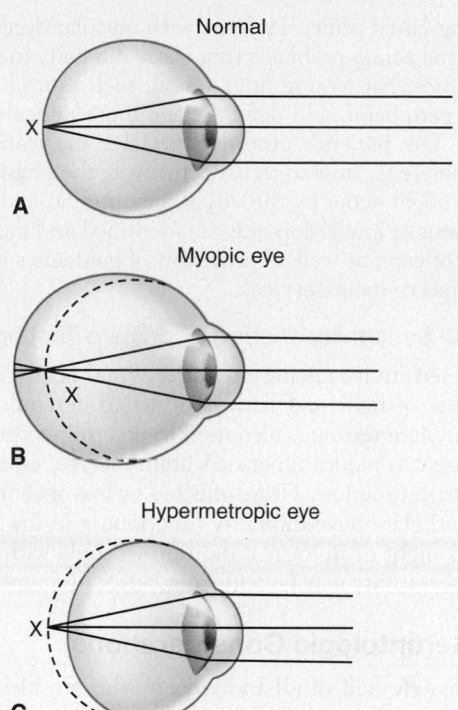

Figure 58-5 • Eyeball shape determines visual acuity in refractive errors. **A.** Normal eye. **B.** Myopic eye. **C.** Hypermetropic eye.

Vision Impairment and Blindness

Vision impairment is defined as having central visual acuity of 20/40 or worse in the better eye with the best possible correction. *Low vision* describes visual impairment that requires the use of devices and strategies to perform visual tasks.

Blindness is having best possible corrected central visual acuity that can range from 20/400 to no light perception. The clinical definition of absolute blindness is the absence of light perception. Legal blindness is a condition of impaired vision and is defined as having central visual acuity of 20/200 or worse in the better eye with the best possible correction or whose widest visual field diameter is 20 degrees or less (Bright Focus Foundation, 2020b). This definition neither equates with functional ability nor classifies the degrees of visual impairment. Legal blindness ranges from an inability to perceive light to having some vision remaining. A person who meets the criteria for legal blindness may be eligible for government financial assistance through disability.

Assessment and Diagnostic Testing

Assessment of vision impairment includes a thorough history and examination of distance and near visual acuity, visual field, contrast sensitivity, glare, color perception, and refraction. Specially designed, low-vision visual acuity charts are used to evaluate patients.

Patient Interview

During history taking, the potential cause and duration of the patient's visual impairment are identified. Patients with retinitis pigmentosa, for example, have a genetic abnormality. Patients with diabetic macular edema typically have fluctuating visual acuity. Patients with macular degeneration have central acuity problems that cause difficulty in performing activities that require finer vision, such as reading. People with peripheral field defects have more difficulties with mobility. The patient's customary ADLs, medication regimen, habits (e.g., smoking), acceptance of the physical limitations brought about by the visual impairment, and realistic expectations of low-vision aids are identified and included in the plan of care, as well as provision of guidelines for safety and referrals to social services.

Contrast-Sensitivity Testing and Glare Testing

Contrast-sensitivity testing measures visual acuity in different degrees of light and dark contrast to determine visual function. Glare testing is also used to determine visual function. Glare can reduce a person's ability to see, especially in patients with cataracts. Those affected by loss of contrast sensitivity and glare have difficulty functioning in low light, or driving at night or in foggy conditions. People with a loss of contrast sensitivity may benefit from better illumination.

 Gerontologic Considerations

Approximately half of all individuals who are identified as legally blind each year are 65 years of age or older (Eliopoulos, 2018). With aging, structural and functional changes occur in the eye (see Chart 58-3). **Presbyopia,** the loss of accommodative power in the lens, interferes with the ability to adequately focus and is the factor responsible for most older

adults requiring some form of corrective lenses (Eliopoulos, 2018). Age-related changes in the eye are summarized in Table 58-1.

Impaired vision is often accompanied by difficulty in performing functional activities. People with visual acuity of 20/80 to 20/100 with a visual field restriction of 60 degrees to greater than 20 degrees can read at a nearly normal level with optical aids. Their visual orientation is near normal but requires increased scanning of the environment (i.e., systematic use of head and eye movements). In a visual acuity range of 20/200 to 20/400 with a 20-degree to greater than 10-degree visual field restriction, the person can read slowly with optical aids.

The most common causes of blindness and visual impairment among adults 40 years and older are diabetic retinopathy, macular degeneration, glaucoma, and cataracts (Centers for Disease Control and Prevention [CDC], 2019). Macular degeneration is more prevalent among Caucasians, whereas glaucoma is more prevalent among African Americans (Eliopoulos, 2018).

Medical Management

Managing vision impairment involves magnification and image enhancement through the use of low-vision aids and strategies, as well as referrals to social services and community agencies. The goals are to optimize the patient's remaining vision and assist the patient to perform customary activities. Table 58-2 presents low-vision aids. Medications are

---

Chart 58-3 · ETHICAL DILEMMA
Should Preservation of Patient Autonomy Threaten the Welfare of Others?

Case Scenario

You work as a staff nurse on a subacute care unit. D.P. is an 85-year-old man who has made daily visits to see his wife who has been a patient on the unit for the past week for daily physical and occupational therapy after having hip surgery. During your morning rounds today, D.P.'s wife tells you that her husband did not visit her yesterday and she is worried about him. After lunch, D.P. arrives on the subacute care unit with a sheepish grin on his face and a bandage on his forehead. When D.P.'s wife tells him that she was worried about him, he replies "Do not worry about me! I got into a fender bender yesterday but I am okay." D.P.'s wife shakes her head and says "Why are you so stubborn? You cannot see well at all anymore and should not be driving!" With tears in his eyes, D.P. says to his wife "But how else would I get here to see you, my sweetheart? Nothing could ever keep me away from you!" Based on previous conversations you have had with D.P. and his wife, you know that they live alone together in a two-bedroom ranch home that they have shared for the past 60 years. They have two adult sons who both live several hundred miles away.

Discussion

In American society, being able to drive is seen as consistent with being able to maintain an independent lifestyle. It is not uncommon for older adults to feel threatened by a possible loss of driving rights. D.P.'s apparent devotion to his wife and inability to identify an acceptable alternative means to visit her seems to be compounding his feelings of vulnerability.

There are some states that require health care providers to report drivers whom they think are impaired and unsafe. As a witness to this verbal exchange between D.P. and his wife, you

may be obligated to investigate this situation further, or be liable for civil or criminal penalties.

Analysis

- Describe the ethical principles that are in conflict in this case (see Chapter 1, Chart 1-7). Is it possible to preserve D.P.'s autonomy while ensuring that neither D.P. nor others are harmed should he continue to drive?
- Regardless of the legal requirements in your state, what are your ethical and moral obligations to D.P., his wife, and to others who may be impacted by D.P.'s driving?
- What resources might you mobilize to be of assistance to you, to D.P., and to D.P.'s wife? It is not uncommon for spouses to neglect their own health needs when their partner becomes ill. You may wish to explore whether D.P. has had a recent focused visual examination, to find whether he has visual deficits amenable to correction. In addition, although D.P.'s children do not live close, D.P. and his wife may have other social support networks that they could tap into to assist them so that D.P. can continue his daily visits with his wife. Local Area Agencies on Aging can also provide a wealth of contacts and support services for older adults that could be explored.

References

Morgan, E. (2018). Driving dilemmas: A guide to driving assessment in primary care. *Clinics in Geriatric Medicine, 34*(1), 107–115.

Resources

See Chapter 1, Chart 1-10 for Steps of an Ethical Analysis and Ethics Resources.

TABLE 58-1 Age-Related Changes in the Eye

External Eye	Structural Change	Functional Change	History and Physical Findings
Eyelids and lacrimal structures	Loss of skin elasticity and orbital fat, decreased muscle tone; wrinkles develop	Lid margins turn in, causing entropion; or lid margins turn out, resulting in ectropion.	Reports of burning, foreign-body sensation, epiphora; injection, inflammation, and ulceration may occur.
Refractive changes; presbyopia	Loss of accommodative power in the lens with age	Reading materials must be held at increasing distance in order to focus.	Patient reports, "Arms are too short!"; need for increased light; reading glasses or bifocals needed.
Cataract	Opacities in the normally crystalline lens	Interference with the focus of a sharp image on the retina.	Patients report increased glare, decreased vision, changes in color values (blue and yellow especially affected).
Posterior vitreous detachment	Liquefaction and shrinkage of vitreous body	May lead to retinal tears and detachment.	Reports light flashes, cobwebs, floaters.
Age-related macular degeneration (AMD)	Drusen (yellowish aging spots in the retina) appear and coalesce in the macula. Abnormal choroidal blood vessels may lead to formation of fibrotic disciform scars in the macula	Central vision is affected; onset is more gradual in dry AMD, more rapid in wet AMD; distortion and loss of central vision may occur.	Reading vision is affected; words may be missing letters, faded areas appear on the page, straight lines may appear wavy; drusen, pigmentary changes in retina; abnormal submacular choroidal vessels.

Adapted from Eliopoulos, C. (2018). *Gerontological nursing* (9th ed.). Philadelphia, PA: Wolters Kluwer.

TABLE 58-2 Activities Affected by Visual Impairment and Suggestions for Low-Vision Aids

Activity	Optical Aids	Nonoptical Aids
Shopping	Hand magnifier	Lighting, color cues
Fixing a snack	Bifocals	Color cues; consistent food storage plan
Eating out	Hand magnifier	Flashlight, portable lamp
Identifying money	Bifocals, hand magnifier	Arrange paper money in wallet compartments
Reading print	High-power spectacle, bifocals, hand magnifier, stand magnifier, closed-circuit television	Lighting, high-contrast print, large print, reading slit
Writing	Hand magnifier	Lighting, bold-tip pen, black ink
Using a telephone	Hand magnifier	Large-print buttons, hand-printed directory Braille phones, picture/photo phones, and talking phones Accessibility settings on smartphones
Crossing streets	Lightweight handheld monoscopes/telescopes	Cane; ask directions
Finding taxis and bus signs	Lightweight handheld monoscopes/telescopes	Ask for assistance
Using ride-sharing services	Lightweight handheld monoscopes/telescopes	Ask for assistance
Reading medication labels	Hand magnifier	Color codes, large print
Reading stove dials	Hand magnifier	Color codes, raised dots
Adjusting the thermostat	Hand magnifier	Enlarged-print model, digital thermostats that can be controlled via voice or apps
Using a computer or electronic tablet	Spectacles	High-contrast color, large-print program. Screen-reader programs convert text on the computer screen to synthesized speech
Reading signs	Spectacles	Move closer
Watching sporting event	Lightweight handheld monoscopes/telescopes	Sit in front rows

Adapted from Pagliuca, L. M., Macêdo-Costa, K. N., Rebouças, C. B., et al. (2014). Validation of the general guidelines of communication between the nurse and the blind. *Revista Brasileira de Enfermagem, 67*(5), 715–721.

prescribed for glaucoma. Ongoing research suggests that gene therapy may replace or be an adjunct to pharmacologic or surgical treatment for ocular disorders in the near future (Jolly, Bridge, & MacLaren, 2019).

Referrals to community agencies may be necessary for patients with low vision who live alone and cannot self-administer their medications. Community agencies, such as the Lighthouse Guild, offer a wide variety of vision and health care services to patients with low vision and blindness.

Nursing Management

Nurses need to be sensitive to the challenges faced by patients with visual impairments. Coping with blindness involves emotional, physical, and social adaptation. The emotional adjustment to blindness or severe visual impairment determines the success of the physical and social adjustments of the patient. Successful emotional adjustment means acceptance of blindness or severe visual impairment.

Promoting Coping

Effective coping may not occur until the patient recognizes the permanence of the low vision or blindness. A patient who is newly visually impaired and their family members undergo the various steps of grieving: denial and shock, anger and protest, restitution, loss resolution, and acceptance. The ability to accept the changes that must come with visual loss and willingness to adapt to those changes influence the successful rehabilitation of the patient with vision loss. Additional aspects to consider are value changes, independence–dependence conflicts, coping with stigma, and learning to function in social settings without visual cues and landmarks.

Promoting Spatial Orientation and Mobility

A person who is blind or severely visually impaired requires strategies for adapting to the environment. ADLs, such as walking to a chair from a bed, require spatial concepts. The person needs to know where they are in relation to the rest of the room, to understand the changes that may occur, and to know how to approach the desired location safely. This requires a collaborative effort between the patient and the responsible adult who serves as the sighted guide. The nurse must assess the degree of physical assistance the person with vision loss requires and communicate this to other health care personnel.

The nurse should be aware of the importance of techniques in providing physical assistance, encouraging independence, and ensuring safety. Strategies for interacting with the patient with vision loss are presented in Chart 58-4. Research supports the use of a validated protocol to educate staff to perform therapeutic communication, deliver services, and minimize communication barriers with patients who are blind (Pagliuca, Macêdo-Costa, Rebouças, et al., 2014). The readiness of the patient and family to learn must be assessed before initiating orientation and mobility training.

Promoting Home, Community-Based, and Transitional Care

The nurse, social worker, family, and others collaborate to assess the patient's home condition and support system. A low vision specialist or occupational therapist should be consulted, particularly for patients for whom identifying and administering medications pose challenges. Referral for vision rehabilitation should be provided for appropriate patients (Shah, Schwartz, Gartner, et al., 2018).

Chart 58-4	Strategies for Interacting with People Who Are Blind or Have Low Vision

- Remember that the only difference between you and people who are blind or have low vision is that they are not able to see through their eyes what you are able to see through yours.
- Do not be uncomfortable when in the company of a person who is blind or has low vision. Talk with the person as you would talk with any other person, honestly and with respect, courtesy, and empathy; do not be concerned about using words like "see" and "look." There is no need to raise your voice unless the person asks you to do so.
- Identify yourself as you approach the person and before you make physical contact. Tell the person your name and your role. If another person approaches, introduce them. When you leave the room, be sure to tell the person that you are leaving and if anyone else remains in the room.
- Keep in mind that it is often appropriate to touch the person's hand or arm lightly to indicate that you are about to speak.
- When talking, face the person and speak directly to them using a normal tone of voice.
- Be specific when communicating direction. Mention a specific distance or use clock cues when possible (e.g., walk left about 2 yards; walk about 20 feet to the right; the telephone is at 2 o'clock). Avoid using phrases such as "over there."
- When you offer to assist someone, allow the person to hold on to your arm just above the elbow and to walk a half step behind you.

- When offering the person a seat, place the person's hand on the back or the arm of the seat.
- When you are about to go up or down a flight of stairs, tell the person and place their hand on the banister.
- Make sure that the environment is free of obstacles; close doors and cabinets so that they are not in the path.
- Offer to read written information, such as a menu.
- If you serve food to the person, use clock cues to specify where everything is on the plate.
- When the person who is blind or has low vision is a patient in a health care facility:
  - Make sure all objects the person will need are close at hand.
  - Identify the location of objects that the person may need (e.g., "The call light is near your right hand"; "The telephone is on the table on the left side of your bed.")
  - Remove obstacles that may be in the person's pathway and could cause a fall.
  - Place all assistive devices that the person uses close at hand; let the person feel the devices so that they know their location.
- Do not distract a service animal unless the owner has given permission.
- Ask the person, "How can I help you?" At some times, the person needs help; at other times, help may not be needed.

Adapted from Pagliuca, L. M., Macêdo-Costa, K. N., Rebouças, C. B., et al. (2014). Validation of the general guidelines of communication between the nurse and the blind. *Revista Brasileira de Enfermagem*, 67(5), 715–721.

Other interventions that are appropriate for some people with visual impairment or blindness include Braille and service animals. There has been an ever-increasing reliance on print magnification technology as well as technology-assisted speech output. However, although the use of Braille may be less important for adults who have already learned language and grammar skills, educators and low vision specialists have continued to advocate that children who are legally blind be given the opportunity to learn Braille.

Guide dogs, also known as service dogs, are dogs that are specially bred, raised, and rigorously trained to assist people who are blind. The guide dog is a constant companion to the person who is blind (also referred to as the animal's handler) and is allowed on airplanes and in restaurants, stores, hotels, and other public places. With the assistance of the guide dog, the person who is blind can be extremely mobile and accomplish normal activities both within and outside of the home and workplace. A dog in harness is a working dog, not a pet. The dog should not be distracted from his job by well-intentioned strangers who want to pet, feed, or play with the animal. The dog's handler should always be consulted before approaching the working guide dog. Most health care facilities have a service animal policy that outlines the responsibilities of the handler with regard to the care of the animal.

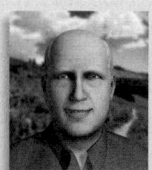

Unfolding Patient Stories: Vernon Watkins • Part 2

Recall from Chapter 14 **Vernon Watkins,** who came to the emergency department with severe abdominal pain and underwent a hemicolectomy for a bowel perforation. During postoperative care the nurse determines that he has poor vision. What measures can the nurse take to maintain a safe environment for a patient with visual impairment? How will the discovery of impaired vision impact the nursing plan of care, discharge planning, and delivery of patient education? Care for Vernon and other patients in a realistic virtual environment: ***vSim** for Nursing* (**thepoint.lww. com/vSimMedicalSurgical**). Practice documenting these patients' care in DocuCare (**thepoint.lww.com/ DocuCareEHR**).

OCULAR MEDICATION ADMINISTRATION

Because medications are often prescribed to treat ocular disorders, nurses must understand the actions of the commonly used medications and effective administration. The main objective of ocular medication delivery is to maximize the amount of medication that reaches the ocular site of action in sufficient concentration to produce a beneficial therapeutic effect. This is determined by the dynamics of ocular pharmacokinetics: absorption, distribution, metabolism, and excretion.

Ocular absorption involves the entry of a medication into the aqueous humor through the different routes of ocular medication administration. The rate and extent of aqueous humor absorption are determined by the characteristics of the medication and the anatomy and physiology of the eye. Natural barriers of absorption that diminish the efficacy of ocular medications include the following:

- *Limited size of the conjunctival sac.* The conjunctival sac can hold only 50 mcL, and any excess is wasted. The volume of one eye drop from commercial topical ocular solutions typically ranges from 20 to 35 mcL.
- *Corneal membrane barriers.* The epithelial, stromal, and endothelial layers are barriers to absorption.
- *Blood–ocular barriers.* Blood–ocular barriers prevent high ocular tissue concentration of most ophthalmic medications because they separate the bloodstream from the ocular tissues and keep foreign substances from entering the eye, thereby limiting a medication's efficacy.
- *Tearing, blinking, and drainage.* Increased tear production and drainage due to ocular irritation or an ocular condition may dilute or wash out an instilled eye drop; blinking expels an instilled eye drop from the conjunctival sac.

Distribution of an ocular medication into the ocular tissues varies by tissue type—the conjunctiva, cornea, lens, iris, ciliary body, and choroids absorb medications to varying degrees. Medications penetrate the corneal epithelium either by intracellular diffusion (passing through the cells) or by intercellular diffusion (passing between the cells). Hydrophilic (water soluble) medications diffuse through the intracellular route, and lipophilic (fat soluble) medications diffuse through the intercellular route. Topical administration usually does not reach the retina in significant concentrations. Because the space between the ciliary process and the lens is small, medication diffusion in the vitreous is slow. When high concentrations of medication in the vitreous are required, intraocular injection is often chosen to bypass the natural ocular anatomic and physiologic barriers (American Society of Ophthalmic Registered Nurses [ASORN], 2013).

Aqueous solutions are most commonly used for the eye. They are the least expensive medications and interfere the least with vision. However, corneal contact time is brief because tears dilute the medication. Ophthalmic ointments have extended retention time in the conjunctival sac and provide a higher concentration than eye drops. The major disadvantage of ointments is the blurred vision that results after application. In general, eyelids and eyelid margins are best treated with ointments. The conjunctiva, limbus, cornea, and anterior chamber are treated most effectively with instilled solutions or suspensions. Subconjunctival injection may be necessary for better absorption in the anterior chamber. If high medication concentrations are required in the posterior chamber, intravitreal injections or systemically absorbed medications are considered. Contact lenses and collagen shields soaked in antibiotic agents are alternative delivery methods for treating corneal infections.

Of all these delivery methods, the topical route of administration—instilled eye drops and applied ointments—remains the most common and widely recommended (ASORN, 2013). Topical instillation, which is the least invasive method, permits self-administration of medication and produces fewer side effects.

Preservatives are commonly used in ocular medications. Benzalkonium chloride, for example, prevents the growth of organisms and enhances the corneal permeability of most medications; however, some patients are allergic to this preservative. This may be suspected even if the patient had never before experienced an allergic reaction to systemic use of the medication in question. Eye drops without preservatives can be prepared by pharmacists.

Common Ocular Medications

Common ocular medications include topical anesthetic, mydriatic, and cycloplegic agents that reduce IOP; anti-infective medications; corticosteroids; nonsteroidal anti-inflammatory drugs (NSAIDs); antiallergy medications; eye irrigants; and lubricants.

Topical Anesthetic Agents

One or two drops of proparacaine hydrochloride and tetracaine hydrochloride are instilled before diagnostic procedures such as tonometry and minor ocular procedures such as removal of sutures or conjunctival or corneal scrapings. Topical anesthetic agents are also used for severe eye pain to allow the patient to open their eyes for examination or treatment (e.g., eye irrigation for chemical burns). Anesthesia occurs within 20 seconds to 1 minute and lasts 10 to 20 minutes.

> ◣ **Quality and Safety Nursing Alert**
>
> *To prevent injury, the nurse educates the patient not to rub the eyes while anesthetized because this may result in damage to the cornea.*

Mydriatic and Cycloplegic Agents

Mydriasis, or pupil dilation, is the main objective of the administration of mydriatics and cycloplegics (see Table 58-3). These two types of medications function differently and are used in combination to achieve the maximal dilation that is needed during surgery and fundus examinations to give the ophthalmologist a better view of the internal eye structures.

Mydriatics potentiate alpha-adrenergic sympathetic effects that result in the relaxation of the ciliary muscle. This causes the pupil to dilate. However, this sympathetic action alone is not enough to sustain mydriasis because of its short duration of action. The strong light used during an eye examination also stimulates miosis (i.e., pupillary contraction). Cycloplegic medications are given to paralyze the iris sphincter.

The patient is educated about the temporary effects of mydriasis on vision, such as glare and the inability to focus properly. The patient may have difficulty reading. The effects of the various mydriatics and cycloplegics can last 3 hours to several days. The patient is advised to wear sunglasses (most eye clinics provide protective sunglasses). The ability to drive depends on the person's age, vision, and comfort level. Some patients can drive safely with the use of sunglasses, whereas others may need to be driven home.

Mydriatic and cycloplegic agents affect the central nervous system. Their effects are most prominent in younger and older adult patients; these patients must be assessed closely for symptoms, such as increased blood pressure, tachycardia, dizziness, ataxia, confusion, disorientation, incoherent speech, and hallucination. These medications are contraindicated in patients with narrow angles or shallow anterior chambers and in patients taking monoamine oxidase inhibitors or tricyclic antidepressants.

Medications Used to Treat Glaucoma

Therapeutic medications for glaucoma are used to lower IOP by decreasing aqueous production or increasing aqueous outflow. Because glaucoma calls for lifetime therapy, the patient must be educated with regard to both the ocular and systemic side effects of the medications. See section on glaucoma later in this chapter.

Anti-Infective Medications

Anti-infective medications include antibiotic, antifungal, and antiviral agents. Most are available as drops, ointments, or subconjunctival or intravitreal injections. Antibiotics

TABLE 58-3 Mydriatics and Cycloplegics			Peak		Recovery Time	
Medication	Available Preparation/ Concentration	Indication/Dosage	Mydriasis (Minutes)	Cycloplegia (Minutes)	Mydriasis	Cycloplegia
atropine	Ointment (0.5–2%) Solutions (0.5–3%)	In uveitis, or after surgery, 2–4 × daily	30–40	60–180	7–10 days	6–12 days
cyclopentolate hydrochloride	Solution (0.5–2%)	Given with mydriatics every 5–10 min × 3 or until the pupils are fully dilated for ophthalmoscopy and surgical procedures	30–60	25–75	1 day	6–24 h
phenylephrine hydrochloride	Solutions (2.5%, 10%)	Given with cycloplegics in pupillary dilation for ophthalmoscopy and surgical procedures every 5–10 min × 3	10–60	—	3–5 h	—
scopolamine hydrobromide	Solution (0.25%)	Same as atropine	20–30	30–60	3–7 days	3–7 days
homatropine	Solution (5–2.5%)	Same as atropine and scopolamine	40–60	30–60	1–3 days	1–3 days

Adapted from Comerford, K. C., & Durkin, M. T. (2020). *Nursing 2020 drug handbook.* Philadelphia, PA: Wolters Kluwer.

include penicillin, cephalosporins, aminoglycosides, and fluoroquinolones. The main antifungal agent is amphotericin B. Side effects of amphotericin are serious and include severe pain, conjunctival necrosis, iritis, and retinal toxicity. Antiviral medications include acyclovir and ganciclovir. They are used to treat ocular infections associated with herpes virus and cytomegalovirus (CMV). Patients receiving ocular anti-infective agents are subject to the same side effects and adverse reactions as those receiving oral or parenteral medications.

Corticosteroids and Nonsteroidal Anti-Inflammatory Drugs

Topical preparations of corticosteroids are commonly used in inflammatory conditions of the eyelids, conjunctiva, cornea, anterior chamber, lens, and uvea. In posterior segment diseases that involve the posterior sclera, retina, and optic nerve, topical agents are less effective and parenteral and oral routes are preferred. When a suspension is prescribed, the patient is instructed to shake the bottle several times to promote mixture of the medication and maximize its therapeutic effect. The most common ocular side effects of long-term topical corticosteroid administration are glaucoma, cataracts, susceptibility to infection, impaired wound healing, mydriasis, and ptosis. High IOP may develop, which is reversible after corticosteroid use is discontinued. To avoid the side effects of corticosteroids, NSAIDs are used as an alternative in controlling inflammatory eye conditions and postoperatively to reduce inflammation.

Antiallergy Medications

Ocular hypersensitivity reactions, such as allergic conjunctivitis, are extremely common. These conditions result primarily from responses to environmental allergens. Most allergens are airborne or carried to the eye by the hand or by other means, although allergic reactions may also be drug induced. Corticosteroids are commonly used as anti-inflammatory and immunosuppressive agents to control ocular hypersensitivity reactions.

Ocular Irrigants and Lubricants

Most irrigating solutions are used to cleanse the external lids to maintain lid hygiene, to irrigate the external corneal surface to regain normal pH (e.g., in chemical burns), to irrigate the corneal surface to eliminate debris, or to inflate the globe intraoperatively. These solutions have various compositions that include sodium, potassium, magnesium, calcium, bicarbonate, glucose, and glutathione (i.e., substance found in the aqueous humor). Sterile irrigating solutions for lid hygiene are available. Irrigating solutions are safe to use with an intact corneal surface; however, the corneal surface should not be irrigated in cases of threatened corneal perforation. For patients with severe corneal ulcer, specific instructions from the ophthalmologist must be obtained regarding whether it is safe to irrigate the corneal surface or just to cleanse the external lids. Although it is good practice to promote hygiene, prevention of complications must be the primary concern. Normal saline solutions are commonly used to irrigate the corneal surface when chemical burns occur.

Lubricants, such as artificial tears, help alleviate corneal irritation, such as dry eye syndrome. Artificial tears are topical preparations of carboxymethylcellulose or hydroxypropyl methylcellulose that are prepared as eye drop solutions, ointments, or ocular inserts (inserted at the lower conjunctival cul-de-sac once each day). The eye drops can be instilled as often as every hour, depending on the severity of symptoms.

Nursing Management

The objectives in administering ocular medications are to ensure proper administration to maximize the therapeutic effects and to ensure the safety of the patient by monitoring for systemic and local side effects (ASORN, 2013). Absorption of eye drops by the nasolacrimal duct is undesirable because of the potential systemic side effects of ocular medications. To diminish systemic absorption and minimize the side effects, it is important to occlude the puncta (see Chart 58-5). This is especially important for patients who are most vulnerable to medication overdose, including older adults; women who are pregnant or lactating; and patients with cardiac, pulmonary, hepatic, or kidney disease. A 5-minute interval between instillation of different types of ocular drops is recommended.

Before the administration of ocular medications, the nurse warns the patient that blurred vision, stinging, and a burning sensation are symptoms that ordinarily occur after instillation and are temporary. Risk for interactions of the ocular medication with other ocular and systemic medications must be emphasized; therefore, a careful patient interview regarding the medications being taken must be obtained.

 Quality and Safety Nursing Alert

To prevent infection, meticulous hand hygiene before and after medication instillation is crucial. In addition, the tip of the eye drop bottle or the ointment tube must never touch any part of the eye, and the medication must be recapped immediately after each use.

If a patient who instills their own medications cannot feel the eye drops when they are instilled, the eye medication may be refrigerated, because a cold drop is easier to detect. A 5-minute interval between successive administrations allows adequate drug retention and absorption. The patient or the caregiver at home should be asked to demonstrate actual eye drop or ointment instillation and punctal occlusion.

GLAUCOMA

The term **glaucoma** is used to refer to a group of ocular conditions characterized by elevated IOP (McMonnies, 2017). If left untreated, the increased IOP damages the optic nerve and nerve fiber layer, but the degree of harm is highly variable (Eliopoulos, 2018). The optic nerve damage is related to the IOP caused by congestion of aqueous humor in the eye. A range of IOPs are considered "normal," but these may also be associated with vision loss in some patients.

Chart
58-5

PATIENT EDUCATION

Instilling Eye Medications

The nurse instructs the patient to:

- Never use eye solutions that have changed colors.
- Perform hand hygiene before and after the procedure.
- Ensure adequate lighting.
- Read the label of the eye medication to verify that it is the correct medication.
- Remove contact lens as needed.
- Assume a comfortable position.
- Avoid touching the tip of the medication container to any part of the eye or face.
- Hold the lower lid down; do not press on the eyeball. Apply gentle pressure to the cheekbone to anchor the finger holding the lid.

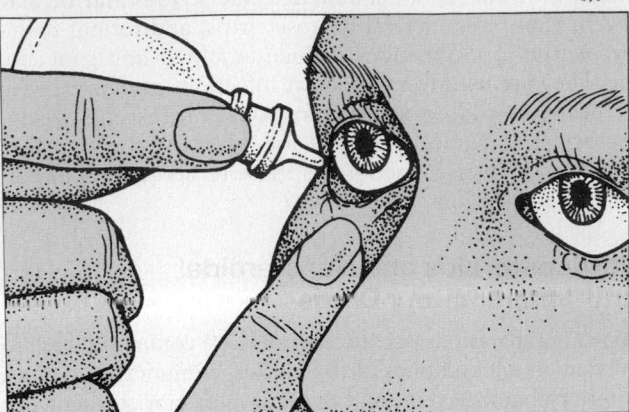

- Instill eye drops before applying ointments.
- Apply a 0.25- to 0.5-inch ribbon of ointment to the lower conjunctival sac.

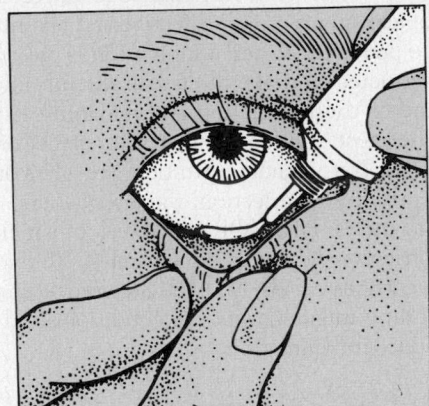

- Keep the eyelids closed, and apply gentle pressure on the inner canthus (punctal occlusion) near the bridge of the nose for 1 or 2 minutes immediately after instilling eye drops.
- Use a clean tissue to gently pat skin to absorb excess eye drops that run onto the cheeks.
- Wait 5 minutes before instilling another eye drop and 10 minutes before instilling another ointment.
- Reinsert contact lens if applicable.

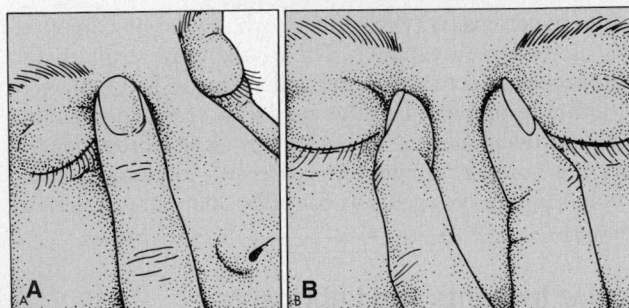

A.

B.

Adapted from American Society of Ophthalmic Registered Nurses (ASORN). (2013). *ASORN recommended practice: Use of multi-dose medications.* San Francisco, CA: Author; Glaucoma Research Foundation. (2020). Eye drop tips. Retrieved on 2/11/2020 at: www.glaucoma.org/treatment/eyedrop-tips.php

Glaucoma is estimated to affect three million Americans, approximately 50% of whom are undiagnosed (Moore et al., 2018). Glaucoma is more prevalent in people older than 40 years, and it is the third most common age-related eye disease in the United States. Chart 58-6 presents the risk factors for glaucoma. There is no cure for glaucoma, but the disease can be controlled (Glaucoma Research Foundation, 2019).

Physiology

Aqueous humor flows between the iris and the lens, nourishing the cornea and lens. Most (90%) of the fluid then flows out of the anterior chamber, draining through the spongy trabecular meshwork into the canal of Schlemm and the episcleral veins (see Fig. 58-6). About 10% of the aqueous fluid exits through the ciliary body into the suprachoroidal space and then drains into the venous circulation of the ciliary body, choroid, and sclera (Norris, 2019). Unimpeded outflow of aqueous fluid depends on an intact drainage system and an open angle (about 45 degrees) between the iris and the cornea. A narrower angle places the iris closer to the trabecular meshwork, diminishing the angle. The amount of aqueous humor produced tends to decrease with age, in systemic diseases such as diabetes, and in ocular inflammatory conditions.

IOP is determined by the rate of aqueous production, the resistance encountered by the aqueous humor as it flows out of the passages, and the venous pressure of the episcleral veins that drain into the anterior ciliary vein. When aqueous fluid production and drainage are in balance, the IOP is between 10 and 21 mm Hg. When aqueous fluid is inhibited from flowing out, pressure builds up within the eye. Fluctuations in IOP occur with time of day, exertion, diet, and medications. IOP tends to increase with blinking, tight lid squeezing, and upward gazing. Systemic conditions such as diabetes and intraocular conditions such as uveitis and retinal detachment have been associated with elevated IOP. Glaucoma may not be recognized in people with thin corneas because measurement of the IOP may be falsely low as a result of this thinness.

Pathophysiology

There are two theories regarding how increased IOP damages the optic nerve in glaucoma. The direct mechanical theory suggests that high IOP damages the retinal layer as it passes through the optic nerve head. The indirect ischemic theory suggests that high IOP compresses the microcirculation in the optic nerve head, resulting in cell injury and death. Some glaucomas appear as exclusively mechanical, and some are exclusively ischemic types. Typically, most cases are a combination of both.

Classification of Glaucoma

There are several types of glaucoma. Forms of glaucoma are identified as wide-angle glaucoma; narrow-angle glaucoma; congenital glaucoma; and glaucoma associated with other conditions, such as developmental anomalies or corticosteroid use. Glaucoma can be primary or secondary, depending on whether associated factors contribute to the rise in IOP. The two common clinical forms of glaucoma in adults are wide- and narrow-angle glaucoma, which are differentiated by the mechanisms that cause impaired aqueous outflow (Norris, 2019). Table 58-4 summarizes the characteristics of the different types of adult glaucoma.

Clinical Manifestations

Glaucoma is often called the "silent thief of sight" because most patients are unaware that they have the disease until

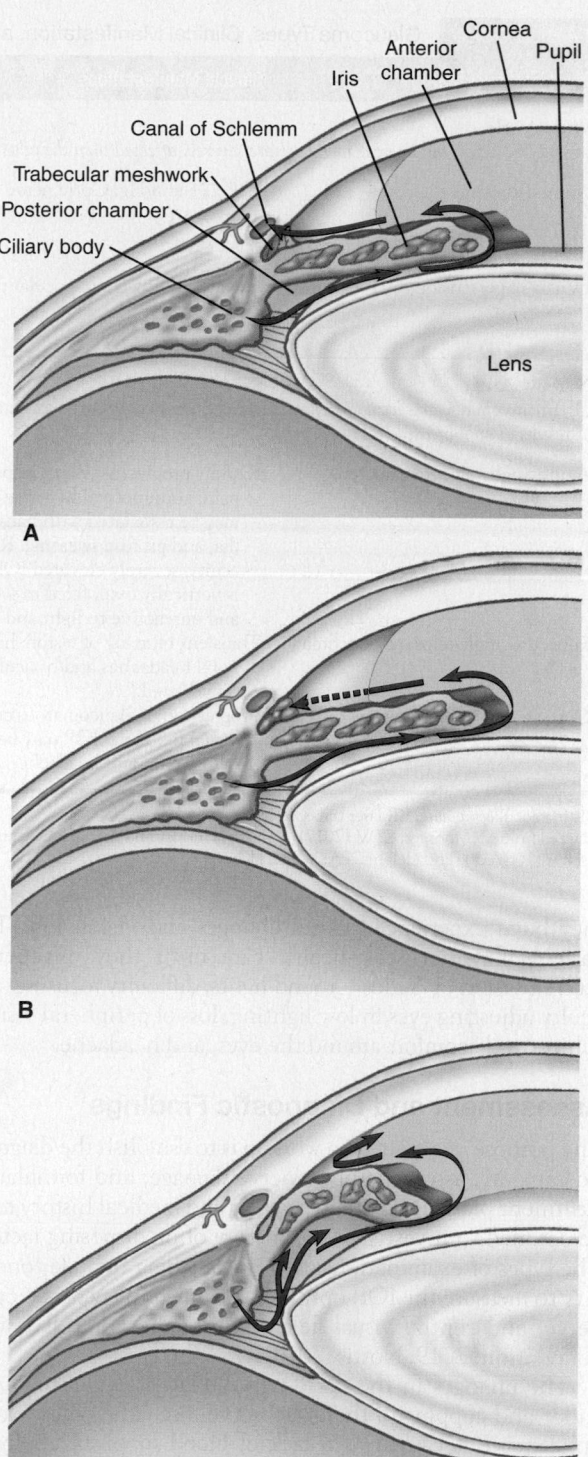

Figure 58-6 • A. Normally, aqueous humor, which is secreted in the posterior chamber, gains access to the anterior chamber by flowing through the pupil. In the angle of the anterior chamber, it passes through the canal of Schlemm into the venous system. **B.** In wide-angle glaucoma, the outflow of aqueous humor is obstructed at the trabecular meshwork. **C.** In narrow-angle glaucoma, the aqueous humor encounters resistance to flow through the pupil. Increased pressure in the posterior chamber produces a forward bowing of the peripheral iris so that the iris blocks the trabecular meshwork. Reprinted with permission from Norris, T. L. (2019). *Porth's pathophysiology: Concepts of altered health states* (10th ed., Fig. 19.11). Philadelphia, PA: Wolters Kluwer.

TABLE 58-4   Glaucoma Types, Clinical Manifestation, and Treatment

Types of Glaucoma	Clinical Manifestations	Treatment
Wide Angle *Usually bilateral, but one eye may be more severely affected than the other. In wide-angle glaucoma, the anterior chamber angle is open and appears normal.*		
Normal-tension glaucoma	IOP ≤21 mm Hg. Optic nerve damage, visual field defects.	If medical treatment is unsuccessful, LT can decrease IOP by 20%. Glaucoma filtering surgery if continued optic nerve damage despite medication therapy and LT.
Ocular hypertension	Elevated IOP. Possible ocular pain or headache.	The best management for normal-tension glaucoma management is yet to be established. Goal is to lower the IOP by at least 30%.
Narrow Angle *Obstruction in aqueous humor outflow due to the complete or partial closure of the angle from the forward shift of the peripheral iris to the trabecula. The obstruction results in an increased IOP.*		
Acute angle–closure glaucoma	Rapidly progressive visual impairment, periocular pain, conjunctival hyperemia, and congestion. Pain may be associated with nausea, vomiting, bradycardia, and profuse sweating. Reduced central visual acuity, severely elevated IOP, corneal edema. Pupil is vertically oval, fixed in a semidilated position, and unreactive to light and accommodation.	Ocular emergency; administration of hyperosmotics, acetazolamide, and topical ocular hypotensive agents. Possible laser iridotomy (incision in the iris) to release blocked aqueous and reduce IOP. Other eye is also treated with pilocarpine eye drops and/or surgical management to avoid a similar spontaneous attack.
Subacute angle–closure glaucoma	Transient blurring of vision, halos around lights; temporal headaches and/or ocular pain; pupil may be semidilated.	Prophylactic peripheral laser iridotomy. Can lead to acute or chronic angle–closure glaucoma if untreated.
Chronic angle–closure glaucoma	Progression of glaucomatous cupping and significant visual field loss; IOP may be normal or elevated; ocular pain and headache.	Management includes laser iridotomy and medications.

IOP, intraocular pressure; LT, laser trabeculoplasty.
Adapted from McMonnies, C. W. (2017). Glaucoma history and risk factors. *Journal of Optometry, 10*(2), 71–78; Norris, T. (2019). *Porth's pathophysiology: Concepts of altered health status* (10th ed.). Philadelphia, PA: Wolters Kluwer.

they have experienced visual changes and vision loss. The patient may not seek health care until they experience blurred vision or "halos" around lights, difficulty focusing, difficulty adjusting eyes in low lighting, loss of peripheral vision, aching or discomfort around the eyes, and headache.

Assessment and Diagnostic Findings

The purpose of a glaucoma workup is to establish the diagnostic category, assess the optic nerve damage, and formulate a treatment plan. The patient's ocular and medical history must be detailed to investigate the history of predisposing factors. The types of examinations used in glaucoma include tonometry to measure the IOP, ophthalmoscopy to inspect the optic nerve, and central visual field testing (Glaucoma Research Foundation, 2019; Norris, 2019).

The changes in the optic nerve related to glaucoma are pallor and cupping of the optic nerve disc. The pallor of the optic nerve is caused by a lack of blood supply. Cupping is characterized by exaggerated bending of the blood vessels as they cross the optic disc, resulting in an enlarged optic cup that appears more basinlike compared with a normal cup. The progression of cupping in glaucoma is caused by the gradual loss of retinal nerve fibers and the loss of blood supply.

As the optic nerve damage increases, visual perception decreases. The localized areas of visual loss (i.e., scotomas) represent loss of retinal sensitivity and nerve fiber damage and are measured and mapped on a graph. In patients with glaucoma, the graph has a distinct pattern that is different from other ocular diseases and is useful in establishing the diagnosis. Figure 58-7 shows the visual changes caused by glaucoma.

Medical Management

The aim of all glaucoma treatment is prevention of optic nerve damage. Lifelong therapy is necessary because glaucoma cannot be cured. Treatment focuses on pharmacologic therapy, laser procedures, surgery, or a combination of these approaches, all of which have potential complications and side effects. The object is to achieve the greatest benefit at the least risk, cost, and inconvenience to the patient. Although treatment cannot reverse optic nerve damage, further damage can be controlled. The goal is to maintain an IOP within a range unlikely to cause further damage (Sheybani, Scott, Samuelson, et al., 2020). The initial target for IOP among

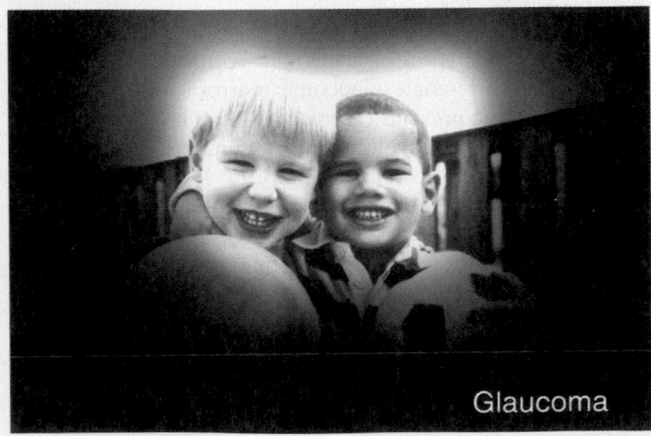

Figure 58-7 • Visual changes associated with glaucoma. Photo courtesy of the National Eye Institute, National Institutes of Health.

TABLE 58-5 Select Medications Used in the Management of Glaucoma

Medication	Action	Side Effects	Nursing Implications
Cholinergics (miotics) (pilocarpine, carbachol intraocular)	Increase aqueous fluid outflow by contracting the ciliary muscle and causing miosis (constriction of the pupil) and opening of trabecular meshwork	Periorbital pain, blurry vision, difficulty seeing in the dark	Caution patients about diminished vision in dimly lit areas. Pilocarpine can be stored at room temperature for up to 8 wks and then should be discarded.
Beta-blockers (timolol maleate)	Decrease aqueous humor production	Can have systemic effects, including bradycardia, exacerbation of pulmonary disease, and hypotension	Contraindicated in patients with asthma, chronic obstructive pulmonary disease, second- or third-degree heart block, bradycardia, or heart failure; educate patients about punctal occlusion to limit systemic effects (see Chart 58-5).
Alpha-adrenergic agonists (apraclonidine, brimonidine)	Decrease aqueous humor production	Eye redness, dry mouth and nasal passages	Educate patients about punctal occlusion to limit systemic effects (see Chart 58-5).
Carbonic anhydrase inhibitors (acetazolamide, dorzolamide)	Decrease aqueous humor production	Oral medications (acetazolamide) are associated with serious side effects, including anaphylactic reactions, electrolyte loss, depression, lethargy, gastrointestinal upset, impotence, and weight loss; side effects of topical form (dorzolamide) include topical allergy	Do not administer to patients with sulfa allergies; monitor electrolyte levels.
Prostaglandin analogues (latanoprost, bimatoprost)	Increase uveoscleral outflow	Darkening of the iris, conjunctival redness, possible rash	Instruct patients to report any side effects.

Adapted from Comerford, K. C., & Durkin, M. T. (2020). *Nursing 2020 drug handbook.* Philadelphia, PA: Wolters Kluwer.

patients with elevated IOP and those with low-tension glaucoma with progressive visual field loss is typically set at 30% lower than the current pressure. The patient is monitored for changes in the appearance of the optic nerve. If there is evidence of progressive damage, the target IOP is again lowered until the optic nerve shows stability.

Pharmacologic Therapy

Medical management of glaucoma relies on systemic and topical ocular medications that lower IOP. Periodic follow-up examinations are essential to monitor IOP, the appearance of the optic nerve, the visual fields, and side effects of medications. Therapy takes into account the patient's health and stage of glaucoma. Comfort, affordability, convenience, lifestyle, and functional ability are factors to consider in the patient's adherence to the medical regimen (Eliopoulos, 2018).

The patient is usually started on the lowest dose of topical medication and then advanced to increased concentrations until the desired IOP level is reached and maintained. Beta-blockers are the preferred initial topical medications because of their efficacy, minimal dosing (can be used once each day), and low cost. One eye is treated first, with the other eye used as a control in determining the efficacy of the medication; once efficacy has been established, treatment of the other eye is started. If the IOP is elevated in both eyes, both are treated. When results are not satisfactory, a new medication is substituted. The main markers of the efficacy of the medication in glaucoma control are lowering of the IOP to the target pressure, stable appearance of the optic nerve head, and the visual field.

Many ocular medications are used to treat glaucoma (see Table 58-5), including miotics, beta-blockers, alpha2-agonists (i.e., adrenergic agents), carbonic anhydrase inhibitors, and prostaglandins. Cholinergics (i.e., miotics) increase the outflow of the aqueous humor by affecting ciliary muscle contraction and pupil constriction, allowing flow through a larger opening between the iris and the trabecular meshwork. Beta-blockers and carbonic anhydrase inhibitors decrease aqueous production. Prostaglandin analogues reduce IOP by increasing aqueous humor outflow (Comerford & Durkin, 2020; Norris, 2019).

Surgical Management

Surgery is reserved for patients in whom pharmacologic treatment has not controlled the IOP. This minimally invasive procedure is specifically designed to improve fluid drainage from the eye to balance IOP. By restoring the eye's natural fluid balance, trabeculectomy surgery stabilizes the optic nerve and minimizes further visual field damage (Sheybani et al., 2020). The surgery is performed through a small incision and does not require creation of a permanent hole in the eye wall or an external filtering bleb or an implant.

In laser trabeculoplasty for glaucoma, a laser beam is applied to the inner surface of the trabecular meshwork to open the intratrabecular spaces and widen the canal of Schlemm, promoting outflow of aqueous humor and decreasing IOP. The procedure is indicated when IOP is inadequately controlled by medications, and it is contraindicated when the trabecular meshwork cannot be fully visualized because of a narrow angle.

In peripheral iridotomy for pupillary block glaucoma, an opening is made in the iris to eliminate the pupillary blockage. Laser iridotomy is contraindicated in patients with corneal edema, which interferes with laser targeting and strength. Potential complications include burns to the cornea, lens, or retina; transient elevated IOP; closure of the iridotomy; uveitis; and blurring.

Filtering procedures for glaucoma are used to create an opening or fistula in the trabecular meshwork to drain aqueous humor from the anterior chamber to the subconjunctival space into a bleb (fluid collection on the outside of the eye), thereby bypassing the usual drainage structures. This allows the aqueous humor to flow and exit by different routes (i.e., absorption by the conjunctival vessels or mixing with tears). Trabeculectomy is the standard filtering technique used to remove part of the trabecular meshwork (Shaw & Lee, 2017). Complications include hemorrhage, an extremely low (hypotony) or extremely elevated IOP, uveitis, cataracts, bleb failure, bleb leak, and **endophthalmitis** (i.e., intraocular infection).

Drainage implants or *shunts* are tubes implanted in the anterior chamber to shunt aqueous humor to the episcleral plate in the conjunctival space. Implants are used when failure has occurred with one or more trabeculectomies in which antifibrotic agents were used. A fibrous capsule develops around the episcleral plate and filters the aqueous humor, thereby regulating the outflow and controlling IOP.

Nursing Management

Nurses in all settings encounter patients with glaucoma. Even patients with long-standing disease and those with glaucoma as a secondary diagnosis should be assessed for knowledge level and adherence to their prescribed therapeutic regimen.

Promoting Home, Community-Based, and Transitional Care

Educating Patients About Self-Care

The medical and surgical management of glaucoma slows the progression of the disease but does not cure it. The lifelong therapeutic regimen mandates patient education. The nature of the disease and the importance of strict adherence to the medication regimen must be included in an individualized education plan. A structured self-management program may increase adherence to the treatment regime. A thorough discussion of the medication program, particularly the interactions of glaucoma-control medications with other medications, is essential. For example, the diuretic effect of acetazolamide may have an additive effect on the diuretic effects of other antihypertensive medications (Comerford & Durkin, 2020). The effects of glaucoma-control medications on vision must also be explained. Miotics and sympathomimetics result in altered focus; therefore, patients need to be cautious in navigating their surroundings. Chart 58-5 presents patient education about instilling eye medications and preventing systemic absorption with punctal occlusion. Chart 58-7 contains additional educational information to review with patients with glaucoma.

Continuing and Transitional Care

Patients with severe glaucoma and impaired function may need referral to home, community-based or transitional

---

Chart 58-7 PATIENT EDUCATION

Managing Glaucoma

The nurse instructs the patient to:

- Know your intraocular pressure measurement and the desired range.
- Be informed about the extent of your vision loss and optic nerve damage.
- Keep a record of your eye pressure measurements and visual field test results to monitor your own progress.
- Review all of your medications (including over-the-counter and herbal medications) with your ophthalmologist, and mention any side effects each time you visit.
- Ask about potential side effects and drug interactions of your eye medications.
- Ask whether generic or less costly forms of your eye medications are available.
- Review the dosing schedule with your ophthalmologist, and inform them if you have trouble following the schedule.
- Participate in the decision-making process. Let your primary provider know what dosing schedule works for you and other preferences regarding your eye care.
- Have the nurse observe you instilling eye medication to determine whether you are administering it properly (see Chart 58-5).
- Be aware that glaucoma medications can cause adverse effects if used inappropriately. Eye drops are to be given as prescribed, not when eyes feel irritated.
- Ask your ophthalmologist to send a report to your primary provider after each appointment.
- Keep all follow-up appointments.

---

services that provide assistance in the home. The loss of peripheral vision impairs mobility the most. These patients also benefit from a referral for low vision and rehabilitation services. Patients who meet the criteria for legal blindness should be offered referrals to agencies that can assist them in obtaining federal assistance.

Reassurance and emotional support are important aspects of care. A lifelong disease involving possible loss of sight has psychological, physical, social, and vocational ramifications. The family must be integrated into the plan of care, and because the disease has a familial tendency, family members should be encouraged to undergo examinations at least once every 2 years to detect glaucoma early.

CATARACTS

A **cataract** is a lens opacity or cloudiness (see Fig. 58-8). Cataracts are responsible for visual disability in 18 million people worldwide (Norris, 2019). By 80 years of age, more than half of all Americans have cataracts. Cataracts are a leading cause of blindness in the world (Prevent Blindness America, 2020).

Pathophysiology

Cataracts can develop in one or both eyes at any age. The three most common types are traumatic, congenital, or senile cataract (Norris, 2019). There are a variety of risk factors, the most common one being age (see Chart 58-8).

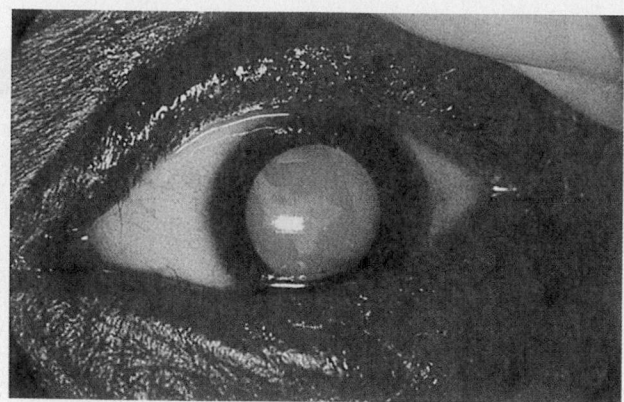

Figure 58-8 • A cataract is a cloudy or opaque lens. On visual inspection, the lens appears gray or milky. Reprinted with permission from Strayer, D. S., Rubin, E., Saffitz, J. E., et al. (2015). *Rubin's pathology: Clinicopathologic foundations of medicine* (7th ed., Fig. 33.2). Philadelphia, PA: Wolters Kluwer.

Clinical Manifestations

Painless, blurry vision is characteristic of cataracts. The person perceives that surroundings are dimmer, as if their glasses need cleaning. Light scattering is common, and the person experiences reduced contrast sensitivity, sensitivity to glare, and reduced visual acuity. Other effects include myopic shift (return of ability to do close work [e.g., reading fine print] without eyeglasses), **astigmatism** (refractive error due to an irregularity in the curvature of the cornea), monocular **diplopia** (double vision), and color changes as lens becomes more brown in color (Eliopoulos, 2018; Shaw & Lee, 2017).

Assessment and Diagnostic Findings

Decreased visual acuity is directly proportionate to cataract density. The Snellen visual acuity test, ophthalmoscopy, and slit-lamp biomicroscopic examination are used to establish the degree of cataract formation. The degree of lens opacity does not always correlate with the patient's functional status. Some patients can perform normal activities despite clinically significant cataracts. Others with less lens opacification have a disproportionate decrease in visual acuity; hence, visual acuity is an imperfect measure of visual impairment.

Medical Management

No nonsurgical treatment (e.g., medications, eye drops, eyeglasses) cures cataracts or prevents age-related cataracts. Optimal medical management is prevention. Patients should be educated by primary providers about risk reduction strategies such as smoking cessation, weight reduction, optimal blood glucose control for patients with diabetes, and should be advised to wear sunglasses outdoors to prevent early cataract formation (Shaw & Lee, 2017).

Surgical Management

In general, if reduced vision from cataract does not interfere with normal activities, surgery may not be needed. In deciding when cataract surgery is to be performed, the patient's functional and visual status should be a primary consideration (Eliopoulos, 2018). Cataract removal is common, with more than one million such surgeries performed in the United

---

Chart 58-8 ⚠ RISK FACTORS
Cataract Formation

Aging

- Accumulation of a yellow-brown pigment due to the breakdown of lens protein
- Clumping or aggregation of lens protein (which leads to light scattering)
- Decreased oxygen uptake
- Decrease in levels of vitamin C, protein, and glutathione (an antioxidant)
- Increase in sodium and calcium
- Loss of lens transparency

Associated Ocular Conditions

- Infection (e.g., herpes zoster, uveitis)
- Myopia
- Retinal detachment and retinal surgery
- Retinitis pigmentosa

Toxic Factors

- Alkaline chemical eye burns, poisoning
- Aspirin use
- Calcium, copper, iron, gold, silver, and mercury, which tend to deposit in the pupillary area of the lens
- Cigarette smoking
- Corticosteroids, especially at high doses and in long-term use
- Ionizing radiation

Nutritional Factors

- Obesity
- Poor nutrition
- Reduced levels of antioxidants

Physical Factors

- Blunt trauma, perforation of the lens with a sharp object or foreign body, electric shock
- Dehydration associated with chronic diarrhea, the use of purgatives in anorexia nervosa, and the use of hyperbaric oxygenation
- Ultraviolet radiation in sunlight and x-ray

Systemic Diseases and Syndromes

- Diabetes
- Disorders related to lipid metabolism
- Down syndrome
- Musculoskeletal disorders
- Renal disorders

Adapted from Norris, T. (2019). *Porth's pathophysiology: Concepts of altered health status* (10th ed.). Philadelphia, PA: Wolters Kluwer; Prevent Blindness. (2020). Know the risk factors for cataract. Retrieved on 2/16/2020 at: www.preventblindness.org/know-risk-factors-cataract

---

States each year (Prevent Blindness America, 2020). Surgery is performed on an outpatient basis and usually takes less than 1 hour, with the patient being discharged in 30 minutes or less afterward. Although complications from cataract surgery are uncommon, they can have significant effects on vision (see Table 58-6). Restoration of visual function through a safe and minimally invasive procedure is the surgical goal, which is achieved with advances in topical anesthesia, smaller wound incision (i.e., clear cornea incision), and lens

TABLE 58-6	Potential Complications of Cataract Surgery	
Complication	**Effects**	**Management and Outcome**
Immediate Preoperative Retrobulbar hemorrhage—can result from retrobulbar infiltration of anesthetic agents if the short ciliary artery is located by the injectia	Increased IOP, proptosis, lid tightness, and subconjunctival hemorrhage with or without edema	Emergent lateral canthotomy (slitting of the canthus) is performed to stop central retinal perfusion when the IOP is dangerously elevated. If this procedure fails to reduce IOP, a puncture of the anterior chamber with removal of fluid is considered. The patient must be closely monitored for at least a few hours. Postponement of cataract surgery for 2–4 wks is advised. Complications such as iris prolapse, vitreous loss, and choroidal hemorrhage could result in a catastrophic visual outcome.
Intraoperative Rupture of the posterior capsule Suprachoroidal (expulsive) hemorrhage—profuse bleeding into the suprachoroidal space	May result in loss of vitreous Extrusion of intraocular contents from the eye or opposition of retinal surfaces	Anterior vitrectomy is required if vitreous loss occurs. Closure of the incision and administration of a hyperosmotic agent to reduce IOP or corticosteroids to reduce intraocular inflammation. Vitrectomy is performed 1–2 wks later. Visual prognosis is poor; some useful vision may be salvaged on rare occasions.
Early Postoperative Acute bacterial endophthalmitis—devastating complication that occurs in about 1 in 1000 cases; the most common causative organisms are *Staphylococcus epidermidis*, *Staphylococcus aureus*, *Pseudomonas*, and *Proteus* species	Characterized by marked visual loss, pain, lid edema, hypopyon, corneal haze, and chemosis	Managed by aggressive antibiotic therapy. Broad-spectrum antibiotics are given while awaiting culture and sensitivity results. Once results are obtained, the appropriate antibiotics are given via intravitreal injection. Corticosteroid therapy is also given.
Toxic anterior segment syndrome—noninfectious inflammation that is a complication of anterior chamber surgery; caused by a toxic agent such as an agent used to sterilize surgical instruments	Corneal edema occurs <24 h after surgery; symptoms include reduced visual acuity and pain	If there is no growth of microorganisms, the treatment is topical steroids alone.
Late Postoperative Suture-related problems	Toxic reactions or mechanical injury from broken or loose sutures	Suture removal relieves the symptoms. Topical corticosteroids are used when the incision is not healed and sutures cannot be removed.
Malposition of the IOL	Results in astigmatism, sensitivity to glare, or appearance of halos	Miotics are used for mild cases, whereas IOL removal and replacement is necessary for severe cases.
Chronic endophthalmitis	Persistent, low-grade inflammation, and granuloma	Corticosteroids and antibiotics are given systemically. If the condition persists, removal of the IOL and capsular bag, vitrectomy, and intravitreal injection of antibiotics are required.
Opacification of the posterior capsule—most common late complication of extracapsular cataract extraction	Visual acuity is diminished	Nd:YAG laser is used to create a hole in the posterior capsule. Blurred vision is cleared immediately.

IOL, intraocular lens; IOP, intraocular pressure; Nd:YAG, Neodymium: yttrium aluminum garnet.
Adapted from Shaw, M., & Lee, A. (2017). *Ophthalmic nursing* (5th ed.). Boca Raton, FL: CRC Press Taylor & Francis Group.

design (i.e., foldable and more accurate intraocular lens [IOL] measurements).

Injection-free topical and intraocular anesthesia, such as 1% lidocaine gel applied to the surface of the eye, eliminates the hazards of regional (retrobulbar and peribulbar) anesthesia, such as ocular perforation, retrobulbar hemorrhage, optic injuries, diplopia, and ptosis, and is ideal for patients receiving anticoagulants. Furthermore, patients can communicate and cooperate during surgery. IV sedation may be used to minimize anxiety and discomfort.

When both eyes have cataracts, one eye is treated first, with at least several weeks, preferably months, separating the two procedures. Because cataract surgery is performed to improve visual functioning, the delay for the other eye gives time for the patient and the surgeon to evaluate whether the results from the first surgery are adequate to preclude the need for a second operation. The delay also provides time for the first eye to recover; if there are any complications, the surgeon may decide to perform the second procedure differently.

Phacoemulsification

In this method of extracapsular cataract surgery, a portion of the anterior capsule is removed, allowing extraction of the lens nucleus and cortex while the posterior capsule and zonular support are left intact. An ultrasonic device is used to liquefy the nucleus and cortex, which are then suctioned out through a tube. An intact zonular–capsular diaphragm provides the needed safe anchor for the posterior chamber IOL. The pupil is dilated to 7 mm or greater (Shaw & Lee, 2017). The surgeon makes a small incision on the upper edge of the cornea and a viscoelastic substance (clear gel) is injected into the space between the cornea and the lens. This prevents the space from collapsing and facilitates insertion of the IOL. Because the incision is smaller than the manual extracapsular cataract extraction, the wound heals more rapidly, and there is early stabilization of refractive error and less astigmatism.

Lens Replacement

After removal of the crystalline lens, the patient is referred to as aphakic (i.e., without lens). The lens, which focuses light on the retina, must be replaced for the patient to see clearly. There are three lens replacement options: aphakic eyeglasses, contact lenses, and IOL implants.

Aphakic glasses, although effective, are rarely used. Objects are magnified by 25%, making them appear closer than they actually are. This magnification creates distortion. Peripheral vision is also limited, and **binocular vision** (i.e., ability of both eyes to focus on one object and fuse the two images into one) is impossible if the other eye is aphakic (without a natural lens).

Contact lenses provide patients with almost normal vision, but because contact lenses need to be removed occasionally, the patient also needs a pair of aphakic glasses. Contact lenses are not advised for patients who have difficulty inserting, removing, and cleaning them. Frequent handling and improper disinfection increase the risk of infection.

Insertion of IOLs during cataract surgery is the most common approach to lens replacement (Eliopoulos, 2018). After cataract extraction, or phacoemulsification, the surgeon implants an IOL. Cataract extraction and posterior chamber IOLs are associated with a relatively low incidence of complications (e.g., eye infection, loss of vitreous humor, slipping of the implant) (Eliopoulos, 2018). IOL implantation is contraindicated in patients with recurrent uveitis, proliferative diabetic retinopathy, neovascular glaucoma, or rubeosis iridis.

Nursing Management

Providing Preoperative Care

The patient with cataracts receives the usual preoperative care for ambulatory surgical patients undergoing eye surgery. The standard battery of preoperative tests (e.g., complete blood count, electrocardiogram, urinalysis) commonly performed for most surgeries is prescribed only if indicated by the patient's medical history.

Alpha-antagonists (particularly tamsulosin, which is used for treatment of enlarged prostate) are known to cause a condition called *intraoperative floppy iris syndrome*. Alpha-antagonists can interfere with pupil dilation during the surgical procedure, resulting in miosis and iris prolapse and leading to complications. Intraoperative floppy iris syndrome can occur even though a patient has stopped taking the drug. The nurse needs to ask patients about a history of taking alpha-antagonists. Surgical team members are then alerted to the risk of this complication (Comerford & Durkin, 2020).

Dilating drops are given prior to surgery. Nurses in the ambulatory surgery setting begin patient education about eye medications (antibiotic, corticosteroid, and anti-inflammatory drops) that will need to be self-administered to prevent postoperative infection and inflammation.

Providing Postoperative Care

Before discharge, the patient receives verbal and written education regarding eye protection, administration of medications, recognition of complications, activities to avoid, and obtaining emergency care (see Chart 58-9). An eye shield is usually worn at night for the first week to avoid injury. The nurse also explains that there should be minimal discomfort after surgery and educates the patient about taking a mild analgesic agent, such as acetaminophen, as needed. Antibiotic, anti-inflammatory, and corticosteroid eye drops or ointments are prescribed postoperatively. Patients prescribed

---

Chart 58-9 HOME CARE CHECKLIST

Intraocular Lens Implant

At the completion of education, the patient and/or caregiver will be able to:

- Name the procedure that was performed and identify any permanent changes in anatomic structure or function as well as changes in ADLs, IADLs, roles, relationships, and spirituality.
- State the name, dose, side effects, frequency, and schedule for all medications.
- Describe ongoing postoperative therapeutic regimen and activities to limit or avoid (e.g., lifting weights, driving a car, engaging in contact sports).
  - Wear glasses or eye shield following surgery as instructed.
  - Always wash hands before touching or cleaning the postoperative eye.
  - Clean postoperative eye with a clean tissue; wipe the closed eye with a single gesture from the inner canthus outward.
  - When bathing or showering, shampoo hair cautiously or seek assistance.
  - Avoid lying on the side of the affected eye the night after surgery.

- Keep activity light (e.g., walking, reading, watching television). Resume the following activities only as directed by the ophthalmologist: driving, sexual activity, unusually strenuous activity.
- Avoid lifting, pushing, or pulling objects heavier than 15 lb.
- Avoid bending or stooping for an extended period.
- Be careful when climbing or descending stairs.
- Describe signs and symptoms of complications (e.g., vision change, continuous flashing lights appear to the affected eye, redness, swelling or increased pain near the eye, change in amount or type of eye drainage, any eye injury, significant pain not relieved by prescribed analgesia).
- Relate how to reach ophthalmologist with questions or complications.
- State time and date of follow-up appointments.
- Identify sources of assistance (e.g., meals, transportation) and support (e.g., friends, relatives, faith community).
- Identify the need for health promotion, disease prevention, and screening activities

ADLs, activities of daily living; IADLs, instrumental activities of daily living.

anti-inflammatory or corticosteroid eye drops are monitored for possible increases in IOP (Phulke, Kaushik, Kaur, et al., 2017).

Promoting Home, Community-Based, and Transitional Care

 Educating Patients About Self-Care

To prevent inadvertent rubbing or poking of the eye, the patient wears a protective eye patch for about the first 24 hours after surgery, followed by eyeglasses worn during the day and an eye shield at night. The nurse educates the patient and family about applying and caring for the eye shield, if one is recommended. Sunglasses should be worn while outdoors during the day because the eye is sensitive to light.

Slight morning discharge, some redness, and a scratchy feeling may be expected for a few days. A clean, damp washcloth may be used to remove slight morning eye discharge. Because cataract surgery increases the risk of retinal detachment, the patient must know to notify the surgeon if new floaters (moving dots) in vision, flashing lights, decrease in vision, pain, or increase in redness occur.

Continuing and Transitional Care

If an eye patch is worn, it is removed after the first follow-up appointment, which should occur within 48 hours of surgery. Nurses should educate patients about the importance of keeping their follow-up appointments, because monitoring of visual status and prompt intervention of postoperative complications enhance good visual outcome. Vision is stabilized when the eye is completely healed, usually within 6 to 12 weeks, when final corrective prescription is completed. Visual correction may still be needed for any remaining refractive errors. Patients who choose multifocal IOLs should be aware that increased night glare and contrast sensitivity may occur.

CORNEAL DISORDERS

Corneal Dystrophies

Corneal dystrophies are inherited as autosomal dominant traits and manifest when the person is about 20 years of age. They are characterized by deposits in the corneal layers. Decreased vision is caused by the irregular corneal surface and corneal deposits. Corneal endothelial decomposition leads to corneal edema and blurring of vision. Persistent edema leads to bullous keratopathy or the formation of blisters that cause pain and discomfort on rupturing. The two main types are keratoconus and Fuchs endothelial dystrophy.

Keratoconus

Keratoconus, the most common type of corneal dystrophy, is characterized by a conical protuberance of the cornea with progressive thinning on protrusion and irregular astigmatism. This hereditary condition has a higher incidence among women. Onset occurs at puberty; the condition may progress for more than 20 years and is bilateral. Corneal scarring occurs in severe cases. Blurred vision is a prominent symptom. Rigid, gas-permeable contact lenses correct irregular astigmatism

and improve vision. Advances in contact lens design have reduced the need for surgery. Penetrating keratoplasty (PKP) is indicated when contact lens correction is no longer effective (Allard & Zetterberg, 2018).

Fuchs Endothelial Dystrophy

Fuchs (pronounced *Fooks*) dystrophy is manifested by a slow death of cells in the endothelial cornea. It affects women more than men and is usually not noted until 50 years of age. Corneal endothelial cell death leads to corneal edema and blurring of vision. Persistent edema leads to bullous keratopathy. A bandage contact lens is used to flatten the bullae, protect the exposed corneal nerve endings, and relieve discomfort. Symptomatic treatments, such as hypertonic drops or ointment (5% sodium chloride), may reduce epithelial edema. Currently, the only cure is a corneal transplant (Moshirfar, Ding, & Shah, 2018).

Corneal Surgeries

Among the surgical procedures used to treat diseased corneal tissue are phototherapeutic keratectomy (PTK), PKP and corneal endothelial transplantation, and Descemet's stripping endothelial keratoplasty (DSEK).

Phototherapeutic Keratectomy

PTK is a laser procedure that is used to treat diseased corneal tissue by removing or reducing corneal opacities and smoothing the anterior corneal surface to improve functional vision. PTK is contraindicated in patients with active herpetic keratitis because the ultraviolet rays may reactivate latent virus. Common side effects are induced hyperopia and stromal haze. Complications are delayed re-epithelialization (particularly in patients with diabetes) and bacterial keratitis. Postoperative management consists of oral analgesic agents for eye pain. Re-epithelialization is promoted with a pressure patch or therapeutic soft contact lens. Antibiotic and corticosteroid ointments and NSAIDs are prescribed postoperatively. Follow-up examinations are required for up to 2 years.

Penetrating Keratoplasty

PKP (corneal transplantation or corneal grafting) involves replacing abnormal host tissue with healthy donor (cadaver) corneal tissue. Common indications are keratoconus, corneal scarring from herpes simplex, keratitis, and chemical burns.

Several factors affect the success of the graft: the condition of the ocular structures (e.g., lids, conjunctiva), quality of the tears, adequacy of blinking, and viability of the donor endothelium. Contraindications for the use of donor tissue are outlined in Chart 58-10.

In PKP, the surgeon determines the graft size before the procedure, and the appropriate size is marked on the surface of the cornea. The surgeon prepares the donor cornea and the recipient bed, removes the diseased cornea, places the donor cornea on the recipient bed, and sutures it in place. Sutures remain in place for 12 to 18 months and are then removed. Potential complications include early graft failure due to poor quality of donor tissue, surgical trauma, acute infection, and persistently increased IOP and late graft failure due to rejection.

<table>
<tr><td>

Chart 58-10

Contraindications to the Use of Donor Tissue for Corneal Transplantation: Donor Characteristics

Systemic Disorders

- Death from unknown cause
- History or suspected history of the following:
  - Acquired immune deficiency syndrome or high risk for human immune deficiency virus infection
  - Creutzfeldt–Jakob disease
  - Eye infection
  - Hepatitis
  - Rabies
  - Systemic infection

Intrinsic Eye Disease

- Disorders of the conjunctiva or corneal surface involving the optical zone of the cornea
- Malignant tumors of anterior segment
- Ocular inflammation
- Retinoblastoma

Other

- Corneal scars
- History of eye trauma
- Previous surgical eye procedures such as corneal graft or LASIK eye surgery

</td></tr>
</table>

Postoperatively, the patient receives mydriatics for 2 weeks and topical corticosteroids for 12 months (daily doses for 6 months and tapered doses thereafter). These mydriatics and corticosteroid drops should be preservative free to prevent a reactive inflammation. Patients typically describe a sensation of postoperative eye discomfort rather than acute pain.

Additional Keratoplasty Surgeries

For many years, PKP was the standard of care for patients with corneal endothelial failure but with poor refractive results. Subsequently, other techniques have been developed. Anterior lamellar keratoplasty (ALK) involves a partial-thickness graft for disorders such as anterior corneal dystrophies or scarring not involving the endothelial portion of the cornea. Deep anterior lamellar keratoplasty (DALK) involves replacement of only anterior corneal layers and not Descemet's membrane or endothelial layers for disorders such as keratoconus. Posterior lamellar keratoplasty (PLK or EK) and DSEK (which replaces only the endothelial layer of the cornea) are procedures indicated for conditions such as Fuchs endothelial dystrophy or bullous keratopathy (Moshirfar et al., 2018). In DSEK, layers of the cornea are dissected and selectively replaced by donor cornea tissue. DSEK offers several advantages, such as less postoperative astigmatism, faster visual recovery, and stronger wound integrity. Theoretically, the risk of rejection is less because less of the patient's tissue is replaced.

Keratoprosthesis

An additional therapeutic option for patients with multiple graft failures or severe corneal disease is keratoprosthesis (artificial cornea; e.g., U.S. Food and Drug Administration [FDA]-approved Boston Keratoprosthesis [KPro] and Alpha-Cor). The design of the keratoprosthesis consists of a central optic core and an outer rim that secures the prosthesis. This procedure has serious potential complications (e.g., glaucoma, endophthalmitis) and requires close follow-up and monitoring (Shalaby Bardan, Al Raqqad, Zarei-Ghanavati, et al., 2018).

Nursing Management

For corneal surgeries, the nurse reinforces instructions regarding visual rehabilitation and visual improvement. A technically successful graft may initially produce disappointing results because the procedure has produced a new optical surface. Only after several months do patients start seeing the natural and true colors of their environment. Correction of a resultant refractive error with eyeglasses or contact lenses determines the final visual outcome. The nurse assesses the patient's support system and their ability to comply with long-term follow-up, which includes frequent clinic visits for several months for tapering of topical corticosteroid therapy, selective suture removal, and ongoing evaluation of the graft site and visual acuity. The nurse also initiates appropriate referrals to community services as indicated.

Because graft failure is an ophthalmic emergency that can occur at any time, the primary goal of nursing care is to educate the patient to identify signs and symptoms of graft failure. The early symptoms are blurred vision, discomfort, tearing, or redness of the eye. Decreased vision results after graft destruction. The patient must contact the ophthalmologist as soon as symptoms occur. Treatment of graft rejection usually involves prompt administration of hourly topical corticosteroids and periocular corticosteroid injections. Systemic immunosuppressive agents may be necessary for severe, resistant cases.

Refractive Surgeries

Refractive surgeries are elective procedures performed to correct refractive errors (myopia or hyperopia) and astigmatism by reshaping the cornea (Gomel, Negari, Frucht-Pery, et al., 2018). Laser vision correction alters the major optical function of the eye and carries risks. Refractive surgery does not alter the normal aging process of the eye. If the reason for the procedure is to meet vision requirements for the patient's occupation, the results must satisfy both the patient and the employer. Precise visual outcome cannot be guaranteed.

The corneal structure must be normal, and the refractive error must be stable. The patient is required to discontinue using contact lenses for a period before the procedure (2 to 3 weeks for soft lenses and 4 weeks for hard lenses). Patients with conditions that are likely to adversely affect corneal wound healing (e.g., corticosteroid use, immunosuppression, elevated IOP) are not good candidates for the procedure. Any superficial eye disease must be diagnosed and fully treated before a refractive procedure.

Patient satisfaction is the ultimate goal; therefore, patient education and counseling about potential risks, complications, and postoperative follow-up are critical. Minimal postoperative care includes topical corticosteroid or NSAID and antibiotic drops.

Laser Vision Correction Photorefractive Keratectomy

Photorefractive keratectomy (PRK) is used to treat myopia and hyperopia with or without astigmatism (Gomel et al., 2018). The excimer laser is applied directly to the cornea according to carefully calculated measurements. For myopia, the relative curvature is decreased; for hyperopia, the relative curvature is increased. A bandage contact lens is placed over the cornea to promote epithelial healing and reduce pain, which is similar to that of a severe corneal abrasion.

Laser-Assisted In Situ Keratomileusis

LASIK involves flattening the anterior curvature of the cornea by removing a stromal lamella or layer. The surgeon creates a corneal flap with a microkeratome, which is an automatic corneal shaper. The surgeon retracts a flap of corneal tissue less than one third the thickness of a human hair to access the corneal stroma and then uses the excimer laser on the stromal bed to reshape the cornea according to calculated measurements (see Fig. 58-9). Data are insufficient to determine whether LASIK or PRK is better at correcting nearsightedness (Gomel et al., 2018). There are few adverse outcomes of either procedure.

Perioperative Complications

Surgically Induced Abnormalities

Corneal surface irregularities can occur after LASIK treatment. These include central islands (central areas of stiffness or elevation), decentered ablations resulting from misalignment of the laser treatment or from involuntary eye movement during laser treatment, and forms of irregular astigmatism. Symptoms of central islands and decentered ablations include monocular diplopia or ghost images, halos, glare, and decreased visual acuity.

Phakic Intraocular Lenses

Increasingly, phakic IOL implantation has been used for patients with moderate to severe myopia (Igarashi, 2019). Phakic IOLs may be used in either the anterior or posterior chamber. The implantation of such devices is reversible because the natural lens is left in place and the normal architecture of the cornea is preserved. This procedure provides more predictable refractive results than procedures that alter the corneal curvature, is safer, and has higher patient satisfaction scores (Igarashi, 2019). Potential complications include cataract, iritis or uveitis, endothelial cell loss, and increased IOP.

Conductive Keratoplasty

Another innovation in refractive surgery for the correction of low to mild hyperopia uses the principles of thermal keratoplasty by applying radiofrequency current to the peripheral cornea using a thin, handheld probe. It does not involve the removal of cornea tissue.

RETINAL DISORDERS

Although the retina is composed of multiple microscopic layers, the two innermost layers—the sensory retina and the retinal pigment epithelium—are most commonly implicated in retinal disorders (Norris, 2019).

Retinal Detachment

Retinal detachment refers to the separation of the retinal pigment epithelium from the neurosensory layer (Norris, 2019). The four types of retinal detachment are rhegmatogenous, traction, a combination of rhegmatogenous and traction, and exudative. *Rhegmatogenous retinal detachment* is the most common form (Liao & Zhu, 2019). In this condition, a hole or tear develops in the sensory retina, allowing some of the liquid vitreous to seep through the sensory retina and detach it from the retinal pigment epithelium (see Fig. 58-10). People at risk for this type of detachment include those with high myopia or those who have aphakia (absence of the natural lens) after cataract surgery. Trauma may also play a role in rhegmatogenous retinal detachment. Between 5% and 10% of all rhegmatogenous retinal detachments are associated with proliferative retinopathy—a retinopathy associated with diabetic neovascularization (see Chapter 46).

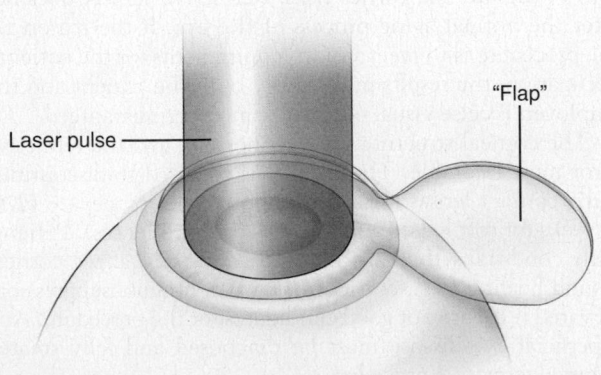

Figure 58-9 • LASIK combines delicate surgical procedures and laser treatment. A flap is surgically created and lifted to one side. A laser is then applied to the cornea to reshape it. With permission from the Wilmer Laser Vision Center, Lutherville, MD.

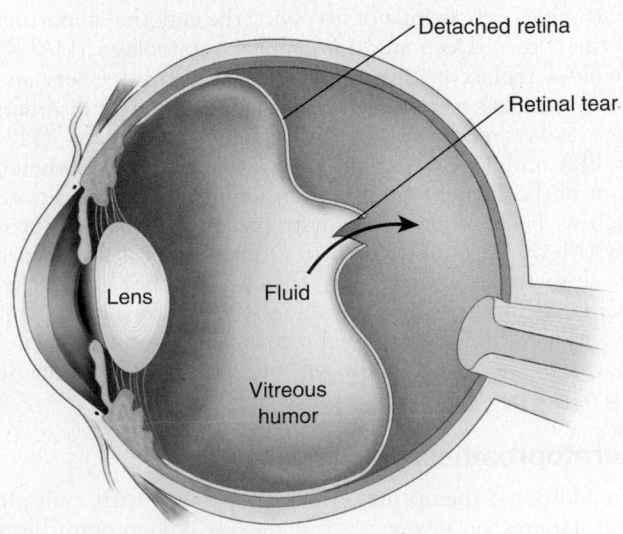

Figure 58-10 • Retinal detachment.

Tension, or a pulling force, is responsible for *traction retinal detachment*. An ophthalmologist must ascertain all of the areas of retinal break and identify and release the scars or bands of fibrous material providing traction on the retina. In general, patients with this condition have developed fibrous scar tissue from conditions such as diabetic retinopathy, vitreous hemorrhage, or the retinopathy of prematurity. The hemorrhages and fibrous proliferation associated with these conditions exert a pulling force on the delicate retina.

Patients can have both rhegmatogenous and traction retinal detachment. *Exudative retinal detachments* are the result of the production of a serous fluid under the retina from the choroid. Conditions such as uveitis and macular degeneration may cause the production of this serous fluid.

Clinical Manifestations

Patients may report the sensation of a shade or curtain coming across the vision of one eye, cobwebs, bright flashing lights, or the sudden onset of a great number of floaters. Patients do not complain of pain but retinal detachment is an ocular emergency, requiring immediate surgical intervention for optimal outcomes.

Assessment and Diagnostic Findings

After visual acuity is determined, the patient must have a dilated fundus examination using an indirect ophthalmoscope as well as slit-lamp biomicroscopy. Stereo fundus photography and fluorescein angiography are commonly used during the evaluation.

Increasingly, optical coherence tomography and ultrasound are used for the complete retinal assessment, especially if the view is obscured by a dense cataract or vitreal hemorrhage. All retinal breaks, all fibrous bands that may be causing traction on the retina, and all degenerative changes must be identified.

Surgical Management

In rhegmatogenous retinal detachment, an attempt is made to surgically reattach the sensory retina to the retinal pigment epithelium. In traction retinal detachment, the source of traction must be removed and the sensory retina reattached. The most commonly used surgical interventions are the scleral buckle and vitrectomy (Park, Lee, & Lee, 2018).

Scleral Buckle

The retinal surgeon compresses the sclera (often with a scleral buckle [see Fig. 58-11] or a silicone band) to indent the scleral wall from the outside of the eye and bring the two retinal layers in contact with each other (Park et al., 2018).

Vitrectomy

A vitrectomy is an intraocular procedure that allows the introduction of a light source through an incision; a second incision serves as the portal for the vitrectomy instrument. The surgeon dissects preretinal membranes under direct visualization while the retina is stabilized by an intraoperative vitreous substitute.

Traction on the retina may be relieved through vitrectomy and may be combined with scleral buckling to repair retinal detachments. A gas bubble, silicone oil, or perfluorocarbon and liquids may be injected into the vitreous cavity to help push the sensory retina up against the retinal pigment epithelium.

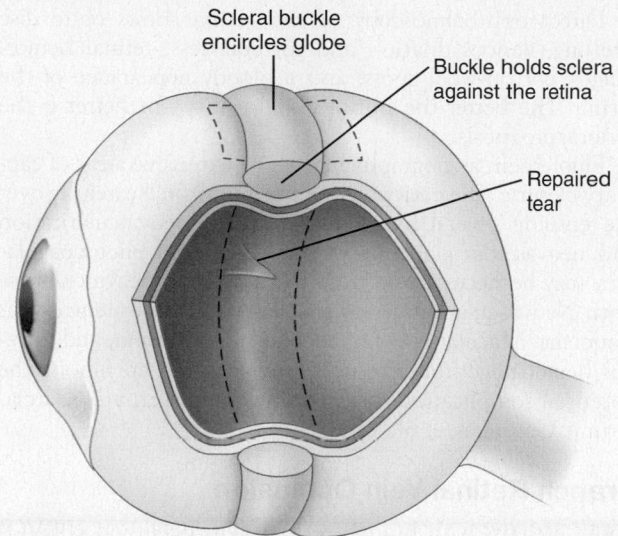

Figure 58-11 • Scleral buckle.

Nursing Management

Nursing management consists of educating the patient and providing supportive care. Postoperative positioning of the patient is critical when a gas bubble is used because the injected bubble must remain in position overlying the area of detachment, providing consistent pressure to reattach the sensory retina. The patient must maintain a prone position that would allow the gas bubble to act as a tamponade for the retinal break (Shaw & Lee, 2017). Patients and family members should be made aware of these needs beforehand so that the patient can be made as comfortable as possible.

In most cases, vitreoretinal procedures are performed on an outpatient basis, and the patient is seen the next day for a follow-up examination. Postoperative complications may include increased IOP, endophthalmitis, retinal detachment, and development of cataracts. Patients must be educated about the signs and symptoms of complications, particularly of increasing IOP and postoperative infection. Contact details for the ophthalmic team are provided and the patient is encouraged to call immediately if complications occur.

Retinal Vascular Disorders

Loss of vision can occur from occlusion of a retinal artery or vein. Such occlusions may result from atherosclerosis, valvular heart disease, venous stasis, hypertension, or increased blood viscosity. Associated risk factors include diabetes, glaucoma, and aging.

Central Retinal Vein Occlusion

Blood supply to and from the ocular fundus is provided by the central retinal artery and vein. Central retinal vein occlusions (CRVOs) are found most often in people older than 50 years. Patients who suffer a CRVO report decreased visual acuity ranging from mild blurring to severely limited.

Direct ophthalmoscopy of the retina shows optic disc swelling, venous dilation and tortuousness, retinal hemorrhages, cotton-wool spots, and a bloody appearance of the retina. The better the initial visual acuity, the better is the general prognosis.

Fluorescein angiography may show extensive areas of capillary closure. The patient should be monitored carefully over the ensuing several months for signs of neovascularization and neovascular glaucoma. Laser panretinal photocoagulation may be necessary to treat the abnormal neovascularization. Neovascularization of the iris may cause neovascular glaucoma. Macular edema, macular nonperfusion, and vitreous hemorrhage from the neovascularization are among the potential complications of CRVO (Schmidt-Erfurth, Garcia-Arumi, Gerendas, et al., 2019).

Branch Retinal Vein Occlusion

Some patients with branch retinal vein occlusion (BRVO) are symptom free, whereas others complain of a sudden loss of vision if the macular area is involved. A more gradual loss of vision may occur if macular edema associated with BRVO develops.

On examination, the ocular fundus appears similar to that found in CRVO. The occlusions generally occur at the arteriovenous crossings. The diagnostic evaluation and follow-up assessments and complications are the same as for CRVO. Associated conditions include glaucoma, systemic hypertension, diabetes, and hyperlipidemia (Schmidt-Erfurth et al., 2019).

Central Retinal Artery Occlusion

Patients with central retinal artery occlusion, a relatively rare disorder that accounts for approximately 1 in 10,000 ophthalmologic visits, present with a sudden loss of vision. Visual acuity is reduced to being able to count the examiner's fingers, or the field of vision is tremendously restricted. A relative afferent pupillary defect is present. Examination of the ocular fundus reveals a pale retina with a cherry-red spot at the fovea. The retinal arteries are thin, and emboli are occasionally seen in the central retinal artery or its branches. Central retinal artery occlusion is a true ocular emergency. Various treatments may include ocular massage, anterior chamber paracentesis, hyperbaric oxygen therapy, topical ocular hypotensive agents, anticoagulation, and intravenous mannitol and acetazolamide. An aggressive stepwise approach may be beneficial, depending on the underlying cause of the occlusion and the amount of time from onset of occlusion to treatment. Most visual loss associated with central retinal artery occlusion is severe and permanent (Schmidt-Erfurth et al., 2019).

Age-Related Macular Degeneration

AMD is the leading cause of irreversible blindness and visual impairment in the world (Bright Focus Foundation, 2020a). AMD is characterized by drusen beneath the retina (see Fig. 58-12). Most people older than 60 years have at least a few small drusen, which are clusters of debris or waste material. When drusen are located in the macular area, they can affect vision. Patients with AMD have a wide range of visual loss,

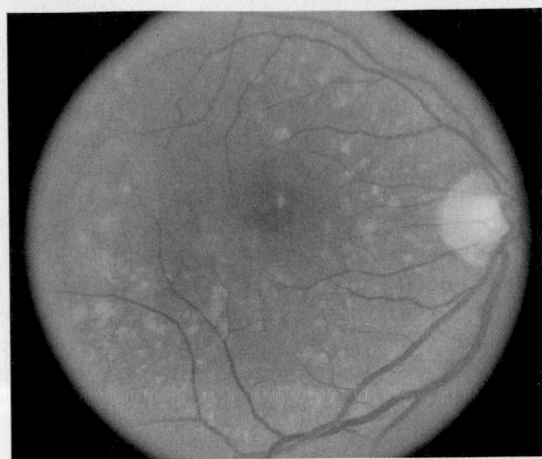

Figure 58-12 • Retina showing drusen and age-related macular degeneration.

but only a small portion experience total blindness. Central vision is generally the most affected, with most patients retaining peripheral vision (see Fig. 58-13). There are two types of AMD: the dry type and the wet type (Bright Focus Foundation, 2020a).

Between 85% and 90% of people with AMD have the dry (nonneovascular, nonexudative) type of the condition, in which the outer layers of the retina slowly break down. With this breakdown comes the appearance of drusen. When the drusen occur outside of the macular area, patients generally have no symptoms. When the drusen occur within the macula, however, there is a gradual blurring of vision that patients may notice when they try to read.

The second type of AMD, the wet (neovascular, exudative) type, may have an abrupt onset and is more damaging to the vision (Bright Focus Foundation, 2020a). Patients report that straight lines appear crooked and distorted or that letters in words appear broken. This effect results from proliferation of abnormal blood vessels growing under the retina, within the choroid layer of the eye, a condition known as choroidal neovascularization. The affected vessels can leak fluid and blood, elevating the retina. Some patients can be treated with laser therapy to stop leakage from these vessels.

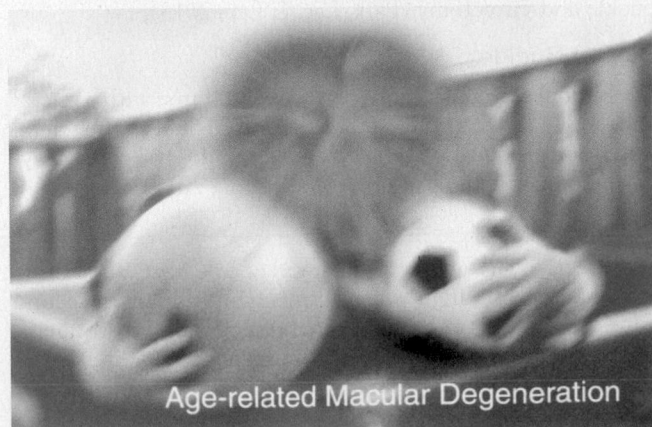

Age-related Macular Degeneration

Figure 58-13 • Visual changes resulting from age-related macular degeneration. Photo courtesy of the National Eye Institute, National Institutes of Health.

Chart 58-11	**PATIENT EDUCATION**
	Education for Patients About Preventing Eye Injuries

The nurse instructs the patient in the following measures to prevent eye injuries:

In and Around the House

- Make sure that all spray nozzles are directed away from yourself before pressing down on the handle.
- Read instructions carefully before using cleaning fluids, detergents, ammonia, or harsh chemicals, and wash hands thoroughly after use.
- Use grease shields on frying pans to decrease spattering.
- Use opaque goggles to avoid burns from sunlamps.
- Wear special goggles to shield the eyes from fumes and splashes when using powerful chemicals.

In the Workshop

- Protect the eyes from flying fragments, fumes, dust particles, sparks, and splashed chemicals by wearing safety glasses.
- Read instructions thoroughly before using tools and chemicals, and follow precautions for their use.

Around Children

- Educate children about the correct way to handle potentially dangerous items, such as scissors and pencils.
- Pay attention to age and maturity level of a child when selecting toys and games, and avoid projectile toys, such as darts and pellet guns.
- Supervise children when they are playing with toys or games that can be dangerous.

In the Garden

- Avoid letting anyone stand at the side of or in front of a moving lawn mower.

- Avoid low-hanging branches.
- Direct pesticide spray can nozzles away from the face.
- Pick up rocks and stones before going over them with the lawn mower (stones can be hurled out of the rotary blades and rebound off curbs or walls, causing severe injury to the eye).

Around the Car

- Put out all smoking materials and matches before opening the hood of the car.
- Take standard safety precautions when using jumper cables (wear goggles; make sure the cars are not touching one another; make sure the jumper cable clamps never touch each other; never lean over the battery when attaching cables; and never attach a cable to the negative terminal of a dead battery).
- Use a flashlight, not a match or lighter, to look at the battery at night.
- Wear goggles when grinding metal or striking metal against metal while performing auto body repair.

In Sports

- Wear protective caps, helmets, or face protectors when appropriate, especially for sports such as ice hockey.
- Wear protective safety glasses, especially for sports such as racquetball, squash, tennis, baseball, and basketball.

Around Fireworks

- Avoid explosive fireworks.
- Avoid standing near others when lighting fireworks.
- Douse firework duds in water instead of attempting to relight them.
- Never allow children to ignite fireworks.
- Wear eyeglasses or safety goggles.

Medical Management

There is no known effective treatment or cure for dry advanced macular degeneration (Bright Focus Foundation, 2020a).

An important component of treatment of wet (neovascular, exudative) AMD targets development and progression of angiogenesis (abnormal blood vessel formation). Vasoproliferation in wet AMD is believed to be caused by an underlying angiogenic stimulus known as vascular endothelial growth factor (VEGF) (Bright Focus Foundation, 2020a). Examples of VEGF inhibitors given by intravitreal injection include ranibizumab and brolucizumab (Bright Focus Foundation, 2020a; Comerford & Durkin, 2020).

Nursing Management

Amsler grids are given to patients to use in their homes to monitor for a sudden onset or distortion of vision. These may provide the earliest sign that macular degeneration is getting worse. Patients should be encouraged to look at these grids, one eye at a time, several times each week with glasses on if needed for corrected near vision. If there is a change in the way the grid appears to the patient (e.g., if the lines or squares appear distorted or faded), the patient should notify the ophthalmologist immediately and should arrange to be seen promptly. There are digital versions of these grids as well that pick up abnormal changes quicker.

Orbital and Ocular Trauma

Whether affecting the eye or the orbit, trauma to the eye and surrounding structures may have devastating consequences for vision. It is preferable to prevent injury rather than treat it. Chart 58-11 details measures to prevent eye injuries.

Orbital Trauma

Injury to the orbit is usually associated with a head injury; hence, the patient's general medical condition must first be stabilized before conducting an ocular examination (Hickey & Strayer, 2020). Only then is the globe assessed for soft tissue injury. During inspection, the face is meticulously assessed for underlying fractures, which should always be suspected in cases of blunt trauma. To establish the extent of ocular injury, visual acuity is assessed as soon as possible, even if it is only a rough estimate. Soft tissue orbital injuries often result in damage to the optic nerve. Major ocular injuries indicated by a soft globe, prolapsing tissue, ruptured globe, and hemorrhage require immediate surgical attention.

Soft Tissue Injury and Hemorrhage

The signs and symptoms of soft tissue injury from blunt or penetrating trauma include tenderness, ecchymosis, lid swelling, **exophthalmos** (abnormal protrusion of the eyeball), and hemorrhage. Closed injuries lead to contusions with subconjunctival hemorrhage, commonly known as a black eye. Blood accumulates in the tissues of the conjunctiva. Hemorrhage may be caused by a soft tissue injury to the eyelid or by an underlying fracture.

Management of soft tissue hemorrhage that does not threaten vision is usually conservative and consists of thorough inspection, cleansing, and repair of wounds. Cold compresses are used in the early phase, followed by warm compresses. Hematomas that appear as swollen, fluctuating areas may be surgically drained or aspirated; if they are causing significant orbital pressure, they may be surgically evacuated.

Orbital Fractures

Orbital fractures are detected by facial x-rays. Depending on the orbital structures involved, orbital fractures can be classified as blowout, zygomatic or tripod, maxillary, midfacial, orbital apex, and orbital roof fractures. Blowout fractures result from compression of soft tissue and the sudden increase in orbital pressure when the force is transmitted to the orbital floor, which is the area of least resistance (McQuillan & Makic, 2020).

The inferior rectus and inferior oblique muscles, with their fat and fascial attachments, or the nerve that courses along the inferior oblique muscle may become entrapped, resulting in enophthalmos (inward displacement of the globe). Computed tomography (CT) scanning can identify the muscle and its auxiliary structures that are entrapped. These fractures are usually caused by the blunt force from a fist or baseball (McQuillan & Makic, 2020).

Orbital roof fractures are dangerous because of potential complications to the brain. Surgical management of these fractures requires a neurosurgeon and an ophthalmologist. The most common indications for surgical intervention are displacement of bone fragments disfiguring the normal facial contours, interference with normal binocular vision caused by extraocular muscle entrapment, interference with mastication in zygomatic fracture, and obstruction of the nasolacrimal duct. Surgery is usually nonemergent, and a period of 10 to 14 days gives the ophthalmologist time to assess ocular function, especially the extraocular muscles and the nasolacrimal duct. Emergency surgical repair is usually not performed unless the globe is displaced into the maxillary sinus. Surgical repair is primarily directed at freeing the entrapped ocular structures and restoring the integrity of the orbital floor.

Foreign Bodies

Foreign bodies that enter the orbit are usually tolerated, except for steel, copper, iron, and vegetable materials such as those from plants or trees, which may cause purulent infection. X-rays and CT scans are used to identify the foreign body. A careful history is important, especially if the foreign body has been in the orbit for a period of time and the incident forgotten. It is important to identify metallic foreign bodies because they prohibit the use of magnetic resonance imaging (MRI) as a diagnostic tool.

After the extent of the orbital damage is assessed, the decision to use conservative treatment or surgical removal is made. In general, orbital foreign bodies are removed if they are superficial and anterior in location; have sharp edges that may affect adjacent orbital structures; or are composed of copper, iron, or vegetable material. Surgical intervention is directed at preventing further ocular injury and maintaining the integrity of the affected areas. Cultures are usually obtained, and the patient is placed on prophylactic IV antibiotic medications that are later changed to an oral route.

Ocular Trauma

Ocular trauma is a leading cause of blindness among children and young adults, especially male trauma victims (Bućan, Matas, Lovrić, et al., 2017). Ocular trauma occurs with occupational injuries (e.g., construction industry), contact sports, weapons (e.g., air guns, BB guns), assaults, motor vehicle crashes (e.g., broken windshields), and explosions (e.g., blast fragments).

There are two types of ocular trauma in which the first response is critical: chemical burn and foreign object in the eye. With a chemical burn, the eye should be immediately irrigated with tap water or normal saline. With a foreign body, no attempt should be made to remove the foreign object. The object should be protected from jarring or movement to prevent further ocular damage. No pressure or patch should be applied to the affected eye. All other traumatic eye injuries should be protected using a patch or shield if available or a stiff paper cup until medical treatment can be obtained (see Fig. 58-14).

Assessment and Diagnostic Findings

A thorough history is obtained, particularly assessing the patient's ocular history, such as pre-injury vision in the affected eye or past ocular surgery. Details related to the injury that help in the diagnosis and assessment of the need for further tests include the nature of the ocular injury (i.e., blunt or penetrating trauma); the type of activity that caused the injury to determine the nature of the force striking the eye; and whether onset of vision loss was sudden, slow, or progressive. For chemical eye burns, the chemical agent must be identified and tested for pH if the agent is available. The corneal surface is examined for foreign bodies, wounds, and abrasions, after which the other external structures of the eye are examined. Pupil size, shape, and light reaction of the pupil of the affected eye are compared with the other eye. Ocular motility (ability of the eyes to move synchronously up, down, right, and left) is also assessed.

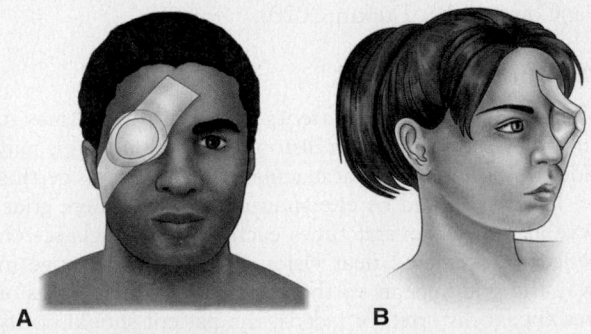

A   **B**

Figure 58-14 • Two kinds of eye patches. **A.** Aluminum shield. **B.** Stiff paper cup shield (innovative substitute when aluminum shield is unavailable).

Medical Management

Splash Injuries

Splash injuries are irrigated with normal saline solution before further evaluation occurs. In cases of a ruptured globe, cycloplegic agents (agents that paralyze the ciliary muscle) or topical antibiotics must be deferred because of potential toxicity to exposed intraocular tissues. Further manipulation of the eye must be avoided until the patient is under general anesthesia. Parenteral, broad-spectrum antibiotics are initiated. Tetanus antitoxin is given, if indicated, as well as analgesic agents. (Tetanus prophylaxis is recommended for full-thickness ocular and skin wounds.) Any topical ophthalmic medication (e.g., anesthetic, dyes) must be sterile.

Foreign Bodies and Corneal Abrasions

After removal of a foreign body from the surface of the eye, an antibiotic ointment is applied and the eye is patched. The eye is examined daily for evidence of infection until the wound is completely healed.

Contact lens wear is a common cause of corneal abrasion. The patient experiences severe pain and **photophobia** (ocular pain on exposure to light). Corneal epithelial defects are treated with antibiotic ointment and, in some instances, a pressure patch to immobilize the eyelids. Topical anesthetic eye drops must not be given to the patient to take home for repeated use after corneal injury because their effects mask further damage, delay healing, and can lead to corneal scarring.

Penetrating Injuries and Contusions of the Eyeball

Sharp penetrating injury or blunt contusion force can rupture the eyeball. When the globe, cornea, and sclera rupture, rapid decompression or herniation of the orbital contents into adjacent sinuses can occur. Blunt traumatic injuries (with an increased incidence of retinal detachment, intraocular tissue avulsion, and herniation) have a worse prognosis than penetrating injuries. Most penetrating injuries result in marked loss of vision with the following signs: hemorrhagic **chemosis** (edema of the conjunctiva), conjunctival laceration, shallow anterior chamber with or without an eccentrically placed pupil, **hyphema** (blood within the anterior chamber), or vitreous hemorrhage.

Hyphema is caused by contusion forces that tear the vessels of the iris and damage the anterior chamber angle. Preventing rebleeding and prolonged increased IOP are the goals of treatment for hyphema. In severe cases, the patient is hospitalized with moderate activity restriction. An eye shield is applied. Topical corticosteroids are prescribed to reduce inflammation. An antifibrinolytic agent (aminocaproic acid) stabilizes clot formation at the site of hemorrhage. Aspirin is contraindicated. A ruptured globe and severe injuries with intraocular hemorrhage require surgical intervention. Vitrectomy is performed for traumatic retinal detachments (Park et al., 2018). Primary **enucleation** (complete removal of the eyeball and part of the optic nerve) is considered only if the globe is irreparable and has no light perception. It is a general rule that enucleation is performed within 2 weeks of the initial injury (in an eye that has no useful vision after sustaining penetrating injury) to prevent the risk of **sympathetic ophthalmia** (an inflammation created in the uninjured eye by the affected eye that can result in blindness of the uninjured eye).

Intraocular Foreign Bodies

A patient who complains of blurred vision and discomfort should be questioned carefully about recent injuries and exposures. Patients may be injured in a number of different situations and experience an intraocular foreign body (IOFB). Precipitating circumstances can include working in construction, striking metal against metal, being involved in a motor vehicle crash with facial injury, a gunshot wound, grinding-wheel work, and explosions.

IOFB is diagnosed and localized by slit-lamp biomicroscopy and indirect ophthalmoscopy, as well as CT or ultrasonography scanning. MRI is contraindicated because most foreign bodies are metallic and magnetic. It is important to determine the composition, size, and location of the IOFB and affected eye structures. Every effort should be made to identify the type of IOFB and whether it is magnetic. Iron, steel, copper, and vegetable matter may cause intense inflammatory reactions. The incidence of endophthalmitis is high. Surgical excision of the foreign body depends on its location and composition and associated ocular injuries. Specially designed IOFB forceps and magnets are used to grasp and remove the foreign body. Any damaged area of the retina is treated to prevent retinal detachment.

Ocular Burns

Alkali, acid, and other chemically active organic substances, such as Mace and tear gas, cause chemical burns. Alkali burns (e.g., lye, ammonia) result in the most severe injury because they penetrate the ocular tissues rapidly and continue to cause long-term damage. Increased IOP also occurs. Acids (e.g., bleach, car batteries, refrigerant) generally cause less damage because the precipitated necrotic tissue proteins form a barrier to further penetration and damage. Chemical burns may appear as superficial punctate keratopathy (i.e., spotty damage to the cornea), subconjunctival hemorrhage, or complete marbleizing of the cornea.

In treating chemical burns, every minute counts. Immediate irrigation with tap water should be started on site before transport of the patient to an emergency department. A brief history and examination are performed. Critical information, if available, is the name of the substance that went into the eye (the actual container is best). Material safety data sheets (MSDSs) should be accessed for reference (see Chapter 68). The corneal surfaces and conjunctival fornices are immediately and copiously irrigated with normal saline or any neutral solution. A local anesthetic is instilled, and a lid speculum is applied to overcome blepharospasm (i.e., spasms of the eyelid muscles that result in closure of the lids). Particulate matter must be removed from the fornices using moistened, cotton-tipped applicators and minimal pressure on the globe. Irrigation continues until the conjunctival pH normalizes (between 7.3 and 7.6). The pH of the corneal surface is checked by placing a pH paper strip in the fornix. Antibiotic agents are instilled, and the eye usually is patched.

The goal of intermediate treatment is to prevent tissue ulceration and promote re-epithelialization of the cornea. Intense lubrication using artificial tears without preservatives (to avoid allergic reactions) is essential. Patching or therapeutic soft lenses may also be used to promote corneal healing, and the patient is closely monitored. Prognosis depends on the type of injury and adequacy of the irrigation immediately after exposure. Long-term treatment consists of two phases: restoration of the ocular surface through grafting procedures and surgical restoration of corneal integrity and optical clarity.

Thermal injury is caused by exposure to a hot object (e.g., curling iron, tobacco, ash), whereas photochemical injury results from ultraviolet irradiation or infrared exposure (e.g., exposure to the reflections from snow, sun gazing, viewing an eclipse of the sun without an adequate filter). These injuries can cause corneal epithelial defect, corneal opacity, conjunctival chemosis and **injection** (congestion of blood vessels), and burns of the eyelids and periocular region. Antibiotic agents and a patch for 24 hours constitute the treatment of mild injuries.

INFECTIOUS AND INFLAMMATORY CONDITIONS

Inflammation and infections of eye structures are common. Table 58-7 summarizes select infections and their treatment.

Dry Eyes

Dry eyes can be caused by decreased tear production or increased tear evaporation, which can be episodic or chronic (Norris, 2019). Decreased tear production (aqueous deficiency) can be caused by systemic disease (Sjögren, connective tissue disease), lacrimal gland obstruction, and systemic drugs (e.g., diuretics, antihistamines, psychotropic drugs). Increased tear evaporation (evaporative dry eye) can be caused by meibomian gland deficiency, lid aperture disorder, vitamin A deficiency, reduced lid blinking rate, preservatives

from topical drugs, ocular surface disease (allergy), and contact lens wear. Risk factors include increasing age, smoking, recent refractive surgery, and postmenopausal status (in women). An increase in the intake of omega-3 fatty acids may be beneficial in reducing the risk (Norris, 2019).

Clinical Manifestations

The most common complaints are photophobia, foreign-body sensation, burning and stinging, redness, and decreased tearing.

Assessment and Diagnostic Findings

Chronic dry eyes may result in chronic conjunctival and corneal irritation that can lead to corneal erosion, scarring, ulceration, thinning, or perforation that can seriously threaten vision. Secondary bacterial infection can occur.

Management

Management of dry eyes requires the cooperation of the patient with a regimen that needs to be followed at home for a long period; otherwise, complete relief of symptoms is unlikely. Instillation of artificial tears during the day and an ointment at night is the usual regimen to hydrate and lubricate the eye and preserve a moist ocular surface. Cyclosporine ophthalmic emulsion is an effective agent that increases tear production and is used once daily. Anti-inflammatory medications are also used, and moisture chambers (e.g., moisture chamber spectacles, swim goggles) may provide additional relief.

Patients may become hypersensitive to chemical preservatives such as benzalkonium chloride and thimerosal. For these patients, preservative-free ophthalmic solutions are

TABLE 58-7	Select Infections and Inflammatory Disorders of Eye Structures	
Disorder	**Description**	**Management**
Hordeolum (stye)	Acute suppurative infection of the glands of the eyelids caused by *Staphylococcus aureus*. The lid is red and edematous with a small collection of pus in the form of an abscess. There is considerable discomfort.	Warm compresses are applied directly to the affected lid area three to four times a day for 10–15 min. If the condition is not improved after 48 h, incision and drainage may be indicated. Application of topical antibiotics may be prescribed thereafter.
Chalazion	Sterile inflammatory process involving chronic granulomatous inflammation of the meibomian glands; can appear as a single granuloma or multiple granulomas in the upper or lower eyelids.	Warm compresses applied three to four times a day for 10–15 min may resolve the inflammation in the early stages. Most often, however, surgical excision is indicated. Corticosteroid injection to the chalazion lesion may be used for smaller lesions.
Blepharitis	Chronic bilateral inflammation of the eyelid margins. There are two types: staphylococcal and seborrheic. Staphylococcal blepharitis is usually ulcerative and is more serious due to the involvement of the base of hair follicles. Permanent scarring can result.	The seborrheic type is chronic and is usually resistant to treatment, but the milder cases may respond to lid hygiene. Staphylococcal blepharitis requires topical antibiotic treatment. Instructions on lid hygiene (to keep the lid margins clean and free of exudates) are given to the patient.
Bacterial keratitis	Infection of the cornea by *S. aureus*, *Streptococcus pneumoniae*, and *Pseudomonas aeruginosa*.	Fortified (high-concentration) antibiotic eye drops are given every 30 min around the clock for the first few days, then every 1–2 h. Systemic antibiotics may be given. Cycloplegics are given to reduce pain caused by ciliary spasm.
Herpes simplex keratitis	Symptoms are severe pain, tearing, and photophobia. The dendritic ulcer has a branching, linear pattern with feathery edges and terminal bulbs at its ends. Herpes simplex keratitis can lead to recurrent stromal keratitis and persist to 12 mo with residual corneal scarring.	Many lesions heal without treatment and residual effects. The treatment goal is to minimize the damaging effect of the inflammatory response and eliminate viral replication within the cornea. Penetrating keratoplasty is indicated for corneal scarring and must be performed when the herpetic disease has been inactive for many months.

Adapted from Shaw, M., & Lee, A. (2017). *Ophthalmic nursing* (5th ed.). Boca Raton, FL: CRC Press Taylor & Francis Group.

used. Management of dry eyes also includes the concurrent treatment of infections, such as chronic blepharitis and acne rosacea, and treating the underlying systemic disease, such as Sjögren syndrome (an autoimmune disease).

Surgical treatment includes punctal occlusion, grafting procedures, and lateral tarsorrhaphy (uniting the edges of the lids). Punctal plugs are made of silicone material for the temporary or permanent occlusion of the puncta. These help to preserve the volume of natural tears and prolong the effects of artificial tears (Norris, 2019).

Conjunctivitis

Conjunctivitis (inflammation of the conjunctiva) is a common ocular disorder worldwide. It is characterized by a pink appearance (hence the common term *pink eye*) because of subconjunctival blood vessel congestion.

Clinical Manifestations

General symptoms include foreign-body sensation, scratching or burning sensation, itching, and photophobia. Conjunctivitis may be unilateral or bilateral, but the infection usually starts in one eye and then spreads to the other eye by hand contact.

Assessment and Diagnostic Findings

The four main clinical features important to evaluate are the type of discharge (watery, mucoid, purulent, or mucopurulent), type of conjunctival reaction (follicular or papillary), presence of pseudomembranes or true membranes, and presence or absence of lymphadenopathy (enlargement of the preauricular and submandibular lymph nodes where the eyelids drain). Pseudomembranes consist of coagulated exudate that adheres to the surface of the inflamed conjunctiva. True membranes form when the exudate adheres to the superficial layer of the conjunctiva, and removal results in bleeding. Follicles are multiple, slightly elevated lesions encircled by tiny blood vessels; they look like grains of rice. Papillae are hyperplastic conjunctival epithelium in numerous projections that are usually seen as a fine mosaic pattern under slit-lamp examination. Diagnosis is based on the distinctive characteristics of ocular signs, acute or chronic presentation, and identification of any precipitating events. Positive results of swab smear preparations and cultures confirm the diagnosis.

Types of Conjunctivitis

Conjunctivitis is classified according to its cause. The major causes are microbial infection, allergy, and irritating toxic stimuli. A wide spectrum of organisms can cause conjunctivitis, including bacteria (e.g., *Chlamydia*), viruses, fungus, and parasites. Conjunctivitis can also result from an existing ocular infection or can be a manifestation of a systemic disease.

Microbial Conjunctivitis

Bacterial Conjunctivitis

Bacterial conjunctivitis can be acute or chronic. The acute type can develop into a chronic condition. Signs and symptoms can vary from mild to severe. Chronic bacterial conjunctivitis is usually seen in patients with lacrimal duct obstruction, chronic dacryocystitis, and chronic blepharitis. The most common causative microorganisms are *Streptococcus pneumoniae, Haemophilus influenzae,* and *Staphylococcus aureus.*

Bacterial conjunctivitis manifests with an acute onset of redness, burning, and discharge. There is papillary formation, conjunctival irritation, and injection in the fornices. The exudates are variable but are usually present on waking in the morning. The eyes may be difficult to open because of adhesions caused by the exudate. Purulent discharge occurs in severe acute bacterial infections, whereas mucopurulent discharge appears in mild cases. In gonococcal conjunctivitis, the symptoms are more acute. The exudate is profuse and purulent, and there is lymphadenopathy. Pseudomembranes may be present.

Trachoma is an infectious disease caused by the bacterium *Chlamydia trachomatis,* an ancient disease and the leading cause of preventable blindness in the world (Norris, 2019). It is prevalent in areas with hot, dry, and dusty climates and in areas with poor living conditions. It is spread by direct contact or by carrier (e.g., insects such as flies and gnats). The onset of trachoma in children is usually insidious, but it can be acute or subacute in adults. The initial symptoms include red inflamed eyes, tearing, photophobia, ocular pain, purulent exudates, preauricular lymphadenopathy, and lid edema. Initial ocular signs include follicular and papillary formations. At the middle stage of the disease, there is an acute inflammation with papillary hypertrophy and follicular necrosis, after which trichiasis and entropion begin to develop. The lashes that are turned in rub against the cornea and, after prolonged irritation, cause corneal erosion and ulceration. The late stage of the disease is characterized by scarred conjunctiva, subepithelial keratitis, abnormal vascularization of the cornea (pannus), and residual scars from the follicles that look like depressions in the conjunctiva (Herbert pits). Severe corneal ulceration can lead to perforation and blindness.

Inclusion conjunctivitis affects sexually active people who have genital chlamydial infection. Transmission is by oral–genital sex or hand-to-eye transmission. Indirect transmission can occur in inadequately chlorinated swimming pools. The eye lesions usually appear a week after exposure and may be associated with a nonspecific urethritis or cervicitis. The discharge is mucopurulent, follicles are present, and there is lymphadenopathy.

Viral Conjunctivitis

Viral conjunctivitis can be acute and chronic. The discharge is watery, and follicles are prominent. Severe cases include pseudomembranes. The common causative organisms are adenovirus and herpes simplex virus. Conjunctivitis caused by adenovirus is highly contagious. The condition is usually preceded by symptoms of upper respiratory infection. Corneal involvement causes extreme photophobia. Symptoms include tearing, redness, and foreign-body sensation that can involve one or both eyes. There is lid edema, ptosis, and conjunctival **hyperemia** (red eyes caused by dilation of blood vessels) (see Fig. 58-15). These signs and symptoms vary from mild to severe. Viral conjunctivitis, although self-limited, tends to last longer than bacterial conjunctivitis.

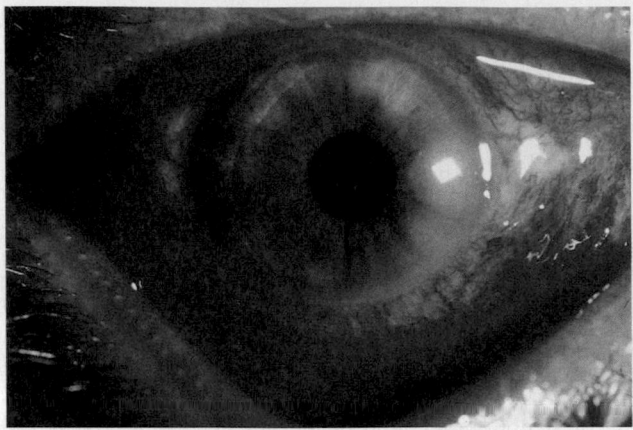

Figure 58-15 • Conjunctival hyperemia in viral conjunctivitis.

Epidemic keratoconjunctivitis is a highly contagious viral conjunctivitis that is easily transmitted from one person to another among household members, schoolchildren, and health care workers. The outbreak of epidemics is seasonal, especially during the summer when people use swimming pools. Epidemic keratoconjunctivitis is most often accompanied by preauricular lymphadenopathy and occasionally periorbital pain. There are marked follicular and papillary formations. This type of conjunctivitis can lead to keratopathy.

Allergic Conjunctivitis

Immunologic or allergic conjunctivitis is a hypersensitivity reaction that occurs as part of allergic rhinitis (hay fever), or it can be an independent allergic reaction. The patient usually has a history of an allergy to pollens and other environmental allergens. There is extreme pruritus, epiphora (excessive secretion of tears), injection, and usually severe photophobia. The stringlike mucoid discharge is usually associated with rubbing the eyes because of severe pruritus. Vernal conjunctivitis is also known as seasonal conjunctivitis because it appears mostly during warm weather. There may be large formations of papillae that have a cobblestone appearance. It is more common in children and young adults. Most affected people have a history of asthma or eczema.

Toxic Conjunctivitis

Chemical conjunctivitis can be the result of medications; chlorine from swimming pools; exposure to toxic fumes among industrial workers; or exposure to other irritants such as smoke, hair sprays, acids, and alkalis.

Medical Management

The management of conjunctivitis depends on the type. Most types of mild and viral conjunctivitis are self-limiting, benign conditions that may not require treatment and laboratory procedures. For more severe cases, topical antibiotic agents, eye drops, or ointments are prescribed. Patients with gonococcal conjunctivitis require urgent antibiotic therapy. If left untreated, this ocular disease can lead to corneal perforation and blindness. The systemic complications can include meningitis and sepsis.

Bacterial Conjunctivitis

Acute bacterial conjunctivitis is almost always self-limiting, lasting 2 weeks if left untreated. If treated with antibiotics, it may last a few days, except for gonococcal and staphylococcal conjunctivitis.

For trachoma, usually broad-spectrum antibiotic agents are given topically and systemically. Surgical management includes the correction of trichiasis to prevent conjunctival scarring.

Adult inclusion conjunctivitis requires 1 week of antibiotics. Prevention of reinfection is important, and affected people and their sexual partners must seek treatment for sexually transmitted infection, if indicated.

Viral Conjunctivitis

Viral conjunctivitis is not responsive to any treatment. Cold compresses may alleviate some symptoms. Viral conjunctivitis, especially epidemic keratoconjunctivitis, is highly contagious. Patients must be made aware of the contagious nature of the disease, and adequate education must be provided (see Chart 58-12).

Proper steps must be taken to avoid health care–associated infections. Frequent hand hygiene and procedures for environmental cleaning and disinfection of equipment used for eye examination must be strictly followed at all times. To prevent spread during outbreaks of conjunctivitis caused by adenovirus, health care facilities must set aside specified areas

---

Chart 58-12

PATIENT EDUCATION

Education for Patients with Viral Conjunctivitis

Viral conjunctivitis is a highly contagious eye infection that can easily spread from one person to another. The symptoms can be alarming but are not serious.

The nurse instructs the patient about this eye condition and the following self-care strategies:

- Be aware that your eyes will look red and will have watery discharge, and your lids will be swollen for about a week.
- Expect to experience eye pain, a sandy sensation in your eye, and sensitivity to light.
- Keep in mind that symptoms will resolve after about 1 week.
- Use lightweight cold compresses over your eyes for about 10 minutes four to five times a day to soothe the pain.
- Use artificial tears for the sandy sensation in your eye and mild pain medications such as acetaminophen.
- Stay at home and do not go outside. You may return to work or school after 7 days, when the redness and discharge have cleared. Obtain a note from your primary provider to return to work or school.
- Do not share towels, linens, makeup, or any items that have come in contact with your eyes.
- Wash your hands thoroughly with soap and water frequently.
- Use a new tissue every time you wipe the discharge from your eye. Dampen the tissue with clean water to clean the outside of the eye.
- Wash your face and take a shower as you normally do.
- Discard all of your makeup articles and do not apply makeup until the infection has resolved.
- Wear dark glasses if bright lights bother you.
- Note if the discharge from your eye turns yellowish and purulent or if your vision changes and return to the primary provider for an examination.

for treating patients diagnosed with or suspected of having conjunctivitis caused by adenovirus. All forms of tonometry must be avoided unless medically indicated. All multidose ophthalmic medications must be discarded at the end of each day or when contaminated. Employees who are infected and others must not be allowed to work or attend school until symptoms have resolved, which can take 3 to 7 days.

Allergic Conjunctivitis

Patients with allergic conjunctivitis, especially recurrent vernal or seasonal conjunctivitis, are usually given corticosteroids in ophthalmic preparations. Depending on the severity of the disease, they may be given oral preparations. The use of vasoconstrictors, such as topical epinephrine solution, cold compresses, ice packs, and cool ventilation usually provide comfort by decreasing swelling.

Toxic Conjunctivitis

For conjunctivitis caused by chemical irritants, the eye must be irrigated immediately and profusely with saline or sterile water.

Uveitis

Uveitis, or inflammation of the uveal tract, can affect the iris, the ciliary body, or the choroid. There are two types of uveitis: nongranulomatous and granulomatous.

The more common form of uveitis is the nongranulomatous type, which manifests as an acute condition with pain, photophobia, and a pattern of conjunctival injection, especially around the cornea. The pupil is small or irregular, and vision is blurred. There may be small, fine precipitates on the posterior corneal surface and cells in the aqueous humor (i.e., cell and flare). If the uveitis is severe, a **hypopyon** (accumulation of inflammatory cells in the anterior chamber of the eye) may develop. The condition may be unilateral or bilateral and may be recurrent. Repeated attacks of nongranulomatous anterior uveitis can cause anterior synechiae (peripheral iris adheres to the cornea and impedes outflow of aqueous humor). Posterior synechiae (adherence of the iris and lens) block aqueous outflow from the posterior chamber. Secondary glaucoma can result from either anterior or posterior synechiae. Cataracts may also occur as a sequela to uveitis.

Granulomatous uveitis can have a more insidious onset and can involve any portion of the uveal tract. It tends to be chronic. Symptoms such as photophobia and pain may be minimal. Vision is markedly and adversely affected. Conjunctival injection is diffuse, and there may be vitreous clouding. In a severe posterior uveitis, such as chorioretinitis, there may be retinal and choroidal hemorrhages.

Medical Management

Because photophobia is a common symptom, patients should wear dark glasses outdoors. Ciliary spasm and synechia are best avoided through mydriasis; cyclopentolate and atropine are commonly used. Local corticosteroid drops instilled four to six times a day are also used to decrease inflammation.

If the uveitis is recurrent, a careful history should be initiated to discover any underlying causes. This evaluation should include a complete history, physical examination, and diagnostic tests, including a complete blood count,

erythrocyte sedimentation rate, antinuclear antibodies, and Venereal Disease Research Laboratory (VDRL) and Lyme disease titers. Underlying causes include autoimmune disorders such as ankylosing spondylitis and sarcoidosis as well as toxoplasmosis, herpes zoster virus, ocular candidiasis, histoplasmosis, herpes simplex virus, tuberculosis, and syphilis.

Orbital Cellulitis

Orbital cellulitis is inflammation of the tissues surrounding the eye that may result from bacterial, fungal, or viral inflammatory conditions of contiguous structures, such as the face, oropharynx, dental structures, or intracranial structures. It can also result from foreign bodies and preexisting ocular infection, such as dacryocystitis and panophthalmitis, or from sepsis. Infection of the sinuses is the most frequent cause. Infection originating in the sinuses can spread easily to the orbit through the thin bony walls and foramina or by means of the interconnecting venous system of the orbit and sinuses. The most common causative organisms are staphylococci and streptococci in adults. The symptoms include pain, eyelid swelling, conjunctival edema, proptosis, and decreased ocular motility. With such edema, optic nerve compression can occur and IOP may increase.

The severe intraorbital tension caused by abscess formation and the impairment of optic nerve function in orbital cellulitis can result in permanent visual loss. Because of the orbit's proximity to the brain, orbital cellulitis can lead to life-threatening complications, such as intracranial abscess and cavernous sinus thrombosis.

Medical Management

Immediate administration of high-dose, broad-spectrum, systemic antibiotics is indicated. Cultures and Gram-stained smears are obtained. Monitoring changes in visual acuity, degree of proptosis, central nervous system function (e.g., nausea, vomiting, fever, cognitive changes), displacement of the globe, extraocular movements, pupillary signs, and the fundus is extremely important. Consultation with an otolaryngologist is necessary, especially when rhinosinusitis is suspected. In the event of abscess formation or progressive loss of vision, surgical drainage of the abscess or sinus is performed. Sinusotomy and antibiotic irrigation are also performed.

ORBITAL AND OCULAR TUMORS

Benign Tumors of the Orbit

Benign tumors can develop from infancy and grow rapidly or slowly and present in later life. Some benign tumors are superficial and are easily identifiable by external presentation, palpation, and x-rays, but some are deep and may require a CT scan to diagnose. There can be significant proptosis, and visual function may be jeopardized. Benign tumors are masses characterized by the lack of infiltration in the surrounding tissues. Examples are cystic dermoid cysts and mucocele, hemangiomas, lymphangiomas, lacrimal tumors, and neurofibromas.

To prevent recurrence, benign masses are excised completely when possible. Excision may be difficult because of the involvement of some portions of the orbital bones, such as deep dermoid cysts, in which dissection of the bone is required. Subtotal resection may be indicated in deep benign tumors that intertwine with other orbital structures, such as optic nerve meningiomas. Complete removal of the tumor may endanger visual function.

Benign Tumors of the Eyelids

There are a wide variety of benign tumors that increase in frequency with age. Nevi may be unpigmented at birth and may enlarge and darken in adolescence or may never acquire any pigment at all. Hemangiomas are vascular capillary tumors that may be bright, superficial, red lesions (formerly known as strawberry angiomas) or bluish and purplish deeper lesions. Milia are small, white, slightly elevated cysts of the eyelid that may occur in multiples. Xanthelasma are yellowish, lipoid deposits on both lids that commonly appear as a result of the aging of the skin or a lipid disorder. Molluscum contagiosum lesions are flat, symmetric growths along the lid margin caused by a virus that can result in conjunctivitis and keratitis if the lesion grows into the conjunctival sac.

Treatment of benign congenital lid lesions is rarely indicated except when visual function is affected. Corticosteroid injection to the hemangioma lesion is usually effective, but surgical excision may be performed. Benign lid lesions usually present aesthetic problems rather than visual function problems. Surgical excision, or electrocautery, is primarily performed for cosmetic reasons, except for cases of molluscum contagiosum, for which surgical intervention is performed to prevent an infectious process that may ensue.

Benign Tumors of the Conjunctiva

Conjunctival nevus, a congenital benign neoplasm, is a flat, slightly elevated, brown spot that becomes pigmented during late childhood or adolescence. This should be differentiated from the pigmented lesion melanosis, which is acquired at middle age and may become melanoma. Keratin- and sebum-containing dermoid cysts are congenital and can be found in the conjunctiva. Dermolipoma is a congenital tumor that manifests as a smooth, rounded growth in the conjunctiva near the lateral canthus. Papillomas are usually soft with irregular surfaces and appear on the lid margins. Treatment consists of surgical excision.

Malignant Tumors of the Orbit

Rhabdomyosarcoma is the most common malignant primary orbital tumor in childhood; it can also develop in older adults (Tang, Zhang, Lu, et al., 2018). The symptoms of rhabdomyosarcoma include sudden painless proptosis of one eye followed by lid swelling, conjunctival chemosis, and impairment of ocular motility. CT or MRI scans of these tumors establish the size, configuration, location, and stage of the disease; delineates the degree of bone destruction; and is useful in estimating the field for radiation therapy. The most common site of metastasis is the lung.

Management of these primary malignant orbital tumors involves three major therapeutic modalities: surgery, radiation therapy, and adjuvant chemotherapy. The degree of orbital destruction is important in planning the surgical approach. Resection often involves removal of the eyeball. The psychological needs of the patient and family are paramount in planning the management approach.

Malignant Tumors of the Eyelid

Basal cell carcinoma is the most common malignant tumor of the eyelid. Squamous cell carcinoma occurs less frequently but is considered the second most common malignant tumor. Melanoma is rare. Malignant eyelid tumors occur more frequently among people with a fair complexion who have a history of chronic exposure to the sun (Norris, 2019).

Basal cell carcinoma appears as a painless nodule that may ulcerate. The lesion is invasive, spreads to the surrounding tissues, and grows slowly but does not metastasize. It usually appears on the lower lid margin near the inner canthus with a pearly white margin. Squamous cell carcinoma of the eyelids may resemble basal cell carcinoma initially because it also grows slowly and painlessly. It tends to ulcerate and invade the surrounding tissues, but it can metastasize to the regional lymph nodes. Melanoma may not be pigmented and can arise from nevi. It spreads to the surrounding tissues and metastasizes to other organs.

Complete excision of these carcinomas is followed by reconstruction with skin grafting if the surgical excision is extensive. The ocular postoperative site and the graft donor site are monitored for bleeding. Donor graft sites may include the buccal mucosa, the thigh, or the abdomen. The patient is referred to an oncologist for evaluation of the need for radiation therapy and monitoring for metastasis. Early diagnosis and surgical management are the basis of a good prognosis. These conditions have life-threatening consequences, and surgical excisions may result in facial disfigurement. Emotional support is an extremely important aspect of nursing management.

Malignant Tumors of the Conjunctiva

Conjunctival carcinoma most often grows in the exposed areas of the conjunctiva. The typical lesions are usually gelatinous and whitish due to keratin formation. They grow gradually, and deep invasion and metastasis are rare. Melanoma is rare but may arise from a preexisting nevus or acquired melanosis during middle age. Squamous cell carcinoma is also rare but invasive.

The management is surgical incision. Some benign tumors and most malignant tumors recur. To avoid recurrences, patients usually undergo radiation therapy and cryotherapy after the excision of malignant tumors. Cosmetic disfigurement may result from extensive excision when deep invasion by the malignant tumor is involved.

Malignant Tumors of the Globe

Ocular melanoma is a rare malignant choroidal tumor sometimes discovered on a retinal examination. In its early stages, it could be mistaken for a nevus. In addition to a complete physical examination to discover any evidence of metastasis (to the liver, lung, and breast), retinal fundus photography, fluorescein angiography, and ultrasonography are performed. The diagnosis is confirmed at biopsy after enucleation.

Tumors are classified according to boundary lines (apical height and basal diameter) as small, medium, or large. Small tumors are generally monitored, whereas medium and large tumors require treatment. Treatment consists of radiation, enucleation, or both. Radiation therapy may be achieved by external beam performed in repeated episodes over several days or through the implantation of a small plaque that contains radioactive iodine (I-125) pellets over the tumor.

SURGICAL PROCEDURES AND ENUCLEATION

Orbital Surgeries

Orbital surgeries may be performed to repair fractures, remove a foreign body, or remove benign or malignant growths. Surgical procedures involving the orbit and lids affect facial appearance, or cosmesis. The goals are to recover and preserve visual function and to maintain the anatomic relationship of the ocular structures to achieve cosmesis. During the repair of orbital fractures, the orbital bones are realigned to follow the anatomic positions of facial structures.

Orbital surgical procedures involve working around delicate structures of the eye, such as the optic nerve, retinal blood vessels, and ocular muscles. Complications of orbital surgical procedures may include blindness as a result of damage to the optic nerve and its blood supply. Sudden pain and loss of vision may indicate intraorbital hemorrhage or compression of the optic nerve. Ptosis and diplopia may result from trauma to the extraocular muscles during the surgical procedure, but these conditions typically resolve after a few weeks.

Prophylaxis with IV antibiotic agents is the usual postoperative regimen after orbital surgery, especially with repair of orbital fractures and intraorbital foreign-body removal. IV corticosteroids may be used if there is concern about optic nerve swelling. Topical ocular antibiotics are typically instilled, and antibiotic ointments are applied externally to the skin suture sites.

For the first 24 to 48 hours postoperatively, ice compresses are applied over the periocular area to decrease periorbital swelling, facial swelling, and hematoma. The head of the patient's bed should be elevated to a comfortable position (30 to 45 degrees).

Discharge education should include information about oral antibiotic agents, instillation of ophthalmic medications, and application of ice compresses.

Enucleation

Enucleation is removal of the eyeball (globe) from the orbit, leaving the muscles and orbital contents intact. It may be surgically performed for the following conditions:

- Injury resulting in prolapse of uveal tissue or loss of light perception
- A blind, painful, deformed, or disfigured eye, usually caused by glaucoma, retinal detachment, or chronic inflammation
- An eye without useful vision that is producing or has produced sympathetic ophthalmia in the other eye
- Intraocular tumors that are untreatable by other means

The procedure for enucleation involves the separation and cutting of each of the ocular muscles and surrounding soft tissue and cutting of the optic nerve from the eyeball. The insertion of an orbital implant typically follows, and the conjunctiva is closed. A large pressure dressing is applied over the area.

Evisceration involves the removal of the intraocular contents through an incision or opening in the cornea or sclera. Evisceration may be surgically performed to treat severe ocular trauma with ruptured globe, severe ocular inflammation, or severe ocular infection. The optic nerve, sclera, extraocular muscles, and sometimes the cornea are left intact. The main advantage of evisceration over enucleation is that the final cosmetic result and motility after fitting the ocular prosthesis are enhanced.

Exenteration is the surgical removal of the entire contents of the orbit, surrounding soft tissue, and most or all of the eyelids. This surgery is indicated in malignancies of the orbit that are life-threatening or when more conservative modalities of treatment have failed or are inappropriate. An example is squamous cell carcinoma of the paranasal sinuses, skin, and conjunctiva with deep orbital involvement. In its most extensive form, exenteration may include the removal of all orbital tissues and resection of the orbital bones.

Ocular Prostheses

Orbital implants and conformers (ocular prostheses usually made of silicone rubber) maintain the shape of the eye after enucleation or evisceration to prevent a contracted, sunken appearance. The temporary conformer is placed over the conjunctival closure after the implantation of an orbital implant. A conformer is placed after the enucleation or evisceration procedure to protect the suture line, maintain the fornices, prevent contracture of the socket in preparation for the ocular prosthesis, and promote the integrity of the eyelids.

All ocular prosthetics have limitations in their motility. There are two designs of eye prostheses. The anophthalmic ocular prostheses are used in the absence of the globe. Scleral shells look just like the anophthalmic prosthesis (see Fig. 58-16) but are thinner and fit over a globe with intact corneal sensation. An eye prosthesis usually lasts about 6 years, depending on the quality of fit, comfort, and cosmetic appearance. When the anophthalmic socket is completely healed, conformers are replaced with prosthetic eyes.

An ocularist is a specially trained and skilled professional who makes prosthetic eyes. After the ophthalmologist is

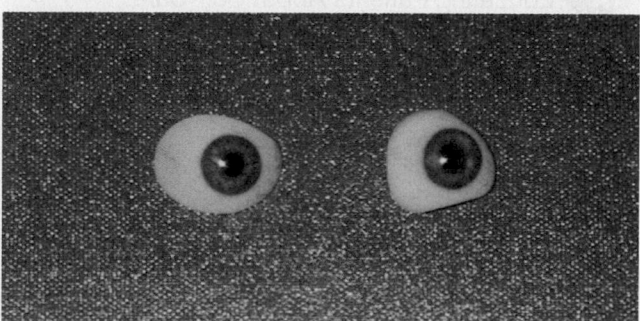

Figure 58-16 • Eye prostheses. **(Left)** Anophthalmic ocular prosthesis. **(Right)** Scleral shell.

satisfied that the anophthalmic socket is completely healed and is ready for prosthetic fitting, the patient is referred to an ocularist. The healing period is usually 6 to 8 weeks. It is advisable for the patient to have a consultation with the ocularist before the fitting. Obtaining accurate information and verbalizing concerns can lessen anxiety about wearing an ocular prosthesis.

Medical Management

Removal of an eye has physical, social, and psychological ramifications for any person. The significance of loss of the eye and vision must be addressed in the plan of care. The patient's preparation should include information about the surgical procedure and placement of orbital implants and conformers and the availability of ocular prosthetics to enhance cosmetic appearance. In some cases, patients may choose to see an ocularist before the surgery to discuss ocular prosthetics.

Nursing Management

Providing Education About Postsurgical and Prosthetic Care

Patients who undergo eye removal need to know that they will usually have a large ocular pressure dressing, which is typically removed after a week, and that an ophthalmic topical antibiotic ointment is applied in the socket three times daily.

After the removal of an eye, there is a loss of depth perception. Patients must be advised to take extra caution in their ambulation and movement to avoid miscalculations that may result in injury. It may take some time to adjust to monocular vision.

The patient must be advised that conformers may inadvertently fall out of the socket. If this happens, the conformer must be washed, wiped dry, and placed back in the socket.

When surgical eye removal is unexpected, such as in severe ocular trauma, leaving no time for the patient and family to prepare for the loss, the nurse's role in providing emotional support is crucial.

Promoting Home, Community-Based, and Transitional Care

The patient with a new prosthetic eye may need referral to home, community-based or transitional services that provide assistance in the home. These patients also benefit from a referral for rehabilitation services.

 Educating Patients About Self-Care

Patients need to be educated about how to insert, remove, and care for the prosthetic eye. Proper hand hygiene must be observed before inserting and removing an ocular prosthesis. A suction cup may be used if there are problems with manual dexterity. Precautions, such as draping a towel over the sink and closing the sink drain, must be taken to avoid loss of the prosthesis. When educating patients or family members, a return demonstration is important to assess the level of understanding and ability to perform the procedure.

Before insertion, the inner punctal or outer lateral aspects and the superior and inferior aspects of the prosthesis must be identified by locating the identifying marks, such as a reddish color in the inner punctal area. For people with low vision, other forms of identifying markers, such as dots or notches, are used. The upper lid is raised high enough to create a space and then the patient learns to slide the prosthesis up, underneath, and behind the upper eyelid. Meanwhile, the patient pulls the lower eyelid down to help put the prosthesis in place and to have its inferior edge fall back gradually to the lower eyelid. The lower eyelid is checked for correct positioning.

To remove the prosthesis, the patient cups one hand on the cheek to catch the prosthesis, places the forefinger of the free hand against the midportion of the lower eyelid, and gazes upward. Gazing upward brings the inferior edge of the prosthesis nearer the inferior eyelid margin. With the finger pushing inward, downward, and laterally against the lower eyelid, the prosthesis slides out into the cupped hand.

Continuing and Transitional Care

An eye prosthesis can be worn and left in place for several months. Hygiene and comfort are usually maintained with daily irrigation of the prosthesis in place with normal saline solution, hard contact lens solution, or artificial tears. In the case of dry eye symptoms, the use of ophthalmic ointment lubricants or oil-based drops, such as vitamin E and mineral oil, can be helpful. Removing crusting and mucus discharge that accumulate overnight is performed with the prosthesis in place. Malpositions may occur when wiping or rubbing the prosthesis in the socket. The prosthesis can be repositioned with the use of clean fingers. Proper wiping of the prosthesis should be a gentle temporal-to-nasal motion to avoid malpositions.

The prosthesis needs to be removed and cleaned when it becomes uncomfortable and when there is increased mucus discharge. The socket should also be rendered free of mucus and inspected for any signs of infection. Any unusual discomfort, irritation, or redness of the globe or eyelids may indicate excessive wear, debris under the shell, or lack of proper hygiene. Any infection or irritation that does not resolve needs medical attention.

OCULAR CONSEQUENCES OF SYSTEMIC DISEASE

Diabetic Retinopathy

Advancements in the treatment of diabetes have enabled patients to have a relatively a normal lifespan, but many have complications of long-term diabetes. One of the most serious complications of diabetes is retinopathy. Patients with diabetes are also at higher risk of cataracts and best practices for glycemic control during cataract surgery are not known (Kiziltoprak, Tekin, Inanc, et al., 2019). See Chapter 46 for a detailed discussion of diabetic retinopathy.

Cytomegalovirus Retinitis

Many ophthalmic complications have been associated with AIDS, and CMV is the most common cause of retinal inflammation in patients with AIDS. Early symptoms of CMV retinitis vary from patient to patient. Some patients complain of floaters or a decrease in peripheral vision. Some have a paracentral or central scotoma, whereas others have fluctuations in vision from macular edema. The retina often becomes thin and atrophic and susceptible to retinal tears and breaks.

CMV retinitis generally takes one of three forms: hemorrhagic, brushfire, or granular. In the hemorrhagic type, large areas of white, necrotic retina may be associated with retinal hemorrhage. In the brushfire type, a yellow-white margin begins at the edge of burned-out atrophic retina. This retinitis expands and, if untreated, involves the entire retina. In the granular type, white granular lesions in the periphery of the retina gradually expand. The white, feathery infiltration of the retina destroys sensory retina and leads to necrosis, optic atrophy, and retinal detachment.

Medical Management

Management of CMV retinitis consists of prescribing the appropriate pharmacologic agent.

Pharmacologic Therapy

Pharmacologic agents available for the treatment of CMV retinitis include ganciclovir, foscarnet, and cidofovir.

Ganciclovir is administered IV, orally, or intravitreously in the acute stage of CMV retinitis. The intravitreous form is available as a 4-mm intraocular implant or insert containing the medication embedded in a polymer-based system that slowly releases the medication. The insert is surgically placed in the posterior segment of the eye, and the medication diffuses locally to the site of the infection over a period of 5 to 8 months before the insert must be replaced. When given systemically, ganciclovir is a very potent medication; it can cause neutropenia, thrombocytopenia, anemia, and elevated serum creatinine levels. The surgically implanted sustained-release insert enables higher concentrations of ganciclovir to reach the CMV retinitis, but there are risks and complications associated with the inserts, including endophthalmitis, retinal detachment, and hypotony.

Foscarnet inhibits viral deoxyribonucleic acid (DNA) replication. It may be the medication of choice when ganciclovir is ineffective. It may be administered by IV or intravitreal injections. The combination of foscarnet and ganciclovir has been more effective than either medication alone. Nephrotoxicity may occur with systemic foscarnet, and renal function must be monitored carefully.

Cidofovir impedes CMV replication and is administered IV. Cidofovir has been shown to delay the progression of CMV retinitis significantly. Nephrotoxicity, proteinuria, and increased serum creatinine levels are significant side effects.

A nucleoside analogue such as zidovudine given in combination with one or more protease inhibitors such as ritonavir in the management of patients with AIDS has led to a major therapeutic success, gradually altering the course of the disease and transforming HIV/AIDS into a chronically manageable disease (Iacob, Iacob, & Jugulete, 2017). The immune system can then recover to a functional level. Some patients develop immune recovery uveitis, characterized by intraocular inflammation, cystoid macular edema, and the formation of epiretinal membranes. Immune recovery uveitis is managed by corticosteroids or by injection of corticosteroids into the sub-Tenon area of the eye.

Hypertension-Related Eye Changes

Long-standing hypertension is associated with atherosclerosis, and retinal changes are evidenced by the development of retinal arteriolar changes, such as tortuousness, narrowing, and a change in light reflex (Weber & Kelley, 2018). Fundoscopic examination reveals a copper or silver coloration of the arterioles and venous compression (arteriovenous nicking) at the arteriolar and venous crossings. Intraretinal hemorrhages from hypertension appear flame shaped because they occur in the nerve fiber layer of the retina.

Hypertension can also occur as an acute consequence of conditions such as pheochromocytoma, acute kidney injury, and pregnancy-induced hypertension. The retinopathy associated with these crisis states is extensive, and the manifestations include cotton-wool spots, retinal hemorrhages, retinal edema, and retinal exudates, often clustered around the macula (Weber & Kelley, 2018).

The choroid is also affected by the profound and abrupt rise in blood pressure and resulting vasoconstriction, and ischemia may result in serious retinal detachments and infarction of the retinal pigment epithelium. Ischemic optic neuropathy and papilledema may also result. Blood pressure in these more severe stages should be lowered in a controlled gradual fashion to avoid ischemia of the optic nerve and brain secondary to a too-rapid fall in blood pressure. See Chapter 27 for further information about hypertension.

CRITICAL THINKING EXERCISES

1 **pcq** You are a home health nurse visiting a 72-year-old male who has a long history of uncontrolled diabetes. He reports that recently he has been having trouble with his vision. Define nursing assessment techniques that are important in evaluating this patient. Describe your nursing priorities of care for a patient with low vision. How would these priorities change if the patient were blind?

2 **ipc** A 45-year-old woman presents to the emergency department complaining she has had progressive loss of vision of her left eye since the morning. She lives alone and is very afraid of going blind. The patient is diagnosed with a retinal detachment and scheduled for surgery. What members of the interdisciplinary team are essential to include? How will you facilitate an interprofessional discussion to develop strategies to decrease her fear?

3 **ebp** An 80-year-old patient reports to you that he has been diagnosed with AMD. What is the evidence base for offering guidelines for managing this condition? What evidence-based educational information can you share? Identify the criteria used to evaluate the strength of the evidence for these practices.

REFERENCES

*Asterisk indicates nursing research.

Books

American Society of Ophthalmic Registered Nurses (ASORN). (2013). *ASORN recommended practice: Use of multi-dose medications.* San Francisco, CA: Author.

Comerford, K. C., & Durkin, M. T. (2020). *Nursing 2020 drug handbook.* Philadelphia, PA: Wolters Kluwer.

Eliopoulos, C. (2018). *Gerontological nursing* (9th ed.). Philadelphia, PA: Wolters Kluwer.

Fischbach, F. T., & Fischbach, M. B. (2018). *A manual of laboratory and diagnostic tests* (10th ed.). Philadelphia, PA: Wolters Kluwer.

Gerstenblith, A. T., & Rabinowitz, M. P. (2017). *The Wills eye manual: Office and emergency room diagnosis and treatment of eye disease* (7th ed.). Philadelphia, PA: Lippincott Williams & Wilkins.

Hickey, J. V., & Strayer, A. L. (2020). *The clinical practice of neurological and neurosurgical nursing* (8th ed.). Philadelphia, PA: Wolters Kluwer.

McQuillan, K. A., & Makic, M. B. (2020). *Trauma nursing: From resuscitation through rehabilitation* (5th ed.). St. Louis, MO: Elsevier.

Moore, K., Dalley, A., & Agur, A. (2018). *Clinically orientated anatomy* (8th ed.). Philadelphia, PA: Wolters Kluwer.

Norris, T. (2019). *Porth's pathophysiology: Concepts of altered health status* (10th ed.). Philadelphia, PA: Wolters Kluwer.

Shaw, M., & Lee, A. (2017). *Ophthalmic nursing* (5th ed.). Boca Raton, FL: CRC Press Taylor & Francis Group.

Strayer, D. S., Rubin, E., Saffitz, J. E., et al. (2015). *Rubin's pathology: Clinicopathologic foundations of medicine* (7th ed.). Philadelphia, PA: Wolters Kluwer.

Weber, J., & Kelley, J. (2018). *Health assessment in nursing* (6th ed.). Philadelphia, PA: Wolters Kluwer.

Journals and Electronic Documents

Allard, K., & Zetterberg, M. (2018). Toric IOL implantation in a patient with keratoconus and previous penetrating keratoplasty: A case report and review of literature. *BMC Ophthalmology, 18*(1), 215.

Bright Focus Foundation. (2020a). Age-related macular degeneration. Retrieved on 1/10/2020 at: www.brightfocus.org/macular

Bright Focus Foundation. (2020b). Eye diseases that can cause legal blindness. Retrieved on 4/1/2020 at: www.brightfocus.org/macular/article/eye-diseases-can-cause-legal-blindness

Bućan, K., Matas, A., Lovrić, J. M., et al. (2017). Epidemiology of ocular trauma in children requiring hospital admission: A 16-year retrospective cohort study. *Journal of Global Health, 7*(1), 010415.

Centers for Disease Control and Prevention (CDC). (2019). Common eye disorders. Retrieved on 12/28/2019 at: www.cdc.gov/visionhealth/basics/ced/index.html

Colour Blind Awareness. (2019). Inherited colour vision deficiency. Retrieved on 11/02/2019 at: www.colourblindawareness.org/colour-blindness/inherited

Glaucoma Research Foundation. (2019). Five common glaucoma tests. Retrieved on 12/16/2019 at: www.glaucoma.org/glaucoma/diagnostic-tests.php

Glaucoma Research Foundation. (2020). Eye drop tips. Retrieved on 2/11/2020 at: www.glaucoma.org/treatment/eyedrop-tips.php

Gomel, N., Negari, S., Frucht-Pery, J., et al. (2018). Predictive factors for efficacy and safety in refractive surgery for myopia. *PLoS One, 13*(12), e0208608.

Iacob, S. A., Iacob, D. G., & Jugulete, G. (2017). Improving the adherence to antiretroviral therapy, a difficult but essential task for a successful HIV treatment—Clinical points of view and practical considerations. *Frontiers in Pharmacology, 8*, 831.

Igarashi, A. (2019). Posterior chamber phakic IOLs vs. LASIK: Benefits and complications. *Expert Review of Ophthalmology, 14*(1), 43–52.

Jolly, J. K., Bridge, H., & MacLaren, R. E. (2019). Outcome measures used in ocular gene therapy trials: A scoping review of current practice. *Frontiers in Pharmacology, 10*, 1076.

Kiziltoprak, H., Tekin, K., Inanc, M., et al. (2019). Cataract in diabetes mellitus. *World Journal of Diabetes, 10*(3), 140–153.

Liao, L., & Zhu, X. H. (2019). Advances in the treatment of rhegmatogenous retinal detachment. *International Journal of Ophthalmology, 12*(4), 660–667.

McMonnies, C. W. (2017). Glaucoma history and risk factors. *Journal of Optometry, 10*(2), 71–78.

Morgan, E. (2018). Driving dilemmas: A guide to driving assessment in primary care. *Clinics in Geriatric Medicine, 34*(1), 107–115.

Moshirfar, M., Ding, Y., & Shah, T. J. (2018). A historical perspective on treatment of Fuchs' Endothelial Dystrophy: We have come a long way. *Journal of Ophthalmic & Vision Research, 13*(3), 339–343.

Norat, P., Soldozy, S., Elsarrag, M., et al. (2019). Application of indocyanine green videoangiography in aneurysm surgery: Evidence, techniques, practical tips. *Frontiers in Surgery, 6*, 34.

*Pagliuca, L. M., Macêdo-Costa, K. N., Rebouças, C. B., et al. (2014). Validation of the general guidelines of communication between the nurse and the blind. *Revista Brasileira de Enfermagem, 67*(5), 715–721.

Park, S. W., Lee, J. J., & Lee, J. E. (2018). Scleral buckling in the management of rhegmatogenous retinal detachment: Patient selection and perspectives. *Clinical Ophthalmology, 12*, 1605–1615.

Phulke, S., Kaushik, S., Kaur, S., et al. (2017). Steroid-induced glaucoma: An avoidable irreversible blindness. *Journal of Current Glaucoma Practice, 11*(2), 67–72.

Prevent Blindness. (2020). Know the risk factors for cataract. Retrieved on 2/16/2020 at: www.preventblindness.org/know-risk-factors-cataract

Schmidt-Erfurth, U., Garcia-Arumi, J., Gerendas, B. S., et al. (2019). Guidelines for the management of retinal vein occlusion by the European Society of Retina Specialists (EURETINA). *Ophthalmologica, 242*(3), 123–162.

Shah, P., Schwartz, S. G., Gartner, S., et al. (2018). Low vision services: A practical guide for the clinician. *Therapeutic Advances in Ophthalmology, 10*, 2515841418776264.

Shalaby Bardan, A., Al Raqqad, N., Zarei-Ghanavati, M., et al. (2018). The role of keratoprostheses. *Eye, 32*(1), 7–8.

Sheybani, A., Scott, R., Samuelson, T. W., et al. (2020). Open-angle glaucoma: Burden of illness, current therapies, and the management of nocturnal IOP variation. *Ophthalmology & Therapy, 9*, 1–14.

Sihota, R., Angmo, D., Ramaswamy, D., et al. (2018). Simplifying "target" intraocular pressure for different stages of primary open-angle glaucoma and primary angle-closure glaucoma. *Indian Journal of Ophthalmology, 66*(4), 495–505.

Singh, M., & Tyagi, S. C. (2018). Genes and genetics in eye diseases: A genomic medicine approach for investigating hereditary and inflammatory ocular disorders. *International Journal of Ophthalmology, 11*(1), 117–134.

Tang, L. Y., Zhang, M. X., Lu, D. H., et al. (2018). The prognosis and effects of local treatment strategies for orbital embryonal rhabdomyosarcoma: A population-based study. *Cancer Management and Research, 10*, 1727–1734.

Resources

American Academy of Ophthalmology, www.aao.org
American Foundation for the Blind (AFB), www.afb.org
American Society of Ophthalmic Registered Nurses (ASORN), www.asorn.org
Foundation Fighting Blindness, www.fightingblindness.org
Glaucoma Research Foundation, www.glaucoma.org
Lighthouse Guild, www.lighthouseguild.org
MAB Community Services, www.mabcommunity.org
Macular Degeneration Foundation, www.eyesight.org
National Diabetes Information Clearinghouse (NDIC), www.niddk.nih.gov/health-information/diabetes
National Eye Institute, www.nei.nih.gov
National Federation of the Blind, www.nfb.org
Prevent Blindness, www.preventblindness.org
Research to Prevent Blindness, www.rpbusa.org

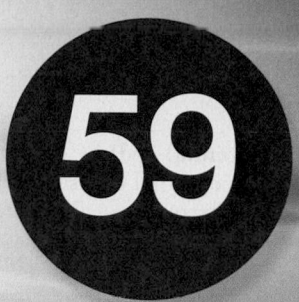

59

Assessment and Management of Patients with Hearing and Balance Disorders

LEARNING OUTCOMES

On completion of this chapter, the learner will be able to:

1. Describe the anatomy and physiology of the ear as well as the methods used to assess hearing and balance disorders.
2. List the manifestations that may be exhibited by a person with hearing and balance disorders.
3. Identify ways to communicate effectively with a person with a hearing disorder, incorporating the differences between Deaf culture and deafness.
4. Differentiate disorders of the external ear from those of the middle ear and inner ear.
5. Compare the various types of surgical procedures used for managing middle ear disorders and appropriate nursing care.
6. Use the nursing process as a framework for care of the patient undergoing mastoid surgery or of the patient with vertigo.
7. Recognize the different types of inner ear disorders, including the clinical manifestations, diagnosis, and management.

NURSING CONCEPTS

Assessment
Communication
Family

Infection
Inflammation
Sensory Perception

Stress

GLOSSARY

acute otitis media: inflammation in the middle ear lasting less than 6 weeks

cholesteatoma: tumor of the middle ear or mastoid, or both, that can destroy structures of the temporal bone

chronic otitis media: repeated episodes of acute otitis media causing irreversible tissue damage

conductive hearing loss: loss of hearing in which efficient sound transmission to the inner ear is interrupted by some obstruction or disease process

Deaf culture: a community that consists of a group of people who are connected by their use of sign language

deafness: partial or complete loss of the ability to hear

dizziness: altered sensation of orientation in space

endolymphatic hydrops: dilation of the endolymphatic space of the inner ear; the pathologic correlate of Ménière's disease

exostoses: small, hard, protrusions in the lower posterior bony portion of the ear canal

external otitis: inflammation of the external auditory canal (*synonym:* otitis externa)

labyrinthitis: inflammation of the labyrinth of the inner ear

Ménière's disease: condition of the inner ear characterized by a triad of symptoms: episodic vertigo, tinnitus, and fluctuating sensorineural hearing loss

middle ear effusion: fluid in the middle ear without evidence of infection

myringotomy: incision in the tympanic membrane (*synonym:* tympanotomy)

nystagmus: involuntary rhythmic eye movement

ossiculoplasty: surgical reconstruction of the middle ear bones to restore hearing

otalgia: sensation of fullness or pain in the ear

otorrhea: drainage from the ear

otosclerosis: a condition characterized by abnormal spongy bone formation around the stapes

presbycusis: progressive hearing loss associated with aging

rhinorrhea: drainage from the nose

sensorineural hearing loss: loss of hearing related to damage to the end organ for hearing or cranial nerve VIII, or both

tinnitus: subjective perception of sound with internal origin; unwanted noises in the head or ear most often described as ringing in the ears

tympanoplasty: surgical repair of the tympanic membrane

vertigo: illusion of movement in which the individual or the surroundings are sensed as moving

The ear is a delicate sensory organ with the dual functions of hearing and balance. The sense of hearing is essential for normal development and maintenance of speech as well as the ability to communicate with others. Balance, or equilibrium, is essential for maintaining body movement, position, and coordination.

The early detection and accurate diagnosis of disorders is necessary for preservation of normal hearing and balance. The diagnosis and treatment of these disorders requires skilled health care professionals such as otolaryngologists, internists, audiologists, and nurses. This chapter provides an overview of the anatomy and physiology of the ear and addresses the general assessment and management of hearing and balance disorders common to adults seen in many health care settings.

ASSESSMENT OF THE EAR

Anatomic and Physiologic Overview

The cranium encloses and protects the brain and surrounding structures, providing attachment for various muscles that control head and jaw movements. The ears are located on either side of the cranium at approximately eye level.

Anatomy of the External Ear

The external ear includes the auricle (pinna) and the external auditory canal (see Fig. 59-1). The external ear is separated from the middle ear by a disc-shaped structure called the *tympanic membrane* (eardrum).

Auricle

The auricle, attached to the side of the head by skin, is composed mainly of cartilage, except for the fat and subcutaneous tissue in the earlobe. The auricle collects the sound waves and directs vibrations into the external auditory canal.

External Auditory Canal

The external auditory canal is approximately 2 to 3 cm long (Norris, 2019). The lateral third is an elastic cartilaginous and dense fibrous framework to which thin skin is attached. The medial two thirds is bone lined with thin skin. The external auditory canal ends at the tympanic membrane.

The skin of the canal contains hair, sebaceous glands, and ceruminous glands, which secrete a brown, waxlike substance called *cerumen* (ear wax). The ear's self-cleaning mechanism moves old skin cells and cerumen to the outer part of the ear.

Just anterior to the external auditory canal is the temporomandibular joint. The head of the mandible can be felt by

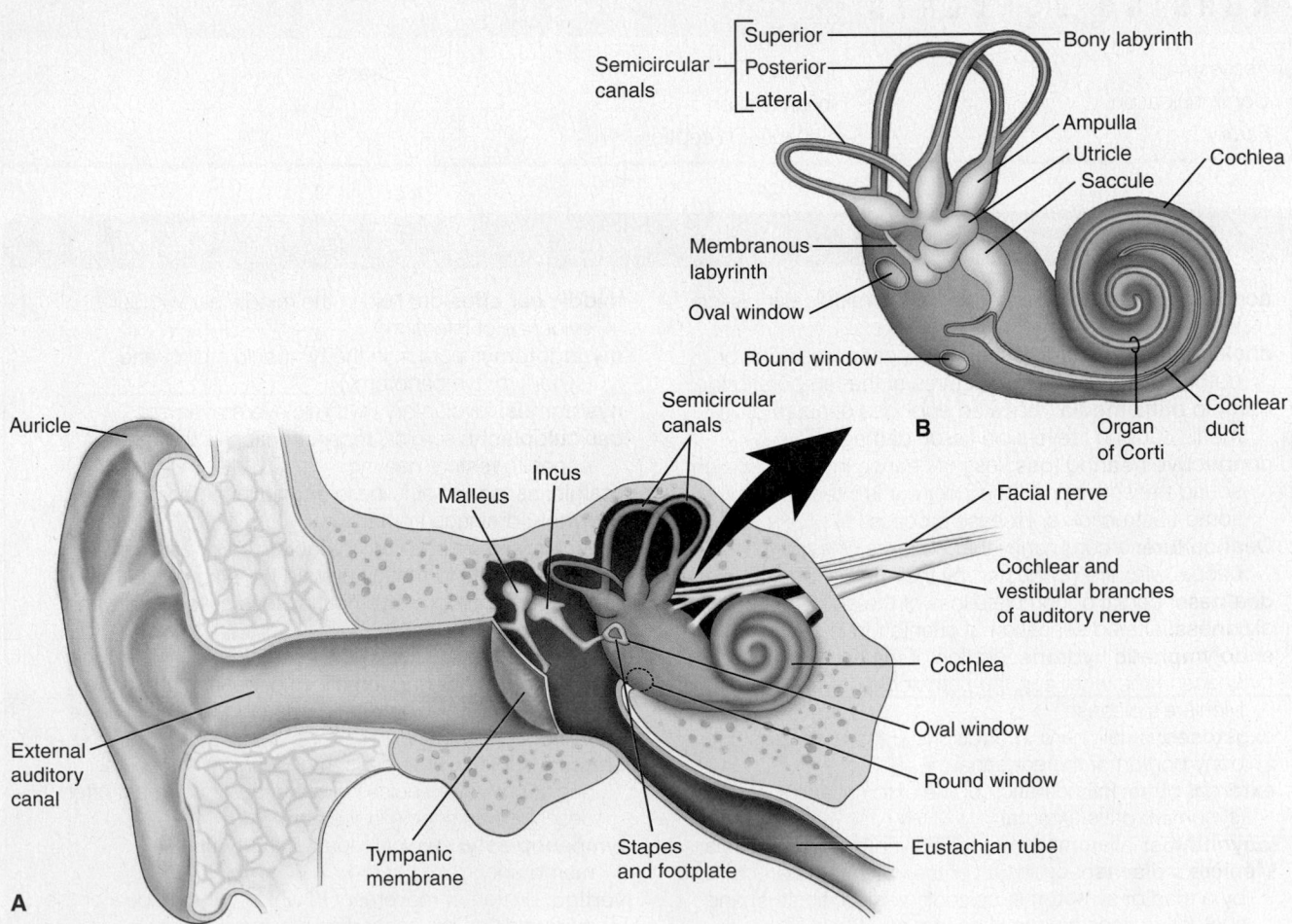

Figure 59-1 • A. Anatomy of the ear. **B.** The inner ear.

placing a fingertip in the external auditory canal while the patient opens and closes the mouth.

Anatomy of the Middle Ear

The middle ear, an air-filled cavity, includes the tympanic membrane laterally and the otic capsule medially. The middle ear cleft lies between the two. The middle ear is connected to the nasopharynx by the eustachian tube and is continuous with air-filled cells in the adjacent mastoid portion of the temporal bone.

The eustachian tube, which is approximately 1 mm wide and 35 mm long, connects the middle ear to the nasopharynx. Normally, the eustachian tube is closed, but it opens by action of the tensor veli palatini muscle when the person performs a Valsalva maneuver, yawns, or swallows. It drains normal and abnormal secretions of the middle ear and equalizes pressure in the middle ear with that of the atmosphere.

Tympanic Membrane

The tympanic membrane (eardrum), about 1 cm in diameter and very thin, is normally pearly gray and translucent (Weber & Kelley, 2018). It consists of three layers of tissue: an outer layer, continuous with the skin of the ear canal; a fibrous middle layer; and an inner mucosal layer, continuous with the lining of the middle ear cavity. Approximately 80% of the tympanic membrane is composed of all three layers and is called the *pars tensa*. The remaining 20% lacks the middle layer and is called the *pars flaccida*. The absence of this fibrous middle layer makes the pars flaccida more vulnerable to pathologic disorders than the pars tensa. Distinguishing landmarks include the annulus, the fibrous border that attaches the eardrum to the temporal bone; the short process of the malleus; the long process of the malleus; the umbo of the malleus, which attaches to the tympanic membrane in the center; the pars flaccida; and the pars tensa (see Fig. 59-2).

The tympanic membrane protects the middle ear and conducts sound vibrations from the external canal to the ossicles.

The sound pressure is magnified 22 times as a result of transmission from a larger area to a smaller one.

Ossicles

The middle ear contains the ossicles, the three smallest bones of the body: the malleus, the incus, and the stapes (Norris, 2019). The ossicles, which are held in place by joints, muscles, and ligaments, assist in the transmission of sound. Two small fenestrae (oval and round windows), located in the medial wall of the middle ear, separate the middle ear from the inner ear. The footplate of the stapes sits in the oval window, secured by a fibrous annulus (ring-shaped structure). The footplate transmits sound to the inner ear. The round window, covered by a thin membrane, provides an exit for sound vibrations (see Fig. 59-1).

Anatomy of the Inner Ear

The inner ear is housed deep within the temporal bone. The organs for hearing (cochlea) and balance (semicircular canals), as well as cranial nerves VII (facial nerve) and VIII (vestibulocochlear nerve), are all part of this complex anatomy (see Fig. 59-1). The cochlea and semicircular canals are housed in the bony labyrinth. The bony labyrinth surrounds and protects the membranous labyrinth, which is bathed in a fluid called *perilymph*.

Membranous Labyrinth

The membranous labyrinth is composed of the utricle, the saccule, the cochlear duct, the semicircular canals, and the organ of Corti, all of which are surrounded by a fluid called *endolymph*. The three semicircular canals—posterior, superior, and lateral, which lie at 90-degree angles to one another—contain sensory receptor organs that are arranged to detect rotational movement. These receptor end organs are stimulated by changes in the rate or direction of a person's movement. The utricle and saccule are involved with linear movements.

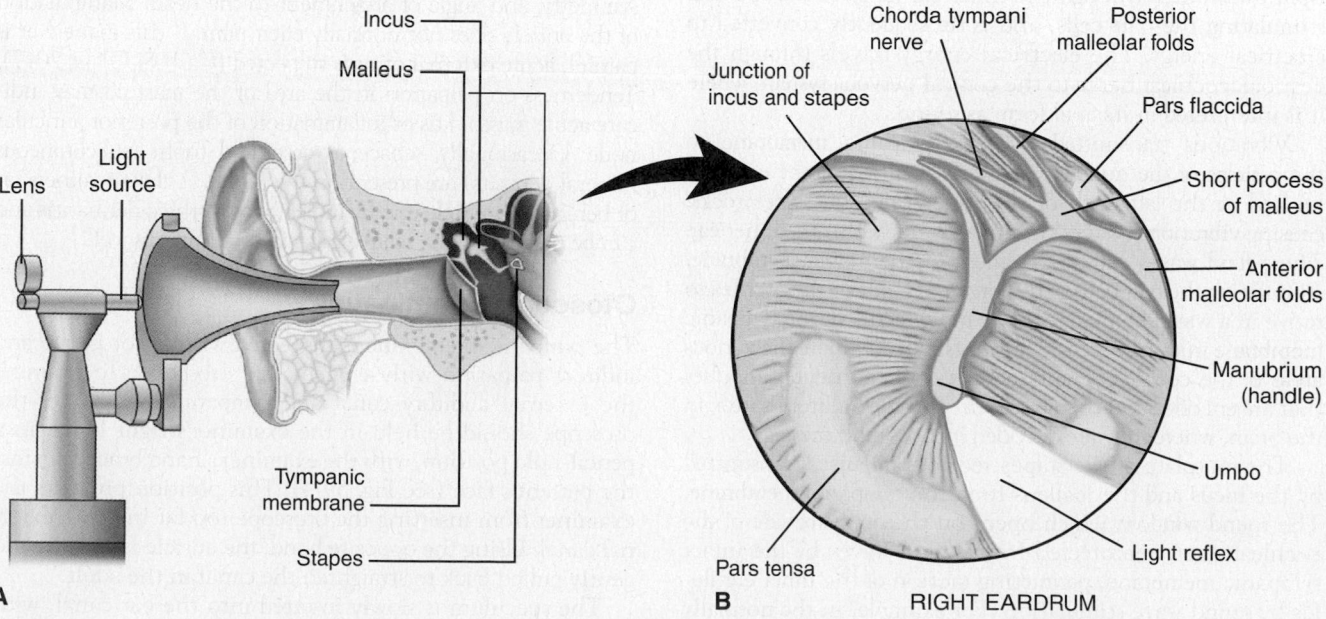

Figure 59-2 • Technique for using the otoscope (**A**) to see the tympanic membrane (**B**).

Organ of Corti

The organ of Corti is housed in the cochlea, a snail-shaped, bony tube about 3.5 cm long with two and a half spiral turns. Membranes separate the cochlear duct (scala media) from the scala vestibuli and the scala tympani from the basilar membrane. The organ of Corti is located on the basilar membrane that stretches from the base to the apex of the cochlea. As sound vibrations enter the perilymph at the oval window and travel along the scala vestibuli, they pass through the scala tympani, enter the cochlear duct, and cause movement of the basilar membrane. The organ of Corti, also referred to as the end organ for hearing, transforms mechanical energy into neural activity and separates sounds into different frequencies. This electrochemical impulse travels through the acoustic nerve to the temporal cortex of the brain to be interpreted as meaningful sound. In the internal auditory canal, the cochlear (acoustic) nerve, arising from the cochlea, joins the vestibular nerve, arising from the semicircular canals, utricle, and saccule, to become the vestibulocochlear nerve (cranial nerve VIII). This canal also houses the facial nerve and the blood supply from the ear to the brain.

Function of the Ears

Hearing

Hearing is conducted over two pathways: air and bone. Sounds transmitted by air conduction travel over the air-filled external and middle ear through vibration of the tympanic membrane and ossicles. Sounds transmitted by bone conduction travel directly through bone to the inner ear, bypassing the tympanic membrane and ossicles. Normally, air conduction is the more efficient pathway.

Sound Conduction and Transmission

Sound enters the ear through the external auditory canal and causes the tympanic membrane to vibrate. These vibrations transmit sound through the lever action of the ossicles to the oval window as mechanical energy. This mechanical energy is then transmitted through the inner ear fluids to the cochlea, stimulating the hair cells, and is subsequently converted to electrical energy. The electrical energy travels through the vestibulocochlear nerve to the central nervous system, where it is interpreted in its final form as sound.

Vibrations transmitted by the tympanic membrane to the ossicles of the middle ear are transmitted to the cochlea, located in the labyrinth of the inner ear. The stapes rocks, causing vibrations (waves) in fluids contained in the inner ear. These fluid waves cause movement of the basilar membrane, stimulating the hair cells of the organ of Corti in the cochlea to move in a wavelike manner. The movements of the tympanic membrane initiate electrical currents that stimulate the various areas of the cochlea. The hair cells generate neural impulses that are encoded and then transferred to the auditory cortex in the brain, where they are decoded into a sound message.

The footplate of the stapes receives impulses transmitted by the incus and the malleus from the tympanic membrane. The round window, which opens on the opposite side of the cochlear duct, is protected from sound waves by the intact tympanic membrane, permitting motion of the inner ear fluids by sound wave stimulation. For example, in the normally intact tympanic membrane, sound waves stimulate the oval window first, and a lag occurs before the terminal effect of the stimulus reaches the round window. However, this lag phase is changed when a perforation of the tympanic membrane allows sound waves to impinge on the oval and round windows simultaneously. This effect cancels the lag and prevents the maximal effect of inner ear fluid motility and its subsequent effect in stimulating the hair cells in the organ of Corti. The result is a reduction in hearing ability (see Fig. 59-3).

Bone conduction occurs by directly stimulating bones of the skull, which send sound to the inner ear. The way in which this occurs can be demonstrated by striking a tuning fork and placing it directly on the skull above the ear. Sound is transmitted to the inner ear.

Balance and Equilibrium

Body balance is maintained by cooperation of muscles and joints of the body (proprioceptive system), the eyes (visual system), and the labyrinth (vestibular system). These areas send their information about equilibrium, or balance, to the brain (cerebellar system) for coordination and perception in the cerebral cortex. The brain obtains its blood supply from the heart and arterial system. A problem in any of these areas, such as arteriosclerosis or impaired vision, can cause a disturbance of balance. The vestibular apparatus of the inner ear provides feedback regarding the movements and the position of the head and body in space.

Assessment

Assessment of hearing and balance involves inspection of the external, middle, and inner ear. Evaluation of gross hearing acuity also is included in every physical examination.

Inspection of the External Ear

Inspection of the external ear is a simple procedure, but it is often overlooked. The external ear is examined by inspection and direct palpation; the auricle and surrounding tissues should be inspected for deformities, lesions, and discharge, as well as size, symmetry, and angle of attachment to the head. Manipulation of the auricle does not normally elicit pain. If this maneuver is painful, acute external otitis is suspected (Cash & Glass, 2017). Tenderness on palpation in the area of the mastoid may indicate acute mastoiditis or inflammation of the posterior auricular node. Occasionally, sebaceous cysts and tophi (subcutaneous mineral deposits) are present on the pinna. A flaky scaliness on or behind the auricle usually indicates seborrheic dermatitis and can be present on the scalp and facial structures as well.

Otoscopic Examination

The tympanic membrane is inspected with an otoscope and indirect palpation with a pneumatic otoscope. To examine the external auditory canal and tympanic membrane, the otoscope should be held in the examiner's right hand, in a pencil-hold position, with the examiner's hand braced against the patient's face (see Fig. 59-4). This position prevents the examiner from inserting the otoscope too far into the external canal. Using the opposite hand, the auricle is grasped and gently pulled back to straighten the canal in the adult.

The speculum is slowly inserted into the ear canal, with the examiner's eye held close to the magnifying lens of the

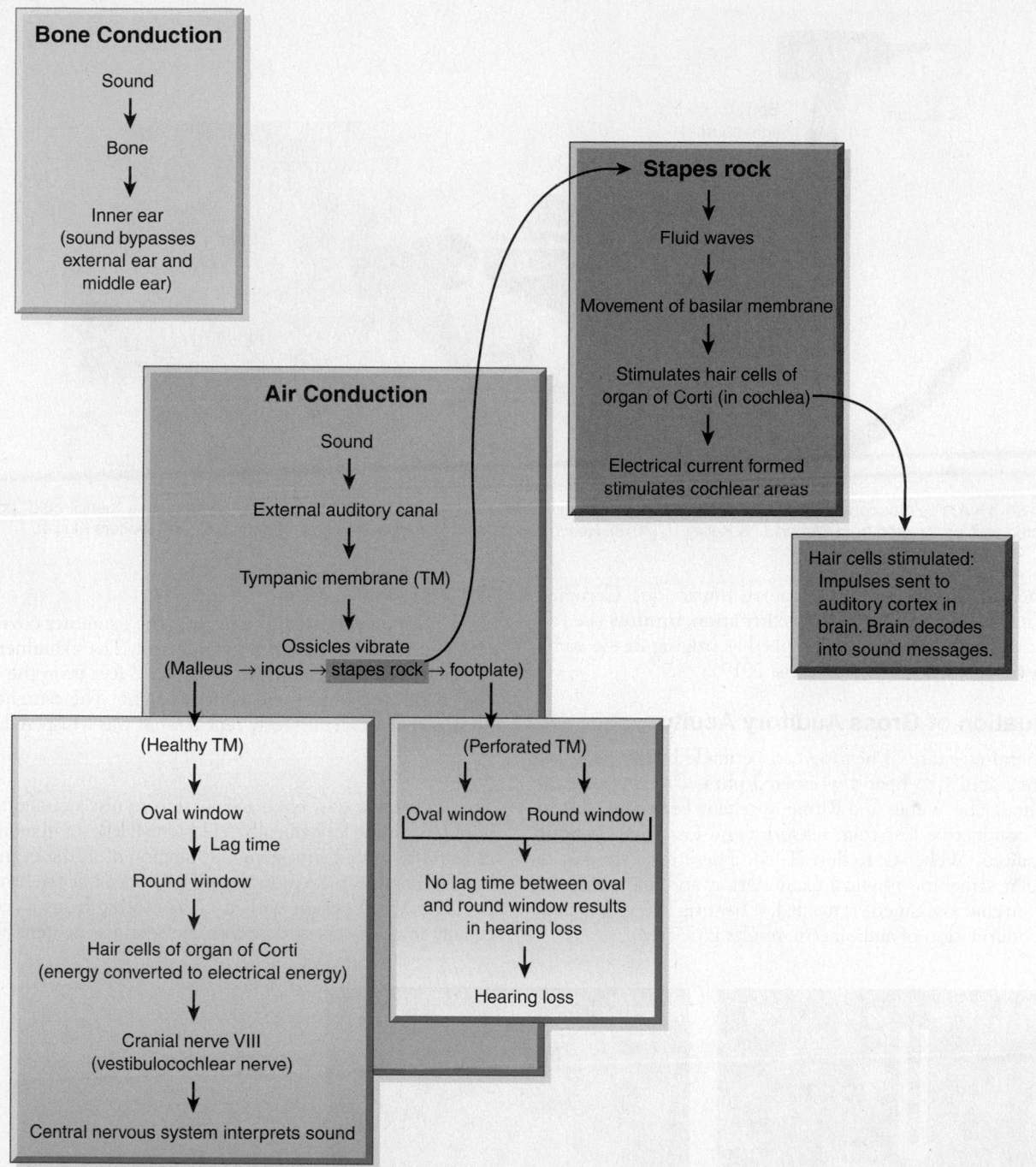

Figure 59-3 • Bone conduction compared to air conduction.

otoscope to visualize the canal and tympanic membrane. The largest speculum that the canal can accommodate (usually 5 mm in an adult) is guided gently down into the canal and slightly forward. Because the distal portion of the canal is bony and covered by a sensitive layer of epithelium, only light pressure can be used without causing pain. The external auditory canal is examined for discharge, inflammation, or a foreign body.

The healthy tympanic membrane is pearly gray and is positioned obliquely at the base of the canal. The following landmarks are identified, if visible (see Fig. 59-2): the pars tensa, the umbo, the manubrium of the malleus, and its short process.

A slow, circular movement of the speculum allows further visualization of the malleolar folds and periphery. The position and color of the membrane and any unusual markings or deviations from normal are documented. Presence of fluid, air bubbles, blood, or masses in the middle ear should also be noted.

Proper otoscopic examination of the external auditory canal and tympanic membrane requires that the canal be free of large amounts of cerumen. Cerumen is normally present in the external canal, and small amounts should not interfere with otoscopic examination. If the tympanic membrane cannot be visualized because of cerumen, the cerumen may be removed using several methods (see later discussion of

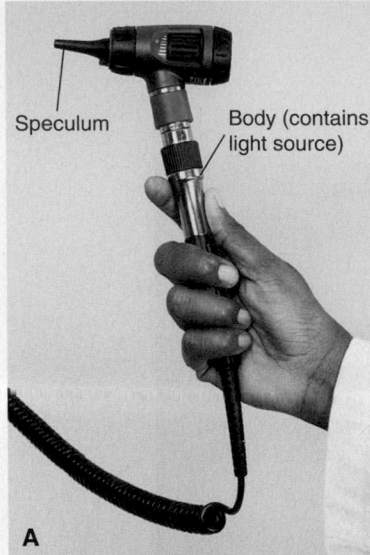

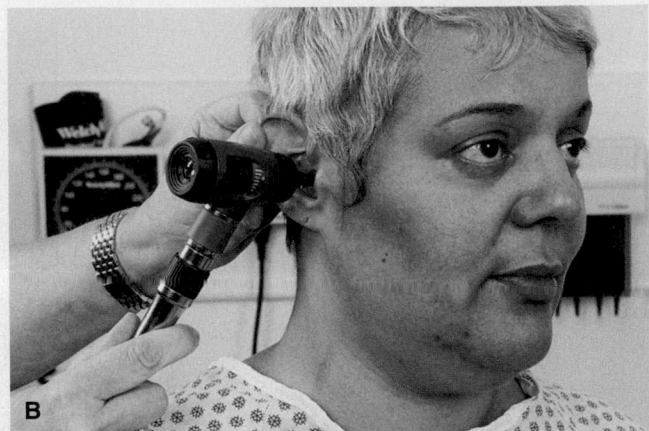

Speculum

Body (contains light source)

A

B

Figure 59-4 • **A.** The otoscope. **B.** Proper technique for examining the ear. Hold the otoscope in the right or left hand, in a "pencil-hold" position. Reprinted with permission from Weber, J., & Kelley, J. (2018). *Health assessment in nursing* (6th ed.). Philadelphia, PA: Wolters Kluwer.

cerumen removal in section Cerumen Impaction). Cerumen buildup is a common cause of local irritation, **tinnitus** (i.e., an unwanted noise commonly described as ringing in the ears), and reversible hearing loss (Norris, 2019).

Evaluation of Gross Auditory Acuity

A general estimate of hearing can be made by assessing the patient's ability to hear a whispered phrase, testing one ear at a time. The Weber and Rinne tests may be used to distinguish conductive loss from sensorineural loss when hearing is impaired (Weber & Kelley, 2018). These tests are part of a regular screening physical examination and are useful if a more specific assessment is needed, if hearing loss is detected, or if confirmation of audiometric results is desired.

Whisper Test

To exclude one ear from the testing, the examiner covers the untested ear with the palm of the hand. The examiner then whispers softly from a distance of 1 or 2 feet from the unoccluded ear and out of the patient's sight. The patient with normal acuity can correctly repeat what was whispered.

Weber Test

The Weber test uses bone conduction to test lateralization of sound. A tuning fork (ideally, 512 Hertz [Hz]), set in motion by grasping it firmly by its stem and tapping it on the examiner's knee or hand, is placed on the patient's head or forehead (see Fig. 59-5A). A person with normal hearing hears the sound equally in both ears or describes the sound as centered in the

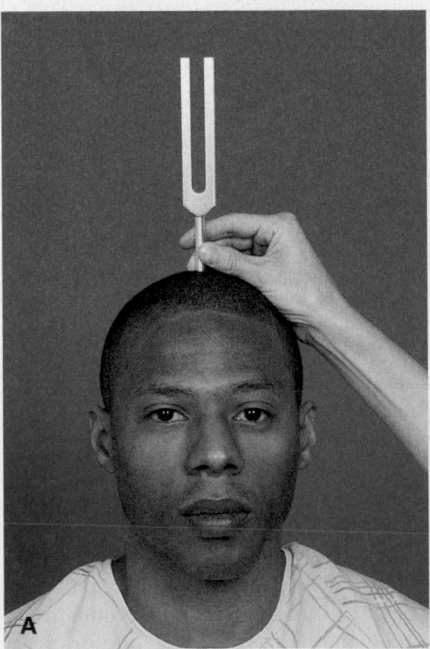

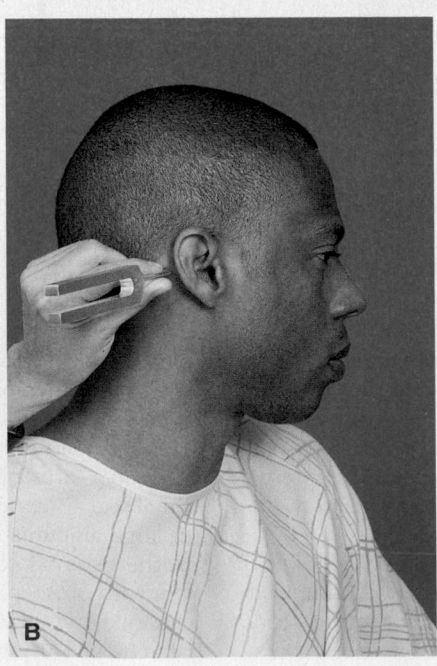

A

B

Figure 59-5 • **A.** The Weber test assesses bone conduction of sound. **B.** The Rinne test assesses both air and bone conduction of sound.

TABLE 59-1	Comparison of Weber and Rinne Tests	
Hearing Status	**Weber**	**Rinne**
Normal hearing	Sound is heard equally in both ears.	Air conduction is audible longer than bone conduction in both ears.
Conductive hearing loss	Sound is heard best in affected ear (hearing loss).	Sound is heard as long or longer in affected ear (hearing loss).
Sensorineural hearing loss	Sound is heard best in normal hearing ear.	Air conduction is audible longer than bone conduction in affected ear.

Adapted from Weber, J., & Kelley, J. (2018). *Health assessment in nursing* (6th ed.). Philadelphia, PA: Wolters Kluwer.

middle of the head. A person with conductive hearing loss, such as from otosclerosis or otitis media, hears the sound better in the affected ear. A person with sensorineural hearing loss, resulting from damage to the cochlear or vestibulocochlear nerve, hears the sound in the better-hearing ear. The Weber test is useful for detecting unilateral hearing loss (see Table 59-1).

Results of the Weber test are used to determine whether the patient has conductive hearing loss (sounds are heard better in the affected ear) or sensorineural hearing loss (sounds are heard better in the normal ear) (see later discussion of hearing loss).

Rinne Test

In the Rinne test (pronounced *rin-ay*), the examiner shifts the stem of a vibrating tuning fork between two positions: 2 inches from the opening of the ear canal (for air conduction) and against the mastoid bone (for bone conduction) (see Fig. 59-5B). As the position changes, the patient is asked to indicate which tone is louder or when the tone is no longer audible.

The Rinne test is useful for distinguishing between conductive and sensorineural hearing loss. A person with normal hearing reports that air-conducted sound is louder than bone-conducted sound. A person with a conductive hearing loss hears bone-conducted sound as long as or longer than air-conducted sound. A person with a sensorineural hearing loss hears air-conducted sound longer than bone-conducted sound.

Cultural Considerations

Deaf culture is distinguished with an uppercase *D*, whereas deafness as an audiologic condition is indicated by a lowercase *d*. In a sociocultural context, Deaf refers to individuals who were born with limited hearing or developed hearing loss before developing a spoken language and who use sign language (e.g., American Sign Language [ASL]) as their primary means of communication (Pendergrass, Newman, Jones, et al., 2019). Core cultural values include a sacred respect for and use of the hands, disassociation from speech, complete acceptance of being Deaf as a normal existence, full access to communication and information sharing, and self-determination (Holcomb, 2013; Padden, 1980).

According to the World Federation of the Deaf (World Federation of the Deaf [WFD], 2020), membership in the Deaf community depends on self-identification, acceptance of other members, and proficiency in a signed language. The Deaf community rejects the term *hearing-impaired* as demeaning and use of this term is discouraged (Holcomb, 2013; Moore & Levitan, 2016). Health professionals should be aware of individual differences and use the appropriate terminology when referring to Deaf, deaf, and people who are hard of hearing. Other appropriate terms used to identify Deaf people include Deaf signers, Deaf ASL users, or culturally Deaf adults.

Deaf and people who are hard of hearing are often hampered by communication barriers and an inadequate level of understanding about their language and culture by the hearing majority (Holcomb, 2013). When communicating with Deaf signers, nurses need to know that one's ability to speak is irrelevant and asking about the details of one's audiologic status is considered rude unless the individual offers this information (Mindess, 2014). Although a person who is deaf may have the ability to speak, it is important to remember that speech benefits the hearing population and the individual is in fact, deaf. As patient advocates, nurses should be mindful of the differences and similarities among Deaf signers, nonsigning deaf, and hard of hearing as well as their own beliefs about these differences and similarities (Lewis & Keele, 2020). See the Nursing Research Profile in Chart 59-1. Although various methods may be necessary, communication should always be based on patient preference.

Diagnostic Evaluation

Many diagnostic procedures are available to measure the auditory and vestibular systems indirectly. These tests are usually performed by a certified audiologist. The nurse educates the patient about the purpose, what to expect, and any possible side effects related to testing. The nurse notes trends in results because they provide information about disease progression as well as the patient's response to therapy.

Audiometry

In detecting hearing loss, audiometry is the single most important diagnostic instrument. Audiometric testing is of two kinds: pure-tone audiometry, in which the sound stimulus consists of a pure or musical tone (the louder the tone before the patient perceives it, the greater the hearing loss), and speech audiometry, in which the spoken word is used to determine the ability to hear and discriminate sounds and words.

When evaluating hearing, three characteristics are important: frequency, pitch, and intensity. *Frequency* refers to the number of sound waves emanating from a source per second, measured as cycles per second, or Hertz. The normal human ear perceives sounds ranging in frequency from 20 to 20,000 Hz. The frequencies from 500 to 2000 Hz are important in understanding everyday speech and are referred to as the speech range or speech frequencies. *Pitch* is the term used to describe frequency; a tone with 100 Hz is considered of low pitch, and a tone of 10,000 Hz is considered of high pitch.

The unit for measuring loudness (*intensity* of sound) is the decibel (dB), the pressure exerted by sound. Hearing loss is measured in decibels—a logarithmic function of intensity that is not easily converted into a percentage. The critical level of loudness is approximately 30 dB. The shuffling of papers in quiet surroundings is about 15 dB; a low conversation, 40 dB; and a jet plane 100 feet away, about 150 dB.

Chart 59-1 NURSING RESEARCH PROFILE
Nurses' Beliefs Toward Deaf and Hard of Hearing Interaction

Lewis, A., & Keele, R. (2020). Development and validation of instrument to measure nurses' beliefs toward Deaf and hard of hearing interaction. *Journal of Nursing Measurement, 28*(2). doi: 10.1891/JNM-D-19-00024

Purpose

Nurse–patient communication has a significant effect on health outcomes and quality of care. Investigating what nurses believe about interacting with Deaf signers, nonsigning deaf, and hard of hearing patients is an important step in minimizing barriers and improving nursing care. The purpose of this research was to develop and test the validity and reliability of an instrument to measure registered nurses' (RNs) beliefs toward interaction with patients who are Deaf signers, nonsigning deaf, and hard of hearing, as well as with certified interpreters.

Design

This study used a quantitative methodologic design.

Findings

Noteworthy findings were associated with the social constructs of power and control. Participant responses strongly indicated the belief that it is acceptable to relinquish the autonomy and self-determination of a Deaf signer, a nonsigning deaf, or a hard of hearing person to a hearing person. This belief is apparent in at least 65% of respondents from three groups of RNs who agreed that "questions or responses for a person who is a Deaf signer, a nonsigning deaf, or hard of hearing should be directed to hearing family members" and at least 60% of respondents from both groups of RNs agreed that "during health care interactions, most Deaf signers prefer to get by without a certified interpreter."

Data collection and analyses resulted in a 25-item D/deaf and Hard of Hearing Interaction Beliefs Scale for Registered Nurses. Psychometric analysis of two separate groups of data concluded that the newly developed scale is a reliable and valid scale to measure nurses' beliefs toward interaction with patients who are either Deaf signers, nonsigning deaf, or hard of hearing. Results of confirmatory factor analysis supported the hypothesized structure of the scale and provided some evidence for its factorial validity.

Nursing Implications

Understanding the beliefs that nurses hold toward interactions with Deaf signers, nonsigning deaf, and hard of hearing persons may shed light on nurses' general beliefs toward individuals who are Deaf signers, nonsigning deaf, and hard of hearing. Furthermore, these beliefs may influence nurses' views about the importance of appropriate and effective interaction with patients who have diverse communication needs. This understanding can lead to the development of standards of practice and organizational policies that reflect federal laws mandating equal communication access for all. Attention to equal communication access can create a nursing culture that views communication diversity not as a barrier, but as an opportunity to open doors and promote every patient's right to autonomy and self-determination.

Sound louder than 80 dB is perceived by the human ear to be harsh and can be damaging to the inner ear. Table 59-2 classifies hearing loss based on decibel level. In surgical treatment of patients with hearing loss, the aim is to improve the hearing level to 30 dB or better within the speech frequencies.

With audiometry, the patient wears earphones and signals to the audiologist when a tone is heard. When the tone is applied directly over the external auditory canal, air conduction is measured. When the stimulus is applied to the mastoid bone, bypassing the conductive mechanism (i.e., the ossicles), nerve conduction is tested. For accuracy, testing is performed in a soundproof room. Responses are plotted on a graph known as an audiogram, which differentiates conductive from sensorineural hearing loss.

TABLE 59-2 Severity of Hearing Loss

Loss in Decibels	Interpretation
0–15	Normal hearing
>15–25	Slight hearing loss
>25–40	Mild hearing loss
>40–55	Moderate hearing loss
>55–70	Moderate to severe hearing loss
>70–90	Severe hearing loss
>90	Profound hearing loss

Tympanogram

A tympanogram, or impedance audiometry, measures middle ear muscle reflex to sound stimulation and compliance of the tympanic membrane by changing the air pressure in a sealed ear canal. Compliance is impaired with middle ear disease.

Auditory Brain Stem Response Audiometry

The auditory brain stem response (ABR) audiometry is a detectable electrical potential from cranial nerve VIII and the ascending auditory pathways of the brain stem in response to sound stimulation. Electrodes are placed on the patient's scalp and on each earlobe (Fischbach & Fischbach, 2018). Acoustic stimuli (e.g., clicks) are made in the ear. The resulting electrophysiologic measurements can determine at which decibel level a patient hears and whether there are any impairments along the nerve pathways (e.g., tumor on cranial nerve VIII). Patients are instructed to wash and rinse their hair prior to this study but to avoid applying any other hair product. ABR audiometry assessment should be used in conjunction with behavioral audiometry for the most accurate results (Bhattacharyya, 2017).

Electronystagmography

Electronystagmography is the measurement and graphic recording of the changes in electrical potentials created by eye movements during spontaneous, positional, or calorically evoked nystagmus (see discussion of nystagmus later in this chapter). It is also used to assess the oculomotor and vestibular systems and their corresponding interaction. It helps to diagnose causes of unilateral hearing loss of unknown origin, vertigo, or tinnitus.

Any vestibular suppressants, such as caffeine and alcohol, are withheld for 48 hours before testing. Medications such as tranquilizers, stimulants, or antivertigo agents are withheld for 5 days before the test (Fischbach & Fischbach, 2018).

Platform Posturography

Platform posturography is recommended for patients with dizziness and balance disorders (American Academy of Otolaryngology—Head and Neck Surgery, 2014). It can be used to determine if a patient's vertigo is worsening or to evaluate a patient's response to treatment. The integration of visual, vestibular, and proprioceptive cues (i.e., sensory integration) with motor response output and coordination of the lower limbs is tested. The patient stands on a platform, surrounded by a screen, and different conditions such as a moving platform with a moving screen or a stationary platform with a moving screen are presented. The responses from the patient are measured and indicate which of the anatomic systems may be impaired. Preparation for the testing is the same as for electronystagmography.

Sinusoidal Harmonic Acceleration

Sinusoidal harmonic acceleration, or a rotary chair, is used to assess the vestibuloocular system by analyzing compensatory eye movements in response to the clockwise and counterclockwise rotation of the chair. Although such testing cannot identify the side of the lesion in unilateral disease, it helps to identify the disease (e.g., Ménière's disease and tumors of the auditory canal) and evaluate the course of recovery. The same patient preparation is required as that for electronystagmography.

Middle Ear Endoscopy

Using instruments called endoscopes that have very small diameters and acute angles, the ear can be examined by an endoscopist specializing in otolaryngology. Middle ear endoscopy is performed safely and effectively as an office procedure to evaluate suspected perilymphatic fistula and new-onset conductive hearing loss, the anatomy of the round window before transtympanic treatment of Ménière's disease, and the tympanic cavity before ear surgery to treat chronic middle ear and mastoid infections.

The tympanic membrane is anesthetized topically for about 10 minutes before the procedure. Then, the external auditory canal is irrigated with sterile normal saline solution. With the aid of a microscope, a tympanotomy is created with a laser beam or a myringotomy knife so that the endoscope can be inserted into the middle ear cavity. Video and photo documentation can be accomplished through the scope.

HEARING LOSS

In the United States, hearing loss has been reported to occur in approximately 2 to 3 of every 1000 births (U.S. Department of Health and Human Services [HHS], 2016). More than half of the 4000 infants born deaf each year have a hereditary disorder associated with genetic sensorineural hearing loss (Antonio, 2018). Genetic syndromes associated with hearing impairment include Waardenburg syndrome, Usher syndrome, Pendred syndrome, and Jervell and Lange-Nielsen syndrome (Antonio, 2018). Chart 59-2 contains

---

Chart 59-2 · GENETICS IN NURSING PRACTICE

Hearing Disorders

Several hearing disorders are associated with genetic mutations and have various patterns of inheritance:

Autosomal dominant:

- Branchiootorenal syndrome
- Neurofibromatosis type 2
- Otosclerosis
- Stickler syndrome
- Waardenburg syndrome

Autosomal recessive:

- Connexin 26 gene hearing loss (majority of cases are recessive; however, there is an autosomal dominant form that occurs less commonly)
- Jervell and Lange-Nielsen syndrome
- Pendred syndrome
- Refsum disease
- Usher syndrome

X-linked syndromic hearing loss:

- Alport syndrome

Nursing Assessments

Refer to Chapter 4, Chart 4-2: Genetics in Nursing Practice: Genetic Aspects of Health Assessment

Family History Assessment Specific to Hearing Loss

- Assess for other family members in several generations with hearing loss (autosomal dominant hearing loss).

- Inquire about genetic relatedness (e.g., individuals who are related, such as first cousins, have a higher chance to share the same recessive genes—autosomal recessive hearing loss).
- Inquire about age at onset of hearing loss.

Patient Assessment Specific to Genetic-Related Hearing Loss

- Assess for:
  - Dizziness
  - Facial numbness or weakness
  - Headaches
  - Tinnitus
- Assess for related genetic conditions, such as vision impairment (e.g., retinitis pigmentosa in Usher syndrome; thyroid disorder in Pendred syndrome).
- Assess for iris, pigment, and hair alterations (white forelock) seen in Waardenburg syndrome.
- Assess for exposure to loud noises (e.g., industrial).
- Assess for presence of rubella, toxoplasmosis, herpes, or cytomegalovirus during pregnancy.
- Determine if patient had taken medications associated with ototoxicity.

Genetics Resources

Genetics of Hearing Loss, www.cdc.gov/ncbddd/hearingloss/genetics.html
Hear-It, www.Hear-it.org/Genetic-hearing-loss
Neurofibromatosis Network, www.nfnetwork.org/
See Chapter 6, Chart 6-7 for components of genetic counseling.

more information about hearing disorders that have a genetic cause. Hearing loss may also be acquired; causes include TORCH infections (TOxoplasmosis, Rubella, Cytomegalovirus, Herpes) during pregnancy as well as trauma or chronic exposure to loud noise (Antonio, 2018). Most hospitals or birthing centers offer universal hearing screenings for newborns after birth and prior to discharge.

Hearing loss occurs in men more often than in women. Approximately 2% of adults between the ages of 45 and 54 years have disabling hearing loss. This percentage increases to 8.5% in the 55 to 64 age group, to 25% of adults in the 65 to 74 age group, and up to 50% for those over 75 years of age (HHS, 2016). Hearing loss is an important health issue; and as people age, hearing screening and treatment are recommended.

Many people are exposed on a daily basis to noise levels that produce high-frequency hearing loss. Occupations such as carpentry, plumbing, and coal mining have the highest risk of noise-induced hearing loss. Wise Ears was developed by the National Institute on Deafness and Other Communication Disorders (NIDCD) and the National Institute for Occupational Safety and Health (NIOSH). It aims to educate the public about noise-induced hearing loss and ways to prevent this hearing loss (NIDCD, 2010).

Conductive hearing loss usually results from an external ear disorder, such as impacted cerumen, or a middle ear disorder, such as otitis media or otosclerosis. In such instances, the efficient transmission of sound by air to the inner ear is interrupted. A **sensorineural hearing loss** involves damage to the cochlea or vestibulocochlear nerve.

Mixed hearing loss and functional hearing loss also may occur. Patients with mixed hearing loss have conductive loss and sensorineural loss, resulting from dysfunction of air and bone conduction. A functional (or psychogenic) hearing loss is nonorganic and unrelated to detectable structural changes in the hearing mechanisms; it is usually a manifestation of an emotional reaction.

Clinical Manifestations

Deafness is the partial or complete loss of the ability to hear. Early manifestations may include tinnitus, increasing inability to hear when in a group, and a need to turn up the volume of the television. Hearing loss can also trigger changes in attitude, the ability to communicate, the awareness of surroundings, and even the ability to protect oneself, thus affecting a person's quality of life. In a classroom, a student with hearing loss may be uninterested and inattentive and have failing grades. A pedestrian with hearing loss may attempt to cross the street and fail to hear an approaching car. People with hearing loss may miss parts of conversations, and may gradually interact with others less, leading to feelings of isolation. Many people are unaware of their gradual hearing loss. Often, it is not the person with the hearing loss but the people with whom they are communicating that recognizes the change (see Chart 59-3).

For various reasons, some people with hearing loss refuse to seek medical attention or wear a hearing aid. They may feel self-conscious about wearing a hearing aid. Other people, however, may feel comfortable asking those with whom they are trying to communicate to let them know whether

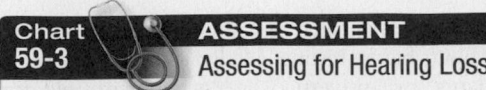

Chart 59-3   **ASSESSMENT**
Assessing for Hearing Loss

The nurse should be alert to the following:

Speech deterioration: The person who slurs words, drops word endings, or produces flat-sounding speech may not be hearing correctly. Hearing guides the voice, both in loudness and in pronunciation.

Fatigue: If a person tires easily when listening to conversation or to a speech, fatigue may be the result of straining to hear. Under these circumstances, a person may become easily irritable.

Indifference: It is easy for the person who cannot hear what others say to become depressed and disinterested in life in general.

Social withdrawal: Not being able to hear what is going on causes a person who is hard of hearing to withdraw from situations that might prove embarrassing.

Insecurity: Lack of self-confidence and fear of mistakes create a feeling of insecurity in many people who are hard of hearing. No one likes to say the wrong thing or do anything that might appear foolish.

Indecision and procrastination: Loss of self-confidence makes it increasingly difficult for a person who is hard of hearing to make decisions.

Suspiciousness: The person who is hard of hearing—who often hears only part of what is being said—may suspect that others are talking about them, or that portions of the conversation are deliberately spoken softly so that they will not hear them.

False pride: The person who is hard of hearing wants to conceal the hearing loss and thus often pretends to be hearing when they actually is not.

Loneliness and unhappiness: Although everyone wishes for quiet now and then, enforced silence can be boring and even somewhat frightening. People with a hearing loss often feel isolated.

Tendency to dominate the conversation: Many people who are hard of hearing tend to dominate the conversation, knowing that as long as it is centered on them and they can control it, they are unlikely to be embarrassed by some mistake.

difficulties in communication exist. The attitudes and behaviors of patients who need hearing assistance should be taken into account when counseling them. The decision to wear a hearing aid is a personal one that is affected by these attitudes and behaviors.

Prevention

Many environmental factors have an adverse effect on the auditory system and with time result in permanent sensorineural hearing loss. The most common is noise. Noise (unwanted and unavoidable sound) has been identified as one of today's environmental hazards. The volume of noise that surrounds us daily has increased into a potentially dangerous source of physical and psychological damage.

Loud, persistent noise has been found to cause constriction of peripheral blood vessels, increased blood pressure and heart rate (because of increased secretion of adrenalin), and increased gastrointestinal activity. Although research is needed to address the overall effects of noise on the human body, a quiet environment is more conducive to peace of mind. A person who is ill feels more at ease when noise is kept to a minimum.

Numerous factors contribute to hearing loss (see Chart 59-4). *Noise-induced hearing loss* refers to hearing loss that follows a long period of exposure to loud noise (e.g., heavy machinery, engines, artillery, rock-band music). *Acoustic trauma* refers to hearing loss caused by a single exposure to an extremely intense noise, such as an explosion. Usually, noise-induced hearing loss occurs at a high frequency (about 4000 Hz). However, with continued noise exposure, the hearing loss can become more severe and include adjacent frequencies. The minimum noise level known to cause noise-induced hearing loss, regardless of duration, is about 85 to 90 dB.

Noise exposure is inherent in many jobs (e.g., mechanics, printers, pilots, flight attendants, musicians) and in hobbies such as woodworking and hunting. Occupational noise level regulations are based on the amount of noise a person is exposed to over an 8-hour work shift, with the maximum legal limits being 85 dB per the NIOSH or 90 dB per the Occupational Safety and Health Administration (OSHA), with a peak sound pressure of 135 dB (Centers for Disease Control and Prevention [CDC], 2018). NIOSH recommends and OSHA requires that workers wear ear protection to prevent noise-induced hearing loss when exposed to noise above the legal limits. Ear protection against noise is the most effective preventive measure available. Hearing loss due to noise is permanent because the hair cells in the organ of Corti are destroyed.

Gerontologic Considerations

With aging, changes occur in the ear that may eventually lead to hearing deficits. Although few changes occur in the external ear, cerumen tends to become harder and drier, posing a greater chance of impaction. In the middle ear, the tympanic membrane may atrophy or become sclerotic. In the inner ear, cells at the base of the cochlea degenerate. A familial predisposition to sensorineural hearing loss is also seen, manifested by inability to hear high-frequency sounds, followed in time by the loss of middle and lower frequencies. The term **presbycusis** is used to describe this progressive hearing loss (Eliopoulos, 2018).

In addition to age-related changes, other factors can affect hearing in the older adult population, such as lifelong exposure to loud noises. Psychogenic factors, other disease processes (e.g., diabetes), and medications may be partially responsible for sensorineural hearing loss. Certain medications, such as aminoglycosides, aspirin, loop diuretics, and platinum-based antineoplastic medications have ototoxic effects when kidney changes result in delayed medication excretion and increased levels of the medications in the blood.

Even with the best health care, people with hearing loss must learn to adjust. Care of older patients includes recognizing emotional reactions related to hearing loss, such as suspicion of others because of an inability to hear adequately; frustration and anger, with repeated statements such as "I didn't hear what you said!"; and feelings of insecurity because of the inability to hear the telephone or alarms. The Americans with Disabilities Act (ADA) of 1990 requires that all emergency services are accessible to people who have text message telephones (teletypewriters [TTYs]). In addition, all 911 centers in the United States must be accessible to people with TTYs.

Depression, isolation, and a decrease in cognitive function can have a negative impact on quality of life in the older adult with hearing loss. Feelings of social isolation, confusion, alterations in daily living activities, and increasing risk of falls have all been associated with hearing loss in older adults (Shukla, Reed, Armstrong, et al., 2019). Hearing loss has also been identified as a factor associated with a significant increase in the risk of hospitalization, readmission, and increased mortality (Hsu, McKee, Roscigno, et al., 2019). Additionally, hearing loss can interfere with relationships due to a loss of communication. A hearing screening is recommended as one component of the physical examination for the older adult when joining Medicare for the first time. "Welcome to Medicare" examinations and annual screenings are also important.

Medical Management

If a hearing loss is permanent or untreatable or if the patient elects not to be treated, aural rehabilitation (discussed at the end of the chapter) may be beneficial.

Nursing Management

Early detection of hearing loss is in the plans for *Healthy People 2030*, and nurses are in a position to assist in meeting this goal if included (Haskins, 2017; HHS, 2017). Another possible objective is for people diagnosed with hearing loss or deafness to use rehabilitation services and supplemental devices to improve communication with hearing people. Resources are available in workplaces and in schools. Questions used to assess for hearing loss may include:

- Have you experienced any hearing loss in the past?
- Are you experiencing any hearing loss now?
- Do your family members think that you are having difficulty hearing or experiencing any hearing loss?

These questions should be included in any routine nursing assessment and referrals made for further evaluation as needed.

Nurses who understand the different types of hearing loss are more successful in adopting a communication style to fit the needs and preferences of each patient. Trying to speak in a loud voice to a person who cannot hear high-frequency sounds only makes understanding more difficult. However, strategies such as talking into the better-hearing ear and using gestures and facial expressions can help (see Chart 59-5).

Communicating with People Who Are Deaf or Have Severe Hearing Loss

For the Person Who Is Hard of Hearing Whose Speech Is Difficult to Understand

- Determine how the person prefers to communicate with others. Do not assume that writing, gestures, or other means are the best or preferred technique.
- Consider if the person uses sign language. Interpreters are available from American Sign Language Services, Inc. (ASLI). These specialists provide the best means of communication, providing accurate, professional services.
- Devote full attention to what the person is saying. Look and listen—do not try to attend to another task while listening.
- Engage the speaker in conversation when it is possible for you to anticipate the replies. This enables you to become accustomed to any peculiarities in speech patterns.
- Try to determine the essential context of what is being said; you can often fill in the details from context.
- Do not try to appear as if you understand if you do not.
- If you cannot understand at all or have serious doubt about your ability to understand what is being said, have the person write the message rather than risk misunderstanding. Having the person repeat the message in speech, after you know its content, also aids you in becoming accustomed to the person's pattern of speech.
- Written communication is an excellent resource. Material should be written at a third-grade level so that the majority of people can understand it.

For the Person Who Is Hard of Hearing Who Speech Reads

- Be aware that speech or lip reading is ineffective because the majority of English sounds are not clearly visible on the lips and even the most proficient lip readers understand less than 30% of verbal communication.
- When speaking, always face the person as directly as possible.
- Make sure that your face is as clearly visible as possible. Locate yourself so that your face is well lighted; avoid being silhouetted against strong light. Do not obscure the person's view of your mouth in any way; avoid talking with any object held in your mouth.
- Be sure that the patient knows the topic or subject before going ahead with what you plan to say. This enables the person to use contextual clues in speech reading.
- Speak slowly and distinctly, pausing more frequently than you would normally.
- If you question whether some important direction or instruction has been understood, check to be certain that the patient has the full meaning of your message.
- If, for any reason, your mouth must be covered (as with a mask), you must direct or instruct the patient, write or communicate the message by another means.

A major issue for many people who are deaf or hard of hearing is that they have other health problems that often do not receive attention, in large part because of communication barriers with their health care providers. To meet the health care needs of these patients, providers are legally obligated to make accommodations for the most effective patient communication and understanding. Providing certified interpreters for those who can communicate through sign language is essential in many situations to ensure effective communication.

During health care and screening procedures, the provider (e.g., dentist, physician, nurse) must be aware that patients who are deaf or hard of hearing are unable to read lips, see a signer, or read written materials in the dark rooms required during some diagnostic tests. The same situation exists if the provider is wearing a mask or is not in sight (e.g., x-ray studies, magnetic resonance imaging [MRI], colonoscopy).

Nurses and other health care providers must work with patients who are deaf or hard of hearing and their families to identify practical and effective means of communication. Nurses can serve as catalysts throughout the health care system to ensure that accommodations are made to meet the communication needs of every patient.

CONDITIONS OF THE EXTERNAL EAR

Cerumen Impaction

Cerumen normally accumulates in the external canal in various amounts and colors. Although wax does not usually need to be removed, impaction occasionally occurs, causing **otalgia** (a sensation of fullness or pain in the ear) with or without a hearing loss. Accumulation of cerumen as a cause of hearing loss is especially significant in older adult patients (Eliopoulos, 2018). Attempts to clear the external auditory canal with matches, hairpins, and other implements are dangerous because trauma to the skin, infection, and damage to the tympanic membrane can occur.

Management

Cerumen can be removed by irrigation, suction, or instrumentation. Unless the patient has a perforated eardrum or an inflamed external ear (i.e., otitis externa), gentle irrigation with warm water usually helps remove impacted cerumen, particularly if it is not tightly packed in the external auditory canal. For successful removal, the water stream must flow behind the obstructing cerumen to move it first laterally and then out of the canal. To prevent injury, the lowest effective pressure should be used. However, if the eardrum behind the impaction is perforated, water can enter the middle ear, producing acute vertigo and infection. If irrigation is unsuccessful, direct visual, mechanical removal can be performed by a trained health care provider on a patient who is cooperative.

> ### Quality and Safety Nursing Alert
>
> *Warm water (never cold or hot) and gentle (not forceful) irrigation should be used to remove cerumen. Irrigation that is too forceful can cause perforation of the tympanic membrane, and ice water causes vomiting.*

Instilling a few drops of warmed glycerin, mineral oil, or half-strength hydrogen peroxide into the ear canal for 30 minutes prior to irrigation can soften cerumen before its removal. Ceruminolytic agents, such as peroxide in glyceryl, are available. The use of any softening solution two or three times a day for several days is generally sufficient. If cerumen cannot be dislodged by these methods, instruments, such as a cerumen curette, aural suction, and a binocular microscope for magnification, can be used. The use of instruments such as a cerumen curette for cerumen removal is reserved for otolaryngologists and nurses with specialized training because of the danger of perforating the tympanic membrane or excoriating the external auditory canal.

Foreign Bodies

Some objects are inserted intentionally into the ear by adults who may have been trying to clean the external canal or relieve itching, or by children who introduce peas, beans, pebbles, toys, and beads. Insects may also enter the ear canal. In either case, the effects may range from no symptoms to profound pain and decreased hearing.

Management

Removing a foreign body from the external auditory canal can be quite challenging. The three standard methods for removing foreign bodies are the same as those for removing cerumen: irrigation, suction, and instrumentation. The contraindications for irrigation are also the same. Foreign vegetable bodies and insects tend to swell; thus, irrigation is contraindicated. Usually, an insect can be dislodged by instilling mineral oil, which will kill the insect and allow it to be removed.

Attempts to remove a foreign body from the external canal may be dangerous in unskilled hands. The object may be pushed completely into the bony portion of the canal, lacerating the skin and perforating the tympanic membrane. In rare circumstances, the foreign body may have to be extracted in the operating room with the patient under general anesthesia.

External Otitis (Otitis Externa)

External otitis (i.e., otitis externa) refers to an inflammation of the external auditory canal. Causes include water in the ear canal (swimmer's ear); trauma to the skin of the ear canal, permitting entrance of organisms into the tissues; and systemic conditions, such as vitamin deficiency and endocrine disorders. Bacterial or fungal infections are most frequently encountered. The most common bacterial pathogens associated with external otitis are *Staphylococcus aureus* and *Pseudomonas* species. The most common fungus isolated in both normal and infected ears is *Aspergillus* (Norris, 2019). External otitis is often caused by a dermatosis such as psoriasis, eczema, or seborrheic dermatitis. Even allergic reactions to hair spray, hair dye, and permanent wave lotions can cause dermatitis, which clears when the offending agent is removed.

Clinical Manifestations

Patients usually report pain; discharge from the external auditory canal; aural tenderness (usually not present in middle ear infections); and occasionally fever, cellulitis, and lymphadenopathy. Other symptoms may include pruritus and hearing loss or a feeling of fullness in the ear. On otoscopic examination, the ear canal is erythematous and edematous. Discharge may be yellow or green and foul smelling. In fungal infections, hairlike black spores may be visible.

Medical Management

The principles of therapy are aimed at relieving the discomfort, reducing the swelling of the ear canal, and eradicating the infection. Patients may require analgesic medications for the first 48 to 96 hours. Treatment most often includes antimicrobial or antifungal otic medications given by dropper at room temperature. In bacterial infection, a combination antibiotic and corticosteroid agent may be used to soothe inflamed tissues (Norris, 2019).

Nursing Management

Nurses should instruct patients not to clean the external auditory canal with cotton-tipped applicators and to avoid events that traumatize the external canal, such as scratching the canal with the fingernail or other objects. Trauma may lead to infection of the canal. Patients should also avoid getting the canal wet when swimming or shampooing the hair. A cotton ball or lamb's wool can be covered in a water-insoluble gel such as petrolatum jelly and placed in the ear as a barrier to the canal getting wet. Infection can be prevented by using antiseptic otic preparations after swimming (e.g., Swim-Ear, Ear Dry), unless there is a history of tympanic membrane perforation or a current ear infection (see Chart 59-6).

Malignant External Otitis

A more serious, although rare, external ear infection is malignant external otitis (temporal bone osteomyelitis). This is a progressive, debilitating, and occasionally fatal infection of the external auditory canal, the surrounding tissue, and the base of the skull. *Pseudomonas aeruginosa* is usually the infecting organism in patients with low resistance to infection (e.g., patients with acquired immune deficiency syndrome (AIDS). Successful treatment includes administration of antibiotics (usually intravenously [IV]) and aggressive local wound care.

Chart 59-6

PATIENT EDUCATION
Prevention of Otitis Externa

The nurse instructs the patient to:

- protect the external canal when swimming, showering, or washing hair. Use ear plugs or place a cotton ball covered in petrolatum jelly in the ear, and wear a swim cap. The external canal may be dried afterward with a hair dryer on low heat.
- place alcohol drops in the external canal to act as an astringent to help prevent infection after water exposure.
- prevent trauma to the external canal. Procedures, foreign objects (e.g., bobby pin), scratching, or any other trauma to the canal that breaks the skin integrity may cause infection.
- be aware that if otitis externa is diagnosed, refrain from any water sport activity for approximately 7 to 10 days to allow the canal to heal completely. Recurrence is highly likely unless you allow the external canal to heal completely.

Standard parenteral antibiotic treatment includes the combination of an antipseudomonal agent and an aminoglycoside, both of which have potentially serious side effects. Because aminoglycosides are nephrotoxic and ototoxic, serum aminoglycoside levels and kidney and auditory function must be monitored during therapy. Local wound care includes limited débridement of the infected tissue, including bone and cartilage, depending on the extent of the infection.

Masses of the External Ear

Exostoses are small, hard, bony protrusions found in the lower posterior bony portion of the ear canal; they usually occur bilaterally. The skin covering the exostosis is normal. It is believed that exostoses are caused by exposure to cold water, as in scuba diving or surfing. The usual treatment, if any, is surgical excision.

Malignant tumors also may occur in the external ear. Most common are basal cell carcinomas on the pinna and squamous cell carcinomas in the ear canal. If untreated, squamous cell carcinoma may spread through the temporal bone, causing facial nerve paralysis and hearing loss. Carcinomas must be treated surgically.

CONDITIONS OF THE MIDDLE EAR

Tympanic Membrane Perforation

Perforation of the tympanic membrane is usually caused by infection or trauma. Sources of trauma include skull fracture, injury from explosion, or a severe blow to the ear. Less frequently, perforation is caused by foreign objects (e.g., cotton-tipped applicators, hairpins, keys) that have been pushed too far into the external auditory canal. In addition to tympanic membrane perforation, injury to the ossicles and even the inner ear may result from this type of trauma. During infection, the tympanic membrane can rupture if the pressure in the middle ear exceeds the atmospheric pressure in the external auditory canal.

Medical Management

Although most tympanic membrane perforations heal spontaneously within weeks after rupture, some may take several months to heal. Some perforations persist because scar tissue grows over the edges of the perforation, preventing extension of the epithelial cells across the margins and final healing. In the case of a head injury or temporal bone fracture, a patient is observed for evidence of cerebrospinal fluid **otorrhea** or **rhinorrhea**—a clear, watery drainage from the ear or nose, respectively. While healing, the ear must be protected from water entering the ear canal.

Surgical Management

Perforations that do not heal on their own may require surgery. The decision to perform a tympanoplasty (see later section in this chapter) is usually based on the need to prevent potential infection from water entering the ear or the desire to improve the patient's hearing. Performed on an outpatient basis, tympanoplasty may involve a variety of surgical techniques. In all techniques, tissue (commonly from the temporalis fascia) is placed across the perforation to allow healing.

Surgery is usually successful in closing the perforation permanently and improving hearing.

Acute Otitis Media

Ear infections can occur at any age; however, they are most commonly seen in children. **Acute otitis media (AOM)** is an acute infection of the middle ear, lasting less than 6 weeks. Pathogens that cause AOM are usually bacterial or viral and enter the middle ear after eustachian tube dysfunction caused by obstruction related to upper respiratory infections, inflammation of surrounding structures (e.g., rhinosinusitis, adenoid hypertrophy), or allergic reactions (e.g., allergic rhinitis) (Norris, 2019). Bacteria can enter the eustachian tube from contaminated secretions in the nasopharynx and the middle ear from a tympanic membrane perforation. A purulent exudate is usually present in the middle ear, resulting in a conductive hearing loss.

Clinical Manifestations

Symptoms of otitis media vary with the severity of the infection. The condition, usually unilateral in adults, may be accompanied by otalgia. The pain is relieved after spontaneous perforation or therapeutic incision of the tympanic membrane. Other symptoms may include drainage from the ear, fever, and hearing loss. Table 59-3 differentiates acute otitis externa from AOM. Risk factors for AOM include younger age, chronic upper respiratory infections, medical conditions that predispose the patient to ear infections (e.g., Down syndrome, cystic fibrosis, cleft palate), and chronic exposure to secondhand cigarette smoke.

Medical Management

The outcome of AOM depends on the efficacy of therapy (the prescribed dose of an oral antibiotic and the duration of

TABLE 59-3	Clinical Features of Otitis	
Feature	**Acute Otitis Externa**	**Acute Otitis Media**
Otorrhea	May or may not be present	Present if tympanic membrane perforates; discharge is profuse
Otalgia	Persistent; may awaken patient at night	Relieved if tympanic membrane ruptures
Aural tenderness	Present on palpation of auricle	Usually absent
Systemic symptoms	Absent	Fever, upper respiratory infection, rhinitis
Edema of external auditory canal	Present	Absent
Tympanic membrane	May appear normal	Erythema, bulging, may be perforated
Hearing loss	Conductive type	Conductive type

Adapted from Weber, J., & Kelley, J. (2018). *Health assessment in nursing* (6th ed.). Philadelphia, PA: Wolters Kluwer.

therapy), the virulence of the bacteria, and the physical status of the patient. With early and appropriate broad-spectrum antibiotic therapy, otitis media may resolve with no serious sequelae. If drainage occurs, an antibiotic otic preparation is usually prescribed. The condition may become subacute (lasting 2 weeks to 3 months) with persistent purulent discharge from the ear. Rarely does permanent hearing loss occur. Secondary complications involving the mastoid and other serious intracranial complications, such as meningitis or brain abscess, although rare, can occur.

Surgical Management

A **myringotomy** (i.e., tympanotomy) is an incision in the tympanic membrane. The tympanic membrane is numbed with a local anesthetic agent such as phenol or by iontophoresis (i.e., in which electrical current flows through a lidocaine and epinephrine solution to numb the ear canal and tympanic membrane). The procedure is painless and takes less than 15 minutes. Under microscopic guidance, an incision is made through the tympanic membrane to relieve pressure and to drain serous or purulent fluid from the middle ear.

Normally, this procedure is unnecessary for treating AOM, but it may be performed if pain persists. Myringotomy also allows the drainage to be analyzed (by culture and sensitivity testing) so that the infecting organism can be identified and appropriate antibiotic therapy prescribed. The incision heals within 24 to 72 hours.

If AOM recurs and there is no contraindication, a ventilating, or pressure-equalizing, tube may be inserted. The ventilating tube, which temporarily takes the place of the eustachian tube in equalizing pressure, is retained for 6 to 18 months. The ventilating tube is then extruded with normal skin migration of the tympanic membrane, with the hole healing in nearly every case. Ventilating tubes are used to treat recurrent episodes of AOM.

Serous Otitis Media

Middle ear effusion, or serous otitis media, involves the presence of fluid, without evidence of active infection, in the middle ear. In theory, this fluid results from a negative pressure in the middle ear caused by eustachian tube obstruction. When this condition occurs in adults, an underlying cause for the eustachian tube dysfunction must be sought. Middle ear effusion is frequently seen in patients after radiation therapy or barotrauma and in patients with eustachian tube dysfunction from a concurrent upper respiratory infection or allergy. Barotrauma results from sudden pressure changes in the middle ear caused by changes in barometric pressure, as in scuba diving or airplane descent. A carcinoma (e.g., nasopharyngeal cancer) obstructing the eustachian tube should be ruled out in adults with persistent unilateral serous otitis media.

Clinical Manifestations

Patients may complain of hearing loss, fullness in the ear or a sensation of congestion, or popping and crackling noises that occur as the eustachian tube attempts to open. The tympanic membrane appears dull on otoscopy, and air bubbles may be visualized in the middle ear. Usually, the audiogram shows a conductive hearing loss.

Management

Serous otitis media need not be treated medically unless infection (i.e., AOM) occurs. If the hearing loss associated with middle ear effusion is significant, a myringotomy can be performed, and a tube may be placed to keep the middle ear ventilated. Corticosteroids in small doses may decrease the edema of the eustachian tube in cases of barotrauma. Decongestants have not proved to be effective. A Valsalva maneuver, which forcibly opens the eustachian tube by increasing nasopharyngeal pressure, may be cautiously performed; this maneuver may cause worsening pain or perforation of the tympanic membrane.

Chronic Otitis Media

Chronic otitis media is recurrent AOM that causes irreversible tissue pathology. Chronic infections of the middle ear damage the tympanic membrane, destroy the ossicles, and involve the mastoid but are rare in developed countries.

Clinical Manifestations

Symptoms may be minimal, with varying degrees of hearing loss and a persistent or intermittent, foul-smelling otorrhea. Pain is not usually experienced, except in cases of acute mastoiditis, when the postauricular area is tender and may be erythematous and edematous. Otoscopic examination may show a perforation, and cholesteatoma can be identified as a white mass behind the tympanic membrane or coming through to the external canal from a perforation.

Cholesteatoma is a cystlike lesion of the external layer of the eardrum into the middle ear. It is generally caused by a chronic retraction pocket of the tympanic membrane, creating a persistently high negative pressure of the middle ear. The skin forms a sac that fills with degenerated skin and sebaceous materials. The sac can attach to the structures of the middle ear, mastoid, or both.

Chronic otitis media can cause chronic mastoiditis and lead to the formation of cholesteatoma. The location will dictate the type of surgery to be performed. If untreated, cholesteatoma will continue to enlarge, possibly causing damage to the facial nerve and horizontal canal and destruction of other surrounding structures.

Cholesteatomas are cystlike lesions of the middle ear (Norris, 2019). They usually do not cause pain; however, if treatment or surgery is delayed, they may burst or destroy the mastoid bone. Cholesteatomas found in older adult patients generally develop in the external canal.

Cholesteatomas may be asymptomatic, or they may cause hearing loss, facial pain and paralysis, tinnitus, or vertigo. Audiometric tests often show a conductive or mixed hearing loss. Based on presenting symptoms, diagnosis may be made by visual examination or by computed tomography (CT) or MRI scan. Therapy includes treatment of the acute infection and surgical removal of the mass to restore hearing.

Medical Management

Local treatment for chronic otitis media consists of careful suctioning of the ear under otoscopic guidance. Instillation of antibiotic drops or application of antibiotic powder is used to treat purulent discharge. Systemic antibiotic agents are prescribed only in cases of acute infection.

Surgical Management

Surgical procedures, including tympanoplasty, ossiculoplasty, and mastoidectomy, are used if medical treatments are ineffective.

Tympanoplasty

The most common surgical procedure for chronic otitis media is **tympanoplasty**, or surgical reconstruction of the tympanic membrane. Reconstruction of the ossicles may also be required. The purposes of a tympanoplasty are to reestablish middle ear function, close the perforation, prevent recurrent infection, and improve hearing.

There are five types of tympanoplasties. The simplest surgical procedure, type I (myringoplasty), is designed to close a perforation in the tympanic membrane. The other procedures, types II through V, involve more extensive repair of middle ear structures. The structures and the degree of involvement can differ, but all tympanoplasty procedures include restoring the continuity of the sound conduction mechanism.

Tympanoplasty is performed through the external auditory canal with a transcanal approach or through a postauricular incision. The contents of the middle ear are carefully inspected, and the ossicular chain (malleus and incus unit) is evaluated. Ossicular interruption is most common in chronic otitis media, but problems of reconstruction can also occur with malformations of the middle ear and ossicular dislocations due to head injuries. Dramatic improvement in hearing can result from closure of a perforation and reestablishment of the ossicles. Surgery is usually performed in an outpatient facility under moderate sedation or general anesthesia.

Ossiculoplasty

Ossiculoplasty is the surgical reconstruction of the middle ear bones to restore hearing. Prostheses made of materials such as Teflon, stainless steel, and hydroxyapatite are used to reconnect the ossicles, thereby reestablishing the sound conduction mechanism. However, the greater the damage, the lower the success rate for restoring normal hearing.

Mastoidectomy

The objectives of mastoid surgery are to remove the cholesteatoma, gain access to diseased structures, and create a dry (noninfected) and healthy ear. If possible, the ossicles are reconstructed during the initial surgical procedure. Occasionally, extensive disease or damage dictates that this be performed as part of a two-stage operation.

A mastoidectomy is usually performed through a postauricular incision. Infection is eliminated by removing the mastoid air cells. A second mastoidectomy may be necessary to check for recurrent or residual cholesteatoma. The hearing mechanism may be reconstructed at this time. The success rate for correcting this conductive hearing loss is approximately 75%. Surgery is usually performed in an outpatient setting. The patient has a mastoid pressure dressing, which can be removed 24 to 48 hours after surgery. Although infrequently injured, the facial nerve, which runs through the middle ear and mastoid, is at some risk for injury during mastoid surgery. As the patient awakens from anesthesia, any evidence of facial paresis should be reported to the primary provider.

NURSING PROCESS

The Patient Undergoing Mastoid Surgery

Although several otologic surgical procedures are performed under moderate sedation, mastoid surgery is performed using general anesthesia.

Assessment

The health history includes a complete description of the ear disorder, including infection, otalgia, otorrhea, hearing loss, and vertigo. Data are collected about the duration and intensity of the disorder, its causes, and previous treatments. Information is obtained about other health problems and all medications that the patient is taking. Medication allergies and family history of ear disease also should be obtained.

Physical assessment addresses erythema, edema, otorrhea, lesions, and characteristics such as odor and color of discharge. The results of the audiogram are reviewed.

Nursing Diagnoses

Based on the assessment data, major nursing diagnoses may include the following:

- Anxiety associated with surgical procedure, potential loss of hearing, potential taste disturbance, and potential loss of facial movement
- Acute pain associated with mastoid surgery
- Risk for infection associated with mastoidectomy; placement of grafts, prostheses, and electrodes; and surgical trauma to surrounding tissues and structures
- Impaired verbal communication associated with ear disorder, surgery, or packing
- Risk for injury associated with impaired balance or vertigo during the immediate postoperative period, dislodgment of the graft or prosthesis, or injury to facial nerve (cranial nerve VII) and chorda tympani nerve
- Lack of knowledge about mastoid disease, surgical procedure, and postoperative care and expectations

Planning and Goals

Major goals of caring for a patient undergoing mastoidectomy include reduction of anxiety, freedom from pain and discomfort, prevention of infection, stable or improved hearing and communication, absence of vertigo and related injury, and increased knowledge regarding the disease, surgical procedure, and postoperative care.

Nursing Interventions

REDUCING ANXIETY

The nurse reinforces the information discussed by the otologic surgeon with the patient, including anesthesia, the location of the incision (postauricular), and expected surgical results (e.g., hearing, balance, taste, facial movement). The patient also is encouraged to discuss any anxieties and concerns about the surgery.

RELIEVING PAIN

Although most patients complain very little about incisional pain after mastoid surgery, they do have some ear discomfort. Aural fullness or pressure after surgery is caused by residual blood or fluid in the middle ear. The prescribed analgesic medication may be taken for the first 24 hours after surgery and then only as needed.

A wick or external auditory canal packing is used if tympanoplasty was performed at the time of the mastoidectomy. For the next 2 to 3 weeks after surgery, the patient may experience sharp, shooting pains intermittently as the eustachian tube opens and allows air to enter the middle ear. Constant, throbbing pain accompanied by fever may indicate infection and should be reported to the primary provider.

PREVENTING INFECTION

Measures are initiated to prevent infection in the operated ear. The external auditory canal wick, or packing, may be impregnated with an antibiotic solution before instillation. Prophylactic antibiotic agents are given as prescribed, and the patient is instructed to prevent water from entering the external auditory canal for 6 weeks. A cotton ball or lamb's wool covered with a water-insoluble substance (e.g., petroleum jelly) and placed loosely in the ear canal usually prevents water from entering the ear canal and should be used when the patient showers or washes their hair, or in any situations in which water may enter the ear canal. The postauricular incision should be kept dry for the first 2 days. Signs of infection such as an elevated temperature and purulent drainage should be reported. Some serosanguineous drainage from the external auditory canal is normal after surgery.

IMPROVING HEARING AND COMMUNICATION

Hearing in the operated ear may be reduced for several weeks because of edema, accumulation of blood and tissue fluid in the middle ear, and dressings or packing. Measures are initiated to improve hearing and communication, such as reducing environmental noise, facing the patient when speaking, speaking clearly and distinctly without shouting, providing good lighting, and using nonverbal clues (e.g., facial expression, pointing, gestures), writing, picture boards, electronic tablets, and other forms of communication. Family members or significant others are instructed about effective ways to communicate with the patient. If the patient uses assistive hearing devices, one can be used in the unaffected ear.

PREVENTING INJURY

Vertigo may occur after mastoid surgery if the semicircular canals or other areas of the inner ear are traumatized. Antiemetic or antivertiginous medications (e.g., antihistamines) can be prescribed if a balance disturbance or vertigo occurs. Safety measures such as assisted ambulation are implemented to prevent falls and injury. The patient is instructed to avoid heavy lifting, straining, exertion, and nose blowing for 2 to 3 weeks after surgery to prevent dislodging the tympanic membrane graft or ossicular prosthesis.

Facial nerve injury is a potential, although rare, complication of mastoid surgery. The patient is instructed to report immediately any evidence of facial nerve (cranial nerve VII) weakness, such as drooping of the mouth on the operated side, slurred speech, decreased sensation, and difficulty swallowing. A more frequent occurrence is a temporary disturbance in the chorda tympani nerve, which is a small branch of the facial nerve that runs through the middle ear. Patients experience

---

Chart 59-7	**PATIENT EDUCATION** Self-Care After Middle Ear or Mastoid Surgery

Postoperative instructions for patients who have had middle ear and mastoid surgery may vary among otolaryngologists. The nurse instructs the patient in the following general guidelines:

- Take antibiotics and other medications as prescribed.
- Avoid nose blowing for 2 to 3 weeks after surgery.
- Sneeze and cough with the mouth open for a few weeks after surgery.
- Avoid heavy lifting (>10 lb), straining, and bending over for a few weeks after surgery.
- Be aware that popping and crackling sensations in the operative ear are normal for approximately 3 to 5 weeks after surgery.
- Note that temporary hearing loss is normal in the operative ear due to fluid, blood, or packing in the ear.
- Report excessive or purulent ear drainage to the physician.
- Avoid getting water in the operative ear for 2 weeks after surgery. You may shampoo the hair 2 to 3 days postoperatively if the ear is protected from water by saturating a cotton ball with petroleum jelly (or some other water-insoluble substance) and loosely placing it in the ear. If the postauricular suture line becomes wet, pat (not rub) the area and cover it with a thin layer of antibiotic ointment.

---

a taste disturbance and dry mouth on the side of surgery for several months until the nerve regenerates.

PROMOTING HOME, COMMUNITY-BASED, AND TRANSITIONAL CARE

Educating Patients About Self-Care. Patients require education about medication therapy, such as analgesic and antivertiginous agents (e.g., antihistamines) prescribed for balance disturbance. Education includes information about the expected effects and potential side effects of the medication. Patients also need instruction about any activity restrictions. Possible complications such as infection, facial nerve weakness, or taste disturbances, including the signs and symptoms to report immediately, are included (see Chart 59-7).

Continuing and Transitional Care. Some patients, particularly older adult patients, who have had mastoid surgery may require the services of a home, community-based, or transitional care nurse for a few days after returning home. However, most people find that assistance from a family member or a friend is sufficient. The caregiver and patient are cautioned that the patient may experience some vertigo and will therefore require help with ambulation to avoid falling. Any symptoms of complications are to be reported promptly to the primary provider. The importance of scheduling and keeping follow-up appointments is also stressed.

Evaluation

Expected patient outcomes may include:

1. Demonstrates reduced anxiety about surgical procedure
   a. Verbalizes and exhibits less stress, tension, and irritability
   b. Verbalizes acceptance of results of surgery and adjustment to possible hearing loss

2. Remains free of discomfort or pain
   a. Exhibits no facial grimacing, moaning, or crying, and reports absence of pain
   b. Uses analgesic agents appropriately
3. Demonstrates no signs or symptoms of infection
   a. Has normal vital signs, including temperature
   b. Demonstrates absence of purulent drainage from the external auditory canal
   c. Describes method for preventing water from contaminating packing
4. Exhibits signs that communication and hearing have stabilized or improved
   a. Describes surgical goal for hearing and judges whether the goal has been met
   b. Verbalizes that hearing has improved
5. Remains free of injury and trauma
   a. Reports absence of vertigo or balance disturbance
   b. Experiences no injury or fall
   c. Avoids activities that can cause dislodgement of graft or prosthesis
   d. Reports no taste disturbance, mouth dryness, or facial weakness
6. Verbalizes the reasons for and methods of care and treatment
   a. Discusses the discharge plan formulated with the nurse with regard to rest periods, medication, and activities permitted and restricted
   b. Lists symptoms that should be reported to the primary provider
   c. Keeps follow-up appointments

Otosclerosis

Otosclerosis involves the stapes and is thought to result from the formation of new, abnormal spongy bone, especially around the oval window, with resulting fixation of the stapes (Norris, 2019). The efficient transmission of sound is prevented because the stapes cannot vibrate and carry the sound as conducted from the malleus and incus to the inner ear. Otosclerosis is more common in women, is a familial condition, and can progress to complete deafness (Eliopoulos, 2018; Norris, 2019).

Clinical Manifestations

Otosclerosis may involve one or both ears and manifests as a progressive conductive or mixed hearing loss. The patient may or may not complain of tinnitus. Otoscopic examination usually reveals a normal tympanic membrane. Bone conduction is better than air conduction on Rinne testing. The audiogram confirms conductive hearing loss or mixed loss, especially in the low frequencies.

Medical Management

The management of otosclerosis can be surgical or medical. Amplification with a hearing aid may help (Norris, 2019).

Surgical Management

One of two surgical procedures may be performed: the stapedectomy or the stapedotomy. A stapedectomy involves removing the stapes superstructure and part of the footplate and inserting a tissue graft and a suitable prosthesis (see Fig. 59-6).

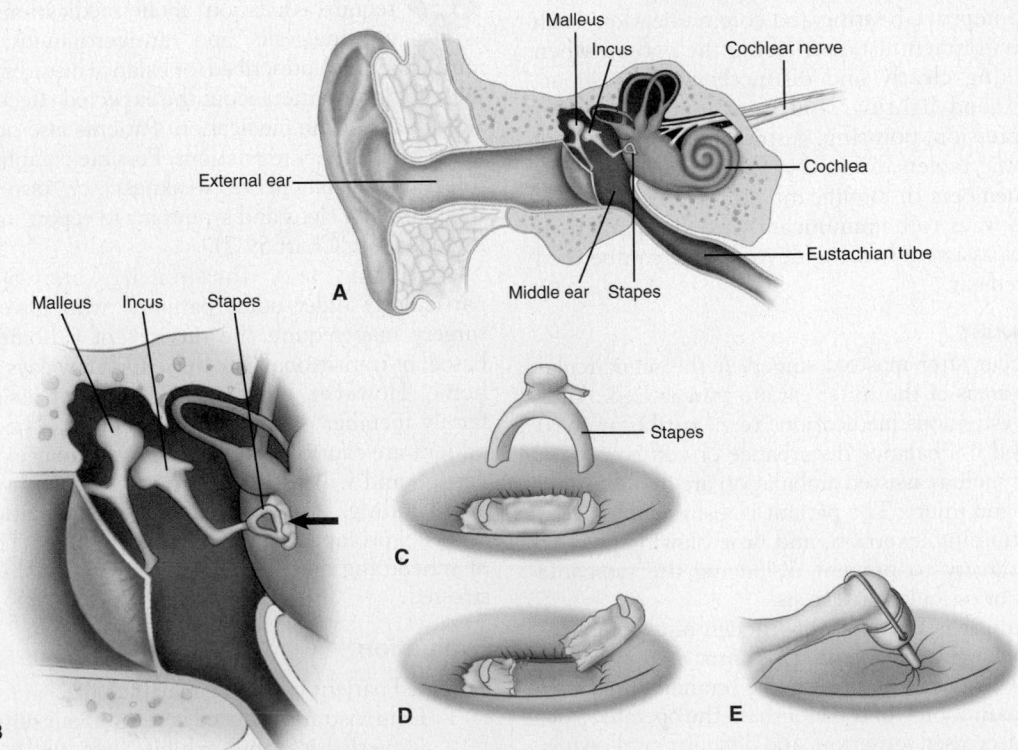

Figure 59-6 • Stapedectomy for otosclerosis. **A.** Normal anatomy. **B.** *Arrow* points to sclerotic process at the foot of the stapes. **C.** Stapes broken away surgically from its diseased base. The hole in the footplate provides an area where an instrument can grasp the plate. **D.** The footplate is removed from its base. Some otosclerotic tissue may remain, and tissue is placed over it. **E.** Robinson stainless steel prosthesis in position.

In a stapedotomy, the surgeon drills a small hole into the stapes, instead of removing it, to hold a prosthesis. In both procedures, the prosthesis bridges the gap between the incus and the inner ear, providing better sound conduction. The majority of patients experience resolution of conductive hearing loss following stapes surgery. The use of sodium fluoride in the postoperative period increases the success rate and hearing ability postoperatively (Norris, 2019). Balance disturbance or true vertigo may occur during the postoperative period for several days. Long-term balance disorders are rare.

Middle Ear Masses

Other than cholesteatoma, masses in the middle ear are rare. Glomus tympanicum is a tumor that arises from Jacobson nerve (in the temporal bone of the skull) and remains limited to the middle ear. On otoscopy, a red blemish on or behind the tympanic membrane is seen. Glomus jugulare tumors are rarely malignant; however, because of their location, treatment may be necessary to relieve symptoms. The treatment is surgical excision, except in patients who are poor surgical candidates, in whom radiation therapy is used.

A facial nerve neuroma is a tumor on cranial nerve VII. These types of tumors are usually not visible on otoscopic examination but are suspected when a patient presents with a facial nerve paresis. X-ray evaluation is used to identify the site of the tumor along the facial nerve. The treatment is surgical removal.

CONDITIONS OF THE INNER EAR

Disorders of balance are common and dizziness may increase the risk of falls (NIDCD, 2018). The term **dizziness** is used frequently by patients and health care providers to describe any altered sensation of orientation in space and is more commonly referred to as lightheadedness (Weber & Kelley, 2018). **Vertigo** is the misperception or illusion of motion of the person or the surroundings. Most patients with vertigo describe a spinning sensation or say they feel as though objects are moving around them. Ataxia is a failure of muscular coordination and may be present in patients with vestibular disease. Syncope, fainting, and loss of consciousness are not forms of vertigo and usually indicate disease in the cardiovascular system.

Nystagmus is an involuntary rhythmic movement of the eyes. Nystagmus occurs normally when a person watches a rapidly moving object (e.g., through the side window of a moving car or train). However, pathologically, it is an ocular disorder associated with vestibular dysfunction. Nystagmus can be horizontal, vertical, or rotary and can be caused by a disorder in the central or peripheral nervous system.

Motion Sickness

Motion sickness is a disturbance of equilibrium caused by a conflict in motion receptor stimuli. For example, it can occur aboard a ship, in a car, while riding on a merry-go-round or swing, or even while viewing virtual motion on a large screen (Brainard & Gresham, 2014).

Clinical Manifestations

The syndrome manifests itself in sweating, pallor, nausea, and vomiting caused by vestibular overstimulation. These manifestations may persist for several hours after the stimulation stops.

Management

Over-the-counter antihistamines such as dimenhydrinate or meclizine may provide some relief of nausea and vomiting by blocking the conduction of the vestibular pathway of the inner ear. Anticholinergic medications, such as scopolamine patches, may also be effective because they antagonize the histamine response. These must be applied 4 hours before exposure to motion and replaced every 3 days (Brainard & Gresham, 2014). Side effects such as dry mouth and drowsiness may occur. Potentially hazardous activities such as driving a car or operating heavy machinery should be avoided if drowsiness occurs.

Ménière's Disease

Ménière's disease is an abnormality in inner ear fluid balance caused by a malabsorption in the endolymphatic sac or a blockage in the endolymphatic duct (NIDCD, 2017b). **Endolymphatic hydrops** (dilation of the endolymphatic space) frequently occurs, causing either increased pressure in the system or rupture of the inner ear membrane, producing symptoms of Ménière's disease (van Steekelenburg, van Weijnen, de Pont, et al., 2020).

Ménière's disease affects 10 to 12 of 1000 people in the United States. It is estimated that there are 615,000 cases in the United States, with approximately 45,500 new cases diagnosed annually (NIDCD, 2017b). More common in adults, onset is generally seen when adults reach their 40s, with symptoms usually beginning between the ages of 20 and 60 years. Ménière's disease appears to be equally common in men and women, and is usually bilateral (Norris, 2019).

Clinical Manifestations

Ménière's disease is characterized by a triad of symptoms: episodic vertigo, tinnitus, and fluctuating sensorineural hearing loss (Luryi, Morse, & Michaelides, 2019). It may also include a feeling of pressure or fullness in the ear and incapacitating vertigo, often accompanied by nausea and vomiting (NIDCD, 2017b). These symptoms range in severity from a minor nuisance to extreme disability, especially if the attacks of vertigo are severe. At the onset of the disease, usually only one or two of the symptoms are manifested.

The disease may be characterized into two subsets: cochlear and vestibular. Cochlear Ménière's disease is recognized as a fluctuating, progressive sensorineural hearing loss associated with tinnitus and aural pressure in the absence of vestibular symptoms or findings. Vestibular Ménière's disease is characterized as the occurrence of episodic vertigo associated with aural pressure but no cochlear symptoms. Patients may experience either cochlear or vestibular disease symptoms at first; however, eventually all of these symptoms develop.

Assessment and Diagnostic Findings

Vertigo is usually the most troublesome complaint related to Ménière's disease. A careful history is taken to determine the frequency, duration, severity, and character of the vertigo attacks. Vertigo may last minutes to hours, possibly accompanied by nausea or vomiting. Diaphoresis and a persistent feeling of imbalance or disequilibrium may awaken patients at night. Some patients report that these feelings last for days. However, they usually feel well between attacks. Hearing loss may fluctuate, with tinnitus and aural pressure waxing and waning with changes in hearing. These feelings may occur during or before attacks, or they may be constant.

Physical examination findings are usually normal, with the exception of those of cranial nerve VIII. Sounds from a tuning fork (Weber test) may lateralize to the ear opposite the hearing loss, the one affected with Ménière's disease. An audiogram typically reveals a sensorineural hearing loss in the affected ear. This can be in the form of a pattern that looks like a hill or mountain. A sensorineural loss in the low frequencies occurs as the disease progresses. The electronystagmogram may be normal or may show reduced vestibular response.

Medical Management

Most patients with Ménière's disease can be successfully treated with diet and medication. Many patients can control their symptoms by adhering to a low-sodium (1000 to 1500 mg/day or less) diet. Chart 59-8 describes dietary guidelines that may be useful in Ménière's disease. The amount of sodium is one of many factors that regulate the balance of fluid within the body. Sodium and fluid retention disrupts the delicate balance between endolymph and perilymph in the inner ear. Psychological evaluation and cognitive therapy may be indicated if a patient is anxious, uncertain, fearful, or depressed (NIDCD, 2017b).

Chart 59-8

PATIENT EDUCATION

Dietary Guidelines for Patients with Ménière's Disease

The nurse instructs the patient to:

- limit foods high in salt or sugar. Be aware of foods with hidden salts and sugars.
- eat meals and snacks at regular intervals to stay hydrated. Missing meals or snacks may alter the fluid level in the inner ear.
- eat fresh fruits, vegetables, and whole grains. Limit the amount of canned, frozen, or processed foods with high sodium content.
- drink plenty of fluids daily. Water, milk, and low-sugar fruit juices are recommended. Limit intake of coffee, tea, and soft drinks. Avoid caffeine because of its diuretic effect.
- limit alcohol intake. Alcohol may change the volume and concentration of the inner ear fluid and may worsen symptoms.
- avoid monosodium glutamate (MSG), which may increase symptoms.
- pay attention to the intake of foods containing potassium (e.g., bananas, tomatoes, oranges) if taking a diuretic that causes potassium loss.
- avoid aspirin and aspirin-containing medications. Aspirin may increase tinnitus and dizziness.

Adapted from National Institute on Deafness and Other Communication Disorders (NIDCD). (2017b). Ménière's disease. Retrieved on 2/22/2020 at: www.nidcd.nih.gov/health/menieres-disease

---

Pharmacologic Therapy

Pharmacologic therapy for Ménière's disease consists of antihistamines, such as meclizine, which shortens the attack (NIDCD, 2017b). Tranquilizers such as diazepam may be used in acute instances to help control vertigo. Antiemetic agents such as promethazine suppositories help control the nausea and vomiting and the vertigo because of their antihistamine effect. Diuretic therapy (e.g., hydrochlorothiazide, triamterene, spironolactone) may relieve symptoms by lowering the pressure in the endolymphatic system (Norris, 2019). Intratympanic injection of gentamicin is used to cause ablation of the vestibular hair cells; however, the risk of significant hearing loss is high (NIDCD, 2017b).

Surgical Management

Although most patients respond well to conservative therapy, some continue to have disabling attacks of vertigo. If these attacks reduce their quality of life, patients may elect to undergo surgery for relief. Surgical procedures include endolymphatic sac procedures and vestibular nerve section (NIDCD, 2017b). However, hearing loss, tinnitus, and aural fullness may continue, because the surgical treatment of Ménière's disease is aimed at eliminating the attacks of vertigo.

Endolymphatic Sac Decompression

Endolymphatic sac decompression, or shunting, theoretically equalizes the pressure in the endolymphatic space. A shunt or drain is inserted in the endolymphatic sac through a postauricular incision. This procedure is favored by many otolaryngologists as a first-line surgical approach to treat the vertigo of Ménière's disease because it is relatively simple and safe and can be performed on an outpatient basis.

Vestibular Nerve Sectioning

Vestibular nerve sectioning provides the greatest success rate (approximately 98%) in eliminating the attacks of vertigo. It can be performed by a translabyrinthine approach (i.e., through the hearing mechanism) or in a manner that can conserve hearing (i.e., suboccipital or middle cranial fossa), depending on the degree of hearing loss. Most patients with incapacitating Ménière's disease have little or no effective hearing. Cutting the nerve prevents the brain from receiving input from the semicircular canals. This procedure may require a brief hospital stay. A plan of nursing care for the patient with vertigo is presented in Chart 59-9.

Benign Paroxysmal Positional Vertigo

Benign paroxysmal positional vertigo is a brief period of incapacitating vertigo that occurs when the position of the patient's head is changed with respect to gravity, typically by placing the head back with the affected ear turned down (Muñoz, Moreno, Balboa, et al., 2019; NIDCD, 2017b). The onset is sudden and followed by a predisposition for positional vertigo, usually for hours to weeks but occasionally for months or years.

Benign paroxysmal positional vertigo is thought to be due to the disruption of debris within the semicircular canal. This debris is formed from small crystals of calcium carbonate from the inner ear structure (the utricle). This is frequently stimulated by head trauma, infection, or other events. In severe cases, vertigo may easily be induced by any head movement.

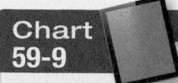

Chart 59-9

PLAN OF NURSING CARE
Care of the Patient with Vertigo

NURSING DIAGNOSIS: Risk for fall-related injury associated with impaired balance, gait disturbance, and vertigo
GOAL: Remains free of physical trauma associated with imbalance and falls

Nursing Interventions	Rationale	Expected Outcomes
1. Assess for balance disturbance or vertigo, including history, onset, description of attacks, duration, frequency, and any associated ear symptoms (hearing loss, tinnitus, aural fullness).	1. Health history provides basis for interventions.	• Experiences no physical trauma due to balance disturbance • Visual and proprioceptive risks identified
2. Perform examination for nystagmus, positive Romberg, and inability to perform tandem Romberg.	2. Peripheral vestibular disorders cause these signs and symptoms.	• Activity level increases • Performs exercises as prescribed
3. Assess extent of disability (i.e., visual acuity and proprioceptive deficits) in relation to activities of daily living.	3. Extent of disability indicates risk of falling. Balance depends on visual, vestibular, and proprioceptive systems.	• Takes prescribed medications appropriately
4. Instruct or reinforce vestibular/balance therapy as prescribed.	4. Exercises hasten labyrinthine compensation, which may decrease vertigo and gait disturbance.	• Assumes safe position when vertigo is present • Keeps head still when vertigo is present
5. Administer, or educate about administration of, antivertiginous medications or vestibular sedation medication; instruct patient about side effects.	5. Alleviates acute symptoms of vertigo.	• Identifies a characteristic fullness or sense of pressure in the ear as occurring before an attack occurs
6. Encourage patient to sit down and restrict activity when dizzy.	6. Decreases possibility of falling and injury.	• Reports measures that help reduce vertigo
7. Place pillow on each side of head to restrict movement.	7. Movement aggravates vertigo.	• Home environment free of hazards
8. Assist patient in identifying aura that suggests an impending attack.	8. Recognition of aura may trigger the need to take medication before an attack occurs, thereby minimizing the severity of effects.	• Has adapted home environment or uses rehabilitative devices to reduce risk of falling
9. Recommend that the patient keep eyes open and stare straight ahead when lying down and experiencing vertigo.	9. Sensation of vertigo decreases and motion decelerates if eyes are kept in a fixed position.	
10. Help identify hazards or use rehabilitative devices in home environment.	10. Adaptation of home environment can reduce risk of falls.	

NURSING DIAGNOSIS: Risk for negative quality of life associated with unpredictability of vertigo
GOAL: Modifies lifestyle to decrease disability and exert maximum control and independence within limits posed by chronic vertigo

Nursing Interventions	Rationale	Expected Outcomes
1. Encourage patient to identify personal strengths and roles that can still be fulfilled.	1. Maximizes sense of regaining control and independence.	• Exerts maximum control of environment and independence within limits imposed by vertigo
2. Provide information about vertigo and what to expect.	2. Reduces fear and anxiety.	• Is informed about condition
3. Include family and significant others in rehabilitative process.	3. Perceived beliefs of significant others are important for patient's adherence to medical regimen.	• Family and significant others are included in rehabilitation process
4. Encourage patient to maintain sense of control by making decisions and assuming more responsibility for care.	4. Reinforces positive psychological and social outcomes.	• Uses strengths and potentials to engage in the most independent and constructive lifestyle

NURSING DIAGNOSIS: Risk for hypovolaemia associated with increased fluid output, altered intake, and medications
GOAL: Maintains normal fluid and electrolyte balance

Nursing Interventions	Rationale	Expected Outcomes
1. Assess, or have patient assess, intake and output (including emesis, liquid stools, urine, and diaphoresis). Monitor laboratory values of electrolytes.	1. Accurate records provide basis for fluid replacement.	• Laboratory values within normal limits
2. Assess indicators of dehydration, including blood pressure (orthostasis), pulse, skin turgor, mucous membranes, and level of consciousness.	2. Prompt recognition of dehydration allows early intervention.	• Alert and oriented; vital signs within normal limits, skin turgor normal; electrolytes normal • Mucous membranes are moist
3. Encourage oral fluids as tolerated; discourage beverages containing caffeine (a vestibular stimulant).	3. Oral replacement is begun as soon as possible to replace losses.	• Vomiting has stopped; usual oral intake is resumed

(continued on page 1956)

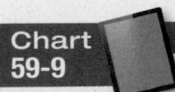

PLAN OF NURSING CARE (continued)
Care of the Patient with Vertigo

Chart 59-9

Nursing Interventions	Rationale	Expected Outcomes
4. Administer, or educate about administration of, antiemetic medications as prescribed and needed. Educate patient about side effects.	4. Antiemetic medications reduce nausea and vomiting, reducing fluid losses and improving oral intake.	

NURSING DIAGNOSIS: Anxiety associated with threat of, or change in, health status and disability effects of vertigo
GOAL: Experiences less or no anxiety

Nursing Interventions	Rationale	Expected Outcomes
1. Assess level of anxiety. Help patient identify coping skills used successfully in the past. 2. Provide information about vertigo and its treatment. 3. Encourage patient to discuss anxieties and explore concerns about vertigo attacks. 4. Educate patient about stress management techniques or make appropriate referral. 5. Provide comfort measures and avoid stress-producing activities. 6. Instruct patient in aspects of treatment regimen.	1. Guides therapeutic interventions and participation in self-care. Past coping skills can relieve anxiety. 2. Increased knowledge helps to decrease anxiety. 3. Promotes awareness and understanding of relationship between anxiety level and behavior. 4. Improved stress management can reduce the frequency and severity of some vertiginous attacks. 5. Stressful situations may exacerbate symptoms of the condition. 6. Patient knowledge helps to decrease anxiety.	• Fear and anxiety about attacks of vertigo reduced or eliminated • Acquires knowledge and skills to deal with vertigo • Feels less tension, apprehension, and uncertainty • Uses stress management techniques when needed • Avoids upsetting encounters • Repeats instructions given and verbalizes understanding of treatments

NURSING DIAGNOSIS: Impaired self feeding, impaired ability to perform hygiene, impaired ability to dress, and impaired self toileting associated with labyrinth dysfunction and episodes of vertigo
GOAL: Able to care for self

Nursing Interventions	Rationale	Expected Outcomes
1. Administer, or educate about administration of, antiemetic and other prescribed medications to relieve nausea and vomiting associated with vertigo. 2. Encourage patient to perform self-care when free of vertigo. 3. Review diet with patient and caregivers. Offer fluids as necessary.	1. Antiemetic and sedative-type medications depress stimuli in the cerebellum. 2. Spacing activities is important because episodes of vertigo vary in occurrence. 3. Sodium restriction helps improve an inner ear fluid imbalance in some patients, thereby decreasing vertigo. Fluids help prevent dehydration.	• Carries out necessary functions during symptom-free periods and takes medications to relieve nausea, vomiting, or vertigo • Carries out daily activities • Accepts dietary plan and reports its effectiveness • Drinks fluids in sufficient amounts

NURSING DIAGNOSIS: Risk for powerlessness associated with illness regimen and feeling helpless in certain situations due to vertigo/balance disturbance
GOAL: Experiences increased sense of control over life and activities despite vertigo/balance disturbance

Nursing Interventions	Rationale	Expected Outcomes
1. Assess patient's needs, values, attitudes, and readiness to initiate activities. 2. Provide opportunities for patient to express feelings about self and illness. 3. Help patient identify previous coping behaviors that were successful.	1. Involving patient in planning activities and care enhances potential for mastery. 2. Expressing feelings increases understanding of individual coping styles and defense mechanisms. 3. Awareness increases understanding of stressors that trigger feeling of powerlessness. Awareness of past successes enhances self-confidence.	• Does not restrict activities unnecessarily due to vertigo • Verbalizes positive feelings about own ability to achieve a sense of power and control • Identifies previous successful coping behaviors

The vertigo is usually accompanied by nausea and vomiting; however, hearing loss does not generally occur.

Bed rest is recommended for patients with acute symptoms. Repositioning techniques can be used to treat vertigo. The canalith repositioning procedure is commonly used (Bhattacharyya, Gubbels, Schwartz, et al., 2017). This noninvasive procedure, which involves quick movements of the body, rearranges the debris in the canal. The procedure is performed by placing the patient in a sitting position, turning the head to a 45-degree angle on the affected side, and then quickly moving the patient to the supine position. The procedure is safe, inexpensive, and easy to perform.

Patients with acute vertigo may be treated with meclizine for 1 to 2 weeks. After this time, the meclizine is stopped and the patient is reassessed. Patients who continue to have severe positional vertigo may be premedicated with prochlorperazine 1 hour before the canalith repositioning procedure is performed.

Vestibular rehabilitation can be used in the management of vestibular disorders. This strategy promotes active use of the vestibular system through an interdisciplinary team approach, including medical and nursing care, stress management, biofeedback, vocational rehabilitation, and physical therapy. A physical therapist prescribes balance exercises that help the brain compensate for the impairment to the balance system.

Tinnitus

Tinnitus may be a symptom of an underlying disorder of the ear that is associated with hearing loss or it may be benign. This condition affects approximately 25 million people in the United States and is most prevalent in adults (NIDCD, 2017c). The severity of tinnitus may range from mild to severe. Patients describe tinnitus as a roaring, buzzing, or hissing sound in one or both ears. Numerous factors may contribute to the development of tinnitus, including several ototoxic substances (see Chart 59-10). Underlying disorders that contribute to tinnitus may include cardiovascular disease, thyroid disease, hyperlipidemia, vitamin B_{12} deficiency, psychological disorders (e.g., depression, anxiety), fibromyalgia, otologic disorders (Ménière's disease, acoustic neuroma), and neurologic disorders (head injury, multiple sclerosis).

A physical examination should be performed to determine the cause of tinnitus. Diagnostic testing determines if hearing loss is present. An audiograph speech discrimination test or a tympanogram may be used to help determine the cause. Some forms of tinnitus are irreversible; therefore, patients may need education and counseling about ways of adjusting to their treatment and dealing with tinnitus in the future.

Labyrinthitis

Labyrinthitis, an inflammation of the labyrinth of the inner ear, can be bacterial or viral in origin. Bacterial labyrinthitis is rare because of antibiotic therapy, but it sometimes occurs as a complication of otitis media. The infection can spread to the inner ear by penetrating the membranes of the oval or round windows. Viral labyrinthitis is a common diagnosis, but little is known about this disorder, which affects hearing and balance. The most common viral causes are mumps, rubella, rubeola, and influenza. Viral illnesses of the upper respiratory tract and herpetiform disorders of the facial and acoustic nerves (i.e., Ramsay Hunt syndrome) also cause labyrinthitis.

Clinical Manifestations

Labyrinthitis is characterized by a sudden onset of incapacitating vertigo, usually with nausea and vomiting, various degrees of hearing loss, and possibly tinnitus. The first episode is usually the worst; subsequent attacks, which usually occur over a period of several weeks to months, are less severe.

Management

Treatment of bacterial labyrinthitis includes IV antibiotic therapy, fluid replacement, and administration of an antihistamine (e.g., meclizine) and antiemetic medications. Treatment of viral labyrinthitis is based on the patient's symptoms.

Ototoxicity

A variety of medications may have adverse effects on the cochlea, vestibular apparatus, or cranial nerve VIII. All but a few, such as aspirin and quinine, cause irreversible hearing loss. Aspirin toxicity can produce bilateral tinnitus. IV medications, especially the aminoglycosides, are a common cause of ototoxicity, because they destroy the hair cells in the organ of Corti (see Chart 59-10). Antineoplastic agents also cause hair cell death in the cochlea, which can lead to hearing loss (Mudd, 2019). These medications can be found in the body several months later; side effects are dose dependent, with higher doses causing increased ototoxicity. Therefore, hearing loss may occur at any time, even several months after the last dose of the medication was given.

To prevent loss of hearing or balance, patients receiving potentially ototoxic medications should be counseled about their side effects. These medications should be used with caution in individuals that are at high risk for complications, such as children, older adults, patients who are pregnant, patients with kidney or liver problems, and patients with current hearing disorders. Blood levels of the medications should be monitored, and patients receiving long-term IV antibiotics should be monitored with an audiogram twice each week during therapy.

Acoustic Neuroma

Acoustic neuromas, also referred to as vestibular schwannomas, are slow-growing, benign tumors of cranial nerve VIII, usually arising from the Schwann cells of the vestibular portion of the nerve. Acoustic tumors typically arise within the internal auditory canal and extend into the cerebellopontine angle to press on the brain stem, possibly destroying the vestibular nerve. Most acoustic neuromas are unilateral, except in von Recklinghausen disease (neurofibromatosis type 2), in which bilateral tumors occur (Norris, 2019).

Chart 59-10

Select Ototoxic Substances

- **Aminoglycoside antibiotic agents:** amikacin, gentamicin, kanamycin, netilmicin, neomycin, streptomycin, tobramycin
- **Anti-inflammatory agents:** salicylates (aspirin), indomethacin
- **Antimalarial agents:** quinine, chloroquine
- **Chemicals:** alcohol, arsenic
- **Chemotherapeutic (antineoplastic) agents:** cisplatin, nitrogen mustard, carboplatin
- **Loop diuretic agents:** ethacrynic acid, furosemide, acetazolamide, torsemide, azosemide, ozolinone, indacrinone, piretanide
- **Metals:** gold, mercury, lead
- **Other antibiotic agents:** erythromycin, azithromycin, clarithromycin, minocycline, polymyxin B, vancomycin

Adapted from Mudd, P. (2019). Ototoxicity. *Medscape.* Retrieved on 3/7/2020 at: emedicine.medscape.com/article/857679-overview

Acoustic neuromas develop in one of every 100,000 people in the United States per year (NIDCD, 2017d). These neuromas account for 8% of all intracranial tumors and seem to occur with equal frequency in men and women at any age, although most occur during middle age (Carlson, Tveiten, Driscoll, et al., 2015).

Assessment and Diagnostic Findings

The most common assessment findings of patients with acoustic neuromas are unilateral tinnitus and hearing loss with or without vertigo or balance disturbance. It is important to identify asymmetry in audiovestibular test results so that further workup can be performed to rule out an acoustic neuroma. Although conflicting data exist, the only known risk factor for acoustic neuroma is cell phone usage (Park, Vernick, & Ramakrishna, 2019). An MRI scan with a contrast agent (i.e., gadolinium or gadopentetate) is the imaging study of choice. If the patient is claustrophobic or cannot undergo an MRI scan for other reasons, or if the scan is unavailable, a CT scan with contrast dye is performed. However, MRI is more sensitive than CT in delineating a small tumor.

Management

Three options for managing an acoustic neuroma include: (1) surgical removal, (2) radiation, and (3) observation (Carlson et al., 2015; NIDCD, 2017d). Conservative treatment and routine monitoring are recommended for patients with tumors less than 1.5 cm and for those who are older. For patients who are at low risk, surgical removal of the acoustic tumor is the treatment of choice because these tumors do not respond well to radiation or chemotherapy. Because treatment of acoustic tumors crosses several specialties, the interdisciplinary treatment approach involves a neurologist and a neurosurgeon. The objective of the surgery is to remove the tumor while preserving facial nerve function. Most acoustic tumors have damaged the cochlear portion of cranial nerve VIII resulting in hearing loss. In these patients, surgery is performed using a translabyrinthine approach, and the hearing mechanism is destroyed. If hearing is still good before surgery, a suboccipital or middle cranial fossa approach to removing the tumor may be used. This procedure exposes the lateral third of the internal auditory canal and preserves hearing (Park et al., 2019).

Potential complications of surgery include facial nerve paralysis, cerebrospinal fluid leakage, meningitis, and cerebral edema. Death from acoustic neuroma surgery is rare (Park et al., 2019).

AURAL REHABILITATION

If hearing loss is permanent or cannot be treated by medical or surgical means or if the patient elects not to undergo surgery, aural rehabilitation may be beneficial. The purpose of aural rehabilitation is to maximize the communication skills of the person with hearing loss. Aural rehabilitation includes auditory training, speech reading, speech training, and the use of hearing aids and hearing guide dogs.

Auditory training emphasizes listening skills, so the person with hearing loss practices concentrating on the speaker. Speech reading (also known as lip reading) can help fill the gaps left by missed or misheard words. The goals of speech training are to conserve, develop, and prevent deterioration of current communication skills.

It is important to identify the type of hearing loss so that rehabilitative efforts can be appropriate for each individual. Surgical correction may be all that is necessary to treat and improve a conductive hearing loss by eliminating the cause of the hearing loss. Advances in hearing aid technology have greatly improved amplification for patients with sensorineural hearing loss.

Hearing Aids

A hearing aid is a device through which speech and environmental sounds are received by a microphone, converted to electrical signals, amplified, and reconverted to acoustic signals. Many aids available for sensorineural hearing loss depress the low frequencies, or tones, and enhance hearing for the high frequencies. A general guideline for assessing the patient's need for a hearing aid is a hearing loss exceeding 30 dB in the range of 500 to 2000 Hz in the better-hearing ear.

A hearing aid makes sounds louder, but it does not improve a patient's ability to discriminate words or understand speech. People who have low discrimination scores (i.e., 20%) on audiograms may derive little benefit from a hearing aid. Hearing aids amplify all sounds, including background noise, which may be particularly disturbing to the first-time wearer. Chart 59-11 identifies additional problems associated with hearing aid use. Computerized hearing aids are available to compensate for background noise or allow amplification at certain programmed frequencies rather than at all frequencies. Occasionally, depending on the type of hearing loss, binaural

---

Chart 59-11 Hearing Aid Problems

Whistling Noise

- Loose ear mold
- Improperly made
- Improperly worn
- Worn out

Improper Aid Selection

- Too much power required in aid, with inadequate separation between microphone and receiver
- Open mold used inappropriately
- Inadequate amplification
- Dead batteries
- Cerumen in ear
- Cerumen or other material in mold
- Wires or tubing disconnected from aid
- Aid turned off or volume too low
- Improper mold
- Improper aid for degree of loss

Pain From Mold

- Improperly fitted mold
- Ear skin or cartilage infection
- Middle ear infection
- Ear tumor
- Unrelated conditions of the temporomandibular joint, throat, or larynx

Chart
59-12

PATIENT EDUCATION

Tips for Hearing Aid Care

The nurse instructs the patient how to clean a hearing aid, check for malfunctions, and recognize complications:

Cleaning

- Keep in mind that the ear mold is the only part of the hearing aid that may be washed frequently.
- Wash the ear mold daily with soap and water.
- Allow the ear mold to dry completely before it is snapped into the receiver.
- Clean the cannula with a small pipe cleaner–like device.
- Note that properly caring for the ear device and keeping the ear canal clean and dry can prevent complications.

Checking for Malfunctions

- Be aware that inadequate amplification, a whistling noise, or pain from the mold can occur when a hearing aid is not functioning properly.
- Check for malfunctions:
  - Is the switch on properly?
  - Are the batteries charged and positioned correctly?
  - Is the ear mold clogged with cerumen? Ear wax can be easily removed with pin, pipe cleaner, or wax loop.
- Notify the hearing aid dealer if the hearing aid is still not working properly.
- Keep in mind that if the unit requires extended time for repair, the dealer may lend you a hearing aid until the repair can be accomplished.

Recognizing Complications

- Understand that common medical complications include external otitis media and pressure injury in the external auditory canal. Signs and symptoms of these infections include painful ear, especially when the external ear is touched; canal swelling; redness; difficulty hearing; pain radiating to the jaw area; and fever.
- Notify your health care provider for evaluation if any of these symptoms are present. You may need medication to treat infection, pain, or both.

aids (i.e., one for each ear) may be indicated. Chart 59-12 provides tips for hearing aid care.

A hearing aid should be fitted according to the patient's needs (e.g., type of hearing loss, manual dexterity, and preference), rather than brand name, by a certified audiologist licensed to dispense hearing aids. Many states have consumer protection laws that allow the hearing aid to be returned after a trial use if the patient is not completely satisfied. In addition, to protect the health and safety of people with hearing loss, the U.S. Food and Drug Administration (FDA) has established certain regulations. A medical evaluation of the hearing loss by a physician must be obtained within 6 months before the purchase of a hearing aid. However, the written statement from a physician may be waived if the patient (a fully informed adult 18 years or older) signs a document to this effect. Health care professionals who dispense hearing aids are required to refer prospective users to a physician if any of the following otologic conditions are evident:

- Visible congenital or traumatic deformity of the ear
- Active drainage from the ear within the previous 90 days

- Sudden or rapidly progressive hearing loss within the previous 90 days
- Complaints of dizziness or tinnitus
- Unilateral hearing loss that has occurred suddenly or within the previous 90 days
- Audiometric air–bone gap of 15 dB or more at 500, 1000, and 2000 Hz
- Significant accumulation of cerumen or a foreign body in the external auditory canal
- Pain or discomfort in the ear

A user instruction brochure is provided with every hearing aid device. In this brochure, the following information is presented:

- Notification that good health practice requires a medical evaluation before purchasing a hearing aid
- Notification that any of the otologic conditions listed previously should be investigated by a physician before purchase of a hearing aid
- Instructions for proper use, maintenance, and care of the hearing aid, as well as instructions for replacing or recharging the batteries
- Repair service information
- Description of avoidable conditions that could damage the hearing aid
- List of any known side effects that may warrant physician consultation (e.g., skin irritation, accelerated cerumen accumulation)

The evolution in technology has led to the availability of many smaller and more effective devices as well as different options and features of hearing aids (FDA, 2018a) (see Chart 59-13). The majority of hearing aids sold today are behind-the-ear, in-the-ear, or in-the-canal types (see Table 59-4). One model is the Lyric, which is placed in the ear canal just 4 mm from the tympanic membrane. Its volume is controlled by a magnet, and when its batteries no longer function (1 to 4 months), a physician can remove it with the magnet and reinsert a new device. This device does not have many of the problems (e.g., feedback noise, overamplification of background noise) associated with other hearing aids, and

Chart
59-13

Options and Features of Hearing Aids to Consider

- *T-Coil:* May improve hearing on the telephone by switching the settings from normal to telephone setting. This feature also assists in amplifying voices when the patient is in larger areas, such as theaters, auditoriums, and gymnasiums. Background noise may be toned down to adequately hear close conversation.
- *Directional Microphone:* Useful in environments with a lot of background noise and activity. The microphone may be directed toward the speaker and amplifies conversation while diminishing background noise.
- *Direct Audio Input:* Allows direct connection from a remote microphone or an FM assistive listening system to devices such as a computer, television, or stereo.
- *Feedback Suppression:* Suppresses whistling feedback noise.

Adapted from U.S. Food and Drug Administration. (2018a). Medical devices: Types of hearing aids. Retrieved on 2/22/2020 at: www.fda.gov/medical-devices/hearing-aids/types-hearing-aids

TABLE 59-4	Hearing Aids	
Site (Range of Hearing Loss)	Advantages	Disadvantages
Body, usually on the trunk (mild–profound)	Separation of receiver and microphone prevents acoustic feedback, allowing high amplification; generally used in a school setting	Bulky; requires long wire, which may be cosmetically displeasing; some loss of high-frequency response
Behind the ear (mild–profound)	Economical; powerful, with no long wires; easily used by children—adapts easily as the child grows, with only the ear mold needing replacement	Large size
In the ear (mild–moderately severe)	One-piece custom fit to contour of ear; no tubes or cords; miniature microphone located in the ear, which is a more natural placement; more cosmetically appealing due to easy concealment	Smaller size limits output; patients who have arthritis or cannot perform tasks requiring good manual dexterity may have difficulty with the small size of aid or battery; can require more repair than the behind-the-ear aid
In the canal (mild–moderately severe)	Same as in-the-ear aids; less visible, so more cosmetically pleasing	Even smaller than in-the-ear aids; requires good manual dexterity and good vision

it does not involve the expense and uncertainty of surgical procedures. However, Lyric is not an option if the ear canal is too narrow to accommodate the device.

Implanted Hearing Devices

There are several types of implanted hearing devices, ranging from implantable to semi-implantable devices (FDA, 2018b).

Bone conduction devices, which transmit sound through the skull to the inner ear, are used in patients with a conductive hearing loss if a hearing aid is contraindicated (e.g., those with chronic infection). The device is implanted postauricularly under the skin into the skull, and an external device—worn above the ear, not in the canal—transmits the sound through the skin. There are two types of implantable hearing aids. The bone-anchored hearing aid (BAHA) is implanted behind the ear in the mastoid area. The middle ear implant (MEI) is implanted in the middle ear cavity. The BAHA is used for conductive or mixed hearing loss, whereas the MEI is used for sensorineural hearing loss (FDA, 2018b).

The implantable middle ear hearing device (IMEHD) comes in two styles: piezoelectric and electromagnetic, which are partially or totally implanted. Patients must be 18 years or older, must be diagnosed with mild to severe sensorineural loss, and must have tried other conventional devices with poor results to be considered candidates for this type of device. The implantable device has several advantages—for example, it may eliminate feedback, achieve good cosmetic results, and allow the patient to perform most preferred leisure activities (e.g., dancing, swimming). Disadvantages are that this device is expensive, necessitates surgery, requires periodic recharging of batteries, and has unpredictable power output (FDA, 2018b).

The FDA has also approved the semi-implantable Vibrant Soundbridge (electromagnetic) and the total implantable Envoy Esteem (piezoelectric) devices. The Vibrant Soundbridge has an external device attached to the postauricular bone that transmits sound to the magnet in the middle ear that is attached to the long process of the incus. The magnet surrounds the long axis of the stapes, which in turn vibrates and sound is heard. The Envoy Esteem works similarly to the natural ear. The piezoelectric transducer is located at the head of the incus, which sends a signal that is amplified, filtered, and then converted back to a vibration signal. This vibration is delivered by the driver (piezoelectric transducer) and attached to the stapes capitulum; then, via the stapes bone, the inner ear receives the signal and is converted into a nerve impulse and translated into sound by the brain. The incus is removed prior to insertion of this device to prevent feedback from the sensor. Clinical trials reported that in best-fit aided conditions, speech reception thresholds improved from 41.2 dB to 29.4 dB and word recognition score at 50 dB hearing level improved from best-fit aided of 46.3% to 68.9% with the Envoy Esteem (Kraus, Shohet, & Catalano, 2011). A 5-year follow-up study of the same group found that word recognition scores were improved by 17%; word recognition score at 50 dB hearing level improved in 49%, and remained the same in 41%; and speech reception threshold improved at every annual follow-up (Shohet, Kraus, Catalano, et al., 2018).

A cochlear implant is an auditory prosthesis used for people with profound sensorineural hearing loss bilaterally who do not benefit from conventional hearing aids. The cochlear implant directly stimulates the auditory nerve and has made it possible for people who have severe hearing loss or who are deaf to hear sound (NIDCD, 2017a). The hearing loss may be congenital or acquired. An implant does not restore normal hearing; rather, it helps the person detect medium to loud environmental sounds and conversation. The implant provides stimulation directly to the auditory nerve, bypassing the nonfunctioning hair cells of the inner ear. The microphone and signal processor, worn outside the body, transmit electrical stimuli to the implanted electrodes. The electrical signals stimulate the auditory nerve fibers and then the brain, where they are interpreted.

Worldwide, more than 324,200 people have received cochlear implants. In the United States, approximately 58,000 adults and 38,000 children have received cochlear implants (NIDCD, 2017a). Studies report that older adult patients with cochlear implants experience improved understanding of speech and better cognition. Patients with cochlear implants were also noted to have more social interactions with others and improved quality of life. Research has reported that hearing improvement with a cochlear implant delays the occurrence as well as the progression of dementia (Sarant, Harris, Busby, et al., 2019). Candidates for a cochlear implant, who are usually at least 1 year of age, are selected after careful screening by otologic history, physical examination, audiologic testing,

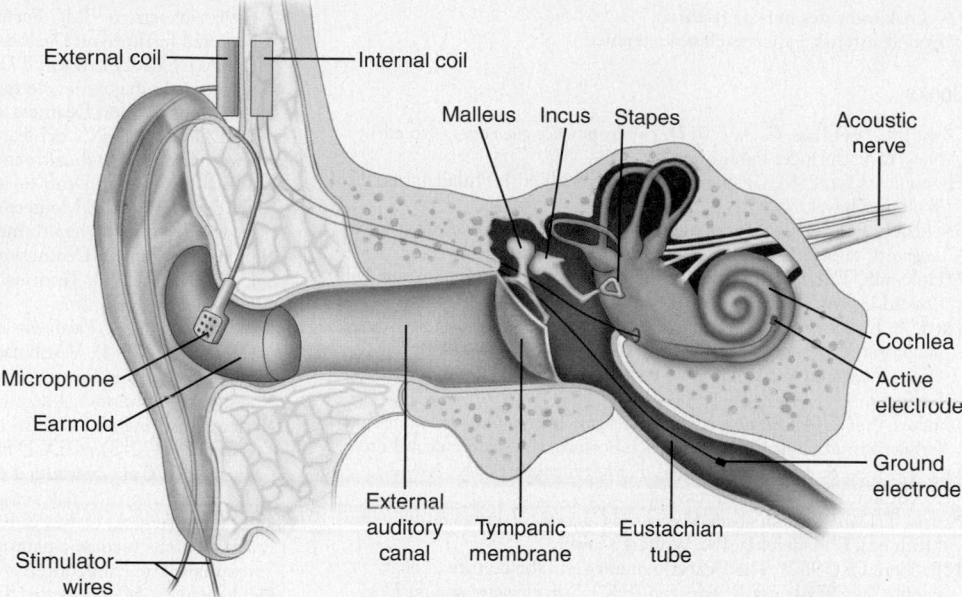

Figure 59-7 • The cochlear implant. The internal coil has a stranded electrode lead. The electrode is inserted through the round window into the scala tympani of the cochlea. The external coil (the transmitter) is held in alignment with the internal coil (the receiver) by a magnet. The microphone receives the sound. The stimulator wire receives the signal after it has been filtered, adjusted, and modified so that the sound is at a comfortable level for the patient. Sound is passed by the external transmitter to the inner coil receiver by magnetic conduction and is then carried by the electrode to the cochlea.

x-rays, and psychological testing. Criteria for choosing adults who may benefit from a cochlear implant include:

- Profound sensorineural hearing loss in both ears
- Inability to hear and recognize speech well with hearing aids
- No medical contraindication to a cochlear implant or general anesthesia
- Indications that being able to hear would enhance the patient's life

The surgery involves implanting a small receiver in the temporal bone through a postauricular incision and placing electrodes into the inner ear (see Fig. 59-7). The microphone and transmitter are worn on an external unit. The patient undergoes extensive cochlear rehabilitation with the multidisciplinary team, which includes an audiologist and speech pathologist. Several months may be needed to learn to interpret the sounds heard. Children and adults who lost their hearing before they learned to speak take much longer to acquire speech. There are wide variations of success with cochlear implants, and there is also controversy about their use, especially among the Deaf community. Patients who have had a cochlear implant are cautioned that an MRI scan will inactivate the implant; MRI should be used only when there is no other diagnostic option.

Hearing Guide Dogs

Specially trained dogs (service dogs) are available to assist the person with a hearing loss. People who live alone are eligible to apply for a dog trained by International Hearing Dog, Inc. The dog reacts to the sound of a telephone, a doorbell, an alarm clock, a baby's cry, a knock at the door, a smoke alarm, or an intruder. The dog alerts its master by physical contact; the dog then runs to the source of the noise. In public, the dog positions itself between the person who is deaf or has severe hearing loss and any potential hazard that the person cannot hear, such as an oncoming vehicle or a loud, hostile person.

A certified hearing guide dog is legally permitted access to public transportation, public eating places, and stores, including food markets.

CRITICAL THINKING EXERCISES

1 **ebp** A 65-year-old woman visits the clinic where you work for a routine well-woman examination. She mentions that her friend was recently diagnosed with hearing loss and fitted for a hearing aid. She has no perceived hearing loss, but she wonders whether she needs a hearing aid. What evidence-based recommendations would you make for this patient about hearing loss screening and diagnosis? What is the strength of the evidence for your recommendations?

2 **pg** A 40-year-old man has complained of hearing loss that has gradually worsened over the past few months. He has difficulty hearing the television and having a telephone conversation. After seeing the primary provider today, he was diagnosed with cerumen impaction. Discuss how you will educate the patient about the diagnosis of cerumen impaction. What is your priority for care of this patient? Give your rationale.

3 **ipc** A 54-year-old man had a cochlear implant placed 5 years ago and has been admitted to the medical-surgical unit due to implant malfunction. Develop a plan of action for communicating with this patient. What should you know about cochlear implants to communicate effectively with the patient? What environmental conditions should be considered to promote patient safety and well-being? Which members of the health care team should be informed about this patient's communication needs?

REFERENCES

*Asterisk indicates nursing research.
**Double asterisk indicates classic reference.

Books

Cash, J. C., & Glass, C. A. (2017). *Family practice guidelines* (4th ed.). New York: Springer Publishing.

Eliopoulos, C. (2018). *Gerontological nursing* (9th ed.). Philadelphia, PA: Wolters Kluwer.

Fischbach, F. T., & Fischbach, M. A. (2018). *A manual of laboratory and diagnostic tests* (10th ed.). Philadelphia, PA: Wolters Kluwer.

**Holcomb, T. K. (2013). *Introduction to American Deaf culture*. New York: Oxford University Press.

Luryi, A. L., Morse, E., & Michaelides, E. (2019). Pathophysiology and diagnosis of Meniere's disease. In S. Babu, C. Schutt, & D. Bojrab (Eds.). *Diagnosis and treatment of vestibular disorders*. Cham, Switzerland: Springer.

Mindess, A. (2014). *Reading between the signs: Intercultural communication for sign language interpreters* (3rd ed.). Boston, MA: Intercultural Press.

Moore, M. S., & Levitan, L. (2016). *For hearing people only* (4th ed.). Rochester, NY: Deaf Life Press.

Norris, T. (2019). *Porth's pathophysiology: Concepts of altered health status* (10th ed) Philadelphia, PA: Wolters Kluwer.

**Padden, C. (1980). The Deaf community and the culture of deaf people. In C. Baker & R. Battison (Eds.). *Sign language and the Deaf community: Essays in honor of William C. Stokoe*. Silver Spring, MD: National Association of the Deaf.

Weber, J., & Kelley, J. (2018). *Health assessment in nursing* (6th ed.). Philadelphia, PA: Wolters Kluwer.

Journals and Electronic Documents

American Academy of Otolaryngology—Head and Neck Surgery. (2014). Position statement: Posturography. Retrieved on 1/16/2020 at: www.entnet.org/content/position-statement-posturography

Antonio, S. (2018). Genetic sensorineural hearing loss clinical presentation. Retrieved on 1/16/2020 at: www.emedicine.medscape.com/article/855875-clinical

Bhattacharyya, N. (2019). Auditory brainstem response auditometry. Retrieved on 1/16/2020 at: www.emedicine.medscape.com/article/836277-overview

Bhattacharyya, N., Gubbels, S. P., Schwartz, S. R., et al. (2017). Clinical practice guideline: Benign paroxysmal positional vertigo (update) executive summary. *Otolaryngology–Head and Neck Surgery*, 156(3), 403–416. Retrieved on 3/7/2020 at: www.doi.org/10.1177%2F0194599816689660

Brainard, A., & Gresham, C. (2014). Prevention and treatment of motion sickness. *American Family Physician*, 90(1), 41–46.

Carlson, M. L., Tveiten, O. V., Driscoll, C. L., et al. (2015). Long-term quality of life in patients with vestibular schwannoma: An international multicenter cross-sectional study comparing microsurgery, stereotactic radiosurgery, observation, and nontumor controls. *Journal of Neurosurgery*, 122(4), 833–842.

Centers for Disease Control and Prevention (CDC). (2018). The National Institute for Occupational Safety and Health (NIOSH). Noise and hearing loss prevention. Retrieved on 2/15/2020 at: www.cdc.gov/niosh/topics/noise/reducenoiseexposure/regsguidance.html

Haskins, J. (2017). Healthy People 2030 to create objectives for health of nation: Process underway for next 10-year plan. *The Nation's Health*, 47(6), 1–14.

Hsu, A. K., McKee, M., Roscigno, C., et al. (2019). Associations among hearing loss, hospitalization, readmission and mortality in older adults: A systematic review. *Geriatric Nursing*, 40(4), 367–379.

Kraus, E. M., Shohet, J. A., & Catalano, P. J. (2011). Envoy Esteem totally implantable hearing system: Phase 2 trial, 1-year hearing results. *Otolaryngology–Head and Neck Surgery*, 145(1), 100–109.

*Lewis, A., & Keele, B. (2020). Development and validation of instrument to measure nurses' beliefs toward Deaf and hard of hearing interaction. *Journal of Nursing Measurement*, 28(2). doi: 10.1891/JNM-D-19-00024

Mudd, P. (2019). Ototoxicity. Retrieved on 3/7/2020 at: www.emedicine.medscape.com/article/857679-overview

Muñoz, R. C., Moreno, J. L. B., Balboa, I. V., et al. (2019). Disability perceived by primary care patients with posterior canal benign paroxysmal positional vertigo. *BMC Family Practice*, 20(1), 156.

**National Institute on Deafness and Other Communication Disorders (NIDCD). (2010). WISE EARS. Update. Retrieved on 1/16/2020 at: www.nidcd.nih.gov/newsletter/2001/summer/wise-ears-update

National Institute on Deafness and Other Communication Disorders (NIDCD). (2017a). Cochlear implants. Retrieved on 2/22/2020 at: www.nidcd.nih.gov/health/cochlear-implants

National Institute on Deafness and Other Communication Disorders (NIDCD). (2017b). Ménière's disease. Retrieved on 2/22/2020 at: www.nidcd.nih.gov/health/menieres-disease

National Institute on Deafness and Other Communication Disorders (NIDCD). (2017c). Tinnitus. Retrieved on 2/22/2020 at: www.nidcd.nih.gov/health/tinnitus

National Institute on Deafness and Other Communication Disorders (NIDCD). (2017d). Vestibular schwannoma (acoustic neuroma) and neurofibromatosis. Retrieved on 2/23/2020 at: www.nidcd.nih.gov/health/vestibular-schwannoma-acoustic-neuroma-and-neurofibromatosis #ref1

National Institute on Deafness and Other Communication Disorders (NIDCD). (2018). NIDCD fact sheet: Balance disorders. Retrieved on 2/22/2020 at: www.nidcd.nih.gov/staticresources/health/balance-disorders

Park, J. K., Vernick, D. M., & Ramakrishna, N. (2019). Vestibular schwannoma (acoustic neuroma). *UpToDate*. Retrieved on 2/23/20 at: www.uptodate.com/contents/vestibular-schwannoma-acoustic-neuroma

Pendergrass, K. M., Newman, S. D., Jones, E., et al. (2019). Deaf: A concept analysis from a cultural perspective using the Wilson method of concept analysis development. *Clinical Nursing Research*, 28(1), 79–93.

Sarant, J., Harris, D., Busby, P., et al. (2019). The effect of cochlear implants on cognitive function in older adults: Initial baseline and 18-month follow up results for a prospective international longitudinal study. *Frontiers in Neuroscience*, 13, 789. doi: 10.3389/fnins.2019.00789

Shohet, J. A., Kraus, E. M., Catalano, P. J., et al. (2018). Totally implantable hearing system: Five-year hearing results. *The Larygoscope*, 128(1), 210–216.

Shukla, A., Reed, N., Armstrong, N. M., et al. (2019). Hearing loss, hearing aid use, and depressive symptoms in older adults—Findings from the Atherosclerosis Risk in Communities Neurocognitive Study (ARIC-NCS). *The Journals of Gerontology: Series B*, doi: 10.1093/geronb/gbz128

U.S. Department of Health & Human Services (HHS). (2016). National Institute on Deafness and Other Communication Disorders: Quick statistics about hearing. Retrieved on 1/16/2020 at: www.nidcd.nih.gov/health/statistics/quick-statistics-hearing

U.S. Department of Health and Human Services (HHS). (2017). *Healthy People 2030*. Retrieved on 7/15/2019 at: www.healthypeople.gov/2020/About-Healthy-People/Development-Healthy-People-2030/framework

U.S. Food and Drug Administration. (2018a). Medical devices: Types of hearing aids. Retrieved on 2/22/2020 at: www.fda.gov/medical-devices/hearing-aids/types-hearing-aids

U.S. Food and Drug Administration. (2018b). Medical devices: Other products and devices to improve hearing. Retrieved on 2/23/2020 at: www.fda.gov/medical-devices/hearing-aids/other-products-and-devices-improve-hearing

van Steekelenburg, J. M., van Weijnen, A., de Pont, L. M. H., et al. (2020). Value of endolymphatic hydrops and perilymph signal intensity in suspected Ménière's disease. *American Journal of Neuroradiology*, 41(3), 529–534

World Federation of the Deaf (WFD). (2020). *International Week of the Deaf 2020*. Retrieved on 8/17/2020 at: www.wfdeaf.org/ get-involved/wfd-events/international-week-deaf/internationalweekofthedeaf/

Resources

Acoustic Neuroma Association (ANA), www.anausa.org

Alexander Graham Bell Association for the Deaf and Hard of Hearing, www.agbell.org

American Academy of Audiology, www.audiology.org

American Academy of Facial Plastic and Reconstructive Surgery, www.aafprs.org

American Academy of Otolaryngology—Head and Neck Surgery, www.entnet.org

American Board of Audiology, www.boardofaudiology.org

American Cochlear Implant Alliance (ACI Alliance), www.acialliance.org
American Speech-Language-Hearing Association, www.asha.org
American Tinnitus Association (ATA), www.ata.org
Association of Late-Deafened Adults, Inc. (ALDA), www.alda.org
Association of Medical Professionals with Hearing Losses (AMPHL), www.amphl.org
Center for Hearing and Communication, www.chchearing.org
Hearing Health Foundation, www.hearinghealthfoundation.org
Hearing Loss Association of America (HLAA), www.hearingloss.org
International Federation of Hard of Hearing People (IFHOH), www.ifhoh.org

International Hearing Dog, Inc., www.hearingdog.org
National Association of the Deaf (NAD), www.nad.org
National Black Deaf Advocates (NBDA), www.nbda.org
National Cued Speech Association (NCSA), www.cuedspeech.org
National Institute on Deafness and Other Communication Disorders (NIDCD), National Institutes of Health, www.nidcd.nih.gov
Society of Otorhinolaryngology and Head-Neck Nurses, www.sohnnurse.com
Usher Syndrome Coalition, www.usher-syndrome.org
Vestibular Disorders Association, www.vestibular.org
World Federation of the Deaf (WFD), www.wfdeaf.org

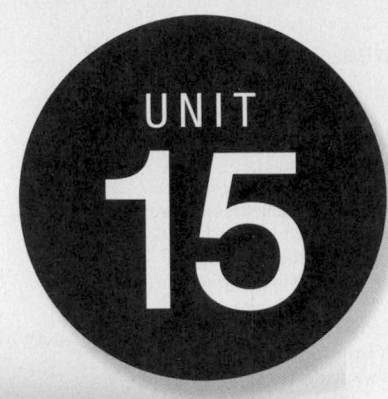

Neurologic Function

Case Study DEVELOPING A TEAM-BASED PLAN OF CARE

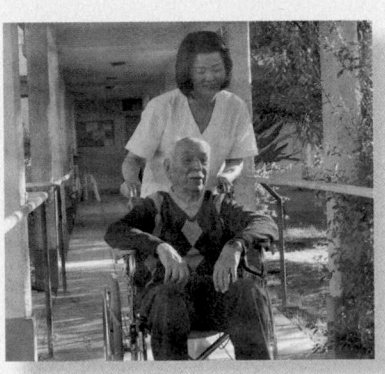

Y ou are the nurse caring for a 70-year-old man with Parkinson's disease who was recently admitted to the skilled nursing facility where you work. The patient was diagnosed with Parkinson's disease 5 years ago but has only recently had a significant decline in function. He can no longer dress himself because he lacks the ability to control fine motor movements in his hands. In addition, he has lost 10 lb in the past 3 months as a result of difficulty feeding himself because of the constant tremors. The patient's wife has reported feeling exhausted prior to her husband's admission; she had not been sleeping well due to her husband having nightmares and trying to get up during the night. You form a task force to help develop a plan of care that is focused on increasing the patient's functionality so that he might be discharged home. Specifically, you invite a staff nutritionist, pharmacist, physical therapist, occupational therapist, and social worker to work with you in developing the plan of care for this patient.

QSEN Competency Focus: Teamwork and Collaboration

The complexities inherent in today's health care system challenge nurses to demonstrate integration of specific interdisciplinary core competencies. These competencies are aimed at ensuring the delivery of safe, quality patient care (Institute of Medicine, 2003). The Quality and Safety Education for Nurses project (Cronenwett, Sherwood, Barnsteiner, et al., 2007; QSEN, 2020) provides a framework for the knowledge, skills, and attitudes (KSAs) required for nurses to demonstrate competency in these key areas, which include *patient-centered care*, *interdisciplinary teamwork and collaboration*, *evidence-based practice*, *quality improvement*, *safety*, and *informatics.*

Teamwork and Collaboration Definition: Function effectively within nursing and interprofessional teams, fostering open communication, mutual respect, and shared decision-making to achieve quality patient care.

SELECT PRE-LICENSURE KSAs	APPLICATION AND REFLECTION
Knowledge	
Describe scopes of practice and roles of health care team members Describe strategies for identifying and managing overlaps in team member roles and accountabilities Recognize contributions of other individuals and groups in helping patient/family achieve health goals	How can you help the patient and his wife identify health goals to manage his Parkinson's disease? Based upon your knowledge of their scopes of practice, identify why you decided which team members to include when you formed the task force. Identify the contributions of the different members of the team in meeting the patient's and wife's goals.
Skills	
Assume role of team member or leader based on the situation Initiate requests for help when appropriate to situation Clarify roles and accountabilities under conditions of potential overlap in team member functioning Integrate the contributions of others who play a role in helping patient/family achieve health goals	What skills will you need to assume the role of team leader and advocate for the needs of both the patient and his wife? What subjective and objective assessment criteria can you use to determine which team members need to be consulted for which specific problem or to help the patient and his wife meet specific goals? Once the consults have been made, what is your role in ensuring that the plan of care for this patient is being implemented?
Attitudes	
Value the perspectives and expertise of all health team members Respect the centrality of the patient/family as core members of any health care team Respect the unique attributes that members bring to a team, including variations in professional orientations and accountabilities	How will you demonstrate to the patient and his wife the value of the various team members? How can team members ensure respect for each other? How will each member of the team maintain accountability for the plan of care?

Cronenwett, L., Sherwood, G., Barnsteiner, J., et al. (2007). Quality and safety education for nurses. *Nursing Outlook*, *55*(3), 122–131; Institute of Medicine. (2003). *Health professions education: A bridge to quality*. Washington, DC: National Academies Press; QSEN Institute. (2020). *QSEN competencies: Definitions and pre-licensure KSAs; Teamwork and collaboration*. Retrieved on 8/15/2020 at: qsen.org/competencies/pre-licensure-ksas/#teamwork_collaboration

60 Assessment of Neurologic Function

Nurses in many practice settings encounter patients with altered neurologic function. Disorders of the nervous system can occur at any time during the lifespan and can vary from mild, self-limiting symptoms to devastating, life-threatening disorders. Nurses must be skilled in the general assessment of neurologic function and be able to focus on specific areas as needed. Assessment requires knowledge of the anatomy and physiology of the nervous system and an understanding of the

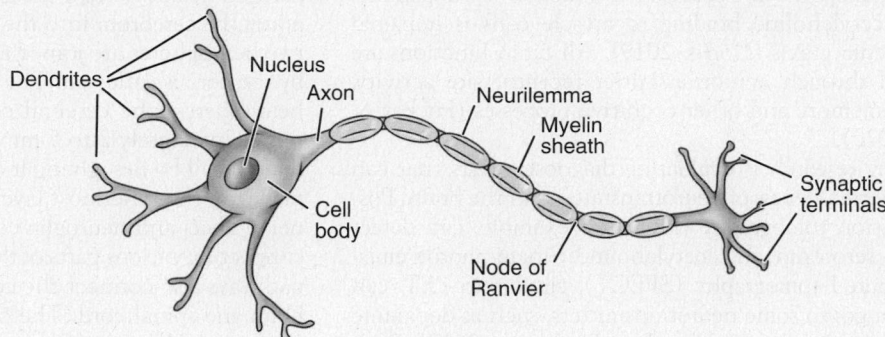

Figure 60-1 • Neuron.

array of tests and procedures used to diagnose neurologic disorders. Knowledge about the nursing implications and interventions related to assessment and diagnostic testing is also essential.

Anatomic and Physiologic Overview

The nervous system consists of two major parts: the central nervous system (CNS), including the brain and spinal cord, and the peripheral nervous system, which includes the cranial nerves, spinal nerves, and autonomic nervous system. The function of the nervous system is to control motor, sensory, autonomic, cognitive, and behavioral activities. The brain itself contains more than 100 billion cells that link the motor and sensory pathways, monitor the body's processes, respond to the internal and external environment, maintain homeostasis, and direct all psychological, biologic, and physical activity through complex chemical and electrical messages (Klein & Stewart-Amidei, 2017).

Cells of the Nervous System

The basic functional unit of the brain is the neuron (see Fig. 60-1). It is composed of dendrites, a cell body, and an axon. The **dendrites** are branch-type structures for receiving electrochemical messages. The **axon** is a long projection that carries electrical impulses away from the cell body. Some axons have a myelinated sheath that increases speed of conduction. Nerve cell bodies occurring in clusters are called *ganglia* or *nuclei*. A cluster of cell bodies with the same function is called a *center* (e.g., the respiratory center). Neurons are supported, protected, and nourished by glial cells, which are 50 times greater in number than neurons (Hickey & Strayer, 2020).

Neurotransmitters

Neurotransmitters communicate messages from one neuron to another or from a neuron to a target cell, such as muscle or endocrine cells. Neurotransmitters are manufactured and stored in synaptic vesicles. As an electrical action potential moves along the axon and reaches the nerve terminal, neurotransmitters are released into the synapse. The neurotransmitter is transported across the synapse, binding to receptors on the postsynaptic cell membrane. A neurotransmitter can either excite or inhibit activity of the target cell. Usually, multiple neurotransmitters are at work in the neural synapse. The source and action of major neurotransmitters are described in Table 60-1. Once released, enzymes either destroy the neurotransmitter or reabsorb it into the neuron for future use.

Many neurologic disorders are due, at least in part, to an imbalance in neurotransmitters. For example, Parkinson's

TABLE 60-1	Major Neurotransmitters	
Neurotransmitter	**Source**	**Action**
Acetylcholine (major transmitter of the parasympathetic nervous system)	Neurons in many areas of the brain; autonomic nervous system	Usually excitatory; parasympathetic effects sometimes inhibitory (stimulation of heart by vagal nerve)
Serotonin	Brain stem, hypothalamus, dorsal horn of the spinal cord	Inhibitory; helps control mood and sleep, inhibits pain pathways
Dopamine	Neurons on the substantia nigra and basal ganglia	Usually inhibitory; affects behavior (attention, emotions) and fine movement
Norepinephrine (major transmitter of the sympathetic nervous system)	Brain stem, hypothalamus, postganglionic neurons of the sympathetic nervous system	Usually excitatory; affects mood and overall activity
Gamma-aminobutyric acid	Nerve terminals of the spinal cord, cerebellum, basal ganglia, some cortical areas	Inhibitory
Enkephalin, endorphin	Nerve terminals in the spine, brain stem, thalamus and hypothalamus, pituitary gland	Excitatory; pleasurable sensation, inhibits pain transmission

Adapted from Norris, T. L. (2019). *Porth's pathophysiology: Concepts of altered health state* (10th ed.). Philadelphia, PA: Wolters Kluwer.

disease develops from decreased availability of dopamine, whereas acetylcholine binding to muscle cells is impaired in myasthenia gravis (Norris, 2019). All brain functions are modulated through neurotransmitter receptor site activity, including memory and other cognitive processes (Hickey & Strayer, 2020).

Ongoing research is evaluating diagnostic tests that can detect abnormal levels of neurotransmitters in the brain. Positron emission tomography (PET), for example, can detect dopamine, serotonin, and acetylcholine. Single-photon emission computed tomography (SPECT), similar to PET, can detect changes in some neurotransmitters, such as dopamine in Parkinson's disease (Fischbach & Fischbach, 2018). Both PET and SPECT are discussed in more detail later in this chapter.

The Central Nervous System

The CNS consists of the brain and the spinal cord.

The Brain

The brain accounts for approximately 2% of the total-body weight; in an average young adult, the brain weighs approximately 1400 g, whereas in an average older adult, the brain weighs approximately 1200 g (Hickey & Strayer, 2020). The brain is divided into three major areas: the cerebrum, the brain stem, and the cerebellum. The cerebrum is composed of two hemispheres, the thalamus, the hypothalamus, and the basal ganglia. The brain stem includes the midbrain, pons, and medulla. The cerebellum is located under the cerebrum and behind the brain stem (see Fig. 60-2).

Cerebrum

The outside surface of the hemispheres has a wrinkled appearance that is the result of many folded layers or convolutions called *gyri*, which increase the surface area of the brain, accounting for the high level of activity carried out by such a small-appearing organ. Between each gyrus is a sulcus or fissure that serves as an anatomic division. In between the

cerebral hemispheres is the great longitudinal fissure that separates the cerebrum into the right and left hemispheres. The two hemispheres are joined at the lower portion of the fissure by the corpus callosum. The external or outer portion of the hemispheres (the cerebral cortex) is made up of gray matter approximately 2 to 5 mm in depth; it contains billions of neuron cell bodies, giving it a gray appearance. White matter makes up the innermost layer and is composed of myelinated nerve fibers and neuroglia cells that form tracts or pathways connecting various parts of the brain with one another. These pathways also connect the cortex with lower portions of the brain and spinal cord. The cerebral hemispheres are divided into pairs of lobes as follows (see Fig. 60-2):

- *Frontal*—the largest lobe, located in the front of the brain. The major functions of this lobe are concentration, abstract thought, information storage or memory, and motor function. It contains Broca area, which is in the left hemisphere and is critical for motor control of speech. The frontal lobe is also responsible in large part for a person's affect, judgment, personality, and inhibitions (Hickey & Strayer, 2020).
- *Parietal*—a predominantly sensory lobe posterior to the frontal lobe. This lobe analyzes sensory information and relays the interpretation of this information to other cortical areas and is essential to a person's awareness of body position in space, size and shape discrimination, and right–left orientation (Hickey & Strayer, 2020).
- *Temporal*—located inferior to the frontal and parietal lobes, this lobe contains the auditory receptive areas and plays a role in memory of sound and understanding of language and music.
- *Occipital*—located posterior to the parietal lobe, this lobe is responsible for visual interpretation and memory.

The corpus callosum (see Fig. 60-3), a thick collection of nerve fibers that connects the two hemispheres of the brain, is responsible for the transmission of information from one side of the brain to the other. Information transferred includes sensation, memory, and learned discrimination. Right-handed people and some left-handed people have cerebral

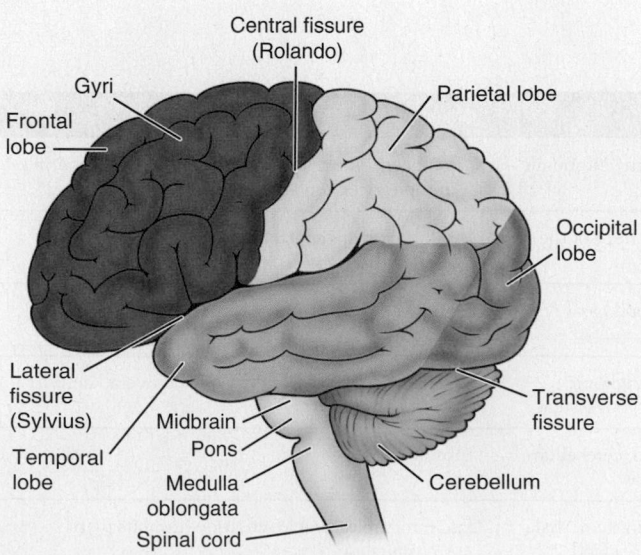

Figure 60-2 • View of the external surface of the brain showing lobes, cerebellum, and brain stem.

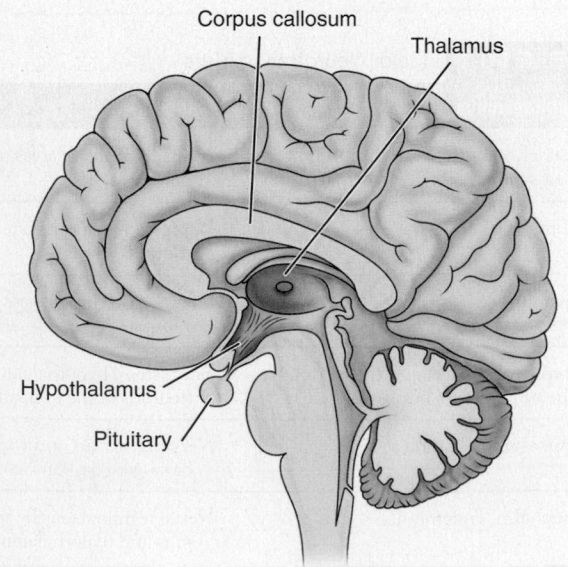

Figure 60-3 • Medial view of the brain.

dominance on the left side of the brain for verbal, linguistic, arithmetic, calculation, and analytic functions. The nondominant hemisphere is responsible for geometric, spatial, visual, pattern, and musical functions. Nuclei for cranial nerves I and II are also located in the cerebrum.

The thalami lie on either side of the third ventricle and act primarily as a relay station for all sensation except smell. All memory, sensation, and pain impulses pass through this section of the brain. The hypothalamus (see Fig. 60-3) is located anterior and inferior to the thalamus, and beneath and lateral to the third ventricle. The infundibulum of the hypothalamus connects it to the posterior pituitary gland. The hypothalamus plays an important role in the endocrine system because it regulates the pituitary secretion of hormones that influence metabolism, reproduction, stress response, and urine production. It works with the pituitary to maintain fluid balance through hormonal release and maintains temperature regulation by promoting vasoconstriction or vasodilatation. In addition, the hypothalamus is the site of the hunger center and is involved in appetite control. It contains centers that regulate the sleep–wake cycle, blood pressure, aggressive and sexual behavior, and emotional responses (e.g., blushing, rage, depression, panic, fear). The hypothalamus also controls and regulates the autonomic nervous system. The optic chiasm (the point at which the two optic tracts cross) and the mammillary bodies (involved in olfactory reflexes and emotional response to odors) are also found in this area.

The basal ganglia are masses of nuclei located deep in the cerebral hemispheres that are responsible for control of fine motor movements, including those of the hands and lower extremities.

Brain Stem

The brain stem consists of the midbrain, pons, and medulla oblongata (see Fig. 60-2). The midbrain connects the pons and the cerebellum with the cerebral hemispheres; it contains sensory and motor pathways and serves as the center for auditory and visual reflexes. Cranial nerves III and IV originate in the midbrain. The pons is situated in front of the cerebellum between the midbrain and the medulla and is a bridge between the two halves of the cerebellum, and between the medulla and the midbrain. Cranial nerves V through VIII originate in the pons. The pons also contains motor and sensory pathways. Portions of the pons help regulate respiration.

Motor fibers from the brain to the spinal cord and sensory fibers from the spinal cord to the brain are in the medulla. Most of these fibers cross, or decussate, at this level. Cranial nerves IX through XII originate in the medulla. Reflex centers for respiration, blood pressure, heart rate, coughing, vomiting, swallowing, and sneezing are also located in the medulla. The reticular formation, responsible for arousal and the sleep–wake cycle, begins in the medulla and connects with numerous higher structures.

Cerebellum

The cerebellum is posterior to the midbrain and pons, and below the occipital lobe (see Fig. 60-2). The cerebellum integrates sensory information to provide smooth coordinated movement. It controls fine movement, balance, and **position (postural) sense** or proprioception (awareness of position of extremities without looking at them).

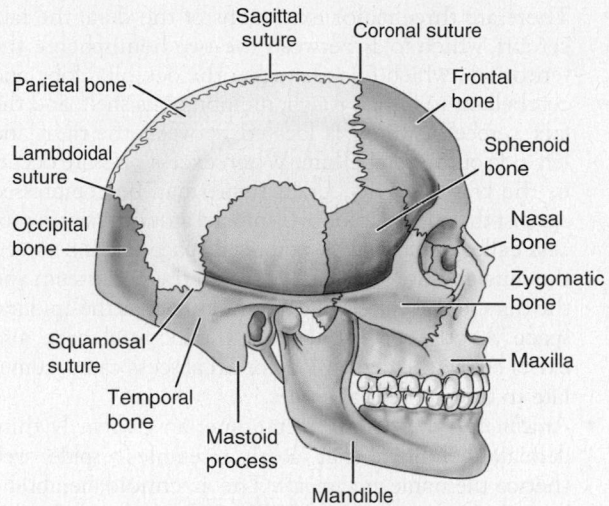

Figure 60-4 • Bones and sutures of the skull.

Structures Protecting the Brain

The brain is contained in the rigid skull, which protects it from injury. The major bones of the skull are the frontal, temporal, parietal, occipital, and sphenoid bones. These bones join at the suture lines (see Fig. 60-4) and form the base of the skull. Indentations in the skull base are known as fossae. The anterior fossa contains the frontal lobe, the middle fossa contains the temporal lobe, and the posterior fossa contains the cerebellum and brain stem.

The meninges (fibrous connective tissues that cover the brain and spinal cord) provide protection, support, and nourishment. The layers of the meninges are the dura mater, arachnoid, and pia mater (see Fig. 60-5):

- *Dura mater*—the outermost layer; covers the brain and the spinal cord. It is tough, thick, inelastic, fibrous, and gray.

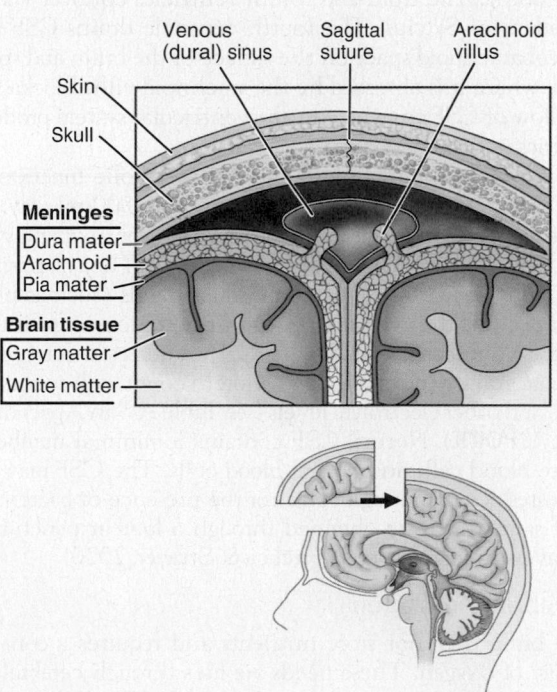

Figure 60-5 • Meninges and related structures.

There are three major extensions of the dura: the falx cerebri, which folds between the two hemispheres; the tentorium, which folds between the occipital lobe and cerebellum to form a tough, membranous shelf; and the falx cerebelli, which is located between the right and left side of the cerebellum. When excess pressure occurs in the cranial cavity, brain tissue may be compressed against these dural folds or displaced around them, a process called *herniation*. A potential space exists between the dura and the skull, and between the periosteum and the dura in the vertebral column, known as the epidural space. Another potential space, the subdural space, also exists below the dura. Blood or an abscess can accumulate in these potential spaces.

- *Arachnoid*—the middle membrane; an extremely thin, delicate membrane that closely resembles a spider web (hence the name *arachnoid*). The arachnoid membrane has cerebrospinal fluid (CSF) in the space below it, known as the subarachnoid space. This membrane has arachnoid villi, which are unique finger-like projections that absorb CSF into the venous system. When blood or bacteria enter the subarachnoid space, the villi become obstructed and *communicating* hydrocephalus (increased size of ventricles) may result.
- *Pia mater*—the innermost, thin, transparent layer that hugs the brain closely and extends into every fold of the brain's surface.

Cerebrospinal Fluid

CSF is a clear and colorless fluid that is produced in the choroid plexus of the ventricles and circulates around the surface of the brain and the spinal cord. There are four ventricles: the right and left lateral and the third and fourth ventricles. The two lateral ventricles open into the third ventricle at the interventricular foramen (also known as the foramen of Monro). The third and fourth ventricles connect via the aqueduct of Sylvius. The fourth ventricle drains CSF into the subarachnoid space on the surface of the brain and spinal cord, where it is absorbed by the arachnoid villi. Blockage of the flow of CSF anywhere in the ventricular system produces *obstructive* hydrocephalus.

CSF is important in immune and metabolic functions in the brain. It is produced at a rate of about 500 mL/day; the ventricles and subarachnoid space contain approximately 125 to 150 mL of fluid (Hickey & Strayer, 2020). The composition of CSF is similar to other extracellular fluids (such as blood plasma), but the concentrations of the various constituents differ. A laboratory analysis of CSF indicates color (clear), specific gravity (normal 1.007), protein count, cell count, glucose, and other electrolyte levels (see Table A-5 in Appendix A on thePoint). Normal CSF contains a minimal number of white blood cells and no red blood cells. The CSF may also be tested for immunoglobulins or the presence of bacteria. A CSF sample may be obtained through a lumbar puncture or intraventricular catheter (Hickey & Strayer, 2020).

Cerebral Circulation

The brain does not store nutrients and requires a constant supply of oxygen. These needs are met through cerebral circulation; the brain receives approximately 15% of the cardiac output, or 750 mL per minute of blood flow. Brain circulation

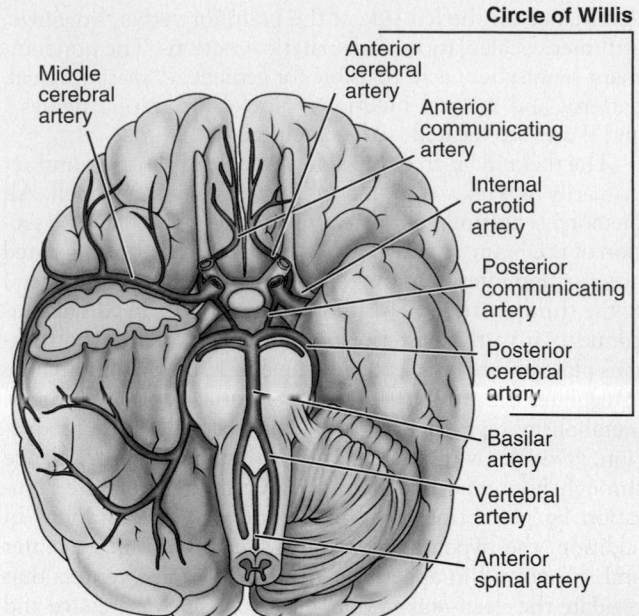

Figure 60-6 • Arterial blood supply of the brain, including the circle of Willis, as viewed from the ventral surface.

is unique in several aspects. First, arterial and venous vessels are not parallel as in other organs in the body; this is due in part to the role the venous system plays in CSF absorption. Second, the brain has collateral circulation through the circle of Willis (see later discussion), allowing blood flow to be redirected on demand. Third, blood vessels in the brain have two rather than three layers, which may make them more prone to rupture when weakened or under pressure.

Arteries

Arterial blood supply to the anterior brain originates from the common carotid artery, which is the first bifurcation of the aorta. The internal carotid arteries arise at the bifurcation of the common carotid. Branches of the internal carotid arteries (the anterior and middle cerebral arteries) and their connections (the anterior and posterior communicating arteries) form the circle of Willis (see Fig. 60-6).

The vertebral arteries branch from the subclavian arteries to supply most of the posterior circulation of the brain. At the level of the brain stem, the vertebral arteries join to form the basilar artery. The basilar artery divides to form the two branches of the posterior cerebral arteries. Functionally, the posterior and anterior portions of the circulation usually remain separate. However, the circle of Willis can provide collateral circulation through communicating arteries if one of the vessels supplying it becomes occluded or is ligated.

The bifurcations along the circle of Willis are frequent sites of aneurysm formation. Aneurysms are outpouchings of the blood vessel due to vessel wall weakness. Aneurysms can rupture and cause a hemorrhagic stroke. See Chapter 62 for a more detailed discussion of aneurysms.

Veins

Venous drainage for the brain does not follow the arterial circulation as in other body structures. The veins reach the brain's surface, join larger veins, and then cross the subarachnoid space and empty into the dural sinuses, which are the vascular channels embedded in the dura (see Fig. 60-5). The network of the sinuses carries venous outflow from the brain and empties into the internal jugular veins, returning the blood to the heart. Cerebral veins are unique, because unlike other veins in the body, they do not have valves to prevent blood from flowing backward and depend on both gravity and blood pressure for flow.

Blood–Brain Barrier

The CNS is inaccessible to many substances that circulate in the blood plasma (e.g., dyes, medications, antibiotic agents) because of the blood–brain barrier. This barrier is formed by the endothelial cells of the brain's capillaries, which form continuous tight junctions, creating a barrier to macromolecules and many compounds. All substances entering the CSF must filter through the capillary endothelial cells and astrocytes. The blood–brain barrier has a protective function but can be altered by trauma, cerebral edema, and cerebral hypoxemia; this has implications for treatment and selection of medications for CNS disorders (Hickey & Strayer, 2020).

The Spinal Cord

The spinal cord is continuous with the medulla, extending from the cerebral hemispheres and serving as the connection between the brain and the periphery. Approximately 45 cm (18 inches) long and about the thickness of a finger, it extends from the foramen magnum at the base of the skull to the lower border of the first lumbar vertebra, where it tapers to a fibrous band called the *conus medullaris.* Continuing below the second lumbar space are the nerve roots that extend beyond the conus, which are called the *cauda equina* because they resemble a horse's tail. Meninges surround the spinal cord.

In a cross-sectional view, the spinal cord has an H-shaped central core of nerve cell bodies (gray matter) surrounded by ascending and descending tracts (white matter) (see Fig. 60-7). The lower portion of the H is broader than the upper portion and corresponds to the anterior horns. The anterior horns contain cells with fibers that form the anterior (motor) root and are essential for the voluntary and reflex activity of the muscles they innervate. The thinner posterior (upper

horns) portion contains cells with fibers that enter over the posterior (sensory) root and thus serve as a relay station in the sensory/reflex pathway.

The thoracic region of the spinal cord has a projection from each side at the crossbar of the H-shaped structure of gray matter called the *lateral horn.* It contains the cells that give rise to the autonomic fibers of the sympathetic division. The fibers leave the spinal cord through the anterior roots in the thoracic and upper lumbar segments.

The Spinal Tracts

The white matter of the spinal cord is composed of myelinated and unmyelinated nerve fibers. The fast-conducting myelinated fibers form bundles; fiber bundles with a common function are called *tracts*.

There are six ascending tracts (see Fig. 60-7). Two tracts, known as the fasciculus cuneatus and gracilis or the posterior columns, conduct sensations of deep touch, pressure, vibration, position, and passive motion from the same side of the body. Before reaching the cerebral cortex, these fibers cross to the opposite side in the medulla. The anterior and posterior spinocerebellar tracts conduct sensory impulses from muscle spindles, providing necessary input for coordinated muscle contraction. They ascend uncrossed and terminate in the cerebellum. The anterior and lateral spinothalamic tracts are responsible for conduction of pain, temperature, proprioception, fine touch, and vibratory sense from the upper body to the brain. They cross to the opposite side of the cord and then ascend to the brain, terminating in the thalamus (Klein & Stewart-Amidei, 2017).

There are eight descending tracts (see Fig. 60-7). The anterior and lateral corticospinal tracts conduct motor impulses to the anterior horn cells from the opposite side of the brain, cross in the medulla, and control voluntary muscle activity. The three vestibulospinal tracts descend uncrossed and are involved in some autonomic functions (sweating, pupil dilation, and circulation) and involuntary muscle control. The corticobulbar tract conducts impulses responsible for voluntary head and facial muscle movement and crosses at the level of the brain stem. The rubrospinal and reticulospinal tracts conduct impulses involved with involuntary muscle movement.

Vertebral Column

The bones of the vertebral column surround and protect the spinal cord and normally consist of 7 cervical, 12 thoracic, and 5 lumbar vertebrae, as well as the sacrum (a fused mass of 5 vertebrae) and terminate in the coccyx. Nerve roots exit from the vertebral column through the intervertebral foramina (openings). The vertebrae are separated by discs, except for the first and second cervical, the sacral, and the coccygeal vertebrae. Each vertebra has a ventral solid body and a dorsal segment or arch, which is posterior to the body. The arch is composed of two pedicles and two laminae supporting seven processes. The vertebral body, arch, pedicles, and laminae all encase and protect the spinal cord.

The Peripheral Nervous System

The peripheral nervous system includes the cranial nerves, the spinal nerves, and the autonomic nervous system.

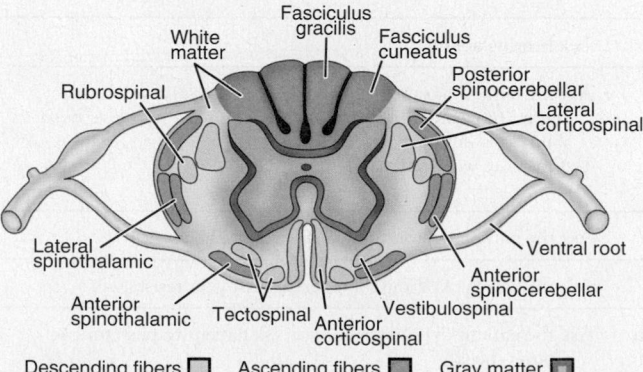

Figure 60-7 • Cross-sectional diagram of the spinal cord showing major spinal tracts.

Cranial Nerves

Twelve pairs of cranial nerves emerge from the lower surface of the brain and pass through openings in the base of the skull. Three cranial nerves are entirely sensory (I, II, VIII), five are motor (III, IV, VI, XI, and XII), and four are mixed sensory and motor (V, VII, IX, and X). The cranial nerves are numbered in the order in which they arise from the brain (see Fig. 60-8). The cranial nerves innervate the head, neck, and special sense structures. Table 60-2 provides a summary of the cranial nerves.

Spinal Nerves

The spinal cord is composed of 31 pairs of spinal nerves: 8 cervical, 12 thoracic, 5 lumbar, 5 sacral, and 1 coccygeal. Each spinal nerve has a ventral root and a dorsal root. The dorsal roots are sensory and transmit sensory impulses from specific areas of the body known as dermatomes (see Fig. 60-9) to the dorsal horn ganglia. The sensory fiber may be somatic, carrying information about pain, temperature, touch, and position sense (proprioception) from the tendons, joints, and body surfaces; or visceral, carrying information from the internal organs.

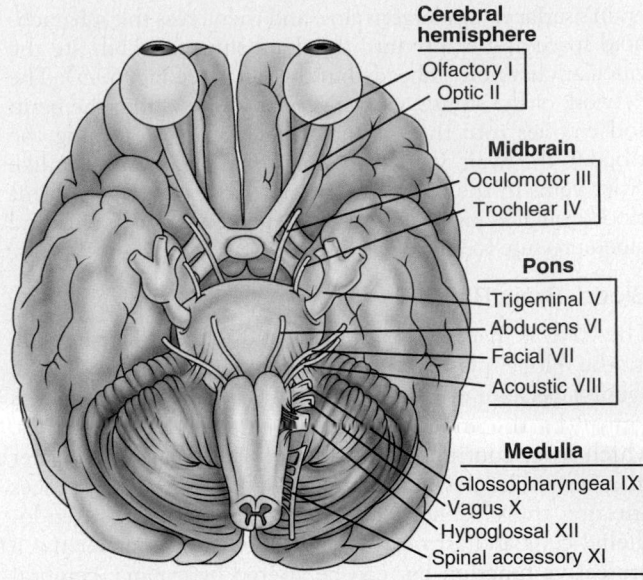

Figure 60-8 • Diagram of the base of the brain showing location of the cranial nerves.

TABLE 60-2	Summary of Cranial Nerves		
Nerve (Number)	**Type**	**Functions**	**Methods for Examining Nerve**
Olfactory (I)	Sensory	Sense of smell	Test each nostril for smell reception with various agents and interpretation
Optic (II)	Sensory	Sense of vision	Test vision for acuity and visual fields
Oculomotor (III)	Motor Raise eyelids	Pupil constriction Test pupillary reaction to light and ability to open and close eyelids	
Trochlear (IV)	Motor/pro-prioceptor	Downward, inward eye movement	Test for downward and inward movement of the eye
Trigeminal (V)	Motor Sensory	Jaw movements—chewing and mastication Sensation on the face and neck	Ask patient to open and clench jaws while you palpate the jaw muscles Test face and neck for pain sensations, light touch, and temperature
Abducens (VI)	Motor	Lateral movement of the eyes	Test ocular movement in all directions
Facial (VII)	Motor Sensory	Muscles of the face Sense of taste on the anterior two thirds of the tongue	Ask the patient to raise eyebrows, smile, show teeth, and puff out cheeks Test for the taste sensation with various agents
Acoustic (VIII)	Sensory	Sense of hearing	Test hearing ability
Glossopharyngeal (IX)	Motor Sensory	Pharyngeal movement and swallowing Sense of taste on the posterior one third of the tongue	Ask the patient to say "ah," and have patient yawn to observe upward movement of the soft palate; elicit gag response; note ability to swallow Test for taste with various agents
Vagus (X)	Motor/sensory	Swallowing and speaking	Ask the patient to swallow and speak; note hoarseness
Accessory (XI)	Motor/sensory	Movement of shoulder muscles	Ask the patient to shrug shoulders against your resistance
Hypoglossal (XII)	Motor	Movement of the tongue; strength of the tongue	Ask the patient to protrude tongue; ask patient to push tongue against cheek

Reprinted with permission from Taylor, C., Lynn, P., & Bartlett, J. L. (2019). *Fundamentals of nursing: The art and science of person-centered care* (9th ed., Table 26-6). Philadelphia, PA: Wolters Kluwer.

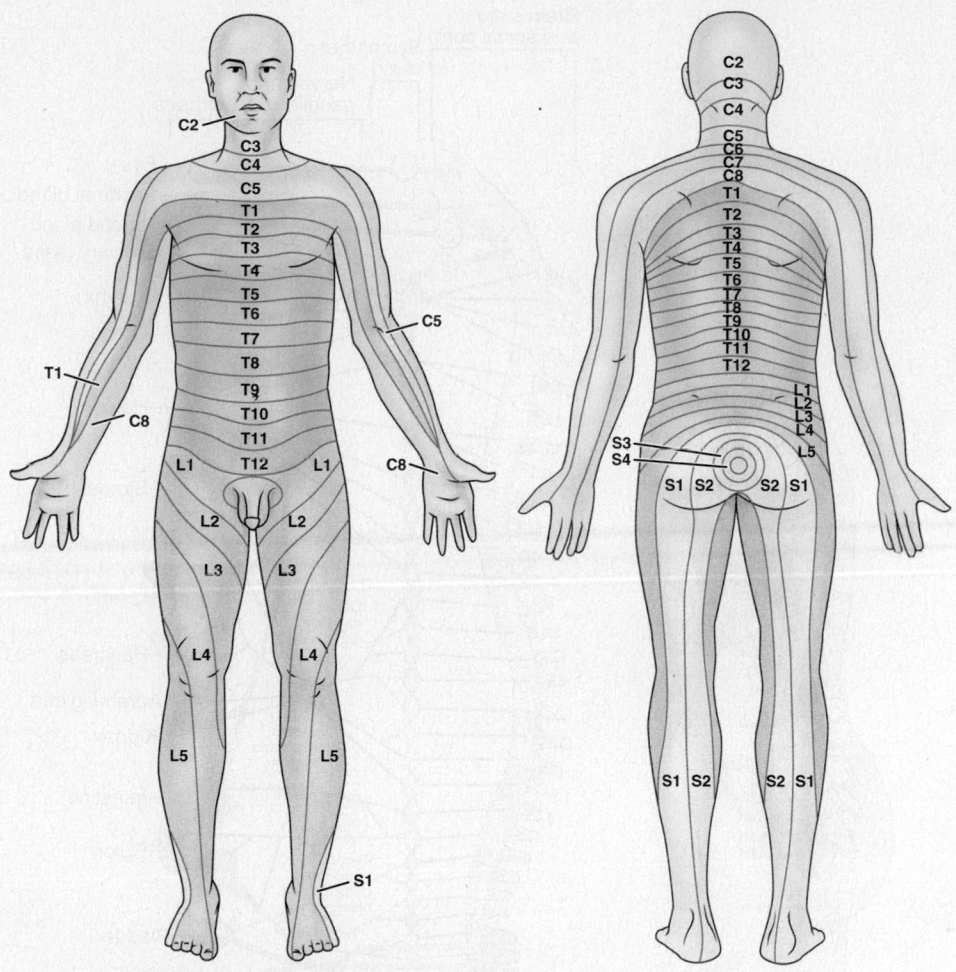

Figure 60-9 • Dermatome distribution.

The ventral roots are motor and transmit impulses from the spinal cord to the body; these fibers are also either somatic or visceral. The visceral fibers include autonomic fibers that control the cardiac muscles and glandular secretions.

Autonomic Nervous System

The **autonomic nervous system** regulates the activities of internal organs such as the heart, lungs, blood vessels, digestive organs, and glands (see Fig. 60-10). Maintenance and restoration of internal homeostasis is largely the responsibility of the autonomic nervous system. There are two major divisions: the **sympathetic nervous system**, with predominantly excitatory responses (i.e., the "fight-or-flight" response), and the parasympathetic nervous system, which controls mostly visceral functions.

The autonomic nervous system innervates most body organs. Although usually considered part of the peripheral nervous system, this system is regulated by centers in the spinal cord, brain stem, and hypothalamus.

The hypothalamus is the major subcortical center for the regulation of autonomic activities, serving an inhibitory–excitatory role. The hypothalamus has connections that link the autonomic system with the thalamus, the cortex, the olfactory apparatus, and the pituitary gland. Located here are the mechanisms for the control of visceral and somatic reactions that were originally important for defense or attack and are associated with emotional states (e.g., fear, anger, anxiety); for the control of metabolic processes, including fat, carbohydrate, and water metabolism; for the regulation of body temperature, arterial pressure, and all muscular and glandular activities of the gastrointestinal tract; for control of genital functions; and for the sleep cycle.

The autonomic nervous system is separated into the anatomically and functionally distinct sympathetic and parasympathetic divisions. Most of the tissues and the organs under autonomic control are innervated by both systems. For example, the parasympathetic division causes contraction (stimulation) of the urinary bladder muscles and a decrease (inhibition) in heart rate, whereas the sympathetic division produces relaxation (inhibition) of the urinary bladder and an increase (stimulation) in the rate and force of the heartbeat. Table 60-3 compares the sympathetic and the parasympathetic effects on the different systems of the body.

Sympathetic Nervous System

The sympathetic division of the autonomic nervous system is best known for its role in the body's fight-or-flight response. Under stress from either physical or emotional causes, sympathetic impulses increase greatly. As a result, the bronchioles dilate for easier gas exchange; the heart's contractions

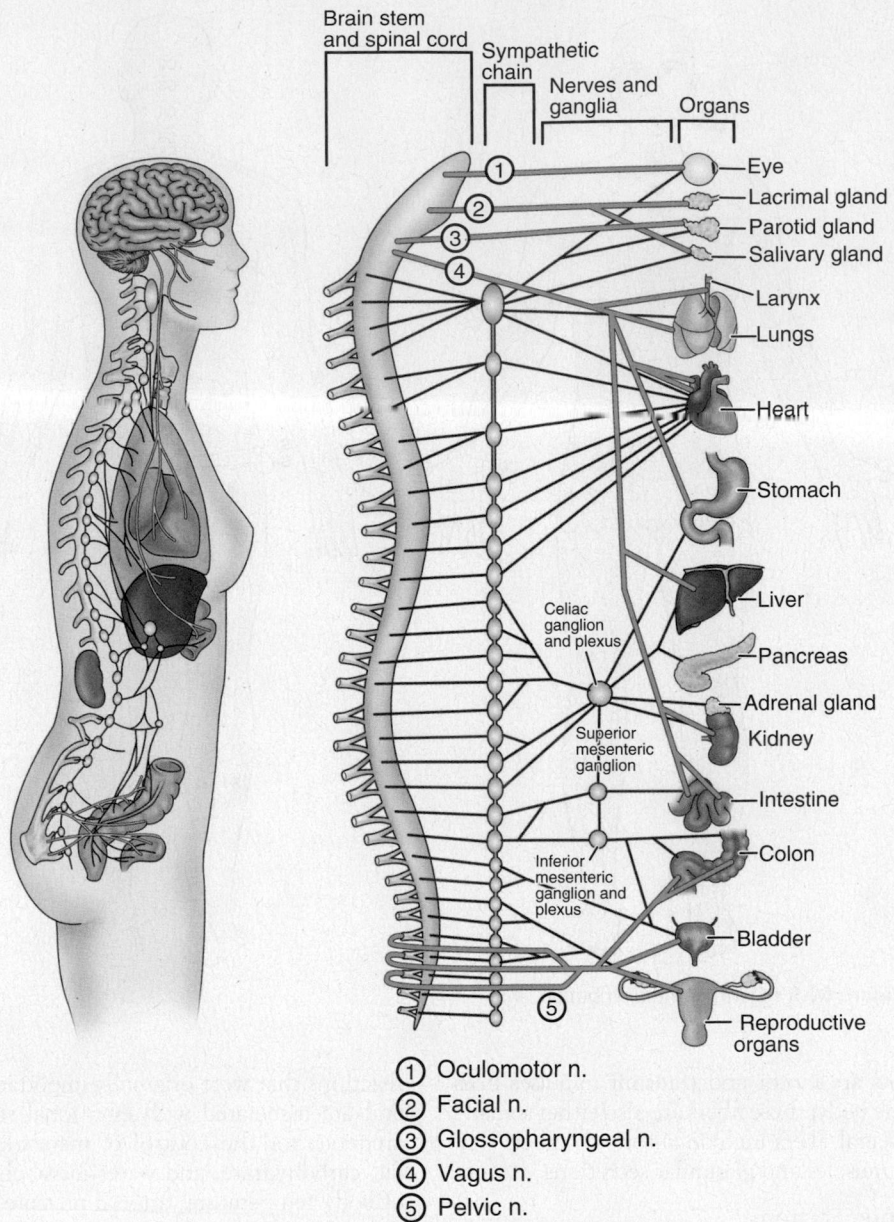

Brain stem
and spinal cord
Sympathetic
chain
Nerves and
ganglia
Organs

① ——— Eye
② ——— Lacrimal gland
③ ——— Parotid gland
——— Salivary gland
④ ——— Larynx
——— Lungs
——— Heart
——— Stomach
Celiac
ganglion
and plexus ——— Liver
——— Pancreas
——— Adrenal gland
Superior
mesenteric
ganglion ——— Kidney
——— Intestine
——— Colon
Inferior
mesenteric
ganglion and
plexus ——— Bladder
⑤ ——— Reproductive
organs

① Oculomotor n.
② Facial n.
③ Glossopharyngeal n.
④ Vagus n.
⑤ Pelvic n.

Figure 60-10 • Anatomy of the autonomic nervous system.

are stronger and faster; the arteries to the heart and voluntary muscles dilate, carrying more blood to these organs; peripheral blood vessels constrict, making the skin feel cool but shunting blood to essential organs; the pupils dilate; the liver releases glucose for quick energy; peristalsis slows; hair stands on end; and perspiration increases. The main sympathetic neurotransmitter is norepinephrine (noradrenaline). A sympathetic discharge releases epinephrine (adrenalin)—hence, the term *adrenergic* is often used to refer to this division.

Sympathetic neurons are located primarily in the thoracic and lumbar segments of the spinal cord, and their axons, or the preganglionic fibers, emerge by way of anterior nerve roots from the eighth cervical or first thoracic segment to the second or third lumbar segment. A short distance from the cord, these fibers diverge to join a chain, composed of 22 linked ganglia, that extends the entire

length of the spinal column, adjacent to the vertebral bodies on both sides. Some form multiple synapses with nerve cells within the chain. Others traverse the chain without making connections or losing continuity to join large "prevertebral" ganglia in the thorax, the abdomen, or the pelvis or one of the "terminal" ganglia in the vicinity of an organ, such as the bladder or the rectum at the end of the colon (see Fig. 60-10). Postganglionic nerve fibers originating in the sympathetic chain rejoin the spinal nerves that supply the extremities and are distributed to blood vessels, sweat glands, and smooth muscle tissue in the skin. Postganglionic fibers from the prevertebral plexuses (e.g., the cardiac, pulmonary, splanchnic, pelvic plexuses) supply structures in the head and neck, thorax, abdomen, and pelvis, respectively, having been joined in these plexuses by fibers from the parasympathetic division.

TABLE 60-3	Effects of the Autonomic Nervous System	
Structure or Activity	Parasympathetic Effects	Sympathetic Effects
Pupil of the Eye	Constricted	Dilated
Circulatory System		
Rate and force of heartbeat	Decreased	Increased
Blood vessels		
In heart muscle	Constricted	Dilated
In skeletal muscle	[a]	Dilated
In abdominal viscera and the skin	[a]	Constricted
Blood pressure	Decreased	Increased
Respiratory System		
Bronchioles	Constricted	Dilated
Rate of breathing	Decreased	Increased
Gastrointestinal System		
Peristaltic movements of digestive tube	Increased	Decreased
Muscular sphincters of digestive tube	Relaxed	Contracted
Secretion of salivary glands	Thin, watery saliva	Thick, viscid saliva
Secretions of stomach, intestine, and pancreas	Increased	[a]
Conversion of liver glycogen to glucose	[a]	Increased
Genitourinary System		
Urinary bladder		
Muscle walls	Contracted	Relaxed
Sphincters	Relaxed	Contracted
Muscles of the uterus	Relaxed; variable	Contracted under some conditions; varies with menstrual cycle and pregnancy
Blood vessels of external genitalia	Dilated	[a]
Integumentary System		
Secretion of sweat	[a]	Increased
Pilomotor muscles	[a]	Contracted (goose flesh)
Adrenal Medulla	[a]	Secretion of epinephrine and norepinephrine

[a]No direct effect.
Adapted from Hickey, J. V., & Strayer, A. L. (2020). *The clinical practice of neurological and neurosurgical nursing* (8th ed.). Philadelphia, PA: Wolters Kluwer.

The adrenal glands, kidneys, liver, spleen, stomach, and duodenum are under the control of the giant celiac plexus, commonly known as the solar plexus. This receives its sympathetic nerve components by way of the three splanchnic nerves, composed of preganglionic fibers from nine segments of the spinal cord (T4 to L1), and is joined by the vagus nerve, representing the parasympathetic division. From the celiac plexus, fibers of both divisions travel along the course of blood vessels to their target organs.

Certain syndromes are distinctive to the sympathetic nervous system. For example, sympathetic storm is a syndrome associated with changes in level of consciousness, altered vital signs, diaphoresis, and agitation that may result from hypothalamic stimulation of the sympathetic nervous system following traumatic brain injury (Fischbach & Fischbach, 2018).

Parasympathetic Nervous System

The **parasympathetic nervous system** functions as the dominant controller for most visceral functions; the primary neurotransmitter is acetylcholine. During quiet, nonstressful conditions, impulses from parasympathetic fibers (cholinergic) predominate. The fibers of the parasympathetic system are located in two sections: one in the brain stem and the other from spinal segments below L2. Because of the location of these fibers, the parasympathetic system is referred to as the craniosacral division, as distinct from the thoracolumbar (sympathetic) division of the autonomic nervous system.

The parasympathetic nerves arise from the midbrain and the medulla oblongata. Fibers from cells in the midbrain travel with the third oculomotor nerve to the ciliary ganglia, where postganglionic fibers of this division are joined by those of the sympathetic system, creating controlled opposition, with a delicate balance always maintained between the two systems.

Motor and Sensory Pathways of the Nervous System

Motor pathways within the CNS are responsible for voluntary, involuntary, and coordination of movement. Sensory pathways receive, integrate, and transmit a wide variety of sensations within the CNS.

Motor Pathways

The corticospinal tract begins in the motor cortex, a vertical band within each frontal lobe, and controls voluntary movements of the body. The exact locations within the brain at which the voluntary movements of the muscles of the face, thumb, hand, arm, trunk, and leg originate are known (see Fig. 60-11). To initiate movement, these particular cells must

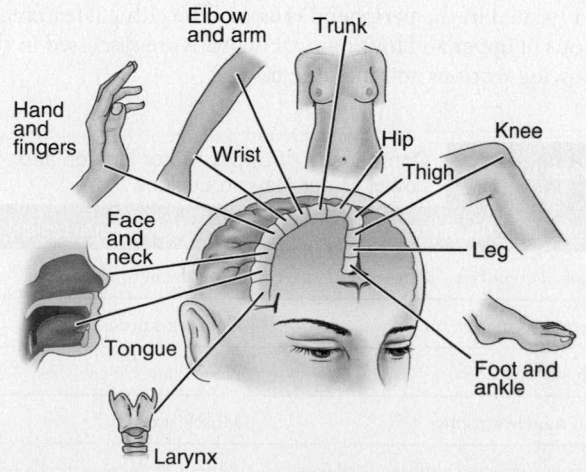

Figure 60-11 • Diagrammatic representation of the cerebrum showing locations for control of motor movement of various parts of the body.

send the stimulus along their fibers. Stimulation of these cells with an electric current also results in muscle contraction. En route to the pons, the motor fibers converge into a tight bundle known as the internal capsule. A comparatively small injury to the internal capsule results in a more severe paralysis than does a larger injury to the cortex itself.

At the medulla, the corticospinal tracts cross to the opposite side, continuing to the anterior horn of the spinal cord, in proximity to a motor nerve cell. Until this point, neurons are known as upper motor neurons. As they connect to motor fibers of the spinal nerves, they become lower motor neurons. The lower motor neurons receive the impulse in the posterior part of the cord and run to the myoneural junction located in the peripheral muscle.

Involuntary motor activity is also possible and is mediated through reflex arcs. Synaptic connections between anterior horn cells and sensory fibers that have entered adjacent or neighboring segments of the spinal cord serve as protective mechanisms. These connections are seen during deep tendon reflex testing.

Upper and Lower Motor Neurons

The voluntary motor system consists of two groups of neurons: upper motor neurons and lower motor neurons. Upper motor neurons originate in the cerebral cortex, the cerebellum, and the brain stem. Their fibers make up the descending motor pathways, are located entirely within the CNS, and modulate the activity of the lower motor neurons. Lower motor neurons are located either in the anterior horn of the spinal cord gray matter or within cranial nerve nuclei in the brain stem. Axons of lower motor neurons in both sites extend through peripheral nerves and terminate in skeletal muscle. Lower motor neurons are located in both the CNS and the peripheral nervous system.

The motor pathways from the brain to the spinal cord, as well as from the cerebrum to the brain stem, are formed by upper motor neurons. They begin in the cortex of one side of the brain, descend through the internal capsule, cross to the opposite side in the brain stem, descend through the corticospinal tract, and synapse with the lower motor neurons in the cord. The lower motor neurons receive the impulse in the posterior part of the cord and run to the myoneural junction located in the peripheral muscle. The clinical features of lesions of upper and lower motor neurons are discussed in the following sections and in Table 60-4.

TABLE 60-4	Comparison of Upper Motor Neuron and Lower Motor Neuron Lesions	
Upper Motor Neuron Lesions	**Lower Motor Neuron Lesions**
Loss of voluntary control	Loss of voluntary control
Increased muscle tone	Decreased muscle tone
Muscle spasticity	Flaccid muscle paralysis
No muscle atrophy	Muscle atrophy
Hyperactive and abnormal reflexes	Absent or decreased reflexes

Adapted from Hickey, J. V., & Strayer, A. L. (2020). *The clinical practice of neurological and neurosurgical nursing* (8th ed.). Philadelphia, PA: Wolters Kluwer.

Upper Motor Neuron Lesions

Upper motor neuron lesions can involve the motor cortex, the internal capsule, the spinal cord gray matter, and other structures of the brain through which the corticospinal tract descends. If the upper motor neurons are damaged or destroyed, as frequently occur with stroke or spinal cord injury, paralysis (loss of voluntary movement) results. However, because the inhibitory influences of intact upper motor neurons are impaired, **reflex** (involuntary) movements are uninhibited, and hence hyperactive deep tendon reflexes, diminished or absent superficial reflexes, and pathologic reflexes such as a Babinski response occur. Severe leg spasms can occur as the result of an upper motor neuron lesion; the spasms result from the preserved reflex arc, which lacks inhibition along the spinal cord below the level of injury. There is little or no muscle atrophy, and muscles remain permanently tense, exhibiting spastic paralysis.

Paralysis associated with upper motor neuron lesions can affect a whole extremity, both extremities, or an entire half of the body. *Hemiplegia* (paralysis of an arm and leg on the same side of the body) can be the result of an upper motor neuron lesion. If hemorrhage, an embolus, or a thrombus destroys the fibers from the motor area in the internal capsule, the arm and the leg of the opposite side become stiff, weak, or paralyzed, and the reflexes are hyperactive. If both legs are paralyzed, the condition is called *paraplegia*. If all four extremities are paralyzed, the condition is called *tetraplegia* (quadriplegia). See Chapter 63 for additional discussion of these disorders.

Lower Motor Neuron Lesions

A patient is considered to have lower motor neuron damage if a motor nerve is damaged between the spinal cord and muscle. The result of lower motor neuron damage is muscle paralysis. Reflexes are lost, and the muscle becomes flaccid (limp) and atrophied from disuse. If the patient has injured the spinal trunk and it can heal, the use of muscles connected to that section of the spinal cord may be regained. However, if the anterior horn motor cells are destroyed, the nerves cannot regenerate, and the muscles are never useful again.

Flaccid paralysis and atrophy of the affected muscles are the principal signs of lower motor neuron disease. Lower motor neuron lesions can be the result of trauma, infection (poliomyelitis), toxins, vascular disorders, congenital malformations, degenerative processes, and neoplasms. Compression of nerve roots by herniated intervertebral discs is a common cause of lower motor neuron dysfunction.

Coordination of Movement

The motor system is complex, and motor function depends not only on the integrity of the corticospinal tracts but also on other pathways from the basal ganglia and cerebellum that control and coordinate voluntary motor function. The smoothness, accuracy, and strength that characterize the muscular movements of a normal person are attributable to the influence of the cerebellum and the basal ganglia.

Through the action of the cerebellum, the contractions of opposing muscle groups are adjusted in relation to each other to maximal mechanical advantage; muscle contractions can be sustained evenly at the desired tension and without significant fluctuation, and reciprocal movements can be reproduced at high and constant speed, in stereotyped fashion and with relatively little effort.

The basal ganglia play an important role in planning and coordinating motor movements and posture. Complex neural connections link the basal ganglia with the cerebral cortex. The major effect of these structures is to inhibit unwanted muscular activity.

Impaired cerebellar function, which may occur as a result of an intracranial injury or some type of an expanding mass (e.g., a hemorrhage, an abscess, or a tumor), results in loss of muscle tone, weakness, and fatigue. Depending on the area of the brain affected, the patient has different motor symptoms or responses. The patient may demonstrate abnormal flexion, abnormal extension, or flaccid posturing. **Flaccidity** (lack of muscle tone) preceded by abnormal posturing in a patient with cerebral injury indicates severe neurologic impairment, which may herald brain death (Klein & Stewart-Amidei, 2017; Posner, Saper, Schiff, et al., 2019). See Chapter 61, Figure 61-1 for further explanation of posturing.

Destruction or dysfunction of the basal ganglia leads not to paralysis but to muscle rigidity, disturbances of posture, and difficulty initiating or changing movement. The patient tends to have involuntary movements. These may take the form of coarse tremors, most often in the upper extremities, particularly in the distal portions; athetosis, which is movement of a slow, squirming, writhing, twisting type; or chorea, marked by spasmodic, purposeless, irregular, uncoordinated motions of the trunk and the extremities, and facial grimacing. Disorders affecting basal ganglia activity include Parkinson's and Huntington diseases (see Chapter 65).

Sensory System Function
Receiving Sensory Impulses

Afferent impulses travel from their points of origin to their destinations in the cerebral cortex via the ascending pathways directly, or they may cross at the level of the spinal cord or in the medulla, depending on the type of sensation carried. Knowledge of these pathways is important for neurologic assessment and for understanding symptoms and their relationship to various lesions.

Sensory impulses convey sensations of heat, cold, and pain; position; and vibration. The axons enter the spinal cord by way of the posterior root, specifically in the posterior gray columns of the spinal cord, where they connect with the cells of secondary neurons. Pain and temperature fibers (located in the spinothalamic tract) cross immediately to the opposite side of the cord and course upward to the thalamus. Fibers carrying sensations of touch, light pressure, and localization do not connect immediately with the second neuron but ascend the cord for a variable distance before entering the gray matter and completing this connection. The axon of the secondary neuron traverses the cord, crosses in the medulla, and proceeds upward to the thalamus.

Position and vibratory sensations are produced by stimuli arising from muscles, joints, and bones. These stimuli are conveyed, uncrossed, all the way to the brain stem by the axon of the primary neuron. In the medulla, synaptic connections are made with cells of the secondary neurons, whose axons cross to the opposite side and then proceed to the thalamus.

Integrating Sensory Impulses

The thalamus integrates all sensory impulses except olfaction. It plays a role in the conscious awareness of pain and the recognition of variation in temperature and touch. The thalamus is responsible for the sense of movement and position as well as the ability to recognize the size, shape, and quality of objects. Sensory information is relayed from the thalamus to the parietal lobe for interpretation.

Sensory Losses

Destruction of a sensory nerve results in total loss of sensation in its area of distribution (see Fig. 60-9). Lesions affecting the posterior spinal nerve roots may impair tactile sensation, causing intermittent severe pain that is referred to their areas of distribution. Destruction of the spinal cord yields complete anesthesia below the level of injury. Selective destruction or degeneration of the posterior columns of the spinal cord is responsible for a loss of position and vibratory sense in segments distal to the lesion, without loss of touch, pain, or temperature perception. A cyst in the center of the spinal cord causes dissociation of sensation—loss of pain at the level of the lesion. This occurs because the fibers carrying pain and temperature cross within the cord immediately on entering; thus, any lesion that divides the cord longitudinally divides these fibers. Other sensory fibers ascend the cord for variable distances, some even to the medulla, before crossing, thereby bypassing the lesion and avoiding destruction. Lesions in the thalamus or parietal lobe result in impaired touch, pain, temperature, and proprioceptive sensations.

Assessment of the Nervous System

An assessment of the nervous system involves conducting a health history and physical assessment.

Health History

An important aspect of the neurologic assessment is the history of the present illness. The initial interview provides an excellent opportunity to systematically explore the patient's current condition and related events while simultaneously observing overall appearance, mental status, posture, movement, and affect. Depending on the patient's condition, the nurse may need to rely on yes-or-no answers to questions, a review of the medical record, input from witnesses or the family, or a combination of these.

Neurologic disorders may be stable or progressive, characterized by symptom-free periods as well as fluctuations in symptoms. The health history therefore includes details about the onset, character, severity, location, duration, and frequency of symptoms and signs; associated complaints; precipitating, aggravating, and relieving factors; progression, remission, and exacerbation; and the presence or absence of similar symptoms among family members.

Common Symptoms

The symptoms of neurologic disorders are as varied as the disease processes. Symptoms may be subtle or intense, fluctuating or permanent, inconvenient or devastating. This chapter discusses the most common signs and symptoms associated with neurologic disease; the relationship of specific signs and symptoms to a disorder is presented in later chapters in this unit.

Pain

Pain is considered an unpleasant sensory perception and emotional experience associated with actual or potential tissue damage or described in terms of such damage. Pain is therefore considered multidimensional and entirely subjective. Pain can be acute or chronic. In general, acute pain lasts for a relatively short period of time and remits as the pathology resolves. In neurologic disease, acute pain may be associated with brain hemorrhage, spinal disc disease (Jarvis, 2020), or trigeminal neuralgia. In contrast, chronic or persistent pain extends for long periods of time and may represent a broader pathology. This type of pain can occur with many degenerative and chronic neurologic conditions (e.g., multiple sclerosis). See Chapter 9 for a more detailed discussion of pain.

Seizures

Seizures are the result of abnormal electrical discharges in the cerebral cortex, which then manifest as an alteration in sensation, behavior, movement, perception, or consciousness. The alteration may be short, such as in a blank stare that lasts only a second, or of longer duration, such as a tonic–clonic grand mal seizure that can last several minutes. The seizure activity reflects the area of the brain affected. Seizures can occur as isolated events, such as when induced by a high fever, alcohol or drug withdrawal, or hypoglycemia. A seizure may also be the first obvious sign of a brain lesion (Hickey & Strayer, 2020).

Dizziness and Vertigo

Dizziness is an abnormal sensation of imbalance or movement. It is common in the older adult and a common complaint encountered by health professionals (Jarvis, 2020). Dizziness can have a variety of causes, including viral syndromes, hot weather, roller-coaster rides, and middle ear infections, to name a few. One difficulty confronting health care providers when assessing dizziness is the vague and varied terms that patients use to describe the sensation.

About 50% of all patients with dizziness have **vertigo**, or the illusion of movement in which the individual or the surroundings are sensed as moving, usually as rotation (Jarvis, 2020). Vertigo is usually a manifestation of vestibular dysfunction. It can be so severe as to result in spatial disorientation, lightheadedness, loss of equilibrium (staggering), and nausea and vomiting.

Visual Disturbances

Visual defects that cause people to seek health care can range from the decreased visual acuity associated with aging to sudden blindness caused by glaucoma. Normal vision depends on functioning visual pathways through the retina and optic chiasm and the radiations into the visual cortex in the occipital lobes. Lesions of the eye itself (e.g., cataract), lesions along the pathway (e.g., tumor), or lesions in the visual cortex (e.g., stroke) interfere with normal visual acuity. Abnormalities of eye movement (as in the nystagmus associated with multiple sclerosis) can also compromise vision by causing diplopia or double vision. See Chapter 58 for a more detailed discussion of disorders that affect vision.

Muscle Weakness

Muscle weakness is a common manifestation of neurologic disease. It frequently coexists with other symptoms of disease and can affect a variety of muscles, causing a wide range of disability. Weakness can be sudden and permanent, as in stroke, or progressive, as in neuromuscular diseases such as amyotrophic lateral sclerosis. Any muscle group can be affected.

Abnormal Sensation

Abnormal sensation is a neurologic manifestation of both central and peripheral nervous system disease. Altered sensation can affect small or large areas of the body. It is frequently associated with weakness or pain and is potentially disabling. Lack of sensation places a person at risk for falls and injury.

Past Health, Family, and Social History

The nurse may inquire about any family history of genetic diseases (see Chart 60-1). A review of the medical history, including a system-by-system evaluation, is part of the health history. The nurse should be aware of any history of trauma or falls that may have involved the head or spinal cord. Questions regarding the use of alcohol, medications, and illicit drugs are also relevant. The history-taking portion of the neurologic assessment is critical and, in many cases of neurologic disease, leads to an accurate diagnosis.

Physical Assessment

The neurologic examination is a systematic process that includes a variety of clinical tests, observations, and assessments designed to evaluate the neurologic status of a complex system. Many neurologic rating scales exist (Herndon, 2006), and some of the more common ones are discussed in this chapter.

The brain and spinal cord cannot be examined as directly as other systems of the body. Therefore, much of the neurologic examination is an indirect evaluation that assesses the function of the specific body part or parts controlled by the nervous system. A neurologic assessment is divided into five components: consciousness and cognition, cranial nerves, motor system, sensory system, and reflexes. One or more components may become the priority assessment, depending on the patient's condition. For example, motor, sensory, and reflex assessments are the priority in patients with spinal injury, whereas in a patient who is comatose, the cranial nerves and level of consciousness become the priority.

Assessing Consciousness and Cognition

Cerebral abnormalities may cause disturbances in mental status, intellectual functioning, thought content, and emotional status. There may also be alterations in language abilities as well as lifestyle. The examiner must also be aware of the patient's overall level of consciousness and any changes over time (Posner et al., 2019).

The examiner records and reports specific observations regarding mental status, intellectual function, thought content, and emotional status, all of which permit comparison by others over time. Alterations should be described in specific and nonjudgmental terms. The use of terms such as "inappropriate" or "demented" is avoided, because they often mean

Chart 60-1 GENETICS IN NURSING PRACTICE

Neurologic Disorders

Several neurologic disorders are associated with genetic abnormalities. Neurologic impairment is noted with many other genetic illnesses. Some examples include:

Autosomal Dominant:

- Cerebral arteriopathy
- Familial Alzheimer's disease
- Huntington disease
- Myotonic dystrophies
- Neurofibromatosis
- Von Hippel–Lindau syndrome

Autosomal Recessive:

- Canavan disease
- Familial dysautonomia
- Friedreich ataxia

X Linked:

- Duchenne muscular dystrophy
- Fragile X syndrome

Inheritance pattern is not distinct; however, there is a genetic predisposition for the disease:

- Amyotrophic lateral sclerosis (ALS)
- Epilepsy
- Neural tube defects (e.g., spina bifida, anencephaly)
- Parkinson's disease
- Tourette syndrome

Other genetic disorders that also impact the neurologic system:

- Bipolar disease
- Down syndrome
- Phenylketonuria (PKU)
- Schizophrenia
- Tay–Sachs disease
- Tuberous sclerosis complex

Nursing Assessments

Refer to Chapter 4, Chart 4-2: Genetics in Nursing Practice: Genetic Aspects of Health Assessment

Family History Assessment Specific to Neurologic Disorders

- Assess for other similarly affected relatives with neurologic impairment.
- Inquire about age of onset (e.g., present at birth—spina bifida; developed in childhood—Duchenne muscular dystrophy; developed in adulthood—Huntington disease, Alzheimer's disease, ALS).
- Inquire about the presence of related conditions such as intellectual disability or learning disabilities (neurofibromatosis type 1).

Patient Assessment

- Assess for the presence of other physical features suggestive of an underlying genetic condition, such as skin lesions seen in neurofibromatosis (*café-au-lait* spots).
- Assess attention span, and the presence of hyperactivity or withdrawn behavior.
- Assess for other congenital abnormalities (e.g., cardiac, ocular).
- Inspect for presence of freckles in the axillary or inguinal areas.
- Assess for presence of uncoordinated movement of extremities, muscle twitching, or history of seizures.
- Assess for poor or hyperactive muscle tone.
- Assess for episodes of forgetfulness or uncharacteristic changes in behavior or mood.
- Inspect for disproportionate facial features (fragile X or Down syndrome).
- Observe for presence of "tics" or uncontrolled body movement.
- Ask about history of seizures or head trauma.

Genetics Resources

Epilepsy Foundation, www.epilepsy.com/learn/diagnosis/genetic-testing
Huntington's Disease Society of America, hdsa.org
Muscular Dystrophy Association, www.mda.org
See Chapter 6, Chart 6-7 for components of genetic counseling.

---

different things to different people and are therefore not useful when describing behavior. Analysis and the conclusions that may be drawn from these findings usually depend on the examiner's knowledge of neuroanatomy, neurophysiology, and neuropathology.

Mental Status

An assessment of mental status begins by observing the patient's appearance and behavior, noting dress, grooming, and personal hygiene. Posture, gestures, movements, and facial expressions often provide important information about the patient. Does the patient appear to be aware of and interact with the surroundings?

Assessing orientation to time, place, and person assists in evaluating mental status. Does the patient know what day it is, what year it is, and the name of the president of the United States? Is the patient aware of where they are? Is the patient aware of who the examiner is and of their purpose for being in the room? Assessment of immediate and remote memory is also important. Is the capacity for immediate memory intact?

Intellectual Function

A person with an average intelligence quotient (IQ) can repeat seven digits without faltering and can recite five digits backward. The examiner might ask the patient to count backward from 100 or to subtract 7 from 100, then 7 from that, and so forth (referred to as serial 7s). The capacity to interpret well-known proverbs tests abstract reasoning, which is a higher intellectual function—for example, does the patient know what is meant by "a stitch in time saves nine"? The intellectual function of patients with damage to the frontal cortex appears intact until one or more tests of intellectual capacity are performed. Questions designed to assess this capacity might include the ability to recognize similarities—for example, how are a mouse and dog or pen and pencil alike? Can the patient make judgments about situations—for example, if the patient arrives home without a house key, what alternatives are there?

Thought Content

During the interview, it is important to assess the patient's thought content. Are the patient's thoughts spontaneous, natural, clear, relevant, and coherent? Does the patient have any fixed ideas, illusions, or preoccupations? What are their insights into these thoughts? Preoccupation with death or morbid events, hallucinations, and paranoid ideation are examples of unusual thoughts or perceptions that require further evaluation.

Emotional Status

An assessment of consciousness and cognition also includes the patient's emotional status. Is the patient's affect (external manifestation of mood) natural and even, or irritable and angry, anxious, apathetic or flat, or euphoric? Does their mood fluctuate normally, or does the patient unpredictably swing from joy to sadness during the interview? Is affect appropriate to words and thought content? Are verbal communications consistent with nonverbal cues?

Language Ability

The person with normal neurologic function can understand and communicate in spoken and written language. Does the patient answer questions appropriately? Can they read a sentence from a newspaper and explain its meaning? Can the patient write their name or copy a simple figure that the examiner has drawn? A deficiency in language function is called *aphasia*. Different types of aphasia result from injury to different parts of the brain (see Table 60-5). See Chapter 62 for a detailed discussion of aphasia.

Impact on Lifestyle

The nurse assesses the impact of any impairment on the patient's lifestyle. Issues to consider include the limitations imposed on the patient by any cognitive deficit and the patient's role in society, including family and community roles. The plan of care that the nurse develops needs to address and support adaptation to the neurologic deficit and continued function to the extent possible within the patient's support system.

Level of Consciousness

Consciousness is the patient's wakefulness and ability to respond to the environment. Level of consciousness is the most sensitive indicator of neurologic function. To assess level of consciousness, the examiner observes for alertness and ability to follow commands.

If the patient is not alert or able to follow commands, the examiner observes for eye opening; verbal response and motor response to stimuli, if any; and the type of stimuli needed to obtain a response. Noxious stimuli should be used first, then

TABLE 60-5	Types of Aphasia and Region of Brain Involved
Type of Aphasia	**Brain Area Involved**
Auditory receptive	Temporal lobe
Visual receptive	Parietal and occipital area
Expressive speaking	Inferior–posterior frontal areas
Expressive writing	Posterior frontal area

Adapted from Norris, T. L. (2019). *Porth's pathophysiology: Concepts of altered health state* (10th ed.). Philadelphia, PA: Wolters Kluwer.

painful stimuli if no response is observed. In the patient with decreased level of consciousness, motor and cranial nerve functions become the priority assessments, because abnormalities can indicate the area of involvement in the absence of responsiveness. See Chapter 61 for further discussion of changes in level of consciousness.

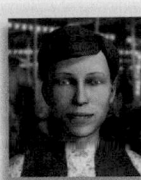

Unfolding Patient Stories: Marilyn Hughes • Part 2

Recall from Chapter 37 **Marilyn Hughes,** who came to the hospital after falling on icy stairs. She sustained a left midshaft tibia–fibula fracture, which requires surgery. Her husband informs the nurse that she also hit her head and did not respond to him for a short time after the fall. Describe the neurologic assessment performed by the nurse. Why should the nurse report this information promptly to the health care team?

Care for Marilyn and other patients in a realistic virtual environment: *vSim for Nursing* (**thepoint.lww.com/vSimMedicalSurgical**). Practice documenting these patients' care in DocuCare (**thepoint.lww.com/DocuCareEHR**).

Examining the Cranial Nerves

Cranial nerves are assessed when level of consciousness is decreased, with brain stem pathology, or in the presence of peripheral nervous system disease (Weber & Kelley, 2018). Right and left cranial nerve functions are compared throughout the examination.

See Table 60-2 for methods of examining the cranial nerves.

Examining the Motor System

Motor Ability

A thorough examination of the motor system includes an assessment of muscle size and tone as well as strength, coordination, and balance. The patient is instructed to walk across the room, if possible, while the examiner observes posture and gait. The muscles are inspected, and palpated if necessary, for their size and symmetry. Any evidence of atrophy or involuntary movements (tremors, tics) is noted. Muscle tone (the tension present in a muscle at rest) is evaluated by palpating various muscle groups at rest and during passive movement. Resistance to these movements is assessed and documented. Abnormalities in tone include **spasticity** (increased muscle tone), **rigidity** (resistance to passive stretch), and flaccidity.

Muscle Strength

Assessing the patient's ability to flex or extend the extremities against resistance tests muscle strength. The function of an individual muscle or group of muscles is evaluated by placing the muscle at a disadvantage. The quadriceps, for example, is a powerful muscle responsible for straightening the leg. Once the leg is straightened, it is exceedingly difficult for the examiner to flex the knee. If the knee is flexed and the patient is asked to straighten the leg against resistance, weakness can be elicited. The evaluation of muscle strength compares the sides of the body to each other. For example, the right upper extremity is compared to the left upper extremity. Subtle differences in strength may be evaluated by testing for drift. For example, both arms are out in front of the patient with palms up; drift is seen as pronation of the palm, indicating a subtle weakness that may not have been detected on the resistance examination.

Clinicians use a 5-point scale to rate muscle strength. A 5 indicates full power of contraction against gravity and resistance or normal muscle strength; 4 indicates fair but not full strength against gravity and a moderate amount of resistance or slight weakness; 3 indicates just sufficient strength to overcome the force of gravity or moderate weakness; 2 indicates the ability to move but not to overcome the force of gravity or severe weakness; 1 indicates minimal contractile power (weak muscle contraction can be palpated but no movement is noted) or very severe weakness; and 0 indicates no movement (Jarvis, 2020).

 Concept Mastery Alert

> When recording muscle strength, a stick figure is used as a precise form to document findings. The five-point scale is used to rate and record distal and proximal strength in both upper and lower extremities. Figure 60-12 provides further details.

Assessment of muscle strength may be as detailed as necessary. One may quickly test the strength of the proximal muscles of the upper and lower extremities, always assessing both sides by comparing one side to the other. The strength of the finer muscles that control the function of the hand (hand grasp) and the foot (dorsiflexion and plantar flexion) can then be assessed.

Balance and Coordination

Cerebellar and basal ganglia influence on the motor system is reflected in balance control and coordination. Coordination

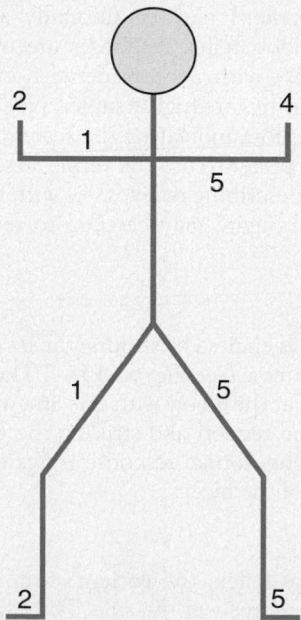

Figure 60-12 • A stick figure may be used to record muscle strength.

in the hands and upper extremities is tested by having the patient perform rapid, alternating movements and point-to-point testing. First, the patient is instructed to pat their thigh as fast as possible with each hand separately. Then, the patient is instructed to alternately pronate and supinate the hand as rapidly as possible. Last, the patient is asked to touch each of the fingers with the thumb in a consecutive motion. Speed, symmetry, and degree of difficulty are noted. Point-to-point testing is accomplished by having the patient touch the examiner's extended finger and then their own nose. This is repeated several times.

Coordination in the lower extremities is tested by having the patient run the heel down the anterior surface of the tibia of the other leg. Each leg is tested in turn. **Ataxia** is an incoordination of voluntary muscle action, particularly of the muscle groups used in activities such as walking or reaching for objects. Tremors (rhythmic, involuntary movements) noted at rest or during movement suggest a problem in the anatomic areas responsible for balance and coordination.

The **Romberg test** is a screening test for balance that can be done with the patient seated or standing. The patient can be seated or stand with feet together and arms at the side, first with eyes open and then with both eyes closed for 20 seconds (Weber & Kelley, 2018). The examiner stands close to support the standing patient if they begin to fall. Slight swaying is normal, but a loss of balance is abnormal and is considered a positive Romberg test. Additional cerebellar tests for balance in the patient who is ambulatory include hopping in place, alternating knee bends, and heel-to-toe walking (both forward and backward).

Examining the Sensory System

The sensory system is even more complex than the motor system, because sensory modalities are more widespread throughout the central and peripheral nervous systems. The sensory examination is largely subjective and requires the cooperation of the patient. The examiner should be familiar with dermatomes that represent the distribution of the peripheral nerves that arise from the spinal cord (see Fig. 60-9) (Jarvis, 2020).

Assessment of the sensory system involves tests for tactile sensation, superficial pain, temperature, vibration, and position sense (proprioception). During the sensory assessment, the patient's eyes are closed. Simple directions and reassurance that the examiner will not hurt or startle the patient encourage the cooperation of the patient.

Tactile sensation is assessed by lightly touching a cotton wisp or fingertip to corresponding areas on each side of the body. The sensitivity of proximal parts of the extremities is compared with that of distal parts, and the right and left sides are compared.

Pain and temperature sensations are transmitted together in the lateral part of the spinal cord, so it is unnecessary to test for temperature sense in most circumstances. Determining the patient's sensitivity to a sharp object can assess superficial pain perception. However, pain sensation is usually reserved for patients who do not respond to or cannot discriminate touch stimulation. The patient is asked to differentiate between the sharp and dull ends of a broken wooden cotton swab or tongue blade; using a safety pin is inadvisable because it breaks the integrity of the skin. Both the sharp and dull sides of the object are applied with equal intensity at all times, and the two sides are compared. In the patient with an altered level of consciousness alternative methods of assessing pain may need to be used (Poulsen, Brix, Andersen, et al., 2016).

Vibration and proprioception are transmitted together in the posterior part of the spinal cord. Vibration may be evaluated through the use of a low-frequency (128 or 256 Hz) tuning fork. The handle of the vibrating fork is placed against a bony prominence, and the patient is asked if a sensation is felt; the patient is then instructed to signal the examiner when the sensation ceases. Common locations used to test for vibratory sense include the distal joint of the great toe and the proximal thumb joint. If the patient does not perceive the vibrations at the distal bony prominences, the examiner progresses upward with the tuning fork until the patient perceives the vibrations. As with all measurements of sensation, a side-to-side comparison is made.

Position sense or proprioception may be determined by asking the patient to close both eyes and indicate, as the great toe or index finger is alternately moved up and down, in which direction movement has taken place. Vibration and position sense are often lost together, frequently in circumstances in which all other sensation remains intact.

Integration of sensation in the brain is evaluated by testing two-point discrimination. When the patient is touched with two sharp objects simultaneously, are they perceived as two or as one? If touched simultaneously on opposite sides of the body, the patient should normally report being touched in two places. If only one site is reported, the one not being recognized is said to demonstrate extinction. Another test of higher cortical sensory ability is tactile identification. The patient is instructed to close both eyes and identify an object (e.g., key, coin) that is placed in one hand by the examiner; inability to identify an object by touch is known as tactile agnosia or astereognosis. **Agnosia** is the general loss of ability to recognize objects through a particular sensory system. The patient can also be shown a familiar object and asked to identify it by name; inability to identify a visualized object is known as visual agnosia. Each of these dysfunctions implicates a different part of the brain (see Table 60-6).

Decreased or absent sensations occur with problems anywhere along the sensory pathway. Sensory deficits resulting from peripheral neuropathy or spinal cord injury follow anatomic dermatomes. Destructive lesions of the brain may affect sensation on an entire side of the body. Stroke affecting

a portion of the sensory cortex will produce altered sensory discrimination.

Examining the Reflexes

Reflexes are involuntary contractions of muscles or muscle groups in response to a stimulus. Reflexes are classified as deep tendon, superficial, or pathologic. Testing reflexes enables the examiner to assess involuntary reflex arcs that depend on the presence of afferent stretch receptors, spinal or brain stem synapses, efferent motor fibers, and a variety of modifying influences from higher levels.

Deep Tendon Reflexes

A reflex hammer is used to elicit a deep tendon reflex. The handle of the hammer is held loosely between the thumb and index finger, allowing a full swinging motion. The wrist motion is similar to that used during percussion. The extremity is positioned so that the tendon is slightly stretched. This requires a sound knowledge of the location of muscles and their tendon attachments. The tendon is then struck briskly (see Fig. 60-13), and the response is compared with that on the opposite side of the body. A wide variation in reflex response may be considered normal; however, it is more important that the reflexes be symmetrically equivalent. When the comparison is made, both sides should be equivalently relaxed, and each tendon struck with equal force.

Valid findings depend on several factors: proper use of the reflex hammer, proper positioning of the extremity, and a patient who is relaxed (Jarvis, 2020). If the reflexes are symmetrically diminished or absent, the examiner may use isometric contraction of other muscle groups to increase reflex activity. For example, if lower extremity reflexes are diminished or absent, the patient is instructed to lock the fingers together and pull in opposite directions. Having the patient clench the jaw or press the heels against the floor or examining table may similarly elicit more reliable biceps, triceps, and brachioradialis reflexes.

The absence of reflexes is significant, although ankle jerks (Achilles reflex) may be normally absent in older adults. Deep tendon reflex responses are often graded on a scale of 0 to 4+, with 2+ considered normal (see Chart 60-2) but scale ratings are highly subjective. Findings can be recorded as a fraction, indicating the scale range (e.g., 2/4). Some examiners prefer to use the terms *present*, *absent*, and *diminished* when describing reflexes. As with muscle strength recording, a stick figure may be used to record numerical findings.

Biceps Reflex

The biceps reflex is elicited by striking the biceps tendon over a slightly flexed elbow (see Fig. 60-13A). The examiner supports the forearm at the elbow with one arm while placing the thumb against the tendon and striking the thumb with the reflex hammer. The normal response is flexion at the elbow and contraction of the biceps.

Triceps Reflex

To elicit a triceps reflex, the patient's arm is flexed at the elbow and hanging freely at the side. The examiner supports the patient's arm and identifies the triceps tendon by palpating 2.5 to 5 cm (1 to 2 inches) above the elbow. A direct blow

TABLE 60-6	Types of Agnosia and Corresponding Sites of Lesions
Type of Agnosia	**Affected Cerebral Area**
Visual	Occipital lobe
Auditory	Temporal lobe (lateral and superior portions)
Tactile	Parietal lobe
Body parts and relationships	Parietal lobe (posteroinferior regions)

Adapted from Norris, T. L. (2019). *Porth's pathophysiology: Concepts of altered health state* (10th ed.). Philadelphia, PA: Wolters Kluwer.

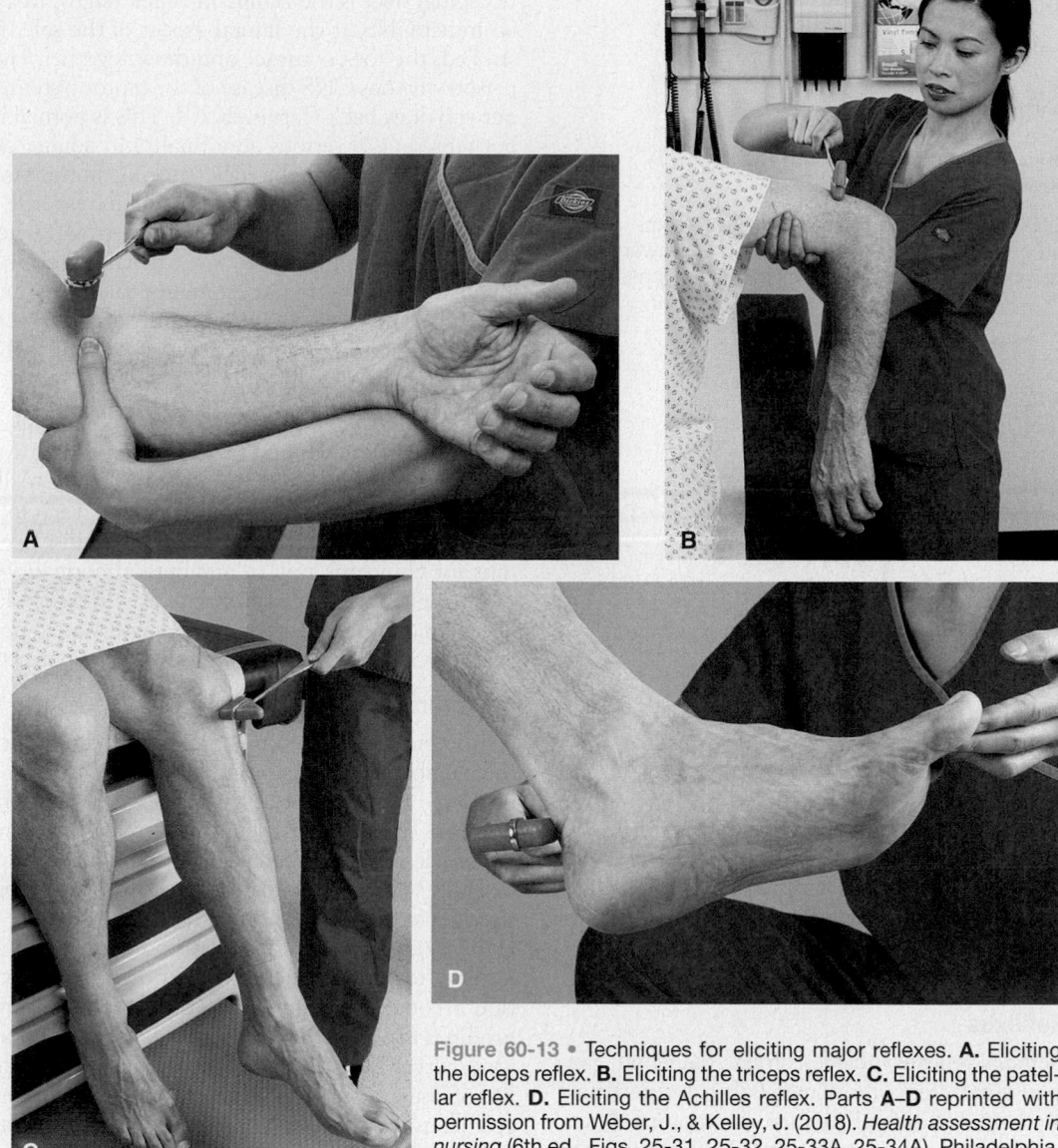

Figure 60-13 • Techniques for eliciting major reflexes. **A.** Eliciting the biceps reflex. **B.** Eliciting the triceps reflex. **C.** Eliciting the patellar reflex. **D.** Eliciting the Achilles reflex. Parts **A–D** reprinted with permission from Weber, J., & Kelley, J. (2018). *Health assessment in nursing* (6th ed., Figs. 25-31, 25-32, 25-33A, 25-34A). Philadelphia, PA: Lippincott Williams & Wilkins.

on the tendon (see Fig. 60-13B) normally produces contraction of the triceps muscle and extension of the elbow.

Brachioradialis Reflex

With the patient's forearm resting on the lap or across the abdomen, the brachioradialis reflex is assessed. A gentle strike of the hammer 2.5 to 5 cm (1 to 2 inches) above the wrist results in flexion and supination of the forearm (Jarvis, 2020).

Patellar Reflex

The patellar reflex is elicited by striking the patellar tendon just below the patella. The patient may be in a sitting or a lying position. If the patient is supine, the examiner supports the legs to facilitate relaxation of the muscles (see Fig. 60-13C). Contractions of the quadriceps and knee extension are normal responses.

Achilles Reflex

To elicit an Achilles reflex, the foot is dorsiflexed at the ankle and the hammer strikes the stretched Achilles tendon (see Fig. 60-13D). This reflex normally produces plantar flexion. If the examiner cannot elicit the ankle reflex and suspects that the patient cannot relax, the patient is instructed to kneel on a chair or similar elevated, flat surface. This position places the ankles in dorsiflexion and reduces any muscle tension in the gastrocnemius. The Achilles tendons are struck in turn, and plantar flexion is usually demonstrated (Jarvis, 2020).

Clonus

When reflexes are hyperactive, a movement called **clonus** may be elicited. If the foot is abruptly dorsiflexed, it may continue to "beat" two or three times before it settles into a position of rest. Occasionally with CNS system disease, this

Chart 60-2 **Documenting Reflexes**

Deep tendon reflexes are graded on a scale of 0–4:

0 No response
1+ Diminished (hypoactive)
2+ Normal
3+ Increased (may be interpreted as normal)
4+ Hyperactive (hyperreflexia)

The deep tendon responses and plantar reflexes are commonly recorded on stick figures. The arrow points downward if the plantar response is normal and upward if the response is abnormal.

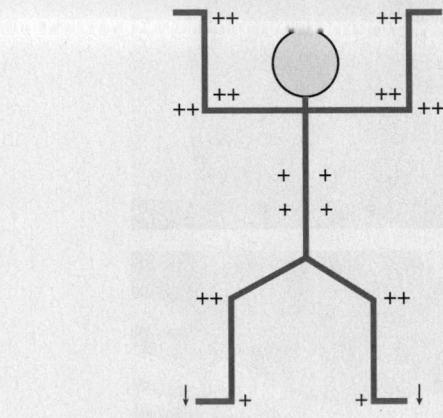

activity persists, and the foot does not come to rest while the tendon is being stretched but persists in repetitive activity. The unsustained clonus associated with normal but hyperactive reflexes is not considered pathologic. Sustained clonus always indicates the presence of CNS disease and requires further evaluation.

Superficial Reflexes

The major superficial reflexes include corneal, palpebral, gag, upper/lower abdominal, cremasteric (men only), and perianal. These reflexes are graded differently than the motor reflexes and are noted to be present (+) or absent (−). Of these, only the corneal, gag, and plantar reflexes are commonly tested.

The corneal reflex is tested carefully using a clean wisp of cotton and lightly touching the outer corner of each eye on the sclera. The reflex is present if the action elicits a blink. A stroke or brain injury might result in loss of this reflex, either unilaterally or bilaterally. Loss of this reflex indicates the need for eye protection and possible lubrication to prevent corneal damage.

The gag reflex is elicited by gently touching the back of the pharynx with a cotton-tipped applicator, first on one side of the uvula and then the other. Positive response is an equal elevation of the uvula and "gag" with stimulation. Absent response on one or both sides can be seen following a stroke and requires careful evaluation and treatment of the resultant swallowing dysfunction to prevent aspiration of food and fluids.

Pathologic Reflexes

Pathologic reflexes are seen in the presence of neurologic disease; they often represent emergence of earlier reflexes that disappeared with maturity of the nervous system. A pathologic reflex indicative of CNS disease affecting the corticospinal tract is the **Babinski reflex (sign)**. In a person with an intact CNS, if the lateral aspect of the sole of the foot is stroked, the toes contract and draw together. However, in a person who has CNS disease of the motor system, the toes fan out and draw back (Jarvis, 2020). This is normal in newborns but represents a serious abnormality in adults. Other pathologic reflexes include the suck (sucking motions in response to touching the lips), snout (lip pursing in response to touching the lips), palmar (grasp in response to stroking the palm), and palmomental (contraction of the facial muscle in response to stimulation of the thenar eminence near the thumb) reflexes in adults. These reflexes often signify progressive nervous system degeneration (Klein & Stewart-Amidei, 2017).

 Gerontologic Considerations

During the normal aging process, the nervous system undergoes many changes and is more vulnerable to illness. Age-related changes in the nervous system vary in degree and must be distinguished from those due to disease. It is important for clinicians not to attribute abnormality or dysfunction to aging without appropriate investigation. For example, although diminished strength and agility are a normal part of aging, localized weakness can only be attributed to disease.

Structural and Physiologic Changes

As the brain ages, neurons are lost, leading to a decrease in the number of synapses and neurotransmitters. This results in slowed nerve conduction and response time. Brain weight decreases, and the ventricle size increases to maintain cranial volume leading to a decreased brain volume. These changes in brain volume accelerate even in healthy people between the ages of 60 and 70 years (Battaglini, Gentile, Luchetti, et al., 2019). Cerebral blood flow and metabolism are reduced, leading to slower mental functions. Temperature regulation becomes less efficient. In the peripheral nervous system, myelin is lost, resulting in a decrease in conduction velocity in some nerves. Visual and auditory nerves degenerate, leading to loss of visual acuity and hearing. Taste buds atrophy, and nerve cell fibers in the olfactory bulb degenerate (Jarvis, 2020). Nerve cells in the vestibular system of the inner ear, cerebellum, and proprioceptive pathways also degenerate, leading to balance difficulties. Deep tendon reflexes can be decreased or in some cases absent. Hypothalamic function is modified such that stage IV sleep is reduced. There is an overall slowing of autonomic nervous system responses. Pupillary responses are reduced or may not appear at all in the presence of cataracts.

Motor Alterations

Reduced nerve input into muscle contributes to an overall reduction in muscle bulk, with atrophy most easily noted in the hands. Changes in motor function often result in decreased strength and agility, with increased reaction time. Gait is often slowed and wide based. These changes can create difficulties in maintaining balance, predisposing the older person to falls.

Sensory Alterations

Tactile sensation is dulled in the older adult due to a decrease in the number of sensory receptors. There may be difficulty in identifying objects by touch, because fewer tactile cues are received from the bottom of the feet and the person may become confused about body position and location.

Sensitivity to glare, decreased peripheral vision, and a constricted visual field occur due to degeneration of visual pathways, resulting in disorientation, especially at night when there is little or no light in the room. Because the older adult takes longer to recover visual sensitivity when moving from a light to dark area, nightlights and a safe and familiar arrangement of furniture are essential.

Loss of hearing can contribute to confusion, anxiety, disorientation, misinterpretation of the environment, feelings of inadequacy, and social isolation. A decreased sense of taste and smell may contribute to weight loss and disinterest in food. A decreased sense of smell may present a safety hazard, because older adults living alone may be unable to detect household gas leaks or fires. Smoke and carbon monoxide detectors—important in every residence—are critical for the older adult.

Temperature Regulation and Pain Perception

The older adult patient may feel cold more readily than heat and may require extra covering when in bed; a room temperature somewhat higher than usual may be desirable. Reaction to painful stimuli may be decreased with age. Because pain is an important warning signal, caution must be used when hot or cold packs are used. The older patient may be burned or suffer frostbite before being aware of any discomfort. Complaints of pain such as abdominal discomfort or chest pain may be more serious than the patient's perception might indicate and thus require careful evaluation. In older adults, two common pain syndromes that affect the neurologic system are diabetic and postherpetic neuropathies. These frequently occur due to the high rate of these comorbid conditions in older adults. See Chapter 46 for a discussion of diabetic neuropathy.

Mental Status

Although mental processing time decreases with age, memory, language, and judgment capacities remain intact. Change in mental status should never be assumed to be a normal part of aging. **Delirium** is an acute confused state that begins with disorientation and if not recognized and treated early can progress to changes in level of consciousness, irreversible brain damage, and sometimes death. Older age is a risk, but delirium is also seen in patients who have underlying CNS damage or are experiencing an acute condition such as infection, adverse medication reaction, or dehydration. Drug toxicity and depression may produce impairment of attention and memory and should be evaluated as a possible cause of mental status change. Assessment with validated screening tool leads to improved detection of delirium (Smulter, Lingehall, Gustafson, et al., 2019). The Confusion Assessment Method (CAM) is a commonly used screening tool (Inouye, van Dyck, Alessi, et al., 1990) (see Chapter 8, Chart 8-7). Delirium must be differentiated from dementia, which is a chronic and irreversible deterioration of cognitive status. See Chapter 61, Table 61-4 for further discussion of delirium and dementia.

Nursing Implications

Nursing care for patients with age-related changes to the nervous system and for patients with long-term neurologic disability who are aging should include the modifications described previously. In addition, the consequences of any neurologic deficit and its impact on overall function such as activities of daily living, the use of assistive devices, and individual coping should be assessed and considered in planning patient care. Fall risk must be evaluated and fall prevention measures instituted for the patient who is hospitalized as well as in the home.

The nurse must understand the altered responses and the changing needs of the older adult patient before providing education. Visual and hearing deficits require adaptations in activities such as preoperative education, diet therapy, and education about new medications. When using visual materials for education or menu selection, adequate lighting without glare, contrasting colors, and large print are used to offset visual difficulties caused by rigidity and opacity of the lens in the eye and slower pupillary reaction. Procedures and preparations needed for diagnostic tests are explained, taking into account the possibility of impaired hearing and slowed responses in the older adult. Even with hearing loss, the older adult patient often hears adequately if the speaker uses a low-pitched, clear voice; shouting only makes it harder for the patient to understand the speaker. Providing auditory and visual cues aids understanding; if the patient has a significant hearing or visual loss, assistive devices, a signer, an interpreter, or a translator may be needed.

Providing education at an unrushed pace and using reinforcement enhance learning and retention. Material should be short, concise, and concrete. Vocabulary is matched to the patient's ability, and terms are clearly defined. The older adult patient requires adequate time to receive and respond to stimuli, learn, and react. These measures allow comprehension, memory, and formation of association and concepts.

Diagnostic Evaluation

A wide range of diagnostic studies may be performed in patients with altered neurologic function. The nurse should educate the patient about the purpose, what to expect, and any possible side effects related to these examinations prior to testing. Women who are premenopausal are advised to practice effective contraception before and for several days after any diagnostic procedure using contrast, and the woman who is breast-feeding is instructed to stop for the time period recommended by the nuclear medicine department (Pagana & Pagana, 2018). The nurse should note trends in results, because they provide information about disease progression as well as the patient's response to therapy.

Computed Tomography Scanning

Computed tomography (CT) scanning uses a narrow x-ray beam to scan body parts in successive layers. The images provide cross-sectional views of the brain, distinguishing differences in tissue densities of the skull, cortex, subcortical structures, and ventricles. An intravenous (IV) contrast agent may be used to highlight differences further. The brightness of each slice of the brain in the final image is proportional to the degree to which it absorbs x-rays. The image is displayed on an oscilloscope or television monitor and is photographed and stored digitally (Fischbach & Fischbach, 2018). CT scanning is usually performed first without contrast material and then with IV contrast, if needed. The patient lies on an adjustable table with the head in a headrest while the scanning system rotates around the head and produces cross-sectional images. The patient must lie with the head held perfectly still without talking or moving the face, because head motion distorts the image. CT scanning is quick and painless and uses a small amount of radiation to produce images; it has a high degree of sensitivity for detecting lesions.

Brain lesions have a different tissue density from the surrounding normal brain tissue. Abnormalities detected on brain CT include tumor or other masses, infarction, hemorrhage, displacement of the ventricles, and cortical atrophy (Fischbach & Fischbach, 2018). CT angiography allows visualization of blood vessels; in some situations, this eliminates the need for formal angiography. Whole-body CT scanners allow cross-sections of the spinal cord to be visualized. The injection of a water-soluble iodinated contrast agent into the subarachnoid space through lumbar puncture improves the visualization of the spinal and intracranial contents on these images. The CT scan, along with magnetic resonance imaging (MRI), has largely replaced myelography as a diagnostic procedure for the diagnosis of herniated lumbar discs.

Nursing Interventions

Essential nursing interventions include preparation for the procedure and patient monitoring. Preparation includes educating the patient about the need to lie quietly throughout the procedure. A review of relaxation techniques may be helpful for patients with claustrophobia. Sedation can be used if agitation, restlessness, or confusion interferes with a successful study. Ongoing patient monitoring during sedation is necessary. If a contrast agent is used, the patient must be assessed before the CT scan for an iodine/shellfish allergy, because the contrast agent used may be iodine based. Kidney function must also be evaluated because the contrast material is cleared through the kidneys. A suitable IV line for contrast injection and a period of fasting (usually 4 hours) are required prior to the study. Patients who receive an IV contrast agent are monitored during and after the procedure for allergic reactions and changes in kidney function (Fischbach & Fischbach, 2018). Fluid intake is also encouraged after IV contrast to facilitate contrast clearance through the kidney.

Magnetic Resonance Imaging

MRI uses a powerful magnetic field to obtain images of different areas of the body. The magnetic field causes the hydrogen nuclei (protons) within the body to align like small magnets in a magnetic field. In combination with radiofrequency pulses, the protons emit signals, which are converted to images. An MRI scan can be performed with or without a contrast agent and can identify a cerebral abnormality earlier and more clearly than other diagnostic tests (Fischbach & Fischbach, 2018). It can provide information about the chemical changes within cells, allowing the clinician to monitor a tumor's response to treatment. It is particularly useful in the diagnosis of brain tumor, stroke, and multiple sclerosis and does not involve ionizing radiation. An MRI scan may take an hour or longer to complete, so its use in emergency situations is limited.

Several MRI applications allow imaging of brain blood flow and metabolism via special imaging techniques added to the MRI. Such techniques include diffusion-weighted imaging (DWI), perfusion-weighted imaging (PWI), magnetic resonance spectroscopy, and fluid attenuation inversion recovery (FLAIR) (Fischbach & Fischbach, 2018). Magnetic resonance angiography (MRA) allows separate visualization of the cerebral vasculature without the administration of an arterial contrast agent. Both MRI and CT images are used as tools to plan and direct surgical intervention.

Nursing Interventions

Patient preparation includes providing education and obtaining an adequate history. Ferromagnetic substances in the body may become dislodged by the magnet, so history of working with metal fragments must be reviewed. Patients with any type of cardiac implantable electronic device need to be screened to see if it is safe for the patient to undergo any type of MRI (Indik, Gimbel, Abe, et al., 2017). The patient is assessed for implants containing metal (e.g., aneurysm clips, orthopedic hardware, artificial heart valves, intrauterine devices). These objects could malfunction, be dislodged, or heat up as they absorb energy. Cochlear implants will be inactivated by MRI; therefore, other imaging procedures are considered. A complete list of metal compatibility may be found on MRI manufacturer Web sites.

Before the patient enters the room where the MRI is to be performed, all metal objects and credit cards (the magnetic field can erase them) must be removed. This includes medication patches that have a metal backing and metallic lead wires; these can cause burns if not removed (Fischbach & Fischbach, 2018). No metal objects may be brought into the room where the MRI is located; this includes oxygen tanks, IV poles, ventilators, or even stethoscopes. The magnetic field generated by the unit is so strong that any metal-containing items will be strongly attracted and literally can be pulled away with such force that they fly like projectiles toward the magnet. There is a risk of severe injury and death. Further, damage to expensive equipment may occur.

> ### ▶ Quality and Safety Nursing Alert
>
> *For patient safety, the nurse prevents any patient care equipment containing metal or metal parts (e.g., portable oxygen tanks, wheelchairs) from entering the room where the MRI is located. The nurse also assesses for and removes any medication patches with foil backing (such as nicotine patches) that may cause a burn while an MRI scan is being performed.*

For the MRI, the patient lies with the head in a frame on a flat platform that is moved into a tube housing the magnet (see Fig. 60-14). The tube is narrow; people with a wide girth may not fit into the scanner. Patients who are unable to lie flat will not be able to tolerate an MRI. The scanning process is painless, but the patient hears loud thumping of the magnetic coils as the magnetic field is being pulsed. Patients may experience claustrophobia while inside the narrow tube; sedation may be prescribed in these circumstances. "Open" MRI machines are less claustrophobic than the other devices and are available in many locations. However, the images

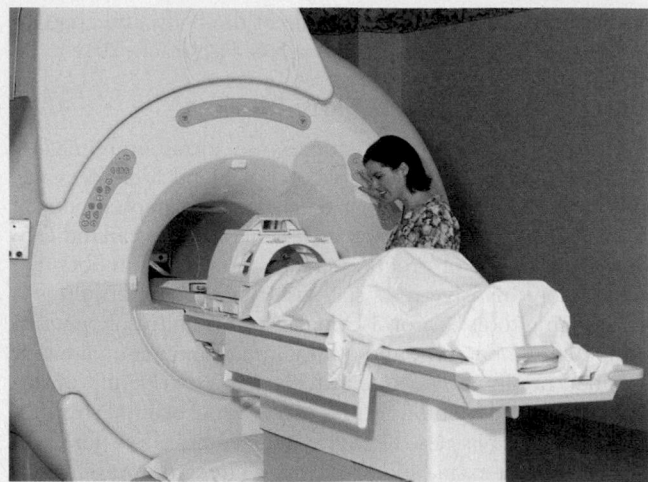

Figure 60-14 • Technician explains what to expect during a magnetic resonance imaging procedure.

produced on these machines are sometimes not so detailed, and traditional devices are preferred for accurate diagnosis. The patient may be educated about the use of relaxation techniques while in the scanner. The patient is informed that it will be possible to talk to the staff during the scan through a microphone inside the scanner (Fischbach & Fischbach, 2018).

Positron Emission Tomography

PET is a computer-based nuclear imaging technique that produces images of actual organ functioning. The patient either inhales a radioactive gas or is injected with a radioactive substance that emits positively charged particles. When these positrons combine with negatively charged electrons (normally found in the body's cells), the resultant gamma rays can be detected by a scanning device that produces a series of two-dimensional views at various levels of the brain. This information is integrated by a computer and gives a composite picture of the brain at work.

PET permits the measurement of blood flow, tissue composition, and brain metabolism and thus indirectly evaluates brain function. The brain is one of the most metabolically active organs, consuming 80% of the glucose the body uses (Hickey & Strayer, 2020). PET measures this activity in specific areas of the brain and can detect changes in glucose use.

PET is useful in showing metabolic changes in the brain (Alzheimer's disease), locating lesions (brain tumor, epileptogenic lesions), identifying blood flow and oxygen metabolism in patients with strokes, distinguishing tumor from areas of necrosis, and revealing biochemical abnormalities associated with mental illness. The isotopes used have a very short half-life and are expensive to produce, requiring specialized equipment for production. Improvement in the scanning procedure and production of isotopes, as well as the advent of reimbursement by third-party payers, has increased the clinical applications of PET studies.

Nursing Interventions

Key nursing interventions include patient preparation, which involves explaining the test and educating the patient about inhalation techniques and the sensations (e.g.,

dizziness, lightheadedness, headache) that may occur. The IV injection of the radioactive substance produces similar side effects. Relaxation exercises may reduce anxiety during the test.

Single-Photon Emission Computed Tomography

SPECT is a three-dimensional imaging technique that uses radionuclides and instruments to detect single photons. It is a perfusion study that captures a moment of cerebral blood flow at the time of injection of a radionuclide. Gamma photons are emitted from a radiopharmaceutical agent given to the patient and are detected by a rotating gamma camera or cameras; the image is sent to a minicomputer. This approach allows areas behind overlying structures or background to be viewed, greatly increasing the contrast between normal and abnormal tissue. It is relatively inexpensive, and the duration is similar to that of a CT scan.

SPECT is useful in detecting the extent and location of abnormally perfused areas of the brain, thus allowing detection, localization, and sizing of stroke (before it is visible by CT scan); localization of seizure foci in epilepsy; detection of tumor progression (Fischbach & Fischbach, 2018); and evaluation of perfusion before and after neurosurgical procedures.

Nursing Interventions

The nursing interventions for SPECT primarily include patient preparation and patient monitoring. Providing education about what to expect before the test can allay anxiety and ensure patient cooperation during the test. Pregnancy and breast-feeding are contraindications to SPECT.

The nurse may need to accompany and monitor the patient during transport to the nuclear medicine department for the scan. Patients are monitored during and after the procedure for allergic reactions to the radiopharmaceutical agent.

Cerebral Angiography

Cerebral angiography is an x-ray study of the cerebral circulation with a contrast agent injected into a selected artery. A valuable tool in investigating vascular disease or anomalies, it is used to determine vessel patency, identify presence of collateral circulation, and provide detail on vascular anomalies that can be used in planning interventions. With the advent of additional imaging techniques, formal cerebral angiography is less frequently performed.

Cerebral angiograms are performed by threading a catheter through the femoral artery in the groin or the radial artery of the wrist and up to the desired vessel. Alternatively, direct puncture of the carotid artery may be performed. X-ray images are obtained as the contrast agent flows through the vessels; the carotid and vertebral arterial systems are visualized, as well as venous drainage. Arterial access may also be used for interventional procedures, such as placing coils in an aneurysm or arteriovenous malformation.

Nursing Interventions

Prior to the angiography, the patient's blood urea nitrogen and creatinine should be checked to ensure the kidneys will be able to excrete the contrast agent. The patient should be well hydrated, and clear liquids are usually permitted up to the time of the test. The patient is instructed to void immediately before the test, and locations of the appropriate peripheral pulses are marked with a felt-tip pen. The patient is instructed to remain immobile during the angiogram process and is told to expect a brief feeling of warmth in the face, behind the eyes, or in the jaw, teeth, tongue, and lips, and a metallic taste when the contrast agent is injected.

When the femoral artery is selected for access, the hair in the groin is clipped and prepared and a local anesthetic agent is given to minimize pain at the insertion site and to reduce arterial spasm. A catheter is introduced into the femoral artery, flushed with heparinized saline, and filled with contrast agent. When the radial artery is selected for access, the wrist will be prepared and accessed using medications to relax and dilate the vessel to allow the catheter to pass (Mason, Shah, Tamis-Holland, et al., 2018). Fluoroscopy is used to guide the catheter to the appropriate vessels. Neurologic assessment is conducted during and immediately following cerebral angiography to observe for embolism or arterial dissection that may occur during the test. Signs of these complications include new onset of alterations in the level of consciousness, weakness on one side of the body, motor or sensory deficits, and speech disturbances.

Nursing care after cerebral angiography includes observation of the injection site for bleeding or hematoma formation (a localized collection of blood). Because a hematoma at the puncture site or embolization to a distal artery affects peripheral pulses, the peripheral pulses that were marked prior to the test are monitored frequently. The color and temperature of the involved extremity are assessed to detect possible embolism (Fischbach & Fischbach, 2018; Mason et al., 2018). Fluids are encouraged to facilitate clearance of the contrast through the kidney. The nurse also monitors for an allergic reaction to the contrast agent, as well as hypotension if vasodilatory medications were used to facilitate a radial approach (Mason et al., 2018).

Myelography

A myelogram is an x-ray of the spinal subarachnoid space taken after the injection of a contrast agent into the spinal subarachnoid space through a lumbar puncture. The water-based contrast agent disperses upward through the CSF to outline the spinal subarachnoid space and shows any distortion of the spinal cord or spinal dural sac caused by tumors, cysts, herniated vertebral discs, or other lesions. Myelography is often followed by CT scanning (Fischbach & Fischbach, 2018).

Nursing Interventions

The patient is educated about what to expect during the procedure and made aware that changes in position may be made during the procedure. After myelography, the patient lies in bed with the head of the bed elevated 30 to 45 degrees. The patient is advised to remain in bed in the recommended position for 4 to 24 hours after testing. Drinking liberal amounts of fluid for rehydration and replacement of CSF may decrease the incidence of post–lumbar puncture headache. The blood pressure, pulse, respiratory rate, and temperature are monitored, as well as the patient's ability to void. Complications that may occur include nausea, vomiting, headache, fever, stiff

neck, seizures, paralysis of one side of the body, and changes in level of consciousness (Fischbach & Fischbach, 2018).

Noninvasive Carotid Flow Studies

Noninvasive carotid flow studies use ultrasound imagery and Doppler measurements of arterial blood flow to evaluate carotid and deep orbital circulation. The graph produced indicates blood velocity. Increased blood velocity can indicate stenosis or partial obstruction. These tests are often obtained before more invasive tests such as arteriography or are used as screening tools. Carotid Doppler, carotid ultrasonography, oculoplethysmography, and ophthalmodynamometry are four common noninvasive vascular techniques that permit evaluation of arterial blood flow and detection of arterial stenosis, occlusion, and plaques. These vascular studies allow noninvasive imaging of extra- and intracranial circulation (Fischbach & Fischbach, 2018).

Transcranial Doppler

Transcranial Doppler uses the same noninvasive techniques as carotid flow studies but records the blood flow velocities of the intracranial vessels. Arterial flow velocities can be measured through thin areas of the temporal and occipital bones of the skull. A handheld Doppler probe emits a pulsed beam; the signal is reflected by the moving red blood cells within the blood vessels. Transcranial Doppler is a noninvasive technique that is helpful in assessing vasospasm (a complication following subarachnoid hemorrhage), altered cerebral blood flow found in occlusive vascular disease, other cerebral pathologies, and brain death.

Nursing Interventions

When a carotid flow study or transcranial Doppler is scheduled, the procedure is described to the patient. The patient is informed that this is a noninvasive test, that a handheld transducer will be placed over the neck and the orbits of the eyes, and that a water-soluble gel or lubricant is used on the transducer (Fischbach & Fischbach, 2018). Either of these two low-risk tests can be performed at the patient's bedside.

Electroencephalography

An electroencephalogram (EEG) represents a record of the electrical activity generated in the brain (Hickey & Strayer, 2020). It is obtained through electrodes applied on the scalp or through microelectrodes placed within the brain tissue. It provides an assessment of cerebral electrical activity. It is useful for diagnosing and evaluating seizure disorders, coma, or organic brain syndrome. Tumors, brain abscesses, blood clots, and infection may cause abnormal patterns in electrical activity. The EEG is also used in making a determination of brain death.

Electrodes are applied to the scalp to record the electrical activity in various regions of the brain. The amplified activity of the neurons between any two of these electrodes is recorded on continuously moving paper; this record is called the encephalogram.

For a baseline recording, the patient lies quietly with both eyes closed. The patient may be asked to hyperventilate for 3 to 4 minutes or to look at a bright, flashing light for photic stimulation. These activation procedures are performed to

---

Chart 60-3

NURSING RESEARCH PROFILE
Electroencephalographic Patterns During Nursing Interventions in Neurointensive Care

Elf, K., Carlsson, T., Santeliz Rivas, L., et al. (2019). Electroencephalographic patterns during common nursing interventions in neurointensive care: A descriptive pilot study. *Journal of Neuroscience Nursing, 51*(1), 10–15.

Purpose

The purpose of this study was to identify changes on electroencephalography (EEG) during standard neurointensive nursing care.

Design

The study was a descriptive pilot study using a convenience sample of patients admitted to the neurointensive care unit with impaired consciousness due to a neurosurgical condition. The sample included 12 participants, with a mean age of 65 years with diagnoses of subarachnoid hemorrhage, intracerebral hemorrhage, acute subdural hematoma, meningitis, ischemic infarction, or traumatic brain injury. All participants were mechanically ventilated, with continuous sedations and intracranial monitoring. The study design included the monitoring of simultaneous continuous EEG and video recording. The nursing interventions

monitored included airway suctioning, repositioning, and when professionally touched for assessment of hygienic interventions.

Findings

Four participants had seizure activity during four nursing interventions (0.4% of nursing interventions); one participant had stimulus-induced rhythmic discharges during an intervention. All 12 participants showed muscle artifacts during 353 nursing interventions (36.3%), which may be a sign of stress. Muscle artifacts happened during all types of nursing interventions but occurred most often when more than one intervention was performed.

Nursing Implications

Patients with neuroscience disorders in intensive care undergo many stressors, and the results of this study indicate that nursing interventions may cause stress in patients. Oral care, repositioning, suctioning, and hygienic care may cause stress. Nurses should be mindful of the comfort of the patient with a neuroscience disorder when delivering care at the bedside and consider shorter and fewer interventions in patients who are sensitive.

---

evoke abnormal electrical discharges, such as seizure potentials. A sleep EEG may be recorded after sedation because some abnormal brain waves are seen only when the patient is asleep. If the epileptogenic area is inaccessible to conventional scalp electrodes, nasopharyngeal electrodes may be used.

Depth recording of EEG is performed by introducing electrodes stereotactically (radiologically placed using instrumentation) into a target area of the brain, as indicated by the patient's seizure pattern and scalp EEG. It is used to identify patients who may benefit from surgical excision of epileptogenic foci. Special transsphenoidal, mandibular, and nasopharyngeal electrodes can be used, and video recording combined with EEG monitoring and telemetry is used in hospital settings to capture epileptiform abnormalities and their sequelae. Some epilepsy centers provide long-term ambulatory EEG monitoring with portable recording devices. Some evidence suggests that continuous EEG may be a useful tool for nurses planning interventions in patients who are critically ill (Elf, Carlsson, Santeliz Rivas, et al., 2019). See the Nursing Research Profile in Chart 60-3.

Nursing Interventions

To increase the chances of recording seizure activity, it is sometimes recommended that the patient be deprived of sleep the night before the EEG. Anticonvulsant agents, tranquilizers, stimulants, and depressants should be withheld 24 to 48 hours before an EEG, because these medications can alter the EEG wave patterns or mask the abnormal wave patterns of seizure disorders (Pagana & Pagana, 2018). Coffee, tea, chocolate, and cola drinks are omitted from the meal before the test because of their stimulating effect. However, the meal itself is not omitted, because an altered blood glucose level can cause changes in brain wave patterns.

The patient is informed that the standard EEG takes 45 to 60 minutes; a sleep EEG requires 12 hours. The patient is assured that the procedure does not cause an electric shock

and that the EEG is a diagnostic test, not a form of treatment. An EEG requires the patient to lie quietly during the test. Sedation is not advisable, because it may lower the seizure threshold in patients with a seizure disorder and it alters brain wave activity in all patients. The nurse needs to check the prescription regarding the administration of anticonvulsant medication prior to testing.

Routine EEGs use a water-soluble lubricant for electrode contact, which can be wiped off and removed by shampooing later. Sleep EEGs involve the use of collodion glue for electrode contact, which requires acetone for removal.

Electromyography

An electromyogram (EMG) is obtained by inserting needle electrodes into the skeletal muscles to measure changes in the electrical potential of the muscles (Pagana & Pagana, 2018). The electrical potentials are shown on an oscilloscope and amplified so that both the sound and appearance of the waves can be analyzed and compared simultaneously.

An EMG is useful in determining the presence of neuromuscular disorders and myopathies. It helps distinguish weakness due to neuropathy (functional or pathologic changes in the peripheral nervous system) from weakness resulting from other causes.

Nursing Interventions

The procedure is explained, and the patient is warned to expect a sensation similar to that of an intramuscular injection as the needle is inserted into the muscle. The muscles examined may ache for a short time after the procedure.

Nerve Conduction Studies

Nerve conduction studies are performed by stimulating a peripheral nerve at several points along its course and recording the muscle action potential or the sensory action potential that results. Surface or needle electrodes are placed on the skin over the nerve to stimulate the nerve fibers. This test is useful in the study of peripheral neuropathies and is often included as part of the EMG.

Evoked Potential Studies

Evoked potential studies involve application of an external stimulus to specific peripheral sensory receptors with subsequent measurement of the electrical potential generated. Electrical changes are detected with the aid of computerized devices that extract the signal, display it on an oscilloscope, and store the data on magnetic tape or disc. In neurologic diagnosis, they reflect nerve conduction times in the peripheral nervous system. In clinical practice, the visual, auditory, and somatosensory systems are most often tested.

In visual evoked responses, the patient looks at a visual stimulus (flashing lights, a checkerboard pattern on a screen). The average of several hundred stimuli is recorded by EEG leads placed over the occipital lobe. The transit time from the retina to the occipital area is measured using computer-averaging methods.

Brainstem auditory evoked responses (BAERs) are measured by applying an auditory stimulus (repetitive auditory click) and measuring the transit time via the brain stem into the cortex. Specific lesions in the auditory pathway modify or delay the response. BAERs may be used in the diagnosis of brain stem abnormalities and in determination of brain death.

In somatosensory evoked responses (SERs), the peripheral nerves are stimulated (electrical stimulation through skin electrodes) and the transit time along the spinal cord to the cortex is measured and recorded from scalp electrodes. SERs are used to detect deficits in spinal cord or peripheral nerve conduction and to monitor spinal cord function during surgical procedures. It is also useful in the diagnosis of demyelinating diseases, such as multiple sclerosis and polyneuropathies, where nerve conduction is slowed.

Nursing Interventions

The nurse explains the procedure and reassures the patient and encourages him or her to relax. The patient is advised to remain perfectly still throughout the recording to prevent artifacts (signals not generated by the brain) that interfere with the recording and interpretation of the test.

Lumbar Puncture and Examination of Cerebrospinal Fluid

A lumbar puncture (spinal tap) is carried out by inserting a needle into the lumbar subarachnoid space to withdraw CSF (Schreiber, 2019). The test may be performed to obtain CSF for examination, to measure and reduce CSF pressure, to determine the presence or absence of blood in the CSF, and to administer medications intrathecally (into the spinal canal).

The needle is inserted into the subarachnoid space in the widest intervertebral spaces; between the second and third, the third and fourth, or fourth and fifth lumbar vertebrae (Schreiber, 2019). Because the spinal cord ends at the first lumbar vertebra, insertion of the needle below the level of the second lumbar vertebra prevents puncture of the spinal cord.

A lumbar puncture may be risky in the presence of an intracranial mass lesion because intraspinal pressure is decreased by removal of CSF, and the brain may herniate downward through the foramen magnum. A successful lumbar puncture requires that the patient be relaxed; a patient who is anxious is tense, and this may artificially alter the pressure reading. The nurse may be asked to assist with a lumbar puncture.

 For the procedural guidelines for assisting with a lumbar puncture, go to **thepoint.lww.com/Brunner15e**.

Cerebrospinal Fluid Analysis

The CSF should be clear and colorless. Pink, blood-tinged, or grossly bloody CSF may indicate a subarachnoid hemorrhage. The CSF may be bloody initially because of local trauma but becomes clearer as more fluid is drained (Hickey & Strayer, 2020; Schreiber, 2019). Specimens are obtained for cell count, culture, glucose, protein, and other tests as indicated. The specimens should be sent to the inhibitor laboratory immediately because changes will take place and alter the result if the specimens are allowed to stand. See Table A-5 in Appendix A on thePoint for the normal values of CSF.

Post–Lumbar Puncture Headache

A post–lumbar puncture headache, ranging from mild to severe, may occur a few hours to several days after the procedure. It is a throbbing bifrontal or occipital headache that is dull and deep in character. It is particularly severe on sitting or standing but lessens or disappears when the patient lies down.

The headache is caused by CSF leakage at the puncture site (Schreiber, 2019). The fluid continues to escape into the tissues by way of the needle track from the spinal canal. As a result of a leak, the supply of CSF in the cranium is depleted to a point at which it is insufficient to maintain proper mechanical stabilization of the brain. When the patient assumes an upright position, tension and stretching of the venous sinuses and pain-sensitive structures occur.

Post–lumbar puncture headache may be avoided if a small-gauge needle (22 gauge) is used (Hickey & Strayer, 2020). A post–lumbar puncture headache is usually managed with analgesic agents, encouraging hydration, ingestion of caffeine, and lying supine (Schreiber, 2019).

Other Complications of Lumbar Puncture

Herniation of the intracranial contents, spinal epidural abscess, spinal epidural hematoma, and meningitis are rare but serious complications of lumbar puncture. Other complications include temporary voiding problems, slight elevation of temperature, backache or spasms, and stiffness of the neck.

Promoting Home, Community-Based, and Transitional Care

 Educating Patients About Self-Care

Many diagnostic tests are carried out in short-procedure units or outpatient testing settings or units. As a result, family members often provide the postprocedure care. Therefore, the patient and family must receive adequate education about precautions to take after the procedure, complications to watch for, and steps to take if complications occur. Because many patients undergoing neurologic diagnostic studies are older adults or have neurologic deficits, provisions must be made to ensure that transportation, postprocedure care, and appropriate monitoring are available.

Continuing and Transitional Care

Contacting the patient and family after diagnostic testing enables the nurse to determine whether they have any questions about the procedure or whether the patient had any untoward results. Education is reinforced and the patient and family are reminded to make and keep follow-up appointments. Patients, family members, and health care providers are focused on the immediate needs, issues, or deficits that necessitated the diagnostic testing.

CRITICAL THINKING EXERCISES

1 **pg** Identify the priorities, approach, and techniques you would use to perform a neurologic assessment on a 32-year-old patient with headaches. How will your priorities, approaches, and techniques differ if the patient has a visual impairment, is hard of hearing, or has lower extremity weakness?

2 **ebp** A 60-year-old patient is scheduled for an MRI scan and tells you he has a pacemaker. What resources would you use to identify whether it is safe for this patient to undergo MRI? What is the evidence base for these practices? Identify the criteria used to evaluate the strength of the evidence for these practices.

REFERENCES

*Asterisk indicates nursing research.
**Double asterisk indicates classic reference.

Books

Fischbach, F. T., & Fischbach, M. A. (2018). *Nurse's quick reference to common laboratory and diagnostic tests* (7th ed.). Philadelphia, PA: Wolters Kluwer.
**Herndon, R. M. (2006). *Handbook of neurologic rating scales* (2nd ed.). New York: Demos Medical Publishing.
Hickey, J. V., & Strayer, A. L. (2020). *The clinical practice of neurological and neurosurgical nursing* (8th ed.). Philadelphia, PA: Wolters Kluwer.

Jarvis, C. (2020). *Physical examination and health assessment* (8th ed.). Philadelphia, PA: Saunders.
Klein, D. G., & Stewart-Amidei, C. (2017). Nervous system alterations. In M. L. Sole, D. G. Klein, & M. J. Moseley (Eds.). *Introduction to critical care nursing* (7th ed.). St. Louis, MO: Elsevier Saunders.
Norris, T. L. (2019). *Porth's pathophysiology: Concepts of altered health state* (10th ed.). Philadelphia, PA: Wolters Kluwer.
Pagana, K. D., & Pagana, T. J. (2018). *Manual of diagnostic and laboratory tests* (6th ed.). St. Louis, MO: Mosby Elsevier.
Posner, J. B., Saper, C. B., Schiff, N. D., et al. (2019). *Plum and Posner's diagnosis of stupor and coma* (5th ed.). Oxford, UK: Oxford University Press.
Weber, J., & Kelley, J. (2018). *Health assessment in nursing* (6th ed.). Philadelphia, PA: Wolters Kluwer.

Journals and Electronic Documents

Battaglini, M., Gentile, G., Luchetti, L., et al. (2019). Lifespan normative data on rates of brain volume changes. *Neurobiology of Aging, 81,* 30–37
*Elf, K., Carlsson, T., Santeliz Rivas, L., et al. (2019). Electroencephalographic patterns during common nursing interventions in neurointensive care: A descriptive pilot study. *Journal of Neuroscience Nursing, 51*(1), 10–15.
Indik, J. H., Gimbel, J. R., Abe, H., et al. (2017). 2017 HRS expert consensus statement on magnetic resonance imaging and radiation exposure in patients with cardiovascular implantable electronic devices. *Heart Rhythm, 14*(7), e97–e153.
**Inouye, S. K., van Dyck, C. H., Alessi, C. A., et al. (1990). Clarifying confusion: The confusion assessment method. A new method for detection of delirium. *Annals of Internal Medicine, 113*(12), 941–948.
Mason, P. J., Shah, B., Tamis-Holland, J. E., et al. (2018). An update on radial artery access and best practices for transradial coronary angiography and intervention in acute coronary syndrome: A scientific statement from the American Heart Association. *Circulation: Cardiovascular Interventions, 11*(9), e000035.
*Poulsen, I., Brix, P., Andersen, S., et al. (2016). Pain assessment scale for patients with disorders of consciousness: A preliminary validation study. *Journal of Neuroscience Nursing, 48*(3), 124–131.
Schreiber, M. L. (2019). Lumbar puncture. *MedSurg Nursing, 28*(6), 402–404.
Smulter, N., Lingehall, H. C., Gustafson, Y., et al. (2019). The use of a screening scale improves the recognition of delirium in older patients after cardiac surgery—A retrospective observational study. *Journal of Clinical Nursing, 28*(11–12), 2309–2318.

Resources

American Headache Society, www.americanheadachesociety.org
American Stroke Association, www.stroke.org
Brain Trauma Foundation, www.braintrauma.org
Epilepsy Foundation, www.epilepsy.com
Harvard Health Publications, Harvard Medical School Office of Public Affairs, www.health.harvard.edu/diagnostic-tests/#brain
National Headache Foundation, www.headaches.org

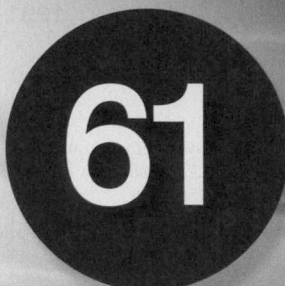

61

Management of Patients with Neurologic Dysfunction

LEARNING OUTCOMES

On completion of this chapter, the learner will be able to:

1. Describe the causes, clinical manifestations, and medical management of various neurologic dysfunctions.
2. Use the nursing process as a framework for care of the patient with altered level of consciousness.
3. Identify the early and late clinical manifestations of increased intracranial pressure and apply the nursing process as a framework for care of the patient with increased intracranial pressure.
4. Compare and contrast the indications for intracranial or transsphenoidal surgery and use the nursing process as a framework for care of the patient undergoing intracranial or transsphenoidal surgery.
5. Explain the various types and causes of seizures and develop a plan of care for the patient experiencing seizures.
6. Recognize the causes, clinical manifestations, and medical and nursing management of the patient experiencing various types of headaches.

NURSING CONCEPTS

Comfort

Development

Family

Health, Wellness, and Illness

Infection

Intracranial Regulation

Mobility

Patient Education

GLOSSARY

akinetic mutism: unresponsiveness to the environment; the patient makes no movement or sound but sometimes opens the eyes

altered level of consciousness (LOC): when a patient is not oriented, does not follow commands, or needs persistent stimuli to achieve a state of alertness

brain death: irreversible loss of all functions of the entire brain, including the brain stem

coma: prolonged state of unconsciousness

craniectomy: a surgical procedure that involves removal of a portion of the skull

craniotomy: a surgical procedure that involves entry into the cranial vault

Cushing's response: the brain's attempt to restore blood flow by increasing arterial pressure to overcome the increased intracranial pressure (*synonym:* Cushing's reflex)

decerebration: an abnormal body posture associated with severe brain injury, characterized by extreme extension of the upper and lower extremities

decortication: an abnormal posture associated with severe brain injury, characterized by abnormal flexion of the upper extremities and extension of the lower extremities

delirium: an acute, confused state that begins with disorientation and if not recognized and treated early can progress to changes in level of consciousness, irreversible brain damage, and sometimes death

dementia: broad term for a syndrome characterized by a general decline in higher brain functioning, such as reasoning, with a pattern of eventual decline in the ability to perform even basic activities of daily living, such as toileting and eating

epilepsy: at least two unprovoked seizures occurring more than 24 hours apart

herniation: abnormal protrusion of tissue through a defect or natural opening

intracranial pressure (ICP): pressure exerted by the volume of the intracranial contents within the cranial vault

locked-in syndrome: condition resulting from a lesion in the pons in which the patient lacks all distal motor activity (paralysis) but cognition is intact

migraine: a severe, unrelenting headache often accompanied by symptoms such as nausea, vomiting, and visual disturbances

minimally conscious state: a state in which the patient demonstrates awareness but cannot communicate thoughts or feelings

Monro–Kellie hypothesis: theory that states that due to limited space for expansion within the skull, an increase in any one of the cranial contents—brain tissue, blood, or cerebrospinal fluid (CSF)—causes a change in the volume of the others (*synonym:* Monro–Kellie doctrine)

persistent vegetative state: condition in which the patient is wakeful but devoid of conscious content, without cognitive or affective mental function

primary headache: a headache for which no specific organic cause can be found

pseudobulbar affect: emotional disturbance characterized by uncontrollable episodes of crying or laughing, or other emotional displays

secondary headache: headache identified as a symptom of another organic disorder (e.g., brain tumor, hypertension)

seizures: paroxysmal transient disturbance of the brain resulting from a discharge of abnormal electrical activity

status epilepticus: episode in which the patient experiences multiple seizures with no recovery time in between

Sudden Unexpected Death in Epilepsy (SUDEP): non-traumatic, nondrowning unexpected death of patient with epilepsy

transsphenoidal: surgical approach to the pituitary via the sphenoid sinuses

This chapter presents an overview of care of the patient with an altered level of consciousness (LOC); the patient with increased intracranial pressure (ICP); and the patient who is undergoing neurosurgical procedures, experiencing seizures, or experiencing headaches. Some of the disorders in this chapter, such as headaches and seizures, may be symptoms of dysfunction in another body system. Alternatively, headaches and seizures can be symptoms of a disruption of the neurologic system. These disorders can also be diagnosed at times as "idiopathic," or without an identifiable cause. The commonalities of these disorders are often the behaviors and needs of the patient and the approaches nurses use to support the patient.

The central nervous system (CNS) contains a vast network of neurons that control the body's vital functions. However, this system is vulnerable, and its optimal function depends on several key factors. First, the neurologic system relies on its structural integrity for support and homeostasis, but this integrity may be disrupted. Examples of structural disruption include head injury, brain tumor, intracranial hemorrhage, infection, and stroke. As brain tissue expands in the inflexible cranium, **intracranial pressure (ICP)** (pressure exerted by the volume of the intracranial contents within the cranial vault) rises, and cerebral perfusion is impaired. Further expansion places pressure on vital centers, which can cause permanent neurologic deficits or lead to brain death.

Second, the neurologic system relies on the body's ability to maintain a homeostatic environment. It requires the delivery of the essential elements of oxygen and glucose, as well as filtration of substrates that are toxic to the neurons. The functions of the neurologic system may be decreased or absent because of the effect of toxic substrates or the body's inability to provide essential substrates. Sepsis, hypovolemia, myocardial infarction, cardiopulmonary arrest, hypoglycemia, electrolyte imbalance, drug and/or alcohol overdose, encephalopathy, and ketoacidosis are examples of such circumstances. Some conditions can be treated and reversed; others result in permanent neurologic deficits and disabilities.

Although the specialty of neuroscience nursing requires an understanding of neuroanatomy, neurophysiology, neurodiagnostic testing, critical-care nursing, and rehabilitation nursing, nurses in all settings care for patients with neurologic disorders (Hickey & Strayer, 2020). Ongoing assessment of the patient's neurologic function and health needs, identification of problems, mutual goal setting, development and implementation of care plans (including education,

counseling, and coordinating activities), and evaluation of the outcomes of care are nursing actions integral to the recovery of the patient. The nurse also collaborates with other members of the health care team to provide essential care, offer a variety of solutions to problems, help the patient and family gain control of their lives, and explore the educational and supportive resources available in the community. The goals are to achieve as high a level of function as possible and to enhance the quality of life for the patient with neurologic impairment and their family.

ALTERED LEVEL OF CONSCIOUSNESS

An **altered level of consciousness (LOC)** is present when the patient is not oriented, does not follow commands, or needs persistent stimuli to achieve a state of alertness. LOC is gauged on a continuum, with a normal state of alertness and full cognition (consciousness) on one end and coma on the other end. **Coma** is a clinical state of unarousable unresponsiveness in which there are no purposeful responses to internal or external stimuli, although nonpurposeful responses to painful stimuli and brain stem reflexes may be present. The usual duration of coma is variable. **Akinetic mutism** is a state of unresponsiveness to the environment in which the patient makes no voluntary movement. **Persistent vegetative state** is a condition in which the patient who is unresponsive resumes sleep–wake cycles after coma but is devoid of cognitive or affective mental function. A **minimally conscious state** differs from persistent vegetative state in that the patient has inconsistent but reproducible signs of awareness (Rohaut, Eliseyev, & Claassen, 2019). **Locked-in syndrome** results from a lesion affecting the pons and results in paralysis and the inability to speak, but vertical eye movements and lid elevation remain intact and are used to indicate responsiveness. The level of responsiveness and consciousness is the most important indicator of the patient's condition (Owen, 2019).

Pathophysiology

Altered LOC is not a disorder itself; rather, it is a result of multiple pathophysiologic phenomena. The cause may be neurologic (head injury, stroke), toxicologic (drug overdose, alcohol intoxication), or metabolic (hepatic or kidney injury, diabetic ketoacidosis).

The underlying cause of neurologic dysfunction is disruption in the cells of the nervous system, neurotransmitters, or brain anatomy (see Chapter 60). Disruptions result from cellular edema or other mechanisms, such as disruption of chemical transmission at receptor sites by antibodies.

Intact anatomic structures of the brain are needed for normal function. The two hemispheres of the cerebrum must communicate, via an intact corpus callosum, and the lobes of the brain (frontal, parietal, temporal, and occipital) must communicate and coordinate their specific functions (see Chapter 60). Other anatomic structures of importance are the cerebellum and the brain stem. The cerebellum has both excitatory and inhibitory actions and is largely responsible for coordination of movement. The brain stem contains areas that control the heart rate, respiration, and blood pressure. Disruptions in the anatomic structures result from trauma, edema, pressure from tumors, or other mechanisms, such as an increase or decrease in the circulation of blood or CSF.

Clinical Manifestations

Alterations in LOC occur along a continuum, and the clinical manifestations depend on where the patient is on this continuum. As the patient's state of alertness and consciousness decreases, changes occur in the pupillary response, eye opening response, verbal response, and motor response. However, initial alterations in LOC may be reflected by subtle behavioral changes, such as restlessness or increased anxiety. The pupils, normally round and quickly reactive to light, become sluggish (response is slower); as the patient becomes comatose, the pupils become fixed (no response to light). The patient in a coma does not open the eyes to voice or command, respond verbally, or move the extremities in response to a request to do so.

Assessment and Diagnostic Findings

The patient with an altered LOC is at risk for alterations in every body system. A complete assessment is performed, with particular attention to the neurologic system. The neurologic examination should be as complete as the LOC allows. It includes an evaluation of mental status, cranial nerve function, cerebellar function (balance and coordination), reflexes, and motor and sensory function. LOC, a sensitive indicator of neurologic function, is assessed based on the criteria in the Glasgow Coma Scale: eye opening, verbal response, and motor response (Hickey & Strayer, 2020). The patient's responses are rated on a scale from 3 to 15. A score of 3 indicates severe impairment of neurologic function, brain death, or pharmacologic inhibition of the neurologic response. A score of 15 indicates that the patient is fully responsive (see Chapter 63, Chart 63-4).

If the patient is comatose and has localized signs such as abnormal pupillary and motor responses, it is assumed that neurologic disease is present until proven otherwise. If the patient is comatose but pupillary light reflexes are preserved, a toxic or metabolic disorder is suspected. Common diagnostic procedures used to identify the cause of unconsciousness include computed tomography (CT) scanning, perfusion CT (PCT), magnetic resonance imaging (MRI), magnetic resonance spectroscopy (MRS), and electroencephalography (EEG). Additional procedures include positron emission tomography (PET) and single-photon emission computed tomography (SPECT) (see Chapter 60). Ongoing research confirms EEG, MRI, and PET as important technologies in determining brain function through the evaluation of metabolic and electrical activity (Rohaut et al., 2019). Laboratory tests include analysis of blood glucose, electrolytes, serum ammonia, and liver function tests; blood urea nitrogen (BUN) levels; serum osmolality; calcium level; and partial thromboplastin and prothrombin times. Other studies may be used to evaluate serum ketones, alcohol and drug concentrations, and arterial blood gases.

Medical Management

The first priority of treatment for the patient with altered LOC is to obtain and maintain a patent airway. The patient may be orally or nasally intubated, or a tracheostomy may be performed. Until the ability of the patient to breathe is determined, a mechanical ventilator is used to maintain adequate oxygenation and ventilation. The circulatory status (blood pressure, heart rate) is monitored to ensure adequate perfusion to the body and brain. An intravenous (IV) catheter is inserted to provide access for IV fluids and medications. Neurologic care focuses on the specific neurologic pathology, if known. Nutritional support, via a feeding tube or a gastrostomy tube, is initiated as soon as possible. In addition to measures designed to determine and treat the underlying causes of altered LOC, other medical interventions are aimed at pharmacologic management and prevention of complications.

NURSING PROCESS

The Patient with an Altered Level of Consciousness

Assessment

Assessment of the patient with an altered LOC often starts with assessing the verbal response through determining the patient's orientation to time, person, and place. Patients are asked to identify the day, date, or season of the year, as well as where they are or the clinicians, family members, or visitors present. Other questions such as "Who is the president?" or "What is the next holiday?" may be helpful in determining the patient's processing of information. Verbal response cannot be evaluated if the patient is intubated or has a tracheostomy, and this should be clearly documented.

Alertness is measured by the patient's ability to open the eyes spontaneously or in response to a vocal or noxious stimulus (pressure or pain). Patients with severe neurologic dysfunction cannot do this. The nurse assesses for periorbital edema (swelling around the eyes) or trauma, which may prevent the patient from opening the eyes, and documents any such condition that interferes with eye opening.

Motor response includes spontaneous, purposeful movement (e.g., the awake patient can move all four extremities with equal strength on command), movement only in response to painful stimuli, or abnormal posturing. If the patient is not responding to commands, the motor response is tested by applying a painful stimulus (firm but gentle pressure) to the nail bed or by squeezing a muscle. If the patient attempts to push away or withdraw, the response is recorded

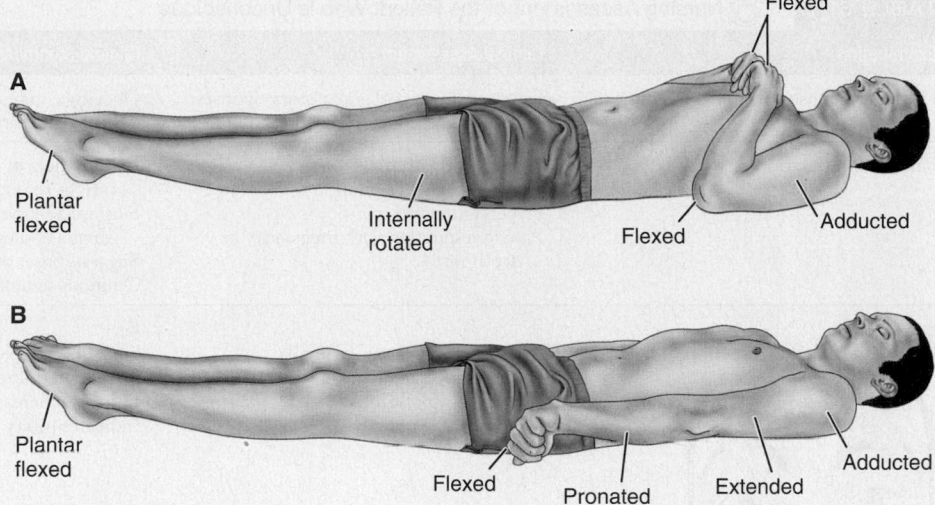

Figure 61-1 • Abnormal posture response to stimuli. **A.** Decorticate posturing and flexion of the upper extremities, internal rotation of the lower extremities, and plantar flexion of the feet. **B.** Decerebrate posturing, involving extension and outward rotation of upper extremities and plantar flexion of the feet. Adapted from Posner, J. B., Saper, C. B., Schiff, N. D., et al. (2007). *Plum and Posner's diagnosis of stupor and coma* (4th ed.). Oxford, UK: Oxford University Press.

as purposeful or appropriate ("Patient withdraws to painful stimulus"). This response is considered purposeful if the patient can cross the midline from one side of the body to the other in response to a painful stimulus. An inappropriate or nonpurposeful response is random and aimless. Posturing may be decorticate or decerebrate (see Fig. 61-1). The most severe neurologic impairment results in flaccidity. The motor response cannot be elicited or assessed when the patient has been given pharmacologic paralyzing agents (i.e., neuromuscular-blocking agents).

In addition to LOC, the nurse monitors parameters such as respiratory status, eye signs, and reflexes on an ongoing basis. Table 61-1 summarizes the assessment and the clinical significance of the findings. Body functions (circulation, respiration, elimination, fluid and electrolyte balance) are examined in a systematic and ongoing manner.

Diagnosis

NURSING DIAGNOSES

Based on the assessment data, major nursing diagnoses may include the following:

- Impaired breathing due to neurologic impairment
- Risk for injury associated with lack of adaptive and defensive resources due to decreased LOC
- Risk for hypovolemia associated with inability to take fluids by mouth
- Risk for impaired nutritional intake associated with inability to ingest nutrients to meet metabolic needs
- Impaired oral mucous membrane integrity associated with mouth breathing, absence of pharyngeal reflex, and altered fluid intake
- Risk for impaired skin integrity associated with prolonged immobility
- Risk for injury associated with diminished or absent corneal reflex
- Impaired thermoregulation associated with damage to hypothalamic center
- Impaired urination associated with altered impairment in neurologic sensing and control
- Bowel incontinence associated with impairment in neurologic sensing and control and also associated with changes in nutritional delivery methods

- Impaired health maintenance associated with neurologic impairment
- Interrupted family process associated with health crisis

COLLABORATIVE PROBLEMS/POTENTIAL COMPLICATIONS

Potential complications may include the following:

- Respiratory distress or failure
- Pneumonia
- Aspiration
- Pressure injury
- Venous thromboembolism (VTE)
- Contractures

Planning and Goals

The patient with altered LOC is subject to all of the complications associated with immobility. Therefore, the goals of care for the patient with altered LOC include normalization of breathing, protection from injury, attainment of fluid volume balance, maintenance of nutritional needs, achievement of intact oral mucous membranes, maintenance of normal skin integrity, absence of corneal injury, attainment of effective thermoregulation, and effective urinary elimination. Additional goals include bowel continence, restoration of health maintenance, maintenance of intact family or support system, and absence of complications.

Because the protective reflexes of the patient who is unconscious are impaired, the quality of nursing care provided may mean the difference between life and death. The nurse must assume responsibility for the patient until the basic reflexes (coughing, blinking, and swallowing) return and the patient becomes conscious and oriented. Therefore, the major nursing goal is to compensate for the absence of these protective reflexes.

Nursing Interventions

ACHIEVING AN ADEQUATE BREATHING PATTERN

The most important consideration in managing the patient with altered LOC is to establish an adequate airway and ensure normalization of the breathing pattern. Obstruction of the airway is a risk because the epiglottis and tongue may relax, occluding the oropharynx, or the patient may aspirate vomitus or nasopharyngeal secretions.

TABLE 61-1 Nursing Assessment of the Patient Who Is Unconscious

Examination	Clinical Assessment	Clinical Significance
Level of responsiveness or consciousness	Eye opening; verbal and motor responses; pupils (size, equality, reaction to light)	Obeying commands is a favorable response and demonstrates a return to consciousness
Pattern of respiration	Respiratory pattern Cheyne–Stokes respiration Hyperventilation Ataxic respiration with irregularity in depth/rate	Disturbances of respiratory center of brain may result in various respiratory patterns Suggests lesions deep in both hemispheres; area of basal ganglia and upper brain stem Suggests onset of metabolic problem or brain stem damage Ominous sign of damage to medullary center
Eyes Pupils (size, equality, reaction to light) 	Equal, normally reactive pupils Equal or unequal diameter Progressive dilation Fixed dilated pupils	Suggests that coma is toxic or metabolic in origin Helps determine location of lesion Indicates increasing intracranial pressure Indicates injury at level of midbrain
Eye movements	Normally, eyes should move from side to side	Functional and structural integrity of brain stem is assessed by inspection of extraocular movements; usually absent in deep coma
Corneal reflex 	When cornea is touched with a wisp of clean cotton, blink response is normal	Tests cranial nerves V and VII; helps determine location of lesion if unilateral; absent in deep coma
Facial symmetry	Asymmetry (sagging, decrease in wrinkles)	Sign of paralysis
Swallowing reflex	Drooling versus spontaneous swallowing	Absent in coma Paralysis of cranial nerves X and XII
Neck	Stiff neck Absence of spontaneous neck movement	Subarachnoid hemorrhage, meningitis Fracture or dislocation of cervical spine
Response of extremity to noxious stimuli	Firm pressure on a joint of the upper and lower extremities Observe spontaneous movements	Asymmetric response in paralysis Absent in deep coma
Deep tendon reflexes	Tap patellar and biceps tendons	Brisk response may have localizing value. Asymmetric response in paralysis Absent in deep coma
Pathologic reflexes 	Firm pressure with blunt object on sole of foot, moving along lateral margin and crossing to the ball of foot	Flexion of the toes, especially the great toe, is normal except in newborn Dorsiflexion of toes (especially great toe) indicates contralateral pathology of corticospinal tract (Babinski reflex) Helps determine location of lesion in brain
Abnormal posture	Observation for posturing (spontaneous or in response to noxious stimuli) Flaccidity with absence of motor response Decorticate posture (flexion and internal rotation of forearms and hands) Decerebrate posture (extension and external rotation)	Deep extensive brain lesion Seen with cerebral hemisphere pathology and metabolic depression of brain function Decerebrate posturing indicates deeper and more severe dysfunction than does decorticate posturing; implies brain pathology; poor prognostic sign

The accumulation of secretions in the pharynx presents a serious problem. Because the patient cannot swallow and lacks pharyngeal reflexes, these secretions must be removed to eliminate the danger of aspiration. Elevating the head of the bed to 30 degrees helps prevent aspiration. Positioning the patient in a lateral or semiprone position also helps because it allows the jaw and tongue to fall forward, thus promoting drainage of secretions.

Positioning alone is not always adequate, however. Suctioning and oral hygiene may be required. Suctioning is performed to remove secretions from the posterior pharynx and upper trachea. Before and after suctioning, the patient is adequately ventilated to prevent hypoxia (Hickey & Strayer, 2020). Chest physiotherapy and postural drainage may be initiated to promote pulmonary hygiene, unless contraindicated by the patient's underlying condition. The chest should be auscultated at least every 8 hours to detect adventitious breath sounds or absence of breath sounds.

Despite these measures, or because of the severity of impairment, the patient with altered LOC often requires intubation and mechanical ventilation. Nursing actions for the patient who is mechanically ventilated include maintaining the patency of the endotracheal tube or tracheostomy, providing frequent oral care, monitoring arterial blood gas measurements, and maintaining ventilator settings (see Chapter 19).

PROTECTING THE PATIENT

For the protection of the patient, side rails are padded. Two rails are kept in the raised position during the day and three at night; however, raising all four side rails is considered a restraint by The Joint Commission if the intent is to limit the patient's mobility. Care should be taken to prevent injury from invasive lines and equipment, and other potential sources of injury should be identified, such as restraints, tight dressings, environmental irritants, damp bedding or dressings, and tubes and drains.

Protection also includes ensuring the patient's dignity during altered LOC. Simple measures such as providing privacy and speaking to the patient during nursing care activities preserve the patient's dignity. Not speaking negatively about the patient's condition or prognosis is also important, because patients in a coma may be able to hear. The patient who is comatose has an increased need for advocacy, and the nurse is responsible for seeing that these advocacy needs are met.

> ### ► Quality and Safety Nursing Alert
>
> *If the patient begins to emerge from unconsciousness, every measure that is available and appropriate for calming and quieting the patient should be used. Any form of restraint is likely to be countered with resistance, leading to self-injury or to a dangerous increase in ICP. Therefore, physical restraints are avoided, if possible; a written prescription must be obtained if their use is essential for the patient's well-being.*

MAINTAINING FLUID BALANCE AND MANAGING NUTRITIONAL NEEDS

Hydration status is assessed by examining tissue turgor and mucous membranes, assessing intake and output trends, and analyzing laboratory data. Fluid needs are met initially by administering the required IV fluids. However, IV solutions (and blood component therapy) for patients with intracranial conditions must be given slowly. If they are given too rapidly, they can increase ICP. The quantity of fluids given may be restricted to minimize the possibility of cerebral edema.

If the patient does not recover quickly and sufficiently enough to take adequate fluids and calories by mouth, a feeding or gastrostomy tube will be inserted for the administration of fluids and enteral feedings. Research suggests that patients fed within 48 hours of injury have improved outcomes over those in whom nutrition is delayed (Lucke-Wold, Logsdon, Nguyen, et al., 2018).

PROVIDING MOUTH CARE

The mouth is inspected for dryness, inflammation, and crusting. The patient who is unconscious requires careful oral care, because there is a risk of parotitis if the mouth is not kept scrupulously clean. The mouth is cleansed and rinsed carefully to remove secretions and crusts and to keep the mucous membranes moist. A thin coating of petrolatum on the lips prevents drying, cracking, and encrustations. If the patient has an endotracheal tube, the tube should be moved to the opposite side of the mouth daily to prevent ulceration of the mouth and lips. If the patient is intubated and mechanically ventilated, good oral care is also necessary. Research suggests that comprehensive mouth care with antiseptic such as chlorhexidine and head of bed elevation decreases ventilator-associated pneumonia and improves the oral health in patients who are intubated (Malhan, Usman, Trehan, et al., 2019).

MAINTAINING SKIN AND JOINT INTEGRITY

Preventing skin breakdown requires continuing nursing assessment and intervention. Special attention is given to patients who are unconscious, because they cannot respond to external stimuli. Assessment includes a regular schedule of turning to avoid pressure, which can cause breakdown and necrosis of the skin. Turning also provides kinesthetic (sensation of movement), proprioceptive (awareness of position), and vestibular (equilibrium) stimulation. After turning, the patient is carefully repositioned to prevent ischemic necrosis over pressure areas. Dragging or pulling the patient up in bed must be avoided, because this creates a shearing force and friction on the skin surface.

Maintaining correct body position is important; equally important is passive exercise of the extremities to prevent contractures. The use of splints or foam boots aids in the prevention of footdrop and eliminates the pressure of bedding on the toes. The use of trochanter rolls to support the hip joints keeps the legs in proper alignment. The arms are in abduction, the fingers lightly flexed, and the hands in slight supination. The heels of the feet are assessed for pressure areas. Specialty beds, such as fluidized or low–air-loss beds, may be used to decrease pressure on bony prominences (Hickey & Strayer, 2020).

PRESERVING CORNEAL INTEGRITY

Some patients who are unconscious have their eyes open and have inadequate or absent corneal reflexes. The cornea may become irritated, dry, or scratched, leading to ulceration. The eyes may be cleansed with cotton balls moistened with sterile normal saline to remove debris and discharge. Artificial tears or methylcellulose may be prescribed to provide lubrication.

Periorbital edema often occurs after cranial surgery. If cold compresses are prescribed, care must be exerted to avoid contact with the cornea. Eye patches should be used cautiously because of the potential for corneal abrasion from contact with the patch; eye shields may provide eye protection with less risk of injury.

MAINTAINING BODY TEMPERATURE

High fever in the patient who is unconscious may be caused by infection of the respiratory or urinary tract, drug reactions, or damage to the hypothalamic temperature-regulating center. A slight elevation of temperature may be caused by dehydration. The environment can be adjusted, depending on the patient's condition, to promote a normal body temperature. If body temperature is elevated, a minimum amount of bedding is used. The room may be cooled to 18.3°C (65°F). However, if the patient is an older adult and does not have an elevated temperature, a warmer environment is needed.

Because of damage to the temperature-regulating center in the brain or severe intracranial infection, patients who are unconscious often develop very high temperatures. Such temperature elevations must be controlled, because the increased metabolic demands of the brain can exceed cerebral circulation and oxygen delivery, potentially resulting in cerebral deterioration (Hickey & Strayer, 2020). Studies suggest that hyperthermia may contribute to poor outcome after brain injury but not through a decreased brain oxygen level (Rincon, 2018). Persistent hyperthermia with no identified clinical source of infection indicates brain stem damage and a poor prognosis.

Quality and Safety Nursing Alert

The body temperature of a patient who is unconscious is never taken by mouth. Rectal, tympanic (if not contraindicated), or core temperature measurement is preferred to the less accurate axillary temperature.

Strategies for reducing fever include:
- Removing all bedding over the patient (with the possible exception of a light sheet, towel, or small drape)
- Administering acetaminophen or ibuprofen as prescribed
- Giving cool sponge baths
- Using a hypothermia blanket
- Monitoring temperature frequently to assess the patient's response to the therapy and to prevent an excessive decrease in temperature and shivering

PREVENTING URINARY RETENTION

The patient with an altered LOC is often incontinent or has urinary retention. The bladder is palpated or scanned at intervals to determine whether urinary retention is present, because a full bladder may be an overlooked cause of overflow incontinence. A portable bladder ultrasound instrument is a useful tool in bladder management and retraining programs.

If the patient is not voiding, a program of intermittent catheterization should be devised in order to reduce the patient's risk of urinary tract infection. A catheter may be inserted during the acute phase of illness to monitor urinary output. Because catheters are a major cause of urinary tract infection, the patient is observed for fever and cloudy urine. The area around the urethral orifice is inspected for drainage and cleansed routinely. The urinary catheter is usually removed if the patient has a stable cardiovascular system and if no diuresis, sepsis, or voiding dysfunction existed before the onset of coma. Although many patients who are unconscious urinate spontaneously after catheter removal, the bladder should be scanned with a portable bladder ultrasound device periodically for urinary retention (see Chapter 47, Fig. 47-8).

An external catheter (condom catheter) for the male patient and absorbent pads or female incontinence device for the female patient can be used for patients who are unconscious and can urinate spontaneously, although involuntarily. As soon as consciousness is regained, a bladder training program is initiated (Hickey & Strayer, 2020). The patient who is incontinent is monitored frequently for skin irritation and skin breakdown. Appropriate skin care is implemented to prevent these complications.

PROMOTING BOWEL FUNCTION

The abdomen is assessed for distention by listening for bowel sounds and measuring the girth of the abdomen with a tape measure. There is a risk of diarrhea from infection, antibiotic agents, and hyperosmolar fluids. Frequent loose stools may also occur with fecal impaction. Commercial fecal collection bags are available for patients with fecal incontinence (see Chapter 41, Fig. 41-1).

Immobility and lack of dietary fiber can cause constipation. The nurse monitors the number and consistency of bowel movements and performs a rectal examination for signs of fecal impaction. Stool softeners may be prescribed and can be given with tube feedings. To facilitate bowel emptying, a glycerin suppository or bowel stimulant may be indicated. The patient may require an enema routinely to empty the lower colon.

RESTORING HEALTH MAINTENANCE

Once increased ICP is not a problem, the nurse assists the patient and family to restore the health of the patient who is unconscious. This involves using auditory, visual, olfactory, gustatory, tactile, and kinesthetic activities to stimulate the patient emerging from coma (Gattuta, Coralo, Lo Buono, et al., 2018). Efforts are made to restore the sense of daily rhythm by maintaining usual day and night patterns for activity and sleep. The nurse touches and talks to the patient and encourages family members and friends to do so. Communication is extremely important and includes touching the patient and spending enough time with the patient to become sensitive to their needs. It is also important to avoid making any negative comments about the patient's status or prognosis in the patient's presence.

The nurse orients the patient to time and place at least once every 8 hours. Sounds from the patient's usual environment may be introduced using a recording. Family members can read to the patient from a favorite book and may suggest radio and television programs that the patient previously enjoyed as a means of enriching the environment and providing familiar input.

When arousing from coma, many patients experience a period of agitation, indicating that they are becoming more aware of their surroundings but still cannot react or communicate in an appropriate fashion. Although this is disturbing for many family members, it is actually a positive clinical sign. At this time, it is necessary to minimize stimulation by limiting background noises, having only one person speak to the patient at a time, giving the patient a longer period of time to respond, and allowing for frequent rest or quiet times. After the patient has regained consciousness, recordings of family or social events may assist the patient in recognizing family and friends and allow them to experience missed events.

Programs of sensory stimulation for patients with brain injury have been developed in an effort to improve outcomes. Although these are controversial programs with inconsistent results, some support the concept of providing structured neurostimulation (Hickey & Strayer, 2020).

MEETING THE FAMILY'S NEEDS

The family of the patient with altered LOC may be thrown into a sudden state of crisis and go through the process of severe anxiety, denial, anger, remorse, grief, and reconciliation. Depending on the disorder that caused the altered LOC and the extent of the patient's recovery, the family may be unprepared for the changes in the cognitive and physical status of their loved one. If the patient has significant residual deficits, the family may require considerable time, assistance, and support to come to terms with these changes. To help family members mobilize resources and coping skills, the nurse reinforces and clarifies information about the patient's condition, encourages the family to be involved in care, and listens to and encourages sharing of feelings and concerns while supporting decision making about management and placement after hospitalization. Families may benefit from participation in support services offered through the hospital, rehabilitation facility, or community organizations.

The family may need to face the death of their loved one. The patient with a neurologic disorder is often pronounced brain dead before the heart stops beating. The term **brain death** describes irreversible loss of all functions of the entire brain and absence of brain stem reflexes (Milliken & Uveges, 2020). The term may be misleading to the family because, although brain function has ceased, the patient appears to be alive, with the heart rate and blood pressure sustained by vasoactive medications and breathing continued by mechanical ventilation. When discussing a patient who is brain dead with family members, it is important to provide accurate, timely, understandable, and consistent information. See Chapter 13 for discussion of end-of-life care.

MONITORING AND MANAGING POTENTIAL COMPLICATIONS

Pneumonia, aspiration, and respiratory failure are potential complications in any patient who has a depressed LOC and who cannot protect the airway or turn, cough, and take deep breaths. The longer the period of unconsciousness, the greater the risk of pulmonary complications.

Vital signs and respiratory function are monitored closely to detect any signs of respiratory failure or distress. Complete blood count and arterial blood gas measurements are assessed to determine whether there are adequate red blood cells to carry oxygen and whether ventilation is effective. Chest physiotherapy and suctioning are initiated to prevent respiratory complications such as pneumonia. Oral care interventions are performed for patients receiving mechanical ventilation to maintain oral health and decrease the incidence of

pneumonia (Malhan et al., 2019). If pneumonia develops, cultures are obtained to identify the organism so that appropriate antibiotic agents can be given.

The patient with altered LOC is monitored closely for evidence of impaired skin integrity, and strategies to prevent skin breakdown and pressure injuries are continued through all phases of care, including hospitalization, rehabilitation, and home care. Factors that contribute to impaired skin integrity (e.g., incontinence, inadequate dietary intake, pressure on bony prominences, edema) are addressed. If pressure injuries develop, strategies to promote healing are undertaken. Care is taken to prevent bacterial contamination of pressure injuries, which may lead to sepsis and septic shock. See Chapter 56 for assessment and management of pressure injuries.

The patient should also be monitored for signs and symptoms of VTE, which may manifest as a deep vein thrombosis (DVT) or pulmonary embolism (PE). Prophylaxis with subcutaneous heparin or low-molecular-weight heparin (dalteparin, danaparoid) as well as anti-embolism stockings or pneumatic compression devices are prescribed according to the patient's risk factors for thrombosis and bleeding (Galan, Egea-Guerrero, Diaz, et al., 2016). The nurse observes for signs and symptoms of DVT or PE.

Patients with a prolonged decrease in LOC are at risk for developing contractures. During acute care, the patient is turned every 2 hours and passive range of motion performed at least twice a day. Splints, provided by occupational therapy, are applied to the hands and feet in a rotating manner to maintain functional joint alignment. Hand splints have been reported to be safe and beneficial for patients in decreasing spasticity and improving hand opening (Khan, Amatya, Bensmail, et al., 2019).

Evaluation

Expected patient outcomes may include:

1. Attains optimal breathing pattern
2. Experiences no injuries
3. Attains or maintains adequate fluid balance and nutritional status
   a. Has no clinical signs or symptoms of dehydration
   b. Demonstrates normal range of serum electrolytes
   c. Has no clinical signs or symptoms of overhydration or malnutrition
4. Achieves healthy oral mucous membranes
5. Maintains intact skin
6. Has no corneal injury
7. Attains or maintains thermoregulation
8. Has no urinary retention
9. Has no diarrhea or fecal impaction
10. Receives appropriate sensory stimulation
11. Has family members who cope with crisis
    a. Verbalize fears and concerns
    b. Participate in patient's care and provide sensory stimulation by talking and touching
12. Is free of complications
    a. Has arterial blood gas values or oxygen saturation levels within normal range
    b. Displays no signs or symptoms of pneumonia
    c. Exhibits intact skin over pressure areas
    d. Does not develop VTE such as DVT or PE

INCREASED INTRACRANIAL PRESSURE

The rigid cranial vault contains brain tissue (1400 g), blood (75 mL), and CSF (75 mL). The volume and pressure of these three components are usually in a state of equilibrium and produce the ICP. ICP is usually measured in the lateral ventricles, with the normal pressure being 0 to 10 mm Hg, and 15 mm Hg being the upper limit of normal (Hickey & Strayer, 2020).

The **Monro–Kellie hypothesis,** also known as the Monro–Kellie doctrine, explains the dynamic equilibrium of cranial contents. The hypothesis states that because of the limited space for expansion within the skull, an increase in any one of the components causes a change in the volume of the others (Witherspoon & Ashby, 2017). Because brain tissue has limited space to expand, compensation typically is accomplished by displacing or shifting CSF, increasing the absorption or diminishing the production of CSF, or decreasing cerebral blood volume. Without such changes, ICP begins to rise. Under normal circumstances, minor changes in blood volume and CSF volume occur constantly as a result of alterations in intrathoracic pressure (coughing, sneezing, straining), posture, blood pressure, and systemic oxygen and carbon dioxide levels.

Pathophysiology

Increased ICP affects many patients with acute neurologic conditions because pathologic conditions alter the relationship between intracranial volume and ICP. Although elevated ICP is most commonly associated with head injury, it also may be seen as a secondary effect in other conditions, such as brain tumors, subarachnoid hemorrhage, and toxic and viral encephalopathies. Increased ICP from any cause decreases cerebral perfusion, stimulates further edema (swelling), and may shift brain tissue, resulting in herniation—a dire and frequently fatal event.

Decreased Cerebral Blood Flow

Increased ICP may reduce cerebral blood flow, resulting in ischemia and cell death. In the early stages of cerebral ischemia, the vasomotor centers are stimulated and the systemic pressure rises to maintain cerebral blood flow. Usually, this is accompanied by a slow bounding pulse and respiratory irregularities. These changes in blood pressure, pulse, and respiration are important clinically because they suggest increased ICP.

The concentration of carbon dioxide in the blood and in the brain tissue also plays a role in the regulation of cerebral blood flow. An increase in the partial pressure of arterial carbon dioxide ($PaCO_2$) causes cerebral vasodilation, leading to increased cerebral blood flow and increased ICP. A decrease in $PaCO_2$ has a vasoconstrictive effect, limiting blood flow to the brain. Decreased venous outflow may also increase cerebral blood volume, thus raising ICP.

Cerebral Edema

Cerebral edema or swelling is defined as an abnormal accumulation of water or fluid in the intracellular space, extracellular space, or both, associated with an increase in the volume of brain tissue. Edema can occur in the gray, white, or interstitial matter. As brain tissue swells within the rigid skull, several mechanisms attempt to compensate for the increasing ICP. These compensatory mechanisms include autoregulation as well as decreased production and flow of CSF. **Autoregulation** refers to the brain's ability to change the diameter of its blood vessels to maintain a constant cerebral blood flow during alterations in systemic blood pressure. This mechanism can be impaired in patients who are experiencing a pathologic and sustained increase in ICP.

Cerebral Response to Increased Intracranial Pressure

As ICP rises, compensatory mechanisms in the brain work to maintain blood flow and prevent tissue damage. The brain can maintain a steady perfusion pressure if the arterial systolic blood pressure is 50 to 150 mm Hg and the ICP is less than 40 mm Hg. Changes in ICP are closely linked with cerebral perfusion pressure (CPP). The CPP is calculated by subtracting the ICP from the mean arterial pressure (MAP). For example, if the MAP is 100 mm Hg and the ICP is 15 mm Hg, then the CPP is 85 mm Hg. The normal CPP is 70 to 100 mm Hg (Hickey & Strayer, 2020). As ICP rises and the autoregulatory mechanism of the brain is overwhelmed, the CPP can increase to greater than 100 mm Hg or decrease to less than 50 mm Hg. Patients with a CPP of less than 50 mm Hg experience irreversible neurologic damage. Therefore, the CPP must be maintained at 70 to 80 mm Hg to ensure adequate blood flow to the brain. If ICP is equal to MAP, cerebral circulation ceases.

A clinical phenomenon known as the **Cushing's response** (also called Cushing's reflex) is seen when cerebral blood flow decreases significantly. When ischemic, the vasomotor center triggers an increase in arterial pressure in an effort to overcome the increased ICP. A sympathetically mediated response causes an increase in the systolic blood pressure with a widening of the pulse pressure and cardiac slowing. This response is seen clinically as an increase in systolic blood pressure, widening of the pulse pressure, and reflex slowing of the heart rate. It is a late sign requiring immediate intervention; however, perfusion may be recoverable if the Cushing's response is treated rapidly.

At a certain point, the brain's ability to autoregulate becomes ineffective and decompensation (ischemia and infarction) begins. When this occurs, the patient exhibits significant changes in mental status and vital signs. The bradycardia, hypertension, and bradypnea associated with this deterioration are known as Cushing's triad, which is a grave sign. At this point, herniation of the brain stem and occlusion of the cerebral blood flow occur if therapeutic intervention is not initiated. **Herniation** refers to the shifting of brain tissue from an area of high pressure to an area of lower pressure (see Fig. 61-2). The herniated tissue exerts pressure on the brain area into which it has shifted, which interferes with the blood supply in that area. Cessation of cerebral blood flow results in cerebral ischemia, infarction, and brain death.

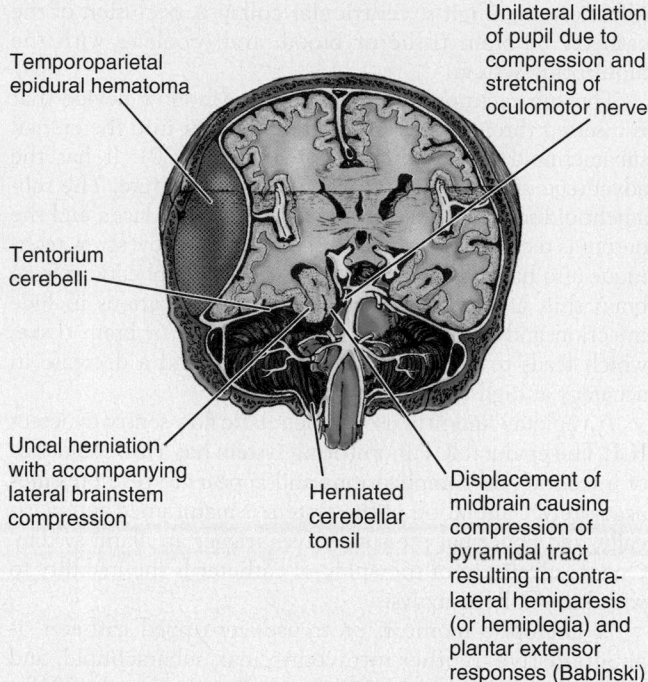

Temporoparietal
epidural hematoma

Unilateral dilation
of pupil due to
compression and
stretching of
oculomotor nerve

Tentorium
cerebelli

Uncal herniation
with accompanying
lateral brainstem
compression

Herniated
cerebellar
tonsil

Displacement of
midbrain causing
compression of
pyramidal tract
resulting in contra-
lateral hemiparesis
(or hemiplegia) and
plantar extensor
responses (Babinski)

Figure 61-2 • Cross-section of the brain showing herniation of part of the temporal lobe through the tentorium as a result of a temporo-parietal epidural hematoma. Reprinted with permission from Kintzel, K. C. (1977). *Advanced concepts in clinical nursing.* Philadelphia, PA: J. B. Lippincott.

Clinical Manifestations

If ICP increases to the point at which the brain's ability to adjust has reached its limits, neural function is impaired; this may be manifested at first by clinical changes in LOC and later by abnormal respiratory and vasomotor responses.

> ◣ *Quality and Safety Nursing Alert*
>
> *The earliest sign of increasing ICP is a change in LOC. Agitation, slowing of speech, and delay in response to verbal suggestions may be early indicators.*

Any sudden change in the patient's condition, such as restlessness (without apparent cause), confusion, or increasing drowsiness, has neurologic significance. These signs may result from compression of the brain due to swelling from hemorrhage or edema, an expanding intracranial lesion (hematoma or tumor), or a combination of both.

As ICP increases, the patient becomes stuporous, reacting only to loud or painful stimuli. At this stage, serious impairment of brain circulation is probably taking place, and immediate intervention is required. As neurologic function deteriorates further, the patient becomes comatose and exhibits abnormal motor responses in the form of **decortication** (abnormal flexion of the upper extremities and extension of the lower extremities), **decerebration** (extreme extension of the upper and lower extremities),

or flaccidity (see Fig. 61-1). If the coma is profound and irreversible with no known confounding factors, brain stem reflexes are absent, and respirations are impaired or absent, the patient may be evaluated for brain death (Milliken & Uveges, 2020).

Assessment and Diagnostic Findings

The diagnostic studies used to determine the underlying cause of increased ICP are discussed in detail in Chapter 60. The most common diagnostic tests are CT scanning and MRI. The patient may also undergo cerebral angiography, PET, or SPECT. Transcranial Doppler studies provide information about cerebral blood flow. The patient with increased ICP may also undergo electrophysiologic monitoring to observe cerebral blood flow indirectly. Evoked potential monitoring measures the electrical potentials produced by nerve tissue in response to external stimulation (auditory, visual, or sensory). Lumbar puncture is avoided in patients with increased ICP, because the sudden release of pressure in the lumbar area can cause the brain to herniate (Hickey & Strayer, 2020). See Chapter 60 for further discussion of lumbar puncture and other diagnostic tests.

Complications

Complications of increased ICP include brain stem herniation, diabetes insipidus, and syndrome of inappropriate antidiuretic hormone (SIADH).

Brain stem herniation results from an excessive increase in ICP in which the pressure builds in the cranial vault and the brain tissue presses down on the brain stem. This increasing pressure on the brain stem results in cessation of blood flow to the brain, leading to irreversible brain anoxia and brain death.

Neurogenic diabetes insipidus is the result of decreased secretion of antidiuretic hormone (ADH). The patient has excessive urine output, decreased urine osmolality, and serum hyperosmolarity (Tudor & Thompson, 2019). Therapy consists of administration of fluids, electrolyte replacement, and administration of a synthetic vasopressin (desmopressin). See Chapters 10 and 45 for a discussion of diabetes insipidus.

SIADH is the result of increased secretion of ADH. The patient becomes volume overloaded, urine output diminishes, and serum sodium concentration becomes dilute. Treatment of SIADH includes fluid restriction (less than 800 mL/day with no free water), which is usually sufficient to correct the hyponatremia. In severe cases, careful administration of a 3% hypertonic saline solution may be therapeutic (Hickey & Strayer, 2020). The change in serum sodium concentration should not exceed a correction rate of approximately 1.3 mEq/L/h. See Chapters 10 and 45 for further discussion of SIADH.

Medical Management

Increased ICP is a true emergency and must be treated promptly. Invasive monitoring of ICP is an important component of management. Immediate management to relieve increased ICP requires decreasing cerebral edema, lowering the volume of CSF, or decreasing cerebral blood volume while maintaining cerebral perfusion. These goals are accomplished by administering osmotic diuretics, restricting fluids, draining CSF, controlling fever, maintaining systemic blood pressure and oxygenation, and reducing cellular metabolic demands. See Chapter 63 for a discussion of the management of increased ICP.

Monitoring Intracranial Pressure and Cerebral Oxygenation

The purposes of ICP monitoring are to identify increased pressure early in its course (before cerebral damage occurs), to quantify the degree of elevation, to initiate appropriate treatment, to provide access to CSF for sampling and drainage, and to evaluate the effectiveness of treatment. ICP can be monitored with the use of an intraventricular catheter (ventriculostomy), a subarachnoid bolt, an epidural or subdural catheter, or a fiberoptic transducer–tipped catheter placed in the subdural space or in the ventricle (see Fig. 61-3).

When a ventriculostomy or intraventricular catheter monitoring device is used for monitoring ICP, a fine-bore catheter is inserted into a lateral ventricle, preferably in the nondominant hemisphere of the brain (Hickey & Strayer, 2020). The catheter is connected by a fluid-filled system to a transducer, which records the pressure in the form of an electrical impulse. In addition to obtaining continuous ICP recordings, the ventricular catheter allows CSF to drain, particularly during acute increases in pressure. The ventriculostomy can also be used to drain blood from the ventricle. Continuous drainage of CSF under pressure control is an effective method of treating intracranial hypertension. Another advantage of a ventricular catheter is access for the intraventricular administration of medications and the occasional instillation of air or a contrast agent for ventriculography. Complications associated with its use include infection, meningitis, ventricular collapse, occlusion of the catheter by brain tissue or blood, and problems with the monitoring system.

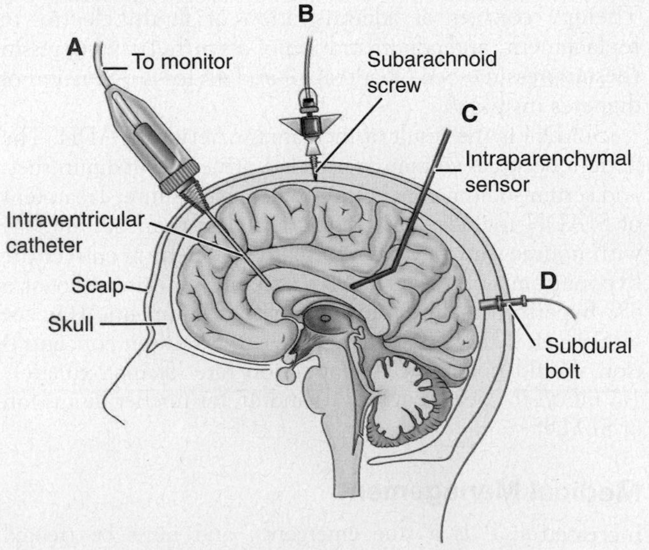

The subarachnoid screw or bolt is a hollow device that is inserted through the skull and dura mater into the cranial subarachnoid space (Hickey & Strayer, 2020). It has the advantage of not requiring a ventricular puncture. The subarachnoid screw is attached to a pressure transducer, and the output is recorded on an oscilloscope. The hollow screw technique also has the advantage of avoiding complications from brain shift and small ventricle size. Complications include infection and blockage of the screw by clot or brain tissue, which leads to a loss of pressure tracing and a decrease in accuracy at high ICP readings.

An epidural monitor uses a pneumatic flow sensor to detect ICP. The epidural ICP monitoring system has a low incidence of infection and complications and appears to read pressures accurately. Calibration of the system is maintained automatically, and abnormal pressure waves trigger an alarm system. One disadvantage of the epidural catheter is the inability to withdraw CSF for analysis.

A fiberoptic monitor, or transducer-tipped catheter, is an alternative to other intraventricular, subarachnoid, and subdural systems (Al-Mufti, Smith, Lander, et al., 2018). The miniature transducer reflects pressure changes, which are converted to electrical signals in an amplifier and displayed on a digital monitor. The catheter can be inserted into the ventricle, subarachnoid space, subdural space, or brain parenchyma or under a bone flap. If inserted into the ventricle, it can also be used in conjunction with a CSF drainage device.

Interpreting Intracranial Pressure Waveforms

Waves of high pressure and troughs of relatively normal pressure indicate changes in ICP. Waveforms are captured and recorded on an oscilloscope. These waves have been classified as A waves (plateau waves), B waves, and C waves (see Fig. 61-4). The plateau waves (A waves) are transient, paroxysmal, recurring elevations of ICP that may last 5 to

Figure 61-3 • Intracranial pressure monitoring. A device may be placed in the ventricle (**A**), the subarachnoid space (**B**), the intraparenchymal space (**C**), or the subdural space (**D**).

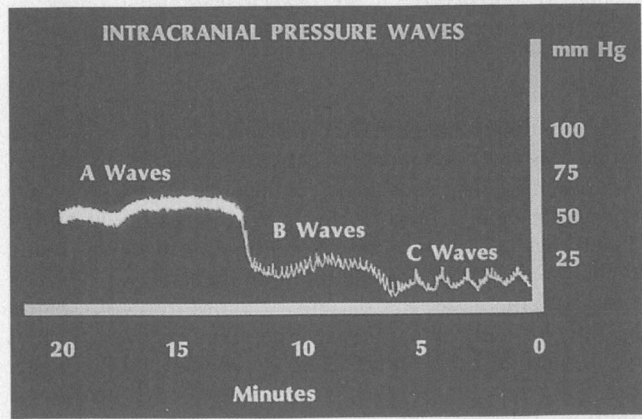

Figure 61-4 • Intracranial pressure waves. Composite diagram of A (plateau) waves, which indicate cerebral ischemia; B waves, which indicate intracranial hypertension and variations in the respiratory cycle; and C waves, which relate to variations in systemic arterial pressure and respirations.

20 minutes and range in amplitude from 40 to 100 mm Hg (Al-Mufti et al., 2018). Plateau waves have clinical significance and indicate changes in vascular volume within the intracranial compartment that are beginning to compromise cerebral perfusion. The A waves may increase in amplitude and frequency, reflecting cerebral ischemia and brain damage that can occur before overt signs and symptoms of raised ICP are seen clinically. B waves are shorter (30 seconds to 2 minutes) and have smaller amplitude (up to 50 mm Hg). They have less clinical significance, but if seen in a series in a patient with depressed consciousness, they may precede the appearance of A waves. B waves may be seen in patients with intracranial hypertension and decreased intracranial compliance. C waves are small, rhythmic oscillations with frequencies of 4 to 8 per minute and appear to be related to rhythmic variations of the systemic arterial blood pressure and respirations (Hickey & Strayer, 2020).

Other Neurologic Monitoring Systems

Another trend in neurologic monitoring is microdialysis of the patient with a brain injury (Zhou & Kalanuria, 2018). Cortical probes are placed near the injured area and are used to measure levels of glutamate, lactate, pyruvate, and glucose, substances that reflect the metabolic function of the brain. Some researchers theorize that direct measurements of glucose and energy by-products in the brain will lead to better management of these patients. Although cerebral microdialysis has reduced the mortality of patients who are brain injured, more study is needed to link it to improved outcomes (Zhou & Kalanuria, 2018).

An additional trend is monitoring of cerebral oxygenation through monitoring of the oxygen saturation in the jugular venous bulb ($SjvO_2$) or via a catheter in the brain. Cerebral oxygenation is thought to be important because changes in cerebral perfusion may reflect an increase in ICP. Readings taken from a catheter residing in the jugular outflow tract allow for a comparison of arterial and venous oxygen saturation, and the balance of cerebral oxygen supply and demand is demonstrated. Venous jugular desaturations can reflect early cerebral ischemia, alerting the clinician before an increase in ICP occurs. Minimizing cerebral desaturations can potentially improve outcomes. This type of monitoring is now widely available and has been successfully used to identify secondary brain insults. A limiting factor is that this saturation reflects overall perfusion of the brain rather than that of a specific injured area (Al-Mufti et al., 2018).

Another method of measuring cerebral oxygenation and temperature is by inserting a fiberoptic catheter into the brain matter. The most common system is Licox (see Fig. 61-5). The system includes a monitor with a screen for the display of oxygen and temperature values and cables that connect to the monitoring probes in the brain (Hickey & Strayer, 2020).

Decreasing Cerebral Edema

Osmotic diuretics such as mannitol and hypertonic saline (3%) may be administered to decrease fluid in the brain tissue and reduce cerebral edema (Witherspoon & Ashby, 2017).

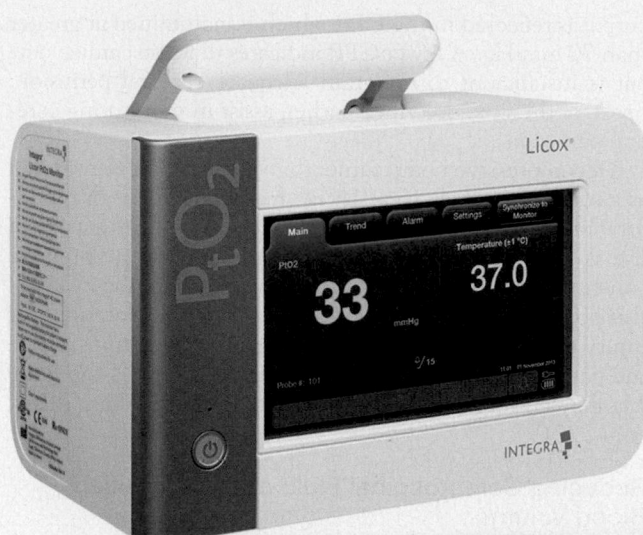

Figure 61-5 • The Licox brain tissue oxygen monitor. Permission granted by Integra LifeSciences Corporation, Princeton, New Jersey, USA.

These agents act by drawing water across intact membranes, thereby reducing the volume of the brain and extracellular fluid. An indwelling urinary catheter is usually inserted to monitor urinary output and to manage the resulting diuresis. If the patient is receiving osmotic diuretics, serum osmolality and electrolytes should be determined to assess hydration status. If a brain tumor is the cause of the increased ICP, corticosteroids (e.g., dexamethasone) help reduce the edema surrounding the tumor.

Another method for decreasing cerebral edema is fluid restriction (Hickey & Strayer, 2020). Limiting overall fluid intake leads to dehydration and hemoconcentration, which draws fluid across the osmotic gradient and decreases cerebral edema. Conversely, overhydration of the patient with increased ICP is avoided, because it increases cerebral edema.

Researchers have long hypothesized that lowering body temperature would decrease cerebral edema by reducing the oxygen and metabolic requirements of the brain, thus protecting the brain from continued ischemia. If body metabolism can be reduced by lowering the body temperature, the collateral circulation in the brain may be able to provide an adequate blood supply to the brain. The effect of hypothermia on ICP requires more study; thus far, induced hypothermia has not consistently been shown to be beneficial for patients with brain injury. Inducing and maintaining hypothermia is a major clinical treatment and requires knowledge and skilled nursing observation and management. The type and length of rewarming techniques after hypothermia may also be factors in the outcome of patients with neurologic injuries (Rincon, 2018).

Maintaining Cerebral Perfusion

Cardiac output may be manipulated to provide adequate perfusion to the brain. Improvements in cardiac output are made using fluid volume and inotropic agents such as dobutamine and norepinephrine. The effectiveness of the cardiac output is reflected in the CPP, which is maintained at greater than 70 mm Hg. A lower CPP indicates that the cardiac output is insufficient to maintain adequate cerebral perfusion. $SjvO_2$ and Licox, described earlier, assist in monitoring cerebral perfusion.

Decompressive hemicraniectomy may also be considered as a surgical strategy to assist in the management of refractory intracranial hypertension. The removal of a part of the skull allows the brain to expand without the pressure constraints exerted by the cranial vault. Complications of this procedure include infection and increased potential for injury to the unprotected underlying brain structures. Once the patient is no longer at risk for increased ICP, the bone flap may be surgically replaced (Hutchinson, Kolias, Tajsic, et al., 2019).

Reducing Cerebrospinal Fluid and Intracranial Blood Volume

CSF drainage is frequently performed, because the removal of CSF with a ventriculostomy drain can dramatically reduce ICP and restore CPP. Caution should be used in draining CSF, however, because excessive drainage may result in collapse of the ventricles and herniation. The reduction in $PaCO_2$ may result in hypoxia, ischemia, and an increase in cerebral lactate levels. Maintaining the $PaCO_2$ at greater than 30 mm Hg may prove beneficial (Hickey & Strayer, 2020).

Controlling Fever

Preventing a temperature elevation is critical, because fever increases cerebral metabolism and the rate at which cerebral edema forms. Strategies to reduce body temperature include administration of antipyretic medications, as prescribed, and the use of a hypothermia blanket. Additional strategies for reducing fever were discussed previously in the Nursing Process section on altered LOC. The patient's temperature is monitored closely, and the patient is observed for shivering, which should be avoided because it is associated with increased oxygen consumption, increased levels of circulating catecholamines, and increased vasoconstriction. Shivering is associated with decreased levels of brain oxygenation; however, the association between shivering and neurologic outcome is unknown.

Maintaining Oxygenation and Reducing Metabolic Demands

Arterial blood gases and pulse oximetry are monitored to ensure that systemic oxygenation remains optimal. Metabolic demands may be reduced through the administration of high doses of barbiturates if the patient is unresponsive to conventional treatment. The mechanism by which barbiturates decrease ICP and protect the brain is uncertain, but the resultant comatose state is thought to reduce the metabolic requirements of the brain, thus providing cerebral protection.

Another method of reducing cellular metabolic demand and improving oxygenation is the administration of medications causing sedation. The patient who receives these agents cannot move; this decreases the metabolic demands and results in a decrease in cerebral oxygen demand. The patient

cannot respond to or report pain either. The most common agents used for sedation are pentobarbital, thiopental, propofol, and dexmedetomidine (Opdenakker, Vanstraelen, De Sloovere, et al., 2019).

If sedative agents are used, the ability to perform serial neurologic assessments is lost. Therefore, other monitoring tools are needed to assess the patient's status and response to therapy. Important parameters that must be assessed include ICP, blood pressure, heart rate, respiratory rate, and the patient's response to ventilator therapy (e.g., patient-ventilator dyssynchrony; see Chapter 19). The level of pharmacologic paralysis is adjusted based on serum levels of the medications given and the assessed parameters. Potential complications of these medications include hypotension caused by decreased sympathetic tone and myocardial depression.

Patients receiving high doses of barbiturates or pharmacologic sedatives require continuous cardiac monitoring, endotracheal intubation, mechanical ventilation, and arterial pressure monitoring, as well as ICP monitoring.

NURSING PROCESS

The Patient with Increased Intracranial Pressure

Assessment

Initial assessment of the patient with increased ICP includes obtaining a history of events leading to the present illness and the pertinent past medical history. It is usually necessary to obtain this information from family or friends. The neurologic examination should be as complete as the patient's condition allows. It includes an evaluation of mental status, LOC, cranial nerve function, cerebellar function (balance and coordination), reflexes, and motor and sensory function. Because the patient is critically ill, ongoing assessment is more focused, including pupil checks, assessment of selected cranial nerves, frequent measurements of vital signs and ICP, and the use of the Glasgow Coma Scale (see Table 61-1).

Diagnosis

NURSING DIAGNOSES

Based on the assessment data, major nursing diagnoses include the following:

- Impaired breathing associated with neurologic dysfunction (brain stem compression, structural displacement)
- Risk for ineffective tissue perfusion associated with the effects of increased ICP
- Hypovolemia associated with fluid restriction
- Risk for infection associated with ICP monitoring system (fiberoptic or intraventricular catheter)

Other relevant nursing diagnoses are included in the earlier section on altered LOC.

COLLABORATIVE PROBLEMS/POTENTIAL COMPLICATIONS

Potential complications may include the following:

- Brain stem herniation
- Diabetes insipidus
- SIADH

Planning and Goals

The goals for the patient include normalization of respiration, adequate cerebral tissue perfusion through reduction in ICP, restoration of fluid balance, absence of infection, and absence of complications.

Nursing Interventions

ACHIEVING AN ADEQUATE BREATHING PATTERN

In order to normalize breathing it is essential to maintain the airway. The patency of the airway is assessed. Secretions that are obstructing the airway must be suctioned with care, because transient elevations of ICP occur with suctioning (Hickey & Strayer, 2020). Hypoxia caused by poor oxygenation leads to cerebral ischemia and edema. Coughing is discouraged because it increases ICP. The lung fields are auscultated at least every 8 hours to determine the presence of adventitious sounds or any areas of congestion. Elevating the head of the bed may aid in clearing secretions and improve venous drainage of the brain.

The patient must be monitored for respiratory irregularities. Increased pressure on the frontal lobes or deep midline structures may result in Cheyne–Stokes respirations, whereas pressure in the midbrain can cause hyperventilation. If the lower portion of the brain stem (the pons and medulla) is involved, respirations become irregular and eventually cease.

There is ongoing controversy about the use of hyperventilation therapy in traumatic brain injury. This therapy is used in some circumstances to reduce ICP by causing cerebral vasoconstriction and a decrease in cerebral blood volume. The nurse collaborates with the respiratory therapist in monitoring the $PaCO_2$, which is usually maintained at less than 30 mm Hg. Employing hyperventilation should follow guidelines for management of TBI as it involves risk of cerebral vasoconstriction and ischemia (Saherwala, Bader, Stutzman, et al., 2018). Patients undergoing hyperventilation therapy also benefit from multimodality monitoring to determine the overall effect of this therapy on brain perfusion (Hickey & Strayer, 2020).

A neurologic observation record (see Fig. 61-6) is maintained, and all observations are made in relation to the patient's baseline condition. Repeated assessments of the patient are made (sometimes minute by minute) so that improvement or deterioration may be noted immediately. If the patient's condition deteriorates, the primary provider is notified emergently and preparations are made for surgical intervention.

OPTIMIZING CEREBRAL TISSUE PERFUSION

In addition to ongoing nursing assessment, strategies are initiated to reduce factors contributing to the elevation of ICP (see Table 61-2).

Proper positioning helps reduce ICP. The patient's head is kept in a neutral (midline) position, maintained with the use of a cervical collar if necessary, to promote venous drainage. Elevation of the head is maintained at 30 to 45 degrees unless contraindicated. Extreme rotation of the neck and flexion of the neck are avoided, because compression or distortion of the jugular veins increases ICP. Extreme hip flexion is also avoided, because this position causes an increase in intra-abdominal and intrathoracic pressures, which can produce an increase in ICP. Relatively minor changes in position can significantly affect ICP. If monitoring reveals that turning the patient raises ICP, rotating beds, turning sheets, and holding the patient's head during turning may minimize the stimuli that increase ICP. Research suggests that patient response to position change is highly variable and requires close hemodynamic monitoring and individualized care (Hickey & Strayer, 2020).

The Valsalva maneuver, which can be produced by straining at defecation or even moving in bed, raises ICP and is to be avoided. Stool softeners may be prescribed. If the patient is alert and able to eat, a diet high in fiber may be indicated. Abdominal distention, which increases intra-abdominal and intrathoracic pressure and ICP, should be noted. Enemas and cathartics are avoided if possible. When moving or being turned in bed, the patient can be instructed to exhale (which opens the glottis) to avoid the Valsalva maneuver.

Mechanical ventilation presents unique problems for the patient with increased ICP. Before suctioning, the patient should be preoxygenated and briefly hyperventilated using 100% oxygen on the ventilator. Suctioning should not last longer than 15 seconds. High levels of positive end-expiratory pressure (PEEP) must be utilized cautiously, because they may decrease venous return to the heart and decrease venous drainage from the brain through increased intrathoracic pressure (Hickey & Strayer, 2020).

Activities that increase ICP, as indicated by changes in waveforms, should be avoided if possible. Spacing of nursing interventions may prevent transient increases in ICP. During nursing interventions, the ICP should not increase above 25 mm Hg, and it should return to baseline levels within 5 minutes. Patients with increased ICP should not demonstrate a significant increase in pressure or change in the ICP waveform. Patients with the potential for a significant increase in ICP may need sedation before initiation of nursing activities (Hickey & Strayer, 2020).

Emotional stress and frequent arousal from sleep are avoided. A calm atmosphere is maintained. Environmental stimuli (e.g., noise, conversation) should be minimal.

MAINTAINING NEGATIVE FLUID BALANCE

The administration of osmotic and loop diuretics is part of the treatment protocol to reduce ICP. Corticosteroids may be used to reduce cerebral edema (except when it results from trauma), and fluids may be restricted. All of these treatment modalities promote dehydration.

Skin turgor, mucous membranes, urine output, and serum and urine osmolality are monitored to assess fluid status. If IV fluids are prescribed, the nurse ensures that they are given at a slow to moderate rate with an IV infusion pump, to prevent too-rapid administration and avoid overhydration. For the patient receiving mannitol, the nurse observes for the possible development of heart failure and pulmonary edema. The intent of treatment is to promote a shift of fluid from the intracellular to the intravascular compartment and to control cerebral edema. However, this shift of fluid volume to the intravascular compartment may overwhelm the ability of the myocardium to increase workload sufficient to meet these demands, which may cause failure and pulmonary edema.

For patients undergoing dehydrating procedures, vital signs, including blood pressure, must be monitored to assess fluid

(text continued on page 2008)

NURSING NEUROLOGIC CRITICAL CARE FLOWSHEET

ADDRESSOGRAPH

	Date												
	Time												
	Initials												
Level of orientation (✓)	Person												
	Place												
	Date and time												
	No orientation												
Awakens to (✓)	Voice												
	Touch												
	Noxious stimuli												
	Painful stimuli												
	No response												
Best verbal response (✓)	Clear and appropriate												
	Clear and inappropriate												
	Difficulty speaking*												
	Perseveration												
	Aphasic expressive (non-fluent)												
	Aphasic receptive (fluent)												
	Sounds no speech												
	No verbal response												
	ETT/TRACH												
Best motor response (✓)	Moves all extremities purposefully												
	Withdraws and lifts to painful stimuli												
	Moves to painful stimuli												
	Decorticates (spinal reflex)												
	Decerebrates (spinal reflex)												
	No motor response												
Best motor strength upper extremities (✓)	No drifts (R/L)	R L	R L	R L	R L	R L	R L	R L	R L	R L	R L	R L	R L
	Drift (R/L)	R L	R L	R L	R L	R L	R L	R L	R L	R L	R L	R L	R L
	Can only lift forearm (R/L)	R L	R L	R L	R L	R L	R L	R L	R L	R L	R L	R L	R L
	Trace movement of hand or arm (R/L)	R L	R L	R L	R L	R L	R L	R L	R L	R L	R L	R L	R L
	Trace movement of fingers only (R/L)	R L	R L	R L	R L	R L	R L	R L	R L	R L	R L	R L	R L
	No motor response (R/L)	R L	R L	R L	R L	R L	R L	R L	R L	R L	R L	R L	R L
Best strength lower extremities (✓)	Raises leg off bed (R/L)	R L	R L	R L	R L	R L	R L	R L	R L	R L	R L	R L	R L
	Drags heel on bed and lifts knee (R/L)	R L	R L	R L	R L	R L	R L	R L	R L	R L	R L	R L	R L
	Trace movement of foot or leg (R/L)	R L	R L	R L	R L	R L	R L	R L	R L	R L	R L	R L	R L
	Trace movement of toes only (R/L)	R L	R L	R L	R L	R L	R L	R L	R L	R L	R L	R L	R L
	No response (R/L)	R L	R L	R L	R L	R L	R L	R L	R L	R L	R L	R L	R L
Seizure activity (✓)	No seizure activity												
	With loss of consciousness*												
	Without loss of consciousness*												
Ataxia (✓)	Gross ataxia												
	Fine motor ataxia												
	Does not apply												
ICP monitoring	Ventriculostomy mL												
	ICP mm Hg												
	Not applicable												

***= FURTHER DOCUMENTATION IS REQUIRED TO VALIDATE ASSESSMENT**

Figure 61-6 • A neurologic assessment flowsheet. The nurse fills these out online now in most institutions.

PUPIL GAUGE (mm)

2	3	4	5	6

7	8	9

B=Brisk, S=Sluggish, F=Fixed

		ADDRESSOGRAPH											
	Date												
	Time												
	Initials												
Incision +/−	Dry and intact												
	Drainage												
Pupils: refer to above gauge (✓) (+)=Present (−)=Absent	Size (R/L)	R L	R L	R L	R L	R L	R L	R L	R L	R L	R L	R L	R L
	Regular (R/L)	R L	R L	R L	R L	R L	R L	R L	R L	R L	R L	R L	R L
	Irregular* (R/L)	R L	R L	R L	R L	R L	R L	R L	R L	R L	R L	R L	R L
	Reaction (R/L) (B) - (S) - (F)	R L	R L	R L	R L	R L	R L	R L	R L	R L	R L	R L	R L
	Ptosis (R/L) (+) (−)	R L	R L	R L	R L	R L	R L	R L	R L	R L	R L	R L	R L
	Gaze preference (R/L) (+)* (−)	R L	R L	R L	R L	R L	R L	R L	R L	R L	R L	R L	R L
Meningeal signs (+)=Present (−)=Absent	Headache												
	Nuchal rigidity												
	Photophobia												
Visual fields (+)=Present (−)=Absent* NA=Not applicable	Right upper outer												
	Right lower outer												
	Left upper outer												
	Left lower outer												
Nystagmus (+)=Present (−)=Absent	Lateral (R/L)	R L	R L	R L	R L	R L	R L	R L	R L	R L	R L	R L	R L
	Vertical (R/L)	R L	R L	R L	R L	R L	R L	R L	R L	R L	R L	R L	R L
Cranial nerves (+)=Present (−)=Absent	III, IV, VI, Extraocular movements												
	VII – Peripheral facial droop (R/L)	R L	R L	R L	R L	R L	R L	R L	R L	R L	R L	R L	R L
	XII – Tongue deviation (R/L)	R L	R L	R L	R L	R L	R L	R L	R L	R L	R L	R L	R L
	IX – Gag reflex												
	V, VII – Corneal reflex (R/L)	R L	R L	R L	R L	R L	R L	R L	R L	R L	R L	R L	R L
	X, IX – Cough reflex												
	Doll's eyes if appropriate												
Follows commands	Two step verbal command												
	One step verbal command												
	Unable to follow command												

*= FURTHER DOCUMENTATION IS REQUIRED TO VALIDATE ASSESSMENT

Initials	Signature	Title	Initials	Signature	Title

Figure 61-6 • (Continued)

TABLE 61-2	Increased Intracranial Pressure and Interventions

Factor	Physiology	Interventions	Rationale
Cerebral edema	Can be caused by contusion, tumor, or abscess; water intoxication (hypo-osmolality); alteration in the blood–brain barrier (protein leaks into the tissue, causing water to follow).	Administer osmotic diuretics as prescribed (monitor serum osmolality). Maintain head of bed elevation at 30 degrees. Maintain alignment of the head.	Promotes venous return. Prevents impairment of venous return through the jugular veins.
Hypoxia	A decrease in PaO_2 to <60 mm Hg causes cerebral vasodilation.	Maintain PaO_2 >60 mm Hg. Maintain oxygen therapy. Monitor arterial blood gas values. Suction when needed. Maintain a patent airway.	Prevents hypoxia and vasodilation.
Hypercapnia (elevated $PaCO_2$)	Causes vasodilation.	Maintain $PaCO_2$ (normally 35–45 mm Hg) by establishing ventilation.	Normalizing $PaCO_2$ minimizes vasodilation and thus reduces the cerebral blood volume.
Impaired venous return	Increases the cerebral blood volume.	Maintain head alignment. Elevate head of bed 30 degrees.	Hyperextension, rotation, or hyperflexion of the neck causes decreased venous return.
Increase in intrathoracic or abdominal pressure	An increase in these pressures due to coughing, PEEP, or Valsalva maneuver causes a decrease in venous return.	Monitor arterial blood gas values, and keep PEEP as low as possible. Provide humidified oxygen. Administer stool softeners as prescribed.	To keep secretions loose and easy to suction or expectorate. Soft bowel movements will prevent straining or Valsalva maneuver.

$PaCO_2$, partial pressure of arterial carbon dioxide; PaO_2, partial pressure of arterial oxygen; PEEP, positive end-expiratory pressure.
Adapted from Hickey, J. V., & Strayer, A. L. (2020). *The clinical practice of neurological & neurosurgical nursing* (8th ed.). Philadelphia, PA: Wolters Kluwer.

---

volume status. An indwelling urinary catheter is inserted to permit assessment of renal function and fluid status. During the acute phase, urine output is monitored hourly. An output greater than 200 mL/h for 2 consecutive hours may indicate the onset of diabetes insipidus (Hickey & Strayer, 2020). These patients need careful oral hygiene, because mouth dryness occurs with dehydration. Frequently rinsing the mouth with nondrying solutions, lubricating the lips, and removing encrustations relieve dryness and promote comfort.

PREVENTING INFECTION

The risk of infection is greatest when ICP is monitored with an intraventricular catheter and increases with the duration of the monitoring. Most health care facilities have written protocols for managing these systems and maintaining their sterility; strict adherence to the protocols is essential.

Aseptic technique must be used when managing the system and changing the ventricular drainage bag. The drainage system is also checked for loose connections, because they can cause leakage and contamination of the CSF as well as inaccurate readings of ICP. The nurse observes the character of the CSF drainage and reports increasing cloudiness or blood. The patient is monitored for signs and symptoms of meningitis: fever, chills, nuchal (neck) rigidity, and increasing or persistent headache. See Chapter 64 for a discussion of meningitis.

MONITORING AND MANAGING POTENTIAL COMPLICATIONS

The primary complication of increased ICP is brain herniation resulting in death (see Fig. 61-2). Nursing management focuses on detecting early signs of increasing ICP, because medical interventions are usually ineffective once later signs develop (Hickey & Strayer, 2020). Frequent neurologic assessments and documentation and analysis of trends will reveal the subtle changes that may indicate increasing ICP.

Detecting Indications of Increasing Intracranial Pressure. The nurse assesses for and immediately reports any signs or symptoms of increasing ICP (see Chart 61-1). The focus is on detecting early signs of increasing ICP.

Monitoring Intracranial Pressure. Because clinical assessment is not always a reliable guide in recognizing increased ICP, especially in patients who are comatose, monitoring of ICP and cerebral oxygenation is an essential part of management. ICP is monitored closely for continuous elevation or significant increase over baseline. The trend of ICP measurements over time is an important indication of the patient's underlying status. Vital signs are assessed when an increase in ICP is noted (Hickey & Strayer, 2020).

Careful attention to aseptic technique is needed when handling any part of the monitoring system (Hickey & Strayer, 2020). The insertion site is inspected for signs of infection. Temperature, pulse, and respirations are closely monitored for systemic signs of infection (Rincon, 2018). All connections and stopcocks are checked for leaks, because even small leaks can distort pressure readings and lead to infection (Hickey & Strayer, 2020).

When ICP is monitored with a fluid system, the transducer is calibrated at a particular reference point, usually 2.5 cm (1 inch) above the ear with the patient in the supine position; this point corresponds to the level of the foramen of Monro (see Fig. 61-7). CSF pressure readings depend on the patient's position. For subsequent pressure readings, the head should be in the same position relative to the transducer. Fiberoptic catheters are calibrated before insertion and do not require further referencing; they do not require the head of the bed to be at a specific position to obtain an accurate reading.

Detecting Increasing Intracranial Pressure (ICP)

Early Signs and Symptoms of Increasing ICP

- *Disorientation, restlessness, increased respiratory effort, purposeless movements, and mental confusion.* These are early clinical indications of increasing ICP because the brain cells responsible for cognition are extremely sensitive to decreased oxygenation.
- *Pupillary changes and impaired extraocular movements.* These occur as the increasing pressure displaces the brain against the oculomotor and optic nerves (cranial nerves II, III, IV, and VI), which arise from the midbrain and brain stem (see Chapter 60).
- *Weakness in one extremity or on one side of the body.* This occurs as increasing ICP compresses the pyramidal tracts.
- *Headache that is constant, increasing in intensity, and aggravated by movement or straining.* This occurs as increasing ICP causes pressure and stretching of venous and arterial vessels in the base of the brain.

Later Signs and Symptoms of Increasing ICP

- The level of consciousness continues to deteriorate until the patient is comatose (Glasgow Coma Scale score ≤8).
- The pulse rate and respiratory rate decrease or become erratic, and the blood pressure and temperature increase. The pulse pressure (the difference between the systolic and diastolic pressures) widens. The pulse fluctuates rapidly, varying from bradycardia to tachycardia.
- Altered respiratory patterns develop, including Cheyne–Stokes breathing (rhythmic waxing and waning of rate and depth of respirations alternating with brief periods of apnea) and ataxic breathing (irregular breathing with a random sequence of deep and shallow breaths).
- Projectile vomiting may occur with increased pressure on the reflex center in the medulla.
- Hemiplegia or decorticate or decerebrate posturing may develop as pressure on the brain stem increases; bilateral flaccidity occurs before death.
- Loss of brain stem reflexes, including pupillary, corneal, gag, and swallowing reflexes, is an ominous sign of approaching death.

Adapted from Hickey, J. V., & Strayer, A. L. (2020). *The clinical practice of neurological & neurosurgical nursing* (8th ed.). Philadelphia, PA: Wolters Kluwer.

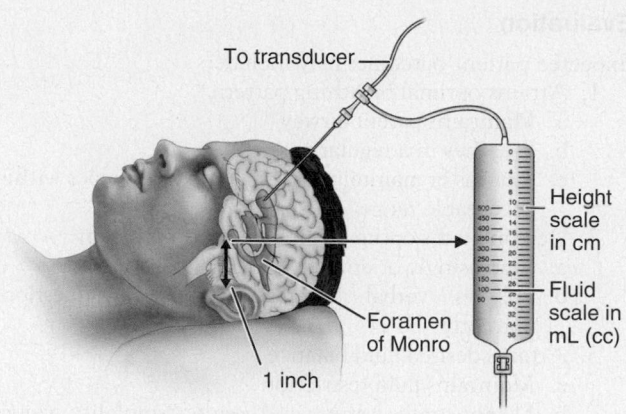

Figure 61-7 • Location of the foramen of Monro for calibration of the intracranial pressure monitoring system.

When technology is associated with patient management, the nurse must be certain that the technologic equipment is functioning properly and used correctly (Liu, Griffith, Jang, et al., 2020) (see the Nursing Research Profile in Chart 61-2). The most important concern must be the patient to whom equipment is attached. The patient and family must be informed about the technology and the goals of its use. The patient's response is monitored, and appropriate comfort measures are implemented to ensure that the patient's stress is minimized.

ICP measurement is only one parameter; repeated neurologic checks and clinical examinations remain important measures. Astute observation, comparison of findings with previous observations, and interventions can assist in preventing life-threatening ICP elevations.

Monitoring for secondary complications. The nurse also assesses for complications of increased ICP, including diabetes insipidus and SIADH (see Chapters 10 and 45). Urine output should be monitored closely. Diabetes insipidus requires fluid and electrolyte replacement, along with the administration of vasopressin, to replace and slow the urine output. Serum electrolyte levels are monitored for imbalances. SIADH requires fluid restriction and monitoring of serum electrolyte levels.

NURSING RESEARCH PROFILE
Aspects of Intracranial Pressure Monitoring

Liu, X., Griffith, M., Jang, H., et al. (2020). Intracranial pressure monitoring via external ventricular drain: Are we waiting long enough before recording the real value? *Journal of Neuroscience Nursing, 52*(1), 37–42.

Purpose

The purpose of this study of intracranial pressure (ICP) recordings was to obtain an insight into how well the intermittent external ventricular drain (EVD) clamping procedure is performed for ICP documentation.

Design

This was a retrospective analysis of ICP recordings. For each recording of ICP, the mean and standard deviation were calculated. The duration of EVD closure, time interval between two adjacent EVD closures, and the total number of EVD closures were calculated for each patient. An algorithm to evaluate whether ICP reached a new equilibrium before the EVD was reopened for drainage was developed. The percentage of EVD closures that reached the equilibrium was calculated.

Findings

Data were obtained from 107 patients with subarachnoid hemorrhage who had 32,755 EVD closures in total. Only 65.9% of openings lasted less than 1 minute and 16.3% lasted longer than 5 minutes. The median duration of each EVD closure was 25 seconds. Only 22.9% of EVD closures reached ICP equilibrium before EVD reopening.

Nursing Implications

This research provides evidence for the need to properly train and provide a standard guideline for bedside nurses to correctly obtain and document ICP. Nurses working in settings where ICP is monitored need to work on clear guidelines that specify the need to wait the required time when opening and closing an EVD in order to get an accurate reading.

Evaluation

Expected patient outcomes may include:

1. Attains optimal breathing pattern
   a. Maintains patent airway
   b. Breathes in a regular pattern
   c. Attains or maintains arterial blood gas values within acceptable range
2. Demonstrates optimal cerebral tissue perfusion
   a. Increasingly oriented to time, place, and person
   b. Follows verbal commands; answers questions correctly
3. Attains desired fluid balance
   a. Maintains fluid restriction
   b. Demonstrates serum and urine osmolality values within acceptable range
4. Has no signs or symptoms of infection
   a. Has no fever
   b. Shows no redness, swelling, or drainage at arterial, IV, and urinary catheter sites
   c. Has no redness, swelling, or purulent drainage from invasive intracranial monitoring device
5. Absence of complications
   a. Has ICP values that remain within normal limits
   b. Demonstrates urine output and serum electrolyte levels within acceptable limits

 INTRACRANIAL SURGERY

A **craniotomy** involves opening the skull surgically to gain access to intracranial structures. This procedure is performed to remove a tumor, relieve elevated ICP, evacuate a blood clot, or control hemorrhage. The surgeon cuts the skull to create a bony flap, which can be repositioned after surgery and held in place by periosteal or wire sutures. One of two approaches through the skull is used: above the tentorium (supratentorial craniotomy) into the supratentorial compartment, or below the tentorium into the infratentorial (posterior fossa) compartment. A third approach, the **transsphenoidal** approach (through the mouth and nasal sinuses) is often used to gain access to the pituitary gland (Hickey & Strayer, 2020). Table 61-3 compares these three different surgical approaches.

Alternatively, intracranial structures may be approached through burr holes (see Fig. 61-8), which are circular openings made in the skull by either a hand drill or an automatic craniotome (which has a self-controlled system to stop the drill when the bone is penetrated). Burr holes may be used to determine the presence of cerebral swelling and injury and the size and position of the ventricles. They are also a means of evacuating an intracranial hematoma or abscess and for making a bone flap in the skull that allows access to the

TABLE 61-3	Comparison of Cranial Surgical Approaches	
Supratentorial	**Infratentorial**	**Transsphenoidal**

Pituitary tumor
Tip of forceps

Site of Surgery Above the tentorium	Below the tentorium, brain stem	Sella turcica and pituitary region
Incision Location Incision is made above the area to be operated on; usually located behind the hairline.	Incision is made at the nape of the neck, around the occipital lobe.	Incision is made beneath the upper lip to gain access into the nasal cavity.
Select Nursing Interventions Maintain head of bed elevated at 30 degrees, with neck in neutral alignment. Position patient on either side or back. (Avoid positioning patient on operative side if a large tumor has been removed.)	Maintain neck in straight alignment. Avoid flexion of the neck to prevent possible tearing of the suture line. Position the patient on either side. (Check surgeon's preference for positioning of patient.)	Maintain nasal packing in place and reinforce as needed. Instruct patient to avoid blowing the nose. Provide oral care according to institutional procedure. Keep head of bed elevated to promote venous drainage and drainage from the surgical site.

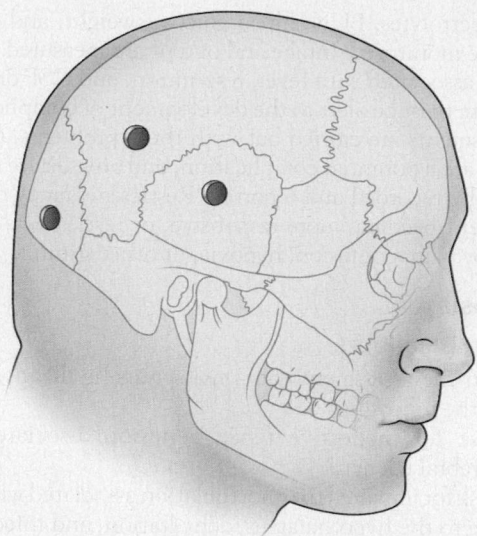

Figure 61-8 • Burr holes may be used in neurosurgical procedures to make a bone flap in the skull, to aspirate a brain abscess, or to evacuate a hematoma.

ventricles for decompression, ventriculography, or shunting procedures. Other cranial procedures include **craniectomy** (excision of a portion of the skull) and cranioplasty (repair of a cranial defect using a plastic or metal plate).

Supratentorial and Infratentorial Approaches

Preoperative Management

Medical Management

Preoperative diagnostic procedures may include a CT scan to demonstrate the lesion and show the degree of surrounding brain edema, the ventricular size, and the displacement. An MRI scan provides information similar to that of a CT scan with improved tissue contrast, resolution, and anatomic definition. Cerebral angiography may be used to study a tumor's blood supply or obtain information about vascular lesions. Transcranial Doppler flow studies are used to evaluate the blood flow within intracranial blood vessels.

Patients may be prescribed an anticonvulsant medication such as phenytoin, levetiracetam, or a phenytoin metabolite (fosphenytoin sodium) before surgery to reduce the risk of postoperative **seizures** (paroxysmal transient disturbance of the brain resulting from a discharge of abnormal electrical activity) (Comerford & Durkin, 2020). Recent research suggests that anticonvulsant medications should not be used routinely, but only when the patient experiences seizures (Mirian, Pedersen, Sabers, et al., 2019). Before surgery, corticosteroids such as dexamethasone may be given to reduce cerebral edema if the patient has a brain tumor. Fluids may be restricted. A hyperosmotic agent (mannitol) and a diuretic agent such as furosemide may be administered IV immediately before and sometimes during surgery if the patient tends to retain fluid, as do many who have intracranial dysfunction. Antibiotic agents may be given if there is a chance of cerebral contamination; diazepam or lorazepam may be prescribed before surgery to allay anxiety.

Nursing Management

The preoperative assessment serves as a baseline against which postoperative status and recovery are compared. This assessment includes evaluating the LOC and responsiveness to stimuli and identifying any neurologic deficits, such as paralysis, visual dysfunction, alterations in personality or speech, and bladder and bowel disorders. Baseline distal and proximal motor strength in both upper and lower extremities is tested and recorded. See Chapter 60 for a discussion of the testing of motor function.

The patient's and family's understanding of and reactions to the anticipated surgical procedure and its possible sequelae are assessed, as is the availability of support systems for the patient and family. Adequate preparation for surgery, with attention to the patient's physical and emotional status, can reduce the risk of anxiety, fear, and postoperative complications. The patient is assessed for neurologic deficits and their potential impact after surgery. For motor deficits or weakness or paralysis of the arms or legs, trochanter rolls are applied to the extremities, and the feet are positioned against a footboard or the ankles are supported in a neutral position with orthotic boots. A patient who can ambulate is encouraged to do so. If the patient is aphasic, writing materials or picture and word cards showing the bedpan, glass of water, blanket, and other frequently used items may help improve communication.

Preparation of the patient and family includes providing education about what to expect during and after surgery. The patient should plan to shower and wash their hair prior to surgery using the preferred cleansing solution. Hair is removed with the use of clippers and the surgical site prepared immediately before surgery (usually in the operating room), and IV antibiotics are given 1 hour prior to the incision to decrease the chance of infection (American Association of Neuroscience Nurses [AANN], 2016b). An indwelling urinary catheter is inserted in the operating room to drain the bladder during the administration of diuretic agents and to permit monitoring of urinary output. The patient may have an arterial line placed for monitoring of pressures after surgery. The large head dressing applied after surgery may impair hearing temporarily. Vision may be limited if the eyes are swollen shut. If a tracheostomy or endotracheal tube remains in place, the patient will be unable to speak until the tube is removed, so an alternative method of communication must be established.

An altered cognitive state may make the patient unaware of the impending surgery. Even so, encouragement and attention to the patient's needs are necessary. Whatever the state of awareness of the patient, the family needs reassurance and support, because they usually recognize the seriousness of brain surgery.

Postoperative Management

Postoperatively, an arterial line may be in place to monitor and manage blood pressure. The patient may be intubated and may receive supplemental oxygen therapy. Ongoing postoperative management is aimed at detecting and reducing cerebral edema, relieving pain and preventing seizures, and monitoring ICP and neurologic status.

Reducing Cerebral Edema

Medications to reduce cerebral edema include mannitol, which increases serum osmolality and draws free water from areas of the brain (with an intact blood–brain barrier). The fluid is then excreted by osmotic diuresis. Dexamethasone may be administered IV every 6 hours for 24 to 72 hours; the route is changed to oral as soon as possible, and the dosage is typically tapered over 5 to 7 days; some patients may require an extended taper (Comerford & Durkin, 2020).

Relieving Pain and Preventing Seizures

Acetaminophen is usually prescribed for temperatures exceeding 37.5°C (99.6°F) (Rincon, 2018) and for mild pain. The patient usually has a headache after a craniotomy as a result of stretching and irritation of nerves in the scalp during surgery. Codeine, administered IV or orally, is often sufficient to relieve headache. Morphine sulfate may also be used in the management of postoperative pain in patients who have undergone a craniotomy with the goal of a patient reporting acceptable pain level (AANN, 2016b).

Anticonvulsant medication (phenytoin, levetiracetam) is often prescribed prophylactically for patients who have undergone supratentorial craniotomy because of the high risk of seizures after these procedures (Hickey & Strayer, 2020). Serum levels are monitored to check that the medication levels are within the therapeutic range.

Monitoring Intracranial Pressure

A patient undergoing intracranial surgery may have an ICP or cerebral oxygenation monitor inserted during surgery. Strict adherence to written protocols for managing these systems is essential, as discussed earlier, for preventing infection and managing ICP. The system is removed after the ICP or cerebral oxygenation is normal and stable. The neurosurgeon must be notified immediately if the system is not functioning.

NURSING PROCESS

The Patient Who Has Undergone Intracranial Surgery

Assessment

After surgery, the frequency of postoperative monitoring is based on the patient's clinical status. Assessing respiratory function is essential, because even a small degree of hypoxia can increase cerebral ischemia. The respiratory rate and pattern are monitored, and arterial blood gas values are assessed frequently. Fluctuations in vital signs are carefully monitored and documented, because they may indicate increased ICP. The patient's temperature is measured to assess for hyperthermia secondary to infection or damage to the hypothalamus. Neurologic checks are made frequently to detect increased ICP resulting from cerebral edema or bleeding. A change in LOC or response to stimuli may be the first sign of increasing ICP.

The surgical dressing is inspected for evidence of bleeding and CSF drainage. The incision is monitored for redness, tenderness, bulging, separation, or foul odor. Sodium retention may occur in the immediate postoperative period. Serum and urine electrolytes, BUN, blood glucose, weight, and clinical status are monitored. Intake and output are measured in view of losses associated with fever, respiration, and CSF drainage. The nurse must be alert to the development of complications; all assessments are carried out with these problems in mind. Seizures are a potential complication, and any seizure activity is carefully recorded and reported. Restlessness may occur as the patient becomes more responsive, or restlessness may be caused by pain, confusion, hypoxia, or other stimuli.

Diagnosis

NURSING DIAGNOSES

Based on the assessment data, major nursing diagnoses may include the following:

- Risk for ineffective tissue perfusion associated with cerebral edema
- Risk for impaired thermoregulation associated with damage to the hypothalamus, dehydration, and infection
- Impaired gas exchange associated with hypoventilation, aspiration, and immobility
- Difficulty coping associated with sensory perception changes due to periorbital edema, head dressing, endotracheal tube, and effects of ICP
- Disturbed body image associated with change in appearance or physical disabilities

Other nursing diagnoses may include impaired communication (aphasia) associated with insult to brain tissue and high risk for impaired skin integrity associated with immobility, pressure, and incontinence; impaired mobility associated with a neurologic deficit secondary to the neurosurgical procedure or to the underlying disorder may also occur.

COLLABORATIVE PROBLEMS/POTENTIAL COMPLICATIONS

Potential complications may include the following:

- Increased ICP
- Bleeding and hypovolemic shock
- Fluid and electrolyte disturbances
- Infection
- CSF leak
- Seizures

Planning and Goals

The major goals for the patient include maintaining or restoring neurologic homeostasis to improve cerebral tissue perfusion, adequate thermoregulation, normal ventilation and gas exchange, ability to cope with sensory deprivation, adaptation to changes in body image, and absence of complications.

Nursing Interventions

MAINTAINING CEREBRAL TISSUE PERFUSION

Attention to the patient's respiratory status is essential, because even slight decreases in the oxygen level (hypoxia) or slight increases in the carbon dioxide level (hypercarbia) can affect cerebral perfusion, the clinical course, and the patient's outcome. The endotracheal tube is left in place until the patient shows signs of awakening and has adequate spontaneous ventilation, as evaluated clinically and by arterial blood gas analysis. Secondary brain damage can result from impaired cerebral oxygenation.

Some degree of cerebral edema occurs after brain surgery; it tends to peak 24 to 36 hours after surgery, potentially producing decreased responsiveness on the second postoperative day. The control of cerebral edema was discussed earlier. Nursing strategies used to control factors that may raise ICP were presented in the previous Nursing Process section on increased ICP. Intraventricular drainage is carefully monitored, using strict asepsis when any part of the system is handled.

Vital signs and neurologic status (LOC and responsiveness, pupillary and motor responses) are assessed every 15 to 60 minutes. Extreme head rotation is avoided, because this raises ICP. After supratentorial surgery, the patient is placed on their back or side (on the unoperated side if a large lesion was removed) with one pillow under the head. The head of the bed may be elevated 30 degrees, depending on the level of the ICP and the neurosurgeon's preference. After posterior fossa (infratentorial) surgery, the patient is kept flat on one side (off the back) with the head on a small, firm pillow. The patient may be turned on either side, keeping the neck in a neutral position. When the patient is being turned, the body should be turned as a unit to prevent placing strain on the incision and possibly tearing the sutures. The head of the bed may be elevated slowly as tolerated by the patient.

The patient's position is changed every 2 hours, and skin care is given frequently. During position changes, care is taken to prevent disruption of the ICP monitoring system. A turning sheet or lift sling placed under the patient's head to midthigh makes it easier to move and turn the patient safely.

REGULATING TEMPERATURE

Moderate temperature elevation can be expected after intracranial surgery because of the reaction to blood at the operative site or in the subarachnoid space. Injury to the hypothalamic centers that regulate body temperature can occur during surgery. Fever is treated vigorously to combat the effect of an elevated temperature on brain metabolism and function.

Nursing interventions include monitoring the patient's temperature and using the following measures to reduce body temperature: removing blankets, placing ice packs, and administering prescribed antipyretics to reduce fever (Rincon, 2018).

Conversely, hypothermia may be seen after lengthy neurosurgical procedures. Therefore, frequent measurements of rectal temperatures are necessary. Rewarming should occur slowly to prevent shivering, which increases cellular oxygen demands.

IMPROVING GAS EXCHANGE

The patient undergoing neurosurgery is at risk for impaired gas exchange and pulmonary infections due to immobility, immunosuppression, decreased LOC, and fluid restriction. Immobility compromises the respiratory system by causing pooling and stasis of secretions in dependent areas and the development of atelectasis. The patient whose fluid intake is restricted may be more vulnerable to atelectasis as a result of inability to expectorate thickened secretions. Pneumonia can develop due to aspiration and restricted mobility.

Repositioning the patient every 2 hours helps to mobilize pulmonary secretions and prevent stasis. After the patient regains consciousness, additional measures to expand collapsed alveoli can be instituted, such as yawning, sighing, deep breathing, incentive spirometry, and coughing (unless contraindicated). If necessary, the oropharynx and trachea are suctioned to remove secretions that cannot be raised by coughing; however, coughing and suctioning increase ICP. Therefore, suctioning should be used cautiously. Increasing the humidity in the oxygen delivery system may help to loosen secretions. The nurse and the respiratory therapist work together to monitor the effects of chest physiotherapy.

COPING WITH SENSORY DEPRIVATION

Periorbital edema is a common consequence of intracranial surgery, because fluid drains into the dependent periorbital areas when the patient has been positioned in a prone position during surgery. A hematoma may form under the scalp and spread down to the orbit, producing an area of ecchymosis (black eye).

Before surgery, the patient and family should be informed that one or both eyes may be edematous temporarily after surgery. After surgery, elevating the head of the bed (if not contraindicated) and applying cold compresses over the eyes will help reduce the edema. The surgeon is notified if periorbital edema increases significantly, because this may indicate that a postoperative clot is developing or that there is increasing ICP and poor venous drainage. Health care personnel should announce their presence when entering the room to avoid startling the patient whose vision is impaired due to periorbital edema or neurologic deficits.

Additional factors that can affect sensation include a bulky head dressing, the presence of an endotracheal tube, and effects of increased ICP. The first postoperative dressing change is usually performed by the neurosurgeon. In the absence of bleeding or a CSF leak, every effort is made to minimize the size of the head dressing. If the patient requires an endotracheal tube for mechanical ventilation, every effort is made to extubate the patient as soon as clinical signs indicate it is possible. The patient is monitored closely for the effects of elevated ICP.

ENHANCING SELF-IMAGE

The patient is encouraged to verbalize feelings and frustrations about any change in appearance. Nursing support is based on the patient's reactions and feelings. Factual information may need to be provided if the patient has misconceptions about puffiness about the face, periorbital bruising, and hair loss. Attention to grooming, the use of the patient's own clothing, and covering the head with a turban (and later a wig until hair growth occurs) are encouraged. Social interaction with close friends, family, and hospital personnel may increase the patient's sense of self-worth.

The family and social support system can be of assistance while the patient recovers from surgery.

MONITORING AND MANAGING POTENTIAL COMPLICATIONS

The nurse must be vigilant for complications that may develop within hours of surgery and require close collaboration with the neurosurgeon. These include increased ICP, bleeding and hypovolemic shock, altered fluid and electrolyte balance (e.g., water intoxication, diabetes insipidus), infection, identification of a CSF leak, and seizures.

Monitoring for Increased Intracranial Pressure and Bleeding. Increased ICP and bleeding are life-threatening to the patient who has undergone intracranial surgery. The following points must be kept in mind when caring for any patient who has undergone such surgery:

- An increase in blood pressure and decrease in pulse with respiratory failure may indicate increased ICP.
- An accumulation of blood under the bone flap (extradural, subdural, or intracerebral hematoma) may pose a threat to life. A clot must be suspected in any patient who does not awaken as expected or whose condition deteriorates. An intracranial hematoma is suspected if the patient has any new postoperative neurologic deficits (especially a dilated pupil on the operative side). In these circumstances, the patient is returned to the operating room immediately for evacuation of the clot, if indicated.
- Cerebral edema, infarction, metabolic disturbances, and hydrocephalus are conditions that may mimic the clinical manifestations of a clot.

The patient is monitored closely for indicators of complications, and early signs and trends in clinical status are reported to the surgeon. Treatments are initiated promptly, and the nurse assists in evaluating the patient's response to treatment. The nurse also provides support to the patient and family.

> ▶ **Quality and Safety Nursing Alert**
>
> *If signs and symptoms of increased ICP occur, efforts to decrease the ICP are initiated: alignment of the head in a neutral position without flexion to promote venous drainage, elevation of the head of the bed to 30 degrees (when prescribed), administration of mannitol (an osmotic diuretic), and possible administration of pharmacologic paralyzing agents.*

Managing Fluid and Electrolyte Disturbances. Fluid and electrolyte imbalances may occur because of the patient's underlying condition and its management or as complications of surgery. These disturbances can contribute to the development of cerebral edema.

The postoperative fluid regimen depends on the type of neurosurgical procedure and is determined on an individual basis. The volume and composition of fluids are adjusted based on daily serum electrolyte values, along with fluid intake and output. Fluids may have to be restricted in patients with cerebral edema.

Oral fluids are usually resumed after the first 24 hours. The presence of gag and swallowing reflexes must be checked before initiation of oral fluids. Some patients with posterior fossa tumors have impaired swallowing, so fluids may need to be given by alternative routes. The patient should be observed for signs and symptoms of nausea and vomiting as the diet is progressed (AANN, 2016b).

Patients undergoing surgery for brain tumors often receive large doses of corticosteroids and are at risk for hyperglycemia. Serum glucose levels are measured every 4 to 6 hours, and sliding scale insulin is prescribed as needed. These patients are prone to stress ulcers, so histamine-2 receptor antagonists (H_2 blockers) or proton pump inhibitors are prescribed to suppress the secretion of gastric acid. Patients also are monitored for bleeding and assessed for gastric pain.

If the surgical site is near to (or causes edema to) the pituitary gland and hypothalamus, the patient may develop symptoms of diabetes insipidus, which is characterized by excessive urinary output, elevated serum osmolality, decreased urine osmolality, hypernatremia, and a low urine specific gravity. The urine specific gravity is measured hourly, and fluid intake and output are monitored. Fluid replacement must compensate for urine output, and serum potassium levels must be monitored.

SIADH, which results in water retention with hyponatremia and serum hypo-osmolality, occurs in a wide variety of CNS disorders (e.g., brain tumor, head trauma) causing fluid disturbances. Nursing management includes careful intake and output measurements, specific gravity determinations of urine, and monitoring of serum and urine electrolyte levels while following directives for fluid restriction. SIADH is usually self-limited.

Preventing Infection. The patient undergoing neurosurgery is at risk for infection associated with the neurosurgical procedure (brain exposure, bone exposure, wound hematomas) and the presence of IV and arterial lines for fluid administration and monitoring. Risk for infection is increased in patients who undergo lengthy intracranial operations and in those who have external ventricular drains in place.

The dressing is often stained with blood in the immediate postoperative period. Because blood is an excellent culture medium for bacteria, the dressing is reinforced with sterile pads so that contamination and infection are avoided. A heavily stained or displaced dressing should be reported immediately. A drain is sometimes placed in the craniotomy incision to facilitate drainage.

After suboccipital surgical procedures, CSF may leak through the incision. This complication is dangerous because of the possibility of meningitis. After a suboccipital craniotomy, the patient is instructed to avoid coughing, sneezing, or nose blowing, which can cause CSF leakage by creating increased pressure on the operative site.

> ▶ **Quality and Safety Nursing Alert**
>
> *Any sudden discharge of fluid from a cranial incision is reported at once, because a large leak often requires surgical repair. Attention should be paid to the patient who complains of a salty taste or "postnasal drip," because this can be caused by CSF trickling down the throat.*

Aseptic technique is used when handling dressings, drainage systems, and IV and arterial lines. The patient is monitored carefully for signs and symptoms of infection, and cultures are obtained if infection is suspected. Appropriate antibiotic agents are given as prescribed. Other causes of infection in the patient undergoing intracranial surgery, such as pneumonia and urinary tract infections, are similar to those in other patients postoperatively.

Monitoring for Seizure Activity. Seizures may occur as complications after any intracranial neurosurgical procedure. Preventing seizures is essential to avoid further cerebral edema. Administering the prescribed anticonvulsant medication before and after surgery may prevent the development of seizures in subsequent months and years. **Status epilepticus** (prolonged seizures without recovery of consciousness in the intervals between seizures) may occur after craniotomy and also may be related to the development of complications (hematoma, ischemia). The management of status epilepticus is described later in this chapter.

Monitoring and Managing Other Complications. Other complications may occur during the first 2 weeks or later and may compromise the patient's recovery. The most important of these are VTE (DVT, PE), pulmonary and urinary tract infection, and pressure injuries. Most of these complications may be avoided with frequent changes of position, adequate suctioning of secretions, thrombosis prophylaxis, early removal of indwelling urinary catheter, early ambulation, and skin care.

PROMOTING HOME, COMMUNITY-BASED, AND TRANSITIONAL CARE

Educating Patients About Self-Care. The recovery at home of a patient who has had neurosurgery depends on the extent of the surgical procedure and its success. The patient's strengths as well as limitations are assessed and explained to the family, along with the family's part in promoting recovery. Because administration of postoperative medication is a priority, the patient and family are educated to use a check-off system, pill boxes, and alarms to ensure that the medication is taken as prescribed.

The patient and family are educated about what to expect after intracranial surgery (see Chart 61-3). Dietary restrictions usually are not required unless another health problem necessitates a special diet. Although showering or tub bathing is permitted, the scalp should be kept dry until all sutures have been removed, unless the primary provider has specific wound care instructions. A clean scarf or cap may be worn until a wig or hairpiece is purchased. If skull bone has been removed, a protective helmet may be prescribed. The patient may require rehabilitation, depending on the postoperative level of function. The patient may require physical therapy for residual weakness and mobility issues. An occupational therapist is consulted to assist with self-care issues. If the patient has aphasia, speech therapy may be necessary.

Continuing and Transitional Care. The patient is discharged from the hospital as soon as possible. Patients with severe motor deficits require extensive physical therapy and rehabilitation. Those with postoperative cognitive and speech impairments require psychological evaluation, speech therapy, and rehabilitation. The nurse collaborates with the primary provider and other health care professionals during hospitalization and home or transitional care to achieve as complete a rehabilitation as possible and to assist the patient in living with residual disability.

If tumor, injury, or disease makes the prognosis poor, care is directed toward making the patient as comfortable as possible. With return of the tumor or cerebral compression, the patient becomes less alert and aware. Other possible consequences include paralysis, blindness, and seizures. The home health nurse, hospice nurse, and social worker collaborate with the family to plan for additional services or placement of the patient in an extended care facility (see the Cerebral Metastases section in Chapter 65). The patient and family are encouraged to discuss end-of-life preferences for care; the patient's end-of-life preferences must be respected (see Chapter 13). The nurse involved in home and continuing care of patients after cranial surgery also should remind patients and family members of the need for health promotion activities and recommended health screening.

Evaluation

Expected patient outcomes may include:
1. Achieves optimal cerebral tissue perfusion
   a. Opens eyes on request; uses recognizable words, progressing to normal speech
   b. Obeys commands with appropriate motor responses
2. Maintains normal body temperature
   a. Registers normal body temperature
3. Has normal gas exchange
   a. Has arterial blood gas values within normal ranges
   b. Breathes easily; lung sounds clear without adventitious sounds
   c. Takes deep breaths and changes position as directed
4. Copes with sensory deprivation
5. Demonstrates improving self-concept
   a. Pays attention to grooming
   b. Visits and interacts with others

Chart 61-3

HOME CARE CHECKLIST

Discharge After Intracranial Surgery

At the completion of education, the patient and/or caregiver will be able to:

- Name the procedure that was performed, any complications that occurred, and identify any permanent changes in anatomic structure or function as well as changes in ADLs, IADLs, roles, relationships, and spirituality.
- Identify interventions and strategies (e.g., durable medical equipment, adaptive equipment) used in recovery period.
- Describe ongoing postoperative therapeutic regimen, including diet and activities to perform (e.g., walking and breathing exercises) and to limit or avoid (e.g., lifting weights, driving a car, contact sports).
- State the name, dose, side effects, frequency, and schedule for all medications.
- State how to obtain medical supplies and carry out dressing changes, wound care, and other prescribed regimens.

- Identify durable medical equipment needs, proper usage, and maintenance necessary for safe utilization.
- Describe signs and symptoms of complications.
- State time and date of follow-up appointments.
- Relate how to reach primary provider with questions or complications.
- Identify community resources for peer and caregiver/family support:
  - Identify sources of support (e.g., friends, relatives, faith community).
  - Identify the contact details for support services for patients and their caregivers/families.
- Identify the need for health promotion (e.g., weight reduction, smoking cessation, stress management), disease prevention and screening activities.

ADL, activities of daily living; IADL, instrumental activities of daily living.

6. Exhibits absence of complications
   a. Exhibits ICP within normal range
   b. Has minimal bleeding at surgical site; surgical incision healing without evidence of infection
   c. Shows fluid balance and electrolyte levels within desired ranges
   d. Exhibits no evidence of seizures

Transsphenoidal Approach

Tumors within the sella turcica and small adenomas of the pituitary can be removed through a transsphenoidal approach (see Table 61-3). Although an otorhinolaryngologist may make the initial opening, the neurosurgeon completes the opening into the sphenoidal sinus and exposes the floor of the sella. Microsurgical techniques provide improved illumination, magnification, and visualization so that nearby vital structures can be avoided.

The transsphenoidal approach offers direct access to the sella turcica with minimal risk of trauma and hemorrhage (Hickey & Strayer, 2020). It avoids many of the risks of craniotomy, and the postoperative discomfort is similar to that of other transnasal surgical procedures. It may also be used for pituitary ablation (destruction) in patients with metastatic breast or prostatic cancer.

Complications

Manipulation of the posterior pituitary gland during surgery may produce transient diabetes insipidus of several days' duration (Hickey & Strayer, 2020). It is treated with vasopressin but occasionally persists. Other complications include CSF leakage, visual disturbances, postoperative meningitis, pneumocephalus (air in the intracranial cavity), and SIADH (see Chapter 45).

Preoperative Management

Medical Management

The preoperative evaluation includes a series of endocrine tests, rhinologic evaluation (to assess the status of the sinuses and nasal cavity), and neuroradiologic studies. Funduscopic examination and visual field determinations are performed, because the most serious effect of pituitary tumor is localized pressure on the optic nerve or chiasm. In addition, the nasopharyngeal secretions are cultured, because a sinus infection is a contraindication to an intracranial procedure using this approach. Corticosteroids may be given before and after surgery, because the surgery involves removal of the pituitary, which is the source of adrenocorticotropic hormone (ACTH). Antibiotic agents may or may not be given prophylactically.

Nursing Management

The patient is educated in deep breathing techniques before surgery. In addition, the patient is instructed that after the surgery, they will need to avoid vigorous coughing, blowing the nose, sucking through a straw, or sneezing, because these actions may place increased pressure at the surgical site and cause a CSF leak (Hickey & Strayer, 2020).

Postoperative Management

Medical Management

Because the procedure disrupts the oral and nasal mucous membranes, management focuses on preventing infection and promoting healing. Medications include antimicrobial agents (which are continued until the nasal packing inserted at the time of surgery is removed), corticosteroids, analgesic agents for discomfort, and agents for the control of diabetes insipidus, if necessary (Hickey & Strayer, 2020).

Nursing Management

Vital signs are measured to monitor hemodynamic, cardiac, and ventilatory status. Because of the anatomic proximity of the pituitary gland to the optic chiasm, visual acuity and visual fields are assessed at regular intervals. One method is to ask the patient to count the number of fingers held up by the nurse. Evidence of decreasing visual acuity suggests an expanding hematoma.

The head of the bed is raised to decrease pressure on the sella turcica and to promote normal drainage. The patient is cautioned against blowing the nose or engaging in any activity that raises ICP, such as bending over or straining during urination or defecation.

Intake and output are measured as a guide to fluid and electrolyte replacement and to assess for diabetes insipidus. The urine specific gravity, serum sodium, and serum osmolality are measured and evaluated regularly. Daily weight is monitored. Fluids are usually given after nausea ceases, and the patient then progresses to a regular diet.

The nasal packing inserted during surgery is checked frequently for blood or CSF drainage. The major discomfort is related to the nasal packing and to mouth dryness and thirst caused by mouth breathing. Oral care is provided every 4 hours or more frequently. Usually, the teeth are not brushed until the incision above the teeth has healed. Warm saline mouth rinses and the use of a cool mist vaporizer are helpful. Petrolatum is soothing when applied to the lips. The packing is removed in 3 to 4 days, and only then can the area around the nares be cleaned with the prescribed solution to remove crusted blood and moisten the mucous membranes (Hickey & Strayer, 2020).

Home care considerations include advising the patient to use a room humidifier to keep the mucous membranes moist and to soothe irritation. The head of the bed is elevated at 30 degrees for at least 2 weeks after surgery. The patient is cautioned against blowing the nose or sneezing for at least 1 month, or as directed by their surgeon (Hickey & Strayer, 2020).

OTHER NEUROLOGIC DYSFUNCTIONS

Three other types of neurologic dysfunctions the nurse should be aware of include delirium, dementia, and pseudobulbar affect.

Delirium

Delirium, often called *acute confusional state*, begins with disorientation and if not recognized and treated can progress to changes in LOC, irreversible brain damage, and sometimes death. In fact, up to 80% of patients in intensive care units are affected, and the presence of delirium triples in-hospital mortality rates (Mulkey, Hardin, Munro, et al., 2019). Delirium is disturbing for the affected patient and their family, associated with worse outcomes, and a significant increase in medical care costs (Devlin, Skrobik, Gelinas, et al., 2018; Mulkey et al., 2019).

Careful clinical assessment is essential because delirium is sometimes mistaken for dementia and the two conditions may overlap; Table 61-4 compares dementia and delirium. It helps to know an individual patient's usual mental status and whether the changes noted are long term, which probably represents dementia, or are abrupt in onset, which is more likely delirium.

There are numerous risk factors for delirium. Risk factors that are modifiable include the use of medications such as benzodiazepines and the administration of blood transfusions (Devlin et al., 2018). Nonmodifiable risk factors include age, presence of dementia, prior coma, as well as recent emergency surgery or trauma (Devlin et al., 2018). Older adults are particularly vulnerable to acute confusion if they are in a debilitated health state or take multiple medications.

Nurses must recognize the symptoms of delirium and report them immediately. The Confusion Assessment Method (CAM) is a commonly used screening tool (Devlin et al., 2018; Inouye, van Dyck, Alessi, et al., 1990). (See Chapter 8, Chart 8-7.) Because of the acute and unexpected onset of symptoms, it is recommended that all patients who are critically ill receive routine screening for delirium at prescribed intervals (Devlin et al., 2018). If the delirium goes unrecognized and the underlying cause is not treated, permanent, irreversible brain damage or death can follow.

The most effective approach is prevention. Strategies include providing therapeutic activities for cognitive impairment, reorienting the patient as needed, ensuring early mobilization, controlling pain, minimizing the use of psychoactive drugs, preventing sleep deprivation, enhancing communication methods (particularly eyeglasses and hearing aids) for vision and hearing impairment, maintaining oxygen levels and fluid and electrolyte balance, and preventing surgical complications (Eliopoulos, 2018). Including the family in therapeutic activities, as appropriate, is encouraged but more research is needed to validate the effect of families (Devlin et al., 2018). There is some research evidence for the use of bright light therapy to reduce delirium in patients who are critically ill (Devlin et al., 2018).

Once delirium occurs, treatment of the underlying cause is most important. Therapeutic interventions vary depending on the cause. Delirium increases the risk of falls; therefore, management of patient safety and behavioral problems is essential. Because medication interactions and toxicity are often implicated, the nurse should alert the prescriber about any nonessential medications that could be discontinued. Nutritional and fluid intake should be supervised and monitored. The environment should be quiet and calm. To increase function and comfort, the nurse provides familiar environmental cues and encourages family members or friends to touch and talk to the patient (see Fig. 61-9). The nurse should provide for sleep hygiene measures in addition to assessing for and managing pain (Bennett, 2019). Ongoing mental status assessments using prior mental cognitive status as a baseline are helpful in evaluating responses to treatment

and upon admission to a hospital or extended care facility. If the underlying problem is adequately treated, the patient often returns to baseline within several days.

Dementia

The cognitive, functional, and behavioral changes that characterize dementia eventually destroy a person's ability to function. The symptoms are usually subtle in onset and often progress slowly until they are obvious and devastating. Dementia in older adults is typically caused by some degree of neurodegeneration (Gale, Acar, & Daffner, 2018). The most common type of **dementia** is Alzheimer's disease (AD) (see Chapter 8 for discussion of AD). AD alone or in conjunction with other dementing disorders accounts for up to 75% of older adults with dementia (Hickey & Strayer, 2020). Other non-Alzheimer's dementias include degenerative, vascular, neoplastic, demyelinating, infectious, inflammatory, toxic, metabolic, and psychiatric disorders. It is important to identify reversible dementia, which occurs when pathologic conditions masquerade as dementia.

Pseudobulbar Affect

The condition known as **pseudobulbar affect** involves inappropriate or exaggerated emotional expression, usually episodes of laughing or crying. It is associated with brain injury (e.g., stroke, traumatic brain injury, multiple sclerosis [MS], amyotrophic lateral sclerosis [ALS], AD, Parkinson's disease). The term "pseudobulbar" refers to damage that occurs in the corticobulbar tracts in the brain (see Chapter 60). The emotional outbursts can cause embarrassment, anxiety, and depression, and often impair quality of life (Hickey & Strayer, 2020).

Older adults with pseudobulbar affect can respond appropriately to treatment. Initial management involves evaluation and recognition that this condition can coexist with mood disorders, such as depression, although crying in these patients should not be considered indicative of depression. Pharmacology studies have reported effective management with dextromethorphan hydrobromide and quinidine sulfate in patients with ALS, MS, stroke, TBI, and dementia (Comerford & Durkin, 2020; Hakimi & Maurer, 2018).

SEIZURE DISORDERS

Seizures are episodes of abnormal motor, sensory, autonomic, or psychic activity (or a combination of these) that result from sudden excessive discharge from cerebral neurons (Hickey & Strayer, 2020). A localized area or all of the brain may be involved. The International League Against Epilepsy (ILAE) has defined **epilepsy** as more than one unprovoked seizure (Fisher, Cross, French, et al., 2017). The ILAE differentiates between three main seizure types: focal onset, generalized onset, and unknown onset seizures (see Chart 61-4). Focal (or partial) seizures are thought to originate within a localized area of the brain. Generalized seizures occur in and rapidly engage bilaterally distributed networks. Unknown onset seizures can be described as "unclassified," so termed because of incomplete data surrounding the event, but they may also

TABLE 61-4 Summary of Differences Between Dementia and Delirium

	Dementia		Delirium
	Alzheimer's Disease (AD)	Vascular (Multi-Infarct) Dementia	
Etiology	Early onset (familial, genetic [chromosomes 14, 19, 21]) Late-onset sporadic—etiology unknown	Cardiovascular (CV) disease Cerebrovascular disease Hypertension	Medication toxicity and interactions; acute disease; trauma; chronic disease exacerbation Fluid and electrolyte disorders
Risk factors	Advanced age; genetics	Preexisting CV disease	Preexisting cognitive impairment
Occurrence	75% of dementias	10–20% of dementias	Up to 80% among hospitalized people
Onset	Slow	Often abrupt Follows a stroke or transient ischemic attack	Rapid, acute onset A harbinger of acute medical illness
Age of onset	Early-onset AD: 40–65 yrs Late-onset AD: 65+ yrs Most commonly: 85+ yrs	Most commonly 50–70 yrs	Any age, although predominantly in older adults
Gender	Males and females equally	Predominantly males	Males and females equally
Course	Chronic, irreversible; progressive, regular, downhill	Chronic, irreversible Fluctuating, stepwise progression	Acute onset Hypoalert—hypoactive Hyperalert—hyperactive Mixed hypo–hyper
Duration	2–20 yrs	Variable; years	Lasts 1 day to 1 mo
Symptom progress	Onset insidious: *Early*—mild and subtle *Middle and late*—intensified Progression to death (infection or malnutrition)	Depends on location of infarct and success of treatment; death attributed to underlying CV disease	Symptoms are fully reversible with adequate treatment; can progress to chronicity or death if underlying condition is ignored
Mood	Depression common	Labile: mood swings	Variable
Speech/language	Speech remains intact until late in disease: *Early*—mild anomia (cannot name objects); deficits progress until speech lacks meaning; echoes and repeats words and sounds; mutism *Early*—no motor deficits	May have speech deficit/aphasia depending on location of lesion	Fluctuating; often cannot concentrate long enough to speak May be somnolent
Physical signs	*Middle*—apraxia (cannot perform purposeful movement) *Late*—Dysarthria (impaired speech) *End stage*—loss of all voluntary activity; positive neurologic signs	According to location of lesion: focal neurologic signs, seizures Commonly exhibits motor deficits	Signs and symptoms of underlying disease
Orientation	Becomes lost in familiar places (topographic disorientation) Has difficulty drawing three-dimensional objects (visual and spatial disorientation) Disorientation to time, place, and person—with disease progression		May fluctuate between lucidity and complete disorientation to time, place, and person
Memory	Loss is an early sign of dementia; loss of recent memory is soon followed by progressive decline in recent and remote memory		Impaired recent and remote memory; may fluctuate between lucidity and confusion
Personality	Apathy, indifference, irritability: *Early disease*—social behavior intact; hides cognitive deficits *Advanced disease*—disengages from activity and relationships; suspicious; paranoid delusions caused by memory loss; aggressive; catastrophic reactions		Fluctuating; cannot focus attention to converse; alarmed by symptoms (when lucid); hallucinations; paranoid
Functional status, activities of daily living	Poor judgment in everyday activities; has progressive decline in ability to handle money, use telephone, use computer and other electronic devices, function in home and workplace		Impaired
Attention span	Distractible; short attention span		Highly impaired; cannot maintain or shift attention
Psychomotor activity	Wandering, hyperactivity, pacing, restlessness, agitation		Variable; alternates between high agitation, hyperactivity, restlessness, and lethargy
Sleep–wake cycle	Often impaired; wandering and agitation at nighttime		Takes brief naps throughout day and night

Adapted from Devlin, J. W., Skrobik, Y., Gelinas, C., et al. (2018). Clinical practice guidelines for the prevention and management of pain, agitation/sedation, delirium, immobility, and sleep disruption in adult patients in the ICU. *Critical Care Medicine, 46*(9), e825–e873; Hickey, J. V., & Strayer, A. L. (2020). *The clinical practice of neurological & neurosurgical nursing* (8th ed.). Philadelphia, PA: Wolters Kluwer.

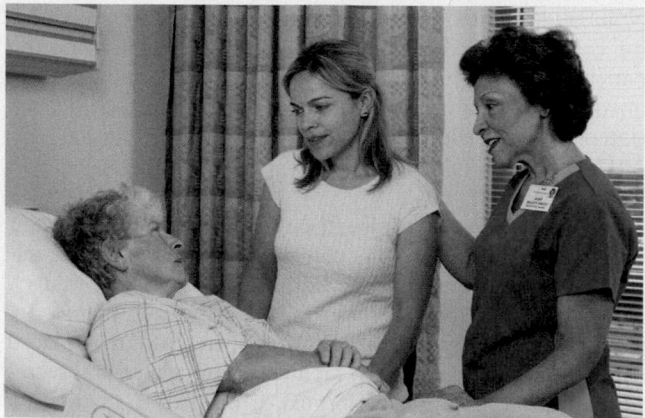

Figure 61-9 • Talking to family members may increase the comfort of patients with delirium.

be described from their clinical features (Fisher et al., 2017). Seizures may also be characterized as "provoked," or related to acute, reversible conditions such as structural, metabolic, immune, infectious, or unknown etiologies.

Pathophysiology

The underlying cause is an electrical disturbance (arrhythmia) in the nerve cells in one section of the brain; these cells emit abnormal, recurring, uncontrolled electrical discharges. The characteristic seizure is a manifestation of this excessive neuronal discharge. Associated loss of consciousness, excess movement or loss of muscle tone or movement, and disturbances of behavior, mood, sensation, and perception may also occur.

Chart 61-4

Classification of Seizures: 2017 Basic Scheme

Focal

- Motor
- Nonmotor
- Awareness
  - Aware
  - Impaired awareness
  - Unknown awareness

Generalized

- Motor
- Absence

Unknown

- Motor
- Nonmotor
- Awareness
  - Aware
  - Impaired awareness
  - Unknown awareness
- Unclassified

Adapted from Fisher, R., Cross, H., French, J., et al. (2017). Operational classification of seizure types by the International League Against Epilepsy (ILAE). Retrieved on 5/25/2020 at: www.ilae.org/files/dmfile/Operational-Classification–Fisher_et_al-2017-Epilepsia.pdf

---

The specific causes of seizures are varied and can be categorized as genetic, due to a structural or metabolic condition, or the cause may be yet unknown etiologies (Fisher et al., 2017).

Causes of seizures include:

- Allergies
- Brain tumor
- Cerebrovascular disease
- CNS infections
- Drug and alcohol withdrawal
- Fever (childhood)
- Head injury
- Hypertension
- Hypoxemia of any cause, including vascular insufficiency
- Metabolic and toxic conditions (e.g., kidney injury, hyponatremia, hypocalcemia, hypoglycemia, pesticide exposure)

Clinical Manifestations

Depending on the location of the discharging neurons, seizures may range from a simple staring episode (generalized absence seizure) to prolonged convulsive movements with loss of consciousness.

The initial pattern of the seizures indicates the region of the brain in which the seizure originates (see Chart 61-4). Only a finger or hand may shake, or the mouth may jerk uncontrollably. The person may talk unintelligibly; may be dizzy; and may experience unusual or unpleasant sights, sounds, odors, or tastes, but without loss of consciousness (Hickey & Strayer, 2020).

Generalized seizures often involve both hemispheres of the brain, causing both sides of the body to react. Intense rigidity of the entire body may occur, followed by alternating muscle relaxation and contraction (generalized tonic–clonic contraction). The simultaneous contractions of the diaphragm and chest muscles may produce a characteristic epileptic cry. The tongue is often chewed, and the patient can be incontinent of urine and feces. After 1 or 2 minutes, the convulsive movements begin to subside; the patient relaxes and lies in deep coma, breathing noisily. The respirations at this point are chiefly abdominal. In the postictal state (after the seizure), the patient is often confused and hard to arouse and may sleep for hours. Many patients report headache, sore muscles, fatigue, and depression (AANN, 2016a). Other generalized seizures may be absence types of seizures (Hickey & Strayer, 2020).

Focal seizures are subdivided into events characterized by both motor and nonmotor symptoms. There may be an impairment of consciousness or awareness or other dyscognitive features, localization, and progression of symptoms (Fisher et al., 2017).

Assessment and Diagnostic Findings

The diagnostic assessment is aimed at determining the type of seizures, their frequency and severity, and the factors that precipitate them. A developmental history is taken, including events of pregnancy and childbirth, to seek evidence of preexisting injury. The patient is also questioned about illnesses or head injuries that may have affected the brain. In addition to physical and neurologic evaluations, diagnostic examinations include biochemical, hematologic, and serologic studies. MRI is used to detect structural lesions such as focal abnormalities, cerebrovascular abnormalities, and cerebral degenerative changes (AANN, 2016a).

The EEG furnishes diagnostic evidence for a substantial proportion of patients with epilepsy and assists in classifying the type of seizure. Abnormalities in the EEG usually continue between seizures or, if not apparent, may be elicited by hyperventilation or during sleep (AANN, 2016a). Microelectrodes (depth electrodes) can be inserted deep in the brain to probe the action of single brain cells. Some people with clinical seizures have normal EEGs, whereas others who have never had seizures have abnormal EEGs. Telemetry and computerized equipment are used to monitor electrical brain activity while the patient pursues their normal activities and to store the readings on computer tapes for analysis. Video recording of seizures taken simultaneously with EEG telemetry is useful in determining the type of seizure as well as its duration and magnitude (Hickey & Strayer, 2020).

SPECT is an additional tool that is sometimes used in the diagnostic workup. It is useful for identifying the epileptogenic zone so that the area in the brain giving rise to seizures can be removed surgically (AANN, 2016a).

Nursing Management

During a Seizure

A major responsibility of the nurse is to observe and record the sequence of signs. The nature of the seizure usually indicates the type of treatment required (AANN, 2016a). Before and during a seizure, the patient is assessed and the following items are documented:

- Circumstances before the seizure (visual, auditory, or olfactory stimuli; tactile stimuli; emotional or psychological disturbances; sleep; hyperventilation)
- Occurrence of an aura (a premonitory or warning sensation, which can be visual, auditory, or olfactory)
- First thing the patient does in the seizure—where the movements or the stiffness begins, conjugate gaze position, and the position of the head at the beginning of the seizure. This information gives clues to the location of the seizure origin in the brain. (In recording, it is important to state whether the beginning of the seizure was observed.)
- Type of movements in the part of the body involved
- Areas of the body involved (turn back bedding to expose patient)
- Size of both pupils and whether the eyes are open
- Whether the eyes or head are turned to one side
- Presence or absence of automatisms (involuntary motor activity, such as lip smacking or repeated swallowing)
- Incontinence of urine or stool
- Duration of each phase of the seizure
- Unconsciousness, if present, and its duration
- Any obvious paralysis or weakness of arms or legs after the seizure
- Inability to speak after the seizure
- Movements at the end of the seizure
- Whether or not the patient sleeps afterward
- Cognitive status (confused or not confused) after the seizure

In addition to providing data about the seizure, nursing care is directed at preventing injury and supporting the patient, not only physically but also psychologically. Consequences such as anxiety, embarrassment, fatigue, and depression can be devastating to the patient.

After a Seizure

After a patient has a seizure, the nurse's role is to document the events leading to and occurring during and after the seizure and to prevent complications (e.g., aspiration, injury). The patient is at risk for hypoxia, vomiting, and pulmonary aspiration. To prevent complications, the patient is placed in the side-lying position to facilitate drainage of oral secretions, and suctioning is performed, if needed, to maintain a patent airway and prevent aspiration (see Chart 61-5). Seizure precautions are maintained, including having available functioning suction equipment with a suction catheter. The bed is placed in a low position with two to three side rails up and padded, if necessary, to prevent injury to the patient. The floor may be padded as an additional safety measure. The patient may be drowsy and may wish to sleep after the seizure; they may not remember events leading up to the seizure and for a short time thereafter.

The Epilepsies

Epilepsy is a group of syndromes characterized by unprovoked, recurring seizures (AANN, 2016a). Epileptic syndromes are classified by specific patterns of clinical features, including age at onset, family history, and seizure type. Epilepsy can be primary (idiopathic) or secondary (when the cause is known and the epilepsy is a symptom of another underlying condition, such as a brain tumor).

Epilepsy affects an estimated 3% of people during their lifetime, and most forms of epilepsy occur in children and older adults (Hickey & Strayer, 2020). The improved treatment for cerebrovascular disorders, head injuries, brain tumors, meningitis, and encephalitis has increased the number of patients at risk for seizures after recovery from these conditions. In addition, advances in EEG have aided in the diagnosis of epilepsy. The general public has been educated about epilepsy, which has reduced the stigma associated with it; as a result, more people are willing to acknowledge that they have epilepsy.

Although some evidence suggests that susceptibility to some types of epilepsy may be inherited, the cause of seizures in many people is idiopathic (unknown). Epilepsy can follow birth trauma, asphyxia neonatorum, head injuries, some infectious diseases (bacterial, viral, parasitic), toxicity (carbon monoxide and lead poisoning), circulatory problems, fever, metabolic and nutritional disorders, or drug or alcohol intoxication. It is also associated with brain tumors, abscesses, and congenital malformations.

Pathophysiology

Messages from the body are carried by the neurons (nerve cells) of the brain by discharges of electrochemical energy that sweep along them. These impulses occur in bursts whenever a nerve cell has a task to perform. Sometimes, these cells or groups of cells continue firing after a task is finished. During the period of unwanted discharges, parts of the

Chart 61-5 Care of the Patient During and After a Seizure

Nursing Care During a Seizure

- Provide privacy, and protect the patient from curious onlookers. (The patient who has an aura may have time to seek a safe, private place.)
- Ease the patient to the floor, if possible.
- Protect the head with a pad to prevent injury (from striking a hard surface).
- Loosen constrictive clothing and remove eyeglasses.
- Push aside any furniture that may injure the patient during the seizure.
- If the patient is in bed, remove pillows and raise side rails.
- *Do not attempt to pry open jaws that are clenched in a spasm or attempt to insert anything in the mouth during a seizure. Broken teeth and injury to the lips and tongue may result from such an action.*

- Do not attempt to restrain the patient during the seizure, because muscular contractions are strong and restraint can produce injury.
- If possible, place the patient on one side with head flexed forward, which allows the tongue to fall forward and facilitates drainage of saliva and mucus. If suction is available, use it if necessary to clear secretions.

Nursing Care After the Seizure

- Keep the patient on one side to prevent aspiration. Make sure the airway is patent.
- On awakening, reorient the patient to the environment.
- If the patient is confused or wandering, guide the patient gently to a bed or chair.
- If the patient becomes agitated after a seizure (postictal), stay a distance away, but close enough to prevent injury until the patient is fully aware.

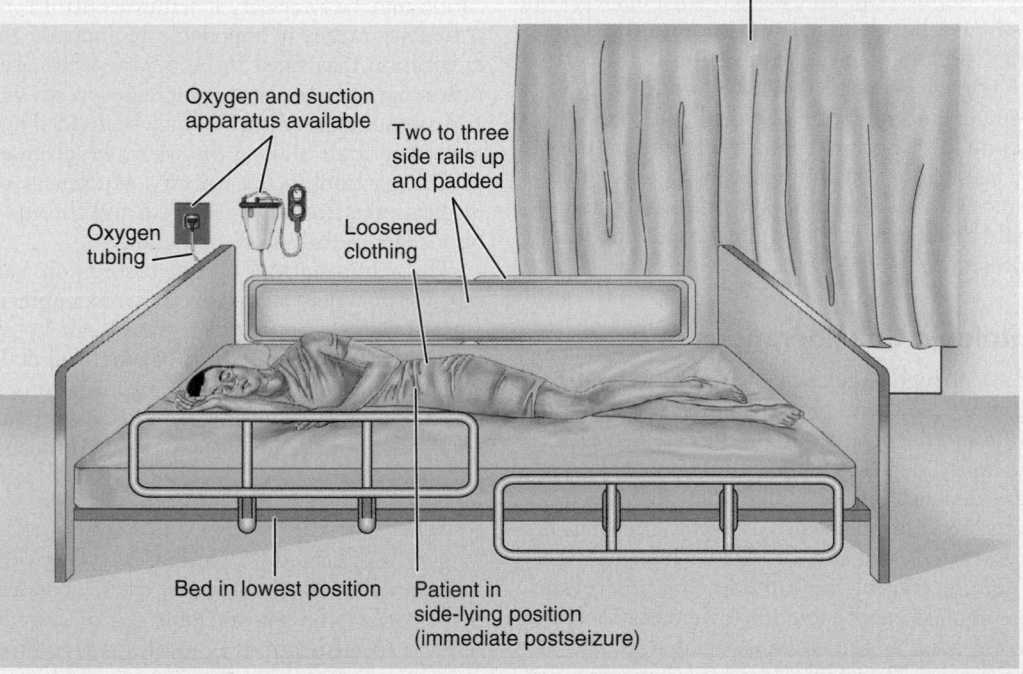

Privacy provided as soon as possible

Oxygen and suction apparatus available

Two to three side rails up and padded

Oxygen tubing

Loosened clothing

Bed in lowest position

Patient in side-lying position (immediate postseizure)

Adapted from American Association of Neuroscience Nurses (AANN). (2016a). *Care of adults and children with seizures and epilepsy: AANN clinical practice guideline series.* Chicago, IL: Author.

body controlled by the errant cells may perform erratically. Resultant dysfunction ranges from mild to incapacitating and often causes loss of consciousness (Hickey & Strayer, 2020). If these uncontrolled, abnormal discharges occur repeatedly, a person is said to have an epileptic syndrome. Epilepsy is not associated with intellectual level. People who have epilepsy without other brain or nervous system disabilities fall within the same intelligence ranges as the overall population. Epilepsy is not synonymous with intellectual or developmental disabilities, but many people who have these types of disabilities, because of serious neurologic damage, also have epilepsy.

Patients with epilepsy, particularly those with generalized events that are medically refractory, are at serious risk for **Sudden Unexpected Death in Epilepsy (SUDEP),** defined as nontraumatic, nondrowning unexpected death of a patient with epilepsy. These events may be witnessed or unwitnessed and postmortem examination reveals no anatomic or toxicologic cause of death. Cardiac and respiratory abnormalities have been implicated in these deaths. SUDEP may or may not be related to a seizure event (Barot & Nei, 2019).

Epilepsy in Women

More than one million American women have epilepsy, and they face particular needs associated with the syndrome. Women with epilepsy often note an increase in seizure frequency during menses; this has been linked to the increase in sex hormones that alter the excitability of neurons in the cerebral cortex. The effectiveness of contraceptives is decreased by anticonvulsant medications. Therefore, patients should be encouraged to discuss family planning with their primary provider and to obtain preconception counseling if they are considering childbearing (Stephen, Harden, Tomson, et al., 2019).

Women of childbearing age who have epilepsy require special care and guidance before, during, and after pregnancy. Many women note a change in the pattern of seizure activity during pregnancy. The risk of congenital fetal anomaly is two to three times higher in women with epilepsy. Maternal seizures, anticonvulsant medications, and genetic predisposition all contribute to possible malformations. Women who take certain anticonvulsant medications for epilepsy are at risk and need careful monitoring, including blood studies to detect the level of anticonvulsant medications taken throughout pregnancy. Mothers who are at high risk (teenagers, women with histories of difficult deliveries, women who use illicit drugs [e.g., "crack" cocaine, heroin], and women with diabetes or hypertension) should be identified and monitored closely during pregnancy, because damage to the fetus during pregnancy and delivery can increase the risk of epilepsy. All of these issues need further study (Stephen et al., 2019).

Because of bone loss associated with the long-term use of anticonvulsant medications, patients receiving anticonvulsant agents should be assessed for low bone mass and osteoporosis. They should be educated about strategies to reduce their risks of osteoporosis (AANN, 2016a).

 ## Gerontologic Considerations

Older adults have a high incidence of new-onset epilepsy (Hickey & Strayer, 2020). Cerebrovascular disease is the leading cause of seizures in the older adult but they are also associated with head injury, dementia, infection, alcoholism, and aging. Treatment depends on the underlying cause. Because many older adults have chronic health problems, they may be taking other medications that can interact with medications prescribed for seizure control. In addition, the absorption, distribution, metabolism, and excretion of medications are altered in the older adult as a result of age-related changes in renal and liver function. Therefore, older adult patients must be monitored closely for adverse and toxic effects of anticonvulsant medications and for osteoporosis.

Prevention

Society-wide efforts are the key to prevention of epilepsy. Head injury is one of the main causes of epilepsy that can be prevented. Through highway safety programs and occupational safety precautions, lives can be saved and epilepsy due to head injury prevented; these programs are discussed in Chapter 63.

Medical Management

The management of epilepsy is individualized to meet the needs of each patient and not just to manage and prevent seizures. Management differs from patient to patient, because some forms of epilepsy arise from brain damage and others result from altered brain chemistry.

Pharmacologic Therapy

Many medications are available to control seizures, although the exact mechanisms of action are unknown. The objective is to achieve seizure control with minimal side effects. Medication therapy controls—rather than cures—seizures. Medications are selected on the basis of the type of seizure being treated and the effectiveness and safety of the medications. If properly prescribed and taken, medications control seizures in 70% to 80% of patients with seizures. However, 20% of patients with generalized seizures and 30% of those with focal seizures do not demonstrate improvement with any prescribed medication or may be unable to tolerate the side effects of medications (AANN, 2016a). Table 61-5 lists select anticonvulsant medications.

Treatment usually starts with a single medication. The starting dose and the rate at which the dosage is increased depend on the occurrence of side effects. The medication levels in the blood are monitored, because the rate of drug absorption varies among patients. Changing to another medication may be necessary if seizure control is not achieved or if toxicity makes it impossible to increase the dosage. The medication may need to be adjusted because of concurrent illness, weight changes, or increases in stress. Side effects of anticonvulsant medications may be divided into three groups: idiosyncratic or allergic disorders, which manifest primarily as skin reactions; acute toxicity, which may occur when the medication is initially prescribed; and chronic toxicity, which occurs late in the course of therapy.

The manifestations of drug toxicity are variable, and any organ system may be involved. For example, gingival hyperplasia (swollen and tender gums) can be associated with long-term use of phenytoin (Comerford & Durkin, 2020). Periodic physical and dental examinations and laboratory tests are performed for patients receiving medications that are known to have hematopoietic, genitourinary, or hepatic effects.

Surgical Management

Surgery is indicated for patients whose epilepsy results from intracranial tumors, abscesses, cysts, or vascular anomalies. Some patients have intractable seizure disorders that do not respond to medication. A focal atrophic process may occur secondary to trauma, inflammation, stroke, or anoxia. If the seizures originate in a reasonably well-circumscribed area of the brain that can be excised without producing significant neurologic deficits, the removal of the area generating the seizures may produce long-term control and improvement (AANN, 2016a).

This type of neurosurgery has been aided by several advances, including microsurgical techniques, EEGs with depth electrodes, improved illumination and hemostasis, and the introduction of neuroleptanalgesic agents (droperidol and fentanyl). These techniques, combined with the use of local anesthetic agents, enable the neurosurgeon to perform surgery on an alert and cooperative patient. Using special testing devices, electrocortical mapping, and the patient's responses to stimulation, the boundaries of the epileptogenic focus (i.e., abnormal area of the brain) are determined. Any abnormal epileptogenic focus is then excised (AANN, 2016a). Resection surgery significantly reduces the incidence of seizures in patients with refractory epilepsy.

TABLE 61-5 Select Anticonvulsant Medications

Medication	Dose-Related Side Effects	Toxic Effects
carbamazepine	Dizziness, drowsiness, unsteadiness, nausea and vomiting, diplopia, mild leukopenia	Severe skin rash, blood dyscrasias, hepatitis
clonazepam	Drowsiness, behavior changes, headache, hirsutism, alopecia, palpitations	Hepatotoxicity, thrombocytopenia, bone marrow failure, ataxia
ethosuximide	Nausea and vomiting, headache, gastric distress	Skin rash, blood dyscrasias, hepatitis, systemic lupus erythematosus
felbamate	Cognitive impairments, insomnia, nausea, headache, fatigue	Aplastic anemia, hepatotoxicity
gabapentin	Dizziness, drowsiness, somnolence, fatigue, ataxia, weight gain, nausea	Leukopenia, hepatotoxicity
lamotrigine	Drowsiness, tremor, nausea, ataxia, dizziness, headache, weight gain	Severe rash (Stevens–Johnson syndrome)
levetiracetam	Somnolence, dizziness, fatigue	Unknown
oxcarbazepine	Dizziness, somnolence, double vision, fatigue, nausea, vomiting, loss of coordination, abnormal vision, abdominal pain, tremor, abnormal gait	Hepatotoxicity
phenobarbital	Sedation, irritability, diplopia, ataxia	Skin rash, anemia
phenytoin	Visual problems, hirsutism, gingival hyperplasia, arrhythmias, dysarthria, nystagmus	Severe skin reaction, peripheral neuropathy, ataxia, drowsiness, blood dyscrasias
primidone	Lethargy, irritability, diplopia, ataxia, impotence	Skin rash
tiagabine	Dizziness, fatigue, nervousness, tremor, difficulty concentrating, dysarthria, weak or buckling knees, abdominal pain	Unknown
topiramate	Fatigue, somnolence, confusion, ataxia, anorexia, depression, weight loss	Nephrolithiasis
valproate	Nausea and vomiting, weight gain, hair loss, tremor, menstrual irregularities	Hepatotoxicity, skin rash, blood dyscrasias, nephritis
zonisamide	Somnolence, dizziness, anorexia, headache, nausea, agitation, rash	Leukopenia, hepatotoxicity

Adapted from Comerford, K. C., & Durkin, M. T. (2020). *Nursing 2020 drug handbook.* Philadelphia, PA: Wolters Kluwer.

When seizures are refractory to medication in adolescents and adults with focal seizures, a vagal nerve stimulator (VNS) may be implanted under the clavicle. The device is connected to the vagus nerve in the cervical area, where it delivers electrical signals to the brain to control and reduce seizure activity. An external programming system is used by the primary provider to change stimulator settings (Tzadok, Harush, Nissenkorn, et al., 2019). Patients can activate the stimulator with a magnet at the time of a seizure or aura. Some patients report that use of the VNS diminishes the severity or duration of the seizure. Complications such as infection, cardiac arrhythmias, hoarseness, cough, and laryngeal spasm can occur with the use of this device (AANN, 2016a).

Another surgical option for patients with refractory seizure activity is the responsive neurostimulation system (RNS). This is a surgically implanted device with electrodes that sense and record brain electrical activity. Electrodes deliver an electrical stimulation to the location of seizure origination within the brain. The RNS works by interrupting brainwave activity before a clinical seizure can occur (Wong, Mani, & Danish, 2019).

For patients with well-defined or anatomically deep epileptogenic lesions, MRI-guided stereotactic laser interstitial thermal therapy (LiTT) offers a less invasive treatment option. This treatment involves computer-assisted placement of a laser probe into the brain and delivery of heat therapy. Decisions about epilepsy surgery are complex, and these patients should be referred to epilepsy centers for further evaluation (Crepeau & Sirven, 2017).

More research is needed to determine the effects of the various surgical approaches on complication rates, quality of life, anxiety, and depression, all of which are issues for patients with epilepsy.

NURSING PROCESS

The Patient with Epilepsy

Assessment

The nurse elicits information about the patient's seizure history. The patient is asked about the factors or events that may precipitate the seizures. Alcohol intake is documented. The nurse determines whether the patient has an aura before an epileptic seizure, which may indicate the origin of the seizure (e.g., seeing a flashing light may indicate that the seizure originated in the occipital lobe). Observation and assessment during and after a seizure assist in identifying the type of seizure and its management.

The effects of epilepsy on the patient's lifestyle are assessed (AANN, 2016a). What limitations are imposed by the seizure disorder? Does the patient participate in any recreational activities? Have any social contacts? Is the patient working, and is it a positive or stressful experience? What coping mechanisms are used?

Diagnosis

NURSING DIAGNOSES

Based on the assessment data, major nursing diagnoses may include the following:

- Risk for injury associated with seizure activity
- Fear associated with the possibility of seizures
- Difficulty coping associated with stresses imposed by epilepsy
- Lack of knowledge associated with epilepsy and anticonvulsant medications

COLLABORATIVE PROBLEMS/POTENTIAL COMPLICATIONS

The major potential complications for patients with epilepsy are status epilepticus and medication side effects (toxicity).

Planning and Goals

The major goals for the patient may include prevention of injury, control of seizures, achievement of a satisfactory psychosocial adjustment, acquisition of knowledge and understanding about the condition, and absence of complications.

Nursing Interventions

PREVENTING INJURY

Injury prevention for the patient with seizures is a priority. Patients for whom seizure precautions are instituted should have pads applied to the side rails while in bed. Steps to prevent or minimize injury are presented in Chart 61-5.

REDUCING FEAR OF SEIZURES

Fear that a seizure may occur unexpectedly can be reduced by the patient's adherence to the prescribed treatment regimen. Cooperation of the patient and family and their trust in the prescribed regimen are essential for control of seizures. The nurse emphasizes that the prescribed anticonvulsant medication must be taken on a continuing basis and that drug dependence or addiction does not occur. Periodic monitoring is necessary to ensure the adequacy of the treatment regimen, to prevent side effects, and to monitor for drug resistance (Hickey & Strayer, 2020).

In an effort to control seizures, factors that may precipitate them are identified, such as emotional disturbances, new environmental stressors, onset of menstruation in female patients, or fever (AANN, 2016a). The patient is encouraged to follow a regular and moderate routine in lifestyle, diet (avoiding excessive stimulants), exercise, and rest (sleep deprivation may lower the seizure threshold). Moderate activity is therapeutic, but excessive exercise should be avoided. An additional dietary intervention, referred to as the ketogenic diet or the Modified Atkins diet, may be helpful for control of seizures in some patients. This high-protein, low-carbohydrate, high-fat diet is most effective in children whose seizures have not been controlled with two anticonvulsant medications and has shown some success in adults with poor seizure control. Dietary therapy is not without risk and requires close monitoring and medical follow-up for possible side effects of

therapy such as hyperlipidemia, malnutrition, weight loss, and osteoporosis (Crepeau & Sirven, 2017).

Photic stimulation (e.g., bright flickering lights, television viewing) may precipitate seizures; wearing dark glasses or covering one eye may be preventive. Tension states (anxiety, frustration) induce seizures in some patients. Classes in stress management may be of value. Because seizures are known to occur with alcohol intake, alcoholic beverages should be avoided.

IMPROVING COPING MECHANISMS

The social, psychological, and behavioral problems that frequently accompany epilepsy can be more of a disability than the actual seizures. Epilepsy may be accompanied by feelings of stigmatization, alienation, depression, and uncertainty (Hickey & Strayer, 2020). The patient must cope with the constant fear of a seizure and the psychological consequences (AANN, 2016a). Children with epilepsy may be ostracized and excluded from school and peer activities. These problems are compounded during adolescence and add to the challenges of dating, not being able to drive, and feeling different from other people. Adults face these problems in addition to the burden of finding employment, concerns about relationships and childbearing, insurance problems, and legal barriers. Substance use disorders may complicate matters. Family reactions may vary from outright rejection of the person with epilepsy to overprotection.

Counseling assists the patient and family to understand the condition and the limitations it imposes. Social and recreational opportunities are necessary for good mental health. Nurses can improve the quality of life for patients with epilepsy by educating them and their families about symptoms and their management (AANN, 2016a).

 PROVIDING PATIENT AND FAMILY EDUCATION

Perhaps the most valuable facets of care contributed by the nurse to the person with epilepsy are education and efforts to modify the attitudes of the patient and family toward the disorder. The person who experiences seizures may consider every seizure a potential source of humiliation and shame. This may result in anxiety, depression, hostility, and secrecy on the part of the patient and family. Ongoing education and encouragement should be given to patients to enable them to overcome these reactions. The patient with epilepsy should carry an emergency medical identification card or wear a medical information bracelet. The patient and family need to be educated about medications as well as care during a seizure.

MONITORING AND MANAGING POTENTIAL COMPLICATIONS

Status epilepticus is the major potential complication and is described later in this chapter. Another complication is the toxicity of medications. The patient and family are educated about side effects and are given specific guidelines to assess and report signs and symptoms that indicate medication overdose. Anticonvulsant medications require careful monitoring for therapeutic levels. The patient should plan to have serum drug levels assessed at regular intervals. Many known drug interactions occur with anticonvulsant medications. A complete pharmacologic profile should be reviewed with the patient to avoid interactions that either potentiate or inhibit the effectiveness of the medications.

> ### ▶ Quality and Safety Nursing Alert
>
> *Patients with epilepsy are at risk for status epilepticus from having their medication regimen interrupted.*

PROMOTING HOME, COMMUNITY-BASED, AND TRANSITIONAL CARE

Educating Patients About Self-Care. Thorough oral hygiene after each meal, gum massage, daily flossing, and regular dental care are essential to prevent or control gingival hyperplasia in patients receiving phenytoin. The patient is also educated to inform all health care providers of the medication being taken, because of the possibility of drug interactions. An individualized comprehensive education plan is needed to assist the patient and family to adjust to this chronic disorder. Written patient education materials must be appropriate for the patient's reading level and must be provided in alternative formats if warranted.

Continuing and Transitional Care. Because epilepsy can be lifelong, health promotion is important. See Chart 61-6 for health promotion strategies for the patient with epilepsy.

For many patients with epilepsy, overcoming employment problems is a challenge. State vocational rehabilitation agencies can provide information about job training. The

Chart 61-6 🍎 HEALTH PROMOTION
Strategies for the Patient with Epilepsy

- Take anticonvulsant medications daily as prescribed to keep the drug level constant to prevent seizures. Never discontinue medications, even if there is no seizure activity.
- Keep a medication and seizure record (in electronic or paper format), noting when medications are taken and any seizure activity.
- Notify the primary provider if unable to take medications due to illness.
- Have anticonvulsant medication serum levels checked regularly. When testing is prescribed, report to the laboratory for blood sampling before taking morning medication.
- Avoid activities that require alertness and coordination (driving, operating machinery) until after the effects of the medication have been evaluated.
- Report signs of toxicity so that dosage can be adjusted. Common signs include drowsiness, lethargy, dizziness, difficulty walking, hyperactivity, confusion, inappropriate sleep, and visual disturbances.
- Avoid over-the-counter medications unless approved by the primary provider.
- Carry a medical alert bracelet or identification card specifying the name of the anticonvulsant medication and primary provider.
- Avoid seizure triggers, such as alcoholic beverages, electrical shocks, stress, caffeine, constipation, fever, hyperventilation, and hypoglycemia.
- Take showers rather than tub baths to avoid drowning if seizure occurs; never swim alone.
- Exercise in moderation in a temperature-controlled environment to avoid excessive heat.
- Develop regular sleep patterns to minimize fatigue and insomnia.
- Be aware of and use the Epilepsy Foundation of America (EFA) special services, including help in obtaining medications, vocational rehabilitation, and coping with epilepsy.

EFA has a training and placement service. If seizures are not well controlled, information about sheltered workshops or home employment programs may be obtained. Federal and state agencies and federal legislation may be of assistance to people with epilepsy who experience job discrimination. As a result of the Americans With Disabilities Act, the number of employers who knowingly hire people with epilepsy is increasing, but barriers to employment still exist.

Patients who have uncontrollable seizures accompanied by psychological and social difficulties should be referred as early as possible to a comprehensive epilepsy center where continuous audio–video and EEG monitoring, specialized treatment, and rehabilitation services are available (AANN, 2016a). Patients and their families need to be reminded of the importance of participating in health promotion activities and recommended health screenings to promote a healthy lifestyle. Genetic and preconception counseling is advised.

Evaluation

Expected patient outcomes may include:
1. Sustains no injury during seizure activity
   a. Adheres to treatment regimen and identifies the hazards of stopping the medication
   b. Can identify appropriate care during seizure; caregivers can do so as well
2. Indicates a decrease in fear
3. Displays effective individual coping
4. Exhibits knowledge and understanding of epilepsy
   a. Identifies the side effects of medications
   b. Avoids factors or situations that may precipitate seizures (e.g., flickering lights, hyperventilation, alcohol)
   c. Follows a healthy lifestyle by getting adequate sleep and eating meals at regular times to avoid hypoglycemia
5. Absence of complications

Status Epilepticus

Status epilepticus (acute prolonged seizure activity) can be defined as a seizure lasting 5 minutes or longer or serial seizures occurring without full recovery of consciousness between attacks (Hickey & Strayer, 2020). The term has been broadened to include continuous clinical or electrical seizures (on EEG) lasting at least 30 minutes, even without impairment of consciousness. It is considered a medical emergency. Status epilepticus produces cumulative effects. Vigorous muscular contractions impose a heavy metabolic demand and can interfere with respirations. Some respiratory arrest at the height of each seizure produces venous congestion and hypoxia of the brain. Repeated episodes of cerebral anoxia and edema may lead to irreversible and fatal brain damage. Factors that precipitate status epilepticus include interruption of anticonvulsant medication, fever, concurrent infection, or other illness.

Medical Management

The goals of treatment are to stop the seizures as quickly as possible, to ensure adequate cerebral oxygenation, and to maintain the patient in a seizure-free state. An airway and adequate oxygenation are established. If the patient remains unconscious and unresponsive, an endotracheal tube is inserted. IV diazepam, lorazepam, or fosphenytoin is given slowly in an attempt to halt seizures immediately. Other medications (phenytoin, phenobarbital) are given later to maintain a seizure-free state.

An IV line is established, and blood samples are obtained to monitor serum electrolytes, glucose, and phenytoin levels. EEG monitoring may be useful in determining the nature of the seizure activity. Vital signs and neurologic signs are monitored on a continuing basis. An IV infusion of dextrose is given if the seizure is caused by hypoglycemia. If initial treatment is unsuccessful, general anesthesia with a short-acting barbiturate may be used. The serum concentration of the anticonvulsant medication is measured, because a low level suggests that the patient was not taking the medication or that the dosage was too low. Cardiac involvement or respiratory depression may be life-threatening. The potential for postictal cerebral edema also exists.

Nursing Management

The nurse initiates ongoing assessment and monitoring of respiratory and cardiac function because of the risk for delayed depression of respiration and blood pressure secondary to administration of anticonvulsant medications and sedatives to halt the seizures. Nursing assessment also includes monitoring and documenting the seizure activity and the patient's responsiveness.

The patient is turned to a side-lying position, if possible, to assist in draining pharyngeal secretions. Suction equipment must be available because of the risk of aspiration. The IV line is closely monitored, because it may become dislodged during seizures.

A person who has received long-term anticonvulsant therapy has a significant risk for fractures resulting from bone disease (osteoporosis, osteomalacia, and hyperparathyroidism), which is a side effect of therapy (Comerford & Durkin, 2020). Therefore, during seizures, the patient is protected from injury with the use of seizure precautions and is monitored closely. The patient having seizures can inadvertently injure nearby people, so nurses should protect themselves. Additional nursing interventions for the person having seizures are presented in Chart 61-5.

HEADACHE

Headache, or cephalalgia, is one of the most common of all human physical complaints. Headache is a symptom rather than a disease entity; it may indicate organic disease (neurologic or other disease), a stress response, vasodilation (migraine), skeletal muscle tension (tension headache), or a combination of factors. A **primary headache** is one for which no organic cause can be identified. This type of headache includes migraine, tension-type, and cluster headaches (Hickey & Strayer, 2020). Cranial arteritis is another common cause of headache. A classification of headaches was issued first by the Headache Classification Committee of the International Headache Society (IHS) in 1988. The IHS revised the headache classification in 2018; an abbreviated list is shown in Chart 61-7.

Chart 61-7 **International Headache Society Classification of Headache**

- Migraine
- Tension-type headache
- Trigeminal autonomic cephalalgias
- Other primary disorders
- Headache attributed to trauma or injury to the head and/or neck
- Headache attributed to cranial or cervical vascular disorder
- Headache attributed to nonvascular intracranial disorder
- Headache attributed to a substance or its withdrawal
- Headache attributed to infection
- Headache attributed to disorder of homeostasis
- Headache or facial pain attributed to disorder of cranium, neck, eyes, ears, nose, sinuses, teeth, mouth, or other facial or cranial structures
- Headache attributed to psychiatric disorder
- Painful cranial neuropathies and other facial pains
- Other headache disorders

Adapted from Headache Classification Committee of the International Headache Society (IHS). (2018). *The International Classification of Headache Disorders*, 3rd edition. *Cephalalgia*, *38*(1), 1–211.

Migraine is a complex of symptoms characterized by periodic and recurrent attacks of severe headache lasting from hours to days in adults. The cause of migraine has not been clearly demonstrated, but it is primarily a vascular disturbance that has a strong familial tendency. The typical time of onset is at puberty, and the incidence is higher in women than men (Hickey & Strayer, 2020).

There are many subtypes of migraine headache, including migraine with and without aura. Most patients have migraine without an aura. *Tension-type headaches* tend to be chronic and less severe and are probably the most common type of headache. *Trigeminal autonomic cephalalgias* include cluster headaches and paroxysmal hemicrania. Cluster headaches are relatively uncommon and seen more frequently in men than in women (Norris, 2019). Types of headaches not subsumed under these categories fall into the *other primary headache* group and include headaches triggered by cough, exertion, and sexual activity (IHS, 2018).

Cranial arteritis is a cause of headache in the older population, reaching its greatest incidence in those older than 70 years of age. Inflammation of the cranial arteries is characterized by a severe headache localized in the region of the temporal arteries. The inflammation may be generalized (in which case cranial arteritis is part of a vascular disease) or focal (in which case only the cranial arteries are involved).

A **secondary headache** is a symptom associated with other causes, such as a brain tumor, an aneurysm, or lumbar puncture. Although most headaches do not indicate serious disease, persistent headaches require further investigation. Serious disorders related to headache include brain tumors, subarachnoid hemorrhage, stroke, severe hypertension, meningitis, and head injuries.

Pathophysiology

The cerebral signs and symptoms of migraine result from a hyperexcitable brain that is susceptible to a phenomenon known as cortical spreading depression, a wave of depolarization over the cerebral cortex, cerebellum, and hippocampus. This depolarization activates inflammatory neuropeptides and other neurotransmitters (including serotonin), resulting in the stimulation of meningeal nociceptors. Vascular changes, inflammation, and a continuation of pain signal stimulation occur (Goadsby & Holland, 2019). The initial phase of this process is known as the premonitory phase and may include light, sound, and smell sensitivity. If treatment is initiated at this point, the migraine may be fully terminated. As the attack progresses, central sensitization occurs, and the migraine becomes much harder to treat.

Attacks can be triggered by hormonal changes associated with menstrual cycles, bright lights, stress, depression, sleep deprivation, fatigue, or odors. Certain foods containing tyramine (aged cheese, red wine, beer), monosodium glutamate, and chocolate may be food triggers (Hickey & Strayer, 2020). The use of oral contraceptives may be associated with increased frequency and severity of attacks in some women.

Emotional or physical stress may cause contraction of the muscles in the neck and scalp, resulting in tension headache. The pathophysiology of cluster headache is not fully understood. One theory is that it is caused by dilation of orbital and nearby extracranial arteries. Cranial arteritis is thought to represent an immune vasculitis in which immune complexes are deposited within the walls of affected blood vessels, producing vascular injury and inflammation. A biopsy may be performed on the involved artery to make the diagnosis.

Clinical Manifestations

Migraine

The migraine with aura can be divided into four phases: premonitory, aura, the headache, and recovery (headache termination and postdrome).

Premonitory Phase

The premonitory phase is experienced by more than 80% of adult migraine sufferers, with symptoms that occur hours to days before a migraine headache. Symptoms may include depression, irritability, feeling cold, food cravings, anorexia, change in activity level, increased urination, diarrhea, or constipation. Patients may experience the same prodrome with each migraine headache. A current theory regarding premonitory symptoms is that they involve the neurotransmitter dopamine.

Aura Phase

An aura may be a variable feature for patients who experience migraines and can be seen in about 30% of patients (Goadsby & Holland, 2019). An aura is characterized by focal neurologic symptoms. Visual disturbances (i.e., light flashes and bright spots) are most common and may be hemianopic (affecting only half of the visual field). Other symptoms that may follow include numbness and tingling of the lips, face, or hands; mild confusion; slight weakness of an extremity; drowsiness; and dizziness.

This period of aura was thought to correspond to the phenomenon of cortical spreading depression that is associated with reduced metabolic demand in abnormally functioning neurons. This can be associated with decreased blood

flow; however, cerebral blood flow studies performed during migraine headaches demonstrate that although changes in blood vessels occur during phases of migraine, cerebral blood flow is not the main abnormality. In fact, some studies suggest that the aura and headache phases may occur simultaneously (Goadsby & Holland, 2019).

Headache Phase

Migraine headache is severe and incapacitating and is often associated with photophobia (light sensitivity), phonophobia (sound sensitivity), or allodynia (abnormal perception of innocuous stimuli) (Goadsby & Holland, 2019). Research differs in the role of vascular changes (either vasodilatory or vasoconstrictive) with respect to migraine pathophysiology and the experience of migraine headache. Symptoms of migraine can also include nausea and vomiting.

Postdrome Phase

In the postdrome phase, the pain gradually subsides, but patients may experience tiredness, weakness, cognitive difficulties, and mood changes for hours to days. Muscle contraction in the neck and scalp is common, with associated muscle ache and localized tenderness. Physical exertion may exacerbate the headache pain. During this postheadache phase, patients may sleep for extended periods.

Other Headache Types

The tension-type headache is characterized by a steady, constant feeling of pressure that usually begins in the forehead, temple, or back of the neck. It is often bandlike or may be described as "a weight on top of my head."

Cluster headaches are unilateral and come in clusters of one to eight daily, with excruciating pain localized to the eye and orbit and radiating to the facial and temporal regions. The pain is accompanied by watering of the eye and nasal congestion. Each attack lasts 15 minutes to 3 hours and may have a crescendo–decrescendo pattern (Hickey & Strayer, 2020). The headache is often described as penetrating.

Cranial arteritis often begins with general manifestations, such as fatigue, malaise, weight loss, and fever. Clinical manifestations associated with inflammation (heat, redness, swelling, tenderness, or pain over the involved artery) usually are present. Sometimes a tender, swollen, or nodular temporal artery is visible. Visual problems are caused by ischemia of the involved structures.

Assessment and Diagnostic Findings

The diagnostic evaluation includes a detailed history, a physical assessment of the head and neck, and a complete neurologic examination. Headaches may manifest differently in the same person over the course of a lifetime, and the same type of headache may manifest differently from patient to patient. The health history focuses on assessing the headache itself, with emphasis on the factors that precipitate or provoke it. The patient is asked to describe the headache in their own words.

Because headache is often the presenting symptom of a wider variety of physiologic and psychological disturbances, a general health history is an essential component of the patient database. Therefore, questions addressed in the health history should cover major medical and surgical illness as well as a body systems review.

The medication history can provide insight into the patient's overall health status and indicate medications that may be provoking headaches. Antihypertensive agents, diuretic medications, anti-inflammatory agents, and mono-amine oxidase (MAO) inhibitors are a few of the categories of medications that can provoke headaches. Daily use of over-the-counter or prescribed pain medications for 8 to 10 days out of a month can lead to a chronic headache due to medication overuse (Comerford & Durkin, 2020). Emotional factors can play a role in precipitating headaches. Stress is thought to be a major initiating factor in migraine headaches; therefore, sleep patterns, level of stress, recreational interests, appetite, emotional problems, and family stressors are relevant. There is a strong familial tendency for headache disorders, and a positive family history may help in making a diagnosis.

A direct relationship may exist between exposure to toxic substances and headache. Careful questioning may uncover chemicals to which a worker has been exposed. Under the Right-to-Know Law, employees have access to the material safety data sheets (commonly referred to as MSDSs) for all substances with which they come in contact in the workplace (see Chapter 68). The occupational history also includes assessment of the workplace as a possible source of stress and for a possible ergonomic basis of muscle strain and headache.

A complete description of the headache itself is crucial. The nurse reviews the age at onset of headaches; this particular headache's frequency, location, and duration; the type of pain; factors that relieve and precipitate the event; and associated symptoms (Starling, 2018). The data obtained should include the patient's own words about the headache in response to the following questions:

- What is the location? Is it unilateral or bilateral? Does it radiate?
- What is the quality—dull, aching, steady, boring, burning, intermittent, continuous, paroxysmal?
- How many headaches occur during a given period of time?
- What are the precipitating factors, if any—environmental (e.g., sunlight, weather change), foods, exertion, other?
- What makes the headache worse (e.g., coughing, straining)?
- What time (day or night) does it occur?
- How long does a typical headache last?
- Are there any associated symptoms, such as facial pain, lacrimation (excessive tearing), or scotomas (blind spots in the field of vision)?
- What usually relieves the headache (aspirin, nonsteroidal anti-inflammatory drugs [NSAIDs], ergot preparation, food, heat, rest, neck massage)?
- Does nausea, vomiting, weakness, or numbness in the extremities accompany the headache?
- Does the headache interfere with daily activities?
- Do you have any allergies?
- Do you have insomnia, poor appetite, loss of energy?
- Is there a family history of headache?
- What is the relationship of the headache to your lifestyle or physical or emotional stress?
- What medications are you taking?

Diagnostic testing often is not helpful in the investigation of headache, because usually there are few objective findings.

In patients who demonstrate abnormalities on the neurologic examination, CT scan, cerebral angiography, or MRI scan may be used to detect underlying causes, such as tumor or aneurysm. Electromyography (EMG) may reveal a sustained contraction of the neck, scalp, or facial muscles. Laboratory tests may include complete blood count, erythrocyte sedimentation rate, electrolytes, glucose, creatinine, and thyroid hormone levels.

Prevention

Prevention begins by having the patient avoid specific triggers that are known to initiate the headache syndrome. Preventive medical management of migraine involves the daily use of one or more agents that are thought to block the physiologic events leading to an attack. Treatment regimens vary greatly, as do patient responses; therefore, close monitoring is indicated.

Alcohol, nitrites, vasodilators, and histamines may precipitate cluster headaches. Elimination of these factors helps prevent the headaches.

Medical Management

Therapy for migraine headache is divided into abortive (symptomatic) and preventive approaches. The abortive approach, best used in those patients who have less frequent attacks, is aimed at relieving or limiting a headache at the onset or while it is in progress. The preventive approach is used in patients who experience more frequent attacks at regular or predictable intervals and may have a medical condition that precludes the use of abortive therapies (Starling, 2018). Medical management of migraine during pregnancy and lactation includes nonpharmacologic strategies in addition to safe medication practices. Nonpharmacologic treatments include mainly avoidance of triggers (Hickey & Strayer, 2020) (see Chart 61-8). Noninvasive neuromodulation devices may also provide some relief with minimal side effects (Tepper, 2019).

The triptans, which are serotonin receptor agonists, are the most specific antimigraine agents available. These agents

---

Chart 61-8

PATIENT EDUCATION

Migraine Headaches

The nurse instructs the patient to:

- Be aware of the definition of migraine headaches along with the characteristics and manifestations.
- Recognize triggers of migraine headaches and how to avoid such triggers as:
  - Foods that contain tyramine, such as chocolate, cheese, coffee, dairy products
  - Dietary habits that result in long periods between meals
  - Menstruation and ovulation (caused by hormone fluctuation)
  - Alcohol (causes vasodilation of blood vessels)
  - Fatigue and fluctuations in sleep patterns
- Develop and use a paper or electronic headache diary.
- Implement stress management and lifestyle changes to minimize the frequency of headaches.
- Ensure correct pharmacologic management: acute therapy and prophylaxis to include medication regimen and side effects.
- Use comfort measures during headache attacks, such as resting in a quiet and dark environment, applying cold compresses to the painful area, and elevating the head.
- Seek out resources for education and support, such as the National Headache Foundation.

cause vasoconstriction, reduce inflammation, and may reduce pain transmission. The triptans in routine clinical use include sumatriptan, naratriptan, rizatriptan, zolmitriptan, almotriptan, eletriptan, and frovatriptan (Comerford & Durkin, 2020). Many of the triptan medications are available in a variety of formulations, such as nasal sprays, inhalers, conventional tablet, disintegrating tablet, suppositories, or injections. The nasal sprays may be useful for patients experiencing nausea and vomiting (Tepper, 2019).

The triptans are considered first-line treatment of the management of moderate to severe migraine pain. Best results are achieved with early use of triptans; oral dosing takes effect within 20 to 60 minutes of taking the drug and if needed may be repeated in 2 to 4 hours. Triptans are contraindicated in patients with ischemic heart disease. Careful administration and dosing instructions to patients are important to prevent adverse reactions such as increased blood pressure, drowsiness, muscle pain, sweating, and anxiety. Interactions are possible if the medication is taken in conjunction with St. John's wort (Comerford & Durkin, 2020).

Ergotamine preparations (taken orally, sublingually, subcutaneously, intramuscularly, by rectum, or by inhalation) may be effective in aborting the headache if taken early in the migraine process. They are low in cost. Ergotamine tartrate acts on smooth muscle, causing prolonged constriction of the cranial blood vessels. Each patient's dosage is based on individual needs. Side effects include aching muscles, paresthesias (numbness and tingling), nausea, and vomiting. Pretreatment with antiemetic agents may be required. None of the triptan medications should be taken concurrently with medications containing ergotamine because of the potential for a prolonged vasoactive reaction (Comerford & Durkin, 2020).

Other nonspecific medications are also used in the treatment of migraine and include NSAIDs, antispasmodic agents, and neuroleptics. Neuroleptic agents can be used alone or in conjunction with triptans and/or NSAIDs (Tepper, 2019).

Prophylactic treatment of migraine includes the use of beta-blockers, antiepileptics, antidepressants, angiotensin-converting enzyme (ACE) inhibitors, and angiotensin receptor blockers. Calcitonin gene–related peptides (CGRPs) have been found in increased levels in patients with migraine, and three CGRP monoclonal antibodies have been approved by the U.S. Food and Drug Administration (FDA) for migraine prevention: erenumab, fremanezumab, and galcanezumab (Hickey & Strayer, 2020).

The medical management of an acute attack of cluster headaches may include 100% oxygen by facemask for 15 minutes, subcutaneous sumatriptan, or intranasal zolmitriptan (Hickey & Strayer, 2020).

The medical management of cranial arteritis consists of early administration of a corticosteroid to prevent the possibility of loss of vision due to vascular occlusion or rupture of the involved artery (Starling, 2018). The patient is instructed not to stop the medication abruptly, because this can lead to relapse. Analgesic agents are prescribed for comfort.

Nursing Management

When migraine or the other types of headaches have been diagnosed, the goal of nursing management is pain relief. It is reasonable to try nonpharmacologic interventions first, but the use of medications should not be delayed. The first priority is to treat the acute event of the headache and the second is to prevent recurrent episodes. Prevention involves patient education regarding precipitating factors, possible lifestyle or habit changes that may be helpful, and pharmacologic measures.

Relieving Pain

Individualized treatment depends on the type of headache and differs for migraine, cluster headaches, cranial arteritis, and tension headache. Nursing care is directed toward treatment of the acute episode. A migraine or a cluster headache in the early phase requires abortive medication therapy instituted as soon as possible. Some headaches can be prevented if the appropriate medications are taken before the onset of pain. Nursing care during an attack includes comfort measures such as a quiet, dark environment; elevation of the head of the bed to 30 degrees; and symptomatic treatment (i.e., administration of antiemetic medication) (Hickey & Strayer, 2020).

Symptomatic pain relief for tension headache may be obtained by application of local heat or massage. Additional strategies may include administration of analgesic agents, antidepressant medications, and muscle relaxants.

Promoting Home, Community-Based, and Transitional Care

 Educating Patients About Self-Care

Headaches, especially migraines, are more likely to occur when the patient is ill, overly tired, or stressed. Nonpharmacologic therapies are important and include patient education about the type of headache, its mechanism (if known), and appropriate changes in lifestyle to avoid triggers. Regular sleep, meals, exercise, relaxation, and avoidance of dietary triggers may be helpful in avoiding headaches (Starling, 2018).

The patient with tension headaches needs education and reassurance that the headache is not the result of a brain tumor or other intracranial disorder. Stress reduction techniques, such as biofeedback, exercise programs, and meditation, are examples of nonpharmacologic therapies that may prove helpful. The patient and family need to be educated about the importance of following the prescribed treatment regimen for headache and keeping follow-up appointments. In addition, the patient is reminded of the importance of participating in health promotion activities and recommended health screenings to promote a healthy lifestyle. Chart 61-8 presents educational topics for the patient with migraine headaches.

Continuing and Transitional Care

The National Headache Foundation (see the Resources section) provides a list of clinics in the United States and the names of primary providers who specialize in headache and who are members of the American Headache Society.

CRITICAL THINKING EXERCISES

1 **PQ** A patient is admitted to your unit for a supratentorial cranial procedure. Identify the nursing priorities before, during, and after the procedure. What are the priorities for patient and caregiver education in preparation for discharge?

2 **ebp** As a member of your unit's practice council, you are working on identifying interventions to assess and manage delirium. Using your knowledge of evidence-based practice guidelines, list the most important assessments and interventions for nurses to implement. Compare and contrast the options supported by the guidelines.

3 **ipc** You are a nurse working in an outpatient neurology clinic. A 28-year-old woman is newly diagnosed with epilepsy. What nursing and interprofessional assessments are indicated? What interventions, including patient education, will you implement? What interprofessional referrals would be appropriate?

REFERENCES

*Asterisk indicates nursing research.
**Double asterisk indicates classic reference.

Books

American Association of Neuroscience Nurses (AANN). (2016a). *Care of adults and children with seizures and epilepsy: AANN clinical practice guideline series.* Chicago, IL: Author.

American Association of Neuroscience Nurses (AANN). (2016b). *Care of the adult patient with a brain tumor: AANN clinical practice guideline series.* Chicago, IL: Author.

Comerford, K. C., & Durkin, M. T. (2020). *Nursing 2020 drug handbook.* Philadelphia, PA: Wolters Kluwer.

Eliopoulos, C. (2018). *Gerontological nursing* (9th ed.). Philadelphia, PA: Wolters Kluwer.

Hickey, J. V., & Strayer, A. L. (2020). *The clinical practice of neurological & neurosurgical nursing* (8th ed.). Philadelphia, PA: Wolters Kluwer.

Norris, T. L. (2019). *Porth's pathophysiology: Concepts of altered health states* (10th ed.). Philadelphia, PA: Wolters Kluwer.

Journals and Electronic Documents

Al-Mufti, F., Smith, B., Lander, M., et al. (2018). Novel minimally invasive multi-modality monitoring in neurocritical care. *Journal of the Neurological Sciences, 390,* 184–192.

Barot, N., & Nei, M. (2019). Autonomic aspects of sudden unexpected death in epilepsy (SUDEP). *Clinical Autonomic Research, 29*(2), 151–160.

Bennett, C. (2019). Caring for patients with delirium. *Nursing, 49*(9), 17–20.

Crepeau, A., & Sirven, J. (2017). Management of adult onset seizures. *Mayo Clinic Proceedings, 92*(2), 306–318.

Devlin, J. W., Skrobik, Y., Gelinas, C., et al. (2018). Clinical practice guidelines for the prevention and management of pain, agitation/sedation, delirium, immobility, and sleep disruption in adult patients in the ICU. *Critical Care Medicine, 46*(9), e825–e873.

Fisher, R., Cross, H., French, J., et al. (2017). Operational classification of seizure types by the International League Against Epilepsy (ILAE). Retrieved on 5/25/2020 at: www.ilae.org/files/dmfile/Operational-Classification–Fisher_et_al-2017-Epilepsia.pdf

Galan, L., Egea-Guerrero, J., Diaz, M., et al. (2016). The effectiveness and safety of pharmacological prophylaxis against venous thromboembolism in patients with moderate to severe traumatic brain injury: A systematic review and meta-analysis. *Journal of Trauma and Acute Care Surgery, 81*(3), 567–574.

Gale, S., Acar, D., & Daffner, K. (2018). Dementia. *American Journal of Medicine, 131*(10), 1161–1169.

Gattuta, E., Coralo, F., Lo Buono, V., et al. (2018). Techniques of cognitive rehabilitation in patients with disorders of consciousness: A systematic review. *Neurological Sciences, 39,* 641–645.

Goadsby, P., & Holland, P. (2019). An update: Pathophysiology of migraine. *Neurology Clinics, 37*(4), 651–671.

Hakimi, M., & Maurer, C. (2018). Pseudobulbar affect in parkinsonian disorders: A review. *Journal of Movement Disorders, 12*(1), 14–21.

Headache Classification Committee of the International Headache Society (IHS). (2018). *The International Classification of Headache Disorders,* 3rd edition. *Cephalalgia, 38*(1), 1–211.

Hutchinson, P., Kolias, A., Tajsic, T., et al. (2019). Consensus statement from the International Consensus Meeting on the role of decompressive craniectomy in the management of traumatic brain injury. *Acta Neurochirurgicaq, 161*(7), 1261–1274.

**Inouye, S. K., van Dyck, C. H., Alessi, C. A., et al. (1990). Clarifying confusion: The confusion assessment method. *Annals of Internal Medicine, 113*(12), 941–948.

Khan, F., Amatya, B., Bensmail, D., et al. (2019). Non-pharmacological interventions for spasticity in adults: An overview of systematic reviews. *Annals of Physical and Rehabilitation Medicine, 62*(4), 265–273.

*Liu, X., Griffith, M., Jang, H., et al. (2020). Intracranial pressure monitoring via external ventricular drain: Are we waiting long enough before recording the real value? *Journal of Neuroscience Nursing, 52*(1), 37–42.

Lucke-Wold, B., Logodon, A., Nguyen, L., et al. (2018). Supplements, nutrition, and alternative therapies for the treatment of traumatic brain injury. *Nutritional Neuroscience, 21*(2), 79–91.

Malhan, N., Usman, M., Trehan, N., et al. (2019). Oral care and ventilator-associated pneumonia. *American Journal of Therapeutics, 26*(5), 604–607.

Milliken, A., & Uveges, M. (2020). Brain death: History, updates, and implications for nurses. *American Journal of Nursing, 120*(3), 32–38.

Mirian, C., Pedersen, M., Sabers, A., et al. (2019). Antiepileptic drugs as prophylaxis for de novo brain tumour-related epilepsy after craniotomy: A systematic review and meta-analysis of harm and benefits. *Journal of Neurology, Neurosurgery, and Psychiatry, 90*(5), 599–607.

Mulkey, M. A., Hardin, S. R., Munro, C. L., et al. (2019). Methods of identifying delirium: A research protocol. *Research in Nursing and Health, 42*(4), 246–255.

Opdenakker, O., Vanstraelen, A., De Sloovere, V., et al. (2019). Sedatives in neurocritical care: An update on pharmacological agents and modes of sedation. *Current Opinion in Critical Care, 25*(2), 97–104.

Owen, A. (2019). The search for consciousness. *Neuron, 102*(3), 526–528.

Rincon, F. (2018). Targeted temperature management in brain injured patients. *Neurosurgical Clinics of North America, 29*(2), 231–253.

Rohaut, B., Eliseyev, A., & Claassen, J. (2019). Uncovering consciousness in unresponsive ICU patients: Technical, medical and ethical considerations. *Critical Care, 23*(1), 1–9.

*Saherwala, A., Bader, M., Stutzman, S., et al. (2018). Increasing adherence to brain trauma foundation guidelines for hospital care of patients with traumatic brain injury. *Critical Care Nurse, 38*(1), e11–e20.

Starling, A. L. (2018). Diagnosis and management of headache in older adults. *Mayo Clinic Proceedings, 93*(2), 252–262.

Stephen, L. J., Harden, C., Tomson, T., et al. (2019). Management of epilepsy in women. *Lancet Neurology, 18*(5), 481–491.

Tepper, S. (2019). Acute treatment of migraine. *Neurology Clinics, 37*(4), 727–742.

Tudor, R., & Thompson, C. (2019). Posterior pituitary dysfunction following traumatic brain injury: Review. *Pituitary, 22*(3), 296–304.

Tzadok, M., Harush, A., Nissenkorn, A., et al. (2019). Clinical outcomes of closed-loop vagal nerve stimulation in patients with refractory epilepsy. *European Journal of Epilepsy, 71,* 140–144.

Witherspoon, B., & Ashby, N. E. (2017). The use of mannitol and hypertonic saline therapies in patients with elevated intracranial pressure. *Nursing Clinics of North America, 52*(2), 249–260.

Wong, S., Mani, R., & Danish, S. (2019). Comparison and selection of current implantable anti-epileptic devices. *Neurotherapeutics, 16*(2), 369–380.

Zhou, T., & Kalanuria, A. (2018). Cerebral microdialysis in neurocritical care. *Current Neurology and Neuroscience Reports, 18,* 101. doi.org/10.1007/s11910-018-0915-6

Resources

American Headache Society, www.americanheadachesociety.org
Brain Injury Association, www.biausa.org
Brain Trauma Foundation (BTF), www.braintrauma.org
Epilepsy Foundation, www.epilepsy.com
Hydrocephalus Association, www.hydroassoc.org
National Headache Foundation, www.headaches.org

62

Management of Patients with Cerebrovascular Disorders

LEARNING OUTCOMES

On completion of this chapter, the learner will be able to:

1. Describe the incidence of, risk factors and preventive measures for, and impact of cerebrovascular disorders.
2. Compare the various types of cerebrovascular disorders: their causes, clinical manifestations, and medical management.
3. Explain the principles of nursing management as they relate to the care of a patient in the acute stage of an ischemic stroke.
4. Use the nursing process as a framework for care of the patient recovering from an ischemic stroke or from a hemorrhagic stroke.
5. Discuss essential elements for family education and preparation for home care of the patient who has had a stroke.

NURSING CONCEPTS

Family	Intracranial Regulation	Perfusion
Functional Ability	Patient Education	Sensory Perception

GLOSSARY

agnosia: loss of ability to recognize objects through a particular sensory system; may be visual, auditory, or tactile

aneurysm: a weakening or bulge in an arterial wall

aphasia: inability to express oneself or to understand language

apraxia: inability to perform previously learned purposeful motor acts on a voluntary basis

dysarthria: defects of articulation due to neurologic causes

dysphagia: difficulty swallowing

expressive aphasia: inability to express oneself; often associated with damage to the left frontal lobe area

hemianopsia: blindness of half of the field of vision in one or both eyes

hemiparesis: weakness of one side of the body, or part of it, due to an injury in the motor area of the brain

hemiplegia: paralysis of one side of the body, or part of it, due to an injury in the motor area of the brain

infarction: tissue necrosis in an area deprived of blood supply

penumbra region: area of low cerebral blood flow

receptive aphasia: inability to understand what someone else is saying; often associated with damage to the temporal lobe area

Cerebrovascular disorder is an umbrella term that refers to a functional abnormality of the central nervous system (CNS) that occurs when the blood supply to the brain is disrupted. Stroke is the primary cerebrovascular disorder in the United States, and while it dropped from the fourth to the fifth leading cause of death, it is still a leading cause of serious, long-term disability. Approximately 795,000 people experience a stroke each year in the United States. Approximately 610,000 of these are new strokes, and 185,000 are recurrent strokes (Virani, Alonso, Benjamin, et al., 2020). About 7 million Americans over the age of 20 who have survived a stroke are alive today. The financial impact of stroke is profound,

with estimated direct and indirect costs of $45.5 billion from 2014 to 2015 (Virani et al., 2020).

Strokes can be divided into two major categories: ischemic (approximately 87%), in which vascular occlusion and significant hypoperfusion occur, and hemorrhagic (approximately 13%), in which there is extravasation of blood into the brain or subarachnoid space (Hickey & Strayer, 2020; Virani et al., 2020). Although there are some similarities between the two types of stroke, differences exist in etiology, pathophysiology, medical management, surgical management, and nursing care. Table 62-1 compares ischemic and hemorrhagic strokes.

TABLE 62-1	Comparison of Major Types of Stroke		
Types of Stroke	**Causes**	**Main Presenting Symptoms**	**Functional Recovery**
Ischemic	• Large artery thrombosis • Small penetrating artery thrombosis • Cardiogenic embolic • Cryptogenic (no known cause) • Other	• Numbness or weakness of the face, arm, or leg, especially on one side of the body, aphasia, vision loss (homonymous hemianopsia)	Majority of recovery made in the first 3–6 mo, slower steps toward recovery may be made up to 1 yr and beyond with therapy.
Hemorrhagic	• Intracerebral hemorrhage • Subarachnoid hemorrhage • Cerebral aneurysm • Arteriovenous malformation	• "Worst headache of my life" • Decreased level of consciousness • Seizure	Slower recovery, typically left with more disability.

Adapted from Hickey, J. V., & Strayer, A. L. (2020). *The clinical practice of neurological & neurosurgical nursing* (8th ed.). Philadelphia, PA: Lippincott Williams & Wilkins.

Ischemic Stroke

An ischemic stroke, formerly referred to as a cerebrovascular accident or "brain attack," is a sudden loss of function resulting from disruption of the blood supply to a part of the brain. The term *brain attack* has been used to suggest to health care practitioners and the public that a stroke is an urgent health care issue similar to a heart attack. The only U.S. Food and Drug Administration (FDA)-approved thrombolytic therapy has a treatment window of 3 hours after the onset of a stroke, and scientific statements have endorsed its expanded use for up to 4.5 hours (Del Zoppo, Saver, Jauch, et al., 2009; Powers, Rabinstein, Ackerson, et al., 2019). Although the time frame for treatment has expanded, urgency is needed on the part of the public and health care practitioners for rapid transport of the patient to a hospital for assessment and administration of the medication.

Ischemic strokes are subdivided into five different types based on the cause: large artery thrombotic strokes (20%), small penetrating artery thrombotic strokes (25%), cardiogenic embolic strokes (20%), cryptogenic strokes (30%), and others (5%) (see Table 62-1). Large artery thrombotic strokes are caused by atherosclerotic plaques in the large blood vessels of the brain. Thrombus formation and occlusion at the site of the atherosclerosis result in ischemia and **infarction** (tissue necrosis in an area deprived of blood supply) (Hickey & Strayer, 2020).

Small penetrating artery thrombotic strokes affect one or more vessels and are a common type of ischemic stroke. Small artery thrombotic strokes are also called *lacunar strokes* because of the cavity that is created after the death of infarcted brain tissue (Hickey & Strayer, 2020).

Cardiogenic embolic strokes are associated with cardiac arrhythmias, usually atrial fibrillation. Embolic strokes can also be associated with valvular heart disease and thrombi in the left ventricle. Emboli originate from the heart and circulate to the cerebral vasculature, most commonly the left middle cerebral artery, resulting in a stroke. Embolic strokes may be prevented by the use of anticoagulation therapy in patients with atrial fibrillation.

The last two classifications of ischemic strokes are cryptogenic strokes, which have no known cause, and strokes from other causes, such as illicit drug use (cocaine), coagulopathies, migraine/vasospasm, or spontaneous dissection of the carotid or vertebral arteries.

COVID-19 Considerations

Severe acute respiratory syndrome coronavirus 2 (SARS-CoV-2) is a community-acquired coronavirus whose primary pathologic evolution occurs within the respiratory system; however, due to abnormal blood clotting, one of the manifestations of coronavirus disease 2019 (COVID-19) can be ischemic stroke (Wadman, Couzin-Frankel, Kaiser, et al., 2020). The increase in blood clots in patients with COVID-19 is associated with laboratory findings of high D-dimer levels (Wadman et al., 2020). Case reports of patients who have had strokes and COVID-19 reveal that many are younger than 50 years of age and that the strokes occur in the large blood vessels of the brain, resulting in severe neurologic deficits (see later discussion) (Oxley, Mocco, Majidi, et al., 2020).

Pathophysiology

In an ischemic brain attack, there is disruption of the cerebral blood flow due to obstruction of a blood vessel. This disruption in blood flow initiates a complex series of cellular metabolic events referred to as the ischemic cascade (see Fig. 62-1).

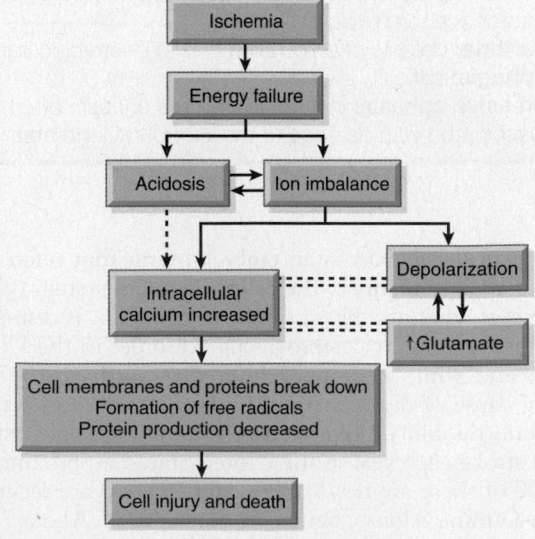

Figure 62-1 • Some of the processes contributing to ischemic brain cell injury.

The ischemic cascade begins when cerebral blood flow decreases to less than 25 mL per 100 g of blood per minute. At this point, neurons are no longer able to maintain aerobic respiration. The mitochondria must then switch to anaerobic respiration, which generates large amounts of lactic acid, causing a change in the pH. This switch to the less efficient anaerobic respiration also renders the neuron incapable of producing sufficient quantities of adenosine triphosphate (ATP) to fuel the depolarization processes. The membrane pumps that maintain electrolyte balance begin to fail, and the cells cease to function.

Early in the cascade, an area of low cerebral blood flow, referred to as the **penumbra region**, exists around the area of infarction. The penumbra region is ischemic brain tissue that may be salvaged with timely intervention. The ischemic cascade threatens cells in the penumbra because membrane depolarization of the cell wall leads to an increase in intracellular calcium and the release of glutamate. The influx of calcium and the release of glutamate, if continued, activate a number of damaging pathways that result in the destruction of the cell membrane, the release of more calcium and glutamate, vasoconstriction, and the generation of free radicals. These processes enlarge the area of infarction into the penumbra, extending the stroke. A person experiencing a stroke typically loses 1.9 million neurons each minute that a stroke is not treated, and the ischemic brain ages 3.6 years each hour without treatment (Saver, 2006).

Each step in the ischemic cascade represents an opportunity for intervention to limit the extent of secondary brain damage caused by a stroke. The penumbra area may be revitalized by administration of tissue plasminogen activator (t-PA). Medications that protect the brain from secondary injury are called *neuroprotectants*. A number of clinical trials have focused on neuroprotective medications and strategies to improve stroke recovery and survival; so far, none have shown positive results (Powers et al., 2019).

Clinical Manifestations

An ischemic stroke can cause a wide variety of neurologic deficits, depending on the location of the lesion (which blood vessels are obstructed), the size of the area of inadequate perfusion, and the amount of collateral (secondary or accessory) blood flow. See Chapter 60 for discussion of anatomy and brain blood supply. The patient may present with any of the following signs or symptoms:

- Numbness or weakness of the face, arm, or leg, especially on one side of the body
- Confusion or change in mental status
- Trouble speaking or understanding speech
- Visual disturbances
- Difficulty walking, dizziness, or loss of balance or coordination
- Sudden severe headache

Motor, sensory, cranial nerve, cognitive, and other functions may be disrupted. Table 62-2 reviews the neurologic deficits frequently seen in patients with stroke. Table 62-3 compares the symptoms and behaviors seen in right hemispheric stroke with those seen in left hemispheric stroke.

Motor Loss

A stroke is an upper motor neuron lesion and results in loss of voluntary control over motor movements. Because the upper motor neurons decussate (cross), a disturbance of voluntary motor control on one side of the body may reflect damage to the upper motor neurons on the opposite side of the brain. The most common motor dysfunction is **hemiplegia** (paralysis of one side of the body, or part of it) caused by a lesion of the opposite side of the brain. **Hemiparesis**, or weakness of one side of the body, or part of it, is another sign. The concept of upper and lower motor neuron lesions is described in more detail in Chapter 60, Table 60-4.

In the early stage of stroke, the initial clinical features may be flaccid paralysis and loss of or decrease in the deep tendon reflexes. When these deep reflexes reappear (usually by 48 hours), increased tone is observed along with spasticity (abnormal increase in muscle tone) of the extremities on the affected side.

Communication Loss

Other brain functions affected by stroke are language and communication. In fact, stroke is the most common cause of **aphasia** (inability to express oneself or to understand language). The following are dysfunctions of language and communication:

- **Dysarthria** (difficulty in speaking) or dysphasia (impaired speech), caused by paralysis of the muscles responsible for producing speech
- Aphasia, which can be **expressive aphasia** (inability to express oneself), **receptive aphasia** (inability to understand language), or global (mixed) aphasia (see Chapter 60, Table 60-5)
- **Apraxia** (inability to perform a previously learned action), as may be seen when a patient makes verbal substitutions for desired syllables or words

Perceptual Disturbances

Perception is the ability to interpret sensation. Stroke can result in visual–perceptual dysfunctions, disturbances in visual–spatial relations, and sensory loss.

Visual–perceptual dysfunctions are caused by disturbances of the primary sensory pathways between the eye and visual cortex. Homonymous **hemianopsia** (blindness in half of the visual field in one or both eyes) may occur from stroke and may be temporary or permanent. The affected side of vision corresponds to the paralyzed side of the body.

Disturbances in visual–spatial relations (perceiving the relationship of two or more objects in spatial areas) are frequently seen in patients with right hemispheric damage.

Sensory Loss

Sensory losses from stroke may be mild, such as a slight impairment of touch, or more severe, with loss of proprioception (ability to perceive the position and motion of body parts) as well as difficulty in interpreting visual, tactile, and auditory stimuli. An **agnosia** is the loss of the ability to recognize objects through a particular sensory system; it may be visual, auditory, or tactile (see Chapter 60, Table 60-6).

Cognitive Impairment and Psychological Effects

If damage has occurred to the frontal lobe, learning capacity, memory, or other higher cortical intellectual functions may be impaired. Such dysfunction may be reflected in a limited attention span, difficulties in comprehension, forgetfulness,

TABLE 62-2	Neurologic Deficits of Stroke: Manifestations and Nursing Implications	
Neurologic Deficit	**Manifestation**	**Nursing Implications/Patient Education Applications**
Visual Field Deficits		
Homonymous hemianopsia (loss of half of the visual field)	• Unaware of persons or objects on side of visual loss • Neglect of one side of the body • Difficulty judging distances	Place objects within intact field of vision. Approach the patient from side of intact field of vision. Instruct/remind the patient to turn head in the direction of visual loss to compensate for loss of visual field. Encourage the use of eyeglasses if available. When educating the patient, do so within patient's intact visual field.
Loss of peripheral vision	• Difficulty seeing at night • Unaware of objects or the borders of objects	Place objects in center of patient's intact visual field. Encourage the use of a cane or other object to identify objects in the periphery of the visual field. Ensure that the patient's driving ability is evaluated.
Diplopia	• Double vision	Explain to the patient the location of an object when placing it near the patient. Consistently place patient care items in the same location.
Motor Deficits		
Hemiparesis	• Weakness of the face, arm, and leg on the same side (due to a lesion in the opposite hemisphere)	Place objects within the patient's reach on the nonaffected side. Instruct the patient to exercise and increase the strength on the unaffected side.
Hemiplegia	• Paralysis of the face, arm, and leg on the same side (due to a lesion in the opposite hemisphere)	Encourage the patient to provide range-of-motion exercises to the affected side. Reposition the patient every 2 h. Maintain body alignment in functional position. Exercise unaffected limb to increase mobility, strength, and use.
Ataxia	• Staggering, unsteady gait • Unable to keep feet together; needs a broad base to stand	Support patient during the initial ambulation phase. Provide supportive device for ambulation (walker, cane). Instruct the patient not to walk without assistance or supportive device.
Dysarthria	• Difficulty in forming words	Provide the patient with alternative methods of communicating. Allow the patient sufficient time to respond to verbal communication. Support patient and family to alleviate frustration related to difficulty in communicating.
Dysphagia	• Difficulty in swallowing	Test the patient's pharyngeal reflexes before offering food or fluids. Assist the patient with meals. Place food on the unaffected side of the mouth. Allow ample time to eat.
Sensory Deficits		
Paresthesia (occurs on the side opposite the lesion)	• Sensation of numbness, tingling, or a "pins and needles" sensation • Difficulty with proprioception	Instruct patient that sensation may be altered. Provide range of motion to affected areas and apply corrective devices as needed. If numbness is present, protect the affected areas from injury and burns.
Verbal Deficits		
Expressive aphasia	• Unable to form words that are understandable; may be able to speak in single-word responses	Encourage patient to repeat sounds of the alphabet. Explore the patient's ability to write as an alternative means of communication.
Receptive aphasia	• Unable to comprehend the spoken word; can speak but may not make sense	Speak clearly and in an unhurried manner to assist the patient in forming the sounds. Explore the patient's ability to read as an alternative means of communication.
Global (mixed) aphasia	• Combination of both receptive and expressive aphasia	Speak clearly and in simple sentences; use gestures or pictures when able. Establish alternative means of communication.
Cognitive Deficits	• Short- and long-term memory loss • Decreased attention span • Impaired ability to concentrate • Poor abstract reasoning • Altered judgment	Reorient patient to time, place, and situation frequently. Use verbal and auditory cues to orient patient. Provide familiar objects (family photographs, favorite objects). Use noncomplicated language. Match visual tasks with a verbal cue; holding a toothbrush, simulate brushing of teeth while saying, "I would like you to brush your teeth now." Minimize distracting noises and views when providing education to the patient. Repeat and reinforce instructions frequently.
Emotional Deficits	• Loss of self-control • Emotional lability • Decreased tolerance to stressful situations • Depression • Withdrawal • Fear, hostility, and anger • Feelings of isolation	Support patient during uncontrollable outbursts. Discuss with the patient and family that the outbursts are due to the disease process. Encourage patient to participate in group activity. Provide stimulation for the patient. Control stressful situations, if possible. Provide a safe environment. Encourage patient to express feelings and frustrations related to disease process.

Adapted from Hickey, J. V., & Strayer, A. L. (2020). *The clinical practice of neurological & neurosurgical nursing* (8th ed.). Philadelphia, PA: Lippincott Williams & Wilkins.

TABLE 62-3	Comparison of Left and Right Hemispheric Strokes	
Left Hemispheric Stroke	**Right Hemispheric Stroke**	
Paralysis or weakness on right side of body	Paralysis or weakness on left side of body	
Right visual field deficit	Left visual field deficit	
Aphasia (expressive, receptive, or global)	Spatial–perceptual deficits	
Altered intellectual ability	Increased distractibility	
Slow, cautious behavior	Impulsive behavior and poor judgment Lack of awareness of deficits	

Adapted from Hickey, J. V., & Strayer, A. L. (2020). *The clinical practice of neurological & neurosurgical nursing* (8th ed.). Philadelphia, PA: Lippincott Williams & Wilkins.

and a lack of motivation. These changes can cause the patient to become easily frustrated during rehabilitation. Depression is common and may be exaggerated by the patient's natural response to this catastrophic event. Emotional lability, hostility, frustration, resentment, lack of cooperation, and other psychological problems may occur.

Assessment and Diagnostic Findings

Any patient with neurologic deficits needs a careful history eliciting the last time the patient was seen well and a rapid focused physical and neurologic examination. Initial assessment focuses on airway patency, which may be compromised by loss of gag or cough reflexes and altered respiratory pattern; cardiovascular status (including blood pressure, cardiac rhythm and rate, carotid bruit); and gross neurologic deficits.

Patients may present to the acute care facility with temporary neurologic symptoms. A transient ischemic attack (TIA) is a neurologic deficit that completely resolves in 24 hours (most last less than 1 hour). A TIA is manifested by a sudden loss of motor, sensory, or visual function. The symptoms result from temporary ischemia (impairment of blood flow) to a specific region of the brain; however, when brain imaging is performed, there is no evidence of ischemia. A TIA may serve as a warning of impending stroke. Approximately 3% to 15% of all strokes are preceded by a TIA and occur within the first 90 days after the TIA (Hickey & Strayer, 2020; Johnston, Easton, Farrant, et al., 2018). Lack of evaluation and treatment of a patient who has experienced previous TIAs may result in a stroke and irreversible deficits.

The initial diagnostic test for a stroke is a noncontrast computed tomography (CT) scan. This should be initiated within 20 minutes from the time the patient presents to the emergency department (ED) to determine if the event is ischemic or hemorrhagic, as the type of stroke determines treatment (Powers et al., 2019). Some cities now have mobile stroke units (an ambulance with a CT scanner) that can rapidly make this important distinction and can begin acute medical management. Further diagnostic workup for ischemic stroke involves attempting to identify the source of the thrombi or emboli and to determine if the patient would benefit from mechanical intervention (clot removal). Studies may include CT angiography or CT perfusion; magnetic resonance imaging (MRI)

and magnetic resonance angiography of the brain and neck vessels; transcranial Doppler flow studies; and transthoracic or transesophageal echocardiography (Hickey & Strayer, 2020; Powers et al., 2019). A 12-lead electrocardiogram (ECG) and a carotid ultrasound are other standard tests.

Prevention

Primary prevention of ischemic stroke remains the best approach. A healthy lifestyle including not smoking, engaging in physical activity (at least 40 minutes a day, 3 to 4 days a week), maintaining a healthy weight, and following a healthy diet (including modest alcohol consumption), can reduce the risk of having a stroke (Virani et al., 2020). Specific diets that have decreased risk of stroke include the Dietary Approaches to Stop Hypertension (DASH) diet (high in fruits and vegetables, moderate in low-fat dairy products, and low in animal protein), the Mediterranean diet (supplemented with nuts), and overall diets that are rich in fruits and vegetables. Research findings suggest that low-dose aspirin may lower the risk of a first stroke for those who are at risk (Meschia, Bushnell, Boden-Albala, et al., 2014).

Stroke risk screenings are an ideal opportunity to lower stroke risk by identifying people or groups of people who are at high risk for stroke and by educating patients and the community about recognition and prevention of stroke. Stroke screenings are usually coordinated and run by nurses. Age, gender, and race are well-known nonmodifiable risk factors for stroke. High-risk groups include people older than 55 years, and the incidence of stroke more than doubles in each successive decade. Men have a higher age-adjusted rate of stroke than that of women in younger and middle age, but that difference narrows in the oldest age groups, in which the rate in women is almost equal to or sometimes even higher than in men. Each year, 55,000 more women than men have a stroke. Compared to Caucasian Americans, African Americans and some Hispanic/Latino Americans have a higher incidence of stroke and higher mortality (Virani et al., 2020).

There are many risk factors for ischemic stroke (see Chart 62-1). For people who are at high risk, interventions that alter modifiable factors, such as treating hypertension and stopping smoking, reduce stroke risk (Meschia et al., 2014).

> **Chart 62-1** ⚠ **MODIFIABLE RISK FACTORS**
> Ischemic Stroke
>
> - Asymptomatic carotid stenosis
> - Atrial fibrillation
> - Diabetes (associated with accelerated atherogenesis)
> - Dyslipidemia
> - Excessive alcohol consumption
> - Hypercoagulable states
> - Hypertension (controlling hypertension, the major risk factor, is the key to preventing stroke)
> - Migraine
> - Obesity
> - Sedentary lifestyle
> - Sleep apnea
> - Smoking
>
> Adapted from Meschia, J. F., Bushnell, C., Boden-Albala, B., et al. (2014). Guidelines for the primary prevention of stroke: A statement for healthcare professionals from the American Heart Association/American Stroke Association. *Stroke, 45*(12), 3754–3832.

Additional treatable conditions that increase risk of stroke include sickle cell diseases, cardiomyopathy (ischemic and nonischemic), and valvular heart disease (e.g., endocarditis, prosthetic heart valves). Lesser known and potentially modifiable risk factors for stroke are migraine (especially migraine with aura), sleep apnea, and inherited and acquired hypercoagulable states. Chronic inflammatory conditions that have been associated with an increased risk of stroke are systemic lupus erythematosus and rheumatoid arthritis (Norris, 2019).

Several methods of preventing recurrent stroke have been identified for patients with TIAs or ischemic stroke. Patients with moderate to severe carotid stenosis are treated with carotid endarterectomy (CEA) or carotid angioplasty and stenting. In patients with atrial fibrillation, which increases the risk of emboli, administration of an anticoagulant that inhibits clot formation may prevent both thrombotic and embolic strokes (Kernan, Ovbiagele, Black, et al., 2014).

Medical Management

Patients who have experienced a TIA or stroke should have medical management for secondary prevention. Those with atrial fibrillation (or cardioembolic strokes) are treated with dose-adjusted warfarin with a target international normalized ratio (INR) of 2 to 3. Other anticoagulants that may be prescribed as alternative drugs include dabigatran, apixaban, edoxaban, or rivaroxaban, unless they are contraindicated. These drugs are also known as direct oral anticoagulants (DOACs). If anticoagulants are contraindicated, aspirin alone is the best option, although the addition of clopidogrel to aspirin is also a reasonable therapy (Kernan et al., 2014).

Platelet-inhibiting medications, including aspirin, extended-release dipyridamole plus aspirin, and clopidogrel decrease the incidence of cerebral infarction in patients who have experienced TIAs and stroke from suspected embolic or thrombotic causes. The specific medication that is used is based on the patient's health history. If the patient has had a minor ischemic stroke or what is considered a TIA with a high risk of having stroke, and they did not receive thrombolytic therapy, they may receive two platelet-inhibiting medications (dual antiplatelet therapy). Typically this is clopidogrel and aspirin, and can be taken for a period of 21 to 90 days after the stroke or TIA (Powers et al., 2019).

Research suggests that medications known as statins reduce coronary events and ischemic strokes. The most current stroke prevention guideline now includes the recommendation of a statin even if the low-density lipoprotein (LDL) cholesterol is below 100 mg/dL and there is no evidence of atherosclerotic cardiovascular disease (coronary artery disease/myocardial infarction, hypertensive heart disease and peripheral arterial disease) (Kernan et al., 2014). The FDA has included indications for statin medications, such as atorvastatin and simvastatin, to include secondary stroke prevention.

After the acute stroke period, antihypertensive medications are also used, if indicated, for secondary stroke prevention. Preferred drugs include angiotensin-converting enzyme (ACE) inhibitors and diuretics, or a combination of both (Kernan et al., 2014).

Medical management of acute ischemic stroke needs to include consideration for endovascular treatment (Powers et al., 2019). The FDA has approved several devices that open the blocked artery and restore blood flow to the brain. These devices are used by specialists in the endovascular suite.

Thrombolytic Therapy

Thrombolytic agents are used to treat ischemic stroke by dissolving the blood clot that is blocking blood flow to the brain. Recombinant t-PA is a genetically engineered form of t-PA (a thrombolytic substance made naturally by the body) (Comerford & Durkin, 2020). It works by binding to fibrin and converting plasminogen to plasmin, which stimulates fibrinolysis of the clot. Rapid diagnosis of stroke and initiation of thrombolytic therapy (within 3 hours) in patients with ischemic stroke leads to a decrease in the size of the stroke and an overall improvement in functional outcome after 3 months (National Institute of Neurological Disorders and Stroke [NINDS], 1995). The goal is for intravenous (IV) t-PA to be given within 45 minutes of the patient arriving to the ED (Powers et al., 2019).

Mechanical intervention (e.g., mechanical thrombectomy, endovascular thrombectomy, intra-arterial mechanical thrombectomy) can be used with t-PA or as an alternative to IV administration (Amatangelo & Thomas, 2019). Intra-arterial mechanical thrombectomy allows for higher concentrations of the drug to be given directly to the clot, and the time window for treatment may be extended up to 24 hours in patients that meet specific criteria (Powers et al., 2019). Those not eligible for IV delivery may be eligible for intra-arterial delivery, and these methods may also be combined. Treatment using intra-arterial delivery must occur in specialized centers with access to emergent cerebral angiogram and interventional operating rooms/suites (Powers et al., 2019). Ongoing clinical trials continue to investigate the efficacy of other thrombolytic agents.

To realize the full potential of early intervention, community education directed at recognizing the symptoms of stroke and obtaining appropriate emergency care is necessary to ensure rapid transport to a hospital and initiation of therapy within the recommended 3-hour period (which may be extended up to 4.5 hours) (Del Zoppo et al., 2009; Powers et al., 2019). Delays make the patient ineligible for therapies, because revascularization of necrotic tissue (which develops after 3 hours) increases the risk of cerebral edema and hemorrhage.

Endovascular Therapy

It is now recommended that patients with acute ischemic stroke receive endovascular therapy and medical management with a stent retriever if they meet specific criteria (Powers et al., 2019). All of the following criteria need to be met:

- Prestroke status of no deficits
- Acute ischemic stroke receiving IV t-PA within 4.5 hours of onset according to guidelines from professional medical societies
- Causative occlusion of the internal carotid artery or middle cerebral artery segment
- Age ≥18 years
- National Institutes of Health Stroke Scale (NIHSS) score of ≥6 (see later discussion)
- An Alberta Stroke Program Evaluation of Computed Tomography (ASPECT) score of ≥6 (a radiologic assessment of the CT scan), and treatment can be initiated (groin puncture) within 6 hours of symptom onset

Patients eligible for t-PA should receive IV t-PA even if endovascular treatments are being considered (Powers et al., 2019). Thrombolytic therapy should not be delayed.

Enhancing Prompt Diagnosis

After being notified by emergency medical service personnel, the ED contacts the appropriate staff (neurologist, neuroradiologist, radiology department, nursing staff, ECG, and laboratory technicians) and informs them of the patient's imminent arrival at the hospital. Many institutions have acute stroke teams that respond rapidly, ensuring that treatment occurs within the allotted period. This may be called a Code Stroke.

Initial management requires the definitive diagnosis of an ischemic stroke by brain imaging and a careful history to determine whether the patient meets the criteria for t-PA therapy (see Chart 62-2). The goal is that diagnostic results from imaging are completed within 25 minutes of the patient's arrival to the ED. Some of the contraindications for thrombolytic therapy include symptom onset greater than 3 hours before admission (expanded to 4.5 hours), a patient who is anticoagulated (with an INR above 1.7), or a patient who has recently had any type of significant intracranial pathology (e.g., previous stroke, head injury, trauma) in the last 3 months.

Before receiving t-PA, the patient is assessed using the NIHSS, a standardized assessment tool that helps evaluate stroke severity (see Table 62-4). Total NIHSS scores range from 0 (normal) to 42 (severe stroke). Certification in the

---

Chart 62-2 — Eligibility Criteria for Tissue Plasminogen Activator Administration

- Age ≥18 years
- Clinical diagnosis of ischemic stroke
- Systolic blood pressure ≤185 mm Hg; diastolic ≤110 mm Hg
- No minor (nondisabling) stroke
- Prothrombin time ≤15 seconds or international normalized ratio ≤1.7 (if taking an anticoagulant, the same guidance is used)
- Not received low-molecular weight heparin during the past 24 hours
- Platelet count ≥100,000/mm³
- No symptoms consistent with infective endocarditis
- No prior intracranial hemorrhage
- No subarachnoid hemorrhage
- No stroke, serious head trauma, or intracranial surgery within 3 months
- No gastrointestinal bleeding within 21 days, or gastrointestinal malignancy

Some of these are relative contraindications (the provider administering the medication needs to weigh the risks and benefits of the therapy). There are more stringent t-PA administration guidelines for patients with stroke symptoms that began 3 to 4.5 hours ago and also for those whose symptoms began longer than 4.5 hours ago or for whom time of onset is unclear, coupled with specific MRI findings. Specific guidance also exists for patients taking thrombin inhibitors or factor Xa inhibitors.

Adapted from Powers, W. J., Rabinstein, A. A., Ackerson, T., et al. (2019). Guidelines for the early management of patients with acute ischemic stroke: 2019 update to the 2018 guidelines for the early management of acute ischemic stroke: A guideline for healthcare professionals from the American Heart association/American Stroke Association. *Stroke, 50*(12), e344–e418.

---

administration of the scale is recommended and is available for nurses and other health care professionals.

Dosage and Administration

The patient is weighed to determine the dose of t-PA. Typically, two or more IV sites are established prior to administration of t-PA (one for the t-PA and the other for administration of IV fluids). The dosage for t-PA is 0.9 mg/kg, with a maximum dose of 90 mg. Ten percent of the calculated dose is given as an IV bolus over 1 minute. The remaining dose (90%) is given IV over 1 hour via an infusion pump (Comerford & Durkin, 2020; Hickey & Strayer, 2020; Powers et al., 2019).

The patient is admitted to the intensive care unit or an acute stroke unit, where continuous cardiac monitoring and frequent neurologic assessments are conducted (Amatangelo & Thomas, 2019). Vital signs are obtained frequently, with particular attention to blood pressure (with the goal of lowering the risk of intracranial hemorrhage) and temperature. An example of a standard protocol would be to obtain vital signs every 15 minutes for the first 2 hours, every 30 minutes for the next 6 hours, then every hour until 24 hours after treatment. Blood pressure should be maintained with the systolic pressure less than 185 mm Hg and the diastolic pressure less than 110 mm Hg (Powers et al., 2019). Fever needs to be treated. Airway management is instituted based on the patient's clinical condition and arterial blood gas values.

Side Effects

Once it is determined that the patient is a candidate for t-PA therapy, no anticoagulant or platelet inhibiting medications (e.g., aspirin, clopidogrel) are given for the next 24 hours. Bleeding is the most common side effect of t-PA administration, and the patient is closely monitored for any bleeding (IV insertion sites, urinary catheter site, endotracheal tube, nasogastric tube, urine, stool, emesis, other secretions). A 24-hour delay in placement of nasogastric tubes, urinary catheters, and intra-arterial pressure catheters is recommended. Intracranial bleeding is a major complication that occurred in approximately 6.4% of patients in the initial t-PA study (NINDS, 1995). A number of factors are associated with the occurrence of symptomatic intracranial bleeding: age greater than 70 years, baseline NIHSS score greater than 20, serum glucose concentration 300 mg/dL or higher, and edema or mass effect observed on the patient's initial CT scan (NINDS, 1995).

Therapy for Patients with Ischemic Stroke Not Receiving Tissue Plasminogen Activator

Not all patients are candidates for t-PA therapy. In some centers, other treatments may include anticoagulant administration (IV heparin or low–molecular-weight heparin). Because of the risks associated with urgent anticoagulation, their general use is not recommended for patients with acute ischemic stroke (Powers et al., 2019).

Careful maintenance of cerebral hemodynamics to maintain cerebral perfusion is extremely important after a stroke. Increased intracranial pressure (ICP) from brain edema and associated complications may occur after a large ischemic stroke. Interventions during this period include measures to reduce ICP, such as administering an osmotic diuretic (e.g., mannitol)

TABLE 62-4	Summary of National Institutes of Health Stroke Scale (NIHSS)	
Category	**Description**	**Score**
1a. LOC	Alert	0
	Arousable by minor stimulation	1
	Obtunded, strong stimulation to attend	2
	Unresponsive, or reflexive responses only	3
1b. LOC questions (month, age)	Answers both correctly	0
	Answers one correctly	1
	Both incorrect	2
1c. LOC commands (open, close eyes; make fist, let go)	Obeys both correctly	0
	Obeys one correctly	1
	Both incorrect	2
2. Best gaze (eyes open—patient follows examiner's finger or face)	Normal	0
	Partial gaze palsy	1
	Forced deviation	2
3. Visual (introduce visual stimulus/threat to patient's visual field quadrants)	No visual loss	0
	Partial hemianopsia	1
	Complete hemianopsia	2
	Bilateral hemianopsia	3
4. Facial palsy (show teeth, raise eyebrows, and squeeze eyes shut)	Normal	0
	Minor	1
	Partial	2
	Complete	3
5a. Motor; arm—left (elevate extremity to 90 degrees and score drift/movement)	No drift	0
	Drift but maintains in air	1
	Unable to maintain in air	2
	No effort against gravity	3
	No movement	4
	Amputation, joint fusion (explain)	N/A
5b. Motor; arm—right (elevate extremity to 90 degrees and score drift/movement)	No drift	0
	Drift but maintains in air	1
	Unable to maintain in air	2
	No effort against gravity	3
	No movement	4
	Amputation, joint fusion (explain)	N/A
6a. Motor; leg—left (elevate extremity to 30 degrees and score drift/movement)	No drift	0
	Drift but maintains in air	1
	Unable to maintain in air	2
	No effort against gravity	3
	No movement	4
	Amputation, joint fusion (explain)	N/A
6b. Motor; leg—right (elevate extremity to 30 degrees and score drift/movement)	No drift	0
	Drift but maintains in air	1
	Unable to maintain in air	2
	No effort against gravity	3
	No movement	4
	Amputation, joint fusion (explain)	N/A
7. Limb ataxia (finger-to-nose and heel-to-shin testing)	Absent	0
	Present in one limb	1
	Present in two limbs	2
8. Sensory (pinprick to face, arm, trunk, and leg—compare side to side)	Normal	0
	Mild to moderate loss	1
	Severe to total loss	2
9. Best language (name items, describe a picture, and read sentences)	No aphasia	0
	Mild to moderate aphasia	1
	Severe aphasia	2
	Mute	3
10. Dysarthria (evaluate speech clarity by having patient repeat words)	Normal	0
	Mild to moderate dysarthria	1
	Severe dysarthria, mostly unintelligible or worse	2
	Intubated or other physical barrier	N/A
11. Extinction and inattention (use information from prior testing to score)	No abnormality	0
	Visual, tactile, auditory, or other extinction to bilateral simultaneous stimulation	1
		2
	Profound hemiattention or extinction to more than one modality	
Total score		——

LOC, level of consciousness; N/A, not applicable.
Adapted from the version available at the National Institute of Neurological Disorders and Stroke (NINDS). (n.d.). *NIH stroke scale*. Bethesda, MD: National Institutes of Health. Retrieved on 3/8/2020 at: www.ninds.nih.gov/sites/default/files/NIH_Stroke_Scale_Booklet.pdf. It is recommended that the full scale with all instructions be used.

to those that are declining clinically. Other treatment measures include the following (Powers et al., 2019):

- Providing supplemental oxygen if oxygen saturation is below 95%
- Elevation of the head of the bed to 30 degrees to assist the patient in handling oral secretions and decrease ICP
- Possible hemicraniectomy for increased ICP from brain edema in a very large stroke
- Intubation with an endotracheal tube to establish a patent airway, if necessary
- Continuous hemodynamic monitoring (the goals for blood pressure in the first 24 hours after a stroke remain controversial for a patient who has not received thrombolytic therapy; antihypertensive treatment may be given to lower the blood pressure by 15% if the systolic blood pressure exceeds 220 mm Hg or the diastolic blood pressure exceeds 120 mm Hg)
- Frequent neurologic assessments to determine if the stroke is evolving and if other acute complications are developing (such complications may include seizures, bleeding from anticoagulation, or medication-induced bradycardia, which can result in hypotension and subsequent decreases in cardiac output and cerebral perfusion pressure)
- Monitoring for the development of fever (elevated temperature in the first 24 hours after stroke has been associated with increased in-hospital mortality)
- Monitoring of blood glucose and management with sliding scale insulin to keep levels in the range of 140 to 180 mg/dL

Managing Potential Complications

Adequate cerebral blood flow is essential for cerebral oxygenation. If cerebral blood flow is inadequate, the amount of oxygen supplied to the brain will decrease, and tissue ischemia will result. Adequate oxygenation begins with pulmonary care, maintenance of a patent airway, and administration of supplemental oxygen as needed. The importance of adequate gas exchange in these patients cannot be overemphasized, because many patients are at risk for aspiration pneumonia.

Other potential complications after a stroke include urinary tract infections, cardiac arrhythmias (ventricular ectopy, tachycardia, and heart blocks), and complications of immobility. Hyperglycemia has been associated with poor neurologic outcomes in acute stroke; therefore, blood glucose levels are monitored and hypoglycemia avoided as well (Powers et al., 2019).

Surgical Prevention of Ischemic Stroke

One surgical procedure for select patients with TIAs and mild stroke is CEA. A CEA is the removal of an atherosclerotic plaque or thrombus from the carotid artery to prevent stroke in patients with occlusive disease of the extracranial cerebral arteries (see Fig. 62-2). This surgery is indicated for patients with symptoms of TIA or mild stroke (or those without symptoms) who are found to have severe (70% to 99%) carotid artery stenosis or moderate (50% to 69%) stenosis with other significant risk factors.

Carotid artery stenting (CAS), with or without angioplasty, is a less invasive procedure that is used for treatment of carotid stenosis. This procedure has less discomfort for the

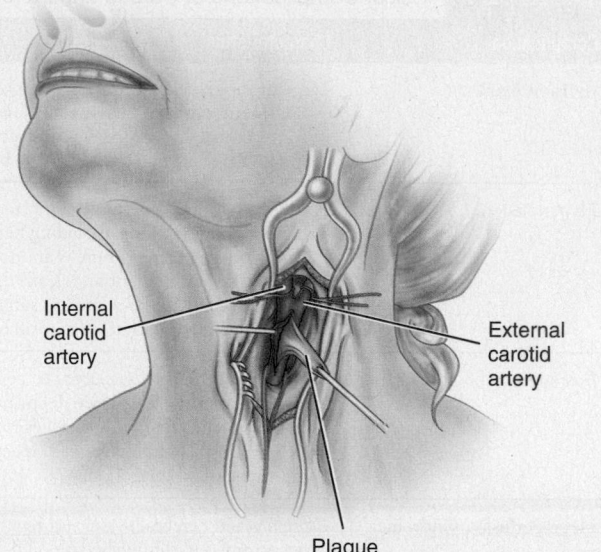

Figure 62-2 • Plaque, a potential source of emboli in transient ischemic attack and stroke, is surgically removed from the carotid artery.

patient and a shorter recovery time than CEA. Age can be considered when deciding which procedure will be best for the patient. For patients older than 70 years, CEA demonstrated improved outcomes in research studies; for those who were younger, outcomes between CAS and CEA were similar when comparing procedure complications (Kernan et al., 2014).

 Nursing Management

The main complications of CEA are stroke, cranial nerve injuries, infection or hematoma at the incision, and carotid artery disruption. It is important to maintain adequate blood pressure levels in the immediate postoperative period. Blood pressure instability is common, and lasts 12 to 24 hours after the procedure (Hickey & Strayer, 2020). Hypotension is avoided to prevent cerebral ischemia and thrombosis. Uncontrolled hypertension may precipitate cerebral hemorrhage, edema, hemorrhage at the surgical incision, or disruption of the arterial reconstruction. Medications are used to reduce the blood pressure to previous levels. Close cardiac monitoring is necessary, because these patients frequently have concomitant coronary artery disease.

After CEA, a neurologic observation record (see Chapter 61, Fig. 61-6) is used to monitor and document assessment parameters for all body systems, with particular attention to neurologic status. The primary provider is notified immediately if a neurologic deficit develops. Formation of a thrombus at the site of the endarterectomy is suspected if there is a sudden new onset of neurologic deficits, such as weakness on one side of the body. The patient should be prepared for repeat endarterectomy.

Difficulty in swallowing, hoarseness, or other signs of cranial nerve dysfunction must be assessed. Cranial nerve injury is the most common complication following CEA. The nurse focuses on assessment of the following cranial nerves: facial (VII), glossopharyngeal (IX), vagus (X), spinal accessory

TABLE 62-5	Select Complications of Carotid Endarterectomy (CEA) and Nursing Interventions	
Complication	**Characteristics**	**Nursing Interventions**
Incision hematoma	Large or rapidly expanding hematomas require emergency treatment. Risks include tracheal deviation and airway compromise. If the airway is obstructed by the hematoma, the incision may be opened at the bedside.	Monitor neck discomfort and wound expansion. Report swelling, subjective feelings of pressure in the neck, difficulty breathing.
Hypertension	Poorly controlled hypertension increases the risk of postoperative complications, including hematoma and hyperperfusion syndrome. There is an increased incidence of neurologic impairment and death due to intracerebral hemorrhage. May be related to surgically induced abnormalities (manipulation) of carotid baroreceptor sensitivity.	Keep in mind that risk is highest in the first 48 h after surgery. Check blood pressure frequently, and report deviations from baseline. Administer medications, as prescribed, to reduce hypertension. Observe for and report new onset of neurologic deficits.
Postoperative hypotension	Treated with fluids (if suspected to be related to hypovolemia) and low-dose phenylephrine infusion (if occurs in normovolemia). Usually resolves in 24–48 h. Patients with hypotension should have serial electrocardiograms to rule out myocardial infarction.	Monitor blood pressure and observe for signs and symptoms of hypotension.
Hyperperfusion syndrome	Occurs when cerebral vessel autoregulation fails. Arteries accustomed to diminished blood flow may be permanently dilated; increased blood flow after endarterectomy coupled with insufficient vasoconstriction leads to capillary bed damage, edema, and hemorrhage. Typically occurs within 2 wks of surgery.	Observe for severe unilateral headache improved by sitting upright or standing. Monitor for any changes in level of consciousness or confusion.
Intracerebral hemorrhage	Occurs infrequently but is often fatal or results in serious neurologic impairment. Can occur secondary to hyperperfusion syndrome. Increased risk with advanced age, hypertension, presence of high-grade stenosis, poor collateral flow, and slow flow in the region of the middle cerebral artery.	Monitor neurologic status, and report any changes in mental status or neurologic functioning immediately.

Adapted from Rich, K., Treat-Jacobson, D., DeVeaux, T., et al; Society for Vascular Nursing Practice and Research Committee. (2017). Society for Vascular Nursing-carotid endarterectomy (CEA) updated nursing clinical practice guideline. *Journal of Vascular Nursing, 35*(2), 90–111.

(XI), and hypoglossal (XII). Some edema in the neck after surgery is expected; however, extensive edema and hematoma formation can obstruct the airway. Emergency airway supplies, including those needed for a tracheostomy, must be available (Rich, Treat-Jacobson, DeVeaux, et al., 2017). Table 62-5 provides more information about potential complications of carotid surgery.

Management after carotid stenting also requires monitoring of neurologic status and evaluation for hematoma formation (at the catheterization site). Cardiac monitoring is necessary with assessment for bilateral pulses distal to the catheterization site. Typically, patients are discharged the day after stenting if there are no complications (Rich et al., 2017).

NURSING PROCESS

The Patient Recovering from an Ischemic Stroke

The acute phase of an ischemic stroke may last 1 to 3 days, but ongoing monitoring of all body systems is essential as long as the patient requires care. The patient who has had a stroke is at risk for multiple complications, including deconditioning and other musculoskeletal problems, swallowing difficulties, bowel and bladder dysfunction, inability to perform self-care, and skin breakdown. Nursing management focuses on the prompt initiation of rehabilitation for any deficits.

Assessment

During the acute phase, a neurologic flow sheet is maintained to provide data about the following important measures of the patient's clinical status:

- Decrease in level of consciousness or responsiveness as evidenced by movement, resistance to changes of position, and response to stimulation; orientation to time, place, and person
- Change in vital signs with particular attention to blood pressure and temperature; maintenance of both within desired parameters
- Presence or absence of voluntary or involuntary movements of the extremities, muscle tone and strength, body posture, and position of the head
- Eye opening, comparative size of pupils and pupillary reactions to light, and ocular position
- Color of the face and extremities; temperature and moisture of the skin
- Quality and rates of pulse and respiration; arterial blood gas values as indicated, body temperature, and arterial pressure
- Ability to speak
- Volume of fluids ingested or given; volume of urine excreted each 24 hours
- Presence of bleeding
- Monitoring of continuous oxygen saturation
- Monitoring blood glucose

After the acute phase, the nurse assesses mental status (memory, attention span, perception, orientation, affect, speech/language), sensation/perception (the patient may have decreased awareness of pain and temperature), motor control (upper and lower extremity movement), swallowing ability, nutritional and hydration status, skin integrity, activity tolerance, and bowel and bladder function. Ongoing nursing assessment continues to focus on any impairment of function in the patient's daily activities, because the quality of life after stroke is closely related to the patient's functional status.

Diagnosis

NURSING DIAGNOSES

Based on the assessment data, major nursing diagnoses may include the following:

- Impaired mobility associated with hemiparesis, loss of balance and coordination, spasticity, and brain injury
- Acute pain (painful shoulder) associated with hemiplegia and disuse
- Impaired ability to perform hygiene, impaired self-toileting, impaired ability to dress, impaired self-feeding associated with stroke sequelae
- Discomfort associated with altered sensory reception, transmission, or integration
- Impaired swallowing
- Impaired urination associated with flaccid bladder, detrusor instability, confusion, or difficulty in communicating
- Constipation associated with change in mental status or difficulty communicating
- Acute confusion associated with brain infarction
- Impaired verbal communication associated with brain damage
- Risk for impaired skin integrity associated with to hemiparesis, hemiplegia, or decreased mobility
- Impaired family process associated with catastrophic illness and caregiving burdens
- Impaired sexual functioning associated with neurologic deficits or fear of failure

COLLABORATIVE PROBLEMS/POTENTIAL COMPLICATIONS

Potential complications may include the following:

- Decreased cerebral blood flow due to increased ICP
- Inadequate oxygen delivery to the brain
- Pneumonia
- Seizure

Planning and Goals

Although rehabilitation begins on the day the patient has the stroke, the process is intensified during convalescence and requires a coordinated team effort. It is helpful for the team to know what the patient was like before the stroke: their illnesses, abilities, mental and emotional state, behavioral characteristics, and activities of daily living. It is also helpful for clinicians to be knowledgeable about the relative importance of predictors of stroke outcome (age, NIHSS score, and level of consciousness at the time of admission) in order to provide survivors of stroke and their families with realistic goals (Powers et al., 2019).

The major goals for the patient (and family) may include improved mobility, avoidance of shoulder pain, achievement of self-care, relief of discomfort, prevention of aspiration, continence of bowel and bladder, decreasing confusion,

achieving a form of communication, maintaining skin integrity, restored family functioning, improved sexual function, and absence of complications.

Nursing Interventions

Nursing care has a significant impact on the patient's recovery. Often, many body systems are impaired as a result of the stroke, and conscientious care and timely interventions can prevent debilitating complications. During and after the acute phase, nursing interventions focus on the whole person. In addition to providing physical care, the nurse encourages and fosters recovery by listening to the patient and asking questions to elicit the meaning of the stroke experience.

IMPROVING MOBILITY AND PREVENTING JOINT DEFORMITIES

A patient with hemiplegia has unilateral paralysis (paralysis on one side). When control of the voluntary muscles is lost, the strong flexor muscles exert control over the extensors. The arm tends to adduct (adductor muscles are stronger than abductors) and rotate internally. The elbow and the wrist tend to flex, the affected leg tends to rotate externally at the hip joint and flex at the knee, and the foot at the ankle joint supinates and tends toward plantar flexion.

Correct positioning is important to prevent contractures; measures are used to relieve pressure, assist in maintaining good body alignment, and prevent compressive neuropathies, especially of the ulnar and peroneal nerves. Because flexor muscles are stronger than extensor muscles, a splint applied at night to the affected extremity may prevent flexion and maintain correct positioning during sleep.

Preventing Shoulder Adduction. To prevent adduction of the affected shoulder while the patient is in bed, a pillow is placed in the axilla when there is limited external rotation; this keeps the arm away from the chest. A pillow is placed under the arm, and the arm is placed in a neutral (slightly flexed) position, with distal joints positioned higher than the more proximal joints (i.e., the elbow is positioned higher than the shoulder and the wrist higher than the elbow). This helps to prevent edema and the resultant joint fibrosis that will limit range of motion if the patient regains control of the arm (see Fig. 62-3).

Positioning the Hand and Fingers. The fingers are positioned so that they are barely flexed. The hand is placed in slight supination (palm faces upward), which is its most functional position. If the upper extremity is flaccid, a splint can be used to support the wrist and hand in a functional position. If the upper extremity is spastic, a hand roll is not used, because

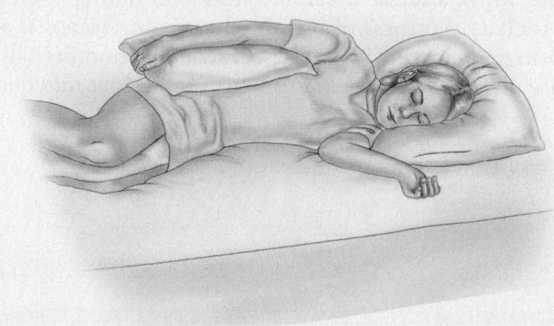

Figure 62-3 • Correct positioning to prevent shoulder adduction.

it stimulates the grasp reflex. In this instance, a dorsal wrist splint is useful in allowing the palm to be free of pressure. Every effort is made to prevent hand edema.

Spasticity, particularly in the hand, can be a disabling complication after stroke. Botulinum toxin type A injected intramuscularly into wrist and finger muscles has been shown to be effective in reducing this spasticity (although the effect is temporary, typically lasting 2 to 4 months). This treatment is also effective for treating lower limb spasticity (Sun, Chen, Fu, et al., 2019). Other treatments for spasticity may include stretching, splinting (in select patients), and oral medications such as baclofen and tizanidine (Teasell, Salbach, Foley, et al., 2020).

Changing Positions. The patient's position should be changed every 2 hours. To place a patient in a lateral (side-lying) position, a pillow is placed between the legs before the patient is turned. To promote venous return and prevent edema, the upper thigh should not be acutely flexed. The patient may be turned from side to side, but if sensation is impaired, the amount of time spent on the affected side should be limited.

If possible, the patient is placed in a prone position for 15 to 30 minutes several times a day. A small pillow or a support is placed under the pelvis, extending from the level of the umbilicus to the upper third of the thigh (see Fig. 62-4). This position helps promote hyperextension of the hip joints, which is essential for normal gait and helps prevent knee and hip flexion contractures. The prone position also helps drain bronchial secretions and prevents contractural deformities of the shoulders and knees. During positioning, it is important to reduce pressure and change position frequently to prevent pressure injuries.

Establishing an Exercise Program. The affected extremities are exercised passively and put through a full range of motion four or five times a day to maintain joint mobility, regain motor control, prevent contractures in the paralyzed extremity, prevent further deterioration of the neuromuscular system, and enhance circulation. Exercise is helpful in preventing venous stasis, which may predispose the patient to venous thromboembolism (VTE). VTE includes deep vein thrombosis (DVT) and pulmonary embolism (PE).

Repetition of an activity forms new pathways in the CNS and therefore encourages new patterns of motion. At first, the extremities are usually flaccid. If tightness occurs in any area, the range-of-motion exercises should be performed more frequently.

The patient is observed for signs and symptoms that may indicate PE or excessive cardiac workload during exercise; these include shortness of breath, chest pain, cyanosis, and increasing pulse rate with exercise. Frequent short periods of exercise always are preferable to longer periods at infrequent intervals. Regularity in exercise is most important. Improvement in muscle strength and maintenance of range of motion can be achieved only through daily exercise.

The patient is encouraged and reminded to exercise the unaffected side at intervals throughout the day. It is helpful to develop a written schedule to remind the patient of the exercise activities. The nurse supervises and supports the patient during these activities. The patient can be instructed to put the unaffected leg under the affected one to assist in moving it when turning and exercising. Flexibility, strengthening, coordination, endurance, and balancing exercises prepare the patient for ambulation. Quadriceps muscle setting and gluteal setting exercises (see Chapter 37, Chart 37-4) are started early to improve the muscle strength needed for walking; these are performed at least five times daily for 10 minutes at a time.

Preparing for Ambulation. As soon as possible, the patient is assisted out of bed and an active rehabilitation program is started. The patient is first educated to maintain balance while sitting and then to learn to balance while standing. If the patient has difficulty in achieving standing balance, a tilt table, which slowly brings the patient to an upright position, can be used. Tilt tables are especially helpful for patients who have been on bed rest for prolonged periods and have orthostatic blood pressure changes.

If the patient needs a wheelchair, the folding type with hand brakes is the most practical because it allows the patient to manipulate the chair. The chair should be low enough to allow the patient to propel it with the uninvolved foot and narrow enough to permit it to be used at home. When the patient is transferred from the wheelchair, the brakes must be applied and locked on both sides of the chair.

The patient is usually ready to walk as soon as standing balance is achieved. Parallel bars are useful in these first efforts. A chair or wheelchair should be readily available in case the patient suddenly becomes fatigued or feels dizzy.

The training periods for ambulation should be short and frequent. As the patient gains strength and confidence, an adjustable cane can be used for support. In general, a three- or four-pronged cane provides a stable support in the early phases of rehabilitation.

PREVENTING SHOULDER PAIN

The incidence of shoulder pain after stroke can vary widely, but has been measured to be as high as 84% (Zhou, Li, Lu, et al., 2018). That pain may prevent patients from learning new skills and affect their quality of life. Shoulder function is essential in achieving balance and performing transfers and self-care activities. Problems that can occur include rotator cuff disorders, spasticity of the shoulder muscles, painful shoulder, subluxation of the shoulder, and shoulder–hand syndrome. Development of a condition known as central pain syndrome may also contribute to the development of shoulder pain after a stroke.

A flaccid shoulder joint may be overstretched by the use of excessive force in turning the patient or from overstrenuous arm and shoulder movement. To prevent shoulder pain, the nurse should never lift the patient by the flaccid shoulder or pull on the affected arm or shoulder. Overhead pulleys should also be avoided. If the arm is paralyzed, subluxation (incomplete dislocation) at the shoulder can occur as a result

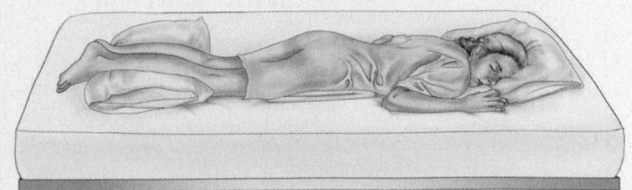

Figure 62-4 • Prone position with pillow support helps prevent hip flexion.

of overstretching of the joint capsule and musculature by the force of gravity when the patient sits or stands in the early stages after a stroke. This results in severe pain. Shoulder–hand syndrome (painful shoulder and generalized swelling of the hand) can cause a frozen shoulder and ultimately atrophy of subcutaneous tissues. When a shoulder becomes stiff, it is usually painful.

Many shoulder problems can be prevented by proper patient movement and positioning. The flaccid arm is positioned on a table or with pillows while the patient is seated. A sling maybe worn on the flaccid arm when the patient first becomes ambulatory, to prevent the paralyzed upper extremity from dangling without support. Range-of-motion exercises are important in preventing painful shoulder. Overstrenuous arm movements are avoided. The patient is instructed to interlace the fingers, place the palms together, and push the clasped hands slowly forward to bring the scapulae forward; the patient then raises both hands above the head. This is repeated throughout the day. The patient is instructed to flex the affected wrist at intervals and move all the joints of the affected fingers. The patient is encouraged to touch, stroke, rub, and look at both hands. Pushing the heel of the hand firmly down on a surface is useful. Elevation of the arm and hand is also important in preventing dependent edema of the hand. Patients with continuing pain after attempted movement and positioning may require the addition of analgesia to their treatment program. Other treatments may include injections to the shoulder joint with corticosteroid medications or botulinum toxin type A, shoulder taping/strapping, acupuncture, electrical stimulation, heat or ice, and soft tissue massage (Teasell et al., 2020; Treister, Hatch, Cramer, et al., 2017).

Medications are often helpful in the management of post-stroke pain. The medications that are used include amitriptyline, gabapentin, lamotrigine, and pregabalin (Teasell et al., 2020; Treister et al., 2017).

ENHANCING SELF-CARE

As soon as the patient can sit up, they are encouraged to participate in personal hygiene activities. The patient is helped to set realistic goals; if feasible, a new task is added daily. The first step is to carry out all self-care activities on the unaffected side. Such activities as combing the hair, brushing the teeth, shaving with an electric razor, bathing, and eating can be carried out with one hand and should be encouraged. Although the patient may feel awkward at first, these motor skills can be learned by repetition, and the unaffected side will become stronger with use. The nurse must be sure that the patient does not neglect the affected side. Assistive devices will help make up for some of the patient's deficits (see Chart 62-3). A small towel is easier to control while drying after bathing, and boxed paper tissues are easier to use than a roll of toilet tissue.

Return of functional ability is important to the patient recovering after a stroke. An early baseline assessment of functional ability with an instrument such as the Functional Independence Measure (FIM™) is important in team planning and goal setting for the patient. The FIM™ is a widely used instrument in stroke rehabilitation and provides valuable information about motor, social, and cognitive function. The patient's morale may improve if ambulatory activities are carried out in street clothes. The family is instructed to bring in clothing that is preferably a size larger than that usually

---

Chart 62-3 · Assistive Devices to Enhance Self-Care After Stroke

Bathing and Grooming Devices

- Electric razors with head at 90 degrees to handle
- Grab bars, nonskid mats, handheld shower heads
- Long-handled bath sponge
- Shower and tub seats, stationary or on wheels

Dressing Aids

- Elastic shoelaces
- Long-handled shoehorn
- Velcro closures

Eating Devices

- Nonskid mats to stabilize plates
- Plate guards to prevent food from being pushed off plate
- Wide-grip utensils to accommodate a weak grasp

Mobility Aids

- Canes, walkers, wheelchairs
- Transfer devices such as transfer boards and belts

Toileting Aids

- Grab bars next to toilet
- Raised toilet seat

---

worn. Clothing fitted with front or side fasteners or Velcro closures is the most suitable. The patient has better balance if most of the dressing activities are carried out while seated.

Perceptual problems may make it difficult for the patient to dress without assistance because of an inability to match the clothing to the body parts. To assist the patient, the nurse can take steps to keep the environment organized and uncluttered, because the patient with a perceptual problem is easily distracted. The clothing is placed on the affected side in the order in which the garments are to be put on. The use of a large mirror while dressing promotes the patient's awareness of what they are putting on the affected side. The patient has to make many compensatory movements when dressing; these can produce fatigue and painful twisting of the intercostal muscles. Support and encouragement are provided to prevent the patient from becoming overly fatigued and discouraged. Even with intensive training, not all patients can achieve independence in dressing.

ADJUSTING TO PHYSICAL CHANGES

Patients with a decreased field of vision should be approached on the side where visual perception is intact. All visual stimuli (e.g., clock, calendar, television) should be placed on this side. The patient can be educated to turn the head in the direction of the defective visual field to compensate for this loss. The nurse should make eye contact with the patient and draw their attention to the affected side by encouraging the patient to move the head. The nurse may also want to stand at a position that encourages the patient to move or turn to visualize who is in the room. Increasing the natural or artificial lighting in the room and providing eyeglasses are important aids to increasing vision.

The patient with homonymous hemianopsia turns away from the affected side of the body and tends to neglect that side and the space on that side; this is known as amorphosynthesis. In such instances, the patient cannot see food on half of the tray, and only half of the room is visible. It is important for the nurse to constantly remind the patient of the other side of the body; to maintain alignment of the extremities; and, if possible, to place the extremities where the patient can see them.

ASSISTING WITH NUTRITION

Stroke can result in **dysphagia** (difficulty swallowing) due to impaired function of the mouth, tongue, palate, larynx, pharynx, or upper esophagus. Patients must be observed for paroxysms of coughing, food dribbling out of or pooling in one side of the mouth, food retained for long periods in the mouth, or nasal regurgitation when swallowing liquids. Swallowing difficulties place the patient at risk for aspiration, pneumonia, dehydration, and malnutrition.

A swallow assessment should be performed as soon as possible after the patient's arrival to the ED (preferably within 4 to 24 hours). This is done before allowing any oral intake. A speech therapist will evaluate the patient's swallowing ability, but an assessment may also be done by the nurse using a validated and reliable assessment tool (Stroke Foundation, 2019).

If swallowing function is partially impaired, it may return over time, or the patient may be educated in alternative swallowing techniques, advised to take smaller boluses of food, and educated about types of foods that are easier to swallow. The patient may be started on a thick liquid or pureed diet, because these foods are easier to swallow than thin liquids. Having the patient sit upright, preferably out of bed in a chair, and instructing them to tuck the chin toward the chest as they swallow will help prevent aspiration. The diet may be advanced as the patient becomes more proficient at swallowing. If the patient cannot resume oral intake, a gastrointestinal feeding tube is placed for ongoing tube feedings and medication administration.

Enteral tubes can be either nasogastric (placed in the stomach) or nasoenteral (placed in the duodenum) to reduce the risk of aspiration. Nursing responsibilities in feeding include elevating the head of the bed at least 30 degrees to prevent aspiration, checking the position of the tube before feeding, ensuring that the cuff of the tracheostomy tube (if in place) is inflated, and giving the tube feeding slowly. The feeding tube is aspirated periodically to ensure that the feedings are passing through the gastrointestinal tract. Retained or residual feedings increase the risk of aspiration. Patients with retained feedings may benefit from the placement of a gastrostomy tube or a percutaneous endoscopic gastrostomy (PEG) tube. In a patient with a feeding tube, the tube should be placed in the duodenum to reduce the risk of aspiration. For long-term feedings, a gastrostomy tube is preferred (see Chapter 39).

ATTAINING BLADDER AND BOWEL CONTROL

After a stroke, the patient may have transient urinary incontinence due to confusion, inability to communicate needs, and inability to use the urinal or bedpan because of impaired motor and postural control. Occasionally after a stroke, the bladder becomes atonic, with impaired sensation in response to bladder filling. Sometimes, control of the external urinary sphincter is lost or diminished. During this period, intermittent catheterization with sterile technique is carried out.

After muscle tone increases and deep tendon reflexes return, bladder tone increases and spasticity of the bladder may develop. Because the patient's sense of awareness is clouded, persistent urinary incontinence or urinary retention may be symptomatic of bilateral brain damage. The voiding pattern is analyzed, and the urinal or bedpan is offered on this pattern or schedule. The upright posture and standing position are helpful for male patients during this aspect of rehabilitation.

Patients may have problems with bowel control, particularly constipation. Unless contraindicated, a high-fiber diet and adequate fluid intake (2 to 3 L/day) should be provided, and a regular time (usually after breakfast) should be established for toileting.

IMPROVING THOUGHT PROCESSES

After a stroke, the patient may have problems with cognitive, behavioral, and emotional deficits related to brain damage. However, in many instances, a considerable degree of function can be recovered, because not all areas of the brain are equally damaged; some remain more intact and functional than others.

After assessment that delineates the patient's deficits, the neuropsychologist, in collaboration with the primary provider, psychiatrist, nurse, and other professionals, structures a training program using cognitive-perceptual retraining, visual imagery, reality orientation, and cueing procedures to compensate for losses. Specific techniques used maybe conventional, computer-assisted, or virtual reality based.

The role of the nurse is supportive. The nurse reviews the results of neuropsychological testing; observes the patient's performance and progress; gives positive feedback; and, most importantly, conveys an attitude of confidence and hope. Interventions capitalize on the patient's strengths and remaining abilities while attempting to improve performance of affected functions. Other interventions are similar to those for improving cognitive functioning after a head injury (see Chapter 63).

IMPROVING COMMUNICATION

Aphasia, which impairs the ability to express oneself and to understand what is being said, may become apparent in various ways. The cortical area that is responsible for integrating the myriad pathways required for the comprehension and formulation of language is called *Broca area*. It is located in a convolution adjoining the middle cerebral artery. This area is responsible for control of the combinations of muscular movements needed to speak each word. Broca area is so close to the left motor area that a disturbance in the motor area often affects the speech area. This is why so many patients who are paralyzed on the right side (due to damage or injury to the left side of the brain) cannot speak, whereas those paralyzed on the left side are less likely to have speech disturbances.

The speech therapist assesses the communication needs of the patient who has had a stroke, describes the precise deficit, and suggests the best overall method of communication. Most language intervention strategies can be tailored for the individual patient. The patient is expected to take an active part in establishing goals.

A person with aphasia may become depressed. The inability to talk on the telephone, text, answer a question, or participate in conversation often causes anger, frustration, fear of the future, and hopelessness. Nursing interventions include strategies to make the atmosphere conducive to communication.

This includes being sensitive to the patient's reactions and needs and responding to them in an appropriate manner while always treating the patient as an adult. The nurse provides strong emotional support and understanding to allay anxiety and frustration.

A common pitfall is for the nurse or other health care team member to complete the thoughts or sentences of the patient. This should be avoided, because it causes the patient to become more frustrated at not being allowed to speak and may deter efforts to practice putting thoughts together and completing sentences. A consistent schedule, routines, and repetition help the patient to function despite significant deficits. A written copy of the daily schedule, a folder of personal information (birth date, address, names of relatives), checklists, and recorded lists help improve the patient's memory and concentration. The patient may also benefit from a communication board (electronic or written), which has pictures of common needs and phrases. The board may be translated into any language.

When talking with the patient, it is important for the nurse to gain the patient's attention, speak slowly, and keep the language of instruction consistent. One instruction is given at a time, and time is allowed for the patient to process what has been said. The use of gestures may enhance comprehension. Speaking is thinking out loud, and the emphasis is on thinking. Listening and sorting out incoming messages require mental effort; the patient must struggle against mental inertia and needs time to organize a response.

In working with the patient with aphasia, the nurse must remember to talk to the patient during care activities. This provides social contact for the patient. Chart 62-4 describes points to keep in mind when communicating with the patient with aphasia.

MAINTAINING SKIN INTEGRITY

The patient who has had a stroke may be at risk for skin and tissue breakdown because of altered sensation and inability to respond to pressure and discomfort by turning and moving. Preventing skin and tissue breakdown requires frequent assessment of the skin, with emphasis on bony areas and dependent parts of the body. During the acute phase, a specialty bed (e.g., low air-loss bed) may be used until the patient can move independently or assist in moving.

A regular turning schedule (e.g., every 2 hours) is adhered to, even if pressure-relieving devices are used to prevent tissue and skin breakdown. When the patient is positioned or turned, care must be used to minimize shear and friction forces, which cause damage to tissues and predispose the skin to breakdown.

The patient's skin must be kept clean and dry; gentle massage of healthy (nonreddened) skin and adequate nutrition are other factors that help to maintain skin and tissue integrity.

IMPROVING FAMILY COPING

Family members play an important role in the patient's recovery. Family members are encouraged to participate in counseling and to use support systems that will help with the emotional and physical stress of caring for the patient. Involving others in the patient's care and providing education about stress management techniques and methods for maintaining personal health also facilitate family coping.

The family may have difficulty accepting the patient's disability and may be unrealistic in their expectations. They are given information about the expected outcomes and are counseled to avoid doing activities that the patient is able to do. They are assured that their love and interest are part of the patient's therapy.

The family needs to be informed that the rehabilitation of the patient with hemiplegia requires many months and that progress may be slow. The gains made by the patient in the hospital or rehabilitation unit must be maintained. All caregivers should approach the patient with a supportive and optimistic attitude, focusing on the patient's remaining abilities. The rehabilitation team, the medical and nursing team, the patient, and the family must all be involved in developing attainable goals for the patient at home.

Most relatives of patients with stroke handle the physical changes better than the emotional aspects of care. The family should be prepared to expect occasional episodes of emotional lability. The patient may laugh or cry easily or without cause (pseudobulbar affect) and may be irritable and demanding or depressed and confused. The nurse can explain to the family that the patient's laughter does not necessarily connote happiness, nor does crying reflect sadness, and that emotional lability usually improves with time.

Family-centered care involves seeing patients and family caregivers as a one unit. Nurses can assess caregivers' strengths and ability to provide care. This assessment should be a continual process because needs change throughout the hospitalization period and rehabilitation stay. Providing information about community resources, respite care and adult day care, and mental health issues (for the patient who has had a stroke and for caregivers) will help with the transition to home.

HELPING THE PATIENT COPE WITH SEXUAL DYSFUNCTION

Sexual functioning can be profoundly altered by stroke. Although research in this area of stroke management is limited, it appears that patients who have had a stroke consider sexual function important, and many have sexual dysfunction. Sexual dysfunction after stroke is multifactorial. There may be medical reasons for the dysfunction (neurologic and cognitive deficits, previous diseases, medications) as well as various psychosocial factors, including depression. A stroke is such a catastrophic illness that the patient experiences loss

---

Chart 62-4

Communicating with the Patient with Aphasia

- Face the patient and establish eye contact.
- Speak in a clear, unhurried manner, and normal tone of voice.
- Use short phrases, and pause between phrases to allow the patient time to understand what is being said.
- Limit conversation to practical and concrete matters.
- Use gestures, pictures, objects, and writing.
- As the patient uses and handles an object, say what the object is. It helps to match the words with the object or action.
- Be consistent in using the same words and gestures each time you give instructions or ask a question.
- Keep extraneous noises and sounds to a minimum. Too much background noise can distract the patient or make it difficult to sort out the message being spoken.

of self-esteem and value as a sexual being. These psychosocial factors play an important role in determining sexual drive, activity, and satisfaction after a stroke.

Nurses in the rehabilitation setting play a crucial role in beginning a dialogue between the patient and their partner about sexuality after a stroke. In-depth assessments to determine sexual history before and after the stroke should be followed by appropriate interventions. Interventions for the patient and partner focus on providing relevant information, education, reassurance, adjustment of medications, counseling regarding coping skills, suggestions for alternative sexual positions, and a means of sexual expression and satisfaction.

MONITORING AND MANAGING POTENTIAL COMPLICATIONS

Decreased cerebral blood flow due to increased ICP, leading to inadequate oxygen delivery to the brain, seizures, and pneumonia are potential complications in any patient who has had an ischemic stroke. The more severe the stroke (i.e., the higher the NIHSS), the greater the risk of complications.

During the acute phase of care, a neurologic flow sheet (see Chapter 61, Fig. 61-6) is used to monitor and document assessment parameters. Changes in blood pressure, pulse, and respiration are important clinically because they suggest increased ICP and are reported immediately. If signs and symptoms of pneumonia develop, cultures are obtained to identify the organism so that appropriate antibiotic agents can be given.

PROMOTING HOME, COMMUNITY-BASED, AND TRANSITIONAL CARE

Educating Patients About Self-Care. Patient and family education is a fundamental component of stroke recovery. The nurse provides education about stroke, its causes and prevention, and the rehabilitation process. In both acute care and rehabilitation facilities, the focus is on educating the patient to resume as much self-care as possible. This may entail using assistive devices or modifying the home environment to help the patient live with a disability.

An occupational therapist may be helpful in assessing the home environment and recommending modifications to help the patient become more independent. For example, a shower is more convenient than a tub for the patient with hemiplegia because most patients do not gain sufficient strength to get up and down from a tub. Sitting on a stool of medium height with rubber suction tips allows the patient to wash with greater ease. A long-handled bath brush with a soap container is helpful to the patient who has only one functional hand. If a shower is not available, a stool may be placed in the tub and a portable shower hose attached to the faucet. Hand rails may be attached alongside the bathtub and the toilet. Other assistive devices include special utensils for eating, grooming, dressing, and writing (see Chart 62-3).

A program of physical therapy can be beneficial, whether it takes place in the home or in an outpatient program. Constraint-induced movement therapy has been used in stroke rehabilitation and involves constraint of the less affected upper limb, and intensely training the more affected limb. Robotic-assisted therapy uses sensorimotor training of the upper limb. This method allows patients to train without the presence of a therapist. Other techniques may include using virtual reality and video game applications, functional/neuromuscular/transcutaneous electrical nerve stimulation, transcranial magnetic stimulation, and ambulation with body weight support and treadmill training to assist with recovery (Veteran's Administration/Department of Defense, The Management of Stroke Rehabilitation Work Group, 2019).

CONTINUING AND TRANSITIONAL CARE

A variety of transitional care models are being used in patients with stroke. Some evidence supports positive outcomes using transitional care but more research and standardization of interventions is needed for confirmation. One model currently being investigated is a person-centered model. This model includes a telephone call at 2, 30, and 60 days after discharge. Calls are conducted either by a nurse or an advanced practice provider. Patients are also seen in the outpatient clinic within 2 weeks after discharge (Bushnell, Duncan, Lycan, et al., 2018). Depending on the specific neurologic deficits resulting from the stroke, the patient at home may require the services of a number of health care professionals. The nurse often coordinates the care of the patient at home and considers the many educational needs of caregivers and patients. The family (often the spouse) requires education as well as assistance in planning and providing care.

The family is advised that the patient may tire easily, may become irritable and upset by small events, and may be less interested in events than expected. Emotional problems associated with stroke are often related to speech dysfunction and the frustrations of being unable to communicate. A speech therapist allows the family to be involved and gives the family practical instructions to help the patient between therapy sessions.

Depression is a common and serious problem (increases mortality) in the patient who has had a stroke. Approximately one third of patients who have had a stroke will suffer from depression (Virani et al., 2020). Risk factors include gender (more prevalent in women), a history of depression, cognitive or physical impairment, anxiety, aphasia and stroke severity (Villa, Ferrari, & Moretti, 2018). Because the length of hospital stays has shortened, depression may not be identified in the acute setting. Nurses in all care settings should identify patients who may be at risk for depression or who show depressive symptoms. In the home or in the rehabilitation setting, nurses may be involved in coordinating care and referring patients and family to appropriate resources. The family can help by continuing to support the patient and by giving positive reinforcement for the progress that is being made. Antidepressant therapy may be prescribed, and may help with recovery from stroke (Elzib, Pawloski, Ding, et al., 2019).

Community-based stroke support groups may allow the patient and family to learn from others with similar problems and to share their experiences. Support groups take the form of in-person meetings as well as Internet-based support programs. The patient is encouraged to continue hobbies and recreational and leisure interests and to maintain contact with friends to prevent social isolation. All nurses coming in contact with the patient should encourage the patient to keep active, adhere to the exercise program, and remain as self-sufficient as possible.

Chart 62-5 NURSING RESEARCH PROFILE
Early Identification of Depression in Caregivers of Stroke Survivors

Byun, E., Evans, L., Sommers, M., et al. (2019). Depressive symptoms in caregivers immediately after stroke. *Topics in Stroke Rehabilitation*, *26*(3), 187–194.

Purpose

In the early weeks post stroke, caregivers face many challenges and increased stress related to caring for a stroke survivor. Recognizing those caregivers most at risk for developing depression early after hospital discharge may lead to decreased symptoms and improved health and quality of life for caregivers. The long-term health of caregivers of stroke survivors is significant; poor health can impact their ability to serve in the capacity of caregiver. The purpose of this study was to identify characteristics of caregivers and stroke survivors associated with caregiver depressive symptoms in the early weeks following a family member's stroke.

Design

This study used a prospective, longitudinal exploratory design. The participants were a convenience sample of 63 caregivers of older adult stroke survivors who had been diagnosed with a new or recurrent ischemic or hemorrhagic stroke within the past 2 weeks. They were recruited from urban acute care settings. Caregivers were enrolled in the study by 2 weeks post stroke (T1) and then revisited 4 weeks later (T2). Symptoms of depression were measured using the Patient Health Questionnaire (PHQ-9). The PHQ-9 is a 9-item scale used as a screening tool for major and minor depression. Uncertainty, stress, coping capacity, social support, chronic illness, and sociodemographic information were measured. Perceived stress was measured with the Perceived Stress Scale. Physiologic stress was measured by salivary cortisol levels measured upon waking and in the evening. The stroke survivor's functional status was measured using the Barthel Index, a 10-item scale measuring functional status. Sociodemographic information and clinical characteristics (severity of stroke,

description of stroke, presence of communication disability, and days post stroke) of the stroke survivors were also collected.

Findings

This study began with 63 caregivers enrolled. By the second time point evaluation (T2), 13 stroke survivors had died, 3 caregivers withdrew from the study, and 7 more were lost to follow-up. A total of 40 caregivers completed the second time point evaluation (T2). Ages of caregivers ranged from 30 to 89 years (mean 56.92 years). Ages of stroke survivors ranged from 65 to 95 years (mean 75.92 years). More than half (57%) of caregivers had at least mild depressive symptoms in the early weeks of caregiving. Six weeks after the stroke, 40% continued to have depressive symptoms. About 30% had at least moderate depressive symptoms at both time points (T1 and T2). Greater depressive symptoms were correlated with elevated salivary cortisol levels in the evening but not with levels upon waking. Characteristics associated with more depressive symptoms across the first 6 weeks post stroke included caregiver uncertainty, perceived stress, coping, social support, race, income, time spent in caregiving, and stroke survivor race and functional status.

Nursing Implications

This study found that depressive symptoms in this sample of caregivers were common in the early weeks of caregiving. It is important for nurses to understand the caregiving experience and the risk in both patients and caregivers for developing depression. Clearly identifying characteristics that are associated with caregivers developing depression can help with earlier recognition of those at risk. If these caregivers receive appropriate interventions and additional support soon after hospital discharge, they may experience decreased depressive symptoms and improved quality of life. Nurses should be involved in the discharge process to home and can help caregivers adjust and be prepared for their new role and challenges.

The nurse should recognize the potential effects of caregiving on the family. Not all families have the adaptive coping skills and adequate psychological functioning necessary for the long-term care of another person. The patient's spouse may be older, with their own health concerns; in some instances, the patient may have been the provider of care to the spouse. A spouse may have to take on new roles and responsibilities in the relationship and around the home. Spouses may also feel a sense of loss (of freedom and leisure time as well as of the marital relationship) and may experience social isolation and financial burdens. Depression is common in caregivers of patients who have survived a stroke, with rates globally documented as approximately 40% (Loh, Tan, Zhang, et al., 2017). Nurses should assess caregivers for signs and symptoms of depression (Byun, Evans, Sommers, et al., 2019). See the Nursing Research Profile in Chart 62-5.

Caregivers may require reminders to attend to their own health concerns and well-being. Even healthy caregivers may find it difficult to maintain a schedule that includes being available around the clock. The nurse encourages the family to arrange for respite care services (planned short-term care to relieve the family from having to provide continuous 24-hour care), which may be available from an adult day care center. Some hospitals also offer weekend respite care that

can provide caregivers with needed time for themselves. The nurse involved in home and continuing care also needs to remind the patient and family of the need for respite care as well as continuing health promotion and screening practices.

Evaluation

Expected patient outcomes may include:
1. Achieves improved mobility
   a. Avoids deformities (contractures and footdrop)
   b. Participates in prescribed exercise program
   c. Achieves sitting balance
   d. Uses unaffected side to compensate for loss of function of hemiplegic side
2. Reports absence of shoulder pain
   a. Demonstrates shoulder mobility; exercises shoulder
   b. Elevates arm and hand at intervals
3. Achieves self-care; performs hygiene care; uses adaptive equipment
4. Demonstrates techniques to compensate for the discomfort of sensory deficits, such as turning the head to see people or objects
5. Demonstrates safe swallowing
6. Achieves usual pattern of bowel and bladder elimination
7. Participates in cognitive improvement program

8. Demonstrates improved communication
9. Maintains intact skin without breakdown
   a. Demonstrates skin turgor within normal limits
   b. Participates in turning and positioning activities
10. Family members demonstrate a positive attitude and coping mechanisms
    a. Encourage patient in exercise program
    b. Take an active part in rehabilitation process
    c. Contact respite care programs or arrange for other family members to assume some responsibilities for care
11. Develops alternative approaches to sexual expression
12. Absence of complications
    a. Has ICP values that remain within normal limits
    b. Has no signs and symptoms of pneumonia

Hemorrhagic Stroke

Hemorrhagic strokes are primarily caused by intracerebral (10%) and subarachnoid hemorrhage (3%) and are caused by bleeding into the brain tissue, the ventricles, or the subarachnoid space (Norris, 2019). Primary intracerebral hemorrhage from a spontaneous rupture of small vessels accounts for approximately 80% of hemorrhagic strokes and is caused chiefly by uncontrolled hypertension. Subarachnoid hemorrhage results from a ruptured intracranial aneurysm (discussed later in this chapter) (Hickey & Strayer, 2020; Virani et al., 2020).

A common cause of primary intracerebral hemorrhage in the older adult is cerebral amyloid angiopathy, which involves damage caused by the deposit of beta-amyloid protein in the small- and medium-sized blood vessels of the brain. Cerebral amyloid angiopathy makes these blood vessels fragile and prone to bleeding. Secondary intracerebral hemorrhage is associated with arteriovenous malformations (AVMs), trauma, intracranial neoplasms, or certain medications (e.g., anticoagulants, cocaine, or amphetamines). The mortality rate has been reported to be as high as 50% after an intracranial hemorrhage (Hickey & Strayer, 2020; Norris, 2019). Patients who survive the acute phase of care usually have more severe deficits and a longer recovery phase compared to those with ischemic stroke.

Pathophysiology

The pathophysiology of hemorrhagic stroke depends on the cause and underlying type of cerebrovascular disorder. Symptoms are produced when a primary hemorrhage, aneurysm, or AVM presses on nearby cranial nerves or brain tissue or, more dramatically, when an aneurysm or AVM ruptures, causing subarachnoid hemorrhage (hemorrhage into the cranial subarachnoid space). Normal brain metabolism is disrupted by the brain's exposure to blood; by an increase in ICP resulting from the sudden entry of blood into the subarachnoid space, which compresses and injures brain tissue; or by secondary ischemia of the brain resulting from the reduced perfusion pressure and vasospasm that frequently accompany subarachnoid hemorrhage.

Intracerebral Hemorrhage

An intracerebral hemorrhage, or bleeding into the brain tissue, is most common in patients with hypertension and cerebral atherosclerosis, because degenerative changes from these diseases cause rupture of the blood vessel. An intracerebral hemorrhage may also result from certain types of arterial pathology, trauma, brain tumors, and the use of medications (e.g., anticoagulants, amphetamines, and cocaine).

Bleeding related to hypertension occurs most commonly in the deeper structures of the brain (basal ganglia and thalamus); it occurs less frequently in the brainstem (mostly the pons) and cerebellum (Hickey & Strayer, 2020). Bleeding in the outer cerebral lobes (lobar hemorrhages) in those 75 or older can be related to cerebral amyloid angiopathy and is frequently in the frontal and parietal lobes. Occasionally, the bleeding ruptures the wall of the lateral ventricle and causes intraventricular hemorrhage, which is associated with poor outcomes and death (Hickey & Strayer, 2020)).

Intracranial (Cerebral) Aneurysm

An intracranial (cerebral) **aneurysm** is a dilation of the walls of a cerebral artery that develops as a result of weakness in the arterial wall. The cause of aneurysms is unknown, although research is ongoing. An aneurysm may be due to atherosclerosis, which results in a defect in the vessel wall with subsequent weakness of the wall; a congenital defect of the vessel wall; hypertensive vascular disease; head trauma; or advancing age.

Any artery within the brain can be the site of a cerebral aneurysm, but these lesions usually occur at the bifurcations of the large arteries at the circle of Willis (see Fig. 62-5). The cerebral arteries most commonly affected by an aneurysm are the internal carotid artery, anterior cerebral artery, anterior communicating artery, posterior communicating artery, posterior cerebral artery, and middle cerebral artery. Multiple cerebral aneurysms are not uncommon.

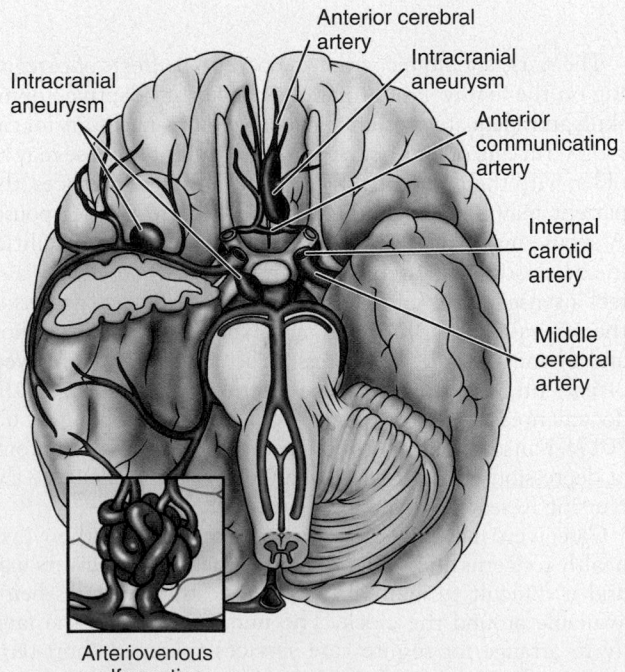

Figure 62-5 • Common sites of intracranial aneurysms and an arteriovenous malformation.

Arteriovenous Malformations

Most AVMs are caused by an abnormality in embryonal development that leads to a tangle of arteries and veins in the brain that lacks a capillary bed (see Fig. 62-5). The absence of a capillary bed leads to dilation of the arteries and veins and eventual rupture. AVM is a common cause of hemorrhagic stroke in young people (Hickey & Strayer, 2020).

Subarachnoid Hemorrhage

A subarachnoid hemorrhage (hemorrhage into the subarachnoid space) may occur as a result of an AVM, intracranial aneurysm, trauma, or hypertension. The most common causes are a leaking aneurysm in the area of the circle of Willis and a congenital AVM of the brain (Hickey & Strayer, 2020).

Clinical Manifestations

The patient with a hemorrhagic stroke can present with a wide variety of neurologic deficits, similar to the patient with ischemic stroke. The conscious patient most commonly reports a severe headache. A comprehensive assessment reveals the extent of the neurologic deficits. Many of the same motor, sensory, cranial nerve, cognitive, and other functions that are disrupted after ischemic stroke are also altered after a hemorrhagic stroke. Table 62-2 reviews the neurologic deficits frequently seen in patients who have had a stroke. Table 62-3 compares the symptoms seen in right hemispheric stroke with those seen in left hemispheric stroke. Other symptoms that may be observed more frequently in patients with acute intracerebral hemorrhage (compared with ischemic stroke) are nausea or vomiting, headache, an early sudden change in level of consciousness (confusion to coma), and possibly seizures.

In addition to the neurologic deficits (similar to those of ischemic stroke), the patient with an intracranial aneurysm or AVM may have some unique clinical manifestations. Rupture of an aneurysm or AVM usually produces a sudden, unusually severe headache and often loss of consciousness for a variable period of time. There may be pain and rigidity of the back of the neck (nuchal rigidity) and spine due to meningeal irritation. Visual disturbances (visual loss, diplopia, ptosis) occur if the aneurysm is adjacent to the oculomotor nerve. Tinnitus, dizziness, photophobia (visual intolerance of light), nausea or vomiting, and hemiparesis may also occur.

At times, an aneurysm or AVM leaks blood, leading to the formation of a clot that seals the site of rupture. In this instance, the patient may show little neurologic deficit. In other cases, severe bleeding occurs, resulting in cerebral damage, followed rapidly by coma and death.

Prognosis depends on the neurologic condition of the patient, the patient's age, associated diseases, and the extent and location of the hemorrhage or intracranial aneurysm. Subarachnoid hemorrhage from an aneurysm is a catastrophic event with significant morbidity and mortality.

Assessment and Diagnostic Findings

Any patient with suspected stroke should undergo a CT scan or MRI scan to determine the type of stroke, the size and location of the hematoma, and the presence or absence of ventricular blood and hydrocephalus. Because hemorrhagic stroke is an emergency, CT scan is usually obtained first because it can be done rapidly. Cerebral angiography using the conventional method or a CT angiography confirms the diagnosis of an intracranial aneurysm or AVM. These tests show the location and size of the lesion and provide information about the affected arteries, veins, adjoining vessels, and vascular branches. Lumbar puncture may be performed if there is no evidence of increased ICP, the CT scan results are negative, and subarachnoid hemorrhage must be confirmed. Lumbar puncture in the presence of increased ICP could result in brainstem herniation or rebleeding.

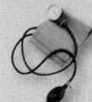 For the procedural guidelines for assisting with a lumbar puncture, go to **thepoint.lww.com/ Brunner15e**.

When diagnosing a hemorrhagic stroke in a patient younger than 40 years, some clinicians obtain a toxicology screen for illicit drug use.

Prevention

Primary prevention of hemorrhagic stroke is the best approach and includes managing hypertension and ameliorating other significant risk factors. Control of hypertension can reduce the risk of hemorrhagic stroke. Additional risk factors are increased age, male gender, certain ethnicities (Latino, African American, and Japanese) and moderate or excessive alcohol intake (Hickey & Strayer, 2020). Stroke risk screenings provide an ideal opportunity to lower hemorrhagic stroke risk by identifying individuals or groups at high risk and educating patients and the community about recognition and prevention.

Complications

Potential complications of hemorrhagic stroke include rebleeding or hematoma expansion; cerebral vasospasm resulting in cerebral ischemia; acute hydrocephalus, which results when free blood obstructs the reabsorption of cerebrospinal fluid (CSF) by the arachnoid villi; and seizures.

Cerebral Hypoxia and Decreased Blood Flow

Immediate complications of a hemorrhagic stroke include cerebral hypoxia, decreased cerebral blood flow, and extension of the area of injury. Providing adequate oxygenation of blood to the brain minimizes cerebral hypoxia. Brain function depends on delivery of oxygen to the tissues. Administering supplemental oxygen and maintaining the hemoglobin and hematocrit at acceptable levels will assist in maintaining tissue oxygenation.

Cerebral blood flow depends on the blood pressure, cardiac output, and integrity of cerebral blood vessels. Adequate hydration (IV fluids) must be ensured to reduce blood viscosity and improve cerebral blood flow. Extremes of hypertension or hypotension need to be avoided to prevent changes in cerebral blood flow and the potential for extending the area of injury.

A seizure can also compromise cerebral blood flow, resulting in further injury to the brain. Observing for seizure activity and initiating appropriate treatment are important components of care after a hemorrhagic stroke.

Vasospasm

The development of cerebral vasospasm (narrowing of the lumen of the involved cranial blood vessel) is a serious complication of subarachnoid hemorrhage and is a leading cause of morbidity and mortality in those who survive the initial subarachnoid hemorrhage. The mechanism responsible for vasospasm is not clear, but it is associated with increasing amounts of blood in the subarachnoid cisterns and cerebral fissures, as visualized by CT scan. Monitoring for vasospasm may be performed through the use of bedside transcranial Doppler ultrasonography or follow-up cerebral angiography (Connolly, Rabinstein, Carhuapoma, et al., 2012; Wilson, Ashcroft, & Troiani, 2019).

Vasospasm most frequently occurs 7 to 8 days after initial hemorrhage (American Association of Neuroscience Nurses [AANN], 2018), when the clot undergoes lysis (dissolution), and the chance of rebleeding is increased. It leads to increased vascular resistance, which impedes cerebral blood flow and causes brain ischemia (delayed cerebral ischemia) and infarction. Vasospasm can also occur 3 to 14 days after subarachnoid hemorrhage (Hickey & Strayer, 2020). Vasospasm is likely not the only factor that plays a role in the development of delayed cerebral ischemia. The signs and symptoms reflect the areas of the brain involved. Vasospasm is often heralded by a worsening headache, a decrease in level of consciousness (confusion, lethargy, and disorientation), or a new focal neurologic deficit (aphasia, hemiparesis).

Management of vasospasm remains difficult and controversial. It is believed that early surgery to clip the aneurysm prevents rebleeding and that removal of blood from the basal cisterns around the major cerebral arteries may prevent vasospasm.

Medication may be effective in the treatment and prevention of vasospasm. Based on the theory that vasospasm is caused by an increased influx of calcium into the cell, medication therapy may be used either to block or antagonize this action, or to prevent or reverse the action of vasospasm if already present. Nimodipine is the most studied calcium channel blocker for prevention of vasospasm in subarachnoid hemorrhage. Current guidelines recommend that nimodipine be prescribed for all patients with subarachnoid hemorrhage (Connolly et al., 2012). This is currently the only drug approved by the FDA for the prevention and treatment of vasospasm in subarachnoid hemorrhage.

Another therapy for vasospasm and the resulting delayed cerebral ischemia, referred to as triple-H therapy, is aimed at minimizing the deleterious effects of the associated cerebral ischemia and includes (1) fluid volume expanders (hypervolemia), (2) induced arterial hypertension, and (3) hemodilution. However, current research and guidelines now endorse euvolemia to prevent delayed cerebral ischemia and induced arterial hypertension for treatment of delayed cerebral ischemia (Connolly et al., 2012).

Increased Intracranial Pressure

An increase in ICP can occur after either an ischemic or a hemorrhagic stroke but almost always follows a subarachnoid hemorrhage, usually because of disturbed circulation of CSF caused by blood in the basal cisterns. Neurologic assessments are performed frequently, and if there is evidence of deterioration from increased ICP (due to cerebral edema, herniation, hydrocephalus, or vasospasm), CSF drainage may be instituted by ventricular catheter drainage (Hemphill, Greenberg, Anderson, et al., 2015). Mannitol may be administered to reduce ICP. When mannitol is used as a long-term measure to control ICP, dehydration and disturbances in electrolyte balance (hyponatremia or hypernatremia; hypokalemia or hyperkalemia) may occur. Mannitol pulls water out of the brain tissue by osmosis and reduces total body water through diuresis. The patient's fluid balance is monitored continuously and is assessed for signs of dehydration and for rebound elevation of ICP. Other interventions may include elevating the head of the bed to 30 to 45 degrees, avoidance of hyperglycemia and hypoglycemia, sedation, and use of hypertonic saline in a variety of concentrations (e.g., 3%, 7.5%, or 23%) (Hickey & Strayer, 2020).

Hypertension

Hypertension is the most common cause of intracerebral hemorrhage, and its treatment is critical. Specific goals for blood pressure management, which are individualized for each patient, remain controversial. Blood pressure goals may depend on the presence of increased ICP. Guidelines for management of intracerebral hemorrhage recommend early blood pressure lowering (if the systolic blood pressure is between 150 and 220 mm Hg) to a goal systolic of 140 mm Hg, and report that lowering blood pressure can be effective for improving patient outcomes. If systolic blood pressure is above 220 mm Hg, IV continuous infusions of antihypertensive agents may be prescribed (Hemphill et al., 2015). Nicardipine is one agent that may be used as a continuous IV infusion. Labetalol and hydralazine are other examples of medications that may be given as an IV bolus. During the administration of antihypertensive agents, hemodynamic monitoring is important to detect and avoid a precipitous drop in blood pressure, which can produce brain ischemia. Stool softeners are used to prevent straining, which can elevate the blood pressure.

Medical Management

The goals of medical treatment for hemorrhagic stroke are to allow the brain to recover from the initial insult (bleeding), to prevent or minimize the risk of rebleeding, and to prevent or treat complications. Management may consist of bed rest with sedation to prevent agitation and stress, management of vasospasm, and surgical or medical treatment to prevent rebleeding. If the bleeding is caused by anticoagulation with warfarin, the INR may be corrected with fresh-frozen plasma and vitamin K or prothrombin complex concentrations. Reversing the anticoagulation effect of DOACs requires use of an antidote. Idarucizumab is a medication that was approved for reversing dabigatran and andexanet alfa; it is an antidote for patients treated with rivaroxaban and apixaban; both are factor Xa inhibitors (Cordonnier, Demchuk, Ziai, et al., 2018). If seizures occur, they are treated with anti-epileptic drugs such as levetiracetam or phenytoin. Hyperglycemia should also be treated, and hypoglycemia is avoided. Intermittent pneumatic compression devices should be used starting on the first day of the hospital admission to prevent DVT. If the patient is not mobile after 1 to 4 days from the onset of the hemorrhage and there is documentation of the bleeding ceasing, then DVT prevention medications (low-molecular-weight heparin or unfractionated heparin) may be prescribed (Hemphill et al., 2015). Analgesic agents may be prescribed for head and neck pain. Fever should be treated with acetaminophen and devices such as cooling blankets. After discharge, most patients will require antihypertensive medications to decrease their risk of another intracerebral hemorrhage.

Surgical Management

In many cases, a primary intracerebral hemorrhage is not treated surgically. However, if the patient is showing signs of worsening neurologic examination, increased ICP, or signs of brainstem compression, then surgical evacuation is recommended for the patient with a cerebellar hemorrhage (Hemphill et al., 2015). Surgical evacuation is most frequently accomplished via a craniotomy (see Chapter 61). Minimally invasive surgical techniques have also been investigated.

The patient with an intracranial aneurysm is prepared for surgical intervention as soon as their condition is considered stable. Surgical treatment of the patient with an unruptured aneurysm is an option. The goal of surgery is to prevent bleeding in an unruptured aneurysm or further bleeding in an already ruptured aneurysm. This objective is accomplished by isolating the aneurysm from its circulation or by strengthening the arterial wall. An aneurysm may be excluded from the cerebral circulation by means of a ligature or a clip across its neck. If this is not anatomically possible, the aneurysm can be reinforced by wrapping it with some substance to provide support and induce scarring.

Advances in technology have led to the introduction of interventional neuroradiology for the treatment of aneurysms. These techniques are now being used more frequently. Endovascular techniques may be used in select patients to occlude the blood flow from the artery that feeds the aneurysm with coils, liquid embolic agents, or other techniques to occlude the aneurysm itself. If the aneurysm is very large or very wide at its neck, a stent-like device made of a very fine mesh may be used to divert the blood flow away from the aneurysm. The determination of which technique should be used is based on many factors (characteristics of the patient and aneurysm) and is made by experienced endovascular specialists (Connolly et al., 2012; Thompson, Brown, Amin-Hanjani, et al., 2015).

Postoperative complications are rare but can occur. Potential complications include psychological symptoms (disorientation, amnesia, Korsakoff syndrome), intraoperative embolization or artery rupture, postoperative artery occlusion, fluid and electrolyte disturbances (from dysfunction of the neurohypophyseal system), and gastrointestinal bleeding. Complications post procedurally may also include bleeding, hematoma, vascular complications, allergic reactions, and stroke.

NURSING PROCESS

The Patient with a Hemorrhagic Stroke

Assessment

A complete neurologic assessment is performed initially and includes evaluation for the following:
- Altered level of consciousness
- Sluggish pupillary reaction
- Motor and sensory dysfunction
- Cranial nerve deficits (extraocular eye movements, facial droop, presence of ptosis)
- Speech difficulties and visual disturbance

- Headache and nuchal rigidity or other neurologic deficits

All patients should be monitored in the intensive care unit after an intracerebral or subarachnoid hemorrhage. Neurologic assessment findings are documented and reported as indicated. The frequency of these assessments varies depending on the patient's condition. Any changes in the patient's condition require reassessment and thorough documentation; changes should be reported immediately.

 Concept Mastery Alert

Alteration in level of consciousness often is the earliest sign of deterioration in a patient with a hemorrhagic stroke. Because nurses have the most frequent contact with patients, they are in the best position to detect subtle changes. Drowsiness and slight slurring of speech may be early signs that the level of consciousness is deteriorating.

Diagnosis

NURSING DIAGNOSES

Based on the assessment data, major nursing diagnoses may include the following:
- Risk for ineffective tissue perfusion associated with bleeding or vasospasm
- Anxiety associated with illness or medically imposed restrictions (aneurysm precautions)

COLLABORATIVE PROBLEMS/POTENTIAL COMPLICATIONS

Potential complications may include the following:
- Vasospasm
- Seizures
- Hydrocephalus
- Rebleeding
- Hyponatremia

Planning and Goals

The goals for the patient may include improved cerebral tissue perfusion, relief of anxiety, and the absence of complications.

Nursing Interventions

OPTIMIZING CEREBRAL TISSUE PERFUSION

The patient is closely monitored for neurologic deterioration resulting from recurrent bleeding, increasing ICP, or vasospasm. A neurologic flow record is maintained. The blood pressure, pulse, level of consciousness (an indicator of cerebral perfusion), pupillary responses, and motor function are checked hourly. Respiratory status is monitored, because a reduction in oxygen in areas of the brain with impaired autoregulation increases the chances of a cerebral infarction. Any changes are reported immediately.

Implementing Aneurysm Precautions. Cerebral aneurysm precautions are implemented for the patient with a diagnosis of aneurysm (prior to any intervention) to provide a nonstimulating environment, prevent increases in ICP, and prevent further bleeding. The patient is placed on bed rest in a quiet, nonstressful environment, because activity, pain, and anxiety are thought to elevate the blood pressure, which may increase the risk for bleeding. Visitors may be restricted (AANN, 2018).

The head of the bed is elevated 30 to 45 degrees to promote venous drainage and decrease ICP. Any activity that suddenly increases the blood pressure or obstructs venous return is avoided. This includes the Valsalva maneuver, straining, forceful sneezing, pushing oneself up in bed, and acute flexion or rotation of the head and neck (which compromises the jugular veins). Stool softeners and mild laxatives are prescribed. Both prevent constipation, which can cause an increase in ICP. Dim lighting is helpful, because photophobia is common. The purpose of aneurysm precautions should be thoroughly explained to both the patient (if possible) and family. Intermittent pneumatic compression devices and unfractionated heparin or low-molecular weight heparin are prescribed to decrease the incidence of DVT resulting from immobility. The legs are observed for signs and symptoms of DVT (tenderness, redness, swelling, warmth, and edema), and abnormal findings are reported.

Relieving Anxiety

Sensory stimulation is kept to a minimum for patients on aneurysm precautions. For patients who are awake, alert, and oriented, an explanation of the restrictions helps reduce the patient's sense of isolation. Reality orientation is provided to help maintain orientation.

Keeping the patient well informed of the plan of care provides reassurance and helps minimize anxiety. Appropriate reassurance also helps relieve the patient's fears and anxiety. The family also requires information and support.

Monitoring and Managing Potential Complications

Vasospasm. The patient is assessed for signs of possible vasospasm: intensified headaches, a decrease in level of responsiveness (confusion, disorientation, lethargy), or evidence of aphasia or partial paralysis. These signs may develop several days after surgery or on the initiation of treatment and must be reported immediately. The calcium channel blocker nimodipine should be given for prevention of vasospasm, and fluid volume expanders in the form of triple-H therapy may be prescribed as well (Connolly et al., 2012).

Seizures. Seizure precautions are maintained for every patient who may be at risk for seizure activity. Should a seizure occur, maintaining the airway and preventing injury are the primary goals. Medication therapy is initiated at this time (see Chapter 61).

Hydrocephalus. Blood in the subarachnoid space or ventricles impedes the circulation of CSF, resulting in hydrocephalus. A CT scan that indicates dilated ventricles confirms the diagnosis. Hydrocephalus can occur within the first 24 hours (acute) after subarachnoid hemorrhage or several days (subacute) to several weeks (delayed) later. Symptoms vary according to the time of onset and may be nonspecific. Acute hydrocephalus is characterized by sudden onset of stupor or coma and is managed with a ventriculostomy drain to decrease ICP. Symptoms of subacute and delayed hydrocephalus include gradual onset of drowsiness, behavioral changes, and ataxic gait. A ventriculoperitoneal shunt is surgically placed to treat chronic hydrocephalus. Changes in patient responsiveness are reported immediately.

Rebleeding. The rate of recurrent hemorrhage is approximately 1% to 5% per patient per year after intracerebral hemorrhage (Hemphill et al., 2015). Hypertension is the most serious and modifiable risk factor, which shows the importance of appropriate antihypertensive treatment.

Aneurysm rebleeding is the highest during the first 2 to 12 hours after the initial hemorrhage (Connolly et al., 2012) and is considered a major complication. Symptoms of rebleeding include sudden severe headache, nausea, vomiting, decreased level of consciousness, and neurologic deficit. Rebleeding is confirmed by CT scan. Blood pressure is carefully maintained with medications. The most effective preventive treatment is to secure the aneurysm if the patient is a candidate for surgery or endovascular treatment.

Hyponatremia. After subarachnoid hemorrhage, hyponatremia is found in 30% to 50% of patients (Wilson et al., 2019). Hyponatremia has been found to be associated with the onset of vasospasm (Connolly et al., 2012). Laboratory data must be checked frequently, and hyponatremia (defined as a serum sodium concentration less than 135 mEq/L) must be identified as early as possible. The patient's primary provider needs to be notified of a low serum sodium level that has persisted for 24 hours or longer. The patient is then evaluated for syndrome of inappropriate antidiuretic hormone (SIADH) or cerebral salt-wasting syndrome. SIADH is described in Chapter 10. Cerebral salt-wasting syndrome occurs when the kidneys are unable to conserve sodium and volume depletion results. The treatment most often is the use of IV hypertonic 3% saline.

Promoting Home, Community-Based, and Transitional Care

Educating Patients About Self-Care. The patient and family are provided with education that will enable them to cooperate with the care and restrictions required during the acute phase of hemorrhagic stroke and to prepare them to return home. Patient and family education includes information about the causes of hemorrhagic stroke and its possible consequences. In addition, the patient and family are informed about the medical treatments that are implemented, including surgical intervention if warranted, and the importance of interventions taken to prevent and detect complications (i.e., aneurysm precautions, close monitoring of the patient). Depending on the presence and severity of neurologic impairment and other complications resulting from the stroke, the patient may be transferred to a rehabilitation unit or center for additional patient and family education about strategies to regain self-care ability. Education addresses the use of assistive devices or modification of the home environment to help the patient live with the disability. Modifications of the home may be required to provide a safe environment.

Continuing and Transitional Care. The acute and rehabilitation phase of care focuses on obvious needs, issues, and deficits for the patient with a hemorrhagic stroke. The patient and family are reminded of the importance of following recommendations to prevent further hemorrhagic stroke and keeping follow-up appointments with health care providers for monitoring of risk factors. Referral for home, community-based, or transitional care may be warranted to assess the home environment and the ability of the patient and to ensure that the patient and family are able to manage at home. Home visits provide opportunities to monitor the physical and psychological status of the patient and the ability of the family to cope with any alterations in the patient's status. In addition, the home health nurse reminds the patient and family of the importance of continuing health promotion and screening practices. Chart 62-6 lists education for the patient recovering from a stroke.

HOME CARE CHECKLIST

Chart 62-6

The Patient Recovering from a Stroke

At the completion of education, the patient and/or caregiver will be able to:

- State the impact of the stroke on physiologic functioning, ADLs, IADLs, roles, relationships, and spirituality.
- State names, dose, side effects, frequency and schedule for all medications.
- State how to contact all members of the treatment team (e.g., health care providers, home care professionals, rehabilitation team, and durable medical equipment and supply vendor).
- State changes in lifestyle (e.g., diet, ADLs, IADLs, activity) necessary for recovery and health maintenance as applicable.
  - Demonstrate environmental modifications and adaptive techniques for accomplishing activities of daily living.
  - Demonstrate home exercises, the use of splints or orthotics, proper positioning, and frequent repositioning.
  - Identify safety measures to prevent falls.
  - Identify holistic interventions for pain management (e.g., positioning, distraction).
  - Describe procedures for maintaining skin integrity.
  - Demonstrate indwelling catheter care, if applicable. Describe a bowel and bladder elimination program as appropriate.
  - Verbalize dietary adjustments (e.g., thickened liquids, pureed diet, small frequent meals) during recovery.
  - Demonstrate swallowing techniques or care of enteral feeding tube.

- Identify psychosocial consequences of stroke (e.g., depression, emotional lability, frustration, fatigue) and appropriate interventions.
- Discuss measures to prevent subsequent strokes.
- Identify potential complications and discuss measures to prevent them (blood clots, aspiration, pneumonia, urinary tract infection, fecal impaction, skin breakdown, contracture).
- Relate how to reach primary provider with questions or complications.
- State time and date of follow-up medical appointments, therapy, and testing.
- Identify resources and other sources of support (e.g., friends, relatives, faith community).
- Identify the contact details for support services for patients and their caregivers/families.
- Identify the need for health promotion, disease prevention, and screening activities.
- Identify appropriate recreational or diversional activities.

Resources

See Chapter 2, Chart 2-6 for additional information about durable medical equipment and Chapter 7, Chart 7-6: Home Care Checklist: Managing Chronic Illness and Disability at Home.

ADLs, activities of daily living; IADLs, instrumental activities of daily living.

Evaluation

Expected patient outcomes may include:

1. Demonstrates stable neurologic status and vital signs and respiratory patterns within normal limits
   a. Is alert and oriented to time, place, and person
   b. Demonstrates understandable speech patterns and stable cognitive processes
   c. Demonstrates usual and equal strength, movement, and sensation of all four extremities
   d. Exhibits deep tendon reflexes and pupillary responses within normal limits
2. Exhibits reduced anxiety level
   a. States rationale for aneurysm precautions
   b. Exhibits clear thought processes
   c. Is less restless
   d. Exhibits absence of physiologic indicators of anxiety (e.g., has vital signs within normal limits; usual respiratory rate; absence of excessive, fast speech)
3. Is free of complications
   a. Exhibits absence of vasospasm
   b. Exhibits vital signs within normal limits and is without seizures
   c. Verbalizes understanding of seizure precautions
   d. Exhibits intact mental, motor, and sensory status
   e. Reports no visual changes

Veterans Considerations

Each year, an estimated 15,000 veterans are hospitalized with a stroke-related diagnosis; of these, between 15% and 30% have severe impairment while 40% have some type of functional limitation (Veteran's Administration/Department of Defense, The Management of Stroke Rehabilitation Work Group, 2019). Care for the veteran who has had a stroke takes place in a variety of settings. There are 33 primary stroke centers, 32 limited hours stroke centers, 43 supporting stroke facilities, and 45 acute rehabilitation facilities within the Department of Veterans Affairs. Nurses who work with patients who have had strokes should be aware of these systems as they may need to assist the veteran and their family to facilitate transfer or referral to facilities that can best meet their health care needs.

CRITICAL THINKING EXERCISES

1 **PCS** A 61-year-old woman arrived in the ED and is being evaluated for suspected stroke. Her family reports that they last saw her normal 2 hours ago. What steps can you take to ensure rapid evaluation and treatment? What are your priorities for her care? If she is found to be eligible for t-PA and/or intra-arterial thrombolysis, how will your priorities change?

2 **IPEC** You are caring for a patient who experienced an ischemic stroke and now has visual loss (homonymous hemianopsia). What nursing interventions can be implemented at the bedside to assist the patient with this visual deficit? What education can be provided to the patient when they are ready for discharge, and what other disciplines would you collaborate with to ensure that the patient is safely discharged to home? What are the specific roles and responsibilities of those other professionals?

3 `ebp` A 74-year-old male patient has experienced a large left hemispheric ischemic stroke. He has just arrived to the nursing unit from the ED and you are his nurse. Your initial assessment reveals that he has a fever, and a finger stick is performed and shows an elevated blood glucose. Evaluate the strength of the evidence surrounding elevated temperature and elevated blood glucose in acute stroke. Is there any evidence supporting the use of hypothermia in acute stroke?

REFERENCES

*Asterisk indicates nursing research.
**Double asterisk indicates classic reference.

Books

American Association of Neuroscience Nurses (AANN). (2018). *Guide to the care of the patient with aneurysmal subarachnoid hemorrhage: AANN clinical practice guideline series.* Glenview, IL: Author.

Comerford, K. C., & Durkin, M. A. (2020). *Nursing 2020 drug handbook* (40th ed.). Philadelphia, PA: Wolters Kluwer.

Hickey, J. V., & Strayer, A. L. (2020). *The clinical practice of neurological & neurosurgical nursing* (8th ed.). Philadelphia, PA: Lippincott Williams & Wilkins.

Norris, T. L. (2019). *Porth's pathophysiology: Concepts of altered health state* (10th ed.). Philadelphia, PA: Wolters Kluwer.

Stroke Foundation. (2019). Clinical Guidelines for Stroke Management (Australian)—Chapter 3 of 8: Acute medical and surgical management. v7.0. Retrieved on 11/6/2019 at: informme.org.au/en/Guidelines/Clinical-Guidelines-for-Stroke-Management

Journals and Electronic Documents

Amatangelo, M. P., & Thomas, S. B. (2019). Priority nursing interventions caring for the stroke patient. *Critical Care Nursing Clinics of North America, 32*(1), 67–84.

Bushnell, C. D., Duncan, P. W., Lycan, S. L., et al. (2018). A person-centered approach to poststroke care: The COMprehensive post-acute stroke services model. *Journal of the American Geriatrics Society, 66*(5), 1025–1030.

*Byun, E., Evans, L., Sommers, M., et al. (2019). Depressive symptoms in caregivers immediately after stroke. *Topics in Stroke Rehabilitation, 26*(3), 187–194.

Connolly, E., Rabinstein, A., Carhuapoma, J., et al. (2012). Guidelines for the management of aneurysmal subarachnoid hemorrhage: A guideline for healthcare professionals from the American Heart Association/American Stroke Association. *Stroke, 43*(6), 1711–1737.

Cordonnier, C., Demchuk, A., Ziai, W., et al. (2018). Intracerebral haemorrhage: Current approaches to acute management. *Lancet, 392*(10154), 1257–1268.

**Del Zoppo, G. J., Saver, J. L., Jauch, E. C., et al; American Heart Association Stroke Council. (2009). Expansion of the time window for treatment of acute ischemic stroke with intravenous tissue plasminogen activator: A science advisory from the American Heart Association/American Stroke Association. *Stroke, 40*(8), 2945–2948.

Elzib, H., Pawloski, J., Ding, Y., et al. (2019). Antidepressant pharmacotherapy and poststroke motor rehabilitation: A review of neurophysiologic mechanisms and clinical relevance. *Brain Circulation, 5*(2), 62–67.

Hemphill, J. C., Greenberg, S. M., Anderson, C. S., et al. (2015). Guidelines for the management of spontaneous intracerebral hemorrhage: A guideline for healthcare professionals from the American Heart Association/American Stroke Association. *Stroke, 46*(7), 2032–2060.

Johnston, S. C., Easton, J. D., Farrant, M., et al; Clinical Research Collaboration, Neurological Emergencies Treatment Trials Network, and the POINT Investigators. (2018). Clopidogrel and aspirin in acute ischemic stroke and high-risk TIA. *The New England Journal of Medicine, 379*(3), 215–225.

Kernan, W. N., Ovbiagele, B., Black, H. R., et al. (2014). Guidelines for the prevention of stroke in patients with stroke and transient ischemic attack: A guideline for healthcare professionals from the American Heart Association/American Stroke Association. *Stroke, 45*(7), 2160–2236.

Loh, A. Z., Tan, J. S., Zhang, M. W., et al. (2017). The global prevalence of anxiety and depressive symptoms among caregivers of stroke survivors. *Journal of the American Medical Directors Association, 18*(2), 111–116.

Meschia, J. F., Bushnell, C., Boden-Albala, B., et al. (2014). Guidelines for the primary prevention of stroke: A statement for healthcare professionals from the American Heart Association/American Stroke Association. *Stroke, 45*(12), 3754–3832.

**National Institute of Neurologic Disorders and Stroke rt-PA Stroke Study Group. (1995). Tissue plasminogen activator for acute ischemic stroke. *The New England Journal of Medicine, 333*(24), 1581–1587.

National Institute of Neurological Disorders and Stroke (NINDS). (n.d.). NIH Stroke Scale. National Institutes of Health. National Institutes of Health Stroke Scale. Retrieved on 3/8/2020 at: www.ninds.nih.gov/sites/default/files/NIH_Stroke_Scale_Booklet.pdf

Oxley, T. J., Mocco, J., Majidi, S., et al. (2020). Large-vessel stroke as presenting feature of COVID-19 in the young. *The New England Journal of Medicine, 382*(20), e60. doi:10.1056/NEJMc2009987

Powers, W. J., Rabinstein, A. A., Ackerson, T., et al. (2019). Guidelines for the early management of patients with acute ischemic stroke: 2019 update to the 2018 guidelines for the early management of acute ischemic stroke: A guideline for healthcare professionals from the American Heart association/American Stroke Association. *Stroke, 50*(12), e344–e418.

Rich, K., Treat-Jacobson, D., DeVeaux, T., et al. (2017). Society for Vascular Nursing-carotid endarterectomy (CEA) updated nursing clinical practice guideline. *Journal of Vascular Nursing, 35*(2), 90–111.

**Saver, J. L. (2006). Time is brain quantified. *Stroke, 37*(1), 263–266.

Sun, L., Chen, R., Fu, C., et al. (2019). Efficacy and safety of botulinum toxin type A for limb spasticity after stroke: A meta-analysis of randomized controlled trials. *BioMed Research International.* doi:10.1155/2019/8329306

Teasell, R., Salbach, N. M., Foley, N., et al. (2020). Canadian stroke best practice recommendations: Rehabilitation, recovery, and community participation following stroke. Part one: Rehabilitation and recovery following stroke; 6th edition update 2019. *International Journal of Stroke, 15*(7), 763–788. doi:10.1177/1747493019897843

Thompson, B. G., Brown, R. J., Amin-Hanjani, S., et al. (2015). Guidelines for the management of patients with unruptured intracranial aneurysms: A guideline for healthcare professionals from the American Heart Association/American Stroke Association. *Stroke, 46*(8), 2368–2400.

Treister, A. K., Hatch, M. N., Cramer, S. C., et al. (2017). Demystifying poststroke pain: From etiology to treatment. *Physical Medicine and Rehabilitation, 9*(1), 63–75.

Veteran's Administration/Department of Defense, The Management of Stroke Rehabilitation Work Group. (2019). VA/DoD Clinical practice guideline for the management of stroke rehabilitation. Version 4.0. Retrieved on 3/9/2020 at: www.healthquality.va.gov/guidelines/Rehab/stroke/VADoDStrokeRehabCPGFinal8292019.pdf

Villa, R. F., Ferrari, F., & Moretti, A. (2018). Post-stroke depression: Mechanisms and pharmacological treatment. *Pharmacology & Therapeutics, 184*(2018), 131–144.

Virani, S. S., Alonso, A., Benjamin, E. J., et al. (2020). Heart disease and stroke statistics—2020 update: A report from the American Heart Association. *Circulation, 141*(9), e139–e596.

Wadman, M., Couzin-Frankel, J., Kaiser, J., et al. (2020). A rampage through the body. *Science, 386*(6489), 356–360.

Wilson, S. E., Ashcraft, S., & Troiani, L. (2019). Aneurysmal subarachnoid hemorrhage: Management by the advanced practice provider. *The Journal for Nurse Practitioners, 15*(8), 553–558.

Zhou, M., Li, F., Lu, W., et al. (2018). Efficiency of neuromuscular electrical stimulation and transcutaneous nerve stimulation on hemiplegic shoulder pain: A randomized controlled trial. *Archives of Physical Medicine and Rehabilitation, 99*(9), 1730–1739.

Resources

American Stroke Association, a Division of the American Heart Association, www.stroke.org

Brain Attack Coalition, www.brainattackcoalition.org

National Aphasia Association, www.aphasia.org

National Institute of Neurological Disorders and Stroke, www.ninds.nih.gov

63

Management of Patients with Neurologic Trauma

GLOSSARY

autonomic dysreflexia: a life-threatening emergency in patients with spinal cord injury that causes a hypertensive emergency (*synonym:* autonomic hyperreflexia)

complete spinal cord lesion: a condition that involves total loss of sensation and voluntary muscle control below the lesion

concussion: a temporary loss of neurologic function with no apparent structural damage to the brain

contusion: bruising of the brain surface

incomplete spinal cord lesion: a condition in which there is preservation of the sensory or motor fibers, or both, below the lesion

neurogenic bladder: bladder dysfunction that results from a disorder or dysfunction of the nervous system; may result in either urinary retention or bladder overactivity

paraplegia: paralysis of the lower extremities with dysfunction of the bowel and bladder from a lesion in the thoracic, lumbar, or sacral region of the spinal cord

primary injury: initial damage to the brain that results from the traumatic event

secondary injury: an insult to the brain subsequent to the original traumatic event

spinal cord injury (SCI): an injury to the spinal cord, vertebral column, supporting soft tissue, or intervertebral discs caused by trauma

tetraplegia: varying degrees of paralysis of both arms and legs, with dysfunction of bowel and bladder from a lesion of the cervical segments of the spinal cord; formerly called *quadriplegia*

transection: severing of the spinal cord; transection can be complete (all the way through the cord) or incomplete (partially through)

traumatic brain injury: an injury to the skull or brain that is severe enough to interfere with normal functioning (*synonym:* craniocerebral trauma)

traumatic brain injury, closed (blunt): occurs when the head accelerates and then rapidly decelerates or collides with another object and brain tissue is damaged, but there is no opening through the skull and dura

traumatic brain injury, open (penetrating): occurs when an object penetrates the skull, enters the brain, and damages the soft brain tissue in its path (penetrating injury), or when blunt trauma to the head is so severe that it opens the scalp, skull, and dura to expose the brain

Trauma involving the central nervous system can be life-threatening. Even if not life-threatening, brain and spinal cord injury (SCI) may result in major physical and psychological dysfunction and can alter the patient's life completely. Neurologic trauma affects the patient, the family, the health care system, and the society as a whole because of its major sequelae and the costs of acute and long-term care of patients with trauma to the brain and spinal cord.

Head Injuries

Head injury is a broad classification that encompasses any damage to the head as a result of trauma. A head injury does not necessarily mean a brain injury is present. **Traumatic brain injury** (TBI) or craniocerebral trauma describes an injury that is the result of an external force and is of sufficient magnitude to interfere with daily life and prompts the seeking of treatment.

The Centers for Disease Control and Prevention (CDC) estimates that there are 2.9 million emergency department (ED) visits in the United States each year, the majority of which are for a mild TBI (CDC, 2019). As a result of TBI, approximately 56,800 people die (contributing to about 30% of all injury-related deaths), 288,000 are hospitalized, and 80,000 to 90,000 will have long-term disability (CDC, 2019; Hickey & Strayer, 2020). Approximately 78% of patients are treated in the ED and released (Williamson & Rajajee, 2018). The most common causes of TBIs are falls (48%), motor vehicle crashes (14%), being struck by objects (15%), and assaults (10%). Children up to 4 years of age, adolescents 15 to 19 years, and adults 65 years and older are most likely to sustain a TBI. In every age group, TBI rates are higher for males than for females (Hickey & Strayer, 2020). An estimated 5.3 million people are living with a TBI-related disability, producing an annual economic impact of approximately $76.5 billion due to medical expenses and the cost of lost productivity (CDC, 2019). The best approach to head injury is prevention (see Chart 63-1).

Chart 63-1 • HEALTH PROMOTION

Preventing Head and Spinal Cord Injuries

- Advise drivers to obey traffic laws and to avoid speeding or driving when under the influence of drugs or alcohol.
- Advise all drivers and passengers to wear seat belts and shoulder harnesses. Children younger than 12 years should use an age/size-appropriate system in the back seat.
- Caution passengers against riding in the back of pickup trucks.
- Advise motorcyclists, scooter riders, bicyclists, skateboarders, and roller skaters to wear helmets.
- Promote educational programs that are directed toward violence and suicide prevention in the community.
- Provide water safety instruction.
- Educate patients about steps that can be taken to prevent falls, particularly in older adults.
- Advise athletes to use protective devices. Recommend that coaches be educated in proper coaching techniques.
- Advise owners of firearms to keep them locked in a secure area where children cannot access them.

Pathophysiology

Damage to the brain from traumatic injury takes two forms: primary injury and secondary injury. **Primary injury** is defined as the consequence of direct contact to the head/brain during the instant of initial injury, causing extracranial focal injuries (e.g., contusions, lacerations, external hematomas, and skull fractures), as well as possible focal brain injuries from sudden movement of the brain within the cranial vault (e.g., subdural hematomas [SDHs], concussion, diffuse axonal injury [DAI]). The greatest opportunity for decreasing TBI is the implementation of prevention strategies (see Chart 63-1).

Secondary injury evolves over the ensuing hours and days after the initial injury and results from inadequate delivery of glucose and oxygen to the cells. Identification, prevention, and treatment of secondary injury are the main foci of early management of severe TBI. Contributors to this process include intracranial pathologic processes such as intracranial hemorrhage, cerebral edema, intracranial hypertension, hyperemia, seizures, and vasospasm (Hickey & Strayer, 2020; Kaur & Sharma, 2018). Systemic effects from hypotension, hyperthermia, hypoxia, hypercarbia, infection, electrolyte imbalances, and anemia can also be factors which add to the complex biochemical, metabolic, and inflammatory changes that further compromise an injured brain (Hickey & Strayer, 2020).

The Monro–Kellie hypothesis, also known as the Monro–Kellie doctrine, explains the dynamic equilibrium of cranial contents. The cranial vault contains three main components: brain, blood, and cerebrospinal fluid (CSF). According to the Monro–Kellie hypothesis, the cranial vault is a closed system, and if one of the three components increases in volume, at least one of the other two must decrease in volume or the pressure will increase. Any bleeding or swelling within the skull increases the volume of contents within the skull and therefore causes increased intracranial pressure (ICP) (see Chapter 61). If the pressure increases enough, it can cause displacement of the brain through or against the rigid structures of the skull. This causes restriction of blood flow to the brain, decreasing oxygen delivery and waste removal. Cells within the brain become anoxic and cannot metabolize properly, producing ischemia, infarction, irreversible brain damage, and eventually brain death (see Fig. 63-1).

Scalp Injury

Isolated scalp trauma is generally classified as a minor injury. Because its many blood vessels constrict poorly, the scalp bleeds profusely when injured. Trauma may result in an abrasion (brush wound), contusion, laceration, or subgaleal hematoma (hematoma beneath the layers of tissue of the scalp) (Hickey & Strayer, 2020). A large avulsion (tearing away) of the scalp may be potentially life-threatening and is a true emergency. Diagnosis of a scalp injury is based on physical examination, inspection, and palpation. Scalp wounds are potential portals of entry for organisms that cause intracranial infections. Therefore, the area is irrigated before the laceration is sutured to remove foreign material and to reduce the risk for infection (Hollander, 2019). Subgaleal hematomas usually reabsorb and do not require any specific treatment.

Skull Fractures

A skull fracture is a break in the continuity of the skull caused by forceful trauma. It may occur with or without damage to

Physiology/Pathophysiology

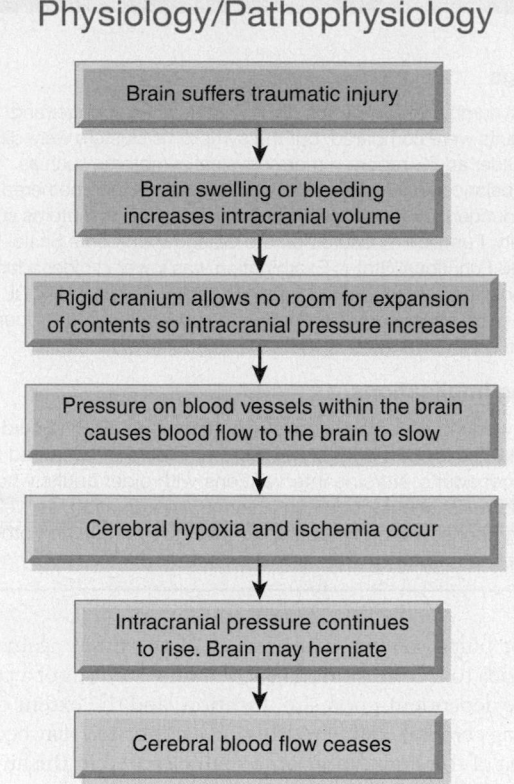

Figure 63-1 • Pathophysiology of traumatic brain injury.

the brain. Skull fractures are classified by type and location. Types include linear, comminuted, and depressed skull fractures, whereas location fractures include frontal, temporal, and basal skull fractures. A simple (linear) fracture is a break in the continuity of the bone. A comminuted skull fracture refers to a splintered or multiple fracture line. Depressed skull fractures occur when the bones of the skull are forcefully displaced downward and can vary from a slight depression to bones of the skull being splintered and embedded within brain tissue. A fracture of the base of the skull is referred to as a basal skull fracture (Hickey & Strayer, 2020). A fracture may be open, indicating a scalp laceration or tear in the dura (e.g., from a bullet or an ice pick), or closed, in which case the dura is intact.

Clinical Manifestations

Symptoms, apart from those of the local injury, depend on the severity and the anatomic location of the underlying brain injury. Persistent, localized pain usually suggests that a fracture is present. Fractures of the cranial vault may or may not produce swelling in the region of the fracture. Fractures of the base of the skull tend to traverse the paranasal sinus of the frontal bone or the middle ear located in the temporal bone. Therefore, they frequently produce hemorrhage from the nose, pharynx, or ears, and blood may appear under the conjunctiva. An area of ecchymosis (bruising) may be seen over the mastoid (Battle sign). Basal skull fractures are suspected when CSF escapes from the ears (CSF otorrhea) and the nose (CSF rhinorrhea). Drainage of CSF is a serious problem, because meningeal infection can occur if organisms gain access to the cranial contents via the nose, ear, or sinus through a tear in the dura.

 Veterans Considerations

Military personnel in combat roles are at increased risk for TBI, with a prevalence rate ranging from 15% to 23% (Turgoose & Murphy, 2018). A common cause of TBI in a veteran is a combat-related blast injury from various forms of improvised explosive devices. Unlike TBI in the civilian population, which causes a primary and secondary injury, TBI in the military population causes four levels of injury (Chapman & Diaz-Arrastia, 2014). The primary injury is due to the atmospheric overpressure followed by underpressure or vacuum. The secondary injury occurs when objects are placed in motion (shrapnel) by the blast, hitting the service member. Tertiary injury occurs when the service member is thrown by the blast and hits their head against the ground, a wall, or other solid surface. Quaternary injury involves other injuries from the blast, such as burns and crush injuries. At this time, there is no evidence to suggest significant differences between a blast injury and a blunt brain injury. Magnetic resonance imaging (MRI) studies do not indicate any microstructural differences. It appears there are no cognitive differences either. Treatment options for a veteran with TBI are the same as those for a civilian with TBI; however, veterans can have complex needs, especially those with multiple injuries.

Assessment and Diagnostic Findings

A computed tomography (CT) scan can be used to diagnose a skull fracture. The ease with which a diagnosis of skull fracture is made depends on the site of the fracture. If a fracture is found on CT scan, there is always the question of associated brain injury, and an MRI scan provides better resolution and clearer pictures of the injured area (Hickey & Strayer, 2020).

 Gerontologic Considerations

Older patients with head injuries differ from those who are younger in terms of etiology of injury, higher mortality rates, longer lengths of hospital stay, and worse functional outcomes (Thompson, Rivara, & Wang, 2020) (see the Nursing Research Profile in Chart 63-2). Neurologic assessment can be challenging, as the older adult patient with a TBI can have hearing or visual deficits or preexisting dementia or cognitive issues, making establishment of a neurologic baseline difficult. The most common causes of injury in older adult patients are falls and motor vehicle crashes. Approximately 81% of all TBIs among adults aged 65 years and older result from falls (CDC, 2019). Physiologic changes related to aging may place the older adult at increased risk for injury, alter the type and severity of injury that occurs, or lead to complications.

Several factors place older adults at increased risk for hematomas. Brain weight decreases, the dura becomes more adherent to the skull, and reaction times slow with increasing age (Battaglini, Gentile, Luchetti, et al., 2019). Also, many older adults take aspirin and anticoagulant agents as part of routine management of chronic conditions.

Medical Management

Nondepressed skull fractures generally do not require surgical treatment; however, close observation of the patient is essential. Nursing personnel may observe the patient in the hospital, but if no underlying brain injury is present, the patient

Chart 63-2

NURSING RESEARCH PROFILE

Head Injury in Older Adults

Thompson, H. J., Rivara, F. P., & Wang, J. (2020). Symptoms, function, and outcomes in the first year after mild-moderate traumatic brain injury. *Journal of Neuroscience Nursing, 52*(2), 46–52.

Purpose

Older adults have higher rates of emergency department (ED) visits, hospitalization, and death for traumatic brain injury (TBI) compared to younger adults. The purpose of this study was to describe and compare the injury trajectory at 1 year for older and younger adults who had a TBI.

Design

This was a prospective longitudinal cohort study of 33 adults who had a mild to moderate TBI. Participants were recruited in the ED and followed for 1 year. Data were collected on symptoms, function using the Glasgow Outcome Scale-Extended Functional Status Examination, and health-related quality of life (HRQOL) for 1 week, then at 1, 3, 6, and 12 months after the injury.

Findings

The total number of symptoms did not differ when younger and older adults were compared, but the symptoms clusters were different. Older adults reported more physical symptoms such as fatigue, balance and coordination problems, and being bothered by noise. Younger adults reported more psychological symptoms such as anxiety. Function measured on the Glasgow Outcome Scale-Extended Functional Status Examination was lower in older adults at 1 year post injury compared to younger adults. Physical HRQOL was lower in older adults consistently over the year compared to younger adults. In contrast, mental HRQOL was higher in older adults.

Nursing Implications

Nurses working with older adults, who have had a TBI should know that they report different symptoms clusters compared to younger adults. Nursing interventions with older adults who have had a TBI should focus on balance, coordination, as well as energy conservation measures to minimize fatigue and other measures to reduce environmental noises.

---

may be allowed to return home. If the patient is discharged home, specific instructions must be given to the family (see later discussion of concussion).

Depressed skull fractures usually require surgery with elevation of the skull and débridement, usually within 24 hours of injury. Skull fractures can be a combination of open, compound, closed, or simple. Associated injuries include concurrent scalp laceration, dural tears, and brain injury directly below the fracture from compression of the tissue below the bony injury and from lacerations produced by the bony fragments (Hickey & Strayer, 2020).

Brain Injury

The most important consideration in any head injury is whether the brain is injured. Even seemingly minor injury can cause significant brain damage secondary to obstructed blood flow and decreased tissue perfusion. The brain cannot store oxygen or glucose to any significant degree. Because the cerebral cells need an uninterrupted blood supply to obtain these nutrients, irreversible brain damage and cell death occur if the blood supply is interrupted for even a few minutes. A **traumatic brain injury, closed (blunt)** occurs when the head accelerates and then rapidly decelerates or collides with another object (e.g., a wall, the dashboard of a car) and brain tissue is damaged but there is no opening through the skull and dura. A **traumatic brain injury, open (penetrating)** occurs when an object penetrates the skull, enters the brain, and damages the soft brain tissue in its path or when blunt trauma to the head is so severe that it opens the scalp, skull, and dura to expose the brain.

Types of Brain Injury

Injuries to the brain can be focal or diffuse. Focal injuries include contusions and several types of hematomas. Concussions and DAI are the major diffuse injuries (Hickey & Strayer, 2020).

Contusion

In cerebral **contusion**, the brain is bruised and damaged in a specific area because of severe acceleration–deceleration force or blunt trauma. The impact of the brain against the skull leads to a contusion. Clinical manifestations of a contusion are dependent upon size, location, and the extent of surrounding cerebral edema. Although a contusion may occur in any area of the brain, most are usually located in the anterior portions of the frontal and temporal lobes, around the sylvian fissure, and at the orbital areas; less commonly, contusions are located at the parietal and occipital areas.

Contusions can be characterized by loss of consciousness associated with stupor and confusion. The effects of injury, particularly hemorrhage and edema, peak after about 18 to 36 hours. These effects, which can cause secondary effects resulting in an increased ICP and possible herniation syndromes, are most pronounced in temporal lobe contusions. Patients are most often managed medically with interventions directed toward prevention of additional insults. Deep contusions are more often associated with hemorrhage and destruction of the reticular activating fibers, altering arousal (Hickey & Strayer, 2020).

Intracranial Hemorrhage

Hematomas are collections of blood in the brain that may be epidural (above the dura), subdural (below the dura), or intracerebral (within the brain) (see Fig. 63-2). Major symptoms are frequently delayed until the hematoma is large enough to cause distortion of the brain and increased ICP. The signs and symptoms of cerebral ischemia resulting from compression by a hematoma are variable and depend on the speed with which vital areas are affected and the area that is injured. A rapidly developing hematoma, even if small, may be fatal, whereas a larger but slowly developing one may allow compensation for increases in ICP.

Epidural Hematoma

After a head injury, blood may collect in the epidural (extradural) space between the skull and the dura mater. This can result from a skull fracture that causes a rupture or laceration of the middle meningeal artery, the artery that runs between the dura and the skull inferior to a thin portion of temporal bone. Hemorrhage from this artery causes rapid pressure in the brain.

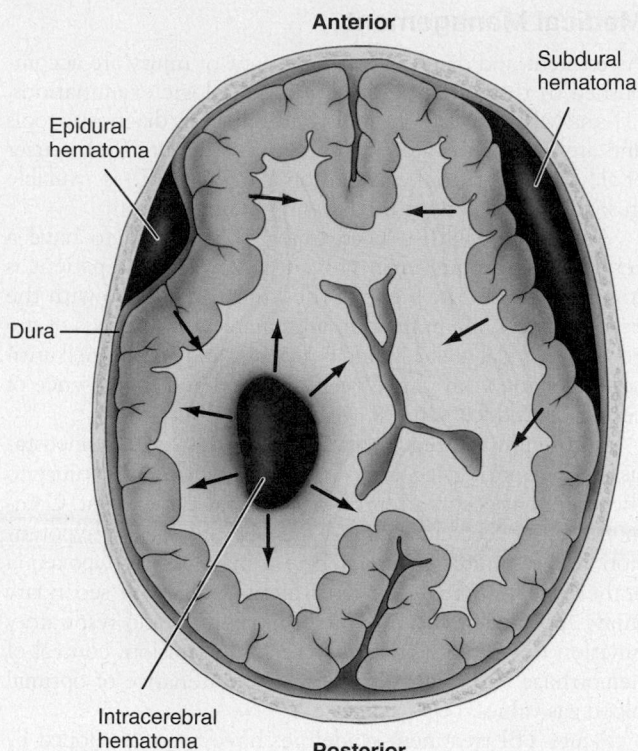

Anterior

Subdural
hematoma

Epidural
hematoma

Dura

Intracerebral
hematoma

Posterior

Figure 63-2 • Location of epidural, subdural, and intracerebral hematomas.

Epidural hematomas (EDHs) account for approximately 2.7% to 4% of traumatic head injuries (Hickey & Strayer, 2020).

Symptoms are caused by the expanding hematoma. EDHs are often characterized by a brief loss of consciousness, followed by a lucid interval in which the patient is awake and conversant. During this lucid interval, compensation for the expanding hematoma takes place by rapid absorption of CSF and decreased intravascular volume, both of which help to maintain the ICP within normal limits. When these mechanisms can no longer compensate, even a small increase in the volume of the blood clot produces a marked elevation in ICP. The patient then becomes increasingly restless, agitated, and confused as the condition progresses to coma. Then, often suddenly, signs of herniation appear (usually deterioration of consciousness and signs of focal neurologic deficits, such as dilation and fixation of a pupil or paralysis of an extremity), and the patient's condition deteriorates rapidly. The most common type of herniation syndrome associated with an EDH is uncal herniation causing pressure on the midbrain (Hickey & Strayer, 2020).

An EDH is considered an extreme emergency; marked neurologic deficit or even respiratory arrest can occur within minutes. Treatment consists of making openings through the skull (burr holes; see Chapter 61, Fig. 61-8) to decrease ICP emergently, remove the clot, and control the bleeding. A craniotomy may be required to remove the clot and control the bleeding. A drain is usually inserted after creation of burr holes or a craniotomy to prevent reaccumulation of blood.

Subdural Hematoma (SDH)

An SDH is a collection of blood between the dura and the brain, a space normally occupied by a thin cushion of fluid. The most common cause is trauma, but it can also occur as a result of coagulopathies or rupture of an aneurysm. An SDH is more frequently venous in origin and is caused by the rupture of small vessels that bridge the subdural space (Vacca & Argento, 2018). SDHs may be acute or chronic depending on the size of the involved vessel and the amount of bleeding in the CT scan.

Acute SDH

An acute SDH is usually caused by some kind of head injury, typically a fall. Signs and symptoms include changes in the level of consciousness (LOC), pupillary signs, and hemiparesis. There may be minor or even no symptoms with small collections of blood. Coma, increasing blood pressure, decreasing heart rate, and slowing respiratory rate are all signs of a rapidly expanding mass requiring immediate intervention.

If the patient can be transported rapidly to the hospital, an immediate craniotomy is performed to open the dura, allowing the subdural clot to be evacuated. Successful outcome also depends on the control of ICP and careful monitoring of respiratory function (see Chapter 61). The mortality rate for patients with acute SDH is high because of associated brain damage (Hickey & Strayer, 2020).

Chronic SDH

A chronic SDH can develop from seemingly minor head injuries and is seen most frequently in older adults who are prone to this type of head injury due to brain atrophy, which is a consequence of the aging process (Vacca & Argento, 2018). Seemingly minor head trauma may produce enough impact to shift the brain contents abnormally. The time between injury and onset of symptoms can be lengthy (e.g., 3 weeks to months), so the actual injury may be forgotten.

A chronic SDH can resemble other conditions—for example, it may be mistaken for a stroke. The bleeding is less profuse, but compression of the intracranial contents still occurs. The blood within the brain changes in character in 2 to 4 days, becoming thicker and darker. In a few weeks, the clot breaks down and has the color and consistency of motor oil. Eventually, calcification or ossification of the clot takes place. The brain adapts to this foreign body invasion, and the clinical signs and symptoms fluctuate. Symptoms include severe headache, which tends to come and go; alternating focal neurologic signs; personality changes; mental deterioration; and focal seizures (Vacca & Argento, 2018).

The treatment for a chronic SDH consists of surgical evaluation for evacuation of the clot. Consideration must be made for reversal of coagulopathies and iatrogenic anticoagulation (Vacca & Argento, 2018). The operative procedure may be carried out through multiple burr holes, or a craniotomy may be performed for a sizable subdural mass that cannot be suctioned or drained through burr holes.

Intracerebral Hemorrhage and Hematoma

Intracerebral hemorrhage is bleeding into the parenchyma of the brain. It is commonly seen in head injuries when force is exerted to the head over a small area (e.g., missile injuries, bullet wounds, stab injuries). These hemorrhages within the brain may also result from the following:

- Systemic hypertension, which causes degeneration and rupture of a vessel
- Rupture of an aneurysm
- Vascular anomalies

- Intracranial tumors
- Bleeding disorders such as leukemia, hemophilia, aplastic anemia, and thrombocytopenia
- Complications of anticoagulant therapy

Nontraumatic causes of intracerebral hemorrhage are discussed in Chapter 62.

The onset may be insidious, beginning with the development of neurologic deficits, followed by headache. Management includes supportive care; control of ICP; and careful administration of fluids, electrolytes, and antihypertensive medications. Surgical intervention by craniotomy or craniectomy permits removal of the blood clot and control of hemorrhage but may not be possible because of the inaccessible location of the bleeding or the lack of a clearly circumscribed area of blood that can be removed.

Concussion

A **concussion** is a temporary loss of neurologic function with no apparent structural damage to the brain. Of the 1.7 million TBIs that occur in the United States each year, it is estimated that approximately 80% of them are concussions, also referred to as "mild TBI" (CDC, 2019). The mechanism of injury is usually blunt trauma from an acceleration–deceleration force, a direct blow, or a blast injury. If brain tissue in the frontal lobe is affected, the patient may exhibit bizarre irrational behavior, whereas involvement of the temporal lobe can produce temporary amnesia or disorientation.

The duration of mental status abnormalities is an indicator of the grade of the concussion. The patient is discharged from the hospital or ED once they return to baseline after a concussion. Monitoring includes observing the patient for a decrease in LOC, worsening headache, dizziness, seizures, abnormal pupil response, vomiting, irritability, slurred speech, and numbness or weakness in the arms or legs (Silverberg, Iaccarino, Panenka, et al., 2020). The occurrence of these symptoms is a red flag indicating the need for further intervention. Recovery may appear complete, but long-term sequelae are possible and repeat injuries are common.

Repeated concussive incidents can lead to a syndrome known as chronic traumatic encephalopathy. This syndrome has been recognized in those participating in contact sports such as football and boxing. The presentation is similar to Alzheimer's disease, characterized by personality changes, memory impairment, and speech and gait disturbances. Imaging findings show gross cerebral, particularly temporal lobe, atrophy (Hickey & Strayer, 2020; Turk & Budson, 2019).

Diffuse Axonal Injury (DAI)

DAI results from widespread shearing and rotational forces that produce damage throughout the brain—to axons in the cerebral hemispheres, corpus callosum, and brain stem. The injured area may be diffuse with no identifiable focal lesion. DAI is associated with prolonged traumatic coma; it is more serious and is associated with a poorer prognosis than a focal lesion. The patient with DAI in severe head trauma experiences no lucid interval, immediate coma, decorticate and decerebrate posturing (see Chapter 61, Fig. 61-1), and global cerebral edema. Diagnosis is made by clinical signs in conjunction with a CT or MRI scan (Schweitzer, Niogi, Whitlow, et al., 2019). Recovery depends on the severity of the axonal injury.

Medical Management

Assessment and diagnosis of the extent of injury are accomplished by the initial physical and neurologic examinations. CT and MRI scans are the main neuroimaging diagnostic tools and are useful in evaluating the brain structure (Schweitzer et al., 2019). Positron emission tomography (PET) is available in some trauma centers for assessing brain function.

Any patient with a head injury is presumed to have a cervical spine injury until proven otherwise. The patient is transported from the scene of the injury on a board with the head and neck maintained in alignment with the axis of the body. A cervical collar should be applied and maintained until cervical spine x-rays have been obtained and the absence of cervical SCI documented.

All therapy is directed toward preserving brain homeostasis and preventing secondary brain injury, which is injury to the brain that occurs after the original traumatic event. Common causes of secondary injury are cerebral edema, hypotension, and respiratory depression that may lead to hypoxemia and electrolyte imbalance. Treatments to prevent secondary injury include stabilization of cardiovascular and respiratory function to maintain adequate cerebral perfusion, control of hemorrhage and hypovolemia, and maintenance of optimal blood gas values.

Acute TBI treatment guidelines have been developed by the Brain Trauma Foundation. Adherence to these treatment guidelines may subsequently improve patient care and outcomes (Saherwala, Bader, Stutzman, et al., 2018).

 Treatment of Increased Intracranial Pressure

As the damaged brain swells with edema or as blood collects within the brain, an increase in ICP occurs; this requires aggressive treatment (see Chapter 61 for a discussion on the relationship between ICP and cerebral perfusion pressure [CPP]). If the ICP remains elevated, it can decrease the CPP. Initial management is based on preventing secondary injury and maintaining adequate cerebral oxygenation (Sacco & Delibert, 2018).

Surgery is required for evacuation of blood clots, débridement and elevation of depressed fractures of the skull, and suture of severe scalp lacerations. ICP is monitored closely; if increased, it is managed by maintaining adequate oxygenation, elevating the head of the bed, and maintaining normal blood volume (McCafferty, Neal, Marshall, et al., 2018). Devices to monitor ICP or drain CSF can be inserted during surgery or at the bedside using aseptic technique. The patient is cared for in the intensive care unit (ICU), where expert nursing care and medical treatment are readily available.

Supportive Measures

Treatment also includes ventilatory support, seizure prevention, fluid and electrolyte maintenance, nutritional support, and management of pain and anxiety. Patients who are comatose are intubated and mechanically ventilated to ensure adequate oxygenation and protect the airway.

Because seizures can occur after head injury and can cause secondary brain damage from hypoxia, anticonvulsant agents may be given. If the patient is very agitated, benzodiazepines are the most commonly used sedative agents which do not affect cerebral blood flow or ICP. Lorazepam and midazolam are frequently used but have active metabolites that may

Chart 63-3 ETHICAL DILEMMA
How Can Advocacy Be Assured for a Patient Who Is Undocumented and Incapacitated?

Case Scenario

J.S. is a 24-year-old man who is undocumented and undomiciled. He was brought to the hospital by ambulance after falling from a 20-foot-high scaffold at a construction site 2 days ago. You are J.S.'s nurse in the intensive care unit (ICU). According to J.S.'s assigned medical social worker, a coworker on the work site where J.S. fell followed him to the hospital post injury. Information gathered from the coworker included that J.S. was working as a day laborer and was sending money to his parents in Honduras. J.S. reportedly speaks no English and only some Spanish; his primary language is native Honduran Moskitu. Despite aggressive interventions, including emergent craniotomy, ventriculostomy placement, and endotracheal intubation and mechanical ventilation, J.S. has remained unresponsive to all stimuli since admission to the ICU, with a current Glasgow Coma Scale score of 3. The consulting neurologist has opined that J.S. will not recover from his traumatic brain injury, and that he will either succumb to his injuries or remain in a persistent vegetative state (see Chapter 61). The state where you work has a provision that two physicians may decide to withdraw life-sustaining therapy for patients who are unbefriended (i.e., without next of kin/surrogates) and decisionally incapacitated such as J.S. The attending physician intensivist assigned to J.S. tells you during her rounds that she intends to consult with another intensivist colleague so that J.S. is extubated, and wants you to prepare to assist them. You ask the intensivist if attempts should be made to find J.S.'s parents to get their permission to withdraw treatment. The intensivist says to you "How are we supposed to find them? And even if we do locate them, they do not speak English, and maybe they do not understand Spanish, either. How can we tell them what has happened and get them on board? For heaven's sake, we are not doing this man any favors by letting him linger like this!"

Discussion

People from socioeconomically disadvantaged groups and those who are racial and ethnic minorities are at greater risk for morbidity and mortality than those who are socioeconomically secure and White. No group is at greater risk for suffering health disparities than those who are undocumented and undomiciled. Patients who are undocumented will typically forego seeking treatment for anything other than a dire health emergency, as they typically are uninsured, not eligible for assistance programs, and risk deportation by seeing a health care provider.

Analysis

- Describe the ethical principles that are in conflict in this case (see Chapter 1, Chart 1-7). Assume that the intensivist believes she is advocating for what is best for J.S. by withdrawing life support. What dangers might be inherent in this type of paternalistic attitude (i.e., *I know what is best for the patient*)?
- How might it be possible to ascertain what J.S.'s wishes would be if he were not incapacitated? Is trying to determine this futile and needlessly prolonging his suffering?
- What resources might you mobilize to be of assistance to you, to J.S., and to J.S.'s parents in Honduras? Do J.S.'s parents have the right to know what has happened to their son? What if his parents are found, and want J.S. to continue life-sustaining treatments? Can they legitimately make that decision on his behalf?

References

Fins, J. J., & Real de Asúa, D. (2019). North of home: Obligations to families of undocumented patients. *Hastings Center Report*, *49*(1), 12–14.
Radtke, K. & Matzo, M. (2017). Liberty and justice for all: When an unauthorized immigrant suffers a brain injury, who decides when treatment is withdrawn? *American Journal of Nursing*, *117*(11), 52–56.

Resources

See Chapter 1, Chart 1-10 for Steps of an Ethical Analysis and Ethics Resources.

---

cause prolonged sedation, making it difficult to conduct a neurologic assessment. Propofol, a sedative–hypnotic agent that is supplied in an intralipid emulsion for intravenous (IV) use, is the sedative of choice. It is an ultrashort-acting, rapid-onset drug with elimination half-life of less than an hour. It has a major advantage of being titratable to its desired clinical effect but still provides the opportunity for an accurate neurologic assessment (Hickey & Strayer, 2020). A nasogastric tube may be inserted, because reduced gastric motility and reverse peristalsis are associated with head injury, making regurgitation and aspiration common in the first few hours.

Brain Death

When a patient has sustained a severe head injury incompatible with life, the patient is a potential organ donor. The nurse may assist in the clinical examination for determination of brain death and in the process of organ procurement. The three cardinal signs of brain death on clinical examination are coma, the absence of brain stem reflexes, and apnea. Adjunctive tests, such as cerebral blood flow studies, electroencephalogram (EEG), transcranial Doppler, and brain stem auditory-evoked potential, are often used to confirm brain death (Hickey & Strayer, 2020). The health care team provides information to the family and assists them with the decision-making process about end-of-life care (see the section Supporting Family Coping and Chart 63-3).

NURSING PROCESS

The Patient with a Traumatic Brain Injury

Assessment

Depending on the patient's neurologic status, the nurse may elicit information from the patient, from the family, or from witnesses or emergency rescue personnel. Although all usual baseline data may not be collected initially, the immediate health history should include the following questions:

- When did the injury occur?
- What caused the injury? A high-velocity missile? An object striking the head? A fall?
- What was the direction and force of the blow?

A history of unconsciousness or amnesia after a head injury indicates a significant degree of brain damage, and changes that occur minutes to hours after the initial injury can reflect recovery or indicate the development of secondary brain damage. The nurse should determine if there was a loss of consciousness, the duration of the unconscious period, and if the patient could be aroused.

In addition to asking questions that establish the nature of the injury and the patient's condition immediately after the injury, the nurse examines the patient thoroughly. This assessment includes determining the patient's LOC using the Glasgow Coma Scale (GCS) and assessing the patient's response to tactile stimuli (if unconscious), pupillary response to light, corneal and gag reflexes, and motor function (Teasdale & Jennett, 1974). The GCS (see Chart 63-4) is based on the three criteria of eye opening, verbal responses, and motor responses to verbal commands or painful stimuli. It is particularly useful for monitoring changes during the acute phase, the first few days after a head injury. It does not take the place of an indepth neurologic assessment.

Detailed assessments are made initially and at frequent intervals throughout the acute phase of care (Hickey & Strayer, 2020). Monitoring of ICP is crucial to decision making for patients with neurologic injuries, yet research findings indicate that proper training and a standard guideline is necessary to correctly document ICP (Liu, Griffith, Jang, et al., 2020) (see the Nursing Research Profile in Chapter 61, Chart 61-2). Baseline and ongoing assessments are critical in nursing assessment of the patient with brain injury, whose condition can worsen dramatically and irrevocably if subtle signs are overlooked (Sacco & Davis, 2019; Urden, Stacy, & Lough, 2018). More information on assessment is provided in the following sections and in Figure 63-3 and Table 63-1.

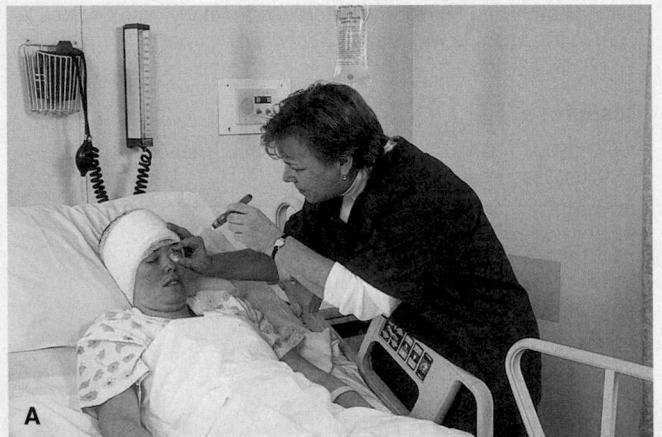
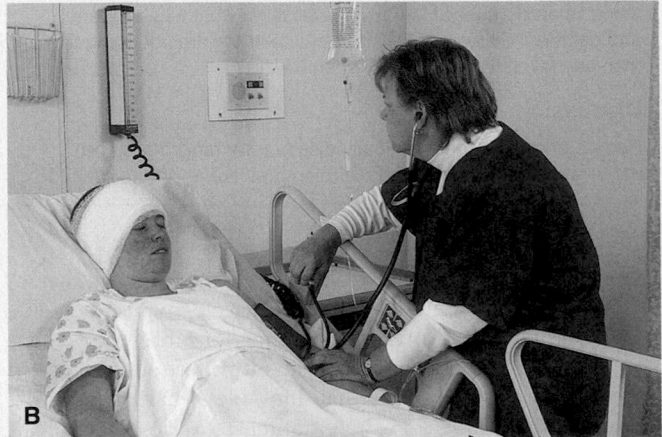
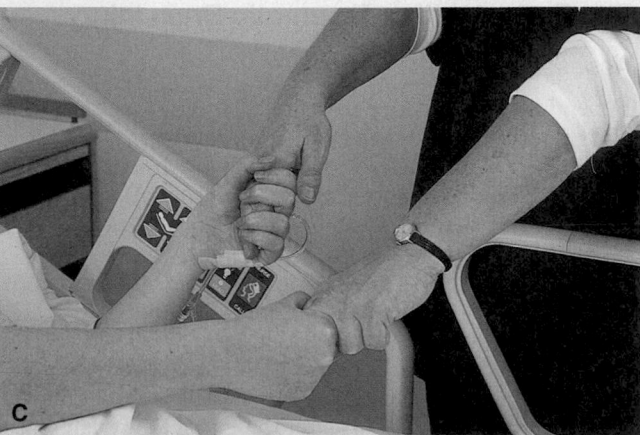
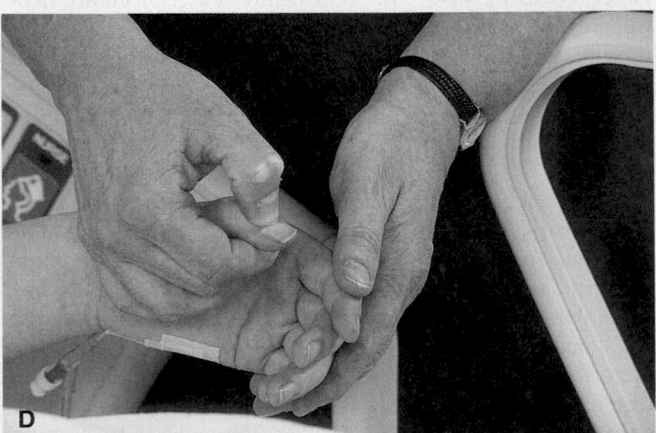

Figure 63-3 • Assessment parameters for the patient with a head injury include eye opening and responsiveness (**A**), vital signs (**B**), and motor response reflected in hand strength or response to painful stimulus (**C, D**). Photos by B. Proud.

TABLE 63-1 Multisystem Assessment Measures for the Patient with Traumatic Brain Injury

System-Specific Considerations	Assessment Data
Neurologic System • Severe TBI results in unconsciousness and alters many neurologic functions. • All body functions must be supported. • Increased ICP and herniation syndromes are life-threatening. • Measures are instituted to control elevated ICP.	• Assessment of neurologic status • Assessment for signs and symptoms of ICP elevation • Calculation of cerebral perfusion pressure if ICP monitor is in place • Monitoring of anticonvulsant medication blood levels
Respiratory System • Complete or partial airway obstruction will compromise the oxygen supply to the brain. • An altered respiratory pattern can result in cerebral hypoxia. • A short period of apnea at the moment of impact can result in spotty atelectasis. • Systemic disturbances from head injury can cause hypoxemia. • Brain injury can alter brain stem respiratory function. • Shunting of blood to the lungs as a result of a sympathetic discharge at the time of injury can cause neurogenic pulmonary edema.	• Assessment of respiratory function: • Auscultate chest for breath sounds • Note the respiratory pattern, if possible (not possible if a ventilator is being used) • Note the respiratory rate • Note whether the cough reflex is intact • Arterial blood gas levels • Complete blood count • Chest x-ray studies • Sputum cultures • Oxygen saturation using pulse oximetry
Cardiovascular System • The patient may develop cardiac arrhythmias, tachycardia, or bradycardia. • The patient may develop hypotension or hypertension. • Because of immobility and unconsciousness, the patient is at high risk for DVT and PE. • Fluid and electrolyte imbalance can be related to several problems including alterations in antidiuretic hormone secretion, the stress response, or fluid restriction. • Specific conditions may occur: • Diabetes insipidus • Syndrome of inappropriate secretion of antidiuretic hormone • Electrolyte imbalance • Hyperglycemic hyperosmolar syndrome.	• Assessment of vital signs • Monitoring for cardiac arrhythmias • Assessment for venous thromboembolism including PE and DVT • Electrocardiogram • Electrolyte studies • Blood coagulation studies • Blood glucose level • Blood acetone level • Blood osmolality • Urine-specific gravity
Gastrointestinal System • Injury to the GI tract can result in paralytic ileus. • Constipation can result from bed rest, NPO status, fluid restriction, and opioids given for pain control. • Bowel incontinence is related to the patient's unconscious state or altered mental state.	• Assessment of abdomen for bowel sounds and distention • Monitoring for decreased hemoglobin
Metabolic (Nutritional) System • The patient receives all fluids IV for the first few days until the GI tract is functioning. • A nutritional consultation is initiated within the first 24–48 h; parenteral or enteral nutrition may be started.	• Assessment of fluid and electrolyte balance • Recording of weight, if possible • Hematocrit • Electrolyte studies
Genitourinary System • Fluid restriction or the use of diuretic agents can alter the amount of urinary output. • Urinary incontinence is related to the patient's unconscious state.	• Intake and output record
Musculoskeletal System • Immobility contributes to musculoskeletal changes. • Decerebrate or decorticate posturing makes proper positioning difficult (see Chapter 61, Fig. 61-1).	• Assessment of range of motion of joints and development of deformities or spasticity
Integumentary System (Skin and Mucous Membranes) • Immobility secondary to TBI and unconsciousness contributes to the development of pressure areas and skin breakdown. • Intubation causes irritation of the mucous membrane and deterioration of oral health.	• Assessment of skin integrity and character • Assessment of oral mucous membrane and oral health of the skin
Psychological/Emotional Response • The patient with TBI is unconscious. • The family needs emotional support to deal with the crisis.	• Alternative methods of assessment for pain are indicated in the patient who is unconscious • Collection of information about the family and the role within the family of the person with head injury • Assessment of the family to determine how functional it was before the injury occurred

DVT, deep vein thrombosis; GI, gastrointestinal; ICP, intracranial pressure; IV, intravenous; NPO, nothing by mouth; PE, pulmonary embolism; TBI, traumatic brain injury.
Adapted from Hickey, J. V., & Strayer, A. (2020). *The clinical practice of neurological & neurosurgical nursing* (8th ed.). Philadelphia, PA: Wolters Kluwer.

Diagnosis

NURSING DIAGNOSES

Based on the assessment data, major nursing diagnoses may include the following:

- Impaired airway clearance and impaired gas exchange associated with brain injury
- Risk for ineffective tissue perfusion associated with increased ICP, decreased CPP, and possible seizures
- Hypovolemia associated with decreased LOC and hormonal dysfunction
- Impaired nutritional status associated with increased metabolic demands, fluid restriction, and inadequate intake
- Risk for injury (self-directed and directed at others) associated with seizures, disorientation, restlessness, or brain damage
- Risk for impaired thermoregulation associated with damaged temperature-regulating mechanisms in the brain
- Risk for impaired skin integrity associated with bed rest, hemiparesis, hemiplegia, immobility, or restlessness
- Difficulty coping associated with brain injury
- Impaired sleep associated with brain injury and frequent neurologic checks
- Risk for impaired family coping associated with unresponsiveness of patient, unpredictability of outcome, prolonged recovery period, and the patient's residual physical disability and emotional deficit
- Lack of knowledge about brain injury, recovery, and the rehabilitation process

The nursing diagnoses for the patient who is unconscious and the patient with increased ICP also apply (see Chapter 61).

COLLABORATIVE PROBLEMS/POTENTIAL COMPLICATIONS

Potential complications may include the following:

- Decreased cerebral perfusion
- Cerebral edema and herniation
- Impaired oxygenation and ventilation
- Impaired fluid, electrolyte, and nutritional balance
- Risk for posttraumatic seizures

Planning and Goals

The goals for the patient may include maintenance of a patent airway, adequate CPP, fluid and electrolyte balance, adequate nutritional status, prevention of secondary injury, maintenance of body temperature within normal limits, maintenance of skin integrity, improvement of coping, prevention of sleep deprivation, effective family coping, increased knowledge about the rehabilitation process, and absence of complications.

Nursing Interventions

The nursing interventions for the patient with a TBI are extensive and diverse. They include making nursing assessments, setting priorities for nursing interventions, anticipating needs and complications, and initiating rehabilitation.

MAINTAINING THE AIRWAY

One of the most important nursing goals in the management of head injury is to establish and maintain an adequate airway.

The brain is extremely sensitive to hypoxia, and a neurologic deficit can worsen if the patient is hypoxic. Therapy is directed toward maintaining optimal oxygenation to preserve cerebral function. An obstructed airway causes carbon dioxide retention and hypoventilation, which can produce cerebral vessel dilation and increased ICP (Urden et al., 2018).

Interventions to ensure an adequate exchange of air are discussed in Chapter 61 and include the following (Hickey & Strayer, 2020):

- Maintaining the patient who is unconscious in a position that facilitates drainage of oral secretions, with the head of the bed elevated about 30 degrees to decrease intracranial venous pressure
- Establishing effective suctioning procedures (pulmonary secretions produce coughing and straining, which increase ICP)
- Guarding against aspiration and respiratory insufficiency
- Closely monitoring arterial blood gas values to assess the adequacy of ventilation. The goal is to keep blood gas values within normal limits to ensure adequate cerebral blood flow
- Monitoring the patient who is receiving mechanical ventilation for pulmonary complications such as acute respiratory distress syndrome and pneumonia

The patient who is intubated is at high risk for ventilator-associated pneumonia and providing good oral hygiene can help prevent this complication (Gallagher, 2017).

MONITORING NEUROLOGIC FUNCTION

Patients with severe TBI are admitted to the ICU for close assessment and monitoring (cardiac monitoring, pulse oximetry, invasive arterial blood pressure monitoring, end-tidal CO_2, and temperature monitoring). Parameters are assessed initially and as frequently as the patient's condition requires. As soon as the initial assessment is made, the use of a neurologic observational flow record is started and maintained. The importance of ongoing assessment and monitoring of the patient with brain injury cannot be overstated.

Level of Consciousness. The GCS is used to assess LOC at regular intervals, because changes in the LOC precede all other changes in vital and neurologic signs. The patient's best responses to predetermined stimuli are recorded (see Chart 63-4). Each response is scored (the greater the number, the better the functioning), and the sum of these scores gives an indication of the severity of coma and a prediction of possible outcome. The lowest score is 3 (least responsive); the highest is 15 (most responsive). A GCS score between 3 and 8 is generally accepted as indicating a severe head injury (Hickey & Strayer, 2020).

 Concept Mastery Alert

The GCS is considered the most sensitive indicator of a lapse in neurologic functioning in patients with TBI and is often the earliest sign of acute change in ICP.

Vital Signs. Although a change in LOC is the most sensitive neurologic indication of deterioration of the patient's condition, vital signs are also monitored at frequent intervals to assess the intracranial status. Table 63-1 depicts the general assessment parameters for the patient with a head injury.

Signs of increasing ICP include bradycardia (slowing of the heart rate), increasing systolic blood pressure, and widening pulse pressure (Cushing's reflex). As brain compression increases, respirations become rapid, the blood pressure may decrease, and the pulse slows further. This is an ominous development, as is a rapid fluctuation of vital signs (Hickey & Strayer, 2020). The temperature is maintained at less than 38°C (100.4°F) (Young & Prescott, 2019). Tachycardia and arterial hypotension may indicate that bleeding is occurring elsewhere in the body.

 Concept Mastery Alert

In a patient with a head injury, a rapid increase in body temperature is regarded as unfavorable because hyperthermia increases the metabolic demands of the brain and may indicate brain stem damage—a poor prognostic sign.

Motor Function. Motor function is assessed frequently by observing spontaneous movements, asking the patient to raise and lower the extremities, and comparing the strength and equality of the upper and lower extremities at periodic intervals. To assess upper extremity strength, the nurse instructs the patient to squeeze the examiner's fingers tightly. The nurse assesses lower extremity motor strength by placing the hands on the soles of the patient's feet and asking the patient to push down against the examiner's hands. Examination of the motor system is discussed in more detail in Chapter 60. The presence or absence of spontaneous movement of each extremity is also noted, and speech and eye signs are assessed.

If the patient does not demonstrate spontaneous movement, responses to painful stimuli are assessed (Hickey & Strayer, 2020). Motor response to pain is assessed by applying a central stimulus, such as pinching the pectoralis major muscle, to determine the patient's best response. Peripheral stimulation may provide inaccurate assessment data because it may result in a reflex movement rather than a voluntary motor response. Abnormal responses (lack of motor response; extension responses) are associated with a poorer prognosis.

Other Neurologic Signs. The size and equality of the pupils and their reaction to light need to be continuously assessed. A unilaterally dilated and poorly responding pupil may indicate a developing hematoma, with subsequent pressure on the third cranial nerve due to shifting of the brain. If both pupils become fixed and dilated, this indicates acute injury and intrinsic damage to the upper brain stem and is a poor prognostic sign (Hickey & Strayer, 2020).

The patient with a head injury may develop deficits such as anosmia (lack of sense of smell), eye movement abnormalities, aphasia, memory deficits, and posttraumatic seizures or epilepsy. Patients may be left with residual psychological deficits (impulsiveness; emotional lability; or uninhibited, aggressive behaviors) and, as a consequence of the impairment, may lack insight into their emotional responses.

MONITORING FLUID AND ELECTROLYTE BALANCE
Brain damage can produce metabolic and hormonal dysfunctions. The monitoring of serum electrolyte levels is important, especially in patients receiving osmotic diuretics, those with syndrome of inappropriate antidiuretic hormone (SIADH) secretion, and those with posttraumatic diabetes insipidus.

Serial studies of blood and urine electrolytes and osmolality are carried out because head injuries may be accompanied by disorders of sodium regulation. Hyponatremia is common after head injury due to shifts in extracellular fluid, electrolytes, and volume. Hyperglycemia, for example, can cause an increase in extracellular fluid that lowers sodium. Hypernatremia may also occur as a result of sodium retention that may last several days, followed by sodium diuresis. Increasing lethargy, confusion, and seizures may be the result of electrolyte imbalance.

Endocrine function is evaluated by monitoring serum electrolytes, blood glucose values, and intake and output. Urine is tested regularly for acetone. A record of daily weights is maintained, especially if the patient has hypothalamic involvement and is at risk for the development of diabetes insipidus.

PROMOTING ADEQUATE NUTRITION
Head injury results in metabolic changes that increase calorie consumption and nitrogen excretion. Protein demand increases. Early initiation of nutritional therapy has been shown to improve outcomes in patients with head injury. Patients with brain injury are assumed to be catabolic, and nutritional support consultation should be considered as soon as the patient is admitted. Parenteral nutrition via a central line or enteral feedings given via a nasogastric or nasojejunal feeding tube should be considered, though enteral is the preferred route (Hickey & Strayer, 2020). If CSF rhinorrhea occurs or if there is any suspicion of disruption to the skull base, an oral feeding tube should be inserted instead of a nasal tube.

Laboratory values should be monitored closely in patients receiving parenteral nutrition. Elevating the head of the bed can help prevent distention, regurgitation, and aspiration. A continuous-drip infusion or pump may be used to regulate the feeding. Enteral or parenteral feedings are usually continued until the swallowing reflex returns and the patient can meet caloric requirements orally. See Chapter 39 for the principles and technique of enteral feedings.

PREVENTING INJURY
Often, as the patient emerges from coma, a period of lethargy and stupor is followed by a period of agitation. Each phase is variable and depends on the person, the location of the injury, the depth and duration of coma, and the patient's age. Restlessness may be caused by hypoxia, fever, pain, or a full bladder. It may indicate injury to the brain but may also be a sign that the patient is regaining consciousness. (Some restlessness may be beneficial because the lungs and extremities are exercised.) Agitation may also be the result of discomfort from catheters, IV lines, restraints, and repeated neurologic checks. Alternatives to restraints must be used whenever possible.

Strategies to prevent injury include the following:
- Assessing the patient to ensure that oxygenation is adequate, and the bladder is not distended. Dressings and casts are checked for constriction
- Using padded side rails or wrapping the patient's hands in mitts to protect the patient from self-injury and dislodging of tubes. Restraints are used judiciously because straining against them can increase ICP or cause other injury. Enclosed or floor-level specialty beds may be indicated

- Avoiding opioids as a means of controlling restlessness, because they depress respiration, constrict the pupils, and alter responsiveness
- Reducing environmental stimuli by keeping the room quiet, limiting visitors, speaking calmly, and providing frequent orientation information (e.g., explaining where the patient is and what is being done)
- Providing adequate lighting to prevent visual hallucinations
- Minimizing disruption of the patient's sleep–wake cycles
- Lubricating the patient's skin with oil or emollient lotion to prevent irritation due to rubbing against the sheet
- Using an external sheath catheter for a male patient if incontinence occurs. Because prolonged use of an indwelling catheter inevitably produces infection, the patient may be placed on an intermittent catheterization schedule.

MAINTAINING THERMOREGULATION

Fever in the patient with a TBI can be the result of damage to the hypothalamus, cerebral irritation from hemorrhage, or infection. The nurse monitors the patient's temperature every 2 to 4 hours. If the temperature increases, efforts are made to identify the cause and to control it using acetaminophen and cooling devices to maintain normothermia. Cooling devices should be used with caution so as not to induce shivering, which increases ICP. If infection is suspected, potential sites of infection are cultured, and antibiotic agents are prescribed and administered. Research about therapeutic hypothermia for patients with TBI suggests there is no clear evidence to guide therapy (Watson, Shepherd, Rhodes, et al., 2018; Weng, Yang, Huang, et al., 2018).

MAINTAINING SKIN INTEGRITY

Patients with TBI often require assistance in turning and positioning because of immobility or unconsciousness. Prolonged pressure on the tissues decreases circulation and leads to tissue necrosis. Potential areas of breakdown need to be identified early to avoid the development of pressure injuries. Specific nursing measures include the following:

- Assessing all body surfaces and documenting skin integrity every 8 hours
- Turning and repositioning the patient every 2 hours
- Providing skin care every 4 hours
- Assisting the patient to get out of bed to a chair three times a day

IMPROVING COPING

Although many patients with head injury survive because of resuscitative and supportive technology, they frequently have ineffective coping due to cognitive sequelae. Cognitive impairment includes memory deficits; decreased ability to focus and sustain attention to a task (distractibility); impulsivity; egocentricity; and slowness in thinking, perceiving, communicating, reading, and writing. Psychiatric, emotional, and relationship problems develop in many patients after head injury. Resulting psychosocial, behavioral, emotional, and cognitive impairments are devastating to the family as well as to the patient (Oyesanya, Arulselvam, Thompson, et al., 2019).

These problems require collaboration among many disciplines. A neuropsychologist (specialist in evaluating and treating cognitive problems) plans a program and initiates therapy or counseling to help the patient reach maximal potential. Cognitive rehabilitation activities help the patient devise new problem-solving strategies. The retraining is carried out over an extended period and may include the use of sensory stimulation and reinforcement, behavior modification, reality orientation, computer training programs, and video games. Assistance from many disciplines is necessary during this phase of recovery. Even if intellectual ability does not improve, social and behavioral abilities may improve.

The patient recovering from a TBI may experience fluctuations in the level of cognitive function, with orientation, attention, and memory frequently affected. Many types of sensory stimulation programs have been tried, and research on these programs is ongoing (Hickey & Strayer, 2020). When pushed to a level greater than the impaired cortical functioning allows, the patient may show symptoms of fatigue, anger, and stress (headache, dizziness). The Rancho Los Amigos Scale: Levels of Cognitive Functioning is frequently used to assess cognitive function and evaluate ongoing recovery from head injury. Progress through the levels of cognitive function can vary widely for individual patients (Hagen, Malkmus, & Durham, 1972). Nursing management and a description of each level are included in Table 63-2.

PREVENTING SLEEP PATTERN DISTURBANCE

Patients who require frequent monitoring of neurologic status may experience sleep deprivation as they are awakened hourly for assessment of LOC. To allow the patient longer times of uninterrupted sleep and rest, the nurse can group nursing care activities so that the patient is disturbed less frequently. Environmental noise is decreased, and the room lights are dimmed. Measures to increase comfort may promote sleep and rest (Giusti, Tuteri, & Mirella, 2016).

SUPPORTING FAMILY COPING

Having a loved one sustain a TBI produces a great deal of stress in the family. This stress can result from the patient's physical and emotional deficits, the unpredictable outcome, and altered family relationships. Families report difficulties in coping with changes in the patient's temperament, behavior, and personality (Oyesanya et al., 2019). Such changes are associated with disruption in family cohesion, loss of leisure pursuits, and loss of work capacity, as well as social isolation of the caretaker. The family may experience marital disruption, anger, grief, guilt, and denial in recurring cycles.

To promote effective coping, the nurse can ask the family how the patient is different now, what has been lost, and what is most difficult about coping with this situation. Helpful interventions include providing family members with accurate and honest information and encouraging them to continue to set well-defined short-term goals. Family counseling helps address the family members' acute feelings of loss and helplessness and gives them guidance for the management of inappropriate behaviors. Support groups help the family members share problems, develop insight, gain information, network, and gain assistance in maintaining realistic expectations, hope, and a good quality of life (Oyesanya et al., 2019).

The Brain Injury Association of America (see the Resources section) serves as a clearinghouse for information and resources for patients with head injuries and their families, including specific information on coma, rehabilitation, behavioral consequences of head injury, and family issues.

TABLE 63-2	Rancho Los Amigos Scale: Levels of Cognitive Function	
Cognitive Level	**Description**	**Nursing Management**
For levels I–III, the key approach is to *provide stimulation*.		
I: No response	Completely unresponsive to all stimuli, including painful stimuli	Multiple modalities of sensory input should be used. Examples are listed here, but management should be individualized and expanded based on available materials and patient preferences (determined by obtaining information from the family).
II: Generalized response	Nonpurposeful response; responds to pain but in a nonpurposeful manner	*Olfactory:* Perfumes, flowers, shaving lotion. *Visual:* Family pictures, card, personal items.
III: Localized response	Responses more focused—withdraws to pain; turns toward sound; follows moving objects that pass within the visual field; pulls on sources of discomfort (e.g., tubes, restraints); may follow simple commands but inconsistently and in a delayed manner	*Auditory:* Radio, television, recordings of family voices or favorite recordings, talking to patient (nurse, family members). The nurse should tell patient what is going to be done, discuss the environment, provide encouragement. *Tactile:* Touching of skin, rubbing various textures on skin. *Movement:* Range-of-motion exercises, turning, repositioning, the use of water mattress.
For levels IV–VI, the key approach is to *provide structure*.		
IV: Confused, agitated response	Alert, hyperactive state in which patient responds to internal confusion/agitation; behavior nonpurposeful in relation to the environment; aggressive, bizarre behavior common	For level IV, which lasts 2–4 wks, interventions are directed at decreasing agitation, increasing environmental awareness, and promoting safety. • Approach patient in a calm manner, and use a soft voice. • Screen patient from environmental stimuli (e.g., sounds, sights); provide a quiet, controlled environment. • Remove devices that contribute to agitation (e.g., tubes), if possible. • Functional goals cannot be set because the patient is unable to cooperate.
V: Confused, inappropriate response	When agitation occurs, it is the result of external rather than internal stimuli; focused attention is difficult; memory is severely impaired; responses are fragmented and inappropriate to the situation; there is no carryover of learning from one situation to the other	For levels V and VI, interventions are directed at decreasing confusion, improving cognitive function, and improving independence in performing ADLs. • Provide supervision. • Use repetition and cues to educate about ADLs. Focus the patient's attention, and help to increase their concentration. • Help the patient organize activities. • Clarify misinformation and reorient when confused. • Provide a consistent, predictable schedule (e.g., post daily schedule on large poster board).
VI: Confused, appropriate response	Follows simple directions consistently but is inconsistently oriented to time and place; short-term memory worse than long-term memory; can perform some ADLs	
For levels VII–X, the key approach is *integration into the community*.		
VII: Automatic, appropriate response	Appropriately responsive and oriented within the hospital setting; needs little supervision in ADLs; some carryover of learning; patient has superficial insight into disability; has decreased judgment and problem-solving abilities; lacks realistic planning for future	For levels VII–X, interventions are directed at increasing the patient's ability to function with minimal or no supervision in the community. • Reduce environmental structure. • Help the patient plan for adapting ADLs for self into the home environment. • Discuss and adapt home-living skills (e.g., cleaning, cooking) to patient's ability. • Provide standby assistance, as needed, for ADLs and home-living skills.
VIII: Purposeful, appropriate	Alert, oriented, intact memory; has realistic goals for the future. Able to complete familiar tasks for 1 h in a distracting environment; overestimates or underestimates abilities, argumentative, easily frustrated, self-centered; uncharacteristically dependent/independent	
IX: Purposeful, appropriate	Independently shifts back and forth between tasks and completes them accurately for at least 2 consecutive hours; uses assistive memory devices to recall schedule and activities; aware of and acknowledges impairments and disability when they interfere with task completion; depression may continue; may be easily irritable and have a low frustration tolerance	• Provide assistance on request for adapting ADLs and home-living skills.
X: Purposeful, appropriate	Able to handle multiple tasks simultaneously in all environments but may require periodic breaks; independently initiates and carries out familiar and unfamiliar tasks but may require more than usual amount of time or compensatory strategies to complete them; accurately estimates abilities and independently adjusts to task demands; periodic periods of depression may occur; irritability and low frustration tolerance when sick, fatigued, or under stress	• Monitor for signs and symptoms of depression. • Help the patient plan, anticipate concerns, and solve problems.

ADLs, activities of daily living.
Adapted from Los Amigos Research and Education Institute, Inc., & Downey, C. A. (2002). Used with permission.

This organization can provide names of facilities and professionals who work with patients with head injuries and can assist families in organizing local support groups.

Many patients with severe head injury die of their injuries, and many of those who survive experience long-term disability that prevents them from resuming their previous roles and functions. During the most acute phase of injury, family members need factual information and support from the health care team.

Many patients with severe head injuries that result in brain death are young and otherwise healthy and are therefore considered for organ donation. Family members of patients with such injuries need support during this extremely stressful time and assistance in making decisions to end life support and permit donation of organs. They need to know that the patient who is brain dead and whose respiratory and cardiovascular systems are maintained through life support is not going to survive and that the severe head injury, not the removal of the patient's organs or the removal of life support, is the cause of the patient's death. Bereavement counselors and members of the organ procurement team are often immensely helpful to family members in making decisions about organ donation and in helping them cope with stress.

MONITORING AND MANAGING POTENTIAL COMPLICATIONS

Decreased Cerebral Perfusion Pressure. Maintenance of adequate CPP is important to prevent serious complications of head injury due to decreased cerebral perfusion. Adequate CPP is greater than 50 mm Hg. If CPP falls below a patient's threshold, a vasodilating cascade occurs, causing the volume of blood to increase inside the brain, which causes ICP to increase. Measures to maintain adequate CPP are essential because a decrease in CPP can impair cerebral perfusion and cause brain hypoxia and ischemia, leading to permanent brain damage. Once the threshold CPP is reached, vasoconstriction of the cerebral blood vessels occurs, causing ICP to decrease. Therapy (e.g., elevation of the head of the bed, increased IV fluids, CSF drainage) is directed toward decreasing cerebral edema and increasing venous outflow from the brain. Systemic hypotension, which causes vasoconstriction and a significant decrease in CPP, is treated with increased IV fluids or vasopressors (Livesay, McNett, Keller, et al., 2017).

Cerebral Edema and Herniation. The patient with a head injury is at risk for additional complications such as increased ICP and brain stem herniation. Cerebral edema is the most common cause of increased ICP in the patient with a head injury, with the swelling peaking approximately 48 to 72 hours after injury. Bleeding also may increase the volume of contents within the rigid, closed compartment of the skull, causing increased ICP and herniation of the brain stem and resulting in irreversible brain anoxia and brain death (Hickey & Strayer, 2020; Vijay & Jaison, 2019). ICP is measured continuously and nursing interventions such as turning and suctioning have been associated with variation in the ICP (Olson, Parcon, Santos, et al., 2017). Measures to control ICP are listed in Chart 63-5 and discussed in Chapter 61.

Impaired Oxygenation and Ventilation. Impaired oxygenation and ventilation may require mechanical ventilatory support. The patient must be monitored for a patent airway, altered breathing patterns, and hypoxemia and pneumonia. Interventions may include endotracheal

---

Chart 63-5 Controlling ICP in Patients with Severe Brain Injury

- Elevate the head of the bed as prescribed.
- Maintain the patient's head and neck in neutral alignment (no twisting or flexing the neck).
- Initiate measures to prevent the Valsalva maneuver (e.g., stool softeners).
- Maintain body temperature within normal limits.
- Administer oxygen (O_2) to maintain partial pressure of arterial oxygen (PaO_2) >90 mm Hg.
- Maintain fluid balance with normal saline solution.
- Avoid noxious stimuli (e.g., excessive suctioning, painful procedures).
- Administer sedation to reduce agitation.
- Maintain cerebral perfusion pressure of 60–70 mm Hg.

Adapted from Hickey, J. V., & Strayer, A. (2020). *The clinical practice of neurological & neurosurgical nursing.* (8th ed.). Philadelphia, PA: Wolters Kluwer.

---

intubation, mechanical ventilation, and positive end-expiratory pressure. See Chapters 19 and 61 for a detailed discussion on these topics.

Impaired Fluid, Electrolyte, and Nutritional Balance. Fluid, electrolyte, and nutritional imbalances are common in the patient with a head injury. Common imbalances include hyponatremia, which is often associated with SIADH (see Chapters 10 and 45), hypokalemia, and hyperglycemia. Modifications in fluid intake with tube feedings or IV fluids, including hypertonic saline, may be necessary to treat these imbalances (Hickey & Strayer, 2020). Insulin administration may be prescribed to treat hyperglycemia; blood glucose levels are maintained between 80 and 160 mg/dL (Vijay & Jaison, 2019).

Undernutrition is also a common problem in response to the increased metabolic needs associated with severe head injury. Decisions about early feeding should be individualized; options include IV hyperalimentation or placement of a feeding tube (jejunal or gastric). Caloric expenditure can increase up to 120% to 140% with TBI, requiring close monitoring of nutritional status, with a higher concentration of protein if tolerated (Quintard & Ichai, 2018).

Posttraumatic Seizures. Patients with head injury are at an increased risk for posttraumatic seizures. Posttraumatic seizures are classified as immediate (within 24 hours after injury), early (within 1 to 7 days after injury), or late (more than 7 days after injury) (Hickey & Strayer, 2020). Seizure prophylaxis is the practice of administering anticonvulsant medications to patients with head injury to prevent seizures. It is important to prevent posttraumatic seizures, especially in the immediate and early phases of recovery, because seizures may increase ICP and decrease oxygenation (Chartrain, Yaeger, Feng, et al., 2017; Zaman, Dubiel, Driver, et al., 2017). However, many anticonvulsant medications impair cognitive performance and can prolong the duration of rehabilitation. Therefore, the overall benefits of these medications must be weighed against their side effects. Research evidence supports the use of prophylactic anticonvulsant agents to prevent immediate and early seizures after head injury, but not for prevention

Chart 63-6 — HOME CARE CHECKLIST
The Patient with a TBI

At the completion of education, the patient and/or caregiver will be able to:

- State the impact of TBI and treatment on physiologic functioning, ADLs, IADLs, roles, relationships, and spirituality.
- State the purpose, dose, route, schedule, side effects, and precautions for prescribed medications.
- State how to contact all members of the treatment team (e.g., health care providers, home care professionals, rehabilitation team, and durable medical equipment and supply vendor).
- State changes in lifestyle (e.g., ADLs, IADLs, activity) necessary for recovery and health maintenance, as applicable.
  - Demonstrate safe techniques to assist patient with self-care, hygiene, and ambulation.
  - Demonstrate safe techniques for eating, feeding patient, or assisting patient with eating.
  - Identify the need for close monitoring of behavior due to changes in cognitive functioning.
  - Describe strategies for reinforcing positive behaviors.
  - Describe household modifications needed to ensure safe environment for the patient.
- Explain the need for monitoring for changes in neurologic status and for complications.

- Identify changes in neurologic status and signs and symptoms of complications (e.g., pneumonia, urinary tract infection, meningitis) that should be reported to the neurosurgeon or nurse.
- Relate how to reach primary provider with questions or complications.
- State the importance of continuing follow-up by health care team.
- State time and date of follow-up medical appointments, therapy, and testing.
- Identify sources of support (e.g., friends, relatives, faith community).
- Identify the contact details for support services for patients and their caregivers/families.
- Identify the need for health-promotion, disease prevention, and screening activities.

Resources

See Chapter 7, Chart 7-6 Home Care Checklist: Managing Chronic Illness and Disability at Home.

ADL, activities of daily living; IADL, instrumental activities of daily living; TBI, traumatic brain injury.

---

of late seizures (Chartrain et al., 2017; Zaman et al., 2017). See Chapter 61 for the nursing management of seizures.

PROMOTING HOME, COMMUNITY-BASED, AND TRANSITIONAL CARE

Educating Patients About Self-Care. Education early in the course of head injury often focuses on reinforcing information given to the family about the patient's condition and prognosis. As the patient's status and expected outcome change over time, family education may focus on interpretation and explanation of changes in the patient's physical and psychological responses.

Once the patient's physical status allows discharge to home, a rehabilitation center, or a subacute care facility, the patient and family are educated about limitations that can be expected and complications that may occur. The nurse explains to the patient and family, verbally and in writing, how to monitor for complications that merit contacting the primary provider. Depending on the patient's prognosis and physical and cognitive status, the patient may be included in education about self-care management strategies.

If the patient is at risk for late posttraumatic seizures, anticonvulsant medications may be prescribed at discharge. The patient and family require education about the side effects of these medications and the importance of continuing to take them as prescribed.

Continuing and Transitional Care. The rehabilitation phase of care for the patient with a TBI begins at hospital admission. Admission to the rehabilitation unit is a milestone in a patient's recovery and requires intense work by the patient to complete the daily schedule of therapies. The goals of rehabilitation are to maximize the patient's ability to return to their highest level of functioning and to their home and the community, address concerns before discharge for a smooth transition to home or rehabilitation, and promote independence with adaptation to deficits. The patient is encouraged to continue the rehabilitation program after discharge, because improvement in status may continue 3 or more years after injury. Changes in the patient with a TBI and the effects of long-term rehabilitation on the family and their coping abilities need ongoing assessment. Continued education and support of the patient and family are essential as their needs and the patient's status change. Education to address with the family of the patient who is about to return home is described in Chart 63-6.

Depending on status, the patient is encouraged to return to usual activities gradually. Referral to support groups and to the Brain Injury Association of America may be warranted (see the Resources section).

During the acute and rehabilitation phases of care, the focus of education is on obvious needs, issues, deficits, and complications. Complications after TBI include infections (e.g., pneumonia, urinary tract infection [UTI], sepsis, wound infection, osteomyelitis, meningitis, ventriculitis, brain abscess) and heterotopic ossification (painful bone overgrowth in weight-bearing joints).

The nurse reminds the patient and family of the need for continuing health promotion and screening practices after the initial phase of care. Patients who have not been involved in these practices in the past are educated about their importance and are referred to appropriate health care providers.

Evaluation

Expected patient outcomes may include:

1. Attains or maintains effective airway clearance, ventilation, and brain oxygenation
   a. Achieves blood gas values within normal limits and has breath sounds clear on auscultation
   b. Mobilizes and clears secretions

2. Achieves satisfactory fluid and electrolyte balance
   a. Demonstrates serum electrolytes within normal limits
   b. Has no clinical signs of dehydration or overhydration
3. Attains adequate nutritional status
   a. Is free of gastric distention and vomiting
   b. Shows minimal weight loss
4. Avoids injury
   a. Shows lessening agitation and restlessness
   b. Is oriented to person, place, and time
5. Maintains body temperature within normal limits
   a. Absence of fever
   b. Absence of hypothermia
6. Demonstrates intact skin integrity
   a. Exhibits no redness or breaks in skin integrity
   b. Exhibits no pressure injuries
7. Shows improvement in coping
8. Demonstrates usual sleep–wake cycle
9. Family demonstrates adaptive family processes
   a. Joins support group
   b. Shares feelings with appropriate health care personnel
   c. Makes end-of-life decisions, if needed
10. Demonstrates absence of complications
    a. Demonstrates ICP within normal limits
    b. Exhibits vital signs and body temperature within normal limits and increases orientation to person, place, and time
11. Experiences no posttraumatic seizures
    a. Takes anticonvulsant medications as prescribed
    b. Identifies side effects/adverse effects of anticonvulsant medications
12. Participates in rehabilitation process as indicated for patient and family members
    a. Takes active role in identifying rehabilitation goals and participating in recommended patient care activities
    b. Prepares for discharge

Spinal Cord Injury (SCI)

Spinal cord injury (SCI), an injury to the spinal cord, vertebral column, supporting soft tissue, or intervertebral discs caused by trauma is a major health disorder. In the United States, approximately 294,000 persons are living with an SCI. An estimated 17,810 new cases occur annually; common causes are motor vehicle crashes, falls, violence (predominantly gunshot wounds), and sports-related injuries (National Spinal Cord Injury Statistical Center [NSCISC], 2020). Males account for 78% of patients with SCI. The average age of injury is 43 years of age (NSCISC, 2020). The indirect cost for the care of patients with SCI averages about $77,701 per patient per year in 2019 dollars (NSCISC, 2020).

The predominant risk factors for SCI include younger age, male gender, and alcohol and illicit drug abuse. The frequency with which these risk factors are associated with SCI serves to emphasize the importance of primary prevention. The same interventions suggested earlier in this chapter for head injury prevention help decrease the incidence of SCI (see Chart 63-1). Life expectancy continues to increase for people with SCI because of improved health care but remains slightly lower than for those without SCI. The major causes of death are pneumonia, pulmonary embolism (PE), and sepsis (Hickey & Strayer, 2020).

Paraplegia (paralysis of the lower body) and **tetraplegia** (paralysis of all four extremities; formerly called *quadriplegia*) can occur, with incomplete tetraplegia being the most frequently occurring injury, followed by complete paraplegia, complete tetraplegia, and incomplete paraplegia.

Pathophysiology

Damage in SCI ranges from transient concussion (from which the patient fully recovers) to contusion, laceration, and compression of the spinal cord tissue (either alone or in combination), to complete **transection** (severing) of the spinal cord (which renders the patient paralyzed below the level of the injury). The vertebrae most frequently involved are the fifth, sixth, and seventh cervical vertebrae (C5–C7), the 12th thoracic vertebra (T12), and the first lumbar vertebra (L1). These vertebrae are most susceptible because there is a greater range of mobility in the vertebral column in these areas (Hickey & Strayer, 2020).

SCI can be separated into two categories: primary injuries and secondary injuries. Primary injuries are the result of the initial insult or trauma and are usually permanent. Secondary injuries resulting from SCI include edema and hemorrhage (Venkatesh, Ghosh, Mullick, et al., 2019). The secondary injury is a major concern for critical-care nurses. Early treatment is essential to prevent partial damage from becoming total and permanent.

Veterans Considerations

Veterans account for a large proportion of those living with SCI (Gary, Cao, Burns, et al., 2020). Veterans who have suffered an SCI are significantly older and predominantly male compared to civilians with SCI (Furlan, Kurban, & Craven, 2019). However, the level of injury, severity, mechanisms of injury, and need for mechanical ventilation after the SCI are all similar to civilians (Furlan et al., 2019). Veterans with war-related SCIs are predominantly young, White, and male; they have commonly sustained thoracic, severe, SCI caused by gunshot or explosion; and they often have at least one other bodily injury in addition to SCI (Furlan, Gulasingam, & Craven, 2017). Differences between veterans and civilians with SCI may influence adjustment and functional outcomes. For example, factors such as the high rates of posttraumatic stress syndrome, the need to accommodate to civilian life, and the burden of not being able to serve increase the risk for poorer health and unhealthy behaviors, mental health problems, and substance use disorder (Gary et al., 2020). Veterans with SCI have higher cognitive function, social integration, self-perceived independence, and social support, as well as less pain and fewer secondary impairments than civilians with SCI. They also have better physical independence and mobility (Gary et al., 2020). Among civilians, there is a greater likelihood of employment post SCI for non-Hispanic White men with a college education. However, veterans with SCI lesions higher in the spinal cord are less likely to be employed.

Clinical Manifestations

Manifestations of SCI depend on the type and level of injury (see Chart 63-7). The type of injury refers to the extent of

Chart 63-7 Effects of Spinal Cord Injuries

Central Cord Syndrome

- *Characteristics*: Motor deficits (in the upper extremities compared to the lower extremities; sensory loss varies but is more pronounced in the upper extremities); bowel/bladder dysfunction is variable, or function may be completely preserved.
- *Cause*: Injury or edema of the central cord, usually of the cervical area. May be caused by hyperextension injuries.

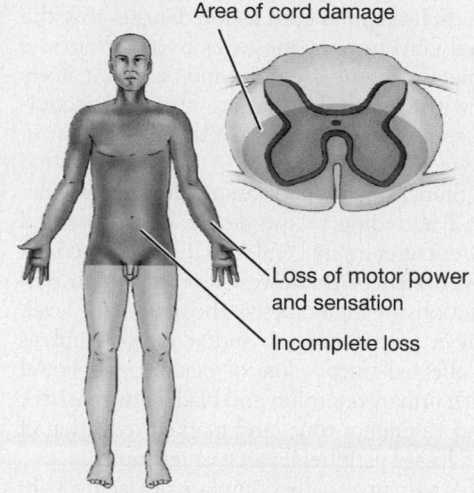

Central cord syndrome

Anterior Cord Syndrome

- *Characteristics*: Loss of pain, temperature, and motor function is noted below the level of the lesion; light touch, position, and vibration sensation remain intact.
- *Cause*: The syndrome may be caused by acute disc herniation or hyperflexion injuries associated with fracture/dislocation of vertebra. It may also occur as a result of injury to the anterior spinal artery, which supplies the anterior two thirds of the spinal cord.

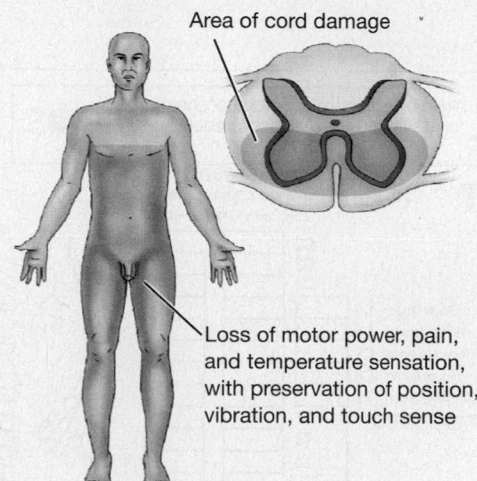

Anterior cord syndrome

Lateral Cord Syndrome (Brown-Séquard Syndrome)

- *Characteristics*: Ipsilateral paralysis or paresis is noted, together with ipsilateral loss of touch, pressure, and vibration and contralateral loss of pain and temperature.
- *Cause*: The lesion is caused by a transverse hemisection of the cord (half of the cord is transected from north to south), usually as a result of a knife or missile injury, fracture/dislocation of a unilateral articular process, or possibly an acute ruptured disc.

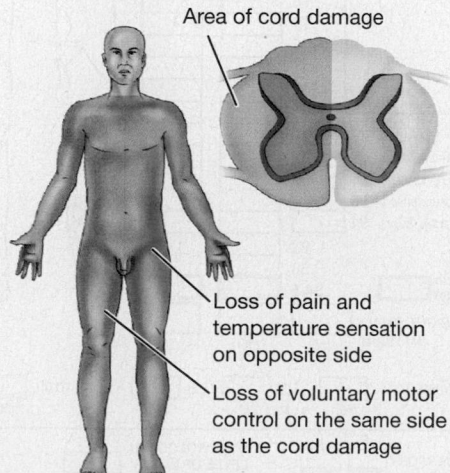

Brown-Séquard syndrome

Adapted from Hickey, J. V., & Strayer, A. (2020). *The clinical practice of neurological & neurosurgical nursing* (8th ed.). Philadelphia, PA: Wolters Kluwer.

injury to the spinal cord itself. A **complete spinal cord lesion** signifies loss of both sensory and voluntary motor communication from the brain to the periphery, resulting in paraplegia or tetraplegia. **Incomplete spinal cord lesion** denotes that the ability of the spinal cord to relay messages to and from the brain is not completely absent. Sensory and/or motor fibers are preserved below the lesion. Injuries are classified according to the area of spinal cord damage: central, lateral, anterior, or peripheral (see Chart 63-7).

The American Spinal Injury Association (ASIA) provides classification of SCI according to the degree of sensory and motor function present after injury (ASIA, 2019; see Fig. 63-4). The neurologic level refers to the lowest level at which sensory and motor functions are intact. Below the neurologic level, there may be total or partial, sensory and/or motor paralysis (dependent upon affected tracts), loss of bladder and bowel control (usually with urinary retention and bladder distention), loss of sweating and vasomotor tone, and marked reduction of blood pressure from loss of peripheral vascular resistance.

If conscious, the patient usually complains of acute pain in the back or neck, which may radiate along the involved nerve. However, absence of pain does not rule out spinal injury, and a careful assessment of the spine should be conducted if there has been a significant force and mechanism of injury (i.e., concomitant head injury).

Respiratory dysfunction is related to the level of injury. The muscles contributing to respiration are the diaphragm (C4), intercostals (T1–T6), and abdominals (T6–T12). Injuries at C4 or above (causing paralysis of the diaphragm) often will require ventilator support, since acute respiratory failure is a leading cause of death (Hickey & Strayer, 2020). Injuries of T12 and above will have impact on respiratory function. Functional abilities by level of injury are described in Table 63-3.

Assessment and Diagnostic Findings

A detailed neurologic examination is performed. Diagnostic x-rays (lateral cervical spine x-rays) and CT scanning are usually performed initially. An MRI scan may be ordered as a further workup if a ligamentous injury is suspected, because significant spinal cord damage may exist even in the absence of

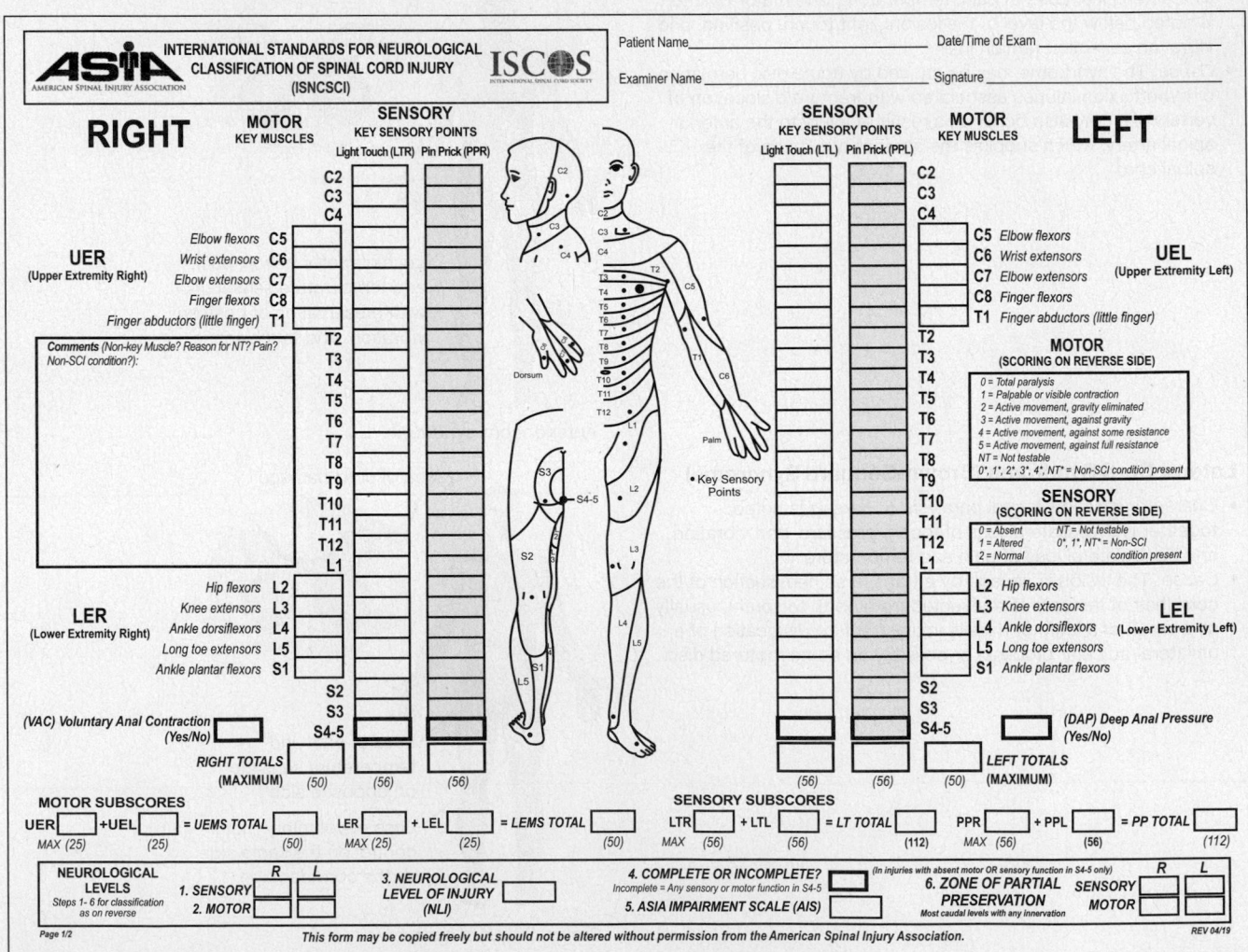

Figure 63-4 • Worksheet for the classification of SCI. From the American Spinal Injury Association International Standards Committee: International Standards for Neurological Classification of Spinal Cord Injury. Retrieved on 3/03/2021 at: https://asia-spinalinjury.org/wp-content/uploads/2019/10/ASIA-ISCOS-Worksheet_10.2019_PRINT-Page-1-2.pdf. © 2021 American Spinal Injury Association. Reprinted with permission.

Muscle Function Grading

0 = Total paralysis

1 = Palpable or visible contraction

2 = Active movement, full range of motion (ROM) with gravity eliminated

3 = Active movement, full ROM against gravity

4 = Active movement, full ROM against gravity and moderate resistance in a muscle specific position

5 = (Normal) active movement, full ROM against gravity and full resistance in a functional muscle position expected from an otherwise unimpaired person

NT = Not testable (i.e. due to immobilization, severe pain such that the patient cannot be graded, amputation of limb, or contracture of > 50% of the normal ROM)

0*, 1*, 2*, 3*, 4*, NT* = Non-SCI condition present [a]

Sensory Grading

0 = Absent   1 = Altered, either decreased/impaired sensation or hypersensitivity

2 = Normal   NT = Not testable

0*, 1*, NT* = Non-SCI condition present [a]

[a] Note: Abnormal motor and sensory scores should be tagged with a '*' to indicate an impairment due to a non-SCI condition. The non-SCI condition should be explained in the comments box together with information about how the score is rated for classification purposes (at least normal / not normal for classification).

When to Test Non-Key Muscles:

In a patient with an apparent AIS B classification, non-key muscle functions more than 3 levels below the motor level on each side should be tested to most accurately classify the injury (differentiate between AIS B and C).

Movement	Root level
Shoulder: Flexion, extension, adbuction, adduction, internal and external rotation **Elbow:** Supination	C5
Elbow: Pronation **Wrist:** Flexion	C6
Finger: Flexion at proximal joint, extension **Thumb:** Flexion, extension and abduction in plane of thumb	C7
Finger: Flexion at MCP joint **Thumb:** Opposition, adduction and abduction perpendicular to palm	C8
Finger: Abduction of the index finger	T1
Hip: Adduction	L2
Hip: External rotation	L3
Hip: Extension, abduction, internal rotation **Knee:** Flexion **Ankle:** Inversion and eversion **Toe:** MP and IP extension	L4
Hallux and Toe: DIP and PIP flexion and abduction	L5
Hallux: Adduction	S1

ASIA Impairment Scale (AIS)

A = Complete. No sensory or motor function is preserved in the sacral segments S4-5.

B = Sensory Incomplete. Sensory but not motor function is preserved below the neurological level and includes the sacral segments S4-5 (light touch or pin prick at S4-5 or deep anal pressure) AND no motor function is preserved more than three levels below the motor level on either side of the body.

C = Motor Incomplete. Motor function is preserved at the most caudal sacral segments for voluntary anal contraction (VAC) OR the patient meets the criteria for sensory incomplete status (sensory function preserved at the most caudal sacral segments S4-5 by LT, PP or DAP), and has some sparing of motor function more than three levels below the ipsilateral motor level on either side of the body. (This includes key or non-key muscle functions to determine motor incomplete status.) For AIS C – less than half of key muscle functions below the single NLI have a muscle grade ≥ 3.

D = Motor Incomplete. Motor incomplete status as defined above, with at least half (half or more) of key muscle functions below the single NLI having a muscle grade ≥ 3.

E = Normal. If sensation and motor function as tested with the ISNCSCI are graded as normal in all segments, and the patient had prior deficits, then the AIS grade is E. Someone without an initial SCI does not receive an AIS grade.

Using ND: To document the sensory, motor and NLI levels, the ASIA Impairment Scale grade, and/or the zone of partial preservation (ZPP) when they are unable to be determined based on the examination results.

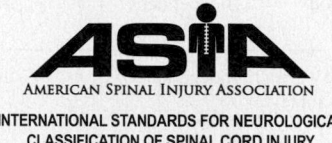

AMERICAN SPINAL INJURY ASSOCIATION

INTERNATIONAL STANDARDS FOR NEUROLOGICAL CLASSIFICATION OF SPINAL CORD INJURY

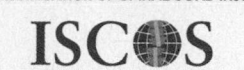

INTERNATIONAL SPINAL CORD SOCIETY

Page 2/2

Steps in Classification

The following order is recommended for determining the classification of individuals with SCI.

1. Determine sensory levels for right and left sides.
The sensory level is the most caudal, intact dermatome for both pin prick and light touch sensation.

2. Determine motor levels for right and left sides.
Defined by the lowest key muscle function that has a grade of at least 3 (on supine testing), providing the key muscle functions represented by segments above that level are judged to be intact (graded as a 5).
Note: in regions where there is no myotome to test, the motor level is presumed to be the same as the sensory level, if testable motor function above that level is also normal.

3. Determine the neurological level of injury (NLI).
This refers to the most caudal segment of the cord with intact sensation and antigravity (3 or more) muscle function strength, provided that there is normal (intact) sensory and motor function rostrally respectively.
The NLI is the most cephalad of the sensory and motor levels determined in steps 1 and 2.

4. Determine whether the injury is Complete or Incomplete.
(i.e. absence or presence of sacral sparing)
If voluntary anal contraction = **No** AND all S4-5 sensory scores = 0 AND deep anal pressure = **No**, then injury is **Complete**.
Otherwise, injury is **Incomplete**.

5. Determine ASIA Impairment Scale (AIS) Grade.
  Is injury <u>Complete</u>?   If YES, AIS=A

  NO ↓

  Is injury <u>Motor Complete</u>? If YES, AIS=B

  NO ↓   (No=voluntary anal contraction OR motor function more than three levels below the <u>motor level</u> on a given side, if the patient has sensory incomplete classification)

  Are <u>at least</u> half (half or more) of the key muscles below the <u>neurological level of injury</u> graded 3 or better?

  NO ↓   **YES** ↓

  AIS=C   AIS=D

If sensation and motor function is normal in all segments, AIS=E
Note: AIS E is used in follow-up testing when an individual with a documented SCI has recovered normal function. If at initial testing no deficits are found, the individual is neurologically intact and the ASIA Impairment Scale does not apply.

6. Determine the zone of partial preservation (ZPP).
The ZPP is used only in injuries with absent motor (no VAC) OR sensory function (no DAP, no LT and no PP sensation) in the lowest sacral segments S4-5, and refers to those dermatomes and myotomes caudal to the sensory and motor levels that remain partially innervated. With sacral sparing of sensory function, the sensory ZPP is not applicable and therefore "NA" is recorded in the block of the worksheet. Accordingly, if VAC is present, the motor ZPP is not applicable and is noted as "NA".

Figure 63-4 • *(Continued)*

bony injury (Hickey & Strayer, 2020). If an MRI scan is contraindicated, a myelogram may be used to visualize the spinal axis. An assessment is made for other injuries because spinal trauma often is accompanied by concomitant injuries, commonly to the head and chest. Continuous electrocardiographic monitoring may be indicated if an SCI is suspected, because bradycardia (slow heart rate) and asystole (cardiac standstill) are common in patients with acute spinal cord injuries.

Emergency Management

The immediate management at the scene of the injury is critical because improper handling of the patient can cause further damage and loss of neurologic function. Any patient who is involved in a motor vehicle crash, a diving or contact sports injury, a fall, or any direct trauma to the head and neck must be considered to have SCI until such an injury is ruled out. Initial care must include a rapid assessment, immobilization, extrication, and stabilization or control of life-threatening injuries, and transportation to the most appropriate medical facility. Immediate transportation to a trauma center with the capacity to manage major neurologic trauma is then necessary (Hickey & Strayer, 2020).

At the scene of the injury, the patient must be immobilized on a spinal (back) board, with the head and neck maintained in a neutral position, to prevent an incomplete injury from becoming complete. One member of the team must assume control of the patient's head to prevent flexion, rotation, or extension; this is done by placing the hands on both sides of the patient's head at about ear level to limit movement and maintain alignment while a spinal board and cervical immobilizing device is applied. If possible, at least four people should slide the patient carefully onto a board for transfer to the hospital. Head blocks should also be considered, as they will further limit any neck movement. Any twisting movement may irreversibly damage the spinal cord by causing bony fragment or disc movement or exacerbating ligamentous injury, causing further instability.

The patient is referred to a regional spinal injury or trauma center because of the multidisciplinary personnel and support services required to counteract the destructive changes that occur in the first 24 hours after injury. During treatment in the emergency and x-ray departments, the patient is kept on the transfer board. The patient must always be maintained in an extended position. No part of the body should be twisted or turned, and the patient is not allowed to sit up. Once the

TABLE 63-3	Functional Abilities by Level of Spinal Cord Injury			
Injury Level	**Segmental Sensorimotor Function**	**Dressing, Eating**	**Elimination**	**Mobility**[a]
C1	Little or no sensation or control of head and neck; no diaphragm control; requires continuous ventilation	Dependent	Dependent	Limited. Voice or sip-n-puff controlled electric wheelchair
C2–C3	Head and neck sensation; some neck control; independent of mechanical ventilation for short periods	Dependent	Dependent	Same as for C1
C4	Good head and neck sensation and motor control; some shoulder elevation; diaphragm movement	Dependent; may be able to eat with adaptive sling	Dependent	Limited to voice, mouth, head, chin, or shoulder-controlled electric wheelchair
C5	Full head and neck control; shoulder strength; elbow flexion	Independent with assistance	Maximal assistance	Electric or modified manual wheelchair, needs transfer assistance
C6	Fully innervated shoulder; wrist extension or dorsiflexion	Independent or with minimal assistance	Independent or with minimal assistance	Independent in transfers and wheelchair
C7–C8	Full elbow extension; wrist plantar flexion; some finger control	Independent	Independent	Independent; manual wheelchair
T1–T5	Full-hand and finger control; use of intercostal and thoracic muscles	Independent	Independent	Independent; manual wheelchair
T6–T10	Abdominal muscle control, partial to good balance with trunk muscles	Independent	Independent	Independent; manual wheelchair
T11–L5	Hip flexors, hip abductors (L1–L3); knee extension (L2–L4); knee flexion; and ankle dorsiflexion (L4–L5)	Independent	Independent	Short distance to full ambulation with assistance
S1–S5	Full leg, foot, and ankle control; innervation of perineal muscles for bowel, bladder, and sexual function (S2–S4)	Independent	Normal to impaired bowel and bladder function	Ambulate independently with or without assistance

[a]Assistance refers to adaptive equipment, setup, or physical assistance.
Adapted from Hickey, J. V., & Strayer, A. (2020). *The clinical practice of neurological & neurosurgical nursing* (8th ed.). Philadelphia, PA: Wolters Kluwer.

extent of the injury has been determined, the patient may be placed on a rotating specialty bed or in a cervical collar (see Fig. 63-5). Later, if SCI and bone instability have been ruled out, the patient may be moved to a conventional bed or the collar may be removed without harm. If a specialty bed is needed but not available, the patient should be placed in a cervical collar and on a firm mattress.

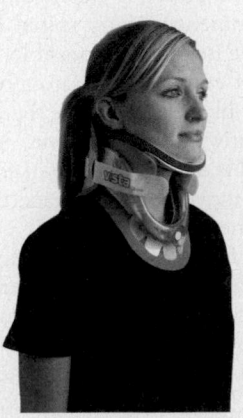

Figure 63-5 • Cervical collar. Used with permission from Aspen Medical Products.

Medical Management (Acute Phase)

The goals of management are to prevent secondary injury, to observe for symptoms of progressive neurologic deficits, and to prevent complications. The patient is resuscitated as necessary, and oxygenation and cardiovascular stability are maintained. SCI is a devastating event; new treatment methods and medications are continually being investigated for the acute and chronic phases of care (Venkatesh et al., 2019).

Pharmacologic Therapy

Administration of high-dose IV corticosteroids (methylprednisolone sodium succinate) in the first 24 or 48 hours is controversial. The validity of studies has been questioned based on critical analysis of the original and additional data. As a result, there is now a consensus that corticosteroids may offer only a slight benefit. Corticosteroids are no longer considered the standard of care for acute SCI, although some centers continue to use corticosteroid protocols (Hickey & Strayer, 2020).

Respiratory Therapy

Oxygen is given to maintain a high partial pressure of arterial oxygen (PaO_2), because hypoxemia can create or worsen a neurologic deficit of the spinal cord. If endotracheal intubation is necessary, extreme care is taken to avoid flexing or extending the patient's neck, which can result in extension of a cervical injury.

In high cervical spine injuries, spinal cord innervation to the phrenic nerve, which stimulates the diaphragm, is lost. Diaphragmatic pacing (electrical stimulation of the phrenic nerve) attempts to stimulate the diaphragm to help the patient breathe. Intramuscular diaphragmatic pacing is currently in the clinical trial phase for the patient with a high cervical injury. This is implanted via laparoscopic surgery, usually after the acute phase.

Skeletal Fracture Reduction and Traction

Management of SCI requires immobilization and reduction of dislocations (restoration of preinjury position) and stabilization of the vertebral column. This can be accomplished by surgical or nonsurgical interventions; both aim to prevent new or worsening neurologic damage.

Cervical fractures can be reduced, and the cervical spine aligned with some form of skeletal traction, such as with skeletal tongs or with the use of the halo device. Traction is applied to the skeletal traction device by weights (ensuring the weights are unencumbered); the amount depends on the size of the patient and the degree of fracture displacement. The traction force is exerted along the longitudinal axis of the vertebral bodies, with the patient's neck in a neutral position. The traction is then gradually increased by adding more weights. As the amount of traction is increased, the spaces between the intervertebral discs widen and the vertebrae are given a chance to slip back into position. Reduction usually occurs after correct alignment has been restored. Once reduction is achieved, as verified by cervical spine x-rays and neurologic examination, the weights are gradually removed until the amount of weight needed to maintain the alignment is identified. Traction is sometimes supplemented with manual manipulation of the neck by a surgeon, to help achieve realignment of the vertebral bodies.

A halo device may be used initially with traction or may be applied after removal of the tongs. It consists of a titanium or stainless-steel halo ring that is fixed to the skull by four pins, which are inserted into the outer table of the skull. The ring is attached to a removable halo vest, a device that suspends the weight of the unit circumferentially around the chest. A frame connects the ring to the chest. Halo devices provide immobilization of the cervical spine while allowing early ambulation (see Fig. 63-6) for patients with adequate function.

Thoracic and lumbar injuries are usually treated with surgical intervention, followed by immobilization with a fitted brace. Traction is often not indicated either before or after surgery, due to the relative stability of the spine in these regions.

> ### ◤ Quality and Safety Nursing Alert
>
> *The patient's vital organ functions and body defenses must be supported and maintained until spinal and neurogenic shock abates and the neurologic system has recovered from the traumatic insult; this can take up to 4 months.*

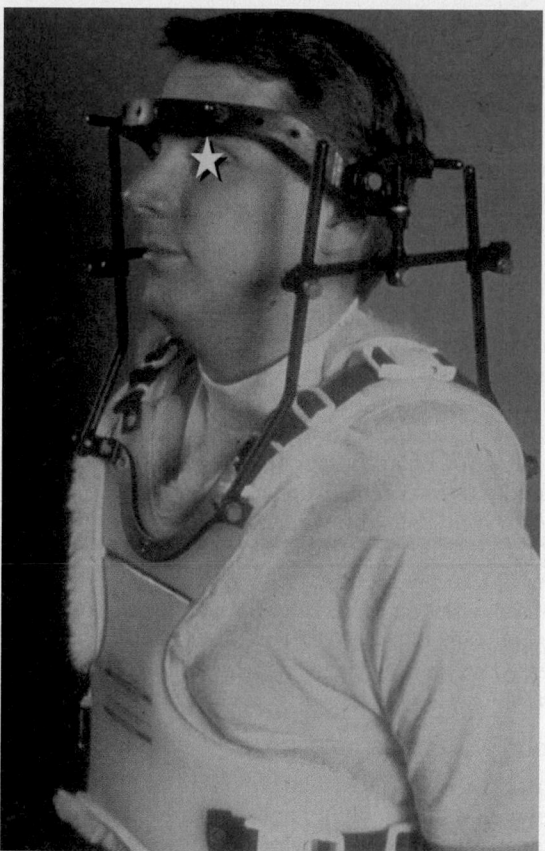

Figure 63-6 • Halo and vest for cervical and thoracic injuries. Adapted from Schwartz, E. D., Adam, E., & Flander, S. (2007). *Spinal trauma: Imaging, diagnosis, and management.* Philadelphia, PA: Lippincott Williams & Wilkins.

Surgical Management

Surgery is indicated in any of the following situations:
- Compression of the cord is evident.
- The injury results in a fragmented or unstable vertebral body.
- The injury involves a wound that penetrates the cord.
- Bony fragments are in the spinal canal.
- The patient's neurologic status is deteriorating.

Early surgical stabilization may improve the clinical outcome of patients compared to surgery performed later during the clinical course. The goals of surgical treatment are to preserve neurologic function by removing pressure from the spinal cord and to provide stability.

Management of Acute Complications of Spinal Cord Injury

Spinal and Neurogenic Shock

The spinal shock associated with SCI reflects a sudden depression of reflex activity in the spinal cord, called areflexia, that occurs below the level of injury. The muscles innervated by the part of the spinal cord segment below the level of the lesion are without sensation, paralyzed, and flaccid, and the reflexes are absent. Blood pressure may be decreased, and the patient may be bradycardic. Hypotension and shock can further damage the spinal cord; therefore, the mean arterial pressure (MAP) should be maintained at

85 mm Hg or higher during the hyperacute phase. The reflexes that initiate bladder and bowel function are affected. Bowel distention and paralytic ileus can be caused by depression of the reflexes and are treated with intestinal decompression by insertion of a nasogastric tube. A paralytic ileus most often occurs within the first 2 to 3 days after SCI and resolves within 3 to 7 days.

Neurogenic shock develops as a result of the loss of autonomic nervous system function below the level of the lesion. The vital organs are affected, causing decreases in blood pressure, heart rate, and cardiac output, as well as venous pooling in the extremities and peripheral vasodilation (Volski & Ackerman, 2020). In addition, the patient does not perspire in the paralyzed portions of the body, because sympathetic activity is blocked; therefore, close observation is required for early detection of an abrupt onset of fever. See Chapter 11 for further discussion on neurogenic shock.

With injuries to the cervical and upper thoracic spinal cord, innervation to the major accessory muscles of respiration is lost and respiratory problems develop. These include decreased vital capacity, retention of secretions, increased partial pressure of arterial carbon dioxide ($PaCO_2$) levels and decreased oxygen levels, respiratory failure, and pulmonary edema.

Venous Thromboembolism

The risk for venous thromboembolism (VTE) is a potential complication of immobility and occurs in patients with SCI at the same rate as those having had other types of traumatic injuries (Wang, Strayer, Harris, et al., 2017). Patients who develop VTE are at high risk for both deep vein thrombosis (DVT) and PE due to immobility, flaccidity, and decreased vasomotor tone (Wang et al., 2017).

Manifestations of PE include pleuritic chest pain, anxiety, shortness of breath, and abnormal blood gas values (increased $PaCO_2$ and decreased PaO_2). A fatal PE has been reported in up to 2% of patients with SCI within the first 3 months after injury (Hickey & Strayer, 2020).

Low-dose anticoagulation therapy usually is initiated to prevent DVT and PE, along with the use of anti-embolism stockings or sequential pneumatic compression devices (SCDs). In some cases, permanent indwelling filters may be placed prophylactically in the vena cava to prevent emboli (dislodged clots) from migrating to the lungs and causing PE. Prevention continues into the rehabilitation and chronic phases of SCI care (Abrams & Wakasa, 2019). See Chapter 26 for further discussion on VTE.

> **▶ Quality and Safety Nursing Alert**
>
> *The calves or thighs of a patient who is immobile should never be massaged because of the danger of dislodging an undetected thromboembolus.*

Other Complications

In addition to the respiratory complications (respiratory failure, pneumonia) and autonomic dysreflexia, other complications that may occur include pressure injuries and infection (urinary, respiratory, and local infection at the skeletal traction pin sites).

NURSING PROCESS

The Patient with Acute Spinal Cord Injury

Assessment

The patient's breathing pattern and the strength of the cough are assessed, and the lungs are auscultated, because paralysis of the diaphragm, in addition to abdominal and respiratory muscles, diminishes coughing and makes clearing of bronchial and pharyngeal secretions difficult. Reduced excursion of the chest also results.

The patient is monitored closely for any changes in motor or sensory function and for symptoms of progressive neurologic damage. In the early stages of SCI, determining whether the cord has been severed may not be possible, because signs and symptoms of cord edema are indistinguishable from those of cord transection. Edema of the spinal cord may occur with any severe cord injury and may further compromise spinal cord function.

Motor and sensory functions are assessed through careful neurologic examination. These findings are recorded on a flow sheet so that changes in the baseline neurologic status can be monitored closely and accurately. The ASIA classification is commonly used to describe the level of function for patients with SCI (see Fig. 63-4). Chart 63-7 also gives examples of the effects of altered spinal cord function. At the minimum:

- Motor ability is tested by asking the patient to spread the fingers, squeeze the examiner's hand, and move the toes or turn the feet.
- Sensation is evaluated by gently pinching the skin or touching it lightly with an object such as a tongue blade, starting at shoulder level and working down both sides of the extremities. The patient should have both eyes closed so that the examination reveals true findings, not what the patient hopes to feel. The patient is asked where the sensation is felt.
- Any decrease in neurologic function is reported immediately.

The patient is also assessed for spinal shock, which is a complete loss of all reflex, motor, sensory, and autonomic activity below the level of the lesion that causes bladder paralysis and distention. The lower abdomen is palpated for signs of urinary retention and overdistention of the bladder. Further assessment is made for gastric dilation and paralytic ileus caused by an atonic bowel, a result of autonomic disruption.

Temperature is monitored because the patient may have periods of hyperthermia as a result of altered temperature control, which is due to the inability to perspire related to autonomic disruption. Body temperature becomes dependent on surroundings (poikilothermia).

Diagnosis

NURSING DIAGNOSES

Based on the assessment data, major nursing diagnoses may include the following:

- Impaired breathing associated with weakness or paralysis of diaphragm, abdominal, and intercostal muscles
- Impaired airway clearance associated with muscle weakness and inability to clear secretions

- Impaired mobility in bed and impaired mobility associated with motor and sensory impairments
- Risk for injury associated with motor and sensory impairment
- Risk for impaired skin integrity associated with immobility and sensory loss
- Urinary retention associated with inability to void spontaneously
- Constipation associated with presence of atonic bowel as a result of autonomic disruption
- Acute pain associated with treatment and prolonged immobility
- Autonomic dysreflexia associated with uninhibited sympathetic response of the nervous system following SCI

COLLABORATIVE PROBLEMS/POTENTIAL COMPLICATIONS

Potential complications may include the following:
- VTE
- Orthostatic hypotension

Planning and Goals

The goals for the patient may include improved breathing pattern and airway clearance, improved mobility, prevention of injury due to sensory impairment, maintenance of skin integrity, relief of urinary retention, improved bowel function, decreasing pain, early recognition of autonomic dysreflexia, and absence of complications.

Nursing Interventions

PROMOTING ADEQUATE BREATHING AND AIRWAY CLEARANCE

Possible impending respiratory failure is detected by observing the patient, measuring vital capacity, monitoring oxygen saturation through pulse oximetry, and monitoring arterial blood gases. Early and vigorous attention to clearing bronchial and pharyngeal secretions can prevent retention of secretions and atelectasis. Suctioning may be indicated but should be used with caution to avoid stimulating the vagus nerve and producing bradycardia and cardiac arrest.

If the patient cannot cough effectively because of decreased inspiratory volume and inability to generate sufficient expiratory pressure, chest physiotherapy and assisted coughing may be indicated. Specific breathing exercises are supervised by the nurse to increase the strength and endurance of the inspiratory muscles, particularly the diaphragm. Assisted coughing promotes clearing of secretions from the upper respiratory tract and is similar to the use of abdominal thrusts to clear an airway. Assisted coughing can be more effective than traditional suctioning because traditional suctioning clears the right mainstem bronchus, whereas sites for atelectasis and pneumonia are most commonly in the left lower lung lobe (Wang et al., 2017). Proper humidification and hydration are important to prevent secretions from becoming thick and difficult to remove even with coughing. The patient is assessed for signs of respiratory infection (e.g., cough, fever, dyspnea). Ascending edema of the spinal cord in the acute phase may cause respiratory difficulty that requires immediate intervention. Therefore, the patient's respiratory status must be monitored closely.

IMPROVING MOBILITY

Proper body alignment is maintained at all times. If not on a specialized rotating bed, the patient should not be turned until the primary provider has indicated that it is safe to do so. Once safe for movement, the patient is repositioned frequently and is assisted out of bed as soon as the spinal column is stabilized. Various types of splints are used to prevent footdrop, which can often occur. When used, the splints are removed and reapplied every 2 hours. Trochanter rolls, applied from the crest of the ilium to the midthigh of both legs, help prevent external rotation of the hip joints. Patients with lesions above the midthoracic level have loss of sympathetic control of peripheral vasoconstrictor activity, leading to hypotension. These patients may tolerate changes in position poorly and require monitoring of blood pressure when positions are changed.

Contractures can develop rapidly with immobility and muscle paralysis. A joint that is immobilized too long becomes fixed as a result of contractures of the tendon and joint capsule. Atrophy of the extremities results from disuse. Contractures and other complications may be prevented by range-of-motion exercises that help preserve joint motion and stimulate circulation. Passive range-of-motion exercises should be implemented as soon as possible after the injury. Toes, metatarsals, ankles, knees, and hips should be put through a full range of motion at least four, or ideally five, times daily.

For most patients who have a cervical fracture without neurologic deficit, reduction in traction followed by rigid immobilization for 6 to 8 weeks restores skeletal integrity. These patients are allowed to move gradually to an erect position. A neck brace or molded collar is applied when the patient is mobilized after traction is removed (see Fig. 63-5).

PREVENTING INJURY DUE TO SENSORY AND PERCEPTUAL ALTERATIONS

The nurse assists the patient to compensate for sensory and perceptual alterations that occur with SCI. The intact senses above the level of the injury are stimulated through touch, aromas, flavorful food and beverages, conversation, and music. Additional strategies include the following:

- Providing glasses to enable the patient to see from the supine position
- Encouraging the use of hearing aids, if indicated, to enable the patient to hear conversations and environmental sounds
- Providing emotional support to the patient and family
- Educating the patient and family about strategies to compensate for, or cope with, sensory deficits

MAINTAINING SKIN INTEGRITY

Pressure injuries are a significant complication of SCI. They may begin within hours of an acute SCI where pressure is continuous and where the peripheral circulation is inadequate as a result of spinal shock and a recumbent position. It is important to move the patient from the backboard as soon as possible and inspect the skin. In addition, patients who wear cervical collars for prolonged periods may develop breakdown from the pressure of the collar under the chin, on the shoulders, and at the occiput. Pressure injury can add substantially to the personal and economic costs of living with SCI.

The most effective approach to addressing this costly complication of SCI is prevention. The patient's position is changed at least every 2 hours. Turning not only assists in the prevention of pressure injuries but also prevents pooling of blood and edema in the dependent areas. Careful inspection of the skin is made each time the patient is turned. The skin over the pressure points is assessed for redness or breaks; the perineum is checked for soilage, and the catheter is observed for adequate drainage. The patient's general body alignment and comfort are assessed. Special attention should be given to pressure areas in contact with the transfer board.

In addition, the patient's skin should be kept clean by washing with a mild soap, rinsing well, and blotting dry. Pressure-sensitive areas should be kept well lubricated and soft with oil or emollient lotion. The patient is educated about the danger of pressure injuries and is encouraged to take control and make decisions about appropriate skin care. See Chapter 56 for other aspects of care and prevention of pressure injuries.

MAINTAINING URINARY ELIMINATION

Immediately after SCI, the urinary bladder becomes atonic and cannot contract by reflex activity. Urinary retention is the immediate result. During the initial acute phase, a urinary catheter is inserted; however, prompt discontinuation is advised due to high risk for catheter-associated urinary tract infection (CAUTI). Once discontinued, the patient has no sensation of bladder distention and overstretching of the bladder and detrusor muscle may occur, delaying the return of bladder function.

Intermittent catheterization is carried out to avoid overdistention of the bladder and high risk for UTI due to retention of urine. At an early stage, family members are shown how to carry out intermittent catheterization and are encouraged to participate in this facet of care, because they will be involved in long-term follow-up and must be able to recognize complications so that treatment can be instituted.

The patient is educated to record fluid intake, voiding pattern, amounts of residual urine after voiding, characteristics of urine, and any unusual sensations that may occur. The management of a **neurogenic bladder** (bladder dysfunction that results from a disorder or dysfunction of the nervous system) is addressed during the rehabilitation phase of care. The types of neurogenic bladder differ according to which motor or sensory pathways are disrupted (Hickey & Strayer, 2020).

External catheters (condom catheters) and leg bags to collect spontaneous voidings are useful for male patients with reflex or total incontinence. The appropriate design and size must be chosen for maximal success, and the patient or caregiver must be taught how to apply the condom catheter and how to provide daily hygiene including skin inspection. Instruction on emptying the leg bag must also be provided, and modifications can be made for patients with limited hand dexterity.

IMPROVING BOWEL FUNCTION

Immediately after SCI, a paralytic ileus usually develops as a result of neurogenic paralysis of the bowel; therefore, a nasogastric tube is often required to relieve distention and to prevent vomiting and aspiration (Stoffel, Van der Aa, Wittmann, et al., 2018).

Bowel activity usually returns within the first week. With the intake of nutrition, it is important to establish a bowel program. A bowel program can help to control bowel movements by establishing a pattern of planned evacuation. The nurse administers prescribed combinations of stool softeners, stimulant laxatives, bulking laxatives, and rectal laxatives along with rectal stimulation, to counteract the effects of immobility and analgesic agents (Stoffel et al., 2018).

PROVIDING COMFORT MEASURES: THE PATIENT IN TRACTION WITH TONGS OR HALO VEST

A patient who has had pins, tongs, or calipers placed for cervical stabilization may have a headache or discomfort for several days after the pins are inserted. Patients initially may be bothered by the rather startling appearance of these devices, but usually they readily adapt to it because the device provides comfort for the unstable neck (see Fig. 63·6). The patient may complain of being caged in and of noise created by any object coming in contact with the frame of a halo device, but they can be reassured that adaptation will occur.

The areas around the four pin sites of a halo device are cleaned at least daily and observed for redness, drainage, and pain. The pins are observed for loosening, which may contribute to infection. If one of the pins becomes detached, the head is stabilized in a neutral position by one person, while another notifies the primary provider. A torque screwdriver should be readily available in case the screws on the frame need tightening.

The skin under the halo vest is inspected for excessive perspiration, redness, and skin blistering, especially on the bony prominences. The vest is opened at the sides to allow the torso to be washed. The liner of the vest should not become wet, because dampness causes skin excoriation. Powder is not used inside the vest, because it may contribute to the development of pressure injuries. The liner should be changed periodically to promote hygiene and good skin care. If the patient is to be discharged with the vest, detailed instructions must be given to the family, with time allowed for them to demonstrate the necessary skills of halo vest care (see Chart 63-8).

RECOGNIZING AUTONOMIC DYSREFLEXIA

Autonomic dysreflexia, also known as autonomic hyperreflexia, is an acute life-threatening emergency that occurs as a result of exaggerated autonomic responses to stimuli that are harmless in people without SCI. It occurs only after spinal shock has resolved. This syndrome is characterized by a severe, pounding headache with paroxysmal hypertension, profuse diaphoresis above the spinal level of the lesion (most often of the forehead), nausea, nasal congestion, and bradycardia. It occurs among patients with cord lesions above T6 (the sympathetic visceral outflow level) after spinal shock has subsided. The sudden increase in blood pressure may cause retinal hemorrhage, hemorrhagic stroke, myocardial infarction, or seizures (Hickey & Strayer, 2020). A number of stimuli may trigger this reflex: distended bladder (the most common cause); distention or contraction of the visceral organs, especially the bowel (from constipation, impaction); or stimulation of the skin (tactile, pain, thermal stimuli, pressure injury). Because this is an emergency situation, the objectives are to remove the triggering stimulus and to avoid the possibility of serious complications (Eldahan & Rabchevsky, 2018).

The following measures are carried out:
- The patient is placed immediately in a sitting position to lower the blood pressure.

Chart 63-8 HOME CARE CHECKLIST
The Patient with a Halo Vest

At the completion of education, the patient and/or caregiver will be able to:

- Name the procedure that was performed and identify any permanent changes in anatomic structure or function as well as changes in ADLs, IADLs, roles, relationships, and spirituality.
  - Describe the rationale for the use of the halo vest.
- State how to contact all members of the treatment team (e.g., health care providers, home care professionals, rehabilitation team, and durable medical equipment and supply vendor).
- State changes in lifestyle (e.g., diet, ADLs, IADLs, activity) necessary for recovery and health maintenance, as applicable.
  - Demonstrate safe techniques to assist the patient with self-care, hygiene, and ambulation.
  - Demonstrate assessment of frame, traction, tongs, and pins.
  - Demonstrate pin care using correct technique.
  - Demonstrate care of skin, including assessment (e.g., reddened or irritated areas, breakdown).
  - Identify signs and symptoms of infection.
  - Explain the reasons for and the method for changing the vest liner.

- Identify holistic measures of pain management.
- Identify signs and symptoms of complications (e.g., venous thromboembolism, respiratory impairment, urinary tract infection).
- Describe emergency measures if respiratory or other complications develop while the patient is in the halo vest or if the frame becomes dislodged.
- Relate how to reach primary provider with questions or complications.
- State time and date of follow-up medical appointments, therapy, and testing.
- Identify sources of support (e.g., friends, relatives, faith community).
- Identify the contact details for support services for patients and their caregivers/families.
- Identify the need for health-promotion, disease prevention, and screening activities.

ADLs, activities of daily living; IADLs, instrumental activities of daily living.

- Rapid assessment is performed to identify and alleviate the cause.
- The bladder is emptied immediately via a urinary catheter. If an indwelling catheter is not patent, it is irrigated or replaced with another catheter.
- The rectum is examined for a fecal mass. If present, a topical anesthetic agent is inserted 10 to 15 minutes before the mass is removed, because visceral distention or contraction can cause autonomic dysreflexia.
- The skin is examined for any areas of pressure, irritation, or broken skin.
- Any other stimulus that could be the triggering event, such as an object next to the skin or a draft of cold air, must be removed.
- If these measures do not relieve the hypertension and excruciating headache, antihypertensive medications may be prescribed and given slowly by the IV route.
- The medical record is labeled with a clearly visible indicator concerning the risk for autonomic dysreflexia.
- The patient is instructed about prevention and management measures.
- Any patient with a lesion above the T6 segment is informed that such an episode is possible and may occur even many years after the initial injury.

MONITORING AND MANAGING POTENTIAL COMPLICATIONS

Patients are at high risk for VTE after SCI. The patient must be assessed for symptoms of VTE including DVT and PE. Chest pain, shortness of breath, and changes in arterial blood gas values must be reported promptly to the primary provider. The circumferences of the thighs and calves are measured and recorded daily; further diagnostic studies are performed if a significant increase is noted. Patients remain at high risk for thrombophlebitis for several months after the initial injury. Patients with paraplegia or tetraplegia are at increased risk for the rest of their lives. Immobilization and the associated venous stasis, as well as varying degrees of autonomic disruption, contribute to the high risk and susceptibility for DVT.

Anticoagulation should be initiated within 72 hours of injury and continued for at least 3 months (Abrams & Wakasa, 2019). The use of low-molecular-weight heparin or low-dose unfractionated heparin may be followed by long-term oral anticoagulation (i.e., warfarin). Additional measures such as range-of-motion exercises, anti-embolism stockings, and adequate hydration are important preventive measures. SCDs may also be used to reduce venous pooling and promote venous return. It is also important to avoid external pressure on the lower extremities that may result from flexion of the knees while the patient is in bed.

Orthostatic Hypotension. For the first 2 weeks after SCI, the blood pressure tends to be unstable and can be quite low. It gradually returns to preinjury levels, but periodic episodes of severe orthostatic hypotension frequently interfere with efforts to mobilize the patient. Interruption in the reflex arcs that normally produce vasoconstriction in the upright position, coupled with vasodilation and pooling in abdominal and lower extremity vessels, can result in hypotension. Orthostatic hypotension is a particularly common problem for patients with lesions above T7. In some patients with tetraplegia, even slight elevations of the head can result in blood pressure dysregulation.

A number of techniques can be used to reduce the frequency of hypotensive episodes. Close monitoring of vital signs before and during position changes is essential. Optimization of fluid status and vasopressor medication can be used to treat the profound vasodilation. Anti-embolism stockings should be applied to improve venous return from the lower extremities. Abdominal binders may also be used to encourage venous return and provide diaphragmatic support when the patient is upright (Abrams & Wakasa, 2019). Activity should be planned in advance, and adequate time should be allowed for a slow progression of position changes from recumbent to sitting and upright. Tilt tables frequently are helpful in assisting patients to make this transition.

PROMOTING HOME, COMMUNITY-BASED, AND TRANSITIONAL CARE

Educating Patients About Self-Care. In most cases, patients with SCI (i.e., patients with tetraplegia or paraplegia) need long-term rehabilitation. The process begins during hospitalization as acute symptoms begin to subside or come under better control and the overall deficits and long-term effects of the injury become clear. The goals begin to shift from merely surviving the injury to learning strategies necessary to cope with the alterations that the injury imposes on activities of daily living (ADLs). The emphasis shifts from ensuring that the patient is stable and free of complications to specific assessment and planning designed to meet the patient's rehabilitation needs. Patient education may initially focus on the injury and its effects on mobility; dressing; and bowel, bladder, and sexual function. As the patient and family acknowledge the consequences of the injury and the resulting disability, the focus of education broadens to address issues necessary for carrying out the tasks of daily living and taking charge of their lives. Education must begin in the acute phase and continue throughout rehabilitation and the patient's entire life as changes occur, the patient ages, and problems arise.

Caring for the patient with SCI at home may at first seem a daunting task to the family. They will require dedicated nursing support to gradually assume full care of the patient. Although maintaining function and preventing complications will remain important, goals regarding self-care and preparation for discharge will assist in a smooth transition to rehabilitation and eventually to the community.

Continuing and Transitional Care. The goal of the rehabilitation process is independence. The nurse becomes a support to both the patient and the family, assisting them to assume responsibility for increasing aspects of patient care and management. Care for the patient with SCI involves members of all health care disciplines, which may include nursing, medicine, rehabilitation, respiratory therapy, physical and occupational therapy, case management, and social services. The nurse often serves as a coordinator of the management team and as a liaison with rehabilitation centers and home care agencies.

There are many challenges in providing care to the patient with SCI; meeting their psychological needs can be particularly challenging (Bibi, Rasmussen, & McLiesh, 2018). The patient and family often require assistance in dealing with the psychological impact of the injury and its consequences; referral to a psychiatric clinical nurse specialist or other mental health care professional often is helpful. Therapeutic horseback riding may help increase balance, muscle strength, and self-esteem (Stergiou, Tzoufi, Ntzani, et al., 2017).

The nurse should reassure female patients with SCI that pregnancy is not contraindicated and fertility is relatively unaffected, but that pregnant women with acute or chronic SCI pose unique management challenges. The normal physiologic changes of pregnancy may predispose women with SCI to many potentially life-threatening complications, including autonomic dysreflexia, pyelonephritis, respiratory insufficiency, thrombophlebitis, PE, and unattended delivery.

Preconception assessment and counseling are strongly recommended to ensure that the woman is in optimal health and to increase the likelihood of an uneventful pregnancy and healthy outcomes (Crane, Doody, Schiff, et al., 2019).

As more patients survive acute SCI, they face the changes associated with aging with a disability. Three common secondary health problems experienced by persons living with SCI include chronic pain, spasticity, and depression (Abrams & Wakasa, 2019). Education in the home and community focuses on health promotion and addresses the need to minimize risk factors (e.g., tobacco use, substance use disorder, obesity). Routine health-screening and preventive services are needed for the older adult with SCI for early detection of secondary health problems. Home health nurses and others who have contact with patients with SCI are in a position to educate patients about healthy lifestyles, remind them of the need for health screenings, and make referrals as appropriate. Assisting patients to identify accessible health care providers, clinical facilities, and imaging centers may increase the likelihood that they will participate in health screening.

Evaluation

Expected patient outcomes may include:

1. Demonstrates improvement in gas exchange and clearance of secretions, as evidenced by normal breath sounds on auscultation
   a. Breathes easily without shortness of breath
   b. Performs hourly deep breathing exercises, coughs effectively, and clears pulmonary secretions
   c. Is free of respiratory infection (e.g., has temperature, respiratory rate, and pulse within normal limits; breath sounds clear to auscultation; absence of purulent sputum)
2. Moves within limits of the dysfunction and demonstrates completion of exercises within functional limitations
3. Avoids injury due to sensory, motor, and perceptual alterations
   a. Uses assistive devices (e.g., glasses, hearing aids, electronic devices) as indicated
   b. Describes sensory, motor, and perceptual alterations as a consequence of injury
4. Demonstrates optimal skin integrity
   a. Exhibits normal skin turgor; skin is free of reddened areas or breaks
   b. Participates in skin care and monitoring procedures within functional limitations
5. Regains urinary bladder function
   a. Exhibits no signs of UTI (e.g., has temperature within normal limits; voids clear, dilute urine)
   b. Has adequate fluid intake
   c. Participates in bladder training program within functional limitations
6. Regains bowel function
   a. Reports regular pattern of bowel movement
   b. Consumes adequate dietary fiber and oral fluids
   c. Participates in bowel training program within functional limitations
7. Reports absence of pain and discomfort

8. Recognizes manifestations of autonomic dysreflexia if they occur (e.g., headache, diaphoresis, nasal congestion, bradycardia, or diaphoresis)
9. Is free of complications
   a. Demonstrates no signs of thrombophlebitis, DVT, or PE
   b. Maintains blood pressure within normal limits
   c. Reports no lightheadedness with position changes

Medical Management of Long-Term Complications of SCI

The patient faces a lifetime disability, requiring ongoing follow-up and care. The expertise of a number of health professionals including physicians (specifically a physiatrist), rehabilitation nurses, occupational therapists, physical therapists, psychologists, social workers, rehabilitation engineers, and vocational counselors, is necessary at different times as the need arises.

The patient with an SCI has a shorter life expectancy compared to those who have not had an SCI (Abrams & Wakasa, 2019). As patients with SCI age, they have many of the same medical problems as others. In addition, they face the threat of complications associated with their disability (Hickey & Strayer, 2020). Usually, patients are encouraged to follow-up at an outpatient spinal cord clinic when complications and other issues arise. Lifetime care includes assessment of the urinary tract at prescribed intervals because there is the likelihood of continuing alteration in detrusor and sphincter function, and the patient is prone to UTI (Abrams & Wakasa, 2019).

Long-term problems and complications of SCI include disuse syndrome, autonomic dysreflexia (discussed earlier), bladder and kidney infections, spasticity, and depression (Abrams & Wakasa, 2019). Pressure injuries with potential complications of sepsis, osteomyelitis, and fistulas occur in about 10% of patients. Spasticity may be particularly disabling. Heterotopic ossification (overgrowth of bone) in the hips, knees, shoulders, and elbows occurs in many patients after SCI. Spasticity and heterotopic ossification are painful and can produce a loss of range of motion (Abrams & Wakasa, 2019). Management includes observing for and addressing any alteration in physiologic status and psychological outlook, as well as the prevention and treatment of long-term complications. The nursing role involves emphasizing the need for vigilance in self-assessment and care.

NURSING PROCESS

The Patient with Tetraplegia or Paraplegia

Assessment

Assessment focuses on the patient's general condition, complications, and how the patient is managing at that particular point in time. A head-to-toe assessment and review of systems should be part of the database, with emphasis on the areas that are prone to problems in this population. A thorough inspection of all areas of the skin for redness or breakdown is critical. The nurse reviews the established bowel and bladder program with the patient, because the program must continue uninterrupted. Patients with tetraplegia or paraplegia have varying degrees of loss of motor power, deep and superficial sensation, vasomotor control, bladder and bowel control, and sexual function. They are faced with potential complications related to immobility, skin breakdown and pressure injuries, recurring UTIs, and contractures. Knowledge about these particular issues can further guide the assessment in any setting. Nurses in all settings, including home care, must be aware of these potential complications in the lifetime management of these patients.

An understanding of the emotional and psychological responses to tetraplegia or paraplegia is achieved by observing the responses and behaviors of the patient and family and by listening to their concerns (Bailey, Gammage, van Ingen, et al., 2017). Documenting these assessments and reviewing the plan with the entire team on a regular basis provide insight into how both the patient and the family are coping with the changes in lifestyle and body functioning. Additional information frequently can be gathered from the social worker or psychiatric/mental health worker.

It takes time for the patient and family to comprehend the magnitude of the disability. They may go through stages of grief, including shock, disbelief, denial, anger, depression, and acceptance. During the acute phase of the injury, denial can be a protective mechanism to shield the patient from the acute reality of what has happened. As the patient realizes the permanent nature of paraplegia or tetraplegia, the grieving process may be prolonged and all-encompassing because of the recognition that long-held plans and expectations are interrupted or permanently altered. A period of depression often follows as the patient experiences a loss of self-esteem in areas of self-identity, sexual functioning, and social and emotional roles. Exploration and assessment of these issues can assist in developing a meaningful plan of care.

Diagnosis

NURSING DIAGNOSES

Based on the assessment data, major nursing diagnoses may include the following:
- Impaired mobility in bed and impaired mobility associated with loss of motor function
- Risk for disuse
- Risk for impaired skin integrity associated with permanent sensory loss and immobility
- Urinary retention associated with level of injury
- Constipation associated with effects of spinal cord disruption
- Impaired sexual functioning associated with neurologic dysfunction
- Difficulty coping associated with impact of disability on daily living
- Lack of knowledge about requirements for long-term management

COLLABORATIVE PROBLEMS/POTENTIAL COMPLICATIONS

Potential complications may include the following:
- Spasticity
- Infection and sepsis

Planning and Goals

The goals for the patient may include attainment of some form of mobility; maintenance of healthy, intact skin; achievement of bladder management without infection; achievement of bowel control; achievement of sexual expression; strengthening of coping mechanisms; knowledge of long-term management; and absence of complications.

Nursing Interventions

The patient requires extensive rehabilitation, which is less difficult if appropriate nursing management has been carried out during the acute phase of the injury or illness. Nursing care is one of the key factors determining the success of the rehabilitation program. The main objective is for the patient to live as independently as possible in the home and community.

INCREASING MOBILITY

Exercise Programs. The unaffected parts of the body are built up to optimal strength to promote maximum self-care. The muscles of the hands, arms, shoulders, chest, spine, abdomen, and neck must be strengthened in the patient with paraplegia, because they must bear full weight on these muscles to ambulate. The triceps and the latissimus dorsi are important muscles used in crutch walking. The muscles of the abdomen and the back also are necessary for balance and for maintaining the upright position.

To strengthen these muscles, the patient can do push-ups when in a prone position and sit-ups when in a sitting position. Extending the arms while holding weights (traction weights can be used) also develops muscle strength. Squeezing rubber balls or crumbling newspaper promotes hand strength.

With encouragement from all members of the rehabilitation team, the patient with paraplegia can develop the increased exercise tolerance needed for gait training and ambulation activities. The importance of maintaining cardiovascular fitness is stressed to the patient. Alternative exercises to increase the heart rate to target levels must be designed within the patient's abilities.

Mobilization. After the spine is stable enough to allow the patient to assume an upright posture, mobilization activities are initiated. A brace or vest may be used, depending on the level of the lesion. The sooner muscles are used, the less chance there is of disuse atrophy. The earlier the patient is brought to a standing position, the less opportunity there is for osteoporotic changes to take place in the long bones. Weight bearing also reduces the possibility of renal calculi and enhances many other metabolic processes.

Braces and crutches enable some patients with paraplegia to ambulate for short distances. Ambulation using crutches requires a high expenditure of energy. Motorized wheelchairs and specially equipped vans can provide greater independence and mobility for patients with high-level SCI or other lesions. Every effort should be made to encourage the patient to be as mobile and active as possible.

Long-term risks include altered body composition, a decrease in lean body mass, decreased bone mineral density, and increased body mass index (BMI). Patients are at high risk for obesity due to high fat intake combined with decreased physical activity (Silveira, Winter, Clark, et al., 2019). This puts patients at higher risk for developing comorbid conditions such as diabetes and cardiovascular diseases. Patients benefit from nutrition counseling to prevent these secondary complications. For those who are overweight or who have obesity, weight-loss programs must be designed to accommodate the dietary and physical activity barriers that are unique to this population.

PREVENTING DISUSE SYNDROME

Patients are at high risk for development of contractures as a result of disuse syndrome due to the musculoskeletal system changes (atrophy) brought about by the loss of motor and sensory functions below the level of injury. Range-of-motion exercises must be provided at least four times a day, and care is taken to stretch the Achilles tendon with exercises, to prevent footdrop. The patient is repositioned frequently and is maintained in proper body alignment whether in bed or in a wheelchair.

Contractures can complicate day-to-day care, increasing the difficulty of positioning and decreasing mobility. A number of surgical procedures have been tried, with varying degrees of success. These techniques are used if more conservative approaches fail, but the best treatment is prevention.

PROMOTING SKIN INTEGRITY

Because these patients spend a great portion of their lives in wheelchairs, pressure injuries are an ever-present threat. Contributing factors are permanent sensory loss over pressure areas; immobility, which makes relief of pressure difficult; trauma from bumps (against the wheelchair, toilet, furniture, and so forth) that cause unnoticed abrasions and wounds; loss of protective function of the skin from excoriation and maceration due to excessive perspiration and possible incontinence; and poor general health (anemia, diabetes), leading to poor tissue perfusion. See Chapter 56 for discussion on the prevention and management of pressure injuries.

The person with tetraplegia or paraplegia must take responsibility for monitoring (or directing monitoring) of their skin status. This involves relieving pressure and not remaining in any position for longer than 2 hours, in addition to ensuring that the skin receives meticulous attention and cleansing. The patient is educated that pressure injuries develop over bony prominences that are exposed to unrelieved pressure in the sitting and lying positions. The most vulnerable areas are identified. The patient with paraplegia is instructed to use mirrors, if possible, to inspect these areas morning and night, observing for redness, slight edema, or any abrasions. While in bed, the patient should turn at 2-hour intervals and then inspect the skin again for redness that does not fade on pressure. The bottom sheet should be checked for wetness and for creases. The patient with tetraplegia or paraplegia, who cannot perform these activities, is encouraged to direct others to check these areas and prevent pressure injuries from developing.

The patient is educated to relieve pressure while in the wheelchair by doing push-ups, leaning from side to side to relieve ischial pressure, and tilting forward while leaning on a table. The caregiver for the patient with tetraplegia will need to perform these activities if the patient cannot do so independently. A wheelchair cushion is prescribed to meet individual needs, which may change in time with changes in posture, weight, and skin tolerance. A referral can be made to a rehabilitation engineer, who can measure pressure levels while the patient is sitting and then tailor the cushion and other necessary aids and assistive devices to the patient's needs.

The diet for the patient with tetraplegia or paraplegia should be high in protein, vitamins, and calories to ensure minimal wasting of muscle and the maintenance of healthy skin, and high in fluids to maintain well-functioning kidneys. Excessive weight gain and obesity should be avoided because they further limit mobility.

IMPROVING BLADDER MANAGEMENT

The effect of the spinal cord lesion on the bladder depends on the level of injury, the degree of cord damage, and the length of time after injury. A patient with tetraplegia or paraplegia usually has either a reflex or a nonreflex bladder. Both bladder types increase the risk for UTI.

The nurse emphasizes the importance of maintaining an adequate flow of urine by encouraging a fluid intake of about 2.5 L daily. The patient should empty the bladder frequently so that there is minimal residual urine and should pay attention to personal hygiene, because infection of the bladder and kidneys almost always occurs by the ascending route. The perineum must be kept clean and dry, and attention must be given to the perianal skin after defecation. Underwear should be cotton (which is more absorbent) and should be changed at least once a day.

If an external catheter (condom catheter) is used, the sheath is removed nightly; the penis is cleansed to remove urine and is dried carefully, because warm urine on the periurethral skin promotes the growth of bacteria. Attention also is given to the collection bag. The nurse emphasizes the importance of monitoring for signs of UTI: cloudy, foul-smelling urine or hematuria (blood in the urine); fever; or chills.

The female patient who cannot achieve reflex bladder control or self-catheterization may need to wear pads or waterproof undergarments. Surgical intervention may be indicated in some patients to create a urinary diversion.

ESTABLISHING BOWEL CONTROL

The objective of a bowel training program is to establish bowel evacuation through reflex conditioning. If the SCI occurs above the sacral segments or nerve roots and there is reflex activity, the anal sphincter may be massaged (digital stimulation) to stimulate defecation. If the cord lesion involves the sacral segment or nerve roots, anal massage is not performed because the anus may be relaxed and lack tone. Massage is also contraindicated if there is spasticity of the anal sphincter. The anal sphincter is massaged by inserting a gloved finger (which has been adequately lubricated) 2.5 to 3.7 cm (1 to 1.5 inches) into the rectum and moving it in a circular motion or from side to side. It soon becomes apparent which area triggers the defecation response. This procedure should be performed at regular time intervals (usually every 48 hours), after a meal, and at a time that will be convenient for the patient at home (Schmelzer, Daniels, & Baird, 2018). The patient is educated about the symptoms of impaction (frequent loose stools; constipation) and is cautioned to watch for hemorrhoids. A diet with sufficient fluids and fiber is essential to developing a successful bowel training program, avoiding constipation, and decreasing the risk for autonomic dysreflexia.

COUNSELING ON SEXUAL EXPRESSION

Many patients with tetraplegia and paraplegia can have some form of meaningful sexual relationship, although modifications are necessary. The patient and partner benefit from counseling about the range of sexual expression possible, special techniques and positions, exploration of body sensations offering sensual feelings, and urinary and bowel hygiene as related to sexual activity. For men with erectile failure, penile prostheses enable them to have and sustain an erection, and medications for erectile dysfunction may be helpful. Sildenafil, vardenafil, and tadalafil, for example, are oral smooth muscle relaxants that cause blood to flow into the penis, resulting in an erection (see Chapter 53). Patients who are sexually active should undergo counseling in birth control methods, as some methods (e.g., oral contraceptives) may increase risks for complications such as VTE (Hickey & Strayer, 2020).

Sexual education and counseling services are included in the rehabilitation services at spinal centers. Small group meetings in which patients can share their feelings, receive information, and discuss sexual concerns and practical aspects are helpful in producing effective attitudes and adjustments.

ENHANCING COPING MECHANISMS

The impact of the disability and loss becomes marked when the patient returns home. Each time something new enters the patient's life (e.g., a new relationship, going to work), the patient is reminded anew of their limitations. Grief reactions and depression are common.

To work through depression, the patient must have some hope for relief in the future. The nurse can encourage the patient to feel confident in their ability to achieve self-care and relative independence. The role of the nurse ranges from caretaker during the acute phase to educator, counselor, and facilitator as the patient gains mobility and independence.

The patient's disability affects not only the patient but also the entire family. In many cases, family therapy is helpful in working through issues as they arise. Adjustment to the disability leads to the development of realistic goals for the future, making the best of the abilities that are left intact, and reinvesting in other activities and relationships. Rejection of the disability causes self-destructive neglect and nonadherence to the therapeutic program, which leads to more frustration and depression. Crises for which interventions may be sought include social, psychological, marital, sexual, and psychiatric problems. The family usually requires counseling, social services, and other support systems to help them cope with the changes in their lifestyle and socioeconomic status.

A major goal of nursing management is to help the patient overcome their sense of futility and to encourage the patient in the emotional adjustment that must be made before they are willing to venture into the outside world. However, an excessively sympathetic attitude on the part of the nurse may cause the patient to develop an overdependence that defeats the purpose of the entire rehabilitation program. The patient is educated and assisted when necessary, but the nurse should avoid performing activities that the patient can do independently with a little effort. This approach to care more than repays itself in the satisfaction of seeing a patient, who is completely demoralized and helpless, become independent and find meaning in a newly emerging lifestyle.

MONITORING AND MANAGING POTENTIAL COMPLICATIONS

Spasticity. Muscle spasticity can be a problematic complication of tetraplegia and paraplegia. Flexor or extensor spasms occur below the level of the spinal cord lesion and can interfere with the rehabilitation process, ADLs, and quality of life (Abrams & Wakasa, 2019). Spasticity results from an imbalance between the facilitatory and inhibitory effects on neurons that exist normally. The area of the cord distal to the site of injury or lesion becomes disconnected from the higher inhibitory centers located in the brain, so facilitatory impulses, which originate from muscles, skin, and ligaments, predominate.

Spasticity is defined as a condition of increased muscle tone in a muscle that is weak. Initial resistance to stretching is quickly followed by sudden relaxation. The stimulus that precipitates spasm can be obvious, such as movement or a position change, or subtle, such as a slight jarring of the wheelchair. Most patients with tetraplegia or paraplegia have some degree of spasticity. Because it increases muscle tone, some degree of spasticity can be beneficial in patients who are weak (Abrams & Wakasa, 2019). With SCI, the onset of spasticity usually occurs from a few weeks to 6 months after the injury. The same muscles that are flaccid during the period of spinal shock develop spasticity during recovery. The intensity of spasticity tends to peak approximately 2 years after the injury, after which the spasms tend to regress.

Management of spasticity is based on the severity of symptoms and the degree of incapacitation. Botulinum toxin injections, as well as the antispasmodic medication baclofen, available in an oral and an intrathecal form, may be indicated (Comerford & Durkin, 2020). Oral medications such as diazepam, dantrolene, and tizanidine help control spasms by decreasing sympathetic outflow from the central nervous system. Other forms of adjunctive therapy include oral and transdermal forms of clonidine (Hickey & Strayer, 2020). All of the antispasmodic medications cause drowsiness, weakness, and vertigo in some patients. Passive range-of-motion exercises and frequent turning and repositioning are helpful, because stiffness tends to increase spasticity. These activities also are essential in the prevention of contractures, pressure injuries, and bowel and bladder dysfunction.

Infection and Sepsis. Patients with tetraplegia and paraplegia are at increased risk for infection and sepsis from a variety of sources: urinary tract, respiratory tract, and pressure injuries. Sepsis remains a major cause of complications and death in these patients. Prevention of infection and sepsis is essential through maintenance of skin integrity, complete emptying of the bladder at regular intervals, and prevention of urinary and fecal incontinence. The risk for respiratory infection can be decreased by avoiding contact with people who have symptoms of respiratory infection, performing coughing and deep breathing exercises to prevent pooling of respiratory secretions, receiving yearly influenza vaccines, and giving up smoking. A high-protein diet is important in maintaining an adequate immune system, as is avoiding factors that may reduce immune system function, such as excessive stress, drug abuse, and excessive alcohol intake.

If infection occurs, the patient requires thorough assessment and prompt treatment. Antibiotic therapy and adequate hydration, in addition to local measures (depending on the site of infection), are initiated immediately.

UTIs are minimized or prevented by aseptic technique in catheter management, adequate hydration, a bladder training program, and prevention of overdistention of the bladder and urinary stasis.

Skin breakdown and infection are prevented by the maintenance of a turning schedule; frequent back care; regular assessment of all skin areas; regular cleaning and lubrication of the skin; passive range-of-motion exercise to prevent contractures; pressure relief over broken skin areas, bony prominences, and heels; and wrinkle-free bed linen.

Pulmonary infections are managed and prevented by frequent coughing, turning, and deep breathing exercises and chest physiotherapy; aggressive respiratory care and suctioning of the airway if a tracheostomy is present; assisted coughing as needed; and adequate hydration.

Infections of any kind can be life-threatening. Aggressive nursing interventions are key to prevention, detection, and early management.

PROMOTING HOME, COMMUNITY-BASED, AND TRANSITIONAL CARE

Educating Patients About Self-Care. Patients with tetraplegia or paraplegia are at risk for complications for the rest of their lives. Therefore, a major aspect of nursing care is educating the patient and family about these complications and about strategies to minimize risks. UTIs, contractures, infected pressure injuries, and sepsis may necessitate hospitalization. Other late complications that may occur include lower extremity edema, joint contractures, respiratory dysfunction, and pain. To avoid these and other complications, the patient and family members are educated about skin care, catheter care, range-of-motion exercises, breathing exercises, and other care techniques. Education is initiated as soon as possible and extends into the rehabilitation or long-term care facility and home. In all aspects of care, it is important for the nurse and patient to set mutual goals and discuss the tasks the patient is capable of doing independently and which tasks the patient needs assistance to complete. See Chart 63-9 for a summary of education points for managing a therapeutic regimen at home.

Continuing and Transitional Care. Referral for home care is often appropriate for assessment of the home setting, patient education, and evaluation of the patient's physical and emotional status. During visits by the nurse, education about strategies to prevent or minimize potential complications is reinforced. The home environment is assessed for adequacy of care and for safety. Environmental modifications are made, and specialized equipment is obtained, ideally before the patient goes home.

The nurse also assesses the patient's and the family's adherence to recommendations and their use of coping strategies. The use of inappropriate coping strategies (e.g., drug and alcohol use) is assessed, and referrals to counseling are made for the patient and family. Appropriate and effective coping strategies are reinforced. The nurse reviews previous education and determines the need for further physical or psychological assistance. The patient's self-esteem and body image may be extremely poor at this time. Because people with high levels of social support often report feelings of well-being despite major physical disability, it is beneficial for the nurse to assess and promote further development of the support system and effective coping strategies for each patient. Caregivers and peer mentors play a critical role in helping patients feel less dependent, experience feelings of freedom, and reintegrate into the community (Gassaway, Jones, Sweatman, et al., 2017).

Chart 63-9 HOME CARE CHECKLIST
Avoiding Complications of SCI

At the completion of education, the patient and/or caregiver will be able to:

- State the impact of SCI and treatment on physiologic functioning, ADLs, IADLs, roles, relationships, and spirituality.
- State the purpose, dose, route, schedule, side effects, and precautions for prescribed medications.
- State how to contact all members of the treatment team (e.g., health care providers, home care professionals, and durable medical equipment and supply vendor).
- State what types of environmental and safety changes or supports are needed for optimum functioning in the home.
- Demonstrate skin care:
  - Inspect bony prominences every morning and evening.
  - Identify stage I pressure injury and actions to take if present.
  - Change dressings for stage II to IV pressure injuries.
  - State dietary requirements to promote healing of pressure injuries.
  - Demonstrate pressure relief at prescribed intervals.
  - State sitting schedule and demonstrate weight lifts in wheelchair.
  - Demonstrate adherence to bed turning schedule, bed positioning, and the use of bridging techniques.
  - Apply and wear protective boots at prescribed times.
  - Demonstrate correct wheelchair sitting posture.
  - Demonstrate techniques to avoid friction and shear in bed.
  - Demonstrate proper hygiene to maintain skin integrity.
- Demonstrate bladder care:
  - State schedule for voiding, toileting, and catheterization.
  - Identify relationship of fluid intake to voiding and catheterization schedule.
  - Demonstrate clean self-intermittent catheterization and care of catheterization equipment.
  - Demonstrate indwelling catheter care.
  - Demonstrate application of external condom catheter.
  - Demonstrate application, emptying, and cleaning of urinary drainage bag.
  - Demonstrate application of incontinence pads and performance of perineal hygiene.
  - State signs and symptoms of urinary tract infection.
  - State signs and symptoms of urinary catheter blockage.
- Demonstrate bowel care:
  - State optimum dietary intake to promote evacuation.
  - Describe medication regimen for bowel care (drug names, schedule, and dosage).
  - Identify schedule for optimum bowel evacuation.

- Demonstrate techniques to increase intraabdominal pressure; Valsalva maneuver; abdominal massage; leaning forward.
- Demonstrate techniques to stimulate bowel movements: ingesting warm liquids; digital stimulation; insertion of suppositories.
- Demonstrate optimum position for bowel evacuation: on toilet with knees higher than hips; left side in bed with knees flexed and head of bed elevated 30 to 45 degrees.
- Identify complications and corrective strategies for bowel retraining: constipation, impaction, diarrhea, hemorrhoids, rectal bleeding, anal tears.
- Identify community resources for peer and caregiver/family support:
  - Identify sources of support (e.g., friends, relatives, faith community).
  - Identify contact details of support services for people with disability and their caregivers/families.
- Demonstrate how to access transportation:
  - Identify locations of wheelchair accessibility for public buses or trains.
  - Identify contact details for private wheelchair van.
  - Contact Division of Motor Vehicles for handicapped parking permit.
  - Contact Division of Motor Vehicles for driving test when appropriate.
  - Identify resources for adapting private vehicle with hand controls or wheelchair lift.
- Identify vocational rehabilitation resources:
  - State the contact details for vocational rehabilitation services.
  - Identify educational opportunities that may lead to future employment.
- Identify community resources for recreation:
  - State local recreation centers that offer programs for people with disability.
  - Identify leisure activities that can be pursued in the community.
  - State how to reach primary provider with questions or if complications arise.
  - State follow-up schedule.
  - Identify the need for health promotion, disease prevention, and screening activities.

ADL, activities of daily living; IADL, instrumental activities of daily living; SCI, spinal cord injury.

The patient requires continuing, lifelong follow-up by the primary provider, physical therapist, and other rehabilitation team members, because the neurologic deficit is usually permanent and new deficits, complications, and secondary conditions can develop. These require prompt attention before they take their toll in additional physical impairment, time, morale, and financial costs. Research suggests that education and peer mentoring may decrease complications following SCI (Abrams & Wakasa, 2019; Gassaway et al., 2017). The local counselor for the Office of Vocational Rehabilitation works with the patient with respect to job placement or additional educational or vocational training. The nurse is in a good position to remind patients and family members of the need for continuing health promotion and screening

practices. Referral to accessible health care providers and imaging centers is important in health promotion and health screening. See Chapter 7 for more information on chronic illness and disability.

Evaluation

Expected patient outcomes may include:

1. Attains maximum form of mobility
2. Contractures do not develop
3. Maintains healthy, intact skin
4. Achieves bladder control, absence of UTI
5. Achieves bowel control
6. Reports sexual satisfaction
7. Shows improved adaptation to environment and others

8. Exhibits reduction in spasticity
   a. Reports understanding of the precipitating factors
   b. Uses measures to reduce spasticity
9. Describes long-term management required
10. Exhibits absence of complications

CRITICAL THINKING EXERCISES

1 **ebp** You are caring for a 27-year-old woman who was involved in a motor vehicle crash. Her CT scan of the head revealed a left subdural hematoma. The Glasgow Coma Scale was 10, pupils were reactive bilaterally, and she moved all four extremities. She had no difficulties with airway control or respirations. What evidence-based nursing interventions will you implement in your care of this patient? Identify the criteria used to evaluate the strength of the evidence for these practices.

2 **pq** A 32-year-old man fell off his 10-speed bicycle, hitting the side of his head on the pavement, losing consciousness. He woke up in the emergency department confused and complained of a headache. His CT scan of the head revealed a right epidural hematoma. He was taken to the operating room for a craniotomy. What are your priority neurological assessments for this patient postoperatively? What are your priority nursing interventions to control intracranial pressure?

3 **ipc** A 22-year-old man, on a dare from his friends, attempted a backward flip from a 20-feett-high rocky cliff into shallow water that was less than 6-feet deep. He struck his back on a large protruding rock before entering the water and sustained a C-5 hyperextension injury to his neck. Upon arrival to the ED, his vital signs are stable but he is flaccid in all extremities with no sensation below nipple line. Which members of the interdisciplinary team do you anticipate will provide care for this patient? What steps will the interdisciplinary team take to address the patient's health care needs?

REFERENCES

*Asterisk indicates nursing research.
**Double asterisk indicates classic reference.

Books

Comerford, K. C., & Durkin, D. T. (2020). *Nursing 2020 drug handbook.* Philadelphia, PA: Wolters Kluwer.

Hickey, J. V., & Strayer, A. L. (2020). *The clinical practice of neurological & neurosurgical nursing* (8th ed.). Philadelphia, PA: Wolters Kluwer.

Quintard, H., & Ichai, C. (2018). Brain injury and nutrition. In M. Berger (Ed.). *Critical care nutrition therapy for non-nutritionists.* Switzerland: Springer.

Urden, L. D., Stacy, K. M., & Lough, M. E. (2018). *Critical care nursing* (8th ed.). Maryland Heights, MO: Elsevier.

Volski, A., & Ackerman, D. (2020). *Neurogenic Shock. In Clinical management of shock—The science and art of physiological restoration.* London, UK: IntechOpen.

Wang, M., Strayer, A., Harris, O., et al. (2017). *Handbook of neurosurgery, neurology, and spinal medicine for nurses and advanced practice health professional.* New York: Routledge.

Journals and Electronic Documents

Abrams, G. M., & Wakasa, M. (2019). Chronic complications of spinal cord injury and disease. *UpToDate.* Retrieved on 4/27/2020 at: www.uptodate.com/contents/chronic-complications-of-spinal-cord-injury-and-disease

American Spinal Injury Association (ASIA). (2019). International standards for neurological classification of spinal cord injury. Retrieved on 4/27/2020 at: asia-spinalinjury.org/wp-content/uploads/2019/10/ASIA-ISCOS-Worksheet_10.2019_PRINT-Page-1-2.pdf

*Bailey, K. A., Gammage, K. L., van Ingen, C., et al. (2017). "My body was my temple": A narrative revealing body image experiences following treatment of a spinal cord injury. *Disability and Rehabilitation,* 39(18), 1886–1892.

Battaglini, M., Gentile, G., Luchetti, L., et al. (2019). Lifespan normative data on rates of brain volume changes. *Neurobiology of Aging,* 81(2019), 30–37.

*Bibi, S., Rasmussen, P., & McLiesh, P. (2018). The lived experience: Nurses' experience of caring for patients with a traumatic spinal cord injury. *International Journal of Orthopaedic and Trauma Nursing,* 30(8), 31–38.

Centers for Disease Control and Prevention (CDC). (2019). Injury prevention & control: Traumatic brain injury & concussion. Retrieved on 4/27/2020 at: www.cdc.gov/traumaticbraininjury/get_the_facts.html

Chapman, J. C., & Diaz-Arrastia, R. (2014). Military traumatic brain injury: A review. *Alzheimer's & Dementia,* 10(3 Suppl), S97–S104.

Chartrain, A. G., Yaeger, K., Feng, R., et al. (2017). Antiepileptics for post-traumatic seizure prophylaxis after traumatic brain injury. *Current Pharmaceutical Design,* 23(42), 6428–6444.

Crane, D. A., Doody, D. R., Schiff, M. A., et al. (2019). Pregnancy outcomes in women with spinal cord injuries: A population-based study. *American Academy of Physical Medicine and Rehabilitation,* 11(8), 795–806.

Eldahan, K. C., & Rabchevsky, A. G. (2018). Autonomic dysreflexia after spinal cord injury: Systemic pathophysiology and methods of management. *Autonomic Neuroscience: Basic and Clinical,* 209(1), 59–70.

Fins, J. J., & Real de Asúa, D. (2019). North of home: Obligations to families of undocumented patients. *Hastings Center Report,* 49(1), 12–14.

Furlan, J. C., Gulasingam, S., & Craven, B. C. (2017). The health economics of the spinal cord injury or disease among veterans of war: A systematic review. *The Journal of Spinal Cord Medicine,* 40(6), 649–664.

Furlan, J. C., Kurban, D., & Craven, B. C. (2019). Traumatic spinal cord injury in military personnel versus civilians: A propensity score-matched cohort study. *BMJ Military Health.* 166(E):e57–e62.

Gallagher, J. (2017). Prevention of ventilator-associated pneumonia in adults. *Critical Care Nurse,* 37(3), e22–e25.

Gary, K. W., Cao, Y., Burns, S. P., et al. (2020). Employment, health outcomes, and life satisfaction after spinal cord injury: Comparison of veterans and nonveterans. *Spinal Cord,* 58(1), 3–10.

*Gassaway, J., Jones, M. L., Sweatman, W. M., et al. (2017). Effects of peer mentoring on self-efficacy and hospital readmission after inpatient rehabilitation of individuals with spinal cord injury: A randomized controlled trial. *Archives of Physical Medicine and Rehabilitation,* 98(8), 1526–1534.e2.

*Giusti, G. D., Tuteri, D., & Mirella, G. (2016). Nursing interactions with intensive care unit patients affected by sleep deprivation: An observational study. *Dimensions of Critical Care Nursing,* 35(3), 154–159.

**Hagen, C., Malkmus, D., & Durham, P. (1972). *The Rancho levels of cognitive functioning scale.* Downey, CA: Communication Disorders Service, Rancho Los Amigos Hospital. Revised 11/15/74 by: Danese Malkmus and Kathryn Stenderup.

Hollander, J. E. (2019). Assessment and management of scalp lacerations. *UpToDate.* Retrieved on 3/7/2020 at: www.uptodate.com/contents/assessment-and-management-of-scalp-lacerations

Kaur, P., & Sharma, S. (2018). Recent advances in pathophysiology of traumatic brain injury. *Current Neuropharmacology,* 16(8), 1224–1238.

*Liu, X., Griffith, M., Jang, H. J., et al. (2020). Intracranial pressure monitoring via external ventricular drain: Are we waiting long enough before recording the real value? *Journal of Neuroscience Nursing,* 52(1), 37–42.

Livesay, S. L., McNett, M. M., Keller, M., et al. (2017). Challenges of cerebral perfusion pressure measurement. *Journal of Neuroscience Nursing, 49*(6), 372–376.

McCafferty, R. R., Neal, C. J., Marshall, S. A., et al. (2018). Neurosurgery and medical management of severe head injury. *Military Medicine, 183*(suppl_2), 67–72.

National Spinal Cord Injury Statistical Center (NSCISC). (2020). Spinal Cord Injury (SCI) facts and figures at a glance. Retrieved on 4/27/2020 at: nscisc.uab.edu/Public/Facts%20and%20Figures%202020.pdf

*Olson, D. M., Parcon, C., Santos, A., et al. (2017). A novel approach to explore how nursing care affects intracranial pressure. *American Journal of Critical Care, 26*(2), 136–139.

*Oyesanya, T. O., Arulselvam, K., Thompson, N., et al. (2019). Health, wellness, and safety concerns of persons with moderate-to-severe traumatic brain injury and their family caregivers: A qualitative content analysis. *Disability and Rehabilitation.* doi: 10.1080/09638288.2019.1638456

Radtke, K., & Matzo, M. (2017). Liberty and justice for all: When an unauthorized immigrant suffers a brain injury, who decides when treatment is withdrawn? *The American Journal of Nursing, 117*(11), 52–56.

Sacco, T. L., & Delibert, S. A. (2018). Management of intracranial pressure Part I: Pharmacologic interventions. *Dimensions of Critical Care Nursing, 37*(3), 120–129.

Sacco, T. L., & Davis, J. G. (2019). Management of intracranial pressure Part II: Nonpharmacologic interventions. *Dimensions of Critical Care Nursing, 38*(2), 61–69.

*Saherwala, A. A., Bader, M. K., Stutzman, S. E., et al. (2018). Increasing adherence to brain trauma foundation guidelines for hospital care of patients with traumatic brain injury. *Critical Care Nurse, 38*(1), e11–e20.

*Schmelzer, M., Daniels, G., & Baird, B. (2018). Bowel control strategies used by veterans with long-standing spinal cord injuries. *Rehabilitation Nursing, 43*(5), 245–254.

Schweitzer, A. D., Niogi, S. N., Whitlow, C. T., et al. (2019). Traumatic brain injury: Imaging patterns and complications. *Radiographics, 39*(6), 1571–1595.

Silveira, S. L., Winter, L. L., Clark, R., et al. (2019). Baseline dietary intake of individuals with spinal cord injury who are overweight or obese. *Journal of the Academy of Nutrition and Dietetics, 119*(2), 301–309.

Silverberg, N. D., Iaccarino, M. A., Panenka, W. J., et al. (2020). Management of concussion and mild traumatic brain injury: A synthesis of practice guidelines. *Archives of Physical Medicine and Rehabilitation, 101*(2), 382–393.

Stergiou, A., Tzoufi, M., Ntzani, E., et al. (2017). Therapeutic effects of horseback riding interventions: A systematic review and meta-analysis. *American Journal of Physical Medicine and Rehabilitation, 96*(10), 717–725.

Stoffel, J. T., Van der Aa, F., Wittmann, D., et al. (2018). Neurogenic bowel management for the adult spinal cord injury patient. *World Journal of Urology, 36*(10), 1587–1592.

**Teasdale, G., & Jennett, B. (1974). Assessment of coma and impaired consciousness. A practical scale. *Lancet, 2*(7872), 81–84.

*Thompson, H. J., Rivara, F. P., & Wang, J. (2020). Effect of age on longitudinal changes in symptoms, function, and outcome in the first year after mild-moderate traumatic brain injury. *Journal of Neuroscience Nursing, 52*(2), 46–52.

Turgoose, D., & Murphy, D. (2018). A review of traumatic brain injury in military veterans: Current issues and understanding. *Open Access Journal of Neurology & Neurosurgery, 7*(3), 1–3.

Turk, K. W., & Budson, A. E. (2019). Chronic traumatic encephalopathy. *Continuum (Minneapolis, Minn.), 25*(1), 187–207.

Vacca, V. M. Jr, & Argento, I. (2018). Chronic subdural hematoma: A common complexity. *Nursing, 48*(5), 24–31.

Venkatesh, K., Ghosh, S. K., Mullick, M., et al. (2019). Spinal cord injury: Pathophysiology, treatment strategies, associated challenges, and future implications. *Cell and Tissue Research, 377*(2), 125–151.

Vijay, V. R., & Jaison, J. (2019). Treatment approaches in intracranial hypertension: A review. *Journal of Nursing Science and Practice, 6*(3), 2249–4758.

Watson, H. I., Shepherd, A. A., Rhodes, J. K. J., et al. (2018). Revisited: A systematic review of therapeutic hypothermia for adult patients following traumatic brain injury. *Critical Care Medicine, 46*(6), 972–979.

Weng, W. J., Yang, C., Huang, X-J., et al. (2018). Effects of brain temperature on the outcome of patients with traumatic brain injury: A prospective observational study. *Journal of Neurotrauma, 36*(7), 1168–1174.

Williamson, C., & Rajajee, V. (2018). Traumatic brain injury: Epidemiology, classification and pathophysiology. *UpToDate.* Retrieved on 3/7/2020 at: www.uptodate.com/contents/traumatic-brain-injury-epidemiology-classification-and-pathophysiology

Young, P. J., & Prescott, H. C. (2019). When less is more in the active management of elevated body temperature of ICU patients. *Intensive Care Medicine, 45*(9), 1275–1278.

Zaman, A., Dubiel, R., Driver, S., et al. (2017). Seizure prophylaxis guidelines following traumatic brain injury: An evaluation of compliance. *Journal of Head Trauma Rehabilitation, 32*(2), E13–E17.

Resources

American Academy of Spinal Cord Injury Professionals, Inc., www.academyscipro.org
American Association of Neuroscience Nurses (AANN), www.aann.org
Association of Rehabilitation Nurses (ARN), www.rehabnurse.org
Brain Injury Association of America, www.biausa.org
Brain Trauma Foundation, www.braintrauma.org
Neurocritical Care Society (NCS), www.neurocriticalcare.org
Paralyzed Veterans of America, www.pva.org
United Spinal Association, www.spinalcord.org
World Federation of Neuroscience Nursing (WFNN), wfnn.org

64

Management of Patients with Neurologic Infections, Autoimmune Disorders, and Neuropathies

The diverse group of neurologic disorders that make up infectious and autoimmune disorders and cranial and peripheral neuropathies presents unique challenges for nursing care. The nurse who cares for patients with these disorders must have a clear understanding of the pathophysiology, diagnostic testing, medical and nursing care, and rehabilitation processes. Some of the issues nurses must help patients and families confront include adaptation to the effects of the disease, potential changes in family dynamics, and end-of-life issues.

INFECTIOUS NEUROLOGIC DISORDERS

The infectious disorders of the nervous system include meningitis, brain abscesses, various types of encephalitis,

Creutzfeldt–Jakob disease (CJD), and variant Creutzfeldt–Jakob disease (vCJD). The clinical manifestations, assessment and diagnostic findings, as well as the medical and nursing management, are related to the specific infectious process.

Meningitis

Meningitis is inflammation of the meninges, which cover and protect the brain and spinal cord. The two main types of meningitis are bacterial and viral (Norris, 2019). Meningitis can be the main reason a patient is hospitalized, or it can develop during hospitalization; it is classified as septic or aseptic. Septic meningitis is caused by bacteria. The bacteria *Streptococcus pneumoniae* and *Neisseria meningitidis* are responsible for

80% to 90% of cases of bacterial meningitis in adults (Hickey & Strayer, 2020). In aseptic meningitis, the cause is viral or secondary to cancer or having a weakened immune system, such as in human immunodeficiency virus (HIV). The most common causative agents are the enteroviruses (Norris, 2019). Aseptic meningitis occurs more frequently in the summer and early fall.

First-year college students and members of the military who have not been vaccinated are at higher risk for meningococcal meningitis. Although infections occur year-round, the peak incidence is in the winter and early spring. Factors that increase the risk of bacterial meningitis include tobacco use and viral upper respiratory infection, because they increase the amount of droplet production. Otitis media and mastoiditis increase the risk of bacterial meningitis, because the bacteria can cross the epithelial membrane and enter the subarachnoid space. People with immune system deficiencies are also at greater risk for development of bacterial meningitis (Norris, 2019).

Pathophysiology

Meningeal infections generally originate in one of two ways: through the bloodstream as a consequence of other infections or by direct spread, such as might occur after a traumatic injury to the facial bones or secondary to invasive procedures.

Once the causative organism enters the bloodstream, it crosses the blood–brain barrier and proliferates in the cerebrospinal fluid (CSF). The host immune response stimulates the release of cell wall fragments and lipopolysaccharides, facilitating inflammation of the subarachnoid and pia mater. Because the cranial vault contains little room for expansion, the inflammation may cause increased intracranial pressure (ICP). CSF circulates through the subarachnoid space, where inflammatory cellular materials from the affected meningeal tissue enter and accumulate.

The prognosis for bacterial meningitis depends on the causative organism, the severity of the infection and illness, and the timeliness of treatment. The *N. meningitidis* bacterium results in an acute fulminant presentation approximately 10% of the time. This presentation may include adrenal damage, circulatory collapse, and widespread hemorrhages (Waterhouse–Friderichsen syndrome) (Hickey & Strayer, 2020). This syndrome is the result of endothelial damage and vascular necrosis caused by the bacteria.

Clinical Manifestations

Headache along with fever and chills are frequent initial symptoms. Fever tends to remain high throughout the course of the illness. The headache is usually either steady or throbbing and very severe as a result of meningeal irritation. Older adults may have mental status changes and focal neurologic deficits (Mount & Boyle, 2017). Meningeal irritation results in a number of other well-recognized signs common to all types of meningitis (Norris, 2019; Weber & Kelley, 2018):

- *Neck immobility:* Nuchal rigidity (a stiff and painful neck) can be an early sign, and any attempts at flexion of the head are difficult because of spasms in the muscles of the neck. Usually, the neck is supple, and the patient can easily bend the head and neck forward.
- *Positive Kernig sign:* When the patient is lying with the thigh flexed on the abdomen, the leg cannot be

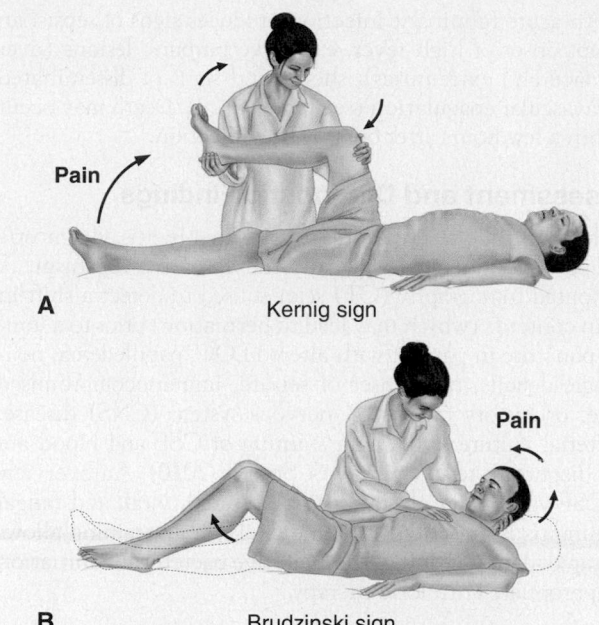

Figure 64-1 • Testing for meningeal irritation. **A.** Kernig sign. Flex the patient's leg at both the hip and knee and then straighten the knee. **B.** Brudzinski sign. As the neck is flexed, watch the hips and knees for a reaction.

completely extended (see Fig. 64-1A). When Kernig sign is bilateral, meningeal irritation is suspected.
- *Positive Brudzinski sign:* When the patient's neck is flexed (after ruling out cervical trauma or injury), flexion of the knees and hips is produced; when the lower extremity of one side is passively flexed, a similar movement is seen in the opposite extremity (see Fig. 64-1B). Brudzinski sign is a more sensitive indicator of meningeal irritation than Kernig sign.
- *Photophobia (extreme sensitivity to light):* This finding is common due to irritation of the meninges, especially around the diaphragm sellae.
- A rash can be a striking feature of *meningococcal meningitidis* infection, occurring in about half of patients with this type of meningitis. Skin lesions develop, ranging from a petechial rash with purpuric lesions to large areas of ecchymosis.

Disorientation and memory impairment are common early in the course of the illness. The changes depend on the severity of the infection as well as the individual response to the physiologic processes. Behavioral manifestations are also common. As the illness progresses, lethargy, unresponsiveness, and coma may develop.

Seizures can occur and are the result of areas of irritability in the brain. ICP increases secondary to diffuse brain swelling or hydrocephalus (Hickey & Strayer, 2020). The initial signs of increased ICP include decreased level of consciousness (LOC) and focal motor deficits. If ICP is not controlled, the uncus of the temporal lobe may herniate through the tentorium, causing pressure on the brainstem. Brainstem herniation is a life-threatening event that causes cranial nerve dysfunction and depresses the centers of vital functions, such as the medulla. See Chapter 61 for discussion of the patient with a change in LOC or increased ICP.

An acute fulminant infection produces signs of sepsis: an abrupt onset of high fever, extensive purpuric lesions (over the face and extremities), shock, and signs of disseminated intravascular coagulation (see Chapter 29). Death may occur within a few hours after onset of the infection.

Assessment and Diagnostic Findings

If the clinical presentation suggests meningitis, diagnostic testing is conducted to identify the causative organism. A computed tomography (CT) scan is used to detect a shift in brain contents (which may lead to herniation) prior to a lumbar puncture in patient with altered LOC, papilledema, neurologic deficits, new onset of seizure, immunocompromised state, or history of central nervous system (CNS) disease. Bacterial culture and Gram staining of CSF and blood are key diagnostic tests (Hickey & Strayer, 2020). An overview of CSF values and alterations in bacterial, viral, and fungal meningitis is presented in Table 64-1. Gram staining allows for rapid identification of the causative bacteria and initiation of appropriate antibiotic therapy.

Prevention

The Advisory Committee on Immunization Practices of the Centers for Disease Control and Prevention (CDC) recommends that the meningococcal conjugated vaccine be given to youth at 11 to 12 years of age, with a booster dose at 16 years of age (CDC, 2020).

People in close contact with patients with meningococcal meningitis should be treated with antimicrobial chemoprophylaxis using rifampin, ciprofloxacin, or ceftriaxone. Therapy should be started within 24 hours after exposure because a delay limits the effectiveness of the prophylaxis. Vaccination should also be considered as an adjunct to antibiotic chemoprophylaxis for anyone living with a person who develops meningococcal infection. Vaccination against *Haemophilus influenzae* and *S. pneumoniae* should be encouraged for children and adults who are at-risk (CDC, 2020).

Medical Management

Successful outcomes depend on the early administration of an antibiotic agent that crosses the blood–brain barrier into the subarachnoid space in sufficient concentration to halt the multiplication of bacteria. Penicillin G in combination with one of the cephalosporins (e.g., ceftriaxone, cefotaxime) is most often administered intravenously (IV), emergently with suspected bacterial meningitis (Hickey & Strayer, 2020).

Dexamethasone has been shown to be beneficial as adjunct therapy in the treatment of acute bacterial meningitis and in pneumococcal meningitis if it is given before or concurrently with the first dose of antibiotic and every 6 hours for the next 4 days. Research suggests that dexamethasone improves the outcome in adults and does not increase the risk of gastrointestinal bleeding (Hickey & Strayer, 2020).

Dehydration and shock are treated with fluid volume expanders. Seizures, which may occur early in the course of the disease, are treated with anticonvulsant medications. Increased ICP is treated as necessary (see Chapter 61).

 ## Nursing Management

The patient with meningitis is critically ill; therefore, many of the nursing interventions are collaborative with the physician, respiratory therapist, and other members of the health care team. The patient's safety and well-being depend on sound nursing judgment. Most patients will need the following nursing interventions:

- Instituting infection control precautions until 24 hours after initiation of antibiotic therapy (oral and nasal discharge is considered infectious)
- Assisting with pain management due to overall body aches and neck pain
- Assisting with getting rest in a quiet, darkened room
- Implementing interventions to treat the elevated temperature, such as antipyretic agents and cooling blankets
- Encouraging the patient to stay hydrated either orally or peripherally
- Ensuring close neurologic monitoring (see Chapter 61)

Neurologic status and vital signs are continually assessed. Pulse oximetry and arterial blood gas values are used to quickly identify the need for respiratory support if increasing ICP compromises the brainstem. Insertion of a cuffed endotracheal tube (or tracheotomy) and mechanical ventilation may be necessary to maintain adequate tissue oxygenation.

Blood pressure (usually monitored using an arterial line) is assessed for early manifestations of shock, which precedes cardiac or respiratory failure. Rapid IV fluid replacement may be prescribed, but care is taken to prevent fluid overload. Fever also increases the workload of the heart and cerebral metabolism. ICP will increase in response to increased cerebral

TABLE 64-1	Cerebrospinal Fluid Values Diagnostic for Meningitis		
Parameter	**Normal CSF**	**Bacterial Meningitis**	**Viral Meningitis**
Opening pressure (mm H_2O)	100–180	Elevated >180	Variable
Leukocyte count (white blood cell/mm³)	0–5	Increased 100–5000	Increased 50–1000
Neutrophils (%)	0	≥80	<40
Protein (mg/dL)	15–50	Elevated 100–500	Normal or slightly increased
Glucose (mg/dL)	40–80; 0.6 times blood glucose level	<40; <0.4 times blood glucose level	Normal

CSF, cerebrospinal fluid.
Adapted from Hickey, J. V., & Strayer, A. L. (2020). *The clinical practice of neurological & neurosurgical nursing* (8th ed.). Philadelphia, PA: Wolters Kluwer.

metabolic demands. Therefore, measures are taken to reduce body temperature as quickly as possible.

Other important components of nursing care include the following measures:

- Protecting the patient from injury secondary to seizure activity or altered LOC
- Monitoring daily body weight; serum electrolytes; and urine volume, specific gravity, and osmolality, especially if syndrome of inappropriate antidiuretic hormone (SIADH) is suspected
- Preventing complications associated with immobility, such as pressure injury and pneumonia

Any sudden, critical illness can be devastating to the family. Because the patient's condition is often critical and the prognosis guarded, the family needs to be informed about the patient's condition. Periodic family visits are essential to facilitate coping of the patient and family. An important aspect of the nurse's role is to support the family and assist them in identifying others who can be supportive to them during the crisis (Hickey & Strayer, 2020).

Promoting Home, Community-Based, and Transitional Care

After the patient has achieved physiologic homeostasis and has demonstrated achievement of major health care goals, rehabilitation continues either in a rehabilitation facility, skilled nursing facility, or at home. Continued support and evaluation by the nurse are essential.

Because patients may have been critically ill and focused on the most obvious needs and issues, the nurse reminds the patient and family about the importance of continuing health promotion and screening practices, such as regular physical examinations and appropriate diagnostic screening tests.

Brain Abscess

Brain abscesses account for less than 1% of space-occupying brain lesions in the United States (Hickey & Strayer, 2020). Brain abscesses are rare in people who are immunocompetent; they are more frequently diagnosed in people who are immunosuppressed as a result of an underlying disease or the use of immunosuppressive medications.

Pathophysiology

A brain abscess is a collection of infectious material within the tissue of the brain. Bacteria are the most common causative organisms. The most common predisposing conditions for abscesses among adults who are immunocompetent are otitis media and rhinosinusitis. It is estimated that 40% of brain abscesses are otogenic in origin (Hickey & Strayer, 2020). An abscess can result from intracranial surgery, penetrating head injury, or tongue piercing. Organisms causing brain abscess may reach the brain by hematologic spread from the lungs, gums, tongue, or heart, or from a wound or intra-abdominal infection.

Clinical Manifestations

The clinical manifestations of a brain abscess result from alterations in intracranial dynamics (edema, brain shift), infection, or the location of the abscess. Headache, usually worse in the morning, is the most prevalent symptom. Mental status changes may occur. Fever is present 53% of the time (Sonneville, Ruimy, Benzonana, et al., 2017). Vomiting and focal neurologic deficits occur as well. Focal deficits including weakness and decreasing vision reflect the area of brain that is involved. As the abscess expands, symptoms of increased ICP such as decreasing LOC and seizures occur (Hickey & Strayer, 2020).

Assessment and Diagnostic Findings

The baseline neurologic examination may reveal a variety of signs and symptoms based on the location of the abscess (see Chart 64-1). Neuroimaging with CT scanning with contrast is used most often to identify the size and location of the abscess. Cerebritis is a small infection in the brain that can progress to an abscess if not detected or treated. Aspiration of the abscess, guided by CT or MRI, is often used to culture and identify the infectious organism. MRI is the preferred study, because it provides higher resolution of the lesion and assists with identification of additional lesions if present (Sonneville et al., 2017). Blood cultures are obtained if the abscess is believed to arise from a distant source.

Medical Management

Treatment is aimed at controlling increased ICP, draining the abscess, and providing antimicrobial therapy directed at the abscess and the main source of infection. Large IV doses of antibiotic agents are given to penetrate the blood–brain barrier and reach the abscess. The choice of the specific antibiotic medication is based on culture and sensitivity testing and directed at the causative organism. Antibiotics should be started as soon as possible; the initial antibiotic started typically is ceftriaxone combined with metronidazole, which will be adjusted based on the culture and sensitivity results (Brouwer & van de Beek, 2017). A stereotactic guided aspiration may be used to drain the abscess and identify the causative organism. Surgical excision is not the preferred method, except in cases where the abscess is large and multi-lobulated

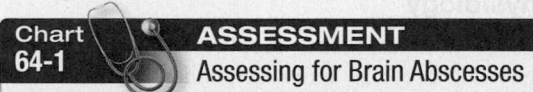

Chart 64-1

ASSESSMENT

Assessing for Brain Abscesses

Be alert to the following signs and symptoms of brain abscess:

Frontal Lobe

- Expressive aphasia (inability to express oneself)
- Frontal headache
- Hemiparesis (weakness on one side of the body)
- Seizures

Temporal Lobe

- Changes in vision
- Facial weakness
- Localized headache
- Receptive aphasia (inability to understand language)

Cerebellar Abscess

- Ataxia
- Nystagmus (rhythmic, involuntary movements of the eye)
- Occipital headache

(Sonneville et al., 2017). Corticosteroids may be prescribed to help reduce the inflammatory cerebral edema if the patient shows evidence of an increasing neurologic deficit. Anticonvulsant medications may be prescribed to prevent or treat seizures (see Chapter 61).

Nursing Management

Nursing care focuses on continuing to assess the neurologic status, administering medications, assessing the response to treatment, and providing supportive care.

Ongoing neurologic assessment alerts the nurse to changes in ICP, which may indicate a need for more aggressive intervention. The nurse also assesses and documents the responses to medications. Blood laboratory test results, specifically blood glucose and serum potassium levels, are closely monitored when corticosteroids are prescribed (Comerford & Durkin, 2020). Administration of insulin or electrolyte replacement may be required to return these values to within normal limits.

Patient safety is another key nursing responsibility. Injury may result from decreased LOC or falls related to motor weakness or seizures.

The patient with a brain abscess is very ill, with neurologic deficits, such as **hemiplegia** (paralysis of one side of the body, or part of it), **hemiparesis** (weakness of one side of the body, or part of it), seizures, visual deficits, and cranial nerve palsies that may persist after treatment. The nurse must assess the family's ability to express distress at the patient's condition, cope with the patient's illness and deficits, and obtain support. Treatment has improved and 70% of patients have no or minimal permanent neurologic deficits, but more research is needed on long-term function (Brouwer & van de Beek, 2017).

Herpes Simplex Encephalitis

Encephalitis is an acute inflammatory process of the brain tissue. The herpes simplex virus (HSV) is the most common cause of acute encephalitis in the United States, accounting for 10% to 15% of cases of encephalitis (Hickey & Strayer, 2020).

Pathophysiology

The pathology of encephalitis involves local necrotizing hemorrhage that becomes more generalized, followed by edema. There is also progressive deterioration of nerve cell bodies (Norris, 2019).

Clinical Manifestations

The initial symptoms of herpes simplex encephalitis include fever, headache, confusion, and hallucinations. Focal neurologic symptoms reflect the areas of cerebral inflammation and necrosis and include fever, headache, behavioral changes, focal seizures, dysphasia, hemiparesis, and altered LOC (Norris, 2019).

Assessment and Diagnostic Findings

Neuroimaging studies, such as electroencephalography (EEG), and CSF examination are used to diagnose encephalitis. MRI is used to detect inflammation that shows up as hyperintense (bright) areas (see Fig. 64-2). The EEG shows diffuse slowing or focal changes in the temporal lobe in the

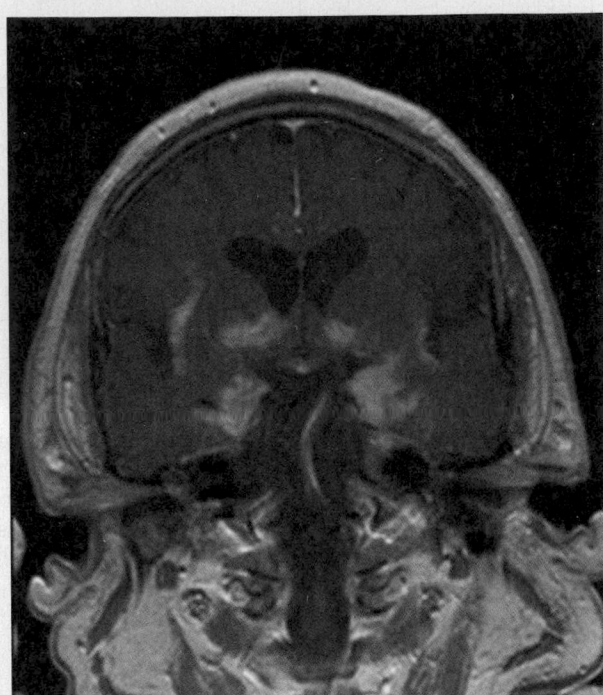

Figure 64-2 • Herpes simplex virus encephalitis. Coronal view, MRI scan. Note bilateral hyperintensity (bright) areas indicative of inflammation. Reprinted with permission from Hickey, J. V., & Strayer, A. L. (2020). *The clinical practice of neurological & neurosurgical nursing* (8th ed., Fig. 28-4C). Philadelphia, PA: Wolters Kluwer.

majority of patients. Lumbar puncture often reveals a high opening pressure, glucose within normal limits, and high protein levels in CSF samples (see Table 64-1). The polymerase chain reaction (PCR) is the standard test for early diagnosis of herpes simplex encephalitis. PCR identifies the deoxyribonucleic acid (DNA) bands of HSV-1 in the CSF with 95% sensitivity and 99% specificity rates (Hickey & Strayer, 2020).

Medical Management

The antiviral agent acyclovir is the medication of choice in the treatment for HSV (Hickey & Strayer, 2020). Early administration of an antiviral agent (usually well tolerated) improves the prognosis associated with HSV. The mode of action is inhibition of viral DNA replication. To prevent relapse, treatment should continue for up to 3 weeks. Slow IV administration over 1 hour prevents crystallization of the medication in the urine. The usual dose of acyclovir is decreased if the patient has a history of renal insufficiency.

Nursing Management

Assessment of neurologic function is key to monitoring the progression of disease. Comfort measures to reduce headache include dimming the lights, limiting noise and visitors, grouping nursing interventions, and administering analgesic agents. Opioid analgesic medications may mask neurologic symptoms; therefore, they are used cautiously. Seizures and altered LOC require care directed at injury prevention and safety. Nursing care addressing patient and family anxieties is ongoing throughout the illness. Monitoring of blood chemistry test results and urinary output alert the nurse to the presence of renal complications related to antiviral therapy.

Arthropod-Borne Virus Encephalitis

Arthropod-borne viruses, or arboviruses, are maintained in nature through biologic transmission between susceptible vertebrate hosts by blood feeding arthropods (mosquitoes, psychodids, ceratopogonids, and ticks). Arthropod vectors transmit several types of viruses that cause encephalitis. The main vector in North America is the mosquito. Arbovirus infection (transmitted by arthropod vectors) occurs in specific geographic areas during the summer and fall. In the United States, there are five main arboviral encephalitides: eastern equine encephalitis, western equine encephalitis, St. Louis encephalitis, La Crosse encephalitis, and West Nile virus encephalitis (Hickey & Strayer, 2020).

Pathophysiology

Viral replication occurs at the site of the mosquito bite. The host immune response attempts to control viral replication. If the immune response is inadequate, viremia will ensue. The virus gains access to the CNS via the olfactory tract, resulting in encephalitis. It spreads from neuron to neuron, predominantly affecting the cortical gray matter, the brainstem, and the thalamus. Meningeal exudates compound the clinical presentation by irritating the meninges and increasing ICP.

Clinical Manifestations

St. Louis and West Nile virus encephalitis most commonly affect adults. An arboviral encephalitis occurs along a continuum with some cases having only flulike symptoms (i.e., headache and fever) but others progressing to specific neurologic manifestations that vary depending on the viral type (Hickey & Strayer, 2020). A unique clinical feature of arboviral encephalitis is SIADH with hyponatremia. Onset of symptoms is abrupt with fever, headache, dizziness, nausea, and malaise. If the disease spreads to the CNS, symptoms include stiff neck, confusion, dizziness, and tremors. Coma can occur in severe cases, and mortality increases with age. Eastern equine encephalitis has the highest mortality rate at 50% (Hickey & Strayer, 2020).

Assessment and Diagnostic Findings

Arboviral infections are seasonal. Preliminary diagnosis is based on clinical presentation and location and dates of recent travel because certain viruses are endemic to certain geographic locales. Neuroimaging and CSF evaluation are useful in the diagnosis of encephalitis. The MRI scan demonstrates inflammation of the basal ganglia in cases of St. Louis encephalitis and inflammation in the periventricular area in cases of West Nile encephalitis. EEG can identify abnormal brain waves, which can help identify some viral infections.

Medical Management

No specific medication for arboviral encephalitis exists; therefore, treatment is supportive and symptom management is key (Hickey & Strayer, 2020). Controlling elevated ICP is a critical component of care in cases with neurologic manifestations.

Nursing Management

Many patients, particularly those with only fever and headache, are treated on an outpatient basis. If the patient is very ill, hospitalization may be required. The nurse carefully assesses neurologic status and identifies improvement or deterioration in the patient's condition. See Chapter 61 for management of the patient with increased ICP. Injury prevention is key in light of the potential for falls or seizures. Any encephalitis that progresses may result in death or lifelong residual health issues such as neurologic deficits and seizures. The family will need support and education to cope with these residual issues. The nurse may need to mobilize community support services for the patient and family, because the recovery may be long.

Public education addressing the prevention of arboviral encephalitis is a key nursing role. Clothing that provides coverage and insect repellents containing 20% to 35% diethyltoluamide (DEET) should be used on exposed clothing and skin in high-risk areas to decrease mosquito and tick bites (Hickey & Strayer, 2020). Remaining indoors at dawn and dusk when mosquito activity is highest is recommended. Screens should be in good repair in the home, and standing water should be removed. All cases of arboviral encephalitis must be reported to the local health department.

Creutzfeldt–Jakob and Variant Creutzfeldt–Jakob Diseases

CJD and vCJD belong to a group of degenerative, infectious neurologic disorders called *transmissible spongiform encephalopathies* (TSE). CJD is rare and has no identifiable cause. vCJD, the human variation of bovine spongiform encephalopathy (BSE) (mad cow disease), results from ingesting meat infected with prions. **Prions,** which cause TSEs, are pathogens smaller than a virus that are resistant to standard methods of disinfection and sterilization (Garcia, 2019). Although CJD and vCJD have distinct clinical features, one characteristic they share is a lack of CNS inflammation. CJD may lie dormant for decades before causing neurologic degeneration. The incubation period of vCJD seems to be shorter (less than 10 years). In both diseases, the symptoms are progressive, there is no definitive treatment, and the outcome is fatal often within 1 year of symptom onset (Hickey & Strayer, 2020).

Almost all cases of vCJD have been reported in the United Kingdom, with a smaller number of cases being identified in 10 other countries worldwide. The risk of vCJD in the United States is thought to be low, because cattle are fed primarily with soy-derived feed as opposed to feed containing animal parts.

Pathophysiology

The prion is a unique pathogen because it lacks nucleic acid, which enables the organism to withstand conventional means of disinfection and sterilization (Garcia, 2019). In both CJD and vCJD, the prion crosses the blood–brain barrier and is deposited in brain tissue and causes degeneration of brain tissue (Hickey & Strayer, 2020). Cell death occurs, and spongiform changes (spongy vacuoles) are produced in the brain. The spongiform vacuoles are surrounded by amyloid plaque.

There are three major forms of CJD (Manthorpe & Simcock, 2019). Approximately 85% of cases appear sporadically, hence this form is called sporadic CJD. The incidence is 1 case per 1 million people. Sporadic CJD occurs spontaneously with no risk factors. The second form is familial or hereditary CJD, and this type accounts for 5% to 10% of cases. The third type is acquired CJD. This form is transmitted by contaminated brain, tissue, or neurosurgical instruments and accounts for less than 1% of cases (World Health Organization [WHO]. n.d.).

The prion exists in lymphoid tissue and blood in both vCJD and CJD. Both prion diseases are believed to be bloodborne. No method is available to screen blood for infectivity. For this reason, the American Red Cross does not accept blood donation from anyone who has stayed more than 3 months in the United Kingdom (UK) between 1980 and 1996 or has received a blood transfusion in France or the UK at any time between 1980 and the present (Miller, Grima, & Plonowski, 2020).

Clinical Manifestations

CJD and vCJD have several clinically distinct features. Psychiatric symptoms occur early in vCJD, whereas they are a late symptom in CJD. The mean age at onset of vCJD is 27 years, whereas the mean age for CJD onset is 65 years. The presenting symptoms of vCJD include affective symptoms (i.e., behavioral changes), sensory disturbance, and limb pain. Muscle spasms and rigidity, dysarthria (difficulty speaking), incoordination, cognitive impairment, and sleep disturbances follow. Patients with sporadic CJD present with mental deterioration, **ataxia** (inability to coordinate movements), and visual disturbance. Memory loss, involuntary movement, paralysis, and mutism occur as the disease progresses. After clinical presentation, people with vCJD survive an average of 14 months; those with CJD survive for less than 1 year (Manthorpe & Simcock, 2019).

Assessment and Diagnostic Findings

Brain biopsy, the only way to confirm diagnosis, is not recommended (Hickey & Strayer, 2020). The three diagnostic tests currently used in suspicious clinical presentations to support the diagnosis of CJD are immunologic assessment, EEG, and MRI scanning. Immunologic assessment of CSF detects a protein kinase inhibitor referred to as 14–3–3 (Hickey & Strayer, 2020). The presence of this inhibitor indicates neuronal cell death, which is not specific to CJD but does support the diagnosis. The EEG reveals a characteristic pattern over the duration of the disease. After initial slowing, the EEG shows periodic activity. Later in the course of the disease, the EEG shows burst suppressions characterized by periodic spikes alternating with slow periods. The MRI scan demonstrates symmetric or unilateral hyperintense signals arising from the basal ganglia.

Medical Management

After the onset of specific neurologic symptoms, progression of disease occurs quickly. There is no effective treatment for CJD or vCJD. The care of the patient is supportive and palliative. Goals of the interprofessional care team include prevention of injury related to immobility and dementia, promotion of patient comfort, and provision of support and education for the family.

Nursing Management

The nursing care of patients is primarily supportive and palliative. Psychological and emotional support of the patient and family throughout the course of the illness is needed. Care extends to providing for a dignified death and supporting the family through the processes of grief and loss. Hospice services are appropriate either at home or at an inpatient facility. See Chapter 13 for an in-depth discussion of end-of-life issues.

Prevention of disease transmission is an important part of nursing care. Although patient isolation is not necessary, the use of standard precautions is important. Institutional protocols are followed for handling of brain, spinal cord, pituitary gland, and eye tissue; and for exposure and decontamination of equipment. If surgery is necessary, it is recommended that disposable instruments be used and then incinerated, because conventional methods of sterilization do not destroy the prion (Hickey & Strayer, 2020). If disposable instruments cannot be used, stringent sterilization methods such as the use of bleach for cleaning and extended sterilization time for instruments should be used (Garcia, 2019).

AUTOIMMUNE PROCESSES

Autoimmune nervous system disorders include multiple sclerosis (MS), myasthenia gravis, and Guillain–Barré syndrome (GBS).

Multiple Sclerosis

MS is an immune-mediated, progressive demyelinating disease of the CNS. Demyelination refers to the destruction of myelin—the fatty and protein material that surrounds certain nerve fibers in the brain and spinal cord; it results in impaired transmission of nerve impulses (see Fig. 64-3). MS

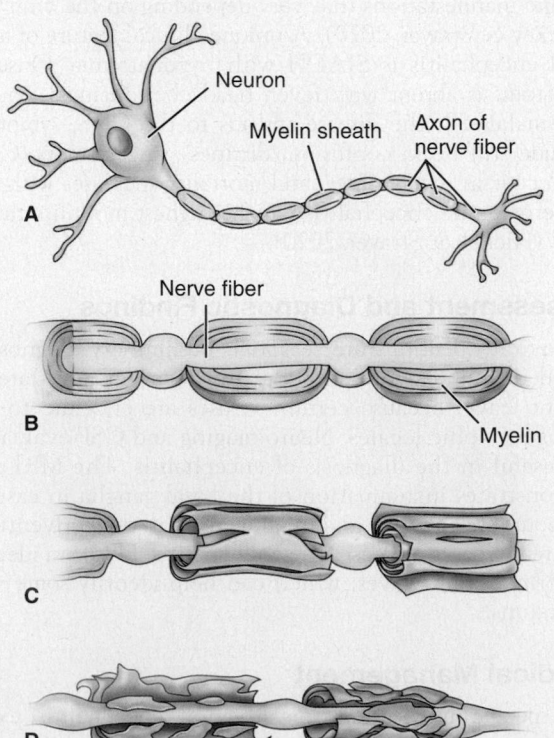

Figure 64-3 • The process of demyelination. **A, B.** A normal nerve cell and axon with myelin. **C, D.** The slow disintegration of myelin, resulting in a disruption in axon function.

affects nearly 400,000 people in the United States (Hickey & Strayer, 2020; Norris, 2019). MS may occur at any age, but the age of peak onset is between 20 and 50 years; it affects women three times more than men (Hickey & Strayer, 2020).

The cause of MS is unknown and is an area of ongoing research. Autoimmune activity results in demyelination, but the sensitized antigen has not been identified. Multiple factors play a role in the initiation of the immune process. Geographic prevalence is highest in Europe, New Zealand, southern Australia, the northern United States, and southern Canada. MS is less prevalent in Asians. There is a greater frequency in northern colder latitudes (Hickey & Strayer, 2020).

MS is considered to have many risks, including genetic factors. It has not been found to be genetically transmitted but there have been 200 genetic variations related to MS (Hickey & Strayer, 2020). A specific virus capable of initiating the autoimmune response has not been identified. It is believed that DNA on the virus mimics the amino acid sequence of myelin, resulting in an immune system cross-reaction in the presence of a defective immune system. Environmental risks include obesity, lack of vitamin D exposure, and a high salt diet in the teenage years (Hickey & Strayer, 2020).

There are several acute and subacute forms of MS. Less severe forms include radiologically isolated syndrome (RIS) and clinically isolated syndrome (CIS). RIS consists of MS-like lesions that are identified on MRI in the absence of clinical signs and symptoms. Approximately one third of patients are diagnosed with MS within 5 years of the identification of an incidental lesion on MRI (Coyle, 2019). CIS is the presence of acute or subacute clinical findings for at least 24 hours (Coyle, 2019).

The four main clinical forms are remitting-relapsing (RRMS), secondary progressive, primary progressive (PPMS), and progressive-relapsing (Bradshaw & Houtchens, 2018).

Pathophysiology

Sensitized T and B lymphocytes cross the blood–brain barrier; their function is to check the CNS for antigens and then leave. In MS, sensitized T cells remain in the CNS and promote the infiltration of other agents that damage the immune system. The immune system attack leads to inflammation that destroys mostly the white matter of the CNS myelin (which insulates the axon and speeds the conduction of impulses along the axon) and the oligodendroglial cells that produce myelin in the CNS (Norris, 2019).

Demyelination interrupts the flow of nerve impulses and results in a variety of manifestations, depending on the nerves affected. Plaques appear on demyelinated axons, further interrupting the transmission of impulses. Demyelinated axons are scattered irregularly throughout the CNS. The areas most frequently affected are the optic nerves, chiasm, and tracts; the cerebrum; the brainstem and cerebellum; and the spinal cord (Norris, 2019). The axons themselves begin to degenerate, resulting in permanent and irreversible damage.

Clinical Manifestations

The course of MS assumes many different patterns. In some patients, the disease follows a benign course, and symptoms are so mild that the patient does not seek health care or treatment. The patient with RIS will have no symptoms, while the typical presentation of CIS includes unilateral optic neuritis, focal symptoms, or partial myelopathy (Coyle, 2019).

Approximately 85% of patients have RRMS (Coyle, 2019). With each relapse, recovery is usually complete; however, residual deficits may occur and accumulate over time, contributing to functional decline. Over time, most patients with RRMS move to the secondary progressive form, in which disease progression occurs with or without relapses. Approximately 15% of patients have PPMS, in which disabling symptoms steadily increase, with rare plateaus and temporary minor improvement. PPMS may result in quadriparesis, cognitive dysfunction, visual loss, and brainstem syndromes (Coyle, 2019). The least common presentation (about 5% of cases) is progressive-relapsing, which is characterized by relapses with continuous disabling progression between exacerbations (Coyle, 2019; Norris, 2019). The signs and symptoms of MS are varied and multiple, reflecting the location of the lesion (plaque) or combination of lesions. Physical, emotional, and cognitive symptoms impact the quality of life (Debska, Milaniak, & Skorupska-Krol, 2020; Kalb, Feinstein, Rohrig, et al., 2019). Fatigue, depression, weakness, numbness, difficulty in coordination, loss of balance, spasticity, and pain are all common (Norris, 2019). Visual disturbances due to lesions in the optic nerves or their connections may include blurring of vision, **diplopia** (double vision, or the awareness of two images of the same object occurring in one or both eyes), scotoma (patchy blindness), and total blindness.

Fatigue affects most people with MS and is often the most disabling symptom (Newland, Lorenz, Smith, et al., 2019). Heat, depression, anemia, deconditioning, and medication may contribute to fatigue. Avoiding hot temperatures, effective treatment of depression and anemia, a change in medication, as well as occupational and physical therapies may help manage fatigue (Coyle, 2019).

Pain is another common symptom of MS. Lesions on the sensory pathways cause pain. Additional sensory manifestations include paresthesias, dysesthesias, and proprioception loss. Many people with MS need daily analgesic medications. In some cases, pain is managed with opioids, anticonvulsant medications, or antidepressants. Rarely, surgery may be needed to interrupt pain pathways.

Among women who are perimenopausal, those with MS are more likely to have pain related to osteoporosis. In addition to estrogen loss, immobility and corticosteroid therapy play a role in the development of osteoporosis among women with MS. Bone mineral density testing is recommended for this high-risk group. See Chapter 36 for a discussion of the diagnosis of and treatment for osteoporosis.

Spasticity is characterized by muscle hypertonicity with increased resistance to stretch often associated with weakness, increased deep tendon reflexes, and diminished superficial reflexes. It occurs in 90% of patients with MS, most often in the lower extremities, and can include loss of the abdominal reflexes. Spasticity results from involvement of the pyramidal tracts, the main motor pathways of the spinal cord. Cognitive and psychosocial problems may reflect frontal or parietal lobe involvement. Some degree of cognitive change (e.g., memory loss, decreased concentration) occurs in about half of patients, but severe cognitive changes with dementia (progressive organic mental disorder) are rare.

Involvement of the cerebellum or basal ganglia can produce ataxia and tremor. Loss of the control connections between the cortex and the basal ganglia may occur and cause emotional lability and euphoria. Bladder, bowel, and sexual dysfunctions are common. Additional complications include urinary tract infections (UTIs), constipation, pressure injury, contracture deformities, dependent pedal edema, pneumonia, and osteoporosis. Emotional, social, marital, economic, and vocational problems may also occur.

Exacerbations and remissions are characteristic of MS. During exacerbations, new symptoms appear and existing ones worsen; during remissions, symptoms decrease or disappear. Relapses may be associated with emotional and physical stress.

 ## Gerontologic Considerations

The life expectancy for patients with MS is 7 to 14 years shorter than patients without MS (Coyle, 2019). Those diagnosed with secondary progressive disease live an average of 38 years after onset. Older adult patients with MS have specific physical and psychosocial challenges. They may have chronic health problems, for which they may be taking additional medications that could interact with medications prescribed for MS. The absorption, distribution, metabolism, and excretion of medications are altered in the older adult as a result of age-related changes in kidney and liver functions. Therefore, older adult patients must be monitored closely for adverse and toxic effects of MS medications and for osteoporosis (particularly if corticosteroids have been used frequently to treat exacerbations). The cost of medications may lead to poor adherence to the prescribed regimen in older adult patients on fixed incomes.

Older adult patients with MS are particularly concerned about increasing disability, family burden, marital concern, and the possible future need for nursing home care. Immobility resulting in fewer social opportunities contributes to loneliness and depression. In addition to functional loss, the physical challenges experienced by older adults with MS include spasticity, pain, bladder dysfunction, impaired sleep, and an increased need for assistance with self-care.

Assessment and Diagnostic Findings

The diagnosis of MS is based on clinical, imaging, and laboratory findings. An important component is the presence of plaques in the CNS disseminated in space and over time observed on MRI scans with no better explanation for the clinical presentation (Thompson, Banwell, Barkhof, et al., 2018). Additional criteria are detailed in Table 64-2. Electrophoresis of CSF identifies the presence of oligoclonal banding (several bands of immunoglobulin G bonded together, indicating an immune system abnormality) (Thompson et al., 2018). Evoked potential studies can help define the extent of the disease process and monitor changes (Coyle, 2019). Underlying bladder dysfunction is diagnosed by urodynamic studies. Neuropsychological testing may be indicated to assess cognitive impairment. A sexual history helps identify changes in sexual function.

Medical Management

There is no cure for MS. An individual treatment program is indicated to relieve symptoms and provide continuing support, particularly for patients with cognitive changes, who may need more structure and support. The goals of treatment are to delay the progression of the disease, manage chronic symptoms, and treat acute exacerbations. Common symptoms

TABLE 64-2	The 2017 McDonald Criteria for Diagnosis of Multiple Sclerosis in Patients with an Attack at Onset	
	Number of Lesions with Objective Clinical Evidence	**Additional Data Needed for a Diagnosis of Multiple Sclerosis**
≥2 clinical attacks	≥2	None[a]
≥2 clinical attacks	1 (as well as clear-cut historical evidence of a previous attack involving a lesion in a distinct anatomical location[b])	None[a]
≥2 clinical attacks	1	Dissemination in space demonstrated by an additional clinical attack implicating a different CNS site or by MRI
1 clinical attack	≥2	Dissemination in time demonstrated by an additional clinical attack or by MRI OR demonstration of CSF-specific oligoclonal bands[c]
1 clinical attack	1	Dissemination in space demonstrated by an additional clinical attack implicating a different CNS site or by MRI AND Dissemination in time demonstrated by an additional clinical attack or by MRI OR demonstration of CSF-specific oligoclonal bands[c]

If the 2017 McDonald Criteria are fulfilled and there is no better explanation for the clinical presentation, the diagnosis is multiple sclerosis. If multiple sclerosis is suspected by virtue of a clinically isolated syndrome but the 2017 McDonald Criteria are not completely met, the diagnosis is possible multiple sclerosis. If another diagnosis arises during the evaluation that better explains the clinical presentation, the diagnosis is not multiple sclerosis.

[a]No additional tests are required to demonstrate dissemination in space and time. However, unless MRI is not possible, brain MRI should be obtained in all patients in whom the diagnosis of multiple sclerosis is being considered. In addition, spinal cord MRI or CSF examination should be considered in patients with insufficient clinical and MRI evidence supporting multiple sclerosis, with a presentation other than a typical clinically isolated syndrome, or with atypical features. If imaging or other tests (e.g., CSF) are undertaken and are negative, caution needs to be taken before making a diagnosis of multiple sclerosis, and alternative diagnoses should be considered.

[b]Clinical diagnosis based on objective clinical findings for two attacks is most secure. Reasonable historical evidence for one past attack, in the absence of documented objective neurologic findings, can include historical events with symptoms and evolution characteristic for a previous inflammatory demyelinating attack; at least one attack, however, must be supported by objective findings. In the absence of residual objective evidence, caution is needed.

[c]The presence of CSF-specific oligoclonal bands does not demonstrate dissemination in time per se but can substitute for the requirement for demonstration of this measure.

Adapted from Thompson, A., Banwell, B., Barkhof, F., et al. (2018). Diagnosis of multiple sclerosis: 2017 revisions of the McDonald criteria. *The Lancet Neurology, 17*(2), 162–173. Copyright 2018, with permission from Elsevier.

requiring intervention include ataxia, bladder dysfunction, depression, fatigue, and spasticity. Management includes pharmacologic and nonpharmacologic strategies.

Pharmacologic Therapy

Medications prescribed for MS include those for disease modification and those for symptom management. Disease-modifying therapies delay disease progression in many forms of MS (Rae-Grant, Day, Marrie, et al., 2018). Many types of medications are used for symptom management in MS.

Disease-Modifying Therapies

In the past decade, the number of disease-modifying therapies has increased dramatically (Bradshaw & Houtchens, 2018). The key concept of disease-modifying therapies is to reduce the frequency of relapse, the duration of relapse, and the number and size of plaques observed on MRI in RRMS; however, these therapies are not effective in PPMS (Hickey & Strayer, 2020). There is debate about whether to use disease-modifying therapies in patients with RIS to prevent future disease progression to MS (Coyle, 2019; Rae-Grant et al., 2018).

Interferon beta-1a and interferon beta-1b are administered subcutaneously every other day. Another preparation of interferon beta-1a may be given intramuscularly once a week and pegylated interferon beta-1a can be given subcutaneously every 14 days. Side effects of all interferon-beta medications include flulike symptoms, increased liver function tests, leukopenia, headache, depression, and skin necrosis (Coyle, 2019). For optimal control of disability, disease-modifying medications should be started early in the course of the disease (Rae-Grant et al., 2018).

Glatiramer acetate also reduces the rate of relapse in RRMS and is administered subcutaneously daily. It has some adverse effects, such as injection-site reactions and flushing, but these are usually self-limiting to a few minutes. There are no monitoring parameters (Bradshaw & Houtchens, 2018).

Teriflunomide, fingolimod, and dimethyl fumarate are oral disease-modifying therapies that may be better tolerated by the patient who has difficulty with injection reactions. These medications have significantly reduced relapse rates in several types of MS (Bradshaw & Houtchens, 2018). Ocrelizumab has a 6% annual relapse reduction rate in patients with PPMS (Bradshaw & Houtchens, 2018).

IV methylprednisolone, used to treat acute exacerbations, shortens the duration of relapse but has not been found to have long-term benefit (Bradshaw & Houtchens, 2018). It exerts anti-inflammatory effects by acting on T cells and cytokines. The medication is given as 1 g IV daily for 3 to 5 days, followed by an oral taper of prednisone. Side effects include mood swings, weight gain, and electrolyte imbalances (Comerford & Durkin, 2020).

The medication mitoxantrone is given via IV infusion every 3 months. Mitoxantrone can reduce the frequency of clinical relapses in patients with secondary progressive or worsening RRMS. Patients must be very closely monitored for side effects (i.e., cardiac toxicity), and there is a maximum lifetime dose that can be given (Hickey & Strayer, 2020).

Symptom Management

Medications are also prescribed for management of specific symptoms. Baclofen, a gamma-aminobutyric acid agonist, is the medication of choice for treating spasticity. It can be given orally or by intrathecal injection for severe spasticity (Hickey & Strayer, 2020). Benzodiazepines (e.g., diazepam), tizanidine, and dantrolene may also be used to treat spasticity and improve motor function (Hickey & Strayer, 2020). Patients with disabling spasms and contractures may require nerve blocks or surgical intervention. Fatigue that interferes with activities of daily living (ADLs) may be treated with amantadine, pemoline, or dalfampridine. Ataxia is a chronic problem most resistant to treatment. Medications used to treat ataxia include beta-adrenergic blockers (e.g., propranolol), the anticonvulsant agent gabapentin, and benzodiazepines (e.g., clonazepam).

Bladder and bowel problems are often difficult for patients, and a variety of medications (anticholinergic agents, alpha-adrenergic blockers, antispasmodic agents) may be prescribed. Nonpharmacologic strategies also assist in establishing effective bowel and bladder elimination.

UTI may be superimposed on the underlying neurologic dysfunction. Increased fluid intake and good perineal care help reduce the risk of UTI. Antibiotic agents are prescribed when appropriate. See Chapter 49 for further discussion of UTI management.

NURSING PROCESS

The Patient with MS

Assessment

Nursing assessment addresses neurologic deficits and the impact of the disease on the patient and family. The patient's mobility and balance are observed to determine whether there is risk of falling. Assessment of function is carried out both when the patient is well rested and when fatigued. The patient is assessed for weakness, spasticity, visual impairment, incontinence, and disorders of swallowing and speech. Additional areas of assessment include how MS has affected the patient's quality of life, how the patient is coping, adherence to the prescribed medication regimen, and what the patient would like to improve (Debska et al., 2020; Newland et al., 2019).

Diagnosis

NURSING DIAGNOSES

Based on the assessment data, major nursing diagnoses may include the following:

- Impaired mobility associated with weakness, muscle paresis, spasticity, increased weight
- Risk for fall associated with sensory and visual impairment, lower extremity weakness
- Fatigue associated with insufficient energy
- Difficulty coping associated with uncertainty of course of MS

COLLABORATIVE PROBLEMS/POTENTIAL COMPLICATIONS

Potential complications may include the following:

- Constipation or fecal incontinence (see Chapter 41)
- Communication issues and potential for aspiration related to cranial nerve involvement (see cranial nerve discussion later in this chapter)
- Cognitive changes

- Managing therapies at home related to physical, psychological, and social limits imposed by MS
- Changes in sexuality
- Urinary incontinence (see Chapter 49)

Planning and Goals

The major goals for the patient may include promotion of physical mobility, avoidance of falls, decreasing fatigue, development of coping strategies, and absence of complications.

Nursing Interventions

An individualized program of physical, occupational, and speech-language therapy, rehabilitation, and education is combined with emotional support. An educational plan of care is developed to enable the person with MS to deal with the physiologic, social, and psychological problems that accompany chronic disease. The presence of depression, pain, fatigue, and walking difficulty all decrease physical activity. Assisting patients with management of these symptoms may help increase the level of physical activity and overall sense of well-being.

PROMOTING PHYSICAL MOBILITY

Relaxation and coordination exercises promote muscle efficiency. Progressive resistive exercises are used to strengthen weak muscles, because diminishing muscle strength is often significant in MS.

Exercise. Walking improves the gait, particularly the problem of loss of position sense of the legs and feet. If certain muscle groups are irreversibly affected, other muscles can be trained to compensate. Instruction in the use of assistive devices may be needed to ensure their safe and correct use.

Minimizing Spasticity and Contractures. Muscle spasticity is common and, in its later stages, is characterized by severe adductor spasm of the hips with flexor spasm of the hips and knees. Without relief, fibrous contractures of these joints occur. Warm packs may be beneficial, but hot baths should be avoided because of risk of burn injury secondary to sensory loss and increasing symptoms that may occur with elevation of the body temperature. Exposure to extreme cold is avoided as this may increase spasticity.

Daily exercises for muscle stretching are prescribed to minimize joint contractures. Special attention is given to the hamstrings, gastrocnemius muscles, hip adductors, biceps, and wrist and finger flexors. Muscle spasticity is common and interferes with usual function. Application of prescribed orthotics may help maintain a functional position and reduce contractures. A stretch–hold–relax routine is helpful for relaxing and treating muscle spasticity. Swimming and stationary bicycling are useful, and progressive weight bearing can relieve spasticity in the legs. The patient should not be hurried in any of these activities, because this often increases spasticity.

Activity and Rest. The patient is encouraged to work and exercise to a point just short of fatigue. Very strenuous physical exercise is not advisable, because it raises the body temperature and may aggravate symptoms. The patient is advised to take frequent short rest periods. Exposure to heat increases fatigue and muscle weakness, so air conditioning is recommended in at least one room.

Nutrition. Similar to the population at large, many patients with MS are overweight or have obesity. Contributing factors include the use of corticosteroids for exacerbations of symptoms and mobility impairments as a result of the disease. Interventions to promote healthy eating and weight reduction need to take into account that fatigue and mobility impairments are barriers to engagement in nutritional behaviors for people with MS. Nurses also need to be certain to include family members in interventions and nutrition education, because they are often the gatekeepers for food preparation and selection. Additional strategies include avoidance of alcohol and cigarette smoking.

PREVENTING FALLS

If motor dysfunction causes problems of incoordination and clumsiness, or if ataxia is apparent, then the patient is at risk for falls. To overcome this risk, the patient is instructed to walk with feet apart to widen the base of support and to increase walking stability. If loss of position sense occurs, the patient is instructed to watch their feet while walking. Gait training may require assistive devices (walker, cane, braces, crutches, parallel bars) and instruction about their use by a physical therapist. If the gait remains inefficient, a wheelchair or motorized scooter may be the solution. The occupational therapist is a valuable resource person in suggesting and securing aids to promote independence. If incoordination is a problem and tremor of the upper extremities occurs when voluntary movement is attempted (intention tremor), weighted wrist weights or neuromodulation devices may be used. The patient is trained in transfer and ADLs.

Because sensory loss may occur in addition to motor loss, pressure injuries are a continuing threat to skin integrity. The need to use a wheelchair continuously increases the risk. See Chapter 56 for a discussion of the prevention and treatment of pressure injury.

MANAGING FATIGUE

Fatigue is a common symptom reported in 60% to 90% of those with MS, but the etiology remains unclear. It is often the most disabling symptom and the most common reason patients cease employment (Hickey & Strayer, 2020; Newland et al., 2019). Many factors contribute to fatigue and the nurse helps the patient identify risks and ameliorate those that lead to fatigue. Research that identified the relationships among MS-related symptoms, sleep hygiene behaviors, and sleep quality in adults with MS who report fatigue suggests that decreasing the use of electronic devices prior to sleep can improve sleep quality and lessen fatigue (Newland et al., 2019). See the Nursing Research Profile in Chart 64-2.

STRENGTHENING COPING MECHANISMS

The diagnosis of MS is distressing to the patient and family. They need to know that no two patients with MS have identical symptoms or courses of illness. Although some patients do experience significant disability, others have a near-normal lifespan with minimal disability. Some families, however, face acute frustrations and problems. MS affects people who are often in an early stage of life and concerned about career and family responsibilities. Family conflict, disintegration, separation, and divorce are not uncommon. Often, young family members assume the responsibility of caring for a parent with MS. Nursing interventions in this area include assisting patients and families to manage or reduce stress and making appropriate referrals for counseling and support to minimize the adverse effects of dealing with chronic illness.

Chart 64-2	**NURSING RESEARCH PROFILE**
	The Relationship Between MS and Sleep

Newland, P., Lorenz, R. A., Smith, J. M., et al. (2019). The relationship among multiple sclerosis-related symptoms, sleep quality, and sleep hygiene behaviors. *Journal of Neuroscience Nursing*, 51(1), 37–42.

Purpose

Fatigue is common among those with MS and has a negative impact on many aspects of their lives. The purpose of this study was to examine the relationships among MS-related symptoms, sleep hygiene behaviors, and sleep quality in adults with MS who report fatigue.

Design

This was a descriptive correlational study with a convenience sample of 39 community dwelling adults with MS. Data were collected about demographic characteristics. Measures used to collect data included the revised MS-Related Symptom Scale, the patient self-report version of the Expanded Disability Status Scale, a single item sleep quality scale, the Pittsburgh

Sleep Quality Index (PSQI), and a sleep behavior self-rating scale.

Findings

The mean age of participants was 45 years; 80% reported having RRMS and 20% reported PPMS. High levels of forgetfulness, anxiety, and difficulty concentrating were significantly correlated with poor sleep quality. Fatigue was higher in those who used electronic devices around bedtime and practiced poor sleep hygiene behaviors. Pain, a frequent symptom in those with MS, was not significantly related to sleep quality.

Nursing Implications

Nurses working with patients with MS should incorporate interventions for symptoms, particularly forgetfulness, anxiety, and difficulty concentrating, as they significantly impact sleep. Education should include the recommendation to remove electronic devices from the bedroom, and to restrict the use of technology in the hours prior to sleep.

The nurse, mindful of these complex problems, initiates home care and coordinates a network of services, including social services, speech therapy, physical therapy, and homemaker services. To strengthen the patient's coping skills, as much information as possible is provided. Patients need a list of available assistive devices, services, and resources.

Coping through problem solving involves helping the patient define the problem and develop alternatives for its management. Planning carefully, maintaining flexibility, and preserving a hopeful attitude are useful for psychological and physical adaptation.

MONITORING AND MANAGING POTENTIAL COMPLICATIONS

Complications that can occur with MS are caused by damage to the myelin in the CNS. The nurse monitors for the presence of cognitive changes, how the patient is able to manage at home, or changes in sexuality. Cognitive changes or inability to manage prescribed therapies at home may be due to psychological effects of MS. The patient is monitored for the risk of suicide as 50% of patients with MS experience major depression and the suicide rate is twice that of the general population (Kalb et al., 2019).

PROMOTING HOME, COMMUNITY-BASED, AND TRANSITIONAL CARE

Educating Patients About Self-Care. As the disease progresses, the patient and family need to learn new strategies to maintain optimal independence. Educating about self-care techniques may be initiated in the hospital or clinic setting and reinforced in the home. Self-care education may address the use of assistive devices, self-catheterization, and administration of medications that affect the course of the disease or treat complications. An education plan that addresses intramuscular or subcutaneous administration of medications (including side effects) is developed for the patient and their family or caregiver. The patient and family are educated about exercises that enable the patient to continue some form of activity or that maintain or improve function (see Chart 64-3).

Continuing and Transitional Care. After discharge, the nurse often provides education and reinforcement of new interventions in the patient's home. Nurses in the home setting assess for changes in the patient's physical and emotional status; provide physical care to the patient if required; coordinate outpatient services and resources; and encourage health promotion, appropriate health screenings, and adaptation. Modifications that allow independence in the home should be implemented (e.g., assistive eating devices, raised toilet seat, bathing aids, telephone modifications, long-handled comb, tongs, modified clothing).

If changes in the disease or its course are noted, the nurse encourages the patient to contact the primary provider, because treatment of an acute exacerbation or new problem may be indicated. Continuing health care and follow-up are recommended.

The patient with MS is encouraged to contact the local chapter of the National MS Society for services, publications, and contact with others who have MS (see the Resources section). Local chapters also provide direct services to patients. Through group interaction, the patient has an opportunity to meet others with similar problems, share experiences, and learn self-help methods.

Evaluation

Expected patient outcomes may include:
1. Improves physical mobility
    a. Participates in gait training and rehabilitation program
    b. Establishes a balanced program of rest and exercise
    c. Uses assistive devices correctly and safely
2. Is free of falls
    a. Monitors self and environment for falls risk factors
    b. Asks for assistance when necessary
3. Reports decreased level of fatigue
    a. Identifies strategies to decrease fatigue
    b. Maintains appropriate sleep hygiene behaviors

Chart
64-3

HOME CARE CHECKLIST

The Patient with MS

At the completion of education, the patient and/or caregiver will be able to:

- State the impact of MS and treatment on physiologic function- ing, ADLs, IADLs, roles, relationships, and spirituality.
- State the purpose, dose, route, schedule, side effects, and pre- cautions for prescribed medications.
  - Demonstrate correct techniques of administering injectable medications, if prescribed.
- State how to contact all members of the treatment team (e.g., health care providers, home care professionals, and durable medical equipment and supply vendor).
- State changes in lifestyle (e.g., exercise, activity) necessary to maintain health.
  - Demonstrate environmental modifications and adaptive techniques for accomplishing activities of daily living.
  - Identify strategies to manage symptoms (pain, cognitive responses, dysphagia, tremors, visual disturbances).
  - State how to prevent complications (e.g., pressure injury, pneumonia, depression).
  - Identify coping strategies.
  - Identify ways to minimize fatigue.
  - Explain how to prevent injury.

- Identify optimal nutritional intake; consider weight reduction as indicated if patient is overweight or has obesity.
- State ways to promote sexual function.
- Discuss ways to manage bowel and bladder function.
- Name benefits of exercise and physical activity.
- Identify ways to minimize immobility and spasticity.
- Relate how to reach primary provider with questions or complications.
- State time and date of follow-up medical appointments, therapy, and testing.
- Identify sources of support (e.g., friends, relatives, faith community).
- Identify the contact details for support services for patients and their caregivers/families (e.g., National MS Society, MS support services).
- Identify the need for health promotion, disease prevention, and screening activities.

Resources

See Chapter 7, Chart 7-9: Home Care Checklist: Managing Chronic Illness for additional information.

ADLs, activities of daily living; IADLs, instrumental activities of daily living; MS, multiple sclerosis.

4. Demonstrates effective coping strategies
   a. Maintains sense of control
   b. Modifies lifestyle to fit goals and limitations
   c. Verbalizes desire to pursue goals and developmental tasks of adulthood
   d. Demonstrates healthy social interactions
   e. Participates in meaningful activities
5. Understands ways to avoid complications and is free of complications
6. Explains reasons for measures to prevent complications

Myasthenia Gravis

Myasthenia gravis, an autoimmune disorder affecting the myo- neural junction, is characterized by varying degrees of weakness of the voluntary muscles. It is uncommon, with an incidence

between 9 and 30 in 1 million people in the United States (Hickey & Strayer, 2020). It occurs more often in women dur- ing the second and third decades of life; however, after age 50, it is more common in men (Hickey & Strayer, 2020).

Pathophysiology

Normally, a chemical impulse precipitates the release of ace- tylcholine from vesicles on the nerve terminal at the myo- neural junction. The acetylcholine attaches to receptor sites on the motor endplate and stimulates muscle contraction. Continuous binding of acetylcholine to the receptor site is required for muscular contraction to be sustained.

In myasthenia gravis, antibodies directed at the acetyl- choline receptor sites impair transmission of impulses across the myoneural junction. Therefore, fewer receptors are avail- able for stimulation, resulting in voluntary muscle weakness that escalates with continued activity (see Fig. 64-4). These

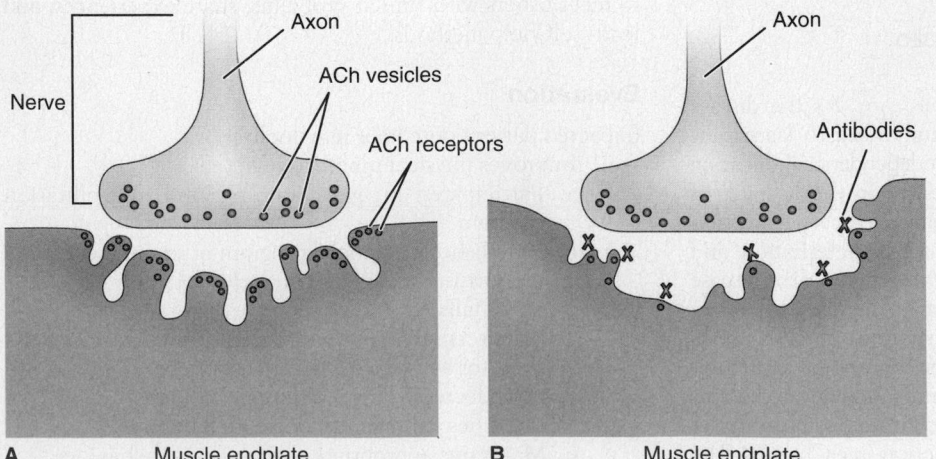

Figure 64-4 • Myasthenia gravis. A. Usual acetylcholine (ACh) receptor site. **B.** ACh receptor site in myasthenia gravis.

antibodies are found in 85% of people with myasthenia gravis (Hickey & Strayer, 2020). Of people with myasthenia gravis, most have either thymic hyperplasia or a thymic tumor, and the thymus gland is believed to be the site of antibody production. In patients who are acetylcholine receptor antibody negative, other antibodies appear to target a protein in the myoneural junction (Hickey & Strayer, 2020).

Clinical Manifestations

The clinical manifestation of myasthenia gravis is highly variable. There are two clinical types: ocular and generalized. In the ocular form, only the eye muscles are involved. Diplopia and **ptosis** (drooping of the eyelids) are common (Hickey & Strayer, 2020). In the generalized form, patients experience weakness of the muscles of the face and throat (bulbar symptoms), limbs, and respiratory weakness. Weakness of the facial muscles results in a bland facial expression. Laryngeal involvement produces **dysphonia** (voice impairment) and **dysphagia** (difficulty swallowing), which increases the risk of choking and aspiration. Generalized weakness affects all extremities and may involve the intercostal muscles, resulting in decreasing vital capacity and respiratory failure. When this occurs, the patient is in a myasthenic crisis (National Institute of Neurological Disorders and Stroke [NINDS], 2020). Myasthenia gravis is purely a motor disorder with no effect on sensation or coordination.

Assessment and Diagnostic Findings

A common test used to diagnose myasthenia gravis is the acetylcholinesterase inhibitor test. It is performed by administering edrophonium chloride IV; 30 seconds after injection, facial muscle weakness and ptosis should resolve for about 5 minutes (Hickey & Strayer, 2020). Immediate improvement in muscle strength after administration of this agent represents a positive test and usually confirms the diagnosis. Atropine should be available to control potential side effects of this medication, which include bradycardia, asystole, bronchoconstriction, sweating, and cramping.

Another study, the ice test, is indicated in patients who have cardiac conditions or asthma. With this test, an ice pack is held over the patient's eyes for 1 minute; the ptosis should temporarily resolve in a patient with myasthenia gravis (Hickey & Strayer, 2020).

Several blood tests for acetylcholine antibodies are also used to confirm the diagnosis (Hickey & Strayer, 2020). Repetitive nerve stimulation (RNS) demonstrates a decrease in successive action potentials. A single-fiber electromyography (EMG) detects a delay or failure of neuromuscular transmission and is about 99% sensitive in confirming the diagnosis of myasthenia gravis (Hickey & Strayer, 2020). This is an uncomfortable test for the patient.

The thymus gland, a site of acetylcholine receptor antibody production, may be enlarged in myasthenia gravis and may be identified by MRI scan.

Medical Management

Management of myasthenia gravis is directed at improving function and reducing and removing circulating antibodies. Therapeutic modalities include administration of anticholinesterase medications and immunosuppressive therapy, intravenous immune globulin (IVIG), therapeutic plasma exchange, and thymectomy. There is no cure for myasthenia gravis; treatments do not stop the production of the acetylcholine receptor antibodies.

Pharmacologic Therapy

Pyridostigmine bromide, an anticholinesterase medication, is the first line of therapy (Hickey & Strayer, 2020). It provides symptomatic relief by inhibiting the breakdown of acetylcholine and increasing the relative concentration of available acetylcholine at the neuromuscular junction. The dosage is gradually increased to a daily maximum and is given in divided doses (usually four times a day). Adverse effects of anticholinesterase medications include diarrhea, abdominal cramps, and/or excessive saliva (Comerford & Durkin, 2020). Pyridostigmine tends to have fewer side effects than other anticholinesterase medications.

If pyridostigmine bromide does not improve muscle strength and control fatigue, the next agents used are the immunomodulating drugs. The goal of immunosuppressive therapy is to reduce production of the antibody. Corticosteroids suppress the patient's immune response, decreasing the amount of antibody production, and this correlates with clinical improvement. An initial dose of prednisone is given daily and maintained for 1 to 2 months; as symptoms improve, the medication is tapered (Hickey & Strayer, 2020). As the corticosteroid medications take effect, the dosage of anticholinesterase medication can usually be lowered. Cytotoxic medications are used to treat myasthenia gravis if there is inadequate response to steroids. Azathioprine inhibits T lymphocytes and B-cell proliferation and reduces acetylcholine receptor antibody levels. Therapeutic effects may not be evident for 3 to 12 months. Leukopenia and hepatotoxicity are serious adverse effects, so monthly evaluation of liver enzymes and white blood cell count is necessary.

IVIG can be used to treat exacerbations; however, in select patients, it is used on a long-term adjunctive basis. IVIG treatment involves the administration of pooled human gamma-globulin and improvement occurs in a few days to a week (Hickey & Strayer, 2020). The effects of IVIG typically last only about 28 days after infusion, and complications include headache, migraine exacerbation, aseptic meningitis, and flulike symptoms (Vitiello, Emmi, Silvestri, et al., 2019).

A number of medications are contraindicated for patients with myasthenia gravis because they exacerbate the symptoms. The primary provider and the patient should weigh risks and benefits before any new medications are prescribed. Procaine should be avoided, and the patient's dentist is informed of the diagnosis of myasthenia gravis.

Therapeutic Plasma Exchange

A technique called therapeutic plasma exchange, formerly referred to as plasmapheresis, is used to treat exacerbations. The patient's plasma and plasma components are removed through a centrally placed large-bore double-lumen catheter. The blood cells and antibody-containing plasma are separated, after which the cells and a plasma substitute are reinfused. Temporary reduction in the level of circulating antibodies is provided with therapeutic plasma exchange. A typical course consists of daily or alternate-day treatment, and the number of treatments is determined by the patient's response (Hickey & Strayer, 2020)

 ### Surgical Management

Thymectomy (surgical removal of the thymus gland) can produce antigen-specific immunosuppression and result in clinical improvement. Optimal outcomes of the surgery are in patients younger than 60 years who have had myasthenia gravis diagnosed within the past 3 years. It is the only treatment that can result in complete remission, which occurs in approximately 35% of patients (Hickey & Strayer, 2020). A course of preoperative IVIG or therapeutic plasma exchange decreases the time needed for postoperative mechanical ventilation. The entire thymus gland must be removed for optimal clinical outcomes.

A thymectomy should be performed at a designated center with a surgical and anesthesia staff experienced in the perioperative management of those with myasthenia gravis (Hickey & Strayer, 2020). After surgery, the patient is monitored in an intensive care unit, with special attention to respiratory function. The patient is weaned from mechanical ventilation after thorough respiratory assessment. After the thymus gland is removed, it may take up to 3 years for the patient to benefit from the procedure because of the long life of circulating T cells. Thymectomy is considered an elective surgery and best performed when the clinical course of the disease is stable for optimal outcomes (Hickey & Strayer, 2020).

 ## Complications

A myasthenic crisis is an exacerbation of the disease process characterized by severe generalized muscle weakness and respiratory and bulbar weakness that may result in respiratory failure. Crisis may result from disease exacerbation or a specific precipitating event. The most common precipitator is respiratory infection; others include medication change, surgery, pregnancy, and medications that exacerbate myasthenia. A cholinergic crisis caused by overmedication with cholinesterase inhibitors is rare (Hickey & Strayer, 2020).

Neuromuscular respiratory failure is the critical complication in myasthenic and cholinergic crises. Respiratory muscle and bulbar weakness combine to cause respiratory compromise. Weak respiratory muscles do not support inhalation. An inadequate cough and an impaired gag reflex, caused by bulbar weakness, result in poor airway clearance. A downward trend of two respiratory function tests, the negative inspiratory force and vital capacity, is the first clinical sign of respiratory compromise.

Endotracheal intubation and mechanical ventilation may be needed (see Chapter 19). Noninvasive positive-pressure ventilation uses an external device in the form of a vest that provides respiratory support without endotracheal intubation. Cholinesterase inhibitors are stopped when respiratory failure occurs and gradually restarted after the patient demonstrates improvement with a course of therapeutic plasma exchange or IVIG. Nutritional support may be needed if the patient is intubated for a long period or swallowing ability is affected (see Chapter 39).

Nursing Management

Because myasthenia gravis is a chronic disease and most patients are seen on an outpatient basis, much of the nursing care focuses on patient and family education. Educational topics for outpatient self-care include medication management, energy conservation, strategies to help with ocular manifestations, and prevention and management of complications.

Medication management is a crucial component of ongoing care. Understanding the actions of the medications and taking them on schedule is emphasized, as are the consequences of delaying medication and the signs and symptoms of myasthenic and cholinergic crises. The patient can determine the best times for daily dosing by keeping a diary to determine fluctuation of symptoms and to learn when the medication is wearing off. The medication schedule can then be manipulated to maximize strength throughout the day.

 > ### Quality and Safety Nursing Alert
>
> *Maintenance of stable blood levels of anticholinesterase medications is imperative to stabilize muscle strength. Therefore, the anticholinesterase medications must be given on time. Any delay in administration of medications may exacerbate muscle weakness and make it impossible for the patient to take medications orally.*

Regular administration of IVIG or subcutaneous immunoglobulin may be prescribed. The patient and family are educated about managing immunoglobulin therapy.

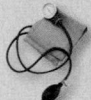 For the procedural guidelines for management of IVIG, go to **thepoint.lww.com/Brunner15e**.

The patient is also educated about strategies to conserve energy. To do this, the nurse helps the patient identify the optimal times for rest throughout the day. If the patient lives in a two-story home, the nurse can suggest that frequently used items (e.g., hygiene products, cleaning products, snacks) be kept on each floor to minimize travel between floors. The patient is encouraged to apply for a handicapped license plate to minimize walking from parking spaces and to schedule activities to coincide with peak energy and strength levels. Using consistent routines, scheduling periods of rest, monitoring for depression, maintaining good sleep patterns, and incorporating interventions to conserve energy are all strategies to reduce fatigue (Hickey & Strayer, 2020).

To minimize the risk of aspiration, mealtimes should coincide with the peak effects of anticholinesterase medication. In addition, rest before meals is encouraged to reduce muscle fatigue. The patient is advised to sit upright during meals, with the neck slightly flexed to facilitate swallowing. Soft foods in gravy or sauces can be swallowed more easily. Eating larger meals in the morning and smaller meals in the evening is another good strategy. Supplemental feedings may be helpful to ensure adequate nutrition.

If choking occurs frequently, the patient should be evaluated by a speech-language pathologist for formal dietary and mechanical techniques to avoid aspiration. Suction should be available at home, with the patient and family instructed in its use.

Impaired vision results from ptosis of one or both eyelids, decreased eye movement, or double vision. To prevent corneal damage when the eyelids do not close completely, the patient is instructed to tape the eyes closed for short intervals and to regularly instill artificial tears. Patients who wear eyeglasses can have "crutches" attached to help lift the eyelids. Patching of one eye or wearing prism glasses can help with double vision.

The patient is reminded of the importance of maintaining health promotion practices and following health care screening recommendations. Factors that exacerbate symptoms and potentially cause crisis should be noted and avoided: emotional stress, infections (particularly respiratory infections), vigorous physical activity, some medications, and high environmental temperature. The Myasthenia Gravis Foundation of America provides support services and educational materials for patients, families, and health care providers (see the Resources section).

 Myasthenic Crisis

Respiratory distress and varying degrees of dysphagia, dysarthria, eyelid ptosis, diplopia, and prominent muscle weakness are symptoms of myasthenic crisis. The patient is placed in an intensive care unit for constant monitoring because of associated intense and sudden fluctuations in clinical condition.

Providing ventilatory assistance takes precedence in the immediate management of the patient with myasthenic crisis. Ongoing assessment for respiratory failure is essential. The nurse assesses the respiratory rate, depth, and breath sounds and monitors pulmonary function parameters (vital capacity and negative inspiratory force) to detect pulmonary problems before respiratory dysfunction progresses. Blood is drawn for arterial blood gas analysis. Endotracheal intubation and mechanical ventilation may be needed (see Chapter 19).

If the abdominal, intercostal, and pharyngeal muscles are severely weak, the patient cannot cough, take deep breaths, or clear secretions. Chest physiotherapy, including postural drainage to mobilize secretions and suctioning to remove secretions, may have to be performed frequently. (Postural drainage should not be performed for 30 minutes after feeding.)

Assessment strategies and supportive measures include the following:

- Arterial blood gases, serum electrolytes, input and output, and daily weight are monitored.
- If the patient cannot swallow, enteral tube feedings may be prescribed (see Chapter 39).
- Sedative and tranquilizing agents are avoided, because they aggravate hypoxia and hypercapnia and can cause respiratory and cardiac depression.

Guillain–Barré Syndrome

Guillain–Barré Syndrome (GBS), also known as acute idiopathic polyneuritis, is an autoimmune attack on the peripheral nerve myelin. The result is acute, rapid segmental demyelination of peripheral nerves and some cranial nerves, producing ascending weakness with dyskinesia (inability to execute voluntary movements), hyporeflexia, and **paresthesias** (a sensation of numbness, tingling, or a "pins and needles" sensation). An antecedent event (most often a viral infection) precipitates clinical presentation in approximately 60% to 70% of cases (CDC, 2019). *Campylobacter jejuni* (implicated in 40% of cases in the United States), cytomegalovirus, Epstein–Barr

virus, *Mycoplasma pneumoniae*, *H. influenzae*, and Zika virus are the most common infectious agents that are associated with the development of GBS.

There are several subtypes of GBS (Malek & Salameh, 2019). With the most well-known type, the patient experiences weakness in the lower extremities, which progresses upward and has the potential for respiratory failure. The second type is purely motor with no altered sensation. A third type, called descending GBS, is much more difficult to diagnose; it mostly affects the head and neck muscles. The rarest type is the Miller–Fisher variant (see discussion later in this chapter) (NINDS, 2018b).

The annual incidence of GBS is 1 to 2 cases per 100,000 people, and it affects males and females equally. Death occurs in 5% to 10% of cases, resulting from respiratory failure, autonomic dysfunction, sepsis, or pulmonary embolism (PE) (Hickey & Strayer, 2020). Seventy percent of patients with GBS experience full recovery. The remaining 30% can have disability ranging from minor to major (NINDS, 2018b).

Pathophysiology

GBS is the result of a cell-mediated and humoral immune attack on peripheral nerve myelin proteins that causes inflammatory demyelination. The best-accepted theory of cause is molecular mimicry, in which an infectious organism contains an amino acid that mimics the peripheral nerve myelin protein. The immune system cannot distinguish between the two proteins and attacks and destroys peripheral nerve myelin. The exact location of the immune attack within the peripheral nervous system is the ganglioside GM1b. With the autoimmune attack, there is an influx of macrophages and other immune-mediated agents that attack myelin and cause inflammation and destruction, interruption of nerve conduction, and axonal loss (NINDS, 2018b).

Myelin is a complex substance that covers nerves, providing insulation and speeding the conduction of impulses from the cell body to the dendrites. The cell that produces myelin in the peripheral nervous system is the Schwann cell. In GBS, the Schwann cell can be spared, allowing for remyelination in the recovery phase of the disease. If damage has occurred to the axons, then regrowth is required and takes months or years and is often incomplete (NINDS, 2018b).

Clinical Manifestations

GBS typically begins with muscle weakness and diminished reflexes of the lower extremities. Hyporeflexia and weakness may progress to tetraplegia. Demyelination of the nerves that innervate the diaphragm and intercostal muscles results in neuromuscular respiratory failure. Sensory symptoms include paresthesias of the hands and feet and pain related to the demyelination of sensory fibers.

The antecedent event usually occurs 1 to 3 weeks before symptoms begin. Weakness usually begins in the legs and may progress upward. Maximum weakness (the plateau) varies in length but usually includes neuromuscular respiratory failure and bulbar weakness. GBS progresses to peak severity typically within 2 weeks and no longer than 4 weeks. If progression is longer, then the patient is classified as having chronic inflammatory demyelinating polyneuropathy (Hickey & Strayer, 2020). Any residual symptoms are permanent and reflect axonal damage from demyelination.

Cranial nerve demyelination can result in a variety of clinical manifestations. Optic nerve demyelination may result in blindness. Bulbar muscle weakness related to demyelination of the glossopharyngeal and vagus nerves results in the inability to swallow or clear secretions. Vagus nerve demyelination results in autonomic dysfunction, manifested by instability of the cardiovascular system. The presentation is variable and may include tachycardia, bradycardia, hypertension, or orthostatic hypotension. The symptoms of autonomic dysfunction occur and resolve rapidly. GBS does not affect cognitive function or LOC.

Although the classic clinical features include areflexia and ascending weakness, variations in the clinical presentation occurs. There may be a sensory presentation, with progressive sensory symptoms; an atypical axonal destruction; or the Miller–Fisher variant, which includes paralysis of the ocular muscles, ataxia, and areflexia (Malek & Salameh, 2019; NINDS, 2018b).

Assessment and Diagnostic Findings

The patient presents with symmetric weakness, diminished reflexes, and upward progression of motor weakness. A history of a viral illness in the previous few weeks suggests the diagnosis. Changes in vital capacity and negative inspiratory force are assessed to identify impending neuromuscular respiratory failure. Serum laboratory tests are not useful in the diagnosis. However, elevated protein levels are detected in CSF evaluation, without an increase in other cells. Electrophysiology studies demonstrate a progressive loss of nerve conduction velocity (Malek & Salameh, 2019).

Medical Management

Because of the possibility of rapid progression and neuromuscular respiratory failure, GBS is a medical emergency that may require management in an intensive care unit. After baseline values are identified, assessment of changes in muscle strength and respiratory function alert the clinician to the physical and respiratory needs of the patient. Respiratory therapy or mechanical ventilation may be necessary to support pulmonary function and adequate oxygenation. Some clinicians recommend elective intubation before the onset of extreme respiratory muscle fatigue. Emergent intubation may result in autonomic dysfunction, and mechanical ventilation may be required for an extended period. The patient is weaned from mechanical ventilation after the respiratory muscles can again support spontaneous respiration and maintain adequate tissue oxygenation.

Other interventions are aimed at preventing the complications of immobility. These may include the use of anticoagulant agents and sequential compression boots to prevent venous thromboembolism (VTE), including deep vein thrombosis (DVT) and PE.

Therapeutic plasma exchange and IVIG are used to directly affect the peripheral nerve myelin antibody level. Both therapies decrease circulating antibody levels and reduce the amount of time the patient is immobilized and dependent on mechanical ventilation. The cardiovascular risks posed by autonomic dysfunction require continuous electrocardiographic (ECG) monitoring. Tachycardia and hypertension are treated with short-acting medications such as alpha-adrenergic blocking agents. The use of short-acting

agents is important, because autonomic dysfunction is very labile. Hypotension is managed by increasing the amount of IV fluid administered.

NURSING PROCESS
The Patient with GBS

Assessment

Ongoing assessment for disease progression is critical. The patient is monitored for life-threatening complications (respiratory failure, cardiac arrhythmias, VTE [including DVT or PE]) so that appropriate interventions can be initiated. Because of the threat to the patient in this sudden, potentially life-threatening disease, the nurse must assess the patient's and family's ability to cope and their use of coping strategies.

Diagnosis

NURSING DIAGNOSES

Based on the assessment data, major nursing diagnoses may include the following:

- Impaired breathing associated with rapidly progressive weakness and impending respiratory failure
- Impaired mobility associated with paralysis
- Impaired nutritional intake associated with inability to swallow
- Impaired verbal communication associated with cranial nerve dysfunction
- Anxiety associated with loss of control and paralysis
- Fatigue associated with physical deconditioning and stressors

COLLABORATIVE PROBLEMS/POTENTIAL COMPLICATIONS

Potential complications may include the following:

- Respiratory failure
- Autonomic dysfunction

Planning and Goals

The major goals for the patient may include improved respiratory function, increased mobility, improved nutritional status, effective communication, decreased anxiety, decreased fatigue, and absence of complications.

Nursing Interventions

MAINTAINING RESPIRATORY FUNCTION

Respiratory function can be maximized with incentive spirometry and chest physiotherapy. Monitoring for changes in vital capacity and negative inspiratory force is key to early intervention for neuromuscular respiratory failure. Mechanical ventilation is required if the vital capacity falls, making spontaneous breathing impossible and tissue oxygenation inadequate.

The potential need for mechanical ventilation should be discussed with the patient and family on admission to provide time for psychological preparation and decision making. Intubation and mechanical ventilation result in less anxiety if they are initiated on a nonemergency basis to a patient who has been well informed. The patient may require mechanical ventilation for a long period. See Chapter 19 for the nursing management of the patient requiring mechanical ventilation.

Bulbar weakness that impairs the ability to swallow and clear secretions is another factor in the development of respiratory failure in the patient with GBS. Suctioning may be needed to maintain a clear airway.

The nurse assesses the blood pressure and heart rate frequently to identify autonomic dysfunction so that interventions can be initiated quickly if needed. Medications are given or a temporary pacemaker placed for clinically significant bradycardia.

ENHANCING PHYSICAL MOBILITY

Nursing interventions to enhance physical mobility and prevent the complications of immobility are key to the function and survival of patients. The paralyzed extremities are supported in functional positions, and passive range-of-motion exercises are performed at least twice daily. DVT and PE are threats to the patient who is paralyzed. Nursing interventions are aimed at preventing VTE. Range-of-motion exercises, position changes, anticoagulation, the use of anti-embolism stockings and sequential compression boots, and adequate hydration decrease the risk of VTE.

Padding may be placed over bony prominences, such as the elbows and heels, to reduce the risk of pressure injury. The need for frequent position changes cannot be overemphasized. The nurse evaluates laboratory test results that may indicate malnutrition or dehydration, both of which increase the risk of pressure injury and decrease mobility. The nurse collaborates with the primary provider and dietitian to develop a plan to meet the patient's nutritional and hydration needs.

PROVIDING ADEQUATE NUTRITION

Paralytic ileus may result from insufficient parasympathetic activity. In this event, the nurse administers IV fluids and parenteral nutrition as a supplement and monitors for the return of bowel sounds. If the patient cannot swallow because of bulbar paralysis (immobility of muscles), a gastrostomy tube may be placed to administer nutrients. The nurse carefully assesses the return of the gag reflex and bowel sounds before resuming oral nutrition.

IMPROVING COMMUNICATION

Because of paralysis, the patient cannot talk, laugh, or cry and therefore has no method for communicating needs or expressing emotion. Although the patient may be unable to speak, cognition is completely intact. Establishing some form of communication with picture cards or an eye blink system provides a means of communication. Collaboration with the speech therapist may be helpful in developing a communication mechanism that is most effective for a specific patient.

DECREASING ANXIETY

The patient and family are faced with a sudden, potentially life-threatening disease; therefore, their levels of anxiety may be high. The impact of disease on the family depends on the patient's role within the family. Referral to a support group may provide information and support to the patient and family.

The family may feel helpless in caring for the patient. Mechanical ventilation and monitoring devices may frighten and intimidate them. Family members often want to participate in physical care; with education and support by the nurse, they should be allowed and encouraged to do so.

In addition the patient may experience isolation, loneliness, lack of control, and fear. Nursing interventions that increase the patient's sense of control include providing information about the condition, emphasizing a positive appraisal of coping resources, and providing education about relaxation exercises and distraction techniques. The positive attitude and atmosphere of the multidisciplinary team are important to promote a sense of well-being.

Diversional activities are encouraged to decrease loneliness and isolation. Encouraging visitors (when possible), engaging visitors or volunteers to read to the patient, listening to musical recordings or audiobooks, assisting with audio visual communication with friends and family through a phone or electronic device, and watching television or movies are ways to alleviate the patient's sense of isolation.

REDUCING FATIGUE

The disease process increases disability and dependence on others for simple activities of living. As the patient begins to recover and regains the ability to perform activities on their own, they will find increased rest is needed to maintain this independence. The patient may need only a little help at the beginning of the day, but as the day progresses may require more assistance. Too much exertion will result in fatigue. The patient will need assistance learning how to pace their daily activities to incorporate periods of rest, both physically and mentally. The nurse can help identify activities that are physically demanding, assess the amount of sleep the patient is getting and needs, assist the patient and family to ensure time for self-care, and provide education about healthy eating to maintain strength.

MONITORING AND MANAGING POTENTIAL COMPLICATIONS

Thorough assessment of respiratory function at regular and frequent intervals is essential, because respiratory insufficiency and subsequent failure due to weakness or paralysis of the intercostal muscles and diaphragm may develop quickly. Respiratory failure is the major cause of mortality, although rare. In addition to the respiratory rate and the quality of respirations, vital capacity is monitored frequently and at regular intervals so that respiratory insufficiency can be anticipated. Decreasing vital capacity with associated muscle weakness indicates impending respiratory failure. Signs and symptoms include breathlessness while speaking, shallow and irregular breathing, the use of accessory muscles, tachycardia, weak cough, and changes in respiratory pattern.

Other complications include cardiac arrhythmias (which necessitate ECG monitoring), transient hypertension, orthostatic hypotension, DVT, PE, urinary retention, and other threats to any patient who is immobilized and paralyzed. These complications require monitoring and attention to prevent them and prompt treatment if indicated.

PROMOTING HOME, COMMUNITY-BASED, AND TRANSITIONAL CARE

Educating Patients About Self-Care. Patients with GBS and their families are usually frightened by the sudden onset of life-threatening symptoms and their severity. Therefore, educating the patient and family about the disorder and its generally favorable prognosis is important (see Chart 64-4).

During the acute phase of the illness, the patient and family are educated about strategies that can be implemented to minimize the effects of immobility and other complications. As function begins to return, family members and other home care providers are educated about care of the patient and their role in the rehabilitation process. Preparation for discharge is an interdisciplinary effort requiring family or caregiver education by all team members, including the nurse, physician, occupational and physical therapists, speech therapist, and respiratory therapist.

Continuing and Transitional Care. Most patients with GBS experience complete recovery. Patients who have experienced total or prolonged paralysis require intensive rehabilitation; the extent depends on the patient's needs. Approaches include a comprehensive inpatient program if deficits are significant, an outpatient program if the patient can travel by car, or a home program of physical and occupational therapy. The recovery phase may be long and requires patience as well as involvement on the part of the patient and family.

During acute care, the focus is on immediate issues and deficits. The nurse needs to remind or educate patients and family members of the need for continuing health promotion and screening practices after this initial phase of care.

Evaluation

Expected patient outcomes may include the following:

1. Maintains effective respirations and airway clearance
   a. Has clear breath sounds on auscultation
   b. Demonstrates gradual improvement in respiratory function
   c. Breathes spontaneously
   d. Has vital capacity within normal range
   e. Exhibits arterial blood gases and pulse oximetry within normal limits
2. Shows increasing mobility
   a. Regains use of extremities
   b. Participates in rehabilitation program
   c. Demonstrates no contractures and minimal muscle atrophy
3. Receives adequate nutrition and hydration
   a. Consumes diet adequate to meet nutritional needs
   b. Swallows without aspiration
4. Demonstrates recovery of speech
   a. Communicates needs through alternative strategies
   b. Practices exercises recommended by the speech therapist
5. Shows less anxiety
6. Experiences fewer episodes of fatigue
   a. Verbalizes a plan to reduce fatigue and increase energy
   b. Takes rest periods during the day
   c. Identifies activities with higher importance during periods of high energy
7. Has absence of complications
   a. Maintains intact skin integrity
   b. Does not develop VTE
   c. Voids without difficulty

CRANIAL NERVE DISORDERS

Because the brainstem and cranial nerves involve vital motor, sensory, and autonomic functions of the body, these nerves may be affected by conditions arising primarily within these structures or in secondary extension from adjacent disease processes. The cranial nerves are examined separately and in sequence (see Chapter 60, Table 60-2). Some cranial nerve deficits can be detected by observing the patient's face, eye movements, speech, and swallowing. EMG is used to investigate motor and sensory dysfunction. An MRI scan is used to obtain images of the cranial nerves and brainstem. An overview of disorders that may affect each of the cranial nerves, including clinical manifestations and nursing interventions, is presented in Table 64-3. The following discussion centers on

TABLE 64-3 Disorders of Cranial Nerves

Disorder	Clinical Manifestations	Nursing Interventions
Olfactory Nerve—I Head trauma Intracranial tumor Intracranial surgery	Unilateral or bilateral anosmia (temporary or persistent) Diminished taste for food	Assess sense of smell Assess for cerebrospinal fluid rhinorrhea if patient has sustained head trauma
Optic Nerve—II Optic neuritis Increased intracranial pressure Pituitary tumor	Lesions of optic tract producing homonymous hemianopsia	Assess visual acuity Restructure environment to prevent injuries Educate patient to accommodate for visual loss
Oculomotor Nerve—III		Assess extraocular movement and for nonreactive pupil
Trochlear Nerve—IV		Assess extraocular movement and for nonreactive pupil
Abducens Nerve—VI Vascular Brainstem ischemia Hemorrhage and infarction Neoplasm Trauma Infection	Dilation of pupil with loss of light reflex on one side Impairment of ocular movement Diplopia Gaze palsies Ptosis of eyelid	Assess extraocular movement and for nonreactive pupil
Trigeminal Nerve—V Trigeminal neuralgia Head trauma Cerebellopontine lesion Sinus tract tumor and metastatic disease Compression of trigeminal root by tumor or blood vessel	Pain in face Diminished or loss of corneal reflex Chewing dysfunction	Assess for pain and triggering mechanisms for pain Assess for difficulty in chewing Discuss trigger zones and pain precipitants with patient Protect cornea from abrasion Ensure good oral hygiene Educate patient about medication regimen
Facial Nerve—VII Bell palsy Facial nerve tumor Intracranial lesion Herpes zoster	Facial dysfunction; weakness and paralysis Hemifacial spasm Diminished or absent taste Pain	Recognize facial paralysis as emergency; refer for treatment as soon as possible Discuss protective care for eyes Select easily chewed foods; patient should eat and drink from unaffected side of mouth Emphasize importance of oral hygiene Provide emotional support for changed appearance of face
Vestibulocochlear Nerve—VIII Tumors and acoustic neuroma Vascular compression of nerve Ménière syndrome	Tinnitus Vertigo Hearing difficulties	Assess pattern of vertigo Provide for safety measures to prevent falls Ensure that patient can maintain balance before ambulating Caution patient to change positions slowly Assist with ambulation Encourage the use of assistive devices
Glossopharyngeal Nerve—IX Glossopharyngeal neuralgia from neurovascular compression of cranial nerves IX and X Trauma Inflammatory conditions Tumor Vertebral artery aneurysms	Pain at base of tongue Difficulty in swallowing Loss of gag reflex Palatal, pharyngeal, and laryngeal paralysis	Assess for paroxysmal pain in throat, decreased or absent swallowing, and gag and cough reflexes Monitor for dysphagia, aspiration, and nasal dysarthric speech. Position patient upright for eating or tube feeding
Vagus Nerve—X Spastic palsy of larynx; bulbar paralysis; high vagal paralysis Guillain–Barré syndrome Vagal body tumors Nerve paralysis from malignancy, surgical trauma such as carotid endarterectomy	Voice changes (temporary or permanent hoarseness) Vocal paralysis Dysphagia	Assess for airway obstruction/provide airway management Prevent aspiration Support patient having voice reconstruction procedures
Spinal Accessory Nerve—XI Spinal cord disorder Amyotrophic lateral sclerosis Trauma Guillain–Barré syndrome	Drooping of affected shoulder with limited shoulder movement Weakness or paralysis of head rotation, flexion, extension; shoulder elevation	Support patient undergoing diagnostic tests

(continued on page 2108)

TABLE 64-3	Disorders of Cranial Nerves (continued)	
Disorder	**Clinical Manifestations**	**Nursing Interventions**

Hypoglossal Nerve—XII
Medullary lesions
Amyotrophic lateral sclerosis
Polio and motor system disease, which
  may destroy hypoglossal nuclei
Multiple sclerosis
Trauma
	Abnormal movements of tongue
	Weakness or paralysis of tongue muscles
	Difficulty in talking, chewing, and
	  swallowing
		Observe swallowing ability
		Observe speech pattern
		Be aware of swallowing or vocal difficulties
		Prepare for alternative feeding methods (tube feeding) to
		  maintain nutrition

Adapted from Hickey, J. V., & Strayer, A. L. (2020). *The clinical practice of neurological & neurosurgical nursing* (8th ed.). Philadelphia, PA: Wolters Kluwer.

the most common disorders of the cranial nerves: trigeminal neuralgia, a condition affecting the fifth cranial nerve, and Bell palsy, caused by involvement of the seventh cranial nerve.

Trigeminal Neuralgia

Trigeminal neuralgia, formerly known as *tic douloureux*, is a condition of the fifth cranial nerve that is characterized by paroxysms of sudden pain in the area innervated by any of the three branches of the nerve (Hickey & Strayer, 2020; see Fig. 64-5). The pain ends as abruptly as it starts and is described as a unilateral shooting and stabbing or burning sensation. The unilateral nature of the pain is an important feature. Associated involuntary contraction of the facial muscles can cause sudden closing of the eye or twitching of the mouth, hence the former name *tic douloureux* (painful twitch). Although the cause is not certain, it is thought to be demyelination of axons in the trigeminal ganglion, root, and nerve by pressing vessels or a demyelinating disease such as MS (Hickey & Strayer, 2020).

Trigeminal neuralgia occurs most often as people age, most commonly between the fifth and sixth decade of life. It is more common in women and in people with MS compared to the general population (Hickey & Strayer, 2020). Patients who develop trigeminal neuralgia before age 50 years should

be evaluated for the coexistence of MS, because trigeminal neuralgia occurs more often in patients with MS (Hickey & Strayer, 2020). Pain-free intervals may be measured in terms of minutes, hours, days, or longer. With advancing years, the painful episodes tend to become more frequent and agonizing. The patient lives in constant fear of attacks.

Paroxysms can occur with any stimulation of the terminals of the affected nerve branches, such as washing the face, shaving, brushing the teeth, eating, and drinking. A draft of cold air or direct pressure against the nerve trunk may also cause pain. Certain areas are called *trigger points* because the slightest touch immediately starts a paroxysm or episode. To avoid stimulating these areas, patients with trigeminal neuralgia try not to touch or wash their faces, shave, chew, or do anything else that might cause an attack. These behaviors are a clue to the diagnosis.

Medical Management

Pharmacologic Therapy

Anticonvulsant agents, such as carbamazepine, relieve pain in most patients with trigeminal neuralgia by reducing the transmission of impulses at certain nerve terminals. Carbamazepine is taken with meals. Serum levels must be monitored to avoid toxicity in patients who require high doses to control the pain. Side effects include nausea, dizziness, drowsiness, and aplastic anemia (Hickey & Strayer, 2020). The patient is monitored for bone marrow depression during long-term therapy. Gabapentin and baclofen are also used for pain control. If pain control is still not achieved, phenytoin may be used as adjunctive therapy.

Surgical Management

If pharmacologic management fails to relieve pain, a number of surgical options are available. Although these procedures may relieve facial pain for a few years, recurrence is possible (Hickey & Strayer, 2020). The choice of procedure depends on the patient's preference and health status. The procedures are designed to either decompress the nerve and save nerve function, or to damage the nerve and destroy nerve function to keep it from malfunctioning (Hickey & Strayer, 2020).

Microvascular Decompression of the Trigeminal Nerve

An intracranial approach is used to relieve the contact between the cerebral vessel and the trigeminal nerve root entry. With the aid of an operating microscope, the artery loop is lifted from the nerve to relieve the pressure, and a small prosthetic device is inserted to prevent recurrence of impingement on

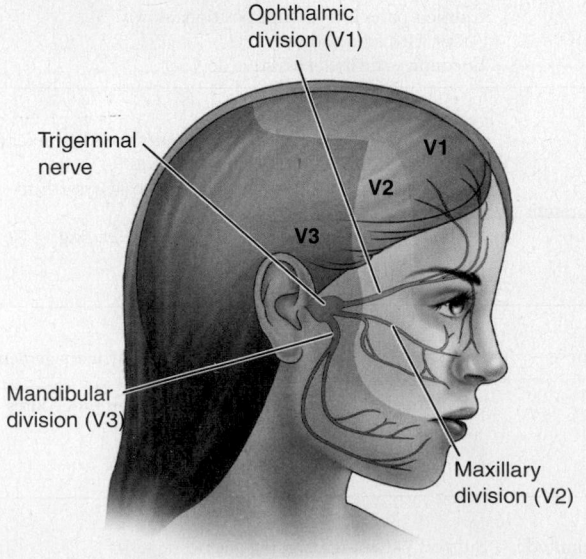

Figure 64-5 • Distribution of trigeminal nerve branches—the fifth cranial nerve.

the nerve. The postoperative management is the same as for other intracranial surgeries (see Chapter 61).

Radiofrequency Thermal Coagulation

Percutaneous radiofrequency produces a thermal lesion on the trigeminal nerve. Although immediate pain relief is experienced, dysesthesia of the face and loss of the corneal reflex may occur. MRI is used for identification of the trigeminal nerve followed by gamma knife radiosurgery. Gamma knife radiosurgery is a noninvasive method of delivering focused radiation to the trigeminal nerve (Obermann, 2019).

Percutaneous Balloon Microcompression

Percutaneous balloon microcompression disrupts large myelinated fibers in all three branches of the trigeminal nerve. After its placement, the balloon is filled with a contrast material for fluoroscopic identification. The balloon compresses the nerve root for 1 minute and provides microvascular decompression (Hickey & Strayer, 2020).

Nursing Management

Preventing Pain

Preoperative management of a patient with trigeminal neuralgia occurs mostly on an outpatient basis and includes recognizing factors that may aggravate excruciating facial pain, such as food that is too hot or too cold or jarring of the patient's bed or chair. Even washing the face, combing the hair, or brushing the teeth may produce acute pain. The nurse can assist the patient in preventing or reducing this pain by providing education about preventive strategies. Providing cotton pads and room temperature water for washing the face, instructing the patient to rinse with mouthwash after eating if toothbrushing causes pain, and performing personal hygiene during pain-free intervals are all effective strategies. The patient is instructed to take food and fluids at room temperature, to chew on the unaffected side, and to ingest soft foods. The nurse recognizes that anxiety, depression, and insomnia often accompany chronic painful conditions and uses appropriate interventions and referrals. See Chapter 9 for management of patients with chronic pain.

Providing Postoperative Care

Postoperative neurologic assessments are conducted to evaluate the patient for facial motor and sensory deficits in each of the three branches of the trigeminal nerve. If the surgery results in sensory deficits to the affected side of the face, the patient is instructed not to rub the eye because the pain of a resulting injury will not be detected. The eye is assessed for irritation or redness. Artificial tears may be prescribed to prevent dryness in the affected eye. The patient is cautioned not to chew on the affected side until numbness has diminished. The patient is observed carefully for any difficulty in eating or swallowing foods of different consistencies.

Bell's Palsy

Bell's palsy (idiopathic facial paralysis) is caused by unilateral inflammation of the seventh cranial nerve, which results in weakness or paralysis of the facial muscles on the affected side (see Fig. 64-6). Although the cause is unknown, theories

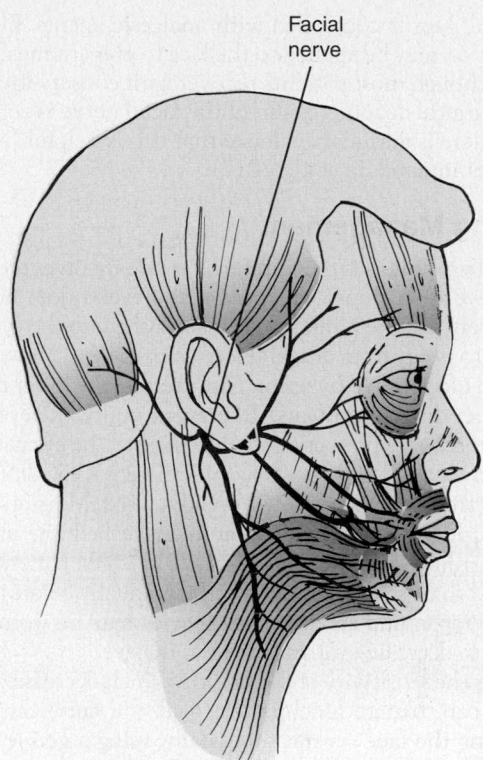

Figure 64-6 • Distribution of the facial nerve—the seventh cranial nerve.

include reactivation of a dormant viral infection (herpes simplex, herpes zoster) or autoimmune syndromes (NINDS, 2018a). Those most commonly affected with Bell's palsy are between the ages of 15 and 45 years (Hickey & Strayer, 2020).

Bell's palsy may be a type of pressure paralysis. The inflamed, edematous nerve becomes compressed to the point of damage, or its blood supply is occluded, producing ischemic necrosis of the nerve. The face is distorted from paralysis of the facial muscles which ranges in severity. Other symptoms may include drooping of the mouth, drooling, excessive lacrimation (tearing), and the patient may experience painful sensations in the face, behind the ear, and in the eye (NINDS, 2018a). The patient may also experience speech difficulties and may be unable to eat on the affected side because of weakness or paralysis of the facial muscles. The majority of patients recover completely and Bell's palsy rarely recurs (Somasundara, Sullivan, & Cheesbrough, 2017).

Medical Management

The objectives of treatment are to maintain the muscle tone of the face and to prevent or minimize denervation. The patient should be reassured that no stroke has occurred and that spontaneous recovery occurs within 3 to 5 weeks in most patients.

Corticosteroid therapy (prednisone) may be prescribed to reduce inflammation and edema; this reduces vascular compression and permits restoration of blood circulation to the nerve. Early administration of corticosteroid therapy, started within 72 hours of symptom onset, is highly effective in diminishing the severity of the disease, relieving the pain, and preventing or minimizing denervation (NINDS, 2018a).

Facial pain is controlled with analgesic agents. Electrical stimulation may be applied to the face to prevent muscle atrophy. Although most patients recover with conservative treatment, surgical decompression of the facial nerve is controversial as there is minimal evidence that this is helpful (NINDS, 2018a; Somasundara et al., 2017).

Nursing Management

While the paralysis is present, nursing care involves protection of the eye from injury. Frequently, the eyelid does not close completely and the blink reflex is diminished, so the eye is vulnerable to injury from dust and foreign particles. Corneal irritation and ulceration may occur. Distortion of the lower lid alters the proper drainage of tears. To prevent injury, the eye should be covered with a protective shield at night. The eye patch may abrade the cornea, however, because there is some difficulty in keeping the partially paralyzed eyelids closed. Moisturizing eye drops during the day and eye ointment at bedtime may help prevent injury (Somasundara et al., 2017). The patient can be educated to close the paralyzed eyelid manually before going to sleep. Wraparound sunglasses or goggles may be worn during the day to decrease evaporation from the eye.

After the sensitivity of the nerve to touch decreases and the patient can tolerate touching the face, the nurse can suggest massaging the face several times daily, using a gentle upward motion, to maintain muscle tone. Facial exercises, such as wrinkling the forehead, blowing out the cheeks, and whistling, may be performed with the aid of a mirror to prevent muscle atrophy. Exposure of the face to cold and drafts is avoided.

DISORDERS OF THE PERIPHERAL NERVOUS SYSTEM

Peripheral Neuropathies

A peripheral **neuropathy** (disorder of the nervous system) is a disorder affecting the peripheral motor and sensory nerves. Peripheral nerves connect the spinal cord and brain to all other organs. They transmit motor impulses from the brain and relay sensory impulses to the brain. Peripheral neuropathies are characterized by bilateral and symmetric disturbance of function, usually beginning in the feet and hands. The most common cause of peripheral neuropathy is diabetes with poor glycemic control (Hickey & Strayer, 2020). Many drugs, such as antineoplastic agents, also cause peripheral neuropathies (Hickey & Strayer, 2020). The major symptoms of peripheral nerve disorders are loss of sensation, muscle atrophy, weakness, diminished reflexes, pain, and paresthesia of the extremities.

Peripheral nerve disorders are diagnosed by history, physical examination, and electrodiagnostic studies such as EEG. The diagnosis of peripheral neuropathy in the older adult population is challenging because many symptoms, such as decreased reflexes, can be associated with the normal aging process (Eliopoulos, 2018).

No specific treatment exists for peripheral neuropathy. Elimination or control of the cause may slow progression. Patients with peripheral neuropathy are at risk for falls, thermal injuries, and skin breakdown. The plan of care includes inspection of the lower extremities for skin breakdown. Assistive devices such as a walker or cane may decrease the risk of falls. Bathwater temperature is checked to avoid thermal injury. Footwear should be accurately sized. Driving may be limited or eliminated, thereby disrupting the patient's sense of independence.

Mononeuropathy

Mononeuropathy is limited to a single peripheral nerve and its branches. It arises when the trunk of the nerve is compressed or entrapped (as in carpal tunnel syndrome), traumatized (as when bruised by a blow), overstretched (as in joint dislocation), punctured by a needle used to inject a drug or damaged by the drugs thus injected, or inflamed because an adjacent infectious process extends to the nerve trunk. Mononeuropathy is frequently seen in patients with diabetes.

Pain is seldom a major symptom of mononeuropathy when the condition is due to trauma, but in patients with complicating inflammatory conditions such as arthritis, pain is prominent. Pain is increased with all body movements that tend to stretch, strain, or cause pressure on the injured nerve and sudden jarring of the body (e.g., from coughing or sneezing). The skin in the areas supplied by nerves that are injured or diseased may become reddened and glossy, the subcutaneous tissue may become edematous, and the nails and hair in this area are altered. Chemical injuries to a nerve trunk, such as those caused by drugs injected into or near it, are often permanent.

The objective of treatment of mononeuropathy is to remove the cause, if possible (e.g., freeing the compressed nerve). Local corticosteroid injections may reduce inflammation and the pressure on the nerve. Aspirin or codeine may be used to relieve pain. Chronic pain can be treated with neuropathic pain medications such as gabapentin (Comerford & Durkin, 2020).

Nursing care involves protection of the affected limb or area from injury, as well as appropriate patient education about mononeuropathy and its treatment. The nurse assesses the impact of pain and weakness on the patient's quality of life and suggests interventions to cope with concerns the patient expresses (Girach, Julian, Varrassi, et al., 2019). Referrals to physical therapy for exercises to prevent muscle wasting and to occupational therapy to evaluate for splints that may help with appropriate positioning may be warranted.

CRITICAL THINKING EXERCISES

1 **ipc** You are participating in morning rounds in the ICU where you work. The team is discussing a patient who has been assigned to you for the day, a 20-year-old woman admitted last night with meningitis. What members of the interprofessional care team are essential to include in the care of this patient? How will you, as this patient's nurse, facilitate an interprofessional discussion to help facilitate her recovery?

2 **pq** You are caring for a 60-year-old man with a recent diagnosis of CJD. His wife of 30 years visits every day. What are the priorities for care of this patient? What will be your priorities when educating this patient and his wife?

3 ebp In the outpatient clinic where you work, a woman with a new diagnosis of MS received treatment and is back to her baseline function. She tells you that she has been "cured." What evidence-based education would you provide the patient about potential triggers that may cause a return of symptoms?

REFERENCES

*Asterisk indicates nursing research.

Books

Comerford, K. C., & Durkin, M. T. (2020). *Nursing 2020 drug handbook.* Philadelphia, PA: Wolters Kluwer.

Eliopoulos, C. (2018). *Gerontological nursing* (9th ed.). Philadelphia, PA: Wolters Kluwer.

Hickey, J. V., & Strayer, A. L. (2020). *The clinical practice of neurological & neurosurgical nursing* (8th ed.). Philadelphia, PA: Wolters Kluwer.

Norris, T. L. (2019). *Porth's pathophysiology: Concepts of altered health status* (10th ed.). Philadelphia, PA: Wolters Kluwer.

Weber, J. R., & Kelley, J. H. (2018). *Health assessment in nursing* (6th ed.). Philadelphia, PA: Wolters Kluwer.

Journals and Electronic Documents

Bradshaw, M., & Houtchens, M. (2018). Neurology board review multiple sclerosis. *Neurology Reviews.* Retrieved on 10/3/2020 at: www.neurologyreviews-digital.com/neurologyreviews/ms_board_review_supp_0618/MobilePagedArticle.action?articleId=1397400#articleId1397400

Brouwer, M., & van de Beek, D. (2017). Epidemiology, diagnosis, and treatment of brain abscesses. *Current Opinion in Infectious Diseases, 30*(1), 129–134.

Centers for Disease Control and Prevention (CDC). (2019). *Guillain-Barré Syndrome.* Retrieved on 9/21/2020 at: www.cdc.gov/campylobacter/guillain-barre.html

Centers for Disease Control and Prevention (CDC). (2020). *Recommended adult immunization schedule—United States, 2020.* Retrieved on 6/27/2020 at: www.cdc.gov/vaccines/schedules/hcp/adult.html

Coyle, P. (2019). Diagnosing and managing multiple sclerosis: A personalized approach. *Neurology Reviews.* Retrieved on 10/3/2020 at: www.globalacademycme.com/cme/neurology/diagnosing-and-managing-multiple-sclerosis/diagnosing-and-managing-multiple-sclerosis/page/0/1

*Debska, G., Milaniak, I., & Skorupska-Krol, A. (2020). The quality of life as a predictor of social support for multiple sclerosis patients and caregivers. *Journal of Neuroscience Nursing, 52*(3), 106–111.

Garcia, S. (2019). High-level disinfection and sterilization. *American Nurse Today, 14*(7), 15–17.

Girach, A., Julian, T., Varrassi, G., et al. (2019). Quality of life in painful peripheral neuropathies: A systematic review. *Pain Research and Management, 2019.* doi:10.1155/2019/2091960

Kalb, R., Feinstein, A., Rohrig, A., et al. (2019). Depression and suicidality in multiple sclerosis: Red flags, management strategies, and ethical considerations. *Current Neurology and Neuroscience Reports, 19* (77). doi:10.1007/s11910-019-0992-1

Malek, E., & Salameh, J. (2019). Guillain-Barré syndrome. *Seminars in Neurology, 39*(5), 489–595.

Manthorpe, J., & Simcock, P. (2019). The role of social work in supporting people affected by Creutzfeldt-Jakob Disease (CJD): A scoping review. *British Journal of Social Work, 49,* 1798–1816.

Miller, Y., Grima, K., & Plonowski, M. (2020). Eligibilty reference manual. American Red Cross. Retrieved on 9/28/2020 at: www.redcrossblood.org/donate-blood/how-to-donate/eligibility-requirements/eligibility-criteria-alphabetical/eligibility-reference-material.html

Mount, H., & Boyle, S. (2017). Aseptic and bacterial meningitis: Evaluation, treatment, and prevention. *American Family Physician, 96*(5), 314–322.

National Institute of Neurological Disorders and Stroke (NINDS). (2018a). Bell's palsy fact sheet. Retrieved on 9/21/2020 at: www.ninds.nih.gov/Disorders/Patient-Caregiver-Education/Fact-Sheets/Bells-Palsy-Fact-Sheet

National Institute of Neurological Disorders and Stroke (NINDS). (2018b). Guillain-Barré syndrome fact sheet. Retrieved on 10/3/2020 at: www.ninds.nih.gov/Disorders/Patient-Caregiver-Education/Fact-Sheets/Guillain-Barr%C3%A9-Syndrome-Fact-Sheet

National Institute of Neurological Disorders and Stroke (NINDS). (2020). Myasthenia gravis fact sheet. Retrieved on 10/3/2020 at: www.ninds.nih.gov/Disorders/Patient-Caregiver-Education/Fact-Sheets/Myasthenia-Gravis-Fact-Sheet

*Newland, P., Lorenz, R. A., Smith, J. M., et al. (2019). The relationship among multiple sclerosis-related symptoms, sleep quality, and sleep hygiene behaviors. *Journal of Neuroscience Nursing, 51*(1), 37–42.

Obermann, M. (2019). Recent advances in understanding/managing trigeminal neuralgia. *F1000 Research, 8.* doi:10.12688/f1000research.16092.1

Rae-Grant, A., Day, G. S., Marrie, R. A., et al. (2018). Practice guideline recommendations summary: Disease-modifying therapies for adults with multiple sclerosis. *Neurology, 90*(17), 777–788.

Somasundara, D., Sullivan, F., & Cheesbrough, G. (2017). Management of Bell's palsy. *Australian Prescriber, 40*(3), 94–97.

Sonneville, R., Ruimy, R., Benzonana, N., et al. (2017). An update on bacterial brain abscess in immunocompetent patients. *Clinical Microbiology and Infection, 23*(9), 614–620.

Thompson, A., Banwell, B., Barkhof, F., et al. (2018). Diagnosis of multiple sclerosis: 2017 revisions of the McDonald criteria. *The Lancet Neurology, 17*(2), 162–173.

Vitiello, G., Emmi, G., Silvestri, E., et al. (2019). Intravenous immunoglobulin therapy: A snapshot for the internist. *Internal and Emergency Medicine, 14*(7), 1041–1049.

World Health Organization (WHO). (n.d.). Creutzfeldt-Jakob disease (CJD) and variant CJD (VCJD). Retrieved on 10/3/2020 at: www.who.int/zoonoses/diseases/Creutzfeldt.pdf

Resources

Creutzfeldt–Jakob Disease Foundation, www.cjdfoundation.org
Guillain–Barré Syndrome Foundation International, www.gbs-cidp.org
Myasthenia Gravis Foundation of America (MGFA), www.myasthenia.org
National Multiple Sclerosis Society, www.nationalmssociety.org
The Foundation for Neuropathy, www.foundationforpn.org

65

Management of Patients with Oncologic or Degenerative Neurologic Disorders

The occurrence of oncologic or degenerative disease processes in the neurologic system produces a unique set of nursing challenges. Thus, nurses who care for patients with these disorders must have a clear understanding of the pathophysiology, diagnostic testing, medical and nursing care, and rehabilitation processes. Nurses provide care for patients with oncologic or degenerative disease processes in many inpatient and outpatient settings. Oncologic disorders include brain and spinal cord tumors. Degenerative neurologic disorders include Parkinson's disease (PD), Huntington disease, amyotrophic lateral sclerosis (ALS), muscular dystrophies,

and degenerative disc disease. Post-polio syndrome (PPS) is thought to be degenerative in nature and is included in this chapter.

ONCOLOGIC DISORDERS OF THE BRAIN AND SPINAL CORD

There are many types of brain and spinal cord tumors, each with its own biology, prognosis, and treatment options. Because of the unique anatomy and physiology, tumors of the central nervous system (CNS) are challenging to diagnose and treat.

Brain Tumors

A brain tumor occupies space within the skull, growing as a spherical mass or diffusely infiltrating tissue. The effects of brain tumors are caused by inflammation, compression, and infiltration of tissue. A variety of physiologic changes result, causing any or all of the following pathophysiologic events (Hickey & Strayer, 2020):

- Increased intracranial pressure (ICP) and cerebral edema
- Focal neurologic signs such as headache
- Seizure activity
- Hydrocephalus
- Altered pituitary function

Neoplastic lesions in the brain ultimately cause death by increasing ICP and impairing vital functions, such as respiration.

There are over 100 types of brain tumors with an estimated 78,000 new cases each year. These include 25,000 malignant and 53,000 nonmalignant brain tumors (American Association of Neuroscience Nurses [AANN], 2016). Brain tumors are classified as primary or secondary. Primary brain tumors originate from cells within the brain. In adults, most primary brain tumors originate from glial cells (cells that make up the structure and support system of the brain and spinal cord) and are supratentorial (located above the covering of the cerebellum). Primary tumors progress locally, rarely metastasize outside the CNS, and have a 5-year survival rate of 33.4% (Garcia, Slone, Dolecek, et al., 2019).

Developed countries have a higher incidence of primary brain tumors, with rates of 5.1 per 100,000 compared to 3.0 per 100,000 in less developed countries. This is most likely due to more frequent diagnosis with improved imaging modalities. Although many risk factors have been investigated, exposure to ionizing radiation is the only known modifiable risk factor (AANN, 2016). Many genetic factors and genetic syndromes (such as neurofibromatosis) are associated with brain tumor risk in families (AANN, 2016).

Secondary, or metastatic, brain tumors develop from structures outside the brain and are twice as common as primary brain tumors (AANN, 2016). Metastatic lesions to the brain can occur from the lung, breast, lower gastrointestinal tract, pancreas, kidney, and skin (melanomas) neoplasms. Single or multiple metastases may occur, and brain metastases may be found at any time during the disease course, even at initial diagnosis of the primary disease. Patient survival rates from primary brain cancers are improving, however, the incidence of brain metastases is increasing (AANN, 2016).

The highest incidence of brain tumors in adults occurs in the fifth through seventh decades of life (Young, Chmura, Wainwright, et al., 2017). There is a slight male predominance in the incidence of malignant brain tumors.

Types of Primary Brain Tumors

Brain tumors may be classified into several groups: those arising from the coverings of the brain (e.g., dural meningioma), those developing in or on the cranial nerves (e.g., acoustic neuroma), those originating within brain tissue (e.g., glioma),

---

Chart 65-1 Classification of Brain Tumors in Adults

I. Intracerebral Tumors
  A. Gliomas—infiltrate any portion of the brain; most common type of brain tumor
    1. Astrocytomas (grades I and II)
    2. Glioblastoma (astrocytoma grades III and IV)
    3. Oligodendroglioma (low and high grades)
    4. Ependymoma (grades I to IV)
    5. Medulloblastoma
II. Tumors Arising From Supporting Structures
  A. Meningiomas
  B. Neuromas (acoustic neuroma, schwannoma)
  C. Pituitary adenomas
III. Developmental Tumors
  A. Angiomas
  B. Dermoid, epidermoid, teratoma, craniopharyngioma
IV. Metastatic Lesions

Adapted from Hickey, J. V., & Strayer, A. L. (2020). *The clinical practice of neurological and neurosurgical nursing* (8th ed.). Philadelphia, PA: Wolters Kluwer.

---

and metastatic lesions originating elsewhere in the body. Tumors of the pituitary and pineal glands and of cerebral blood vessels are also types of brain tumors. Relevant clinical considerations include the location and the histologic character of the tumor. About 70% of the time tumors are benign but even benign tumors, such as colloid cysts, can occur in vital areas and can grow large enough to have serious effects (Hickey & Strayer, 2020). See Chart 65-1 for the classification of brain tumors.

Gliomas

In adults, gliomas (principally astrocytoma) account for approximately 25% of symptomatic primary brain tumors. Glial tumors, the most common type of intracerebral brain neoplasm, are divided into many categories (McFaline-Figueroa & Lee, 2018). Astrocytomas, arising from astrocytic cells, are the most common type of glioma and are graded from I to IV, indicating the degree of malignancy (McFaline-Figueroa & Lee, 2018). The grade is based on cellular density, cell mitosis, and degree of differentiation from the original cell type. Grades III and IV tumors are known as glioblastomas and have little resemblance to the original cell type. Astrocytomas infiltrate into the surrounding neural connective tissue and therefore cannot be totally removed without causing considerable damage to vital structures.

Oligodendroglial tumors, arising from oligodendroglial cells, represent about 1.4% of gliomas (Hickey & Strayer, 2020). Most oligodendrogliomas occur in adults aged 50 to 60, are found in men more often than in women, and are categorized as low or high grade (anaplastic) (Young et al., 2017). The histologic distinction between astrocytomas and oligodendrogliomas is difficult to make but is important, because oligodendrogliomas are more sensitive than astrocytomas to chemotherapy. Tumors originating from ependymal cells, another type of glial cell, are known as ependymomas and are more common in children than adults. Glial tumors may be treated with a combination of surgery, radiation therapy, and chemotherapy, depending on specific cell and patient characteristics as well as the location of the tumor (Young et al., 2017).

Meningiomas

Meningiomas, which represent 37% of all primary brain tumors, are common benign encapsulated tumors of arachnoid cells on the meninges (McFaline-Figueroa & Lee, 2018). They are slow growing, occur most often in middle-aged adults, and are more common in women. Meningiomas often occur in areas proximal to the venous sinuses. Manifestations depend on the area involved and are often the result of compression rather than invasion of brain tissue. Preferred treatment for symptomatic lesions is surgery with complete removal or partial dissection, although radiation therapy may be useful for some patients. Metastasis is rare with meningiomas but benign meningiomas may be challenging to remove surgically without causing neurologic deficits if the tumor is located at the base of the skull or surrounds the optic nerve, or in the rare case if the tumor is invasive. Multiple meningiomas may occur with neurofibromatosis type 2 (Euskirchen & Peyre, 2018).

Acoustic Neuromas

Acoustic neuromas account for 16% of brain tumors, with men and women equally affected, and occur most commonly in the fifth decade of life (Hong & Moliterno, 2019).

An acoustic neuroma is a tumor of the eighth cranial nerve—the cranial nerve most responsible for hearing and balance. It usually arises just within the internal auditory meatus, where it frequently expands before filling the cerebellopontine recess. An acoustic neuroma may grow slowly and attain considerable size before it is diagnosed. The patient usually experiences loss of hearing, tinnitus, and episodes of vertigo and staggering gait. As the tumor becomes larger, painful sensations of the face may occur on the same side as a result of the tumor's compression of the fifth cranial nerve (Hong & Moliterno, 2019). Many acoustic neuromas are benign and can be managed conservatively. Many that continue to grow can be surgically removed and have a good prognosis (see Chapter 59). Some acoustic neuromas may be suitable for stereotactic radiotherapy rather than open craniotomy. Stereotactic radiotherapy is discussed later in this chapter.

Pituitary Adenomas

Pituitary tumors account for about 16% of all primary brain tumors (AANN, 2016). They can occur at any age but are more common in older adults. Women are affected more often than men, particularly during the childbearing years. Pituitary tumors are rarely malignant but cause symptoms as a result of pressure on adjacent structures or hormonal changes (Jang, Oh, Lee, et al., 2020).

Pressure Effects of Pituitary Adenomas

Pressure from a pituitary adenoma may be exerted on the optic nerves, optic chiasm, or optic tracts or on the hypothalamus or the third ventricle if the tumor invades the cavernous sinuses or expands into the sphenoid bone. These pressure effects produce headache, visual dysfunction, hypothalamic disorders (disorders of sleep, appetite, temperature, and emotions), increased ICP, and enlargement and erosion of the sella turcica (Donovan & Welch, 2018; Jang et al., 2020; Molitch, 2017).

Hormonal Effects of Pituitary Adenomas

Functioning pituitary tumors can produce one or more hormones normally produced by the anterior pituitary. Hormonal hypersecretion is caused only by pituitary adenomas (Molitch, 2017). Many adenomas (50%) secrete an excess amount of hormone including prolactin (prolactinomas), growth hormone (GH) producing acromegaly in adults, adrenocorticotropic hormone (ACTH) resulting in Cushing's disease, or thyroid-stimulating hormone (TSH) (Molitch, 2017). Adenomas that secrete TSH or follicle-stimulating hormone and luteinizing hormone occur infrequently, whereas adenomas that produce both GH and prolactin are relatively common.

The female patient whose pituitary gland is secreting excessive quantities of prolactin presents with amenorrhea or galactorrhea (excessive or spontaneous flow of milk). Male patients with prolactinomas may present with impotence and hypogonadism. Acromegaly, caused by excess GH, produces enlargement of the hands and feet, distortion of the facial features, and pressure on peripheral nerves (entrapment syndromes). The clinical features of Cushing's disease, a condition associated with prolonged overproduction of cortisol, occur with excessive production of ACTH. Manifestations include a form of obesity with redistribution of fat to the facial, supraclavicular, and abdominal areas; hypertension; purple striae and ecchymoses; osteoporosis; elevated blood glucose levels; and emotional disorders. See Chapter 45 for a discussion of endocrine disorders resulting from these tumors.

Gerontologic Considerations

The incidence of all brain tumors increases with age (Young et al., 2017). Intracranial tumors can produce personality changes, confusion, speech dysfunction, or disturbances of gait. In older adult patients, early signs and symptoms of intracranial tumors can be easily overlooked or incorrectly attributed to cognitive and neurologic changes associated with normal aging (Eliopoulos, 2018). Neurologic signs and symptoms in the older adult must be carefully evaluated, because brain metastases occur in patients with a history of prior cancer. Regardless of the age of the patient or the decision to proceed or not with treatment, the nurse provides supportive care. Researchers have reported that the degree of frailty influences clinical outcomes of older adult patients undergoing surgery for brain tumor resection (Harland, Wang, Gunaydin, et al., 2020). Patients identified as moderately frail or frail are at increased risk for a longer length of hospital stay and tend to require discharge to a long-term care facility rather than home (Harland et al., 2020).

Clinical Manifestations

Brain tumors can produce both focal or generalized neurologic signs and symptoms. Generalized symptoms reflect increased ICP, and the most common focal or specific signs and symptoms result from tumors that interfere with functions in specific brain regions. Figure 65-1 indicates common brain tumor sites.

Increased Intracranial Pressure

As discussed in Chapter 61, the skull is a rigid compartment containing essential noncompressible contents: brain matter, intravascular blood, and cerebrospinal fluid (CSF). The Monro-Kellie hypothesis or doctrine explains the dynamic equilibrium of the cranial contents. According to this hypothesis, if any one of these skull components increases in volume,

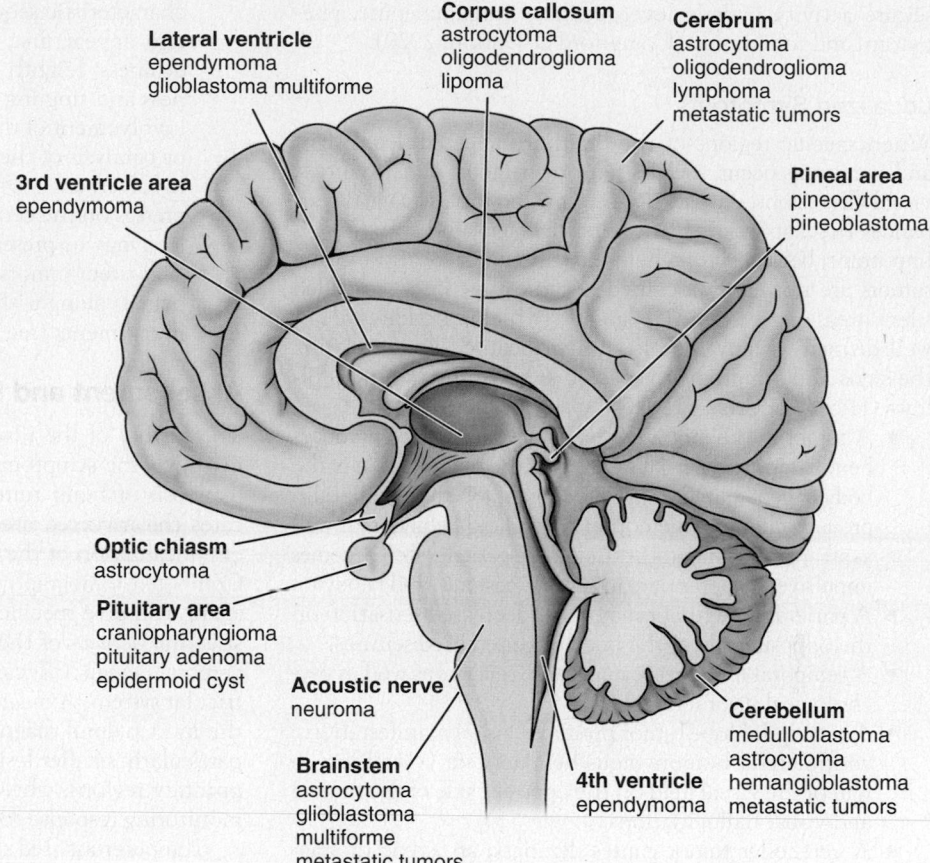

Figure 65-1 • Common brain tumor sites.

ICP increases unless one of the other components decreases in volume. Consequently, any change in volume occupied by the brain (as occurs with disorders such as brain tumor or cerebral edema) produces signs and symptoms of increased ICP (Witherspoon & Ashby, 2017).

The enlarging tumor and its associating edema disrupts the equilibrium between the brain, blood, and CSF. As the tumor grows, compensatory adjustments may occur through compression of intracranial veins, reduction of CSF volume (by increased absorption or decreased production), a modest decrease in cerebral blood flow, or reduction of intra- and extracellular brain tissue mass. When these compensatory mechanisms fail, the patient develops signs and symptoms of increased ICP, most often including headache, nausea with or without vomiting, and **papilledema** (swelling of the optic nerve) (Hickey & Strayer, 2020). Personality changes and a variety of focal deficits, including motor, sensory, and cranial nerve dysfunction, are common.

Headache

One third of patients with brain tumors report headache as an early symptom (Hickey & Strayer, 2020). Headache is most commonly reported in the early morning and is made worse by coughing, straining, or sudden movement (Norris, 2019). It is thought to be caused by the tumor invading, compressing, or distorting the pain-sensitive structures or by edema that accompanies the tumor. The headaches may be generalized or localized to the site of the tumor. As the edema increases, headache is generally bifrontal or bioccipital regardless of the tumor location (Hickey & Strayer, 2020).

Vomiting

Vomiting, seldom related to food intake, is usually the result of irritation of the vagal centers in the medulla (Hickey & Strayer, 2020). Forceful vomiting is described as projectile vomiting. Headache may be relieved by vomiting.

Visual Disturbances

The tumor itself or the surrounding edema can compress the third cranial nerve, causing optic disc swelling or papilledema. This limits the visual acuity along the visual pathway, mildly or profoundly, as diplopia (double vision), hemianopsia (visual field deficits), or varying levels of blindness (Jang et al., 2020).

Seizures

Seizures are common in patients with brain tumors either initially or throughout their disease process (McFaline-Figueroa & Lee, 2018). Seizures may be focal or generalized. Tumors of the frontal, parietal, and temporal lobes carry the greatest risk of seizures; seizures are unusual with brainstem or cerebellar tumors. See Chapter 61 for discussion about seizures and related management.

If not the initial presentation, seizures can be a result of metabolic factors (electrolyte imbalances, liver failure or kidney disease, radiation or chemotherapy side effects), structural causes (parenchymal metastases, leptomeningeal disease, dural metastases) or a new hemorrhage, thrombosis, or development of meningitis (Hickey & Strayer, 2020). If the patient presents with a seizure, then anticonvulsant drugs are prescribed. Medications with the best evidence for controlling seizure activity include levetiracetam, carbamazepine, phenytoin, and zonisamide (Comerford & Durkin, 2020).

Localized Symptoms

When specific regions of the brain are affected, local signs and symptoms occur, such as sensory or motor abnormalities, visual alterations, alterations in cognition, or language disturbances (e.g., aphasia). Identifying the signs and symptoms is important, because it can help identify tumor location. Some tumors are not easily localized because they lie in so-called silent areas of the brain (i.e., areas in which functions are not well defined). Many tumors can be localized by correlating the signs and symptoms to specific areas in the brain, as follows (Hickey & Strayer, 2020).

- A tumor in the motor cortex of the frontal lobe produces hemiparesis and partial seizures on the opposite side of the body or generalized seizures. A frontal lobe tumor may also produce changes in emotional state and behavior, as well as an apathetic mental attitude. The patient often becomes impulsive, inappropriate in speech, gestures, and behavior.
- A parietal lobe tumor may cause decreased sensation on the opposite side of the body or generalized seizures.
- A temporal lobe tumor may cause seizures as well as psychological disorders.
- An occipital lobe tumor produces visual manifestations: contralateral homonymous hemianopsia (visual loss in half of the visual field on the opposite side of the tumor) and visual hallucinations.
- A cerebellar tumor causes dizziness; an ataxic or staggering gait with a tendency to fall toward the side of the lesion; marked muscle incoordination; and nystagmus (involuntary rhythmic eye movements), usually in the horizontal direction.
- A cerebellopontine angle tumor usually originates in the sheath of the acoustic nerve and gives rise to a characteristic sequence of symptoms. Tinnitus and vertigo appear first, soon followed by progressive nerve deafness (eighth cranial nerve dysfunction). Numbness and tingling of the face and tongue occur (due to involvement of the fifth cranial nerve). Later, weakness or paralysis of the face develops (seventh cranial nerve involvement). Finally, because the enlarging tumor presses on the cerebellum, abnormalities in motor function may be present.
- Brainstem tumors may be associated with cranial nerve deficits along with complex motor and sensory function impairments (see Chapter 64, Table 64-3).

Assessment and Diagnostic Findings

The history of the illness, the manner, and the time frame in which the symptoms evolved are key components in the diagnosis of brain tumors. A neurologic examination indicates the involved areas of the CNS. To assist in the precise localization of the lesion, a battery of tests is performed. Computed tomography (CT) scans, enhanced by a contrast agent, can give specific information concerning the number, size, and density of the lesions, and the extent of secondary cerebral edema. CT can provide information about the ventricular system. A magnetic resonance imaging (MRI) scan is the most helpful diagnostic tool for detecting brain tumors, particularly smaller lesions, and tumors in the brainstem and pituitary regions, where bone is thick. MRI is also useful in monitoring response to treatment.

Computer-assisted stereotactic (three-dimensional) biopsy is used to diagnose deep-seated brain tumors and to provide a basis for treatment and prognosis. Stereotactic approaches involve the use of a three-dimensional frame that allows very precise localization of the tumor; a stereotactic frame and multiple imaging studies (x-rays, CT scans, or MRIs) are used to localize the tumor and verify its position (see Fig. 65-2).

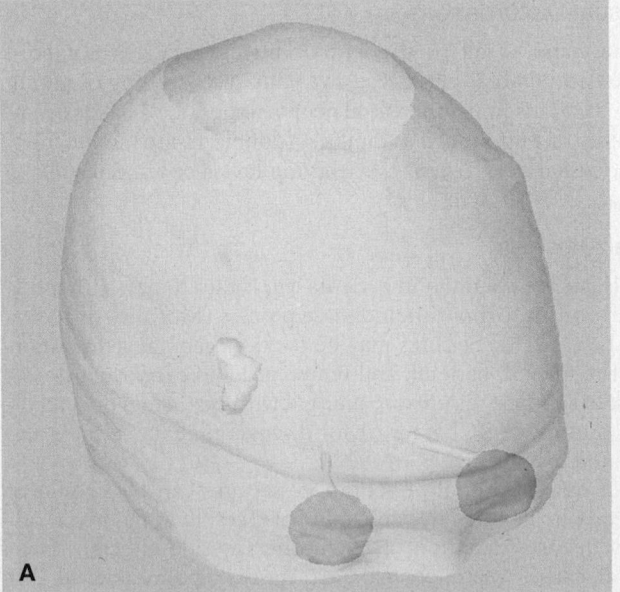
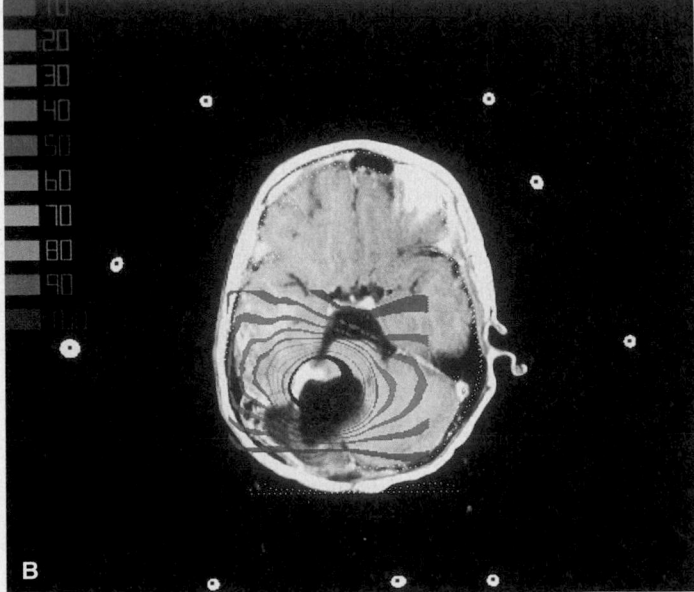

Figure 65-2 • A. Using stereotactic or "brain-mapping" guided approach, a three-dimensional computer image fuses the computed tomography image and magnetic resonance image to pinpoint the exact location of the brain tumor. This low-grade astrocytoma is localized adjacent to the brainstem, is inoperable, and is treated with radiation. Note the optic chasm and optic nerves. **B.** Computerized image of the prescribed radiation dose.

Brain-mapping technology helps determine the proximity of diseased areas of the brain to structures essential for normal brain function.

Positron emission tomography (PET) is used to supplement MRI scanning in many centers. On PET scans, low-grade tumors are associated with hypometabolism, and high-grade tumors show hypermetabolism. This information can be useful in making treatment decisions (Achrol, Rennert, Anders, et al., 2019). An electroencephalogram can detect abnormal brain waves in regions occupied by or adjacent to tumor; it is used to evaluate temporal lobe seizures and to assist in ruling out other disorders. Cytologic studies of the CSF may be performed to detect malignant cells as CNS tumors can shed cells into the CSF resulting in metastasis.

Medical Management

A variety of medical management approaches, including surgery, chemotherapy, and external-beam radiation therapy, are used alone or in combination (AANN, 2016; Hickey & Strayer, 2020). A relatively new treatment option for glioblastomas is tumor-treating fields. This device provides alternating electric field therapy that disrupts the mitotic process and is worn on the head (McFaline-Figueroa & Lee, 2018). The main side effect is skin irritation.

Secreting tumors may be treated with medications that suppress hormones. Nonfunctioning tumors may have no effect on pituitary function or may suppress hormone production and release. Hormone replacement may be necessary for these patients to restore normal endocrine function. The management of brain tumors is complex and requires an interdisciplinary approach to care to optimize patient outcomes (Achrol et al., 2019).

Surgical Management

The objective of surgical management is to remove as much tumor as possible without increasing the neurologic deficit (paralysis, blindness), or to relieve symptoms by partial removal (decompression). Surgery also provides the opportunity to biopsy tissue to establish a definitive diagnosis. A variety of surgical approaches may be used; the specific approach depends on the type of tumor, its location, and its accessibility. Conventional surgical approaches require a craniotomy (incision into the skull). See Chapter 61 for a discussion of care of the patient who has undergone a craniotomy. This approach is used in patients with meningiomas, acoustic neuromas, cystic astrocytomas of the cerebellum, colloid cysts of the third ventricle, congenital tumors such as dermoid cyst, and some of the granulomas. With improved imaging techniques and the availability of the operating microscope and microsurgical instrumentation, even large tumors can be removed through a relatively small craniotomy. For patients with malignant glioma, complete removal of the tumor and cure are not possible, but the rationale for resection includes relief of ICP, removal of any necrotic tissue, and reduction in the bulk of the tumor, which theoretically leaves behind fewer cells to become resistant to radiation or chemotherapy. Most pituitary adenomas are treated by transsphenoidal microsurgical removal (see Chapter 61), and the remainder of tumors that cannot be removed completely are treated by radiation (Hickey & Strayer, 2020).

Radiation Therapy

Radiation therapy—the cornerstone of treatment for many brain tumors—decreases the incidence of recurrence of incompletely resected tumors (AANN, 2016). Gamma radiation is delivered via an external beam to the tumor in multiple fractions. Brachytherapy (the surgical implantation of radiation sources to deliver high doses at a short distance) is an option for some types of tumors depending on their location. It is usually used as an adjunct to conventional radiation therapy or as a rescue measure for recurrent disease. Radioisotopes such as iodine 131 (^{131}I) are used to minimize effects on surrounding brain tissue.

Stereotactic procedures may be performed using a linear accelerator or gamma knife to perform radiosurgery (Hickey & Strayer, 2020). These procedures allow treatment of deep, inaccessible tumors, often in a single session. Precise localization of the tumor is accomplished by the stereotactic approach and by minute measurements and precise positioning of the patient. Multiple narrow beams then deliver a very high dose of radiation. An advantage of this method is that no surgical incision is needed. Disadvantages include the lag time between treatment and the desired result as well as the potential for developing radiation necrosis (AANN, 2016).

Chemotherapy

Chemotherapy may be used in conjunction with radiation therapy, or as the sole therapy, with the goal of increasing survival time. The greatest challenge in chemotherapy of brain tumors is that the blood–brain barrier prevents drugs from getting to the tumor in effective doses without causing systemic toxicity (AANN, 2016).

Malignant glioma is usually treated with 6 weeks of oral temozolomide during radiation therapy, followed by 6 to 12 months of oral temozolomide. Low-grade gliomas may be treated with 6 months of oral temozolomide alone. Temozolomide is an oral chemotherapy that crosses the blood–brain barrier (McFaline-Figueroa & Lee, 2018). Several other chemotherapy agents are used alone or in combination depending on the type of tumor.

Autologous bone marrow transplantation is used in some patients who will receive chemotherapy or radiation therapy, because it can "rescue" the patient from the bone marrow toxicity associated with high doses of chemotherapy and radiation. A fraction of the patient's bone marrow is aspirated, usually from the iliac crest, and stored. The patient receives large doses of chemotherapy or radiation therapy to destroy large numbers of malignant cells. The marrow is then reinfused intravenously after treatment is completed. See Chapter 12 for discussion of bone marrow transplant.

Pharmacologic Therapy

Corticosteroids are useful in relieving headache and alterations in level of consciousness. Corticosteroids such as dexamethasone are thought to reduce inflammation and edema around tumors (AANN, 2016). Other medications used include osmotic diuretics (e.g., mannitol and hypertonic saline) to decrease the fluid content of the brain, which leads to a decrease in ICP. Anticonvulsant medications are used to treat and control seizures (Comerford & Durkin, 2020).

Nursing Management

The characteristics of headache, when present, should be assessed. Upright positioning and pain medications may be useful in managing pain; nurses should evaluate the effectiveness of pain management interventions (Ijzerman-Korevaar, Snijers, Saskia, et al., 2018). Even if seizure history is absent, the patient and family should be educated about the possibility of seizure and the need to adhere to prophylactic anticonvulsant medications, if prescribed. The patient with a brain tumor may be at increased risk for aspiration as a result of cranial nerve dysfunction. Medications to alleviate nausea and to prevent vomiting should be considered (Ijzerman-Korevaar et al., 2018). Preoperatively, the gag reflex and ability to swallow are evaluated. In patients with diminished gag response, care includes educating the patient to direct food and fluids toward the unaffected side, having the patient sit upright to eat, offering a semisoft diet, and having suction readily available. The effects of increased ICP caused by the tumor mass are reviewed in Chapter 61. The nurse performs neurologic checks; monitors vital signs; maintains a neurologic observation record (see Chapter 61, Fig. 61-6); spaces nursing interventions to prevent rapid increase in ICP; and reorients the patient when necessary to person, time, and place. The use of corticosteroids to control headache and neurologic symptoms requires astute nursing assessment and intervention because many adverse effects can occur, including hyperglycemia, electrolyte abnormalities, and muscle weakness (see Chapter 45, Table 45-3). Patients with changes in cognition caused by their lesion require frequent reorientation and the use of orienting devices (e.g., personal possessions, photographs, lists, a clock), supervision of and assistance with self-care, and ongoing monitoring and intervention for prevention of injury. Patients with seizures are carefully monitored and protected from injury. Motor function is checked at intervals because specific motor deficits may occur, depending on the tumor's location. When muscle weakness is present, an interprofessional approach, including the nurse and physical and occupational therapists, can be used to preserve muscle strength, promote range of motion, and facilitate independence in self-care. Sensory disturbances are assessed and any area of numbness should be protected from injury. Speech is evaluated, and patients with speech deficits can be educated to use alternative forms of communication. Eye movement and pupillary size and reaction may be affected by cranial nerve involvement. Fatigue is common during therapy; efforts should be made to conserve energy and promote rest.

The psychosocial effects on family caregivers of a family member who has brain metastases may be significant (Ketcher, Otto, & Reblin, 2020). Caregivers should be included in the plan of care.

The nursing process for patients undergoing neurosurgery is discussed in Chapter 61. The patient's functional abilities should be reassessed postoperatively, because changes can occur.

Cerebral Metastases

A significant number of patients with cancer experience neurologic deficits caused by metastasis to the nervous system, which can include the brain, CSF, and meninges. Metastatic lesions to the brain are more common than primary brain tumors and have an associated 2-year survival rate of less than 10% (Achrol et al., 2019). The high number of metastatic brain tumors is clinically important, as more patients with all forms of cancer live longer because of improved therapies. Neurologic signs and symptoms include headache, gait disturbances, visual impairment, personality changes, altered mentation (memory loss and confusion), focal weakness, paralysis, aphasia, and seizures (McFaline-Figueroa & Lee, 2018). These signs and symptoms can be devastating to both patient and family. Metastases to the CSF and meninges, known as leptomeningeal metastases, can produce symptoms of headache and isolated cranial nerve deficits.

Medical Management

The treatment of metastatic nervous system cancer is palliative and involves eliminating or reducing serious symptoms. Even when palliation is the goal, distressing signs and symptoms can be relieved, thereby improving the quality of life for both patient and family (McFaline-Figueroa & Lee, 2018). Patients with intracerebral metastases who are not treated have a poor prognosis with a limited survival time. The therapeutic options include whole brain radiation therapy (the foundation of treatment) for multiple metastases or stereotactic radiosurgery for up to three sites of metastases. Surgery may be considered for a single symptomatic metastasis. Systemic chemotherapy directed at the primary cancer may be ineffective in crossing the blood–brain barrier, but chemotherapy that crosses this barrier may be added. Intrathecal chemotherapy, with direct injection of chemotherapy agents into the CSF of the brain or spinal canal, may be useful in persons with metastases (Song, Li, Yin, et al., 2018). Some combination of these treatments is usually the optimal method.

Pain can be a significant problem and is managed by means of a stepped progression in the doses and type of analgesic agents needed for relief. If the patient has severe pain, morphine can be infused into the epidural or subarachnoid space through a spinal needle and a catheter placed as near as possible to the spinal segment where the pain is projected. Small doses of morphine are given at prescribed intervals (see Chapter 9).

NURSING PROCESS

The Patient with Nervous System Metastases or Primary Brain Tumor

Assessment

The nursing assessment includes a baseline neurologic examination and focuses on how the patient is functioning, moving, and walking; adapting to weakness or paralysis and to loss of vision and speech; and dealing with seizures. Assessment addresses symptoms that cause distress to the patient and affect the quality of life, including pain, respiratory problems, bowel and bladder disorders, and sleep disturbances, as well as impairment of skin integrity, fluid balance, and temperature regulation (Hickey & Strayer, 2020). Nutritional status is assessed, because cachexia and cancer-related anorexia-cachexia syndrome are common (see Chapter 12).

The nurse takes a dietary history to assess food intake, intolerance, and preferences. Calculation of body mass index can confirm the loss of subcutaneous fat and lean body mass (see

Chapter 4). Biochemical measurements are reviewed to assess the degree of malnutrition, impaired cellular immunity, and electrolyte balance (normal laboratory values are found in Appendix A on thePoint). A dietitian assists in determining the caloric needs of the patient.

The nurse works with other members of the health care team to assess the impact of the illness on the family in terms of home care, altered relationships, financial problems, time pressures, and family problems. This information is important in helping family members cope with the diagnosis and the changes associated with it.

Diagnosis

NURSING DIAGNOSES

Based on the assessment data, major nursing diagnoses may include the following:

- Impaired self-feeding, impaired ability to perform hygiene, impaired ability to dress, and impaired self-toileting associated with loss or impairment of motor and sensory functions and decreased cognitive abilities
- Impaired nutritional status associated with cachexia due to treatment and tumor effects, decreased nutritional intake, and malabsorption
- Impaired nutritional status associated with increased nutritional intake and impaired metabolism
- Anxiety associated with uncertainty, change in appearance, or altered lifestyle
- Interrupted family process associated with situational crisis imposed by the care of the person with a terminal illness

COLLABORATIVE PROBLEMS/POTENTIAL COMPLICATIONS

Potential complications may include the following:
- Seizures (see Chapter 61)
- Headaches (see Chapter 61)

Planning and Goals

The goals for the patient include compensating for self-care deficits, improving nutrition, reducing anxiety, enhancing family coping skills, and absence of complications.

Nursing Interventions

COMPENSATING FOR SELF-CARE DEFICITS

The patient may have difficulty participating in goal setting depending on the tumor location and if cognitive function is affected. The nurse encourages the family to assist the patient to be as independent as possible for as long as possible (Hickey & Strayer, 2020). Increasing assistance with self-care activities is to be expected. Because the patient with nervous system metastasis and the family live with uncertainty, they are encouraged to plan for each day and to make the most of each day. The tasks and challenges are to assist the patient to find useful coping mechanisms, adaptations, and compensations for solving problems that arise. Use of an interprofessional health care team is helpful. An individualized exercise program helps maintain strength, endurance, and range of motion. Eventually, referral for home or hospice care may be necessary (see Chapter 13).

IMPROVING NUTRITION

Patients with nausea, vomiting, diarrhea, breathlessness, and pain are rarely interested in eating. These symptoms are managed or controlled through assessment, planning, and care.

The nurse educates the family about how to position the patient for comfort and safety during meals. A dietician may help with alternative food choices that are easily tolerated. Meals are planned for times when the patient is rested and in less distress from pain or the effects of treatment.

The patient needs to be clean, comfortable, and free of pain for meals in an environment that is as attractive as possible. Oral hygiene before meals helps to improve appetite. Offensive sights, sounds, and odors are eliminated. Creative strategies may be required to make food more palatable, provide enough fluids, and increase opportunities for socialization during meals. The family may be asked to keep a log of daily weights and to record the quantity of food eaten to determine the daily calorie count. Dietary supplements, if acceptable to the patient, can be provided to meet increased caloric needs. If the patient is not interested in most usual foods, those foods preferred by the patient should be offered. When the patient shows marked deterioration as a result of tumor growth and effects, some other form of nutritional support (e.g., tube feeding, parenteral nutrition) may be indicated if consistent with the patient's end-of-life preferences (AANN, 2016) (see Chapter 39 for discussion of tube feeding and Chapter 41 for discussion of parenteral nutrition). Nursing interventions include assessing the patency of the central and intravenous lines or feeding tube, monitoring the insertion site for infection, checking the infusion rate, monitoring intake and output, and changing the intravenous tubing and dressing. Family members are instructed in these techniques if they will be providing care at home. Parenteral nutrition can be provided at home if indicated. The patient's quality of life may guide the selection, initiation, maintenance, and discontinuation of nutritional support. The nurse and family should not place too much emphasis on eating or on discussions about food, because the patient may not desire aggressive nutritional intervention. The subsequent course of action must be congruent with the wishes and choices of the patient and family.

Increased appetite may occur in patients receiving steroids and may result in weight gain as well as hyperglycemia. Patients and family members should be instructed to monitor weight and blood glucose (if appropriate), as well as maintain a healthy diet with caloric intake appropriate to patient needs.

RELIEVING ANXIETY

Patients may be restless, with changing moods that may include intense depression, euphoria, paranoia, and severe anxiety. The patient's response to a life-threatening illness reflects their pattern of reaction to other crisis situations. Serious illness imposes additional strains that often bring other unresolved problems to light. The patient's own coping strategies can help deal with anxious and depressed feelings. Health care providers need to be sensitive to the patient and caregivers' concerns and fears (Ketcher et al., 2020).

Patients need the opportunity to exercise some control over their situation. A sense of mastery can be gained as they learn to understand the disease and its treatment and how to deal with their feelings. Researchers have reported that resilience positively influences problem-based coping strategies (Liang, Liu, Lu, et al., 2020). The presence of family, friends, a spiritual advisor, and health care professionals may be supportive. Brain tumor support services may provide a feeling of meaning and strength (see the Resources section).

Spending time with patients allows them time to talk and to communicate their fears and concerns. Open communication and acknowledgment of fears are often therapeutic. Touch is also a form of communication. These patients need reassurance that continuing care will be provided and that they will not be abandoned. If a patient's emotional reactions are very intense or prolonged, additional help from a spiritual advisor, social worker, or mental health professional may be indicated.

ENHANCING FAMILY PROCESSES

The family needs to be reassured that their loved one is receiving optimal care and that attention will be paid to the patient's changing symptoms and concerns. If the patient can no longer carry out self-care, the family and additional support systems (social worker, home health aide, home health nurse, hospice nurse) may be needed. Assessment and education of family caregivers about neurologic and cognitive symptoms is necessary, acute, and challenging (Boele, Terhorst, Prince, et al., 2019). Investigating resources that are available may decrease the burden on the caregivers. These efforts improve the psychosocial well-being of the patient and family caregivers (Boele et al., 2019; Ketcher et al., 2020).

PROMOTING HOME, COMMUNITY-BASED, AND TRANSITIONAL CARE

Educating Patients About Self-Care. The patient and family often have major responsibility for care at home. Caregivers may struggle with a new "normal" while their support systems fluctuate as their relationship with the patient they are caring for is strengthened, maintained, or strained (Ketcher et al., 2020). In addition to the psychological aspect, education includes pain management strategies, prevention of complications related to treatment strategies, and methods to ensure adequate fluid and food intake (see Chart 65-2). Educational needs of the patient and family regarding care priorities are likely to change as the disease progresses; the nurse should assess the changing needs of the patient and the family and inform them about resources and services early and frequently to assist them (see the Resources section).

Continuing and Transitional Care. Home health services are valuable resources that should be made available to the patient and the family early in the course of an illness. Anticipating needs before they occur can assist in smooth initiation of services. Home health focuses on the areas of symptom and pain control, assistance in self-care, control of treatment complications, and administration of specific forms of treatment (e.g., parenteral nutrition). The nurse assesses pain management, respiratory status, complications of the disorder and its treatment, and the patient's cognitive and emotional status. In addition, the nurse assesses the family's ability to perform necessary care and notifies the primary provider about changing needs or complications, if indicated.

Steps to initiate hospice care, including discussion of hospice care as an option, should not be postponed until death is imminent for the patient with a metastasis or high-grade tumor. Exploration of hospice care as an option should be initiated at a time when hospice services can provide support and care to the patient and family consistent with their end-of-life decisions and can assist in allowing death with dignity. See Chapter 13 for in-depth discussion of end-of-life care.

Evaluation

Expected patient outcomes may include:

1. Engages in self-care activities to extent possible
   a. Uses assistive devices or accepts assistance as needed
   b. Schedules periodic rest periods to permit maximal participation in self-care
2. Maintains as optimal a nutritional status as possible
   a. Eats and accepts food within limits of condition and preferences

---

Chart 65-2	HOME CARE CHECKLIST

The Patient with Nervous System Metastases or Primary Brain Tumor

At the completion of education, the patient and/or caregiver will be able to:

- State effects of the tumor according to its type and location in the brain or spinal cord.
- State the impact of the tumor and treatment on physiologic functioning, ADLs, IADLs, roles, relationships, and spirituality.
  - Describe goals and side effects of treatment and suggested management approaches.
- State the name, dose, side effects, frequency, and schedule for all medications.
  - When indicated, use nonpharmacologic pain management techniques in addition to prescribed pharmacologic methods.
- State how to contact all members of the treatment team (e.g., health care providers, home care professionals, and durable medical equipment and supply vendor).
- State changes in lifestyle (e.g., nutritional needs, ADL assistance) necessary to maintain health.
- Identify coping strategies, such as:
  - Taking control, setting daily goals, and staying positive
  - Participating in rehabilitation to improve self-care

- Engaging in relaxation techniques
- Utilizing family support
- Contacting support services (e.g., American Brain Tumor Association)
  - Participating in faith community/religious practices
- Identify community resources, including palliative care, home health service, or hospice, as appropriate.
- List complications of medications/therapeutic regimen necessitating a call to the nurse or primary provider.
- List complications of medications/therapeutic regimen necessitating a visit to the emergency department.
- Relate how to reach primary provider with questions or complications.
- State time and date of follow-up medical appointments, therapy, and testing.

Resources

See Chapter 12, Chart 12-10: Home Care Checklist: The Patient Receiving Care for an Oncologic Disorder.

ADLs, activities of daily living; IADLs, instrumental activities of daily living.

b. Accepts alternative methods of providing nutrition if indicated
3. Reports being less anxious
   a. Is less restless and is sleeping better
   b. Verbalizes concerns and fears
   c. Participates in activities of personal importance
4. Family members seek help as needed
   a. Demonstrate ability to bathe, feed, and care for the patient and participate in pain management and prevention of complications
   b. Express feelings and concerns to appropriate health professionals
   c. Discuss and seek hospice care as needed
5. Understands ways to avoid complications and is free of complications
   a. Explains reasons for measures to prevent complications
   b. Seizures and headaches are controlled to the extent possible

Spinal Cord Tumors

Tumors within the spinal canal are classified according to their anatomic relation to the spinal cord (Hickey & Strayer, 2020). They include intramedullary lesions (within the spinal cord), extramedullary-intradural lesions (within or under the spinal dura), and extramedullary-extradural lesions (outside the dural membrane). Primary tumors are usually intramedullary, consisting of astrocytoma or ependymoma; meningiomas can occur as extramedullary-intradural lesions (Epstein, 2018). Secondary tumors are far more common and are usually extramedullary-extradural lesions. Tumors that occur within the spinal canal or exert pressure on it cause symptoms ranging from localized or shooting pains, weakness, and loss of reflexes below the tumor level to progressive loss of motor function and paralysis. Usually, sharp pain occurs in the area innervated by the spinal roots that arise from the cord in the region of the tumor. In addition, increasing sensory deficits develop below the level of the lesion. Loss of bowel and bladder function is common.

Assessment and Diagnostic Findings

Neurologic examination and diagnostic studies are used to make the diagnosis. Neurologic examination focuses on assessing pain and identifying loss of reflexes, sensation, or motor function. Helpful diagnostic studies include CT scans, MRI scans, and biopsy. The MRI scan is the most commonly used and the most sensitive diagnostic tool (Hickey & Strayer, 2020) and it is particularly helpful in detecting epidural spinal cord compression and metastases (Kaplow & Iyere, 2016).

Medical Management

Treatment of specific intraspinal tumors depends on the type and location of the tumor, the presenting symptoms, and the patient's physical status. Surgical intervention is the primary treatment for most spinal cord tumors followed by chemotherapy and radiation therapy.

Extramedullary-extradural spinal cord compression occurs in 5% to 7% of patients who die of cancer and is considered a neurologic emergency (Kaplow & Iyere, 2016). For the patient with spinal cord compression resulting from metastatic cancer (most commonly from breast, prostate, or lung), high-dose dexamethasone combined with radiation therapy is effective in relieving pain (see Chapter 12 for a discussion of care of the patient with spinal cord compression). Palliative care may be an option for the medical management of some patients. Chemotherapy specific to the tumor type may be considered (AANN, 2016).

Surgical Management

Tumor removal is desirable but not always possible. The goal is to remove as much tumor as possible while sparing uninvolved portions of the spinal cord. Sudden decrease or loss of motor, sensory, and bowel and bladder function indicates the need for emergent surgery to reestablish function and protect the cord from further damage (Hickey & Strayer, 2020). Microsurgical techniques have improved the prognosis for patients with intramedullary tumors. Extramedullary-intradural tumors may be completely resected. Prognosis is related to the degree of neurologic impairment at the time of surgery, the speed with which symptoms occurred, and the origin of the tumor. Patients with extensive neurologic deficits before surgery are less likely to regain full functional recovery after successful tumor removal.

Nursing Management

Providing Preoperative Care

The objectives of preoperative care include recognition of neurologic changes through ongoing assessments, pain control, and management of altered activities of daily living (ADLs) resulting from sensory and motor deficits and bowel and bladder dysfunction. The nurse assesses for weakness, muscle wasting, spasticity, sensory changes, bowel and bladder dysfunction, and potential respiratory problems, especially if a cervical tumor is present. The patient is also evaluated for coagulation deficiencies. A history of anticoagulation medication use is obtained and reported, because the use of these may impede hemostasis postoperatively. The patient is educated about breathing exercises, and they are demonstrated preoperatively. Postoperative pain management strategies are discussed with the patient before surgery.

Assessing the Patient After Surgery

The patient is monitored for deterioration in status with frequent and targeted assessments of vital signs and neurologic examinations (Hickey & Strayer, 2020). A sudden onset of neurologic deficit is an ominous sign and may be due to spinal cord ischemia or infarction. Frequent neurologic checks are carried out, with emphasis on movement, strength, and sensation of the upper and lower extremities. Assessment of sensory function involves pinching the skin of the arms, legs, and trunk to determine if there is loss of feeling and, if so, at what level. Vital signs are monitored at regular intervals to detect and treat potential complications early (Hemmer, 2018).

Managing Pain

The prescribed pain medication should be given in adequate amounts and at appropriate intervals to relieve pain and prevent its recurrence. Pain is the hallmark of spinal metastasis.

Patients with sensory root involvement may suffer excruciating pain, which requires effective pain management.

The bed is usually kept flat initially. The nurse turns the patient as a unit, keeping shoulders and hips aligned and the back straight (also referred to as logrolling) (see discussion later in chapter). The side-lying position is usually the most comfortable, because this position imposes the least pressure on the surgical site. Placement of a pillow between the knees of the patient in a side-lying position helps to prevent extreme knee flexion.

Monitoring and Managing Potential Complications

If the tumor was in the cervical area, respiratory compromise due to postoperative edema may occur (Kaplow & Iyere, 2016). The nurse monitors the patient for asymmetric chest movement, abdominal breathing, and abnormal breath sounds. For a high cervical lesion, the endotracheal tube remains in place until adequate respiratory function is ensured. The patient is encouraged to perform deep-breathing and coughing exercises.

The area over the bladder is palpated or a bladder scan performed to assess for urinary retention (see Chapter 47, Fig. 47-8). The nurse also monitors for incontinence, because urinary dysfunction usually implies significant decompensation of spinal cord function. An intake and output record is maintained. In addition, the abdomen is auscultated for bowel sounds.

Staining of the dressing may indicate leakage of CSF from the surgical site, which may lead to serious infection or to an inflammatory reaction in the surrounding tissues that can cause severe pain in the postoperative period. Bulging at the incision may indicate contained CSF leak. The site should be monitored for increasing bulging, known as pseudomeningocele, which may require surgical repair (Alattar, Hirshman, McCutcheon, et al., 2018; Hickey & Strayer, 2020).

Promoting Home, Community-Based, and Transitional Care

 Educating Patients About Self-Care

In preparation for discharge, the patient is assessed for the ability to function independently in the home and for the availability of resources such as family members to assist in caregiving. Patients with residual sensory involvement are cautioned about the dangers of extremes in temperature. They should be educated about the dangers of heating devices (e.g., hot water bottles, heating pads, space heaters) as their sensory integration may be impaired, causing them to lose the ability to detect dangerous stimulations and to react appropriately. The patient is educated to check skin integrity daily. Patients with impaired motor function related to motor weakness or paralysis may require training in ADLs and safe use of assistive devices, such as a cane, walker, or wheelchair. The patient and family members are educated about pain management strategies, bowel and bladder management, and assessment for signs and symptoms that should be reported promptly (see Chart 65-2).

Continuing and Transitional Care

Referral for inpatient or outpatient rehabilitation may be warranted to improve self-care abilities. A consultation for home, community-based, or transitional care may be indicated and provides the nurse with the opportunity to assess the patient's physical and psychological status and the patient's and family's ability to adhere to recommended management strategies. During the home visit, the nurse determines whether changes in neurologic function have occurred. The patient's respiratory status and nutritional status are assessed. The adequacy of pain management is assessed, and modifications are made to ensure adequate pain relief. The need for hospice services or placement in an extended care facility is discussed with the patient and family if warranted, and the patient is asked about preferences for end-of-life care. In addition, social workers may be consulted to assist the patient and family members in identifying support services that can provide help in coping with the disease process (Hickey & Strayer, 2020).

DEGENERATIVE DISORDERS

Disorders of the central and peripheral nervous system that are **neurodegenerative** (leading to deterioration of normal cells or function of the nervous system) are characterized by the slow onset of signs and symptoms. Patients are managed at home for as long as possible and are admitted to the acute care setting for exacerbations, treatments, and surgical interventions as needed.

Parkinson's Disease

PD is a slowly progressing neurologic movement disorder that eventually leads to disability. It affects about 1 million patients who are hospitalized in the United States each year (Moore, Smith, & Cho, 2017). The disease affects men more often than women. Symptoms usually first appear in the fifth decade of life; however, cases have been diagnosed as early as 30 years of age. The degenerative or idiopathic form of PD is the most common; there is also a secondary form with a known or suspected cause. Although the cause of most cases is unknown, research suggests a multifactorial combination of age, environment, and heredity (AANN, 2019).

Pathophysiology

PD is associated with decreased levels of dopamine resulting from degeneration of dopamine storage cells in the substantia nigra in the basal ganglia region of the brain (see Fig. 65-3). Fibers or neuronal pathways project from the substantia nigra to the corpus striatum, where neurotransmitters are vital to the control of complex body movements. Through the neurotransmitters acetylcholine (excitatory) and dopamine (inhibitory), striatal neurons relay messages to the higher motor centers that control and refine motor movements. The loss of dopamine stores in this area of the brain results in more excitatory neurotransmitters than inhibitory neurotransmitters, leading to an imbalance that affects voluntary movement (Hickey & Strayer, 2020).

Clinical symptoms do not appear until 60% of the pigmented neurons are lost and the striatal dopamine level is decreased by 80%. Cellular degeneration impairs the extrapyramidal tracts that control semiautomatic functions and coordinated movements; motor cells of the motor cortex and the pyramidal tracts are not affected. Researchers are working

Physiology/Pathophysiology

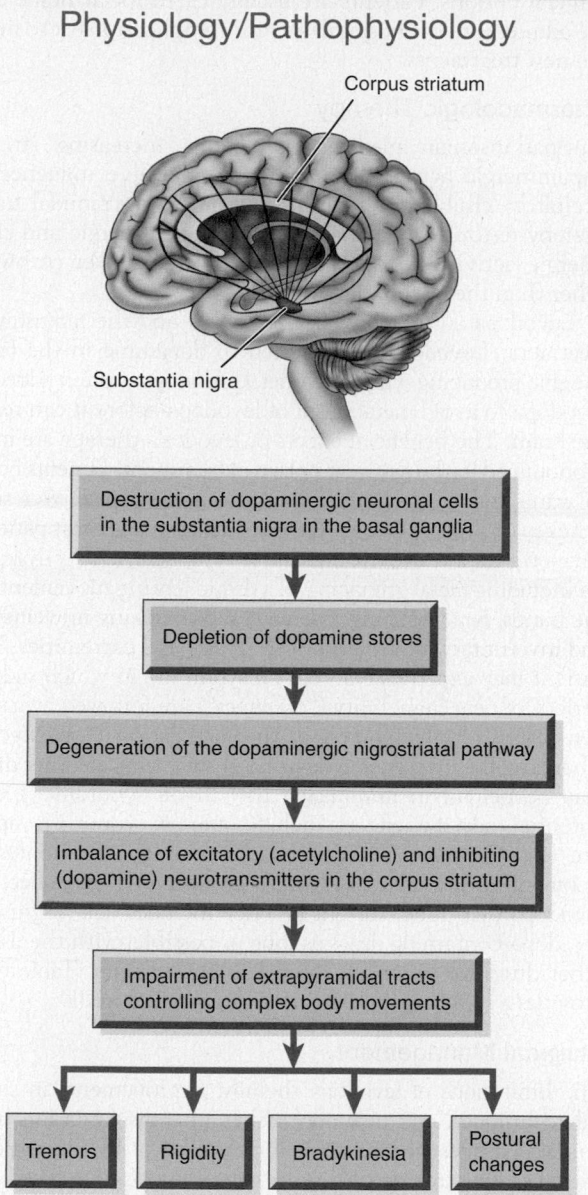

Figure 65-3 • Pathophysiology of Parkinson's disease. The nuclei in the substantia nigra project fibers to the corpus striatum. The nerve fibers carry dopamine to the corpus striatum. The loss of dopamine nerve cells from the brain's substantia nigra is thought to be responsible for the symptoms of Parkinson's disease.

on uncovering the exact mechanism of neurodegeneration. Current theories suggest a combined and complicated interweaving of both environmental and genetic factors that affect numerous fundamental cellular processes. Fifteen percent of early PD cases are associated with multiple genetic mutations (Poewe, Seppi, Tanner, et al., 2017). Ongoing research includes recognition of biomarkers and development of individualized treatment options (Poewe et al., 2017).

Clinical Manifestations

PD has a gradual onset, and symptoms progress slowly over a chronic, prolonged course. The cardinal signs are tremor, rigidity, bradykinesia/akinesia, and postural instability

(Hickey & Strayer, 2020). Two major subtypes of PD are tremor dominant (most other symptoms are absent) and non-tremor dominant (akinetic-rigid and postural instability).

Tremor

Although symptoms are variable, a slow, unilateral resting tremor is present in the majority of patients at the time of diagnosis. Resting tremor characteristically disappears with purposeful movement and during sleep but is evident when the extremities are motionless or at rest. The tremor may manifest as a rhythmic, slow turning motion (pronation–supination) of the forearm and the hand and a motion of the thumb against the fingers as if rolling a pill between the fingers.

Rigidity

Resistance to passive limb movement characterizes muscle rigidity. Passive movement of an extremity may cause the limb to move in jerky increments, referred to as lead-pipe or cogwheel movements. Involuntary stiffness of the passive extremity increases when another extremity is engaged in voluntary active movement. Stiffness of the arms, legs, face, and posture are common. Early in the disease, the patient may complain of shoulder pain due to rigidity (Hickey & Strayer, 2020).

Bradykinesia

A common feature of PD is **bradykinesia**, which refers to the overall slowing of active movement (Bronner & Korczyn, 2017). Patients may also take longer to complete activities and have difficulty initiating movement, such as rising from a sitting position or turning in bed.

Postural Instability

The patient commonly develops postural and gait problems. Due to a loss of postural reflexes, the patient stands with the head bent forward and walks with a propulsive gait. The posture is caused by the forward flexion of the neck, hips, knees, and elbows. The patient may walk faster and faster, trying to move the feet forward under the body's center of gravity (shuffling gait). Difficulty in pivoting causes loss of balance, either forward (propulsion) or backward (retropulsion). Gait impairment and postural instability place the patient at increased risk for falls (Hickey & Strayer, 2020).

Other Manifestations

The effect of PD on the basal ganglia often produces autonomic symptoms that include excessive and uncontrolled sweating, drooling, paroxysmal flushing, orthostatic hypotension, gastric and urinary retention, constipation, and sexual dysfunction (Bronner & Korczyn, 2017). Dysphagia is a substantial problem, with more than 50% of patients reporting choking as well as vision and olfactory changes (AANN, 2019). Neurogenic orthostatic hypotension occurs in 30% to 50% of patients with PD (Sin & Khemani, 2020).

Psychiatric changes include depression, anxiety, dementia, delirium, hallucinations, and psychosis. Depression and anxiety are common; whether these are reactions to the disorder or related to a biochemical abnormality is uncertain (AANN, 2019). Stress, medications, and depression contribute to the cognitive changes of diminished executive functions, attention difficulties, decreased thinking, and word-finding challenges. More than 80% of patients with a 20-year disease duration of PD experience **dementia,** a broad term for a syndrome characterized by a general decline in higher brain functioning, such as reasoning, with a pattern of eventual decline in ability to perform even basic ADLs, such as toileting and eating (Gale, Acar, & Daffner, 2018). In addition, auditory and visual hallucinations have been reported in people with PD and may be associated with depression, dementia, lack of sleep, or adverse effects of medications.

Hypokinesia (abnormally diminished movement) is also common and may appear after the tremor. The freezing phenomenon refers to a transient inability to perform active movement and is thought to be an extreme form of bradykinesia. The patient tends to shuffle and exhibits a decreased arm swing as well. As dexterity declines, micrographia (small handwriting) develops. The face becomes increasingly masklike and expressionless, and the frequency of blinking decreases. **Dysphonia** (voice impairment or altered voice production) may occur as a result of weakness and incoordination of the muscles responsible for speech. In many cases, the patient develops dysphagia, begins to drool, and is at risk for choking and aspiration (AANN, 2019).

Complications associated with PD are common and are typically related to disorders of movement. As the disease progresses, patients are at risk for respiratory and urinary tract infection, skin breakdown, and injury from falls. The adverse effects of medications used to treat the symptoms are associated with numerous complications such as **dyskinesia** (impaired ability to execute voluntary movements) or orthostatic hypotension.

Assessment and Diagnostic Findings

Although laboratory tests and imaging studies are not helpful to the provider in diagnosing PD, ongoing research with PET and single-photon emission CT scanning has been helpful in understanding the disease and advancing treatment. Currently, the disease is diagnosed clinically from the patient's history and the presence of two of the four cardinal manifestations: tremor, rigidity, bradykinesia, and postural changes.

Early diagnosis can be challenging because patients rarely are able to pinpoint when the symptoms started. Often, a family member notices a change such as stooped posture; a stiff arm; a slight limp; tremor; or slow, small handwriting. The medical history, presenting symptoms, neurologic examination, and response to pharmacologic management are carefully evaluated when making the diagnosis. Diagnosis is often confirmed by a positive response to a levodopa trial (Hickey & Strayer, 2020).

The Revised Movement Disorder Society Unified Parkinson Disease Rating Scale (MDS-UPDRS) is a helpful assessment tool as it measures the disease progression including motor and nonmotor symptoms, and includes treatment complications (AANN, 2019).

Medical Management

Treatment is directed toward controlling symptoms and maintaining functional independence, because no medical or surgical approaches in current use prevent disease progression (AANN, 2019). Care is individualized for each patient based on presenting symptoms and social, occupational, and emotional needs. Pharmacologic management is the mainstay of treatment, although advances in research have led to more surgical options. Patients are usually cared for at home and are admitted to the hospital only for complications or to initiate new treatments.

Pharmacologic Therapy

Antiparkinsonian medications act by increasing striatal dopaminergic activity; reducing the excessive influence of excitatory cholinergic neurons on the extrapyramidal tract, thereby restoring a balance between dopaminergic and cholinergic activities; or acting on neurotransmitter pathways other than the dopaminergic pathway.

Levodopa is the most effective agent and the mainstay of treatment. Levodopa is converted to dopamine in the basal ganglia, producing symptom relief. Carbidopa is often added to levodopa to avoid metabolism of levodopa before it can reach the brain. The beneficial effects of levodopa therapy are most pronounced in the first year or two of treatment. Benefits begin to wane and adverse effects become more severe over time (Hickey & Strayer, 2020). Within 5 to 10 years, most patients develop a response to the medication characterized by dyskinesia including facial grimacing, rhythmic jerking movements of the hands, head bobbing, chewing and smacking movements, and involuntary movements of the trunk and extremities. The patient may experience an on–off syndrome in which sudden periods of near immobility ("off effect") are followed by a sudden return of effectiveness of the medication ("on effect"). Changing the drug dosing regimen or switching to other drugs may be helpful in minimizing the on–off syndrome. Other potential adverse effects include nausea, vomiting, appetite loss, decreased BP, dystonia, dyskinesia, and confusion (Comerford & Durkin, 2020). To minimize adverse effects of levodopa over time, current practice includes delaying use of levodopa-containing drugs as long as possible, with the use of other drugs for symptom control in the interim. Table 65-1 provides a summary of select medications used in PD.

Surgical Management

The limitations of levodopa therapy, improvements in surgical techniques, and new approaches in transplantation have renewed interest in the surgical treatment of PD. In patients with disabling tremor, rigidity, or severe levodopa-induced dyskinesia, surgery may be considered. Although surgery provides symptom relief in select patients, it has not been shown to alter the course of the disease or to produce permanent improvement.

Stereotactic Procedures

Thalamotomy and pallidotomy are ablative procedures that were formerly used to relieve symptoms of PD such as tremors. However, these procedures permanently destroy brain tissue and are rarely used today. Deep brain stimulation (DBS) has largely replaced ablative procedures in the surgical treatment of PD. DBS involves surgical implantation of an electrode into the brain in either the globus pallidus or subthalamic nucleus. Stimulation of these areas may increase dopamine release or block anticholinergic release, thereby improving tremor and rigidity. Levodopa medication dose may be able to be reduced, thus improving dyskinesias.

Patients eligible for DBS are those who have responded to levodopa but are impaired by dyskinesias, have had the disease for at least 5 years, and are disabled by tremor. Patients with dementia and atypical PD are usually not considered for surgical

TABLE 65-1 Select Medications Used to Treat Parkinson's Disease		
Medications	**Indications and Therapeutic Effects**	**Common Side Effects**
Anticholinergic Agents		
trihexyphenidyl hydrochloride	Control of tremor in patients with early-onset disease	Blurred vision, flushing, rash, constipation, urinary retention, and acute confusional states
benztropine mesylate	Counteract the action of acetylcholine	Contraindicated in patients with narrow-angle glaucoma
Antiviral Agent		
amantadine hydrochloride	Reduce rigidity, tremor, bradykinesia, and postural changes in early Parkinson's disease (PD)	Psychiatric disturbances (mood changes, confusion, depression, hallucinations), lower extremity edema, nausea, epigastric distress, urinary retention, headache, and visual impairment
Dopamine Agonists		
bromocriptine mesylate	Early PD as well as secondary drug therapy after carbidopa or levodopa loses effectiveness	Nausea, vomiting, diarrhea, lightheadedness, hypotension, impotence, and psychiatric effects
pergolide		
Nonergot Derivatives		
ropinirole hydrochloride	Early stages of PD	May cause drowsiness or dizziness
pramipexole		
Monoamine Oxidase-Inhibitors		
selegiline	Inhibit dopamine breakdown	Agitation, dizziness, nausea, headache, rhinitis, back pain, stomatitis, orthostatic hypotension, insomnia
rasagiline		
Catechol-O-Methyltransferase Inhibitors		
entacapone	Increase the duration of action of carbidopa or levodopa	Abdominal pain, back pain, constipation, nausea, diarrhea, blood in urine
tolcapone	Reduce motor fluctuations in patients with advanced PD	

Adapted from Moore, D. J., Smith, B. M., & Cho, M. H. (2017). Managing meditations for hospital patients with Parkinson disease. *American Nurse Today, 12*(1), 9–12.

procedures. PD rating scales and specific neurologic tests are used to identify patients who are eligible. Surgical treatment typically occurs 10 to 13 years after diagnosis (AANN, 2019).

A CT or MRI scan is used to localize the appropriate surgical site in the brain. Then, the patient's head is positioned in a stereotactic frame (see Fig. 65-4). After the surgeon makes an incision in the skin and a burr hole, an electrode is passed through to the target area to the subthalamic nuclei or globus pallidus. The desired response of the patient to the electrical stimulation (i.e., a decrease in rigidity) is used to confirm electrode placement. Electrode placement is completed on one side of the brain at a time; bilateral electrodes are usually placed (AANN, 2019). Electrodes are then connected to a pulse generator that is implanted in a subcutaneous subclavicular or abdominal pouch (see Fig. 65-5). The battery-powered

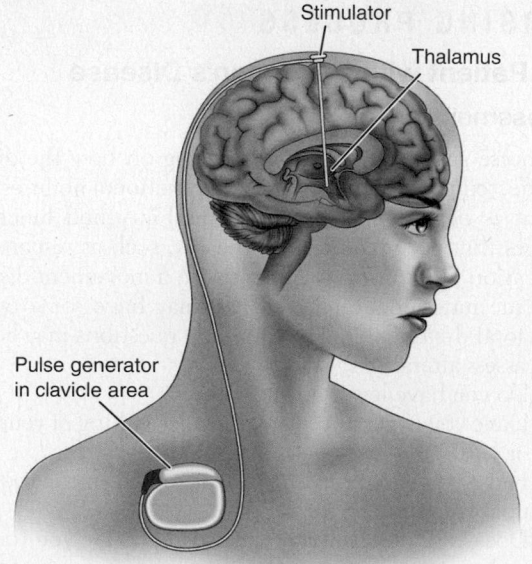

Stimulator

Thalamus

Pulse generator in clavicle area

Figure 65-4 • A stereotactic frame is applied to a patient's head in preparation for deep brain stimulation. The frame provides external points of reference.

Figure 65-5 • Deep brain stimulation is provided by a pulse generator surgically implanted in a pouch beneath the clavicle. The generator sends high-frequency electrical impulses to the thalamus, thereby blocking the nerve pathways associated with tremors in Parkinson's disease.

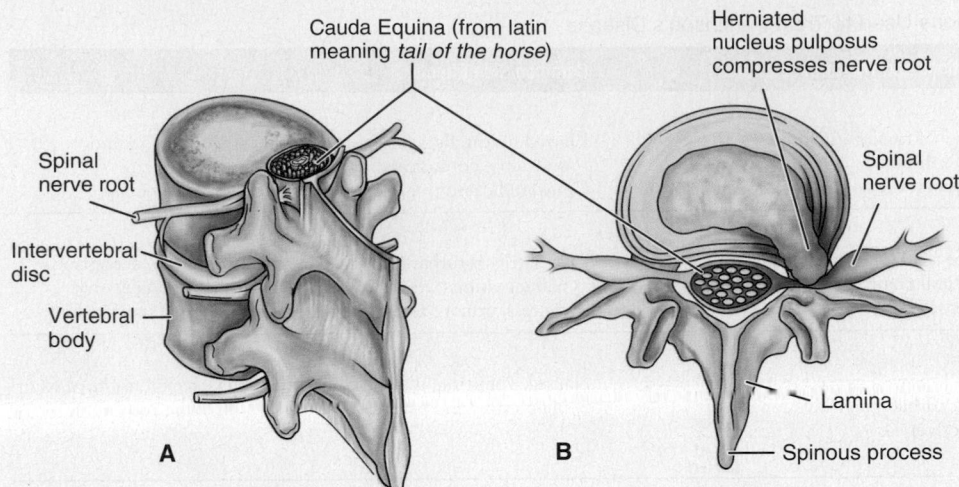

Figure 65-6 • A. Normal lumbar spine vertebrae, invertebral discs, and spinal nerve root. **B.** Ruptured vertebral disc.

Labels: Cauda Equina (from latin meaning *tail of the horse*); Spinal nerve root; Intervertebral disc; Vertebral body; **A**; Herniated nucleus pulposus compresses nerve root; Spinal nerve root; Lamina; Spinous process; **B**

pulse generator sends high-frequency electrical impulses through a wire placed under the skin to a lead anchored to the skull (see Fig. 65-6). These devices are not without complications that can result from both the surgical procedure needed for implantation (e.g., weakness, paresthesias, confusion, hemorrhage) and the device itself (e.g., infection, lead leakage) (Hickey & Strayer, 2020).

Neural Transplantation

Ongoing research is exploring transplantation of porcine neuronal cells, human fetal cells, and stem cells to replace degenerated striatal cells (Kirkeby, Parmar, & Barker, 2017). Legal, ethical, and political concerns surrounding the use of fetal brain cells and stem cells have limited the exploration of these procedures.

NURSING PROCESS

The Patient with Parkinson's Disease

Assessment

The nurse gathers information focusing on how the disease has affected the patient's ADLs and functional abilities. The patient is observed for degree of disability and functional changes that occur throughout the day, such as responses to medication. Almost every patient with a movement disorder has some functional alteration and may have some type of behavioral dysfunction. The following questions may be useful to assess alterations:

- Do you have leg or arm stiffness?
- Have you experienced any irregular jerking of your arms or legs?
- Have you ever been "frozen" or rooted to the spot and unable to move?
- Does your mouth water excessively? Have you (or others) noticed yourself grimacing or making faces or chewing movements?
- What specific activities do you have difficulty doing?
- Have you had any recent falls?

During this assessment, the nurse observes the patient for quality of speech, loss of facial expression, swallowing deficits

(drooling, poor head control, coughing), tremors, slowness of movement, weakness, forward posture, rigidity, evidence of mental slowness, and confusion. PD symptoms, as well as side effects of medications, put these patients at high risk for falls; therefore, a fall risk assessment should be conducted (Hickey & Strayer, 2020).

Diagnosis

NURSING DIAGNOSES

Based on the assessment data, major nursing diagnoses may include the following:

- Impaired mobility associated with muscle rigidity and postural impairment
- Impaired self-feeding, impaired ability to dress, impaired ability to perform hygiene, impaired self-toileting associated with tremor and muscle rigidity
- Constipation associated with medication and reduced activity
- Impaired nutritional intake associated with tremor, slowness in eating, difficulty in chewing and swallowing
- Impaired verbal communication associated with decreased speech volume, slowness of speech, inability to move facial muscles
- Difficulty coping associated with depression and dysfunction due to disease progression

COLLABORATIVE PROBLEMS/POTENTIAL COMPLICATIONS

Potential complications may include the following:

- Sleep disturbances
- Psychiatric disturbances

Planning and Goals

The goals for the patient may include improving functional mobility, maintaining independence in ADLs, achieving adequate bowel elimination, attaining and maintaining acceptable nutritional status, achieving effective communication, and developing positive coping mechanisms.

Nursing Interventions

IMPROVING MOBILITY

A progressive program of daily exercise will increase muscle strength, improve coordination and dexterity, reduce muscular rigidity, and prevent contractures that occur when muscles are not used (Hickey & Strayer, 2020). Walking, riding a stationary bicycle, swimming, and gardening are all exercises that help maintain joint mobility. Stretching (stretch–hold–relax) and range-of-motion exercises promote joint flexibility. Postural exercises are important to counter the tendency of the head and neck to be drawn forward and down. A physical therapist may be helpful in developing an individualized exercise program and can provide instruction to the patient and caregiver on exercising safely. Faithful adherence to an exercise and walking program helps delay the progress of the disease. Warm baths and massage, in addition to passive and active exercises, help relax muscles and relieve painful muscle spasms that accompany rigidity.

Balance may be adversely affected because of the rigidity of the arms (arm swinging is necessary in normal walking). Special walking techniques must be learned to offset the shuffling gait and the tendency to lean forward. The patient is educated to concentrate on walking erect, to watch the horizon, and to use a wide-based gait (i.e., walking with the feet separated). A conscious effort must be made to swing the arms, raise the feet while walking, and use a heel–toe placement of the feet with long strides. The patient is advised to practice walking to marching music or to the sound of a ticking metronome, because this provides sensory reinforcement. Performing breathing exercises while walking provides additional movement of the ribcage and aerates larger parts of the lungs. Frequent rest periods aid in preventing frustration and fatigue.

ENHANCING SELF-CARE ACTIVITIES

Encouraging, educating, and supporting the patient during ADLs promote self-care (Hickey & Strayer, 2020). Environmental modifications are necessary to compensate for functional disability. Patients may have severe mobility problems that make normal activities impossible. Adaptive or assistive devices may be useful. A hospital bed at home with bedside rails, an over-bed frame with a trapeze, or a rope tied to the foot of the bed can provide assistance in pulling up without help. An occupational therapist can evaluate the patient's needs in the home, make recommendations regarding adaptive devices, and educate the patient and caregiver how to improvise.

IMPROVING BOWEL ELIMINATION

The patient may have severe problems with constipation. Among the factors causing constipation are weakness of the muscles used in defecation, lack of exercise, inadequate fluid intake, and decreased autonomic nervous system activity. The medications used for the treatment of the disease also inhibit normal intestinal secretions. A regular bowel routine may be established by encouraging the patient to follow a regular time pattern, consciously increase fluid intake, and eat foods with moderate fiber content. Laxatives should be avoided. Psyllium, for example, decreases constipation but carries the risk of bowel obstruction (Comerford & Durkin, 2020). A raised toilet seat is useful because the patient has difficulty in moving from a standing to a sitting position. Additional time may be needed for the patient to navigate to the toilet due to gait disturbances.

IMPROVING NUTRITION

Patients may have difficulty maintaining their weight. Eating becomes a very slow process, requiring concentration due to a dry mouth from medications and difficulty chewing and swallowing. These patients are at risk for aspiration because of impaired swallowing and the accumulation of saliva. They may be unaware that they are aspirating; subsequently, pneumonia may develop (Aslam, Simpson, Baugh, et al., 2019).

Monitoring weight on a weekly basis indicates whether caloric intake is adequate. Supplemental feedings increase caloric intake. As the disease progresses, a nasogastric or percutaneous endoscopic gastrostomy (PEG) tube may be necessary to maintain adequate nutrition. A consultation with dietitian may be indicated.

ENHANCING SWALLOWING

Swallowing difficulties and choking are common in PD, leading to aspiration and pneumonia. To offset the aspiration risk, the patient should sit in an upright position during mealtime (Aslam et al., 2019). A semisolid diet with thick liquids is easier to swallow than solids; thin liquids should be avoided. The patient is instructed to think through the swallowing sequence, place the food on the tongue, close the lips and teeth, lift the tongue up and then back, and swallow. The patient is encouraged to chew first on one side of the mouth and then on the other. To control the buildup of saliva, the patient is reminded to hold the head upright and make a conscious effort to swallow. Massaging the facial and neck muscles before meals may be beneficial.

ENCOURAGING THE USE OF ASSISTIVE DEVICES

An electric warming tray keeps food hot and allows the patient to rest during the prolonged time that it may take to eat. Special utensils also assist at mealtime. A plate that is stabilized, a nonspill cup, and eating utensils with built-up handles are useful self-help devices. The occupational therapist can assist in identifying appropriate adaptive devices.

IMPROVING COMMUNICATION

Speech disorders are present in most patients with PD. The low-pitched, monotonous, soft speech of patients requires that they make a conscious effort to speak slowly, with deliberate attention to what they are saying. The patient is reminded to face the listener, exaggerate the pronunciation of words, speak in short sentences, and take a few deep breaths before speaking. A speech therapist may be helpful in designing speech improvement exercises and assisting the family and health care personnel to develop and use a method of communication that meets the patient's needs. A small electronic amplifier is helpful if the patient has difficulty being heard.

SUPPORTING COPING ABILITIES

Support can be given by encouraging the patient and pointing out that activities will be maintained through active participation. Patients with PD can become socially and emotionally withdrawn. It is best if patients are active participants in their therapeutic program, including social and recreational events.

Patients often feel embarrassed, apathetic, inadequate, bored, and lonely. In part, these feelings may result from physical slowness and the great effort that even small tasks require. The patient is assisted and encouraged to set achievable goals (e.g., improvement of mobility). Every effort should be made to encourage patients to carry out the tasks involved in meeting their own daily needs and to remain independent. Doing things for the patient merely to save time undermines the basic goal of improving coping abilities and promoting a positive self-concept.

MONITORING AND MANAGING POTENTIAL COMPLICATIONS

A planned program of activity throughout the day prevents too much daytime sleeping as well as disinterest and apathy. When sleep disturbances occur, several interventions can improve sleep, including limiting caffeine intake before bedtime and assessing for nocturia.

The patient with PD is monitored regularly for signs and symptoms of depression. An interprofessional approach with a combination of physiotherapy, psychotherapy, medication therapy, and support group participation is used to treat depression when diagnosed (Hickey & Strayer, 2020).

The patient in late stages of PD is particularly at risk for psychiatric disturbances such as hallucinations, psychosis, and paranoid delusions (Hickey & Strayer, 2020). Interventions to manage psychiatric disturbances include low doses of antipsychotic drugs, minimizing medications with psychiatric side effects (see Table 65-1), and avoidance of dopamine depleting medications (Hickey & Strayer, 2020). Patients and their caregivers benefit from an interprofessional approach to care when psychiatric disturbances are present.

PROMOTING HOME, COMMUNITY-BASED, OR TRANSITIONAL CARE

Educating Patients About Self-Care. Patient and family education is important in the management of PD. The needs depend on the severity of symptoms and the stage of the disease. Care must be taken not to overwhelm the patient and family with too much information early in the disease process. Ongoing assessment, intervention, and evaluation of the patient and family's adaptations and education requirements are necessary with every encounter. The strategies to promote health include a clear explanation of the disease and the goal of assisting the patient to remain functionally independent as long as possible (see Chart 65-3). The patient and family must be educated about the effects and side effects of medications and about the importance of reporting side effects to the primary provider. Nurses in the home help patients and their families enhance self-management and quality of life.

Continuing and Transitional Care. Family members and partners often serve as caregivers, with home, community-based, or transitional services available to assist in meeting health care needs as the disease progresses. The caregiver may be under considerable stress from living with and caring for a person with a significant disability. Providing information about treatment and care helps anticipate future needs. The caregiver is included in the plan and may be advised to learn stress reduction techniques, to include others in the caregiving process, to obtain periodic relief from responsibilities, and to have a yearly health assessment. Allowing family members and partners to express feelings of frustration, anger, and guilt is often helpful to them.

The patient should be evaluated in the home for adaptation and safety needs and adherence to the plan of care. In the advanced stages, patients usually enter long-term care facilities. Periodically, admission to an acute care facility may be necessary for changes in medical management or treatment of complications. Nurses provide support, education, and monitoring of patients over the course of the illness.

Chart 65-3 — HEALTH PROMOTION
Strategies for the Patient with PD

To promote optimal health, the nurse works closely with the patient and family to ensure that they understand:

- How PD and its treatment impact physiologic functioning, ADLs, IADLs, roles, relationships, and spirituality
- The importance of adhering to the prescribed medication regimen; including knowing the purpose, dose, route, schedule, side effects, and precautions for all medications
- How and when to contact all members of the treatment team (e.g., health care providers, home care professionals, and durable medical equipment and supply vendors)
- Specific types of environmental and safety changes or support that will allow optimum functioning in the home
- The risk of falls/injury and how to implement fall prevention and adaptive measures in the home

In addition, the nurse advises the patient and family about lifestyle changes that are necessary to maintain health and promote self-care and independence. These include:

- Ensuring nutritional needs, including adhering to dietary restrictions, managing dysphagia, and preventing aspiration
- Promoting speech and communication skills: speech exercises, communication techniques, breathing exercises
- Managing constipation: fluid intake, bowel routine
- Managing urinary problems: functional incontinence, retention (indwelling urinary catheter care, suprapubic catheter care)
- Avoiding the effects of immobility and promoting the advantages of preventive care: skin breakdown (frequent turning, pressure release, skin care), pneumonia (deep breathing, movement), contractures (range-of-motion exercises)
- Promoting the benefits of a daily exercise program
- Ensuring safe walking and balancing
- Using appropriate coping mechanisms and diversional activities

ADLs, activities of daily living; IADLs, instrumental activities of daily living; PD, Parkinson's disease.

The nurse involved in home and continuing care educates the patient and family members about the importance of addressing health promotion needs such as screening for hypertension and stroke risk assessments in this predominantly older adult population. Patients are referred to appropriate health care providers. Information is available from both the Parkinson's Foundation and the American Parkinson Disease Association (see the Resources section).

Evaluation

Expected patient outcomes may include:
1. Strives toward improved mobility
   a. Participates in exercise program daily
   b. Walks with wide base of support; exaggerates arm swinging when walking
   c. Takes medications as prescribed
2. Progresses toward self-care
   a. Allows time for self-care activities
   b. Uses self-help devices
3. Maintains bowel function
   a. Consumes adequate fluid
   b. Increases dietary intake of fiber
   c. Reports regular pattern of bowel function
4. Attains improved nutritional status
   a. Swallows without aspiration
   b. Takes time while eating

5. Achieves a method of communication
   a. Communicates needs
   b. Practices speech exercises
6. Copes with effects of PD
   a. Sets realistic goals
   b. Demonstrates persistence in meaningful activities
   c. Verbalizes feelings to appropriate person

Huntington Disease

Huntington disease is a chronic, progressive, hereditary disease of the nervous system that results in progressive involuntary choreiform movement and dementia. The disease affects approximately 1 in 10,000 men or women of all races at midlife. Every person has the gene that causes Huntington disease; however, only those who inherit the expansion of the gene will develop the disease and pass it onto their children. Because it is transmitted by an autosomal dominant gene, each child of a parent with Huntington disease has a 50% risk of inheriting the disorder (Smedley & Coulson, 2019).

A genetic mutation in Huntington disease, the presence of a repeat in the Huntington gene (*HTT*), has been identified (Smedley & Coulson, 2019). Genetic testing can identify people who will develop this disease but cannot predict timing of disease onset. Although the gene was mapped in 1983, patients may choose not to be tested because of concerns about employment and health care discrimination. People of childbearing age with a family history of Huntington disease often seek information about their risk of disease transmission. Genetic counseling is crucial, and patients and their families may require long-term psychological counseling and emotional, financial, and legal support (see Chapter 6).

Pathophysiology

The basic pathology involves premature death of cells in the striatum (caudate and putamen) of the basal ganglia, the region deep within the brain that is involved in the control of movement. Cells also are lost in the cortex, the region of the brain associated with thinking, memory, perception, judgment, and behavior, and in the cerebellum, the area that coordinates voluntary muscle activity. Why the protein destroys only certain brain cells is unknown, but several theories have been proposed to explain the phenomenon. One possible theory is that glutamine, a building block for protein, abnormally collects in the cell nucleus, causing cell death (McColgan & Tabrizi, 2017).

Clinical Manifestations

This condition is characterized by a triad of symptoms that includes motor dysfunction (the most prominent is **chorea**, or rapid, jerky, involuntary, purposeless movements); cognitive impairment (problems with attention and emotion recognition); and behavioral features, such as apathy and blunted affect (McColgan & Tabrizi, 2017). As the disease progresses, constant writhing, twisting, and uncontrollable movements may involve the entire body. These motions are devoid of purpose or rhythm, although patients may try to turn them into purposeful movement. All of the body musculature is involved. Facial movements produce tics and grimaces.

Speech becomes slurred, hesitant, often explosive, and eventually unintelligible. Chewing and swallowing are difficult, and there is a constant danger of choking and aspiration. Choreiform movements persist during sleep but are diminished (Mestre & Shannon, 2017).

As with speech, the gait becomes disorganized to the point that ambulation eventually is impossible. Although independent ambulation should be encouraged for as long as possible, a wheelchair usually becomes necessary. Eventually, the patient is confined to bed when the chorea interferes with walking, sitting, and all other activities. Bladder and bowel control are lost.

Cognitive impairment, such as problems with attention or recognizing emotions, occurs early on; in later stages, marked dementia is present. Initially, the patient is aware that the disease is responsible for the myriad dysfunctions that are occurring.

The behavioral changes may be more devastating to the patient and family than the abnormal movements. Personality changes may result in nervous, irritable, or impatient behaviors. In the early stages, patients are particularly subject to uncontrollable fits of anger, profound and often suicidal depression, apathy, anxiety, psychosis, or euphoria. Judgment and memory are impaired, and dementia eventually ensues (Mestre & Shannon, 2017). Hallucinations, delusions, and paranoid thinking may precede the appearance of disjointed movements. Emotional and cognitive symptoms often become less acute as the disease progresses (Mestre & Shannon, 2017).

Onset usually occurs between 35 and 45 years of age, although about 10% of patients are children. The disease progresses slowly. Despite a ravenous appetite, patients usually become emaciated and exhausted. Patients succumb in 10 to 20 years to heart failure, pneumonia, or infection, or as a result of a fall or choking (Mestre & Shannon, 2017).

Assessment and Diagnostic Findings

The diagnosis is made based on the clinical presentation of characteristic symptoms, a positive family history, and the known presence of the genetic marker cytosine-adenine-guanine (CAG) repeating on the Huntington gene (HTT) (Smedley & Coulson, 2019). CT or MRI scans show symmetrical striatal atrophy before motor symptoms appear (Urrutia, 2019).

Medical Management

No treatment halts or reverses the underlying process; therefore, the focus is on optimizing quality of life with available medication and supportive treatment. Patients experience the most benefit when they have integrated expertise of a Huntington disease multidisciplinary team (Urrutia, 2019). The only medication that is approved by the U.S. Food and Drug Administration to treat the symptom of chorea is tetrabenazine (Comerford & Durkin, 2020).

Benzodiazepines and neuroleptic drugs have also been reported to control chorea. Motor signs must be assessed and evaluated on an ongoing basis so that optimal therapeutic drug levels can be reached. Akathisia (motor restlessness) in the patient who is overmedicated is dangerous because it may be mistaken for the restless fidgeting of the illness and consequently may be overlooked. In certain types of the disease, hypokinetic motor impairment resembles PD. In patients who present with rigidity, some temporary benefit may be obtained from antiparkinson medications, such as levodopa.

Selective serotonin reuptake inhibitors and tricyclic antidepressants have been recommended for control of psychiatric symptoms. The threat of suicide is present particularly early in the course of the disease. Psychotic symptoms usually respond to antipsychotic medications. Psychotherapy aimed at allaying anxiety and reducing stress may be beneficial. Nurses must look beyond the disease to focus on the patient's needs and capabilities (see Chart 65-4).

Promoting Home, Community-Based, and Transitional Care

 Educating Patients About Self-Care

The needs of the patient and family for education depend on the nature and severity of the physical, cognitive, and psychological changes experienced by the patient. The patient and family members are educated about the medications prescribed and about signs indicating a need for change in medication or dosage. The educational plan addresses strategies to manage symptoms such as chorea, swallowing problems, limitations in ambulation, memory loss, irritability, depression, and loss of bowel and bladder function. Consultation with a speech therapist may be indicated to assist in identifying alternative communication strategies if speech is affected. A PEG tube may be considered for nutritional support later in the disease (Eliopoulos, 2018).

Continuing and Transitional Care

A program combining medical, nursing, psychological, social, occupational, speech, and physical rehabilitation services and palliative care is needed to help the patient and family cope with this severely disabling illness. Huntington disease exacts

---

Chart 65-4 Care of the Patient with Huntington Disease

Nursing Diagnosis: Risk for injury from falls and possible skin breakdown (pressure injury abrasions), resulting from constant movement

Nursing Interventions

Pad the sides and head of the bed; ensure that the patient can see over the sides of bed.
Use padded heel and elbow protectors.
Keep the skin meticulously clean.
Apply emollient cleansing agent and skin lotion as needed.
Use soft sheets and bedding.
Have patient wear football padding or other forms of padding.
Encourage ambulation with assistance to maintain muscle tone.
Secure the patient (only if necessary) in bed or chair with padded protective devices, making sure that they are loosened frequently.

Nursing Diagnosis: Impaired nutritional intake due to inadequate ingestion and dehydration resulting from swallowing or chewing disorders and danger of choking or aspirating food

Nursing Interventions

Administer phenothiazines (chlorpromazine) as prescribed before meals (calms some patients).
Talk to the patient before mealtime to promote relaxation; use mealtime for social interaction. Provide undivided attention and help the patient enjoy the mealtime experience.
Use a warming tray to keep food warm.
Learn the position that is best for *this* patient. Keep patient as close to upright as possible while feeding. Stabilize patient's head gently with one hand while feeding.
Show the food, explain what the foods are, and temperature (e.g., whether hot or cold).
Encircle the patient with one arm and get as close as possible to provide stability and support while feeding. Use pillows and wedges for additional support.
Do not interpret stiffness, turning away, or sudden turning of the head as rejection; these are uncontrollable choreiform movements.
For feeding, use a long-handled spoon (iced tea spoon). Place spoon on middle of tongue and exert slight pressure.
Place bite-sized food between patient's teeth. Serve stews, casseroles, and thick liquids.
Disregard messiness, and treat the person with dignity.

Wait for the patient to chew and swallow before introducing another spoonful. Make sure that bite-sized food is small.
Give between-meal feedings. Constant movement expends more calories. Patients often have voracious appetites, particularly for sweets.
Use blenderized meals if patient cannot chew; do not repeatedly give the same strained baby foods. Gradually introduce increased textures and consistencies to the diet.

For swallowing difficulties:

Apply gentle deep pressure around the patient's mouth.
Rub fingers in circles on the patient's cheeks and then down each side of the patient's throat.
Develop skill in the abdominal thrust (to be used in the event of choking).

Nursing Diagnosis: Impaired verbal communication from excessive grimacing and unintelligible speech

Nursing Interventions

Read to the patient.
Employ biofeedback and relaxation therapy to reduce stress.
Consult with speech therapist to help maintain and prolong communication abilities.
Try to devise a communication system, perhaps using cards with words or pictures of familiar objects, before verbal communication becomes too difficult. Patients can indicate correct card by hitting it with hand, grunting, or blinking the eyes.
Learn how this particular patient expresses needs and wants—particularly nonverbal messages (widening of eyes, responses).
Patients can understand even if unable to speak. Do not isolate patients by ceasing to communicate with them.

Nursing Diagnosis: Acute confusion and impaired socialisation

Nursing Interventions

Reorient the patient after awakening.
Have clock, calendar, and wall posters in view to assist in orientation.
Use every opportunity for one-to-one contact.
Use music for relaxation.
Have the patient wear a medical identification bracelet.
Keep the patient in the social mainstream.
Recruit and train volunteers for social interaction. Role-model appropriate and creative interactions.
Do not abandon a patient because the disease is terminal. Patients are *living* until the end.

enormous emotional, physical, social, and financial tolls on every member of the family. The family needs supportive care as they adjust to the impact of the illness. Regular follow-up visits help allay the fear of abandonment.

Home care assistance, day care centers, respite care, and eventually skilled long-term care can assist the patient and family in coping with the constant strain of the illness. Although the relentless progression of the disease cannot be halted, families can benefit from supportive care. Planning for end-of-life care should occur early in the disease (see Chapter 13).

Voluntary organizations can be major aids to families and have been largely responsible for bringing the illness to national attention. The Huntington Disease Society of America helps patients and families by providing information, referrals, family and public education, and support for research (see the Resources section).

Amyotrophic Lateral Sclerosis

ALS is a disease of unknown cause in which there is a loss of motor neurons (nerve cells controlling muscles) in the anterior horns of the spinal cord and the motor nuclei of the lower brainstem. It is often referred to as Lou Gehrig disease, after the famous baseball player who suffered from the disease. As motor neuron cells die, the muscle fibers that they supply undergo atrophic changes. Neuronal degeneration may occur in both the upper and lower motor neuron systems (see Chapter 60). The leading theory held by researchers is that overexcitation of nerve cells by the neurotransmitter glutamate results in cell injury and neuronal degeneration. Risk factors are noted in Chart 65-5.

ALS most commonly occurs between 40 and 60 years of age and affects all social, racial, and ethnic backgrounds, with men being affected at slightly higher rates than women. The majority of cases of ALS arise sporadically, but 5% to 10% of cases are familial ALS resulting from an autosomal dominant trait carried by one parent. Familial ALS occurs 10 years earlier than the ALS average, and those afflicted tend to have a shorter life span (Hardiman, Al-Chalabi, Chio, et al., 2017).

Clinical Manifestations

Clinical manifestations depend on the location of the affected motor neurons, because specific neurons activate specific muscle fibers. The chief symptoms are fatigue, progressive muscle weakness, cramps, fasciculations (twitching), and lack of coordination. Loss of motor neurons in the anterior horns of the spinal cord results in progressive weakness and atrophy

---

Chart 65-5 ⚠️ **RISK FACTORS**
Amyotrophic Lateral Sclerosis

- Age
- Autoimmune disease
- Environmental exposures to toxins
- Family history
- Smoking
- Viral infections

Adapted from Vacca, V. M. (2020). Amyotrophic lateral sclerosis: Nursing care and considerations. *Nursing, 50*(6), 32–39.

---

of the muscles of the arms, trunk, or legs. Spasticity usually is present, and the deep tendon stretch reflexes become brisk and overactive. Usually, the function of the anal and bladder sphincters remains intact, because the spinal nerves that control muscles of the rectum and urinary bladder are not affected.

In about 25% of patients, weakness starts in the muscles supplied by the cranial nerves, and difficulty in talking, swallowing, and ultimately breathing occurs (Conde, Martin, & Winck, 2019; Vacca, 2020). When the patient ingests liquids, soft palate and upper esophageal weakness cause the liquid to be regurgitated through the nose. Weakness of the posterior tongue and palate impairs the ability to laugh, cough, or even blow the nose. If bulbar muscles are impaired, speaking and swallowing are progressively difficult, and aspiration becomes a risk. The voice assumes a nasal sound, and articulation becomes so disrupted that speech is unintelligible. Some emotional lability may be present. It was traditionally believed that ALS spared cognitive function, but it is now recognized that some patients experience cognitive impairment.

The prognosis generally is based on the area of CNS involvement and the speed with which the disease progresses. Eventually, respiratory function is compromised (Conde et al., 2019). Death usually occurs as a result of infection, respiratory insufficiency, or aspiration.

Assessment and Diagnostic Findings

ALS is diagnosed on the basis of the signs and symptoms, because no clinical or laboratory tests are specific to this disease. Electromyography and muscle biopsy studies of the affected muscles indicate reduction in the number of functioning motor units. An MRI scan may show high signal intensity in the corticospinal tracts; this differentiates ALS from a multifocal motor neuropathy. Neuropsychological testing can assist in assessment and diagnosis (Hickey & Strayer, 2020).

Management

No cure exists for ALS (Vacca, 2020). The main focus of medical and nursing management is on interventions to maintain or improve function, well-being, and quality of life. Because ALS is a progressive disease, the therapeutic needs are different than those of patients with acute processes. Insurance carriers tend to limit the number of therapy sessions, but with early integration into ALS clinics, alliances are developed for future contact with therapists familiar with the disease process (Hogden, Foley, Henderson, et al., 2017).

Two drugs are used to treat ALS, riluzole and edaravone (Vacca, 2020). The precise action of these drugs is not clear, but both are considered disease modifying treatments for ALS (Vacca, 2020).

Symptomatic treatment and rehabilitative measures are used to support the patient and improve the quality of life. Baclofen, dantrolene sodium, or diazepam may be useful for patients troubled by spasticity, which causes pain and interferes with self-care. Modafinil may be used for fatigue, and additional medications may be added to manage the pain, depression, drooling, and constipation that often accompany the disease. Research suggests that greater functional impairment is associated with greater depressive symptoms;

consequently, managing depression helps to maintain a better quality of life (Soofi, Bello-Haas, Kho, et al., 2018). Many clinical trials and an ALS registry contribute to the ongoing study of this devastating disease (Vacca, 2020).

Most patients with ALS are managed at home and in the community, with hospitalization for acute problems. The most common reasons for hospitalization are dehydration and malnutrition, pneumonia, and respiratory failure; recognizing these problems at an early stage in the illness allows for the development of preventive strategies. End-of-life issues include pain, dyspnea, and delirium (Hickey & Strayer, 2020).

Mechanical ventilation (using negative-pressure ventilators) is an option if alveolar hypoventilation develops. Noninvasive positive-pressure ventilation is also an option. The use of noninvasive positive-pressure ventilation is particularly helpful at night and postpones the decision about whether to undergo a tracheotomy for long-term mechanical ventilation (Conde et al., 2019). A patient experiencing aspiration and swallowing difficulties may require enteral feeding. A PEG tube is inserted before the forced vital capacity drops below 50% of the predicted value. The tube can be safely placed in patients who are using noninvasive positive-pressure ventilation for ventilatory support (Hickey & Strayer, 2020).

Decisions about life support measures are made by the patient and family and should be based on a thorough understanding of the disease, the prognosis, and the implications of initiating such therapy. Patients are encouraged to complete an advance directive to preserve their autonomy in decision making. See Chapter 13 for additional discussion of end-of-life care.

The ALS Association has broad programs of research funding, patient and clinical services, patient information and support, and medical and public information (see the Resources section). The *ALS Association Newsletter* is a source of practical information.

Muscular Dystrophies

The muscular dystrophies are a group of incurable muscle disorders characterized by progressive weakening and wasting of the skeletal or voluntary muscles with 30 different types to date. Most of these diseases are inherited. Duchenne muscular dystrophy, the most common and severe type, occurs in 1 of every 3500 male births (Norris, 2019). The pathologic features include degeneration and loss of muscle fibers, variation in muscle fiber size, phagocytosis and regeneration, and replacement of muscle tissue by connective tissue. The common characteristics of these diseases include varying degrees of muscle wasting and weakness and abnormal elevation in serum levels of muscle enzymes. Differences among these diseases center on the genetic pattern of inheritance, the muscles involved, the age at onset, and the rate of disease progression. The symptoms can be diverse and may include muscle stiffness or weakness, decreased respiratory reserve, or cardiomyopathy. Prognosis depends on the type of muscular dystrophy. Regardless of age of onset, this disease varies in progression (Birnkrant, Bushby, Bann, et al., 2018b). The unique needs of these patients, who in the past did not live to adulthood, must be addressed, as they are living longer because of better supportive care and the emergence of disease modifying therapies (Birnkrant et al., 2018b; Trout, Case, Clemens, et al., 2018).

Medical Management

Treatment of the muscular dystrophies focuses on supportive care and prevention of complications in the absence of a cure (Birnkrant et al., 2018b). The goal of supportive management is to keep the patient active and functioning as normally as possible and to minimize functional deterioration. An individualized therapeutic exercise program is prescribed to prevent muscle tightness, contractures, and disuse atrophy. Night splints and stretching exercises are used to delay contractures of the joints, especially the ankles, knees, and hips. Braces may compensate for muscle weakness.

Spinal deformity is a severe problem. Weakness of trunk muscles and spinal collapse occur almost routinely in patients with severe neuromuscular disease. To help prevent spinal deformity, the patient is fitted with an orthotic jacket to improve sitting stability and reduce trunk deformity. This measure also supports cardiovascular status. In time, spinal fusion is performed to maintain spinal stability. Other procedures may be carried out to correct deformities.

Compromised pulmonary function may result either from progression of the disease or from deformity of the thorax secondary to severe scoliosis (Norris, 2019; Trout et al., 2018). Upper respiratory infections and fractures from falls must be vigorously treated in a way that minimizes immobilization because joint contractures become worse when the patient's activities are more restricted than usual.

Other difficulties may manifest in relation to the underlying disease. Weakness of the facial muscles makes it difficult to attend to dental hygiene and to speak clearly, and impairs the ability to swallow safely (Birnkrant, Bushby, Bann, et al., 2018a). Gastrointestinal tract problems may include gastric dilation, rectal prolapse, and fecal impaction. Finally, cardiomyopathy appears to be a common complication in all forms of muscular dystrophy (Birnkrant et al., 2018a).

Genetic counseling is advised for parents and siblings of the patient because of the genetic nature of this disease. The Muscular Dystrophy Association (MDA) works to combat neuromuscular disease through research, programs of patient services and clinical care, and professional and public education (see the Resources section).

Nursing Management

The goals of the patient and the nurse are to maintain function at optimal levels and to enhance the quality of life. Therefore, the patient's physical requirements, which are considerable, are addressed without losing sight of emotional and developmental needs. The patient and family are actively involved in decision making, including end-of-life decisions (see Chapter 13).

During hospitalization for treatment of complications, the knowledge and expertise of the patient and family members responsible for caregiving in the home are assessed. Because the patient and family caregivers often have developed caregiving strategies that work effectively for them, these strategies need to be acknowledged and accepted, and provisions must be made to ensure that they are maintained during hospitalization (Birnkrant et al., 2018b).

Families of adolescents and young adults with muscular dystrophy need assistance to shift the focus of care from pediatric to adult care and to understand the usual disease course (Lindsay, Cagliostro, & McAdam, 2019; Trout et al., 2018). Nursing goals include assisting the adolescent to make the transition to adult values and expectations while providing age-appropriate ongoing care. The nurse may need to help build the confidence of an older adolescent or adult patient by encouraging them to pursue job training to become economically independent. Other nursing interventions might include guidance in accessing adult health care and finding appropriate programs in sex education.

Promoting Home, Community-Based, and Transitional Care

 Educating Patients About Self-Care

Management goals are addressed in special rehabilitation programs or in the patient's home and community. Therefore, the patient and family require information and education about the disorder, its anticipated course, and care and management strategies that will optimize the patient's growth and development and physical and psychological status. Members of a variety of health-related disciplines are involved in patient and family education; recommendations are communicated to all members of the health care team so that they may work toward common goals.

Continuing and Transitional Care

Both the neuromuscular disease and the associated deformities may progress in adolescence and adulthood. Self-help and assistive devices can aid in maintaining maximum independence. These devices, recommended by physical and occupational therapists, often become necessary as more muscle groups are affected.

The family is instructed to monitor the patient for respiratory problems, because respiratory infection and cardiac failure are the most common causes of death. As respiratory difficulties develop, patients and their families need information regarding respiratory support. Options currently exist that can provide ventilatory support (e.g., negative-pressure devices, positive-pressure ventilators) while allowing mobility (Birnkrant et al., 2018a). Patients can remain relatively independent in a wheelchair, for example, while being maintained on a ventilator at home for many years.

The patient is encouraged to continue with range-of-motion exercises to prevent contractures, which are particularly disabling. Practical adaptations must be made, however, to cope with the effects of chronic neuromuscular disability. The patient at various stages of the disease may require a manual or an electric wheelchair, gait aids, upper and lower extremity and spinal orthotics, seating systems, bathroom equipment, lifts, ramps, and additional assistive devices, all of which require a team approach. The nurse assesses how the patient and family are managing, makes referrals, and coordinates the activities of the physical therapist, occupational therapist, and social services.

Patients who express concerns about increasing disability and dependence on others, as well as significant deterioration in health-related quality of life, benefit from an interprofessional approach to care (Trout et al., 2018). The patient is faced with a progressive loss of function, leading eventually to death. Feelings of helplessness and powerlessness are common. Each functional loss is accompanied by grief and mourning. The patient and family are assessed for depression, anger, or denial. The patient and family are assisted and encouraged to address decisions about end-of-life options before their need arises (see Chapter 13).

A psychiatric nurse clinician or other mental health professional may assist the patient to cope and adapt to the disease. By understanding and addressing clinical concerns that are important for patients and their families, while at the same time assessing caregiver knowledge and burden during every encounter, the nurse provides a hopeful, supportive, and nurturing environment.

Degenerative Disc Disease

Low back pain is the second most common neurologic disorder in the United States, with one quarter of all adults reporting recent (within 3 months) back pain (Hickey & Strayer, 2020). It is frequently associated with depression, anxiety, smoking, alcohol abuse, obesity, and stress; and it is the most common reason for missed work and decreased productivity while at work (Ramanathan, Hibbert, Wiles, et al., 2018). Low back pain results in significant economic costs to patients, their families, and society. Acute pain lasts less than 3 months, whereas chronic pain has a duration of 3 months or longer. Approximately 90% of patients with low back pain recover spontaneously within 4 to 6 weeks (Hickey & Strayer, 2020). See Chapter 36, Chart 36-2 for further discussion of strategies to prevent acute low back pain.

Pathophysiology

The intervertebral disc is a cartilaginous plate that forms a cushion between the vertebral bodies (see Fig. 65-6A). This tough, fibrous material is incorporated in a capsule. A ball-like cushion in the center of the disc is called the *nucleus pulposus*. In herniation of the intervertebral disc (ruptured disc), the nucleus of the disc protrudes into the annulus (the fibrous ring around the disc), with subsequent nerve compression (Norris, 2019). Protrusion or rupture of the nucleus pulposus usually is preceded by degenerative changes that occur with aging. Loss of protein polysaccharides in the disc decreases the water content of the nucleus pulposus. The development of radiating cracks in the annulus weakens resistance to nucleus herniation. After trauma (falls and repeated minor stresses such as lifting incorrectly), the cartilage may be injured.

For most patients, the immediate symptoms of trauma are short-lived, and those resulting from injury to the disc do not appear for months or years. Disc degeneration pushes the capsule back into the spinal canal. It could also rupture and allow the nucleus pulposus to be pushed back against the dural sac or against a spinal nerve as it emerges from the spinal column (see Fig. 65-6B). This disease of the spinal root produces pain and extreme sensitivity to touch due to radiculopathy (pressure in the area of distribution of the involved nerve endings). Continued pressure may produce degenerative changes in the involved nerve, such as changes in sensation and deep tendon reflexes.

Gerontologic Considerations

Low back pain is commonly reported in older adults (Eliopoulos, 2018). Degenerative disc disease is also prevalent among older adults, but age alone should not exclude a patient from undergoing lumbar fusion if indicated (Badhiwala, Karmur, Hachem, et al., 2019). Researchers studied a group of 2238 patients ($n = 1119$, age <70; $n = 1119$, age ≥70) who underwent spinal fusion. The groups were balanced for factors including sex, race, diabetes, hypertension, congestive heart failure, smoking, chronic steroid use, type of fusion, and number of levels (see later discussion). Rates of all complications were similar between younger and older age groups, except urinary tract infection, which was more frequent among the ≥70 age group (OR 2.32, $p = .009$). Those in the older age group were more likely to be discharged to a rehabilitation or skilled care facility, rather than directly home (Badhiwala et al., 2019).

Clinical Manifestations

A herniated disc with accompanying pain may occur in any portion of the spine: cervical, thoracic (rare), or lumbar. The clinical manifestations depend on the location, the rate of development (acute or chronic), and the effect on the surrounding structures. Functional limitations are the main manifestation reported by patients. Researchers also report that pain intensity in patients with low back pain has a direct effect on ADLs and sleep quality (Kose, Tastan, Temiz, et al., 2019).

Assessment and Diagnostic Findings

A thorough health history and physical examination are important to rule out potentially serious conditions that may manifest as low back pain, including fracture, tumor, infection, or cauda equina syndrome (Hickey & Strayer, 2020).

The MRI scan has become the diagnostic tool of choice for localizing even small disc protrusions, particularly for lumbar spine disease. If the clinical symptoms are not consistent with the pathology seen on MRI, CT scanning and myelography are performed. A neurologic examination is carried out to determine whether reflex, sensory, or motor impairment from root compression is present and to provide a baseline for future assessment. Electromyography may be used to localize the specific spinal nerve roots involved. See Chapter 36, Chart 36-1 for a summary of additional diagnostic studies that may be used to evaluate low back pain.

Medical Management

Herniations of the cervical and the lumbar discs occur most commonly and are usually managed conservatively with medication and physical therapy or exercise (Hickey & Strayer, 2020). Surgery is sometimes necessary.

Surgical Management

Surgical excision of a herniated disc is performed if there is evidence of a progressing neurologic deficit (muscle weakness and atrophy, loss of sensory and motor function, loss of sphincter control) and radicular pain (pain that follows the dermatomal distribution [see Chapter 60, Fig. 60-9]

of the compressed nerve) that are unresponsive to conservative management. The goal of surgical treatment is to reduce the pressure on the nerve root to relieve pain and reverse neurologic deficits. Microsurgical techniques make it possible to remove only the amount of tissue that is necessary, which preserves the integrity of normal tissue better and imposes less trauma on the body. During these procedures, spinal cord function can be monitored electrophysiologically.

Some of the surgical techniques available include (Hickey & Strayer, 2020):

- *Microdiscectomy*: Removal of herniated or extruded fragments of intervertebral disc material
- *Laminectomy*: Removal of the bone between the spinal process and facet pedicle junction to expose the neural elements in the spinal canal; this allows the surgeon to inspect the spinal canal, identify and remove pathologic tissue, and relieve compression of the cord and roots
- *Hemilaminectomy*: Removal of part of the lamina and part of the posterior arch of the vertebra
- *Partial laminectomy or laminotomy*: Creation of a hole in the lamina of a vertebra
- *Discectomy with fusion*: Fusion of the vertebral spinous process with a bone graft (from iliac crest or bone bank), with the object of spinal fusion being to bridge over the defective disc to stabilize the spine and reduce the rate of recurrence
- *Foraminotomy*: Enlargement of the intervertebral foramen to increase the space for exit of a spinal nerve, resulting in reduced pain, compression, and edema

Herniation of a Cervical Intervertebral Disc

The cervical spine is subjected to stresses that result from disc degeneration (due to aging, improper body mechanics) and **spondylosis** (degenerative changes occurring in a disc and adjacent vertebral bodies). Cervical disc degeneration may lead to lesions that can cause damage to the spinal cord and its roots (Hickey & Strayer, 2020).

Clinical Manifestations

A cervical disc herniation usually occurs at the C5–C6 or C6–C7 interspaces and compresses a unilateral nerve root (Hickey & Strayer, 2020). Pain and stiffness may occur in the neck, the top of the shoulders, and the region of the scapulae. Patients sometimes interpret these signs as symptoms of heart trouble or bursitis. Pain may also occur in the arm and hand, accompanied by **paresthesia** (numbness, tingling, or a "pins and needles" sensation) of the upper extremity. Cervical MRI usually confirms the diagnosis. Occasionally, the disc herniates centrally onto the spinal cord, causing Lhermitte syndrome, an electriclike shock sensation in the extremities or spine with neck flexion or straining, and myelopathy (bilateral arm and leg weakness). Myelopathy indicates compression of the spinal cord. The patient may exhibit a decrease in fine motor skills, difficulty with ambulation, difficulty with bowel and bladder control, and respiratory impairment if compression has occurred high in the cervical spine (Hemmer, 2018).

Medical Management

The goals of treatment are to rest and immobilize the cervical spine to give the soft tissues time to heal and to reduce inflammation in the supporting tissues and the affected nerve roots in the cervical spine (Hickey & Strayer, 2020). It also reduces inflammation and edema in soft tissues around the disc, relieving pressure on the nerve roots. Proper positioning on a firm mattress may bring dramatic relief from pain.

The cervical spine may be rested and immobilized by a cervical collar, cervical traction, or a brace. A collar allows maximal opening of the intervertebral foramina and holds the head in a neutral or slightly flexed position. The patient may have to wear the collar 24 hours a day during the acute phase. The skin under the collar is inspected for irritation. After the patient is free of pain, cervical isometric exercises are started to strengthen the neck muscles.

Pharmacologic Therapy

Analgesic agents (nonsteroidal anti-inflammatory drugs [NSAIDs], acetaminophen/oxycodone, or acetaminophen/hydrocodone) are prescribed during the acute phase to relieve pain, and sedative agents may be given to control the anxiety that is often associated with cervical disc disease. Muscle relaxants (cyclobenzaprine, methocarbamol, metaxalone) are prescribed for less than 1 week to interrupt muscle spasm and to promote comfort (Hickey & Strayer, 2020). NSAIDs (aspirin, ibuprofen, naproxen) or corticosteroids are prescribed to treat the inflammation and swelling that usually occurs in the affected nerve roots and supporting tissues. Occasionally, a corticosteroid is injected into the epidural space for relief of radicular pain. NSAIDs are given with food to prevent gastrointestinal irritation (Comerford & Durkin, 2020). Hot, moist compresses (for 10 to 20 minutes) applied to the back of the neck several times daily increase blood flow to the muscles and help relax the patient and reduce muscle spasm.

Surgical Management

Surgical excision of the herniated disc may be necessary if there is a significant neurologic deficit, progression of the deficit, evidence of cord compression, or pain that either worsens or fails to improve. A cervical discectomy, with or without fusion, may be performed to alleviate symptoms. An anterior surgical approach may be used through a transverse incision to remove disc material that has herniated into the spinal canal and foramina, or a posterior approach may be used at the appropriate level of the cervical spine. Potential complications with the anterior approach include carotid or vertebral artery injury, recurrent laryngeal nerve dysfunction, esophageal perforation, and airway obstruction (Hickey & Strayer, 2020). Complications of the posterior approach include damage to the nerve root or the spinal cord due to retraction or contusion of either of these structures, resulting in weakness of muscles supplied by the nerve root or cord.

Microsurgery, such as endoscopic microdiscectomy, may be performed in select patients through a small incision, using magnification techniques. This usually results in less tissue trauma and pain, and patients consequently have a shorter length of hospital stay compared with those who have conventional surgery (Hickey & Strayer, 2020).

NURSING PROCESS

The Patient Undergoing a Cervical Discectomy

Assessment

The patient is asked about past injuries to the neck, such as whiplash injury, because unresolved trauma can cause persistent discomfort, pain and tenderness, and symptoms of arthritis in the injured joint of the cervical spine. Assessment includes determining the onset, location, and radiation of pain and assessing for paresthesias, limited movement, and diminished function of the neck, shoulders, and upper extremities. It is important to determine whether the symptoms are bilateral; with large herniations, bilateral symptoms may be caused by cord compression. The area around the cervical spine is palpated to assess muscle tone and tenderness. Range of motion in the neck and shoulders is evaluated.

The patient is asked about any health issues that may influence the postoperative course and quality of life. It is also important to assess mood and stress levels. The nurse determines the patient's need for information about the surgical procedure and reinforces what the primary provider has explained. Strategies for pain management are discussed with the patient (Hickey & Strayer, 2020).

Diagnosis

NURSING DIAGNOSES

Based on the assessment data, major nursing diagnoses may include the following:

- Acute pain associated with the surgical procedure
- Impaired mobility associated with the postoperative surgical regimen
- Lack of knowledge about the postoperative course and home care management

COLLABORATIVE PROBLEMS/POTENTIAL COMPLICATIONS

Potential complications may include the following:

- Hematoma at the surgical site, resulting in cord compression and neurologic deficit
- Recurrent or persistent pain after surgery

Planning and Goals

The goals for the patient may include relief of pain, improved mobility, increased knowledge and self-care ability, and prevention of complications.

Nursing Interventions

RELIEVING PAIN

Incisional pain is expected. Radicular pain improves over time as the nerve recovers. If the patient has had a bone fusion with bone removed from the iliac crest, considerable pain may be experienced at the donor site. Interventions consist of monitoring the donor site for hematoma formation, administering the prescribed postoperative analgesic agent, positioning for comfort, and reassuring the patient that the pain can be relieved. If the patient experiences a sudden increase in pain, extrusion of the graft may have occurred, requiring reoperation. A sudden increase in pain should be promptly reported to the surgeon (Lall, 2018).

The patient may experience a sore throat, hoarseness, and dysphagia due to temporary edema. These symptoms are relieved by throat lozenges, voice rest, and humidification. A pureed diet may be given if the patient has dysphagia.

IMPROVING MOBILITY

Postoperatively, a cervical collar (neck orthosis) may be worn, which contributes to limited neck motion and altered mobility. The patient is instructed to turn the body instead of the neck when looking from side to side. The neck should be kept in a neutral (midline) position. The patient is assisted during position changes to make sure that the head, shoulders, and thorax are kept aligned. When assisting the patient to a sitting position, the nurse supports the patient's neck and shoulders. To increase stability, the patient should wear shoes when ambulating. The patient is encouraged not to lift more than 10 pounds.

MONITORING AND MANAGING POTENTIAL COMPLICATIONS

The patient is evaluated for bleeding and hematoma formation by assessing for swelling, excessive pressure in the neck, or severe pain in the incision area. The dressing is inspected for serosanguineous drainage, which suggests a dural leak. If this occurs, meningitis is a threat. A complaint of headache requires careful evaluation. Neurologic checks are made for swallowing deficits and upper and lower extremity weakness, because cord compression may produce rapid or delayed onset of paralysis (Hickey & Strayer, 2020). The patient who has had an anterior cervical discectomy is also assessed for a sudden return of radicular (spinal nerve root) pain, which may indicate instability of the spine (Hemmer, 2018).

Throughout the postoperative course, the patient is monitored frequently to detect any signs of respiratory difficulty, because retractors used during surgery may injure the laryngeal nerve, resulting in hoarseness and the inability to cough effectively and clear pulmonary secretions. In addition, the blood pressure and pulse are monitored to evaluate cardiovascular status and optimal circulation to the surgical site.

Bleeding at the surgical site and subsequent hematoma formation may occur. Severe localized pain not relieved by analgesic agents should be reported. A change in neurologic status (motor or sensory function) should be reported promptly, because it suggests hematoma formation that may necessitate surgery to prevent irreversible motor and sensory deficits (Hickey & Strayer, 2020).

PROMOTING HOME, COMMUNITY-BASED, AND TRANSITIONAL CARE

Educating Patients About Self-Care. The patient's length of hospital stay is likely to be short; therefore, the patient and family should understand the care that is important for a smooth recovery. A cervical collar, if prescribed, is usually worn for about 6 weeks. The patient is educated in the use and care of the cervical collar. The patient will need to alternate tasks that involve minimal body movement (e.g., reading) with tasks that require greater body movement.

The patient is educated about strategies to manage the incision and to manage pain, and about signs and symptoms that may indicate complications that should be reported to the primary provider. The nurse assesses the patient's understanding of these management strategies, limitations, and recommendations. In addition, the nurse assists the patient in identifying strategies to cope with ADLs (e.g., self-care, child care) and minimize risks to the surgical site (see Chart 65-6). A discharge educational plan is developed collaboratively by members of the health care team to decrease the risk of recurrent disc herniation. Topics include those previously discussed as well as proper body mechanics, maintenance of optimal weight, proper exercise techniques, and modifications in activity.

Continuing and Transitional Care. The patient is instructed to see the primary provider at prescribed intervals so that the provider can document the disappearance of old symptoms and assess the range of motion of the neck. Recurrent or persistent pain may occur despite removal of the offending disc or disc fragments. Patients who undergo discectomy usually have consented to surgery after prolonged pain; they have often undergone repeated courses of ineffective conservative management and previous surgeries to relieve the pain. Therefore, the recurrence or persistence of symptoms postoperatively, including pain and sensory deficits, is often discouraging for the patient and family. The patient who experiences recurrence of symptoms requires emotional support and understanding. In addition, the patient is assisted in modifying activities and in considering options for subsequent treatment. The nurse educates the patient and family members about the need to participate in health-promotion and health-screening practices.

Evaluation

Expected patient outcomes may include:

1. Reports decreasing frequency and severity of pain
2. Demonstrates improved mobility
   a. Demonstrates progressive participation in self-care activities
   b. Identifies prescribed activity limitations and restrictions
   c. Demonstrates proper body mechanics
3. Is knowledgeable about postoperative course, medications, and home care management
   a. Lists the signs and symptoms to be reported postoperatively
   b. Identifies dose, action, and potential side effects of medications
   c. Identifies appropriate home care management activities and any restrictions
4. Has absence of complications
   a. Reports no increase in incision pain or sensory symptoms
   b. Demonstrates normal findings on neurologic assessment

Herniation of a Lumbar Disc

Most lumbar disc herniations occur at the L5–S1 region (Hickey & Strayer, 2020). A herniated lumbar disc produces low back pain accompanied by varying degrees of sensory and motor impairment.

Chart 65-6   HOME CARE CHECKLIST

The Patient with Cervical Discectomy and Cervical Collar

At the completion of education, the patient and/or caregiver will be able to:

- Name the procedure that was performed and identify any permanent changes in anatomic structure or function as well as changes in ADLs, IADLs, roles, relationships, and spirituality.
- Identify interventions and strategies (e.g., durable medical equipment, adaptive equipment) used in adapting to any permanent changes in structure or function to promote safety and optimum functioning.
  - Use adequate mattress and chair support.
- State the name, dose, side effects, frequency, and schedule for all medications.
  - Describe nonpharmacologic interventions for pain relief used in conjunction to prescribed pain relief preparations.
- State how to obtain medical supplies and carry out dressing changes, wound care, and other prescribed regimens.
- State how to contact all members of the treatment team (e.g., health care providers, home care professionals, and durable medical equipment and supply vendor).
- Describe ongoing postoperative therapeutic regimen, including diet and activities to perform (e.g., exercises) and to limit or avoid (e.g., lifting, stair climbing, driving a car) during rehabilitation.
- Describe care for the surgical incision site.
  - Keep staples or sutures clean and dry and cover with dry dressing.
- Demonstrate proper body mechanics and prescribed exercise techniques.
  - Describe how to modify activity for optimum functioning.
  - Avoid sitting or standing for more than 30 minutes.
  - Avoid twisting, flexing, extending, or rotating the neck.
  - Avoid sleeping in a prone position or the use of pillows to minimize neck flexion in bed; keep head in a neutral position.
  - Wear low-heeled shoes.
  - Place a wrinkle-free silk scarf under the collar to increase comfort.

- **For men:** Shave without twisting or moving the neck. This may be done with help while lying flat or sitting. Remove only the front part of the collar for shaving.
- Practice stress reduction and relaxation techniques.
- Care of the cervical collar:
  - Wear the collar at all times until directed otherwise by the primary provider.
  - Wash the neck under the collar twice a day with mild soap.
  - Keep the neck still while the collar is open.
  - With the assistance of a helper, wash the neck in steps.
  - Lie flat and supine.
  - Open the Velcro tabs on each side of the collar and remove its front portion.
  - Gently wash and dry the neck.
  - Replace the front part of the collar and refasten the tabs.
  - Turn to one side with a thin pillow under the head.
  - Open one tab.
  - Gently wash and dry the back of the neck. Refasten the tab.
  - Turn to the other side and wash and dry this side. Refasten the tab.
- Notify primary provider if any signs or symptoms of infection occur, such as fever, redness or irritation, drainage, increased pain.
- Relate how to reach primary provider with questions or complications.
- State time and date of follow-up medical appointments, therapy, and testing.
- Identify sources of support for patient and caregivers (e.g., friends, relatives, faith community).
- Identify the contact details for support services for patients and their caregivers/families.
- Identify the need for health promotion, disease prevention, and screening activities.

ADLs, activities of daily living; IADLs, instrumental activities of daily living.

Clinical Manifestations

The patient complains of low back pain with muscle spasm and **sciatica** (pain and tenderness that radiates along the sciatic nerve that runs through the thigh and leg). Pain is aggravated by actions that increase intraspinal fluid pressure, such as bending, lifting, or straining (as in sneezing or coughing), and usually is relieved by bed rest. There is often some type of postural deformity, because pain causes an alteration of the normal spinal mechanics. If the patient lies on the back and attempts to raise a leg in a straight position, pain radiates into the leg; this maneuver, called the *straight-leg raising test*, stretches the sciatic nerve. Additional signs include muscle weakness, alterations in tendon reflexes, and sensory loss.

Assessment and Diagnostic Findings

The diagnosis of lumbar disc disease is based on the history and physical findings, specifically the location, quality, severity of pain, and the use of imaging techniques such as MRI and CT scans as well as myelography.

Medical Management

The objectives of treatment are to relieve pain, slow disease progression, and increase the patient's functional ability. Bed rest is discouraged because it may weaken muscles, but activities that exacerbate pain should be avoided.

Because muscle spasm is prominent during the acute phase, muscle relaxants are used. NSAIDs and systemic corticosteroids may be given to counter the inflammation and swelling that usually occurs in the supporting tissues and the affected nerve roots. Moist heat and massage help relax muscles. Strategies for increasing the patient's functional ability include weight reduction, physical therapy, and biofeedback. Exercises, prescribed by physical therapy, can help strengthen back muscles and decrease pain (Hickey & Strayer, 2020). See Chapter 9 for descriptions of nursing interventions for the patient with pain.

Surgical Management

In the lumbar region, surgical treatment includes lumbar disc excision through a posterolateral laminotomy and the techniques of microdiscectomy and percutaneous discectomy. In microdiscectomy, an operating microscope is used to visualize the offending disc and compressed nerve roots; it permits a small incision (2.5 cm [1 inch]) and minimal blood loss and takes about 30 minutes of operating time. In general, the length of hospital stay is short, and the patient makes a rapid recovery. Several minimally invasive techniques in spinal surgery have led to improved patient outcomes and lower hospital costs (Hickey & Strayer, 2020).

A patient undergoing a disc procedure at one level of the vertebral column may have a degenerative process at other levels. A herniation relapse may occur at the same level or elsewhere, so the patient may become a candidate for another disc procedure. Arachnoiditis (inflammation of the arachnoid membrane) may occur after surgery (and after myelography); it involves an insidious onset of diffuse, frequently burning pain in the lower back, radiating into the buttocks. Disc excision can leave adhesions and scarring around the spinal nerves and dura, which then produce inflammatory changes that create chronic neuritis and neurofibrosis. Disc surgery may relieve pressure on the spinal nerves, but it does not reverse the effects of neural injury and scarring and the pain that results. Failed disc syndrome (recurrence of sciatica after lumbar discectomy) remains a cause of disability (Hickey & Strayer, 2020).

Nursing Management

Providing Preoperative Care

Most patients fear surgery on any part of the spine and therefore need explanations about the surgery and reassurance that it will not weaken the back. When data are being collected for the health history, any reports of pain, paresthesia, or muscle spasm are recorded to provide a baseline for comparison after surgery. Health issues that may influence the postoperative course and quality of life (e.g., fatigue, mood, stress, patient expectations, smoking) are important to assess. Preoperative assessment also includes an evaluation of movement of the extremities as well as bladder and bowel function (Hickey & Strayer, 2020). To facilitate the postoperative turning procedure, the patient is instructed to turn as a unit (called logrolling) as part of the preoperative preparation. Before surgery, the patient is also encouraged to take deep breaths, cough, and perform muscle setting exercises to maintain muscle tone.

Research suggests that the use of motivational interviewing helps build self-confidence with self-care management of symptoms in the postoperative period (Scheffel, Amidei, & Fitzgerald, 2019). See the Nursing Research Profile in Chart 65-7.

Assessing the Patient After Surgery

After lumbar disc excision, vital signs are checked frequently and the wound is inspected for hemorrhage, because vascular injury is a complication of disc surgery. Because postoperative neurologic deficits may occur from nerve root injury, the sensation and motor strength of the lower extremities are evaluated at specified intervals, along with the color and temperature of the legs and sensation of the toes. It is important to assess for urinary retention, which is another sign of neurologic deterioration (Hickey & Strayer, 2020). In discectomy with fusion, the patient has an additional surgical incision if bone fragments were taken from the iliac crest or fibula to serve as wedges in the spine. The recovery period is longer for patients who undergo discectomy with spinal fusion, because bony union must take place.

Positioning the Patient

To position the patient, a pillow is placed under the head, and the knee rest is elevated slightly to relax the back muscles. When the patient is lying on one side, however, extreme knee flexion must be avoided. The patient is encouraged to move from side to side to relieve pressure and is reassured that no injury will result from moving. When the patient is ready to turn, the bed is placed in a flat position and a pillow is placed

---

Chart 65-7 · NURSING RESEARCH PROFILE

Improving Confidence with Self-Care Management

Scheffel, K., Amidei, C., & Fitzgerald, K. A. (2019). Motivational interviewing: Improving confidence with self-care management in postoperative thoracolumbar spine patients. *Journal of Neuroscience Nursing, 51*(3), 113–117.

Purpose

Patients undergoing spine surgery often lack confidence in self-care management of symptoms such as pain, lack of sleep, depression, and immobility. The purpose of this study was to examine whether a targeted motivational interview would improve confidence with self-care management of symptoms following spine surgery.

Design

This pilot study used a quasi-experimental, one group, pretest–posttest design with 15 participants who were undergoing spine surgery. The two main instruments used to gather data included the 10-item Oswestry Disability Index (ODI) and the Health Confidence Index (HCI).

Findings

Paired sample t-tests of the pre- and postintervention scores on both the ODI and HCI showed statistically significant differences. The HCI showed a statistically significant increase in scores with mean preintervention scores of 6.73 (SD = 2.12) and mean postintervention scores of 8.73 (SD = 1.43) indicating a significant increase in confidence in self-care of symptom-related disability.

Nursing Implications

Motivational interviewing is an effective strategy for implementing health promoting behaviors. This study adds evidence that motivational interviewing is a strategy nurses can use to improve patients' confidence in self-care management of symptoms following spine surgery.

between the patient's legs. The patient turns as a unit (log-rolls) without twisting the back.

To get out of bed, the patient lies on one side while pushing up to a sitting position. At the same time, the nurse or family member eases the patient's legs over the side of the bed. Coming to a sitting or standing posture is accomplished in one long, smooth motion. Most patients walk to the bathroom on the same day as the surgery. Sitting is discouraged except for defecation.

Promoting Home, Community-Based, and Transitional Care

 Educating Patients About Self-Care

The patient is instructed to increase activity gradually, as tolerated, because it takes up to 6 weeks for the ligaments to heal. Excessive activity may result in spasm of the paraspinal muscles (Hickey & Strayer, 2020).

Activities that produce flexion strain on the spine (e.g., driving a car) should be avoided until healing has taken place. Heat may be applied to the back to relax muscle spasms. Scheduled rest periods are important, and the patient is advised to avoid heavy work for 2 to 3 months after surgery. Exercises are prescribed to strengthen the abdominal and erector spinal muscles. A back brace or corset may be necessary if back pain persists.

Continuing and Transitional Care

Referral for inpatient or outpatient rehabilitation may be warranted to improve self-care abilities after medical or surgical treatment for herniation of a lumbar disc. A home care referral may be indicated and provides the nurse with the opportunity to assess the patient's physical and psychological status, as well as their ability to adhere to recommended management strategies. During the home visit, the nurse determines whether changes in neurologic function have occurred. The adequacy of pain management is assessed, and modifications are made to ensure adequate pain relief (Hickey & Strayer, 2020).

Post-Polio Syndrome

Polio has mostly been eradicated globally due to concerted vaccination efforts. However, people who survived the polio epidemic of the 1940s and 1950s, many of whom are now older adults, are developing new symptoms of weakness, fatigue, and musculoskeletal pain identified as PPS. This phenomenon, which occurs at least 15 years after the polio exposure, affects 15 to 20 million people worldwide (Shing, Chipika, Finegan, et al., 2019). Men and women appear to be equally at risk for this condition.

Pathophysiology

The exact cause of PPS is not known, but researchers suspect that with aging or muscle overuse, the neurons not destroyed by the poliovirus continue generating axon sprouts (Shing et al., 2019). These new terminal axon sprouts reinnervate the affected muscles after the initial insult but may become more vulnerable as the body ages.

Assessment and Diagnostic Findings

No specific diagnostic test exists for PPS. Clinical diagnosis is made on the basis of the history and physical examination and exclusion of other medical conditions that could be causing the new symptoms. Patients report a history of paralytic poliomyelitis followed by partial or complete recovery of function, with a plateau of function and then the recurrence of symptoms. Signs and symptoms may occur decades after the original onset of poliomyelitis (Shing et al., 2019).

Management

No specific medical or surgical treatment is available for this syndrome, and therefore nurses play a pivotal role in the team approach to assisting patients and families in dealing with the symptoms of progressive loss of muscle strength and significant fatigue (Shing et al., 2019; Pastuszak, Stepien, Tomczykiewicz, et al., 2017). Pain and weakness may be improved with infusion of intravenous immunoglobulin (Shing et al., 2019).

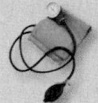 For the procedural guidelines for managing immunoglobulin therapy, go to **thepoint.lww. com/Brunner15e**.

Nursing interventions are aimed at maintaining the patient's strength as well as physical, psychological, and social well-being. Other health care professionals who may assist in patient care include physical, occupational, speech, and respiratory therapists; social workers; and chaplains.

The patient needs to plan and coordinate activities to conserve energy and reduce fatigue. Rest periods should be planned and assistive devices used to reduce weakness and fatigue. Important activities should be planned for the morning, because fatigue often increases in the afternoon and evening.

Pain in muscles and joints may be a problem. Nonpharmacologic techniques such as the application of heat and cold are appropriate, because older adults may not tolerate or may react to medications, particularly when they are taking multiple medications (Eliopoulos, 2018).

Maintaining a balance between adequate nutritional intake and avoiding excess calories that can lead to obesity is a challenge in this group of patients who are sedentary. Pulmonary hygiene and adequate fluid intake can help with airway management. Several interventions can improve sleep, including limiting caffeine intake before bedtime and assessing for nocturia. The patient may need to be evaluated for obstructive sleep apnea. Supportive ventilation may be appropriate, with continuous positive airway pressure if sleep apnea is a problem (see Chapter 18).

Bone density testing in patients with PPS has revealed low bone mass and osteoporosis. Therefore, the importance of identifying risks, preventing falls, and treating osteoporosis must be discussed with patients and families. Families also need to be made aware of the possibility of changes in individual and family relationships due to the many symptoms of PPS. The nurse also needs to remind patients and family members of the need for health-promotion activities and health screening (Shing et al., 2019).

CRITICAL THINKING EXERCISES

1 `ebp` A 64-year-old man has been admitted to the unit where you work after having a seizure and has been newly diagnosed with a brain tumor. Identify the evidence-based practices for the management of brain tumors. Describe the evidence base for the practices that you have identified and the criteria used to evaluate the strength of that evidence. Identify the health-promotion activities you would recommend to this patient and the rationale for your recommendations.

2 `pq` You are caring for a 55-year-old woman newly diagnosed with Parkinson's disease. Assess and prioritize the patient's physiologic and psychosocial needs. What nursing interventions and actions would you suggest to assist in managing the treatment of and coping with Parkinson's disease? How would this be different if the patient lives alone?

3 `ipc` You are participating in morning rounds on the surgery unit where you work. The team is discussing one of the patients who has been assigned to you for the day, a 75-year-old man admitted yesterday following a lumbar disc excision. What members of the interprofessional care team should be included in the care of this patient? How will you, as this patient's nurse, facilitate an interprofessional discussion to assist with his discharge?

REFERENCES

*Asterisk indicates nursing research.

Books

American Association of Neuroscience Nurses (AANN). (2016). *Care of the adult patient with a brain tumor: AANN clinical practice guideline series.* Chicago, IL: Author.

American Association of Neuroscience Nurses (AANN). (2019). *Evidence-based strategies for care of the patient with movement disorders and deep brain stimulation: AANN clinical practice guideline series.* Chicago, IL: Author.

Comerford, K. C., & Durkin, M. T. (2020). *Nursing 2020 drug handbook.* Philadelphia, PA: Wolters Kluwer.

Eliopoulos, C. (2018). *Gerontological nursing* (9th ed.). Philadelphia, PA: Wolters Kluwer.

Hickey, J. V., & Strayer, A. L. (2020). *The clinical practice of neurological and neurosurgical nursing* (8th ed.). Philadelphia, PA: Wolters Kluwer.

Norris, T. L. (2019). *Porth's pathophysiology: Concepts of altered health states* (10th ed.). Philadelphia, PA: Wolters Kluwer.

Journals and Electronic Documents

Achrol, A. S., Rennert, R. C., Anders, C., et al. (2019). Brain metastases. *Nature Reviews. Disease Primers, 5*(1), 1–26.

Alattar, A. A., Hirshman, B. R., McCutcheon, B. A., et al. (2018). Risk factors for readmission with cerebrospinal fluid leakage within 30 days of vestibular schwannoma surgery. *Neurosurgery, 82*(5), 630–637.

Aslam, S., Simpson, E., Baugh, M., et al. (2019). Interventions to minimize complications in hospitalized patients with Parkinson disease. *Neurology: Clinical Practice, 10*(1), 23–28.

Badhiwala, J. H., Karmur, B. S., Hachem, L. D., et al. (2019). The effect of older age on the perioperative outcomes of spinal fusion surgery in patients with lumbar degenerative disc disease with spondylolisthesis: A propensity score-matched analysis. *Neurosurgery, 87*(4), 672–878.

Battie, M. C., Joshi, A. B., & Gibbons, L. E. (2019). Degenerative disc disease: What is in a name? *Spine, 44*(21), 1523–1529.

Birnkrant, D. J., Bushby, K., Bann, C. M., et al. (2018a). Diagnosis and management of Duchenne muscular dystrophy, part 2: Respiratory, cardiac, bone health, and orthopaedic movement. *The Lancet. Neurology, 17*(4), 347–361.

Birnkrant, D. J., Bushby, K., Bann, C. M., et al. (2018b). Diagnosis and management of Duchenne muscular dystrophy, part 3: Primary care, emergency management, psychosocial care, and transitions of care across the lifespan. *The Lancet. Neurology, 17*(3), 445–455.

*Boele, F. W., Terhorst, L., Prince, J., et al. (2019). Psychometric evaluation of the caregiver needs screen in neuro-oncology family caregivers. *Journal of Nursing Measurement, 27*(2), 162–176.

Bronner, G., & Korczyn, A. D. (2017). The role of sex therapy in the management of patients with Parkinson's disease. *Movement Disorders Clinical Practice, 5*(1), 6–13.

Conde, B., Martins, N., & Winck, J. C. (2019). Ventilatory support outcomes in amyotrophic lateral sclerosis (ALS) patients. *Neuropsychiatry, 9*(2), 2228–2236.

Donovan, L. E., & Welch, M. R. (2018). Headaches in patients with pituitary tumors: A clinical conundrum. *Current Pain and Headache Reports, 22*(8), 57. doi.org/10.1007/s11916-018-0709-1

Epstein, N. E. (2018). Nursing review of spinal meningiomas. *Surgical Neurology International, 9*(41). doi:10.4103/sni.sni_408_17

Euskirchen, P., & Peyre, M. (2018). Management of meningiomas. *Neuro-Oncology Quarterly Medical Review, 47*(11-12), e247–254.

Gale, S., Acar, D., & Daffner, K. (2018). Dementia. *American Journal of Medicine, 131*(10), 1161–1169.

Garcia, C., Slone, S., Dolecek, T., et al. (2019). Primary brain and central nervous system tumor treatment and survival in the United States 2004–2014. *Neuroncology, 144*(1), 179–191.

Hardiman, O., Al-Chalabi, A., Chio, A., et al. (2017). Amyotrophic lateral sclerosis. *Nature Reviews. Disease Primers, 3,* 17071. doi.org/10.1038/nrdp.2017.71

Harland, T. A., Wang, M., Gunaydin, D., et al. (2020). Frailty as a predictor of neurosurgical outcomes in brain tumor patients. *World Neurosurgery, 133,* e813–e818. doi.org/10.1016/j.wneu. 2019.10.010

Hemmer, C. (2018). Surgical complications associated with cervical spine surgery. *Orthopedic Nursing, 37*(6), 348–354.

Hogden, A., Foley, G., Henderson, R. D., et al. (2017). Amyotrophic lateral sclerosis: Improving care with a multidisciplinary approach. *Journal of Multidisciplinary Healthcare, 10,* 205–215.

Hong, C. S., & Moliterno, J. (2019). The patient-centered approach: A review of the literature and its application for acoustic neuromas. *Journal of Neurological Surgery. Part B, 81*(3), 280–286.

Ijzerman-Korevaar, M., Snijers, T. J., Saskia, C. C. M. T., et al. (2018). Symptom monitoring in glioma patients: Development of the Edmonton Symptom Assessment System Glioma Module. *Journal of Neuroscience Nursing, 50*(6), 381–387.

*Jang, M. K., Oh, E. G., Lee, H., et al. (2020). Postoperative symptoms and quality of life in pituitary macroadenomas patients. *The Journal of Neuroscience Nursing, 52*(1), 30–36.

Kaplow, R., & Iyere, K. (2016). Understanding spinal cord compression. *Nursing, 46*(9), 44–51.

*Ketcher, D., Otto, A. K., & Reblin, M. (2020). Caregivers of patients with brain metastases: A description of caregiving responsibilities and psychosocial well-being. *Journal of Neuroscience Nursing, 52*(3), 112–116.

Kirkeby, A., Parmar, M., & Barker, R. A. (2017). Strategies for bringing stem cell-derived dopamine neurons to the clinic: A European approach (STEM-PD). *Progress in Brain Research, 230,* 191–212.

*Kose, G., Tastan, S., Temiz, N. C., et al. (2019). The effect of low back pain on daily activities and sleep quality in patients with lumbar disc herniation: A pilot study. *The journal of Neuroscience Nursing, 51*(4), 184–189.

Lall, M. P. (2018). Nursing care of the patient undergoing lumbar spinal fusion. *Journal of Nursing Education and Practice, 8*(5), 44–52.

*Liang, S. Y., Liu, H. C., Lu, Y. Y., et al. (2020). The influence of resilience on the coping strategies in patients with primary brain tumors. *Asian Nursing Research, 14*(1), 50–55.

Lindsay, S., Cagliostro, E., & McAdam, L. (2019). Meaningful occupations of young adults with muscular dystrophy and other neuromuscular disorders. *Canadian Journal of Occupational Therapy, 86*(4), 277–288.

McColgan, P., & Tabrizi, S. J. (2017). Huntington's disease: A clinical review. *European Journal of Neurology, 25*(1), 24–34.

McFaline-Figueroa, J. R., & Lee, E. Q. (2018). Brain tumors. *The American Journal of Medicine, 131*(8), 875–882.

Mestre, T. A., & Shannon, K. (2017). Huntington disease care: From the past to the present, to the future. *Parkinsonism and Related Disorders, 44,* 114–118.

Molitch, M. E. (2017). Diagnosis and treatment of pituitary adenomas: A review. *JAMA, 317*(5), 516–524.

Moore, D. J., Smith, B. M., & Cho, M. H. (2017). Managing meditations for hospital patients with Parkinson disease. *American Nurse Today, 12*(1), 9–12.

Pastuszak, Z., Stepien, A., Tomczykiewicz, K., et al. (2017). Post-polio syndrome: Cases report and review of literature. *Polish Journal of Neurology and Neurosurgery, 51*(2017), 140–145.

Poewe, W., Seppi, K., Tanner, C. M., et al. (2017). Parkinson disease. *Nature Reviews Disease Primers, 3,* 1713. doi:10.1038/nrdp.2017.13

Ramanathan, S., Hibbert, P., Wiles, L., et al. (2018). What is the association between the presence of comorbidities and the appropriateness of care for low back? A population-based medical record review study. *BMC Musculoskeletal Disorders, 19*(391), 1–9.

*Scheffel, K., Amidei, C. & Fitzgerald, K. A. (2019). Motivational interviewing: Improving confidence with self-care management in postoperative thoracolumbar spine patients. *Journal of Neuroscience Nursing, 51*(3), 113–117.

Shing, L. H. S., Chipika, R. H., Finegan, E., et al. (2019). Post-polio syndrome: More than just a lower motor neuron disease. *Frontiers in Neurology, 10,* 773. doi:10.3389/fneur.2019.00773

Sin, M., & Khemani, P. (2020). Neurogenic orthostatic hypotension: An underrecognized complication of Parkinson disease. *Journal of Neuroscience Nurses, 52*(5), 230–233.

Smedley, R. M., & Coulson, N. S. (2019). Genetic testing for Huntington's disease: A thematic analysis of online support community messages. *Journal of Health Psychology,* 1–15. doi:10.1177/1359105319826340

Song, L., Li, Q., Yin, R., et al. (2018). Choriocarcinoma with brain metastasis after term pregnancy. *Medicine, 97*(42), e12904.

Soofi, A. Y., Bello-Haas, D. V., Kho, M. E., et al. (2018). The impact of rehabilitative interventions on quality of life: A qualitative evidence synthesis of personal experiences of individuals with amyotrophic lateral sclerosis. *Quality of Life Research, 27*(4), 845–856.

Trout, C. J., Case, L. E., Clemens, P. R., et al. (2018). A transition toolkit for Duchenne Muscular Dystrophy. *Pediatrics, 142*(Suppl 2), S110–S117.

Urrutia, N. L. (2019). Adult-onset Huntington disease an update. *Nursing, 49*(7), 37–43.

Vacca, V. M. (2020). Amyotrophic lateral sclerosis: Nursing care and considerations. *Nursing, 50*(6), 32–39.

Witherspoon, B., & Ashby, N. E. (2017). The use of mannitol and hypertonic saline therapies in patients with elevated intracranial pressure. *Nursing Clinics of North America, 52*(2), 249–260.

Young, J. S., Chmura, C. J., Wainwright, D. A., et al. (2017). Management of glioblastoma in elderly patients. *Journal of Neurological Sciences, 380,* 250–255.

Resources

ALS Association, www.alsa.org

American Association of Neuroscience Nurses, www.aann.org

American Brain Tumor Association, www.abta.org

American Parkinson Disease Association, www.apdaparkinson.org

Family Caregiver Alliance, www.caregiver.org

Huntington's Disease Society of American, www.hdsa.org

Muscular Dystrophy Association, www.mda.org

National Brain Tumor Society, www.braintumor.org

Parkinson's Foundation, www.parkinson.org

Spinal Cord Tumor Association, INC, www.spinalcordtumor.org

The Michael J. Fox Foundation, www.michaeljfox.org

Acute Community-Based Challenges

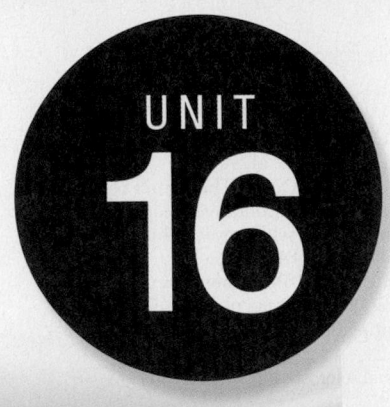

Case Study

USING EVIDENCE-BASED PRACTICES FOR EFFECTIVE CARE DURING A NOVEL VIRUS OUTBREAK

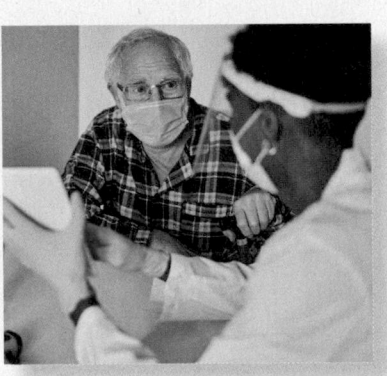

Y̲ou are a home health nurse in an urban community. The Centers for Disease Control and Prevention (CDC) has informed the agency where you work that there is an outbreak within your community of a novel respiratory virus that is implicated in causing pneumonia and acute respiratory failure. You know that when a novel virus begins to circulate among a population that universally has no immunity, some groups will be at greater risk of contracting the virus than others. You are worried about the patients you routinely care for as they have multiple comorbidities, likely placing them at higher risk. How will you find and integrate the best current evidence with clinical expertise, while also respecting patient and family preferences and values for delivery of optimal health care during a novel virus outbreak?

QSEN Competency Focus: Evidence-Based Practice

The complexities inherent in today's health care system challenge nurses to demonstrate integration of specific interdisciplinary core competencies. These competencies are aimed at ensuring the delivery of safe, quality patient care (Institute of Medicine, 2003). The Quality and Safety Education for Nurses project (Cronenwett, Sherwood, Barnsteiner, et al., 2007; QSEN, 2020) provides a framework for the knowledge, skills, and attitudes (KSAs) required for nurses to demonstrate competency in these key areas, which include *patient-centered care*, *interdisciplinary teamwork and collaboration*, *evidence-based practice*, *quality improvement*, *safety*, and *informatics*.

Evidence-Based Practice Definition: Integrate best current evidence with clinical expertise and patient/family preferences and values for delivery of optimal health care.

SELECT PRE-LICENSURE KSAs	APPLICATION AND REFLECTION
Knowledge	
Explain the role of evidence in determining best clinical practice	Which federal, state, and local sources will you use to identify an evolving evidence base around an outbreak of a novel virus? How will you judge the strength and the relevance of the evidence you locate?
Describe how the strength and relevance of available evidence influences the choice of interventions in provision of patient-centered care	Describe how utilizing evidence-based education will help to increase the knowledge that a given patient will have regarding care during a pandemic.
Skills	
Read original research and evidence reports related to area of practice	Discuss what evidence you would use to guide your practice during an outbreak of a novel virus.
Locate evidence reports related to clinical practice topics and guidelines	According to the evidence-based literature, what are effective infection control techniques for patients of different ages and with various comorbidities during a novel viral outbreak?
Attitudes	
Acknowledge own limitations in knowledge and clinical expertise before determining when to deviate from evidence-based best practices	Reflect on how it would feel to have a novel viral outbreak impose restrictions on your life. How does a novel viral outbreak have the potential to impact the daily lives of patients with comorbidities?

Cronenwett, L., Sherwood, G., Barnsteiner, J., et al. (2007). Quality and safety education for nurses. *Nursing Outlook, 55*(3), 122–131; Institute of Medicine. (2003). *Health professions education: A bridge to quality*. Washington, DC: National Academies Press; QSEN Institute. (2020). *QSEN Competencies: Definitions and pre-licensure KSAs; Evidence-based practice*. Retrieved on 8/15/2020 at: qsen.org/competencies/pre-licensure-ksas/#evidence-based_practice

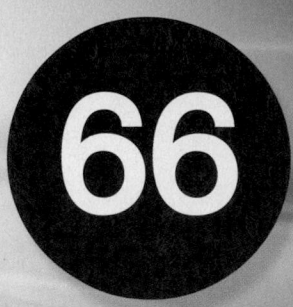

66

Management of Patients with Infectious Diseases

LEARNING OUTCOMES

On completion of this chapter, the learner will be able to:

1. Differentiate between the concepts of colonization, infection, and disease.
2. Identify federal, state, and local resources available to the nurse seeking information about infectious diseases and discuss the benefits of recommended vaccines for health care workers and patients.
3. Compare and contrast standard and transmission-based precautions and discuss the elements of each of these prevention methods.
4. Describe the concept and the nursing management of patients with emerging infectious diseases.
5. Use the nursing process as a framework for care of the patient with a sexually transmitted infection or with an infectious disease.

NURSING CONCEPTS

Cellular Regulation

Family

Fluids and Electrolytes

Infection

Patient Education

Safety

Sexuality

Thermoregulation

GLOSSARY

bacteremia: laboratory-confirmed presence of bacteria in the bloodstream

carrier: person who has a pathogen without apparent signs and symptoms; one who is able to transmit an infection to others

colonization: the presence of microorganisms in or on a host, without host interference or interaction and without eliciting symptoms in the host

coronavirus disease 2019 (COVID-19): a disease caused by the virus SARS-CoV-2

emerging infectious diseases: human infectious diseases with an increased incidence within the past two decades, or with a potential to increase in the near future

epidemic: a widespread outbreak of a specific infectious disease from a single source within a community or population that exceeds anticipated levels of impact

health care–associated infection (HAI): an infection not present or incubating at the time of admission to the health care setting; this term has replaced the term *nosocomial infection*

host: an organism that provides living conditions to support a microorganism

immune: person with protection from a previous infection or vaccination who resists reinfection when re-exposed to the same agent

incubation period: time between contact and onset of signs and symptoms

infection: condition in which the host interacts physiologically and immunologically with a microorganism

infectious disease: any disease caused by the growth of pathogenic microbes in the body that may or may not be communicable

latency: time interval after primary infection when a microorganism lives within the host without producing clinical evidence of disease

methicillin-resistant *Staphylococcus aureus* (MRSA): *Staphylococcus aureus* bacterium that is not susceptible to extended-penicillin antibiotic formulas, such as methicillin, oxacillin, or nafcillin; MRSA may occur in a health care or community setting

normal flora: persistent nonpathogenic organisms colonizing a host

outbreak: the occurrence of a disease within a population that exceeds normal expectations

pandemic: an epidemic that spreads across multiple countries or continents

reservoir: any person, plant, animal, substance, or location that provides living conditions for microorganisms and that enables further dispersal of the organism

severe acute respiratory syndrome coronavirus 2 (SARS-CoV-2): the virus that causes COVID-19

standard precautions: strategy of assuming all patients may carry infectious agents and using appropriate barrier precautions for all health care worker–patient interactions

susceptible: not possessing immunity to a particular pathogen

transient flora: organisms that have been recently acquired and are likely to be shed in a relatively short period

transmission-based precautions: precautions used in addition to standard precautions when contagious or epidemiologically significant organisms are recognized; the three types of transmission-based precautions are airborne, droplet, and contact precautions

vancomycin-resistant *Enterococcus* (VRE): *Enterococcus* bacterium that is not susceptible to the antibiotic vancomycin

virulence: degree of pathogenicity of an organism

An **infectious disease** is any disease caused by the growth of pathogenic microbes in the body. It may or may not be communicable (i.e., contagious). Although modern science had controlled, eradicated, or decreased the incidence of many infectious diseases, emerging novel pathogens continue to plague the globe, taxing economic and social resources, and proving hazardous to the health and well-being of patients, families, communities, and cultural systems. Examples of such threatening infectious diseases are presented in this chapter. Other infectious diseases are discussed in the appropriate chapters (e.g., see Chapter 19 for information on tuberculosis [TB]). It is important to understand infectious causes and the treatment of contagious, serious, common infections as well as emerging noncommon infections. Table 66-1 presents select infectious diseases, their causative organisms, mode of transmission, and usual **incubation period** (time between contact and development of the first signs and symptoms).

The nurse plays an important role in infection control and prevention. Educating patients may decrease their risk of becoming infected or may decrease the sequelae of infection. Using appropriate barrier precautions, observing prudent hand hygiene, and ensuring aseptic care of intravenous (IV) catheters and other invasive equipment also assists in reducing infections.

The Infectious Process

The Chain of Infection

A complete chain of events is necessary for infection to occur. Six elements are necessary, including a causative organism, a reservoir of available organisms, a portal of exit from the reservoir, a mode of transmission from the reservoir to the **host** (an organism that provides living conditions to support a microorganism) and a mode of entry into a susceptible host.

Nurses must clearly understand the elements of the chain of infection in order to identify points at which they can intervene to interrupt the chain, thus protecting patients, themselves, and others from infectious diseases. Figure 66-1 illustrates these concepts.

Causative Organism

The types of microorganisms that cause infections are bacteria, rickettsiae, viruses, protozoa, fungi, and helminths.

Reservoir

Reservoir is the term used for any person, plant, animal, substance, or location that provides nourishment for microorganisms and enables further dispersal of the organism. Infections may be prevented by eliminating the causative organisms from the reservoir.

Portal of Exit

The organism must have a portal of exit from a reservoir. An infected host must shed organisms to another or to the environment for transmission to occur. Organisms exit through the respiratory tract, the gastrointestinal tract, the genitourinary tract, or the blood.

Route of Transmission

A route of transmission is necessary to connect the infectious source with its new host. Organisms may be transmitted through food intake, sexual contact, skin-to-skin contact, percutaneous injection, or infectious particles carried in the air. A person who carries or transmits a pathogen but does not have apparent signs and symptoms of infection is called a **carrier**.

Specific organisms require specific routes of transmission for infection to occur. For example, *Mycobacterium tuberculosis* is almost always transmitted by the airborne route. Health care providers do not "carry" *M. tuberculosis* bacteria on their hands or clothing. In contrast, bacteria such as *Staphylococcus aureus* are easily transmitted from patient to patient on the hands of health care providers. Some organisms cause infection through several routes. For example, the virus **severe acute respiratory syndrome coronavirus 2 (SARS-CoV-2)**, the virus that causes the **coronavirus disease 2019 (COVID-19)**, is highly contagious (see discussion later in this chapter). When appropriate, the nurse explains routes of disease transmission to patients.

Susceptible Host

For infection to occur, the host must be **susceptible** (not possessing immunity to a pathogen). Previous infection or vaccine administration may render the host **immune** (not susceptible) to further infection with an agent. Although exposure to potentially infectious microorganisms occurs essentially on a constant basis, people have complex immune systems that generally prevent infection from occurring. A person who is immunosuppressed has much greater susceptibility to infection than a healthy person.

Portal of Entry

A portal of entry is needed for the organism to gain access to the host. Again, specific organisms may require specific portals of entry for infection to occur. For example, airborne *M. tuberculosis* does not cause disease when it settles on the skin of an exposed host; the only entry route for *M. tuberculosis*

(*text continued on page 2148*)

TABLE 66-1 Select Infectious Diseases, Causative Organisms, Modes of Transmission, and Usual Incubation Periods

Disease or Condition	Organism	Usual Mode of Transmission	Approximate Incubation Period (Infection to First Symptom)
Acquired immune deficiency syndrome (AIDS)	Human immune deficiency virus (HIV)	Sexual; percutaneous; perinatal	Variable. Median of 10 yrs without effective therapy
Anthrax	*Bacillus anthracis*	Airborne, contact, or ingestion	1–43 days (inhalation) 5–7 days (cutaneous) 1–6 days (gastrointestinal)
Chancroid	*Haemophilus ducreyi*	Sexual	3–5 days
Chickenpox	Varicella zoster	Airborne or contact	10–21 days
Coronavirus disease 2019 (COVID-19)	Severe acute respiratory syndrome coronavirus 2 (SARS-CoV-2)	Droplet and contact are principal modes In some situations, may be aerosolized	2–14 days
Cytomegalovirus infection	Cytomegalovirus	Transfusion and transplantation; sexual; perinatal	Highly variable: 3–8 wks after transfusion, 3–12 wks after delivery of newborn
Diarrheal disease (common causes)	*Campylobacter* species	Ingestion of contaminated food	2–5 days
	Clostridioides difficile	Fecal–oral	Variable; over 2 days
	Salmonella species	Ingestion of contaminated food or drink	12–36 h
	Shigella species	Ingestion of contaminated food or drink; direct contact with carrier	1–3 days
	Yersinia species	Ingestion of contaminated food or drink; direct contact with carrier	3–7 days
Ebola	Ebola virus	Contact with blood or body fluids	2–21 days
Gonorrhea	*Neisseria gonorrhoeae*	Sexual; perinatal	1–14 days
Hand, foot, and mouth disease	Coxsackievirus	Direct contact with nose and throat secretions and with feces of people who are infected	3–5 days
Hantavirus pulmonary syndrome	Sin Nombre virus	Contact (direct or indirect) with rodents	2 days to 6 wks
Hepatitis, foodborne	Hepatitis A virus	Ingestion of contaminated food or drink; direct contact with carrier	14–42 days
	Hepatitis E virus	Ingestion of contaminated food or drink; direct contact with carrier	15–65 days
Hepatitis, bloodborne	Hepatitis B virus	Sexual; perinatal; percutaneous	45–180 days
	Hepatitis C virus	Sexual; perinatal; percutaneous	15 days to 6 mo
Herpes simplex	Human herpes viruses 1 and 2	Contact with mucous membrane secretions	2–12 days
Histoplasmosis	*Histoplasma capsulatum*	Inhalation of airborne spores	3–17 days
Hookworm disease	*Necator americanus; Ancylostoma duodenale*	Contact with soil contaminated with human feces	A few weeks to many months
Impetigo	*Staphylococcus aureus, Streptococcus pyogenes*	Contact with carrier or with patient's soiled towels or combs	4–10 days
Influenza	Influenza virus A, B, or C	Droplet spread	24–72 h
Legionnaires disease	*Legionella pneumophila*	Airborne from water source	2–10 days
Lyme disease	*Borrelia burgdorferi*	Tick bite	3–32 days
Lymphogranuloma venereum	*Chlamydia trachomatis*	Sexual	Weeks to years
Malaria	*Plasmodium vivax; Plasmodium malariae; Plasmodium falciparum; Plasmodium ovale*	Bite from *Anopheles* species mosquito	9–40 days

TABLE 66-1 Select Infectious Diseases, Causative Organisms, Modes of Transmission, and Usual Incubation Periods (continued)

Disease or Condition	Organism	Usual Mode of Transmission	Approximate Incubation Period (Infection to First Symptom)
Marburg hemorrhagic fever	Marburg virus	Unknown route of transmission from animals to humans; person-to-person by droplets and direct contact	5–15 days
Meningococcal meningitis or bacteremia	*Neisseria meningitidis*	Contact with pharyngeal secretions; perhaps airborne	2–10 days
Mononucleosis	Epstein–Barr virus	Contact with pharyngeal secretions	4–6 wks
Mycobacterial diseases (non-tuberculosis *Mycobacterium* species)	*Mycobacterium avium; Mycobacterium kansasii; Mycobacterium fortuitum; Mycobacterium gordonae;* other *Mycobacterium* species	Variable; probably contact with soil, water, or other environmental source; none is person-to-person transmissible	Variable
Norovirus	Norovirus	Fecal–oral by food or water or by person-to-person spread	10–48 h
Pediculosis	*Pediculus humanus capitis* (head louse); *Pthiriasis pubis* (crab louse)	Direct or indirect contact	1–2 wks
Pertussis (whooping cough)	*Bordetella pertussis*	Contact with respiratory droplets	7–10 days
Pinworm disease	*Enterobius vermicularis*	Direct contact with egg-contaminated articles	1–2-mo life cycle; often takes months of infection before recognition
Pneumocystis jirovecii pneumonia	*Pneumocystis jirovecii*	Unknown; not transmitted person to person	Infants: 1–2 mo; adults: unclear
Pneumococcal pneumonia	*Streptococcus pneumoniae*	Droplet spread	Probably 1–3 days
Rabies	Rabies virus	Bite from rabid animal	3–8 wks
Respiratory syncytial disease	Respiratory syncytial virus	Self-inoculation by mouth or nose after contact with infectious respiratory secretions	1–10 days
Rocky Mountain spotted fever	*Rickettsia rickettsii*	Bite from infected tick	2–21 days
Roseola infantum	Human herpes virus 6	Saliva	10–15 days
Rotavirus gastroenteritis	Rotavirus	Fecal–oral route	24–72 h
Rubella	Rubella virus	Droplet spread; direct contact	14–21 days
Scabies	*Sarcoptes scabiei*	Direct skin contact	2–6 wks
Smallpox (Eradicated since 1980)	Variola major and minor	Airborne droplets and contact	7–17 days
Syphilis	*Treponema pallidum*	Sexual; perinatal	10 days to 12 wks
Tetanus	*Clostridium tetani*	Puncture wound	3–21 days
Tinea (ringworm)	*Microsporum* species; *Trichophyton* species	Direct and indirect contact with lesions	4–10 days
Trichinosis	*Trichinella spiralis*	Ingestion of insufficiently cooked foods, especially pork and beef	8–15 days
Tuberculosis	*Mycobacterium tuberculosis*	Airborne	2–10 wks to the formation of primary lesion
West Nile virus	West Nile virus	Bite of infected mosquitoes; from transfusions and transplants; perinatal	2–14 days
Zika virus	Zika virus	Bite of infected *Aedes* mosquitoes	3–14 days

Adapted from Centers for Disease Control and Prevention. (2015). In Hamborsky, J., Kroger, A., & Wolfe, S. (Eds.). *Epidemiology and prevention of vaccine-preventable diseases* (13th ed.). Washington, DC: Public Health Foundation; Krow-Lucal, E. R., Biggerstaff, B. J., & Staples, J. E. (2017). Estimated incubation period for Zika virus disease. *Emerging Infectious Diseases, 23*(5), 841–845.

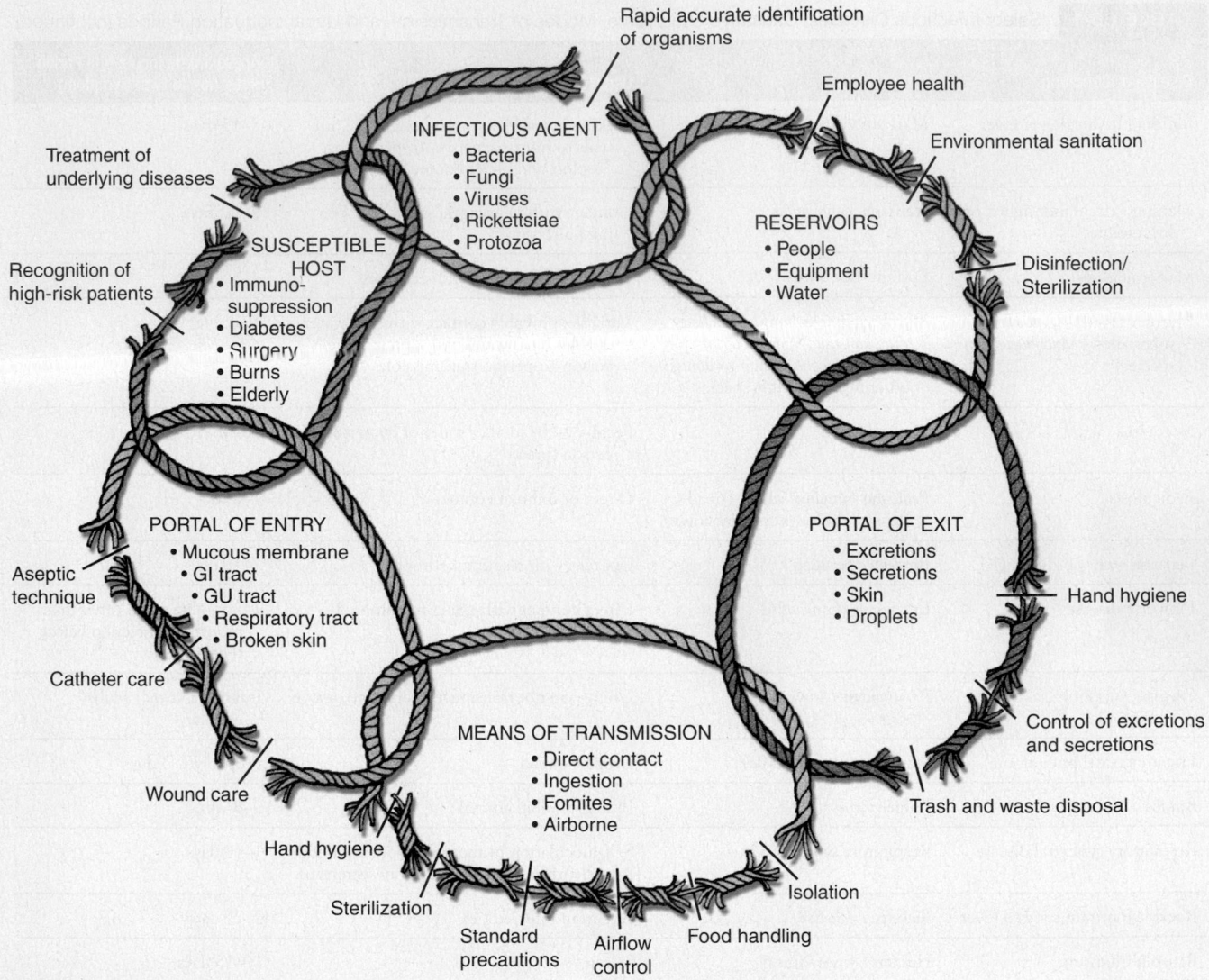

Figure 66-1 • Health care workers' interventions used to break the chain of infection transmission.

is through the respiratory tract. The portal of entry for the SARS-CoV-2 virus is respiratory; however, the virus can remain airborne indoors for hours, accumulate over time, and can travel in airflows over distances greater than 6 feet (Prather, Wang, & Schooley, 2020).

Colonization, Infection, and Infectious Disease

Relatively few anatomic sites (e.g., brain, blood, bone, heart, vascular system) are sterile. Bacteria found throughout the body usually provide beneficial **normal flora** (nonpathogenic organisms colonizing a host) to compete with potential pathogens, to facilitate digestion, or to work in other ways symbiotically with the host.

Colonization

The term **colonization** is used to describe the presence of microorganisms without host interference or interaction. Organisms reported in microbiology test results often reflect colonization rather than infection. The patient's health care

team must interpret microbiology test results accurately to ensure appropriate treatment.

Infection

Infection indicates a host interaction with an organism. A patient colonized with *S. aureus* may have staphylococci on the skin without any skin interruption or irritation. However, if the patient has an incision, *S. aureus* entering the wound can induce an immune system reaction of local inflammation and migration of white cells to the site. Clinical evidence of redness, heat, and pain and laboratory evidence of white blood cells in the wound specimen smear suggest infection. In this situation, the host identifies the staphylococci as *foreign*. Infection is recognized by the host reaction (manifested by signs and symptoms) and by laboratory-based evidence of white blood cell reaction and microbiologic organism identification.

Infectious Disease

Infectious disease is the state in which the infected host displays a decline in wellness due to the infection. When the

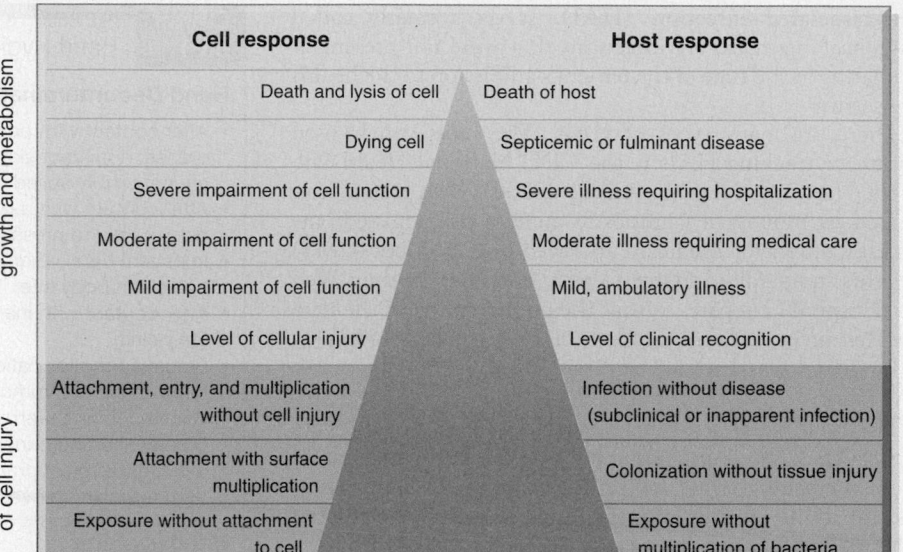

Figure 66-2 • Biologic spectrum of response to bacterial infection at the cellular level (*left*) and of the intact host (*right*). Redrawn from Evans, A. S., & Brachman, P. S. (1998). *Bacterial infections in humans: Epidemiology and control* (3rd ed., p. 40). New York: Plenum.

host interacts immunologically with an organism but remains symptom free, the definition of infectious disease has not been met. For example, most people who are infected with M. *tuberculosis* have no symptoms. This is considered **latency,** or the time interval after primary infection when a microorganism lives within the host without producing clinical evidence of disease. The severity of an infectious disease ranges from mild to life-threatening (Norris, 2019). Figure 66-2 depicts the range of response to bacterial infection at the cellular and host level.

The primary source of information about most bacterial infections is the microbiology laboratory report, which should be viewed as a tool to be used along with clinical indicators to determine if a patient is colonized or infected. Microbiology reports from clinical specimens usually show three components: the smear and stain, the culture and organism identification, and the antimicrobial susceptibility (i.e., sensitivity). As a marker for the likelihood of infection, the smear and stain generally provide the most helpful information because they describe the mix of cells present at the anatomic site at the time of specimen collection. Culture and sensitivity results specify which organisms are recognized and which antibiotic agents actively affect the bacteria.

Infection Control and Prevention

The World Health Organization (WHO) and the Centers for Disease Control and Prevention (CDC) are the principal agencies involved in setting guidelines about infection prevention. The impact of infectious diseases changes over time as microorganisms mutate, as human behavior patterns shift, or as therapeutic options change. The CDC provides timely recommendations about many of the situations that a nurse may face when caring for or educating a patient with an infectious disease and routinely publishes recommendations, guidelines, and summaries. Through its Internet site and its weekly journal, the *Morbidity and Mortality Weekly Report (MMWR),* the CDC reports significant cases, **outbreaks** (the occurrence of a disease within a population that exceeds

normal expectations), environmental hazards, or other public health problems. Examples of important CDC guidelines and summaries include *Immunization Schedules* (CDC, 2020b) and *Interim Infection Prevention and Control Recommendations for Healthcare Personnel During the COVID-19 Pandemic* (CDC, 2020c).

Nurses serve important roles in preventing the transfer of organisms given their frequent encounters with patients and families. It is essential for the nurse to model appropriate and effective hand hygiene practices in all aspects of patient care. Nurses can also help reduce hand-to-hand spread of organisms by serving as patient advocates. The nurse should observe the hand hygiene activities of other professionals and alert them to lapses in technique that are observed. Nurses need to educate patients and their families to feel comfortable in reminding health care workers to perform hand hygiene before patient contact.

This chapter summarizes several aspects of infectious diseases. However, the field of infection control and prevention changes rapidly. The COVID-19 **pandemic** provides a striking example of how a new infectious agent can place new expectations and responsibilities on health care workers, including nurses. A pandemic is an **epidemic** (an outbreak of infectious disease within a population that exceeds anticipated levels of impact) that spreads across multiple countries or continents. The COVID-19 crisis created unprecedented challenges with health care systems modifying everyday practices, and making administrative system wide changes. Nurses carried out complex care, simultaneously adapting to frequent changes in protocols, therapies, and other day-to-day routines, while also providing direction and support for stressed patients and family members. See Chapter 68 for discussion of moral distress during the COVID-19 pandemic.

Preventing Infection in Health Care Settings

The prevention of infection in the health care setting focuses upon following the appropriate standard and transmission-based precautions as well as reducing the risk of a **health** care–associated infection (HAI). HAIs, formerly called *nosocomial infections*, are infections that were not present or incubating at the time of the patient's admission to the health care setting.

There are many types of HAIs. The most widely used system for tracking HAIs is the CDC National Healthcare Safety Network (NHSN) (CDC, 2020d). The system can be used by individual facilities to analyze risk-adjusted outcomes. Centers for Medicare and Medicaid Services (CMS) uses this standardized source to post outcomes on their Web site, Hospital Compare, so that the public can view the data (see Resources section). CMS also uses these data for imposing financial penalties for facilities who have less favorable HAI rates.

The NHSN has reporting systems for several health care facility types. These include acute care facilities, ambulatory care centers, long-term care facilities, outpatient dialysis centers, inpatient rehabilitation facilities, inpatient psychiatric facilities, and home dialysis facilities (CDC, 2020d).

Isolation Precautions

Isolation precautions are guidelines created to prevent transmission of microorganisms in health care facilities. The Healthcare Infection Control Practices Advisory Committee (HICPAC) of the CDC recommends two tiers of isolation precautions. The first tier, called **standard precautions**, is designed for the care of *all* patients and is the primary strategy for preventing HAIs. The second tier, called **transmission-based precautions**, is designed for care of patients with known or suspected infectious diseases spread by airborne, droplet, or contact routes. In addition, Occupational Safety and Health Administration (OSHA) regulations are followed to prevent exposure to bloodborne pathogens and hazardous substances (Occupational Safety and Health Administration [OSHA], 2012).

Standard Precautions

The basis of standard precautions is that all patients are colonized or infected with microorganisms, whether or not there are signs or symptoms, and that a uniform level of caution should be used in the care of all patients. The health care worker should use additional barriers in the form of personal protective equipment (PPE), including gloves, masks, eye protection, and cover gowns, depending on the expected degree of exposure to patient excretions or secretions. The elements of standard precautions include appropriate hand hygiene, the use of PPE, proper handling of patient care equipment and linen, environmental control, prevention of injury from sharps devices, and patient room assignments within health care facilities. Hand hygiene, glove use, needlestick prevention, and avoidance of splash or spray of body fluids are discussed in the following sections. See Chapter 32, Chart 32-5 for a description of standard precautions.

Hand Hygiene

The most frequent cause of bacterial transmission in health care institutions is spread of microorganisms by the hands of health care workers. Health care workers should perform hand hygiene frequently during patient care. Chart 66-1 describes the indications for different hand hygiene methods (CDC, 2002).

Chart 66-1 **Hand Hygiene Methods**

Hand Decontamination with Alcohol-Based Product

- After contact with body fluids, excretions, mucous membranes, nonintact skin, or wound dressings; as long as hands are not visibly soiled
- After contact with a patient's intact skin (e.g., after taking pulse or blood pressure or lifting a patient)
- In patient care, when moving from a contaminated body site to a clean body site
- After contact with inanimate objects in the patient's immediate vicinity
- Before caring for patients with severe neutropenia or other forms of severe immune suppression
- Before donning sterile gloves when inserting central catheters
- Before inserting urinary catheters or other devices that do not require a surgical procedure
- After removing gloves

Handwashing

- When hands are visibly dirty or contaminated with biologic material from patient care
- When health care workers do not tolerate waterless alcohol product

Adapted from Centers for Disease Control and Prevention (CDC). (2002). Guideline for hand hygiene in health care settings. *MMWR. Morbidity and Mortality Weekly Report, 51*(RR 16), 1–56.

When hands are visibly dirty or contaminated with biologic material from patient care, the worker should wash hands with soap and water. In intensive care units and other locations in which virulent or resistant organisms are likely to be present, antimicrobial agents (e.g., chlorhexidine gluconate, iodophor, chloroxylenol) may be used. Effective handwashing requires at least *20 seconds of vigorous scrubbing*, with special attention to the area around nail beds and between fingers, where there is a high bacterial load. Hands should be thoroughly rinsed after washing (CDC, 2002).

If hands are not visibly soiled, health care providers are encouraged to use alcohol-based, waterless antiseptic agents for routine hand decontamination. These solutions are superior to soap or antimicrobial handwashing agents in their speed of action and effectiveness against most microorganisms. Because they are formulated with emollients, they are usually better tolerated than other agents, and because they can be used without sinks and towels, health care workers may be more adherent with their use. Nurses working in home health care or other settings where they are relatively mobile should carry pocket-sized containers of alcohol-based solutions. The spore form of the bacterium *Clostridioides difficile* is resistant to alcohol and other hand disinfectants; therefore, the use of gloves and handwashing (soap and water for physical removal) are required when *C. difficile* has been identified (CDC, 2019c).

Normal skin flora usually include relatively benign coagulase-negative staphylococci or diphtheroids. Health care workers may temporarily carry more potentially pathogenic bacteria such as *S. aureus* or *Pseudomonas aeruginosa*. This temporary carriage is considered **transient flora** which will likely be shed with hand hygiene and natural skin degeneration over time.

Hand hygiene decreases bacterial transmission to patients by reducing bacterial load on health care workers' hands. The Joint Commission includes hand hygiene as one of the National Patient Safety Goals and focuses on this behavior in surveys of health care facilities (The Joint Commission, 2021). All health care settings should have mechanisms to measure and improve adherence with hand hygiene by all personnel who care for patients (Schierhorn, 2019).

Artificial fingernails or nail extenders have been epidemiologically linked to several significant infection outbreaks and therefore should not be worn when providing patient care. Natural nails should be kept less than 0.6 cm (0.25 inch) long, and nail polish should be removed when chipped because it can support increased bacterial growth (CDC, 2002).

Glove Use

Gloves provide an effective barrier for hands from the microflora associated with patient care. Gloves should be worn when a health care worker has contact with any patient secretions or excretions and must be discarded after each patient care contact. Because microbial organisms colonizing health care workers' hands can proliferate in the warm, moist environment provided by gloves, hands must be washed or disinfected after gloves are removed. As patient advocates, nurses have an important role in promoting hand hygiene and glove use by other hospital workers, such as laboratory personnel, technicians, physicians, and others who have contact with patients.

Compared with vinyl gloves, latex or nitrile gloves are preferred because they resist puncture better and provide greater comfort and fit. Improvements in latex gloves have reduced the incidence of latex hypersensitivity, but some workers continue to experience local skin irritation or more severe reactions, including generalized dermatitis, conjunctivitis, asthma, angioedema, and anaphylaxis (see Chapter 33). The nurse who experiences irritation or an allergic reaction associated with exposure to latex should report symptoms to an occupational health specialist or a primary provider and avoid latex-based products.

Needlestick Prevention

The most important aspect of reducing the risk of bloodborne infection is avoidance of percutaneous injury. Extreme care is essential in all situations in which needles, scalpels, and other sharp objects are handled. Used needles should not be recapped. Instead, they are placed directly into puncture-resistant containers close to where they are used. If a situation dictates that a needle must be recapped, the nurse must use a mechanical device to hold the cap or use a one-handed approach to decrease the likelihood of skin puncture. OSHA requires use of needleless devices and other instruments designed to prevent injury from sharps when appropriate (OSHA, 2012).

Avoidance of Splash and Spray

When the health care professional is involved in an activity in which body fluids may be sprayed or splashed, appropriate barriers must be used. If a splash to the face may occur, goggles and a facemask are warranted. If the health care worker is involved in a procedure in which clothing may be contaminated with biologic material, a cover gown should be worn (CDC, 2007).

Transmission-Based Precautions

Reducing the risk of HAIs requires specific preventive activities in addition to implementing standard precautions. Some microbes are so contagious or epidemiologically important that, in addition to standard precautions, a second tier of precautions—transmission-based precautions—should be used when such organisms have been identified. Transmission-based categories are airborne, droplet, and contact precautions (CDC, 2007). As the term implies, the precautions are based on the routes of transmission. Diseases spread by very small respiratory particles that are suspended as aerosol require airborne precautions, those spread by larger respiratory droplets require droplet precautions, and those spread by touch require contact precautions.

Airborne precautions are required for patients with presumed or proven pulmonary TB, varicella, or other airborne pathogens such as COVID-19. When hospitalized, patients should be in airborne infection isolation rooms, engineered to provide negative air pressure, rapid turnover of air, and air either highly filtered or exhausted directly to the outside. If a facility does not have negative pressure rooms available, portable high-efficiency particular air (HEPA) filters may be used. Health care providers should wear an N95 respirator (i.e., protective mask) (see Chapter 68, Fig. 68-1) at all times while in the patient's room. The nurse should be able to validate room negative pressure by reading a pressure manometer placed outside the room or by witnessing that a tissue held at the gap between the door and the floor will be pulled toward the room.

Droplet precautions are used for organisms such as influenza or meningococcus that can be transmitted by close contact with respiratory or pharyngeal secretions. When caring for a patient requiring droplet precautions, the nurse should wear a facemask within 3 to 6 feet of the patient; however, because the risk of transmission is limited to close contact, the door may remain open.

Contact precautions are used for organisms that are spread by skin-to-skin contact, such as antibiotic-resistant organisms or *C. difficile*. Contact precautions are designed to emphasize cautious technique and the use of barriers. When possible, the patient requiring contact isolation is placed in a private room to facilitate hand hygiene and decreased environmental contamination. Masks are not needed, and doors do not need to be closed (see Chart 66-2).

COVID-19 Considerations

Guidelines for preventing transmission of COVID-19 in health care facilities include using a combination of all the transmission-based precautions and adding other prevention elements, such as increased use of PPE, enhanced cleaning, and adjusted visitor policies (CDC, 2020c). The SARS-CoV-2 virus is primarily transmitted by close contact to droplets and aerosol and by touching contaminated surfaces, with subsequent self-infection when touching the face. In most social interactions, the virus appears to be spread from droplets from the infected person to another. In the health care setting, airborne transmission can occur when aerosol-generating procedures are conducted. Procedures such as intubation, extubation, suctioning, and administering nebulized medication can mechanically aerosolize droplets so that infective particles can be inhaled. Similar transmission may

Chart 66-2 Summary of Types of Precautions and Patients Requiring the Precautions

Standard Precautions

Use standard precautions for the care of all patients.

Airborne Precautions

In addition to standard precautions, use airborne precautions for patients known or suspected to have serious illnesses transmitted by airborne droplet nuclei. Examples of such illnesses include:

- Measles
- Varicella (including disseminated zoster)[a]
- Tuberculosis

Airborne precautions are also used when performing aerosol generating procedures for patients with coronavirus disease 2019 (COVID-19) (along with a focus on droplet and contact precautions).

Droplet Precautions

In addition to standard precautions, use droplet precautions for patients known or suspected to have serious illnesses transmitted by large particle droplets. Examples of such illnesses include:

- Invasive *Haemophilus influenzae* type b disease, including meningitis, pneumonia, epiglottitis, and sepsis
- Invasive *Neisseria meningitidis* disease, including meningitis, pneumonia, and sepsis
- Other serious bacterial respiratory infections spread by droplet transmission, including:
  - Diphtheria (pharyngeal)
  - Primary atypical pneumonia (*Mycoplasma pneumoniae*)
  - Pertussis
  - Pneumonic plague
  - Streptococcal (group A) pharyngitis, pneumonia, or scarlet fever in infants and young children
- Serious viral infections spread by droplet transmission, including:
  - COVID-19 (along with contact precautions; and airborne precautions during aerosol-generating procedures)
  - Adenovirus[a]

- Influenza
- Mumps
- Parvovirus B19
- Rubella

Contact Precautions

In addition to standard precautions, use contact precautions for patients known or suspected to have serious illnesses easily transmitted by direct patient contact or by contact with items in the patient's environment. Examples of such illnesses include:

- Gastrointestinal, respiratory, skin, or wound infections or colonization with multidrug-resistant bacteria judged by the infection control program, based on current state, regional, or national recommendations, to be of special clinical and epidemiologic significance
- Enteric infections with a low infectious dose or prolonged environmental survival, including:
  - *Clostridioides difficile*
  - For patients who are diapered or incontinent: enterohemorrhagic *Escherichia coli* O157:H7, *Shigella* species, hepatitis A, or rotavirus
- Respiratory syncytial virus, parainfluenza virus, or enteroviral infections in infants and young children
- Skin infections that are highly contagious or that may occur on dry skin, including:
  - Diphtheria (cutaneous)
  - Herpes simplex virus (neonatal or mucocutaneous)
  - Impetigo
  - Major (noncontained) abscesses, cellulitis, or pressure injuries
  - Pediculosis
  - Scabies
  - Staphylococcal furunculosis in infants and young children
- Zoster (disseminated or in the immunocompromised host)[a]
- Viral and hemorrhagic conjunctivitis
- Viral hemorrhagic infections (Ebola, Lassa, or Marburg)

[a]Certain infections require more than one type of precaution.
Adapted from Centers for Disease Control and Prevention (CDC). (2007). 2007 *Guideline for isolation precautions: Preventing transmission of infectious agents in healthcare settings.* Retrieved on 3/13/2020 at: www.cdc.gov/hicpac/2007ip/2007ip_part1.html; Centers for Disease Control and Prevention (CDC). (2020c). Interim infection prevention and control recommendations for healthcare personnel during the coronavirus disease 2019 (COVID-19) pandemic. Retrieved on 7/17/2020 at: www.cdc.gov/coronavirus/2019-ncov/hcp/infection-control-recommendations.html

be possible with other close contact, such as may be required in the care of a patient infected with COVID-19. Due to COVID-19's **virulence** (degree of pathogenicity of an organism), contagiousness, and lack of treatment, guidelines advise facilities to use a combination of droplet, airborne, and contact precautions (CDC, 2020c). See discussion later in this chapter.

To protect against potential airborne transmission, health care workers in close contact with patients infected with COVID-19 were advised to use N95 respirators or powered air-purified respirators (PAPRs) (CDC, 2020c). When there is not an adequate supply of such devices to use for all patients with confirmed or suspected COVID-19 infection, a system should be designed to prioritize their use for aerosol-generating procedures. Some health care facilities have been able to reprocess N95s to expand their availability (CDC, 2020e). See Chapter 56 for recommendations for preventing and treating occupationally induced dermatologic conditions

during the COVID-19 pandemic (American Academy of Dermatology [AAD], 2020).

Gowns and gloves are worn to prevent transmission by contact. Health care workers must carefully put on, use, and safely take off PPE. Using the correct sequence for putting on and taking off PPE is especially important with SARS-CoV-2 as well as other highly contagious or virulent pathogens. The recommended sequence for putting on and safely removing PPE is outlined in Chart 66-3.

Specific Organisms with HAI Potential

Prior to the COVID-19 crisis, the WHO and CDC had focused increased attention on HAIs, which have also received increased focus from The Joint Commission, the Institute for Healthcare Improvement (IHI), and Medicare. HAI rates for each hospital are posted on the Hospital Compare Web site (see the Resources section). The Hospital Compare site also reports on some infections where the actual

Chart 66-3 Use of Personal Protective Equipment (PPE) When Caring for the Patient with Suspected or Confirmed COVID-19

Donning (Putting on the Gear)

More than one donning method may be acceptable. Training and practice using your health care facility's procedure is critical. Below is one example of donning.

1. **Identify and gather the proper PPE to don.** Ensure choice of gown size is correct (based on training).
2. **Perform hand hygiene using hand sanitizer.**
3. **Put on isolation gown.** Tie all of the ties on the gown. Assistance may be needed by another HCP.
4. **Put on NIOSH-approved N95 filtering facepiece respirator or higher (use a facemask if a respirator is not available).** If the respirator has a nosepiece, it should be fitted to the nose with both hands, not bent or tented. Do not pinch the nosepiece with one hand. Respirator/facemask should be extended under chin. Both your mouth and nose should be protected. Do not wear respirator/facemask under your chin or store in scrubs pocket between patients.[a]
   a. **Respirator:** Respirator straps should be placed on crown of head (top strap) and base of neck (bottom strap). Perform a user seal check each time you put on the respirator.
   b. **Facemask:** Mask ties should be secured on crown of head (top tie) and base of neck (bottom tie). If mask has loops, hook them appropriately around your ears.
5. **Put on face shield or goggles.** When wearing an N95 respirator or half facepiece elastomeric respirator, select the proper eye protection to ensure that the respirator does not interfere with the correct positioning of the eye protection, and the eye protection does not affect the fit or seal of the respirator. Face shields provide full face coverage. Goggles also provide excellent protection for eyes, but fogging is common.
6. **Put on gloves.** Gloves should cover the cuff (wrist) of gown.
7. **HCP may now enter patient room.**

Doffing (Taking Off the Gear)

More than one doffing method may be acceptable. Training and practice using your health care facility's procedure is critical. Below is one example of doffing.

1. **Remove gloves.** Ensure glove removal does not cause additional contamination of hands. Gloves can be removed using more than one technique (e.g., glove-in-glove or bird beak).
2. **Remove gown.** Untie all ties (or unsnap all buttons). Some gown ties can be broken rather than untied. Do so in gentle manner, avoiding a forceful movement. Reach up to the shoulders and carefully pull gown down and away from the body. Rolling the gown down is an acceptable approach. Dispose in trash receptacle.[a]
3. **HCP may now exit patient room.**
4. **Perform hand hygiene.**
5. **Remove face shield or goggles.** Carefully remove face shield or goggles by grabbing the strap and pulling upwards and away from head. Do not touch the front of face shield or goggles.
6. **Remove and discard respirator (or facemask if used instead of respirator).[a]** Do not touch the front of the respirator or facemask.
   a. **Respirator:** Remove the bottom strap by touching only the strap and bring it carefully over the head. Grasp the top strap and bring it carefully over the head, and then pull the respirator away from the face without touching the front of the respirator.
   b. **Facemask:** Carefully untie (or unhook from the ears) and pull away from face without touching the front.
7. **Perform hand hygiene after removing the respirator/facemask** and before putting it on again if your workplace is practicing reuse.

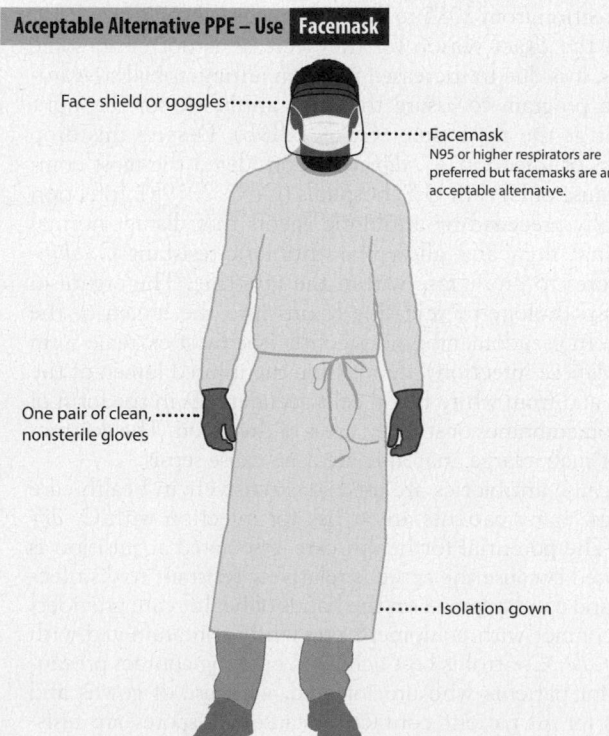

Preferred PPE – Use N95 or Higher Respirator

Face shield or goggles ·········

········ N95 or higher respirator
When respirators are not available, use the best available alternative, like a facemask.

One pair of clean, ········ nonsterile gloves

········ Isolation gown

Acceptable Alternative PPE – Use Facemask

Face shield or goggles ·········

········ Facemask
N95 or higher respirators are preferred but facemasks are an acceptable alternative.

One pair of clean, ········ nonsterile gloves

········ Isolation gown

[a]Facilities implementing reuse or extended use of PPE will need to adjust their donning and doffing procedures to accommodate those practices.
Reprinted from Centers for Disease Control and Prevention (CDC). COVID-19 Factsheets. Retrieved on 2/16/2021 at: www.cdc.gov/coronavirus/2019-ncov/downloads/A_FS_HCP_COVID19_PPE.pdf

acquisition location is difficult to determine. For example, Hospital Compare shows rates for C. *difficile*, considering any case first diagnosed after the third day of hospitalization as a hospital onset case.

Antibiotic-Resistant Organisms

Extensive use of antibiotic agents in agriculture and health care has led to a growing prevalence of organisms with fewer effective antibiotics. Approximately 3 million people develop antibiotic-resistant infections in the United States each year, and approximately 35,000 die from these infections (CDC, 2019a). Bacteria that most commonly develop resistance include P. *aeruginosa* (resistant to fluoroquinolone antibiotics, carbapenems), *Acinetobacter* species (resistant to many antibiotics, including carbapenems), and both *Klebsiella pneumoniae* and *Escherichia coli* (resistant to extended-spectrum beta-lactam antibiotics).

Concerns about antibiotic-resistant organisms and the loss of effective antibiotic therapy for serious infections have grown. The Joint Commission National Patient Safety Goals include requirements to have a program to analyze and reduce antibiotic resistant-infections (The Joint Commission, 2021). The CDC provides explanations about the causes of multiple drug resistant organisms, current efforts to control them, estimates of incidence, and mortality rates for significant pathogens (CDC, 2019a).

Clostridioides difficile

C. *difficile* is a spore-forming bacterium that has significant HAI potential. An especially virulent strain has affected health care facilities throughout North America in the past several years. After marked increases in the first decade after 2000, a 29% decrease in the rate of hospital-onset C. *difficile* infection from 2015 to 2018 was recorded (CDC, 2019b). While the exact reason for the decrease is not clear, some believe it is due to increased focus on antimicrobial stewardship, a program to assure the right antibiotic for the right patient at the right time (CDC, 2019b). Despite this drop in rates of infection, C. *difficile* is considered the most common cause of HAI in U.S. hospitals (CDC, 2019b). Infection is usually preceded by antibiotic agents that disrupt normal intestinal flora and allow the antibiotic-resistant C. *difficile* spores to proliferate within the intestine. The organism causes pathology by releasing toxins into the lumen of the bowel. In pseudomembranous colitis (the most extreme form of C. *difficile* infection), debris from the injured lumen of the bowel and from white blood cells accumulates in the form of pseudomembranes or studded areas of the colon. The destruction of such a large anatomic area can cause sepsis.

Because antibiotics are used so extensively in health care settings, many patients are at risk for infection with C. *difficile*. The potential for health care–associated acquisition is increased because the spore is relatively resistant to disinfectants and can be spread on the hands of health care providers after contact with equipment previously contaminated with C. *difficile*. Control is best achieved by using contact precautions for patients who are infected, with use of gowns and gloves for all patient contact. Because the spores are resistant to alcohol, waterless hand products are not as effective as handwashing with soap and water for use in hand hygiene. Bleach-based cleaning products are optimal because bleach can kill spores, whereas other cleaning agents often do not. Frequently touched equipment, such as overbed tables and side rails, should be cleaned daily and whenever visibly soiled. IV poles and other peripheral items should be cleaned when the patient is discharged (CDC, 2019c).

Methicillin-Resistant *Staphylococcus aureus*

Methicillin-resistant *Staphylococcus aureus* (MRSA), a common human pathogen, refers to S. *aureus* that is resistant to methicillin or its comparable pharmaceutical agents, oxacillin and nafcillin. Soon after penicillin was discovered in the 1940s, S. *aureus* became all but universally penicillin resistant. Alternative therapies in the form of cephalosporins and synthetic penicillin solutions such as methicillin were introduced. During the late 1970s, MRSA became increasingly more prevalent, as transmission within hospitals and nursing homes was well documented.

Health Care–Associated MRSA. Health care providers transmit MRSA to patients easily because S. *aureus* has an affinity for skin colonization. The patient who is colonized with MRSA has an increased probability of developing an infection with MRSA, especially when invasive procedures (e.g., IV therapy, respiratory therapy, surgery) are performed. Such infections are characterized as healthcare-associated methicillin-resistant *Staphylococcus aureus* (HA-MRSA). HA-MRSA may persist as normal flora in the patient for an extended time. The patient who is colonized also serves as a reservoir for MRSA transmission to others. In recent years, the incidence of invasive HA-MRSA has decreased (Kourtis, Hatfield, Baggs, et al., 2019). Although the exact reasons for the decline are unknown, it is likely that infection control efforts (especially those focused on reduction of bloodstream infections) and declining lengths of hospital stay (therefore decreasing exposure within health care agencies) are important factors.

Community-Associated MRSA. New strains of MRSA have caused infections and outbreaks in children, members of sports teams, and prison inmates, and in other people who had no apparent health care exposure. These community-associated methicillin-resistant *Staphylococcus aureus* (CA-MRSA) infections are typically caused by strains of S. *aureus* that are molecularly distinct from HA-MRSA. The CA-MRSA strains typically produce more toxins than HA-MRSA and localized skin and soft tissue infections, and can lead to necrotizing fasciitis or **bacteremia** (laboratory-confirmed presence of bacteria in the bloodstream). Often, skin symptoms are initially mistaken for insect or spider bites (Kourtis et al., 2019). CA-MRSA infections have resulted in serious skin and soft tissue infections; pneumonia; and, in rare cases, death.

Control of MRSA in Health Care Facilities. Nurses must be prepared to educate patients and their families about the definitions of colonization and infection. The CDC recommends contact precautions for patients with MRSA colonization or infection (CDC, 2007). That guidance has become increasingly controversial as some research has reported that contact precautions may not decrease the acquisition of new infections (Renaudin, Llorens, Goetz, et al., 2017). In facilities that use contact precautions for MRSA, nurses must explain the reason for isolation to patients and their families.

Vancomycin and linezolid are typically the preferred treatment options for serious MRSA infection. However, there is concern that MRSA will eventually become resistant to even these medications because they are used so frequently.

Multidrug Resistant Enterobacteriaceae

A group of gram-negative organisms called Enterobacteriaceae, organisms associated with gastrointestinal colonization, are becoming resistant to multiple classes of antibiotics. Clinically important Enterobacteriaceae include *E. coli* and *Klebsiella* species, among others. Some produce enzymes known as extended spectrum beta-lactamases that disrupt the efficacy of some common antibiotics including penicillins and cephalosporins (Comerford & Durkin, 2020). Extended spectrum beta-lactamases infections increased by approximately 50% between 2012 and 2017 and were identified in the community and all health care settings (CDC, 2019a).

Carbapenem antibiotics can be used for extended spectrum beta-lactamases infections. However, some of these bacteria have also developed resistance to carbapenem antibiotics. These carbapenem-resistant Enterobacteriaceae (CRE) organisms are very difficult to treat. Among patients who are hospitalized and infected with CRE organisms, the mortality rate is approximately 50% (CDC, 2020f).

Patients with extended spectrum beta-lactam resistance or carbapenem resistance should be isolated, using contact precautions. If multiple patients with CRE on one unit within a facility are identified, or if there is other evidence of transmission, additional prevention steps should be implemented. These steps include dedicating personnel to solely care for these groups of patients, conducting cultures of other patients in the unit or service, and enhanced investigation of new cases (CDC, 2020f).

Candida Auris

Candida auris is a multi-drug resistant fungus, a yeast species that is difficult to identify in the laboratory, and difficult to remove with hospital disinfectants. It has caused outbreaks in acute care and long-term care settings. Between 2017 and 2018, reported cases increased by over 300% (CDC, 2019c). Although a patient can have an asymptomatic colonization, it can also cause bloodstream and other serious infections, with mortality rates approaching 30% (CDC, 2019c).

Patients with *C. auris* colonization or infection should be placed in contact precautions and should be reported to local health departments. When multiple patients are diagnosed with *C. auris*, an investigation should include culturing to detect other patients in the unit or area close to the patient with confirmed *C. auris* who also may be colonized (CDC, 2019c).

Vancomycin-Resistant *Enterococcus*

Vancomycin-resistant *Enterococcus* (VRE) refers to *Enterococcus* bacterium that is resistant to the antibiotic vancomycin; it is the second most frequently isolated source of HAIs in the United States. This gram-positive bacterium can produce significant disease when it infects blood, wounds, or the urinary tract (CDC, 2019a).

Enterococcus has several traits that make it an easily transmittable HAI organism. It is a part of the normal flora of the gastrointestinal tract; it is bile resistant and able to withstand harsh anatomic sites, such as the intestine; and it persists well on the hands of health care providers and on environmental objects.

Enterococcus is a relatively antimicrobial-resistant organism at baseline; thus, therapy is limited to penicillin formulations (e.g., ampicillin), vancomycin in combination with an aminoglycoside (e.g., gentamicin), or linezolid. VRE colonization and infection may serve as a reservoir of vancomycin-resistant coded genes that may be transferred to the more virulent *S. aureus*. The two most frequently cultured enterococcal species are *Enterococcus faecalis* (approximately 7% resistant) and *Enterococcus faecium* (CDC, 2019a).

Health Care–Associated Bloodstream Infections

Any vascular catheter can serve as the source for a bloodstream infection. Central lines (vascular catheters where the tip ends in or near the heart) are more likely to be associated with bloodstream infection. Central line–associated bloodstream infections (CLABSIs) add an estimated average cost of $50,000 per hospital stay and increase the risk of mortality by an estimated threefold (Agency for Healthcare Research and Quality [AHRQ], 2017). Increasingly, long-term central catheters are used to provide IV therapy to patients who are hospitalized as well as to patients in long-term care facilities, patients in clinics, and patients receiving home health care. In all instances, the nurse must use appropriate care to reduce the risk of bacteremia and to be alert to signs of its presence.

The recommended bundle approach for preventing CLABSIs includes hand hygiene; maximal barrier precautions; chlorhexidine skin antisepsis; optimal catheter site selection, with avoidance of the femoral vein for central venous access in adult patients; and daily review of line necessity with prompt removal of unnecessary lines (see Chapter 11, Chart 11-2).

Preventing Infection in the Community

The CDC as well as state and local public health departments share responsibility for prevention and control of infection in the community. Methods of infection prevention include sanitation techniques (e.g., water purification, disposal of sewage and other potentially infectious materials), regulated health practices (e.g., the handling, storage, packaging, and preparation of food by institutions), and immunization programs.

Most infections occur in the community, out of health care settings. Nurses working in schools or public health facilities educate patients and the public to reduce the incidence of influenza, foodborne infections, and other infections. Local epidemics and pandemics are the most significant type of community-acquired infections.

Pandemics are usually caused by novel viruses which begin to circulate among a population that universally has no immunity. The epidemiologic definition of a pandemic, based on the degree of spread, has often been used socially to instead convey disaster. In recent centuries, significant pandemics have included the 1918 influenza pandemic, the pandemic in the 1980s and 1990s caused by the then-novel human immune deficiency virus (HIV), the 2009 H1N1 influenza pandemic, and most recently the 2019–2021 COVID-19 pandemic (see the discussion of COVID-19 later in this chapter).

Novel virus based pandemics can be catastrophic compared with other anticipated public health problems because they last longer than other emergency events, often occur in "waves," have the potential to deplete the available health care workforce, and reduce the supply of medical equipment because of their widespread nature. The frequency and severity of pandemics cannot be accurately predicted, but models suggest that even a medium-intensity pandemic can quickly overwhelm the existing health care infrastructure (CDC, 2016).

The COVID-19 pandemic has changed many previous infection prevention practices as well as the way health care is delivered. Some clinicians have proposed that just as the crisis caused by the HIV pandemic led to sweeping changes in the delivery of health care that included the use of Standard Precautions, the COVID-19 crisis may lead to the use of Universal Pandemic Precautions (Weber, Babcock, Hayden, et al., 2020). These new precautions would have individual implications, as all health care workers would universally use masks and eye protection during patient care (Weber et al., 2020). Health care facilities would increase the screening and isolation for patients with symptoms of possible viral disease (Weber et al., 2020). Such an approach would likely protect workers from exposure to SARS-CoV-2 in anticipated future waves and would protect from other pathogens spread through a contact and droplet route.

Nurses play a crucial role during a pandemic as they provide care while themselves becoming potentially exposed. During these times, nurses demonstrate the importance of following standard precautions and transmission-based precautions. With COVID-19 and other pandemics, critically important PPE supplies as well as lifesaving equipment and drugs can become scarce. As the extreme burden on nurses caring for patients with COVID-19 quickly became evident, formalized recommendations to improve nurse education, to add occupational prevention measures, and to include a nursing perspective in national planning were drafted (Veenema, Meyer, Bell, et al., 2020).

Vaccination Programs

The goal of vaccination programs is to use wide-scale efforts to prevent specific infectious diseases from occurring in a population. Public health decisions about vaccination efforts are complex. Risks and benefits for the person and the community must be evaluated in terms of morbidity, mortality, and financial cost and benefit. Successful vaccine programs have reduced the incidence of many infectious diseases in the United States. (See later section COVID-19 Vaccines for further details of that program.)

Vaccines are suspensions of antigen preparations that are intended to produce a human immune response to protect the host from future encounters with the organism. Because no vaccine is completely safe for all recipients, contraindications on package inserts of a vaccine and CDC "Vaccine Information Statements" must be heeded. These documents provide details about studied experiences with allergy and other complications and provide crucial information about refrigeration, storage, dosage, and administration.

The recommended immunization schedules are revised by the CDC as epidemiologic evidence warrants. The two principal schedules are for children and adults (CDC, 2020b). Variations to the recommended immunization schedule should be made on a case-by-case basis, depending on the patient's risk factors as well as likely exposures. An annual influenza vaccine is recommended for all people 6 months or older, unless contraindicated. Health care workers should be immune to measles, mumps, rubella, pertussis, tetanus, hepatitis B, and varicella.

The CDC provides information about individual vaccines and vaccine-preventable diseases (see the Resources section). Advice about optimal vaccinations for travelers is available at the CDC and WHO Web sites as well.

The incidence of vaccine-preventable diseases, such as measles, mumps, rubella, and diphtheria, is affected by immigration from developing countries. Vaccine campaigns in developing countries are often financially and logistically constrained, and immigrants from such areas may be more likely than U.S. residents to be unprotected. Individual and epidemic risks are reduced when vaccination campaigns reach all communities.

Reporting Problems with Vaccines

Nurses should ask adult vaccine recipients to provide information about any problems encountered after vaccination. If a patient reports problems after receiving a vaccination, a Vaccine Adverse Event Reporting System (VAERS) form must be completed with the following information: type of vaccine received, timing of vaccination, onset of the adverse event, current illnesses or medication, history of adverse events after vaccination, and demographic information about the recipient. Forms can be submitted online (see the Resources section).

Contraindications to Vaccines

As a general rule, multiple vaccines may be given at the same visit and separating the dosing by time is not indicated. If they must be given on separate visits, it is then wise to separate by at least 4 weeks so that there is no immune reaction interfering with the response to the second vaccine (CDC, 2020b). Patients who have developed anaphylaxis or other moderate or severe sequelae after a previous dose should not receive further doses. Some live vaccines (e.g., varicella, MMR [against measles, mumps, and rubella], yellow fever) are contraindicated for people who are severely immunosuppressed or pregnant. All decisions about vaccination should be made by the patient's primary provider after careful review of vaccine-specific contraindications.

Common Vaccines

Measles, Mumps, and Rubella Vaccine

Since the time of licensing of the MMR vaccines, endemic rubeola (measles) has been eliminated in the United States, and mumps and rubella have decreased substantially. To maintain this effective public health strategy, routine MMR vaccination should be given to children at 12 to 15 months of age, with repeat dosing at 4 to 6 years of age. Adults who have not received the MMR vaccine should receive one to two doses (CDC, 2020b).

Patients should be advised that fever, transient lymphadenopathy, or hypersensitivity reaction might occur following an MMR vaccination. The risk of side effects is greater in vaccine recipients who have not previously received the vaccine than in those who have received repeat doses. Antipyretic agents may be used to decrease the risk of fever.

Varicella (Chickenpox) Vaccine and Zoster (Shingles) Vaccine

Varicella zoster virus (VZV) causes chickenpox and herpes zoster. In its natural state, VZV often attacks children, causing disseminated disease in the form of chickenpox. The severity of chickenpox may be increased among adolescents, adults, pregnant women, and those who are immune compromised (CDC, 2020b). Transmission occurs by the airborne and contact routes. With rare exception, varicella infects a person only once. The incubation period is about 2 weeks (range, 10 to 21 days). During a prodrome of general malaise (often noticed about 2 days before the rash develops), the newly infected host is capable of transmitting the virus to other susceptible contacts. Typically, the vesicular, pustular rash spreads rapidly from few to many lesions in a matter of hours. New lesions continue to form for 2 to 3 days and appear at different stages throughout this time. By the fourth symptomatic day, the lesions begin to dry, and new lesions usually do not develop. Fever is common during the 4 to 6 days of rash progression. When the lesions have crusted, the patient is no longer contagious.

The varicella vaccine is effective in preventing chickenpox in approximately 70% to 90% of people who receive two doses of vaccine. The vaccine is also available as part of MMRV, a formulation providing a combined vaccine for measles, mumps, rubella, and varicella. The vaccine should not be given to those who have severely depressed immune function, are pregnant, have moderate or severe concurrent illnesses, or have demonstrated allergy to varicella vaccine (CDC, 2019a).

Herpes zoster, also known as shingles, is a painful, localized rash caused by recurrent VZV. Vesicles occur along single associated nerve groups. VZV may be transmitted from the rash of those with shingles to people who are susceptible to varicella; the new varicella infections are manifested as chickenpox, not shingles. It is estimated that more than 30% of people over age 60 will develop shingles. A new vaccine was approved in 2017 and is recommended for people older than age 50 as it reduces the risk of shingles by approximately 90% (CDC, 2020b).

Influenza Vaccine

Influenza is an acute viral respiratory disease that predictably and periodically causes epidemics and pandemics. Epidemics occur every 2 to 3 years, with a highly variable degree of severity. An estimated 12,000 to 61,000 deaths per year since 2010 have been associated with influenza or its sequelae (i.e., pneumonia, cardiopulmonary collapse). Older adults are more susceptible to influenza, and the incidence of the disease in the United States is increasing as the number of older adults increases (CDC, 2020i).

Each year, different influenza vaccine formulations are released and are based on predictions of what strains will likely circulate. The CDC recommends that everyone over the age of 6 months get an annual influenza vaccine. There are now many flu vaccine options. Trivalent vaccines are composed of three strains (two type A influenza and one type B influenza) or quadrivalent, composed of four strains (two of type A and two of type B). The formulations can be given as an injection or as a nasal spray. There are different strengths for different age groups and different formulations available for those with egg allergy (CDC, 2020i).

Although the effectiveness of the vaccine varies from year to year, the vaccine reduces the risk of illness from flu by 50% to 60% overall when the circulating strains are included in the vaccine that year. The vaccine is less effective in preventing illness in older adults but reduces hospitalization and mortality in that age group (CDC, 2020i).

Human Papillomavirus Vaccine

Human Papillomavirus (HPV) is the most prevalent of all sexually transmitted viruses and is the principal cause of cervical cancer (see Chapter 51) (CDC, 2020q). It can also cause reproductive organ and oropharyngeal cancers. HPV vaccination at age 11 or 12 is recommended for both males and females. The vaccines are administered in a series according to CDC guidelines. The vaccine is not recommended for those with a history of hypersensitivity to any vaccine component, those with a history of anaphylactic latex allergy, or for women who are pregnant (Meites, Szilagyi, Chesson, et al., 2019).

Planning for a Pandemic

The U.S. Department of Health and Human Services has published pandemic plans that are updated and revised as new threats are recognized and new containment strategies are developed. The plans address federal, state, and local responsibilities, and the need for coordination with the WHO and other international partnerships and agencies (Homeland Security Council, 2006). These plans encourage all health care institutions to have their own pandemic plans and to test the components of the plans regularly.

Home-Based Care of the Patient with an Infectious Disease

The nurse who cares for the patient with an infectious disease in the home should provide information about infection risk prevention to the patient, the family, and the caregiver (see Chart 66-4). Recognizing that a health history may not identify all active or latent infections, the caregiver should carefully follow standard precautions in the home. The nurse should establish a work environment that facilitates hand hygiene and aseptic technique.

Family caregivers should receive an annual influenza vaccine. This is especially true if the caregiver or the patient is older than 50 years, has underlying cardiac or pulmonary disease, or has underlying immunosuppression.

Patients requiring home care are often people with immunosuppression from underlying conditions, such as HIV infection or cancer, or those who have treatment-induced immunosuppression, as occurs with many antineoplastic agents. Careful assessment for signs of infection is important.

Reducing Risk to the Patient

Equipment Care

All caregivers must pay careful attention to disinfection and aseptic technique while providing care and using medical equipment. Catheter-related sepsis should be suspected in a patient who has unexplained fever, redness, swelling, and drainage around a vascular catheter insertion site. Indwelling urinary catheters should be discontinued whenever possible,

---

Chart 66-4

HOME CARE CHECKLIST

Prevention of Infection in the Home Care Setting

At the completion of education, the patient and/or caregiver will be able to:

- State the impact of infectious disease and treatment on physiologic functioning, ADLs, IADLs, roles, relationships, and spirituality.
- State the need for infection risk prevention for the patient (preventing recurrence or new infections), caregivers, and family in the home.
  - Verbalize the route of transmission for agent of infection.
- State the purpose, dose, route, schedule, side effects, and precautions for prescribed medications.
  - Adhere to antibiotic regimen (patient) or completion of vaccination series (patient and caregiver).
- State how to contact all members of the treatment team (e.g., health care providers, home care professionals, and durable medical equipment and supply vendor).
- State changes in lifestyle (e.g., diet, activity) or home environment necessary to decrease risk for infection.
  - Perform satisfactory hand hygiene technique, oral hygiene, total body hygiene, and maintain skin integrity (patient).
  - Ensure thorough hand hygiene (alcohol-based disinfectant or handwashing) after care (family/caregiver).
  - Avoid contact with someone who has a known infectious disease.
  - Cook all foods thoroughly and store meat, poultry, and fish products separately from other food groups.
  - Use separate eating utensils and towels.
  - Demonstrate aseptic technique in the care of technical equipment such as IV catheter and indwelling urinary catheter.

- Identify signs and symptoms of infection to report to the primary provider, such as fever; chills; wet or dry cough; breathing problems; white patches in the mouth; swollen glands; nausea; vomiting; persistent abdominal pain; persistent diarrhea; problems with urination or changes in the character of the urine; red, swollen, or draining wounds; sores or lesions on the body; persistent vaginal discharge with or without itching; and severe fatigue.
- Demonstrate how to monitor for signs of infection.
- Describe to whom, how, and when to report signs of infection.
- Describe appropriate actions to take should infection occur.
- Relate how to reach primary provider with questions or complications.
- State time and date of follow-up medical appointments, therapy, and testing.
- Identify sources of support (e.g., friends, relatives, faith community).
- Identify the contact details for support services for patients and their caregivers/families.
- Identify the need for health-promotion, disease prevention, and screening activities.

Resources

See Chapter 29, Chart 29-7: Home Care Checklist: The Patient at Risk for Infection for additional information.

ADLs, activities of daily living; IADLs, instrumental activities of daily living; IV, intravenous.

---

because each day of use increases the risk of infection. The nurse should promptly report signs of urinary tract infection or generalized sepsis to the patient's primary provider.

Patient Education

When assessing the risk of infection in the home environment of the patient who is immunosuppressed, it is important to realize that intrinsic colonizing bacteria and latent viral infections present a greater risk than do extrinsic environmental contaminants. The nurse should reassure the patient and family that their home needs to be clean but not sterile. Family members seldom need to use masks, gowns, or other elements of PPE. Commonsense approaches to cleanliness and risk reduction are helpful.

For patients with neutropenia or T-cell dysfunction (e.g., patients with acquired immune deficiency syndrome [AIDS]), it is wise to restrict visits of people with potentially contagious illnesses. The patient who is immunosuppressed is vulnerable to acquiring bacterial infection with enteric pathogens from food; therefore, family members should be reminded about the need to follow recommendations for hygiene, storage, and safe cooking times and temperatures.

Reducing Risk to Household Members

Establishing reasonable barriers to infection transmission in the household is an important part of home care. The route of transmission of the organism in question must first be determined. The nurse can then educate household members about strategies to reduce their risk of becoming infected. If the patient has active pulmonary TB, the public health department should be contacted to provide screening and treatment for family members. If the patient has herpes zoster, family members who have had varicella vaccine or who have previously had chickenpox are considered immune and need no precautions. However, if a family member is immunosuppressed or otherwise susceptible to varicella, maintaining physical separation is an important strategy during the time when the patient has draining lesions. When the patient is infected with enteric organisms, the family should be reassured that common household disinfectants are effective in controlling environmental contamination.

Family members who assist in the care of a patient with a bloodborne infection such as HIV or hepatitis C can prevent transmission by carefully handling any sharp objects that are contaminated with blood. Family education may include discussion about the need for caution when shaving the patient, performing dressing changes, or administering any IV or injected medication. To collect and dispose of used needles, syringes, and vascular access equipment, the family should use containers designed for sharps disposal. With the exception of TB, the opportunistic infections associated with AIDS do not usually pose a risk to the healthy family member. Family members should be reassured that dishes are safe to use after being washed with hot water and that linens and clothing are safe to use after being washed in a hot water cycle.

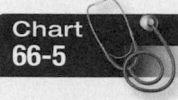

Chart 66-5 ASSESSMENT
Assessing for Infectious Disease

The nurse should ask the patient the following questions:

- Do you have a history of previous or recurrent infections?
- Have you had fever? How high has your temperature been? Is your temperature constant, or does it rise and fall? Has fever been associated with chills? Have you taken any medication to relieve fever?
- Do you have a cough? Is the cough chronic or acute? Is it associated with shortness of breath? Does the cough produce sputum? Is the sputum bloody? Have you had a tuberculin skin test recently or blood test to detect tuberculosis (TB)? If so, what were the results? Have you been given isoniazid prophylaxis for TB infection? Have you been treated for TB in the past?
- Do you have pain? Where is the pain? What is the nature of the pain? Do you have a sore throat, headache, myalgias, or arthralgias? Is there pain on urination or other activity?
- Do you have any swelling? Is there drainage associated with the swelling? Is the swollen area warm to the touch?
- Do you have a draining lesion? Is the drainage associated with trauma or a previous procedure? Is the drainage pus or clear? Does the drainage have an odor?
- Do you have diarrhea, vomiting, or abdominal pain?
- Do you have a rash? What is the nature of the rash—is it flat, raised, red, crusted, weeping, or lacelike? Have you taken

medications that could have induced the rash? Have you been exposed to another person with an identified infectious disease or rash?
- What is your vaccination history? Are your immunizations up-to-date?
- Have you had an insect or animal bite? Have you had an animal scratch or other exposure to pets, farm animals, or experimental animals?
- What medications do you use? Have you taken antibiotic agents recently or long term? Are you being treated with corticosteroids, immunosuppressive agents, or chemotherapy?
- Have you been treated for other infectious diseases in the past? Have you been hospitalized for infectious diseases?
- If sexual history is pertinent: Have you had sexual exposure to another person with a known sexually transmitted infection (STI)? Have you been treated for STIs in the past? Are you pregnant, or have you recently been pregnant? Have you been tested for human immune deficiency virus (HIV)?
- Have you traveled abroad, including developing countries? What was the immunization or antimicrobial prophylaxis used for protection while you were traveling?
- What is your occupation? What are your recreational activities? Hobbies?

Nursing Management

Assessment

Symptoms of infectious diseases vary significantly for different diseases and different people. For some infections, visible symptoms such as rash, redness, or swelling provide early warnings of infection. In other infections, such as TB and HIV, asymptomatic latency is prolonged, and infection must be determined through diagnostic procedures.

A careful history along with a review of the patient's medical record will determine current symptoms and underlying conditions. Chart 66-5 outlines questions the nurse should ask when obtaining a health history.

Physical examination may reveal signs of infection. Generalized signs of chronic infection may include significant weight loss or pallor associated with anemia of chronic diseases. Acute infection may manifest with fever, chills, lymphadenopathy, or rash. Localized signs vary by source of infection. Purulent drainage, pain, edema, and redness are strongly associated with localized infection. Cough and shortness of breath may be caused by influenza, pneumonia, or TB, as well as many noninfectious causes.

Nursing Interventions

Preventing Infection Transmission

Preventing the spread of infection requires an understanding of the usual routes of transmission of the organism. The patient in a health care facility may pose a contagious risk to others if the disease is easily spread (such as *C. difficile*) or is spread through an airborne route (such as TB). In these situations, strict adherence to isolation measures is important to reduce the opportunity for spread. Preventing transmission of organisms from patient to patient requires participation of all members of the health care team. Recent research also

highlights the importance of the inpatient environment for potential reservoirs for organisms that cause HAIs (Cohen, Spirito, Liu, et al., 2019). See the Nursing Research Profile in Chart 66-6.

Quality and Safety Nursing Alert

It is imperative that nurses disinfect their hands before and after contact with patients in any setting and after performing a potentially hand-contaminating activity. Hands must be disinfected each time gloves are removed.

Educating About the Infectious Process

The first step in preventing the spread of infections is diagnosis. The nurse can educate the patient to understand the diagnosis and to adhere to the treatment regimen. Infectious diseases often seem mysterious and are frequently socially stigmatizing. Patient education requires empathy and sensitivity. Some infections must be reported to public health officials for contact tracing and complete follow-up. Nurses are key to educating patients about guidelines for preventing transmission of infectious diseases such as COVID-19 in the community (see later discussion in this chapter).

The nurse must stress the importance of immunization to parents of young children and to others for whom vaccines are recommended, such as older adults or those who are immunosuppressed or have chronic illness or disability. Nurses should recognize their personal responsibility to receive the hepatitis B vaccine and an annual influenza vaccine to reduce potential transmission to themselves and vulnerable patient groups. Most recently, the nurse has a professional responsibility to be

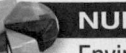

Chart 66-6 NURSING RESEARCH PROFILE

Environmental Concerns for Possible Inpatient Transmission of Bacterial Pathogens

Cohen, B., Spirito, C. M., Liu, J., et al. (2019). Concurrent detection of bacterial pathogens in hospital roommates. *Nursing Research, 68*(1), 80–83.

Purpose

The inpatient environment is a potential reservoir for organisms. The purpose of this study was to determine the incidence of concurrent detection of bacterial pathogens among hospital roommates.

Design

The study was a retrospective analysis using administrative and clinical data collected from four inpatient facilities in New York City between 2006 and 2012. A computerized algorithm identified the presence of concurrent organisms among roommates, defined as two patients sharing a room for at least 1 day and having a first positive culture for that organism within 3 days following cohabitation.

Findings

A total of 741,271 patient admissions were included in the analysis. The algorithm identified 373 valid concurrent detection events among roommates. Among these events, 158 (42%) were pairs in which the patients' first positive cultures were drawn after they were no longer sharing a room but within 3 days of cohabitation. In 144 pairs (39%), the first positive cultures were drawn while the patients were still sharing a room but on different days. In the remaining 71 pairs (19%), the patients' positive cultures were drawn while they were sharing a room on the same day.

Nursing Implications

This study illustrates the important role nurses play in planning and implementing interventions to reduce bioburden in the inpatient environment, particularly in patient rooms. Nurses need to pay attention to the methods used for environmental decontamination as part of a comprehensive approach to infection prevention in hospitals. In particular, nurses may be able to improve environmental decontamination by identifying frequently missed surfaces or equipment that require attention from environmental services teams.

---

vaccinated for COVID-19 and to advocate for all professional and personal contacts to receive the vaccine at the first available opportunity.

Controlling Fever and Accompanying Discomforts

Fever must always be investigated to determine the source. Fever may potentiate beneficial functions in the syndrome of reactions known as *acute-phase reaction*. These reactions include changes in liver protein synthesis; alterations in serum metals, such as iron; and increased production of certain classes of white blood cells and other cells of the immune system (Norris, 2019). Most fevers are physiologically controlled so that the temperature remains below 41°C (105.8°F). However, severe fever may cause complications. Even mild fevers accompanied by fatigue, chills, and diaphoresis are often uncomfortable for the patient. Whether fever is treated or untreated, adequate fluid intake is important during febrile episodes. See Chapter 19 for management of fever in the patient with COVID-19.

> ⚑ *Quality and Safety Nursing Alert*
>
> *Because fever is a key symptom, outpatients with fever should be instructed to obtain accurate temperature readings. Frequently, family caregivers know that a patient has warm skin but do not take a temperature reading. Body temperature information can be very helpful in adjusting therapy or in reevaluating a preliminary diagnosis.*

Monitoring and Managing Potential Complications

The patient with a rapidly progressive infectious disease should have vital signs and level of consciousness closely monitored. Results from radiologic and laboratory diagnostics (microbiologic, parasitologic, immunologic, hematologic, cytologic, etc.) must be interpreted in the context of other clinical findings to assess the course of the infectious disease.

Antibiotic therapy is frequently complex, and modifications are necessary because of drug susceptibility test results and disease progression. To rapidly ensure therapeutic blood levels, antibiotic therapy should be initiated as soon as it is prescribed rather than waiting until routine medication scheduling times. Chart 66-7 describes nursing interventions for infection.

Diarrheal Diseases

Worldwide, diarrheal diseases are a significant cause of mortality, especially for children (CDC, 2020j). In the United States, the epidemiology of diarrheal diseases changes continually. Water disinfection, pasteurization, and appropriate food packaging have decreased the incidence of diseases such as typhoid and cholera. However, importation of foreign foods, environmental and ecologic changes, and changes in diagnostic test modalities have led to recognition of new trends and outbreaks.

Transmission

The portal of entry of diarrheal pathogens is oral ingestion. Although food is far from sterile, the high acidity of the stomach and the antibody-producing cells of the small bowel generally decrease the potential of pathogens. Infection can occur when the infectious dose is high enough or if the acidic digestive environment is neutralized. Decreased gastric acidity with disruption of normal bowel flora (as occurs after surgery), the use of antimicrobial agents, and other causes of immune suppression decrease intestinal defenses.

Causes

There are many viral, bacterial, and parasitic causes of diarrheal diseases. The most significant viral cause of diarrhea is the *Calicivirus* (often called *Norovirus*, a virus associated with outbreaks in long-term care facilities and cruise ships) (CDC, 2020k). Common causes of bacterial infection include

(text continued on page 2165)

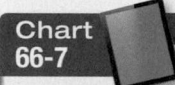

PLAN OF NURSING CARE

Chart 66-7

Care of the Patient with an Infectious Disease

NURSING DIAGNOSIS: Risk for infection
GOAL: Prevention of infection

Nursing Interventions	Rationale	Expected Outcomes
1. Prevent patient-to-patient infection spread.	1. Organisms that are spread through an airborne route or are very contagious through direct contact can be transmitted in a health care setting.	• No evidence of patient-to-patient transmission of infection
a. Provide isolation according to CDC guidelines and standard precautions.	a. CDC isolation strategies are developed to reduce the likelihood of transmission from patients who are infected to others.	• No evidence of transmission via health care workers • No occupationally acquired infections in nurses and other health care workers • No evidence of transmission due to contaminated equipment
b. Ensure that patients with airborne infections remain in private rooms during hospital stay. If they must leave their rooms, arrangements should be made to decrease the likelihood of contact with others. Rooms should be ventilated according to CDC criteria. Personal protective equipment that includes N95 respirators should be worn as indicated.	b. Engineering controls are important in the prevention of airborne diseases. The N95 respirator is the minimal level of personal protection for tuberculosis (TB) control. The "N" indicates the filter resistance to oil aerosols; the "95" indicates that the respirator has 95% effectiveness in filtering test particles.	• Absence of bacteremia and sepsis • Absence of urinary tract infections • Absence of pneumonia
c. Ensure that patients with highly transmissible, nonairborne organisms such as *C. difficile* and *Shigella* species are physically separated from other patients if hygiene or institutional policy dictates.	c. Increased prevention strategies are needed when the organism has high epidemic potential.	
d. Identify areas needing environmental decontamination.	d. Prevents patient-to-patient spread	
2. Prevent health care workers' transfer of organisms from patient to patient.	2. Transfer of organisms on the hands of health care workers is a common route of transmission. Hospital organisms colonizing the hands of health care workers may be virulent.	
a. Perform hand hygiene (by handwashing or by using alcohol-based solution) consistently and thoroughly, disinfecting hands before and after each patient contact, and after procedures that offer contamination risk while caring for an individual patient.	a. Hand hygiene is important in reducing transient flora on outer epidermal layers of skin. Alcohol-based hand disinfectants are effective methods to reduce transient flora.	
b. Use gloves when handling any body fluid from any patient. Change gloves between patient care activities, and disinfect hands after gloves are removed.	b. Gloves provide effective barrier protection. Gloves quickly become contaminated and then become a potential vehicle for the transfer of organisms between patients. Microflora on hands are likely to proliferate while gloves are worn.	
c. Avoid wearing artificial fingernails or extenders when providing patient care. Keep natural nails less than ¼ inch long and remove nail polish when chipped.	c. Artificial fingernails and extenders harbor microorganisms.	
d. Monitor the hand hygiene and glove use behaviors of health care professionals caring for the patient.	d. Poor adherence to hand hygiene among health care workers has been well documented and should be anticipated. It is important for the nurse (as the patient's advocate) to communicate protective behavior.	

(continued on page 2162)

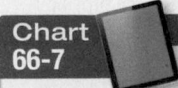

Chart 66-7

PLAN OF NURSING CARE (continued)
Care of the Patient with an Infectious Disease

Nursing Interventions	Rationale	Expected Outcomes
3. Prevent transmission of infection from patient to health care worker.	**3.** Health care workers may acquire infections occupationally due to close contact with patients.	
a. Avoid risk of infection with TB.	**a.** The most important element in the reduction of TB is early identification. Many of the symptoms of TB are subtle and may be first observed by the nurse who has prolonged contact with the patient.	
1. Participate in the early identification of patients with active disease. Patients will be asked about risk factors, symptoms, previous exposure, and status of tuberculin skin test or other rapid tests.	**1.** Identification of patients at risk can help to prevent exposure.	
2. Expedite diagnostic workup with chest x-ray, sputum analysis for organisms, and administration of TB testing as appropriate.	**2.** Confirmation of diagnosis facilitates development of an appropriate treatment plan, including prevention of spread of infection.	
3. Maintain engineering controls. Keep the patient in a private room with a closed door.	**3.** Confining airflow to the immediate vicinity of the patient and exhausting air to the outside reduces the likelihood of transmission to health care workers in areas outside of the patient room.	
4. Use protection in isolation room or when participating in procedures that are likely to generate cough, such as suctioning, intubation, or administering nebulized medications.	**4.** N95 respirators are designed to reduce health care workers' risk.	
b. Avoid risk of transmission of bloodborne diseases such as hepatitis B, hepatitis C, and the human immune deficiency virus.	**b.** Health care workers can contract bloodborne diseases via percutaneous injury such as needlestick or by contact with blood or body fluids to mucous membranes, such as eyes and mouth.	
1. Get hepatitis B vaccination.	**1.** Hepatitis B vaccine should be given to reduce risk from this contagious bloodborne virus.	
2. Use standard precautions as defined by the CDC (see Chapter 32, Chart 32-5).	**2.** Standard precautions are based on the recognition that most patients are not identified as infected by physical assessment or history taking. Health care workers must assume that all patients may be infected with bloodborne or other infection and must use barrier precautions appropriately for *all* patients.	
3. Use "needleless" syringes and other injury-preventing devices.	**3.** The use of injury-preventing devices decreases risk of transmission of bloodborne diseases.	
c. Avoid risk of airborne diseases.	**c.** Influenza vaccine is recommended for health care workers to reduce the likelihood of transmission in health care settings where patients who are immunocompromised can be exposed.	
1. Receive influenza vaccination annually.		
2. Get vaccinated or produce proof of immunity to measles, mumps, rubella, and varicella.		

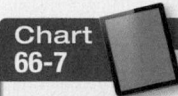

Chart 66-7

PLAN OF NURSING CARE (continued)

Care of the Patient with an Infectious Disease

Nursing Interventions	Rationale	Expected Outcomes
4. Prevent patient exposure to contaminated medical equipment.	4. Technologic advances offer increased opportunity for invasive procedures. Equipment may be complex and difficult to clean.	
a. Ensure that equipment being inserted through intact skin is sterilized between patient uses.	a. Sterilization renders equipment free of all microorganisms.	
b. Ensure that equipment that has contact with mucous membranes is sterilized or receives "high-level disinfection" between patient uses.	b. High-level disinfection renders an object free of all microorganisms with the possible exception of spore-producing organisms.	
c. Ensure that equipment used against intact skin is thoroughly cleaned and receives "low-level disinfection" between patient uses.	c. The disinfection goal for low-level disinfection is to reduce the load of microorganisms to a level that is not threatening to the host with intact skin.	
5. Follow established guidelines for the routine removal and replacement of IV devices.	5. Indwelling IV devices can serve as a conduit for organisms to migrate into the bloodstream.	
6. Remove urinary catheters at the earliest time possible.	6. The risk of urinary tract infections is directly proportional to the length of time that a urinary catheter remains in place.	
7. Remove endotracheal and nasogastric tubes as soon as possible.	7. The risk for pneumonia is increased as the use of indwelling equipment increases.	

NURSING DIAGNOSIS: Lack of knowledge about disease, cause of infection, and preventive measures
GOAL: Acquisition of knowledge about the infectious process

Nursing Interventions	Rationale	Expected Outcomes
1. Listen carefully to what the patient says about illness and previous treatment.	1. Listening facilitates detection of misunderstanding and misinformation and provides opportunity for education.	• Patient actively participates in treatment • Patient adheres to infection control measures
2. Provide pertinent explanations about: a. Organism and route of transmission b. Treatment goals c. Follow-up schedule d. Prevention of transmission to others	2. Knowledge about specific diagnoses and treatments may promote adherence.	
3. Allow opportunities for questions and discussions.	3. The patient's questions indicate issues that need clarification.	
4. Educate the patient and family about: a. Prophylaxis or immunization, if recommended b. Community resources, if necessary c. Means of preventing transmission within the home	4. Understanding of the risks and precautions associated with an infectious disease may reduce the opportunity for further spread.	

NURSING DIAGNOSIS: Fever
GOAL: Return to normal body temperature

Nursing Interventions	Rationale	Expected Outcomes
1. Monitor temperature, pulse, and respirations at regular intervals.	1. Graph fever curve to help evaluate when fever occurs, how long it lasts, and whether it responds to therapy.	• Body temperature within normal limits • Maintenance of fluid and electrolyte balance
2. Administer antipyretic agents as prescribed.	2. Prompt treatment will improve outcomes.	

(continued on page 2164)

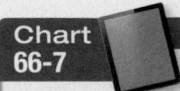

Chart 66-7

PLAN OF NURSING CARE (continued)
Care of the Patient with an Infectious Disease

COLLABORATIVE PROBLEMS: Potential complications include bacteremia or sepsis, septic shock, dehydration, and abscess formation

GOAL: Absence of complications

Nursing Interventions	Rationale	Expected Outcomes
Bacteremia, Sepsis		
1. Assess patient for evidence of infection at any location and monitor laboratory results for indicators of infection.	1. Vigilance for bacterial or fungal infection at any site promotes early recognition and treatment and reduces the likelihood of secondary infections.	• No episode of infection • Effective treatment for identified bacterial and fungal infections without progression to bloodstream infection
2. Assess treatment effectiveness of all identified infections.	2. The natural course of some infections may be rapid unless antibiotic agents are given promptly.	• Early improvement in septic course
3. Administer antibiotic agents as prescribed with first dose given at the earliest time possible.	3. Prompt treatment will improve outcomes.	
Septic Shock		

1. Routinely, and as warranted, monitor vital signs for patients with recognized infections and for patients who are severely immunosuppressed at risk for shock. In particular, be alert to signs of:
a. Fever
b. Tachycardia (>90 bpm)
c. Tachypnea (>20 breaths/min)
d. Evidence of decreased perfusion or dysfunction of vital organs in the form of:
  1. Change in mental status
  2. Hypoxemia as measured by arterial blood gases
  3. Elevated lactate levels
  4. Urine output (<0.5 mL/kg/h within 6 hours)
	1. Early recognition of the signs and prompt treatment of impending shock may reduce the associated severity or mortality.	• Absence of symptoms of septic shock
		• Hemodynamic and respiratory status within normal range

2. Administer antibiotic agents, fluid replacement, vasopressors, and oxygen as prescribed.	2. Therapeutic maintenance of hemodynamic and respiratory status is necessary until infection is effectively treated with an antimicrobial regimen.	
Dehydration		
1. Assess for dehydration (thirst, dryness of mucous membranes, loss of skin turgor, reduced peripheral pulses, urine output <400 mL in 24 hours or <0.5 mL/kg/h over 6 hours).	1. Signs of dehydration provide a basis for fluid replacement and suggest possible further complications of circulatory collapse.	• Attains fluid balance (output approximates intake: body weight unchanged) • Mucous membranes appear moist; normal skin turgor • Serum electrolytes within normal limits
2. Monitor weight.	2. Rapid changes in weight indicate fluid volume changes.	
3. Monitor intake and output and serum electrolyte levels.	3. Dehydration produces a deficit in some electrolytes. Decreased urine production may indicate hypovolemia and decreased renal perfusion.	
4. Replace fluids as needed. If the patient can tolerate oral fluids, offer fluids every 2–4 hours. Administer IV fluids as prescribed.	4. When possible, oral hydration is preferable because the patient can select the beverage, control the rate and interval of replacement, and care for self at home. In addition, the risks associated with vascular devices are avoided. If IV fluid is required, IV solutions are selected to facilitate intestinal reabsorption of fluid and electrolytes.	

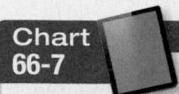

Chart 66-7 — PLAN OF NURSING CARE (continued)
Care of the Patient with an Infectious Disease

Nursing Interventions	Rationale	Expected Outcomes
Abscess Formation		
1. Assess vascular access sites, wound sites, pressure injuries, and other appropriate sites for apparent collections of purulent material.	1. Collections of purulent material often require drainage before antimicrobial therapy is effective.	• Absence of abscess • Takes antibiotic agents as prescribed
2. Assess the patient who has had abdominal surgery or trauma to abdominal area for localized signs of intra-abdominal abscess. These signs include: a. Low-grade fever b. Elevated peripheral white blood cell count c. Localized pain d. Abdominal tenderness e. Visible or palpable mass f. Postoperative diarrhea g. GI bleeding	2. Intra-abdominal abscess formation is most common following traumatic or surgical disruption of the GI tract. Signs are often initially subtle.	
3. Assess patient who has had percutaneous abscess drainage to determine whether drainage has been successful. Be alert to all of the previously mentioned signs and symptoms.	3. After percutaneous drainage, recurrent or persistent signs of abscess may indicate the need for surgical treatment.	
4. Administer antibiotic agents as prescribed.	4. Antibiotic agents, along with drainage, are the most important elements of intra-abdominal abscess management.	

CDC, Centers for Disease Control and Prevention; GI, gastrointestinal; IV, intravenous; TB, tuberculosis.

Campylobacter, Salmonella, Shigella, and *E. coli.* A common parasitic infection of importance is *Giardia.* Diarrheal disease may also be caused by *Vibrio cholera.*

Calicivirus (Norovirus)

Calicivirus, which is often referred to as the *Norovirus,* is the most common cause of foodborne illness and gastroenteritis in the United States. Onset of illness is usually acute, with vomiting and watery diarrhea that generally last for approximately 2 days. Most outbreaks occur between November and April. Dehydration is the most common complication. *Calicivirus* has been associated with large diarrheal outbreaks in schools, day care centers, cruise ships, long-term care facilities, and hospitals (CDC, 2020k).

Calicivirus is transmitted easily from person to person by direct contact and by ingesting contaminated food. Waterborne outbreaks have been associated with sewage-contaminated wells and contaminated swimming pools. Although people with *Calicivirus* infection typically recover within 2 to 3 days, they may continue to transmit the virus to others for approximately 2 more weeks (CDC, 2020k).

Caliciviruses can withstand environmental extremes of heat or cold and are resistant to chemical disinfection, which are significant reasons for their epidemic potential. Control of *Calicivirus* in health care facilities requires a coordinated program to make decisions about isolation, environmental disinfection diagnosis method, and coordination with public health officials. Contact precautions should be used when caring for patients with incontinence and during outbreaks of the virus. Workers should wear masks if they are cleaning heavily soiled areas or caring for a patient who is actively vomiting. The CDC recommends disinfecting surfaces with a freshly prepared bleach solution, with 5 to 25 tablespoons of bleach per gallon of water, or other product that is approved by the Environmental Protection Agency (EPA) for *Norovirus* disinfection (CDC, 2020k).

Campylobacter Infections

Campylobacter species are frequent causes of diarrheal disease in the United States (CDC, 2020l). The bacterium, which is abundant in animal foods, is especially common in poultry but can also be found in beef and pork. Direct person-to-person transmission appears to be less common than it is for other enteric pathogens, such as *Shigella.*

Cooking and storing food at appropriate temperatures protect against *Campylobacter* infection. Kitchen utensils used in meat preparation must be kept away from other food to prevent transmission from *Campylobacter* and other foodborne organisms (CDC, 2020l).

After a person is infected, the bacterium directly attacks the lumen of the intestine and may cause disease through enterotoxin release. Symptoms can range from mild abdominal cramping and minimal diarrhea to severe disease with profuse watery bloody diarrhea and debilitating abdominal cramping. Antimicrobial therapy is recommended only for patients who are seriously ill (CDC, 2020l).

Salmonella Infection

Salmonella is a gram-negative bacillus with many species, including the very pathogenic *Salmonella typhi* (cause of typhoid fever). Of the nontyphi species, most organisms are prevalent in animal food sources, especially eggs and chicken. However, the bacteria also can contaminate other meats, nuts, produce, and processed foods (CDC, 2020m).

Salmonella infections produce variable symptoms, including an asymptomatic carrier state, gastroenteritis, and systemic infection. Diarrhea with gastroenteritis is common. Disseminated disease and bacteremia, sometimes accompanied by diarrhea, occur less often.

The person with *Salmonella*-caused diarrhea will seldom transmit infections to others. Hand hygiene is imperative after any contact with a person with *Salmonella* diarrhea. Although patients with systemic salmonellosis require antimicrobial therapy, those with gastroenteritis only are not usually treated, because antibiotic use may increase the period of time that the patient carries the bacteria while not improving the clinical outcome.

Shigella Infection

Shigella species are gram-negative organisms that invade the lumen of the intestine and can cause severe watery (sometimes bloody) diarrhea and disseminated disease. *Shigella* species are spread through the fecal–oral route, with easy transmission from one person to another. *Shigella* exhibits a high level of virulence, as infection with very few bacteria can cause disease. Because transmission occurs easily with improper hygiene, it is not surprising that *Shigella* organisms disproportionately affect pediatric populations. Disease in the very young may infrequently be complicated by pulmonary or neurologic symptoms.

Antimicrobial therapy should be instituted early. Frequently, initial therapy choices must be altered when final microbiologic testing reveals the organism's sensitivity (Williams & Berkley, 2018).

Escherichia coli

E. coli is the most common aerobic organism colonizing the large bowel. When *E. coli* bacteria are cultured from fecal specimens, the results usually reflect normal flora. However, certain strains of *E. coli* with increased virulence have been responsible for significant outbreaks of diarrheal disease in recent years. These more pathologic strains are subgrouped as Shiga toxin–producing *Escherichia coli* (STEC) because of their production of enterotoxins. STEC strains often cause choleralike disease, with rapid, severe dehydration and an increased risk of death.

Several outbreaks of STEC have been linked to the ingestion of undercooked beef and to vegetables that have been contaminated by animal wastewater (Shane, Mody, Crump, et al., 2017). This bacterium lives in the intestines of cattle and can be introduced into meat at the time of slaughter. Prevention of disease from STEC strains is aimed at educating the public to wash fruits and vegetables thoroughly, to separate foods during preparation, and to use a food thermometer to assure meat has been cooked thoroughly (CDC, 2020n).

Giardia lamblia

Transmission of the protozoan *Giardia lamblia* occurs when food or drink is contaminated with viable cysts of the organism. People often become infected while traveling to endemic areas or by drinking contaminated water from mountain streams within the United States. The organism can be transmitted by close contact, such as occurs in day care settings. Transmission by sexual contact has also been documented.

Frequently, the infection goes unnoticed. Infection is often recognized more easily in children than in adults. In extreme cases, the patient may experience abdominal pain and chronic diarrhea, usually described as containing mucus and fat but not blood. Microscopic examination of stool specimens reveals the trophozoite or cyst stages of the parasitic life cycle.

The CDC recommends metronidazole to treat *Giardia* (CDC, 2020o). Patients with *Giardia* infections should be instructed that the organism can be easily transmitted in family or group settings. Personal hygiene measures should be reinforced, and those who travel or camp where water is not treated and filtered should be advised to avoid local water supplies unless water is purified before drinking or using it in cooking.

Vibrio Cholerae

Cholera is rare in the United States but remains a significant infectious cause of death worldwide. The causative organism is transmitted by contaminated food or water. Cases in the United States have been from contaminated shellfish found in the Gulf of Mexico or from contaminated shellfish brought into the United States by visitors. Cholera causes disease with a very rapid onset of copious diarrhea in which up to 1 L of fluid per hour can be lost. Dehydration, with subsequent cardiopulmonary collapse, may cause rapid progression from onset of signs and symptoms to death. Rehydration efforts should be vigorous and sustained. If oral rehydration cannot be accomplished, the patient may need IV fluid replacement (CDC, 2018).

Cholera should be suspected in patients who have watery diarrhea after eating shellfish harvested from the Gulf of Mexico. Confirmation of the causative organism can be made by stool culture. It is imperative that all cases are reported to local and state public health authorities.

NURSING PROCESS

The Patient with Infectious Diarrhea

Assessment

The most important element of assessment in the patient with diarrhea is to determine hydration status. The goal of rehydration is to correct the dehydration. Assessment includes evaluation for thirst, dryness of oral mucous membranes, sunken eyes, a weakened pulse, and loss of skin turgor. Careful observation for these signs is especially important in cases of rapidly dehydrating diseases (most notably cholera) and in younger children.

Intake and output measurements are crucial in determining fluid balance. Liquid stool should be measured and recorded, along with the frequency of stools. It is important to note the consistency and appearance of stool as key indicators of the type and severity of the diarrheal disease. The presence of mucus or blood should also be documented.

When conducting a health history, the nurse asks the patient what they have eaten recently and about recent travel, treatment with antibiotics, and potential exposure to others with diarrheal disease. Frequently, patients attribute symptoms to the most recent meal eaten. However, because the incubation period for most diarrheal conditions is longer than the time interval between meals, the nurse must obtain detailed information about the meal preceding the illness as well as all food intake in the previous 3 to 4 days. When eliciting this kind of history, it is helpful to ask the patient to list every food tasted. The nurse also asks if the patient is employed in a food preparation service, because the local public health departments should be notified about any person with infectious diarrhea who works in the food industry.

Diagnosis

NURSING DIAGNOSES

Based on the assessment data, nursing diagnoses may include the following:

- Hypovolemia associated with fluid lost through diarrhea
- Lack of knowledge about the infection and the risk of transmission to others

COLLABORATIVE PROBLEMS/POTENTIAL COMPLICATIONS

Potential complications may include the following:

- Bacteremia
- Hypovolemic shock

Planning and Goals

The most important goals are maintenance of fluid and electrolyte balance, increased knowledge about the disease and risk of transmission, and absence of complications.

Nursing Interventions

CORRECTING DEHYDRATION ASSOCIATED WITH DIARRHEA

The patient is assessed to determine the degree of dehydration and the amount and route of rehydration needed. Oral rehydration therapy is a strategy used to reduce the severe complications of diarrheal disease regardless of causative agent. It is inexpensive and effective for most patients, but it is often underused due to some cultural beliefs worldwide discouraging oral intake during episodes of diarrhea. The WHO and the United Nations Children's Emergency Fund (UNICEF) recommend zinc replacement and oral rehydration salts (ORS) solution for the treatment of children and adults with dehydration and electrolyte imbalance associated with cholera and other forms of diarrheal disease. Commercial ORS preparations are available and should be mixed with clean, safe water. When the ORS preparations are not available, salted vegetable soup or chicken soup can be used for fluid replacement. The ORS formula contains (in grams per liter) (CDC, 2018):

- sodium chloride: 2.6
- glucose (anhydrous): 13.5
- potassium chloride: 1.5
- trisodium citrate (dihydrate): 2.9

The most important consideration is to provide more fluid than normal. Sports drinks do not replace fluid losses correctly and should not be used, unless they are the only fluid that is available or tolerated (CDC, 2018).

Mild Dehydration. The patient exhibits dry oral mucous membranes of the mouth and increased thirst. The rehydration goal at this level of dehydration is to deliver about 50 mL of ORS per 1 kg of weight over a 4-hour interval (CDC, 2018).

Moderate Dehydration. Common findings are sunken eyes, loss of skin turgor, increased thirst, and dry oral mucous membranes. The rehydration goal at this level of dehydration is to deliver about 100 mL/kg of ORS over 4 hours.

Severe Dehydration. The patient with severe dehydration shows signs of shock (i.e., rapid thready pulse, cyanosis, cold extremities, rapid breathing, lethargy, or coma; see Chapter 11) and should receive IV replacement until hemodynamic and mental status return to normal. When improvement is evident, the patient can be treated with ORS.

ADMINISTERING REHYDRATION THERAPY

Because diarrheal episodes are often accompanied by vomiting, rehydration and refeeding can be difficult. Oral rehydration therapy should be delivered frequently in small amounts. When patients are persistently vomiting, they often require frequent administration of fluids by spoonfuls. IV therapy is necessary for the patient who is severely dehydrated or in shock.

It is important for children and adults with acute diarrheal symptoms to maintain caloric intake. As soon as dehydration has been corrected, an age-appropriate, unrestricted diet is allowed. Recommended foods include starches, cereals, yogurt, fruits, and vegetables. Foods that are high in simple sugars, such as undiluted apple juice or gelatin, should be avoided (CDC, 2018).

INCREASING KNOWLEDGE AND PREVENTING SPREAD OF INFECTION

Public health nurses, school nurses, and others who are involved in patient education should emphasize principles of safe food preparation, with special attention to meat, poultry, and fish preparation and cooking as follows (CDC, 2020p):

- Fish and whole cuts of meat must reach a temperature of 145°F (63°C).
- Ground meat must reach 160°F (71°C).
- Leftovers and poultry (both ground or whole cut) must reach 165°F (74°C).
- Before and after food preparation, all food should be maintained at temperatures below 40°F (5°C) or above 140°F (60°C).

In planning events that involve food preparation for groups of people, it is important to ensure adequate provision for proper storage and reheating to temperature thresholds. It is also important to use different surfaces, knives, and other equipment for raw meat, poultry, and fish and to keep these items separate from other foods.

Diarrheal diseases discussed in this section must be reported to local or state health departments. The goal of reporting is to provide information for determining incidence trends and promptly identifying any restaurants or other food preparation establishments that may have served contaminated food.

In both homes and health care delivery settings, good hygiene and principles of standard precautions should be emphasized.

MONITORING AND MANAGING POTENTIAL COMPLICATIONS

Bacteremia. *E. coli*, *Salmonella*, and *Shigella* are organisms that can enter the bloodstream and disseminate to other organs. Blood cultures are necessary for the patient who is acutely febrile with diarrhea. If initial smear results reveal gram-negative organisms, antibiotic therapy is instituted.

Hypovolemic Shock. Shock associated with diarrheal diseases demands accurate intake and output assessment and vigorous fluid replacement. In rare instances, patients with severe fluid imbalance require intensive care nursing support with aggressive hemodynamic monitoring (see Chapter 11).

Evaluation

Expected patient outcomes may include:
1. Attains fluid balance
   a. Output approximates intake.
   b. Mucous membranes appear moist.
   c. Skin turgor is normal.
   d. Adequate amounts of fluids and calories are ingested.
   e. Absence of vomiting.
   f. Stools are of normal color and consistency.
2. Acquires knowledge and understanding about infectious diarrhea and transmission potential
   a. Takes proper precautions to prevent spread of infection to others.
   b. Describes principles and techniques of safe food storage, preparation, and cooking.
3. Absence of complications
   a. Temperature is within normal range.
   b. Blood culture reports are negative.
   c. Fluid balance is achieved.

Sexually Transmitted Infections

Sexually transmitted infections (STIs) are diseases acquired through sexual contact with a person who is infected. Select STIs and their routes of transmission are included in Table 66-1. Infections caused by organisms not generally considered STIs can also be transmitted during sexual contact—for example, *G. lamblia,* usually associated with contaminated water, can be transmitted through sexual exposure. STIs are sometimes called sexually transmitted diseases (STDs) as well.

STIs are the most common infectious diseases in the United States and are epidemic in most parts of the world. Portals of entry of STI-causing microorganisms and sites of infection include the skin and mucosal linings of the urethra, cervix, vagina, rectum, and oropharynx.

More than 2 million STIs are reported among Americans annually. However, many infections go undiagnosed or unreported, so surveillance data underestimate true incidence. Surveillance reliability is diminished when public health departments are underfunded, and when some populations have decreased access to care (CDC, 2020q).

Education about prevention of STIs includes information about risk factors and behaviors that can lead to infection. Using straightforward language and personal testimonials for targeted audiences (e.g., people who want information about protecting themselves) and conducting presentations with trusted establishments (e.g., churches, health care facilities) are the recommended educational strategies. Included in this education is information about the relative value of condoms in reducing the risk of infection. The use of condoms to provide a protective barrier from transmission of STI-related organisms has been broadly promoted, especially since the recognition of HIV/AIDS. At first referred to as a method to ensure *safe sex,* the use of condoms has been shown to reduce but not eliminate the risk of transmission of HIV and other STIs. Thus, the term *safer sex* more appropriately connotes the public health message to be used when promoting the use of condoms. See Chapter 32 for most information about AIDS and HIV.

STIs provide a unique set of challenges for nurses, physicians, and public health officials. Because of perceived stigma and possible threat to emotional relationships, people with symptoms of STIs are often reluctant to seek health care in a timely fashion. STIs may progress without symptoms, and a delay in diagnosis and treatment is potentially harmful because the risk of complications for the person who is infected and the risk of transmission to others increase over time.

Infection with one STI suggests the possibility of infection with other diseases as well. After one STI is identified, diagnostic evaluation for others should be conducted. The possibility of HIV infection should be pursued when any STI is diagnosed.

Syphilis

Syphilis is an acute and chronic infectious disease caused by the spirochete *Treponema pallidum.* It is acquired through sexual contact or may be congenital in origin. The rates of primary and secondary syphilis have been on the rise, with a 15% increase between 2017 and 2018 (CDC, 2020q).

Stages of Syphilis

The course of untreated syphilis can be divided into three stages: primary, secondary, and tertiary. These stages reflect the time from infection and the clinical manifestations observed in that period and are the basis for treatment decisions.

Primary syphilis occurs 2 to 3 weeks after initial inoculation with the organism. Painless lesions at the site of infection, called chancres, usually resolve spontaneously within 3 to 12 weeks, with or without treatment (Norris, 2019).

Secondary syphilis occurs by hematogenous spread leading to generalized infection. The rash of secondary syphilis occurs from 1 week to 6 months after the chancre (Norris, 2019). Transmission can occur through contact with these lesions. Generalized signs of infection may include lymphadenopathy, arthritis, meningitis, hair loss, fever, malaise, and weight loss.

After the secondary stage, there is a period of latency, when the person who is infected has no signs or symptoms of syphilis. Latency can be interrupted by a recurrence of secondary syphilis symptoms (Norris, 2019).

Tertiary syphilis is the final stage in the natural history of the disease. It is estimated that between 20% and 40% of those infected do not exhibit signs and symptoms in this final stage. Tertiary syphilis may present as a slowly progressive inflammatory disease with the potential to affect multiple organs. The most common manifestations at this level are aortitis and neurosyphilis, as evidenced by dementia, psychosis, paresis, stroke, or meningitis (Norris, 2019).

Assessment and Diagnostic Findings

Because syphilis shares symptoms with many diseases, clinical history and laboratory evaluation are important. The conclusive diagnosis of syphilis can be made by direct identification of the spirochete obtained from the chancre lesions of primary syphilis. Serologic tests used in the diagnosis of secondary and tertiary syphilis require clinical correlation in interpretation. The serologic tests are summarized as follows (O'Bryne, 2019):

- *Nontreponemal* or *reagin tests*, such as the Venereal Disease Research Laboratory (VDRL) or the rapid plasma reagin circle test (RPR-CT), are generally used for screening and diagnosis. After adequate therapy, the test result is expected to decrease quantitatively until it is read as negative, usually about 2 years after therapy is completed.
- *Treponemal tests*, such as the fluorescent treponemal antibody absorption (FTA-ABS) test and the microhemagglutination test for *Treponema pallidum* (MHA-TP), are used to verify that the screening test did not represent a false-positive result. Positive results usually are positive for life and therefore are not appropriate to determine therapeutic effectiveness

Medical Management

Treatment of all stages of syphilis is administration of antibiotic medications. Penicillin G benzathine is the medication of choice for early syphilis or early latent syphilis of less than 1 year's duration. It is given by intramuscular injection at a single session. Patients with late latent or latent syphilis of unknown duration should receive three injections at 1-week intervals. Patients who are allergic to penicillin are usually treated with doxycycline. The patient treated with penicillin is monitored for 30 minutes after the injection to observe for a possible allergic reaction (CDC, 2020s).

Treatment guidelines established by the CDC are updated on a regular basis. Recommendations provide special guidelines for treatment in the setting of pregnancy, allergy, HIV infection, pediatric infection, congenital infection, and neurosyphilis. The CDC Web site, "Sexually Transmitted Diseases," provides a link to the most recent guidelines as well as additional information about drug shortages and other concurrent treatment considerations. The Web site also regularly updates guidance about how to modify usual STI/STD screening and treatment care during the COVID-19 pandemic (CDC, 2020s).

Nursing Management

Syphilis is a reportable communicable disease. In any health care facility, a mechanism must be in place to ensure that all patients who are diagnosed are reported to the state or local public health department to ensure community follow-up. The public health department is responsible for identification of sexual contacts, contact notification, and contact screening.

Lesions of primary and secondary syphilis may be highly infective. Gloves are worn when direct contact with lesions is likely, and hand hygiene is performed after gloves are removed. Isolation in a private room is not required (see Chart 66-8).

Chlamydia trachomatis and *Neisseria gonorrhoeae* Infections

Chlamydia trachomatis and *Neisseria gonorrhoeae* are the most commonly reported infectious diseases in the United States. Coinfection with *C. trachomatis* often occurs in patients infected with *N. gonorrhoeae*. The greatest risk of

---

Chart 66-8

PATIENT EDUCATION

Preventing the Spread of Syphilis

The nurse instructs the patient to:

- Complete the full course of therapy if multiple penicillin injections are required.
- Refrain from sexual contact with previous or current partners until the partners have been treated.
- Be aware that if you have primary or secondary syphilis, skin lesions and other sequelae of infection will improve with proper treatment, and serology eventually will reflect cure.
- Recognize that condoms significantly reduce the risk of transmission of syphilis and other STIs.
- Be aware that having multiple sexual partners increases the risk of acquiring syphilis and other STIs.

STIs, sexually transmitted infections.

C. trachomatis infection occurs in young women between 15 and 24 years of age (CDC, 2020q, 2020r).

Clinical Manifestations

Both *C. trachomatis* and *N. gonorrhoeae* infections frequently do not cause symptoms in women. When symptoms are present, mucopurulent cervicitis with exudates in the endocervical canal is the most frequent finding. Women with gonorrhea can also present with symptoms of urinary tract infection or vaginitis. See Chapter 51 for more in-depth coverage of STIs in women.

Although men are more likely than women to have symptoms when infected, infection with *N. gonorrhoeae* or *C. trachomatis* can be asymptomatic. When symptoms are present, they may include burning during urination and penile discharge. Patients with *N. gonorrhoeae* infection may also report painful, swollen testicles (CDC, 2020q, 2020r).

Complications

In women, pelvic inflammatory disease (PID), ectopic pregnancy, endometritis, and infertility are possible complications of either *N. gonorrhoeae* or *C. trachomatis* infection. In men, epididymitis, a painful disease that may lead to infertility, may result from infection with either bacterium. In both men and women, arthritis or bloodstream infection may be caused by *N. gonorrhoeae* (CDC, 2020q, 2020r).

Assessment and Diagnostic Findings

The patient is assessed for fever, discharge (urethral, vaginal, or rectal), and signs of arthritis. Diagnostic methods used in *N. gonorrhoeae* infection include Gram stain (appropriate only for male urethral samples), culture, and nucleic acid amplification tests (NAATs). Gram stain and the direct fluorescent antibody test can be used in chlamydia. NAATs are also available for *C. trachomatis*. In the female patient, samples are obtained from the endocervix, anal canal, and pharynx. In the male patient, specimens are obtained from the urethra, anal canal, and pharynx. Because *N. gonorrhoeae* organisms are susceptible to environmental changes, specimens for culture must be delivered to the laboratory immediately after they are obtained.

Because as many as 70% of chlamydial infections are asymptomatic, the CDC recommends *Chlamydia* testing for all women who are pregnant. Annual testing is also recommended for women younger than 25 years who are sexually active, and for women over 25 years who have a new sexual partner or multiple partners (CDC, 2020q, 2020r).

Medical Management

Because patients are often coinfected with both gonorrhea and chlamydia, dual therapy is recommended, even if only gonorrhea has been laboratory proven (CDC, 2020r). The CDC guidelines should be used to determine alternative therapy for the patient who is pregnant or allergic or who has a complicated chlamydial infection. The CDC updates STI therapy recommendations regularly because of growing challenges with bacterial antibiotic resistance patterns and drug shortages (CDC, 2020r).

Although the number of resistant strains of gonorrhea has increased, that is not the reason for the use of combination antibiotic therapy. Such therapy is prescribed in order to treat both gonorrhea and chlamydia, because many patients with gonorrhea have a coexisting chlamydial infection.

Patients with uncomplicated gonorrhea who are treated with CDC-recommended therapy do not routinely need to return for a proof-of-cure visit. If the patient reports a new episode of symptoms or tests are positive for gonorrhea again, the most likely explanation is reinfection rather than treatment failure. Serologic testing for syphilis and HIV should be offered to patients with gonorrhea or chlamydia, because any STI increases the risk of other STIs (CDC, 2020r).

Nursing Management

Gonorrhea and chlamydia are reportable communicable diseases. In any health care facility, a mechanism should be in place to ensure that all patients who are diagnosed are reported to the local public health department to ensure follow-up of the patient. The public health department also is responsible for interviewing the patient to identify sexual contacts so that contact notification and screening can be initiated.

The target group for preventive patient education about gonorrhea and chlamydia is the adolescent and young adult population. Along with reinforcing the importance of abstinence, when appropriate, education should address postponing the age of initial sexual exposure, limiting the number of sexual partners, and using condoms for barrier protection. Young women and those who are pregnant should also be instructed about the importance of routine screening for chlamydia.

NURSING PROCESS

The Patient with a Sexually Transmitted Infection

Assessment

The patient should be asked to describe the onset and progression of symptoms and to characterize any lesions by location and by describing drainage, if present. Brief explanations of why the information is needed are often helpful. Clarification of terms may be necessary if either the patient or nurse uses words that are unfamiliar to the other.

Protecting confidentiality is important when discussing sexual issues. When a detailed sexual history is necessary, it is important to respect the patient's right to privacy. When obtaining a sexual history, the CDC recommends the following systematic interview of key areas, the "five Ps": partners, prevention of pregnancy, protection from STIs, practices, and past history of STIs.

Asking specific information about sexual contacts usually should be done only when the nurse is part of a team that will conduct partner notification. The nurse should describe to the patient the public health notification process and resources that are available to assist sexual partners or infants and children.

During the physical examination, the examiner looks for rashes, lesions, drainage, discharge, or swelling. Inguinal nodes are palpated to elicit tenderness and to assess swelling. Women are examined for abdominal or uterine tenderness. The mouth and throat are examined for signs of inflammation or exudate. The nurse wears gloves while examining the mucous membranes, and gloves are changed and replaced after vaginal or rectal examination.

Diagnosis

NURSING DIAGNOSES

Based on assessment data, major nursing diagnoses may include the following:

- Lack of knowledge about the disease and risk for spread of infection and reinfection
- Anxiety associated with anticipated stigmatization and to prognosis and complications
- Impaired ability to manage regime associated with integrating a therapeutic regimen for treatment

COLLABORATIVE PROBLEMS/POTENTIAL COMPLICATIONS

Potential complications may include the following:

- Ectopic pregnancy
- Infertility
- Transmission of infection to fetus, resulting in congenital abnormalities and other outcomes
- Neurosyphilis
- Gonococcal meningitis
- Gonococcal arthritis
- Syphilitic aortitis
- HIV-related complications

Planning and Goals

Major goals are increased patient understanding of the natural history and treatment of the infection, reduction in anxiety, increased adherence with therapeutic and preventive goals, and absence of complications.

Nursing Interventions

INCREASING KNOWLEDGE AND PREVENTING SPREAD OF DISEASE

Education about STIs and prevention of the spread to others are often accomplished simultaneously. The patient who is infected should be told what the causative organism is and should receive an explanation of the usual course of the infection (including the interval of potential communicability to others) and possible complications. The nurse should stress the importance of following therapy as prescribed and the need to report any side effects or symptom progression. Discussion should emphasize that the same behaviors that led to infection with one STI increase the risk of infection with other STIs, including HIV. Methods used to contact sexual partners should be discussed. The patient should understand that until the partner has been treated, continued sexual exposure to the same person may lead to reinfection.

Target groups for preventive patient education about STIs include the adolescent and young adult populations. Along with reinforcing the importance of abstinence, when appropriate, education should address postponing the age of initial sexual exposure, limiting the number of sexual partners, and using condoms for barrier protection. The use of condoms reduces but does not eliminate the risk of transmission of HIV and other STIs.

REDUCING ANXIETY

When appropriate, the patient is encouraged to discuss anxieties and fear associated with the diagnosis, treatment, or prognosis. By individualizing education, factual information applied to specific needs may offer reassurance. Patients may need help in planning discussion with partners. If the patient is especially apprehensive about this aspect, referral to a social worker or other specialist may be appropriate. For example, such support is especially important when the patient has newly diagnosed HIV infection. Patients with HIV may benefit from programs that combine support, education, counseling, and therapeutic goals. Such programs are designed to offer coordinated care throughout the course of disease progression.

INCREASING ADHERENCE

In group settings (e.g., an outpatient obstetric setting) or in a one-to-one setting, open discussion about STI information facilitates patient education. Discomfort can be reduced by factual explanation of causes, consequences, treatments, prevention, and responsibilities. Because most communities have expanded STI prevention resources, referrals to appropriate agencies can complement individual educational efforts and ensure that later questions or uncertainties can be addressed by experts.

MONITORING AND MANAGING POTENTIAL COMPLICATIONS

Infertility and Increased Risk of Ectopic Pregnancy. STIs may lead to PID and increased risk of ectopic pregnancy and infertility. See Chapters 50 and 51 for additional information.

Congenital Infections. All STIs can be transmitted to infants in utero or at the time of birth. Complications of congenital infection can range from localized infection (e.g., throat infection with *N. gonorrhoeae*), to congenital abnormalities (e.g., stunting of growth or deafness from congenital syphilis), and to life-threatening disease (e.g., congenital herpes simplex virus).

Neurosyphilis, Gonococcal Meningitis, Gonococcal Arthritis, and Syphilitic Aortitis. STIs can cause disseminated infection. The central nervous system may be infected, as seen in cases of neurosyphilis or gonococcal meningitis. Gonorrhea that infects the skeletal system may result in gonococcal arthritis. Syphilis can infect the cardiovascular system by forming vegetative lesions on the mitral or aortic valves (CDC, 2020s).

Human Immune Deficiency Virus–Related Complications. HIV infection, if untreated, leads to the profound immunosuppression that is characteristic of AIDS.

Complications of HIV infection include many opportunistic infections, including those due to *Pneumocystis jirovecii, Cryptococcus neoformans*, cytomegalovirus, and *Mycobacterium avium* (see Chapter 32).

Evaluation

Expected patient outcomes may include:
1. Exhibits knowledge about STIs and their transmission
2. Demonstrates a less anxious demeanor
   a. Discusses anxieties and goals for treatment
   b. Inspects self for lesions, rashes, and discharge
   c. Accepts support, education, and counseling when indicated
   d. Assists with sharing information about infection with sexual partners
   e. Discusses risk reduction behaviors and safer sex practices
3. Adheres to treatment
4. Achieves effective treatment
5. Reports for follow-up examinations if necessary
6. Absence of complications

Emerging Infectious Diseases

As defined by the CDC, **emerging infectious diseases** are human diseases of infectious origin that have increased within the past two decades or that are likely to increase in the near future. Examples of emerging infectious diseases presented here include COVID-19, Zika virus, West Nile virus, Ebola virus disease, Legionnaires disease, and pertussis. Bioterrorism agents such as anthrax and plague are also considered emerging infectious diseases because a bioterrorist act would introduce a new mode of transmission for these agents. Other examples, covered earlier in this chapter, include novel influenza viruses, CRE, and *C. auris*.

Infectious diseases may begin anywhere in the world; therefore, epidemiologists worldwide collaborate to share information about the detection of new diseases, their clinical presentations, laboratory identification methods, and possible treatments. In the United States, the CDC is the central agency for this coordination. The CDC collaborates with numerous agencies, including other U.S. government agencies (such as the National Institutes of Health [NIH] and Food and Drug Administration [FDA]) as well as the WHO and other international agencies, faith-based agencies, nongovernmental organizations, and businesses throughout the world. Elaborate disease surveillance and reporting methods are established with the goal of early detection and control of actual and potential epidemics and pandemics (CDC, 2017).

Many factors contribute to newly emerging or re-emerging infectious diseases. These include travel, globalization of food supply and central processing of food, population growth, increased urban crowding, population movements (e.g., those that result from war, famine, or human-made or natural disasters), ecologic changes, human behavior (e.g., risky sexual behavior, IV/injection drug use), antimicrobial resistance, and breakdown in public health measures.

Emerging infectious diseases are important from an epidemiologic standpoint because their incidence is not stable. When the pattern of disease in a community is not well understood in the medical-scientific community, patients, families, and others in the community often become alarmed about these diseases. During times of increased concern about bioterrorism, whether triggered by actual events or by hoaxes, nurses have responsibility to rationally separate facts from fears. In discussions with patients and other caregivers, it is important to keep the focus on what is known and to clarify the plan for diagnosis, treatment, and containment.

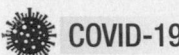 ## COVID-19

The COVID-19 pandemic began in Wuhan, China, in late 2019. As research into the novel pathogen responsible for the 2019–2021 global pandemic progresses, new information about the pathogenesis, risks, clinical manifestations, and management of patients infected with SARS-CoV-2 continues to emerge. Of those individuals in the United States diagnosed with COVID-19, the case fatality rate is estimated to be 5.6% (Johns Hopkins University & Medicine Coronavirus Resource Center, 2020).

Pathophysiology

COVID-19 transmission occurs through virus-laden droplets and aerosols exhaled by an infected host while breathing, speaking, coughing, and sneezing (Prather, Wang, & Schooley, 2020). SARS-CoV-2 gains entry into host cells through the angiotensin-converting enzyme 2 (ACE2) cellular surface receptors (see Chapter 27, Fig. 27-2) (Vaduganathan, Vardeny, Michel, et al., 2020). In addition, the aerosols of SARS-CoV-2 can accumulate, remain infectious in indoor air for hours, and can be inhaled deep into the lungs (Prather et al., 2020). The virus multiplies rapidly within an infected host and, unless checked by the immune system, symptoms begin with a week of transmission (Prather et al., 2020).

Risk Factors

Individuals of any age, gender, and ethnicity can be at risk for infection; however, adults 65 years of age and older, and those who reside in long-term care or skilled nursing facilities are at higher risk of death from COVID-19 (NIH COVID-19 Treatment Guidelines Panel, 2020). Some studies suggest that men with COVID-19 have a higher fatality rate compared to women (Chen, Zhou, Dong, et al., 2020; Deng, Yin, Chen, et al., 2020). While information on risk continues to evolve, Chart 66-9 lists the demonstrated and possible risk factors for COVID-19 in adults. Having a history of several chronic diseases, particularly if the diseases are not properly managed, appears to be associated with higher risk of severe disease and death (CDC, 2020g; CDC, 2020h). Patients who are immunosuppressed for a variety of reasons (e.g., active neoplasm, organ transplant recipient) are also thought to be at higher risk of dying from COVID-19 (CDC, 2020g; CDC, 2020h; NIH COVID-19 Treatment Guidelines Panel, 2020).

Clinical Manifestations

COVID-19 clinical manifestations occur on a wide spectrum, from mild symptoms that can be managed at home to severe illness with manifestations that can cause multisystem morbid complications requiring care in an ICU setting. While primarily respiratory in nature, mild COVID-19 manifestations

---

Chart 66-9 ⚠ **RISK FACTORS**
Development of Severe Illness due to COVID-19 in Adults

Increased Risk Demonstrated

- Cancer
- Chronic kidney disease
- COPD
- Down Syndrome
- Heart failure, coronary artery disease, or cardiomyopathy
- Immunocompromised state from solid organ transplant
- Obesity (body mass index [BMI] of 30 kg/m² or higher but ≤40 kg/m²)
- Severe obesity (BMI ≥40 kg/m²)
- Pregnancy
- Sickle cell disease
- Smoking
- Type 2 diabetes

Possible Increased Risk

- Asthma (moderate-to-severe)
- Cerebrovascular disease
- Cystic fibrosis
- Dementia
- Hypertension
- Immunocompromised state from blood or bone marrow transplant, immune deficiencies, HIV, use of corticosteroids, or use of other immune weakening medicines
- Liver disease
- Overweight (BMI ≥25 kg/m², but ≤30 kg/m²)
- Pulmonary fibrosis
- Thalassemia
- Type 1 diabetes

COPD, chronic obstructive pulmonary disease.
Adapted from Centers for Disease Control and Prevention (CDC). (2020g). Interim clinical guidance for management of patients with confirmed coronavirus disease (COVID-19). Retrieved on 7/24/2020 at: www.cdc.gov/coronavirus/2019-ncov/hcp/clinical-guidance-management-patients.html; Centers for Disease Control and Prevention (CDC). (2020h). COVID-19: People with certain medical conditions. Retrieved on 7/24/2020 at: www.cdc.gov/coronavirus/2019-ncov/need-extra-precautions/people-with-medical-conditions.html

---

may include fever, nonproductive cough, sore throat, fatigue, myalgias (muscle aches), nasal congestion, nausea, vomiting, diarrhea, anosmia (loss of smell), and ageusia (loss of taste) (Cascella, Rajnik, Cuomo, et al., 2020; Kim & Gandhi, 2020). See Chapter 19 for further discussion of the spectrum of clinical manifestations in the patient with COVID-19.

Medical Management

Patients with mild symptoms, about 80% of patients, can be managed at home (Cascella et al., 2020; Kim & Gandhi, 2020). Those with severe illness are hospitalized (Kim & Gandhi, 2020). See Chapter 19 for further discussion of medical management of the patient with mild, moderate, and severe COVID-19 infection.

Nasopharyngeal samples are the recommended method of diagnosing SARS-CoV-2 (NIH COVID-19 Treatment Guidelines Panel, 2020). Those testing people for possible infection with SARS-CoV-2 either work with their state, tribal, local, and territorial health departments to coordinate testing through public health laboratories, or with commercial or clinical laboratories using molecular and antigen tests. The type of specimen collected is based on the test being used and the specific manufacturer instructions (CDC, 2020a).

Ideally, the diagnosis of COVID-19 is confirmed by patient self-administration of bilateral nasal swabbing for viral antigen or nucleic acid. Self-swabbing minimizes the risk of person-to-person transmission of respiratory droplets. The act of patient self-swabbing should be observed by a health care provider whenever possible to assure it is performed properly (CDC, 2020a).

COVID-19 Vaccines

Operation Warp Speed was an unprecedented response to the study of safety and efficacy of new vaccine platforms never before used in humans (Castells & Phillips, 2020). Two SARS-CoV-2 mRNA vaccines were authorized for emergency use in the United States in December of 2020, less than a year after the SARS-CoV-2 sequence was discovered (Castells & Phillips, 2020). Both vaccines require 2 doses for efficacy, the second dose of the Pfizer-BioNTech 21 days after the first dose, and the Moderna mRNA 28 days later. Early reports indicated the Pfizer-BioNTech vaccine had an anaphylaxis rate of 1 in 100,000 compared with a rate of 1 in 1,000,000 for other vaccines (Castells & Phillips, 2020). Ongoing efforts are needed by nurses and all health care workers to maintain a proactive response to support public confidence and reduce vaccine hesitancy. Anaphylaxis is a treatable reaction that requires early recognition and an appropriate and timely response (see Chapter 33). A VAERS form must be completed for any adverse reaction and can be submitted online (see the Resources section). Nurses should be vaccinated for COVID-19 and should advocate for all of their professional and personal contacts receiving the vaccine at the first available opportunity.

Nursing Management

Nursing management of the patient with COVID-19 mirrors that of medical management. The majority of patients with known or suspected mild COVID-19 may be managed on an outpatient basis within their homes, which conserves hospital resources and diminishes the likelihood of exposure to others, including health care workers (Kim & Gandhi, 2020). Few medications are used to either treat COVID-19 or to mitigate its effects in patients with mild disease who are managed at home; thus, care is largely supportive. The nursing management of patients with mild COVID-19 mirrors that of other viral respiratory illnesses.

Patients with moderate or severe COVID-19 are most often managed in the hospital setting. Health care workers are at increased risk for acquiring COVID-19 and should wear complete PPE as discussed earlier in this chapter (CDC, 2020c). See Chapter 19 for further discussion of nursing management of the patient with mild, moderate, and severe COVID-19 infection. Supportive care for a patient, whether at home or in the hospital setting, requires very careful use of infection control measures and psychological support for the patient and family.

Early in the COVID-19 pandemic, important measures were recommended by the CDC to help mitigate the spread of SARS-CoV-2. Nurses should provide education to help patients and their families implement these measures to help slow viral transmission. One measure is to wear a mask with 2 or more layers of breathable fabric that snugly covers the nose and mouth; this type of mask should be worn in public places to help patients and families protect themselves and others (Prather et al., 2020). One study of mask usage reported that among 139 clients exposed to two symptomatic hair stylists with confirmed COVID-19, while both the stylists and the clients wore face masks, no symptomatic secondary cases were identified (Hendrix, Walde, Findley, et al., 2020). Another important practice is to 'socially distance' by remaining at least 6 feet apart from others and avoiding crowds. The nurse should also encourage frequent handwashing with at least 20 seconds of scrubbing, rinsing, and drying after washing (CDC, 2002). If handwashing is not possible, then hand sanitizer with at least 60% alcohol should be used.

Zika Virus

The Zika virus was first discovered as a pathogen in monkeys in the Zika Forest of Uganda in the 1940s; it was found to cause human disease in the 1950s. The epidemiologic pattern changed as the first large outbreak in humans did not occur until 2007 in Micronesia. The disease was not seen in the Western Hemisphere until July 2015, when a large outbreak began in Brazil. Within the next year, infections were noted in countries throughout the Americas and Pacific Islands (WHO, 2016).

The incubation period for Zika virus disease is estimated to be between 3 and 14 days (Krow-Lucal, Biggerstaff, & Staples, 2017). Among patients who are symptomatic, most have self-limiting illness of 2 to 7 days duration with mild fever, rash, headache, conjunctivitis, or joint and muscle pain. Zika has been associated with microcephaly and other congenital abnormalities in infants of some women infected with Zika during pregnancy. The virus can also cause Guillain–Barré syndrome, a condition with nerve and muscle weakness that often quickly progresses to a paralysis (WHO, 2016).

Zika is primarily transmitted through bites of infected mosquitos from the *Aedes* genus. Sustained outbreaks have been more common in tropical areas where these mosquitos thrive. The *Aedes* mosquito is also the carrier of other mosquito-borne viruses such as dengue, chikungunya, and yellow fever. Unlike these other mosquito-borne diseases, Zika can also be transmitted through sexual transmission. This combination of transmission routes makes prevention efforts especially challenging. People can travel to epidemic areas, and later, as asymptomatic infected carriers, transmit the virus to their sexual partners. Because of the concern about congenital infection, women who are pregnant are advised to avoid travel to endemic areas and to use abstinence or safer sex methods if their sexual partners have traveled to such regions. Similarly, couples with exposure to areas where there is ongoing transmission are counseled in contraceptive options (CDC, 2020s).

West Nile Virus

The West Nile virus was first recognized in the 1930s in Africa and was first seen in humans in the United States in 1999. Those infected have a range of presentations. Approximately

20% of people who are infected have a mild disease called *West Nile fever*. These patients usually experience headache, fever, and a persistent fatigue that may continue for several months. In these patients, fewer than 1% of infections develop into more serious disease, which is characterized by severe neuroinvasive illness, meningitis, encephalitis, and paralysis or poliomyelitis. The mortality rate for people with neuroinvasive diseases is approximately 10% (CDC, 2020t).

The incubation period (i.e., from mosquito bite to onset of symptoms) is between 2 and 14 days. Currently, there is no treatment for West Nile virus infection. Medical and nursing management consists of fluid replacement, airway management, and supportive nursing care when meningitis or symptoms are present.

Birds are the natural reservoir for the virus, and since 1999, the population of infected birds in the United States has increased steadily. Mosquitoes become infected when feeding on birds and can transmit the virus to animals and humans. Human-to-human transmission of West Nile virus is very rare; however, transplacental mother-to-infant transmission and blood transfusion or organ transplant transmission have rarely occurred (CDC, 2020t).

Ebola Virus Disease

The first human outbreak of Ebola virus disease occurred in 1976. For decades, the virus maintained a pattern of sporadic outbreaks in remote African villages, followed by intervening periods without any recognized cases worldwide. In 2014, the virus broke this pattern and rampaged through the West African countries Liberia, Guinea, and Sierra Leone, with secondary cases in other countries in Africa, Europe, and the United States with approximately 28,600 cases (CDC, 2020u). Between 2017 and 2020, several significant outbreaks occurred in the Republic of the Congo, with an estimated 3400 cases (CDC, 2020u).

Pathophysiology

Ebola is spread through direct contact with blood or body fluids (urine, vomit, feces, saliva, sweat, semen, and breast milk) from the person who is ill from the virus and possibly from contact with semen of a man who has recovered from Ebola. It is not spread through air, water, or insect bite. In Africa, it may occasionally be spread by handling infected bats or infected wild animals that are sometimes hunted for food. Ebola virus is only detected in blood after the patient becomes symptomatic and viral levels rise significantly as the disease progresses (CDC, 2020u).

The incubation period from exposure to first symptoms ranges from 2 to 21 days. If there are no symptoms by 21 days after exposure, there is essentially no risk of developing Ebola. Patients are not contagious to others before symptoms occur. Thorough identification of Ebola contacts and careful symptom monitoring can prevent subsequent waves of transmission (CDC, 2020u).

Clinical Manifestations

The initial clinical manifestations include high fever, muscle aches, and fatigue. Between the third and fifth symptomatic day, the patient often develops severe diarrhea, abdominal pain, and vomiting. Patients are at great risk for severe dehydration at this point as many produce over 5 L of liquid stool per day. This stage can persist for a week or more, and many patients develop hemodynamic shock (see Chapter 11). Patients may also show increasing neurologic symptoms during that period, such as confusion, agitation, delirium, or encephalitis. Approximately 5% will develop bleeding or hemorrhage, a very poor prognostic indicator. Patients who do not die during the first 2 weeks of the disease are likely to survive (CDC, 2020u).

Medical Management

No therapies have been approved for Ebola, but two antiviral treatments are under investigation (CDC, 2020u). Treatment is largely supportive maintenance of the circulatory and respiratory systems. It is likely that the patient who is infected will need ventilator and dialysis support during the acute phase of illness (CDC, 2020u).

Ebola Vaccines

In late 2019, the FDA approved the first Ebola vaccine effective at reducing the incidence of the Zaire strain of Ebola. The vaccine is approved for adults 18 years and older. Patient education is important as potential recipients should be informed that the vaccine has not shown protection for strains other than the Zaire strain, and adverse reactions (including anaphylaxis) have been reported (U.S. FDA, 2019).

Nursing Management

Nursing management mirrors that of medical management and is largely supportive. Supportive care for a patient with such a devastating disease requires very careful use of infection control measures and psychological support for the patient and family.

Health care workers are at increased risk for acquiring Ebola because they may have contact with body fluids or equipment contaminated from exposure to body fluids. Because patients with Ebola emit abundant viral particles in body fluids, especially in vomit and diarrhea, the patient should be promptly isolated in a private room, away from other patients. Health care workers should wear complete PPE. Systems must be set up so that an observer guides each worker to meticulously don PPE before direct contact with a patient who is infected to ensure that all equipment is worn correctly. After a worker has direct contact with a patient who is infected, an observer should direct careful doffing (removal) of PPE to ensure that no exposure occurs in the process. (See Chart 66-3 and Resources section for more information on donning and doffing PPE.) Equipment used for the patient with Ebola virus should be used solely for that patient and should be disposed of after use. If equipment must be reused, it should be sterilized or scrupulously cleaned with a bleach-based solution before reuse. Care for the patient with Ebola requires hospitals and transport systems to develop plans to coordinate staffing, supply maintenance, handling of waste, and communication with the public (WHO, 2020). Because care for Ebola patients is so complex, during a time of increased risks, communities are encouraged to assign some facilities as the designated facilities for Ebola care. Other facilities will have the responsibility to carefully screen patients with suspected Ebola and to cautiously transport them to a designated Ebola care facility.

Legionnaires Disease

Legionnaires disease is a multisystem illness that usually includes pneumonia and is caused by the gram-negative bacterium *Legionella pneumophila*. Named after an outbreak among people attending a convention of the American Legion in 1976, its potential to cause outbreaks has been demonstrated repeatedly in hospitals and other settings. It continues to be considered an emerging infectious disease because there are new patterns in recent years. There are approximately 5000 new cases each year (CDC, 2020v).

Legionella organisms are found in many man-made and naturally occurring water sources. Although the organisms may initially be introduced to the plumbing system in low numbers, growth is enhanced by water storage, sediment, temperatures ranging from 25°C to 42°C (77°F to 108°F), and certain amoebae frequently present in water that can support intracellular growth of legionellae. Because incidence appears to increase in the summer and autumn months, vacation-related exposure to hotel or cruise ship plumbing and air-conditioning systems, whirlpool spas, and decorative fountains may be the causative risk (Soda, Barskey, Shah, et al., 2017).

Pathophysiology

Legionella pneumophila is transmitted by the aerosolized route from an environmental source to a person's respiratory tract. In hospitals, patients may be exposed to aerosols created by cooling towers, water exposure from in-room plumbing, and respiratory therapy equipment. Person-to-person transmission does not occur. Because underlying medical conditions can increase host susceptibility and subsequent severity of disease, and because hospital plumbing systems are often very complex, outbreaks occur in hospitals more frequently than at other centers within the community. The mortality rate for Legionnaires disease may be as high as 10%; for those who acquire the disease while in a health care facility, the rate is approximately 25% (Soda et al., 2017).

Risk Factors

Risk factors for *Legionella* infection include diseases that lead to severe immunosuppression, such as AIDS, hematologic malignancy, end-stage kidney disease, or the use of immunosuppressive agents. Other factors associated with increased risk include diabetes, smoking, exposure to whirlpool spas, and recent travel (CDC, 2020v; Soda et al., 2017).

Clinical Manifestations

The lungs are the principal organs of infection; however, other organs may also be involved. The incubation period ranges from 2 to 10 days. Early symptoms may include malaise, myalgias, headache, and dry cough. The patient develops increasing pulmonary symptoms, including productive cough, dyspnea, and chest pain. Patients are usually febrile,

and body temperatures may reach or exceed 39.4°C (103°F). Diarrhea and other gastrointestinal symptoms are common. In severe cases, multiorgan involvement and failure may follow (CDC, 2020v).

Assessment and Diagnostic Findings

The diagnostic approach generally involves using information obtained from the history, physical examination, x-rays, laboratory findings, and assessment of therapeutic effectiveness. Chest x-ray abnormalities may vary in severity and in location within the lungs. Laboratory tests available for the diagnosis of *Legionella* include culture or tests that detect either antigen or antibody. The most frequently used test is the urinary antigen. The greatest limitation of the test is that it detects only one subgroup of one of the several species of *Legionella*. The CDC recommends using multiple tests when Legionnaires disease is suspected because none of the tests is completely accurate (CDC, 2020v).

Medical Management

The antibiotic agents of choice are azithromycin or a fluoroquinolone such as moxifloxacin. The antibiotic doxycycline may also be used (CDC, 2020v).

Nursing Management

The nursing management described for the patient with any pneumonia (see Chapter 19) should form the basis of care for the patient with *Legionella* pneumonia. Isolation is not required because *Legionella* is not transmitted between humans. Legionellosis should be reported to public health authorities. When the patient has acquired the infection in a health care facility, water sampling should be performed to determine if the water supply is contaminated and to verify eradication after water treatment.

Pertussis

Pertussis, also known as whooping cough, a common childhood disease in the pre-vaccine era, is an example of a disease that has re-emerged. Incidence rates declined until the 1980s, when rates for all age groups began to increase steadily for the next three decades, peaking in 2012 and plateauing in the following years (CDC, 2020w).

Pertussis is caused by the bacterium *Bordetella pertussis*. It is highly contagious, and patients usually present to health care professionals with a paroxysmal (sudden) cough that is accompanied by a characteristic whoop—a high-pitched noise heard when inhaling.

Pathophysiology

B. pertussis is transmitted by droplets. The bacteria easily attach to pharyngeal epithelial cells, where they release a number of antigens, toxins, and other substances that trigger the immune system. Because most of the disease manifestations are caused by this immune reaction, patients are usually contagious only early in the disease (when the bacteria are still present) and not during the protracted period of cough (when the immune reaction is causing the pathology).

Clinical Manifestations

Pertussis causes a range of respiratory symptoms, with cough being the most frequent. It is generally most severe for infants who have not yet been vaccinated. Pneumonia is the most common consequence of infection, but the disease can also lead to seizures, encephalopathy, and, rarely, death. People who have been vaccinated seldom have severe disease (CDC, 2020w).

Assessment and Diagnostic Findings

Most diagnoses of pertussis are made, at least initially, without laboratory confirmation. The clinical case definition, unless there is a preexisting condition to explain the symptoms, is a new cough lasting at least 2 weeks with inspiratory whoop or vomiting after cough. Laboratory confirmation can be made by clinical culture or by polymerase chain reaction assay for *B. pertussis*. Serologic testing, although less reliable, can also strengthen the diagnostic suspicion. The best source for a culture is a nasopharyngeal specimen obtained by swab or aspirate (CDC, 2020w).

Medical Management

Early treatment for pertussis is important to prevent complications. The antibiotic agents of choice are azithromycin, erythromycin, or clarithromycin (Comerford & Durkin, 2020). The antibiotic trimethoprim sulfamethoxazole may also be used (CDC, 2020w). Close contacts of a patient with proven or suspected pertussis should receive prophylaxis with one of these agents to reduce the risk of disease.

Nursing Management

Patients who are hospitalized with pertussis should be isolated in droplet precautions until they have received 5 days of appropriate therapy. Household members should receive antimicrobial prophylaxis and should be advised to report any symptoms of an upper respiratory infection.

Immunization is an important element of pertussis prevention. There are two acellular formulations of pertussis vaccine; both are combinations of diphtheria and pertussis. The pediatric formula, called DTaP, is designed for children between 2 months and 6 years. The teen and adult formulation, called Tdap, contains a decreased amount of the diphtheria element. Tdap should be given to children over 11 years, all adults every 10 years, and pregnant women early in pregnancy (CDC, 2020w). All adults who are around infants under 12 months on a regular basis should be vaccinated to reduce the risk of transmitting pertussis.

Travel and Immigration

Travel, trade, migration, and wars have led to many epidemics throughout history. The potential for epidemics is greatest when travelers and immigrants introduce microorganisms to which the host population has little or no immunity. Examples of important epidemics in the Western Hemisphere have included yellow fever, malaria, hookworm, leprosy, smallpox, measles, mumps, and syphilis. The COVID-19 pandemic demonstrates how global travel contributes to a rapidly occurring epidemic.

In the United States, an infrastructure with enforced vaccination, clean water, and insect and rodent control decreases the risk that epidemics will progress even when travel may introduce exotic microorganisms. The CDC maintains an active surveillance system to monitor and halt the incidence of many diseases prospectively. However, the 2016 experience with Zika virus reinforced knowledge that insect transmission can lead to significant outbreaks. Insects can infest cargo; in addition, travelers who may have been exposed abroad to insect-borne infections may then serve as reservoirs for further disease spread. For example, concern grows that vector-borne diseases such as dengue and malaria may increase in the United States as mosquitoes can transmit disease locally when a reservoir of infected humans is established.

Immigration and Acquired Immune Deficiency Syndrome

The fact that AIDS reached pandemic proportions less than a decade after its recognition attests to the efficiency of world travel in spreading disease. Such rapid transmission rates are especially dramatic because HIV essentially requires intimate contact between two people through sexual activity or sharing blood through needles (see Chapter 32).

Immigration and Tuberculosis

Immigration has long been an important influence in the epidemiology of TB in the United States. In 2017, the year with the lowest total of new TB cases in the United States since the 1950s, 70% of those reported were individuals who were foreign-born. The incidence among those who are foreign-born has been increasing steadily (CDC, 2020x). Multi-drug resistance is also more prevalent in cases among those who are foreign-born because the bacille Calmette–Guérin (BCG) vaccine is used in many countries. After receiving BCG, people often have some degree of tuberculin skin test reactivity for a prolonged time, thus making the diagnosis of TB infection challenging.

The QuantiFERON-TB Gold (QFT-G) test is an enzyme-linked immunosorbent assay (ELISA) that detects the release of interferon-gamma by white blood cells when the blood of a patient with TB is incubated with peptides similar to those in M. *tuberculosis*. The results of the QFT-G test are available in less than 24 hours and are not affected by prior vaccination with BCG. See Chapter 19 for more detailed discussion.

Immigration and Vector-Borne Diseases

Malaria and dengue are diseases that cause significant morbidity and mortality throughout the developing world. These diseases may be introduced to the United States via travel, immigration, or commerce with approximately 2000 cases each year (CDC, 2020y). Malaria and dengue are caused by microorganisms that can be spread to humans by mosquitoes in the United States that thrive in tropical zones and breed in stagnant water sources. Although malaria was eradicated in the United States in the 1950s, limited local outbreaks have occurred regularly when mosquitoes acquire the bacteria from a person recently traveling from an area in which malaria is endemic and transmit it to a small number of people.

Similarly, an increase of dengue virus in the Caribbean has caused concern that outbreaks may occur in the United States (CDC, 2020y).

CRITICAL THINKING EXERCISES

1 `ebp` The community clinic where you work has had an increase in STIs in the last 6 months. Identify how STIs occur. What evidence-based strategies could be used in the community to decrease the incidence of STIs? Identify the criteria used to evaluate the strength of the evidence for the practices you identify.

2 `pq` You are a home health nurse making a home visit for a 75-year-old patient with multiple medical conditions who has recently been discharged from the hospital following an ICU stay of 10 days for COVID-19. What are your priorities for providing information about infection prevention to the patient, the family, and the caregiver?

3 `ipc` You are serving on a committee to address pandemic preparation. What members of the interprofessional care team should be included in this committee? What methods should the team offer to address possible shortages of PPE? What methods could be used to provide prophylaxis or vaccines, if they are available?

REFERENCES

*Asterisk indicates nursing research.
**Double asterisk indicates classic reference.

Books

Centers for Disease Control and Prevention. (2015). In Hamborsky, J., Kroger, A., & Wolfe, S. (Eds.). *Epidemiology and prevention of vaccine-preventable diseases* (13th ed.). Washington D.C.: Public Health Foundation.

Comerford, K. C., & Durkin, M. A. (2020). *Nursing 2020 drug handbook* (40th ed.). Philadelphia, PA: Wolters Kluwer.

Norris, T. L. (2019). *Porth's pathophysiology: Concepts of altered health states* (10th ed.). Philadelphia, PA: Wolters Kluwer.

Schierhorn, C. (2019). *Healthcare worker safety checklists: Protecting those who serve.* Chicago, IL: The Joint Commission.

Journals and Electronic Documents

Agency for Healthcare Research and Quality (AHRQ). (2017). Estimating the additional hospital inpatient cost and mortality associated with selected hospital-acquired conditions. Retrieved on 3/16/2020 at: www.ahrq.gov/hai/pfp/haccost2017-results.html

American Academy of Dermatology (AAD). (2020). Preventing and treating occupationally induced dermatologic-conditions during COVID-19. Retrieved on 10/16/2020 at: assets.ctfassets.net/1ny4yoiyrq ia/1evNAmDqSmw6w9dhozuJGZ/303efdeff53db6e0347df52c65baf4bc/ OCC_Derm_Conditions_V11_30Apr2020.pdf

Cascella, M., Rajnik, M., Cuomo, A., et al. (2020). Features, evaluation, and treatment of coronavirus (COVID-19). *StatPearls.* Treasure Island, FL: StatPearls Publishing. Retrieved on 6/9/2020 at: www.ncbi.nlm.nih. gov/books/NBK554776/

Castells, M. C., & Phillips, E. J. (2021). Maintaining safety with SARS CoV-2 vaccines. *The New England Journal of Medicine, 384*(7), 643–649.

**Centers for Disease Control and Prevention (CDC). (2002). Guideline for hand hygiene in health care settings. MMWR. *Morbidity and Mortality Weekly Report, 51*(RR 16), 1–56.

**Centers for Disease Control and Prevention (CDC). (2007). Guideline for isolation precautions: Preventing transmission of infectious agents in healthcare settings (2007). Retrieved on 3/13/2020 at: www.cdc.gov/ hicpac/2007ip/2007ip_part1.html

Centers for Disease Control and Prevention (CDC). (2016). Healthcare system preparedness and response. Retrieved on 7/24/2020 at: www. cdc.gov/flu/pandemic-resources/planning-preparedness/healthcare-preparedness-response.html

Centers for Disease Control and Prevention (CDC). (2017). Global Health: CDC's global health partnerships. Retrieved on 8/4/2020 at: www.cdc.gov/globalhealth/partnerships.htm

Centers for Disease Control and Prevention (CDC). (2018). Cholera—*Vibrio cholerae infection.* Retrieved on 3/19/2020 at: www.cdc/cholera/ treatment/rehydration-therapy.html

Centers for Disease Control and Prevention (CDC). (2019a). Antibiotic resistance threats in the United States, 2019. Retrieved on 3/12/2020 at: www.cdc.gov/drugresistance/Biggest-Threats.html

Centers for Disease Control and Prevention (CDC). (2019b). 2018 National and state healthcare-associated infections progress report. Retrieved on 3/12/2020 at: www.cdc.gov/hai/data/portal/progress-report. html#Executive

Centers for Disease Control and Prevention (CDC). (2019c). FAQs for clinicians about C. diff. Retrieved on 3/12/2020 at: www.cdc.gov/cdiff/ clinicians/faq.html#anchor_1529601824235

Centers for Disease Control and Prevention (CDC). (2020a). Interim guidelines for collecting and handling clinical specimens for COVID-19 testing. Retrieved on 12/15/2020 at: www.cdc.gov/coronavirus/2019-nCoV/lab/guidelines-clinical-specimens.html#collecting

Centers for Disease Control and Prevention (CDC). (2020b). Immunization schedules. Retrieved on 3/16/2020 at: www.cdc.gov/vaccines/ schedules

Centers for Disease Control and Prevention (CDC). (2020c). Interim infection prevention and control recommendations for healthcare personnel during the coronavirus disease 2019 (COVID-19) pandemic. Retrieved on 7/17/2020 at: www.cdc.gov/coronavirus/2019-ncov/hcp/ infection-control-recommendations.html

Centers for Disease Control and Prevention (CDC). (2020d). National Healthcare Safety Network (NHSN). Retrieved on 3/14/2020 at: www. cdc.gov/nhsn/index.html

Centers for Disease Control and Prevention (CDC). (2020e). Strategies for optimizing the supply of N95 respirators. Retrieved on 7/18/2020 at: www.cdc.gov/coronavirus/2019-ncov/hcp/respirators-strategy/index. html

Centers for Disease Control and Prevention (CDC). (2020f). Healthcare associated infections - Clinicians: Information about CRE. Retrieved on 3/13/2020 at: www.cdc.gov/hai/organisms/cre/cre-clinicians.html

Centers for Disease Control and Prevention (CDC). (2020g). Interim clinical guidance for management of patients with confirmed coronavirus disease (COVID-19). Retrieved on 7/24/2020 at: www.cdc.gov/ coronavirus/2019-ncov/hcp/clinical-guidance-management-patients. html

Centers for Disease Control and Prevention (CDC). (2020h). COVID-19: People with certain medical conditions. Retrieved on 7/24/2020 at: www.cdc.gov/coronavirus/2019-ncov/need-extra-precautions/people-with-medical-conditions.html

Centers for Disease Control and Prevention (CDC). (2020i). Influenza (Flu). Retrieved on 3/17/2020 at: www.cdc.gov/flu

Centers for Disease Control and Prevention (CDC). (2020j). Global water, sanitation, & hygiene (WASH): Global diarrhea burden. Retrieved on 3/19/2020 at: www.cdc.gov/healthywater/global/diarrhea-burden.html

Centers for Disease Control and Prevention (CDC). (2020k). Preventing Norovirus infection. Retrieved on 3/18/2020 at: www.cdc.gov/norovirus/ about

Centers for Disease Control and Prevention (CDC). (2020l). *Campylobacter* (Campylobacteriosis): Information for health professionals. Retrieved on 3/18/2020 at: www.cdc.gov/campylobacter/technical.html

Centers for Disease Control and Prevention (CDC). (2020m). *Salmonella* and food. Retrieved on 3/18/2020 at: www.cdc.gov/features/salmonella-food/index.html

Centers for Disease Control and Prevention (CDC). (2020n). *E. coli* (*Escherichia coli*): Prevention. Retrieved on 3/18/2020 at: www.cdc.gov/ ecoli/ecoli-prevention.html

Centers for Disease Control and Prevention (CDC). (2020o). Parasites—*Giardia.* Retrieved on 3/18/2020 at: www.cdc.gov/parasites/giardia/ index.html

Centers for Disease Control and Prevention (CDC). (2020p). Food Safety: Keep food safe. Retrieved on 3/18/2020 at: www.cdc.gov/foodsafety/keep-food-safe.html

Centers for Disease Control and Prevention (CDC). (2020q). Sexually transmitted disease surveillance, 2018 National profile. Retrieved on 3/18/2020 at: www.cdc.gov/std/stats18/natoverview.htm

Centers for Disease Control and Prevention (CDC). (2020r). Sexually transmitted diseases (STDs). Retrieved on 8/4/2020 at: www.cdc.gov/std/treatment/default.htm

Centers for Disease Control and Prevention (CDC). (2020s). Zika and pregnancy: Women and their partners trying to become pregnant. Retrieved on 3/18/2020 at: www.cdc.gov/pregnancy/zika/women-and-their-partners.html

Centers for Disease Control and Prevention (CDC). (2020t). West Nile virus. Retrieved on 3/20/2020 at: www.cdc.gov/westnile/index.html

Centers for Disease Control and Prevention (CDC). (2020u). Ebola (Ebola virus disease). Retrieved on 3/20/2020 at: www.cdc.gov/vhf/ebola/index.html

Centers for Disease Control and Prevention (CDC). (2020v). *Legionella* (Legionnaires' disease and pontiac fever). Retrieved on 3/20/2020 at: www.cdc.gov/legionella/

Centers for Disease Control and Prevention (CDC). (2020w). Pertussis (Whooping cough). Retrieved on 3/21/2020 at: www.cdc.gov/pertussis/

Centers for Disease Control and Prevention (CDC). (2020x). Immigrant and refugee health; Domestic tuberculosis guidelines. Retrieved on 3/22/2020 at: www.cdc.gov/immigrantrefugeehealth/guidelines/domestic/tuberculosis-guidelines.html

Centers for Disease Control and Prevention (CDC). (2020y). *Malaria; Malaria and travelers for US residents.* Retrieved on 3/22/2020 at: www.cdc.gov/malaria/about/faqs.html

Chen, N., Zhou, M., Dong, X., et al. (2020). Epidemiological and clinical characteristics of 99 cases of 2019 novel coronavirus pneumonia in Wuhan, China: A descriptive study. *Lancet, 395*(10223), 507–513.

*Cohen, C., Spirito, C. M., Liu, J., et al. (2019). Concurrent detection of bacterial pathogens in hospital roommates. *Nursing Research, 68*(1), 80–83.

Deng, G., Yin, M., Chen, X., et al. (2020). Clinical determinants for fatality of 44,672 patients with COVID-19. *Critical Care, 24*(1), 179. Published online on 4/28/2020. doi:org/10.1186/s13054-020-02902-w

Hendrix, M. J., Walde, C., Findley, K., et al. (2020). Absence of apparent transmission of SARS-CoV-2 from two stylists after exposure at a hair salon with a universal face covering policy—Springfield, Missouri, May 2020. MMWR. *Morbidity and Mortality Weekly Report, 69*(28), 930–932.

**Homeland Security Council. (2006). National strategy for pandemic influenza: Implementation plan. Retrieved on 7/24/2020 at: www.cdc.gov/flu/pandemic-resources/pdf/pandemic-influenza-implementation.pdf

Johns Hopkins University & Medicine Coronavirus Resource Center. (2020). Maps and trends: Mortality analyses. Retrieved on 6/12/2020 at: coronavirus.jhu.edu/data/mortality

Kim, A. Y., & Gandhi, R. T. (2020). COVID-19: Management in hospitalized adults. *UpToDate.* Retrieved on 6/4/2020 at: www.uptodate.com/contents/coronavirus-disease-2019-covid-19-management-in-hospitalized-adults

Kourtis, A. P., Hatfield, K., Baggs, J., et al. (2019). Vital signs: Epidemiology and recent trends in methicillin-resistant and in methicillin-susceptible Staphylococcus aureus bloodstream infections—United States. MMWR. *Morbidity & Mortality Weekly Report, 68*(9), 214–219.

Krow-Lucal, E. R., Biggerstaff, B. J., & Staples, J. (2017). Estimated incubation period for Zika virus disease. *Emerging Infectious Diseases, 23*(5), 841–845.

Meites, E., Szilagyi, P., Chesson, H., et al. (2019). Human papillomavirus vaccination for adults: Updated recommendations of the Advisory Committee on Immunization Practices. MMWR. *Morbidity & Mortality Weekly Report, 68*(32), 698–702. Retrieved on 7/26/2020 at: www.cdc.gov/mmwr/volumes/68/wr/pdfs/mm6832a3-H.pdf

National Institutes of Health (NIH) COVID-19 Treatment Guidelines Panel. (2020). Coronavirus disease 2019 (COVID-19) treatment guidelines. Retrieved on 7/21/2020 at: www.covid19treatmentguidelines.nih.gov/

O'Bryne, P. (2019). Practice; Clinical updates: Syphilis. *BMJ, 365,* l4159. Retrieved on 8/3/2020 at: www.bmj.com/content/365/bmj.l4159

**Occupational Safety and Health Administration (OSHA). (2012). Bloodborne pathogens. Retrieved on 3/11/2020 at: www.osha.gov/pls/oshaweb/owadisp.show_document?p_table=STANDARDS&p_id=10051

*Prather, K. A., Wang, C. C., & Schooley, R. T. (2020). Reducing transmission of SARS-CoV-2. *Science, 68*(6498), 1422–1424.

Renaudin, L., Llorens, M., Goetz, C., et al. (2017). Impact of discontinuing contact precautions for MRSA and ESBLE in an intensive care unit: A prospective noninferiority before and after study. *Infection Control and Hospital Epidemiology, 38*(11), 1342–1350.

Shane, A. L., Mody, R. K., Crup, J. A., et al. (2017). Infectious Diseases Society of America clinical practice guidelines for the diagnosis and management of infectious diarrhea. *Clinical Infectious Diseases, 65*(12), e45–e80

Soda, E. A., Barskey, A. E., Shah, P. P., et al. (2017). Vital signs: Health care-associated Legionnaires' disease surveillance data from 20 states and a large metropolitan area—United States, 2015. MMWR. *Morbidity and Mortality Weekly Report, 66*(22), 584–589.

The Joint Commission. (2021). 2021 National Patient Safety Goals. Retrieved on 12/22/2020 at: www.jointcommission.org

U.S. Food and Drug Administration (FDA). (2019). FDA news release, December 19, 2019: First FDA-approved vaccine for the prevention of Ebola virus disease, marking a critical milestone in public health preparedness and response. Retrieved on 3/20/2020 at: www.fda.gov/NewsEvents/Newsroom/PressAnnouncements/ucm335891.htm

Vaduganathan, M., Vardeny, O., Michel, T., et al. (2020). Renin-angiotensin-aldosterone system inhibitors in patients with COVID-19. *The New England Journal of Medicine, 282*(17), 1653–1659.

Veenema, T. G., Meyer, D., Bell, S., et al. (2020). Recommendations for improving national nurse preparedness for pandemic response: Early lessons from COVID-19. Retrieved on 7/17/2020 at: www.centerforhealthsecurity.org/our-work/publications/recommendations-for-improving-national-nurse-preparedness-for-pandemic-response—early-lessons-from-covid-19

Weber, D. J., Babcock, H., Hayden M. K., et al. (2020). Universal pandemic precautions—an idea ripe for the times. *Infection Control and Hospital Epidemiology, 41*(11), 1321–1322.

Williams, P. C. M., & Berkley, J. A. (2018). Guidelines for the treatment of dysentery (shigellosis): A systematic review of the evidence. *Paediatrics and International Child Health, 38*(Supp 1), S50–S65.

World Health Organization (WHO). (2016). *Zika virus disease.* Retrieved on 3/11/2020 at: www.who.int/topics/zika/en/

World Health Organization (WHO). (2020). *Ebola virus disease.* Retrieved on 8/11/2020 at: www.who.int/mediacentre/factsheets. www-cdc-gov/coronavirus/2019-ncov/your-health/need-to-know.html

Resources

American Public Health Association (APHA), www.apha.org

Association for Professionals in Infection Control and Epidemiology (APIC), www.apic.org

Centers for Disease Control and Prevention (CDC) (includes video demonstrations of donning and doffing PPE), www.cdc.gov

Hospital Compare, www.medicare.gov/hospitalcompare

Infectious Diseases Society of America (IDSA), www.idsociety.org

Johns Hopkins University & Medicine, Coronavirus Resource Center, coronavirus.jhu.edu

National Foundation for Infectious Diseases (NFID), www.nfid.org

National Institute of Allergy and Infectious Diseases (NIAID), www.niaid.nih.gov

Occupational Safety and Health Administration (OSHA), www.osha.gov

Society for Healthcare Epidemiology of America (SHEA), www.shea-online.org

Vaccine Adverse Event Reporting System (VAERS), www.vaers.hhs.gov

World Health Organization (WHO), www.who.int/en/

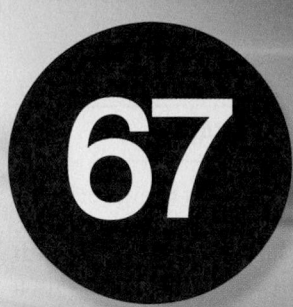

67 Emergency Nursing

The term *emergency management* traditionally refers to care given to patients with urgent and critical needs. However, because many people lack access to health care, the emergency department (ED) is used frequently for nonurgent problems. Therefore, the philosophy of emergency management has broadened to include the concept that an emergency is whatever the patient or the family considers it to be.

The emergency nurse has had specialized education, training, and expertise in assessing and identifying patients' health problems in crisis situations. In addition, the emergency nurse establishes priorities, monitors, and continuously assesses patients who are acutely ill and injured, supports and attends to families, supervises allied health personnel, and educates patients and families within a time-limited, high-pressured care environment. Nursing interventions are accomplished interdependently, in consultation with or under the direction of a physician or advanced practitioner such as a nurse practitioner or physician assistant. The roles of nursing and medicine are complementary in an emergency situation. Appropriate nursing and medical interventions are anticipated based on assessment data. Members of the ED staff work as a team in performing the highly technical, hands-on skills required to care for patients in emergency situations (Emergency Nurses Association [ENA], 2020a).

People seek emergency care for serious life-threatening conditions, such as cardiac arrhythmias, acute coronary syndrome, acute heart failure, pulmonary edema, and stroke. Priorities for managing these cardiac and other conditions are discussed in Chapters 22, 23, 25, and 62. Emergency management of trauma and conditions not found elsewhere in this book are discussed in this chapter. Facts about ED visits in the United States are presented in Chart 67-1.

Chart 67-1	Facts About Emergency Department Visits—2017

In 2017, there were 139 million visits to emergency departments (EDs); 40 million were as a result of an injury. Additional relevant statistics included the following:

- The most common reasons for ED visits were abdominal pain, chest pain, cough, and fever.
- Most patients had health insurance, with only 16% of patients without insurance.
- Approximately 14.5% of patients arrived at the ED by ambulance.
- 14.5 million visits resulted in admission; of these, 2 million required admission to an intensive care unit (ICU).
- Injuries and poisonings accounted for 18.9% of all ED visits.
- The leading causes of injuries were unintentional, totaling 68.2% of injury admissions, with falls and motor vehicle collisions making up 32% of these.
- Nearly 40% of patients were seen by a provider in less than 15 minutes after arrival to the ED.

Adapted from Rui, P., & Kang, K. (2017). National Hospital Ambulatory Medical Care Survey: 2017 emergency department summary tables. National Center for Health Statistics. Retrieved on 4/20/2020 at: www.cdc.gov/nchs/data/nhamcs/web_tables/2017_ed_web_tables-508.pdf

ISSUES IN EMERGENCY NURSING CARE

Emergency nursing is demanding because of the diversity of conditions and situations that present unique challenges. These challenges include legal issues, occupational health and safety risks for ED staff, and the challenge of providing holistic care in the context of a fast-paced, technology-driven environment in which serious illness and death are encountered on a daily basis. Another dimension of emergency nursing is providing nursing care in disasters. Disasters result in mass casualty incidents that ensue after natural disasters (e.g., earthquakes, tsunamis); from exposure to pathogens during outbreaks, epidemics, and pandemics; from human-made unintentional disasters (e.g., bridge collapse, train crash); or from weapons of terror (e.g., blast, biologic, chemical, radiologic terroristic events) (see Chapter 68).

Documentation of Consent and Privacy

Consent to examine and treat the patient is part of the ED record. The patient needs to give consent for invasive procedures (e.g., angiography, lumbar puncture) unless they are unconscious or in a critical condition and unable to make decisions. If the patient is unconscious and brought to the ED without family or friends, this fact must be documented. Monitoring of the patient's condition, as well as all instituted treatments and the times at which they were performed, must be documented. After treatment, a notation is made on the record about the patient's condition, response to the treatment, and condition at discharge or transfer and about instructions given to the patient and family for follow-up care.

The patient is also provided with a statement of the privacy policy of the health care agency, according to federal law. Patients involved in violent events can be provided with an alias, and access to the electronic health record (EHR) is limited to protect the privacy of the patient. A patient may also request extra privacy by limiting access to their room and by choosing not to receive phone calls, mail, flowers, other gifts, or certain visitors. These practices relate to the federally mandated privacy policy stipulated in the Health Insurance Portability and Accountability Act (HIPAA).

According to the Emergency Medical Treatment and Active Labor Act (EMTALA), every ED with a Medicare provider agreement must perform a medical screening examination on all patients arriving with an emergency medical complaint if their acute signs and symptoms could result in serious injury or death if left untreated. EDs are also required to provide treatment aimed at stabilizing each patient's condition. If the patient must be transferred to another facility, the patient's consent for transfer should be obtained, if possible. In addition, acceptance by the receiving facility and primary provider must be obtained, and an appropriate method of transfer for the patient should be secured. Documentation of assessment and treatment must be sent with the patient upon transfer (ENA, 2020a).

Limiting Exposure to Health Risks

ED staff are at an increased risk for exposure to communicable diseases through blood, respiratory droplets, or other body fluids. This risk for exposure to any communicable disease is further compounded because of the common use of a multitude of invasive treatments for patients in the ED (e.g., suturing, wound débridement, aerosol generating procedures). This increased risk had been apparent for many years because of increasing numbers of people infected with hepatitis, human immune deficiency virus (HIV), and tuberculosis; however, these risks became magnified because of concerns of infecting ED staff with severe acute respiratory syndrome coronavirus 2 (SARS-CoV-2), the virus responsible for the pandemic of coronavirus disease 2019 (COVID-19); see following discussion.

The potential for exposure to highly contagious organisms, hazardous chemicals or gases, and radiation related to acts of terrorism or natural or human-engineered disasters presents additional risks to ED staff. See Chapter 68 for information about decontamination procedures.

> **Quality and Safety Nursing Alert**
>
> *To limit the risk of exposure to airborne diseases, early identification and strict adherence to transmission-based precautions for patients who are potentially infected and contagious is crucial.*

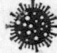 **COVID-19 Considerations**

In response to the COVID-19 pandemic, all emergency health care providers must adhere strictly to standard precautions for minimizing exposure, because not all patients who are infected with SARS-CoV-2 are symptomatic. Universal screening measures should be implemented upon arrival to the ED for all ED staff, patients, and visitors/family members (assuming that their presence in the ED is not prohibited). Patients and visitors/family members should wear their own mask or face coverings as tolerated, and if they do not have them, they should be provided upon their arrival to the ED. ED staff should wear facemasks at all times while in the hospital. In general, cloth masks, bandanas, and scarves are not considered suitable masks for use by health care workers (ENA, 2020b). Health care workers, patients, and visitors all need to be educated on the importance of hand hygiene and social distancing (Centers for Disease Control and Prevention [CDC], 2020a).

The ENA (2020b) issued a statement that all emergency nurses providing direct care for patients with suspected or confirmed COVID-19 must be provided the appropriate level of personal protective equipment (PPE) to safely care for these patients. The PPE provided to emergency nurses in this situation should meet standards set by the National Institute for Occupational Safety and Health (NIOSH) (see Chapter 66 for further discussion of PPE); N95 respirators, which include a facemask that seals firmly to the face and that filters at least 95% of airborne particles, are recommended over other less effective masks or face coverings (CDC, 2020b).

Violence in the Emergency Department

Not only do ED staff members encounter patients who may be violent because of the effects of substance use disorder (SUD), injury, or other emergencies, they may also encounter other violent situations. Patients and families waiting for assistance may be emotionally volatile. Often, ED waiting rooms are the sites where feelings of dissatisfaction, fear, and anger are channeled violently. EDs assign security officers to the area and have installed silent alarm systems or metal detectors to identify weapons in order to protect patients, families, and staff. Safety is the first priority.

Patients and family members under the influence of illicit drugs or alcohol, or who may have psychiatric disorders, including delirium or dementia, or who may be influenced by social situations such as gang membership, are at risk for committing a violent act, whether intentional or not (CDC, 2019a). The environment of the ED, including being subjected to long wait times and at times crowded conditions, may also increase their risk of committing violent events. Physical threats are most often accompanied by verbal abuse, which is the most common type of violence (Copeland & Henry, 2017). Although not a typical occurrence, a patient or family member may come to the ED armed. To avoid angry confrontations, members of gangs and families who are feuding need to be separated in the ED, in the waiting room, and later in the inpatient nursing unit. Nurses and other personnel must be prepared to deal with these circumstances. The ED should be locked against entry if security is questionable.

Patients who are violent or potentially violent must be vigilantly monitored by the ED staff. Care must be taken to avoid injury. Patients from prison and those who are under guard need to be handcuffed to the bed and appropriately assessed to ensure the safety of hospital staff and other patients. The emergency nurse must understand how to employ safe use of restraints. The Joint Commission has strict standards regarding documentation of the reason, monitoring for safety, and ensuring the dignity of the patient who is restrained. Precautions to be taken to avoid injury include the following situations (ENA 2020a; Ziaei, Massoudifar, Rajabpour-Sanati, et al., 2018):

- For prisoners, the hand or ankle restraint (handcuff) is never released, and a guard is always present in the room.
- A mask can be placed on the patient to prevent spitting or biting, if a mask is not already being used.
- Nonrestraint techniques should be tried when possible—for example, talking with the patient, minimizing environmental stimulation.
- Physical restraints are used on any patient who is violent only as needed and, if used, should be humanely and professionally given; nonetheless, the staff should be cognizant that the patient could head-butt, even if restrained.
- Distance should be maintained from the patient to avoid grabbing; staff should not wear items that can be grabbed by the patient, such as dangling jewelry and stethoscopes. Furthermore, distance should be maintained between the patient and the door so that an escape route for the staff member is preserved.
- Objects should not be left within patient reach; even an intravenous (IV) line spike can become a tool of violence if the patient is determined.
- Courses on safety (de-escalation and physical restraint techniques) assist the staff with preparing for various violent situations.

In the case of gunfire in the ED, self-protection is a priority. There is no advantage to protecting others if health care providers are injured. Security officers and police must gain control of the situation first, and then care is provided to the injured.

Providing Holistic Care

Patients and families experiencing sudden injury or illness are often overwhelmed by anxiety because they have not had time to adapt to the crisis. They experience real and terrifying fear of death, mutilation, immobilization, and other assaults on their personal identity and bodily integrity. When confronted with trauma, severe disfigurement, severe illness, or sudden death, the family experiences several stages of crisis. The stages begin with anxiety and progress through denial, remorse and guilt, anger, grief, and reconciliation. The initial goal for the patient and family is anxiety reduction, a prerequisite to effective and appropriate coping. During this stressful time, safety is of primary importance. Close observation and preplanning are essential and security personnel are stationed nearby in the event that a patient or family member responds to stress with physical violence.

Assessment of the patient and family's psychological function includes evaluating emotional expression, degree of anxiety, and cognitive functioning. Possible nursing diagnoses include:

- Anxiety or death anxiety associated with uncertain potential outcomes of the illness or trauma
- Difficulty coping associated with acute situational crisis

Possible nursing diagnoses for the family include:

- Family grief
- Interrupted family process
- Impaired or risk for impaired family coping associated with acute situational crises

Patient-Focused Interventions

Clinicians caring for the patient should act confidently and competently to relieve anxiety and promote a sense of security. Explanations should be given that the patient can understand. Human contact and reassuring words reduce the panic of the person who is severely injured or ill and aid in dispelling fear of the unknown.

The patient who is unconscious should be treated as if conscious—that is, the patient should be touched, called by name, and provided an explanation of every procedure that is performed. As the patient regains consciousness, the nurse should orient the patient by stating their name, the date, and the location. This basic information should be provided repeatedly, as needed, in a reassuring way.

Ensuring patient safety is a major focus in clinical practice settings. Some of the most common **sentinel events** (unanticipated events that result in patient harm) in the ED include delays to care and medication errors. Common root causes for these sentinel events revolve around nurse staffing patterns, patient volume, and specialty availability. Solutions to patient safety issues in the ED include ensuring optimal nurse staffing, pharmacy presence, and rapid diagnostics turnaround times to minimize wait time to diagnosis and fostering teamwork and support by leadership. All errors should be reported and investigated even if a patient was not harmed. In this way, future injury or death may be avoided (The Joint Commission, 2020).

Family-Focused Interventions

The family is kept informed about where the patient is, how they are doing, and the care that is being given. Encouraging family members to stay with the patient, when possible, also helps alleviate their anxieties. In many facilities, family presence during resuscitation is permitted to assist the family to cope through this difficult time. Many family members respond very well to this approach. Research has indicated that families view emergency professionals favorably when a family member was resuscitated. They view their role as supportive and protective of the patient. Allowing family presence in the critical care areas of the hospital, whenever possible, enhances the family role and builds trust in the caregivers (Toronto & LaRocco, 2019). The presence of a family facilitator, who is trained to provide support to family members, is vital to the success of a family presence program (ENA, 2017). Additional interventions are based on the assessment of the stage of crisis that the family is experiencing. Measures to help family members cope with sudden death are presented in Chart 67-2.

Chart 67-2 **Helping Family Members Cope with Sudden Death**

When able to do so, the nurse takes the following actions:

- Take the family to a private place.
- Talk to the family together so that they can grieve together and hear the information given together.
- Reassure the family that everything possible was done; inform them of the treatment rendered.
- Avoid using euphemisms such as "passed on." Show the family that you care by touching, offering coffee, water, and the services of a chaplain.
- Encourage family members to support each other and to express emotions freely (grief, loss, anger, helplessness, tears, disbelief).
- Avoid giving sedation to family members; this may mask or delay the grieving process, which is necessary to achieve emotional equilibrium and to prevent prolonged depression.
- Encourage the family to view the body if they wish; this action helps to integrate the loss. Cover disfigured and injured areas before the family sees the body. Go with the family and do not leave them alone. Show acceptance by touching the body to give the family "permission" to touch.
- Spend time with the family, listening to them and identifying any needs that they may have for which the nursing staff can be helpful.
- Allow family members to talk about the deceased and what the person meant to them; this permits ventilation of feelings of loss. Encourage the family to talk about events preceding admission to the emergency department. Do not challenge initial feelings of anger or denial.
- Avoid volunteering unnecessary information (e.g., the patient was drinking).

Note: These interventions might not be advisable or permitted if "social distancing" prohibitions are in place, such as those prohibitions implemented to thwart transmission of severe acute respiratory coronavirus 2 (SARS-CoV-2) infection during the coronavirus disease (COVID-19) pandemic.

Anxiety and Denial

During these crises, family members are encouraged to recognize and talk about their feelings of anxiety. Asking questions is encouraged. Honest answers given at the level of the family's understanding must be provided. Although denial is an ego-defense mechanism that protects individuals from recognizing painful and disturbing aspects of reality, prolonged denial is not encouraged or supported. The family must be prepared for the reality of what has happened and what may come (Ocak & Avsarogullari, 2019).

Remorse and Guilt

Expressions of remorse and guilt are common, with family members accusing themselves (or each other) of negligence or minor omissions. Family members are urged to verbalize their feelings to help them cope appropriately.

Anger

Expressions of anger, common in crisis situations, are a way of handling anxiety and fear. Anger is frequently directed by the family at the patient, but it is also often expressed toward the physician, the nurse, or admitting personnel. The therapeutic approach is to allow the anger to be expressed and to assist the family members to identify their feelings of frustration.

Grief

Grief is a complex emotional response to anticipated or actual loss. The key nursing intervention is to help family members work through their grief and to support their coping mechanisms, letting them know that it is normal and acceptable for them to cry, feel pain, and express loss. The hospital chaplain and social services staff serve as invaluable members of the team when assisting families to work through their grief (see Chapter 13).

Caring for Emergency Personnel

Concerted efforts have been made to focus on the needs of the ED staff, especially after serious and stressful events (ENA, 2020a). Events can range from a local trauma case involving children; to treating someone known to the emergency worker, such as a colleague or family member; to a more complex natural disaster or mass casualty incident. It is important to remember that all staff members may not necessarily respond in the same way; an event that is stressful to one person may not be as stressful to another. Compassion fatigue may result from continuous exposure to suffering and injury, and energy is expended on a daily basis. Fatigue occurs when the affected staff members cannot replenish energy stores (Schmidt & Haglund, 2017). In addition, because stress is a daily occurrence in the ED, staff may not recognize the personal effect of any one event or the cumulative effect of day-to-day crisis interventions. ED leadership should be aware of staff coping patterns and support systems, patterns of interactions between staff members, staff members' health problems, including addiction, and appropriately assist with identifying behaviors caused by workplace stress. The availability of nonjudgmental counseling is essential to promoting a healthy staff.

After serious events, critical incident stress management (CISM) is useful to critique individual and group performance and to facilitate healthy coping. Optimally, this consists of three steps: defusing, debriefing, and follow-up. Defusing occurs immediately after the critical incident. During this session, affected staff are encouraged to discuss their feelings about the incident, are reassured that negative reactions and feelings are normal but that these diminish over time, and are given contact information so that they may talk to someone if they have disturbing symptoms (e.g., sleeplessness, excessive worry). Debriefing typically occurs 1 to 10 days after the critical incident. Debriefing sessions follow a format similar to the initial defusing session; however, during these sessions, participating staff are encouraged to discuss their feelings about the incident and are again reassured that their negative reactions and feelings are normal and that their negative feelings will diminish over time. At the end of these sessions, participants should have a feeling of closure and be able to resume their professional roles at an emotional level commensurate to that prior to the critical incident. Some staff may require further professional follow-up, however. Follow-up may occur after the debriefing session is completed for those participants who have persistent negative symptoms and may consist of continued individual or group counseling and therapy (Schmidt & Haglund, 2017).

 ## COVID-19 Considerations

Holistic, patient-centered care remains a top priority in EDs, even during disaster situations such as the COVID-19 pandemic. It is also a top priority that emergency nurses have the mechanisms and support to properly manage their heightened stress during such situations. Assuring holistic care of patients and families and supporting the emotional well-being of emergency staff pose unique challenges during such disasters as the COVID-19 pandemic.

In particular, regulations and mitigation strategies enforced in response to the COVID-19 pandemic prohibit family and visitor presence during hospitalizations in geographic regions experiencing an upswing in confirmed cases in order to keep patients, family members, and health care workers safe (Hart, Turnbull, Oppenheim, et al., 2020). Family presence and visitation policies are adapted in efforts to maintain open communication and family involvement in patient care. These adaptive strategies rely heavily on technology, which include the use of smartphones and computers, and require stable Internet connection and technologic literacy. Barriers exist for patients and families who either lack technologic literacy or who come from socioeconomically disadvantaged backgrounds, which preclude their ability to be able to tap into engaging in virtual conversations (Hart et al., 2020).

During these difficult times, ED staff are encouraged to develop a communication plan with family members, designating one person as the point of contact, ensuring that contact person has adequate access to technology, and identifying and eliminating any barriers to effective communication. Videoconferencing can be used when possible, particularly during end-of-life situations (Hart et al., 2020). The use of support teams that includes pastoral care, palliative care, and behavioral health should be mobilized to assist in the grieving process (Hart et al., 2020).

The emotional burden experienced by emergency nurses on the frontlines of the COVID-19 pandemic has been reported to be greatly magnified. Emergency nurses reportedly experienced fear as they faced a shortage of PPE, emotional and physical exhaustion, and ongoing stress. In some cases, nurses were the only persons physically present with patients who were severely ill and provided the only source of distant communication between patients and their family members. Confronted with not being able to provide the care for patients as they would have done under nonpandemic conditions, many emergency nurses experienced moral distress. Moral distress can be disruptive to emotional health; symptoms may include "self-criticism, intense feelings of shame, guilt, or disgust and may contribute to depression or post-traumatic stress disorder" (American Psychiatric Nurses Association, 2020, p. 1). Although the ultimate long-term impact of COVID-19 on the health of emergency nurses is not known at this time, supportive strategies must be implemented in order to preserve the health care workforce that has experienced severe stress as a consequence of COVID-19 (The Joint Commission, 2020).

EMERGENCY NURSING AND THE CONTINUUM OF CARE

A key principle underlying emergency care is that the patient is rapidly assessed, treated, and referred to the appropriate setting for ongoing care. This makes the ED a temporary point on the continuum of care. In 2017, only 10.4% of patients who received care in an ED in the United States were admitted to the hospital, which means emergency nurses must plan and facilitate the patient's safe discharge and follow-up care in the home, community, and the transitional care environment (CDC, 2017a).

Discharge Planning

Before discharge, instructions for continuing care are given to the patient and to the family or significant others, if possible. A variety of formats are used including verbal, written, or video instructions; research findings suggest that video instructions are well received by patients and family members (Wilkin, 2020). Many EDs have preprinted standard instruction sheets for the more common conditions (e.g., concussion), which can then be individualized. Discharge instructions should be available in commonly used languages. A language interpreter should be used as necessary to provide instructions in any format.

Instructions should include information about prescribed medications, treatments, diet, activity, and when to contact a health care provider or schedule follow-up appointments. Discharge planning is the "teachable moment" for the patient, providing the opportunity to present injury prevention or smoking cessation strategies, alcohol counseling opportunities, and more. It is imperative that instructions are written legibly, use simple language, and are clear in their important points. When providing discharge instructions, the nurse also considers any special needs the patient may have related to hearing or visual impairments. Alternative formats of instruction (e.g., large print, Braille, audiotape, online videoclips) should be available to meet the needs of patients with hearing or visual impairments.

Community and Transitional Services

Before discharge, some patients require the services of a social worker to help them meet continuing health care needs. Home health care resources may be contacted before discharge to arrange services. This is particularly important for patients who may need assistance, such as those who are older adults or those with disability. Identifying continuing health care needs and making arrangements for meeting these needs can prevent return visits to the ED or readmission to the hospital.

For patients who are returning to long-term care facilities and for those who already rely on community agencies for continuing health care, communication about the patient's condition and any changes in health care needs that have occurred must be provided to the appropriate facilities or agencies. This communication is essential to promote continuity of care and to ensure ongoing care that meets the patient's changing health care needs.

Many patients who utilize EDs have health problems that are nonurgent. Moreover, some patients return repeatedly to the ED with nonurgent problems (ENA, 2019). It is posited that patients who present to the ED with nonurgent problems do so because there is a dearth of outpatient health care resources to fill their needs. In order to fill these gaps, some areas of the United States, particularly rural areas, are offering mobile integrated health-community paramedicine programs. Emergency medical system (EMS) personnel provide in-home visits, without emergency calls, to identify needs and provide education and in-home care. If necessary, they can also transport patients to the ED. These programs have decreased unnecessary EMS calls (ENA, 2019).

Gerontologic Considerations

The ED is a common point of entry into the health care system for patients 65 years and older. The CDC (2017b) reports that 32% of ED visits by patients older than 65 years resulted in hospital admission. As age increases, the percentage of admissions increases. Of these admissions, 17% were related to trauma, primarily falls (CDC, 2017b). Older adult patients typically arrive with one or more presenting conditions. Nonspecific symptoms, such as weakness and fatigue, episodes of falling, incontinence, and change in mental status, may be manifestations of acute, potentially life-threatening illness in the older person. Emergencies in this age group may be more difficult to manage because older adult patients may have an atypical presentation, an altered response to treatment, a greater risk of developing complications, or a combination of these factors.

The older adult patient may perceive the emergency as a crisis signaling the end of an independent lifestyle or even death. The nurse should give attention to the patient's feelings of anxiety and fear (Cortez, 2018).

The older adult patient may have limited sources of social and financial support during times of crises. The nurse should assess the psychosocial resources of the patient (and of the caregiver, if necessary) and anticipate discharge needs.

Referrals for support services (e.g., to the social service department or a gerontologic nurse specialist) may be necessary.

 ## Obesity Considerations

The growing rate of obesity in the United States has implications for treating patients with obesity within the ED, in terms of stocking appropriately sized equipment, gowns, and stretchers; ensuring that equipment (e.g., computed tomography [CT] scanners) is able to handle a greater weight capacity; and recognizing specific disorders and complications that may occur in these patients. For instance, research suggests that increased mortality is associated with the degree of obesity (ENA, 2020a). Other considerations in ED management of patients with obesity include an understanding that it is generally more challenging to insert IV lines and airways. Ventilation also can be a challenge from the increased weight of the chest wall and the increased incidence of hypoventilation and sleep apnea among patients with obesity. Special consideration must be taken with lipophilic medications, as they take longer to clear from the larger volume of adipose tissue. Weight-based medications must be calculated carefully using ideal body mass. X-rays may be difficult to visualize because of poor penetration (Richardson & Harris, 2018).

Complications that patients with obesity are more prone to experience during hospitalization include respiratory failure, acute kidney injury (AKI), pneumonia, deep vein thrombosis, and pressure injuries. Patients with severe obesity who have femur fractures have a significantly higher risk of death, as well as a higher risk of acute respiratory distress syndrome (ARDS) and sepsis than patients of normal weight (Richardson & Harris, 2018). Although many of these complications do not occur until later in the hospital stay, some preventive measures (e.g., encouraging turning, coughing, and deep-breathing exercises to prevent atelectasis) may be initiated in the ED. Functional recovery time is extended in patients with obesity, resulting in longer lengths of stay and increased hospital costs. Initiating prevention measures in the ED, such as early backboard removal and providing early preventive respiratory care, are targeted to improve recovery time (Richardson & Harris, 2018). Arranging transfers of patients with obesity must also take into consideration the availability of appropriately sized equipment.

PRINCIPLES OF EMERGENCY CARE

By definition, emergency care is care that must be rendered without delay. In an ED, several patients with diverse health problems—some life-threatening, some not—may present to the ED simultaneously. One of the first principles of emergency care is triage.

Triage

The word **triage** comes from the French word *trier*, meaning "to sort." In the daily routine of the ED, triage is used to sort patients into groups based on the severity of their health problems and the immediacy with which these problems must be treated.

A basic and widely used triage system that had been in use for many years utilized three categories: emergent, urgent, and nonurgent. In this system, emergent patients had the highest priority, urgent patients had serious health problems but not immediately life-threatening ones, and nonurgent patients had episodic illnesses.

A comprehensive, valid, and reliable five-level triage severity rating system that recognizes that EDs are used for both emergency and routine health care is also used. The increased number of triage levels assists the triage nurse to more precisely determine the needs of the patient and the urgency for treatment. Systems that meet these criteria for validity and reliability that are commonly used in the United States are the Emergency Severity Index (ESI) and the Canadian Triage and Acuity Scale (CTAS). The ESI assigns patients into five levels, from level 1 (most urgent) to level 5 (least urgent). With the ESI, patients are assigned to triage levels based on both their acuity and their anticipated resource needs (Soontorn, Sitthimongkol, Thosingha, et al., 2018). The CTAS system's five levels include time parameters that guide how frequently patients must be reassessed by either a nurse or provider. Patients assigned to the *resuscitation* category must receive continuous nursing surveillance, those in the *emergent* category must be reassessed at least every 15 minutes, patients in the *urgent* category must be reassessed at least every 30 minutes, patients in the *less urgent* category must be reassessed at least every 60 minutes, and those in the *nonurgent* category must be reassessed at least every 120 minutes. The goal of all triage is rapid assessment and decision making, preferably under 5 minutes (ENA, 2020a).

Although the ESI and the CTAS are valid and reliable triage severity rating systems, many EDs in the United States have high patient volumes and slow flow. Patients arriving at the ED may experience bottlenecks at triage. To further refine the system, triage bypass moves an incoming patient directly to a bed if open beds are available in the ED. This reduces patient waiting time; the receiving nurse performs the initial assessment and vital signs. In team triage (or provider in triage [PIT]), the triage nurse works with the physician or nurse practitioner or physician assistant within the triage area itself. Team triage can move patients to diagnostics and possibly discharge without full admission to the ED. Both of these additional triage concepts decrease wait time for treatment and improve flow in the ED (ENA, 2020a). The flow of patients within the ED needs to be as efficient as possible so that wait times are diminished, and so that flow is conducive for EMS agencies and for true emergencies.

Triage is an advanced skill. Emergency nurses spend many hours learning to classify different illnesses and injuries to ensure that patients most in need of care do not needlessly wait. Protocols may be followed to initiate laboratory or x-ray studies while the patient is in the triage area. Collaborative protocols are developed and used by the triage nurse based on their level of experience (ENA, 2018a). Nurses in the triage area collect additional crucial baseline data: full vital signs including pain assessment, history of the current event and past medical history, neurologic assessment findings, weight, allergies (especially to latex and medications), intimate partner violence screening, and necessary diagnostic data. Asking questions is key to appropriate triage decisions. The following questions reflect the minimum information that should be obtained from the patient or from the person who accompanied the patient to the ED (so long as that person is not suspected of abuse or neglect; see later discussion) and then are documented (ENA, 2020a):

- What were the circumstances, precipitating events, location, and time of the injury or illness?
- When did the symptoms appear?
- Was the patient unconscious after the injury or onset of illness?
- How did the patient get to the ED?
- What was the health status of the patient before the injury or illness?
- Is there a history of medical illness or previous surgeries? A history of admissions to the hospital?
- Is the patient currently taking any medications, especially hormones, insulin, digitalis, or anticoagulants? Is the patient using any complementary or alternative therapies such as herbology, naturopathy, Reiki, massage, or acupuncture?
- Does the patient have any allergies, especially to latex, medications, eggs, or nuts?
- Does the patient use tobacco products or recreational drugs? How frequently? What type? When was the last time they were used?
- Does the patient have any fears? Does the patient feel in danger or in an unsafe situation?
- When was the last meal eaten? (This is important if general anesthesia is to be given or if the patient is unconscious.)
- When was the last menstrual period?
- Is the patient under a provider's care? What is the name and contact information for the provider?
- What was the date of the patient's most recent tetanus immunization?

In addition to the collection of initial vital signs and medical history, triage consists of providing basic first aid, which may include application of ice, bleeding control, and basic wound care, as well as initiating protocol-based prescriptions (e.g., x-rays, administering antipyretic or mild analgesic agents, obtaining an electrocardiogram [ECG] or urinalysis, removing sutures). The triage nurse also is responsible for and monitors the waiting area, maintains a safe environment, reassesses patients who are waiting, and is the initial liaison to the families of patients.

Routine ED triage protocols differ significantly from the triage protocols used in disasters and mass casualty incidents (field triage). Routine triage directs all available resources to the patients who are most critically ill, regardless of potential outcome. In field triage (or hospital triage during a disaster), scarce resources must be used to benefit the most people possible (ENA, 2020a). This distinction affects triage decisions (see Chapter 68).

✱ COVID-19 Considerations

In response to the COVID-19 pandemic, it is important to decrease the spread of infection and properly screen and triage all patients presenting to the ED for infection with or exposure to SARS-CoV-2. All patients should enter the ED with a face covering, which may be cloth, and maintain social distance restrictions away from other patients of 6 feet, if possible. If possible, patients should monitor their own temperature prior to arrival to the ED and notify the ED staff if they

are experiencing any of the signs and symptoms of COVID-19. These include (CDC, 2020c):

- Fever or chills
- Cough
- Shortness of breath or difficulty breathing
- Fatigue
- Muscle or body aches
- Headache
- New loss of taste or smell
- Sore throat
- Congestion or runny nose
- Nausea or vomiting
- Diarrhea

It is also important that all patients who present to the ED are screened to find if they have traveled to areas with a high prevalence of COVID-19, or been exposed to others suspected or known to be infected with SARS-CoV-2 within the last 2 weeks. Patients who are asymptomatic and without any possible exposure within the past 2 weeks should be triaged to a designated area away from those patients who are symptomatic or were likely exposed (CDC, 2020c).

Assess and Intervene

For the patient assigned to an urgent or higher triage category, stabilization, provision of critical treatments, and prompt transfer to the appropriate setting (intensive care unit, operating room, general care unit) are the priorities of emergency care. Although treatment is initiated in the ED, ongoing definitive treatment of the underlying problem is provided in other settings, and the sooner the patient is stabilized and moved to that area, the better the outcome.

A systematic approach to effectively establishing and treating health priorities is the primary survey/secondary survey approach. The **primary survey** focuses on stabilizing life-threatening conditions. The ED staff work collaboratively and follow the ABCDE (Airway, Breathing, Circulation, Disability, Exposure) method:

- Establish a patent airway.
- Provide adequate ventilation, employing resuscitation measures when necessary. Patients who have experienced trauma must have the cervical spine protected and chest injuries assessed first, immediately after the airway is established.
- Evaluate and restore cardiac output by controlling hemorrhage, preventing and treating shock, and maintaining or restoring effective circulation. This includes the prevention and management of hypothermia. In addition, peripheral pulses are examined, and any immediate closed reductions of fractures or dislocations are performed if an extremity is pulseless.
- Determine neurologic disability by assessing neurologic function using the Glasgow Coma Scale (GCS) (see Chapter 63, Chart 63-4) and a motor and sensory evaluation of the spine (see Chapter 60, Fig. 60-9). A quick neurologic assessment may be performed using the AVPU mnemonic:
  - A—alert. Is the patient alert and responsive?
  - V—verbal. Does the patient respond to verbal stimuli?
  - P—pain. Does the patient respond only to painful stimuli?

- *U*—unresponsive. Is the patient unresponsive to all stimuli, including pain?
- Undress the patient quickly but gently so that any wounds or areas of injury are identified; this may entail cutting away articles of clothing (ENA, 2020a).

After these priorities have been addressed, the ED team proceeds with the **secondary survey**. This includes the following:

- Complete health history, including the history of the current event
- Head-to-toe assessment (includes a reassessment of airway and breathing parameters and vital signs)
- Diagnostic and laboratory testing
- Insertion or application of monitoring devices such as ECG electrodes, arterial lines, or urinary catheters
- Splinting of suspected fractures
- Cleansing, closure, and dressing of wounds
- Performance of other necessary interventions based on the patient's condition

Once the patient has been assessed, stabilized, and tested, appropriate medical and nursing diagnoses are formulated, initial important treatment is started, and plans for the proper disposition of the patient are made (ENA, 2020a). Many emergent and urgent conditions and priority emergency interventions are discussed in detail in the remaining sections of this chapter.

In addition to the management of the illness or injury, the ED nurse must also focus on providing comfort and emotional support to the patient and family. Included in this is pain management. Effective pain management must be instituted early and should include rapid-acting agents that result in minimal sedation so that the patient can continue to interact with the staff for ongoing assessment. Moderate sedation can help facilitate short procedures in the ED; the patient will not remember the procedure later. The patient is closely monitored during the procedure and then rapidly awakens when it is complete (see Chapter 15).

It is essential that family crisis intervention services are available for families of patients in the ED. Even if a patient's condition is not emergent, the situation may be perceived as such by the family. Every family needs attention and support. The chaplain and social worker may be available to assist with interventions.

AIRWAY OBSTRUCTION

Acute upper airway obstruction is a life-threatening medical emergency.

Pathophysiology

The airway may be partially or completely occluded. Partial obstruction of the airway can lead to progressive hypoxia, hypercarbia, and respiratory and cardiac arrest. If the airway is completely obstructed, permanent brain injury or death will occur within 3 to 5 minutes secondary to hypoxia. Air movement is absent in the presence of complete airway obstruction. Oxygen saturation of the blood decreases rapidly because obstruction of the airway prevents entry of air into the lungs. Oxygen deficit occurs in the brain, resulting in unconsciousness, with death following rapidly.

Upper airway obstruction has a number of causes, including aspiration of foreign bodies, anaphylaxis, viral or bacterial infection, trauma, and inhalation or chemical burns. For older adult patients, especially those in extended care facilities, sedative and hypnotic medications, diseases affecting motor coordination (e.g., Parkinson's disease), and mental dysfunction (e.g., dementia, intellectual disability) are risk factors for asphyxiation by food. As patients age, atrophy of the posterior pharynx occurs, resulting in aspiration or difficulty swallowing. In adults, aspiration of a bolus of meat is the most common cause of airway obstruction. Peritonsillar abscesses, epiglottitis, and other acute infectious processes of the posterior pharynx can also result in airway obstruction. The most common causes of airway obstruction are from an allergic reaction (i.e., causing laryngospasm), infection, or angioedema (ENA, 2020a).

Clinical Manifestations

Typically, a person with a foreign-body airway obstruction cannot speak, breathe, or cough. The patient may clutch the neck between the thumb and fingers (i.e., universal distress signal). Other common signs and symptoms include choking, apprehensive appearance, refusing to lie flat, inspiratory and expiratory stridor, labored breathing, the use of accessory muscles (suprasternal and intercostal retraction), flaring nostrils, increasing anxiety, restlessness, and confusion. Cyanosis and loss of consciousness, which develop as hypoxia worsens, are late signs. Action must be taken before these manifestations develop, if possible, or immediately if the patient has already exhibited these signs.

Assessment and Diagnostic Findings

Assessment of the patient who has a foreign object occluding the airway may involve simply asking the person whether they are choking and require help. If the person is unconscious, inspection of the oropharynx may reveal the offending object. X-rays, laryngoscopy, or bronchoscopy also may be performed. Oxygen supplementation should be considered immediately.

Management

If the patient can breathe and cough spontaneously, a partial obstruction should be suspected. The patient is encouraged to cough forcefully and to persist with spontaneous coughing and breathing efforts as long as good air exchange exists. There may be some wheezing between coughs. If the patient demonstrates a weak, ineffective cough, high-pitched noise while inhaling, increased respiratory difficulty, or cyanosis, the patient should be managed as if there were complete airway obstruction.

After the obstruction is removed, rescue breathing is initiated. If the patient has no pulse, cardiac compressions are instituted. These measures provide oxygen to the brain, heart, and other vital organs until definitive medical treatment can restore and support normal heart and ventilatory activity (ENA, 2020a). See Chapter 25 for review of current CPR guidelines.

Establishing an Airway

Establishing an airway may be as simple as repositioning the patient's head to prevent the tongue from obstructing the pharynx. Alternatively, other maneuvers, such as the head-tilt/chin-lift maneuver, the jaw-thrust maneuver, or insertion of specialized equipment, may be needed to open the airway, remove a foreign body, or maintain the airway. In all maneuvers, the cervical spine must be protected from injury. After these maneuvers are performed, the patient is assessed for breathing by watching for chest movement and listening and feeling for air movement. In such a case, nursing diagnoses would include impaired airway clearance associated with obstruction of the airway by the tongue, an object, or fluids (blood, saliva) and impaired breathing associated with airway obstruction or injury.

An oropharyngeal airway is a semicircular tube or tube-like plastic device that is inserted over the back of the tongue into the lower posterior pharynx in a patient who is breathing spontaneously but who is unconscious. This type of airway prevents the tongue from falling back against the posterior pharynx and obstructing the airway. It also allows health care providers to suction secretions. The nasopharyngeal airway provides the same airway access but is inserted through the nares. With an airway in place the patient may breathe spontaneously. If breathing is ineffective or absent, bag-valve-mask ventilation is necessary (Atanelov & Rebstock, 2020).

> ### ◣ Quality and Safety Nursing Alert
>
> *In the case of potential facial trauma or basal skull fracture, the nasopharyngeal airway should not be used because it could enter the brain cavity instead of the pharynx.*

Endotracheal Intubation

The purpose of endotracheal intubation is to establish and maintain the airway in patients with respiratory insufficiency or hypoxia. Endotracheal intubation is indicated to establish an airway for a patient who cannot be adequately ventilated with an oropharyngeal or nasopharyngeal airway, bypass an upper airway obstruction, prevent aspiration, permit connection of the patient to a resuscitation bag or mechanical ventilator, or facilitate the removal of tracheobronchial secretions (see Fig. 67-1).

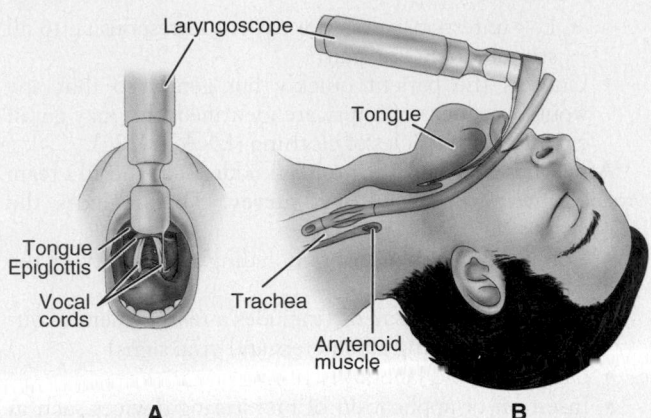

A **B**

Figure 67-1 • Endotracheal intubation in a patient without a cervical spine injury. **A.** The primary glottic landmarks for tracheal intubation as visualized with proper placement of the laryngoscope. **B.** Positioning the endotracheal tube.

Because of the level of skill required, endotracheal intubation is performed only by those who have had extensive training. These may include physicians, nurse anesthetists, respiratory therapists, flight nurses, and nurse practitioners. However, the emergency nurse commonly assists with intubation.

Rapid sequence intubation may be indicated, which provides management of the patient in a situation similar to that in the operating room. Medications used to facilitate rapid sequence intubation include a sedative, an analgesic, and a neuromuscular blockade agent; these are usually given by the provider performing the intubation.

Intubation with a King Tube or Laryngeal Mask Airway

If the patient is not hospitalized and cannot be intubated in the field, emergency medical personnel may insert a King Tube, which rapidly provides pharyngeal ventilation. When the tube is inserted into the trachea, it functions like an endotracheal tube (see Fig. 67-2).

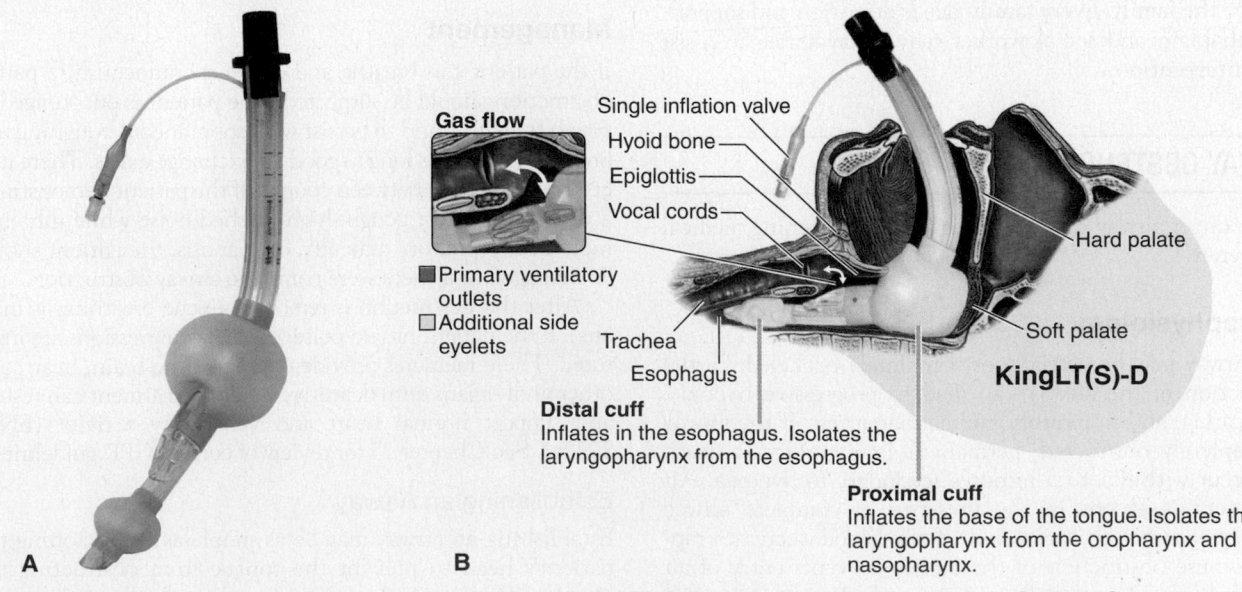

A **B**

Figure 67-2 • King Tube (**A**) correctly placed in esophageal position (**B**). Reprinted with permission from King Systems Corporation, Noblesville, Indiana.

The two balloons that surround the tube are inflated after the tube is inserted. One balloon is large and occludes the oropharynx. This permits ventilation by forcing air through the larynx. The smaller balloon is inflated with air and occludes the esophagus at a site distal to the glottis. Breath sounds are auscultated after balloon inflation to make sure that the oropharyngeal balloon (or cuff) does not obstruct the glottis. One variant type of King Tube is designed so that a gastric tube may also be passed for suction. If it is difficult to establish an airway, a laryngeal mask airway (LMA) may be inserted as an interim airway device. The design of the LMA provides a "mask" in the subglottic airway with a cuff inflated within the esophagus. It allows easy insertion for rapid airway control until a more definitive airway can be placed. Some LMAs also permit removal of secretions from the esophagus (Bosson & Gordon, 2018) (see Chapter 15, Fig. 15-4A).

Cricothyroidotomy

Cricothyroidotomy is the opening of the cricothyroid membrane to establish an airway. This procedure is used in emergency situations in which endotracheal intubation is either not possible or contraindicated, as in airway obstruction from extensive maxillofacial trauma, cervical spine injuries, laryngospasm, laryngeal edema (after an allergic reaction or extubation), hemorrhage into neck tissue, or obstruction of the larynx. A cricothyroidotomy is replaced with a formal tracheostomy when the patient is able to tolerate this procedure.

Maintaining Ventilation

After the airway is determined to be unobstructed, the nurse must ensure that ventilation is adequate by checking for equal bilateral breath sounds. Satisfactory management of ventilations may prevent hypoxia and hypercapnia. The nurse must quickly assess for absent or diminished breath sounds, open chest wounds, and difficulty delivering artificial breaths for the patient. The nurse should monitor pulse oximetry, capnography, and arterial blood gases if the patient requires airway or ventilatory assistance. A tension pneumothorax can mimic hypovolemia, so ventilatory assessment precedes assessment for hemorrhage. A pneumothorax (both simple and tension) or sucking (open) chest wound is managed with a chest tube and occlusion of the sucking wound; immediate relief of increasing positive intrathoracic pressure and maintenance of adequate ventilation should occur (see Chapter 19).

HEMORRHAGE

Stopping bleeding is essential to the care and survival of patients in an emergency or disaster situation. Hemorrhage that results in the reduction of circulating blood volume is a main cause of shock. Minor bleeding, which is usually venous, generally stops spontaneously unless the patient has a bleeding disorder or has been taking anticoagulant agents. Internal hemorrhage can hide in many anatomic spaces and compartments, resulting in shock without external evidence of hemorrhage. The internal spaces and compartments that are capable of housing large amounts of blood include the retroperitoneum, pelvis, chest, and thighs (ENA, 2020a).

The patient is assessed for signs and symptoms of shock: cool, moist skin (resulting from poor peripheral perfusion), decreasing blood pressure, increasing heart rate, delayed capillary refill, and decreasing urine volume (see Chapter 11). The goals of emergency management are to control the bleeding, maintain adequate circulating blood volume for tissue oxygenation, and prevent shock. Patients who hemorrhage are at risk for cardiac arrest caused by hypovolemia with secondary anoxia. Nursing interventions are carried out collaboratively with other members of the emergency health care team (ENA, 2020a).

Management

Fluid Replacement

Whenever a patient is hemorrhaging—whether externally or internally—a loss of circulating blood results in a fluid volume deficit and decreased cardiac output. Therefore, fluid replacement is imperative to maintain circulation. Typically, two large-gauge IV catheters are inserted, preferably in an uninjured extremity, to provide a means for fluid and blood replacement. Blood samples are obtained for analysis, typing, and cross-matching. Replacement fluids are given as prescribed, depending on clinical estimates of the type and volume of fluid lost. Replacement fluids may include isotonic electrolyte solutions (e.g., lactated Ringer's, normal saline), colloids, and blood component therapy.

Packed red blood cells are infused when there is massive blood loss, which may also necessitate transfusion of other blood components, including platelets and clotting factors (ENA, 2020a). See Chapter 28 for full discussion of blood component therapy indications and treatment.

> ◤ **Quality and Safety Nursing Alert**
>
> *The infusion rate is determined by the severity of the blood loss and the clinical evidence of hypovolemia. Blood replacement therapy that involves transfusing several units of blood products should be given via warmer when possible, because administration of large amounts of blood that has been refrigerated has a core cooling effect that may lead to cardiac arrest and coagulopathy.*

Control of External Hemorrhage

If a patient is hemorrhaging externally (e.g., from a wound), a rapid physical assessment is performed as the patient's clothing is cut away in an attempt to identify the area of hemorrhage. Direct, firm pressure is applied over the bleeding area or the involved artery at a site that is proximal to the wound (see Fig. 67-3). Most bleeding can be stopped or at least controlled by application of direct pressure. Otherwise, unchecked arterial bleeding can result in death. A firm pressure dressing is applied, and the injured part is elevated to stop venous and capillary bleeding, if possible. If the injured area is an extremity, the extremity is immobilized to control blood loss.

A tourniquet is applied to an extremity when the external hemorrhage cannot be controlled in any other way and until surgery can be performed. The tourniquet is applied just proximal to the wound and tied tightly enough to

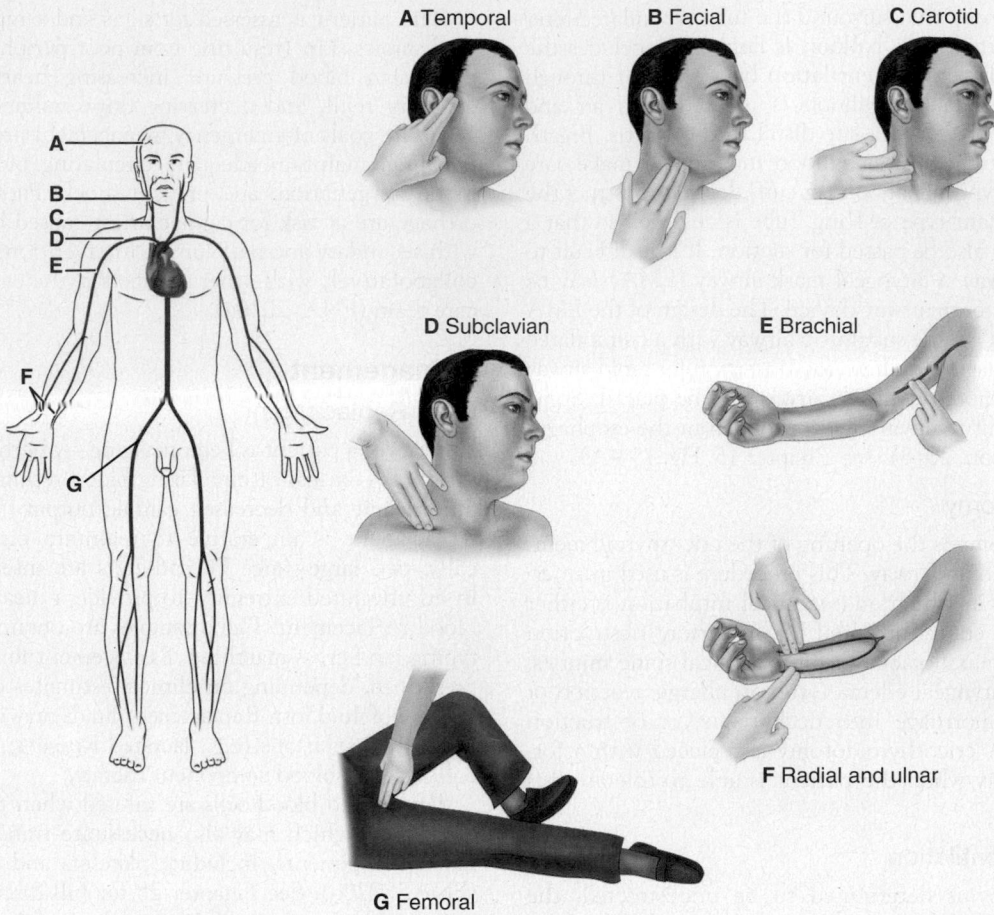

A Temporal **B** Facial **C** Carotid

D Subclavian **E** Brachial

F Radial and ulnar

G Femoral

Figure 67-3 • Pressure points for control of hemorrhage.

control arterial blood flow. The tourniquet is labeled with the date and time it was applied. If the patient has suffered a traumatic amputation with uncontrollable hemorrhage, the tourniquet remains in place until the patient is in the operating room. Time of tourniquet application and removal should be documented. Tourniquet placement among military personnel with battle-associated trauma has demonstrated clear mortality reduction, although it occasionally has led to amputation or fasciotomy (Cornelius, Campbell, & McGauly, 2017).

Control of Internal Hemorrhage

If the patient shows no external signs of bleeding but exhibits tachycardia, falling blood pressure, thirst, apprehension, cool and moist skin, or delayed capillary refill, internal hemorrhage is suspected. Typically, packed red blood cells, plasma, and platelets are given at a rapid rate, and the patient is prepared for more definitive treatment (e.g., surgery, pharmacologic therapy). In addition, arterial blood gas specimens are obtained to evaluate pulmonary function and tissue perfusion and to establish baseline hemodynamic parameters, which are then used as an index for determining the amount of fluid replacement the patient can tolerate and the response to therapy. The patient is maintained in the supine position and monitored closely until hemodynamic or circulatory parameters improve, or until they are transported to the operating room or intensive care unit.

HYPOVOLEMIC SHOCK

Shock is a condition in which there is loss of effective circulating blood volume. Inadequate organ and tissue perfusion follows, ultimately resulting in cellular metabolic derangements. In any emergency situation, the onset of shock should be anticipated by immediately assessing all people who are injured. The underlying cause of shock (hypovolemic, cardiogenic, neurogenic, anaphylactic, or septic) must be determined. Of these, hypovolemia is the most common cause. See Chapter 11 for further discussion of management of hypovolemic shock.

WOUNDS

Wounds involving injury to soft tissues can vary from minor tears to severe crushing injuries. The types of wounds that may occur are defined in Chart 67-3. The main goal of treatment is to restore the physical integrity and function of the injured tissue while minimizing scarring and preventing infection. Proper documentation of the characteristics of the wound, using precise descriptions and correct terminology, is essential. Such information may be needed in the future for forensic evidence. Photographs are helpful because they provide an accurate, visible depiction of the wound. Photographs

Chart 67-3	Definition of Terms: Wounds

Abrasion: denuded skin
Avulsion: tearing away of tissue from supporting structures
Cut: incision of the skin with well-defined edges, usually longer than deep
Ecchymosis/contusion: blood trapped under the surface of the skin
Hematoma: tumorlike mass of blood trapped under the skin
Laceration: skin tear with irregular edges and vein bridging
Patterned: wound representing the outline of the object (e.g., steering wheel) causing the wound
Stab: incision of the skin with well-defined edges, usually caused by a sharp instrument; a stab wound is typically deeper than long

also become important for exigent wounds (i.e., wounds that will eventually heal). Patients experiencing intimate partner violence (IPV) or trauma may need the photographs later to visually describe the extent of injury.

Determining *when* and *how* the wound occurred is important because a treatment delay increases infection risk. Using aseptic technique, the clinician inspects the wound to determine the extent of damage to underlying structures or the presence of a foreign body. Sensory, motor, and vascular function is evaluated for changes that might indicate complications.

Management

Wound Cleansing

Hair around the wound may be clipped (only as directed) if it is anticipated that the hair will interfere with wound closure. Typically, the area around the wound is cleansed with normal saline solution or a polymer agent (e.g., Shur-Clens). The antibacterial agent povidone-iodine should not be allowed to get deep into the wound without thorough rinsing. Povidone-iodine is used only for the initial cleansing because it injures exposed and healthy tissue, resulting in further tissue damage (ENA, 2020a).

If indicated, the area is infiltrated with a local intradermal anesthetic through the wound margins or by regional block. Patients with soft tissue injuries usually have localized pain at the site of injury. The nurse then assists with cleaning and débriding the wound. The wound is irrigated gently and copiously with sterile isotonic saline solution to remove surface dirt. Devitalized tissue and foreign matter are removed because they impede healing and may promote infection. Any small bleeding vessels are clamped, tied, or cauterized. After wound treatment, a nonadherent dressing is applied to protect the wound and to serve as a splint and as a reminder to the patient that the area is injured.

Primary Closure

The decision to suture a wound depends on the nature of the wound, the time since the injury was sustained, the degree of contamination, and the vascularity of tissues. If primary closure is indicated, the wound is sutured or stapled, usually by the emergency provider, with the patient receiving either local anesthesia or moderate sedation (see Chapter 15). Wound closure begins when subcutaneous fat is brought together loosely with a few sutures to close off the dead space. The subcuticular layer is then closed, and finally the epidermis is closed. Sutures are placed near the wound edge, with the skin edges leveled carefully to promote optimal healing. Instead of sutures, sterile strips of reinforced microporous tape or a bonding agent (skin glue) may be used to close clean, superficial wounds (ENA, 2020a).

Delayed Primary Closure

Delayed primary closure may be indicated if tissue has been lost or there is a high potential for infection. A thin layer of gauze (to ensure drainage and prevent pooling of exudate), covered by an occlusive dressing, may be used. The wound is splinted in a functional position to prevent motion and decrease the possibility of contracture.

If there are no signs of suppuration (formation of purulent drainage), the wound may be sutured (with the patient receiving a local anesthetic). The use of antibiotic agents to prevent infection depends on factors such as how the injury occurred, the age of the wound, and the risk of contamination. The site is immobilized and elevated to limit accumulation of fluid in the interstitial spaces of the wound.

Tetanus prophylaxis is given as prescribed, based on the condition of the wound and the patient's immunization status. If the patient's last tetanus booster was given more than 5 years ago, or if the patient's immunization status is unknown, a tetanus booster must be given (ENA, 2020a). The patient is educated about signs and symptoms of infection and is instructed to contact the primary provider or clinic if there is sudden or persistent pain, fever or chills, bleeding, rapid swelling, foul odor, drainage, or redness surrounding the wound.

TRAUMA

Trauma (an unintentional or intentional wound or injury inflicted on the body from a mechanism against which the body cannot protect itself) is the fourth leading cause of death in the United States. Trauma is the leading cause of death in children and in adults younger than 44 years. The incidence is increasing in adults older than 44 years. SUD is often implicated as a factor in both blunt and penetrating trauma (ENA, 2020a).

Collection of Forensic Evidence

In assessing and managing any patient with an emergency condition, but especially the patient experiencing trauma, meticulous documentation is essential. Included in documentation are descriptions of all wounds, mechanism of injury, time of events, and collection of evidence. In trauma care, the nurse must be exceedingly careful with all potential evidence, handling and documenting it properly.

The basics of care management for patients with traumatic injury include an understanding that trauma in any patient (living or dead) has potential legal or forensic science implications if criminal activity is suspected. Hence, proper management from both a medical and forensic evidence perspective is essential.

When clothing is removed from the patient who has experienced trauma, the nurse must be careful not to cut through or disrupt any tears, holes, blood stains, or dirt present on the clothing if criminal activity is suspected. Each piece of clothing should be placed in an individual paper bag. Plastic bags are not used because they retain moisture; moisture may promote mold and mildew formation, which can destroy evidence. If the clothing is wet, it should be hung to dry. Clothing should not be given to families. Valuables should be inventoried and either placed in the hospital safe or clearly documented to which family member they were given. If a police officer is present to collect clothing or any other items from the patient, each item is labeled and the transfer of custody to the officer, the officer's name, the date, and the time are documented. Evidence cannot be left unattended in the room; a formal chain of custody must be maintained for the evidence to be valid and useful for legal purposes (ENA, 2020a).

All deaths of patients who experienced trauma are reported to the medical examiner. If suicide or homicide is suspected in a patient who experienced trauma, the medical examiner examines the body on site or has the body moved to the coroner's office for autopsy. All tubes and lines must remain in place. The patient's hands must be covered with paper bags to protect evidence on the hands or under the fingernails. In the patient who has survived trauma, tissue specimens may be swabbed from the hands and nails as potential evidence. Photographs of wounds or clothing are essential and should include a reference ruler in one photo and another without the ruler.

Documentation should also include any statements made by the patient in the patient's own words and surrounded by quotation marks. A chain of evidence is essential. If the patient's case is reviewed in a court of law in the future, clear documentation assists the judicial process and helps to identify the activities that occurred in the ED.

Injury Prevention

Any discussion of trauma management must address injury prevention. A component of the emergency nurse's daily role is to provide injury prevention information to every patient with whom there is contact, including patients admitted for reasons other than injury (ENA, 2020a). The only way to reduce the incidence of trauma is through prevention.

There are three components of injury prevention. The first is education. Providing information and materials to help prevent violence and to maintain safety at home and in vehicles is important. Involvement in local injury prevention organizations, nursing organizations, and health fairs promotes wellness and safety. In practice, nursing and other health care professionals should avoid using the word *accident,* because trauma events are *preventable* and should be viewed as such rather than as "fate" or "happenstance." Responsibility and accountability must be assigned to traumatic incidents, particularly because of the high rate of trauma recidivism (repeated trauma). People who are at risk for trauma and trauma recidivism should be identified and provided with education and counseling directed toward altering risky behaviors and preventing further trauma (ENA, 2020a).

The second component of injury prevention is legislation. Nurses should be actively involved in safety legislation at the local, state, and federal levels. Such legislation is meant to provide universal safety measures, not to infringe on rights.

The third component is automatic protection. Airbags and automotive design are included in this category. These mechanisms provide for safety without requiring personal intervention.

Emergency nurses may develop injury prevention programs using a focus similar to the ABCDE approach used in the primary survey in trauma care. In this case, however (ENA, 2020a):

- A—describes *assessment* of the community for common injury mechanisms
- B—is used to describe *building* a coalition of key community members
- C—refers to *communicating* awareness of the trauma mechanisms and risks prevalent in the local community
- D—stands for *developing* and implementing interventions, which may be educational or legislative
- E—refers to *evaluating* the injury prevention program soon after it is launched, which may result in either continuation or revision of the program

Multiple Trauma

Multiple trauma is caused by a single catastrophic event that causes life-threatening injuries to at least two distinct organs or organ systems. Mortality in patients with multiple trauma is related to the severity of the injuries, the number of systems and organs involved, and the severity of each injury alone and in combination. Patients with single-system trauma can also have life-threatening or very severe traumatic injuries. Immediately after injury from major trauma, including multiple trauma or severe single-system trauma, the body is hypermetabolic and severely stressed. In addition, major trauma can cause hypothermia, acidosis, and coagulopathy, sometimes called the *triad of death* because each of these factors is associated with increased mortality (Saqe-Rockoff, Schubert, Ciardiello, et al., 2018).

Assessment and Diagnostic Findings

External evidence of trauma may be sparse or absent. Patients with multiple trauma should be assumed to have a spinal cord injury until it is proven otherwise. The injury regarded as the least significant in appearance may be the most lethal. For example, the pelvic fracture not identified until an x-ray is obtained may cause rapid and massive hemorrhage into the pelvic cavity, but an obvious amputation of the arm may have already stopped bleeding from the body's normal response of vasoconstriction.

Management

The goals of treatment are to determine the extent of injuries and to establish priorities of treatment. Any injury interfering with a vital physiologic function (e.g., airway, breathing, circulation) is an immediate threat to life and has the highest priority for immediate treatment. Essential lifesaving procedures are performed simultaneously by the emergency team. As soon as the patient is resuscitated, clothes are removed or cut off and a rapid physical assessment is performed. Transfer from field management to the ED must be orderly and controlled, with attention and silence given to listen to the verbal report from EMS personnel. Treatment in a trauma center

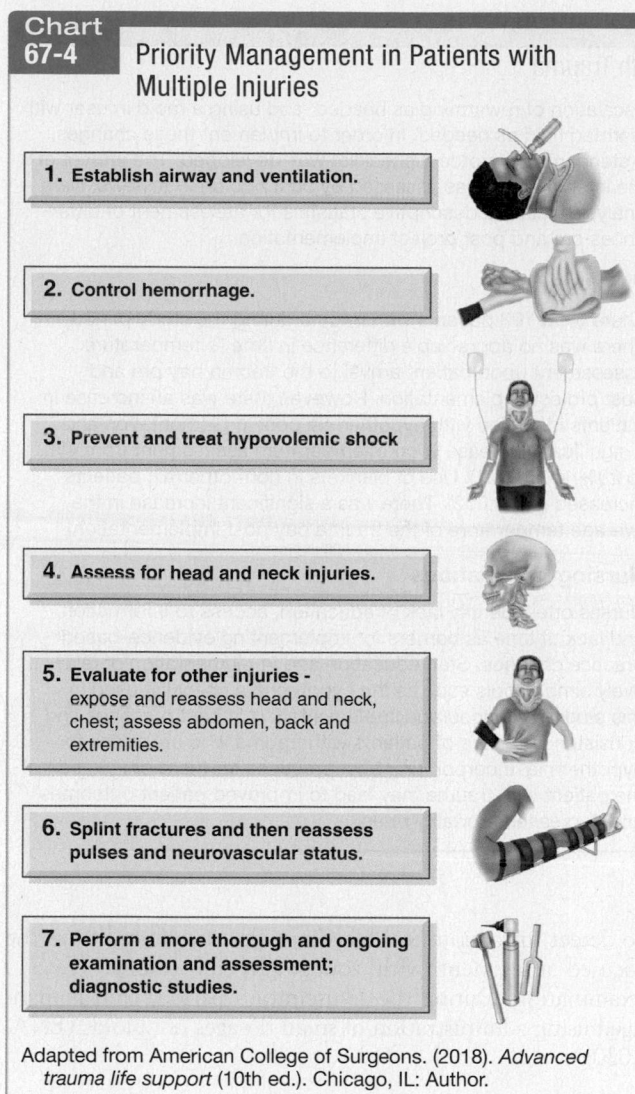

Chart 67-4

Priority Management in Patients with Multiple Injuries

1. **Establish airway and ventilation.**

2. **Control hemorrhage.**

3. **Prevent and treat hypovolemic shock**

4. **Assess for head and neck injuries.**

5. **Evaluate for other injuries -** expose and reassess head and neck, chest; assess abdomen, back and extremities.

6. **Splint fractures and then reassess pulses and neurovascular status.**

7. **Perform a more thorough and ongoing examination and assessment; diagnostic studies.**

Adapted from American College of Surgeons. (2018). *Advanced trauma life support* (10th ed.). Chicago, IL: Author.

is appropriate for patients experiencing major trauma. Treatment priorities are presented in Chart 67-4.

A trauma alert is typically activated for patients with major trauma who present to trauma centers. Trauma alert activations are based upon specific criteria that are established by the individual institution. The trauma alert mobilizes the designated members of the trauma team, whose composition varies depending upon the size of the hospital and availability of its resources and staff (Dehli, Uleberg, & Wisborg, 2018). Common members of the trauma team include a trauma surgeon, trauma emergency nurse, x-ray technician, and nursing assistant. An advanced practice nurse and a chaplain may also be included as members of the trauma team (Crawford, 2019). The trauma emergency nurse typically is responsible for assessing and monitoring the patient, ensuring/maintaining airway and IV access, administering prescribed medications, collecting laboratory specimens, and documenting activities and the patient's subsequent responses.

In addition to managing the treatment priorities described in Chart 67-4, the trauma emergency nurse must implement interventions that can mitigate the effects of hypothermia. In some trauma centers, the ambient temperature in the trauma

bay where the patient with major trauma is treated is kept higher than normal (e.g., 26°C [78.8°F]). Any wet clothing is removed and warm blankets may be applied. IV fluids may be warmed while they are infusing. See the Nursing Research Profile in Chart 67-5.

Large volumes of IV crystalloids might need to be infused to manage the effects of hypovolemia (see Chapter 11); however, normal saline can exacerbate the metabolic acidosis that ensues. Therefore, the preferred IV crystalloid solution is typically lactated Ringer's. However, large volumes of any crystalloid solution may also dilute the presence of clotting factors, causing coagulopathy. Therefore, the patient with major trauma is judiciously managed with crystalloid IV fluids as needed. Blood component therapy may be required (see Chapter 28). The trauma team is responsible for continuously monitoring the patient's hemodynamic status as well as the temperature of the patient and the ambient environment in order to reduce the risks of the deadly trio of hypothermia, acidosis, and coagulopathy (Saqe-Rockoff et al., 2018).

Intra-Abdominal Injuries

Intra-abdominal injuries are categorized as penetrating or blunt trauma. *Penetrating* abdominal injuries (i.e., gunshot wounds, stab wounds) are serious and usually require surgery. Penetrating abdominal trauma results in a high incidence of injury to hollow organs, particularly the small bowel. The liver is the most frequently injured solid organ due to its size and anterior placement in the right upper quadrant of the abdomen. In gunshot wounds, the most important prognostic factor is the velocity at which the missile enters the body. High-velocity missiles (bullets) produce extensive tissue damage. All abdominal gunshot wounds that cross the peritoneum require surgical exploration. On the other hand, some stab wounds may be managed nonoperatively due to low velocity and less penetration of the implement (i.e., weapon) (ENA, 2020a).

Blunt trauma to the abdomen may result from motor vehicle crashes, falls, blows, or explosions. Blunt trauma is commonly associated with extra-abdominal injuries to the chest, head, or extremities. Patients with blunt trauma pose a challenge because injuries may be difficult to detect. The incidence of delayed and trauma-related complications is greater than for penetrating injuries. This is especially true of blunt injuries involving the liver, kidneys, spleen, or blood vessels, which can lead to massive blood loss into the peritoneal cavity (ENA, 2020a).

Assessment and Diagnostic Findings

As the history of the traumatic event is obtained, the abdomen is inspected as a part of the secondary survey for obvious signs of injury, including penetrating injuries, bruises, and abrasions. Abdominal assessment continues with auscultation of bowel sounds to provide baseline data from which changes can be noted. Absence of bowel sounds may be an early sign of intraperitoneal involvement, although stress can also decrease or halt peristalsis and thus bowel sounds. Further abdominal assessment may reveal progressive abdominal distention, involuntary guarding, tenderness, pain, muscular rigidity, or rebound tenderness along with changes in bowel

NURSING RESEARCH PROFILE

Chart 67-5

Improving Thermoregulation for Patients with Trauma

Saqe-Rockoff, A., Schubert, F. D., Ciardiello, A., et al. (2018). Improving thermoregulation for trauma patients in the emergency department: An evidence-based practice project. *Journal of Trauma Nursing*, 25(1), 14–20.

Purpose

Research indicates there is a strong association between increased mortality in patients with trauma and hypothermia. Therefore, hypothermia is an important modifiable risk factor for patients with trauma. A variety of rewarming methods currently exist and are utilized with varying degrees of success. Gaps in emergency nursing practice include the assessment of temperature as well as limited personnel knowledge regarding the management of patients with hypothermia and the utilization of rewarming techniques.

Design

The setting was a 450 bed Level I trauma center with more than 75,000 annual ED visits. The project goals were to decrease time to temperature assessment upon patient arrival to the trauma bay and to improve use of best practice rewarming methods among patients with trauma. The research team utilized the Iowa Model of Evidence-Based Practice to provide a framework for the evaluation of current practice and implementation of best practices. Practice changes that were instituted on patients with trauma during the study period included providing warmed blankets, ensuring regulated standardized trauma bay temperature, assessing patient temperature on arrival with appropriate

escalation of rewarming as needed, and using a rapid infuser with warmed fluid as needed. In order to implement these changes, a standardized protocol checklist was developed. The impact of the interventions was assessed by *post hoc* chart reviews. Data analysis included descriptive statistics for assessment of differences pre and post project implementation.

Findings

There were 193 patients with trauma during the study period. There was no appreciable difference in time to temperature assessment upon patient arrival to the trauma bay pre and post project implementation. However, there was an increase in patients identified with hypothermia post implementation and a significant increase in core temperature assessment from 4% to 23% ($p < 0.001$). Use of blankets in normothermic patients increased ($p = 0.002$). There was a significant increase in the average temperature of the trauma bay post implementation.

Nursing Implications

Nurses often identify lack of education, access to information, and lack of time as barriers for implementing evidence-based practice changes. Staff education and implementation of relatively simple tools such as the hypothermia checklist used in this study can encourage implementation of best practices and consistency of care of patients with trauma who are at risk for hypothermia. Incorporating best practices for thermoregulation of the patient with trauma may lead to improved patient outcomes and decreased mortality rates.

---

sounds, all of which are signs of peritoneal irritation. Hypotension and signs and symptoms of shock may also be noted. In addition, the chest and other body systems are assessed for injuries that frequently accompany intra-abdominal injuries (ENA, 2020a).

Laboratory studies that aid in assessment include the following:

- Serial hemoglobin and hematocrit levels to evaluate trends reflecting the presence or absence of bleeding
- Lactate to determine acidosis and need for continued resuscitation
- Arterial blood gas (ABG) for pH (acidosis), base deficit for resuscitation evaluation, and ventilation parameters ($PaCO_2$, PaO_2)
- International normalized ratio (INR) to identify coagulopathy or presence of pharmacologically induced anticoagulation
- White blood cell (WBC) count to detect elevation (generally associated with trauma)

Internal Hemorrhage

Hemorrhage frequently accompanies abdominal injury, especially if the liver or spleen has been traumatized. Therefore, the patient is assessed continuously for signs and symptoms of external and internal bleeding. The front of the body, flanks, and back are inspected for bluish discoloration, asymmetry, abrasion, and contusion. Abdominal CT scans permit detailed evaluation of abdominal contents and retroperitoneal examination. Abdominal ultrasounds can be used to rapidly assess patients who are hemodynamically unstable

to detect intraperitoneal bleeding. This is referred to as the focused assessment with sonography for trauma (FAST) examination. During the resuscitation period, pain is managed using administration of small dosages of opioids (ENA, 2020a).

> **Quality and Safety Nursing Alert**
>
> *The location of pain can indicate certain types of intra-abdominal injuries. Pain in the left shoulder is common in a patient with bleeding from a ruptured spleen, whereas pain in the right shoulder can result from laceration of the liver.*

Intraperitoneal Injury

The abdomen is assessed for tenderness, rebound tenderness, guarding, rigidity, spasm, increasing distention, and pain. Referred pain is a significant finding because it suggests intraperitoneal injury. To determine if there is intraperitoneal injury and bleeding, the patient is usually prepared for diagnostic procedures, such as diagnostic peritoneal lavage (DPL), abdominal ultrasonography, or abdominal CT scanning. DPL, although no longer the standard diagnostic study used to evaluate a traumatized abdomen, remains a viable backup procedure that is easily performed and is very useful during mass casualty incidents when CT scanners may not be readily available. DPL involves the instillation of 1 L of warmed lactated Ringer's or normal saline solution into the abdominal cavity. After a minimum of 400 mL has been returned, a fluid specimen is sent to the laboratory for analysis. Positive laboratory findings include a red blood cell count greater than 100,000/mm^3; a WBC count greater than 500/mm^3; or the presence of bile, feces, or food (ENA, 2020a).

Genitourinary Injury

A focused genitourinary examination, which typically includes a rectal and vaginal examination, is performed to determine any injury to the pelvis, bladder, urethra, vagina, or intestinal wall. In the male patient, a high-riding prostate gland (abnormal position) discovered during a rectal examination indicates a potential urethral injury. A digital vaginal examination is performed on female patients to determine if there is an open pelvic fracture that has torn the vagina (ENA, 2020a).

> ◣ *Quality and Safety Nursing Alert*
>
> *To decompress the bladder and monitor urine output in a patient with a genitourinary injury, an indwelling catheter is inserted after a rectal examination has been completed, not before the examination. In addition, urethral catheter insertion when a possible urethral injury is present is contraindicated; a urology consultation and further evaluation of the urethra are required.*

Management

As indicated by the patient's condition, resuscitation procedures (restoration of airway, breathing, and circulation) are initiated as described previously.

With blunt trauma, the patient is kept on a stretcher to immobilize the spine. If the patient has been placed on a backboard, it should be removed as early as possible to prevent skin breakdown. Cervical spine immobilization is maintained until cervical x-rays have been obtained and cervical spine injury has been ruled out. Likewise, once the backboard is removed, logrolling can be used to protect the spine until x-rays are obtained and confirm that there is no evidence of injuries.

Knowing the mechanism of injury (e.g., penetrating force from a gunshot or knife, blunt force from a blow) is essential to determining the type of management needed. All wounds are located, counted, and documented. If abdominal viscera protrude, the area is covered with sterile, moist saline dressings to keep the viscera from drying.

Typically, oral fluids are withheld in anticipation of surgery, and the stomach contents are aspirated with an orogastric tube to reduce the risk of aspiration and to decompress the stomach in preparation for diagnostic procedures.

Trauma predisposes the patient to infection by disruption of mechanical barriers, exposure to exogenous bacteria from the environment at the time of injury, aspiration of vomitus, and diagnostic and therapeutic procedures (hospital-acquired infection). Tetanus prophylaxis and broad-spectrum antibiotics are given as prescribed.

Throughout the stay in the ED, the patient's condition is continuously monitored for changes. If there is continuing evidence of shock, blood loss, free air under the diaphragm, evisceration, hematuria, severe head injury, musculoskeletal injury, or suspected or known abdominal injury, the patient is rapidly transported to surgery. In most cases, blunt liver and spleen injuries are managed nonsurgically. The goal for the management of all patients who have experienced trauma is to minimize the length of stay in the ED. The patient should be moved to the definitive destination quickly so that care and rehabilitation can continue (ENA, 2020a).

Crush Injuries

Crush injuries occur when a person is caught between opposing forces (e.g., run over by a moving vehicle, crushed between two cars, crushed under a collapsed building).

Assessment and Diagnostic Findings

The patient is observed for the following:

- Hypovolemic shock resulting from extravasation of blood and plasma into injured tissues after compression has been released (see Chapter 11)
- Spinal cord injury (see Chapter 63)
- Erythema and blistering of skin (see Chapter 56)
- Fractures (usually an extremity) (see Chapter 37)
- AKI (e.g., acute tubular necrosis [ATN]) (see Chapter 48)

Management

In conjunction with maintaining the airway, breathing, and circulation, the patient is observed for AKI. Injury to the back can cause renal trauma. Severe muscular damage may cause **rhabdomyolysis**, a toxic syndrome caused by a release of myoglobin from ischemic skeletal muscle, resulting in ATN. See Chapter 48 for the treatment of AKI, renal trauma, and ATN. Rhabdomyolysis may also result from major burns (see Chapter 57), heat stroke, and abuse of illicit drugs, in addition to crush injuries (see later discussions). The classic triad of clinical manifestations suggestive of rhabdomyolysis includes myalgias (muscle cramps), generalized muscle weakness, and darkened urine. The serum creatine kinase (CK) is monitored as the most sensitive indicator of rhabdomyolysis; levels in excess of 6000 IU/L are considered diagnostic (Atias-Varon, Sherman, Yanovich, et al., 2017). In addition to treatment aimed at preventing or treating ATN, major soft tissue injuries are splinted promptly to control bleeding and pain. The serum lactic acid level is monitored; a decrease to less than 2.0 mmol/L is an indication of successful resuscitation (Nicks, McGinnism, Borron, et al., 2018).

If an extremity is injured, it is elevated to relieve swelling and pressure. If compartment syndrome develops, the physician may perform a **fasciotomy** (i.e., surgical incision to the level of the fascia) to restore neurovascular function (see Chapter 37). Medications for pain and anxiety are then given as prescribed, and the patient is quickly transported to the operating suite for wound débridement and fracture repair. A hyperbaric oxygen chamber (if available) may be used to hyperoxygenate crushed tissue, if indicated.

Fractures

Immediate appropriate management of a fracture may determine the patient's eventual outcome and may mean the difference between recovery and disability. When the patient is being examined for fracture, the body part is handled gently and as little as possible. Clothing is cut off to visualize the affected body part. Assessment is conducted for pain over or near a bone, swelling (from blood, lymph, and exudate infiltrating the tissue), and circulatory disturbance. The patient is assessed for ecchymosis, tenderness, and crepitation (see Chapter 37). The nurse must remember that the patient may have multiple fractures accompanied by head, chest, spine, or abdominal injuries.

Management

Immediate attention is given to the patient's general condition. Assessment of airway, breathing, and circulation (which includes pulses in the extremities) is conducted. The patient is also evaluated for neurologic or abdominal injuries before the extremity is treated, unless a pulseless extremity is detected.

If a pulseless extremity is identified, repositioning of the extremity to proper alignment is required. If the pulseless extremity involves a fractured femur, Hare traction (a portable in-line traction device) may be applied to assist with alignment. If repositioning is ineffective in restoring the pulse, a rapid total-body assessment must be completed, followed by transfer of the patient to the operating room for arteriography and possible arterial repair versus amputation.

After the initial evaluation has been completed, all injuries identified are evaluated and treated. The fractured body part is inspected. Using a systematic head-to-toe approach, the nurse inspects the entire body, observing for lacerations, swelling, and deformities, including angulation (bending), shortening, rotation, and asymmetry. All peripheral pulses, especially those distal to the fractured extremity, are palpated. The extremity is also assessed for coolness, blanching, and decreased sensation and motor function, which are indicative of injury to the extremity's neurovascular supply.

A splint is applied before the patient is moved. Splinting immobilizes the joint at a site distal and proximal to the fracture, relieves pain, restores or improves circulation, prevents further tissue injury, and prevents a closed fracture from becoming an open one. To splint an extremity, one hand is placed distal to the fracture and some traction is applied while the other hand is placed beneath the fracture for support. The splints should extend beyond the joints adjacent to the fracture. Upper extremities must be splinted in a functional position. If the fracture is open, a moist, sterile dressing is applied.

After splinting, the vascular status of the extremity is checked by assessing color, temperature, pulse, and blanching of the nail bed. In addition, the patient is assessed for neurovascular compromise if pain or pressure is reported. See Chapter 37 for a complete description of fracture management (ENA, 2020a).

ENVIRONMENTAL EMERGENCIES

Emergencies that can occur due to environmental factors include heat related illnesses, including the extremes of heat stroke, frostbite, and hypothermia; nonfatal drowning; decompression sickness; animal, human, and insect bites.

Heat-Induced Illnesses

Heat-induced illnesses may range in severity from mild and self-limiting to life-threatening emergencies. The most

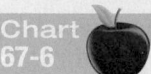

Chart 67-6 HEALTH PROMOTION

Preventing Heat-Induced Illnesses

The nurse provides the following advice for the patient treated for heat-induced illness:

- Avoid immediate re-exposure to high temperatures; hypersensitivity to high temperatures may remain for a considerable time.
- Maintain adequate fluid intake, wear loose clothing, and reduce activity in hot weather.
- Monitor fluid losses and weight loss during workout activities or exercise and replace fluids and electrolytes.
- Use a gradual approach to physical conditioning, allowing sufficient time for return to baseline temperature.
- Plan outdoor activities to avoid the hottest part of the day (between 10 AM and 2 PM).

For older patients living in urban settings with high environmental temperatures:

- The nurse directs these patients to places where air conditioning is available (e.g., shopping mall, library, church) and advises them that fans alone are not adequate to prevent heat-induced illness.

serious of these—heat stroke—is an acute medical emergency caused by failure of the heat-regulating mechanisms of the body. It is the inability to maintain cardiac output in the face of moderately high body temperatures and is associated with dehydration. The most common cause of heat stroke is nonexertional, prolonged exposure to an environmental temperature of greater than 39.2°C (102.5°F), although a heat index of greater than 35°C (95°F) is associated with increased mortality (ENA, 2020a). It usually occurs during extended heat waves, especially when they are accompanied by high humidity. Exertional heat stroke is caused by strenuous physical activity that occurs in a hot environment (ENA, 2020a).

People at risk for nonexertional heat stroke are those not acclimatized to heat, those who are older or very young, those unable to care for themselves, those with chronic and debilitating diseases, and those taking certain medications (e.g., major tranquilizers, anticholinergics, diuretics, beta-blockers) (ENA, 2020a; Tintinalli, Stapczyski, Ma, et al., 2020). Older adults, the very young, people with mental illness, and people with chronic diseases have the highest rates of mortality (CDC, 2017a). Exertional heat stroke occurs in healthy individuals during sports or work activities (e.g., exercising in extreme heat and humidity). Hyperthermia results because of inadequate heat loss. Strategies used to prevent heat-induced illnesses are reviewed in Chart 67-6.

Less severe forms of heat-induced illnesses include heat exhaustion and heat illness or heat cramps. The causes of heat exhaustion are the same as for heat stroke. Heat illness is caused by a loss of electrolytes, typically during strenuous physical activity in a hot environment (ENA, 2020a).

 ### Gerontologic Considerations

Most heat-related deaths occur in older adults because their circulatory systems are unable to compensate for stress imposed by heat. Older adults have a decreased ability to perspire as well as a decreased ability to vasodilate and vasoconstrict. They have less subcutaneous tissue, a decreased thirst mechanism, and a diminished ability to concentrate urine to compensate for heat. Many older adults do not drink adequate amounts of fluid, partly because of fear of incontinence, and thus have a greater risk of heat stroke. In addition, many older adults fear being victims of crime, so even if their residence lacks air conditioning, they tend to keep windows closed despite high temperatures and humidity levels (ENA, 2020a).

Assessment and Diagnostic Findings

Heat stroke, whether the cause is exertional or nonexertional, causes thermal injury at the cellular level, resulting in coagulopathies and widespread damage to the heart, liver, and kidneys. Recent patient history reveals exposure to elevated ambient temperature or excessive exercise during extreme heat. When assessing the patient, the nurse notes the following symptoms: profound central nervous system (CNS) dysfunction (manifested by confusion, delirium, bizarre behavior, coma, seizures); elevated body temperature (40.6°C [105°F] or higher); hot, dry skin; and usually anhidrosis (absence of sweating), tachypnea, hypotension, and tachycardia. The patient with heat exhaustion, on the other hand, may exhibit similarly high body temperatures accompanied by headaches, anxiety, syncope, profuse diaphoresis, gooseflesh, and orthostasis. The cardinal manifestations of heat illness include muscle cramps, particularly in the shoulders, abdomen, and lower extremities; profound diaphoresis; and profound thirst (ENA, 2020a).

Management

The main goal is to reduce the high body temperature as quickly as possible, because mortality in heat stroke or morbid progression to heat stroke with less serious forms of heat-induced illnesses is directly related to the duration of hyperthermia. For the patient with heat stroke, simultaneous treatment focuses on stabilizing oxygenation using the CABs (Circulation, Airway, and Breathing) of basic life support. This includes establishing IV access for fluid administration.

After the patient's clothing is removed, the core (internal) temperature is reduced to 39°C (102°F) as rapidly as possible, preferably within 1 hour. One or more of the following methods may be used as prescribed (ENA, 2020a):

- Cool sheets and towels or continuous sponging with cool water
- Ice applied to the neck, groin, chest, and axillae while spraying with tepid water
- Cooling blankets
- Immersion of the patient in a cold water bath is the optimal method for cooling (if available)

During cooling procedures, an electric fan is positioned so that it blows on the patient to augment heat dissipation by convection and evaporation. The patient's temperature is constantly monitored with a thermistor placed in the rectum, bladder, or esophagus to evaluate core temperature. Caution is used to avoid hypothermia and to prevent hyperthermia, which may recur spontaneously within 3 to 4 hours. The cooling process should stop at 38°C (100.4°F) in order to avoid iatrogenic hypothermia (ENA, 2020a).

Throughout treatment, the patient's status is monitored carefully, including vital signs, ECG findings (for possible myocardial ischemia, myocardial infarction, and arrhythmias), central venous pressure (CVP), and level of responsiveness, all of which may change with rapid alterations in body temperature. A seizure may be followed by recurrence of hyperthermia. To meet tissue needs exaggerated by the hypermetabolic condition, 100% oxygen is given. Endotracheal intubation and mechanical ventilation to support failing cardiopulmonary systems may be required.

IV infusion therapy of normal saline or lactated Ringer's solution is initiated as directed to replace fluid losses and maintain adequate circulation. Fluids are given carefully because of the dangers of myocardial injury from high body temperature and poor kidney function. Cooling redistributes fluid volume from the periphery to the core.

Urine output is also measured frequently, because ATN may occur as a complication of heat stroke from rhabdomyolysis (see previous discussion). Blood specimens are obtained for serial testing to detect bleeding disorders, such as disseminated intravascular coagulation (DIC), and for serial enzyme studies to estimate thermal hypoxic injury to the liver, heart, and muscle tissue. Permanent liver, cardiac, and CNS damage may occur.

Additional supportive care may include dialysis for AKI, anticonvulsant medications to control seizures, potassium for hypokalemia, and sodium bicarbonate to correct metabolic acidosis. Benzodiazepines such as diazepam may be prescribed to suppress seizure activity, while a phenothiazine such as chlorpromazine may be prescribed to suppress shivering (Tintinalli et al., 2020).

Patients with heat exhaustion or heat illness may be managed less aggressively. These patients should lie supine in a cool environment. Patients with heat exhaustion may require IV fluids but may also take oral fluids, if they are tolerated. Patients with heat illness are given oral sodium supplements and oral electrolyte solutions (ENA, 2020a). Patients who have experienced a heat-induced illness should receive education to prevent another heat-related illness (see Chart 67-6).

Frostbite

Frostbite is trauma from exposure to freezing temperatures and freezing of the intracellular fluid and fluids in the intercellular spaces. It results in cellular and vascular damage. Frostbite can result in venous stasis and thrombosis. Body parts most frequently affected by frostbite include the feet, hands, nose, and ears. Frostbite ranges from first degree (redness and erythema) to fourth degree (full-depth tissue destruction) (ENA, 2020a).

Assessment and Diagnostic Findings

A frozen extremity may be hard, cold, and insensitive to touch and may appear white or mottled blue-white. The extent of injury from exposure to cold is not always initially known. The patient history should include environmental temperature, duration of exposure, clothing worn, humidity, and the presence of wet conditions (ENA, 2020a).

Management

The goal of management is to restore normal body temperature. Constrictive clothing and jewelry that could impair circulation are removed. Wet clothing is removed as rapidly as possible. If the lower extremities are involved, the patient should not be allowed to ambulate as this may exacerbate tissue damage (CDC, 2019b).

Controlled yet rapid rewarming is instituted. Frozen extremities are usually placed in a 37°C to 40°C (98.6°F to 104°F) circulating bath for 30- to 40-minute spans. This treatment is repeated until circulation is effectively restored. Early rewarming appears to decrease the amount of ultimate tissue loss. During rewarming, an analgesic for pain is given as prescribed, because the rewarming process may be very painful. To avoid further mechanical injury, the body part is not handled. Massage is contraindicated.

Once rewarmed, the part is protected from further injury and is elevated to help control swelling. Sterile gauze or cotton is placed between affected fingers or toes to prevent maceration, and a bulky dressing is placed on the extremity. A foot cradle may be used to prevent contact with bedclothes if the feet are involved. Hemorrhagic blebs, which may develop 1 hour to a few days after rewarming, are left intact and not ruptured. Nonhemorrhagic blisters are débrided to decrease the inflammatory mediators found in the blister fluid.

A physical assessment is conducted with rewarming to observe for concomitant injury, such as soft tissue injury, dehydration, alcohol intoxication, or fat embolism. Problems such as hyperkalemia (e.g., from release of potassium in the damaged cells) and hypovolemia, which occur frequently in people with frostbite, are corrected. Risk of infection is also great; therefore, aseptic technique is used during dressing changes, and tetanus prophylaxis is given as indicated. Nonsteroidal anti-inflammatory drugs (NSAIDs) are prescribed for their anti-inflammatory effects and to control pain (ENA, 2020a).

Additional measures that may be carried out when appropriate after emergency stabilization measures have been instituted include the following:

- Whirlpool bath for the affected body parts to aid circulation and débridement of necrotic tissue to help prevent infection
- Escharotomy (incision through the eschar) to prevent further tissue damage, to allow for normal circulation, and to permit joint motion
- Fasciotomy to treat compartment syndrome

After rewarming, hourly active motion of any affected digits is encouraged to promote maximal restoration of function and to prevent contractures (Mayo Clinic, 2019). Discharge instructions also include encouraging the patient to avoid tobacco, alcohol, and caffeine because of their vasoconstrictive effects, which further reduce the already deficient blood supply to injured tissues.

Hypothermia

Hypothermia is a condition in which the core (internal) temperature is 35°C (95°F) or less as a result of exposure to cold or an inability to maintain body temperature in the absence of low ambient temperatures. Urban hypothermia (extreme exposure to cold in an urban setting) is associated with a high mortality rate; older adults, infants, people with concurrent illnesses, and those who are homeless are particularly susceptible. Alcohol ingestion increases susceptibility because it causes systemic vasodilation. Some medications (e.g., phenothiazines) or medical conditions (e.g., hypothyroidism,

spinal cord injury) decrease the ability to shiver, hampering the body's innate ability to generate body heat. Fatigue and sleep deprivation are also associated with the development of hypothermia. Heat loss of 2% is normal but increases with exposure. Wet clothing accelerates heat loss, and immersion in cold water increases heat loss by 25% (ENA, 2020a). Victims of trauma are also at risk for hypothermia resulting from treatment with cold fluids, unwarmed oxygen, and exposure during examination. The patient may also have frostbite, but hypothermia takes precedence in treatment.

Assessment and Diagnostic Findings

Hypothermia leads to physiologic changes in all organ systems. There is progressive deterioration, with apathy, poor judgment, ataxia, dysarthria, drowsiness, pulmonary edema, acid–base abnormalities, coagulopathy, and eventual coma. Shivering may be suppressed at a temperature of less than 32.2°C (90°F), because the body's self-warming mechanisms become ineffective. Cardiac output and blood pressure may be so weak that peripheral pulses become undetectable. Cardiac arrhythmias may also occur. Other physiologic abnormalities include hypoxemia and acidosis (ENA, 2020a).

Management

Management consists of removal of wet clothing, continuous monitoring, rewarming, and supportive care.

Monitoring

The CABs of basic life support are a priority. The patient's vital signs, CVP, urine output, arterial blood gas levels, blood chemistry determinations (blood urea nitrogen [BUN], creatinine, glucose, electrolytes), and chest x-rays are evaluated frequently. Core body temperature is monitored with an esophageal, bladder, or rectal thermistor. Continuous ECG monitoring is performed, because cold-induced myocardial irritability leads to conduction disturbances, especially ventricular fibrillation. An arterial line is inserted and maintained to record blood pressure and to facilitate blood sampling.

Rewarming

Rewarming methods include active internal (core) rewarming and passive (spontaneous) or active external rewarming (Higginson, 2018).

Active internal rewarming methods are used for moderate to severe hypothermia (less than 28°C to 32.2°C [82.5°F to 90°F]) and include cardiopulmonary bypass, warm fluid administration, warmed humidified oxygen by ventilator, and warmed peritoneal lavage. Monitoring for ventricular fibrillation as the patient's temperature increases from 31°C to 32°C (88°F to 90°F) is essential.

Passive or active external rewarming is used for mild hypothermia (32.2°C to 35°C [90°F to 95°F]). Passive external rewarming uses over-the-bed heaters to the extremities and increases blood flow to the acidotic, anaerobic extremities. The cold blood from peripheral tissues has high lactic acid levels. As this blood returns to the core, it causes a significant drop in the core temperature (i.e., core temperature afterdrop) and can potentially cause cardiac arrhythmias and electrolyte disturbances. Active external rewarming uses forced-air warming blankets. Care must be taken to prevent extremity burn from these devices, because the patient may not have effective sensation to feel the burn.

Supportive Care

Supportive care during rewarming includes the following as directed (ENA, 2020a):

- External cardiac compression (typically performed only as directed in patients with temperatures higher than 31°C [88°F])
- Defibrillation of ventricular fibrillation. A patient whose temperature is less than 32°C (90°F) experiences spontaneous ventricular fibrillation if moved or touched. Defibrillation is ineffective in patients with temperatures lower than 31°C (88°F); therefore, the patient must be rewarmed first.
- Mechanical ventilation with positive end-expiratory pressure (PEEP) and heated humidified oxygen to maintain tissue oxygenation
- Administration of warmed IV fluids to correct hypotension and to maintain urine output and core rewarming, as described previously
- Administration of sodium bicarbonate to correct metabolic acidosis if necessary
- Administration of antiarrhythmic medications
- Insertion of an indwelling urinary catheter to monitor urinary output and kidney function

Nonfatal Drowning

Nonfatal drowning is defined as survival for at least 24 hours after submersion that caused a respiratory arrest. The most common consequence is hypoxemia. Children under 5 years of age and those over the age of 85 have the highest risk of drowning. An estimated 320,000 drownings occur throughout the world annually, accounting for 7% of global mortality from unintentional injury (World Health Organization [WHO], 2020). Drowning and nonfatal drowning can be prevented by avoiding rip currents offshore; approximately 85% of shore drownings involve a rip current. Pool drownings can be prevented by surrounding the pool with fencing, a self-latching/closing gate, and providing swimming lessons. Supervision near water is still the best prevention measure. When boating, a personal flotation device (PFD), even for swimmers, prevents drowning events. Approximately 50% of nonfatal drownings require hospital admission for management (WHO, 2020).

Factors associated with drowning and nonfatal drowning include alcohol ingestion, inability to swim, diving injuries, hypothermia, and exhaustion. The majority of drowning events occur in pools, lakes, and bathtubs. Suicide by drowning rarely occurs in pools and rarely involves alcohol (WHO, 2020).

Efforts to save the patient should not be abandoned prematurely. Successful resuscitation with full neurologic recovery has occurred in patients who have experienced nonfatal drowning after prolonged submersion in cold water (Parenteau, Stockinger, Hughes, et al., 2018). This is possible because of a decrease in metabolic demands and the diving reflex. The nonfatal drowning process involves the onset of hypoxia, hypercapnia, bradycardia, and arrhythmias. If there is a violent struggle associated with the nonfatal drowning

episode, exercise-induced acidosis and tachypnea can result in aspiration. Hypoxia and acidosis cause eventual apnea and loss of consciousness. When the victim loses consciousness and makes a final effort to breathe, the terminal gasp occurs. Water then moves passively into the airways prior to death.

After resuscitation, hypoxia and acidosis are the major complications experienced by a person who has experienced nonfatal drowning; immediate intervention in the ED is essential. Resultant pathophysiologic changes and pulmonary injury depend on the type of fluid (fresh or salt water) and the volume aspirated. Freshwater aspiration results in a loss of surfactant and, therefore, an inability to expand the lungs. Saltwater aspiration leads to pulmonary edema from the osmotic effects of the salt within the lungs. If a person survives submersion, ARDS, resulting in hypoxia, hypercarbia, and respiratory or metabolic acidosis, can occur (ENA, 2020a).

Management

Therapeutic goals include maintaining cerebral perfusion and adequate oxygenation to prevent further damage to vital organs. Cardiopulmonary resuscitation is the factor with the greatest influence on survival. The most important priority in resuscitation is to manage the hypoxia, acidosis, and hypothermia. Prevention and management of hypoxia are accomplished by ensuring an adequate airway and respiration, thus improving ventilation (which helps correct respiratory acidosis) and oxygenation. Arterial blood gases are monitored to evaluate oxygen, carbon dioxide, bicarbonate levels, and pH. These parameters determine the type of ventilatory support needed. The use of endotracheal intubation with PEEP improves oxygenation, prevents aspiration, and corrects intrapulmonary shunting and ventilation–perfusion abnormalities (caused by aspiration of water). If the patient is breathing spontaneously, supplemental oxygen may be given by mask. However, an endotracheal tube is necessary if the patient does not breathe spontaneously.

Because of submersion, the patient is usually hypothermic. A rectal probe or other core measurement device is used to determine the degree of hypothermia. Prescribed rewarming procedures (e.g., extracorporeal warming, warmed peritoneal dialysis, inhalation of warm aerosolized oxygen, torso warming) are started during resuscitation. The choice of warming method is determined by the severity and duration of hypothermia and available resources. Intravascular volume expansion and inotropic agents are used to treat hypotension and impaired tissue perfusion. ECG monitoring is initiated, because arrhythmias frequently occur. An indwelling urinary catheter is inserted to measure urine output. Hypothermia and accompanying metabolic acidosis may compromise kidney function. Nasogastric intubation is used to decompress the stomach and to prevent the patient from aspirating gastric contents.

Even if the patient appears healthy, close monitoring continues with serial vital signs, serial arterial blood gas values, ECG monitoring, intracranial pressure assessments, serum electrolyte levels, intake and output, and serial chest x-rays. After a nonfatal drowning, the patient is at risk for complications such as hypoxic or ischemic cerebral injury, ARDS, and life-threatening cardiac arrest. The patient is also at heightened risk for aspiration; vomiting frequently occurs in patients requiring rescue breathing and in up to 86% of patients requiring CPR (ENA, 2020a).

Decompression Sickness

Decompression sickness, also known as "the bends," occurs in patients who have engaged in diving (lake/ocean diving), high-altitude flying, or flying in commercial aircraft within 24 hours after diving. It occurs relatively infrequently in the United States, but its effects can be hazardous. Being aware of decompression sickness and assessing the patient properly ensures appropriate management and results in decreased morbidity.

Decompression sickness results from formation of nitrogen bubbles that occur with rapid changes in atmospheric pressure. They may occur in joint or muscle spaces, resulting in musculoskeletal pain, numbness, or hypesthesia. More significantly, nitrogen bubbles can become air emboli in the bloodstream and thereby produce stroke, paralysis, or death. Taking a rapid history about the events preceding the onset of symptoms is essential (Tintinalli et al., 2020).

Assessment and Diagnostic Findings

To identify decompression sickness, a detailed history is obtained from the patient or diving partner. Evidence of rapid ascent, loss of air in the tank, buddy breathing, recent alcohol intake or lack of sleep, or a flight within 24 hours after diving suggests possible decompression sickness. Some patients describe a perfect dive yet still have the signs and symptoms of decompression sickness, in which case they must receive treatment for the condition.

Signs and symptoms include joint or extremity pain, numbness, hypesthesia, and loss of range of motion. Neurologic symptoms mimicking those of a stroke or spinal cord injury can indicate an air embolus. Cardiopulmonary arrest can also occur in severe cases and is usually fatal. Any neurologic symptoms should be rapidly assessed. All patients with decompression sickness need rapid transfer to a hyperbaric chamber (ENA, 2020a).

Management

A patent airway and adequate ventilation are established, as described previously, and 100% oxygen is given throughout treatment and transport. A chest x-ray is obtained to identify aspiration, and at least one IV line is started with lactated Ringer's or normal saline solution. Research findings suggest that among patients requiring air transport (e.g., helicopter), oxygen saturations and symptoms improve when both oxygen and IV fluids are given. If air transport is required, the aircraft should remain at low altitude (i.e., below 300 m [approximately 1000 feet]) (Holleran, Wolfe, & Frakes, 2018).

The cardiopulmonary and neurologic systems are supported as needed. If an air embolus is suspected, the head of the bed should be lowered. If the patient's wet clothing is still present, it is removed. The patient is kept warm. Transfer to the closest hyperbaric chamber for treatment is initiated. However, the patient who is awake and alert without central neurologic deficits may be able to travel by ground ambulance or by automobile, depending on the severity of symptoms. Throughout treatment, the patient is continually assessed, and changes are

documented. If aspiration is suspected, antibiotic agents and other treatment may be prescribed (ENA, 2020a).

Animal and Human Bites

Bites are a common reason for visits to the ED. Dog bites constitute 80% to 90% of these bites and are responsible for the majority of deaths from bites by a nonvenomous animal (Tintinalli et al., 2020). Cat bites have a high risk of infection because of the presence of *Pasteurella* in their saliva. All animal bites must be reported to public health authorities, which must provide follow-up screening of the offending animal for rabies. If the animal cannot be located and rabies vaccination verified, rabies prophylaxis for the person who has been bitten must be instituted (ENA, 2020a).

Human bites are frequently associated with rapes, sexual assaults, or other forms of battery. The human mouth contains more bacteria than that of most other animals, so a high risk of bite-related infection exists. Depending on the circumstances surrounding the event, the victim may delay seeking treatment. The ED nurse should inspect any bitten tissue for pus, erythema, or necrosis. A health care provider should take photographs, which can be used as evidence in criminal and legal proceedings. Guidelines for collecting forensic evidence for photographing with and without a measuring device should be followed. Cleansing with soap and water is then necessary, followed by the administration of antibiotics and tetanus toxoid as prescribed (Tintinalli et al., 2020).

Snakebites

Venomous (poisonous) snakes caused more than 2000 of the 6000 snakebites in the United States annually (Tintinalli et al., 2020). Across the globe, between 4.5 and 5.4 million people get bitten by snakes each year, with 81,000 to 138,000 dying from complications (WHO, 2019). Children between 1 and 9 years of age are the most likely victims. The greatest number of bites occurs during the daylight hours and early evening of the summer months. The most frequent poisonous snakebite in the United States occurs from Crotalidae, otherwise called pit vipers, such as water moccasins, copperheads, and rattlesnakes. The most common site is the upper extremity (ENA, 2020a). Of pit viper bites, 75% to 80% result in **envenomation** (injection of a poisonous material by sting, spine, bite, or other means); the rest result in what are called *dry bites* (Tintinalli et al., 2020). Venomous snakebites are medical emergencies.

Nineteen different species of venomous snakes are found in various regions within the United States. Nurses should be familiar with the types of snakes common to the geographic region in which they practice. However, the exotic pet industry sells atypical snakes as "pets." Because of this, venomous snakes such as cobras and asps may be found outside of their native region.

Clinical Manifestations

Snake venom consists primarily of proteins and has a broad range of physiologic effects. It may affect multiple organ systems, especially the neurologic, cardiovascular, and respiratory systems.

Classic clinical signs of envenomation are edema, ecchymosis, and hemorrhagic bullae, leading to necrosis at the site of envenomation. Symptoms include lymph node tenderness, nausea, vomiting, numbness, and a metallic taste in the mouth. Without decisive treatment, these clinical manifestations may progress to include fasciculations, hypotension, paresthesias, seizures, and coma (ENA, 2020a).

Management

Initial first aid at the site of the snakebite includes having the person lie down, removing constrictive items such as rings, providing warmth, cleansing the wound, covering the wound with a light sterile dressing, and immobilizing the injured body part below the level of the heart. CABs are the priorities of care. Ice, incision and suction, or a tourniquet is *not* applied. Tetanus and analgesia should be given as necessary. Initial evaluation in the ED is performed quickly and includes information about the following (Tintinalli et al., 2020):

- Whether the snake was venomous or nonvenomous; discourage bringing the snake for identification—even a dead snake's venom is poisonous. Do *not* handle any snake brought to the ED. If the snake is transported to the ED, caution should be taken because the snake is frequently in a stunned, not dead, state. The bite reflex can remain intact for up to 90 minutes after the death of the snake.
- Where and when the bite occurred and the circumstances of the bite.
- Sequence of events, signs, and symptoms (fang punctures, pain, edema, and erythema of the bite and nearby tissues).
- Severity of poisonous effects. Call the local poison control phone number to gain access to information about an exotic snakebite presentation and management, as necessary. The poison control center may also be able to assist with retrieving antivenin for these particular species.
- Vital signs.
- Circumference of the bitten extremity or area at several points. The circumference of the extremity that was bitten is compared with the circumference of the opposite extremity.
- Laboratory data (complete blood count, urinalysis, and coagulation studies).

The course and prognosis of snakebite injuries depend on the kind and amount of venom injected; where on the body the bite occurred; and the general health, age, and size of the patient. There is no one specific protocol for treatment of snakebites. In general, ice, tourniquets, heparin, and corticosteroids are not used during the acute stage. Corticosteroids are contraindicated in the first 6 to 8 hours after the bite because they may depress antibody production and hinder the action of **antivenin** (antitoxin manufactured from the snake venom and used to treat snakebites).

Parenteral fluids may be used to treat hypotension. If vasopressors are used to treat hypotension, their use should be short term. Surgical exploration of the bite is rarely indicated. Typically, the patient is observed closely for at least 6 hours. The patient is *never* left unattended.

Administration of Antivenin

Although envenomation does not always occur, it should always be suspected with snakebites. An assessment of progressive signs and symptoms is essential before considering administration of antivenin, which is most effective if given within 4 hours and no greater than 12 hours after the snakebite. The decision to administer antivenin depends on worsening tissue injury and evidence of systemic and coagulopathic symptoms. Rattlesnakes are more likely to cause coagulation abnormalities as well as more systemic effects. Coagulation abnormalities are not restricted to severe envenomation (Tintinalli et al., 2020).

The most readily available antivenin in the United States is Crotalidae polyvalent immune Fab antivenom (FabAV or CroFab). The dose depends on the type of snake and the estimated severity of the bite. Indications for antivenin depend on the progression of symptoms, including coagulopathy and systemic reaction (ENA, 2020a).

Crotalidae polyvalent immune Fab antivenom does not require pretesting (i.e., skin sensitivity screening for an allergic reaction; see Chapter 33), albeit monitoring for a hypersensitivity reaction is still necessary. Outside of the United States, however, other antivenin formulas that may be commercially available may still result in severe serum sickness. If the dose exceeds 10 vials, serum sickness will most likely occur. Serum sickness is a type of hypersensitivity response that results in fever, arthralgias, pruritus, lymphadenopathy, and proteinuria and can progress to neuropathies (ENA, 2020a). However, FabAV must be given cautiously to patients receiving anticoagulation therapy. Administration of FabAV may result in a recurring coagulopathy. The dosage and administration of FabAV are different from previously manufactured types of antivenin and should be reviewed carefully before the medication is given.

Before administering antivenin and every 15 minutes thereafter, the circumference of the affected part is measured. Premedication with diphenhydramine or cimetidine may be indicated, because these antihistamines may decrease the allergic response to antivenin. Antivenin is given as an IV infusion whenever possible, although intramuscular administration can be used.

Depending on the severity of the snakebite, the antivenin is diluted in 500 to 1000 mL of normal saline solution. The infusion is started slowly, and the rate is increased after 10 minutes if there is no reaction. The total dose should be infused during the first 4 to 6 hours after the bite. The initial dose is repeated until symptoms decrease, after which time the circumference of the affected part should be measured every 30 to 60 minutes for the next 48 hours to detect symptoms of compartment syndrome (swelling, loss of pulse, increased pain, and paresthesias) (ENA, 2020a).

There is no limit to the number of antivenin vials that can be given. The decision to continue to administer vials is based upon patient symptoms. Consultation with a snakebite expert is essential at this point; this consultant may be identified and found through contacting the Poison Control Center (see the Resources section) or a local zoo reptile center. The most common cause of allergic reaction to the antivenin is too-rapid infusion. Reactions may consist of a feeling of fullness in the face, urticaria, pruritus, malaise, and apprehension. These symptoms may be followed by tachycardia, shortness of breath, hypotension, and shock. In this situation, the infusion should be stopped immediately and IV diphenhydramine given. Vasopressors are used for patients in shock, and resuscitation equipment must be on standby while antivenin is infusing. It is important to note that serum sickness (hypersensitivity) can occur within the first few weeks after discharge. The patient and the patient's family members should be educated about the clinical manifestations of serum sickness (i.e., fever; rash starting on the chest and spreading to the back; arthralgia; gastrointestinal [GI] disturbances [e.g., nausea, vomiting, diarrhea, abdominal pain], and headache) and return to the ED if they occur (Tintinalli et al., 2020).

Spider Bites

There are two venomous spiders found in the United States that may interact with humans: the brown recluse and the black widow. Both are usually found in dark places such as closets, woodpiles, and attics, as well as in shoes (ENA, 2020a).

Brown recluse spider bites are painless. Systemic effects such as fever and chills, nausea and vomiting, malaise, and joint pain develop within 24 to 72 hours. The site of the bite may appear reddish to purple in color within 2 to 8 hours after the bite. Necrosis occurs in the next 2 to 4 days in approximately 10% of cases. The center of the bite may become necrotic, and surgical débridement may be necessary. Wound care consists of cleansing with soap and water, and hyperbaric oxygen treatments may be helpful. Most wounds heal within 2 to 3 months (ENA, 2020a; Tintinalli et al., 2020).

Black widow spider bites feel like pinpricks. Systemic effects usually occur within 30 minutes—much more rapidly than with brown recluse spider bites. Signs and symptoms include abdominal rigidity, nausea and vomiting, hypertension, tachycardia, and paresthesias. Severe pain also develops within 60 minutes and increases over 1 to 2 days. Treatment involves application of ice to the site to decrease swelling and discomfort, along with elevation and assessment of tetanus immunization status. Analgesic agents and benzodiazepines may relieve muscle spasms. Cardiopulmonary monitoring is essential. Antivenin is effective for severe black widow spider bites. This antivenin is horse serum based; therefore, testing for sensitivity must be performed prior to administration (ENA, 2020a).

Tick Bites

Tick bites are common in many areas of the United States, and they usually occur in grassy or wooded areas. It is important to learn the place where the bite occurred as well as the location of the bite on the body. The tick bite itself is not usually the problem; rather, it is the pathogen transmitted by the tick that can cause serious disease. Ticks can carry diseases such as Rocky Mountain spotted fever, tularemia, west Nile virus, and Lyme disease.

Ticks transmit pathogens through their saliva; therefore, the earlier the tick is removed, the better the prognosis. The tick should be removed with tweezers using a straight upward pull (see Fig. 67-4), and the patient should be informed of the signs and symptoms of diseases carried by ticks, especially if the patient lives in or has visited an area endemic for tick-related diseases (e.g., Lyme disease) (ENA, 2020a).

Lyme disease has three stages. Stage I may present with erythema migrans (a classic "bull's-eye" rash) that typically

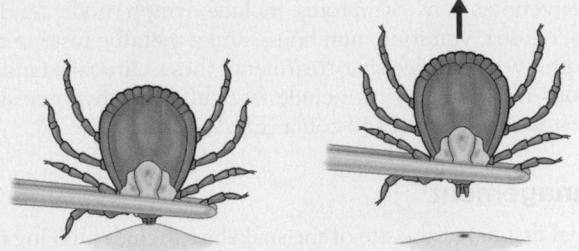

Figure 67-4 • Removal of tick with tweezers using a straight upward pull.

can be found in the axilla, groin, or thigh area and that appears within 4 weeks after the tick bite, with a peak manifestation time of 7 days after the bite. Classically, this rash is at least 5 cm in diameter with bright red borders. It is accompanied by flulike signs and symptoms that may include chills, fever, myalgia, fatigue, and headache. Without treatment, the rash subsides within 3 to 4 weeks. However, the rash and flulike manifestations can be significantly reduced within days if prompt treatment with antibiotic agents (e.g., doxycycline) is initiated. If antibiotics are not given, stage II Lyme disease may present within 4 to 10 weeks following the tick bite and may manifest with joint pain, memory loss, poor motor coordination, adenopathy, and cardiac abnormalities. Facial nerve palsy is the most common manifestation of stage II Lyme disease (Tintinalli et al., 2020). Stage III can begin anywhere from weeks to more than a year after the bite and has serious long-term chronic sequelae, including arthritis, neuropathy, myalgia, and myocarditis. Even after appropriate treatment with antibiotics, 10% to 20% of patients may experience long-term effects including fatigue and arthralgias; some experience neurologic symptoms that may persist for over 10 years (Tintinalli et al., 2020).

POISONING

A poison is any substance that, when ingested, inhaled, absorbed, applied to the skin, or produced within the body in relatively small amounts, injures the body by its chemical action. Poisoning from inhalation and ingestion of toxic materials, both intentional and unintentional, constitutes a major health hazard and an emergency situation. Emergency treatment is initiated with the following goals:

- Removal or inactivation of the poison before it is absorbed
- Provision of supportive care in maintaining vital organ function
- Administration of a specific antidote to neutralize a specific poison
- Implementation of treatment that hastens the elimination of the absorbed poison

Ingested (Swallowed) Poisons

Swallowed poisons may be corrosive. **Corrosive poisons** include alkaline and acid agents that can cause tissue destruction after coming in contact with mucous membranes. Alkaline products include lye, drain cleaners, toilet bowl cleaners, bleach, nonphosphate detergents, oven cleaners, and button batteries (batteries used to power watches, calculators, hearing aids, or cameras). Acid products include toilet bowl cleaners, pool cleaners, metal cleaners, rust removers, and battery acid.

Control of the airway, ventilation, and oxygenation are essential. In the absence of cerebral or renal damage, the patient's prognosis depends largely on successful management of respiration and circulation. Measures are instituted to stabilize cardiovascular and other body functions. ECG, vital signs, and neurologic status are monitored closely for changes. Shock may result from the cardiodepressant action of the substance ingested, from venous pooling in the lower extremities, or from reduced circulating blood volume resulting from increased capillary permeability (see Chapter 11). An indwelling urinary catheter is inserted to monitor kidney function. Blood specimens are obtained to determine the concentration of drug or poison (ENA, 2020a).

Efforts are made to determine what substance was ingested; the amount; the time since ingestion; signs and symptoms, such as pain or burning sensations, any evidence of redness or burn in the mouth or throat, pain on swallowing or an inability to swallow, vomiting, or drooling; age and weight of the patient; and pertinent health history.

> ### Quality and Safety Nursing Alert
>
> The local poison control center should be called if an unknown toxic agent has been taken or if it is necessary to identify an antidote for a known toxic agent.

Measures are instituted to remove the toxin or decrease its absorption. If there is a specific chemical or physiologic antagonist (antidote), it is given as early as possible to reverse or diminish the effects of the toxin. If this measure is ineffective, procedures may be initiated to remove or dilute the ingested substance. These procedures include administration of multiple doses of activated charcoal, dialysis, or hemoperfusion. Hemoperfusion involves detoxification of the blood by processing it through an extracorporeal circuit and an adsorbent cartridge containing charcoal or resin, after which the cleansed blood is returned to the patient (ENA, 2020a).

The patient who has ingested a corrosive poison, which can be a strong acid or alkaline substance, is given water or milk to drink for dilution. However, dilution is not attempted if the patient has acute airway edema or obstruction; potential for vomiting; or if there is clinical evidence of esophageal, gastric, or intestinal burn or perforation. The following gastric emptying procedures may be used as prescribed:

- Gastric lavage for the patient who is obtunded is only useful within 1 hour of ingestion, for sustained-release substances, or massive life-threatening amounts of a substance; however, complications of aspiration and stomach or esophageal perforation outweigh its usefulness. If performed, gastric aspirate is saved and sent to the laboratory for testing (toxicology screens).
- Activated charcoal administration if the poison is one that is absorbed by charcoal; given orally or by nasogastric tube, it is effective in small intermittent doses to decrease vomiting. It should be diluted as a slurry so that

it is easier to drink or pass through the nasogastric tube. Activated charcoal absorbs most commonly ingested poisons except corrosives, heavy metals and hydrocarbons, iron, and lithium.

Cathartics, which had traditionally accompanied the use of activated charcoal, are rarely indicated because they can result in severe electrolyte imbalances, diarrhea, and hypovolemia (ENA, 2020a). Furthermore, syrup of ipecac to induce vomiting in the patient who is alert is not recommended due to the risk of aspiration and should *never* be used with corrosive poisons or with petroleum distillates (e.g., lubricating oil, fuel oil) or further corrosive damage to the upper airway and pharyngeal structures may occur.

> ### Quality and Safety Nursing Alert
>
> Vomiting is never induced after ingestion of caustic substances (acid or alkaline) or petroleum distillates.

Throughout detoxification, the patient's vital signs, CVP, and fluid and electrolyte balance are monitored closely. Hypotension and cardiac arrhythmias are possible. Seizures are also possible because of CNS stimulation from the poison or from oxygen deprivation. If the patient complains of pain, analgesic agents are given cautiously. Severe pain causes vasomotor collapse and reflex inhibition of normal physiologic functions.

After the patient's condition has stabilized and discharge is imminent, written material should be given to the patient indicating the signs and symptoms of potential problems related to the poison ingested and signs or symptoms requiring evaluation by a health care provider. If poisoning was determined to be a suicide or self-harm attempt, a psychiatric consultation should be requested before the patient is discharged. In cases of inadvertent poison ingestion, poison prevention and home poison-proofing instructions should be provided to the patient and family.

Carbon Monoxide Poisoning

Carbon monoxide poisoning may occur as a result of industrial or household incidents or attempted suicide. It is the most common cause of fatality from poisoning and is frequently under-reported to poison control centers or misdiagnosed (Tintinalli et al., 2020). Carbon monoxide exerts its toxic effect by binding to circulating hemoglobin and thereby reducing the oxygen-carrying capacity of the blood. Hemoglobin absorbs carbon monoxide 200 times more readily than it absorbs oxygen. Carbon monoxide–bound hemoglobin, called **carboxyhemoglobin**, does not transport oxygen.

Clinical Manifestations

Because the CNS has a critical need for oxygen, CNS symptoms predominate with carbon monoxide toxicity. A person with carbon monoxide poisoning may appear intoxicated (from cerebral hypoxia). Other signs and symptoms include headache, muscular weakness, palpitation, dizziness, and confusion, which can progress rapidly to coma. Skin color, which can range from pink or cherry-red to cyanotic and pale, is not a reliable sign. Pulse oximetry may reveal a high hemoglobin saturation, which may be deceiving, since the hemoglobin molecule is saturated with carbon monoxide rather than oxygen (ENA, 2020a).

Management

Exposure to carbon monoxide requires immediate treatment. Goals of management are to reverse cerebral and myocardial hypoxia and to hasten elimination of carbon monoxide. Whenever a patient inhales a poison, the following general measures apply:

- Move the patient to fresh air immediately, if possible.
- Open all doors and windows.
- Loosen all tight clothing.
- Initiate traditional cardiopulmonary resuscitation.
- Prevent chilling; wrap the patient in blankets.
- Keep the patient as quiet as possible.
- Do not give alcohol in any form or permit the patient to smoke.

In addition, for the patient with carbon monoxide poisoning, carboxyhemoglobin levels are analyzed on arrival at the ED and before treatment with oxygen if possible. To reverse hypoxia and accelerate the elimination of carbon monoxide, 100% oxygen is given at atmospheric or preferably hyperbaric pressures. Oxygen is given until the carboxyhemoglobin level is less than 5%. The patient is monitored continuously. Psychoses, spastic paralysis, ataxia, visual disturbances, and deterioration of mental status and behavior may persist after resuscitation and may be symptoms of permanent brain damage (Tintinalli et al., 2020).

When unintentional carbon monoxide poisoning occurs, the health department should be contacted so that the dwelling or building in question can be inspected. A psychiatric consultation is warranted if it has been determined that the poisoning was a suicide attempt.

Skin Contamination Poisoning (Chemical Burns)

Skin contamination injuries from exposure to chemicals are challenging because of the large number of possible offending agents with diverse actions and metabolic effects. The severity of a chemical burn is determined by the mechanism of action, the penetrating strength and concentration, and the amount and duration of exposure of the skin to the chemical. A wet chemical should be removed as soon as possible with copious amounts of water. Dry substances should be gently brushed off the skin before the area is flushed (ENA, 2020a). The skin should be flushed with a constant stream of cool water as the patient's clothing is removed. The skin of health care personnel assisting the patient should be appropriately protected if the burn is extensive or if the agent is significantly toxic or still present. Prolonged lavage with generous amounts of tepid water is important. The decontamination shower (deluge) in the ED is the optimal place for total body flushing. The staff attending the patient should wear proper PPE to prevent cross-contamination (Veenema, 2019).

Attempts to determine the identity and characteristics of the chemical agent are necessary in order to specify future treatment. The standard burn treatment appropriate for the size and location of the wound (antimicrobial treatment,

débridement, tetanus prophylaxis, antidote administration as prescribed) is instituted (ENA, 2020a) (see Chapter 57). The patient may require plastic surgery for further wound management. The patient is instructed to have the affected area reexamined at 24 and 72 hours and in 7 days because of the risk of underestimating the extent and depth of these types of injuries.

Food Poisoning

Food poisoning is a sudden illness that occurs after ingestion of contaminated food or drink. Botulism is a serious form of food poisoning that requires continual surveillance (see Chapter 68, Table 68-6). Assessment questions for patients with suspected food poisoning are discussed in Chart 67-7.

The key to treatment is determining the source and type of food poisoning. If possible, the suspected food should be brought to the medical facility and a history obtained from the patient or family.

Food, gastric contents, vomitus, serum, and feces are collected for examination. The patient's respirations, level of consciousness (LOC), blood pressure and hemodynamic status, and muscular activity are monitored closely. Measures are instituted to support the respiratory system. Death from respiratory paralysis can occur with botulism, fish poisoning, and some other food poisonings.

Because large volumes of electrolytes and water are lost by vomiting and diarrhea, fluid and electrolyte status should be assessed. Severe vomiting produces alkalosis, and severe diarrhea produces acidosis. Hypovolemic shock may also occur from severe fluid and electrolyte losses. The patient is assessed for signs and symptoms of fluid and electrolyte imbalances, including lethargy, rapid pulse rate, fever, oliguria, anuria, hypotension, and delirium. Baseline weight and serum electrolyte levels are obtained for future comparisons.

Measures to control nausea are also important to prevent vomiting, which could exacerbate fluid and electrolyte imbalances. An antiemetic medication is given parenterally as prescribed if the patient cannot tolerate fluids or medications by mouth (Tintinalli et al., 2020). For mild nausea, the patient

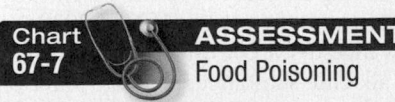

Chart 67-7	**ASSESSMENT** Food Poisoning

Use the following questions to elicit information about the circumstances surrounding the possibility of food poisoning:

- How soon after eating did the symptoms occur? (Immediate onset suggests chemical, plant, or animal poisoning.)
- What was eaten in the previous meal? Did the food have an unusual odor or taste? (Most foods causing bacterial poisoning *do not* have unusual odor or taste.)
- Did anyone else become ill from eating the same food?
- Did vomiting occur? What was the appearance of the vomitus?
- Did diarrhea occur? (Diarrhea is usually absent with botulism and with shellfish or other fish poisoning.)
- Are any neurologic symptoms present? (These occur in botulism and in chemical, plant, and animal poisoning.)
- Does the patient have a fever? (Fever is characteristic in salmonella, ingestion of fava beans, and some fish poisoning.)

is encouraged to take sips of weak tea, carbonated drinks, or tap water. After nausea and vomiting subside, clear liquids are usually prescribed for 12 to 24 hours, and the diet is gradually progressed to a low-residue, bland diet.

SUBSTANCE USE DISORDER (SUD)

SUD is the misuse of specific substances, such as drugs or alcohol, to alter mood or behavior. Drug abuse is the use of drugs for other than legitimate medical purposes. People who abuse drugs often take a variety of drugs simultaneously (such as alcohol, barbiturates, opioids, and tranquilizers), and the combination may have additive and addictive effects.

"Rave parties" are large-scale parties attended by hundreds of people involved in illicit drug use. At these events, one of the most commonly used drugs is 3,4-methylenedioxymeth-amphetamine (MDMA), or Ecstasy, a methamphetamine-based drug that users believe produces a "harmless high." ED nurses should be aware of rave parties in their geographic area so that they can prepare for a potential influx of patients who abuse this drug (ENA, 2020a). Others may combine Ecstasy with sildenafil; this drug combination is nicknamed "sextasy."

Spice is a synthetic cannabinoid sold commercially as a smoking mixture under the names "spice," "incense," or "K2." Its chemical structure and effects are similar to marijuana, targeting the same receptor sites in the brain. Spice is sold with variable concentrations and unregulated potency (National Institute on Drug Abuse, 2018).

Bath salts are synthetic stimulants similar to Ecstasy known as "mephedrone," "drone," or "MCAT." Their effects are similar to amphetamines, MDMA, and cocaine. Although bath salts are most commonly swallowed or snorted, they may also be smoked or injected; the method of intake affects the severity and duration of effects (Table 67-1). The structural formula 3,4-methylenedioxypyrovalerone (MDPV) is the most common type of bath salt abused (ENA, 2020a).

Abuse of various inhalants (see Table 67-1) has also increased in popularity; these products generally result more often in cravings than withdrawal when their use is stopped. The method of inhalation varies with the product chosen and requires several deep inhalations to reach euphoria. Methods include sniffing or snorting by directly inhaling the fumes. "Bagging" (sniffing from a bag) or "huffing" (sniffing from a rag or cloth) provide the greatest concentration; "dusting" is another method that delivers the inhalant by directly spraying it into the nostrils. Long-term use results in cortical atrophy and brain stem dysfunction, in addition to cardiomyopathy and emphysema like abnormalities of the lung. Significant others or parents may report that the patient has had poor school or work performance or attendance, weight loss, poor hygiene, fatigue, nosebleeds, and decreased appetite (National Institute on Drug Abuse, 2020).

Clinical manifestations vary with the substance used, but the underlying principles of management are essentially the same. Table 67-1 identifies commonly abused drugs, listing their clinical manifestations and therapeutic management. Treatment goals for a patient with a drug overdose are to support the respiratory and cardiovascular functions, to enhance clearance of the agent, and to provide for safety of the patient and staff. People who abuse IV/injection drugs are at increased risk for HIV infection, acquired immune deficiency syndrome, hepatitis B and C, and tetanus.

Cannabis remains popular, available, and in some states, is now legal. A newer method of cannabis abuse is butane honey oil (BHO) or "dabs." BHO is created at home by heating cannabis with butane to strip the chemical from the plant, which is then heated further to remove the butane. It may be further distilled to "shatter" by being placed in a vacuum to remove any residual butane. The product results in a "dab" which can then be inhaled. Butane in the presence of an ignition source can result in explosion and fire resulting in chemical and thermal burns (National Institute on Drug Abuse, 2019).

Acute Alcohol Intoxication

Alcohol is a psychotropic drug that affects mood, judgment, behavior, concentration, and consciousness. Many people who drink heavily are young adults or those older than 60 years. There is a high prevalence of alcoholism among patients presenting to the ED for management; up to 31% have histories of SUD with alcohol. Among patients who present to the ED with various injuries, up to 50% may have histories of SUD with alcohol (ENA, 2020a). Because patients with SUD from alcohol return frequently to the ED, they present a challenge to the health professionals who care for them. The CDC advocates routine screening for SUD with alcohol in all outpatient settings, including EDs. Therefore, screenings, brief interventions, and referral to treatment (SBIRT) for patients presenting with suspected SUD with alcohol are recommended. All level I and II verified trauma centers are required to provide this service. SBIRT is considered cost-effective in saving quality of life-years lost and preventing the morbid consequences of continued SUD with alcohol (American College of Emergency Physicians [ACEP], 2017).

Alcohol, or ethanol, is a multisystem toxin and CNS depressant that causes drowsiness, impaired coordination, slurring of speech, sudden mood changes, aggression, belligerence, grandiosity, and uninhibited behavior. In excess, it can also cause stupor and eventually coma and death (i.e., alcohol poisoning). Frequently, underage minors and college students arrive at the ED with alcohol poisoning from binge drinking.

In the ED, the patient who is intoxicated with alcohol or who presents with alcohol poisoning is assessed for head injury, hypoglycemia (which mimics intoxication), and other health problems. Possible nursing diagnoses include impaired breathing associated with CNS depression and impaired impulse control associated with severe intoxication from alcohol.

Treatment involves detoxification of the acute poisoning, recovery, and rehabilitation. Commonly, the patient uses mechanisms of denial and defensiveness. The nurse should approach the patient in a nonjudgmental manner, using a firm, consistent, and accepting attitude. Speaking in a calm and slow manner is helpful because alcohol interferes with thought processes. If the patient appears intoxicated, hypoxia, hypovolemia, and neurologic impairment must be ruled out before it is assumed that the patient is intoxicated. Typically, a blood specimen is obtained for analysis of the blood alcohol level.

(text continued on page 2210)

TABLE 67-1	Emergency Management of Patients with Drug Overdose	
Drug	**Clinical Manifestations**	**Therapeutic Management**
Cocaine *Routes may include:* • Intranasally ("snorting")—inhaled into nostrils through straws • By smoking ("freebasing")—cocaine hydrochloride dissolved in ether to yield a pure cocaine alkaloid base ("crack," "rocks"); smoking in a small pipe delivers large quantities of cocaine to lungs. • IV • Polysubstance (cocaine and heroin)	Cocaine is a CNS stimulant that can cause: • Increased heart rate and blood pressure • Hyperpyrexia • Seizures • Sluggish, dilated pupillary response • Muscle rigidity • Increased energy, agitation, aggression • Ventricular arrhythmias • Intense euphoria, then anxiety, sadness, insomnia, and sexual indifference • Cocaine hallucinations with delusions • Psychosis with extreme paranoia and ideas of persecution • Hypervigilance Chronic psychotic symptoms may persist. Overall psychotic symptoms are short-lived compared to methamphetamines	1. Maintain airway and provide respiratory support. 2. Control seizures. 3. Monitor cardiovascular effects; have antiarrhythmic drugs and defibrillator available. 4. Treat for hyperthermia. 5. If cocaine was ingested, evacuate stomach contents and use activated charcoal to treat. Whole bowel irrigation may be necessary to treat body packers ("mules"). 6. Refer for psychiatric evaluation and treatment in an inpatient unit that eliminates access to the drug. Include drug rehabilitation counseling.
Opioids Heroin Opium or paregoric Morphine, codeine, semisynthetic derivatives: oxycodone, methadone, meperidine, tramadol, fentanyl	Acute intoxication (overdose) can result in: • Pinpoint pupils (may be dilated with severe hypoxia) • Decreased blood pressure • Marked respiratory depression/arrest • Pulmonary edema • Stupor → coma • Seizures Fresh needle marks along course of any superficial vein Skin abscesses (from "popping")	1. Support respiratory and cardiovascular functions. 2. Establish IV lines; obtain blood for chemical and toxicologic analysis. Patient may be given bolus of glucose to eliminate possibility of hypoglycemia. 3. Administer narcotic antagonist (naloxone hydrochloride IV, IM) as prescribed to reverse severe respiratory depression and coma. 4. Continue to monitor level of responsiveness and respirations, pulse, and blood pressure. Duration of action of naloxone hydrochloride is shorter than that of heroin; repeated dosages may be necessary. 5. Send urine for analysis; opioids can be detected in urine. 6. Obtain an ECG. 7. Do not leave patient unattended; they may lapse back into coma rapidly. Clinical status may change from minute to minute. Hemodialysis may be indicated for severe drug intoxication. Activated charcoal may be considered if opioids were taken orally and if the patient is alert. 8. Monitor for pulmonary edema, which is frequently seen in patients who abuse/overdose on narcotics. 9. Refer patient for psychiatric and drug rehabilitation evaluation before discharge.

Barbiturates
Pentobarbital, secobarbital, amobarbital, gamma-hydroxybutyrate (GHB, "liquid Ecstasy")
	Acute intoxication (may mimic alcohol intoxication):
	• Respiratory depression
	• Flushed face
	• Decreased pulse rate; decreased blood pressure
	• Increasing nystagmus (to vertical and horizontal gaze)
	• Sluggish pupils
	• Lack of convergence of eyes
	• Depressed deep tendon reflexes
	• Decreasing mental alertness
	• Difficulty in speaking
	• Poor motor coordination and flaccid muscles
	• Coma, death
	GHB:
	• Sexual disinhibition
	• Amnesia, myoclonus, agitation
	• Overdoses when mixed with alcohol
		1. Maintain airway and provide respiratory support.
		2. Endotracheal intubation or tracheostomy is considered if there is any doubt about the adequacy of airway exchange.
		  a. Check airway frequently.
		  b. Perform suctioning as necessary.
		3. Support cardiovascular and respiratory functions; most deaths result from respiratory depression or shock.
		4. Start infusion through large-gauge needle or IV catheter to support blood pressure; coma and dehydration result in hypotension and respond to infusion of IV fluids with elevation of blood pressure.
		5. Evacuate stomach contents or lavage if within 1 h of ingestion to prevent absorption; repeated doses of activated charcoal may be given.
		6. Assist with hemodialysis for patient with severe overdose.
		7. Maintain neurologic and vital sign flow sheet.
		8. Patient awakening from overdose may demonstrate combative behavior.
		9. Refer for psychiatric and drug rehabilitation consultation to evaluate suicide potential and drug abuse.

TABLE 67-1	Emergency Management of Patients with Drug Overdose (continued)	
Drug	**Clinical Manifestations**	**Therapeutic Management**

Inhalants

Amyl nitrate
Freon
Propane
Trichloroethylene
Gasoline
Perchloroethylene
Toluene (metallic paint spray)
Helium
Canned air
Hand sanitizer
Routes may include:
- Sniffing/snorting—direct inhalation of fumes
- "Bagging"—sniff from a bag
- "Huffing"—sniff from a rag/cloth
- "Dusting"—direct spray into the nostrils

Effects mimic those of alcohol, with dizziness and imbalance:
- Euphoria, headache, disinhibition, altered level of consciousness to coma
- Renal, hepatic, and cardiac toxicity
- Aplastic anemia
- Fetal growth retardation
- Respiratory depression, arrest from CNS depression
- Vasodilation
- Nosebleeding
- Vertical and horizontal nystagmus
- Lack of convergence of eyes
- Sluggish pupils
- Temperature fluctuations
- Circumoral red spots/rash
- Air embolus

1. Provide airway support, ventilation, and oxygen.
2. Treat cardiac arrhythmias and hypotension.
3. Provide advanced cardiac life support as needed.
4. Monitor for profound hypotension when amyl nitrate is combined with MDMA and sildenafil or with anesthetic agents.
5. Monitor for hypertension when volatile solvents are used.

Amphetamine-Type Drugs (pep pills, "uppers," "speed," "crystal meth")

amphetamine
dextroamphetamine
methamphetamine ("speed")
3,4-methylenedioxymethamphetamine (MDMA) ("Ecstasy," "Adam")[a]
3,4-methylenedioxy-N-ethylamphetamine (MDEA) ("Eve")
3,4-methylenedioxyamphetamine (MDA); methylphenidate "ice," "rocks," "crystal meth"
3,4-methylenedioxypyrovalerone (MDPV) or 4-methylmethcathinone; "Bath salts" (synthetic stimulant)

- Nausea, vomiting, anorexia
- Palpitations, tachycardia
- Increased blood pressure
- Tachypnea, anxiety
- Nervousness
- Diaphoresis, mydriasis
- Repetitive or stereotyped behavior
- Irritability, insomnia, agitation
- Visual misperceptions, auditory hallucinations
- Fearfulness, anxiety, depression, hostility, paranoia
- Hyperactivity, rapid speech, euphoria, hyperalertness
- Decreased inhibition
- Seizures, coma, hyperthermia
- Cardiovascular collapse
- Rhabdomyolysis
- MDMA is both a hallucinogenic and a stimulant.
- MDPV and 4-methylmethcathinone effects last >24 h.

1. Provide airway support, ventilation, cardiac monitoring; insert IV line.
2. Use GI evacuation in cases of oral overdose; activated charcoal, gastric lavage if within 1 h of ingestion.
3. Keep in calm, cool, quiet environment; elevated temperature potentiates amphetamine toxicity. Maintain normothermia, cooling the patient as necessary.
4. Administer small doses of diazepam (IV) or haloperidol as prescribed for CNS and muscular hyperactivity.
5. Administer appropriate pharmacologic therapy as prescribed for severe hypertension and ventricular arrhythmias.
6. Treat seizures with benzodiazepines (e.g., diazepam) as prescribed.
7. Treat sympathetic stimulation with beta-blocker agents as prescribed.
8. Try to communicate with patient if delusions or hallucinations are present.
9. Place in a protective environment (preferably psychiatric security room with video monitoring) to observe for suicide attempt.
10. Refer for psychiatric and drug rehabilitation evaluation.

Hallucinogens or Psychedelic-Type Drugs

Lysergic acid diethylamide (LSD)
Phencyclidine HCl (PCP, "angel dust")
Mescaline, psilocybin
Ketamine ("special K")
Synthetic cannabinoids ("spice," "incense," "K2")
Butane honey oil (BHo)—"dabs," "shatter"

- Nystagmus
- Pupil dilation
- Mild hypertension
- Marked confusion bordering on panic
- Incoherence, hyperactivity
- Withdrawn
- Combative behavior; delirium, mania, self-injury (lasts 6–12 h)
- Hallucinations, body image distortion
- Hypertension, hyperthermia, acute kidney injury
- Flashback—recurrence of LSD-like state without having taken the drug; may occur weeks or months after drug was taken
- Ketamine—"out-of-body" experience; increased aggressiveness
- Manufacturing can result in burns

1. Evaluate and maintain patient's circulation, airway, and breathing.
2. Determine by urine or serum drug screen whether the patient has ingested hallucinogenic drug or has a toxic psychosis.
3. Try to communicate with and reassure the patient.
   a. "Talking down" involves understanding the process through which the patient is proceeding and helping the patient overcome fears while establishing contact with reality.
   b. Remind the patient that fear is common with this problem.
   c. Reassure the patient that they are not losing their mind but are experiencing the effect of drugs and that this will wear off.
   d. Instruct the patient to keep the eyes open; this reduces the intensity of reaction.
   e. Reduce sensory stimuli by minimizing noise, lights, movement, tactile stimulation.

(continued on page 2208)

TABLE 67-1	Emergency Management of Patients with Drug Overdose (continued)	
Drug	**Clinical Manifestations**	**Therapeutic Management**

		4. Sedate the patient as prescribed if hyperactivity cannot be controlled; diazepam or a barbiturate may be prescribed.
		5. Search for evidence of trauma; patients who use hallucinogens have a tendency to "act out" their hallucinations.
		6. Manage seizures with benzodiazepines (e.g., diazepam) as necessary.
		7. Observe patient closely; patient's behavior may become hazardous. Have safety officers stationed near the patient's room.
		8. Monitor for hypertensive crisis if patient has prolonged psychosis due to drug ingestion.
		9. Place patient in a protected environment under proper medical supervision to prevent self-inflicted bodily harm.
		Management for Phencyclidine Abuse
		1. Place patient in a calm, supportive environment to minimize stimuli; protect from self-injury.
		2. Avoid talking down.
		3. Do not leave patient unobserved. Treat symptoms as they occur.
		   a. Drug effects are unpredictable and prolonged.
		   b. Symptoms are likely to exacerbate; patient becomes out of control.
		4. Refer all patients in this category for psychiatric and drug evaluation/rehabilitation.

Drugs Producing Sedation, Intoxication, or Psychological and Physical Dependence (nonbarbiturate sedatives)		

diazepam
chlordiazepoxide
oxazepam
lorazepam
midazolam
flunitrazepam ("roofies," "date rape drug")[a]
	Seizures, coma, circulatory collapse, death
	Acute intoxication:
	• Respiratory depression
	• Decreasing mental alertness
	• Confusion
	• Slurred speech, decreased blood pressure
	• Ataxia
	• Pulmonary edema
	• Coma, death
	Flunitrazepam:
	• Disinhibition with antegrade amnesia
	• Weakness and unsteadiness with impaired judgment
	• Powerlessness
		1. Endotracheal tube is inserted as a precaution; use assisted ventilation to stabilize and correct respiratory depression. Observe for sudden apnea and laryngeal spasm.
		2. Assess for hypotension.
		   a. Insert indwelling urinary catheter for patient who is comatose; decreased urinary volume is an index of reduced renal flow associated with reduced intravascular volume or vascular collapse.
		   b. Start volume expansion with saline or dextrose as prescribed.
		3. Evacuate stomach contents; lavage (if within 1 h of ingestion); activated charcoal.
		4. Start ECG monitoring. Observe for arrhythmias.
		5. Administer flumazenil, a benzodiazepine antagonist (reversal agent).
		6. Refer patient for psychiatric evaluation (potential suicide intent).

Salicylate Poisoning Aspirin (present in compound analgesic tablets) • Toxic levels (150–200 mg/kg body weight) • Chronic toxicity (occurs in older adults due to decreased kidney function) • Long-term intoxication (>100 mg/kg/day for more than 2 days)	• Restlessness • Tinnitus, deafness • Blurring of vision • Hyperpnea • Hyperpyrexia • Sweating • Epigastric pain, vomiting • Dehydration • Respiratory alkalosis and metabolic acidosis • Disorientation, coma • Cardiovascular collapse • Coagulopathy	1. Treat respiratory depression. 2. Induce gastric emptying by lavage (if within 1 h after ingestion). 3. Give activated charcoal to adsorb aspirin. 4. Support patient with IV infusions as prescribed to establish hydration and correct electrolyte imbalances, including administration of sodium bicarbonate. 5. Enhance elimination of salicylates as directed by forced diuresis, alkalinization of urine, peritoneal dialysis, or hemodialysis, according to severity of intoxication. 6. Monitor serum salicylate level for efficacy of treatment. 7. Administer specific prescribed pharmacologic agent for bleeding and other problems. 8. Recognize that concretions formed in the gut may result in prolonged exposure as they are digested. 9. Refer patient for psychiatric evaluation (potential suicide intent). 10. Monitor thromboelastography for platelet function.

TABLE 67-1	Emergency Management of Patients with Drug Overdose (continued)	
Drug	**Clinical Manifestations**	**Therapeutic Management**
Acetaminophen (present in prescription and nonprescription analgesics, antipyretics, and cold remedies) • Toxic levels (≥140 mg/kg body weight)	Lethargy to encephalopathy and death GI upset, diaphoresis Right upper quadrant pain Abnormal liver function tests, prolonged prothrombin time, increased bilirubin, disseminated intravascular coagulation Hepatomegaly leading to liver failure Metabolic acidosis Hypoglycemia Stage I—within 24 h; GI irritation, possible metabolic acidosis and coma if severe ingestion Stage II—24–48 h; monitor liver and coagulation studies. Stage III—after 48 h; hepatic encephalopathy/jaundice, vomiting, right upper quadrant pain, coagulopathy, hypoglycemia, acute kidney injury	1. Maintain airway. 2. Obtain acetaminophen level. 3. Laboratory studies—liver function tests, prothrombin time/partial thromboplastin time, complete blood count, blood urea nitrogen, creatinine. 4. Lavage (if within 1 h after ingestion); activated charcoal. 5. Prepare for possible hemodialysis, which clears acetaminophen but does not halt liver damage. 6. Administer NAC as soon as possible. NAC replenishes essential liver enzymes and requires a total of 18 doses every 4 h. Charcoal absorbs NAC; do not administer together. Repeat NAC dose if patient vomits. 7. Refer patient for psychiatric evaluation (potential suicide intent).
Tricyclic Antidepressants amitriptyline doxepin nortriptyline imipramine	Arrhythmia: ventricular fibrillation/tachycardia, sinus tachycardia Hypotension Pulmonary edema, hypoxemia, acidosis Confusion, agitation, coma Visual hallucinations Clonus, tremors, hyperactive reflexes, nystagmus, myoclonic jerking Seizures Blurred vision, flushing, hyperthermia	1. Provide airway support, ventilation, cardiac monitoring; insert IV line with normal saline solution. 2. If within 1–2 h after overdose, insert a nasogastric tube and instill activated charcoal every 4 h × 3. 3. Administer a sodium bicarbonate drip to decrease arrhythmias; the alkaline environment increases the protein binding of the metabolite. Synchronized cardioversion may be indicated with some arrhythmias refractory to sodium bicarbonate. Torsades de pointes should be treated with IV magnesium sulfate. 4. Administer vasopressors. 5. Manage seizure activity with benzodiazepines (e.g., diazepam) as necessary. 6. Refer patient for psychiatric evaluation for potential suicide intent and evaluation of medication regimen for effectiveness.
Selective Serotonin Reuptake Inhibitors and Other Antidepressants trazodone fluoxetine paroxetine sertraline venlafaxine escitalopram bupropion	Decreased level of consciousness, confusion Respiratory depression Increased heart rate Serotonin syndrome may occur if the SSRI was taken in conjunction with dextromethorphan or meperidine Agitation, seizures Hyperthermia, diaphoresis Hypertension, headache, shivering, "goose flesh," cardiac arrhythmias, loss of consciousness	1. Administer activated charcoal with possibly whole bowel irrigation if a sustained-release medication was taken. 2. Use seizure precautions and administer benzodiazepines (e.g., diazepam) as prescribed.
Anabolic Steroids "roids," "juice," methandrostenolone, stanozolol, nandrolone Synthetic testosterone	Increase in LDL, decrease in HDL Alter carbohydrate metabolism Hyponatremia, hypokalemia Hypocalcemia/osteoporosis Mood swings/violent behaviors Invincibility, depression, potential for suicide attempts Memory loss, cognitive disability Immunosuppression Used to bulk up muscles, so skeletal muscle hypertrophy is a common manifestation.	1. Provide supportive therapy appropriate to patient's emotional manifestations. 2. Protect the patient from self-harm/harming others. 3. Encourage the patient to stop use; refer patient for psychiatric evaluation.

→, precedes; CNS, central nervous system; ECG, electrocardiogram; GI, gastrointestinal; HDL, high-density lipoprotein; IM, intramuscular; IV, intravenous; LDL, low-density lipoprotein; NAC, N-acetylcysteine; SSRI, selective serotonin reuptake inhibitor.
[a]Polydrug use at "rave clubs" frequently involves MDMA, alcohol, amphetamines, LSD, and sometimes dextromethorphan. Terms such as "Ecstasy" may refer to flunitrazepam, GHB, ephedrine, and/or caffeine, in addition to MDMA.
Adapted from Emergency Nurses Association (ENA). (2020a). *Sheehy's manual of emergency care* (8th ed.). St. Louis, MO: Mosby; Tintinalli, J. E., Stapczyski, J. S., Ma, O. J., et al. (2020). *Tintinalli's emergency medicine manual* (9th ed.). New York: McGraw-Hill Medical.

If drowsy, the patient should be allowed to sleep off the state of alcoholic intoxication. During this time, maintenance of a patent airway and observation for symptoms of CNS depression are essential. The patient should be kept warm with blankets. On the other hand, if the patient is noisy or belligerent, sedation may be necessary. If sedation is used, the patient should be monitored carefully for hypotension and decreased LOC.

In addition, the patient is examined for alcohol withdrawal delirium and for injuries and organic disease (such as head injury, seizures, pulmonary infections, hypoglycemia, and nutritional deficiencies) that may be masked by alcoholic intoxication. People with alcoholism suffer more injuries than the general population. Acute alcohol intoxication is the cause of trauma for many patients without alcoholism as well. Pulmonary infections are also more common in patients with alcoholism, resulting from respiratory depression, an impaired defense system, and a tendency toward aspiration of gastric contents. The patient may show little increase in temperature or WBC count. The patient may be hospitalized or admitted to a detoxification center in an effort to examine problems underlying SUD (ENA, 2020a).

Alcohol Withdrawal Syndrome

Alcohol withdrawal syndrome is an acute toxic state that occurs as a result of sudden cessation of alcohol intake after a bout of heavy drinking or, more typically, after prolonged intake of alcohol. Severity of symptoms depends on how much alcohol was ingested and for how long. Delirium tremens, the most severe form of alcohol withdrawal syndrome, may be precipitated by acute injury or infection (e.g., pneumonia, pancreatitis, hepatitis). Delirium tremens is a life-threatening condition and carries a high mortality rate if untreated (Moore, Fuehrlein, & Rosenheck, 2017).

Patients with alcohol withdrawal syndrome show signs of anxiety, uncontrollable fear, tremor, irritability, agitation, insomnia, and incontinence. Usually, all vital signs are elevated in the alcoholic toxic state. Approximately 5% of patients with alcohol withdrawal syndrome experience delirium tremens, which manifest with visual, tactile, olfactory, and auditory hallucinations that often are terrifying; the patient exhibits agitation. Autonomic overactivity occurs and is evidenced by tachycardia, hypertension, dilated pupils, hyperthermia, and profuse perspiration. Classically, delirium tremens commence within approximately 48 to 96 hours after the last drink of alcohol (Hoffman & Weinhouse, 2020).

The goals of management for alcohol withdrawal syndrome are to give adequate sedation and support to allow the patient to rest and recover without danger of injury or peripheral vascular collapse. A physical examination is performed to identify pre-existing or contributing illnesses or injuries (e.g., head injury, pneumonia). A drug history is obtained to elicit information that may facilitate adjustment of any sedative requirements. Baseline blood pressure is determined, because the patient's subsequent treatment may depend on blood pressure changes.

Usually, the patient is sedated as directed with a sufficient dosage of benzodiazepines to establish and maintain sedation, which reduces agitation, prevents exhaustion, prevents seizures, and promotes sleep. The patient should be calm, able to respond, and able to maintain an airway safely on their own. A variety of medications and combinations of medications are used (e.g., chlordiazepoxide, lorazepam, and clonidine). Haloperidol, esmolol, or midazolam may be given for delirium tremens. Dosages are adjusted according to the patient's symptoms (agitation, anxiety) and blood pressure response (ENA, 2020a).

The patient is placed in a calm, nonstressful environment (usually a private room) and observed closely. The room remains lighted to minimize the potential for illusions (visual misrepresentations) and hallucinations. Homicidal or suicidal responses may result from hallucinations. Closet and bathroom doors are closed to eliminate shadows. A staff member is designated to stay with the patient as much as possible. The presence of another person has a reassuring and calming effect, which helps the patient maintain contact with reality. To orient the patient to reality, any illusions are explained.

> ### ▶ Quality and Safety Nursing Alert
>
> *Restraints are used as prescribed, if necessary, if the patient is aggressive or violent, but only when other alternatives have been unsuccessful. The patient who is restrained must be watched continuously on a one-on-one basis by an ED staff member. The least restrictive device that will prevent injury to the patient or others is used. Caution is taken to ensure that restraints are applied properly and that they are not impairing circulation to any part of the patient's body or interfering with respirations. Restraints should be used in tandem with verbal intervention to calm the patient and promote adherence. Restraints must be released according to protocol. Physical observation (e.g., skin integrity, circulatory status, respiratory status) is ongoing, and the patient's response is documented.*

Fluid losses may result from GI losses (vomiting), profuse perspiration, and hyperventilation. In addition, the patient may be dehydrated as a result of alcohol's effect of decreasing antidiuretic hormone. The oral or IV route is used to restore fluid and electrolyte balance.

Temperature, pulse, respiration, and blood pressure are recorded frequently (every 30 minutes with delirium tremens) to monitor for peripheral circulatory collapse or hyperthermia (the two most serious complications).

Frequently seen complications include infections (e.g., pneumonia), trauma, hepatic failure, hypoglycemia, and cardiovascular problems. Hypoglycemia may accompany alcohol withdrawal syndrome because alcohol depletes liver glycogen stores and impairs gluconeogenesis; many patients with alcoholism also are malnourished. Parenteral dextrose may be prescribed if the liver glycogen level is depleted. Orange juice, sports drinks, or other sources of carbohydrates are given to stabilize the blood glucose level and counteract tremulousness. Supplemental vitamin therapy and a high-protein diet are provided as prescribed to counteract nutritional deficits. The patient should be referred to an alcoholic treatment center for follow-up care and rehabilitation.

VIOLENCE, ABUSE, AND NEGLECT

EDs are often the first place where victims of family violence, abuse, or neglect go to seek help.

Family Violence, Abuse, and Neglect

In the United States, about 1 in 4 women and nearly 1 in 10 men have experienced sexual violence, physical violence, and/or stalking by an intimate partner during their lifetime. Over 43 million women and 38 million men have experienced psychological aggression by an intimate partner (CDC, 2019c). IPV may include physical violence, sexual violence, stalking, psychological aggression, neglect, financial abuse, or intimidation by a former or intimate partner (ENA, 2018b). It is important to recognize that IPV does occur in all cultures and populations; these may include teenagers, older adults, and heterosexual, transgender, and same sex couples (ENA, 2018b).

Those who have been subjected to IPV have significantly higher rates of visits to the ED than the general population. Because patients subjected to IPV often have contact first with nurses in the health care system, ED nurses must be vigilant in their assessments of both women and men who present with injuries that may be consistent with IPV (Herzog, Maina, & Maposa, 2019). In addition, ED nurses must be aware that men and women with disability are at higher risk of domestic violence and abuse than people without disability and should include questions that screen for IPV in their evaluations (see Chapter 50, Chart 50-3).

Gerontologic Considerations

It is estimated that more than 1 in 10 adults 70 years or older (14%) have been abused or neglected, a type of IPV called *elder abuse* (Rosay & Mulford, 2017). The majority of elder abuse is perpetrated by family members (National Center on Elder Abuse, 2017). Elder abuse takes many forms, including physical, sexual, emotional, and verbal abuse; neglect; violation of personal rights; abandonment; and financial abuse (ENA, 2020a).

Clinical Manifestations

When people who have been abused seek treatment, they may present with physical injuries or health problems such as anxiety, insomnia, or GI symptoms related to stress. The possibility of IPV should be investigated whenever a person presents with multiple injuries that are in various stages of healing, when injuries are unexplained, and when the explanation does not fit the physical picture (see Chart 67-8). The possibility of neglect should be investigated whenever a person who is dependent shows evidence of inattention to hygiene, to nutrition, or to know medical needs (e.g., unfilled medication prescriptions, missed appointments with health care providers). In the ED, the most common physical injuries seen are unexplained bruises, lacerations, abrasions, head injuries, or fractures. The most common clinical manifestations of neglect are malnutrition and dehydration (ENA, 2020a).

Assessment and Diagnostic Findings

Nurses in EDs are in an ideal position to provide early detection and interventions for victims of IPV. This requires an acute awareness of the signs of possible IPV, including abuse, maltreatment, and neglect. Nurses must be skilled in interviewing techniques that are likely to elicit accurate

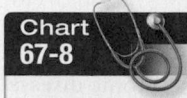

Chart 67-8

ASSESSMENT

Assessing for Abuse, Maltreatment, and Neglect

The following questions may be helpful when assessing a patient for abuse, maltreatment, and neglect:

- I noticed that you have a number of bruises. Can you tell me how they happened? Has anyone hurt you?
- You seem frightened. Has anyone ever hurt you?
- Patients sometimes tell me that they have been hurt by someone at home or at work. Could this be happening to you?
- Are you afraid of anyone at home or work, or of anyone with whom you come in contact?
- Has anyone failed to help you to take care of yourself when you needed help?
- Has anyone prevented you from seeing friends or other people whom you wish to see?
- Have you signed any papers that you did not understand or did not wish to sign?
- Has anyone forced you to sign papers against your will?
- Has anyone forced you to engage in sexual activities within the past year?
- Has anyone prevented you from using an assistive device (e.g., wheelchair, walker) within the past year?
- Has anyone you depend on refused to help you take your medicine, bathe, groom, or eat within the past year?

information. A careful history is crucial in the screening process. Asking questions in private—away from others—may be helpful in eliciting information about abuse, maltreatment, and neglect. Nurses need to be aware that women may withhold directly answering questions regarding IPV in fear of retaliation, loss of children, and retribution against the children (Herzog et al., 2019).

Whenever evidence leads the nurse to suspect abuse or neglect, an evaluation with careful documentation of descriptions of events and drawings or photographs of injuries is important, because the medical record may be used as part of a legal proceeding. Assessment of the patient's general appearance and interactions with significant others, an examination of the entire surface area of the body, and a mental status examination are crucial.

Management

The aims of IPV screening include earlier identification of patients who have been abused and prevention of continued abusive events, including homicide (ENA, 2018b). Whenever abuse, maltreatment, or neglect is suspected, the health care provider's main concern should be the safety and welfare of the patient. Treatment focuses on the consequences of the abuse, violence, or neglect and on prevention of further injury. Protocols of most EDs require that a multidisciplinary approach be used. Nurses, physicians, social workers, and community agencies work collaboratively to develop and implement a plan for meeting the patient's needs.

If the patient is in immediate danger, they should be separated from the person who is abusive or neglectful whenever possible. Referral to a shelter may be the most appropriate action, but many shelters are inaccessible to people with mobility limitations.

When abuse or neglect is the result of stress experienced by a caregiver who is no longer able to cope with the burden of caring for an older adult or a person with chronic disease or a disability, respite services may be necessary. Support groups may be helpful to these caregivers. When mental illness of the person who is abusive or neglectful is responsible for the situation, alternative living arrangements may be required.

Nurses must be mindful that competent adults are free to accept or refuse the help that is offered to them. Some patients insist on remaining in the home environment where the abuse or neglect is occurring. The wishes of patients who are competent and not cognitively impaired should be respected. However, all possible alternatives, available resources, and safety plans should be explored with the patient.

Mandatory reporting laws in most states require health care workers to report suspected abuse of children or older adults to an official agency, usually Child or Adult Protective Services. All that is required for reporting is the suspicion of abuse; the health care worker is not required to prove abuse or neglect. Likewise, health care workers who report suspected abuse are immune from civil or criminal liability if the report is made in good faith. Subsequent home visits resulting from the report of suspected abuse are a part of gathering information about the patient in the home environment. In addition, many states have resource hotlines for use by health care workers and by patients who seek answers to questions about abuse and neglect (ENA, 2020a).

Sexual Assault

The definition of *rape* is forced sexual acts, especially if these acts involve vaginal or anal penetration. Attempted rape may include verbal threats of rape (ENA, 2020a). Perpetrators and victims may be either male or female. Rape crisis centers offer support and education and help people who have been sexually assaulted through the subsequent police investigation and courtroom experience.

The manner in which the patient is received and treated in the ED is important to their future psychological well-being. Crisis intervention should begin when the patient enters the health care facility. The patient should be seen immediately. Most hospitals have a written protocol that addresses the patient's physical and emotional needs as well as collection of forensic evidence.

In many states, the emergency nurse has the opportunity to become trained as a sexual assault nurse examiner (SANE). Preparing for this role requires specific training in forensic evidence collection, history taking, documentation, and ways to approach the patient and family. Specialized training also includes learning proper photographic methods and the use of colposcopy. Colposcopy facilitates assessment by magnifying tissues and looking for evidence of microtrauma. Evidence is collected through photography, videography, and analysis of specimens. Another tool useful to the SANE is the light-staining microscope, which enables the examiner to identify motile and nonmotile sperm and infectious organisms. This tool saves time and also enhances assessment. The SANE complements the ED staff and can spend more time with both the patient and police officers investigating the incident (ENA, 2020a).

Assessment and Diagnostic Findings

The patient's reaction to rape has been termed *rape trauma syndrome* and is seen as an acute stress reaction to a life-threatening situation. The nurse performing the assessment is aware that the patient may go through several phases of psychological reactions, which have been described as follows (ENA, 2020a):

- An acute disorganization phase, which may manifest as an expressed state in which shock, disbelief, fear, guilt, humiliation, anger, and other such emotions are encountered or as a controlled state in which feelings are masked or hidden and the victim appears composed.
- A phase of denial and unwillingness to talk about the incident, followed by a phase of heightened anxiety, fear, flashbacks, sleep disturbances, hyperalertness, and psychosomatic reactions that is consistent with PTSD (see later discussion).
- A phase of reorganization, in which the incident is put into perspective. Some victims never fully recover and go on to develop chronic stress disorders and phobias.

Management

The goals of management are to provide support, to reduce the patient's emotional trauma, and to gather available evidence for possible legal proceedings. All of the interventions are aimed at encouraging the patient to gain a sense of control over their life.

Throughout the patient's stay in the ED, the patient's privacy and sensitivity must be respected. The patient may exhibit a wide range of emotional reactions, such as hysteria, stoicism, or feelings of being overwhelmed. Support and caring are crucial. The patient should be reassured that anxiety is natural and asked whether a person who can provide support may be called. Appropriate support is available from professional and community resources. The National Sexual Assault Hotline (see the Resources section, under the Rape, Abuse, and Incest National Network) will automatically route the patient to the nearest assault or crisis intervention center for services, as needed. The patient should never be left alone.

Physical Examination

A written, witnessed informed consent must be obtained from the patient (or parent or guardian if the patient is a minor) for examination, for taking of photographs, and for release of findings to police. A history is obtained only if the patient has not already talked to a police officer, social worker, or crisis intervention worker. The patient should not be asked to repeat the history. Any history of the event that is obtained should be recorded in the patient's own words. The patient is asked whether they have bathed, douched, brushed their teeth, changed clothes, urinated, or defecated since the attack, because these actions may alter interpretation of subsequent findings. The time of admission, time of examination, date and time of the alleged rape, and the patient's emotional state and general appearance (including any evidence of trauma, such as discoloration, bruises, lacerations, secretions, or torn and bloody clothing) are documented. If the patient has no recollection of the event, drugs that induce retrograde amnesia may have been involved, such as alcohol, ketamine, gamma-hydroxybutyrate, benzodiazepines, or fluni-trazepam. Urine drug test must be completed within 96 hours of the event to capture the presence of these drugs. Emesis can also be collected for testing (ENA, 2020a).

For the physical examination, the patient is helped to undress and is draped properly. Each item of clothing is placed in a separate paper bag. As noted previously, plastic bags are not used in order to avoid possible destruction of evidence from mold or mildew formation. The bags are labeled and given to appropriate law enforcement authorities.

The patient is examined (from head to toe) for injuries, especially injuries to the head, neck, breasts, thighs, back, and buttocks. Body diagrams and photographs aid in documenting the evidence of trauma. The physical examination focuses on the following:

- External evidence of trauma (bruises, contusions, lacerations, stab wounds)
- Dried semen stains (appearing as crusted, flaking areas) on the patient's body or clothes
- Broken fingernails and body tissue and foreign materials under nails (if found, samples are taken)
- Oral examination, including a specimen of saliva and cultures of gum and tooth areas

Pelvic and rectal examinations are also performed. The perineum and other areas are examined with a Wood lamp or other filtered ultraviolet light. Areas that appear fluorescent may indicate semen stains. The color and consistency of any discharge present is noted. A water-moistened, rather than lubricated, vaginal speculum is used for the examination. Lubricant contains chemicals that may interfere with later forensic testing of specimens and acid phosphatase determinations. The rectum is examined for signs of trauma, blood, and semen. During the examination, the patient should be advised of the nature and necessity of each procedure and given the rationale for each (ENA, 2020a).

Specimen Collection

During the physical examination, numerous laboratory specimens may be collected, including the following:

- Vaginal aspirate, examined for presence or absence of motile and nonmotile sperm.
- Secretions (obtained with a sterile swab) from the vaginal pool for acid phosphatase, blood group antigen of semen, and precipitin test against human sperm and blood.
- Separate smears from the oral, vaginal, and anal areas.
- Culture of body orifices for gonorrhea.
- Blood serum for syphilis and HIV testing and deoxyribonucleic acid (DNA) analysis. A sample of serum for syphilis may be frozen and saved for future testing.
- Pregnancy test if there is a possibility that the female patient may be pregnant.
- Any foreign material (leaves, grass, dirt), which is placed in a clean envelope.
- Pubic hair samples obtained by combing or trimming. Several pubic hairs with follicles are placed in separate containers and identified as the patient's hair.

To preserve the chain of evidence, each specimen is labeled with the name of the patient, the date and time of collection, the body area from which the specimen was obtained, and the names of personnel collecting specimens. The specimens are then given to a designated person (e.g., crime laboratory technician), and an itemized receipt is obtained (ENA, 2020a).

Treating Potential Consequences of Rape

After the initial physical examination is completed and specimens have been obtained, any associated injuries are treated as indicated. The patient is given the option of prophylaxis against sexually transmitted infections (STIs) (also referred to as sexually transmitted disease [STDs]). Ceftriaxone given intramuscularly with 1% lidocaine may be prescribed as prophylaxis for gonorrhea. In addition, a single oral dose of metronidazole and either a single oral dose of azithromycin or a 7-day oral regimen of doxycycline may be prescribed as prophylaxis for syphilis and chlamydia (ENA, 2020a).

Antipregnancy measures may be considered if the patient is a female of childbearing age. A postcoital contraceptive medication, such as an oral contraceptive medication that contains levonorgestrel and ethinyl estradiol, may be prescribed after a pregnancy test. To promote effectiveness, the contraceptive medication should be given within 12 to 24 hours and no later than 72 hours after penile-vaginal intercourse. The 21-day package is prescribed so that the patient does not mistakenly take the inert tablets included in the 28-day package. An antiemetic agent may be given as prescribed to decrease discomfort from side effects. A cleansing douche, mouthwash, and fresh clothing are usually offered.

Follow-Up Care

The patient is informed of counseling services to prevent long-term psychological effects. Counseling services should be made available to both the patient and the family. A referral is made to the National Sexual Assault Hotline (see the Resources section) or directly to a local crisis intervention center. Appointments for follow-up surveillance for pregnancy and for STI and HIV testing also are made (ENA, 2020a).

The patient is encouraged to return to their previous level of functioning as soon as possible. When leaving the ED, the patient should be accompanied by a family member or friend.

Human Trafficking

Human trafficking is a type of modern-day slavery and one of the fastest growing global health issues. Human trafficking is defined as the exploitation of individuals with the use of force, fraud, coercion, or deception (ENA, 2018c; Roney & Villano, 2020). In 2016, an estimated 40.3 million people were trafficked; 1 in 4 of these were children, with nearly 25 million people involved in forced labor (ENA, 2018c). In the United States in 2018, over 23,078 contacts used the National Human Trafficking Hotline, which was a 25% increase compared to 2017 (Polaris Project, National Human Trafficking Hotline, 2018). People subjected to human trafficking have limited access to health care, and the ED may be the only access point to identify their situation (ENA, 2018c).

A victim of trafficking may present to the ED with injury, accompanied by a significantly older boyfriend or travel partner. The victim may have a history of being a chronic runaway, or of homelessness, and of self-mutilation. Common behaviors exhibited by these patients may include cowering or deferring to the person accompanying them, who may appear controlling, and appearing frightened or agitated. The patient may have a special mark/tattoo present, poor dentition, and multiple injuries in various stages of healing. Common physical complaints include injuries, poor healing or poorly healed old injuries, abdominal pain, dizziness, headaches, rashes, or sores. Patients may demonstrate addiction, panic attacks, impulse control, hostility, and suicidal ideation (Roney & Villano, 2020).

The ED nurse may be well positioned to offer an opportunity for the patient to speak, alone without an accompanying companion, who could be a perpetrator of abuse. Targeted, appropriate questions may include asking patients if they are in control of their own money; whether or not they are able to come and go as they please; and who is the person or persons accompanying them (ENA, 2020a). Patients may decline assistance. The National Human Trafficking Hotline may be tapped into as a resource (see the Resources section).

PSYCHIATRIC EMERGENCIES

A psychiatric emergency is an urgent, serious disturbance of behavior, affect, or thought that makes the patient unable to cope with life situations and interpersonal relationships. A patient presenting with a psychiatric emergency may display overactive or violent, underactive or depressed, or suicidal behaviors.

The most important concern of the ED personnel is determining whether the patient is at risk for injuring self or others. The aim is to try to maintain the patient's self-esteem (and life, if necessary) while providing care. Determining whether the patient is under psychiatric care is important so that contact can be made with the therapist or provider who works with the patient.

Patients Who Are Overactive

Patients who display disturbed, uncooperative, and paranoid behavior and those who feel anxious and panicky may be prone to assaultive and destructive impulses and abnormal social behavior. Intense nervousness, depression, and crying are evident in some patients. Disturbed and noisy behavior may be exacerbated or compounded by alcohol or drug intoxication.

A reliable source for obtaining an accurate history is needed to identify events leading to the crisis. Past mental illness, hospitalizations, injuries, serious illnesses, the use of alcohol or drugs, crises in interpersonal relationships, or intrapsychic conflicts are explored. Because abnormal thoughts and behavior may be manifestations of an underlying physical disorder, such as hypoglycemia, drug or alcohol toxicity, a stroke, a seizure disorder, or head injury, a physical assessment is also performed.

The immediate goal is to gain control of the situation. If the patient is potentially violent, security or police should be nearby. Restraints are used as a last resort and only as prescribed. Approaching the patient with a composed, confident, and firm manner is therapeutic and has a calming effect. Helpful interventions include the following:

- Introduce yourself by name.
- Tell the patient, "I am here to help you."
- Repeat the patient's name from time to time.
- Speak in one-thought sentences, and be consistent.
- Give the patient space and time to slow down.
- Show interest in, listen to, and encourage the patient to talk about personal thoughts and feelings.
- Offer appropriate and honest explanations.

A psychotropic agent (e.g., one that exerts an effect on the mind) may be prescribed for emergency management of functional psychosis. However, a patient with a personality disorder should not be treated with psychotropic medications, and psychotropic medications should not be used if the patient's behavior results from the use of hallucinogens (e.g., lysergic acid diethylamide [LSD]).

Agents such as chlorpromazine and haloperidol act specifically against psychotic symptoms of thought fragmentation and perceptual and behavioral aberrations. The initial dose depends on the patient's body weight and the severity of the symptoms. After administration of the initial dose, the patient is observed closely to determine the degree of change in psychotic behavior. Subsequent doses depend on the patient's response. Typically, after stabilization, the patient is transferred to an inpatient psychiatric unit, or psychiatric outpatient treatment is arranged (ENA, 2020a).

Patients with Posttraumatic Stress Disorder (PTSD)

PTSD is the development of characteristic symptoms after a psychologically stressful event that is considered outside the range of normal human experience (e.g., rape, combat, motor vehicle crash, natural catastrophe, terrorist attack). Symptoms of this disorder include intrusive thoughts and dreams, phobic avoidance reaction (avoidance of activities that arouse recollection of the traumatic event), heightened vigilance, exaggerated startle reaction, generalized anxiety, and societal withdrawal. PTSD may be acute, chronic, or delayed. PTSD often presents as multiple readmissions to the ED for minor or recurring complaints without evidence of injury.

Veterans Considerations

Veterans are known to be at heightened risk of PTSD, particularly if they served in combat situations. It is estimated that between 11% and 20% of veterans who served during Operation Iraqi Freedom (2003–2011) and Operation Enduring Freedom (2001–2014) have had PTSD symptoms in a given year. Furthermore, 12% of veterans who served during the Persian Gulf War (1991) have had PTSD symptoms in a given year, while approximately 30% of veterans who served during the Vietnam War (1962–1973) have had PTSD symptoms at some point in their lifetime. In addition, veterans of any era may have been subjected to sexual assault or sexual harassment during their time in service, which may have resulted in military sexual trauma (MST), a specific type of PTSD. Approximately 23% of female veterans have been sexually assaulted while serving, while 55% of female veterans and 38% of male veterans have been subjected to sexual harassment while serving. In response to these statistics, the U.S. Department of Veterans Affairs (DVA) has sponsored a National Center for PTSD, which provides resources and hotlines to help veterans effectively deal with the effects of PTSD (see the Resources section) (DVA, 2020).

Patients Who Are Underactive or Depressed

In the ED, depression may be seen as the main condition bringing the patient to the health care facility, or it may be masked by anxiety and somatic complaints. The person who is depressed has a mood disturbance. Any patient who is depressed may be at risk for suicide. Most suicide attempts are expressions of extreme distress, not bids for attention (ENA, 2020a).

The patient must be screened regarding any attempts or thoughts of suicide. Questions such as "Have you ever thought about taking your own life?" may be helpful. In general, the patient is relieved to have an opportunity to discuss personal feelings. The emergency nurse's responsibility when caring for a patient with depression is to maintain a high suspicion for the diagnosis, especially for those populations at risk (see following discussion) (ENA, 2020a).

Patients Who Are Suicidal

Attempted suicide is an act that stems from depression (e.g., loss of a loved one, loss of body integrity or status, poor self-image) and can be viewed as a cry for help and intervention. Males are at greater risk of successfully committing suicide than females, who attempt suicide more often (ENA, 2020a). Others at risk are older adults; young adults; people who are enduring unusual loss or stress; those who are unemployed, divorced, widowed, or living alone; those showing signs of significant depression (e.g., weight loss, sleep disturbances, somatic complaints, suicidal preoccupation); and those with a history of a previous suicide attempt, suicide in the family, or psychiatric illness.

Being aware of people at risk and assessing for specific factors that predispose a person to suicide are key management strategies. Specific signs and symptoms of potential suicide include the following:

- Communication of suicidal intent, such as preoccupation with death or speaking of someone else's suicide (e.g., "I'm tired of living." "I've put my affairs in order." "I'm better off dead." "I'm a burden to my family.")
- History of a previous suicide attempt, with risk being much greater in these cases
- Family history of suicide
- Loss of a parent at an early age
- Specific plan for suicide
- A means to carry out the plan

Emergency management focuses on treating the consequences of the suicide attempt (e.g., gunshot wound, drug overdose) and preventing further self-injury. A patient who has made a suicidal attempt may do so again. Crisis intervention is used to determine suicidal potential, to discover areas of depression and conflict, to find out about the patient's support system, and to determine whether hospitalization or psychiatric referral is necessary. Depending on the patient's potential for suicide, the patient may be admitted to the intensive care unit, referred for follow-up care, or admitted to the psychiatric unit.

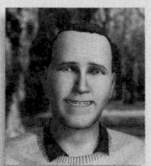
CRITICAL THINKING EXERCISES

1 `ebp` A 48-year-old male arrived in the ED via ambulance. EMS personnel report that the patient was fishing when his boat overturned in a lake. He was in the water for at least 15 minutes before someone was able to get to him. The patient was initially unresponsive but was resuscitated by EMS en route to the hospital. His current body temperature is 34°C (93°F). What evidence-based interventions, including methods of rewarming, are indicated? What additional supportive care will be required? Explain the rationale and levels of support for these methods of treatment.

2 `ipc` A 19-year-old female college student arrives in the ED accompanied by her friend. She had just been at a party and states an acquaintance she knew forced her to have intercourse against her will. She is tearful and shaking and she appears to have some visible bruising. What priority nursing actions should be taken? What resources will need to be utilized in her care? Who should be consulted for the patient and what type of consent must she provide? Detail the steps that will be taken as you begin to care for this patient. What follow-up care will this patient need?

3 `pq` A 32-year-old female was brought to the ED by her fiancé. He states he had been working on a faulty hot water heater in the basement most of the day; when he came upstairs, the patient voiced complaints of a headache that had begun about 2 hours ago. He brought her to the ED when she began to complain of dizziness, palpitations, and she seemed to become increasingly confused. What questions would you include in your assessment? Explain the management of this patient and additional care that would be required. What concerns would you have for her fiancé?

REFERENCES

*Asterisk indicates nursing research.

Books

American College of Surgeons. (2018). *Advanced trauma life support* (10th ed.). Chicago, IL: Author.

Atanelov, Z., & Rebstock, S. E. (2020) Nasopharyngeal airway. *StatPearls [Internet]*. Treasure Island, FL: StatPearls Publishing. Retrieved on 4/6/2020 at: www.ncbi.nlm.nih.gov/books/NBK513220/

Emergency Nurses Association (ENA). (2017). *Emergency nursing scope and standards of practice* (2nd ed.). Des Plaines, IL: Author.

Emergency Nurses Association (ENA). (2020a). *Sheehy's manual of emergency care* (7th ed.). St. Louis, MO: Mosby.

Holleran, R., Wolfe, A., & Frakes, M. (2018). *Patient transport: Principles & practice* (5th ed.). St. Louis, MO: Elsevier.

Tintinalli, J. E., Stapczyski, J. S., Ma, O. J., et al. (2020). *Tintinalli's emergency medicine manual* (9th ed.). New York: McGraw-Hill Medical.

Veenema, T. G. (2019). *Disaster nursing and emergency preparedness* (4th ed.). New York: Springer.

Journals and Electronic Documents

American College of Emergency Physicians (ACEP). (2017). Alcohol screening in the emergency department. Retrieved on 4/13/2020 at: www.acep.org/patient-care/policy-statements/alcohol-screening-in-the-emergency-department/

American Psychiatric Nurses Association. (2020). Managing stress and self-care during COVID-19: Information for nurses. Retrieved on 6/30/2020 at: www.apna.org/i4a/pages/index.cfm?pageid=6685

Atias-Varon, D., Sherman, H., Yanovich, R., et al. (2017). Rhabdomyolysis after crawling military training. *Military Medicine, 182*(7), e1948–e1952.

Bosson, N., & Gordon, G. (2018). Laryngeal mask airway. *Medscape*. Retrieved on 4/6/2020 at: emedicine.medscape.com/article/82527-overview

Centers for Disease Control and Prevention (CDC) National Center for Health Statistics. (2017a). Emergency department visits, data for the US. Retrieved on 4/6/2020 at: www.cdc.gov/nchs/fastats/emergency-department.htm

Centers for Disease Control and Prevention (CDC). (2017b). Emergency department visits for injury and illness among adults aged 65 and over: United States, 2012–2013. *NCHS Data Brief, 272*. Retrieved on 3/6/2020 at: www.cdc.gov/nchs/products/databriefs/db272.htm

Centers for Disease Control and Prevention (CDC) National Institute for Occupational Safety and Health. (2019a). Workplace violence prevention for nurses. CDC Course No. WB2908- NIOSH Pub. No. 2013-155. Retrieved on 4/3/2020 at: www.cdc.gov/niosh/topics/violence/training_nurses.html

Centers for Disease Control and Prevention (CDC). (2019b). Natural disasters and severe weather. Prevent hypothermia and frostbite. Retrieved on 7/3/2020 at: www.cdc.gov/disasters/winter/staysafe/hypothermia.html

Centers for Disease Control and Prevention (CDC). (2019c). Violence prevention. Retrieved on 4/13/2020 at: www.cdc.gov/violenceprevention/intimatepartnerviolence/fastfact.html

Centers for Disease Control and Prevention (CDC). (2020a). Interim infection prevention and control recommendations for healthcare personnel during the coronavirus disease 2019 (COVID-19) pandemic. Retrieved on 7/3/2020 at: www.cdc.gov/coronavirus/2019-ncov/hcp/infection-control-recommendations.html

Centers for Disease Control and Prevention (CDC). (2020b). Proper N95 respirator use for respiratory protection preparedness. Retrieved on 6/30/2020 at: blogs.cdc.gov/niosh-science-blog/2020/03/16/n95-preparedness/

Centers for Disease Control and Prevention (CDC). (2020c). Coronavirus 2019 (COVID-19). Screening and triage at intake. Screening dialysis patients for COVID-19. Retrieved on 7/3/2020 at: www.cdc.gov/coronavirus/2019-ncov/hcp/dialysis/screening.html

Copeland, D., & Henry, M. (2017). Workplace violence and perceptions of safety among emergency department staff members: Experiences, expectations, tolerance, reporting, and recommendations. *Journal of Trauma Nursing, 24*(2), 65–77.

Cornelius, B., Campbell, R., & McGauly, P. (2017). Tourniquets in trauma care: A review of application. *Journal of Trauma Nursing, 24*(3), 203–207.

Cortez, R. (2018). Geriatric trauma protocol. *Journal of Trauma Nursing, 25*(4), 218–226.

Crawford, C. C. (2019). Addition of advanced practice registered nurses to the trauma team: An integrative systematic review of literature. *Journal of Trauma Nursing, 26*(3), 141–146.

Dehli, T., Uleberg, O., & Wisborg, T. (2018). Trauma team activation—common rules, common gain. *Acta Anaesthesiologica Scandinavica, 62*(2), 144–146.

Emergency Nurses Association (ENA). (2018a). Position statement: Triage qualifications and competency. Retrieved on 4/1/2020 at: www.ena.org/docs/default-source/resource-library/practice-resources/position-statements/triagequalificationscompetency

Emergency Nurses Association (ENA). (2018b). Joint position statement: Intimate partner violence. Retrieved on 4/13/2020 at: www.ena.org/docs/default-source/resource-library/practice-resources/position-statements/joint-statements/intimatepartnerviolence.pdf?sfvrsn=4cdd3d4d_8

Emergency Nurses Association (ENA). (2018c). Position statement. Human trafficking awareness in the emergency care setting. Retrieved on 4/14/2020 at: www.ena.org/docs/default-source/resource-library/practice-resources/position-statements/humantraffickingpatientawareness.pdf?sfvrsn=cd0ad835_14

Emergency Nurses Association (ENA). (2019). Emergency nursing interface with mobile integrated health (MIH) and community paramedicine (CP) programs position statement. Retrieved on 4/6/2020 at: www.ena.org/docs/default-source/resource-library/practice-resources/position-statements/interfacemihandcp.pdf?sfvrsn=16bec1ae_14

Emergency Nurses Association (ENA). (2020b). ENA statement on emergency nurse protection during COVID-19 pandemic. Retrieved on 7/29/2020 at: www.ena.org/press-room/2020/03/27/ena-statement-on-emergency-nurse-protection-during-covid-19-pandemic

Hart, J. L., Turnbull, A. E., Oppenheim, I. M., et al. (2020). Family-centered care during the COVID-19 era. *Journal of Pain and Symptom Management, 60*(2), e93–e97.

*Herzog, T., Maina, G., & Maposa, S. (2019). Translating clinical experience into action: Developing an educational protocol to improve intimate partner violence screening by emergency department nurses. *Canadian Journal of Emergency Nursing, 42*(1), 12–15.

Higginson, R. (2018). Causes of hypothermia and the use of patient-rewarming techniques. *The British Journal of Nursing, 27*(21), 1222–1224.

Hoffman, R. S., & Weinhouse, G. L. (2020). Management of moderate and severe alcohol withdrawal syndromes. *UpToDate*. Retrieved on 9/27/2020 at: www.uptodate.com/contents/management-of-moderate-and-severe-alcohol-withdrawal-syndromes

Mayo Clinic. (2019). Frostbite, diagnosis and treatment. Retrieved on 4/10/2020 at: www.mayoclinic.org/diseases-conditions/frostbite/diagnosis-treatment/drc-20372661

Moore, D. T., Fuehrlein, B. S., & Rosenheck, R. A. (2017). Delirium tremens and alcohol withdrawal nationally in the Veterans Health Administration. *The American Journal on Addictions, 26*(7), 722–730.

National Center on Elder Abuse. (2017). Statistics and data. Retrieved on 4/13/2020 at: ncea.acl.gov/What-We-Do/Research/Statistics-and-Data.aspx#perpetrators

National Institute on Drug Abuse; Advancing Addiction Science. (2018). Synthetic cannabinoids (K2/Spice). Retrieved on 4/13/2020 at: www.drugabuse.gov/publications/drugfacts/synthetic-cannabinoids-k2spice

National Institute on Drug Abuse; Advancing Addiction Science. (2019). Marijuana. Retrieved on 4/13/2020 at: www.drugabuse.gov/publications/drugfacts/marijuana#mjextracts

National Institute on Drug Abuse; Advancing Addiction Science. (2020). Inhalants. Retrieved on 4/13/2020 at: www.drugabuse.gov/publications/drugfacts/inhalants

Nicks, B., McGinnism, H., Borron, S., et al. (2018). Acute lactic acidosis. *Medscape*. Retrieved on 4/10/2020 at: emedicine.medscape.com/article/768159-overview

Ocak, U., & Avsarogullari, L. (2019). Expectations and needs of relatives of critically ill patients in the emergency department. *Hong Kong Journal of Emergency Medicine, 26*(6), 328–335.

Parenteau, M., Stockinger, Z., Hughes, S., et al. (2018). Drowning management. *Military Medicine, 183*(suppl_2), 172–179.

Polaris Project, National Human Trafficking Hotline. (2018). Statistics. Retrieved on 4/14/2020 at: humantraffickinghotline.org/sites/default/files/Polaris_National_Hotline_2018_Statistics_Fact_Sheet.pdf

Richardson, S., & Harris, S. (2018). Managing the bariatric patient in the ED setting. *Emergency Nurse New Zealand*, November, P9–P15.

Roney, L. N., & Villano, C. E. (2020). Recognizing victims of a hidden crime: Human trafficking victims in your pediatric trauma bay. *Journal of Trauma Nursing*, 27(1), 37–41.

Rosay, A. B., & Mulford, C. F. (2017). Prevalence estimates and correlates of elder abuse in the United States: The national intimate partner and sexual violence survey. *Journal of Elder Abuse and Neglect*, 29(1), 1–14.

Rui, P., & Kang, K. (2017). National Hospital Ambulatory Medical Care Survey: 2017 emergency department summary tables. National Center for Health Statistics. Retrieved on 4/21/2020 at: www.cdc.gov/nchs/data/nhamcs/web_tables/2017_ed_web_tables-508.pdf

*Saqe-Rockoff, A., Schubert, F. D., Ciardiello, A., et al. (2018). Improving thermoregulation for trauma patients in the emergency department: An evidence-based practice project. *Journal of Trauma Nursing*, 25(1), 14–20.

Schmidt, M., & Haglund, K. (2017). Debrief in emergency departments to improve compassion fatigue and promote resiliency. *Journal of Trauma Nursing*, 24(5), 317–322.

*Soontorn, T., Sitthimongkol, Y., Thosingha, O., et al. (2018). Factors influencing the accuracy of triage by registered nurses in trauma patients. *Pacific Rim International Journal of Nursing Research*, 22(2), 120–130.

The Joint Commission. (2020). Sentinel event policy and procedures. Retrieved on 4/6/2020 at: www.jointcommission.org/resources/patient-safety-topics/sentinel-event/sentinel-event-policy-and-procedures/

Toronto, C. E., & LaRocco, S. A. (2019). Family perception of and experience with family presence during cardiopulmonary resuscitation: An integrative review. *Journal of Clinical Nursing*, 28(1-2), 32–46.

United States Department of Veterans Affairs (DVA). (2020). How common is PTSD in veterans? Retrieved on 10/21/2020 at: www.ptsd.va.gov/understand/common/common_veterans.asp

*Wilkin, Z. L. (2020). Effects of video discharge instructions on patient understanding: A prospective, randomized trial. *Advanced Emergency Nursing Journal*, 42(1), 71–78.

World Health Organization (WHO). (2019). Snakebite. Retrieved on 4/10/2020 at: www.who.int/health-topics/snakebite#tab=tab_1

World Health Organization (WHO). (2020). Drowning. Retrieved on 4/10/2020 at: www.who.int/news-room/fact-sheets/detail/drowning

Ziaei, M., Massoudifar, A., Rajabpour-Sanati, A., et al. (2018). Management of violence and aggression in emergency environment: A narrative review of 200 related articles. *Advanced Journal of Emergency Medicine*, 3(1), e7.

Resources

American Association of Poison Control Centers (AAPCC), www.aapcc.org

American College of Emergency Physicians (ACEP), www.acep.org

American College of Surgeons (ACS), Injury Prevention and Control, www.facs.org/quality-programs/trauma/ipc

American Heart Association, www.heart.org

American Trauma Society (ATS), www.amtrauma.org/default.aspx

American Red Cross, Prepare for Emergencies, www.redcross.org/get-help/prepare-for-emergencies/types-of-emergencies

Divers Alert Network (DAN), www.diversalertnetwork.org

Emergency Nurses Association (ENA), www.ena.org

National Capital Poison, Poison Control Center, poison.org

National Center on Elder Abuse (NCEA), ncea.acl.gov

National Center for Health Statistics (NCHS), cdc.gov/nchs/

National Human Trafficking Hotline, www.humantraffickinghotline.org

National Institute on Drug Abuse, www.drugabuse.gov

National Safety Council, nsc.org

Rape, Abuse, and Incest National Network (RAINN), National Sexual Assault Hotline, rainn.org

Society of Trauma Nurses (STN), traumanurses.org

United States Department of Veterans Affairs PTSD: National Center for PTSD, www.ptsd.va.gov/understand/common/common_veterans.asp

68 Disaster Nursing

LEARNING OUTCOMES

On completion of this chapter, the learner will be able to:

1. Describe the types of disasters that the nurse may encounter as a member of the health care team.
2. Identify essential components of an emergency operations plan and disaster preparedness including personal protection and decontamination procedures.

3. Discuss how triage in a disaster differs from triage in an emergency department.
4. Explain clinical manifestations and treatment of injuries and illnesses resulting from natural disasters, from outbreaks, epidemics, and pandemics, and from various weapons of terror (blast, biologic, chemical, and radiologic events).

NURSING CONCEPTS

Health Care Systems   Managing Care   Safety

GLOSSARY

biologic weapon: a biologic agent that is used to spread disease among the general population or the military

chemical weapon: a chemical agent that is used to cause disability and mortality in the general population or the military

decontamination: process of removing, or rendering harmless, contaminants that have accumulated on personnel, patients, and equipment

disaster: a sudden disruption or event that interrupts the functioning of a community

disaster nursing: adaptation of nursing knowledge and skills to recognize and meet the health needs of individuals during times of crises

epidemic: a widespread outbreak of a specific infectious disease from a single source within a community or population that exceeds anticipated levels of impact

mass casualty incident (MCI): situation in which the number of casualties exceeds the number of available resources

material safety data sheet (MSDS): provides information to employees and health care providers regarding specific chemical agents; includes chemical name, physical

data, chemical ingredients, fire and explosive hazard data, health and reactive data, spill or leak procedures, special protection information, and special precautions (*synonym:* the Workers' Right to Know)

natural disaster: a natural event such as a tornado, hurricane, flood, or earthquake that results in significant damage and loss of life

outbreak: the occurrence of a disease within a population that exceeds normal expectations

pandemic: an epidemic that spreads across multiple countries or continents

personal protective equipment (PPE): equipment beyond standard precautions; may include different levels of equipment to provide complete protection, depending on the nature of the suspected biologic, chemical, or radiologic agent

radiologic weapon: byproducts of radiation contamination that are used to cause morbidity and mortality in the general population or the military

terrorism: unlawful, systematic use of violence or threats of violence against people in order to coerce or intimidate

weapons of mass destruction (WMD): weapons used to cause widespread death and destruction

Health care facilities must be prepared for any type of disaster. A **disaster** is a sudden disruption or event that interrupts the functioning of a community (Veenema, 2019). This chapter focuses on disaster preparedness and the role of the nurse in

preparing for and responding to disasters. **Disaster nursing** requires the adaptation of nursing knowledge and skills to recognize and meet the health and emotional needs of individuals during such times of crises known as disasters. Nurses serve on the frontline in providing care during a disaster or health crisis; they are called upon to work through difficult situations, sometimes with limited resources. They must utilize innovative thinking, lead effective coordination efforts, and clearly communicate the needs of their patients as well as their own personal needs (Veenema, 2019). Nursing responsibilities include preparing for and managing patients harmed by the effects of all disasters, including natural disasters, outbreaks, epidemics, and pandemics, as well as injuries and illnesses that can occur after biologic, chemical, and nuclear or radiation incidents, which may result from attacks of terrorism. Information about the process that nurses should follow in order to respond to these emergencies is applicable to other types of disasters as well.

Disaster Planning

The possibility and reality of mass casualties associated with disasters is not new to human history. Historically, communities that anticipated and devised plans to deal with the effects of disasters had better morbidity and mortality rates than those that did not. Within the United States, a plan that adheres to guidelines devised by the National Incident Management System (NIMS), which is directed by the U.S. Department of Homeland Security Federal Emergency Management Agency (FEMA), is essential for every community and facility. The preparation based on the NIMS guidelines is effective for terrorist events; **terrorism** is the unlawful, systematic use of violence or threats of violence against people in order to coerce or intimidate. NIMS guidelines are also followed for any other disaster situation, including natural disasters, outbreaks, epidemics, and pandemics. **Natural disasters** are caused by environmental forces including storms, floods, fires, earthquakes, and similar forces of nature that result in significant damage or loss of life (Veenema, 2019). Airplane crashes, train crashes, and toxic substance spills are other disasters that can result in mass casualties and tax the resources of health care facilities and their communities.

Federal, State, and Local Responses to Disasters

Many resources are available at the federal, state, and local levels to assist in the management of disasters, mass casualty incidents, public health crises, and emergencies. A **mass casualty incident (MCI)** is defined as any incident that causes a large number of casualties to the extent that necessary resources become too scarce (Veenema, 2019). When resources to care for casualties become scarce, the greatest good for the greatest number of patients becomes the mode of operation. Local communities must be prepared to act in isolation (i.e., called *sustainability planning*) and provide competent care for up to 5 days before federal or other state resources may become available (FEMA, 2019).

Disasters are categorized by type based upon anticipated use of resources and incident duration. A list of local resources with specific instructions about how and when to contact these agencies or organizations should be readily available to local disaster planning committees and frequently reviewed by those committees for necessary updates.

A disaster response strategy cannot succeed without appropriate physical assets and staff trained and prepared to carry out the plan. Assets such as increased security; stockpiles of equipment and medications; and planning, drills, and training are essential (Veenema, 2019). Hazard vulnerability assessments should be performed to identify potential and actual threats that involve a particular facility or community. Mutual aid agreements among various communities must take these vulnerabilities into account. Successful execution of a response plan is based on knowledge, confidence, and readiness.

Federal Agencies

The National Health Security Strategy was designed to protect the health of all citizens of the United States in the event of any large-scale MCI or disaster (Veenema, 2019). This national strategy aims to prioritize the use of limited resources and to ensure a rapid coordinated response by the entire affected community so that the maximum number of lives are saved, property is preserved and protected, and basic health care needs are met in the aftermath of any incident that results in mass casualties (FEMA, 2019). State authorities must request federal assistance with resources through appropriate government channels. A request for federal resources generally is made when local resources have become or are expected to become depleted.

Federal agencies that may provide resources in response to an MCI or a disaster include the Department of Health and Human Service (HHS), the Department of Defense, and the Department of Homeland Security (see Table 68-1). Each of these federal departments oversees hundreds of agencies that may respond to MCIs.

Nurses may be called upon to volunteer to provide support to select agencies or programs set up to respond to an MCI or a disaster. For example, Disaster Medical Assistance Teams (DMATs) organize voluntary medical personnel who can set up and staff a field hospital; DMATs are located across the country. Teams deploy with enough personnel, supplies, and equipment to be self-sufficient for 72 hours at a fixed or temporary medical site. During MCIs, team responsibilities may include triage, providing medical care despite adverse conditions, and preparing patients for evacuation (Veenema, 2019).

The Department of Homeland Security, through the National Terrorism Advisory System (NTAS), designates a level of security threat that is intended to alert the country to credible threats of terrorism. The NTAS notes two levels of terrorism threats, which include *bulletins* and *alerts*. An NTAS bulletin describes trends and developments in threats of terrorism; whereas, an NTAS alert more fully warns of a credible threat of terrorism within the United States. The NTAS alerts may be more specifically designated as an *elevated alert*, meaning that there is indeed a credible alert posted, or an *imminent alert*, meaning that there is a specific pending threat of terrorism within the United States (Department of Homeland Security [NTAS], 2019).

Additional support during disasters is available from the American Red Cross, which provides support systems and shelters as needed. A nongovernment, nonprofit agency, the American Red Cross mobilizes support for those in need

TABLE 68-1	Select U.S. Federal Agencies Involved in Disaster Response
Agency and Website	**Responsibilities**
Centers for Disease Control and Prevention (CDC) www.cdc.gov	Primary agency for disease prevention; controls activities and provides backup support to state and local health departments.
Department of Health and Human Service (HHS) www.hhs.gov	Primary agency for coordinating health, medical, and health-related social services under the federal emergency response plan.
Department of Defense (DoD) www.defense.gov	The armed service branches of DoD including the Army, Air Force, Coast Guard, Marine Corps, Navy, and National Guard, are the frontline military defense against acts of war and terrorist threats.
Department of Homeland Security www.dhs.gov	Develops and coordinates a comprehensive national strategy to strengthen federal, state, and local counterterrorism efforts.
Food and Drug Administration (FDA) www.fda.gov/home	Responsible for protecting the public health by ensuring the safety, efficacy, and security of human and veterinary drugs, biologic products, and medical devices; and by ensuring the safety of the food supply, cosmetics, and products that emit radiation
National Disaster Medical System (NDMS) www.phe.gov/ Preparedness/responders/ ndms/Pages/default.aspx	A multiagency system that supports and manages the coordination of medical responses to major emergencies and federally declared disasters that works in collaboration with public and private entities. NDMS is designed to care for victims of any incident that exceeds the capability of the state, regional, or federal health care system.Includes teams such as: • Disaster Medical Assistance Teams (DMATs) • Disaster Mortuary Operational Response Team (DMORTs) • Veterinary Medical Assistance Teams (VMATs) • National Medical Response Teams for Weapons of Mass Destruction (NMRTs)
U.S. Public Health Service (USPHS) www.usphs.gov/	A division of HHS that works to preserve and protect the public health of the nation. The USPHS consists of physicians, nurses, dentists, veterinarians, scientists, engineers, and other professionals who work in a variety of governmental agencies that promote the safety of the nation.

because of the effects of disasters through training and mobilizing volunteers.

 COVID-19 Considerations

In response to the coronavirus disease 2019 (COVID-19) pandemic, the Centers for Disease Control and Prevention (CDC) has provided an abundance of education addressing safety measures to combat the virus and precautions for populations at risk and offered regulatory guidance. These important regulations have informed government decisions enacted to ensure the safety of individuals during the pandemic (CDC, 2020a).

In addition to these measures, the Food and Drug Administration (FDA) accelerated the review of diagnostic tests to mitigate the spread of the virus. The FDA was responsible for ensuring that testing methods would provide both accurate and reliable results (FDA, 2020). Congress enacted an Emergency Use Authorization (EUA) that relaxed regulations and ultimately increased the availability of tests. The FDA then revised their standard procedures to allow for laboratory testing prior to FDA validation assessment, an unprecedented policy change that also allowed for increased testing capabilities (FDA, 2020).

State and Local Agencies

State and local resources that might be mobilized in response to a disaster may include branches of the CDC or American Red Cross, poison control centers, and other local volunteer organizations. The Metropolitan Medical Response Team Systems are local teams of health care providers located in cities considered possible terrorist targets who are funded for specialty responses. Many state and federal task forces have been developed to assist in the development and improvement of civilian medical response to chemical and biologic terrorism.

Most cities and all states have an Office of Emergency Management (OEM) or Office of Emergency Services (OES). The OEM/OES coordinates the disaster relief efforts at the state and local levels. The OEM/OES is responsible for providing interagency coordination during an emergency. It maintains a corps of emergency management personnel, including a leader, responders, planners, and administrative and support staff (Toner, 2017).

State and local governments play the primary role in the management of public health emergencies, such as the COVID-19 pandemic, until a request is made by a state that federal assistance is needed (Veenema, 2019). The Public Health Service (PHS) and FEMA are the two federal agencies that coordinate these efforts. In response to the COVID-19 pandemic, FEMA partnered with HHS to ensure adequacy of medical supplies and testing sites (FEMA, 2020a).

The Incident Command System

The Incident Command System (ICS) is a federally mandated command structure that coordinates personnel, facilities, equipment, and communication in any emergency situation. The ICS is the center of operations for organization, planning, and transport of patients in the event of a specific local MCI. Successful incident management requires equipment compatibility, effective communication, adequate distribution of resources, and clear differentiation of members' roles. The ICS ensures that any hazardous substances used during an MCI are identified promptly and that appropriate **personal protective equipment (PPE)** is distributed. PPE describes the use of equipment beyond standard precautions and may include different levels of protection, depending on the nature of the suspected biologic, chemical, or radiologic event (see later discussion). In addition to these responsibilities, the ICS is also responsible for determining when an MCI has ended (Veenema, 2019).

The Hospital Incident Command System (HICS) is a modification of the ICS that is used by both hospitals and law enforcement agencies. The HICS incident commander is the hospital emergency preparedness coordinator who oversees and coordinates all efforts surrounding the event. The HICS team includes a safety officer, public information officer, liaison officer, operations chief, logistics chief, planning chief, and finance chief. Each team member has a specific responsibility and communicates directly back to the incident commander (Veenema, 2019).

Hospital Emergency Preparedness Plans

Health care facilities are required by the Joint Commission to create a plan for emergency preparedness and to practice this plan with all employees at least twice a year. In general, these plans are developed by the facility's safety/disaster management committee and are overseen by an administrative liaison (California Hospital Association, 2017).

Before the basic emergency operations plan (EOP) can be developed, the planning committee of the health care facility evaluates characteristics of the community to identify the likely types of natural and man-made disasters that might occur. This hazard vulnerability analysis process is the responsibility of the local health care facility and its safety committee, safety officer, or emergency department (ED) manager. This information can be gathered by questioning local law enforcement, fire departments, and emergency medical systems and assessing the patterns of local train traffic, automobile traffic, and flood, earthquake, tornado, or hurricane activity. Consideration is also given to possible MCIs that could arise because of the community's proximity to chemical plants, nuclear facilities, or military bases. Federal, judicial, or financial buildings, schools, and any places where large groups of people gather can be considered high-risk areas (Veenema, 2019).

The emergency preparedness planning committee must have a realistic understanding of its resources. The goal of each health care institution is to remain self-sufficient to provide and sustain core services without the support of external assistance for at least 96 hours from the inception of the incident; ideally, this self-sufficiency should last for 7 days (Veenema, 2019). The committee might also outline how staff would triage and assign priority to patients when resources are limited (e.g., when ventilators are in short supply). Multiple factors influence a facility's ability to respond effectively to a sudden influx of patients who are injured or sick, and the committee must anticipate various scenarios to improve its preparedness.

 COVID-19 Considerations

As the incidence of COVID-19 cases in the United States continued to rise at a rapid pace during the early phases of this pandemic, political leaders began to encourage physical distancing among individuals to slow the rate of transmission; this practice became known as social distancing. The goal of social distancing was to attempt to flatten the curve of new infections, thereby avoiding a surge of demand on the health care system. However, the effects of social distancing were not enough to decrease the burden experienced by many U.S. hospitals in key geographic areas, such as New York City and New Orleans. Hospitals in these areas reported shortages of key equipment needed to care for patients who were critically ill, including ventilators and PPE for medical staff (Ranney, Griffeth, & Jha, 2020).

Insufficient PPE (e.g., respirators, face shields, gowns, hand and equipment sanitizer) for frontline health care workers resulted not only in exposures to severe acute respiratory syndrome coronavirus 2 (SARS-CoV-2), but also in the deaths of health care workers from COVID-19. In response to these shortages, health care providers made pleas to government officials to try to secure adequate PPE for their frontline workers (Ranney et al., 2020). On February 4, 2020, the HHS Secretary declared the EUA of respiratory protective devices, which authorized the use of additional respiratory protective devices. During this time, the FDA provided frequent updates to manufacturers, facilities, and local and state jurisdictions to increase the production of respirators and additional PPE (CDC, 2020a).

On April 8, 2020, the FEMA COVID-19 Supply Chain Task Force developed a four-step plan to preserve critical resources for medical use. The four steps included preservation, acceleration, expansion, and allocation (FEMA, 2020b). The shortage of critical medical supplies became a global crisis. In the United States, the Defense Production Act (DPA) allowed the president to direct private companies to produce equipment needed for a national emergency. A crucial role for the government is to coordinate efforts to ensure that areas that have been impacted the most are receiving needed equipment and supplies. As U.S. health care facilities continued to care for the growing number of patients hospitalized and critically ill with COVID-19, government officials worked to secure essential equipment needed to care for patients and ensure the safety of their workforce (Ranney et al., 2020).

Components of the Emergency Operations Plan

The principles of emergency management must be a part of the EOP design and include a comprehensive plan for tackling all potential and actual hazards. The main goal is the protection of the community. The EOP should be integrated with local, state, and federal government plans and coordinated with the private sector and volunteers. It must be coordinated in advance to achieve a single common purpose; yet the plan must be flexible enough to adapt to any potential disaster. Essential components of the EOP include the following (California Hospital Association, 2017):

- *Activation response:* The EOP activation response of a health care facility defines where, how, and when the response is initiated.

- *Internal/external communication plan:* Communication is critical for all parties involved, including communication to and from the prehospital arena.
- *Plan for coordinated patient care:* A response is planned for organized patient care into and out of the facility, including transfers from within the hospital to other facilities. The site of the disaster can determine where the greater number of patients may self-refer.
- *Security plans:* A coordinated security plan involving facility and community agencies is key to the control of an otherwise chaotic situation.
- *Identification of external resources:* Resources outside the facility are identified, including local, state, and federal resources and information about how to activate these resources.
- *Plan for people management and traffic flow:* "People management" includes strategies to manage the patients, the public, the media, and the personnel. Specific areas are assigned, and a designated person is delegated to manage each of these groups.
- *Data management strategy:* A data management plan for every aspect of the disaster will save time at every step. A backup system for documenting, tracking, and staffing is developed if the facility utilizes an electronic health record.
- *Demobilization response:* Deactivation of the response is as important as activation; resources should not be unnecessarily exhausted. The person who decides when the facility resumes daily activities is clearly identified. Any possible residual effects of a disaster must be considered before this decision is made.
- *After action report or corrective plan:* Facilities often see increased volumes of patients 3 months or more after an incident. Postincident response must include a critique and a debriefing for all parties involved, immediately and again at a later date.
- *Plan for practice drills:* Practice drills that include community participation allow for troubleshooting any issues before a real-life incident occurs.
- *Anticipated resources:* Food and water must be available for staff, families, and others who may be at the facility for an extended period.
- *MCI planning:* MCI planning includes such issues as planning for mass fatalities and morgue readiness.
- *Education plan for all of the above:* A strong education plan for all personnel regarding each step of the plan allows for improved readiness and additional input for fine-tuning the EOP.

As noted previously, hospitals are required to periodically hold disaster drills. Results from these drills can identify flaws within the EOP as well as unanticipated needs prior to any real disaster situation. Evidence indicates that full-scale regional exercises that coordinate responses from both hospitals and emergency medical services (EMS) are the most effective drills because they clearly identify breakdowns in communication (FEMA, 2019).

Initiating the Emergency Operations Plan

Notification of a disaster situation to a health care facility varies with each situation. In general, the notification to the facility comes from outside sources unless the initial incident occurred at the facility. The disaster activation plan should clearly state how the EOP is to be initiated. If communication is functioning, field incident command will give notice of the approximate number of patients who are arriving, although the number of patients who are self-referring will not be known (Tintinalli, Ma, Yealy, et al., 2020).

 COVID-19 Considerations

In response to the COVID-19 pandemic, the CDC provided evidence-based guidance for maintaining the EOP for all health care facilities, which provided guidance for staff, patients, and visitors. The guidelines were developed to minimize the spread of the virus within the community and to ensure all hospital staff were trained, equipped, and capable of executing these mitigation practices (CDC, 2020b).

Identifying Patients and Documenting Patient Information

Patient tracking is a critical component of casualty management. Disaster tags, which are numbered and include triage priority, name, address, age, location and description of injuries, and treatments or medications given, are used to communicate patient information. The tag should be securely placed on the patient and remain with the patient at all times. The tag number and the patient's name, if known, are recorded in a disaster log. The log is used by the command center to track patients, assign beds, and provide families with information.

Triage

Triage is the sorting of patients to determine the priority of their health care needs and the proper site for treatment. In nondisaster situations, health care workers assign a high priority and allocate the most resources to those who are the most critically ill (see Chapter 67). For example, under ordinary circumstances, a young adult who has a chest injury and is in cardiac arrest would receive advanced cardiopulmonary resuscitation, including medications, chest tubes, intravenous (IV) fluids, blood, and possibly emergency surgery in an effort to restore life. However, in a disaster, when health care providers are faced with a large number of casualties, the fundamental principle guiding resource allocation is to do the greatest good for the greatest number of people. Decisions are based on the likelihood of survival and consumption of available resources. Therefore, this same patient, and others with conditions associated with a high mortality rate, will be assigned as a low triage priority in a disaster situation, even if the person is conscious. Although this may sound uncaring, from an ethical standpoint the expenditure of limited resources on people with a low chance of survival, and denial of those resources to others with serious but treatable conditions, cannot be justified.

The triage officer rapidly assesses those injured at the disaster scene. Patients are immediately tagged and transported or given lifesaving interventions. One person performs the initial triage while other EMS personnel perform immediate lifesaving measures (e.g., intubation) and transport patients. Although EMS personnel carry out initial field triage, secondary and continuous triage at all subsequent levels of care is essential (Tintinalli et al., 2020).

TABLE 68-2	Triage Categories During a Mass Casualty Incident			
Triage Category		Priority	Color	Typical Conditions
Immediate: Injuries are life-threatening but survivable with minimal intervention. Individuals in this group can progress rapidly to expectant if treatment is delayed.		1	Red	Sucking chest wound, airway obstruction secondary to mechanical cause, shock, hemothorax, tension pneumothorax, asphyxia, unstable chest and abdominal wounds, incomplete amputations, open fractures of long bones, and second/third-degree burns of 15–40% total body surface area
Delayed: Injuries are significant and require medical care but can wait hours without threat to life or limb. Individuals in this group receive treatment only after immediate casualties are treated.		2	Yellow	Stable abdominal wounds without evidence of significant hemorrhage; soft tissue injuries; maxillofacial wounds without airway compromise; vascular injuries with adequate collateral circulation; genitourinary tract disruption; fractures requiring open reduction, débridement, and external fixation; most eye and central nervous system injuries
Minimal: Injuries are minor, and treatment can be delayed hours to days. Individuals in this group should be moved away from the main triage area.		3	Green	Upper extremity fractures, minor burns, sprains, small lacerations without significant bleeding, behavioral disorders or psychological disturbances
Expectant: Injuries are extensive, and chances of survival are unlikely even with definitive care. Persons in this group should be separated from other casualties, but not abandoned. Comfort measures should be provided when possible.		4	Black	Patients who are unresponsive with penetrating head wounds, high spinal cord injuries, wounds involving multiple anatomic sites and organs, second/third-degree burns in excess of 60% of body surface area, seizures or vomiting within 24 h after radiation exposure, profound shock with multiple injuries, agonal respirations, no pulse, no blood pressure, pupils fixed and dilated

Adapted from Tintinalli, J. E., Ma, O. J., Yealy, D., et al. (2020). *Tintinalli's emergency medicine manual: A comprehensive study guide* (9th ed.). New York: McGraw-Hill Medical.

It is important that an experienced ED provider is positioned at the entrance to provide primary triage at the acute care facility. Traffic control within the facility is one of the most important components of managing the disaster and resources (Veenema, 2019). The triage area may be outside the entry or just at the door of the ED. This facilitates the triage of all patients—those arriving by medical transport and those who walk into the ED. Some patients who have already been seen in the field may be reclassified in the triage area based on their current presentation.

Triage categories separate patients according to the severity of injury. A common triage method is the use of a special color-coded tagging system so that the triage category is immediately obvious. This system consists of four colors: red, yellow, green, and black. Each color signifies a different level of priority. Table 68-2 describes each category and gives examples of how different injuries would be classified (see Chapter 67). Alternative triage systems exclusively for MCI have also been designed. One triage system that has gained support in the United States and is used for mass casualty transport is the SALT (Sort, Assess, Lifesaving interventions, Treatment/Transport) system. It instructs the providers to quickly "Sort" casualties by assessing a patient's ability to follow commands, then to individually "Assess" casualties to rapidly apply "Lifesaving interventions," and assign a priority for "Treatment and/or Transport." SALT triage was developed to allow for rapid evaluation and sorting of patients of any age, injured in any type of event (Veenema, 2019).

Managing Internal Problems

The American Red Cross has developed a basic survival/shelter resource kit; however, each facility must determine its supply lists based on its own needs assessment. The EOP committee should determine the top 10 critical medications used during normal day-to-day operations and then anticipate which other medications may be required in a disaster or in an MCI. For example, the health care facility might plan to have available a stockpile of antidotes (e.g., cyanide kits) or antibiotics used in treating biologic agents. Information should be available about stocking or restocking any of the basic and special supplies, how those supplies are requested, and the time required to receive those supplies.

Communicating with the Media and Family

Communication is a key component of disaster management. Communication within the vast team of disaster responders is paramount; however, effective, informative communication with the media and worried family members is also crucial.

Managing Media Requests for Information

Although the media have an obligation to report the news and can play a positive role in communication, reporters and newscasters and their support teams can compromise operations and patient confidentiality. The disaster plan should include a clearly defined process for managing all media requests, including social media, and include a designated spokesperson, the public information officer, a site for the dissemination of information (away from patient care areas), and a regular schedule for providing updates.

The EOP helps prevent the release of contradictory or inaccurate information. Initial statements should focus on current efforts and what is being done to better understand the scope and impact of the situation. Information about casualties should not be released. Security staff should not allow media personnel access to patient care areas. However, media resources may be mobilized to notify the general population when disease containment is needed in case of an epidemic or the potential for one, including the location of shelters, necessity of quarantines, and point of dispensing units in the case of bioterrorism (Veenema, 2019).

Caring for Families

Friends and family members converging on the scene must be cared for by the facility. The public information officer's role is to provide direction for the families and provide them with information as it becomes available. They may be feeling intense anxiety, shock, or grief and should be provided with information and updates about their loved ones as soon as possible and regularly thereafter. They should not be in the triage or treatment areas but in a designated area staffed by available social workers, counselors, therapists, or clergy. Access to this area should be controlled to prevent families from being disturbed. Information regarding loved ones can also be obtained at this time, which assists in identification of both the injured and the deceased.

There may be times during a disaster situation such as an outbreak, epidemic, or pandemic that health care facilities must restrict visitation or access to the hospital. Health care organizations and nurses who typically pride themselves on providing patient- and family-centered care may be forced to prohibit visitors from accompanying loved ones to the hospital in order to reduce the spread of a virus or other infectious diseases which could be potentially fatal to visitors who are living with chronic health conditions. The health care team, which may be organized by the nurse, is responsible for developing a clear communication plan that designates a primary point of contact and eliminates barriers to communication (Hart, Turnbull, Oppenheim, et al., 2020). To keep families informed and encourage interactions among patients and their support network, hospitals have relied heavily on using technology during these disaster situations (e.g., FaceTime™, Google Hangouts™, Skype™, Zoom™). Some patients and their families may come from socioeconomically disadvantaged backgrounds and not have access to computer systems and associated software that can facilitate remote conversations. An adequate plan addresses the needs of families who may be socioeconomically disadvantaged and puts into effect plans that can meet their needs (Hart et al., 2020).

COVID-19 Considerations

In response to the COVID-19 pandemic, many U.S. hospitals restricted visitors and family members from entering the hospitals for the health and safety of visitors, patients, and employees. The CDC provided strict visitation guidelines for health care facilities in order to reduce the risk of transmission and combat the lack of PPE. Many hospitals restricted visitors in all inpatient locations, behavioral health units, EDs, and ambulatory procedure units. Many elective procedures were cancelled (see Chapter 52, Chart 52-4). One support person was permitted to be with the obstetric patient during labor, delivery, and postpartum care. When possible, the identified support person was to remain with the patient for the duration of the admission. Temporary visitation may have been granted for patients in extenuating circumstances (e.g., imminent death), or for specific populations who required extra support, including patients with developmental disability or cognitive impairment. Facilities were encouraged to identify alternative methods for patients and families to communicate and interact, including the use of technology as described previously (CDC, 2020c).

Chart 68-1 discusses cultural variables to consider when coping with disaster-related injuries and death.

The Nurse's Role in Disaster Response Plans

Nurses make up the largest component of the health care workforce across the globe (Veenema, 2019). The role of the

---

> **Chart 68-1** | **Cultural Considerations**
>
> Any disaster or mass casualty incident can be expected to involve members of diverse religious, ethnic, and cultural groups or may be targeted at and predominately affect a specific religious or ethnic group. Health care providers likewise include members of all religious, ethnic, and cultural backgrounds and should bear in mind that victims may have needs relating to the following:
>
> - Family roles and extended family importance
> - Language difficulties that increase fears and frustrations
> - Privacy
> - Rituals about handling the dead
> - Specific religious practices related to medical treatment, hygiene, or diet
> - Specific places/times for prayer
> - Timing of funeral services
> - Travel and visa restrictions limiting access to one's country of origin, family, work, or educational opportunities.
>
> Some religious communities have plans for emergencies and disasters, and local hospitals should integrate these plans to the extent possible into their emergency operations plans.

---

nurse during a disaster varies. Nurses may be asked to perform duties outside their areas of expertise and may take on responsibilities normally held by physicians or advanced practice nurses. For example, a critical care nurse may intubate a patient or even insert a chest tube. A nurse may perform wound débridement or suturing. A nurse may serve as the triage officer. In these situations, it is imperative that nurses strive to maximize patient safety and be aware of state regulations related to nursing practice (American Nurses Association [ANA], 2017; Casey, 2017).

Although the exact role of a nurse in disaster management depends on the specific needs of the facility at the time, it should be clear which nurse or physician is in charge of a given patient care area and which procedures each individual nurse may or may not perform. Assistance can be obtained through the HICS, and nonmedical personnel can provide services where possible. Nurses may be asked to delegate care to others, including students, staff assisting from other institutions, or volunteers. This process requires the nurse to rapidly assess the skills of those who are available to assist in patient care. Nurses must continue to emphasize patient safety and delegate appropriately. As the availability of coworkers, clinical experts, or support services may be limited, nurses may need to rely more upon their own competence or the collective competence of a new team (ANA, 2020).

During a disaster, nurses may feel a tension between maintaining traditional patient-centered approaches to care, which aim to achieve the maximum good for individual patients, and the need for public-focused approaches, which prioritize fair resource allocation during crisis conditions. A public health approach to ethics can provide nurses guidance in balancing this tension. "Public health emergencies require clinicians to change their practice, including in some situations, acting to prioritize the community above the individual in fairly allocating scarce resources" (Berlinger, Wynia, Powell, et al., 2020, p. 1). Nurses should remember that nursing

Chart 68-2 ETHICAL DILEMMA
Who Receives a Mechanical Ventilator When They Are Scarce Commodities During a Pandemic?

Case Scenario

You are a staff nurse who works in an emergency department (ED) in a university-affiliated hospital. Your community is in the midst of a surge of positive cases of coronavirus disease 2019 (COVID-19), and all ICU beds are filled with patients with COVID-19. For the past 12 hours, there have been no mechanical ventilators available for patients who are admitted and who are in severe respiratory distress until a patient who is intubated dies in the ICU, freeing up a ventilator. Currently, there are two patients waiting in the ED who would be intubated and mechanically ventilated if ventilators were available. Both patients have no significant medical or surgical history, are of normal weight, are nonsmokers, and take no prescription medications. One of these patients is T.C., a 55-year-old woman who is a cashier at a supermarket. The other patient is E.W., a 22-year-old female nursing student. Since both T.C. and E.W. are considered to be equivalent in terms of purported benefits of mechanical ventilation, the hospital's predetermined randomization protocol is implemented to determine who receives the ventilator. T.C. is selected to receive ventilatory support. As E.W.'s primary nurse, you question why T.C. is selected over E.W. and wonder if E.W.'s younger age and presumably longer lifespan and her chosen field of work as a future nurse should have given her preferential advantages over T.C. in receiving ventilatory support.

Discussion

During times of crises with scarcity of critical resources, protocols must be devised to assure that scarce resources are allocated in a fair and just manner. Most hospitals in the United States devised such contingency protocols in response to the COVID-19 pandemic. These protocols were devised to maximize potential benefits to society and ensure fair and equitable access to needed resources. In order to ensure fairness, patients eligible to receive resources may not face discrimination because of ethnic origin or race, socioeconomic status, sexual orientation, gender, or age.

Analysis

- Describe the ethical principles that are in conflict in this case (see Chapter 1, Chart 1-7). Patient autonomy is typically the preeminent ethical principle in all but crises situations. How can you ensure that E.W.'s dignity may be preserved despite these trying circumstances? Presumably, E.W.'s age can mean that she has more years of life ahead of her than T.C. Should this give her an advantage over T.C.? Should purported benefits to therapy be quantified by projecting years of productive life?

- Frontline health care workers are triaged to receive some benefits before others during pandemics (e.g., priority for vaccinations). E.W. is not a frontline worker. However, she is a nursing student and could be a future frontline worker. There are some who may argue that while E.W. could be a future frontline worker, that T.C., as a supermarket cashier, is already functioning as an essential worker. Should either one of them be given preferential consideration for receiving ventilatory support due to their current or potential designation as frontline workers? Why or why not?

- What resources may be available to assist you in reconciling this distressing rationing situation in your ED? How can you ensure that just and fair decisions are being made for your patients and for the people you serve within your community?

References

Baumrucker, S. J., Carter, G., Adkins, R. W., et al. (2020). Ethics roundtable: Distribution of critical care resources in the setting of a COVID-19 surge. *American Journal of Hospice and Palliative Care Medicine, 37*(12), 1096–1101.

Resources

See Chapter 1, Chart 1-10 for Steps of an Ethical Analysis and Ethics Resources.

---

care in a disaster focuses on essential care from a perspective of what is best for all patients (see Chart 68-2). In addition, acquiring knowledge of the hospital disaster plan, participating in drills, and honing competencies related to disaster management are essential (Casey, 2017). Nurse leaders and administrators should be cognizant of potential security issues and assess and plan for surge capacity capability and inhouse resources such as water, supplies, pharmaceuticals, and generator power. They also should predetermine means to evacuate the hospital if necessary, including identifying an ultimate destination or destinations. The hospital must plan for shortages of all kinds—staff, medications, water/food, and equipment (Veenema, 2019).

New settings and atypical roles for nurses arise during a disaster—for example, the nurse may provide shelter care in a temporary housing area or bereavement support and assistance with identification of deceased loved ones. People may require crisis intervention, or the nurse may participate in counseling other staff members and in critical incident stress management (CISM). Special care may be warranted for at-risk populations during a disaster (see Chart 68-3).

Considering Ethical Conflicts

Disasters can present a disparity between the resources of the health care agency and the needs of those affected

Chart 68-3 Caring for People with Disability During a Disaster

When a disaster occurs, the multiple agencies involved attempt to provide food, water, and shelter to all those affected. People with disability have specific needs that require attention. It is recommended that people with disability have a personal support network to check on them after a disaster and to provide needed assistance. They should also have a backup system and an evacuation plan. Agencies need to be aware that service animals are also affected during a disaster and may be brought to shelters with their companions.

Evacuation assistance is imperative for people with disability. Directions to personal equipment (e.g., communication aids, medications, oxygen) should be available to rescue personnel. In a rapid evacuation, mobility devices, oxygen, suction, and medications will be needed at the shelters. Special efforts to keep those with vision or hearing impairment informed should be implemented. People skilled in sign language are also valuable resources during a disaster. The American Red Cross and the National Organization on Disability provide information on their websites for disaster preparedness for people with disability (see the Resources section).

Adapted from Centers for Disease Control and Prevention (CDC). (2018a). *Preparedness and safety messaging for hurricanes, flooding, and similar disasters*. Retrieved on 3/1/2020 at: www.cdc.gov/cpr/readiness/00_docs/CDC_Hurricanes_PreparednessSafetyMessaging_July2018_508.pdf

by the disaster (Leider, DeBruin, Reynolds, et al., 2017). This generates ethical dilemmas for nurses and other health care providers. Issues include conflicts related to the following:

- Assisted suicide
- Confidentiality
- Consent
- Duty
- Futile therapy
- Rationing care
- Resuscitation

Nurses may find it difficult to not provide care to the dying or to withhold information to avoid spreading fear and panic. Clinical scenarios that are unimaginable in normal circumstances confront the nurse in extreme instances. Other ethical dilemmas may arise out of health care providers' instincts for self-protection and protection of their families.

Nurses can plan for the ethical dilemmas they will face during disasters by establishing a framework for evaluating ethical questions before they arise and by identifying and exploring possible responses to difficult clinical situations. They can consider how the fundamental ethical principles of autonomy, nonmaleficence, beneficence, and distributive justice will influence their decisions and care in disaster response (Ram-Tiktin, 2017) (see Chapter 1).

 COVID-19 Considerations

The COVID-19 crisis has created unprecedented challenges and ethical issues for frontline health care professionals, including insufficient supplies of PPE, shortages of lifesaving equipment, compromised standards of care, and conflicts between professional duties and personal health and safety concerns. As a result, many nurses and other health care providers have been at risk for or experienced moral distress (Altman, 2020). Examples of ethical issues related to COVID-19 included:

- Strictly limited hospital visitation policies that hampered nurses from involving families in care decisions
- Isolation measures that resulted in patients dying without family physically present
- Dire situations in which patients could have been denied potentially lifesaving therapies due to shortages and triaged care

The Code of Ethics for Nurses highlights the importance of providing safe, quality patient care. However, nurses also have an obligation to self-care and to providing support to their own families. Nurses may worry that they will cause harm to a loved one and struggle with how to balance their professional responsibilities with their personal commitments (Johns Hopkins University [JHU], 2020). These equally important obligations contribute to conflicts during pandemics when nurses must care for critically ill infectious patients, often under extreme circumstances that may include an insufficiency and inadequacy of resources and uncontained contagion. During pandemics, nurses must decide how much care they can provide to others while also taking care of themselves. They must be supported in these crucial decisions by the systems in which they provide care and by society (ANA, 2020). Nurses may struggle with the call to volunteer and respond in a pandemic. According to a policy statement drafted by the ANA (2020) in response to the COVID-19

pandemic, nurses may choose not to respond for the following reasons:

- Being a member of a vulnerable group
- Safety concerns related to a lack of PPE or inadequate testing
- Inadequate support to meet personal or family needs
- Concerns regarding professional and legal protection for providing nursing care

Organizational support for the nurse must be assured. Nurses must continue to advocate for systems and protocols that protect their ethical obligations as nurses, as well as ensure equity and fairness to all concerned in times of pandemics (ANA, 2020) (see Ethical Dilemmas in Chart 68-2, and in Chapter 19, Chart 19 7, and Chapter 18, Chart 18 9).

Managing Behavioral Issues

Disasters by nature are stressful and life-changing experiences which may cause adverse psychological effects, social disruption, and increased risks for vulnerable populations, including violence and abuse (Sloand, Killion, Yarandi, et al., 2017). Although most individuals function well during a disaster, both people and communities suffer immediate and sometimes long-term psychological trauma that most often relates to fear and anxiety (Veenema, 2019). Common responses to disaster include:

- Anxiety
- Compassion fatigue
- Depression
- Impaired performance
- Interpersonal conflicts
- Posttraumatic stress disorder
- Somatization (fatigue, general malaise, headaches, gastrointestinal disturbances, skin rashes)
- Substance use disorder (SUD)

Factors that influence a person's response to disaster include the degree and nature of the exposure to the disaster; loss of friends, family members, and pets; existing coping strategies; available resources and support; and the personal meaning attached to the event. Other factors, such as loss of home and valued possessions, extended exposure to danger, and exposure to toxic contamination, also influence response and increase the risk of adjustment problems. Those exposed to the dead and injured, those endangered by the event, older adults, children, emergency first responders, and health care personnel caring for victims are considered to be at higher risk for emotional sequelae. A person's normal response to stress and bereavement will also affect their response after a disaster (Emergency Nurses Association [ENA], 2020).

Nurses can assist victims of disaster through active listening and providing emotional support, giving information, and referring patients to therapists or social workers. Experience has shown that few victims of disaster seek these services, and early intervention minimizes psychological consequences. Nurses can also discourage victims from subjecting themselves to repeated exposure to the event through media replays and news articles, as well as encourage them to return to normal activities and social roles when appropriate (ENA, 2020).

Critical Incident Stress Management

CISM is an approach to preventing and treating the emotional trauma that can affect emergency responders as a consequence of their jobs and that can also occur to anyone involved in a disaster or MCI. CISM is handled by teams, which are available to the OEM. There are 350 such teams in the United States. All branches of emergency services have CISM teams, as do the military and civilian industries (e.g., airline industry).

Components of a management plan include education (preparedness) before an incident occurs about critical incident stress and coping strategies; field support (ensuring that staff get adequate rest, food, and fluids, and rotating workloads) during an incident; and defusings, debriefings, demobilization, supportive services to the family and follow-up care after the incident (Kalanlar, 2019; Veenema, 2019) (see Chapter 67 for further discussion on CISM).

Preparedness and Response

Preparedness and response planning are essential to identify risks of disasters and minimize the negative impact of potential disasters on individuals and communities.

Recognition and Awareness

Preparedness for disasters includes devising specific community contingency plans that prepare residents, particularly those who are vulnerable (e.g., older adults, people with disability) for access to necessary life-sustaining resources and for evacuation, as necessary. Preparedness also includes an awareness of the potential for covert use of **weapons of mass destruction (WMD)** (i.e., weapons used to cause widespread death and destruction), self-protection, and early detection, containment, or decontamination of substances and agents that may affect others by secondary exposure. The strength of many toxins, mobility of many members of society, and long incubation periods for some organisms and diseases can result in an epidemic that can quickly and silently spread across the entire country. For example, a formerly healthy person with a rapid onset of pneumonia and respiratory failure can have an ominous illness, such as COVID-19.

Nurses should have a heightened awareness of trends that may suggest deliberate dispersal of toxic or infectious agents or the onset of an outbreak, epidemic, or pandemic that may include the following:

- An unusual increase in the number of people seeking care for fever, respiratory, or gastrointestinal symptoms
- Clusters of patients who present with the same unusual illness from a single location. For example, clusters can be from a specific geographic location, such as a city, or from a single sporting or entertainment event or social gathering (e.g., wedding, funeral)
- A large number of fatalities, especially when death occurs within 72 hours after hospital admission
- Any increase in disease incidence in a normally healthy population. These cases should be reported to the state health department and to the CDC

If any of these trends are noted, a targeted patient history is taken in an attempt to identify the possible agent involved. This history includes an occupational, work, and environmental assessment, in addition to the regular admission history. An exposure history contains, at a minimum, information about current and past exposures to possible hazards and an assessment of the patient's typical day and any deviations in routines. The work history includes, at a minimum, a description of all previous jobs, including short-term, seasonal, and part-time employment and any military service. The environmental history includes an assessment of present and previous home locations, water supply, and any hobbies, to name a few factors. The admission history should include such information as recent travel, especially international travel, and contact with others who have been ill or have recently died of a fatal illness. This is just a brief review of the history that may need to be obtained to identify an exposure agent (Veenema, 2019).

In all cases, unusual trends, suspicions, or findings are reported to the appropriate resources in the facility and to proper authorities in the community. Resources can include the infection control department, the state health department, the CDC, the local poison control center, various internet sites, and **material safety data sheets (MSDS)** (see the Resources section). The MSDS provides information to employees and health care providers regarding specific chemical agents; it includes the chemical name, physical data, chemical ingredients, fire and explosive hazard data, health and reactive data, spill or leak procedures, special protection information, and special precautions. Reporting furnishes data elements to those agencies responsible for epidemiology and response. Reporting also allows for sharing of information among facilities and jurisdictions and can help determine the source of infections or exposure and prevent further exposures and even deaths (Occupational Safety and Health Administration [OSHA], 2012).

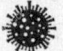 **COVID-19 Considerations**

Patterns of illness can continue to evolve during outbreaks, epidemics, and pandemics that involve novel pathogens. For instance, at the beginning of the COVID-19 pandemic, it was thought that children could not become infected with SARS-CoV-2; however, as the virus continued to spread, it became clear that the number of children infected was, in fact, equivalent to the rate of infection in adults. The majority of children who were infected, however, experienced much milder symptoms. It was only after cases in New York City peaked and began to decline that pediatricians began to see a new pattern in which dozens of children exposed to COVID-19 were becoming extremely ill, yet presented with different symptoms than adults. The CDC (2020d) began to warn of multisystem inflammatory syndrome in children (MIS-C), a condition which causes inflammatory changes to a variety of organs, including the heart, lungs, kidneys, brain, skin, eyes, or gastrointestinal organs. The cause remains unknown, but many of the children with MIS-C had been infected with SARS-CoV-2 or had been exposed to someone who had the virus. MIS-C can be serious and even deadly without prompt medical care (CDC, 2020d).

Personal Protective Equipment (PPE)

Another component of preparedness and response involves the protection of the health care provider by additional PPE. Chemical or biologic agents and radiation are silent killers and are generally colorless and odorless. The purpose of PPE is to shield health care workers from the chemical, physical, biologic, and radiologic hazards that may exist when caring for patients who have been contaminated or who can spread contagion. The U.S. Environmental Protection Agency

---

Chart 68-4

NURSING RESEARCH PROFILE
Whole-Process Training to Improve Use of Personal Protective Equipment

Tan, W., Ye, Y., Yang, Y., et al. (2020). Whole-process emergency training of personal protective equipment helps healthcare workers against COVID-19. *Journal of Occupational and Environmental Medicine, 62*(6). 420–423.

Purpose

Health care workers are at increased risk of exposure to the pathogen that causes coronavirus disease 2019 (COVID-19). Without proper knowledge of the donning and doffing of personal protective equipment (PPE), health care professionals are more susceptible to infection, illness, and possibly death. The purpose of this study was to evaluate the effectiveness of a three-phase training program on the proper use of PPE for health care workers in China.

Design

This study was developed in a hospital system in Beijing, China, where health care workers were caring for patients who had a known or suspected diagnosis of COVID-19. Qualified instructors and training assistants developed an educational program on appropriate use of PPE (e.g., hats, N95 respirators, goggles, face shields, shoe covers, and protective coveralls) across various areas of workflow (e.g., clean, possibly contaminated, contaminated). Teaching strategies included lecture and demonstration by faculty, followed by simulation, which allowed participants to practice what they had learned prior to being evaluated in phase three. Program developers established scoring criteria to evaluate the effectiveness of participants' performance. Two researchers independently scored participants on a variety of

predetermined outcomes (e.g., proficiency levels) before and after the training sessions. Paired *t* tests were used to analyze differences in scores before and after the educational session. Prior to conducting large-scale training and evaluation, researchers conducted an experimental or pilot study using a smaller number of participants.

Findings

Thirty-eight health care workers participated in the initial experimental training, including 31 nurses. Significant differences were found between pre- and posttest scores. Almost three quarters of the participants (73.68%) did not pass the pretest. However, 100% were successful following the educational program. Subsequently, 263 health care workers participated in the large-scale training, including 225 nurses; posttest scores were also significantly improved in this sample. Participants struggled the most with the use of N95 respirators and protective coveralls.

Nursing Implications

Multimodal educational programs, which include simulation have the potential to provide critical educational experiences for nurses that assist in keeping them safe and reducing the transmission of life-threatening viruses. Simulation enables experts to guide health care workers during an extremely stressful time and allows learners to practice the skills they need to protect themselves, their coworkers, and their patients. Such programs are essential in preparing an educated workforce to be ready to face the next pandemic or crisis.

(EPA) has divided protective clothing and respiratory protection into the following four categories, levels A through D:

- *Level A* protection is worn when the highest level of respiratory, skin, eye, and mucous membrane protection is required. This includes a self-contained breathing apparatus (SCBA) and a fully encapsulating, vapor-tight, chemical-resistant suit with chemical-resistant gloves and boots.
- *Level B* protection requires the highest level of respiratory protection but a lesser level of skin and eye protection than with level A situations. This level of protection includes the SCBA and a chemical-resistant suit, but the suit is not vapor tight.
- *Level C* protection requires an air-purified respirator, which uses filters or sorbent materials to remove harmful substances from the air. A chemical-resistant coverall with splash hood, chemical-resistant gloves, and boots are included in level C protection.
- *Level D* protection is the typical work uniform and is used for nuisance contamination only; it does not provide adequate protection in cases in which respiratory or skin threats are present. Other PPE such as gloves or mask may be required based on the situation.

Levels C and D PPE are the levels most often used in hospital facilities. Protective equipment must be donned before contact with a patient who has been contaminated. The acute care facility's standard precaution PPE (level D) generally is not adequate for protection from a patient who has been chemically, biologically, or radiologically contaminated. Level C PPE is adequate for the average patient exposure.

The health care provider must use equipment that is capable of providing protection against the agent involved. This may mean using a splash suit along with a full-face positive- or negative-pressure respirator (a filter-type gas mask) or even an SCBA for medical personnel in the field.

No single PPE is capable of protecting against all hazards. Under no circumstances should responders wear any PPE without proper training, practice, and fit testing of respirator masks as necessary (OSHA, 2017). See the Nursing Research Profile in Chart 68-4.

N95 respirator masks are used to reduce the nurse's exposure to particles, which include small-particle aerosols and large droplets (see Fig. 68-1). The mask filters out at least

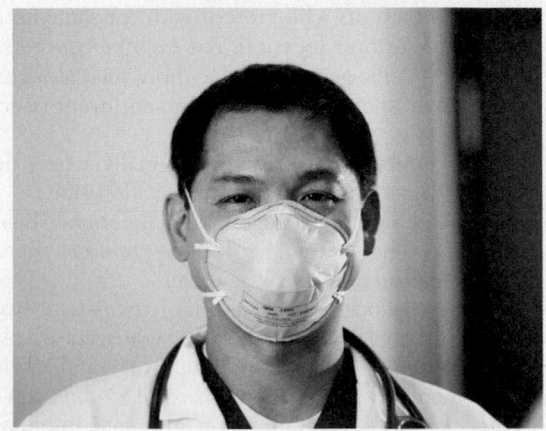

Figure 68-1 • N95 respirator. Courtesy of 3M Health Care.

95% of airborne particles and, in ideal situations, should be discarded after each patient encounter or aerosol-generating procedure. The mask should be discarded when it becomes damaged or deformed, no longer forms an effective seal to the face, becomes wet or visibly dirty, breathing becomes difficult, or it becomes contaminated with blood, respiratory or nasal secretions, or other bodily fluid (CDC, 2020e). Alternatively, a regular surgical mask provides the nurse protection against large droplets, splashes or sprays, bodily or other hazardous fluids, and protects the patient from the nurse's respiratory emissions. This mask does not require a tight seal, does not provide the wearer with a reliable level of protection from inhaling smaller airborne particles, and is not considered respiratory protection. Ideally, surgical masks should also be discarded after each patient encounter (CDC, 2020e). The CDC provides guidance to health care facilities regarding when it is appropriate to wear an N95 respirator mask versus a regular surgical mask during patient encounters. The N95 respirator mask must be evaluated, tested, and approved for the individual prior to wearing per facility policy and procedures.

Decontamination

Decontamination, the process of removing accumulated contaminants or rendering them harmless, is critical to the health and safety of health care providers by preventing secondary contamination. The decontamination plan should establish procedures and educate employees about decontamination procedures, identify the equipment needed and methods to be used, and establish methods for disposal of contaminated materials (Veenema, 2019).

Although many principles and theories surround decontamination of a patient, authorities agree that to be effective,

decontamination must include a minimum of two steps. First step is the removal of the patient's clothing and jewelry and then rinsing the patient with water. Depending on the type of exposure, this step alone can remove a large amount of the contamination and decrease secondary contamination. The second step consists of a thorough soap-and-water wash and rinse. The hospital must be prepared to perform additional decontamination prior to entry into the facility. The hospital personnel may also treat "walking wounded" who did not receive any decontamination at the scene (Tintinalli et al., 2020).

 Quality and Safety Nursing Alert

When patients arrive at the facility after being assessed and treated by a prehospital provider, it should not be assumed that they have been thoroughly decontaminated.

Natural Disasters

Natural disasters may result in mass casualties. Natural disasters can occur anywhere at any time and include events such as tornadoes, hurricanes, floods, avalanches, tidal waves (e.g., tsunamis), earthquakes, and volcanic eruptions (see Table 68-3). In the event of a natural disaster, loss of communications, potable water, and electricity is usually the greatest obstacle to a well-coordinated emergency response, and preparatory planning is essential. Wireless technology (e.g., cellular phones, computers, other communication devices) may not be functional (Tintinalli et al., 2020).

The majority of the immediate casualties are trauma related. These mass casualties require the trauma system to provide triage, transport of patients (in poor weather and road conditions), and management within the trauma centers.

TABLE 68-3	Select Natural Disasters
Event	**Issues and Injuries**
Earthquakes	Associated with multiple aftershocks, tsunamis Buildings require tethering in earthquake-prone areas *Injuries:* Physical injury; dehydration; pulmonary problems
Flooding	Can accompany other natural disasters Results in home and community destruction *Injuries:* Nonfatal drowning/drowning (e.g., people swept away in currents); waterborne and vector-borne diseases (e.g., shigellosis, *Escherichia coli* infection, hepatitis A, giardiasis, leptospirosis, malaria, plague, dengue fever); physical injury from debris
Hurricanes	Cause flooding (see previous discussion) and tornadoes (see later discussion) Failure to evacuate Food and water safety *Injuries:* From recovery activities (e.g., chainsaws), stress-related disorders, and GI and other vector-borne diseases; physical injury; bites from traumatized pets
Tornadoes	Minimal warning, fast moving (approximately 30 mph and travel approximately 20 km) Massive destruction, shelter loss *Injuries:* Physical injury; blastlike effects from pressure (see discussion of blast injuries in text)
Tsunamis	As with flooding (see above) but with much more rapid onset resulting in immediate large volume of water on land *Injuries:* Physical injury from debris; vector-borne diseases (see the Flooding section); cholera
Volcanic eruptions	Hazards from lava, openings in ground, gases, ash up to a 20-mile radius *Injuries:* Acid rain; toxic gases result in inhalation injury; physical injury

GI, gastrointestinal.
Adapted from Veenema, T. G. (2019). *Disaster nursing and emergency preparedness* (4th ed.). New York: Springer.

Most patients usually begin arriving within an hour of the event. However, the "walking wounded" may not seek care for 5 days to 2 weeks after the event or may seek care for injuries received during cleanup activities. Casualties arrive at hospitals in three waves. The first wave consists of people who are minimally (generally) injured who arrive of their own accord. The second wave consists of patients who are severely injured. The third wave consists of patients who are injured and who arrive after they are discovered by rescuers. For example, in the event of earthquakes, rescuers may find injured patients in collapsed buildings; the majority of fatalities from injuries in this case primarily involve the head and chest (Veenema, 2019).

Excessive exposure to the natural elements and the need for food and water (by both patients and emergency responders) are critical issues. Without cover (e.g., buildings may be unsafe or destroyed) or potable water (e.g., water may be either contaminated or unavailable), injuries from exposure to heat, cold, or contaminated food or water can occur. Safety equipment that protects rescue workers from injury, exposure, and potentially dangerous animals (e.g., snakes, alligators, spiders) must be readily available. Rescue workers may also injure themselves in the process of extrication or cleanup (e.g., chain saws, building collapse). Hypothermia can occur rapidly in workers who are exposed to water at temperatures of 23.9°C (75°F) or less. As is true during all disasters, mental health workers and shelters are needed throughout the community. Veterinary assistance is also essential because pets are frequently abandoned and injured. In addition, emergency response workers must be prepared to treat the most common ailments experienced after exposure to a specific natural disaster. For instance, pulmonary problems peak with earthquakes and volcanic eruptions because of the increased particulate matter in the air (Veenema, 2019).

In some instances, early warning systems have assisted in decreasing the number of deaths from tornadoes and hurricanes. Even with the advent of early warning systems, some people are unable or unwilling to leave prior to the occurrence of the natural disaster.

When buildings collapse, rapid response to identify and remove trapped victims is the only means of improving survivability. Water-damaged buildings are not safe and require extensive examination before experts can ensure safe occupancy. Larger-scale issues that can cause significant later morbidity and mortality include the absence of water purification, waste removal, removal of human and animal remains, and vector control. Removal or disposal of biologic, chemical, and nuclear agents must also be considered (Tintinalli et al., 2020).

Outbreaks, Epidemics, and Pandemics

An **outbreak** is the occurrence of a disease within a population that exceeds normal expectations. Outbreaks can be classified as communicable disease outbreaks, outbreaks caused by exposure to chemicals or toxins, and outbreaks from unknown sources. An outbreak may be transmitted via persons, animals, or from the environment (WHO, 2020b).

An **epidemic** is a widespread outbreak of a specific infectious disease from a single source within a community or population that exceeds anticipated levels of impact. An epidemic exists when new cases exceed the expected incidence of that disease. The rate and transmission of the infectious disease is dependent on multiple factors which include preexisting levels of the disease in the community, environmental changes that occurred as a result of the disease, population density and displacement, disruption of utilities, interruption of health services, and public sanitation. In order for a true epidemic to occur, there must be a vulnerable population, the presence of a disease agent, and a mechanism that supports large-scale transmission (Veenema, 2019). During an epidemic, there is a need to respond quickly and intentionally as catastrophic loss of human life and economic devastation may occur. Epidemics may be deemed an emergency if any of the following characteristics are present (Veenema, 2019):

- Large number of cases projected to occur
- Disease leads to serious disability or death
- Disease threatens to cause social or economic disruption
- Officials are unable to manage resources adequately due to the surge in cases. This includes sufficient number of trained personnel, necessary supplies and equipment (e.g., vaccines, medications, testing equipment, etc.)
- Risk to transmit the disease internationally

A **pandemic** is an epidemic that spreads across multiple countries or continents. There are many more individuals affected and greater number of deaths associated with pandemics than epidemics. In March 2020, the World Health Organization (WHO) characterized COVID-19 as a pandemic (WHO, 2020a).

Communicable disease outbreaks, which may eventually lead to epidemics or pandemics, are investigated through public health surveillance and the monitoring of clusters of illnesses. Interviews, questionnaires, and home visits may be beneficial when people are experiencing the same symptoms of illness (CDC, 2018b). It is imperative to identify the source of the illness and institute measures for the containment of the outbreak. An outbreak is over when the numbers of new cases fall below the number of normally expected cases (CDC, 2018b).

Weapons of Terror

Geopolitical forces and interests and the availability of destructive technology have brought the possibility of more terrorist events to our doorstep. Terrorism involves the systematic use of violence to create feelings of fear. Examples include the destruction of the World Trade Center towers and the damage to the Pentagon on September 11, 2001; the Boston Marathon bombing on April 15, 2013; and the coordinated series of terrorist attacks in Paris on November 13, 2015; in Brussels on March 22, 2016; and the London attacks on Westminster Bridge and Parliament on June 3, 2017. Over 26,445 deaths had occurred in 2017 from terrorism-related violence; over the last decade, deaths across the world from terrorism ranged from a low of 7827 in 2010 to a high of 44,490, in 2014 (Ritchie, Hasell, Appel, et al., 2020). Terrorists have become increasingly sophisticated, organized, and therefore effective. It is no longer a question of *whether* a terrorist event will again lead to mass casualties, but *when* such an event will occur. The U.S. Department of Homeland Security was created after the attacks of September 11, 2001, to coordinate federal and state efforts to combat terrorist activity.

Terrorists preferentially use WMD which may leverage the use of blasts or biologic, chemical, or radiologic agents. Although terrorist events are not everyday events, they can occur at any facility, and every nurse needs to know the basics of caring for patients who have been affected.

Blast Injury

A blast may result from terrorism but can also occur anywhere at any time if the right (or wrong) circumstances come together (e.g., welding inside of a tank that formerly contained tar but was not properly cleaned can result in an explosion as well as severe tar burns to the worker).

Types of Explosive Devices

The bomb most commonly utilized by terrorists is the pipe bomb, which contains low-velocity explosives and may also contain nails or other implements that cause more damage when the explosive ignites. Another type of commonly used explosive device is the Molotov cocktail, which uses a common flammable liquid such as gasoline in a glass bottle and a source of ignition, such as a rag. This forms a simple yet effective incendiary device. Other types of explosive devices include fertilizer bombs and dirty bombs, which include a radioactive source that spreads radiation after the initial blast (Durakovic, 2017).

Hazards following a bombing include secondary devices (set to explode at a predetermined time, typically after the arrival of rescue personnel); building collapse; contamination from biologic, chemical, or radiologic weapons; and the presence of terrorists among the patients and bystanders. The entire scene of the bombing is a crime scene and is treated as such. Triage of patients involved in a bombing is the same as for all other disasters, with a heightened awareness that serious internal injuries from the blast wave may not be immediately evident.

Physical Injuries

Distance from the blast, whether the blast space was enclosed, composition of the explosive, whether a building collapsed, and the efficiency of medical resources available after the blast all affect patient outcomes after a blast injury. The actual blast that occurs during the initial seconds of the bombing or explosion causes a pressure wave or primary blast wave. Injuries can result from the impact of the explosion, the primary blast wave, or shrapnel (i.e., debris from the bomb). The majority of injuries are caused by the primary blast wave (Tintinalli et al., 2020). A blast wave has four effects. These include spalling, which refers to the pressure wave itself; implosion, which refers to rupture of organs from entrapped gases; shearing, which refers to the blast response of different body tissues, dependent on their density; and irreversible work, which refers to the presence of forces that exceed the tensile strength of an organ or tissue. If the blast occurs in an enclosed space, the wave has the opportunity to be reflected and thus amplified (Veenema, 2019). The various phases of blasts and related injuries are detailed in Table 68-4.

Blast Lung

Blast lung results from the blast wave as it passes through air-filled lungs. The result is hemorrhage and tearing of the lung, ventilation–perfusion mismatch, and possible air emboli. Typical signs and symptoms include dyspnea, hypoxia, tachypnea or apnea (depending on severity), cough, chest pain, and hemodynamic instability. Management involves providing respiratory support that includes administration of supplemental oxygen with nonrebreathing mask but may also require endotracheal intubation and mechanical ventilation. If a hemothorax or pneumothorax is present, a chest tube must be inserted to re-expand the lung. In the event of an air embolus, the patient should be immediately placed in the prone, left lateral position to prevent migration of the embolus and will require emergent treatment in a hyperbaric chamber (Tintinalli et al., 2020). Complications following blast lung can include respiratory failure as well as acute respiratory distress syndrome (ARDS) (see Chapter 19).

Tympanic Membrane Rupture

Tympanic membrane (TM) rupture is the most frequent injury after subjection to a pressure wave because TM is the

TABLE 68-4	Phases of Blasts and Associated Common Injuries
Phase of Blast Injury	**Common Injuries**
Primary: Results from initial blast or air wave.	Affects primarily air-filled organs: Tympanic membrane rupture, middle ear injury—permanent deafness may occur Pulmonary—pneumothorax, pulmonary contusions, air embolus Head injuries, including concussion, other severe brain injuries Abdominal hollow organ perforation, hemorrhage
Secondary: Results from debris from the scene or shrapnel from the bomb that act as projectiles	Penetrating trunk, skin, and soft tissue injuries Fractures, traumatic amputations
Tertiary: Results from pressure wave that causes the victim to be thrown	Head injuries Fractures, including skull
Quaternary: Results from preexisting conditions exacerbated by the force of the blast or by postblast injury complications	Severe injuries with complex injury patterns—burns, crush injuries, head injuries Common preexisting conditions that become exacerbated—COPD, asthma, cardiac conditions, diabetes, and hypertension

COPD, chronic obstructive pulmonary disease.
Adapted from Jorolemon, M. R., Lopez, R. A., & Krywko, D. M. (2019). Blast injuries. In *StatPearls [Internet]*. Treasure Island, FL: StatPearls Publishing. Retrieved on 3/27/2020 at: www.ncbi.nlm.nih.gov/books/NBK430914/

body's most sensitive organ to pressure. There is an increased incidence of TM rupture when a blast occurs in close proximity to the patient and when it occurs in an enclosed space. Signs and symptoms include hearing loss, tinnitus, pain, dizziness, and otorrhea (Jorolemon, Lopez, & Krywko, 2019). The majority of TM ruptures heal spontaneously. Approximately 5% of patients with TM rupture from a blast will require hearing aids, whereas the majority will suffer only mild high-frequency hearing loss (ENA, 2019). Other ear injuries may include ossicular disruption and impaction of foreign bodies.

Abdominal and Head Injuries

Blast abdomen may be evidenced by abdominal hemorrhage and internal organ injury. The typical signs and symptoms of internal abdominal injury can include pain, guarding, rebound tenderness, rectal bleeding, nausea, and vomiting (Jorolemon et al., 2019) (see Chapter 67).

Head injuries are typically minor, but those that are severe result in the majority of postblast deaths. These injuries can occur without a direct blow to the head and may result from the blast itself, building collapse, or flying debris. Concussions commonly occur post blast, and the usual follow-up evaluation and treatment for postconcussive syndrome is indicated (see Chapter 63). Approximately 30% of head injuries involve vascular structures (e.g., arteriovenous fistula, pseudoaneurysm, or dissection) (Veenema, 2019).

Special Populations

Special populations may have different blast-associated risks. For instance, older adults are particularly susceptible to bone fractures because they tend to have decreased bone density. They also tend to have more preexisting morbid conditions that may be exacerbated by the explosion. Patients who are pregnant are particularly susceptible to placental shear forces that may result in abruptio placentae. People with mobility disability may have difficulty extricating themselves from the site of the blast (CDC, 2018a).

Biologic Weapons

Biologic weapons are weapons that spread disease among the general population or the military. They can be used for sabotage, such as food or water contamination with a small target area or may be used by global terrorists with intentions to spread fear and disruption of daily life (Tintinalli et al., 2020).

Effects of Biologic Weapons

Biologic weapons are easily obtained and easily disseminated and can result in significant mortality and morbidity (see Table 68-5). The potential use of biologic weapons calls for continuous increased surveillance by health departments and an increased index of suspicion by clinicians. Many biologic weapons result in signs and symptoms similar to those of common disease processes. Appropriate management of a biologic threat includes rapid recognition of the potential weapon; the use of proper PPE; decontamination, isolation, or quarantine of patients who are infected when appropriate; and the administration of appropriate vaccinations, antidotes, or medications to people at risk.

Biologic weapons are delivered in either a liquid or a dry state, applied to foods or water, or vaporized for inhalation

TABLE 68-5	Categories of Biologic Weapons	
Category	Mortality and Morbidity	Examples of Biologic Agents That May Be Weaponized
Category A	High mortality	*Bacillus anthracis* (anthrax) *Clostridium botulinum* (botulism) *Francisella tularensis* (tularemia) Viral hemorrhagic fevers (e.g., dengue, Ebola) *Variola* (i.e., smallpox) *Yersinia pestis* (plague)
Category B	Low mortality, moderate morbidity	*Brucella* species (brucellosis) *Coxiella burnetii* (Q fever) *Staphylococcus aureus*, *Vibrio* species (food poisoning) *Rickettsia typhi* (typhus) Arboviruses (viral encephalitis) *Cryptosporidium parvum* (cryptosporidiosis)
Category C	Low mortality, low morbidity	Hantavirus

Adapted from Veenema, T. G. (2019). *Disaster nursing and emergency preparedness* (4th ed.). New York: Springer.

or direct contact. Vaporization may be accomplished through spray or explosives loaded with the weapon. Because of increase in travel by people in industrialized nations, a biologic weapon could be released in one city and affect people in other cities thousands of miles away. The vector can be an insect, animal, or person, or there may be direct contact with the weapon itself.

Two of the biologic agents most likely to be used or weaponized are discussed in the next section. Table 68-6 describes other easily weaponized biologic agents.

Types of Biologic Weapons

Anthrax

Anthrax is recognized as the most likely weaponized biologic agent available and has been recognized as a highly debilitating agent for centuries. *Bacillus anthracis* is a naturally occurring gram-positive, encapsulated rod-shaped bacterium that lives in the soil in the spore state throughout the world. The bacterium sporulates (i.e., is liberated) when exposed to air and is infective only in the spore form. Contact with infected animal products (raw meat) or inhalation of the spores results in infection. Cattle and other herbivores are vaccinated against anthrax to prevent transmission through contaminated meat. As an aerosol, anthrax is odorless and invisible and can travel a great distance before disseminating; hence, the site of release and the site of infection can be miles apart (ENA, 2020).

Clinical Manifestations

Anthrax is caused by replicating bacteria that release toxin, resulting in hemorrhage, edema, and necrosis. There are three main methods of infection: skin contact, gastrointestinal ingestion, and inhalation. Approximate incubation periods are 5 to 7 days (cutaneous), 1 to 6 days (gastrointestinal), and 1 to 43 days (inhalation). Skin lesions (the most common infection) cause edema with pruritus and macule or papule

TABLE 68-6 Select Examples of Biologic Agents That Can Be Used as Weapons

Agent/Organism	Contagion	Decontamination and Protective Equipment	Signs and Symptoms	Treatment (Mortality Rate)
Botulism—*Clostridium botulinum:* Botulinum blocks acetyl-choline-containing vesicles from fusing with the terminal membranes of the motor neuron end plate, resulting in a flaccid paralysis.	Direct contact Not contagious through human-to-human contact	Any skin exposure to the botulinum toxin can be treated with soap and water or a 0.1% hypochlorite solution. Standard precautions are used when treating patients with botulism.	*Gastrointestinal botulism:* Abdominal cramps, nausea, vomiting, and diarrhea *Inhalation botulism:* Fever; symmetric descending flaccid paralysis with multiple cranial nerve palsies. *Classic signs and symptoms include* diplopia, dysphagia, dry mouth, lack of fever, and alert mental status. *Other possible symptoms include* ptosis of the eyelids, blurred vision, enlarged sluggish pupils, dysarthria, and dysphonia. *Mortality secondary to:* Airway obstruction and inadequate tidal volume.	Supportive ventilatory therapy is necessary if respiratory infection occurs. Aminoglycosides and clindamycin are contraindicated because they exacerbate neuromuscular blockage. Equine antitoxin is used to minimize subsequent nerve damage. There is a 2% rate of anaphylaxis to the antitoxin; therefore, diphenhydramine and epinephrine must be immediately available for use. Supportive care—mechanical ventilation, nutrition, fluids, prevention of complications. (Mortality rate = 5%)
Plague—*Yersinia pestis:* nonsporulating, gram-negative coccobacillus. The bacterium causes destruction and necrosis of the lymph nodes.	Contagious *Bubonic plague:* Transmitted through flea bites with no person-to-person transmission *Pneumonic plague:* Transmitted through respiratory droplet contact	Isolation barrier precautions with full-face respirators; the patient should wear a mask. Rooms should receive a terminal cleaning. Clothing and linens with body fluids on them should be cleaned with the usual disinfectant. Routine precautions should be used in the case of death.	*Bubonic plague:* Sudden fever and chills, weakness, a swollen and tender lymph node (bubo) in the groin, axilla, or cervical area. The resultant bacteremia progresses to septicemia from the endotoxin and, finally, shock and death. *Primary septicemic plague:* Disseminated intravascular coagulation, necrosis of small vessels, purpura, and gangrene of the digits and nose (black death). *Pneumonic plague:* Severe bronchospasm, chest pain, dyspnea, cough, and hemoptysis. There is a 100% mortality associated with pneumonic plague if not treated within the first 24 h.	Streptomycin or gentamicin for 10–14 days. Start within 12–24 h. Tetracycline or doxycycline is an acceptable alternative if an aminoglycoside cannot be given. People with close contact exposure (<2 m) require prophylaxis with doxycycline for 7 days. (Mortality rate = 50%)
Tularemia—*Francisella tularensis:* Gram-negative, coccobacillus, one of the most infectious bacteria known.	Direct contact with infected animals or aerosolized as a bioterror weapon; bites Not contagious through human-to-human contact Found in Oklahoma, Missouri, Arkansas	Standard barrier precautions. Clothing and linens should be laundered under the usual hospital protocol.	*Initial:* Abrupt onset of fever, fatigue, chills, headache, lower backache, malaise, rigor, coryza, dry cough, and sore throat without adenopathy. Nausea and vomiting or diarrhea possible. *As disease progresses:* Sweating, fever, progressive weakness, anorexia, and weight loss demonstrate continued illness. *Mortality secondary to:* Pneumonitis (if inhalation is the source) with copious watery or purulent sputum, hemoptysis, respiratory insufficiency, sepsis, and shock.	Streptomycin or gentamicin/aminoglycoside for 10–14 days. Inhalation tularemia must be treated within 48 h of onset. In mass casualty situations, doxycycline or ciprofloxacin is recommended. For persons exposed to tularemia, tetracycline or doxycycline is recommended for 14 days. (Mortality rate = 2%)

Adapted from Emergency Nurses Association. (2020). *Sheehy's emergency nursing: Principles and practice* (7th ed.). St. Louis, MO: Elsevier Mosby; Emergency Nurses Association. (2019). *Trauma nursing core course* (8th ed.). Chicago: Author; and Veenema, T. G. (2019). *Disaster nursing and emergency preparedness* (4th ed.). New York: Springer.

formation, resulting in ulceration with 1- to 3-mm vesicles. A painless eschar develops, which falls off in 1 to 2 weeks (ENA, 2020).

Ingestion of anthrax results in fever, nausea and vomiting, abdominal pain, bloody diarrhea, and occasionally ascites. If severe diarrhea develops, decreased intravascular volume becomes the major treatment concern. The bacterium targets the terminal ileum and cecum. Sepsis can occur (ENA, 2020).

Inhaling anthrax results in severe clinical manifestations. Its symptoms mimic those of the flu, and usually treatment is sought only when the second stage of severe respiratory distress occurs. Antibiotic therapy does not halt the progress of the disease. Inhaled anthrax can incubate for up to 60 days, making it difficult to identify its source. Initial signs and symptoms include cough, headache, fever, vomiting, chills, weakness, mild chest discomfort, dyspnea, and syncope without rhinorrhea or nasal congestion. Most patients have a brief recovery period followed by the second stage within 1 to 3 days, characterized by fever, severe respiratory distress, stridor, hypoxia, cyanosis, diaphoresis, hypotension, and shock. These patients require optimization of oxygenation, correction of electrolyte imbalances, and ventilatory and hemodynamic support. More than 50% of these patients have hemorrhagic mediastinitis on a chest x-ray (a hallmark sign). Inhalation anthrax may progress to include meningitis with subarachnoid hemorrhage. Death results approximately 24 to 36 hours after the onset of severe respiratory distress. The mortality rate approaches 100% (ENA, 2020).

Management

At present, anthrax is penicillin sensitive; however, strains of penicillin-resistant anthrax are thought to exist. Recommended treatment includes penicillin, ciprofloxacin, levofloxacin, and doxycycline (ENA, 2020). If antibiotic treatment begins within 24 hours after exposure, death can be prevented. In a mass casualty situation, treatment with ciprofloxacin or doxycycline is recommended, because these easily given oral antibiotic agents are stockpiled and there should be sufficient dosages to fully treat many patients who have been anthrax-exposed. Treatment is continued for 60 days. For patients who have been directly exposed to anthrax but have no signs and symptoms of disease, ciprofloxacin or doxycycline is used for prophylaxis for 60 days (U.S. Department of Health and Human Services, 2018).

Standard precautions are needed when caring for a patient infected with anthrax. The patient is not contagious, and the disease cannot spread from person to person. Equipment should be cleaned using standard hospital disinfectant. After death, cremation is recommended because the spores can survive for decades and represent a threat to morticians and forensic medicine personnel. A vaccination, which includes six doses is available for the Department of Defense, and the CDC is in the process of developing a civilian vaccination protocol (ENA, 2020).

Smallpox

Smallpox (variola) is classified as a deoxyribonucleic acid (DNA) virus. It has an incubation period that ranges from 7 to 17 days. It is extremely contagious and spread by direct contact, by contact with clothing or linens, or by droplets from person to person only after the fever has decreased and the rash phase has begun (ENA, 2020). Aerosolization of the virus would result in widespread dissemination.

The WHO declared eradication of smallpox in 1977 and stopped worldwide vaccination in 1980. In the United States, the last child was vaccinated in 1972. Therefore, a large portion of the current population has no immunity to the virus. A smallpox vaccination plan, introduced in 2003, proposed that a designated number of ED staff receive the first vaccinations to ensure that ED staff would be immunized in the event of a smallpox outbreak. The government estimated that 0.1% of those people receiving the vaccine would have serious side effects. Of these, approximately 4% would have life-threatening complications, and 0.1% would die. Currently, only people with a high likelihood of exposure to smallpox are encouraged to receive the vaccination (CDC, 2017).

Clinical Manifestations

Signs and symptoms of smallpox infection include high fever, malaise, headache, backache, and prostration. After 1 to 2 days, a maculopapular rash appears, evolving at the same rate, beginning on the face, mouth, pharynx, and forearms. Only then does the rash progress to the trunk and become vesicular to pustular (Veenema, 2019). There is a large amount of virus in the saliva and pustules. The person remains contagious until the rash crusts over and falls off (ENA, 2020). There are two forms of smallpox: variola major and variola minor. Variola major is more common, results in a higher fever and more extensive rash, and has a 30% case fatality rate (i.e., the likelihood of fatality per case diagnosed). Hemorrhagic smallpox, a subtype of variola major, includes all of the above signs and symptoms plus a dusky erythema and petechiae leading to frank hemorrhage of the skin and mucous membranes, and it results in death by day 5 or 6 (Veenema, 2019).

Management

Treatment includes supportive care with antibiotic agents for any additional infection. Antivirals and immune globulin may aid in treatment; however, vaccination remains the most effective method of prevention (ENA, 2020). The patient should be isolated in a negative-pressure environment, using strict airborne and contact precautions. Laundry and biologic wastes should be autoclaved before being washed with hot water and bleach. Standard decontamination of the room is effective. All people who have household or face-to-face contact with the patient after the fever begins should be vaccinated within 4 days to prevent infection and death. A patient with a temperature of 38°C (101°F) or higher within 17 days after exposure must be placed in isolation. Cremation is preferred for all deaths, because the virus can survive in scabs for up to 13 years (Veenema, 2019).

Chemical Weapons

Chemical weapons may be used as agents in warfare or for terrorist purposes. These are overt agents whose effects are more apparent and occur more quickly than those caused by biologic weapons (see Table 68-7). Poisonous exposure to everyday chemicals also may occur; the same management principles discussed later apply when patients are exposed to these chemical agents when not used as weapons. Typical exposures in these instances include industrial chemicals, gasoline, turpentine, kerosene, and insecticides (ENA, 2019).

Characteristics of Chemicals

Volatility

Volatility is the tendency for a chemical to become vapor. The most common volatile agents are phosgene and cyanide. Most chemicals are heavier than air, except for hydrogen cyanide. Therefore, in the presence of most chemicals, people

TABLE 68-7	Common Chemical Agents		
Agent	**Action**	**Signs and Symptoms**	**Decontamination and Treatment**
Nerve Agents Sarin Soman	Inhibition of cholinesterase	Increased secretions (salivation, lacrimation, emesis, urination), gastrointestinal motility, diarrhea, bronchospasm	Soap and water Supportive care Benzodiazepines Pralidoxime Atropine
Blood Agent Cyanide	Inhibition of aerobic metabolism	Inhalation—tachypnea, tachycardia, coma, seizures; bright red skin; can progress to respiratory arrest, respiratory failure, cardiac arrest, death	Soap and water Sodium nitrite Sodium thiocyanate Amyl nitrate Hydroxocobalamin
Vesicant Agents Lewisite Sulfur mustard Nitrogen mustard Phosgene	Blistering agents	Superficial to partial-thickness burn with vesicles that coalesce; conjunctivitis, nasal irritation	Soap and water Blot; do not rub dry
Pulmonary Agents Phosgene Chlorine	Separation of alveoli from capillary bed	Pulmonary edema, bronchospasm, chest tightness, burning sensation, blurry vision; phosgene can result in pain then blisters followed by partial to full-thickness burn	Copious flushing Move to fresh air—away from gases Airway management Ventilatory support Bronchoscopy

Adapted from Emergency Nurses Association. (2020). *Sheehy's manual of emergency care: Principles and practice* (7th ed.). St. Louis, MO: Elsevier Mosby; Emergency Nurses Association. (2019). *Trauma nursing core course* (8th ed.). Chicago: Author; and Veenema, T. G. (2019). *Disaster nursing and emergency preparedness* (4th ed.). New York: Springer.

should stand up to avoid heavy exposure (because the chemical will sink toward the floor or ground).

Persistence

Persistence means that the chemical is less likely to vaporize and disperse. More volatile chemicals do not evaporate very quickly. Most industrial chemicals (e.g., cyanide) are not very persistent. Weaponized agents (chemicals developed as weapons by the military or terrorists [e.g., mustard gas]) are more likely than industrial chemicals to penetrate the skin and mucous membranes and cause secondary exposure.

Toxicity

Toxicity is the potential of an agent to cause injury to the body. The median lethal dose (LD_{50}) is the amount of the chemical that will cause death in 50% of those who are exposed. For example, cyanogen chloride has the highest LD_{50}, twice that of hydrogen cyanide and eight times higher than sulfur mustard (OSHA, 2012). The median effective dose (ED_{50}) is the amount of the chemical that will cause signs and symptoms in 50% of those who are exposed. The concentration time (CT) is the concentration released multiplied by the time exposed (in milligrams per minute). For example, if 1000 mg of a chemical is released and the time a person is exposed to this amount of chemical is 10 minutes, then the CT would be 10,000 mg/min.

Latency

Latency is the time from absorption to the appearance of signs and symptoms. Sulfur mustards and pulmonary agents have the longest latency, whereas other vesicants, nerve agents, and cyanide produce signs and symptoms within seconds.

Limiting Exposure

Evacuation is essential, as is removal of the person's clothing and decontamination as close to the scene as possible and before transport of the person who has been exposed. Soap and water are effective means of decontamination in most cases. Staff involved in decontamination efforts must wear PPE and contain and dispose of the runoff after decontamination procedures (ENA, 2020).

Types of Chemicals

Vesicants

Vesicants are chemicals that cause blistering and result in burning, conjunctivitis, bronchitis, pneumonia, hematopoietic suppression, and death. Examples of vesicants include lewisite, phosgene, nitrogen mustard, and sulfur mustard. In World War I and in the Iran–Iraq conflict of 1980 to 1988, vesicants were used to disable opponents. Vesicants were the main incapacitating agents, resulting in minimal (less than 5%) death but large numbers of injuries (Veenema, 2019). Liquid sulfur mustard was the most frequently used vesicant in these conflicts.

Clinical Manifestations

The initial presentation after exposure to a vesicant is similar to that of a large superficial to partial-thickness burn in the warm and moist areas of the body (i.e., perineum, axillae, antecubital spaces). There is stinging and erythema for approximately 24 hours, followed by pruritus, painful burning, and small vesicle formation after 2 to 18 hours. These vesicles can coalesce into large, fluid-filled bullae. Lewisite and phosgene result in immediate pain after exposure. Tissue damage occurs within minutes (Veenema, 2019).

If the eyes are exposed, there will be pain, photophobia, lacrimation, and decreased vision. This progresses to conjunctivitis, blepharospasm, corneal ulcer, and corneal edema.

Respiratory effects are more serious and often are the cause of mortality with vesicant exposure. Manifestations may include dyspnea, necrosis of large airway mucosa with sloughing, chemical pneumonitis, pulmonary edema, and ARDS which may lead to respiratory failure and death (Veenema, 2019). Gastrointestinal exposure may cause nausea and vomiting, leukopenia, and upper gastrointestinal bleeding.

Management

Appropriate decontamination includes soap and water. Scrubbing and the use of hypochlorite solutions should be avoided because they increase penetration. Once the substance has penetrated, it cannot be removed. Eye exposure requires copious irrigation. For respiratory exposure, intubation and bronchoscopy to remove necrotic tissue are essential. With lewisite exposure, dimercaprol is administered IV for systemic toxicity and topically for skin lesions. All persons with sulfur mustard exposures should be monitored for 24 hours for latent (delayed) effects (ENA, 2020).

Nerve Agents

The most toxic agents in existence are the nerve agents such as sarin, soman, tabun, and VX. They are inexpensive, effective in small quantities, and easily dispersed. In the liquid form, nerve agents evaporate into a colorless, odorless vapor. Organophosphates (pesticides) are similar in nature to the nerve agents used in warfare and are readily available in the farming industry (ENA, 2020).

Nerve agents can be inhaled or absorbed percutaneously or subcutaneously. These agents bond with acetylcholinesterase so that acetylcholine is not inactivated; the adverse result is hyperstimulation (continuous stimulation) of the nerve endings. Carbamates, which are insecticides originally extracted from the Calabar bean, are derivatives of carbamic acid; they are nerve agents that specifically inhibit acetylcholinesterase for several hours and then spontaneously become unbound from the acetylcholinesterase. However, organophosphates require the formation of new enzyme (acetylcholinesterase) before nervous system function can be restored.

A very small drop of a nerve agent is enough to result in sweating and twitching at the site of exposure. A larger amount results in more systemic symptoms. Effects can begin anywhere from 30 minutes up to 18 hours after exposure. The more common organophosphates and carbamates (e.g., sevin, malathion) that are used in agriculture result in less severe symptoms than do those used in warfare or in terrorist attacks. In an ordinary situation (e.g., nonwarfare, nonterrorist attack situation), a patient could arrive at the ED having been unintentionally exposed to organophosphates or intentionally exposed to these agents in a suicidal attempt (ENA, 2020).

Clinical Manifestations

Signs and symptoms of nerve gas exposure are those of cholinergic crisis and include bilateral miosis, visual disturbances, increased gastrointestinal motility, nausea and vomiting, diarrhea, substernal spasm, indigestion, bradycardia and atrioventricular block, bronchoconstriction, laryngeal spasm, weakness, fasciculations, and incontinence. The patient must be examined in a dark area to truly identify miosis. Neurologic responses include insomnia, forgetfulness, impaired judgment, depression, and irritability. A lethal dose results in loss of consciousness, seizures, copious secretions, fasciculations, flaccid muscles, and apnea (ENA, 2019).

Management

Decontamination with copious amounts of soap and water or saline solution for 8 to 20 minutes is essential. The water is blotted off, not wiped off, the skin. Wiping may have the unintended effect of rubbing more of the agent into the skin. Fresh 0.5% hypochlorite solution (bleach) can also be used. The airway is maintained, and suctioning is frequently required. Plastic airway equipment should not be used, because plastic will absorb sarin gas and may result in continued exposure to the agent.

Atropine 2 to 4 mg is administered by IV, followed by 2 mg every 3 to 8 minutes for up to 24 hours of treatment. Alternatively, IV atropine 1 to 2 mg per hour may be given until clear signs of anticholinergic activity have returned (decreased secretions, tachycardia, and decreased gastrointestinal motility). Another medication that may serve as an antidote is pralidoxime, which allows cholinesterase to become active against acetylcholine. Pralidoxime 1 to 2 g in 100 to 150 mL of normal saline solution is given over 15 to 30 minutes. Pralidoxime has no effect on secretions and may have any of the following side effects: hypertension, tachycardia, weakness, dizziness, blurred vision, and diplopia. Diazepam or other benzodiazepines are used to control seizures, to decrease fasciculations, and to alleviate apprehension and agitation (ENA, 2020).

Blood Agents

Blood agents such as hydrogen cyanide and cyanogen chloride have a direct effect on cellular metabolism, resulting in asphyxiation through alterations in hemoglobin. Cyanide is an agent that has profound systemic effects. It is commonly used in the mining of gold and silver and in the plastics and dye industries.

A cyanide release is often associated with the odor of bitter almonds. In house fires, cyanide is released during the combustion of plastics, rugs, silk, furniture, and other construction materials. There is a significant correlation between blood cyanide and carbon monoxide levels in patients who survive fires, and in some cases, the cause of death is cyanide poisoning (Veenema, 2019).

Clinical Manifestations

Cyanide can be ingested, inhaled, or absorbed through the skin and mucous membranes. Cyanide is protein bound and inhibits aerobic metabolism, leading to respiratory muscle failure, respiratory arrest, cardiac arrest, and death. Its inhalation results in flushing, tachypnea, tachycardia, nonspecific neurologic symptoms, stupor, coma, and seizure preceding respiratory arrest (ENA, 2019).

Management

Rapid administration of amyl nitrate, sodium nitrite, and sodium thiosulfate is essential to the successful management of cyanide exposure. First, the patient is intubated and placed on a ventilator. Next, amyl nitrate pearls are crushed and placed in the ventilator reservoir to induce methemoglobinemia. Cyanide has a 20% to 25% higher affinity for methemoglobin than it does for hemoglobin; it binds methemoglobin to form either cyanomethemoglobin or sulfmethemoglobin. The cyanomethemoglobin is then detoxified in the liver by the enzyme rhodanese. Next, IV sodium nitrite is given to induce the rapid formation of methemoglobin. IV sodium thiosulfate is then given; it has a higher affinity for cyanide than methemoglobin and stimulates the conversion of cyanide to sodium thiocyanate, which can be excreted by the kidneys (ENA, 2019). Although they may be lifesaving, these emergency medications do have side effects—sodium nitrite can result in severe hypotension, and thiocyanate can cause vomiting, psychosis, arthralgia, and myalgia.

The production of methemoglobin is contraindicated in patients with smoke inhalation, because they already have decreased oxygen-carrying capacity secondary to the carboxyhemoglobin produced by smoke inhalation. In facilities where a hyperbaric chamber is available, it may be used to provide oxygenation while the previously discussed therapies are initiated. An alternative suggested treatment for cyanide poisoning is hydroxocobalamin (vitamin B_{12a}). Hydroxocobalamin binds with cyanide to form cyanocobalamin (vitamin B_{12}). It must be administered IV in large doses (Tintinalli et al., 2020). Administration of hydroxocobalamin can result in a transient pink discoloration of mucous membranes, skin, and urine. In high doses, tachycardia and hypertension can occur, but they usually resolve within 48 hours.

Pulmonary Agents

Pulmonary agents such as phosgene and chlorine destroy the pulmonary membrane that separates the alveolus from the capillary bed, disrupting alveolar–capillary oxygen transport mechanisms. Capillary leakage results in fluid-filled alveoli. Phosgene and chlorine both vaporize rapidly causing this pulmonary injury. Phosgene has the odor of freshly mown hay.

Signs and symptoms include pulmonary edema with shortness of breath, especially during exertion. An initial hacking cough is followed by frothy sputum production. A particulate air filter mask is the only protection required to protect health care personnel. Phosgene does not injure the eyes. In a review of a chlorine spill in South Carolina that exposed 155 patients, the most useful tool for identifying worsening symptoms was the pulse oximeter. Ordinary triage systems did not predict the severity of exposure (Veenema, 2019).

Nuclear Radiation Exposure

The threat of nuclear warfare or exposure to a radiologic weapon is very real with the availability of nuclear material and easily concealed simple devices, such as the so-called dirty bomb, for dispersal. A dirty bomb is a conventional explosive (e.g., dynamite) that is packaged with radioactive material that scatters when the bomb is detonated. It disperses radioactive material and may be called a **radiologic weapon**, but it is not a nuclear weapon, which uses a complex nuclear fission reaction that is thousands of times more devastating than the dirty bomb (Durakovic, 2017).

Sources of radioactive material include not only nuclear weapons but also reactors and simple radioactive samples, such as weapons-grade plutonium or uranium, freshly spent nuclear fuel, or medical supplies (e.g., radium, certain cesium isotopes) used in cancer treatments and radiology. Exposure to a large number of people can be accomplished by placing a radioactive sample in a public place. Thousands may be exposed this way; some may be immediately affected, and others may require health monitoring for many years to assess long-term effects (Durakovic, 2017).

Any terrorist act or unintentional radiation release can be sizable and may require the entire hospital and prehospital staff to be prepared, recognize signs and symptoms of exposure, and rapidly treat victims without contamination of personnel, visitors, patients, or the facility itself.

Types of Radiation

Atoms consist of protons, neutrons, and electrons. The protons and neutrons are in balance in the nucleus. The protons repel each other because they are all positively charged. The number of protons is specific for each element in the periodic table. There is a specific ratio of protons and neutrons for each different atom, and the result is element stability. When an element is radioactive, there is an imbalance in the nucleus, resulting from an excess of neutrons.

To achieve stability, a radioactive nuclide can eject particles until the most stable number (an even number) of protons and neutrons exists. A proton can become a neutron by ejecting a positron; conversely, a neutron can become a proton by ejecting a negative electron. An alpha particle is released when two protons and two electrons are ejected (beta particles are electrons).

Alpha particles cannot penetrate the skin. A thin layer of paper or clothing is all that is necessary to protect the skin from alpha radiation. However, this low-level radiation can enter the body through inhalation, ingestion, or injection (open wound). Only localized damage occurs.

Beta particles have the ability to moderately penetrate the skin to the layer in which skin cells are being produced. This high-energy radiation can cause skin damage if the skin is exposed for a prolonged period and can cause injury if beta particles penetrate the skin.

Gamma radiation is a short-wavelength electromagnetic energy that is emitted when there is excess core nucleus energy. Gamma particles are penetrating. Therefore, it is difficult to shield against gamma radiation. X-rays are an example of gamma radiation. Gamma radiation often accompanies both alpha particle and beta particle emission (Tintinalli et al., 2020).

Measurement and Detection

Radiation is measured in several different units. The *rad* is the basic unit of measurement. A rad is equivalent to 0.01 J of energy per kilogram of tissue. To determine the damaging effect of the rad, a conversion to the *rem* (roentgen equivalents man) is necessary. The rem reflects the type of radiation absorbed and the potential for damage. For example, 200,000 mrem results in mild radiation sickness (1 rem = 1000 mrem) (Tintinalli et al., 2020). Typical natural yearly exposure for a person is 360 mrem. Another important concept is *half-life*. The half-life of a radioactive product is the time it takes to lose half of its radioactivity.

The only way to detect radiation is through a device that determines the exposure per minute. There are various devices for this purpose. The Geiger counter (or Geiger–Müller survey meter) can measure background radiation quickly through detection of gamma radiation and some beta radiation. With high-level radiation, the Geiger counter may underestimate exposure. Other devices include the ionization chamber survey meter, alpha monitors, and dose rate meters (ENA, 2020). Personal dosimeters are simple tools that identify radiation exposure and are worn by radiology personnel every day.

Exposure

Exposure is affected by time, distance, and shielding. The longer a person is within the radiation area, the higher the exposure. In addition, the larger the amount of radioactive material in the area, the greater the exposure. The farther away the person is from the radiation source, the lower the exposure. Shielding from the radiation source also decreases exposure.

Three types of radiation-induced injury can occur: external irradiation, contamination with radioactive materials, and incorporation of radioactive material into body cells, tissues, or organs (ENA, 2020):

- *External irradiation* exposure occurs when all or part of the body is exposed to radiation that penetrates or passes completely through the body. In this type of exposure, the person is not radioactive and does not require special isolation or decontamination measures. Irradiation does not necessarily constitute a medical emergency.
- *Contamination* occurs when the body is exposed to radioactive gases, liquids, or solids either externally or internally. If internal, the contaminant can be deposited within the body. Contamination requires immediate medical management to prevent incorporation.
- *Incorporation* is the actual uptake of radioactive material into the cells, tissues, and susceptible organs. The organs involved are usually the kidneys, bones, liver, and thyroid.

Sequelae of contamination and incorporation can occur days to years later. The thyroid gland can be largely protected from radiation exposure by administration of stable iodine (potassium iodide) before or promptly after the intake of radioactive iodine. Priorities in the treatment of any type of radiation exposure are always treatment for life-threatening injuries and illnesses first, followed by measures to limit exposure, contamination control, and finally decontamination (Tintinalli et al., 2020).

Decontamination

Hospital and community disaster plans should be in effect when managing a radiation disaster. Access restriction is essential to prevent contamination of other areas of the hospital. Triage outside the hospital is the most effective means of preventing contamination of the facility itself. Floors are covered to prevent tracking of contaminants throughout the treatment areas. Strict isolation precautions should be in effect. All air ducts and vents must be sealed to prevent spread. Waste is controlled through double-bagging and the use of plastic-lined containers outside of the facility. All radiation-contaminated waste must be disposed of in appropriate color-coded yellow and magenta canisters.

Staff are required to wear protective clothing, such as water-resistant gowns, two pairs of gloves, masks, caps, goggles, and booties. Dosimetry devices should be worn by all staff members participating in patient care. The radiation safety officer in the hospital should be notified immediately to assist with surveys (using a radiation survey meter) of the incoming patients and to provide dosimeters to all staff personnel involved in direct care of patients who have been exposed. There is minimal risk to staff if the patients are properly surveyed and decontaminated.

Each patient arriving at the hospital should first be surveyed with the radiation survey meter for external contamination and then directed toward the decontamination area as needed. The majority of patients can be safely decontaminated with soap and water. Decontamination occurs outside of the ED with a shower, collection pool, tarp, and collection containers for patient belongings, as well as soap, towels, and disposable paper gowns for patients. Water runoff needs to be contained. Patients who are uninjured can perform self-decontamination with handheld showers. After the patient has showered, a resurvey is conducted to determine whether the radioactive contaminants have been removed. Additional washings should occur until the patient is free of contamination. It is important to ensure that during showers, previously clean areas are not contaminated with runoff from the washed contaminated areas (e.g., hair should be washed in a position that protects the body from contamination). Wounds are irrigated and then covered with a water-resistant dressing prior to total body decontamination.

Internal contamination or incorporation requires decontamination through catharsis, gastric lavage with chelating agents (agents that bind with radioactive substances and are then excreted), or both. Samples of urine, feces, and vomitus are surveyed to determine internal contamination levels. Biologic samples are taken through nasal and throat swabs, and a complete blood count with differential is obtained (Tintinalli et al., 2020).

Acute Radiation Syndrome

Acute radiation syndrome (ARS) can occur after exposure to radiation. It is the dose, rather than the source, that determines whether ARS develops. Factors that determine whether the patient's response to exposure will result in ARS include a high dose (minimum 100 rad) and rate of radiation with total body exposure and penetrating-type radiation. Age, medical history, and genetics also affect the outcome after exposure. The course is predictable. Table 68-8 identifies the phases of ARS.

Each body system is affected differently in ARS. Systems with cells that rapidly reproduce are most commonly affected. The hematopoietic system is the first system affected and serves as an indicator of the severity of radiation exposure (Veenema, 2019). A predictor of outcome is the absolute lymphocyte count at 48 hours after exposure. A significant exposure would be indicated by blood lymphocyte counts of 300 to 1200/mm^3. Barrier precautions should be implemented to protect the patient from infection. Neutrophils decrease within 1 week, platelets decrease

TABLE 68-8	Phases of Effects of Acute Radiation Syndrome	
Phase	**Time of Occurrence**	**Signs and Symptoms**
Prodromal phase (presenting symptoms)	48–72 h after exposure	Nausea, vomiting, loss of appetite, diarrhea, fatigue High-dose radiation—fever, respiratory distress, and increased excitability
Latent phase (a symptom-free period)	After resolution of prodromal phase; can last up to 3 wks With high-dose radiation, latent period is shorter	Decreasing lymphocytes, leukocytes, thrombocytes, red blood cells
Manifest illness phase	After latent period phase	Infection, fluid and electrolyte imbalance, bleeding, diarrhea, shock, and altered level of consciousness
Recovery phase OR	After manifest illness phase	Can take weeks to months for full recovery
Death	After manifest illness phase	Increased intracranial pressure is a sign of impending death

Adapted from Centers for Disease Control and Prevention (CDC). (2018c). *Acute radiation syndrome: A fact sheet for clinicians.* Retrieved on 3/1/2020 at: www.emergency.cdc.gov/radiation/arsphysicianfactsheet.asp

within 2 weeks, and red blood cells decrease within 3 weeks. Hemorrhagic complications including fever and sepsis are common.

The gastrointestinal system, with its rapidly reproducing cells, is also readily affected by radiation. Doses of radiation required to produce symptoms are approximately 600 rad or higher. The gastrointestinal symptoms usually occur at the same time as the changes in the hematopoietic system. Nausea and vomiting occur within 2 hours after exposure. Sepsis, fluid and electrolyte imbalance, and opportunistic infections can occur as complications. An ominous sign is the presence of high fever and bloody diarrhea; these typically appear on day 10 after exposure (ENA, 2019).

The central nervous system is affected when the dose exceeds 1000 rad (ENA, 2019). The symptoms occur when damage to the blood vessels of the brain results in fluid leakage. Signs and symptoms include cerebral edema; nausea; vomiting; headache; and increased intracranial pressure, which heralds a poor outcome and imminent death. Central nervous system injury with this amount of exposure is irreversible and occurs before hematopoietic or gastrointestinal system symptoms appear. Cardiovascular collapse is usually seen in conjunction with these injuries.

Skin effects can also indicate the dose of radiation exposure. With an exposure of 600 to 1000 rad, erythema occurs; it can disappear within hours and then reappear. The patient who has been exposed must be evaluated hourly for the presence of erythema. With exposures greater than 1000 rad, desquamation (radiation dermatitis) of the skin occurs. Necrosis becomes evident within a few days to months at doses greater than 5000 rad (CDC, 2018c).

Secondary injury can occur when the radiation exposure occurs during a traumatic event such as a blast or burn. Trauma in addition to radiation exposure increases patient mortality. Attention must first be directed toward the primary assessment for trauma. Airway, breathing, circulation, and fracture reduction require immediate attention. All definitive treatments must occur within the first 48 hours. Thereafter, all surgical procedures should be delayed for 2 to 3 months because of the potential for delayed wound healing and the possible development of opportunistic infections several weeks after exposure (Veenema, 2019).

Survival

There are three categories of predicted survival after radiation exposure: probable, possible, and improbable. Triage of victims at the scene, after decontamination, is conducted using the routine system for disaster triage. Presenting signs and symptoms determine the potential for survival and therefore the category of predicted survival during triage.

Probable survivors have either no initial symptoms or only minimal symptoms (e.g., nausea and vomiting), or these symptoms resolve within a few hours. These patients should have a complete blood count drawn and may be discharged with instructions to return if any symptoms recur.

Possible survivors present with nausea and vomiting that persist for 24 to 48 hours. They experience a latent period, during which leukopenia, thrombocytopenia, and lymphocytopenia occur. Barrier precautions and protective isolation are implemented if the patient's lymphocyte count is less than 1200/mm³. Supportive treatment includes administration of blood products, prevention of infection, and provision of enhanced nutrition.

Improbable survivors have received more than 800 rad of total-body penetrating irradiation. People in this group demonstrate an acute onset of vomiting, bloody diarrhea, and shock. Any neurologic symptoms suggest a lethal dose of radiation (ENA, 2019). These patients still require decontamination to prevent further contamination of the area and of others. Personal protection is essential, because it is virtually impossible to fully decontaminate these patients; all of their internal organs have been irradiated. The survival time is variable; however, death usually occurs swiftly due to shock. If there are no neurologic symptoms, patients may be alert and oriented, similar to a patient with extensive burns. In a mass casualty situation, these patients would be triaged into the black category, where they will receive comfort measures and emotional support. If it is not a mass casualty situation, aggressive fluid and electrolyte therapies are essential.

CRITICAL THINKING EXERCISES

1 pq You are one of the several nurses volunteering at a music festival. You suddenly hear a loud explosion and hundreds of attendees are screaming and scattering in all directions. You see people are bleeding and notice that some individuals are on the ground not moving. You know you need to organize efforts and provide care. What are the priority actions you should take in order to ensure the safety of yourself and others on the scene? How will information be communicated to the community? What strategies will you utilize in this situation to triage those who have been impacted? As EMS arrive, who will have priority to be transported to the hospital?

2 ebp You are working in the emergency department and caring for a patient who complains of a fever for the past 2 days, cough, shortness of breath, severe fatigue, and loss of appetite. You are concerned that this patient may have COVID-19. Identify the immediate precautions that you will need to implement when providing care for this patient. When conducting an assessment, what questions will you ask this patient? Discuss the education you will provide the patient and family to reduce the potential transmission of SARS-CoV-2 and the evidence-based resources you will use to support this education.

REFERENCES

*Asterisk indicates nursing research.
**Double asterisk indicates classic reference.

Books

Emergency Nurses Association (ENA). (2019). *Trauma nursing core course* (8th ed.). Chicago: Emergency Nurses Association.
Emergency Nurses Association (ENA). (2020). *Sheehy's emergency nursing: Principles and practice* (7th ed.). St. Louis, MO: Elsevier Mosby.
Jorolemon M. R., Lopez, R. A., & Krywko, D. M. (2019). Blast injuries. In *StatPearls [Internet]*. Treasure Island, FL: StatPearls Publishing. Retrieved on 3/27/2020 at: www.ncbi.nlm.nih.gov/books/NBK430914/
Tintinalli, J. E., Ma, O. J., Yealy, D. M., et al. (2020). *Tintinalli's emergency medicine: A comprehensive study guide* (9th ed.). New York: McGraw-Hill Medical.
Veenema, T. G. (2019). *Disaster nursing and emergency preparedness* (4th ed.). New York: Springer.

Journals and Electronic Documents

Altman, M. (2020). Facing moral distress during the COVID-19 crisis. American Association of Critical-Care Nurses (Blog). Retrieved on 5/21/2020 at: www.aacn.org/blog/facing-moral-distress-during-the-covid-19-crisis
American Nurses Association (ANA). (2017). Who will be there? Ethics, the law, and a nurse's duty to respond in a disaster. Retrieved on 5/21/2020 at: www.nursingworld.org/~4af058/globalassets/docs/ana/ethics/who-will-be-there_disaster-preparedness_2017.pdf
American Nurses Association (ANA). (2020). Nurses, ethics and the response to the COVID-19 pandemic. Retrieved on 5/21/2020 at: www.nursingworld.org/~495c6c/globalassets/practiceandpolicy/work-environment/health--safety/coronavirus/nurses-ethics-and-the-response-to-the-covid-19-pandemic.pdf
Baumrucker, S. J., Carter, G., Adkins, R. W., et al. (2020). Ethics roundtable: Distribution of critical care resources in the setting of a COVID-19 surge. *American Journal of Hospice and Palliative Care, 37*(12), 1096–1101.

Berlinger, N., Wynia, M., Powell, T., et al. (2020). Ethical framework for health care institutions & guidelines for institutional ethics services responding to the coronavirus pandemic. Retrieved on 5/23/2020 at: www.thehastingscenter.org/ethicalframeworkcovid19/
California Hospital Association. (2017). Emergency preparedness; preparing hospitals for disasters. Emergency Operation Plan (EOP). Retrieved on 3/1/2020 at: www.calhospitalprepare.org/emergency-operations-plan
Casey, D. (2017). Ethics, law, and policy. Ethical considerations during disaster. *Med Surg Nursing, 26*(6), 411–413.
Centers for Disease Control and Prevention (CDC). (2017). Smallpox: Who should get vaccination. Retrieved on 3/1/2020 at: www.cdc.gov/smallpox/vaccine-basics/who-gets-vaccination.html
Centers for Disease Control and Prevention (CDC). (2018a). Preparedness and safety messaging for hurricanes, flooding, and similar disasters. Retrieved on 3/1/2020 at: www.cdc.gov/cpr/readiness/00_docs/CDC_Hurricanes_PreparednessSafetyMessaging_July2018_508.pdf
Centers for Disease Control and Prevention (CDC). (2018b). Foodborne outbreaks. Retrieved on 8/1/2020 at: www.cdc.gov/foodsafety/outbreaks/investigating-outbreaks/investigations/index.html
Centers for Disease Control and Prevention (CDC). (2018c). Acute radiation syndrome: A fact sheet for clinicians. Retrieved on 3/1/2020 at: www.emergency.cdc.gov/radiation/arsphysicianfactsheet.asp
Centers for Disease Control and Prevention (CDC). (2020a). CDC in action: Working 24/7 to stop the threat of COVID-19. Retrieved on 7/7/2020 at: www.cdc.gov/budget/documents/covid-19/CDC-247-Response-to-COVID-19-fact-sheet.pdf
Centers for Disease Control and Prevention (CDC). (2020b). Strategies to optimize the supply of PPE and equipment. Retrieved on 5/20/2020 at: www.cdc.gov/coronavirus/2019-ncov/hcp/ppe-strategy/index.html
Centers for Disease Control and Prevention (CDC). (2020c). Management of visitors to healthcare facilities in the context of COVID-19: Non-US healthcare settings. Retrieved on 5/20/2020 at: www.cdc.gov/coronavirus/2019-ncov/hcp/non-us-settings/hcf-visitors.html
Centers for Disease Control and Prevention (CDC). (2020d). For parents: Multisystem inflammatory syndrome in children (MIS-C) associated with COVID-19. Retrieved on 5/21/2020 at: www.cdc.gov/coronavirus/2019-ncov/daily-life-coping/children/mis-c.html
Centers for Disease Control and Prevention (CDC). (2020e). Personal protective equipment: Questions and answers. Retrieved on 5/21/2020 at: www.cdc.gov/coronavirus/2019-ncov/hcp/respirator-use-faq.html
Durakovic, A. (2017). Medical effects of a transuranic "dirty bomb". *Military Medicine, 182*(3–4), 1591–1595.
Hart, J. L., Turnbull, A. E., Oppenheim, I. M., et al. (2020). Family-centered care during the COVID-19 era. *Journal of Pain and Symptom Management, 60*(2), e93–e97.
Johns Hopkins University (JHU). (2020). In fight against COVID-19, nurses face high-stakes decisions, moral distress. Retrieved on 5/20/2020 at: https://hub.jhu.edu/2020/04/06/covid-nursing-cynda-rushton-qa/
*Kalanlar, B. (2019). The challenges and opportunities of disaster nursing education in Turkey. *Journal of Trauma Nursing, 26*(3), 164–170.
Leider, J. P., DeBruin, D., Reynolds, N., et al. (2017). Ethical guidance for disaster response, specifically around crisis standards of care: A systematic review. *American Journal of Public Health, 107*(9), e1–e9.
Occupational Safety and Health Administration. (2017). Section VIII: Chapter 1. Chemical protective clothing. In OSHA technical manual. Retrieved on 3/1/2020 at: www.osha.gov/dts/osta/otm/otm_viii/otm_viii_1.html
**Occupational Safety and Health Administration. (2012). Hazard communication standard: Safety data sheets. Retrieved on 3/1/2020 at: www.osha.gov/Publications/OSHA3514.html
Ram-Tiktin, E. (2017). Ethical considerations of triage following natural disasters: The IDF experience in Haiti as a case study. *Bioethics, 31*(6), 467–475.
Ranney, M. L., Griffeth, V., & Jha, A. K. (2020). Critical supply shortages—the need for ventilators and personal protective equipment during the Covid-19 pandemic. *New England Journal of Medicine, 382*(18), e41.
Ritchie, H., Hasell, J., Appel, C., et al. (2020). Terrorism. Retrieved on 2/25/2020 at: ourworldindata.org/terrorism.
*Sloand, E., Killion, C., Yarandi, H., et al. (2017). Experiences of violence and abuse among internally displaced adolescent girls following a natural disaster. *Journal of Advanced Nursing, 73*(12), 3200–3208.
*Tan, W., Ye, Y., Yang, Y., et al. (2020). Whole-process emergency training of personal protective equipment helps healthcare workers against

COVID-19: Design and effect. *Journal of Occupational and Environmental Medicine*, 62(6), 420–423.

Toner, E. (2017). Healthcare preparedness: Saving lives. *Health Security*, 15(1), 8–11.

U.S. Department of Health and Human Services, Food and Drug Administration [FDA], Center for Drug Evaluation and Research [CDER]. (2018). *Anthrax: Developing drugs for prophylaxis of inhalational anthrax: Guidance for Industry*. Retrieved on 3/1/2020 at: www.fda.gov/media/71320/download

U.S. Department of Homeland Security Federal Emergency Management Agency (FEMA). (2019). Hazardous materials incidents, guidance for state, local, tribal, territorial and private sector partners. Retrieved on 3/12/2020 at: www.fema.gov/media-library-data/1566393023589-8134367aaf67f65c7a159453c0b8c27b/Hazardous_Materials_Incidents.pdf

U.S. Department of Homeland Security Federal Emergency Management Agency (FEMA). (2020a). Supporting patients and healthcare workers. Retrieved July 7, 2020 at: www.fema.gov/coronavirus/patients-healthcare

U.S. Department of Homeland Security Federal Emergency Management Agency (FEMA). (2020b). FEMA COVID-19 Supply chain task force: Supply chain stabilization. Retrieved on 5/20/2020 at: www.fema.gov/news-release/2020/04/08/fema-covid-19-supply-chain-task-force-supply-chain-stabilization

U.S. Department of Homeland Security National Terrorism Advisory System (NTAS). (2019). NTAS frequently asked questions. Retrieved on 3/1/2020 at: www.dhs.gov/ntas-frequently-asked-questions

U.S. Food and Drug Administration (FDA). (2018). What we do. Retrieved on 5/1/2020 at: www.fda.gov/about-fda/what-we-do

U.S. Food and Drug Administration (FDA). (2020). FDA statement: Coronavirus (COVID-19) update: FDA expedites review of diagnostic tests to combat COVID-19. Retrieved on 5/21/2020 at: www.fda.gov/news-events/press-announcements/coronavirus-covid-19-update-fda-expedites-review-diagnostic-tests-combat-covid-19

World Health Organization (WHO). (2020a). Q&A on coronavirus (COVID-19). Retrieved on 5/22/2020 at: www.who.int/emergencies/diseases/novel-coronavirus-2019/question-and-answers-hub/q-a-detail/q-a-coronaviruses

World Health Organization (WHO). (2020b). Environment, climate change, and health, disease outbreaks. Retrieved on 8/1/2020 at: www.who.int/teams/environment-climate-change-and-health/emergencies/disease-outbreaks/

Resources

Agency for Toxic Substances and Disease Registry, www.atsdr.cdc.gov

American Red Cross, Beat Disaster with Preparedness, www.redcross.org/news/article/Beat-Disaster-with-Preparedness

Centers for Disease Control and Prevention (CDC, Coronavirus (COVID-19)), www.cdc.gov/coronavirus/2019-nCoV/index.html?cid = EPR-homepage

Centers for Disease Control and Prevention (CDC), Emergency Preparedness and Response, www.emergency.cdc.gov

Federal Emergency Management Agency (FEMA), www.fema.gov

Global Terrorism Database, www.start.umd.edu/gtd

Johns Hopkins University & Medicine, www.coronavirus.jhu.edu/map.html

National Organization on Disability, www.nod.org

Prevent Epidemics, www.preventepidemics.org

Resolve to Save Lives: An Initiative of Vital Strategies, www.resolvetosavelives.org

U.S. Department of Homeland Security, www.dhs.gov

World Health Organization (WHO). Q&A on Coronavirus (COVID-19), www.who.int/emergencies/diseases/novel-coronavirus-2019/question-and-answers-hub/q-a-detail/q-a-coronaviruses

World Health Organization, www.who.int

Index